国家出版基金项目
NATIONAL PUBLICATION FOUNDATION

"十三五"国家重点图书出版规划项目
天津市重点出版扶持项目

Textbook of Organ Transplantation

Volume 1

器官移植学

上 卷

〔美〕艾伦·D. 柯克　等　主编
朱继业　徐　骁　李　照　主译

天津出版传媒集团
天津科技翻译出版有限公司

著作权合同登记号:图字:02 - 2016 - 05

图书在版编目(CIP)数据

器官移植学 / (美)艾伦·D. 柯克(Allan D. Kirk)等主编;朱继业,徐骁,李照主译. —天津:天津科技翻译出版有限公司,2020. 3
书名原文:Textbook of Organ Transplantation
ISBN 978 - 7 - 5433 - 4014 - 5

Ⅰ.①器… Ⅱ.①艾… ②朱… ③徐… ④李… Ⅲ.①器官移植 Ⅳ.①R617

中国版本图书馆 CIP 数据核字(2020)第 039496 号

授权单位:John Wiley & Sons Limited
出　　版:天津科技翻译出版有限公司
出 版 人:刘子媛
地　　址:天津市南开区白堤路 244 号
邮政编码:300192
电　　话:022 - 87894896
传　　真:022 - 87895650
网　　址:www. tsttpc. com
印　　刷:山东临沂新华印刷物流集团有限责任公司
发　　行:全国新华书店
版本记录:889mm × 1194mm　16 开本　119 印张　3600 千字
2020 年 3 月第 1 版　2020 年 3 月第 1 次印刷
定价:680. 00 元(上下卷)

(如有印装问题,可与出版社调换)

译者名单

主　译　朱继业　徐　骁　李　照

译校者　（按姓氏汉语拼音排序）

陈　峻　陈俊丽　陈康辰　程　倩　崔　笑　董思依　高　峰
高鹏骥　郭海军　郭颂一　郭靖珩　韩威力　胡士华　胡志平
焦守斐　柯庆宏　李　博　李　照　李仕进　李勇剑　林丽丹
林天雨　凌　琪　刘　鹏　刘　晓　刘以俊　刘原兴　刘治坤
马慧云　毛雨鸽　倪彦彬　倪一鸣　彭　鹏　秋宇典　沈　恬
汪　洋　王辉杭　王建国　王思奇　王亚洲　危荣沥　魏绪勇
文　雪　吴建永　奚　斌　肖增丽　谢文勇　向　骁　徐　骁
许庭珉　荀晓冬　杨　帆　杨崇威　杨梦凡　杨墨丹　禹　琛
张　超　张长坤　张大方　张龙辉　张云凯　赵海格　郑骏楠
周舒扬　朱凤雪　朱继业　卓建勇

主编名单

Allan D. Kirk, MD, PhD, FACS

Professor and Chairman, Department of Surgery
Duke University School of Medicine;
Surgeon-in-Chief for Duke University Health System
Duke University Medical Center
Durham, NC, USA

Stuart J. Knechtle, MD

Professor of Surgery
Emory University School of Medicine
Atlanta, GA, USA

Christian P. Larsen, MD, DPhil

Dean - Emory School of Medicine
Surgeon-in-Chief Emory Healthcare
Emory University
Atlanta, GA, USA

Joren C. Madsen, MD, DPhil

Professor of Surgery
W. Gerald and Patricia R. Austen
Distinguished Scholar in Cardiac Surgery
Massachusetts General Hospital
Boston, MA, USA

Thomas C. Pearson, MD

Emory Transplant Center
Emory University School of Medicine
Atlanta, GA, USA

Steven A. Webber, MBChB, MRCP

James C. Overall Professor and Chair, Department of Pediatrics
Monroe Carell Jr. Children's Hospital at Vanderbilt
Vanderbilt University School of Medicine
Nashville, TN, USA

编者名单

Michael Abecassis, MD, MBA
J. Roscoe Miller Distinguished Professor
Department of Surgery and Microbiology-Immunology
Chief, Division of Organ Transplantation
Founding Director, Comprehensive Transplant Center
Northwestern University Feinberg School of Medicine
Chicago, IL, USA

Kareem M. Abu-Elmagd, MD, PhD, FACS
Professor of Surgery
Department of Surgery
Transplant Division
Intestinal Rehabilitation and Transplantation Center
University of Pittsburgh Medical Center
Pittsburgh, PA, USA

Andrew B. Adams, MD, PhD
Assistant Professor of Surgery
Emory Transplant Center
Emory University School of Medicine
Atlanta, GA, USA

Avinash Agarwal, MD, FACS
Assistant Professor of Surgery
Department of Surgery, University of Virginia
Charlottesville, VA, USA

Maria-Luisa Alegre, MD, PhD
Professor of Medicine
University of Chicago
Chicago, IL, USA

Rita R. Alloway, PharmD, FCCP
Research Professor of Medicine
Director, Transplant Clinical Research
Director, Transplant Pharmacy PGY 2 Residency and Fellowship
University of Cincinnati
Cincinnati, OH, USA

Winston A. Ally, PharmD, BCPS
Pharmacy Clinical Coordinator
Solid Organ Transplantation
Director, PGY-2 Solid Organ Transplant Pharmacy Residency
Department of Pharmacy Services
University of Virginia Health System
Charlottesville, VA;
Clinical Assistant Professor
Department of Pharmacotherapy and Outcomes Science
Virginia Commonwealth University School of Pharmacy
Richmond, VA, USA

Estella M. Alonso, MD
Professor of Pediatrics
Department of Pediatrics
Northwestern University Feinberg School of Medicine
Medical Director of Hepatology and Liver Transplantation
Ann and Robert H. Lurie Children's Hospital of Chicago
Chicago, IL, USA

Sandra Amaral, MD, MHS
Co-Director, Pediatric Kidney Transplant Program
Assistant Professor, University of Pennsylvania
The Children's Hospital of Philadelphia
Philadelphia, PA, USA

Douglas J. Anderson, MD
Senior Resident
Department of Surgery
Emory University School of Medicine
Atlanta, GA, USA

Vincent T. Armenti, MD, PhD
Principal Investigator
National Transplantation Pregnancy Registry (NTPR)
Gift of Life Institute
Philadelphia, PA;
Professor of Anatomy and Surgery
University of Central Florida College of Medicine
Orlando, FL, USA

Todd L. Astor, MD
Assistant Professor of Medicine, Harvard Medical School
Medical Director, Lung and Heart-Lung Transplant Program
Pulmonary and Critical Care Unit
Massachusetts General Hospital
Boston, MA, USA

Robin K. Avery, MD
Professor of Medicine
Johns Hopkins University School of Medicine
Infectious Disease Division
Johns Hopkins Hospital
Baltimore, MD, USA

David A. Axelrod, MD, MBA
Section Chief, Solid Organ Transplant Surgery
Dartmouth Hitchcock Medical Center
Lebanon, NH, USA

Agnes M. Azimzadeh, PhD
Assistant Professor of Surgery
University of Maryland School of Medicine
Baltimore, MD, USA

Raul Badell, MD
Chief Resident
Department of Surgery
Emory University School of Medicine
Atlanta, GA, USA

Remzi Bag, MD
McKelvey Scholar
The McKelvey Center for Lung Transplantation
Assistant Professor of Medicine, Pulmonary, Allergy and Critical Care
Emory University School of Medicine
Atlanta, GA, USA

William M. Baldwin III, MD, PhD
Staff, Department of Immunology
Cleveland Clinic
Cleveland, OH, USA

Erik R. Barthel, MD, PhD
Resident in General Surgery
Harbor-UCLA Medical Center
UCLA David Geffen School of Medicine
Los Angeles, CA, USA

Stephen T. Bartlett, MD
Peter Angelos Distinguished Professor and Chairman
Department of Surgery
University of Maryland School of Medicine
Surgeon-in-Chief, University of Maryland Medical System
Baltimore, MD, USA

Lokesh Bathla, MD
Transplant Surgeon
Methodist Specialty and Transplant Hospital
San Antonio, TX, USA

Julia B. Becker, MD
Fellow in Pulmonary and Critical Care Medicine
University of Chicago
Chicago, IL, USA

Lorraine E. Bell, MDCM, FRCPC
Associate Professor of Pediatrics, McGill University
Director, Pediatric Renal Transplant Programme
Director, Pediatric Transition to Adult Care
Montreal Children's Hospital-McGill University Health Centre
Montreal, QC, Canada

Jennifer Berumen, MD
Chief Resident, General Surgery
UC San Diego
La Jolla, CA, USA

Oriol Bestard
Renal Transplant Unit
Nephrology Department
University Hospital of Bellvitge
University of Barcelona
Barcelona, Spain

Arvind Bhimaraj, MD, MPH, FACC
Assistant Professor of Medicine
Weill Cornell Medical College, NY;
Department of Cardiology
Methodist DeBakey Heart & Vascular Center
Houston Methodist Hospital
Houston, TX, USA

Adam W. Bingaman, MD, PhD
Director, Live Donor and Incompatible Kidney Transplant Programs
Methodist Specialty and Transplant Hospital
San Antonio, TX, USA

Roy D. Bloom, MD
Professor of Medicine
Perelman School of Medicine
University of Pennsylvania
Medical Director
Penn Kidney Pancreas Transplant Program
Philadelphia, PA, USA

Emily A. Blumberg, MD
Professor of Medicine
Perelman School of Medicine
University of Pennsylvania
Philadelphia, PA, USA

J. Andrew Bradley, PhD, FRCS
Professor of Surgery
University of Cambridge
Cambridge, UK

Gerald Brandacher, MD
Associate Professor of Surgery (PAR)
Scientific Director
Reconstructive Transplantation Program
Department of Plastic and Reconstructive Surgery
Johns Hopkins University School of Medicine
Baltimore, MD, USA

Robert A. Bray, PhD
Professor of Pathology
Co-Director, Histocompatibility and Molecular Immunogenetics Laboratory
Department of Pathology
Emory University Hospital
Atlanta, GA, USA

Daniel C. Brennan, MD
Professor of Medicine
Director, Transplant Nephrology
Washington University in St. Louis
School of Medicine
St. Louis, MO, USA

Lori E. Brigham, MBA
President and CEO
Washington Regional Transplant Community
Annandale, VA, USA

Jonathan S. Bromberg, MD, PhD
Professor of Surgery and Microbiology and Immunology
University of Maryland School of Medicine
Baltimore, MD, USA

Kimberly A. Brown, MD
Chief, Gastroenterology and Hepatology
Henry Ford Hospital
Detroit, MI, USA

John C. Bucuvalas
Professor of Pediatrics
Associate Medical Director, Pediatric Liver Care Center
Cincinnati Children's Hospital Medical Center
Cincinnati, OH, USA

Deborah Budge, MD
Associate Director
UTAH Cardiac Transplant Program
Intermountain Medical Center
Salt Lake City, UT, USA

Andrew Bushell, DPhil
Senior Scientist and University Research Lecturer
Transplantation Research Immunology Group
Nuffield Department of Surgical Sciences
John Radcliffe Hospital
Oxford, UK

Chris J. Callaghan, PhD, FRCS
Consultant Transplant and Vascular Access Surgeon
Guy's Hospital
London, UK

Sir Roy Y. Calne, FRS
Emeritus Professor of Surgery
Cambridge University
Cambridge, UK;
Visiting Professor
National University of Singapore
Singapore

Esther-Marie Carmichael, MT(ASCP), CLS, PHM, BSc
Quality Assurance Manager
Keck Hospital of USC, Transplant Institute
Los Angeles, CA, USA

Kelly Carter, MS, RN, NE-BC
Virginia Commonwealth University Health System
Medical College of Virginia Hospitals
Nurse Manager
Pauley Heart Center
Richmond, VA, USA

J. Michael Cecka, PhD
Emeritus Professor
Department of Pathology and Laboratory Medicine;
Director, Clinical Research
UCLA Immunogenetics Center
David Geffen School of Medicine
University of California, Los Angeles
Los Angeles, CA, USA

Linda C. Cendales, MD
Associate Professor of Surgery
Division of Plastic and Reconstructive Surgery and Division of Transplantation (dual appointment)
Director, Vascularized Composite Allotransplantation
Duke University Medical Center
Durham, NC, USA

Ashtar Chami, MD
Assistant Professor of Medicine
Emory Transplant Center
Emory University School of Medicine
Atlanta, GA, USA

Jeremy Chapman, MD, FRCP
Director, Renal Medicine
Centre for Transplant and Renal Research
Westmead Milennium Institute
Sydney University
Westmead Hospital
Westmead, NSW, Australia

Ali H. Charafeddine, MD
General Surgery Resident
Montefiore Medical Centre
Albert Einstein College of Medicine
Bronx, New York, NY, USA

Serban Constantinescu, MD, PhD
Medical Director, Kidney Transplant Program
Associate Professor of Medicine
Temple University School of Medicine
Philadelphia, PA, USA

Damon S. Cooney, MD, PhD
Assistant Professor of Plastic Surgery
Department of Plastic and Reconstructive Surgery
Johns Hopkins University School of Medicine
Baltimore, MD, USA

Matthew Cooper, MD
Associate Professor of Surgery
Medstar Georgetown Transplant Institute
Georgetown University School of Medicine
Washington, DC, USA

Jack G. Copeland, MD
Professor of Cardiothoracic Surgery
Director of Cardiac Transplantation and Mechanical Circulatory Support
UC San Diego
La Jolla, CA, USA

Hannah Copeland, MD
Chief Resident, General Surgery
UC San Diego
La Jolla, CA, USA

A. Benedict Cosimi, MD
Claude E. Welch Distinguished Professor of Surgery
Harvard Medical School
Chief Emeritus
Division of Transplantation
Massachusetts General Hospital
Boston, MA, USA

Guilherme Costa, MD, FACS
Assistant Professor of Surgery
Department of Surgery
University of Pittsburgh
Pittsburgh, PA, USA

Peter J. Cowan, PhD
Professor, Immunology Research Centre
St Vincent's Hospital Melbourne;
Department of Medicine
University of Melbourne
Melbourne, VIC, Australia

John M. Craig, MD
Clinical Assistant Professor of Surgery
University of Tennessee Health Science Center
Baptist Memorial Hospital
Memphis, TN, USA

Josep M. Cruzado
Renal Transplant Unit
Nephrology department.
University Hospital of Bellvitge
University of Barcelona
Barcelona, Spain

Marcelo Cypel, MD, MSc
Assistant Professor of Surgery
Toronto Lung Transplant Program
University Health Network
University of Toronto
Toronto, ON, Canada

Anthony M. D'Alessandro, MD
Professor of Surgery
Director of Liver Transplantation
University of Wisconsin School of Medicine and Public Health
Madison, WI, USA

Gabriel M. Danovitch, MD
Professor of Medicine, Division of Nephrology
Medical Director, Kidney Transplant Program
Department of Medicine
David Geffen School of Medicine at UCLA
Los Angeles, CA, USA

Anthony J.F. d'Apice, MD, MBBS
Professor
Immunology Research Centre
St Vincent's Hospital Melbourne;
Department of Medicine
University of Melbourne
Melbourne, VIC, Australia

R. Duane Davis, MD, MBA
Director of Transplantation
Professor of Surgery
Duke University Medical School and Medical Center
Durham, NC, USA

John M. Davison, MD
Professor Emeritus and Consultant Obstetrician
Institute of Cellular Medicine
Newcastle University
Newcastle upon Tyne, UK

Rowena Delos Santos, MD
Assistant Professor of Medicine
Renal Division
Washington University in St. Louis
St. Louis, MO, USA

Sacha A. De Serres, MD, SM, FRCPC
Research Fellow, Brigham and Women's Hospital and Harvard Medical School
Boston, MA;
Assistant Professor of Medicine
Universite Laval
Quebec, QC, Canada

Patrick G. Dean, MD
Assistant Professor of Surgery
Division of Transplant Surgery
Mayo Clinic
Rochester, MN, USA

Francis L. Delmonico, MD
President, The Transplantation Society;
World Health Organization
Advisory for Human Transplantation;
Professor of Surgery
Harvard Medical School
Massachusetts General Hospital
Transplant Center
Boston, MA;
Medical Director
New England Organ Bank
Waltham, MA, USA

Anthony J. Demetris, MD
Starzl Professor of Liver and Transplant Pathology
Director, Division of Liver and Transplant Pathology
Department of Pathology
University of Pittsburgh Medical Center
Pittsburgh, PA, USA

Yaozhong Ding, PhD
Associate Professor (retired)
Department of Surgery
University of Maryland School of Medicine
Baltimore, MD, USA

Cinthia B. Drachenberg, MD
Professor of Pathology
Director, Electron Microscopy Laboratory
University of Maryland School of Medicine
Baltimore, MD, USA

Regina Eady
Research Data Informatics Analyst, Senior
Emory University
Atlanta, GA, USA

Bijan Eghtesad, MD
Professor of Surgery
Director, Fellowship Program
Hepato-Pancreato-Biliary/Liver Transplantation Surgery
Cleveland Clinic
Cleveland, OH, USA

Howard J. Eisen, MD
Thomas J. Vischer Professor of Medicine
Chief, Division of Cardiology
Drexel University College of Medicine
Philadelphia, PA, USA

Robert Ettenger, MD
Professor of Pediatrics
Division of Nephrology
Department of Pediatrics
David Geffen School of Medicine at UCLA;
Director of Pediatric Renal Transplant Program
Director, Pediatric Nephrology Fellowship Program
Mattel Children's Hospital, UCLA
Los Angeles, CA, USA

Richard Eliot Fagley, MD
Anesthesiologist and Intensivist
Virginia Mason Medical Center
Seattle, WA, USA

Robert L. Fairchild, PhD
Staff, Department of Immunology
Cleveland Clinic
Cleveland, OH, USA

Konrad S. Famulski, PhD, DSc
Faculty Service Officer
Manager and Lead in Transcriptomics
Alberta Transplant Applied Genomics Centre
Department of Medicine
Division of Nephrology and Transplant Immunology
Edmonton, AB, Canada

Ji Fan, MD
Instructor of Clinical Surgery
University of Miami Miller School of Medicine
Miami Transplant Institute
Miami, FL, USA

Myriam Farah, MD, FRCPC
Clinical Assistant Professor
Division of Nephrology
University of British Columbia
Vancouver, BC, Canada

Douglas G. Farmer, MD
Professor of Surgery
Director, Intestinal Transplant Program
Surgical Director, Pediatric Liver Transplant Program
Dumont-UCLA Transplant Center
David Geffen School of Medicine at UCLA
Los Angeles, CA, USA

Albert Faro, MD
Associate Professor of Pediatrics
Division of Pediatric Allergy, Immunology and Pulmonary Medicine
Washington University School of Medicine
St. Louis, MO, USA

Alton Brad Farris III, MD
Assistant Professor
Director, Laboratory of Nephropathology and Electron Microscopy
Emory University
Atlanta, GA, USA

Carol Farver, MD, MS
Section Head, Surgical Pathology
Director, Pulmonary Pathology
Pathology and Laboratory Medicine Institute
Cleveland Clinic
Cleveland, OH, USA

Sandy Feng, MD, PhD
Professor of Surgery
Division of Transplant Surgery
University of California, San Francisco
San Francisco, CA, USA

Thomas Fishbein, MD
Executive Director, Georgetown Transplant Institute
Professor of Surgery
Georgetown University School of Medicine
Washington DC, USA

Jay A. Fishman, MD
Associate Director
MGH Transplantation Center;
Director, Transplant Infectious Disease &
Compromised Host Program
Massachusetts General Hospital;
Professor of Medicine
Harvard Medical School
Boston, MA, USA

Rachel C. Forbes, MD, MBA
Assistant Professor of Surgery
Division of Kidney and Pancreas Transplantation
Department of Surgery
Vanderbilt University
Nashville, TN, USA

Mandy L. Ford, PhD
Assistant Professor
Emory Transplant Center
Department of Surgery
Emory University
Atlanta, GA, USA

Richard N. Formica Jr, MD
Associate Professor of Medicine and Surgery
Director, Transplant Nephrology
Medical Director of Adult and Pediatric Kidney
Transplantation
Medical Director of Pancreas Transplantation
Yale University School of Medicine
New Haven, CT, USA

O.H. Frazier, MD
Chief, Transplant Services
Chief, Center for Cardiac Support
Director, Cullen Cardiovascular Research Laboratory
Texas Heart Institute
Houston, TX, USA

Richard Freeman, MD
Professor of Surgery
Dartmouth Hitchcock Medical Center
Lebanon, NH, USA

Alessandrina M. Freitas, MD, MPH
Resident in General Surgery
Department of Surgery
Emory University School of Medicine
Research Fellow
Vascularized Composite Allotransplantation
Emory Transplant Center
Atlanta, GA, USA

John Fung, MD, PhD
Professor of Surgery
Cleveland Clinic Lerner College of Medicine
Case Western Reserve University;
Chairman of Digestive Disease Institute
Cleveland Clinic
Cleveland, OH, USA

Jennifer Garcia, MD
Assistant Professor of Clinical Pediatrics
Division of Gastroenterology, Hepatology, and
Nutrition
University of Miami Miller School of Medicine
Miami Transplant Institute
Miami, FL, USA

Sireesha Garikipati, MD
Fellow in Cardiology
University of Texas Medical Branch
Galveston, TX, USA

Edward R. Garrity Jr, MD, MBA
Professor of Medicine
Vice Chair for Clinical Operations
The University of Chicago Medical Center
Chicago, IL, USA

Robert S. Gaston, MD
Co-Director, Comprehensive Transplant Institute
Robert G. Luke Endowed Chair in Transplant
Nephrology
University of Alabama at Birmingham
Birmingham, AL, USA

Howard M. Gebel, PhD
Professor of Pathology
Co-Director, Histocompatibility and Molecular
Immunogenetics Laboratory
Department of Pathology
Emory University Hospital
Atlanta, GA, USA

Donna George, MS, RN, NEA-BC
Transplant Administrator & Nursing Director
The Hume-Lee Transplant Center
Virginia Commonwealth University Health System
Medical College of Virginia Hospitals
Richmond, VA, USA

John S. Gill, MD, MS, FRCP(C)
Associate Professor, Nephrology
Division of Nephrology
University of British Columbia
St. Paul's Hospital
Vancouver, BC, Canada

Alexandra K. Glazier, JD, MPH
Chair, UNOS Ethics Committee;
Vice-President and General Counsel
New England Organ Bank
Waltham, MA, USA

Denis Glotz
Department of Nephrology and Kidney
Transplantation and Research Unit INSERM U940
Hopital Saint Louis
Paris, France

Veronica Gomez-Lobo, MD
Director of Pediatric and Adolescent Obstetrics and
Gynecology
MedStar Washington Hospital Center and Children's
National Medical Center
Professor of Clinical Obstetrics and Gynecology
Department of Pediatrics, Georgetown University
Washington, DC, USA

Jeremy Goodman, MD, FACS
Assistant Professor of Surgery
Division of Transplant Surgery
University of Alabama at Birmingham
Birmingham, AL, USA

Chad R. Gordon, DO
Assistant Professor of Surgery
Department of Plastic and Reconstructive Surgery
Johns Hopkins University School of Medicine
Baltimore, MD, USA

Michael Green, MD, MPH
Professor of Pediatrics, Surgery and Clinical and
Translational Science
University of Pittsburgh School of Medicine
Division of Infectious Diseases
Children's Hospital of Pittsburgh
Pittsburgh, PA, USA

Bartley P. Griffith, MD
Thomas E. and Alice Marie Hales
Distinguished Professor in Transplantation
University of Maryland School of Medicine
Division of Cardiac Surgery
Baltimore, MD, USA

Tracy C. Grikscheit, MD, FACS
Assistant Professor of Surgery
Children's Hospital Los Angeles
Division of Pediatric Surgery
Keck University of Southern California School of
Medicine
Los Angeles, CA, USA

Josep M. Grinyó, MD
Chief of Nephrology
University Hospital of Bellvitge
University of Barcelona
Barcelona, Spain

Lakshman Gunaratnam
Assistant Professor of Medicine, Microbiology &
Immunology
University of Western Ontario
London, ON, Canada

Susan Gunderson, BSN, MHA
Chief Executive Officer
LifeSource
St. Paul, MN, USA

Divya Gupta, MD
Assistant Professor of Medicine
Division of Cardiology
Advanced Heart Failure and Transplant
Emory University School of Medicine
Atlanta, GA, USA

Philip F. Halloran, MD, PhD
Director
Alberta Transplant Applied Genomics Centre
University of Alberta
Edmonton, AB, Canada

Jenny E. Han
Assistant Professor, Division of Pulmonary and Critical Care Medicine
Department of Medicine
Emory University School of Medicine
Atlanta, GA, USA

Steven I. Hanish, MD
Assistant Professor of Surgery
Emory University School of Medicine
Atlanta, GA, USA

Douglas W. Hanto, MD, PhD
Associate Dean for Continuing Medical Education
Continuing Medical Education Office
Professor of Surgery
Washington University School of Medicine in St. Louis
St. Louis, MO, USA

Karen L. Hardinger, PharmD, BCPS
Clinical Professor of Pharmacy Practice
University of Missouri – Kansas City
School of Pharmacy
Kansas City, MO, USA

William Harmon, MD
Professor of Pediatrics
Harvard Medical School;
Pediatric Nephrology
President, Physicians' Organization
Boston Children's Hospital
Boston, MA, USA

Matt Hartwig, MD
Assistant Professor of Surgery
Duke University
Durham, NC, USA

Koji Hashimoto, MD, PhD
Assistant Professor of Surgery
Cleveland Clinic Lerner College of Medicine
Case Western Reserve University;
Digestive Disease Institute
Cleveland Clinic
Cleveland, OH, USA

Peggy B. Hasley, MD, MHSc
Associate Professor of Internal Medicine
Associate Program Director for Ambulatory Medicine
Director, Generalist Track
University of Pittsburgh Medical Center
Pittsburgh, PA, USA

Steven Head, MS
Director
Microarray and Next Generation Sequencing Core Laboratories
The Scripps Research Institute
La Jolla, CA, USA

Timm Heinbokel
Division of Transplant Surgery and Transplant Surgery Research Laboratory
Brigham and Women's Hospital
Harvard Medical School, Boston, MA;
Institute of Medical Immunology
Charité – Universitätsmedizin Berlin
Berlin, Germany

Peter Heining, PhD
Senior Toxicologist
Novartis Pharmaceuticals Corporation
East Hanover, NJ, USA

Lorna K. Henderson, MBChB, MRCP, PhD
Transplant Fellow
National Pancreas Transplant Unit
University of Sydney at Westmead Hospital
Westmead, NSW, Australia

Mitchell L. Henry, MD
Professor of Surgery
Chief, Division of Transplantation
Department of Surgery
The Ohio State University
Columbus, OH, USA

Joanna Hester, PhD
Senior Scientist
Transplantation Research Immunology Group
Nuffield Department of Surgical Sciences
John Radcliffe Hospital
Oxford, UK

J. Mark Hexham, PhD, MSc
Clinical Research Director
Novartis Pharmaceuticals Corporation
East Hanover, NJ, USA

Naim Issa, MD
Assistant Professor of Medicine
Transplant Nephrologist
Division of Renal Diseases and Hypertension
Department of Medicine
University of Minnesota
Minneapolis, MN, USA

Pamala A. Jacobson, PharmD
Associate Professor
University of Minnesota, College of Pharmacy
Minneapolis, MN, USA

Anthony M. Jevnikar, MD, MSc
Professor of Medicine, Surgery, Microbiology & Immunology
Co-Director Multi Organ Transplant Program
University of Western Ontario
London, ON, Canada

Maryl R. Johnson, MD
Professor of Medicine
Medical Director, Heart Failure and Transplantation
University of Wisconsin School of Medicine and Public Health
Madison, WI, USA

Guido Junge, MD, MBA
Vice President and Global Therapeutic Area Head
Infectious Disease and Transplantation
Novartis Pharma AG
Basel, Switzerland

Elizabeth A. Kallenborn, MSN, RN, CCTC
Clinical Manager
Liver Transplant and Hepatology
Thomas E. Starzl Transplantation Institute
University of Pittsburgh Medical Center
Pittsburgh, PA, USA

Bruce Kaplan, MD
Professor of Medicine, Microbiology, Molecular Genetics and Immunology
University of Kansas Medical Center
Kansas, MO, USA;
Adjunct Professor of Medicine
Alberta Applied Genomics and Transplant Center
University of Alberta, Canada

Dixon B. Kaufman, MD, PhD
Ray Owen Professor and Chair
Division of Transplantation
University of Wisconsin School of Medicine and Public Health
Madison, WI, USA

Daniel Kaul, MD
Associate Professor of Medicine
Director, Transplant Infectious Diseases
Division of Infectious Disease
University of Michigan School of Medicine
Ann Arbor, MI, USA

Tatsuo Kawai, MD, PhD
Associate Professor of Surgery
Harvard Medical School
A. Benedict Cosimi Endowed Chair in Transplant Surgery
Massachusetts General Hospital
Boston MA, USA

Marwan Kazimi, MD
Director
Multivisceral and Intestinal Transplantation Program
Division of Transplant Surgery
Transplant Institute
Henry Ford Hospital
Detroit, MI, USA

Desmond Barry Keenan, PhD, MBA
Research Director and Technical Fellow
Closed Loop Development
Medtronic Diabetes
Northridge, CA, USA

Shaf Keshavjee, MD, MSc, FRCSC, FACS
Surgeon-in-Chief, University Health Network
Professor, Division of Thoracic Surgery
Director, Toronto Lung Transplant Program
University of Toronto
Toronto, ON, Canada

Zain Khalpey, MD, PhD, MRCS(Eng)
Surgical Director of Heart Transplant and Mechanical Circulatory Support
Distinguished Tony Marnell Chair in Cardiothoracic Surgery
Surgical Director of Regenerative Medicine
Associate Professor of Surgery
Physiological Sciences & Biomedical Engineering
University of Arizona
Tucson, AZ, USA

Michael S. Kiernan, MD, MS
Assistant Professor of Medicine
Medical Director, Ventricular Assist Device Program
Tufts University School of Medicine
Boston, MA, USA

S. Joseph Kim
Division of Nephrology
Toronto General Hospital;
University Health Network and the Institute for Health Policy, Management and Evaluation
Faculty of Medicine
University of Toronto
Toronto, ON, Canada

Allan D. Kirk, MD, PhD, FACS
Professor and Chairman, Department of Surgery
Duke University School of Medicine;
Surgeon-in-Chief for Duke University Health System
Duke University Medical Center
Durham, NC, USA

Michelle M. Kittleson, MD, PhD
Assistant Clinical Professor of Medicine, UCLA
Director, Heart Failure Research
Director, Post-Graduate Education in Heart Failure and Transplantation
Cedars-Sinai Heart Institute
Los Angeles, CA, USA

Andrew Klein, MD, MBA, FACS
Director, Comprehensive Transplant Center
Esther and Mark Schulman Chair of Surgery and Transplant Medicine
Professor and Vice Chair
Department of Surgery
Cedars-Sinai Medical Center
Los Angeles, CA, USA

Christina L.M. Klein, MD
Assistant Professor of Medicine
Medical Director, Pancreas Transplant
Director, High Risk Kidney Transplant
Washington University in St. Louis
St. Louis, MO, USA

Stuart J. Knechtle, MD
Professor of Surgery
Emory University School of Medicine
Atlanta, GA, USA

Jon A. Kobashigawa, MD
DSL/Thomas D. Gordon Chair in Heart Transplantation Medicine
Director, Advanced Heart Disease Section
Director, Heart Transplant Program
Cedars-Sinai Heart Institute
Los Angeles, CA, USA

Chatchai Kreepala, MD
Clinical and Research Fellow
Alberta Transplant Applied Genomics Centre
Department of Medicine
Division of Nephrology and Transplant Immunology
University of Alberta
Edmonton, AB, Canada

Jill C. Krisl, PharmD
Transplant Pharmacy Fellow
Department of Surgery
Division of Transplantation
University of Cincinnati
Academic Health Center
Cincinnati, OH, USA

Aleksandra Kukla, MD
Assistant Professor of Medicine
Transplant Nephrologist;
Medical Director of Pancreas Transpant Program
Division of Renal Diseases and Hypertension
Department of Medicine
University of Minnesota
Minneapolis, MN, USA

Sunil M. Kurian, PhD
Staff Scientist
Laboratory of Functional Genomics
Department of Molecular and Experimental Medicine
The Scripps Research Institute
La Jolla, CA, USA

Keren Ladin, PhD, MSc
Director
Research on Ethics, Aging, and Community Health
Tufts University;
Assistant Professor
Department of Occupational Therapy
Tufts University
Medford, MA;
Department of Public Health and Community Medicine
Tufts University School of Medicine
Boston, MA, USA

Alan Langnas
Chief, Section of Transplant Surgery
University of Nebraska Medical Center
Omaha, NE, USA

Dianne LaPointe Rudow, ANP-BC, DNP, CCTC
Associate Professor
Department of Health Evidence and Policy
Director, Zweig Family Center for Living Donation
Medical Director of Liver and Kidney Donor Program
Recanati/Miller Transplant Institute
The Mount Sinai Medical Center
New York, NY, USA

Christian P. Larsen, MD, DPhil
Dean – Emory School of Medicine
Surgeon-in-Chief Emory Healthcare
Emory University
Atlanta, GA, USA

E. Clinton Lawrence, MD
Director, Andrew J. McKelvey Lung Transplant Center
Emory Transplant Center
Emory University Hospital;
Augustus J. McKelvey Professor of Lung Transplantation Medicine
Emory University School of Medicine
Department of Medicine
Division of Pulmonary, Allergy and Critical Care Medicine
Emory University
Atlanta, GA, USA

Daniel J. Lebovitz, MD
Associate Director, Critical Care
Akron Children's Hospital
Akron, OH;
Director, PICU
MetroHealth Medical Center
Cleveland OH;
Medical Director
Lifebanc
Cleveland, OH, USA

Sung-Gyu Lee
Professor of Surgery
Hepato-Biliary Surgery and Liver Transplantation
Department of Surgery
Asan Medical Center
University of Ulsan College of Medicine
Seoul, Korea

W.P. Andrew Lee, MD
The Milton T Edgerton, MD, Professor and Chairman
Department of Plastic and Reconstructive Surgery
Johns Hopkins University School of Medicine
Baltimore, MD, USA

Soyoung Lee, MD
Research Fellow
Massachusetts General Hospital
Boston, MA, USA

Jason R. Lees, PhD
Assistant Professor
Department of Microbiology and Immunology
Uniformed Services of Health Sciences
Bethesda, MD, USA

Carmen Lefaucheur
Department of Nephrology and Kidney Transplantation and Research Unit INSERM U940
Hopital Saint Louis
Paris, France

Henri G.D. Leuvenink, PhD
Associate Professor
Principle Investigator, Experimental Transplantation
Surgical Research Laboratory
Department of Surgery
University Medical Center Groningen
Groningen, The Netherlands

Matthew H. Levine, MD, PhD
Assistant Professor of Surgery
Division of Transplant Surgery
Perelman School of Medicine
University of Pennsylvania
Philadelphia, PA, USA

Xian C. Li, MD, PhD, ASCI
Director
Immunobiology & Transplantation Research
Houston Methodist Hospital
Texas Medical Center
Houston, Texas

Sundus A. Lodhi, MD,
Assistant Professor
Transplant Nephrology
Emory University
Atlanta, GA, USA

Marc I. Lorber, MD
Sr. Vice President and Chief Medical Officer
XenoLung Clinical Development
Lung Biotechnology, Inc
United Therapeutics Corporation
Silver Spring, MD, USA

Richard S. Luskin, MPA
President and CEO
New England Organ Bank
Waltham, MA, USA

G. Marshall Lyon, MD, MMSc
Associate Professor of Medicine
Director of Transplant Infectious Disease
Emory University School of Medicine
Atlanta, GA, USA

Joren C. Madsen, MD, DPhil
Professor of Surgery
W. Gerald and Patricia R. Austen
Distinguished Scholar in Cardiac Surgery
Massachusetts General Hospital
Boston, MA, USA

Joseph F. Magliocca, MD
Assistant Professor of Surgery
Emory University School of Medicine
Atlanta, GA, USA

Sayeed Malek, MD
Clinical Director, Division of Transplant Surgery
Brigham and Women's Hospital
Harvard Medical School
Boston, MA, USA

Roslyn B. Mannon, MD
Professor of Medicine and Surgery
University of Alabama at Birmingham
Birmingham, AL, USA

James F. Markmann, MD, PhD
Professor of Surgery
Harvard Medical School;
Chief, Division of Transplantation
Massachusetts General Hospital
Boston, MA, USA

Benjamin M. Martin, MD
Senior Resident, Department of Surgery
Emory University School of Medicine
Atlanta, GA, USA

Paulo Martins, MD, PhD
Instructor, Harvard Medical School
Clinical Fellow, Massachusetts General Hospital
Boston, MA, USA

Allan B. Massie, PhD
Department of Surgery
Johns Hopkins School of Medicine
Baltimore, MD, USA

Virginia A. McBride, RN, MPH
President
AMVAT Consulting
Grand Junction, CO, USA

Kenneth R. McCurry, MD
Staff Surgeon
CCF
Cleveland Clinic
Cleveland, OH, USA

Gwen McNatt, MS, RN, CNN, FNP-BC
Director, Operations
Kovler Organ Transplantation Center and Infectious Disease
Northwestern Memorial Hospital
Chicago, IL, USA

Mandeep R. Mehra, MD
Brigham and Women's Hospital
Harvard Medical School
Boston, MA, USA

Aneesh K. Mehta, MD
Assistant Professor of Medicine
Assistant Director of Transplant Infectious Diseases
Emory University School of Medicine
Atlanta, GA, USA

Edward A. Meister, PhD
College of Medicine
Division of Nephrology
University of Arizona
Tucson, AZ, USA

Michael H. Mengel, MD
Associate Professor
University of Alberta
Edmonton, AB, Canada

Diana Metes, MD
Associate Professor of Surgery and Immunology
Starzl Transplantation Institute
Department of Surgery and Department of Immunology
University of Pittsburgh School of Medicine
Pittsburgh, PA, USA

Charles M. Miller, MD
Professor of Surgery
Cleveland Clinic Lerner College of Medicine
Case Western Reserve University;
Director, Liver Transplant Program
Digestive Disease Institute
Cleveland Clinic
Cleveland, OH, USA

Marta I. Minervini, MD
Assistant Professor of Pathology
Department of Pathology
University of Pittsburgh Medical Center
Pittsburgh, PA, USA

Saeed Mohammad, MD, MS
Assistant Professor
Department of Pediatrics
Northwestern University Feinberg School of Medicine
Ann and Robert H. Lurie Children's Hospital of Chicago
Chicago, IL, USA

Deok-Bog Moon
Professor of Surgery
Hepato-Biliary Surgery and Liver Transplantation
Department of Surgery
Asan Medical Center
University of Ulsan College of Medicine
Seoul, Korea

Christian Morath, MD
Department of Medicine
Division of Nephrology and Hypertension
University of Heidelberg
Heidelberg, Germany

Michael J. Moritz, MD
Chief, Transplant Services
Lehigh Valley Health Network
Allentown, PA;
Professor of Surgery
University of South Florida
Morsani College of Medicine
Tampa, FL, USA

Tim Morris
Director, Research Informatics
Research and Woodruff Health Sciences IT
Emory University
Atlanta, GA, USA

Cathi L. Murphey, PhD
Director, Histocompatibility and Immunogenetics Laboratory
Southwest Immunodiagnostics, Inc.
San Antonio, TX, USA

Michael A. Nalesnik, MD
Professor of Pathology
Department of Pathology
University of Pittsburgh Medical Center
Pittsburgh, PA, USA

Jung-Man Namgoong
Clinical Instructor of Surgery
Hepato-Biliary Surgery and Liver Transplantation
Department of Surgery
Asan Medical Center
University of Ulsan College of Medicine
Seoul, Korea

Brian J. Nankivell, MD, PhD, FRACP
Transplant Physician
Department of Renal Medicine
Westmead Hospital
Sydney, NSW, Australia

Peter Neuhaus, MD, PhD
Chairman of General, Visceral, and Transplantation Surgery
Experimental Surgery and Regenerative Medicine
Charité – Campus Virchow, Universitätsmedizin Berlin
Berlin, Germany

David C. Neujahr, MD
Medical Director
Andrew McKelvey Adult Lung Transplant Program
Emory University Transplant Center
Assistant Professor of Medicine, Pulmonary, Allergy and Critical Care
Emory University School of Medicine
Atlanta, GA, USA

Kenneth A. Newell, MD, PhD
Professor of Surgery
Emory Transplant Center
Emory University School of Medicine
Atlanta, GA, USA

Silke Niederhaus, MD
Assistant Professor of Surgery
University of Maryland Medical System
Division of Transplantation
Baltimore, MD, USA

Seigo Nishida, MD
Department of Surgery, Division of Transplantation
University of Miami
Miami, FL, USA

Douglas J. Norman, MD
Professor of Medicine
Director, Transplant Medicine
Director, Laboratory of Immunogenetics and Transplantation
Oregon Health & Science University
Portland, OR, USA

Rupert Oberhuber, MD
Division of Transplant Surgery and Transplant Surgery Research Laboratory
Brigham and Women's Hospital
Harvard Medical School
Boston, MA;
Department of Visceral, Transplant and Thoracic Surgery
Medical University of Innsbruck
Innsbruck, Austria

Philip J. O'Connell, MBBS, PhD, FRACP
Professor and Director of Transplantation
University of Sydney at Westmead Hospital
Sydney, NSW, Australia

Jon S. Odorico, MD, FACS
Professor of Surgery
Director, Pancreas Transplantation
Co-director, Islet Transplantation
University of Wisconsin School of Medicine and Public Health
Madison, WI, USA

John G. O'Grady, MD, FRCPI
Professor of Hepatology
Institute of Liver Studies
King's College Hospital
London, UK

Linda Ohler, MSN, RN, CCTC, FAAN
Quality and Compliance Manager
Georgetown Transplant Institute
Georgetown University Hospital
Washington, DC, USA

Toshihiro Okamoto, MD, PhD
Department of Thoracic and Cardiovascular Surgery, Heart and Vascular Institute
Cleveland Clinic
Cleveland, OH, USA

Marc J. Overcash
Deputy Chief Information Officer
Assistant Dean, Information Technology
Emory University School of Medicine
Atlanta, GA, USA

Eugenia K. Page, MD
Surgical Resident
Emory University School of Medicine
Atlanta, GA, USA

John C. Papadimitriou, MD, PhD
Professor of Pathology
Director, Surgical Pathology
University of Maryland School of Medicine
Baltimore, MD, USA

Samir Parekh, MD
Assistant Professor of Medicine
Transplant Hepatology Fellowship Director
Emory University School of Medicine
The Emory Transplant Center
Atlanta, GA, USA

Steven M. Parnis, BS
Assistant Director, Center for Technology Development
Texas Heart Institute
Houston, TX, USA

Stephen Pastan, MD
Medical Director, Kidney and Pancreas Transplant Program
Emory Transplant Center
Associate Professor of Medicine
Emory University School of Medicine
Atlanta, GA, USA

Jignesh K. Patel, MD, PhD
Medical Director, Heart Transplant Program
Cedars-Sinai Heart Institute
Los Angeles, CA, USA

Thomas C. Pearson, MD, DPhil
Livingston Professor of Surgery
Emory University School of Medicine;
Executive Director
Director, Kidney Transplant Program
Emory Transplant Center
Atlanta, GA, USA

Alice Peng, MD
Associate Professor of Medicine
Medical Director
Pancreas Transplantation Program
Cedars-Sinai Medical Center
Los Angeles, CA, USA

Phuong-Chi T. Pham, MD
Professor of Medicine
David Geffen School of Medicine at UCLA
Olive View-UCLA-Medical Center
Chief, Division of Nephrology and Hypertension
Director, UCLA-OVMC Nephrology Training Program
Sylmar, CA, USA

Phuong-Thu T. Pham, MD
Professor of Medicine
David Geffen School of Medicine at UCLA
Department of Medicine, Nephrology Division
Director, Outpatient Services
Kidney Transplant Program
Los Angeles, CA, USA

Nicole A. Pilch, PharmD, MSCR, BCPS
Residency Program Director, PGY-2 Transplant Residency Program
Clinical Specialist, Solid Organ Transplantation
Clinical Assistant Professor, Department of Pharmacy and Clinical Sciences
South Carolina College of Pharmacy – MUSC Campus
Medical University of South Carolina
Department of Pharmacy Services
Charleston, SC, USA

Rutger J. Ploeg, MD, PhD, FRCS
Professor of Transplant Biology
University of Oxford;
Professor of Transplant Surgery
University of Groningen;
Honorary Consultant Transplant Surgeon
OUH NHS Trust
Nuffield Department of Surgical Sciences
Oxford, UK

Jennifer M. Porter, Esq
Partner, Gurne Porter, PLLC
Washington, DC, USA

Luke Preczewski
Administrative Director
Comprehensive Transplant Center
Northwestern University Feinberg School of Medicine
Chicago, IL, USA

Timothy L. Pruett, MD
John S. Najarian Clinical Chair
Professor of Surgery and Internal Medicine
University of Minnesota
Minneapolis, MN, USA

Cristiano Quintini, MD
Assistant Professor of Surgery
Cleveland Clinic Lerner College of Medicine
Case Western Reserve University
Liver Transplant Program
Digestive Disease Institute
Cleveland Clinic
Cleveland, OH, USA

Giorgio Raimondi, PhD
Department of Plastic and Reconstructive Surgery
Johns Hopkins School of Medicine
Baltimore, MD, USA

Raja Rajalingam, PhD
Professor of Clinical Surgery
Director of Immunogenetics and Transplantation Laboratory
University of California, San Francisco
San Francisco, CA, USA

Parmjeet Randhawa, MD
Professor of Pathology
Department of Pathology
University of Pittsburgh Medical Center
Pittsburgh, PA, USA

Nathanael Raschzok, MD
General, Visceral, and Transplantation Surgery
Experimental Surgery and Regenerative Medicine
Universitätsmedizin Berlin
Berlin, Germany

Elaine F. Reed, PhD
Professor
Department of Pathology and Laboratory Medicine;
Director, UCLA Immunogenetics Center
David Geffen School of Medicine
University of California, Los Angeles
Los Angeles, CA, USA

John Adam Reich, MD
Instructor of Anesthesiology
Tufts University
Staff Anesthesiologist
Director, Post Anesthesia Care Unit
Tufts Medical Center
Boston, MA, USA

Scott A. Reule, MD
Nephrology Fellow
Division of Renal Diseases and Hypertension
Department of Medicine
University of Minnesota
Minneapolis, MN, USA

Camillo Ricordi, MD
Stacy Joy Goodman Professor of Surgery
Director, Cell Transplant Center and Diabetes Research Institute
University of Miami
Miami, FL, USA

E. Rene Rodriguez, MD
Professor of Pathology
Director, Cardiovascular Pathology
Director, Autopsy Pathology
Department of Anatomic Pathology/L25
The Cleveland Clinic
Cleveland, OH, USA

Christin C. Rogers, PharmD, FCCP, BCPS
Clinical Pharmacy Coordinator – Solid Organ Transplant
Beth Israel Deaconess Medical Center
Boston, MA, USA

Erin Rubin, MD
Associate Professor of Pathology
Department of Pathology
University of Pittsburgh Medical Center
Pittsburgh, PA, USA

Phillip Ruiz Jr, MD, PhD
Professor of Pathology and Surgery
Medical Director, Transplant Laboratories
University of Miami Miller School of Medicine
Miami, FL, USA

David H. Sachs, MD
Scientific Director, Transplantation Biology Research Center
Massachusetts General Hospital;
Paul S Russel/Warner-Lambert Professor of Surgery
Harvard Medical School
Boston, MA, USA

Daniel R. Salomon, MD
Professor, Department of Molecular and Experimental Medicine
Program Medical Director, Scripps Center for Organ Transplantation
The Scripps Research Institute
La Jolla, CA, USA

Alberto Sánchez-Fueyo, MD, PhD
Institute of Liver Studies
School of Medicine
King's College London
Denmark Hill
London, UK

Chandrasekar Santhanakrishnan, MD
Assistant Professor of Clinical Surgery
Division of Transplant Surgery
Department of Surgery
University of California Davis Medical Center
Sacramento, CA, USA

Eizaburo Sasatomi, MD, PhD
Assistant Professor of Pathology
Department of Pathology
University of Pittsburgh Medical Center
Pittsburgh, PA, USA

Igor M. Sauer, MD
Chairman of Research
General, Visceral, and Transplantation Surgery
Experimental Surgery and Regenerative Medicine
Charité – Campus Virchow, Universitätsmedizin Berlin
Berlin, Germany

Deirdre Sawinski, MD
Assistant Professor of Medicine
Department of Medicine
University of Pennsylvania Perelman School of Medicine
Philadelphia, PA, USA

Birgit Sawitzki
Institute of Medical Immunology
Charite University Medicine
Berlin, Germany

Franz Schaefer, MD
Professor of Pediatrics
Center for Pediatrics and Adolescent Medicine
University of Heidelberg
Heidelberg, Germany

Margaret Schaeffer, MS, MSHA, RN
Virginia Commonwealth University Health System
Medical College of Virginia Hospitals
Nurse Manager
Hume-Lee Transplant Center
Richmond, VA, USA

Peter Schemmer, MD, MBA
Department of Surgery
Division of Visceral and Transplantation Surgery
University of Heidelberg
Heidelberg, Germany

Stefan Schneeberger, MD
Department of Visceral, Transplant and Thoracic Surgery
Innsbruck Medical University
Innsbruck, Austria;
Department of Plastic and Reconstructive Surgery
Johns Hopkins University School of Medicine
Baltimore, MD, USA

Jesse D. Schold, PhD
Associate Staff
Department of Quantitative Health Sciences
Cleveland Clinic
Cleveland, OH, USA

Kristine S. Schonder, PharmD
Assistant Professor
Pharmacy and Therapeutics
Clinical Pharmacist, Transplant
University of Pittsburgh School of Pharmacy
Thomas E. Starzl Transplantation Institute
Pittsburgh, PA, USA

Kathy Schwab, RN, BSN, CCTC
Compliance Coordinator
Mayo Clinic
Rochester, MN, USA

Dorry L. Segev, MD, PhD
Associate Vice Chair of Research
Associate Professor of Surgery
Associate Professor of Epidemiology
Johns Hopkins University
Baltimore, MD, USA

Gennaro Selvaggi, MD
Associate Professor of Clinical Surgery
University of Miami Miller School of Medicine
Miami Transplant Institute
Miami, FL, USA

Keyur B. Shah, MD
Virginia Commonwealth University;
Medical College of Virginia Hospital
Richmond, VA, USA

A.M. James Shapiro, MD, PhD, FRCS(Eng), FRCSC, MSM, DSc, FRS(Canada)
Canada Research Chair in Transplantation Surgery and Regenerative Medicine
Director, Clinical Islet Transplant Program
University of Alberta
Edmonton, AB, Canada

Ron Shapiro, MD
Professor of Surgery
Robert J. Corry Chair in Transplantation Surgery
University of Pittsburgh Medical Center
Thomas E. Starzl Transplantation Institute
Pittsburgh, PA, USA

Chris Shay-Downer, RN, BSN, CCTC
Transplant & Cardiac Program Director
BioScrip, Inc.
Elmsford, NY, USA

Jaimie T. Shores
Assistant Professor of Plastic Surgery
Department of Plastic and Reconstructive Surgery
Johns Hopkins University School of Medicine
Baltimore, MD, USA

William D. Simmons, RPh
US Medical
Novartis Pharmaceuticals Corporation
Madison, WI, USA

Daniel B. Sims, MD
Assistant Professor
Montefiore Medical Center
Albert Einstein College of Medicine
Bronx, NY, USA

Alan Slade, PharmD
Translational Medicine Director, Transplantation
Novartis Pharmaceuticals Corporation
East Hanover, NJ, USA

Richard G. Smith, MSEE
Director, Marshall Foundation Artificial Heart Laboratory
University Medical Center
Tucson, AZ, USA

Andrew L. Smith, MD
Professor of Medicine
Medical Director, Heart Failure and Transplantation
Division of Cardiology
Emory University School of Medicine
Atlanta, GA, USA

Lonnie D. Smith, PharmD
Manager, Department of Solid Organ Transplant
Director, PGY-2 Pharmacy Residency – Transplant
University of Utah Hospitals and Clinics
Salt Lake City, UT, USA

Mark Schnitzler, PhD
Professor
St. Louis University School of Medicine
St. Louis, MO, USA

Hans W. Sollinger, MD, PhD
Folkert Belzer Professor
Division of Transplantation
University of Wisconsin School of Medicine and Public Health
Madison, WI, USA

Lisa G. Sorensen, PhD
Assistant Professor of Clinical Psychiatry and Behavioral Sciences
Northwestern University Feinberg School of Medicine;
Ann and Robert H. Lurie Children's Hospital of Chicago
Chicago, IL, USA

James R. Spivey, MD
Associate Professor of Medicine and Surgery
Director of Hepatology
Medical Director, Liver Transplantation
Emory University School of Medicine
The Emory Transplant Center
Atlanta, GA, USA

Mark D. Stegall
Professor of Surgery and Immunology
Mayo Clinic
Rochester, MN, USA

Josef Stehlik, MD, MPH
Associate Professor of Medicine
University of Utah School of Medicine
Salt Lake City, UT, USA

Garry M. Steil, PhD
Research Scientist, Division of Medicine Critical Care
Boston Children's Hospital;
Assistant Professor of Pediatrics
Harvard Medical School
Boston, MA, USA

Neema Stephens, MD
Assistant Professor
Transplant Nephrology
University of Texas – San Antonio
San Antonio, TX, USA

Peter G. Stock, MD, PhD
Division of Transplant Surgery
University of California, San Francisco
San Francisco, CA, USA

Margaret L. Stuber, MD
Assistant Dean of Student Affairs for Career Development and Well-Being
Vice Chair for Education in Psychiatry
Daniel X. Freedman Professor, Psychiatry and Biobehavioral Sciences
David Geffen School of Medicine at UCLA
Los Angeles, CA, USA

Charles A. Su, BS
Graduate Student
Department of Immunology
Cleveland Clinic
Cleveland, OH, USA

Ram M. Subramanian
Assistant Professor of Medicine and Surgery
Emory University School of Medicine
Atlanta, GA, USA

Stuart C. Sweet, MD, PhD
W. McKim Marriott Professor of Pediatrics
Division of Pediatric Allergy, Immunology and Pulmonary Medicine
Washington University School of Medicine
St. Louis, MO, USA

David J. Taber, PharmD, BCPS
Assistant Professor
Division of Transplant Surgery
Department of Surgery
Medical University of South Carolina
Charleston, SC, USA

Carmela D. Tan, MD
Assistant Professor
Department of Anatomic Pathology
The Cleveland Clinic
Cleveland, OH, USA

Akin Tekin, MD
Assistant Professor of Clinical Surgery
University of Miami Miller School of Medicine
Miami Transplant Institute
Miami, FL, USA

Paul I. Terasaki, PhD
Professor Emeritus
University of California, Los Angeles;
Terasaki Foundation
Los Angeles, CA, USA

Angus W. Thomson, PhD, DSc
Distinguished Professor of Surgery and Immunology
Starzl Transplantation Institute;
Department of Surgery and Department of Immunology
University of Pittsburgh School of Medicine
Pittsburgh, PA, USA

Eric M. Tichy, PharmD, FCCP, BCPS
Clinical Pharmacy Specialist
Solid Organ Transplant
Director, PGY-2 Residency – Transplant
Yale-New Haven Hospital
Department of Pharmacy
New Haven, CT, USA

Paul L. Tso, MD
Associate Professor of Surgery
Emory University School of Medicine
Atlanta, GA, USA

Stefan G. Tullius, MD, PhD, FACS
Professor of Surgery, Harvard Medical School
Chief, Division of Transplant Surgery & Director,
Transplant Surgery Research Laboratory,
Brigham and Women's Hospital
Boston, MA, USA

Nicole A. Turgeon, MD, FACS
Assistant Professor of Surgery
Emory University Hospital
Atlanta, GA, USA

Alexandra P. Turner, MD
Abdominal Transplant Fellow
Emory Transplant Center
Department of Surgery
Emory University School of Medicine
Atlanta, GA, USA

Heth R. Turnquist, PhD
Assistant Professor of Surgery and Immunology
Starzl Transplantation Institute
Department of Surgery and Department of Immunology
University of Pittsburgh School of Medicine
Pittsburgh, PA, USA

Andreas Tzakis, MD, PhD, Dhc
Director of Liver and Kidney Transplant
Cleveland Clinic Florida
Weston, FL, USA

Simon Urschel, MD
Assistant Professor of Pediatrics and Immunology
Department of Pediatrics
Alberta Transplant Institute
University of Alberta
Edmonton, AB, Canada

Parsia A. Vagefi, MD
Division of Transplant Surgery
Massachusetts General Hospital;
Harvard Medical School
Boston, MA, USA

Anna Valujskikh, PhD
Associate Staff, Department of Immunology
Cleveland Clinic
Cleveland, OH, USA

Ronald G. Van Valen
Sr. Global Program
Regulatory Director/Transplantation
Novartis Pharmaceuticals
East Hanover, NJ, USA

Robert S. Venick, MD
Assistant Professor of Pediatrics
David Geffen School of Medicine at UCLA
Los Angeles, CA, USA

Flavio Vincenti, MD
Professor of Clinical Medicine
University of California
San Francisco, CA, USA

Gus J. Vlahakes, MD
Professor of Surgery
Massachusetts General Hospital
Boston, MA, USA

Philip Y. Wai, MD
Assistant Professor of Surgery
Division of Intra-abdominal Transplantation
Department of Surgery
Loyola University Medical Center
Maywood, IL, USA

W. Dean Wallace, MD
Associate Professor
Chief, Pulmonary Pathology
Department of Pathology and Laboratory Medicine
David Geffen School of Medicine at UCLA
Los Angeles, CA, USA

Candace Wang, MD
Novartis Pharmaceuticals Corporation
East Hanover, NJ, USA

Rui Wang
The Transplant Institute and Center for Transplant Outcomes and Quality Improvement
Beth Israel Deaconess Medical Center;
Harvard Medical School
Boston, MA, USA

Claire A. Watkins, MD, MS
Resident Physician in Cardiothoracic Surgery
University of Maryland School of Medicine
Division of Cardiac Surgery
Baltimore, MD, USA

Melissa Watson, MD
Clinical Fellow
Abdominal Multiorgan Transplantation Surgery
Cleveland Clinic
Cleveland, OH, USA

Jeff Weaver, MBA
Director, Data Solutions
Research and Woodruff Health Sciences IT
Emory University
Atlanta, GA, USA

Steven A. Webber, MBChB, MRCP
James C. Overall Professor and Chair
Department of Pediatrics
Vanderbilt University School of Medicine
Nashville, TN, USA

Allison B. Webber, MD
Assistant Clinical Professor of Medicine
University of California
San Francisco, CA, USA

Lori J. West, MD, DPhil, FRCPC
Professor of Pediatrics, Surgery and Immunology
Department of Pediatrics
Alberta Transplant Institute
University of Alberta
Edmonton, AB, Canada

David Wheeler, RRT
Anesthesia Institute
Cleveland Clinic
Cleveland, OH, USA

Marissa B. Wilck, MBChB
Assistant Professor
Department of Medicine
University of Pennsylvania
Philadelphia, PA, USA

Kathryn J. Wood, DPhil
Professor of Immunology
Transplantation Research Immunology Group
Nuffield Department of Surgical Sciences
John Radcliffe Hospital
Oxford, UK

E. Steve Woodle, MD, FACS
William A. Altemeier Chair in Surgery
Professor of Surgery
Director, Division of Transplantation
Director, Isreal Penn International Tranasplant Tumor Registry
University of Cincinnati
Cincinnati, OH, USA

Jiangnan Xu, MD
Associate Professor
Capital Medical University
Beijing, China

Heidi Yeh, MD
Surgical Director
Pediatric Transplantation;
Instructor, Harvard Medical School
Assistant in Surgery, Massachusetts General Hospital
Boston, MA, USA

Jonathan C. Yeung, MD, PhD
Fellow in Thoracic Surgery
Toronto Lung Transplant Program
University Health Network
University of Toronto
Toronto, ON, Canada

Melissa Y. Yeung, MD, FRCPC
Instructor in Medicine
Transplantation Research Center
Brigham and Women's Hospital and Harvard Medical School
Boston, MA, USA

Martin G. Zeier, MD, FASN
Head, Division of Nephrology
Heidelberg University Hospital
Heidelberg, Germany

Qiuheng Zhang, PhD
Assistant Professor
Department of Pathology and Laboratory Medicine;
Associate Director
UCLA Immunogenetics Center
David Geffen School of Medicin,
University of California, Los Angeles
Los Angeles, CA, USA

Shelley Zomak, RN MS CCTC
Unit Director, Cardiothoracic Transplant
University of Pittsburgh Medical Center
Pittsburgh, PA, USA

中文版序言

经历半个多世纪的探索与发展，在全球范围内，以心脏、肝脏、肾脏等大器官移植为代表的器官移植技术已经挽救了近百万罹患各类终末期疾病患者的生命，器官移植技术已经成为治疗终末期器官衰竭的最佳手段。在我国器官移植工作者数十载孜孜以求的不懈努力下，中国器官移植无论在实施数量还是临床疗效方面，都取得了令国人鼓舞、国际瞩目的巨大成就，成千上万的终末期疾病患者获得了新生。为了更好地推进健康中国建设，一个重大且亟待解决的现实问题摆在我们面前：我们应当为器官移植事业的人才培养做些什么？要培养未来一流的临床医生、医学科学家，必须以一流的医学教育作为基础。

因此，编撰一本适应当前器官移植教育教学需求的《器官移植学》教材是人才培养的要求、国家的需求、时代的需求。

由美国 Wiley Blackwell 出版社出版的 *Textbook of Organ Transplantation* 一书内容新颖、丰富，紧跟科学技术前沿，不仅涵盖医学专业领域知识，还包括相关移植国家政策的介绍与解读，是国际移植学术界经典的参考用书，广受好评。此书的中文版由北京大学人民医院朱继业教授和浙江大学医学院附属第一医院徐骁教授领衔翻译，50余位移植临床、教学和科研一线且经验丰富的专家学者共同努力，同心同德，群策群力，在尊重原文的前提下，灵活解读，用词精准，文笔简练，使读者更易于理解与阅读。因此，我相信本书不仅可作为器官移植专科医师的培训教材，也是研究生科研与创新的参考书，更是广大奋战于器官移植一线工作者的工具书，同时也可为国家器官移植相关政策制定与修改提供重要借鉴。

器官移植学是生物医学学科领域中一门年轻活跃、发展迅速的新兴学科。随着分子生物学与基因工程技术逐步介入移植及其相关研究领域，器官移植面临着前所未有的挑战与机遇。我能为此书作序，感到十分的荣幸，愿借此书以启发广大从事器官移植专业的医务工作者们，更好地服务于健康中国建设。

中国工程院院士
中华医学会副会长
中国医师协会副会长
鄭樹森

中文版前言

器官移植作为20世纪最伟大的医学成果之一，经过半个多世纪的发展，已经成为终末期器官功能衰竭患者的有效治疗手段。我国器官移植始于20世纪70年代，几经波折，但经过老一辈移植工作者的不懈努力，目前已经发展成为世界器官移植第二大国，其数量和质量都居于国际领先水平。由黄洁夫部长推动的器官移植改革已经使得国际社会彻底接受和承认中国在器官移植领域所取得的成就，我国提出的器官捐献的“中国模式”、肝癌肝移植的“杭州标准”已经被世界所认同，中国正以崭新的姿态站在世界器官移植的舞台上。

器官移植学是一门新兴学科，涉及多个学科的交叉和融合，新概念和新技术不断涌现，为了更好地与国际移植学界接轨，培养我国优秀的器官移植人才，特组织工作在移植一线的专家学者翻译了此部由美国艾伦·D.柯克等教授所著的《器官移植学》上下卷。

本书内容全面丰富，除了囊括了器官移植历史、基础理论、手术技术、术后管理、器官分配等各个方面，同时还涵盖了移植伦理、移植研究设计、移植政策制定等非临床相关内容，是一本不可多得的器官移植教学参考书。

由于时间仓促和水平有限，本书翻译过程中难免有疏漏之处，恳请广大读者给予批评指正。

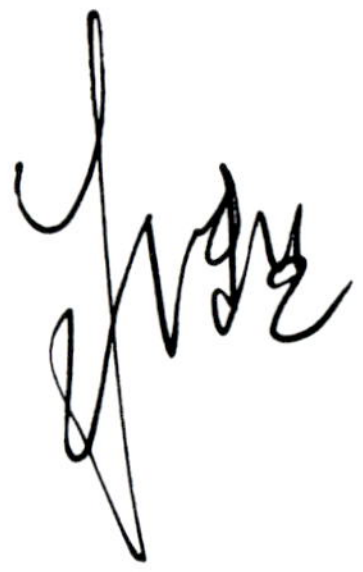

目　录

上卷

下卷

第 1 篇

历史/前言

前　言

Allan D. Kirk

要了解器官移植,就等于要了解所有的现代医学,而开展器官移植就要全面理解现代医疗所带来的根本挑战。

尽管本书介绍的内容会因为这个领域日新月异的发展而出现一些偏差,但并没有夸大其词。实际上,客观来讲,很少有认真的医学生会为他们所坚持的原则进行争辩。

最基本的医学诊断即活着或死亡。在很大程度上,对死亡的客观确定是由于器官捐赠的伦理需要,脑死亡概念和临床器官捐献也密不可分,而且,移植医师必须比任何领域的人都了解这些标准。同样,除了知道什么构成了活的个体,专业的移植工作者还会通过客观阐述我们仅作为人体的一部分来重新定义我们是谁。从功利主义角度来讲,我们身体的大部分是可替换的。实际上,这个概念在器官移植中是经验性的,密切相关的移植工作者比其他专业医生更有发言权。在更微观的水平上,移植工作者(为了避免混淆科学家、外科医师、非外科医师等所有在器官移植领域的工作人员而创造的一个专业术语)是把人的生物学特性——分子组织相容性作为移植工具。对于器官捐献来讲,通过移植研究提出的基本的生物学特性和脑死亡概念同等重要。显然,相比其他领域的专家,移植工作者更经常应用这些生物学特性去解决伦理问题的难点,还要处理每天实际面对的关于利益、争议和效用的问题。

除了上述的高级概念,移植的综合诊疗在医疗实践的日常工作中也应运而生,并确定了其核心地位。移植一直用来治疗终末期疾病,而所讨论的疾病的病因可能是器官特异性的,而任何器官疾病达到终末期都需要进行移植。因此,移植工作者不得不化整为零地看待一个患者。暴发性肝功能衰竭的患者很少发生严重的脑、心、肺或肾功能障碍。决定纠正潜在的肝功能衰竭时,移植工作者必须先严格判定这些系统的功能,然后才能进行手术,而不能只是关注于一个器官。同样,鉴于移植后免疫调节治疗的复杂性,移植工作者需要起到类似于保健与康复相关亚专业的作用。由于需要参与延长受者寿命的免疫治疗,器官移植者对长期健康维护的理解要远超于其他亚专业的专家。对于移植外科医师来讲,要比普通外科医师更精通对糖尿病和高血压的药物治疗,更了解手术相关并发症及切口愈合。另外,接受移植的患者也可能和普通患者一样患有相同疾病,但是器官移植接受者患任何疾病都可能在一定程度上涉及器官移植。移植事业的发展,成功推动器官移植成为所有相关专业的核心。如果没有移植相关的基础知识,不能认为自己是一个真正的专科医师,包括心内科、内分泌科、消化科、肝病科、肾内科、儿科、呼吸科或者外科。

移植药理学同样推动了药理学的发展。免疫抑制治疗的概念源自移植治疗,临床上首次将单克隆抗体和生物工程应用于移植。移植药理学较少用到,但是长期服务于移植事业的临床药师也需要掌握。

事实证明,通过移植的方法可以促进医疗保健的不断发展。如同首次移植成功所述,移植需要多学科合作,从一开始,外科医师、内科医师、护士、综合医疗保健人员和基础研究的科学家共同组成的团队超过了其他的医学领域,移植不是成了一个团队,而是自始至终都是一个团队从而成为促进医疗服务向前发展的榜样。在更高层次的水平,很久以前采用的移植医疗服务方法现在依然很流行:保健网络、定额付款计划、支付协议、公私合作,移植的分配方法在过去的几十年已经进行了更新,医学的其他领域会再次期望移植作为数据源构建健康服务模型。

同样,移植已经演示了通过记录地区或国家层面的数据来描绘未来的客观方法。捐献者的有限可用性和疾病治疗的生死存亡,毫无疑问地刺激着人们探索并发展该领域。虽然其他领域可能在基本的约束(短缺和严重程度)上有不同的看法,但移植临床数据库模型对其他医学领域有很多可借鉴之处。移植所积极报道的并发症,为癌症、感染性疾病、代谢综合征等很多疾病的生物学方面带来了启示。基础生理学也已经从器官替代的实验中获得了难以估计的发展。

总之,教材内容的广度和深度,要覆盖器官移植的所有方向是一项艰巨的任务。但是,没有什么比移植本身面临的挑战更多了:以一个人的心脏替换另一个人的心脏,免疫治疗,合理分配稀缺的捐献器官,支付所有费用……

因此,本书的核心内容并非包含一切或达到最大的深度,而是要合理地阐明移植工作者的大部分工作。章节的安排可能是医师所期望的顺序。首先提出基础概念,从必要的发展史和一般性科学概念到移植相关生物学和同种免疫、免疫调节的基本原则。其次,所有的移植都离不开供体,展开了手术前、手术及手术后三部分临床相关内容。每一部分的章节都包含主要的系统器官:肾、肝、心脏、肺、胰腺和胰岛、小肠和多器官联合、区域性选择、血管复合移植。在术前的部分中,有器官功能达到终末期的重症患者进行复杂治疗相关的具体章节,包括重症特级护理和人工生命支持设备。手术的部分介绍了重要的手术技术,明确了做任何事情都有很多种方法。其目标是为外科医师在起始阶段提供基本要点并帮助他们合理理解手术过程。术后部分主要内容为具体的器官移植后管理,包括急性和慢性治疗问题,对免疫治疗及其后续问题、特殊感染和恶性并发症也提供了足够关注。排斥的诊断作为术后患者最关心的核心问题,有以下两种方法:用该器官明确的组织病理学或者该器官的临床治疗优势诊断。该部分以当前每一种器官移植远期预后结束。

如上所述,目前移植相关的基础设施和组织需求、道德原则和管理指南是广大医疗社区遇到的特殊问题。因此,术中的几个部分阐述了这些问题,不仅要教授学生学习移植方面特殊的知识,即"怎么解决问题",还要给学生示例在其他领域可能怎么做。

本书的总体目标是合理呈现当代移植复杂性的各个方面。希望这样的参考书在某些时候能够派上用场。对于本科生、医学生、住院医师或者进修医师来说,本书会成为帮助他们在移植事业中拓宽视野、开拓进取的助手。对于从事等待患者的护理、移植后随访的非移植专业人员,如心内科、内分泌科、消化科、肝病科、肾内科、呼吸科等医师来讲,本书会提供足够的随访相关知识,以及明确何时转诊比较明智。实际上,有两章内容是直接介绍社区医师所关注的问题。对于真正的移植工作者,当碰到移植中不常见的问题时,这些知识是不可或缺的,比如肾移植患者的心脏移植,基础研究科学家想要的临床信息,帮助理解某主题相关原始文献中某一篇译文的背景知识等。最后,对于移植单位或医院管理者来说,本书可以提供大量的移植主题信息以帮助组织管理移植中心,了解来自临床移植实践的边际收益和风险。

从某种程度上来讲,由于内容多、范围广,第1版出版过程较缓慢。在某些时候,会选择实用性而非完整性,也希望一直如此。本书不能取代原始文献的作用,但是会成为理解原始文献的重要信息。我们正在尝试通过把教科书直接链接到原始文献,尤其是Wiley-Blackwell出版的杂志,来提高将来的水准,希望本书可以成为一个新的范例。

第 1 章
临床器官移植简史

Sir Roy Y. Calne

引言

移植是20世纪最有远见和影响力的医学成就之一。由于20世纪早期的技术进步和理论基础,移植在技术上的可行性激发了少数有远见的研究者基于临床需求对其生理障碍的认真研究。从他们对移植物排斥的遗传和免疫基础的描述以及第一次移植手术的开创性工作中，移植的临床实践迅速成为临床护理结构的交织,不仅从实际的角度,也成为高级医疗实践中巨大可能性和挑战的一个例子。在如今的医疗工作中,很多理所当然的概念,如免疫抑制、单克隆抗体的应用、死亡概念的界定等,都起源于移植。很多现在的伦理困境也可以追溯到移植带来的这些问题。

移植发展史是很多移植相关书籍的主题，重要在于突出学科发展至今的主要贡献，而科学和医学因目标相同而紧密结合就是一个典型的例子。本章会以合适的方法向读者介绍该领域的历史，需要的时候会涉及更多决定性的工作和本书的其他章节。通常情况下，是以器官移植为主题进行重点介绍，本书中更多详细的历史性事件会放在各个章节中单独介绍。

移植外科的概念

器官移植的概念是一个外科概念，建立在对器官的解剖学和生理学的基础上，以保持器官的存活和发挥其生物学作用。像替换这种直观概念可以追溯到几百年之前。在20世纪早期,一些欧洲国家的学者进行了认真的探索，其成果促进了以肾为主要目标的器官移植。肾衰竭是一种相对常见的致命性疾病,肾的生理学功能研究较为透彻,解剖关系非常明确。重要的是,一个功能正常的肾脏足够维持患者的身体健康。肾脏在解剖学吻合了动脉、静脉和输尿管,足够保证其维持生理功能。神经、淋巴和筋膜毗邻关系也很重要,但不是必要的。在20世纪初期,Alexis Carrel(图1.1)设计了一种吻合血管的方法[1]，并凭借此技术获得了1912年的诺贝尔医学奖。由于无灌注时间延长会导致不可逆的缺血性损伤，倘若在短时间内恢复动脉灌注、静脉流出,肾脏就是有功能的,Carrel自己用该技术展示了肾脏是可以摘取和移植的。

Carrel和Guthrie在猫和狗身上证实了该技术的可行性，并且发现把肾脏从动物的体内转移到该动物身体的其他部位后,被转移的肾脏可以长期存活,并且可以切除该动物对侧的肾脏[2]。但是,把一个动物的肾脏移植给另外一个动物,在短期的功能正常化之后,必然会出现功能衰竭。Carrel虽然记录了该发现,但是当时却没能解释这种目前被我们称为“同种异体移植肾脏”的快速功能衰竭[3]。为患者进行肾移植的首次报道引起了很多外科医师和历史学者的争论。曾有关于将人类肾脏或动物肾脏移植到人肱血管或股血管的描述,在Francis Moore博士的著作《移植》中[4],有对这些早期发现及失败案例的热烈讨论，但其肾功能都不能长期维持。后来人们才发现,由Carrel和Guthrie积累的经验及程序是不成熟的。

移植生物学

在20世纪四五十年代，丹麦的Morten Simonsen和伦敦的William Dempster分别描述了本质上和Carrel及Guthrie的实验类似的研究，并确定通过自体移植可以使器官功能维持更长时间。但是,同种异体移植试验普遍成功不了，并且他们发现来自同一个供体的第二次移植在同一受者体内立刻就会失去功能。这些发现是Simonsen和Dempster多年辛勤研究的巅峰之

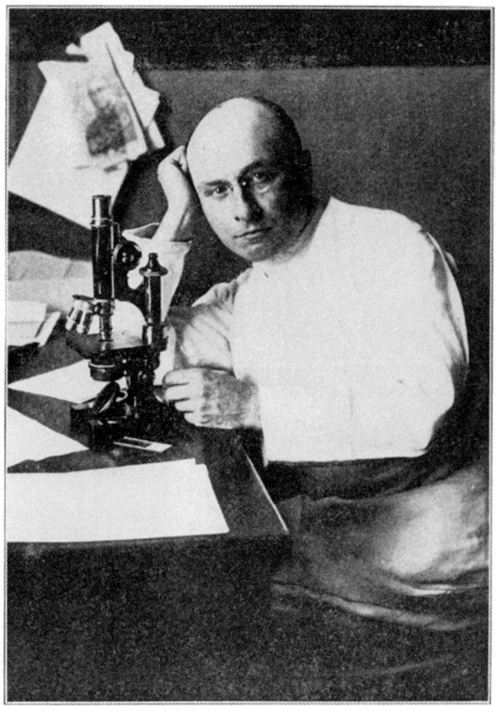

(A)

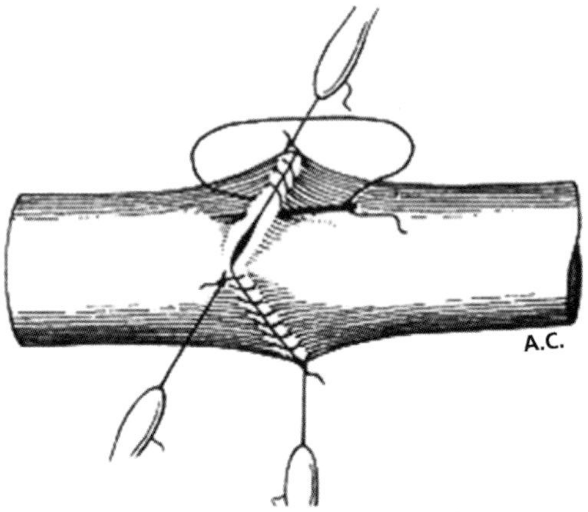

(B)

图 1.1 (A)Alexis Carrel 因发明了血管吻合(B)方法被普遍认为是移植外科之父,并在 1912 年被授予诺贝尔医学奖。

作，他们也报道了同种异体肾移植受体中肾上腺皮质激素的应用。他们都描述了同种异体肾移植时的组织学变化,肾皮质被大量中性粒细胞、巨噬细胞、淋巴细胞、嗜酸性粒细胞和浆细胞所浸润,这些炎症反应是伴随着肾坏死出现的。Simonsen 和 Dempster 都认为,这些细胞来自移植器官,是一种移植物抗宿主反应[5,6]。但随后,Porter 和 Calne 通过同位素标记的方法发现这些炎症细胞是来自于受体[7]。

在 Simonsen 和 Dempster 正在进行犬科同种异体肾移植实验的时候,Peter Medawar(图 1.2)和他的团队也在研究鼠和兔的皮肤移植排斥反应的生物学。第一组移植在几天之后发生白细胞浸润,移植物在 7~10 天之后发生坏死。来自同一供体的第二组移植会立刻出现坏死，未曾形成新的微循环，被称为“无效移植”。Medawar 团队证实，皮肤移植排斥的免疫特性毋庸置疑[8],从他们的实验可以推测,同卵双胞胎之间的肾移植会与同卵双胞胎之间的皮肤移植类似，事实证明这样的手术效果是令人满意的，且不会发生任何排斥反应。以此为基础,Medawar 团队明确表示,同卵和非同卵的牛双胞胎之间进行皮肤移植会有相反的结果。但令他们吃惊的是，当非同卵双胞胎牛之间以同卵双胞胎牛的方式进行皮肤移植时,结果却令人失望[9]。他们开始关注到 Ray Owen 关于牛的非同卵双胞胎的研究,发现牛的非同卵双胞胎作为健康的动物，经常会有不同类型的血[10]。这相当于同一个人有一部分 A 型红细胞,还有一部分 B 型红细胞,由于天然抗体的存在,这显然是不会出现的。由于和神秘的拥有不同物种器官的古希腊动物(图 1.3)有奇特的相似之处,Owen 把这种非同寻常的红细胞群称为“嵌合型”。

然后,Medawar 与他的同事 Billingham 和 Brent 一起用近交系小鼠设计了一系列对照实验。很多同胞兄妹交配后产生的同源个体被称为近交系，皮肤移植可以在近交系小鼠之间进行。但是从一个近交系小鼠皮肤移植至另一个近交系小鼠则会产生排斥反应，后来这被称为“同种异体排斥”。

以在牛双胞胎上的研究为基础,Medawar 团队克服了一些技术难题，发现把一个近交系小鼠的细胞注射到另一个近交系小鼠的胎儿体内，出现了一些幸存者,后来被称为同源组织的移植耐受(图 1.2B)[11]。后来,他们发现,这种耐受在新出生的动物身上也可以出现,虽然面临的技术挑战仍然严峻,但已经不需要针对胎儿进行操作。“适应性免疫学耐受”的发现是免疫学

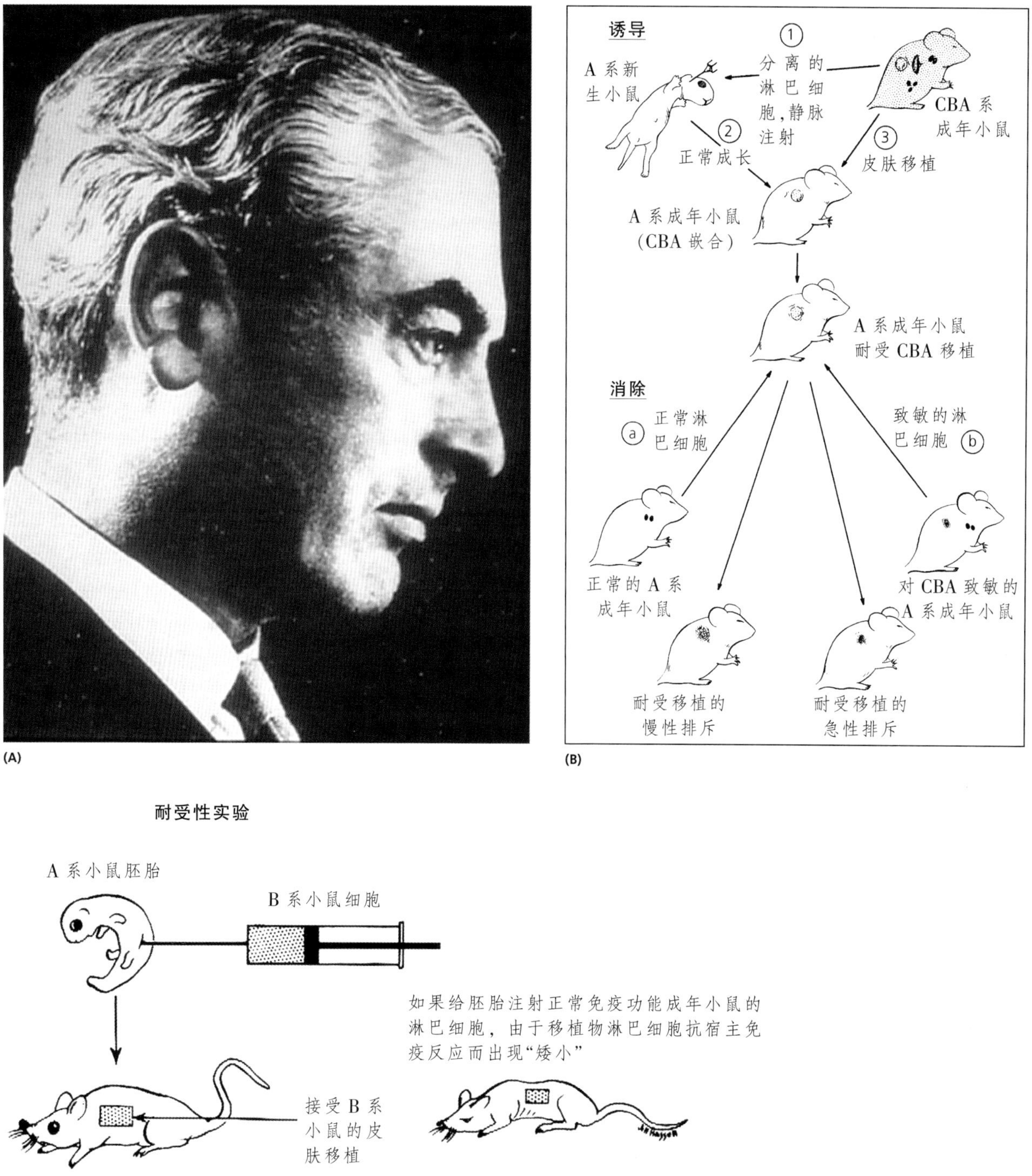

图 1.2　(A)Peter Medawar 因其研究适应性免疫耐受的生物学原理(B)而获得了 1960 年的诺贝尔医学奖。(C)移植物抗宿主反应诱发“矮小病”的机制阐述。

发展的基本前提，被授予了诺贝尔医学奖，并提出了一个实际问题：成人的免疫系统是否可以像胎儿般拥有可塑性，即使随后免疫系统会恢复功能，至少可以暂时性地允许进行移植。Medawar 团队的另一项重要发现是当供体含有淋巴细胞时，会出现供体排斥宿主的反应，引起一种称为“矮小病”的消耗性疾病(图 1.2C)[12]。后来证实，这种移植物抗宿主反应在骨髓移植中，显得尤为重要，在部分器官移植中，如肝移植会伴随供肝带入很多淋巴细胞，也是如此。

到 20 世纪 50 年代早期，David Hume 通过将肾动脉及肾静脉吻合到受体的股血管，并进行输尿管皮肤造口的方式开展了一些临床肾移植[13]，虽然没有刻意

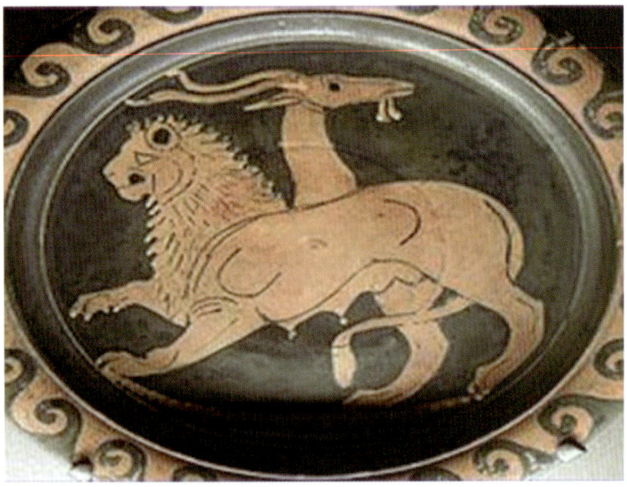

图 1.3 嵌合体:《荷马史诗》所描述的希腊神话中的一种动物,融合了狮子、蛇和山羊,是移植的象征。

降低受体的免疫功能,但一些移植物确实存活了下来,甚至有一例持续了约5个月时间都能产生尿液。出现肾衰竭的时候,人们发现了细胞浸润现象,并且出现了后来被称为“慢性同种异体排斥反应”的典型性严重小动脉狭窄。研究者怀疑,人类肾移植比动物实验中观察到的排斥反应更轻,可能是由于他们都患有尿毒症,尿毒症通常情况下会使人变得虚弱,但是可能同时也削弱了正常的免疫系统。

同一时代,在波士顿彼得·本特·布利格汉姆医院,外科的 Francis Moore 和内科的 George Torn 两位教授也在进行实验研究。外科实验室主任由整形外科医师 Joseph Murray(图 1.4)担任,他在面部严重畸形的外科矫正领域有很深的造诣,他把他的技术应用于实验室,并在狗身上改进了肾移植技术,将肾动脉和肾静脉同髂血管进行吻合,并把输尿管植入了膀胱,避免了输尿管造瘘方法的逆行性感染带来的不利影响。1953年,Rene Kuss 教授在巴黎使用骨盆内肾移植方法进行了母亲向儿子捐献肾脏的移植手术,肾功能维持了23天[14]。在手术技术发展的过程中,这是一个重要的进步。

早期临床实践

1954 年,一例肾衰竭患者被转诊给了肾病专家 Merrill 教授,他致力于通过同卵双胞胎间的肾移植提高成功率,患者原来的主管医师推荐道:“您会对这个患者感兴趣的,因为他是同卵双胞胎之一,应该和您的研究相关。”经过伦理方面和同卵双胞胎方面的评估(双向皮肤移植评估法),Murray 教授和他的团队在彼得·本特·布利格汉姆医院开展了第一例同卵双胞胎肾移植并取得了惊人的成功(图 1.5)[15]。该手术证明,和动物实验一样,如果能够避免免疫排斥,手术可以为受者提供优质的远期疗效,并且单侧肾切除不会造成远期危害。由于该贡献及其后续研究,Joseph Murray 于1990年被授予了诺贝尔医学奖。首例双胞胎捐赠者健康地存活了50余年,成为关于活体捐赠安全性随访研究的前沿。

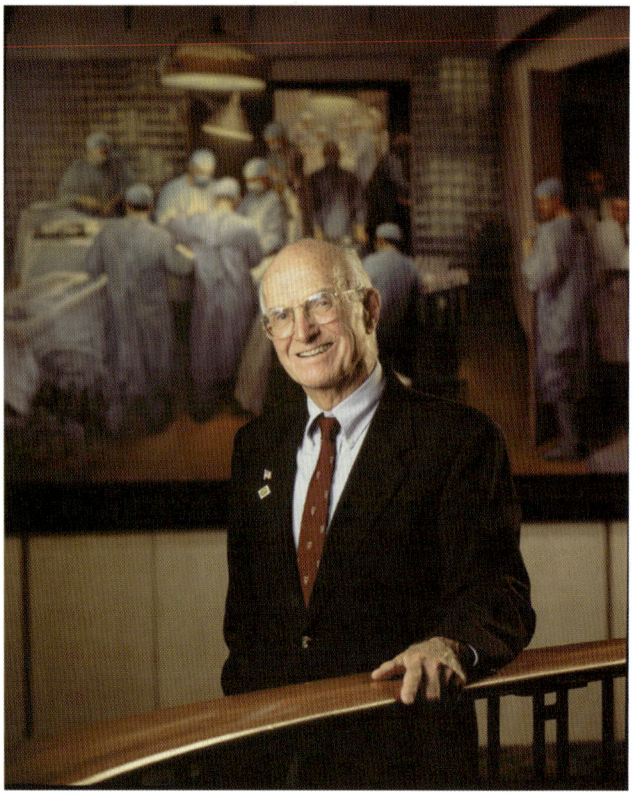

图 1.4 Joseph Murray 站在描绘了他的重大成就(首次肾移植成功)的画像前,他获得了1990年的诺贝尔医学奖。(Photograph reproduced from *American Journal of Transplantation*, January 2013, with permission from John Wiley & Sons.)

在某种情况下,即使是来自双胞胎供肾的移植,也会由于受者自身免疫性疾病导致移植肾功能衰竭,从而引起死亡[16]。这样的情况促进了削弱受者免疫功能方法的研究。骨髓移植的研究发现,啮齿类动物会由于接受致死剂量X线照射而出现免疫功能缺陷,但是可以通过注射同系动物骨髓的方法获救。静脉注射的骨髓细胞将迁移至受者的骨髓,不仅能够成为造血成分,还

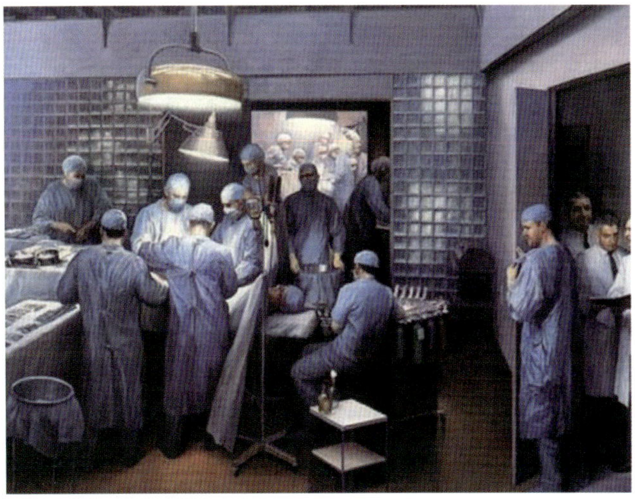

图 1.5 《首次肾移植成功》画作于 1996 年由 Joel Babb 绘成，珍藏于弗朗西斯的哈佛医学图书馆中。

可以形成淋巴结和脾脏的淋巴细胞，修复免疫功能[17]。如果是非自体骨髓，将面临移植失败，即使部分存活，也会出现致命性的移植物抗宿主排斥反应。后来，骨髓移植发展到应用轻度非消融条件作用对受体进行治疗而不是全身照射的方法，疗效比较成功，即使是移植物抗宿主反应也被用来作为治疗白血病的手段[18,19]。

全身辐射后进行骨髓移植实验和临床的成功给肾移植的受体带来了希望。在狗身上的结果令人鼓舞[20]，但是除了彼得·本特·布利格汉姆医院和巴黎的两对非同卵双胞胎间的肾移植之外，所有全身 X 线照射的尝试都以惨痛的失败而告终，非但没能控制排斥反应，还导致患者在晚期出现了严重的脓毒症[21,22]。为了继续临床研究，并减轻全身放射治疗的毒性，斯坦福的 Slavin 和 Strober[23]采用了对脾脏和淋巴器官进行重复小剂量照射的方法(详见第 76 章)。

在 20 世纪 50 年代后期，大家意识到对肾移植受体需要提供更优质的方法来保证其安全。用来治疗白血病的药物 6-巯基嘌呤可以使兔对外来抗原不产生抗体，这个研究成果是一个重要暗示。1959 年，Schwartz 和 Dameshek 发表了该研究结果，并认为停用 6-巯基嘌呤后，该作用会持续存在，并称其为“药物诱导免疫耐受”[24]。于是，在伦敦和里士满开展了对 6-巯基嘌呤的研究，研究者将其作为免疫抑制剂用在同种异体肾移植的狗身上，延长了该同种异体移植的存活时间，并没有出现免疫耐受，其疗效已经明显优于全身接受 X 线放射的方法[25,26]。但是，由于免疫功能被严重削弱，引起了较高的感染发生率。Hitchings 和 Elion 认为，一些实验室合成的 6-巯基嘌呤值得一试，有可能会比 6-巯基嘌呤有更好的治疗指标。实验证明，其中的硫唑嘌呤略优于 6-巯基嘌呤，并成了彼得·本特·布利格汉姆医院开展系列动物实验和临床免疫抑制治疗时期的指定用药[27]。最初的临床试验结果令人失望，直到治疗中加入了类固醇，在不相关的同种异体移植中才出现了成功的案例[28]。目前，硫唑嘌呤仍然被用于移植的免疫抑制治疗，在第 98 章中将有详细介绍。

Medawar 和 Dempster 曾经对类固醇激素进行过研究，但是单用的效果并不好，和硫唑嘌呤联合应用之后获得了较好的疗效。Tom Starzl 在丹佛详细记录了同种异体肾移植中的应用成果。Goodwin 已经证明，应用口服的类固醇可以在同种异体肾移植发生急性排斥反应时使其暂时恢复功能[29,30]。

通过每日监测患者状态，并调整药物剂量，尝试探索既能预防排斥反应又能避免重度毒性反应的合理剂量，使得同种异体肾移植 1 年内约 50%可维持功能，但是一旦失败，将给患者、家属及手术医师带来极大负担。然而，在这一时期，斯坦福的 Lower 和 Shumway 开展了心脏移植实验技术[31]。此外，丹佛的 Starzl 和波士顿彼得·本特·布利格汉姆医院的 Francis Moore 成功开展了肝脏移植[32,33]。莫斯科的 Demikov 开展了头和四肢移植的实验，在那个时候，这个实验与其说是要应用于临床还不如说是出于外科医师的好奇心[34]。

很显然，非双胞胎的近亲之间进行移植效果要优于无血缘的供体。Dausset、Payne、Van Rood 和 Terasaki 逐渐阐明了移植群体差异的理论基础[35-38]。从血细胞中分离出的人类白细胞抗原(HLA)可以通过产生抗红细胞抗体避免急性移植物无功能。第 3 章将详细介绍这一划时代的发现——HLA。

1963 年，Starzl 进行了第 1 例临床肝移植[39]，但是早期移植失败和患者死亡导致其工作被迫中止，直到 1967 年 Barnard 进行第 1 例心脏移植，他才重新踏上肝移植项目的征程。第 1 例儿童心脏移植将在第 115 章中详述[40,41]。医学史上，媒体对心脏移植的空前热衷导致其发展走向歧途，全世界的外科医师都企图通过临床心脏移植加入“移植俱乐部”，但由于其中大多数医师对移植生物学和免疫抑制治疗知识掌握并不详尽，这样的状况令人担忧。

虽然应用了硫唑嘌呤和类固醇，但心脏移植和肝脏移植的疗效仍不容乐观,不过一些患者结果却很好。为了提高免疫抑制疗效,研究者也使用了很多其他药物和方法,包括胸导管淋巴液体外引流、供肾和循环血液体外照射等。这些方法都失败了,但是人们发现提高抗人淋巴细胞抗体的概念是充满希望的。在爱丁堡,Woodruff 及其同事在证实鼠抗淋巴细胞血清延长皮肤移植存活的有效性之后,率先开展了在器官移植方面的实验[42]。这种抗淋巴细胞抗体是多克隆抗体,也就是说可以和很多种不同抗原反应,由被注射淋巴细胞或者胸腺细胞的另外一个物种产生,比如马或兔。这些抗体较难纯化,因此每一批的疗效和毒性都不同,但是有些疗效很显著,在第 98 章有详细描述,临床上仍然在用精炼的兔抗人胸腺细胞抗体[43]。

当代免疫治疗

1978 年,瑞士巴塞尔山德瑞实验室的免疫学家 Borel 阐述了一种被作为抗生素研究的真菌环素——环孢素在抑制免疫功能中的疗效[44],其抗生素性能较差,但是小鼠皮肤移植实验证实,其无论在体外还是体内,抑制免疫功能活性均令人印象深刻。以 Borel 的研究成果为基础,我们和伦敦诺斯威克公园医院的研究者将环孢素应用在了小鼠同种异体异位心脏移植中,发现疗效极好[45,46]。我们又把环孢素应用在犬的同种异体肾移植和猪的同种异体原位心脏移植中,在这些物种以及后来兔的研究中,环孢素都表现出了强力的免疫抑制疗效,且少有副作用[47]。但是当其首次被应用于临床肾移植时,却表现出了明显的肾毒性,这是在动物实验中不曾出现的毒性[48]。后来证实,第一次临床试验是按照之前动物实验剂量进行治疗,剂量过大引起了明显的肾毒性。实践证明,环孢素的应用是里程碑式的进步,使同种异体肾移植的 1 年健康生存率从 50%提高到了 80%,这个疗效的提高改变了之前人们对药物治疗在器官移植中所起作用的怀疑态度。之前,全世界范围内大约只有 10 家单位进行临床器官移植,在引入环孢素之后,1 年之内就有超过上千个中心,捐献器官的突然短缺引起了前所未有的关注。第 17 章将详细介绍环孢素的作用机制,并讲解所有移植相关的特殊用药。

日本的 Ochiai 证实,藤泽公司开发的链霉菌源化合物他克莫司能够以低剂量延长移植物生存时间[49]。经过早期不同物种的同种异体器官移植实验之后,他克莫司被用在了临床器官移植中,匹兹堡的 Starzl 团队进行了详细的研究[50]。和环孢素相比,他克莫司虽然有相似的肾毒性,但是却不会出现环孢素引起的多毛症等其他副作用。

生产单克隆抗体的 Kohler 和 Millstein 于 1975 年提供了一种单分子靶向药物[51]。伴随着 OKT3,一种鼠源性特异性抗 CD3 阳性 T 细胞单克隆抗体的研发,这很快就被应用在了移植领域。该药起效快,药效短,特异性降低外周血 T 细胞,可以用来治疗急性排斥反应[52]。1986 年,OKT3 成为首种被批准应用于任何人类疾病的单克隆抗体,其副作用可以被特异性抗鼠抗体所消除。但是,随着更多其他的耐受性治疗方法的出现,OKT3 逐渐退出了市场,总之,OKT3 成了医学上单克隆抗体治疗保证的象征性概念。人源化是指通过基因工程使抗体和人体结构结合更紧密从而避免抗体疗效下降,随着达利珠单抗的发明,人源化的概念也被引入到了移植治疗中[53]。和 OKT3 一样,一种全新的治疗药物通过移植首次应用于临床。在当代临床实践中,该药物也已经退出舞台,但是在医疗中,人们发现了它们其他的用途(详见第 99 章)。这方面的概念主要来自 Waldmann 和 Winter 的研究,他们发明了人源性特种淋巴细胞的单克隆抗体 Campath 1H 或者阿伦珠单抗,这是一种特别强效的抗淋巴细胞抗体,几乎可以在几个小时之内完全清除循环中的淋巴细胞[54]。该药的产生起初是用来治疗慢性淋巴细胞性白血病的,后来发现其用于临床肾移植患者时可以作为有效的诱导剂,能使免疫功能持续抑制在很低的水平,从而消除了维持治疗药物的大多数副作用。以低剂量维持的耐受性抗淋巴细胞诱导治疗,并非总能达到耐受,但可能已经是目前器官移植受体最合理的治疗方法[55,56]。

早期猪的肝移植和后来啮齿类的肝移植实验表明,肝移植很少发生比其他组织移植更严重的排斥反应,甚至受体动物可以出现不接受免疫抑制治疗的长期术后耐受。移植肝通常要经过生物化学和组织学反应,但是可以自然康复[57–59]。这些发现是基于匹兹堡拒不配合医师进行免疫移植治疗患者“实验”的理论基础,这些不接受免疫抑制治疗的肝移植患者中的一部分存活时间超过了 20 年,毫无疑问,他们可以被认为是术后耐受。在第 76 章中将讨论因为感染或为了观察停用免疫抑制药物后是否出现耐受的患者出现的不同预后，一些没有恶化的患者无限期地接受了移植物，但是另外一些则出现了排斥反应而不得不再次接受免疫抑制治疗。对于器官移植受者来说，即使是剂量很低的免疫抑制药物也很重要，如果停用，将会出现难以逆转的急性排斥反应[60,61]。

以成功的小鼠实验为基础，研究者对一种更合理的趋向免疫抑制的方法已经研究了很多年，外来组织在受体免疫系统中不仅能够识别并排斥表面抗原，还能联合抗原提呈细胞传递第二信号给免疫反应细胞。关于第二信号的研究已经非常详尽，在第11章将会详细介绍第二信号敲出、共刺激信号等多种实验方法，其应用于临床研究的成果令人鼓舞[62]。

伦理挑战

在过去的50年，器官移植从理论上或者在想象中存在、发展至全面开展临床治疗，经过了很长一段路程，现在依然有很多生物学上的困难需要研究和克服，特别是器官移植后疾病复发、肾功能损伤、钙调磷酸酶抑制剂相关性糖尿病、感染和恶性肿瘤，尤其是淋巴瘤和皮肤癌。器官移植令人头疼的种种特性已经逐渐显露，也出现了很多预防和治疗副作用的方法。实际上，正是由于对这些困境的深入了解才形成了当代移植临床应用的基本理论知识，这也是本书中多数章节的内容。器官移植的成功也提出了一些伦理问题，其实已经出现了成堆的问题，也是早期器官移植先驱们所难以想象的问题，本书中有专门的章节进行讨论（第136~139章）。随着器官移植的发展，需求不断增加，但是器官捐献量却并未同步增长。任何国家都没有足够的死者捐献器官供给移植。实际上，公共舆论并不支持死者捐献器官，也不支持政府投资于公共教育的基础设施或者对潜在捐献者进行重症监护的医疗设备。曾经，西班牙各种死者捐献器官超过每百万人口30例，是最成功的国家，但是随着头部外伤治疗的改善和道路交通事故的减少，捐献器官数量已经减少了[63,64]。第53章会详细介绍该部分内容。

从同卵双胞胎之间的器官捐献开始，活体器官捐献已经广泛应用。通常情况下，直系或非直系亲属之间进行肾移植或者父母捐献肝脏移植给子女符合伦理要求，但是如果超出了这些关系的器官捐献，会面临很大的器官捐献伦理问题（详见第138章）。如果患者的家庭成员或者朋友被施压，让其捐献，他们可能会迫于压力而接受，或者因为拒绝而感觉到内疚。供者和受者对捐献的态度因身份而不同。纽约的一位外科医师为其妻子捐献了一个肾脏，后来他们离婚了，考虑其无私的捐献，法院判给他一笔可观的损伤赔偿[65]。成人活体捐献肝脏移植给另一位成人将面对难以预知的风险，很可能会延长供者患病时间，而且可能会导致供者失业甚至因器官捐献手术而死亡，这些足以使供者充分考虑其将要面临的风险。据报道，有5例部分肝脏捐献的供者在术后出现了肝功能衰竭，其中4例死亡，仅有1例通过肝移植存活下来。有钱人可能会非法购买器官，但是很少出现有钱人捐献器官给贫穷的受体[66]。

伦理问题不是轻而易举能够克服的，但是首先要有明确的规定。20世纪60年代中期，研究者试图将动物器官移植给人类，在新奥尔良、丹佛、里士满、弗吉尼亚都有证据确凿的肾移植报道，以及一些其他异种器官移植的零星报道。除了新奥尔良记录到一例接受黑猩猩肾移植的患者活了9个月之外，没有长期存活的案例，且都逐渐发生了慢性排斥反应[67]。在研究异种移植反应和克服障碍方面，人们已经投入了大量的精力，在第12章会有该话题的深入探讨。然而，尽管进行了大量昂贵的实验，每一个困难都像是越野赛中的障碍，但必须克服了第一个才能看清下一个。目前，我们不知道前方还有多少障碍，路漫漫其修远兮，吾将上下而求索。

总结

在不到60年的短暂时间里，移植已经由因好奇心而开展的简单实验发展成多数器官终末期疾病的救命手段，过程也越来越规范，其成功已经越来越值得期待。短期内，即使能够克服移植相关的外科技术难题和免疫学治疗的困难，我们也仍将面临器官短缺的问题，这也是现任器官移植协会不得不向公众及政府坦白的事实，因为不是每一个人都能从器官移植中获益，也不是每一个人都能支持该项工作，尤其是在一些发展相对落后的国家。通过这本综合性的图书，读者会了解到移植领域的历史发展，通过本书的简要概述，可以发现一些划时代的事件。当代器官移植消耗巨大，从基础生物学到人类的基本道德问题，希望我们能够发现生命的线索。移植学者们将会承担起该领域赋予他们的使命,不断开拓进取。

(张龙辉 译 李照 校)

参考文献

1. Carrel A. La technique operatoire des anastomosis vasculaires et al transplantation des visceres. Lyon Medical. 1902;99:859–864.
2. Carrel A, Guthrie CC. Successful transplantation of both kidneys from a dog into a bitch with removal of both normal kidneys from the latter. Science. 1906; 23:394–395.
3. Carrel J. The ultimate results of double nephrectomy and replantation of one kidney. Journal of Experimental Medicine. 1911;14:124.
4. Moore FD. Transplant—The Give and Take of Tissue Transplantation. Philadelphia: Saunders; 1964.
5. Simonsen M. Biological incompatibility in kidney transplantation in dogs. Acta Pathologica et Microbiologica Scandinavica. 1953;32:1–84.
6. Dempster WJ. Kidney homotransplantion. British Journal of Surgery. 1953;40:447.
7. Porter KA, Calne RY. Origins of the infiltrating cells in skin and kidney homografts. Transplantation Bulletin. 1960;26:458.
8. Gibson T, Medawar PB. The fate of skin homografts in man. Journal of Anatomy. 1943;77:299–310.
9. Anderson D, Billingham RE, Lampkin GH, et al. The use of skin grafting to distinguish between monzygotic and dizygotic twins in cattle. Heredity. 1951;5:379–397.
10. Owen RD. Immunogenetic consequences of vascular anastomosis between bovine twins. Science. 1945;102:400.
11. Billingham RE, Brent L, Medawar PB. Actively acquired tolerance of foreign cells. Nature. 1953;172:603–606.
12. Billingham RE, Brent L. A simple method for inducing tolerance of skin homografts in mice. Transplantation Bulletin. 1957;4:67.
13. Hume DM, Merrill JP, Miller BF. Experiences with renal homotransplantations in the human: report of nine cases. Journal of Clinical Investigation. 1955; 34:327–382.
14. Kuss R, Teinturier J, Milliez P. Quelques essays de greffe rein chex l'homme. Memoires. Academie de Chirurgie. 1951;77:755–768.
15. Merrill JP, Murray JE, Harrison JE, et al. Successful homotransplantations of the human kidney between identical twins. JAMA: Journal of the American Medical Association. 1956;160:277–282.
16. Dixon FJ, McPhaul JJ Jnr, Lerner R. Recurrence of glomerulonephritis in the transplanted kidney. Archives of Internal Medicine. 1969;123:554–557.
17. Lorenz E, Uphoff D, Reed R, et al. Modification of irradiation injury in mice and guinea pigs by bone marrow rejection. Journal of the National Cancer Institute 1951;12:197–201.
18. Storb R, Wagner R, Conq YO, et al. Allogeneic stem cell transplantation: clinical research and practice. Blood. 1997;89:3048–3054.
19. Slavin S, Nagler A, Naparstek E, et al. The mystique of hepatic tolerogenicity: an epiphany. Blood. 1998;91:756.
20. Mannick JA, Lochte HL, Ashley CA, et al. A functioning kidney homotransplant in the dog. Surgery. 1959;46:821.
21. Merrill JP, Murray JE, Harrison JH, et al. Successful homotransplantation of the kidney between non-identical twins. New England Journal of Medicine. 1960; 262:1251–1260.
22. Kuss R, Legrain M, Mathe G, et al. Etude de quatre cas d'irradiation totale par le cobalt radioactive. (A des doses respectives de 250, 400 et 600 rads). Prealable a une transplantation renale allogenique. Revue Francaise d'Etudes Cliniques et Biologiques. 1962;7:1028–1047.
23. Slavin S, Strober S. Induction of allograft tolerance after total lymphoid irradiation (TLI): development of suppressor cells of the mixed leucocyte reaction (MLR). Journal of Immunology. 1979;123:942–946.
24. Schwartz R, Damashek W. Drug induced immunologic tolerance. Nature. 1959;183:1682–1683.
25. Calne RY. The rejection of renal homografts. Inhibition in dogs by using 6-mercaptopurine. Lancet. 1960;1:417–418.
26. Zukoski CF, Lee HM, Hume DM. The prolongation of functional survival of canine renal homografts by 6-mercaptopurine. Surgical Forum. 1960;11:470.
27. Calne RY. Inhibition of the rejection of renal homografts in dogs by purine analogues. Transplantation Bulletin. 1961;28:445–461.
28. Murray JE, Merrill JP, Harrison JH, et al. Prolonged survival of human kidney homografts by immunosuppressive drug therapy. New England Journal of Medicine. 1963;268:1315–1323.
29. Goodwin WE, Kaufman JJ, Mims MM, et al. Human renal transplantation. I. Clinical experiences with six cases of renal transplantation. Journal of Urology. 1963;89:13.
30. Starzl TE, Marchioro TL, Waddell WR. The reversal of rejection in human renal homografts with subsequent development of homograft tolerance. Surgery, Gynecology and Obstetrics. 1963;117:385–395.
31. Lower RR, Stofer RC, Shumway NE. Homovital transplantation of the heart. Journal of Thoracic Imaging. 1961;41:196–204.
32. Starzl TE, Kaupp HA Jr, Brock DR, et al. Reconstructive problems in canine liver homotransplantations with special reference to the postoperative role of hepatic venous flow. Surgery, Gynecology and Obstetrics. 1960;111:733.
33. Moore FD, Smith LL, Burnap TK, et al. One-stage homotransplantations of the liver following total hepatectomy in dogs. Transplantation Bulletin. 1959;6: 103–107.
34. Demikhov VP. Transplantation of the Head. Experimental Transplantation of Vital Organs. New York, NY: Consultant's Bureau; 1962.
35. Dausset J. Iso-leucoanticorps and blood transfusion. Acta Haematologica Basel. 1958;20:156–166.
36. Payne R, Rolfs MR. Fetomaternal leukocyte incompatibility. Journal of Clinical Investigation. 1958;37:1756–1763.
37. Van Rood JJ, Van Leeuwen A, Eernisse JG. Leukocyte antibodies in sera of pregnant women. Vox Sanguinis. 1959;4:427–444.
38. Terasaki PI, McClelland JD. Microdroplet assay of human serum cytotoxins. Nature. 1964;204:998–1000.
39. Starzl TE, Marchioro TL, Von Kaulla KN, et al. Homotransplantation of the liver in humans. Surgery, Gynecology and Obstetrics. 1963;117:659–676.
40. Starzl TE, Porter KA, Brettschneider L, et al. Clinical and pathologic observations after orthotopic transplantation of the human liver. Surgery, Gynecology and Obstetrics. 1969;128:327.
41. Barnard CN. The operation. A human cardiac transplant: an interim report of a successful operation performed at Groote Schuur Hospital, Cape Town. South African Medical Journal. Suid-Afrikaanse Tydskrif vir Geneeskunde. 1967;41:1271–1274.
42. Woodruff MFA, Anderson NF. Effect of lymphocyte depletion by thoracic duct fistula and administration of antilymphocyte serum on the survival of skin homografts in rats. Nature. 1963;200:702.
43. Starzl TE, Marchioro TL, Porter KA, et al. The use of heterologous antilymphoid agents in canine renal homotransplantation. Surgery, Gynecology and Obstetrics. 1967;124:301–318.
44. Borel JF, Feurer C, Gubler HU, et al. Biological effects of cyclosporine A: A new antilymphocytic agent. Agents and Actions. 1976;6:468–475.
45. Kostakis AJ, White DJG, Calne RY. Toxic effects in the use of cyclosporine A in alchoholic solution as an immunosuppressant of rat heart allografts. IRCS Medical Science [Microform]. 1977;5:280.
46. Green CJ, Alison AC. Extensive prolongation of rabbit kidney allograft survival after short-term cyclosporine A treatment. Lancet. 1978;1:1182.
47. Calne RY, White DJG, Rolles K, et al. Prolonged survival of pig orthotopic heart grafts treated with cyclosporin. Lancet. 1978;1(8075):1183–1185.
48. Calne RY, Rolles K, White DJG, et al. Cyclosporin A initially as the only immunosuppressant in 34 recipients of cadaveric organs: 32 kidneys, 2 pancreases, and 2 livers. Lancet. 1979;2:1033–1036.
49. Ochiai T, Nagata M, Nakajima K. Studies of the effect of FK506 on renal allografts in the beagle dog. Transplantation. 1987;44:7334–7738.
50. Starzl TE, Todo S, Fung J, et al. FK506 for liver, kidney, and pancreas transplantation. Lancet. 1989;2:1000–1004.
51. Kohler G, Milstein C. Continuous cultures of fused cells secreting antibody of predefined specificity. Nature. 1975;256:495–497.
52. The Ortho Multicenter Transplant Study Group. A randomized clinical trial of OKT3 monoclonal antibody for acute rejection of cadaveric renal transplants. New England Journal of Medicine. 1985;313:337–342.
53. Vincenti F, Kirkman R, Light S, et al. Interleukin-2-receptor blockade with daclizumab to prevent acute rejection in renal transplantation. Daclizumab Triple Therapy Study Group. New England Journal of Medicine. 1998;338:161–165.
54. Hale G, Dyer MJS, Clark MR, et al. Remission indication in non-Hodgkin lymphoma with reshaped human monoclonal antibody campath 1H. Lancet. 1988;2:1394–1399.
55. Calne RY, Friend PJ, Moffatt S, et al. Prope tolerance, perioperative campath IH, and low-dose cyclosporin monotherapy in renal allograft recipients. Lancet. 1998;351:1701–1702.
56. Calne RY, Watson CJE. Some observations on prope tolerance. Current Opinion in Organ Transplantation. 2011;16:353–358.
57. Calne RY, Sells RA, Pena JR, et al. Induction of immunological tolerance by porcine liver allografts. Nature. 1969;223:472–476.
58. Zimmermann FA, Butcher GW, Davies HS, et al. Techniques for orthotopic liver transplantation in the rat and some studies of the immunologic responses to fully

allogeneic liver grafts. Transplantation Proceedings. 1979;11:571–577.
59. Kamada N, Calne RY, Wight DGD, et al. Orthotopic rat liver transplantation after long-term preservation by continuous perfusion with fluorocarbon emulsion. Transplantation. 1980;30:43–48.
60. Mazariegos GV. Immunosuppression withdrawal after liver transplantation: what are the next steps. Transplantation. 2011;91:697–699.
61. Woodruff M. Nothing Venture Nothing Win. Edinburgh: Scottish Academic Press; 1996.
62. Vincenti F, Charpentier B, Vanrenterghem Y, et al. A Phase III study of belatacept-based immunosuppression regimens v. cyclosporin in renal transplant recipients. American Journal of Transplantation. 2010;10:535–546.
63. Blanca M, Gonzalez I, Natividad C, et al. Mean age of organ donors, Spain. Transplantation. 1996;61:1119.
64. International Summit on Transplant Tourism and Organ Trafficking. Declaration of Istanbul on Organ Trafficking and Transplant Tourism. Clinical Journal of the American Society of Nephrology. 2008;3:1227–1231.
65. Foster P. Chinese teen sells his kidney for an iPad 2. Daily Telegraph. 2011.
66. McShane L. Long Island doctor Ruichard Batista to estranged wife: give me my kidney back or $1.5M. Daily News, New York, January 07, 2008.
67. Ringe B, Xiao G, Sass DA, et al. Rescue of a living donor with liver transplantion. American Journal of Transplantation. 2008;8:1557.
68. Reemtsma K. Renal transplantation from nonhuman primates to man. Annals of the New York Academy of Sciences. 1969;162:412–418.

第 2 篇

移植生物学

第 2 章 免疫生理学概论

Hēth R. Turnquist, Giorgio Raimondi, Diana Metes, Angus W. Thomson

引言

理解个体对移植器官的应答反应，需要总体上对免疫系统及免疫系统在维持生理稳态中的作用有基本的理解。事实上，重要的是认识到移植引起的同源性或者异源性免疫是由与器官移植完全没有关系的选择性压力进化过程所介导的，移植特异性反应主要源自机体在众多环境病原体和威胁个体的病理因素中维持稳定的系统。人体持续地暴露于如病毒、细菌、真菌、原生动物和寄生虫等各种病原体中，如果没有进行预防接种或者机体被动防御启动，这些病原体将引起感染性疾病甚至宿主死亡。除此以外，日常体力活动常可引起机体不同程度的创伤性损伤，相关的组织损伤必须得到适当的处理才能维持正常的生理功能。为了应对这些外界刺激，体内免疫系统进化出了完整的应对机制，包括全身的屏障机制、一系列反应灵敏的造血细胞和一套特异性效应分子。

虽然研究免疫系统的免疫学普遍被认为是一门现代科学[1]，但它历史久远，在其历史长河中，医生和科学家一直在研究免疫系统在健康和疾病中的作用。早在公元元年，古罗马人塞尔苏斯在 *De medicina* 中记载，热、肿、痛、红是由我们身体对损伤的炎性反应所引起的。在近代历史中，我们弄清了很多构成免疫反应的细胞、分子和免疫应答反应过程。随着对免疫学理解的不断加深，我们对免疫系统在正常组织器官生理功能方面作用的认识也在不断加深。随着对生理、病理和治疗性免疫应答反应理解的深化，我们也在进行转化方面的尝试以改善机体状况。对移植物、移植免疫应答的研究及这一过程的调控机制（移植免疫学）已经成为学术研究的热门领域，并在临床应用上获得成功。在本章，我们主要对分子、细胞免疫学进行大体框架性介绍，以帮助在后续更专业和更具体的章节更好地理解移植特异性免疫机制。这也将有助于理解贯穿本书的移植免疫学文献所需的通用词汇。现代优秀的免疫学书籍[1,2]已经详细阐述了针对异物及病原体保护性免疫反应的核心概念，以及不利的免疫反应，又称免疫病理学。

全身防御屏障和防御因素

防御屏障组织，如皮肤和黏液/呼吸道纤毛上皮作为抵抗多数病原体的一线屏障（图 2.1A）。同时，胃肠道和泌尿生殖道的低 pH 环境对于大多数生物是无法生存的，易受侵袭的部位（如眼结膜和口腔）受到抗菌酶的保护，如溶菌酶、β 防御素或磷脂酶 A。这些屏障组织还可以被机体共生的细菌或微生物群落所黏附，以“挤压”病原组织生存空间的方式预防病原体感染。在消化道黏膜，这些屏障还扮演着调控免疫活性的角色[3]。

免疫系统组织和器官

淋巴器官可分类为中枢性淋巴器官和外周性淋巴器官（图 2.1B）。中枢性淋巴器官特指骨髓和胸腺，是淋巴细胞发育的部位。人类骨髓的造血区域每天产生约 5000 亿血细胞，所生产的不同造血细胞用于组成机体的先天和获得性免疫系统（图 2.1C）。骨髓和胸腺所组成的中枢性淋巴器官不仅参与淋巴细胞的生产，还可以进行淋巴细胞的筛选。所谓筛选，指的是细胞与机体内的细胞环境适度作用以维持机体稳态并防止自身免

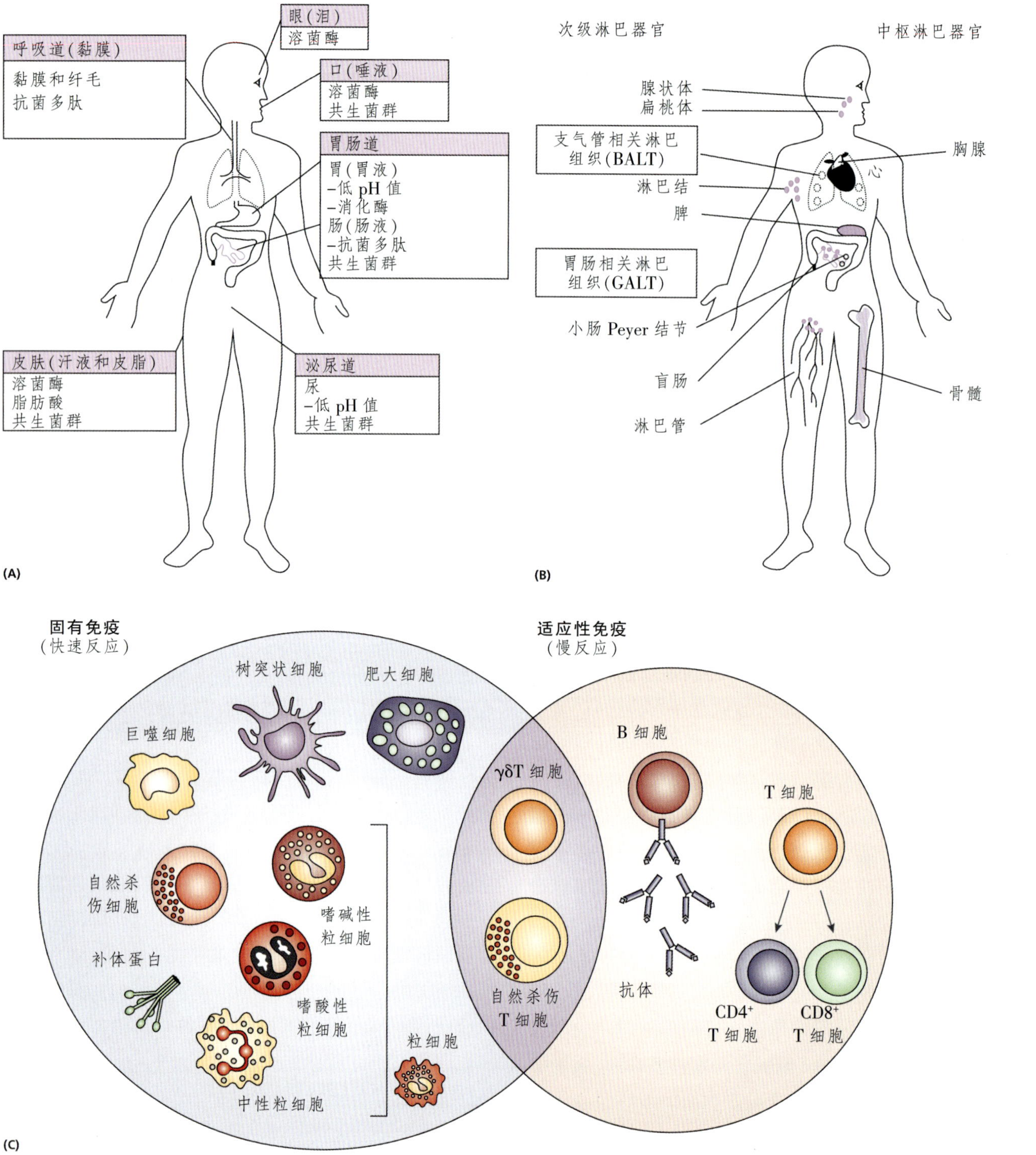

图 2.1 免疫系统组成。(A,B) Reprinted from Keogan MT, Wallace EM, and O'Leary P (2006), Concise Clinical Immunology for Healthcare Professionals. Figure 1.2.1 page 9, and Figure 1.3.2, page 16, with permission from Taylor and Francis Books[103].(C)Reprinted by permission from Macmillan Publishers Ltd: Dranoff G, Cytokines in cancer pathogenesis and cancer therapy Nature Reviews Cancer 2004, 4: 11–22, copyright (2004)[104].

疫反应。胸腺为造血干细胞前体向 T 细胞发育提供了适合的环境,不仅如此,胸腺基质细胞还可以作用于筛选功能性和自身耐受性 T 细胞。因此,胸腺在维持自身免疫耐受(中枢性耐受,见下文)方面有着十分重要的意义。

外周淋巴器官是汇集组织间液或者淋巴液的场

所，这些液体的主要成分是含有侵入病原体成分的血浆。这些病原体的成分(或者称为抗原)可以激活特异性免疫应答反应。同样,包括淋巴结、脾脏等外周及其他区域淋巴组织的外周淋巴器官是沟通固有免疫细胞和适应性免疫细胞的重要纽带，而这些区域也是绝大多数免疫反应开始的地方。淋巴系统由一系列参与机体细胞外液体再循环系统的血管所连接，在这一系统中淋巴液汇集并输送到淋巴结,并重新回流入血。

固有免疫和适应性免疫系统细胞

虽然前面所提到的全身性屏障和保护物质在阻止病原体从暴露部位侵入时十分有效,但特异性的造血细胞可以特异性强化抵御病原体的反应,这些白细胞在血液中循环和淋巴系统中巡视、观察、监视包括移植器官在内的外周组织(图 2.1C)。白细胞在伤口愈合和修复组织损伤方面也发挥重要的作用。

白细胞根据功能特征和细胞膜表面表达的独特受体可归为两类免疫系统:一类是固有免疫,一类是适应性免疫。除此之外,正如其他著作所描述的[4],固有免疫细胞和适应性免疫细胞之间还存在着一些重要的区别。总体来说,固有免疫细胞能够发现病原体及局部组织损伤，在结合单个激活信号受体的情况下即可进行反应。这与特异性免疫细胞不同,它需要由其他免疫细胞所引起的多重放大的信号激活才能获得完全的免疫性。尤为重要的是,通过这些信号的激活,适应性免疫细胞通过增殖分化并克隆特定抗原的识别能力，不断放大后续的免疫反应。另一项重要的区别是适应性免疫细胞在接受刺激并分离后，可持续在体内存在很长一段时间,并保持对特异性抗原的记忆性反应能力(见下文)。通过它的作用,当再次遇到相同的抗原时,机体将产生更迅速和强烈的应答反应。固有免疫细胞生存周期短,由于不能克隆增殖,即使再次接触相同抗原,出现的应对反应无论时间还是强度都和第一次接触相差无几。但是在移植免疫反应过程中,固有免疫细胞和适应性免疫细胞相互之间密切合作，因此很难分清二者在此反应过程中各自的功能和在免疫应答中的作用。不仅如此,证据显示固有免疫细胞和适应性免疫细胞间的交互作用对于免疫系统的产生和调控作用很大。因此纯粹的固有免疫或者适应性免疫应答概念可能理论意义大于实际意义。

固有免疫细胞

固有免疫细胞被认为在宿主抵抗不同病原体的过程中不断进化,是公认的抵御细菌、真菌、寄生虫的第一道防线[5]。属于固有免疫系统的炎性细胞主要有粒细胞和吞噬细胞,在类型识别受体(PRR)检测到病原体相关分子类型(PAMPS[4,6])和内源性损伤相关分子类型后(DAMPS[7]),病原体迅速激活这些细胞。与适应性免疫一个重要的不同点是,固有免疫细胞是非克隆性的,同一种系的细胞表现出相同的种系编码受体。固有免疫细胞中的白细胞细胞质中含有抗微生物物质、酶和免疫调节成分。可进行如下分类,第一类为粒细胞:中性粒细胞、嗜酸性粒细胞、嗜碱性粒细胞和肥大细胞。第二类是具有获得并选择性处理外源性物质能力的细胞,包括:单核细胞、巨噬细胞、树突状细胞(DC),也称为单核吞噬细胞[8,9]。第三类是具有某些特异性免疫特征的细胞,如具有特定疾病免疫功能的 γδ T 细胞[10]和 NK 细胞[11],这类细胞可以在没有预先致敏的情况下直接杀死病毒感染的细胞或肿瘤细胞。第 7 章将详细讨论固有免疫的移植特异性免疫机制。

粒细胞

通常，粒细胞在感知入侵病原体或局部炎性刺激后激活,快速释放出细胞和胞质性免疫介质,可以直接杀伤病原体,促进局部炎症和免疫反应。

中性粒细胞

中性粒细胞囊括了循环内白细胞的大部分，在参与病原体侵入反应和组织损伤中发挥了极为重要的作用[12]。中性粒细胞所表达的细胞膜受体和分子使得它们可以感受并迁移到感染和炎性反应区域。一般来说，作为首先到达的免疫细胞，中性粒细胞通过吞噬或者摄取补体调理作用(见下文)对微生物及损伤组织发挥作用。通过释放含有具有抗菌作用的活性氧(ROS)和细胞毒性物质颗粒,以及一系列炎性介质,中性粒细胞能够影响固有和特异性免疫细胞而放大局部的固有免疫反应和适应性免疫反应。中性粒细胞还可以发挥重要的促进炎症缓解和损伤修复的作用。

肥大细胞、嗜酸性粒细胞和嗜碱性粒细胞

肥大细胞在体内数量很少但寿命较长，主要存在于外周组织特别是神经支配和富含血管的区域[13]。激活肥大细胞可以使其释放含有组胺的颗粒，组胺可以增加血管的通透性并刺激局部神经。肥大细胞还可以产生脂质衍生的花生酸信使，调节周围环境并促进其他免疫细胞的炎性趋化作用。嗜酸性粒细胞和嗜碱性粒细胞都是血液中存量稀少的颗粒细胞，通过释放组胺、肝素、细胞因子，主要是IL-4和趋化物，参与过敏反应和抗寄生虫的反应[14,15]。

自然杀伤(NK)细胞

自然杀伤细胞是一类具有细胞毒性的固有免疫细胞，主要作用是清除异常细胞[16,17]。NK细胞与相关的NK T细胞是异质性的淋巴细胞，主要作用为清除病原体感染细胞和异常细胞。它们通过归属于免疫球蛋白样受体和C型凝集素受体家族的种系编码的细胞表面受体监测外周组织，通过受体的调控，能够抑制或者增强NK细胞的细胞毒作用。

单核吞噬细胞

吞噬作用是指细胞主动摄入超过0.5μm的大颗粒过程，是由中性粒细胞和一系列被称为单核吞噬细胞如单核细胞、巨噬细胞、树突状细胞的固有免疫细胞所完成的。单核细胞、巨噬细胞、树突状细胞和中性粒细胞一样是专门的吞噬细胞。在体内，绝大多数吞噬反应都是由它们完成的[18]。单核吞噬细胞不仅通过吞噬作用清理病原体，而且通过这一过程对抗原进行摄取、处理，并将其提呈给适应性免疫细胞[19]。

单核吞噬细胞另外的一些必要特性使得单核吞噬细胞不仅可以作为吞噬效应细胞，还可以作为核心的免疫前哨，协调固有免疫与适应性免疫反应。单核细胞、巨噬细胞特别是树突状细胞可以获取、处理抗原，并将其提呈给特异性T淋巴细胞识别并引发必要的免疫反应。如此，巨噬细胞和树突状细胞被认为是专门的抗原提呈细胞(APC)。关于抗原处理和提呈的过程将在下面详细说明。

单核细胞、巨噬细胞和树突状细胞如同其他固有免疫细胞一样表达不同种系编码的环境感知受体。这些类型识别受体使得细胞能够感受到外源性病原体所释放的病原体相关分子类型[4]，以及局部组织损伤和细胞死亡所释放的损伤相关分子类型[20,21]，如已有深入研究的Toll样受体(TLR)[22]、细胞因子受体、C型凝集素受体、NOD类受体和RIG-I样受体[23]。激活受体可以引导单核吞噬细胞的激活和分化过程，从而引发不同促炎髓系细胞精准地协调后续的适应性免疫反应，特别是能够识别APC所提呈抗原的T细胞。在静态环境以及缺乏刺激的情况下，单核吞噬细胞被称为“未成熟”的APC细胞，同时以致敏原耐受的方式抑制提呈抗原对T细胞的激活反应。

树突状细胞(DC)

一般来说，树突状细胞是$CD34^+$造血干细胞来源的一类细胞，在体内含量非常稀少，散在分布，具有迁移特性[24-27]。它们从外周组织如皮肤或其他非淋巴组织转运抗原，将其提呈给外周淋巴器官中的T细胞。DC特别擅长抗原获取、处理并提呈给表达特异受体的少数T细胞，这些受体可识别结合于主要组织相容性复合体(MHC)分子的抗原多肽。

树突状细胞按类型、定位和功能可分为多个亚型(即，经典的迁移性树突状细胞、淋巴组织定植的树突状细胞、炎性树突状细胞和浆细胞样树突状细胞)[28,29]。经典的迁移性树突状细胞位于非淋巴器官中，主要根据其CD11c、CD11b，或者CD103表达不同分为上皮朗格汉斯细胞(LC)和小肠黏膜内、肺或者肾脏树突状细胞，它们能够启动T细胞免疫[30-32]。其一般特征是能够通过输入性的淋巴管从外周淋巴组织向引流淋巴结迁移。在此过程，迁移性树突状细胞不仅可以逐渐发育成熟，而且可以将外周获得抗原运送到淋巴结中，在这里抗原将被传递给此处的树突状细胞(抗原的交叉提呈)。除此之外，近期研究表明，可再生的幼稚T细胞与迁移性树突状细胞的相互作用也可以发生在外周组织中(非淋巴组织)，这种相互作用可以进一步提升T细胞激活的数目和程度[33]。淋巴组织定植树突状细胞，如$CD4^+$、$CD8^+$或者双阴性树突状细胞只出现在淋巴器官中，由淋巴器官的前体细胞分化而来[34,35]。浆细胞样树突状细胞(pDC)作为重要的抗病毒细胞因子如Ⅰ型干扰素(IFN)的分泌宿主，主要由经典的迁移性和淋巴定植树突状细胞分化而来[36]。除了迁移性、淋巴定植性和浆细胞样树突状细胞外，炎性树突状细胞在炎症反应的情况下也可以从外周和次级淋巴器官中的

单核细胞转化而来[37]。

树突状细胞重要的免疫调节功能

通常，树突状细胞的基本作用是将来自外周组织比如皮肤或者非淋巴组织的抗原，传递给位于外周淋巴器官负责免疫监视的 T 细胞[24,38]。更为重要的是，树突状细胞根据机体内的情况需要，既可以促进也可以抑制活化的 T 细胞免疫反应。

在非淋巴组织中，如能进行器官移植的脏器（肾、心、肝和胰腺），树突状细胞以未成熟的抗原提呈细胞形式存在[39-42]。新分离出的树突状细胞，其膜表面少有表达来自共显性遗传基因的高度多元化的表面蛋白-MHC 分子，T 细胞对抗原的识别及活化作用必须通过 MHC 实现（见第 5 章），因此 MHC 对 T 细胞免疫具有极为重要的作用。抗原提呈细胞特别是树突状细胞可以通过吞噬或者受体介导的细胞吞噬作用有效地摄取抗原，在一个专门的胞内空间中处理抗原。将与细胞表面 MHC 分子结合的抗原来源多肽提呈给 T 细胞[43]（图 2.2）。APC 细胞的 MHC Ⅱ类分子复合物与 $CD4^+$的 T 细胞相互作用，APC 表面的 MHC Ⅰ类分子复合物则与 $CD8^+$的 T 细胞相互作用。MHC Ⅰ类分子所提呈的抗原来源多肽主要来源于病原体细胞内成分，并被胞浆蛋白酶所降解。而 MHC Ⅱ类分子复合物所提呈的多肽则主要来自细胞外成分，在溶酶体小室内降解[44,45]。一项将两种提呈方式结合的方式称为交互提呈，包括 MHC Ⅰ类分子将外源性抗原提呈给 $CD8^+$ T 细胞的方式，或者通过自噬（一种细胞通过溶酶体机制降解自身组成部分的过程）方式降解外源性胞浆蛋白，通过 MHC Ⅱ类分子将抗原提呈给 $CD4^+$ T 细胞[46,47]。在抗原提呈细胞中，由于树突状细胞具有精确表达 T 细胞共刺激和细胞内的黏附分子，以及能够分泌促炎细胞因子启动天然 T 细胞的作用，因此被公认为专门的抗原提呈细胞[43]。巨噬细胞和活化的 B 淋巴细胞亦可以通过 MHC Ⅱ类分子提呈抗原，但在启动天然 T 细胞作用方面效果不明显。未成熟树突状细胞即使没有外源刺激，也可以通过环境感受受体（如 TLR）敏锐地感知局部变化，探测病原体相关分子类型（PAMPS）或损伤相关分子类

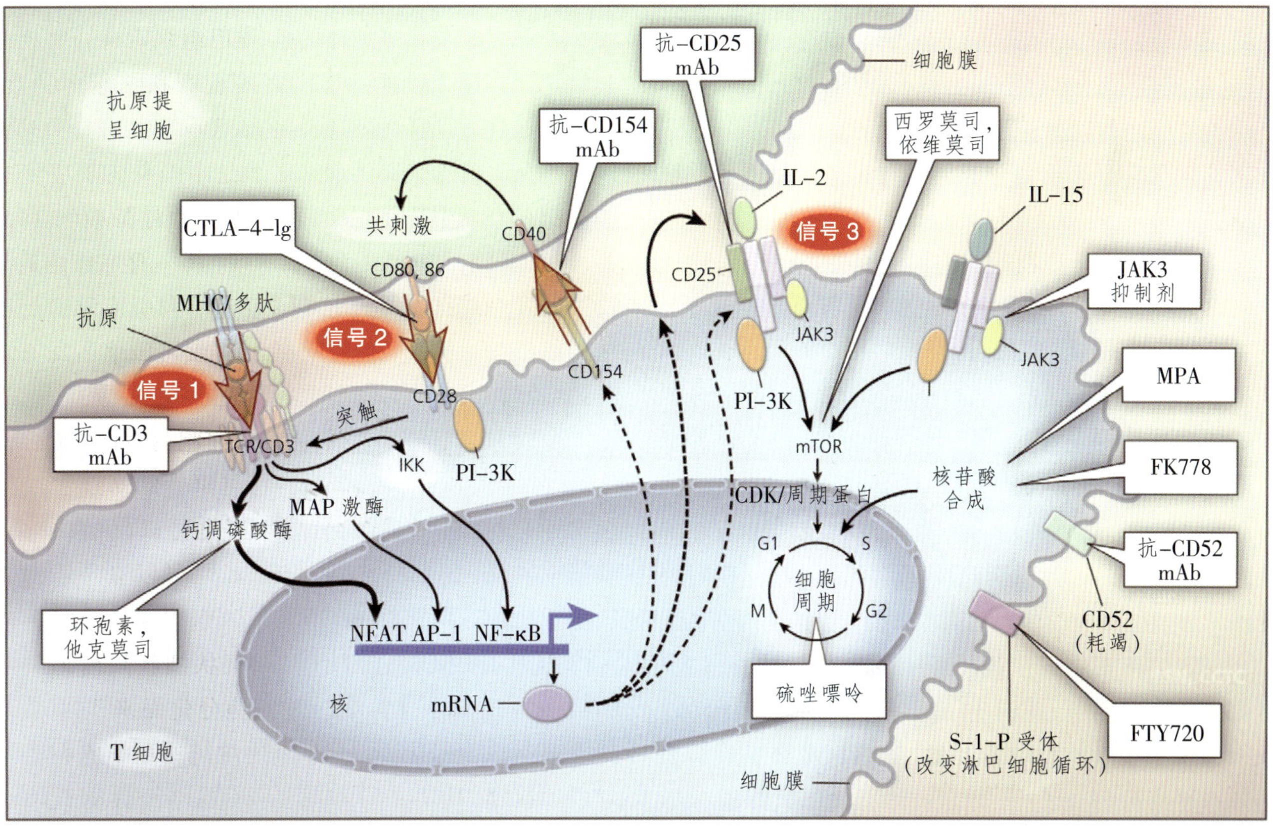

图 2.2　抗原提呈细胞与 T 细胞作用。描绘了三个参与激活 T 细胞的信号通路。From Halloran PF. Immunosuppressive Drugs for Kidney Transplantation. NEJM 2004 351: 2715-19. Copyright © 2004 Massachusetts Medical Society. Reprinted with permission from Massachusetts Medical Society[105].

型(DAMPS),指示局部危险,可直接激活树突状细胞成熟的信号通路,包括上调共刺激分子和分泌具有生物学活性的促炎蛋白促进免疫反应。

巨噬细胞

与树突状细胞类似,巨噬细胞具有高度的可塑性,是从单核细胞起源,经过环境和细胞的共同作用,获得有不同分子和功能类型的一种抗原提呈细胞[48]。它们通过感知感染物或者应激、伤害反应进行组织监视[49]。通过前面所提到的种系编码的环境感知类型识别受体而发挥作用。这些参与受体启动一系列复杂的过程被称为细胞内和细胞外激活。激活的巨噬细胞能够进行吞噬和抗原处理,根据激活程度的不同表达不同水平的MHCⅡ类和共刺激分子。与树突状细胞类似,活化的巨噬细胞也是专门的抗原提呈细胞,能够将有效的抗原提呈给T细胞。但它们之间存在一个重要的区别,虽然两种细胞都可以将抗原提呈给初始状态T细胞,但只有树突状细胞能够有效地向天然T细胞提呈抗原(如下)[25]。因此,在应对抗原或者移植物的免疫反应中,由树突状细胞所提呈的抗原是启动强烈的适应性免疫反应所必需的,而广泛存在于炎症组织的巨噬细胞,通过整合来自初始T细胞和炎症环境的信号,在适应性免疫反应和固有免疫反应之间调整。

除了对病原体相关分子类型和损伤相关分子类型的反应不同外,巨噬细胞还能够通过与完全分化的效应T细胞反应和接触特别的细胞因子而分化成不同的功能状态。巨噬细胞可以通过经典或者选择性方式被激活为M1或者M2型[50]。M1巨噬细胞可针对细胞内微生物和肿瘤发挥作用[51],M2巨噬细胞异质性更高,可包裹并清除细胞外的寄生虫,处理1型炎症反应,以及促进组织修复和重塑。当然,M2型巨噬细胞也可以发挥免疫调控和促进肿瘤进展的作用。M1和M2巨噬细胞不仅在功能上存在差异,而且根据其生物活性不同而表达不同的受体和酶。M1巨噬细胞表达高水平的炎性细胞因子(IL-12、IL-23、TNF、IL-1β和IL-6)和趋化因子(CXCL9、CXCL10、CXCL11、CCL2、CCL3、CCL4、CCL5和CXCL2),以及参与活性氧和NO生成的酶[51]。M2巨噬细胞虽然表达低水平的炎症介质,但却高表达IL-10、甘露糖和半乳糖受体。尤为重要的是,在小鼠体内,M2巨噬细胞表达的精氨酸酶1可以通过抑制NO的产生路径(通过诱导性NO合成酶),合成在组织修复和纤维化中发挥作用的鸟氨酸和多聚氨基酸。

虽然通过对M1/M2型简单地划分有助于理解巨噬细胞在免疫反应中的核心作用,但近期研究表明,巨噬细胞其实并不适合被这样机械地划分。因为它们会根据不同的组织、刺激和炎性状态而表达些许不同的炎性谱。此外,通过研究发现了巨噬细胞在免疫反应不同阶段所发挥的新功能,提出了如“清除性巨噬细胞”和“调节性巨噬细胞”的分类,进一步确定了这类细胞的复杂性和多样的功能活性[52]。

适应性免疫细胞

适应性免疫细胞包括T细胞和B细胞,在细胞表面表达不同类型的抗原受体,称为T细胞受体和B细胞受体。遵循同源重组基因(RAG1和RAG2)编码的区域特异性重排机制对基因进行重排,而形成T细胞和B细胞抗原受体的特异性决定域(可变的)[53]。由随机过程产生的T细胞和B细胞受体抗原检测区域使适应性免疫细胞具有对任意抗原进行识别和进行免疫应答的能力。除了来源于病原体的抗原,这些抗原中还包括自身抗原,因此未成熟的T细胞和B细胞必须经历选择性成熟过程,以清除具有自身免疫性和潜在自身免疫性的T细胞。骨髓来源的前体T细胞迁移入胸腺,在那里筛选出具有识别功能而没有自身免疫性的T细胞,释放至外周。B细胞在骨髓产生后继续在骨髓间质细胞的帮助下发育为成熟B细胞。更多关于T细胞和B细胞筛选的细节过程将在免疫耐受部分详述(见下文)。第5章和第6章将讲述这些细胞之间的关系和移植免疫。

T细胞免疫生物学

除了根据T细胞受体进行鉴别外,也可以通过T细胞膜表达的CD3分子进行鉴别,CD3也是T细胞受体信号中重要的组成部分[54](图2.2)。根据细胞膜表达CD4或者CD8的不同,T细胞被分为两大不同类别。CD4和CD8作为T细胞受体的共同受体,对识别抗原至关重要。与此相似,根据CD4和CD8可将T细胞划分为适应性免疫反应中重要的T细胞亚群。通常来说,$CD4^+$和$CD8^+$T淋巴细胞的功能并不重叠,可以在宿主防御性免疫反应中相互协作。

T 细胞通过 TCR 识别 MHC 抗原

T 细胞上的 CD4 或 CD8 分子与 TCR 异二聚体的 CD3 和 α/β 以及 γ/δ 链结合，构成了 T 细胞检测的信号传导体系。这些集合的 T 细胞表面蛋白，CD4 或者 CD8/CD3/TCR 组成了 T 细胞受体复合物[55]。正如前面所提到的，T 细胞通过 T 细胞受体复合物监视外周组织和细胞，发现潜在的病原体/外源性抗原。它们接收来自其他细胞尤其是 APC 细胞膜表面的 MHC 分子传递的信号信息。CD8⁺ T 细胞识别 MHC Ⅰ类分子形式的多肽，而 CD4⁺ T 细胞则识别 MHC Ⅱ类分子上的抗原。在上述两种情况下，T 细胞共同受体 CD4 或 CD8 加强 T 细胞受体与 MHC 分子间的相互作用。T 细胞受体与 MHC 分子间的相互作用，彰显出其特异性或者同源性的多肽抗原，引发信号传导通路关键分子，包括 ζ 链相关蛋白激酶 70(ZAP70)、脾脏络氨酸激酶(Syk)、细胞外信号调节激酶 1/2(ERK1/2)、磷脂肌醇-3 激酶/丝氨酸/苏氨酸激酶 Akt(PI3K/AKT)，以及激活细胞核因子通路(NFAT)的磷酸化，操控下游转录因子表达、染色体重塑和细胞骨架重建[56,57]。T 细胞受体信号所引发的效果还包括效应性功能，如引起细胞因子分泌和对目标细胞的溶解作用。

CD8⁺ T 细胞

CD8⁺ T 细胞又称为细胞毒性 T 细胞，被认为是清除感染细胞内病原体的初级效应细胞。细胞毒性 T 细胞通过释放多种细胞因子、小分子信号影响免疫细胞、其他类型细胞(见后面的细胞因子章节)，以及破坏靶细胞的细胞毒物质。这些细胞毒物质包括可以通过激活促凋亡途径引起细胞死亡的颗粒酶、丝氨酸蛋白酶，以及帮助颗粒酶进入目的细胞的穿孔蛋白[58]。此外，激活的 CD8⁺ T 细胞表达 FasL(CD95L)，通过启动膜表面表达(Fas)CD95 的目标细胞凋亡[59]。

CD4⁺ T 细胞

CD4⁺ T 细胞，又称为 T 辅助细胞，在启动外周淋巴组织中的免疫反应中具有重要的意义。它们通过释放细胞因子和表达免疫调节表面分子将信号提呈给效应细胞和记忆性 CD8⁺阳性 T 细胞、B 细胞或者其他免疫细胞(如 APC 细胞)。并且，在外周组织中，CD4⁺ T 细胞可以释放趋化因子吸引其他免疫细胞以放大免疫反应或者施加直接的效应性作用。效应性 T 辅助细胞是特异性 T 细胞和 B 细胞反应的重要调控因子，也是固有性免疫反应的协调细胞。T 辅助细胞的细胞因子产物、表面分子和特异性转录因子常被用来对 T 辅助细胞进行不同功能亚型区分(图 2.3)(后文的细胞因子谱和 T 辅助细胞极化章节有详细说明[60])。

激活 T 细胞需要抗原提呈细胞的共刺激作用

在初始 T 细胞激活的过程中，共刺激分子的作用对 T 细胞的生长、增殖和极化十分重要(图 2.2)(见第 5 章)。树突状细胞通过膜表面表达的 CD80 和 CD86，识别 CD28(初始 T 细胞持续表达共刺激分子)后，初始 T 细胞上调高亲和力 IL-2 受体 α 链(CD25)和 CD40L(CD154)表达，同时还表达抗凋亡 Bcl-xL 分子，并激活西罗莫司(mTOR，曾被称为西罗莫司哺乳动物靶标)通路，从而启动 T 细胞增殖[61]。除此之外，激活的 T 细胞上的诱导 CD40L 通过结合树突状细胞表面的 CD40 进一步促进树突状细胞激活(上调 MHC、共刺激分子和炎性细胞因子的分泌)，并增强同源性 T 细胞的信号识别能力[62]。或者，初始 T 细胞在没有共刺激的情况下，与未成熟抗原提呈细胞的同源性 MHC 抗原接触后，对产生相同 MHC 抗原的细胞不再产生应答和排斥[63]。

细胞因子环境和 Th 细胞极化

局部细胞因子环境可以影响 T 细胞的极化和细胞系的分化。信号传导激活转录因子(STAT)分子特征是感受外界细胞因子环境，继而支配 T 细胞所表达的转录因子(图 2.3)、细胞因子类型和处理的病原体种类，并抑制其他 T 细胞不适宜的细胞因子表达。

特别是，Th1 细胞表达 TGF-β，分泌 IL-2、IFN-γ 和 TNF，并处理细胞内病原体[64]。STAT4 和 STAT1 是非常重要的信号分子，接受来自 IL-12 和 IFN-γ 信号的激活，进一步诱导 TGF-β 释放，维持 Th1 功能，抑制其他转录因子如 GATA-3、ROR-γt 和 Bcl-6，继而分别抑制 IL-4、IL-17 和 IL-21 合成。Th2 细胞表达转录因子 GATA-3，分泌 IL4、IL-5、IL-10 和 IL-13 并控制细胞外感染和蠕虫感染[65]。STAT3 和 STAT6 进一步促进 Th2 细胞再生和初始 T 细胞向其分化，抑制 Th1 和 Th17 细胞产生。Th17 细胞表达 ROR-γt 和 IL-17，预防来自细胞外的细菌和真菌感染。IL-6 和 IL-23 可以通过激活

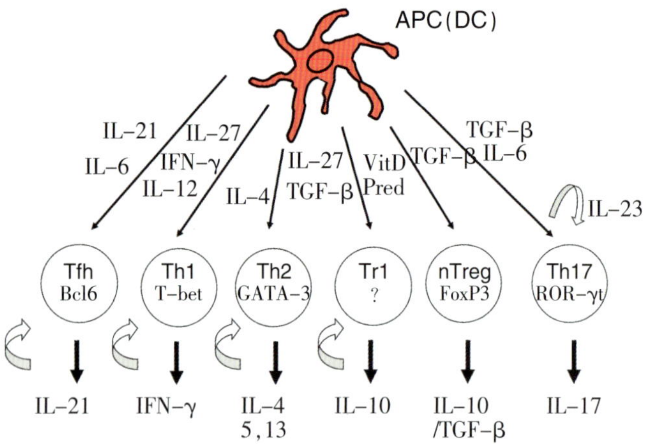

图 2.3 初始T细胞多极分化为不同的辅助性T细胞亚群。T细胞分化的命运决定于树突状细胞(抗原提呈细胞)传递给T细胞的细胞因子指令(信号3),还有抗原类型指令(信号1)和共刺激因子特性的指令(信号2)。这些信号被Th细胞释放的细胞因子强化(正性反馈机制),图示为每种辅助性T细胞亚群的细胞因子指令和关键转录因子。

STAT3引起ROR-γt驱动Th17细胞反应[66]。滤泡T细胞(Tfh)分泌IL-21并且辅助B细胞功能,对免疫球蛋白转变和抗体产生至关重要[67]。Tfh细胞还可以表达受STAT3、IL-6和IL-21调控的Bcl-6[68]。Th22和Th9是新近发现的T细胞亚族,但其重要性仍有争议[69,70]。

在人和小鼠中已经发现了一些抑制其他T细胞抗原特异性免疫反应(CD8和CD4反应)的T细胞亚型[71-74]。这些细胞被称为调节性T细胞(Treg)。天然产生的Treg细胞具有表达IL-2受体α链 (IL-2R;CD25)和转录因子Foxp3的特点,见后面的免疫耐受章节。关于调节性T细胞在移植中作用的讨论详见第5章和第8章。

T细胞的可塑性

在以上部分讨论了不同的Th细胞亚群及其不同的免疫学功能,由于其所具有的稳定性和遗传性特征,在传统上被认为是固定"种系"[75,76]。但是,最近的一些报道推翻了这一定律,并提出T细胞亚群可塑性的直接证据,说明后天性的调控可以激活负责转录复合物特征继而拓展T细胞的类型[77]。接下来,以GATA-3/Th2细胞为例,在淋巴细胞性脉络丛脑膜炎病毒(LCMV)感染的情况下,可以转变为GATA-3^+/T-β^+和IL-4/IFN-γ亚型[78]。ROR-γt/IL-17细胞可以在自身免疫模型中转变成ROR-γt^+/T-β和IL-17^+/IFN-γ^+细胞[79]。同样,Tfh细胞不仅表达IL-21和Bcl-6,这些细胞还可以分泌Th1、Th2和Th17[80]。如同下游细胞效应反馈功能一样,T细胞亚型的可塑性和稳定性之间转换关系的阐明,需要关于转录因子、细胞染色体和基因表达间关系的更多探索研究。

B细胞免疫生物学

对哺乳动物来说,并没有一个像胸腺那样供T细胞发育的独立器官供B细胞发育使用。但B细胞却可以在多个组织如肝脏、骨髓和脾脏中发育。虽然在免疫功能方面区别很大,但T细胞和B细胞间也存在很多相似之处,比如发育、受体结构、免疫耐受机制和激活信号。其中最为重要的证据来自T细胞受体所属的基因家族,是同一种免疫球蛋白超基因家族。B细胞所特异性表达的免疫球蛋白家族是包括T细胞受体在内的一大类重要的免疫性基因。分泌型免疫球蛋白产物是人体免疫的基础——抗体。膜黏附免疫球蛋白基因产物是与T细胞受体相类似的B细胞抗原结合受体。B细胞发育、筛选、清除或者对自身细胞免疫性失活的过程与T细胞类似,在此不做更详尽的说明。B细胞有两个特别重要的独有成熟途径:同型转变和亲和力成熟或者体细胞突变。关于这些过程中的移植特异性成分将在第6章进行详述。

同型转化

共有5种类型的免疫球蛋白(同种类型):根据其免疫球蛋白重链区域ξ、δ、γ、ε或者α的不同,分为IgM、IgD、IgG、IgE和IgA。成熟的天然B细胞在膜表面表达IgM和IgD,这也是B细胞唯一表达的超过一种的免疫球蛋白类型。IgM和IgD都可以发挥B细胞受体的功能识别抗原。B细胞在激活同型转变后,可分泌任意一种IgG,通常包括的亚型有(小鼠IgG1、IgG2a/c、IgG2b、IgG3,在人类则包括IgG1、IgG2、IgG3、IgG4),IgE或者IgA,并可进一步分化和增殖。

体细胞高频突变和亲和性成熟

在对一种抗原获得免疫后,B细胞在免疫球蛋白基因位点上发生体细胞点突变。体细胞突变的目的是重新更新免疫球蛋白谱系。突变过程本质是随机的。因此,一些突变的免疫球蛋白基因具有较为恒定的抗原亲和力,而另一些则具有或高或低的抗原亲和性。由于B细胞的扩增、成熟和生存需要依赖抗原的持续刺激,这些 B 细胞的自身突变使得具有高亲和力的免疫球蛋白基因具有更多的生存优势。这是免疫反应中的亲和性不断成熟的结果。

B 细胞激活

非依赖 T 细胞抗原

通常来说，B 细胞需要在 T 细胞的作用下对抗原产生反应（见下文）。但是，仍有一小部分抗原含有重复抗原决定簇序列，对于跨膜免疫球蛋白亲和力很高。这些抗原主要是细菌壳多糖，其抗原传递过程则不需要 T 细胞参与。这些抗原被称为非依赖 T 细胞抗原。

同源性相互作用引起共刺激信号

绝大多数 B 细胞抗原可能并不能与免疫球蛋白广泛地相互作用，因此激活 B 细胞主要靠自身。这一过程主要依赖 T 细胞，B 细胞同源互助。在这种情况下，抗原结合 B 细胞表面的免疫球蛋白并内化，然后将 B 细胞 MHC Ⅱ 类分子提呈给 $CD4^+$ T 细胞。活化 T 细胞与 B 细胞接触，启动活化过程，同时也使得 B 细胞表面受体 CD40 与 T 细胞表面的配体结合（CD40L、CD154）。信号通过 CD40 与 T 细胞启动的细胞因子协同作用而激活 B 细胞。

抗体分泌

在适当的激活和信号转导后，以前未成熟的 B 细胞分泌 IgM 并向两个方向分化：发育成记忆性细胞或者分化成分泌抗体的浆细胞。后一种分化方向常合并自体突变和同型转化分泌 IgA、IgG 或者 IgE，而一些浆细胞则不能进行类型转化和分泌 IgM。这项过程常需要持续 2~3 周，在一个未经免疫的动物体内，初始的抗体反应是 IgM，接下来转变成 IgG 和 IgA。抗体依据其类型的不同发挥不同的作用。这些机制包括补体结合作用、调理素作用及结晶片段受体阳性（FcR）细胞的吞噬作用。通过细胞介导的细胞毒作用进行调理素溶解（即天然效应细胞杀灭抗体附着的细胞），引发嗜酸性粒细胞脱颗粒作用。

补体系统

补体系统（图 2.4）是一套复杂的作用于目的细胞的系统，包括蛋白水解酶、调节蛋白和裂解酶[81,82]。可分为三个部分引起 C3 激活，这对细菌抗原的调理作用非常重要。C3b 片段激活膜攻击复合物 （MAC）（C5、C6、C7、C8、C9）引起膜的破坏，导致作用细胞的渗透性裂解[83]。

激活通路包括三条称为“经典”的激活通路，“凝集素结合”以及“替代性”途径，经典的补体途径激活包括第一个补体成分 C1 的结合，吸引 IgM 或者 IgG 抗体结合成抗原抗体复合物。激活的 C1 是蛋白水解酶，C1 酯酵素能够将经典途径中的 C4 和 C2 补体分解成多个片段。C4b 与 C2a 复合物是一种丝氨酸蛋白酶，可以酶切 C3，将其裂解为 C3a 和 C3b。凝集素途径通过甘露糖结合凝集素途径相关的丝氨酸蛋白酶 （MASP）与 C2a 切割 C4b，接下来将 C3 分裂为 C3a 和 C3b。C3 还可以被替代性途径的转化酶所酶切。在抗原抗体复合物、细菌、LPS 和其他激活物的作用下，通过选择性通路转化酶对 C3 进行酶切。在这条通路中，当因子 B 与 C3b 结合后，因子 D 可以对前者进行水解。C3bBb 复合物形成后成为替代性途径中 C3 的转化酶。C3b 可被多种类型细胞表面受体识别，如巨噬细胞和 B 细胞。C3b 与抗体包被的细菌结合是巨噬细胞识别 C3b 受体，启动吞噬作用的开始。另一方面，C3b 对参与造成细胞水解的膜攻击复合物 （MAC） 的补体反应终末产物（C5、C9）至关重要。C5b-C9 复合物负责补体对细胞膜的作用。

除了在补体系统中的调理作用和酶解物的作用，在补体反应中的激活过程产生的一些补体成分（C3a、C5a）也是炎症反应的有效介质。C3a 结合肥大细胞和碱性粒细胞表面受体引起组胺的释放，激发过敏反应。C5a 还是中性粒细胞和单核细胞的趋化物[84]。更多关于补体在移植排斥反应作用的内容可以参见近期的几篇综述[85,86]（见第 7 章）。

细胞因子

细胞因子是一种多肽类物质，由有核细胞产生，可以对造血细胞和其他细胞施加多效调控作用，参与宿主抵抗和修复作用。细胞因子包括淋巴细胞驱动或者单核细胞驱动因子、造血生长因子（克隆刺激因子）、结缔组织生长因子和趋化因子。更多关于细胞因子生物学和作用的信息见参考文献 87。绝大多数细胞因子通

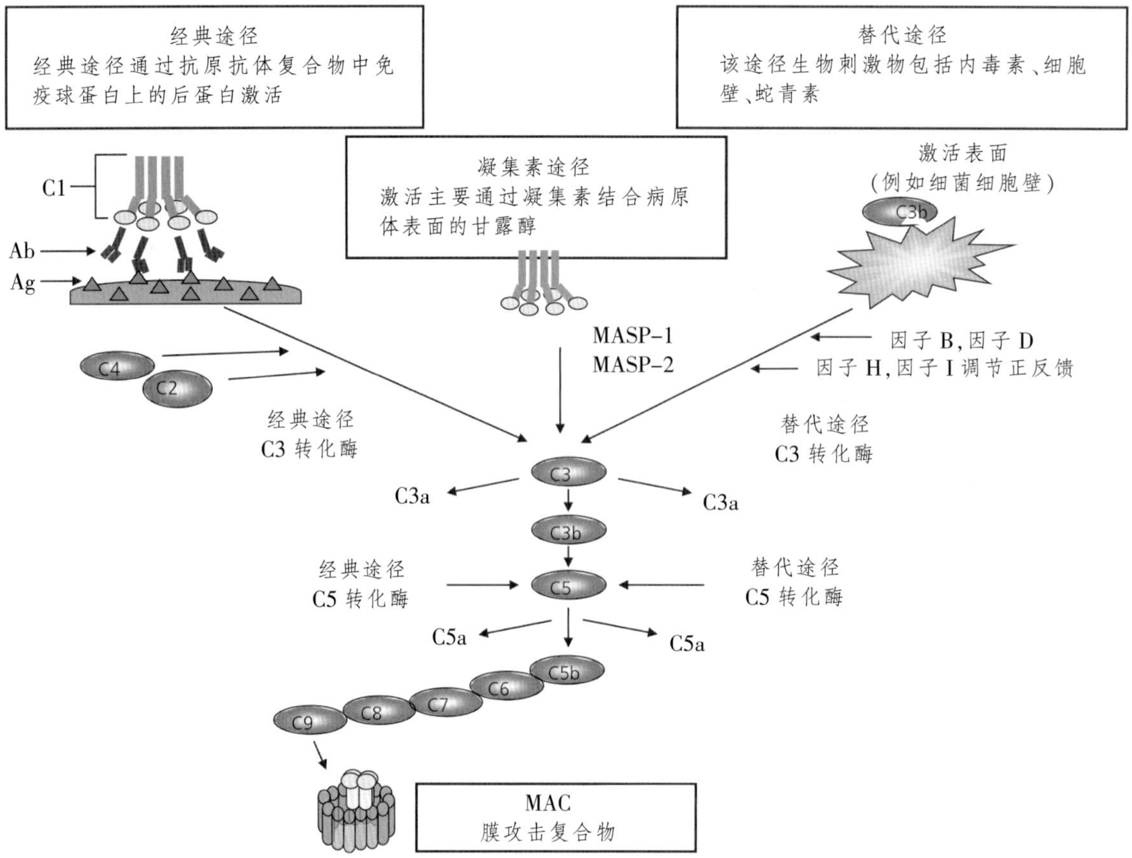

图 2.4 补体激活途径,补体激活主要通过三条途径激活:经典途径(主要由抗体抗原复合物启动)、替代途径和凝集素途径。三条途径均需要C3转化酶参与。最终形成膜攻击复合物(MAC),通过破坏细胞膜介导细胞裂解。

过局部或者短距离发挥自分泌或者外分泌细胞信号作用,当然也有例外情况,它们偶然进入循环并启动系统反应。细胞因子一般并不持续产生,主要在应对威胁组织的危险信号时产生,其功能在于通过损伤控制,促进组织修复,调控内在宿主防御和免疫系统维持内环境稳定性。细胞因子作用强大,一般在pM至nM级浓度发挥作用,它们的特征见表2.1。

多种细胞因子现在已归入白介素家族(IL)(如IL-1曾被称为单核细胞驱动淋巴细胞激活因子),其他的则保留过去的名称[如IFN-a/β、TNF、淋巴毒素(LT-α和LT-β)、转化生长因子(TGF-β)、白细胞抑制因子(LIF)、多数的集落刺激因子等]。曾用名表示过去众多功能作用中的一种(通常是首次被认识到的)。白介素是内容很宽泛的学术用语,目前白介素家族已经增长到35个成员,对它们的研究涉及分子生物学和炎症以及免疫学功能。类似的细胞因子的结构特征使得人们将其归类为"家族"(表2.2),比如细胞因子TNF家族、IL-1和TGF-β家族。炎性趋化因子及其受体(见表2.1)家族被指定分为四种亚型,主要包括CXC、C、CX3C和CC,按连续数字排列。

细胞因子的结构及类型特征

一些细胞因子家族的蛋白质序列具有高度同源性,比如所有的IFN-α/β家族成员在氨基酸序列至少30%同源。在其他一些情况下,当序列相差较大时,则主要靠相似的三维空间结构进行区别。这一类型的例子就是IL-2/IL-4家族。此家族成员具有相似排列的4个a-螺旋结构。尽管有些细胞因子结构差异很大,但它们因共用相同的受体而具有类似的功能。这适用于IL-1α和IL-1β以及TNF和LT,它们使用共享和非共享的受体。细胞因子共享受体链。比如,IL-2、4、7、9、15和21识别IL-2γR。IL-6受体的gp130链可以被IL-6、IL-11、LIF及其他细胞因子所识别。TNF家族可以结合TNFR受体类似物。包括TNF、LTα、LTβ复合物、Fas链、CD70、CD40L、CD30L、神经生长因子及其他。β链家族可以被IL-3、IL-5和GM-CSF共同识别。IL-8和

表 2.1　细胞因子特征

- 多数是结构简单的多肽或者糖蛋白 ≤30 kDa
- 一般情况下产量很低或没有；主要被刺激因子在转录或者翻译水平调控
- 细胞因子参与作用时间短暂，主要通过自分泌和旁分泌作用，不通过内分泌作用
- 细胞因子结合特异性、高亲和力的细胞膜受体(10^{-12}~10^{-9}MKd)
- 多数细胞因子作用取决于目标细胞的基因表达方式。细胞因子作用可促进或者抑制细胞增殖、分化状态的改变和(或)功能的改变
- 一般单个细胞因子的作用比较宽泛多样，至少部分细胞因子可以作用于造血细胞

趋化因子家族成员可以识别同源性的 G 蛋白偶联受体类似物。同 TGF-β 家庭类似，IFN-α、β、ω、γ 和 IL-10 受体具有同源性。IL-12 和 IL-18 具有类似的活性，它们的受体也可能相关。

细胞因子的重要性

细胞因子是防御过程的主要协调者，因此，在宿主对外源性和内源性损伤的反应、修复、自我稳态维持等过程中发挥核心作用。它们可以介导宿主对组织损伤、微生物侵犯、肿瘤，及细胞和组织移植的免疫反应。尤为重要的是微生物病原体可以产生细胞因子的变异体(如病毒性 IL-10)，细胞因子受体和趋化因子的拮抗物继而逆转宿主炎症和免疫防御。清除这些有害物可以降低这些病毒的致病性。更为敏感的检测方式可以检测到这些物质，而血液中低水平的细胞因子则与血浆中的不同附着蛋白相关。这可能也说明了细胞因子是机体在普通环境中对许多非病原体性刺激产生的反应。检测和定量疾病不同阶段的细胞因子水平可以作为疾病诊断的重要工具。除此之外，治疗性使用不同药物剂量的细胞因子已经应用于一系列感染性疾病、自身免疫性疾病和恶性肿瘤的治疗中。这也促进了对细胞因子拮抗剂抗炎作用性能(如 TNFR)的评估。

表 2.2　根据细胞因子的结构特征将其分类

家族	代表成员
IL-2/IL-4	IL-2
	IL-4
	IL-5
	GM-CSF
IL-6/IL-12	IL-6
	IL-12*
干扰素-α/β	IFN-α(多种亚型)
	IFN-β
	IFN-ω
	IFN-τ
肿瘤坏死因子	TNF-α
	LT-α(TNF-β)
	LT-β
	Fas 配体
	CD40 配体
	TRAIL
IL-10	IL-10
	IL-19
	IL-20
	IL-22
IL-17	IL-17
	IL-25
IL-1	IL-1α
	IL-1β
	IL-1R 拮抗剂
	IL-18
TGF-β	TGF-β
	骨形成蛋白
	抑制素
	激活素
趋化因子	CXC 亚家族(CXCL1-16)
	CC 亚家族(CCL1-28)
	C 亚家族(CL1/淋巴细胞趋化因子)
	CX3C 亚家族(CX3CL1/重组人膜结合型趋化因子)

*IL-12 是一种异二聚体结构，其中一个亚单位在结构上与 IL-6 相类似。另一个结构与 IL-6 受体细胞膜外片段相类似(α 链)。TRAIL, TNFR 凋亡诱导配体；LT，淋巴毒素。

协同和拮抗作用

细胞因子既可以作用于周围环境，也可以被环境所影响，尤其当其他生物活性因子(如细胞因子、激素、生长因子、前列腺素、微生物产物等)出现或消失时。在一般情况下，细胞通常很少只受一种细胞因子的作用。也就是说，细胞通常受多种细胞因子和其他生物学活性因子的影响，所引起的生物学活动实际上反映了不同因子在一起的协同和拮抗作用。表 2.3 总结了细胞因子作用的典型特征。

表 2.3 细胞因子作用特征

作用	特征
多效性	多种作用细胞和功能
冗余性	多种细胞因子具有相似功能
协同性/拮抗性	将细胞同时暴露于一种细胞因子，可能引起完全不同性质的反应（如 IFN-γ 和 TNF-α 的协同性）
细胞因子反应链	细胞因子可能促进或者抑制另一种细胞因子的分泌
受体相互调控性	细胞因子可能促进或者抑制另一种细胞因子或生长因子受体的表达
受体信号交互传导	一种细胞因子可能增强或者抑制另一种细胞因子或生长因子所介导的信号

细胞因子的刺激和抑制特性

细胞因子一项重要的特性就是它们具有刺激和抑制其他细胞因子产生的能力。因此，许多细胞因子的作用是间接的，主要是由于其他细胞因子量的变化导致的生物学反应改变。一个关于此类间接反应的例子是，IL-1 通过刺激 IL-2 表达促进鼠胸腺细胞有丝分裂的作用，IL-2 是直接刺激胸腺细胞增殖的实际效应分子。IL-1 刺激 IL-2 表达继而作用于 T 细胞增殖是许多其他细胞因子作用的典型化过程。另一个例子就是 IL-12 对 IFN-γ 的刺激作用。激活的抗原提呈细胞表达 IL-12，刺激 T 细胞和 NK 细胞分泌 IFN-γ，IL-12 是 IFN-γ 表达主要的调控物。IL-25 刺激 T 细胞分泌 IL-4、IL-5 和 IL-13。

目前对于细胞因子的报道主要集中在刺激分泌作用，但细胞因子也具有抑制其他细胞因子分泌的能力。IL-10 通过 Th1 和单核细胞/巨噬细胞/DC 细胞抑制细胞因子表达。TGF-β 的多种抗炎和抑炎作用主要由于它可以抑制 T 细胞和 APC 细胞产生细胞因子的作用。一个关于多个细胞因子共同参与促进和抑制作用的例子是对极化 Th1 和 Th2 细胞的发育作用。Th1 细胞分泌 IL-2 和 IFN-γ，能够有效地激活细胞免疫反应，促进细胞内病原体的清除。与此相对，Th2 细胞分泌 IL-4、IL-5、IL-10 和 IL-13，促进抗体反应，主要是通过 IgE 的产生引起过敏反应。在此过程中主要的调控物是 IL-12，促进 IFN-γ 表达和 Th1 细胞发育。

冗余和多效性

细胞因子作用广泛的冗余性和多效性导致难以预测细胞因子在活体内作用的独特性和必要性。特定基因干扰技术的不断发展，极大地帮助我们弄清了细胞因子是如何在宿主体内产生作用的。但是，仍有很多最终决定细胞因子在活体内整体作用的复杂机制需要了解。

免疫耐受

T 细胞和 B 细胞对宿主抵御病原体侵入和复制过程非常有效，但同时它们也可以攻击宿主。这些风险来源于个体发生过程中产生 T 细胞和 B 细胞抗原受体（TCR，BCR）的机制。如上所述，这些受体通过结合 T 细胞受体和抗体位点 V、D 和 J 片段而产生。出现的谱系包括多源性的 V 片段和包括能够结合自身蛋白来源抗原的受体。因此就需要多个检查位点以阻止自身反应性淋巴细胞的产生和功能作用[88]。淋巴细胞是终身持续产生的，因此需要终身对此进行控制。

虽然耐受促进机制是紧密结合的整体，共同发挥作用，但是仍可以划分为两类：①控制淋巴细胞发育的检查点，通常指的是“中枢性耐受”；②影响完全发育的淋巴细胞活性的检查点或称“外周耐受”。理解耐受机制是理解如何治疗和观察免疫受体的关键一步。第 11 章将对移植耐受的机制进行深入讨论。这对理解为什么免疫抑制药物可以阻断淋巴细胞激活，还可以抑制耐受引起的内源性程序改变非常重要。所以要对它们未来的应用前景进行仔细地考虑。

T 细胞中枢性耐受

在胸腺内 T 细胞发育过程中，自发性 T 细胞受体片段重组过程只有在新形成的 T 细胞受体结合到胸腺内配体时才会停止[89]。由 T 细胞受体和 CD4 受体共同连接产生了强大的正性选择信号，引导其向 CD4 辅助细胞系方向分化，而 T 细胞受体与 CD8 共受体连接产生了较弱和（或）较短信号，引导其向 CD8 细胞毒细胞方向分化。过于强烈的信号可导致参与其中的胸腺细胞发生凋亡，通常指的是负性选择。当抗原出现在胸腺髓质时，可导致胸腺细胞被清除。这不禁让人疑惑：对组织特异性抗原的耐受是如何产生的。外周组织特异性抗原出现在胸腺内,可能来自外周抗原提呈细胞(树突状细胞和B细胞)的迁移,还可能来自胸腺上皮细胞通过最新发现的表达于淋巴髓质中的转录因子Aire(自身免疫调节)所促进的随机抗原表达。

并不是所有能够特异性识别自身抗原的胸腺细胞都会被清除。高亲和力的T细胞受体与配体结合可以引起T调节细胞的产生,从而在淋巴细胞激活的情况下维持免疫耐受。这一点会使得中枢性和外周性免疫耐受的区别并不明显,使我们对每种作用机制的理解更加深入。

T细胞外周免疫耐受

当T细胞受体对自身蛋白低度亲和时,或者当它们具有高度亲和组织特异性的抗原(在胸腺中表达数目不足)时,自身免疫性T细胞可以逃过负性筛选。对于这些T细胞,免疫耐受主要依靠外周机制[90]。

忽略

识别自身MHC复合物的阻碍在于将潜在的自身免疫性T细胞从表达特异抗原的间质细胞中分离出来。天然T细胞从血液中循环至次级淋巴器官、输出淋巴组织,然后再重新回流至血液中。因此,天然T细胞可以从非淋巴外周组织中分离,并且遇到可以表达高浓度组织特异性抗原的概率变得更高。这些特异性运送初始T细胞的过程促进了对组织特异性抗原的(无意识)忽略过程。

清除与失能

如同早期所发现的,激活T细胞需要通过T细胞受体、同步共刺激分子和成熟抗原提呈细胞所共同参与作用的信号整合。这种苛刻的要求为维持免疫耐受设立了一个重要的调控节点[91,92]。在缺乏共刺激因素的情况下,T细胞在识别目标抗原时,将会启动一个无效的激活过程,使得其后续繁殖细胞被清除。这个过程将激活自杀程序引入T细胞分化过程中,也就是通常所说的凋亡机制。有趣的是,不是所有参与反应的细胞在缺乏共刺激的情况下面对抗原后都会被清除。在无效的T细胞激活过程中,其余的细胞进入功能失活状态,称之为失能。与凋亡类似,失能是对一个激活和抑制的特异性基因进行精确调控的程序所引起的,失能细胞的主要特征在于它们对T细胞受体与抗原结合反应失能,即使在共刺激存在的情况下,依然不会进行反应。虽然凋亡过程的优势已被证实,但是为什么循环中失能细胞还会持续存在仍并不完全清楚。失能细胞存在的优点有两个:第一,确保能够识别不同的抗原(病原体),并能紧密结合存活的细胞,在需要时通过逆转细胞免疫功能不足的状态,维持效应细胞的数目。第二,失能细胞还可以进入调节性细胞的群体中,参加调控其他自身反应性淋巴细胞的激活(见下文)。

调节性T细胞

如前所述,T淋巴细胞发育特征除了通过选择潜在效应细胞攻击目标外,还具有调节激活免疫系统能力的T细胞,称之为调节T细胞(见第8章)[93]。最初其标记为$CD25^+CD4^+$ T细胞,随后发现可以特异性表达转录因子Foxp3,这些细胞通常表现出与普通T细胞亚群截然不同的功能。如果功能失调,可导致自身免疫性疾病。越来越多的证据显示,调节T细胞可以调控几乎所有生理或者病理适应性免疫反应。成年动物的胸腺可以持续地产生天然调节性T细胞。对它们的筛选倾向于被高亲和力和自反应性T细胞受体所诱导,但还有很多具体情况并不清楚。在循环中,这种细胞被设定用来控制各种涉及自身抗原的免疫反应中。这是通过多重机制共同作用的[94]。比如调节性T细胞能够与抗原提呈细胞相互作用,并削弱提呈和T细胞刺激功能,抑制天然T细胞的激活和增殖能力,控制完全分化的效应T细胞的杀伤功能。几种抑制机制以协同互补的方式发挥作用。

调节性T细胞涉及各个免疫反应过程,比如低水平的自身免疫性反应常发生在以下情况,由于病原体感染所引起的组织破坏后,树突状细胞发生激活,将自身抗原提呈给自身反应性T细胞。调节T细胞主动聚集至炎症反应部位,被激活,抑制自身反应性T细胞,因此阻止自身免疫反应进展至慢性自身免疫性疾病。

除了胸腺可以产生天然调节T细胞外,外周的初始T细胞也可以被诱导上调Foxp3表达并获得调节T细胞的功能。越来越多的证据显示,被诱导的调节T细胞还可以出现在小肠等部位。虽然并不清楚诱导$Foxp3^+$调节T细胞对全身免疫耐受有多大作用,但是可以预测其确实发挥了补充性的作用,缺乏天然和诱导$Fox3^+$调节T细胞与严重自身免疫性疾病有关。

另一个参与免疫耐受相关机制的是B细胞，它除了具有效应细胞的功能还具有调节细胞的功能[95,96]。虽然对调节性B细胞(Bregs)的首次描述可追溯到多年以前，但最近发现它们是以IL-10分泌型B细胞的亚群出现在小鼠体内，在人体内相对应的细胞具有调控T细胞和B细胞参与炎症反应的作用。

B细胞中枢性耐受

B细胞分为三类不同细胞系：B1a、B1b和B2细胞。B1细胞以非依赖T细胞的方式发挥作用,并产生针对病原菌和寄生虫等非固有免疫应答的抗体。而B2细胞在T细胞的生发中心激活,参与适应性免疫反应。这些互补性行为降低了对B细胞不同阶段发育以及激活控制潜在自身反应抗体产物对多种信号通路作用的要求[89,97]。

据估计，超过半数新合成的B细胞受体能够结合自身抗原。但是,并非所有能够结合自身抗原的B细胞受体都对机体有害。例如,一部分B细胞受体对自身抗原亲和力较低,并不会激活自身免疫反应,而对外源性抗原结合能力强而具有保护力。这进一步降低了清除或者控制有害的自身免疫性B细胞的复杂性。

成熟B1和B2细胞只有在通过检测点后才出现，这些检测点评估抗原亲和力(亲和性和密度)及B细胞受体信号激活阈值途径以增强自身耐受。在骨髓中B细胞前体形成过程中(或胎肝),相当数量的细胞被阻滞在发育过程中。目前仍不清楚,这种对前体B细胞受体的阴性筛选究竟有多少是通过结合自身抗原进行,多少是由于功能受体形成障碍所致。不幸的是，关于中枢性B细胞耐受的自身抗原提呈模式目前知之甚少。在人类B细胞发育过程中,部分自身反应细胞在从前体B细胞到成熟B细胞转化过程中消亡,为自身反应性确定一个额外的检测点需要更多的研究。而关于非成熟B细胞方面的争议很少(在啮齿动物和人类中都已证实)。在这一阶段,自身反应性B细胞受体可以通过“受体编辑”的方式灭活,即通过抗原结合引起抗体基因序列的重排。同时将具有自身反应性的B细胞同步清除，这一过程导致自身反应细胞作用特异性的改变。

B细胞外周耐受

骨髓中B细胞发育过程在通过检测点时允许10%的新产生的非成熟B细胞发育为过渡细胞(先是T1然后是T2细胞)。虽然这一过程十分有效,但是这些机制并不能清除所有潜在的自身反应性B细胞，因为这些过渡细胞在向脾脏迁徙，在那里它们将接触到骨髓中不存在的外周自身抗原。与抗原的高度亲和性,使得B细胞在T1阶段即被清除,与此相对,当亲和力不高或者很低时,将引起过敏反应。这一状态被归纳为B细胞受体信号的脱敏,抑制机体反应,使得抗原提呈能力和抗体产生能力缺失，减少B细胞生存因子的消耗。此外，剩余的过渡性B细胞与成熟性初始B细胞类似，在T细胞的辅助下，对自身抗原和重排的外源性抗原适度反应。不管它们的特异性如何,在缺乏T细胞辅助作用(或选择性共刺激信号通路)的情况下,刺激后的过渡B细胞将在2~3天内消亡。

与T细胞不同,B细胞一旦成熟,在抗原刺激后其生发中心中可变序列基因发生体细胞超突变，进一步拓展其受体特异性作用的范围。这将不可避免地引起细胞表达自身抗体受体,并需要额外的调控机制。生发中心环境在阻止成熟天然B细胞自身反应作用范围扩大中扮演着关键角色。这代表了一种微环境,过度突变的B细胞根据其亲和力进行阳性筛选，而依据局部抗原提呈树突状细胞和Tfh细胞结合位点的竞争造成的自身反应性进行负性筛选。与过渡性B细胞相似,生发中心B细胞在抗原接触后如不能接收到来自Tfh细胞的生存信号,将被清除。

免疫记忆

当免疫系统再次或者序贯接受同一外来物的刺激后,淋巴细胞系统快速激活(B细胞和T细胞),清除外源性物质,这一现象被称为免疫记忆[98]。

T细胞记忆

如前所述,T细胞和抗原提呈细胞相互作用,促进T细胞分化为效应性T细胞。在生理条件下,这些效应细胞(包括CD4系列和CD8细胞毒T细胞)快速清除激发抗原，参与反应的效应细胞数目在一周内达到顶峰。约90%的效应细胞在1~2周的收缩期内消亡,其余的成为长期存活的记忆性T细胞。这些记忆性细胞与初始T细胞在种类和功能上不同，主要的特征在于当再次接触同一刺激后，在很低的阈值就可以快速再次激活[99]。最近,人们认识到初始T细胞和记忆性T细胞在同种异体排斥反应中存在的差异具有十分重要的意义。这一观点将在第9章进行深入探讨。记忆性细胞也具有异质性,目前认为至少存在两种分类[100]:效应性T细胞(Tem细胞)和中枢性T细胞(Tcm细胞)。Tem细胞表达的宿主受体可以促使其迁移至炎症的非淋巴组织区域,在TCR的作用下,数小时后可产生一系列杀菌性细胞因子。与此相对,Tcm细胞通过T细胞受体激活后,虽然可以分泌IL-2细胞,进行广泛的增殖并获得效应性细胞因子参与,但并不立即产生典型的效应性细胞因子。它可以通过表达如CD62L和CCR7受体促进细胞向淋巴结和黏膜淋巴组织迁移。因此,有人假设Tcm细胞可以在这些区域内循环往复,并引发新Tcm细胞产生继发性反应。

这些特征表明,在连续或间断接触抗原后,Tem和Tcm细胞产生具有明显本质和数量区别的不同免疫反应。这将使得继发性免疫反应更强、更快、更灵敏,在继发刺激物多样化的情况下也更为有效。

B细胞记忆

如上所述,B细胞激活包括生发中心的选择过程(受到APC细胞以及活化T细胞所构建环境的作用),导致反应细胞的"亲和性成熟"。在这以后,一些B细胞分化成为抗体,分泌浆细胞,其他的细胞成为记忆性B细胞(Bmem细胞)[101,102]。这些Bmem细胞停止分裂,进入一个长期的稳定静息期。这与T细胞的记忆反应很像,Bmem细胞可以调控继发性体液反应的不同特性。这些反应可以在非常短的时间内发生(继发性一般在3~5天,而初次反应一般在7~10天),并具有大量抗体产生和持续时间长的特点。除此之外,再次应答还有分泌高度特异抗体(由于初始亲和力成熟的过程)和出现IgM外同类型抗体(主要是IgG、IgA、IgE)的特点。这样可以对以前接触过的病原体相关众多抗原迅速发生反应,并在多个部位发生作用。

总结

免疫学整体上构成了理解个体如何在海量病原体和威胁内环境稳定的环境中生存的过程。也是机体保持健康的基石,它与器官移植技术背道而驰,其免疫调节作用对于现代器官移植技术的成功与挑战具有重大意义。通过对本章的阅读,读者应该认识到生理性免疫过程中存在大量交互作用的因子,需要对其进行约束控制才能维持移植物耐受存活,是实现自身免疫耐受的重要方式。因此,移植专家和临床医师应该认识到过度抑制免疫功能的后果,努力在抑制与上调之间调控免疫系统。

致谢

编者的工作得到了美国国立卫生研究院基金R01 AI67541、U01 AI51698、U01 AI91197(AWT)、R01 HL97603(DM)、R00 HL97155(HRT)和美国移植基础科学院发展基金资助。

(崔笑 译 王思奇 李照 校)

参考文献

1. Janeway CA, Travers P, Walport M, et al. Immunobiology: The Immune System in Health and Disease, 5th Edition. New York: Garland Science; 2001.
2. Male D, Brostoff J, Roth D, et al. Immunology, 7th Edition. Philadelphia: Elsevier Health Sciences; 2012.
3. Guarner F, Malagelada JR. Gut flora in health and disease. Lancet. 2003;361:512-519.
4. Janeway CA Jr, Medzhitov R. Innate immune recognition. Annual Review of Immunology. 2002;20:197-216.
5. Beutler B. Innate immunity: an overview. Molecular Immunology. 2004;40:845-859.
6. Medzhitov R, Janeway CA Jr. Innate immunity: the virtues of a nonclonal system of recognition. Cell. 1997;91:295-298.
7. Bianchi ME. DAMPs, PAMPs and alarmins: all we need to know about danger. Journal of Leukocyte Biology. 2007;81:1-5.
8. Chow A, Brown BD, Merad M. Studying the mononuclear phagocyte system in the molecular age. Nature Reviews. Immunology. 2011;11:788-798.
9. Geissmann F, Manz MG, Jung S, et al. Development of monocytes, macrophages, and dendritic cells. Science. 2010;327:656-661.
10. Brenner MB, Strominger JL, Krangel MS. The gamma delta T cell receptor. Advances in Immunology. 1988;43:133-192.
11. Herberman RB. Natural killer cells. Progress in Clinical and Biological Research. 1989;288:161-167.
12. Mantovani A, Cassatella MA, Costantini C, et al. Neutrophils in the activation and regulation of innate and adaptive immunity. Nature Reviews. Immunology. 2011;11:519-531.
13. Kunder CA, St John AL, Abraham SN. Mast cell modulation of the vascular and lymphatic endothelium. Blood. 2011;118:5383-5393.
14. Karasuyama H, Mukai K, Tsujimura Y, et al. Newly discovered roles for basophils: a neglected minority gains new respect. Nature Reviews. Immunology. 2009;9:9-13.
15. Kita H. Eosinophils: multifaceted biological properties and roles in health and disease. Immunological Reviews. 2011;242:161-177.
16. Vivier E, Tomasello E, Baratin M, et al. Functions of natural killer cells. Nature Immunology. 2008;9:503-510.
17. Tsirigotis PD, Resnick IB, Shapira MY. The role of natural killer cells in hematopoietic stem cell transplantation. Annals of Medicine. 2012;44:130-145.
18. Rabinovitch M. Professional and non-professional phagocytes: an introduction. Trends in Cell Biology. 1995;5:85-87.
19. Savina A, Amigorena S. Phagocytosis and antigen presentation in dendritic cells. Immunological Reviews. 2007;219:143-156.
20. Gallucci S, Lolkema M, Matzinger P. Natural adjuvants: endogenous activators of

dendritic cells. Nature Medicine. 1999;5:1249–1255.
21. Chen GY, Nunez G. Sterile inflammation: sensing and reacting to damage. Nature Reviews. Immunology. 2010;10:826–837.
22. Beutler BA. TLRs and innate immunity. Blood. 2009;113:1399–1407.
23. Kawai T, Akira S. Toll-like receptors and their crosstalk with other innate receptors in infection and immunity. Immunity. 2011;34:637–650.
24. Steinman RM, Hawiger D, Nussenzweig MC. Tolerogenic dendritic cells. Annual Review of Immunology. 2003;21:685–711.
25. Banchereau J, Briere F, Caux C, et al. Immunobiology of dendritic cells. Annual Review of Immunology. 2000;18:767–811.
26. Lotze MT, Thomson AW, editors. Dendritic Cells: Biology and Clinical Applications. London, San Diego: Academic Press; 2001: 1–794.
27. Morelli AE, Thomson AW. Dendritic cells: regulators of alloimmunity and opportunities for tolerance induction. Immunological Reviews. 2003;196: 125–146.
28. Steinman RM, Idoyaga J. Features of the dendritic cell lineage. Immunological Reviews. 2010;234:5–17.
29. Heath WR, Carbone FR. Dendritic cell subsets in primary and secondary T cell responses at body surfaces. Nature Immunology. 2009;10:1237–1244.
30. Poulin LF, Henri S, de Bovis B, et al. The dermis contains langerin+ dendritic cells that develop and function independently of epidermal Langerhans cells. Journal of Experimental Medicine. 2007;204:3119–3131.
31. Coombes JL, Powrie F. Dendritic cells in intestinal immune regulation. Nature Reviews. Immunology. 2008;8:435–446.
32. Moltedo B, Li W, Yount JS, et al. Unique type I interferon responses determine the functional fate of migratory lung dendritic cells during influenza virus infection. PLoS Pathogens. 2011;7:e1002345.
33. Allenspach EJ, Lemos MP, Porrett PM, et al. Migratory and lymphoid-resident dendritic cells cooperate to efficiently prime naive CD4 T cells. Immunity. 2008;29:795–806.
34. Vremec D, Shortman K. Dendritic cell subtypes in mouse lymphoid organs: cross-correlation of surface markers, changes with incubation, and differences among thymus, spleen, and lymph nodes. Journal of Immunology. 1997; 159:565–573.
35. Steinman RM, Pack M, Inaba K. Dendritic cells in the T-cell areas of lymphoid organs. Immunological Reviews. 1997;156:25–37.
36. Liu Y-J. IPC: Professional Type 1 interferon-producing cells and plasmacytoid dendritic cell precursors. Annual Review of Immunology. 2005;23: 275–306.
37. Dominguez PM, Ardavin C. Differentiation and function of mouse monocyte-derived dendritic cells in steady state and inflammation. Immunological Reviews. 2010;234:90–104.
38. Banchereau J, Steinman RM. Dendritic cells and the control of immunity. Nature. 1998;392:245–252.
39. Austyn JM, Hankins DF, Larsen CP, et al. Isolation and characterization of dendritic cells from mouse heart and kidney. Journal of Immunology. 1994;152:2401–2410.
40. Larsen CP, Ritchie SC, Hendrix R, et al. Regulation of immunostimulatory function and costimulatory molecule (B7-1 and B7-2) expression on murine dendritic cells. Journal of Immunology. 1994;152:5208–5219.
41. Woo J, Lu L, Rao AS, et al. Isolation, phenotype, and allostimulatory activity of mouse liver dendritic cells. Transplantation. 1994;58:484–491.
42. Coates PT, Duncan FJ, Colvin BL, et al. In vivo-mobilized kidney dendritic cells are functionally immature, subvert alloreactive T-cell responses, and prolong organ allograft survival. Transplantation. 2004;77:1080–1089.
43. Mellman I, Steinman RM. Dendritic cells: specialized and regulated antigen processing machines. Cell. 2001;106:255–258.
44. Purcell AW, Elliott T. Molecular machinations of the MHC-I peptide loading complex. Current Opinion in Immunology. 2008;20:75–81.
45. Trombetta ES, Ebersold M, Garrett W, et al. Activation of lysosomal function during dendritic cell maturation. Science. 2003;299:1400–1403.
46. Bevan MJ. Cross-priming for a secondary cytotoxic response to minor H antigens with H-2 congenic cells which do not cross-react in the cytotoxic assay. Journal of Experimental Medicine. 1976;143:1283–1288.
47. Munz C. Selective macroautophagy for immunity. Immunity. 2010;32:298–299.
48. Gordon S, Taylor PR. Monocyte and macrophage heterogeneity. Nature Reviews. Immunology. 2005;5:953–964.
49. Mosser DM, Edwards JP. Exploring the full spectrum of macrophage activation. Nature Reviews. Immunology. 2008;8:958–969.
50. Mege JL, Mehraj V, Capo C. Macrophage polarization and bacterial infections. Current Opinion in Infectious Diseases. 2011;24:230–234.
51. Mantovani A, Sica A, Locati M. Macrophage polarization comes of age. Immunity. 2005;23:344–346.
52. Stables MJ, Shah S, Camon EB, et al. Transcriptomic analyses of murine resolution-phase macrophages. Blood. 2011;118:e192–e208.
53. Chen J, Shinkai Y, Young F, et al. Probing immune functions in RAG-deficient mice. Current Opinion in Immunology. 1994;6:313–319.
54. Davis MM, Bjorkman PJ. T-cell antigen receptor genes and T-cell recognition. Nature. 1988;334:395–402.
55. Weiss A, Littman DR. Signal transduction by lymphocyte antigen receptors. Cell. 1994;76:263–274.
56. Lin J, Weiss A. T cell receptor signalling. Journal of Cell Science. 2001;114:243–244.
57. Smith-Garvin JE, Koretzky GA, Jordan MS. T cell activation. Annual Review of Immunology. 2009;27:591–619.
58. Cullen SP, Martin SJ. Mechanisms of granule-dependent killing. Cell Death and Differentiation. 2008;15:251–262.
59. Harty JT, Tvinnereim AR, White DW. CD8+ T cell effector mechanisms in resistance to infection. Annual Review of Immunology. 2000;18:275–308.
60. Wan YY, Flavell RA. How diverse—CD4 effector T cells and their functions. Journal of Molecular Cell Biology. 2009;1:20–36.
61. Greenwald RJ, Freeman GJ, Sharpe AH. The B7 family revisited. Annual Review of Immunology. 2005;23:515–548.
62. van Kooten C, Banchereau J. Immune regulation by CD40-CD40-L interactions. Frontiers in Bioscience. 1997;2:d1–d11.
63. Schwartz RH. T cell anergy. Annual Review of Immunology. 2003;21:305–334.
64. Abbas AK, Murphy KM, Sher A. Functional diversity of helper T lymphocytes. Nature. 1996;383:787–793.
65. Mowen KA, Glimcher LH. Signaling pathways in Th2 development. Immunological Reviews. 2004;202:203–222.
66. Bettelli E, Carrier Y, Gao W, et al. Reciprocal developmental pathways for the generation of pathogenic effector TH17 and regulatory T cells. Nature. 2006;441:235–238.
67. Crotty S. Follicular helper CD4 T cells (TFH). Annual Review of Immunology. 2011;29:621–663.
68. Fazilleau N, Mark L, McHeyzer-Williams LJ, et al. Follicular helper T cells: lineage and location. Immunity. 2009;30:324–335.
69. Duhen T, Geiger R, Jarrossay D, et al. Production of interleukin 22 but not interleukin 17 by a subset of human skin-homing memory T cells. Nature Immunology. 2009;10:857–863.
70. Veldhoen M, Hocking RJ, Atkins CJ, et al. TGFbeta in the context of an inflammatory cytokine milieu supports de novo differentiation of IL-17-producing T cells. Immunity. 2006;24:179–189.
71. Sakaguchi S, Sakaguchi N, Asano M, et al. Immunologic self-tolerance maintained by activated T cells expressing IL-2 receptor alpha-chains (CD25). Breakdown of a single mechanism of self-tolerance causes various autoimmune diseases. Journal of Immunology. 1995;155:1151–1164.
72. Asano M, Toda M, Sakaguchi N, et al. Autoimmune disease as a consequence of developmental abnormality of a T cell subpopulation. Journal of Experimental Medicine. 1996;184:387–396.
73. Sakaguchi S, Sakaguchi N, Shimizu J, et al. Immunologic tolerance maintained by CD25+ CD4+ regulatory T cells: their common role in controlling autoimmunity, tumor immunity, and transplantation tolerance. Immunological Reviews. 2001;182:18–32.
74. Shevach EM. CD4+ CD25+ suppressor T cells: more questions than answers. Nature Reviews. Immunology. 2002;2:389–400.
75. Mosmann TR, Coffman RL. TH1 and TH2 cells: different patterns of lymphokine secretion lead to different functional properties. Annual Review of Immunology. 1989;7:145–173.
76. Szabo SJ, Sullivan BM, Peng SL, et al. Molecular mechanisms regulating Th1 immune responses. Annual Review of Immunology. 2003;21:713–758.
77. Nakayamada S, Takahashi H, Kanno Y, et al. Helper T cell diversity and plasticity. Current Opinion in Immunology. 2012;24:297–302.
78. Hegazy AN, Peine M, Helmstetter C, et al. Interferons direct Th2 cell reprogramming to generate a stable GATA-3(+)T-bet(+) cell subset with combined Th2 and Th1 cell functions. Immunity. 2010;32:116–128.
79. Nistala K, Adams S, Cambrook H, et al. Th17 plasticity in human autoimmune arthritis is driven by the inflammatory environment. Proceedings of the National Academy of Sciences of the United States of America. 2010;107: 14751–14756.
80. Reinhardt RL, Liang HE, Locksley RM. Cytokine-secreting follicular T cells shape the antibody repertoire. Nature Immunology. 2009;10:385–393.
81. Walport MJ. Complement. First of two parts. New England Journal of Medicine. 2001;344:1058–1066.
82. Zipfel PF, Skerka C. Complement regulators and inhibitory proteins. Nature Reviews. Immunology. 2009;9:729–740.
83. Alper CA. A history of complement genetics. Experimental and Clinical Immunogenetics. 1998;15:203–212.
84. Carroll MV, Sim RB. Complement in health and disease. Advanced Drug Deliv-

ery Reviews. 2011;63:965–975.
85. Baldwin WM, Ota H, Rodriguez ER. Complement in transplant rejection: diagnostic and mechanistic considerations. Springer Seminars in Immunopathology. 2003;25:181–197.
86. Sacks SH, Zhou W. The role of complement in the early immune response to transplantation. Nature Reviews. Immunology. 2012;12:431–442.
87. Thomson AW, Lotze ML, editors. The Cytokine Handbook, 4th edition. Vols. 1–2, Boston: Academic Press; 2004.
88. von Boehmer H, Melchers F. Checkpoints in lymphocyte development and autoimmune disease. Nature Immunology. 2010;11:14–20.
89. Hogquist KA, Baldwin TA, Jameson SC. Central tolerance: learning self-control in the thymus. Nature Reviews. Immunology. 2005;5:772–782.
90. Mueller DL. Mechanisms maintaining peripheral tolerance. Nature Immunology. 2010;11:21–27.
91. Choi S, Schwartz RH. Molecular mechanisms for adaptive tolerance and other T cell anergy models. Seminars in Immunology. 2007;19:140–152.
92. Wells AD. New insights into the molecular basis of T cell anergy: anergy factors, avoidance sensors, and epigenetic imprinting. Journal of Immunology. 2009;182:7331–7341.
93. Wing K, Sakaguchi S. Regulatory T cells exert checks and balances on self tolerance and autoimmunity. Nature Immunology. 2010;11:7–13.
94. Vignali DA, Collison LW, Workman CJ. How regulatory T cells work. Nature Reviews. Immunology. 2008;8:523–532.
95. Lund FE, Randall TD. Effector and regulatory B cells: modulators of CD4(+) T cell immunity. Nature Reviews. Immunology. 2010;10:236–247.
96. Bouaziz JD, Yanaba K, Tedder TF. Regulatory B cells as inhibitors of immune responses and inflammation. Immunological Reviews. 2008;224:201–214.
97. Basten A, Silveira PA. B-cell tolerance: mechanisms and implications. Current Opinion in Immunology. 2010;22:566–574.
98. Ahmed R, Gray D. Immunological memory and protective immunity: understanding their relation. Science. 1996;272:54–60.
99. Jameson SC, Masopust D. Diversity in T cell memory: an embarrassment of riches. Immunity. 2009;31:859–871.
100. Sallusto F, Geginat J, Lanzavecchia A. Central memory and effector memory T cell subsets: function, generation, and maintenance. Annual Review of Immunology. 2004;22:745–763.
101. Tangye SG, Tarlinton DM. Memory B cells: effectors of long-lived immune responses. European Journal of Immunology. 2009;39:2065–2075.
102. Good-Jacobson KL, Shlomchik MJ. Plasticity and heterogeneity in the generation of memory B cells and long-lived plasma cells: the influence of germinal center interactions and dynamics. Journal of Immunology. 2010;185:3117–3125.
103. Keogan MT, Wallace EM, O'Leary P. Concise Clinical Immunology for Healthcare Professionals. Abingdon, UK: Routledge; 2006.
104. Dranoff G. Cytokines in cancer pathogenesis and cancer therapy. Nature Reviews Cancer. 2004;4:11–22.
105. Halloran PF. Immunosuppressive drugs for kidney transplantation. New England Journal of Medicine. 2004;351:2715–2719.

第 3 章

移植抗原：HLA 的发现历史

Paul I. Terasaki

引言

器官移植临床实践中最重要的成果之一是，发现主要组织相容性复合物(MHC)，被称为 HLA，位于第 6 号染色体上。组织相容类型，指的是 MHC 对于供体和受体的配对，在方法学确立后，已经成为器官移植中的规范，同种免疫反应被认为是由此区域的多态性所引起的严重反应。事实上，针对 HLA 多态性的同种抗体是目前进行器官分配的基本衡量标准，作为同种免疫器官损伤的标志指标也逐渐被认可。这一章讲述了在理解和认识 HLA 过程中的重要事件，并且对读者从根源理解移植生物学的概念具有重要作用。在第 1 章中，专门回忆了临床移植的恢宏历史，在后面的一些章节(如第 36 章和第 89 章)现代组织相容性实验和同种抗体实验也有专门介绍。

早期研究

20 世纪 50 年代后期，临床肾脏移植的出现推动了 HLA 的发展，当 Joseph Murray 和 David Hume 首次进行人类肾脏移植时[1,2]，关于人类实验的相关科学证据相当缺乏。动物的皮肤移植物[3]和狗的移植肾脏[4]仅能存活数周。Peter Gorer 和 George Snell[5]发现了组织相容系统的存在，它决定了移植物是否可以被受体接纳。其也被称为"H-2"系统，在人类体内存在着相类似的系统。但如何证明人类组织相容系统的存在则是一个挑战。

在 ABO 血型发现后[6]，红细胞抗原的检测已经众所周知。研究人员认为，从白细胞着手是弄清组织相容性的最佳途径。因为有多次输血经历的患者发生输血反应意味着抗体可能参与其中，Peter Miesher[7]和其同事借鉴处理红细胞的方法，将细胞凝集来研究白细胞抗原。Jean Dausset，巴黎的一个血库工作人员，发现三个患者的抗体有类似反应。这项发现提出了第一个白细胞抗原类型，称之为 MAC[8]。Johannes van Rood 也在荷兰的一家血库工作，他在怀孕女性体内白细胞凝集抗体中寻找其特异性[9]。最初，凝集实验的主要问题是不够可靠，重复性差，原因是处理粒细胞很困难。为了解决这一问题，Van Rood 想到了使用计算机来分类复杂反应，并鉴别出 4a、4b 特异物[10]。同时，斯坦福大学的 Rose Payne 与 Walter 和 Julia Bodmer 合作，也在致力于研究孕妇血液中的白细胞凝集抗体[11]，并发现两种抗原簇，称之为 LA1 和 LA2[12]。

研究者意识到，需要对组织分型方法取得共识。1964 年，Bernard Amos 在杜克大学举办了第一次组织相容性协作会议，来对研究方法进行比较[13]。5 个实验室使用的是白细胞凝集实验，一或两个实验室使用混合凝集、补体结合、间接球蛋白消耗、混合淋巴细胞培养和微淋巴细胞毒性实验[14]。在 1965 年，Van Rood 在荷兰举办了第二次协作会议，这次 10 个实验室使用了白细胞凝集实验，只有 Ruggero Ceppellini 和我们实验室使用了微细胞毒实验(图 3.1)[15]。最为重要的是，我们已经能够相互比较不同实验室所鉴定的组织分类结果。我们开始检视我们所拥有的标本，共鉴定出 10 种类型[15]。在不同实验室中的工作仍在进行着，两年后的 1967 年，第三次组织相容性协作会议由 Ceppellini 在 Torino 主办，有 16 个实验室参加[16]。会议中，我们将其分为 11 个家族，首次得以发现能够产生这些反应的一个独立系统或者基因位点。

在这次会议之后，WHO 举行的一次会议规定了命名方法[17]。Amos 总结道，参会人员争论的主题是将该系统命名为 Dausset 建议的"Hu"，还是命名为 Payne 和 Bodmers 建议的"LA"[18]。最后，我取了个折中的方案，将

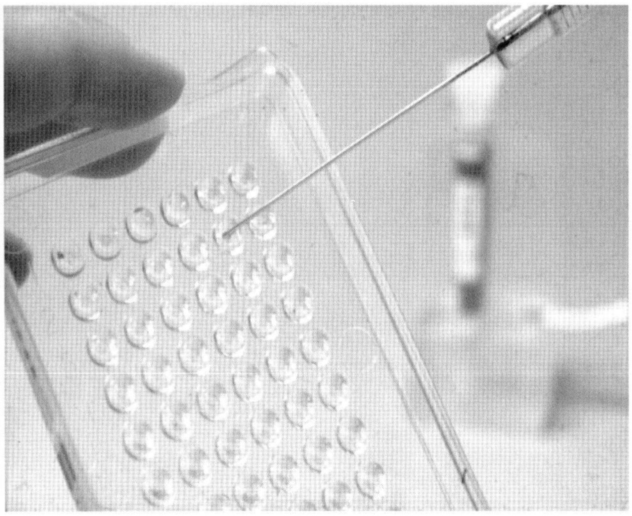

图 3.1　微淋巴毒性实验检测在 1964 年被引入。它利用 0.0001mL 的抗体血清、0.001mL 的淋巴细胞和 0.005mL 的兔补体。在每个皿中加入油滴防止挥发,在连续加入试剂的过程中不需要反复开闭盒盖,因为油密度小,总是浮在最上层(来自编者的个人经验)。

其称为"HLA",Dausset 发现的第一个抗原被称为 HLA2,而 Payne 和 Bodmer 发现的 LA1 被称为 HLA1。在会议之后,正式以"人类白细胞抗原"进行命名,而不是根据习惯以它的起源作为命名。

现已确定 13 种抗原,合并为一类,HLA 系统的基本原则是在 1967 年确立的,距第一次研讨会仅 3 年。Flemming Kissmeyer-Nielsen 提供的证据证实,这个系统有两个部分:A 和 B 位点[19]。1970 年,在 UCLA 举行的第四次协作会议上,微细胞毒性实验[20]被采纳为国际标准。这一方法在以后的会议中一直得到认可。1970 年,15 个实验室交换使用了 116 个血清,通过微细胞毒实验,多达 298 个家族可以被检测,我们最终检测出 27 个特异性标记[21]。

值得注意的是,在这期间,Baruj Benacerraf 使用半抗原聚合多聚赖氨酸对远亲动物进行了同种抗原免疫实验。他观察到免疫反应并不一致,并且可以定位到一个称之为免疫反应基因的基因位点上,这与 MHC 概念一致。

在 1975 年法国埃维昂第五次协作会议上,Dausset 揭示了 HLA 在人类学研究中的重要应用。根据不同的地理区域分类,一张世界范围内 HLA 特异性分布频率的图表被构建出来[22]。鉴别出许多重要的种族,不同的国家中家族相关特异性也被发现。比如,主要出现在高加索人种中的 B8 在苏格兰人中出现比例大约为 30%,在法国人中约 20%,在意大利人中约 10%,而在中东国家的高加索人中约为 5%。

由于 HLA 在人群中极大的多样性,故可将 HLA 应用于亲子鉴定:因为来自父辈的染色体是独一无二的,所以父亲几乎可以百分之百被鉴定出来[23]。当鉴定出两个异卵双胞胎有不同的父亲时,也就意味着发生了小组织分型[24]。

HLA C 位点抗原的存在在丹麦奥尔胡斯第六次会议中得到确认[25],DR 抗原位点则是在牛津举行的第七次会议中被认可[26]。在洛杉矶举行的第 8 次会议上,共 78 个位点被定义完成[27]。从那时起,7 次更为国际化的会议(每 2~3 年举行一次)进一步定义了 HLA 特异性。主要的变化是来自 DNA 技术的引进,从那时起共有超过 5000 个 HLA 特异性位点被定义出来。

那时,在 UCLA 组织分类实验室,我们发现了将白细胞培养超过两周的方法,开始在国际间进行细胞交换(1974 年)[28]。每个月在国际实验室间交换 4 种细胞,进行盲测,以确定它们的种类。这有助于在国际范围内建立 HLA 分类标准。这种每个月的国际间细胞交换持续到了 40 多年后的今天。

1980 年,诺贝尔生理或医学奖被授予 Jean Dausset、George Snell 和 Baruj Benacerraf,以表彰他们发现了受基因调控的细胞膜表面免疫反应的结构(图 3.2)。由 Terasaki 编辑的 10 篇回顾 HLA 发现历史的文章已于 1990 年在 UCLA 出版。

HLA 与疾病

几乎目前每种已知疾病都被进行了 HLA 分类,以了解其特异性结构是否与相应的疾病相关。这在 70 年代尤为火热。在 1985 年我们编写了一本概要,收录了关于超过 540 种疾病研究的 4000 篇已出版论文[29]。在这么多的研究论文中,具有临床应用价值的极少,只有用 B27 来诊断强直性脊柱炎[30,31]的研究被广泛应用。DR52 和 DQ1 与发作性睡病高度相关[32],但是这一相关性并没被应用于临床。自身免疫病已被证明与 DR3 和 DQ2 有关[29],但这一相关性确实没有太多临床应用性。关于 HLA 与免疫应答基因相关,并因此与许多疾病相关的理念并没有证据证实。有人推测,HLA 分子和其他多种感染性疾病的分子具有相近的氨基酸序列,但是

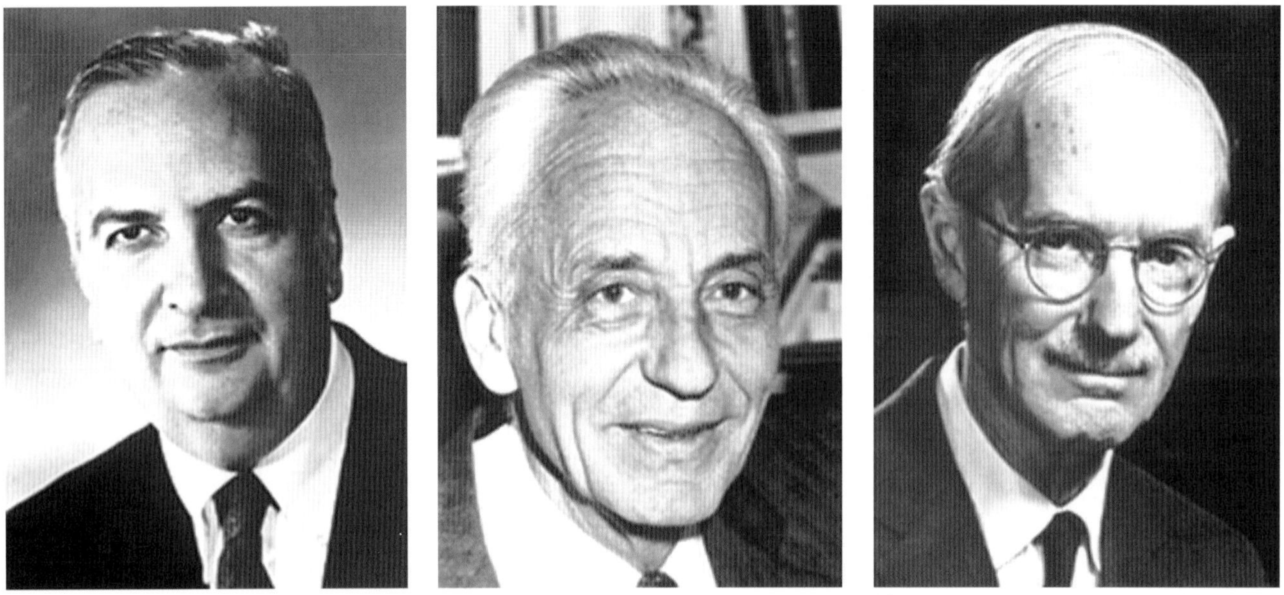

图 3.2 1980 年度诺贝尔生理学或医学奖获得者：(A)Baruj Benacerraf，(B)Jean Dausset，(C)George Snell，他们发现了受基因调控的细胞膜表面免疫反应的结构。(From the Nobel Foundation: The Nobel Prize in Physiology or Medicine 1980. Nobelprize.org. 3 Apr 2013. http://www.nobelprize.org/nobel_prizes/medicine/laureates/1980/)

HLA 与病原体的相似性并没有普遍性。HLA 与阿巴卡韦治疗的副反应相关[33]，这为 HLA 的应用前景提出了新的方向。但总的来说，起初对 HLA 与多种疾病明确相关的希望确实落空了。

HLA 与移植

HLA 在医学中的重要作用在移植中得到了体现。在 UCLA，我们再次认识到，只有对来自其他移植中心的患者进行检测，才能得出有意义的移植结果——以评价供体和受体组织分型匹配效果——因为每个移植中心能做的移植数量很少。从 1964 年起，我们建立了一个邮寄血样的系统[34]，这样即使远在巴黎的移植物也可以被分析[35]。之所以能够做到，是由于我们是以可存活数天的淋巴细胞为研究目标。这一项目使得我们能够以领先其他实验室的方式记录组织分型的有效性。我们检测了来自 18 个中心的供体和受体血样本。并在 1968 年首次报道了 HLA 一致亲属的肾脏移植器官的存活率最高[36]。

接下来，我们发现了一个非常不同的情况。当我们积攒的病例越来越多的时候，我们发现不匹配的器官也能运行得很好，这与人们的预期恰恰相反。接下来，我在 1970 年 9 月的荷兰海牙国际器官移植大会上介绍了这一发现[37]。这给我们带来了一场风暴，因为在“科学”的背景下，这可能是不正确的，只有匹配很好的患者才能获得更好的移植器官功能。在这个关键的时候，NIH 开始资助我们的研究，并在海牙会议后 3 个月内召开了一次大型委员会议，并且访问了我们的中心，这在 Thomas Starzl 的著作 *The Puzzle People* 中也有提及[38]。我们与 NIH 的协议在 1971 年终止，在海牙会议 6 个月之后。另外，Dausset 在 1 月份于巴黎召开了一个全部组织分型的临时会议，以否定我们的海牙声明。实验结果在不断汇总，他们希望证明是我们错了。这些分析从未被发表，主要原因是不能驳斥我们的观点。接下来，更明确的组织分型文章被发表在 1971 年出版的 *Transplant Proceedings* 第 3 卷中，如 Dausset 和 Rapaport 所强调的那样，每个作者都认为我们的分析出了问题[39]。图 3.3 展示了那张在海牙会议上给我们惹来大麻烦的幻灯片。X 轴是患者的临床分型，A 代表最好，F 代表失败，N 代表非适应性免疫失败。Y 轴是 HLA 的匹配程度，D 代表最差。值得注意的是，许多不匹配的患者移植效果还不错。右图显示 1987—1995 年间联合器官共享网络(UNOS)肾移植登记处的信息。与我们的数据一致，不匹配的患者效果很好，匹配的患者效果也很好，但是数量相对较小。

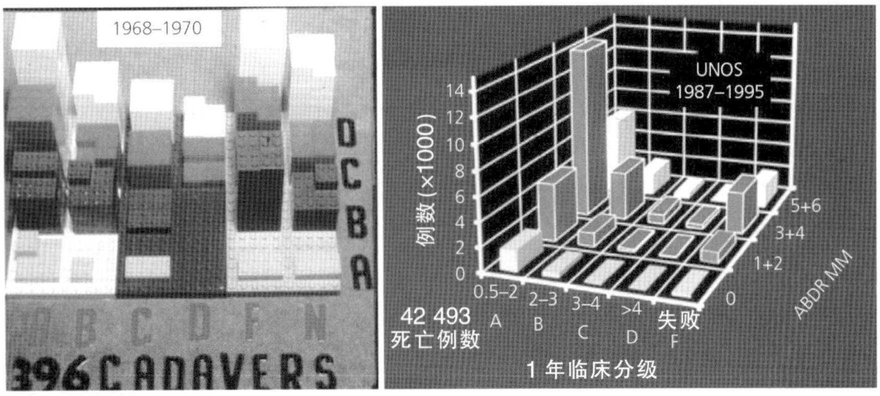

图 3.3 图示两个时期的临床分型（X 轴）与 HLA 匹配分级（Y 轴）相关性。左图是在 1970 年海牙国际移植大会上展示的关于 1968—1970 年间肾移植的结果。请注意，虽然许多严重匹配不良的移植物功能不佳，但也有很多不完全匹配的移植物效果却很好，临床评分是 A 级。右图显示了相同的不完全匹配的移植物在移植术后 17 年依然功能良好。同一时期完全匹配的移植物很少，移植后效果也很好（来自编者个人数据）。

组织分型机构的不安和困惑是可以理解的。对于任何具有科学背景的人来说，HLA 不匹配将导致早期失败都是显而易见的。正如早期那些使用动物皮肤移植但患者只能存活数周的免疫学者会被 Hume 和Murray 进行的人类肾脏移植所震惊一样，科学家推论，不匹配的移植物不能正常运行。值得注意的是，机体内 HLA 体系的极端多样性常意味着绝大多数患者与无血缘关系的已故供体之间区别很大。但 Starzl 并没有反对推翻“科学”理论的这一行为。当他发现不匹配患者一样可以获得好的效果后，他认为 HLA 匹配系统并不会成为进行器官移植的障碍。事实上，他承认当他决定忽略 HLA 分型时，他对肝移植的尝试才得以实现。他是第一位尝试这条路的外科医师。后来其他人迅速跟进，HLA 分型开始得到了坏名声。

与此同时，骨髓移植研究开始了，第一例成功的移植案例是在患者与 HLA 分型匹配的供体间进行的[40]。Donnall Thomas 开始了他的研究项目：纳入了大批骨髓移植患者，所有的移植均是依据 HLA 分型。但找到除了近亲骨髓捐赠者外的捐赠者是最主要的问题，因为无血缘关系的捐赠者很难与患者在 HLA 分型上匹配。骨髓供体项目在海军的资助下起始于 1987 年，作为一个国家级项目，其目的是为了对无血缘关系的供体进行 HLA 分型，并建立 HLA 匹配的患者登记系统。当我们把已知 HLA 等位位点增加到超过 5000 种时，这项工作变得非常困难。目前，在国家骨髓捐赠项目中登记的有超过 950 万名自愿捐献者，在全世界范围内这一数字超过 1600 万。

HLA 分型对实体器官而言则完全不同，虽然在初期 HLA 匹配名声不佳，因为不匹配一样有良好的效果。但随着免疫抑制水平的进步，医师们开始认识到精准的匹配移植效果最佳[36]。当我们发现不匹配患者效果也很好时，我们从 1971 年开始进行肾移植登记，以找出哪些因素可以影响移植后器官存活。与此目标相伴而来的是，UCLA 登记也成为追溯 HLA 匹配效果的最重要资源之一[41]。为了克服获得良好匹配过程中的困难，我们设计了一种简单的冷储存办法，实现了向远距离受者运送匹配肾脏的可能[42]。这个完全匹配项目由 UNOS 所资助，在 1988 年报道了首批接受完全匹配肾脏移植的 88 例患者，并进一步将人群扩大[43]。从那以后，超过 21 000 例肾脏通过 UNOS 分配系统在国内分配给完全匹配的患者，通过数据分析 HLA 匹配效果，患者在接受精确匹配的肾脏后生存率最高[44]，而那些非匹配位点多的患者，通常预后最差。但是，非匹配肾脏与完全匹配肾脏在功能作用上几乎一样。多项对美国数据进行的研究显示出类似的结果，不匹配的程度与预后结果并没有显著相关。这项研究迫使 UNOS 在 1995 年和 2003 年分别终止了 A 和 B 位点的优先分配权。政策的变化没有影响移植患者的总体预后[45]。

目前，HLA 匹配对于骨髓移植是非常必要的，但对实体器官移植则意义有限。只有通过国家登记系统和肾脏远距离运输，才有可能获得肾脏的良好匹配，这种良好匹配的数量仅占全美死后器官捐赠的 14%。

HLA 抗体

HLA 抗体的作用方式与 HLA 匹配完全不同。如前所述，只有通过抗体才能定义 HLA 系统。除了用作试剂外，抗体在评估移植物结局方面的重要性也日益增加。移植受体的抗体直接作用于供体的抗原，从而引起肾脏的超急性排斥反应[46]。除此之外，在移植前，受体内的抗体水平可以确定机体预致敏状态，这种状态常伴有早期器官衰竭的风险[47]。在术前，需要判断受体的特异性抗体情况，避免具有该特异抗原的供体捐献。使用了超过 30 年的方法是将预输入细胞与受体血清混合检测。通过这一反应，在计算机的辅助下我们可以判断抗体的特异性。但是有一个问题，由于细胞具有 A、B、C 和 DR 抗原，判断哪种抗原与抗体发生反应比较困难，这可能导致器官的不准确分配。只有在重组细胞外层附着一种单独抗原的情况下，才能准确判别特异性位点[48]。这些技术将在第 89 章详细描述。

在过去的 10 年，HLA 抗体在移植手术中的作用越来越受到重视，因为它们被认为是器官排斥的最主要原因[49]。支持这一结论的证据逐渐增多：几乎所有发生肾脏排斥反应的患者体内都会检出抗体[50]；在排斥的肾脏中可以检出抗体[51]；那些曾经在移植后出现抗体的患者将比未出现的患者器官衰竭的概率更高[52]，这对移植肾脏（图 3.4）[53-56]、心脏[57-59]、肺脏[60,61]、肝脏[62]和胰腺[63,64]的患者同样适用。最重要的是，发生肾脏排斥的患者在发生肾脏排斥之前均可以检测到抗体。这些因素符合由 Bradford Hill 和 Richard Doll 提出的 9 项标准，构成了从相关到因果的联系[65]。因此，我们推断 HLA 抗体与器官排斥间存在因果关系[66]。近来，越来越多证据显示，在抗体介导的急性排斥反应中，体内抗体发生消耗的患者比没有发生抗体浓度减少的患者预后更好[67-69]。这一发现出现在那些发生急性排斥反应而组织学变化发生逆转的患者中。并且，在肾或肺移植物发生功能衰竭之前清除抗体可以改善器官功能和预后[70]。通过移除抗体组分可以提高移植器官的功能状态，最终证明 HLA 可以引起移植器官排斥，而且可能是移植失败的主要原因。

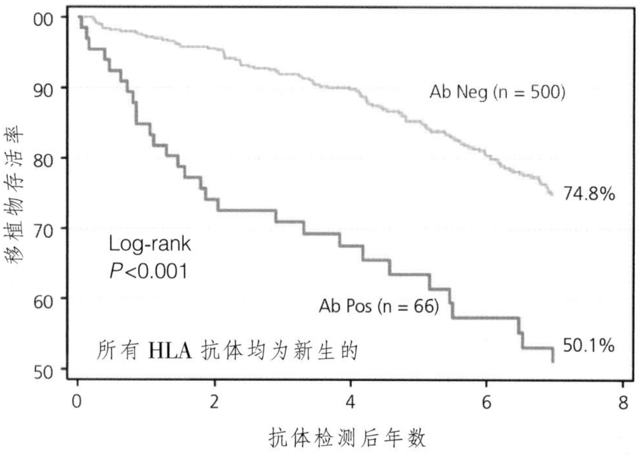

图 3.4 在 2002 年，作为国际组织相容协作会议的一部分，研究者对具有良好肾脏功能的肾移植患者（n=566）进行了检测，根据 HLA 抗体不同分为阴性组和阳性组。经过 8 年的随访，抗体阳性的患者发生器官排斥的概率显著高于阴性组（来自编者个人数据）。

总结

HLA 是人类主要的组织相容性位点，从 1967 年被首次命名后，发生了一段引人入胜的历史。在这 44 年里，HLA 是目前已知最具多样性的系统，共有超过 5000 种类型获得确认。这一多样性使得无血缘关系的骨髓移植极度困难。在非血缘性供体与受体之间，多数实体器官如心脏、肝脏和肺获得匹配的可能性也非常渺茫。所以，移植医师不得不忽略 HLA 配型，而更多地依赖于提升免疫抑制水平。即使在肾脏移植中使用健康的非血缘性活体器官，也显示 HLA 系统可以基本被忽略。但是，现在证据越来越清楚地表明，即使开始不匹配可以被忽略，但是其中一定数量的患者会形成针对不匹配器官的抗体。这些移植物特异性抗体将会与移植器官发生反应，造成移植器官排斥而丧失功能。近期研究发现，清除这些抗体将延长移植物的寿命，非常有力地证明：抗体造成了移植物的排斥。HLA 系统的作用在开始时并不明显，但它对移植的作用至关重要。

（崔笑 译 王思奇 李照 校）

参考文献

1. Hume DM, Merrill JP, Miller BF, et al. Experiences with renal homotransplantation in the human: report of nine cases. Journal of Clinical Investigation. 1955;34:327.
2. Dammin GJ, Couch NP, Murray JE. Prolonged survival of skin homografts in uremic patients. Annals of the New York Academy of Sciences. 1957;64:967.
3. Billingham RE, Krohn PL, Medawar PB. Effect of cortisone on survival of skin homografts in rabbits. British Medical Journal. 1951;1(4716):1157.

4. Dempster WJ. The homotransplantations of kidneys in dogs. British Journal of Surgery. 1953;40:477.
5. Gorer PA, Lyman S, Snell GD. Studies on the genetic and antigenetic basis of tumor transplantation. Linkage between a histocompatibility gene and "fused" in mice. Proceedings of the Royal Society of London. Series B. Biological Sciences. 1948; 135:499.
6. Landsteiner K. Zur kenntnis der antitermentativen, lytischen und agglutinierenden Wirkungen des Blutserums und der Lymphe. Zentralblatt für Bakteriologie Parasitenkund und Infectionskrankheiten. 1900;27:357.
7. Miescher P, Fauconnet M. Mise en evidence de differents groupes leucocytaires chez l'homme. Schweizerische Medizinische Wochenschrift. 1954;84:597.
8. Dausset J. Iso-leuco-anticorps. Acta haematologica. 1958;20:156.
9. Van Rood JJ, Eernisse JG, Van Leeuwen A. Leucocyte antibodies in sera from pregnant women. Nature. 1958;181:1735.
10. Van Rood JJ, Van Leeuwen A. Leukocyte grouping. A method and its application. Journal of Clinical Investigation. 1963;42:1382.
11. Payne R, Rolfs MR. Fetomaternal leukocyte incompatibility. Journal of Clinical Investigation. 1958;37:1756.
12. Payne R, Tripp M, Weigle J, et al. A new leukocyte isoantigen system in man. Cold Spring Harbor Symposium on Quantitative Biology. 1964;29:285.
13. Amos DB, editor. Workshop on Histocompatibility testing. In: Histocompatibility testing publication 1229. Washington, DC: National Academy of Science-National Research Council; 1965.
14. Terasaki PI, McClelland JD. Microdroplet assay of human serum cytotoxins. Nature. 1964;204:998.
15. Balner H, Cleton FJ, Eernisse JG, editors. Histocompatibility Testing, 1965. Copenhagen: Munksgaard; 1965.
16. Ceppellini R, Curtoni ES, Mattiuz PL, et al. Genetics of leukocyte antigens: a family study of segregation and linkage. In: Curtoni E, Mattiuz PL, Tosi RM, editors. Histocompatibility Testing 1967. Copenhagen: Munksgaard; 1967: 149–187.
17. Walford RL. First meeting WHO leukocyte nomenclature committee, New York, Sept 1968. In: Terasaki PI, editor. History of HLA: Ten Recollections. Los Angeles, CA: UCLA tissue Typing Lab; 1990: 121.
18. Amos DB. The 1991 nomenclature report. Human Immunology. 1992;34:1.
19. Kissmeyer-Nielsen F, Svejgaard A, Ahrons S, et al. Crossing-over within the HL-A system. Nature. 1969;224:75.
20. Mittal KK, Mickey MR, Singal DP, et al. Serotyping for homotransplantation. XVIII. Refinement of microdroplet lymphocyte cytotoxicity test. Transplantation. 1968;6:913–927.
21. Terasaki PI. Histocompatibility Testing 1970. Report of 4th International Histocompatibility Workshop and Conference. Los Angeles, CA, USA; Jan 1970.
22. Dausset J. Histocompatibility Testing 1972. Report of 5th International Histocompatibility Workshop and Conference. Evian, France; May 1972.
23. Terasaki PI. Resolution by HLA testing of 1000 paternity cases not excluded by ABO testing. Journal of Family Law. 1977;16:543–557.
24. Terasaki PI, Gjertson D, Bernoco D, et al. Twins with two different fathers identified by HLA. New England Journal of Medicine. 1978;299:590.
25. Kissmeyer-Nielsen F. Histocompatibility Testing 1975. Report of 6th International Histocompatibility Workshop and Conference. Copenhagen: Munksgaard; June 1975.
26. Bodmer WF, Batchelor JR, Bodmer JG, et al. Histocompatibility Testing 1977. Report of 7th International Histocompatibility Workshop and Conference. Oxford, England. Copenhagen: Munksgaard; Sept 1977.
27. Terasaki PI. Histocompatibility Testing 1980. Report of 8th International Histocompatibility Workshop and Conference. Los Angeles, CA; Feb 1980.
28. Loon J, Takemura S, Terasaki PI. Ten-year progress report of the International Cell Exchange. Tissue Antigens. 1984;24:215.
29. Tiwari JL, Terasaki PI. HLA and Disease Associations. New York, NY: Springer-Verlag; 1985.
30. Schlosstein L, Terasaki PI, Bluestone R, et al. High association of an HL-A antigen, W27, with ankylosing spondylitis. New England Journal of Medicine. 1973;288:704.
31. Brewerton DA, Hart FD, Nicholls A, et al. Ankylosing spondylitis and HL-A 27. Lancet. 1973;1(7809):904.
32. Matsuki K, Juji T, Tokunaga K, et al. Human histocompatibility leukocyte antigen (HLA) haplotype frequencies estimated from the data on HLA class I, II, and III antigens in 111 Japanese narcoleptics. Journal of Clinical Investigation. 1985;76:2078.
33. Mallal S, Phillips E, Carosi G, et al. HLA-B*5701 screening for hypersensitivity to abacavir. New England Journal of Medicine. 2008;358:568.
34. Uhse HG, Terasaki PI. Transport of lymphocytes for typing. Transplantation. 1969;8:311.
35. Terasaki PI, Vredevoe DL, Mickey MR. Serotyping for homotransplantation. X. Survival of 196 grafted kidneys subsequent to typing. Transplantation. 1967;5:1057.
36. Singal DP, Mickey MR, Terasaki PI. Serotyping for homotransplantation. XXIII. Analysis of kidney transplants from parental versus sibling donors. Transplantation. 1968;7:246.
37. Mickey MR, Kreisler M, Albert ED, et al. Analysis of HL-A incompatibility in human renal transplants. Tissue Antigens. 1971;1:57.
38. Starzl TE. The Puzzle People: Memoirs of a Transplant Surgeon. Pittsburgh, PA: University of Pittsburgh Press; 2003.
39. Dausset J, Rapaport FT. Current problems in analysis of results of renal transplantation in man. Transplantation Proceedings. 1971;3:979.
40. Thomas ED, Storb R, Clift RA, et al. Bone-marrow transplantation (second of two parts). New England Journal of Medicine. 1975;292:895.
41. Opelz G, Mickey MR, Terasaki PI. Identification of unresponsive kidney-transplant recipients. Lancet. 1972;1(7756):868.
42. Collins GM, Bravo-Shugarman M, Terasaki PI. Kidney preservation for transportation. Initial perfusion and 30 hours' ice storage. Lancet. 1969;2(7632): 1219–1222.
43. Takemoto S, Terasaki PI, Cecka JM, et al. Survival of nationally shared, HLA-matched kidney transplants from cadaveric donors. The UNOS Scientific Renal Transplant Registry. New England Journal of Medicine. 1992;327:834.
44. Burlingham WJ, Munoz del Rio A, Lorentzen D, et al. HLA-A, -B, and -DR zero-mismatched kidneys shipped to the University of Wisconsin, Madison, 1993-2006: superior graft survival despite longer preservation time. Transplantation. 2010;90:312.
45. Ashby VB, Port FK, Wolfe RA, et al. Transplanting kidneys without points for HLA-B matching: consequences of the policy change. American Journal of Transplantation. 2011;11:1712–1718.
46. Patel R, Terasaki PI. Significance of the positive crossmatch test in kidney transplantation. New England Journal of Medicine. 1969;280:735.
47. Terasaki PI, Mickey MR, Kreisler M. Presensitization and kidney transplant failures. Postgraduate Medical Journal. 1971;47:89.
48. Pei R, Lee JH, Shih NJ, et al. Single human leukocyte antigen flow cytometry beads for accurate identification of human leukocyte antigen antibody specificities. Transplantation. 2003;75:43.
49. Terasaki PI. Humoral theory of transplantation. American Journal of Transplantation. 2003;3:665.
50. El-Awar N, Terasaki PI, Lazda V, et al. Almost all patients who are waiting for a regraft of a kidney transplant have anti-HLA antibodies. Transplantation Proceedings. 2002;34:2531.
51. Zou Y, Heinemann FM, Grosse-Wilde H, et al. Detection of anti-MICA antibodies in patients awaiting kidney transplantation, during the post-transplant course, and in eluates from rejected kidney allografts by Luminex flow cytometry. Human Immunology. 2006;67:230.
52. Terasaki PI, Ozawa M, Castro R. Four-year follow-up of a prospective trial of HLA and MICA antibodies on kidney graft survival. American Journal of Transplantation. 2007;7:408.
53. Lachmann N, Terasaki PI, Budde K, et al. Anti-human leukocyte antigen and donor-specific antibodies detected by luminex posttransplant serve as biomarkers for chronic rejection of renal allografts. Transplantation. 2009;87:1505.
54. Ntokou IA, Iniotaki AG, Kontou EN, et al. Long-term follow up for anti-HLA donor specific antibodies postrenal transplantation: high immunogenicity of HLA class II graft molecules. Transplant International. 2011;24:1084.
55. Lee PC, Zhu L, Terasaki PI, et al. HLA-specific antibodies developed in the first year posttransplant are predictive of chronic rejection and renal graft loss. Transplantation. 2009;88:568.
56. Kimball PM, Baker MA, Wagner MB, et al. Surveillance of alloantibodies after transplantation identifies the risk of chronic rejection. Kidney International. 2011;79:1131.
57. Smith JD, Banner NR, Hamour IM, et al. De novo donor HLA-specific antibodies after heart transplantation are an independent predictor of poor patient survival. American Journal of Transplantation. 2011;11:312.
58. Kaczmarek I, Deutsch MA, Kauke T, et al. Donor-specific HLA alloantibodies: long-term impact on cardiac allograft vasculopathy and mortality after heart transplant. Experimental and Clinical Transplantation. 2008;6:229.
59. Morales-Buenrostro LE, Castro R, Terasaki PI. A single human leukocyte antigen-antibody test after heart or lung transplantation is predictive of survival. Transplantation. 2008;85:478.
60. Angaswamy N, Saini D, Ramachandran S, et al. Development of antibodies to human leukocyte antigen precedes development of antibodies to major histocompatibility class I-related chain A and are significantly associated with development of chronic rejection after human lung transplantation. Human Immunology. 2010;71:560.
61. Paantjens AW, van de Graaf EA, Kwakkel-van Erp JM, et al. The induction of IgM and IgG antibodies against HLA or MICA after lung transplantation. Pulmonary Medicine. 2011;2011:432169.
62. O'Leary JG, Kaneku H, Susskind BM, et al. High mean fluorescence intensity donor-specific anti-HLA antibodies associated with chronic rejection post liver transplant. American Journal of Transplantation. 2011;11:1868.
63. Cantarovich D, De Amicis S, Akl A, et al. Posttransplant donor-specific anti-HLA antibodies negatively impact pancreas transplantation outcome. American Journal

of Transplantation. 2011;12:2737.
64. de Kort H, Munivenkatappa RB, Berger SP, et al. Pancreas allograft biopsies with positive C4d staining and anti-donor antibodies related to worse outcome for patients. American Journal of Transplantation. 2010;10:1669.
65. Hill AB. The environment and disease: association or causation? Proceedings of the Royal Society of Medicine. 1965;58:295.
66. Terasaki PI, Cai J. Human leukocyte antigen antibodies and chronic rejection: from association to causation. Transplantation. 2008;86:377.
67. Everly MJ, Everly JJ, Arend LJ, et al. Reducing de novo donor-specific antibody levels during acute rejection diminishes renal allograft loss. American Journal of Transplantation. 2009;9:1063.
68. Lefaucheur C, Nochy D, Andrade J, et al. Comparison of combination plasmapheresis/IVIg/anti-CD20 versus high-dose IVIg in the treatment of antibody-mediated rejection. American Journal of Transplantation. 2009;9:1099.
69. Everly MJ, Rebellato LM, Ozawa M, et al. Beyond histology: lowering human leukocyte antigen antibody to improve renal allograft survival in acute rejection. Transplantation. 2010;89:962.
70. Hachem RR, Yusen RD, Meyers BF, et al. Anti-human leukocyte antigen antibodies and preemptive antibody-directed therapy after lung transplantation. Journal of Heart and Lung Transplantation. 2010;29:973.

第 4 章
移植抗原生物学

Raja Rajalingam, Qiuheng Zhang, J. Michael Cecka, Elaine F. Reed

引言

从一个个体到另一个个体的器官或组织的移植，因供体和受体之间存在不同的抗原而引起破坏性免疫应答反应，因而十分困难。这些移植或组织相容性抗原具有不同的类型，比较复杂，会对移植过程产生影响。例如，主要的血型抗原 A 和 B 与这些抗原呈阴性的人体内的天然抗体反应并引起即时反应。它们的作用范围有限，可以通过供体和受体匹配来避免。然而，主要组织相容性复合物抗原是移植更具挑战性的障碍。除了从父母那里继承同一组 HLA 抗原的兄弟姐妹之外，人类白细胞抗原（HLA）的不相容性是无法避免的。极其多态的 HLA 抗原本身在正常的免疫应答中起着关键作用，个体之间的相似性和差异性允许由于直接和间接抗原呈递而产生的同种免疫应答。因此，对异体暴露的免疫应答可能比针对少量外源或移植物抗原的免疫应答要强很多倍，并且需要终身抑制免疫系统以防止移植物破坏。在本章中，我们将描述人类主要移植抗原 HLA 的生物学、遗传学、结构和功能。我们还将描述那些被认为在同种免疫中起作用的非 HLA 抗原。本章内容与第 36 章和第 89 章相关，这两章分别详细介绍了检测 HLA 差异和 HLA 特异性抗体的方法。由于对 HLA 的了解对于理解同种异体免疫至关重要，因此我们回顾了移植的历史，并在第 3 章中有详细介绍。

主要组织相容性复合物（MHC）的遗传学

人类的 MHC 基因位于 6 号染色体短臂上的 5 兆碱基区[1,2]。人类 MHC 基因包含 224 个基因座，并且由于其高基因密度而与人类基因组的其他区域相区别。预测将近 57%的 MHC 基因（128 个基因）被表达，并且 40%的表达基因具有已知的免疫功能。图 4.1 显示了人类 MHC 主要基因的示意图。传统上分为三个不同的非重叠区域，从着丝粒到端粒分别指定为Ⅱ、Ⅲ和Ⅰ区。

MHC Ⅰ类

该簇包含编码具有相似结构但性质不同的蛋白质的三组基因。经典的Ⅰ类基因（或Ⅰa 类）包括三种高度多态性基因（*HLA-A*、*HLA-B* 和 *HLA-C*），其编码 HLA Ⅰ类分子的跨膜 α 链（重链）。α 链表达为异二聚体以及非共价结合的轻链 β_2-微球蛋白（β_2m），其由位于 15 号染色体上的非多态非 MHC 基因产生。所有三种Ⅰa 分子分布在所有有核细胞的表面。

非经典Ⅰ类基因（或Ⅰb 类）包括编码功能分子（*HLA-E*、*HLA-F* 和 *HLA-G*）的三个基因和不表达属于该类的蛋白质的 12 个假基因。Ⅰb 类分子与Ⅰa 类产物序列高度相似，与 β_2m 结构相关，但其在属性上有所不同：一是Ⅰb 类分子的表达仅限于某些细胞类型；其次，Ⅰb 类分子显示有限的多态性。

类似Ⅰ类基因（或Ⅰc 类）包括 7 个 MHC Ⅰ类相关链（MIC）基因，其中仅两个（*MICA* 和 *MICB*）编码功能分子，其余为假基因。MIC 蛋白与 HLA Ⅰ类分子在结构上相关，但是不能形成三分子复合物，因为它们不与 β_2m 结合，也不能形成多肽呈递给 T 细胞。MIC 基因的表达主要限于成纤维细胞和上皮细胞，而在其他细胞类型中受到应激诱导。与Ⅰb 类基因相反，*MICA* 和 *MICB* 基因都是高度多态的。

HLA Ⅰ类基因包含 8 个外显子，每个外显子编码不同的结构域：外显子-1（前导肽）、外显子-2（α1 结构域）、外显子-3（α2 结构域）、外显子-4（α3 结构域）、外显子-5（跨膜区）和外显子 6-8（短细胞质尾）。

MHC Ⅱ类

Ⅱ类簇包含编码经典（HLA-DR、HLA-DQ 和 HLA-DP）和非经典（HLA-DM 和 HLA-DO）Ⅱ类分子的基因。Ⅱ类分子是 α 和 β 链的异源二聚体，每条链由 MHC 区域中的不同基因编码（α 链由基因 A 编码，β 链由基因 B 编码）（图 4.1 和图 4.2）。HLA Ⅱ类基因包含 7 个外显子，每个外显子编码不同的结构域：外显子-1（前导肽）、外显子-2（α1 或 β1 结构域）、外显子-3（α2 或 β2 结构域）、外显子-4（跨膜区）和外显子 5~7（短细胞质尾）。与经典的Ⅱ类基因不同，非经典的Ⅱ类基因产物不在细胞表面表达，而是参与经典Ⅱ类分子上的肽加载。

HLA-DR 区含有单一单态性 DRA 基因和多个多态性 DRB 基因。已经鉴定了 9 个不同的 DRB 基因，其中 4 个（*DRB1*、*DRB3*、*DRB4* 和 *DRB5*）具有功能性和多态性，编码特定Ⅱ类分子的 β 链，5 个是非功能性假基因（*DRB2*、*DRB6*、*DRB7*、*DRB8* 和 *DRB9*）。DRB 基因的数目和类型是通过单体型而变化的，具有 5 种不同的基因内容单元型：DR1 组、DR8 组、DR51 组、DR52 组和 DR53 组（图 4.1）。所有 5 种单体型携带 *DRB1* 基因，但 DR51、DR52 和 DR53 组单倍型含有额外的功能性 DRB 基因（分别为 *DRB5*、*DRB3* 或 *DRB4*），因此 DR51、DR52 和 DR53 组单倍型表达两种 DR 分子，一种来自 *DRB1*（β 链）和 DRA 基因（α 链），另一种来自 *DRB5*、*DRB3* 或 *DRB4* 基因（β 链）和 DRA 基因（α 链）（图 4.2）。

DQ 区包含 5 个基因（*DQA1*、*DQA2*、*DQB1*、*DQB2* 和 *DQB3*），其中只有 *DQA1* 和 *DQB1* 分别编码功能蛋白 α 和 β 链，它们一起在细胞表面形成 DQ 异源二聚体（图 4.2）。与 DR 基因相反，*DQA1* 和 *DQB1* 基因都是多态的，因此通过不同的“顺式”和“反式”链组合产生额外的多态性，产生 4 种不同的 DQ 异源二聚体。DP 区包含两个 DPA 基因（*DPA1* 和 *DPA2*）和两个 DPB 基因（*DPB1* 和 *DPB2*），其中只有 *DPA1* 和 *DPB1* 有功能。与 DQ 基因一样，*DPA1* 和 *DPB1* 基因都是多态的，因此可以通过不同的“顺式”和“反式”组合产生 4 种不同的 DP 异二聚体。

MHC Ⅱ类区域包括产物参与抗原加工和运输的几个非 HLA 基因，例如蛋白酶体相关序列（*PSMB8* 和 *PSMB9*）的基因和抗原转运蛋白（*TAP1* 和 *TAP2*）基因。

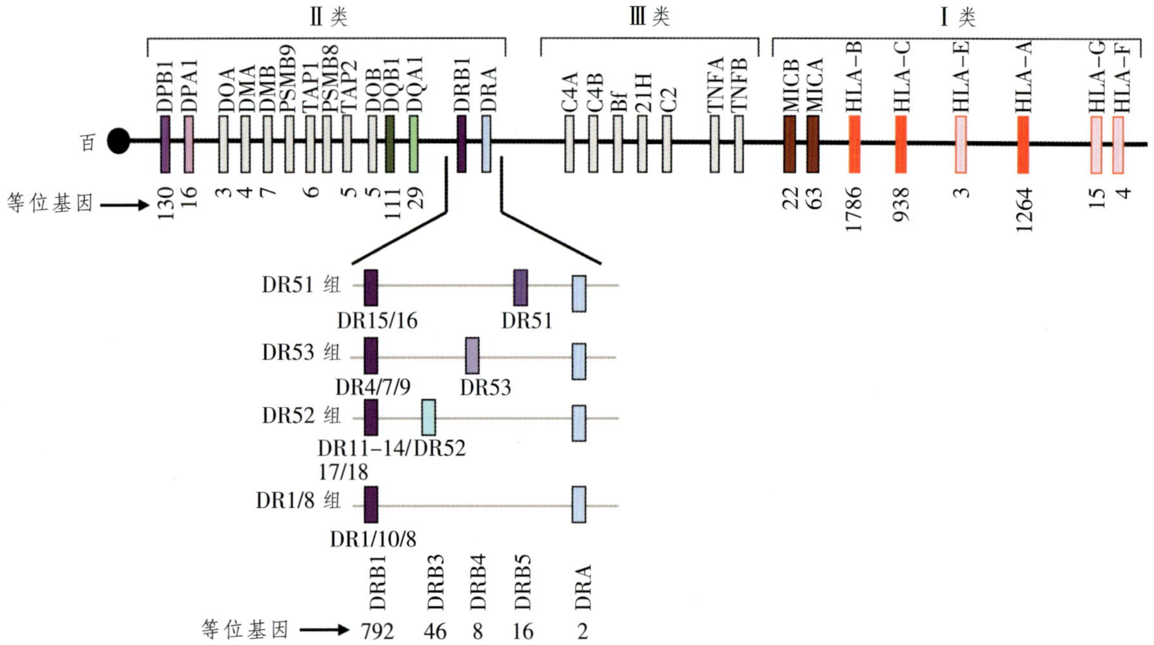

图 4.1 人类主要组织相容性复合物（MHC）的基因组图谱。包含 3 个非重叠区域的第 6 号染色体上的人类 MHC 示意图：Ⅰ类、Ⅱ类和Ⅲ类。着丝点（圆圈）和主要的 MHC 基因（框）按顺序表示，但未按比例绘制。指出了Ⅱ类 DR 区中 DRB 基因含量的单倍型差异。由各功能性 DRB 基因编码的血清学特异性被提供在适当的基因座下方。各基因座下显示不同等位基因的数目（Source：IMGT/HLA database, Release 3.6, October 2011; http://www.ebi.ac.uk/imgt/hla/stats.html）。分布在Ⅰ类（*HLA-H*，*-J*，*-K*，*-L*，*-N*，*-P*，*-S*，*-T*，*-U*，*-V*，*-W*，*-X*，*-Y*，*MICC*，*MICD* 和 *MICE*）和Ⅱ类（*HLA-Z*，*DRB2*，*DRB6*，*DRB7*，*DRB8*，*DRB9*，*DQA2*，*DQB2*，*DQB3*，*DPA2*，*DPA3* 和 *DPB2*）区域的非功能性 HLA 基因片段（伪基因）未显示。

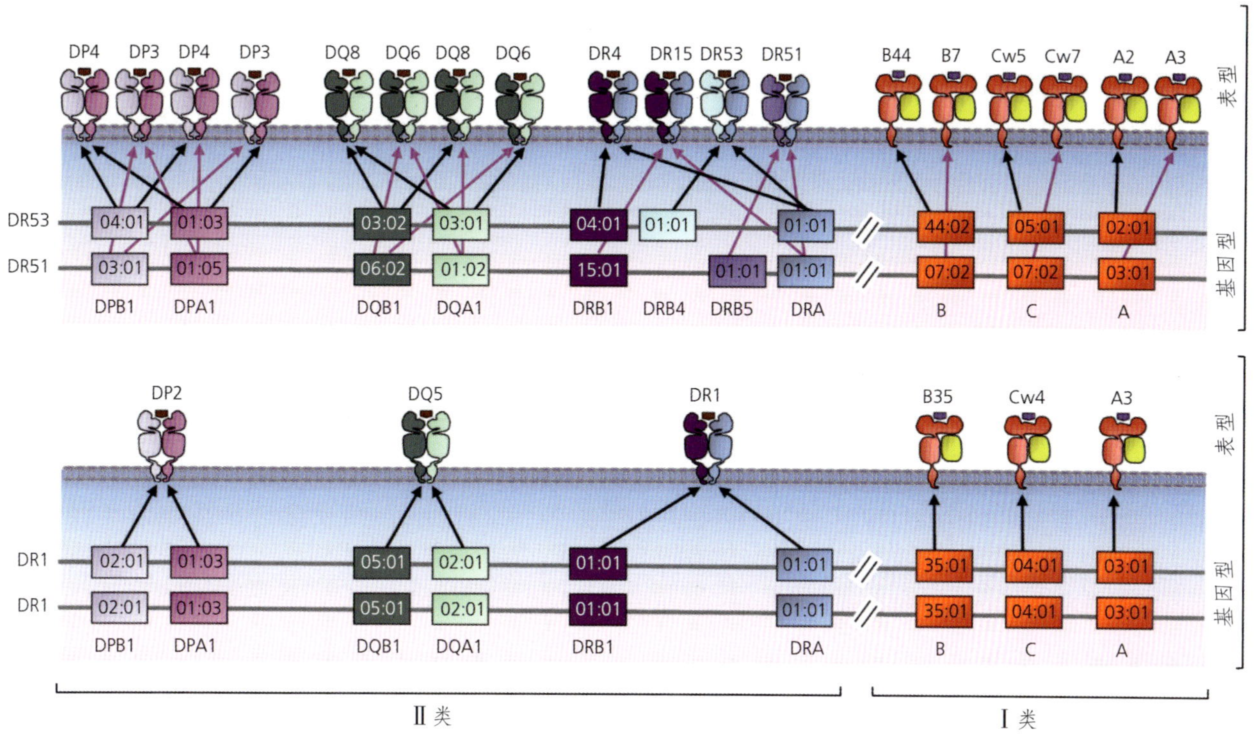

图 4.2　即使在两个兄弟姐妹之间,HLA 分子的数量和类型也可能大不相同。图示在同一家族内的两个兄弟间不同的 HLA 基因型和表型。兄弟 1 携带两个在所有经典 HLA 基因(HLA-A * 03:01,B * 35:01,C * 04:01,DRB1 * 01:01,DRA * 01:01,DQB1 * 05:01,DQA1 * 02:01,DPB1 * 02:01 和 DPA1 * 01:03)中相同的 DR1-群单元型(一个来自母亲,另一个来自父亲),因此在每个基因座(A1,B27,Cw7,DR1,DQ5 和 DP4)共有 6 种不同的 HLA 分子。相反,兄弟 2 携带在每个基因座(A2,A3,B7,B44,Cw5,Cw7,DR4,DR15,DR51,DR53,DQ6,DQ8,DP3 和 DP4)处显示不同等位基因的 DR53 和 DR51 单倍型,共有 18 种不同的 HLA 分子。

PSMB8 和 *PSMB9* 是Ⅰ类相关蛋白酶体的 IFN-γ 诱导的亚基,其产生Ⅰ类蛋白所需的抗原肽,以呈递给 CTL。*TAP1* 和 *TAP2* 是参与肽从细胞质转运到内质网的 ATP 结合盒基因超家族的成员。

MHC Ⅲ类

Ⅲ类簇包含与 HLA 基因没有结构或功能相关性的基因。大量的Ⅲ类区域基因编码参与抗原加工和呈递分子、补体系统和炎性过程。Ⅲ类区域还包括几个没有鉴定出免疫功能的基因。

HLA 多态性的性质

HLA 基因编码区中的多数多态性对应于与抗原肽或 T 细胞受体相互作用的氨基酸位置[3]。HLA Ⅰ类多态性在重链的前 180 个氨基酸中占优势,在 α 和(或)β 链的前 90~95 个氨基酸中发现Ⅱ类多态性[4]。编码这些多态性残基的基因的外显子或区段是Ⅰ类的外显子 2 和 3,Ⅱ类基因的外显子 2。基于 DNA 的 HLA 分型方法针对这些高度多态性的区域[5]。对 HLA 等位基因的比较揭示了同一基因座的等位基因之间重组事件的结果的特征性模式,这大概是由阳性达尔文选择所引起的,以促进 HLA 结合抗原肽库的多样性[6]。

每个等位基因都是与其他等位基因共享序列基序的混合物,因此大多数替换是由同一基因座的两个或多个 HLA 等位基因共享的(图 4.3)。序列多态性的拼凑模式可能是通过重组和基因转换的节段性交换产生的[7]。多态性的共同拼凑模式使 HLA 分型以及 HLA 抗体鉴定复杂化。由于给定基因座的两个区别序列与同一基因座的其他等位基因的广泛共享,通常不可能使用现有技术明确地分配实际等位基因对,而只能执行额外的分层测试来排除一些等位基因组合。在 IMGT/HLA 数据库(<http://www.ebi.ac.uk/imgt/hla/ambig.html>)中,提供了所有等位基因组合的列表,为官方认可的 HLA 序列提供了一个数据库。

```
AA 位置          10         20         30         40         50         60         70         80         90
A*01:01 GSHSMRYFFT SVSRPGRGEP RFIAVGYVDD TQFVRFDSDA ASQKMEPRAP WIEQEGPEYW DQETRNMKAH SQTDRANLGT LRGYYNQSED G
A*02:01 ---------- ---------- ---------- ---------- ---R------ ---------- -G---KV--- ---H-VD--- ---------A -
A*03:01 ---------- ---------- ---------- ---------- ---R------ ---------- ------V--Q -----VD--- ---------A -
A*11:01 --------Y- ---------- ---------- ---------- ---R------ ---------- ------V--Q -----VD--- ---------- -
A*23:01 --------S- ---------- ---------- ---------- ---R------ ---------- -E--GKV--- -----E--RI ALR------A -
A*24:02 --------S- ---------- ---------- ---------- ---R------ ---------- -E--GKV--- -----E--RI ALR------A -
A*25:01 --------Y- ---------- ---------- ---------- ---R------ ---------- -RN---V--- -----ES-RI ALR------- -
A*26:01 --------Y- ---------- ---------- ---------- ---R------ ---------- -RN---V--- ---------- ---------- -
A*29:01 --------T- ---------- ---------- ---------- ---R------ ---------- -LQ---V--Q ---------- ---------A -
A*30:01 --------S- ------S--- ---------- ---------- ---R------ -----R---- ------V--Q -----VD--- ---------A -
A*31:01 --------T- ---------- ---------- ---------- ---R------ -----R---- ------V--- --I--VD--- ---------A -
A*32:01 ---------- ---------- ---------- ---------- ---R------ ---------- ------V--- -----ES-RI ALR------A -
A*33:01 --------T- ---------- ---------- ---------- ---R------ ---------- -RN---V--- --I--VD--- ---------A -
A*34:01 --------Y- ---------- ---------- ---------- ---R------ ---------- -RN--KV--Q -----VD--- ---------- -
A*36:01 ---------- ---------- ---------- ---------- ---------- ---------- ---------- ---------- ---------- -
A*43:01 --------Y- ---------- ---------- ---------- ---R------ ---------- -LQ---V--- ---------- ---------- -
A*66:01 --------Y- ---------- ---------- ---------- ---R------ ---------- -RN---V--Q -----VD--- ---------- -
A*68:01 --------Y- ---------- ---------- ---------- ---R------ ---------- -RN---V--Q -----VD--- ---------A -
A*68:01 --------Y- ---------- ---------- ---------- ---R------ ---------- -RN---V--Q -----VD--- ---------A -
A*69:01 --------Y- ---------- ---------- ---------- ---R------ ---------- -RN---V--Q -----VD--- ---------A -
A*74:01 ---------- ---------- ---------- ---------- ---R------ ---------- ------V--- -----VD--- ---------A -
A*80:01 ---------- ---------- ---------- S--Q------ ---R------ -----E---- -E----V--- ---N------ ---------- -

AA 位置        100        110        120        130        140        150        160        170        180
A*01:01 SHTIQIMYG CDVGPDGRFL RGYRQDAYDG KDYIALNEDL RSWTAADMAA QITKRKWEAV HAAEQRRVYL EGRCVDGLRR YLENGKETLQ RT
A*02:01 ---V-R--- ----S-W--- ---H-Y---- ------K--- ---------- -T--H----A -V---L-A-- --T--EW--- ---------- --
A*03:01 --------- ----S----- ---------- ---------- ---------- ---------A -E---L-A-- D-T--EW--- ---------- --
A*11:01 --------- ---------- ---------- ---------- ---------- ---------A -----Q-A-- -----EW--- ---------- --
A*23:01 ---L-M-F- ----S----- ---H-Y---- ------K--- ---------- ---Q-----A RV---L-A-- --T------- ---------- --
A*24:02 ---L-M-F- ----S----- ---H-Y---- ------K--- ---------- ---------A -V---Q-A-- --T------- ---------- --
A*25:01 -----R--- ---------- ---Q------ ---------- ---------- ---Q----TA -E---W-A-- -----EW--- ---------- --
A*26:01 -----R--- ---------- ---Q------ ---------- ---------- ---Q----TA -E---W-A-- -----EW--- ---------- --
A*29:01 -----M--- -H--S----- ---------- ---------- ---------- ---Q-----A RV---L-A-- --T--EW--- ---------- --
A*30:01 --------- ----S----- ---E-H---- ---------- ---------- ---Q-----A RW---L-A-- --T--EW--- ---------- --
A*31:01 -----M--- ----S----- ---Q------ ---------- ---------- ---Q-----A RV---L-A-- --T--EW--- ---------- --
A*32:01 -----M--- --------L- ---Q------ ---------- ---------- ---Q-----A RV---L-A-- --T--EW--- ---------- --
A*33:01 -----M--- ----S----- ---Q------ ---------- ---------- ---Q-----A RV---L-A-- --T--EW--- H--------- --
A*34:01 -----R--- ---------- ---Q------ ---------- ---------- ---Q----TA -E---W-A-- --T--EW--- ---------- --
A*36:01 --------- ---------- ---------- ---------- ---------- ---------- ---------- --T--EW--- ---------- --
A*43:01 -----R--- ---------- ---Q------ ---------- ---------- ---Q----TA -E---W-A-- -----EW--- ---------- --
A*66:01 -----R--- ---------- ---Q------ ---------- ---------- ---Q----TA -E---W-A-- -----EW--- ---------- --
A*68:01 -----M--- ----S----- ---------- ------K--- ---------- -T--H----A -V---W-A-- --T--EW--- ---------- --
A*68:01 -----M--- ----S----- ---------- ------K--- ---------- -T--H----A -V---W-A-- --T--EW--- ---------- --
A*69:01 ---V-R--- ----S-W--- ---H-Y---- ------K--- ---------- -T--H----A -V---L-A-- --T--EW--- ---------- --
A*74:01 -----M--- --------L- ---Q------ ---------- ---------- ---Q-----A RV---L-A-- --T--EW--- ---------- --
A*80:01 --------- ----S----- ---------- ---------- ---------- ---------A RR---L-A-- --E------- ---------- --
```

图 4.3 HLA 序列多态性。代表主要抗原组的常见 HLA-A 同种异型的 α1(上图)和 α2(下图)结构域的氨基酸序列。HLA-A * 01:01 是上面列出的参考序列,参照相同的其他等位基因的氨基酸位置显示为连字符(-)。标准单字母代码表示与参考序列的氨基酸差异。大部分的替代是由不止一个序列共享的。阴影标识构成 HLA-A25,A26,A34,A43 和 A66 多个同种异体共有的表位氨基酸。

人类 HLA 的多样性

作为二倍体,人类具有 MHC 基因复合体的两个拷贝,一个父系起源和一个母系起源。由于 HLA 基因具有高度的多态性,因此个体内每个 HLA 基因的等位基因几乎总是不同的(杂合的)[8]。因为两个 HLA 等位基因在细胞表面上表达水平相当(共显性表达),所以人类可以在其细胞表面上表达的 HLA 分子的数目和类型不同。例如,携带 *HLA-A*、*B*、*C*、*DRB1*、*DRA*、*DQB1*、*DQA1*、*DPB1* 和 *DPA1* 单倍型的两个 DR1-群单体型(一个来自母亲,另一个来自父亲)可以在这些位点(例如 A1,B27,Cw7,DR1,DQ5 和 DP4 总共 6 个不同的 HLA 分子)表达单一的 HLA 类型(图 4.2,兄弟 1)。相反,携带在所有 HLA 基因座上展示不同等位基因的 DR53 和 DR51 单元型的同胞可以表达两种 HLA-A 分子、两种 HLA-B 分子、两种 HLA-Cw 分子、4 种 HLA-DR 分子、4 种 HLA-DQ 分子和 4 种 HLA-DP 分子(18 种不同的 HLA 分子)(图 4.2,兄弟 2)。由于孟德尔遗传的结果,如果他们的父母携带以下单倍型,在这对兄弟中出现的这种极端多样性发生率为 25%:母亲有 DR51 和 DR1,父亲有 DR53 和 DR1。

一些 HLA 基因有 1000 多个等位基因,其单体型组合在人群中具有广泛的多样性(图 4.1)[9]。多态性如此之高，以至于在混合群体（非同系交配）中没有两个个体具有完全相同的一组 MHC 基因和分子。如此高度的多态性在某个体和人群之间都是重要的。在个体内，由于可用于呈递给 T 细胞的病毒肽的组成部分减少，重复（纯合 HLA 等位基因）遗传可能导致不能抵抗慢性病毒感染。杂合子优势（超过显性选择）的假设认为，在 HLA 位点杂合的个体能够提供从纯合体到免疫系统的范围更广的抗原肽，从而增强免疫监视[10]。Ⅰ型基因座（A，B 和 C）的最大 HLA 杂合性在感染人免疫缺陷病毒 1 型（HIV-1）的患者中可延迟适应性免疫缺陷综合征（AIDS）发病，而对于一个或多个基因座纯合的个体感染病毒会迅速发展至死亡[11]。因此，预测过度选择将有利于肽结合特异性范围最大的个体。

在人群水平上，HLA 多态性提供了限制流行病原体传播的机制，否则这种病原体可能在整个宿主群体中无限制地繁殖。人群中存在许多不同的等位基因，确保总是至少有少数具有特定 HLA 分子（稀有或新的等位基因）的个体能够加载适当的肽，以发展适当的免疫反应克服病原体，从而使群体在大流行中幸存下来。罕见等位基因优势（频率依赖性选择）的原理是，具有罕见（例如新的）MHC 等位基因的个体可以更好地响应不同的病原体变体，从而在病原体普遍存在的群体中赋予该个体优势[12]。这种频率依赖性选择可能已经导致冈比亚人群中暴露于疟疾的 HLA-B*53 频率增加。同样，HLA-B54 几乎全部在日本和邻近的亚洲国家被发现，HLA-A74 在黑人中很常见，但在其他人群中非常罕见。因此，在给定的人群中，随着时间的推移，似乎选择了不同的 HLA 等位基因亚型，并且维持的等位基因总数在人群中是不同的[13,14]。此外，美洲原住民等人群可能经历了重大变故，导致 HLA 等位基因多样性有限[15]。连锁不平衡是一种邻近 HLA 基因座的等位基因一起被遗传的机会比预期要多的现象。例如，如果人群中 HLA-A1 和 HLA-B8 分别以 16%和 10%的频率出现，那么发现它们的概率应该是 1.6%。然而，HLA-A1-B8 组合的实际发生率显著高于预测发生率（约 8%）。正向选择被认为是对单体型进行操作，并且所连接的基因座赋予宿主选择性优势[16]。

HLA 命名

由于从血清学分型（定义抗原）到 DNA 分型（定义等位基因）的变化导致了一些冲突，HLA 命名可能十分艰难[9]。HLA 抗原按抗血清鉴定的顺序命名。通常可以将特异性细化为抗体“分裂”抗原特异性为两种或更多种新的特异性，通常鉴定相关抗原家族内的等位基因或等位基因组。较常见的 HLA 抗原通常具有较低的数目，如 A2 或 B7，新的或不常见的 HLA 抗原具有较高的数目。例如，HLA-B40 随后被分成两组，重新命名为 B60 和 B61。在此基础上构建的标准 DNA 命名法包括四个区域（例如，HLA-A*02:01:01:01），描述了由结肠分离抗原，等位基因组和指定沉默取代（不会导致蛋白质的变化），以及非编码区域的差异[9]。在临床上，在等位基因水平（HLA-A * 02:01）报道了造血干细胞移植的 HLA 分型，并且在抗原水平（HLA-A2）报道了用于实体器官移植的 HLA 分型。后者通常是星号后的前两位，但由于 DNA 命名法使用的是与核苷酸序列相似性相关的等位基因，也有一些例外[17]。B*15:01 对应 B62 抗原，B*15:02 对应 B75，B*40:01 对应 B60，以及 B*40:02 对应 B61。同样，对于 HLA Ⅱ类等位基因，DRB1*03:01 对应 DR17 抗原，DRB1*03:02 对应 DR18，DQB1*03:01 对应 DQ7，DQB1*03:02 对应 DQ8，以及 DQB1*03:03 对应 DQ9。在每种情况下，等位基因都对应于亲本抗原的分裂。

HLA 抗原决定簇和交叉反应的结构基础

HLA 多态性的局限性和有时重叠的性质（见图 4.3）导致其具有一系列同种异体抗原结构的分子，其范围从那些与单个等位基因独特相关的分子到相关 HLA 分子共有的分子。对单一 HLA 同种异体抗原（通过妊娠、输血或同种异体移植物）的免疫可导致针对免疫抗原共享序列基序（称为表位）的一系列 HLA 抗原的抗体产生。从附着于微球体的纯化的 HLA 抗原吸附和洗脱的抗体显示出与 HLA 分子的反应性模式，HLA 分子与映射到 HLA 分子结构区域并可能影响抗体结合位点的特定共有氨基酸相关[18]。这些抗原属于由特定抗体定义的交叉反应基团（CREG）。例如，针对 HLA-A25 抗原的免疫可导致抗 HLA-A25、A26、A34、A43 和 A66 的抗体，其在位点 9（酪氨酸）和位点 149（苏氨酸）处共享氨基酸，而在其他 HLA 抗原的相同位点处无此氨基酸。

HLA分子结构和功能

HLA Ⅰ类和Ⅱ类分子在它们的结构、表达的细胞、处理抗原的来源以及它们相互作用的T细胞功能上有所不同。

HLA Ⅰ类分子结构

HLA Ⅰ类分子(A,B和C)是由12kD β2-微球蛋白($β_2m$)轻链非共价结合32kD α链组成的异二聚体跨膜蛋白(图4.4)。α链由3个片段(α1、α2和α3)组成，每个片段长度约90个氨基酸。X线晶体学研究表明，α1和α2区域折叠在一起形成一个单一的结构，是两个片段α1螺旋镶嵌在一个八链β团上[19]。α1和α2的折叠形成结合自身肽和非自身肽的裂隙。HLA Ⅰ类分子的肽结合裂隙长约25Å,并且容纳长度为8~11个氨基酸的小肽。

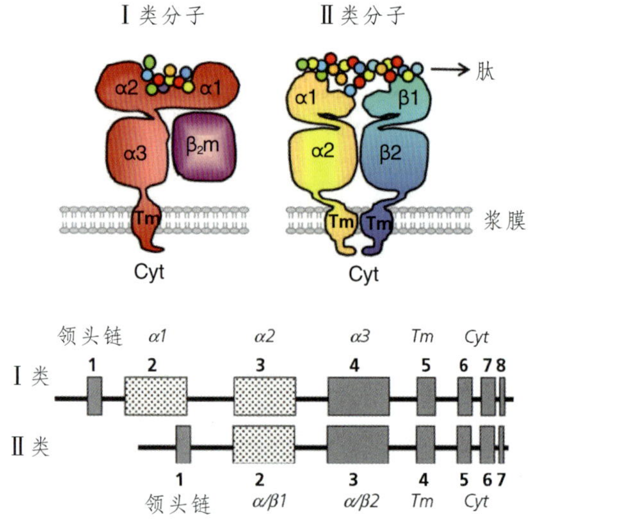

图4.4 图示HLA蛋白(上图)和基因(下图)的结构组织。HLA Ⅰ类分子是与非MHC基因(位于染色体15中)非共价结合的跨膜重链α(由*HLA-A*、*-B*或*-C*基因编码)的异二聚体,其编码光$β_2$-微球蛋白($β_2m$)链,不跨越胞膜。α链折叠成三个结构域:α1、α2和α3。α1和α2结构域形成抗原结合沟。HLA Ⅱ类分子由两个跨膜糖蛋白链α(由*DRA*、*DQA1*或*DPA1*编码)和β(由*DRB1*、*DQB1*或*DPB1*编码)组成。每条链有两个结构域,两条链形成一个类似于HLA Ⅰ类分子的紧密的四结构域结构。Ⅱ类分子的α1和β1结构域形成肽结合裂口。Ⅰ类基因包含8个外显子(以框表示),而Ⅱ类基因包含7个外显子。每个外显子编码的蛋白质结构域以斜体显示。Ⅰ类外显子2和3以及Ⅱ类基因(斑点框)的外显子2编码多态性抗原结合结构域。Reproduced from Grody WW,Nakamura RM,Kiechle FL,Strom C (2010)*Molecular Diagnostics:Techniques and Applications for the Clinical Laboratory*,with permission from Elsevier. Copyright©2010,Elsevier [115].

Ⅰ类的α3结构域与$β_2m$非共价结合,这对分子在细胞表面必须正确折叠。α3结构域还含有与T细胞上的CD8分子结合的高度保守的α3免疫球蛋白样结构域[20]。分子的羧基末端含有由41个氨基酸残基组成的疏水跨膜区和由27个残基组成的短细胞质尾。Ⅰ类分子的稳定表达需要组装由Ⅰ类α链、$β_2m$和结合的自身或非自身肽形成的三分子复合物。

HLA Ⅱ类分子结构

HLA Ⅱ类分子DR、DQ和DP是由包含32~34kD的α链和29~32kD的β链的两条跨膜糖蛋白链组成的异二聚体(图4.4)。α2和β2折叠形成肽结合裂缝[21]。多态性残基主要位于α1和β1结构域，并参与肽结合以及与T细胞受体的相互作用。Ⅱ类肽结合沟的末端是开放的,因此可以容纳30个残基或更长更大的肽[22,23]。Ⅱ类α2结构域中的一个环作为CD4分子的对接位点。α2和β2结构域的羧基末端由短的疏水性跨膜区域组成,其将分子锚定在质膜中,随后是短的亲水性细胞质尾部。

肽结合HLA Ⅰ类和Ⅱ类分子的结构基础

与HLA Ⅰ类和Ⅱ类分子结合的多肽是由多肽中的特异氨基酸残基和互补氨基酸残基的相互作用所引导的,互补氨基形成了裂隙底部的β链和裂隙侧面的α螺旋。主要在Ⅰ类分子的α1和α2结构域中发现的多态性和Ⅱ类分子的α1和β1结构域形成肽结合口袋。多态性氨基酸侧链改变了HLA抗原的表面电荷、疏水性、大小和形状,并决定着特定的肽是否会与裂缝结合[24,25]。适合这些肽的残基被称为锚定残基。广泛的多态性改变了每个HLA Ⅰ类和Ⅱ类等位基因的肽结合特征,使得每个等位基因结合一组独特的肽。与Ⅰ类分子结合的肽长度一般为8~10个氨基酸。将肽的氨基端和羧基端埋入裂缝中，并通过一系列氢键与保守的重链残基结合。与Ⅱ类分子结合的肽较长(10~30个氨基酸),并且以延伸的构象连接,肽的末端悬挂在裂缝的边缘上[21]。肽是否结合给定的Ⅰ类等位基因是由形成抗原结合裂隙的锚定残基的氨基酸侧链决定的。因此,可被特定HLA Ⅰ类等位基因结合的肽组通常具有共同的“序列基序”。以下几个网站有关于肽结合基序和算法的有用信息，能够预测特定的肽结合 HLA 分子，包括：http://www.ashi-hla.org/，http://www.ebi.ac.uk/imgt/hla/，http://www-bimas.cit.nih.gov/molbio/hla_bind/index.shtml 和 http://www.syfpeithi.de/.

抗原处理和提呈

抗原处理和提呈是抗原呈递细胞以淋巴细胞可识别的形式在细胞表面表达抗原的方式。在第 2 章中我们已经深入地讨论过促进抗原提呈的细胞过程和表面分子。抗原处理包括蛋白质片段化(蛋白水解)，片段与 HLA 抗原的结合以及肽-HLA 复合物在细胞表面的表达，使它们可以被 T 细胞上的 T 细胞受体(TCR)识别。HLA Ⅰ类和Ⅱ类分子以不同的方式处理和提呈抗原。HLA Ⅰ类分子呈现在细胞胞质中产生的外来和自身肽(图 4.5)[26]，而 HLA Ⅱ类分子主要但不限于细胞外来源的蛋白抗原(图 4.6)[27-29]。

HLA Ⅰ类提呈的肽的主要来源是由蛋白酶体将内源性蛋白质加工成多肽(图 4.5)[30]。蛋白酶体是由在细胞的细胞质中发现的大量蛋白酶复合物组成的[31]。蛋白酶体由 14 个具有广泛蛋白水解活性的亚基组成，并且具有将细胞质蛋白质降解成肽的功能。针对蛋白酶体进行降解的蛋白质需要首先与被称为泛素蛋白的小蛋白质共价连接[32]。然后，将蛋白质展开，去除泛素，并将蛋白质在蛋白酶体中降解成多种肽。有趣的是，两种蛋白酶体亚基 PSMB9 和 PSMB8 编码在Ⅱ类区域内，它们的活性特异性地被促炎细胞因子如 INF-γ 所启动[33]。因此，INF-γ 激活的免疫细胞表达被称为“免疫蛋白酶体”的变体蛋白酶体，其特征在于独特的催化亚基。与标准蛋白酶体相比，免疫蛋白酶体具有更强的催化活性。最近的研究表明，这种免疫蛋白酶体的活性增强可以防止在炎症过程中降解底物的积累[34]。

在 HLA Ⅰ类分子上加载肽是一个高度协调的过程，涉及存在于内质网(ER)中的数个伴侣蛋白质[35,36](图 4.5)。在 HLA Ⅰ类分子的重链合成之后，其靶向 ER，在这里与 ER 伴侣蛋白钙连接蛋白和 Grp78 结合。这些分子伴侣参与将Ⅰ类分子的多肽插入 ER 的内腔室，并引发重链折叠和链内二硫键形成。从钙连接蛋白解离后，Ⅰ类重链与 β_2m 结合并与直系同源伴侣蛋白钙

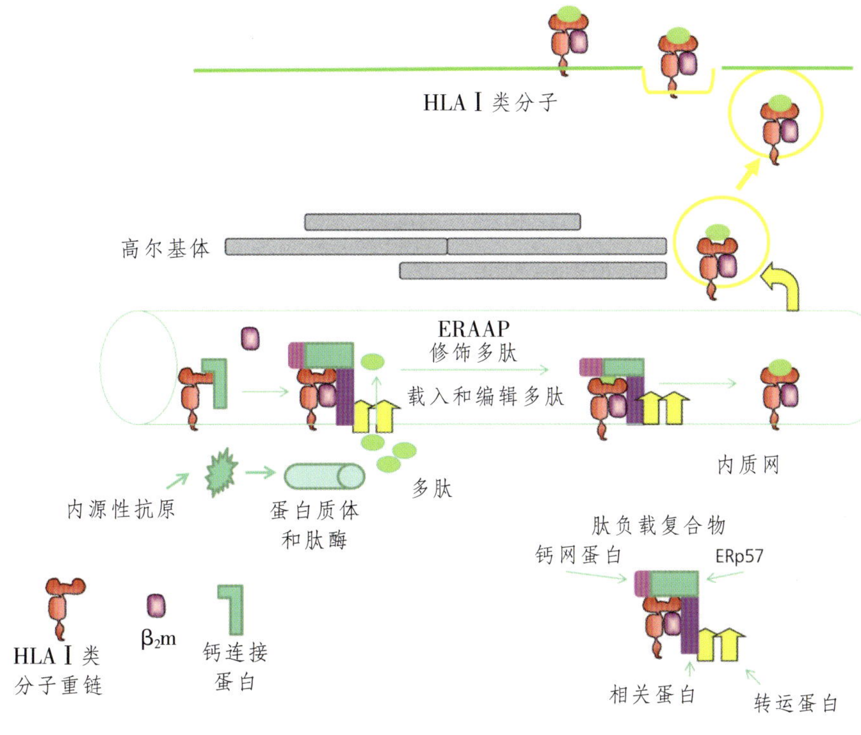

图 4.5　MHC Ⅰ类分子肽加工和呈现的示意图。MHC Ⅰ类重链与 β_2m 聚集并被募集到内质网中的肽负载复合物。MHC Ⅰ类分子最初与分子伴侣钙连接蛋白结合，触发折叠和二硫键形成。从钙连接蛋白解离后，Ⅰ类重链与 β_2m 结合并与伴侣蛋白钙网蛋白结合，掺入肽负载复合物中。肽负载复合物含有与抗原加工相关的转运蛋白(TAP1 和 TAP2)的两个亚基、跨膜糖蛋白相关蛋白、钙网蛋白和 ERp57。肽通过 TAP1 和 TAP2 分子转运到内质网中。相关蛋白可促进肽装载和 ERAAP 功能，在其与 MHC Ⅰ类分子结合之前和之后在其氨基末端修剪肽。然后将肽-MHC Ⅰ类分子输出到细胞表面。

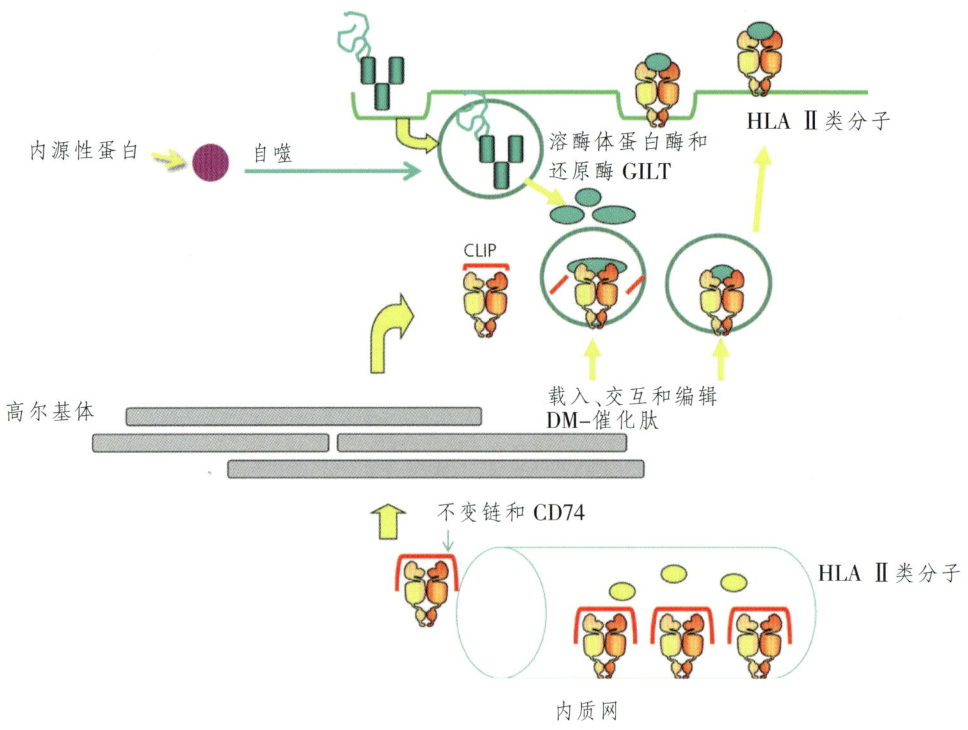

图 4.6　MHC Ⅱ类分子肽加工和呈现的示意图。MHC Ⅱ类分子在含有内涵体靶向信号的不变链(Ii)的内质网中聚集。在内涵体室中，Ii 被切割，仅留下占据肽结合裂缝的较小片段 CLIP。外源蛋白被内化到内涵体通路中，它们的解折叠和片段化由二硫化物还原酶 GILT 和溶酶体蛋白酶催化。HLA-DM 催化 CLIP 的释放，接着肽片段结合和交换。HLA-DM 编辑运输到细胞表面的肽-MHC Ⅱ复合物。

网蛋白结合，被并入肽负载复合物中。肽负载复合物负责将最佳肽加载到 MHC Ⅰ类分子上。肽负载复合物含有与抗原加工有关的转运蛋白(TAP1 和 TAP2)、跨膜糖蛋白相关蛋白、可溶性内质网伴侣蛋白钙网蛋白和可溶性巯基氧化还原酶 ERp57 的两个亚基[35]。肽通过 TAP1 和 TAP2 分子转运到内质网中。TAP 基因编码在 MHC 的Ⅱ类区域内，与 *PSMB9* 和 *PSMB8* 基因连接[37]。TAP 与内质网膜的细胞质侧多肽和位于腔表面的Ⅰ类分子结合。在内质网中，肽可以通过 ERAAP(或 ERAP1)修饰(如果需要的话)至需要的 8~10 个氨基酸的长度以结合Ⅰ类分子，ERAAP(或 ERAP1)是专门的内质网相关氨基酶，其识别肽羧基末端和修剪氨基末端，产生长度为 8~10 个残基的肽[38]。被称为 Tapasin 相关蛋白的 TAP 相关糖蛋白也被编码在 MHC 中，并且可促进内质网中Ⅰ类分子的肽装载作用[39]。Tapasin 相关蛋白将 HLA Ⅰ类分子与伴侣分子伴侣和巯基氧化还原酶 ERp57 的 TAP 分子连接起来，它们一起形成肽负载复合物[39,40]。Tapasin 相关蛋白稳定空的Ⅰ类二聚体，将其保留在内质网中，直到通过肽加载复合物加载肽。HLA Ⅰ类分子可以依赖于或不依赖于蛋白酶的肽负载[40]。

与Ⅰ类分子结合的肽的主要组成成分包括来源于细胞内胞质产物的蛋白酶体降解的多种蛋白质(包括 HLA 分子本身)。然而，有专门的细胞，特别是巨噬细胞和树突状细胞(DC)，可以捕获细胞外抗原，并通过一个称为交叉提呈的过程将这些抗原提呈给 CD8 T 细胞[41]。在交叉提呈期间，通常认为内质网的元件被并入吞噬体和内涵体中。交叉提呈对于提呈来自无病毒感染 DC 的多肽是重要的[42]。交叉提呈也涉及对 DC 中不合成的自身蛋白质的耐受性。

HLA Ⅱ类分子提呈在细胞内体室中产生的肽(图 4.6)。由Ⅱ类分子提呈的许多肽来源于外源抗原，但它们也可以通过自噬过程从细胞质中获得[43-45]。外源性抗原被内化，然后转运到溶酶体和包含半胱氨酸蛋白酶、组织蛋白酶 L 和组织蛋白酶 S 等蛋白水解酶的内涵体[35]。Ⅱ类分子在内质网中与称为不变链(Ii)或 CD74 的蛋白质组装在一起。不变链阻断肽被装载到内质网中的Ⅱ类分子上，并伴随着新合成的Ⅱ类分子进入 MCII(一个特殊的发生肽加载的内涵体室)[46]。在酸化的 MCII 区室中,不变链由组织蛋白酶介导的蛋白水解降解[47]以产生Ⅱ类相关不变链肽或 CLIP[48]。CLIP 结合到Ⅱ类分子的裂缝,裂缝内部被保护而免于降解。CLIP 需要被去除, 以便使裂缝可以被细胞外蛋白质产生的肽所接近。HLA-DMA 和 HLA-DMB 在Ⅱ类区域内编码,起到催化 CLIP 的解离作用,并促进肽在载体的内吞作用[49,50]。DM 的功能是确保肽和编辑复合物的有效结合, 从而增加 HLA Ⅱ类稳定的肽结合剂的效果[51]。DM 的活性可以通过另一个 HLA Ⅱ类编码蛋白进一步修饰,称为 HLA-DO,它可以作为肽编辑器,通过改变 DM 介导的 MHC Ⅱ类负载的最佳 pH 值到更酸性的条件[52]。与Ⅱ类分子结合的肽由被称为组织蛋白酶的蛋白酶产生, 其存在于内涵体室中。有趣的是, 不同的 APC 使用的组织蛋白酶库存在差异,这可能影响产生肽的性质[53]。另外一种被称为 γ-干扰素诱导的溶酶体巯基还原酶或 GILT 的溶酶体加工酶已经被鉴定用于提呈具有二硫键的一些抗原[54]。克雷斯韦尔实验室的研究表明,GILT 对 MHC Ⅰ类分子上病毒抗原子集的提呈也是重要的[55]。

细胞质和膜细胞蛋白也可以作为细胞蛋白正常转化的结果进入抗原提呈的Ⅱ类途径, 该过程被称为自噬。在这个途径中,细胞质蛋白质被捕获在称为自噬体的内质网衍生的囊泡中,这些囊泡与溶酶体融合,细胞质蛋白被降解, 并且可以像来自外源抗原的肽一样递送到Ⅱ类分子[56](图 4.6)。自我蛋白质的加工和表达被认为在中枢耐受诱导过程中发挥重要的作用[57]。除了耐受性诱导之外,研究还表明,一些病毒抗原可以通过Ⅱ类分子在细胞内进行交叉提呈[45],这一机制对于防止病毒病原体可能是十分重要的。

HLAⅠ类和Ⅱ类分子的差异表达

HLAⅠ类和Ⅱ类分子在细胞中具有不同的分布,这反映了识别它们的 T 细胞的不同效应功能。HLAⅠ类分子将来自细胞内病原体(通常是病毒)的肽呈递给 $CD8^+$细胞毒性 T 细胞, 其专门杀死它们特异识别的任何细胞[58]。Ⅰ类分子在所有有核细胞上组成表达。Ⅰ类分子的广泛表达与提呈细胞内病原体如病毒的Ⅰ类分子的功能相关联。相比之下,HLA Ⅱ类分子将来自细胞外抗原的肽提呈给 CD4 T 细胞, 继而调节免疫系统的其他效应细胞的活化。因此,HLA Ⅱ类分子通常在专职抗原提呈细胞上发现,包括 B 淋巴细胞、树突状细胞和巨噬细胞。包括 INF-α、INF-β、INF-γ 和肿瘤坏死因子 α(TNF-α)在内的细胞因子可增加Ⅰ类分子的表达水平。Ⅱ类分子表达被 INF-γ 增强。细胞因子通过增加基因转录的速率来增加 HLAⅠ类和Ⅱ类的表达。该作用由细胞因子激活的转录因子与 HLAⅠ类和Ⅱ类基因的启动子区域中的调控 DNA 序列的结合介导。HLA Ⅱ类分子的表达在许多细胞类型(包括 T 细胞)中对细胞因子的应答都是可诱导的。Ⅱ类基因的转录受到主要调控因子的控制, 该因子被称为 MHC-Ⅱ反式激活因子(CIITA)[59]。驱动编码Ⅱ类反式激活因子的基因表达的三个独立启动子的差异激活最终决定了 MHC Ⅱ类基因表达的精确调节模式。除增加Ⅰ类和Ⅱ类基因及 $β_2m$ 的转录外,INF-γ 还增加 TAP 的蛋白酶体和亚基的转录。

HLAⅠb 类分子

HLA-E、F、G 和 Hfe(HLA-H)分子是 MHC 区域内编码的非经典Ⅰ类分子[60]。这些分子与 $β_2m$ 结合并具有限制性多态性并结合有限的一组肽。HLA-E 在大多数组织中被转录。HLA-E 具有有限的多态性, 只有 9 个等位基因(3 种蛋白质变体)。它具有一个结合裂隙,其中包含一组来自 HLA-A、B、C 和 G 分子的信号序列的肽段。HLA-E 结合自然杀伤(NK)细胞上的 CD94-NKG2A / C 受体并调节 NK 细胞功能[61]。

HLA-G 具有有限的组织表达, 主要在包括滋养层、胸腺和角膜的免疫特异性位点表达[62]。在可溶性形式中,HLA-G 被认为可以抑制母体对胎儿的免疫反应。HLA-G 肽的表达受限于一些细胞内蛋白质的纳米肽。HLA-G 与白细胞 Ig 样抑制性受体(LIR-1 和 LIR-2)和 KIR2DL4 受体相互作用。HLA-F 是细胞内蛋白质而不是膜蛋白质,其功能尚不完善。

HFE 基因是与 $β_2m$ 结合而表达的Ⅰ类基因。*HFE* 不结合肽, 而是充当转铁蛋白受体的结合位点以将铁运输穿过细胞膜。具有 *HFE* 基因突变的个体(酪氨酸 282)缺乏 *HFE* 的表达,并且不能提供铁吸收的负面反馈, 这将导致血色素沉着症。这是一种铁超载的疾病,与血清中铁水平升高和肝脏等器官的沉积有关。

HLA 介导的信号传导

HLA 分子的交联在淋巴细胞、内皮细胞(EC)和平滑肌细胞(SMC)中诱导信号传导。HLAⅠ或Ⅱ与 B 细胞、T细胞或抗原提呈细胞中的抗体的交联导致程序性细胞死亡或活化和增殖[63]。导致免疫细胞死亡或增殖的途径有常见的第二信使，包括细胞内钙、PLC、PKC和Src家族激酶[64-67]。抗MHC Ⅰ类抗体也能诱导人主动脉EC[68-71]和气道上皮细胞的增殖[72,73]，表明同种抗体可能导致慢性同种异体移植物排斥和移植血管病变(TV)[74]。

HLA Ⅰ类分子与抗体的交联引起HLA Ⅰ与整合素亚基β4之间的分子关联，随后激活细胞内信号，导致细胞存活、增殖和迁移(图4.7)[75,76]。在Ⅰ类分子的抗体连接后，酪氨酸激酶Src被磷酸化[77]。Src是一种重要的信号传导物，它具有调节细胞骨架改变、迁移、有丝分裂发生、细胞周期进程和细胞存活等功能。接下来，黏着斑激酶(FAK)磷酸化促进Src家族激酶复合形成[71,77,78]，达到最大的激酶活性。然后，FAK促进桩蛋白(一种参与黏着斑形成的衔接蛋白)磷酸化，其将信号分子募集到细胞中的特定区室。FAK和桩蛋白激活的一个主要功能性结果是细胞骨架重排和黏着斑的形成或稳定[77,78]，这在调节内皮通透性以及信号转导中是重要的[79]。HLA Ⅰ连接激活磷脂酰肌醇3激酶(PI3K)并募集3-磷酸肌醇依赖性蛋白激酶(PDK1)和Akt到膜上。Akt通过激活mTOR途径促进细胞增殖。mTOR存在于细胞中的两个复合物中。mTOR复合物1(mTORC1)调节核糖体生物合成和蛋白质合成，其由mTOR、raptor和GβL组成。mTOR复合体2(mTORC2)包括mTOR、Sin1、GβL和rictor，其参与细胞骨架调节和Akt反馈[80]。HLA Ⅰ连接后，mTOR被磷酸化并形成活化下游靶标的信号复合物，包括S6激酶、S6核糖体蛋白和4E-BP1。此外，RhoA在HLA Ⅰ类连接之后与应激纤维形成和细胞骨架重组相关的方式迅速转移至细胞膜[69]。这些信号级联改变了HLA Ⅰ类连接后的细胞骨架，与涉及mTOR活化的细胞增殖途径有关[71,80]。特别是，由rictor、Sin1和GβL组成的mTORC2已经显示出通过其刺激F-肌动蛋白应力纤维、桩蛋白、RhoA、Rac1、Cdc42和PKCα来调节细胞骨架的作用。

用低剂量的HLA Ⅰ抗体刺激EC促进细胞存活和抗凋亡[81-84]。HLA Ⅰ交联引起促凋亡蛋白Bad的磷酸化，导致其通过14-3-3蛋白从线粒体中螯合(图4.7)[85]。这

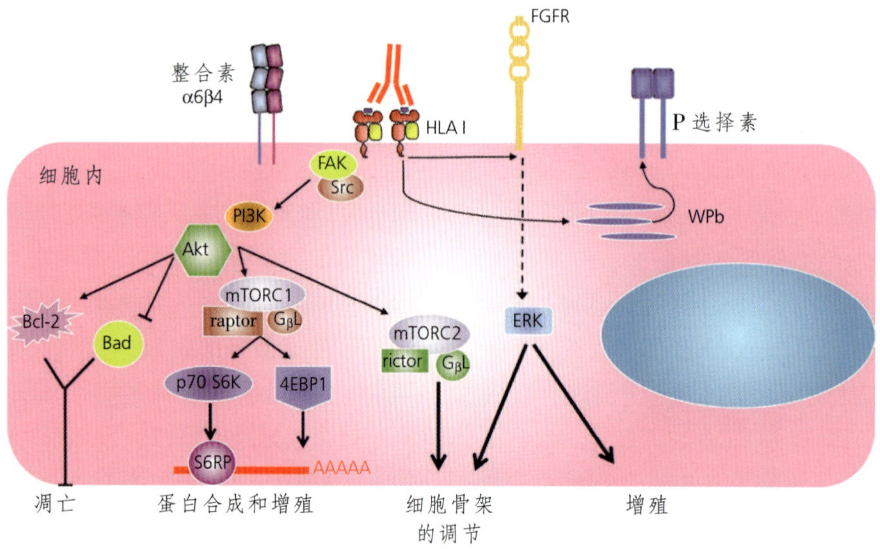

图4.7 抗体交联HLA Ⅰ类分子诱导细胞生长、骨架调节和抗细胞死亡等信号传导途径。在内皮上结合HLA Ⅰ后，成纤维细胞生长因子受体(FGFR)的细胞表面表达迅速增加，支持增加的细胞对生长因子的敏感性和增加的ERK激活。Src和FAK被激活，导致PI3K/Akt轴的激活。FAK也是细胞骨架的重要调节剂，支持黏着斑。PI3K依赖性激活Akt，导致抗凋亡和生长信号。Akt影响凋亡调节因子，抑制促凋亡因子Bad和增加抗凋亡因子Bcl-2和Bcl-xL的水平。这些作用导致细胞对诸如补体激活等信号的死亡抵抗。Akt还可以靶向西罗莫司(mTOR)的哺乳动物靶标，其存在于两种不同的复合物中：mTOR复合物1(mTORC1)和mTOR复合物2(mTORC2)。mTOR复合物1触发S6激酶和S6RP激活，蛋白质在蛋白质合成期间是必需的。另外，mTORC1调节4EBP-1以增加mRNA的翻译。相反，mTOR复合体2作用于下游细胞骨架调节剂以控制肌动蛋白细胞骨架的组织。通过抗体交联HLA Ⅰ后，内皮细胞显示显著的应激纤维和黏着斑，这些事件依赖于mTORC2。mTORC2为Akt提供了积极的反馈。最后，HLA Ⅰ抗体触发含有血管性血友病因子和P选择素的内皮细胞囊泡的快速动员。这种胞吐作用导致细胞表面P选择素增加，从而启动白细胞募集级联反应。

些 Bcl 家族成员通过调节线粒体膜通透性来阻止程序性细胞死亡，从而防止胱天蛋白酶的激活。循环中有 DSA 的同种异体心脏和肾脏移植患者的移植物中，以及发生 AMR 的同种异体小鼠心脏移植物中都发现 Bcl-2 表达增高，在体内证实了这一现象[84,86]。其他抗细胞凋亡的基因，包括血红素加氧酶 1 在 HLA Ⅰ连接后上调[83,87]。

对 EC 增殖途径的进一步研究揭示，在Ⅰ类连接之后，成纤维细胞生长因子受体(FGFR)细胞表面表达被上调(图 4.7)[70,88]。增加的 FGFR 表达与增加的 bFGF 配体结合和通过 MAPK 途径增加的细胞增殖有关。这些数据表明，FGFR 的上调和由此产生的细胞增殖是Ⅰ类诱导的 FAK/肌动蛋白依赖性细胞增殖途径的替代途径。

除了细胞存活和增殖信号之外，抗 HLA Ⅰ抗体还通过诱导内皮中的黏附分子而引起白细胞募集(图 4.7)。HLA 与抗体的结合导致称为 Weibel-Palade 小体的内皮囊泡的释放和 P 选择素快速提呈，其可促进白细胞黏附[89]。大鼠心脏同种异体移植慢性排斥反应的研究显示，内膜中 P 选择素表达增加和内膜增厚相关[90,91]。

杀伤细胞免疫球蛋白样受体(KIR)

除了抗原提呈细胞毒性 T 细胞，HLA Ⅰ类分子同时也作为 NK 细胞受体的配体。NK 细胞占正常人外周血单核细胞部分的 5%~25%。历史上，NK 细胞被认为是固有免疫的组成部分(参见附加讨论固有免疫的第 7 章)，因为它们内在的自发杀伤不需要靶细胞的 HLA 和结合肽的任何限制。现在很清楚，NK 细胞应用高度特异性和复杂的靶细胞识别受体系统，通过整合由广泛常规生殖系统编码基因家族的大量抑制性和活化性受体触发的信号来进行调节[92]。

KIR 被认为是参与人类 NK 细胞发育和功能的关键受体。已经鉴定了 14 种不同的 KIR 受体，其中 7 种是抑制型，而另一些则是活化型受体。在与不同的 HLA Ⅰ类配体(HLA-A、B 和 C)结合后，抑制性 KIR 受体抑制 NK 细胞反应性。当激活的 KIR 受体感觉到在靶细胞上表达的未知配体时，会刺激 NK 细胞反应性，例如与 HLA Ⅰ类分子(例如 MICA 和 MICB)结构相关的“自我诱导”“自我改变”(负载有外源肽的 HLA Ⅰ类分子)或编码“非自身”(与感染相关的分子、肿瘤转化和同种异体移植抗原)的病原体。KIR 位点是高度多态性的，并且定位于染色体 19.KIR，和 HLA 基因家族独立分离，产生表达 KIR 受体的许多个体，它们缺乏 HLA Ⅰ类配体，反之亦然，造成人类多样性的 KIR-HLA 基因组合，其中一些已经与某些疾病的易感性相关[93]。

因为 NK 细胞可以自发地提供效应器功能，所以它们不会攻击周围的健康细胞。为了防止这种有害的自身免疫应答，NK 细胞至少有一种抑制性受体与自我 HLA Ⅰ类分子结合[94]。抑制性 KIR 受体与同源 HLA Ⅰ类配体的相互作用进一步限定了 NK 细胞能力的阈值[95]。HLA Ⅰ类分子在正常健康细胞中的大量表达为 NK 细胞的多种抑制性受体提供配体，并且因此使健康的细胞变得对 NK 细胞攻击耐受。由于某些病毒感染、肿瘤转化或其他形式的应激，导致 HLA Ⅰ类表达的下调减轻了对 NK 细胞的抑制作用，允许 NK 细胞消除这些不健康的靶细胞，这种现象最初被描述为“自我迷失”假设[96]。

在同种异体移植环境中，即使在与 HLA 相容的移植物(但不是与 HLA-A、B、C 相同的移植物)中，表达抑制受体的受体 NK 细胞在缺乏相应的抑制受体的 HLA Ⅰ类配体的同种异体移植细胞中也能被激活[97]。van Bergen 及其同事的一项研究显示，受体抑制型 KIR 受体的供体 HLA Ⅰ类配体的缺失与 HLA-A、B、DR 相容性肾移植中移植物的长期存活率降低有关[98,99]。Kunert 等人[100]发现，接受者基因型的抑制性受体数量较多，与肾功能稳定的患者之间存在联系。Vampa 等人[101]发现，携带更多活化 KIR 基因的受体比携带更少活化 KIR 基因的受体可触发更多的 NK 细胞毒性。这些研究提供的证据表明，抑制 NK 细胞活性对于改善肾移植物的存活可能是重要的。

非 HLA 移植抗原

尽管对 HLA 抗原的免疫应答在同种异体移植排斥反应中起着核心作用，但有证据表明，非 HLA 抗原也参与了急性和慢性排斥反应的发病机制，并使实体器官移植的长期移植存活率降低[102]。虽然许多这些非 HLA 抗原保留并不明确，但大多数是除 MICA 抗原以外的自身抗原[103,104]，并通常牵涉与移植物功能障碍相关的抗体。主要抗原靶标在同种异体移植物的细胞上表达，包括内皮和上皮细胞。抗内皮细胞抗体(AECA)代表包含 IgM 和 IgG 亚类的异质性抗体组，并针对各种抗原决定簇[105]。其他自身抗原包括心脏中的波形蛋白和心肌肌球蛋白(CM)[106,107]、肺部胶原V(Col V)和K-α1微管蛋白[108,109]、肾移植中集聚蛋白和血管紧张素Ⅱ受体Ⅰ型(AT1)[110,111],它们已被确定为具有较差移植结果的免疫靶标。移植受体中这些自身抗体的发病机制已经通过几种方式被证实:①体外诱导细胞损伤;②在动物模型中被动转移时引起移植排斥反应;③通过血浆置换或免疫抑制剂去除导致疾病临床症状的改善。

与针对难以接近的细胞内抗原的抗体相比,针对胞外抗原的抗体的发病机制更容易理解。然而,在移植过程中,冷缺血再灌注损伤引起的组织损伤和移植手术引起的炎症可能通过直接和间接的同种识别途径激活抗供体同种免疫,导致细胞内的抗原从损伤的细胞内释放。这些同种异体抗原可通过间接识别途径提呈宿主T细胞以产生自体反应性细胞和体液免疫应答。间接同种免疫反应一旦开始,就可以扩散到主要靶抗原内的附加决定簇,称为分子内表位扩散。用自身抗原重复刺激 $CD4^+$ T细胞可能超过自身耐受的阈值并导致自身抗体诱导的 $CD4^+$ T细胞的发展。这种移植后自身免疫可导致移植失败。已经证明,将抗MHCⅠ类抗体注入小鼠的肺部引发了 $CD4^+$ T细胞驱动的自身反应性,IL-1β和TNF-α的产生,以及抗自体抗原K-α1微管蛋白抗体和胶原蛋白V的产生[112]。

抗MICA抗体

MICA由高度多态性基因编码,至少有63个位于MHCⅠ类区域的等位基因[113]。MICA抗原具有限制的组织分布,并在上皮、内皮、角质形成细胞和成纤维细胞上表达。MICA基因含有热休克反应元件(HRE)启动子,其表达水平可以响应缺血再灌注损伤所介导的细胞应激和细胞因子如IL-2、IL-4和IL-15的作用。MICA作为NK细胞活化NKG2D受体和T细胞亚群的配体。MICA既不结合 $β_2m$ 也不结合肽。

针对MICA的同种抗体与肾脏和心脏移植的急性和慢性血管排斥有关。在一项大型多中心研究中,对MICA的预致敏与HLA匹配良好的肾移植受者的移植物丢失增加相关。MICA抗体可介导对内皮细胞的补体依赖性细胞毒性,表明这些抗体可引起补体介导的同种异体移植物的损伤[114]。然而,大多数关于MICA在移植中起作用的研究报道都是间接的,因为抗体的供体特异性未被确定。

总结

主要组织相容性复合物(MHC)是存在于所有脊椎动物物种中的紧密连锁的基因组。MHC编码与抗原提呈有关的免疫系统相关的多种蛋白质,肽转运蛋白分子TAP1和2(催化和调节肽交换的分子),补体成分C2、C4和B因子,细胞因子TNF-α和TNF-β,热休克蛋白70-1和2,21-羟化酶(参与类固醇代谢),以及其他不太明确的产物和调节元件。作为主要移植抗原的人类HLAⅠ类和Ⅱ类细胞表面抗原由人类MHC编码。

一些MHC基因具有显著的多态性。人类已经鉴定了超过10 000个HLA-A、-B、-C、-DR、-DQ和DP等位基因,这些等位基因编码至少有100种是可以经血清学检测的抗原。多样性是由一些有趣和新颖的遗传机制产生的,很可能是通过适应病原体和疾病而选择的。

每个个体都以严格的孟德尔方式继承独特的MHCⅠ类和Ⅱ类分子群,A和DQB1之间的交叉频率大约<1%。同样在HLA-A、-B、-C、-DR和-DQ位点匹配的概率是25%。

MHC分子通过将来自蛋白质抗原的肽以特定受体的形式提呈给T细胞而在免疫应答中起关键作用。CD8和CD4细胞表面分子的亲和性分别通过Ⅰ类和Ⅱ类MHC分子将肽从细胞内蛋白质提呈给 $CD8^+$ T细胞和 $CD4^+$ T细胞。细胞内蛋白质肽被加载到内质网中的MHCⅠ类分子的裂隙中,而Ⅱ类MHC分子的裂隙在ER中被保护,但随后在胞质内囊泡中被来自细胞外蛋白质的肽加载。

同种异体HLA分子引起T细胞和B细胞免疫应答。抗体可识别一系列结构特征(表位),这些结构特征(表位)是独特的,但因HLA抗原共享可导致交叉反应。

其他非HLA抗原也可作为移植抗原,包括细胞外不正常表达的隐匿性抗原和自身抗原,其中大多数可能通过直接或间接提呈HLA分子刺激受体免疫系统。HLA分子也是自然杀伤细胞的配体,代表了它们在临床移植中同样发挥重要的作用。

致谢

本章编写得到了美国国立过敏和传染病研究所RO1A042819（E.F.R.）、美国国立卫生研究院(NIH) U01AI077821(E.F.R.)和美国国立心肺和血液研究所RO1HL090995(E.F.R.)的资助。

（胡士华 译 王思奇 李照 校）

参考文献

1. The MHC Sequencing Consortium. Complete sequence and gene map of a human major histocompatibility complex. The MHC sequencing consortium. Nature. 1999;401:921–923.
2. Horton R, Wilming L, Rand V, et al. Gene map of the extended human MHC. Nature Reviews. Genetics. 2004;5:889–899.
3. Parham P, Adams EJ, Arnett KL. The origins of HLA-A,B,C polymorphism. Immunological Reviews. 1995;143:141–180.
4. Parham P, Lomen CE, Lawlor DA, et al. Nature of polymorphism in HLA-A, -B, and -C molecules. Proceedings of the National Academy of Sciences of the United States of America. 1988;85:4005–4009.
5. Erlich HA, Opelz G, Hansen J. HLA DNA typing and transplantation. Immunity. 2001;14:347–356.
6. Prugnolle F, Manica A, Charpentier M, et al. Pathogen-driven selection and worldwide HLA class I diversity. Current Biology. 2005;15:1022–1027.
7. Erlich HA, Gyllensten UB. The evolution of allelic diversity at the primate major histocompatibility complex class II loci. Human Immunology. 1991;30: 110–118.
8. Parham P, Ohta T. Population biology of antigen presentation by MHC class I molecules. Science. 1996;272:67–74.
9. Marsh SG, Albert ED, Bodmer WF, et al. Nomenclature for factors of the HLA system, 2010. Tissue Antigens. 2011;75:291–455.
10. Doherty PC, Zinkernagel RM. Enhanced immunological surveillance in mice heterozygous at the H-2 gene complex. Nature. 1975;256:50–52.
11. Carrington M, Nelson GW, Martin MP, et al. HLA and HIV-1: heterozygote advantage and B*35-Cw*04 disadvantage. Science. 1999;283:1748–1752.
12. Trachtenberg E, Korber B, Sollars C, et al. Advantage of rare HLA supertype in HIV disease progression. Nature Medicine. 2003;9:928–935.
13. Erlich HA, Bergstrom TF, Stoneking M, et al. HLA sequence polymorphism and the origin of humans. Science. 1996;274:1552–1554.
14. Middleton D, Menchaca L, Rood H, et al. New allele frequency database: http://www.allelefrequencies.net. Tissue Antigens. 2003;61:403–407.
15. Belich MP, Madrigal JA, Hildebrand WH, et al. Unusual HLA-B alleles in two tribes of Brazilian Indians. Nature. 1992;357:326–329.
16. de Bakker PI, McVean G, Sabeti PC, et al. A high-resolution HLA and SNP haplotype map for disease association studies in the extended human MHC. Nature Genetics. 2006;38:1166–1172.
17. Schreuder GM, Hurley CK, Marsh SG, et al. HLA dictionary 2004: summary of HLA-A, -B, -C, -DRB1/3/4/5, -DQB1 alleles and their association with serologically defined HLA-A, -B, -C, -DR, and -DQ antigens. Human Immunology. 2005;66:170–210.
18. El-Awar N, Lee JH, Tarsitani C, et al. HLA class I epitopes: recognition of binding sites by mAbs or eluted alloantibody confirmed with single recombinant antigens. Human Immunology. 2007;68:170–180.
19. Bjorkman PJ, Saper MA, Samraoui B, et al. The foreign antigen binding site and T cell recognition regions of class I histocompatibility antigens. Nature. 1987;329:512–518.
20. Gao GF, Tormo J, Gerth UC, et al. Crystal structure of the complex between human CD8alpha(alpha) and HLA-A2. Nature. 1997;387:630–634.
21. Brown JH, Jardetzky TS, Gorga JC, et al. Three-dimensional structure of the human class II histocompatibility antigen HLA-DR1. Nature. 1993;364:33–39.
22. Garboczi DN, Madden DR, Wiley DC. Five viral peptide-HLA-A2 co-crystals. Simultaneous space group determination and X-ray data collection. Journal of Molecular Biology. 1994;239:581–587.
23. Reinherz EL, Tan K, Tang L, et al. The crystal structure of a T cell receptor in complex with peptide and MHC class II. Science. 1999;286:1913–1921.
24. Garrett TP, Saper MA, Bjorkman PJ, et al. Specificity pockets for the side chains of peptide antigens in HLA-Aw68. Nature. 1989;342:692–696.
25. Rammensee HG, Falk K, Rotzschke O. Peptides naturally presented by MHC class I molecules. Annual Review of Immunology. 1993;11:213–244.
26. Rammensee HG. Chemistry of peptides associated with MHC class I and class II molecules. Current Opinion in Immunology. 1995;7:85–96.
27. Chicz RM, Urban RG, Gorga JC, et al. Specificity and promiscuity among naturally processed peptides bound to HLA-DR alleles. Journal of Experimental Medicine. 1993;178:27–47.
28. Cresswell P. Assembly, transport, and function of MHC class II molecules. Annual Review of Immunology. 1994;12:259–293.
29. Unanue ER. Perspective on antigen processing and presentation. Immunological Reviews. 2002;185:86–102.
30. Shastri N, Schwab S, Serwold T. Producing nature's gene-chips: the generation of peptides for display by MHC class I molecules. Annual Review of Immunology. 2002;20:463–493.
31. Rivett AJ, Hearn AR. Proteasome function in antigen presentation: immunoproteasome complexes, Peptide production, and interactions with viral proteins. Current Protein and Peptide Science. 2004;5:153–161.
32. Kloetzel PM, Ossendorp F. Proteasome and peptidase function in MHC-class-I-mediated antigen presentation. Current Opinion in Immunology. 2004;16: 76–81.
33. Pamer E, Cresswell P. Mechanisms of MHC class I–restricted antigen processing. Annual Review of Immunology. 1998;16:323–358.
34. Seifert U, Bialy LP, Ebstein F, et al. Immunoproteasomes preserve protein homeostasis upon interferon-induced oxidative stress. Cell. 2010;142:613–624.
35. Cresswell P, Ackerman AL, Giodini A, et al. Mechanisms of MHC class I-restricted antigen processing and cross-presentation. Immunological Reviews. 2005;207: 145–157.
36. Purcell AW, Elliott T. Molecular machinations of the MHC-I peptide loading complex. Current Opinion in Immunology. 2008;20:75–81.
37. McCluskey J, Rossjohn J, Purcell AW. TAP genes and immunity. Current Opinion in Immunology. 2004;16:651–659.
38. Serwold T, Gonzalez F, Kim J, et al. ERAAP customizes peptides for MHC class I molecules in the endoplasmic reticulum. Nature. 2002;419:480–483.
39. Cresswell P, Bangia N, Dick T, et al. The nature of the MHC class I peptide loading complex. Immunological Reviews. 1999;172:21–28.
40. Williams A, Peh CA, Elliott T. The cell biology of MHC class I antigen presentation. Tissue Antigens. 2002;59:3–17.
41. Ackerman AL, Kyritsis C, Tampe R, et al. Early phagosomes in dendritic cells form a cellular compartment sufficient for cross presentation of exogenous antigens. Proceedings of the National Academy of Sciences of the United States of America. 2003;100:12889–12894.
42. Carbone FR, Heath WR. The role of dendritic cell subsets in immunity to viruses. Current Opinion in Immunology. 2003;15:416–420.
43. Brooks AG, McCluskey J. Class II-restricted presentation of a hen egg lysozyme determinant derived from endogenous antigen sequestered in the cytoplasm or endoplasmic reticulum of the antigen presenting cells. Journal of Immunology. 1993;150:3690–3697.
44. Gueguen M, Long EO. Presentation of a cytosolic antigen by major histocompatibility complex class II molecules requires a long-lived form of the antigen. Proceedings of the National Academy of Sciences of the United States of America. 1996;93:14692–14697.
45. Jacobson S, Sekaly RP, Jacobson CL, et al. HLA class II-restricted presentation of cytoplasmic measles virus antigens to cytotoxic T cells. Journal of Virology. 1989;63:1756–1762.
46. Anderson HA, Bergstralh DT, Kawamura T, et al. Phosphorylation of the invariant chain by protein kinase C regulates MHC class II trafficking to antigen-processing compartments. Journal of Immunology. 1999;163:5435–5443.
47. Nakagawa TY, Rudensky AY. The role of lysosomal proteinases in MHC class II-mediated antigen processing and presentation. Immunological Reviews. 1999;172:121–129.
48. Chapman HA. Endosomal proteolysis and MHC class II function. Current Opinion in Immunology. 1998;10:93–102.
49. Brocke P, Garbi N, Momburg F, et al. HLA-DM, HLA-DO and tapasin: functional similarities and differences. Current Opinion in Immunology. 2002;14:22–29.
50. Castellino F, Zappacosta F, Coligan JE, et al. Large protein fragments as substrates for endocytic antigen capture by MHC class II molecules. Journal of Immunology. 1998;161:4048–4057.
51. Grotenbreg GM, Nicholson MJ, Fowler KD, et al. Empty class II major histocompatibility complex created by peptide photolysis establishes the role of DM in peptide association. Journal of Biological Chemistry. 2007;282:21425–21436.
52. van den Hoorn T, Paul P, Jongsma ML, et al. Routes to manipulate MHC class II antigen presentation. Current Opinion in Immunology. 2011;23:88–95.

53. Honey K, Rudensky AY. Lysosomal cysteine proteases regulate antigen presentation. Nature Reviews. Immunology. 2003;3:472–482.
54. Maric M, Arunachalam B, Phan UT, et al. Defective antigen processing in GILT-free mice. Science. 2001;294:1361–1365.
55. Singh R, Cresswell P. Defective cross-presentation of viral antigens in GILT-free mice. Science. 2010;328:1394–1398.
56. Munz C. Antigen processing via autophagy—not only for MHC class II presentation anymore? Current Opinion in Immunology. 2010;22:89–93.
57. Im JS, Arora P, Bricard G, et al. Kinetics and cellular site of glycolipid loading control the outcome of natural killer T cell activation. Immunity. 2009;30:888–898.
58. Zinkernagel RM, Doherty PC. Restriction of in vitro T cell-mediated cytotoxicity in lymphocytic choriomeningitis within a syngeneic or semiallogeneic system. Nature. 1974;248:701–702.
59. Reith W, LeibundGut-Landmann S, Waldburger JM. Regulation of MHC class II gene expression by the class II transactivator. Nature Reviews. Immunology. 2005;5:793–806.
60. Hofstetter AR, Sullivan LC, Lukacher AE, et al. Diverse roles of non-diverse molecules: MHC class Ib molecules in host defense and control of autoimmunity. Current Opinion in Immunology. 2011;23:104–110.
61. Sullivan LC, Clements CS, Rossjohn J, et al. The major histocompatibility complex class Ib molecule HLA-E at the interface between innate and adaptive immunity. Tissue Antigens. 2008;72:415–424.
62. Carosella ED, LeMaoult J. HLA-G: a look back, a look forward. Cellular and Molecular Life Sciences. 2011;68:337–340.
63. Truman JP, Choqueux C, Charron D, et al. HLA class II molecule signal transduction leads to either apoptosis or activation via two different pathways. Cellular Immunology. 1996;172:149–157.
64. Haylett RS, Koch N, Rink L. MHC class II molecules activate NFAT and the ERK group of MAPK through distinct signaling pathways in B cells. European Journal of Immunology. 2009;39:1947–1955.
65. Rich T, Lawler SE, Lord JM, et al. HLA class II-induced translocation of PKC alpha and PKC beta II isoforms is abrogated following truncation of DR beta cytoplasmic domains. Journal of Immunology. 1997;159:3792–3798.
66. Skov S. Intracellular signal transduction mediated by ligation of MHC class I molecules. Tissue Antigens. 1998;51:215–223.
67. Skov S, Bregenholt S, Claesson MH. MHC class I ligation of human T cells activates the ZAP70 and p56lck tyrosine kinases, leads to an alternative phenotype of the TCR/CD3 zeta-chain, and induces apoptosis. Journal of Immunology. 1997;158:3189–3196.
68. Bieri M, Oroszlan M, Farkas A, et al. Anti-HLA I antibodies induce VEGF production by endothelial cells, which increases proliferation and paracellular permeability. International Journal of Biochemistry and Cell Biology. 2009;41: 2422–2430.
69. Coupel S, Leboeuf F, Boulday G, et al. RhoA activation mediates phosphatidylinositol 3-kinase-dependent proliferation of human vascular endothelial cells: an alloimmune mechanism of chronic allograft nephropathy. Journal of the American Society of Nephrology. 2004;15:2429–2439.
70. Harris PE, Bian H, Reed EF. Induction of high affinity fibroblast growth factor receptor expression and proliferation in human endothelial cells by anti-HLA antibodies: a possible mechanism for transplant atherosclerosis. Journal of Immunology. 1997;159:5697–5704.
71. Jin YP, Korin Y, Zhang X, et al. RNA interference elucidates the role of focal adhesion kinase in HLA class I-mediated focal adhesion complex formation and proliferation in human endothelial cells. Journal of Immunology. 2007;178: 7911–7922.
72. Jaramillo A, Smith CR, Maruyama T, et al. Anti-HLA class I antibody binding to airway epithelial cells induces production of fibrogenic growth factors and apoptotic cell death: a possible mechanism for bronchiolitis obliterans syndrome. Human Immunology. 2003;64:521–529.
73. Reznik SI, Jaramillo A, Zhang L, et al. Anti-HLA antibody binding to hla class I molecules induces proliferation of airway epithelial cells: a potential mechanism for bronchiolitis obliterans syndrome. Journal of Thoracic and Cardiovascular Surgery. 2000;119:39–45.
74. Li F, Atz ME, Reed EF. Human leukocyte antigen antibodies in chronic transplant vasculopathy-mechanisms and pathways. Current Opinion in Immunology. 2009;21:557–562.
75. Valenzuela NM, Reed EF. The link between major histocompatibility complex antibodies and cell proliferation. Transplantation Reviews (Orlando, Fla.). 2011;25:154–166.
76. Zhang X, Rozengurt E, Reed EF. HLA class I molecules partner with integrin beta4 to stimulate endothelial cell proliferation and migration. Science Signaling. 2010;3:ra85.
77. Jin YP, Singh RP, Du ZY, et al. Ligation of HLA class I molecules on endothelial cells induces phosphorylation of Src, paxillin, and focal adhesion kinase in an actin-dependent manner. Journal of Immunology. 2002;168:5415–5423.
78. Lepin EJ, Jin YP, Barwe SP, et al. HLA class I signal transduction is dependent on Rho GTPase and ROK. Biochemical and Biophysical Research Communications. 2004;323:213–217.
79. Ziegler ME, Souda P, Jin YP, et al. Characterization of the endothelial cell cytoskeleton following HLA class I ligation. PLoS ONE. 2012;7:e29472.
80. Jindra PT, Jin YP, Rozengurt E, et al. HLA class I antibody-mediated endothelial cell proliferation via the mTOR pathway. Journal of Immunology. 2008; 180:2357–2366.
81. Atz ME, Reed EF. Role of anti-MHC class I antibody in facilitating transplant accommodation. Critical Reviews in Immunology. 2008;28:485–511.
82. Iwasaki K, Miwa Y, Haneda M, et al. Significance of HLA class I antibody-induced antioxidant gene expression for endothelial cell protection against complement attack. Biochemical and Biophysical Research Communications. 2010;391:1210–1215.
83. Narayanan K, Jaramillo A, Phelan DL, et al. Pre-exposure to sub-saturating concentrations of HLA class I antibodies confers resistance to endothelial cells against antibody complement-mediated lysis by regulating Bad through the phosphatidylinositol 3-kinase/Akt pathway. European Journal of Immunology. 2004;34:2303–2312.
84. Salama AD, Delikouras A, Pusey CD, et al. Transplant accommodation in highly sensitized patients: a potential role for Bcl-xL and alloantibody. American Journal of Transplantation. 2001;1:260–269.
85. Jin YP, Fishbein MC, Said JW, et al. Anti-HLA class I antibody-mediated activation of the PI3K/Akt signaling pathway and induction of Bcl-2 and Bcl-xL expression in endothelial cells. Human Immunology. 2004;65:291–302.
86. Jindra PT, Hsueh A, Hong L, et al. Anti-MHC class I antibody activation of proliferation and survival signaling in murine cardiac allografts. Journal of Immunology. 2008;180:2214–2224.
87. Narayanan K, Jendrisak MD, Phelan DL, et al. HLA class I antibody mediated accommodation of endothelial cells via the activation of PI3K/cAMP dependent PKA pathway. Transplant Immunology. 2006;15:187–197.
88. Bian H, Harris PE, Reed EF. Ligation of HLA class I molecules on smooth muscle cells with anti-HLA antibodies induces tyrosine phosphorylation, fibroblast growth factor receptor expression and cell proliferation. International Immunology. 1998;10:1315–1323.
89. Yamakuchi M, Kirkiles-Smith NC, Ferlito M, et al. Antibody to human leukocyte antigen triggers endothelial exocytosis. Proceedings of the National Academy of Sciences of the United States of America. 2007;104:1301–1306.
90. Koskinen PK. Lemstrom KB. Adhesion molecule P-selectin and vascular cell adhesion molecule-1 in enhanced heart allograft arteriosclerosis in the rat. Circulation. 1997;95:191–196.
91. Phillips JW, Barringhaus KG, Sanders JM, et al. Single injection of P-selectin or P-selectin glycoprotein ligand-1 monoclonal antibody blocks neointima formation after arterial injury in apolipoprotein E-deficient mice. Circulation. 2003;107:2244–2249.
92. Rajalingam R. Killer cell immunoglobulin-like receptors influence the innate and adaptive immune responses. Iranian Journal of Immunology. 2007;4: 61–78.
93. Khakoo SI, Carrington M. KIR and disease: a model system or system of models? Immunological Reviews. 2006;214:186–201.
94. Valiante NM, Uhrberg M, Shilling HG, et al. Functionally and structurally distinct NK cell receptor repertoires in the peripheral blood of two human donors. Immunity. 1997;7:739–751.
95. Kim S, Poursine-Laurent J, Truscott SM, et al. Licensing of natural killer cells by host major histocompatibility complex class I molecules. Nature. 2005;436: 709–713.
96. Ljunggren HG, Karre K. In search of the 'missing self': MHC molecules and NK cell recognition. Immunology Today. 1990;11:237–244.
97. Rajalingam R. Variable interactions of recipient killer cell immunoglobulin-like receptors with self and allogenic human leukocyte antigen class I ligands may influence the outcome of solid organ transplants. Current Opinion in Organ Transplantation. 2008;13:430–437.
98. van Bergen J, Thompson A, Haasnoot GW, et al. KIR-ligand mismatches are associated with reduced long-term graft survival in HLA-compatible kidney transplantation. American Journal of Transplantation. 2011;11:1959–1964.
99. Rajalingam R, Gebel HM. KIR-HLA mismatching in human renal allograft transplantation: emergence of a new concept. American Journal of Transplantation. 2011;11:1771–1772.
100. Kunert K, Seiler M, Mashreghi MF, et al. KIR/HLA ligand incompatibility in kidney transplantation. Transplantation. 2007;84:1527–1533.
101. Vampa ML, Norman PJ, Burnapp L, et al. Natural killer-cell activity after human renal transplantation in relation to killer immunoglobulin-like receptors and human leukocyte antigen mismatch. Transplantation. 2003;76:1220–1228.

102. Zhang Q, Reed EF. Non-MHC antigenic targets of the humoral immune response in transplantation. Current Opinion in Immunology. 2010;22:682–688.
103. Zhang Q, Cecka JM, Gjertson DW, et al. HLA and MICA: targets of antibody-mediated rejection in heart transplantation. Transplantation. 2011;91:1153–1158.
104. Zou Y, Stastny P, Susal C, et al. Antibodies against MICA antigens and kidney-transplant rejection. New England Journal of Medicine. 2007;357:1293–1300.
105. Bordron A, Revelen R, D'Arbonneau F, et al. Functional heterogeneity of anti-endothelial cell antibodies. Clinical and Experimental Immunology. 2001;124:492–501.
106. Jurcevic S, Ainsworth ME, Pomerance A, et al. Antivimentin antibodies are an independent predictor of transplant-associated coronary artery disease after cardiac transplantation. Transplantation. 2001;71:886–892.
107. Tanaka M, Zwierzchoniewska M, Mokhtari GK, et al. Progression of alloresponse and tissue-specific immunity during graft coronary artery disease. American Journal of Transplantation. 2005;5:1286–1296.
108. Burlingham WJ, Love RB, Jankowska-Gan E, et al. IL-17-dependent cellular immunity to collagen type V predisposes to obliterative bronchiolitis in human lung transplants. Journal of Clinical Investigation. 2007;117:3498–3506.
109. Goers TA, Ramachandran S, Aloush A, et al. De novo production of K-alpha1 tubulin-specific antibodies: role in chronic lung allograft rejection. Journal of Immunology. 2008;180:4487–4494.
110. Dragun D, Muller DN, Brasen JH, et al. Angiotensin II type 1-receptor activating antibodies in renal-allograft rejection. New England Journal of Medicine. 2005;352:558–569.
111. Joosten SA, Sijpkens YW, van Ham V, et al. Antibody response against the glomerular basement membrane protein agrin in patients with transplant glomerulopathy. American Journal of Transplantation. 2005;5:383–393.
112. Fukami N, Ramachandran S, Saini D, et al. Antibodies to MHC class I induce autoimmunity: role in the pathogenesis of chronic rejection. Journal of Immunology. 2009;182:309–318.
113. Zwirner NW, Marcos CY, Mirbaha F, et al. Identification of MICA as a new polymorphic alloantigen recognized by antibodies in sera of organ transplant recipients. Human Immunology. 2000;61:917–924.
114. Zou Y, Mirbaha F, Lazaro A, et al. MICA is a target for complement-dependent cytotoxicity with mouse monoclonal antibodies and human alloantibodies. Human Immunology. 2002;63:30–39.
115. Rajalingam R, Cecka M, Reed EF. Molecular HLA typing methods used in clinical laboratories. In: Grody WW, Nakamura RM, Kiechle FL, Strom C, editors. Molecular Diagnostics: Techniques and Applications for the Clinical Laboratory. Boston, MA: Elsevier; 2010.

第5章 适应性免疫之细胞免疫机制

Maria-Luisa Alegre

引言

遗传上不同个体之间移植的器官以T细胞依赖性方式被排斥。宿主T细胞识别来自相同物种内的移植器官抗原的能力被称为同种异体识别，并且在不存在一定程度的免疫修饰的情况下导致受体T细胞活化、增殖和分化,获得效应细胞的功能,迁移到同种异体移植物内,以及最终破坏移植物。固有免疫细胞对于初始呈递同种异体抗原至外周淋巴器官中的初始T细胞是必需的，并且在移植物中也可以通过效应T细胞激活并且通过分泌炎性因子而破坏移植。此外,活化的T细胞可以帮助B细胞产生同种异体抗体，驱动体液免疫机制,也可以损害移植物。在本章中,我们将讨论同种异体识别和T细胞依赖同种异体移植排斥的关键特征。体液免疫的细节可以在第6章中找到。本章将集中于直接涉及T细胞介导的移植物破坏的机制；关于生理性细胞免疫的讨论见第2章。细胞介导的排斥的组织学和临床表现细节见组织病理学综合征（移植排斥和复发性疾病的组织病理学综合征部分）和移植物排斥的临床诊断与管理（临床同种异体移植排斥综合征:诊断和管理部分)。

同种抗原的T细胞识别:直接、半直接和间接呈递

T细胞表达一种T细胞受体(TCR),其可以结合由位于MHC分子槽中的肽形成的复合体,所述MHC分子自身在抗原呈递细胞(APC)的表面表达。T细胞在胸腺中发育，使得它们的TCR可以识别自体MHC复合物,其呈现源自内源自身蛋白的肽,其中$CD8^+$ T细胞识别MHCⅠ类（人类中的HLA-A、B和C),$CD4^+$ T细胞识别MHCⅡ类(HLA-DR、DP、DQ)。MHC抗原的详细描述可见第4章。具有高亲和力的识别自身肽/MHC(pMHC)的TCR胸腺细胞在阴性选择的过程中消除,这降低了能够介导自身免疫反应的T细胞的频率,而具有对自身pMHC足够的亲和力以触发存活途径,但不足以导致完全激活的胸腺细胞被保留下来。相反,不能结合自身pMHC的胸腺细胞则被清除。因此,填充身体的成熟T细胞“限制性”地识别自身MHC分子。当这些分子呈现出胸腺外的内源自身肽的正常阵列时,结合的T细胞既接收到生存信号又不被激活或增殖[1]。这些T细胞中的每一种都具有被给定的“外源”同源肽完全活化的能力。这些“外源肽”可以取代自身MHC分子上的内源肽,并且可以起源于感染性生物体、体细胞突变的蛋白质或同种异体细胞。在自身MHC分子背景下,同种异体肽(衍生自同种异体MHC分子或来自供体和受体非MHC蛋白质之间称为次要抗原的多态性变异)的呈递称为间接呈递,并且需要宿主APC识别来自吞噬作用、胞饮作用或者内吞作用的濒死供体细胞(图5.1)。

令人惊讶的是，尽管胸腺选择性产生具有受自身MHC分子限制的TCR的T细胞，但是许多T细胞也可以结合同种异体MHC分子,可能是因为没有在胸腺中消除识别同种异体反应的T细胞，因为同种异体MHC分子在胸腺中不表达。事实上,虽然在10^6个T细胞中只有大约1个可识别给定自身MHC等位基因上的“外源”抗原,但据估计,1%~10%的T细胞可直接参与同种异体MHC分子[2]。这种高前体频率最初使科学家假设T细胞可以以不同于自身MHC分子的方式结合同种异体MHC分子,可能仅接触MHC残基,因此允许每个MHC等位基因上出现多个肽。然而,对已经解决的少数TCR/p/同种-MHC晶体结构的分析(见下文)表明,相互作用是肽依赖性的[3]。第9章将进一步讨

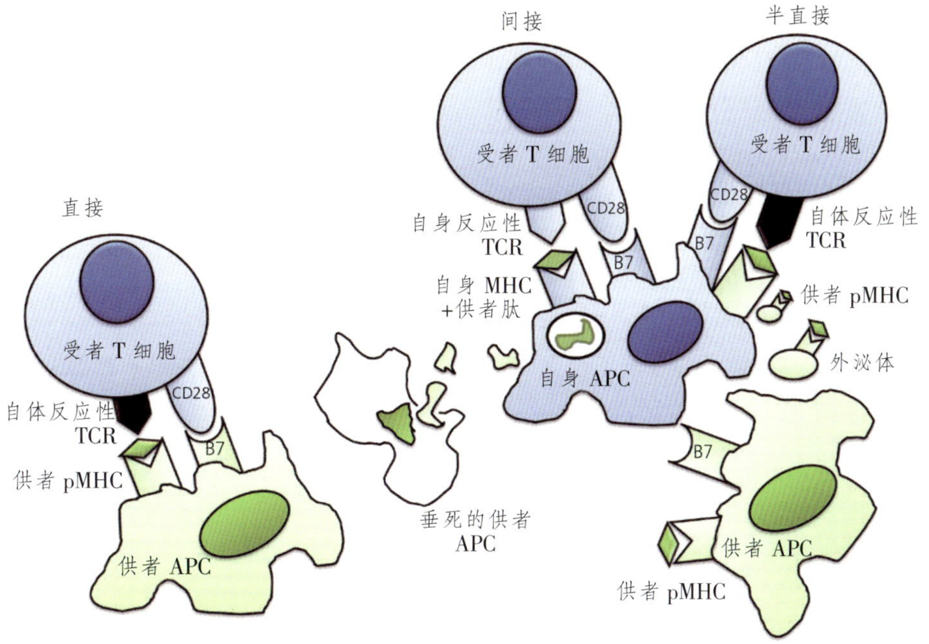

图 5.1　同种异体识别的类型。基于其 TCR 对自身 MHC 分子识别的限制，在胸腺中选择 T 细胞。然而，一部分 T 细胞也可以通过同种异体和自身 MHC /肽复合物之间的交叉反应或通过不同的 TCR/MHC 停靠位点识别同种异体 MHC 分子/供体肽。移植后，这些 T 细胞可以直接在供体 APC 或实质细胞的表面上识别同种异体 MHC(直接识别)。另外，含有供体 MHC 的完整膜的片段可以在细胞-细胞接触或细胞-内体接触之后与受体 APC 的膜融合，使得 T 细胞可以识别受体 APC 上的完整供体 MHC(半定向呈递)。最后，垂死移植物的细胞片段可以由受体 APC 摄取，并且衍自供体和受体之间不同的多态性蛋白质的同种异体肽可以通过自身 MHC 分子呈递(间接呈递)。这些机制可以全部应用于 $CD4^+$ T 细胞识别供体或受体 MHC Ⅱ类和 $CD8^+$ T 细胞识别供体或受体。

论构成人的同种免疫谱系的受体配体相互作用谱。MHC 分子具有高度多态性，在人群中有数百个 MHC 等位基因，并且每个人能够表达高达 6 个 MHC Ⅰ类和 6 个 MHC Ⅱ类等位基因(第 6 对染色体上各有 3 个；参见第 4 章)。因为每个 MHC 等位基因都可以呈现许多内源性肽，所以可以识别具有特定同种异体 MHC 等位基因的特定肽的 T 细胞组合加起来呈现了非常大的数目，这就可能解释具有直接同种异体反应的 T 细胞的高频率。

通过宿主 T 细胞对供体肽/供体 MHC 分子的直接同位素识别可以发生在移植器官中含有的供体 APC 上(直接呈递)，或者发生在将完整膜的片段从供体细胞转移到受体 APC 上之后 (半直接呈递)(图 5.1)(见第 2 章)[4]。后者可以作为宿主和供体细胞之间的细胞-细胞接触的结果或通过与宿主 APC 质膜融合的供体外来体的转移而发生。传统上，MHC Ⅰ类分子被描述为主要提呈来源于细胞溶质蛋白的肽，其通过与抗原加工相关的转运(TAP)到内质网，MHC Ⅱ类则呈递来源于胞外蛋白的肽，其由吞噬作用、胞饮作用或胞吞作用递送至内溶酶体。然而，现在清楚的是，MHC Ⅰ类分子提呈细胞外蛋白质，MHC Ⅱ类分子呈递细胞质蛋白。自噬过程中产生的核小体可向溶酶体途经传递细胞内细胞质抗原，从而产生Ⅱ类表达[5,6]，而细胞外吞噬体物可以通过未完全解释的机制从细胞器渗出到细胞质中，并且可用于蛋白酶体加工、TAP 易位和Ⅰ类呈现[7]。这些途径进一步拓宽了用于直接和间接 T 细胞同种异体识别的可能的肽库。

TCR 对同种异体抗原结构性识别

TCR 包含形成三个高度可变的互补决定区(CDR)的 α 和 β 链，其负责与肽和 MHC 分子上的氨基酸残基接触。近年来，人们对自 MHC 抑制培养的 T 细胞如何直接识别同种异体 MHC 进行了积极的研究。这项研究的主要障碍是，天然存在于 MHC 分子上的内源性肽通常是未知的，并且可以来自供体蛋白质组内的任何地方。只有少数具有自身 pMHC 和同种异体 pMHC 已知配体的 TCR 已经被共结晶并直接比较[8]。一些结构揭示了分子拟态，利用TCR和pMHC的可塑性（诱导拟合）优化同种异体肽/同种异型MHC复合物模拟外源肽/自身MHC的构象。其他结构已经证明了TCR对自身MHC和同种异体MHC复合物的独特接合策略，但是在这两种情况下，都包括与肽和MHC分子本身的接触。报告进一步证明，同种异体反应性受内源性肽库的限制，表明同种异体识别是肽依赖和肽特异的，如自身MHC常规识别外源肽[9]。这还表明，由于α链等位排除失败（1%~8%的T细胞库）而表达两种不同特异性TCR的T细胞具有更强的同种异体反应性[10]（见第9章）。由于同种识别规则得到了更好的定义，故可以预测宿主T细胞对供体pMHC的交叉反应性，以帮助选择具有较低潜力的最佳供体来激活受体T细胞。

T细胞的共刺激和分化

除了需要TCR结合，初始T细胞（T细胞致敏）仅当在额外的表面分子即共刺激受体同时结合到TCR时可以启动完全激活[11]。初始T细胞上仅有少量共刺激受体表达，CD28是其中主要的一个。CD28是在APC上表达的CD80（B7-1）和CD86（B7-2）配体的受体，并且在炎症条件下，在APC和一些实质细胞上进一步上调。已经显示在TCR结合期间阻断CD28可导致T细胞凋亡或随后不应答于再刺激，称为T细胞无反应的状态。这些发现导致药物阿巴西普和贝拉西普的应用，其可以结合CD80和CD86并防止这些配体参与活化CD28，因此可显著减少T细胞的致敏。贝拉西普在2011年被批准作为肾移植的免疫抑制药物。这些试剂可防止移植后同种异体反应性T细胞的活化，导致它们的凋亡或无反应性，而不影响在贝拉西普治疗时不涉及TCR的其他特异性T细胞。

在T细胞活化后，T细胞上调许多额外的共刺激受体，包括免疫球蛋白超家族的成员，例如ICOS和TNF受体家族，例如4-1BB和OX40，以及T细胞免疫球蛋白黏蛋白（TIM）家族[12]。活化的T细胞也上调CD40L（CD154），它是TNF家族成员，集结APC上的TNFR家族成员CD40并驱动APC表达更高水平的MHC、CD80和CD86，并产生细胞因子。许多共刺激分子在初始T细胞分化为效应细胞和记忆细胞后仍然表达，使得先前活化的T细胞比初始活化的T细胞更难以抑制，因为这些受体可以降低T细胞活化的阈值。这些共刺激受体的配体在APC上表达，其中一些可以在实质细胞，例如上皮和内皮细胞中上调。

共刺激受体的表达除了能促进T细胞活化外，有的亦可以抑制或终止T细胞活化，所以有时也称为共刺激抑制性受体。这些包括CTLA-4（以比CD28高的亲和力结合CD80和CD86）、PD-1（结合PDL1和PDL2）、BTLA（结合HVEM）、LAG3（结合MHC Ⅱ类），以及T细胞上尚未鉴定的新近描述的受体，包括B7-H4、B7S3、BTNL2和VISTA的APC上的配体。所有这些抑制性受体都是免疫球蛋白超家族的成员，并且它们的诱导对于抑制T细胞应答是必需的，因为缺乏这些分子的动物会出现各种程度的淋巴增殖和自身免疫病，其中CTLA-4缺陷是致死的。这些受体的配体在APC和一些实质细胞上表达。

刺激后，初始T细胞产生IL-2，并将其用作自分泌生长因子进行增殖。此外，根据它们在繁殖期间遇到的细胞因子，它们可以分化为各种类型的效应T细胞，通过它们分泌的细胞因子谱来区分（图5.2）。$CD4^+$ T细胞通常被称为T辅助细胞（Th），而$CD8^+$ T细胞通常被称为细胞毒性T细胞（Tc）（参见第2章）。暴露于IL-12的活化T细胞将分化成主要产生IFN-γ的效应T细胞，并被称为Th1/Tc1，而与IL-4的相遇将驱动产生IL-4、IL-5、IL-10和IL-13的Th2/Tc2细胞的分化，并且暴露于TGF-β和IL-6将导致产生IL-17A（IL-17）、IL-17F和IL-22的Th17/Tc17细胞的分化[13,14]。效应T细胞的这些细胞因子各自独特地作用于特定的病原体，Th1细胞在消除细胞内病原体中起主要作用，Th2细胞对寄生虫起作用，Th17细胞对细胞外微生物起重要作用。在一些情况下，这些细胞也可以变得致病，Th1和Th17细胞与自身免疫相关，Th2细胞与哮喘和过敏相关。在移植中，急性同种异体移植排斥主要与产生IFN-γ的Th1/Tc1细胞的存在相关，同时IL-17的存在在排斥同种异体移植物和Th2细胞中越来越受到认可，并且已经显示Th2细胞和Th2细胞因子能够驱动排斥反应。

增殖和分化后，T细胞经历收缩期，其中大多数发生凋亡或细胞周期停滞作为终止免疫应答的手段，其余T细胞获得记忆特征。在移植中，转移记忆T细胞至免疫缺陷小鼠比那些接受初始T细胞的小鼠可以更快产生动力学抑制即同种异体移植物排斥反应[15]。重要的是，对微生物的先前免疫应答导致病原体特异性记

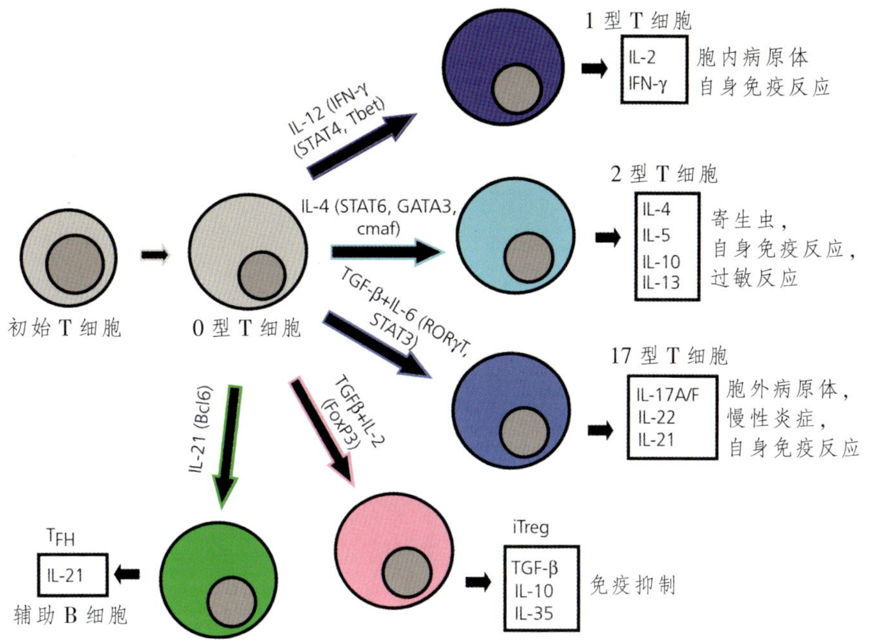

图 5.2 T 细胞分化途径。如图所示，一旦激活，基于各种细胞因子作用和转录因子的功能，T 细胞可以被驱使分化成各种功能表型。一般来说，采用经典模式，T 细胞有五种主要类型：Th-1、Th-2、Th-17、诱导的 T 调节细胞（iTreg）和 T 滤泡辅助细胞（Tfh）。

忆 T 细胞的产生，其中一些，如初始 T 细胞，也可以发生同种异体免疫排斥反应[16]。这些记忆细胞对常规免疫抑制治疗较不敏感，并且是接受同种异体移植物的重要障碍（见第 9 章）。

除了传统的 $CD4^+$和 $CD8^+$ T 细胞之外，$CD4^+$ T 细胞的一个子集已经被显示表达转录因子 Foxp3 并且缺乏产生 IL-2 的能力。相反，这些细胞在体外和体内抑制传统 T 细胞的功能，并且现在被称为调节性 T 细胞（Treg）（见第 8 章）[17]。Treg 是维持 T 细胞体内稳态和防止自身免疫所必需的，因为在 Treg 缺乏的小鼠或在成年后 Treg 被永久消除的小鼠中，会因淋巴细胞增殖和自身免疫疾病而迅速死亡。已知在人类中因 *Foxp3* 基因突变致其功能丧失的先天性疾病称为 IPEX 综合征，并且类似地导致自身免疫病。目前已经描述了两种类型的 $Foxp3^+$ Treg，第一种在胸腺中发育，如传统 T 细胞，通常被称为天然 Treg（nTreg）。第二种类型在 TGF-β 和 IL-2 或视黄酸的存在下在体外或体内激活的成熟天然 T 细胞中发育而来，被称为诱导或适应性 Treg（iTreg）。小鼠和人类中 5%~10%的 $CD4^+$ T 细胞形成 Treg。nTreg 和 iTreg 都可以抑制免疫反应，并且已经显示两者都是维持 T 细胞稳态所必需的，至少在小鼠中是如此[18]。在移植中，已经显示 iTreg 可以在共刺激阻断后被诱导[19]，并且 nTreg 和 iTreg 可以在成功移植的同种异体胰岛移植物中被观察到[20]。然而，各亚群对控制急性或慢性排斥反应的相对重要性仍有待确定。因为 nTregs 和 iTregs 都表达 CD4、Foxp3、高水平 CD25 和低水平 CD127，区分它们仍然具有挑战性。据报道，nTregs 比 iTregs 表达更高水平的转录因子 Helios[21]，虽然这仍然有争议，但和 nTregs 相比，iTregs 的 *Foxp3* 基因内的特定位点甲基化水平更低，即部分甲基化[22,23]。

因为 iTreg 可以在体外从 PBMC 产生并扩展到非常大的数量，临床试验正在探索将 iTreg 过继转移入移植受体的安全性和有效性。骨髓移植的初步试验显示，欧洲和美国，移植物抗宿主病（GVHD）减少，实体器官移植试验已经开始[24]。

固有免疫信号影响 T 细胞反应

激活后，APC 可分泌有助于形成 T 细胞分化的细胞因子。因为免疫系统进化可以抵抗感染，识别存在于微生物中的分子模式的受体在驱动 APC 激活和桥接先天和适应性免疫中作用关键（见第 2 章）。病原相关分子模式（PAMP）包括内毒素、鞭毛蛋白、蛋白聚糖、非甲基化 CpG 基序、双链 RNA 和其他[25]。这些 PAMP 可以结合在 APC 的质膜和内体膜上表达的 Toll 样受体（TLR），但也可以结合在 T 细胞和一些实质细胞上[26]。

TLR在APC中的接合导致共刺激配体的上调,从而促进它们向T细胞呈递抗原，以及产生如Ⅰ型IFN、IL-1、TNF、IL-6和IL-12等细胞因子。如上所述,基于对感染生物的适当反应，这些细胞因子定义了活化T细胞将经历的分化类型,IL-12促进Th1分化、IL-6促进Th17分化。重要的是,在无菌炎症期间产生的分子模式因子，例如在缺血和再灌注期间由同种异体移植物所经历的,也可以通过直接连接它们或将这些TLR敏化至最小浓度的微生物配体来激活一些TLR，主要是TLR2和TLR4[27]。在移植的背景下,已经描述了一些损伤相关分子模式(DAMP)作为佐剂来增加同种异体反应,HMGB1、热休克蛋白(HSP)和透明质酸都已显示可增强同种异体反应性[25]。此外,据报道,触珠蛋白——一种急性期蛋白在移植组织中上调，缺乏触珠蛋白的皮肤在移植后的小鼠中表现出生存期延长，其中一半以上的动物长期保留其移植物[28]。这些数据表明,通过减少供体器官TLR信号传导的局部治疗可能有益于移植。

重要的是,一些TLR在T细胞本身表达,包括传统的T细胞和Treg。TLR在常规T细胞中的参与已显示可促进T细胞活化和T细胞存活[29],而他们在Treg中的参与可以根据情况增强或防止它们的抑制功能,可能通过影响表观遗传调节*Foxp3*基因[30-36]。在小鼠移植中,TLR的参与已经显示可以阻止小鼠通过共刺激阻断治疗阻止诱导移植耐受，并驱动同种异体反应性T细胞分化成Th1和Th17表型，同时抑制IL-6和IL-17恢复移植物的存活[37-39]。这些数据表明,这些先天受体感受到损伤或感染可以塑造同种异体移植T细胞的同种异体反应类型，并通过不同的效应机制促进T细胞依赖性排斥[40,41]。目前,科学家正在考虑将这些炎症途径作为新的治疗靶点来辅助产生移植耐受。

TLR并不是可以感受损伤和病原体的唯一受体。另一种类型的膜结合受体——C型凝集素受体(CLR)可以吸引真菌和细菌PAMP并触发炎症细胞因子如TNF和IL-6的产生。迄今描述的其他受体都是细胞溶质的并且包括能感知各种PAMP、颗粒物质、晶体和其他无菌炎症因子的NOD样受体(NLR),以诱导炎性小体或炎症细胞因子下游的IL-1产生，以及感知RNA的RIG-I样受体(RLR)和感知DNA的受体,两者都能触发Ⅰ型IFN产生(和一些DNA-感受体的IL-1)。这些受体对同种免疫的影响仍有待确定,但可能的是,濒死的供体细胞将触发好几种这些途径，从而增强同种异体反应性。

移植后,T细胞将在哪里致敏?

移植物中的供体实质细胞全部表达MHCⅠ类,因此可以被具有直接同种异体反应性的宿主CD8⁺ T细胞识别。内皮和一些暴露于缺血和再灌注应激的上皮细胞可上调MHC Ⅱ类分子,因此可被具有直接同种异体反应性的宿主CD4⁺ T细胞识别。然而,与同样表达MHC Ⅱ类分子的专职APC（例如活化的树突细胞、巨噬细胞和B细胞)不同,大多数实质细胞不表达共刺激配体,因此不能活化T细胞,因为T细胞,特别是在它们的初始状态下，需要在TCR连接时共刺激受体如CD28的参与才能够产生免疫应答。因此,大多数具有直接同种异体反应性的T细胞的激活被认为最初是由移植物携带的供体APC所触发,并且通常称为载客白细胞。Lafferty和同事在20世纪70年代进行的研究表明，通过体外培养从供体组织中消除人白细胞显著降低了其免疫原性[42]。已知供体APC移植到引流的外周淋巴器官、脾脏和淋巴结中,由T细胞巡查以寻找其同源抗原。此外，接受濒死的供体细胞或膜的受体APC也迁移到外周淋巴器官以间接或半间接地呈递同种异体抗原。然而,如前所述,直接识别同种异体抗原的T细胞的前体频率高于具有间接同种异体识别的T细胞的前体频率,使得人们认为移植后通过供体APC直接活化同种异体反应性T细胞被认为是移植后T细胞活化的主要途径。由于供体APC的半衰期短,所以间接途径的同种异体识别随时间变得更占优势，因此可能在急性排斥和慢性排斥的后期发作中起作用。通过使用导致淋巴结发生的遗传突变小鼠（Aly/Aly小鼠)进行外科脾切除术(见第14章)证明了外周淋巴器官对同种异体反应性T细胞引发和移植物排斥是必需的。Aly/Aly小鼠不能排斥同种异体皮肤移植,而缺乏淋巴结和脾的小鼠不能排斥血管化心脏移植[43,44]。有趣的是,淋巴结似乎是协同刺激阻断疗法诱导移植耐受所必需的[45],表明T细胞活化可以在引发部位中止,并具有长期的后果。

重要的是,移植幼稚的T细胞到脾切除的Aly/Aly小鼠必须需要外周淋巴器官，而移植记忆T细胞转移会导致回忆反应，因为它们的增殖和排斥无须淋巴结和脾[46]。记忆细胞的这种性质增强了它们的免疫抑制挑战，因为它们可能在直接进入移植物之前就已造成损伤，比之前更难以抑制。

效应阶段的同种异体反应：T细胞到移植物

一旦启动，初始T细胞便开始增殖、分化和获得效应器功能。它们在淋巴结的出口受鞘氨醇-1磷酸(S1P)受体调节，并且药物FTY720介导的S1P1激动活性已经在实验中显示可以捕获胸腺、淋巴结和派伊尔淋巴结中的淋巴细胞[47]，尽管在试验剂量下使用FTY720并没有显示免疫抑制功效。一旦进入循环中，效应T细胞被认为响应于趋化因子梯度而进入炎症组织，尽管当趋化因子信号传导被阻断时，移植物浸润和急性排斥仍然可能发生，并且将T细胞募集到特定移植器官的确切趋化因子或产生这些趋化因子的细胞还不明确[48]。在缺血再灌注后浸润同种异体移植物的中性粒细胞已显示可促进CD8+ T细胞募集到同种异体移植物中，并且多形核细胞的耗竭可与刺激阻断治疗协同作用以预防小鼠心脏同种异体移植物的排斥[49]，提示减少急性移植物浸润的一种途径。

在考虑效应T细胞是如何识别移植部位的同种异体抗原和触发移植损伤时（图5.3），需要分别考虑CD4+和CD8+ T细胞直接与间接同种异体识别。具有直接同种异体识别的CD8+ T细胞应当能够在所有成核移植细胞上使用同种异体抗原，因为它们都表达MHC Ⅰ类。已经证实CD8+ T细胞可以被同种异体内皮细胞活化，并且供体MHC Ⅰ类仅存在于小鼠的非造血细胞时，心脏移植物可被排斥[50]。这些结果表明，脉管系统中同种异体抗原的识别对于CD8+ T细胞直接进入移植物以及随后杀死实质细胞是必需的，或者CD8+ T细

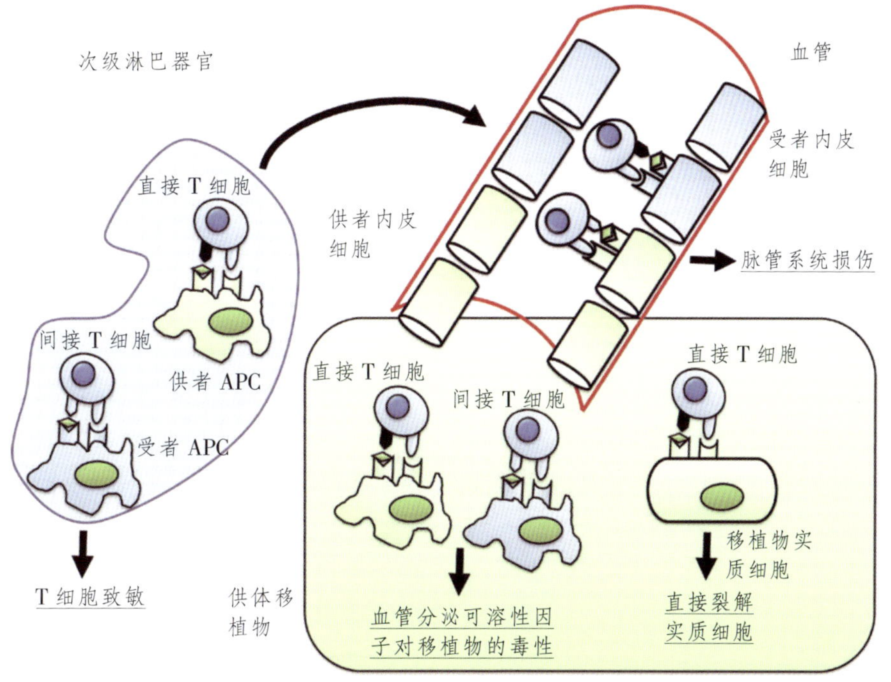

图5.3　T细胞介导的同种异体移植排斥的机制。具有直接和间接同种异体反应性的T细胞可分别由供体和受体APC中在次级淋巴器官中引发。一旦活化，这些T细胞增殖、分化，获得效应子功能，并通过传出淋巴管迁移至血流。在到达移植物后，同种异体反应性T细胞可以识别在移植物中呈递外源肽或供体内皮细胞的受体内皮细胞，并且可以介导对脉管系统的损害，因此损害器官。同种异体抗原在内皮细胞上的识别也可以促进其募集或进入同种异体移植物。浸润移植物的T细胞可识别供体或受体APC呈递肽。这可能导致T细胞和APC的活化以分泌可能损伤移植物的炎性因子。或者，具有直接同种异体反应性的T细胞还可识别实质细胞并通过Fas信号传导或穿孔素和颗粒酶细胞毒性导致其死亡。在一些情况下，CD4+ T细胞或CD8+ T细胞可以独立地足以排斥移植物；在其他情况下，活化的CD4+ T细胞可以帮助活化的CD8+ T细胞发展其效应子功能。在稳定的同种异体移植中，内皮和实质细胞可能不再表达共刺激配体，并且它们的相遇可能导致T细胞死亡或失活以延续耐受性，而不是T细胞活化和排斥发作。具有直接和间接特异性的Treg也可以在第二淋巴器官中的引发阶段和移植物中的效应阶段起到抑制同种异体反应的作用。

胞可以损伤血管内皮细胞，导致由营养物剥夺引起的下游移植物损伤或血栓栓塞事件。

MHC Ⅱ类的表达比 MHC Ⅰ类的表达更受限制，仅有树突状细胞、巨噬细胞、B 细胞、活化的内皮细胞和一些上皮细胞表达它。因此，具有直接识别同种异体能力的 $CD4^+$ T 细胞在移植物中获得同种异体抗原应当更有限。对于小鼠，在心脏同种异体移植物中，供体 MHC Ⅱ类的表达已经足够用于 CD4 介导的排斥，无须宿主 MHC Ⅱ类分子参与[51]。此外，供体造血细胞上的Ⅱ类比内皮细胞更重要[52]。不完全清楚的是，移植物中供体造血细胞的集结是如何促使 $CD4^+$ T 细胞移植物排斥的，原本认为 T 细胞可以激活供体 APC 以产生对移植物中的实质细胞有毒性的炎症因子。一旦供体 APC 离开移植物，因协同刺激不同，$CD4^+$ T 细胞与Ⅱ类分子实质细胞的相互作用可能会导致它们失活或死亡，或转变为 Th2 表型。事实上，在移植后直接途径的反应性 T 细胞的频率随时间降低[4]。

T 细胞与间接同种异体识别也可以在同种异体移植排斥中发挥作用。对于具有间接异源性的 $CD8^+$ T 细胞被激活，它们需要遇到宿主细胞呈递衍生自供体 MHC 或其他多态性蛋白质的肽，其可能通过吞噬供体细胞的吞噬作用获得，供体蛋白逃避内体进入胞质 TAP /内质网状/自身 MHC Ⅰ类途径。内皮细胞能够以这种方式交叉呈递供体抗原[53]。已经使用对由宿主MHC Ⅰ类($H-2^b$)呈递的并且不能识别供体 MHC($H-2^k$)的雄性抗原特异性的 TCR 转基因 $CD8^+$ T 细胞揭示间接 $CD8^+$细胞在同种异体中的致病作用的证据。只有当血管系统表达自体 MHC 分子时[54]，这些 T 细胞以不依赖于 IFN-γ 的方式显示排斥供体皮肤移植。然而，间接 $CD8^+$ T 细胞在完全错配的心脏同种异体移植模型中没有影响[55]，因此当直接识别途径也正在运作时，这种途径的影响受到质疑。

间接识别 $CD4^+$ T 细胞的作用已通过使用对由宿主 MHC Ⅱ类分子呈递的雄性抗原特异性的 TCR 转基因 T 细胞得到了解决。通过使用来自具有不能将抗原呈递给转基因 $CD4^+$ T 细胞的不同 MHC 等位基因的雄性小鼠的心脏同种异体移植物，人们发现逐渐替代移植物中的供体内皮细胞的宿主内皮细胞，可以激活间接 $CD4^+$ T 细胞诱导移植物血管病变和慢性排斥反应[56]。总的来说，所有这些研究均强调内皮细胞的重要免疫功能，如 APC 或作为效应 T 细胞的靶标。内皮细胞还可以作为同种异体抗体和固有免疫细胞的靶标，使其成为急性和慢性排斥的中心参与者，在未来的研究中值得特别关注[57]。B 细胞对于间接启动 $CD4^+$ T 细胞也很重要，因为限制于 B 细胞区室的 MHC Ⅱ类缺乏可以导致同种异体反应性 $CD4^+$ T 细胞的活化减少，进而减少同种异体抗体的产生并延长同种异体心脏移植的小鼠存活[58]。

Treg 的 TCR 也可以与同种异体抗原具有直接和间接反应性，但是已经显示具有间接特异性的 Treg 在体内具有更大的抑制同种异体反应的能力[59]。有趣的是，Treg 在同种异体反应中的抑制功能已经显示出依赖于由 Treg 产生的 IFN-γ[60]，这与先前报道的 IFN-γ 依赖性信号转导的移植耐受性相一致[61]。因此，IFN-γ 可以是双刃细胞因子，在 Th1/Tc1 细胞的发病机制中很重要，但在 Treg 的免疫抑制功能中也很重要。在稳定的肾移植患者中已经证实了 Treg 对间接同种异体反应的主要抑制作用，因为 PBMC 中 Treg 的消耗会导致增强的 HLA-DR 特异性肽的 IFN-γ 产生[62]。Treg 抑制间接同种异体反应的能力将它们良好地定位于控制慢性排斥，其可能更多地依赖于在客体白细胞死亡之后间接呈递同种异体抗原。事实上，据报道，在含有发炎性纤维化的肾移植患者活检中存在更多数量的 Treg 与更好的同种异体移植物存活相关[63]。此外，具有间接特异性的 Treg 已经在大鼠中显示可抑制同种异体抗体在体内生产[64]，已知其有助于慢性排斥。

在移植后 Treg 生物学中另一个重要的考虑因素是它们是否能抑制外周淋巴器官中的 T 细胞启动和同种异体移植中的效应 T 细胞应答。研究表明，Treg 可以从血液中迁移到发炎的同种异体胰岛移植物，然后返回引流淋巴结，并防止树突状细胞迁移到外周淋巴器官[65]。因此，Treg 可以减少初始同种异体反应性，T 细胞启动和帮助诱导免疫耐受。此外，已显示在共刺激阻断后，Treg 在同种异体移植物中累积，并且近来研究表明，其在移植位点的持续抑制对于感染性移植耐受是必需的，所谓感染性移植耐受是指新效应 T 细胞的同源抗原是由 APC 表达的而 APC 也存在于现有 Tregs 中，那么新的效应 T 细胞就会变成 iTregs。当然，这些 APC 也能将同源抗原提呈给现有的 Treg[66,67]。这些数据表明 Treg 也参与维持移植耐受。

效应 T 细胞：Th1、Th2、Th17 和细胞毒性 T 细胞

不同器官的排斥提示有不同的 T 细胞亚群参与，至少在鼠模型中是这样的(见第 14 章)。值得注意的一个有趣的现象是：虽然在移植心脏排斥反应中浸润的 T 细胞大多数是 $CD8^+$ T 细胞，但是心脏同种异体移植排斥可以在无 $CD8^+$ T 细胞而仅有 $CD4^+$ T 细胞的情况下发生，这表明Ⅱ类分子在移植物中表达已经足以使 $CD4^+$ T 细胞介导排斥，并且提示除细胞溶解外可能有其他替代性排斥机制，因为许多 $CD4^+$ T 细胞不含有细胞毒性颗粒。然而，当 $CD4^+$ T 细胞应答的强度降低时，例如在 CD28 缺陷的小鼠中，急性排斥变得依赖于 $CD4^+$和 $CD8^+$ T 细胞，强调 $CD8^+$ T 细胞参与的重要性，特别是在免疫抑制条件下[68]。

据报道，胰腺胰岛的排斥依赖于 $CD4^+$或 $CD8^+$ T 细胞，这取决于所使用的菌株组合。类似地，$CD4^+$或 $CD8^+$ T 细胞足以驱动皮肤和肠同种异体移植排斥。原因可能是强烈激活了 $CD8^+$ T 细胞，与朗格汉斯细胞一样，消除了它们对 $CD4^+$ T 细胞辅助其激活的需要。然而，$CD4^+$ T 细胞的帮助可能是记忆 $CD8^+$ T 细胞产生同种异体反应所必需的[69]。

不同的效应细胞表型，如 Th1、Th2 和 Th17，在同种异体移植排斥反应中的相对重要性仍然是一个争论的焦点。IFN-γ 的产生最常与同种异体移植排斥相关，T-bet 是 Th1/Tc1 细胞的标志性转录因子，可在来自接受急性排斥的肾移植受体的活检中检测到[70]。然而，缺乏 IFN-γ 的小鼠在同种异体移植物排斥中没有受损，反而在同种异体移植物中出现耐受[61,71,72]，且在缺乏 STAT4 (IL-12 下游的转录因子）的小鼠中，Th1 分化是有缺陷的，也不会发生同种异体移植的排斥[73,74]。相反的，有报道称，在没有排斥反应的患者血清中检测到高浓度的 IFN-γ[75]。重要的是，除了 Th1/Tc1 细胞外，IFN-γ 和 T-bet 也可以由许多其他类型细胞表达，例如 NK 细胞、Treg 甚至树突状细胞，这使得即使在混合淋巴细胞反应中检测该细胞因子，也不一定就等同于 Th1 同种异体反应。

鉴于最近的发现，Th17 细胞在许多病理过程中得到仔细探究，移植排斥也不例外。已经在经历急性或慢性排斥的许多同种异体移植物中鉴定出了 IL-17 表达，并且在肾脏的尿沉渣中发现了 IL-17mRNA[63,76-79]。最初显示，阻断 IL-17 可延长大鼠心脏同种异体移植物的存活率[80]。在小鼠模型中，Th17/Tc17 细胞的致病作用主要在缺乏 T-bet 的动物中得到证明，所述动物在一种模型中以 Tc17 依赖性方式对协同刺激阻断疗法诱导移植耐受产生抗性，或者发展成 Th17 依赖的加速血管病变模型[81,82]。在野生型小鼠中，TLR 激动剂在移植时的信号传导也显示增加 IL-6 产生和加重 IL-6/IL-17 依赖的同种异体移植物排斥[38]。这与对被感染的凋亡细胞的吞噬作用相一致，即通过摄取凋亡物质产生 TGF-β 并通过刺激 TLR 产生 IL-6，这是 Th17 细胞在体内可能不同的临床情况[83]。另外，已报道移植损伤后自体抗原(例如胶原 V 或微管蛋白)的暴露导致在动物和人类同种异体移植物上具有病理学后果的自身免疫 Th17 细胞[84-88]。重要的是，一些 T 细胞可以共同产生 IFN-γ 和 IL-17，并且可以构成特别致病的 T 细胞亚群。值得注意的是，终末分化为效应 Th 和 Tc 表型可能不像最初认为的那样，并且细胞可以保留多能性和可塑性以根据环境转化为其他表型[89]，重要的是在移植受者体内监测 T 细胞功能，因为 T 细胞会随时间调整免疫抑制策略，进而改变同种异体的反应性。

记忆 $CD8^+$ T 细胞是进入同种异体移植物和启动移植物排斥的第一种细胞[90]，使得这条重要通路被抑制。效应物和记忆 $CD8^+$ T 细胞在同种异体移植排斥中的致病作用最常归因于其产生 IFN-γ 和通过其穿孔素和含颗粒酶的颗粒或通过 FasL(CD95L)上调裂解靶细胞的能力，其可以通过集结靶细胞上促凋亡分子 Fas (CD95)来杀死靶细胞[91,92]。在小鼠中，已经显示 FasL 和穿孔素对移植的胰岛发挥急性排斥是足够而且必然的[93]，其中 $CD8^+$ T 细胞自身分泌的 IFN-γ 也是急性排斥发生的关键因素[94]。穿孔素和颗粒酶在慢性排斥反应中也很重要，敲除了的小鼠显示内皮细胞凋亡减少和随后的同种异体移植血管病变减少[95,96]。重要的是，Treg 也表达粒酶 B，并通过裂解 $CD4^+$ T 细胞而发挥其抑制功能[97]。与这一观察一致的是，在 $Foxp3^+$细胞中颗粒酶 B 的表达对于在小鼠中诱导皮肤同种异体移植物耐受是必需的[98]，提示效应途径可以具有相反的结果，这取决于它们表达在何种细胞内。

治疗应用

由于同种异体移植排斥是绝对 T 细胞依赖性的，

免疫抑制策略集中在预防T细胞反应上。靶向的途径将在第17章中深入讨论。大多数现有的免疫抑制剂，如钙调神经磷酸酶抑制剂或DNA合成抑制剂，都试图降低T细胞活化和增殖，并且不诱导移植耐受。诱导耐受性的实验目的在于删除同种异体反应性T细胞（使用消耗性抗体，照射或基因编辑[99]），或者内在（通过共刺激阻断或使用致耐受性APC的免疫治疗）或外在地诱导其失活（增强Treg，骨髓衍生的抑制细胞，间充质干细胞或其他细胞的抑制能力）[99,100]。有趣的是，mTOR抑制可以促进iTreg分化，同时阻止Th1、Th2和Th17细胞的分化[101]，使得西罗莫司在移植中成为一种有吸引力的药物，虽然它也被证明可低剂量促进记忆$CD8^+$ T细胞反应[102,103]。因为T细胞的缺失可以矛盾地促进残余T细胞的增殖以填充空间，并且获得记忆细胞特征（即抵抗诱导免疫耐受）[104]，因此，部分缺失与诱导无能的组合和（或）抑制残留T细胞可能是更合理的诱导耐受的方法。

总结

T细胞及其生物学特性仍然是移植生物学的核心，并且对涉及T细胞介导的同种异体识别机制的了解仍然是临床移植实践的基础。T细胞的功能性作用使其成为所有急性细胞同种异体移植排斥的基本临床综合征，并且也是大多数抗体介导的排斥形式的核心。鉴于T细胞在保护性免疫中发挥的关键作用，这一生物学特性也会继续影响移植受者长期管理的感染和恶性并发症。

致谢

感谢米歇尔·米勒对本章的批判性阅读和编辑。MLA的移植免疫学研究由R01 AI052352和AI071080资助支持。

（胡士华 译 王思奇 程倩 校）

参考文献

1. Germain RN, Stefanova I, Dorfman J. Self-recognition and the regulation of $CD4^+$ T cell survival. Advances in Experimental Medicine and Biology. 2002;512:97–105.
2. Suchin EJ, Langmuir PB, Palmer E, et al. Quantifying the frequency of alloreactive T cells *in vivo*: new answers to an old question. Journal of Immunology. 2001;166:973–981.
3. Felix NJ, Allen PM. Specificity of T-cell alloreactivity. Nature Reviews Immunology. 2007;7:942–953.
4. Safinia N, Afzali B, Atalar K, et al. T-cell alloimmunity and chronic allograft dysfunction. Kidney International Supplement. 2010;78:S2–12.
5. Paludan C, Schmid D, Landthaler M, et al. Endogenous MHC class II processing of a viral nuclear antigen after autophagy. Science. 2005;307:593–596.
6. Zhou D, Li P, Lin Y, et al. Lamp-2a facilitates MHC class II presentation of cytoplasmic antigens. Immunity. 2005;22:571–581.
7. Ackerman AL, Giodini A, Cresswell P. A role for the endoplasmic reticulum protein retrotranslocation machinery during crosspresentation by dendritic cells. Immunity. 2006;25:607–617.
8. Gras S, Kjer-Nielsen L, Chen Z, et al. The structural bases of direct T-cell allorecognition: implications for T-cell-mediated transplant rejection. Immunology and Cell Biology. 2011;89:388–395.
9. Morris GP, Ni PP, Allen PM. Alloreactivity is limited by the endogenous peptide repertoire. Proceedings of the National Academy of Sciences of the United States of America. 2011;108:3695–3700.
10. Morris GP, Allen PM. Cutting edge: highly alloreactive dual TCR T cells play a dominant role in graft-versus-host disease. Journal of Immunology. 2009;182:6639–6643.
11. Li XC, Rothstein DM, Sayegh MH. Costimulatory pathways in transplantation: challenges and new developments. Immunological Reviews. 2009;229:271–293.
12. Yeung MY, McGrath M, Najafian N. The emerging role of the TIM molecules in transplantation. American Journal of Transplantation. 2012, 2011;11:2019.
13. Atalar K, Afzali B, Lord G, et al. Relative roles of Th1 and Th17 effector cells in allograft rejection. Current Opinion in Organ Transplantation. 2009;14:23–29.
14. Tay SS, Plain KM, Bishop GA. Role of IL-4 and Th2 responses in allograft rejection and tolerance. Current Opinion in Organ Transplantation. 2009;14:16–22.
15. Valujskikh A, Li XC. Memory T cells and their exhaustive differentiation in allograft tolerance and rejection. Current Opinion in Organ Transplantation. 2011;19:19.
16. Macedo C, Orkis EA, Popescu I, et al. Contribution of naive and memory T-cell populations to the human alloimmune response. American Journal of Transplantation. 2009;9:2057–2066.
17. Wieckiewicz J, Goto R, Wood KJ. T regulatory cells and the control of alloimmunity: from characterisation to clinical application. Current Opinion in Immunology. 2010;22:662–668.
18. Haribhai D, Williams JB, Jia S, et al. A requisite role for induced regulatory T cells in tolerance based on expanding antigen receptor diversity. Immunity. 2011;35:109–122.
19. Ochando JC, Homma C, Yang Y, et al. Alloantigen-presenting plasmacytoid dendritic cells mediate tolerance to vascularized grafts. Nature Immunology. 2006;7:652–662.
20. Fan Z, Spencer JA, Lu Y, et al. *In vivo* tracking of 'color-coded' effector, natural and induced regulatory T cells in the allograft response. Nature Medicine. 2010;16:718–722.
21. Thornton AM, Korty PE, Tran DQ, et al. Expression of Helios, an Ikaros transcription factor family member, differentiates thymic-derived from peripherally induced Foxp3+ T regulatory cells. Journal of Immunology. 2010;184:3433–3441.
22. Floess S, Freyer J, Siewert C, et al. Epigenetic control of the Foxp3 locus in regulatory T cells. PLoS Biology. 2007;5:e38.
23. Lal G, Zhang N, van der Touw W, et al. Epigenetic regulation of Foxp3 expression in regulatory T cells by DNA methylation. Journal of Immunology. 2009;182:259–273.
24. Schlieer U, Streitz M, Sawitzki B. Tregs: application for solid-organ transplantation. Current Opinion in Organ Transplantation. 2011;1:1.
25. Alegre ML, Chong AS. Toll-like receptors (TLRs) in transplantation. Frontiers in Bioscience. 2009;1:36–43.
26. Alegre ML, Leemans J, Le Moine A, et al. The multiple facets of toll-like receptors in transplantation biology. Transplantation. 2008;86:1–9.
27. Rock KL, Latz E, Ontiveros F, et al. The sterile inflammatory response. Annual Review of Immunology. 2010;28:321–342.
28. Shen H, Song Y, Colangelo CM, et al. Haptoglobin activates innate immunity to enhance acute transplant rejection in mice. Journal of Clinical Investigation. 2012;122:383–387.
29. Gelman AE, LaRosa DF, Zhang J, et al. The adaptor molecule MyD88 activates PI-3 kinase signaling in $CD4^+$ T cells and enables CpG oligodeoxynucleotide-mediated costimulation. Immunity. 2006;25:783–793.
30. Crellin NK, Garcia RV, Hadisfar O, et al. Human $CD4^+$ T cells express TLR5 and its ligand flagellin enhances the suppressive capacity and expression of FOXP3 in $CD4^+CD25^+$ T regulatory cells. Journal of Immunology. 2005;175:8051–8059.
31. Dai J, Liu B, Ngoi SM, et al. TLR4 hyperresponsiveness via cell surface expression

of heat shock protein gp96 potentiates suppressive function of regulatory T cells. Journal of Immunology. 2007;178:3219–3225.
32. Caramalho I, Lopes-Carvalho T, Ostler D, et al. Regulatory T cells selectively express toll-like receptors and are activated by lipopolysaccharide. Journal of Experimental Medicine. 2003;197:403–411.
33. Peng G, Guo Z, Kiniwa Y, et al. Toll-like receptor 8-mediated reversal of $CD4^+$ regulatory T cell function. Science. 2005;309:1380–1384.
34. Sutmuller RP, den Brok MH, Kramer M, et al. Toll-like receptor 2 controls expansion and function of regulatory T cells. Journal of Clinical Investigation. 2006;19:19.
35. Oberg HH, Juricke M, Kabelitz D, et al. Regulation of T cell activation by TLR ligands. European Journal of Cell Biology. 2011;90:582–592.
36. Lal G, Yin N, Xu J, et al. Distinct inflammatory signals have physiologically divergent effects on epigenetic regulation of Foxp3 expression and Treg function. American Journal of Transplantation. 2011;11:203–214.
37. Porrett PM, Yuan X, LaRosa DF, et al. Mechanisms underlying blockade of allograft acceptance by TLR ligands. Journal of Immunology. 2008;181:1692–1699.
38. Chen L, Ahmed E, Wang T, et al. TLR signals promote IL-6/IL-17-dependent transplant rejection. Journal of Immunology. 2009;182:6217–6225.
39. Chen L, Wang T, Zhou P, et al. TLR engagement prevents transplantation tolerance. American Journal of Transplantation. 2006;6:2282–2291.
40. Alegre ML, Goldstein DR, Chong AS. TLR signaling in transplantation. Current Opinions in Organ Transplantation. 2009;13:358–365.
41. Ahmed EB, Daniels M, Alegre ML, et al. Bacterial infections, alloimmunity, and transplantation tolerance. Transplantation Reviews. 2011;25:27–35.
42. Lafferty KJ, Prowse SJ, Simeonovic CJ, et al. Immunobiology of tissue transplantation: a return to the passenger leukocyte concept. Annual Review of Immunology. 1983;1:143–173.
43. Lakkis FG, Arakelov A, Konieczny BT, et al. Immunologic 'ignorance' of vascularized organ transplants in the absence of secondary lymphoid tissue. Nature Medicine. 2000;6:686–688.
44. Ng YH, Chalasani G. Role of secondary lymphoid tissues in primary and memory T-cell responses to a transplanted organ. Transplantation Reviews (Orlando, Fla.). 2010;24:32–41.
45. Ochando JC, Yopp AC, Yang Y, et al. Lymph node occupancy is required for the peripheral development of alloantigen-specific $Foxp3^+$ regulatory T cells. Journal of Immunology. 2005;174:6993–7005.
46. Chalasani G, Dai Z, Konieczny BT, et al. Recall and propagation of allospecific memory T cells independent of secondary lymphoid organs. Proceedings of the National Academy of Sciences of the United States of America. 2002;99: 6175–6180.
47. Rosen H, Sanna G, Alfonso C. Egress: a receptor-regulated step in lymphocyte trafficking. Immunological Reviews. 2003;195:160–177.
48. Schenk AD, Rosenblum JM, Fairchild RL. Chemokine-directed strategies to attenuate allograft rejection. Clinics in Laboratory Medicine. 2008;28:441–454, vii.
49. El-Sawy T, Belperio JA, Strieter RM, et al. Inhibition of polymorphonuclear leukocyte-mediated graft damage synergizes with short-term costimulatory blockade to prevent cardiac allograft rejection. Circulation. 2005;112:320–331.
50. Kreisel D, Krupnick AS, Gelman AE, et al. Non-hematopoietic allograft cells directly activate $CD8^+$ T cells and trigger acute rejection: an alternative mechanism of allorecognition. Nature Medicine. 2002;8:233–239.
51. Pietra BA, Wiseman A, Bolwerk A, et al. CD4 T cell-mediated cardiac allograft rejection requires donor but not host MHC class II. Journal of Clinical Investigation. 2000;106:1003–1010.
52. Kreisel D, Krasinskas AM, Krupnick AS, et al. Vascular endothelium does not activate $CD4^+$ direct allorecognition in graft rejection. Journal of Immunology. 2004;173:3027–3034.
53. Bagai R, Valujskikh A, Canaday DH, et al. Mouse endothelial cells cross-present lymphocyte-derived antigen on class I MHC via a TAP1- and proteasome-dependent pathway. Journal of Immunology. 2005;174:7711–7715.
54. Valujskikh A, Lantz O, Celli S, et al. Cross-primed $CD8(^+)$ T cells mediate graft rejection via a distinct effector pathway. Nature Immunology. 2002;3:844–851.
55. Valujskikh A, Zhang Q, Heeger PS. CD8 T cells specific for a donor-derived, self-restricted transplant antigen are nonpathogenic bystanders after vascularized heart transplantation in mice. Journal of Immunology. 2006;176:2190–2196.
56. Kapessidou Y, Habran C, Buonocore S, et al. The replacement of graft endothelium by recipient-type cells conditions allograft rejection mediated by indirect pathway $CD4^+$ T cells. Transplantation. 2006;82:582–591.
57. Taflin C, Charron D, Glotz D, et al. Immunological function of the endothelial cell within the setting of organ transplantation. Immunology Letters. 2011; 139:1–6.
58. Noorchashm H, Reed AJ, Rostami SY, et al. B cell-mediated antigen presentation is required for the pathogenesis of acute cardiac allograft rejection. Journal of Immunology. 2006;177:7715–7722.
59. Sanchez-Fueyo A, Domenig CM, Mariat C, et al. Influence of direct and indirect allorecognition pathways on $CD4^+CD25^+$ regulatory T-cell function in transplantation. Transplant International. 2007;20:534–541.
60. Sawitzki B, Kingsley CI, Oliveira V, et al. IFN-gamma production by alloantigen-reactive regulatory T cells is important for their regulatory function in vivo. Journal of Experimental Medicine. 2005;201:1925–1935.
61. Konieczny BT, Dai Z, Elwood ET, et al. IFN-gamma is critical for long-term allograft survival induced by blocking the CD28 and CD40 ligand T cell costimulation pathways. Journal of Immunology. 1998;160:2059–2064.
62. Salama AD, Najafian N, Clarkson MR, et al. Regulatory $CD25^+$ T cells in human kidney transplant recipients. Journal of the American Society of Nephrology. 2003;14:1643–1651.
63. Zuber J, Brodin-Sartorius A, Lapidus N, et al. FOXP3-enriched infiltrates associated with better outcome in renal allografts with inflamed fibrosis. Nephrology, Dialysis, Transplantation. 2009;24:3847–3854.
64. Callaghan CJ, Rouhani FJ, Negus MC, et al. Abrogation of antibody-mediated allograft rejection by regulatory CD4 T cells with indirect allospecificity. Journal of Immunology. 2007;178:2221–2228.
65. Zhang N, Schröppel B, Lal G, et al. Regulatory T cells sequentially migrate from inflamed tissues to draining lymph nodes to suppress the alloimmune response. Immunity. 2009;30:458–469.
66. Lee I, Wang L, Wells AD, et al. Recruitment of $Foxp3^+$ T regulatory cells mediating allograft tolerance depends on the CCR4 chemokine receptor. Journal of Experimental Medicine. 2005;201:1037–1044.
67. Kendal AR, Chen Y, Regateiro FS, et al. Sustained suppression by $Foxp3^+$ regulatory T cells is vital for infectious transplantation tolerance. Journal of Experimental Medicine. 2011;208:2043–2053.
68. Szot GL, Zhou P, Rulifson I, et al. Different mechanisms of cardiac allograft rejection in wildtype and CD28-deficient mice. American Journal of Transplantation. 2001;1:38–46.
69. Zhai Y, Wang Y, Wu Z, et al. Defective alloreactive CD8 T cell function and memory response in allograft recipients in the absence of CD4 help. Journal of Immunology. 2007;179:4529–4534.
70. Hoffmann SC, Hale DA, Kleiner DE, et al. Functionally significant renal allograft rejection is defined by transcriptional criteria. American Journal of Transplantation. 2005;5:573–581.
71. Saleem S, Konieczny BT, Lowry RP, et al. Acute rejection of vascularized heart allografts in the absence of IFNgamma. Transplantation. 1996;62:1908–1911.
72. Miura M, El-Sawy T, Fairchild RL. Neutrophils mediate parenchymal tissue necrosis and accelerate the rejection of complete major histocompatibility complex-disparate cardiac allografts in the absence of interferon-gamma. American Journal of Pathology. 2003;162:509–519.
73. Koglin J, Glysing-Jensen T, Gadiraju S, et al. Attenuated cardiac allograft vasculopathy in mice with targeted deletion of the transcription factor STAT4. Circulation. 2000;101:1034–1039.
74. Zhou P, Szot GL, Guo Z, et al. Role of STAT4 and STAT6 signaling in allograft rejection and CTLA4-Ig-mediated tolerance. Journal of Immunology. 2000; 165:5580–5587.
75. Daniel V, Naujokat C, Sadeghi M, et al. Association of high IFN-gamma plasma levels with low B-cell counts in renal transplant recipients with stable long-term graft function. Clinical Transplantation. 2010;24:281–289.
76. Antonysamy MA, Fanslow WC, Fu F, et al. Evidence for a role of IL-17 in organ allograft rejection: IL-17 promotes the functional differentiation of dendritic cell progenitors. Journal of Immunology. 1999;162:577–584.
77. Hsieh HG, Loong CC, Lui WY, et al. IL-17 expression as a possible predictive parameter for subclinical renal allograft rejection. Transplant International. 2001;14:287–298.
78. Loong CC, Hsieh HG, Lui WY, et al. Evidence for the early involvement of interleukin 17 in human and experimental renal allograft rejection. Journal of Pathology. 2002;197:322–332.
79. Van Kooten C, Boonstra JG, Paape ME, et al. Interleukin-17 activates human renal epithelial cells *in vitro* and is expressed during renal allograft rejection. Journal of the American Society of Nephrology. 1998;9:1526–1534.
80. Tang JL, Subbotin VM, Antonysamy MA, et al. Interleukin-17 antagonism inhibits acute but not chronic vascular rejection. Transplantation. 2001;72:348–350.
81. Burrell BE, Csencsits K, Lu G, et al. $CD8^+$ Th17 mediate costimulation blockade-resistant allograft rejection in T-bet-deficient mice. Journal of Immunology. 2008;181:3906–3914.
82. Yuan X, Paez-Cortez J, Schmitt-Knosalla I, et al. A novel role of CD4 Th17 cells in mediating cardiac allograft rejection and vasculopathy. Journal of Experimental Medicine. 2008;205:3133–3144.
83. Torchinsky MB, Garaude J, Martin AP, et al. Innate immune recognition of infected apoptotic cells directs T(H)17 cell differentiation. Nature. 2009; 458:78–82.
84. Yoshida S, Haque A, Mizobuchi T, et al. Anti-type V collagen lymphocytes that

express IL-17 and IL-23 induce rejection pathology in fresh and well-healed lung transplants. American Journal of Transplantation. 2006;6:724–735.

85. Bharat A, Narayanan K, Street T, et al. Early posttransplant inflammation promotes the development of alloimmunity and chronic human lung allograft rejection. Transplantation. 2007;83:150–158.
86. Burlingham WJ, Love RB, Jankowska-Gan E, et al. IL-17-dependent cellular immunity to collagen type V predisposes to obliterative bronchiolitis in human lung transplants. Journal of Clinical Investigation. 2007;117:3498–3506.
87. Bobadilla JL, Love RB, Jankowska-Gan E, et al. Th-17, monokines, collagen type V, and primary graft dysfunction in lung transplantation. American Journal of Respiratory and Critical Care Medicine. 2008;177:660–668.
88. Saini D, Weber J, Ramachandran S, et al. Alloimmunity-induced autoimmunity as a potential mechanism in the pathogenesis of chronic rejection of human lung allografts. Journal of Heart and Lung Transplantation. 2011;30:624–631.
89. Ashoor IF, Najafian N. Rejection and regulation: a tight balance. Current Opinion in Organ Transplantation. 2011;9:9.
90. Schenk AD, Nozaki T, Rabant M, et al. Donor-reactive CD8 memory T cells infiltrate cardiac allografts within 24-h posttransplant in naive recipients. American Journal of Transplantation. 2008;8:1652–1661.
91. Clayberger C. Cytolytic molecules in rejection. Current Opinion in Organ Transplantation. 2009;14:30–33.
92. Choy JC. Granzymes and perforin in solid organ transplant rejection. Cell Death and Differentiation. 2010;17:567–576.
93. Sleater M, Diamond AS, Gill RG. Islet allograft rejection by contact-dependent $CD8^+$ T cells: perforin and FasL play alternate but obligatory roles. American Journal of Transplantation. 2007;7:1927–1933.
94. Diamond AS, Gill RG. An essential contribution by IFN-gamma to $CD8^+$ T cell-mediated rejection of pancreatic islet allografts. Journal of Immunology. 2000;165:247–255.
95. Choy JC, Kerjner A, Wong BW, et al. Perforin mediates endothelial cell death and resultant transplant vascular disease in cardiac allografts. American Journal of Pathology. 2004;165:127–133.
96. Choy JC, Cruz RP, Kerjner A, et al. Granzyme B induces endothelial cell apoptosis and contributes to the development of transplant vascular disease. American Journal of Transplantation. 2005;5:494–499.
97. Gondek DC, Lu LF, Quezada SA, et al. Cutting edge: contact-mediated suppression by $CD4^+CD25^+$ regulatory cells involves a granzyme B-dependent, perforin-independent mechanism. Journal of Immunology. 2005;174:1783–1786.
98. Gondek DC, Devries V, Nowak EC, et al. Transplantation survival is maintained by granzyme B^+ regulatory cells and adaptive regulatory T cells. Journal of Immunology. 2008;181:4752–4760.
99. Watson D, Hu M, Zhang GY, et al. Tolerance induction by removal of alloreactive T cells: in-vivo and pruning strategies. Current Opinion in Organ Transplantation. 2009;14:357–363.
100. Morelli AE, Thomson AW. Tolerogenic dendritic cells and the quest for transplant tolerance. Nature Reviews Immunology. 2007;7:610–621.
101. Kole TP, Zheng Y, Delgoffe GM, et al. The mTOR kinase differentially regulates effector and regulatory T cell lineage commitment. Immunity. 2009;30: 832–844.
102. Araki K, Turner AP, Shaffer VO, et al. mTOR regulates memory CD8 T-cell differentiation. Nature. 2009;460:108–112.
103. Powell JD, Delgoffe GM. The mammalian target of rapamycin: linking T cell differentiation, function, and metabolism. Immunity. 2010;33:301–311.
104. Wu Z, Bensinger SJ, Zhang J, et al. Homeostatic proliferation is a barrier to transplantation tolerance. Nature Medicine. 2004;10:87–92.

第 6 章 适应性免疫之体液免疫机制

William M. Baldwin III, Robert L. Fairchild

引言

免疫学的体液机制包括液体相反应物,如抗体、补体、凝血因子和细胞因子,作为适应性免疫应答的一部分。抗体具有抗原特异性受体,而补体和细胞因子是固有免疫系统的抗原非特异性介质。所有这些介质也可以与固有免疫系统的细胞,特别是血小板、粒细胞、单核细胞/巨噬细胞和 NK 细胞接合。这些天然的细胞和体液介质可以放大和修改抗体介导的损伤。结果,体液免疫介质引起的同种异体移植物破坏范围从超急性到急性再到慢性排斥。在本章中,我们将首先分别考虑体液介质,然后讨论抗体和介质与受体和供体细胞之间的相互作用,就是这些相互作用介导了同种异体移植的组织损伤。本章将重点介绍直接涉及移植物破坏的机制,可以在第 2 章中找到关于生理性体液免疫的更多讨论。抗体介导排斥反应的组织学和临床表现见器官特定章节中组织病理学综合征(移植排斥和复发性疾病的组织病理学综合征)和移植排斥的临床诊断和管理(临床同种异体移植排斥综合征:诊断和管理)。

抗体

抗体的结构和功能由多种因素决定,所有因素均随着免疫反应的进行而改变。对同种异体移植物的新抗体应答开始于低水平的 IgM 抗体,随后是数量和质量增加的 IgG 抗体。虽然 IgM 和 IgG 共享免疫球蛋白的基本元件,即与恒定片段(可结晶片段或 Fc)连接的两个抗原结合片段(Fab),但是关键结构的差异产生不同的功能(图 6.1)(见第 2 章)。例如,IgM 抗体的单个 Fab 以低亲和力结合抗原,但是由 IgM 五聚体结构中的 10 个相同的 Fab 产生的组合亲和力高达 10^7 倍。IgM 的五聚体结构还通过将 5 个 Fc 连接在一起而促进补体的活化。

随着免疫应答的进行,抗体从 IgM 切换到 IgG,其通过突变和选择过程致亲和力成熟。这导致 IgG 抗体的 Fab 具有越来越高的亲和力。随着时间进展,单体 IgG 同种抗体的亲和力超过五聚体 IgM 的亲和力。转换到 IgG 给免疫应答带来了几个新的维度。较小的(约 150kD)单体 IgG 比非常大的五聚体 IgM(900kD)更容易穿过毛细血管和静脉屏障,使得几乎一半的 IgG 存在于间质和淋巴区室中。IgG 亚类的进化增加了功能多样性。人类有四个亚类的 IgG,具有不同的 Fc 结构,从而使功能多样化。IgG1 和 IgG3 比 IgG2 能更有效地激活补体,并且 IgG4 不激活补体。类似地,每个亚类对白细胞上的 Fc 受体(FcR)具有不同的结合亲和力。通过由大多数白细胞群体表达的 IgG Fc(FcγR)的多种类型的受体,功能范围进一步增加[1]。相反,一种 IgM 特异性 FcμR 被鉴定,其由 T 和 B 淋巴细胞表达[2]。小鼠和人类的白细胞表达具有不同亲和力并递送刺激或抑制信号的 FcγR 家族。小鼠和人类都具有一个高亲和力的 FcγR(FcγRI)和多个低至中等亲和力能够启动激活信号的 FcγR,以及一个低至中等亲和力的 FcγR(FcγRIIB),其在细胞质的结构域含有负调节性免疫受体酪氨酸基抑制基序(ITIM)。

重要的是要记住抗体是糖蛋白,并且抗体上的蛋白质和碳水化合物部分都有助于其功能的发挥。蛋白质结构决定碳水化合物侧链的数量和位置。所有 IgG 和 IgM 抗体在 Fc 上都有糖基化位点,并且碳水化合物侧链可以改变 Fc 与补体和 FcR 的相互作用[3]。此外,少数抗体在 Fab 区中具有糖基化位点,其可以显著改变抗原抗体结合。

目前,免疫球蛋白糖基化存在几个重要的分支。首先,已知在药物治疗的患者中,年龄、性别或是否怀孕[4-7]

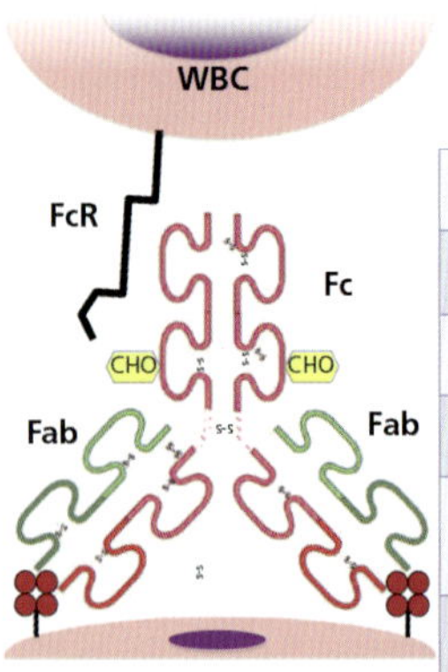

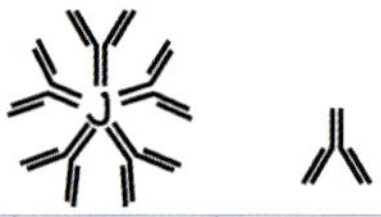

	IgM	IgG
亚型	无	1,2,3,4
激活 C	+++	0~+++
FcR	有限	多样
半衰期	5 天	7(G3)~23 天
功能	天然,早期	亲和力成熟

图 6.1 图示重链(粉红色)和轻链(绿色)具有恒定区(浅色)和可变区(黑色)的基本 IgG 抗体结构。木瓜蛋白酶将铰链区中的 IgG(检查)切割成三个片段:一个 Fc(可结晶片段)和两个 Fab(片段抗原结合)。Fc 上的糖基化位点由黄色六边形指示。右表比较了 IgM 和 IgG 抗体的重要功能。

的患者中发生的糖基化变化也不同,而这可改变抗体对移植物的反应结果。第二,Ravetch 和同事[8]通过改变免疫球蛋白的糖基化,使之产生更多具有免疫调节抑制功能的静脉内免疫球蛋白(IVIg)。

已经开发了许多机制来检测移植物特异性同种异体抗体。这些内容将在第 89 章中讨论。

抗原

抗原是决定抗体介导的免疫结果的关键因素。影响抗体功能的抗原变量包括结构和分布。所有血管内皮细胞上的高浓度 MHC Ⅰ类抗原为抗体紧密结合提供了最佳靶标以激活补体并使白细胞上高亲和力和低亲和力的 FcR 集结于白细胞。MHC Ⅱ类抗原在内皮细胞上的表达较不均匀于白细胞。在人类中,例如,MHC Ⅱ类抗原在心脏中的所有血管内皮上组成型表达,但仅限于肾脏毛细血管和静脉。然而,在缺血再灌注期间和炎症部位,MHC 抗原的表达则增加。关于 MHC 的深入讨论可以在第 4 章中找到。

与 MHC 抗原一样,主要血型抗原 A 和 B 以高浓度在内皮细胞上表达。然而,MHC 和血型抗原之间不同[9]。A 和 B 抗原是末端碳水化合物表位,其可以连接到与四种不同的核心糖链,进而脂质或蛋白质形成糖脂或糖蛋白。已显示 A 和 B 表位与各种膜糖蛋白以及由内皮细胞释放的可溶性蛋白质,例如 von Willebrand 因子(vWf)共价连接[10,11]。

作为抗体介导排斥的潜在重要靶标的其他抗原,包括 MICA(主要组织相容性复合体Ⅰ类相关链 A)、次要同种异体抗原和自身抗原仍在研究中[12]。与 MHC 抗原不同,这些抗原以低浓度在细胞内位置表达,或作为在正常条件下不暴露的隐蔽表位表达。因此,在静止条件下,这些抗原可能不是抗体的最佳靶标。然而,与移植(供体的脑死亡、缺血-再灌注损伤和手术创伤)或随后的排斥或感染相关的炎症可以上调这些抗原的表达,以增加其对抗体介导排斥的易感性。作为这种相互作用的实例,已有研究表明,MICA 抗体的产生往往是抗体对 HLA 反应的结果[13]。

补体

当高浓度的抗体结合同种异体细胞时,完全补体级联可以通过经典途径或凝集素途径激活,这取决于具有可变末端糖的 Fc 碳水化合物侧链的结构(见第 2 章和第 7 章)。与大多数血清糖蛋白相反,只有少数人 IgG 碳水化合物具有末端唾液酸。相反,这些侧链的分支经常以半乳糖残基终止以增加 C1q[14]的结合,这是经典途径的引发剂。抗体糖基化的变化是自身免疫疾病的众所周知的方面[15]。缺乏末端唾液酸和半乳糖的抗体(称为 G0 抗体)具有暴露的末端 N-乙酰葡糖胺(GlcNAc)残基。甘露糖结合凝集素(MBL)——凝集素途径的起始子,与 G0 抗体上的 GlcNAc 亲和结合。已经证实,G0 自身抗体通过凝集素途径在人和小鼠中激活补体[14]。在小鼠中,G0 IgG 水平在自身免疫倾向的小鼠中较高,并随着年龄和非特异性炎症刺激而增加[16]。在人类中,末端糖残基的异质性取决于某些疾病、药物治疗、年龄和性别[4-7]。

C1 和 MBL 都需要两个或多个相邻的 IgM 或 IgG 的 Fc 区用于有效地结合和激活。这允许结合的 C1(即 C1r 和 C1s) 或 MBL (MBL 相关的丝氨酸蛋白酶;MASP)的酶亚单位开始一系列酶促步骤,其可以通过生产越来越多具有生物活性的“裂解”产物来显著扩增和多样化免疫应答[17](图 6.2)。补充级联的细节在第 2 章中已有综述。简而言之,C4 首先被切割成两个片段——C4a 和 C4b。小 C4a 片段是可溶性介体,较大的 C4b 含有硫酯基团。该硫酯可与其最接近的蛋白质或碳水化合物上的羟基或氨基形成共价键。第一个酶促

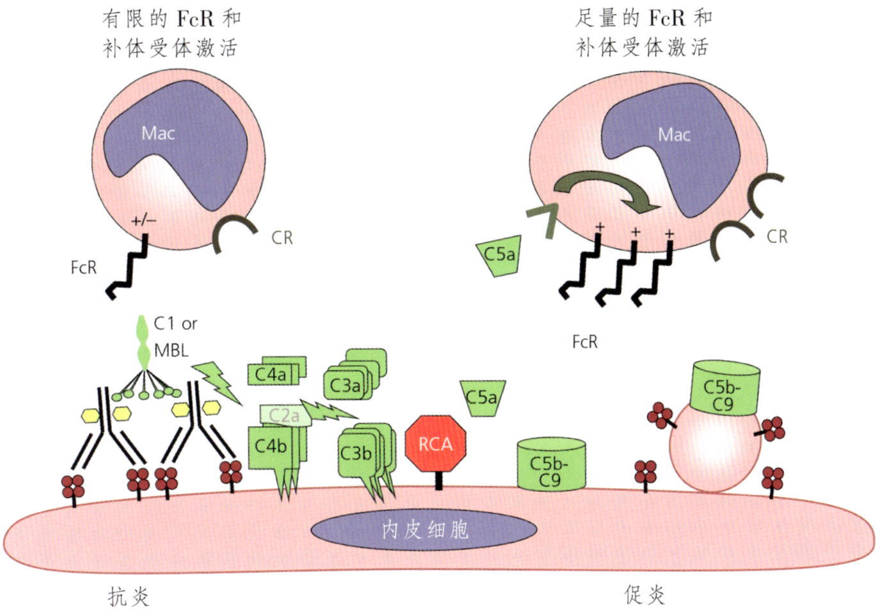

图 6.2 图示通过抗体激活补体使炎症反应增加的原理。具有 Fc 受体(例如中性粒细胞和巨噬细胞)的白细胞可以被与抗原结合的抗体刺激。Fc 受体与 IgG 相互作用的强度取决于抗体上的碳水化合物侧链(黄色六边形)。IgG 上的碳水化合物侧链也与经典和凝集素补体途径的第一组分相互作用。需要至少两个紧密间隔的 IgG 抗体来启动一个 C1 或 MBL 分子的结合。C1 或 MBL 可酶促切割 C4 的许多分子,产生可共价结合至细胞膜的 C4b。C4b 锚定经典转化酶(C4b 和 C2a 的复合物),其切割大量 C3 生成 C3b(其可共价结合组织)和 C3a(其为中性粒细胞和巨噬细胞的化学吸引剂)。C3b 结合 C4bC2a 形成经典 C5 转化酶,将 C5 切割成 C5a 和 C5b。C5b 启动膜攻击复合物(MAC; C5b–C9)的形成。C3 和 C5 转化酶都是补体活化(RCA)的几种调节剂的靶标。结果,内皮裂解在 AMR 中不广泛,但是溶解量的 MAC 可以刺激内皮细胞产生细胞因子,表达黏附分子,并脱落含有违规 MAC 的微粒。C5a 是关键的炎症介质,因为它是中性粒细胞和巨噬细胞的极有力的化学引诱物,并且它还引起巨噬细胞上调刺激性 Fc RIII 以及下调 IgG 的抑制性 Fc RIIB。这些受体使巨噬细胞对抗体更加响应并补充分裂产物。(Reproduced with permission from reference [17].)

步骤可以导致显著扩增,其中约 25 个分子的 C4b 结合在激活抗体上或附近[18]。在更下游,C4b 用作 C2 的附着位点,然后被 C1s 切割,以产生 C2a,C2a 保持与 C4b 缔合。C4bC2a 复合物是将中心补体成分 C3 切割成两个片段 C3a 和 C3b 的经典途径 C3 转化酶。小的 C3a 片段是流体相血管活性介质,其可以结合附近的内皮细胞或肥大细胞上的 C3a 受体(C3aR)。较大的片段 C3b 在结构上与 C4b 同源并含有可共价结合的硫酯基团。C3b 与 C4b 相比具有相似但更广泛的功能。像 C4b 一样,它是具有补体受体 1(CR1; CD35)的细胞的配体。另外,C3b 可以结合补体旁路途径的因子 B 并且参与替代途径,其作为扩增环,导致更多的 C3 分裂产物(图 6.3)。作为经典和扩增途径的结果,对于每个 C1 或 MBL,约 250 个 C3b 片段可以沉积在靶细胞上。

与相邻补体分裂产物结合,C3b 可形成经典和替代性 C5 转化酶(分别为 C4bC2aC3b 和 C3bBbC3b),其将 C5 切割成 C5a 和 C5b。正是在这一点上,补体级联加强其促炎作用[19]。作为催化剂,小片段 C5a 在数量上比 C3a 更有效,并且可使巨噬细胞极化为促炎功能。如图 6.2 所示,较大的片段 C5b 启动补体(C5b–C9)的末端组分装配成孔形成结构,膜攻击复合体(MAC)。如下所述,MAC 即使在溶血浓度下,也可改变内皮细胞功能。

补体是对损伤的固有免疫应答的关键组分。关于这方面作用的其他细节见第 7 章。

补体调节

毫不奇怪的是,这种强效效应分子的进展几乎每一步都受到高度调节。然而,不同的调节分子可以改变不同方向的免疫应答。补体的调节对于理解抗体介导的排斥和作为调节补体系统的潜在治疗干预具有非常重要的意义。

调节开始于用 C1 抑制剂(丝氨酸蛋白酶抑制剂丝氨酸蛋白酶超家族)补体激活的初始步骤。它提供了捕

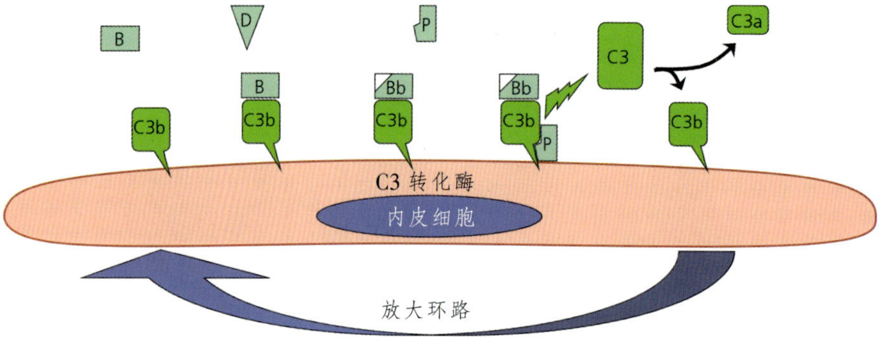

图 6.3 一旦 C3b 连接到细胞膜上,便可以充当放大环的中枢,其中旁路途径产生更多的 C3b。在该过程中,C3b 用作因子 B(B)的锚,然后被因子 D(D)切割,以形成 C3 转化酶 C3bBb。备解素(P)与该复合物结合并稳定该酶。这种稳定的酶复合物具有增加的半衰期,以将更多的 C3 切割成 C3b 并产生长寿命反馈回路。

获丝氨酸蛋白酶的底物，包括 C1r、C1s 和 MASP 的底物。这使得非酶 C1q 或 MBL 结合抗体。在组织损伤的情况下,C1q 和 MBL 对通过清道夫巨噬细胞清除凋亡小体和避免自身免疫是至关重要的[20,21]。有可能通过 C1q 受体巨噬细胞的接合在同种异体移植中也具有有益效果。事实上,Bishop 和同事报道,同种异体移植物被 C1q 缺陷小鼠更快地排斥[22]。

作为丝氨酸蛋白酶抑制剂,C1 抑制剂具有对移植物潜在有益的额外效果。这包括激肽释放酶和凝血系统的抑制[23]。最近的研究表明,C1 抑制剂可以与内皮细胞上的选择素结合,并干扰白细胞滚动[24]。

大多数补体调节剂聚焦于 C4b 和 C3b。许多这些调节剂由各种数量高度保守的短共有重复组成，并且是位于染色体 1 上的补体激活(RCA)基因簇的调节子成员(图 6.4A)。通常,这些调节剂通过两种机制起作用:转化酶的解离和辅助因子功能(图 6.4B)。C4 结合

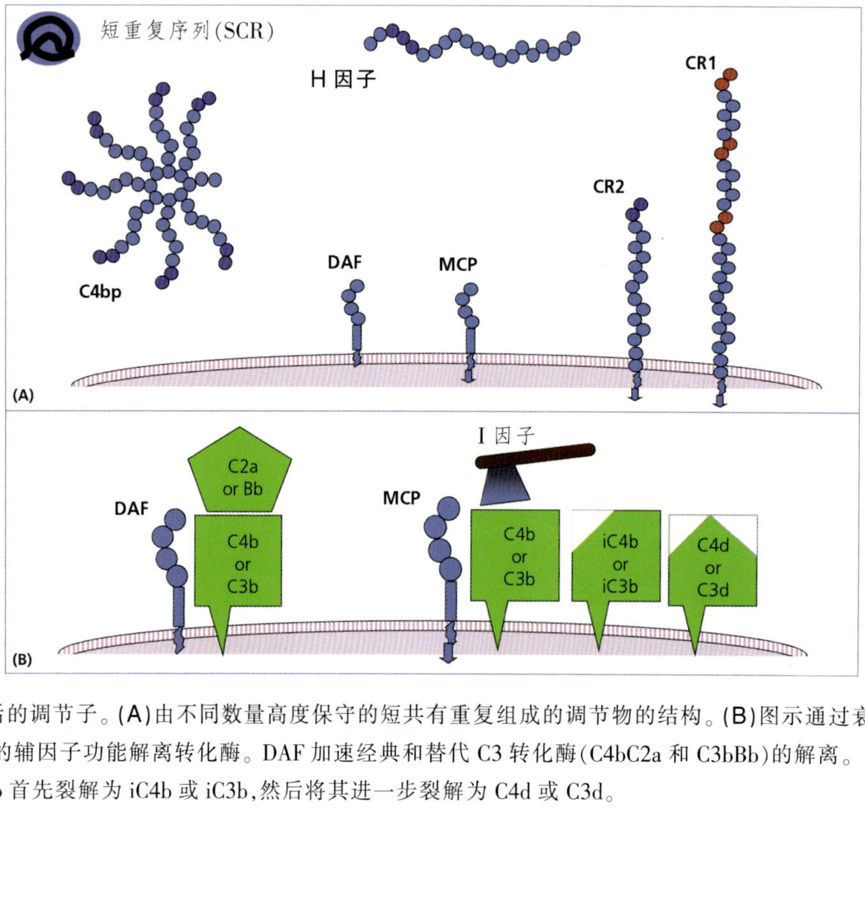

图 6.4 图示补体激活的调节子。(A)由不同数量高度保守的短共有重复组成的调节物的结构。(B)图示通过衰变加速因子(DAF)和膜辅因子蛋白(MCP)的辅因子功能解离转化酶。DAF 加速经典和替代 C3 转化酶(C4bC2a 和 C3bBb)的解离。 MCP 作为酶因子 I 的辅因子,将 C4b 或 C3b 首先裂解为 iC4b 或 iC3b,然后将其进一步裂解为 C4d 或 C3d。

蛋白(C4bp)和衰变加速因子(DAF; CD55)加速 C2a 从 C4b 的解离并缩短该 C3 转化酶的半衰期。相比之下,膜辅因子蛋白(MCP; CD46)作为酶因子 I 的辅因子,首先将 C4b 或 C3b 切割成 iC4b 或 iC3b, 然后将其进一步裂解为 C4d 或 C3d。C4bp、因子 H 和补体受体 1 (CR1; CD35)也作为因子 I 的辅因子起作用(图 6.4A)。末端补体组分受到保护素(CD59)的调节,其可防止 C9 与 C5b-C8 的缔合。

补体介质和调节剂之间的平衡对炎症有反应。IL-1、IL-6、IL-8 和 TNF 刺激肝脏产生急性期蛋白, 其中包括补体成分和调节物。MBL、C3、因子 B、C5、C1 抑制剂和 C4bp 等肝脏产物随着炎症细胞因子的反应增加。在炎症局部位置,巨噬细胞和某些实质细胞特别是上皮细胞可以产生补体成分[25-27]。这被内皮细胞表面上补体调节剂的上调抵消。特别地,已经证明,在一些肾脏和心脏移植物中,在抗体介导的排斥期间 DAF 被上调[28,29]。

当中等水平的补体被激活时, 调节剂的表达足以防止同种异体移植物中大多数细胞的裂解。然而,高水平的抗体可以压倒调节分子并引起内皮细胞的裂解,表现为超急性排斥。缺乏裂解的情况下,一系列可能的结果取决于所产生的裂解产物的平衡。

治疗干预可以在不同的步骤中调节补体的激活。C5 被认为是导致严重炎症的临界点。因此,已经开发了阻断 C5 切割的单克隆抗体,可溶性 C5a 受体和 C5a 受体的拮抗剂,并且已应用于临床的不同阶段[19]。已经证明人源化抗 C5 抗体依库丽单抗在患者中抑制抗体介导的排斥[30]。

人类 C1 抑制剂目前正在进行肾移植受者的临床试验。这种方法是有吸引力的,因为它抑制 C1 和 MBL 的酶组分,但不干扰 C1q 和 MBL 的凋亡清除机制。C1 抑制剂对激肽释放酶和凝血系统的额外作用[23]也可能有益于移植受者。

人类与远距离系统发生物种(例如猪)之间的不相容性显著混淆异种移植。关于补充调节和预先形成的抗体的深入讨论,因为涉及异种移植可以在第 12 章中找到。

细胞

除了补体分裂产物的沉积, 在急性体液排斥中观察到的病理变化还包括内皮细胞活化和粒细胞或单核细胞着边[31,32]。这些反应可通过抗体对每种细胞类型的直接和间接影响预测。器官移植的血管内皮细胞是抗体的第一个可用靶标。当抗体交联内皮细胞上的 MHC 抗原时,Von Willebrand 因子和 P-选择蛋白在几分钟内从 Weibel-Palade 储存颗粒中胞吐[33]。这导致血小板黏附和活化, 由于大量血小板和由血小板释放的多种多样的介质而定量和定性地延长了炎症[34,35]。与移植特别相关的是趋化因子和作用于中性粒细胞、巨噬细胞和 T 细胞的配体。包括存储在血小板的 α 粒子中的 IL-8、PF4(CXCL4)、RANTES(CCL5)、P-选择蛋白和 CD40L(CD154)。抗体激活内皮细胞通过补体激活产物增强, 补体激活产物从连续更有效的过敏毒素(C4a, C3a 和 C5a)开始并进展到 MAC。过敏毒素通过结合内皮细胞和肥大细胞上的特异性受体增加血管通透性[19]。最后,MAC 在亚溶解型 C5b,甚至不完全组装的 MAC(C5b-C8)中导致钙流量激活内皮细胞[36-38]。这会导致细胞收缩和预先形成的黏附分子的胞吐作用。在炎症细胞因子例如 IL-1α 和 TNF 的存在下, 由 MAC 活化的内皮细胞合成中性粒细胞和单核细胞(IL-8 和 MCP-1;CCL2)的趋化因子,并上调黏附分子(P-选择蛋白、E-选择蛋白和 ICAM-1)用于白细胞浸润。抗体和 MAC 独立地诱导内皮细胞产生生长因子(PDGF 和 FGF)并增殖,与慢性排斥相关[39-41]。与红细胞不同,有核细胞通过快速脱落或嵌入包含 MAC 的膜进行反应[42,43],但是这释放了潜在的抗原性微泡, 其可以被获得并呈递以启动或扩增适应性免疫应答。

中性粒细胞和巨噬细胞是抗体介导排斥的特征性参与者,它们都表达多种 Fc 和补体受体。这些受体具有交互作用,其通过 C5aR 和 FcR 做了最好的说明。除了是中性粒细胞和巨噬细胞的极强的化学引诱剂,C5a 还可引起巨噬细胞上调调节刺激性 FcγRⅢ 和下调 IgG 的抑制性 FcγRⅡB[44],使巨噬细胞对抗体更强响应。类似地,通过 FcR 的刺激导致巨噬细胞产生更多的补体[45]。

虽然单核细胞和巨噬细胞与排斥相关, 但它们具有广泛的功能,从促炎性、促纤维性到抗炎性[46-48]。相对于 T 细胞巨噬细胞的这些亚群被充分地定义。在这种情况下, 来自 Th1 或 NK 细胞的 IFNγ 和 TNF 刺激促炎(或 M1)巨噬细胞产生 IL-12、IL-1 和 IL-6(见第 2 章)。相反,促纤维(或 M2)巨噬细胞响应于来自 Th2 细胞的 IL-4 而产生,并且特征性地产生 TGFβ 和结缔组织生长因子(CTGF)。最后,抗炎(或调节)巨噬细胞应答并产生IL-10。

已发现缺血性损伤第一波引起炎症巨噬细胞，随后是伤口愈合巨噬细胞[48,49]。在不同体液免疫介质作用下浸润同种异体移植物的巨噬细胞尚未被鉴定。然而，最适合的类比是通过C5aR和刺激性FcR的活化使巨噬细胞偏向炎症。在光谱的另一端将是在没有末端补体活化的情况下由早期补体成分刺激的巨噬细胞。如补体部分所讨论的，已知C1q或MBL介导巨噬细胞可去除凋亡泡而不引起炎症或纤维化[50-54]。

体液免疫排斥的类别

关于体液免疫排斥表现的概念由具有超活性排斥的原始灾难性经历支配。随着越来越复杂的检测抗体和探测活检方法的发展，关于体液免疫更微妙的影响的概念已经发生演变。

超急性排斥反应

在超急性排斥中，高水平的抗体激活足够的补体以超过所有的调节障碍，并发生血管内皮细胞的显著裂解。这种血管完整性的破坏导致出血和血栓形成。大量的补体分裂产物也吸引并激活代表超急性排斥的许多中性粒细胞。Patel和Terasaki于1969年发表的一篇具有里程碑意义的出版物[55]中描述并验证了预先形成的抗体的血清学测试。这一革命性实现的历史详见第3章。该试验在约30%的患者中检出了抗体。超过1/3的具有抗体的患者对于供体特异性抗体(DSA)是交叉匹配阳性的。在80%的DSA患者中发生超急性排斥，15%的患者在移植物上未表达抗原的抗体。在接受第二次移植的患者中，超急性排斥反应发生非常频繁(约41%)。到1974年，Mel Williams在一篇关于David Hume的纪念研讨会上报告说，交叉匹配试验消除了24名第二次移植患者一系列的超急性排斥反应[56]。

急性排斥

补体激活的量取决于抗体的滴度和类别以及靶抗原的密度。移植后由幼稚或记忆B细胞产生的同种异体抗体不会立即达到高效价。低水平的抗体将导致更少的补体激活，这样可以更好地被多种调节机制调节。

当足够的补体被激活，C3转化酶的调节被操控并且形成大量的C5转化酶时，则体液排斥的全貌被发现。这包括由于血管通透性增加，C4和C3分裂产物(C4d和C3d)沉积以及中性粒细胞和巨噬细胞边缘化和浸润引起的水肿。病理学家专家组一致认同在肾脏、心脏和胰腺移植中抗体介导的排斥的基本现象[57-59]。单核细胞和巨噬细胞的通用标记常用于定义单核浸润。当然不区分巨噬细胞的亚型。

当由于抗体滴度低、补体激活抗体的不同混合物或抗体对抗原低密度表达使得补体激活较少时，病理学发现不太明显。急性移植物功能障碍已被描述为缺乏C4d[60]。这些病例有时被归因于抗体的补体依赖性作用。也可能出现在具有某些少量补体调节剂的患者中。例如，低水平的循环因子H允许替代C3转化酶具有更长的半衰期，这将使得少量的C4活化通过不适当调节的扩增回路引起显著的C3和C5产生。在用针对因子H的阻断抗体治疗的动物中和在具有功能因子H突变的人类中已经证明了正常因子H功能在防止C3过度活化中的重要性[61]。膜结合补体调节剂的表达也很关键[62]。在炎症细胞因子应答中上调的DAF在肾移植和心脏移植抗体介导的排斥的一些情况下以较低水平表达[28,29]。这将有望延长C3转化酶的功能并导致更多的C3活化。

相反，已经在一些活检中发现C4d，其没有显示任何其他体液排斥的证据。已经证实，在没有炎症和移植物功能障碍的情况下，与C4d沉积相关的供体特异性HLA的抗体代表亚临床排斥[63]。在非人类的灵长类动物模型中，这些发现可以早于慢性排斥证据几个月出现[64]。

慢性排斥

临床上，体液免疫应答与肾移植中的慢性排斥有关[65]。肾移植活检中的循环DSA和C4d沉积与肾小球病的最终发展相关。然而，慢性肾小球病比C4d沉积更加普遍。Sis及其同事已经注意到在没有可证实的C4d沉积物的情况下，在分子水平上内皮干扰的高发病率，并且这种内皮损伤的分子特征与慢性移植物衰竭相关[66,67]。这可以部分反映选择性过程，因为激活可被检测量的补体的高滴度抗体将导致急性移植物功能障碍。较低的抗体滴度可引起可促成慢性血管变化的内皮细胞和平滑肌细胞的补体依赖性应答。包括成纤维细胞生长因子(FGF)受体的上调和增殖增加[68]。低水平的抗体和补体激活也可以刺激内皮细胞内吞或胞吐其质膜的掺杂部分[42,43]。实验动物模型已经证明，大量共价结合的补体分裂产物(C4d 和 C3d)可以在供体特异性抗体消除后3~5天内减少至不可检测的水平[69]。

免疫耐受和适应

与主要血型抗原A和B不相容的肾移植提供了对体液免疫应答的两种非炎性结果的观点：调节和耐受。针对A和B抗原的抗体与针对HLA的抗体不同，因为“天然”血凝素抗体在生命的第一年中发展，可能是响应于定殖肠道的细菌上的交叉反应性碳水化合物抗原。超急性或急性排斥可以通过在移植前和移植后第一周耗尽接受者中的天然抗体来避免。在这个关键时期之后，抗体的重新产生确实导致C4d在管周毛细血管中沉积，但通常是在没有白细胞边缘化或移植物功能障碍的情况下发生[70,71]。移植物对抗体和补体的表观弹性称为调节。适应的几个方面相对于体液免疫应答是有指导意义的。第一个涉及抗体滴度。当抗体滴度高且抗体在移植前没有耗尽时，对A和B血型抗原的抗体可以引起超急性排斥[72]。与适应性相关的复发性抗体应答通常逐渐发展并且仅获得较低滴度。具有>64滴度的血凝素的发展与排斥的发生相关[73]。其次，为了使移植物适应，在术后当移植物由于缺血再灌注和外科创伤经历非特异性炎症时维持抗体消耗。最后，碳水化合物血型抗原的生物化学性质可能是关键的。A和B抗原可以与内皮细胞释放的可溶性蛋白(例如vWf)以及肾内的各种膜蛋白结合[10,11]，这一事实可能会改变抗体分布和补体活化的关键方面。在调节中观察到的补体激活的典型标志物，即C4d和C3d，是因子Ⅰ调节的终产物。这些分裂产物不一定表明非常促炎的C5和MAC已经被激活。早期补体组分的许多活化产物，特别是C1q和iC3b，都具有抗炎作用。如补充部分所述，C1q对于去除凋亡小体而不刺激炎症或抗原呈递是至关重要的。类似地，当iC3b与抗原呈递细胞上的CR3(CD11b / CD18)相互作用时，促炎细胞因子IL-1β、IL-6、IL-12和TNF的产生和分泌减少[74-76]。CR3也可以在T细胞内上调，并且该补体受体的交联抑制T细胞增殖和IL-2释放[77]。

尚不清楚是否可通过C1q或iC3b的活性实现对血型抗原或HLA的耐受性。当然，在存在针对HLA的抗体的情况下适应的病例明显不如那些血型不相容移植的病例稳定。然而，当把ABO血型不相容的心脏在出生后6个月内成功移植到婴儿中时，可以实现对ABO不相容的同种异体移植物的长期耐受。这些移植物诱导了对供体血型的耐受性，这一点可以通过缺乏能够产生供体血型抗原的抗体B细胞来证明[78]。供体抗原保持在移植物内皮上表达，但受体B细胞不产生针对供体血型抗原的抗体，而抗体确实正常发展成非供体血型抗原。长期以来，这些患者中有少数已经被报道会对供体血型抗原产生抗体[79]，但这些抗体可以识别附着于用于血细胞凝集测定中红细胞表达的碳水化合物骨架的A和B表位，而不是移植物内皮[80]。

总结

体液免疫包括广泛的相互依赖的介质、调节剂、受体和细胞，其可以产生从超急性至急性排斥的破坏性病理变化。在光谱的另一端，体液免疫可能与慢性变化甚至下调组织损伤相关。近年来，对移植物破坏的体液机制的看法已经显著改善。其未来的挑战将是找到控制这些过程的方法，以避免它们以移植物特异性方式产生作用。

(胡士华 译 程倩 校)

参考文献

1. Nimmerjahn F, Ravetch JV. Fcgamma receptors as regulators of immune responses. Nature Reviews. Immunology. 2008;8:34-47.
2. Kubagawa H, Oka S, Kubagawa Y, et al. Identity of the elusive IgM Fc receptor (FcmuR) in humans. Journal of Experimental Medicine. 2009;206:2779-2793.
3. Arnold JN, Wormald MR, Sim RB, et al. The impact of glycosylation on the biological function and structure of human immunoglobulins. Annual Review of Immunology. 2007;25:21-50.
4. Axford JS, Sumar N, Alavi A, et al. Changes in normal glycosylation mechanisms in autoimmune rheumatic disease. Journal of Clinical Investigation. 1992;89:1021-1031.
5. Mesko B, Poliska S, Szamosi S, et al. Peripheral blood gene expression and IgG glycosylation profiles as markers of tocilizumab treatment in rheumatoid arthritis. Journal of Rheumatology. 2012;39:916-928.
6. Wang J, Balog CI, Stavenhagen K, et al. Fc-glycosylation of IgG1 is modulated by B-cell stimuli. Molecular and Cellular Proteomics. 2011;10:M110.004655.
7. Pucic M, Muzinic A, Novokmet M, et al. Changes in plasma and IgG N-glycome during childhood and adolescence. Glycobiology. 2012;22:975-982.
8. Anthony RM, Kobayashi T, Wermeling F, et al. Intravenous gammaglobulin suppresses inflammation through a novel T(H)2 pathway. Nature. 2011;475:110-113.
9. King KE, Warren DS, Samaniego-Picota M, et al. Antibody, complement and accommodation in ABO-incompatible transplants. Current Opinion in Immunology. 2004;16:545-549.
10. Matsui T, Shimoyama T, Matsumoto M, et al. ABO blood group antigens on human plasma von Willebrand factor after ABO-mismatched bone marrow transplantation. Blood. 1999;94:2895-2900.
11. Tasaki M, Yoshida Y, Miyamoto M, et al. Identification and characterization of major proteins carrying ABO blood group antigens in the human kidney. Transplantation. 2009;87:1125-1133.

12. Smith JD, Brunner VM, Jigjidsuren S, et al. Lack of effect of MICA antibodies on graft survival following heart transplantation. American Journal of Transplantation. 2009;9:1912–1919.
13. Nath DS, Angaswamy N, Basha HI, et al. Donor-specific antibodies to human leukocyte antigens are associated with and precede antibodies to major histocompatibility complex class I-related chain A in antibody-mediated rejection and cardiac allograft vasculopathy after human cardiac transplantation. Human Immunology. 2010;71:1191–1196.
14. Nimmerjahn F, Anthony RM, Ravetch JV. Agalactosylated IgG antibodies depend on cellular Fc receptors for in vivo activity. Proceedings of the National Academy of Sciences of the United States of America. 2007;104:8433–8437.
15. Malhotra R, Wormald MR, Rudd PM, et al. Glycosylation changes of IgG associated with rheumatoid arthritis can activate complement via the mannose-binding protein. Nature Medicine. 1995;1:237–243.
16. Bodman KB, Hutchings PR, Jeddi PA, et al. IgG glycosylation in autoimmune-prone strains of mice. Clinical and Experimental Immunology. 1994;95:103–107.
17. Baldwin WM 3rd, Halushka MK, Valujskikh A, et al. B cells in cardiac transplants: from clinical questions to experimental models. Seminars in Immunology. 2011;24:122–130.
18. Ollert MW, Kadlec JV, David K, et al. Antibody-mediated complement activation on nucleated cells. A quantitative analysis of the individual reaction steps. Journal of Immunology. 1994;153:2213–2221.
19. Woodruff TM, Nandakumar KS, Tedesco F. Inhibiting the C5-C5a receptor axis. Molecular Immunology. 2011;48:1631–1642.
20. Cortes-Hernandez J, Fossati-Jimack L, Petry F, et al. Restoration of C1q levels by bone marrow transplantation attenuates autoimmune disease associated with C1q deficiency in mice. European Journal of Immunology. 2004;34:3713–3722.
21. Botto M, Dell'Agnola C, Bygrave AE, et al. Homozygous C1q deficiency causes glomerulonephritis associated with multiple apoptotic bodies. Nature Genetics. 1998;19:56–59.
22. Csencsits K, Burrell BE, Lu G, et al. The classical complement pathway in transplantation: unanticipated protective effects of C1q and role in inductive antibody therapy. American Journal of Transplantation. 2008;8:1622–1630.
23. Davis AE 3rd, Lu F, Mejia P. C1 inhibitor, a multi-functional serine protease inhibitor. Thrombosis and Haemostasis. 2010;104:886–893.
24. Cai S, Dole VS, Bergmeier W, et al. A direct role for C1 inhibitor in regulation of leukocyte adhesion. Journal of Immunology. 2005;174:6462–6466.
25. Brooimans RA, Stegmann AP, van Dorp WT, et al. Interleukin 2 mediates stimulation of complement C3 biosynthesis in human proximal tubular epithelial cells. Journal of Clinical Investigation. 1991;88:379–384.
26. Seelen MA, Brooimans RA, van der Woude FJ, et al. IFN-gamma mediates stimulation of complement C4 biosynthesis in human proximal tubular epithelial cells. Kidney International. 1993;44:50–57.
27. Pratt JR, Basheer SA, Sacks SH. Local synthesis of complement component C3 regulates acute renal transplant rejection. Nature Medicine. 2002;8:582–587.
28. Brodsky SV, Nadasdy GM, Pelletier R, et al. Expression of the decay-accelerating factor (CD55) in renal transplants–a possible prediction marker of allograft survival. Transplantation. 2009;88:457–464.
29. Tan CD, Sokos GG, Pidwell DJ, et al. Correlation of donor-specific antibodies, complement and its regulators with graft dysfunction in cardiac antibody-mediated rejection. American Journal of Transplantation. 2009;9:2075–2084.
30. Stegall MD, Diwan T, Raghavaiah S, et al. Terminal complement inhibition decreases antibody-mediated rejection in sensitized renal transplant recipients. American Journal of Transplantation. 2011;11:2405–2413.
31. Lones MA, Czer LS, Trento A, et al. Clinical-pathologic features of humoral rejection in cardiac allografts: a study in 81 consecutive patients. Journal of Heart and Lung Transplantation. 1995;14:151–162.
32. Magil AB, Tinckam K. Monocytes and peritubular capillary C4d deposition in acute renal allograft rejection. Kidney International. 2003;63:1888–1893.
33. Yamakuchi M, Kirkiles-Smith NC, Ferlito M, et al. Antibody to human leukocyte antigen triggers endothelial exocytosis. Proceedings of the National Academy of Sciences of the United States of America. 2007;104:1301–1306.
34. Morrell CN, Sun H, Swaim AM, et al. Platelets, an inflammatory force in transplantation. American Journal of Transplantation. 2007;7:2447–2454.
35. Kuo HH, Morrell CN, Baldwin WM 3rd. Alloantibody induced platelet responses in transplants: potent mediators in small packages. Human Immunology. 2012;73:1233–1238.
36. Hattori R, Hamilton KK, McEver RP, et al. Complement proteins C5b-9 induce secretion of high molecular weight multimers of endothelial von Willebrand factor and translocation of granule membrane protein GMP-140 to the cell surface. Journal of Biological Chemistry. 1989;264:9053–9060.
37. Saadi S, Platt JL. Transient perturbation of endothelial integrity induced by natural antibodies and complement. Journal of Experimental Medicine. 1995;181:21–31.
38. Kilgore KS, Flory CM, Miller BF, et al. The membrane attack complex of complement induces interleukin-8 and monocyte chemoattractant protein-1 secretion from human umbilical vein endothelial cells. American Journal of Pathology. 1996;149:953–961.
39. Benzaquen LR, Nicholson-Weller A, Halperin JA. Terminal complement proteins C5b-9 release basic fibroblast growth factor and platelet-derived growth factor from endothelial cells. Journal of Experimental Medicine. 1994;179:985–992.
40. Harris PE, Bian H, Reed EF. Induction of high affinity fibroblast growth factor receptor expression and proliferation in human endothelial cells by anti-HLA antibodies: a possible mechanism for transplant atherosclerosis. Journal of Immunology. 1997;159:5697–5704.
41. Bian H, Reed EF. Alloantibody-mediated class I signal transduction in endothelial cells and smooth muscle cells: enhancement by IFN-gamma and TNF-alpha. Journal of Immunology. 1999;163:1010–1018.
42. Pilzer D, Gasser O, Moskovich O, et al. Emission of membrane vesicles: roles in complement resistance, immunity and cancer. Springer Seminars in Immunopathology. 2005;27:375–387.
43. Moskovich O, Fishelson Z. Live cell imaging of outward and inward vesiculation induced by the complement c5b-9 complex. Journal of Biological Chemistry. 2007;282:29977–29986.
44. Godau J, Heller T, Hawlisch H, et al. C5a initiates the inflammatory cascade in immune complex peritonitis. Journal of Immunology. 2004;173:3437–3445.
45. Kumar V, Ali SR, Konrad S, et al. Cell-derived anaphylatoxins as key mediators of antibody-dependent type II autoimmunity in mice. Journal of Clinical Investigation. 2006;116:512–520.
46. Mosser DM, Edwards JP. Exploring the full spectrum of macrophage activation. Nature Reviews. Immunology. 2008;8:958–969.
47. Anders HJ, Ryu M. Renal microenvironments and macrophage phenotypes determine progression or resolution of renal inflammation and fibrosis. Kidney International. 2011;80:915–925.
48. Lee S, Huen S, Nishio H, et al. Distinct macrophage phenotypes contribute to kidney injury and repair. Journal of the American Society of Nephrology. 2011;22:317–326.
49. Nahrendorf M, Swirski FK, Aikawa E, et al. The healing myocardium sequentially mobilizes two monocyte subsets with divergent and complementary functions. Journal of Experimental Medicine. 2007;204:3037–3047.
50. Korb LC, Ahearn JM. C1q binds directly and specifically to surface blebs of apoptotic human keratinocytes: complement deficiency and systemic lupus erythematosus revisited. Journal of Immunology. 1997;158:4525–4528.
51. Navratil JS, Watkins SC, Wisnieski JJ, et al. The globular heads of C1q specifically recognize surface blebs of apoptotic vascular endothelial cells. Journal of Immunology. 2001;166:3231–3239.
52. Ogden CA, deCathelineau A, Hoffmann PR, et al. C1q and mannose binding lectin engagement of cell surface calreticulin and cd91 initiates macropinocytosis and uptake of apoptotic cells. Journal of Experimental Medicine. 2001;194:781–796.
53. Nauta AJ, Castellano G, Xu W, et al. Opsonization with C1q and mannose-binding lectin targets apoptotic cells to dendritic cells. Journal of Immunology. 2004;173:3044–3050.
54. Benoit ME, Clarke EV, Morgado P, et al. Complement protein C1q directs macrophage polarization and limits inflammasome activity during the uptake of apoptotic cells. Journal of Immunology. 2012;188:5682–5693.
55. Patel R, Terasaki PI. Significance of the positive crossmatch test in kidney transplantation. New England Journal of Medicine. 1969;280:735–739.
56. Williams GM. Clinical aspects of allograft rejection. Transplantation Proceedings. 1974;6 (4 Suppl. 1):71–77.
57. Racusen LC, Colvin RB, Solez K, et al. Antibody-mediated rejection criteria - an addition to the banff 97 classification of renal allograft rejection. American Journal of Transplantation. 2003;3:708–714.
58. Berry GJ, Angelini A, Burke MM, et al. The ISHLT working formulation for pathologic diagnosis of antibody-mediated rejection in heart transplantation: evolution and current status (2005–2011). Journal of Heart and Lung Transplantation. 2011;30:601–611.
59. Drachenberg CB, Torrealba JR, Nankivell BJ, et al. Guidelines for the diagnosis of antibody-mediated rejection in pancreas allografts-updated Banff grading schema. American Journal of Transplantation. 2011;11:1792–1802.
60. Fishbein MC, Kobashigawa J. Biopsy-negative cardiac transplant rejection: etiology, diagnosis, and therapy. Current Opinion in Cardiology. 2004;19:166–169.
61. Noone D, Al-Matrafi J, Tinckam K, et al. Antibody mediated rejection associated with complement factor H-related protein 3/1 deficiency successfully treated with eculizumab. American Journal of Transplantation. 2012;12:2546–2553.
62. Cruzado JM, de Cordoba SR, Melilli E, et al. Successful renal transplantation in a patient with atypical hemolytic uremic syndrome carrying mutations in both factor I and MCP. American Journal of Transplantation. 2009;9:1477–1483.
63. Colvin RB, Smith RN. Antibody-mediated organ-allograft rejection. Nature Reviews. Immunology. 2005;5:807–817.
64. Smith RN, Kawai T, Boskovic S, et al. Four stages and lack of stable accommodation in chronic alloantibody-mediated renal allograft rejection in Cynomolgus monkeys. American Journal of Transplantation. 2008;8:1662–1672.
65. Gaston RS, Cecka JM, Kasiske BL, et al. Evidence for antibody-mediated injury as

a major determinant of late kidney allograft failure. Transplantation. 2010;90: 68–74.
66. Sis B, Jhangri GS, Bunnag S, et al. Endothelial gene expression in kidney transplants with alloantibody indicates antibody-mediated damage despite lack of C4d staining. American Journal of Transplantation. 2009;9:2312–2323.
67. Sis B, Jhangri GS, Riopel J, et al. A new diagnostic algorithm for antibody-mediated microcirculation inflammation in kidney transplants. American Journal of Transplantation. 2012;12:1168–1179.
68. Zhang X, Rozengurt E, Reed EF. HLA class I molecules partner with integrin beta4 to stimulate endothelial cell proliferation and migration. Science Signaling. 2010;3:ra85.
69. Minami K, Murata K, Lee C-Y, et al. C4d deposition and clearance in cardiac transplants correlates with alloantibody levels and rejection in rats. American Journal of Transplantation. 2006;6:923–932.
70. Platt JL. C4d and the fate of organ allografts. Journal of the American Society of Nephrology. 2002;13:2417–2419.
71. Haas M, Rahman MH, Racusen LC, et al. C4d and C3d staining in biopsies of ABO- and HLA-incompatible renal allografts: correlation with histologic findings. American Journal of Transplantation. 2006;6:1829–1840.
72. Starzl TE, Marchioro TL, Holmes JH, et al. Renal homografts in patients with major donor-recipient blood group incompatibilities. Surgery. 1964;55:195–200.
73. Tobian AA, Shirey RS, Montgomery RA, et al. ABO antibody titer and risk of antibody-mediated rejection in ABO-incompatible renal transplantation. American Journal of Transplantation. 2010;10:1247–1253.
74. Verbovetski I, Bychkov H, Trahtemberg U, et al. Opsonization of apoptotic cells by autologous iC3b facilitates clearance by immature dendritic cells, down-regulates DR and CD86, and up-regulates CC chemokine receptor 7. Journal of Experimental Medicine. 2002;196:1553–1561.
75. Morelli AE, Larregina AT, Shufesky WJ, et al. Internalization of circulating apoptotic cells by splenic marginal zone dendritic cells: dependence on complement receptors and effect on cytokine production. Blood. 2003;101:611–620.
76. Amarilyo G, Verbovetski I, Atallah M, et al. iC3b-opsonized apoptotic cells mediate a distinct anti-inflammatory response and transcriptional NF-kappaB-dependent blockade. European Journal of Immunology. 2010;40:699–709.
77. Wagner C, Hansch GM, Stegmaier S, et al. The complement receptor 3, CR3 (CD11b/CD18), on T lymphocytes: activation-dependent up-regulation and regulatory function. European Journal of Immunology. 2001;31:1173–1180.
78. Fan X, Ang A, Pollock-Barziv SM, et al. Donor-specific B-cell tolerance after ABO-incompatible infant heart transplantation. Nature Medicine. 2004;10:1227–1233.
79. Conway J, Manlhiot C, Allain-Rooney T, et al. Development of donor-specific isohemagglutinins following pediatric ABO-incompatible heart transplantation. American Journal of Transplantation. 2012;12:888–895.
80. Jeyakanthan M, West LJ. Donor-specific isohemagglutinins: measuring the unknown. American Journal of Transplantation. 2012;12:803–805.

第 7 章
固有免疫

Melissa Y. Yeung, Sacha A. De Serres, Xian C. Li

引言

固有免疫是免疫的一个关键组成部分，并与适应性免疫系统一起形成一个复杂的系统，保护我们免受无数的病原体侵入。固有免疫系统还通过消除癌性和应激细胞来促进组织内稳态。先天性反应由固有免疫细胞进行，包括树突状细胞(DC)、巨噬细胞、单核细胞、自然杀伤(NK)细胞、中性粒细胞、肥大细胞和嗜酸性粒细胞。与适应性免疫系统的细胞，即T和B细胞相反，固有免疫细胞不具有直接识别外来抗原的机体重排的细胞表面受体。相反，它们表达过多的模式识别受体，接合保守的病原体片段、危险信号和受损的细胞产物；它们还表达补体产物、抗体和不断检测“自体”或“丢失的自体”以控制细胞反应的其他非多形性活化和抑制性受体。这些特征允许固有免疫细胞形成第一道防线，并且还会影响适应性免疫应答的开始、持续时间和特征。

历史上，移植研究主要集中在适应性免疫系统的细胞，特别是参与移植物损伤的T细胞。实验观察发现，组织和器官移植通常在同种异体移植受者中T细胞不存在时长期存活。最近，固有免疫细胞对移植结果(排斥或接受)的贡献越来越受到重视[1-3]。固有免疫细胞可被微生物产物或来自受损移植物的内源性配体(报警蛋白)活化，一些先天细胞可以直接响应同种异体移植物。这样的细胞通过多种机制影响移植结果，包括改变T细胞活化程序。在各种情况下，根据环境和耐受方案，固有免疫细胞与排斥或保护同种异体移植物密切相关，还有助于广泛的移植物损伤。因此，固有免疫细胞通常是同种免疫的重要贡献者，要想成功诱导移植耐受性，需要在移植后更好地理解和合理靶向此类细胞。在本章中，我们将回顾固有免疫系统中的关键细胞和分子途径，详细说明固有免疫系统如何对同种异体移植物做出反应，并总结移植环境中固有免疫系统治疗靶向的挑战和机遇。本章将补充第5章和第6章的内容，分别涉及适应性免疫反应的细胞和体液成分。

固有免疫系统

固有免疫系统由多种细胞类型、分子传感器、细胞表面活化和抑制性受体以及可溶性介质组成。下面详细讨论系统中的关键元件。

树突状细胞

树突状细胞(DC)是免疫系统中的稀有细胞类型，约占总淋巴样细胞的1%。它们广泛分布在体内，并且通过从细胞体中伸出的树突而在形态学上得到鉴定(参见第2章)。树突状细胞由骨髓前体形成，并且基于解剖位置、表面标记物和成熟状态，它们可以分为各种子集[4,5]。淋巴组织中的DC称为淋巴组织驻留DC，而在其他位点的DC通常称为间质DC。表型上，DC表达β整联蛋白CD11c，并且与其他表面标记物组合，它们可以进一步分为骨髓DC（$CD11c^+CD11b^+CD205^-$），淋巴样DC（$CD11c^+$ $CD11b^-CD205^+$）和浆细胞样DC $^+B220^+$ PDCA$^+$)。因此，尽管高度专业化但DC仍是极端异质的，并且不同的DC亚型在体内执行不同的功能。早期研究表明，各种DC亚类位于淋巴组织中的不同位置，并且在其趋化因子、趋化因子受体和归巢受体的表达中表现出显著的差异。它们也在激活后分泌不同的细胞因子，随后产生不同的细胞因子环境以分化适应性T细胞。例如，浆细胞样DC产生大量的Ⅰ型干扰素，而骨髓DC在激活后分泌高水平的IL–12。

DC的主要功能是吞噬、加工和向适应性免疫系统的细胞呈递外来抗原。然而，DC是非常动态的，它们的表型和功能可以通过各种机制进行调节。它们可以表达令人难以置信的复杂阵列的 toll 样受体（见下文），允许它们对微生物产物或内源性组织产物(统称为“危险信号”)做出反应;它们能够产生并且也响应过多的炎性细胞因子。这些反应通常会导致 DC 进一步增殖和成熟,如通过细胞表面上 MHC 分子和 T 细胞共刺激分子(例如 CD80、CD86、CD40 和 OX40 配体等)的高表达所反映。在这个过程中,DC 通常转化为在适应性免疫细胞活化中高度有效的抗原呈递细胞(APC)(见第 6 章)。因此,根据是否存在“危险信号”,DC 可以保持休眠细胞的状态或变得完全活化,并且有证据表明,静息和活化的 DC 可以在体内执行不同的功能。活化的 DC 可有效触发免疫激活，而静息的 DC 可能需要通过激活和支持调节细胞来实现免疫耐受[6]。在幼稚小鼠中 DC 的遗传消融导致广泛的自身免疫疾病,表明 DC 不仅对于强大的免疫而且对于耐受性和免疫稳定都是必要的[7]。因此,DC 提供了先天性和适应性免疫系统之间的基本联系；它们也很好地定位免疫和免疫耐受之间的界面。

单核细胞和巨噬细胞

单核细胞和巨噬细胞是具有许多特殊特征的单核吞噬细胞。单核细胞从骨髓前体细胞发育而来,驻留在血液中，并且在炎症触发时，它们迅速渗透到炎症部位,在那里成熟为巨噬细胞[8]。在一些器官中,巨噬细胞获得额外的组织特异性特征并且成为器官的完整细胞组分，例如肝脏中的库普弗细胞和脑中的神经胶质细胞。在人类中,单核细胞构成血液中外周循环白细胞的 5%~10%。虽然单核细胞和巨噬细胞密切相关,但它们可以通过不同的表面标记来区分。例如，单核细胞是 CD11b^{高}和 F4/80^{-}，并且它们表达低水平的 MHC Ⅱ类和 CD80、CD86、CD40 共刺激分子。相反,巨噬细胞是 CD11b^{高}和 F4/80^{+}，并且还具有高水平的表面 MHC Ⅱ类、CD80、CD86 和 CD40 分子。除了在炎症部位分化为巨噬细胞外，单核细胞还在选择的模型中原位分化成骨髓 DC。此外,CD14^{+} CD16^{-}单核细胞在吞噬作用方面高度有效，并且可以产生高水平的炎症细胞因子,而 CD14^{低} CD16^{+}单核细胞表达 MHC Ⅱ类分子,并且在抗原呈递中高度有效[8]。此外,使用活体显微镜直接检查血液中单核细胞的研究揭示了其额外的复杂性。例如，Ly6C^{-}GR1^{-}单核细胞巡逻血管壁,并且在外渗后分化成Ⅱ型(M2)巨噬细胞(见下文),而 Ly6C^{+} GR1^{+}单核细胞分化为树突状细胞样细胞或产生Ⅰ型巨噬细胞(M1)[9]。

巨噬细胞是炎症部位的主要细胞浸润物，它们主要作为 APC 和炎症细胞起作用[10]。巨噬细胞有效吞噬外来实体，然后将抗原表位呈递给 T 细胞以启动适应性免疫。它们还产生以及响应大量的炎症细胞因子,从而进一步扩增它们的吞噬作用和 APC 功能。类似于 DC，巨噬细胞也由多个表型和功能不同的子集组成。刺激巨噬细胞的细胞因子环境在巨噬细胞的极化中起决定性作用。例如,在富含 IFN-γ、TNF-α 或 IL-12 的环境中，巨噬细胞极化为Ⅰ型巨噬细胞或 M1 巨噬细胞。M1 巨噬细胞是高度炎症细胞,促进 Th1 诱导,主要通过产生活性氧和 TNF 表现出细胞杀伤活性[11]。另一方面，Ⅱ型巨噬细胞或 M2 巨噬细胞在富含 IL-4 的环境中产生,M2 巨噬细胞表现出免疫调节功能并促进伤口愈合[12,13]。机制上,IL-4 刺激巨噬细胞中的精氨酸酶活性,将精氨酸转化为鸟氨酸,导致胶原产生增加和伤口愈合。M2 巨噬细胞还可产生抑制 T 细胞活化的抑制性细胞因子 IL-10、TGF-β 和前列腺素 E2。M1 和 M2 巨噬细胞可能代表相当广泛的巨噬细胞功能谱的极端，但它们强调了巨噬细胞的可塑性和环境因素在确定巨噬细胞功能中的重要性[14]。

此外，在某些条件下，一些巨噬细胞可能成为 Foxp3^{+} Tregs 的有效诱导剂,间接促进免疫调节的 PD-L1 的表达(见第 5 章)[15,16],而其他促进免疫调节并通过分化成骨髓来源的抑制细胞(MDSC),这是一种具有强效免疫抑制性质的细胞[17]产生耐受性。最后,有新发现的证据表明，巨噬细胞可以产生同种异体反应和直接响应同种[18]或异种抗原[19],虽然这种同种异体反应的确切分子基础仍有待定义。

自然杀伤细胞

自然杀伤(NK)细胞是固有免疫系统中的主要细胞类型,代表血液中的第三大淋巴细胞群(除了 T 细胞和 B 细胞)。NK 细胞在血液、脾脏、淋巴结和其他淋巴组织中表现良好,它们也大量存在于非淋巴部位,特别是在肝和肺中[20]。NK 细胞存在于炎症部位的细胞浸润中,它们与其他固有和适应性免疫细胞相互作用。

成熟的 NK 细胞显示出显著的细胞溶解活性,它们容易杀死靶细胞且不会引发先前的抗原，其与自适应 T 细胞形成鲜明对比。靶细胞杀伤主要由穿孔素和颗粒酶的释放介导，穿孔素和颗粒酶紧密填充在NK细胞内作为大的预形成颗粒，并且NK细胞的靶细胞识别触发快速脱粒和靶细胞凋亡。NK细胞在刺激后也产生大量细胞因子，并且这些细胞因子包括促炎（例如IFN-γ、TNF）和抗炎细胞因子（例如IL-10、TGF-β），因此对免疫反应的性质产生不同影响。

NK细胞的一个关键特征是它们表达的细胞表面受体具有多样性，这些受体共同控制NK细胞的发育，教育和效应子功能（图7.1）。从功能上，NK受体分为激活受体和抑制受体[21,22]。激活受体包括小鼠的天然细胞毒性受体或NCR（NKp46、NKp44和NKp30），c型凝集素样Ly49受体（例如Ly49H和Ly49D）和人类的杀伤免疫球蛋白样受体（KIR）和NKG2家族受体（NKG2C）。某些NK亚群也表达作为激活受体的CD16和CD27。在小鼠中，抑制性NK受体属于Ly49家族（例如Ly49C、Ly49G和Ly49I），而人类NK细胞表达KIR家族的抑制性受体，包括KIR2DL1、KIR2DL2、KIR2DL3、KIR3DL1和KIR3DL2。在人类和小鼠中，NK细胞也表达异二聚体抑制性受体NKG2A-CD94。除了少数例外，大多数NK活化受体在其细胞质结构域中缺乏信号基序。相反，它们募集衔接分子DAP10、DAP12、CD3ζ或FcεR-Iγ以转导激活信号。相比之下，抑制性NK受体直接通过其细胞质尾部的免疫受体酪氨酸抑制基序（ITIM）在发送信号。可以预见，这种NK受体的配体是非常多样的，其包括病原体、多态性MHC Ⅰ类分子或Ⅰ类相关分子受损或应激细胞上的从头诱导分子。

许多NK生物学都涉及抑制性受体。如上所述，抑制性受体的配体是自身MHC Ⅰ类分子，并且通过NK抑制性受体的自身MHC Ⅰ类的结合防止自我破坏并确保自身耐受性。这样的NK细胞也被选中经历进一步成熟成为针对非自身靶目标的功能性杀伤剂。这个特征是在发育中获得的，通常被称为“NK教育”或“NK许可”[23]。外周中的大多数成熟NK细胞表达至少一种抑制性受体，因此是完全许可的。个体NK细胞表

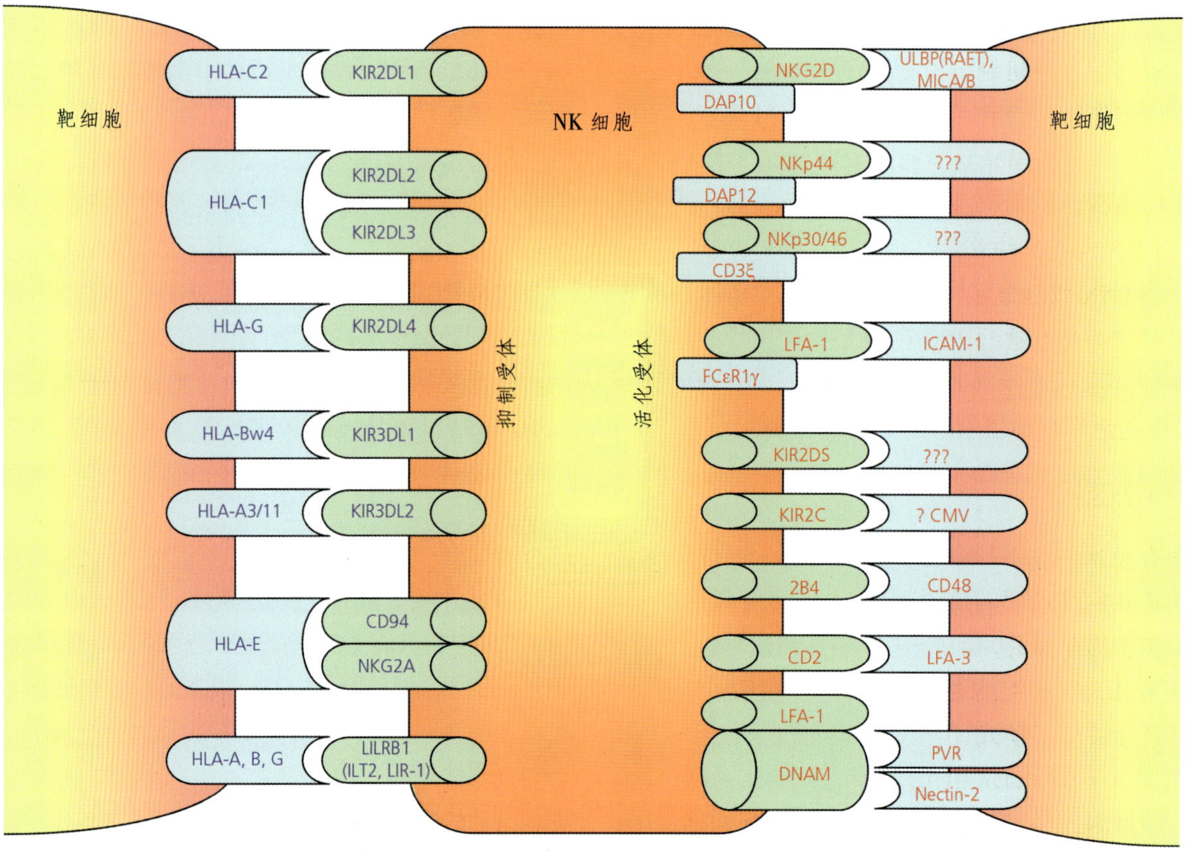

图7.1 人类NK细胞表达多种活化和抑制性受体。人类NK细胞上的NK受体可以分为激活受体和抑制受体。抑制受体的配体是自身MHC Ⅰ类分子，而激活受体的配体包括病原体、一些MHC分子和在应激或损伤的细胞上的诱导表面分子。来自激活和抑制受体的信号共同控制NK细胞的功能。

达的抑制性受体越多,它们对靶细胞的杀伤潜力越大。那些不能表达抑制性受体的 NK 细胞是无能的或无活力的(未经许可的 NK 细胞)。因此,在遇到缺失或具有下调的自身 MHC Ⅰ类分子的靶细胞时,NK 细胞将释放其强有力的杀伤活性。这在某些情况下也适用于移植(骨髓和实体器官移植)中 MHC Ⅰ型错配的靶细胞[24,25],在这种情况下 NK 介导的杀伤被称为“自我识别缺失”[26]。然而,在大多数情况下,NK 细胞不断地调查周围环境,整合来自激活和抑制受体的信号,然后确定它们的行动。因此,如果使用多个激活受体,这样的激活受体可以超越抑制信号以启动 NK 介导的靶细胞杀伤。例如,除了自身 MHC Ⅰ类之外,损伤和应激的细胞通常表达 NK 激活受体的多种配体,因此通常被 NK 细胞杀死,这种过程也称为“诱导自我识别”。

实质上,NK 细胞受抑制和激活信号的平衡控制,最终结果由一系列信号决定。在生理条件下,抑制性信号占优势。在病毒感染的情况下,不表达抑制性受体的 NK 细胞(未经许可的 NK 细胞)比表达抑制性受体 NK 细胞反应更好。此外,NK 许可是一个动态和连续的过程,以这种方式成熟的 NK 细胞可以重新接受教育[27]。另外,不同的调节机制可以在控制 NK 细胞产生细胞因子方面起作用。NK 细胞的多样性和可塑性表明它们在免疫反应中的作用是复杂的。

证据表明,NK 细胞可能具有适应性免疫的一些特征,特别是免疫记忆的获得。小鼠模型中的精细研究表明,激活后 NK 细胞显示出类似于 $CD8^+$ T 细胞的扩增和收缩模式,并且这些 NK 细胞以增加的频率持续存在,在继发性再激发后响应增加的幅度和动力学[28]。关于 NK 细胞记忆在移植中的意义了解很少。

固有传感器

固有免疫细胞对病原体和组织损伤有强烈反应,这是由最初称为模式识别受体或 PRR 的一系列复杂的分子传感器介导的。这些传感器分子识别来自细菌、分枝杆菌、DNA 和 RNA 病毒、真菌和原生动物的保守的病原体相关分子模式(PAMP),它们还可识别被称为损伤相关分子模式(DAMP)或报警蛋白的受损或受应激的自体细胞结构,这些结构的示例包括热休克蛋白、肽聚糖、高迁移率组盒染色体蛋白 1(HMGB1)、硫酸肝素、葡萄糖调节蛋白、纤维蛋白原、透明质酸和核苷酸片段(见第 2 章)。通过相应配体与这些先天传感器的结合引起免疫和炎症基因的激活,其产物驱动免疫应答以消除侵入的病原体或促进组织修复[29]。

到目前为止,已鉴定出三个家族的固有传感器,每个家族包括许多成员(图 7.2)。Toll 样受体或 TLR 是迄今为止研究最多的家族[30]。其他两个家族包括 NOD 样受体(NLR)[31]和 RIG 样受体(RLR)[32]。TLR 家族由至少 13 个成员组成,除了与内体膜相关的细胞内受体 TLR3、TLR7、TLR8 和 TLR9 之外,其余的是由细胞外结构域、跨膜结构域和细胞内结构域组成的跨膜受体。细胞外结构域包含参与配体结合的多个富含亮氨酸的重复基序(LRR),细胞内结构域信号、激活 NF-κB 转录因子的 MyD88 依赖性通路或刺激Ⅰ型干扰素的 TRIF 依赖性通路[33]。与膜锚定的 TLR 相反,NLR 是由参与配体结合、寡聚化和信号传导的多个功能结构域组成的游离胞质蛋白。在 NLR 家族中有 23 个成员,但 NOD1、NOD2、NALP1-3 和 Ipaf 是研究最多的。NOD1 和 NOD2 激活 NF-κB,随后表达强烈的炎症细胞因子,包括前 IL-1β 和前 IL-18。NALP1-3、Ipaf 形成炎性小体并激活半胱天冬酶 1 和半胱天冬酶 5,导致活性 IL-1β 和 IL-18 的加工和生产[30]。RLR 是一种有趣的先天传感器家族,它们类似于 NLR 的细胞质蛋白。与细胞内 TLR(TLR3、TLR7、TLR8 和 TLR9)相似,RLR 刺激 NF-κB 活化和Ⅰ型干扰素产生。然而,RLR 在细胞质中感知病毒核酸,而细胞内 TLR 在核内体间室识别病毒产物[32]。此外,RLR 广泛表达于固有免疫细胞,对Ⅰ型干扰素的反应迅速上调。总之,这些传感器分子家族提供了针对病原体和组织损伤的非凡的预警系统。

TLR、NLR 和 RLR 对病原体的应答有一定的特异性。TLR 识别细胞外和细胞内病原体,并且单个 TLR 响应不同的实体。NLR 检测细胞内细菌衍生产物,而 RLR 检测细胞内病毒核酸。这些受体还彼此相互作用以触发最佳反应,如 NOD1-2 和 NALP1-3 在活性 IL-1 和 IL-18 的生成中相互作用。这些受体的刺激导致固有免疫细胞的激活、有效的促炎细胞因子的产生、DC 的成熟和适应性免疫的启动。因此,先天传感器起着连接先天和自适应反应的关键作用(见第 5 章)。

补体

补体是固有免疫系统的组成部分,由许多血清蛋白(C1~C9)组成(图 7.3)。血清补体主要在肝脏中产生,研究表明,其他组织和细胞也在局部产生补体。补

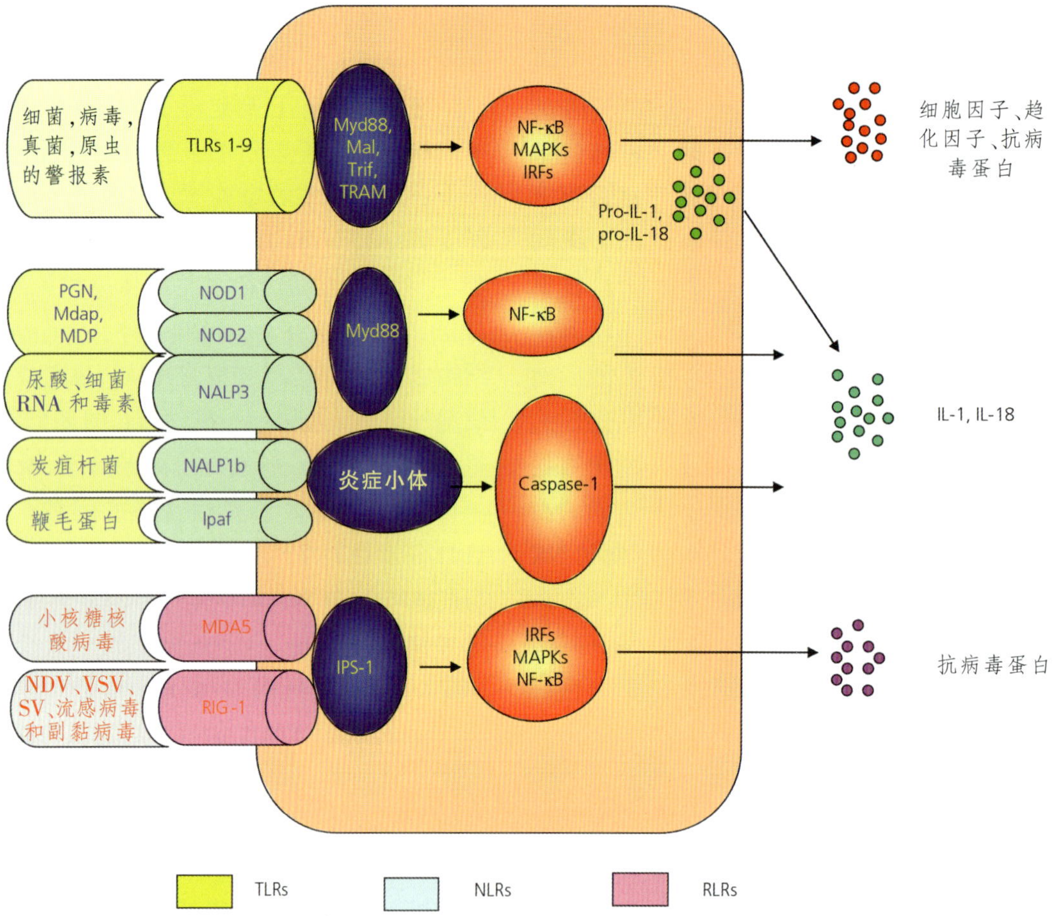

图 7.2 由固有免疫细胞表达的分子传感器。固有传感器大致分为三个家族，包括跨膜受体和细胞内受体。它们对来自受损细胞的病原体产物和内源性配体起反应，具有一定程度的特异性。它们一起提供了一个特别的预警系统来检测和响应“危险信号”。

体激活受到正负调节剂的严格控制[34]。补体激活的三种不同途径在第2章中进行了综述。

补体激活的经典途径是抗体介导血管损伤的主要效应机制。然而，包括缺血再灌注损伤在内的其他炎症反应中，补体产物可另外作为“危险信号”起作用，并通过作为化学引诱剂辅助T细胞启动。补体活化可以被多种调节蛋白抑制。衰变加速因子(DAF，CD55)是一种细胞表面分子，其加速C3转化酶的衰变，从而阻止补体级联的放大和下游膜攻击复合物的形成[35]。其他抑制性蛋白包括CD46和CD59。由于它们的调节特性，这种抑制性蛋白质已经被作为靶标以预防补体介导的移植物损伤，包括缺血再灌注损伤，这将在下面讨论。

除介导细胞裂解、化学吸引和先天细胞活化外，补体的作用最近已显著扩大，包括T细胞活化的共刺激[36,37]和DC的成熟[38]。T细胞和DC可以产生补体组分，并且还表达C3a和C5a的受体。这两种细胞类型都利用补体途径发挥最佳功能。在这种情况下，原位产生的补体而非全身补体至关重要[39]。类似地，移植物衍生的补体已经显示在移植后有助于移植物损伤[40]。

对移植物的固有免疫反应

免疫系统以显著不同的方式响应于同种异体移植，从缺血再灌注损伤到排斥，最终到耐受诱导，并且先天臂密切参与所有过程，从而严重影响移植的结果。

缺血再灌注损伤(IRI)

在实体器官移植中，手术创伤、移植物缺血、保存和再灌注是手术的组成部分，其不可避免地导致组织损伤。缺血时代谢供应和需求的不平衡还将导致严重的移植物内缺氧和血管功能障碍，导致进一步的移植物损伤。损伤或受损的移植物组分首先通过多种途径移动固有免疫细胞，所述途径导致组织炎症、活性氧物质(ROS)和促炎细胞因子的产生、APC活化，并且最终

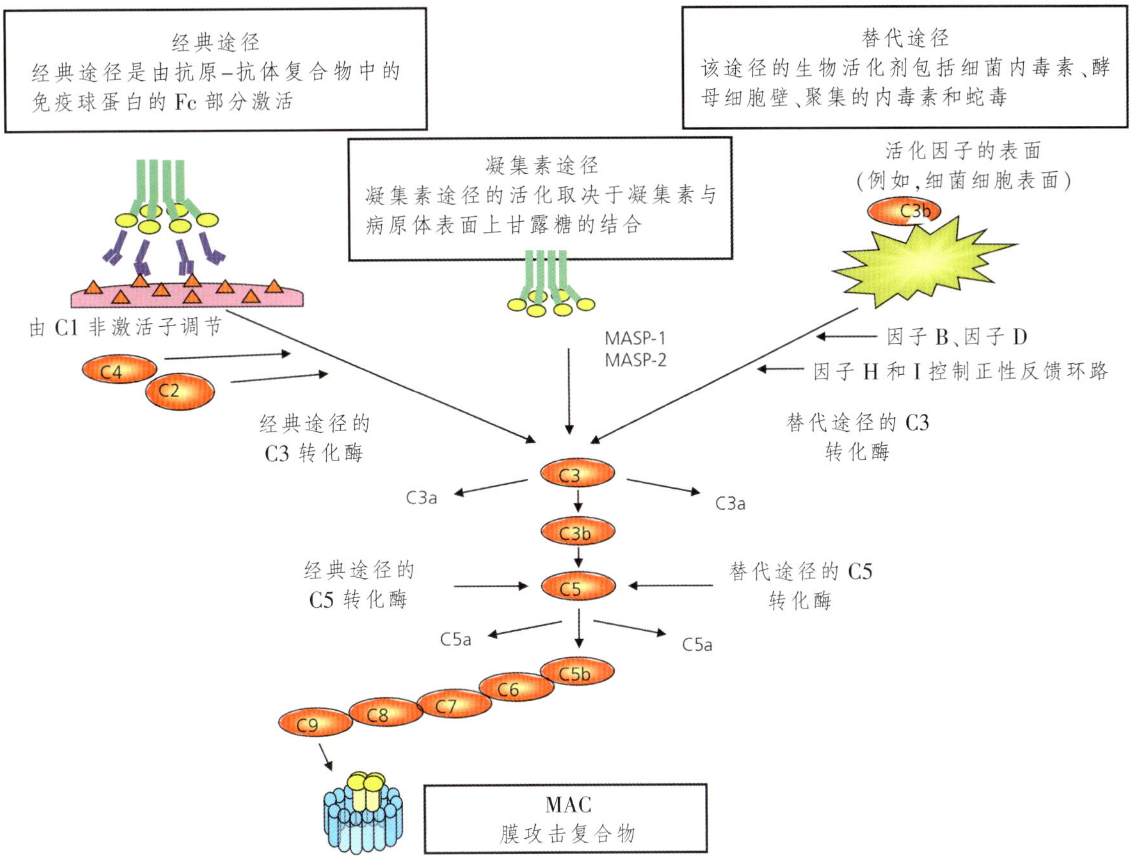

图 7.3 图示补体激活途径。补体激活由三种途径介导:经典途径(由抗原–抗体复合物介导)、替代途径和凝集素途径启动。所有途径集中于 C3 转化酶的活化,最终形成膜攻击复合物(MAC),其通过破坏细胞膜来介导细胞裂解。

导致移植物损失的更大风险。该过程涉及几乎所有固有免疫细胞、分子传感器和途径。

移植缺血再灌注损伤(IRI)引发单核细胞、巨噬细胞、中性粒细胞和 NK 细胞以及某些记忆 T 细胞迅速流入移植物。IRI 还会动员移植物间质 DC 和宿主 DC 的迁移。这种大规模的细胞浸润可能是对有效的炎性细胞因子、趋化因子和补体产物的反应,为细胞反应的协作、激活和扩增创造了理想的基础。在这种情况下,关键过程包括:①来自受损细胞的 DAMP 刺激 TLR;②通过活化的先天细胞产生额外的炎性细胞毒性细胞因子和 ROS;③能够诱导适应性反应的 APC 的成熟;④在其他健康细胞上诱导应激标记,这些细胞被 NK 细胞识别并引发 NK 介导的杀伤。所有这些反应都已在临床前模型中进行了广泛研究,并且某些途径正成为进一步临床开发的有吸引力的治疗靶点。例如,受损细胞释放大量核蛋白 HMGB1,其与 TLR2、TLR4 或 RAGE 结合以激活先天免疫细胞。因此,缺乏 TLR4、MyD88 和(或)TRIF 的小鼠免受 IRI 的影响[41]。同样,在肝脏 IRI 和心肌梗死模型中,TLR4 缺陷小鼠的组织损伤程度显著降低[42,43]。在细胞水平,用脂质体氯磷酸盐消耗巨噬细胞或抑制它们向移植物的运输减弱了组织的损伤。此外,在肾 IRI 模型中,白喉毒素 CD11c–DTR 小鼠肾脏 DC 的消耗可防止会导致肾功能不全的肾小管细胞坏死[44]。此外,在缺血再灌注后 NK 细胞通过识别诱导分子 Rae–1 易杀伤肾小管上皮细胞,NK 缺陷或抗体介导的 NK 耗竭可防止肾脏 IR 损伤[45]。这些发现为支持先天免疫系统在移植 IRI 中的重要性提供了坚实的证据。

补体还有助于缺血再灌注损伤,并且使用眼镜蛇毒因子抑制补体的开创性研究证明可减轻 IRI[46]。其他研究显示了 IRI 中各种补体成分的重要性[47]。例如,在各种动物模型中,补体受体 1、补体受体相关基因 Y、C1 酯酶、C3[48]、C5[49]、因子 B 和降解加速因子(DAF)[35,50]都涉及 IRI。实际上,在再灌注之前用抑制 C3 转化酶的 DAF 治疗小鼠,保护它们免受 IRI[51]。这种保护作用是由于补体激活和促炎细胞因子释放的减少。尽管源自肝脏的血清补体负责抗体引发介导的损伤，但似乎移植物衍生的补体也有助于IRI[40,52]。在鼠模型中已经显示，当移植C3缺陷肾脏时，具有正常血清补体水平的受体显示出移植物存活期延长。此外，这些移植物移植到同基因受体阻止IRI[53]。局部补体对组织损伤重要性的进一步证据来自研究，其中移植物内皮上补体调节蛋白DAF的过表达减少移植后IRI的程度[54]。

急性排斥

在大多数情况下，固有免疫细胞虽然具有各种效应机制，但不直接介导急性和完全同种异体移植排斥本身。然而，固有免疫细胞基本上参与适应性T细胞程序的控制，因此间接影响排斥反应的性质。固有免疫系统的这一方面在移植结果中起重要作用，并且越来越受到人们的赞赏。

移植物为固有免疫系统提供了理想的环境。IRI产生的"危险信号"刺激有效的促炎细胞因子如IL-1、IL-6、TNF和趋化因子(例如MIP-1α、MIP-1β、MCP-1、IP-10、RANTES等)，其动员移植间质DC并且介导宿主单核细胞、巨噬细胞、中性粒细胞和宿主DC以及适应性T细胞和B细胞的快速流入(见第2章)。浸润移植物的先天细胞在活化后产生另外的炎性细胞因子和趋化因子，进一步扩增移植物中的炎性环境。这种丰富的炎症环境驱动APC的增殖和成熟，包括在细胞表面上调MHCⅠ类、Ⅱ类分子和诱导共刺激分子(CD80、CD86、CD40、OX40L等)。成熟的APC有效地使T细胞和B细胞启动排斥反应[55]。因此，固有免疫细胞与适应性T细胞和B细胞配合以介导急性排斥。换句话说，适应性免疫细胞需要活化和成熟的APC来呈递同种异体抗原以触发它们的活化。这种移植物排斥的相互依赖性在一些临床前动物模型中显示。在次要的同种异体抗原错配的小鼠模型(男性对女性皮肤移植)中，适配子分子MyD88的遗传缺陷(其防止TLR信号传导并因此阻止APC的成熟)导致不确定的皮肤移植物存活[56]。在更严格的环境中，MyD88和TRIF的缺乏延长了MHC错配同种异体移植物的存活[57]。这些发现还突出了先天传感器在APC成熟和同种异体移植排斥中的重要性。

在急性排斥期间，存在APC，尤其是DC的相互迁移。宿主DC可以渗透移植的移植物，并且移植物DC可以归于宿主的引流淋巴结。这些途径在移植中的相对重要性是一个持续争论的问题，但是任一途径都可以引发急性排斥。尽管供体DC和宿主DC表达的同种异体抗原与T细胞不同，但是参与驱动它们活化和成熟的机制相同(即先天传感器，促炎细胞因子)，这允许它们最佳地结合T细胞。一些固有免疫细胞，例如巨噬细胞和NK细胞，一旦获得效应子功能，可显著促成急性排斥反应的破坏阶段。巨噬细胞长期以来在人肾移植的同种异体移植活检和动物模型中被鉴定，它们在通过免疫组织化学染色检测的浸润性白细胞中占40%~60%[58]，CD68是最常用于检测人巨噬细胞的胞内溶菌酶相关糖蛋白。还有观察发现，巨噬细胞浸润也见于伴有内皮炎或内膜动脉炎的急性血管排斥[59]。从急性排斥的动物模型观察，探索了巨噬细胞清除或拮抗作用[60–62]，显然这些细胞是针对同种异体移植物的急性反应的关键组分。这一结论也得到临床研究的支持。其中T细胞已经应用于阿仑单抗耗尽的肾同种异体移植受者中，在外周T细胞计数极低的情况下发生急性移植排斥，并且通常与单核细胞的大量浸润相关[63]。类似地，在使用阿仑单抗或胸腺球蛋白的肠移植中观察到嗜酸性粒细胞驱动的急性排斥反应[64]。沿着同一条线，NK细胞也有助于急性排斥。例如，在CD28KO小鼠中，NKG2D(NK细胞激活受体)抗体介导的阻断可显著延长心脏移植物存活[65]，表明NK细胞促进排斥反应[66]。此外，如果NK细胞被IL-15激活，它们本身能够在不存在T或B淋巴细胞的情况下介导急性排斥反应[67]。

在先天分子中，补体在同种异体移植排斥中具有独特的作用。在诱导补体活化的移植模型中，移植物破坏的速度令人难以置信(可以在数小时内)，并且是不可逆的。在这种情况下，移植排斥通常涉及血管内皮损伤、血液凝固和激活先天细胞而没有适应性T细胞的参与。最好的例子是由抗供体同种异体抗体引发的体液排斥或急性抗体介导的排斥(AMR)(见第6章)[68]。抗供体抗体(主要是抗供体HLA分子、ABO抗原和内皮抗原)与移植物中的供体抗原形成免疫复合物，通过经典途径激活补体级联。该过程是稳定的，由C1的活化引发，并且导致MAC(C5b~C9复合物)的形成，化学引诱物C3a和C5a的产生，并且因此导致移植物中大量细胞死亡、内移发炎和广泛的血液凝固。此外，最近的研究表明，T细胞和APC自身产生补体成分，并且还表达选择的补体元件的受体(例如C3a和C5a的受体)。因此，它们可以通过影响APC的成熟和在同种异体抗原刺激下T细胞活化的共刺激，使局部产生的补体发挥最佳作用[52,69]。此外，C3aR和C5aR在APC上的结合诱导先天细胞因子(IL-12、IL-23)的释放和上调共刺激分子，再次放大T效应物应答[37,39]。这提供了先天分子如何增强移植环境中适应性免疫应答的另一个实例。补体在同种异体反应性T细胞免疫和IRI中的作用至少部分解释了缺乏C3的鼠肾同种异体移植物显示出长期存活的事实[40]，而缺乏DAF的那些肾脏同种异体移植物结果更差[70]。

慢性排斥

慢性同种异体移植排斥主要涉及移植物血管系统[71,72]。在形态上，慢性排斥的特征在于同心的内膜增生和最终的血管闭塞，并且该损伤影响移植物中的所有大小血管。此外，广泛的移植物间质性纤维化通常伴随血管变化。这些特征对于移植是独特的，因此也称为移植血管病变。与急性排斥相比，慢性排斥发生反应需要更长的时间，并且通常发生在患者移植后几年。这已成为阻碍临床长期移植成功的主要原因。慢性排斥的确切机制仍然是难以捉摸的，但是目前的观点是慢性排斥可能是移植物损伤和长期重塑的表现，期间免疫和非免疫都受到影响。重要的是，目前的研究已表明先天性免疫机制在慢性移植排斥的发病机制中的重要性。

慢性排斥有明显的特征。与急性排斥相反，固有免疫细胞(主要是单核细胞和巨噬细胞)主导病变中的细胞浸润，并且也经常检测到同种抗体和补体沉积。此外，分子谱研究经常显示慢性病变中的持续组织炎症，如多种炎症细胞因子的高表达所示。因此，可以想到由固有细胞、通路和固有分子传感器驱动的组织损伤可显著促进移植血管病变的发展。

TLR信号与动脉粥样硬化的发展密切相关，动脉粥样硬化是慢性同种异体移植血管病变的标志[73,74]。最近，在完全不匹配的小鼠肾移植模型中，已发现TLR2、TLR4和衔接蛋白MyD88、TRIF是慢性排斥的关键介质[75]。此外，在具有同种异体移植物内皮功能障碍证据的心脏移植患者中，TLR4表达和分泌作为TLR信号传导的下游靶标IL-12和TNF的水平高于没有内皮功能障碍的心脏受体[76]表明，先天传感器参与细胞激活。在细胞水平，巨噬细胞浸润心脏同种异体移植物，并在慢性排斥的动物模型中造成移植血管病变[77]。在这个模型中，使用角叉菜胶部分消耗巨噬细胞降低了慢性血管病变的严重性。这独立于吞噬作用，因为用钆治疗会抑制吞噬作用，对疾病的严重性没有影响。在另一项研究中，使用腺病毒策略靶向巨噬细胞功能改善了间质性纤维化和肾小管萎缩(IF/TA)的大鼠模型中同种异体移植物功能障碍的组织学特征[78]。单核细胞/巨噬细胞在化学引诱物、秘密生长因子和促纤维化细胞因子如TGF-β和IL-13的影响下浸润受损的同种异体移植实质[12]。它们还可以直接分化为纤维细胞[79]，从而促进细胞外基质蛋白的合成，并刺激管状上皮细胞转变为成纤维细胞[12]。在人类移植受者，早期活检标本中巨噬细胞的存在预示着IF/TA的发展[80,81]。

针对HLA、MHCⅠ类多肽相关序列A(MICA)、自身抗原和内皮抗原的循环同种抗体的存在增加了长期移植物损伤的风险[82,83]。由移植物损伤中同种抗体启动的效应器应答主要涉及先天途径。最重要的是补体的激活。事实上，在人类的肾移植中，慢性排斥中所见的肾小球病和动脉疾病与移植物中的C4d沉积密切相关，支持补体活化在慢性移植物损伤中的作用[68]。在动物模型中，C6缺陷影响补体级联的终末膜攻击复合物的形成，降低了移植物动脉硬化的严重性和发病率[84]。研究还证明了在慢性肾移植物损伤中局部衍生的补体(而不是全身补体)的重要性。例如，当移植到野生型受体中时，C3缺陷肾移植物对阿霉素诱导的肾小管损伤具有抗性[85]。在C3a受体缺陷小鼠中，阿霉素诱导较少的肾损伤，间质1型胶原和α-平滑肌肌动蛋白的表达较低。通过移植物来源的补体损伤也被认为影响人类的长期移植结果。

有些情况下，同种异体抗体诱导的慢性同种异体移植物排斥仍然可以独立于补体而产生，研究发现，NK细胞是驱动慢性移植物损伤的关键效应细胞[86]。在心脏移植的小鼠模型中，移植受体对于T细胞和B细胞[即重组酶激活基因(RAG)缺陷小鼠]是有缺陷的，将供体同种异体抗体输注到移植受体中可诱导突出的同种异体移植血管病变。使用非补体结合异体抗体或补体激活缺陷的受体小鼠观察到类似的发现。这表明抗体介导的移植血管病变仍然可以通过补体依赖性途径发生。事实上，在临床上有一些肾移植患者在没有C4d沉积的情况下发生动脉病变或肾小球病变[87]，再次支持了非补体依赖机制。有趣的是，NK细胞被确定为移植血管病变中独立于补体的关键介质，因为NK细胞的消耗或移植受体NK细胞的缺乏完全阻止了供体同种异体抗体诱导的慢性排斥反应的发生[86]。另一个观察是,在MHC相容的肾移植患者队列中,供体和受体之间的KIR错配(其产生同种异体反应性NK细胞)与最差的移植结果相关,因此间接地表明,NK细胞在临床慢性移植物损失中的作用[88]。这些研究结果提示人们关注固有免疫细胞和慢性同种异体移植排斥的机制。

移植接受或提示耐受

移植耐受是积极获得的状态，其中对同种异体移植物的细胞病变反应缺失，而对病原体的细胞致病反应保存良好。重要的是,这种耐受状态可以维持稳定而无须延长的免疫抑制。这在第11章中将进行深入讨论。传统上,固有免疫系统的细胞被认为是免疫应答的启动子,因此与排斥相关。然而,新的数据显示,这种细胞也可能是诱导和维持移植耐受性所必需的。

移植耐受的关键原则是促进效应T细胞的死亡和刺激调节细胞(见第8章)[89]。固有免疫细胞和途径可以对耐受诱导过程的两个臂产生显著影响(图7.4)。例如,DC不仅需要强大的免疫力,而且还需要耐受性,因为在初始小鼠体内缺失CD11c^{+}DC会降低耐受性并诱导广泛的自身免疫[7]。这一发现导致"耐受性DC"在耐受性诱导中的特性和应用。事实上,DC以几种不同的方式促进耐受性。成熟DC可以在增殖暴发后驱动细胞病变效应T细胞的细胞凋亡缺失；DC的亚类也介导Foxp3^{+} Treg的诱导或天然Treg的内环境稳定。此外,DC，特别是CD8^{+} DC，它们表达的DEC205、Clec9A、CD36、Tim-1和Tim-4[90-92]对凋亡细胞的吞噬非常有效,并且凋亡细胞的清除是维持耐受性的关键过程[93]。此外,同种异体凋亡细胞的吞噬作用抑制DC成熟,其下调同种异体刺激功能,同时促进Treg细胞[94]。因此,作为细胞治疗方法的"致耐受性DC"在移植耐受中仍具有希望。

其他先天细胞类型在耐受性诱导中表现出相似的特征。在某些情况下,单核细胞/巨噬细胞可以发挥有助于维持外周耐受性的有效的抗炎和免疫抑制效应。例如,活化的M2巨噬细胞或调节巨噬细胞(Mreg,参见第2章）能够分泌抗炎细胞因子，例如IL-10和TGF-β，参与逐渐减少的免疫应答和移植物炎症的消

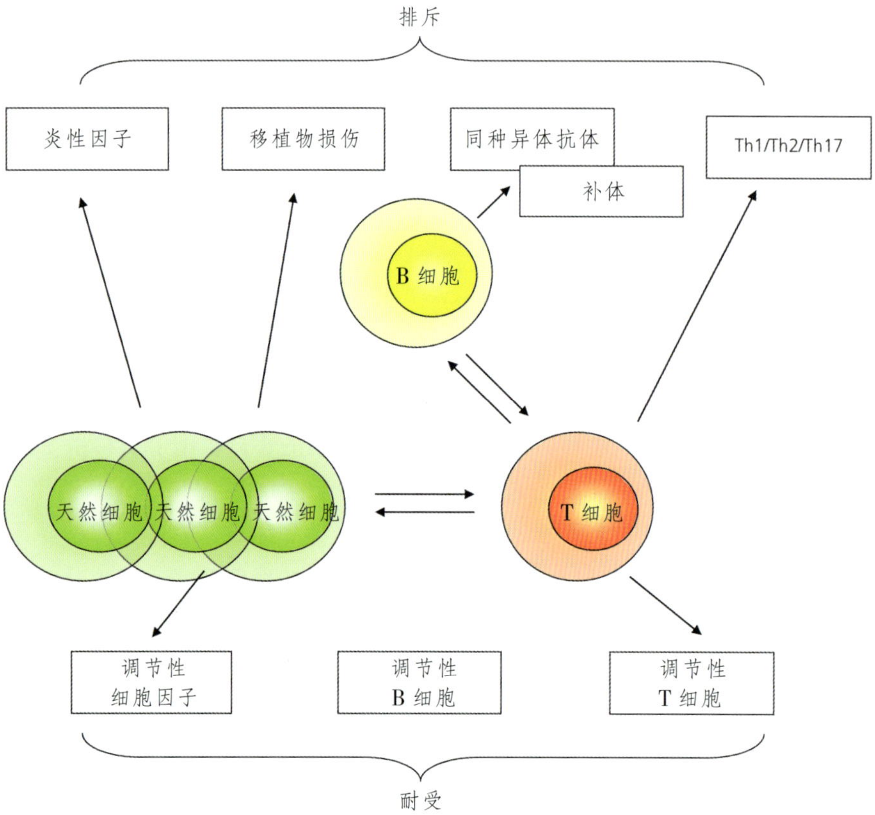

图7.4 固有和适应性免疫细胞在移植中的相互作用。固有免疫细胞类似于其自适应对应物,根据环境、模型和耐受性治疗,通过多种机制调节移植物排斥和耐受诱导。

退[12]。事实上，一些研究表明，过继转移 Mreg 可以改善实验性自身免疫性脑炎（多发性硬化的小鼠模型）的诱导，并通过诱导和扩大 Foxp3+ Treg 预防自身免疫性结肠炎[16]。另外，在人肾移植受者群体中过继转移供体来源的 Mreg 可显著减少免疫抑制药物的使用[95]。类似地，NK 细胞也采用不同的机制来促进移植耐受。NK 细胞由“缺失的自我识别”引导，可以消除移植物衍生的同种异体 DC，从而通过抗原呈递的直接途径减少 T 细胞引发[25]。NK 细胞杀伤供体细胞有利于间接抗原呈递，其牵涉耐受性诱导。此外，一些 NK 细胞通过 IL-10 依赖性机制表现出调节功能，并通过倾向于调节平衡来促进耐受[96]。

固有免疫细胞在移植环境中的显著二分法（排斥与耐受）最有可能是与环境无关的，因为不同的细胞亚群可以根据其成熟状态和与环境的相互作用而发挥不同的效应。例如，在许多情况下，NK 细胞可以是致耐受性的。然而，IL-15 信号通路使 NK 进一步成熟促进排斥反应。M1 巨噬细胞是促炎的，M2 巨噬细胞是免疫抑制的。此外，TLR 信号介导 DC 和单核细胞在排斥中的成熟。然而，Treg 也表达某些 TLR，并且 TLR 刺激可以增加 Treg 的抑制性质，从而促进耐受性。先天性途径的环境依赖性功能和先天性免疫细胞的环境依赖性调节是控制同种异体移植物免疫应答的主要挑战。

总结

总之，固有免疫的细胞在缺血再灌注损伤后早期被激活，并参与动物模型和人类的急性和慢性排斥的发病机制。一个重大的挑战是在移植环境中对体内固有免疫细胞不同亚群之间的复杂相互作用了解甚少。此外，先天性和适应性免疫之间的动态串扰使得我们必须进一步理解用于耐受诱导目的的两个臂。

致谢

感谢刘文涛博士协助准备图片。M.Y.Yeung 获得了美国心脏协会的教师转移补助金。X.C. Li 获得美国国立卫生研究院资助。

（胡士华 译　程倩 校）

参考文献

1. Murphy SP, Porrett PM, Turka LA. Innate immunity in transplant tolerance and rejection. Immunological Reviews. 2011;241:39–48.
2. Liu W, Li XC. An overview on non-T cell pathways in transplant rejection and tolerance. Current Opinion in Organ Transplantation. 2010;15:422–426.
3. LaRosa DF, Rahman AH, Turka LA. The innate immune system in allograft rejection and tolerance. Journal of Immunology. 2007;178:7503–7509.
4. Coquerelle C, Moser M. DC subsets in positive and negative regulation of immunity. Immunological Reviews. 2010;234:317–334.
5. Ueno H, Schmitt N, Klechevsky E, et al. Harnessing human dendritic cell subsets for medicine. Immunological Reviews. 2010;234:199–212.
6. Morelli AE, Thomson AW. Tolerogenic dendritic cells and the quest for transplant tolerance. Nature Reviews Immunology. 2007;7:610–621.
7. Ohnmacht C, Pullner A, King SBS, et al. Constitutive ablation of dendritic cells breaks self-tolerance of CD4 T cells and results in spontaneous fatal autoimmunity. Journal of Experimental Medicine. 2009;206:549–559.
8. Gordon S, Taylor PR. Monocyte and macrophage heterogeneity. Nature Reviews Immunology. 2005;5:953–964.
9. Auffray C, Fogg D, Garfa M, et al. Monitoring of blood vessels and tissues by a population of monocytes with patrolling behavior. Science. 2007;317:666–670.
10. Murray PJ, Wynn TA. Protective and pathogenic functions of macrophage subsets. Nature Reviews Immunology. 2011;11:723–737.
11. Serbina NV, Salazar-Mather TP, Biron CA, et al. TNF/iNOS-producing dendritic cells mediate innate immune defense against bacterial infection. Immunity. 2003;19:59–70.
12. Ricardo SD, Van Goor H, Eddy AA. Macrophage diversity in renal injury and repair. Journal of Clinical Investigation. 2008;118:3522–3530.
13. Wynn TA. Fibrotic disease and the TH1/TH2 paradigm. Nature Reviews Immunology. 2004;4:583–594.
14. Biswas SK, Mantovani A. Macrophage plasticity and interaction with lymphocyte subsets: cancer as a paradigm. Nature Immunology. 2010;11:889–896.
15. Denning TL, Wang YC, Patel SR, et al. Lamina propria macrophages and dendritic cells differentially induce regulatory and interleukin 17-producing T cell responses. Nature Immunology. 2007;8:1086–1094.
16. Brem-Exner BG, Sattler C, Hutchinson JA, et al. Macrophages driven to a novel state of activation have anti-inflammatory properties in mice. Journal of Immunology. 2008;180:335–349.
17. Allavena P, Sica A, Garlanda C, et al. The Yin-Yang of tumor-associated macrophages in neoplastic progression and immune surveillance. Immunological Reviews. 2008;222:155–161.
18. Liu W, Xiao X, Demirci G, et al. Innate NK cells and macrophages recognize and reject allogeneic nonself in vivo via different mechanisms. Journal of Immunology. 2012;188:2703–2711.
19. Fox A, Mountford J, Braakhuis A, et al. Innate and adaptive immune responses to nonvascular xenografts: evidence that macrophages are direct effectors of xenograft rejection. Journal of Immunology. 2001;166:2133–2140.
20. Shi FD, Ljunggren HG, La Cava A, et al. Organ-specific features of natural killer cells. Nature Reviews Immunology. 2011;11:658–671.
21. Lanier LL. NK cell recognition. Annual Review of Immunology. 2005;23:225–274.
22. Lanier LL. Up on the tightrope: natural killer cell activation and inhibition. Nature Immunology. 2008;9:495–502.
23. Elliott JM, Yokoyama WM. Unifying concepts of MHC-dependent natural killer cell education. Trends in Immunology. 2011;32:364–372.
24. Ruggeri L, Capanni M, Urbani E, et al. Effectiveness of donor natural killer cell alloreactivity in mismatched hematopoietic transplants. Science. 2002;295:2097–2100.
25. Yu G, Xu X, Vu MD, et al. NK cells promote transplant tolerance by killing donor antigen-presenting cells. Journal of Experimental Medicine. 2006;203:1851–1858.
26. Kroemer A, Edtinger K, Li XC. The innate NK cells in transplant rejection and tolerance induction. Current Opinion in Organ Transplantation. 2008;13:339–343.
27. Sun JC. Re-educating natural killer cells. Journal of Experimental Medicine. 2010;207:2049–2052.
28. Sun JC, Beilke JN, Lanier LL. Adaptive immune features of natural killer cells. Nature. 2009;457:557–561.
29. Kawai T, Akira S. The role of pattern-recognition receptors in innate immunity: update on toll-like receptors. Nature Immunology. 2010;11:373–384.
30. Iwasaki A, Medzhitov R. Toll-like receptor control of the adaptive immune

responses. Nature Immunology. 2004;5:987–995.
31. Elinav E, Strowig T, Henao-Mejia J, et al. Regulation of the antimicrobial response by NLR proteins. Immunity. 2011;34:665–679.
32. Kato H, Takahasi K, Fujita T. RIG-I-like receptors: cytoplasmic sensors for non-self RNA. Immunological Reviews. 2011;243:91–98.
33. O'Neill LAJ, Bowie AG. The family of five: TIR-domain-containing adaptors in Toll-like receptor signalling. Nature Reviews Immunology. 2007;7:353–364.
34. Zipfel PF, Skerka C. Complement regulators and inhibitory proteins. Nature Reviews Immunology. 2009;9:729–740.
35. Medof ME, Kinoshita T, Nussenzweig V. Inhibition of complement activation on the surface of cells after incorporation of decay-accelerating factor (DAF) into their membranes. Journal of Experimental Medicine. 1984;160:1558–1578.
36. Heeger PS, Lalli PN, Lin F, et al. Decay-accelerating factor modulates induction of T cell immunity. Journal of Experimental Medicine. 2005;201:1523–1530.
37. Lalli PN, Strainic MG, Yang M, et al. Locally produced C5a binds to T cell expressed C5aR to enhance effector T-cell expansion by limiting antigen-induced apoptosis. Blood. 2008;112:1759–1766.
38. Castellano G, Woltman AM, Nauta AJ, et al. Maturation of dendritic cells abrogates C1q production in vivo and in vitro. Blood. 2004;103:3813–3820.
39. Strainic MG, Liu J, Huang D, et al. Locally produced complement fragments C5a and C3a provide both costimulatory and survival signals to naive $CD4^+$ T cells. Immunity. 2008;28:425–435.
40. Pratt JR, Basheer SA, Sacks SH. Local synthesis of complement component C3 regulates acute renal transplant rejection. Nature Medicine. 2002;8:582–587.
41. Shigeoka AA, Holscher TD, King AJ, et al. TLR2 is constitutively expressed within the kidney and participates in ischemic renal injury through both myD88-dependent and -independent pathways. Journal of Immunology. 2007;178: 6252–6258.
42. Zhai Y, Shen XD, O'Connell R, et al. Cutting edge: TLR4 activation mediates liver ischemia/reperfusion inflammatory response via IFN regulatory factor 3-dependent MyD88-independent pathway. Journal of Immunology. 2004; 173:7115–7119.
43. Chong AJ, Shimamoto A, Hampton CR, et al. Toll-like receptor 4 mediates ischemia/reperfusion injury of the heart. Journal of Thoracic and Cardiovascular Surgery. 2004;128:170–179.
44. Li L, Okusa MD. Macrophages, dendritic cells, and kidney ischemia-reperfusion injury. Seminars in Nephrology. 2010;30:268–277.
45. Zhang ZX, Wang S, Huang X, et al. NK cells induce apoptosis in tubular epithelial cells and contribute to renal ischemia-reperfusion injury. Journal of Immunology. 2008;181:7489–7498.
46. Maroko PR, Carpenter CB, Chiariello M, et al. Reduction by cobra venom factor of myocardial necrosis after coronary artery occlusion. Journal of Clinical Investigation. 1978;61:661–670.
47. Diepenhorst GMP, Van Gulik TM, Hack CE. Complement-mediated ischemia-reperfusion injury: lessons learned from animal and clinical studies. Annals of Surgery. 2009;249:889–899.
48. Brown KM, Kondeatis E, Vaughan RW, et al. Influence of donor C3 allotype on late renal-transplantation outcome. New England Journal of Medicine. 2006; 354:2014–2023.
49. Zhou W, Farrar CA, Abe K, et al. Predominant role for C5b-9 in renal ischemia/reperfusion injury. Journal of Clinical Investigation. 2000;105:1363–1371.
50. Yamada K, Miwa T, Liu J, et al. Critical protection from renal ischemia reperfusion injury by CD55 and CD59. Journal of Immunology. 2004;172:3869–3875.
51. Lu X, Li Y, Simovic MO, et al. Decay-accelerating factor attenuates c-reactive protein-potentiated tissue injury after mesenteric ischemia/reperfusion. Journal of Surgical Research. 2011;167:e103–e115.
52. Zhou W, Medof ME, Heeger PS, et al. Graft-derived complement as a mediator of transplant injury. Current Opinion in Immunology. 2007;19:569–576.
53. Farrar CA, Zhou W, Lin T, et al. Local extravascular pool of C3 is a determinant of postischemic acute renal failure. FASEB Journal. 2006;20:217–226.
54. Pratt JR, Jones ME, Dong J, et al. Nontransgenic hyperexpression of a complement regulator in donor kidney modulates transplant ischemia/reperfusion damage, acute rejection, and chronic nephropathy. American Journal of Pathology. 2003;163:1457–1465.
55. Li XC, Rothstein DM, Sayegh MH. Costimulatory pathways in transplantation: challenges and new developments. Immunological Reviews. 2009;229:271–293.
56. Goldstein DR, Tesar BM, Akira S, et al. Critical role of the Toll-like receptor signal adaptor protein MyD88 in acute allograft rejection. Journal of Clinical Investigation. 2003;111:1571–1578.
57. McKay D, Shigeoka A, Rubinstein M, et al. Simultaneous deletion of MyD88 and Trif delays major histocompatibility and minor antigen mismatch allograft rejection. European Journal of Immunology. 2006;36:1994–2002.
58. Hancock WW, Thomson NM, Atkins RC. Composition of interstitial cellular infiltrate identified by monoclonal antibodies in renal biopsies of rejecting human renal allografts. Transplantation. 1983;35:458–463.
59. Matheson PJ, Dittmer ID, Beaumont BW, et al. The macrophage is the predominant inflammatory cell in renal allograft intimal arteritis. Transplantation. 2005;79:1658–1662.
60. Gao W, Topham PS, King JA, et al. Targeting of the chemokine receptor CCR1 suppresses development of acute and chronic cardiac allograft rejection. Journal of Clinical Investigation. 2000;105:35–44.
61. Jose MD, Ikezumi Y, Van Rooijen N, et al. Macrophages act as effectors of tissue damage in acute renal allograft rejection. Transplantation. 2003;76:1015–1022.
62. Qi F, Adair A, Ferenbach D, et al. Depletion of cells of monocyte lineage prevents loss of renal microvasculature in murine kidney transplantation. Transplantation. 2008;86:1267–1274.
63. Kirk AD, Hale DA, Mannon RB, et al. Results from a human renal allograft tolerance trial evaluating the humanized CD52-specific monoclonal antibody alemtuzumab (Campath-1H). Transplantation. 2003;76:120–129.
64. Wu T, Bond G, Martin D, et al. Histopathologic characteristics of human intestine allograft acute rejection in patients pretreated with thymoglobulin or alemtuzumab. American Journal of Gastroenterology. 2006;101:1617–1624.
65. Kim J, Chang CK, Hayden T, et al. The activating immunoreceptor NKG2D and its ligands are involved in allograft transplant rejection. Journal of Immunology. 2007;179:6416–6420.
66. Degli-Esposti MA, Smyth MJ. Close encounters of different kinds: dendritic cells and NK cells take centre stage. Nature Reviews Immunology. 2005;5: 112–124.
67. Kroemer A, Xiao X, Degauque N, et al. The innate NK cells, allograft rejection, and a key role for IL-15. Journal of Immunology. 2008;180:7818–7826.
68. Colvin RB. Antibody-mediated renal allograft rejection: diagnosis and pathogenesis. Journal of the American Society of Nephrology. 2007;18:1046–1056.
69. Raedler H, Heeger PS. Complement regulation of T-cell alloimmunity. Current Opinion in Organ Transplantation. 2011;16:54–60.
70. Pavlov V, Raedler H, Yuan S, et al. Donor deficiency of decay-accelerating factor accelerates murine T cell-mediated cardiac allograft rejection. Journal of Immunology. 2008;181:4580–4589.
71. Solez K, Colvin RB, Racusen LC, et al. Banff 07 classification of renal allograft pathology: updates and future directions. American Journal of Transplantation. 2008;8:753–760.
72. Racusen LC, Regele H. The pathology of chronic allograft dysfunction. Kidney International. 2010;78(Suppl. 119):S27–S32.
73. Michelsen KS, Doherty TM, Shah PK, et al. TLR signaling: an emerging bridge from innate immunity to atherogenesis. Journal of Immunology. 2004;173: 5901–5907.
74. Mann DL. The emerging role of innate immunity in the heart and vascular system: for whom the cell tolls. Circulation Research. 2011;108:1133–1145.
75. Wang S, Schmaderer C, Kiss E, et al. Recipient Toll-like receptors contribute to chronic graft dysfunction by both MyD88- and TRIF-dependent signaling. Disease Models and Mechanisms. 2010;3:92–103.
76. Methe H, Zimmer E, Grimm C, et al. Evidence for a role of toll-like receptor 4 in development of chronic allograft rejection after cardiac transplantation. Transplantation. 2004;78:1324–1331.
77. Kitchens WH, Chase CM, Uehara S, et al. Macrophage depletion suppresses cardiac allograft vasculopathy in mice. American Journal of Transplantation. 2007;7:2675–2682.
78. Yang J, Reutzel-Selke A, Steier C, et al. Targeting of macrophage activity by adenovirus-mediated intragraft overexpression of TNFRp55-Ig, IL-12p40, and vIL-10 ameliorates adenovirus-mediated chronic graft injury, whereas stimulation of macrophages by overexpression of IFN-(gamma) accelerates chronic graft injury in a rat renal allograft model. Journal of the American Society of Nephrology. 2003;14:214–225.
79. Niedermeier M, Reich B, Gomez MR, et al. $CD4^+$ T cells control the differentiation of $Gr1^+$ monocytes into fibrocytes. Proceedings of the National Academy of Sciences of the United States of America. 2009;106:17892–17897.
80. Pilmore HL, Painter DM, Bishop GA, et al. Early up-regulation of macrophages and myofibroblasts: a new marker for development of chronic renal allograft rejection. Transplantation. 2000;69:2658–2662.
81. Jevnikar AM, Mannon RB. Late kidney allograft loss: what we know about it, and what we can do about it. Clinical Journal of the American Society of Nephrology: CJASN. 2008;3(Suppl. 2):S56–S67.
82. Einecke G, Sis B, Reeve J, et al. Antibody-mediated microcirculation injury is the major cause of late kidney transplant failure. American Journal of Transplantation. 2009;9:2520–2531.
83. Gaston RS, Cecka JM, Kasiske BL, et al. Evidence for antibody-mediated injury as a Major determinant of late kidney allograft failure. Transplantation. 2010; 90:68–74.
84. Qian Z, Hu W, Liu J, et al. Accelerated graft arteriosclerosis in cardiac transplants. Transplantation. 2001;72:900–906.
85. Sheerin NS, Risley P, Abe K, et al. Synthesis of complement protein C3 in the kidney is an important mediator of local tissue injury. FASEB Journal. 2008; 22:1065–1072.

86. Hirohashi T, Chase CM, Della Pelle P, et al. A novel pathway of chronic allograft rejection mediated by NK cells and alloantibody. American Journal of Transplantation. 2012;12:313–321.
87. Sis B, Campbell PM, Mueller T, et al. Transplant glomerulopathy, late antibody-mediated rejection and the ABCD tetrad in kidney allograft biopsies for cause. American Journal of Transplantation. 2007;7:1743–1752.
88. Van Bergen J, Thompson A, Haasnoot GW, et al. KIR-ligand mismatches are associated with reduced long-term graft survival in HLA-compatible kidney transplantation. American Journal of Transplantation. 2011;11:1959–1964.
89. Li XC, Strom TB, Turka LA, et al. T cell death and transplantation tolerance. Immunity. 2001;14:407–416.
90. Schulz O, Reis E, Sousa C. Cross-presentation of cell-associated antigens by CD8(alpha)$^+$ dendritic cells is attributable to their ability to internalize dead cells. Immunology. 2002;107:183–189.
91. Iyoda T, Shimoyama S, Liu K, et al. The CD8$^+$ dendritic cell subset selectively endocytoses dying cells in culture and in vivo. Journal of Experimental Medicine. 2002;195:1289–1302.
92. Schnorrer P, Behrens GMN, Wilson NS, et al. The dominant role of CD8$^+$ dendritic cells in cross-presentation is not dictated by antigen capture. Proceedings of the National Academy of Sciences of the United States of America. 2006; 103:10729–10734.
93. Savill J, Fadok V. Corpse clearance defines the meaning of cell death. Nature. 2000;407:784–788.
94. Morelli AE, Larregina AT. Apoptotic cell-based therapies against transplant rejection: role of recipient's dendritic cells. Apoptosis. 2010;15:1083–1097.
95. Hutchinson JA, Riquelme P, Sawitzki B, et al. Cutting edge: immunological consequences and trafficking of human regulatory macrophages administered to renal transplant recipients. Journal of Immunology. 2011;187:2072–2078.
96. Deniz G, Erten G, Kucuksezer UC, et al. Regulatory NK Cells Suppress Antigen-Specific T Cell Responses. Journal of Immunology. 2008;180:850–857.

第 8 章

免疫调节机制

Kathryn J. Wood, Andrew Bushell, Joanna Hester

引言

在白细胞亚群中，大部分引起移植物损害的排斥反应的细胞也同样在管控免疫耐受反应中起作用[1]。在某些情况下，调节细胞包括一些特殊的亚群，这些亚群被选择为或分化成为具有功能性调控和抑制能力的细胞。在其他情况下，与异体组织或者淋巴组织一同出现的微环境将使得在该位置的免疫反应得到控制。在移植研究中，无论是在引起排斥和移植的细胞、器官以及组织破坏的免疫反应中，还是在对这些意料之外的激进免疫反应控制中，T 细胞经常扮演着中心角色。然而，其他粒细胞亚群同样具有这两种能力。以 B 细胞为例，其在进行抗体分泌的同时也调节着 B 细胞的生成；树突状细胞也同时具有刺激免疫反应和诱导免疫耐受的双向功能[2]。在本章中，我们将同时对能被免疫系统应用于预防非预期的免疫反应的免疫调节机制和一些能进行异体免疫反应调节的不同的细胞群进行回顾。虽然对这些机制的具体操纵仍然是未来的潜力，但是在确定常规免疫抑制剂的最终效果方面，调控可能发挥重要作用，并且在实验和临床实践中可以影响移植接受和排斥的平衡。本章的讨论补充了第 11 章所述的宽容机制。

细胞死亡

可以识别和响应自身抗原或移植后供体异体抗原的淋巴细胞的死亡或被删除是一种非常有效的在免疫细胞谱中消除具有损害移植物潜力的淋巴细胞的机制，以此来创造出无免疫反应性或者免疫耐受。T 细胞和 B 细胞都可以从细胞谱中以如下方式删除。

中央型异体抗原反应性 T 细胞删除

免疫系统通过消除或删除表达 T 细胞受体的 T 细胞来重塑 T 细胞谱系的能力是胸腺内 T 细胞发育过程的关键部分，此类 T 细胞将来可能无用或可能对受体产生危险。T 细胞前体在骨髓中由造血干细胞分化而来，后迁移至胸腺。进入胸腺后，这些祖细胞开始重新排列其 T 细胞受体(TCR)基因并经历胸腺程序性的筛选。该过程涉及一系列复杂的事件，其中表达完整 αβTCR 的 $CD4^+$ $CD8^+$胸腺细胞离开胸腺之前经历了阳性和阴性筛选，以成熟单阳性(仅表达 CD4 或 CD8)T 细胞移入外周。阳性选择的过程识别或选择表达对自身肽主要组织相容性复合物(pMHC)具有足够高亲和力的 TCR 的 T 细胞，使得细胞接收到存活信号。表达没有亲和力的自身 pMHC 复合物的 TCR 的 T 细胞未被选择并通过凋亡过程而死亡。对自身 pMHC 复合物具有很高亲和力并因此可以与周围组织表达的自身抗原反应的 TCR 的细胞在被称为阴性筛选的过程中被删除。通过这些机制，能够识别与对宿主免疫系统潜在有用的外源肽结合的自身 MHC 分子的 T 细胞得到维持并填充外周系统，同时确保大部分危险的自身或自身反应性 T 细胞被消除。

为了确保 T 细胞的阴性筛选尽可能完整，从而降低自身免疫性疾病的可能性，在胸腺中必须存在或表达一个大范围的自身 pMHC 复合物。由于一些蛋白质仅在外周表达，该过程需要一种特殊的机制，并由自身免疫调节蛋白(AIRE)控制。AIRE 是一种转录调节因子，其能促进编码胸腺中很大一部分 mRNA 转录产物大量合成不同的蛋白质，而此类 mRNA 通常仅在外周的组织中表达。以这种方式，在胸腺中进行选择的 T 细胞将会遇到大范围的自身 pMHC 复合物。重要的是，

AIRE 中的突变可能会损害其功能,因此胸腺中自身反应性 T 细胞的删除将会受到影响。AIRE 功能缺陷导致自身反应性 T 细胞出现在外周,可以攻击特定器官,导致自身免疫疾病[3]。该系统非常敏感,胸腺中仅有一个 AIRE 诱导的多肽缺失将导致自身免疫[4]。

虽然 AIRE 非常有效地确保在胸腺中表达广泛的 pMHC 复合物,但是阴性选择的过程仍然不完整,因此对宿主可能有害的一些 T 细胞可能会逃避阴性筛选并存在于外周免疫谱系中。为了防止对宿主的伤害,免疫系统已经开发了一种故障安全机制来控制非需求的 T 细胞活性,这一机制通过在胸腺中选择所谓的胸腺或天然存在的调节性 T 细胞(nTreg)来完成[5]。这种选择过程允许 T 细胞具有中间体,而不是高亲和力的自身 pMHC 复合物来表达转录因子 Foxp3[6]。选择后,Treg 迁移到其他 T 细胞的周边,在这些细胞中,它们可以控制任何潜在有害的自身反应性 T 细胞。

中央型耐受现象(比如非需求 T 细胞的删除)的开拓促进了移植耐受概念的引入。中央型异体反应性 T 细胞的删除已经通过经胸腺内注射直接递送同种异体抗原进入胸腺[7,8],以及在实验模型中建立同种异体混合骨髓嵌合体来实现[9]。这些研究提供的证据表明,可以利用胸腺中抗原反应性细胞的删除机制来促进手术移植耐受。

外源缺失的同种异体抗原反应性 T 细胞活化诱导的细胞死亡或免疫耗竭

通过活化诱导细胞死亡(AICD)的抗原反应性 T 细胞的凋亡是控制免疫反应性的另一种机制。AICD 是 T 细胞在周边细胞死亡的过程[10]。通过 TCR 进行再刺激后,许多不同的分子,包括 CD95(FAS)、肿瘤坏死因子受体 1(TNFR1)和肿瘤坏死因子相关的凋亡诱导配体受体(TRAILR),可以根据情况在 AICD 中发挥作用,引发一系列复杂的信号事件,最终导致胱天蛋白酶激活、DNA 断裂、细胞骨架降解和细胞死亡。

同种异体抗原反应性 B 细胞的删除

B 细胞从所有组成中的消除也是一种确保在骨髓进入外周期之前,骨髓中清除多反应性和能结合自身抗原的 B 细胞的机制。由于免疫球蛋白基因的重排是随机发生的,以使尽可能多的外源蛋白质和碳水化合物抗原被识别,所以不可避免地导致表达可识别自身抗原的 B 细胞受体(BCR)的 B 细胞的产生。虽然有所不同,但估计高达 70%的未成熟 B 细胞产生自身反应。通过受体编辑消除了 1/3 的这些未成熟 B 细胞,由此新的基因重排导致可与现有重链配对的替代轻链的产生,从而改变表达 BCR 的抗原识别性质。当未成熟的 B 细胞识别具有高亲和力的自身抗原时,其迅速内化抗原并经历一段发育停滞。不能表达淋巴结归巢受体,如 CD62 配体(CD62L),并且不诱导 B 细胞活化因子(BAFF)的受体,即 B 细胞存活所需的细胞因子。此外,重组酶激活基因保持接通,这允许通过编辑轻链来替代 B 细胞受体(BCR)。如果不能表达非自身反应性受体,任何经历该过程的 B 细胞将在 1~2 天后死亡。通过该途径的死亡不需要 FAS,部分是由于 Bcl-2 相互作用的细胞死亡介质(Bim)的抗原诱导表达,其抑制 Bcl-2 家族的 B 细胞存活蛋白。

受体编辑是一种机制,可用于删除能识别供体同种异体抗体的未成熟 B 细胞,特别是在白细胞消耗或诱导混合嵌合体后以及当器官移植给婴儿时。

如果受体编辑不能消除所有产生的自身反应性 B 细胞,则通过与自身抗原的相互作用触发表达高度自反应性受体的残留未成熟 B 细胞。已经使用免疫球蛋白转基因小鼠研究了这种控制或调节机制,并且获得的数据表明,当它们识别的抗原是膜结合时,B 细胞被有效地删除。发现该过程的效率取决于未成熟 B 细胞遇到相关自身抗原的可能性,因此其效率与抗原密度或频率明显相关。

能够从移植受体的所有组成部分识别供体同种异体抗原的 B 细胞的缺失是在移植中可以利用的机制。当认定的抗原以高剂量存在时,这种调节机制是最有效的。ABO 不相容的心脏同种异体移植物的婴儿受者已被证明能够删除心脏移植物上出现的血型抗原产生抗体的 B 细胞[11]。如果所实现的嵌合水平足以确保 B 细胞遇到供体细胞,那么导致供体和受体骨髓共存的混合嵌合现象也应使得供体反应性 B 细胞被删除[12]。

无反应性

无反应性是用于描述淋巴细胞功能失活的术语,导致细胞变得难以治疗或对进一步刺激无反应。生物反应的特征在于生化变化,导致响应细胞发生一定程度的发育停滞,并且当它们重新遇到其同源抗原时,激活阈值增加。控制免疫反应性的这种机制适用于T细胞和B细胞，并且可能在某些环境中有助于可以发挥作用以控制移植后同种异体抗原免疫反应性的机制。然而，重要的是，要注意无反应是无感应性的可逆状态。

T细胞无反应

鉴于与结合相关的pMHC复合物(信号1)和T细胞及抗原呈递细胞(APC)上的分子之间的配体－受体相互作用,外部T细胞被激活,统称为共刺激途径(信号2)。在体外,在没有共刺激的情况下,抗原识别(即相关的pMHC复合物的TCR连接)已经显示出可诱导T细胞无反应性[13]。在抗原识别时,没有通过CD28共刺激被证明对于在这些体外系统中诱导T细胞无反应性至关重要。在体内,T细胞无反应的诱导也显示依赖于CTLA-4(CD152)的连接。

随着对共刺激途径的了解不断发展，已经清楚的是,其他配体-受体相互作用也可能有助于T细胞无反应性的发育和(或)维持。共刺激分子编程死亡1(PD-1)在无能T细胞和一些组织中高度表达,并且与其配体PDL-1的相互作用也已被证明参与T细胞的诱导和可能的维持无能。因此,在体外和体内,T细胞无反应性可以由于没有正确的附加共刺激信号而连接TCR引起,导致T细胞活化过程的衰减,从而限制T细胞响应的能力。

B细胞无反应

如上所述,T细胞的中枢B细胞耐受机制也不完整。因此，自身反应性B细胞可以逃避骨髓的中枢耐受,并出现在外周。以较低亲和力通过BCR结合其同源抗原的外周自身反应性B细胞变为无反应性。这是由于当B细胞长期暴露于低水平的抗原时，细胞内信号传导改变[14]。在实验模型中,已经在B细胞中证明了B细胞无反应性,其结合低亲和力的可溶性抗原。

在正常的异质B细胞谱中，结合自身抗原的无能B细胞以及再结合外源抗原的初始滤泡B细胞定位于次级淋巴器官的T细胞区域。在没有T细胞帮助和激活无能B细胞中的其他信号通路的情况下，这些细胞在1~5天内死亡。相比之下,当幼稚B细胞在T细胞存在下接触抗原时,有助于它们与CD4细胞合作并分化成抗体分泌的浆细胞。

已经发现,通过Toll样受体(TLR)配体的共刺激被阻断在无能B细胞中。在移植后的早期阶段,这可能是有帮助的,已明确TLR被存在于移植的器官或组织中的受损细胞激活并有助于排斥过程。在移植后,保持低亲和力显然也是有利的,同种异体反应性B细胞处于无能状态，以防止它们在移植后分泌供体特异性抗体(DSA)。仍在寻找实现这一目标的方法。有趣的是,免疫抑制剂,如环孢菌素A(CsA)在预防抗体介导的慢性同种异体移植物排斥反应方面并不特别有效[15],其中已经鉴定了经历慢性排斥反应的同种异体移植物中的B细胞簇[16]。这种缺乏有效性可能是由于CsA不能模拟在无能B细胞中发生的信号事件。

免疫调节

作为诱导和维持免疫反应性或对自身抗原的耐受性的策略，缺失和无反应性是不完全或不稳定的。因此,免疫系统开发了许多故障安全机制,以确保尽管在外围存在自身反应性T细胞和B细胞，但仍然保持耐受性。这些相同的故障安全机制,包括能够控制任何潜在的自身反应性淋巴细胞的调节或抑制细胞的群体,可以用于控制移植后对同种异体抗原的免疫应答。

调节性T细胞

已经描述了具有调节活性的许多不同类型的T细胞,包括:$CD4^+$ T细胞[17,18]、$CD8^+$ T细胞[19-21]、$CD4^-CD8^-$双阴性T细胞[22]、NKT细胞[23]和γδT细胞[24]。由于对具有调节功能的$CD4^+$ T细胞迄今已进行了更深入的研究,本章的这一部分将重点关注这一调控细胞群体。

$CD25^+$ $FOXP3^+$ T调节细胞(Treg)可以通过两种不同的发育途径产生。首先,如上所述,胸腺来源或天然存在的(nTreg)在胸腺中分化,并且被认为主要用于抑制对自身抗原的反应并因此防止自身免疫疾病。这方面的证据来自对具有罕见遗传缺陷的患者以及具有天然存在或遗传工程缺陷的小鼠的研究。例如,在免疫失调、多发性内分泌疾病、肠病、X连锁(IPEX)综合征的患者中观察到导致自身免疫的深刻免疫失调。已经发现IPEX患者在基因编码因子叉头基因P3(*FOXP3*)[25,26]中有一个点突变，这是T细胞调控的主基因，导致体外Treg活性的功能受损[27]。Scurfy小鼠也具有*foxp3*和相关免疫特征的突变[28]。第二,当$CD4^+$ T细胞在外周的耐受性微环境中遇到抗原时，例如当未成熟树突状细胞(DC)或免疫抑制细胞因子存在抗原时，$CD4^+$ T 细胞分化为“适应性”抗原诱导的 Treg(iTreg)[6]。在移植的背景下，可以认为这种途径可能是移植后产生供体异体抗原反应性 Treg 的更重要的途径[29]。有趣的是，尽管其起源不同，但 nTreg 和 iTreg 均依赖于 FOXP3 的高水平转录抑制功能的持续表达(图 8.1)。

重要的是，移植提供了 T 细胞体内抑制或免疫调节的一些最早的证据。来自新生儿耐受性研究的数据表明，除了供体反应性细胞缺失外，还有其他机制[30,31]。后来，一个明确的迹象表明，长期免疫抑制的同种异体移植物长期存活(称为手术移植耐受性的状态)涉及 T 细胞的存在，具有调节初始同种异体反应性 T 细胞功能的能力，从而防止对新鲜移植物的排斥反应[32,33]。随后发现，这种形式的细胞调节与 $CD4^+$ T 细胞相关，Hall 及其同事首先提出 CD25 可能是鉴定具有调节活性的 $CD4^+$ T 细胞的有用标记[34]。在大鼠肾同种异体移植模型中获得了相似的数据，其中通过供体特异性输血诱导操作耐受性[35,36]。作为表达高水平 CD25 的 $CD4^+$ T 细胞可以调节排斥的直接证据，Hara 及其同事发现，来自耐受动物的 $CD4^+$ $CD25^+$ T 细胞的共转移导致 80% 用幼稚 CBA 效应 T 细胞重建的免疫缺陷小鼠皮肤移植物存活率不确定[37]。

在没有任何先前暴露于同种异体抗原的情况下，nTreg 数量通常不足以阻止完全同种异体(MHC +次要

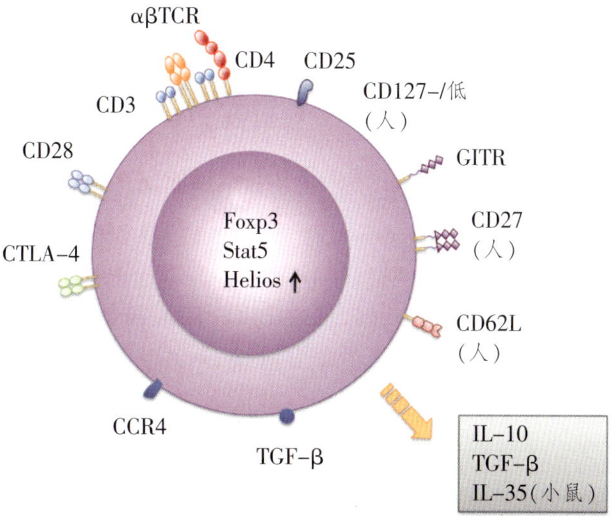

图 8.1 调节性 T 细胞的特定标记。图中显示具有特定调节潜能的 T 细胞的胞内转录特征、细胞表面分子及特定细胞因子。

组织相容性抗原不匹配)移植物的排斥，因为存在于能够对移植物产生破坏性反应的谱系中的 T 细胞频率远远超过 nTreg 的数量，因此排斥发生[37]。在不存在免疫抑制的情况下，nTreg 不能防止同种异体移植物破坏的事实并不意味着细胞不起作用。然而，在这种情况下，排斥和调节之间的平衡反对调节，因为任何 Treg 存在的抑制活性都被效应 T 细胞介导的破坏性反应所压倒。在接受者中，存在先前存在的供体同种抗原反应性记忆 T 细胞也可以压倒免疫调节，因为记忆细胞的激活动力学非常快，除非在反应开始时存在非常多数量的 Treg，否则平衡排斥与监管之间的显著推动有利于排斥[38]。重要的是，移植物破坏和接受之间的这种关键平衡可以以多种方式转移，特别是通过采用增加相对频率和(或)活化状态的策略，并因此促进 Treg 的功能活性，然后可以在移植前或移植后的早期对供体同种异体抗原产生反应[39,40]，或抑制或降低效应细胞的活性。

虽然观察到具有长期存活的同种异体移植物的小鼠含有同种异体抗原反应性 $CD25^+$ Treg 的群体是重要的，但是这些实验不能区分由诱导策略本身产生的 Treg 和仅通过存在接受的同种异体移植物产生的 Treg。在开发潜在的临床方法方面，重要的是要明确归纳策略，最终导致长期的操作容忍能驱使 Treg 发展独立于移植物本身。数据显示，在不存在移植的情况下暴露于同种异体抗原可导致在许多研究中获得 $CD4^+$ $CD25^+$ Treg 的诱导。例如，当用供体同种异体抗原与非消耗性抗 CD4 组合治疗 28 天后，从小鼠中分离出 $CD4^+$ $CD25^+$时，这些细胞阻止了敏感的过继转移模型中测试皮肤移植物的排斥反应[41]。重要的是，对于从幼稚小鼠中分离的类似群体或仅用抗 CD4 或 DST 处理的小鼠，没有观察到对受试移植物的保护，表明如果接受者暴露于移植前，由 $CD25^+$ Treg 介导的耐受能够在体内诱导条件允许下给予同种异体抗原。此外，据报道，即使同种异体移植物本身已被拒绝[42]，单独存在的同种异体移植物也可以导致具有调控特性的 T 细胞的发育，从而保护移植物免受排斥反应[43]。这两个实例都证实，具有调节活性的 T 细胞可以在同种异体抗原存在的情况下和(或)注射同种异体抗原的情况下被诱导，并且这些细胞可以有助于控制随后对体内同种异体抗原的反应。

正在研究的另一个重要问题是，可以控制同种异体

移植排斥功能的Treg功能在哪里最有效,以及在体内何处可以发现或检测到它们。有证据表明,移植后Treg功能随时间而变化位置。在移植后的早期反应中,Treg已被证明在引流淋巴结中存在且功能上有活性,而在移植后过程中的晚期,Treg已被证明在同种异体移植物内起作用用[44]。事实上越来越多的证据表明,免疫调节的重要部位在同种异体移植物本身内,Treg功能可以创造出一种允许控制的环境[45,46]。此外,将Treg重新暴露于组织中的抗原可能使它们变为更有效的抑制因子,因此在控制排斥反应方面更有效[47]。

尽管许多工作已经证明,Treg可以控制对同种异体抗原的反应,但是大多数研究已经使用体外测定或实验模型,由此将细胞过继转移到免疫缺陷受体中,其中同种异体移植排斥是由相对数量较少的效应T细胞驱动的,在体内可以发现完整免疫谱的数量。可以说,临床应用这个方法的一个更相关的问题是Treg在完整的免疫系统中发挥什么作用?在移植中,Treg特异性失活可以表明,在上述抗CD4 / DST耐受诱导模型中,原发性心脏同种异体移植物在正常的、淋巴结丰富的受体中的存活也明确依赖于受耐受诱导方案驱动的iTreg[48]。这些数据表明,确实可以提高非淋巴细胞移植患者Tregs的功能。

调节性B细胞

在20世纪80年代,首先描述了具有抑制小鼠自身免疫性疾病发展能力的B细胞。尽管已经描述了一些异质性,但调节性B细胞(Breg)表达高水平的CD1d、CD21、CD24和IgM以及中等水平的CD19,表明Breg可能存在不同的子集[49](图8.2)。具有调节活性的B细胞的特征之一是其分泌IL-10的能力。似乎需要CD40来刺激IL-10产生,并且据报道,其对于Breg的活化是必需的,使得它们能够显示其功能活性并抑制Th1分化。有研究表明,调节性B细胞和T细胞之间存在联系,Breg是Treg的有效产生者。Breg已经在老鼠和人类中被描述过。小鼠Breg表达T细胞Ig结构域和黏蛋白结构域蛋白1(Tim 1)[50]。人类调节性B细胞与其小鼠对应物(包括未成熟表型)共享一些性质,并且包含总B细胞池的一小部分。

在移植中,只有间接证据表明Breg可能在控制同种异体抗原的免疫应答方面发挥作用。有趣的是,在没有免疫抑制的情况下,在具有功能性移植物的肾移植

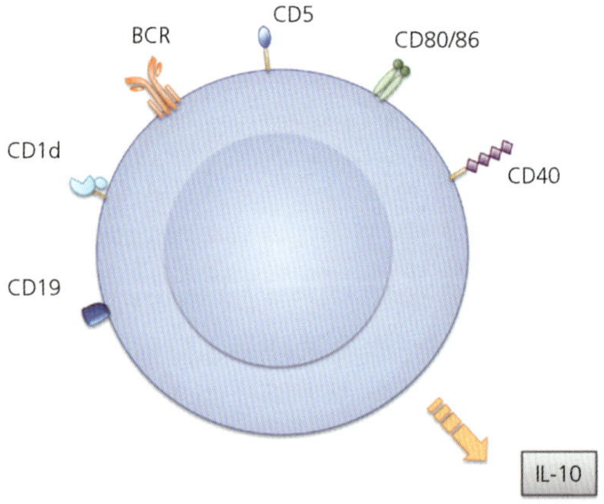

图8.2 调节性B细胞的特征性标记。图中显示了由特定调节潜能的B细胞所表达的细胞表面分子及特定细胞因子。

受者中,发现B细胞特征与供体同种异体抗体的这种操作耐受状态相关[51,52]。在单独的长期免疫抑制肾移植受体群体中鉴定出了一个独特的,但也是B细胞主导的耐受性标志物[53]。

目前关于Breg在移植中作用的实验研究有限。在长期肾移植耐受的大鼠模型中,可观察到外周和内在基因表达从IgG到IgM的变化,以及移植物中出现IgM^+,而不是IgG^+ B细胞簇[54]。在小鼠中,B细胞的Tim-1连接诱导具有调节活性的Tim-1^+ B细胞[50],这表明,增加体内Breg数量的潜在治疗策略还需要更多的工作来确定和表征Breg在调节同种异体免疫应答方面的贡献以及与DSA生产的关系[55]。

树突状细胞

DC是免疫反应的激活/引发的核心,但矛盾的是它们也可以促进耐受性的发展[1,56,57]。最初,在细胞表面表达低水平的MHC Ⅱ类和共刺激分子的未成熟骨髓DC被鉴定为具有诱导T细胞耐受能力的DC的主要形式。相比之下,表达更高水平的MHC和共刺激分子的成熟骨髓DC被发现能最有效地提供T细胞应答。然而,随后成熟DC也被证明具有诱导耐受性的能力,因此,DC的成熟状态与其致耐受性潜力之间的关系现在不被认为是决定DC刺激的重要因素或抑制同种异体免疫反应的发展。

有许多研究表明,DC可以促进对实体器官同种异体移植物和骨髓移植物的耐受性[56]。例如,在移植MHC不匹配的心脏同种异体移植物前7天单次注射供体来源的DC,以供体特异性方式延长[58]或无限期延长生存

期[59]。通过免疫调节剂的共同给药如共刺激阻断可以增强DC的潜在致耐受性作用[60]。具有低共刺激能力的“激活性”或“调节性”DC也可以在移植前7天使用，以保护MHC错配的皮肤移植物免于排斥反应[61]和小鼠避免致死性急性移植物宿主病[62]。

浆细胞样DC(pDC)可以说是可以影响免疫反应调节过程的最具特征性的DC亚型。pDC最初由其响应于病毒分泌大量Ⅰ型干扰素的能力定义，并且在保护个体免受无害抗原的炎症反应方面发挥重要作用，但是现在也已经显示出能够诱导人类调节T体外细胞。这些调节性细胞产生大量的IL-10，少量IFN-γ，但不产生IL-4、IL-5或转化生长因子(TGF)-β[63]。非淋巴组织pDC，例如存在于气道、肠道和肝脏中的pDC在调节黏膜免疫中起重要作用，并且对于吸收或摄取的抗原耐受性的发展至关重要。

pDC用于促进耐受性的分子机制是复杂的[64]，包括可以促进Foxp3$^+$ Treg分化的证据。在移植模型中，耐受pDC可以在同种异体移植物中获得同种异体抗原，然后通过血液迁移到外周淋巴结转移，从而诱导CCR4$^+$ CD4$^+$ CD25$^+$ Foxp3$^+$ Treg的产生[65]。重要的是，在免疫抑制治疗不存在的情况下，移植前7天输注供体衍生的pDC能够延长随后的心脏同种异体移植物存活(9~22天)[66]，但是这种作用被抗CD154mAb给药显著增强[67]。在小鼠中，pre-pDC似乎是促成造血干细胞移植和诱导同种异体受体中供体特异性皮肤移植耐受的主要细胞类型[63]。通过联合使用DC和共刺激阻滞可能是迄今为止确定的最有希望的方法。

骨髓源性抑制细胞

骨髓源性抑制细胞(MDSC)已经与许多抑制功能相关，包括抗原特异性和非特异性。这些包括先天免疫调节、T细胞活化和肿瘤免疫。MDSC是在炎症免疫反应期间可以在组织中积累的异源祖细胞群。MDSC的扩增和激活受到存在于相同微环境中其他细胞产生的因子的调节；涉及的其他细胞类型包括基质细胞、活化的T细胞和肿瘤中的肿瘤细胞本身。

已经在小鼠和人类中描述了许多MDSC子集[68](图8.3，从参考文献[69]中总结的数据改编而来)。尽管存在异质性，但常见的表型标志物包括小鼠中的Gr1和CD11b，以及人类的CD33、CD11b、CD34和低水平的MHCⅡ类。活化的MDSC通过诱导一氧化氮合酶1(诱导一氧化氮生成)和精氨酸酶1(消耗精氨酸)等机制体外抑制T细胞、B细胞和NK细胞的增殖和细胞因子产生。这两种途径都可以诱导抑制细胞功能的几种机制。MDSC也似乎能够修饰T细胞分化途径，据报道，它们促进Treg分化。

在实验模型中，MDSC可以在同种异体抗原诱导耐受中发挥作用。例如，在循环白细胞中不表达MHCⅡ类的小鼠中不能诱导移植耐受性。这一发现符合受体MHCⅡ类$^+$细胞诱导同种抗原耐受性的要求[70]。此外，已经报道了有关CD11b$^+$ CD115$^+$ Gr1$^+$单核细胞对小鼠心脏同种异体移植物的耐受性作用的直接证据的数据[71]，而在大鼠中，肾脏中表达iNOS的MDSC的证据已有报道[72]。

调节性巨噬细胞

在活化的功能结果方面，巨噬细胞天生具有可塑性。经典活化的巨噬细胞是高度促炎症的，并且是响应于TLR的连接产生的，导致炎性信号级联的激活和炎性细胞因子的产生，包括肿瘤坏死因子-α和IL-1β。或者，暴露于细胞因子IL-4诱导的活化巨噬细胞促炎症效果较弱，并且在一些环境中可以产生调节免疫应答的微环境，否则这些免疫应答对它们所在的组织是有害的[73]。调节性巨噬细胞可能代表另外的群体，它不同于其他两种形式，其主要生理作用是抑制炎症免疫应答并防止与长期经典巨噬细胞活化相关的免疫病理学[74]。

调节性巨噬细胞通常与两种配体(例如TLR和免疫复合物)共同刺激后产生大量的IL-10。它们不表达精氨酸酶，并且不依赖于STAT6信号传导，或者是活化的巨噬细胞。目前，尚未建立稳定或方便的特异性调节性巨噬细胞的表面标志物(图8.4[75])。在组织中，调节性巨噬细胞在解剖学上被定位于与淋巴细胞相互作用，因此有证据表明，这些细胞可以影响彼此的活性。在体外，调节性巨噬细胞是高效的APC，可诱导由Th2细胞因子产生主导的高度极化的抗原特异性T细胞应答。

从外周血分离的人类调节性巨噬细胞具有调节对同种异体抗原免疫应答的能力，并且在先导研究中已经通过静脉注射应用于活体供体肾移植受体[76]。

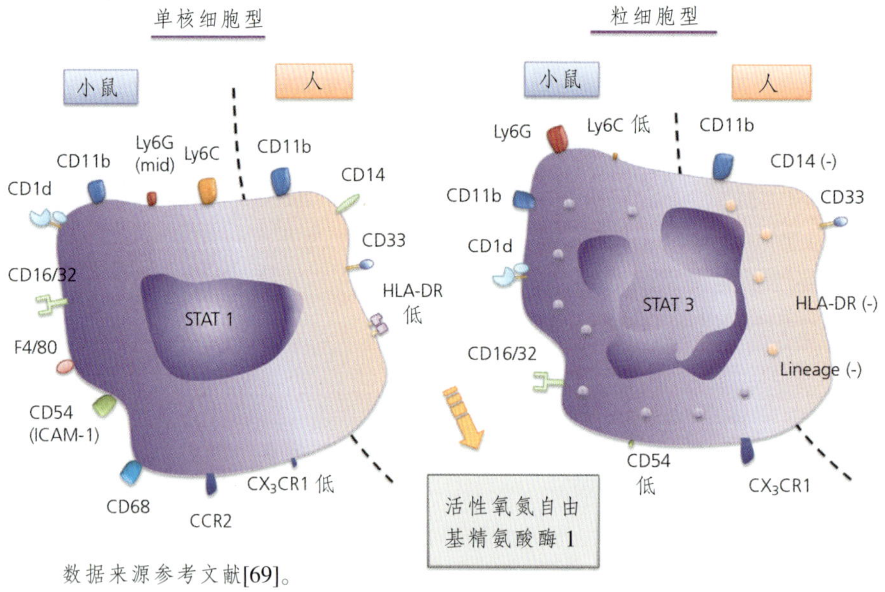

数据来源参考文献[69]。

图 8.3 骨髓源性抑制细胞的特征性标记。图中显示具有特定调节潜能的骨髓源性抑制细胞(左,单核细胞型;右,粒细胞型)的细胞内转录特征,细胞表面分子及特征性细胞因子蛋白。

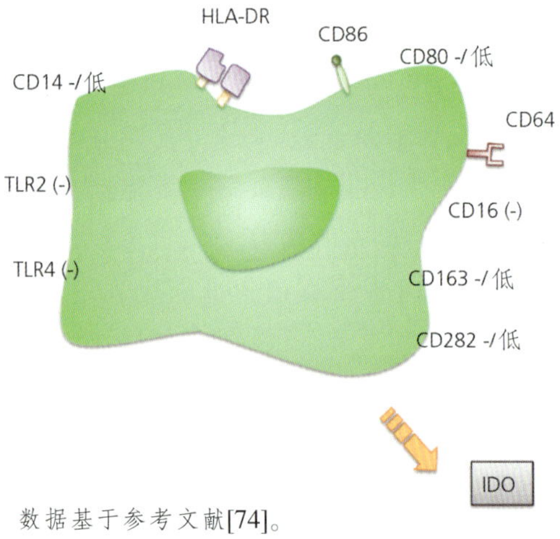

数据基于参考文献[74]。

图 8.4 人调节性巨噬细胞的特征性标记。图中显示有特定调节潜能的人巨噬细胞的表面分子标记及特征性蛋白。

忽略

可以说，有助于维持外周耐受的最简单的机制是自身抗原的T细胞忽略。在这种情况下,自身反应性T细胞逃避胸腺内的阴性选择并进入外周，但是这样的T细胞被阻止访问表达其同源肽的位点，或者它们从未看到足够的肽以使其克服激活阈值[77]。在移植中,很难设想这种机制如何以持续的方式有效地调节同种异体免疫应答。

小结

免疫调节是一个复杂的过程,涉及多种机制,通常有多种细胞类型共同作用来控制免疫反应。这些过程是避免不必要的免疫反应和限制所需免疫反应的外周作用所必需的。虽然没有准确地操纵这些机制的方法,但它们无疑在确定同种异体移植物的最终命运方面发挥作用，并且在将来精细管理同种异体免疫应答中将变得越来越重要。

(汪洋 译 李照 校)

参考文献

1. Wood KJ, Goto R. Mechanisms of rejection: current perspectives. Transplantation. 2012;93:1–10.
2. Wood KJ, Bushell A, Hester J. Regulatory immune cells in transplantation. Nature Reviews. Immunology. 2012;12:417–430.
3. Mathis D, Benoist C. Aire. Annual Review of Immunology. 2009;27:287–312.
4. Metzger TC, Anderson MS. Control of central and peripheral tolerance by Aire. Immunological Reviews. 2011;241:89–103.
5. Wing K, Sakaguchi S. Regulatory T cells exert checks and balances on self tolerance and autoimmunity. Nature Immunology. 2010;11:7–13.
6. Josefowicz SZ, Rudensky A. Control of regulatory T cell lineage commitment and maintenance. Immunity. 2009;30:616–625.

7. Posselt AM, Barker CF, Tomaszewski JE, et al. Induction of donor-specific unresponsiveness by intrathymic islet transplantation. Science. 1990;249:1293–1295.
8. Jones N, Fluck N, Mellor A, et al. Deletion of alloantigen-reactive thymocytes as a mechanism of adult transplantation tolerance induction following intrathymic antigen administration. European Journal of Immunology. 1997;27:1591–1600.
9. Sykes M. Hematopoietic cell transplantation for tolerance induction: animal models to clinical trials. Transplantation. 2009;87:309–316.
10. Krammer PH, Arnold R, Lavrik IN. Life and death in peripheral T cells. Nature Reviews. Immunology. 2007;7:532–542.
11. Fan X, Ang A, Pollock-Barziv S, et al. Donor-specific B-cell tolerance after ABO-incompatible infant heart transplantation. Nature Medicine. 2004;10:1227–1233.
12. Sykes M. Mixed chimerism and transplant tolerance. Immunity. 2001;14: 417–424.
13. Jenkins MK, Pardoll DM, Mizuguchi J, et al. T-cell unresponsiveness in vivo and in vitro: fine specificity of induction and molecular characterization of the unresponsive state. Immunological Reviews. 1987;95:113–135.
14. Yarkoni Y, Getahun A, Cambier JC. Molecular underpinning of B-cell anergy. Immunological Reviews. 2010;237:249–263.
15. Rose ML. Activation of autoimmune B cells and chronic rejection. Transplantation. 2005;79:S22–S24.
16. Thaunat O. Pathophysiologic significance of B-cell clusters in chronically rejected grafts. Transplantation. 2011;92:121–126.
17. Wood KJ, Sakaguchi S. Regulatory T cells in transplantation tolerance. Nature Reviews. Immunology. 2003;3:199–210.
18. Sakaguchi S, Miyara M, Costantino CM, et al. FOXP3+ regulatory T cells in the human immune system. Nature Reviews. Immunology. 2010;10:490–500.
19. Reibke R, Garbi N, Ganss R, et al. CD8+ regulatory T cells generated by neonatal recognition of peripheral self-antigen. Proceedings of the National Academy of Sciences of the United States of America. 2006;103:15142–15147.
20. Vlad G, Cortesini R, Suciu-Foca N. CD8+ T suppressor cells and the ILT3 master switch. Human Immunology. 2008;69:681–686.
21. Li XL, Ménoret S, Bezie S, et al. Mechanism and localization of CD8 regulatory T cells in a heart transplant model of tolerance. Journal of Immunology. 2010; 185:823–833.
22. Thomson C, Lee B, Zhang L. Double-negative regulatory T cells. Immunologic Research. 2006;35:163–177.
23. Monteiro M, Almeida CF, Caridade M, et al. Identification of regulatory Foxp3+ invariant NKT cells induced by TGF-β. Journal of Immunology. 2010;185: 2157–2163.
24. Hayday A, Tigelaar R. Immunoregulation in the tissues by gammadelta T cells. Nature Reviews. Immunology. 2003;3:233–242.
25. Bennett CL, Christie F, Ramsdell F, et al. The immune dysregulation, polyendocrinopathy, enteropathy, X-linked syndrome (IPEX) is caused by mutations of FOXP3. Nature Genetics. 2001;27:20–21.
26. Kobayashi I, Shiari R, Yamada M, et al. Novel mutations of FOXP3 in two Japanese patients with immune dysregulation, polyendocrinopathy, enteropathy, X linked syndrome (IPEX). Journal of Medical Genetics. 2001;38:874–876.
27. Bacchetta R, Passerini L, Gambineri E, et al. Defective regulatory and effector T cell functions in patients with FOXP3 mutations. Journal of Clinical Investigation. 2006;116:1713–1722.
28. Ramsdell F. Foxp3 and natural regulatory T cells: key to a cell lineage? Immunity. 2003;19:165–168.
29. Wood KJ, Bushell A, Jones ND. Immunologic unresponsiveness to alloantigen in vivo: a role for regulatory T cells. Immunological Reviews. 2011;241:119–132.
30. Billingham RE, Brent L, Medawar PB. Actively acquired tolerance of foreign cells. Nature. 1953;172:603–606.
31. Wood KJ, Bushell AR, Jones ND. The discovery of immunological tolerance: now more than just a laboratory solution. Journal of Immunology. 2010;184:3–4.
32. Hall BM, Jelbart ME, Dorsch SE. Suppressor T cells in rats with prolonged cardiac allograft survival after treatment with cyclosporine. Transplantation. 1984;37: 595–600.
33. Hall B, Jelbart M, Gurley K, et al. Specific unresponsiveness in rats with prolonged cardiac allograft survival after treatment with cyclosporine. Mediation of specific suppression by T helper/inducer cells. Journal of Experimental Medicine. 1985;162:1683–1694.
34. Hall B, Pearce N, Gurley K, et al. Specific unresponsiveness in rats with prolonged cardiac allograft survival after treatment with cyclosporine. III. Further characterisation of the CD4+ suppressor cell and its mechanisms of action. Journal of Experimental Medicine. 1990;171:141–157.
35. Quigley RL, Wood KJ, Morris J. Mediation of antigen-induced suppression of renal allograft rejection by a CD4 (W3/25^{+}) T cell. Transplantation. 1989;47:684–688.
36. Quigley RL, Wood KJ, Morris PJ. Transfusion induces blood donor-specific suppressor cells. Journal of Immunology. 1989;142:463.
37. Hara M, Kingsley C, Niimi M, et al. IL-10 is required for regulatory T cells to mediate tolerance to alloantigens in vivo. Journal of Immunology. 2001; 166:3789–3796.
38. Yang J, Brook M, Carvalho-Gaspar M, et al. Allograft rejection mediated by memory T cells is resistant to regulation. Proceedings of the National Academy of Sciences of the United States of America. 2007;104:19954–19959.
39. Graca L, Thompson S, Lin C-Y, et al. Both CD4+CD25+ and CD4+CD25- regulatory cells mediate dominant transplantation tolerance. Journal of Immunology. 2002;168:5558–5565.
40. Francis RS, Feng G, Tha-In T, et al. Induction of transplantation tolerance converts potential effector T cells into graft protective regulatory T cells. European Journal of Immunology. 2011;41:726–738.
41. Kingsley CI, Karim M, Bushell AR, et al. CD25+CD4+ regulatory T cells prevent graft rejection: CTLA-4- and IL-10-dependent immunoregulation of alloresponses. Journal of Immunology. 2002;168:1080–1086.
42. Hamano K, Rawsthorne M, Bushell A, et al. Evidence that the continued presence of the organ graft and not peripheral donor microchimerism is essential for the maintenance of tolerance to alloantigen in anti-CD4 treated recipients. Transplantation. 1996;62:856–860.
43. Tullius S, Nieminen M, Bechstein W, et al. Chronically rejected rat kidney allografts induce donor-specific tolerance. Transplantation. 1997;64:158–161.
44. Carvalho-Gaspar M, Jones ND, Luo S, et al. Location and time-dependent control of rejection by regulatory T cells culminates in a failure to generate memory T cells. Journal of Immunology. 2008;180:6640–6648.
45. Graca L, Cobbold SP, Waldmann H. Identification of regulatory T cells in tolerated allografts. Journal of Experimental Medicine. 2002;195:1641–1646.
46. Kendal AR, Chen Y, Regateiro FS, et al. Sustained suppression by Foxp3+ regulatory T cells is vital for infectious transplantation tolerance. Journal of Experimental Medicine. 2011; 208:2043–2053.
47. Rosenblum MD, Gratz IK, Paw JS, et al. Response to self antigen imprints regulatory memory in tissues. Nature. 2011;480:538–542.
48. Bushell A, Wood KJ. GITR ligation blocks allograft protection by induced CD25+CD4+ regulatory T cells without enhancing effector T-cell function. American Journal of Transplantation. 2007;7:759–768.
49. Mauri C, Blair PA. Regulatory B cells in autoimmunity: developments and controversies. Nature Reviews Rheumatology. 2010;6:636–643.
50. Ding Q, Yeung M, Camirand G, et al. Regulatory B cells are identified by expression of TIM-1 and can be induced through TIM-1 ligation to promote tolerance in mice. Journal of Clinical Investigation. 2011;121:3645–3656.
51. Sagoo P, Perucha E, Sawitzki B, et al. Development of a cross-platform biomarker signature to detect renal transplant tolerance in humans. Journal of Clinical Investigation. 2010;120:1848–1861.
52. Newell KA, Asare A, Kirk AD, et al. Identification of a B cell signature associated with renal transplant tolerance in humans. Journal of Clinical Investigation. 2010;120:1836–1847.
53. Pallier A, Hillion S, Danger R, et al. Patients with drug-free long-term graft function display increased numbers of peripheral B cells with a memory and inhibitory phenotype. Kidney International. 2010;78:503–513.
54. Le Texier L, Thebault P, Lavault A, et al. Long-term allograft tolerance is characterized by the accumulation of B cells exhibiting an inhibited profile. American Journal of Transplantation. 2011;11:429–438.
55. Chong AS, Sciammas R. Matchmaking the B-cell signature of tolerance to regulatory B cells. American Journal of Transplantation. 2011;11:2555–2560.
56. Morelli AE, Thomson AW. Tolerogenic dendritic cells and the quest for transplant tolerance. Nature Reviews. Immunology. 2007;7:610–621.
57. van Kooten C, Lombardi G, Gelderman KA, et al. Dendritic cells as a tool to induce transplantation tolerance: obstacles and opportunities. Transplantation. 2011; 91:2–7.
58. Fu F, Li Y, Qian S, et al. Costimulatory molecule-deficient dendritic cell progenitors (MHC class II^{+}, CD80^{dim}, CD86^{-}) prolong cardiac allograft survival in nonimmunosupressed recipients. Transplantation. 1996;62:659–665.
59. Lutz M, Suri R, Niimi M, et al. Immature dendritic cells generated with low doses of GM-CSF in the absence of IL-4 are maturation resistant and prolong allograft survival in vivo. European Journal of Immunology. 2000;30:1813–1822.
60. Lu L, Li W, Fu F, et al. Blockade of the CD40-CD40 ligand pathway potentiates the capacity of donor-derived dendritic cell progenitors to induce long-term cardiac allograft survival. Transplantation. 1997;64:1808–1815.
61. Roelen D, Schuurhuis D, van den Boogaardt D, et al. Prolongation of skin graft survival by modulation of the alloimmune response with alternatively activated dendritic cells. Transplantation. 2003;76:1608–1615.
62. Sato K, Yamashita N, Yamashita N, et al. Regulatory dendritic cells protect mice from murine acute graft-versus-host disease and leukemia relapse. Immunity. 2003;18:367–379.
63. Gilliet M, Liu Y-J. Generation of human CD8 T regulatory cells by CD40 ligand-activated plasmacytoid dendritic cells. Journal of Experimental Medicine. 2002;195:695–704.
64. Swiecki M, Colonna M. Unraveling the functions of plasmacytoid dendritic cells during viral infections, autoimmunity, and tolerance. Immunological Reviews. 2010;234:142–162.

65. Ochando JC, Homma C, Yang Y, et al. Alloantigen-presenting plasmacytoid dendritic cells mediate tolerance to vascularized grafts. Nature Immunology. 2006;7: 652–662.
66. Abe M, Wang Z, de Creus A, et al. Plasmacytoid dendritic cell precursors induce allogeneic T-cell hyporesponsiveness and prolong heart graft survival. American Journal of Transplantation. 2005;5:1808–1819.
67. Bjorck P, Coates PTH, Wang Z, et al. Promotion of long-term heart allograft survival by combination of mobilized donor plasmacytoid dendritic cells and anti-CD154 monoclonal antibody. Journal of Heart and Lung Transplantation. 2005;24:1118–1120.
68. Boros P, Ochando JC, Chen S-H, et al. Myeloid-derived suppressor cells: natural regulators for transplant tolerance. Human Immunology. 2010;71:1061–1066.
69. Gabrilovich DI, Nagaraj S. Myeloid-derived suppressor cells as regulators of the immune system. Nature Reviews. Immunology. 2009;9:162–174.
70. Yamada A, Chandraker A, Laufer TM, et al. Cutting edge: recipient MHC class II expression is required to achieve long-term survival of murine cardiac allografts after costimulatory blockade. Journal of Immunology. 2001;167:5522–5526.
71. Garcia MR, Ledgerwood L, Yang Y, et al. Monocytic suppressive cells mediate cardiovascular transplantation tolerance in mice. Journal of Clinical Investigation. 2010;120:2486–2496.
72. Dugast A-S, Haudebourg T, Coulon F, et al. Myeloid-derived suppressor cells accumulate in kidney allograft tolerance and specifically suppress effector T cell expansion. Journal of Immunology. 2008;180:7898–7906.
73. Martinez FO, Helming L, Gordon S. Alternative activation of macrophages: an immunologic functional perspective. Annual Review of Immunology. 2009;27: 451–483.
74. Fleming BD, Mosser DM. Regulatory macrophages: setting the threshold for therapy. European Journal of Immunology. 2011;41:2498–2502.
75. Hutchinson JA, Riquelme P, Geissler EK. Human regulatory macrophages as a cell-based medicinal product. Current Opinion in Organ Transplantation. 2012; 17:48–54.
76. Hutchinson JA, Riquelme P, Sawitzki B, et al. Cutting edge: immunological consequences and trafficking of human regulatory macrophages administered to renal transplant recipients. Journal of Immunology. 2011;187:2072–2078.
77. Walker LSK, Abbas AK. The enemy within: keeping self-reactive T cells at bay in the periphery. Nature Reviews. Immunology. 2002;2:11–19.

第 9 章
同种免疫、异种免疫及相关自身免疫的种类

Mandy L. Ford, Andrew B. Adams, Christian P. Larsen

引言

同种异体免疫反应是创伤、细胞损伤和外科移植引起的缺血再灌注损伤等背景下多种效应细胞及其分泌产物对外来人抗原作用的总称。虽然同种异体反应的基本原理在个体之间是相似的，但伴随着同种异体抗原差异的变化以及随时间推移应答者免疫病史的改变，同种异体免疫应答反应大小和性质在不同个体间差异很大。事实上，这些变化被认为对我们理解近交动物和临床移植中观察到的变异性至关重要。在本章中，我们将回顾导致同种异体反应固有变异性的因素，并指明受体的免疫史可以从根本上重塑其同种异体反应潜能的机制。

同种异体反应的谱系

核心的同种异体反应潜力主要依靠三种细胞类型，这些细胞可识别同种异体抗原并启动同种异体免疫反应，它们是自然杀伤(NK)细胞、T 细胞和 B 细胞。对于 B 细胞和 T 细胞，通过识别供体来源的外来抗原被激活，对于 NK 细胞，细胞因自身 MHC 的缺失而被激活。虽然关于移植排斥反应的激活和调停机制的细节已在第 5 章和第 6 章中具体介绍，但需要高度注意的是同种异体反应器的潜能以及同种异体反应免疫应答的强度与频率在个体之间和不同供体之间变化很大。事实上，相比一个确定的供体来说，它在一个单独个体内随着时间的推移而变化。在这种不同程度的同种异体反应背后存在着许多决定因素，其中最显著的是供体和受体之间的 MHC 匹配程度。然而，接受者的免疫系统的特征和功能可能在确定给定供体组织的同种异体反应的量值和性质方面起重要作用。关于上述细胞在同种异体反应中的中心型作用，后文将对其进行分别阐述。

淋巴细胞作为移植后同种异体免疫的效应细胞

如上所述，淋巴细胞的三个主要亚类可以参与移植后的同种异体免疫应答。虽然 NK 细胞介导的排斥反应在实体器官移植中的作用仍然是有争议的[1-5]，这一内容已在第 7 章中深入阐述，但最近的证据表明，受体的传染病史可能会影响 NK 细胞的自然分型[6,7]。具体来说，现在已知尽管 NK 细胞在编码其激活受体的基因中不经历重排，但是在病毒感染期间它们确实经历了克隆扩增过程，这导致产生满足标准的免疫记忆[6,7]。重要的是，这些记忆 NK 细胞已被证明可以介导针对先前遇到的病原体的更强的二级应答[6,7]，这也提高了导致 NK 细胞活化的先前免疫事件增加 NK 介导的对移植屏障的可能性。还需要进一步的工作来评估病毒诱导的 NK 细胞记忆对同种异体免疫的影响。

在等待移植的患者中，先前存在的体液同种异体免疫的谱系得到了较好的阐明，并已在第 6 章中讨论。体液致敏程度是用通道反应性抗体(PRA，在第 36 章深入描述)定义的。以 PRA 评估来自受体的血清抗体反应的流程中在特定的系列通道内使用了 HLA 分子的频率，并以此评估受体经历体液排斥的总体风险。例如，20%的 PRA 提示患者将与 5 个供体中的 1 个不相容。实际上，PRA 值在不同个体中有着广泛的差异，但据估计，大约 30%的透析患者表现出大于 20%的 PRA，这被定义为高度敏感[8]，其中更有一半患者的 PRA>80%[9]。此外，一般认为较高的移植前 PRA 提示了移植后抗体介导的移植物损伤的风险；虽然这与包含了供体特异的同种异体抗体相对应[9]。有趣的是，在潜在的肾移植受者中比较 PRA 和通道反应性 T 细胞应

答的研究表明，移植前异体抗体的水平并不总是与移植前供体反应性T细胞的频率相关，表明T细胞同种异体反应的存在并不常常意味着B细胞致敏，反之亦然[8]。一般来说，同种异体抗体被认为是T细胞依赖性的，但是T细胞可以对加工的抗原产生反应，而同种异体抗体是针对抗原的四级结构的。我们可以理解，这两个过程的谱系是不一样的。未经移植的患者同种异体抗体的起源最常见于通过输血或怀孕隐匿接触同种异体抗原的情况，并且已得到确认的是怀孕前的状态可能会影响同种异体抗体的产生[8]。此外，我们还知道全身性病毒感染可导致多克隆活化和随后的抗体分泌伴与刺激物无关的广泛特异性[10]。虽然这种多克隆抗体是T细胞独立的，而不是生发中心的反应结果(见第2章)，但它含有同种异体反应特异性抗体[10]的潜能。再者，这种机制对观察到的个体体液免疫中异种免疫作用的贡献值得进一步研究。相比之下，鉴于细胞介导的免疫在转移排斥中的主要作用以及关于同种异体反应性T细胞性质的更深入的研究，对T细胞中同种异体免疫的谱系以及外显子的机制还需更多了解，比如纳入环境抗原、病原体和老化等因素对同种异体免疫反应的影响。因此，本章的其余部分将主要侧重于T细胞同种异体免疫。

T细胞谱及其对病原体和同种异体抗原的识别

为了防御不断变化的病原体，哺乳动物免疫系统已经发展出产生极度多样化的受体T细胞谱系的能力，其能够区分在自身MHC背景下呈现的外来肽。虽然多样性的理论上限可能超过1×10^{13}，但估计在小鼠中表达的不同克隆型的实际数量更接近于1×10^{6}，而在人类中为2.5×10^{7}[11]。理论和实验证据表明，具有特定受体的T细胞克隆亚群的种类在小鼠中为100~200，在人类中为1000~4000。对小细胞病毒淋巴细胞性脉络丛脑膜炎病毒（LCMV）的反应研究表明，T细胞前体(定义为在抗原性攻击前小鼠中给定的肽-MHC组合特异性的初始T细胞的数量）响应免疫显性Ⅰ类和Ⅱ类限制性表位具有相似的前体数量范围为每10^5个$CD8^+$或$CD4^+$ T细胞中1~2个[12,13]。

虽然免疫系统没有进化以排斥移植组织，但仍然显而易见的是，针对来自物种内的非遗传相同个体的组织的免疫应答是特别有效的。这至少部分归因于对这种同种异体刺激反应的T细胞的高数量[14-16]。事实上，在实验系统中已经发现，初始个体的T细胞谱系中0.1%~10%能够与由给定的MHC完全不同的供体[14]表达的同种异体抗原反应，这个数字比病毒特异性响应的估计前体数量大2~3个对数[12,13]。通过将上述不同克隆数量的估值与同种异体反应率(~1%)的中间估值相结合，小鼠和人类可分别承载约20 000和250 000个不同的同种异体反应的克隆。因此，对病原体和移植物的反应从初始前体数量的基本不同的范围开始，这一事实可能对T细胞应答的结果具有重大影响。

T细胞前体数量对T细胞行为的影响

高T细胞前体数量是同种异体反应性的标志之一。众所周知，这种高T细胞前体数量从根本上改变了响应T细胞群体的质量。具体来说，Marzo等人的研究显示，初始的T细胞前体数量强烈影响$CD8^+$ T细胞分化的结果，较高的前体数量导致中央记忆$CD8^+$ T细胞的净增加[17]。高T细胞前体的数量也加速了T细胞扩张的动力学[18]，但也矛盾地缩短了初始和记忆T细胞群体的寿命[19]。此外，其他研究者已经发起了一个有趣的观察：高频率的$CD8^+$前体可以将辅助因子依赖性反应转化为辅助性依赖性和独立于CD154的反应[20]，研究已经证明，幼稚$CD4^+$和$CD8^+$ T细胞频率在确定移植后供体反应性T细胞增殖和分化程度以及介导共刺激阻断排斥方面的重要作用[21,22]。具体来说，以非常高频率存在的幼稚T细胞移植前似乎消除了对CD28和CD154介导的共刺激的需求。高前体频率在确定同种异体反应性T细胞应答效能方面的关键作用已在幼稚和记忆T细胞中被证明[23-26]。初始高前体频率反应的同种异体反应性T细胞表现出CD25表达增加，IL-2受体亲和力增加[27]，抑制性受体程序性死亡-1(PD-1)的表达降低[25]，减少了对于$CD4^+$ T细胞帮助的需求[22]，并且必须进行更少的细胞分裂，以达到效应物临界阈值数量，从而介导移植物排斥反应(图9.1)[24]。高频T细胞应答在介导同种异体移植物排斥反应中的主要作用进一步被观察到MHC匹配增加，其减少了同种异体表位的数目，从而减少了该反应中同种异体反应性T细胞克隆的数量，导致5年移植物存活率增加(图9.2)。总之，这些研究表明，高频T细胞反应作为幼稚或记忆同种异体反应性T细胞群体，在介导同种异体移植排斥反应中起重要作用[28]。

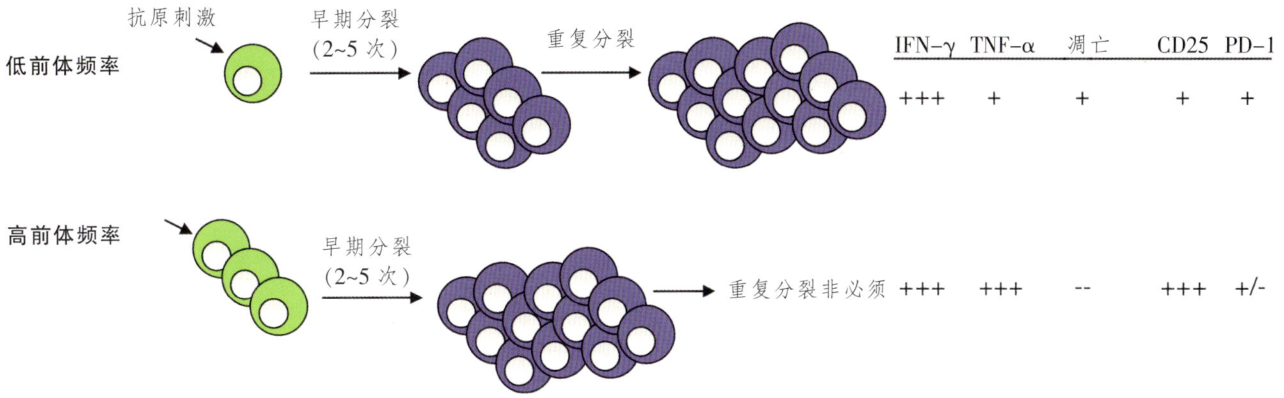

图 9.1　较高前体 T 细胞数量对同种异体 T 细胞免疫反应的影响。起始状态时的低前体细胞数量导致了 T 细胞必须经过更多代数的分裂来达到关键的同种异体效应细胞数并以此介导移植物排斥反应，而起始状态的前体细胞数较高时，T 细胞到达关键细胞数的分裂代数较少。此外，高前体细胞数量分化而来的 T 细胞内包含更多的高质量双细胞因子分泌细胞，并且其凋亡细胞数量更少，CD25 表达增加，而 IL-2 表达减少。

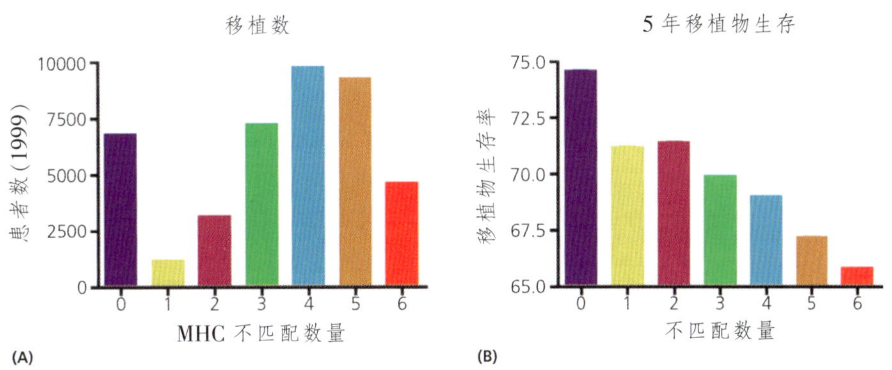

图 9.2　MHC 分子配型对肾脏同种异体移植物的 5 年存活率的影响。(A)图示接受死亡供体、扩大标准供体(ECD)肾同种异体移植在 0、1、2、3、4、5 和 6 MHC 位点不匹配的移植术后 5 年供体死亡率。(B)A 图中接受 0~6 MHC 位点不匹配的肾移植的患者数量。数据来源于 2006 年 OPTN/SRTR 年度报告[118]。

同种异体反应的分子基础

在过去半个世纪的研究期间，这种高的前体频率已经导致人们猜测同种识别与一种标称抗原的 TCR 识别有本质上的不同。这种高前体频率的分子基础是什么？早期研究提出，由于进化选择的种系编码的 TCR 基因片段与 MHC 分子结合的可能性，或许在不存在阴性选择的情况下，TCR 以肽独立的方式连接 MHC。如果所有同种异体反应性 TCR 可以结合同种异体 MHC，而不管所呈现的特定肽，这可能导致非常高的前体频率。然而，同种异体感染的肽独立性不能通过与其配体接触的异种特异性 TCR 的晶体结构来支持。这些研究揭示了相同的正交取向，其中 TCR CDR3 区域与 MHC 肽结合槽接触[29]。随后的研究已经证明了肽对同种异体反应的依赖性[30,31]。尽管很高的同种异体反应性前体频率部分来自给定的供体衍生的 APC 所呈现的大量异位表达，但还有另一个可能导致高同种异体反应前体频率的因素，即同种异体反应性 T 细胞克隆的多特异性。这在研究探索同种异体反应性 $CD4^+$ T 细胞多肽：MHC 复合物的特异性的开创性研究中得到证实，作者发现同种异体反应性 T 细胞具有对不共享序列同源性的多个不同肽表位产生反应的固有倾向[32]。在 $CD8^+$人 T 细胞克隆中进行了类似的观察，因为当人类 T 细胞用自身 MHC 上存在的单个肿瘤抗原引发时，可以预料到响应的 T 细胞克隆对于特定的抗原是高度特异性的[33]。然而，引人注目的是，当 T 细胞群体用同种异体 MHC 呈递的肿瘤抗原引发时，反应性 T 细胞克隆不仅识别免疫抗原，而且还能识别出广泛的不同肽表位[33]。总之，这些数据表明，相对于常规T细胞的同种异体反应性T细胞的多特异性，这是允许它们对许多不相关的肽序列做出反应的性质，从而增加T细胞克隆被招募到给定的抗供体反应中的频率[30]。

异源免疫：病原体暴露与同种异体反应的相互作用

数十年来进行的许多研究记录了预先存在的病原体免疫力影响同种异体反应的能力，这种现象被称为异源免疫。在绝大多数情况下，病原体暴露的作用是增强细胞同种异体免疫应答，并且在某些情况下可能会导致移植排斥反应(图9.3)。在广泛的描述中，存在两种潜在的机制，通过该机制病原体暴露可以增加同种异体免疫：①同种异体反应性T细胞的抗原依赖性活化；②同时移植的设置中抗原独立扩增的同种异体免疫。因此，虽然早期研究记录了病原体介导的同种异体增生的现象[34]，但是他们未能区分这两个假设，作为对观察结果的解释。然而，最近出现的新的实验证据认为真正的分子模拟鉴定可能是对异源免疫应答中观察到的同种异体反应的一种潜在解释[35,36]。我们将在后文分别考虑这些异源免疫机制。

记忆间同种异体反应的证据

由于个体所面临的一套特定的免疫挑战，一个特定个体的免疫系统在此人的一生中发生了根本改变。对环境抗原、病毒和细菌的反应从根本上改变了T细胞和B细胞谱系的组成和特征。已知当实验室小鼠只含有2%~10%抗原经历的记忆T细胞[37]时，大约50%的成年人的外周T细胞室是$CD45RO^{+}$ $CD45RA^{-}$记忆T细胞[38]，结果在宿主的生命中感染和响应多种药剂。这些记忆T细胞在其表型、功能、运送模式和最佳记忆反应的要求方面具有很大的异质性[39]。但在正常健康未感染个体的这些记忆T区内是否存在同种异体反应性？多年来，在记忆性T细胞群体中，同种异体反应克隆的相对表达有相当大的争议[38,40]。这个重要的问题首先是使用涉及脐带血衍生的T细胞制剂的方法，其可以显示含有非常少的记忆T细胞[38]，并且随后使用基于ELISPOT的实验来鉴定哪些能够快速产生干扰素(IFN)-γ，以响应同种异体抗原的短暂刺激，这是T细胞记忆的标志[41]。最近，已经使用多色流式细胞术技术来识别和分类幼稚($CD45RO^{+}$ $CD62L^{-}$)、中央记忆($CD45RO^{+}$ $CD62L^{+}$)、效应记忆($CD45RO^{+}$ $CD62L^{-}$)和末端效应记忆($CD45RO^{-}$ $CD62L^{-}$)$CD4^{+}$及$CD8^{+}$ T细胞区室内的细胞，并评估这些亚群内同种异体反应性T细胞的前体频率[42]。这些数据表明，不同的T细胞亚型中，同种异体反应性可能不同。例如，当使用增殖作为同种异体活性的量度时，与记忆$CD8^{+}$ T细胞相比，在幼稚亚组中检测到较高的同种异体反应性T细胞的前体频率，但与幼稚$CD8^{+}$ T细胞相比，当使用穿孔素或

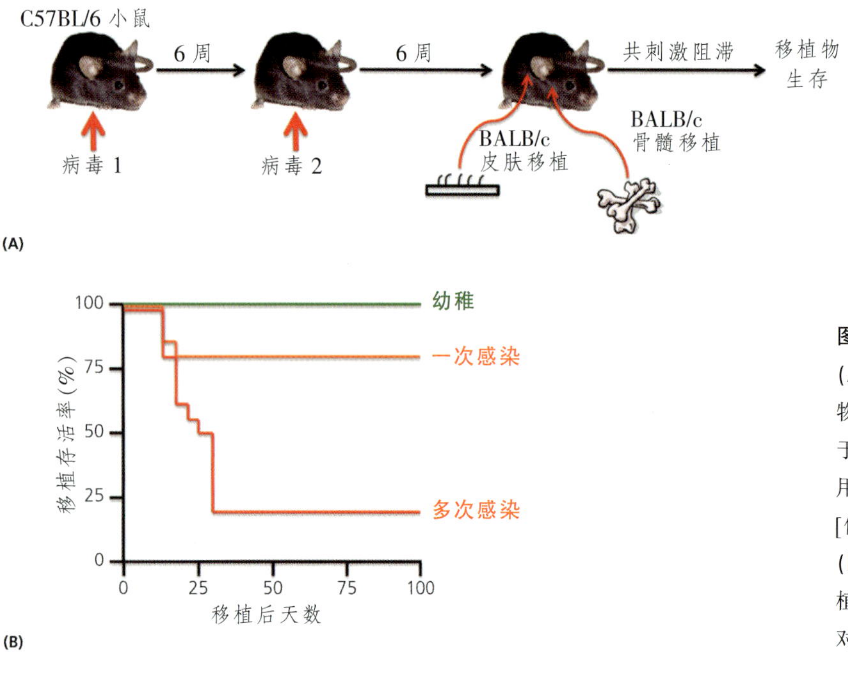

图9.3 病原体诱导的异源免疫的实验证据[23]。(A)用于证明病毒病原体暴露对同种异体移植物存活的影响的实验设计。将小鼠连续暴露于各种病毒病原体并使其抵抗感染。然后使用基于共刺激阻断的免疫抑制方案进行移植[例如皮肤和(或)骨髓]，并观察移植物存活。(B)在多次感染后接受移植动物的同种异体移植物存活率低于那些未经感染或病毒感染相对较少的动物。

颗粒酶表达作为读数时，CD8⁺ Tem 似乎含有较高的同种异体反应性 T 细胞的前体频率[42]。因此，重要的是考虑到，尽管事实上同种异体反应性 T 细胞克隆的频率可能在幼稚和记忆 T 细胞间室之间具有可比性，但同种异体抗原识别的免疫表现可能非常不同，并对移植物有潜在的深远影响。在这方面，确定对于移植物破坏最关键的同种异体反应性 T 细胞的精确效应子功能仍然是一个重要的目标。

异源免疫和产生同种异体反应性 T 细胞记忆

供体反应性记忆 T 细胞可以通过多种独立机制产生(图 9.4)，它们许多(如果不是全部)可能在个体移植受体中发挥作用。异种记忆 T 细胞通常可以分为三个主要来源：①在用同种异体抗原致敏后产生的“传统”供体反应性记忆 T 细胞(即先前的移植、输血或怀孕)；

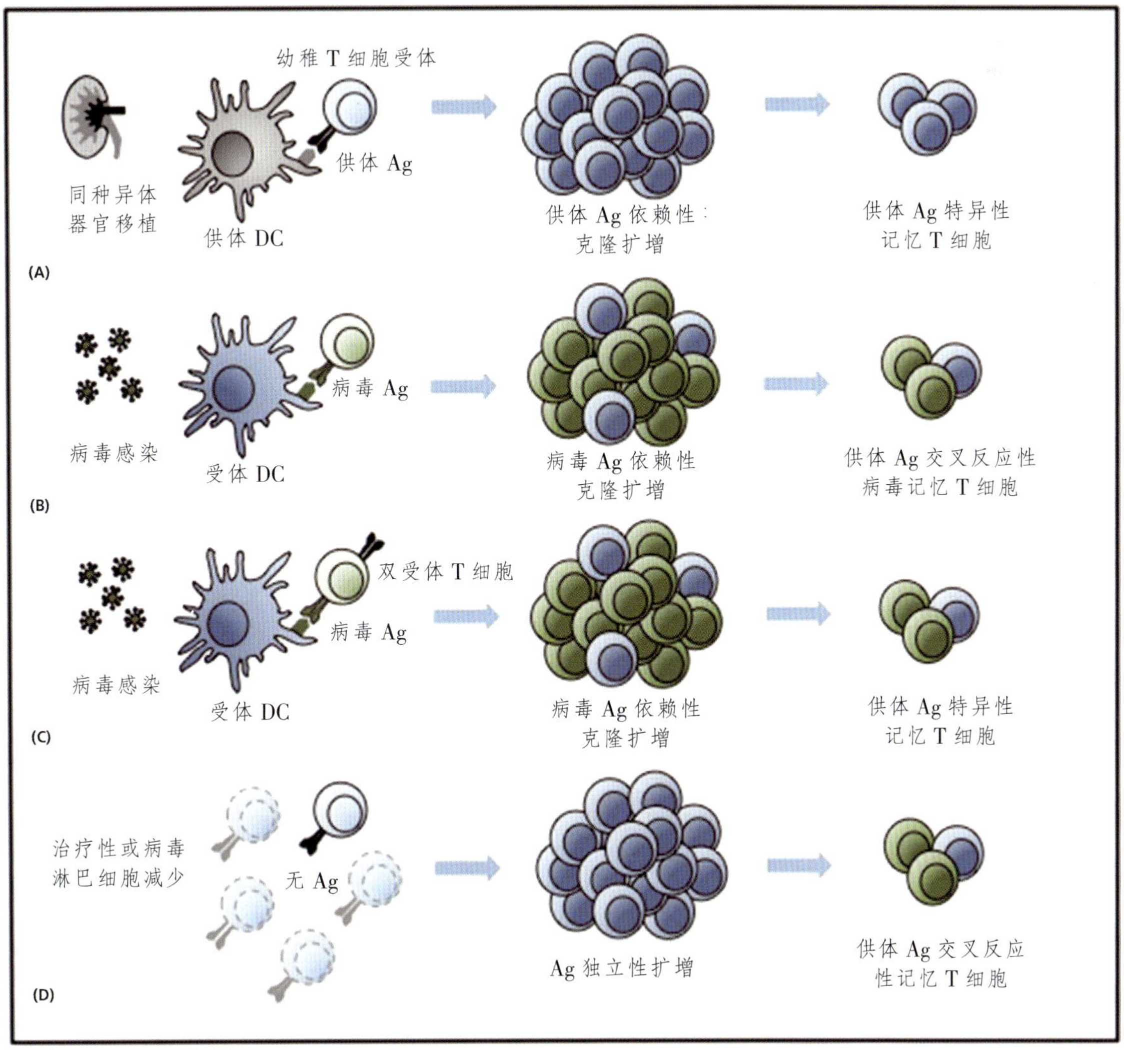

图 9.4　可能出现供体-反应性记忆 T 细胞的机制。可通过至少四种独立机制产生同种异体反应性记忆 T 细胞。(A)“传统的”供体-反应性记忆可能通过先前移植、输血或怀孕形式的同种抗原致敏而产生。(B)同种异体反应性记忆 T 细胞可以在引发记忆 T 细胞致敏的病原体衍生抗原后产生，由于其 TCR 的退化性质而与同种异体抗原交叉反应。(C)同种异体反应性记忆 T 细胞也可能在双受体 T 细胞活化后出现。这些细胞具有一种非同种异体抗原的受体特征，并且当被非同种异体抗原激活时，导致记忆 T 细胞。如果这些细胞携带同种异体反应的第二受体，它们可能作为记忆 T 细胞对同种抗原产生反应。(D)同种异体反应性记忆 T 细胞也可以在病毒或药理学诱导的淋巴细胞减少后通过稳态重建产生。浅蓝色和绿色 T 细胞代表幼稚 T 细胞。克隆扩增和记忆 T 细胞群包含病原体反应性(绿色)和同种异体反应性(蓝色)细胞的组合。Ag，抗原；DC，树突状细胞。Reproduced from Krummey SM and Ford ML. Heterogeneity within T Cell Memory: Implications for Transplant Tolerance, 2012. Frontiers in Immunology. 3:36. Epub 2012 Mar 1. PMCID: PMC3342058[119]. With permission from Frontiers subject to a Creative Commons Attribution License(http://creativecommons.org/licenses/by/3.0/)。

②通过抗原非依赖性机制产生的记忆T细胞；③暴露于非同种异体抗体后引发的交互反应性记忆T细胞。首先，在先前同种异体移植物失败的情况下产生供体反应性记忆T细胞(图9.4)。来自两个实验模型[43,44]和临床患者[41]的证据一致证明了先前移植物失败的受试者结果较差,与“第二组”排斥一致。同种异体反应记忆T细胞也可能在怀孕期间出现,此时(尽管存在多个免疫机制在胎儿/母亲界面上起作用以促进胎儿的耐受性）这个女性可以对抗胎儿携带的父系抗原[45]。关于输血后的非致敏化,已经证实通过血小板输注产生的免疫力足以在随后的小鼠接受者的骨髓移植中诱导排斥反应[46]。由于肝移植受者的早期血小板输注率特别高，这些数据表明高输血的移植受者可能存在记忆性T细胞介导的移植排斥风险增加。

可能引起同种异体反应记忆性T细胞的第二种机制是宿主中存在淋巴细胞的情况(图9.4)。在这些条件下,幼稚$CD4^+$和$CD8^+$同种异体反应前体可诱导经历抗原依赖性,但内稳态增殖依赖于IL-7且随后分化为记忆T细胞[47,48]。Turka及其同事的开创性研究证实了这一现象，这表明初级淋巴细胞群体转移到T细胞和B细胞缺陷型严重联合免疫缺陷(SCID)受体中,抗体诱导的鼠移植受体中淋巴细胞的消耗，导致外周T细胞间室与记忆T细胞的快速重建[49]。这些发现的临床意义在于,揭示了在被病毒病原体如HIV感染之后、在用干扰素治疗HCV之后以及将治疗性消耗T细胞用于治疗自身免疫或移植后发生淋巴细胞减少的事实[50]。来自基础免疫学文献的研究表明,由淋巴细胞减少引起的“假记忆”T细胞随后发生稳态重建具有记忆性T细胞的表型和功能特征，并且在二次激活期间表现为记忆性T细胞[47,48]。因此,淋巴细胞减少诱导的免疫记忆基本上与通过抗原依赖性机制产生的真实记忆无法区分。在稳态扩张后产生的记忆细胞也被证明是移植耐受诱导的障碍,后文将进一步讨论[49]。

接下来，同种异体反应记忆T细胞理论上可以在双重受体T细胞的先前激活之后产生(图9.4),这是常常被忽视的机制。同种异体反应性双受体记忆T细胞可以在两种不同的TCR(一种特异于同种异体抗原,一种特异于病原体或其他非同种异体抗原）共存于同一T细胞的情况下产生。如果该T细胞遇到其特异性的非同种异体抗原,则其将被激活并分化成记忆T细胞。如果在某个未来的时间内，相同的T细胞经由第二受体遇到其同源同种异体抗原，则其将以与之前没有遇到的同种异体抗原一样的记忆性T细胞的动力学和活化阈值做出反应。双重受体T细胞存在于小鼠或男性中的证据是什么？虽然由于TCR基因等位基因排除的原理,绝大多数外周T细胞和表达单个α和单个β链，但已经显示高达30%的成熟外周人T细胞和高达8%的蛋白质在mRNA水平表达第二个α链[51]。鉴于这些双重受体T细胞的存在,这些细胞具有同种异体活性并因此可能有助于同种异体移植排斥的证据是什么？对移植物抗宿主病(GVHD)的鼠模型进行的研究表明,与非同种异体反应性T细胞间室相比,在同种异体反应性T细胞间室中观察到更高频率的双受体$CD4^+$ T细胞[52]。然而，这些细胞在GVHD或实体器官移植排斥反应中在小鼠和人体中的确切作用仍有待充分阐明。

存在由于TCR交叉反应性而导致的同种异体反应记忆

除了上述机制之外，小鼠和人类系统都有证据表明,在称为异源免疫的过程中,同种异体反应记忆T细胞产生在先前暴露于非同种异体抗体之后[23,53,54]。例如，在某些情况下，已知微生物病原体活化抗原特异性T细胞，然后与同种异体组织交叉反应并导致移植排斥反应[36,53,55-57]。由于TCR具有识别一系列相关肽:MHC配体的结合[58-60]的固有能力,当病毒特异性记忆T细胞上的TCR与同种异体抗原相互作用时会出现这种现象。事实上,据估计,单个TCR可以识别多达10^6个不同的配体,并且T细胞谱的计算分析表明,这种高度的TCR交叉反应性实际上完全覆盖多数潜在的可能由病原体或其他外来抗原产生的肽表位[11]。实验数据表明,病原体来源的表位移植物来源的表位之间存在这种交叉反应性：这个结论是源于受HLA-B8限制的EBV-EBNA3A特异性的$CD8^+$ T细胞对与HLA-B44络合的不相关自肽具有交叉反应性[55-57,61]。病毒和异位表达之间的交叉反应也在其他几个实例中得到证实，其中包括HLA-DR3所示的破伤风类毒素表位特异性$CD4^+$ T细胞与同种异体MHC分子HLA-DR4交叉反应的事实[62],以及由HLA-A2与同种异体MHC分子HLA-B44交叉反应的特异性的单纯疱疹病毒(HSV)-VP13/14的T细胞[63]。如上所述,与标称抗原特异性的细胞相比,同种异体反应性T细胞也被证明是更混杂的或具有增加的“多特异性”[30,31]。通过晶体学研究进一步证实了这种同种异体反应性T细胞的“多特异性”，该晶体学研究调查了EBV-EBNA3A/HLA-B08限制性TCR与HLA-B44分子观察到的交叉反应的分子机制[35]，发现单个单克隆TCR与两个离散的、无关的同源异体肽：MHC复合物几乎相同。此外，本研究的作者提出了诱导拟合模型来解释异基因的TCR识别，因为病毒和异构体需要与TCR连接以获得相同的构象[35,64]。因此，病原体引发的记忆T细胞与同种异体抗原交叉反应的生物化学机制已经明确证明异源免疫可以在分子模拟水平上起作用，部分由同种异体反应性T细胞克隆的内在混杂性质促进。

因此，这些非常具体的实例证实了分子模拟作为潜在的异源免疫机制的存在，但确切地说，在人类中病原体引起的配体反应性记忆T细胞究竟有多常见？2010年的研究显示，同种异体抗原的交叉反应性病原体特异性T细胞克隆实际上是很常见的。使用MHC四聚体进行T细胞系的FACS纯化和潜在病毒病原体EBV和CMV的特异性克隆，研究者测试了所得细胞对大片HLA型抗原呈递细胞的反应性。有趣的是，80%的$CD8^+$ T细胞系和45%的病原体衍生的抗原特异性$CD8^+$ T细胞克隆与至少一个MHC等位基因分配交叉反应[65]。在这项研究中，病原体和同种异体反应都可以通过单个TCR赋予，从而在分子模拟水平上证明了TCR交叉反应性，排除了双重受体T细胞[65]。此外，在病例报道中包括水痘带状疱疹病毒疫苗在内，已经证明了病原体感染或免疫增强同种免疫的潜力可促进同种异体反应性T细胞的产生[66]。这些研究表明，病原体引起的交叉反应性T细胞记忆并不罕见，因此可能对临床移植的结果具有深远影响[67]。具体来说，如果单个T细胞库内的大部分记忆T细胞克隆具有内在的同种异体活性，并且单个个体具有数千万的记忆性T细胞克隆，那么重要的是不仅简单地询问供体反应性记忆T细胞是否存在于任何给定的个体中，还要确定其存在的程度、频率、表型和在功能上对长期移植物存活构成威胁的程度。以这种方式，先前的个体患者的免疫和感染史从根本上塑造了移植受者的同种异体免疫。

特异性供体/受体组合影响同种异体反应性T细胞记忆的程度

鉴于记忆性T细胞之间存在同种异体活性，之前已经假设由于记忆T细胞的活化阈值较低，许多不同的同种异体抗原可能能够刺激记忆T细胞，并且接受者具有高频率的同种异体反应记忆T细胞，可能会对更广泛的潜在捐赠者表现出敏感性。然而，虽然同种异体反应性TCR具有内在的交叉反应性，但是使用病毒特异性人类记忆T细胞克隆的上述研究证明这种交叉反应性通常限于单个HLA等位基因[65]。因此，虽然现在已经有几项研究表明记忆中存在同种异体反应性，但供体反应性记忆T细胞的程度似乎高度依赖于所测试的供体组织。例如，在2007年的研究中，来自11个不同非人灵长类动物的$CD8^+$记忆T细胞用表达14种不同HLA分子的一组细胞进行刺激，结果表明供体反应性$CD8^+$记忆T细胞前体在个体记忆中的频率T细胞间隔跨越超过40倍的范围，这取决于异型刺激器的HLA类型[68]。相当惊人的发现是，前体频率跨越远远大于初始的同种异体反应性T细胞观察到的范围，这一发现可能意味着供体反应记忆T细胞前体频率的广泛范围不是由于这些动物的同种异体反应性T细胞谱系，而是由于其免疫学历史的差异而导致同种异体反应性T细胞克隆的差异扩增[68]。

旁观者活化对同种异体免疫和移植排斥反应的影响

前面讨论的研究结论性地证明，通过TCR交叉反应性产生同种异体反应记忆T细胞是一种重要的机制，通过该机制，先前的病原体感染可导致同种异体免疫增加。然而，病原体感染也可以通过所谓的“旁观者激活”，一种与抗原无关的过程来影响同种异体免疫。基于相对于移植时间的感染的类型和时间，旁观者激活的作用是可变的。具体来说，同时感染急性病毒（LCMV阿姆斯特朗）或细菌（单核细胞增多性李斯特菌）的鼠移植受体可导致增强的同种异体免疫，更高度分化的同种异体反应性，加速同种异体移植排斥并丧失耐受诱导[69,70]。然而，已经确定耐受后的LCMV阿姆斯特朗感染对维持移植物存活没有影响[69]，而李斯特菌感染在100%受体中以IFN-β和IL-6依赖方式引起耐受性丧失并促使移植物排斥[71]。有趣的是，另一种细菌感染——金黄色葡萄球菌，不能破坏建立的耐受性[71]。此外，李斯特菌的先前感染对随后的耐药诱导没有影响，而先前感染的LCMV阿姆斯特朗在约7%的受体中消除了耐受诱导[72]。相比之下，对于先前感染过LCMV克隆13或人类Epstein-Barr病毒（EBV）的鼠同源物的移植受体，这两种病毒都能在宿主体内存活，并且可能在基线或病毒发生期间诱发一些低水平的炎症再次激活，100%的接受者完全抑制耐受诱导[72,73]。另一个例子是，在小鼠多瘤病毒(一种感染肾脏的人类BK病毒)感染实验中，病原体相关的炎症功能增强了同种免疫反应，导致多瘤病毒相关性肾病(PVAN)的实验模型[74]影响一些移植受者。在小鼠模型中，多瘤病毒感染导致异基因而非同基因移植肾丧失[74]，伴随同种异体抗原特异性 CD8+ T 细胞增加[74]。在该系统中，病毒特异性 T 细胞与同种异体表型的 TCR 交叉反应性未能被检测到，这表明多瘤病毒感染引起的炎性环境增加促进了与抗原无关的同种异体反应性 T 细胞克隆的活化和分化。随后的研究证实了这一假说，其中具有非常高病毒载量的免疫缺陷型动物无法承受移植物损失，这提示移植物衰竭的非感染性病因[75]。实际上，是过继转移的同种异体反应物，而不是多瘤病毒特异性 T 细胞导致移植物损失[75]。总之，在特定病毒或细菌感染后建立的炎症环境可以以不依赖抗原的方式深刻地影响同种异体免疫应答的强度和结果[76]。这种现象的机制可能涉及特定感染因子通过诱导细胞因子如 IL-6 和Ⅰ型干扰素[71,77]的辅助作用而激活先天免疫应答的能力(见第 7 章)(TLR)[78]或其他与病原体相关的分子模式(PAMP)受体，以授权异源表达树突状细胞[79,80]。

衰老和同种异体反应免疫能力

同样的免疫也可能受到年龄的影响[81]。衰老的免疫系统因记忆性 T 细胞，特别是 Tem 细胞的频率增加而增加[82,83]，许多研究已经表明同种异体移植排斥反应在老年小鼠中动力学较慢[84,85]。这种延迟排斥是由于 T 细胞反应的改变，因为老年同种异体反应性 T 细胞过继转移到年轻的 T 细胞缺陷型宿主中仍然导致延迟的排斥动力学，而过敏性转移年轻的同种异体反应性 T 细胞进入老年 T 细胞则不会[85]。然而，衰老似乎并不影响供体来源的 DC 在实验模型中启动同种异体免疫反应的能力[85]。实验模型中的这些发现得到临床观察的支持，接受者年龄与急性排斥发生率降低有关[86-90]，但捐赠者年龄与急性排斥发生率增加有关[86]。此外，潜伏性病毒感染，特别是 CMV 诱导通气性 T 细胞应答，可以实现老年个体外周 CD8+ T 细胞间室的 50%~80%的频率[91-95]，这种现象可能具有“挤出”同种异体反应性 T 细胞的作用。因此，以这些方式，潜伏病毒感染的衰老和相关影响可能对同种异体反应器的免疫能力产生深远的影响。

预先存在的自身免疫对同种异体反应的影响

同种异体反应性也可能受到先前存在的器官特异性或全身性自身免疫的影响，这通常是首先需要移植的潜在疾病。反复自身免疫可以在肾脏、肝脏和胰岛或胰腺移植中表现出来。进行肾移植的患者可能具有并发的自身免疫病症，如狼疮、Goodpasture 病、IgA 肾病等，导致肾移植前肾小球性肾炎[96,97]。在肝移植方面，有三种主要的自身免疫性疾病，移植是潜在的最终治疗选择：原发性胆汁性肝硬化、原发性硬化性胆管炎和自身免疫性肝炎。复发性疾病发生在高达 20%~40%的由于这些适应证而接受原位肝移植的受者中，最常见于移植后第二年或第三年[98]。潜在自身免疫被认为是在维持免疫抑制减少后发生的，其特征在于肝功能检查异常和肝活检后淋巴细胞浸润[98]。最后，1 型糖尿病患者可能会接受肾脏、肾/胰腺联合或胰岛移植。总体而言，移植自身免疫性适应证的受体可能会增加急性排斥的风险[99]，控制复发性自身免疫性疾病通常需要增加免疫抑制，以减轻自身反应性淋巴细胞的存活和(或)功能。

由于交叉反应性自身反应性 T 细胞或自身抗体而引起的同种异体反应性增加

基础自身免疫可能通过三种不同的机制影响同种异体反应。首先，具有预先存在的自身免疫的患者通常具有对自身抗原特异性的效应物或记忆 T 细胞和(或)抗体，其可以在供体组织的环境中识别这些抗原，从而介导移植物的破坏。例如，对肾小球抗原特异性的循环自身抗体的存在可直接导致患有 IgA 肾病和 Goodpasture 病患者的肾移植损伤[96,97]。此外，众所周知，胰岛同种异体移植物的Ⅰ型糖尿病受体具有记忆，甚至可能活化效应子，针对导致 β 细胞破坏的自身免疫应答之后持续的 β 细胞抗原的 T 细胞已经消退。鉴于存在非常良好的 1 型糖尿病小鼠模型，已经进行了广泛的工作以探索预先存在的 β 细胞特异性 T 细胞应答对糖尿病患者的胰岛同种异体移植物存活的影响和对各种免疫抑制方案的反应性。例如，在通过 β 细胞抗原特异性 T 细胞的外周激活自发发展 1 型糖尿病的 NOD 小鼠中，用 CTLA-4Ig[100]、抗 CD154[101]或抗 LFA-1[102]防止胰岛炎和明显的糖尿病发作。然而，将延迟治疗推迟到疾病已经建立之后（大多数研究中大于9~10周龄）并不能抑制疾病进程[100,101]。因此，这些结果表明，对抑制新生抗原特异性T细胞反应有效的疗法可能延长非自身免疫接受者的胰岛同种异体移植物或异种移植物存活，但几乎不能减少预先存在的β细胞1型糖尿病患者的特异性T细胞应答。

在这方面，具有预先存在的自身免疫的患者可能表现为预敏性患者，因为与同种抗原交叉反应的这些效应物/记忆T细胞和器官特异性抗体可能使其对免疫抑制更难治。这一点引发了有关MHC匹配在具有预先存在的自身免疫的移植受体中的重要性的有趣问题，因为紧密的MHC匹配可能增加复发性自身免疫的可能性，这是由于预先存在的自身反应性T细胞群体在匹配良好的同种异体MHC的背景下识别自身抗原的可能性增加。相比之下，MHC不协调移植物和更大程度的异种移植物可能不太容易受到复发性自身免疫的影响，这是由于不一致MHC分子中自身反应性TCR识别自身抗原的可能性降低。

第二，由潜在的自身免疫引起的炎症状态的存在可以增强移植后更具侵袭性的同种异体免疫反应的产生。例如，狼疮性肾炎和IgA肾病患者的抗核抗体的TLR连接和DC活化的存在可以增强这些受体中的新生同种异体免疫反应[96,97]。此外，由这些先前存在的自身免疫疾病引起的血管周围补体沉积也可以促进肾移植后抗体介导的排斥反应的发展[96,97]。

第三，导致发展自身免疫倾向的遗传因素也可能使给定的移植受体更有可能发展侵袭性的同种异体免疫。这在小鼠模型的研究中是最好的，在小鼠模型中，遗传易感发展为自身免疫的小鼠，包括SJL和C57BL/6(其发展为实验性自身免疫性脑脊髓炎)和NOD(其发展为1型糖尿病)也表现出更具攻击性的同种异体免疫反应和较少受到许多治疗干预[103]。总之，观察到自身免疫接受者同种异体移植排斥发生率增加的机制可能是多因素的。解释上述机制的具体贡献与观察到的患者临床排斥反应增加的原因仍然是一个重要的目标。

针对同种异体反应和自身反应性T细胞记忆的治疗干预

无论上述机制中哪一种移植物特异性记忆T细胞出现，由于其活化阈值降低，这些细胞都可能会对长期同种异体移植物存活产生负面影响。例如，使用标准钙调神经磷酸酶抑制剂的免疫抑制[41]或实验性耐受诱导方案[104]的研究已经观察到供体反应性记忆T细胞前体频率(短暂的体外再刺激后通过IFN-γ产生测量)与增加急性排斥的风险。然而，同种异体反应记忆T细胞反应的体外分析显示，他克莫司对同种异体反应记忆T细胞增殖有强烈的抑制作用[105]。鉴于与使用钙调神经磷酸酶抑制相关的已知毒性[106]，鉴定和治疗靶向替代途径以抑制同种异体反应记忆T细胞回忆反应是一个重要的调查领域。此外，目前人们普遍认为记忆性$CD8^+$ T细胞能够抵抗CD28共刺激阻断的作用，这可能部分是由于在Ⅱ期和Ⅲ期临床试验中，与环孢素相比，使用CD28受体阻滞剂贝拉西普治疗的患者[107]急性排斥反应发生率和严重程度增加[108-110]。

在实验系统中已经确定了其他几种对于同种异体反应记忆性T细胞应答很重要的途径（图9.5)(见第18章)。例如，Vu等在鼠移植系统中证明，应阻断OX40，而不是ICOS、CD70或41BB与CD28或CD40阻断相结合以介导移植物排斥[111]。然而，其他研究发现抗CD70可以抑制缺乏淋巴结的小鼠记忆细胞介导的排斥反应[112]。此外，可诱导的共刺激分子(ICOS,CD278)的阻断已显示可有效抑制移植物浸润记忆T细胞的效应功能[113]。

限制记忆T细胞致病性的另一个潜在策略可能是阻断其进入移植组织的能力。研究表明，LFA-1和VLA-4的拮抗作用均为促进白细胞进入发炎组织的整联蛋白，在实验模型中，抑制记忆T细胞浸润到供者组织中，并与共刺激阻断协同作用抑制记忆T细胞介导的移植物排斥[114,115]。此外，Kirk及其同事报道，靶向CD2/LFA-3的黏附途径消除了$CD2^{hi}$ Tem细胞介导CD28共刺激阻断排斥反应的能力。最后，记忆T细胞可能至少部分易受调节性T细胞的影响，特别是当其诱导嗜中性粒细胞迁移到同种异体移植物的能力同时被阻断时[116,117]。

总结

总之，移植受体的被动免疫史深刻地影响了移植前同种异体免疫的数量和质量，在许多情况下对移植物存活有直接的影响。鉴定和量化移植受体中相同抗

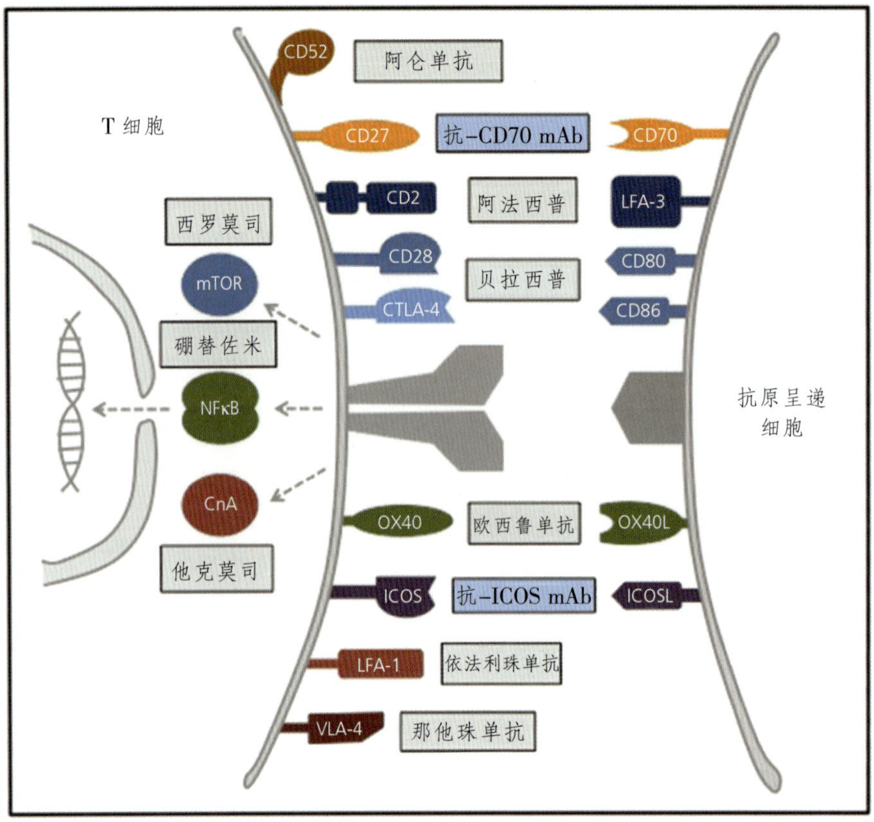

图 9.5 用于抑制同种异体反应性记忆 T 细胞反应的当前和实验性治疗靶标。鉴于供体-反应性记忆 T 细胞可以通过先前的致敏、异源免疫和自身免疫而产生的事实，正在开发治疗剂以特异性地靶向同种异体反应性记忆 T 细胞。其中包括：阿仑单抗，抗 CD52 单克隆抗体；阿法西普，LFA-3 Ig 融合蛋白；抗 OX40L mAb，抗 OX40 配体单克隆抗体；欧西鲁单抗，抗 OX40 单克隆抗体；依法利珠单抗，抗 LFA-1 单克隆抗体；那他珠单抗，抗 VLA-4 单克隆抗体；硼替佐米，蛋白酶抑制剂；西罗莫司，哺乳动物西罗莫司靶蛋白（mTOR）途径抑制剂；以及他克莫司，钙调神经磷酸酶 A（CnA）-NFAT 途径抑制剂。Reproduced from Krummey SM and Ford ML. Heterogeneity within T Cell Memory: Implications for Transplant Tolerance, 2012. Frontiers in Immunology. 3:36. Epub 2012 Mar 1. PMCID: PMC3342058[119]. With permission from Frontiers subject to a Creative Commons Attribution License (http://creativecommons.org/licenses/by/3.0/).。

体相对强度的免疫学参数可能为免疫抑制的定制提供参考，使感染性并发症降到最低，并最大限度改善移植后患者健康状况。

（汪洋 译 李照 校）

参考文献

1. Beilke JN, Kuhl NR, Van Kaer L, et al. NK cells promote islet allograft tolerance via a perforin-dependent mechanism. Nature Medicine. 2005;11:1059–1065.
2. Kean LS, Hamby K, Koehn B, et al. NK cells mediate costimulation blockade-resistant rejection of allogeneic stem cells during nonmyeloablative transplantation. American Journal of Transplantation. 2006;6:292–304.
3. Kitchens WH, Chase CM, Uehara S, et al. Macrophage depletion suppresses cardiac allograft vasculopathy in mice. American Journal of Transplantation. 2007;7:2675–2682.
4. Kitchens WH, Uehara S, Chase CM, et al. The changing role of natural killer cells in solid organ rejection and tolerance. Transplantation. 2006;81:811–817.
5. Uehara S, Chase CM, Kitchens WH, et al. NK cells can trigger allograft vasculopathy: the role of hybrid resistance in solid organ allografts. Journal of Immunology. 2005;175:3424–3430.
6. Sun JC, Beilke JN, Lanier LL. Adaptive immune features of natural killer cells. Nature. 2009;457:557–561.
7. Sun JC, Beilke JN, Lanier LL. Immune memory redefined: characterizing the longevity of natural killer cells. Immunological Reviews. 2010;236:83–94.
8. Poggio ED, Clemente M, Hricik DE, et al. Panel of reactive T cells as a measurement of primed cellular alloimmunity in kidney transplant candidates. Journal of the American Society of Nephrology. 2006;17:564–572.
9. Bray RA, Nolen JD, Larsen C, et al. Transplanting the highly sensitized patient: the Emory algorithm. American Journal of Transplantation. 2006;6:2307–2315.
10. Verdonck E, Pfau CJ, Gonzalez MD, et al. Influence of viral infection on anti-erythrocyte autoantibody response after immunization of mice with rat red blood cells. Autoimmunity. 1994;17:73–81.
11. Nikolich-Zugich J, Slifka MK, Messaoudi I. The many important facets of T-cell repertoire diversity. Nature Reviews. Immunology. 2004;4:123–132.
12. Blattman JN, Antia R, Sourdive DJ, et al. Estimating the precursor frequency of naive antigen-specific CD8 T cells. Journal of Experimental Medicine. 2002;195:657–664.
13. Whitmire JK, Benning N, Whitton JL. Precursor frequency, nonlinear proliferation, and functional maturation of virus-specific CD4+ T cells. Journal of Immunology. 2006;176:3028–3036.
14. Suchin EJ, Langmuir PB, Palmer E, et al. Quantifying the frequency of alloreac-

tive T cells in vivo: new answers to an old question. Journal of Immunology. 2001;166:973–981.
15. Matesic D, Valujskikh A, Pearlman E, et al. Type 2 immune deviation has differential effects on alloreactive CD4+ and CD8+ T cells. Journal of Immunology. 1998;161:5236–5244.
16. Lindahl KF, Wilson DB. Histocompatibility antigen-activated cytotoxic T lymphocytes. II. Estimates of the frequency and specificity of precursors. Journal of Experimental Medicine. 1977;145:508–522.
17. Marzo AL, Klonowski KD, Le Bon A, et al. Initial T cell frequency dictates memory CD8+ T cell lineage commitment. Nature Immunology. 2005;6:793–799.
18. Badovinac VP, Haring JS, Harty JT. Initial T cell receptor transgenic cell precursor frequency dictates critical aspects of the CD8(+) T cell response to infection. Immunity. 2007;26:827–841.
19. Hataye J, Moon JJ, Khoruts A, et al. Naive and memory CD4+ T cell survival controlled by clonal abundance. Science. 2006;312:114–116.
20. Mintern JD, Davey GM, Belz GT, et al. Cutting edge: precursor frequency affects the helper dependence of cytotoxic T cells. Journal of Immunology. 2002;168:977–980.
21. Ford ML, Koehn BH, Wagener ME, et al. Antigen-specific precursor frequency impacts T cell proliferation, differentiation, and requirement for costimulation. Journal of Experimental Medicine. 2007;204:299–309.
22. Ford ML, Wagener ME, Hanna SS, et al. A critical precursor frequency of donor-reactive CD4+ T cell help is required for CD8+ T cell-mediated CD28/CD154-independent rejection. Journal of Immunology. 2008;180:7203–7211.
23. Adams AB, Williams MA, Jones TR, et al. Heterologous immunity provides a potent barrier to transplantation tolerance. Journal of Clinical Investigation. 2003;111:1887–1895.
24. Ford ML, Koehn BH, Wagener ME, et al. Antigen-specific precursor frequency impacts T cell proliferation, differentiation, and requirement for costimulation. Journal of Experimental Medicine. 2007;204:299–309.
25. Koehn BH, Ford ML I., Ferrer R, et al. PD-1-dependent mechanisms maintain peripheral tolerance of donor-reactive CD8+ T cells to transplanted tissue. Journal of Immunology. 2008;181:5313–5322.
26. Floyd TL, Orr SB, Coley SM, et al. High-frequency alloreactive T cells augment effector function of low-frequency CD8+ T-cell responses under CD28/CD154 blockade. Transplantation. 2010;89:1208–1217.
27. Ford ML, Stempora LL, Larsen CP. CD28 blockade induces division-dependent downregulation of interleukin-2 receptor alpha. Transplant Immunology. 2011; 24:94–99.
28. Ford ML, Kirk AD, Larsen CP. Donor-reactive T-cell stimulation history and precursor frequency: barriers to tolerance induction. Transplantation. 2009;87: S69–S74.
29. Reiser JB, Darnault C, Guimezanes A, et al. Crystal structure of a T cell receptor bound to an allogeneic MHC molecule. Nature Immunology. 2000;1:291–297.
30. Felix NJ, Allen PM. Specificity of T-cell alloreactivity. Nature Reviews. Immunology. 2007;7:942–953.
31. Felix NJ, Donermeyer DL, Horvath S, et al. Alloreactive T cells respond specifically to multiple distinct peptide-MHC complexes. Nature Immunology. 2007;8:388–397.
32. Feldman HI, Kobrin S, Wasserstein A. Hemodialysis vascular access morbidity. Journal of the American Society of Nephrology. 1996;7:523–535.
33. Falkenburg WJ, Melenhorst JJ, van de Meent M, et al. Allogeneic HLA-A*02-restricted WT1-specific T cells from mismatched donors are highly reactive but show off-target promiscuity. Journal of Immunology. 2011;187:2824–2833.
34. Adams AB, Pearson TC, Larsen CP. Heterologous immunity: an overlooked barrier to tolerance. Immunological Reviews. 2003;196:147–160.
35. Macdonald WA, Chen Z, Gras S, et al. T cell allorecognition via molecular mimicry. Immunity. 2009;31:897–908.
36. Brehm MA, Daniels KA, Priyadharshini B, et al. Allografts stimulate cross-reactive virus-specific memory CD8 T cells with private specificity. American Journal of Transplantation. 2010;10:1738–1748.
37. Schenk AD, Nozaki T, Rabant M, et al. Donor-reactive CD8 memory T cells infiltrate cardiac allografts within 24-h posttransplant in naive recipients. American Journal of Transplantation. 2008;8:1652–1661.
38. Lombardi G, Sidhu S, Daly M, et al. Are primary alloresponses truly primary? International Immunology. 1990;2:9–13.
39. Jameson SC, Masopust D. Diversity in T cell memory: an embarrassment of riches. Immunity. 2009;31:859–871.
40. Lechler R, Batchelor R, Lombardi G. The relationship between MHC restricted and allospecific T cell recognition. Immunology Letters. 1991;29:41–50.
41. Heeger PS, Greenspan NS, Kuhlenschmidt S, et al. Pretransplant frequency of donor-specific, IFN-gamma-producing lymphocytes is a manifestation of immunologic memory and correlates with the risk of posttransplant rejection episodes. Journal of Immunology. 1999;163:2267–2275.
42. Macedo C, Orkis EA, Popescu I, et al. Contribution of naive and memory T-cell populations to the human alloimmune response. American Journal of Transplantation. 2009;9:2057–2066.
43. Valujskikh A, Pantenburg B, Heeger PS. Primed allospecific T cells prevent the effects of costimulatory blockade on prolonged cardiac allograft survival in mice. American Journal of Transplantation. 2002;2:501–509.
44. Zhai Y, Meng L, Gao F, et al. Allograft rejection by primed/memory CD8+ T cells is CD154 blockade resistant: therapeutic implications for sensitized transplant recipients. Journal of Immunology. 2002;169:4667–4673.
45. van Halteren AG, Jankowska-Gan E, Joosten A, et al. Naturally acquired tolerance and sensitization to minor histocompatibility antigens in healthy family members. Blood. 2009;114:2263–2272.
46. Patel SR, Cadwell CM, Medford A, et al. Transfusion of minor histocompatibility antigen-mismatched platelets induces rejection of bone marrow transplants in mice. Journal of Clinical Investigation. 2009;119:2787–2794.
47. Goldrath AW, Bogatzki LY, Bevan MJ. Naive T cells transiently acquire a memory-like phenotype during homeostasis-driven proliferation. Journal of Experimental Medicine. 2000;192:557–564.
48. Murali-Krishna K, Ahmed R. Cutting edge: naive T cells masquerading as memory cells. Journal of Immunology. 2000;165:1733–1737.
49. Wu Z, Bensinger SJ, Zhang J, et al. Homeostatic proliferation is a barrier to transplantation tolerance. Nature Medicine. 2004;10:87–92.
50. Sener A, Tang AL, Farber DL. Memory T-cell predominance following T-cell depletional therapy derives from homeostatic expansion of naive T cells. American Journal of Transplantation. 2009;9:2615–2623.
51. Padovan E, Casorati G, Dellabona P, et al. Expression of two T cell receptor alpha chains: dual receptor T cells. Science. 1993;262:422–424.
52. Morris GP, Allen PM. Cutting edge: highly alloreactive dual TCR T cells play a dominant role in graft-versus-host disease. Journal of Immunology. 2009;182: 6639–6643.
53. Pantenburg B, Heinzel F, Das L, et al. T cells primed by Leishmania major infection cross-react with alloantigens and alter the course of allograft rejection. Journal of Immunology. 2002;169:3686–3693.
54. Brehm MA, Markees TG, Daniels KA, et al. Direct visualization of cross-reactive effector and memory allo-specific CD8 T cells generated in response to viral infections. Journal of Immunology. 2003;170:4077–4086.
55. Burrows SR, Khanna R, Burrows JM, et al. An alloresponse in humans is dominated by cytotoxic T lymphocytes (CTL) cross-reactive with a single Epstein-Barr virus CTL epitope: implications for graft-versus-host disease. Journal of Experimental Medicine. 1994;179:1155–1161.
56. Burrows SR, Silins SL, Khanna R, et al. Cross-reactive memory T cells for Epstein-Barr virus augment the alloresponse to common human leukocyte antigens: degenerate recognition of major histocompatibility complex-bound peptide by T cells and its role in alloreactivity. European Journal of Immunology. 1997;27:1726–1736.
57. Burrows SR, Silins SL, Moss DJ, et al. T cell receptor repertoire for a viral epitope in humans is diversified by tolerance to a background major histocompatibility complex antigen. Journal of Experimental Medicine. 1995;182:1703–1715.
58. Evavold BD, Sloan-Lancaster J, Allen PM. Tickling the TCR: selective T-cell functions stimulated by altered peptide ligands. Immunology Today. 1993;14: 602–609.
59. Sloan-Lancaster J, Allen PM. Altered peptide ligand-induced partial T cell activation: molecular mechanisms and role in T cell biology. Annual Review of Immunology. 1996;14:1–27.
60. Ford ML, Evavold BD. Degenerate recognition of T cell epitopes: impact of T cell receptor reserve and stability of peptide:MHC complexes. Molecular Immunology. 2004;40:1019–1025.
61. D'Orsogna LJ, Roelen DL, van der Meer-Prins EM, et al. Tissue specificity of cross-reactive allogeneic responses by EBV EBNA3A-specific memory T cells. Transplantation. 2011;91:494–500.
62. Umetsu DT, Yunis EJ, Matsui Y, et al. HLA-DR-4-associated alloreactivity of an HLA-DR-3-restricted human tetanus toxoid-specific T cell clone: inhibition of both reactivities by an alloantiserum. European Journal of Immunology. 1985;15:356–361.
63. Koelle DM, Chen HB, McClurkan CM, et al. Herpes simplex virus type 2-specific CD8 cytotoxic T lymphocyte cross-reactivity against prevalent HLA class I alleles. Blood. 2002;99:3844–3847.
64. Beddoe T, Chen Z, Clements CS, et al. Antigen ligation triggers a conformational change within the constant domain of the alphabeta T cell receptor. Immunity. 2009;30:777–788.
65. Amir AL, D'Orsogna LJ, Roelen DL, et al. Allo-HLA reactivity of virus-specific memory T-cells is common. Blood. 2010;115:3146–3157.
66. D'Orsogna LJ, van Besouw NM, van der Meer-Prins EM, et al. Vaccine-induced allo-HLA-reactive memory T cells in a kidney transplantation candidate. Transplantation. 2011;91:645–651.
67. D'Orsogna LJ, Roelen DL, Doxiadis II, et al. Alloreactivity from human viral specific memory T-cells. Transplant Immunology. 2010;23:149–155.

68. Nadazdin O, Boskovic S, Murakami T, et al. Phenotype, distribution and alloreactive properties of memory T cells from cynomolgus monkeys. American Journal of Transplantation. 2010;10:1375–1384.
69. Williams MA, Tan JT, Adams AB, et al. Characterization of virus-mediated inhibition of mixed chimerism and allospecific tolerance. Journal of Immunology. 2001;167:4987–4995.
70. Wang T, Chen L, Ahmed E, et al. Prevention of allograft tolerance by bacterial infection with Listeria monocytogenes. Journal of Immunology. 2008;180:5991–5999.
71. Wang T, Ahmed EB, Chen L, et al. Infection with the intracellular bacterium, Listeria monocytogenes, overrides established tolerance in a mouse cardiac allograft model. American Journal of Transplantation. 2010;10:1524–1533.
72. Williams MA, Onami TM, Adams AB, et al. Cutting edge: persistent viral infection prevents tolerance induction and escapes immune control following CD28/CD40 blockade-based regimen. Journal of Immunology. 2002;169:5387–5391.
73. Stapler D, Lee ED, Selvaraj SA, et al. Expansion of effector memory TCR Vbeta4+ CD8+ T cells is associated with latent infection-mediated resistance to transplantation tolerance. Journal of Immunology. 2008;180:3190–3200.
74. Han Lee ED, Kemball CC, Wang J, et al. A mouse model for polyomavirus-associated nephropathy of kidney transplants. American Journal of Transplantation. 2006;6:913–922.
75. Albrecht JA, Dong Y, Wang J, et al. Adaptive immunity rather than viral cytopathology mediates polyomavirus-associated nephropathy in mice. American Journal of Transplantation. 2012;12:1419–1428.
76. Ahmed EB, Daniels M, Alegre ML, et al. Bacterial infections, alloimmunity, and transplantation tolerance. Transplantation Reviews (Orlando, Fla.). 2011;25:27–35.
77. Ahmed EB, Wang T, Daniels M, et al. IL-6 induced by Staphylococcus aureus infection prevents the induction of skin allograft acceptance in mice. American Journal of Transplantation. 2011;11:936–946.
78. Porrett PM, Yuan X, LaRosa DF, et al. Mechanisms underlying blockade of allograft acceptance by TLR ligands. Journal of Immunology. 2008;181:1692–1699.
79. Alegre ML, Goldstein DR, Chong AS. Toll-like receptor signaling in transplantation. Current Opinion in Organ Transplantation. 2008;13:358–365.
80. Alegre ML, Leemans J, Le Moine A, et al. The multiple facets of toll-like receptors in transplantation biology. Transplantation. 2008;86:1–9.
81. Martins PN, Pratschke J, Pascher A, et al. Age and immune response in organ transplantation. Transplantation. 2005;79:127–132.
82. Miller RA. The aging immune system: primer and prospectus. Science. 1996;273:70–74.
83. Yung RL. Changes in immune function with age. Rheumatic Diseases Clinics of North America. 2000;26:455–473.
84. Rosenberg AS, Sechler JM, Horvath JA, et al. Assessment of alloreactive T cell subpopulations of aged mice in vivo. CD4+ but not CD8+ T cell-mediated rejection response declines with advanced age. European Journal of Immunology. 1994;24:1312–1316.
85. Shen H, Tesar BM, Du W, et al. Aging impairs recipient T cell intrinsic and extrinsic factors in response to transplantation. PLoS ONE. 2009;4:e4097.
86. Tullius SG, Milford E. Kidney allocation and the aging immune response. New England Journal of Medicine. 2011;364:1369–1370.
87. Tullius SG, Tran H, Guleria I, et al. The combination of donor and recipient age is critical in determining host immunoresponsiveness and renal transplant outcome. Annals of Surgery. 2010;252:662–674.
88. Collins BH, Pirsch JD, Becker YT, et al. Long-term results of liver transplantation in older patients 60 years of age and older. Transplantation. 2000;70:780–783.
89. Pirsch JD, Kalayoglu M, D'Alessandro AM, et al. Orthotopic liver transplantation in patients 60 years of age and older. Transplantation. 1991;51:431–433.
90. Pirsch JD, Stratta RJ, Armbrust MJ, et al. Cadaveric renal transplantation with cyclosporine in patients more than 60 years of age. Transplantation. 1989;47:259–261.
91. Karrer U, Mekker A, Wanke K, et al. Cytomegalovirus and immune senescence: culprit or innocent bystander? Experimental Gerontology. 2009;44:689–694.
92. Karrer U, Sierro S, Wagner M, et al. Memory inflation: continuous accumulation of antiviral CD8+ T cells over time. Journal of Immunology. 2003;170:2022–2029.
93. Karrer U, Wagner M, Sierro S, et al. Expansion of protective CD8+ T-cell responses driven by recombinant cytomegaloviruses. Journal of Virology. 2004;78:2255–2264.
94. Munks MW, Cho KS, Pinto AK, et al. Four distinct patterns of memory CD8 T cell responses to chronic murine cytomegalovirus infection. Journal of Immunology. 2006;177:450–458.
95. Munks MW, Gold MC, Zajac AL, et al. Genome-wide analysis reveals a highly diverse CD8 T cell response to murine cytomegalovirus. Journal of Immunology. 2006;176:3760–3766.
96. Ponticelli C, Coppo R, Salvadori M. Glomerular diseases and transplantation: similarities in pathogenetic mechanisms and treatment options. Nephrology, Dialysis, Transplantation. 2011;26:35–41.
97. Ponticelli C, Salvadori M, Coppo R. The kidney, a victim and culprit of autoimmune and alloimmune responses. Nephron Clinical Practice. 2011;119:c200–c204.
98. O'Grady J. The immunoreactive patient: rejection and autoimmune disease. Liver Transplantation. 2011;17(Suppl. 3):S29–S33.
99. Rowe IA, Webb K, Gunson BK, et al. The impact of disease recurrence on graft survival following liver transplantation: a single centre experience. Transplant International. 2008;21:459–465.
100. Lenschow DJ, Ho SC, Sattar H, et al. Differential effects of anti-B7-1 and anti-B7-2 monoclonal antibody treatment on the development of diabetes in the nonobese diabetic mouse. Journal of Experimental Medicine. 1995;181:1145–1155.
101. Balasa B, Krahl T, Patstone G, et al. CD40 ligand-CD40 interactions are necessary for the initiation of insulitis and diabetes in nonobese diabetic mice. Journal of Immunology. 1997;159:4620–4627.
102. Nicolls MR, Coulombe M, Yang H, et al. Anti-LFA-1 Therapy Induces Long-Term Islet Allograft Acceptance in the Absence of IFN-gamma or IL-4. Journal of Immunology. 2000;164:3627–3634.
103. Williams MA, Trambley J, Ha J, et al. Genetic characterization of strain differences in the ability to mediate CD40/CD28-independent rejection of skin allografts. Journal of Immunology. 2000;165:6849–6857.
104. Nadazdin O, Boskovic S, Murakami T, et al. Host alloreactive memory T cells influence tolerance to kidney allografts in nonhuman primates. Science Translational Medicine. 2011;3:86ra51.
105. Pearl JP, Parris J, Hale DA, et al. Immunocompetent T-cells with a memory-like phenotype are the dominant cell type following antibody-mediated T-cell depletion. American Journal of Transplantation. 2005;5:465–474.
106. Halloran PF. Immunosuppressive drugs for kidney transplantation. New England Journal of Medicine. 2004;351:2715–2729.
107. Larsen CP, Pearson TC, Adams AB, et al. Rational development of LEA29Y (belatacept), a high-affinity variant of CTLA4-Ig with potent immunosuppressive properties. American Journal of Transplantation. 2005;5:443–453.
108. Vincenti F, Larsen C, Durrbach A, et al. Costimulation blockade with belatacept in renal transplantation. New England Journal of Medicine. 2005;353:770–781.
109. Vincenti F, Charpentier B, Vanrenterghem Y, et al. A phase III study of belatacept-based immunosuppression regimens versus cyclosporine in renal transplant recipients (BENEFIT Study). American Journal of Transplantation. 2010;10:535–546.
110. Durrbach A, Pestana JM, Pearson T, et al. A phase III study of belatacept versus cyclosporine in kidney transplants from extended criteria donors (BENEFIT-EXT Study). American Journal of Transplantation. 2010;10:547–557.
111. Vu MD, Clarkson MR, Yagita H, et al. Critical, but conditional, role of OX40 in memory T cell-mediated rejection. Journal of Immunology. 2006;176:1394–1401.
112. Yamada A, Salama AD, Sho M, et al. CD70 signaling is critical for CD28-independent CD8+ T cell-mediated alloimmune responses in vivo. Journal of Immunology. 2005;174:1357–1364.
113. Schenk AD, Gorbacheva V, Rabant M, et al. Effector functions of donor-reactive CD8 memory T cells are dependent on ICOS induced during division in cardiac grafts. American Journal of Transplantation. 2009;9:64–73.
114. Setoguchi K, Schenk A, Ishii D, et al. Anti-lymphocyte function-associated antigen-1 (LFA-1) monoclonal antibody prevents graft-infiltrating CD8 memory T cells early post-transplant. American Journal of Transplantation. 2009;9:209.
115. Kitchens WH, Haridas D, Wagener ME, et al. Integrin antagonists prevent costimulatory blockade-resistant transplant rejection by CD8+ memory T cells. American Journal of Transplantation. 2012;12:69–80.
116. Yang J, Brook MO, Carvalho-Gaspar M, et al. Allograft rejection mediated by memory T cells is resistant to regulation. Proceedings of the National Academy of Sciences of the United States of America. 2007;104:19954–19959.
117. Jones ND, Brook MO, Carvalho-Gaspar M, et al. Regulatory T cells can prevent memory CD8+ T-cell-mediated rejection following polymorphonuclear cell depletion. European Journal of Immunology. 2010;40:3107–3116.
118. Organ Procurement and Transplantation Network (OPTN) and Scientific Registry of Transplant Recipients (SRTR). OPTN/SRTR 2006 Annual Data Report. Rockville, MD: Department of Health and Human Services, Health Resources and Services Administration, Healthcare Systems Bureau, Division of Transplantation; 2007.
119. Krummey SM, Ford ML. Heterogeneity within T cell memory: implications for transplant tolerance. Frontiers in Immunology. 2012;3:36.

第 10 章

移植物损伤和再生的基本概念：组织损伤、组织质量和受体因素

Chatchai Kreepala, Konrad S. Famulski, Philip F. Halloran

前言和定义

谁看到过风？不管你还是我都没看到过，但是当树被吹得弯腰时，风正在经过。

Christina Rossetti, 1830—1894

损伤就像风一样。我们认为它的作用是：功能障碍、炎症、组织学变化和"损伤修复反应"的分子变化。但这些是对组织中伤口反应的表现，而不是有害物质的直接后果。这个概念是每个组织都有一个程序化的伤口修复反应，有它自身的创伤修复形式、高度组织和定型。这种反应的程度告诉我们最近是否发生了损伤。大多数功能障碍是由于损伤修复所必需的组织去分化：在一台机器工作时难以修复它。本章的主要内容如表 10.1 所示。

十年前，我们回顾了延迟移植功能(DGF)的问题[1]，并将从那时起开始专注于新知识。在此期间，供体衰老/组织质量和受体衰老以及并发症已经逐渐显现出更严重的问题，心脏死亡器官捐献(DCD)供体的使用引入了急性损伤新的水平。然而，不断改进交叉配型和对早期抗体介导排斥(ABMR)的识别[2]已经大大消除了未检测到的致敏和免疫介导的 DGF 的影响，除非决定移植配型阳性的器官(表 10.2)。同种异体抗体致敏化的后果和临床方法将在第 68 章和第 89 章中具体讨论。这需要结

表 10.1　急性损伤、组织质量/老化和受体老化/合并症：延迟移植物功能三联症和扩大标准的供体悖论

1."延迟移植物功能≠急性肾功能损伤"：临床上观察到的早期移植功能异常是一个需要鉴别的复杂诊断，包括梗死、技术原因和早期抗体介导的排斥反应

2.急性肾损伤
- 急性肾损伤常能恢复，很少有晚期并发症，但是如果程度严重的话，偶尔也可见功能不能完全恢复
- 急性肾损伤触发了复杂的损伤修复模式(创伤愈合)，包括实质、间质、微循环和炎症细胞，涉及很多分子学改变
- 急性肾损伤中的炎症是创伤愈合中固有存在的并且可能不会引起扩大的损伤
- 急性肾损伤不增加免疫原性和 MHC 配型不匹配的排斥反应

3.质量/年龄
- 老龄的脑死亡供体经常要比患者的年龄更"老"，多因为年龄相关的疾病，例如高血压
- 老龄器官较小(实质丧失)并且剩余组织也会"老化"：比较脆弱，修复能力受损

4.受体年龄是一个被低估的较强相关因素，因为存在的合并症(如左室功能异常)很难被发现

5.扩大标准供体的困扰：组织老化/质量和受体老化/合并症的相互作用
- 扩大标准供肾的预后很大程度上受到将它们分配给高风险受者这个策略影响，这种分配政策将低风险的器官分配给年轻没有合并症的受体，而高风险的器官自然就分配给了高风险的受体，使得风险很难分开，即一些供体风险其实就是受体的风险

6.一旦器官拥有功能，移植物存活率不受早期功能影响。大部分肾衰竭是由于以下疾病：抗体介导的排斥反应、患者不依从导致的排斥反应、疾病复发和其他疾病(BK 病毒、PTLD 等)

7.动物模型易误导并且被认为是不可靠的

8.对登记注册数据的分析是有用的，但是必须认识到其内在的局限性

表 10.2 延迟移植物功能:生物学因素、预后和潜在干预

生物学因素	早期表型	晚期功能,如1年GFR	晚期功能恶化并发展到衰竭,大部分导致移植受者死亡或者移植后疾病(抗体介导的排斥反应、患者不依从导致的排斥反应、疾病复发和其他疾病、BK病毒、PTLD等)	潜在的干预手段
肾脏质量(年龄、高血压、糖尿病等)、受体年龄、合并症	"延迟移植物功能恢复" "缓慢移植物功能恢复" 组织学	晚期功能减退	一般不会发展为功能丧失	选择;分配
LVEF	影像学改变 活检中的急性肾损伤分子信号	患者存活率 移植物存活率 没有明显的功能丧失,除非受者有内在疾病	一般不会发展为功能丧失	选择;分配
急性肾损伤: 脑死亡 低血压 器官切取 保存 器官植入 植入后		急性肾损伤本身可以导致肾单元永久损伤并且不能恢复	不会发展为功能丧失	预防急性肾损伤 处理肾损伤来允许恢复 目前没有治疗

合三个因素考虑:急性损伤、组织老化和受体因素。本章重点介绍这三个因素间的关系,以肾移植为例,但这些原则与所有移植有关。因为功能性标记物(如肌酐)的便利可用性和活检的可及性,已经证明肾脏有助于我们了解急性损伤和恢复,同时支持系统(透析)的可用性使患者在严重功能障碍期间可以存活,最终恢复。

急性肾损伤(AKI)本身可引起不可逆转的变化(特别是严重时会导致梗死),但一旦恢复,通常对长期移植物存活影响相对较小。活检研究表明,晚期移植物丢失主要是由于受体死亡和移植后发生的肾衰竭:ABMR,不依从导致的排斥反应,原发性疾病复发,BK等[3]。因此,一旦考虑到如供体衰老和受体共同发病/衰老的因素时,恢复正常功能的AKI通常不是延迟移植物丢失的风险因素[4,5]。例如,在潜在的标准供体(SCD)中,供体晚期肌酐升高不是晚期移植物丢失的危险因素[6]。同样,长时间的冷缺血(CIT)也会增加DGF的发生率,但对这些因素校正的它长期疗效没有影响[7]。即使在扩大标准供体(ECD)的肾移植中,冷缺血时间对晚期移植物存活的影响也很小或没有[8]。

脑损伤和脑死亡对所有组织造成应激,包括脑死亡后捐献(DBD)的重度血流动力学和内分泌代谢紊乱,也许激素和其他因素通过严重的脑损伤释放到循环中[9]。脑死亡导致Cushing反射的初始高动力阶段——对下丘脑缺血的反应,导致交感神经兴奋增加、收缩压升高、脉压升高和心动过缓。由于儿茶酚胺作用使全身血管阻力增加,这种高动力反应将在短时间内出现,功能上降低左心室输出,随后心脏功能受损和多器官功能障碍[10]。此外,下丘脑-垂体-肾上腺轴会有变化,导致抗利尿激素(ADH)、皮质醇和甲状腺激素的消耗。ADH生产不足可导致中枢性尿崩症,导致低渗多尿[尿量>3L/d或>5mL/(kg·h)][11]和高钠血症(血清钠>145mEq/L,血浆渗透压>295mosmol/kg)[11]。证据表明,肾上腺功能不全与基础皮质醇水平较低和对ACTH刺激的反应失衡是脑死亡后常见的。此外,脑死亡后也可以发现"甲状腺功能低下症状"(游离T3低,但TSH正常)。为了抵消上述所有的影响,使用去氨加压素(或加压素)、甲基泼尼松龙和碘塞罗宁或左甲状腺素进行三联疗法,可以在死亡供体中促进血流动力学稳定。因此,理论上对于具有充足容量的心血管循环不稳定性的情况使用高剂量的血管活性剂是有用的[12]。然而,还缺少证明这种治疗方法有效的证据[12-14]。

脑损伤可以通过循环障碍(局部缺血)和可能的体

液因子如细胞因子损伤肾脏,但是这种细胞因子是否可引起肾内皮或实质损伤是没有证据的。脑损伤诱导炎症反应,可能通过 NF-κB 活化介导,导致胶质细胞中的 IL-6 产生,随后将 IL-6 释放到全身循环中。有丝分裂原激活的蛋白激酶(MAP 激酶)可能参与全身性炎症信号的过程,导致肾脏局部变化类似于急性期反应[9,15]。

由于动脉手术引起的手术后血管痉挛和由于灌注不足,第三间隔和左心室功能差引起的低血压,都会导致肾缺血损伤,尽管它们难以在数据上被发现。因此,供体肾脏带来损伤和应激,可从脑死亡开始,在手术后继续。此外,采取一些措施来保护其他器官,减少容量以保护心脏并预防肺水肿,可能会对肾脏产生不利影响。最终许多影响汇聚在一起造成组织损伤,这可能比简单的氧缺乏(缺氧)和低灌注(缺血)更复杂。

器官移植的挑战之一是,评估已经受到慢性损伤(如老化和疾病)和急性损伤的器官,并将其移植到有合并症的老年受体中,并在损伤修复期间进行支持治疗来获得好的预后。这就造成了 ECD 的悖论:避免将年老的器官分配给年轻人的临床必要性,以及不断增长的老年人器官等待名单和巨大的器官需求,将急性损伤、供受体老龄化以及并发症之间联系在一起。此外,这三个问题可能有协同效应而不是简单的叠加:老年受体左心室射血分数差,由于老化和 AKI 具有高阻力,难以灌注移植肾。需要对与生物学上的供体老化/组织质量和术后器官功能预测之间的关系有一个新的认识和可靠的监测:人口学因素和活检组织学与术后恢复过程相关,但实际上预测能力差[16-20]。

定义

急性肾损伤(AKI)在这里被定义为由应激如缺血或毒素引起的表型变化,包括反映对损伤(伤口愈合)反应的分子变化。AKI 表现为功能障碍,但还有其他原因导致的功能障碍,包括一些不诱发实质损伤的纯血管舒缩状态,例如 ACE 抑制剂的影响和钙调神经磷酸酶抑制剂(CNI)的血管收缩作用。根据这里所使用的定义,AKI 意味着可逆的伤害。更严重的缺血形式可以诱发梗死:斑块状皮质坏死、完全皮质坏死或全身梗死。AKI 专门排除了用于鉴别诊断的这些病因,如动静脉吻合口的破坏、肾动脉狭窄和输尿管梗阻等。

损伤修复反应是由损伤引起的组织中转录物的变化,是一种组织反应。损伤修复反应最佳评估办法是通过活组织检查(分子评估)[21,22],但可以通过尿液或血液中的生物标志物推断,至少一部分是由肾脏损伤诱导的基因产物。许多用于移植的生物标志物来源于肾 AKI 中使用的生物标志物,但需要在移植环境中进行验证和校准。

损伤修复反应的策略是:

1.稳定局部保护宿主。

2.如果可能,将组织恢复到之前的状态。

3.如果不可能恢复以前的状态,则实现最佳的稳定状态(例如萎缩-纤维化)。

4.激活炎症/固有免疫以进行宿主防御和修复。

移植物功能延迟(DGF)定义为在移植后任何原因导致的肾脏功能严重损害。DGF 的原因包括吻合问题、皮质坏死、输尿管梗阻和抗体介导的排斥反应以及 AKI。因此,DGF 不是 AKI 的同义词。登记表分析中的常规是将 DGF 定义为第一周的任何透析,因为这些数据可以由注册管理机构轻松收集,但临床定义非常宽泛。DGF 可以通过许多功能评估来进行临床定义:尿量、GFR 评估、影像学或透析依赖。但是要认识到,一些受体本身的肾脏还有残留肾功能,即使移植肾没有功能,也不一定要依赖透析,因此可能不满足 DGF 的透析依赖性定义。

移植物功能缓慢(SGF)被定义为任何原因导致的不符合 DGF 标准的早期功能障碍。SGF 与 DGF 密切相关,并且通常标志着 AKI 并表现为典型的损伤修复反应,但比透析依赖性肾脏中所见的程度更轻[1]。患者有尿量,同种异体移植物功能受损,但无须透析。移植后第一周血清肌酐可能升高,然后缓慢下降,反映出缺乏稳定状态。一些有用的指标包括移植后第 5 天或第 7 天的血清肌酐>3mg/dL[23];或受体血清肌酐在移植后第 7 天降低 70%以下(与移植前的透析前水平相比)[24]。然而,不依赖透析是 SGF 所有定义的一部分,但是否需要透析的决定在某种程度上比较武断。

实际上,功能是连续变化的,静止孤立地看数据会丢失很多信息。DGF 是 SGF 的延续,移植的每个肾脏都有一定程度的损伤,正如在活体供体的小鼠肾脏同种移植物中所显示的那样[22]。因此,通过干预将 DGF 转化为 SGF(例如动脉灌注)可能不代表移植组织状态的任何重大变化[1]。

原发性无功能(PNF)被定义为未能达到足够的同种异体移植功能以避免透析。因此,这是一个回顾性的诊断，应该进行分解，以表明病因是ABMR、手术并发症或者通常在3个月的观察后无法从明显的AKI恢复[25]。当研究人员描述DGF时，重要的是要知道它们是否包括PNF，以及如何排除它们。

移植物缺血时间是指从器官冷却或血管夹闭到器官植入后血管开放的时间。它可以分为三个时期：热缺血时间(WIT)、冷缺血时间(CIT)和吻合时间。WIT是指从心脏停搏（心脏死亡后捐献的情况，见下文）或从肾动脉夹闭时（在脑死亡后捐献或活体捐献的情况下）直到器官冷保存的时间。CIT是指器官用保存液（器官采集后）冷却到血管吻合开放血流的时间[26]。记录血管吻合所需的时间也很有用，当准确记录时，它是DGF的强大预测因子[27]。

扩大标准供体(ECD)**和ECD悖论**：ECD，如移植受者科学登记中心3所定义的，是指60岁以上的死亡捐赠者或年龄在50~59岁之间，以下三个标准中至少符合两个的捐赠者：①移植前血肌酐>1.5mg/dL；②高血压病史；③脑血管因素引起脑死亡[28]。具有良好特征的肾脏不符合ECD的定义，称为标准供体(SCD)肾脏。

ECD肾脏移植物损失风险比SCD肾脏大1.7倍[28]，但这部分原因可能是由于受者具有合并症和ECD悖论（将ECD肾脏分配给高风险的老年人政策）。由于受者的合并症难以在数据库中获取（例如左心室功能障碍），因此ECD悖论高估了ECD供者问题的影响，并低估了老年受体问题。

边缘供肾(MDK)不仅描述了ECD中供体的质量，而且还包括其定义中的临床损伤变量。一般来说，MDK是指具有一种或多种以下移植前因素的肾脏：供体年龄>55岁，高血压/糖尿病病史长于10年，心脏死亡后捐献(DCD)或冷缺血时间长于36小时[29]。然而，有些人认为传播传染病和(或)恶性肿瘤的风险、活检组织学（肾小球硬化和间质性纤维化）和移植前肾功能等是MDK的标准[28]。以这种方式，MDK可以描述生存和死亡的供体，而ECD只适用于死亡供体[30]。不符合MDK标准的器官称为理想供体肾(IDK)或最佳供体肾。

因此，ECD的定义是基于年龄和年龄相关并发症，而MDK包括其他风险。我们将把讨论只限于ECD。有关ECD捐赠的其他临床问题可参见第53章。

心脏死亡后捐献(DCD)**或非心脏跳动供体**(NHBD)：DCD是指明显不可逆循环停止后的捐赠，导致长时间的热缺血和器官损伤。与已经宣布脑死亡并且心脏仍在跳动（脑死亡后的捐献，DBD）的死亡供体相反，DCD的器官应激更大。

在马斯特里赫特举行的DCD捐献国际研讨会提出了5类DCD捐献者[31]：

Ⅰ在医院外死亡/心脏骤停。

Ⅱ复苏后死亡（医院外）尝试未成功。

Ⅲ等待心脏骤停（脑死亡后的情况，主动照护，特别是肌力药物或呼吸机停止）。

Ⅳ心脏骤停，而脑死亡（脑死亡申报过程中或器官恢复前心脏骤停的情况）。

Ⅴ在医院住院患者意外心跳停搏。

另一种基于循环死亡时间的简化分类方法在临床实践中得到应用。它们分为“不受控制的DCD供体”和“受控DCD供体”。不受控制的DCD是指在转院前或转院期间突然和意外死亡的捐献者，或住院患者的心血管复苏不成功。这对应于马斯特里赫特分类的Ⅰ、Ⅱ或Ⅴ类的捐助者。同时，受控DCD对应于马斯特列赫特分类的Ⅲ或Ⅳ类供体，是指由于终止生命支持即将到来的心脏死亡，在脑死亡申报过程中的心脏骤停或在器官获取之前在手术室发生的心搏骤停[32]。不受控制的DCD具有脑和心脏死亡的不确定时间，并且它们将具有更长的WIT。另一方面，受控DCD具有潜在的更短的WIT，并且DGF和PNF发生率较低[32]。

DCD供肾的移植效果通过与DBD供肾比较短期和长期移植物功能来进行评估。结果表明，与DBD肾(17%~39%)相比，DCD中DGF的发生率(40%~80%)[33-36]明显升高[33-36]。在DCD肾中，PNF的发生率也高达15%~25%[37]，而据报道DBD肾PNF发生率为2%~6%[34,38]。然而，DCD和DBD肾脏的长期移植功能（1年和5年）、GFR下降的斜率和移植物存活率相似[33-36]。这表明DCD肾中的器官亚损伤可恢复并达到DBD肾功能。

DCD肾结果的主要问题是PNF或由于各种程度的梗死，从局灶性皮质坏死到肾小球梗死所导致的长期功能损害。使用DCD肾脏，特别是Ⅰ类和Ⅱ类的器官时，可以通过检测来识别不可逆损伤的器官，因为梗死等变化需要过一段时间才能显现。可用的检测包括近端肾小管细胞的酶学指标，如谷胱甘肽-S-转移酶(GST)，其在DCD肾脏中会明显升高。然而，这种测试是否适用于DCD供体评估还不清楚，因为DCD中的器官损伤与器官获取时间相隔很近，损伤带来的指标变化没有时间显现（参见“AKI生物标志物在临床中有用吗?")。有关 DCD 捐献的其他讨论可参见第 22 章。

人口研究经验—— 移植物延迟功能的原因和后果

DGF 代表急性损伤、预先存在的老化和受体老化之间的复杂相互作用,包括 ECD 悖论。这种复杂性不能在实验动物中进行研究,因为与人体组织相比,衰老涉及哪些物种的过程不同。一般来说,对移植物 AKI 的理解是从现有的种群研究中,从非移植肾 AKI 和衰老研究以及实验模型中得来的,解释推论非常保守,存在明显缺陷[39,40]。与这些早期研究相比,现在越来越强调供受体的老龄化以及 ECD 的使用。

移植和非移植肾脏缺血后的损伤修复反应相似。支持这一点的一个例子是两种疾病状态下常见肾脏损伤生物标志物的发现[41,42](参见"AKI 生物标志物在临床中有用吗?")。然而,肾移植中的损伤修复反应可以通过组织持续/处理(例如低温储存,器官保存溶液和搏动性机器灌注)以及供体和受体复合风险因素来改变。

肾移植中 DGF 相关的许多特点在 1990 年之前被阐述。在 0~4℃的低温储存仍被用于降低缺血过程中的组织代谢率。然而,低温技术需要使用保护溶液来保护器官免受缺血性损伤。基于缺血的生物学变化开发的保存方案,目的在于:

1.通过最小化细胞外和细胞内腔隙之间的渗透梯度来预防细胞水肿[43]。

2.通过提供氧自由基清除剂和缓冲液来维持生理 pH 值,延迟细胞破坏[43]。

3.通过达到正确的钾(K^+)浓度来最大限度地提高器官功能,以防止由于细胞外 K^+的高浓度导致的细胞去极化和细胞 ATP 的减少[44,45]。这导致了 UW 液(威斯康星大学)和 HTK(组氨酸、色氨酸和酮戊二酸)等溶液的开发。然而,比较 UW 和 HTK 使用的研究未能在解决方案之间显示移植物或患者生存的差异[46]。

搏动式机器灌注与冷保存相比观察到的 DGF 发生减少,但对生存率影响不大[47]。一些研究报道的长期生存差异可能是由于变量间的偶然不平衡造成的[48]。

损伤、炎症、DGF 和结局之间的关系是复杂的。损伤引起炎症改变,其可以模拟 T 细胞介导的排斥(TCMR)并且可能被曲解[49]。因此,AKI 可以产生肾小管炎、间质炎症和可能的内皮损伤("v 病变")[49]。在过去,由于交叉配型不合,使得免疫因素扮演了一定角色[50],而现在,只有在交叉配型阳性时而刻意移植时这些因素才是重要的。在敏感性肾移植受者中对早期 ABMR 的识别,将其作为不同于 TCMR 和 AKI 的综合征[51]和交叉匹配的进展在很大程度上消除了由于未确定的 ABMR 引起的 DGF。由于免疫因素或组织质量(老年供体)造成的 DGF 与长期预后不佳有关,而纯 AKI 则没有,例如 CIT [1]。例如,来自一个供体的配对肾的研究表明,当有 DGF 时,两个肾通常均表现不佳,强调供体相关因子的重要性,而不是 DGF 表型本身[52]。

DGF 表型与长期的移植物和患者生存率降低有关,但其关联不能被解读为"直接后果"[53]。观察到的早期功能障碍(DGF 或 SGF)[54]包括许多负相关变量,与晚期移植物和患者存活明显相关,但不是 DGF 或 SGF 的后果,例如 ECD 悖论。这些关联使改善早期功能的干预措施影响晚期预后的假定复杂化[53]:GFR 从 5 增加到 10 可能意味着还没达到 DGF 的定义,但这实际上并不是肾实质损伤状态的主要改变,由于 ECD 悖论并没有改变受者的风险。

与影响组织质量和受体健康的变量不同,一旦肾脏恢复,DGF 对移植物就没有长期影响[4,5]。CIT 就是一个例子。影响功能性移植物生存多因素分析表明,尽管 CIT 是 DGF 的强大危险因素,但并不是移植物存活的独立危险因素[7]。从 2000—2009 年间从国家移植受体科学登记处分析的配对 DBD 肾移植数据表明,配对供体移植物存活类似,与有无 DGF 无关。这些结果表明,延后的 CIT 导致的 DGF 对移植长期预后的影响有限[7]。来自其他配对肾脏分析的经验显示,许多受体特征与 DGF 相关:受体性别(男性)、非裔美国人、肥胖、糖尿病、HLA 不匹配、等候名单上的持续时间以及存在一组反应性抗体(超过 10%)。

虽然临床医生希望更好地管理改良的受者和移植风险因素(如肥胖、等待时间和 CIT)将减少 DGF 的发生,但是干预的效果通常令人失望。例如,通过简单地减少时间并不能减少合并症(例如缺血性心脏病)[55]。灌注应该优于冷保存,但其对观察到的早期可逆性移植物功能障碍的影响相当有限,不伴随晚期移植物生存或功能的改善[56,57]。

AKI 可能不介导晚期移植物恶化

由于 2005 年以来使用前瞻性组织活检,晚期移植物丢失的原因已经被人们更好地认识 。行活检的晚期肾脏移植物丢失的主要原因是 ABMR （有时因非依从性导致更加复杂）和复发性疾病，较少部分是由于多瘤病毒肾病和其他原因引起的[3,58,59]。换句话说，晚期恶化是由于疾病而不是神秘的纤维化[60]。没有病因的萎缩-纤维化是常见的，因为在具有广泛萎缩-纤维化的肾脏中容易错过疾病诊断，但这并不意味着原发性纤维化过程。

供体年龄与受体年龄以及和 ECD 悖论的相互作用

供体和受体年龄均影响同种异体肾移植物存活：晚期同种异体移植物衰竭的风险通过供体和受体年龄之间的相互作用而增加。供体衰老无疑是重要的：肾脏损失细胞/组织要素（例如肾脏质量和功能的丧失，即肾单位和 GFR）[61]。我们发现在植入后肾活检中测量的 AKI 分子仅预测肾脏的早期功能（表现为 DGF），但组织质量/老化会影响移植肾早期和晚期功能[4]，受供体年龄和老化相关疾病的影响。

供体组织老化/质量和受体老化/合并症在移植物存活中的作用是复杂的[4]。ECD 悖论意味着来自年轻捐献者的理想肾脏通常被分配给年轻接受者以最大化效用[62]。因此，老年捐赠者有更多的合并症，但是这在登记系统中并不能被显示。最有可能发生 DGF 的老年肾脏被选择性地给予最高风险的接受者（图 10.1）。人群研究中 AKI、供体年龄、受者年龄和移植物存活之间的关系[63,64]必须被谨慎解释，因为来自老年捐赠者的高风险肾脏与年龄较大的伴有合并症的受者之间有强烈的关联。

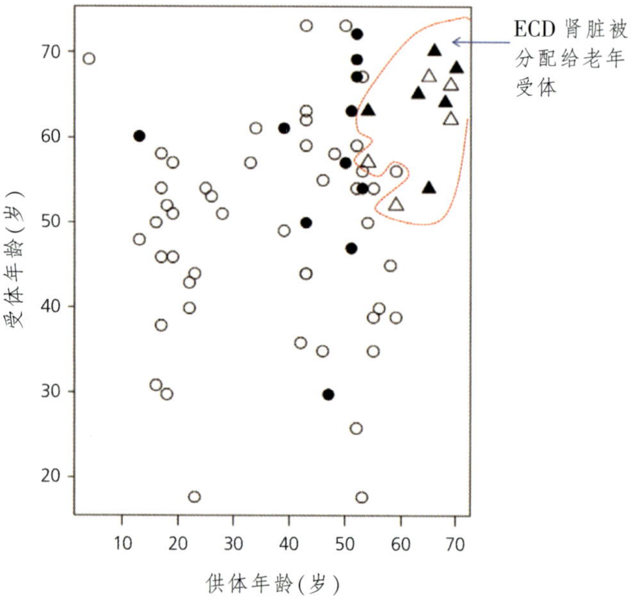

标记：○=SCD 早期移植物功能，●=SCD 移植物功能，△=ECD 早期移植物功能，▲=ECD 移植物功能，SCD-标准供体，ECD-扩大标准供体。

图 10.1 ECD 悖论。来自年轻捐赠者的理想肾脏通常分配给年轻受者。同时，分配给年龄较大受者的老年捐赠者移植的早期功能障碍风险很高。因此，早期移植物功能障碍（DGF 或 SGF）的解释被供体和受体年龄之间的关系所混淆。

老年受者的移植生存率最低[65]，主要是因为可预见的功能性移植物死亡。然而，受者的合并疾病和入住 ICU 也是移植物存活的危险因素，并可能损害免疫抑制治疗。因此，有合并症的受者不仅增加了患者死亡的风险，而且增加了因合并疾病导致的移植物衰竭风险。

接受老年供体肾脏的年轻受体的移植物衰竭与接受年轻供体肾脏的年轻受体相比有增加（相对危险度=1.97；P=0.001）[66]，尽管其原因尚不清楚。老年供体肾脏的受体具有较差的移植功能，这可能对年轻受体具有更大的负面影响（即与老年受体相比，其心血管相关发病率和死亡率的风险增加，预期寿命较长）。一些证据表明，肾功能不全是冠状动脉疾病、充血性心力衰竭和高血压的独立风险[67-70]，尽管不清楚是否在 Framingham 风险[71]后肾功能是独立危险因素[71]。然而，给予年轻受体老年肾脏的决定可能受到受体的医疗风险驱动。

由于移植受体具有比在等候名单上的患者更多的生存和生活质量优势，因此器官短缺迫使临床医生进行 ECD 移植。认识到老年供体肾对移植物存活的不利影响，使用年轻器官对年轻受体优先配置是可以理解的，从而改善移植物和患者的生存。这种做法的合理性、效用和公平性超出了本章的范围。老年供体组织和老年受体年龄的问题是强烈相关并且可能相互作用的，例如来自 ECD 的高耐药性肾脏可能在左心室射血分数降低的老年受体中灌注不良。

总而言之，必须考虑捐献者的年龄（特别是死亡捐献者的年龄）。

1.年轻的成年肾脏对于年轻人或老年人都是最好的。“老供老”移植[72]有利于老年肾脏的充分利用，但对于老年患者来说，虽然效果通常优于透析，但也并不理想。

2.年龄较大供体的肾脏应该分配（不丢弃），但对年轻受体来说不是一个很好的解决方案，导致 ECD 悖论。

3.衰老的表型包括功能性物质的损失和剩余组织

的衰老变化，这可能表现为脆性（“伤害性”）和损伤修复不良。

衰老生物学不是线性的

时间对人体组织的影响包括生长发育和衰老。理想的捐赠者不应是婴儿，而是一个年轻的成年人，因此是 U 形风险分布。基于肾脏特征表现出失败风险的经验衍生方程［例如 Schold [73] 和肾脏供体风险指数（KDRI）[74]］都包括捐赠者年龄，但表示为描述 U 形分布的复杂方程式。衰老对移植物的复杂影响反映了移植物质量[75]、体细胞衰老[76]、血管阻力、功能、易受损伤和修复潜力等因素。对于这个讨论，当年轻人完成成长和发育时，老龄化便开始了。

实验模型

实验模型的教训和限制

小型和大型的动物模型可能会产生误导，因为它们不能模拟人类观察到的风险，例如组织质量/衰老和受体因素。但老龄化和体细胞衰老的生物学在人类和小动物中不同。因此，在 AKI 的大鼠和小鼠模型中产生有益效果的干预措施很少转化为成功的人体试验。

基于小动物模型的一个强有力的假设是“炎症”是有害的。事实上炎症是伤口修复的关键。实验模型的操作在这方面可能是误导性的：由操作实验动物产生的许多概念无法转化为人类的应用。尽管在大鼠和小鼠中，损伤有时会引起长期的肾脏恶化，但是这涉及这些模型独特的与人类无关的过程，例如局灶性肾小球硬化。此外，与普遍的假设相反，没有证据证明伤害倾向于排斥；在大多数情况下，排斥和损伤是叠加的（参见 AKI 的临床治疗）。

组织和器官水平的损伤修复生物学

肾单位具有蠕虫样结构，其发育及维持稳态过程中的程序样运转、反馈以及调节的过程相当复杂，比如肾血流动力学等。而自动调节是通过肌原性拉伸受体反应和肾小球反馈相互作用介导的维持肾血浆流量（RPF）和 GFR 恒定在某一范围的动脉血压机制[77]。

由肾小球滤过中断引起的流体柱运动停止改变了肾原发性纤毛的功能（另一种肾小管运动感受器）[78]。通过这些肾小管的流体运动向肾上皮细胞提供信号，以维持其正常的分化状态。肾原发性纤毛感觉流体流动的能力也对肾损伤和修复期间的上皮分化具有重要作用。它们包含运动感应机械感受器样蛋白（如多丝丝霉素），在细胞外环境的变化从纤毛转移到细胞内环境中起重要作用，导致上皮细胞分化、增殖、迁移和黏附的调节[78]。

动脉血流停止导致细胞立即氧剥夺（即代谢产物积累的缺氧），还有许多其他影响，例如柱塞在毛细血管和小管内流体的运动中断。在肾脏中，与内皮层和髓质相比，动脉血液输送的减少导致外皮层相对较大的缺血。（因此，在相对严重的缺血后，皮质坏死的边缘可能延伸至外皮层。）血流量的严重下降导致高能量磷酸盐消耗，并且随后不能维持细胞膜上的生理离子梯度。ATP 耗尽导致 ATP 依赖的运输泵停止，导致线粒体肿胀和外膜破裂，释放细胞色素 c 和细胞凋亡诱导因子（AIF），其也参与凋亡的启动[79]。

在缺血性肾损伤后，细胞死亡坏死和凋亡的模式主要取决于损伤的严重程度和细胞类型的耐药性。坏死组织学特征在于膜完整性丧失，细胞质肿胀和细胞破碎，通常发生在严重损伤后[80]。细胞凋亡的特征在于细胞质和核收缩[80]。细胞凋亡在不太严重的损伤后占主导地位，并导致凋亡细胞的形成，这些细胞被吞噬作用迅速清除。该过程是通过来自促细胞凋亡蛋白（Bax 和 Bid）响应于细胞应激和（或）促凋亡细胞因子的信号启动的[81]。

在调节因子中，促细胞凋亡转录因子 p53 已被证明在 mRNA 和蛋白质水平上被诱导。通过 pifithrin-α 抑制 p53 的缺血诱导的软骨细胞易位。然而，pifithrin-α 在人类中不太可能是治疗考虑因素，因为 p53 依赖性凋亡的全身抑制可能促进其他器官系统中受损或突变携带细胞的存活[81,82]。

受损的肾小管上皮细胞通过分泌趋化因子（例如 CXCL1）、细胞因子（例如 IL6 和 IL18）和其他炎性介质[83]产生反应，并表达 ITGB6，其激活与细胞外基质结合的潜伏性 TGF-β[84-86]。AKI 的炎症可能是伤口修复的一个组成部分，但通常被认为是损伤的延伸——通常被称为“适应不良”，或称“有害”。实际上，受伤的组织会自动增加伤口的感觉。将早期炎症变化概念化为对创伤的稳定，清除碎片和寻找感染的先天免疫机制的激活更为合适。在小鼠肾移植同种移植物中，巨噬细胞在第一周累积[87]，持续数周后减少。它们有许多潜在的作用,例如清除碎片。效应记忆T细胞也累积在损伤的组织中,但其作用不明确。

与AKI相关的组织学变化在肾脏的皮质神经结合处最为明显。人类缺血性AKI的一些形态特征包括:①近端管再生,失去毛边;②斑块远端肾小管坏死;③再生;④着色(血红素)颗粒状铸件;⑤炎症和⑥直肠中的有核细胞[88]。与AKI的天然肾组织学相比,AKI移植的肾被认为具有较少的管状截面,偶尔有完整管状横截面的坏死,以及较少的管状去分化和再生。此外,可能有较多的草酸钙晶体、微钙化和等量空泡化(有时可能反映钙调磷酸酶抑制剂的毒性)。老年供体中的动脉透明化和动脉纤维性内膜增厚增加,因此与DGF相关[89],但与年龄关联可能更强。一般来说,移植肾活检中老化的组织学变化与移植结果相关,但不能可靠地预测移植结果。通过超声检查可以检测到AKI的肾脏回声引起的皮质回归和肾脏损伤,可能反映水肿,但这一特征是非特异性的[90,91]。

在用AKI移植肾的指征活检中,存在与GFR抑制相关的特征性AKI转录本变化,而与称为"急性肾小管损伤"的管状变化无关(见下文)[21]。

因此,损伤修复反应可能不会对组织造成额外的压力,而仅仅是伤口中的炎症对受伤组织产生的压力,也是程序的一个组成部分。肾小管细胞继续经历修复、迁移和增殖,并重新尝试建立细胞和小管完整性。随着细胞分化的持续和细胞及器官功能恢复,GFR开始改善[92]。一些形态学变化持续到恢复期,与功能无关,而随着功能恢复,单侧管状上皮细胞的毛刷边界变化和脱离逐渐消退[93,94]。

肾细胞损伤的反应与肾单位的反应相结合。肾单位最好被概念化为拥有情报系统,接收信息并回应一系列潜在的反应,包括:

1.暂时关闭,无伤口修复反应,例如纯血管舒缩功能障碍;

2.临时停机,有伤口修复反应,使机体恢复质量标准;

3.永久性关闭,萎缩性纤维化和肾小球全球性硬化,可能最终消失。

图10.2描述了随着时间的推移讨论的过程。

AKI的分子变化

肾的损伤修复反应类似于伤口修复,上皮和基质重塑是恢复体内平衡所必需的。实际上,肾脏再生/修复过程与肾癌具有一些特征[81,95-99],包括细胞外基质组分的细胞生长和增殖的合成。(癌症被称为"不愈合的伤口"。)炎症级联由介质如促炎细胞因子例如TNF-α、IL-6和TGF-β引发[83,100]。这种损伤修复反应的主要元素是实质的去分化,实质的修复和胚胎程序的外观,基质的重塑和微循环,以及细胞循环的波浪和炎症。

虽然大多数功能障碍是由于大量去分化,而不是细胞死亡,但是伴随着这种过程有各种形式的细胞死亡。细胞死亡有几种类型:凋亡、自噬和坏死,并且可能导致任何这些损伤。然而,细胞死亡可能更多仅仅是伤害造成的直接原因:它可能是损伤修复过程的一部分,对损伤的组织元件的重塑至关重要。细胞凋亡在胚胎发育程序中至关重要,有时可能是这些发展计划重组损伤后组织重建的一部分[101]。

实验移植模型:与肾脏同种移植物损伤相关的基因表达谱

移植诱导的AKI可以在啮齿动物肾脏同种异体移植中建模[22]。损伤修复诱导的转录本(IRIT)在小鼠肾脏移植中反映同种异体移植不同类型的损伤(即早、中、晚期)[22]。早期IRIT反映了系统性影响(伤口,麻醉),中期和晚期IRIT代表上皮的局部应激变化,使人想起天然肾脏的ATN损伤(图10.3)。在同种异体移植物中,IRIT表达谱(早期、中期和晚期IRIT)最初与同种异体移植物相似,但由于TCMR[101],差异较大。

与应激反应、肾脏发育、细胞周期和ECM过程相关的转录丰富了中期和晚期IRIT表达谱。与中期IRIT相比,与胚胎肾和输尿管芽发育相关的转录被表达过多,而在晚期IRIT以及ECM组分和TGFβ1/纤维形成相关转录物中,间质相关转录物突出。

对基因表达移植后时间过程的详细检查表明,同种异体移植物显示轻度但复杂的活性损伤修复反应和丧失上皮特征(KT1、KT2),伴有炎症特征(QCAT、GRIT、QCMAT和AMAT)。在第7天ATN中观察到类似的变化(图10.4)[102,103]。值得注意的是,主动的损伤修复反应伴随有继发性炎症反应,在没有排斥反应的情况下,IFNG作用和巨噬细胞功能尤为重要。然而,随着愈合过程的继续,它们的表达恢复正常。

同种异体移植物(图10.4)显示了同种异体移植物的所有特征,但第3天后逐渐积累更多的T细胞和巨

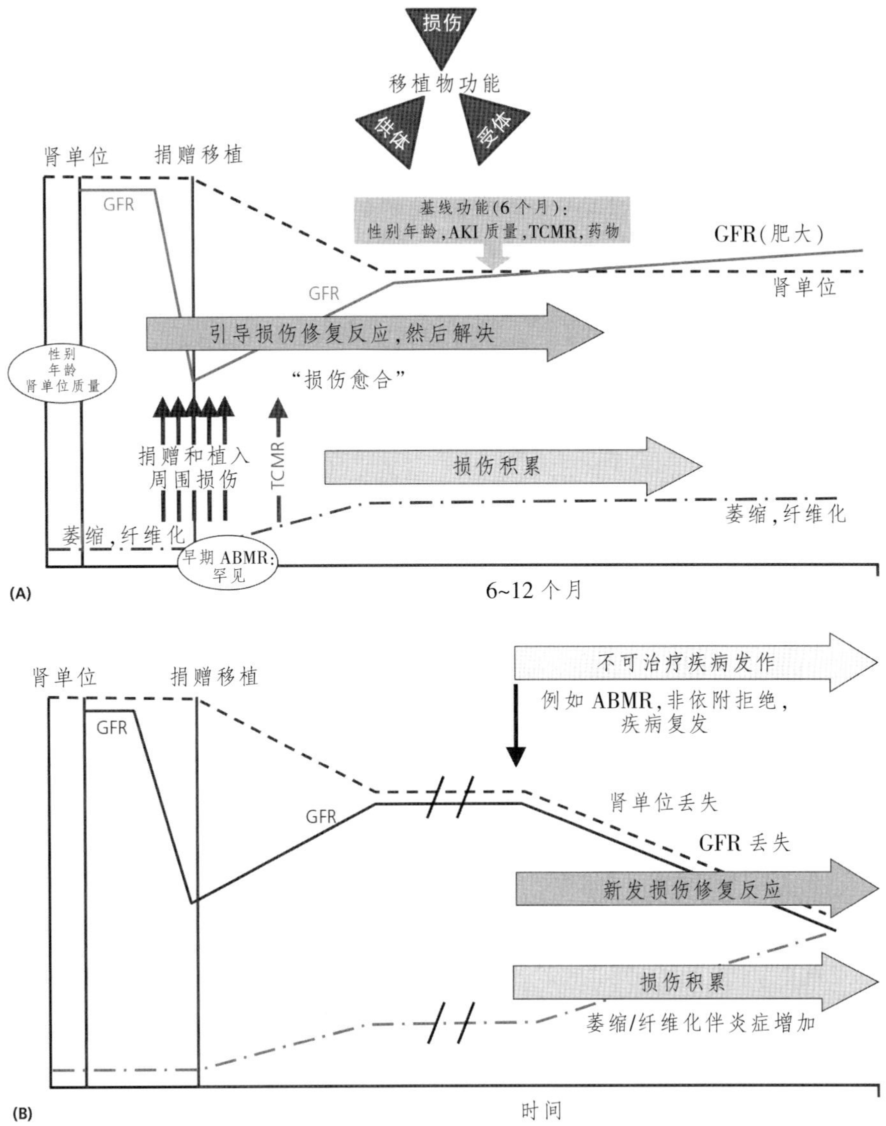

图 10.2　概念化肾脏移植的时间过程。(A)早期移植期的应激诱导损伤修复反应。肾脏移植的大多数变化反映了与捐赠和植入相关的损伤的解决,以及 AKI、TCMR 和药物毒性期间的损伤,随后稳定。损伤是在伤口修复反应和后来肾单位丢失的情况下暂时发生的。肾单位的损失是由损伤引起的,而不是由损伤修复反应引起的。伤口修复反应具有适应性和自我限制性,如伤口愈合,早期伤害不会引发无情的恶化,但主动伤害-修复反应通常会留下至少一些永久性的伤害负担。(B)尽管早期受伤,但肾脏移植在出现疾病之前一直保持稳定。出现功能障碍晚期(>1 年)的肾脏通常可能表现出新的疾病。此外,应始终将不依从问题视为必须纠正以防止遗失的条件。不应将早期恶化解释为早期远程伤害的结果。萎缩瘢痕形成反映了损伤修复反应的失败,使受损组织恢复到以前的状态。

噬细胞转录物,并伴有积极的损伤修复反应(中期和晚期),ENDAT 和 KT 降低,与出现的情况相吻合。间质浸润然后排斥。重要的是,这项研究表明,在用 TCMR 排斥同种异体移植物中,中间和晚期 IRIT 的表达增加与 T 细胞细胞毒性分子、B 细胞或免疫球蛋白无关。因此,TCMR 的机制似乎涉及对肾单位固有的损伤修复反应的触发。

单核细胞-巨噬细胞-树突状细胞群体(MMDC)的积累和激活是复杂的,并且与损伤的程度和类型密切相关[104]。MMDC 群体在炎症、吞噬作用、对损伤的反应以及组织重塑中具有许多潜在的作用[105]。在损伤修复反应中有两种巨噬细胞活化表型。经典的巨噬细胞激活(CMA)本质上是由 IFNG 驱动的,而替代性的巨噬细胞激活(AMA)更为复杂。AMA 通常在体外由 IL4 和 IL13 建模[106],但也可以由激活素 A 驱动[105,107]。每个都在针对某些病原体的先天反应中起作用。由于 AMA

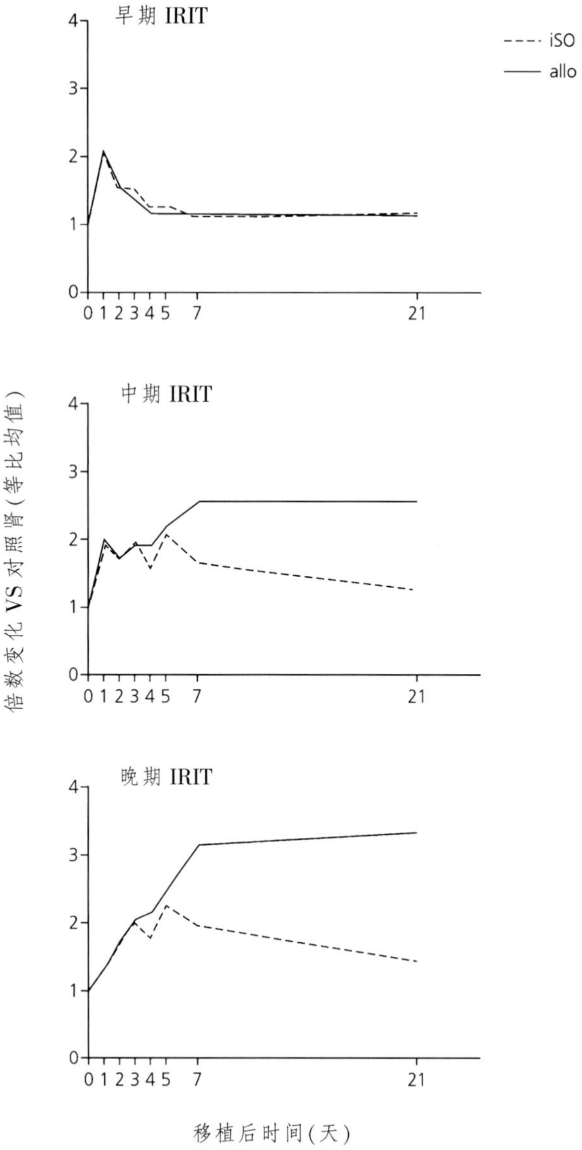

图 10.3 小鼠同种异体和同基因移植物中损伤修复反应的异质性。损伤和修复诱导的转录物(IRIT)的表达时间过程:早期 IRIT、中期 IRIT 和晚期 IRIT。虚线表示等值线，实线表示同种异体。早期 IRIT 在第 1 天显示出瞬时峰值,并且在同种异体和同基因异体中均被诱导。他们代表麻醉和创伤的系统性影响。中期和晚期 IRIT 在等位基因的第 1~5 天显示出广泛的表达峰值,然后降低。在同种异体中,中期特别是晚期 IRIT 的表达在移植后第 5 天显著升高。(Reproduced from Famulski et al. 2007 [22], with permission from John Wiley and Sons Ltd.)

特征与组织损伤[108]和损伤后组织重塑[109]密切相关,因此引起了研究者极大的兴趣。在人类群体中的严重 AKI 中可以看到 IFNG 效应和替代性巨噬细胞激活的综合表达，但它可能是由于组织损伤而定量表达 TCMR[21]。

人类肾移植中 AKI 相关的分子变化

移植后活检

我们检测了移植后进行的活检组织中的基因表达与肾功能的关系[21],重点关注了移植后早期(前 6 周内)进行的伴随 AKI 的肾脏组织活检，并排除了具有早期排斥反应组织学证据或特定疾病的病例。肾活检时提示功能较差(eGFR),但 6 个月后就恢复了功能。

我们确定了 AKI 信号的前 30 名候选基因 (表 10.3),提供了组织发育和癌症,特别是侵袭性和转移性癌症以及纤维化的损伤修复反应(对伤口的反应)中的定型机制。AKI 信号与 GFR 和 AKI 表型良好相关，而 AKI 的组织学变化与肾功能或表型无关。因此,具有早期 AKI 的肾移植代表了非免疫损伤的成功修复,并且其转录本反映了在肾脏恢复过程中发生的主动损伤修复反应的快照[110]。

令人惊讶的是,AKI 信号是受损和患病的肾实质的一般特征,因此可在移植后晚期的移植物中检测到。晚期移植物的损伤信号是纤维化、炎症或胶原基因表达的未来移植物损失更好的预测因子。AKI 信号至少 19 个单独基因可预测未来的移植物损失[111]。因此,在可逆性损伤中定义的急性损伤信号存在于许多进行性疾病中,作为实质性痛苦的反映。AKI 信号与失败风险的关联由诱导损伤决定，即可治疗或自我限制及不可治愈或持续。因此,造成移植进展困难主要是由疾病引起的持续的实质损伤而非纤维化。

移植物活检

植入肾脏的局部和全身反应都具有早期的 DGF 表型。此外,DGF 的高发生率与损伤修复反应(IRIT)和炎症相关的基因表达相关[112]。

如 DBD 肾所示,AKI 信号对于植入活检中的 DGF 具有预测价值[113]。与具有良好功能的肾脏相比,肾脏 AKI 信号得分明显高于未来功能差的肾脏。活体供肾和对照肾 AKI 信号得分最低。

在一些报道中,在植入时检测炎症与移植后临床结果相关，但炎症是具有斑块性瘢痕形成的老年肾脏的特征。因此,这些报道需要确认,以适应 ECD 捐助者、高危患者和 ECD 悖论等因素。非裔美国人受体种族、死亡

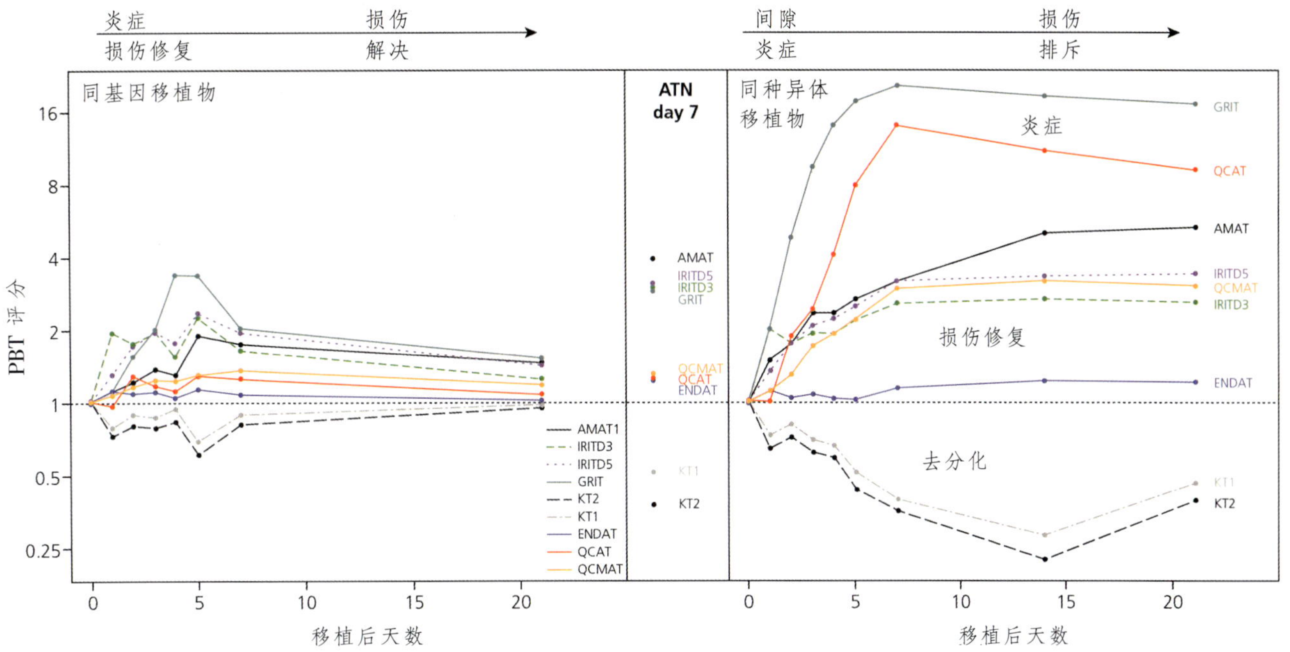

图 10.4　基于发病机制的转录组表达的时间过程表明在炎症、损伤修复反应和组织去除之间的密切关系。T 细胞介导的排斥(右)触发与同基因移植物(左)中相同的损伤修复(AKI)反应。当伤害在同种异体中消退时，炎症、损伤反应和组织去分化减弱。然而，在高度炎症状态中(同种异体移植物)，损伤反应和组织去分化是显著且连续的。请注意，缺血性损伤(ATN)表现出与同种异体移植相似的损伤反应。AKI-QCAT，效应器/效应器记忆 T 细胞负荷；AMAT1，激活的巨噬细胞；ENDAT，微循环(内皮细胞)对损伤的反应；GRIT，干扰素-γ 对组织和炎症细胞的影响；IRIT3，损伤和修复诱导的转录物在损伤修复反应期间，在第 3 天在小鼠异位症中达到峰值(中期)；IRIT5，损伤和修复诱导的转录物在损伤修复反应期间，在第 5 天在小鼠异位症中达到峰值(晚期)；KT1，在损伤修复反应期间减少的实质转录物；KT2，在损伤修复反应期间减少的溶质载体转录物。QCMAT，巨噬细胞负荷。((Reproduced from Halloran et al. 2010 [101], with permission from John Wiley and Sons Ltd.)

后捐赠、捐赠者年龄增加、移植前 3 个月出现急性排斥反应、HLA 不匹配程度、CD25 增加和 BCL2L1 基因表达降低都是移植后 6 个月移植肾功能不良(血清肌酐≥2.0mg/dL)的预测因素[114]。在一项研究中，高 CD3 和低血小板内皮细胞黏附分子(PECAM)与更差的 2 年同种异体移植功能相关，而高 TNF-α 可预测死亡检测和整体 2 年移植物存活率较差[4]，但是调整临床变量后，基因表达谱中没有一个与移植后 3 年或 4 年的独特临床结果相关。

分子数据不支持移植中纯 AKI 导致长期移植结果差的观念。注册数据中 DGF 肾损伤的长期存活不是纯 AKI 的影响，这是不可取的，但本质上是可逆的。

AKI 中的一些关键问题

炎症是否增加/延长损伤的发生率及持续时间？

有人怀疑，作为肾脏损伤反应的一部分，炎症细胞有助于组织损伤。因此，许多研究者试图操纵损伤反应来减轻实验移植模型的损伤。目前，没有人类的证据表明，器官受损后数分钟、数小时或数天内炎症细胞产生损伤。正如在任何伤口愈合部位一样，这些细胞存在并且可能已被招募，因为它们在愈合反应中具有益处。伤口愈合是多细胞生物体中如此重要的程序，难以改善，并且来自干预的明显表型“益处”可能在其他模型或诊所中不可重复，或与另一时间的不良事件相关。然而，鉴于对炎性细胞的强烈兴趣，研究者可能会继续在器官受损的情况下努力操纵伤口愈合。

损伤是否增加免疫原性和 TCMR 或 ABMR？

在缺血再灌注损伤模型中，AKI 诱导促炎细胞分化[115]，这增加了 MHC 的表达，从而增加了肾的“抗原性”，但是这是否增加了 MHC 的“免疫原性”尚不明确。ABMR 也可以伪装成 DGF 和早期 AKI。然而，AKI 和 DGF 尚未显示出可诱导从头 HLA 抗体形成和 ABMR。

DGF 表型具有许多协变量(供体年龄、受体年龄、

表 10.3 按 AKI 活检与原始方案活检的倍数变化排序的与 AKI 相关的前 30 个基因

基因*(缩写)	基因全称	倍数变化:AKI 移植肾脏对比正常肾脏	AKI 移植物活检样本与 eGFR校准后的值†	是否对 AKI 表型具有提示意义(AUC≥0.7)	是否对未来移植失功能有提示意义
ITGB6	整合素,β6	7.9	−0.69	是	是
SERPINA3	丝氨酸(或半胱氨酸)蛋白酶抑制剂,进化枝 A3	6.1	−0.71	是	
MTND6	NADH 脱氢酶,亚基 6(复合体 1)	5.6	−0.51	是	
OLFM4	嗅觉素 4	5.5	−0.74	是	
PTX3	Pentaxin 相关基因,可快速诱导 IL-1 beta	5.3	−0.58	是	
LCN2	脂蛋白 2(致癌基因 24p3)	4.3	−0.57	是	是
VCAN	硫酸软骨素蛋白聚糖 2	4.1	−0.35‡	是	是
LTF	乳运铁蛋白	4.1	−0.63	是	是
SLPI	分泌型白细胞蛋白酶抑制剂(抗清蛋白酶)	4.1	−0.70	是	是
ADAMTS1	是一种整合素样金属蛋白酶(溶血素类型)血小板反应蛋白 1 型	4.0	−0.64	是	
MEGF11	多个 EGF 样结构域	3.8	−0.68	是	是
CDH6	钙黏着蛋白 6,类型 2,K-钙黏着蛋白(胎肾)	3.7	−0.72	是	是
PI15	肽酶抑制剂 15	3.6	−0.40	是	
FCGR3A	IgG 的 Fc 片段,低亲和力Ⅲa,(CD16)的受体	3.4	−0.30‡	是	是
NNMT	烟酰胺 N-甲基转移酶	3.3	−0.56	是	是
S100A8	S100 钙结合蛋白 A8(钙蛋白 A)	3.2	−0.11‡	是	
SOD2	超氧化物歧化酶 2,线粒体的	3.2	−0.61	是	是
ITGB3	整合素,β3(血小板糖蛋白Ⅲa,抗原 CD61)	3.0	−0.74	是	是
NFKBIZ	κB 轻核多肽的核因子,B 细胞抑制剂 zeta 中的基因增强子	3.0	−0.67	是	是
AKAP12	A 激酶(PRKA)锚蛋白	3.0	−0.60	是	是
VMP1	可能是大鼠液泡膜蛋白 1 的直系同源基因	2.9	−0.71	是	是
ADAM9	整合素和金属蛋白酶结构域 9	2.9	−0.57	是	
PTPRC	蛋白酪氨酸磷酸酶,受体类型,C	2.9	−0.53	是	是
FOS	v-fos FBJ 鼠骨肉瘤病毒致癌基因同源物	2.9	−0.48	是	
OSMR	制抑素 M 受体	2.8	−0.80	是	是
C9orf71	染色体 9 开放阅读框 71	2.8	−0.41	是	
EGR1	早期生长响应 1	2.8	−0.48	是	
CTSS	组织蛋白酶 S	2.7	−0.50	是	是
RARRES1	维 A 酸受体响应剂(他扎罗汀诱导的)1	2.7	−0.55	是	是
EVI2A	生态病毒整合站点 2A	2.7	−0.32‡	是	是

* 显示了非冗余和注释的基因。如果每个基因有多个转录本,则选择倍数变化最高的一个。

† 活检时基因表达与 eGFR 的 Spearman 相关性被认为是显著的,$P<0.05$。

‡ P 值没有意义。

脑死亡、致敏等),使其难以解释。DGF 表型与 TCMR 的更多组织学诊断相关[116],但由于损伤诱导的小管炎和间质浸润,这些可能是假阳性,因为肾脏与 DGF 的活检比具有良好功能的肾脏更为频繁。肾脏与 AKI 表型的方案活组织检查显示出类似于排斥反应的炎症频率增加[117],因为损伤引起间质炎症和小管炎,甚至可能是内皮炎(v-病变)[49],所有这些都会造成假阳性 TCMR 诊断。存在于协议活组织检查中的炎症,其中一些称为

"亚临床排斥反应",其实主要是 AKI 的反映[118]。此外,排斥并非主要由供体组织的特征决定。与 DGF 相关的排斥概念可能是由于大量活组织检查造成的观察性假象。

衰老和与体细胞衰老相关的器官损伤

老年供体年龄是 DGF 的一个问题,GFR 的长期损害是一个问题,在这里与 DGF 有关。器官年龄较老是早期器官功能障碍的主要决定因素,也是导致器官丢弃的主要问题。此外,ECD 悖论规定,来自老年捐赠者的器官被投入高危人群中,使得受益人死亡和并发症伴随着与捐赠者年龄相关的复杂关联。供者对于活体,来自老年捐赠者的肾脏表现良好,除了预期的 GFR 下降。然而,高血压或肾脏疾病的活体供体通常被排除在外。(一些中心接受具有良好控制的高血压的肾脏供体,且没有任何损伤证据。)

在死亡供体中,高血压持续时间是移植物存活的独立危险因素。与供体-年龄匹配对照组相比,3 年移植物存活率较低(65%对 75%,高血压≥10 年相对危险度=1.36,P=0.001)[20](但再次,必须考虑 ECD 悖论)。高血压和糖尿病对移植结果的负面影响可能是严重程度和持续时间的问题,例如供体高血压持续时间> 10 年。

来自植入前活组织检查的组织学损伤,包括肾小球硬化、间质和纤维化以及小动脉的纤维性内膜增厚对于移植器官功能超过供者老化和人口统计学方程的预测价值有疑问,导致一些人认为不应进行活组织检查以评价老化和(或)质量[119]。此外,大多数已发表的评估组织质量评估方法的研究缺乏适当的验证[119]。

如何处理 ECD 肾脏的问题没有简单的答案:将两个移植到一个受者中,两个移植到两个受者中,或者两个都丢弃[120]。将两个老年捐赠者的肾脏移植到一个接受者的做法并没有得到很好的证据支持:没有任何试验将两个肾脏随机移植到一个接受者中,而是将其移植到单个接受者身上。对于单次 ECD 肾移植,双肾移植的结果研究通常发现双肾移植患者和移植物存活率与单肾移植相似(分别为 95%和 90%)[121,122]。鉴于捐助者短缺,ECD 肾脏应该以单肾移植(分为两个接受者),而不是将其移植给一个接受者,如果可能的话,尽管双肾移植给同一患者优于丢弃两个肾脏。

这就将老化的生物学提到了理解器官移植表现和器官损伤的议程上。实质上,问题在于老旧的器官"较小",它们已经失去了功能性的质量,而剩下的细胞是"老"的,它们更脆弱,容易受到伤害[123]。在脑死亡后供体充分发挥功能的老年肾脏比年轻器官显示出更多的 DGF。老年捐赠人群质量上有差异,有更多高血压性血管疾病,因此在器官质量上有第二个问题,即死亡前的更为先进的变化。相反,可以选择同龄的活体供体来避免高血压疾病,避免肾功能不全。这些选择不能在死亡的捐赠者中进行,而评估非常有限。

衰老的分子变化包括端粒,TP53 和线粒体中进行的 DNA 损伤[124]。由于细胞经历衰老,其线粒体功能受损,导致蛋白质、脂质和 DNA 修饰[125],包括糖基化[126]。

体细胞衰老有两个主要理论[127]:端粒缩短理论[128]和 P16INK4A(cyclindependent kinase inhibitor 2A,CDKN2A)理论[129]。端粒是染色体的末端,它们随细胞复制而缩短,因为末端不能在细胞复制中完全再生。问题是体细胞中没有端粒酶。

在实验动物如大鼠和小鼠中,端粒非常长,并且不随年龄显著缩短。在人类和系统发育程度较高的动物中,端粒短缩并随着年龄增长。在某一点上,它们限制和引起 DNA 损伤反应[130,131]。这是有益的,因为它保持体细胞免于过度复制,从而起到抗癌的作用。事实上,任何癌症必须通过诸如重新表达端粒酶或 TP53 失活等策略来找到绕过体细胞衰老机制的方法。

体细胞进入衰老时使用的主要细胞周期调节因子是 CDKN2A。CDKN2A 在培养物中的体细胞中表达,例如成纤维细胞,因为它们经历复制诱导的捕获。体细胞具有有限数量的周期,这被称为"Hayflick 限制"。Hayflick 限制是由端粒缩短引起的。培养细胞的其他限制包括氧化应激,其损害细胞的许多方面。当细胞进入复制性阻滞时,它们表达 CDKN2A,作为细胞周期的不可逆抑制剂。表观遗传因素也有助于老化过程和 CDKN2A 表达[132-134]。许多研究表明,复制衰老发生在人、小鼠和大鼠肾脏中。这些问题已经被审查[76,135]。移植肾活检中的细胞衰老是术后器官功能的预测[136]。

体细胞衰老标记作为移植时器官生物学年龄的测量尚未得到证实,比时间年龄本身提供更多的信息。供体年龄强烈地预测了头几周的损伤和功能。为了在移植时使用端粒长度或 CDKN2A 测量,为了评估器官的真实年龄,必须表明这些测量值优于人口统计学因素。以复合加权方程式表示的常用风险指数(Schold,

KDRI)受捐赠者年龄的强烈影响。

体细胞衰老是器官存活的一个因素吗?

器官移植的应激诱导复制和氧化应激，进一步增加由预先存在的衰老造成的体细胞衰老。因此,如染色所示，具有广泛萎缩和纤维化的器官表现出高水平的CDKN2A表达。此外,表达模式异常,并且在萎缩性小管细胞质以及细胞核中非常广泛。CDKN2A在肾移植和天然肾脏中的表达与器官功能受损有关，并支持伴随衰老的一些细胞衰老变化也会导致由于损伤和疾病引起的应激[4]。此外,植入研究[4]表明,只有供体年龄和与体内相关的组织学(特别是间质性纤维化)与长期移植物功能有关。这表明体细胞衰老是器官存活的一个因素。然而,本研究还发现,植入时的损伤/缺血应激与长期功能无关[137]。

体细胞衰老机制能否被忽视或药物治疗?

应考虑暂时中止我们的一些抗癌控制措施以确保其在急性损伤中的额外复制能力[138],但必须衡量潜在的风险。体细胞衰老机制与癌症防御之间有一个联系:不患癌症的代价是体内细胞不是不朽的。诱导端粒酶阻止端粒缩短和绕过CDKN2A的尝试理论上对给予细胞额外的复制能力是有吸引力的。在CDKN2A敲除小鼠中有一些令人鼓舞的结果，但是人们必须关心绕过体细胞作为癌症防御的限制。在整个动物水平和器官中,可能会有绕过端粒酶机制或CDKN2A机制的后果和风险。

AKI临床治疗

AKI生物标志物在临床中有用吗?

研究已经检验了使用分子工具与AKI诊断相关的目的，在功能紊乱发作之前较为理想。如前所述,AKI分子变化的功能分类揭示了免疫和防御反应、配体介导的信号传导、细胞增殖和分化以及凋亡的变化。一些基因上调,但一些基因在AKI后下调[139,140]。例如,IL-6和IL-18的表达升高(炎性生物标志物)以及HAVCR1(KIM-1)的表达,其是由凋亡细胞激励的信号的受体。同时,GGT和SLC9A3可能由于上皮的去分化而下调。检测到AKI的生物标志物作为尿液或血液中的产物[4]或作为人类肾脏中的mRNA表达[110]。大多数候选标记物最初在天然肾脏疾病中发现,随后在人类移植后A-KI中发现(表10.4)。

在移植肾中,移植后AKI中前30个上调基因是预测AKI的潜在标志物[4]。此外,响应于损伤,HAVCR1和IL-18在肾组织中升高，表明作为肾损伤的生物标志物的潜在作用。AKI的分子标志物也已在植入前活检中进行了研究。结果表明,AKI信号(OSMR、SOD2、NNMT、ITGB6、CTSS、ITGB3 CDH6、LCN2、SLPI和VCAN)的个体基因成员也显示DGF在植入时显著的重新启动能力(曲线下面积AUC>0.7)[141]。

在DCD肾脏中,乳酸脱氢酶(LDH)水平已被评估为损伤程度的指标[142]。然而,LDH不常用,因为它不是肾组织特异性的(也可以从受损的红细胞中释放)。在目前的实践中,更广泛地使用基于谷胱甘肽-S-转移酶(GST)和α-GST同位酶的活力标志物,近端肾小管细胞的溶酶体蛋白质。这些与热缺血时间相关，在DCD肾脏中明显增加,这将永远不会起作用[110]。然而,没有单一的生物标志物是AKI的理想标志物，其应该具有预测损伤表型的能力,对肾脏是独一无二的,容易在损伤早期检测,具有高度准确性、敏感性和特异性,并且价格便宜[4]。

前30名AKI转录本中的许多转录本使用衍生的移植物衰竭的分子风险评分分类,如NMMT、ITGB6和VCAN [143]。这表明在持续性进行性疾病的背景下也存在急性应激引起的实质和基质反应。AKI和进行性疾病的分子变化之间的关联强调需要确定扰乱实质的侵袭性过程[144,145],并成为临床进展的重要工具[146]。AKI信号在具有进行性疾病的肾移植中的突出性，例如ABMR,对潜在的治疗具有令人鼓舞的影响。如果进展是由于原发性疾病的持续影响造成的结果，如果造成疾病的伤害被禁止,那么疾病的进展也将停止。如果进展是自主的继发过程,例如功能障碍性纤维化(或FS-GS,如啮齿动物),则有必要治疗原发性疾病和继发自主进程。

特别是负责对ECD肾脏使用做出决定的临床医师将通过器官衰老/质量的新测试来帮助,无论是基于活组织检查或体液检查。我们已经分析了除了临床风险(例如捐赠者年龄)外,植入活组织检查中的AKI信号是否可作为未来肾功能不良的预测因子。将放射活

表 10.4 AKI 研究中报道的潜在生物标志

生物标志名称	基因名称	被检测样本	分子功能	生物学过程	研究类型
中性粒细胞明胶酶相关的脂蛋白(NGAL)	*LCN2* 别名:*NGAL*	血清、尿液	铁离子结合 转运蛋白活性	凋亡的调控 先天免疫应答 铁载体的转运	原发 AKI 肾移植术后 AKI
γ-谷氨酰转肽酶(γGT)(γ-GGT1)	*GGT* 别名:*GGT1*	尿液	酰基转移酶活性 γ-谷氨酰转移酶活性 蛋白结合	谷胱甘肽的生物合成过程	原发 AKI
钠/氢交换剂 3(Na(+)/ H(+)交换剂 3)	*SLC9A3* 别名:*NHE3*	尿液	钠:氢反转运活性	离子转运	原发 AKI
白介素 6(IL-6)[B 细胞刺激因子 2(BSF-2)] 杂交瘤生长因子干扰素 β-2 [IFN-β-2)]	*IL-6* 别名:*IFNB2*	血清	细胞因子活性 生长因子活性 IL-6 受体结合	急性期炎性反应	原发 AKI 肾移植术后 AKI
肾脏损伤分子 1(KIM-1) 甲型肝炎病毒细胞受体 1 同源物(HAVcr-1)	*HAVCR1* 别名:*KIM-1*	尿液	受体活性	宿主-病毒反应	原发 AKI 肾移植术后 AKI
白介素 18(IL-18)(干扰素 γ 诱导因子)	*IL-18* 别名:*IGIF*	血清、尿液	细胞因子活性 信号传感器活性	T-辅助者 1 型免疫反应 血管生成 细胞间信号 粒细胞巨噬细胞集落刺激因子的生物合成过程 干扰素-γ 的生物合成过程 IL-2、IL-13、IL-17 生物合成过程 NK T 细胞的正向调节，活化的 T 细胞增殖 积极调控组织重塑调控细胞黏附	原发 AKI 肾移植术后 AKI

检中的 AKI 信号添加到人口学风险评分(如肾脏捐赠者风险指数)中优于单独使用组织学或临床风险[147,148]。体液中的生物标志物是否将反映组织中的分子变化并且允许 AKI 的定量估计仍有待观察。

AKI 治疗:失败的教训

已经研究了许多药剂和实验化合物用于潜在预防或治疗 AKI,但在随后的临床试验中几乎全部失败(如表 10.5 所示)。实验模型中管理伤害的策略是以三个要点为依据的:

1.通过改善肾血管流量或减少修复肾小管组织中的氧需求来增加向受伤的肾组织的氧输送;

2.通过抑制或消除促炎细胞因子、自由基氧、凋亡、黏附分子的表达或白细胞功能来减少炎症;

3.通过生长因子或间充质干细胞治疗增强肾小管再生。

这些模式会让人产生误解。事实上,AKI 模型的干预措施在预测人类干预方面基本上没有取得任何成功。红细胞生成素对于 AKI 的治疗就是一个例子,实验模型表明有效[149],但临床试验却失败了[150]。

也许现在是改变这种模式的时候了,但是,即使我们不知道为什么,在啮齿动物组织中"改善"功能的干预措施现在似乎不太可能改善人体组织的结局。这些啮齿动物模型中的许多功能障碍实际上是由于与成年人中看到的不同的事件 (从人的观点来看是一个无关紧要的事件),其中损伤、供体衰老和受体发病率的问题非常复杂。

话虽如此, 但在诊所中治疗甚至预防 AKI 是很难

表 10.5 预防和治疗缺血性 AKI 的临床试验结果

干预方式	药物/干预方式分类	基本原理	实验室试验(动物研究)结果	临床试验(人体研究)结果
目的:增加向受伤肾脏组织的氧气输送				
多巴胺	血管扩张药	扩张血管	预防和治疗[158-160]	未受益[161-163]
非诺多泮	血管扩张药	扩张血管	预防和治疗[163]	未受益[164,165]
呋塞米	利尿剂	降低肾小管氧合需求	治疗[166-168]	未受益[169-171]
血红氧,一氧化碳释放化合物和胆红素	血管扩张药/抗氧化剂	1.扩张血管 2.清除过氧自由基并抑制脂质过氧化	预防和治疗[172,173]	缺少临床试验
内皮素拮抗剂	血管扩张药	扩张血管	预防和治疗[174]	缺少临床试验
心房肽	血管扩张药	收缩输入小动脉,同时收缩输出小动脉	预防和治疗[175]	未受益[176]
远程缺血预调控	操作	短暂性非致死性缺血器官的血流再灌注机制可保护另一器官或组织免于随后发生的致死性缺血和再灌注(AKI)		未受益[177](NCT00975702 试验的实际收益将在2012年底完成)
目的:通过抑制或消除肌蛋白原性细胞因子、自由基氧物种、凋亡、黏附分子表达或白细胞功能来减少氨基糖化				
甘露醇	利尿剂	自由基清除剂	预防[178]	无益于防御 AKI[179-181]
他汀类	抗炎症反应	他汀类药物可诱导内皮一氧化氮合酶的细胞蓄积;抑制募集在黏附细胞中的黏附分子和趋化因子的表达;抑制促凝血因子的表达并改善血小板高反应性涉及他汀类药物的细胞作用的途径/因素包括胆固醇生物合成途径,Ras/Rho,核因子-κB 和激活蛋白-1 介导的蛋白促动途径,以及核因子,如过氧化物酶体增殖物激活受体和 Kruppel 样因子 2	预防[182]	临床数据不足(缺少 RCT[183])
碱性磷酸酶	抗炎症反应/杀菌	碱性磷酸酶(AP)减弱脂多糖解毒的反应,并可能预防败血症期间的器官损伤 抑制肾脏诱导型 NO 合酶的上调,从而导致 NO 代谢产物的产生减少	治疗[184]	临床数据不足(缺乏 RCT[185,186])
N-乙酰半胱氨酸(NAC)	抗氧化剂	减少氧自由基	预防和治疗[187-189]	无益于防御 AKI[190,191]
半胱天冬酶抑制剂	抗凋亡/坏死	胱天蛋白酶的抑制	预防和治疗[192,193]	缺乏临床试验
二甲胺四环素	抗凋亡/坏死	抑制 p53 和 BAX	预防[82,194]	缺乏临床试验
p53 抑制剂	抗凋亡/坏死	抑制 p53	预防与治疗[195]	缺乏临床试验
PARP 抑制剂	抗凋亡/坏死	抑制聚 ADP-核糖聚合酶(PARP)活化	治疗[196]	缺乏临床试验
可溶性血栓调节蛋白	杀菌	下调 VCAM-1,ICAM-1,E-选择素	预防[197]	治疗无益[198,199]
丙酮酸乙酯	杀菌	抑制肿瘤坏死因子-α(TNF-α),下调 iNOS	治疗[200]	无益于防御 AKI[201] 治疗无益[202]
活性蛋白 C	杀菌	下调 VCAM-1,ICAM-1,E-选择素	治疗[201]	

(待续)

表 10.5(续)

干预方式	药物/干预方式分类	基本原理	实验室试验(动物研究)结果	临床试验(人体研究)结果
磷酸鞘氨醇类似物(FTY720)	抗免疫/免疫抑制	1. S1P1R 的直接激活导致淋巴细胞(B 和 T 细胞)从循环可逆性重新分布到次级淋巴组织,从而远离修饰部位 2. 通过激活有丝分裂原活化的蛋白激酶/细胞外调节激酶(MEK/ERK)和磷脂酰肌醇 3-激酶(PI3K)/Akt 信号传导,防止细胞凋亡	预防[203,204]	无益于防御 AKI [205]
α 促黑激素	抗炎症反应	抑制白细胞促炎症细胞因子,抑制 iNOS	治疗[206,207]	缺乏临床试验
IL10	抗炎症反应	抑制白细胞中促炎症细胞因子,抑制 iNOS	治疗[208]	缺乏临床试验
过氧化酶增生物(PRAP)激活受体	抗炎症反应	过氧化酶增生物(PPAR)激活受体抑制 NF-κB,并下调 VCAM-1 表达	预防[209,210]	缺乏临床试验
诱导型一氧化氮合酶抑制剂	抗炎症反应	抑制 iNOS	治疗[211]	治疗无益[212]
目的:通过生长因子或间充质干细胞疗法促进肾小管再生				
红细胞生成素	生长因子	下调 NF-κB 和激活蛋白 1(AP-1)	预防和治疗[148,213,214]	缺乏临床试验
干细胞生长因子	生长因子	肝细胞生长因子(HGF)是许多细胞类型(包括肾小管)的有效再生因子,具有促有丝分裂、运动发生和形态发生活性。在缺血性 ARF HGF 通过抑制 TNF 介导的内皮 ICAM-1 诱导来调节中性粒细胞-内皮相互作用后,HGF 及其受体的肾表达 c-met 增加。HGF 还能够抑制 E-选择素的重新诱导,E-选择素是白细胞与内皮细胞黏附的另一个关键分子	预防和治疗[215-217]	缺乏临床试验
胰岛素样生长因子	生长因子	IGF-1R 信号传导也可以激活磷脂酰肌醇 3 激酶(P13-K),进而激活蛋白激酶 B(PKB/Akt),后者还可以防止细胞凋亡。这些途径都集中在对半胱天冬酶特别是半胱天冬酶 3 的抑制上,而半胱天冬酶 3 则被阻止执行凋亡引发的聚腺苷二磷酸核糖聚合酶(PARP)裂解,并被阻止降解钙黏蛋白(部分钙黏蛋白细胞黏附系统)	预防和治疗[218,219]	治疗无益[220]
干细胞	操作	在实验室中扩增成年间充质干细胞或鉴定因子,然后在受伤时将其重新引入受体以促进肾小管细胞增殖	预防和治疗[221-223]	缺乏临床试验

的,因为很多严重的损伤发生在器官移除前的捐赠者,难以预防。此外,AKI临床试验中成功治疗的主要限制是AKI生物学和实质重塑的复杂性。直接针对细胞周期进行干预,从而抗癌防御引起了对安全和不利影响的担忧。损伤修复过程与癌症途径密切相关,绕过体细胞衰老也绕过了诸如端粒缩短和CDKN2A等机制,这是我们抗癌防御的一部分。在通过暂停这些机制修改或"改进"维修过程的努力时,必须牢记这一点。未来的策略可能需要针对更具体的疾病途径的药物,而不是广泛的治疗,但重要的是预测操纵修复机制的后果。

损伤修复伤口愈合是每个组织中的一个显著程序,我们在临床上改善自然程序方面收获很少,即使在加速无菌手术伤口的愈合方面。这不应该是沮丧的根源,只需认识到在分子水平上对这一领域的研究仍然具有挑战性。

高风险早期同种异体移植功能障碍的管理

减少和管理AKI的详细策略超出了本章的范围,但显然包括捐赠者和接受者ICU护理的一般原则,例如用于维持器官的中枢静脉压8~10cmH_2O的晶体或胶体的液体置换灌注,同时避免过度水合[5,151]。其他预移植、受体导向的治疗(如用一氧化碳缺血预处理[152])、血管扩张剂(如内皮素受体拮抗剂,选择性腺苷A1受体拮抗剂和钙通道阻断剂)[153-155]尚未在临床研究中得到证实用于治疗同种异体移植AKI[152-155]。

钙调神经磷酸酶抑制剂(CNI,环孢菌素和他克莫司)至少部分是由剂量依赖性的可逆性肾小球前血管收缩,减少肾血流量和GFR而导致肾毒性。它们可能很少诱导DGF,但可以延长恢复时间[156],并使功能障碍的管理和解释复杂化。许多临床医生延迟引入CNI,通常使用抗体诱导,这在早期同种异体移植物功能障碍患者中更难诊断[156]。比较移植后早期和延迟CNI起始的研究已经发现,在早期或延迟的CNI起始方案中,DGF、急性排斥反应、移植物衰竭和肾功能的发生率相似[157]。已经提出以西罗莫司抑制剂(mTORi)为基础的方案(西罗莫司和依维莫司)的哺乳动物靶标作为CNI的替代物,但它们会延迟损伤修复并延长DGF的恢复。根据现有的信息,抗体诱导的组合方案,CNI的最小化剂量以及霉酚酸酯和类固醇的使用通常用于接受早期功能障碍或高表达早期功能障碍的肾脏的患者。

小结

临床观察到的早期移植物功能障碍(DGF或SGF)的鉴别诊断较为复杂,包括梗死、技术问题和ABMR。DGF的原因包括吻合问题、皮质坏死、输尿管梗阻和抗体介导的排斥反应以及AKI。AKI在这里被定义为由缺血或毒素的应激引起的可逆表型变化,包括反映对损伤(伤口愈合)反应的分子变化。因此,DGF不是AKI的同义词。AKI通常可以恢复且很少出现后期并发症。然而,偶尔严重的AKI后不能达到充分的功能恢复。AKI中的炎症是伤口愈合中固有的,可能不会"延长"损伤。同种异体移植功能受以下三联征的影响:供体因子(组织老化/质量),植入时的损伤和受体老化/共病相互作用。ECD肾脏的结果会由于将其分配给高风险受体(ECD悖论)而受到很大影响。AKI模型的干预措施在临床上基本没有取得任何成功。也许这是由于我们在成年人中看到的情况、损伤、供体老化和受体发病的问题如此复杂。在通过暂停这些机制修改或"改进"修复过程时,必须牢记这一点。未来的策略可能需要针对具体疾病的药物,而不是广泛的治疗,但重要的是预测操纵修复机制的后果。

(汪洋 译 李照 校)

参考文献

1. Halloran PF, Hunsicker LG. Delayed graft function: state of the art, November 10-11, 2000. Summit meeting, Scottsdale, Arizona, USA. American Journal of Transplantation. 2001;1:115-120.
2. Halloran PF. The clinical importance of alloantibody-mediated rejection. American Journal of Transplantation. 2003;3:639-640.
3. Sellares J, De Freitas D, Mengel M, et al. Understanding the causes of kidney transplant failure: the dominant role of antibody-mediated rejection and non-adherence. American Journal of Transplantation. 2012;12:388-399.
4. Kreepala C, Reeve J, Chang J, et al. Adding molecular assessment to KDRI increases the predictive power of pretransplant deceased kidney donor risk assessment. American Journal of Transplantation. 2012;12:62.
5. Siedlecki A, Irish W, Brennan DC. Delayed graft function in the kidney transplant. American Journal of Transplantation. 2011;11:2279-2296.
6. Kayler LK, Garzon P, Magliocca J, et al. Outcomes and utilization of kidneys from deceased donors with acute kidney injury. American Journal of Transplantation. 2009;9:367-373.
7. Kayler LK, Srinivas TR, Schold JD. Influence of CIT-induced DGF on kidney transplant outcomes. American Journal of Transplantation. 2011;11:2657-2664.
8. Kayler LK, Magliocca J, Zendejas I, et al. Impact of cold ischemia time on graft survival among ECD transplant recipients: a paired kidney analysis. American Journal of Transplantation. 2011;11:2647-2656.
9. Bouma HR, Ploeg RJ, Schuurs TA. Signal transduction pathways involved in brain death-induced renal injury. American Journal of Transplantation. 2009;9:989-997.
10. Weymann A, Schmack B, Szabó G. Pathophysiological consequences of brain death. Applied Cardiopulmonary Pathophysiology. 2011;15:184-190.

11. Rose B, Post T. Hyperosmolol States-Hypernatremia. Clinical Physiology of Acid-Base and Electrolyte Disorders, 5th ed. New York: McGraw-Hill; 2001: 751–754.
12. Wood KE, Becker BN, McCartney JG, et al. Care of the potential organ donor. New England Journal of Medicine. 2004;351:2730–2739.
13. Howlett TA, Keogh AM, Perry L, et al. Anterior and posterior pituitary function in brain-stem-dead donors: a possible role for hormonal replacement therapy. Transplantation. 1989;47:828–834.
14. Powner DJ, Hendrich A, Lagler RG, et al. Hormonal changes in brain dead patients. Critical Care Medicine. 1990;18:702–708.
15. Westendorp WH, Leuvenink HG, Ploeg RJ. Brain death induced renal injury. Current Opinion in Organ Transplantation. 2011;16:151–156.
16. Sung RS, Christensen LL, Leichtman AB, et al. Determinants of discard of expanded criteria donor kidneys: impact of biopsy and machine perfusion. American Journal of Transplantation. 2008;8:783–792.
17. Mengel M, Sis B. An appeal for zero-time biopsies in renal transplantation. American Journal of Transplantation. 2008;8:2181–2182.
18. Edwards EB, Posner MP, Maluf DG, et al. Reasons for non-use of recovered kidneys: the effect of donor glomerulosclerosis and creatinine clearance on graft survival. Transplantation. 2004;77:1411–1415.
19. Gaber LW, Moore LW, Alloway RR, et al. Glomerulosclerosis as a determinant of posttransplant function of older donor renal allografts. Transplantation. 1999;60:334–339.
20. Mueller TF, Solez K, Mas V. Assessment of kidney organ quality and prediction of outcome at time of transplantation. Seminars in Immunopathology. 2011;33:185–199.
21. Famulski KS, de Freitas DG, Kreepala C, et al. Molecular phenotypes of acute kidney injury in human kidney transplants. Journal of the American Society of Nephrology. 2012;23:948–958.
22. Famulski KS, Broderick G, Hay K, et al. Transcriptome analysis reveals heterogeneity in the injury response of kidney transplants. American Journal of Transplantation. 2007;7:2483–2495.
23. Humar A, Ramcharan T, Kandaswamy R, et al. Risk factors for slow graft function after kidney transplants: a multivariate analysis. Clinical Transplantation. 2002;16:425–429.
24. Gueutin V, Ficheux M, Chatelet V, et al. Hydration status of patients with end-stage renal disease after kidney transplantation. Clinical Transplantation. 2011;25:E656–E663.
25. Stevens RB, Skorupa JY, Rigley TH, et al. Increased primary non-function in transplanted deceased-donor kidneys flushed with histidine-tryptophan-ketoglutarate solution. American Journal of Transplantation. 2009;9:1055–1062.
26. Prasad GS, Ninan CN, Devasia A, et al. Is Euro-Collins better than ringer lactate in live related donor renal transplantation? Indian Journal of Urology. 2007;23:265–269.
27. Sandid MS, Assi MA, Hall S. Intraoperative hypotension and prolonged operative time as risk factors for slow graft function in kidney transplant recipients. Clinical Transplantation. 2006;20:762–768.
28. Metzger RA, Delmonico FL, Feng S, et al. Expanded criteria donors for kidney transplantation. American Journal of Transplantation. 2003;3(Suppl. 4): 114–125.
29. Ojo AO, Hanson JA, Meier-Kriesche HU, et al. Survival in recipients of marginal cadaveric donor kidneys compared with other recipients and wait-listed transplant candidates. Journal of the American Society of Nephrology. 2001;12: 589–597.
30. Gopalakrishnan G, Gourabathini SP. Marginal kidney donor. Indian Journal of Urology. 2007;23:286–293.
31. Kootstra G, van Heurn E. Non-heartbeating donation of kidneys for transplantation. Nature Clinical Practice. Nephrology. 2007;3:154–163.
32. Sanchez-Fructuoso AI, Prats D, Torrente J, et al. Renal transplantation from non-heart beating donors: a promising alternative to enlarge the donor pool. Journal of the American Society of Nephrology. 2000;11:350–358.
33. Weber M, Dindo D, Demartines N, et al. Kidney transplantation from donors without a heartbeat. New England Journal of Medicine. 2002;347:248–255.
34. Gok MA, Buckley PE, Shenton BK, et al. Long-term renal function in kidneys from non-heart-beating donors: a single-center experience. Transplantation. 2002;74:664–669.
35. Sudhindran S, Pettigrew GJ, Drain A, et al. Outcome of transplantation using kidneys from controlled (Maastricht category 3) non-heart-beating donors. Clinical Transplantation. 2003;17:93–100.
36. Chapman J, Bock A, Dussol B, et al. Follow-up after renal transplantation with organs from donors after cardiac death. Transplant International. 2006;19: 715–719.
37. Hoogland ER, Snoeijs MG, van Heurn LW. DCD kidney transplantation: results and measures to improve outcome. Current Opinion in Organ Transplantation. 2010;15:177–182.
38. Weber CL, Rush DN, Jeffery JR, et al. Kidney transplantation outcomes in Canadian aboriginals. American Journal of Transplantation. 2006;6:1875–1881.
39. Woo YM, Pereira BJ, Gill JS. Chronic kidney disease progression in native and transplant kidneys. Current Opinion in Nephrology and Hypertension. 2004;13:607–611.
40. Hall IE, Parikh CR. Human models to evaluate urinary biomarkers of kidney injury. Clinical Journal of the American Society of Nephrology. 2010;5: 2141–2143.
41. Perry TE, Muehlschlegel JD, Liu KY, et al. Plasma neutrophil gelatinase-associated lipocalin and acute postoperative kidney injury in adult cardiac surgical patients. Anesthesia and Analgesia. 2010;110:1541–1547.
42. Du Y, Zappitelli M, Mian A, et al. Urinary biomarkers to detect acute kidney injury in the pediatric emergency center. Pediatric Nephrology (Berlin, Germany). 2011;26:267–274.
43. Toledo-Pereyra LH, Palma-Vargas JM, Toledo AH. Kidney preservation. In: Toledo-Pereyra LH, editor. Organ preservation for Transplantation, 3rd ed. Austin, TX.: Landes Bioscience; 2010: 124–142.
44. Hauet T, Eugene M. A new approach in organ preservation: potential role of new polymers. Kidney International. 2008;74:998–1003.
45. Jawdeh BG, Rabb H. Delayed kidney allograft function - what does it tell us about acute kidney injury? Contributions to Nephrology. 2011;174:173–181.
46. Agarwal A, Murdock P, Fridell JA. Comparison of histidine-tryptophan ketoglutarate solution and University of Wisconsin solution in prolonged cold preservation of kidney allografts. Transplantation. 2006;81:480–482.
47. Halloran P, Aprile M, Robinette M, et al. A randomized prospective trial of cold storage versus pulsatile perfusion for cadaver kidney preservation. Transplantation Proceedings. 1985;17:1471–1473.
48. Wight J, Chilcott J, Holmes M, et al. The clinical and cost-effectiveness of pulsatile machine perfusion versus cold storage of kidneys for transplantation retrieved from heart-beating and non-heart-beating donors. Health Technology Assessment. 2003;7:1–94.
49. Shoskes DA, Parfrey NA, Halloran PF. Increased major histocompatibility complex antigen expression in unilateral ischemic acute tubular-necrosis in the mouse. Transplantation. 1990;49:201–207.
50. Halloran P, Aprile M. Factors influencing early renal function in cadaver kidney transplants. A case-control study. Transplantation. 1988;45:122–127.
51. Halloran PF, Wadgymar A, Ritchie S, et al. The significance of the anti-class I antibody response. I. Clinical and pathologic features of anti-class I-mediated rejection. Transplantation. 1990;49:85–91.
52. Gourishankar S, Jhangri GS, Cockfield SM, et al. Donor tissue characteristics influence cadaver kidney transplant function and graft survival but not rejection. Journal of the American Society of Nephrology. 2003;14:493–499.
53. Halloran PF, Aprile MA, Farewell V, et al. Early function as the principal correlate of graft survival. A multivariate analysis of 200 cadaveric renal transplants treated with a protocol incorporating antilymphocyte globulin and cyclosporine. Transplantation. 1988;46:223–228.
54. Humar A, Johnson EM, Payne WD, et al. Effect of initial slow graft function on renal allograft rejection and survival. Clinical Transplantation. 1997;11: 623–627.
55. Doshi MD, Garg N, Reese PP, et al. Recipient risk factors associated with delayed graft function: a paired kidney analysis. Transplantation. 2011;91:666–671.
56. Halloran PF, Aprile M. A randomized prospective trial of cold storage versus pulsatile perfusion for cadaver kidney preservation. Transplantation. 1987;43: 827–832.
57. Ciancio G, Gaynor JJ, Sageshima J, et al. Machine perfusion following static cold storage preservation in kidney transplantation: donor-matched pair analysis of the prognostic impact of longer pump time. Transplant International. 2012;25: 34–40.
58. Einecke G, Sis B, Reeve J, et al. Antibody-mediated microcirculation injury is the major cause of late kidney transplant failure. American Journal of Transplantation. 2009;9:2520–2531.
59. Gaston RS, Cecka JM, Kasiske BL, et al. Evidence for antibody-mediated injury as a major determinant of late kidney allograft failure. Transplantation. 2010;90:68–74.
60. Sellares J, de Freitas DG, Mengel M, et al. Inflammation lesions in kidney transplant biopsies: association with survival is due to the underlying diseases. American Journal of Transplantation. 2011;11:489–499.
61. Epstein M. Aging and the kidney. Journal of the American Society of Nephrology. 1996;7:1106–1122.
62. Lim WH, Chang S, Chadban S, et al. Donor-recipient age matching improves years of graft function in deceased-donor kidney transplantation. Nephrology, Dialysis, Transplantation. 2010;25:3082–3089.
63. Moreso F, Seron D, Gil-Vernet S, et al. Donor age and delayed graft function as predictors of renal allograft survival in rejection-free patients. Nephrology, Dialysis, Transplantation. 1999;14:930–935.
64. Noppakun K, Cosio FG, Dean PG, et al. Living donor age and kidney transplant

outcomes. American Journal of Transplantation. 2011;11:1279–1286.
65. Tullius SG, Tran H, Guleria I, et al. The combination of donor and recipient age is critical in determining host immunoresponsiveness and renal transplant outcome. Annals of Surgery. 2010;252:662–674.
66. Waiser J, Schreiber M, Budde K, et al. Age-matching in renal transplantation. Nephrology, Dialysis, Transplantation. 2000;15:696–700.
67. Di AE, Chowdhury R, Sarwar N, et al. Chronic kidney disease and risk of major cardiovascular disease and non-vascular mortality: prospective population based cohort study. BMJ (Clinical Research Ed.). 2010;341:c4986.
68. Anavekar NS, McMurray JJ, Velazquez EJ, et al. Relation between renal dysfunction and cardiovascular outcomes after myocardial infarction. New England Journal of Medicine. 2004;351:1285–1295.
69. Smith GL, Lichtman JH, Bracken MB, et al. Renal impairment and outcomes in heart failure: systematic review and meta-analysis. Journal of the American College of Cardiology. 2006;47:1987–1996.
70. Rahman M, Pressel S, Davis BR, et al. Cardiovascular outcomes in high-risk hypertensive patients stratified by baseline glomerular filtration rate. Annals of Internal Medicine. 2006;144:172–180.
71. Dawber TR, Meadors GF, Moore FE Jr. Epidemiological approaches to heart disease: the Framingham Study. American Journal of Public Health and the Nation's Health. 1951;41:279–281.
72. Gill J, Bunnapradist S, Danovitch GM, et al. Outcomes of kidney transplantation from older living donors to older recipients. American Journal of Kidney Diseases. 2008;52:541–552.
73. Schold JD, Kaplan B, Baliga RS, et al. The broad spectrum of quality in deceased donor kidneys. American Journal of Transplantation. 2005;5:757–765.
74. Rao PS, Schaubel DE, Guidinger MK, et al. A comprehensive risk quantification score for deceased donor kidneys: the kidney donor risk index. Transplantation. 2009;88:231–236.
75. Hubbard WJ, Dashti N. Aging and transplantation – a topic for biomedicine or bioethics? Aging and Disease. 2011;2:181–185.
76. Melk A, Schmidt BMW, Braun H, et al. Effects of donor age and cell senescence on kidney allograft survival. American Journal of Transplantation. 2009;9: 114–123.
77. Schnermann J, Briggs JP, Weber PC. Tubuloglomerular feedback, prostaglandins, and angiotensin in the autoregulation of glomerular filtration rate. Kidney International. 1984;25:53–64.
78. Verghese E, Ricardo SD, Weidenfeld R, et al. Renal primary cilia lengthen after acute tubular necrosis. Journal of the American Society of Nephrology. 2009;20:2147–2153.
79. Singaravelu K, Padanilam BJ. p53 target Siva regulates apoptosis in ischemic kidneys. American Journal of Physiology. Renal Physiology. 2011;300: F1130–F1141.
80. Olsen S, Burdick JF, Keown PA, et al. Primary acute renal failure ("acute tubular necrosis") in the transplanted kidney: morphology and pathogenesis. Medicine (Baltimore). 1989;68:173–187.
81. Devarajan P. Update on mechanisms of ischemic acute kidney injury. Journal of the American Society of Nephrology. 2006;17:1503–1520.
82. Kelly KJ, Plotkin Z, Vulgamott SL, et al. P53 mediates the apoptotic response to GTP depletion after renal ischemia-reperfusion: protective role of a p53 inhibitor. Journal of the American Society of Nephrology. 2003;14:128–138.
83. Akcay A, Nguyen Q, Edelstein CL. Mediators of inflammation in acute kidney injury. Mediators of Inflammation. 2009;2009:137072.
84. Nishimura SL. Integrin-mediated transforming growth factor-beta activation, a potential therapeutic target in fibrogenic disorders. American Journal of Pathology. 2009;175:1362–1370.
85. Hahm K, Lukashev ME, Luo Y, et al. alpha v beta 6 integrin regulates renal fibrosis and inflammation in Alport mouse. American Journal of Pathology. 2007;170: 110–125.
86. Einecke G, Mengel M, Hidalgo LG, et al. The early course of renal allograft rejection: Defining the time when rejection begins. American Journal of Transplantation. 2009;9:483–493.
87. Molitoris BA. Acute kidney injury. In: Goldman L, editor. Cecil Medicine, 23rd edition. Philadelphia, PA: Saunders Elsevier; 2007: 862–865.
88. Solez K. The pathology and pathogenesis of human "acute tubular necrosis". In: Solez KWA, editor. Acute Renal Failure: Correlations Between Morphology and Function (Kidney Disease). New York, NY: Marcel Dekker Inc; 1984: 3–12.
89. Matignon M, Desvaux D, Noel LH, et al. Arteriolar hyalinization predicts delayed graft function in deceased donor renal transplantation. Transplantation. 2008;86:1002–1005.
90. Rajiah P, Lim YY, Taylor P. Renal transplant imaging and complications. Abdominal Imaging. 2006;31:735–746.
91. American College of Radiology. ACR Appropriateness Criteria of renal failure. National Guideline Clearinghouse; 2008.
92. Solez K, D'Agostini RJ, Stawowy L, et al. Beneficial effect of propranolol in a histologically appropriate model of postischemic acute renal failure. American Journal of Pathology. 1977;88:163–192.
93. Riss J, Khanna C, Koo S, et al. Cancers as wounds that do not heal: differences and similarities between renal regeneration/repair and renal cell carcinoma. Cancer Research. 2006;66:7216–7224.
94. Venkatachalam MA, Griffin KA, Lan RP, et al. Acute kidney injury: a springboard for progression in chronic kidney disease. American Journal of Physiology. Renal Physiology. 2010;298:F1078–F1094.
95. Bonventre JV, Zuk A. Ischemic acute renal failure: an inflammatory disease? Kidney International. 2004;66:480–485.
96. Friedewald JJ, Rabb H. Inflammatory cells in ischemic acute renal failure. Kidney International. 2004;66:486–491.
97. Ramesh G, Reeves WB. Inflammatory cytokines in acute renal failure. Kidney International. Supplement. 2004;91:S56–S61.
98. Kielar ML, John R, Bennett M, et al. Maladaptive role of IL-6 in ischemic acute renal failure. Journal of the American Society of Nephrology. 2005;16: 3315–3325.
99. Simmons EM, Himmelfarb J, Sezer MT, et al. Plasma cytokine levels predict mortality in patients with acute renal failure. Kidney International. 2004;65: 1357–1365.
100. Bonventre JV. Mechanisms of acute kidney injury and repair. In: Jorres A, Ronco C, Kellum JA, editors. Management of Acute Kidney Problems. Berlin: Springer; 2010: 13–20.
101. Halloran PF, de Freitas DG, Einecke G, et al. The molecular phenotype of kidney transplants. American Journal of Transplantation. 2010;10:2215–2222.
102. Famulski KS, Sis B, Billesberger L, et al. Interferon-gamma and donor MHC class I control alternative macrophage activation and activin expression in rejecting kidney allografts: a shift in the Th1-Th2 paradigm. American Journal of Transplantation. 2008;8:547–556.
103. Famulski KS, Kayser D, Einecke G, et al. Alternative macrophage activation-associated transcripts in T-cell-mediated rejection of mouse kidney allografts. American Journal of Transplantation. 2010;10:490–497.
104. Wyburn KR, Jose MD, Wu H, et al. The role of macrophages in allograft rejection. Transplantation. 2005;80:1641–1647.
105. Gordon S, Martinez FO. Alternative activation of macrophages: mechanism and functions. Immunity. 2007;32:593–604.
106. Ogawa K, Funaba M, Chen Y, et al. Activin A functions as a Th2 cytokine in the promotion of the alternative activation of macrophages. Journal of Immunology. 2006;177:6787–6794.
107. Martinez FO, Helming L, Gordon S. Alternative activation of macrophages: an immunologic functional perspective. Annual Review of Immunology. 2009;27: 451–483.
108. Wynn TA. Fibrotic disease and the T(H)1/T(H)2 paradigm. Nature Reviews. Immunology. 2004;4:583–594.
109. Famulski KS, Einecke G, Sis B, et al. Defining the canonical form of T-cell-mediated rejection in human kidney transplants. American Journal of Transplantation. 2010;10:810–820.
110. Famulski K, de Freitas DG, Kreepala C, et al. The acute kidney injury signal is induced in kidney transplants by chronic diseases and predicts progression to failure. American Journal of Transplantation. 2012;12(s3):385.
111. Mueller TF, Reeve J, Jhangri GS, et al. The transcriptome of the implant biopsy identifies donor kidneys at increased risk of delayed graft function. American Journal of Transplantation. 2008;8:78–85.
112. Kreepala C, Reeve J, Chang J, et al. The acute kidney injury signal in deceased donor kidneys at the time of transplantation predicts early function better than histopathology risk scores. American Journal of Transplantation. 2012;12(s3):224.
113. Avihingsanon Y, Ma N, Pavlakis M, et al. On the intraoperative molecular status of renal allografts after vascular reperfusion and clinical outcomes. Journal of the American Society of Nephrology. 2005;16:1542–1548.
114. Bodonyi-Kovacs G, Putheti P, Marino M, et al. Gene expression profiling of the donor kidney at the time of transplantation predicts clinical outcomes 2 years after transplantation. Human Immunology. 2010;71:451–455.
115. Mengel M, Chang J, Kayser D, et al. The molecular phenotype of six-week protocol biopsies from human renal allografts: reflections of prior injury but not future course. American Journal of Transplantation. 2011;11:708–718.
116. Kazi J, Mubarak M. Pathology of renal transplantation. In: Mubarak M, editor. Topics in Renal Biopsy and Pathology. Rijeka: InTech; 2012: 159–180.
117. Wilkinson A. Protocol transplant biopsies: are they really needed? Clinical Journal of the American Society of Nephrology. 2006;1:130–137.
118. Ojo AO, Leichtman AB, Punch JD, et al. Impact of pre-existing donor hypertension and diabetes mellitus on cadaveric renal transplant outcomes. American Journal of Kidney Diseases. 2000;36:153–159.
119. Shapiro R, Halloran PF, Delmonico FL, et al. The 'two, one, zero' decision: what to do with suboptimal deceased donor kidneys. American Journal of Transplantation. 2010;10:1959–1960.
120. Ekser B, Furian L, Broggiato A, et al. Technical aspects of unilateral dual kidney transplantation from expanded criteria donors: experience of 100 patients. Amer-

ican Journal of Transplantation. 2010;10:2000–2007.
121. Westhoff JH, Schildhorn C, Jacobi C, et al. Telomere shortening reduces regenerative capacity after acute kidney injury. Journal of the American Society of Nephrology. 2010;21:327–336.
122. Anderson S, Eldadah B, Halter JB, et al. Acute kidney injury in older adults. Journal of the American Society of Nephrology. 2011;22:28–38.
123. Sahin E, DePinho RA. Axis of ageing: telomeres, p53 and mitochondria. Nature Reviews. Molecular Cell Biology. 2012;13:397–404.
124. Lenaz G. Mitochondria and reactive oxygen species. Which role in physiology and pathology? Advances in Experimental Medicine and Biology. 2012;942: 93–136.
125. Negre-Salvayre A, Coatrieux C, Ingueneau C, et al. Advanced lipid peroxidation end products in oxidative damage to proteins. Potential role in diseases and therapeutic prospects for the inhibitors. British Journal of Pharmacology. 2008;153:6–20.
126. Halloran PF, Melk A. Renal senescence, cellular senescence, and their relevance to nephrology and transplantation. Advances in Nephrology From the Necker Hospital. 2001;31:273–283.
127. Melk A, Ramassar V, Helms LM, et al. Telomere shortening in kidneys with age. Journal of the American Society of Nephrology. 2000;11:444–453.
128. Melk A, Schmidt BM, Takeuchi O, et al. Expression of p16INK4a and other cell cycle regulator and senescence associated genes in aging human kidney. Kidney International. 2004;65:510–520.
129. Famulski KS, Halloran PF. Molecular events in kidney ageing. Current Opinion in Nephrology and Hypertension. 2005;14:243–248.
130. Katada S, Imhof A, Sassone-Corsi P. Connecting threads: epigenetics and metabolism. Cell. 2012;148:24–28.
131. Rando TA, Chang HY. Aging, rejuvenation and epigenetic reprogramming: resetting the aging clock. Cell. 2012;148:46–57.
132. Shiels PG. Improving precision in investigating aging: why telomeres can cause problems. Journals of Gerontology. Series A, Biological Sciences and Medical Sciences. 2010;65:789–791.
133. Lee DH, Wolstein JM, Pudasaini B, et al. INK4a deletion results in improved kidney regeneration and decreased capillary rarefaction after ischemia reperfusion injury. American Journal of Physiology. Renal Physiology. 2012; 302:F183–F191.
134. Naesens M. Replicative senescence in kidney aging, renal disease, and renal transplantation. Discovery Medicine. 2011;11:65–75.
135. McGlynn LM, Stevenson K, Lamb K, et al. Cellular senescence in pretransplant renal biopsies predicts postoperative organ function. Aging Cell. 2009;8:45–51.
136. Melk A, Schmidt BM, Vongwiwatana A, et al. Increased expression of senescence-associated cell cycle inhibitor p16INK4a in deteriorating renal transplants and diseased native kidney. American Journal of Transplantation. 2005;5: 1375–1382.
137. Chan CH, Gao Y, Moten A, et al. Novel ARF/p53-independent senescence pathways in cancer repression. Journal of Molecular Medicine (Berlin, Germany). 2011;89:857–867.
138. Perco P, Pleban C, Kainz A, et al. Gene expression and biomarkers in renal transplant ischemia reperfusion injury. Transplant International. 2007;20:2–11.
139. Siew ED, Ware LB, Ikizler TA. Biological markers of acute kidney injury. Journal of the American Society of Nephrology. 2011;22:810–820.
140. Coca SG, Yalavarthy R, Concato J, et al. Biomarkers for the diagnosis and risk stratification of acute kidney injury: a systematic review. Kidney International. 2008;73:1008–1016.
141. Daemen JH, Heineman E, Kootstra G. Viability assessment of non-heart-beating donor kidneys during machine preservation. Transplantation Proceedings. 1995;27:2906–2907.
142. Gok MA, Pelsers M, Glatz JF, et al. Use of two biomarkers of renal ischemia to assess machine-perfused non-heart-beating donor kidneys. Clinical Chemistry. 2003;49:172–175.
143. Famulski KS, Reeve J, de Freitas DG, et al. Kidney transplants with progressing chronic kidney diseases express high levels of acute kidney injury transcripts. American Journal of Transplantation. 2013;13:634–644.
144. Akalin E, O'Connell PJ. Genomics of chronic allograft injury. Kidney International. Supplement. 2010;119:S33–S37.
145. Mannon RB. Immune monitoring and biomarkers to predict chronic allograft dysfunction. Kidney International. Supplement. 2010;119:S59–S65.
146. Molitoris BA, Melnikov VY, Okusa MD, et al. Technology insight: biomarker development in acute kidney injury–what can we anticipate? Nature Clinical Practice. Nephrology. 2008;4:154–165.
147. Johnson DW, Pat B, Vesey DA, et al. Delayed administration of darbepoetin or erythropoietin protects against ischemic acute renal injury and failure. Kidney International. 2006;69:1806–1813.
148. Sharples EJ, Patel N, Brown P, et al. Erythropoietin protects the kidney against the injury and dysfunction caused by ischemia-reperfusion. Journal of the American Society of Nephrology. 2004;15:2115–2124.
149. Endre ZH, Walker RJ, Pickering JW, et al. Early intervention with erythropoietin does not affect the outcome of acute kidney injury (the EARLYARF trial). Kidney International. 2010;77:1020–1030.
150. Shoskes DA, Halloran PF. Delayed graft function in renal transplantation: etiology, management and long-term significance. Journal of Urology. 1996;155: 1831–1840.
151. Bacchi G, Buscaroli A, Fusari M, et al. The influence of intraoperative central venous pressure on delayed graft function in renal transplantation: a single-center experience. Transplantation Proceedings. 2010;42:3387–3391.
152. Hanto DW, Maki T, Yoon MH, et al. Intraoperative administration of inhaled carbon monoxide reduces delayed graft function in kidney allografts in Swine. American Journal of Transplantation. 2010;10:2421–2430.
153. Neuhofer W, Pittrow D. Role of endothelin and endothelin receptor antagonists in renal disease. European Journal of Clinical Investigation. 2006;36(Suppl. 3):78–88.
154. Kuypers DR, Neumayer HH, Fritsche L, et al. Calcium channel blockade and preservation of renal graft function in cyclosporine-treated recipients: a prospective randomized placebo-controlled 2-year study. Transplantation. 2004;78:1204–1211.
155. Slawsky MT, Givertz MM. Rolofylline: a selective adenosine 1 receptor antagonist for the treatment of heart failure. Expert Opinion on Pharmacotherapy. 2009; 10:311–322.
156. Shoskes DA, Shahed AR, Kim S. Delayed graft function. Influence on outcome and strategies for prevention. Urologic Clinics of North America. 2001;28: 721–732.
157. Li G, Xu J, Wang P, et al. Catecholamines regulate the activity, secretion, and synthesis of renalase. Circulation. 2008;117:1277–1282.
158. Bellomo R, Chapman M, Finfer S, et al. Low-dose dopamine in patients with early renal dysfunction: a placebo-controlled randomised trial. Australian and New Zealand Intensive Care Society (ANZICS) Clinical Trials Group. Lancet. 2000;356:2139–2143.
159. Lauschke A, Teichgraber UK, Frei U, et al. 'Low-dose' dopamine worsens renal perfusion in patients with acute renal failure. Kidney International. 2006; 69:1669–1674.
160. Friedrich JO, Adhikari N, Herridge MS, et al. Meta-analysis: low-dose dopamine increases urine output but does not prevent renal dysfunction or death. Annals of Internal Medicine. 2005;142:510–524.
161. Halpenny M, Markos F, Snow HM, et al. Effects of prophylactic fenoldopam infusion on renal blood flow and renal tubular function during acute hypovolemia in anesthetized dogs. Critical Care Medicine. 2001;29:855–860.
162. Aravindan N, Samuels J, Riedel B, et al. Fenoldopam improves corticomedullary oxygen delivery and attenuates angiogenesis gene expression in acute ischemic renal injury. Kidney and Blood Pressure Research. 2006;29:165–174.
163. Tumlin JA, Finkel KW, Murray PT, et al. Fenoldopam mesylate in early acute tubular necrosis: a randomized, double-blind, placebo-controlled clinical trial. American Journal of Kidney Diseases. 2005;46:26–34.
164. Aravindan N, Shaw A. Effect of furosemide infusion on renal hemodynamics and angiogenesis gene expression in acute renal ischemia/reperfusion. Renal Failure. 2006;28:25–35.
165. Aravindan N, Aravindan S, Riedel BJ, et al. Furosemide prevents apoptosis and associated gene expression in a rat model of surgical ischemic acute renal failure. Renal Failure. 2007;29:399–407.
166. van der Voort PH, Boerma EC, Koopmans M, et al. Furosemide does not improve renal recovery after hemofiltration for acute renal failure in critically ill patients: a double blind randomized controlled trial. Critical Care Medicine. 2009; 37:533–538.
167. Cantarovich F, Rangoonwala B, Lorenz H, et al. High-dose furosemide for established ARF: a prospective, randomized, double-blind, placebo-controlled, multicenter trial. American Journal of Kidney Diseases. 2004;44:402–409.
168. Mehta RL, Pascual MT, Soroko S, et al. Diuretics, mortality, and nonrecovery of renal function in acute renal failure. JAMA. 2002;288:2547–2553.
169. Vera T, Henegar JR, Drummond HA, et al. Protective effect of carbon monoxide-releasing compounds in ischemia-induced acute renal failure. Journal of the American Society of Nephrology. 2005;16:950–958.
170. Adin CA, Croker BP, Agarwal A. Protective effects of exogenous bilirubin on ischemia-reperfusion injury in the isolated, perfused rat kidney. American Journal of Physiology. Renal Physiology. 2005;288:F778–F784.
171. Nakao A, Neto JS, Kanno S, et al. Protection against ischemia/reperfusion injury in cardiac and renal transplantation with carbon monoxide, biliverdin and both. American Journal of Transplantation. 2005;5:282–291.
172. Birck R, Knoll T, Braun C, et al. Improvement of postischemic acute renal failure with the novel orally active endothelin-A receptor antagonist LU 135252 in the rat. Journal of Cardiovascular Pharmacology. 1998;32:80–86.
173. Wilhelm SM, Stowe NT, Robinson AV, et al. The use of the endothelin receptor antagonist, tezosentan, before or after renal ischemia protects renal function.

Transplantation. 2001;71:211–216.
174. Schiffrin EL, Turgeon A, Tremblay J, et al. Effects of ANP, angiotensin, vasopressin, and endothelin on ANP receptors in cultured rat vascular smooth muscle cells. American Journal of Physiology. 1991;260:H58–H65.
175. Allgren RL, Marbury TC, Rahman SN, et al. Anaritide in acute tubular necrosis. New England Journal of Medicine. 1997;336:828–834.
176. Choi YS, Shim JK, Kim JC, et al. Effect of remote ischemic preconditioning on renal dysfunction after complex valvular heart surgery: a randomized controlled trial. Journal of Thoracic and Cardiovascular Surgery. 2011;142: 148–154.
177. Zager RA, Foerder C, Bredl C. The influence of mannitol on myoglobinuric acute renal failure: functional, biochemical, and morphological assessments. Journal of the American Society of Nephrology. 1991;2:848–855.
178. Ip-Yam PC, Murphy S, Baines M, et al. Renal function and proteinuria after cardiopulmonary bypass: the effects of temperature and mannitol. Anesthesia and Analgesia. 1994;78:842–847.
179. Sabbatini M, Pisani A, Uccello F, et al. Atorvastatin improves the course of ischemic acute renal failure in aging rats. Journal of the American Society of Nephrology. 2004;15:901–909.
180. Yasuda H, Yuen PS, Hu X, et al. Simvastatin improves sepsis-induced mortality and acute kidney injury via renal vascular effects. Kidney International. 2006;69:1535–1542.
181. Gueler F, Rong S, Park JK, et al. Postischemic acute renal failure is reduced by short-term statin treatment in a rat model. Journal of the American Society of Nephrology. 2002;13:2288–2298.
182. Molnar AO, Coca SG, Devereaux PJ, et al. Statin use associates with a lower incidence of acute kidney injury after major elective surgery. Journal of the American Society of Nephrology. 2011;22:939–946.
183. Su F, Brands R, Wang Z, et al. Beneficial effects of alkaline phosphatase in septic shock. Critical Care Medicine. 2006;34:2182–2187.
184. Heemskerk S, Masereeuw R, Moesker O, et al. Alkaline phosphatase treatment improves renal function in severe sepsis or septic shock patients. Critical Care Medicine. 2009;37:417–423, e1.
185. Nitescu N, Ricksten SE, Marcussen N, et al. N-acetylcysteine attenuates kidney injury in rats subjected to renal ischaemia-reperfusion. Nephrology, Dialysis, Transplantation. 2006;21:1240–1247.
186. Conesa EL, Valero F, Nadal JC, et al. N-acetyl-L-cysteine improves renal medullary hypoperfusion in acute renal failure. American Journal of Physiology. Regulatory Integrative and Comparative Physiology. 2001;281:R730–R737.
187. Adabag AS, Ishani A, Bloomfield HE, et al. Efficacy of N-acetylcysteine in preventing renal injury after heart surgery: a systematic review of randomized trials. European Heart Journal. 2009;30:1910–1917.
188. Baker WL, Anglade MW, Baker EL, et al. Use of N-acetylcysteine to reduce post-cardiothoracic surgery complications: a meta-analysis. European Journal of Cardio-Thoracic Surgery. 2009;35:521–527.
189. Ho KM, Morgan DJ. Meta-analysis of N-acetylcysteine to prevent acute renal failure after major surgery. American Journal of Kidney Diseases. 2009;53: 33–40.
190. Melnikov VY, Faubel S, Siegmund B, et al. Neutrophil-independent mechanisms of caspase-1- and IL-18-mediated ischemic acute tubular necrosis in mice. Journal of Clinical Investigation. 2002;110:1083–1091.
191. Tiwari MM, Brock RW, Megyesi JK, et al. Disruption of renal peritubular blood flow in lipopolysaccharide-induced renal failure: role of nitric oxide and caspases. American Journal of Physiology. Renal Physiology. 2005;289:F1324–F1332.
192. Sutton TA, Kelly KJ, Mang HE, et al. Minocycline reduces renal microvascular leakage in a rat model of ischemic renal injury. American Journal of Physiology. Renal Physiology. 2005;288:F91–F97.
193. Kelly KJ, Sutton TA, Weathered N, et al. Minocycline inhibits apoptosis and inflammation in a rat model of ischemic renal injury. American Journal of Physiology. Renal Physiology. 2004;287:F760–F766.
194. Kelly KJ, Plotkin Z, Dagher PC. Guanosine supplementation reduces apoptosis and protects renal function in the setting of ischemic injury. Journal of Clinical Investigation. 2001;108:1291–1298.
195. Chatterjee PK, Chatterjee BE, Pedersen H, et al. 5-Aminoisoquinolinone reduces renal injury and dysfunction caused by experimental ischemia/reperfusion. Kidney International. 2004;65:499–509.
196. Sharfuddin AA, Sandoval RM, Berg DT, et al. Soluble thrombomodulin protects ischemic kidneys. Journal of the American Society of Nephrology. 2009;20: 524–534.
197. Yamakawa K, Fujimi S, Mohri T, et al. Treatment effects of recombinant human soluble thrombomodulin in patients with severe sepsis: a historical control study. Critical Care (London, England). 2011;15:R123.
198. Ulloa L, Ochani M, Yang H, et al. Ethyl pyruvate prevents lethality in mice with established lethal sepsis and systemic inflammation. Proceedings of the National Academy of Sciences of the United States of America. 2002;99:12351–12356.
199. Miyaji T, Hu X, Yuen PS, et al. Ethyl pyruvate decreases sepsis-induced acute renal failure and multiple organ damage in aged mice. Kidney International. 2003;64:1620–1631.
200. Bennett-Guerrero E, Swaminathan M, Grigore AM, et al. A phase II multicenter double-blind placebo-controlled study of ethyl pyruvate in high-risk patients undergoing cardiac surgery with cardiopulmonary bypass. Journal of Cardiothoracic and Vascular Anesthesia. 2009;23:324–329.
201. Mizutani A, Okajima K, Uchiba M, et al. Activated protein C reduces ischemia/reperfusion-induced renal injury in rats by inhibiting leukocyte activation. Blood. 2000;95:3781–3787.
202. Marti-Carvajal AJ, Sola I, Lathyris D, et al. Human recombinant activated protein C for severe sepsis. Cochrane Database of Systematic Reviews. 2011;(4): CD004388.
203. Bajwa A, Jo SK, Ye H, et al. Activation of sphingosine-1-phosphate 1 receptor in the proximal tubule protects against ischemia-reperfusion injury. Journal of the American Society of Nephrology. 2010;21:955–965.
204. Lien YH, Yong KC, Cho C, et al. S1P(1)-selective agonist, SEW2871, ameliorates ischemic acute renal failure. Kidney International. 2006;69:1601–1608.
205. Tedesco-Silva H, Lorber MI, Foster CE, et al. FTY720 and everolimus in de novo renal transplant patients at risk for delayed graft function: results of an exploratory one-yr multicenter study. Clinical Transplantation. 2009;23:589–599.
206. Chiao H, Kohda Y, McLeroy P, et al. Alpha-melanocyte-stimulating hormone protects against renal injury after ischemia in mice and rats. Journal of Clinical Investigation. 1997;99:1165–1172.
207. Simmons MN, Subramanian V, Crouzet S, et al. Alpha-melanocyte stimulating hormone analogue AP214 protects against ischemia induced acute kidney injury in a porcine surgical model. Journal of Urology. 2010;183:1625–1629.
208. Deng J, Kohda Y, Chiao H, et al. Interleukin-10 inhibits ischemic and cisplatin-induced acute renal injury. Kidney International. 2001;60:2118–2128.
209. Li S, Gokden N, Okusa MD, et al. Anti-inflammatory effect of fibrate protects from cisplatin-induced ARF. American Journal of Physiology. Renal Physiology. 2005;289:F469–F480.
210. Patel NS, di Paola R, Mazzon E, et al. Peroxisome proliferator-activated receptor-alpha contributes to the resolution of inflammation after renal ischemia/reperfusion injury. Journal of Pharmacology and Experimental Therapeutics. 2009;328:635–643.
211. Noiri E, Peresleni T, Miller F, et al. In vivo targeting of inducible NO synthase with oligodeoxynucleotides protects rat kidney against ischemia. Journal of Clinical Investigation. 1996;97:2377–2383.
212. Watson D, Grover R, Anzueto A, et al. Cardiovascular effects of the nitric oxide synthase inhibitor NG-methyl-L-arginine hydrochloride (546C88) in patients with septic shock: results of a randomized, double-blind, placebo-controlled multicenter study (study no. 144-002). Critical Care Medicine. 2004;32:13–20.
213. Patel NS, Sharples EJ, Cuzzocrea S, et al. Pretreatment with EPO reduces the injury and dysfunction caused by ischemia/reperfusion in the mouse kidney in vivo. Kidney International. 2004;66:983–989.
214. Spandou E, Tsouchnikas I, Karkavelas G, et al. Erythropoietin attenuates renal injury in experimental acute renal failure ischaemic/reperfusion model. Nephrology, Dialysis, Transplantation. 2006;21:330–336.
215. Fiaschi-Taesch NM, Santos S, Reddy V, et al. Prevention of acute ischemic renal failure by targeted delivery of growth factors to the proximal tubule in transgenic mice: the efficacy of parathyroid hormone-related protein and hepatocyte growth factor. Journal of the American Society of Nephrology. 2004;15:112–125.
216. Mizuno S, Nakamura T. Prevention of neutrophil extravasation by hepatocyte growth factor leads to attenuations of tubular apoptosis and renal dysfunction in mouse ischemic kidneys. American Journal of Pathology. 2005;166:1895–1905.
217. Vijayan A, Martin DR, Sadow JL, et al. Hepatocyte growth factor inhibits apoptosis after ischemic renal injury in rats. American Journal of Kidney Diseases. 2001;38:274–278.
218. Goes N, Urmson J, Vincent D, et al. Effect of recombinant human insulin-like growth factor-1 on the inflammatory response to acute renal injury. Journal of the American Society of Nephrology. 1996;7:710–720.
219. Daemen MARC, van't Veer C, Denecker G, et al. Inhibition of apoptosis induced by ischemia-reperfusion prevents inflammation. Journal of Clinical Investigation. 1999;104:541–549.
220. Hirschberg R, Kopple J, Lipsett P, et al. Multicenter clinical trial of recombinant human insulin-like growth factor I in patients with acute renal failure. Kidney International. 1999;55:2423–2432.
221. Bi B, Schmitt R, Israilova M, et al. Stromal cells protect against acute tubular injury via an endocrine effect. Journal of the American Society of Nephrology. 2007;18:2486–2496.
222. Broekema M, Harmsen MC, Koerts JA, et al. Determinants of tubular bone marrow-derived cell engraftment after renal ischemia/reperfusion in rats. Kidney International. 2005;68:2572–2581.
223. Lange C, Togel F, Ittrich H, et al. Administered mesenchymal stem cells enhance recovery from ischemia/reperfusion-induced acute renal failure in rats. Kidney International. 2005;68:1613–1617.

第 11 章 同种移植耐受的机制

Raul Badell, Allan D. Kirk

引言

在过去的60年里,临床器官移植逐渐从预后极差的试验性治疗成功发展为大多数终末期患者的标准治疗方案。然而,尽管大部分器官移植术后一年生存率可达90%,对于急性排斥的控制也较为乐观,但这一领域的发展仍然面临诸多障碍,例如移植物缺失和免疫抑制毒性相关的发病率和死亡率[1]。慢性免疫抑制及其所带来的副作用表明,器官移植进入了一个获益日益降低的阶段,持续免疫抑制会将移植存活率降至最低,并最大限度地增加死亡率。因此,想要提高移植的存活率,就必须探索出提高免疫耐受的治疗方案,以及增强机体对移植物免疫适应能力的辅助治疗方法,而不是抑制体内的免疫反应。

免疫耐受,也就是既能维持同种异体移植物功能,又不产生免疫抑制,是长期以来同种移植术所追求的目标。在特定情况下,极少数移植受者能避免免疫抑制而不出现明显的临床症状[2,3]。事实上,曾有文献报道过一些肾脏移植后达到免疫耐受的患者[4-7],而经过严格筛选的肝移植受者中也有高达20%的人成功避免了免疫抑制[8-13]。这些特例表明,免疫耐受是可以实现但又是十分偶然的,如何提前可靠地诱导持久免疫耐受仍然是一大难题。

尽管免疫耐受在临床上很罕见,但却很容易在动物试验模型中实现。人们开始越来越多地探索同种异体排斥和耐受的根本免疫机制,例如在啮齿类动物以及更高级的动物(包括猪[14,15]、狗[16-18]、灵长类动物[19,20])体内,免疫耐受都得以成功实现,并且越来越有规律。然而,动物模型中的成功并不能可靠地转移至人类体内。事实上,人类免疫耐受最初是发生在依从性欠佳或者因为并发症停药的患者身上的[21],但从中可以观察到一些共性问题。我们知道,免疫耐受随着时间推移会逐渐增强,在移植晚期发生频率越来越高。移植器官可能需要一些修复能力,因此年轻的供体器官和增生能力强的器官(如肝脏)更受欢迎,同时也说明,在移植早期,免疫系统可能会对移植物造成损伤。更低的MHC错配度有助于诱导免疫耐受,这表明供体特异性前体细胞频率的降低是有益的。然而,预测免疫耐受的可靠方法尚未出现[22],而中断免疫抑制治疗可能带来诱发排斥的风险,所以即使对于情况稳定的受体,也禁止中断免疫抑制。部分患者可能已经产生了免疫耐受,但由于缺乏评估病情的可靠方法,仍需维持免疫抑制治疗。因此,想在临床上实现免疫耐受,就需要探索在出现耐受时能及时进行识别的方法。

本章将概述诱导和维持免疫耐受的主要机制:嵌合体、耗竭、共刺激阻断和免疫调节,并介绍B细胞相关的免疫耐受机制。其中,会强调可转移的治疗性试验,并提供可以解释相关临床试验的思维框架,对于免疫耐受的进一步思考以及对相关临床试验的详细评论见第76章。

概念解析

1953年,Billingham、Brent和Medawar发表了他们里程碑式的发现,其中指出,免疫耐受可以在试验情况下被人为诱导[23],随之诞生了移植免疫学的原则,并为这一领域的所有重要研究奠定了基础。他们发现,给处于子宫内胎儿时期的小鼠注射供者的同种抗原,成年后其中2/5对于供体特异性的皮肤移植都不会产生排斥。此外,给免疫耐受的小鼠被动输注致敏淋巴细胞,将会导致对该皮肤移植的迅速排斥。其余3/5无免疫耐受的小鼠对皮肤移植产生了排斥,其中2/5是在移植后早期,另外1/5出现在移植很长时间之后。通过这一发现，Medawar 得出了一些预测性结论，一直沿用于当今的移植耐受理念。

Medawar 总结，免疫耐受的产生并不具备“全或无”的特征，每种程度的耐受都可能出现，甚至只是让移植物保留了几天的完整性。事实上，免疫并不是一种“全或无”的现象，而是一种免疫应答的范围，涵盖了从排斥到耐受。随后，人们发现生理免疫需要上下信号通路，来增强或抑制效应应答，从而提高免疫应答的适应性。正如 Medawar 的试验所示，人类免疫耐受可以实现，但大部分同种移植的自然转归是免疫排斥，这表明在器官移植中，机体状态更倾向于攻击性免疫应答。这并不是说无法诱导免疫耐受的“完美风暴”，而是表明免疫排斥是由多因素联合导致的，包括高前体细胞频率、再灌注损伤和移植物适应性免疫记忆的建立（将在后文进行阐述）。免疫排斥甚至可能出现于诱导耐受的患者，因为顾名思义，一个健全的免疫系统必须保持适应环境变化的能力，从而维持其动态特性，而该特性正是由数不胜数的动态变化所决定的[21]。从本质上而言，免疫耐受是可观察但不可预测的，而且在大部分诱导免疫耐受的机体内，并不是无法确定的，除非受者的免疫系统发生了本质的改变。

Medawar 还宣称，免疫耐受的实现具有个体免疫特异性。也就是说，对于某一供体移植物耐受的小鼠仍保持有对于另一供体移植物的排斥能力。这种特异性对任何免疫耐受的维持都很重要，因为从本质上而言，任何低反应性都会出现系统免疫抑制的状态，而任何免疫反应在临床上最特异的表现就是感染中毒性休克。抗原抗体的特异性结合必须在正确的环境下出现，才能保持免疫耐受和免疫反应的平衡[24]。抗原适应性免疫耐受的发展有助于维持机体的保护性机制，以及对其他抗原和有害病原体的应答能力。

最后，Medawar 总结，免疫耐受的实现是由于宿主免疫应答的特异性损伤，宿主自身始终保持有移植物介导的适应性免疫应答的能力，直到对其产生耐受。换句话说，移植物排斥或耐受是由免疫系统对供体抗原的反应决定的，而不是对供体抗原的免疫忽视或由免疫耐受的宿主引起的抗原特性改变。人们往往误认为免疫耐受是一种无免疫应答的状态，而实际上它最确切的定义是有害免疫应答的缺失，但仍然存在免疫应答，这意味着免疫应答活性可以增强或阻断移植物耐受。机体内必须存在抗原识别，但应避免产生攻击性免疫反应。免疫耐受过程中，并不是抗原识别缺失了，而是识别后的结果发生了改变，也就是说，改变的是翻译过程，而非识别过程。

Medawar 在 60 多年前总结的概念至今仍在影响人们对免疫耐受机制的理解。免疫耐受具有同种抗原特异性，是免疫应答和免疫调节联合作用的结果，而免疫应答可以在移植后任何时间引起免疫排斥。尽管从理论上来说，保护性免疫应答的维持依赖于对同种免疫应答的选择性抑制，但同种免疫和保护性免疫应答之间必然存在某些交叉重叠。例如，免疫耐受和免疫应答的共存取决于大量交叉反应的存在，在这些反应中，供体特异性细胞以十分随机的方式分布，从而得以消除供同种免疫应答，同时避免干扰病原适应性免疫应答（图 11.1）。由于这是一个随机过程，一些交叉反应细胞可能会受到影响，使机体丧失病原适应性免疫应答，但大多数情况下，该免疫应答能得以保留。

成功诱导真正的免疫耐受需要将同种抗原引入受体，从而打破免疫排斥，建立起新的免疫耐受平衡。初始抗原暴露可以破坏供体适应性免疫应答，这一过程需要激活足量效应细胞来弥补，因为后者可以建立有助于同种免疫耐受的代偿性免疫应答。目前，诱导免疫耐受的主要策略包括嵌合体、淋巴细胞耗竭和共刺激阻断，以及新出现的免疫调节技术——B 细胞靶向治疗。这些方法的目的在于通过中枢或周围免疫耐受机制改变免疫应答，本质上是改变了次级淋巴组织胸腺的环境，有助于建立免疫耐受（图 11.2）。考虑到人类免疫应答的复杂性，同时又需要控制整体的免疫反应，在临床上建立免疫耐受可能需要联合使用多种免疫调节

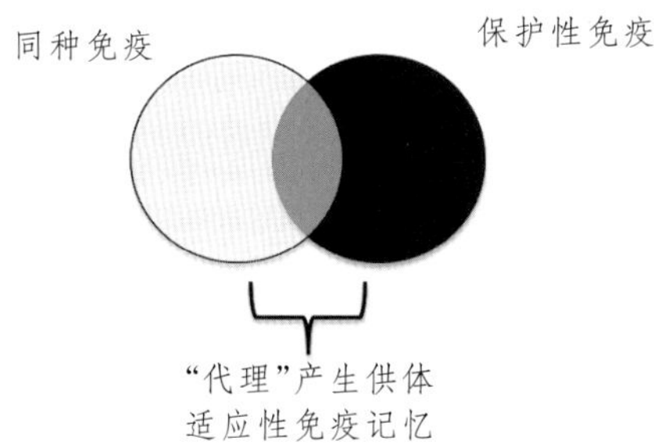

图 11.1 同种免疫和保护性免疫之间的关系。同种免疫和保护性免疫应答之间必然存在某些交叉重叠，这就通过“代理”产生了供体适应性免疫记忆。在这种情况下，对同种免疫应答的选择性抑制可能会消除病原适应性免疫应答，而保护性免疫的维持依赖于交叉反应的供体适应性免疫细胞的随机分布，从而有助于免疫耐受和免疫应答的共存。

策略,而不是单独使用其中某一种。事实上,通过下面对免疫机制的讨论,人们会发现,这些方法在实际应用过程中,往往都需要联合多种不同的机制(例如,通过T细胞耗竭和共刺激阻断来产生嵌合体)。

嵌合体

造血干细胞处于不同环境下，可以通过两种途径发挥功能：作为消耗性同种抗原驱动抗原诱导的细胞死亡(AICD),或者移植诱导嵌合体。前者是一种外周机制,目的在于通过共刺激阻断等机制引起AICD(详见相关章节),从而选择性清除同种T细胞。而后者是一种中枢机制（需要依靠胸腺或其他初级淋巴器官),通过供体造血干细胞的移植,完成受体的骨髓替换。两者的目的都在于诱导移植耐受。

完全嵌合体通常出现于骨髓移植(BMT)中,受体体内所有骨髓驱动的细胞都被清除并由供体细胞所取代。这种造血细胞移植的形式为同种免疫耐受提供了理想的环境，例如血液系统恶性肿瘤患者在骨髓移植后出现了肾衰竭，随后进行的肾移植将不再需要免疫抑制[25]。然而,骨髓移植会增加严重感染和移植物抗宿主反应的发病率,并且远远多于标准免疫抑制方案,这就阻碍了骨髓移植被用于器官移植时免疫耐受的诱导。为了以最小的发病率达到同样的疗效,研究者们研究出了混合嵌合体[26,27]。通过使用非骨髓移植的预处理方案,避免了完全破坏受体的造血系统。在混合嵌合体中,受体骨髓大部分得以保留,但被进行了修饰,使得供体和受体的造血成分在其中得以共存[28]。

最初的验证试验是对小鼠进行致死剂量的全身放射[26,29],随后诞生了更多可转移的非骨髓抑制技术[30],如T细胞耗竭和局部胸腺放射，这些方法都成功建立了混合嵌合体和供者适应性免疫耐受。随后在猪[31,32]和NHP模型[33,34]中也取得了类似的成功,这扩展了非骨髓抑制预处理方案的应用范围。不久之后,在人体内也成功诱导了淋巴造血嵌合体，建立了实体器官免疫耐受[35]。在这些试验中,通过避免某段时间内供体骨髓排斥,输注的造血细胞进入受体的胸腺和骨髓,有助于供体特异性T细胞和B细胞的中枢清除[29,36]。这种非骨髓抑制的方案毒性更少,保留了免疫系统功能,降低了移植物抗宿主反应的风险。然而,它依赖于严格的早期预处理方案,包括T细胞耗竭、一过性持续免疫抑制,以及胸腺或全淋巴组织放射,从而避免骨髓排斥[35,37]。

有趣的是，尽管在最初的鼠类试验中需要建立稳定的混合嵌合体,但在灵长类和人类试验中,在没有嵌合体的情况下仍然可以建立免疫耐受表型。因此,我们仍不清楚,在人体内哪种机制是最主要的。在小鼠中,供体适应性免疫耐受需要稳定的嵌合体，并长期通过中枢胸腺内的克隆清除来维持，而不是外周免疫抑制或失效能,因为在缺乏供体抗原时,供体适应性免疫耐受的缺失是依赖于胸腺的[38]。基于共刺激阻断的治疗方案已成功应用于建立混合嵌合体和免疫耐受，并可以不依赖于T细胞耗竭和骨髓细胞清除[39,40]。为了建立混合嵌合体,除了外周T细胞免疫耐受,胸腺内T细胞清除也有助于长期维持耐受状态,而在这一模型中,免疫调节细胞并未发挥重要作用[41,42]。然而,在其他小鼠模型中，用共刺激阻断作为同种骨髓移植的预处理方案,结果T细胞耗竭不完全,并提前出现了供体特异性T细胞,在这种情况下,外周免疫调节机制也参与了长期免疫耐受的维持[36,43]。

相比于小鼠模型中稳定的混合嵌合体,NHP中通过类似方案联合脾切除所建立的多向嵌合体只是一过性的[33]。然而,在这一方案的重要试验中,受体并未排斥其同种移植物,并建立了供体适应性免疫耐受。所有未接受脾切除的受体都出现了同种抗体介导的免疫排斥[44],这表明体液免疫是免疫耐受的一大障碍。用共刺激阻断(抗CD154)代替脾切除后,长期存活率得以提高,稳定的嵌合体也得以保留[45]。嵌合体缺失后免疫耐受仍可长期稳定存在,这说明在灵长类动物体内,外周机制可能与免疫耐受的维持有关。此外,在多发性骨髓瘤合并终末期肾病的患者体内,进行HLA一致的骨髓和肾脏移植[46],尽管造血嵌合体缺失,仍然可以建立持续的肾移植耐受，这也说明除了小鼠体内的中枢清除以外,还存在着免疫耐受的外周机制。体外试验表明,嵌合体丢失后仍然存在抗同种反应和$CD25^+$ $CD4^+$ T细胞的富集，这些机制都与人体内免疫耐受的调节机制有关[47]。

2008年,Kawai等人第一次发表了未持续免疫抑制的HLA不同的同种移植[48]。通过不同的预处理方案和供者骨髓融合,4/5的活体肾移植受者都中断了免疫抑制治疗，并在2年内未出现免疫排斥。在小鼠实验中，建立嵌合体是试验成功必不可少的步骤，相比之下,类似于之前的NHP试验,本次试验也并未建立稳

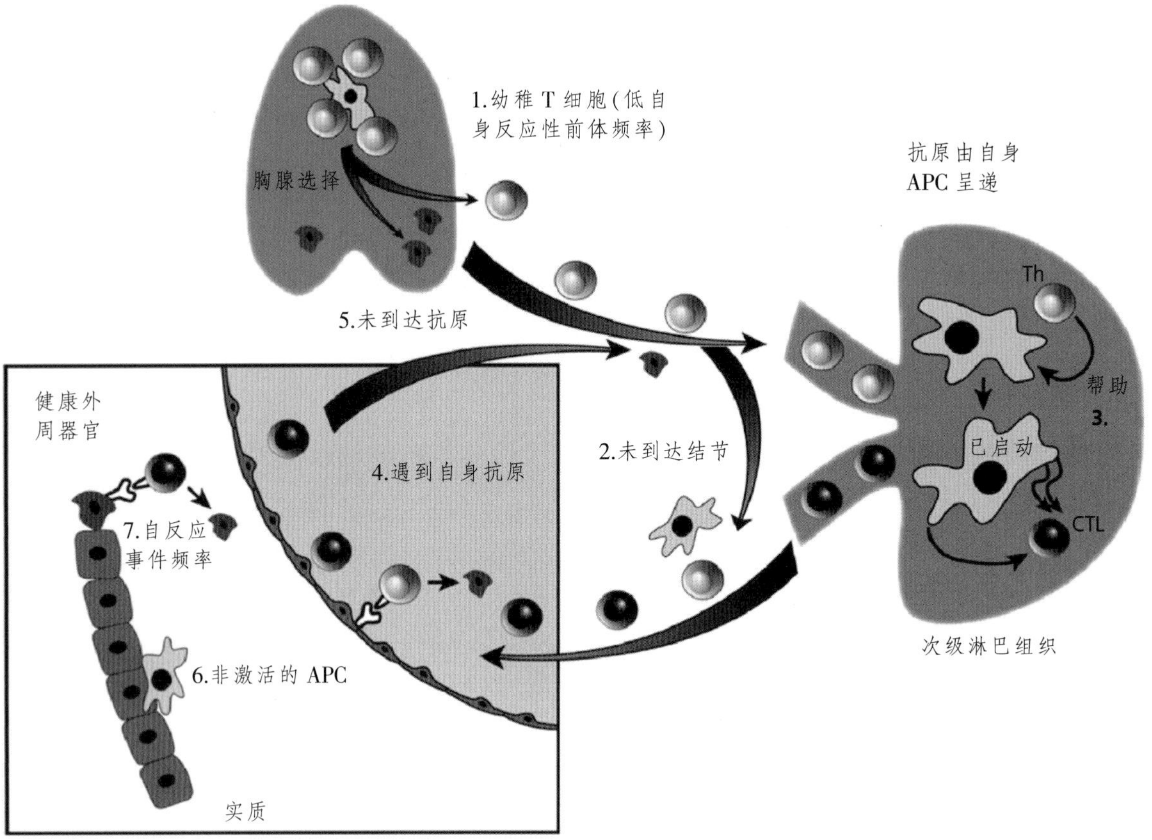
1.幼稚T细胞(低自
身反应性前体频率)
胸腺选择
抗原由自身
APC呈递
Th
5.未到达抗原
健康外
周器官
帮助
3.
2.未到达结节
4.遇到自身抗原
已启动
7.自反应
事件频率
CTL
6.非激活的APC
次级淋巴组织
实质

(A)

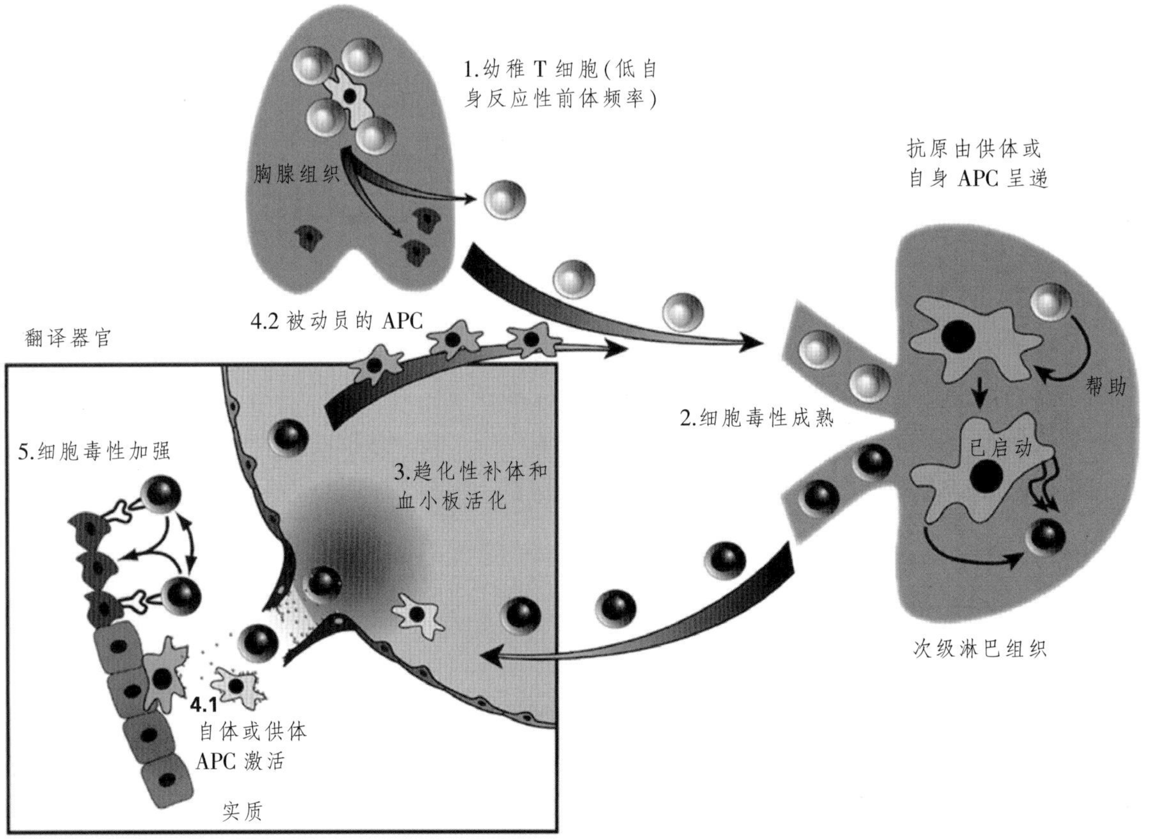
1.幼稚T细胞(低自
身反应性前体频率)
胸腺组织
抗原由供体或
自身APC呈递
4.2 被动员的APC
翻译器官
帮助
2.细胞毒性成熟
5.细胞毒性加强
已启动
3.趋化性补体和
血小板活化
4.1
自体或供体
APC激活
次级淋巴组织
实质

(B)

定的混合嵌合体。4 位患者产生了体液免疫并发症，这一结果强调了 B 细胞的重要作用，但我们对该作用目前知之甚少。有趣的是，这些肾移植患者体内 Foxp3 高表达，这表明调节 T 细胞在免疫耐受的维持中也发挥了一定作用。

一些其他试验证明嵌合体和免疫耐受有一定关系。Scandling 等人报道，在经历了 HLA 一致的骨髓和肾脏移植的患者中，有 1/3 存在稳定的混合嵌合体，并成功建立了免疫耐受[49]。Alexander 等人报道了一位 HLA 不匹配的肝移植受者，在未接受骨髓干细胞移植的情况下，自发建立了多系嵌合体和免疫耐受，在移植后出现了淋巴细胞减少症和感染并发症[50]。尽管存在这些有意义的试验结果，但尚未出现真正的单独免疫耐受方案[51]。关于嵌合体和免疫耐受的各种报道，其相通之处仅仅在于，在初始抗原暴露后，机体都出现了持续的淋巴细胞减少症。因此，在淋巴细胞减少和再生过程中，淋巴细胞的具体变化仍有待于进一步试验以深入理解(详见下文“免疫耗竭”部分)。

在器官移植领域，嵌合体的诱导维持和免疫耐受之间的真正关系仍然是未解之谜。人们普遍认为，微嵌合体(供体细胞<1%的嵌合体)和大嵌合体(供体细胞>1%的嵌合体)差别很大，并且是移植受体本身的特性，而并非免疫耐受的产生机制[52]。同样重要的是，移植受体本身就是嵌合体，因为位于受体体内的移植器官就是由大量供体抗原所组成的。人们还不清楚，在实体器官本身就具备大量造血细胞抗原的情况下，为何造血细胞在这一过程中仍然如此重要。但无论如何，在造血干细胞移植联合肾移植的动物试验及临床方案中，稳定大嵌合体存在与否都是一个很重要的变量。尽管 NHP 不同于小鼠，似乎不需要靠长期稳定的大嵌合体来维持器官移植后的免疫耐受，但这种情况还是可以在人体内观察到[48-50]。在西北大学和路易斯维尔大学的一项试验中，在肾移植受体体内通过骨髓干细胞移植进行了非骨髓抑制的预处理，并成功建立了全嵌合体和免疫耐受[53]。该试验组在 HLA 不一致的骨髓干细胞和肾移植患者体内也建立了稳定嵌合体，并发现 T 细胞嵌合体和建立稳定的供体嵌合体有关，并可使受体在中断免疫抑制治疗后仍然保持完整的肾脏功能。此外，Ramakrishnan 等人近期报道，在 NHP 模型中，稳定的全血细胞(非 T、B 细胞)嵌合体的建立有利于长期免疫耐受的维持[54]。该试验强调了在缺乏 T 细胞嵌合体的情况下，多系嵌合体有助于同种移植肾脏功能的长期维持。因此，通过小鼠试验可以发现，人们有必要探索可再生的稳定多系嵌合体的建立方案。

尽管基于混合嵌合体产生了上述一系列临床治疗方案，但嵌合体不存在时也可以建立免疫耐受，而它存在时也能出现免疫排斥。在不同动物模型中，诱导免疫耐受的方法和机制都不尽相同。在小鼠中，可以实现完全 T 细胞耗竭，混合嵌合体能长期存在，免疫耐受主要依靠中枢克隆清除。这种耐受的维持不依赖于器官移植物的存在，当移植物被移除后仍可持续存在。在猴和人类中，T 细胞耗竭并不完全，而且尽管在骨髓干细胞移植早期有中枢清除的参与，但当外周嵌合体消失后，免疫耐受的维持主要依靠供者器官的存在，并且外周调节

图 11.2　自身免疫耐受(A)和克服诱导免疫耐受(B)的机制。(A)(1)通过胸腺选择，幼稚 T 细胞池发生改变，以正确识别自身 MHC。这导致了自体反应性 T 细胞频率与供体特异性 T 细胞频率的比值降低。(2 和 3)由于抗原呈递主要在次级淋巴组织完成，极少数逃逸阴性选择的自体反应 T 细胞在其中随机分布，并与外周活化的抗原呈递细胞(APC)结合，因此在次级淋巴组织中自身抗原的呈递极其罕见。(4)一旦自体反应 T 细胞成功被自身抗原激活，由于缺乏内皮细胞活化和趋化信号，它们迁移到靶器官的频率也是很低并且很随机的。偶尔会有未活化的 T 细胞不需要 APC 即可在外周与自身抗体结合，这就会产生共刺激作用，导致 T 细胞失效能或细胞凋亡。(5)未能结合抗原的活化 T 细胞最终会走向凋亡。(B)(1)通过胸腺选择，若幼稚 T 细胞池内供体特异性前体细胞频率较高，会使得任何 T 细胞活化过程几乎都产生明显的免疫应答。通过嵌合体和(或)供体特异性淋巴细胞耗竭，可将供体抗原引入受体胸腺，可以中和这一免疫反应机制。(2)在次级淋巴组织内，通过自身或供体表型的 APC 进行自体抗原呈递，高频的供体特异性 T 细胞有利于这一过程的实现，同时嵌合体和(或)淋巴细胞耗竭也可以控制这一过程的进行。共刺激阻断可能会与 T 细胞-APC 衔接相互影响，通过诱导 T 细胞失效能或凋亡组织 T 细胞活化。(3)受损内皮是血小板结合和代偿反应的作用场所，由此可激活内皮细胞和启动趋化信号，募集淋巴细胞与供体抗原结合。控制缺血和再灌注损伤的措施以及细胞黏附都会削弱这一同种免疫应答。(4)活化的血小板结合 APC，从而使其迁移到局部次级淋巴组织，产生共刺激阻断，阻止 T 细胞活化。(5)由于高前体细胞频率和趋化作用，足量的细胞毒性淋巴细胞进入靶器官，在富含炎症因子(如 IL-2)的环境中引起免疫排斥。免疫耗竭和共刺激阻断抑制了这一反应，并阻断了有利于细胞毒性 T 细胞发挥作用的环境形成。图中未呈现免疫调节和 B 细胞作用机制。

T细胞的供体适应性免疫应答也发挥了重要作用。

过去几十年中，人们通过骨髓移植诱导嵌合体和免疫耐受，并且意识到了理解其机制的必要性。然而，在人类和灵长类体内，嵌合体尚未成为预示成功的标志，而不同于T细胞反应的抗体反应也有待于进一步理解(详见“B细胞”部分)。上述关于嵌合体和免疫耐受的关系强调了个体免疫耐受诱导方案之间存在相互依赖关系，如何联合使用这些方案最可能诱导真正的免疫耐受仍有待进一步研究。

免疫耗竭

对同种免疫相关的淋巴组织进行靶向放射治疗，已经成为动物[16,55-57]和人类[58-60]移植后控制免疫应答的一种策略。单独进行淋巴组织放射可以清除活化的T细胞，但最近更多地作为免疫抑制方案，被用于骨髓移植和随后的混合嵌合体[60]。作为一种移植前预处理方案，淋巴细胞放射可以在嵌合体和非嵌合体内诱导免疫耐受，然而移植后的放射并不能诱导嵌合体或免疫耐受[61]。

耗竭耐受策略目的都在于控制供体特异性T细胞前体细胞频率，1%~10%的外周T细胞可以识别同种抗原[62,63]，这远远超过了识别自身抗原的T细胞数量。淋巴细胞单克隆或多克隆抗体的耗竭预期将成为非特异性降低前体细胞频率的策略，这将使得外周机制在免疫耐受中发挥作用，同时降低移植损伤的风险。$CD4^+$和$CD8^+$抗原特异性前体细胞频率会影响T细胞的增殖、分化和免疫应答的总体效能[64,65]。然而，相关代偿反应包括免疫耗竭、血细胞再生等，也会影响免疫应答的特征，产生相对活化的免疫表型[66]。这些概念已在第9章详细介绍。目前为止，抗体耗竭已经在临床上被用于诱导免疫耐受和急性排斥的急救[67]。抗体耗竭的有效性使耗竭策略具有理论可行性，但随后人们认识到免疫耗竭类型的复杂性，因此如何将其正确用于免疫耐受仍有待考证。据相关文献报道，正确认识每种免疫耗竭策略的独特性是极其重要的。

1997年，Knechtle等人报道了在NHP体内，通过CD3适应性免疫毒素进行T细胞耗竭，能延长肾移植存活时间，并诱导5/6的受体出现供体皮肤移植耐受，尽管也存在皮肤移植的排斥反应[68]。在该实验之前，通过耗竭兔抗胸腺细胞球蛋白(ATG)，可以促进免疫耐受，但仅仅是在联合骨髓移植的情况下[69,70]。相比于ATG和T细胞放射，免疫毒素可以单独促进免疫耐受，无论在外周循环还是淋巴结内，它都可以提高T细胞选择性和T细胞溶解的有效性[33,71]。有趣的是，尽管啮齿类动物试验表明，受体胸腺内存在供体MHCⅠ类或Ⅱ类分子抗原，可以联合抗T细胞治疗，促进免疫耐受[72-74]，但向胸腺内输注供体淋巴细胞并没有致耐受性效应。

尽管免疫毒素有望成为独立致耐受性因素，但随后的试验证明它被用于免疫诱导的辅助治疗效果更佳。移植前单独使用免疫毒素，可以提高同种移植存活率，在至少1/3受体体内诱导免疫耐受，但在移植后(与临床更相关)联合脱氧精胍菌素或吗替麦考酚酯(MMF)，比单独使用免疫毒素诱导的免疫耐受时间更长[75]。在接受免疫毒素治疗的NHP体内，相关机制研究发现，供体特异性细胞毒性T细胞的前体频率和免疫应答都受到了抑制，但混合淋巴细胞反应和同种抗体的产生均未受到影响[76,77]。相关组织学和血清学研究发现，同种抗体介导的肾小球和动脉损伤联合炎症因子INF-γ和IL-2[78]，可以致敏早期T细胞，促进抗体介导的移植损伤。移植后接受免疫毒素治疗的动物也可以产生供体特异性抗体反应，进一步证明体液免疫机制与免疫耐受诱导的失败有关，而这也是B细胞抑制剂脱氧精胍菌素成功应用的原理所在，该药联合激素或免疫毒素可以在NHP体内有效诱导免疫耐受[79]。

这些与CD3适应性免疫毒素有关的临床前试验奠定了T细胞耗竭治疗的基础，在移植同时使用该方案可以促进长期免疫耐受的形成。Calne等人在人类肾脏移植受者体内，通过使用阿仑单抗-1H(一种CD52抗体)耗竭T细胞和B细胞，并联合环孢霉素维持低剂量的免疫抑制状态，诱导免疫耐受[80,81]。随后的临床随机对照实验证实，阿仑单抗可以诱导免疫耗竭，随后维持低剂量的免疫抑制，避免排斥反应，从而达到免疫耐受状态[82,83]。该试验组指出，在任何方案的指导下，人为诱导免疫耐受都是十分困难的，因为供体和受体的器官组织存在巨大的不匹配性，而固有免疫活性以及对于打破免疫耐受的感染和过敏反应的敏感性也存在着巨大差异。因此，他们建立了近乎免疫耐受的试验模型，通过低剂量的免疫抑制剂维持免疫耐受状态[84]。尽管这个临床试验结果很容易为人所接受，但相关机制是与免疫耐受有关，还是仅仅与有效的免疫抑制有关，还不得而知。无论如何，通过达到阿仑单抗等抗体的最高浓度，可以实现淋巴细胞耗竭，但这一策略并不能单独诱导免疫耐受。也有其他试验试图推翻这一结论，让活体肾移植受者在移植前接受大剂量的阿仑单抗治疗，以彻底清除外周血和次级淋巴组织中的 T 细胞[85]。尽管在治疗后出现了淋巴细胞减少症，但本试验的所有患者仍然都产生了免疫排斥，而该排斥反应主要以移植物内单核细胞（不是淋巴细胞）浸润为特征。这些数据表明，在免疫排斥中，尽管实现了淋巴细胞耗竭，但非淋巴细胞群也发挥了重要作用，也可能只需要极少量 T 细胞即可引发免疫排斥反应。本试验还得出了另外一个重要结论，非特异性多克隆清除并不是均一性的，因为记忆 T 细胞对于这种清除具有相对抵抗性[86]。然而，这些细胞对钙调磷酸酶抑制剂十分敏感，部分解释了基于钙调磷酸酶的免疫耐受诱导试验的有效性。此外，耗竭后剩余的 T 细胞会增殖达到平衡状态，这也是诱导免疫耐受的一大障碍[66,87]。在接受阿仑单抗治疗的肾移植患者体内，B 细胞也参与了免疫耗竭抵抗相关的排斥反应，这与机体 BAFF（一种维持 B 细胞稳态的因子）水平的提高有关[88]。因此，充分的免疫耗竭并不能单独诱导免疫耐受。

关于免疫耗竭的研究让我们意识到了对发展免疫耐受方案至关重要的机制。我们知道同种移植物功能障碍不仅仅是由 T 细胞的毒性所决定的，而免疫耗竭对巨噬细胞、T 细胞和 B 细胞有不一致的影响。耗竭前免疫反应状态的不同（记忆细胞与幼稚细胞比值），以及不同的稳态扩展动力学都可能影响免疫耗竭的最终效果。总体而言，淋巴细胞耗竭常被视作其他诱导耐受方案的组成部分，而对许多患者来说，它确实可以减少维持耐受所需的免疫抑制剂量。对于免疫耗竭策略的研究有助于在器官移植中改善诱导免疫耐受的策略。

共刺激阻断

1975 年，Lafferty 和 Cunningham 提出了关于 T 细胞激活的双信号假说，这说明免疫应答在特定环境下可以促进免疫耐受，而并非仅仅是强制进行抗原破坏[89]。这一概念上的突破奠定了随后几十年研究工作的基础，人们不断通过试验证实，共刺激阻断可以诱导免疫耐受[90–93]。共刺激阻断的原理在于，适应性免疫应答需要两条信号才能达到最佳活化状态[94]。当缺少其中一条辅助信号时，抗原刺激会引起免疫细胞失效能或凋亡。因此通过抗原暴露活化信号 1，再抑制信号 2 或共刺激信号，可以以抗原特异性的方式清除免疫细胞。在临床前模型中，共刺激阻断有助于促进免疫耐受，特别是当遇到外周抗原时，无论是移植物本身[95–98]还是融合的造血细胞[99]，同时，该方法也被用于促进嵌合体形成[45,100]。这一模型随后被修饰成为包含"信号 3"的模型[101]，后者是细胞因子诱导的信号，并且可以控制免疫细胞激活后的级联放大反应。

人们越来越意识到，共刺激信号对于 T 细胞活化、增殖、分化极其重要，于是进行了大量关于共刺激分子的研究，同时也研究其在促进供体特异性 T 细胞反应和移植后促进免疫耐受的机制。在众多报道的共刺激通路中[102]，描述得最清晰也可能最重要的就是 TNF：TNFR 家族中的 CD40 和 CD154（CD40L）以及免疫球蛋白超家族中的 CD80（B7-1）/CD86（B7-2）和 CD28。这些分子发挥作用的确切机制还未完全为人所知，但通过基因敲除小鼠、单克隆抗体或融合蛋白抑制这些信号，可以对免疫应答产生重要影响[103]。

Lenschow 等人最初报道了 CTLA4Ig，这是一种 CTLA4 的可溶性融合蛋白，可以结合 B7 分子，阻断小鼠体内的胰岛排斥反应，诱导供者适应性免疫耐受[104]。随后，人们通过抗 CD154 抗体，阻断 CD40：CD154 通路，从而取得了类似的小鼠胰岛移植的成功[105]。不久，Larsen 等人发现，在严格控制条件的小鼠体内，皮肤和心脏移植后的长期耐受需要同时阻断 CD28 和 CD40，而不是单独阻断其中一条[95]。在特定鼠类移植模型中，通过阻断 CD28 和 CD40 共刺激信号诱导免疫耐受的方案，随后被复制到了 NHP 身上[96,97,106]，但在大型动物临床前模型中可以持续诱导免疫耐受的方案是否可以用于临床仍有待进一步考证[19,20,107]。此外，在人类肾脏移植中，一项关于人源化 CD154 特异性抗体的研究发现，5/7 的患者发生了免疫排斥，这使人们开始重新思考这一策略的有效性[108]。

造成鼠类、灵长类和人类模型中结果差异的原因还不甚明了，但可能部分在于人类免疫系统的复杂性增加，并且相比于试验动物，人类长期暴露于不同的环境中[19,20,107]。尽管还未完全理解，但进一步的试验仍然证实了阻碍共刺激阻断诱导免疫耐受的障碍[102,109]。其中包括某系共刺激信号的双重活化和调节效应，以及由记忆 T 细胞介导的不同免疫反应[110]，相关细节详见第 9 章。

CTLA4 比 CD28 更容易结合 CD80 和 CD86，并且

可以产生竞争性抑制作用,这就造成了 B7 共刺激阻断诱导免疫耐受的第一大障碍[111,112]。由于 B7 阻断可能抑制不同的信号通路,通过修饰 T 细胞共刺激作用来建立免疫耐受,要比单独阻断初始活化共刺激信号复杂得多。因此,不难发现,单独阻断 CD28:B7 既不能在鼠类移植模型也不能在 NHP 模型中诱导免疫耐受[20,113]。阻断 CD40:CD154 通路也有其局限性,尽管最初曾研制出 CD154 特异性抗体,但 NHP 和人类模型中的血栓并发症让人们几乎放弃了 CD154 信号通路的靶向治疗[108,114]。幸运的是,临床前试验证实[115-119],选择性阻断 CD40 有一定疗效,而 CD40 特异性靶向药物正处于临床研究阶段[120]。然而,CD40:CD154 的研究表明,尽管共刺激分子通常被认为对 T 细胞有一定作用,但受体-配体结合所引起的都是双向效应,会造成明显的免疫和非免疫后果。在共刺激阻断的同时,倘若无意中阻断了负性调节通路或非 T 细胞和非免疫作用,都可能对诱导免疫耐受造成负面影响。

阻断 T 细胞共刺激通路,可以抑制移植后幼稚的供体特异性 T 细胞产生免疫反应,但供体激活的记忆 T 细胞有时会对移植后长期存活以及诱导免疫耐受造成无法逾越的障碍(图 11.3)[109]。记忆 T 细胞会排斥同种移植物,这一过程不依赖于刺激淋巴器官[121],并对许多介入治疗都具有抵抗能力[86,122],其中就包括共刺激阻断[110,123-125]。此外,在移植后存在共刺激信号的情况下,$CD4^+$和 $CD8^+$的前体细胞频率决定了 T 细胞介导免疫排斥的能力[64,65]。最近,研究表明,在 NHP 肾移植模型中,高频供体特异性记忆 T 细胞会削弱免疫耐受[126]。因此,在移植受者体内,高频记忆 T 细胞可能不需要共

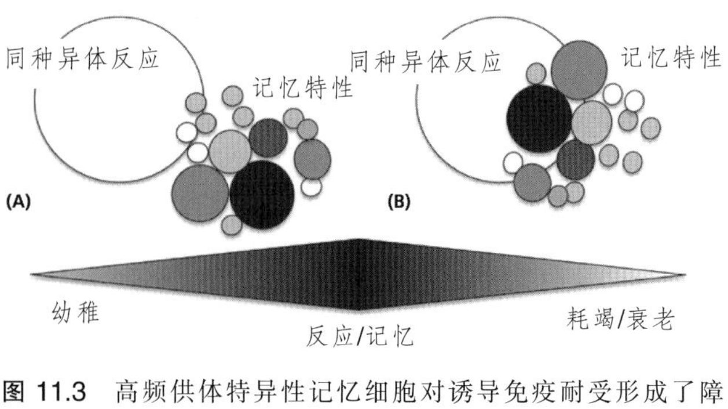

图 11.3 高频供体特异性记忆细胞对诱导免疫耐受形成了障碍。在图(A)中,低频同种记忆反应有助于诱导免疫耐受,因为共刺激阻断可以有效抑制供体特异性幼稚 T 细胞的应答。相反,在图(B)中,高频供体特异性记忆细胞是共刺激阻断诱导耐受的一大障碍。

刺激信号,从而介导了抵抗共刺激阻断的移植排斥,并阻碍了免疫耐受的形成[109,127]。

对于通过共刺激阻断诱导移植后免疫耐受来说,共刺激通路的复杂性既提供了机会,也带来了挑战。共刺激分子从多方面调节了同种免疫应答,从最初的幼稚 T 细胞到记忆 T 细胞和调节 T 细胞的形成,并具有正性和负性双重作用,可以增强或削弱抗原特异性 T 细胞反应。目前较为清楚的是,正如其他免疫抑制方法一样,单独使用共刺激阻断并不能成功建立免疫耐受。然而,随着最近贝拉西普[128](一种用于临床的高效 CTLA4Ig)的出现,共刺激阻断可以被列入临床治疗方案,并在人类身上进行测试。正如淋巴细胞耗竭抗体一样,临床有效性将会鼓舞人们探索更多理论上可行的治疗方案。

通过靶向 T 细胞共刺激阻断,临床上出现了一些可选方案来实现免疫耐受。负性共刺激分子提供了抑制或阻断免疫应答的生理方法,从而诱导免疫耐受。研究得最深入的是 CTLA4,因为许多试验证明,它在免疫调节中发挥重要作用[129],并且其信号通路对于诱导免疫耐受是必不可少的[130-132],而通过增强 CTLA4 信号通路的治疗方案可能会诱导内源性免疫耐受。此外,在 NHP 肾脏和胰岛移植模型中,选择性抑制记忆 T 细胞联合共刺激阻断,可以成功中和这一共刺激耐受细胞群体,预防移植排斥反应的发生[133,134]。在啮齿类动物模型中,靶向阻断许多其他共刺激分子可将免疫抑制效应放大数倍。然而,具体罗列每种共刺激阻断已经超出了本章的范围,相关的其他途径将会在别处扩展介绍[93,102,109,135,136]。

最近一段时间,共刺激阻断的应用发生了一些变化,从最初的免疫耐受诱导工具,发展成了维持免疫耐受的一线药物,并且不依赖于 CNI 药物[92]。在肾移植中,通过使用 CD28 阻断剂贝拉希普取得了鼓舞人心的实验结果[128,137,138],这意味着在未来,共刺激阻断可能成为诱导移植后免疫耐受的治疗方案的一部分。

免疫调节

正如 Peter Medawar 早期预测的“主动获得的免疫耐受”一样,免疫耐受的机制可能是可逆的,不断受到新出现的效应细胞和炎症因子的威胁,同时也受到整体炎症环境和抗原暴露的影响。因此,理论上而言,主动免疫抑制机制可能在维持免疫耐受中发挥一定作

用。为了移植后的存活以及诱导免疫耐受,控制固有免疫和适应性免疫是极其重要的。免疫细胞促进免疫排斥还是耐受取决于细胞初始的状态和机体目前的情况。尽管白细胞群体(如巨噬细胞、树突状细胞、B 细胞和 T 细胞)可以介导移植后组织损伤,它们也可以促进移植物存活和免疫耐受[139]。关于其调控机制详见第 8 章。

20 年前的早期试验证实,在特定环境下,$CD4^+$ T 细胞可以抑制免疫应答损伤[140-143]。小鼠试验表明,在未接受免疫抑制药物治疗但长期免疫耐受的小鼠体内[144,145],存在主动抑制移植物排斥反应的 T 细胞,若将该细胞群体输注给其他小鼠模型,可以诱导供体适应性免疫耐受[146]。随后人们发现,这种形式的免疫细胞调节与表达 CD25 的 $CD4^+$ T 细胞有关,CD25 是 IL-2 受体的 α 链[147-149],而 $CD4^+$ $CD25^+$的 T 细胞可以抑制 T 细胞增殖[150]。最后,小鼠试验表明在诱导 $CD4^+$T 细胞转变为调节 T 细胞过程中,还需要转录因子 Foxp3[151-153]。在肝移植和肾移植受体的循环系统和免疫耐受器官内,这些调节细胞的数量都大大增加了[154-159]。

$CD8^+$ T 细胞[160-162]、CD4-CD8-T 细胞[163]、自然杀伤细胞[164]以及 γδT 细胞[165]以及许多新发现的 T 细胞群体都有免疫调节活性,但 $CD4^+CD25^{hi}Foxp3^+$调节 T 细胞(Tregs)仍然是试验结果最佳的调节细胞。它们可以维持对自身抗原的免疫耐受,通过负反馈机制控制免疫反应[166]。Treg 既是通过胸腺中枢选择自然存在的细胞[167],又可以在外周免疫耐受环境中,通过外周抗原诱导并分化为诱导 Treg[168]。人们已经发现了调节 T 细胞抑制免疫应答的多种细胞机制[169],其中包括直接细胞接触抑制效应 T 细胞增殖[170],以及诱导靶细胞(如抗原提呈细胞 APC)溶解或细胞周期捕获和凋亡[171-173]。调节 T 细胞也能通过旁分泌调节直接诱导免疫抑制,主要通过分泌抑制性细胞因子 IL-10、TGF-β 和 IL-35[148,174],或者消耗增殖性细胞因子 IL-2[150,175]。此外,Treg 上表达的 CTLA4 可以阻断 T 细胞活化所需的共刺激信号,由于 CD80/CD86 比 CD28 具有更高的亲和力,可以通过 CD80/CD86 介导的 APC 内吲哚胺 2,3-过氧化酶的活化来抑制 T 细胞增殖[176]。

移植后早期的同种抗原暴露时,通常没有足够的 Treg 抑制免疫排斥,这部分是由于存在高频供者特异性 T 细胞[122]。这种不平衡有利于同种 T 细胞的激活,从而使免疫反应倾向于移植物破坏方向。然而,如果控制了早期的同种免疫反应,在长期抗原刺激下,Treg 细胞就可以在外周被激活或者由胸腺细胞演变而来,因此,理论上而言,免疫反应就倾向于免疫调节过程[177-179]。免疫破坏和免疫调节之间存在平衡关系,这就使人们可以通过抑制效应 T 细胞活性,或者增加供体特异性 Treg 的相对数量或免疫活性来控制免疫应答,从而有利于诱导免疫耐受[180-183]。

非 T 细胞免疫调节细胞可能在同种免疫耐受中发挥重要的介导作用。人们发现,在免疫耐受的肾移植受者体内,B 细胞相关的基因呈高表达量,这使人们开始关注 B 细胞介导的免疫耐受[184-186]。人类调节 B 细胞 $CD19^+$ $CD24^{hi}CD38^{hi}$ 可以分泌促调节细胞因子 IL-10[187-190],但其在同种免疫中的确切作用还不得而知。调节性巨噬细胞具有特异的形态、细胞表型以及抑制 T 细胞增殖的能力,同时,巨噬细胞也分泌 IL-10,这表明其可能会抑制促炎症性弥漫免疫应答[190,191]。尽管树突状细胞在抗原特异性 T 细胞的产生过程中发挥重要作用,但其也被证明可以促进免疫耐受的形成[192,193]。

有利于保护移植物和诱导免疫耐受的,可能是由以上几种免疫调节细胞介导的总体相互作用,而不是其中某种细胞的单独效应。Wood 等人发现[194],可能在免疫应答早期,固有免疫应答使定向造血干细胞聚集于移植物内,从而启动了免疫调节反应,并为调节性巨噬细胞和树突状细胞的形成创造了有利的微环境。当活化的 T 细胞返回次级淋巴组织时,在胸腺驱动 Treg 和调节性 B 细胞的辅助下,这种致耐受性微环境可以诱导外周 Treg 的产生。这些过程都依赖于免疫抑制治疗的辅助,因为后者可以将免疫平衡从移植物破坏转变为免疫耐受,只有在免疫耐受环境中,同种抗原适应性免疫调节机制才可能成熟和完善。

能否通过免疫调节机制诱导免疫耐受的关键在于,目前的免疫抑制方案对体内效应细胞的作用,以及能否产生免疫调节细胞群体,因为后者是非常多变的,并且依赖于免疫抑制剂使用的时间和联合方式。例如,通过阿仑单抗诱导的淋巴细胞耗竭,可以减少效应细胞数量,使调节细胞得以再生,有助于预防免疫排斥[195-197]。另一方面,CNI 和抗增殖药物(如 MMF)的维持治疗可以同时抑制效应细胞和调节细胞。抗 CD-25 抗体对 Treg 的作用是有争议的,而西罗莫司在体外可以促进 Treg 增殖,在体内则会增强其功能[198,199]。相关数据表明,CTLA4Ig 会使 Treg 依赖的移植模型预后变差,因为其阻断了 CTLA4 介导的 T 细胞活化抑制作用[200-202]。

因此,不同免疫抑制方案之间存在相互矛盾,而在使用免疫调节机制诱导耐受时,也必须要考虑到这一点。

基于临床前动物试验的结果[203,204],免疫调节治疗在临床上的应用正在努力实践中,并且不断尝试向受者输注 Treg 细胞联合或不联合各种不同的免疫抑制剂。尽管试验结果乐观,但向受者输注 Treg 细胞在临床上的应用受到了一定限制,因为其在体内的频率很低,这就需要在体外分离扩增 Treg 细胞[205]。其方案包括扩增自然 Treg 细胞,从前体细胞诱导适应性 Treg 细胞,以及通过异位基因表达产生 Treg 细胞[206]。目前的临床实践仍然局限于骨髓移植细胞,但即将开展的欧盟"ONE Study"计划建议使用免疫调节细胞[207-209],包括在活体肾移植受者体内扩增其自身的天然 Treg 细胞。尽管如此,将 Treg 细胞治疗初步用于临床肝移植仍然是前景可观的,并且为未来实体器官移植奠定了基础。

B 细胞

以往人们认为,T 细胞是同种异体移植物排斥反应的罪魁祸首,但现在人们已意识到,同种抗体介导的体液机制在抗体介导的排斥反应(AMR)中的重要性亦不可忽视[210,211]。AMR 的机制已在第 6 章深入讨论过。2%~10%的排斥反应可以用 AMR 来解释,而在致敏的患者群体中这一比例更高[212]。AMR 的特征是供体特异性抗体的形成[213]和组织病理学上补体的沉积[214],它还和同种异体移植后长期生存率不佳有关。近些年越来越多的证据显示,抗体依赖性和非抗体依赖性 B 细胞介导的免疫应答是同种异体移植耐受发展的重大障碍。

我们关于 B 细胞耐受机制的很多知识,都来源于对自身免疫中 B 细胞的研究[215,216]。V(D)J 基因的重组使得 B 细胞受体随机募集,这产生了巨大的受体多样性,进而导致了最多达 20%~50%的自身反应性[217-219]。生理学上自我耐受的达成有中枢和外周两种途径:中枢性耐受倾向于通过克隆删除和受体编辑,清除高亲和力自身反应 B 细胞[220-222]。自身抗原刺激自身反应性 B 细胞受体,导致受体内化以及 B 细胞成熟抑制[223,224]。此外,自身反应性细胞的死亡可归因于促凋亡因子(如 BCL2 样蛋白 11)的升高和 B 细胞生存蛋白的抑制。有些自身免疫性 B 细胞可以躲过克隆删除,其 V(D)J 的重组使得 RAG 基因持续表达,进而发生受体编辑以及出现新的受体组合,这种结果让这些细胞得以抵抗自身免疫作用[225-227]。外周性耐受的机制包括逃脱了中枢性耐受的低亲和力过渡期 B 细胞,正如前文所述,通过提高兴奋阈值和激活自身反应性 B 细胞固有调控途径的分子机制产生无应答[228,229]。为了维持外周 B 细胞数量的稳定,低亲和力自身反应性 B 细胞还可以在新出现的非固有 B 细胞机制影响下,被克隆性地忽略[230],正如 TNFSF13B 对有限的卵泡生长因子的竞争那样[231]。对 B 细胞生理性调控的中枢和外周机制的研究将引领 B 细胞耐受手段的发展。

现阶段对于 AMR 的 B 细胞靶向治疗,并不能有效地控制 B 细胞依赖性效应器的免疫反应。有些患者处于低丙种球蛋白状态,机体出于维持稳态的目的,抗体代偿性合成,这限制了这些患者血浆置换时非选择性同种抗体的清除,此外有些患者因服用抑制剂如利妥昔单抗(抗 CD20)、硼替佐米(蛋白酶和浆细胞抑制剂)、依库丽单抗(抗 C5)等导致普遍体液抑制,考虑到安全问题,它们并不能提供稳定的免疫抑制[232-234]。因此,我们亟须发展新的 B 细胞耐受疗法,但与 T 细胞相似,相比于动物实验,B 细胞的耐受难以在人体条件下成功诱导。尽管如此,在获取同种异体移植免疫耐受的 B 细胞方面,动物实验的观察结果亦可作为现代临床策略发展的基石[19,20,235]。

在共用胎盘循环的牛和注射同种异体抗原的鼠胚胎实验中,研究者们观察到了新生期耐受[236],这可能是由同种异体反应 B 细胞的克隆删除引起的。人类不同血型的单绒毛膜异卵双胞胎,在子宫内便已对对方的血型产生了新生期耐受[237]。类似的 B 细胞耐受的机制可能有助于婴儿 ABO 血型不相容移植的成功,因为婴儿 5~6 个月才开始产生 ABO 特异性的抗体,所以他们发生超急性同种异体移植物排斥的可能性较低[238]。婴儿的 ABO 血型不相容的心脏移植已成功实施,并未出现超急性排斥反应或其他 ABO 血型不相容相关问题[239]。这种现象的原因似乎与同种异体抗原出现时 ABO 特异性的 B 细胞一过性缺失有关,因为在移植了 ABO 血型不相容的心脏的受者身上,研究者发现了特异性的 B 细胞重新出现,而这些细胞与先前的 ABO 血型抗原决定簇并不匹配[240]。因此,相比于涉及中枢性机制的新生期耐受,同种异体移植耐受似乎需要外周的抗原来刺激。这一方面更多的治疗手段见第 112 章。

2004 年一项对于 ABO 血型不相容的心脏移植受者的研究显示,对供者血型抗原的 B 细胞耐受可自发发生[241]。即使这些受者并未产生对供者 HLA 的耐受，但对供者血型抗原的 B 细胞耐受的出现，是对人类获得新生期耐受的首次描述。ABO 血型不相容的移植术已在肾移植和肝移植中进行了尝试[242,243]，其中 1 岁以下儿童受者的成功率最高[244,245]。对婴儿耐受机制的深入理解，将会有力推动成人同种异体移植中 B 细胞耐受获取策略的发展。

B 细胞在混合嵌合体治疗中的角色仍不明确。多向造血干细胞的混合嵌合与 T 细胞、B 细胞对供者移植物的中枢调控耐受有关[246]。在上文提及的一项混合嵌合体研究中[48]，5 名肾移植患者中的 4 名获得了免疫耐受，但其中一位受者因急性 AMR 出现了移植物损伤，另有两位尽管有短暂的嵌合，但也发现了同种异体抗体，这提示我们免疫耐受可与 B 细胞对供者一定水平的抗体反应共存。虽然一过性嵌合和 B 细胞介导耐受间的联系还未明确，但若达成了一过性嵌合，长期耐受的原因似乎就不仅仅是克隆删除了。因此对人类来说，或许 B 细胞还可以通过其他外周途径诱导免疫耐受。

淋巴细胞的消耗非特异地减少了 T 细胞和 B 细胞的同种异体抗原特异的前体数量。然而，浆细胞及一些抵抗淋巴细胞消耗疗法的 B 细胞，可能会给同种异体移植耐受的诱导带来障碍[85,247]。虽然消耗疗法已在大体上降低了排斥率，但它对 B 细胞耐受的影响却未被评估过。事实上，一些消耗剂可能与 AMR 比例的增加有关[248,249]，因为为了达到稳态而激活的 T 细胞可能反倒会促进 T 细胞介导 B 细胞产生抗体。因此，既往认为的局部 B 细胞消耗会导致 B 细胞功能下调以及 AMR 发生减少的这一概念，可能其理论基础就存在纰漏，且值得我们更深入地研究。

此外，T 细胞和 B 细胞的大量消耗可能与 TNFSF13B 生成的增加有关[88]，它是 B 细胞生存、成熟、分化方面重要的细胞因子[250-252]。TNFSF13B 生成的增加可能是因替代减少的淋巴细胞而产生的稳态压力所致，这种变化可能会导致一组矛盾：当出现 B 细胞淋巴球减少症时，B 细胞反而激活。以 TNFSF13B 为靶点调控 B 细胞稳态和生存，对移植耐受有潜在的重要影响。例如，使用 TNFSF13B 抑制剂后，B 细胞克隆的消除和控制下的粒子数再增可能会促进移植耐受的诱导，因为暴露于供体抗原下时，这些新生 B 细胞能够经历耐受性机制的诱导。

一篇探索机制的研究分析了 25 位自愿接受肾脏移植受者的免疫耐受网络中外周淋巴细胞基因表达情况[184]。相比于使用免疫抑制剂后移植物功能稳定的患者组以及健康对照组，免疫耐受患者的基因表达提示移植耐受与 B 细胞分化相关的多个基因的高表达密切相关。这些 B 细胞相关的基因或“B 细胞信号”，由自发耐受的肾移植受者幼稚和过渡期 B 细胞数目升高，以及尿沉渣细胞中 CD20mRNA 的上调组成。相似地，欧盟的一项研究[185]大致筛选出了 11 名肾移植术后移植耐受的受者，研究包括有移植损伤表现的免疫抑制的受者和健康对照两个人群。该研究发现，相较于其他患者，耐受患者外周血有更高水平的 B 细胞相关基因。这些结果提示，在移植耐受的肾移植受者中，B 细胞在调控同种免疫反应方面扮演着重要角色。

总结

长期的免疫抑制仍是移植领域的一项重要任务，这使得免疫耐受成为改善移植长期预后的热点话题。排斥反应是一种整体的表型，它受多个相互联系的通路影响，为获得供者特异的耐受，这些通路都应被抑制。因此整合应用本章所述的现有策略，最可能实现长期免疫耐受的诱导。虽然嵌合体方案目的性强且已获得了早期成功，迄今未出现与稳定嵌合体相关的不良反应，但学术界仍未提出任一可被证实的治疗方案。淋巴细胞耗竭本身并不会导致耐受，但可能会通过增强免疫力的方式改变内稳态。共刺激通路阻断对免疫反应有明确而重要的影响，但这些影响的主要对象在于幼稚的免疫应答。虽然 CD28：B7 通路阻断已以贝拉西普的形式用于临床，但若要以其作为耐受原，那么相应的辅助治疗亦不可或缺。在未来的耐受研究方面，适应性免疫调控和 B 细胞机制将注定占据越来越重要的地位。随着人工诱导的移植耐受越来越多，同步进展的临床工作对它的鉴定与研究将会为移植耐受的机制研究提供线索。

（毛雨鸽　张超　译　李照　校）

参考文献

1. Lodhi SA, Lamb KE, Meier-Kriesche HU. Solid organ allograft survival improvement in the United States: the long-term does not mirror the dramatic short-term success. American Journal of Transplantation. 2011;11:1226–1235.
2. Orlando G, Soker S, Wood K. Operational tolerance after liver transplantation.

Journal of Hepatology. 2009;50:1247–1257.
3. Orlando G, Hematti P, Stratta RJ, et al. Clinical operational tolerance after renal transplantation: current status and future challenges. Annals of Surgery. 2010;252:915–928.
4. Owens ML, Maxwell JG, Goodnight J, et al. Discontinuance of immunosuppression in renal transplant patients. Archives of Surgery. 1975;110:1450–1451.
5. Uehling DT, Hussey JL, Weinstein AB, et al. Cessation of immunosuppression after renal transplantation. Surgery. 1976;79:278–282.
6. Starzl TE, Murase N, Demetris AJ, et al. Lessons of organ-induced tolerance learned from historical clinical experience. Transplantation. 2004;77:926–929.
7. Roussey-Kesler G, Giral M, Moreau A, et al. Clinical operational tolerance after kidney transplantation. American Journal of Transplantation. 2006;6:736–746.
8. Mazariegos GV, Reyes J, Marino IR, et al. Weaning of immunosuppression in liver transplant recipients. Transplantation. 1997;63:243–249.
9. Devlin J, Doherty D, Thomson L, et al. Defining the outcome of immunosuppression withdrawal after liver transplantation. Hepatology (Baltimore, Md.). 1998;27:926–933.
10. Girlanda R, Rela M, Williams R, et al. Long-term outcome of immunosuppression withdrawal after liver transplantation. Transplantation Proceedings. 2005; 37:1708–1709.
11. Lerut J, Sanchez-Fueyo A. An appraisal of tolerance in liver transplantation. American Journal of Transplantation. 2006;6:1774–1780.
12. Sanchez-Fueyo A. Hot-topic debate on tolerance: immunosuppression withdrawal. Liver Transplantation. 2011;17(Suppl. 3):S69–S73.
13. Feng S, Ekong UD, Lobritto SJ, et al. Complete immunosuppression withdrawal and subsequent allograft function among pediatric recipients of parental living donor liver transplants. JAMA. 2012;307:283–293.
14. Calne RY, Sells RA, Pena JR, et al. Induction of immunological tolerance by porcine liver allografts. Nature. 1969;223:472–476.
15. Horner BM, Cina RA, Wikiel KJ, et al. Predictors of organ allograft tolerance following hematopoietic cell transplantation. American Journal of Transplantation. 2006;6:2894–2902.
16. Strober S, Modry DL, Hoppe RT, et al. Induction of specific unresponsiveness to heart allografts in mongrel dogs treated with total lymphoid irradiation and antithymocyte globulin. Journal of Immunology. 1984;132:1013–1018.
17. Storb R, Yu C, Wagner JL, et al. Stable mixed hematopoietic chimerism in DLA-identical littermate dogs given sublethal total body irradiation before and pharmacological immunosuppression after marrow transplantation. Blood. 1997; 89:3048–3054.
18. Kuhr CS, Allen MD, Junghanss C, et al. Tolerance to vascularized kidney grafts in canine mixed hematopoietic chimeras. Transplantation. 2002;73:1487–1492.
19. Kirk AD. Crossing the bridge: large animal models in translational transplantation research. Immunological Reviews. 2003;196:176–196.
20. Kean LS, Gangappa S, Pearson TC, et al. Transplant tolerance in non-human primates: progress, current challenges and unmet needs. American Journal of Transplantation. 2006;6:884–893.
21. Kirk AD. Meteorology and tolerance. American Journal of Transplantation. 2006;6:645–646.
22. Newell KA, Larsen CP. Tolerance assays: measuring the unknown. Transplantation. 2006;81:1503–1509.
23. Billingham RE, Brent L, Medawar PB. Actively acquired tolerance of foreign cells. Nature. 1953;172:603–606.
24. Preston E, Kirk AD. Context-based therapy: a conceptual framework for transplantation tolerance. Transplantation Reviews. 2002;16:142–162.
25. Dey B, Sykes M, Spitzer TR. Outcomes of recipients of both bone marrow and solid organ transplants. A review. Medicine. 1998;77:355–369.
26. Ildstad ST, Sachs DH. Reconstitution with syngeneic plus allogeneic or xenogeneic bone marrow leads to specific acceptance of allografts or xenografts. Nature. 1984;307:168–170.
27. Sykes M, Szot GL, Swenson KA, et al. Induction of high levels of allogeneic hematopoietic reconstitution and donor-specific tolerance without myelosuppressive conditioning. Nature Medicine. 1997;3:783–787.
28. Sykes M. Mixed chimerism and transplant tolerance. Immunity. 2001;14: 417–424.
29. Ildstad ST, Wren SM, Bluestone JA, et al. Characterization of mixed allogeneic chimeras. Immunocompetence, in vitro reactivity, and genetic specificity of tolerance. Journal of Experimental Medicine. 1985;162:231–244.
30. Sharabi Y, Sachs DH. Mixed chimerism and permanent specific transplantation tolerance induced by a nonlethal preparative regimen. Journal of Experimental Medicine. 1989;169:493–502.
31. Huang CA, Fuchimoto Y, Scheier-Dolberg R, et al. Stable mixed chimerism and tolerance using a nonmyeloablative preparative regimen in a large-animal model. Journal of Clinical Investigation. 2000;105:173–181.
32. Fuchimoto Y, Huang CA, Yamada K, et al. Mixed chimerism and tolerance without whole body irradiation in a large animal model. Journal of Clinical Investigation. 2000;105:1779–1789.
33. Kawai T, Cosimi AB, Colvin RB, et al. Mixed allogeneic chimerism and renal allograft tolerance in cynomolgus monkeys. Transplantation. 1995;59:256–262.
34. Kimikawa M, Kawai T, Sachs DH, et al. Mixed chimerism and transplantation tolerance induced by a nonlethal preparative regimen in cynomolgus monkeys. Transplantation Proceedings. 1997;29:1218.
35. Spitzer TR, Delmonico F, Tolkoff-Rubin N, et al. Combined histocompatibility leukocyte antigen-matched donor bone marrow and renal transplantation for multiple myeloma with end stage renal disease: the induction of allograft tolerance through mixed lymphohematopoietic chimerism. Transplantation. 1999;68:480–484.
36. Domenig C, Sanchez-Fueyo A, Kurtz J, et al. Roles of deletion and regulation in creating mixed chimerism and allograft tolerance using a nonlymphoablative irradiation-free protocol. Journal of Immunology. 2005;175:51–60.
37. Millan MT, Shizuru JA, Hoffmann P, et al. Mixed chimerism and immunosuppressive drug withdrawal after HLA-mismatched kidney and hematopoietic progenitor transplantation. Transplantation. 2002;73:1386–1391.
38. Khan A, Tomita Y, Sykes M. Thymic dependence of loss of tolerance in mixed allogeneic bone marrow chimeras after depletion of donor antigen. Peripheral mechanisms do not contribute to maintenance of tolerance. Transplantation. 1996;62:380–387.
39. Wekerle T, Sayegh MH, Hill J, et al. Extrathymic T cell deletion and allogeneic stem cell engraftment induced with costimulatory blockade is followed by central T cell tolerance. Journal of Experimental Medicine. 1998;187:2037–2044.
40. Wekerle T, Kurtz J, Ito H, et al. Allogeneic bone marrow transplantation with costimulatory blockade induces macrochimerism and tolerance without cytoreductive host treatment. Nature Medicine. 2000;6:464–469.
41. Kurtz J, Shaffer J, Lie A, et al. Mechanisms of early peripheral CD4 T-cell tolerance induction by anti-CD154 monoclonal antibody and allogeneic bone marrow transplantation: evidence for anergy and deletion but not regulatory cells. Blood. 2004;103:4336–4343.
42. Fehr T, Takeuchi Y, Kurtz J, et al. Early regulation of CD8 T cell alloreactivity by $CD4^+CD25^-$ T cells in recipients of anti-CD154 antibody and allogeneic BMT is followed by rapid peripheral deletion of donor-reactive $CD8^+$ T cells, precluding a role for sustained regulation. European Journal of Immunology. 2005; 35:2679–2690.
43. Bigenzahn S, Blaha P, Koporc Z, et al. The role of non-deletional tolerance mechanisms in a murine model of mixed chimerism with costimulation blockade. American Journal of Transplantation. 2005;5:1237–1247.
44. Kawai T, Poncelet A, Sachs DH, et al. Long-term outcome and alloantibody production in a non-myeloablative regimen for induction of renal allograft tolerance. Transplantation. 1999;68:1767–1775.
45. Kawai T, Sogawa H, Boskovic S, et al. CD154 blockade for induction of mixed chimerism and prolonged renal allograft survival in nonhuman primates. American Journal of Transplantation. 2004;4:1391–1398.
46. Buhler LH, Spitzer TR, Sykes M, et al. Induction of kidney allograft tolerance after transient lymphohematopoietic chimerism in patients with multiple myeloma and end-stage renal disease. Transplantation. 2002;74:1405–1409.
47. Fudaba Y, Spitzer TR, Shaffer J, et al. Myeloma responses and tolerance following combined kidney and nonmyeloablative marrow transplantation: in vivo and in vitro analyses. American Journal of Transplantation. 2006;6:2121–2133.
48. Kawai T, Cosimi AB, Spitzer TR, et al. HLA-mismatched renal transplantation without maintenance immunosuppression. New England Journal of Medicine. 2008;358:353–361.
49. Scandling JD, Busque S, Dejbakhsh-Jones S, et al. Tolerance and chimerism after renal and hematopoietic-cell transplantation. New England Journal of Medicine. 2008;358:362–368.
50. Alexander SI, Smith N, Hu M, et al. Chimerism and tolerance in a recipient of a deceased-donor liver transplant. New England Journal of Medicine. 2008; 358:369–374.
51. Kirk AD. Clinical tolerance 2008. Transplantation. 2009;87:953–955.
52. Wekerle T, Sykes M. Mixed chimerism and transplantation tolerance. Annual Review of Medicine. 2001;52:353–370.
53. Leventhal J, Abecassis M, Miller J, et al. Chimerism and tolerance without GVHD or engraftment syndrome in HLA-mismatched combined kidney and hematopoietic stem cell transplantation. Science Translational Medicine. 2012;4:124ra28.
54. Ramakrishnan SK, Page A, Farris AB 3rd, et al. Evidence for kidney rejection after combined bone marrow and renal transplantation despite ongoing whole-blood chimerism in rhesus macaques. American Journal of Transplantation. 2012;12:1755–1764.
55. Slavin S, Strober S, Fuks Z, et al. Induction of specific tissue transplantation tolerance using fractionated total lymphoid irradiation in adult mice: long-term survival of allogeneic bone marrow and skin grafts. Journal of Experimental Medicine. 1977;146:34–48.
56. Myburgh JA, Smit JA, Hill RR, et al. Transplantation tolerance in primates fol-

lowing total lymphoid irradiation and allogeneic bone marrow injection II. Renal allografts. Transplantation. 1980;29:405–408.
57. Raaf J, Bryan C, Monden M, et al. Bone marrow and renal transplantation in canine recipients prepared by total lymphoid irradiation. Transplantation Proceedings. 1981;13:429–433.
58. Levin B, Hoppe RT, Collins G, et al. Treatment of cadaveric renal transplant recipients with total lymphoid irradiation, antithymocyte globulin, and low-dose prednisone. Lancet. 1985;2(8468):1321–1325.
59. Strober S, Dhillon M, Schubert M, et al. Acquired immune tolerance to cadaveric renal allografts. A study of three patients treated with total lymphoid irradiation. New England Journal of Medicine. 1989;321:28–33.
60. Strober S, Benike C, Krishnaswamy S, et al. Clinical transplantation tolerance twelve years after prospective withdrawal of immunosuppressive drugs: studies of chimerism and anti-donor reactivity. Transplantation. 2000;69:1549–1554.
61. Strober S, Lowsky RJ, Shizuru JA, et al. Approaches to transplantation tolerance in humans. Transplantation. 2004;77:932–936.
62. Ford WL, Atkins RC. The proportion of lymphocytes capable of recognizing strong transplantation antigens in vivo. Advances in Experimental Medicine and Biology. 1973;29:255–262.
63. Suchin EJ, Langmuir PB, Palmer E, et al. Quantifying the frequency of alloreactive T cells in vivo: new answers to an old question. Journal of Immunology. 2001;166:973–981.
64. Ford ML, Koehn BH, Wagener ME, et al. Antigen-specific precursor frequency impacts T cell proliferation, differentiation, and requirement for costimulation. Journal of Experimental Medicine. 2007;204:299–309.
65. Ford ML, Wagener ME, Hanna SS, et al. A critical precursor frequency of donor-reactive $CD4^+$ T cell help is required for $CD8^+$ T cell-mediated CD28/CD154-independent rejection. Journal of Immunology. 2008;180:7203–7211.
66. Wu Z, Bensinger SJ, Zhang J, et al. Homeostatic proliferation is a barrier to transplantation tolerance. Nature Medicine. 2004;10:87–92.
67. Kirk AD. Induction immunosuppression. Transplantation. 2006;82:593–602.
68. Knechtle SJ, Vargo D, Fechner J, et al. FN18-CRM9 immunotoxin promotes tolerance in primate renal allografts. Transplantation. 1997;63:1–6.
69. Thomas FT, Carver FM, Foil MB, et al. Long-term incompatible kidney survival in outbred higher primates without chronic immunosuppression. Annals of Surgery. 1983;198:370–378.
70. Thomas JM, Verbanac KM, Smith JP, et al. The facilitating effect of one-DR antigen sharing in renal allograft tolerance induced by donor bone marrow in rhesus monkeys. Transplantation. 1995;59:245–255.
71. Neville DM Jr, Scharff J, Hu HZ, et al. A new reagent for the induction of T-cell depletion, anti-CD3-CRM9. Journal of Immunotherapy with Emphasis on Tumor Immunology. 1996;19:85–92.
72. Goss JA, Nakafusa Y, Flye MW. MHC class II presenting cells are necessary for the induction of intrathymic tolerance. Annals of Surgery. 1993;217:492–499. discussion 9–501.
73. Oluwole SF, Chowdhury NC, Jin MX, et al. Induction of transplantation tolerance to rat cardiac allografts by intrathymic inoculation of allogeneic soluble peptides. Transplantation. 1993;56:1523–1527.
74. Knechtle SJ, Wang J, Jiao S, et al. Induction of specific tolerance by intrathymic injection of recipient muscle cells transfected with donor class I major histocompatibility complex. Transplantation. 1994;57:990–996.
75. Knechtle SJ. Treatment with immunotoxin. Philosophical Transactions of the Royal Society of London. Series B, Biological Sciences. 2001;356:681–689.
76. Fechner JH Jr, Vargo DJ, Geissler EK, et al. Mechanisms of tolerance induced by an immunotoxin against CD3 epsilon in a rhesus kidney allograft model. Transplantation Proceedings. 1997;29:1158.
77. Fechner JH Jr, Vargo DJ, Geissler EK, et al. Split tolerance induced by immunotoxin in a rhesus kidney allograft model. Transplantation. 1997;63: 1339–1345.
78. Armstrong N, Buckley P, Oberley T, et al. Analysis of primate renal allografts after T-cell depletion with anti-CD3-CRM9. Transplantation. 1998;66:5–13.
79. Thomas JM, Contreras JL, Jiang XL, et al. Peritransplant tolerance induction in macaques: early events reflecting the unique synergy between immunotoxin and deoxyspergualin. Transplantation. 1999;68:1660–1673.
80. Calne R, Friend P, Moffatt S, et al. Prope tolerance, perioperative campath 1H, and low-dose cyclosporin monotherapy in renal allograft recipients. Lancet. 1998;351:1701–1702.
81. Calne R, Moffatt SD, Friend PJ, et al. Campath IH allows low-dose cyclosporine monotherapy in 31 cadaveric renal allograft recipients. Transplantation. 1999; 68:1613–1616.
82. Vathsala A, Ona ET, Tan SY, et al. Randomized trial of alemtuzumab for prevention of graft rejection and preservation of renal function after kidney transplantation. Transplantation. 2005;80:765–774.
83. Margreiter R, Klempnauer J, Neuhaus P, et al. Alemtuzumab (Campath-1H) and tacrolimus monotherapy after renal transplantation: results of a prospective randomized trial. American Journal of Transplantation. 2008;8:1480–1485.
84. Calne RY. Prope tolerance—the future of organ transplantation from the laboratory to the clinic. Transplant Immunology. 2004;13:83–86.
85. Kirk AD, Hale DA, Mannon RB, et al. Results from a human renal allograft tolerance trial evaluating the humanized CD52-specific monoclonal antibody alemtuzumab (CAMPATH-1H). Transplantation. 2003;76:120–129.
86. Pearl JP, Parris J, Hale DA, et al. Immunocompetent T-cells with a memory-like phenotype are the dominant cell type following antibody-mediated T-cell depletion. American Journal of Transplantation. 2005;5:465–474.
87. Neujahr DC, Chen C, Huang X, et al. Accelerated memory cell homeostasis during T cell depletion and approaches to overcome it. Journal of Immunology. 2006;176:4632–4639.
88. Bloom D, Chang Z, Pauly K, et al. BAFF is increased in renal transplant patients following treatment with alemtuzumab. American Journal of Transplantation. 2009;9:1835–1845.
89. Lafferty KJ, Cunningham AJ. A new analysis of allogeneic interactions. Australian Journal of Experimental Biology and Medical Science. 1975;53:27–42.
90. Gudmundsdottir H, Turka LA. T cell costimulatory blockade: new therapies for transplant rejection. Journal of the American Society of Nephrology. 1999;10: 1356–1365.
91. Harlan DM, Kirk AD. The future of organ and tissue transplantation: can T-cell costimulatory pathway modifiers revolutionize the prevention of graft rejection? JAMA. 1999;282:1076–1082.
92. Larsen CP, Knechtle SJ, Adams A, et al. A new look at blockade of T-cell costimulation: a therapeutic strategy for long-term maintenance immunosuppression. American Journal of Transplantation. 2006;6:876–883.
93. Alegre ML, Najafian N. Costimulatory molecules as targets for the induction of transplantation tolerance. Current Molecular Medicine. 2006;6:843–857.
94. Cunningham AJ, Lafferty KJ. A simple conservative explanation of the H-2 restriction of interactions between lymphocytes. Scandinavian Journal of Immunology. 1977;6:1–6.
95. Larsen CP, Elwood ET, Alexander DZ, et al. Long-term acceptance of skin and cardiac allografts after blocking CD40 and CD28 pathways. Nature. 1996; 381:434–438.
96. Kirk AD, Harlan DM, Armstrong NN, et al. CTLA4-Ig and anti-CD40 ligand prevent renal allograft rejection in primates. Proceedings of the National Academy of Sciences of the United States of America. 1997;94:8789–8794.
97. Kirk AD, Burkly LC, Batty DS, et al. Treatment with humanized monoclonal antibody against CD154 prevents acute renal allograft rejection in nonhuman primates. Nature Medicine. 1999;5:686–693.
98. Kirk AD, Tadaki DK, Celniker A, et al. Induction therapy with monoclonal antibodies specific for CD80 and CD86 delays the onset of acute renal allograft rejection in non-human primates. Transplantation. 2001;72:377–384.
99. Preston EH, Xu H, Dhanireddy KK, et al. IDEC-131 (anti-CD154), sirolimus and donor-specific transfusion facilitate operational tolerance in non-human primates. American Journal of Transplantation. 2005;5:1032–1041.
100. Kean LS, Adams AB, Strobert E, et al. Induction of chimerism in rhesus macaques through stem cell transplant and costimulation blockade-based immunosuppression. American Journal of Transplantation. 2007;7:320–335.
101. Mescher MF, Curtsinger JM, Agarwal P, et al. Signals required for programming effector and memory development by $CD8^+$ T cells. Immunological Reviews. 2006;211:81–92.
102. Li XC, Rothstein DM, Sayegh MH. Costimulatory pathways in transplantation: challenges and new developments. Immunological Reviews. 2009;229:271–293.
103. Salama AD, Sayegh MH. Challenges for the translation of T cell costimulatory blockade therapies to the clinic. Expert Opinion on Biological Therapy. 2002;2: 453–457.
104. Lenschow DJ, Zeng Y, Thistlethwaite JR, et al. Long-term survival of xenogeneic pancreatic islet grafts induced by CTLA4Ig. Science. 1992;257:789–792.
105. Parker DC, Greiner DL, Phillips NE, et al. Survival of mouse pancreatic islet allografts in recipients treated with allogeneic small lymphocytes and antibody to CD40 ligand. Proceedings of the National Academy of Sciences of the United States of America. 1995;92:9560–9564.
106. Kenyon NS, Chatzipetrou M, Masetti M, et al. Long-term survival and function of intrahepatic islet allografts in rhesus monkeys treated with humanized anti-CD154. Proceedings of the National Academy of Sciences of the United States of America. 1999;96:8132–8137.
107. Jonker M, Ossevoort Ma, Vierboom M. Blocking the CD80 and CD86 costimulation molecules: lessons to be learned from animal models. Transplantation. 2002;73(1 Suppl.):S23–S26.
108. Kirk AD, Knechtle SJ, Sollinger HW, et al. Preliminary results of the use of humanized anti-CD154 in human renal allotransplantation. American Journal of Transplantation. 2001;1(S1):191.

109. Ford ML, Larsen CP. Translating costimulation blockade to the clinic: lessons learned from three pathways. Immunological Reviews. 2009;229:294–306.
110. Adams AB, Williams MA, Jones TR, et al. Heterologous immunity provides a potent barrier to transplantation tolerance. Journal of Clinical Investigation. 2003;111:1887–1895.
111. Linsley PS, Brady W, Urnes M, et al. CTLA-4 is a second receptor for the B cell activation antigen B7. Journal of Experimental Medicine. 1991;174:561–569.
112. Sharpe AH, Freeman GJ. The B7-CD28 superfamily. Nature Reviews Immunology. 2002;2:116–126.
113. Lechler RI, Sykes M, Thomson AW, et al. Organ transplantation—how much of the promise has been realized? Nature Medicine. 2005;11:605–613.
114. Kawai T, Andrews D, Colvin RB, et al. Thromboembolic complications after treatment with monoclonal antibody against CD40 ligand. Nature Medicine. 2000;6:114.
115. Pearson TC, Trambley J, Odom K, et al. Anti-CD40 therapy extends renal allograft survival in rhesus macaques. Transplantation. 2002;74:933–940.
116. Haanstra KG, Ringers J, Sick EA, et al. Prevention of kidney allograft rejection using anti-CD40 and anti-CD86 in primates. Transplantation. 2003;75: 637–643.
117. Imai A, Suzuki T, Sugitani A, et al. A novel fully human anti-CD40 monoclonal antibody, 4D11, for kidney transplantation in cynomolgus monkeys. Transplantation. 2007;84:1020–1028.
118. Gilson CR, Milas Z, Gangappa S, et al. Anti-CD40 monoclonal antibody synergizes with CTLA4-Ig in promoting long-term graft survival in murine models of transplantation. Journal of Immunology. 2009;183:1625–1635.
119. Badell IR, Thompson PW, Turner AP, et al. Nondepleting anti-CD40-based therapy prolongs allograft survival in nonhuman primates. American Journal of Transplantation. 2012;12:126–135.
120. Kirk AD. 4D11: the second mouse? American Journal of Transplantation. 2009;9:1701–1702.
121. Chalasani G, Dai Z, Konieczny BT, et al. Recall and propagation of allospecific memory T cells independent of secondary lymphoid organs. Proceedings of the National Academy of Sciences of the United States of America. 2002;99: 6175–6180.
122. Yang J, Brook MO, Carvalho-Gaspar M, et al. Allograft rejection mediated by memory T cells is resistant to regulation. Proceedings of the National Academy of Sciences of the United States of America. 2007;104:19954–19959.
123. Valujskikh A, Pantenburg B, Heeger PS. Primed allospecific T cells prevent the effects of costimulatory blockade on prolonged cardiac allograft survival in mice. American Journal of Transplantation. 2002;2:501–509.
124. Pantenburg B, Heinzel F, Das L, et al. T cells primed by Leishmania major infection cross-react with alloantigens and alter the course of allograft rejection. Journal of Immunology. 2002;169:3686–3693.
125. Zhai Y, Meng L, Gao F, et al. Allograft rejection by primed/memory $CD8^+$ T cells is CD154 blockade resistant: therapeutic implications for sensitized transplant recipients. Journal of Immunology. 2002;169:4667–4673.
126. Nadazdin O, Boskovic S, Murakami T, et al. Host alloreactive memory T cells influence tolerance to kidney allografts in nonhuman primates. Science Translational Medicine. 2011;3:86ra51.
127. Ford ML, Larsen CP. Transplantation tolerance: memories that haunt us. Science Translational Medicine. 2011;3:86ps22.
128. Vincenti F, Larsen C, Durrbach A, et al. Costimulation blockade with belatacept in renal transplantation. New England Journal of Medicine. 2005;353:770–781.
129. Wing K, Onishi Y, Prieto-Martin P, et al. CTLA-4 control over $Foxp3^+$ regulatory T cell function. Science. 2008;322:271–275.
130. Judge TA, Wu Z, Zheng XG, et al. The role of CD80, CD86, and CTLA4 in alloimmune responses and the induction of long-term allograft survival. Journal of Immunology. 1999;162:1947–1951.
131. Zheng XX, Markees TG, Hancock WW, et al. CTLA4 signals are required to optimally induce allograft tolerance with combined donor-specific transfusion and anti-CD154 monoclonal antibody treatment. Journal of Immunology. 1999;162:4983–4990.
132. Taylor PA, Lees CJ, Waldmann H, et al. Requirements for the promotion of allogeneic engraftment by anti-CD154 (anti-CD40L) monoclonal antibody under nonmyeloablative conditions. Blood. 2001;98:467–474.
133. Weaver TA, Charafeddine AH, Agarwal A, et al. Alefacept promotes costimulation blockade based allograft survival in nonhuman primates. Nature Medicine. 2009;15:746–749.
134. Badell IR, Russell MC, Thompson PW, et al. LFA-1-specific therapy prolongs allograft survival in rhesus macaques. Journal of Clinical Investigation. 2010;120:4520–4531.
135. Clarkson MR, Sayegh MH. T-cell costimulatory pathways in allograft rejection and tolerance. Transplantation. 2005;80:555–563.
136. Pilat N, Sayegh MH, Wekerle T. Costimulatory pathways in transplantation. Seminars in Immunology. 2011;23:293–303.
137. Vincenti F, Charpentier B, Vanrenterghem Y, et al. A phase III study of belatacept-based immunosuppression regimens versus cyclosporine in renal transplant recipients (BENEFIT study). American Journal of Transplantation. 2010;10: 535–546.
138. Vincenti F, Larsen CP, Alberu J, et al. Three-year outcomes from BENEFIT, a randomized, active-controlled, parallel-group study in adult kidney transplant recipients. American Journal of Transplantation. 2012;12:210–217.
139. Wood KJ, Goto R. Mechanisms of rejection: current perspectives. Transplantation. 2012;93:1–10.
140. Sakaguchi S, Takahashi T, Nishizuka Y. Study on cellular events in post-thymectomy autoimmune oophoritis in mice. II. Requirement of Lyt-1 cells in normal female mice for the prevention of oophoritis. Journal of Experimental Medicine. 1982;156:1577–1586.
141. Hall BM, Jelbart ME, Gurley KE, et al. Specific unresponsiveness in rats with prolonged cardiac allograft survival after treatment with cyclosporine. Mediation of specific suppression by T helper/inducer cells. Journal of Experimental Medicine. 1985;162:1683–1694.
142. Kong YM, Giraldo AA, Waldmann H, et al. Resistance to experimental autoimmune thyroiditis: $L3T4^+$ cells as mediators of both thyroglobulin-activated and TSH-induced suppression. Clinical Immunology and Immunopathology. 1989;51:38–54.
143. Powrie F, Mason D. OX-22high CD4+ T cells induce wasting disease with multiple organ pathology: prevention by the OX-22low subset. Journal of Experimental Medicine. 1990;172:1701–1708.
144. Hall BM, Jelbart ME, Dorsch SE. Suppressor T cells in rats with prolonged cardiac allograft survival after treatment with cyclosporine. Transplantation. 1984;37: 595–600.
145. Qin S, Cobbold SP, Pope H, et al. "Infectious" transplantation tolerance. Science. 1993;259:974–977.
146. Hall BM, Pearce NW, Gurley KE, et al. Specific unresponsiveness in rats with prolonged cardiac allograft survival after treatment with cyclosporine. III. Further characterization of the CD4+ suppressor cell and its mechanisms of action. Journal of Experimental Medicine. 1990;171:141–157.
147. Sakaguchi S, Sakaguchi N, Asano M, et al. Immunologic self-tolerance maintained by activated T cells expressing IL-2 receptor alpha-chains (CD25). Breakdown of a single mechanism of self-tolerance causes various autoimmune diseases. Journal of Immunology. 1995;155:1151–1164.
148. Hara M, Kingsley CI, Niimi M, et al. IL-10 is required for regulatory T cells to mediate tolerance to alloantigens in vivo. Journal of Immunology. 2001; 166:3789–3796.
149. Taylor PA, Lees CJ, Blazar BR. The infusion of ex vivo activated and expanded $CD4^+CD25^+$ immune regulatory cells inhibits graft-versus-host disease lethality. Blood. 2002;99:3493–3499.
150. Thornton AM, Shevach EM. $CD4^+CD25^+$ immunoregulatory T cells suppress polyclonal T cell activation in vitro by inhibiting interleukin 2 production. Journal of Experimental Medicine. 1998;188:287–296.
151. Hori S, Nomura T, Sakaguchi S. Control of regulatory T cell development by the transcription factor Foxp3. Science. 2003;299:1057–1061.
152. Khattri R, Cox T, Yasayko SA, et al. An essential role for Scurfin in $CD4^+CD25^+$ T regulatory cells. Nature Immunology. 2003;4:337–342.
153. Fontenot JD, Gavin MA, Rudensky AY. Foxp3 programs the development and function of CD4+CD25+ regulatory T cells. Nature Immunology. 2003;4: 330–336.
154. Li Y, Koshiba T, Yoshizawa A, et al. Analyses of peripheral blood mononuclear cells in operational tolerance after pediatric living donor liver transplantation. American Journal of Transplantation. 2004;4:2118–2125.
155. Yoshizawa A, Ito A, Li Y, et al. The roles of CD25+CD4+ regulatory T cells in operational tolerance after living donor liver transplantation. Transplantation Proceedings. 2005;37:37–39.
156. Martinez-Llordella M, Puig-Pey I, Orlando G, et al. Multiparameter immune profiling of operational tolerance in liver transplantation. American Journal of Transplantation. 2007;7:309–319.
157. Vlad G, Ho EK, Vasilescu ER, et al. Anti-CD25 treatment and FOXP3-positive regulatory T cells in heart transplantation. Transplant Immunology. 2007;18: 13–21.
158. Akl A, Jones ND, Rogers N, et al. An investigation to assess the potential of $CD25^{high}CD4^+$ T cells to regulate responses to donor alloantigens in clinically stable renal transplant recipients. Transplant International. 2008;21: 65–73.
159. Li Y, Zhao X, Cheng D, et al. The presence of Foxp3 expressing T cells within grafts of tolerant human liver transplant recipients. Transplantation. 2008;86: 1837–1843.
160. Reibke R, Garbi N, Ganss R, et al. $CD8^+$ regulatory T cells generated by neonatal recognition of peripheral self-antigen. Proceedings of the National Academy of Sciences of the United States of America. 2006;103:15142–15147.

161. Vlad G, Cortesini R, Suciu-Foca N. CD8$^+$ T suppressor cells and the ILT3 master switch. Human Immunology. 2008;69:681–686.
162. Li XL, Menoret S, Bezie S, et al. Mechanism and localization of CD8 regulatory T cells in a heart transplant model of tolerance. Journal of Immunology. 2010;185:823–833.
163. Thomson CW, Lee BP, Zhang L. Double-negative regulatory T cells: non-conventional regulators. Immunologic Research. 2006;35:163–178.
164. Monteiro M, Almeida CF, Caridade M, et al. Identification of regulatory Foxp3$^+$ invariant NKT cells induced by TGF-β. Journal of Immunology. 2010; 185:2157–2163.
165. Hayday A, Tigelaar R. Immunoregulation in the tissues by γδ T cells. Nature Reviews Immunology. 2003;3:233–242.
166. Wood KJ, Sakaguchi S. Regulatory T cells in transplantation tolerance. Nature Reviews Immunology. 2003;3:199–210.
167. Sakaguchi S, Miyara M, Costantino CM, et al. FOXP3$^+$ regulatory T cells in the human immune system. Nature Reviews Immunology. 2010;10:490–500.
168. Josefowicz SZ, Rudensky A. Control of regulatory T cell lineage commitment and maintenance. Immunity. 2009;30:616–625.
169. Yamaguchi T, Wing JB, Sakaguchi S. Two modes of immune suppression by Foxp3$^+$ regulatory T cells under inflammatory or non-inflammatory conditions. Seminars in Immunology. 2011;23:424–430.
170. Shevach EM. Mechanisms of Foxp3$^+$ T regulatory cell-mediated suppression. Immunity. 2009;30:636–645.
171. Grossman WJ, Verbsky JW, Barchet W, et al. Human T regulatory cells can use the perforin pathway to cause autologous target cell death. Immunity. 2004;21: 589–601.
172. Gondek DC, Lu LF, Quezada SA, et al. Cutting edge: contact-mediated suppression by CD4$^+$CD25$^+$ regulatory cells involves a granzyme B-dependent, perforin-independent mechanism. Journal of Immunology. 2005;174: 1783–1786.
173. Garin MI, Chu CC, Golshayan D, et al. Galectin-1: a key effector of regulation mediated by CD4$^+$CD25$^+$ T cells. Blood. 2007;109:2058–2065.
174. Kingsley CI, Karim M, Bushell AR, et al. CD25$^+$CD4$^+$ regulatory T cells prevent graft rejection: CTLA-4- and IL-10-dependent immunoregulation of allore-sponses. Journal of Immunology. 2002;168:1080–1086.
175. Pandiyan P, Zheng L, Ishihara S, et al. CD4$^+$CD25$^+$Foxp3$^+$ regulatory T cells induce cytokine deprivation-mediated apoptosis of effector CD4$^+$ T cells. Nature Immunology. 2007;8:1353–1362.
176. Grohmann U, Orabona C, Fallarino F, et al. CTLA-4-Ig regulates tryptophan catabolism in vivo. Nature Immunology. 2002;3:1097–1101.
177. Hamano K, Rawsthorne MA, Bushell AR, et al. Evidence that the continued presence of the organ graft and not peripheral donor microchimerism is essential for maintenance of tolerance to alloantigen in vivo in anti-CD4 treated recipients. Transplantation. 1996;62:856–860.
178. Tullius SG, Nieminen M, Bechstein WO, et al. Chronically rejected rat kidney allografts induce donor-specific tolerance. Transplantation. 1997;64: 158–161.
179. Steger U, Kingsley CI, Karim M, et al. CD25+CD4+ regulatory T cells develop in mice not only during spontaneous acceptance of liver allografts but also after acute allograft rejection. Transplantation. 2006;82:1202–1209.
180. Graca L, Thompson S, Lin CY, et al. Both CD4$^+$CD25$^+$ and CD4$^-$CD25$^+$ regulatory cells mediate dominant transplantation tolerance. Journal of Immunology. 2002;168:5558–5565.
181. Feng G, Wood KJ, Bushell A. Interferon-γ conditioning ex vivo generates CD25+CD62L+Foxp3+ regulatory T cells that prevent allograft rejection: potential avenues for cellular therapy. Transplantation. 2008;86:578–589.
182. Francis RS, Feng G, Tha-In T, et al. Induction of transplantation tolerance converts potential effector T cells into graft-protective regulatory T cells. European Journal of Immunology. 2011;41:726–738.
183. Feng G, Nadig SN, Backdahl L, et al. Functional regulatory T cells produced by inhibiting cyclic nucleotide phosphodiesterase type 3 prevent allograft rejection. Science Translational Medicine. 2011;3:83ra40.
184. Newell KA, Asare A, Kirk AD, et al. Identification of a B cell signature associated with renal transplant tolerance in humans. Journal of Clinical Investigation. 2010;120:1836–1847.
185. Sagoo P, Perucha E, Sawitzki B, et al. Development of a cross-platform biomarker signature to detect renal transplant tolerance in humans. Journal of Clinical Investigation. 2010;120:1848–1861.
186. Pallier A, Hillion S, Danger R, et al. Patients with drug-free long-term graft function display increased numbers of peripheral B cells with a memory and inhibitory phenotype. Kidney International. 2010;78:503–513.
187. Fillatreau S, Sweenie CH, McGeachy MJ, et al. B cells regulate autoimmunity by provision of IL-10. Nature Immunology. 2002;3:944–950.
188. Mauri C, Gray D, Mushtaq N, et al. Prevention of arthritis by interleukin 10-producing B cells. Journal of Experimental Medicine. 2003;197:489–501.
189. Fillatreau S, Gray D, Anderton SM. Not always the bad guys: B cells as regulators of autoimmune pathology. Nature Reviews Immunology. 2008;8:391–397.
190. Fleming BD, Mosser DM. Regulatory macrophages: setting the threshold for therapy. European Journal of Immunology. 2011;41:2498–2502.
191. Murray PJ, Wynn TA. Protective and pathogenic functions of macrophage subsets. Nature Reviews Immunology. 2011;11:723–737.
192. Morelli AE, Thomson AW. Tolerogenic dendritic cells and the quest for transplant tolerance. Nature Reviews Immunology. 2007;7:610–621.
193. van Kooten C, Lombardi G, Gelderman KA, et al. Dendritic cells as a tool to induce transplantation tolerance: obstacles and opportunities. Transplantation. 2011;91:2–7.
194. Wood KJ, Bushell A, Hester J. Regulatory immune cells in transplantation. Nature Reviews Immunology. 2012;12:417–430.
195. Bloom DD, Chang Z, Fechner JH, et al. CD4$^+$ CD25$^+$ FOXP3$^+$ regulatory T cells increase de novo in kidney transplant patients after immunodepletion with Campath-1H. American Journal of Transplantation. 2008;8:793–802.
196. Hester J, Mills N, Shankar S, et al. Th17 cells in alemtuzumab-treated patients: the effect of long-term maintenance immunosuppressive therapy. Transplantation. 2011;91:744–750.
197. Heidt S, Hester J, Shankar S, et al. B cell repopulation after alemtuzumab induction-transient increase in transitional B cells and long-term dominance of naïve B cells. American Journal of Transplantation. 2012;12:1784–1792.
198. Battaglia M, Stabilini A, Migliavacca B, et al. Rapamycin promotes expansion of functional CD4$^+$CD25$^+$FOXP3$^+$ regulatory T cells of both healthy subjects and type 1 diabetic patients. Journal of Immunology. 2006;177:8338–8347.
199. Hester J, Schiopu A, Nadig SN, et al. Low-dose rapamycin treatment increases the ability of human regulatory T cells to inhibit transplant arteriosclerosis in vivo. American Journal of Transplantation. 2012;12:2008–2016.
200. Riella LV, Liu T, Yang J, et al. Deleterious effect of CTLA4-Ig on a Treg-dependent transplant model. American Journal of Transplantation. 2012;12:846–855.
201. Charbonnier LM, Vokaer B, Lemaitre PH, et al. CTLA4-Ig restores rejection of MHC class-II mismatched allografts by disabling IL-2-expanded regulatory T cells. American Journal of Transplantation. 2012;12:2313–2321.
202. Maltzman JS. Costimulation blockade-a double-edged sword? American Journal of Transplantation. 2012;12:2269–2270.
203. Nadig SN, Wieckiewicz J, Wu DC, et al. In vivo prevention of transplant arteriosclerosis by ex vivo-expanded human regulatory T cells. Nature Medicine. 2010;16:809–813.
204. Sagoo P, Ali N, Garg G, et al. Human regulatory T cells with alloantigen specificity are more potent inhibitors of alloimmune skin graft damage than polyclonal regulatory T cells. Science Translational Medicine. 2011;3:83ra42.
205. Issa F, Schiopu A, Wood KJ. Role of T cells in graft rejection and transplantation tolerance. Expert Review of Clinical Immunology. 2010;6:155–169.
206. McMurchy AN, Bushell A, Levings MK, et al. Moving to tolerance: clinical application of T regulatory cells. Seminars in Immunology. 2011;23: 304–313.
207. Trzonkowski P, Bieniaszewska M, Juscinska J, et al. First-in-man clinical results of the treatment of patients with graft versus host disease with human ex vivo expanded CD4+CD25+CD127- T regulatory cells. Clinical Immunology (Orlando, Fla.). 2009;133:22–26.
208. Di Ianni M, Falzetti F, Carotti A, et al. Tregs prevent GVHD and promote immune reconstitution in HLA-haploidentical transplantation. Blood. 2011; 117:3921–3928.
209. Brunstein CG, Miller JS, Cao Q, et al. Infusion of ex vivo expanded T regulatory cells in adults transplanted with umbilical cord blood: safety profile and detection kinetics. Blood. 2011;117:1061–1070.
210. Vongwiwatana A, Tasanarong A, Hidalgo LG, et al. The role of B cells and alloantibody in the host response to human organ allografts. Immunological Reviews. 2003;196:197–218.
211. Colvin RB, Smith RN. Antibody-mediated organ-allograft rejection. Nature Reviews Immunology. 2005;5:807–817.
212. Moll S, Pascual M. Humoral rejection of organ allografts. American Journal of Transplantation. 2005;5:2611–2618.
213. Feucht HE. Significance of donor-specific antibodies in acute rejection. Transplantation Proceedings. 2005;37:3693–3694.
214. Feucht HE, Mihatsch MJ. Diagnostic value of C4d in renal biopsies. Current Opinion in Nephrology and Hypertension. 2005;14:592–598.
215. Goodnow CC, Sprent J, Fazekas de St Groth B, et al. Cellular and genetic mechanisms of self tolerance and autoimmunity. Nature. 2005;435:590–597.
216. Shlomchik MJ. Sites and stages of autoreactive B cell activation and regulation. Immunity. 2008;28:18–28.
217. Pelanda R, Schwers S, Sonoda E, et al. Receptor editing in a transgenic mouse model: site, efficiency, and role in B cell tolerance and antibody diversification. Immunity. 1997;7:765–775.
218. Wardemann H, Yurasov S, Schaefer A, et al. Predominant autoantibody produc-

tion by early human B cell precursors. Science. 2003;301:1374–1377.
219. Nemazee D. Receptor editing in lymphocyte development and central tolerance. Nature Reviews Immunology. 2006;6:728–740.
220. Goodnow CC, Crosbie J, Adelstein S, et al. Altered immunoglobulin expression and functional silencing of self-reactive B lymphocytes in transgenic mice. Nature. 1988;334:676–682.
221. Nemazee DA, Burki K. Clonal deletion of B lymphocytes in a transgenic mouse bearing anti-MHC class I antibody genes. Nature. 1989;337:562–566.
222. Hartley SB, Cooke MP, Fulcher DA, et al. Elimination of self-reactive B lymphocytes proceeds in two stages: arrested development and cell death. Cell. 1993;72:325–335.
223. Lang J, Arnold B, Hammerling G, et al. Enforced Bcl-2 expression inhibits antigen-mediated clonal elimination of peripheral B cells in an antigen dose-dependent manner and promotes receptor editing in autoreactive, immature B cells. Journal of Experimental Medicine. 1997;186:1513–1522.
224. Strasser A, Bouillet P. The control of apoptosis in lymphocyte selection. Immunological Reviews. 2003;193:82–92.
225. Gay D, Saunders T, Camper S, et al. Receptor editing: an approach by autoreactive B cells to escape tolerance. Journal of Experimental Medicine. 1993;177:999–1008.
226. Tiegs SL, Russell DM, Nemazee D. Receptor editing in self-reactive bone marrow B cells. Journal of Experimental Medicine. 1993;177:1009–1020.
227. Casellas R, Shih TA, Kleinewietfeld M, et al. Contribution of receptor editing to the antibody repertoire. Science. 2001;291:1541–1544.
228. Cooke MP, Heath AW, Shokat KM, et al. Immunoglobulin signal transduction guides the specificity of B cell-T cell interactions and is blocked in tolerant self-reactive B cells. Journal of Experimental Medicine. 1994;179:425–438.
229. Lesley R, Xu Y, Kalled SL, et al. Reduced competitiveness of autoantigen-engaged B cells due to increased dependence on BAFF. Immunity. 2004;20:441–453.
230. Aplin BD, Keech CL, de Kauwe AL, et al. Tolerance through indifference: autoreactive B cells to the nuclear antigen La show no evidence of tolerance in a transgenic model. Journal of Immunology. 2003;171:5890–5900.
231. Cyster JG, Hartley SB, Goodnow CC. Competition for follicular niches excludes self-reactive cells from the recirculating B-cell repertoire. Nature. 1994;371:389–395.
232. Vieira CA, Agarwal A, Book BK, et al. Rituximab for reduction of anti-HLA antibodies in patients awaiting renal transplantation: 1. Safety, pharmacodynamics, and pharmacokinetics. Transplantation. 2004;77:542–548.
233. Venetz JP, Pascual M. New treatments for acute humoral rejection of kidney allografts. Expert Opinion on Investigational Drugs. 2007;16:625–633.
234. Sberro-Soussan R, Zuber J, Suberbielle-Boissel C, et al. Bortezomib as the sole post-renal transplantation desensitization agent does not decrease donor-specific anti-HLA antibodies. American Journal of Transplantation. 2010;10:681–686.
235. Baldwin WM 3rd, Valujskikh A, Fairchild RL. Antibody-mediated rejection: emergence of animal models to answer clinical questions. American Journal of Transplantation. 2010;10:1135–1142.
236. Owen RD. Immunogenetic consequences of vascular anastomoses between bovine twins. Science. 1945;102:400–401.
237. Rieben R, Tucci A, Nydegger UE, et al. Self tolerance to human A and B histo-blood group antigens exists at the B cell level and cannot be broken by potent polyclonal B cell activation in vitro. European Journal of Immunology. 1992;22:2713–2717.
238. Fong SW, Qaqundah BY, Taylor WF. Developmental patterns of ABO isoagglutinins in normal children correlated with the effects of age, sex, and maternal isoagglutinins. Transfusion. 1974;14:551–559.
239. West LJ, Pollock-Barziv SM, Dipchand AI, et al. ABO-incompatible heart transplantation in infants. New England Journal of Medicine. 2001;344:793–800.
240. West LJ. Targeting antibody-mediated rejection in the setting of ABO-incompatible infant heart transplantation: graft accommodation vs. B cell tolerance. Current Drug Targets Cardiovascular and Haematological Disorders. 2005;5:223–232.
241. Fan X, Ang A, Pollock-Barziv SM, et al. Donor-specific B-cell tolerance after ABO-incompatible infant heart transplantation. Nature Medicine. 2004;10:1227–1233.
242. Gugenheim J, Samuel D, Reynes M, et al. Liver transplantation across ABO blood group barriers. Lancet. 1990;336:519–523.
243. Stegall MD, Dean PG, Gloor JM. ABO-incompatible kidney transplantation. Transplantation. 2004;78:635–640.
244. Shishido S, Asanuma H, Tajima E, et al. ABO-incompatible living-donor kidney transplantation in children. Transplantation. 2001;72:1037–1042.
245. Egawa H, Oike F, Buhler L, et al. Impact of recipient age on outcome of ABO-incompatible living-donor liver transplantation. Transplantation. 2004;77:403–411.
246. Sykes M. Immune tolerance: mechanisms and application in clinical transplantation. Journal of Internal Medicine. 2007;262:288–310.
247. Ciancio G, Burke GW, Gaynor JJ, et al. The use of Campath-1H as induction therapy in renal transplantation: preliminary results. Transplantation. 2004;78:426–433.
248. Ciancio G, Burke GW 3rd. Alemtuzumab (Campath-1H) in kidney transplantation. American Journal of Transplantation. 2008;8:15–20.
249. Pascual J, Pirsch JD, Odorico JS, et al. Alemtuzumab induction and antibody-mediated kidney rejection after simultaneous pancreas-kidney transplantation. Transplantation. 2009;87:125–132.
250. Crowley JE, Scholz JL, Quinn WJ 3rd, et al. Homeostatic control of B lymphocyte subsets. Immunologic Research. 2008;42:75–83.
251. Treml JF, Hao Y, Stadanlick JE, et al. The BLyS family: toward a molecular understanding of B cell homeostasis. Cell Biochemistry and Biophysics. 2009;53:1–16.
252. Mackay F, Schneider P. Cracking the BAFF code. Nature Reviews Immunology. 2009;9:491–502.

第 12 章
异种免疫

Peter J. Cowan, Anthony J.F. d'Apice

引言

异种移植指跨物种的器官移植。虽然技术上包括所有供体和受体物种的组合，但异种移植的领域几乎已经完全趋向于以猪-人组合作为与临床最相关的组合。人体器官、组织和细胞的短缺限制了当前异体移植术的发展，而临床上以猪作为异种移植的供体有很大的可能解决这个问题。临床上异种移植的主要障碍是对移植物的免疫排斥反应。除非这个主要障碍可以被克服，其他的一些重要问题如生理相容性[1]和感染风险[2]等才能变得无关紧要。

本书的大多数内容都是关于同种异体移植的，当我们脑海中联想到移植免疫时很自然地会关注那些在同种异体移植中至关重要的机制，尤其是细胞和体液的适应性(或获得性)免疫(已在第 5 章、第 6 章分别讨论)。当一个移植物移植到一个非致敏受体当中，免疫应答的第一个明显的迹象是初次排斥反应的出现，一般在一星期后出现，其主要的机制为 T 细胞介导的迟发超敏反应。然而异种移植的表现与上述表现完全不同，我们会注意到初次排斥反应在几分钟之内就会发生。这主要是预先形成的抗体结合及增强的固有免疫应答所导致的。固有免疫系统的元素是同种异体移植及异种移植的共同参与者(参见第 7 章)，但主要参与的是异种移植。由于移植程序相关的组织损伤，同种异体移植物会激活部分固有免疫系统，而异种移植物本身就是一种异源分子的来源，能强有力而快速地激活固有免疫系统。然而，这只是一个复杂故事的开始，异种免疫与同种免疫之间不仅仅只有至关重要的差异之处，也存在许多重要的相似之处。因此，大家将会发现生理免疫学章节（第 2 章）及基本同种异体免疫章节(第 5~7 章)为本章的内容做了补充，尤其是关于异种移植排斥反应的后期形成方面。

对异种免疫机制的探索依赖于一些小型和大型动物模型，每种动物模型各自具有其促成因素，且与临床上猪-人异种移植的相关性也大有不同。由于这些模型的详尽讨论超出了本章的范围，这里的大部分重点将放在猪-非人类灵长类动物(NHP)临床前研究模型上。第 15 章主要概述猪和灵长类大动物模型，本章的讨论对第 15 章内容进行了补充。

猪血管异种移植的排斥反应

阻止实体器官异种移植物的排斥反应就像剥洋葱一样——只有去除上一层，下一层才会暴露。猪心脏和肾脏异种移植物的研究对于理解排斥过程至关重要，因为它们是唯一可以在 NHP 受体中存活超过 1 周的器官。本节主要从心脏和肾脏的猪-NHP 文献中去描述免疫排斥的阶段及机制，以及促进异种移植物长期存活所需采取的措施。

超急性异种移植排斥反应

抗-αGal 抗体和补体：超急性排斥反应的关键介质

超急性排斥反应(HAR)是一个强有力的过程，在这个过程中，猪的移植物在移植到未经治疗的接受者身上后的终末损伤可维持数分钟至数小时（图 12.1)。如同血型 ABO 不相容的同种异体移植物的 HAR 一样，异种移植物的 HAR 是由于供体和受体之间的糖基化差异导致的。大多数物种，包括猪，都会表达一种称为 α1,3-半乳糖基转移酶(也叫 GalT)的糖基转移酶，其合成了糖蛋白和糖脂的末端碳水化合物结构半乳糖-α1,3-半乳糖-β1,4-N-乙酰葡糖胺（Galα1,3-Galβ1,4-

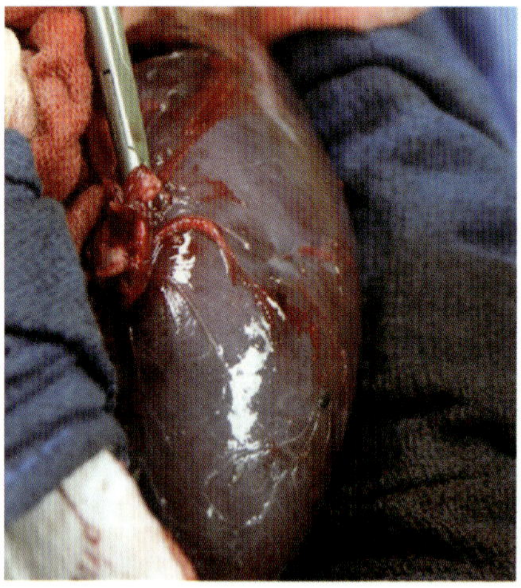

(A)

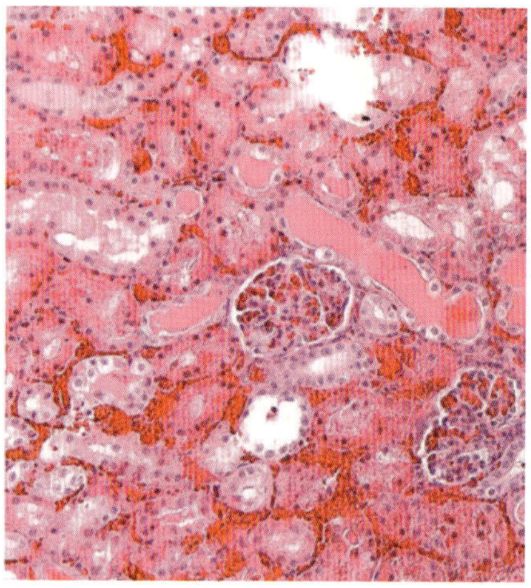

(B)

图 12.1 超急性排斥反应。猪-狒狒肾脏异种移植，移植数分钟后的超级性排斥反应的大体(A)及组织学(B)外观。注意观察血管充血，表明移植物血栓形成，大量出血证据在组织学上表明血管完整性遭到破坏。

GlcNAc)。该部分被称为αGal表位，其与血型B组抗原不同之处仅仅在于其倒数第二个半乳糖上没有结合岩藻糖残基。大多数猪细胞表面都存在大量的αGal，特别是在血管内皮细胞上，其上的αGal估计密度为每个细胞超过1000万个表位[3]。相比之下，由于GalT基因的编码区域的移码和无义突变，人类及其亲缘最近的猿猴和旧大陆猴不表达αGal[4]。持续暴露于肠道细菌上的αGal诱导了这些物种体内抗αGal的IgM和IgG抗体的发展[5]。在人类中，抗αGal由高达1%的B细胞所产生[6]，包括80%预先形成的（“天然”）抗猪IgM[7]，是最丰富的天然形成的IgG[8]。可以推论，所有人类都能对猪血管表面上密集表达的抗原产生高水平的预先形成的细胞毒性抗体，这对猪器官异种移植物来说是毁灭性的打击。

抗αGal IgM抗体结合到异种移植物的血管内皮上激发了补体激活的经典途径，后者继而激活凝血级联反应(图12.2A)。上述过程导致的发病机制在宏观上和微观水平都是惊人的。移植物在再灌注之后不久就会变得斑驳和乌黑，有功能的迹象（如果有的话）迅速消失。HAR的心脏异体移植物的详细组织病理学分析发现，静脉和小静脉血栓是起始事件，随后发生充血、水肿和大量间质性出血的进展[9]。这些特征是HAR的标志。HAR早期阶段的免疫组化分析可见大量沉积的IgM、激活的补体成分、血小板聚集以及P型选择素的表达，但几乎没有内皮细胞裂解或凋亡的证据[10]。总体情况与内皮细胞的Ⅰ型激活一致，后者为蛋白合成非依赖性过程，涉及细胞连接的开放、来自Weibel-Palade小体的血小板配体P选择素的胞吐作用及细胞表面抗凝物质的丢失[11]。异种移植物内皮细胞的Ⅰ型激活的介质为补体的抗体结合与水解活化[12,13]。在超急性免疫反应的后期阶段，可以观察到许多凋亡的内皮细胞[10]，潜在地通过暴露磷脂酰丝氨酸[14]和释放组织因子容受微粒来促进血栓形成[15]。

同源限制和膜补体调节剂：质量与数量？

可以推测，物种之间的不相容性有助于高效地调节HAR中补体的激活。一般来说，补体能有效地溶解来自不同物种的“非自体”细胞而不是“自我”细胞[16]。解释这种被称为同源限制现象的早期假说为：一个物种的膜结合补体调节蛋白(CRP)不能抑制另一个物种的补体[17,18]。与人类一样，猪表达CD46（膜辅助因子蛋白）、CD55（衰变加速因子或DAF）和CD59；也许这些猪CRP不能移植灵长类动物补体的激活可能从一定程度上解释了HAR破坏的快速性。然而，最近的研究表明，同源限制是一个不完整而非普遍的现象。并且猪的三种CRP在调节人类补体与它们的同源类似物上有着类似的功效[19,20]。在自体免疫调节系统存在的情况下，ABO不相容的人类同种异体移植物也可以发生HAR[21]。人类(h)CRP阻止转基因猪异种移植物的HAR的能力可能是由于调节补体能力的总体提高，而不是内源性分子不相容性得到了校正。

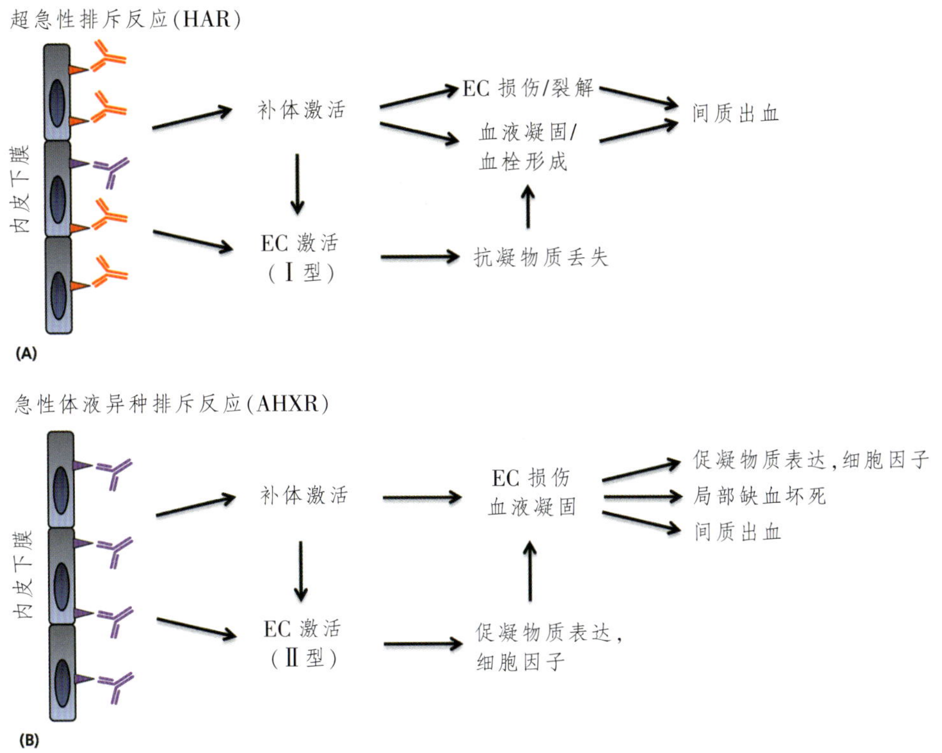

图 12.2 器官异种移植排斥的分期。(A)超急性排斥反应由预先形成的抗-αGal 抗体(红色)与异种移植物内皮细胞(EC)相连接，激活一连串的事件，以血管损伤和大量的间质出血为终点。(B)急性体液异种移植无排斥反应，在此以 GTKO 异种移植物为例，是一个延伸的过程，在此过程中引发的非-Gal 抗体(紫色)的结合驱动内皮环境从抗凝状态转化为促凝状态。

预防 HAR

传统的免疫抑制不是为了处理高水平的预先形成的抗体而设计的，所以对抵抗 HAR 没有效果[22]。一些研究表明，为预防 HAR，受体的治疗需要以其基础组分中的一种或两种为靶点，即补体和抗-αGal 抗体。例如，用眼镜蛇毒因子去除补体的系统治疗可以将心脏异种移植物的排斥反应从不足 1 小时延长至 6 天[23]。类似地，通过免疫吸附清除抗-αGal 抗体可以将肾异种移植物的排斥延迟至平均 7 天，尽管循环中抗-αGal 抗体再次出现时所有的移植物仍会被最终受到排斥[24]。虽然这些方法为 HAR 机制的研究提供了有价值的信息，但从长期来看，它们的实际效益有限，因为它们通常只是起到短暂的保护作用，并且可能损害受者对感染的抵抗力。

在理论上比系统治疗更优的技术是异种移植所独有的技术——供体遗传修饰。在 1994 年，两个研究组率先采用了这种方式，生成了表达 hDAF[25]或 hCD59[26]的转基因猪，随之出现了表达 hCD46[27,28]或 hCRP[29-32]组合的猪。除了罕见的例外情况[33]，不管是否采用其他治疗方法，来自于 hCRP 转基因猪的器官均未引起 HAR[27,28,30,31]。使用特定 hCRP:DAF 和 CD46 是有理论依据的，因为它们可以调节 CD59 的上游补体，CD46 比 DAF 能更有效地调节替代途径[28]，CD59 在膜攻击复合物中有重要作用，凝血酶能通过直接激活 C5 而不受 DAF 和 CD46 的调节[34]。然而，目前尚不清楚哪种 hCRP 或其组合能提供免受 HAR 的最佳补体调节方式。

供体猪遗传工程的第二个重大突破是 GalT 基因的敲除[35-40]。所得到的 GalT 敲除(GTKO)猪缺乏 αGal 表达，但表现得完全正常或可按预期那样产生抗 αGal 抗体[41]。在猪-NHP 模型中，GTKO 肾脏和心脏异种移植物能免于遭受 HAR[42-47]，这暗示了 αGal 在排斥过程中起到了核心作用。

预先形成的非 αGal 决定簇的抗体

尽管抗-αGal 是人类和更高级灵长类动物中主要的天然抗体，但通过培养来自非敏化个体的血清与内皮细胞或来自野生型和 GTKO 猪的单核细胞的外周血，已检测到了具有其他特异性的预先形成的抗体存在[48-51]。已经有人提出,许多这些天然的“非 Gal”抗体只识别在猪中表达的碳水化合物而不识别人类表达的碳水化合物[52],例如 Hanganutziu-Deicher 抗原[53]。预先形成的非 Gal IgG 和 IgM 抗体的滴度差异很大,能够诱导补体依赖性裂解和针对猪细胞的抗体依赖性细胞毒性(ADCC)[50]。然而,GTKO 异种移植物在猪-NHP 模型中的一致生存期超过 24 小时表明,它们在 HAR 中很少发挥作用。

急性体液性异种移植排斥反应

当移植物免受 HAR 后,常规的免疫抑制通常会使猪-NHP 心脏和肾脏异种移植的存活时间延长数天至数周。在这段时间内,大多数异种移植物将被第二种抗体依赖性的途径所排斥,该途径被称为急性体液性异种移植排斥反应(AHXR)(图 12.2B),也被称为急性血管排斥反应(AVR)或迟发性异种移植排斥(DXR)[54-57]。这个排斥阶段可替换的术语反映了对其潜在机制在一定程度上的不确定性,但即使是低水平的抗移植物抗体,其作用似乎也已经很好地确立。AHXR 的免疫病理学和组织病理学征象包括抗体和补体沉积、微血管血栓形成、局灶性缺血性坏死和间质性出血以及从肿胀到严重损伤和凋亡的内皮细胞变化[47,56,58]。还可以观察到血管外周淋巴细胞和巨噬细胞浸润,但通常只有当免疫抑制相对无效时才可见。AHXR 的发生和严重程度因供体的遗传背景[例如 hCRP 转基因和(或)GTKO]、免疫抑制方案甚至器官的类型不同而有所不同。

正如异种移植物内皮细胞的Ⅰ型激活是 HAR 的一部分,Ⅱ型激活是 AHXR 病理生理学的关键因素[59]。Ⅱ型激活是蛋白合成依赖过程,由一系列因素引发,尤其是促炎因子如 TNF-α 和 IL-1[11]。激活机制设计转录因子 NF-kB 和 AP-1 的激活以及随后的促炎蛋白包括趋化分子和黏附分子的表达,结果是细胞因子和白细胞介导的内皮细胞损伤,进而有利于血栓形成[11]。即使不存在补体激活,猪内皮细胞的Ⅱ型激活也可通过结合异种抗体启动[60]。

T 细胞依赖的异种反应

如第 5 章所述,供体抗原可以通过两种途径呈递给受体 T 细胞:直接途径,T 细胞受体(TCR)与供体抗原呈递细胞(APC)上错配的 MHC-肽复合物结合;间接途径,受体 APC 摄取并加工供体分子并将自身 MHC 内的抗原性片段呈现于 TCR 中。同种异体移植 T 细胞反应源于直接呈递和间接呈递的混合,直接途径在急性同种异体排斥中占优势[61]。[第三个途径(半直接表达)对同种异体排斥反应的意义尚不清楚[62]。]相比之下,急性异种移植物排斥反应的平衡似乎更偏向于间接呈递[63,64]。由于损伤,异种移植物会释放大量的猪蛋白质和碳水化合物,为可以通过间接途径呈递的异种抗原表位物质来源。这并不是说直接呈递没有发挥作用——人类 TCR 可以识别猪白细胞抗原(SLA,MHC 的猪当量)[65],体外数据表明猪淋巴细胞可以直接激活人类 T 细胞[66]。T 细胞激活所需的总体刺激非常强大,其中 T 细胞对 B 细胞的帮助对 AHXR 的发展具有重要意义。

导致 AHXR 的抗体与抗原特性

引发抗 αGal 抗体是 αGal 阳性的异种移植物产生 AHXR 反应的主要原因[67]。当 αGal 抗体被中和时,AHXR 可以由非 GAL 抗体或预先形成的高滴度 IgG 或引发的 IgG 和 IgM 所诱导[68,69]。非 Gal 抗体也可导致 GTKO 器官的 AHXR 反应[70]。相关的非 Gal 异种抗原目前还没有明确的定义。候选的碳水化合物异种抗原包括 N-羟乙酰神经氨酸(NeuGc)、N-乙酰神经氨酸(NeuAc)和 T 和 Tn 抗原[71]。另一方面,蛋白质异种抗原的数目可能会达数百甚至数千。几乎所有的猪蛋白质都显示出其与人类同源物不同的氨基酸序列,因此具有潜在的免疫源性。已经在 NHP 和猪异种移植物的受体中检测到了被诱导的非 Gal 抗体应答。一项 NHP 研究表明,被诱导的 GTKO 细胞的非 Gal 抗体是由有限数量的种系祖细胞所编码的,并可能与在结构上和 αGal 相关的碳水化合物表位相结合[48]。在人类受体中,只要异种移植物保留在受体中,针对大量未被识别的猪蛋白质的非 Gal 抗体就会连续产生,并且很明显来自多个 B 细胞克隆[72]。

非 Gal 抗体可能对内皮细胞功能的影响

除了激活内皮细胞和介导 ADCC 外,引发的非 Gal 抗体可能通过干扰关键的血管保护机制来促进 AHXR。一个研究团队通过使用富集了非 Gal IgG 的致敏狒狒血清来筛选猪内皮细胞表达库[73]。非 Gal 的四种靶标经鉴定为参与调节补体(CD46 和 CD59)以及血栓形成/炎症反应(内皮蛋白 C 受体及 CD9)的内皮细胞膜蛋白。尽管没有评估血清抑制这些蛋白质功能的能力,但似乎可以想象,甚至非 Gal 抗体反应可能通过阻断异种内皮细胞的天然防御系统来促进 AHXR。这加强了猪表达相应的人类蛋白质的论据，正如已经表达的 CD46 和 CD59 所做的那样。

预防 AHXR

AGal 的缺失显著延长了心脏和肾脏异种移植物的存活时间[74],但是 GTKO 器官的 AHXR 反应已被证实是极难预防的。能够保护肾脏同种异体移植物的常规免疫抑制不能保护 GTKO 异种移植物,而后者则死于诱导的非 Gal 抗体反应[44]。这一结果突出表明,旨在抑制急性 T 细胞同种异体反应的药物主要涉及直接呈递过程,而对大多数间接的异种排斥反应无效。使用基于阻断剂的方案，特别是使用抗 CD154 已经取得了巨大的成功,GTKO±hCD46 的心脏存活期可长达 8 个月[43,75],而 GTKO 复合肾-胸腺移植物的存活期可达 3 个月[42]。然而，异种移植物在排斥或受体死亡时的免疫组化分析表明,非 Gal 抗体未被这些方案完全否定。可以理解的是,异种移植物背景下独特的分子不相容性(将在以下两个小节中讨论）促进相对低水平的异种反应性抗体不成比例的反应。

固有免疫细胞的作用

正如第 7 章所述，固有免疫的重要组成部分是固有免疫细胞对病原体相关分子模式及损伤相关分子模式(PAMP 和 DAMP)的识别及反应能力,该过程主要通过 Toll 样受体实现[76,77]。无论供体是相同还是不同的物种,移植过程都会产生 DAMP。异种移植与同种移植不同,人类固有免疫细胞可直接把猪细胞识别为外来细胞,这主要是因为细胞表面的糖基化不同所造成的[78,79]。还有证据表明，分子不相容性会影响特定的细胞间相互作用,这将在下面进一步讨论。

NK 细胞

自然杀伤细胞(NK 细胞)通过多种机制损伤和裂解靶细胞。虽然这些细胞在实体器官同种异体移植中的作用尚未得到充分的定义，但数据表明它们在移植过程中被激活，并通过产生炎症细胞因子如干扰素 γ (INF-γ)促进急性排斥反应[80-82]。NK 细胞表达一组激活和抑制性受体，其细胞溶解活性由靶细胞上这些受体和配体之间相互作用的平衡所决定。在人类同种异体移植物中，关键的 NK 受体包括抑制性杀伤细胞免疫球蛋白样受体(KIP)家族及 NKG2A,后者是与自身结合而非同种异体 MHC Ⅰ类分子，激活的 NKG2D 受体可以识别许多在同种异体移植物中上调的“应激”配体[83-85]。

几项体外研究表明，人类 NK 细胞对异种移植物的反应比同种异体移植物的反应更为显著。尽管通过清除 αGal 使得 FcγRIII 介导的 ADCC 显著削弱[86],但由于引发的非 Gal IgG 抗体存在[87],使其仍然是个问题。人 NK 细胞也能直接对猪内皮细胞产生直接的穿孔素/颗粒酶 B 介导的细胞毒性[88]。此外,有证据表明,猪细胞引起了人类 NK 细胞激烈的细胞毒性反应[89]。基因序列分析表明 SLA Ⅰ类分子不会向人类 KIR 和 NKG2A 传递抑制信号[90]。相比之下,几个激活途径是完全可操作的(图 12.3)。人类 NKG2D 有效地结合在猪内皮细胞表达的 ULBP1 上,引发 NK 细胞的细胞毒性[91],并且还可以结合到另外的尚未确定的猪配体上[92]。NKp44 也可从未知的猪配体上传导激活信号[93]。结合到 N-乙酰乳糖胺(NAcLac)和 αGal 的人类 C 型凝集素 NKRP1A 的参与方式尚不清楚[94]。作为 α1,3-半乳糖基转移酶的底物,NAcLac 可能在 GTKO 动物中的水平会增加，但这仅在小鼠[94,95]而不是在猪[96]身上得到了证明。然而,不管 NKRP1A 发挥什么样的作用,异种移植中抑制和激活 NK 信号之间的平衡似乎倾向于激活。

减轻人类 NK 细胞异种排斥反应活性的逻辑遗传策略是通过在猪组织上表达抑制性配体和(或)删除活化配体来改变这种平衡，但由于仍存在许多未知的配体，其数量和多样性使得删除活化配体这个策略更具挑战性，因此在该领域的大多数工作都集中在抑制信号表达方面。这种方法的最先进的例子是继理论研究在体外证明之后[98,99],表达非经典人类 MHC Ⅰ类分子的 HLA-E 转基因猪的产生[97]。由于 HLA-E 可以结合抑制性 NK 受体 NKG2A,并且是同种异体 T 细胞应答的较差的诱导剂,因此得到应用。来自转基因猪的内皮细胞在体外以 NKG2A 依赖的方式被部分保护从而免受人 NK 细胞介导的细胞毒性[97]。确定体内有效性需要将 HLA-E 转化到一个合适的遗传背景中,在这种遗传背景中其他更深层的非免疫机制(如 GTKO±hCRP 转基因)已经被解决。GTKO 供体的使用本身可以减少 NK 细胞的反应,因为一些研究已经证明人 NK 细胞直接识别猪内皮细胞上的αGal,尽管这一说法仍有争议[87]。

巨噬细胞

巨噬细胞浸润是急性抗体介导的肾同种异体移植物排斥反应的常见特征[100],尽管仍缺乏其在排斥过程中直接作用的证据[82]。巨噬细胞表达Fc受体及补体受体，因此可能参与异种移植排斥反应的抗体和补体的依赖机制。已经显示人单核细胞通过半乳凝素-3受体直接识别猪内皮细胞上的αGal[72]。此外,与NK细胞的情况类似，跨物种的分子不相容性可能降低猪细胞激活人巨噬细胞的阈值(图12.3)。SIRPα是高度多态性的巨噬细胞抑制性受体，其识别CD47作为其他细胞上“自身”的标记[101]。在没有功能性SIRPα/ CD47相互作用的情况下,巨噬细胞能够吞噬造血细胞[102]。虽然人类SIRPα被证明可以在体外结合猪CD47[103],但随后的研究表明,这种相互作用不会产生抑制信号,因此不会阻止人类巨噬细胞吞噬猪细胞[104]。与此一致,在体外研究中，人类CD47在猪细胞上的表达抑制了猪细胞被人巨噬细胞吞噬[104],并保护它们免于受到小鼠肿瘤模型的排斥反应[105]。这些结果表明,人类CD47在猪体内的转基因表达可能是防止巨噬细胞介导的异种移植物破坏的有效策略。这种方法可能对于细胞异种移植物如造血干细胞(用于耐受诱导)和胰岛最为有益。

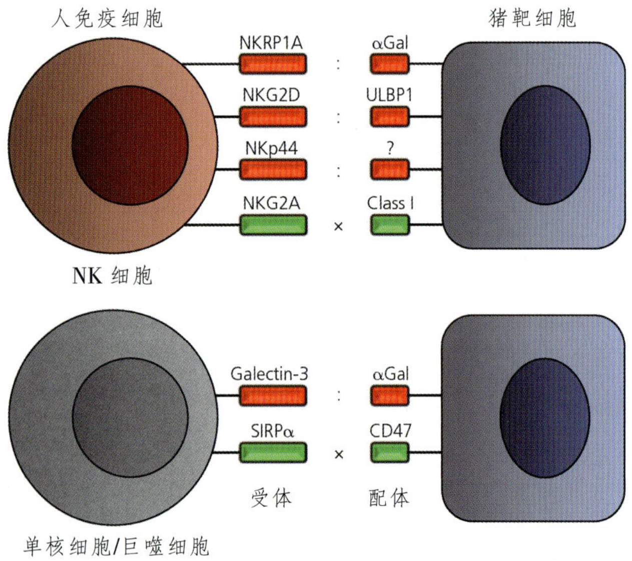

图12.3 人类固有免疫细胞对猪靶细胞的反应性升高。激活受体/配体对(红色)之间的相互作用被保留,而关键的抑制相互作用(绿色)似乎由于分子不相容性而不起作用。

嗜中性粒细胞

嗜中性粒细胞在同种异体移植排斥反应中的作用在很大程度上仍是未知的[82],但是它们在抗体和补体介导的机制下被募集和活化的事实说明了其至少作为次要角色参与了异种移植排斥反应。此外,体外研究表明，人类嗜中性粒细胞在没有抗体和补体的情况下直接识别、黏附并激活猪内皮细胞[106,107]。如果这种相互作用被证明在体内是重要的,那么将难以预防。几乎没有治疗手段可以在不使受体易受机会性感染的情况下控制嗜中性粒细胞的数量和(或)活性。供体进行基因修饰使之能表达人CD47是有益处的,因为已知嗜中性粒细胞与巨噬细胞一样可以表达SIRPα,尽管不相容的人类SIRPα/猪CD47相互作用似乎对于巨噬细胞的激活具有更大的意义。人类嗜中性粒细胞对猪分子的直接识别与删除并不是通过αGal[107],而是通过另一种途径。

凝血功能失调

移植物内皮细胞被一系列机制激活，包括缺血再灌注损伤(IRI)、抗体结合及补体激活[108]。在极端情况下，内皮细胞活化的促凝血效应会导致同种异体移植物损坏。肾脏同种异体移植的并发症之一血栓性微血管病变(TMA)就是一个例子。肾组织中的TMA由免疫抑制药物或急性抗体介导的排斥反应触发，其特征是血管壁增厚和微血管血栓形成[109]。它通常与调节补体激活替代途径的能力降低有关。具有突变的循环替代途径调节因子H和因子I的肾同种异体移植受体触发TMA的风险似乎更高[110]。这不仅反映了补体和凝血途径之间的相互作用，而且还指出了器官异种移植物可能面临的一些独特问题。在异种移植中激活补体的途径比同种异体移植更多且多变，并且已经显示诱导的抗体以猪内皮细胞上表达的补体调节物为靶点[73]。

实际上，尽管在同种异体移植中严重的凝血很罕见,但是在异种移植中相对常见并且较难处理。凝血功能失调是当前器官异种移植的主要挑战之一[74,111-113]。在猪-NHP异种移植物中，被排斥的心脏和肾脏中经常可观察到TMA[114,115]。即使体液反应看上去已经被有效抑制,但TMA仍然会发展并且成为异种移植失败的主要原因[43,45,116]。异种移植物中的TMA通常伴随着消耗性凝血病的发展,表现为血小板减少(通常为重度)、纤维蛋白原浓度下降、D-二聚体和凝血酶-抗凝血酶复合物水平升高及凝血时间延长。凝血障碍在肾脏异种移植受体中很常见[30,117–120]，且只能通过移除移植物治疗[118]。心脏异种移植物的接受者似乎不太容易出现这种情况[121,122]，尽管没有例外[116]。也有人提出，这些不同的结果可能是由于肾脏和心脏异种移植物的内皮中基因反应的差异性造成的，前者的血管性血友病因子(vWF)和P–选择蛋白(有利于血小板沉积)上调，而后者纤溶酶原活化剂抑制剂–1(有利于纤维蛋白沉积)上调[123]。

凝血功能失调也在肺和肝脏异种移植中起主要作用。肺异种移植物的长期功能尚未在猪–NHP 模型中实现。异种抗体、补体激活、肺巨噬细胞、肺内皮脱落的 vWF 和对凝血的控制不良被认为在排斥过程中发挥作用[124,125]。据报道，使用 vWF 缺陷的耗竭巨噬细胞的供体最长存活时间为 4.5 天[126]，但大多数情况下，生存时间以小时为单位[127–129]。即使 GTKO / hDAF 转基因供体的组合以及肺巨噬细胞的消耗也不能使移植物存活期延长超过 2 天[130]。肺异种移植排斥的主要组织学特征是微血管和大血管性血栓形成，嗜中性粒细胞浸润和水肿[126,129]。消耗性凝血病的发展比肾异种移植更加快速和一致，尽管猪肺异种移植物特别容易凝血的原因仍不清楚。

以重度血小板减少症形式出现的凝血病是猪–NHP 肝异种移植的主要问题。由于移植了 GTKO / hCD46 肝脏的狒狒均死亡或不得不在 7 天内进行安乐死，这不是因为排斥反应而是由于移植 1 小时内血小板计数急剧下降导致的出血问题[131]。尸检时，移植物在宏观和微观水平上仅显示斑块性损伤[131,132]，而肝功能相对正常[133]。肝脏中血小板沉积的程度不足以说明血小板减少症的严重程度，而是假定由于血小板活化迅速，随后在循环中形成血小板–白细胞聚集体[134]。在离体灌注研究的基础上提出的一种替代机制是猪肝窦内皮细胞和 Kupffer 细胞以抗体和补体非依赖的方式快速有效地吞噬人血小板[135–137]。

受体血小板和单核细胞表达组织因子

体外和体内研究表明，即使在不存在补体的情况下，抗 αGal 和(或)非 Gal 抗体活化的猪内皮细胞上的组织因子表达也会上调(图 12.4)，有助于血管内凝血和消耗性凝血病的发展[138]。最近，已经有人提出，诱导受体血小板和单核细胞上的组织因子的表达也可能起重要作用。在不存在抗体和补体的情况下，人血小板和

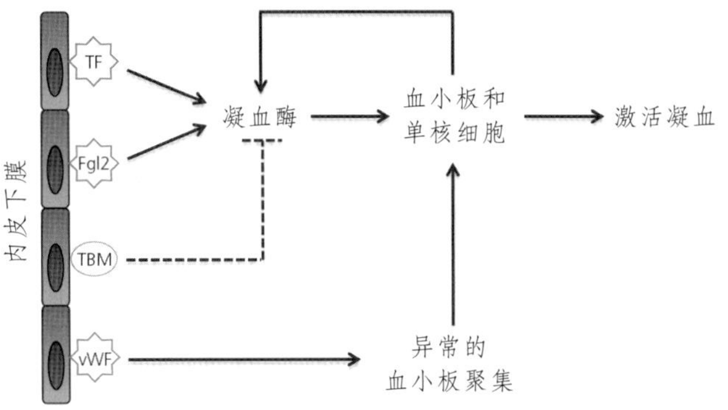

图 12.4 实体器官凝血功能失调的潜在机制。由激活的异种移植物内皮细胞诱导的组织因子(TF)和直接凝血酶原酶 fgl2 的表达驱动了凝血酶的产生，其由猪血栓调节蛋白(TBM)控制不良。此外，人血小板在没有剪切力的情况下对猪血管性血友病因子 vWF 产生应答而聚集，并且通过与猪内皮接触而被激活。

单核细胞仅通过与猪内皮细胞接触来上调组织因子的表达和活性[139]。被排斥的 GTKO 猪–狒狒心脏异种移植物在血栓形成的血管和间质中的受体巨噬细胞上显示了组织因子的表达[116]。对 GTKO/hCD46 猪肾异种移植物的狒狒受体的循环细胞进行时间过程分析，揭示了几个相当明显的阶段：移植后一天内血小板上的组织因子上调，随后出现越来越多的血小板–白细胞聚集体，最后单核细胞表达组织因子，同时伴有血小板减少症和凝血病的其他特征[120]。在尸检时，受体的原始心脏和肝脏中也检测到了组织因子的表达。这些事件在明显缺乏体液应答的情况下发生，导致研究者提出以下假设：①移植后不久，在炎症反应及与异种移植物内皮细胞接触刺激下，血小板被激活且表达组织因子；②单核细胞被凝血酶和(或)黏附到活化血小板上所激活，继而表达组织因子；③受体组织因子的全身暴露导致了消耗性凝血病[120]。然而，其他实验组并没有在 GTKO 肾脏异种移植物受体中发现非常早期且严重的凝血疾病[140]，说明了它可能是模型依赖性的现象而非普遍存在的。

依赖组织分子的凝血：直接促凝血酶原酶活性

猪内皮细胞表达一种称为 fgl2 的酶，其直接将人凝血酶原转化为凝血酶[141](图 12.4)。fgl2 在猪内皮细胞中的表达和活性是通过包括人 TNF–α 在内的促炎细胞因子诱导的[141,142]。被排斥的猪–狒狒肾异种移植物的 fgl2 表达上调，这与小血管和肾小球毛细血管中的纤维蛋白沉积相关[141]。有趣的是，在被排斥的人肾和小

鼠心脏的同种异体移植物中也观察到 fgl2 和纤维蛋白的共定位[143,144]。这表明,在实体器官移植物的急性排斥反应中,fgl2 是一种常见的参与组织因子非依赖性凝血过程的炎症介导机制,尽管应该指出,这一观点并不是普遍存在的[144]。

在凝血与炎症控制中分子的不协调性

凝血和炎症强大的相互关联过程，需要多重水平的调节[145,146]。通过表达一系列调节蛋白,血管内皮维持抗凝和抗炎的表面。组织因子途径抑制剂-1 (TFPI-1 与因子 Xa 和因子 VIIa /组织因子螯合,是凝血起始阶段的主要生理调节因子[147]。抗凝血酶抑制多种凝血丝氨酸蛋白酶,包括因子 Xa 和凝血酶[148]。血栓调节蛋白(TBM)结合凝血酶并改变其特性,从促凝血剂和促炎症基质如纤维蛋白原和蛋白酶激活的受体改变为蛋白 C; 活化蛋白 C(APC)通过失活因子 Va 和 VIIIa 抑制凝血的进展期[149]。内皮蛋白 C 受体(EPCR)通过 TBM /凝血酶复合物增强了 APC 产生,并介导 APC 的许多抗炎和细胞保护作用[150]。TBM 还通过其凝集素样结构域发挥直接的不依赖 APC 的抗炎效应[151,152]。

这些调节剂(TFPIα 和抗凝血酶)中的一些是通过硫酸乙酰肝素蛋白聚糖与内皮细胞表面缔合的循环蛋白质,而其他的是整合的内皮细胞膜蛋白。在移植的器官中,后一组(TFPIβ、TBM 和 EPCR)将作为供体来源的——这在同种异体移植中是不相关的，但是在异种移植中如果调节因子由于物种屏障的原因不能有效地起作用,则可能是至关重要的。20 世纪 90 年代的体外研究中首次突出表明,猪 TFPI 不与人类因子 Xa 结合,这种失败可能引起了异种移植物中不受控制的凝血反应[153,154]。然而最近,在转染细胞中表达的重组形式的猪 TFPI 被证明与人 TFPI 一样可有效地结合并灭活人类 Xa 因子和 VIIa 因子/组织因子[155]。此外,即使存在一定程度的不相容性，也应通过受体衍生的 TFPIα 与异种移植物内皮的结合对其进行一定程度上的校正。

有更多的引人注目的证据表明分子不相容性影响了蛋白 C 途径。猪 TBM 可结合人凝血酶,但是对于人类蛋白 C 的活化是个较差的辅因子，其仅具有人类 TBM 活性的 1%~10%[156-158]。考虑到蛋白 C 途径是微脉管系统中凝血和炎症的关键调节因子[149],并且微血管血栓形成是异种移植物排斥反应的特征[9,58],可以想象这种水平的损伤会对体内产生有害的影响(图 12.4)。人类 TBM 在体外培养的猪内皮细胞中的表达抑制了经典和直接(fgl2)凝血酶原酶活性,延迟了细胞介导的人血浆凝血[143,159]。尽管据报道,猪 EPCR 在体外可以结合人类蛋白 C,但其深入研究较少[160];通过诱导抗体靶向该调节因子[73]可能被证明是比分子不相容性更重要的问题。

在体外定义的另一种不相容性可能促进异种移植物中的血小板黏附和聚集。由于人血小板糖蛋白 Ib (GPIb)与 vWF 的 O-糖基化的 A1 结构域之间的异常相互作用，人血小板在没有剪切应力的情况下与猪 vWF 接触时会自发聚集(图 12.4)[161-163]。这种升高的血小板反应在体内的意义仍是未知的。使用严重 vWF 表达缺陷的供体对猪-狒狒肾异种移植模型中的凝血或移植物存活没有明显影响[164],表明猪 vWF 不是凝血功能失调的主要原因。然而,本研究中受者的唯一治疗手段是在移植之前通过免疫吸附清除天然抗猪抗体。面对随后的体液反应,vWF 缺陷的任何影响都会变得难以区分,而体液反应是非常严重的,并且可在 5 天之内产生对所有移植物的排斥反应[164]。

控制凝血功能失调的途径

短期离体猪器官异种灌注模型中的血管内血栓形成可以通过药理学抗血栓药物来抑制，这些药物包括 APC[165],去氨加压素(可降低 vWF 含量)[166]和替罗非班(一种血小板 GPIIb/IIIa 受体抑制剂)[167]。体外实验表明，他汀类也可能通过阻断活化的猪内皮细胞中组织因子的上调发挥作用[168]。体内抗凝药物更具挑战性,因为剂量必须与出血风险的增加相平衡。猪-NHP 模型已被用于测试许多抗凝血和抗血小板药物，包括华法林、抗凝血酶、APC、肝素、阿司匹林和氯吡格雷[45,169-173]。虽然有证据表明这些研究的益处有限，但可以公平地说，药物治疗不是控制血栓形成和延长异种移植物存活的完整答案[174]。这可能部分反映了 ADCC 等不受抗凝直接作用影响的机制对异种移植物的内皮产生的进行性损伤。

解决凝血问题的最佳前景也许是供体猪的遗传修饰。这个问题已经通过删除 αGal 并表达 hCRP 得到了部分解决,减少了内皮细胞活化和凝血。然而,这些修饰似乎是不完善的,因为在 GTKO±hCRP-转基因异种移植物的狒狒受体中仍然存在凝血功能异常[116,120]。下一个合乎逻辑的步骤是表达人类抗凝血剂和抗血小板分子,以纠正分子不相容性和(或)异种移植物内提供血栓形成的超生理水平的控制。表达人 TFPI 和 TBM 的有益效果已经在小鼠移植模型中得到证实[175,176]。两种蛋白质也已经在转基因猪中表达[168,177-179],但是其体内效价数据尚不可用。

另一种有趣的分子是外源核苷酸酶 CD39,其在血管内皮上起着重要的血栓调节和抗炎作用[180]。CD39 依次将细胞外 ATP 降解成 ADP 和 AMP,然后通过 CD73 水解为腺苷。因此,它可以去除促炎(ATP)和促栓(ADP)信号,同时促进腺苷的产生,对固有和适应性免疫细胞的活性具有普遍的抑制作用[181,182]。像其他几种抗凝血剂/抗炎剂分子一样,包括硫酸乙酰肝素[183]、TBM[184]和 EPCR[185],在炎症过程中 CD39 从内皮上丢失,促进血管损伤[186]。因此,CD39 的过度表达是异种移植方面较有吸引力的前景。使用转基因小鼠的概念验证证明,人类 CD39 的表达可保护心脏和肾脏免受移植相关的血管损伤[187,188]。一项初步报告表明,将人类 CD39 添加到 GTKO / hCRP 转基因背景中并不足以预防猪-狒狒肾异种移植物的 AHXR,尽管据报道 CD39 表达水平较低[189]。

慢性异种移植物排斥反应

慢性异种移植物损伤的报道相对较少,因为很少有器官异种移植物能存活足够长的时间使得这种类型的损伤得以发展。慢性血管病变被认为是慢性同种异体移植物排斥反应的特征性表现,在 GTKO 猪-狒狒心脏异种移植物中可观察到,这些异种移植物的存活时间为 78~179 天[47]。在另一项研究中,在免疫耐受方案下存活 81 天的 GTKO 猪-狒狒肾异种移植物显示出慢性肾小球病的证据,与在临床同种异体移植中所观察到的类似[190]。肾小球病发展的可能原因是不稳定的耐受性诱导、预先形成的非 Gal 抗体所造成的损伤及凝血功能失调。然而,慢性异种移植物排斥的机制可能仍然不清楚,直到更长的存活期达成才可能得出一致结论。

猪胰岛异种移植的排斥反应

猪胰岛异种移植包括广泛的程序,其中可能存在不同的组织来源(胚胎、胎儿、新生儿、年轻、成年),不同的手术途径(门静脉内、肾下囊、腹膜内、皮下、网膜)和不同的免疫保护方法(免疫抑制、包装)。这些因素中的许多都已经在最近的综述中进行了讨论[191,192]。因此,这一节将主要侧重于新生或成年猪胰岛经门静脉移植到 NHP 中,因为这是使用最广泛的模型,最能反映目前临床胰岛移植实践。有关本话题的其他讨论可参见第 15 章。

血液介导的瞬时炎症反应

门静脉内移植使胰岛直接与循环接触,立即引发血栓形成/炎症反应,称为血液介导的瞬时炎症反应(IBMIR)。这种现象首先在同种异体移植中被发现[193],其特征在于补体和凝血系统的快速活化,活化的血小板黏附到胰岛表面,胰岛被血凝块捕获以及活化的嗜中性粒细胞和单核细胞浸润[194]。可能的机制包括天然抗体的结合,组织因子的胰岛表达和诸如 MCP-1 的化学引诱物,血栓形成分子如胶原的暴露,以及缺乏补体和凝血系统的膜调节剂[195-197]。IBMIR 被认为是造成大约一半胰岛同种异体移植物早期破坏的主要因素[198,199]。

IBMIR 在猪-NHP 胰岛异种移植[200-202]和猪-人体外模型中[200,203,204]也有很好的描述。事实上,由于更高水平的天然抗体和对异种细胞的过度活跃的固有免疫应答,IBMIR 可能在异种移植中表现得更严重[205]。在 NHP 中持续逆转糖尿病所需的猪群数量(每千克体重 25 000~100 000 胰岛当量)[206-208]远高于临床同种异体移植中类似效果的人胰岛数量,这样的观察结果支持了上述结论。

猪胰岛异种移植物的急性细胞排斥反应

在 IBMIR 的初始先天性发作中存活的门静脉胰岛异种移植物受到主要依赖于 T 细胞并由 T 细胞介导的适应性免疫应答的攻击[191]。在没有免疫抑制作用的情况下,成年猪的胰岛在 3 天内就会被急性细胞排斥作用所破坏,$CD4^+$和 $CD8^+$ T 细胞和巨噬细胞浸润最为突出[201]。通过 T 细胞靶向免疫抑制(包括共刺激阻断),来自野生型猪的门静脉胰岛异种移植物能够使糖尿病猴子中的胰岛素独立性恢复几个月[206,209,210]。

αGal 在猪胰岛异种移植物排斥反应中的作用

αGal 在猪胰岛 β 细胞上的表达似乎与其成熟度相关,新生猪 β 细胞表达显著,而成年猪 β 细胞几乎没有[211]。除了在残留的污染性非内分泌细胞上表达的

αGal,成年猪胰岛素制剂只含有少量αGal,因此似乎对抗αGal抗体不敏感[191,206]。这一解释得益于GTKO成年胰岛异种移植物的明显生存获益的猪-猴研究,尽管研究数量太小而无法得出明确的结论[207]。相比之下,α-Gal在新生猪胰岛的排斥反应中显然起着重要的作用。来自新生GTKO猪的异种移植物移植成活率更高,并且在糖尿病猴子中比野生型小鼠更少引起肝内炎症[212]。

保护猪胰岛异种移植物的策略

对于有些器官而言,移植益处超过免疫抑制药物副作用的患者比例很小,而胰岛则不同。因此,在胰岛异种移植中制定策略以降低所需的免疫抑制水平甚至完全消除它们至关重要。对于门静脉内胰岛异种移植物,主要目标是保护胰岛免受早期的炎症和血栓形成机制,因为这样可以移植较少的胰岛并减少适应性异种移植免疫的刺激。药理学和遗传学方法的组合可能是必要的。调节补体和凝血的一种治疗方法是低分子量硫酸葡聚糖[203,207]。在遗传方面,αGal的缺失对新生猪胰岛异种移植物具有明显的益处[212],并且hCD46的表达虽然不能防止早期消耗,但能显著延长成年胰岛异种移植物的存活期[207]。设计用于保护器官异种移植物的遗传修饰,如早先描述的各种人抗凝血分子的表达也应该对胰岛异种移植物有益。

诱导耐受是最近另一种已经产生希望的途径。用抗LFA-1、抗-CD154和低剂量西罗莫司治疗的成年猪胰岛移植的糖尿病猴显示异种抗原特异性T细胞耐受性,并维持胰岛素非依赖性的正常血糖超过140天[208]。

保护猪胰岛免受IBMIR和异种免疫应答的另一个策略是将其包裹在基于藻酸盐的化合物中,允许营养物质和胰岛素通过,但阻止抗体和免疫细胞进入。在用微胶囊[213]腹膜内移植或用大包膜装置[214]皮下移植的猴中已经证明了在没有免疫抑制的情况下,封闭的猪胰岛具有长期纠正糖尿病的潜力。新西兰目前正在进行微胶囊化猪胰岛Ⅱ期临床试验,但尚未得出全面的结果。

排斥其他类型的猪异种移植

神经细胞异种移植

在很久以前就有研究提出将猪的多巴胺组织移植到脑中用以治愈帕金森病。在20世纪90年代的临床试验中,12个患者被移植了猪的神经元细胞,其中一半受者接受环孢菌素治疗,另一半受者接受用抗MHC Ⅰ类抗原的单克隆抗体的Fab片段修饰过的移植物[215]。尽管有证据表明部分患者的功能得到提高,但是两个免疫抑制策略都不能阻止免疫排斥的发生,尽管脑是一个相对的免疫豁免器官。相反,一项老鼠的研究表明猪脑神经细胞异种移植可以免受免疫排斥:通过短期CTLA4Ig、抗CD154和抗LFA -1共同刺激和阻断[216]。最近,用帕金森猴子模型移植了猪胎神经组织,该移植物通过一个神经特异性启动子表达了人类CTLA4Ig,通过环孢素、麦考酚质、类固醇抑制免疫。初始数据提示移植延长到了17个月,猴子接受CTLA4Ig的转基因细胞的启动能力也得到了提高,但是对照组没有接受CTLA4Ig的移植物没有该表现[217]。受者在移植后淋巴增生性疾病相对较高的发病率表明,免疫抑制的调节和(或)供体远期基因修饰仍是必需的。

角膜移植

最近有人回顾了猪角膜的异种移植[218,219]。相对较少的猪- NHP角膜异种移植的研究数据表明:角膜异种移植不太可能会引起HAR,可能原因是角膜是无血管组织,移植到了免疫豁免区域,但是通常会在数周至数月内引起大T细胞介导的免疫排斥过程[220-223]。角膜内皮是引起免疫排反应的初级靶点[221],角膜异种移植的去细胞化减少了免疫排斥的发生[223]。aGal和非aGal在角膜异种移植的作用还没被研究清楚,但是aGal在角膜基质细胞和内皮细胞[218]中的表达和非aGal在补体固定抗体[224]中的特异性表明,GTKO±hCRP转基因异种移植可能有幸存优势。

减少免疫抑制负担

系统免疫抑制因为其复杂性和边际效应,是异种移植中的挑战,相对于异体移植而言,异种移植反应更严重。异种移植猪的固态器官不能进入临床实践,除非免疫抑制程度能被减少到可被控制的程度,下面将阐述3条可能的解决方案:

诱导调节

尽管有循环异种抗体和抗体的免疫组化和补体在内皮下沉积的证据,但猪-NHP异种移植常被发现是存活的并且功能正常[67,225,226]。这是一个适应的例子，也是一个未被完全理解的现象，在这个现象中，血管化的器官移植物，不论是同种异体还是异种，都获得了对急性液体反应和排斥的抵抗力[227,228]。关于猪-NHP 模型的适应机制或耐受性知之甚少。其他模型表明尚不致命的移植物损伤是特异性抗体结合的结果，会导致保护通路的激活以抵抗体液免疫。这些通路包括：上调补体调节因子 DAF 和 CD59[229,230]，细胞保护分子例如 A20 和亚铁血红素-1[231]。部分基因策略被设计以抑制猪器官液体排斥例如：hCRP 的表达可能会促进该调节机制的发展。然而目前没有证据表明这是个例，猪-NHP 的异种移植调节仍是难以捉摸的。

诱导耐受

T 细胞介导的异种移植是猪-NHP 固态器官异种移植的巨大障碍。甚至说联合基因修饰供体和加强 T 细胞介导的免疫耐受也没有导致临床应用结果。这趋向于表明诱导 T 细胞耐受（详见第 11 章）对于任何疗法和临床异种移植都是很重要的[232]。两种免疫耐受方法分别是混合嵌合现象和共移植胸腺组织。两种方法都被用于建立人类 T 细胞可以耐受猪异种移植，或高度人源化的老鼠模型[233,234]。猪-NHP 模型更为挑战性的是，稳定的嵌合现象很难达到，即使受体进行了前处理和大量的野生型猪造血干细胞（HSC）应用[235]。没有证据表明异种抗体是 HSC 移植的障碍。GTKO 在受体上的使用通过混合淋巴细胞反应减少了达到相同水平的嵌合水平的细胞数量，延长了细胞低反应性[236]。一项新的研究也使用 GTKO HSC，短暂骨髓嵌合以及对猪细胞的无反应性和受体中非 Gal 抗体反应一致[237]。只有两只移植前高非 Gal 水平的狒狒没有表现出嵌合现象或者猪相关的抗体反应低度活跃，它们在骨髓输入后出现快速免疫排斥猪肾移植[237]。猪 HSC 没有稳定移植的另一个可能原因是巨噬细胞和 NK 细胞的破坏作用，由于前文提到的 SIRPα/CD47 和 KIR/SLA 交叉物种不相容。到底是人 CD47 还是 HLA-E 在受体的表达能够强化嵌合的建立仍需拭目以待。

猪血管化胸腺组织的移植，无论作为胸腺小叶还是胸腺肾（肾异种移植前用自体胸腺组织灌注的肾），都已经获得了更为有希望的结果。原始实验用 αGal 阳性的嵌合肾为血栓形成和 T 细胞介导的低反应性提供了一些体外实验证据，但是异种移植免疫排斥在 30 天之内随着抗-αGal 的生成而发生[238]。GTKO 在受体的应用成功使得狒狒中的嵌合肾记录延长到了 83 天，超过异种移植猪-NHP 模型的生命支持记录[42]。免疫抑制方法包括胸腺切除、脾切除、全身照射（WBI）、抗体介导的 T 细胞消耗、霉酚酸酯、抗 CD154 和低剂量类固醇。不幸的是，这类方法易引起早期术后并发症如感染的发生。几个动物因为功能移植物而死亡，但是免疫组化相对正常，只有少量的排斥现象[42]。提高 WBI 和类固醇，减少早期并发症，总体生存时间从 34 天延长到 51 天，尽管最长生存时间没有延长[140]。调节 T 细胞消耗策略对远期而言没有提高，即使受体的非 Gal 抗体水平很低[239]。但是这些研究提供了一个吸引人的方向——胸腺移植方法，可能是联合嵌合技术，将最终导致异种移植的长期免疫耐受。首先要克服模型的诸多挑战，找到抗-CD154 的代替物，这样才可能成功，但是目前不适用。

移植调节（原位）免疫抑制

对于异种移植新的策略是移植组织分泌免疫抑制蛋白，调节移植物局部微环境。大部分数据支持的局部免疫抑制效率是小型动物同种异体移植模型，包括腺病毒和转基因 CTLA4Ig 的表达[240-243]。猪-NHP 模型相似的数据局限于观察到 CTLA4Ig 的转基因表达似乎被用于长期猪神经元移植到帕金森猴子[217]。需要注意的是，强大而普遍存在的猪 CTLA4Ig 转基因表达导致猪的高死亡率，因为累积了体液免疫[244]。组织限制和（或）调节转基因的表达可能可以解决这个问题。

猪-NHP 模型的局限性

尽管猪-NHP 模型要进入临床必须要有具有普遍有效性[245]，仍需谨记该模型也不是没有限制。首先 NHP 可能会表达猪有而人没有的抗原。例如，NHP 和猪表达 NeuGc，也被称为 Hanganutziu-Deicher 抗原[94,246]，而人类没有相应的抗体[247]。这种抗体的相关性没人会知道，除非有相应的临床实践[248]。第二，NHP 看起来和人相比有一个凝血性更高的表型[249]，这表明当我们解决同种异体移植固态器官移植血栓问题的时候，我们可能把界限设置得过高了。最后，NHP 和人相比，胰岛素依赖性更高，提示需要更大量的猪胰岛细胞来完成该模型的胰岛素独立[250]。这些因素和其他的注意事项导致一些人呼吁尽快开始临床研究[71]。

总结

总体来看,在异种移植进入临床之前,免疫学挑战必须被攻克。异种移植物被糖基化,使其立即被认为是外来的,不仅吸引了大量预先形成的抗体,而且也吸引了先天免疫系统的细胞。大量的蛋白质和碳水化合物的抗原差异引发了一种强大的T细胞异种反应,这似乎与同种异体反应完全不同。此外,异种免疫在一个先天免疫细胞更容易激活的背景下运作,而调控凝血和炎症的几个关键机制因为分子不相容而被抑制。因此,为防止所有的排斥反应而设计的药物对异种反应的效果显著降低,这就不足为奇了。

平衡这些"缺点"的是一种独特而强大的"优势"——通过基因修饰改造供体,去除刺激信号,纠正分子的不兼容性,并加强抗移植的防御能力。即使在目前的猪-NHP模型中进行了相对较少的修饰,但也明显延长了异位和正位心脏异种移植的最长存活时间,分别为8个月[75]和2个月[251],肾脏异种移植延长至3个月[42],胰岛异种移植延长到13个月[207],神经细胞异种移植延长到17个月[217]。一些新的转基因猪正在体内测试中,越来越复杂的方法正在被开发出来[97,252-254],以便更精确和有效地控制猪基因组[255-257]。这些进展以及提高免疫抑制的治疗方案旨在诱导免疫耐受,使人们谨慎但乐观地认为,临床异种移植将成为"下一场医学革命"[74]。

(禹琛 郭靖珩 译 李照 校)

参考文献

1. Ibrahim Z, Busch J, Awwad M, et al. Selected physiologic compatibilities and incompatibilities between human and porcine organ systems. Xenotransplantation. 2006;13:488–499.
2. Meije Y, Tonjes RR, Fishman JA. Retroviral restriction factors and infectious risk in xenotransplantation. American Journal of Transplantation. 2010;10:1511–1516.
3. Macher BA, Galili U. The Galalpha1,3Galbeta1,4GlcNAc-R (alpha-Gal) epitope: a carbohydrate of unique evolution and clinical relevance. Biochimica et Biophysica Acta. 2008;1780:75–88.
4. Larsen RD, Rivera-Marrero CA, Ernst LK, et al. Frameshift and nonsense mutations in a human genomic sequence homologous to a murine UDP-Gal:beta-D-Gal(1,4)-D-GlcNAc alpha(1,3)-galactosyltransferase cDNA. Journal of Biological Chemistry. 1990;265:7055–7061.
5. Galili U, Mandrell RE, Hamadeh RM, et al. Interaction between human natural anti-alpha-galactosyl immunoglobulin G and bacteria of the human flora. Infection and Immunity. 1988;56:1730–1737.
6. Galili U, Anaraki F, Thall A, et al. One percent of human circulating B lymphocytes are capable of producing the natural anti-Gal antibody. Blood. 1993;82:2485–2493.
7. Parker W, Bruno D, Holzknecht ZE, et al. Characterization and affinity isolation of xenoreactive human natural antibodies. Journal of Immunology. 1994;153:3791–3803.
8. Galili U, Rachmilewitz EA, Peleg A, et al. A unique natural human IgG antibody with anti-alpha-galactosyl specificity. Journal of Experimental Medicine. 1984;160:1519–1531.
9. Rose AG, Cooper DK. Venular thrombosis is the key event in the pathogenesis of antibody-mediated cardiac rejection. Xenotransplantation. 2000;7:31–41.
10. Shimizu A, Colvin RB. Pathological features of antibody-mediated rejection. Current Drug Targets. Cardiovascular and Haematological Disorders. 2005;5:199–214.
11. Pober JS, Sessa WC. Evolving functions of endothelial cells in inflammation. Nature Reviews. Immunology. 2007;7:803–815.
12. Saadi S, Platt JL. Transient perturbation of endothelial integrity induced by natural antibodies and complement. Journal of Experimental Medicine. 1995;181:21–31.
13. Palmetshofer A, Robson SC, Bach FH. Tyrosine phosphorylation following lectin mediated endothelial cell stimulation. Xenotransplantation. 1998;5:61–66.
14. Bombeli T, Karsan A, Tait JF, et al. Apoptotic vascular endothelial cells become procoagulant. Blood. 1997;89:2429–2442.
15. Chironi GN, Boulanger CM, Simon A, et al. Endothelial microparticles in diseases. Cell and Tissue Research. 2009;335:143–151.
16. Hansch GM, Hammer CH, Vanguri P, et al. Homologous species restriction in lysis of erythrocytes by terminal complement proteins. Proceedings of the National Academy of Sciences of the United States of America. 1981;78:5118–5121.
17. Atkinson JP, Oglesby TJ, White D, et al. Separation of self from non-self in the complement system: a role for membrane cofactor protein and decay accelerating factor. Clinical and Experimental Immunology. 1991;86(Suppl. 1):27–30.
18. Dalmasso AP, Vercellotti GM, Platt JL, et al. Inhibition of complement-mediated endothelial cell cytotoxicity by decay-accelerating factor. Potential for prevention of xenograft hyperacute rejection. Transplantation. 1991;52:530–533.
19. Morgan BP, Berg CW, Harris CL. "Homologous restriction" in complement lysis: roles of membrane complement regulators. Xenotransplantation. 2005;12:258–265.
20. Fisicaro N, Aminian A, Hinchliffe SJ, et al. The pig analogue of CD59 protects transgenic mouse hearts from injury by human complement. Transplantation. 2000;70:963–968.
21. Starzl TE, Marchioro TL, Holmes JH, et al. The incidence, cause, and significance of immediate and delayed oliguria or anuria after human renal transplantation. Surgery, Gynecology and Obstetrics. 1964;118:819–827.
22. Chen RH, Naficy S, Logan JS, et al. Hearts from transgenic pigs constructed with CD59/DAF genomic clones demonstrate improved survival in primates. Xenotransplantation. 1999;6:194–200.
23. Kobayashi T, Taniguchi S, Neethling FA, et al. Delayed xenograft rejection of pig-to-baboon cardiac transplants after cobra venom factor therapy. Transplantation. 1997;64:1255–1261.
24. Xu Y, Lorf T, Sablinski T, et al. Removal of anti-porcine natural antibodies from human and nonhuman primate plasma in vitro and in vivo by a Galalpha1-3Galbeta1-4betaGlc-X immunoaffinity column. Transplantation. 1998;65:172–179.
25. Cozzi E, Langford GA, Richards A, et al. Expression of human decay accelerating factor in transgenic pigs. Transplantation Proceedings. 1994;26:1402–1403.
26. Fodor WL, Williams BL, Matis LA, et al. Expression of a functional human complement inhibitor in a transgenic pig as a model for the prevention of xenogeneic hyperacute organ rejection. Proceedings of the National Academy of Sciences of the United States of America. 1994;91:11153–11157.
27. Diamond LE, Quinn CM, Martin MJ, et al. A human CD46 transgenic pig model system for the study of discordant xenotransplantation. Transplantation. 2001;71:132–142.
28. Loveland BE, Milland J, Kyriakou P, et al. Characterization of a CD46 transgenic pig and protection of transgenic kidneys against hyperacute rejection in non-immunosuppressed baboons. Xenotransplantation. 2004;11:171–183.
29. Byrne GW, McCurry KR, Martin MJ, et al. Transgenic pigs expressing human CD59 and decay-accelerating factor produce an intrinsic barrier to complement-mediated damage. Transplantation. 1997;63:149–155.
30. Cowan PJ, Aminian A, Barlow H, et al. Renal xenografts from triple-transgenic pigs are not hyperacutely rejected but cause coagulopathy in non-immunosuppressed baboons. Transplantation. 2000;69:2504–2515.
31. Menoret S, Plat M, Blancho G, et al. Characterization of human CD55 and CD59 transgenic pigs and kidney xenotransplantation in the pig-to-baboon combination. Transplantation. 2004;77:1468–1471.
32. Manez R, Lopez-Pelaez E, Centeno A, et al. Transgenic expression in pig hearts of both human decay-accelerating factor and human membrane cofactor protein does not provide an additional benefit to that of human decay-accelerating

factor alone in pig-to-baboon xenotransplantation. Transplantation. 2004;78: 930–933.
33. Lam TT, Hausen B, Boeke-Purkis K, et al. Hyperacute rejection of hDAF-transgenic pig organ xenografts in cynomolgus monkeys: influence of pre-existing anti-pig antibodies and prevention by the alpha GAL glycoconjugate GAS914. Xenotransplantation. 2004;11:517–524.
34. Huber-Lang M, Sarma JV, Zetoune FS, et al. Generation of C5a in the absence of C3: a new complement activation pathway. Nature Medicine. 2006;12:682–687.
35. Dai Y, Vaught TD, Boone J, et al. Targeted disruption of the alpha1,3-galactosyltransferase gene in cloned pigs. Nature Biotechnology. 2002;20: 251–255.
36. Lai L, Kolber-Simonds D, Park KW, et al. Production of alpha-1,3-galactosyltransferase knockout pigs by nuclear transfer cloning. Science. 2002;295:1089–1092.
37. Phelps CJ, Koike C, Vaught TD, et al. Production of alpha 1,3-galactosyltransferase-deficient pigs. Science. 2003;299:411–414.
38. Kolber-Simonds D, Lai L, Watt SR, et al. Production of alpha-1,3-galactosyltransferase null pigs by means of nuclear transfer with fibroblasts bearing loss of heterozygosity mutations. Proceedings of the National Academy of Sciences of the United States of America. 2004;101:7335–7340.
39. Nottle MB, Beebe LF, Harrison SJ, et al. Production of homozygous alpha-1,3-galactosyltransferase knockout pigs by breeding and somatic cell nuclear transfer. Xenotransplantation. 2007;14:339–344.
40. Fujimura T, Takahagi Y, Shigehisa T, et al. Production of alpha 1,3-galactosyltransferase gene-deficient pigs by somatic cell nuclear transfer: a novel selection method for gal alpha 1,3-Gal antigen-deficient cells. Molecular Reproduction and Development. 2008;75:1372–1378.
41. Dor FJ, Tseng YL, Cheng J, et al. alpha1,3-Galactosyltransferase gene-knockout miniature swine produce natural cytotoxic anti-Gal antibodies. Transplantation. 2004;78:15–20.
42. Yamada K, Yazawa K, Shimizu A, et al. Marked prolongation of porcine renal xenograft survival in baboons through the use of alpha1,3-galactosyltransferase gene-knockout donors and the cotransplantation of vascularized thymic tissue. Nature Medicine. 2005;11:32–34.
43. Kuwaki K, Tseng YL, Dor FJ, et al. Heart transplantation in baboons using alpha1,3-galactosyltransferase gene-knockout pigs as donors: initial experience. Nature Medicine. 2005;11:29–31.
44. Chen G, Qian H, Starzl T, et al. Acute rejection is associated with antibodies to non-Gal antigens in baboons using Gal-knockout pig kidneys. Nature Medicine. 2005;11:1295–1298.
45. Tseng YL, Kuwaki K, Dor FJ, et al. alpha1,3-Galactosyltransferase gene-knockout pig heart transplantation in baboons with survival approaching 6 months. Transplantation. 2005;80:1493–1500.
46. Cowan PJ, Salvaris EJ, Crikis S, et al. Gal KO pig renal xenografts are not hyperacutely rejected by non-immunosuppressed baboons. American Journal of Transplantation. 2006;6(s2):1050.
47. Hisashi Y, Yamada K, Kuwaki K, et al. Rejection of cardiac xenografts transplanted from alpha1,3-galactosyltransferase gene-knockout (GalT-KO) pigs to baboons. American Journal of Transplantation. 2008;8:2516–2526.
48. Kiernan K, Harnden I, Gunthart M, et al. The anti-non-gal xenoantibody response to xenoantigens on gal knockout pig cells is encoded by a restricted number of germline progenitors. American Journal of Transplantation. 2008;8: 1829–1839.
49. Saethre M, Baumann BC, Fung M, et al. Characterization of natural human anti-non-gal antibodies and their effect on activation of porcine gal-deficient endothelial cells. Transplantation. 2007;84:244–250.
50. Baumann BC, Stussi G, Huggel K, et al. Reactivity of human natural antibodies to endothelial cells from Galalpha(1,3)Gal-deficient pigs. Transplantation. 2007;83:193–201.
51. Ezzelarab M, Hara H, Busch J, et al. Antibodies directed to pig non-Gal antigens in naive and sensitized baboons. Xenotransplantation. 2006;13:400–407.
52. Ezzelarab M, Ayares D, Cooper DK. Carbohydrates in xenotransplantation. Immunology and Cell Biology. 2005;83:396–404.
53. Morozumi K, Kobayashi T, Usami T, et al. Significance of histochemical expression of Hanganutziu-Deicher antigens in pig, baboon and human tissues. Transplantation Proceedings. 1999;31:942–944.
54. Bach FH, Winkler H, Ferran C, et al. Delayed xenograft rejection. Immunology Today. 1996;17:379–384.
55. Lin SS, Weidner BC, Byrne GW, et al. The role of antibodies in acute vascular rejection of pig-to-baboon cardiac transplants. Journal of Clinical Investigation. 1998;101:1745–1756.
56. Platt JL, Lin SS, McGregor CG. Acute vascular rejection. Xenotransplantation. 1998;5:169–175.
57. Dorling A. Are anti-endothelial cell antibodies a pre-requisite for the acute vascular rejection of xenografts? Xenotransplantation. 2003;10:16–23.
58. Shimizu A, Yamada K. Histopathology of xenografts in pig to non-human primate discordant xenotransplantation. Clinical Transplantation. 2010; 24(Suppl. 22):11–15.
59. Auchincloss H Jr, Sachs DH. Xenogeneic transplantation. Annual Review of Immunology. 1998;16:433–470.
60. Palmetshofer A, Galili U, Dalmasso AP, et al. Alpha-galactosyl epitope-mediated activation of porcine aortic endothelial cells: type II activation. Transplantation. 1998;65:971–978.
61. Bharat A, Mohanakumar T. Allopeptides and the alloimmune response. Cellular Immunology. 2007;248:31–43.
62. Wood KJ, Goto R. Mechanisms of rejection: current perspectives. Transplantation. 2012;93:1–10.
63. Dorling A, Lombardi G, Binns R, et al. Detection of primary direct and indirect human anti-porcine T cell responses using a porcine dendritic cell population. European Journal of Immunology. 1996;26:1378–1387.
64. Tadaki DK, Craighead N, Saini A, et al. Costimulatory molecules are active in the human xenoreactive T-cell response but not in natural killer-mediated cytotoxicity. Transplantation. 2000;70:162–167.
65. Xu XC, Naziruddin B, Sasaki H, et al. Allele-specific and peptide-dependent recognition of swine leukocyte antigen class I by human cytotoxic T-cell clones. Transplantation. 1999;68:473–479.
66. Tadaki DK, Williams A, Lee KP, et al. Porcine CD80: cloning, characterization, and evidence for its role in direct human T-cell activation. Xenotransplantation. 2003;10:252–258.
67. Lin SS, Hanaway MJ, Gonzalez-Stawinski GV, et al. The role of anti-Galalpha1-3Gal antibodies in acute vascular rejection and accommodation of xenografts. Transplantation. 2000;70:1667–1674.
68. Chen G, Sun H, Yang H, et al. The role of anti-non-Gal antibodies in the development of acute humoral xenograft rejection of hDAF transgenic porcine kidneys in baboons receiving anti-Gal antibody neutralization therapy. Transplantation. 2006;81:273–283.
69. Lam TT, Paniagua R, Shivaram G, et al. Anti-non-Gal porcine endothelial cell antibodies in acute humoral xenograft rejection of hDAF-transgenic porcine hearts in cynomolgus monkeys. Xenotransplantation. 2004;11:531–535.
70. Tseng YL, Moran K, Dor FJ, et al. Elicited antibodies in baboons exposed to tissues from alpha1,3-galactosyltransferase gene-knockout pigs. Transplantation. 2006;81:1058–1062.
71. Breimer ME. Gal/non-Gal antigens in pig tissues and human non-Gal antibodies in the GalT-KO era. Xenotransplantation. 2011;18:215–228.
72. Galili U. Induced anti-non gal antibodies in human xenograft recipients. Transplantation. 2012;93:11–16.
73. Byrne GW, Stalboerger PG, Du Z, et al. Identification of new carbohydrate and membrane protein antigens in cardiac xenotransplantation. Transplantation. 2011;91:287–292.
74. Ekser B, Ezzelarab M, Hara H, et al. Clinical xenotransplantation: the next medical revolution? Lancet. 2012;379:672–683.
75. Mohiuddin MM, Corcoran PC, Singh AK, et al. B-cell depletion extends the survival of GTKO.hCD46Tg pig heart xenografts in baboons for up to 8 months. American Journal of Transplantation. 2012;12:763–771.
76. Bianchi ME. DAMPs, PAMPs and alarmins: all we need to know about danger. Journal of Leukocyte Biology. 2007;81:1–5.
77. Prince LR, Whyte MK, Sabroe I, et al. The role of TLRs in neutrophil activation. Current Opinion in Pharmacology. 2011;11:397–403.
78. Artrip JH, Kwiatkowski P, Michler RE, et al. Target cell susceptibility to lysis by human natural killer cells is augmented by alpha(1,3)-galactosyltransferase and reduced by alpha(1, 2)-fucosyltransferase. Journal of Biological Chemistry. 1999;274:10717–10722.
79. Jin R, Greenwald A, Peterson MD, et al. Human monocytes recognize porcine endothelium via the interaction of galectin 3 and alpha-GAL. Journal of Immunology. 2006;177:1289–1295.
80. van der Touw W, Bromberg JS. Natural killer cells and the immune response in solid organ transplantation. American Journal of Transplantation. 2010;10: 1354–1358.
81. Suarez-Alvarez B, Lopez-Vazquez A, Baltar JM, et al. Potential role of NKG2D and its ligands in organ transplantation: new target for immunointervention. American Journal of Transplantation. 2009;9:251–257.
82. Murphy SP, Porrett PM, Turka LA. Innate immunity in transplant tolerance and rejection. Immunological Reviews. 2011;241:39–48.
83. Quiroga I, Salio M, Koo DD, et al. Expression of MHC class I-related Chain B (MICB) molecules on renal transplant biopsies. Transplantation. 2006;81: 1196–1203.
84. Hankey KG, Drachenberg CB, Papadimitriou JC, et al. MIC expression in renal and pancreatic allografts. Transplantation. 2002;73:304–306.
85. Bromberg JS, Heeger PS, Li XC. Evolving paradigms that determine the fate of an allograft. American Journal of Transplantation. 2010;10:1143–1148.

86. Baumann BC, Forte P, Hawley RJ, et al. Lack of galactose-alpha-1,3-galactose expression on porcine endothelial cells prevents complement-induced lysis but not direct xenogeneic NK cytotoxicity. Journal of Immunology. 2004;172: 6460–6467.
87. Schneider MK, Seebach JD. Current cellular innate immune hurdles in pig-to-primate xenotransplantation. Current Opinion in Organ Transplantation 2008;13:171–177.
88. Matter-Reissmann UB, Forte P, Schneider MK, et al. Xenogeneic human NK cytotoxicity against porcine endothelial cells is perforin/granzyme B dependent and not inhibited by Bcl-2 overexpression. Xenotransplantation. 2002;9: 325–337.
89. Li S, Waer M, Billiau AD. Xenotransplantation: role of natural immunity. Transplant Immunology. 2009;21:70–74.
90. Sullivan JA, Oettinger HF, Sachs DH, et al. Analysis of polymorphism in porcine MHC class I genes: alterations in signals recognized by human cytotoxic lymphocytes. Journal of Immunology. 1997;159:2318–2326.
91. Lilienfeld BG, Garcia-Borges C, Crew MD, et al. Porcine UL16-binding protein 1 expressed on the surface of endothelial cells triggers human NK cytotoxicity through NKG2D. Journal of Immunology. 2006;177:2146–2152.
92. Tran PD, Christiansen D, Winterhalter A, et al. Porcine cells express more than one functional ligand for the human lymphocyte activating receptor NKG2D. Xenotransplantation. 2008;15:321–332.
93. Forte P, Lilienfeld BG, Baumann BC, et al. Human NK cytotoxicity against porcine cells is triggered by NKp44 and NKG2D. Journal of Immunology. 2005;175:5463–5470.
94. Christiansen D, Mouhtouris E, Milland J, et al. Recognition of a carbohydrate xenoepitope by human NKRP1A (CD161). Xenotransplantation. 2006;13: 440–446.
95. Shinkel TA, Chen CG, Salvaris E, et al. Changes in cell surface glycosylation in alpha1,3-galactosyltransferase knockout and alpha1,2-fucosyltransferase transgenic mice. Transplantation. 1997;64:197–204.
96. Diswall M, Angstrom J, Schuurman HJ, et al. Studies on glycolipid antigens in small intestine and pancreas from alpha1,3-galactosyltransferase knockout miniature swine. Transplantation. 2007;84:1348–1356.
97. Weiss EH, Lilienfeld BG, Muller S, et al. HLA-E/human beta2-microglobulin transgenic pigs: protection against xenogeneic human anti-pig natural killer cell cytotoxicity. Transplantation. 2009;87:35–43.
98. Crew MD, Cannon MJ, Phanavanh B, et al. An HLA-E single chain trimer inhibits human NK cell reactivity towards porcine cells. Molecular Immunology. 2005;42:1205–1214.
99. Lilienfeld BG, Crew MD, Forte P, et al. Transgenic expression of HLA-E single chain trimer protects porcine endothelial cells against human natural killer cell-mediated cytotoxicity. Xenotransplantation. 2007;14:126–134.
100. Magil AB. Monocytes/macrophages in renal allograft rejection. Transplantation Reviews (Orlando, Fla.). 2009;23:199–208.
101. Barclay AN. Signal regulatory protein alpha (SIRPalpha)/CD47 interaction and function. Current Opinion in Immunology. 2009;21:47–52.
102. Yang YG. CD47 in xenograft rejection and tolerance induction. Xenotransplantation. 2010;17:267–273.
103. Subramanian S, Parthasarathy R, Sen S, et al. Species- and cell type-specific interactions between CD47 and human SIRPalpha. Blood. 2006;107:2548–2556.
104. Ide K, Wang H, Tahara H, et al. Role for CD47-SIRPalpha signaling in xenograft rejection by macrophages. Proceedings of the National Academy of Sciences of the United States of America. 2007;104:5062–5066.
105. Wang C, Wang H, Ide K, et al. Human CD47 expression permits survival of porcine cells in immunodeficient mice that express SIRPalpha capable of binding to human CD47. Cell Transplantation. 2011;20:1915–1920.
106. Cardozo LA, Rouw DB, Ambrose LR, et al. The neutrophil: the unnoticed threat in xenotransplantation? Transplantation. 2004;78:1721–1728.
107. Al-Mohanna F, Saleh S, Parhar RS, et al. Human neutrophil gene expression profiling following xenogeneic encounter with porcine aortic endothelial cells: the occult role of neutrophils in xenograft rejection revealed. Journal of Leukocyte Biology. 2005;78:51–61.
108. Aird WC. Endothelium and allotransplantation. Transplantation. 2006; 82(1 Suppl.):S6–S8.
109. Noris M, Remuzzi G. Thrombotic microangiopathy after kidney transplantation. American Journal of Transplantation. 2010;10:1517–1523.
110. Le Quintrec M, Lionet A, Kamar N, et al. Complement mutation-associated de novo thrombotic microangiopathy following kidney transplantation. American Journal of Transplantation. 2008;8:1694–1701.
111. Cowan PJ, Robson SC, d'Apice AJ. Controlling coagulation dysregulation in xenotransplantation. Current Opinion in Organ Transplantation 2011;16: 214–221.
112. Schmelzle M, Schulte Esch J 2nd, Robson SC. Coagulation, platelet activation and thrombosis in xenotransplantation. Current Opinion in Organ Transplantation 2010;15:212–218.
113. Pierson RN 3rd, Dorling A, Ayares D, et al. Current status of xenotransplantation and prospects for clinical application. Xenotransplantation. 2009;16:263–280.
114. Houser SL, Kuwaki K, Knosalla C, et al. Thrombotic microangiopathy and graft arteriopathy in pig hearts following transplantation into baboons. Xenotransplantation. 2004;11:416–425.
115. Shimizu A, Yamada K, Yamamoto S, et al. Thrombotic microangiopathic glomerulopathy in human decay accelerating factor-transgenic swine-to-baboon kidney xenografts. Journal of the American Society of Nephrology. 2005;16:2732–2745.
116. Ezzelarab M, Garcia B, Azimzadeh A, et al. The innate immune response and activation of coagulation in alpha1,3-galactosyltransferase gene-knockout xenograft recipients. Transplantation. 2009;87:805–812.
117. Ierino FL, Kozlowski T, Siegel JB, et al. Disseminated intravascular coagulation in association with the delayed rejection of pig-to-baboon renal xenografts. Transplantation. 1998;66:1439–1450.
118. Buhler L, Basker M, Alwayn IP, et al. Coagulation and thrombotic disorders associated with pig organ and hematopoietic cell transplantation in nonhuman primates. Transplantation. 2000;70:1323–1331.
119. Cozzi E, Simioni P, Boldrin M, et al. Alterations in the coagulation profile in renal pig-to-monkey xenotransplantation. American Journal of Transplantation. 2004;4:335–345.
120. Lin CC, Ezzelarab M, Shapiro R, et al. Recipient tissue factor expression is associated with consumptive coagulopathy in pig-to-primate kidney xenotransplantation. American Journal of Transplantation. 2010;10:1556–1568.
121. Shimizu A, Hisashi Y, Kuwaki K, et al. Thrombotic microangiopathy associated with humoral rejection of cardiac xenografts from alpha1,3-galactosyltransferase gene-knockout pigs in baboons. American Journal of Pathology. 2008;172: 1471–1481.
122. Bauer A, Postrach J, Thormann M, et al. First experience with heterotopic thoracic pig-to-baboon cardiac xenotransplantation. Xenotransplantation. 2010;17: 243–249.
123. Knosalla C, Yazawa K, Behdad A, et al. Renal and cardiac endothelial heterogeneity impact acute vascular rejection in pig-to-baboon xenotransplantation. American Journal of Transplantation. 2009;9:1006–1016.
124. Cantu E, Parker W, Platt JL, et al. Pulmonary xenotransplantation: rapidly progressing into the unknown. American Journal of Transplantation. 2004;4(Suppl. 6):25–35.
125. Holzknecht ZE, Coombes S, Blocher BA, et al. Immune complex formation after xenotransplantation : evidence of type III as well as type II immune reactions provide clues to pathophysiology. American Journal of Pathology. 2001;158: 627–637.
126. Cantu E, Balsara KR, Li B, et al. Prolonged function of macrophage, von Willebrand factor-deficient porcine pulmonary xenografts. American Journal of Transplantation. 2007;7:66–75.
127. Nguyen BN, Azimzadeh AM, Zhang T, et al. Life-supporting function of genetically modified swine lungs in baboons. Journal of Thoracic and Cardiovascular Surgery. 2007;133:1354–1363.
128. Gaca JG, Lesher A, Aksoy O, et al. The role of the porcine von Willebrand factor: baboon platelet interactions in pulmonary xenotransplantation. Transplantation. 2002;74:1596–1603.
129. Cantu E, Gaca JG, Palestrant D, et al. Depletion of pulmonary intravascular macrophages prevents hyperacute pulmonary xenograft dysfunction. Transplantation. 2006;81:1157–1164.
130. Bush EL, Barbas AS, Holzknecht ZE, et al. Coagulopathy in alpha-galactosyl transferase knockout pulmonary xenotransplants. Xenotransplantation. 2011;18:6–13.
131. Ekser B, Long C, Echeverri GJ, et al. Impact of thrombocytopenia on survival of baboons with genetically modified pig liver transplants: clinical relevance. American Journal of Transplantation. 2010;10:273–285.
132. Ekser B, Klein E, He J, et al. Genetically-engineered pig-to-baboon liver xenotransplantation: histopathology of xenografts and native organs. PLoS ONE. 2012;7:e29720.
133. Ekser B, Echeverri GJ, Hassett AC, et al. Hepatic function after genetically engineered pig liver transplantation in baboons. Transplantation. 2010;90: 483–493.
134. Ezzelarab M, Ekser B, Gridelli B, et al. Thrombocytopenia after pig-to-baboon liver xenotransplantation: where do platelets go? Xenotransplantation. 2011; 18:320–327.
135. Burlak C, Paris LL, Chihara RK, et al. The fate of human platelets perfused through the pig liver: implications for xenotransplantation. Xenotransplantation. 2010;17:350–361.
136. Paris LL, Chihara RK, Reyes LM, et al. ASGR1 expressed by porcine enriched liver sinusoidal endothelial cells mediates human platelet phagocytosis in vitro. Xenotransplantation. 2011;18:245–251.

137. Chihara RK, Paris LL, Reyes LM, et al. Primary porcine Kupffer cell phagocytosis of human platelets involves the CD18 receptor. Transplantation. 2011;92: 739–744.
138. Gollackner B, Goh SK, Qawi I, et al. Acute vascular rejection of xenografts: roles of natural and elicited xenoreactive antibodies in activation of vascular endothelial cells and induction of procoagulant activity. Transplantation. 2004;77: 1735–1741.
139. Lin CC, Chen D, McVey JH, et al. Expression of tissue factor and initiation of clotting by human platelets and monocytes after incubation with porcine endothelial cells. Transplantation. 2008;86:702–709.
140. Griesemer AD, Hirakata A, Shimizu A, et al. Results of gal-knockout porcine thymokidney xenografts. American Journal of Transplantation. 2009;9:2669–2678.
141. Ghanekar A, Mendicino M, Liu H, et al. Endothelial induction of fgl2 contributes to thrombosis during acute vascular xenograft rejection. Journal of Immunology. 2004;172:5693–5701.
142. Miwa Y, Yamamoto K, Onishi A, et al. Potential value of human thrombomodulin and DAF expression for coagulation control in pig-to-human xenotransplantation. Xenotransplantation. 2010;17:26–37.
143. Ning Q, Sun Y, Han M, et al. Role of fibrinogen-like protein 2 prothrombinase/fibroleukin in experimental and human allograft rejection. Journal of Immunology. 2005;174:7403–7411.
144. Hancock WW, Szaba FM, Berggren KN, et al. Intact type 1 immunity and immune-associated coagulative responses in mice lacking IFN gamma-inducible fibrinogen-like protein 2. Proceedings of the National Academy of Sciences of the United States of America. 2004;101:3005–3010.
145. Delvaeye M, Conway EM. Coagulation and innate immune responses: can we view them separately? Blood. 2009;114:2367–2374.
146. Amara U, Flierl MA, Rittirsch D, et al. Molecular intercommunication between the complement and coagulation systems. Journal of Immunology. 2010;185: 5628–5636.
147. Broze GJ Jr, Girard TJ. Tissue factor pathway inhibitor: structure-function. Frontiers in Bioscience. 2012;17:262–280.
148. Rau JC, Beaulieu LM, Huntington JA, et al. Serpins in thrombosis, hemostasis and fibrinolysis. Journal of Thrombosis and Haemostasis. 2007;5(Suppl. 1): 102–115.
149. Esmon CT, Esmon NL. The link between vascular features and thrombosis. Annual Review of Physiology. 2011;73:503–514.
150. Bae JS, Yang L, Rezaie AR. Receptors of the protein C activation and activated protein C signaling pathways are colocalized in lipid rafts of endothelial cells. Proceedings of the National Academy of Sciences of the United States of America. 2007;104:2867–2872.
151. Conway EM, Van de Wouwer M, Pollefeyt S, et al. The lectin-like domain of thrombomodulin confers protection from neutrophil-mediated tissue damage by suppressing adhesion molecule expression via nuclear factor kappaB and mitogen-activated protein kinase pathways. Journal of Experimental Medicine. 2002;196:565–577.
152. Van de Wouwer M, Plaisance S, De Vriese A, et al. The lectin-like domain of thrombomodulin interferes with complement activation and protects against arthritis. Journal of Thrombosis and Haemostasis. 2006;4:1813–1824.
153. Kopp CW, Siegel JB, Hancock WW, et al. Effect of porcine endothelial tissue factor pathway inhibitor on human coagulation factors. Transplantation. 1997; 63:749–758.
154. Kopp CW, Robson SC, Siegel JB, et al. Regulation of monocyte tissue factor activity by allogeneic and xenogeneic endothelial cells. Thrombosis and Haemostasis. 1998;79:529–538.
155. Lee KF, Salvaris EJ, Roussel JC, et al. Recombinant pig TFPI efficiently regulates human tissue factor pathways. Xenotransplantation. 2008;15:191–197.
156. Roussel JC, Moran CJ, Salvaris EJ, et al. Pig thrombomodulin binds human thrombin but is a poor cofactor for activation of human protein C and TAFI. American Journal of Transplantation. 2008;8:1101–1112.
157. Siegel JB, Grey ST, Lesnikoski BA, et al. Xenogeneic endothelial cells activate human prothrombin. Transplantation. 1997;64:888–896.
158. Lawson JH, Daniels LJ, Platt JL. The evaluation of thrombomodulin activity in porcine to human xenotransplantation. Transplantation Proceedings. 1997;29: 884–885.
159. Kopp CW, Grey ST, Siegel JB, et al. Expression of human thrombomodulin cofactor activity in porcine endothelial cells. Transplantation. 1998;66: 244–251.
160. Cowan PJ, d'Apice AJ. Complement activation and coagulation in xenotransplantation. Immunology and Cell Biology. 2009;87:203–208.
161. Mazzucato M, De Marco L, Pradella P, et al. Porcine von Willebrand factor binding to human platelet GPIb induces transmembrane calcium influx. Thrombosis and Haemostasis. 1996;75:655–660.
162. Schulte am Esch J 2nd, Cruz MA, Siegel JB, et al. Activation of human platelets by the membrane-expressed A1 domain of von Willebrand factor. Blood. 1997;90:4425–4437.
163. Schulte Am Esch J 2nd, Robson SC, Knoefel WT, et al. O-linked glycosylation and functional incompatibility of porcine von Willebrand factor for human platelet GPIb receptors. Xenotransplantation. 2005;12:30–37.
164. Meyer C, Wolf P, Romain N, et al. Use of von Willebrand diseased kidney as donor in a pig-to-primate model of xenotransplantation. Transplantation. 1999;67:38–45.
165. Ramackers W, Friedrich L, Tiede A, et al. Effects of pharmacological intervention on coagulopathy and organ function in xenoperfused kidneys. Xenotransplantation. 2008;15:46–55.
166. Kim YT, Lee HJ, Lee SW, et al. Pre-treatment of porcine pulmonary xenograft with desmopressin: a novel strategy to attenuate platelet activation and systemic intravascular coagulation in an ex-vivo model of swine-to-human pulmonary xenotransplantation. Xenotransplantation. 2008;15:27–35.
167. Brandl U, Jockle H, Erhardt M, et al. Reduced fibrin deposition and intravascular thrombosis in hDAF transgenic pig hearts perfused with tirofiban. Transplantation. 2007;84:1667–1676.
168. Lin CC, Ezzelarab M, Hara H, et al. Atorvastatin or transgenic expression of TFPI inhibits coagulation initiated by anti-nonGal IgG binding to porcine aortic endothelial cells. Journal of Thrombosis and Haemostasis. 2010;8: 2001–2010.
169. Byrne GW, Davies WR, Oi K, et al. Increased immunosuppression, not anticoagulation, extends cardiac xenograft survival. Transplantation. 2006;82: 1787–1791.
170. Cowan PJ, Aminian A, Barlow H, et al. Protective effects of recombinant human antithrombin III in pig-to-primate renal xenotransplantation. American Journal of Transplantation. 2002;2:520–525.
171. Kuwaki K, Knosalla C, Dor FJ, et al. Suppression of natural and elicited antibodies in pig-to-baboon heart transplantation using a human anti-human CD154 mAb-based regimen. American Journal of Transplantation. 2004;4:363–372.
172. Cozzi E, Simioni P, Boldrin M, et al. Effects of long-term administration of high-dose recombinant human antithrombin in immunosuppressed primate recipients of porcine xenografts. Transplantation. 2005;80:1501–1510.
173. Simioni P, Boldrin M, Gavasso S, et al. Effects of long-term administration of recombinant human protein C in xenografted primates. Transplantation. 2011;91:161–168.
174. Schmelzle M, Cowan PJ, Robson SC. Which anti-platelet therapies might be beneficial in xenotransplantation? Xenotransplantation. 2011;18:79–87.
175. Chen D, Weber M, McVey JH, et al. Complete inhibition of acute humoral rejection using regulated expression of membrane-tethered anticoagulants on xenograft endothelium. American Journal of Transplantation. 2004;4:1958–1963.
176. Crikis S, Zhang XM, Dezfouli S, et al. Anti-inflammatory and anticoagulant effects of transgenic expression of human thrombomodulin in mice. American Journal of Transplantation. 2010;10:242–250.
177. Lee HJ, Lee BC, Kim YH, et al. Characterization of transgenic pigs that express human decay accelerating factor and cell membrane-tethered human tissue factor pathway inhibitor. Reproduction in Domestic Animals. 2011;46: 325–332.
178. Petersen B, Ramackers W, Tiede A, et al. Pigs transgenic for human thrombomodulin have elevated production of activated protein C. Xenotransplantation. 2009;16:486–495.
179. Aigner B, Klymiuk N, Wolf E. Transgenic pigs for xenotransplantation: selection of promoter sequences for reliable transgene expression. Current Opinion in Organ Transplantation 2010;15:201–206.
180. Kaczmarek E, Koziak K, Sevigny J, et al. Identification and characterization of CD39/vascular ATP diphosphohydrolase. Journal of Biological Chemistry. 1996;271:33116–33122.
181. Kumar V, Sharma A. Adenosine: an endogenous modulator of innate immune system with therapeutic potential. European Journal of Pharmacology. 2009;616: 7–15.
182. Hasko G, Linden J, Cronstein B, et al. Adenosine receptors: therapeutic aspects for inflammatory and immune diseases. Nature Reviews Drug Discovery. 2008; 7:759–770.
183. Platt JL, Vercellotti GM, Lindman BJ, et al. Release of heparan sulfate from endothelial cells. Implications for pathogenesis of hyperacute rejection. Journal of Experimental Medicine. 1990;171:1363–1368.
184. Scaldaferri F, Sans M, Vetrano S, et al. Crucial role of the protein C pathway in governing microvascular inflammation in inflammatory bowel disease. Journal of Clinical Investigation. 2007;117:1951–1960.
185. Menschikowski M, Hagelgans A, Eisenhofer G, et al. Regulation of endothelial protein C receptor shedding by cytokines is mediated through differential activation of MAP kinase signaling pathways. Experimental Cell Research. 2009;315: 2673–2682.

186. Robson SC, Kaczmarek E, Siegel JB, et al. Loss of ATP diphosphohydrolase activity with endothelial cell activation. Journal of Experimental Medicine. 1997; 185:153–163.
187. Dwyer KM, Robson SC, Nandurkar HH, et al. Thromboregulatory manifestations in human CD39 transgenic mice and the implications for thrombotic disease and transplantation. Journal of Clinical Investigation. 2004;113:1440–1446.
188. Crikis S, Lu B, Murray-Segal LM, et al. Transgenic overexpression of CD39 protects against renal ischemia-reperfusion and transplant vascular injury. American Journal of Transplantation. 2010;10:2586–2595.
189. Le Bas-Bernardet S, Tillou X, Poirier N, et al. Xenotransplantation of galactosyltransferase knockout, CD55, CD59, CD39, and fucosyl-transferase transgenic pig kidneys into baboons. Transplantation Proceedings. 2011;43:3426–3430.
190. Shimizu A, Yamada K, Robson SC, et al. Pathologic characteristics of transplanted kidney xenografts. Journal of the American Society of Nephrology. 2012;23: 225–235.
191. Hering BJ, Walawalkar N. Pig-to-nonhuman primate islet xenotransplantation. Transplant Immunology. 2009;21:81–86.
192. Dufrane D, Gianello P. Pig islets for clinical islet xenotransplantation. Current Opinion in Nephrology and Hypertension. 2009;18:495–500.
193. Bennet W, Sundberg B, Groth CG, et al. Incompatibility between human blood and isolated islets of Langerhans: a finding with implications for clinical intraportal islet transplantation? Diabetes. 1999;48:1907–1914.
194. Nilsson B, Ekdahl KN, Korsgren O. Control of instant blood-mediated inflammatory reaction to improve islets of Langerhans engraftment. Current Opinion in Organ Transplantation 2011;16:620–626.
195. Moberg L, Johansson H, Lukinius A, et al. Production of tissue factor by pancreatic islet cells as a trigger of detrimental thrombotic reactions in clinical islet transplantation. Lancet. 2002;360:2039–2045.
196. Piemonti L, Leone BE, Nano R, et al. Human pancreatic islets produce and secrete MCP-1/CCL2: relevance in human islet transplantation. Diabetes. 2002;51: 55–65.
197. Tjernberg J, Ekdahl KN, Lambris JD, et al. Acute antibody-mediated complement activation mediates lysis of pancreatic islets cells and may cause tissue loss in clinical islet transplantation. Transplantation. 2008;85:1193–1199.
198. Eich T, Eriksson O, Lundgren T. Visualization of early engraftment in clinical islet transplantation by positron-emission tomography. New England Journal of Medicine. 2007;356:2754–2755.
199. Eich T, Eriksson O, Sundin A, et al. Positron emission tomography: a real-time tool to quantify early islet engraftment in a preclinical large animal model. Transplantation. 2007;84:893–898.
200. Bennet W, Sundberg B, Lundgren T, et al. Damage to porcine islets of Langerhans after exposure to human blood in vitro, or after intraportal transplantation to cynomologus monkeys: protective effects of sCR1 and heparin. Transplantation. 2000;69:711–719.
201. Kirchhof N, Shibata S, Wijkstrom M, et al. Reversal of diabetes in non-immunosuppressed rhesus macaques by intraportal porcine islet xenografts precedes acute cellular rejection. Xenotransplantation. 2004;11:396–407.
202. Goto M, Tjernberg J, Dufrane D, et al. Dissecting the instant blood-mediated inflammatory reaction in islet xenotransplantation. Xenotransplantation. 2008; 15:225–234.
203. Goto M, Johansson H, Maeda A, et al. Low molecular weight dextran sulfate prevents the instant blood-mediated inflammatory reaction induced by adult porcine islets. Transplantation. 2004;77:741–747.
204. Ji M, Yi S, Smith-Hurst H, et al. The importance of tissue factor expression by porcine NICC in triggering IBMIR in the xenograft setting. Transplantation. 2011;91:841–846.
205. van der Windt DJ, Bottino R, Casu A, et al. Rapid loss of intraportally transplanted islets: an overview of pathophysiology and preventive strategies. Xenotransplantation. 2007;14:288–297.
206. Hering BJ, Wijkstrom M, Graham ML, et al. Prolonged diabetes reversal after intraportal xenotransplantation of wild-type porcine islets in immunosuppressed nonhuman primates. Nature Medicine. 2006;12:301–303.
207. van der Windt DJ, Bottino R, Casu A, et al. Long-term controlled normoglycemia in diabetic non-human primates after transplantation with hCD46 transgenic porcine islets. American Journal of Transplantation. 2009;9:2716–2726.
208. Jung KC, Park CG, Jeon YK, et al. In situ induction of dendritic cell-based T cell tolerance in humanized mice and nonhuman primates. Journal of Experimental Medicine. 2011;208:2477–2488.
209. Cardona K, Milas Z, Strobert E, et al. Engraftment of adult porcine islet xenografts in diabetic nonhuman primates through targeting of costimulation pathways. American Journal of Transplantation. 2007;7:2260–2268.
210. Cardona K, Korbutt GS, Milas Z, et al. Long-term survival of neonatal porcine islets in nonhuman primates by targeting costimulation pathways. Nature Medicine. 2006;12:304–306.
211. Rayat GR, Rajotte RV, Hering BJ, et al. In vitro and in vivo expression of Galalpha-(1,3)Gal on porcine islet cells is age dependent. Journal of Endocrinology. 2003;177:127–135.
212. Thompson P, Badell IR, Lowe M, et al. Islet xenotransplantation using gal-deficient neonatal donors improves engraftment and function. American Journal of Transplantation. 2011;11:2593–2602.
213. Sun Y, Ma X, Zhou D, et al. Normalization of diabetes in spontaneously diabetic cynomologus monkeys by xenografts of microencapsulated porcine islets without immunosuppression. Journal of Clinical Investigation. 1996;98: 1417–1422.
214. Dufrane D, Goebbels RM, Gianello P. Alginate macroencapsulation of pig islets allows correction of streptozotocin-induced diabetes in primates up to 6 months without immunosuppression. Transplantation. 2010;90:1054–1062.
215. Schumacher JM, Ellias SA, Palmer EP, et al. Transplantation of embryonic porcine mesencephalic tissue in patients with PD. Neurology. 2000;54:1042–1050.
216. Larsson LC, Corbascio M, Pearson TC, et al. Induction of operational tolerance to discordant dopaminergic porcine xenografts. Transplantation. 2003;75:1448–1454.
217. Leveque X, Cozzi E, Naveilhan P, et al. Intracerebral xenotransplantation: recent findings and perspectives for local immunosuppression. Current Opinion in Organ Transplantation 2011;16:190–194.
218. Kim MK, Wee WR, Park CG, et al. Xenocorneal transplantation. Current Opinion in Organ Transplantation 2011;16:231–236.
219. Hara H, Cooper DK. Xenotransplantation–the future of corneal transplantation? Cornea. 2011;30:371–378.
220. Amano S, Shimomura N, Kaji Y, et al. Antigenicity of porcine cornea as xenograft. Current Eye Research. 2003;26:313–318.
221. Pan Z, Sun C, Jie Y, et al. WZS-pig is a potential donor alternative in corneal xenotransplantation. Xenotransplantation. 2007;14:603–611.
222. Li A, Pan Z, Jie Y, et al. Comparison of immunogenicity and porcine-to-rhesus lamellar corneal xenografts survival between fresh preserved and dehydrated porcine corneas. Xenotransplantation. 2011;18:46–55.
223. Choi HJ, Kim MK, Lee HJ, et al. Efficacy of pig-to-rhesus lamellar corneal xenotransplantation. Investigative Ophthalmology and Visual Science. 2011;52:6643–6650.
224. Hargrave SL, Mayhew E, Hegde S, et al. Are corneal cells susceptible to antibody-mediated killing in corneal allograft rejection? Transplant Immunology. 2003;11:79–89.
225. Platt JL, Vercellotti GM, Dalmasso AP, et al. Transplantation of discordant xenografts: a review of progress. Immunology Today. 1990;11:450–456; discussion 6-7.
226. Fischel RJ, Matas AJ, Platt JL, et al. Cardiac xenografting in the pig-to-rhesus monkey model: manipulation of antiendothelial antibody prolongs survival. Journal of Heart and Lung Transplantation. 1992;11:965–973; discussion 73-4.
227. Dorling A. Transplant accommodation-are the lessons learned from xenotransplantation pertinent for clinical allotransplantation? American Journal of Transplantation. 2012; 12:545–553.
228. Lynch RJ, Platt JL. Accommodation in renal transplantation: unanswered questions. Current Opinion in Organ Transplantation. 2010;15:481–485.
229. Dalmasso AP, Benson BA, Johnson JS, et al. Resistance against the membrane attack complex of complement induced in porcine endothelial cells with a Gal alpha(1-3)Gal binding lectin: up-regulation of CD59 expression. Journal of Immunology. 2000;164:3764–3773.
230. Ding JW, Zhou T, Ma L, et al. Expression of complement regulatory proteins in accommodated xenografts induced by anti-alpha-Gal IgG1 in a rat-to-mouse model. American Journal of Transplantation. 2008;8:32–40.
231. Lin Y, Soares MP, Sato K, et al. Accommodated xenografts survive in the presence of anti-donor antibodies and complement that precipitate rejection of naive xenografts. Journal of Immunology. 1999;163:2850–2857.
232. Sachs DH, Sykes M, Yamada K. Achieving tolerance in pig-to-primate xenotransplantation: reality or fantasy. Transplant Immunology. 2009;21:101–105.
233. Lan P, Wang L, Diouf B, et al. Induction of human T-cell tolerance to porcine xenoantigens through mixed hematopoietic chimerism. Blood. 2004;103: 3964–3969.
234. Habiro K, Sykes M, Yang YG. Induction of human T-cell tolerance to pig xenoantigens via thymus transplantation in mice with an established human immune system. American Journal of Transplantation. 2009;9:1324–1329.
235. Buhler L, Awwad M, Treter S, et al. Pig hematopoietic cell chimerism in baboons conditioned with a nonmyeloablative regimen and CD154 blockade. Transplantation. 2002;73:12–22.
236. Tseng YL, Dor FJ, Kuwaki K, et al. Bone marrow transplantation from alpha1,3-galactosyltransferase gene-knockout pigs in baboons. Xenotransplantation. 2004;11:361–370.

237. Griesemer A, Liang F, Hirakata A, et al. Occurrence of specific humoral non-responsiveness to swine antigens following administration of GalT-KO bone marrow to baboons. Xenotransplantation. 2010;17:300–312.
238. Barth RN, Yamamoto S, LaMattina JC, et al. Xenogeneic thymokidney and thymic tissue transplantation in a pig-to-baboon model: I. Evidence for pig-specific T-cell unresponsiveness. Transplantation. 2003;75:1615–1624.
239. Nishimura H, Scalea J, Wang Z, et al. First experience with the use of a recombinant CD3 immunotoxin as induction therapy in pig-to-primate xenotransplantation: the effect of T-cell depletion on outcome. Transplantation. 2011;92: 641–647.
240. Londrigan SL, Sutherland RM, Brady JL, et al. In situ protection against islet allograft rejection by CTLA4Ig transduction. Transplantation. 2010;90: 951–957.
241. Akamaru Y, Ito T, Uchikoshi F, et al. Ex vivo and systemic transfer of adenovirus-mediated CTLA4Ig gene combined with a short course of FK506 therapy prolongs islet graft survival. Transplant Immunology. 2003;11:91–100.
242. Laumonier T, Potiron N, Boeffard F, et al. CTLA4Ig adenoviral gene transfer induces long-term islet rat allograft survival, without tolerance, after systemic but not local intragraft expression. Human Gene Therapy. 2003;14:561–575.
243. Sutherland RM, Brady JL, Georgiou HM, et al. Protective effect of CTLA4Ig secreted by transgenic fetal pancreas allografts. Transplantation. 2000;69: 1806–1812.
244. Phelps CJ, Ball SF, Vaught TD, et al. Production and characterization of transgenic pigs expressing porcine CTLA4-Ig. Xenotransplantation. 2009;16:477–485.
245. Hering BJ, Cooper DK, Cozzi E, et al. The International Xenotransplantation Association consensus statement on conditions for undertaking clinical trials of porcine islet products in type 1 diabetes– executive summary. Xenotransplantation. 2009;16:196–202.
246. Miwa Y, Kobayashi T, Nagasaka T, et al. Are N-glycolylneuraminic acid (Hanganutziu-Deicher) antigens important in pig-to-human xenotransplantation? Xenotransplantation. 2004;11:247–253.
247. Taylor RE, Gregg CJ, Padler-Karavani V, et al. Novel mechanism for the generation of human xeno-autoantibodies against the nonhuman sialic acid N-glycolylneuraminic acid. Journal of Experimental Medicine. 2010;207: 1637–1646.
248. Padler-Karavani V, Varki A. Potential impact of the non-human sialic acid N-glycolylneuraminic acid on transplant rejection risk. Xenotransplantation. 2011;18:1–5.
249. Spiezia L, Bertini D, Boldrin M, et al. Reference values for thromboelastometry (ROTEM(R)) in cynomolgus monkeys (Macaca fascicularis). Thrombosis Research. 2010;126:e294–e297.
250. Graham ML, Bellin MD, Papas KK, et al. Species incompatibilities in the pig-to-macaque islet xenotransplant model affect transplant outcome: a comparison with allotransplantation. Xenotransplantation. 2011;18:328–342.
251. Byrne GW, Du Z, Sun Z, et al. Changes in cardiac gene expression after pig-to-primate orthotopic xenotransplantation. Xenotransplantation. 2011;18:14–27.
252. Klose R, Kemter E, Bedke T, et al. Expression of biologically active human TRAIL in transgenic pigs. Transplantation. 2005;80:222–230.
253. Cho B, Koo OJ, Hwang JI, et al. Generation of soluble human tumor necrosis factor-alpha receptor 1-Fc transgenic pig. Transplantation. 2011;92:139–147.
254. Petersen B, Ramackers W, Lucas-Hahn A, et al. Transgenic expression of human heme oxygenase-1 in pigs confers resistance against xenograft rejection during ex vivo perfusion of porcine kidneys. Xenotransplantation. 2011;18: 355–368.
255. Hauschild J, Petersen B, Santiago Y, et al. Efficient generation of a biallelic knock-out in pigs using zinc-finger nucleases. Proceedings of the National Academy of Sciences of the United States of America. 2011;108:12013–12017.
256. Garrels W, Mates L, Holler S, et al. Germline transgenic pigs by Sleeping Beauty transposition in porcine zygotes and targeted integration in the pig genome. PLoS ONE. 2011;6:e23573.
257. Fisicaro N, Londrigan SL, Brady JL, et al. Versatile co-expression of graft-protective proteins using 2A-linked cassettes. Xenotransplantation. 2011;18: 121–130.

第 13 章 同种异体反应性的体外模型

Charles A. Su, Anna Valujskikh, William M. Baldwin III, Robert L. Fairchild

引言

移植必定是一项体内操作。同种异体移植作为终末期心、肺、肝、肾疾病或糖尿病的一项治愈性方法，伴随着复杂炎症反应及排斥移植物的免疫反应。首先，供体器官缺血保存时间的长短，通过在再灌注期间由移植的内皮细胞及移植的其他细胞产生的反应性氧自由基，进一步刺激急性期细胞因子产生的过程，决定了早期炎症的强度[1,2]。第二，这些氧自由基及细胞因子不仅介导了移植组织的直接损伤，也通过刺激白细胞趋化因子，及上调移植内皮细胞上细胞黏附因子表达密切参与到炎症反应，黏附因子具有协同引导先天性免疫成分（如中性粒细胞、单核细胞、巨噬细胞、树突状细胞）至移植物以及它们的激活至表达介导移植组织损伤的功能。第三，这种对异体移植早期炎症先天性应答，其后表达供体异体抗原特异性受体的内源性记忆T细胞浸润，及移植物内记忆T细胞的激活使炎症反应及组织损伤进一步加重[3,4]。这种初始的炎症反应也可激活移植呈递白细胞和初级间质树突状细胞，使其从移植物转移到受体负责异体抗原反应T及B细胞克隆增殖及分化成效应细胞的次级淋巴器官[2,5]。这些初级效应T细胞转移至移植物后被重新激活并表达介导急性和（或）慢性移植组织损伤的功能。这一系列过程在第5章有详细的描述[6]。激活的B细胞表达供体抗原对应的表面免疫球蛋白受体，使它们分化成为抗体生成细胞、成浆细胞或浆细胞，及抗体与移植内皮细胞及其他细胞靶供体抗原结合以多种机制（详见第6章）损伤组织[7,8]。

许多步骤，如缺血再灌注损伤及从固有免疫到供体抗原特异性介导的炎症反应及致移植组织损伤的一系列反应，都需要使用体内模型进行有效的研究，因为这些过程涉及无法使用体外模型模拟的复杂的物质及反应。然而，体外实验提供了许多证据有助于对移植细胞及器官的体内反应进行更深刻的了解。本章将详细描述我们可以通过体外实验了解到同种异体免疫反应的定义及特征中的哪些方面。

刺激同种异体反应性T细胞增殖

最初探究T细胞同种异体反应性机制时，确定了细胞表达同种异体免疫复合物分子来激活并驱动T细胞的体外增殖[9-11]。这项发现促成了杂交淋巴细胞反应（MLR）的发展，其可以验证T细胞对同种异体性刺激细胞的反应过程的存在及强度。这种理论中，原始T细胞与表达Ⅰ级或Ⅱ级同种异体性免疫复合物分子的刺激细胞共同培养。同种异体性刺激细胞通常通过辐射或有丝分裂抑制处理来进行灭活，灭活后就可以更精确地检测到T细胞的激活及增殖。T细胞受体通过$CD4^+$或$CD8^+$应答细胞与Ⅰ级或Ⅱ级同种异体性免疫复合物分子相结合，引发T细胞激活后产生生长因子、初级白细胞介素2及表达生长因子的高敏感性受体。这导致了细胞循环的进程及同种异体性T细胞增殖。此理论中最初检测到了T细胞的增殖，方法是在培养最后24小时加入^3H胸腺嘧啶核苷，之后评估^3H胸腺嘧啶核苷整合入DNA的细胞数量作为细胞增殖的指标。原始T细胞或未接触抗原的T细胞增殖的最佳观察时间是在开始培养后的4~5天，而记忆T细胞的增殖在培养开始后的1~2天就能观察到。

近来，使用^3H胸腺嘧啶核苷来评估T细胞增殖的方法被使用可保留在应答细胞内的荧光染料标记应答 T 细胞的方法所取代，因此最常使用的染料是羟基荧光素琥珀酰亚胺酯(CFSE)[12]。CFSE 是羟基荧光素双乙酸盐琥珀酸亚胺酯(CFDA-SE)的衍生物。非荧光性 CFDA-SE 具有高细胞透过性并可以进入细胞质。细胞内酯酶去除醋酸基团并将分子转化为羟基荧光素衍生物 CFSE,CFSE 通过共价键结合细胞内的赖氨酸残基及其他氨基酸停留在细胞内。当应答 T 细胞分裂时,每经过一个增殖周期,细胞内染料的量在子细胞内就会减半(图 13.1)。因此,不分裂的细胞与可分裂的细胞可以通过流式细胞仪测量 CFSE 稀释的程度区分出来。将应答 T 细胞与自体同源/自体细胞作为刺激物一起进行培养时,加以适当的控制,就能够评估其自然增殖的过程。这不仅对于检测同种异体反应性应答 T 细胞增殖方面是一项重要的进展,而且对于明确完成了几次增殖周期及详细研究不分裂 T 细胞与可分裂 T 细胞的特性也非常重要。Wells 及同事完成了一系列研究[13],使用多克隆 T 细胞受体(TCR)拮抗剂抗 CD3m 抗体来激活 CFSE 标记的 T 细胞,发现 T 细胞进入增殖细胞池的效率是通过 TCR 调节，但加入 CD28 介导的共同刺激后可同时调节应答细胞的效率及分裂周期的次数。另外，这项研究可以联合抗体示踪来检测特异性细胞表面分子,如细胞激活标记物 CD11a、CD44 和(或)CD69,或是细胞内细胞因子产物,因此每个增殖应答周期内的细胞均可以对特异的激活和分化标志物进行研究[14]。CSFE 标记技术已经被广泛地应用在多种动物及人体同种异体抗原诱导的 T 细胞增殖的独立研究中[15-17]。

增殖以外，培养的同种异体刺激细胞激活 T 细胞的功能性特征可以通过多种不同的方法测量。这些方法包括使用酶联免疫吸附测定(ELISA)测算 MLR 培养中上层清液因子产量，或对放射性或 CFSE 标记的同种异体性靶细胞使用细胞溶解法测定。另外,酶联免疫吸附标记(ELISPOT)法可以用来计算同种异体性 T 细胞对同种异体刺激细胞产生应答时产生的特异性细胞因子(图 13.2)。在这种方法中,应答 T 细胞及同种异体刺激细胞将在包裹有需要测定的细胞因子的特异性抗体的滤器中进行培养。经过 24~72 小时的培养,将细胞从滤器上洗脱,并加入所测定细胞因子的第二种抗体,

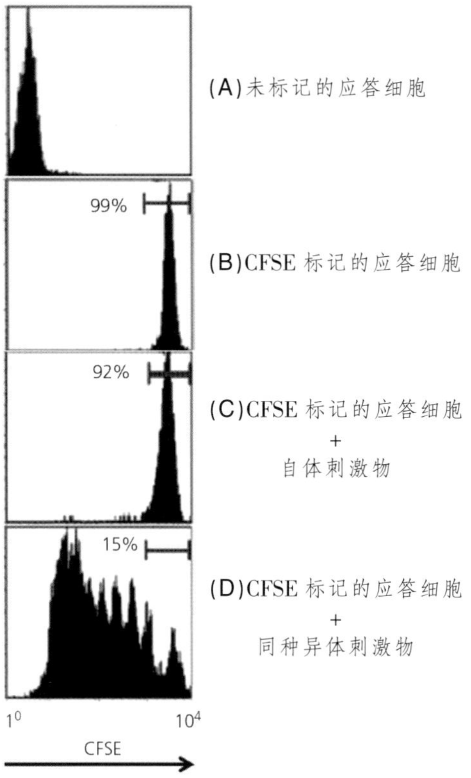

图 13.1 通过体外 CFSE 稀释法检测同种异体反应性 T 细胞的增殖。将等量的未标记(A)或 CFSE 标记(B~D)的应答 T 细胞等分到培养板中。然后用单纯培养基(B)或自体(C)或同种异体刺激细胞(D)对应答 T 细胞进行刺激。培养 3 天后,收获应答细胞,并通过流式细胞仪稀释 CFSE 评估其增殖。

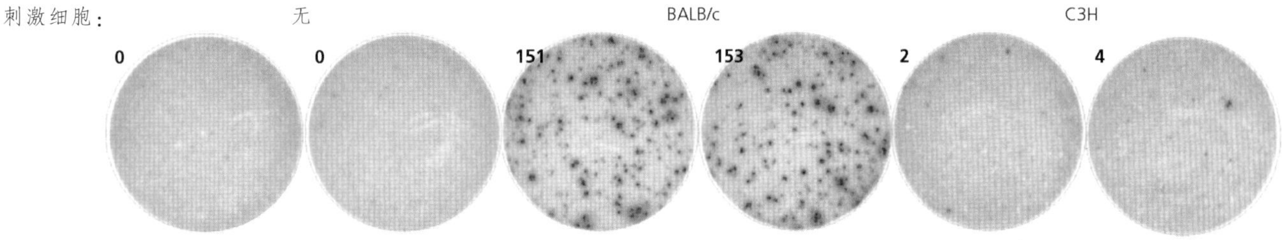

图 13.2 ELISPOT 法。从接受 BALB/c(H-2[d])小鼠心脏同种异体移植的 B6(H-2[b])受体小鼠中分离的脾细胞使用 IFN-γ ELISPOT 法测试其对 BALB/c 小鼠和第三方 SJL(H-2[s])小鼠刺激细胞的回忆反应。两个孔中每个孔铺有 10 万个细胞。数字代表每个孔中的染色位点数量。

例外是若抗体与可将基质转化为一种可被滤器作为一个位点保留的染色剂偶联则使用读数器对标记进行计数，这代表了同种异体T细胞产生特异性细胞因子的数量。这些进展指出，在未进行控制的培养中，同种异体性抗原激活$CD4^+$及$CD8^+$T细胞促进其分化成为产IFN-γ细胞，$CD8^+$T细胞也分化为表达FasL的细胞并可耐受穿孔素或颗粒酶B介导的对同种异体靶细胞的细胞溶解。但是需要重点注意的是，MLR培养的成分可以进行操控，驱使同种异体抗原特异性T细胞表达其他的功能，以下进行详细讨论。

Lafferty和Cunningham[18]的重要研究引出了同种异体T细胞的激活需要两种信号的假说。体内及体外研究为此种假说提供了支持证据，即原始T细胞被激活分化成为表达不同功能细胞的同时需要TCR复合物及现在被称作共刺激分子两者传递的信号[19]。目前已通过体外实验明确了同种异体抗原呈递细胞刺激下，激活（或抑制）同种异体抗原特异性原始T细胞和记忆T细胞的关键性共刺激分子反应。

体外实验研究首先被用在证明单克隆抗人CD28抗体激动剂和抗CD3抗体在激活人T细胞产生IL-2及增殖中的协同作用，进而确定了激活人T细胞需要CD28的刺激[20-22]。后续研究证明，同种异体性人T细胞的激活依赖于CD28-B7（如B7-1/B7-2或CD80/CD86）的相互作用，即转染B7缺陷性同种异体性刺激细胞使其表达CD28的配合基[23]。Peter Linsley及其同事[24]发现了由T细胞表达的另一种B7分子的配合基——CTLA-4，和一种生成的融合蛋白——CTLA-4Ig，可抑制人同种异体反应性T细胞在MLR增殖，及CD4T助手细胞为体外B细胞产生抗体的信号呈递过程。这些研究为Turka及其同事的发现提供了重要的线索，他们证明了CTLA-4Ig可以延长MHC错配的挪威小鼠心脏进行同种异体移植到Lewis小鼠受体的生存期[25]。在20年间，这些初步的体外研究明确了T细胞表达的CD28及CTLA-4的分子结构及特性，以及它们与抗原呈递细胞上CD80/86分子的相互作用，这些发现促进了一种新的修饰过的CTLA-4Ig——贝拉西普的发现，此种物质在改善肾移植患者移植肾预后方面表现出了很好的效果[26,27]。

自从发现了CD28-CD80/86介导的共刺激反应，学者推测还有更多的共刺激腺受体对可疑正向或负向影响同种异体性T细胞的激活[19]。这些T细胞及其抗原呈递细胞上的配体的额外正性或负性共刺激分子的识别和功能，需要使用曾用来探究CD28/CTLA-4分子及相关配体CD80/CD86结构及功能的体外实验进行进一步研究。

同种异体抗原呈递至T细胞

同种异体抗原可被T细胞通过三种呈递通路进行识别，之后诱导增殖、激活标志物的表达及移植物损伤特异性功能的表达[28-32]。根据TCR的特异性，同种异体反应性T细胞可通过直接通路识别供体抗原呈递细胞上的多肽/同种异体性Ⅰ级或Ⅱ级MHC复合物，或通过间接通路识别自身抗原呈递细胞上的MHC复合体呈递的供体同种异体性多肽。在后一种情况中，来源于移植物同种异体性MHC复合物分子的多肽或等位基因变异的其他蛋白，被获取、加工并被宿主或自身抗原呈递细胞呈递。另外，宿主抗原呈递细胞多可通过移植物细胞释放的外含小体获取完整的多肽/同种异体性MHC复合物，外含小体进入细胞膜并通过半直接通路呈递给表达同种异体性多肽/MHC复合物特异性受体的T细胞。

通过直接或间接通路呈递的同种异体抗原特异性T细胞，可以通过多种不同的体外方法进行检测及研究。基本上，这样的方法必须使用纯化T细胞，纯化T细胞会在与适当的抗原呈递细胞及抗原一起培养时发生应答。对于通过直接通路进行应答的同种异体反应性T细胞，此过程仅涉及纯化T细胞与表达同种异体性Ⅰ级和（或）Ⅱ级MHC分子的抗原呈递细胞共同培养，例如与同种异体性供体或同种异体性肿瘤细胞隔离。在监测和（或）测量通过直接通路应答的T细胞时，一起加入纯化的同源性抗原呈递细胞与同种异体性蛋白、多肽、异体移植物的无细胞组织匀浆、来自同种异体性MHC分子或其他靶细胞的同源性多肽。这些培养方法可以像前文讨论过的用来测量应答T细胞的增殖，或是其激活产生可通过ELISA或ELISPOT检测到的细胞因子。通过使用这些体外实验方法来检测从MHC错配的同种异体移植受者分离出的T细胞，Benichou及其同事[31]发现，从移植到急性移植物排斥反应期间分离出的大部分（>90%）同种异体反应性T细胞都是通过直接同种异体抗原呈递通路。

因为后文所述的原因，可应答多肽/同种异体性MHC复合物的T细胞占全部细胞的比例大概是$1/10^4$~

1/10，而可应答自身 MHC 分子呈递的同种异体性多肽的 T 细胞与应答自身 MHC 分子呈递的其他外源性多肽的 T 细胞占总体的比例相同，均小于 $1/10^5$。因此，同种异体反应性 T 细胞通过直接呈递通路应答的强度要远高于间接通路，并且通常主要是由对同种异体移植强而初级的同种免疫应答组成，此反应构成了强效的移植免疫抑制反应。

对于同种异体反应性前体出现频率的分析

供体内重组使用的 α 和 β 链基因片段的数量，以及核酸交叉插入产生的额外的多样性，可以导致在胸腺中产生多于 $1×10^{13}$ 个不同的 α/β TCR 或 T 细胞克隆[33]。大量的 T 细胞克隆保证了个体在面对大多数病原体时的最佳免疫保护能力。除了产生具有广泛多样性的对病原体的保护反应潜力外，必须从整体中筛选去除具有高自体多肽/MHC 复合物反应性的克隆，这样就降低了自身免疫疾病的风险。T 细胞在胸腺中整体发展的过程，结合了高亲和性自身多肽/MHC 复合物的 TCR，诱导信号导致胸腺细胞死亡，防止 T 细胞克隆脱离胸腺并种植在外周 T 细胞群中。这些事件在第 2 章中有详细的描述。或者，胸腺细胞表达无法结合自身多肽/MHC 复合物的 TCR，不被给予细胞生存所需的信号，并且这些“没用的”克隆也从细胞群中移除。只有胸腺细胞表达的 TCR 可以“中度”紧密地结合自身多肽/MHC 复合物，被给予了适当的促进细胞存活的细胞间信号并种植在外周 T 细胞群中。

关于同种异体免疫反应，重点是认识到胸腺细胞的发育过程中，仅会去除对自身多肽/MHC 复合物反应性强的细胞，而不会去除对多肽/同种异体性 MHC 复合物反应性强的细胞。因为 T 细胞受体的进化，赋予了 T 细胞受体天生的对多肽/MHC 复合物的亲和性，被选择与自身多肽/MHC 复合物结合的 TCR 具有对多肽/MHC 复合物的强反应性，并且导致了对在培养及同种异体移植中表达多肽/同种异体性 MHC 复合物的抗原呈递细胞的强大应答。测量大鼠及人类外周 T 细胞群中对明确的同种异体性 MHC 分子发生反应的 T 细胞准确的出现频率，是目前 T 细胞及移植免疫生理学积极研究的领域。之前的研究使用了限制性稀释分析法来研究小鼠和人 $CD4^+$或 $CD8^+$T 细胞的增殖或对明确的同种异体性刺激细胞的细胞毒性测定[34-38]。这些研究进展明确了可应答任何不同的 MHC 单体差异的 T 细胞的概率约为 0.2%~2%。而另一种研究方法使用免疫应答多种蛋白抗原 T 细胞生成的 T 细胞克隆，测试一组结合了不同 MHC 单体的同种异体性抗原呈递细胞能否激活增殖进程，结果显示所有的克隆均有对一种或多种同种异体性刺激细胞的反应性[39]。后来，有学者使用 CFSE 增殖法来测定同种异体性 MHC 分子相关 T 细胞的比例[40,41]。总而言之，同种异体性多肽/MHC 复合物相关 T 细胞的前驱比例比外来多肽/自体 MHC 复合物特异性 T 细胞高 3~4 个数量级，后者通常为 $1:10^5$~$1:10^6$，且此数据与同种异体反应性 T 细胞应答的强度相关。这些内容已在第 9 章详细描述。

这些研究促进了对 T 细胞受体与多肽/同种异体性 MHC 分子在直接同种异体抗原呈递过程中发生的具体内容相关的研究[42]。在此之前，学术界尚不明确 $CD8^+$细胞上的 TCR 异质二聚体蛋白与同种异体性 MHC 分子以多种灵活的方式结合是否与Ⅰ级 MHC 分子的 α 螺旋槽内呈递的多肽无关，或是 T 细胞受体与同种异体性Ⅰ级 MHC 分子的反应也依赖于凹槽内呈递的特异性多肽。早先的晶体学研究指出，T 细胞受体蛋白与多肽/自体Ⅰ级 MHC 复合物的反应过程和它与多肽/同种异体性Ⅰ级 MHC 分子反应时相似，即 T 细胞受体异质二聚体成斜角接触多肽/MHC 复合物平面，之后 T 细胞受体的 CDR3 区域结合多肽[43]。然而，T 细胞受体与多肽/同种异体性Ⅰ级 MHC 复合物间反应时会有更多灵活的对接角度[44]。另外，至少一类可与多肽/自身Ⅱ级 MHC 复合物反应的 T 细胞受体亦可以与同种异体性Ⅰ级及Ⅱ级 MHC 复合物呈递的多肽发生反应（见第 9 章）[45]。目前已将晶体学分析与前文讨论过的 T 细胞激活测定联合起来测定特定的 T 细胞受体，即人 T 细胞上对病毒多肽/HLA-B 分子有反应性且对具有相同结合结构同种异体性多肽/同种异体性 HLA-B 复合物有反应性的受体，表明在一些案例中 TCR 同种异体反应性的结构基础是分子拟态而不是物理上改变 TCR 与多肽/MHC 复合物的结合方式[46]。

原始 T 细胞与记忆 T 细胞对同种异体抗原增殖的比较

单个个体的 T 淋巴细胞库中包括原始 T 细胞和记

忆T细胞,记忆T细胞的比例随着年龄增加,反映了接触抗原经历的积累。移植过程中的原始及记忆T淋巴细胞从功能上、存在空间上及时间上都与平时不同。与原始T细胞不同,记忆T细胞可以再次暴露在相同抗原发起的更快更强的免疫应答,因为记忆T细胞具有更高的效率,可提高对抗原的功能活动性,且对共同刺激要求低[4,47]。尽管原始T淋巴细胞仅分布在次级淋巴器官,记忆T细胞自身也不尽相同,目前已经在人类和啮齿类动物身上发现两个记忆位点。这些位点被标为①主要存在于淋巴组织的中心记忆T细胞;和②存在于淋巴及非淋巴组织中的效应记忆T细胞[48]。重要的是,临床研究指出,记忆T细胞对于免疫抑制治疗造成的T细胞耗竭具有更高的耐受性,因为免疫抑制治疗会显著减少原始T细胞的数量[49,50]。

移植受体体内存在对同种异体性MHC分子具有活性的预存记忆T细胞已经被广泛认识,它被认为是诱导及保持耐受的主要屏障[47]。同种异体特异性记忆T细胞的生成是由于曾暴露于既往移植、输血或者妊娠带来的同种异体抗原。然而,未被既往同种异体抗原致敏过的个体也拥有同种异体反应性记忆T细胞。这些个体中同种异体特异性记忆的产生与直接同种异体抗原暴露无关,其产生被认为是通过异种免疫反应(在第9章中有详细介绍),即记忆T细胞的诱导是通过先前环境暴露完成的,如病毒、细菌及疫苗,然后与无关的抗原——如同种异体抗原发生交叉反应并被激活[51,52]。此原理已经通过小鼠暴露在淋巴性脉络丛脑膜炎病毒(LCMV)及利什曼原虫等病原体的实验中进行了证明[53,54]。对啮齿类动物、非人灵长类动物及人类的体外实验研究为理解原始T细胞如何应答同种异体抗原并分化成为记忆T细胞提供了重要证据。

体外实验研究使用小鼠模型证明了以每一个细胞为基础,抗原特异性记忆T细胞与抗原特异性原始T细胞相比,具有更不严格的激活要求及更强的激活效果。TCR转基因小鼠的发展,即CD4⁺或CD8⁺T细胞表达一种对某个特定的多肽抗原/MHC复合物具有特异性的TCR,使一对一比较对某个特定同种异体抗原具有特异性的记忆T细胞及原始T细胞成为可能。使用这种TCR转基因系统,可发现在体外同源抗原刺激下同种异体抗原特异性CD8⁺记忆T细胞相比原始CD8⁺T细胞激活更迅速,尽管TCR及CD8水平相同[55]。通过ELISA分析培养上清液,发现记忆CD8⁺T细胞相比原始CD8⁺T细胞分泌IFN-γ及IL-2的速度更快且数量更多。另外,体外实验使用铬释放法测量细胞溶解活动时发现记忆CD8⁺T细胞具有明显的细胞溶解性,而原始CD8⁺T细胞则没有[55,56]。原始T细胞需要专门的抗原呈递细胞(APC)——如树突状细胞提供的CD28/B7介导的共同刺激,而记忆细胞可以在没有CD28/B7或者CD40/154通路共同刺激的情况下被完全激活,而且可以更自由地被不同的非专门APC激活——如休眠的B细胞及巨噬细胞[57]。这些发现已经得到体外实验证据支持,记忆同种异体性CD8⁺T细胞可以在与表皮细胞共同培养时被激活、扩增并分化成为细胞毒性T细胞,而原始CD8⁺T细胞则不能[58]。

与实验室小鼠相反,在猴子及人类体内在移植前就存在大量的同种异体反应性记忆T细胞。例如在一项共48只从野外捕捉的猕猴的研究中,记忆T细胞(以表面CD95表达区分)占所有T细胞的将近48%,并均等地分为中枢和效应T细胞[59]。从这些猴子的外周血分离出原始T细胞及记忆T细胞,并通过体外ELISPOT方法计数产细胞因子细胞,来测试这些细胞对同种异体性供体辐照外周血单核细胞的同种异体反应能力。虽然只有少量原始T细胞可进行应答,但预存的内源性记忆T细胞可发生强大的直接同种异体应答,特点是高效分泌IFN-γ及IL-2。另外,与小鼠的研究结果类似,这些体外实验中记忆T细胞产生炎症细胞因子的动力学及总量都明显高于纯化原始T细胞。这些非人灵长类动物数据,通过研究自然生成的内源性同种异体反应性记忆T细胞群体,为记忆T细胞相对于原始T细胞在生理环境下有着更强的动力学及功能提供了证据。

临床上,移植前的患者外周血出现供体反应性记忆T细胞与同种异体移植器官功能延迟恢复及长期预后差相关。与此类细胞出现有关的不良反应在对患者进行观察后有了进一步明确,效应记忆T细胞对T细胞消耗剂如阿仑单抗或兔抗胸腺细胞球蛋白诱导的免疫抑制相对不敏感,而这有效地消耗了原始T细胞[49]。1999年,Heeger及其同事率先利用体外ELISPOT法检测肾移植术前患者外周血中供体特异性产IFN-γ淋巴细胞[60]。ELISPOT法可以在单细胞数量级检测具有免疫启动史的细胞的细胞因子产量,因此可以代表效应/记忆T细胞的供体适应性免疫力。此法检测到的IFN-γ的生成是内源性记忆T细胞的特殊表现,并且发现移植前患者出现这些供体特异性记忆细胞的频率与移植后发生急性排斥的风险明显相关[60,61]。可以使用这种测量方法评估移植前同种异体反应性的强度及预测移植预后，强调了除抗原 MHC 位点错配数量外，预存受体反应性记忆 T 细胞的重要性。尽管如此，通过 ELISPOT 法获得的信息具有临床价值，但是在死亡供体移植的情况下，无法在此方法所需的时间窗内进行测定。

另一种叫作反应性 T 细胞组或是 PRT 的体外方法可作为传统 ELISPOT 法的变种。使用 PRT 法时，检测等待移植患者的外周血 T 细胞对一组同种异体刺激细胞的反应性，而不是检测对供体来源的刺激细胞的反应性。这种同种异体刺激细胞组由数个不同供体的脾细胞产生的 B 细胞系组成，其整体包含了大于 90% 的人 HLA 抗原。患者内源性记忆 T 细胞与各同种异体 B 细胞系共同培养时产生的同种异体反应性应答，可以用 ELISPOT 法计数产生 IFN-γ 的 T 细胞数量，并且移植前 PRT 结果是阳性被发现与甚至在没有体液免疫同种致敏的情况下发生的急性肾移植排斥反应明确相关[62,63]。

体外同种异体反应性 T 细胞的功能发育倾向

除了测定 MHC 同种异体刺激细胞的 T 细胞频率外，此体外方法对于促进同种异体抗原反应性 T 细胞分化为不同的功能表型很有帮助，以便在同种异体反应中测试表达的不同功能造成的影响。

Mossman 及其同事的进一步研究[64,65]表明，在体外激活抗原特异性 $CD4^+T$ 细胞的过程中，T 细胞可分化为产生与延迟型超敏反应相关的 IFN-γ 和淋巴毒素-α(LT-α)(即 1 型细胞因子)的细胞，或是分化为产生与过敏反应相关的 IL-4、IL-5 和 IL-10(即 2 型细胞因子)的细胞，此分化过程取决于在 T 细胞激活培养中的协同因子。鼠 $CD8^+T$ 细胞克隆的体外同种异体抗原激活刺激 IFN-γ 和 LT-α 生成，表明同种异体免疫 $CD8^+$ T 细胞介导的免疫应答可能与延迟型超敏反应相关的功能有重叠[66]。其他实验室的后续研究指出，在抗原呈递细胞膜上产生和（或）表达的因子可使抗原特异性 $CD4^+T$ 细胞倾向于分化成为 Th1 或 Th2 细胞[67,68]。抗原呈递细胞功能依赖性 T 细胞分化为 T1 或 T2 细胞的结果与模型所得一致，模型中抗原呈递细胞激活 $CD4^+T$ 细胞参与细胞介导/延迟型超敏反应时，该免疫位点接收信号以表达包括生成 IL-12 等功能，使分化倾向于 Th1 细胞。类似地，抗原呈递细胞激活 $CD4^+T$ 细胞去参与过敏反应时，将在变应原免疫期间接收信号，诱导产生包括 IL-4 等因子，使分化倾向于 Th2 功能表型[67,68]。在每种情况下，树突细胞来源的信号激活转录因子，转录因子改变反应性 T 细胞的功能分化倾向，其中 T-bet 使其分化为产生 IFN-γ 的 Th1 表型而 GATA-3 使其分化为产生 IL-4 的 Th2 表型[69]。最近，免疫学家发现了 $CD4^+T$ 细胞的其他几个功能亚类，包括表达转录因子 FoxP3 并介导免疫调节的细胞(即 Tregs)以及表达转录因子 RORγT 并产生 IL-17 和 IL-23 的细胞（即 T17）[69]。

关于抗原特异性 $CD4^+T$ 细胞分化趋向的发现促使移植免疫学界去研究不同功能表型的同种异体抗原特异性 T 细胞介导移植物损伤的能力。在加入 IL-2 或 TGF-β 的情况下将纯化的人 $CD4^+T$ 细胞与同种异体刺激细胞共同培养，会促使同种异体反应性 T 细胞成为生成 IL-2 和 IFN-γ 的细胞，而在培养时加入 IL-4、IL-10 或抗 TGF-β 会促使 CD4+T 细胞成为生成 IL-4 和 IL-10 的细胞[70]。Orosz 和 Bishop 通过实验研究了这种 T 细胞功能分化对同种异体移植物预后的影响，比较了体外分化的同种异体反应性 Th1 细胞与 Th2 细胞在小鼠模型中介导排斥反应的能力[71,72]。这些 $CD4^+T$ 细胞与同种异体刺激细胞、适当的细胞因子辅因子和中和抗体共同培养过程中进行分化，随后转移到心脏同种异体移植 SCID 小鼠宿主中。在这些研究中，Th2 细胞与 Th1 细胞等效地介导心脏同种异体移植的快速排斥反应，且同种异体反应性 Th2 细胞介导的排斥伴随着移植物中严重的嗜酸性粒细胞浸润。其他实验室使用相似的方法证明了 Th1 相对 Th2 以不同的组织病理学方式介导移植物排斥的效应功能[73-75]。最近的研究集中于供体反应性 CD^+4 和 $CD8^+T$ 细胞产生 IL-17 以介导同种异体移植物排斥反应的能力，并且已经在实验动物模型和临床移植手术中发现这种细胞引起移植物损伤的能力[76-78]。总体而言，这些研究已经证明了体外分化的 $CD4^+T$ 细胞介导移植损伤的能力，尽管根据移植物内 T 细胞表达的功能不同，造成损伤的具体组织病理学基础可能不同。然而，在同种异体移植受体的同种抗原启动过程中，供体反应性 $CD4^+$和 $CD8^+T$ 细胞应答在很大程度上倾向于产生 IFN-γ 的 Th1 表型，原因很可能是手术造成的组织应激而导致的炎症环境，以及缺血再灌注损伤对移植物的影响。

值得注意的是，许多研究使用了体外方法来诱导T细胞表达对同种异体免疫反应的调节功能[79-81]。这些研究测试了促进分化的各种因素、调节性T细胞的特异性和调节性T细胞表达的抑制同种异体反应性应答的功能。测试调节性T细胞功能的常见体外方法是测量其对同种异体刺激细胞或多克隆有丝分裂原发生应答时抑制同种异体反应性T细胞增殖的能力。这种方法常使用CFSE标记的效应T细胞来评估同种异体反应性T细胞增殖的减少。此外，数个实验室现在正在使用体外方法来培养大量的T调节细胞，用于输注到实验模型和临床移植的胰岛或器官移植受体中[82-85]。

总结

然而，移植仍然是必须在体内进行的步骤，但体外模型一直是研究和阐明免疫系统对同种异体抗体的识别和应答的基本机制的关键工具。体外方法如MLR的发展，对于研究自体多肽/MHC选择的受体T细胞识别同种异体MHC分子的能力非常必要。MLR的修饰及与ELISA和ELISPOT方法联合使用为研究提供了强大的工具，不仅发现了同种异体反应性免疫细胞对同种异体抗原应答而增殖的能力，还发现了其表达包括细胞因子、生长因子和细胞溶解分子等的效应功能，这些功能可导致在体内的移植物损伤和功能障碍。通过使用这种体外模型可获得关于同种异体反应性T细胞应答的知识，其内容已经从移植相关延伸到基础免疫学原理方面，包括免疫细胞的共刺激性需求、原始T细胞和记忆T细胞之间的基础性差异以及各T细胞亚群的发育和分化。重要的是，这样的体外研究不仅为移植中靶向临床治疗提供了新的理解，而且在PRT测定中这些体外工具应用于人体移植之前可有效地评估发生急性排斥的可能性，并在术前评估患者的预后。虽然在过去几十年的移植免疫学研究已经取得了巨大的进展，但手术移植的同种异体器官的免疫反应是一个复杂的过程，许多其他问题仍然没有得到解答。为了充分理解同种异体移植排斥机制和研发靶向治疗方法以改善移植患者预后，体外模型将继续作为必要且宝贵的工具。

（郭颂一 译 李照 校）

参考文献

1. Eltzschig HK, Eckle T. Ischemia and reperfusion-from mechanism to translation. Nature Medicine. 2011;17:1391-1401.
2. Land WG. Emerging role of innate immunity in organ transplantation. Part I: evolution of innate immunity and oxidative allograft injury. Transplantation Reviews. 2012;26:60-72.
3. Schenk AD, Nozaki T, Rabant M, et al. Donor-reactive CD8 memory T cells infiltrate cardiac allografts within 24-h posttransplant in naive recipients. American Journal of Transplantation. 2008;8:1652-1661.
4. Valujskikh A, Baldwin WM III, Fairchild RL. Recent progress and new perspectives in studying T cell responses to allografts. American Journal of Transplantation. 2010;10:1117-1125.
5. Morelli AE, Thomson AW. Tolerogenic dendritic cells and the quest for transplant tolerance. Nature Reviews. Immunology. 2007;7:610-621.
6. Wood KJ, Goto R. Mechanisms of rejection: current perspectives. Transplantation. 2012;93:1-10.
7. Colvin RB, Smith RN. Antibody-mediated organ-allograft rejection. Nature Reviews. Immunology. 2005;5:807-817.
8. Kittleson MM, Kobashigawa JA. Antibody-mediated rejection. Current Opinion in Organ Transplantation. 2012;17:551-557.
9. Bach F, Hirschhorn K. Lymphocyte interaction: a potential histocompatibility test *in vitro*. Science. 1964;143:813-814.
10. Silvers WK, Wison DB, Palm J. Mixed leukocyte reactions and histocompatibility in rats. Science. 1967;155:703-704.
11. Wilson DB, Blyth JL, Nowell PC. Quantitative studies on the mixed lymphocyte interaction in rats. III. Kinetics of response. Journal of Experimental Medicine. 1968;128:1157-1181.
12. Lyons AB. Analysing cell division *in vivo* and *in vitro* using flow cytometric measurement of CFSE dye dilution. Journal of Immunological Methods. 2000;243:147-154.
13. Wells AD, Gudmundsdottir H, Turka LA. Following the fate of individual T cells throughout activation and clonal expansion. Journal of Clinical Investigation. 1997;100:3173-3183.
14. Wells AD, Walsh MC, Sankaran D, et al. T cell effector function and anergy avoidance are quantitatively linked to cell division. Journal of Immunology. 2000;165:2432-2443.
15. Bloom DD, Hu H, Fechner JH, et al. T-lymphocyte alloresponse of Campath-1H-treated kidney transplant patients. Transplantation. 2006;81:81-87.
16. Godfrey WR, Krampf MR, Taylor PA, et al. Ex vivo depletion of alloreactive cells based on CFSE dye dilution, activation antigen selection and dendritic cell stimulation. Blood. 2004;103:1158-1165.
17. Tanaka Y, Ohdan H, Onoe T, et al. Low incidence of acute rejection after living-donor liver transplantation: immunologic analyses by mixed lymphocyte reaction using a carboxyfluorescein diacetate succinimidyl ester labeling technique. Transplantation. 2005;79:1262-1267.
18. Lafferty KJ, Cunningham AJ. A new analysis of allogeneic interactions. Australian Journal of Experimental Biology and Medical Science. 1975;53:27-42.
19. Pilat N, Sayegh M, Wekerle T. Costimulatory pathways in transplantation. Seminars in Immunology. 2011;23:293-303.
20. June CH, Ledbetter JA, Gillespie MM, et al. T-cell proliferation involving the CD28 pathway is associated with cyclosporine-resistant interleukin 2 gene expression. Molecular and Cellular Biology. 1987;7:4472-4481.
21. Lesslauer W, Koning F, Ottenhoff T, et al. T90/44 (9.3 antigen). A cell surface molecule with a function in human T cell activation. European Journal of Immunology. 1986;16:1289-1296.
22. Thompson CB, Lindsten T, Ledbetter JA, et al. C28 activation pathway regulates the production of multiple T-cell-derived lymphokines/cytokines. Proceedings of the National Academy of Sciences of the United States of America. 1989;86:1333-1337.
23. Norton SD, Zuckerman L, Urdahl KB, et al. The CD28 ligand, B7, enhances IL-2 production by providing a costimulatory signal to T cells. Journal of Immunology. 1992;149:1556-1561.
24. Linsley PS, Brady W, Umes M, et al. CTLA-4 is a second receptor for the B cell activation antigen B7. Journal of Experimental Medicine. 1991;174:561-569.
25. Turka LA, Linsley PS, Lin H, et al. T-cell activation by the CD28 ligand B7 is required for cardiac allograft rejection *in vivo*. Proceedings of the National Academy of Sciences of the United States of America. 1992;89:11102-11105.
26. Vincenti F, Larsen C, Durrbach A, et al. Costimulation blockade with Belatacept in renal transplantation. New England Journal of Medicine. 2005;353:770-781.
27. Vincenti F, Larsen CP, Alberu J, et al. Three-year outcomes from BENEFIT, a randomized, active-controlled, parallel-group study in adult kidney transplant recipients. American Journal of Transplantation. 2012;12:210-217.

28. Afzali B, Lombadi G, Lechler RI. Pathways of major histocompatibility complex allorecogntiion. Current Opinion in Organ Transplantation. 2008;13:438–444.
29. Gokmen MR, Lombardi G, Lechler RI. The importance of the indirect pathway of allorecognition in clinical transplantation. Current Opinion in Immunology. 2008;20:568–574.
30. Hornick P. Direct and indirect allorecognition. Methods in Molecular Biology. 2006;333:145–156.
31. Benichou G, Valujskikh A, Heeger PS. Contributions of direct and indirect T cell alloreactivity during allograft rejection in mice. Journal of Immunology. 1999;162:352–358.
32. Heeger PS. T-cell allorecognition and transplant rejection: a summary and update. American Journal of Transplantation. 2003;3:525–533.
33. Nikolich-Zugich J, Slifka MK, Messaoudi I. The many important facets of T-cell repertoire diversity. Nature Reviews. Immunology. 2004;4:123–132.
34. Bishop DK, Orosz CG. Limiting dilution analysis for alloreactive TCGF-secretory T cells. Two related LDA methods that discriminate between unstimulated precursor T cells and *in vivo*-alloactivated T cells. Transplantation. 1989;47:671–677.
35. Lindahl KF, Wilson DB. Histocompatibility antigen-activated cytotoxic T lymphocytes. II. Estimates of the frequency and specificity of precursors. Journal of Experimental Medicine. 1977;145:508–522.
36. Orosz CG, Horstemeyer B, Zinn NE, et al. Development and evaluation of a limiting dilution analysis technique that can discriminate *in vivo* alloactivated cytotoxic T lymphocytes from their naive CTL precursors. Transplantation. 1989;47: 189–194.
37. Sharrock CEM, Man S, Wanachiwanawin W, et al. Analysis of the alloreactive T cell repertoire in man. I. Differences in precursor frequency for cytotoxic T cell responses against allogeneic MHC molecules in unrelated individuals. Transplantation. 1987;43:699–703.
38. Weyand C, Goronzy J, Hammerling GJ. Recognition of polymorphic H-2 domains by T lymphocytes. I. Functional role of different H-2 domains for the generation of alloreactive cytotoxic T lymphocytes and determination of precursor frequencies. Journal of Experimental Medicine. 1981;54:1717–1731.
39. Ashwell JD, Chen C, Schwartz RH. High frequency and nonrandom distribution of alloreactivity in T cell clones selected for recognition of foreign antigen in association with self class II molecules. Journal of Immunology. 1986;136: 389–395.
40. Noorchashm H, Lieu YK, Rostami SY, et al. A direct method for the calculation of alloreactive $CD4^+$ T cell precursor frequency. Transplantation. 1999;67: 1281–1284.
41. Suchin EJ, Langmuir PB, Palmer E, et al. Quantifying the frequency of alloreactive T cells *in vivo*: new answers to old questions. Journal of Immunology. 2001;166: 973–981.
42. Smith C, Miles JJ, Khanna R. Advances in direct T-cell alloreactivity: function, avidity, biophysics and structure. American Journal of Transplantation. 2012;12:15–26.
43. Colf LA, Bankovich AJ, Hanick NA, et al. How a single T cell receptor recognizes both self and foreign MHC. Cell. 2007;129:135–146.
44. Felix NJ, Allen PM. Specificity of T-cell alloreactivity. Nature Reviews. Immunology. 2007;7:942–953.
45. Yin L, Huseby E, Scott-Browne J, et al. A single T cell receptor bound to major histocompatibility complex class I and class II glycoproteins reveals switchable TCR conformers. Immunity. 2011;35:23–33.
46. Macdonald WA, Chen Z, Gras S, et al. T cell allorecognition via molecular mimicry. Immunity. 2009;31:897–908.
47. Valujskikh A. Targeting T-cell memory: where do we stand? Current Opinion in Organ Transplantation. 2008;13:344–349.
48. Lanzavecchia A, Sallusto F. Understanding the generation and function of memory T cell subsets. Current Opinion in Immunology. 2005;17:326–332.
49. Pearl JP, Parris J, Hale DA, et al. Immunocompetent T-cells with a memory-like phenotype are the dominant cell type following antibody-mediated T-cell depletion. American Journal of Transplantation. 2005;5:465–474.
50. Zeevi A, Husain S, Spichty KJ, et al. Recovery of functional memory T cells in lung transplant recipients following induction therapy with alemtuzumab. American Journal of Transplantation. 2007;7:471–475.
51. Ford ML, Larsen CP. Overcoming the memory barrier in tolerance induction: molecular mimicry and functional heterogeneity among pathogen-specific T-cell populations. Current Opinion in Organ Transplantation. 2010;15:405–410.
52. Selin LK, Brehm MA, Naumov YN, et al. Memory of mice and men: $CD8^+$ T-cell cross-reactivity and heterologous immunity. Immunological Reviews. 2006; 211:164–181.
53. Patenburg B, Heinzel F, Das L, et al. T cells primed by Leishmania major infection cross-react with alloantigens and alter the course of allograft rejection. Journal of Immunology. 2002;169:3686–3693.
54. Adams AB, Williams MR, Jones TR, et al. Heterologous immunity provides a potent barrier to transplantation tolerance. Journal of Clinical Investigation. 2003;111:1887–1895.
55. Cho BK, Wang C, Sugawa S, et al. Functional differences between memory and naive CD8 T cells. Proceedings of the National Academy of Sciences of the United States of America. 1999;96:2976–2981.
56. Kedl RM, Mescher MF. Qualitative differences between naive and memory T cells make a major contribution to the more rapid and efficient memory CD8+ T cell response. Journal of Immunology. 1998;161:674–683.
57. Bingaman AW, Farber DL. Memory T cells in transplantation: generation, function, and potential role in rejection. American Journal of Transplantation. 2004;4:846–852.
58. Dengler TJ, Pober JS. Human vascular endothelial cells stimulate memory but not naive $CD8^+$ T cells to differentiate into CTL retaining an early activation phenotype. Journal of Immunology. 2000;164:5146–5155.
59. Nadazdin O, Boskovic S, Murakami T, O'Conner DH, et al. Phenotype, distribution and alloreactive properties of memory T cells from cynomolgus monkeys. American Journal of Transplantation. 2010;10:1375–1384.
60. Heeger PS, Greenspan NS, Kuhlenschmidt S, et al. Pretransplant frequency of donor-specific, IFN-gamma-producing lymphocytes is a manifestation of immunologic memory and correlates with the risk of post-transplant rejection episodes. Journal of Immunology. 1999;163:2267–2275.
61. Augustine JJ, Siu DS, Clemente MJ, et al. Pre-transplant IFN-gamma ELISPOTs are associated with post-transplant renal function in African American renal transplant recipients. American Journal of Transplantation. 2005;5: 1971–1975.
62. Poggio ED, Augustine JJ, Clemente M, et al. Pretransplant cellular alloimmunity as assessed by a panel of reactive T cells assay correlates with acute renal graft rejection. Transplantation. 2007;83:847–852.
63. Poggio ED, Clemente M, Hricik DE, et al. Panel of reactive T cells as a measurement of primed cellular alloimmunity in kidney transplant candidates. Journal of the American Society of Nephrology. 2006;17:564–572.
64. Cher DJ, Mosmann TR. Two types of murine helper T cell clone. II. Delayed-type hypersensitivity is mediated by TH1 clones. Journal of Immunology. 1987;138: 3688–3694.
65. Mosmann TR, Cherwinski H, Bond MW, et al. Two types of murine helper T cell clone. I. Definition according to profiles of lymphokine activities and secreted proteins. Journal of Immunology. 1986;136:2348–2357.
66. Fong TA, Mosmann TA. Alloreactive murine $CD8^+$ T cell clones secrete the Th1 pattern of cytokines. Journal of Immunology. 1990;144:1744–1752.
67. Hsieh CS, Macatonia S, Tripp C, et al. Development of Th1 $CD4^+$ T cells through IL-12 produced by *Listeria*-induced macrophages. Science. 1993;260: 547–549.
68. Seder RA, Gazzinelli R, Sher A, et al. IL-12 acts directly on $CD4^+$ T cells to enhance priming for IFN-γ production and diminishes IL-4 inhibition on such priming. Proceedings of the National Academy of Sciences of the United States of America. 1993;90:10188–10192.
69. Kanno Y, Vahedi G, Hirahara K, et al. Transcriptional and epigenetic control of T helper cell specification: molecular mechanisms underlying commitment and plasticity. Annual Review of Immunology. 2012;30:707–731.
70. Pawelec G, Rehbnein A, Schlotz E, et al. Cytokine modulation of TH1/TH2 phenotype differentiation in directly alloresponsive $CD4^+$ human T cells. Transplantation. 1996;62:1095–1101.
71. Piccotti JR, Chan S, VanBuskirk AM, et al. Are Th2 helper lymphocytes beneficial, deleterious, or irrelevant in promoting allograft survival. Transplantation. 1997;63:619–624.
72. VanBuskirk AM, Wakely ME, Orosz CG. Transfusion of polarized TH2-like cell populations into SCID mouse cardiac allograft recipients results in acute allograft rejection. Transplantation. 1996;62:229–238.
73. Barbara JA, Turvey SE, Kingsley CI, et al. Islet allograft rejection can be mediated by $CD4^+$, alloantigen experienced, direct pathway T cells of TH1 and TH2 cytokine phenotype. Transplantation. 2000;70:1641–1649.
74. Matesic D, Valujskikh A, Pearlman E, et al. Type 2 immune deviation has differential effects on alloreactive $CD4^+$ and $CD8^+$ T cells. Journal of Immunology. 1998;161:5236–5244.
75. Valujskikh A, Matesic D, Gilliam A, et al. T cells reactive to a single immunodominant self-restricted allopeptide induce skin graft rejection in mice. Journal of Clinical Investigation. 1998;101:1398–1407.
76. Burlingham WJ, Love RB, Jankowska-Gan E, et al. IL-17-dependent cellular immunity to collagen type V predisposes to obliterative bronchiolitis in human lung transplants. Journal of Clinical Investigation. 2007;117:3498–3506.
77. Burrell BE, Csencsits K, Lu G, et al. $CD8^+$ Th17 mediate costimulation blockade-resistant allograft rejection in T-bet-deficient mice. Journal of Immunology. 2008;181:3906–3914.
78. Yuan X, Paez-Cortexz J, Schmitt-Knosalla I, et al. A novel role of CD4 Th17 cells in mediating cardiac allograft rejection and vasculopathy. Journal of Experimental Medicine. 2008;205:3133–3144.
79. McMurchy AN, Bushell A, Levings MK, et al. Moving to tolerance: clinical application of T regulatory cells. Seminars in Immunology. 2011;23:304–313.

80. Tang S, Bluestone JA, Kang S-M. CD4^{+}Foxp3^{+} regulatory T cell therapy in transplantation. Journal of Cell Biology. 2012;4:11–21.
81. Wood KJ, Bushell A, Hester J. Regulatory immune cells in transplantation. Nature Reviews. Immunology. 2012;12:417–430.
82. Brennan TV, Tang Q, Liu FC, et al. Requirements for prolongation of allograft survival with regulatory T cell infusion in lymphosufficient hosts. Journal of Surgical Research. 2011;169:e69–e75.
83. Issa F, Hester J, Goto R, et al. Ex vivo-expanded human regulatory T cells prevent the rejection of skin allografts in a humanized mouse model. Transplantation. 2010;90:1321–1327.
84. Nadig SN, Wieckiewicz J, Wu DC, et al. *In vivo* prevention of transplant arteriosclerosis by ex vivo-expanded human regulatory T cells. Nature Medicine. 2010;16:809–813.
85. Sagoo P, Ali N, Garg G, et al. Human regulatory T cells with alloantigen specificity are more potent inhibitors of alloimmune skin graft damage than polyclonal regulatory T cells. Science Translational Medicine. 2011;3:83ra42.

第 14 章

器官移植小型动物模型

Lakshman Gunaratnam, Anthony M. Jevnikar, Roslyn B. Mannon

引言

对人类同种异体免疫的研究可借助动物实验来完成。这些研究不仅提供了练习外科技术的机会，也搭建了研究同种异体免疫损伤机制及免疫抑制方案的平台。之前的研究主要着眼于移植相关损伤的啮齿类动物模型，包括大鼠及小鼠。大鼠模型在血管化及新生血管化环境下免疫应答方面的研究获得了重大进展。因为拥有着对小鼠免疫系统的深刻理解、丰富多样的试剂以及最重要的一点——可对供体及受体进行基因操作，小鼠模型在研究排斥反应的生理过程及先天性免疫损伤方面提供了大量信息。在本章，我们将综述使用移植动物模型的历史，缺血再灌注损伤治疗性干预的生理基础及未来发展，明确同种异体免疫介导损伤模型及减轻此种损伤的方法，并比较小动物模型与大动物模型——包括在人身上使用药物前使用非人类哺乳类动物模型。本章对 13、15、16 章的内容进行了补充，这 3 章分别是体外、大动物及硅芯片移植模型。

建立同种异体免疫损伤模型进行研究时，必须认识到随着移植器官及组织不同，致免疫性也大不相同。抗原呈递的程度及组织抗原特异性与排斥反应应答潜力相关，而同种异体移植物的微环境及与引流淋巴结相同对同种异体应答有重要影响。在啮齿类动物移植模型中，最严重的排斥反应发生在皮肤——一种非血管化移植，致免疫性依次减低分别是心脏、肾脏及胰岛[1,2]。这样的发现在严格的皮肤模型中更为多见，但是在致免疫性更强的器官的较不严格模型中移植物延长存活非常少见。

在建立动物模型时，非常重要的另一点是供体和受体品系。举例来说，取决于受体的品系，小鼠肾移植可以在没有任何免疫抑制的情况下拥有较长的生存期[3]；当供体品系为 Balb/c 品系（$H-2^d$）而受体为 C57BL/6($H-2^d$)时，完全的 MHC 错配不会导致严重的排斥反应，而供体受体相反时则不然。同种异体心脏移植时使用分离的Ⅰ级或Ⅱ级 MHC 错配可导致伴随血管病变的延迟移植排斥反应应答[4]。在使用近系繁殖品系的小动物模型时，对排斥反应及非免疫损伤方面获得了独特的认识，同时了解到这样得出的结果对于远系繁殖的人类来说具有局限性。在后文中，我们将尝试聚焦于每种模型的关键因素以及应用于人身上的潜力。

啮齿类动物实体器官移植模型的改进

移植动物模型的历史非常丰富，充满了事实发现以及奇闻轶事。关于这段历史的详细讨论在第 8 章有所记述。在移植研究中使用实验室啮齿类动物模型得益于内外科水平的进步，小动物器官的操作需要高水平的手术技巧。法国外科医生 Alexis Carrel 开创了血管吻合术，使他完成了首次狗的肾及心脏移植，他也因此于 1912 年获得了诺贝尔奖[5]。19 世纪 30 年代，George Snell 将过去连续的同亲代个体繁殖改良为近系繁殖小鼠，最小化小鼠间基因变异，包括 Medawar 的大鼠皮肤移植。Snell 定义了同种异体免疫的关键性基因——“组织相容性(H)”基因。与 Peter Gorer 一同，Snell 确定了小鼠的此基因主要位点与编码“抗原Ⅱ”的位点相同，也就是组织相容性位点 2 或 H–2。Jean Dausset 通过研究曾接受过输血的患者血清中的抗体，描绘了决定人类 H–2 系统同源体的基因，命名为主要组织相容性复合物或 HLA。小鼠及人类同种异体免疫的研究从此互为补充。1980 年，Snell 及 Dausset 获得诺贝尔奖使这项发现受到了重视。移植相关研究曾有着严格的限制，仅允许使用无繁殖能力的成年动物进行研究,直到第一种抗排斥药物出现。Hitchings 和 Elion 发现了抗代谢药 6-巯基嘌呤(6-MP)及硫唑嘌呤,并在 19 世纪 60 年代问世[6],其后出现了环孢霉素[7,8](见第 17 章)。

啮齿类动物模型的发展与技术 (例如外科技巧)和诊断挑战(例如排斥反应)密切相关,在克服了以上问题后,许多研究者能够利用小动物模型来进行特定器官系统及指定区域的研究。Lacy 在发现了使用胶原酶分离法可从大鼠胰腺获取胰岛细胞后, 在 1967 年进行了首次胰岛移植[9-11]。重要的是,他证明了将胰岛细胞植入大鼠肾被膜下腔隙是一个相对简单的动物模型,可以用来模拟纠正自身免疫性糖尿病代谢性胰岛素生成缺陷或链佐星治疗过的动物。相对于胰岛移植最大的挑战在于分离胰岛细胞,小鼠的实体器官移植模式受限于需要的技术技巧(例如难度依次为心脏<肾脏<肝脏,小肠)。

使用大鼠的啮齿类异位心脏移植模型在 1964 年[12]报道了此手术会导致下肢血流严重受阻并造成了下肢轻瘫或截瘫。一种改良后迅速被采用的小鼠异位移植腹部手术方式使移植器官及受体生存率达到了 90%[13](图 14.1)。因为小鼠腹部心脏移植"非生理的"及"非负荷的"独特心内血流方向,且此模型手术成本低、人力需求相对少以及多种基因型的近系繁殖小鼠品系,此模型被广泛用于免疫耐受的研究。重要的是,心脏相比于其他实质器官(例如肝脏、肾脏)有着较低的自然耐受率,有助于分析有潜力的免疫耐受诱导方案。使用触诊法评估排斥程度从最早被提出一直沿用至今。但是,以从"0"(移植心脏收缩停止)到"4"(移植心脏收缩活跃)来评估心肌收缩力被认为过于主观,对于移植后早期改变不敏感,且对于评估长期移植存活效果较差[13,14]。组织学仍然是临床及实验室诊断心脏排斥的金标准, 但一系列研究表明因为啮齿类动物心脏体积过小所以并不适用[15]。心电生理[16]、磁共振[17]、超声、冠脉造影研究和排斥反应的生化及分子标记物的应用都进一步优化了排斥反应的诊断[18],但也显著提高了复杂性及成本。

小鼠肾脏移植由 Skoskiewicz 和 Russell 在 1973 年首次报道[19],并由 Kalina 和 Zhong[20]进一步完善[21]。但是,此种动物模型仍然受限于细小血管(小鼠肾动脉平均直径为 0.3mm)、外科血管吻合技术困难及更高的技术失败率,开展的移植中心相对于小鼠心脏移植要少。传统观念认为,仅有左肾可以获取作为供体器官,因为右肾静脉较短且与受体腔静脉血管吻合难度大, 所以被认为不适合用来移植。移植器官血管与腹主动脉及腔静脉进行端侧吻合, 泌尿系重建则是将一小块供体膀胱与受体膀胱顶缝合(图 14.2)。鼠类肾脏对缺血再

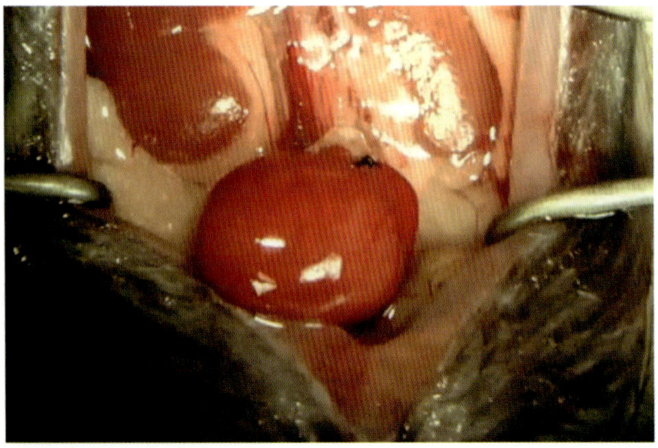

图 14.1 小鼠有血供的异位心脏移植。图示小鼠异体心脏移植置于下方。心脏由主动脉供血,存活时可在体外触诊到搏动。但是静脉还不充盈,因此无心输出量,受体的存活与移植物的存活无关。(Photo courtesy of Jean Kwun.)

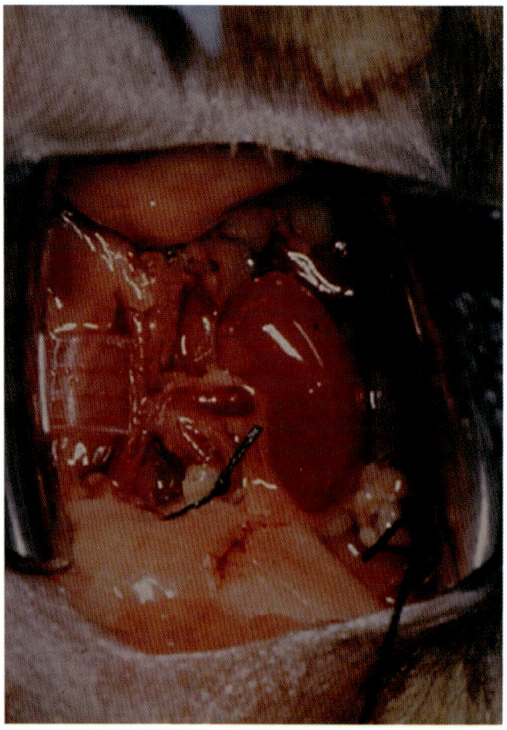

图 14.2 小鼠有血供的肾移植。图示小鼠肾移植的代表性技术--端侧吻合及输尿管-膀胱吻合。若将受体自体肾切除,此模型可作为存活模型,通过血肌酐来评估病情。若自体肾仍保留,此移植物可与生存独立研究。

灌注损伤(IRI)相当敏感，血管吻合及热缺血时间一般限制在 35~40 分钟以内。对双侧肾切除受体(例如生存模型)进行移植可以简化排斥反应的诊断，使用这种方法时较长的热缺血时间及随后移植功能延迟恢复与高死亡率密切相关。或者可以使用二期手术的方法，将原来的右肾保留至第 7 天。这种方法虽然有着较低的死亡率，但可能会对同种异体免疫应答及之后的移植物存活期产生微妙的影响，源于同种异体抗原暴露过程中自身肾中的固有免疫调节因子[22]。虽然免疫排斥可以在生化层面上通过监测血清肌酐水平来观察，但病理学仍然是评价排斥的金标准。这一点对于使用 B6 (H-2^b)作为供体移植到 Balb/c B6(H-2^d)的品系组合的小鼠肾移植自然耐受率将近 30%时十分重要[2,3]。

虽然大鼠心脏及肾脏移植依然是主要的实验啮齿类动物移植模型，但其他器官特殊的生理学及免疫学应答促进了小鼠的几乎全部实质器官移植模型的发展。令人惊讶的是，直到 1991 年 Starzl 的小组才报道了第一例小鼠原位肝移植[23]，基于早先 19 世纪 70 年代描述的大鼠肝移植技术[24-26]。特别是在大鼠模型中，使用低反应性品系如 PVG 或 Dark Agouti(DA)充分认识到了更高的自然肝移植耐受率，可接受完全 MHC 错配的肝脏并存活 100 天以上[27]。

肠和肺脏的移植模型也被证明是在免疫诱导方面具有极大挑战的实体器官移植模型。特定器官对免疫诱导的敏感性的差别体现在有着更多细菌暴露及先天免疫系统激活的器官[28]。Zhong 在 1993 年报道了异位小鼠小肠移植[29,30]。但是这种移植是不具有功能的，因为移植的肠管独立于正常的胃肠道通路，而且因为宿主营养由原来的营养通路提供，所以判定明确的排斥反应的终点也更加困难。这一问题随着 2005 年原位肠移植的发展得以解决[31]。原位肺移植也同样在大鼠[32,33]及小鼠[34,35]模型中被报道。

品系的多样性

小鼠基因操纵这一特有技术使大量的研究受益，操纵供体及受体可以有助于了解免疫应答特定的内容[36]。这些基因操作中包括剔除特定种类的同种异体免疫应答复合物(表 14.1)。关于这些品系及获取途径的详细讨论不在此章讨论范围内，详见参考文献 37。这些品系既可以作为移植供体也可以作为受体，还可以用来测试受体免疫和(或)对供体抗原或蛋白的应答需求。另外还有一系列的基因敲除品系，如删除了细胞因子或者免疫系统关键信号分子。其中包括 Janus 激酶(JAK)，这是一种参与免疫反应及造血组织的无对应受体的酪氨酸激酶。JAK3 缺乏是一种严重的人联合免疫缺陷[38]。基因转写信号换能及激活(STAT)蛋白在免疫应答中被激活，产生大量的细胞因子、生长因子以及激素，并催化特定的靶基因。通过使用缺陷小鼠，可确定 STAT4 及 STAT6 是 Th1 及 Th2 介导的应答反应中所必需的，还为研究实体器官移植同种异体反应性免

表 14.1　有免疫缺陷的转基因小鼠

品系名(缩写)	缺陷	免疫缺陷	情景品系
裸鼠	Fomml 突变	无胸腺、T 细胞耗竭	H-2^d
RAG 缺陷(RAG^+)	VDJ 重组酶缺陷或缺失	缺乏抗原特异性细胞或体液免疫	H-2^b
严重的混合性免费缺陷(SCID)μT 缺陷($μT^{-/-}$)	蛋白激酶、DNA 激酶、催化多肽突变 IgM 膜外显子基因的 μ 链缺失；前 B 细胞上的 IgM 受体缺失	缺乏 B 细胞及 T 细胞，补体激活受损 B 细胞缺乏，体液免疫受损	H-2^b
$β_2$ 微球蛋白缺陷($β_{2m}^{-/-}$)	$β_2$ 微球蛋白基由中断	缺乏完整的 MHCJ 级表达 CD8 T 细胞耗竭	H-2^b
$A^bβ$ 缺陷($A^bβ^{-/-}$)	$A^bβ$ 基因中断	缺乏Ⅱ级表达；CD4 T 细胞耗竭	H-2^b
CD4 缺陷($CD4^{-/-}$)	CD4 基因中断	CD4 T 细胞缺乏	H-2^b
CD8 缺陷($CD8^{-/-}$)	CD8α 基因中断	CD8 T 细胞缺乏	H-2^b
米色鼠(bg^J/bg^J)	自然突变	NK 细胞耗竭；细胞毒 T 细胞及巨噬细胞功能受损	
op/op	骨硬化症	m-CSF 单核细胞耗竭	
IL-2 受体，r 链缺陷($IL2rg^{-/-}$)	IL-2 受体 r 链突变	NK 细胞发育缺陷；IL-s，4，7，9，15 及 21 信号异常	
Prf1 缺陷($Rrf1^{-/-}$)	穿孔素 1 突变	NK 细胞及 $CD8^+$ 淋巴细胞功能缺陷	

疫应答提供了新的工具[39,40](见第5章)。近来,缺乏特定细胞因子的小鼠也被用来研究Th2应答中Th1可能起到的作用[41-46](见第2章)。

总的来说,与大鼠模型相比,小鼠动物模型需要更优秀的显微外科技术,所以仅在不多的实验室中开展。小鼠同种异体移植排斥强度较大鼠模型要小,包括对比MHC错配的程度。而且就像前文中提到的,相比大鼠模型来说,小鼠模型移植存活的可能性更大。然而,小鼠相对较小的体型使其性价比更高,且因为有着大量的基因工程品系可以使用而更利于科学研究。

同种异体免疫损伤模型:急性损伤

急性细胞排斥

随着我们对宿主免疫应答理解的加深,急性细胞排斥成为关键的研究领域。像之前提到的,品系的不同可以导致免疫反应的不同。另外,移植的种类非常重要,微环境也会影响反应的程度。

皮肤移植仍然是技术最简单的移植模型之一。移植的简化便于对免疫调节及机理进行大量研究。皮肤移植在临床前的耐受研究中被用来作为供体特异的低反应性的初步测试。在所有的组织及器官移植中,皮肤移植免疫原性最强,提供了高级别的免疫严密性。但是,此类移植是无血管的,而且可以耐受缺血导致的变性及坏死,这使得移植的皮肤容易受到免疫应答的影响[47]。排斥反应还受到组织特异性抗原的影响,此种抗原是免疫反应的重要目标[48]。另外,皮肤含有专门的抗原呈递细胞(朗格汉斯细胞),这种细胞可以从移植皮肤转移到受体并有效地激活T细胞。最后,移植器官的大小也会对移植排斥造成影响,更多供体组织的量意味着更多的供体APC并影响受体的排斥反应[49]。使用特定的小鼠品系组合进行更加谨慎而详细的研究,比较心脏、胰岛以及皮肤的排斥反应得出以下结论,原有APC或组织特异性抗体的量不影响受体应答中T细胞的量,移植物微环境及大小也与排斥反应的敏感程度无关[50]。Singer和Rosenberg使用皮肤同种异体移植进行了重要研究,为研究CD4和CD8 T细胞在MHC Ⅰ级分子完全错配的小鼠皮肤移植过程中的作用奠定了基础[51]。

使用小鼠肾脏移植来研究排斥反应在之后慢性移植损伤章节中有详细讨论,因为目前已知,不采用免疫抑制时肾脏移植在同样的供体-受体组合情况下与皮肤及心脏移植相比有着较长的生存期。此类动物模型提供了一种研究慢性免疫损伤的平台。近来,肾脏移植模型被用来研究抗体介导损伤以及病毒性肾炎对移植物功能及存活的影响。然而,随着品系改良会发现更急性的排斥反应。确实,C57BL/6品系肾脏移植到完全错配的Balb/c受体会在2周内发生快速的排斥,使用抗CD45RB治疗会减轻排斥反应,进而引起移植及受体生存、组织学层面及肾脏功能改善[52]。只有少数的受体对移植皮肤有低供体特异反应性的同时排斥第三方的皮肤。这一新奇的阻断策略正在非人哺乳类动物身上进行更多的研究,目标是理解反应机制并提供临床前研究平台。

发生抗原结合的位置

另一个仅能使用小鼠模型解释的重要概念是抗原是在什么地方、以何种方式结合。虽然多年来的主流观点认为抗原结合发生在移植物,但目前认识到次级淋巴器官(包括脾脏、淋巴结以及局灶淋巴组织)不仅能提供适合抗原呈递的环境,也能起到发起排斥反应的作用。这些研究使用心脏同种异体移植至野生型小鼠,包括缺乏淋巴结及Peyer结的淋巴细胞人工型(*aly/aly*)小鼠、完全缺乏次级淋巴组织的脾切除后的*aly/aly*小鼠以及无脾脏的*Hox11*$^{-/-}$小鼠。尽管没有淋巴组织或脾,*aly/aly*和*Hox11*$^{-/-}$小鼠对心脏移植发生了排斥,但*aly/aly*小鼠排斥发生的时间相对延后[53]。切除脾脏的*aly/aly*小鼠勉强地耐受了心脏移植,但是无法产生供体特异性抗体。因此有完整血供的同种异体器官移植,在没有次级淋巴器官组织时,无法诱导产生有效的免疫应答。与此相反,皮肤移植没有在*aly/aly*受体身上发生排斥,却在*Hox11*$^{-/-}$小鼠受体中发生了排斥,说明发生免疫反应时抗原存在的位置很重要。这些研究看起来相当有说服力,在切除脾的淋巴细胞毒素α缺陷及β受体缺陷的小鼠(两种没有淋巴结及Peyer结的小鼠)身上发生了对皮肤及心脏移植的有效排斥反应,即使与野生型受体相比动力学上相对延后,也提示了次级淋巴组织并不是同种异体移植排斥反应所必需的[54]。在小肠移植中,带有供体淋巴组织是介导受体免疫应答的重要因素[55]。这些研究指出了在小肠移植中免疫原性的关键因素是供体淋巴结组织,也是介导同种异体移植排斥的最低要求。

同种识别

大量的研究使用小鼠移植模型来明确移植排斥活动中所必须且必要的同种识别过程。起初,因为移植物可发生排斥反应而认为直接识别是唯一的机制。然而,现在已经通过使用皮肤移植后 MHC 分子免疫的大鼠实验,明确了间接通路也可以介导排斥反应[56,57]。在 CD8 T 细胞耗竭的小鼠身上,缺乏 MHC Ⅱ级分子的供体小鼠(I-A^b 缺陷小鼠)器官会迅速发生排斥,且发现 CD4 T 细胞被受体细胞上的Ⅱ级抗原间接呈递的供体多肽所致敏[58]。Steele 及其同事使用 MHC Ⅱ级分子缺陷小鼠或被改造为有完整的 CD4 间室(因为Ⅱ级分子仅在胸腺表达)的Ⅱ级分子缺陷小鼠,发现了间接识别过程是 B 细胞激活及产生同种异体抗体的原因[59]。此通路亦与慢性排斥反应相关,且被认为对当前的免疫抑制治疗耐受性较差[60]。

次级组织相容性抗原

次级组织相容性抗原是来源于多形态的自身蛋白的免疫原性多肽,对于激发排斥反应是必要的[61]。一般认为,供体及受体 MHC 抗原组成的 MHC/多肽复合物,无论是供体直接呈递的还是由受体树突状细胞间接呈递而来,其从本质上来讲是相同的。另外,有小概率可能同种异体反应性 T 细胞识别刺激抗原,导致相对于直接识别介导的排斥过程而言较为缓慢且延后的移植物排斥。典型的次级抗原有男性 H-Y 抗原,它是在小鼠皮肤移植模型上研究得最多的一种抗原。这些研究表明 CD4C MHC Ⅱ级分子限定的辅助 T 细胞与 $CD8^+$ MHC Ⅰ级限定的细胞毒 T 细胞可产生协同作用[62]。使用 IL-17 缺陷小鼠(IL-$17^{-/-}$)作为次级错配皮肤移植的受体,Vokaer 等发现了次级皮肤移植有较长的生存期,而调节 T 细胞可促进一条 Th17 介导的中性粒细胞依赖的移植排斥通路[63]。

移植排斥反应中的 Th 偏差

小鼠模型研究中一个必须考虑的问题就是移植中 Th1 T 细胞与 Th2 T 细胞的比较。Th1 来源的细胞因子被认为通过介导延迟型超敏反应(DTH)和细胞毒反应以及通过抗体依赖的细胞毒反应(ADCC)而促进了排斥反应。另一方面,Th2 细胞因子被认为通过 IgE 生成抗体及非细胞毒性的 IgG 亚类可抑制 DTH 及巨噬细胞激活来防止排斥反应。过去有关细胞因子表达与移植预后的研究支持这些假设。但使用细胞因子敲除小鼠进行的研究发现,免疫的复杂性存在偏差及排斥反应中涉及繁多的细胞因子[64]。例如,IL-2 缺陷小鼠被证明可以完全排斥胰岛同种异体移植及完全错配的心脏同种异体移植[46],提示 Th1 细胞因子对于排斥反应来说不是必需的[65]。另外有趣的是,使用 CTLA4Ig 诱导耐受需要 IL-2 的表达[65]。IL-2 及 IL-4 均敲除的小鼠也可以排斥胰岛及心脏同种异体移植,表明原来通过 IL-2γ 链受体的信号可以通过 IL-15、IL-7 或 IL-9 来介导排斥反应[43]。类似地,使用共刺激阻断剂(CSB)时的长期生存需要 IFN-γ,因为这种治疗方法对 IFN-$\gamma^{-/-}$的受体无效[66]。而且 IFN-$\gamma^{-/-}$小鼠排斥完全错配或Ⅰ级错配的同种异体移植,但却不排斥Ⅱ级错配的移植[67]。因此,虽然 IL-2、IL-4 及 IFN-γ 均参与急性排斥,但它们都不是必需的。在下文中会谈到,Th2 应答与长期移植生存的联系也被考虑得过于简单了,例如事实上 IL-4 在 IL-$2^{-/-}$或 IFN-$\gamma^{-/-}$小鼠中不会造成移植生存延长[45,46,65,66]。总的来说,这些研究举例说明了在小鼠模型的研究中意外发现引出了 Th 对免疫偏差的作用及对移植免疫反应研究的贡献。

Th17 细胞及其在移植排斥和耐受中的功能是近期研究的热点。目前主流观点认为,Th17 细胞是移植耐受前的一道屏障,而且可能有拮抗 Treg 细胞分化的作用。例如,抑制 IL-17 可延长大鼠心脏移植存活期[68],也有研究表明,IL-17 的抑制与大鼠肺移植慢性损伤存在联系[69]。更直接的证据支持来自对 Tbet 缺陷小鼠($Tbet^{-/-}$)的研究,此种小鼠缺乏完整的 Th1 应答,会对心脏移植产生迅速而强烈的排斥反应,此反应与移植物内产生 IL-17 的 CD4 T 细胞相关[70]。类似的是 CSB 对 $Tbet^{-/-}$小鼠无效,与生成 IL-17 的 $CD8^+$T 细胞有关[71]。但是,生成 IL-17 的 T 细胞是否是临床移植免疫损伤中重要的介质仍在讨论中。在激活 Th1 应答过程中,Th17 细胞是否参与了排斥反应仍不明确,以及 Th17 细胞是否对传统免疫抑制治疗有反应也存在矛盾[72]。最后,移植中 Treg 细胞对 Th17 细胞的调控能力如何仍没有答案。

关于 Treg 细胞的功能已经通过动物模型进行了广泛的研究,通常目标是通过:①体外过继转化增殖或②为受体提供适合的内环境来促进抑制同种异体性免疫反应，从而增强此类细胞的活性。既往的研究方法是在体外培养人类CD4 T细胞并予以多克隆刺激，结果显示Treg细胞可以在小鼠嵌合人化动脉移植中抑制血管病变[73]。同一小组的另一种研究方法是通过使用指定培养条件下的供体抗原呈递细胞来刺激受体$CD4^+T$细胞，以扩增同种异体反应性Treg细胞。在这种情况下，Treg细胞可以延长MHC完全错配的小鼠皮肤移植的生存期[74]。类似的，人$CD45RO^-CD25^-CD4^+T$细胞，在相同培养条件下，可以抑制人动脉移植模型中血管病变的发生[75]。存在于骨髓来源树突状细胞中的$FoxP3^+CD25^+CD4^+Treg$细胞进行同种异体抗原特异性的扩增，导致小鼠受体对心脏移植低反应性，但对第三方供体移植没有影响[76]。因此，临床前模型提供了可信的数据表明此方法应用于人体的可行性。

为促进Treg细胞扩增对受体进行操纵成为多个关于耐受诱导研究的焦点（见下文）。这些研究表明了受体免疫抑制对预后影响的重要性。例如，一部分研究涉及使用mTOR抑制剂有益于介导CSB环境下的长期生存[77,78]及人体内Treg细胞的发展[79]，但是这种促进作用不是每次都能被观察到[80]。另外，使用抗淋巴细胞血清及供体胰腺淋巴结细胞对受体小鼠进行处理，导致小鼠$FoxP3^+Tregs$细胞分化增殖并有利于胰岛移植的存活[81]。IL-2或抗IL-2复合体治疗与小鼠$FoxP3^+Tregs$细胞分化增殖相关，与G-CSF治疗一样会引起骨髓来源的抑制细胞扩增，及MHCⅡ级错配的皮肤移植排斥反应的发生明显延迟[82]。这些资料支持着应用于人体的可能性，但是可能难以用实践来支持这些研究方法。值得注意的一点是，近期研究表明对小鼠使用CT-LA4Tg抑制B7/CD28通路可以改变Treg细胞内稳态，且不利于依赖于Treg细胞延长移植物存活的情形[83]。

同种异体移植先天性免疫损伤的机制

NK细胞在急性排斥反应中的作用是研究的热点，在第7章中有专门的叙述。由先天性免疫激发并与适应性免疫共同作用的机制是临床初期及长期管理的关键，因为先天性免疫应答不是免疫抑制治疗的主要关注点。对大鼠的研究发现，NK细胞缺陷不能影响排斥反应的动力学[84,85]。但是，在大鼠心脏移植急性排斥反应中观察到了NK细胞的激活[86]，且特定的亚类可能通过直接识别同种异体抗原的方式参与了小鼠心脏移植的排斥反应[87]。这一点在CD28缺陷（$CD28^{-/-}$）小鼠可以接受抗CD154抗体排斥的心脏移植[88]的实验中得到验证，而NK1.1细胞的消耗可能提高存活率[89]。NKG2D是在NK细胞和CD8 T细胞表面表达的负责激活免疫反应的受体，对其进行阻断可以防止$CD28^{-/-}$受体发生排斥[90]。NK细胞还被发现有着直接介导移植排斥的功能，有证据表明IL-15（一种NK细胞激活细胞因子）参与了RAG敲除小鼠（缺乏B细胞及T细胞）皮肤移植的排斥进程，而没有RAG共有γ链（γc，CD132）缺陷的小鼠也缺乏NK细胞[91]。

巨噬细胞可能也参与了急性移植排斥过程[92]（见第7章），并且多个研究利用小鼠模型来分析这条通路。基因删除CCR1[93]与延长MHCⅠ级、MHCⅡ级分子都错配的小鼠心脏移植生存期相关，删除CCR5[94]与改善MHCⅡ级错配的心脏移植排斥反应有关。在这两种情况中，巨噬细胞的浸润程度都有降低。对受体小鼠使用有抑制巨噬细胞功能的DTCM-戊二酰亚胺进行处理，可以延长完全错配的心脏移植生存期[95]。氯膦酸二钠脂质体是一种可以杀死巨噬细胞的介质，用其进行处理过的大鼠可以改善肾移植功能及减轻炎症反应[96]。转基因CD11b-DTR小鼠一定程度的巨噬细胞消耗导致肾移植炎症反应显著减轻[97]。这些研究发现一起指向了巨噬细胞在急性排斥反应中有促进炎症的作用。

急性抗体介导损伤

抗体介导的排斥反应逐渐被认识到是导致移植失败的原因之一（见第6章）。现在人们认识到抗体介导损伤是延迟移植肾丧失功能的重要原因[98]，也是心脏移植进行性损伤的关键因素[99]，目前迫切需要在动物模型中研究其损伤机制。Colvin和他的同事们基于非人哺乳类动物（NHP）模型探明了发生在人体的一系列事件[100]。在各种小动物模型中，当代的焦点在于小鼠模型，人们用其来研究抗体产生的发病机制、损伤机制、生化标记物以及潜在的治疗性干预措施。

在小鼠身上发生的急性抗体介导的排斥反应（AMR）难以一概而全。接种供体特异性MHC蛋白抗体到$RAG^{-/-}$小鼠不会引起明显的抗体介导损伤反应，且程度与抗体滴定量有关[101]。使用对抗特定的MHC分子的单克隆抗体接种至接受特定供体心脏移植的$RAG^{-/-}$小鼠受体的方法也同样无法诱发严重的损伤反应，但是会出现抗体沉积在毛细血管的表现[102]。

这些接种实验确实提供了一些抗体介导损伤方面

令人感兴趣的概念。但是这种研究存在着限制。使用单克隆抗体的实验集中于研究MHCⅠ级和Ⅱ级分子谁才是此过程的决定因素，而对人类来说此过程中往往是两者组合作用的结果。而在人体晚期移植失败中，抗MHCⅡ级分子抗体是抗体中的主要类型。小鼠MHCⅡ级分子平时在内皮细胞上不表达，仅在发生炎症时才上调表达水平；而人类Ⅱ级蛋白是时常表达的。最后，$RAG^{-/-}$小鼠缺少完整的细胞应答，这一机制可促进B细胞激活，可产生改变移植组织中MHC分子表达的关键细胞因子，并可激活参与排斥反应的其他炎症细胞。

由Bickerstaff和其同事报道的另一种动物模型，使用CCR5敲除小鼠($CCR5^{-/-}$)[101]。在此种模型中，将A/J型小鼠的心脏移植到$CCR5^{-/-}$小鼠会迅速发生排斥，反应伴有极少的细胞浸润，但有明显的C3d补体在移植物大血管及毛细血管的沉积，这些表现符合AMR。供体特异性抗体的量相比野生型受体有着明显的升高，获得性接种这种血清会导致供体特异性的心脏移植产生迅速的体液免疫排斥反应。同样，加重的排斥反应也可见于隔离的Ⅰ级分子分化过程中，而且这种反应明显地依赖于持续生成的抗体而不是细胞毒T细胞[103]。这些结论并不像A/J型小鼠的肾脏移植到$CCR5^{-/-}$小鼠那样具有器官特异性，后者会迅速发生排斥反应并伴随着病理学证据存在抗体的沉积[104]。使用μ-链缺陷、$CCR5^{-/-}$共同缺陷的小鼠作为肾移植的受体来避免排斥反应，以此来研究抗体生成细胞对于介导器官排斥反应的必要性。

虽然这些动物模型重点关注毛细血管内抗原及补体沉积，但排斥反应中也可以见到动脉损伤。使用人系膜动脉插入beige/SCID小鼠腹主动脉，同时接种抗Ⅰ级HLA抗体，可以导致补体沉积及新生内膜形成[105]。这些研究结果很难完全套用到心脏移植上，因为心脏移植过程中有动脉外膜内血管滋养管的破坏，而这种影响在损伤模型的研究中没有进行说明。这些内容在以下慢性抗体介导移植损伤部分有更多讨论。

补体激活

补体的激活在导致内皮损伤过程中起到重要作用，这一现象经检验证明是另一种可减轻抗体介导损伤的潜在传导通路(见第2章及第7章)。而如何抑制补体是动物研究减轻急性损伤的焦点。1995年首次报道了在猪-灵长类异种心脏移植的超急性期排斥模型中，使用抗C5抗体抑制了超急性期排斥的进展，保证了正常的功能及避免病理性损伤[106]。随后，对小鼠进行的研究发现了相似的有益效果。在此动物模型中，Balb/c小鼠先被移植了C3H小鼠的皮肤，7天之后再接受与皮肤移植同品系供体的心脏移植。结果是术后第3天迅速发生了移植物失功能。联合使用低剂量环孢霉素、环磷酰胺及抗C5抗体可以延长移植物存活时间至100天以上，除全身及移植物内出现了抗供体抗体及补体外未见组织学异常，而移植物和受体均出现了免疫学改变，这些是成功的移植耐受所必需的[107]。

使用可溶性补体受体1(sCR1)阻断补体激活后，在预致敏过的超急性期排斥模型上得出了类似的结果。例如Pruitt和Bollinger发现，使用ACI小鼠皮肤预致敏后移植ACI小鼠肾脏的Lewis小鼠受体的血管损伤有所改善[108]。DA小鼠接受使用可溶性补体受体1(sCR1)处理过的Lewis小鼠肾脏后，血管损伤及细胞介导的损伤相对于未处理者都有所减轻[109]。眼镜蛇毒因子可减弱C3补体的活性，也能抑制移植了ACI小鼠心脏的预致敏的Lewis受体发生的超急性期排斥[110]。补体C6终末成分基因缺陷导致心脏移植血管损伤改变。在此模型中，对PVG大鼠($RT1^c$)进行基因操作使小鼠缺乏补体C6，使用皮肤移植进行致敏后再进行ACI小鼠心脏移植。缺乏这种补体终末成分可表现为抗体及细胞介导损伤相对于野生型受体减少[111]。最后，阻断C5转化酶联合CTLA4Ig可以明显地延长错配的小鼠心脏移植的生存期，也有可能阻断T细胞介导的移植排斥反应[112]。因此，在大鼠及小鼠已存在抗体的情况下，无论是肾移植或心脏移植，急性抗体介导的损伤似乎都可通过限制补体传导完全激活的方式减轻。这样话题性的数据支持了目前人体临床试验[113]。

但是值得注意的是，补体早期分子是重要的抗炎症介质。C1q缺乏与自身免疫相关，也许是因为它参与了巨噬细胞清除凋亡小体的过程[114]。因为C1q缺乏小鼠排斥心脏移植的速度比野生型受体更快，证明C1q的缺乏可以改变同种异体免疫应答的过程[115]。这一研究提示了补体早期蛋白具有复杂的功能。

BK多瘤病毒肾病

肾移植中一个令人烦恼的问题就是BK多瘤病毒感染。这种病毒有泌尿生殖上皮选择性，在过度免疫抑制的条件下可能会变成活动性感染或从供体移植物传染到受体。这种感染会引起移植肾内促炎症反应,组织学改变类似急性细胞排斥并伴随移植物失功能[116]。治疗方法首先是撤除免疫抑制，并在一些环境下使用抗病毒治疗，其中如西多福韦的疗效受限于它固有的肾毒性[117]。监测可提高早期发现病情并干预的机会。但是仍然存在着严重的问题，比如理解这一疾病的发病机制、如何干预功能强大的CD8细胞毒T细胞及疾病与预纤维生成反应的关联[118],或是制定新的抗病毒治疗方案。这些问题需要使用动物疾病模型进行更多的研究。

因为BK病毒对人体组织的特异性，想找到一个理想的小动物模型非常困难。曾经有报道在研究新的免疫抑制方案时在猕猴身上发现了与人类相似的BK病毒感染情况[119],其后在松鼠猴身上也有类似发现[120]。近来报道了一种多瘤病毒肾病的小鼠模型[121]。在此研究中,C57BL/6小鼠后足垫皮下接种野生A2型鼠多瘤病毒(Mpy)。感染高峰出现在接种后的第4天,伴随着$CD8^+$细胞毒T细胞的增殖,监测方法是MHCⅠ级分子四聚体中包含病毒多肽表位以及测量经病毒多肽刺激的IFN-γ产量。感染后6个月血中已检测不到病毒,但是包括肾脏在内的一些实质脏器在这个时间点仍然可以检测到病毒的存在。

在这种移植条件下,将C57BL/6($H-2^b$,同系移植物)或者C3H/HeJ小鼠($H-2^k$,异系移植物)的肾脏移植到联合双侧肾病的C57BL/6受体。移植术后第一天MPy急性感染相比未感染组加速了同系肾移植的失败,而对异系移植功能和受体生存均没有影响。检查发现,相比异系移植肾及未感染的受体,感染的同系移植肾有更多的肾小管细胞死亡、更严重的炎症及小肠水肿,还伴随着感染受体肾内病毒载量的升高。另外,抗供体细胞毒T细胞反应也会增强，这种反应会导致同系移植失败。此模型可以提供研究免疫机理及导致人PVN移植失败的病毒相关因素方面的新认识。令人感兴趣的一点是,IFN-γ通过阻断病毒复制及减少病毒蛋白表达来抑制此动物模型中的BK病毒复制[122]。使用小鼠感染模型可以得到大量的关于病毒复制、病毒存续及治疗效果的认识，也可以明确人体同系移植损伤的病理发展机制[123]。这些研究结果虽然提供了丰富的资料,但是并不能准确地模拟人体感染的情况,人体感染病毒有可能在活跃期之前有着数年的潜伏期或者是表现得如同初次感染。

同种异体免疫损伤模型:"慢性"损伤

长期移植存活仍然是所有实体器官移植的难题。此疾病的关键在于移植物纤维化、进行性炎症反应以及血管病变。小动物模型提供了人体条件下的许多独到见解,提供了更多关于治疗方案、生物标记以及病理机制方面的信息[124]。此问题一个关键的理论是寻找合适的动物模型来模拟特定的某一种研究中的人体疾病。

肾脏慢性损伤

对于肾脏来说,晚期移植失败许多年来被称为"慢性排斥",后来称为"慢性移植肾病"("CAN")[125]。这种说法源于其以间质纤维化(IF)及肾小管萎缩(TA)为特点的组织学改变。许多研究者开始推测,即使缺乏组织学诊断证据，以上发现也正是此疾病的本质及晚期移植失败的原因。就结果来说，在目前的临床实践中"CAN"的说法已经没有了,而着重于专注以病理学方法研究IF/TA及功能丧失的原因[126]。因此,寻找理想的动物模型可能仅限于存在IF/TA的模型之中，但是认识到如BK感染或抗体介导损伤为病因时，需要使用更多特定的动物模型。

因为技术相对简单，大鼠模型是最先被建立起来的。如前所述,为提供更加稳定的晚期移植失败的动物模型,品系操作是关键。1969年,White等人第一次报道了使用仅有少数MHC错配的供体可以延长移植物存活[127]。最常用的模型是F344小鼠的器官移植到Lewis小鼠受体,使用低剂量的环孢霉素A[CsA,5mg/(kg·d)]10天进行免疫抑制[128];这样供体和受体的MHCⅠ级和Ⅱ级分子完成匹配伴有少量或没有MHC抗体不一致。移植肾是具有完整血管的，吻合移植输尿管与受体膀胱后异位安置在腹腔内，分期或同期行双侧肾切除保证生存期取决于移植的器官。在移植后的12~16周内,可出现部分或广泛的硬化,伴随着增多的肾小管萎缩、内膜增生及皮质内血管逐渐阻塞。在24周时,肾功能恶化伴随着蛋白尿出现。使用此模型的许多研究强调,出现了促炎症反应包括宿主T细胞及巨噬细胞的激活[128,129]。延长此动物模型中CsA的使用会导致更严重的间质纤维化，而使用麦考酚酯会导致促炎症细胞因子水平的下调[130]。使用CSB类药物,特别是单一剂量的 CTLA4Ig，可以有效降低这种损伤并改善组织学异常[131,132]。此模型中损伤的发展过程可以用单个移植肾的肾单位供应减低来进一步解释，而保留一个原有肾可以减轻蛋白尿及肾小球硬化症[133],证明在此模型中肾单位量不足会促进慢性损伤。但是此类研究低估了此模型中发生的同种异体免疫应答的潜力,特别是低估了体液免疫的功能。

小鼠肾移植的发展受限于显微外科专业技术的需求。主要的操作挑战在于相对较小的血管管径及输尿管吻合,需要成功地进行端端吻合。因为最初建立此模型意在研究肾急性排斥过程，已经明确了这些小鼠模型与大鼠模型相比，皮肤移植也同样会随品系组合发生的不同机制产生不同程度的排斥反应[134]。B10.D2($H-2^d$)小鼠的肾脏移植到 B6AF1($H-2^{b/a}$)小鼠可以得到超过数周的长期存活。一些受体可以在移植后存活一年以上。基于体外实验的理论,在进行提高供体反应性的处理后，这些动物具有供体特异性反应及介导免疫原性损伤的能力,故无法耐受移植[135]。

近期，针对导致低反应性的相关因素及使用此类模型研究更多的慢性排斥的可能性进行了深入研究。Mannon 及其同事发现,小鼠长期存活伴随着移植器官功能差及包括 IF/TA 的慢性免疫损伤的组织学特点[3]。使用供体组织缺乏完整 MHC 分子的Ⅰ级和Ⅱ级 MHC 敲除品系进行研究时中，发现移植失败的机理有一定程度的变化,不管是Ⅰ级分子[136]或是Ⅱ级分子[137]缺失,排斥反应的程度都有所减轻。但是供体 MHC 完全缺失的话,会导致明显的功能改善且 IF/TA 改变减少[137]。这些研究进一步发现了细胞免疫和体液免疫介导慢性移植损伤的共同关键物质。他们还利用肾功能菊粉清除率作为更敏感的损伤评估办法。

许多研究通过验证受体低反应性对肾移植的作用,探究肾脏微环境的作用。一个令人感兴趣的现象是受体 $CD8^+$T 细胞下调细胞表面的 TCR 表达,并有可能影响免疫反应激活[138]。在未使用免疫抑制剂的情况下,移植生存时间超过 60 天,这种自发的免疫耐受现象发生在 DBA/2 小鼠肾脏移植到 C57BL/6 小鼠受体的情况下，此现象被认为与宿主 TGF-β 表达上调而 IL-10 无上调有关[139]。这种表达改变没有出现在迅速发生排斥的相同品系小鼠的心脏移植过程中[140]。此外,这种肾移植组织内会出现 $FoxP3^+$调节 T 细胞浸润(见第 8 章),伴随着 IDO 及调节树突状细胞表达的上调[141]。这些研究提出了受体小鼠免疫调节可使免疫反应更加迅速且持久，这种反应可以延长生存期但仍有持续的免疫反应,可导致表现为 IF/TA 的慢性损伤。

肾脏慢性移植损伤中的治疗性干预

基于其他肾脏疾病的纤维化模型中相关肾素血管紧张素系统(RAS)的资料[142],以及 RAS 激活可刺激成纤维化细胞因子 TGF-β[143],大量研究评估了阻断 RAS 对减轻慢性损伤的作用。这些研究特别使用了上述将 F344 小鼠肾脏移植到 Lewis 大鼠的慢性纤维化及肾小球硬化模型。移植时初次使用血管紧张素受体阻断剂,对尿蛋白减少、肾小球毛细血管压力及肾小球萎缩均有影响[144,145]。促炎症细胞因子及间质炎症也有减轻[144]。这些效果仅出现在使用此药物时，使用其他的药物降低血压时没有出现类似的效果[146]。这些研究指出,RAS 移植可能有益于长期移植失败的治疗，目前已有用于人体的临床治疗方案。

似乎不论损伤是何类型，免疫及非免疫介导损伤的长期并发症均是移植物纤维化及肾小管萎缩。因此,另一种治疗方案是使用抗纤维化药物。此类药物通过刺激基质降解或减慢、停止沉积的方式干扰胶原蛋白形成过程。曾有少数的移植相关临床前研究使用了这些药物并进行了报道[147]。但是其中一些研究结果非常有用。使用 4-脯氨酰羟化酶抑制剂(PHI)来限制活化胶原蛋白链的形成，减轻了小鼠肾移植纤维化模型中的慢性损伤，还伴随着明显的肾功能改善及间质纤维化和炎症的减轻[148]。但是这些药物对肾脏有着更多的影响,包括低氧诱发因子及下游基因的过表达[149],这些物质本身就可以对炎症产生调节作用。

这种方法的限制在于最初的表现不明显，但是使用这些药物时有几个困难。大多数研究在移植后立刻给予治疗以预防纤维化损伤，但是需要所有受体重新接受治疗。在实践中无法在人体身上实现。因为这些药物的毒性非常明显，可造成包括伤口不愈合等影响。PHI 类药物对其他生理通路有着潜在的影响，包括诱导产生红细胞生成素[149]。因此在损伤发展时予以干预更加合理，但是移植受体中纤维化损伤的生物标记仍然是一个谜。最后,促使纤维化的事件不会被这些治疗方案所影响,引出了无偿激活成纤维化及修补的通路,受体的移植器官处于一个不重要的地位。

心脏血管病变

慢性同系移植血管病变是晚期心脏移植失败的主要原因，已经通过使用小鼠心脏同种移植模型进行了大量的研究。这种损伤的组织学特点是内膜增生伴心外膜分支及小血管管腔狭窄。在大鼠中，MHC Ⅰ级分子匹配品系[RT1.A 和(或)RT1.E]异位心脏移植，如自Lewis 大鼠向 Fisher-344 大鼠受体移植，术后生存 30天~120 天左右出现了内膜增生[150,151]。这种组合似乎对于其他 MHC 位点会得出不一样的结论，有证据显示会发生急性排斥及心肌炎症细胞浸润[151,152]。使用 ACI 小鼠供体及(LEW×BN)F_1 受体时，两者 MHC 及非 MHC 抗原均不同，在适度的 CsA 之后移植器官存活 20~50天时出现了动脉内膜纤维化，Cramer 等进行了关于大鼠品系及此组织学变化更详细的研究[153]。同系对照移植相较 MHC Ⅰ级不匹配的品系组合相比有着较少的异常，提示不同水平的急性炎症及内膜纤维化。非 MHC 不匹配品系组合的病变会持续中度到重度的移植排斥反应，伴随心肌纤维化及心肌内中到大动脉同心性肌内膜改变。这些差异表明，动物模型的预后与品系密切相关，血管病变在具有更活跃的急性排斥反应的受体中较不突出，而在 MHC Ⅰ级匹配受体或同系对照中较常见。

这些血管病变的发病机制已被广泛研究。CMV 感染可能介导内皮细胞损伤、血管平滑肌增生及随后的内膜增厚[154,155]。如上所述，早期炎症阶段发生于血管损伤之前，且巨噬细胞起关键作用，响应上皮细胞MHC Ⅱ级分子和 ICAM-1 表达上调[156,157]与相关的上调MCP-1[158]及诱导生成一氧化氮[159]。限制大鼠单核细胞浸润的方法十分有限。在下面讨论的小鼠模型中，在一定限制条件下完成了进一步的成功尝试。

供体特异性抗体参与了大鼠心脏血管病变的发病过程，但是调节 T 细胞应答获得了明显的成功。CSB 通常用于移植后早期，显示出对晚期免疫损伤有着巨大的影响。使用 Lewis 大鼠器官移植到 Fisher-344 大鼠的模型，并在移植后 2 天使用单剂量 CTLA4Ig，出现促炎细胞因子和巨噬细胞相关细胞因子减少以及动脉硬化概率和严重程度降低，移植物存活延长到近70 天[160]，证明 T 细胞活化在慢性损伤发展的早期有着重要的作用。类似的，阻断 CD40-CD154 通路可以减轻这种大鼠模型中急性和慢性损伤而带来移植物的长期存活[161]。通过移植 T 细胞缺失的同种异体骨髓的造血嵌合法也成功减轻了此模型中的慢性损伤，证明这种方法有影响长期预后的潜力[162]。其他成功的策略包括使用基因改造成过表达吲哚胺 2,3-双加氧酶的树突状细胞[163]、口服供体特异性抗原[164]以及使用 HLA-B7分子的 α1 结构域 75~84 残基一致的合成肽治疗[165]。各种方法都可以明显地调节 T 细胞反应和随后的血管病变。然而，尚未进行进一步的临床试验。

移植血管病变的小鼠模型也已被研究，并通过使用基因工程的供体器官和受体提供了一些非常具体的见解。一些动物模型现在已经建立并且效果显著。B10.A 小鼠心脏异位移植到 B10.BR 受体时，在 4~6 周的时间内没有免疫抑制的情况下，移植冠状动脉血管可发生以反复内膜增生为特征的病变[166]。这种组合在 MHC Ⅰ类的 D 和 L 位点上不同，但对于Ⅰ类、Ⅱ类和次要MHC 蛋白的 K 位点是相同的（见第 4 章关于 MHC 分子结构和功能的详细讨论）。在 4~7 周引起血管病变的额外的品系组合包括：移植品系间有独立的 MHC Ⅱ类差异[bm12($H-2^{bm12}$)移植到 C57/BL6($H-2^b$)，bm6($H-2^{bm6}$)移植到 C57/BL6($H-2^b$)]以及供体和受体[129/J($H-2^b$)到 C57BL/6($H-2^b$)]存在的多个非 H-2 差异[4,167]。也可以使用供体和受体之间 MHC 完全错配的组合，但需要辅助免疫调节。例如，将 CBA/CaJ($H-2^k$)品系的心脏移植到 C57BL/6($H-2^b$)品系，将在联合抗 CD4/抗 CD8治疗的覆盖下发生血管病变[168]。长期使用抗 CD4[169]或硝酸镓[170,171]治疗的 DBA($H-2^d$)品系供体到 C57BL/6($H-2^b$)品系的移植也将发生慢性血管病变。硝酸镓是一种免疫调节性半金属元素，通过影响铁运输抑制部分 T 细胞和巨噬细胞激活。在镓治疗下，这些同种异体移植物的长期耐受与受体中 TGF-β 的产生及抑制供体特异性 DTH 反应有关[172]。

研究者使用这些模型进一步评估了同种异体抗体的关键作用。虽然 B10.BR 品系的心脏移植到 B10.A 品系受体没有发生动脉病变，加上多克隆抗供体抗体的被动转移会导致剂量依赖性的冠状动脉病变[173]。也只有加入抗 B10.BR 血清时，B10.BR 小鼠的心脏移植到C.B-17 SCID 小鼠才会导致动脉病变[173]。类似地，B10.BR 小鼠心脏移植到缺乏 B 细胞和 T 细胞的 $RAG^{-/-}$小鼠时，进一步接受单克隆 IgG2a 抗 $H-2K^k$ 的被动转移后也会发生动脉病变[174]，并且该反应依赖于继续使用供体特异性血清。此外，将 IgG2b 抗体被动转移到免疫球蛋白敲除小鼠(C57BL/6 Igh-6)中进行重组可以重现抗体介导的心脏同种异体移植损伤[175]。虽然内膜增厚可能发生在供体特异性抗 MHC Ⅰ类抗体的背景下,但这些反应不依赖于补体结合[176]。这些数据支持在人体内不存在组织学上可检测的补体激活的情况下也可能发生慢性损伤的概念。

研究者使用这些模型对抗原依赖性和非抗原依赖性的排斥机制的贡献进行了评估。在使用 CD8 缺陷型小鼠[177]或通过 CD8 消耗性抗体治疗[168]的 MHC Ⅰ类、Ⅱ类均不匹配的模型中,证实了排斥反应对 CD8 细胞毒性 T 细胞应答的依赖性。共刺激性阻断 CD40-CD154 通路而不是单独阻断 CD28/B7 通路已经证明可以有效地减轻血管病变[178,179],而此反应依赖于品系[180]。先天免疫反应也对此反应有贡献。受体中巨噬细胞消耗角叉菜胶可以减轻 C57BL/6 小鼠移植到(C57BL/6xBalb/c) F_1 小鼠受体时的血管病变,表明巨噬细胞作为一条可能与 B 细胞或 T 细胞免疫无关的最终共同通路中的末效应细胞[181]。由 NK 细胞产生的先天性免疫应答在 CCR4 缺陷型受体[182]、亲代移植到 F_1 受体[183]或遗传缺乏成熟 NK 细胞(γ 链敲除)的小鼠中表现明显[184]。最后,非抗原依赖因子包括氧化应激[185]、黏附分子的上调[186,187]和存在病毒感染[188]。

慢性血管和肾小球损伤也可以由非 MHC 特异性抗体引起,表明与受损组织相关的自身免疫现象。在大鼠模型中,非 MHC 特异性抗体包括心肌肌球蛋白[189]、大鼠心脏同种异体移植失败中的其他非 MHC 抗体[190]、导致 F344 品系移植到 Lewis 受体时肾小球病变的基底膜聚糖及Ⅳ型和Ⅵ型胶原蛋白的抗体[191]以及抗疟疾细胞抗体[192,193]。在小鼠中,波形蛋白的抗体[194]也被认为有致病性。慢性损伤中抗体反应对结构蛋白的作用需要进一步了解。

这些研究突出了血管病变的发展,而 Bishop 及其同事选择研究移植物肥厚和纤维化的发展。他们的研究使用抗 CD4 抗体诱导的 MHC 完全错配的心脏同种异体移植($H-2^b$ 移植到 $H-2^d$),突出了由 IL-6[195]、下游效应子 CTGF[196]和 Th17 细胞[197]介导的新的纤维化通路。这些研究和该模型的使用可能有助于确定炎症介导的心脏肥大中的新型治疗靶点。最后,使用[198]或未使用[199] CSB 治疗的 $IL-17^{-/-}$小鼠心脏同种异体移植中纤维化程度明显降低,表明 IL-17 在慢性损伤发展过程中存在不利作用。

血管同种异体移植——另一种快速动脉硬化动物模型?

作为移植物动脉硬化模型的异位心脏移植的替代方案,许多研究者使用了将动脉"跳跃"移植到受体主动脉的动物模型。该模型可以使用大鼠和小鼠受体。在小鼠模型中,供体受体组合包括 DA($RT1^a$)供体移植到 Wistar Furth($RT1^u$)受体且 1 至 5 个月期间不使用免疫抑制[200],Lewis($RT1^l$)供体移植至 F344($RT1^{lv}$)受体后超过 75 天不使用免疫抑制[201],Brown Norway($RT1^n$)供体移植到 Lewis 受体[202],PVG($RT1^c$)供体移植到 DA($RT1^a$)受体[203]。一般会观察到细胞炎症反应,伴随 T 细胞和巨噬细胞浸润内外膜。目前已经使用鼠类动物模型对这些免疫反应进行了彻底的研究。近期有报道强调了无免疫抑制的情况下 B10.A 供体移植到 C57BL/6 受体在 30 天内发生了血管损伤及平滑肌细胞增殖,进一步证明这种小鼠模型的技术可行性[204]。然而,合理地使用转基因小鼠强调了介导这种炎症性内膜纤维化需要完整的细胞和体液免疫,特别是 B 细胞、巨噬细胞和 $CD8^+T$ 细胞[205]。

虽然这些数据为细胞介导损伤和抗体介导损伤提供了令人感兴趣的线索,而且该模型制作简单,但是这些移植物与完全血管化的同种异体移植物之间存在显著差异。如已经指出的那样,血管滋养血管是存在于动脉外膜中给动脉壁提供营养物质和氧气的微血管网络,此结构在这些移植物中遭到了破坏。缺乏这种生理结构会产生明显影响,而且可能会改变动脉硬化病变的发展,使得得出的结论生物学相关性较差[206]。间质树突状细胞的缺乏也意味着同种异体识别的直接通路的相对缺失,迫使只有间接途径激活受体 T 细胞。这与在血管化器官排斥反应中两种途径均被激活形成对比。这些限制使得该模型在研究移植物动脉硬化时的生物学相关性较差,而完整的器官模型则受到青睐。

闭塞性细支气管炎综合征和肺同种异体移植

过去研究慢性肺损伤机制,即细支气管炎闭塞综合征(BOS)时,受限于小动物模型实用性差。一种常用的方法是异位气管同种异体移植。此模型将一段气管植入受体小鼠的皮下[207]。一般来说,会使用 MHC 不匹配的品系,并在 4 周内使用一些免疫抑制剂,通常为CsA。气管同种异体移植在术后2周发生了上皮细胞损伤和CD4及CD8T细胞浸润,6周时上皮细胞脱落并堵塞管腔,最终在第15周形成致密的胶原性瘢痕[208,209]并伴有大量T细胞细胞因子的释放[210]。免疫反应的严重程度取决于MHC错配及细胞免疫[211]和体液免疫[212]对MHC Ⅰ类抗原的初步免疫应答。进一步的研究发现,上皮细胞是免疫损伤的重要目标,因为上皮再生活跃,提供了可自我更新的抗原来源[213,214]。这种目标性损伤会随着包括CMV在内的病毒感染而进一步加重[215]。TGF-β和IL-13也可以起到促纤维化细胞因子的作用[216,217]。像其他慢性同种异体移植损伤一样,共刺激性阻断可以改善此病变的发展[218]。最后,使用抗CXCL12抑制纤维细胞迁移可以减弱BOS的组织学特征[219]。

这是研究气道损伤的一个简单的模型,没有通气功能的生理被动型模型存在着限制,因此无法概括完整的肺模型。其次,这是一种新生血管移植物,且没有建立微循环,现在这些因素被认为是造成同种异体损伤的关键因素[220]。最后,气管的形态学表现与细支气管不同,无法与原位肺移植术后的小细支气管做比较[221]。因此,一些实验室已经建立了一种完全血管化的大鼠异位肺移植模型,随后建立了相应的小鼠模型。这些模型有着不同的供体和受体品系组合,包括Wistar Kyoto大鼠移植到F-344大鼠[222,223],F-344大鼠移植到Wistar Kyoto大鼠[224],Lewis大鼠移植到F-344大鼠[225],Brown Norway大鼠移植到Lewis大鼠[226,227]。在这些模型中,常常发现T细胞介导的炎症损伤导致纤维化和气道阻塞,可能需要在损伤进展的数月间使用低剂量CsA治疗[226,228,229],但是此发现未见于所有报道[223,230]。额外的危害,包括吸入木炭[226]和病毒及细菌感染[225]可以引发更严重的伤害。这些模型得出的结果不尽相同的原因仍不清楚,但是似乎与手术技术无关。病变可能需要两种损害因素,也可能与供应商提供的实验动物品系变异有关[224]。

目前已经建立了一种更优质的小鼠原位肺移植模型。在这种模型中,MHC不匹配的C57BL/6小鼠供体左肺被移植到Balb/c受体[35]。在术后前7天内观察到了广泛的CD4和CD8 T细胞以及单核细胞的炎症细胞浸润及明显的组织水肿。使用抗CD154 mAb和CTLA4Ig进行双重共刺激阻断治疗导致严重的血管排斥反应伴间质纤维化,而气道上皮保持完整[231]。采取分期肺切除术及适合的供体肺,受者的生存期取决于移植本身及排斥反应中可以量化的功能和组织学特征[232]。在此模型中,排斥反应与次级淋巴器官无关[233]。这些研究证明了老鼠原位肺移植的可行性,并强调了急性排斥反应的可能。进一步改变供体和受体品系的组合进行研究后得出了关于BOS更准确的结果,例如仅有轻微的MHC不匹配的C57BL/10(H-2^b)小鼠的肺移植到C57BL/6受体。移植后2周内迅速发生了BOS表现,可通过中和IL-17A得到改善[234]。在Balb/c移植到C57BL/6受体时结合使用CsA及皮质激素可导致在大约10周急性炎症损伤及排斥反应后发生BOS,但是肺功能测量结果与晚期组织学异常的严重程度无关[235]。在一种外科技术相对困难的模型中进行的研究可能会为损伤介导BOS的发生机制提供新的见解。

免疫抑制剂的毒性

第17章将讨论钙调神经磷酸酶抑制剂CsA作为免疫抑制剂的作用及其作用机制。在其早期临床应用中,发现CsA会介导剂量依赖性肾功能衰竭,这种情况最初见于肾移植受者[236]。随着此药开始广泛使用,其肾脏毒性也在原有肾脏、非肾器官的移植受体以及治疗自身免疫性疾病的患者中得到证实[237]。为验证此临床观察结果,研究者使用大鼠模型对肾毒性进行了详细分析,Sprague Dawley大鼠每天用12.5mg/kg CsA治疗3~10周,出现了肾功能降低以及沿亨利环后上肢发生肾小管变性为组织学特征的“条纹样纤维化”,以及外髓质成纤维细胞增殖和胶原沉积[238]。这些表现会因低钠饮食而加重,而不会受单侧肾切除影响。已经使用了其他大鼠品系进行研究,包括发生了类似反应的Wistar大鼠[239]和PVG大鼠[240],表明这不是品系特有的现象。使用的CsA剂量为5~25mg/(kg·d),持续平均4周[239],几乎每个模型均强调使用低钠饮食来增强血管收缩过程。

使用这种毒性模型的机制研究已经确定了几种关键的介质种类,包括血管紧张素Ⅱ[241-246]。事实上,使用螺内酯[247]或血管紧张素受体阻断剂[242]治疗可以减轻该模型中的肾损伤。类似地,血管收缩类花生酸如血栓素A2[248-252]和白三烯[240,253]表达会在该模型中上调,而抑制这些途径可以改善肾功能及组织学改变。参与此过程的其他分子包括内皮素[254]和一氧化氮[255-257]。

CsA的促纤维化作用与诱导PDGF和TGF-β与

肾脏[239,258-260]以及 CTGF[261]有关。TGF-β 在该模型中功能上的影响已进一步通过用吡非尼酮[262]以及抗 TGF-β 抗体可以治疗 CsA 诱导的纤维化证实[259]。此外,随着血管紧张素Ⅱ的表达与 TGF-β 的诱导有关,几项研究已经证明当血管紧张素途径被拮抗时 TGF-β 的总量会减少[242,263]。HMG-CoA 还原酶治疗还可以减轻此肾毒性模型中肾纤维化及间质炎症[264]。虽然 TGF-β 在此模型中主要与纤维化的发生相关,但是由于 TGF-β 具有较强的免疫调节作用,因此此通路的拮抗剂可能具有意想不到的效果。

因为 CsA 可以介导肾小管损伤,所以在暴露期间发生细胞凋亡并不奇怪。这一点已经在肾毒性大鼠模型中使用 TUNEL 染色法得到了证实[265]。肾毒性大鼠模型中的肾脏也发生了促凋亡基因的上调[266],小鼠模型亦同[267]。逆转这种表达可以作为改善损伤的潜在治疗策略[268-270]。纤维化损伤也可以通过巢蛋白表达来进行额外的调节,这种现象可以在 CsA 肾毒性损伤后的肾脏间质组织中发现[271]。发生损伤时去除巨噬细胞与肾功能的改善及 CsA 治疗后间质坏死的减少相关[272]。

内质网(ER)应激反应在人肾小管上皮细胞体外实验中是一种介导 CsA 损伤的潜在机制[273]。实际上,延长大鼠 CsA 治疗时间与伴随上皮细胞凋亡的 ER 应激反应[274]以及 CsA 治疗后上皮细胞的自噬现象有关[275]。此外,预防内质网发生 CsA 介导的应激反应可以改善大鼠的肾功能并减轻 CsA 毒性的特异性组织学改变[276]。这些研究表明,存在一种新的机制可以作为改善 CsA 介导的肾小管损伤的另一条治疗途径。

虽然大多数关于 CsA 肾毒性机制的数据是通过使用大鼠模型获得的,但也已经有许多使用小鼠模型进行研究的报道。与移植模型类似,小鼠模型有着动物体型较小、遗传操作方便以及对小鼠的免疫应答方面的了解更多及可用试剂更多的优点。然而,小鼠会抵抗这种治疗[277,278],因此需要进行额外的处理。对 ICR 小鼠使用 0.01%低钠饮食联合 CsA 30mg/(kg·d) 皮下注射,在治疗的第 28 天,这些动物发生了 CsA 肾毒性的特征性病变[279]。相比之下,在正常的钠饮食下,即使使用 100mg/(kg·d) 的量进行处理,甚至在治疗 56 天后 CsA 对肾功能或其结构也没有造成影响。肾小管上皮凋亡增加及凋亡蛋白基因表达上调与这种损伤相关[267],此结果与在大鼠模型中观察到的结果非常类似。这些报道提出了另一种研究 CsA 损伤动物模型的可能性。他克莫司与 CsA 相比,所介导的肾毒性是否有差异尚待探究。

移植耐受的小动物模型

动物模型,特别是啮齿类动物模型,为了追求可预测且可靠的移植耐受治疗方案,并可在临床上成功应用,已经被广泛研究了 50 多年。关于耐受机制和临床中耐受原则的讨论可以分别在第 11 章和第 76 章中找到。尽管我们目前关注啮齿动物模型,但移植耐受的研究范围同时包括小型和大型动物模型。事实上,我们对免疫耐受基础的理解很大程度受益于对多物种的综合研究。J.B. Murphy 早在 1914 年就发现外源组织可以在免疫系统不完善的鸡胚绒毛尿囊膜上生长,这种现象可以通过加入成年脾细胞来逆转[280]。R.D.Owen 在 1945 年在大动物实验中获得了移植耐受研究的革命性进展,指出牛异卵双胞胎之间存在红细胞嵌合体嵌合现象。Medawar 的观察结果显示,牛异卵双胞胎通常对彼此的皮肤移植会发生自然的"耐受"[281]。然而,在 1953 年移植耐受与使用小动物(如啮齿类)模型之间的联系已经明确建立,Medawar 的研究小组报告说可以通过过继转移淋巴细胞到小鼠胚胎来建立耐受,随后此小鼠就可以耐受相同供体来源的皮肤移植[282]。

在小动物模型中产生移植耐受往往具有操作上的要求,通常在停止治疗后 100~150 天耐受同种异体移植物。如果该动物不排斥来自同一供体的移植物,但是仍有排斥"第三方"组织或器官的能力,产生的免疫耐受则会更严格。由于小动物实验的技术限制,通常使用供体特异性皮肤移植物作为二次移植进行刺激。因为皮肤移植对排斥最敏感而仍然是检测排斥反应的"金标准",但是皮肤组织与首次移植物在免疫学上有巨大差异。实际上,已经有研究表明,使用可耐受皮肤移植作为检验普遍耐受的标准过于严格,因为引起皮肤移植物排斥所需的 T 细胞数量要比引起心脏排斥所需要的数量小 6000 倍[50]。

虽然在移植研究中使用小动物大大增加了我们对免疫耐受的理解,但显然没有提供揭示耐受现象的决定性证据,也无法成为大型动物(例如猪)、非人灵长类动物(NHP)或临床人体试验的替代品。Medawar 的试验发现了小鼠耐受的机制,即使在 1953 年,在近交系小鼠的移植耐受会受到比他所建立的模型更复杂的因素影响时，Medawar 的发现依然适用，因为移植物存活可能是永久或是暂时的，并且具有高度的品系特异性。此外，Medawar 在小鼠实验中诱导耐受依赖于在胎儿小鼠免疫成熟之前进行同种异体抗原呈递，这种情况在临床上非常少见。然而，他在 20 世纪 50 年代的创新性试验明确表明，改变受体免疫力可以使其获得对成年组织的免疫耐受，并且开启了“免疫调节”的领域。尽管存在局限性，但小动物模型为我们提供了移植耐受方面有价值的见解。先进技术不仅提供了需要在小型和大型动物模型中进行验证的新疗法，还提供了可用于测试特定潜在传导通路或更准确地反映人类系统的独特遗传修饰小鼠模型。

小动物模型在耐受研究中的局限性

毫无疑问，对于移植耐受的认识来自小鼠实验，移植研究已经通过使用基因工程转基因小鼠、基因敲除小鼠和基因诱变小鼠[283-288]以及淋巴细胞膜标记的单克隆抗体探针[289]获得了革命性的进步。然而，与大型远交系动物相比，小型近交系动物似乎更容易达到耐受，甚至强壮的动物模型都似乎比患者更具挑战性。即便是小鼠耐受的生理学基础也十分复杂。在 Medawar 的中枢耐受的经典实验中，值得注意的是，5 只小鼠中只有 3 只在围生期注射供体组织后对皮肤组织产生了耐受，这 3 只小鼠中的 1 只在移植后 75~91 天之间皮肤移植失活[290]。很明显，虽然小动物和啮齿类动物仍然在发现潜在诱导耐受方法十分“经济”，但是存在着复杂的因素会影响应用于人类移植免疫耐受研究的有效性。啮齿类动物的免疫系统与大型动物和某些灵长类动物(表 14.2)不同，区别在于 MHC 组织、与年龄相关的 T 细胞再生能力下降、T 细胞群的多样性、不同调节因子下 B 细胞和 T 细胞发育、细胞因子和趋化因子群的差异、排斥中的细胞毒效应细胞及 T 细胞耗竭法中稳态 T 细胞增殖和记忆 T 细胞的扩增[291-293]。众所周知，通常许多实验用近交小鼠品系代表了极端的免疫学表型，包括相对于 Th2 细胞应答趋向于产生 Th1 细胞[294]。也许最相关的区别是动物的寿命，寿命长的“有抗原经验”的哺乳类动物及人类与寿命短的倾向于“无抗原经验”啮齿类动物相比，会导致原始 T 细胞和记忆 T 细胞及 B 细胞的形成存在差异[290,295-297]。例如，基于 CSB 的耐受诱导疗法在啮齿动物中非常成功，而在具有较高比例记忆细胞的动物中较不敏感[298]。

表 14.2 实验性移植研究中啮齿类动物模型和非人类哺乳类动物模型的比较

比较项目	非人类哺乳类	啮齿类
处理	困难，尤其是体型较大者	相对容易
每只费用	高	低
品系选择	有限	可选种类多
强健度	高	低
转基因模型	不可行	可行
技术性难度	高	低
模拟人类免疫系统	基础类似	基础及适应性
寿命	1~3 年	20~40 年
生理指标解析	复杂	简单
繁殖	容易	非常困难(尚未造成)
试剂选择	有限/非特异性	种类多样/品系特异性
自发性变异	不常见	较少
用于实验性治疗	更高的适应性	较低的适应性
与人体解剖相似	类似	不同
与人体生理相似	类似	不同
营养	配方复杂	配方简单

小动物中的移植耐受

中枢移植耐受

自身反应性 T 细胞和 B 细胞在小鼠和人类的初级淋巴器官即胸腺和骨髓中被灭活[287,299,300]。胸腺对于 T 细胞成熟和通过克隆删除诱导对自身抗原的“中枢”耐受是必需的，而自身反应性 T 细胞可以离开胸腺并且有潜力引起自身免疫性疾病(见第 2 章)。因此，免疫调节是十分必要的，包括“外周耐受”机制，其主要是无功能[301]、外周缺失[302]和可以下调自身反应性细胞活性的调节性 T 细胞和 B 细胞[303,304]。胸腺去除抗原反应性 T 细胞的能力在小鼠胸腺内注射胰岛细胞的实验中得到证实[305]，但是胸腺内同种异体多肽的呈递可能会受限于成年人胸腺退化。供体抗原的短暂存在也可以解释在临床上观察到的心脏移植患者中使用供体细胞时出现的移植保护缺乏现象[306]。

混合的嵌合移植耐受

混合的淋巴造血嵌合体来自经照射的小鼠（及更大的物种)，由 T 细胞耗竭的宿主和供体骨髓的混合物重组而成。中枢耐受的一种形式为宿主和供体淋巴和造血元件在这些受体动物体内终身存在，并且移植的供体组织在没有免疫抑制的情况下被接受[307]。混合的嵌合耐受在小型动物受体中很强大，其可以越过广泛的主要和次要组织相容性抗原屏障接受高免疫原性皮肤和小肠移植[308,309]。从机制上讲，耐受状态包括反应性细胞的去除以及外周调节机制[310-314]。对移植前宿主状态调整的要求，包括亚致死性辐射、使用清髓剂及寿命有限的混合嵌合体，限制了该策略在除患有血液恶性肿瘤并发肾衰竭的特定患者之外的临床应用[315]。混合嵌合体产生T细胞耗竭的单克隆抗体，但局部胸腺照射的效果在小鼠中似乎比非人类灵长类动物更持久，其中嵌合体似乎仅短暂存在[316,317]。啮齿动物模型的研究因此集中在替换有害的调整手段以减少宿主发病率，如高剂量MHC错配骨髓、单次注射抗CD40L和细胞毒T淋巴细胞相关抗原4免疫球蛋白(CTLA-4 Ig)[318]。使用具有免疫调节能力的供体衍生的胚胎干细胞或间充质干细胞有可能提高生成混合嵌合体方法的效率[319-322]。虽然理论上的中央耐受具有吸引力，但是其临床转化的速度很慢，因为作为制作混合造血嵌合体的必要条件，所使用的临床可接受的毒性方案尚未实现。

外周移植耐受

共刺激分子阻断

由于自身抗原反应性细胞可以逃避胸腺灭活，因此存在另外的机制来调节出现在外周具有潜在自身反应性的T细胞的功能。外周耐受是一个泛指的术语，适用于可导致外周自身反应性T细胞的无反应性、缺失或调节细胞抑制的自然发生机制。使用小鼠移植模型的研究对探明外周耐受对同种异体抗体的反应机制很关键，而更重要作用的是研发利用这些机制的临床治疗方案。小鼠中的外周免疫应答可被T细胞和B细胞上的“阻尼”受体减弱，而被共刺激增强。阻尼受体已经在小鼠移植模型中被详细研究，包括许多分子如CTLA-4[323]、T细胞免疫球蛋白黏蛋白家族(TIM)的成员[324]、程序性细胞死亡受体(PD1)及其配体PDL-1[325,326]，以及B细胞、Fc和其他抑制性(ITIM)受体[327,328]。

在实验小鼠模型中，同种抗原识别时阻断CD28-CD80/86共刺激已被证明是诱导外周耐受的一种强而有效的方法。其次重要的共刺激通路是CD40(在APC上发现)/CD40L(CD154)(在T细胞上发现)通路，其在$CD4^+T$细胞应答的过程中起到关键作用[329]。通过CTLA-4传递信号似乎是移植物耐受的必要通路[330]。在小鼠身上发现$CD4^+$ $CD25^+$ T调节细胞可表达组成表面和细胞质的CTLA-4(CD152)[331]，并通过抗CTLA-4抗体阻断CTLA-4而导致同种异体移植皮肤的急性排斥反应[332]。早期研究发现，通过阻断信号1(抗CD4和抗CD8 mAbs)或信号2(抗CD40L或CTLA4Ig)可部分抑制T细胞功能而诱导小鼠中同种异体移植物的长期存活[333]。使用含有与人免疫球蛋白Fc链融合的人CTLA-4细胞外结构域的CTLA-4Ig融合蛋白抑制CD80/CD86(B7)-CD28通路传递的信号被证明在皮肤移植和心脏同种异体移植物中是有效的[334]。使用CTLA-4Ig的实验小鼠模型在近期使用LEA29Y(贝拉西普)修饰的高亲和力CTLA-4Ig融合蛋白对B7:CD28/CTLA4通路的药物治疗研究中很重要，其在2011年被FDA批准用于临床肾脏移植[335-337]。

有辅助方法可以增强CSB在啮齿动物移植模型中的作用。$CD4^+T$细胞似乎比$CD8^+T$细胞对CSB更敏感，在一些小鼠模型中，抑制共刺激分子后的同种异体移植物存活期会因为$CD8^+T$细胞的减少或消耗而延长[291]。在小鼠皮肤同种异体移植模型中，用抗CD40L mAb和供体特异性细胞输注(DST)的治疗可以通过诱导同种异体反应性$CD8^+T$细胞的灭活来延长皮肤移植物的存活[338-341]。CTLA-4Ig治疗也可与注射供体同种异体抗原或抗CD40L抗体联合应用[342]，因为当CSB与供体抗原呈递相结合时，诱导啮齿类动物的耐受状态趋向于更强大。虽然在一些情况下使用钙调神经磷酸酶抑制剂可以阻断CSB诱导的耐受形成[77,343]，但西罗莫司被证明可以增强CSB作用并增加完全主要和次要MHC分子错配的皮肤移植模型的长期耐受概率[77]。虽然CTLA-4和CD40L是小鼠CSB移植研究的主要靶点，但也存在着其他的CSB靶点。在小鼠心脏同种异体移植模型中，缺乏诱导的共刺激分子ICOS($ICOS^{-/-}$)的小鼠表现出移植物存活期延长[344,345]。程序性死亡-1(PD-1)及其配体PDL-1和PDL-2(B7的同源物)已经在小鼠移植中进行了试验。在心脏同种异体移植模型中，使用PDL-1 Ig融合蛋白处理的小鼠表现出同种异体移植物存活期延长，并且在某些情况下永久存活[346]。

T调节细胞

供体适应性免疫调节活动存在于啮齿动物移植受体的淋巴细胞室内，其在移植生物学中的作用在第8章中有详细讨论。抑制剂或调节性T细胞对于在体内诱导和维持供体同种异体抗原的无反应性至关重要：这可能提出了一种用来移植免疫耐受治疗的重要方法。在20世纪70年代，使用小鼠皮肤移植模型提出了淋巴细胞外周调节免疫应答的理论[347-349]。纯化的小鼠脾T淋巴细胞可以在皮肤移植前达到耐受，从而将供体特异性无反应性转移到抗淋巴细胞治疗的二次受体中，这种现象有时是永久性的。关于CD8+"抑制细胞"存在与否的争论，在CD4+T调节细胞存在的有力证据出现后停止。很久之前就发现了短期阻断抗CD4和抗CD8单克隆抗体可以在小鼠皮肤同种异体移植受体中产生"显性"的耐受表现，而这种供体特异性的非反应性可以通过多种淋巴细胞转移到数代之后的原始受体小鼠。这种现象被称为"传染性耐受"[347,350]。然而，传染性耐受的早期研究是在次要组织相容性不匹配的小鼠中进行的，而传染性耐受在有主要遗传差异的小鼠移植中缺乏证据或不成立。

正常人体内的大多数CD4+调节细胞(Treg)是在胸腺中生成的所谓自然T细胞或nTreg细胞。调节性CD4+T细胞也可以通过各种方法诱导(iTreg)产生。已经使用表达CD25(IL-2R alpha)的细胞来更具体地分辨并丰富小鼠中表现出强大调节活性的CD4+T细胞亚群[351]。CD4+ CD25+ T细胞能够在体内调节对同种异体抗原的反应过程，此类细胞可以从经供体特异性输血(DST)和抗CD4单克隆抗体预处理过的小鼠中分离出来[352]。一个CD4+调节T细胞功能关键转录因子的重要之处戏剧性地在使用同源性变异皮屑小鼠的研究中被发现，这种小鼠缺乏叉头转录因子3(Foxp3)。选择性去除CD4+Foxp3+Treg细胞会导致"灾难性的"多系统自身免疫反应[353]。除了Foxp3外，已经发现许多T细胞表达的分子具有调节活性，包括CD62、CD103和GITR[291,351]。同种异体抗原特异性CD4+ CD25+调节T细胞能够阻止由CD4+和CD8+T细胞介导的皮肤移植排斥反应[291]。另外，还明确存在其他调节细胞，包括CD8+、CD8+ CD28+、TCR+ CD4- CD8-("双阴性")和天然杀伤T细胞。因此CD4+ CD25+细胞可能只代表在啮齿类动物移植模型中一类重要的调节细胞[354,355]。在小鼠模型中，调节性T细胞在微环境下对细胞因子具有反应性。IL-10和TGF-β在同种异体抗原特异性CD4+ CD25+调节性T细胞的抑制活动中起关键作用。将从使用抗CD4/DST耐受方案预处理的受体中分离得到的T调节细胞，与原始效应细胞一起接种至T细胞缺陷小鼠时，在使用抗IL-10受体抗体处理时该小鼠无法阻止发生的皮肤移植排斥反应，而在没有进行抗IL-10受体抗体处理时，所有的移植物均被接受[332]。类似地，TGF-β1 mRNA在来自接受使用DST处理过的大鼠的心脏同种异体移植的个体中以高水平表达[356]。

移植微环境在耐受中的作用

越来越明显的证据表明，供体移植物具有与受体免疫应答相互作用或躲避受体免疫应答的能力，以达到接受或增强耐受。在眼前房中的抗原不受免疫系统的攻击，表明组织可以阻止损害性免疫效应系统[357]。自发地接受肝脏和肾脏同种异体移植以及最近在没有添加任何免疫抑制的小鼠中的胚状体的成功，均支持基于组织的保护机制的存在[134,358,359]。在联合移植实验中，供体肾脏不仅需要诱发耐受，还需要能够维持来自同一供体联合移植的心脏的耐受。有趣的是，将CD25+细胞从心肾受体接种至单独心脏受体会产生短期而不是长期的耐受，表明肾脏内Treg细胞在持续学习[22]。包括移植遗传背景、移植实体器官的性质以及并发可增加固有炎症反应的缺血或感染情况在内的因素可能会改变耐受性的发展。实验小鼠模型将需要解决这些因素的影响，以提供可应用于临床移植的数据。

缺血再灌注损伤

组织缺血是实体器官移植无法避免的后果。越来越多的人认识到，在器官采集和植入期间，移植物发生的最初的损伤对移植预后有着重大影响。

冷冻保存的历史

1849年，Loebel试图首次灌注一个孤立的器官[360]。然后在1895年，Langendorf开发了简易的器官灌注装置。Lindbergh和Carrel首先提出低温保存器官，之后为此发明了一个灌注装置。直到1964年，Belzer与Najarian在加利福尼亚大学旧金山分校开始研究低温灌注技术用于死亡捐献者肾脏移植计划[361]。1969年，

Collins 通过使用兔子模型建立了第一个有效的冷冻保存解决方案，帮助将移植实践从急诊手术转变为半择期手术[362,363]。这种解决方案对延长成功的肾脏保存时间有着很大的帮助，但不幸的是这个方案不适用于长时间保存和肝组织[360]。1980 年初，Belzer 和 Southard 开发了威斯康星大学(UW)方案[364]。UW 方案已经进行了一些改进，尽管优于许多其他方案，但仍不适合超过 24 小时的器官储存。不足为奇的是，冷缺血时间是肾移植后延迟移植物功能恢复(DGF)的最重要预测因子[365]。移植到受体后，重建血流(再灌注)通过产生自由基导致组织进一步损伤进而促使 DGF[366]。"温"和"冷"缺血引起的伤害统称为缺血再灌注损伤(IRI)[367]。虽然大多数伴有 DGF 的移植物之后会有可接受范围内的功能，但是这些移植物的长期存活明显不如功能立即恢复的移植物[368]。IRI 会负性影响移植物平均寿命，增加需要再次移植的患者数量，继而加重了供体器官短缺的问题。器官短缺问题促使使用扩大标准的供体；然而，由于其性质，ECD 器官更容易出现 IRI，因此 DGF 更容易发生[369,370]。最近，脉搏灌注的使用已经被证明可以改善肾功能，并且与人类肾脏同种异体移植中移植物存活改善有关[371]。因此，IRI 已经成为实验室移植研究的重点。

冷缺血损伤

目前已经建立了动物模型来进一步研究 IRI 的机制和潜在的治疗方法[372-374]。冷缺血是指器官(例如肾)被摘除、灌洗并在类似于人类移植冷保存条件下的低温下储存[375]。在经过一段时间后，将肾脏重新植入并进行再灌注。在发展出小鼠移植模型和转基因技术之前，冷缺血(肠、心脏、肺、肝和肾)主要使用狗、兔和大鼠进行研究[376-378]。最近，小鼠模型已经超越了所有其他动物模型而作为 IRI 研究的首选。这些实验模型大大促进了我们对冷缺血性损伤机制的认识[360,374,379,380]。特别是动物模型对器官冷保存方案的发展有很大帮助[381]。虽然冷缺血模型很好地模拟人类器官移植的过程，但我们对移植物 IRI 的了解大部分来源于使用热缺血模型的研究[367,382]。尽管事实上，损伤的分布和模式可能与冷缺血-再灌注模型大相径庭。

IRI 的病理生理学

IRI 是一个动态过程，其涉及两个差异明显却又相互关联的损伤阶段：缺血性器官损伤和炎症介导的再灌注损伤。细胞损伤可能源自被动或主动机制。被动机制包括细胞 ATP/GTP 的消耗[383]、细胞内酸中毒及低体温[360,384]。细胞损伤的活动期开始于再灌注，并导致先天免疫和适应性免疫通路的激活[385,386]。IRI 的一个关键特征是活性氧(ROS)的积累，这种现象被认为是由于 IRI 介导的损伤导致的线粒体中电子传递系统的解耦合造成的。尽管多种细胞和分子通路可以减轻和调节组织损伤，但固有免疫和适应性免疫系统之间的相互作用在肝脏 IRI 的发病机制中起着重要的作用。进化模型指出，最开始的缺血再灌注组织损伤通过激活先天免疫机制作为对器官同种异体免疫应答的"佐剂"[386]。

发生缺血损伤的细胞面临两种命运：依赖上皮细胞再生从亚致死性损伤中恢复[387]，或是因细胞凋亡或坏死造成细胞死亡[388-391]。细胞凋亡是 IRI 的共同特征[373-382]。细胞死亡对 IRI 的发病机制非常重要，因为在 IRI 开始时，抑制细胞凋亡通路可以改善组织损伤和限制器官功能障碍[392-397]。令人困惑的是，细胞凋亡被认为是尸体处理中一种免疫沉默的机制[398]。在这种情况下，死亡细胞的"激增"可能会压倒内源性清除机制[399]，使凋亡细胞发生继发性坏死[400,401]。与凋亡细胞不同，坏死的细胞将它们的细胞内容物释放至细胞外环境中，并通过激活先天性免疫反应[386,403,404](见第 7 章)来诱发无菌性炎症反应(SIR)[402]。这个"附带损害"的炎症反应是器官功能障碍的关键因素[405-407]，并且可以被内源性"危险"信号或警报素激发，其中警报素由受侵害、受损伤或是非正常死亡的细胞释放，有提醒免疫系统的功能[408-410]。危险或损害相关分子模式(DAMP)分子是正常细胞或细胞外基质中的成分，它们由细胞损伤或损伤组织中的蛋白酶分别释放[411]。炎症信号可从受损细胞转导，并通过 IL-1R-Myd88 通路引起组织损伤[409]，或是肾脏缺血性损伤中通过 TLR4 通路传递信号[412]而肾上皮细胞可以通过引导肾脏的炎症反应直接参与损伤过程。

IRI 的免疫反应

先天免疫细胞例如 NK 细胞和 NKT 细胞是小鼠肾脏发生 IRI 后早期浸润的细胞中的一部分[413]。虽然 NKT 细胞缺乏重组的 T 细胞受体(TCR)，但这些细胞可以对由非典型 MHC Ⅰ类分子 CD1d(见第 2 章)呈递的脂质、糖脂或高度疏水多肽抗原起反应。阻断 CD1d

分子或耗尽NKT细胞抑或使用NKT细胞缺陷小鼠可以显著减轻小鼠肾脏的缺血性损伤[414]。此外,NK细胞可以触发同源肾小管上皮细胞进行细胞凋亡,并且对NK细胞、T细胞、B细胞缺失小鼠接种NK细胞可能会加重肾脏IRI [415]。去除NK细胞上的CD39分子可使ATP和ADP磷酸水解为AMP,明显减少伴随致热受体的调节,减轻小鼠肝脏的热缺血损伤[416]。综上所述,这些结果表明了NK细胞和NKT细胞对IRI的大致作用。

动物模型已成为用来分析IRI中损伤涉及因素的关键工具(表14.3)。例如,在治疗非肾切除大鼠发生肾缺血之前,使用抗CD11a和抗CD11b进行治疗,可以改善肾功能并减轻炎症反应[417]。现在有压倒性的证据表明T细胞是IRI的直接介质。在CD4和CD8双重缺陷的小鼠发生肾缺血时,与野生型相比,肾功能明显改善、中性粒细胞浸润减少、肾小管萎缩评分明显降低,表明肾脏IRI时T细胞耗竭有着保护作用[418]。类似地,T细胞缺陷小鼠也被保护免受肾脏[419]以及肝脏[420]缺血性损伤,表明需要$CD4^+$T细胞应答介导损伤[420]。对共刺激阻断CD28/B7通路产生的保护作用提供了进一步证据提示T细胞在IRI发病机制中的作用[372,421]。

表14.3 小动物模型研究中缺血再灌注损伤过程中涉及的通路

IRI及修复中的通路	模型	参考文献
髓质中的血流变化	大鼠热IRI	[480,481]
巨噬细胞	小鼠热IRI;siRNA	[482]
B细胞	小鼠热IRI	[483,484]
T细胞	大鼠及小鼠热/冷IRI;NUDE;SCID;$Rag1^{-/-}$;获得转移;$CD4^{-/-}$;$CD8^{-/-}$	[372,420,485-488]
NKT细胞	小鼠热IRI;Jalpha18(-/-)	[489,490]
Toll样受体	小鼠热IRI;$TLR4^{-/-}$	[317,412,423,491]
中性粒细胞	小鼠热IRI	[492]
ICAM-1	小鼠热IRI;$ICAM\text{-}1^{-/-}$	[492]
补体	小鼠热IRI;$Cr1^{-/-}Cr2^{-/-}$	[413,483,493-496]
选择素	小鼠热IRI及小肠移植;P-选择素敲除	[156,497,498]
补充死亡肾小管上皮细胞的细胞来源	小鼠热IRI;细胞演变示踪;骨髓嵌合体	[387,441,442]
凋亡	抑制剂;敲除小鼠	[396,413,499,500]
纤维化	小鼠热IRI;细胞演变示踪	[444,501,502]
缺氧诱导因子	小鼠热/冷IRI;抑制剂;敲除小鼠	[503-506]

靶向IRI

如表14.3所示,IRI的复杂性以及适应性免疫与先天免疫的联系,使IRI超过冷冻储存方案和离体灌注机成为治疗的焦点。我们已经注意到了抗凋亡疗法在限制IRI中的作用。许多研究已经证明,在IRI过程中一氧化碳(CO)有着细胞保护作用,这种现象存在于大鼠肝脏[422,423]、肾脏[424-426]、肺[427]和小肠[428,429]以及其他器官和组织[430]。炎性细胞浸润可以通过将淋巴细胞阻断在次级淋巴器官中来缓解,原理是使用鞘氨醇1磷酸酯类似物防止它们进入缺血器官,这种物质可以诱导小鼠淋巴细胞减少并让它们免于肺[33]和肾脏[431-433]缺血性损伤。腺苷在许多组织中有血管扩张的作用,选择性激活腺苷A2A受体已被证明可以减少心脏、肝脏、脊髓、肺和脑组织损伤[434]。抑制HMG-coA还原酶可以类似地改善小鼠肾脏IRI,因为已知其具有人体安全性,可以作为有效的治疗辅助药物[435]。可降解基质分子的基质金属蛋白酶也参与传播IRI,且对小鼠进行基因删除后,会对IRI产生负面影响[436]。因此,使用基因删除、蛋白质耗竭或受体阻断方法进行的动物研究发现了会导致缺血性组织损伤的分子。

靶向治疗的主要限制之一是其潜在的非特异性和非靶向效果。RNA干扰(RNAi)是一种新兴的治疗方法,它提供了高抑制活性、限制活动持续时间、最小的毒性以及精确性,已经进行了IRI相关研究[437]。例如,目标为可调节肾脏IRI中细胞凋亡的转录因子p53的siRNA,可以减轻小鼠缺血组织损伤[438,439]。这种治疗方案已经进入人体临床试验阶段。将siRNA引入受体的方法中一个很有吸引力的选择是将其添加到移植前的器官保存液中。

肾脏IRI后的组织修复

肾脏有一个显著特征就是其具有损伤后的自我修复能力,但器官恢复的程度取决于损伤的严重程度以及炎症反应的调控水平[440]。肾小管上皮细胞(TEC)的增殖是肾小管修复的一个标志。紧随IRI后损伤期,一般处于休眠期的肾小管细胞进入细胞周期[441]。受损肾脏中细胞再生的起源仍然存在争议,使用来自绿色荧光蛋白转基因小鼠的骨髓嵌合体确定了骨髓来源细胞并未对受缺血性损伤的肾小管上皮恢复起重要作用[442,443]。此外,对特异性肾细胞启动子和小鼠 IRI 模型使用命运追踪技术进行研究已经发现了 TEC 是成年小鼠肾脏 IRI 后肾小管上皮细胞再生的主要细胞来源[387]。当 IRI 程度较轻且局限时,修复通路可以将肾脏恢复至其正常的结构和功能状态。然而,去修复程度更严重的损伤或损伤叠加在基础肾脏疾病之上时,修复过程可导致纤维化及慢性肾脏疾病。在经受严重的损伤之后,近端肾小管细胞反应受到损伤,其增殖反应改变使细胞周期停止于 G2/M 期,导致产生促纤维化因子,包括细胞因子、生长因子和基质蛋白[444,445]。

急性肾损伤的生物标记物——肾脏损伤分子-1(Kim-1)是免疫球蛋白基因超家族的一员,最初是在肾脏 IRI 大鼠模型中被发现的[446]。随后的体外研究表明,它是一种非骨髓来源的磷脂酰丝氨酸受体,可以将上皮细胞转化为半功能的吞噬细胞[447],并在损伤期间通过尿液排出[448]。虽然 Kim-1 不被认为是治疗的靶点,在确定其有潜力作为急性肾损伤的生物标志物的过程中,使用小型啮齿动物模型非常关键,引发了人体介入性试验终点的革新。类似地,由单核细胞产生的 IL-18 已经被认为是另一种潜在的治疗通路,以及急性缺血性损伤的生物标志物[449,450]。

现存 IRI 动物模型的局限性

由于我们对 IRI 理解的加深和成功建立啮齿动物模型,已经将数个方法确定为潜在的临床疗法,但是这些方法都未能进一步转化到临床,特别是应用到急性肾损伤的治疗中。研究难以获得进展可能是由于在建议模型时遇到的以下问题:①动物模型中 IRI 的发病机制通常没有人体中复杂,因为患者常常有多种损伤原因和多个器官功能障碍;②人体发生 IRI 时通常伴随脓毒症,但难以在动物体内建立脓毒症和 IRI 模型;③由于血清肌酐已被用作急性肾损伤发作的生物标志物,所以 IRI 中许多经测试的应用可能太晚了;④因人类受试者的保护问题,为了保护受体以及供体家属和供体的意愿,在供体中测试的治疗方法难以开始进行人体试验。

最广泛使用的实验模型是将肾血管蒂或肾动脉夹闭不同时长随后再灌注。大鼠是模型所用的基础动物品种,但随着转基因技术的出现,过去十年来已经倾向于使用小鼠。不幸的是,这种模型受到很多批评。首先,动物模型中的形态学发现与人“急性肾小管坏死”(ATN)活检标本中的结果不一致[451]。矛盾的是,在经研究的有限的人体活检样本中,仅存在局限性坏死。肾移植中 ATN 的表现与非移植 ATN 非常相似,表现为局限的实质性损伤和明显的肾功能异常[452]。小鼠 IRI 由于实验者的原因结果非常容易发生差异,甚至细微的温度变化也会造成影响。因为低温具有保护作用,而肾脏温度预计会在阻断时下降,若左侧肾脏暴露则更为明显,所以动物体温控制非常重要[453]。小鼠不同品系之间应答也存在差异。此外,我们必须记住人类和动物肾脏有着根本区别。与人类不同,大鼠肾脏具有发育良好的髓质外条和周围的复合维管束,包括 Henle 短循环的细降支,对应着人肾脏中没有内容物的简单维管束。另一方面,啮齿类动物的肾脏是单肾小叶和单侧尿细胞结构,这些都与人体结构相反[454,455]。总体来说,抛开局限性,IRI 的动物模型显著提高了我们对肾损伤的认识。

异种移植

随着同种异体移植的成功和人体器官短缺情况的日益严重,异种器官移植领域重新引起了大家的兴趣。这个话题已在第 12 章详细描述,但一些方面与小动物模型相关,因为异种移植从定义上就是一个物种特异性的尝试。然而,这个领域仍然存在着一些障碍。包括宿主免疫系统对异种移植物的反应、动物组织或器官之间的生理不相容性及人体系统内诸如生长因子和其他蛋白质的相容性,以及将感染因子从供体转移到受体或一般群体的可能性[456]。

物种选择

虽然非人灵长类动物的系统发育和其他物种相比与人类更为接近,但由于伦理问题、将感染跨物种间传染给人类的高风险、育种困难及器官大小不匹配等原因,无法作为合适的器官来源[457]。因为这些原因以及一起实践和生物学方面的原因,猪被认为是人类首选的器官供体。猪器官的大小与人体器官更接近,猪便于大规模繁殖,且易于进行遗传修饰从而强化其作为器官来源的功能[458]。因为猪血糖水平与人类相似,且猪胰岛素在人体中有效，它们也被认为是理想的人类胰岛移植的来源。然而,猪的这些优势被人体异种免疫反应对猪组织格外强烈并出现了巨大免疫障碍这一事实所抵消了。

移植的免疫学屏障

人体异种移植的免疫反应包括体液免疫和细胞免疫系统。由抗体介导的过程包括超急性排斥反应(HAR)和延迟的异种移植排斥反应(DXR),会迅速攻击移植到未经处理的灵长类体内的猪血管化器官[456]。HAR是异种移植的第一道免疫屏障,主要由名为a抗Gal抗体介导，此抗体是针对移植物内皮表达的α键连接的半乳糖残基Gal1α1-3Gal分子的IgM抗体[459]。该抗体自然产生于缺乏与血型抗原抗体相似的免疫清除机制的受体中[460]。此抗原由α1,3-半乳糖基转移酶(α1,3GT)合成,此酶存在于下等哺乳动物和新世界猴子中,但不存在于老世界猴子、猿类和人类中[461]。因此,亲缘关系较远的不同物种作为供体组合,例如猪器官移植到灵长类动物中，再灌注后抗GAL抗体与内皮细胞结合后立即发生补体的激活,导致内皮损伤及随后异种移植物内血栓形成和坏死[461]。而亲缘关系接近的组合,如仓鼠器官移植到大鼠,这种情况下不会产生抗Gal抗体,而在产生抗移植物抗体后补体可能会参与延迟排斥反应[456]。因此,有目的地培育出了α-半乳糖基转移酶基因(GTKO)突变的猪[462,463]。最初的猪GTKO心脏移植至灵长类动物的异种移植没有发生超急性排斥反应,中位生存期为78天[464,465]。其他预防超急性排斥反应的方法包括对接受物种特异性器官如肝脏的受体用体外灌注法免疫吸附异种抗体[466]。

在通过去除抗Gal抗体或抑制补体活化预防HAR发生后,通常会观察到DXR[467]。其特征是移植物中NK细胞、单核细胞和粒细胞浸润,以及内皮细胞中纤维蛋白沉积和血小板聚集的内皮细胞活化[468,469]。而DXR的关键特征是血管内皮细胞激活和上述细胞中的Fc受体通过天然抗体(IgG抗-αGal)介导而激活。在与Fc受体结合时,效应细胞释放其颗粒内容物以介导抗体依赖性细胞毒性（ADCC)。由于其性质,DXR是成功的临床异种移植所面临的关键免疫屏障。

细胞介导的异种移植排斥

异种移植也受细胞免疫介导的排斥影响。异种移植物会引发强烈的抗原特异性T细胞应答，此反应是完成成功的异种移植的重要障碍[470]。由于抗体反应似乎与异种胰岛移植的排斥反应无关，阐明此动物模型中的细胞免疫反应扩大了我们对细胞免疫反应，特别是抗猪类细胞免疫反应的理解[471]。通过加入CSB例如CTLA4Ig或抗CD40L抗体,可明显改善猪异体胰腺存活情况[472]。此外,将猪胚胎胰岛样细胞置入裸鼠肾囊下与置入野生型小鼠相比。炎症损伤会更局限并有所减轻[473],证明胰岛异种移植排斥反应依赖完整的T细胞。支持这一结论的有，最近猪器官移植到非人类灵长类动物[474]和猪器官移植到小鼠[475-478]的研究表明,使用CSB类药物抗CD40L抗体或使用影响多种途径的联合疗法可以改善异种移植生存。

同种免疫应答的靶点是MHC抗原,而对异种移植物的反应可以指向多种分子构成不同的蛋白质和碳水化合物。类似于同种异体T细胞应答,T细胞对异种细胞应答涉及两个不同的通路:直接通路和间接通路[471]。在间接通路中，异种抗原在受体MHC环境下被APC细胞拾取、处理并呈递,且不涉及任何交叉物种信号1和信号2之间的相互作用。另一方面,直接通路是通过受体的CD4和CD8 T细胞与(异种)供体APC的表面上的MHC分子相互作用传递信号。只有当信号1和信号2都匹配时,物种间分子相互作用,才会使生产性的T细胞激活。而在人体中,未接受治疗的受体的抗猪类反应相当强烈[479]。

异种移植的前景

异种移植仍然是解决逐渐上升的器官移植率最可行的办法。使用小动物模型已经发现了这些反应中的一些生物学机制，并且证明了体液免疫和细胞介导的免疫功能都是将异种移植临床应用于人体过程中的巨大阻碍。近期,猪转基因技术的进步和成功使用非人类灵长类动物建立临床前模型，为进入临床阶段燃起了希望[458]。

总结

本章重点介绍了小动物模型在扩展我们对移植免

疫学知识方面起到的许多作用。主要的临床挑战包括晚期移植损伤、抗体介导的损伤和难以达成免疫耐受。表 14.2 重点介绍了小型和大型 NHP 动物模型之间的关键问题及两者的特点。可以操纵小鼠的遗传基因一直是支持其用于研究的关键因素之一。使用同基因标记可以帮助我们在转移种植试验中发现关键免疫组分的特征。可用试剂的种类包括抗体和分子试剂,对基因工程起到了强有力的补充。但是使用这些小动物也有缺点。血管化操作在技术上难度高,仅限于具有熟练掌握显微外科技术的医师的实验室才能完成。在压缩的时间里模拟人体疾病十分困难。免疫反应基础也与人体大不相同,小动物 T 细胞谱缺乏多样性且克隆量小,这不仅会影响免疫反应的强度,也会影响其基础和变异。异源免疫力的作用是另一个关键问题,因为饲养的小鼠不携带病原体,而人类要经常面临免疫原的侵袭。然而,在我们整体的理解中,两种模型都为同种异体免疫提供了重要理解。因此,我们应认为小动物模型对临床治疗有着重要贡献。

(郭颂一 译 李照 校)

参考文献

1. Nash JR, Peters M, Bell PR. Comparative survival of pancreatic islets, heart, kidney, and skin allografts in rats, with and without enhancement. Transplantation. 1977;24:70–73.
2. Zhang Z, Zhu L, Quan D, et al. Pattern of liver, kidney, heart, and intestine allograft rejection in different mouse strain combinations. Transplantation. 1996;62:1267–1272.
3. Mannon RB, Kopp JB, Ruiz P, et al. Chronic rejection of mouse kidney allografts. Kidney International. 1999;55:1935–1944.
4. Russell PS, Chase CM, Winn HJ, et al. Coronary atherosclerosis in transplanted mouse hearts. I. Time course and immunogenetic and immunopathological considerations. American Journal of Pathology. 1994;144:260–274.
5. Carrel A, Guthrie CC. Anastomosis of blood vessels by the patching method and transplantation of the kidney. 1906 [classical article]. Yale Journal of Biology and Medicine. 2001;74:243–247.
6. Muller-Ruchholtz W. Glances at the history of transplantation immunology. Transplantation Proceedings. 1999;31:1443–1451.
7. Calne RY, White DJ, Rolles K, et al. Prolonged survival of pig orthotopic heart grafts treated with cyclosporin A. Lancet. 1978;1:1183–1185.
8. Calne RY, White DJ, Thiru S, et al. Cyclosporin A in patients receiving renal allografts from cadaver donors. Lancet. 1978;2:1323–1327.
9. Kemp CB, Knight MJ, Scharp DW. Transplantation of isolated pancreatic islets into the portal vein of diabetic rats. Nature. 1973;244:447.
10. Lacy PE. The pancreatic beta cell. Structure and function. New England Journal of Medicine. 1967;276:187–195.
11. Lacy PE, Kostianovsky M. Method for the isolation of intact islets of Langerhans from the rat pancreas. Diabetes. 1967;16:35–39.
12. Abbott CP, Lindsey ES, Creech O Jr, et al. A technique for heart transplantation in the rat. Archives of Surgery. 1964;89:645–652.
13. Corry RJ, Winn HJ, Russell PS. Heart transplantation in congenic strains of mice. Transplantation Proceedings. 1973;5:733–735.
14. Corry RJ, Winn HJ, Russell PS. Primarily vascularized allografts of hearts in mice. The role of H-2D, H-2K, and non-H-2 antigens in rejection. Transplantation. 1973;16:343–350.
15. Zhou YQ, Bishay R, Feintuch A, et al. Morphological and functional evaluation of murine heterotopic cardiac grafts using ultrasound biomicroscopy. Ultrasound in Medicine and Biology. 2007;33:870–879.
16. Mottram PL, Smith JA, Mason A, et al. Electrocardiographic monitoring of cardiac transplants in mice. Cardiovascular Research. 1988;22:315–321.
17. Haug CE, Shapiro JI, Cosby RL, et al. 31P nuclear magnetic resonance spectroscopy of heart, heart-lung, and kidney allograft rejection in the rat. Transplantation Proceedings. 1988;20:848–855.
18. Szabo G, Batkai S, Dengler TJ, et al. Systolic and diastolic properties and myocardial blood flow in the heterotopically transplanted rat heart during acute cardiac rejection. World Journal of Surgery. 2001;25:545–552.
19. Skoskiewicz M, Chase C, Winn HJ, et al. Kidney transplants between mice of graded immunogenetic diversity. Transplantation Proceedings. 1973;5:721–725.
20. Kalina SL, Mottram PL. A microsurgical technique for renal transplantation in mice. Australian and New Zealand Journal of Surgery. 1993;63:213–216.
21. Zhang Z, Schlachta C, Duff J, et al. Improved techniques for kidney transplantation in mice. Microsurgery. 1995;16:103–109.
22. Mezrich J, Yamada K, Sachs DH, et al. Regulatory T cells generated by the kidney may mediate the beneficial immune effects of combining kidney with heart transplantation. Surgery. 2004;135:473–478.
23. Qian SG, Fung JJ, Demetris AV, et al. Orthotopic liver transplantation in the mouse. Transplantation. 1991;52:562–564.
24. Kamada N, Calne RY. Orthotopic liver transplantation in the rat. Technique using cuff for portal vein anastomosis and biliary drainage. Transplantation. 1979;28:47–50.
25. Lee S, Charters AC, Chandler JG, et al. A technique for orthotopic liver transplantation in the rat. Transplantation. 1973;16:664–669.
26. Lee S, Charters C, Chandler JG, et al. Prolonged survival after orthotopic liver transplantation in inbred rats. Surgical Forum. 1973;24:381–383.
27. Zimmermann FA, Davies HS, Knoll PP, et al. Orthotopic liver allografts in the rat. The influence of strain combination on the fate of the graft. Transplantation. 1984;37:406–410.
28. Chen L, Wang T, Zhou P, et al. TLR engagement prevents transplantation tolerance. American Journal of Transplantation. 2006;6:2282–2291.
29. Zhang Z, Schlachta C, Garcia B, et al. Intestinal transplantation in different mouse strain combinations. Transplantation Proceedings. 1994;26:1532.
30. Zhong R, Zhang Z, Quan D, et al. Development of a mouse intestinal transplantation model. Microsurgery. 1993;14:141–145.
31. Liu J, Fishbein TM, Bromberg JS, et al. Orthotopic small bowel transplantation in mice. Transplantation. 2005;79:973–976.
32. Mizuta T, Kawaguchi A, Nakahara K, et al. Simplified rat lung transplantation using a cuff technique. Journal of Thoracic and Cardiovascular Surgery. 1989;97:578–581.
33. Okazaki M, Kreisel F, Richardson SB, et al. Sphingosine 1-phosphate inhibits ischemia reperfusion injury following experimental lung transplantation. American Journal of Transplantation. 2007;7:751–758.
34. Krupnick AS, Lin X, Li W, et al. Orthotopic mouse lung transplantation as experimental methodology to study transplant and tumor biology. Nature Protocols. 2009;4:86–93.
35. Okazaki M, Krupnick AS, Kornfeld CG, et al. A mouse model of orthotopic vascularized aerated lung transplantation. American Journal of Transplantation. 2007;7:1672–1679.
36. Mannon RB, Coffman TM. Gene targeting: applications in transplantation research. Kidney International. 1999;56:18–27.
37. Belizario JE. Immunodeficient mouse models: an overview. Open Immunology Journal. 2009;2:79–85.
38. Yamaoka K, Saharinen P, Pesu M, et al. The Janus kinases (Jaks). Genome Biology. 2004;5:253.
39. Akira S. Functional roles of STAT family proteins: lessons from knockout mice. Stem Cells. 1999;17:138–146.
40. Zhou P, Szot GL, Guo Z, et al. Role of STAT4 and STAT6 signaling in allograft rejection and CTLA4-Ig-mediated tolerance. Journal of Immunology. 2000;165:5580–5587.
41. Bishop DK, Chan Wood S, Eichwald EJ, et al. Immunobiology of allograft rejection in the absence of IFN-gamma: CD8+ effector cells develop independently of CD4+ cells and CD40-CD40 ligand interactions. Journal of Immunology. 2001;166:3248–3255.
42. Le Moine A, Flamand V, Demoor FX, et al. Critical roles for IL-4, IL-5, and eosinophils in chronic skin allograft rejection. Journal of Clinical Investigation. 1999;103:1659–1667.
43. Li XC, Roy-Chaudhury P, Hancock WW, et al. IL-2 and IL-4 double knockout mice reject islet allografts: a role for novel T cell growth factors in allograft rejection. Journal of Immunology. 1998;161:890–896.
44. Raisanen-Sokolowski A, Mottram PL, Glysing-Jensen T, et al. Heart transplants in interferon-gamma, interleukin 4, and interleukin 10 knockout mice. Recipient

environment alters graft rejection. Journal of Clinical Investigation. 1997;100: 2449–2456.
45. Saleem S, Konieczny BT, Lowry RP, et al. Acute rejection of vascularized heart allografts in the absence of IFNgamma. Transplantation. 1996;62:1908–1911.
46. Steiger J, Nickerson PW, Steurer W, et al. IL-2 knockout recipient mice reject islet cell allografts. Journal of Immunology. 1995;155:489–498.
47. Medawar PB. The behaviour and fate of skin autografts and skin homografts in rabbits: a report to the War Wounds Committee of the Medical Research Council. Journal of Anatomy. 1944;78:176–199.
48. Steinmuller D. The enigma of skin allograft rejection. Transplantation Reviews. 1998;12:42–57.
49. Sun J, Sheil AG, Wang C, et al. Tolerance to rat liver allografts: IV. Acceptance depends on the quantity of donor tissue and on donor leukocytes. Transplantation. 1996;62:1725–1730.
50. Jones ND, Turvey SE, Van Maurik A, et al. Differential susceptibility of heart, skin, and islet allografts to T cell-mediated rejection. Journal of Immunology. 2001;166:2824–2830.
51. Rosenberg AS, Singer A. Cellular basis of skin allograft rejection: an in vivo model of immune-mediated tissue destruction. Annual Review of Immunology. 1992;10:333–358.
52. Lazarovits AI, Poppema S, Zhang Z, et al. Prevention and reversal of renal allograft rejection by antibody against CD45RB. Nature. 1996;380:717–720.
53. Lakkis FG, Arakelov A, Konieczny BT, et al. Immunologic 'ignorance' of vascularized organ transplants in the absence of secondary lymphoid tissue. Nature Medicine. 2000;6:686–688.
54. Zhou P, Hwang KW, Palucki D, et al. Secondary lymphoid organs are important but not absolutely required for allograft responses. American Journal of Transplantation. 2003;3:259–266.
55. Wang J, Dong Y, Sun JZ, et al. Donor lymphoid organs are a major site of alloreactive T-cell priming following intestinal transplantation. American Journal of Transplantation. 2006;6:2563–2571.
56. Dalchau R, Fangmann J, Fabre JW. Allorecognition of isolated, denatured chains of class I and class II major histocompatibility complex molecules. Evidence for an important role for indirect allorecognition in transplantation. European Journal of Immunology. 1992;22:669–677.
57. Fangmann J, Dalchau R, Fabre JW. Rejection of skin allografts by indirect allorecognition of donor class I major histocompatibility complex peptides. Journal of Experimental Medicine. 1992;175:1521–1529.
58. Lee RS, Grusby MJ, Glimcher LH, et al. Indirect recognition by helper cells can induce donor-specific cytotoxic T lymphocytes in vivo. Journal of Experimental Medicine. 1994;179:865–872.
59. Steele DJ, Laufer TM, Smiley ST, et al. Two levels of help for B cell alloantibody production. Journal of Experimental Medicine. 1996;183:699–703.
60. Vella JP, Spadafora-Ferreira M, Murphy B, et al. Indirect allorecognition of major histocompatibility complex allopeptides in human renal transplant recipients with chronic graft dysfunction. Transplantation. 1997;64:795–800.
61. Simpson E, Scott D, Chandler P. The male-specific histocompatibility antigen, H-Y: a history of transplantation, immune response genes, sex determination and expression cloning. Annual Review of Immunology. 1997;15: 39–61.
62. Cobbold S, Waldmann H. Skin allograft rejection by L3/T4+ and Lyt-2+ T cell subsets. Transplantation. 1986;41:634–639.
63. Vokaer B, Van Rompaey N, Lemaitre PH, et al. Critical role of regulatory T cells in Th17-mediated minor antigen-disparate rejection. Journal of Immunology. 2010;185:3417–3425.
64. Lakkis FG. Role of cytokines in transplantation tolerance: lessons learned from gene-knockout mice. Journal of the American Society of Nephrology. 1998;9: 2361–2367.
65. Dai Z, Konieczny BT, Baddoura FK, et al. Impaired alloantigen-mediated T cell apoptosis and failure to induce long-term allograft survival in IL-2-deficient mice. Journal of Immunology. 1998;161:1659–1663.
66. Konieczny BT, Dai Z, Elwood ET, et al. IFN-gamma is critical for long-term allograft survival induced by blocking the CD28 and CD40 ligand T cell costimulation pathways. Journal of Immunology. 1998;160:2059–2064.
67. Ring GH, Saleem S, Dai Z, et al. Interferon-gamma is necessary for initiating the acute rejection of major histocompatibility complex class II-disparate skin allografts. Transplantation. 1999;67:1362–1365.
68. Antonysamy MA, Fanslow WC, Fu F, et al. Evidence for a role of IL-17 in organ allograft rejection: IL-17 promotes the functional differentiation of dendritic cell progenitors. Journal of Immunology. 1999;162:577–584.
69. Yoshida S, Haque A, Mizobuchi T, et al. Anti-type V collagen lymphocytes that express IL-17 and IL-23 induce rejection pathology in fresh and well-healed lung transplants. American Journal of Transplantation. 2006;6:724–735.
70. Yuan X, Paez-Cortez J, Schmitt-Knosalla I, et al. A novel role of CD4 Th17 cells in mediating cardiac allograft rejection and vasculopathy. Journal of Experimental Medicine. 2008;205:3133–3144.
71. Burrell BE, Csencsits K, Lu G, et al. CD8+ Th17 mediate costimulation blockade-resistant allograft rejection in T-bet-deficient mice. Journal of Immunology. 2008;181:3906–3914.
72. Chadha R, Heidt S, Jones ND, et al. Th17: contributors to allograft rejection and a barrier to the induction of transplantation tolerance? Transplantation. 2011;91:939–945.
73. Nadig SN, Wieckiewicz J, Wu DC, et al. In vivo prevention of transplant arteriosclerosis by ex vivo-expanded human regulatory T cells. Nature Medicine. 2010; 16:809–813.
74. Feng G, Nadig SN, Backdahl L, et al. Functional regulatory T cells produced by inhibiting cyclic nucleotide phosphodiesterase type 3 prevent allograft rejection. Science Translational Medicine. 2011;3:83ra40.
75. Tsang JY, Tanriver Y, Jiang S, et al. Indefinite mouse heart allograft survival in recipient treated with CD4(+)CD25(+) regulatory T cells with indirect allospecificity and short term immunosuppression. Transplant Immunology. 2009;21: 203–209.
76. Xia G, He J, Leventhal JR. Ex vivo-expanded natural CD4+CD25+ regulatory T cells synergize with host T-cell depletion to promote long-term survival of allografts. American Journal of Transplantation. 2008;8:298–306.
77. Li Y, Li XC, Zheng XX, et al. Blocking both signal 1 and signal 2 of T-cell activation prevents apoptosis of alloreactive T cells and induction of peripheral allograft tolerance. Nature Medicine. 1999;5:1298–1302.
78. Li Y, Zheng XX, Li XC, et al. Combined costimulation blockade plus rapamycin but not cyclosporine produces permanent engraftment. Transplantation. 1998;66: 1387–1388.
79. Tang Q, Bluestone JA, Kang SM. CD4(+)Foxp3(+) regulatory T cell therapy in transplantation. Journal of Molecular Cell Biology. 2012;4:11–21.
80. Kim JI, O'Connor MR, Duff PE, et al. Generation of adaptive regulatory T cells by alloantigen is required for some but not all transplant tolerance protocols. Transplantation. 2011;91:707–713.
81. Shi Q, Lees JR, Scott DW, et al. Endogenous expansion of regulatory T cells leads to long-term islet graft survival in diabetic NOD mice. American Journal of Transplantation. 2012;12:1124–1132.
82. Adeegbe D, Serafini P, Bronte V, et al. In vivo induction of myeloid suppressor cells and CD4(+)Foxp3(+) T regulatory cells prolongs skin allograft survival in mice. Cell Transplantation. 2011;20:941–954.
83. Riella LV, Liu T, Yang J, et al. Deleterious effect of CTLA4-Ig on a Treg-dependent transplant model. American Journal of Transplantation. 2012;12:846–855.
84. Heidecke CD, Araujo JL, Kupiec-Weglinski JW, et al. Lack of evidence for an active role for natural killer cells in acute rejection of organ allografts. Transplantation. 1985;40:441–444.
85. Markus PM, van den Brink M, Cai X, et al. Effect of selective depletion of natural killer cells on allograft rejection. Transplantation Proceedings. 1991;23: 178–179.
86. Dresske B, Zhu X, Herwartz C, et al. The time pattern of organ infiltration and distribution of natural killer cells and macrophages in the course of acute graft rejection after allogeneic heart transplantation in the rat. Transplantation Proceedings. 1997;29:1715–1716.
87. McNerney ME, Lee KM, Zhou P, et al. Role of natural killer cell subsets in cardiac allograft rejection. American Journal of Transplantation. 2006;6:505–513.
88. Szot GL, Zhou P, Rulifson I, et al. Different mechanisms of cardiac allograft rejection in wildtype and CD28-deficient mice. American Journal of Transplantation. 2001;1:38–46.
89. Maier S, Tertilt C, Chambron N, et al. Inhibition of natural killer cells results in acceptance of cardiac allografts in CD28−/− mice. Nature Medicine. 2001;7: 557–562.
90. Kim J, Chang CK, Hayden T, et al. The activating immunoreceptor NKG2D and its ligands are involved in allograft transplant rejection. Journal of Immunology. 2007;179:6416–6420.
91. Kroemer A, Xiao X, Degauque N, et al. The innate NK cells, allograft rejection, and a key role for IL-15. Journal of Immunology. 2008;180:7818–7826.
92. Mannon RB. Macrophages: contributors to allograft dysfunction, repair, or innocent bystanders? Current Opinion in Organ Transplantation. 2012;17: 20–25.
93. Gao W, Topham PS, King JA, et al. Targeting of the chemokine receptor CCR1 suppresses development of acute and chronic cardiac allograft rejection. Journal of Clinical Investigation. 2000;105:35–44.
94. Gao W, Faia KL, Csizmadia V, et al. Beneficial effects of targeting CCR5 in allograft recipients. Transplantation. 2001;72:1199–1205.
95. Takeiri M, Tachibana M, Kaneda A, et al. Inhibition of macrophage activation and suppression of graft rejection by DTCM-glutarimide, a novel piperidine derived from the antibiotic 9-methylstreptimidone. Inflammation Research. 2011;60:879–888.

96. Jose MD, Ikezumi Y, van Rooijen N, et al. Macrophages act as effectors of tissue damage in acute renal allograft rejection. Transplantation. 2003;76:1015–1022.
97. Qi F, Adair A, Ferenbach D, et al. Depletion of cells of monocyte lineage prevents loss of renal microvasculature in murine kidney transplantation. Transplantation. 2008;86:1267–1274.
98. Gaston RS, Cecka JM, Kasiske BL, et al. Evidence for antibody-mediated injury as a major determinant of late kidney allograft failure. Transplantation. 2010; 90:68–74.
99. Berry GJ, Angelini A, Burke MM, et al. The ISHLT working formulation for pathologic diagnosis of antibody-mediated rejection in heart transplantation: evolution and current status (2005–2011). Journal of Heart and Lung Transplantation. 2011;30:601–611.
100. Smith RN, Kawai T, Boskovic S, et al. Four stages and lack of stable accommodation in chronic alloantibody-mediated renal allograft rejection in Cynomolgus monkeys. American Journal of Transplantation. 2008;8:1662–1672.
101. Nozaki T, Amano H, Bickerstaff A, et al. Antibody-mediated rejection of cardiac allografts in CCR5-deficient recipients. Journal of Immunology. 2007;179: 5238–5245.
102. Jindra PT, Hsueh A, Hong L, et al. Anti-MHC class I antibody activation of proliferation and survival signaling in murine cardiac allografts. Journal of Immunology. 2008;180:2214–2224.
103. Hattori Y, Bucy RP, Kubota Y, et al. Antibody-mediated rejection of single class I MHC-disparate cardiac allografts. American Journal of Transplantation. 2012;12:2017–2028.
104. Bickerstaff A, Nozaki T, Wang JJ, et al. Acute humoral rejection of renal allografts in CCR5(−/−) recipients. American Journal of Transplantation. 2008;8:557–566.
105. Galvani S, Auge N, Calise D, et al. HLA class I antibodies provoke graft arteriosclerosis in human arteries transplanted into SCID/beige mice. American Journal of Transplantation. 2009;9:2607–2614.
106. Kroshus TJ, Rollins SA, Dalmasso AP, et al. Complement inhibition with an anti-C5 monoclonal antibody prevents acute cardiac tissue injury in an ex vivo model of pig-to-human xenotransplantation. Transplantation. 1995;60:1194–1202.
107. Wang H, Arp J, Liu W, et al. Inhibition of terminal complement components in presensitized transplant recipients prevents antibody-mediated rejection leading to long-term graft survival and accommodation. Journal of Immunology. 2007;179:4451–4463.
108. Pruitt SK, Bollinger RR. The effect of soluble complement receptor type 1 on hyperacute allograft rejection. Journal of Surgical Research. 1991;50:350–355.
109. Pratt JR, Hibbs MJ, Laver AJ, et al. Effects of complement inhibition with soluble complement receptor-1 on vascular injury and inflammation during renal allograft rejection in the rat. American Journal of Pathology. 1996;149:2055–2066.
110. Forbes RD, Pinto-Blonde M, Guttmann RD. The effect of anticomplementary cobra venom factor on hyperacute rat cardiac allograft rejection. Laboratory Investigation. 1978;39:463–470.
111. Brauer RB, Baldwin WM 3rd, Ibrahim S, et al. The contribution of terminal complement components to acute and hyperacute allograft rejection in the rat. Transplantation. 1995;59:288–293.
112. Raedler H, Vieyra MB, Leisman S, et al. Anti-complement component C5 mAb synergizes with CTLA4Ig to inhibit alloreactive T cells and prolong cardiac allograft survival in mice. American Journal of Transplantation. 2011;11: 1397–1406.
113. Woodle ES, Baldwin WM 3rd. Of mice and men: terminal complement inhibition with anti-C5 monoclonal antibodies. American Journal of Transplantation. 2011;11:2277–2278.
114. Nayak A, Ferluga J, Tsolaki AG, et al. The non-classical functions of the classical complement pathway recognition subcomponent C1q. Immunology Letters. 2010;131:139–150.
115. Csencsits K, Burrell BE, Lu G, et al. The classical complement pathway in transplantation: unanticipated protective effects of C1q and role in inductive antibody therapy. American Journal of Transplantation. 2008;8:1622–1630.
116. Ramos E, Drachenberg CB, Wali R, et al. The decade of polyomavirus BK-associated nephropathy: state of affairs. Transplantation. 2009;87:621–630.
117. Johnston O, Jaswal D, Gill JS, et al. Treatment of polyomavirus infection in kidney transplant recipients: a systematic review. Transplantation. 2010;89: 1057–1070.
118. Mannon RB, Hoffmann SC, Kampen RL, et al. Molecular evaluation of BK polyomavirus nephropathy. American Journal of Transplantation. 2005;5: 2883–2893.
119. van Gorder MA, Della Pelle P, Henson JW, et al. Cynomolgus polyoma virus infection: a new member of the polyoma virus family causes interstitial nephritis, ureteritis, and enteritis in immunosuppressed cynomolgus monkeys. American Journal of Pathology. 1999;154:1273–1284.
120. Zaragoza C, Li RM, Fahle GA, et al. Squirrel monkeys support replication of BK virus more efficiently than simian virus 40: an animal model for human BK virus infection. Journal of Virology. 2005;79:1320–1326.
121. Han Lee ED, Kemball CC, Wang J, et al. A mouse model for polyomavirus-associated nephropathy of kidney transplants. American Journal of Transplantation. 2006;6:913–922.
122. Wilson JJ, Lin E, Pack CD, et al. Gamma interferon controls mouse polyomavirus infection in vivo. Journal of Virology. 2011;85:10126–10134.
123. Swanson PA 2nd, Lukacher AE, Szomolanyi-Tsuda E. Immunity to polyomavirus infection: the polyomavirus-mouse model. Seminars in Cancer Biology. 2009;19:244–251.
124. Jevnikar AM, Mannon RB. Late kidney allograft loss: what we know about it, and what we can do about it. Clinical Journal of the American Society of Nephrology. 2008;3(Suppl. 2):S56–S67.
125. Racusen LC, Solez K, Colvin RB, et al. The Banff 97 working classification of renal allograft pathology. Kidney International. 1999;55:713–723.
126. Solez K, Colvin RB, Racusen LC, et al. Banff '05 Meeting Report: differential diagnosis of chronic allograft injury and elimination of chronic allograft nephropathy ('CAN'). American Journal of Transplantation. 2007;7:518–526.
127. White E, Hildemann WH, Mullen Y. Chronic kidney allograft reactions in rats. Transplantation. 1969;8:602–617.
128. Hancock WW, Whitley WD, Baldwin WM 3rd, et al. Cells, cytokines, adhesion molecules, and humoral responses in a rat model of chronic renal allograft rejection. Transplantation Proceedings. 1992;24:2315–2316.
129. Tullius SG, Hancock WW, Heemann U, et al. Reversibility of chronic renal allograft rejection. Critical effect of time after transplantation suggests both host immune dependent and independent phases of progressive injury. Transplantation. 1994;58:93–99.
130. Nadeau KC, Azuma H, Tilney NL. Sequential cytokine expression in renal allografts in rats immunosuppressed with maintenance cyclosporine or mycophenolate mofetil. Transplantation. 1996;62:1363–1366.
131. Azuma H, Chandraker A, Nadeau K, et al. Blockade of T-cell costimulation prevents development of experimental chronic renal allograft rejection. Proceedings of the National Academy of Sciences of the United States of America. 1996;93:12439–12444.
132. Chandraker A, Azuma H, Nadeau K, et al. Late blockade of T cell costimulation interrupts progression of experimental chronic allograft rejection. Journal of Clinical Investigation. 1998;101:2309–2318.
133. Mackenzie HS, Tullius SG, Heemann UW, et al. Nephron supply is a major determinant of long-term renal allograft outcome in rats. Journal of Clinical Investigation. 1994;94:2148–2152.
134. Russell PS, Chase CM, Colvin RB, et al. Kidney transplants in mice. An analysis of the immune status of mice bearing long-term, H-2 incompatible transplants. Journal of Experimental Medicine. 1978;147:1449–1468.
135. Russell PS, Chase CM, Colvin RB, et al. Induced immune destruction of long-surviving, H-2 incompatible kidney transplants in mice. Journal of Experimental Medicine. 1978;147:1469–1486.
136. Coffman T, Geier S, Ibrahim S, et al. Improved renal function in mouse kidney allografts lacking MHC class I antigens. Journal of Immunology. 1993;151: 425–435.
137. Mannon RB, Griffiths R, Ruiz P, et al. Absence of donor MHC antigen expression ameliorates chronic kidney allograft rejection. Kidney International. 2002;62: 290–300.
138. Mannon RB, Kotzin BL, Nataraj C, et al. Downregulation of T cell receptor expression by CD8(+) lymphocytes in kidney allografts. Journal of Clinical Investigation. 1998;101:2517–2527.
139. Bickerstaff AA, Wang JJ, Pelletier RP, et al. Murine renal allografts: spontaneous acceptance is associated with regulated T cell-mediated immunity. Journal of Immunology. 2001;167:4821–4827.
140. Bickerstaff AA, Wang JJ, Pelletier RP, et al. The graft helps to define the character of the alloimmune response. Transplant Immunology. 2002;9: 137–141.
141. Cook CH, Bickerstaff AA, Wang JJ, et al. Spontaneous renal allograft acceptance associated with "regulatory" dendritic cells and IDO. Journal of Immunology. 2008;180:3103–3112.
142. Anderson S, Meyer TW, Rennke HG, et al. Control of glomerular hypertension limits glomerular injury in rats with reduced renal mass. Journal of Clinical Investigation. 1985;76:612–619.
143. Kagami S, Border WA, Miller DE, et al. Angiotensin II stimulates extracellular matrix protein synthesis through induction of transforming growth factor-beta expression in rat glomerular mesangial cells. Journal of Clinical Investigation. 1994;93:2431–2437.
144. Ziai F, Nagano H, Kusaka M, et al. Renal allograft protection with losartan in Fisher-->Lewis rats: hemodynamics, macrophages, and cytokines. Kidney International. 2000;57:2618–2625.
145. Mackenzie HS, Ziai F, Nagano H, et al. Candesartan cilexetil reduces chronic renal allograft injury in Fisher-->Lewis rats. Journal of Hypertension. 1997;15

(Suppl.):S21–S25.
146. Amuchastegui SC, Azzollini N, Mister M, et al. Chronic allograft nephropathy in the rat is improved by angiotensin II receptor blockade but not by calcium channel antagonism. Journal of the American Society of Nephrology. 1998;9:1948–1955.
147. Mannon RB. Therapeutic targets in the treatment of allograft fibrosis. American Journal of Transplantation. 2006;6:867–875.
148. Franceschini N, Cheng O, Zhang X, et al. Inhibition of prolyl-4-hydroxylase ameliorates chronic rejection of mouse kidney allografts. American Journal of Transplantation. 2003;3:396–402.
149. Schofield CJ, Ratcliffe PJ. Oxygen sensing by HIF hydroxylases. Nature Reviews. Molecular Cell Biology. 2004;5:343–354.
150. Laden AM, Sinclair RA. Thickening of arterial intima in rat cardiac allografts. A light and electron microscopic study. American Journal of Pathology. 1971;63:69–84.
151. Adams DH, Tilney NL, Collins JJ Jr, et al. Experimental graft arteriosclerosis. I. The Lewis-to-F-344 allograft model. Transplantation. 1992;53:1115–1119.
152. Lurie KG, Billingham ME, Jamieson SW, et al. Pathogenesis and prevention of graft arteriosclerosis in an experimental heart transplant model. Transplantation. 1981;31:41–47.
153. Cramer DV, Qian SQ, Harnaha J, et al. Cardiac transplantation in the rat. I. The effect of histocompatibility differences on graft arteriosclerosis. Transplantation. 1989;47:414–419.
154. Lemstrom K, Koskinen P, Krogerus L, et al. Cytomegalovirus antigen expression, endothelial cell proliferation, and intimal thickening in rat cardiac allografts after cytomegalovirus infection. Circulation. 1995;92:2594–2604.
155. Lemstrom KB, Bruning JH, Bruggeman CA, et al. Cytomegalovirus infection enhances smooth muscle cell proliferation and intimal thickening of rat aortic allografts. Journal of Clinical Investigation. 1993;92:549–558.
156. Adams DH, Russell ME, Hancock WW, et al. Chronic rejection in experimental cardiac transplantation: studies in the Lewis-F344 model. Immunological Reviews. 1993;134:5–19.
157. Russell ME, Wallace AF, Hancock WW, et al. Upregulation of cytokines associated with macrophage activation in the Lewis-to-F344 rat transplantation model of chronic cardiac rejection. Transplantation. 1995;59:572–578.
158. Russell ME, Adams DH, Wyner LR, et al. Early and persistent induction of monocyte chemoattractant protein 1 in rat cardiac allografts. Proceedings of the National Academy of Sciences of the United States of America. 1993;90:6086–6090.
159. Russell ME, Wallace AF, Wyner LR, et al. Upregulation and modulation of inducible nitric oxide synthase in rat cardiac allografts with chronic rejection and transplant arteriosclerosis. Circulation. 1995;92:457–464.
160. Russell ME, Hancock WW, Akalin E, et al. Chronic cardiac rejection in the LEW to F344 rat model. Blockade of CD28-B7 costimulation by CTLA4Ig modulates T cell and macrophage activation and attenuates arteriosclerosis. Journal of Clinical Investigation. 1996;97:833–838.
161. Yuan X, Dong VM, Coito AJ, et al. A novel CD154 monoclonal antibody in acute and chronic rat vascularized cardiac allograft rejection. Transplantation. 2002;73:1736–1742.
162. Orloff MS, DeMara EM, Coppage ML, et al. Prevention of chronic rejection and graft arteriosclerosis by tolerance induction. Transplantation. 1995;59:282–288.
163. Li J, Meinhardt A, Roehrich ME, et al. Indoleamine 2,3-dioxygenase gene transfer prolongs cardiac allograft survival. American Journal of Physiology, Heart and Circulatory Physiology. 2007;293:H3415–H3423.
164. Hancock WW, Sayegh MH, Kwok CA, et al. Oral, but not intravenous, alloantigen prevents accelerated allograft rejection by selective intragraft Th2 cell activation. Transplantation. 1993;55:1112–1118.
165. Murphy B, Kim KS, Buelow R, et al. Synthetic MHC class I peptide prolongs cardiac survival and attenuates transplant arteriosclerosis in the Lewis-->Fischer 344 model of chronic allograft rejection. Transplantation. 1997;64:14–19.
166. Ardehali A, Billingsley A, Laks H, et al. Experimental cardiac allograft vasculopathy in mice. Journal of Heart and Lung Transplantation. 1993;12:730–735.
167. Fischbein MP, Yun J, Laks H, et al. CD8+ lymphocytes augment chronic rejection in a MHC class II mismatched model. Transplantation. 2001;71:1146–1153.
168. Raisanen-Sokolowski A, Glysing-Jensen T, Mottram PL, et al. Sustained anti-CD4/CD8 treatment blocks inflammatory activation and intimal thickening in mouse heart allografts. Arteriosclerosis, Thrombosis, and Vascular Biology. 1997;17:2115–2122.
169. Orosz CG, Huang EH, Bergese SD, et al. Prevention of acute murine cardiac allograft rejection: anti-CD4 or anti-vascular cell adhesion molecule one monoclonal antibodies block acute rejection but permit persistent graft-reactive alloimmunity and chronic tissue remodelling. Journal of Heart and Lung Transplantation. 1997;16:889–904.
170. Orosz CG, Wakely E, Sedmak DD, et al. Prolonged murine cardiac allograft acceptance: characteristics of persistent active alloimmunity after treatment with gallium nitrate versus anti-CD4 monoclonal antibody. Transplantation. 1997;63:1109–1117.
171. Orosz CG, Wakely E, Bergese SD, et al. Prevention of murine cardiac allograft rejection with gallium nitrate. Comparison with anti-CD4 monoclonal antibody. Transplantation. 1996;61:783–791.
172. Bickerstaff AA, Wang JJ, Xia D, et al. Allograft acceptance despite differential strain-specific induction of TGF-beta/IL-10-mediated immunoregulation. American Journal of Transplantation. 2002;2:819–827.
173. Russell PS, Chase CM, Winn HJ, et al. Coronary atherosclerosis in transplanted mouse hearts. II. Importance of humoral immunity. Journal of Immunology. 1994;152:5135–5141.
174. Uehara S, Chase CM, Cornell LD, et al. Chronic cardiac transplant arteriopathy in mice: relationship of alloantibody, C4d deposition and neointimal fibrosis. American Journal of Transplantation. 2007;7:57–65.
175. Wasowska BA, Qian Z, Cangello DL, et al. Passive transfer of alloantibodies restores acute cardiac rejection in IgKO mice. Transplantation. 2001;71:727–736.
176. Hirohashi T, Uehara S, Chase CM, et al. Complement independent antibody-mediated endarteritis and transplant arteriopathy in mice. American Journal of Transplantation. 2010;10:510–517.
177. Fischbein MP, Yun J, Laks H, et al. Role of CD8+ lymphocytes in chronic rejection of transplanted hearts. Journal of Thoracic and Cardiovascular Surgery. 2002;123:803–809.
178. Fischbein MP, Ardehali A, Yun J, et al. CD40 signaling replaces CD4+ lymphocytes and its blocking prevents chronic rejection of heart transplants. Journal of Immunology. 2000;165:7316–7322.
179. Shimizu K, Schonbeck U, Mach F, et al. Host CD40 ligand deficiency induces long-term allograft survival and donor-specific tolerance in mouse cardiac transplantation but does not prevent graft arteriosclerosis. Journal of Immunology. 2000;165:3506–3518.
180. van Maurik A, Wood KJ, Jones ND. Impact of both donor and recipient strains on cardiac allograft survival after blockade of the CD40-CD154 costimulatory pathway. Transplantation. 2002;74:740–743.
181. Kitchens WH, Chase CM, Uehara S, et al. Macrophage depletion suppresses cardiac allograft vasculopathy in mice. American Journal of Transplantation. 2007;7:2675–2682.
182. Huser N, Tertilt C, Gerauer K, et al. CCR4-deficient mice show prolonged graft survival in a chronic cardiac transplant rejection model. European Journal of Immunology. 2005;35:128–138.
183. Uehara S, Chase CM, Kitchens WH, et al. NK cells can trigger allograft vasculopathy: the role of hybrid resistance in solid organ allografts. Journal of Immunology. 2005;175:3424–3430.
184. Hirohashi T, Chase CM, Della Pelle P, et al. A novel pathway of chronic allograft rejection mediated by NK cells and alloantibody. American Journal of Transplantation. 2012;12:313–321.
185. Hancock WW, Buelow R, Sayegh MH, et al. Antibody-induced transplant arteriosclerosis is prevented by graft expression of anti-oxidant and anti-apoptotic genes. Nature Medicine. 1998;4:1392–1396.
186. Ardehali A, Laks H, Drinkwater DC, et al. Vascular cell adhesion molecule-1 is induced on vascular endothelia and medial smooth muscle cells in experimental cardiac allograft vasculopathy. Circulation. 1995;92:450–456.
187. Okada M, Wang CY, Hwang DW, et al. Transcriptional control of cardiac allograft vasculopathy by early growth response gene-1 (Egr-1). Circulation Research. 2002;91:135–142.
188. Cook CH, Bickerstaff AA, Wang JJ, et al. Disruption of murine cardiac allograft acceptance by latent cytomegalovirus. American Journal of Transplantation. 2009;9:42–53.
189. Rolls HK, Kishimoto K, Dong VM, et al. T-cell response to cardiac myosin persists in the absence of an alloimmune response in recipients with chronic cardiac allograft rejection. Transplantation. 2002;74:1053–1057.
190. Wu GD, Jin YS, Salazar R, et al. Vascular endothelial cell apoptosis induced by anti-donor non-MHC antibodies: a possible injury pathway contributing to chronic allograft rejection. Journal of Heart and Lung Transplantation. 2002;21:1174–1187.
191. Joosten SA, van Dixhoorn MG, Borrias MC, et al. Antibody response against perlecan and collagen types IV and VI in chronic renal allograft rejection in the rat. American Journal of Pathology. 2002;160:1301–1310.
192. Joosten SA, van Ham V, Borrias MC, et al. Antibodies against mesangial cells in a rat model of chronic renal allograft rejection. Nephrology, Dialysis, Transplantation. 2005;20:692–698.
193. Paul LC, Muralidharan J, Muzaffar SA, et al. Antibodies against mesangial cells and their secretory products in chronic renal allograft rejection in the rat. American Journal of Pathology. 1998;152:1209–1223.
194. Mahesh B, Leong HS, Nair KS, et al. Autoimmunity to vimentin potentiates graft

vasculopathy in murine cardiac allografts. Transplantation. 2010;90:4–13.
195. Diaz JA, Booth AJ, Lu G, et al. Critical role for IL-6 in hypertrophy and fibrosis in chronic cardiac allograft rejection. American Journal of Transplantation. 2009;9:1773–1783.
196. Booth AJ, Csencsits-Smith K, Wood SC, et al. Connective tissue growth factor promotes fibrosis downstream of TGFbeta and IL-6 in chronic cardiac allograft rejection. American Journal of Transplantation. 2010;10:220–230.
197. Booth AJ, Bishop DK. TGF-beta, IL-6, IL-17 and CTGF direct multiple pathologies of chronic cardiac allograft rejection. Immunotherapy. 2010;2:511–520.
198. Faust SM, Lu G, Marini BL, et al. Role of T cell TGFbeta signaling and IL-17 in allograft acceptance and fibrosis associated with chronic rejection. Journal of Immunology. 2009;183:7297–7306.
199. Itoh S, Nakae S, Axtell RC, et al. IL-17 contributes to the development of chronic rejection in a murine heart transplant model. Journal of Clinical Immunology. 2010;30:235–240.
200. Mennander A, Paavonen T, Hayry P. Intimal thickening and medial necrosis in allograft arteriosclerosis (chronic rejection) are independently regulated. Arteriosclerosis and Thrombosis. 1993;13:1019–1025.
201. Hancock WW, Shi C, Picard MH, et al. LEW-to-F344 carotid artery allografts: analysis of a rat model of posttransplant vascular injury involving cell-mediated and humoral responses. Transplantation. 1995;60:1565–1572.
202. Motomura N, Lou H, Maurice P, et al. Acceleration of arteriosclerosis of the rat aorta allograft by insulin growth factor-I. Transplantation. 1997;63:932–936.
203. Gohra H, McDonald TO, Verrier ED, et al. Endothelial loss and regeneration in a model of transplant arteriosclerosis. Transplantation. 1995;60:96–102.
204. Shi C, Russell ME, Bianchi C, et al. Murine model of accelerated transplant arteriosclerosis. Circulation Research. 1994;75:199–207.
205. Shi C, Lee WS, He Q, et al. Immunologic basis of transplant-associated arteriosclerosis. Proceedings of the National Academy of Sciences of the United States of America. 1996;93:4051–4056.
206. Mulligan-Kehoe MJ. The vasa vasorum in diseased and nondiseased arteries. American Journal of Physiology, Heart and Circulatory Physiology. 2010;298: H295–H305.
207. Hertz MI, Jessurun J, King MB, et al. Reproduction of the obliterative bronchiolitis lesion after heterotopic transplantation of mouse airways. American Journal of Pathology. 1993;142:1945–1951.
208. Neuringer IP, Mannon RB, Coffman TM, et al. Immune cells in a mouse airway model of obliterative bronchiolitis. American Journal of Respiratory Cell and Molecular Biology. 1998;19:379–386.
209. Kelly KE, Hertz MI, Mueller DL. T-cell and major histocompatibility complex requirements for obliterative airway disease in heterotopically transplanted murine tracheas. Transplantation. 1998;66:764–771.
210. Neuringer IP, Walsh SP, Mannon RB, et al. Enhanced T cell cytokine gene expression in mouse airway obliterative bronchiolitis. Transplantation. 2000;69: 399–405.
211. Chalermskulrat W, Neuringer IP, Brickey WJ, et al. Hierarchical contributions of allorecognition pathways in chronic lung rejection. American Journal of Respiratory and Critical Care Medicine. 2003;167:999–1007.
212. Maruyama, T, Jaramillo A, Narayanan K, et al. Induction of obliterative airway disease by anti-HLA class I antibodies. American Journal of Transplantation. 2005;5:2126–2134.
213. Neuringer IP, Aris RM, Burns KA, et al. Epithelial kinetics in mouse heterotopic tracheal allografts. American Journal of Transplantation. 2002;2:410–419.
214. Qu N, de Haan A, Harmsen MC, et al. Specific immune responses against airway epithelial cells in a transgenic mouse-trachea transplantation model for obliterative airway disease. Transplantation. 2003;76:1022–1028.
215. Kuo E, Bharat A, Shih J, et al. Role of airway epithelial injury in murine orthotopic tracheal allograft rejection. Annals of Thoracic Surgery. 2006;82: 1226–1233.
216. Lama VN, Harada H, Badri LN, et al. Obligatory role for interleukin-13 in obstructive lesion development in airway allografts. American Journal of Pathology. 2006;169:47–60.
217. McKane BW, Fernandez F, Narayanan K, et al. Pirfenidone inhibits obliterative airway disease in a murine heterotopic tracheal transplant model. Transplantation. 2004;77:664–669.
218. Yamada A, Konishi K, Cruz GL, et al. Blocking the CD28-B7 T-cell costimulatory pathway abrogates the development of obliterative bronchiolitis in a murine heterotopic airway model. Transplantation. 2000;69:743–749.
219. Harris DA, Zhao Y, Lapar DJ, et al. Inhibiting CXCL12 blocks fibrocyte migration and differentiation and attenuates bronchiolitis obliterans in a murine heterotopic tracheal transplant model. Journal of Thoracic and Cardiovascular Surgery. 2013;145:854–861.
220. Babu AN, Murakawa T, Thurman JM, et al. Microvascular destruction identifies murine allografts that cannot be rescued from airway fibrosis. Journal of Clinical Investigation. 2007;117:3774–3785.
221. Hyun Sung S, Warnock M, Fang KC, et al. A comparison of rat tracheal transplant models: implantation verses anastomotic techniques for the study of airway rejection. Transplantation. 2002;73:695–700.
222. Okada Y, Zuo XJ, Marchevsky AM, et al. Pre-transplant donor-specific transfusions induce allograft rejection and IL-2 gene expression in the WKY-->F344 functional tolerance model of rat lung transplantation. Transplant Immunology. 1998;6:137–146.
223. Hirt SW, You XM, Moller F, et al. Wottge, HU: development of obliterative bronchiolitis after allogeneic rat lung transplantation: implication of acute rejection and the time point of treatment. Journal of Heart and Lung Transplantation. 1999;18:542–548.
224. Hirschburger M, Greschus S, Kuchenbuch T, et al. Lung transplantation in the Fischer 344-->Wistar Kyoto rat strain combination is not suitable to study bronchiolitis obliterans. Journal of Heart and Lung Transplantation. 2007;26: 390–398.
225. Wiebe K, Fraund S, Steinmuller C, et al. Rat cytomegalovirus and Listeria monocytogenes infection enhance chronic rejection after allogenic rat lung transplantation. Transplant International. 2005;18:1166–1174.
226. Lee AG, Wagner FM, Chen MF, et al. A novel charcoal-induced model of obliterative bronchiolitis-like lesions: implications of chronic nonspecific airway inflammation in the development of posttransplantation obliterative bronchiolitis. Journal of Thoracic and Cardiovascular Surgery. 1998;115:822–827.
227. Jungraithmayr W, Vogt P, Inci I, et al. A model of chronic lung allograft rejection in the rat. European Respiratory Journal. 2010;35:1354–1363.
228. Uyama T, Winter JB, Groen G, et al. Late airway changes caused by chronic rejection in rat lung allografts. Transplantation. 1992;54:809–812.
229. Lee AG, Wagner FM, Giaid A, et al. Immunohistochemical characterization of inflammatory and proliferative events during chronic rejection in rat lung allografts. Transplantation. 1997;64:465–471.
230. Yasufuku K, Heidler KM, Woods KA, et al. Prevention of bronchiolitis obliterans in rat lung allografts by type V collagen-induced oral tolerance. Transplantation. 2002;73:500–505.
231. Okazaki M, Gelman AE, Tietjens JR, et al. Maintenance of airway epithelium in acutely rejected orthotopic vascularized mouse lung transplants. American Journal of Respiratory Cell and Molecular Biology. 2007;37:625–630.
232. Li W, Sugimoto S, Lai J, et al. Orthotopic vascularized right lung transplantation in the mouse. Journal of Thoracic and Cardiovascular Surgery. 2010;139: 1637–1643.
233. Gelman AE, Li W, Richardson SB, et al. Cutting edge: acute lung allograft rejection is independent of secondary lymphoid organs. Journal of Immunology. 2009;182:3969–3973.
234. Fan L, Benson HL, Vittal R, et al. Neutralizing IL-17 prevents obliterative bronchiolitis in murine orthotopic lung transplantation. American Journal of Transplantation. 2011;11:911–922.
235. De Vleeschauwer S, Jungraithmayr W, Wauters S, et al. Chronic rejection pathology after orthotopic lung transplantation in mice: the development of a murine BOS model and its drawbacks. PLoS ONE. 2012;7:e29802.
236. Bennett WM, Norman DJ. Action and toxicity of cyclosporine. Annual Review of Medicine. 1986;37:215–224.
237. Andoh TF, Bennett WM. Chronic cyclosporine nephrotoxicity. Current Opinion in Nephrology and Hypertension. 1998;7:265–270.
238. Rosen S, Greenfeld Z, Brezis M. Chronic cyclosporine-induced nephropathy in the rat. A medullary ray and inner stripe injury. Transplantation. 1990;49: 445–452.
239. Shehata M, Cope GH, Johnson TS, et al. Cyclosporine enhances the expression of TGF-beta in the juxtaglomerular cells of the rat kidney. Kidney International. 1995;48:1487–1496.
240. Butterly DW, Spurney RF, Ruiz P, et al. A role for leukotrienes in cyclosporine nephrotoxicity. Kidney International. 2000;57:2586–2593.
241. Murray BM, Paller MS, Ferris TF. Effect of cyclosporine administration on renal hemodynamics in conscious rats. Kidney International. 1985;28:767–774.
242. Shihab FS, Bennett WM, Tanner AM, et al. Angiotensin II blockade decreases TGF-beta1 and matrix proteins in cyclosporine nephropathy. Kidney International. 1997;52:660–673.
243. Perico N, Benigni A, Bosco E, et al. Acute cyclosporine A nephrotoxicity in rats: which role for renin-angiotensin system and glomerular prostaglandins? Clinical Nephrology. 1986;25(Suppl. 1):S83–S88.
244. Perico N, Zoja C, Benigni A, et al. Effect of short-term cyclosporine administration in rats on renin-angiotensin and thromboxane A2: possible relevance to the reduction in glomerular filtration rate. Journal of Pharmacology and Experimental Therapeutics. 1986;239:229–235.
245. Pichler RH, Franceschini N, Young BA, et al. Pathogenesis of cyclosporine nephropathy: roles of angiotensin II and osteopontin. Journal of the American Society of Nephrology. 1995;6:1186–1196.

246. Yoon HE, Ghee JY, Piao S, et al. Angiotensin II blockade upregulates the expression of Klotho, the anti-ageing gene, in an experimental model of chronic cyclosporine nephropathy. Nephrology, Dialysis, Transplantation. 2011;26: 800–813.
247. Macunluoglu B, Arikan H, Atakan A, et al. Effects of spironolactone in an experimental model of chronic cyclosporine nephrotoxicity. Transplantation Proceedings. 2008;40:273–278.
248. Coffman TM, Carr DR, Yarger WE, et al. Evidence that renal prostaglandin and thromboxane production is stimulated in chronic cyclosporine nephrotoxicity. Transplantation. 1987;43:282–285.
249. Perico N, Benigni A, Zoja C, et al. Functional significance of exaggerated renal thromboxane A2 synthesis induced by cyclosporin A. American Journal of Physiology. 1986;251:F581–F587.
250. Perico N, Rossini M, Imberti O, et al. Thromboxane receptor blockade attenuates chronic cyclosporine nephrotoxicity and improves survival in rats with renal isograft. Journal of the American Society of Nephrology. 1992;2:1398–1404.
251. Rossini M, Belloni A, Remuzzi G, et al. Thromboxane receptor blockade attenuates the toxic effect of cyclosporine in experimental renal transplantation. Circulation. 1990;81:I61–I67; discussion I68.
252. Spurney RF, Mayros SD, Collins D, et al. Thromboxane receptor blockade improves cyclosporine nephrotoxicity in rats. Prostaglandins. 1990;39:135–146.
253. Atakan A, Arikan H, Macunluoglu B, et al. Renal protective effects of leukotriene receptor blockers in an experimental model of cyclosporine nephrotoxicity. Transplantation Proceedings. 2008;40:279–284.
254. Kon V, Hunley TE, Fogo A. Combined antagonism of endothelin A/B receptors links endothelin to vasoconstriction whereas angiotensin II effects fibrosis. Studies in chronic cyclosporine nephrotoxicity in rats. Transplantation. 1995;60:89–95.
255. Andoh TF, Gardner MP, Bennett WM. Protective effects of dietary L-arginine supplementation on chronic cyclosporine nephrotoxicity. Transplantation. 1997;64:1236–1240.
256. Shihab FS, Bennett WM, Isaac J, et al. Nitric oxide modulates vascular endothelial growth factor and receptors in chronic cyclosporine nephrotoxicity. Kidney International. 2003;63:522–533.
257. Shihab FS, Yi H, Bennett WM, et al. Effect of nitric oxide modulation on TGF-beta1 and matrix proteins in chronic cyclosporine nephrotoxicity. Kidney International. 2000;58:1174–1185.
258. Sun BK, Li C, Lim SW, et al. Expression of transforming growth factor-beta-inducible gene-h3 in normal and cyclosporine-treated rat kidney. Journal of Laboratory and Clinical Medicine. 2004;143:175–183.
259. Islam M, Burke JF Jr, McGowan TA, et al. Effect of anti-transforming growth factor-beta antibodies in cyclosporine-induced renal dysfunction. Kidney International. 2001;59:498–506.
260. Shihab FS, Andoh TF, Tanner AM, et al. Sodium depletion enhances fibrosis and the expression of TGF-beta1 and matrix proteins in experimental chronic cyclosporine nephropathy. American Journal of Kidney Diseases. 1997;30: 71–81.
261. Shihab FS, Bennett WM, Yi H, et al. Effect of cyclosporine and sirolimus on the expression of connective tissue growth factor in rat experimental chronic nephrotoxicity. American Journal of Nephrology. 2006;26:400–407.
262. Shihab FS, Bennett WM, Yi H, et al. Pirfenidone treatment decreases transforming growth factor-beta1 and matrix proteins and ameliorates fibrosis in chronic cyclosporine nephrotoxicity. American Journal of Transplantation. 2002;2: 111–119.
263. Sun BK, Li C, Lim SW, et al. Blockade of angiotensin II with losartan attenuates transforming growth factor-beta1 inducible gene-h3 (betaig-h3) expression in a model of chronic cyclosporine nephrotoxicity. Nephron. Experimental Nephrology. 2005;99:e9–e16.
264. Li C, Yang CW, Park JH, et al. Pravastatin treatment attenuates interstitial inflammation and fibrosis in a rat model of chronic cyclosporine-induced nephropathy. American Journal of Physiology. Renal Physiology. 2004;286:F46–F57.
265. Thomas SE, Andoh TF, Pichler RH, et al. Accelerated apoptosis characterizes cyclosporine-associated interstitial fibrosis. Kidney International. 1998;53: 897–908.
266. Shihab FS, Andoh TF, Tanner AM, et al. Expression of apoptosis regulatory genes in chronic cyclosporine nephrotoxicity favors apoptosis. Kidney International. 1999;56:2147–2159.
267. Yang CW, Faulkner GR, Wahba IM, et al. Expression of apoptosis-related genes in chronic cyclosporine nephrotoxicity in mice. American Journal of Transplantation. 2002;2:391–399.
268. Lee SY, Jo SK, Cho WY, et al. The effect of alpha-melanocyte-stimulating hormone on renal tubular cell apoptosis and tubulointerstitial fibrosis in cyclosporine A nephrotoxicity. Transplantation. 2004;78:1756–1764.
269. Li C, Yang CW, Ahn HJ, et al. Colchicine decreases apoptotic cell death in chronic cyclosporine nephrotoxicity. Journal of Laboratory and Clinical Medicine. 2002;139:364–371.
270. Shihab FS, Bennett WM, Yi H, et al. Effect of pirfenidone on apoptosis-regulatory genes in chronic cyclosporine nephrotoxicity. Transplantation. 2005;79: 419–426.
271. Ahn KO, Li C, Lim SW, et al. Infiltration of nestin-expressing cells in interstitial fibrosis in chronic cyclosporine nephropathy. Transplantation. 2008;86: 571–577.
272. Ghee JY, Han DH, Song HK, et al. The role of macrophage in the pathogenesis of chronic cyclosporine-induced nephropathy. Nephrology, Dialysis, Transplantation. 2008;23:4061–4069.
273. Pallet N, Rabant M, Xu-Dubois YC, et al. Response of human renal tubular cells to cyclosporine and sirolimus: a toxicogenomic study. Toxicology and Applied Pharmacology. 2008;229:184–196.
274. Han SW, Li C, Ahn KO, et al. Prolonged endoplasmic reticulum stress induces apoptotic cell death in an experimental model of chronic cyclosporine nephropathy. American Journal of Nephrology. 2008;28:707–714.
275. Pallet N, Bouvier N, Legendre C, et al. Autophagy protects renal tubular cells against cyclosporine toxicity. Autophagy. 2008;4:783–791.
276. Pallet N, Bouvier N, Bendjallabah A, et al. Cyclosporine-induced endoplasmic reticulum stress triggers tubular phenotypic changes and death. American Journal of Transplantation. 2008;8:2283–2296.
277. Masri MA. Comparative study of toxicity and efficacy of cyclosporine, cyclosporine G (OG37), FK 506, and rapamycin in BALB/c mice with fitted skin grafts. Transplantation Proceedings. 1995;27:366.
278. Wolf G, Neilson EG. Increases in levels of collagen types I and IV messenger ribonucleic acid in murine kidneys after treatment with ciclosporin. Nephron. 1992;60:87–91.
279. Andoh TF, Lam TT, Linsdley J, et al. Enhancement of chronic cyclosporine nephrotoxicity by sodium depletion in an experimental mouse model. Nephrology. 1997;3:471–478.
280. Murphy JB. Factors of resistance to heteroplastic tissue-grafting studies in tissue specificity. Journal of Experimental Medicine. 1914;19:513–522.
281. Anderson D, Billingham RE, Lampkin GH, et al. The use of skin grafting to distinguish between monozygotic and dizygotic twins in cattle. Heredity. 1951;5:379–397.
282. Billingham RE, Brent L, Medawar PB. Actively acquired tolerance of foreign cells. Nature. 1953;172:603–606.
283. Goodnow CC, Basten A. Self-tolerance in B lymphocytes. Seminars in Immunology. 1989;1:125–135.
284. Miller JF, Morahan G, Allison J. Immunological tolerance: new approaches using transgenic mice. Immunology Today. 1989;10:53–57.
285. Miller JF, Morahan G, Allison J, et al. A transgenic approach to the study of peripheral T-cell tolerance. Immunological Reviews. 1991;122:103–116.
286. Evans MJ. Potential for genetic manipulation of mammals. Molecular Biology and Medicine. 1989;6:557–565.
287. Schonrich G, Kalinke U, Momburg F, et al. Down-regulation of T cell receptors on self-reactive T cells as a novel mechanism for extrathymic tolerance induction. Cell. 1991;65:293–304.
288. Teh HS, Kishi H, Scott B, et al. Deletion of autospecific T cells in T cell receptor (TCR) transgenic mice spares cells with normal TCR levels and low levels of CD8 molecules. Journal of Experimental Medicine. 1989;169:795–806.
289. Kohler G, Milstein C. Continuous cultures of fused cells secreting antibody of predefined specificity. Nature. 1975;256:495–497.
290. Girlanda R, Kirk AD. Frontiers in nephrology: immune tolerance to allografts in humans. Journal of the American Society of Nephrology. 2007;18:2242–2251.
291. Kingsley CI, Nadig SN, Wood KJ. Transplantation tolerance: lessons from experimental rodent models. Transplant International. 2007;20:828–841.
292. Neujahr DC, Chen C, Huang X, et al. Accelerated memory cell homeostasis during T cell depletion and approaches to overcome it. Journal of Immunology. 2006;176:4632–4639.
293. Wu Z, Bensinger SJ, Zhang J, et al. Homeostatic proliferation is a barrier to transplantation tolerance. Nature Medicine. 2004;10:87–92.
294. Mosmann TR, Coffman RL. TH1 and TH2 cells: different patterns of lymphokine secretion lead to different functional properties. Annual Review of Immunology. 1989;7:145–173.
295. Chong AS, Yin D, Boussy IA. Transplantation tolerance: of mice and men. Graft. 2002;5:127.
296. Lakkis FG, Sayegh MH. Memory T cells: a hurdle to immunologic tolerance. Journal of the American Society of Nephrology. 2003;14:2402–2410.
297. Welsh RM, Selin LK. No one is naive: the significance of heterologous T-cell immunity. Nature Reviews. Immunology. 2002;2:417–426.
298. Valujskikh A, Pantenburg B, Heeger PS. Primed allospecific T cells prevent the effects of costimulatory blockade on prolonged cardiac allograft survival in mice. American Journal of Transplantation. 2002;2:501–509.
299. Dyson PJ, Knight AM, Fairchild S, et al. Genes encoding ligands for deletion of

V beta 11 T cells cosegregate with mammary tumour virus genomes. Nature. 1991;349:531–532.

300. Kappler JW, Roehm N, Marrack P. T cell tolerance by clonal elimination in the thymus. Cell. 1987;49:273–280.
301. Rocha B, Grandien A, Freitas AA. Anergy and exhaustion are independent mechanisms of peripheral T cell tolerance. Journal of Experimental Medicine. 1995;181:993–1003.
302. Wekerle T, Kurtz J, Sayegh M, et al. Peripheral deletion after bone marrow transplantation with costimulatory blockade has features of both activation-induced cell death and passive cell death. Journal of Immunology. 2001;166:2311–2316.
303. Akl A, Luo S, Wood KJ. Induction of transplantation tolerance-the potential of regulatory T cells. Transplant Immunology. 2005;14:225–230.
304. Ding Q, Yeung M, Camirand G, et al. Regulatory B cells are identified by expression of TIM-1 and can be induced through TIM-1 ligation to promote tolerance in mice. Journal of Clinical Investigation. 2011;121:3645–3656.
305. Posselt AM, Barker CF, Tomaszewski JE, et al. Induction of donor-specific unresponsiveness by intrathymic islet transplantation. Science. 1990;249:1293–1295.
306. Remuzzi G, Ferrazzi P, Bontempelli M, et al. Preliminary results of intrathymic injection of donor cells to prevent acute rejection in human heart transplantation. Journal of the American Society of Nephrology. 1995;6:1291–1294.
307. Ildstad ST, Sachs DH. Reconstitution with syngeneic plus allogeneic or xenogeneic bone marrow leads to specific acceptance of allografts or xenografts. Nature. 1984;307:168–170.
308. Kawai T, Sogawa H, Koulmanda M, et al. DS, CK: long-term islet allograft function in the absence of chronic immunosuppression: a case report of a nonhuman primate previously made tolerant to a renal allograft from the same donor. Transplantation. 2001;72:351–354.
309. Sykes M. Mixed chimerism and transplant tolerance. Immunity. 2001;14: 417–424.
310. Sykes M, Sachs DH. Mixed allogeneic chimerism as an approach to transplantation tolerance. Immunology Today. 1988;9:23–27.
311. Wekerle T, Sykes M. Induction of tolerance. Surgery. 2004;135:359–364.
312. Guo Z, Wang J, Dong Y, et al. Long-term survival of intestinal allografts induced by costimulation blockade, busulfan and donor bone marrow infusion. American Journal of Transplantation. 2003;3:1091–1098.
313. Manilay JO, Pearson DA, Sergio JJ, et al. Intrathymic deletion of alloreactive T cells in mixed bone marrow chimeras prepared with a nonmyeloablative conditioning regimen. Transplantation. 1998;66:96–102.
314. Wekerle T, Sayegh MH, Hill J, et al. Extrathymic T cell deletion and allogeneic stem cell engraftment induced with costimulatory blockade is followed by central T cell tolerance. Journal of Experimental Medicine. 1998;187:2037–2044.
315. Fudaba Y, Spitzer TR, Shaffer J, et al. Myeloma responses and tolerance following combined kidney and nonmyeloablative marrow transplantation: in vivo and in vitro analyses. American Journal of Transplantation. 2006;6:2121–2133.
316. Kawai T, Hoshino T, Fujioka S, et al. [Mixed chimerism and immune tolerance induction by low-stress pretreatment before kidney transplantation in monkeys]. Nihon Rinsho Men'eki Gakkai Kaishi. 1995;18:670–674.
317. Kawai T, Sogawa H, Boskovic S, et al. CD154 blockade for induction of mixed chimerism and prolonged renal allograft survival in nonhuman primates. American Journal of Transplantation. 2004;4:1391–1398.
318. Wekerle T, Kurtz J, Ito H, et al. Allogeneic bone marrow transplantation with costimulatory blockade induces macrochimerism and tolerance without cytoreductive host treatment. Nature Medicine. 2000;6:464–469.
319. Inoue S, Popp FC, Koehl GE, et al. Immunomodulatory effects of mesenchymal stem cells in a rat organ transplant model. Transplantation. 2006;81:1589–1595.
320. Bolanos-Meade J, Vogelsang GB. Mesenchymal stem cells and organ transplantation: current status and promising future. Transplantation. 2006;81: 1388–1389.
321. Le Blanc K, Ringden O. Immunobiology of human mesenchymal stem cells and future use in hematopoietic stem cell transplantation. Biology of Blood and Marrow Transplantation. 2005;11:321–334.
322. Fandrich F, Lin X, Chai GX, et al. Preimplantation-stage stem cells induce long-term allogeneic graft acceptance without supplementary host conditioning. Nature Medicine. 2002;8:171–178.
323. Walunas TL, Lenschow DJ, Bakker CY, et al. CTLA-4 can function as a negative regulator of T cell activation. Immunity. 1994;1:405–413.
324. Sanchez-Fueyo A, Tian J, Picarella D, et al. Tim-3 inhibits T helper type 1-mediated auto- and alloimmune responses and promotes immunological tolerance. Nature Immunology. 2003;4:1093–1101.
325. Francisco LM, Salinas VH, Brown KE, et al. PD-L1 regulates the development, maintenance, and function of induced regulatory T cells. Journal of Experimental Medicine. 2009;206:3015–3029.
326. Keir ME, Butte MJ, Freeman GJ, et al. PD-1 and its ligands in tolerance and immunity. Annual Review of Immunology. 2008;26:677–704.
327. Daeron M, Latour S, Malbec O, et al. The same tyrosine-based inhibition motif, in the intracytoplasmic domain of Fc gamma RIIB, regulates negatively BCR-, TCR-, and FcR-dependent cell activation. Immunity. 1995;3:635–646.
328. Van den Herik-Oudijk IE, Capel PJ, van der Bruggen T, et al. Identification of signaling motifs within human Fc gamma RIIa and Fc gamma RIIb isoforms. Blood. 1995;85:2202–2211.
329. van Essen D, Kikutani H, Gray D. CD40 ligand-transduced costimulation of T cells in the development of helper function. Nature. 1995;378:620–623.
330. Zheng XX, Markees TG, Hancock WW, et al. CTLA4 signals are required to optimally induce allograft tolerance with combined donor-specific transfusion and anti-CD154 monoclonal antibody treatment. Journal of Immunology. 1999;162:4983–4990.
331. Read S, Malmstrom V, Powrie F. Cytotoxic T lymphocyte-associated antigen 4 plays an essential role in the function of CD25(+)CD4(+) regulatory cells that control intestinal inflammation. Journal of Experimental Medicine. 2000; 192:295–302.
332. Kingsley CI, Karim M, Bushell AR, et al. CD25+CD4+ regulatory T cells prevent graft rejection: CTLA-4- and IL-10-dependent immunoregulation of alloresponses. Journal of Immunology. 2002;168:1080–1086.
333. Gudmundsdottir H, Turka LA. T cell costimulatory blockade: new therapies for transplant rejection. Journal of the American Society of Nephrology. 1999;10:1356–1365.
334. Larsen CP, Elwood ET, Alexander DZ, et al. Long-term acceptance of skin and cardiac allografts after blocking CD40 and CD28 pathways. Nature. 1996; 381:434–438.
335. Larsen CP, Pearson TC, Adams AB, et al. Rational development of LEA29Y (belatacept), a high-affinity variant of CTLA4-Ig with potent immunosuppressive properties. American Journal of Transplantation. 2005;5:443–453.
336. Vincenti F, Charpentier B, Vanrenterghem Y, et al. A phase III study of belatacept-based immunosuppression regimens versus cyclosporine in renal transplant recipients (BENEFIT study). American Journal of Transplantation. 2010;10: 535–546.
337. Vincenti F, Larsen C, Durrbach A, et al. Costimulation blockade with belatacept in renal transplantation. New England Journal of Medicine. 2005;353:770–781.
338. Honey K, Cobbold SP, Waldmann H. CD40 ligand blockade induces CD4+ T cell tolerance and linked suppression. Journal of Immunology. 1999;163: 4805–4810.
339. Iwakoshi NN, Mordes JP, Markees TG, et al. Treatment of allograft recipients with donor-specific transfusion and anti-CD154 antibody leads to deletion of alloreactive CD8+ T cells and prolonged graft survival in a CTLA4-dependent manner. Journal of Immunology. 2000;164:512–521.
340. Jones ND, Van Maurik A, Hara M, et al. CD40-CD40 ligand-independent activation of CD8+ T cells can trigger allograft rejection. Journal of Immunology. 2000;165:1111–1118.
341. Meng L, Guo Z, Kim O, et al. Blockade of the CD40 pathway fails to prevent CD8 T cell-mediated intestinal allograft rejection. Transplantation Proceedings. 2001;33:418–420.
342. Judge TA, Wu Z, Zheng XG, et al. The role of CD80, CD86, and CTLA4 in alloimmune responses and the induction of long-term allograft survival. Journal of Immunology. 1999;162:1947–1951.
343. Taylor PA, Lees CJ, Wilson JM, et al. Combined effects of calcineurin inhibitors or sirolimus with anti-CD40L mAb on alloengraftment under nonmyeloablative conditions. Blood. 2002;100:3400–3407.
344. Ozkaynak E, Gao W, Shemmeri N, et al. Importance of ICOS-B7RP-1 costimulation in acute and chronic allograft rejection. Nature Immunology. 2001;2: 591–596.
345. Snanoudj R, de Preneuf H, Creput C, et al. Costimulation blockade and its possible future use in clinical transplantation. Transplant International. 2006; 19:693–704.
346. Ozkaynak E, Wang L, Goodearl A, et al. Programmed death-1 targeting can promote allograft survival. Journal of Immunology. 2002;169:6546–6553.
347. Gershon RK, Kondo K. Infectious immunological tolerance. Immunology. 1971;21:903–914.
348. Kilshaw PJ, Brent L, Pinto M. Suppressor T cells in mice made unresponsive to skin allografts. Nature. 1975;255:489–491.
349. Li XC, Turka LA. An update on regulatory T cells in transplant tolerance and rejection. Nature Reviews. Nephrology. 2010;6:577–583.
350. Qin SX, Cobbold S, Benjamin R, et al. Induction of classical transplantation tolerance in the adult. Journal of Experimental Medicine. 1989;169:779–794.
351. Hall BM, Verma ND, Tran GT, et al. Distinct regulatory CD4+T cell subsets; differences between naive and antigen specific T regulatory cells. Current Opinion in Immunology. 2011;23:641–647.
352. Bushell A, Morris PJ, Wood KJ. Transplantation tolerance induced by antigen pretreatment and depleting anti-CD4 antibody depends on CD4+ T cell regulation during the induction phase of the response. European Journal of Immunol-

ogy. 1995;25:2643–2649.

353. Kim JM, Rasmussen JP, Rudensky AY. Regulatory T cells prevent catastrophic autoimmunity throughout the lifespan of mice. Nature Immunology. 2007;8: 191–197.
354. Dugast AS, Vanhove B. Immune regulation by non-lymphoid cells in transplantation. Clinical and Experimental Immunology. 2009;156:25–34.
355. Thomson CW, Lee BP, Zhang L. Double-negative regulatory T cells: non-conventional regulators. Immunologic Research. 2006;35:163–178.
356. Josien R, Douillard P, Guillot C, et al. A critical role for transforming growth factor-beta in donor transfusion-induced allograft tolerance. Journal of Clinical Investigation. 1998;102:1920–1926.
357. Streilein JW, Masli S, Takeuchi M, et al. The eye's view of antigen presentation. Human Immunology. 2002;63:435–443.
358. Calne RY, Sells RA, Pena JR, et al. Induction of immunological tolerance by porcine liver allografts. Nature. 1969;223:472–476.
359. Robertson NJ, Brook FA, Gardner RL, et al. Embryonic stem cell-derived tissues are immunogenic but their inherent immune privilege promotes the induction of tolerance. Proceedings of the National Academy of Sciences of the United States of America. 2007;104:20920–20925.
360. Salahudeen AK. Cold ischemic injury of transplanted kidneys: new insights from experimental studies. American Journal of Physiology. Renal Physiology. 2004;287:F181–F187.
361. Belzer FO, Hoffman RM, Southard JH. Kidney preservation. Surgical Clinics of North America. 1978;58:261–271.
362. Collins GM, Bravo-Shugarman M, Novom S, et al. Kidney preservation for transplantation. I. Twelve-hour storage in rabbits. Transplantation Proceedings. 1969;1:801–807.
363. Collins GM, Bravo-Shugarman M, Terasaki PI. Kidney preservation for transportation. Initial perfusion and 30 hours' ice storage. Lancet. 1969;2: 1219–1222.
364. Belzer FO, Southard JH. Principles of solid-organ preservation by cold storage. Transplantation. 1988;45:673–676.
365. Chatauret N, Thuillier R, Hauet T. Preservation strategies to reduce ischemic injury in kidney transplantation: pharmacological and genetic approaches. Current Opinion in Organ Transplantation. 2011;16:180–187.
366. Hassanain M, Tchervenkov J, Cantarovich M, et al. Delayed graft function has an equally bad impact on deceased donor renal graft survival in both standard criteria donors and expanded criteria donors. Transplantation Proceedings. 2009;41:133–134.
367. Zhai Y, Busuttil RW, Kupiec-Weglinski JW. Liver ischemia and reperfusion injury: new insights into mechanisms of innate-adaptive immune-mediated tissue inflammation. American Journal of Transplantation. 2011;11:1563–1569.
368. Yarlagadda SG, Coca SG, Formica RN, et al. Association between delayed graft function and allograft and patient survival: a systematic review and meta-analysis. Nephrology, Dialysis, Transplantation. 2009;24:1039–1047.
369. Di Cocco P, Orlando G, Rizza V, et al. Kidney transplantation from older donors. Transplantation Proceedings. 2011;43:1033–1035.
370. Timsit MO, Yuan X, Floerchinger B, et al. Consequences of transplant quality on chronic allograft nephropathy. Kidney International. 2010;78 (Suppl. 119): S54–S58.
371. Moers C, Smits JM, Maathuis MH, et al. Machine perfusion or cold storage in deceased-donor kidney transplantation. New England Journal of Medicine. 2009;360:7–19.
372. Chandraker A, Takada M, Nadeau KC, et al. CD28-b7 blockade in organ dysfunction secondary to cold ischemia/reperfusion injury. Kidney International. 1997;52:1678–1684.
373. Salahudeen AK, Joshi M, Jenkins JK. Apoptosis versus necrosis during cold storage and rewarming of human renal proximal tubular cells. Transplantation. 2001;72:798–804.
374. Warnecke G, Sommer SP, Gohrbandt B, et al. Warm or cold ischemia in animal models of lung ischemia-reperfusion injury: is there a difference? Thoracic and Cardiovascular Surgeon. 2004;52:174–179.
375. Ge F, Gong W. Strategies for successfully establishing a kidney transplant in a mouse model. Experimental and Clinical Transplantation. 2011;9:287–294.
376. Fujiwara H, Raju S, Grogan JB, et al. Organ preservation injury in small bowel transplantation. Journal of Investigative Surgery. 1990;3:23–32.
377. Malhorta D, Zhou HZ, Kong YL, et al. Improvement in experimental cardiac preservation based on metabolic considerations. Transplantation. 1991;52: 1004–1008.
378. Stringham JC, Southard JH, Hegge J, et al. Limitations of heart preservation by cold storage. Transplantation. 1992;53:287–294.
379. O'Callaghan JM, Knight SR, Morgan RD, et al. Preservation solutions for static cold storage of kidney allografts: a systematic review and meta-analysis. American Journal of Transplantation. 2012;12:896–906.
380. Shen XD, Gao F, Ke B, et al. Inflammatory responses in a new mouse model of prolonged hepatic cold ischemia followed by arterialized orthotopic liver transplantation. Liver Transplantation. 2005;11:1273–1281.
381. Southard JH, van Gulik TM, Ametani MS, et al. Important components of the UW solution. Transplantation. 1990;49:251–257.
382. Heyman SN, Rosenberger C, Rosen S. Acute kidney injury: lessons from experimental models. Contributions to Nephrology. 2011;169:286–296.
383. Kelly KJ, Plotkin Z, Dagher PC. Guanosine supplementation reduces apoptosis and protects renal function in the setting of ischemic injury. Journal of Clinical Investigation. 2001;108:1291–1298.
384. Salahudeen AK, Huang H, Joshi M, et al. Involvement of the mitochondrial pathway in cold storage and rewarming-associated apoptosis of human renal proximal tubular cells. American Journal of Transplantation. 2003;3:273–280.
385. Huang Y, Rabb H, Womer KL. Ischemia-reperfusion and immediate T cell responses. Cellular Immunology. 2007;248:4–11.
386. LaRosa DF, Rahman AH, Turka LA. The innate immune system in allograft rejection and tolerance. Journal of Immunology. 2007;178:7503–7509.
387. Humphreys BD, Valerius MT, Kobayashi A, et al. Intrinsic epithelial cells repair the kidney after injury. Cell Stem Cell. 2008;2:284–291.
388. Bonegio R, Lieberthal W. Role of apoptosis in the pathogenesis of acute renal failure. Current Opinion in Nephrology and Hypertension. 2002;11: 301–308.
389. Bonventre JV, Weinberg JM. Recent advances in the pathophysiology of ischemic acute renal failure. Journal of the American Society of Nephrology. 2003; 14:2199–2210.
390. Devarajan P. Cellular and molecular derangements in acute tubular necrosis. Current Opinion in Pediatrics. 2005;17:193–199.
391. Devarajan P. Update on mechanisms of ischemic acute kidney injury. Journal of the American Society of Nephrology. 2006;17:1503–1520.
392. Oberbauer R, Rohrmoser M, Regele H, et al. Apoptosis of tubular epithelial cells in donor kidney biopsies predicts early renal allograft function. Journal of the American Society of Nephrology. 1999;10:2006–2013.
393. Perrin C, Ecarnot-Laubriet A, Vergely C, et al. Calpain and caspase-3 inhibitors reduce infarct size and post-ischemic apoptosis in rat heart without modifying contractile recovery. Cellular and Molecular Biology (Noisy-Le-Grand, France). 2003;49:OL497–OL505.
394. Xie J, Guo Q. Apoptosis antagonizing transcription factor protects renal tubule cells against oxidative damage and apoptosis induced by ischemia-reperfusion. Journal of the American Society of Nephrology. 2006;17: 3336–3346.
395. Cursio R, Gugenheim J, Ricci JE, et al. A caspase inhibitor fully protects rats against lethal normothermic liver ischemia by inhibition of liver apoptosis. FASEB Journal. 1999;13:253–261.
396. Daemen MA, van't Veer C, Denecker G, et al. Inhibition of apoptosis induced by ischemia-reperfusion prevents inflammation. Journal of Clinical Investigation. 1999;104:541–549.
397. Mueller TH, Kienle K, Beham A, et al. Caspase 3 inhibition improves survival and reduces early graft injury after ischemia and reperfusion in rat liver transplantation. Transplantation. 2004;78:1267–1273.
398. Fadeel B, Xue D, Kagan V. Programmed cell clearance: molecular regulation of the elimination of apoptotic cell corpses and its role in the resolution of inflammation. Biochemical and Biophysical Research Communications. 2010;396: 7–10.
399. Rovere P, Sabbadini MG, Vallinoto C, et al. Delayed clearance of apoptotic lymphoma cells allows cross-presentation of intracellular antigens by mature dendritic cells. Journal of Leukocyte Biology. 1999;66:345–349.
400. Peter C, Wesselborg S, Herrmann M, et al. Dangerous attraction: phagocyte recruitment and danger signals of apoptotic and necrotic cells. Apoptosis. 2010;15:1007–1028.
401. Thorp EB. Mechanisms of failed apoptotic cell clearance by phagocyte subsets in cardiovascular disease. Apoptosis. 2010;15:1124–1136.
402. Rock KL, Latz E, Ontiveros F, et al. The sterile inflammatory response. Annual Review of Immunology. 2010;28:321–342.
403. Scaffidi P, Misteli T, Bianchi ME. Release of chromatin protein HMGB1 by necrotic cells triggers inflammation. Nature. 2002;418:191–195.
404. Silva MT, do Vale A, dos Santos NM. Secondary necrosis in multicellular animals: an outcome of apoptosis with pathogenic implications. Apoptosis. 2008;13: 463–482.
405. Bolisetty S, Agarwal A. Neutrophils in acute kidney injury: not neutral any more. Kidney International. 2009;75:674–676.
406. Kinsey GR, Li L, Okusa MD. Inflammation in acute kidney injury. Nephron. Experimental Nephrology. 2008;109:e102–e107.
407. Majno G, La Gattuta M, Thompson TE. Cellular death and necrosis: chemical, physical and morphologic changes in rat liver. Virchows Archiv Fur Pathologische Anatomie und Physiologie und fur klinische Medizin. 1960;333: 421–465.

408. Apetoh L, Ghiringhelli F, Tesniere A, et al. The interaction between HMGB1 and TLR4 dictates the outcome of anticancer chemotherapy and radiotherapy. Immunological Reviews. 2007;220:47–59.
409. Chen CJ, Kono H, Golenbock D, et al. Identification of a key pathway required for the sterile inflammatory response triggered by dying cells. Nature Medicine. 2007;13:851–856.
410. Matzinger P. Tolerance, danger, and the extended family. Annual Review of Immunology. 1994;12:991–1045.
411. Walker PD, Kaushal GP, Shah SV. Meprin A, the major matrix degrading enzyme in renal tubules, produces a novel nidogen fragment in vitro and in vivo. Kidney International. 1998;53:1673–1680.
412. Wu H, Chen G, Wyburn KR, et al. TLR4 activation mediates kidney ischemia/reperfusion injury. Journal of Clinical Investigation. 2007;117:2847–2859.
413. Ascon DB, Lopez-Briones S, Liu M, et al. Phenotypic and functional characterization of kidney-infiltrating lymphocytes in renal ischemia reperfusion injury. Journal of Immunology. 2006;177:3380–3387.
414. Li L, Huang L, Sung SS, et al. NKT cell activation mediates neutrophil IFN-gamma production and renal ischemia-reperfusion injury. Journal of Immunology. 2007;178:5899–5911.
415. Zhang ZX, Wang S, Huang X, et al. NK cells induce apoptosis in tubular epithelial cells and contribute to renal ischemia-reperfusion injury. Journal of Immunology. 2008;181:7489–7498.
416. Beldi G, Banz Y, Kroemer A, et al. Deletion of CD39 on natural killer cells attenuates hepatic ischemia/reperfusion injury in mice. Hepatology (Baltimore, Md.). 2010;51:1702–1711.
417. Rabb H, Mendiola CC, Dietz J, et al. Role of CD11a and CD11b in ischemic acute renal failure in rats. American Journal of Physiology. 1994;267:F1052–F1058.
418. Rabb H, Daniels F, O'Donnell M, et al. Pathophysiological role of T lymphocytes in renal ischemia-reperfusion injury in mice. American Journal of Physiology. Renal Physiology. 2000;279:F525–F531.
419. Burne-Taney MJ, Liu M, Baldwin WM, et al. Decreased capacity of immune cells to cause tissue injury mediates kidney ischemic preconditioning. Journal of Immunology. 2006;176:7015–7020.
420. Zwacka RM, Zhang Y, Halldorson J, et al. CD4(+) T-lymphocytes mediate ischemia/reperfusion-induced inflammatory responses in mouse liver. Journal of Clinical Investigation. 1997;100:279–289.
421. Takada M, Chandraker A, Nadeau KC, et al. The role of the B7 costimulatory pathway in experimental cold ischemia/reperfusion injury. Journal of Clinical Investigation. 1997;100:1199–1203.
422. Ikeda A, Ueki S, Nakao A, et al. Liver graft exposure to carbon monoxide during cold storage protects sinusoidal endothelial cells and ameliorates reperfusion injury in rats. Liver Transplantation. 2009;15:1458–1468.
423. Kaizu T, Nakao A, Tsung A, et al. Carbon monoxide inhalation ameliorates cold ischemia/reperfusion injury after rat liver transplantation. Surgery. 2005;138:229–235.
424. Caumartin Y, Stephen J, Deng JP, et al. Carbon monoxide-releasing molecules protect against ischemia-reperfusion injury during kidney transplantation. Kidney International. 2011;79:1080–1089.
425. Neto JS, Nakao A, Kimizuka K, et al. Protection of transplant-induced renal ischemia-reperfusion injury with carbon monoxide. American Journal of Physiology. Renal Physiology. 2004;287:F979–F989.
426. Faleo G, Neto JS, Kohmoto J, et al. Carbon monoxide ameliorates renal cold ischemia-reperfusion injury with an upregulation of vascular endothelial growth factor by activation of hypoxia-inducible factor. Transplantation. 2008;85:1833–1840.
427. Kohmoto J, Nakao A, Stolz DB, et al. Carbon monoxide protects rat lung transplants from ischemia-reperfusion injury via a mechanism involving p38 MAPK pathway. American Journal of Transplantation. 2007;7:2279–2290.
428. Katada K, Bihari A, Mizuguchi S, et al. Carbon monoxide liberated from CO-releasing molecule (CORM-2) attenuates ischemia/reperfusion (I/R)-induced inflammation in the small intestine. Inflammation. 2010;33:92–100.
429. Nakao A, Kimizuka K, Stolz DB, et al. Carbon monoxide inhalation protects rat intestinal grafts from ischemia/reperfusion injury. American Journal of Pathology. 2003;163:1587–1598.
430. Siriussawakul A, Chen LI, Lang JD. Medical gases: a novel strategy for attenuating ischemia-reperfusion injury in organ transplantation? Journal of Transplantation. 2012;2012:819382.
431. Awad AS, Ye H, Huang L, et al. Selective sphingosine 1-phosphate 1 receptor activation reduces ischemia-reperfusion injury in mouse kidney. American Journal of Physiology. Renal Physiology. 2006;290:F1516–F1524.
432. Bajwa A, Jo SK, Ye H, et al. Activation of sphingosine-1-phosphate 1 receptor in the proximal tubule protects against ischemia-reperfusion injury. Journal of the American Society of Nephrology. 2010;21:955–965.
433. Lai LW, Yong KC, Igarashi S, et al. A sphingosine-1-phosphate type 1 receptor agonist inhibits the early T-cell transient following renal ischemia-reperfusion injury. Kidney International. 2007;71:1223–1231.
434. Bajwa A, Kinsey GR, Okusa MD. Immune mechanisms and novel pharmacological therapies of acute kidney injury. Current Drug Targets. 2009;10:1196–1204.
435. Yokota N, O'Donnell M, Daniels F, et al. Protective effect of HMG-CoA reductase inhibitor on experimental renal ischemia-reperfusion injury. American Journal of Nephrology. 2003;23:13–17.
436. Kunugi S, Shimizu A, Kuwahara N, et al. Inhibition of matrix metalloproteinases reduces ischemia-reperfusion acute kidney injury. Laboratory Investigation. 2011;91:170–180.
437. Zhang ZX, Min WP, Jevnikar AM. Use of RNA interference to minimize ischemia reperfusion injury. Transplantation Reviews (Orlando, Fla.). 2012;26:140–155.
438. Molitoris BA, Dagher PC, Sandoval RM, et al. siRNA targeted to p53 attenuates ischemic and cisplatin-induced acute kidney injury. Journal of the American Society of Nephrology. 2009;20:1754–1764.
439. Singaravelu K, Padanilam BJ. p53 target Siva regulates apoptosis in ischemic kidneys. American Journal of Physiology. Renal Physiology. 2011;300:F1130–F1141.
440. Bonventre JV, Yang L. Cellular pathophysiology of ischemic acute kidney injury. Journal of Clinical Investigation. 2011;121:4210–4221.
441. Witzgall R, Brown D, Schwarz C, et al. Localization of proliferating cell nuclear antigen, vimentin, c-Fos, and clusterin in the postischemic kidney. Evidence for a heterogenous genetic response among nephron segments, and a large pool of mitotically active and dedifferentiated cells. Journal of Clinical Investigation. 1994;93:2175–2188.
442. Duffield JS, Park KM, Hsiao LL, et al. Restoration of tubular epithelial cells during repair of the postischemic kidney occurs independently of bone marrow-derived stem cells. Journal of Clinical Investigation. 2005;115:1743–1755.
443. Lin F, Moran A, Igarashi P. Intrarenal cells, not bone marrow-derived cells, are the major source for regeneration in postischemic kidney. Journal of Clinical Investigation. 2005;115:1756–1764.
444. Yang L, Besschetnova TY, Brooks CR, et al. Epithelial cell cycle arrest in G2/M mediates kidney fibrosis after injury. Nature Medicine. 2010;16:535–543, 1p following 143.
445. Yang L, Humphreys BD, Bonventre JV. Pathophysiology of acute kidney injury to chronic kidney disease: maladaptive repair. Contributions to Nephrology. 2011;174:149–155.
446. Ichimura T, Bonventre JV, Bailly V, et al. Kidney injury molecule-1 (KIM-1), a putative epithelial cell adhesion molecule containing a novel immunoglobulin domain, is up-regulated in renal cells after injury. Journal of Biological Chemistry. 1998;273:4135–4142.
447. Ichimura T, Asseldonk EJ, Humphreys BD, et al. Kidney injury molecule-1 is a phosphatidylserine receptor that confers a phagocytic phenotype on epithelial cells. Journal of Clinical Investigation. 2008;118:1657–1668.
448. Bailly V, Zhang Z, Meier W, et al. Shedding of kidney injury molecule-1, a putative adhesion protein involved in renal regeneration. Journal of Biological Chemistry. 2002;277:39739–39748.
449. He Z, Lu L, Altmann C, et al. Interleukin-18 binding protein transgenic mice are protected against ischemic acute kidney injury. American Journal of Physiology. Renal Physiology. 2008;295:F1414–F1421.
450. Wu H, Craft ML, Wang P, et al. IL-18 contributes to renal damage after ischemia-reperfusion. Journal of the American Society of Nephrology. 2008;19:2331–2341.
451. Rosen S, Heyman SN. Difficulties in understanding human "acute tubular necrosis": limited data and flawed animal models. Kidney International. 2001;60:1220–1224.
452. Solez K, Racusen LC, Marcussen N, et al. Morphology of ischemic acute renal failure, normal function, and cyclosporine toxicity in cyclosporine-treated renal allograft recipients. Kidney International. 1993;43:1058–1067.
453. Heyman SN, Lieberthal W, Rogiers P, et al. Animal models of acute tubular necrosis. Current Opinion in Critical Care. 2002;8:526–534.
454. Neal A, Murphy L. A unipapillary kidney by any other name. Medical Journal of Australia. 1983;1:403–404.
455. Peterson JE, Pinckney LE, Rutledge JC, et al. The solitary renal calyx and papilla in human kidneys. Radiology. 1982;144:525–527.
456. Platt JL. Xenotransplantation. Washington, DC: ASM Press; 2001.
457. Yang YG, Sykes M. Xenotransplantation: current status and a perspective on the future. Nature Reviews. Immunology. 2007;7:519–531.
458. Ekser B, Ezzelarab M, Hara H, et al. Clinical xenotransplantation: the next medical revolution? Lancet. 2012;379:672–683.
459. Cooper DK, Koren E, Oriol R. Oligosaccharides and discordant xenotransplantation. Immunological Reviews. 1994;141:31–58.
460. Byrne GW, McGregor CG. Cardiac xenotransplantation: progress and challenges. Current Opinion in Organ Transplantation. 2012;17:148–154.
461. Cowan PJ, d'Apice AJ. Complement activation and coagulation in xenotransplantation. Immunology and Cell Biology. 2009;87:203–208.

462. Dai Y, Vaught TD, Boone J, et al. Targeted disruption of the alpha1,3-galactosyltransferase gene in cloned pigs. Nature Biotechnology. 2002;20:251–255.
463. Phelps CJ, Koike C, Vaught TD, et al. Production of alpha 1,3-galactosyltransferase-deficient pigs. Science. 2003;299:411–414.
464. Kuwaki K, Tseng YL, Dor FJ, et al. Heart transplantation in baboons using alpha1,3-galactosyltransferase gene-knockout pigs as donors: initial experience. Nature Medicine. 2005;11:29–31.
465. Tseng YL, Kuwaki K, Dor FJ, et al. alpha1,3-Galactosyltransferase gene-knockout pig heart transplantation in baboons with survival approaching 6 months. Transplantation. 2005;80:1493–1500.
466. Azimzadeh A, Meyer C, Watier H, et al. Removal of primate xenoreactive natural antibodies by extracorporeal perfusion of pig kidneys and livers. Transplant Immunology. 1998;6:13–22.
467. Bach FH, Winkler H, Ferran C, et al. Delayed xenograft rejection. Immunology Today. 1996;17:379–384.
468. Candinas D, Belliveau S, Koyamada N, et al. T cell independence of macrophage and natural killer cell infiltration, cytokine production, and endothelial activation during delayed xenograft rejection. Transplantation. 1996;62:1920–1927.
469. Chong AS, Shen J, Xiao F, et al. Delayed xenograft rejection in the concordant hamster heart into Lewis rat model. Transplantation. 1996;62:90–96.
470. Le Bas-Bernardet S, Blancho G. Current cellular immunological hurdles in pig-to-primate xenotransplantation. Transplant Immunology. 2009;21:60–64.
471. Scalea J, Hanecamp I, Robson SC, et al. T-cell-mediated immunological barriers to xenotransplantation. Xenotransplantation. 2012;19:23–30.
472. Feng S, Quickel RR, Hollister-Lock J, et al. Prolonged xenograft survival of islets infected with small doses of adenovirus expressing CTLA4Ig. Transplantation. 1999;67:1607–1613.
473. Karlsson-Parra A, Ridderstad A, Wallgren AC, et al. Xenograft rejection of porcine islet-like cell clusters in normal and natural killer cell-depleted mice. Transplantation. 1996;61:1313–1320.
474. Thompson P, Cardona K, Russell M, et al. CD40-specific costimulation blockade enhances neonatal porcine islet survival in nonhuman primates. American Journal of Transplantation. 2011;11:947–957.
475. Arefanian H, Tredget EB, Rajotte RV, et al. Short-term administrations of a combination of anti-LFA-1 and anti-CD154 monoclonal antibodies induce tolerance to neonatal porcine islet xenografts in mice. Diabetes. 2010;59:958–966.
476. Arefanian H, Tredget EB, Rajotte RV, et al. Combination of anti-CD4 with anti-LFA-1 and anti-CD154 monoclonal antibodies promotes long-term survival and function of neonatal porcine islet xenografts in spontaneously diabetic NOD mice. Cell Transplantation. 2007;16:787–798.
477. Jung YS, Jeong JH, Yook S, et al. Surface modification of pancreatic islets using heparin-DOPA conjugate and anti-CD154 mAb for the prolonged survival of intrahepatic transplanted islets in a xenograft model. Biomaterials. 2012;33:295–303.
478. Kumagai-Braesch M, Ekberg H, Wang F, et al. Corbascio, M: anti-LFA-1 improves pig islet xenograft function in diabetic mice when long-term acceptance is induced by CTLA4Ig/anti-CD40L. Transplantation. 2007;83:1259–1267.
479. Schwartz RH. A cell culture model for T lymphocyte clonal anergy. Science. 1990;248:1349–1356.
480. Wolgast M, Karlberg L, Kallskog O, et al. Hemodynamic alterations in ischaemic acute renal failure. Nephron. 1982;31:301–303.
481. Mason J, Torhorst J, Welsch J. Role of the medullary perfusion defect in the pathogenesis of ischemic renal failure. Kidney International. 1984;26:283–293.
482. Day YJ, Huang L, Ye H, et al. Renal ischemia-reperfusion injury and adenosine 2A receptor-mediated tissue protection: role of macrophages. American Journal of Physiology. Renal Physiology. 2005;288:F722–F731.
483. Burne-Taney MJ, Ascon DB, Daniels F, et al. B cell deficiency confers protection from renal ischemia reperfusion injury. Journal of Immunology. 2003;171:3210–3215.
484. Austen WG Jr, Zhang M, Chan R, et al. Murine hindlimb reperfusion injury can be initiated by a self-reactive monoclonal IgM. Surgery. 2004;136:401–406.
485. de Perrot M, Young K, Imai Y, et al. Recipient T cells mediate reperfusion injury after lung transplantation in the rat. Journal of Immunology. 2003;171:4995–5002.
486. Burne MJ, Haq M, Matsuse H, et al. Genetic susceptibility to renal ischemia reperfusion injury revealed in a murine model. Transplantation. 2000;69:1023–1025.
487. Geudens N, Vanaudenaerde BM, Neyrinck AP, et al. The importance of lymphocytes in lung ischemia-reperfusion injury. Transplantation Proceedings. 2007;39:2659–2662.
488. Yang Z, Day YJ, Toufektsian MC, et al. Myocardial infarct-sparing effect of adenosine A2A receptor activation is due to its action on CD4+ T lymphocytes. Circulation. 2006;114:2056–2064.
489. Afzali B, Lechler RI, Hernandez-Fuentes MP. Allorecognition and the alloresponse: clinical implications. Tissue Antigens. 2007;69:545–556.
490. Zhang B, Ramesh G, Uematsu S, et al. TLR4 signaling mediates inflammation and tissue injury in nephrotoxicity. Journal of the American Society of Nephrology. 2008;19:923–932.
491. Zhai Y, Shen XD, O'Connell R, et al. Cutting edge: TLR4 activation mediates liver ischemia/reperfusion inflammatory response via IFN regulatory factor 3-dependent MyD88-independent pathway. Journal of Immunology. 2004;173:7115–7119.
492. Kelly KJ, Williams WW Jr, Colvin RB, et al. Intercellular adhesion molecule-1-deficient mice are protected against ischemic renal injury. Journal of Clinical Investigation. 1996;97:1056–1063.
493. Williams JP, Pechet TT, Weiser MR, et al. Intestinal reperfusion injury is mediated by IgM and complement. Journal of Applied Physiology. 1999;86:938–942.
494. Reid RR, Woodcock S, Shimabukuro-Vornhagen A, et al. Functional activity of natural antibody is altered in Cr2-deficient mice. Journal of Immunology. 2002;169:5433–5440.
495. Fleming SD, Shea-Donohue T, Guthridge JM, et al. Mice deficient in complement receptors 1 and 2 lack a tissue injury-inducing subset of the natural antibody repertoire. Journal of Immunology. 2002;169:2126–2133.
496. Thurman JM, Ljubanovic D, Royer PA, et al. Altered renal tubular expression of the complement inhibitor Crry permits complement activation after ischemia/reperfusion. Journal of Clinical Investigation. 2006;116:357–368.
497. Ma XL, Weyrich AS, Lefer DJ, et al. Monoclonal antibody to L-selectin attenuates neutrophil accumulation and protects ischemic reperfused cat myocardium. Circulation. 1993;88:649–658.
498. Carmody IC, Meng L, Shen XD, et al. P-selectin knockout mice have improved outcomes with both warm ischemia and small bowel transplantation. Transplantation Proceedings. 2004;36:263–264.
499. Ozaki KS, Yoshida J, Ueki S, et al. Carbon monoxide inhibits apoptosis during cold storage and protects kidney grafts donated after cardiac death. Transplant International. 2012;25:107–117.
500. Farber A, Connors JP, Friedlander RM, et al. A specific inhibitor of apoptosis decreases tissue injury after intestinal ischemia-reperfusion in mice. Journal of Vascular Surgery. 1999;30:752–760.
501. Humphreys BD, Lin SL, Kobayashi A, et al. Fate tracing reveals the pericyte and not epithelial origin of myofibroblasts in kidney fibrosis. American Journal of Pathology. 2010;176:85–97.
502. Iwano M, Plieth D, Danoff TM, et al. Evidence that fibroblasts derive from epithelium during tissue fibrosis. Journal of Clinical Investigation. 2002;110:341–350.
503. Natarajan R, Salloum FN, Fisher BJ, et al. Hypoxia inducible factor-1 activation by prolyl 4-hydroxylase-2 gene silencing attenuates myocardial ischemia reperfusion injury. Circulation Research. 2006;98:133–140.
504. Sheldon RA, Osredkar D, Lee CL, et al. HIF-1 alpha-deficient mice have increased brain injury after neonatal hypoxia-ischemia. Developmental Neuroscience. 2009;31:452–458.
505. Bernhardt WM, Gottmann U, Doyon F, et al. Donor treatment with a PHD-inhibitor activating HIFs prevents graft injury and prolongs survival in an allogenic kidney transplant model. Proceedings of the National Academy of Sciences of the United States of America. 2009;106:21276–21281.
506. Kojima I, Tanaka T, Inagi R, et al. Protective role of hypoxia-inducible factor-2alpha against ischemic damage and oxidative stress in the kidney. Journal of the American Society of Nephrology. 2007;18:1218–1226.

第 15 章
器官移植大型动物模型

Douglas J. Anderson, Benjamin M. Martin, Allan D. Kirk, David H. Sachs

引言

1954 年，由 Joseph Murray 博士带领的团队成功地实施了同卵双胞胎之间的肾脏移植手术，开启了现代器官移植的篇章[1]。而早在 1953 年，Billingham、Brent 和 Madawar 就针对同种异体细胞耐受性的获得问题发表了他们具有里程碑意义的研究成果[2]。在过去的 60 年中，站在这些巨人的肩膀上，临床研究者能够看到手术技术、围术期护理以及免疫抑制等方面的显著进步使得患者的预后有了稳定的提高[3,4]。然而，前方依然存在许多挑战。在临床上，我们才刚刚开始实现移植物的持久耐受[5-7]，因此，在大多数情况下，我们仍然要求患者以一种慢性疾病状态交换另一种慢性疾病状态——终生的免疫抑制。当我们继续为了患者利益解决这些问题时，我们必须小心地遵循着从实验室到临床的途径。尽管小鼠模型已经无数次地证明了其在帮助阐明新的生物学和治疗学概念方面的价值，大型动物实验仍然是转化为人类试验的最好选择。本章将对移植中常用的大型动物模型及其各自相对的优势和劣势进行概述，目的在于展示在从理论到治疗的转化过程中大型动物模型所发挥的价值。本章是对第 13 章、第 14 章和第 16 章的补充，这些章节主要讲了移植的体外模型、小型动物体内模型以及移植硅芯片模型。

为什么使用大型动物?

早在 Aristotle 和 Erasistratus 的时代，动物实验就已经是医学进步的重要力量，并且为人类的治疗及技术提供了转化的合理性基础[8]。实际上，使用动物来完善手术技术的历史至少可以追溯到 12 世纪，当时 Ibn Zuhr(Avenzoar)在一只山羊身上实施了气管造口术[9]。尽管人体试验不应该没有创新性，但是除非一种方法已经在模型上试验过，并且至少能有效地去预测计划干预的安全性，否则这个方法就无法为患者提供必要且适当的背景，无法使患者在真正知情的情况下做出有关他们参与研究的决定。通常，动物实验能为人类试验提供基于伦理学的基础。

尽管动物模型往往不能完全预示着一种方案在人类中的成功，但其仍是预测安全与否的最佳手段。免疫和排斥反应的复杂性阻碍了任何一种能够模拟基本免疫应答的体外模型的发展，更谈不上预测免疫应答。因此，动物仍是推进治疗手段转化为临床应用的最佳模型。然而鉴于动物模型不能预测人类治疗效果的所有方面，故应在考虑到这一限制的情况下设计实验并解释实验。

由于现代社会已经认识到动物也有接受人道待遇的权利，指导各类动物实验的伦理原则，尤其是大型动物实验，变得越来越复杂。Tomas Aquinas 断言“动物没有权利”，而这一主张已经不再为社会所接受。虽然他的言论看起来没有什么价值，但更仔细地审视 Aquinas 以人性为中心的人生观后，我们会发现其并没有忽视动物的福利，而是提升了人类的地位，并为动物实验提供了合理的理由[10]。在过去的半个世纪中，动物实验伦理学的现代观点推动了重要的法规的颁布以确保动物的正确使用。伦理动物实验的具体指南可以在“实验动物护理和使用指南”[11] 以及美国实验动物护理协会的出版物中找到[12]。许多学术机构和杂志出版商都要遵守这些准则。减少、替代和优化原则是所有伦理动物实验的核心。动物模型只能在没有合适的替代品的情况下使用，并且所有的技术都应根据动物的福利进行最大程度的改进。使用的动物数量应该是解决实验问题所需的最小值。然而，如果不能解决实验所提出的问题，不做实验才是符合伦理的。因此，减少使用动物的数量却未能达到目的的实验与一个使用了更多的动物的成功实验相比更加不符合伦理。

小鼠动物实验相对于大型动物模型具有几个明显的优势。小鼠的成本相对便宜,但具有充分的生物学相似性,并且其基因操作简单,使其成为通路测定和机制研究的理想选择。相比之下,大型动物模型更加昂贵,除了近亲交配的小型猪之外,其遗传学多样性使其难以进行最终的机制研究。然而,大型动物进行机制研究的不切实际性同时也使它们成为临床前研究的最佳选择。大型动物模型的额外复杂性为实验增加了意想不到的变量,使得这些实验最适用于检查实用性、安全性和普遍成效。但这并不意味着实验不需要测量结果以保持与整体假设一致。关于移植学和免疫学,具体来说,鼠模型有许多潜在的缺点。在无病原体的环境中繁殖的实验小鼠以及4~8周龄的实验小鼠具有的主要是固有免疫系统[13]。这可能解释了为什么许多治疗方法,包括一些容易诱导小鼠耐受的方法,尽管已经在小鼠模型中进行了细致的研究,一旦转移到更为复杂的动物中[14,15],甚至是暴露于病原体的小鼠中却往往失败[16]。与迄今为止所测试过的所有大型动物物种不同,小鼠内皮细胞不会结构性地表达MHCⅡ类抗原,这可能解释了为什么相对于小鼠,大型动物中MHCⅡ类抗原匹配对于移植结果具有更大的重要性[17,18]。用于测试治疗效果的动物所具有的特殊遗传背景也已显示会影响治疗效果[19]。远系繁殖的大型动物模型的遗传多样性和免疫学经验有利于避免上述缺点。因此,在移植术在人类临床试验开始之前,大型动物模型,最常见的是非人灵长类(NHP)动物模型实验已经成为一种必要条件[15,20]。

由于免疫系统极其复杂,当治疗手段转化到用于大型动物模型或随后的人类时,治疗可能会失败。这很少是模型本身的失败,而更可能是由于一个或几个最初并不被重视的关键差异所导致的。药物分布或新陈代谢的差异可能导致一项治疗的明显失败,如果进行了适当的剂量调整,治疗方法可能会相当成功。在现代生物与抗体治疗的时代,特别值得注意的是,分子结构中相对较小的差异可能对药物发挥预期效果的能力产生深远的影响。如前所述,免疫学实验的多样性是大型动物模型的主要优点,并且可以通过异源免疫相互作用对治疗结果产生显著的影响。该实验参数的量化和控制非常具有挑战性。最后,治疗期间对动物的实际护理无法直接复制到临床上。手术模型中的创伤护理往往很困难。对于有意识的动物模型,检测和血管穿刺也是具有挑战性的。笼子设计上的创新允许NHP留置导管,然而这些笼子并不总是可用的,也不是没有缺点的。

大型动物模型的最后一个问题是时间,不仅是指动物的年龄还指生存结果。由于实际原因,被用于实验的动物往往比较年轻,相当于青春期。证据表明,这些年轻动物的T细胞主要是幼稚细胞,随着年龄的增长会慢慢成熟为记忆表型[21-24]。这与绝对年龄相同的人类儿童更为相似,而非构成了大部分临床移植人群的成年人。关于动物模型中的模糊的移植物存活期限,小鼠模型中规定100天作为验收指标,而对于较大的动物常采用几年。尽管与人类相比,这些动物的整体寿命更短,移植物在人类身体中可能预计持续10年甚至更长时间,但是没有证据可以支持移植物存活期应与预期寿命成比例的解释。因此,最好不要将这些研究中的数据解释为移植物更长存活期的象征。

尽管上述所指出的大型动物模型存在挑战和缺点,它们仍然是临床转化中所考虑的预测广泛功效和治疗安全性的最佳指标。

常见的大型动物模型

在移植术中,最常用的大型动物模型有犬、猪以及非人灵长类(NHP)。每种物种在解剖学和生理学都与人类有着足够的相似性,用于本质上同时具有技术性和药理学特性的实验研究。这些物种之间的免疫反应是相似的,均以T细胞网络为基础,对相似组织的主要组织相容性复合物(MHC)产生应答。因此,未经修饰的同种异体移植物排斥反应的组织学以及速度都与人类预期相似。尽管有这些相似之处,这些模型在不同程度上存在着彼此差异及与人类的差异,从而使其不能完全预测临床结果。

在单独讨论每个动物模型之前,可以进行几个概括。药物代谢和吸收可以并且经常在物种之间广泛变化,使得药物反应曲线以及对人类或其他动物模型的毒性难以直接进行转化。然而,在适当调整药物分布后,在大型动物模型与人类之间,大多数药物的生理反应和疗效是相似的。

在移植的人类研究中,供体和受体之间的亲缘程度及MHC匹配程度通常是已知的。虽然人类移植配对之间的MHC匹配程度对结果的相对影响随着被移植器官的不同而变化,但一般来说,匹配度越高,结果越好。对动物模型也可以这样说,但是大型动物的MHC分型通常更困难,因此常被忽略。在动物实验中未能控制可变的MHC差异可能导致实验结果的解释中引入重要的混杂因素。

虽然对MHC遗传学的全面回顾超出了本章的范围,但聚焦于物种之间的差异进行一个基本的回顾还是很值得的。人类MHC结构的深度治疗可以参见第4章。人类MHC也称为人白细胞抗原(HLA),由染色体6p21.3上的260多个基因组成[25]。虽然这些基因中有许多与免疫功能有关,但与抗原呈递有关的且与本节讨论内容有关的基因,包括Ⅰ类分子HLA-A、HLA-B和HLA-C,以及Ⅱ类分子HLA-DP、HLA-DQ和HLA-DR。个体从其父母那里分别遗传一个基因的两个等位基因。这些基因的高度多态性导致群体内HLA分子的广泛多样性。这里提出的3种动物模型中的MHC基因座的整体结构是相似的,尽管有一些重要的遗传差异值得讨论。

犬类MHC,即犬白细胞抗原(DLA),已被透彻地研究。犬MHC位于12号染色体上,含有4种完整的Ⅰ类抗原:DLA-88、DLA-12、DLA-64和DLA-79。Ⅱ类区域包含DLA-DRB1、DLA-DQB1和DLA-DQA,任何一种都具有多态性。另外一个Ⅱ类基因,DLA-DRA,似乎是单态的[26]。由于犬MHC的初步结构已被阐明,通过对各种犬品种进行的大量调查,发现了几个额外的等位基因[27]。已经发现两个高度多态性的卫星标记物,一个接近Ⅰ类基因和Ⅱ类基因座的等位基因并且显示可用于确定家族内DLA单体型遗传,循序选择具有特异性DLA匹配的同窝动物进行移植研究。因为这些标志物不能鉴别特定的基因型,所以它们目前不适用于非相关动物的配对[26]。整个犬基因组的测序已经实现[28],并且通过DLA-DRB1的直接测序来确定等位基因同一性已经投入使用[29],提高了更完整的基因分型,可能改善非亲缘犬的移植研究配对。

猪模型相对于犬和NHP的主要优点在于人们对于猪MHC或猪白细胞抗原(SLA)有更广泛的了解,以及可以通过育种或通过病毒转染来遗传修饰猪。SLA位于第7号染色体上[25],已经定义为3种已知的经典Ⅰ类基因,标记为SLA-3、SLA-2和SLA-1(与先前由血清学定义的SLA A、B、C系列蛋白一致)。Ⅱ类区域也有明确的定义。与DLA类似,SLA-DRA是单态的,而SLADRB、SLA-DQA和SLA-DQB具有高度多态性[30-32]。通过MHC-已知的小型猪的育种,有助于对SLA及其功能重要性的了解,显著增加了猪移植实验的有效性。繁殖猪的便利性使得猪的遗传操作相对简单。这已成为异种器官移植的一个特别的福音,其中已经产生了不表达Gal异种抗原的基因敲除猪[33,34]。额外的基因修饰包括补体调节剂的上调[35,36]。这些转基因猪的使用将在本书的其他部分讨论。

在最新的移植研究中,非人灵长类动物成为受欢迎的大型动物模型,因为具有高度受体特异性的新的生物疗法正在进行测试。虽然猴子不能同系交配达到像小鼠、犬和猪一样的程度,它们也不能算是真正的远系繁殖。用于移植研究的大多数NHP来自有限杂交的专用克隆。直到最近,建立NHP遗传差异的技术还相对有限,主要由混合淋巴细胞反应和DR区域血清学分析或PCR分析组成。为了解恒河猴的MHC结构,前人付出了巨大的努力才得到了现在的成果。恒河猴MHC位于4号染色体上,由于其ⅠA和ⅠB基因(也称为Mamu-A和Mamu-B,恒河猴没有HLA-C同源物)的明显重复,导致其显著大于人类MHC[37]。恒河猴MHCⅡ类基因也是重复的,但是程度较低。这些基因的重复导致每个染色体都表达多达4个Mamu-A基因和14个Mamu-B基因,显著增加了杂合个体的复杂性[37]。此外,克隆方法已经揭示了这些基因是分层表达的,而在人类中则是共显性表达[38],有效地使基于DNA的等位基因特异性的分型在预测MHC分子表达方面无效。最近的两项进展显著提高了我们测定恒河猴亲缘性的能力。第一个是几个DNA微卫星探针的鉴定,能确定几代恒河猴之间的常染色体和性染色体遗传,使得恒河猴育种群体的准确谱系的绘制成为可能。虽然这种方法缺乏MHC等位基因特异性测定,但能够确定完整MHC单体型的遗传。第二大进展是大规模平行焦磷酸测序的发展以实现对MHC表达的综合分析[41]。焦磷酸盐测序能够说明上述恒河猴MHC的极端复杂性。该技术允许在规划移植实验时确定任何动物完整的MHC分型。这两项技术的应用,使得研究者在了解动物之间MHC差异的基础上设计实验,显著提高了结果的有效性。

移植术中的犬模型

犬在手术练习和手术技术的发展中占据了传统地位。因此,犬作为早期移植研究中的主要模型并不奇怪。许多与手术移植相关的技术问题都是在犬模型中得出的。实际上,肾脏[42]、心脏[43]、肝脏[44,45]、肺[46]、肠[47,48]、骨髓[49]、胰腺[50,51]和胰岛移植[52]的早期技术都是在犬模型中进行测试的。在Clane的实验中,声称在犬模型上,免疫抑制首次得到了成功使用[53]。尽管避免在实验中使用驯养动物的社会压力已经减少了犬模型的使用,但是近些年来在心脏[54]、肾脏[55]、胰岛[56]、肝脏[57]和肠道移植[58]方面的研究中,犬模型仍然被使用着。西雅图的Storb研究组一直并继续在实验性骨髓移植中广泛使用犬模型[59,60],他们也将该模型用于器官[61]和复合组织[62]的研究。在实体器官移植研究中,犬的实验已经显著减少,因而犬模型的使用并不认为是广泛存在的,仅在现代生物驱动制度下的转化研究中占有很少的地位。

移植术中的猪模型

由于猪的解剖学和生理学与人类相似,猪模型已经多年作为复杂人类疾病的实验模型。疾病的猪模型可能是自发的、遗传的、诱导的或转基因的。国产猪特别是小型猪常被用于生理学、药理学、毒理学、放射学、手术和器官移植、创伤学、病理学、胚胎学、胃肠冰雪、肾脏学、新生儿手术和心血管研究领域的研究。有几个实验室研究了猪的MHC[31,63-65],并且举办了很多研讨会来实现SLA系统术语的标准化[66-68]。此外,现在有大量可用于猪细胞表面抗原研究的单克隆抗体[69-73],使猪成为细胞群表征与操作的多功能动物模型,仅次于小鼠和人类。

此外,仅有少数几种大型动物的育种特征使得遗传实验成为可能,而猪就是其中之一。猪的产仔量相对较大(3~10个子代),妊娠期较短(114天)。它们大约在6月龄时达到性成熟期,母猪发情周期为3周(与之相比,犬每年只有两次发情期)。这些繁殖特征使得其中一个作者(DHS)的实验室可以在相对较短的时间内培育出MHC纯合子小型猪,并使得分离新的MHC重组体,使其变为纯合子,进行短期回交实验以确定和研究遗传分离成为可能[74-76]。因此,这些小型猪成为唯一一种MHC基因可重现控制的大型动物模型[77]。也因而在评估选择性MHC匹配对排斥和(或)诱导耐受的效果方面非常有用。

目前保留了三系带有纯合子SLA单体型,SLA^{a},SLA^{c}、SLA^{d}以及五系携带SLA内重组单体型(图15.1)。所有的这些系的组织相容性位点不同,大多数与人类移植有关的移植匹配组合都可以采用这种模型去模拟。因此,举个例子,在同一个MHC纯合子群之间的移植相当于HLA相合同胞间的移植,而不同群体之间的移植就相当于死亡捐赠者或HLA不相合同胞间的移植。同样,杂合体配对之间的移植可经选择使之相当于亲代与子代间的移植或一个单体型不匹配的同胞移植。此外,选择SLA^{dd}动物的一个亚系进行进一步的同系繁殖,以产生完全自交系的小型猪。当这个亚系的近交系数达到>94%时,子代之间互相进行皮肤移植没有引起排斥,从而将其定义为大型动物的第一个组织相

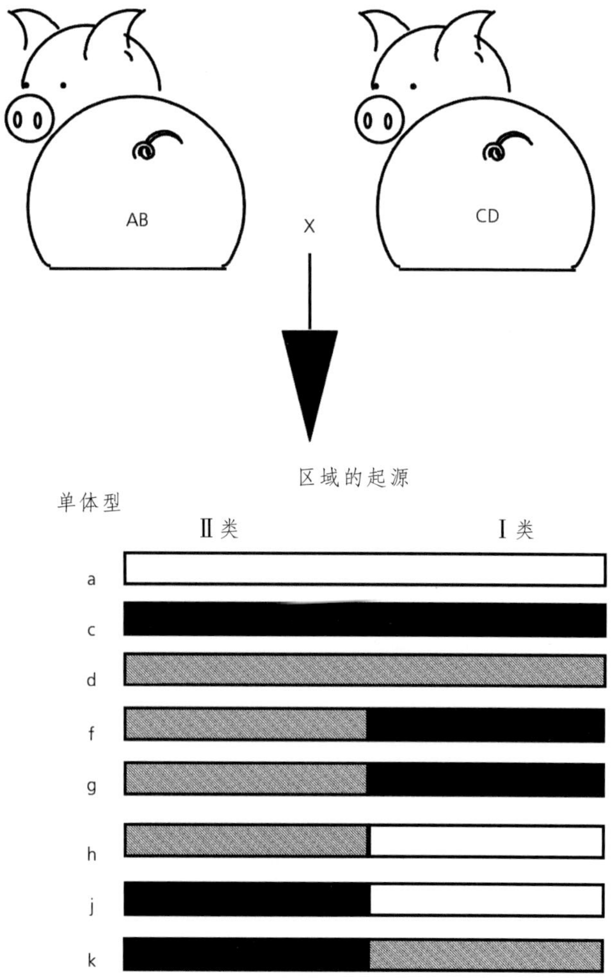

图15.1 小型猪单体型的起源。

容性品种[78]。随后的研究已经利用这些高度近交的动物作为淋巴群过继转移的捐献者，这种尝试在此之前只有在近交啮齿动物模型上实现过[79]。

器官同种异体移植的耐受性研究

小型猪的部分近交系对器官移植排斥和耐受性的研究非常有用。当在选择性 MHC-不匹配的组合中进行自发诱导肾脏同种移植物耐受性的研究时，所有Ⅱ类抗原不匹配的移植物都产生了剧烈的排斥反应[17]。相比之下，当移植物的Ⅱ类抗原匹配而Ⅰ类抗原有一个单体型不同时（例如，$SLA^{gg}\rightarrow SLA^{gd}$，见图 15.1），在约 30%的病例中可观察到自发耐受的诱导，同种异体器官获得长期耐受(>100 天)[17]。Ⅱ类抗原匹配Ⅰ类抗原不匹配的自发接受者，同种异体移植物在术后 2~4周期间表现出明显的排斥危象，随后自发消退并长期维持正常的肾功能。接受了Ⅰ类抗原不匹配的同种异体肾脏的动物并没有忽视移植物上的 MHC 抗原，而是对这些抗原积极地耐受。因此，在排斥危象期间，在受体动物中可以检测到针对供体Ⅰ类抗原的毒性抗体，但这些抗体几乎全是 IgM，说明了正常 IgM 向 IgG 的转变失败，该过程特征性地发生在排斥移植物的动物中。由于从 IgM 到 IgG 的转化通常被认为是依赖于 T 细胞的帮助[80,81]，这些结果表明，在没有足够 T 细胞帮助的情况下，仅仅Ⅰ类抗原不匹配的肾同种异体移植物可能诱导了耐受而非排斥反应。因此假设，并不是免疫系统没有识别出Ⅰ类抗原，肾移植物通过Ⅰ类抗原加上微小差异被受体所接受可能是主动免疫过程诱导的免疫耐受的结果。与该假设一致，与放置在对照动物上的相似的Ⅰ类抗原不匹配的皮肤移植物[(1.67±2.6)天]相比，来自原始肾脏供体的皮肤移植物的存活期显著延长[(31.7±20.4)天]。尽管存活期延长，所有的皮肤移植物最终都会被排斥，这可能是由于皮肤特异性的抗原而非免疫耐受被破坏所导致的，因为并没有出现肾功能的伴随损害，也没有抗Ⅰ类抗原的抗体产生。在此回顾，在这些早期研究中导致免疫耐受的积极进程无疑是调解性 T 细胞的诱导过程，这一假说随后便在该模型的最新研究中得到了证实[82-84]。

为了增加耐受诱导的发生率，随后的研究中，在 2 个单体型Ⅰ类抗原错配，Ⅱ类抗原匹配的肾移植($SLA^{gg}\rightarrow SLA^{dd}$，见图 15.1)中，研究者利用了短期疗程的环孢菌素 A(CyA)治疗。众所周知，这种配对组合下，在没有免疫抑制的情况下，受体会迅速地产生排斥肾脏移植物的反应，而结果却相反，8 个受体均诱导出了长期、特异性的耐受[85]。随后，至少有 50 个被 CyA 处理过的动物都证实了这项成果，所有的动物都表现出了长期耐受。这种移植组合和治疗方案已经成为随后小型猪耐受性研究中的“标准方案”，并在该模型中对耐受机制的研究提供了许多深刻见解[82,86-93]。心脏和肺的同种异体移植耐受性研究也在小型猪模型中进行[94-97]。重要的是，与小鼠的移植耐受性研究的情况不同，基本上所有在猪模型中发现的成果都能被转化到 NHP 上[98-101]，在某些情况下可以转化到临床中[5,101-103]。

移植术中的非人灵长类模型

由于与人类具有高度同源性，非人灵长类作为转化移植研究中最常用的动物群体出现。在具有高度特异性的单克隆抗体和融合蛋白等生物制剂的研究中尤其如此[104]。用于实验的灵长类有狒狒和猕猴，较少使用的有黑猩猩。黑猩猩与人类的同源性最高，曾经在历史场合中为人类作为捐献者[105]。然而，它们的濒危状态和进化地位使人们对黑猩猩研究的伦理性产生怀疑。的确，在 2011 年，NIH 严格限制了设计黑猩猩的新研究。狒狒通常用于异种移植研究，因为它们的体格巨大能够更好地适应猪器官。猕猴(食蟹猕猴、恒河猴和豚尾猴)是使用最普遍的 NHP。由于其体格小，护理相对容易，猕猴是首选实验模型。它们表现出与人类足够的同源性，因此，大多数分子都能交叉反应，除了 CD3 是个例外。猕猴现在作为实验模型几乎用于所有移植领域。

肾移植模型

猕猴中的肾移植相对简单，有些模仿儿科使用的技术。供体和受体在切除和植入期间都需肝素化。供体肾脏在确保血管和输尿管长度足够的情况下离体。虽然供体肾脏双侧都可以使用，但是由于脉管系统的长度，优选左肾。然后供体肾在受体的主动脉和腔静脉靠近分叉的部位吻合，通常吻合在右侧。通常在膀胱后部，输尿管穿过腹膜后间隙之后实施基础输尿管膀胱造口术(图 15.2)，在移植完成之后，以防止真性无尿的任何阶段的发生，受体本来的肾脏需要移除[106,107]。值得注意的是，双侧腹膜后剥离对动物来说是极大的应激。如果可能，在移植之前择期实施左肾的预备性肾切除，这

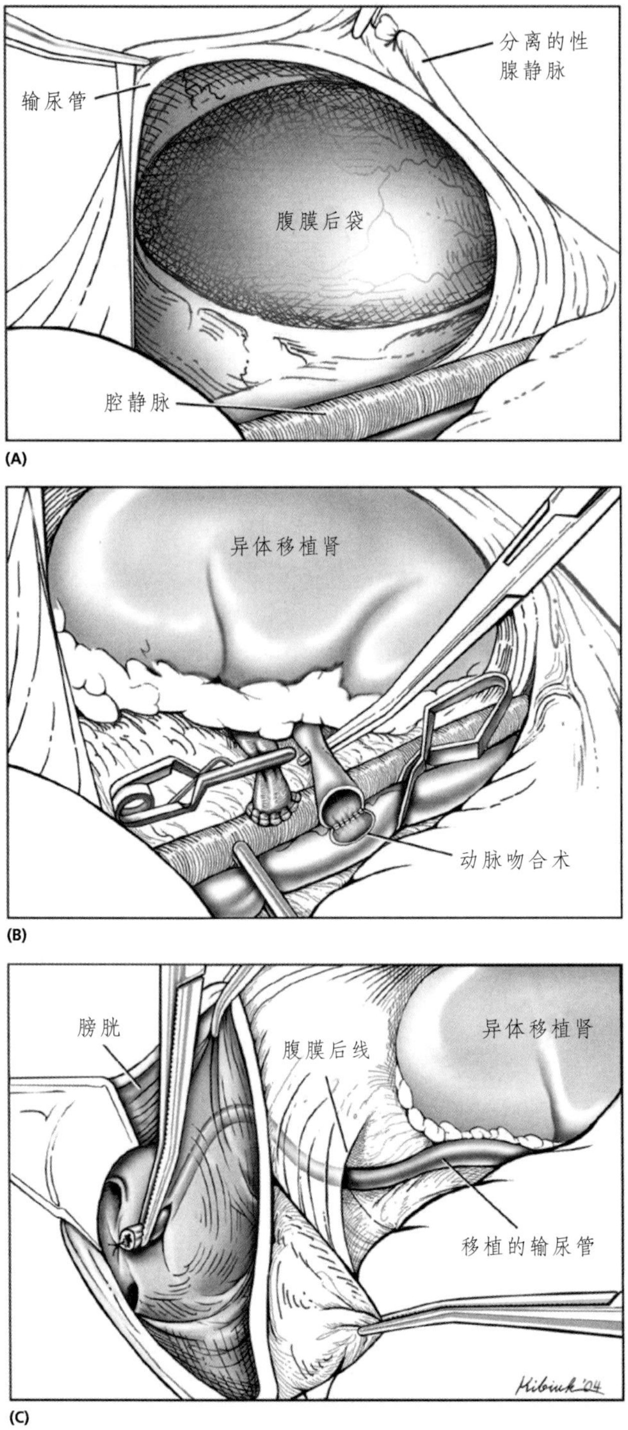

图 15.2 非人灵长类的肾移植术。(A)腹膜后袋是通过将原位输尿管内侧切开并向两侧分离得到的。(B)实施血管吻合术，从静脉开始吻合。(C)肾脏再灌注之后，实施膀胱切开术，从膀胱至先前做的腹膜后袋造一条腹膜后通道。移植的输尿管通过这条通道运送并固定在膀胱内。

样可以使得在移植当天腹膜后剥离仅限于右侧，能使动物更好地耐受。以“多米诺”的方式规划实验，动物首先轮流是捐赠者，然后是受者，将肾切除术后的肾脏用于移植，并最大限度地减少未被移植的器官数量。一般来说，对于动物来讲，移植手术耐受较好且并发症最小往往与输尿管吻合有关。在 Song 等的一项研究中，研究者在食蟹猕猴中进行了 182 例移植术，总并发症发生率为 10.4%。值得注意的是，超过 2/3 的并发症与输尿管吻合有关。在该研究中，输尿管采用的是端-端输尿管吻合术[108]。

皮肤移植模型

NHP 的皮肤移植术已被用于测试许多潜在的免疫抑制方案，包括抗淋巴细胞球蛋白[109]、黏附分子阻断[110]，通过 CD80 阻断共刺激信号[111]及 CD154 阻断[112]。在技术上，除了动物的大小之外，其他动物的皮肤移植术与小鼠模型的皮肤移植术没有什么区别。通常从供体的腹部取得供体移植物，然后种植到受体的背部。灵长类的皮肤移植有一个独特的方面是需要在创伤愈合过程中及之后对移植物进行保护。应使用软垫以维持移植物对下层组织的轻度压力(图 15.3)。此外，动物要佩戴保护性网状夹克以防止移植物在机体修整期间受到损伤。训练动物舒适地穿上夹克需要一个驯化阶段，可能需要几个星期的时间。

胰岛移植模型

胰岛移植的 NHP 模型中不存在非肥胖型糖尿病(NOD)鼠类的替代品。通常通过切除胰腺或更为常见的是静脉内注射链脲佐菌素来实现 NHP 糖尿病。必须在移植前通过测定没有天然 c 肽的产生来确认糖尿病状态。以人类方法相似的方式在移植入糖尿病 NHP 受体之前通过供体胰腺切除术和分离得到异体胰岛组织。胰岛移植过程是通过重力依赖性灌注进入门静脉或肠系膜静脉达到肝内种植，而其他部位如骨髓、肾囊、腹膜腔、网膜和肌肉的种植方法已经或正在探索中[113]。当耳塞训练完成之后，日常禁食及餐后血糖可以很容易地检测，在合适的时机也有助于胰岛素注射。胰岛移植的 NHP 模型在评估基于共刺激基因阻断的方案中起着重要作用，后者包括 CTLA4、CD40 和 CD40L(CD154)[114-120]。

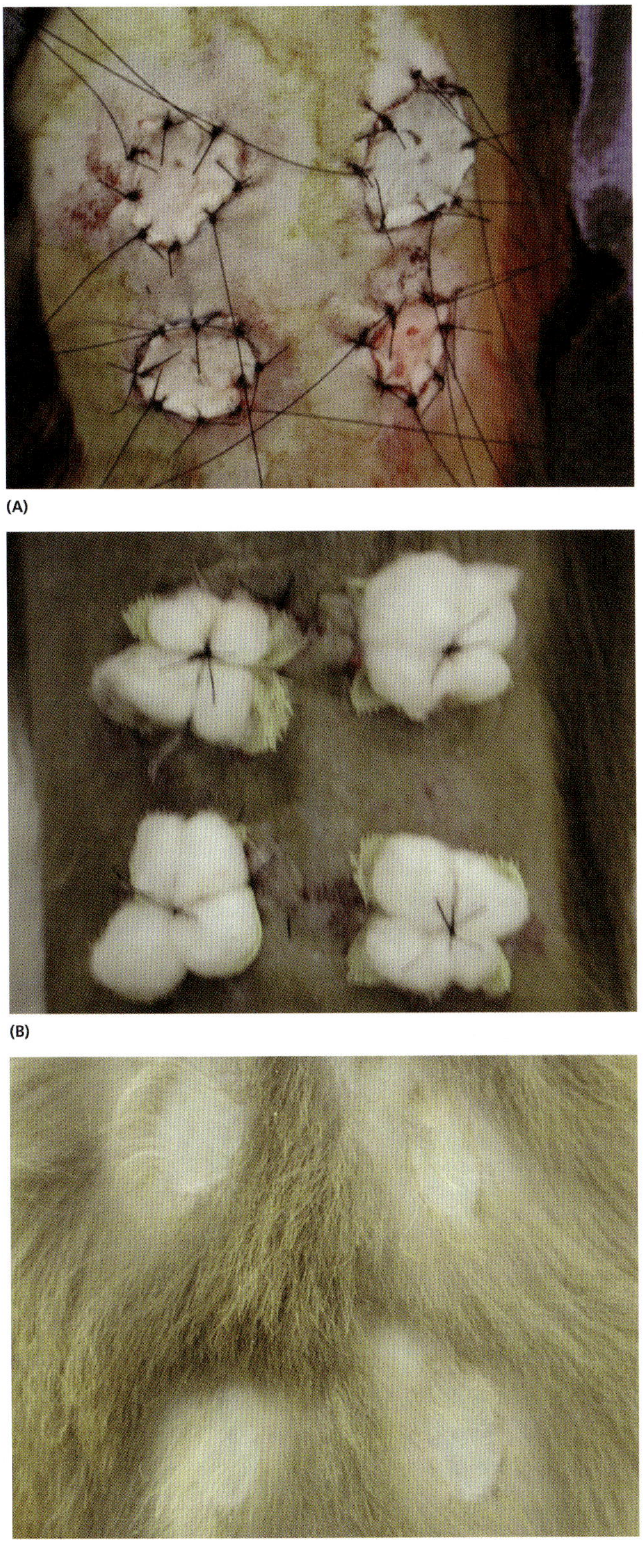

图 15.3　NHP 皮肤移植物上软垫举例。(A)皮肤移植物已经被缝合，留出长线头用以固定软垫。(B)在药用纱布上放置软棉花垫并固定。(C)在移植物愈合到下层组织后，可以移除软垫。

心脏和肺移植模型

非人类灵长类动物较少被用作同种异体心脏和肺移植的模型，尽管每个都有例子[121–123]。异基因心脏移植通常异位移植到动物的腹部，通过触诊或超声来评估收缩功能[124,125]。研究者已经通过测试植入的 EKG 电极用于确定移植物的排斥反应[54]。NHP 中同种异体心脏移植或肺移植相对不常见，与之相反，灵长类动物常常作为异种移植研究中的心脏或肺移植物的受体，我们将在下面简单地进行介绍，更多的细节参见第 12 章。

血管化复合同种异体移植模型

显微技术和免疫抑制的最新进展使复合组织作为功能单位的移植成为可能。这种移植的临床现实化导致了 NHP 模型的发展，用以研究这些移植物的免疫生物学。NHP 中复合移植物的实例是存在的，如狒狒手移植[126]以及将手的桡部移植在恒河猴中[127]。然而，这些移植物可能对存活的受者的功能产生负面影响。Cendales 等开发了一种恒河猴模型，该模型涉及移植含有感觉性骨皮瓣的桡侧前臂皮瓣，包含部分桡骨、股二头肌、前臂内侧和外侧皮神经、掌长肌、桡动脉、头静脉以及覆盖的皮肤[128](图 15.4)。这个模型保留了捐献者与受体双方的功能，允许捐献者和受体两个个体间的“多米诺(连锁式移植手术)”或移植物交换。马里兰大学的一个研究小组利用一部分颌骨、咬肌、上皮、颈总动脉和颈内静脉开发了一种食蟹猕猴面部移植的灵长类动物模型[129,130]。

异种移植模型

第 12 章将详细介绍异种移植的具体内容。下面将介绍与其密切相关的两个特定话题的简单处理。

猪作为异种移植供体

为试图克服移植器官的短缺，目前猪被认为是最有可能作为人类异种移植供体的动物(见第 12 章)。根据定义，异种移植是一种物种特异性的尝试，猪也已经成为大多数临床相关的异种移植实验的主要供体。许多实验室已经通过基因工程培育出了 α-1,3-半乳糖基转移酶基因被破坏的 Gal 基因敲除猪[33,131–133]。先前的主要问题在于东方灵长类和人类血清中存在高水平的针对 Gal 的天然抗体，而这些 Gal 基因敲除猪的细胞

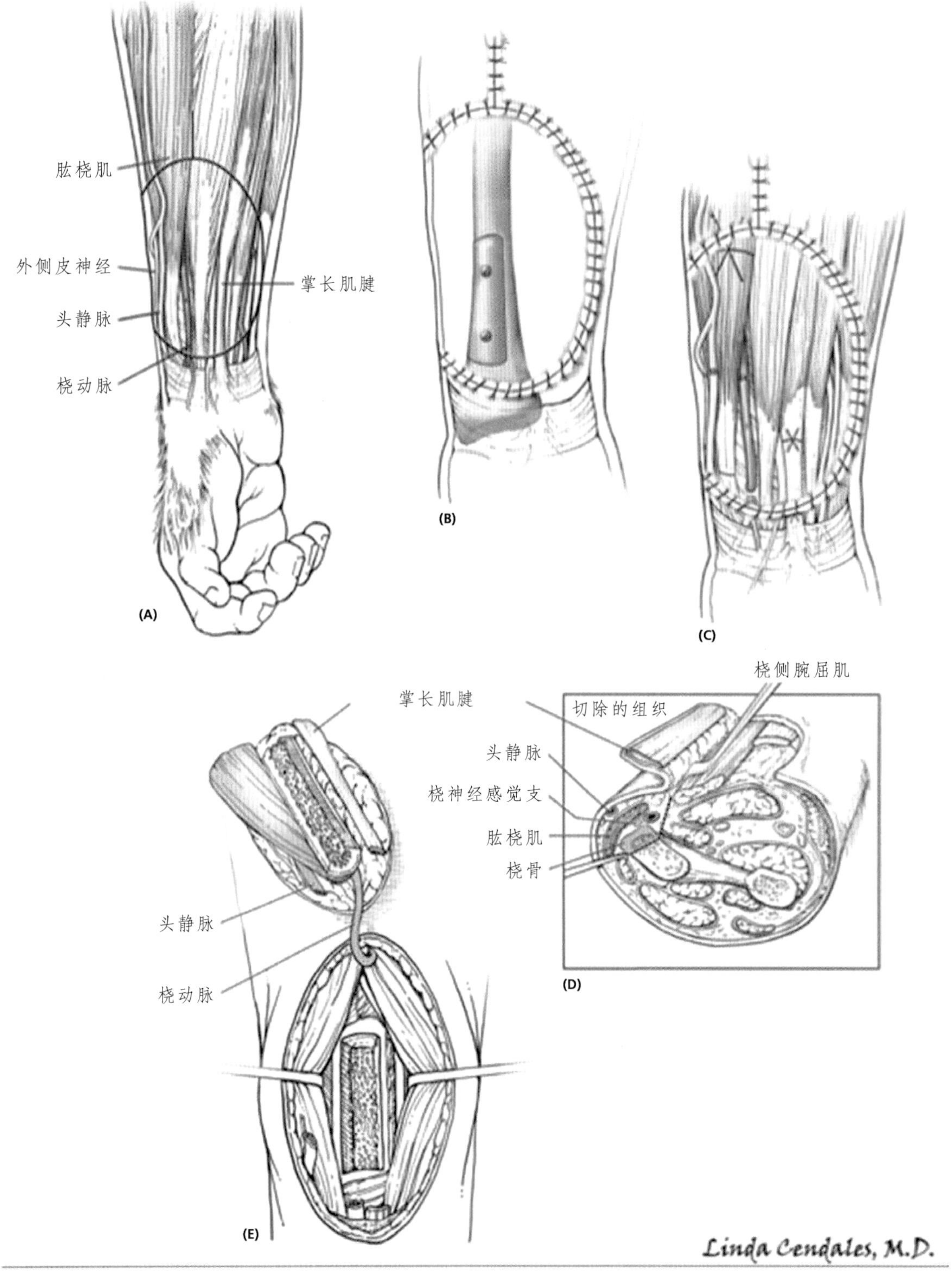

图 15.4 在NHP中的桡侧前臂血管化复合组织同种异体移植物。该皮瓣包括骨骼(视情况选择)、肌肉、肌腱、神经、血管、皮下脂肪和皮肤。(A)带有掌长肌腱的感觉性桡骨前臂骨肌皮瓣的解剖。(B)用螺丝实施桡骨骨折固定术。(C)移植后对掌长肌腱、肱桡肌、头静脉、桡神经感觉支以及桡动脉近端进行解剖学修复。(D)横截面视图。皮瓣的切除从尺侧开始,包括深筋膜及掌长肌腱。(E)皮瓣从近端血管蒂分离。(Reproduced from [128] Cendales LC, Xu H, Bacher J, Eckhaus MA, Kleiner DE, Kirk AD. Composite tissue allotransplantation: Development of a preclinical model in nonhuman primates. Transplantation. 2005 Nov 27;80(10):1447 - 54, with permission from Wolters Kluwer Health.)

表面糖蛋白上不表达普遍存在的 Gal 表位，因而可以避免这一主要问题[134,135]。希望这种遗传修饰以及其他涉及添加转基因的修饰（图 15.5）将最终使猪成为理想的异种供体。

由于体型问题，小型猪可能尤其适合作为潜在的异种供体。这些动物成年体重为 120~140kg。因此，对于任何潜在的人类受体，不论从新生婴儿到成年人，都可以选择合适大小的小型猪作为器官供体。相比之下，家猪成年体重超过 450kg，明显大于器官捐赠所需。使用由最高近交系小型猪衍生出的成纤维细胞系（见上文），通过同源重组的方式破坏 α-1，3-半乳糖基转移酶基因，然后通过核转移产生相应的基因敲除动物（GalT-KO）[132,136]。这些高度近交的 GalT-KO 动物的可用性使得研究者可以进行一系列指导跨越猪-灵长类动物屏障的耐受性诱导研究[137-142]。

胰细胞岛异种移植

细胞异种移植物，主要指胰岛，在血管化异种移植模型中缺乏导致血栓形成调节失常的内皮组分，因此可能是异种移植中的第一个可移植的平台。在大型动物模型中，这些临床前研究主要局限于猪胰岛异种移植的 NHP 模型。由于供体的容易获得性、人类与猪的葡萄糖稳态的相似性，特定的无病原的胰岛主要从猪中获得。其他来源包括牛和非洲鲫鱼。非人灵长类受体是一种用于转化医学的强大模型。与人类相比，非糖尿病食蟹猕猴的空腹血糖更低，胰岛素/c-肽水平更高[143]。对于猪胰岛分离的时间目前存在一些争议——应选择婴儿期、新生儿期或是成人期——因为未成熟胰岛对缺血更耐受[144]。新生猪和成年猪的异体胰岛注射入糖尿病恒河猴体内后，都能够延长胰岛素依赖性的血糖正常持续时间。尽管通过病毒预防的途径保留了恒河猴的先天免疫功能[145-148]。这些功能的发挥依旧需要重要的免疫抑制，包括使用 CD154 特异性的单克隆抗体。如前所述，异种移植必须服从源猪的遗传修饰，并且在使异种移植物细胞化的情况下，进行离体转染。作为预先形成的异种抗体的主要靶点，鉴别 gal 抗原表位 Galα（1，3），Galβ（1，4），GlcNAc-R，使用 gal 缺陷的新生猪供体能够促进胰岛移植和功能[148]。异种适应性免疫方面的新进展将阐明更多基因修饰靶点，可能在不久的将来就能降低对免疫抑制的要求。

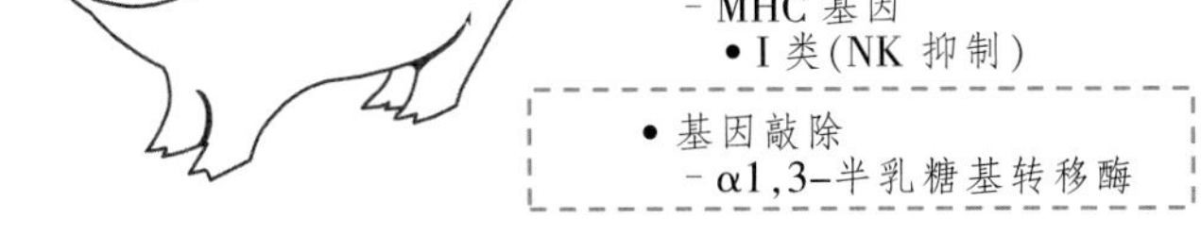

图 15.5　作为异种移植供体的小型猪的基因修饰。

非人灵长类的围术期护理

为 NHP 提供的围术期和随访护理只能类似于人类患者所能获得的护理。常规动物护理以及任何并发症或临床疾病的治疗应与当地兽医协会协商完成。应注意动物的临床状态，因为活动性或食欲的变化可能代表着排斥反应或恶化迹象的早期征象。对于接受肾脏或胰岛移植的受体，以及接受肾毒性免疫抑制剂（如高剂量的钙调神经磷酸酶抑制剂）的动物应监测尿量。术后以及任何临床变化发生都需常规检查血液学研究和血生化。免疫抑制药物有很多使用途径。通常，需要每日给药的药物应通过口服或皮下或肌内注射给药，避免反复镇静。给药不那么频繁的药物也可以静脉输注给药。当血容量不足时，动物被镇静，此时流体可以轻易地经静脉内或皮下给药，而在一些中心会使用特殊的笼子，这种笼子可以在动物有意识的情况下留置尿管以及持续输注。厌食或营养不良的动物可以在镇静的情况下使用胃管补充营养。许多临床上使用的药物，如镇痛药和抗生素也可用于 NHP，但通常需要调整剂量。接受免疫抑制治疗的动物可能会增加感染的风险，在某些情况下需要预防性地治疗。基于 PCR 技术已确认了 CMV 和 EBV 的猕猴同系物。

小分子免疫抑制

已经发现大多数常用的小分子免疫抑制剂在延长大型动物移植物存活期以及在某些情况下的耐受方面有一定的成功。随着新的更特异的靶向治疗已投入测试，了解小分子免疫抑制的现有成果非常重要。

硫唑嘌呤和霉酚酸酯

Calne 用犬模型确立了 6-MP 和硫唑嘌呤在移植中的功效[53]。硫唑嘌呤在临床上的使用是移植史上的一个重要的里程碑，并且直到钙调神经磷酸酶抑制剂发展之前，硫唑嘌呤可能是临床免疫抑制治疗的骨干。在大多数临床方案中基本替代硫唑嘌呤的霉酚酸酯,在犬模型中也被证明是有效的[149,150]。作为大多数临床免疫抑制方案的一部分,在大型动物模型中，霉酚酸酯依然作为联合治疗的一部分被广泛使用和研究。

钙调神经磷酸酶抑制剂

自从引入环孢菌素以来，钙调神经磷酸酶抑制剂已经成为大多数临床免疫移植方案的主干。这一类药物已经在本章讨论的所有 3 种模型中都进行了广泛的研究,并且都被证实有效。在 Clane 等在硫唑嘌呤的研究取得成功之后，他们是最先开始在大型动物中研究环孢菌素的,并且首先发布了他们在犬肾脏模型[151],其次在猪心脏模型中所得到的成果[152]。他克莫司也在犬模型中被广泛研究过,其有效性的证据促进了其发展。然而,值得注意的是,由于其对所研究的犬有高毒性，NHP 中的研究都需要确保转化到人体中的安全性[153]。钙调神经磷酸酶抑制剂如果剂量合适，能够预防犬中的肝脏或肾脏排斥反应，尽管当其不与另一种药物联合使用时常会出现中度排斥反应[151,153-157]。猪能耐受超临界剂量的钙调神经磷酸酶抑制剂而不发生毒性反应,允许肾脏或肝脏移植物耐受性的形成[85,158-162]。环孢菌素也能够在部分 MHC 匹配的恒河猴模型中诱导耐受[163]。钙调神经磷酸酶抑制剂仍是大型动物模型中常用的免疫抑制剂，并且常用于联合治疗或作为新药测试的对照。

mTOR 抑制剂

由于西罗莫司相当低的剂量即能引起肠毒性,其在犬模型中的使用已经被限于联合治疗，通常与钙调神经磷酸酶抑制剂配伍[164]。在猪模型中,西罗莫司将移植物存活期延长到了 60 天，取得了更大的成功[165,166]。然而,在猪模型中,西罗莫司尚未实现耐受性。西罗莫司单药治疗已被证明可以使肾脏移植物在灵长类动物中的存活期延长至 20~30 天而副作用很少[167,168]。有两项研究确定了西罗莫司的血清低值以确保充分的药物传输[169]。西罗莫司和他克莫司的组合具有协同作用,很少有动物在结束免疫抑制之后仍能保持移植物的存活[170]。然而，在他克莫司和西罗莫司组合中加入达昔单抗诱导治疗被证实具有明显的肠毒性[171]。最近研究显示,西罗莫司对 T 调节细胞的抑制活性有正面作用[172],并且现在常在准备 Treg 细胞用于细胞治疗时，与 Tregs 细胞治疗联合使用[173],或作为 Treg 离体细胞扩增期间的引物使用[172]。依维莫司是第二种 mTOR 抑制剂,在大型动物模型中使用较少。NHP 肺移植模型中它与环孢菌素联合使用[122],NHP 胰岛模型中与巴利昔单抗和 FTY720 联合使用,均已被证明有效[174]。

FTY720

FTY720 在猕猴模型[175]和犬模型[176]中单独使用或与钙调神经磷酸酶抑制剂协同使用都能够延长同种异体肾移植物的存活期。在两种模型中,FTY720 对外周淋巴细胞的影响似乎一致，两个模型都表现为外周淋巴细胞显著降低。值得注意的是,在犬的肝脏模型中，FTY720 在较低剂量下更有效[177]。虽然其原因尚不清楚，但这种现象似乎具有物种和器官特异性。该研究也证实了 FTY720 与钙调神经磷酸酶抑制剂联合使用时的协同作用，尽管 FTY720 与他克莫司联合使用时的过度免疫抑制导致了感染。

Sotrastaurin

Sotrastaurin 是一种选择性的蛋白激酶 C 抑制剂，已证明其能在 NHP 肾脏移植模型中延长移植物存活期[178]。研究还发现,Sotrastaurin 还能与许多其他的免疫抑制剂(包括环孢菌素、依维莫司和 FTY720)有协同作用[178,179]。在低于它单独使用时所需的最低剂量时仍能观察到其协同效益。

托法替尼

托法替尼(CP-690550)是 Janus 激酶 3(JAK3)的抑制剂,参与了许多细胞因子受体的下游信号通路。JAK3 蛋白自然发生的失功能性突变导致常染色体重症联合免疫缺陷病。食蟹猕猴肾脏移植受体接受托法替尼治疗后可以将移植物存活期延长至平均 46 天。与多种细胞因子阻断相一致,托法替尼使用期间可以观察到循环系统 NK 和 T 细胞显著减少[180]。

PG490-88

PG490-88 是 PG490(雷公藤内酯)的前体药物,后者是免疫抑制性中草药雷公藤多苷的活性成分。单独使用 PG490-88 或与他克莫司联合使用均可延长犬模型和食蟹猕猴模型中的同种异体肾移植物的存活期[181,182]。

共刺激阻断

共刺激通路阻断是免疫抑制的一种途径,可能诱导免疫耐受。这一方式基于 20 世纪 70 年代的研究工作而形成,当时人们首次认识到,在最佳免疫应答中,除了抗原识别以外,还需要共刺激信号的辅助参与[183,184]。此后进一步的研究工作发现,基于不同刺激,有多种共刺激信号参与免疫应答的精密调控[185]。

尽管在啮齿类动物模型中,共刺激通路阻断可以诱导免疫耐受,但要想在大型动物及远系繁殖模型上重复该结果,目前仍具有一定挑战性[186-188]。这可能是由于有时免疫应答并不完全依赖于共刺激信号,主要见于以下两种情况。第一,存在大量同种反应性免疫细胞的前体细胞[189]。显然,缺乏共刺激信号时,免疫识别过程中会产生其他细胞应答反应[190]。尽管这种反应可能很低效,但存在大量前体细胞时,活化的细胞数量之多可以弥补其低效能而产生有意义的生理反应[191]。第二,存在不依赖于共刺激信号的细胞群体,尤其是免疫记忆细胞[192]。再次免疫时,体内可能储备有大量同种反应性记忆细胞,由于其具有较高的敏感性,且存在异源性相互作用,再次免疫应答很少依赖于共刺激信号。

出于对免疫应答中共刺激信号的关注,人们分离鉴定了大量具有免疫调节能力的受体-配体对[193]。这些分子中,部分可以纳入同一受体家族,包括免疫球蛋白和 TNF 超家族,以及干扰素和 TIM 家族,因此,在不同信号通路之间,也常存在大量串扰。由于共刺激信号通路存在个体差异,而在免疫应答中,分子表达也会不断变化,因此,将共刺激通路阻断用于移植免疫治疗,目前是一个极其复杂的问题,而 NPH 则是研究相关问题的理想大型动物模型[104]。

CD28-B7 阻断

CD28-B7 是目前研究最清楚的共刺激信号通路。T 细胞表面的 CD28 与 B7-1(CD80)和 B7-2(CD86)相互作用提供共刺激信号,激活 T 细胞并分泌 IL-2[194-196]。活化 T 细胞表面的 CTLA4 同时选择性结合这两种受体,其结合具有更高亲和力,并向 T 细胞传导抑制信号,阻断 T 细胞的活化[197]。

用单克隆抗体阻断 CD28 配体,可提高猕猴肾移植后存活率[198]。有 3 个实验室用单克隆抗体分别阻断 CD80/CD86、1F1 以及 3D1,在啮齿类动物和人体模型中均取得了成功。Kirk 等发现,在恒河猴上单用任何一种抗体均可以适度提高肾移植后存活率,而如果使用联合抗体则可以显著提高存活率。但因为这些抗体无法阻断供体特异性同种抗体反应,仍无法诱导免疫耐受[198]。该实验室的另一项试验显示,与抗 CD154 单克隆抗体治疗相比,联合 1F1 和 3D1 共同阻断 CD154 并没有显著提高存活率,但可以延迟同种抗体的形成[199]。在食蟹猴肾移植模型中,Birsan 等将人源化 1F1 和 3D1 抗体及西罗莫司联合用于术后治疗,移植存活率显著高于单用抗体或西罗莫司,不过同样没有达到免疫耐受[200]。Hausen 等所做的第三个试验中,将人源化抗体与环孢霉素或甾体类激素联合使用,两种方式都未影响抗克隆抗体的效能,并且与任何单一治疗相比,CD80/86 阻断联合环孢霉素可显著提高移植存活率[201]。Ossevoort 等分别研究了抗 CD80/86、B7-24 和 1G10 的鼠源抗体克隆:在恒河猴皮肤移植模型中,B7-24 联合环孢霉素仅稍提高移植存活率[202];在肾移植模型中,这些抗体分别与 CD40 阻断或环孢霉素联合使用[203]。其中,CD80/86 阻断可以显著提高存活率,联合 CD40 阻断并未对存活率产生显著影响,但猴抗鼠反应却消失了;而联合环孢素 A 与单用环孢素 A 存活率相当。尽管这些早期试验得到了一些阳性结果,人们仍希望进一步研究 1F1 和 3D1 以指导临床应用。

另一阻断 CD28 信号通路的方式是 CTLA4 受体的可溶形式,即 CTLA4-Ig 融合蛋白。CTLA4-Ig 可以结合两种 B7 配体,因此可阻断 CD28 激活信号通路和 CTLA4 的抑制信号通路。CTLA4-Ig 在啮齿类模型中证实有效,随后进一步用于 NHP 模型的研究[188,204,205]。早期试验仅证实,CTLA4-Ig 联合 CD4 抗体能适度提高胰岛、肾[106]和心脏移植的存活率[207]。随后进一步的研究使贝拉希普应运而生,它与 CTLA4-Ig 仅差 2 个氨基酸,抑制 T 细胞活化的能力却高了 10 倍[208]。作为单克隆抗体,贝拉希普比 CTLA4-Ig 更为优越,而与麦考酚酯和甾体类激素或巴利昔单抗联合使用时更能显著提高移植存活率[208]。该实验室后来还证实,贝拉希普持续治疗联合西罗莫司和巴利昔单抗/抗 CD154 诱导治疗具有更高的效能[146]。Lo 等和 Lowe 等也证实了贝拉希普联合西罗莫司可以提高肾和胰岛移植存活率,同时还确定了具体剂量[168,209]。贝拉希普在 NHP 模型上的成功使得人体临床研究得以开展,2011 年 6 月 FDA 正式批准该药用于临床。

通过 B7-1 和 B7-2 阻断 CD28 信号通路,会同时阻断CTLA4 介导的共同抑制信号,因此,人们开始寻找可特异性阻断 CD28 通路而保留 CTLA4 通路的方法。人们研制了一种针对 CD28 的单克隆抗体 TNG1412,该抗体具有超激动活性,可以选择性扩增调节 T 细胞,从而抑制自身免疫,延长移植术后生存时间[210]。但 TGN1412 一期临床试验导致了灾难性的结果,6 名接受该药治疗的志愿者都并发了严重甚至危及生命的全身炎性反应[211]。人们不得不重新改进抗 CD28 治疗,英国国家生物标准与控制研究所发布了新的试验控制推荐方案,以利于更全面地研究抗体的激动或超激动潜能[212,213]。自 TGN1412 试验以来,人们在灵长类动物体内开展了两次抗 CD28 抗体的试验。第一次利用了单价融合抗体 sc28AT,Poirier 等证实,对于肾移植后的狒狒或者心脏移植后的食蟹猴,sc28AT 联合他克莫司或环孢霉素可以延长其术后生存时间[214]。随后,该实验室在食蟹猴体内进行了 FR104 的药代动力学研究。FR104 是聚二乙醇化的单价抗 CD28 Fab’段抗体,在啮齿类动物上的试验结果较为可观,但人们还未在灵长类动物体内开展过相关移植试验[215]。

CD40-CD154 阻断

CD40-CD154(CD40L)的相互作用在未成熟 T 细胞激活过程中有重要作用[216,217]。然而,不同于 CD28-B7,CD40-CD154 不直接参与 T 细胞激活,而是促进 T 细胞-APC 之间的相互作用:活化的辅助 T 细胞表面的 CD154 和抗原呈递细胞表面的 CD40 结合,极大地提高了 APC 的抗原呈递能力和共刺激潜能,从而激活 $CD8^+$细胞毒性效应 T 细胞[218,219]。它也参与血小板脱颗粒激活 APC 的过程,从而将固有免疫与适应性免疫联系起来[220,222]。因此,阻断 CD40-CD154 可削弱初始呈递信号,从而阻断 T 细胞活化。这一机制也可以说明,CTLA4-Ig 治疗在啮齿类动物比大型动物和人体中效果更显著[14]。

多种灵长类动物模型均证实,针对 CD154 的单克隆抗体 hu5c8 治疗是有效的,其中包括恒河猴肾[223,224]或皮肤移植[112],恒河猴或狒狒胰岛移植[114,115],以及恒河猴心脏移植[225]。不同于以往 1mg/kg 的标准剂量,人们首次采用 20mg/kg 的剂量对一批抗体进行测试,而 hu5c8 恰巧是其中之一。此后人们发现,体内多种细胞都表达 CD154,这就可产生大量竞争结合的配体,而其中血小板可能引发免疫排斥[221]。

hu5c8 并不是唯一拮抗 CD154 的抗体。单克隆抗体 IDEC-131 已被用于 NHP 心脏、皮肤和肾移植模型中,尽管在心脏移植中疗效甚微[121,226,227],但在皮肤和肾移植中,无论单独使用还是与西罗莫司或 DST 联合使用都取得了一定疗效[228,229],即使存在大量记忆细胞反应[230]。相似的,ABI793 在恒河猴和食蟹猴移植模型中也有类似疗效[231,213]。然而,由于阻断血小板表面 CD154 易引起血栓栓塞,人们不得不停止抗 CD154 治疗的临床应用[233]。

CD154 阻断的疗效引发了对于 CD40-CD154 通路的进一步研究,不过关注点转移到了 CD40 分子,因其并不参与止血过程。早期啮齿类动物模型研究结果可观,由此产生了 Chi220,这是一种拮抗 CD40 的嵌合抗体,且仅有受体激动能力[117]。在早期恒河猴肾移植模型中,Chi220 可以将平均生存时间从 7 天延长至 48.5 天。与单独使用 Chi220 相比,联合 CTLA4-Ig 治疗并未显著延长存活时间[234]。随后该实验室在胰岛移植模型中,用更高亲和力的贝拉希普代替了 CTLA4-Ig,效果显著增强[117]。这两次试验中,人们发现 Chi220 会一过性地耗竭 B 细胞,但 2005 年的试验表明,与抗 CD20 抗体利妥昔单抗相比,B 细胞耗竭其实并不完全归因于这两种药物。

由于 B 细胞耗竭作用,抗 CD40 抗体治疗在临床应用上受阻。Badell 等发现了一种不耗竭 B 细胞的抗 CD40 单克隆抗体 3A8[119]。尽管在恒河猴胰岛移植模型中,3A8 可以保持其移植保护功能,但它也有部分激动潜能,且不能完全阻止同种抗体的形成。3A8 不能完全阻断可溶性 CD154 的结合,这就表明完全阻断 CD40-CD154 的结合并不是必需的[118]。该实验室发现,3A8 联合 CTLA4-Ig 和西罗莫司可阻断体液免疫反应,也能延长恒河猴骨髓嵌合模型的生存时间[235]。

人们还研发了许多其他抗 CD40 抗体。部分耗竭 B 细胞的 4D11 可延长食蟹猴肾移植后的存活时间[236,237],

还可抑制脾和淋巴结内生发中心的形成，另一非耗竭性抗 CD40 单抗 ch5D12 中也具有该抑制作用[238]。Lowe 等发现，嵌合抗体 2C10 的结合表位不同于 Chi220 或 3A8[120]，在恒河猴胰岛移植模型中，该抗体联合基础剂量的西罗莫司和巴利昔单抗可以显著延长存活时间。

CD28-B7 和 CD40-CD154 联合阻断

两条共刺激信号通路分别如前所述，而人们对两者的联合阻断也进行了许多研究。最初 Kirk 等发现联合 hu5c8 和 CTLA4-Ig 可以获得显著延长生存时间[106]。然而，之后研究者对两条通路阻断的优化，消除了联合治疗的优势，虽然其可以延迟同时异体抗体的形成[199]。在恒河猴肾移植模型中，Pearson 等联合使用 CTLA4-Ig 和 Chi220（CD40 阻断剂）或 H106（CD154 阻断剂）[234]，尽管有 2 只恒河猴移植后生存时间>100 天，但平均生存时间并未延长。但在胰岛移植模型中，Adams 等用贝拉希普代替了 CTLA4-Ig，并且观察到了显著的增强效应[117]。Haanstra 等联合使用 ch5D12（CD40 抗体）和 CD86 阻断剂，发现与单独使用 CD40 阻断相比，未显著延长生存时间[239]。Ossevoort 等联合 CD80/86 阻断剂和 CD40 阻断剂，未发现显著优势，但观察到了 B 细胞抑制[203]。这些数据表明，CD28-B7 和 CD40-CD154 联合阻断并不能显著延长移植后生存时间，但这两条途径之间的增强效能的确存在，特别是在体液免疫反应中。

其他共刺激和共抑制信号通路

人们还发现了许多其他共刺激和共抑制信号通路，这些通路在同种免疫反应中发挥重要作用，并调节 T 细胞的功能分化[240]，其中包括 OX40-OX40L、PD-1-PDL-1/2、CD27-CD70、ICOS、PD-1 以及 TIM 家族分子。尽管许多信号通路是当下的研究热点，但大部分还未在大型动物上建立移植模型。人们仍需进一步研究这些相互作用，以指导未来的临床治疗。

黏附分子阻断

各种各样的细胞表面分子介导细胞间的黏附作用，其中某些还在免疫系统中发挥特殊作用。除了细胞示踪，一些黏附分子还可稳定免疫突触，为免疫细胞提供共刺激信号。这一部分将综述两对主要的黏附分子及其在移植试验中的作用。

LFA-1

目前为止研究得最清楚的是 LFA-1 及其主要配体 ICAM-1。两者相互作用有助于白细胞黏附于血管壁，迁移通过血管内皮，定植于次级淋巴器官[241-243]。此外，LFA-1 是免疫突触的重要组成部分，稳定 T 细胞和 APC 之间的相互作用[244]，提高 B 细胞抗原呈递能力[245]。LFA-1 和 ICAM-1 的相互作用也可直接传递共刺激信号[246,247]。

LFA-1 在免疫应答中发挥重要作用，因此，人们建立了大量模型研究抗 LFA-1 治疗[247]。早期啮齿类动物试验的结果非常可观，而在食蟹猴皮肤移植[110]和恒河猴心脏移植模型中[248]，生存时间都显著延长。Badell 等将抗 LFA-1 抗体 TS-1/22 用于恒河猴胰岛移植模型，发现联合西罗莫司和巴利昔单抗或贝拉希普治疗，可显著延长移植后生存时间[249]。

但 FLA-1 阻断剂的临床应用面临极大挑战。早期试验没有证实抗 LFA-1 治疗可抑制急性排斥反应[250]，随后试验证实了抗 FLA-1 抗体奥度莫单抗可以阻止胸腺细胞产生免疫球蛋白，从而预防急性排斥反应[251]。此后的临床试验主要研究依法利珠单抗，该药已经获得 FDA 批准用于治疗银屑病。在肾[252]和胰岛[253]移植方面，早期研究结果可观，但随后 4 例银屑病患者并发了进行性多灶性脑白质病，该药不得不被撤出市场。尽管 LFA-1 阻断剂的结果可观，但任何治疗都应将患者的安全置于首位，因此还需要研发特异性更高的抗体，以规避 LFA-1 阻断剂的副作用。

CD2-LFA3

CD2-LFA3 相互作用能增强 T 细胞与 APC 之间的相互作用，但正如 LFA-1 和 ICAM-1 一样，也能传导重要的共刺激信号[254]。Kaplon 等研发了 LFA3 的一种可溶形式，命名为 LFA3TIP，在狒狒心脏移植模型中，该药可将术后生存时间延长约 8 天[255]。另一项研究发现，鼠抗猿 CD2 抗体 LO-CD2b 可明显耗竭 $CD2^+$，从而适度延长狒狒心脏移植后的生存时间[586]。试验证实，类似的抗人 CD2 抗体 LO-CD2a 可预防和逆转人体急性排斥反应[257,258]，此后人们进行了该抗体（商品名为希普利珠单抗）安全性和药代动力学的研究，但有效性仍有待评估[259]。Weaver 等利用融合蛋白阿法赛特（LFA3-Ig）建立了恒河猴肾移植模型[167]。阿法赛特联合 CTLA4-Ig、西罗莫司和DST治疗,可以显著清除记忆细胞,延长移植后生存时间。但该实验室随后发现,用更高亲和力的贝拉希普代替了CTLA4-Ig,并不能发挥类似的增强效能作用[168]。CD2阻断所发挥的具体作用还有待进一步研究。

其他黏附分子

随着对于免疫细胞定植、黏附和迁移机制的理解进一步完善,人们正不断研发相关靶向治疗,并逐渐用于临床前研究。整合素VLA-4就是其中之一,它被阻断后,可减少免疫细胞迁移进入移植组织[260]。早期啮齿类动物研究证实,VLA-4阻断剂联合LFA-1阻断剂[261]或者共刺激信号阻断剂可以获得增强效能[262]。人源化抗VLA-4抗体那他珠单抗已获批用于多发性硬化的治疗,未来也可能被用于移植后免疫抑制。

耗竭方案

正如本章之前所述,有两重障碍限制了大型动物和人体免疫耐受模型的建立:相对较高的前体细胞频率和记忆细胞的敏感性,两者可以通过抗原暴露或异种免疫反应获得。淋巴细胞耗竭可以减少或消除这些障碍,并可辅助建立免疫耐受。然而,必须注意耗竭调节细胞和细胞毒性细胞的相对性。如果耗竭免疫调节细胞,将产生负面影响,这一点将会在下面加以讨论。

胸导管引流

最直观的耗竭免疫细胞的方式是简单将其从循环系统中清除。大部分淋巴液通过胸导管回流至循环系统,这为清除体内淋巴细胞提供了理想场所。1962年,Gowans等证实在大鼠体内,胸导管引流可以起到耗竭和免疫抑制作用[263]。随后的犬类肾移植模型证实,该方法可以适度延长生存时间[264]。但随后人们发现,大鼠模型中的胸导管引流并不适用于人体。尽管该方式可以快速清除淋巴细胞,但至少30天才能达到最大免疫抑制效能[265]。因此,这一方式并未被推广,并很快被无创便捷的药物治疗所取代。1996年,Todo和Starzl带领的科研团队在犬肾移植模型中,通过乳糜管食管瘘再次建立了胸导管引流,将生存时间延长了9~18天[266]。胸导管内引流的优势如前所述,然而其低效性使得这一操作非常不可靠。食管引流的优势在于可以将同种抗原引入胃肠道,从而介导"口服免疫耐受"[267]。Kinukawa等1997年开展的试验未能证实,胸导管引流联合环孢霉素及甾体类激素具有治疗优势[268]。因此,胸导管引流早已成为历史。

多克隆耗竭

淋巴细胞多克隆耗竭是使用抗淋巴细胞免疫球蛋白或血清进行淋巴细胞耗竭。它是第一种被研究出来并应用于大型动物模型的耗竭方案。除了抗淋巴细胞抗体,还有拮抗多种其他细胞表面分子的抗体,特别是黏附分子。因此,这一方案在缺血性损伤中尤为重要,例如尸体捐献者,其激活的内皮细胞为白细胞黏附和迁移提供了合适的界面[269]。

人们已研发出抗胸腺细胞免疫球蛋白,并在大型动物中开展了实验,如犬类、猪类和NHP[270-274]。这些实验的结果具有各自的特异性,因为从某一物种体内提取的抗T细胞多克隆抗体,在其他物种体内可能具有不同的抗原表位范围。这些实验证实了部分有效性,但仍无法达到免疫耐受。在NHP模型中,兔抗胸腺细胞免疫球蛋白(ATG)可延长移植后生存时间至30天[275],但使用剂量明显超过人体剂量,这可能是由于预处理过程中特异性降低[276]。ATG联合全身淋巴结照射(TLI)可以进一步延长生存时间至100天[277]。

由于ATG不能单独诱导免疫耐受,目前主要用于诱导治疗,随后再辅以免疫抑制剂维持治疗。Hirshberg等发现兔ATG和西罗莫司序贯疗法可以延长NHP胰岛移植后生存时间,然而,由于西罗莫司的毒性,生存时间也十分有限[278]。Liu等在该方案中加入了B细胞耗竭剂利妥昔单抗,证实其可以进一步延长胰岛移植术后生存时间[279]。Haanstra等证实ATG诱导的免疫耗竭缩短了免疫排斥时间,如果与共刺激通路阻断剂联合使用,会增加同种抗体的形成,这可能是由于抑制分子CTLA4和调节因子FoxP3水平的降低[280]。此外,Pearl等证实,ATG诱导耗竭之后,移植细胞将具备丰富的记忆表型,减少了活化所需的共刺激信号[230]。

多克隆异种抗体是物种特异性因子,它们高度特异又种类繁多。因此,它们在某一物种体内的作用不可能在另一物种体内涵盖相同的范围,而希望从某一物种体内提取的抗体(如兔体内抗人抗体RATG)在另一物种(如恒河猴)体内发挥同等作用是不可能的。目前,尚没有可在人和动物模型中发挥相同作用的多克隆抗体,所有抗体都需要调整剂量,这就使其具有不同的耗竭范围和阻断作用,以及不同的有效时间。因此,目前还无法建立多克隆因子的大型动物模型。

单克隆抗体制备

单克隆耗竭的目的是清除或包被效应 T 细胞,阻止其发挥免疫功能,同时最大限度减少低特异性多克隆抗体耗竭所带来的全身免疫抑制。大多相关临床前大型动物模型都取材于 NHP,这是由于其体内目标分子高度保守、交叉反应的表位稳定。然而,NHP 并不是唯一选择,Watson 等曾成功研发出针对犬类 CD4、CD8 和 Thy-1 的单克隆抗体,并证实它们可以延长肾移植后的生存时间,特别是在联合使用时[281]。

在单肾移植的狒狒模型中,结合了去甲氧柔红霉素的 CD3 和 CD4 抗体联合 TLI(一种潜在的耗竭治疗)可建立可操控耐受性[282]。如果这种结合抗体不是在移植前单独使用,而是在移植后两周给药,就无法诱导免疫耐受,这表明在移植后早期,免疫调节细胞会发挥重要作用[283]。单独使用 CD4 结合抗体只能适度延长移植后生存时间,而另一种非耗竭性 CD4 抗体 OKT4A 也只能适度延长该时间[284-286],这说明了耗竭作用在建立免疫耐受中的重要性。

广泛耗竭 CD45 阳性细胞是预处理方案的一种,目前正在造血组织移植模型中接受试验,并在犬类体内取得了一定疗效[287]。在啮齿类动物实体器官移植模型中,选择性耗竭 CD45RB 阳性细胞可以延长术后生存时间[288]。在食蟹猴肾移植模型中,Chen 等发现这一方案也可适度延长生存时间[289],其有效性与单克隆抗体治疗和联合他克莫司治疗相当。

尽管目前的研究主要关注 T 细胞耗竭,但 B 细胞耗竭也可以在移植中发挥积极作用。在 NHP 胰岛[279]和心脏[290]移植模型中,抗 CD20 单克隆抗体利妥昔单抗联合其他免疫抑制剂可以延长移植后生存时间。然而,也应注意利妥昔单抗的副作用,一项 NHP 肾移植的模型中,将利妥昔单抗加入 ATG、西罗莫司以及供者骨髓融合治疗中,并未改善生存率,可能是由于接受治疗的动物并发了极高的 SV40 感染率[291]。

本章“共刺激阻断”和“黏附分子阻断”中所提及的部分单克隆抗体,也可通过耗竭作用发挥部分功能。事实上, 抗 CD2 融合蛋白阿法赛特以及抗 CD40 抗体 Chi22 都具有部分耗竭作用[117,168]。除此之外,还有一些耗竭方案正在啮齿类动物模型中开展试验,尚未转移至大型动物模型上。活化因子 LAG3 的耗竭方案在大鼠模型中结果可观[292],并被证实可阻断狒狒体内的迟发型超敏反应[293]。但在恒河猴肾移植模型中,早期研究使用了不同的克隆,疗效极低(该研究数据未发表)。

免疫毒素

在 NHP 模型中,最成功的耗竭因子是免疫毒素(IT),这是一种修饰白喉毒素(CRM9)和 FN18 单克隆抗体的融合蛋白,以灵长类动物 CD3 为靶点[294,295]。由 Knechtle 和 Tomas 带领的试验组分别证实[107,296,297],在灵长类肾移植模型中,移植前免疫毒素治疗可诱导免疫耐受,若联合骨髓融合方案,可适度增加有效性[297]。Thomas 证实了免疫毒素在胰岛异种移植中的有效性[298]。此外,在恒河猴肾移植模型中,免疫毒素还可逆转免疫排斥[299]。

移植过程中的免疫毒素治疗对于促进免疫耐受并不十分有效。这一治疗方案可延长移植后生存时间,抑制细胞排斥,但由于抗供者 IgG 仍然存在,同种抗体造成的移植损伤和免疫排斥仍会出现[300]。经过改进,人们建立了慢性同种移植排斥的模型,灵长类动物移植反应在组织学上与临床样本有许多相似之处,因此该模型是一种罕见并可重复的动物慢性排斥模型[301]。Jonker 等研究了移植后免疫毒素治疗的疗效,发现其联合传统免疫抑制剂如环孢霉素和西罗莫司,可适度延长生存时间[302]。但也应注意这一治疗所带来的高毒性和感染并发症。

由于 FN18-CRM9 免疫毒素的低产量和连锁异质性,人们研发出了重组抗 CD3 免疫毒素[295,303,304]。随后,Page 等在恒河猴肾移植受者体内,用重组免疫毒素和他克莫司,建立了抗体介导的慢性免疫排斥模型[303]。这一模型证实,在接受该药治疗的动物中,100%都产生了新的同种抗体,因此这一模型是可重复的现代抗体介导免疫排斥模型。

免疫毒素也在猪模型中进行过试验,但其特有的神经毒性限制了其继续应用[305],而这一副作用在灵长类动物体内不曾出现[306]。人们进一步研发了不同结构的新型猪免疫毒素,相比于既往药物,该药有效性稍有降低,但在猪体内既能保持 T 细胞耗竭活性,又不具神经毒性[307]。

由于动物实验的成功,免疫耗竭逐渐被应用于人体试验。但由于人体和灵长类动物 CD3 分子的差异，免疫毒素尚不能直接用于临床。其中，CD52 抗体阿仑单抗在人体内可以产生相似的 T 细胞耗竭作用，尽管无法诱导免疫耐受[310]，但可以延长同种移植后生存时间[308,309]。

嵌合体

嵌合体是指受者器官内基因不一致的细胞群，其中部分来自受者本身，部分来自供者。这一定义有别于镶嵌体，后者是指由同一受精卵产生的基因不同的细胞群。由于移植物的存在，所有受者器官都可被认为是嵌合体，但在器官移植领域，“嵌合体”一词特指造血系统嵌合体，因为造血细胞会特异地影响受者的免疫反应。基于嵌合体的治疗主要诱导供者 APC 参与受者的免疫应答以扩展移植免疫耐受的机制[311]。

人们对于免疫耐受的学习始于嵌合体。1945 年，Owen 等首次描述了去生殖器牛体内的红细胞嵌合体，子宫内的胎盘血管吻合使造血祖细胞得以交换，从而产生终生嵌合体[312]。随后，Medawar 的试验组证实，这些牛仅能接受其孪生兄弟姐妹的皮肤移植[313]。此后的研究又进一步证实，嵌合体可在小鼠[2,314]甚至人体体内诱导免疫耐受[5,315-318]。

根据供者细胞在循环系统所有细胞中所占比例，造血嵌合体可以进一步分为全嵌合体、微嵌合体和混合嵌合体。全嵌合体是指供者细胞几乎占循环细胞的 100%，微嵌合体则指供者细胞占循环细胞的比例<1%（仅能通过极其敏感的技术，如 PCR 进行检测）。混合嵌合体是指来自供者细胞所占比例介于可检测(>1%)和不完全(<100%)的中间状态。将骨髓或外周血的造血干细胞植入无移植条件的受者，会引起快速免疫排斥反应，从而导致移植失败或产生微嵌合体。然而，有移植条件的受者需接受大剂量消融治疗，这会产生严重的毒性作用。考虑到移植后免疫抑制的相对安全性和有效性，在临床上广泛推广嵌合体治疗还面临着巨大阻碍，相关治疗方案仍待完善[311]。

微嵌合体

微嵌合体是通过供者特异性普通骨髓移植建立的，无须预处理，目前有许多大型动物和人体模型正在试验其疗效[319-323]。从某种程度而言，几乎所有受者器官都是微嵌合体[324]，但显然不是所有受者都能接受移植。因此，微嵌合体能否诱导免疫耐受，还有待进一步考证[325]。许多试验表明，单独微嵌合体治疗不能显著延长受者生存时间[326-333]。这是由于，尽管受者次级淋巴器官内存在供者抗原，但其浓度不足以诱导免疫耐受。当联合应用其他治疗如共刺激通路阻断时，可以显著延长生存时间[334]。Thomas 等[322]的研究证实，骨髓中存在否决细胞亚群，因此，这些细胞可以消除抗供体细胞毒反应，可能是骨髓输注诱导外周耐受的一种机制。

全嵌合体

为了根除癌细胞，恶性血液病骨髓移植必须建立全嵌合体。以往认为，这种全嵌合体只有在无 GvHD 且 HLA 完全相同的兄弟姐妹间才可实现。然而，随后的研究发现，全嵌合体受者再次接受其供者的肾移植时，可诱导免疫耐受[315,335,336]。接受全骨髓移植的猪[337]和犬[338,339]，经过致死性全身照射，还可接受者其他供者的肾移植，前提是该供者与最初骨髓供者的 MHC 一致。但在诱导耐受过程中，全嵌合体也存在着一些缺点[314]。相比于混合性嵌合体，建立全嵌合体意味着更严格的条件控制和更高的 GvHD 风险。另外，由于胸腺阳性选择细胞和外周 APC 的 MHC 不同，全嵌合体经常会造成免疫无能[340]。因此，全嵌合体治疗方案仍有待改善，特别是在克服 MHC 障碍进行移植时。

混合性嵌合体

以往认为，持久免疫耐受依赖于长期稳定的巨嵌合体。啮齿类动物试验证实持久的中枢耐受需要稳定的嵌合体[341,342]，但大型动物和人体试验表明，仅需要短暂的巨嵌合体[316,343,344]。相反，在 NHP 肾同种移植模型中，尽管建立了稳定的嵌合体，却并未成功诱导免疫耐受[345]。因此，诱导免疫耐受可能需要多系嵌合体[346]，而嵌合体和同种移植耐受之间的明确关系仍有待进一步研究。

Storb 等通过肾移植，建立了犬类混合性嵌合体，其中试验组还接受了亚致死量全身照射联合环孢霉素短疗程治疗，包括/未包括吗替麦考酚酯治疗[61,344,347,348]，结果发现，不是所有受者都可再次接受同供者皮肤移植，这反映了混合性嵌合体可能存在组织特异性[61,344,348]。Storb 等则通过加入 CTLA4-Ig 和 DST[349]，或将照射区域局限于淋巴链[350]，减少了全身照射剂量。这些研究证实，条件化照射可抑制受者的免疫系统，使供者骨髓得以在髓腔内增殖。Tillson 等的试验证实了相似结果[351]，另外还得到两点结论：第一，DLA 同一性和单倍同一性的犬类肾移植后，都可以长期生存，但只有 DLA 同一性者可再次接受同供者皮肤移植；第二，接受其他预处理而未接受骨髓移植的动物也可接受肾移植，这表明嵌合体可能不是必需的预处理方案。

通过 T 细胞耗竭联合/不联合外照射，人们成功建立了小猪混合性嵌合体[87,352]。这些动物可再次接受同供者皮肤移植，但不能接受第三方移植。另外，这些动物往往会并发器官移植后淋巴增殖紊乱性疾病(PTLD)，可能与猪 γ 疱疹病毒有关[353]。进一步的研究发现，在这一模型中，MHC 错配程度和 T 细胞耗竭的增加都是并发 PTLD 的高危因素[354]，而 B 细胞耗竭等预处理可以从本质上降低 PTLD 发生率[355]。在小猪模型中，通过肾、心脏和血管化复合组织移植，都可成功建立嵌合体[97,356,357]。

Boston 试验组建立了食蟹猴一过性混合性嵌合体，经过预处理后，都可再次接受肾移植，该预处理包括照射、骨髓输注、T 细胞耗竭、移植同时脾切除以及移植后短疗程环孢素 A 治疗[99,100]。在大部分实验动物中，混合性嵌合体方案还能预防供者特异性抗体的形成，但环孢素 A 治疗后的活检发现[343]，某些动物仍然具有抗供者免疫活性[99]。类似于小猪模型，这些动物也并发了 PTLD，可能与淋巴隐病毒(LCV)有关[358]。在心脏移植模型中，Kawai 等对这一方案进行了研究，但并未建立完全免疫耐受，移植物最终也因慢性细胞和体液免疫而被排斥和破坏[360]。联合使用 CD154 阻断剂 5C8 可以避免脾切除，但因为一些动物可产生慢性免疫排斥，仍无法建立长期免疫耐受[360]。在大部分灵长类动物中，Kawai 等的治疗方案可诱导免疫耐受，甚至可克服 MHC 障碍而避免造成 GvHD。在 HLA 不匹配的人体肾移植模型中[99,100,360]，人们也首次通过该方案成功诱导了免疫耐受[5]。

在恒河猴混合性免疫耐受模型中[361]，人们以白消安而非外照射进行预处理[361]，并在之后辅以免疫抑制的诱导和维持治疗。前者使用巴利昔单抗，后者使用贝拉希普、西罗莫司和抗 CD154 抗体 H106，这一模型可产生持久的高水平混合性嵌合体(约为 80%，平均持续 145 天)。但停止免疫抑制治疗后，受者很快出现排斥反应，并且骨髓移植后病毒感染率很高[362]。该实验室还研究了 CD40 阻断是否可使受者获益[361]，其预处理方案包括白消安、巴利昔单抗、CTLA4-Ig、西罗莫司和抗 CD40 抗体 3A8，该方案可以促进混合性嵌合体的形成，改善移植预后。但类似于之前的模型，停用免疫抑制药物后，受者也出现了移植物排斥反应，嵌合体随之消失[235]。这些模型均未能明确嵌合体形成后对实体器官移植排斥反应的影响。

通过混合性嵌合体诱导免疫耐受，是少数几个成功从小鼠过渡至大型动物的实验之一，并且可以进行人体试验。但其预处理方案比标准方案毒性大，因此这一途径目前还处于试验阶段。此外，灵长类实验表明，安全问题也不容忽视，包括病毒感染和 PTLD。尽管存在这些缺点，这一方案仍然是极具前景的，对于嵌合体诱导免疫耐受值得进一步深入研究。

总结

本章概述了实体器官移植的主要大型动物模型，讨论了与这些动物有关的技术问题，以及如何延长术后生存时间或建立免疫耐受。由于全面讨论所有相关文献过于冗长，我们只重点讨论有意义的研究进展，以了解目前有关免疫调节的治疗方案。其中某些治疗方式已被广泛应用于临床，而另一些治疗的结果并不可观。关于这种差异的原因是多种多样的，其中有些我们能给出解释，而另一些可能尚不为人所知。尽管存在各种问题，大型动物模型仍然是目前研究人体免疫应答的最佳模型。任何符合伦理的临床试验都必须基于肯定的动物实验结果，而大型动物则是研究治疗方案效果的最佳试验床。

(毛雨鸽 译 李照 校)

参考文献

1. Merrill JP, Murray JE, Harrison JH, et al. Successful homotransplantation of the human kidney between identical twins. Journal of the American Medical Association. 1956;160:277–282.
2. Billingham RE, Brent L, Medawar PB. Actively acquired tolerance of foreign cells. Nature. 1953;172:603–606.
3. Hariharan S, Johnson CP, Bresnahan BA, et al. Improved graft survival after renal transplantation in the United States, 1988 to 1996. New England Journal of Medicine. 2000;342:605–612.
4. Organ Procurement and Transplantation Network (OPTN) and Scientific Registry of Transplant Recipients (SRTR). OPTN/SRTR 2011 Annual Data Report. Rockville, MD: Department of Health and Human Services, Health Resources and Services Administration, Healthcare Systems Bureau, Division of Transplantation; 2012.
5. Kawai T, Cosimi AB, Spitzer TR, et al. HLA-mismatched renal transplantation without maintenance immunosuppression. New England Journal of Medicine. 2008;358:353–361.
6. Scandling JD, Busque S, Dejbakhsh-Jones S, et al. Tolerance and chimerism after

renal and hematopoietic-cell transplantation. New England Journal of Medicine. 2008;358:362–368.
7. Leventhal J, Abecassis M, Miller J, et al. Chimerism and tolerance without GVHD or engraftment syndrome in HLA-mismatched combined kidney and hematopoietic stem cell transplantation. Science Translational Medicine. 2012;4:124ra28.
8. Hajar R. Animal testing and medicine. Heart Views. 2011;12:42.
9. Haddad FS. Ibn Zuhr and experimental tracheostomy and tracheotomy. Journal of the American College of Surgeons. 2004;199:665.
10. Martin J. The rights of man and animal experimentation. Journal of Medical Ethics. 1990;16:160–161.
11. National Research Council. Guide for the Care and Use of Laboratory Animals, 6th ed. Washington, DC: National Academies Press; 2011.
12. Association for Assessment and Accreditation of Laboratory Animal Care. [accessed Dec. 2013]; Available from: http://www.aaalac.org/resources/.
13. Blattman JN, Antia R, Sourdive DJD, et al. Estimating the precursor frequency of naive antigen-specific CD8 T cells. Journal of Experimental Medicine. 2002; 195:657–664.
14. Kirk AD. Crossing the bridge: large animal models in translational transplantation research. Immunological Reviews. 2003;196:176–196.
15. Sachs DH. Tolerance: of mice and men. Journal of Clinical Investigation. 2003;111:1819–1821.
16. Adams AB, Pearson TC, Larsen CP. Heterologous immunity: an overlooked barrier to tolerance. Immunological Reviews. 2003;196:147–160.
17. Pescovitz MD, Thistlethwaite JR, Auchincloss H, et al. Effect of class II antigen matching on renal-allograft survival in miniature swine. Journal of Experimental Medicine. 1984;160:1495–1508.
18. Choo JK, Seebach JD, Nickeleit V, et al. Species differences in the expression of major histocompatibility complex class II antigens on coronary artery endothelium: implications for cell-mediated xenoreactivity. Transplantation. 1997;64: 1315–1322.
19. Williams MA, Trambley J, Ha J, et al. Genetic characterization of strain differences in the ability to mediate CD40/CD28-independent rejection of skin allografts. Journal of Immunology. 2000;165:6849–6857.
20. 't Hart BA, Amor S, Jonker M. Evaluating the validity of animal models for research into therapies for immune-based disorders. Drug Discovery Today. 2004;9:517–524.
21. Nam KH, Akari H, Terao K, et al. Age-dependent remodeling of peripheral blood CD4(+) CD8(+) T lymphocytes in Cynomolgus monkeys. Developmental and Comparative Immunology. 1998;22:239–248.
22. Nam KH, Akari H, Terao K, et al. Age-related changes in major lymphocyte subsets in cynomolgus monkeys. Experimental Animals. 1998;47:159–166.
23. Saalmuller A, Werner T, Fachinger V. T-helper cells from naive to committed. Veterinary Immunology and Immunopathology. 2002;87:137–145.
24. Rodriguez-Carreno MP, Lopez-Fuertes L, Revilla C, et al. Phenotypic characterization of porcine IFN-gamma-producing lymphocytes by flow cytometry. Journal of Immunological Methods. 2002;259:171–179.
25. Kelley J, Walter L, Trowsdale J. Comparative genomics of major histocompatibility complexes. Immunogenetics. 2005;56:683–695.
26. Wagner JL, Burnett RC, Storb R. Organization of the canine major histocompatibility complex: current perspectives. Journal of Heredity. 1999;90:35–38.
27. Kennedy LJ, Barnes A, Short A, et al. Canine DLA diversity: 1. New alleles and haplotypes. Tissue Antigens. 2007;69:272–288.
28. Lindblad-Toh K, Wade CM, Mikkelsen TS, et al. Genome sequence, comparative analysis and haplotype structure of the domestic dog. Nature. 2005;438: 803–819.
29. Wagner JL, Works JD, Storb R. DLA-DRB1 and DLA-DQB1 histocompatibility typing by PCR-SSCP and sequencing. Tissue Antigens. 1998;52:397–401.
30. Chardon P, Renard C, Gaillard C, et al. The porcine major histocompatibility complex and related paralogous regions: a review. Genetics, Selection, Evolution. 2000;32:109.
31. Lunney JK, Pescovitz MD, Sachs DH. The swine major histocompatibility complex: its structure and function. In: Tumbleson ME, editor. Swine in Biomedical Research. New York, NY: Plenum Press; 1986: 1821–1836.
32. Lunney JK, Sachs DH. The swine leukocyte antigen (SLA) complex. In: Bach FH, Auchincloss HJ, editors. Transplantation Immunology. New York, NY: John Wiley & Sons, Inc; 1995: 339–345.
33. Lai L, Kolber-Simonds D, Park K-W, et al. Production of alpha-1,3-galactosyltransferase knockout pigs by nuclear transfer cloning. Science. 2002; 295:1089–1092.
34. Dai Y, Vaught TD, Boone J, et al. Targeted disruption of the alpha1,3-galactosyltransferase gene in cloned pigs. Nature Biotechnology. 2002;20: 251–255.
35. Cowan PJ, Aminian A, Barlow H, et al. Renal xenografts from triple-transgenic pigs are not hyperacutely rejected but cause coagulopathy in non-immunosuppressed baboons. Transplantation. 2000;69:2504–2515.
36. van der Windt DJ, Bottino R, Casu A, et al. Long-term controlled normoglycemia in diabetic non-human primates after transplantation with hCD46 transgenic porcine islets. American Journal of Transplantation. 2009;9: 2716–2726.
37. Kean LS, Singh K, Blazar BR, et al. Nonhuman primate transplant models finally evolve: detailed immunogenetic analysis creates new models and strengthens the old. American Journal of Transplantation. 2012;12:812–819.
38. Otting N, Heijmans CMC, Noort RC, et al. Unparalleled complexity of the MHC class I region in rhesus macaques. Proceedings of the National Academy of Sciences of the United States of America. 2005;102:1626–1631.
39. Andrade MCR, Penedo MCT, Ward T, et al. Determination of genetic status in a closed colony of rhesus monkeys (Macaca mulatta). Primates; Journal of Primatology. 2004;45:183–186.
40. Penedo MCT, Bontrop RE, Heijmans CMC, et al. Microsatellite typing of the rhesus macaque MHC region. Immunogenetics. 2005;57:198–209.
41. Wiseman RW, Karl JA, Bimber BN, et al. Major histocompatibility complex genotyping with massively parallel pyrosequencing. Nature Medicine. 2009;15: 1322–1326.
42. Calne RY, Pegg DE, Pryse-Davies J, et al. Renal preservation by ice-cooling: an experimental study relating to kidney transplantation from cadavers. British Medical Journal. 1963;2(5358):651–655.
43. Barnard MS. Heart transplantation: an experimental review and preliminary research. South African Medical Journal. 1967;41:1260–1262.
44. Busuttil RW, De Carlis LG, Mihaylov PV, et al. The first report of orthotopic liver transplantation in the Western World. American Journal of Transplantation. 2012;12:1385–1387.
45. Brock DR, Starzl TE. Histopathologic alterations associated with the transplanted homologous dog liver. Experimental and Molecular Pathology. 1962;1: 187–203.
46. Slim MS, Yacoubian HD, Simonian SJ, et al. Bilateral reimplantation of canine lungs: anatomical and physiological observations in a long-term survivor. Annals of Thoracic Surgery. 1965;1:755–759.
47. Macalalad FV, Johnson HA, Apostol JV, et al. Survival of intestinal allografts in the dog with and without immunosuppression. Surgical Forum. 1965;16: 224–225.
48. Preston FW, Macalalad F, Graber R, et al. Function and survival of jejunal homotransplants in dogs with and without immunosuppressive treatment. Transplantation. 1965;3:224–229.
49. Winchell HS, Pollycove M, Loughman WD, et al. Autologous bone marrow transplantation studies in dogs irradiated by Y90-DTPA urine-recycling technic. Blood. 1964;23:44–52.
50. Reemtsma K, Lucas JF, Rogers RE, et al. Islet cell function of the transplanted canine pancreas. Annals of Surgery. 1963;158:645–654.
51. De Jode LR, Howard JM. The function of the homotransplanted canine pancreas. British Journal of Surgery. 1966;53:364–371.
52. Kolb E, Ruckert R, Largiadèr F. Intraportal and intrasplenic autotransplantation of pancreatic islets in the dog. European Surgical Research. Europaische Chirurgische Forschung. Recherches Chirurgicales Europeennes. 1977;9: 419–426.
53. Calne RY. The initial study of the immunosuppressive effects of 6-mercaptopurine and azathioprine in organ-transplantation and a few words on cyclosporin-A. World Journal of Surgery. 1982;6:637–640.
54. Horai T, Fumoto H, Saeed D, et al. Novel implantable device to detect cardiac allograft rejection. Circulation. 2009;120(11 Suppl.):S185–S190.
55. Brasile L, Glowacki P, Castracane J, et al. Pretransplant kidney-specific treatment to eliminate the need for systemic immunosuppression. Transplantation. 2010;90:1294–1298.
56. Hefty TR, Kuhr CS, Chong KT, et al. Omental roll-up: a technique for islet engraftment in a large animal model. Journal of Surgical Research. 2010;161: 134–138.
57. Sergi C, Gross W, Mory M, et al. Biliary-type cytokeratin pattern in a canine isolated perfused liver transplantation model. Journal of Surgical Research. 2008;146:164–171.
58. Kim YI, Chung K-Y, So BJ, et al. Mucosal protective effect of PGI2 on canine small bowel auto-transplantation. Transplantation Proceedings. 2012;44: 1169–1170.
59. Ladiges WC, Storb R, Thomas ED. Canine models of bone-marrow transplantation. Laboratory Animal Science. 1990;40:11–15.
60. Chen Y, Kornblit B, Hamlin DK, et al. Durable donor engraftment after radioimmunotherapy using α-emitter astatine-211-labeled anti-CD45 antibody for conditioning in allogeneic hematopoietic cell transplantation. Blood. 2012;119: 1130–1138.
61. Kuhr CS, Yunusov M, Sale G, et al. Long-term tolerance to kidney allografts in a preclinical canine model. Transplantation. 2007;84:545–547.
62. Mathes DW, Noland M, Graves S, et al. A preclinical canine model for composite

tissue transplantation. Journal of Reconstructive Microsurgery. 2010;26: 201–207.
63. Chardon P, Renard C, Vaiman M. The major histocompatibility complex in swine. Immunological Reviews. 1999;167:179–192.
64. Haller GW, Esnaola N, Yamada K, et al. Thymic transplantation across an MHC class I barrier in swine. Journal of Immunology. 1999;163:3785–3792.
65. Kanai TH, Tanioka Y, Tanigawa M, et al. Allelic diversity at class II DRB1 and DQB loci of the pig MHC (SLA). Immunogenetics. 1999;50:295–300.
66. Haverson K, Saalmuller A, Alvarez B, et al. Overview of the third international workshop on swine leukocyte differentiation antigens. Veterinary Immunology and Immunopathology. 2001;80:5–23.
67. Lunney JK, Walker K, Goldman T, et al. Overview of the first international workshop to define swine leukocyte cluster of differentiation (CD) antigens. Veterinary Immunology and Immunopathology. 1994;43:193–206.
68. Saalmuller A, Pauly T, Lunney JK, et al. Overview of the Second International Workshop to define swine cluster of differentiation (CD) antigens. Veterinary Immunology and Immunopathology. 1998;60:207–228.
69. Hammerberg C, Schurig GG. Characterization of monoclonal antibodies directed against swine leukocytes. Veterinary Immunology and Immunopathology. 1986;11:107–121.
70. Huang CA, Lorf T, Arn JS, et al. Characterization of a monoclonal anti-porcine CD3 antibody. Xenotransplantation. 1999;6:201–212.
71. Mulder A, Kardol MJ, Arn JS, et al. Human monoclonal HLA antibodies reveal interspecies crossreactive swine MHC class I epitopes relevant for xenotransplantation. Molecular Immunology. 2010;47:809–815.
72. Pescovitz MD, Lunney JK, Sachs DH. Preparation and characterization of monoclonal antibodies reactive with porcine PBL. Journal of Immunology. 1984;133:368–375.
73. Pescovitz MD, Book BK, Aasted B, et al. Summary of workshop findings for antibodies reacting with porcine T-cells and activation antigens: results from the Second International Swine CD Workshop. Veterinary Immunology and Immunopathology. 1998;60:251–260.
74. Sachs DH, Leight G, Cone J, et al. Transplantation in miniature swine. I. Fixation of the major histocompatibility complex. Transplantation. 1976;22:559–567.
75. Pennington LR, Flye MW, Kirkman RL, et al. Transplantation in miniature swine. X. Evidence for non-SLA-linked immune response gene(s) controlling rejection of SLA-matched kidney allografts. Transplantation. 1981;32:315–320.
76. Pennington LR, Lunney JK, Sachs DH. Transplantation in miniature swine. VIII. Recombination within the major histocompatibility complex of miniature swine. Transplantation. 1981;31:66–71.
77. Sachs DH. MHC homozygous miniature swine. In: Swindle MM, Moody DC, Phillips LD, editors. Swine as Models in Biomedical Research. Ames, IA: Iowa State University Press; 1992: 3–15.
78. Mezrich JD, Haller GW, Arn JS, et al. Histocompatible miniature swine: an inbred large-animal model. Transplantation. 2003;75:904–907.
79. Okumi M, Scalea JR, Gillon BC, et al. The induction of tolerance of renal allografts by adoptive transfer in miniature swine. American Journal of Transplantation. 2013;13:1193–1202.
80. Davie JM, Paul WE. Role of T lymphocytes in the humoral immune response. I. Proliferation of B lymphocytes in thymus-deprived mice. Journal of Immunology. 1974;113:1438–1445.
81. Steele DJ, Laufer TM, Smiley ST, et al. Two levels of help for B cell alloantibody production. Journal of Experimental Medicine. 1996;183:699–703.
82. Griesemer AD, LaMattina JC, Okumi M, et al. Linked suppression across an MHC-mismatched barrier in a miniature swine kidney transplantation model. Journal of Immunology. 2008;181:4027–4036.
83. Ierino FL, Yamada K, Hatch T, et al. Preliminary in vitro evidence for regulatory cells in a miniature swine renal allograft model. Transplantation Proceedings. 1997;29:1165.
84. Mezrich J, Yamada K, Sachs DH, et al. Regulatory T cells generated by the kidney may mediate the beneficial immune effects of combining kidney with heart transplantation. Surgery. 2004;135:473–478.
85. Rosengard BR, Ojikutu CA, Guzzetta PC, et al. Induction of specific tolerance to class-I – disparate renal-allografts in miniature swine with cyclosporine. Transplantation. 1992;54:490–497.
86. Blancho G, Gianello PR, Lorf T, et al. Molecular and cellular events implicated in local tolerance to kidney allografts in miniature swine. Transplantation. 1997;63:26–33.
87. Fuchimoto Y, Huang CA, Yamada K, et al. Mixed chimerism and tolerance without whole body irradiation in a large animal model. Journal of Clinical Investigation. 2000;105:1779–1789.
88. Gianello P, Fishbein JM, Sachs DH. Tolerance to primarily vascularized allografts in miniature swine. Immunological Reviews. 1993;133:19–44.
89. Ierino FL, Yamada K, Hatch T, et al. Peripheral tolerance to class I mismatched renal allografts in miniature swine: donor antigen-activated peripheral blood lymphocytes from tolerant swine inhibit antidonor CTL reactivity. Journal of Immunology. 1999;162:550–559.
90. Mezrich JD, Yamada K, Lee RS, et al. Mechanisms of tolerance induction in the heart/kidney model in miniature swine. Journal of Heart and Lung Transplantation. 2001;20:172–173.
91. Okumi M, Fishbein JM, Griesemer AD, et al. Role of persistence of antigen and indirect recognition in the maintenance of tolerance to renal allografts. Transplantation. 2008;85:270–280.
92. Yamada K, Ierino FL, Gianello PR, et al. Role of the thymus in transplantation tolerance in miniature swine. III. Surgical manipulation of the thymus interferes with stable induction of tolerance to class I-mismatched renal allografts. Transplantation. 1999;67:1112–1119.
93. Yamada K, Mawulawde K, Menard MT, et al. Mechanisms of tolerance induction and prevention of cardiac allograft vasculopathy in miniature swine: the effect of augmentation of donor antigen load. Journal of Thoracic and Cardiovascular Surgery. 2000;119:709–719.
94. Meltzer AJ, Veillette GR, Aoyama A, et al. Donor Brain Death Inhibits Tolerance Induction in Miniature Swine Recipients of Fully MHC-Disparate Pulmonary Allografts. American Journal of Transplant. 2012;12:1290–1295.
95. Mezrich JD, Benjamin LC, Sachs JA, et al. Role of the thymus and kidney graft in the maintenance of tolerance to heart grafts in miniature swine. Transplantation. 2005;79:1663–1673.
96. Schwarze ML, Menard MT, Fuchimoto Y, et al. Mixed hematopoietic chimerism induces long-term tolerance to cardiac allografts in miniature swine. Annals of Thoracic Surgery. 2000;70:131–138.
97. Shoji T, Sahara H, Muniappan A, et al. Operational tolerance to class I disparate lungs can be induced despite pretransplant immunization with class I allopeptides. Transplantation. 2007;84:1467–1473.
98. Cosimi AB, Sachs DH. Mixed chimerism and transplantation tolerance. Transplantation. 2004;77:943–946.
99. Kawai T, Cosimi AB, Colvin RB, et al. Mixed allogeneic chimerism and renal-allograft tolerance in cynomolgus monkeys. Transplantation. 1995;59: 256–262.
100. Kimikawa M, Sachs DH, Colvin RB, et al. Modifications of the conditioning regimen for achieving mixed chimerism and donor-specific tolerance in cynomolgus monkeys. Transplantation. 1997;64:709–716.
101. Sachs DH, Sykes M, Kawai T, et al. Immuno-intervention for the induction of transplantation tolerance through mixed chimerism. Seminars in Immunology. 2011;23:165–173.
102. Kawai T, Cosimi AB, Sachs DH. Preclinical and clinical studies on the induction of renal allograft tolerance through transient mixed chimerism. Current Opinion in Organ Transplantation 2011;16:366–371.
103. Spitzer TR, Sykes M, Tolkoff-Rubin N, et al. Long-term follow-up of recipients of combined human leukocyte antigen-matched bone marrow and kidney transplantation for multiple myeloma with end-stage renal disease. Transplantation. 2011;91:672–676.
104. Kirk AD. Transplantation tolerance: a look at the nonhuman primate literature in the light of modern tolerance theories. Critical Reviews in Immunology. 1999;19:349–388.
105. Reemtsma K. Heterotransplantation. Transplantation Proceedings. 1969;1: 251–255.
106. Kirk AD, Harlan DM, Armstrong NN, et al. CTLA4-Ig and anti-CD40 ligand prevent renal allograft rejection in primates. Proceedings of the National Academy of Sciences of the United States of America. 1997;94:8789–8794.
107. Knechtle SJ, Vargo D, Fechner J, et al. FN18-CRM9 immunotoxin promotes tolerance in primate renal allografts. Transplantation. 1997;63:1–6.
108. Song L, Qi S, Dun H, et al. Surgical complications in kidney transplantation in nonhuman primates. Microsurgery. 2010;30:327–331.
109. Garcia-Rinaldi R, Rossen RD, Sell KW, et al. In vitro binding studies of antihuman lymphocyte globulin: analysis of samples tested for immunosuppression in the primate skin allograft system. Journal of Immunological Methods. 1977;16:313–329.
110. Berlin PJ, Bacher JD, Sharrow SO, et al. Monoclonal antibodies against human T cell adhesion molecules–modulation of immune function in nonhuman primates. Transplantation. 1992;53:840–849.
111. Ossevoort MA, Lorre K, Boon L, et al. Prolonged skin graft survival by administration of anti-CD80 monoclonal antibody with cyclosporin A. Journal of Immunotherapy. 1999;22:381–389.
112. Elster EA, Xu H, Tadaki DK, et al. Treatment with the humanized CD154-specific monoclonal antibody, hu5C8, prevents acute rejection of primary skin allografts in nonhuman primates. Transplantation. 2001;72:1473–1478.
113. Cantarelli E, Piemonti L. Alternative transplantation sites for pancreatic islet grafts. Current Diabetes Reports. 2011;11:364–374.
114. Kenyon NS, Fernandez LA, Lehmann R, et al. Long-term survival and function of intrahepatic islet allografts in baboons treated with humanized anti-CD154.

Diabetes. 1999;48:1473–1481.
115. Kenyon NS, Chatzipetrou M, Masetti M, et al. Long-term survival and function of intrahepatic islet allografts in rhesus monkeys treated with humanized anti-CD154. Proceedings of the National Academy of Sciences of the United States of America. 1999;96:8132–8137.
116. Adams AB, Shirasugi N, Durham MM, et al. Calcineurin inhibitor-free CD28 blockade-based protocol protects allogeneic islets in nonhuman primates. Diabetes. 2002;51:265–270.
117. Adams AB, Shirasugi N, Jones TR, et al. Development of a chimeric anti-CD40 monoclonal antibody that synergizes with LEA29Y to prolong islet allograft survival. Journal of Immunology. 2005;174:542–550.
118. Badell IR, Russell MC, Cardona K, et al. CTLA4Ig prevents alloantibody formation following nonhuman primate islet transplantation using the CD40-specific antibody 3A8. American Journal of Transplantation. 2012;12:1918–1923.
119. Badell IR, Thompson PW, Turner AP, et al. Nondepleting anti-CD40-based therapy prolongs allograft survival in nonhuman primates. American Journal of Transplantation. 2012;12:126–135.
120. Lowe M, Badell IR, Thompson P, et al. A novel monoclonal antibody to CD40 prolongs islet allograft survival. American Journal of Transplantation. 2012;12:2079–2087.
121. Azimzadeh AM, Pfeiffer S, Wu G, et al. Alloimmunity in primate heart recipients with CD154 blockade: evidence for alternative costimulation mechanisms. Transplantation. 2006;81:255–264.
122. Hausen B, Ikonen T, Briffa N, et al. Combined immunosuppression with cyclosporine (neoral) and SDZ RAD in non-human primate lung transplantation: systematic pharmacokinetic-based trials to improve efficacy and tolerability. Transplantation. 2000;69:76–86.
123. Hausen B, Gummert J, Berry GJ, et al. Prevention of acute allograft rejection in nonhuman primate lung transplant recipients: induction with chimeric anti-interleukin-2 receptor monoclonal antibody improves the tolerability and potentiates the immunosuppressive activity of a regimen using low doses of both microemulsion cyclosporine and 40-O-(2-hydroxyethyl)-rapamycin. Transplantation. 2000;69:488–496.
124. Suzuki J, Isobe M, Kawauchi M, et al. Altered expression of matrix metalloproteinases and tissue inhibitors of metalloproteinases in acutely rejected myocardium and coronary arteriosclerosis in cardiac allografts of nonhuman primates. Transplant International. 2000;13:106–113.
125. Li J, Chen G, Ye P, et al. CCR5 blockade in combination with cyclosporine increased cardiac graft survival and generated alternatively activated macrophages in primates. Journal of Immunology. 2011;186:3753–3761.
126. Stark GB, Swartz WM, Narayanan K, et al. Hand transplantation in baboons. Transplantation Proceedings. 1987;19:3968–3971.
127. Hovius SE, Stevens HP, Van Nierop PW, et al. Replantation of the radial side of the hand in the rhesus monkey: anatomical and functional aspects. A preliminary study to composite tissue allografting. Journal of Hand Surgery (Edinburgh, Lothian). 1992;17:651–656.
128. Cendales LC, Xu H, Bacher J, et al. Composite tissue allotransplantation: development of a preclinical model in nonhuman primates. Transplantation. 2005;80:1447–1454.
129. Silverman RP, Banks ND, Detolla LJ, et al. A heterotopic primate model for facial composite tissue transplantation. Annals of Plastic Surgery. 2008;60:209–216.
130. Barth RN, Bluebond-Langner R, Nam A, et al. Facial subunit composite tissue allografts in nonhuman primates: I. Technical and immunosuppressive requirements for prolonged graft survival. Plastic and Reconstructive Surgery. 2009;123:493–501.
131. Nottle MB, Beebe LFS, Harrison SJ, et al. Production of homozygous alpha-1,3-galactosyltransferase knockout pigs by breeding and somatic cell nuclear transfer. Xenotransplantation. 2007;14:339–344.
132. Kolber-Simonds D, Lai L, Watt SR, et al. Production of alpha-1,3-galactosyltransferase null pigs by means of nuclear transfer with fibroblasts bearing loss of heterozygosity mutations. Proceedings of the National Academy of Sciences of the United States of America. 2004;101:7335–7340.
133. Phelps CJ, Koike C, Vaught TD, et al. Production of alpha 1,3-galactosyltransferase-deficient pigs. Science. 2003;299:411–414.
134. Galili U, Wang L, LaTemple DC, et al. The natural anti-Gal antibody. Sub-Cellular Biochemistry. 1999;32:79–106.
135. Galili U, Shohet SB, Kobrin E, et al. Man, apes, and Old World monkeys differ from other mammals in the expression of alpha-galactosyl epitopes on nucleated cells. Journal of Biological Chemistry. 1988;263:17755–17762.
136. Byrne GW, McCurry KR, Martin MJ, et al. Transgenic pigs expressing human CD59 and decay-accelerating factor produce an intrinsic barrier to complement-mediated damage. Transplantation. 1997;63:149–155.
137. Griesemer AD, Hirakata A, Shimizu A, et al. Results of gal-knockout porcine thymokidney xenografts. American Journal of Transplantation. 2009;9:2669–2678.
138. Sachs DH. Pig to primate xenotransplantation: tolerance through mixed chimerism. Xeno. 1995;3:52–55.
139. Barth RN, Yamamoto S, LaMattina JC, et al. Xenogeneic thymokidney and thymic tissue transplantation in a pig-to-baboon model: I. Evidence for pig-specific T-cell unresponsiveness. Transplantation. 2003;75:1615–1624.
140. Ghazi A, Griesemer A, Hirakata A, et al. Specific non-responsiveness to pig in baboons receiving BMT from GalT-KO pigs. American Transplant Congress; 2007.
141. Yamada K, Yazawa K, Shimizu A, et al. Marked prolongation of porcine renal xenograft survival in baboons through the use of alpha1,3-galactosyltransferase gene-knockout donors and the cotransplantation of vascularized thymic tissue. Nature Medicine. 2005;11:32–34.
142. Yamamoto S, Lavelle JM, Vagefi PA, et al. Vascularized thymic lobe transplantation in a pig-to-baboon model: a novel strategy for xenogeneic tolerance induction and T-cell reconstitution. Transplantation. 2005;80:1783–1790.
143. Casu A, Bottino R, Balamurugan AN, et al. Metabolic aspects of pig-to-monkey (Macaca fascicularis) islet transplantation: implications for translation into clinical practice. Diabetologia. 2008;51:120–129.
144. Marigliano M, Bertera S, Grupillo M, et al. Pig-to-nonhuman primates pancreatic islet xenotransplantation: an overview. Current Diabetes Reports. 2011;11:402–412.
145. Hering BJ, Walawalkar N. Pig-to-nonhuman primate islet xenotransplantation. Transplant Immunology. 2009;21:81–86.
146. Cardona K, Korbutt GS, Milas Z, et al. Long-term survival of neonatal porcine islets in nonhuman primates by targeting costimulation pathways. Nature Medicine. 2006;12:304–306.
147. Cardona K, Milas Z, Strobert E, et al. Engraftment of adult porcine islet xenografts in diabetic nonhuman primates through targeting of costimulation pathways. American Journal of Transplantation. 2007;7:2260–2268.
148. Thompson P, Badell IR, Lowe M, et al. Islet xenotransplantation using gal-deficient neonatal donors improves engraftment and function. American Journal of Transplantation. 2011;11:2593–2602.
149. Platz KP, Bechstein WO, Eckhoff DE, et al. Rs-61443 reverses acute allograft-rejection in dogs. Surgery. 1991;110:736–741.
150. Bechstein WO, Schilling M, Steele DM, et al. RS-61443/cyclosporine combination therapy prolongs canine liver allograft survival. Transplantation Proceedings. 1993;25:702–703.
151. Calne RY. Immunosuppression for organ grafting—observations on cyclosporin-A. Immunological Reviews. 1979;46:113–124.
152. Calne RY, White DJG, Rolles K, et al. Prolonged survival of pig orthotopic heart grafts treated with cyclosporin-A. Lancet. 1978;1(8075):1183–1185.
153. Todo S, Ueda Y, Demetris JA, et al. Immunosuppression of canine, monkey, and baboon allografts by FK-506 – with special reference to synergism with other drugs and to tolerance induction. Surgery. 1988;104:239–249.
154. Ochiai T, Nagata M, Nakajima K, et al. Studies of the effects of FK506 on renal allografting in the beagle dog. Transplantation. 1987;44:729–733.
155. Homan WP, French ME, Millard P, et al. Studies on the effects of cyclosporin-a upon renal-allograft rejection in the dog. Surgery. 1980;88:168–173.
156. Toledo-Pereyra LH, Bandlien KO, Mackenzie GH, et al. Orthotopic liver-transplantation – various immunosuppressive regimens to improve survival. American Surgeon 1984;50:258–263.
157. Williams JW, Peters TG, Haggitt R, et al. Cyclosporin-A in orthotopic canine hepatic transplants. Journal of Surgical Research. 1982;32:576–585.
158. Fishbein JM, Rosengard BR, Gianello P, et al. Development of tolerance to class-Ii mismatched renal-transplants after a short-course of cyclosporine therapy in miniature swine. Transplantation. 1994;57:1303–1308.
159. Utsugi R, Barth RN, Lee RS, et al. Induction of transplantation tolerance with a short course of tacrolimus (FK506) I. Rapid and stable tolerance to two-haplotype fully MHC-mismatched kidney allografts in miniature swine. Transplantation. 2001;71:1368–1379.
160. Bom-van Noorloos AA, Visser JJ, Drexhage HA, et al. Cyclosporin A in orthotopic porcine liver transplantation. Long-term survival after short-term treatment. European Surgical Research. 1984;16:329–335.
161. Calne RY, Watson CJE, Brons IGM, et al. Tolerance of porcine renal-allografts induced by donor spleen-cells and seven days treatment with cyclosporine. Transplantation. 1994;57:1433–1435.
162. Oike F, Talpe S, Otsuka M, et al. A 12-day course of FK506 allows long-term acceptance of semi-identical liver allograft in inbred miniature swine. Transplantation. 2000;69:2304–2314.
163. Jonker M, van de Hout Y, Neuhaus P, et al. Complete withdrawal of immunosuppression in kidney allograft recipients—a prospective study in rhesus monkeys. Transplantation. 1998;66:925–927.
164. Ochiai T, Gunji Y, Nagata M, et al. Effects of rapamycin in experimental organ

allografting. Transplantation. 1993;56:15–19.
165. Almond PS, Moss A, Nakhleh RE, et al. Rapamycin—immunosuppression, hyporesponsiveness, and side-effects in a porcine renal-allograft model. Transplantation. 1993;56:275–281.
166. Granger DK, Cromwell JW, Chen SC, et al. Prolongation of renal-allograft survival in a large animal-model by oral rapamycin monotherapy. Transplantation. 1995;59:183–186.
167. Weaver TA, Charafeddine AH, Agarwal A, et al. Alefacept promotes costimulation blockade based allograft survival in nonhuman primates. Nature Medicine. 2009;15:746–749.
168. Lo DJ, Anderson DJ, Weaver TA, et al. Belatacept and sirolimus prolong nonhuman primate renal allograft survival without a requirement for memory T cell depletion. American Journal of Transplantation. 2013;13:320–328.
169. Qi S, Xu D, Peng J, et al. Effect of tacrolimus (FK506) and sirolimus (rapamycin) mono- and combination therapy in prolongation of renal allograft survival in the monkey. Transplantation. 2000;69:1275–1283.
170. Chen H, Peng J, Luo H, et al. Compromised kidney graft rejection response in vervet monkeys after withdrawal of immunosuppressants tacrolimus and sirolimus. Transplantation. 2000;69:1555–1561.
171. Montgomery SP, Mog SR, Xu H, et al. Efficacy and toxicity of a protocol using sirolimus, tacrolimus and daclizumab in a nonhuman primate renal allotransplant model. American Journal of Transplantation. 2002;2:381–385.
172. Singh K, Kozyr N, Stempora L, et al. Regulatory T cells exhibit decreased proliferation but enhanced suppression after pulsing with sirolimus. American Journal of Transplantation. 2012;12:1441–1457.
173. Ma A, Qi S, Song L, et al. Adoptive transfer of CD4+CD25+ regulatory cells combined with low-dose sirolimus and anti-thymocyte globulin delays acute rejection of renal allografts in Cynomolgus monkeys. International Immunopharmacology. 2011;11:618–629.
174. Wijkstrom M, Kenyon NS, Kirchhof N, et al. Islet allograft survival in nonhuman primates immunosuppressed with basiliximab, RAD, and FTY720. Transplantation. 2004;77:827–835.
175. Schuurman HJ, Menninger K, Audet M, et al. Oral efficacy of the new immunomodulator FTY720 in cynomolgus monkey kidney allotransplantation, given alone or in combination with cyclosporine or RAD. Transplantation. 2002;74:951–960.
176. Suzuki T, Jin MB, Shimamura T, et al. A new immunosuppressant, FTY720, in canine kidney transplantation: effect of single-drug, induction and combination treatments. Transplant International. 2004;17:574–584.
177. Furukawa H, Suzuki T, Jin MB, et al. Prolongation of canine liver allograft survival by a novel immunosuppressant, FTY720 – Effect of monotherapy and combined treatment with conventional drugs. Transplantation. 2000;69:235–241.
178. Bigaud M, Wieczorek G, Beerli C, et al. Sotrastaurin (AEB071) alone and in combination with cyclosporine A prolongs survival times of non-human primate recipients of life-supporting kidney allografts. Transplantation. 2012;93:156–164.
179. Bigaud M, Wieczorek G, Preussing E, et al. NVP-AEB071 (AEB), the novel oral inhibitor of protein kinase C (PKC) and early T-cell activation, prolongs nonhuman primates (NHP) kidney allograft survival when combined with everolimus (RAD), ERL080 (ERL) or FTY720 (FTY) without calcineurin inhibitor (CNI). American Journal of Transplantation. 2006;6(Suppl. 2):251–252.
180. Borie DC, Changelian PS, Larson MJ, et al. Immunosuppression by the JAK3 inhibitor CP-690,550 delays rejection and significantly prolongs kidney allograft survival in nonhuman primates. Transplantation. 2005;79:791–801.
181. Wang X, Sun H, Chen G, et al. Immunosuppression with a combination of pg490-88 and a subtherapeutic dose of FK506 in a canine renal allograft model. Transplantation. 2005;79:1537–1544.
182. Chen G, Sun H, Arp J, et al. A synergistic effect between PG490-88 and tacrolimus prolongs renal allograft survival in monkeys. American Journal of Transplantation. 2006;6:714–723.
183. Bretscher P, Cohn M. A theory of self-nonself discrimination. Science. 1970;169:1042–1049.
184. Lafferty KJ, Cunningham AJ. New analysis of allogeneic interactions. Australian Journal of Experimental Biology and Medical Science. 1975;53:27–42.
185. Ford ML, Larsen CP. Translating costimulation blockade to the clinic: lessons learned from three pathways. Immunological Reviews. 2009;229:294–306.
186. Turka LA, Linsley PS, Lin H, et al. T-cell activation by the CD28 ligand-B7 is required for cardiac allograft-rejection in vivo. Proceedings of the National Academy of Sciences of the United States of America. 1992;89:11102–11105.
187. Larsen CP, Elwood ET, Alexander DZ, et al. Long-term acceptance of skin and cardiac allografts after blocking CD40 and CD28 pathways. Nature. 1996;381:434–438.
188. Pearson TC, Alexander DZ, Winn KJ, et al. Transplantation tolerance induced by CTLA4-Ig. Transplantation. 1994;57:1701–1706.
189. Ford ML, Koehn BH, Wagener ME, et al. Antigen-specific precursor frequency impacts T cell proliferation, differentiation, and requirement for costimulation. Journal of Experimental Medicine. 2007;204:299–309.
190. Viola A, Lanzavecchia A. T cell activation determined by T cell receptor number and tunable thresholds. Science. 1996;273:104–106.
191. Germain RN. The art of the probable: system control in the adaptive immune system. Science. 2001;293:240–245.
192. London CA, Lodge MP, Abbas AK. Functional responses and costimulator dependence of memory CD4+ T cells. Journal of Immunology. 2000;164:265–272.
193. Pilat N, Sayegh MH, Wekerle T. Costimulatory pathways in transplantation. Seminars in Immunology. 2011;23:293–303.
194. Salomon B, Bluestone JA. Complexities of CD28/B7: CTLA-4 costimulatory pathways in autoimmunity and transplantation. Annual Review of Immunology. 2001;19:225–252.
195. Howland KC, Ausubel LJ, London CA, et al. The roles of CD28 and CD40 ligand in T cell activation and tolerance. Journal of Immunology. 2000;164:4465–4470.
196. Fraser JD, Irving BA, Crabtree GR, et al. Regulation of interleukin-2 gene enhancer activity by the T cell accessory molecule CD28. Science. 1991;251:313–316.
197. Thompson CB, Allison JP. The emerging role of CTLA-4 as an immune attenuator. Immunity. 1997;7:445–450.
198. Kirk AD, Tadaki DK, Celniker A, et al. Induction therapy with monoclonal antibodies specific for CD80 and CD86 delays the onset of acute renal allograft rejection in non-human primates. Transplantation. 2001;72:377–384.
199. Montgomery SP, Xu H, Tadaki DK, et al. Combination induction therapy with monoclonal antibodies specific for CD80, CD86, and CD154 in nonhuman primate renal transplantation. Transplantation. 2002;74:1365–1369.
200. Birsan T, Hausen B, Higgins JP, et al. Treatment with humanized monoclonal antibodies against CD80 and CD86 combined with sirolimus prolongs renal allograft survival in cynomolgus monkeys. Transplantation. 2003;75:2106–2113.
201. Hausen B, Klupp J, Christians U, et al. Coadministration of either cyclosporine or steroids with humanized monoclonal antibodies against CD80 and CD86 successfully prolong allograft survival after life supporting renal transplantation in cynomolgus monkeys. Transplantation. 2001;72:1128–1137.
202. Ossevoort MA, de Boer M, Lorre K, et al. Blocking of costimulatory pathways using monoclonal antibodies as a new strategy to prevent transplant rejection in a non-human primate model. Transplantation Proceedings. 1998;30:1061–1062.
203. Ossevoort MA, Ringers J, Boon L, et al. Blocking of costimulation prevents kidney graft rejection in rhesus monkeys. Transplantation Proceedings. 1998;30:2165–2166.
204. Akalin E, Chandraker A, Russell ME, et al. CD28-B7 T cell costimulatory blockade by CTLA4Ig in the rat renal allograft model - Inhibition of cell-mediated and humoral immune responses in vivo. Transplantation. 1996;62:1942–1945.
205. Bolling SF, Lin H, Wei RQ, et al. Preventing allograft rejection with CTLA4IG: effect of donor-specific transfusion route or timing. Journal of Heart and Lung Transplantation. 1996;15:928–935.
206. Levisetti MG, Padrid PA, Szot GL, et al. Immunosuppressive effects of human CTLA4Ig in a non-human primate model of allogeneic pancreatic islet transplantation. Journal of Immunology. 1997;159:5187–5191.
207. Krieger NR, Yuh D, McIntyre WB, et al. Prolongation of cardiac graft survival with anti-CD4Ig plus hCTLA4Ig in primates. Journal of Surgical Research. 1998;76:174–178.
208. Larsen CP, Pearson TC, Adams AB, et al. Rational development of LEA29Y (belatacept), a high-affinity variant of CTLA4-Ig with potent immunosuppressive properties. American Journal of Transplantation. 2005;5:443–453.
209. Lowe MC, Badell IR, Turner AP, et al. Belatacept and sirolimus prolong nonhuman primate islet allograft survival: adverse consequences of concomitant alefacept therapy. American Journal of Transplantation. 2013;13:312–319.
210. Beyersdorf N, Gaupp S, Balbach K, et al. Selective targeting of regulatory T cells with CD28 superagonists allows effective therapy of experimental autoimmune encephalomyelitis. Journal of Experimental Medicine. 2005;202:445–455.
211. Suntharalingam G, Perry MR, Ward S, et al. Cytokine storm in a phase 1 trial of the anti-CD28 monoclonal antibody TGN1412. New England Journal of Medicine. 2006;355:1018–1028.
212. Findlay L, Eastwood D, Stebbings R, et al. Improved in vitro methods to predict the in vivo toxicity in man of therapeutic monoclonal antibodies including TGN1412. Journal of Immunological Methods. 2010;352:1–12.
213. Stebbings R, Findlay L, Edwards C, et al. "Cytokine storm" in the phase I trial of monoclonal antibody TGN1412: better understanding the causes to improve preclinical testing of immunotherapeutics. Journal of Immunology. 2007;179:

3325–3331.
214. Poirier N, Azimzadeh AM, Zhang T, et al. Inducing CTLA-4-dependent immune regulation by selective CD28 blockade promotes regulatory T cells in organ transplantation. Science Translational Medicine. 2010;2:17ra10.
215. Poirier N, Mary C, Dilek N, et al. Preclinical efficacy and immunological safety of FR104, an antagonist anti-CD28 monovalent Fab' antibody. American Journal of Transplantation. 2012;12:2630–2640.
216. Larsen CP, Alexander DZ, Hollenbaugh D, et al. CD40-gp39 interactions play a critical role during allograft rejection – Suppression of allograft rejection by blockade of the CD40-gp39 pathway. Transplantation. 1996;61:4–9.
217. Larsen CP, Pearson TC. The CD40 pathway in allograft rejection, acceptance, and tolerance. Current Opinion in Immunology. 1997;9:641–647.
218. Bennett SR, Carbone FR, Karamalis F, et al. Help for cytotoxic-T-cell responses is mediated by CD40 signalling. Nature. 1998;393:478–480.
219. Schoenberger SP, Toes RE, van der Voort EI, et al. T-cell help for cytotoxic T lymphocytes is mediated by CD40-CD40L interactions. Nature. 1998;393:480–483.
220. Henn V, Slupsky JR, Gräfe M, et al. CD40 ligand on activated platelets triggers an inflammatory reaction of endothelial cells. Nature. 1998;391:591–594.
221. Xu H, Zhang X, Mannon RB, et al. Platelet-derived or soluble CD154 induces vascularized allograft rejection independent of cell-bound CD154. Journal of Clinical Investigation. 2006;116:769–774.
222. Charafeddine AH, Kim EJ, Maynard DM, et al. Platelet-derived CD154: ultrastructural localization and clinical correlation in organ transplantation. American Journal of Transplantation. 2012;12:3143–3151.
223. Kirk AD, Burkly LC, Batty DS, et al. Treatment with humanized monoclonal antibody against CD154 prevents acute renal allograft rejection in nonhuman primates. Nature Medicine. 1999;5:686–693.
224. Xu H, Elster E, Batty D, et al. Effects of dose and duration of anti-CD154 antibody therapy in preventing renal allograft rejection in a nonhuman primate model. Transplantation Proceedings. 2001;33:223–224.
225. Pierson RN, Chang AC, Blum MG, et al. Prolongation of primate cardiac allograft survival by treatment with anti-CD40 ligand (CD154) antibody. Transplantation. 1999;68:1800–1805.
226. Pfeiffer S, Iii GLZ, Azimzadeh AM, et al. Monotherapy with anti-CD40 ligand antibody (IDEC 131) for non-human primate allograft heart transplantation. Journal of Heart and Lung Transplantation. 2001;20:250.
227. Pierson RN, Crowe JE, Pfeiffer S, et al. CD40-ligand in primate cardiac allograft and viral immunity. Immunologic Research. 2001;23:253–262.
228. Xu H, Montgomery SP, Preston EH, et al. Studies investigating pretransplant donor-specific blood transfusion, rapamycin, and the CD154-specific antibody IDEC-131 in a nonhuman primate model of skin allotransplantation. Journal of Immunology. 2003;170:2776–2782.
229. Preston EH, Xu H, Dhanireddy KK, et al. IDEC-131 (anti-CD154), sirolimus and donor-specific transfusion facilitate operational tolerance in non-human primates. American Journal of Transplantation. 2005;5:1032–1041.
230. Pearl JP, Xu H, Leopardi F, et al. CD154 blockade, sirolimus, and donor-specific transfusion prevents renal allograft rejection in cynomolgus monkeys despite homeostatic T-cell activation. Transplantation. 2007;83:1219–1225.
231. Kanmaz T, Fechner JJH, Torrealba J, et al. Monotherapy with the novel human anti-CD154 monoclonal antibody ABI793 in rhesus monkey renal transplantation model. Transplantation. 2004;77:914–920.
232. Schuler W, Bigaud M, Brinkmann V, et al. Efficacy and safety of ABI793, a novel human anti-human CD154 monoclonal antibody, in cynomolgus monkey renal allotransplantation. Transplantation. 2004;77:717–726.
233. Kawai T, Andrews D, Colvin R, et al. Thromboembolic complications after treatment with monoclonal antibody against CD40 ligand. Nature Medicine. 2000;6:114.
234. Pearson TC, Trambley J, Odom K, et al. Anti-CD40 therapy extends renal allograft survival in rhesus macaques. Transplantation. 2002;74:933–940.
235. Page A, Srinivasan S, Singh K, et al. CD40 blockade combines with CTLA4Ig and sirolimus to produce mixed chimerism in an MHC-defined rhesus macaque transplant model. American Journal of Transplantation. 2012;12:115–125.
236. Aoyagi T, Yamashita K, Suzuki T, et al. A human anti-CD40 monoclonal antibody, 4D11, for kidney transplantation in cynomolgus monkeys: induction and maintenance therapy. American Journal of Transplantation. 2009;9:1732–1741.
237. Imai A, Suzuki T, Sugitani A, et al. A novel fully human anti-CD40 monoclonal antibody, 4D11, for kidney transplantation in cynomolgus monkeys. Transplantation. 2007;84:1020–1028.
238. de Vos AF, Melief M-J, van Riel D, et al. Antagonist anti-human CD40 antibody inhibits germinal center formation in cynomolgus monkeys. European Journal of Immunology. 2004;34:3446–3455.
239. Haanstra KG, Ringers J, Sick EA, et al. Prevention of kidney allograft rejection using anti-CD40 and anti-CD86 in primates. Transplantation. 2003;75:637–643.
240. Magee CN, Boenisch O, Najafian N. The role of costimulatory molecules in directing the functional differentiation of alloreactive T helper cells. American Journal of Transplantation. 2012;12:2588–2600.
241. Kavanaugh AF, Lightfoot E, Lipsky PE, et al. Role of CD11/CD18 in adhesion and transendothelial migration of T cells. Analysis utilizing CD18-deficient T cell clones. Journal of Immunology. 1991;146:4149–4156.
242. Hamann A, Jablonski-Westrich D, Duijvestijn A, et al. Evidence for an accessory role of LFA-1 in lymphocyte-high endothelium interaction during homing. Journal of Immunology. 1988;140:693–699.
243. Warnock RA, Askari S, Butcher EC, et al. Molecular mechanisms of lymphocyte homing to peripheral lymph nodes. Journal of Experimental Medicine. 1998;187:205–216.
244. Pribila JT, Quale AC, Mueller KL, et al. Integrins and T cell-mediated immunity. Annual Review of Immunology. 2004;22:157–180.
245. Moy VT, Brian AA. Signaling by lymphocyte function-associated antigen 1 (LFA-1) in B cells: enhanced antigen presentation after stimulation through LFA-1. Journal of Experimental Medicine. 1992;175:1–7.
246. Van Seventer GA, Shimizu Y, Horgan KJ, et al. The LFA-1 ligand ICAM-1 provides an important costimulatory signal for T cell receptor-mediated activation of resting T cells. Journal of Immunology. 1990;144:4579–4586.
247. Nicolls MR, Gill RG. LFA-1 (CD11a) as a therapeutic target. American Journal of Transplantation. 2006;6:27–36.
248. Poston RS, Robbins RC, Chan B, et al. Effects of humanized monoclonal antibody to rhesus CD11a in rhesus monkey cardiac allograft recipients. Transplantation. 2000;69:2005–2013.
249. Badell IR, Russell MC, Thompson PW, et al. LFA-1-specific therapy prolongs allograft survival in rhesus macaques. Journal of Clinical Investigation. 2010;120:4520–4531.
250. Le Mauff B, Hourmant M, Rougier JP, et al. Effect of anti-LFA1 (CD11a) monoclonal antibodies in acute rejection in human kidney transplantation. Transplantation. 1991;52:291–296.
251. Hourmant M, Bedrossian J, Durand D, et al. A randomized multicenter trial comparing leukocyte function-associated antigen-1 monoclonal antibody with rabbit antithymocyte globulin as induction treatment in first kidney transplantations. Transplantation. 1996;62:1565–1570.
252. Vincenti F, Mendez R, Pescovitz M, et al. A phase I/II randomized open-label multicenter trial of efalizumab, a humanized anti-CD11a, anti-LFA-1 in renal transplantation. American Journal of Transplantation. 2007;7:1770–1777.
253. Turgeon NA, Avila JG, Cano JA, et al. Experience with a novel efalizumab-based immunosuppressive regimen to facilitate single donor islet cell transplantation. American Journal of Transplantation. 2010;10:2082–2091.
254. Bromberg JS. The biology of CD2: adhesion, transmembrane signal, and regulatory receptor of immunity. Journal of Surgical Research. 1993;54:258–267.
255. Kaplon RJ, Hochman PS, Michler RE, et al. Short course single agent therapy with an LFA-3-IgG1 fusion protein prolongs primate cardiac allograft survival. Transplantation. 1996;61:356–363.
256. Dehoux JP, Talpe S, Dewolf N, et al. Effects on human and nonhuman primate immune response of a new rat anti-CD2 monoclonal antibody. Transplantation. 2000;69:2622–2633.
257. Mourad M, Besse T, Malaise J, et al. BTI-322 for acute rejection after renal transplantation. Transplantation Proceedings. 1997;29:2353.
258. Squifflet JP, Besse T, Malaise J, et al. BTI-322 for induction therapy after renal transplantation: a randomized study. Transplantation Proceedings. 1997;29:317–319.
259. Pruett TL, McGory RW, Wright FH, et al. Safety profile, pharmacokinetics, and pharmacodynamics of siplizumab, a humanized anti-CD2 monoclonal antibody, in renal allograft recipients. Transplantation Proceedings. 2009;41:3655–3661.
260. Hammer MH, Zhai Y, Katori M, et al. Homing of in vitro-generated donor antigen-reactive CD4+ T lymphocytes to renal allografts is alpha 4 beta 1 but not alpha L beta 2 integrin dependent. Journal of Immunology. 2001;166:596–601.
261. Yang H, Issekutz TB, Wright JR. Prolongation of rat islet allograft survival by treatment with monoclonal antibodies against VLA-4 and LFA-1. Transplantation. 1995;60:71–76.
262. Kitchens WH, Haridas D, Wagener ME, et al. Integrin antagonists prevent costimulatory blockade-resistant transplant rejection by CD8(+) memory T cells. American Journal of Transplantation. 2012;12:69–80.
263. Gowans JL, McGregor DD, Cowen DM, et al. Initiation of immune responses by small lymphocytes. Nature. 1962;196:651–655.
264. Singh LM, Vega RE, Makin GS, et al. External thoracic duct fistula and canine renal homograft. JAMA. 1965;191:1009–1011.
265. Starzl TE, Koep LJ, Weil R, et al. Thoracic duct drainage in organ transplantation: will it permit better immunosuppression? Transplantation Proceedings. 1979;11:276–284.
266. Funakoshi Y, Carrieri G, Yagihashi A, et al. Effect of preoperative thoracic duct

drainage on canine kidney transplantation. Journal of Investigative Surgery. 1996;9:359–367.
267. Dumont AE. Thoracic-duct-to-esophagus shunt. Transplantation. 1987;43:320.
268. Kinukawa T, Ono Y, Takeuchi N, et al. Analysis of long-term results in kidney transplantation performed using a rejection-free protocol with cyclosporine and thoracic duct drainage. Transplantation Proceedings. 1997;29:946–947.
269. Hammer C, Thein E. Visualization of the effect of polyclonal antithymocyte globulins on adhesion of leukocytes. Transplantation Proceedings. 2002;34:2486–2487.
270. Braf ZF, Smellie WA, Williams GM, et al. Evaluation of antithymocyte serum in the treatment of canine renal homografts. Surgery, Gynecology and Obstetrics. 1969;129:71–78.
271. White HJ, Symes MO, Golby MS, et al. Observations on the effect of horse anti-pig leucocyte serum in suppressing the rejection of renal allografts in pigs. British Journal of Surgery. 1971;58:859.
272. Gams E, Bornikoel K, Hagl S, et al. Heterotopic allogeneic heart transplantation in dogs. Experimental investigations for early detection of the rejection after immunosuppressive monotherapy with ALS or azathioprine. European Surgical Research. 1973;5:202–215.
273. Shanfield I, Wolf JS, Wren SF, et al. Mechanism of permanent survival of canine renal allografts following a limited course of ALS treatment. Transplantation Proceedings. 1973;5:533–534.
274. Thomas F, Thomas J, Millington M, et al. Species variability in clinical antihuman antithymocyte globulin production: rabbit vs horse AHTG in primate skin graft survival. Surgical Forum. 1973;24:288–290.
275. Thomas JM, Williams EA, Thomas FT, et al. T cell-specific activity in rabbit anti-human thymocyte globulin. Correlation with immunosuppresive activity in non-human primates. Transplantation. 1978;25:97–102.
276. Preville X, Flacher M, LeMauff B, et al. Mechanisms involved in antithymocyte globulin immunosuppressive activity in a nonhuman primate model. Transplantation. 2001;71:460–468.
277. Bieber CP, Jamieson S, Raney A, et al. Cardiac allograft survival in rhesus primates treated with combined total lymphoid irradiation and rabbit anti-thymocyte globulin. Transplantation. 1979;28:347–350.
278. Hirshberg B, Preston EH, Xu H, et al. Rabbit antithymocyte globulin induction and sirolimus monotherapy supports prolonged islet allograft function in a non-human primate islet transplantation model. Transplantation. 2003;76:55–60.
279. Liu C, Noorchashm H, Sutter JA, et al. B lymphocyte–directed immunotherapy promotes long-term islet allograft survival in nonhuman primates. Nature Medicine. 2007;13:1295–1298.
280. Haanstra KG, Sick EA, Ringers J, et al. No synergy between ATG induction and costimulation blockade induced kidney allograft survival in rhesus monkeys. Transplantation. 2006;82:1194–1201.
281. Watson CJE, Cobbold SP, Davies HFS, et al. Immunosuppression of canine renal-allograft recipients by CD4 and CD8 monoclonal-antibodies. Tissue Antigens. 1994;43:155–162.
282. Myburgh JA, Smit JA, Pieterz GA, et al. Tolerance in baboon kidney transplantation with total lymphoid irradiation (TLI) and anti-CD3/CD4-Idarubicin conjugates. Transplantation. 2001;72:1150–1152.
283. Botha JF, Tandon V, Linley W, et al. Prolonged survival of baboon renal allografts using idarubicin-conjugated anti-CD4 monoclonal antibodies. Transplant International. 2000;13(Suppl. 1):S480–S481.
284. Cosimi AB, Delmonico FL, Wright JK, et al. Prolonged survival of nonhuman primate renal allograft recipients treated only with anti-CD4 monoclonal antibody. Surgery. 1990;108:406–413.
285. Wee SL, Stroka DM, Preffer FI, et al. The effects of OKT4A monoclonal antibody on cellular immunity of nonhuman primate renal allograft recipients. Transplantation. 1992;53:501–507.
286. Mourad GJ, Preffer FI, Wee SL, et al. Humanized IgG1 and IgG4 anti-CD4 monoclonal antibodies: effects on lymphocytes in the blood, lymph nodes, and renal allografts in cynomolgus monkeys. Transplantation. 1998;65:632–641.
287. Nakamae H, Kerbauy FR, Wilbur DS, et al. Pilot study of a 213Bismuth-Labeled anti-CD45 mAb as a novel nonmyeloablative conditioning for DLA-haploidentical littermate hematopoietic transplantation. Transplantation. 2010;89:1336–1340.
288. Lazarovits AI, Poppema S, Zhang Z, et al. Prevention and reversal of renal allograft rejection by antibody against CD45RB. Nature. 1996;380:717–720.
289. Chen G, Luke PPW, Yang H, et al. Anti-CD45RB monoclonal antibody prolongs renal allograft survival in cynomolgus monkeys. American Journal of Transplantation. 2007;7:27–37.
290. Kelishadi SS, Azimzadeh AM, Zhang T, et al. Preemptive CD20+ B cell depletion attenuates cardiac allograft vasculopathy in cyclosporine-treated monkeys. Journal of Clinical Investigation. 2010;120:1275.
291. Maki T, Carville A, Stillman IE, et al. SV40 infection associated with rituximab treatment after kidney transplantation in nonhuman primates. Transplantation. 2008;85:893–902.
292. Haudebourg T, Dugast A-S, Coulon F, et al. Depletion of LAG-3 positive cells in cardiac allograft reveals their role in rejection and tolerance. Transplantation. 2007;84:1500–1506.
293. Poirier N, Haudebourg T, Brignone C, et al. Antibody-mediated depletion of lymphocyte-activation gene-3 (LAG-3+)-activated T lymphocytes prevents delayed-type hypersensitivity in non-human primates. Clinical and Experimental Immunology. 2011;164:265–274.
294. Neville DM, Scharff J, Hu HZ, et al. A new reagent for the induction of T-cell depletion, anti-CD3-CRM9. Journal of Immunotherapy. 1996;19:85–92.
295. Ma S, Hu H, Thompson J, et al. Genetic construction and characterization of an anti-monkey CD3 single-chain immunotoxin with a truncated diphtheria toxin. Bioconjugate Chemistry. 1997;8:695–701.
296. Knechtle SJ, Fechner JH, Dong YC, et al. Primate renal transplants using immunotoxin. Surgery. 1998;124:438–446.
297. Thomas JM, Neville DM, Contreras JL, et al. Preclinical studies of allograft tolerance in rhesus monkeys – A novel anti-CD3-immunotoxin given peritransplant with donor bone marrow induces operational tolerance to kidney allografts. Transplantation. 1997;64:124–135.
298. Thomas FT, Ricordi C, Contreras JL, et al. Reversal of naturally occuring diabetes in primates by unmodified islet xenografts without chronic immunosuppression. Transplantation. 1999;67:846–854.
299. Knechtle SJ, Fechner JH, Stavrou S, et al. Reversal of acute allograft rejection using immunotoxin. Transplantation Proceedings. 1998;30:2150–2151.
300. Armstrong N, Buckley P, Oberley T, et al. Analysis of primate renal allografts after T-cell depletion with anti-CD3-CRM9. Transplantation. 1998;66:5–13.
301. Torrealba JR, Fernandez LA, Kanmaz T, et al. Immunotoxin-treated rhesus monkeys: a model for renal allograft chronic rejection. Transplantation. 2003;76:524–530.
302. Jonker M, Ringers J, Ossevoort MA, et al. Long-term kidney graft survival by delayed T cell ablative treatment in rhesus monkeys. Transplantation. 2002;73:874–880.
303. Page EK, Page AJ, Kwun J, et al. Enhanced de novo alloantibody and antibody-mediated injury in rhesus macaques. American Journal of Transplantation. 2012;12:2395–2405.
304. Kim G-B, Wang Z, Liu YY, et al. A fold-back single-chain diabody format enhances the bioactivity of an anti-monkey CD3 recombinant diphtheria toxin-based immunotoxin. Protein Engineering, Design and Selection. 2007;20:425–432.
305. Huang CA, Yamada K, Murphy MC, et al. In vivo T cell depletion in miniature swine using the swine CD3 immunotoxin, pCD3-CRM9. Transplantation. 1999;68:855–860.
306. Gargollo P, Yamada K, Esnaola N, et al. Neuropathy in miniature swine after administration of the mutant diphtheria toxin-based immunotoxin, pCD3-CRM9. Transplantation. 2001;72:818–822.
307. Wang Z, Duran-Struuck R, Crepeau R, et al. Development of a diphtheria toxin based antiporcine CD3 recombinant immunotoxin. Clinical Pharmacology and Therapeutics. 2011;22:2014–2020.
308. Calne R, Friend P, Moffatt S, et al. Prope tolerance, perioperative campath 1H, and low-dose cyclosporin monotherapy in renal allograft recipients. Lancet. 1998;351:1701–1702.
309. Knechtle SJ, Pirsch JD, Fechner JH, et al. Campath-1H induction plus rapamycin monotherapy for renal transplantation: results of a pilot study. American Journal of Transplantation. 2003;3:722–730.
310. Kirk AD, Hale DA, Mannon RB, et al. Results from a human renal allograft tolerance trial evaluating the humanized CD52-specific monoclonal antibody alemtuzumab (CAMPATH-1H). Transplantation. 2003;76:120–129.
311. Pilat N, Wekerle T. Transplantation tolerance through mixed chimerism. Nature Reviews Nephrology. 2010;6:594–605.
312. Owen RD. Immunogenetic consequences of vascular anastomoses between bovine twins. Science. 1945;102:400–401.
313. Billingham RE, Brent L, Medawar PB. Quantitative studies on tissue transplantation immunity .3. Actively acquired tolerance. Philosophical Transactions of the Royal Society of London. Series B, Biological Sciences. 1956;239:357–412.
314. Ildstad ST, Sachs DH. Reconstitution with syngeneic plus allogeneic or xenogeneic bone marrow leads to specific acceptance of allografts or xenografts. Nature. 1984;307:168–170.
315. Sayegh MH, Fine NA, Smith JL, et al. Immunologic tolerance to renal allografts after bone marrow transplants from the same donors. Annals of Internal Medicine. 1991;114:954–955.
316. Spitzer TR, Delmonico F, Tolkoff-Rubin N, et al. Combined histocompatibility leukocyte antigen-matched donor bone marrow and renal transplantation for multiple myeloma with end stage renal disease: the induction of allograft toler-

ance through mixed lymphohematopoietic chimerism. Transplantation. 1999; 68:480-484.
317. Buhler LH, Spitzer TR, Sykes M, et al. Induction of kidney allograft tolerance after transient lymphohematopoietic chimerism in patients with multiple myeloma and end-stage renal disease. Transplantation. 2002;74: 1405-1409.
318. Fudaba Y, Spitzer TR, Shaffer J, et al. Myeloma responses and tolerance following combined kidney and nonmyeloablative marrow transplantation: in vivo and in vitro analyses. American Journal of Transplantation. 2006;6:2121-2133.
319. Thomas FT, Carver FM, Foil MB, et al. Long-term incompatible kidney survival in outbred higher primates without chronic immunosuppression. Annals of Surgery. 1983;198:370-378.
320. Hartner WC, Defazio SR, Maki T, et al. Prolongation of renal-allograft survival in antilymphocyte-serum treated dogs by postoperative injection of density gradient fractionated donor bone-marrow. Transplantation. 1986;42:593-597.
321. Brendel MD, Kong SS, Schachner RD, et al. The influence of donor specific vertebral body derived bone marrow cell infusion on canine islet allograft survival without irradiation conditioning of the recipient. Experimental and Clinical Endocrinology and Diabetes. 1995;103:129-132.
322. Thomas JM, Carver FM, Cunningham PRG, et al. Kidney allograft tolerance in primates without chronic immunosuppression—the role of veto cells. Transplantation. 1991;51:198-207.
323. Gruessner RWG, Zhang KY, Dunning M, et al. Bone marrow augmentation in kidney transplantation: a large animal study. Transplant International. 2001;14:159-169.
324. Starzl TE, Demetris AJ, Trucco M, et al. Systemic chimerism in human female recipients of male livers. Lancet. 1992;340:876-877.
325. Wood K, Sachs DH. Chimerism and transplantation tolerance: cause and effect. Immunology Today. 1996;17:584-587.
326. Fisher RA, Cohen DS, BenEzra JM, et al. Induction of long-term graft tolerance and donor recipient chimerism. Journal of Surgical Research. 1996;60:181-185.
327. Alard P, Matriano JA, Socarras S, et al. Detection of donor-derived cells by polymerase chain reaction in neonatally tolerant mice. Microchimerism fails to predict tolerance. Transplantation. 1995;60:1125-1130.
328. Abu-Elmagd K, Reyes J, Todo S, et al. Clinical intestinal transplantation: new perspectives and immunologic considerations. Journal of the American College of Surgeons. 1998;186:512-525.
329. Devlin J, Doherty D, Thomson L, et al. Defining the outcome of immunosuppression withdrawal after liver transplantation. Hepatology (Baltimore, Md.). 1998;27:926-933.
330. Elwood ET, Larsen CP, Maurer MH, et al. Microchimerism and rejection in clinical transplantation. Lancet. 1997;349:1358-1360.
331. Schlitt HJ, Hundrieser J, Hisanaga M, et al. Patterns of donor-type microchimerism after heart-transplantation. Lancet. 1994;343:1469-1471.
332. Sivasai KSR, Alevy YG, Duffy BF, et al. Peripheral blood microchimerism in human liver and renal transplant recipients—rejection despite donor-specific chimerism. Transplantation. 1997;64:427-432.
333. Suberbielle C, Caillatzucman S, Legendre C, et al. Peripheral microchimerism in long-term cadaveric-kidney allograft recipients. Lancet. 1994;343:1468-1469.
334. Lin H, Bolling SF, Linsley PS, et al. Long-term acceptance of major histocompatibility complex mismatched cardiac allografts induced by CTLA4Ig plus donor-specific transfusion. Journal of Experimental Medicine. 1993;178: 1801-1806.
335. Helg C, Chapuis B, Bolle JF, et al. Renal transplantation without immunosuppression in a host with tolerance induced by allogeneic bone marrow transplantation. Transplantation. 1994;58:1420-1422.
336. Jacobsen N, Taaning E, Ladefoged J, et al. Tolerance to an HLA-B,DR disparate kidney allograft after bone-marrow transplantation from same donor. Lancet. 1994;343:800.
337. Guzzetta PC, Sundt TM, Suzuki T, et al. Induction of kidney-transplantation tolerance across major histocompatibility complex barriers by bone-marrow transplantation in miniature swine. Transplantation. 1991;51:862-866.
338. Rapaport FT, Bachvaroff RJ, Watanabe K, et al. Induction of allogeneic unresponsiveness in adult dogs. Role of non-DLA histocompatibility variables in conditioning the outcome of bone marrow, kidney, and skin transplantation in radiation chimeras. Journal of Clinical Investigation. 1978;61:790-800.
339. Storb R, Weiden PL, Graham TC, et al. Studies of marrow transplantation in dogs. Transplantation Proceedings. 1976;8:545-549.
340. Sykes M. Mixed chimerism and transplant tolerance. Immunity. 2001; 14:417-424.
341. Nomoto K, Yung-Yun K, Omoto K, et al. Tolerance induction in a fully allogeneic combination using anti-T cell receptor-alpha beta monoclonal antibody, low dose irradiation, and donor bone marrow transfusion. Transplantation. 1995; 59:395-401.
342. Sharabi Y, Sachs DH. Mixed chimerism and permanent specific transplantation tolerance induced by a nonlethal preparative regimen. Journal of Experimental Medicine. 1989;169:493-502.
343. Kawai T, Poncelet A, Sachs DH, et al. Long-term outcome and alloantibody production in a non-myeloablative regimen for induction of renal allograft tolerance. Transplantation. 1999;68:1767-1775.
344. Graves SS, Mathes DW, Georges GE, et al. Long-term tolerance to kidney allografts after induced rejection of donor hematopoietic chimerism in a preclinical canine model. Transplantation. 2012;94:562-568.
345. Ramakrishnan SK, Page A, Farris AB, et al. Evidence for kidney rejection after combined bone marrow and renal transplantation despite ongoing whole-blood chimerism in rhesus macaques. American Journal of Transplantation. 2012;12:1755-1764.
346. Horner BM, Cina RA, Wikiel KJ, et al. Predictors of organ allograft tolerance following hematopoietic cell transplantation. American Journal of Transplantation. 2006;6:2894-2902.
347. Storb R, Yu C, Wagner JL, et al. Stable mixed hematopoietic chimerism in DLA-identical littermate dogs given sublethal total body irradiation before and pharmacological immunosuppression after marrow transplantation. Blood. 1997;89:3048-3054.
348. Kuhr CS, Allen MD, Junghanss C, et al. Tolerance to vascularized kidney grafts in canine mixed hematopoietic chimeras. Transplantation. 2002;73:1487-1493.
349. Storb R, Yu C, Zaucha JM, et al. Stable mixed hematopoietic chimerism in dogs given donor antigen, CTLA4Ig, and 100 cGy total body irradiation before and pharmacologic immunosuppression after marrow transplant. Blood. 1999; 94:2523-2529.
350. Storb R, Yu C, Barnett T, et al. Stable mixed hematopoietic chimerism in dog leukocyte antigen-identical littermate dogs given lymph node irradiation before and pharmacologic immunosuppression after marrow transplantation. Blood. 1999;94:1131-1136.
351. Tillson M, Niemeyer GP, Welch JA, et al. Hematopoietic chimerism induces renal and skin allograft tolerance in DLA-identical dogs. Experimental Hematology. 2006;34:1759-1770.
352. Huang CA, Fuchimoto Y, Scheier-Dolberg R, et al. Stable mixed chimerism and tolerance using a nonmyeloablative preparative regimen in a large-animal model. Journal of Clinical Investigation. 2000;105:173-181.
353. Huang CA, Fuchimoto Y, Gleit ZL, et al. Posttransplantation lymphoproliferative disease in miniature swine after allogeneic hematopoietic cell transplantation: similarity to human PTLD and association with a porcine gammaherpesvirus. Blood. 2001;97:1467-1473.
354. Cho PS, Mueller NJ, Cameron AM, et al. Risk factors for the development of post-transplant lymphoproliferative disorder in a large animal model. American Journal of Transplantation. 2004;4:1274-1282.
355. Cina RA, Wikiel KJ, Lee PW, et al. Stable multilineage chimerism without graft versus host disease following nonmyeloablative haploidentical hematopoietic cell transplantation. Transplantation. 2006;81:1677-1685.
356. Fuchimoto Y, Huang CA, Yamada K, et al. Induction of kidney allograft tolerance through mixed chimerism in miniature swine. Transplantation Proceedings. 2001;33:77.
357. Mathes DW, Randolph MA, Bourget JL, et al. Recipient bone marrow engraftment in donor tissue after long-term tolerance to a composite tissue allograft. Transplantation. 2002;73:1880-1885.
358. Schmidtko J, Wang R, Wu C-L, et al. Posttransplant lymphoproliferative disorder associated with an Epstein-Barr-related virus in cynomolgus monkeys. Transplantation. 2002;73:1431-1439.
359. Kawai T, Cosimi AB, Wee SL, et al. Effect of mixed hematopoietic chimerism on cardiac allograft survival in cynomolgus monkeys. Transplantation. 2002;73: 1757-1764.
360. Kawai T, Sogawa H, Boskovic S, et al. CD154 blockade for induction of mixed chimerism and prolonged renal allograft survival in nonhuman primates. American Journal of Transplantation. 2004;4:1391-1398.
361. Kean LS, Adams AB, Strobert E, et al. Induction of chimerism in rhesus macaques through stem cell transplant and costimulation blockade-based immunosuppression. American Journal of Transplantation. 2007;7:320-335.
362. Larsen CP, Page A, Linzie KH, et al. An MHC-defined primate model reveals significant rejection of bone marrow after mixed chimerism induction despite full MHC matching. American Journal of Transplantation. 2010;10:2396-2409.

第 16 章 硅芯片中的移植学前沿:移植研究中应用功能基因组学来研究全局基因表达

Steven Head, Sunil M. Kurian, Daniel R. Salomon

引言

功能基因组学包括四个主要学科及与之关系紧密的学科技术:整体基因表达谱、串联质谱蛋白质组学、遗传学和表观遗传学。本章主要针对以上提到的和整体基因表达谱及其在移植研究中的应用进行讨论。我们将讨论重点放眼于“功能”一词,旨在通过不同基因组学科从“分子”水平了解生物的生老病死。相信读者无疑已经从前文不断提到的“组学”一词中意识到,例如,新兴领域微生物组学或代谢组学等,都有许多信息值得学习和分享。然而,我们同样担心的是,对于该词的一味滥用可能并不能带来更多的实际意义。

首先我们对功能基因组学用生物学术语进行定义(用以体现细胞和组织在分子水平层面的复杂性)。我们认为,这有助于推进人们从细胞和有机体水平了解基础细胞生物学理论,从而进一步了解健康有机体是如何向疾病状态进行转变的。本章是对第 13 章至第 15 章有关体外、小型动物模型、大型动物模型移植研究的进一步补充。这是一种由结果向原因逆推的研究方法。在临床医学方面,我们相信运用功能基因组学是可以阐明疾病的发生、发展和转归的。任何引起个体发病的病因都受多方因素影响,包括基因、环境、个人病史以及治疗选择等。例如,移植排斥反应是在多重均衡机制影响下引发的免疫介导反应,但是这一过程不仅受供体和受体的影响,同时还与受体年龄、免疫学病史、免疫抑制剂的选择和使用时机、个体遗传学以及表观遗传学对于组织损伤的反应、自愈和代偿能力等息息相关。由此可见,逆向推演的功能基因学为生物学和医学设立了全新的视角,相比还原论通过更加简明扼要的理论和规则解释疾病发生机制而言,通过功能基因学解释疾病发生机制是个不小的挑战。

我们相信,功能基因组学将有助于进一步推进早期诊断和治疗的发展进程。虽然我们早前就一直担心个体化医疗已被过度炒作,但是我们同样相信它将会成为未来的发展趋势,将是划时代的一大壮举。我们对此抱有充分信心,是因为在我们的基因组 DNA 中囊括了祖先进化而来的全部生物学信息。如此硕大的人类知识库就像一个巨大的“活着的”搜索引擎,不断地进行创造、分化、维持、防御和治疗。在我们看来,功能基因组学适用于基因组信息的任何一步,从破解 DNA、转录 RNA、再到翻译和修饰蛋白,整个复杂程序的监管和信息通路都可以见到功能基因组学的身影。当功能基因组学作为一个成熟完整的科学体系被应用于揭示整个信息流的全部细节时,我们将会对整个疾病病因有一更加全面的认识,但是我们并不确定在有生之年会对此有所突破。

功能基因组学的实际应用

下面我们将一起回顾目前在移植整体基因表达谱中所涉及的相关技术。我们将向大家讲解每种工具的基本原理。在此过程中,我们还会向大家讲解其在实验设计和数据解释方面的局限性。在充分了解相关信息后,读者便可以更有效地将这些工具应用于有关实验,来解答在医学或临床过程中遇到的诸类问题。

基因表达谱的概念

在细胞核中,DNA 经过激活后将基因组信息流转录至 mRNA。这一层面的信息流需通过基因表达谱进行研究。基因转录的第一个产物称为前体 mRNA[1,2]，它含有 DNA 编码的所有内含子和外显子。而后在前体 mRNA 中内含子的介导下，有超过 100 种不同种类的蛋白质组成多蛋白复合物，进而组装成为剪接体。内含子–外显子所含有的不同序列可以调节剪接体的组装，它借由特定外显子序列，通过对蛋白质进行复杂多样的能量依赖性磷酸化来实现调节的目的。原则上，在细胞中合成蛋白质时，所有前体 mRNA 在转录时都需要拼接在 mRNA 上。目前最大的疑团就是，细胞是如何决定在"何时""何处"进行选择性剪接的，例如，在特定条件下，某些前体 mRNA 中含有的特定外显子就会被放入 mRNA 或者从 mRNA 中移除[3]。实验表明，在免疫介导激活人类 T 细胞和 B 细胞的过程中，会诱导剪接产生大量不同的 mRNA，上调转录表达[4]。我们认为，目前大多数检测基因表达差异性的方法基本上都忽略了这种选择性剪接造成的潜在影响。

经过剪接或选择性剪接于外显子–内含子之间，形成成熟的 mRNA。这些成熟的 mRNA 转录产物又通过能量依赖的方式从核糖体输送至细胞质内进一步翻译称为蛋白质。蛋白质翻译受多个步骤调节，包括核糖体的组装，蛋白质组装时的氨基酸传递，调节 mRNA 转录半衰期的调控通路，如绑定于 RISC 的 miRNA 复合体[5]。十分重要的是，蛋白质的合成同样受 mTOR 复合物的调节，而这些靶蛋白又是例如西罗莫司类免疫抑制剂的作用靶点[6]。整个翻译过程非常复杂。因此，有必要在这里向读者传达一个十分重要的信息：成熟 mRNA 的基因表达谱十分具有启示作用，但是对于实际信息流而言依旧十分有限，而且在细胞中有多个步骤可以参与调节翻译的表达过程。在新方法的辅助下，有助于我们进一步了解整体基因表达谱中的选择性剪接，可谓一大进步。但与此同时，我们还要明辨，在这些全新的知识体系中到底有哪些知识有助于我们理解以上这些复杂的过程，同时还要尽力避免外界诱惑以及在各方压力作用下对于解释原理做出的夸大假设。

基因表达谱的重要性在于，它有助于我们将一种或多种状态（静息与激活、早与晚）进行比较，将在不同表型间（排斥与耐受、病毒感染与急性排斥）进行比较，以及在这种情况下研究单个细胞或者整个组织中究竟是哪些基因直接影响了某蛋白质的合成及功能。通过特定基因分析方式示踪已知分子在整个系统中的作用，例如，炎症、凋亡、肿瘤转化、细胞信号传导、细胞增殖等，同样十分重要。许多公司就此进行发展，以对通路进行定量 PCR 检测为例就获得了无限商机。然而也正因于此，由于整体基因表达谱微芯片或深度 RNA 测序成本的迅速降低，才能够允许我们无偏倚地对基因表达差异进行对比。虽然在各种各样的文献中对于功能性通路的报道层出不穷，但是对于整体分析而言依旧值得我们去进一步探索。芯片的另一个常见应用就是用于发现生物标志物[7,8]。在这里特指可以用于检测在持续性既定状态下出现或与患者表型相关（急性或慢性排斥反应、肝移植再生或功能障碍）的特异性 mRNA[9–12]。

十年间已经有大量基因组学文献在移植方面对小鼠模型和人类患者进行研究，确定了不同的基因表达谱。研究数据囊括了对于正常和排异肾脏、肝脏、心脏和肺组织的活检，以及在不同组织培养基、小动物模型、血细胞亚群（Treg、B 细胞、巨噬细胞）下对不同免疫及炎症细胞、术后耐受肾组织及肝移植术后患者外周血细胞的分析。因此，对于研究某一基因的基因表达而言时，最事半功倍的做法就是首先在公共领域数据库中查询现有文献。在此提供几个较为可靠的数据库，基因表达数据库（Gene Expression Omnibus，GEO）、NIH 国家图书馆医学基因表达数据库（http:// www.ncbi.nlm.nih.gov/geo/）以及欧洲生物信息学研究所的数组快捷档案（http:// www.ebi.ac.uk/arrayexpress/）。另一个较好的数据来源就是在特定领域内搜索独立文献，大部分文章都可以在基因表达数据库中找到专供读者浏览的补充图表，或者这些文献已经收录于以上介绍的这几个数据库之中。这些数据库都是强有力的实验工具，尤其是对于那些具有丰富经验的生物信息学家而言，应该充分善用这一资源。

还有一点重要的是，查询投稿提交指南 MIAME（Minimum Information About a Microarray Experiment）有助于规范实验术语。但是目前尚没有相关机构对这些公共数据进行质量把控。这些实验在数据质量、技术平台、实验方法和实验设计上的一些关键步骤都存在极大差异，而且也并没有在 MIAME 数据库中对关键细节问题进行详细具体的描述。事实上，即便这些上千甚至上百万的数据存在这样那样的问题，也并不意味着这些基础实验就会戛然而止。基于同样态度的研究人员在得到任何结论之前也会查询这些数据库，通过横向和纵向比较试图得到相对谨慎的实验设想和结论。

由此可见,我们认为那些声称通过各种生物信息学工具“挖掘”实验数据进而得到的某些结论可能夸大了其实际意义。相信生物信息学领域专家可能对我们提出的以上观点提出强烈反对。他们相信,通过全新的统计学方法结合对这些实验数据进行深入的挖掘和分析,他们已经成功将实验科学向前推进了一步。对此我们的态度是,不能只信任这些数据库,但是活用数据可以事半功倍。这些数据会经过时间的淘洗去伪存真。

基因表达谱芯片

通过商业芯片可以很轻易地对整体基因表达谱进行解读(表 16.1)。芯片通过在类似玻璃或者塑料斜面等物理表面印刷或合成 DNA 原位互补探针的方式发挥作用[13,14]。芯片上的每个独立位点上都有数以百计的探针,这些位点都是为专门研究某一特定 mRNA 转录产物而特异设计的。因此,你可以借助这些独特的探针通过在不同位点的特异性结合来识别和记录各种不同的 RNA 转录产物。目前通过现有的技术手段,只要应用 96 孔板就可以轻易将整个人类基因组探针位点打印出来。将这些探针移嫁在微珠表面同样可以制作成芯片(例如 Illumina)。各个芯片的工作原理相同,只是在力学和几何学上略有差异。应用这些技术得到的实验结果充分可信而且具有可重复性。

通过在全部样品中选取部分 RNA 转录产物并通过逆转录方式生成互补 cDNA,进而对这些 mRNA 进行定量和定性分析。大多数寡核苷酸芯片通过体外转录的方式用生物素标记 cRNA。这些 cRNA 分子再与芯片上的寡核苷酸探针进行杂交。杂交后,再用荧光分子标记生物素对芯片进行结合染色,最后再进行洗脱。将未结合转录产物洗脱后,在 UV 光照下激发染色芯片,此时记录每个芯片位点上释放的荧光信号,就可以定量地对基因标记的 mRNA 转录产物进行分析了。

得出的数据可以与提供的相关基因表达标定的信号量度进行比较,从而得出标准化的基因表达数据。多年来,我们使用过多种标准化工具进行研究,最近我们已通过 RMA 秩分量归一法对所有数据进行标准化处理[15]。然而,在对数据进行抽样对比前还需要完成一项重要步骤。我们发现,芯片在对极低信号水平进行检测时有明显放大差异表达的倾向。这是因为在对低信号进行标准化处理以及方差分析比较的过程中(见下文),倾向于选择一类数据点较少的信号变化作为参考,从而有可能夸大了信号的实际意义。如果每组数据有数百个芯片,那么这一情况可能不会造成很大影响,但如果数据样本量较小就可能难以避免这一情况的出现。因此通常在实验室中,我们会在对数据进行标准化处理之前先对信号进行筛选,将低信号去除。通常在特定实验中,这些低信号明显低于整个芯片中经过标准化处理的背景信号。虽然与数据本身相关,但在对信号进行 log2 处理后得到的数值,通常范围在 5.64~6.64 之间,相当于对 Affymetrix 芯片数据进行 log10 处理后的 50~100 的数据范围。虽然原理相同,但是如上所述,在除去低表达基因时,要考虑到芯片的背景阈值。

下面,我们对两个或多个不同实验组(例如分类)中的多个独立样本进行分类比较。以 50 例出现急性排斥反应和 50 例移植后功能良好患者行活检为例,这些样本中的不同基因称为差异表达。对芯片背景量进行标准化处理后,针对每个基因对应的数值或信号进行标准化处理后得到的数据就是原始数据。将数据根据实验设计进行分类比较(例如,排斥反应组对比对照组),将阳性变化标记为“上调”,将阴性变化标记为“下调”。差异表达通常被称为“折叠变化”,这是因为在排斥反应组中,选定基因通常出现多次反复上调或下调表现。在生物功能途径中可以通过各种方式研究这些差异表达基因,以探讨其在急性排斥反应中所发挥的作用。但是需要再次强调的是,这些对于差异表达基因的研究方式只是基于目前认知水平而提出的,尚有大量未知领域有待研究。也就是说,即便在一篇文章中提及了在大鼠模型中脑组织中的某一基因功能与生长因子受体信号传导相关,虽然有可能是某些类似的信号因子,但这并不能表明它在活化 B 细胞中起到的作用是相同

表 16.1 商业芯片

Affymetrix
3'IVT 芯片:HG U133 Plus 2.0
外显子探针芯片:人类基因 ST 芯片
全外显子 ST 芯片:人类外显子 ST 芯片
Agilent
基因芯片:SurePrint G3 人类基因表达芯片
全外显子 ST 芯片:SurePrint G3 外显子芯片
Illumia
微珠分析:人类 HT-12 v4 表达微珠分析

的。新一代的研究方式需要通过另一种全新的视角。实验发现，在复杂的数据系统中存在某些协同的表达方式，以此推断这些基因在发挥作用时可能存在某种协调功能。这些基因可能通过几十种不同的生物通路发挥作用，但重点是在既定环境中，这些关联基因在所有的生物通路中发挥作用时是有迹可循的。例如，急性排斥反应时调动T细胞受体反应，同时通过共刺激通路激活细胞因子基因上调，通过同源受体引起靶细胞增殖，不仅可以作用于功能传导途径，同时还可以抑制细胞凋亡。

然后就可以使用多种工具将差异表达基因列表依据功能生物学通路进行绘图，来研究在我们的标本中促进急性排斥反应的机制。读者应该牢记这些绘图工具仅仅建立在目前对基因的认识上，而基因的许多功能仍然有待发现。所以仅仅因为一个研究员关注小鼠大脑中的一个基因功能并宣布它与生长因子受体传递的信号相关，并不意味着其在激活的B细胞中的功能是一样的，但很可能它是某种形式的信号因子。新一代的绘图工具使用了一种大不相同的方法。他们从复杂的数据集中发现协同表达的行为模式，表明成组的基因功能存在某种关联网络。可能有十几个不同的功能各异的通路包含在这样的网络中，而研究者发现所有此网络中相连的基因、所有的功能通路，在特定情况下会以可预见的方式发生变化。例如，急性排斥反应可以引发经由T细胞受体传递的信号，上调一条共刺激通路的功能激活数个细胞因子基因，并通过它们的同源受体传递信号且触发诱导细胞增殖的功能通路，且抑制细胞凋亡。这一连串相关的事件在使用这些新工具时会全部显示在同一个网络中。Cytoscape是新一代的网络绘制工具的一个很好的例子，它是一款可供任何人使用的开源软件(http://www.cytoscape.org)。声称可以从基因表达数据推算出关联的功能通路的具体认识尚言之过早，但是任何研究项目都应该尝试使用这种工具。

差异表达的数据也可以用于制造特殊的生物标记，这种生物标记可以用来诊断活检中是否发生了排斥反应，或告知使用者一些特征，如严重程度或敏感度。分类预测是另一类工具，其采用由同一组样本创建的差异表达基因列表，以预测从不同但相似的对象中获得的一组新样本的分类，例如，急性排斥反应与对照组。这就是我们如何验证这样的基因列表，以及如何开发临床诊断使用的生物标志物，以及制订诊断结果中阳性和阴性预测值（平衡同组中每个样本的假阳性和假阴性分类以正确诊断如急性排斥）的受体操作曲线(ROC)。如前所述，有成千上万个数据点都遵守着实验设计的规则。你仍然需要仔细设计实验，设置适当的变量控制和恰当的各组样品数量，然后重复和验证任何结果。

实验设计：效力、重复、批次和验证

在从全球的表达谱芯片上得出可靠的结论之前都需要考虑统计学效力的问题。现在用于类比较和类预测的工具可以提供具有高统计学意义的候选基因列表。但是，如果研究组没有足够的样本量，那么这些候选基因调用的统计学效力可能非常低，而且在着重于新发现的出版物中往往没有进行解释。作为基于多年计算数组实验的统计学效力的通用指南，我们发现，在基因表达实验中，每组20个样本时可以有85%或以上的效力以检测到1.5或更大的倍数变化。尽管如此，即使一开始具有令人满意的统计学效力，你必须至少使用在临床样本分析设计上规模近似的独立样本队列重复这个实验一次，或是在细胞培养或是基于动物模型的实验中采取相同实验设计的情况下使用另一组生物复制重复这个实验。

不过，也有着用于特定目标的其他途径。例如，在完善的实验系统中的假设生成阶段可以始于少量的微队列作为探索的第一步；例如，每组6个队列通常较为合适。你还是要重复一次实验以确认结果，但你仍然每组只有12个队列。然后，基于高价值候选者的明确列表，使用正交机械型工作设计法来验证你的结果，如敲减你预测的几个对于反应过程关键信号分子，以qPCR或蛋白质磷酸化测量下游基因的改变，或是对细胞增殖或其他一些细胞功能的广泛影响。

批次处理是指对样品进行分组并为实际分析做准备的关键步骤。每当你有不同的技术人员准备总RNA或标记过程中许多步骤之一时，你可能会引入一种我们称为“批次效应”的技术偏倚。每次更改用于标记的套件类型或套件批次时，或购买一组新的队列并实验完成的每一天，都可能会引入批次效应。所以我们大费周章地安排实验，使每个部分都由相同的技术人员以完全相同的方式完成。我们总是随机抽取样品，以使来自不同实验组和对照组的各个样品的日期、队列和试剂都平等分配。我们每天还将 mRNA 库(例如,活化的 T 细胞)至少重复制作 3 次,其处理与其他样品完全一样,但是技术过程不可避免地引入某些数据变异。虽然有统计工具可用于去除硅片中的批次效应,但这些工作会难以避免地减少你可以研究的基因数量以及用于比较的信号的动态范围,从而牺牲了潜在的重要生物学细节。我们坚信,良好的实验设计是最小化批次效应、强调生物学差异的最佳方式,这是整个工作的重点。

最后,我们应该谈谈验证,因为这在审查论文和准过方面经常出现。首先,质疑当代微芯片的技术重复性没有任何意义,因为它们已经建立了成熟的平台间和平台内良好可重复性[16],现在做这种事只是浪费金钱和人力。验证生物重复性才是应该做的。其次,如果前述工作都正确进行,那么要求有基因表达结果明显不同的 qPCR 重复性真的没有任何意义。没有人会要求使用微芯片来确认 qPCR 产生的结果,在正确操作的前提下,我们应当像"信任"qPCR 一样"信任"微芯片的结果。如果微芯片分析没有被正确地完成,则使用 qPCR 不足以挽救结果。所以如果验证是必要的,那么最好的方法是通过不同的方法和技术进行正交验证。例如,如果微芯片证明某个信号通路对于某个实验系统至关重要,那么敲减或过度表达此通路,创建一个记录器结构,显示对下游的影响等将有更大价值,特别是在机械意义上。如果结论涉及临床预后如急性排斥反应,则应参考包括动物模型在内的现有文献,并考虑在平行临床样本上进行质谱法蛋白质组学或在使用细胞或动物的临床预后模型中验证假设(例如,急性排斥组织活检中的 T 细胞活化或蛋白质组学分析)。

通过深度 RNA 测序(RNAseq)进行基因制谱

最新的基因表达谱技术是深度 RNA 测序。这些仪器的工作原理是检测并读出通过接合体固定到载玻片、小珠或电子传感器表面的 mRNA 或 miRNA 转录物的序列。这些技术的详细内容十分复杂,超出了本章的范围[17]。但是基本原理是对从靶细胞或组织获得的各个 mRNA 转录物进行大规模平行测序。因此,上文讨论的代替简单地检测与微芯片上的特异性互补探针杂交的给定 mRNA 序列的量,深 RNA 测序通过一次添加一个碱基,不断循环读出整个捕获的转录物序列,并且检测荧光产生的信号或如带电氢分子释放的信号。大规模是通过在同一个表面上捕获数以百万计的转录物,并在每个周期中并行排序。

mRNA 转录物的相对数量取决于每个 mRNA 在 RNA 库中确定的序列对准或映射到该特定基因从而获得的读数。这项操作在开始时与标记整个 mRNA 转录物非常不同,将其与互补寡核苷酸探针杂交,并读出在微芯片上指定点检测到的荧光信号总量。另一方面,技术发展的本质就是不同于过去。所以,首要的问题就是任何技术获得的数据的实际价值是否存在明显差异。一旦两种技术都准确地提供了总 RNA 池中 mRNA 转录物的相对数量的数值时,就了解所揭示的转录信息的生物学意义而言,两者价值是相同的。深度测序是最新技术的事实并不会使你的数据变得神奇或是赋予其神奇的价值。关键在于了解这些技术的局限性和优点,然后合理地应用这些技术。

用于比较深度测序技术的常用度量单位是"读取长度",如它字面上的意思代表着某一项技术可以在单次字符串读取时获得的最大序列长度(表 16.2)。目前的"短读"仪器可以单次读取到 250 个碱基对,也可以做到单次向基因的两个方向读取同样的距离,被称作双端测序读取。目前的"长读"工具可以单次读取上至 750 碱基对,而几家制造商声称他们可以达到单次读取 1000 碱基对,而且这个数据在不久的将来会更长。虽然这些在描述性文献中听起来很好,但事实上使用深度 RNA 测序进行基因表达谱分析时,单向读取长度为 50~100 碱基对就完全够用了。长度更长的读取及双端测序读取并不是必需的,而且仅会增加成本。然而,

表 16.2　深度测序技术

次世代深度测序(短读)
Illumina HiSeq 2000
SOLid 5500xi
次世代深度测序(长读)
Roche 454 FLX
Pacific Biosciences
"个性化"深度测序平台
Ion Torrent
Illumina MiSeq
Roche 454 Junior

如果你还希望测量选择性剪接的 mRNA 并用于识别不同的外显子,则非常需要双端测序读取 100~150 碱基对,甚至是必需的。

尽管如此,大多数关于实现更大量和更长的读取长度以及越来越强的测序能力的商业炒作都指向 DNA 测序和遗传学。目前的商业竞争是谁能第一个达到仅用 1000 美元或更少的价格提供达到"医学级"准确度标准的完整人类基因组测序,一般认为这个价格将会立刻开启理想中的个体化医疗时代。我们期待着这一技术成果的实现,并认识到它会降低临床上不同患者人群中全基因组的测序门槛。在一个新的领域中拥有更多数据是一件好事。但是仅仅获得更多的数据,即便以每人基因组测序 35 亿个碱基的速度获得数据,不等于突然理解了成功地提供真正的个体化医疗所需的基因生物功能及其对健康和疾病的影响。在解决了功能基因组学领域中那些极为复杂的挑战,或是解读基因组代码中包含的生物学、健康和疾病方面的信息之前,宣称在成功简化测序方面取得了革命性影响只是夸大其词。

深度 RNA 测序的另一个关键指标是"读取深度"。对 RNA 的深度测序得到的数据通过将所给样本的所有读取结果与人类基因组的已知序列匹配,来揭示检测到的读数。作为对成功的 RNAseq 的简易指南,我们的目标是使所有获得的人类基因读数成功比对率达到 75%~80%。基于 RNAseq 的基因表达分析的目的是简单地检测总 RNA 池中某种 mRNA 转录物的存在和相对数量。因此,一条 Illumina HiSeq 2000 通道大约 2 亿读数具有 80%比对率时,可以获得约 1.6 亿个基因组序列读数。如果你从通过仅将测序接合体放在 mRNA 上创建的 RNA 库开始,则可以认为每个读数(例如 1.6 亿个)可以映射到已知人类基因的编码序列作为个体事件。一般认为有任何转录物至少十个读数,就足以有统计学意义证明此转录物是存在的。因此,如果要测量两个不同样本中相同转录物或 miRNA 的相对表达数量,仅需要依赖两个条件(例如,休息与激活,对照与排斥)下检测到的读数数量的差别,就可以检测并定量基因表达的差别。

但是,如果你还想相互比较同一个实验中的多个不同的 mRNA 转录物,那么你必须先要"标准化"的数据。标准化是非常重要的,因为每个 mRNA 长度均不相同。因此,读取到 100 个 5000 碱基对长的基因转录物的概率显著高于读取到 100 个仅 1000 碱基长的 mRNA 的概率。将深度 RNA 测序数据标准化为独立的基因长度产生了术语 FPKM(测序 1 000 000 个片段后映射到外显子每一千个碱基对中片段的数量)[18]。如果你不想只是简单地确认所给基因转录物的存在,并将其变化与其他可以产生功能通路或调节你所研究的基因转录物进行比较,那么这件事就很重要,因为这是你展示最终结果该用的方式。

事实上,一旦建立了标准化基因检测值(FPKM),所有用于分析微芯片基因表达谱的标准工具都可以互换使用深度 RNA 测序表达的数据。这件事在实践中十分重要,因为过去十年为我们建立了一个非常成熟的流程,以及多个用于分析和图像化从微芯片获得的全局基因表达数据的经验证可靠的工具,而不必依靠生物信息学专家来分析你的数据。这些也可以用于深度 RNA 测序产生的数据,对我们所有人来说都是非常重要的。

以此为明确的起点,现在一些深度 RNA 测序所能做到的事情相比微芯片来说都是重大进步。事实上,这些新成果开拓了功能基因组研究的全新领域。例如,将复合型条码已经证明的有效性给予成功测序一组同一条细胞流道上不同样本,我们现在已经熟练地使用深度测序进行 miRNA 分析。此方法的成本计算和可信范围明显优于任何当前可用的商业 miRNA 芯片。我们现在正在利用深层 miRNA 测序进行更多的研究,如同时分析成熟 miRNA 和前体 miRNA (pre-mIR)。因此,miRNA 基因最初被转录以在细胞核中产生初级 miRNA(pri-mIR),然后,该转录物通过 Drosha 和 DGCR8 (例如 Pasha)以特定的茎环结构拼合成为剪切蛋白以被识别。之后 pri-miR 通过一系列能量依赖步骤运输到细胞质中另一种称作导入蛋白 5 的蛋白质。一旦进入细胞质中,由 DICER 和 Argonaut 形成另一种 RNA 剪接复合体以产生成熟的 miRNA,并将其转运到靶 mRNA 转录物。所有这些步骤都受到调节,但我们对其知之甚少。深度测序为推动对此的研究创造了一个新的机会。另一个例子是 RNA 表达谱与遗传变异研究之间的交集。因为深度测序揭示了实际的序列,此成果可用于研究编码转录物(例如,外显子序列)中出现遗传变异。在这项研究中采用的技术,是与将 DNA 进行外显子组捕捉(如全外显子组测序)后使用深度测序技术的基因变异研究相结合。然而,读者应该注意,实验设计中所需的测序深度及检测此类变异的分析管线,与通常基因表达谱中所用的大不相同。最后,该领域的另一个非常惊艳的新方向是长非编码 RNA (lncRNA)的分析。目前,由 ENCODE 联盟(DNA 因子百科;由 NIH 的国家人类基因研究所建立)发布的研究成果中,已经明确 RNA 是由人类基因上许多固有的非编码区域产生,或是由特定基因转录物产生,在后者过程中 NDA 的反义链也被转录, 但是不会编码已知的蛋白质[19]。lncRNA 的功能以及 lncRNA 在应对激活、应激及其他信号时如何调节基因表达和细胞功能的规律尚待发现。

使用深度 RNA 测序进行选择性剪切以及目前的挑战

我们认为, 选择性剪接的研究是移植生物学的下一个重要探索领域之一, 因为这种剪接技术是创造基因组多样性的强大工具, 可以随意地改变细胞的蛋白质组[20]。此外,细胞激活导致选择性剪接基因谱的细胞发生显著改变, 这种改变经表达谱测量后发现,与 mRNA 转录物层次的变化无关。

在我们迄今为止的经验中,通过配对末端读取深度 RNA 测序获得的数据,显著优于用于使用最新一代微芯片选择性剪切所获得的数据。但是,根据我们的经验,选择性剪接需要配对终端读取(通常长度为 100×100)、更深的测序深度(例如,每个流道的样本量更少)以及更为复杂的生物信息学工作来检测外显子转录情况的差异, 这些显著增加了完成单次流程所需的成本和时间。因此,在成本方面,使用 Affymetrix(GeneChip Human Exon 1.0 ST Array) 提供的商业微芯片进行选择性剪切分析经济效益更高, 此微芯片有着目前人类基因组构建中所有已知外显子的探针。而问题在于如何确定数据的质量。在使用这种芯片和深度测序的经验中我们发现, 由芯片检测到的剪接事件中有 25%无法通过测序验证。但仍然有 75%的样本可以被检测到,这些数据足以用来比较两种技术, 正如下面讨论的那样,在比较两种方法时,保持开放性思维非常重要,正确使用每种方法都有价值。我们要提醒读者,微芯片技术也在持续发展。Affymetrix 承诺新一代剪切拼接芯片具有可定制的新型探针, 这项新技术基于对选择性剪切和外显子-内含子交界带了解的不断加深,这可能会缩小或消除今后与配对末端 RNA 深度测序的差距。因此,在进行技术以及实验设计前,读者们应向当地技术基因组的技术专家咨询以获取最新信息。

但是, 选择性剪切也提出了目前所面临的两大挑战。首先,检测外显子的不同用途很难,因为事实并不是简单的某个基因只有一种可能的替代形式, 并简单地以 1:1 的比例共存。大多数基因具有多个不同的转录物(常有 6 个或更多),它们可以以任何比例混合存在,并且在任何特定的时间及条件下,总 RNA 池中都可存在每种已知基因的多种不同转录物 (例如同工型)。而且如果你想要进一步为难自己,在细胞池中不同细胞中的同一基因会有数组不同的转录物亚型,而这些细节我们直到有了单细胞基因表达谱(见后述章节)技术之前都不知道。所以第一个挑战是,选择性剪切需要技术努力和资源。

第二个挑战是理解得到的选择性剪接数据的意义。想要清楚地解释这个挑战,需要先介绍一下目前功能基因学的背景知识。目前在这个领域,如果你正确标准化并检测编码某个蛋白的基因的 mRNA 转录物有显著差异的表达,那么你就能证明这个蛋白的存在。仍然有一些较顽固的研究者喜欢反复提起一个错误的学术观点——“可能存在没有对应蛋白质的转录物”。实际上,现有的 mRNA 制谱和蛋白质组学技术的检测技术、覆盖深度和动态范围的差异解释了为什么很难检测由全 mRNA 表达谱预测到的每一个蛋白质。事实上,当蛋白质组学覆盖深度很深时, 可以检测蛋白质中大部分的细胞蛋白质编码转录组[21]。因此,对转录物提起重视听起来非常有科学意义, 但是要求研究者耗费宝贵的资源和精力去进行平行的蛋白质组学实验, 而这些实验非常耗费精力(例如,蛋白质印迹实验或非定量免疫组织化学实验),并且原始结论提升很少。诚然,如果在设计良好的实验中有一个已知的编码 mRNA 转录物, 通过适当保守地使用最新一代的信息学工具进行数据分析来进行验证,将会得到对应的蛋白质。

然而,对于选择性剪切技术来说,情况完全不同。首先, 许多选择性剪切操作会截断转录物并阻止其翻译为蛋白。但更重要的是,我们对某种选择性剪切改变对蛋白的功能会有什么影响, 以及关于其在细胞内复杂的分子通路中有什么样的作用,都知之甚少。举例来说,我们可以确认在某个特定细胞群或组织内,一个外显子的转录物被剪除 25%后, 观察到这个外显子包含了一种衔接蛋白的结合序列或因激活被磷酸化的酪氨酸。但是目前我们只能猜测在某个情况下,例如,记忆

CD4 细胞的免疫激活过程，这些主要的结构改变对于细胞应答的意义。其次，探究选择性剪切仅是第一步，而且在我们理解在真正的功能和分子层面究竟发生了什么之前都没有重要意义。但毫无疑问的是，选择性剪切可以对蛋白质造成重要的改变，包括蛋白质的功能、在细胞内的位置、与传导通路中其他关键物质复合的能力，或是识别配体的能力，甚至调节 mRNA 转录物的半衰期。透彻地理解移植免疫生理学，并将这些发现与现存的知识整合到一起，是新基因技术创造的重大的科学机遇。

但是，也有一些有建设意义的注意事项。选择性剪切所带来的这些挑战是功能基因组学研究中种种缺陷的一个完美例子；每当通过新技术了解到新的知识时，都会引诱研究者在不考虑会耗费生物学上多少努力的情况下计算大量的数据。然而，通过合理设计的实验和预期，用新技术进行探索分析绝对可以合理地成为必要的第一步；例如，为了证明我们几年前报道过的 T 细胞和 B 细胞激活时，基因转录和选择性剪切变化间的复杂关系[4]。如果没有至少先使用这些新的分析技术建立与我们意欲发展的生物学知识相关的理论可能性，那以综合方式研究选择性剪切的意义何在？但是，一旦建立了这样的概念证据，接下来的一系列实验必须在一定程度上创造新的知识，而对于选择性剪切来说，这并不是个小挑战。只要我们明确知道任何指定的一组实验的目标和相对价值，妥善处理限定条件，不要将使用新奇的新技术与不切实际的知识相混淆，那么这就是科学工作的自然发展过程。

微芯片法与 RNA 深度测序的对比

目前一个非常重要的问题就是应该使用 RNA 深度测序还是微芯片法来进行基因表达分析。答案是“视情况而定”。

RNA 深度测序的灵敏度取决于读取深度。因此，一些专家得出初步结论，通过真正的深度测序，将会发现许多永远不会被微芯片检测到转录物。这就是目前人们认为微芯片“逐渐被淘汰”的开端，RNA 深度测序揭示了全新层次的转录活动。具有讽刺意味的是，这种观点还支持另一个不正确的观点，即 RNA 转录分析需要非常深的测序深度，以便能够检测到这些“隐藏”的转录物，而如此深层次的测序成本是非常昂贵的。通过深层次的 RNA 测序观察到低表达水平的转录物的检测结果是绝对真实的，但是“魔鬼”隐藏在细微之处。当你对如癌细胞系这种特化良好的细胞系统进行足够深层次的测序时，结果发现大多数检测到的低表达水平基因转录实际上可能只是转录噪音，而且这些转录物往往不映射到与正在研究的条件相关且有重要生物意义的通路上[22-24]。事实上这并不令人惊讶，因为我们许多年前已经知道所有的基因组系统都是存在“漏出”的，而因此我们提出了“充满噪音的转录组”的假设。我们最近对活化的人 T 细胞进行了非常深层次的 RNA 测序，以证明这些低表达水平转录物中的大部分在功能意义上确实是“杂音”，提示了这些基因的位置非常接近高转录基因并且在高转录基因的转录隔离子边界内，这解释了“漏出”的原因（稿件已提交）。我们还证明了大多数这些嘈杂的转录物没有被深层次蛋白质组学覆盖范围检测到。此外，随着新型定向测序法的发展，我们还认识到这些低水平转录物中部分来自编码基因的互补链。前面讨论过的推测为调节性 lncRNA 转录物就是一个功能过去被误认定的例子，它实际上功能是编码转录。这些发现造成的一个实际影响是，全基因表达分析不需要非常深层次的 RNA 测序覆盖范围，于是芯片法与深度测序的成本/价值公式突然间发生了巨大变化。

目前，如果你的目标只是简单的全基因表达分析，那么你是选择微芯片法或深度 RNA 测序其实并不重要。这个结论是基于我们最近完成的为器官移植联盟中 NIH 临床试验联盟进行的比较研究得出的（稿件已提交）。此项试验性工作流程中的细节上与以往有很大不同，但得出的 RNA 分析数据基本上是相同的。与最近的热潮相反，深层 RNA 测序并不比最新一代商业用微芯片具有更高的敏感性、特异性或是可重复性。当然，我们无法改变错误的观念，即具有如此潜力的新技术一定具有强大的功能，或者使新项目成为“高精尖”水平就需要使用深度测序。但简单的事实是，最新一代的商业 DNA 微芯片功能非常强大、易于使用、经济效益极高且具有高度的可重复性，可在 2 天内完成 100 个芯片的全自动化吞吐量，并且基本上可以在本地每个核心学术机构或在社区服务性的商业实验室中使用。此外，Scripps 公司的全 RNA 表达微芯片[Affymetrix ST 1.1ST 与深层 RNA 测序（具有 NuGEN 资料库的准备和多路复用的 Illumina HiSeq2000）对比]进行成本对比发现每个样品成本包括人工费后，微芯片法为约 225 美元，而深层测序为约 400 美元/样品。

另一方面,在深度 RNA 测序实验的设计期间就可以控制测序的深度。因此,为了检测拷贝数很低的转录物,可以将检测灵敏度提高到适宜水平。这在复杂的细胞混合物（如移植活组织检查）的情况下可能非常重要，其中正在研究的效应细胞仅占所分析细胞总数中很小一部分。

但是,正如我们之前详细讨论过的,一旦你想要进行比简单的基因表达分析更进一步的研究，情况就会大不相同。深度测序在 miRNA 研究、选择性剪切、遗传变异、lncRNA 和发现新 RNA 形态等方面具有巨大的优势,ENCODE 联盟正在进行此方面的研究。另外,所有技术都在迅速更新这一点也并不令人惊讶。近来已经引入了许多可以产生用于深度 RNA 测序的数据库的商用自动化仪器，并且这些仪器具有相当大的希望可以明显降低进门门槛、时间和人力成本。另一个在迅速发展的深度测序的技术领域，其中具有代表性的就是由 Life Technologies 公司提供的 IonTorrent 仪器,该技术使用新型的固态序列检测方案，可以将测序所需要的时间从目前的 1 周缩短到不到 1 天(http://www.iontorrent.com)。而为了不被淘汰,Illumina 公司已经在其 MiSeq 设备上加入了最新版本的 TruSeq 化学测序,这项技术可以几乎同等程度地缩短运行时间(http://www.illumina.com/systems/miseq.ilmn),并将读取长度增加到 250 个碱基(可以双端模式运行,单次可读取 500 个碱基)。举例来证明这很重要:双端读取覆盖率的显著增加使对整个 VDJ 区域进行测序成为可能,以及分析移植后或输血后由抗原暴露导致的 B 细胞抗体生成中的重组情况的能力。

因此,在作出决定之前,你应该与你的功能基因组学专家以及当地核心实验室的技术专家一起讨论得出实验问题的最佳选择。最后要注意的是,你必须与有经验的技术专家来进行讨论、设计实验并正确地解析结果,否则最好的方法或技术都是没有价值的。仅仅购买仪器是不够的。最终考虑事项应该是专家、工作流程的复杂性、总成本、实验需要的时间和资源以及可用于数据分析的资源。

下一代 qPCR——数码及单细胞 qPCR

正如在新技术的快速发展过程中经常发生的,新发现为旧技术发展带来了新契机,并满足特定技术空缺或要求。对于微芯片和深度测序来说,技术开发的循环也转回了创造新一代的定量 PCR(qPCR)技术。因此,这些新技术也应考虑到 mRNA 转录物分析的实验设计中来。使用微芯片或深度测序来分析 RNA 转录物在鉴别不同环境或临床状态之间相对变化具有很大的作用。而另一个明显的优点是它们可以通过测序实现无偏差、全局表达分析,甚至发现新的 RNA 形态。但这些技术也有一些限制,可以通过 qPCR 来更好地解决。

首先，微芯片以及深度测序不能像 qPCR 一样严格定量,尽管声称 RNA 深度测序是一种“数字表达”数据的形式。如果可以正确地标准化,深度 RNA 测序数据可以横向对比不同条件下单个转录物表达的变化进行高准确度的比较，但是在得出成千上万个基因之间的表达比较结论时，更需要注意数据有同等级别数位及精确度。例如，我们一组由实验室合成的 400 个 miRNA,配置成相同的浓度并将其用作为“阳性”对照组，对我们开发的新的多重深度测序方案进行基准校对测试[25]。然而,并没有像所预测的“数字表达”技术那样,读数接近全部 400 个 miRNA,结果是每种方法获得精确读数都存在差异。我们还不能确定是什么原因导致了这一令人惊讶的结果。

第二，微芯片是基于使用互补的 DNA 或 RNA 探针与标记的 mRNA 杂交捕获目标的,结果在不同序列中不尽相同,创造了数据的多样性,且具有用于筛选表现不佳探针组的潜力。好消息是,RNA 深度测序数据库受这种限制较小。而另一方面,准备 RNA 测序数据库时，有多种酶活性和扩增步骤易受测序内容特异性偏差影响。第三,qPCR 可以在不到 1 小时内完成,而大多数使用芯片和测序方法的研究需要至少 1 天或 2 天的时间才能完成,并有着更高的分析成本。这让 qPCR 在你有明确的想要分析的目标基因的情况下成为成本效益更高的方法,而且在用于功能性通路相关的 qPCR 图谱(例如,Treg 细胞、炎症、细胞凋亡、NFκB 信号传导)时尤其高效。第四,微芯片上杂交捕获法检测 RNA 转录物的灵敏度总是会比 qPCR 检测明显降低。这种限制对深度 RNA 测序来说并不存在。但是,如果足够深层次的测序真的可以检测到几乎所有的转录物,即使其没有生物学功能，我们很好奇究竟需要多少次极高循环数的 PCR 才能检测到该转录物来证明实验中涉及某个通路或基因。

在新基因组学时代，第一个挑战就是使 qPCR 技术能够在一次运行中处理至少数百甚至数千个基因。较早的一个例子是由 Applied Biosystem 公司研发的 qPCR 仪器,打破了 96 孔的瓶颈并创造了 384 孔 qPCR 板(TaqMan 低密度芯片; TLDA)。这些反应可以在仅仅 1μL 体积内完成,可以明显节省试剂成本和时间。我们使用这种技术可以单次验证微芯片获得的 100 个候选基因表达结果,并且最近已经测试了其用于验证选择性剪切技术的效果。然而,最新一代的 ABI qPCR 技术提供了 OpenArray 系统，能够单次运行产生超过 30 000 个数据点,可轻松地完成 1000 个基因的分析。

应用 Wafergen 公司开发的 qPCR 技术开发了一种芯片,可以一次运行 5184 个不同的 qPCR 反应,从而使并行分析 1000 个基因 4 遍成为可能。这种技术也可以在纳升体积内进行，有着自动化高吞吐量工作的巨大潜力。Luminex 公司使用了不同的平台但具有相似的目标,使用其荧光珠技术设计了高通量、多路复用、基于珠粒的 qPCR 方法。这种技术的优点是,声称他们可以在单个珠粒填充的孔内复用多达 500 种不同的 qPCR 测定,使用他们的荧光珠设备 1 天内可以很轻松地对几百或更多不同临床患者样品进行分析。这些技术显示出的能力将会非常重要，因为生物标志物的转录物分析结果被转化为临床诊断,其消耗的成本、人力和时间变得非常重要。读者应该期待这方面的新技术和新公司的持续发展。

由 Fluidigm 公司开发并实施的另一个新的 qPCR 技术平台,称为 BioMark 系统,利用微流体工程技术创建了一个能够在纳升的空间内仅仅几个小时内单次运行中进行 9216 次 qPCR 反应的平台。该系统的 qPCR 采用 ABI 公司的 TaqMan 技术，具有几乎相同的灵敏度和可重复性。第一个主要的优点是在单次运行中可完成的反应数量明显增加。在标准配置中,平台可以对 96 个不同样品(例如,适用于临床生物标志物分析)的 96 个不同的基因、同一样品的 9216 个基因或是可满足 96×96 反应孔格式的基因与样品的任意组合。事实上，微流体工程的设计带来了第二个主要优势，将新 qPCR 技术应用到单细胞基因表达中。此技术的实现是因为 BioMark 仪器中的微流体芯片具有多个可以选择性连接到多个反应位点的并行样本位点。因此,使用其 96×96 芯片设计,研究人员可以在一次运行中对 96 个单个细胞中的 96 个基因逐个进行分析。这种单细胞方法开始揭示复杂细胞混合物中每个不同细胞的区别。这对研究癌细胞混合物非常重要，因为其中单个恶性细胞的行为就可以影响整体预后。

单细胞分析技术能对移植生物学和免疫学的机制了解多少尚待研究。因此,关键问题是,我们的生理学研究究竟是分析单个细胞还是分析包括全部细胞大混合物才能得到更好的结果。如上所述,仅当这些技术成熟可用且研究人员愿意及时投入时间在移植方面开展这些技术时,我们才可以开始提出这些关键问题。

非 PCR 转录物侦测和数字 PCR

虽然我们认识到基于 PCR 的基因检测有着强大的功能和实用性,但 PCR 也存在一些限制。首先,PCR 的表现明显受目标序列的影响,就像 DNA 微芯片使用的 DNA 杂交方法一样，我们也怀疑深层 RNA 测序所需的逐步碱基配对亦是如此。目前,有功能完美的 PCR 引物组,也有对同一靶基因靶序列效果略差的引物组,只因为两个个体间由于遗传或获得性基因差异，导致序列引物结合位点上下游的仅几百个碱基或仅有几个碱基对改变。虽然我们几乎总是可以优化单一反应 PCR 的表现，但当我们想要一次进行数百或数千种不同的 PCR 反应时情况就会很不一样,因此,必须让所有反应在相同的反应条件下进行。其次,为 PCR 灵敏度高付出的代价之一就是以目前的技术不同反应间有较大的差异(往往以对数级别衡量)。这就是为什么 qPCR 反应通常是并行 4 次,并将结果用于计算平均表达数据。第三,完成 PCR 循环的次数越多,因扩增偏差导致靶序列产生差异的风险就越大。因此，真正定量 PCR 方法需要纯化的靶序列（通常是该基因的 cDNA 克隆）的平行对照以及将每个基因精确稀释到各浓度组。这样所需的基因控制变得非常复杂,限制了任何试图达到绝对量化的、高通量的、多基因 qPCR 分析的尝试。事实上,以上讨论的任何“次世代”qPCR 平台都没能克服这些挑战。

PCR 的这一限制的一个解决方案是 Affymetrix 公司的 Panomics Quantigene 系统，此系统没有需要检测的 PCR 扩增,因为单个孔中总共只有 200 个 mRNA 分子。在该技术中,基因特异性捕获探针首先结合到测定孔的底部或 Luminex 珠的表面。将样品加入每个孔中或珠粒混合物中并与捕获探针杂交过夜。在接下来的步骤中,第二组探针结合捕获 RNA 之后加入具有许多酶分子的支链 DNA 探针，当暴露于可溶性底物时就会产生比色或荧光定量。显而易见，这种技术事实上就是 ELISA 法，不过使用了 RNA 探针代替抗体，且靶物质是 RNA 转录物而不是蛋白质。这项技术对于在一次运行中精确分析几百个基因时非常有用，因其定量准确而且可以在 96 孔和 Luminex 珠粒格式使用。用于临床诊断的一个潜在缺点是需要一晚上的杂交步骤，因此，比当前 qPCR 的技术增加了约 1 天的时间。另外，费用上与目前简单的 qPCR 平台相比也不具有竞争力。

另一个 PCR 扩增偏差的解决方案是使用乳液 PCR 的新一代数字 PCR 技术。简单来说，这种技术是生成微小的油滴并稀释输入的总靶 RNA 样品，使得每个液滴中约包含有 1 个 mRNA 转录物。效果上，你已经创建了一个独立的包含单个靶 RNA 的整体，并且进行最多 40 个或更多个 PCR 循环而不存在任何竞争或由不同基因序列的引物对之间的相对差异而产生的偏差。

数字 PCR 的新技术使用微流体工程来建立能够在单次运行中使用微滴或结合微滴微珠进行数千次乳液 PCR 反应的仪器。例如，RainDance Technologies 公司开发了 RainDrop 数字 PCR 系统，可以一次为 8 个不同的样品自动创建 10^7 PL 的乳液 PCR 液滴，然后在单独的仪器上一次检测 96 个样品的扩增情况。该平台在技术上能够使用不同的荧光进行多次重复使用，因此，该平台可以一次分析一个样本中数百个基因或多个样品各 10 个基因。另一种乳液 PCR 仪器是 BioRad 公司的 QX100 Droplet Digital PCR 产品，其具有与 RainDrop 系统类似的工作原理及功能，但是可以每个样品产生约 20 000 滴液滴。从统计学上来看，BioRad 公司认为 20 000 滴可以准确生成用来捕捉所研究的差异表达的数字数据而绰绰有余，这在许多情况下可能是正确的。然而，RainDrop 系统的一个潜在优势是，有了如此多的液滴以供分析，降低初始 RNA 输入浓度不再必要，这可能会明显地优化工作流程。

断言数字 PCR 的功能相比目前所用的微芯片、RNA 深度测序和高通量定量 PCR 技术能达到怎样的水平为时尚早。然而，没有其他的基因表达平台目前真正地实现定量。关键是，如果这种新的数字 PCR 技术完全实现了其“数字化”的承诺，那么我们将有能力一次运行内绝对量化一个细胞在不同实验操控或疾病状态下数千个基因的 mRNA 转录物数量及其变化。这是非常值得关注的。

技术和实验设计

功能基因组学和系统的理论知识必须通过使用多种技术手段进行探求和验证，然后对这些技术得出的结果进行整合，并对结论进行严密地验证才能达到我们的目标。但这些技术每一项都很复杂且在迅速发展。其后果是该技术需要庞大的专业知识才能正确使用。此部分的第一点是，只是将一组样品交给核心实验室、要求使用特定的技术进行实验并返回最终结果的电子表格，听起来很简单但是这并不可行。即使实际上样品是由一批技术专家及其核心技术员来进行实验，科学家们也必须充分了解所选择的技术及其产生的数据。

事实上，这些基因组技术平台从仪器到套件几乎完全由商业生命科学公司主导，这就又增加了另一层炒作、误导、成本和竞争相关的因素。如果你看到广告，你可以每年更改十几次研究方法，并且每次都会得到“保证”新数据将多么好。但这都不是真的，而且研究方法的改变可能会严重破坏你的数据的价值，特别是当你需要比较可能是在 1 年或更长时间内产生的不同阶段的实验数据。因此第二点是，当你制订计划使用功能基因组来解决一个学术目标，你必须关注每一部分实验计划而不只是选择主要仪器平台。样品材料是如何采集、储存、纯化、扩增和标记，甚至选择的试剂盒的制造商对数据完整性的影响都与选择的芯片一样重要。例如，我们总以一种方式来纯化总 RNA，我们都相信这对于 DNA 微芯片“优化”杂交是必要的。直到有一天我们决定现在也想研究 miRNA 时，发现使用这种技术会滤除所有的 miRNA，这使得我们的所有样本都无法用来进行此项研究！

另一点是整合由不同技术得来的数据需要整合使用不同的物理法则获得的数据。例如，假设我们要总结的东西非常基础，就像当 RNA 转录物被上调之后对应的蛋白质的翻译也会上调。得出答案需要整合杂交法 DNA 捕获 DNA 微芯片探针上标记的 RNA 转录物和并用肽质谱法蛋白质组学产生的电离能量介导的发射光谱。因此，我们需要生物信息学专家开发计算方法，找到不同种类的数据的交叉点，才能整合来自多个技术平台的结果。在实践中，这意味着距离真正的进展还需要很长时间、庞大的资源和具有如何正确使用这些工具的具体知识的科学家团队。坦白地说,所有的技术已经成"挡路巨石"。你无法忽视它;而且必须处理掉它。但这绝对会将已经很复杂的科学难题变得更加复杂。人们从本能上往往会拒绝这种挑战,并认为"石头"并不重要,想着"这只是一个愚蠢的东西",或技术会干扰"真正的科学"或"我只是雇用专业人士来运行机器"。这对于功能基因组学来说并不比假装声称你只是聘请移植外科医生来进行手术更有说服力。在制订方案和解释结果的过程中,你必须接受至少一点点所选择的技术的"所有权",因为它们是复杂且不断变化的,这不是一个小小的挑战。

决定价值定位

如果功能基因组学(包括生物上和技术上)的复杂性构成了第一个挑战,第二个挑战就是决定这项工作的价值定位。这些引人注目的生物学新观点需要解决如何将功能基因组学应用于改变医学实践的问题。一个重要的价值定位是,基础和转化学家将以功能基因组学为指导进行次世代细胞或器官的生物学的机制理论研究。这些基础理论知识将来自多个模型系统以及人类受试者。证明工作的合理性对推进对健康和疾病的生物学机制的理解是关键且必要的。良好的科学是一剂良药。但是最终某领域的成功将由我们为患者、家属、卫生保健服务系统、我们的社会所创造的价值定位来决定。我们所有的工作都直接或间接地由这些期望所资助。有很多方法可以从科学创造价值,但最终价值必须被创造。

例如,假设你决定你要了解由B细胞介导的慢性排斥反应的分子基础。我们都认同这是一个非常有价值的目标。然后我们考虑责任的问题。没人能一下就承担如此重大的任务。这项工作需要分散成多个阶段,需要细化,并按阶段提供资金并发布成果。功能基因组学很强大,生物学很复杂,而你选择的临床难题对于医学至关重要,不意味着您可以简单地分析一堆活组织检查标本或血液样本就得出任何有用的答案或提出任何价值定位。在任何新功能基因组学研究计划的制订中,首先要确认你希望研究的内容,以及这些工作将如何贡献真正的价值。请在此技术方面专家的帮助下进行分析。之后你才可以设计并优化你的研究使其成功。

总结

我们相信功能基因组学将推动新的发现。为了创造价值,此发现必须建立在对我们临床移植原则有着务实认识的基础上。如果做到这一点,这将指导移植中生物标志物的发展,并且直接应用到实践以及建立在假设上的移植免疫学、排斥反应和耐受相关的机制研究。但是我们必须认清现实。目前,功能基因组学揭示的细胞生物学和免疫学的复杂内涵将需要大量的研究、培养新一代临床和基础研究员,以及对我们目前的实验设计方法的改进,之后我们才真正成为"宇宙霸主"。

(郭颂一 译 李照 校)

参考文献

1. Brody E, Abelson J. The "spliceosome": yeast pre-messenger RNA associates with a 40S complex in a splicing-dependent reaction. Science. 1985;228: 963-967.
2. Abmayr SM, Reed R, Maniatis T. Identification of a functional mammalian spliceosome containing unspliced pre-mRNA. Proceedings of the National Academy of Sciences of the United States of America. 1988;85:7216-7220.
3. Lopez AJ. Alternative splicing of pre-mRNA: developmental consequences and mechanisms of regulation. Annual Review of Genetics. 1998;32:279-305.
4. Grigoryev YA, Kurian SM, Nakorchevskiy AA, et al. Genome-wide analysis of immune activation in human T and B cells reveals distinct classes of alternatively spliced genes. PLoS ONE. 2009;4:e7906.
5. Fabian MR, Sonenberg N, Filipowicz W. Regulation of mRNA translation and stability by microRNAs. Annual Review of Biochemistry. 2010;79:351-379.
6. Hay N, Sonenberg N. Upstream and downstream of mTOR. Genes and Development 2004;18:1926-1945.
7. Quackenbush J. Microarray analysis and tumor classification. New England Journal of Medicine. 2006;354:2463-2472.
8. Kittleson MM, Hare JM. Molecular signature analysis: using the myocardial transcriptome as a biomarker in cardiovascular disease. Trends in Cardiovascular Medicine. 2005;15:130-138.
9. de Jonge J, Kurian S, Shaked A, et al. Unique early gene expression patterns in human adult-to-adult living donor liver grafts compared to deceased donor grafts. American Journal of Transplantation. 2009;9:758-772.
10. Flechner SM, Kurian SM, Head SR, et al. Kidney transplant rejection and tissue injury by gene profiling of biopsies and peripheral blood lymphocytes. American Journal of Transplantation. 2004;4:1475-1489.
11. Kurian SM, Heilman R, Mondala TS, et al. Biomarkers for early and late stage chronic allograft nephropathy by proteogenomic profiling of peripheral blood. PLoS ONE. 2009;4:e6212.
12. Levitsky J, Salomon DR, Abecassis M, et al. Clinical and plasma proteomic markers correlating with chronic kidney disease after liver transplantation. American Journal of Transplantation. 2011;11:1972-1978.
13. Maskos U, Southern EM. Oligonucleotide hybridizations on glass supports: a novel linker for oligonucleotide synthesis and hybridization properties of oligonucleotides synthesised in situ. Nucleic Acids Research. 1992;20: 1679-1684.
14. Schena M, Shalon D, Davis RW, et al. Quantitative monitoring of gene expression patterns with a complementary DNA microarray. Science. 1995;270: 467-470.
15. Bolstad BM, Irizarry RA, Astrand M, et al. A comparison of normalization

methods for high density oligonucleotide array data based on variance and bias. Bioinformatics (Oxford, England). 2003;19:185–193.
16. Shi L, Reid LH, Jones WD, et al. The MicroArray Quality Control (MAQC) project shows inter- and intraplatform reproducibility of gene expression measurements. Nature Biotechnology. 2006;24:1151–1161.
17. Rizzo JM, Buck MJ. Key principles and clinical applications of "next-generation" DNA sequencing. Cancer Prevention Research. 2012;5:887–900.
18. Mortazavi A, Williams BA, McCue K, et al. Mapping and quantifying mammalian transcriptomes by RNA-Seq. Nature Methods. 2008;5:621–628.
19. ENCODE Project Consortium. A user's guide to the encyclopedia of DNA elements (ENCODE). PLoS Biology. 2011;9:e1001046.
20. Modrek B, Lee C. A genomic view of alternative splicing. Nature Genetics. 2002;30:13–19.
21. Nagaraj N, Wisniewski JR, Geiger T, et al. Deep proteome and transcriptome mapping of a human cancer cell line. Molecular Systems Biology. 2011;7:548.
22. Mercer TR, Gerhardt DJ, Dinger ME, et al. Targeted RNA sequencing reveals the deep complexity of the human transcriptome. Nature Biotechnology. 2012;30: 99–104.
23. van Bakel H, Nislow C, Blencowe BJ, et al. Most "dark matter" transcripts are associated with known genes. PLoS Biology. 2010;8:e1000371.
24. Tarazona S, Garcia-Alcalde F, Dopazo J, et al. Differential expression in RNA-seq: a matter of depth. Genome Research. 2011;21:2213–2223.
25. Van Nieuwerburgh F, Soetaert S, Podshivalova K, et al. Quantitative bias in Illumina TruSeq and a novel post amplification barcoding strategy for multiplexed DNA and small RNA deep sequencing. PLoS ONE. 2011;6:e26969.

免疫调节机制

第 17 章 现有的免疫调控通路

Jason R. Lees, Agnes M. Azimzadeh, Yaozhong Ding, Jiangnan Xu, Jonathan S. Bromberg

引言

随着对免疫介导的排斥反应机制的深入认识以及相应同种异体免疫排斥药物的发展，器官移植已经逐步成为一种卓有成效的标准治疗。虽然所有常用的免疫抑制剂都会破坏生理性免疫过程，并具有脱靶的副作用，但是只要医生理解免疫抑制剂的作用机制并能预测可能发生的副反应，免疫抑制剂仍可以被成功地使用。同样的，免疫抑制剂的副反应可以通过联合应用机制互补的药物来最小化。本章将概述临床常用免疫抑制剂的作用机制。补充章节为第 98 章和第 101 章，将分别详述适应证内及超适应证应用的免疫抑制剂。仍在研究中的免疫抑制剂通路将在第 18 章中介绍。

类固醇类

皮质类固醇，产生于肾上腺皮质，具有广泛的免疫抑制及抗炎作用，是用于免疫抑制的第一类药物的一种[1]。糖皮质激素，包括天然及人工合成的能够激活糖异生的类固醇药物，包括泼尼松和甲泼尼龙，被广泛应用于抑制器官移植排斥反应的免疫抑制方案的一部分[2]。虽然这类药物对于抑制急性排斥反应有效，但是也可能导致一系列并发症甚至死亡。尤其，糖皮质激素可导致心血管疾病、骨代谢异常和升高的感染风险[3]。因此，从 20 世纪 90 年代末期，糖皮质激素在很多免疫抑制诱导及维持方案中被减量、撤除或停药[4]。

结构与生化通路

泼尼松是最常应用的糖皮质激素，在肝脏中代谢为泼尼松龙，是其主要的活性代谢产物。如图 17.1，未结合的类固醇通过细胞膜被动弥散进入细胞，与皮质类固醇结合球蛋白结合的类固醇还能够通过受体介导的转运或者胞吞作用进入细胞[1,5-7]。在胞质溶胶中，类固醇结合并激活糖皮质激素受体，类固醇–糖皮质激素受体二聚体可与不同的基因启动子序列的糖皮质激素应答元件相互作用，以调节免疫基因表达。糖皮质激素能够抑制多条炎性反应通路[1,5]。这些通路可以诱导并

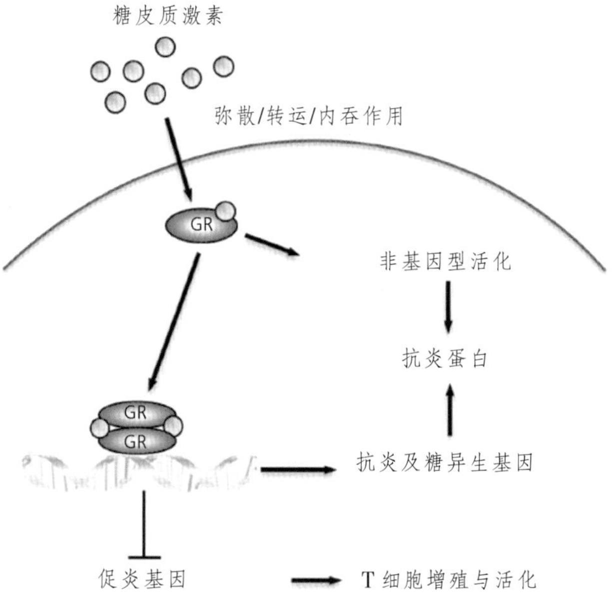

图 17.1 糖皮质激素的作用机制。非结合状态的类固醇被动地通过细胞膜弥散进入细胞，与皮质类固醇结合球蛋白结合的类固醇还能够通过受体介导的转运或者胞吞作用进入细胞。在胞浆中，类固醇与糖皮质激素受体结合，活化的类固醇–糖皮质激素受体二聚体以为进入细胞核，并与靶基因的糖皮质激素应答元件。激活的受体也与特定的转录因子(如 AP-1 和 NF-kB)相互作用，并阻止靶基因的转录。最终结果是减少了促炎细胞因子的产生，淋巴细胞的增殖和细胞转动的变化。

激活膜联蛋白Ⅰ,该分子能够抑制胞质溶胶中的磷脂酶A2α,进而抑制其他促炎性分子。糖皮质激素还可以诱导并激活丝裂原激活蛋白激酶磷酸酶 1,进而抑制丝裂原激活蛋白激酶信号级联炎性反应。糖皮质激素能够直接干扰 NF-κB 信号通路,继而抑制炎性细胞因子、趋化因子、细胞黏附分子、补体因子以及其他炎性介质[5]。因此,糖皮质激素首先阻断促炎性的 Th1 细胞因子,可可能阻断 Th17 细胞因子[8],促进 Th2 细胞因子生成,维持或增加白介素-10 的产生,以有助于移植物存活[9,10]。

细胞靶点

糖皮质激素的作用机制及细胞靶点是高变异性的,且仍未完全阐明。糖皮质激素可诱导 T 淋巴细胞凋亡[11],如上所述机制,可下调多种细胞的细胞因子和黏附分子的基因表达[12,13]。除了由胞浆内的糖皮质激素受体介导的基因起作用(转录活化和转录抑制),糖皮质激素还可抑制非基因机制的免疫反应,包括胞质信号分子与糖皮质激素受体的直接作用,糖皮质激素插入细胞膜,以及激活内皮细胞 NO 合成酶[14-16]。糖皮质激素抗炎的特点包括,抑制前列腺素的合成,稳定溶酶体膜,减少组胺和缓激肽释放,抑制树突细胞抗原递呈,抑制 CD4 T 细胞增殖、迁移和活化[17,18]。

适应性免疫

糖皮质激素可抑制树突细胞的抗原递呈,降低血液循环中 $CD4^+$ T 细胞数量,以及抑制 IL-1 生成和淋巴细胞活化[17,18]。较大的糖皮质激素剂量可抑制 B 细胞生成免疫球蛋白[19,20]。因此,糖皮质激素从多方面抑制适应性免疫。

固有免疫

糖皮质激素减少中性粒细胞向血管外迁移,并能降低其对血管内皮细胞的黏附能力和杀菌能力[19]。糖皮质激素能限制趋化性、吞噬作用、巨噬细胞及其他抗原呈递细胞释放 TNF-α 和 IL-1 等细胞因子,并抑制前列腺素、白三烯和血小板活化因子等炎性介质的表达[19]。因此,糖皮质激素也抑制大量不同的固有免疫机制和效应器。

感染

如上所述,糖皮质激素可同时抑制适应性免疫和固有免疫,因此,与感染风险增加有关。丙型病毒性肝炎加速感染是应用糖皮质激素一个主要问题[21]。糖皮质激素逐渐减量和无类固醇的免疫抑制方案可减少丙肝再感染、巨细胞病毒感染和丙型肝炎复发相关肝纤维化的发生[22-26]。

伤口愈合

巨噬细胞对于伤口愈合是不可缺少的。糖皮质激素可抑制循环中的单核细胞、巨噬细胞的汇集、生长因子和细胞因子的产生以及吞噬作用[27-30],这将对伤口愈合产生不利影响。糖皮质激素还通过延缓上皮再行成、降低成纤维细胞反应、减慢毛细血管增生、抑制胶原合成和伤口成熟,来减慢伤口愈合[27,29,31]。

代谢

糖皮质激素因诱导多种糖异生进程而具有许多不良反应(表 17.1)。糖皮质激素还可导致库欣综合征样改变、高血糖、骨密度降低、股骨头缺血性坏死、白内障、青光眼、皮肤变薄、皮肤脆性、瘀斑、紫纹、高血压、水潴留、肾上腺功能不全和心肌梗死、脑血管病等继发性心血管并发症[20]。

钙调磷酸酶抑制剂

简介

自从引入环孢素 A(CsA)以来,磷酸酶抑制剂(CNI)

表 17.1 糖皮质激素常见并发症

器官/系统	并发症
内分泌与代谢系统	肾上腺功能不全、高血糖、水潴留、小儿生长迟缓
造血系统	白细胞增多症
免疫系统	细菌、真菌、病毒感染,伤口愈合延迟、Ⅳ型超敏反应抑制
消化系统	胃刺激症状、消化性溃疡
心血管系统	高血压、心肌梗死、脑血管疾病
皮肤	皮肤变薄、皮肤脆性、瘀斑、紫纹
运动系统	骨质疏松、股骨头缺血性坏死、肌病
眼	白内障、青光眼
中枢神经系统	睡眠障碍、失眠、欣快感、抑郁症、躁狂症、精神病、强迫症、假性脑瘤
生殖系统	阳痿、月经不调
外貌形态	满月脸、水牛背、向心性肥胖

已经成为移植医学中免疫抑制维持的主流药物[32-34]。CNI通过抑制钙调磷酸酶与其底物-活化T细胞核因子(NFAT)[35-37],来抑制T细胞活性和细胞因子的转录[38-40]。CNI的临床耐受性较好,但是具有肾毒性和胰岛毒性。此外,CNI还与伤口并发症有关,尤其与哺乳动物西罗莫司靶蛋白抑制剂mTOR抑制剂合用时[41]。因此,许多团队近期限制CNI在移植受体中的应用[42-44]。本部分主要介绍CNI的结构、功能及药理学特点。

结构与生化通路

了解钙调磷酸酶及其在免疫调节中的作用,是了解CNI的必备条件。钙调磷酸酶是一种依赖钙的钙调蛋白磷酸酶[45,46]。CNI是含有活性域及自身抑制域的异质二聚体,不含自身抑制域的为突变的钙调磷酸酶,持续具有活性[45,46]。T细胞被细胞表面受体活化,导致细胞内钙浓度增加。钙-钙调蛋白-钙调磷酸酶通路进而激活NFAT[47]。NFAT家族至少由5名成员组成,是一组转录因子,包括编码炎症相关细胞因子和趋化因子的基因(图17.2)[47,48]。仅缺乏该家族2名成员(NFAT1和NFAT2)的小鼠将丧失产生细胞因子的能力[48]。钙激活钙调磷酸酶的磷酸酶活性,进而可去除NFAT调节域的磷酸根。这将启动一系列事件,其中一个核输出信号与Crm1(又名核输出受体)结合,导致NFAT迁移进入细胞核,脱去磷酸根的NFAT为许多重要的免疫基因充当转录因子[48]。

他克莫司(又名FK506)和CsA与细胞内不同的免疫亲和素结合,特别的,CsA与亲环素类结合,他克莫司与FK结合蛋白(FKBP)结合[35]。除了这些差别,这两种药物均通过形成药物依赖的复合物抑制钙调磷酸酶-钙调蛋白来产生免疫抑制作用[35,49]。

细胞靶点

CNI可显著抑制T细胞的增殖和活化,移植医生利用这种效应来抑制抗移植物T细胞反应。CNI尤其是他克莫司,可抑制依赖T细胞的细胞因子合成,包括IL-2,4,5、TNF-α和INF-γ,这些细胞因子的合成需要T细胞的辅助及增殖[50-52]。有趣的是,CNI的T细胞抑制具有种属特异性。此外,CNI可能加强调解性T细胞的功能,尤其在自身免疫性皮肤病中,但仍有争议[53-55]。CNI可作用于成熟及未成熟T细胞,并可抑制阳性选择中双阳性前体细胞发育为$CD4^+$和$CD8^+$单阳性淋巴细胞[56],这可能会增强CNI的免疫抑制功效。

CNI影响B细胞最显著的通路是通过抑制T细胞辅助和免疫球蛋白类别转换[50,57]。因此,CNI对B细胞的效应主要是间接的。在体外研究中,他克莫司或CsA与T细胞、B细胞联合培养,免疫球蛋白的产量下降。但

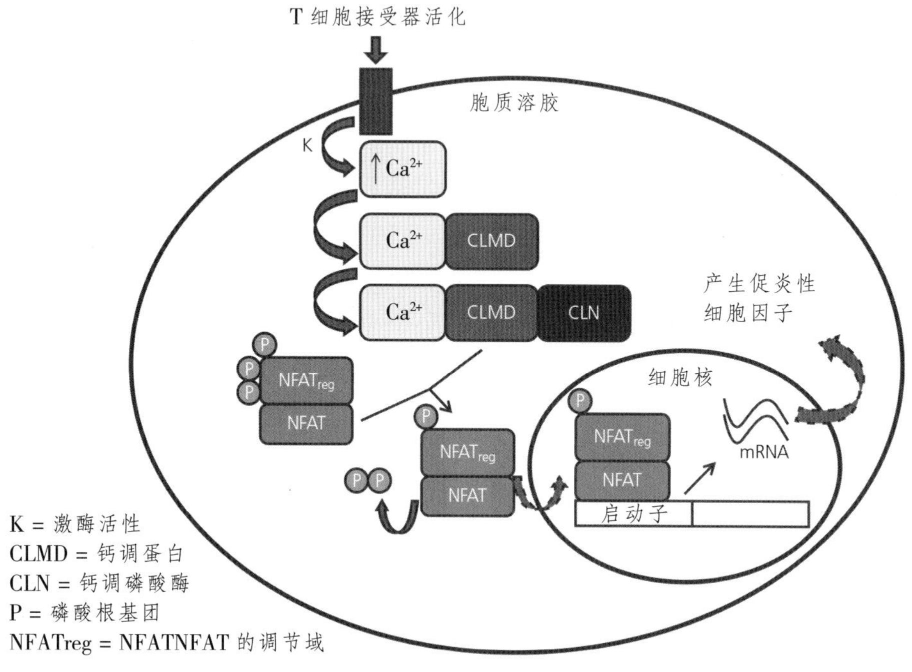

图17.2 T细胞被细胞表面受体活化,导致细胞内钙浓度增加。钙激活钙调磷酸酶的磷酸酶活性,进而可去除NFAT调节域的磷酸根。NFAT然后从细胞质迁移进入细胞核,脱去磷酸根的NFAT为许多重要的免疫基因充当转录因子。

是当去除 T 细胞，他克莫司、CsA 与 B 细胞联合培养时，免疫球蛋白产量未明显下降，他克莫司无法抑制免疫球蛋白的合成，CsA 仅仅轻度抑制免疫球蛋白合成[50]。其他研究提示 CsA 确实可直接作用于 B 细胞。亲环蛋白 B 是 CsA 的细胞内靶点，与蛋白质折叠相关，可能被 CsA 抑制[58]。在 B 细胞中，这种抑制可导致 IgG 生物合成的剂量和时间依赖性下降，在该实验中，CsA 对于 IgG 转录无任何影响，其生物合成下降是由内质网应激导致的[59]。

CNI 还影响中性粒细胞功能。这些效应与血管紧张素Ⅱ已同时在血管损伤的体外模型中被研究。因为血管紧张素Ⅱ上调钙调磷酸酶的活性和合成，并与中性粒细胞在内皮细胞中的活化相关，研究者假设 CsA 可能通过抑制上游事件来降低中性粒细胞活化[60]。在实验中，CsA 可通过抑制 MAPK 和 ERK 通路来降低血管紧张素Ⅱ刺激的中性粒细胞活化，同时，CsA 可抑制 Rac2 的移位[61]，该分子是中性粒细胞细胞质释放促炎性活性氧进入细胞核的分子开关[62]。受损的移位是血管紧张素Ⅱ被抑制的下游效应，而血管紧张素Ⅱ是已知的 Rac2 刺激物。因此，CsA 可抑制血管紧张素Ⅱ刺激的中性粒细胞，该过程极大地依赖于 Rac2 移位[60]。

CNI 还能减少细胞因子产生，例如，减少 T 细胞分泌的 INF-γ。因为 INF-γ 是一种强大的巨噬细胞刺激物，CNI 下调效应包括抑制单核细胞和巨噬细胞。CNI 对单核细胞和巨噬细胞的直接效应可能是有限的[52]。在啮齿类动物的自发性溃疡性结肠炎的研究中，研究者表明他克莫司可抑制肠黏膜 T 细胞而不是单核细胞、巨噬细胞活化，加入 CNI 会导致巨噬细胞活化减少[52]。

对实质细胞的效应

CNI 对于内皮细胞具有已知的毒性[66,64]，这是心脏同种异体移植物血管病变的病理基础。当把牛的主动脉内皮细胞与 CsA 共同培养时，时间与剂量依赖的细胞破坏（最终为细胞溶解）的特点是，洗脱乳酸脱氢酶、前列腺素和血栓素浓度将增加[65]。CsA 对内皮细胞的有害作用可能由于一氧化氮（NO）和内皮素-1（ET-1）的调节变化，这些会降低血管舒张。有趣的是，研究者评估西罗莫司却未观察到 NO 及 ET-1 有同样的变化，西罗莫司是否会导致移植物血管病。因为 NO 及 ET-1 对内皮细胞调节异常导致炎性细胞因子产生，所以研究者设想通过血管内皮生长因子来抑制该调节异常，可能会缓解钙调磷酸酶相关性血管病[66]。的确，在体外的人体内皮细胞模型中，研究者发现当内皮细胞与内皮生长因子 7 共同培养时，CsA 及他克莫司导致的细胞黏附明显减少，因此推断针对此通路可能有利于心脏移植[66]。

CNI 已知具有肾毒性[67,68]，会降低肾小管及肾小球功能，这可能是因为水通道蛋白基因下调导致[69,70]。除了影响尿的生成和收集，CsA 及他克莫司均可能通过胞外信号调节激酶通路（ERK）促进肾间质细胞有丝分裂[71]。结果还提示，CNI 诱发的肾毒性机制是内质网应激和 CD147 上调导致的肾纤维化[58]。

早已报道 CNI 可抑制胰岛功能[72]。CNI 相关性胰岛功能下降，部分因为钙调磷酸酶影响胰岛素释放[73]。当 β 细胞与超治疗剂量的他克莫司或 CsA 共同培养时，两药均可导致稳态条件下基础胰岛素生成下降 48%~69%。此外，他克莫司在超治疗剂量时，可使胰岛素释放减少 61%~87%。他克莫司和 CsA 的致糖尿病作用是由于钙调磷酸酶的抑制和转录因子 SREBP-1c 的胰岛特异性下调，该转录因子可调控胰岛细胞功能。此外，两药均具有细胞毒性，可导致胰岛细胞死亡[72]。

功能性免疫通路（适应性反应、缺血再灌注损伤、感染）

CNI 抑制 T 细胞活化、增殖和下调巨噬细胞活性是其抗排斥反应的基础，但是，因为抑制了适应性免疫及固有免疫，所以 CNI 具有潜在的并发症发生率。在 CsA 与 FK506 毒性对比研究中，CsA 组具有更高的感染风险，并且按照剂量依赖方式具有最高风险的机会性感染[74]。相反，CNI 可能具有与移植无关的免疫学影响，例如，改善局灶及全身缺血以及缺血再灌注损伤[75,76]。改善缺血与 CNI 可以抑制 NO 合成、防止氧化应激[75]、进而减少 DNA 损伤和脂质过氧化有关。基于这些数据和其他数据进行的一项随机对照实验表明，供肝使用 20ng/mL 的他克莫司灌注，与未行灌注的供肝进行对比[77]，研究者发现两组移植物结局无明显差异，但是发现在分子水平，灌注组缺血再灌注损伤减轻[77]。

非免疫功能（代谢、伤口/愈合、肿瘤/增殖）

CNI 与伤口愈合不良、神经毒性、肾毒性、高胆固醇血症、高甘油三酯血症和胆汁淤积有关[67,74,78]。对于伤口愈合，CsA 可减少成纤维细胞源生长因子，尤其是激活素 B。尽管具有其他免疫效应[79]，但 CsA 对成纤维细胞 TGF-β 或整合素-1 几乎没有影响。移植后高脂血症(PTHL)已经被详细阐明。虽然类固醇类与PTHL具有明确联系,但是CNI对PTHL的作用还不清楚[80]。有趣的是,CsA(而非他克莫司)可增加总胆固醇和低密度脂蛋白,移植术后1个月达到峰值[81]。有趣的是,在同一时间点,高密度脂蛋白没有伴随增加[81]。其他团队也观察到类似的结果,他克莫司比CsA更能够提高脂质水平,这可能是因为低密度脂蛋白氧化的改变。神经系统并发症在引入CNI后有据可查[82]。这些效应可能因为:①CNI与细胞内参与其他生理过程的底物结合;②血管收缩;③内皮素生成;④过多的活性氧族的产生。

恶性肿瘤形成也是应用免疫抑制剂的风险之一[84]。肾移植后最常见的恶性肿瘤是皮肤癌和非霍奇金淋巴瘤[84]。肾移植术后3年约7%的患者会罹患皮肤癌。此外,还有大约7%受体发生其他癌症,其中最常见的为非霍奇金淋巴瘤[84]。有趣的是,虽然他克莫司对于抑制免疫排斥反应更加有效,但其并未增加新发癌症概率[85]。虽然移植术后新发癌症可以轻易地归因于免疫抑制剂,但是有些数据也提示肾移植等待患者中癌症患者比例也很高。此外,终末期肾病患者发生的癌症类型与肾移植后新发癌症类型相似。终末期肾病的肿瘤风险可能因为肾毒性导致的基因毒性,进而增加氧化应激[87]。CNI的致癌潜能可能与NF-κB细胞核因子的调节有关,该因子可以调节生长因子和致癌的凋亡机制[88,89]。

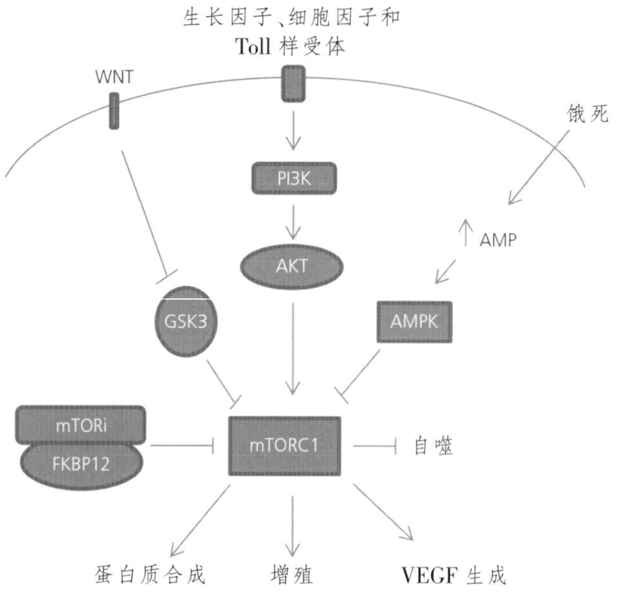

图17.3 mTOR信号通路的激动剂和抑制剂。mTORC1信号复合物的激活后通过增强蛋白质合成来促进细胞生长,通过抑制自噬来促进细胞增殖。同时,mTORC1可诱导其他因子生成,包括VEGF允许组织重塑及修复。mTORi复合物和细胞内蛋白FKBP12可抑制mTORC1的功能。内源性的调节器例如糖原合成酶激酶3(GSK-3)和一磷酸腺苷活化激酶(AMPK)也都阻断mTORC1的活性。通过WNT受体的信号可抑制GSK3的活性,虽然AMPK活性仅由增加的AMP浓度伴随能量消耗而激活。mTORC1能通过AKT激活而激活,这是通过受体识别生长因子、细胞因子和Toll样受体配体(例如脂多糖),激活磷脂酰肌醇-3-激酶(PI3K)信号通路来实现的。

mTOR抑制剂

西罗莫司对于很多类型的细胞增殖的潜在影响导致了对西罗莫司的哺乳动物靶点(mTOR)的阐明。mTOR是一个丝氨酸/苏氨酸蛋白激酶,作为两个不同信号通路(mTORC1和mTORC2)的组成部分,参与调节细胞代谢、活化和增殖等多种通路[90-94]。近期可用的mTOR抑制剂包括西罗莫司和依维莫司,它们能够阻断mTOR活化,包括mTORC1复合物形成以及随后的活性激活,进而阻止分解代谢到合成代谢的转化[90,95]。此外,有证据表明,mTORi能够在一些状况下阻断mTOR2信号通路进而影响细胞功能[96]。总之,目前的mTORi药理学机制表明其对于细胞增殖具有广泛抑制,尤其是由生长因子诱导的增殖[90-94](图17.3)。

虽然mTOR是一个细胞内普遍存在的信号成分,但是与免疫相关的细胞代谢需求明显增加将导致免疫细胞优先依赖mTOR激活来维持免疫细胞的生存和功能。因此,mTORi表现出强大的免疫抑制作用,尤其是与其他免疫抑制路径的靶向药物(例如,吗替麦考酚酯)合用时[97,98]。但是,近期研究表明,抑制mTOR还会导致固有免疫细胞产生更多的炎性细胞因子以及更强的适应性免疫记忆。这些互相矛盾的结果意味着mTOR在免疫中具有多种复杂作用。

细胞靶点

T细胞是参与移植物排斥反应的主要免疫细胞。mTORi降低T细胞增殖的能力是公认的,在mTOR介导的免疫抑制中起到重要作用。T细胞增殖的抑制与G1期细胞周期阻滞以及蛋白质合成的严重减少有关。此外,在mTORi存在时,T细胞的抗原刺激已被证实会导致对随后刺激的低反应性,这被称为免疫无能。最后,最新数据表明mTORi能够影响T细胞迁移,通过将T细胞隔离在淋巴组织中来调节免疫抑制[101]。

mTORi 介导的无反应性诱导与 FoxP3+的调节性 T 细胞(Tregs)的诱导和(或)存活增加有关[102-109]。有证据表明 mTORi 对 FoxP3 表达的重新诱导、T 细胞调节功能、和调节 T 细胞的优先生存具有积极作用[102,107,110,111]。对于后者，建议调节 T 细胞可通过交替的信号通路来调节代谢[110]。总之,这表明了,mTORi 改变了效应细胞向抑制 T 细胞的平衡,有利于抑制 T 细胞。

有趣的是,mTORi 治疗也可增强 T 细胞抗原特异性刺激后的免疫记忆形成。免疫记忆增强已经在多种系统中得到清晰的证实,并且,被认为是移植中诱导淋巴细胞减少后记忆表型细胞积累增强的原因[109,112-115]。

类似 T 细胞,B 细胞似乎是依赖 mTOR 信号来保证效应器功能的发育和生成。有趣的是,研究表明,抑制 mTOR 信号通路[116]和基本的 mTOR 信号通路[117]均可负面影响 B 细胞发育和活性。这些发现表明,在正常情况下,严格控制的 mTOR 信号通路对于 B 细胞是非常重要的。但是,mTORi 与 B 细胞在免疫抑制中相互作用的很多方面仍有待探索。

除了 mTOR 在适应性免疫反应中的重要作用，mTOR 在固有免疫细胞的炎性过程中也扮演重要角色。抑制 mTOR 已被证明可降低循环中中性粒细胞数量，并抑制中性粒细胞的粒细胞巨噬细胞集落刺激因子(GM-CSF)相关的组织迁移[118]。对于树突细胞和单核巨噬细胞等抗原递呈细胞,mTOR 抑制剂的效应是复杂的。监测 mTOR 对树突细胞抗原递呈抑制效应的研究表明,mTOR 激活是树突细胞成熟和进一步活化 T 细胞的必备条件。应用西罗莫司后,在炎性信号存在伴随树突细胞成熟的情况下，树突细胞增加表达 GM-CSF、IL-1 和 IL-4 等共刺激分子的能力下降。mTORi 治疗后导致的树突细胞成熟能力下降已被证实与调节性 T 细胞的生成有关。

相反,mTORi 治疗可以增加树突细胞和单核细胞产生炎性细胞因子,包括 TNF-α、IL-6、IL-12 和 IL-23,并且阻断抗炎因子 IL-10 的产生[119]。而且,mTORi 还可抑制类固醇的免疫抑制作用[120]。因此,mTORi 对于树突细胞和单核细胞具有抗炎及促炎双重作用[121,122]。

最后,实质细胞是炎症的重要组成成分,并且他们也可被 mTORi 调节[123-125]。的确,mTORi 似乎可以调节组织细胞参与炎性反应的能力,明显影响组织破坏、重塑及修复。尤其是 mTORi 已被证实可以降低成纤维细胞对伤口相关生长因子的反应性，抑制细胞更替及伤口愈合[126,127]。这种抑制作用伴随有伤口处 VEGF 生成的减少,伴有血管组织恢复的损失[128]。

适应性免疫

以上介绍的 mTORi 对于免疫系统各部分的作用提示,mTORi 对适应性免疫反应的作用是复杂的。如前所述,mTORi 对淋巴细胞介导的移植物排斥反应具有明显的免疫抑制作用，并且增强了 CD8 T 细胞的免疫记忆[109,112-115]。该发现适用于抗原特异性 T 细胞反应和自我平衡扩张所产生的记忆表型 T 细胞，这两者均可发生于移植中[113]。总之,mTORi 有助于一般的免疫抑制,并且增加感染的易感性,虽然对于特殊的病原体可降低感染风险(详见后面感染章节)。

缺血再灌注炎性反应

一些团队已经发现 mTOR 信号通路对于缺血预适应的保护作用和或胰岛素对缺血再灌注损伤是很重要的。据此,mTORi 会加剧缺血再灌注损伤,并且促进缺血再灌注损伤相关的炎性反应。但是，也有证据表明 mTORi 可能抑制缺血再灌注损伤[129]。因此,需要进一步研究来探明 mTORi 与缺血再灌注损伤之间的确切影响。

感染

有趣的是,mTORi 对 CD8 T 细胞免疫记忆的促进作用[130,131],可缓解免疫抑制相关的移植后淋巴细胞增生性疾病和巨噬细胞感染[132]。因此,虽然 mTORi 像其他免疫抑制剂一样,可导致机会性感染,但是它可以降低受体对特殊病原体的易感性。

代谢

作为细胞代谢的重要成分之一,mTORi 对于代谢和稳态具有重要的病理效应。应用西罗莫司可产生剂量依赖性血脂异常,并可导致心血管并发症[133]。有强烈证据表明,mTORi 增加移植后糖尿病发病率[134,135]。临床前模型研究提示,mTORi 的致糖尿病作用是因为胰岛素敏感度降低和 β 细胞功能破坏或凋亡所致[135]。

伤口/愈合

在伤口愈合过程中,mTORi 对增殖的抑制很强大。应用西罗莫司，会通过影响愈合过程的多个方面而增加手术切口并发症[125,136-138]。

肿瘤/增殖

mTOR 是血管形成和生长因子介导的增殖的重要组成部分。这些功能让 mTORi 可明显降低移植后肿瘤发生率[140,141]。并且,有证据表明 mTORi 诱导的 CD8 T 细胞免疫记忆增强可导致某些环境下的肿瘤控制。目前正在研究 mTORi 用于多种肿瘤的治疗。

嘌呤类似物

嘌呤类似物是一种类似 DNA 和 RNA 重要组分的一种化学物质。嘌呤类似物能通过阻碍 DNA、RNA 和其他核酸及蛋白质的合成，来抑制细胞增殖和免疫反应。硫唑嘌呤(AZA)和 6-巯基嘌呤(6-MP)是广泛用于防止移植排斥反应的免疫抑制剂和抗炎制剂。AZA 和 6-MP 由英国移植先驱 Sir Roy Calne 引入临床。Thomas Starzl 医生引入了移植中 AZA 联合类固醇的概念。AZA 是 6-MP 的前体药物,毒性更低,口服消化后,AZA 代谢为有活性的 6-MP。在嘌呤通路中,其他类似化合物是吗替麦考酚酯(MMF)和霉酚酸(MPA),MPA 是 MMF 的活性代谢产物。通过抑制肌苷一磷酸脱氢酶(IMPDH)，进而抑制鸟嘌呤核苷酸的从头合成,MMF 抑制了细胞增殖。虽然其他细胞可以利用补救途径合成鸟嘌呤核苷酸，但是淋巴细胞依赖肌苷一磷酸脱氢酶进行从头合成,因此,相对于 AZA[142],MMF 是一种更特异和有效的抑制嘌呤合成的药物。结果,近年来许多移植中心使用 MMF 来代替 AZA。

结构与生化通路

如图 17.4,AZA 被吸收后，代谢为活性形式 6-MP,通过 6-硫肌苷-5'-单磷酸盐(6-Thio-IMP),进一步被代谢为 6-硫鸟嘌呤核苷酸(6-TGN)。内源性嘌呤是细胞周期 S 期的必需物质,作为其拮抗剂,6-TGN 可合并入 DNA 和 RNA,因此可直接阻断细胞增殖。对小鼠白血病细胞中 6-MP 的研究表明，细胞死亡是由于 6-TGN 嵌入 DNA 导致 DNA 损伤。6-TGN 还可抑制内源性嘌呤合成,改变 DNA 和 RNA 的合成和功能,因此阻止了细胞尤其是淋巴细胞增殖[142]。对于 MMF,它被代谢为其活性形式 MPA,MPA 作为 IMPDH 的非竞争性抑制剂，通过抑制鸟嘌呤核苷酸从头合成而特异性靶向抑制淋巴细胞增殖[142](图 17.4)。

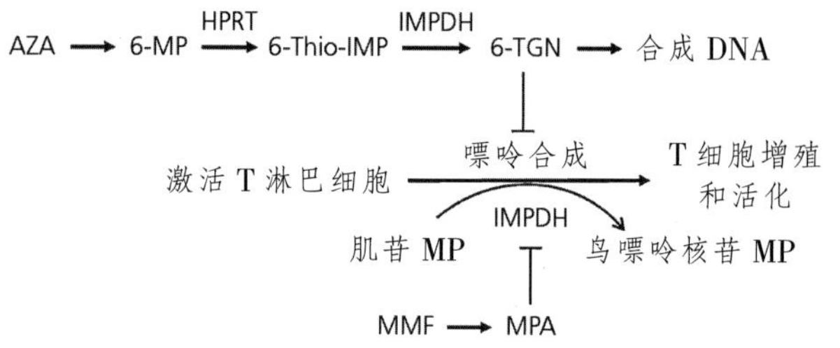

图 17.4 AZA,6-MP 及 MMF 的代谢活动。AZA，硫唑嘌呤;6-MP,6-巯基嘌呤;HPRT,次黄嘌呤核糖核酸转移酶;6-Thio-IMP,6-硫肌苷-5'-单磷酸盐;IMPDH,肌苷一磷酸脱氢酶;MMF,霉酚酸酯;MPA,霉酚酸。

细胞靶点

移植后,受体免疫细胞将对同种异体抗原响应,增殖并启动免疫反应以排斥并破坏移植物。AZA 和 MMF 的主要靶点是细胞增殖,因此,阻止了免疫反应诱导期的淋巴细胞增殖，进而抑制了细胞及体液免疫反应。AZA/6-MP 将 CD8 共刺激信号转变为凋亡信号。特别的,AZA/6-MP 产生了 6-thio-GTP,它与 GTP 结合蛋白 Rac 结合,因此,阻止了 Rac1 的激活,从而阻止 Rac1 调节基因的激活,例如,MEK、NF-κB 和 Bcl-xl,最终导致了细胞凋亡的线粒体途径。还有报道称,6-TG 通过阻断 Vav 对 Rac 蛋白质的活性，阻断了 GTP 酶的激活,干扰了 T 细胞与抗原递呈细胞之间的相互作用,进而阻断了免疫活化[143]。

6-MP 与树突细胞分化之间的相互作用及激活近期得到了验证。结果表明,6-MP 抑制 CD14 前体细胞分化为树突细胞,降低 LPS 诱导的 CD83 表达[144]。因为 CD83 是树突细胞成熟的标记物，它能促进抗原递呈细胞与 T 细胞的交互作用,影响抗原递呈细胞表面的 MHC Ⅱ类分子转化，并能决定 $CD8^+$ T 细胞在免疫反应中存活[145-147],6-MP 下调 CD83 导致异基因和抗原特异性 T 细胞增殖受损。CCR7 对于淋巴结归巢是必须的[144,148],6-MP 能降低其在树突细胞上的表达。这些报道均表明,AZA 也通过调节树突细胞成熟和活化来抑制免疫反应[144]。

MMF 通过 IMPDH 发挥其抗增殖效应,特别是对 T 细胞。IMPDH 的两种亚型已经被证实,活化的 T 细胞可强烈表达Ⅱ型 PMPDH，它对 MPA 的亲和力比Ⅰ型 IMPDH 高 5 倍。MPA 在培养的 MOLT-4 细胞中能将细胞凋亡率从 12%提高到 82%~92%[149],通过触发小鼠和人的凋亡机制来促进加速超级抗原活化的 T 细胞的消除。MPA 抑制 IMPDH 和内源性嘌呤合成，耗尽 GTP，结果干扰甘露糖和岩藻糖转移至淋巴细胞糖蛋白[142]，影响淋巴细胞黏附分子的形成。MPA 降低了人 T 细胞黏附至人内皮细胞，使用 MPA 作用于 T 细胞和内皮细胞将导致进一步导致黏附下降，说明 MPA 还通过内皮细胞影响免疫反应。MMF 明显降低 ICAM-1 和 LFA 的表达，LFA+细胞渗透入不同的移植及炎症模型，这表明 MMF 通过抑制黏附分子表达和免疫细胞迁移抑制免疫反应。

MMF 减少 CD40 和 CD86 的表达，LPS 诱导的 IL-12 合成，这降低了啮齿类树突细胞对同种异体 T 细胞的刺激作用[158]。在人类单核细胞分化培养为树突细胞中，MMF 减少了未成熟树突细胞的数量，诱导凋亡，下调共刺激通路和 CO40、CD54、CD80 和 CD86 等黏附分子的表达降低 TNF-α、IL-10、IL-12 和 IL-18 的产生，抑制同种反应性 T 细胞的刺激[159]。综上所述，这些结果提示 MMF 通过影响树突细胞分化和活化来抑制免疫反应。

MPA 降低单核细胞中 GTP 水平[142]，减少糖蛋白的甘露糖基化和单核细胞黏附于内皮细胞。类似于淋巴细胞的促凋亡效应，MMF 在 THP-1 和 U937 单核细胞系中可诱导细胞凋亡，并在链佐星介导的糖尿病患者中浸润[149,162]。综上所述，这些结果提示 MMF 能直接减弱单核细胞和巨噬细胞的反应。

适应性免疫

如上所述，嘌呤类似物和相关药物可直接抑制淋巴细胞增殖，因此，可通过体液及细胞免疫反应抑制适应性免疫的诱导期。这些化合物还可影响抗原递呈细胞，尤其是许多树突细胞的功能，因此，可干扰淋巴细胞与抗原递呈细胞的交互作用，来抑制适应性免疫反应。

固有免疫

AZA 和 MMF 抑制树突细胞分化、黏附分子表达、成熟以及细胞因子表达，来抑制固有免疫和适应性免疫。此外，MMF 直接诱导单核细胞和巨噬细胞凋亡，以及抑制其迁移并渗透入移植物和炎症位置，进一步提示 MMF 对固有免疫反应的抑制作用。

感染

在移植免疫中，MPA 特异性针对 T 细胞和 B 细胞也增加了感染并发症的风险[163,164]。据报道，相对于AZA，MMF 的移植物存活率更高[165]，但是接受 MMF 治疗的受体因感染导致的再入院率更高[166]。巨细胞病毒感染是 MMF 相关的最常见的感染并发症，这可能是因为相较于 AZA，应用 MMF 者中血清抗巨细胞病毒 IgM 滴度更低[170,171]。应用含有 MMF 免疫抑制方案后[172,174]，还可出现 BK 病毒感染、水痘病毒感染及真菌感染[175,176]。另一方面，有报道称，MMF 可能具有一定的抗微生物作用，包括抗登革热病毒、丙肝病毒、乙肝病毒、肺孢子虫、西尼罗河病毒和黄热病毒[177]。

代谢

MMF 对移植患者的典型副作用是胃肠道作用，包括腹泻、恶心、呕吐和腹部绞痛，这可能因为肠上皮毒性和或免疫抑制引起的轻度肠道感染[178,179]。MMF 还可能具有一定血液系统副作用，包括白细胞减少、贫血、血小板减少和血细胞发育不良[178,180]。泌尿生殖系统副作用，包括尿急、尿频、排尿困难和无菌性脓尿[181-184]。其他副反应例如发热、肌痛、头痛和失眠，以及周围性水肿和高血压等心血管症状[180,185,186]。

单克隆生物制剂

生物制剂是由重组 DNA 技术生产而不是化学合成。生物制剂设计成选择性针对某一关键免疫通路，而不具有化学合成药物的副作用[187,188]。该部分将主要介绍单克隆生物治疗移植排斥反应。Kohler 和 Milstein 因合成预定的特异性抗体，即单克隆抗体而获得诺贝尔奖[189]。单克隆抗体在移植和肿瘤治疗中应用广泛，是生物制剂中的重要成员。

巴利昔单抗和达利珠单抗：抗 IL-2R 抗体

结构与生化通路

IL-2 和 IL-2R 的受体由三个亚基组成：α、β 和 γ 亚基，也分别称作 CD25、CD122 和 CD132。巴利昔单抗（舒莱）和达利珠单抗（赛尼哌）均是针对 CD25 和 IL-2 的强效单克隆抗体[191]。它们被用来防止移植物排斥反应。巴利昔单抗和 IL-2R 已经被研究并建模。巴利昔单抗是人-小鼠嵌合抗体，达利珠单抗是人化的啮齿类抗体，均结合于 IL-2α 链（巴利昔单抗特异性结合于 IL-

2Rα 胞外域),可明显限制免疫反应。达利珠单抗因为经济原因于2009年退出市场,但是,在过去15年的文献中,其数据尤为突出。IL-2是T细胞的产物,同时也是单克隆T细胞增殖的标志[190,191]。此外,IL-2信号通路可正反馈上调CD25的表达,这将导致T细胞的快速活化和增殖[192]。在体内试验中,巴利昔单抗使$CD25^+$ T细胞减少近6周。因为除了抑制性调节T细胞,$CD25^+$还表达于$CD4^+$细胞上,研究者假设巴利昔单抗可能会损伤调节性T细胞的抑制机制[93]。在人类患者中,尽管在应用巴利昔单抗后$CD4^+/CD25^+/FoxP3^+$细胞数量减少,$CD4^+/CD25^+/FoxP3^+$细胞数量却增加。一项评估应用巴利昔单抗T细胞亚群变化的研究得出结论,虽然巴利昔单抗减低了调节性T细胞的数量,但是并未导致其功能下降,巴利昔单抗可能不抑制调节T细胞的致耐受性潜能[193]。其他团队证实,巴利昔单抗并不改变效应T细胞/调节T细胞比率,而兔抗胸腺细胞球蛋白被认为可增加调节T细胞数量[194]。

利妥昔单抗:抗CD20抗体

结构与生化通路

CD20(最初称作B1)在绝大多数成熟B细胞上表达,但却不在早期B前体细胞、活化的抗体分泌细胞和浆细胞上表达[195,196]。利妥昔单抗是一种人源化的嵌合体的抗CD20药物,最初被批准用于复发的惰性淋巴瘤[197,198]。利妥昔单抗目前被用来清除B细胞以控制同种异体抗体反应。利妥昔单抗通过补体依赖的细胞毒性作用(CDC)和抗体依赖细胞介导的细胞毒性作用(ADCC)来清除B细胞。利妥昔单抗诱导的ADCC是通过Fc受体被结合来调节的[199]。对于CDC,利妥昔单抗直接结合于C1q,启动补体级联[199]。有趣的是,地塞米松等类固醇治疗被证明可增强CDC,但是并不增强ADCC[200]。利妥昔单抗也被认为可通过MAPK通路下调IL-20而促使B细胞凋亡。因为浆细胞和高度成熟的抗体分泌细胞几乎不表达CD20,所以利妥昔单抗治疗同种异体抗体反应和体液排斥反应的效果是很有限的。

阿来组单抗:抗CD52抗体

结构与生化通路

阿来组单抗(坎帕斯)针对T细胞、B细胞、巨噬细胞、单核细胞和NK细胞表面的糖蛋白CD52。CD52不在红细胞和造血干细胞表面表达[201]。阿来组单抗最初被批准用于治疗慢性淋巴细胞白血病,但是被移植界采用作为诱导疗法,可广泛快速地清除白细胞,这可能导致钙调磷酸酶抑制剂和类固醇用量降到最小,从而达到免疫耐受状态[202,203]。在一项多中心试验中,阿来组单抗可降低3年内急性排斥反应发生,但也可导致恶性肿瘤的发生[204]。并且,相比于马抗胸腺细胞球蛋白等药物,阿来组单抗可保持更长效的淋巴细胞清除状态,所以可能需要1~2年来恢复正常的外周血白细胞数量及各种白细胞亚群分布。

莫罗单抗:抗CD3抗体

结构与生化通路

莫罗单抗,也称作OKT-3,是一种啮齿类单克隆抗IgG2a抗体。OKT-3的靶点是CD3,是抗原特异性T细胞受体复合物的组分之一,在成熟T细胞和骨髓胸腺细胞表面表达[205]。OKT-3是第一个被批准用于人体的单克隆抗体。因为被其他药物取代,该药于几年前退市,但在移植文献和目前抗体制剂应用理念上仍具有重要意义。其他诱导药物可能降低T细胞数量持续数天或数周,然而CD3数量在停用OKT-3 48h后就开始上升[205]。类似利妥昔单抗[206],OKT-3通过CDC和ADCC起效[206],但是它还通过活化诱导的细胞死亡机制(AICD)和调理素作用来起效[206]。OKT-3还被认为可使T细胞受体从细胞表面脱落,从而使其不再与抗原递呈细胞作用。OKT-3还可能诱导产生长效的克隆无能,模拟免疫缺陷。对于许多其他抗体制剂,T细胞表面受体交联能引起快速大量T细胞活化,并释放细胞因子,导致细胞因子风暴,临床症状表现为高热、心动过速、低血压、血管渗漏和多脏器功能衰竭[207]。

贝拉西普

概念与结构

目前用于移植的生物药物是单克隆抗体,贝拉西普属于一种新型生物制剂。它代表一种重组融合蛋白,对应于偶联于免疫球蛋白框架的T细胞表面受体的溶解形式[208]。并且,贝拉西普是目前用于临床的唯一的针对适应性免疫通路(共刺激通路)的生物制剂。

主要组织相容性复合体(MHC)无关性器官移植的排斥反应是由 T 细胞协调和介导的。共刺激通路可被定义为第二个必需信号,和 T 细胞受体(TCR)与抗原递呈细胞表面的多肽–MHC 复合物介导的第一信号共同传递给 T 细胞(图 17.5)。在体外实验中,如果没有足够的共刺激信号(信号 2),仅通过 TCR 的信号(信号 1)无法产生 T 细胞反应,会导致 T 细胞无能或者低反应性[209,210]。这些发现提示了在自身免疫疾病和移植中阻断病理性免疫反应一种新方法[187,211–213],这也是最近十年的科研热点。许多 T 细胞活化必需的共刺激分子已被发现[214]。在许多移植模型中阻断共刺激通路已经证实,共刺激信号造成了免疫反应的结果,是同种异体免疫的有效免疫调节剂[215–222]。

20 世纪 90 年代对目前最具特点的共刺激受体(CD28)的阐明导致了贝拉西普的研发。细胞毒性 T 细胞抗原–4(CTLA–4)是 T 细胞共刺激受体 CD28 的一种结构性类似物,其与同一 B7 密切结合。由 CTLA–4 的胞外域及人 IgG1 Fc 域(CTLA–4–Ig)组成的重组融合蛋白特异性结合 B7 配体,因此阻断 CD28–B7 交互作用。该阻断在不同的动物模型中被证明是强效的免疫抑制分子[213,215–200]。CTLA4–Ig(阿巴西普)的第一个临床配方是具有一段突变的 Fc 域,被用来治疗类风湿关节炎和银屑病。贝拉西普(LEA29Y)是研发的第二代更高亲和力的用于移植临床试验的突变体[208]。2011 年,美国食品和药物管理局(FDA)批准贝拉西普用(Nulojix)于预防成年人肾移植急性排斥反应。

细胞靶点

贝拉西普的直接的分子靶点 B7–1(CD80)和 B7–2(CD86)在特异性造血细胞(树突细胞、B 细胞、巨噬细胞)上弱表达,并被激活这些细胞成熟为抗原递呈细胞的激活信号(CD40、TLR 激动剂、炎性介质)所上调。B7–1 和 B7–2 代表共刺激受体 CD28 的配体,其表达于所有小鼠和大多数人外周 T 细胞上。

CD28/B7 的 T 细胞活化是关键通路[213]。CD28 T 细

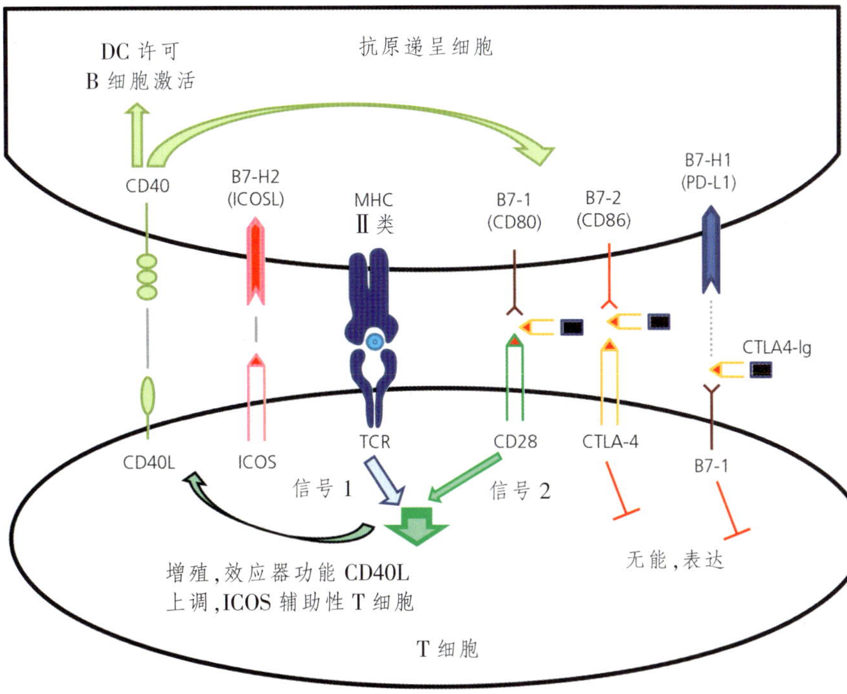

图 17.5 贝拉西普的激活机制。CD28–B7 复合物包含 2 个 B7 配体(CD80 和 CD86)以及两个 T 细胞受体(CD28 和 CTLA–4)。两个 B7 配体能与 CD28 和 CTLA–4 结合。如果 T 细胞与抗原特异性 T 细胞受体(TCR)介导的信号(信号 1)结合,然后,B7–CD28 交互作用产生共刺激信号(信号 2),包括上调 CD40L 和 ICOS 等共刺激分子促进 T 细胞的完全激活以及树突细胞和 B 细胞的交互激活。与此相反,B7–CTLA–4 和 B7–1–PD–L1 交互作用可能通过 T 细胞无能和调节抑制免疫反应。贝拉西普是一种重组的融合蛋白,由 CTLA–4 的胞外域和人 IgG1 Fc 域组成。它与 B7 配体密切结合,进而阻止 B7 与其他受体的交互作用。最终结果是 T 细胞、B 细胞和树突细胞活化下降的免疫抑制状态。

胞受体提供一个信号，与T细胞抗原受体(TCR)协同刺激活化T细胞，使其增殖并分泌细胞因子[223-225](图17.5)。通过增加IL-2的转录和mRNA的稳定性，以及增加抗凋亡蛋白Bcl-XL的表达，共同刺激T细胞扩增。因此，阻断该通路可抑制T细胞增殖，在某些情况下可引起T细胞抗原特异性低反应性、无能或细胞死亡[209,226]。CD28信号还可通过上调细胞因子和趋化因子来调节辅助T细胞分化[227]和迁移[228,229]。CD28信号还增强CD154和ICOS等其他共刺激分子的表达，这些共刺激分子也与T细胞活化有关。因此，在多个体内和体外实验模型中，CTLA4-Ig可抑制T细胞增殖、活化和分化[230-233]。

不同的T细胞亚群对CTLA4-Ig的易感性不同。多年来，人们认为记忆性T细胞不需要CD28/B7衍生的共刺激来产生回忆反应[234]。基于先前的研究结果，记忆性CD4 T细胞在体外被B1缺陷的APC完全激活[235,236]，并且CD28-/-小鼠在记忆性CD8 T细胞对病毒感染的产生或回忆中没有受损[237]。但是，最近证据对该理念产生挑战，啮齿类$CD4^+$和$CD8^+$ T细胞需要CD28同刺激通路来达到最大量的扩增和抗原清除[238-240]，虽然CD28/B7交互作用可以调节某一些但并不是所有的T细胞功能[241]。CTLA4-Ig治疗类风湿关节炎[242]和银屑病[243]等由CD4记忆T细胞驱动的疾病的临床效果[212]，提示CD28/B7通路也可能调节人CD4记忆T细胞介导的免疫反应。但是，人类记忆和效应T细胞亚群不表达CD28已被描述，因此预计对CTLA4-Ig不敏感。此外，应用CTLA4-Ig阻断B7可抑制阳性(CD28/B7)和阴性(CTLA-4/B7和PD-L1/B7)免疫调节信号，这可引起CTLA4-Ig对效应和记忆T细胞产生复杂的影响[250,251]。除了原始和记忆T细胞，CD28和CTLA-4受体也表达在自然的和诱导的调节T细胞上[259]，B7/CD28共刺激对于调节T细胞的稳态是十分重要的[260,261]，CTLA-4调节自然调节T细胞的潜能[262]。CTLA4-Ig因此可改变调节T细胞的稳定状态和数量[262-265]，对接受长期治疗的患者关于其对内源性调节T细胞的影响具有潜在意义。

虽然CD28已经被完全定义为典型T淋巴细胞受体，它还表达于浆细胞表面[266,267]，但是在B细胞的表达受到特别限制[268]。因此，虽然CTLA4-Ig在各种模型中对调节体液反应的影响归因于辅助T细胞和生发中心形成的共刺激[219,220,269]，B系对CD28在控制浆细胞分化和功能方面的内在作用超越生发中心形成在理论上是可能的[268]。

在体外使用CTLA4-Ig治疗巨噬细胞可下调细胞因子的生成[269,270]，在体外CTLA4-Ig能减少巨噬细胞相关基因在大树肾移植模型中的表达[219]。此外，CTLA4-Ig能结合表达于树突细胞上的B7分子，并激活色氨酸分解代谢通路，导致吲哚胺2,3双加氧酶(IDO)产生，这是一种可以分解色氨酸的细胞内酶，可间接抑制淋巴细胞活化和T细胞死亡[271,272]。虽然CTLA4-Ig的临床制剂(阿巴西普和贝拉西普)有突变的Fc域，但是其是否还保持该固有属性仍不明确。

适应性免疫

因为CTLA4-Ig/贝拉西普可调节T细胞活化和T-B和T-APC同源相互作用的共刺激信号，故推测其可强效抑制自身免疫疾病和移植中的病理性适应性免疫反应[230-233]。

缺血再灌注损伤和炎性反应

用CTLA4-Ig阻断T细胞CD28-B7共刺激通路可明显降低T细胞和巨噬细胞在大鼠肾移植模型中的渗透和活化[273]。并且，B7-1参与调节啮齿类动物脓毒症中固有免疫反应，该过程由依赖B7相关NF-κB受体IRAK-M的巨噬细胞/中性粒细胞调控[274]。这些结果提示贝拉西普可能直接作用于固有免疫反应。

感染

相对于其他的免疫抑制治疗，贝拉西普相关的机会性感染风险增加。在肾移植临床试验中，贝拉西普治疗组总感染率类似于环孢素组，但是贝拉西普的结核病和单纯疱疹的感染率较高。

代谢

在一项三期多中心肾移植临床试验中，相对于对照组(标准的环孢素免疫抑制方案)，贝拉西普组非免疫性毒性反应较少(神经毒性、高脂血症和心血管事件)。此外，相对于环孢素组，贝拉西普组血压水平较低[275-277]。

肿瘤/增殖

类似于环孢素，贝拉西普因为其系统性的免疫抑制，发生肿瘤的风险增加。此外，贝拉西普还可导致移植后淋巴组织增生性疾病(PTLD)，主要是中枢神经系统。

结果，EB 病毒血清学阴性或未知者禁用贝拉西普。贝拉西普对肿瘤增殖无直接抑制作用，除非该肿瘤表达 B7。

抗胸腺细胞球蛋白

抗淋巴细胞血清，尤其是抗胸腺细胞血清在移植免疫中具有悠久且辉煌的历史[278-280]。近期，两类抗胸腺细胞 γ 球蛋白(ATG)产品，来自兔(rATG，临床上为即复宁)或者来自马(eATG，临床上为 ATGAM®)，被用于诱导方案和急性排斥反应。两种 ATG 均为纯化的多克隆免疫球蛋白混合物，主要含有从人胸腺细胞免疫动物中提取的 IgG 亚型抗体。直接比较 rATG 和 eATG 表明，在淋巴细胞减少症的诱导和维持，以及防止肾移植急性排斥反应中，rATG 效果更好[281]。

细胞靶点

T 细胞是 ATG 的主要细胞靶点。ATG 识别的分子是极其多样的，包括 T 细胞特异性靶点如 CD3、CD28、CD152 和 T 细胞受体，主要表达于 T 细胞的分子如 CD2、CD4、CD8 和 CD25，以及表达更广泛的蛋白如 CD11a、CD45 和 HLA Ⅰ类和Ⅱ类分子。

ATG 识别 T 细胞后具有多种效应[282-288]。T 细胞耗损是快速的，通过几种不同机制发生，包括补体介导的细胞溶解[285]、受体介导的细胞凋亡[282]和 ADCC[287]。并且，ATG 可通过 CD25 负性调节 T 细胞增殖[289]。ATG 还可通过特异性结合于 T 细胞黏附分子或趋化因子受体来调节 T 细胞迁移[283,290]。ATG 还可增强调节性 T 细胞的发育和积聚[291-294]。这些细胞反过来通过一系列机制负性调节效应 T 细胞功能[295]。

虽然 T 细胞是 ATG 的预定靶点，但是 ATG 还可调控其他细胞。ATG 可消耗 NK 细胞和 B 细胞[296,297]。未被消耗的 NK 细胞活化标记物增多[298]，产生 IFN-γ，但也表现 ADCC 能力下降[299]。

除了作用于淋巴细胞，ATG 还可调控固有免疫细胞，尤其是树突细胞和中性粒细胞。ATG 治疗可导致中性粒细胞短暂活化，随后出现中性粒细胞减少[300]。ATG 可阻断树突细胞针对炎性信号的抗原摄取和细胞成熟，并减少细胞凋亡[301]。

适应性免疫

ATG 可耗尽 $CD4^+$和 $CD8^+$ T 细胞、B 细胞、浆细胞和启动适应性免疫的树突细胞。并且，暴露于 ATG 但侥幸存活的细胞，其功能也受到抑制，涉及抗原递呈与识别、B 细胞辅助、迁移和效应功能。ATG 的这些活动导致效应淋巴细胞大量减少。所有这些 ATG 对白细胞的效应使其成为适应性免疫的有效抑制剂[278,279]。

缺血再灌注炎性反应(IRI)

有证据表明，ATG 大概是通过抑制与 IRI 相关的固有免疫细胞的迁徙及功能活动来抑制 IRI[290]。在 ATG 治疗灵长类动物模型中，内皮黏附分子的数量明显下降。这与促炎细胞因子表达下降有关，表明抑制白细胞迁徙可以降低缺血再灌注相关的炎性反应。

感染

ATG 可增加机会性感染的易感性，尤其是巨细胞病毒感染[302-305]。但是其他团队报道 ATG 增加巨细胞病毒感染风险，其程度与另一种诱导方法相同，表明 ATG 具有全面的免疫抑制作用，其增加感染风险不是 ATG 的固有效应[306]。另一项研究表明，在预防措施下巨细胞病毒感染风险将会消除[307]。

代谢

ATG 与代谢副反应无关，所以它被用于皮质类固醇诱导方案中减轻代谢副反应[308,309]。

肿瘤/增殖

ATG 对肿瘤的发生，尤其是 PTLD 的影响，在多项研究中结果相互矛盾[310-312]。虽然 ATG 对于肿瘤发生的作用不明确，但是联用免疫抑制剂导致的整体免疫抑制状态似乎会增加肿瘤风险[311]。因此，类似免疫诱导中的其他药物，ATG 会增加 PTLD 和其他肿瘤发生的概率[310,311]。

静脉用免疫球蛋白(IVIG)

活体捐献增加了器官的数量，但是发现供体对同种异体抗原的敏感性增加，表现为抗体对 HLA 抗原具有广泛的特异性。此外，移植后出现的抗体介导的排斥反应(AMR)中同种异体抗体已成为肾移植[313,314]、心脏移植和胰腺移植[315]的成功的主要障碍。不幸的是，近期的免疫抑制治疗没有有效针对这种抗体介导的免疫机制。静脉用免疫球蛋白已经在许多抗体介导的自身免疫疾病中取得巨大临床疗效[316-318],近期已经成为移植前免疫诱导的药物之一,以治疗抗体介导的排斥反应[319]。但静脉用免疫球蛋白的疗效仍具有争议，并且其作用机制也未明确[320-322]。静脉用免疫球蛋白也已经成功用于治疗 ABO 血型不合的器官移植[323]。此外,在巨细胞病毒阴性血液制品和更昔洛韦出现之前[324],IVIG 被广泛用于骨髓移植患者病毒感染的治疗或预防治疗，并且在骨髓[325]或器官移植后[326-328]仍偶尔用于治疗感染。

概念与结构

静脉用免疫球蛋白大部分含有大量血浆提取的 IgG，仅仅少量的 IgA 和 IgM。静脉用免疫球蛋白是经过消毒的净化的产品。虽然其疗效明显,但是静脉用免疫球蛋白含有提取自 5000~50 000 名供体的 IgG,这限制了它的产量,增加了费用,并且每一袋 IVIG 可能具有其独特的免疫特点,从而影响其耐受性和效果。

虽然 IVIG 在治疗体液免疫缺陷疾病、自身免疫调节、炎症和器官移植中获得成功,但其作用机制还不明确[329-331]。它的某些机制可能是由于自然抗体或抗独特性抗体的存在[332,333]。静脉用免疫球蛋白直接结合并中和抗原、不同的靶细胞和分子,并阻断补体凝集。除了抗原结合,或 Fab 介导的机制,近期的证据确认了免疫球蛋白 Fc 部分的作用,以及 IVIG 介导的在调节免疫调节中 Fc 多聚体化的作用[334-337]。Fab 与 Fc 依赖的机制并不是互相独立的,它们可能不变地参与不同的病理环境。

细胞靶点

IVIG 能通过与 Fcγ 受体(FcγR)作用直接结合多种细胞。在小鼠中已经发现 4 种不同的 FcγR(FcγRⅠ、FcγRⅡ、FcγRⅢ、FcγRⅣ),在人与猿猴中,同源蛋白质被分为 3 大类(FcγRⅠ、FcγRⅡ、FcγRⅢ),在每个种族中都有其余的变种。不同的造血细胞，包括单核细胞、巨噬细胞、树突细胞、中性粒细胞、肥大细胞、NK 细胞和 NKT 细胞,表达一种或多种 FcγR,但是 FcγR 在 T 细胞中缺失。大多数 FcγR 传递细胞免疫功能的激活信号,例如,吞噬作用和 ADCC。相反,FcγRIIB 作为唯一的 FcγR,是一种免疫受体酪氨酸抑制基序,可抑制细胞免疫反应,并与免疫耐受有关[338-340]。B 细胞仅表达 FcγRⅡB [341,342],B 细胞的活化和生存均由 FcγR 信号调控，这些发现与 IVIG 对体液排斥反应的治疗效果一致。IVIG 还可通过结合于内皮细胞新生的 Fc 受体(FcRn)加速病理性 IgG 抗体的清除[343,344]。

适应性免疫

临床应用 ICIG 主要针对适应性体液免疫反应中的演进(B 细胞和浆细胞)和产物(抗体)。并且,FcγR 存在于不同的造血细胞、调节性 T 细胞[345]和抑制性 T 细胞亚型上,表明 IVIG 对免疫稳态和免疫耐受还具有其他潜在作用。

缺血再灌注损伤和炎性反应

由同种异体抗体调控放大的 IRI 和炎性反应可被 IVIG 间接抑制。此外,因为 IVIG 对其他疾病具有抗炎作用,其对表达 FcγR 的固有免疫细胞也认为具有直接作用[333]。

感染

IVIG 对骨髓移植受体的病毒感染具有预防和治疗作用[324],在骨髓移植[325]和器官移植[326-328]中仍偶尔用于感染。应用 IVIG 和利妥昔单抗抗排斥不增加肾移植的感染风险[347]。但是,人来源的 IVIG 具有潜在的未知感染风险。

代谢

应用 IVIG 治疗抗体介导的排斥反应患者中,可观察到少量但是显著的血栓形成率，这可被更慢的灌注速度和抗血小板和抗凝治疗纠正。IVIG 对动脉粥样硬化的研究提示 IVIG 对代谢具有有益的作用[349]。

肿瘤/增殖

在 IVIG 中的自然抗体可抑制肿瘤生长[350]。但是,由 FcγR 抑制信号调节的免疫抑制可导致肿瘤发生。

总结

现代移植仍需要依赖多种免疫调节药物，根据作用机制和结构，可分为糖皮质激素、钙调磷酸酶抑制剂、mTOR 抑制剂、嘌呤类似物和单克隆、多克隆蛋白制剂。认识到其效应和副反应,这些药物使移植成为可能。当制定临床决策阻止和治疗排斥反应时,读者可参考这些药物的参考文献和本章节所描述的作用机制。

(焦守斐 译 程倩 校)

参考文献

1. Baxter JD. The effects of glucocorticoid therapy. Hospital Practice (Office Ed.). 1992;27:111-114, 115-118, 123 passim.
2. Opelz G, Dohler B, Laux G. Long-term prospective study of steroid withdrawal in kidney and heart transplant recipients. American Journal of Transplantation. 2005;5:720-728.
3. Matas AJ, Kandaswamy R, Gillingham KJ, et al. Prednisone-free maintenance immunosuppression—a 5-year experience. American Journal of Transplantation. 2005;5:2473-2478.
4. Augustine JJ, Hricik DE. Steroid sparing in kidney transplantation: changing paradigms, improving outcomes, and remaining questions. Clinical Journal of the American Society of Nephrology. 2006;1:1080-1089.
5. Rhen T, Cidlowski JA. Antiinflammatory action of glucocorticoids-new mechanisms for old drugs. New England Journal of Medicine. 2005;353:1711-1723.
6. Breuner CW, Orchinik M. Plasma binding proteins as mediators of corticosteroid action in vertebrates. Journal of Endocrinology. 2002;175:99-112.
7. Henley DE, Lightman SL. New insights into corticosteroid-binding globulin and glucocorticoid delivery. Neuroscience. 2011;180:1-8.
8. Almawi WY, Melemedjian OK, Rieder MJ. An alternate mechanism of glucocorticoid anti-proliferative effect: promotion of a Th2 cytokine-secreting profile. Clinical Transplantation. 1999;13:365-374.
9. Chakraborty A, Blum RA, Mis SM, et al. Pharmacokinetic and adrenal interactions of IL-10 and prednisone in healthy volunteers. Journal of Clinical Pharmacology. 1999;39:624-635.
10. Mittal SK, Sharma RK, Gupta A, et al. Increased interleukin-10 production without expansion of CD4+CD25+ T-regulatory cells in early stable renal transplant patients on calcineurin inhibitors. Transplantation. 2009;88:435-441.
11. Herold MJ, McPherson KG, Reichardt HM. Glucocorticoids in T cell apoptosis and function. Cellular and Molecular Life Sciences. 2006;63:60-72.
12. Caramori G, Adcock I. Anti-inflammatory mechanisms of glucocorticoids targeting granulocytes. Current Drug Targets. Inflammation and Allergy. 2005;4:455-463.
13. Tuckermann JP, Kleiman A, McPherson KG, et al. Molecular mechanisms of glucocorticoids in the control of inflammation and lymphocyte apoptosis. Critical Reviews in Clinical Laboratory Sciences. 2005;42:71-104.
14. Buttgereit F, Straub RH, Wehling M, et al. Glucocorticoids in the treatment of rheumatic diseases: an update on the mechanisms of action. Arthritis and Rheumatism. 2004;50:3408-3417.
15. Hafezi-Moghadam A, Simoncini T, Yang Z, et al. Acute cardiovascular protective effects of corticosteroids are mediated by non-transcriptional activation of endothelial nitric oxide synthase. Nature Medicine. 2002;8:473-479.
16. Gold R, Buttgereit F, Toyka KV. Mechanism of action of glucocorticosteroid hormones: possible implications for therapy of neuroimmunological disorders. Journal of Neuroimmunology. 2001;117:1-8.
17. Geissler EK, Schlitt HJ. Immunosuppression for liver transplantation. Gut. 2009;58:452-463.
18. Taylor AL, Watson CJ, Bradley JA. Immunosuppressive agents in solid organ transplantation: mechanisms of action and therapeutic efficacy. Critical Reviews in Oncology. 2005;56:23-46.
19. Segal BH, Sneller MC. Infectious complications of immunosuppressive therapy in patients with rheumatic diseases. Rheumatic Diseases Clinics of North America. 1997;23:219-237.
20. Poetker DM, Reh DD. A comprehensive review of the adverse effects of systemic corticosteroids. Otolaryngologic Clinics of North America. 2010;43:753-768.
21. Henry SD, Metselaar HJ, Van Dijck J, et al. Impact of steroids on hepatitis C virus replication in vivo and in vitro. Annals of the New York Academy of Sciences. 2007;1110:439-447.
22. Vivarelli M, Burra P, La Barba G, et al. Influence of steroids on HCV recurrence after liver transplantation: a prospective study. Journal of Hepatology. 2007;47:793-798.
23. Segev DL, Sozio SM, Shin EJ, et al. Steroid avoidance in liver transplantation: meta-analysis and meta-regression of randomized trials. Liver Transplantation. 2008;14:512-525.
24. Klintmalm GB, Washburn WK, Rudich SM, et al. Corticosteroid-free immunosuppression with daclizumab in HCV(+) liver transplant recipients: 1-year interim results of the HCV-3 study. Liver Transplantation. 2007;13:1521-1531.
25. Llado L, Fabregat J, Castellote J, et al. Impact of immunosuppression without steroids on rejection and hepatitis C virus evolution after liver transplantation: results of a prospective randomized study. Liver Transplantation. 2008;14:1752-1760.
26. Sgourakis G, Radtke A, Fouzas I, et al. Corticosteroid-free immunosuppression in liver transplantation: a meta-analysis and meta-regression of outcomes. Transplant International. 2009;22:892-905.
27. Atkinson JB, Kosi M, Srikanth MS, et al. Growth hormone reverses impaired wound healing in protein-malnourished rats treated with corticosteroids. Journal of Pediatric Surgery. 1992;27:1026-1028.
28. Nguyen H, Lim J, Dresner ML, et al. Effect of local corticosteroids on early inflammatory function in surgical wound of rats. Journal of Foot and Ankle Surgery. 1998;37:313-318.
29. Goforth P, Gudas CJ. Effects of steroids on wound healing: a review of the literature. Journal of Foot Surgery. 1980;19:22-28.
30. Suh DY, Hunt TK, Spencer EM. Insulin-like growth factor-I reverses the impairment of wound healing induced by corticosteroids in rats. Endocrinology. 1992;131:2399-2403.
31. Lenco W, McKnight M, Macdonald AS. Effects of cortisone acetate, methylprednisolone and medroxyprogesterone on wound contracture and epithelization in rabbits. Annals of Surgery. 1975;181:67-73.
32. Jordan ML, Shapiro R, Fung J, et al. Initial studies with FK506 in renal transplantation. Cleveland Clinic Journal of Medicine. 1991;58:444-446.
33. Todo S, Fung JJ, Starzl TE, et al. Single-center experience with primary orthotopic liver transplantation with FK 506 immunosuppression. Annals of Surgery. 1994;220:297-308.
34. Reding R, Wallemacq PE, Lamy ME, et al. Conversion from cyclosporine to FK506 for salvage of immunocompromised pediatric liver allografts. Efficacy, toxicity, and dose regimen in 23 children. Transplantation. 1994;57:93-100.
35. Shaw KT, Ho AM, Raghavan A, et al. Immunosuppressive drugs prevent a rapid dephosphorylation of transcription factor NFAT1 in stimulated immune cells. Proceedings of the National Academy of Sciences of the United States of America 1995;92:11205-11209.
36. Li H, Rao A, Hogan PG. Interaction of calcineurin with substrates and targeting proteins. Trends in Cell Biology. 2011;21:91-103.
37. Halloran PF. Mechanism of action of the calcineurin inhibitors. Transplantation Proceedings. 2001;33:3067-3069.
38. Sharif A, Shabir S, Chand S, et al. Meta-analysis of calcineurin-inhibitor-sparing regimens in kidney transplantation. Journal of the American Society of Nephrology. 2011;22:2107-2118.
39. Casey MJ, Meier-Kriesche HU. Calcineurin inhibitors in kidney transplantation: friend or foe? Current Opinion in Nephrology and Hypertension. 2011;20:610-615.
40. Pham PT, Pham PM, Pham SV, et al. New onset diabetes after transplantation (NODAT): an overview. Diabetes, Metabolic Syndrome and Obesity. 2011;4:175-186.
41. Pengel LH, Liu LQ, Morris PJ. Do wound complications or lymphoceles occur more often in solid organ transplant recipients on mTOR inhibitors? A systematic review of randomized controlled trials. Transplant International. 2011;24:1216-1230.
42. Weir MR, Mulgaonkar S, Chan L, et al. Mycophenolate mofetil-based immunosuppression with sirolimus in renal transplantation: a randomized, controlled Spare-the-Nephron trial. Kidney International. 2011;79:897-907.
43. Busque S, Leventhal J, Brennan DC, et al. Calcineurin-inhibitor-free immunosuppression based on the JAK inhibitor CP-690,550: a pilot study in de novo kidney allograft recipients. American Journal of Transplantation. 2009;9:1936-1945.
44. Shaffer D, Kizilisik AT, Feurer I, et al. Calcineurin inhibitor avoidance versus steroid avoidance following kidney transplantation: postoperative complications. Transplantation Proceedings. 2006;38:3464-3465.
45. Hashimoto Y, Perrino BA, Soderling TR. Identification of an autoinhibitory domain in calcineurin. Journal of Biological Chemistry. 1990;265:1924-1927.
46. Kissinger CR, Parge HE, Knighton DR, et al. Crystal structures of human calcineurin and the human FKBP12-FK506-calcineurin complex. Nature. 1995;378:641-644.
47. Heissmeyer V, Macián F, Im SH, et al. Calcineurin imposes T cell unresponsiveness through targeted proteolysis of signaling proteins. Nature Immunology. 2004;5:255-265.
48. Macian F, López-Rodríguez C, Rao A. Partners in transcription: NFAT and AP-1. Oncogene. 2001;20:2476-2489.
49. Liu J, Farmer JD Jr, Lane WS, et al. Calcineurin is a common target of cyclophilin-cyclosporin A and FKBP-FK506 complexes. Cell. 1991;66:807-815.
50. Heidt S, Roelen DL, Eijsink C,et al. Calcineurin inhibitors affect B cell antibody responses indirectly by interfering with T cell help. Clinical and Experimental

Immunology. 2010;159:199–207.
51. Sakuma S, Higashi Y, Sato N, et al. Tacrolimus suppressed the production of cytokines involved in atopic dermatitis by direct stimulation of human PBMC system. (Comparison with steroids). International Immunopharmacology. 2001; 1:1219–1226.
52. Okada Y, Maeda N, Takakura S, et al. Preventive and therapeutic effects of tacrolimus in an interleukin-10-deficient mouse model of colitis. Inflammation Research. 2011;60:1049–1059.
53. Caproni M, Torchia D, Antiga E, et al. The effects of tacrolimus ointment on regulatory T lymphocytes in atopic dermatitis. Journal of Clinical Immunology. 2006;26:370–375.
54. Levitsky J, Gallon L, Miller J, et al. Allospecific regulatory effects of sirolimus and tacrolimus in the human mixed lymphocyte reaction. Transplantation. 2011; 91:199–206.
55. Vukmanovic-Stejic M, McQuaid A, Birch KE, et al. Relative impact of CD4+CD25+ regulatory T cells and tacrolimus on inhibition of T-cell proliferation in patients with atopic dermatitis. British Journal of Dermatology. 2005; 153:750–757.
56. Kuwata T, Asada A, Ohoka Y, et al. A role of calcineurin in coreceptor regulation during differentiation of Cd4+Cd8+ T cells. Biochemical and Biophysical Research Communications. 1998;247:242–248.
57. Steele DJ, Laufer TM, Smiley ST, et al. Two levels of help for B cell alloantibody production. Journal of Experimental Medicine. 1996;183:699–703.
58. Lamoureux F, Mestre E, Essig M, et al. Quantitative proteomic analysis of cyclosporine-induced toxicity in a human kidney cell line and comparison with tacrolimus. Journal of Proteomics. 2011;75:677–694.
59. Lee J, Choi TG, Ha J, et al. Cyclosporine A suppresses immunoglobulin G biosynthesis via inhibition of cyclophilin B in murine hybridomas and B cells. International Immunopharmacology. 2012;12:42–49.
60. El Bekay R, Alba G, Reyes ME, et al. Rac2 GTPase activation by angiotensin II is modulated by Ca2+/calcineurin and mitogen-activated protein kinases in human neutrophils. Journal of Molecular Endocrinology. 2007;39: 351–363.
61. El Bekay R, Alvarez M, Monteseirin J, et al. Oxidative stress is a critical mediator of the angiotensin II signal in human neutrophils: involvement of mitogen-activated protein kinase, calcineurin, and the transcription factor NF-kappaB. Blood. 2003;102:662–671.
62. Knaus UG, Heyworth PG, Evans T, et al. Regulation of phagocyte oxygen radical production by the GTP-binding protein Rac 2. Science. 1991;254: 1512–1515.
63. Meiser BM, Billingham ME, Morris RE, et al. Effects of cyclosporin, FK506, and rapamycin on graft-vessel disease. Lancet. 1991;338:1297–1298.
64. Zoja C, Furci L, Ghilardi F, et al. Cyclosporin-induced endothelial cell injury. Laboratory Investigation. 1986;55:455–462.
65. Ramzy D, Rao V, Tumiati LC, et al. Role of endothelin-1 and nitric oxide bioavailability in transplant-related vascular injury: comparative effects of rapamycin and cyclosporine. Circulation. 2006;114:214–219.
66. Badiwala MV, Guha D, Tumiati L, et al. Epidermal growth factor-like domain 7 is a novel inhibitor of neutrophil adhesion to coronary artery endothelial cells injured by calcineurin inhibition. Circulation. 2011;124:S197–S203.
67. Myers BD, Sibley R, Newton L, et al. The long-term course of cyclosporine-associated chronic nephropathy. Kidney International. 1988;33:590–600.
68. Scalea JR, Butler CC, Munivenkatappa RB, et al. Pancreas transplant alone as an independent risk factor for the development of renal failure: a retrospective study. Transplantation. 2008;86:1789–1794.
69. Rinschen MM, Klokkers J, Pavenstadt H, et al. Different effects of CsA and FK506 on aquaporin-2 abundance in rat primary cultured collecting duct cells. Pflugers Archiv: European Journal of Physiology. 2011;462:611–622.
70. Busauschina A, Schnuelle P, van der Woude FJ. Cyclosporine nephrotoxicity. Transplantation Proceedings. 2004;36:229S–233S.
71. el Akool S, Gauer S, Osman B, et al. Cyclosporin A and tacrolimus induce renal Erk1/2 pathway via ROS-induced and metalloproteinase-dependent EGF-receptor signaling. Biochemical Pharmacology. 2012;83:286–295.
72. Ozbay LA, Smidt K, Mortensen DM, et al. Cyclosporin and tacrolimus impair insulin secretion and transcriptional regulation in INS-1E beta-cells. British Journal of Pharmacology. 2011;162:136–146.
73. Lawrence MC, Bhatt HS, Easom RA. NFAT regulates insulin gene promoter activity in response to synergistic pathways induced by glucose and glucagon-like peptide-1. Diabetes. 2002;51:691–698.
74. Ekberg H, Bernasconi C, Noldeke J, et al. Cyclosporine, tacrolimus and sirolimus retain their distinct toxicity profiles despite low doses in the Symphony study. Nephrology, Dialysis, Transplantation. 2010;25:2004–2010.
75. Nito C, Ueda M, Inaba T, et al. FK506 ameliorates oxidative damage and protects rat brain following transient focal cerebral ischemia. Neurological Research. 2011;33:881–889.
76. Furuichi Y, Katsuta K, Maeda M, et al. Neuroprotective action of tacrolimus (FK506) in focal and global cerebral ischemia in rodents: dose dependency, therapeutic time window and long-term efficacy. Brain Research. 2003;965: 137–145.
77. Kristo I, Wilflingseder J, Kainz A, et al. Effect of intraportal infusion of tacrolimus on ischaemic reperfusion injury in orthotopic liver transplantation: a randomized controlled trial. Transplant International. 2011;24:912–919.
78. Dandel M, Lehmkuhl HB, Knosalla C, et al. Impact of different long-term maintenance immunosuppressive therapy strategies on patients' outcome after heart transplantation. Transplant Immunology. 2010;23:93–103.
79. Petri JB, Schurk S, Gebauer S, et al. Cyclosporine A delays wound healing and apoptosis and suppresses activin beta-A expression in rats. European Journal of Dermatology. 1998;8:104–113.
80. Pirsch JD, D'Alessandro AM, Sollinger HW, et al. Hyperlipidemia and transplantation: etiologic factors and therapy. Journal of the American Society of Nephrology. 1992;2:S238–S242.
81. Perrea DN, Moulakakis KG, Poulakou MV, et al. Correlation between lipid abnormalities and immunosuppressive therapy in renal transplant recipients with stable renal function. International Urology and Nephrology. 2008;40: 521–527.
82. Martinez Castelao A, Ramos R, Seron D, et al. Effect of cyclosporin and tacrolimus on lipoprotein oxidation after renal transplantation. Nefrologia. 2002;22:364–369.
83. Senzolo M, Ferronato C, Burra P. Neurologic complications after solid organ transplantation. Transplant International. 2009;22:269–278.
84. Kasiske BL, Snyder JJ, Gilbertson DT, et al. Cancer after kidney transplantation in the United States. American Journal of Transplantation. 2004; 4:905–913.
85. Braconnier P, Del Marmol V, Broeders N, et al. Combined introduction of anti-IL2 receptor antibodies, mycophenolic acid and tacrolimus: effect on malignancies after renal transplantation in a single-centre retrospective cohort study. Nephrology, Dialysis, Transplantation. 2012;27:2547–2553.
86. Maisonneuve P, Agodoa L, Gellert R, et al. Cancer in patients on dialysis for end-stage renal disease: an international collaborative study. Lancet. 1999; 354:93–99.
87. Schupp N, Heidland A, Stopper H. Genomic damage in endstage renal disease-contribution of uremic toxins. Toxins (Basel). 2010;2:2340–2358.
88. Romano S, Mallardo M, Romano MF. FKBP51 and the NF-kappaB regulatory pathway in cancer. Current Opinion in Pharmacology. 2011;11: 288–293.
89. Marienfeld R, Neumann M, Chuvpilo S, et al. Cyclosporin A interferes with the inducible degradation of NF-kappa B inhibitors, but not with the processing of p105/NF-kappa B1 in T cells. European Journal of Immunology. 1997;27: 1601–1609.
90. Powell JD, Delgoffe GM. The mammalian target of rapamycin: linking T cell differentiation, function, and metabolism. Immunity. 2010;33:301–311.
91. Weichhart T, Saemann MD. The multiple facets of mTOR in immunity. Trends in Immunology. 2009;30:218–226.
92. Saemann MD, Haidinger M, Hecking M, et al. The multifunctional role of mTOR in innate immunity: implications for transplant immunity. American Journal of Transplantation. 2009;9:2655–2661.
93. Thomson AW, Turnquist HR, Raimondi G. Immunoregulatory functions of mTOR inhibition. Nature Reviews. Immunology. 2009;9:324–337.
94. Schmelzle T, Hall MN. TOR, a central controller of cell growth. Cell. 2000;103:253–262.
95. Wullschleger S, Loewith R, Hall MN. TOR signaling in growth and metabolism. Cell. 2006;124:471–484.
96. Sarbassov DD, Ali SM, Sengupta S, et al. Prolonged rapamycin treatment inhibits mTORC2 assembly and Akt/PKB. Molecular Cell. 2006;22:159–168.
97. Weir MR, Diekmann F, Flechner SM, et al. mTOR inhibition: the learning curve in kidney transplantation. Transplant International. 2010;23:447–460.
98. Halloran PF. Immunosuppressive drugs for kidney transplantation. New England Journal of Medicine. 2004;351:2715–2729.
99. Zheng Y, Collins SL, Lutz MA, et al. A role for mammalian target of rapamycin in regulating T cell activation versus anergy. Journal of Immunology. 2007; 178:2163–2170.
100. Zheng Y, Delgoffe GM, Meyer CF, et al. Anergic T cells are metabolically anergic. Journal of Immunology. 2009;183:6095–6101.
101. Sinclair LV, Finlay D, Feijoo C, et al. Phosphatidylinositol-3-OH kinase and nutrient-sensing mTOR pathways control T lymphocyte trafficking. Nature Immunology. 2008;9:513–521.
102. Valmori D, Tosello V, Souleimanian NE, et al. Rapamycin-mediated enrichment of T cells with regulatory activity in stimulated CD4+ T cell cultures is not due to the selective expansion of naturally occurring regulatory T cells but to the induction of regulatory functions in conventional CD4+ T cells. Journal of

Immunology. 2006;177:944–949.

103. Tresoldi E, Dell'Albani I, Stabilini A, et al. Stability of human rapamycin-expanded CD4+CD25+ T regulatory cells. Haematologica. 2011;96: 1357–1365.

104. Battaglia M, Stabilini A, Migliavacca B, et al. Rapamycin promotes expansion of functional CD4+CD25+FOXP3+ regulatory T cells of both healthy subjects and type 1 diabetic patients. Journal of Immunology. 2006;177:8338–8347.

105. Battaglia M, Stabilini A, Draghici E, et al. Rapamycin and interleukin-10 treatment induces T regulatory type 1 cells that mediate antigen-specific transplantation tolerance. Diabetes. 2006;55:40–49.

106. Battaglia M, Stabilini A, Roncarolo MG. Rapamycin selectively expands CD4+CD25+FoxP3+ regulatory T cells. Blood. 2005;105:4743–4748.

107. Kang J, Huddleston SJ, Fraser JM, et al. De novo induction of antigen-specific CD4+CD25+Foxp3+ regulatory T cells in vivo following systemic antigen administration accompanied by blockade of mTOR. Journal of Leukocyte Biology. 2008;83:1230–1239.

108. Delgoffe GM, Kole TP, Zheng Y, et al. The mTOR kinase differentially regulates effector and regulatory T cell lineage commitment. Immunity. 2009;30: 832–844.

109. Morelon E, Lefrancois N, Besson C, et al. Preferential increase in memory and regulatory subsets during T-lymphocyte immune reconstitution after Thymoglobulin induction therapy with maintenance sirolimus vs cyclosporine. Transplant Immunology. 2010;23:53–58.

110. Basu S, Golovina T, Mikheeva T, et al. Cutting edge: foxp3-mediated induction of pim 2 allows human T regulatory cells to preferentially expand in rapamycin. Journal of Immunology. 2008;180:5794–5798.

111. Procaccini C, De Rosa V, Galgani M, et al. An oscillatory switch in mTOR kinase activity sets regulatory T cell responsiveness. Immunity. 2010;33: 929–941.

112. Vogelbacher R, Meister S, Guckel E, et al. Bortezomib and sirolimus inhibit the chronic active antibody-mediated rejection in experimental renal transplantation in the rat. Nephrology, Dialysis, Transplantation. 2010;25: 3764–3773.

113. Li Q, Rao RR, Araki K, et al. A central role for mTOR kinase in homeostatic proliferation induced CD8+ T cell memory and tumor immunity. Immunity. 2011;34:541–553.

114. Rao RR, Li Q, Odunsi K, et al. The mTOR kinase determines effector versus memory CD8+ T cell fate by regulating the expression of transcription factors T-bet and Eomesodermin. Immunity. 2010;32:67–78.

115. Araki K, Turner AP, Shaffer VO, et al. mTOR regulates memory CD8 T-cell differentiation. Nature. 2009;460:108–112.

116. Zhang S, Readinger JA, DuBois W, et al. Constitutive reductions in mTOR alter cell size, immune cell development, and antibody production. Blood. 2011; 117:1228–1238.

117. Benhamron S, Tirosh B. Direct activation of mTOR in B lymphocytes confers impairment in B-cell maturation and loss of marginal zone B cells. European Journal of Immunology. 2011;41:2390–2396.

118. Gomez-Cambronero J. Rapamycin inhibits GM-CSF-induced neutrophil migration. FEBS Letters. 2003;550:94–100.

119. Weichhart T, Haidinger M, Katholnig K, et al. Inhibition of mTOR blocks the anti-inflammatory effects of glucocorticoids in myeloid immune cells. Blood. 2011;117:4273–4283.

120. Weichhart T, Costantino G, Poglitsch M, et al. The TSC-mTOR signaling pathway regulates the innate inflammatory response. Immunity. 2008;29: 565–577.

121. Fischer R, Turnquist HR, Taner T, et al. Use of rapamycin in the induction of tolerogenic dendritic cells. Handbook of Experimental Pharmacology. 2009;188: 215–232.

122. Haidinger M, Poglitsch M, Geyeregger R, et al. A versatile role of mammalian target of rapamycin in human dendritic cell function and differentiation. Journal of Immunology. 2010;185:3919–3931.

123. Mohacsi PJ, Tuller D, Hulliger B, et al. Different inhibitory effects of immunosuppressive drugs on human and rat aortic smooth muscle and endothelial cell proliferation stimulated by platelet-derived growth factor or endothelial cell growth factor. Journal of Heart and Lung Transplantation. 1997;16: 484–492.

124. Schuler W, Sedrani R, Cottens S, et al. SDZ RAD, a new rapamycin derivative: pharmacological properties in vitro and in vivo. Transplantation. 1997;64: 36–42.

125. Vogelbacher R, Wittmann S, Braun A, et al. The mTOR inhibitor everolimus induces proteinuria and renal deterioration in the remnant kidney model in the rat. Transplantation. 2007;84:1492–1499.

126. Azzola A, Havryk A, Chhajed P, et al. Everolimus and mycophenolate mofetil are potent inhibitors of fibroblast proliferation after lung transplantation. Transplantation. 2004;77:275–280.

127. Salas-Prato M, Assalian A, Mehdi AZ, et al. Inhibition by rapamycin of PDGF- and bFGF-induced human tenon fibroblast proliferation in vitro. Journal of Glaucoma. 1996;5:54–59.

128. Goren I, Muller E, Schiefelbein D, et al. Akt1 controls insulin-driven VEGF biosynthesis from keratinocytes: implications for normal and diabetes-impaired skin repair in mice. Journal of Investigative Dermatology. 2009;129:752–764.

129. Khan S, Salloum F, Das A, et al. Rapamycin confers preconditioning-like protection against ischemia-reperfusion injury in isolated mouse heart and cardiomyocytes. Journal of Molecular and Cellular Cardiology. 2006;41:256–264.

130. Majewski M, Korecka M, Joergensen J, et al. Immunosuppressive TOR kinase inhibitor everolimus (RAD) suppresses growth of cells derived from posttransplant lymphoproliferative disorder at allograft-protecting doses. Transplantation. 2003;75:1710–1717.

131. Krams SM, Martinez OM. Epstein-Barr virus, rapamycin, and host immune responses. Current Opinion in Organ Transplantation. 2008;13:563–568.

132. Webster AC, Lee VW, Chapman JR, et al. Target of rapamycin inhibitors (sirolimus and everolimus) for primary immunosuppression of kidney transplant recipients: a systematic review and meta-analysis of randomized trials. Transplantation. 2006;81:1234–1248.

133. Groth CG, Backman L, Morales JM, et al. Sirolimus (rapamycin)-based therapy in human renal transplantation: similar efficacy and different toxicity compared with cyclosporine. Sirolimus European Renal Transplant Study Group. Transplantation. 1999;67:1036–1042.

134. Johnston O, Rose CL, Webster AC, et al. Sirolimus is associated with new-onset diabetes in kidney transplant recipients. Journal of the American Society of Nephrology. 2008;19:1411–1418.

135. Fraenkel M, Ketzinel-Gilad M, Ariav Y, et al. mTOR inhibition by rapamycin prevents beta-cell adaptation to hyperglycemia and exacerbates the metabolic state in type 2 diabetes. Diabetes. 2008;57:945–957.

136. Valente JF, Hricik D, Weigel K, et al. Comparison of sirolimus vs. mycophenolate mofetil on surgical complications and wound healing in adult kidney transplantation. American Journal of Transplantation. 2003;3:1128–1134.

137. Troppmann C, Pierce JL, Gandhi MM, et al. Higher surgical wound complication rates with sirolimus immunosuppression after kidney transplantation: a matched-pair pilot study. Transplantation. 2003;76:426–429.

138. Dean PG, Lund WJ, Larson TS, et al. Wound-healing complications after kidney transplantation: a prospective, randomized comparison of sirolimus and tacrolimus. Transplantation. 2004;77:1555–1561.

139. Kuppahally S, Al-Khaldi A, Weisshaar D, et al. Wound healing complications with de novo sirolimus versus mycophenolate mofetil-based regimen in cardiac transplant recipients. American Journal of Transplantation. 2006;6: 986–992.

140. Kauffman HM, Cherikh WS, Cheng Y, et al. Maintenance immunosuppression with target-of-rapamycin inhibitors is associated with a reduced incidence of de novo malignancies. Transplantation. 2005;80:883–889.

141. Salgo R, Gossmann J, Schofer H, et al. Switch to a sirolimus-based immunosuppression in long-term renal transplant recipients: reduced rate of (pre-) malignancies and nonmelanoma skin cancer in a prospective, randomized, assessor-blinded, controlled clinical trial. American Journal of Transplantation. 2010;10:1385–1393.

142. Allison AC, Eugui EM. Mycophenolate mofetil and its mechanisms of action. Immunopharmacology. 2000;47:85–118.

143. Poppe D, Tiede I, Fritz G, et al. Azathioprine suppresses ezrin-radixin-moesin-dependent T cell-APC conjugation through inhibition of Vav guanosine exchange activity on Rac proteins. Journal of Immunology. 2006;176: 640–651.

144. Aldinucci A, Biagioli T, Manuelli C, et al. Modulating dendritic cells (DC) from immunogenic to tolerogenic responses: a novel mechanism of AZA/6-MP. Journal of Neuroimmunology. 2010;218:28–35.

145. Lechmann M, Berchtold S, Hauber J, et al. CD83 on dendritic cells: more than just a marker for maturation. Trends in Immunology. 2002;23:273–275.

146. Kuwano Y, Prazma CM, Yazawa N, et al. CD83 influences cell-surface MHC class II expression on B cells and other antigen-presenting cells. International Immunology. 2007;19:977–992.

147. Prazma CM, Tedder TF. Dendritic cell CD83: a therapeutic target or innocent bystander? Immunology Letters. 2008;115:1–8.

148. Aerts-Toegaert C, Heirman C, Tuyaerts S, et al. CD83 expression on dendritic cells and T cells: correlation with effective immune responses. European Journal of Immunology. 2007;37:686–695.

149. Cohn RG, Mirkovich A, Dunlap B, et al. Mycophenolic acid increases apoptosis, lysosomes and lipid droplets in human lymphoid and monocytic cell lines. Transplantation. 1999;68:411–418.

150. Izeradjene K, Revillard JP. Apoptosis of superantigen-activated T cells induced by mycophenolate mofetil treatment. Transplantation. 2001;71:118–125.

151. Nakamura M, Ogawa N, Shalabi A, et al. Positive effect on T-cell regulatory

apoptosis by mycophenolate mofetil. Clinical Transplantation. 2001;15(Suppl. 6): 36–40.
152. Allison AC, Eugui EM. Immunosuppressive and other effects of mycophenolic acid and an ester prodrug, mycophenolate mofetil. Immunological Reviews. 1993;136:5–28.
153. Heemann U, Azuma H, Hamar P, et al. Mycophenolate mofetil inhibits lymphocyte binding and the upregulation of adhesion molecules in acute rejection of rat kidney allografts. Transplant Immunology. 1996;4:64–67.
154. Richter M, Zahn S, Richter H, et al. Reduction of ICAM-1 and LFA-1-positive leukocytes in the perivascular space of arteries under mycophenolate mofetil therapy reduces rat heart transplant vasculopathy. Journal of Heart and Lung Transplantation. 2004;23:1405–1413.
155. Barten MJ, van Gelder T, Gummert JF, et al. Pharmacodynamics of mycophenolate mofetil after heart transplantation: new mechanisms of action and correlations with histologic severity of graft rejection. American Journal of Transplantation. 2002;2:719–732.
156. Muller V, Hamar P, Szabo A, et al. Effect of mycophenolate mofetil on the in vivo infiltration of lymphocytes in the rat remnant kidney. Transplantation Proceedings. 1998;30:982.
157. Jonsson CA, Erlandsson M, Svensson L, et al. Mycophenolate mofetil ameliorates perivascular T lymphocyte inflammation and reduces the double-negative T cell population in SLE-prone MRLlpr/lpr mice. Cellular Immunology. 1999;197: 136–144.
158. Mehling A, Grabbe S, Voskort M, et al. Mycophenolate mofetil impairs the maturation and function of murine dendritic cells. Journal of Immunology. 2000;165:2374–2381.
159. Colic M, Stojic-Vukanic Z, Pavlovic B, et al. Mycophenolate mofetil inhibits differentiation, maturation and allostimulatory function of human monocyte-derived dendritic cells. Clinical and Experimental Immunology. 2003;134: 63–69.
160. Laurent AF, Dumont S, Poindron P, et al. Mycophenolic acid suppresses protein N-linked glycosylation in human monocytes and their adhesion to endothelial cells and to some substrates. Experimental Hematology. 1996; 24:59–67.
161. Glomsda BA, Blaheta RA, Hailer NP. Inhibition of monocyte/endothelial cell interactions and monocyte adhesion molecule expression by the immunosuppressant mycophenolate mofetil. Spinal Cord. 2003;41:610–619.
162. Utimura R, Fujihara CK, Mattar AL, et al. Mycophenolate mofetil prevents the development of glomerular injury in experimental diabetes. Kidney International. 2003;63:209–216.
163. Allison AC, Eugui EM. Mechanisms of action of mycophenolate mofetil in preventing acute and chronic allograft rejection. Transplantation. 2005;80: S181–S190.
164. Eugui EM, Almquist SJ, Muller CD, et al. Lymphocyte-selective cytostatic and immunosuppressive effects of mycophenolic acid in vitro: role of deoxyguanosine nucleotide depletion. Scandinavian Journal of Immunology. 1991;33: 161–173.
165. Hanvesakul R, Kubal C, Jham S, et al. Increased incidence of infections following the late introduction of mycophenolate mofetil in renal transplant recipients. Nephrology, Dialysis, Transplantation. 2008;23:4049–4053.
166. Pourfarziani V, Panahi Y, Assari S, et al. Changing treatment protocol from azathioprine to mycophenolate mofetil: decrease in renal dysfunction, increase in infections. Transplantation Proceedings. 2007;39:1237–1240.
167. Sollinger HW. Mycophenolate mofetil for the prevention of acute rejection in primary cadaveric renal allograft recipients. U.S. Renal Transplant Mycophenolate Mofetil Study Group. Transplantation. 1995;60:225–232.
168. Moreso F, Seron D, Morales JM, et al. Incidence of leukopenia and cytomegalovirus disease in kidney transplants treated with mycophenolate mofetil combined with low cyclosporine and steroid doses. Clinical Transplantation. 1998;12: 198–205.
169. Wang K, Zhang H, Li Y, et al. Safety of mycophenolate mofetil versus azathioprine in renal transplantation: a systematic review. Transplantation Proceedings. 2004;36:2068–2070.
170. Zmonarski SC, Boratynska M, Madziarska K, et al. Mycophenolate mofetil severely depresses antibody response to CMV infection in early posttransplant period. Transplantation Proceedings. 2003;35:2205–2206.
171. Hardwick LL, Savatta SG, Book BK, et al. Effect of mycophenolate mofetil on the Anti-CMV serologic response after renal transplantation. Transplantation Proceedings. 2001;33:1865–1866.
172. Mengel M, Marwedel M, Radermacher J, et al. Incidence of polyomavirus-nephropathy in renal allografts: influence of modern immunosuppressive drugs. Nephrology, Dialysis, Transplantation. 2003;18:1190–1196.
173. Shi Y, Moriyama T, Namba Y, et al. Association of treatment with 15-deoxyspergualin and BK virus nephropathy in kidney allograft recipients. Clinical Transplantation. 2007;21:502–509.
174. Barton TD, Blumberg EA, Doyle A, et al. A prospective cross-sectional study of BK virus infection in non-renal solid organ transplant recipients with chronic renal dysfunction. Transplant Infectious Disease. 2006;8: 102–107.
175. Fehr T, Bossart W, Wahl C, et al. Disseminated varicella infection in adult renal allograft recipients: four cases and a review of the literature. Transplantation. 2002;73:608–611.
176. Meier-Kriesche HU, Friedman G, Jacobs M, et al. Infectious complications in geriatric renal transplant patients: comparison of two immunosuppressive protocols. Transplantation. 1999;68:1496–1502.
177. Ritter ML, Pirofski L. Mycophenolate mofetil: effects on cellular immune subsets, infectious complications, and antimicrobial activity. Transplant Infectious Disease. 2009;11:290–297.
178. Behrend M. Adverse gastrointestinal effects of mycophenolate mofetil: aetiology, incidence and management. Drug Safety: An International Journal of Medical Toxicology and Drug Experience. 2001;24:645–663.
179. Goldblum R. Therapy of rheumatoid arthritis with mycophenolate mofetil. Clinical and Experimental Rheumatology. 1993;11(Suppl. 8):S117–S119.
180. Zwerner J, Fiorentino D. Mycophenolate mofetil. Dermatologic Therapy. 2007;20:229–238.
181. Sterneck M, Fischer L, Gahlemann C, et al. Mycophenolate mofetil for prevention of liver allograft rejection: initial results of a controlled clinical trial. Annals of Transplantation: Quarterly of the Polish Transplantation Society. 2000;5: 43–46.
182. Nogueras F, Espinosa MD, Mansilla A, et al. Mycophenolate mofetil-induced neutropenia in liver transplantation. Transplantation Proceedings. 2005;37: 1509–1511.
183. Asmis LM, Hadaya K, Majno P, et al. Acquired and reversible Pelger-Huet anomaly of polymorphonuclear neutrophils in three transplant patients receiving mycophenolate mofetil therapy. American Journal of Hematology. 2003;73: 244–248.
184. Kennedy GA, Kay TD, Johnson DW, et al. Neutrophil dysplasia characterised by a pseudo-Pelger-Huet anomaly occurring with the use of mycophenolate mofetil and ganciclovir following renal transplantation: a report of five cases. Pathology. 2002;34:263–266.
185. Epinette WW, Parker CM, Jones EL, et al. Mycophenolic acid for psoriasis. A review of pharmacology, long-term efficacy, and safety. Journal of the American Academy of Dermatology. 1987;17:962–971.
186. Szyper-Kravitz M, Sheinberg P, Sidi Y, et al. Hypersensitivity to mycophenolate mofetil in systemic lupus erythematosus: diagnostic measures and successful desensitization. International Archives of Allergy and Immunology. 2005;138: 334–336.
187. Harlan DM, Kirk AD. The future of organ and tissue transplantation: can T-cell costimulatory pathway modifiers revolutionize the prevention of graft rejection? JAMA. 1999;282:1076–1082.
188. Vincenti F. What's in the pipeline? New immunosuppressive drugs in transplantation. American Journal of Transplantation. 2002;2:898–903.
189. Kohler G, Milstein C. Continuous cultures of fused cells secreting antibody of predefined specificity. Nature. 1975;256:495–497.
190. Du J, Yang H, Zhang D, et al. Structural basis for the blockage of IL-2 signaling by therapeutic antibody basiliximab. Journal of Immunology. 2010;184: 1361–1368.
191. Kahan BD, Rajagopalan PR, Hall M. Reduction of the occurrence of acute cellular rejection among renal allograft recipients treated with basiliximab, a chimeric anti-interleukin-2-receptor monoclonal antibody. United States Simulect Renal Study Group. Transplantation. 1999;67:276–284.
192. Smith KA. Interleukin-2: inception, impact, and implications. Science. 1988; 240:1169–1176.
193. Vondran FW, Timrott K, Tross J, et al. Impact of Basiliximab on regulatory T-cells early after kidney transplantation: down-regulation of CD25 by receptor modulation. Transplant International. 2010;23:514–523.
194. Krystufkova E, Sekerkova A, Striz I, et al. Regulatory T cells in kidney transplant recipients: the effect of induction immunosuppression therapy. Nephrology, Dialysis, Transplantation. 2012;27:2576–2582.
195. Rassidakis GZ, Medeiros LJ, Viviani S, et al. CD20 expression in Hodgkin and Reed-Sternberg cells of classical Hodgkin's disease: associations with presenting features and clinical outcome. Journal of Clinical Oncology. 2002;20: 1278–1287.
196. Tedder TF, Streuli M, Schlossman SF, et al. Isolation and structure of a cDNA encoding the B1 (CD20) cell-surface antigen of human B lymphocytes. Proceedings of the National Academy of Sciences of the United States of America. 1988;85:208–212.
197. McLaughlin P, Grillo-Lopez AJ, Link BK, et al. Rituximab chimeric anti-CD20 monoclonal antibody therapy for relapsed indolent lymphoma: half of patients respond to a four-dose treatment program. Journal of Clinical Oncology.

1998;16:2825–2833.
198. Cerny T, Borisch B, Introna M, et al. Mechanism of action of rituximab. Anti-Cancer Drugs. 2002;13(Suppl. 2):S3–S10.
199. Jazirehi AR, Bonavida B. Cellular and molecular signal transduction pathways modulated by rituximab (rituxan, anti-CD20 mAb) in non-Hodgkin's lymphoma: implications in chemosensitization and therapeutic intervention. Oncogene. 2005;24:2121–2143.
200. Vega MI, Huerta-Yepaz S, Garban H, et al. Rituximab inhibits p38 MAPK activity in 2F7 B NHL and decreases IL-10 transcription: pivotal role of p38 MAPK in drug resistance. Oncogene. 2004;23:3530–3540.
201. Reiff A, Shaham B, Weinberg KI, et al. Anti-CD52 antibody-mediated immune ablation with autologous immune recovery for the treatment of refractory juvenile polymyositis. Journal of Clinical Immunology. 2011;31: 615–622.
202. Calne R, Moffatt SD, Friend PJ, et al. Campath IH allows low-dose cyclosporine monotherapy in 31 cadaveric renal allograft recipients. Transplantation. 1999;68:1613–1616.
203. Gallon L, Chhabra D, Skaro AI. T-cell-depleting agents in kidney transplantation: is there a place for alemtuzumab? American Journal of Kidney Diseases. 2012;59:15–18.
204. Hanaway MJ, Woodle ES, Mulgaonkar S, et al. Alemtuzumab induction in renal transplantation. New England Journal of Medicine. 2011;364: 1909–1919.
205. Norman DJ. Mechanisms of action and overview of OKT3. Therapeutic Drug Monitoring. 1995;17:615–620.
206. Bonnefoy-Berard N, Revillard JP. Mechanisms of immunosuppression induced by antithymocyte globulins and OKT3. Journal of Heart and Lung Transplantation. 1996;15:435–442.
207. Hansel TT, Kropshofer H, Singer T, et al. The safety and side effects of monoclonal antibodies. Nature Reviews Drug Discovery. 2010;9:325–338.
208. Larsen CP, Pearson TC, Adams AB, et al. Rational development of LEA29Y (belatacept), a high-affinity variant of CTLA4-Ig with potent immunosuppressive properties. American Journal of Transplantation. 2005;5:443–453.
209. Tan P, Anasetti C, Hansen JA, et al. Induction of alloantigen-specific hyporesponsiveness in human T lymphocytes by blocking interaction of CD28 with its natural ligand B7/BB1. Journal of Experimental Medicine. 1993;177: 165–173.
210. Matzinger P. Friendly and dangerous signals: is the tissue in control? Nature Immunology. 2007;8:11–13.
211. Sayegh MH. Finally, CTLA4Ig graduates to the clinic. Journal of Clinical Investigation. 1999;103:1223–1225.
212. Bluestone JA, St Clair EW, Turka LA. CTLA4Ig: bridging the basic immunology with clinical application. Immunity. 2006;24:233–238.
213. Linsley PS, Nadler SG. The clinical utility of inhibiting CD28-mediated costimulation. Immunological Reviews. 2009;229:307–321.
214. Azimzadeh AM, Lees JR, Ding Y, et al. Immunobiology of transplantation: impact on targets for large and small molecules. Clinical Pharmacology and Therapeutics. 2011;90:229–242.
215. Linsley PS, Wallace PM, Johnson J, et al. Immunosuppression in vivo by a soluble form of the CTLA-4 T cell activation molecule. Science. 1992; 257:792–795.
216. Lin H, Bolling SF, Linsley PS, et al. Long-term acceptance of major histocompatibility complex mismatched cardiac allografts induced by CTLA4Ig plus donor-specific transfusion. Journal of Experimental Medicine. 1993;178: 1801–1806.
217. Larsen CP, Elwood ET, Alexander DZ, et al. Long-term acceptance of skin and cardiac allografts after blocking CD40 and CD28 pathways. Nature. 1996; 381:434–438.
218. Russell ME, Hancock WW, Akalin E, et al. Chronic cardiac rejection in the LEW to F344 rat model. Blockade of CD28-B7 costimulation by CTLA4Ig modulates T cell and macrophage activation and attenuates arteriosclerosis. Journal of Clinical Investigation. 1996;97:833–838.
219. Akalin E, Chandraker A, Russell ME, et al. CD28-B7 T cell costimulatory blockade by CTLA4Ig in the rat renal allograft model: inhibition of cell-mediated and humoral immune responses in vivo. Transplantation. 1996;62:1942–1945.
220. Levisetti MG, Padrid PA, Szot GL, et al. Immunosuppressive effects of human CTLA4Ig in a non-human primate model of allogeneic pancreatic islet transplantation. Journal of Immunology. 1997;159:5187–5191.
221. Kirk AD, Harlan DM, Armstrong NN, et al. CTLA4-Ig and anti-CD40 ligand prevent renal allograft rejection in primates. Proceedings of the National Academy of Sciences of the United States of America. 1997;94:8789–8794.
222. Pierson RN 3rd, Chang AC, Blum MG, et al. Prolongation of primate cardiac allograft survival by treatment with ANTI-CD40 ligand (CD154) antibody. Transplantation. 1999;68:1800–1805.
223. Riley JL, Mao M, Kobayashi S, et al. Modulation of TCR-induced transcriptional profiles by ligation of CD28, ICOS, and CTLA-4 receptors. Proceedings of the National Academy of Sciences of the United States of America. 2002; 99:11790–11795.
224. Diehn M, Alizadeh AA, Rando OJ, et al. Genomic expression programs and the integration of the CD28 costimulatory signal in T cell activation. Proceedings of the National Academy of Sciences of the United States of America. 2002;99:11796–11801.
225. Rudd CE, Taylor A, Schneider H. CD28 and CTLA-4 coreceptor expression and signal transduction. Immunological Reviews. 2009;229:12–26.
226. Harding FA, McArthur JG, Gross JA, et al. CD28-mediated signalling costimulates murine T cells and prevents induction of anergy in T-cell clones. Nature. 1992;356:607–609.
227. Lakkis FG, Konieczny BT, Saleem S, et al. Blocking the CD28-B7 T cell costimulation pathway induces long term cardiac allograft acceptance in the absence of IL-4. Journal of Immunology. 1997;158:2443–2448.
228. Herold KC, Lu J, Rulifson I, et al. Regulation of C-C chemokine production by murine T cells by CD28/B7 costimulation. Journal of Immunology. 1997; 159:4150–4153.
229. Carroll RG, Riley JL, Levine BL, et al. Differential regulation of HIV-1 fusion cofactor expression by CD28 costimulation of CD4+ T cells. Science. 1997; 276:273–276.
230. Wells AD, Gudmundsdottir H, Turka LA. Following the fate of individual T cells throughout activation and clonal expansion. Signals from T cell receptor and CD28 differentially regulate the induction and duration of a proliferative response. Journal of Clinical Investigation. 1997;100:3173–3183.
231. Knoerzer DB, Karr RW, Schwartz BD, et al. Collagen-induced arthritis in the BB rat. Prevention of disease by treatment with CTLA-4-Ig. Journal of Clinical Investigation. 1995;96:987–993.
232. Pearson TC, Alexander DZ, Hendrix R, et al. CTLA4-Ig plus bone marrow induces long-term allograft survival and donor specific unresponsiveness in the murine model. Evidence for hematopoietic chimerism. Transplantation. 1996;61:997–1004.
233. Khoury SJ, Akalin E, Chandraker A, et al. CD28-B7 costimulatory blockade by CTLA4Ig prevents actively induced experimental autoimmune encephalomyelitis and inhibits Th1 but spares Th2 cytokines in the central nervous system. Journal of Immunology. 1995;155:4521–4524.
234. Salomon B, Bluestone JA. Complexities of CD28/B7: CTLA-4 costimulatory pathways in autoimmunity and transplantation. Annual Review of Immunology. 2001;19:225–252.
235. Croft M, Bradley LM, Swain SL. Naive versus memory CD4 T cell response to antigen. Memory cells are less dependent on accessory cell costimulation and can respond to many antigen-presenting cell types including resting B cells. Journal of Immunology. 1994;152:2675–2685.
236. London CA, Lodge MP, Abbas AK. Functional responses and costimulator dependence of memory CD4+ T cells. Journal of Immunology. 2000;164:265–272.
237. Suresh M, Whitmire JK, Harrington LE, et al. Role of CD28-B7 interactions in generation and maintenance of CD8 T cell memory. Journal of Immunology. 2001;167:5565–5573.
238. Boesteanu AC, Katsikis PD. Memory T cells need CD28 costimulation to remember. Seminars in Immunology. 2009;21:69–77.
239. Fuse S, Zhang W, Usherwood EJ. Control of memory CD8+ T cell differentiation by CD80/CD86-CD28 costimulation and restoration by IL-2 during the recall response. Journal of Immunology. 2008;180:1148–1157.
240. Kalland ME, Oberprieler NG, Vang T, et al. T cell-signaling network analysis reveals distinct differences between CD28 and CD2 costimulation responses in various subsets and in the MAPK pathway between resting and activated regulatory T cells. Journal of Immunology. 2011;187:5233–5245.
241. Ndejembi MP, Teijaro JR, Patke DS, et al. Control of memory CD4 T cell recall by the CD28/B7 costimulatory pathway. Journal of Immunology. 2006;177: 7698–7706.
242. Kremer JM, Westhovens R, Leon M, et al. Treatment of rheumatoid arthritis by selective inhibition of T-cell activation with fusion protein CTLA4Ig. New England Journal of Medicine. 2003;349:1907–1915.
243. Abrams JR, Lebwohl MG, Guzzo CA, et al. CTLA4Ig-mediated blockade of T-cell costimulation in patients with psoriasis vulgaris. Journal of Clinical Investigation. 1999;103:1243–1252.
244. Nadazdin O, Boskovic S, Murakami T, et al. Phenotype, distribution and alloreactive properties of memory T cells from cynomolgus monkeys. American Journal of Transplantation. 2010;10:1375–1384.
245. Kitchens WH, Haridas D, Wagener ME, et al. Integrin antagonists prevent costimulatory blockade-resistant transplant rejection by CD8(+) memory T cells. American Journal of Transplantation. 2012;12:69–80.
246. Hodge G, Mukaro V, Reynolds PN, et al. Role of increased CD8/CD28(null) T cells and alternative costimulatory molecules in chronic obstructive pulmonary disease. Clinical and Experimental Immunology. 2011;166:94–102.

247. Strioga M, Pasukoniene V, Characiejus D. CD8+ CD28- and CD8+ CD57+ T cells and their role in health and disease. Immunology. 2011;134: 17–32.
248. Betjes MG, Meijers RW, de Wit LE, et al. A killer on the road: circulating CD4+CD28null T cells as cardiovascular risk factor in ESRD patients. Journal of Nephrology. 2012;25:183–191.
249. Broux B, Pannemans K, Zhang X, et al. CX(3)CR1 drives cytotoxic CD4(+) CD28(-) T cells into the brain of multiple sclerosis patients. Journal of Autoimmunity. 2012;38:10–19.
250. Lo DJ, Weaver TA, Stempora L, et al. Selective targeting of human alloresponsive CD8+ effector memory T cells based on CD2 expression. American Journal of Transplantation. 2011;11:22–33.
251. Scarsi M, Ziglioli T, Airo P. Baseline numbers of circulating CD28-negative T cells may predict clinical response to abatacept in patients with rheumatoid arthritis. Journal of Rheumatology. 2011;38:2105–2111.
252. Krummel MF, Allison JP. Pillars article: CD28 and CTLA-4 have opposing effects on the response of T cells to stimulation. The journal of experimental medicine. 1995. 182: 459–465. Journal of Immunology. 2011;187:3459–3465.
253. Perez VL, Van Parijs L, Biuckians A, et al. Induction of peripheral T cell tolerance in vivo requires CTLA-4 engagement. Immunity. 1997;6:411–417.
254. Issazadeh S, Zhang M, Sayegh MH, et al. Acquired thymic tolerance: role of CTLA4 in the initiation and maintenance of tolerance in a clinically relevant autoimmune disease model. Journal of Immunology. 1999;162: 761–765.
255. Alegre ML, Frauwirth KA, Thompson CB. T-cell regulation by CD28 and CTLA-4. Nature Reviews. Immunology. 2001;1:220–228.
256. Greenwald RJ, Boussiotis VA, Lorsbach RB, et al. CTLA-4 regulates induction of anergy in vivo. Immunity. 2001;14:145–155.
257. Akiyama Y, Shirasugi N, Uchida N, et al. B7/CTLA4 pathway is essential for generating regulatory cells after intratracheal delivery of alloantigen in mice. Transplantation. 2002;74:732–738.
258. Butte MJ, Keir ME, Phamduy TB, et al. Programmed death-1 ligand 1 interacts specifically with the B7-1 costimulatory molecule to inhibit T cell responses. Immunity. 2007;27:111–122.
259. Jonuleit H, Schmitt E. The regulatory T cell family: distinct subsets and their interrelations. Journal of Immunology. 2003;171:6323–6327.
260. Salomon B, Lenschow DJ, Rhee L, et al. B7/CD28 costimulation is essential for the homeostasis of the CD4+CD25+ immunoregulatory T cells that control autoimmune diabetes. Immunity. 2000;12:431–440.
261. Tang AL, Teijaro JR, Njau MN, et al. CTLA4 expression is an indicator and regulator of steady-state CD4+ FoxP3+ T cell homeostasis. Journal of Immunology. 2008;181:1806–1813.
262. Wing K, Onishi Y, Prieto-Martin P, et al. CTLA-4 control over Foxp3+ regulatory T cell function. Science. 2008;322:271–275.
263. Poirier N, Azimzadeh AM, Zhang T, et al. Inducing CTLA-4-dependent immune regulation by selective CD28 blockade promotes regulatory T cells in organ transplantation. Science Translational Medicine. 2010;2:17ra10.
264. Zhang T, Fresnay S, Welty E, et al. Selective CD28 blockade attenuates acute and chronic rejection of murine cardiac allografts in a CTLA-4-dependent manner. American Journal of Transplantation. 2011;11:1599–1609.
265. Yang J, Riella LV, Boenisch O, et al. Paradoxical functions of B7: CD28 costimulation in a MHC class II-mismatched cardiac transplant model. American Journal of Transplantation. 2009;9:2837–2844.
266. Kozbor D, Moretta A, Messner HA, et al. Tp44 molecules involved in antigen-independent T cell activation are expressed on human plasma cells. Journal of Immunology. 1987;138:4128–4132.
267. Rozanski CH, Arens R, Carlson LM, et al. Sustained antibody responses depend on CD28 function in bone marrow-resident plasma cells. Journal of Experimental Medicine. 2011;208:1435–1446.
268. Delogu A, Schebesta A, Sun Q, et al. Gene repression by Pax5 in B cells is essential for blood cell homeostasis and is reversed in plasma cells. Immunity. 2006; 24:269–281.
269. Schaub M, Stadlbauer TH, Sayegh MH. CTLA4Ig: effects on cellular and humoral immunity and macrophage activation. Experimental Nephrology. 1997;5: 370–374.
270. Cutolo M, Soldano S, Montagna P, et al. CTLA4-Ig interacts with cultured synovial macrophages from rheumatoid arthritis patients and downregulates cytokine production. Arthritis Research and Therapy. 2009;11:R176.
271. Grohmann U, Orabona C, Fallarino F, et al. CTLA-4-Ig regulates tryptophan catabolism in vivo. Nature Immunology. 2002;3:1097–1101.
272. Finger EB, Bluestone JA. When ligand becomes receptor–tolerance via B7 signaling on DCs. Nature Immunology. 2002;3:1056–1057.
273. Takada M, Chandraker A, Nadeau KC, et al. The role of the B7 costimulatory pathway in experimental cold ischemia/reperfusion injury. Journal of Clinical Investigation. 1997;100:1199–1203.
274. Nolan A, Kobayashi H, Naveed B, et al. Differential role for CD80 and CD86 in the regulation of the innate immune response in murine polymicrobial sepsis. PLoS ONE. 2009;4:e6600.
275. Vincenti F, Blancho G, Durrbach A, et al. Five-year safety and efficacy of belatacept in renal transplantation. Journal of the American Society of Nephrology. 2010;21:1587–1596.
276. Grinyo J, Charpentier B, Pestana JM, et al. An integrated safety profile analysis of belatacept in kidney transplant recipients. Transplantation. 2010;90: 1521–1527.
277. Vincenti F, Larsen CP, Alberu J, et al. Three-year outcomes from BENEFIT, a randomized, active-controlled, parallel-group study in adult kidney transplant recipients. American Journal of Transplantation. 2012;12:210–217.
278. Gaber AO, Monaco AP, Russell JA, et al. Rabbit antithymocyte globulin (thymoglobulin): 25 years and new frontiers in solid organ transplantation and haematology. Drugs. 2010;70:691–732.
279. Deeks ED, Keating GM. Rabbit antithymocyte globulin (thymoglobulin): a review of its use in the prevention and treatment of acute renal allograft rejection. Drugs. 2009;69:1483–1512.
280. Taber DJ, Weimert NA, Henderson F, et al. Long-term efficacy of induction therapy with anti-interleukin-2 receptor antibodies or thymoglobulin compared with no induction therapy in renal transplantation. Transplantation Proceedings. 2008;40:3401–3407.
281. Hardinger KL, Rhee S, Buchanan P, et al. A prospective, randomized, double-blinded comparison of thymoglobulin versus Atgam for induction immunosuppressive therapy: 10-year results. Transplantation. 2008;86: 947–952.
282. Genestier L, Fournel S, Flacher M, et al. Induction of Fas (Apo-1, CD95)-mediated apoptosis of activated lymphocytes by polyclonal antithymocyte globulins. Blood. 1998;91:2360–2368.
283. Michallet MC, Preville X, Flacher M, et al. Functional antibodies to leukocyte adhesion molecules in antithymocyte globulins. Transplantation. 2003;75: 657–662.
284. Michallet MC, Saltel F, Preville X, et al. Cathepsin-B-dependent apoptosis triggered by antithymocyte globulins: a novel mechanism of T-cell depletion. Blood. 2003;102:3719–3726.
285. Preville X, Flacher M, LeMauff B, et al. Mechanisms involved in antithymocyte globulin immunosuppressive activity in a nonhuman primate model. Transplantation. 2001;71:460–468.
286. LaCorcia G, Swistak M, Lawendowski C, et al. Polyclonal rabbit antithymocyte globulin exhibits consistent immunosuppressive capabilities beyond cell depletion. Transplantation. 2009;87:966–974.
287. van de Linde P, Tysma OM, Medema JP, et al. Mechanisms of antibody immunotherapy on clonal islet reactive T cells. Human Immunology. 2006;67: 264–273.
288. Mohty M. Mechanisms of action of antithymocyte globulin: T-cell depletion and beyond. Leukemia. 2007;21:1387–1394.
289. Bonnefoy-Berard N, Verrier B, Vincent C, et al. Inhibition of CD25 (IL-2R alpha) expression and T-cell proliferation by polyclonal anti-thymocyte globulins. Immunology. 1992;77:61–67.
290. Beiras-Fernandez A, Walther S, Kaczmarek I, et al. In vitro influence of polyclonal anti-thymocyte globulins on leukocyte expression of adhesion molecules. Experimental and Clinical Transplantation. 2005;3:370–374.
291. Lopez M, Clarkson MR, Albin M, et al. A novel mechanism of action for anti-thymocyte globulin: induction of CD4+CD25+Foxp3+ regulatory T cells. Journal of the American Society of Nephrology. 2006;17:2844–2853.
292. Liu Z, Fang Y, Wang X, et al. Upregulation of molecules associated with T-regulatory function by thymoglobulin pretreatment of human CD4+ cells. Transplantation. 2008;86:1419–1426.
293. Minamimura K, Gao W, Maki T. CD4+ regulatory T cells are spared from deletion by antilymphocyte serum, a polyclonal anti-T cell antibody. Journal of Immunology. 2006;176:4125–4132.
294. Feng X, Kajigaya S, Solomou EE, et al. Rabbit ATG but not horse ATG promotes expansion of functional CD4+CD25highFOXP3+ regulatory T cells in vitro. Blood. 2008;111:3675–3683.
295. Shevach EM. From vanilla to 28 flavors: multiple varieties of T regulatory cells. Immunity. 2006;25:195–201.
296. Stauch D, Dernier A, Sarmiento Marchese E, et al. Targeting of natural killer cells by rabbit antithymocyte globulin and campath-1H: similar effects independent of specificity. PLoS ONE. 2009;4:e4709.
297. Zand MS, Vo T, Huggins J, et al. Polyclonal rabbit antithymocyte globulin triggers B-cell and plasma cell apoptosis by multiple pathways. Transplantation. 2005; 79:1507–1515.
298. Dalle JH, Dardari R, Menezes J, et al. Binding of thymoglobulin to natural killer cells leads to cell activation and interferon-gamma production. Transplantation. 2009;87:473–481.

299. Muller C, Schernthaner G, Kovarik J, et al. Natural killer cell activity and antibody-dependent cellular cytotoxicity in patients under various immunosuppressive regimens. Clinical Immunology and Immunopathology. 1987;44:12–19.
300. Turunen AJ, Lindgren L, Salmela KT, et al. Association of graft neutrophil sequestration with delayed graft function in clinical renal transplantation. Transplantation. 2004;77:1821–1826.
301. Naujokat C, Berges C, Fuchs D, et al. Antithymocyte globulins suppress dendritic cell function by multiple mechanisms. Transplantation. 2007;83:485–497.
302. Issa NC, Fishman JA. Infectious complications of antilymphocyte therapies in solid organ transplantation. Clinical Infectious Diseases. 2009;48:772–786.
303. Yoon HS, Lee JH, Choi ES, et al. Cytomegalovirus infection in children who underwent hematopoietic stem cell transplantation at a single center: a retrospective study of the risk factors. Pediatric Transplantation. 2009;13:898–905.
304. Mohty M, Jacot W, Faucher C, et al. Infectious complications following allogeneic HLA-identical sibling transplantation with antithymocyte globulin-based reduced intensity preparative regimen. Leukemia. 2003;17:2168–2177.
305. von Muller L, Schliep C, Storck M, et al. Severe graft rejection, increased immunosuppression, and active CMV infection in renal transplantation. Journal of Medical Virology. 2006;78:394–399.
306. Brennan DC, Schnitzler MA. Long-term results of rabbit antithymocyte globulin and basiliximab induction. New England Journal of Medicine. 2008;359:1736–1738.
307. Opelz G, Dohler B, Ruhenstroth A. Cytomegalovirus prophylaxis and graft outcome in solid organ transplantation: a collaborative transplant study report. American Journal of Transplantation. 2004;4:928–936.
308. Woodle ES, Peddi VR, Tomlanovich S, et al. A prospective, randomized, multicenter study evaluating early corticosteroid withdrawal with Thymoglobulin in living-donor kidney transplantation. Clinical Transplantation. 2010;24:73–83.
309. Eason JD, Loss GE, Blazek J, et al. Steroid-free liver transplantation using rabbit antithymocyte globulin induction: results of a prospective randomized trial. Liver Transplantation. 2001;7:693–697.
310. Opelz G, Dohler B. Lymphomas after solid organ transplantation: a collaborative transplant study report. American Journal of Transplantation. 2004;4:222–230.
311. Kirk AD, Cherikh WS, Ring M, et al. Dissociation of depletional induction and posttransplant lymphoproliferative disease in kidney recipients treated with alemtuzumab. American Journal of Transplantation. 2007;7:2619–2625.
312. Cherikh WS, Kauffman HM, McBride MA, et al. Association of the type of induction immunosuppression with posttransplant lymphoproliferative disorder, graft survival, and patient survival after primary kidney transplantation. Transplantation. 2003;76:1289–1293.
313. Einecke G, Sis B, Reeve J, et al. Antibody-mediated microcirculation injury is the major cause of late kidney transplant failure. American Journal of Transplantation. 2009;9:2520–2531.
314. Kirk AD, Turgeon NA, Iwakoshi NN. B cells and transplantation tolerance. Nature Reviews Nephrology. 2010;6:584–593.
315. Drachenberg CB, Odorico J, Demetris AJ, et al. Banff schema for grading pancreas allograft rejection: working proposal by a multi-disciplinary international consensus panel. American Journal of Transplantation. 2008;8:1237–1249.
316. Clynes R. Protective mechanisms of IVIG. Current Opinion in Immunology. 2007;19:646–651.
317. Kaveri SV, Lacroix-Desmazes S, Bayry J. The antiinflammatory IgG. New England Journal of Medicine. 2008;359:307–309.
318. Imbach P, Lazarus AH, Kuhne T. Intravenous immunoglobulins induce potentially synergistic immunomodulations in autoimmune disorders. Vox Sanguinis. 2010;98:385–394.
319. Jordan SC, Toyoda M, Vo AA. Regulation of immunity and inflammation by intravenous immunoglobulin: relevance to solid organ transplantation. Expert Review of Clinical Immunology. 2011;7:341–348.
320. Hachem RR, Yusen RD, Meyers BF, et al. Anti-human leukocyte antigen antibodies and preemptive antibody-directed therapy after lung transplantation. Journal of Heart and Lung Transplantation. 2010;29:973–980.
321. Rehman S, Meier-Kriesche HU, Scornik J. Use of intravenous immune globulin and rituximab for desensitization of highly human leukocyte antigen-sensitized patients awaiting kidney transplantation. Transplantation. 2010;90:932; author reply 932–933.
322. Kozlowski T, Andreoni K. Limitations of rituximab/IVIg desensitization protocol in kidney transplantation; is this better than a tincture of time? Annals of Transplantation. 2011;16:19–25.
323. Kahwaji J, Vo AA, Jordan SC. ABO blood group incompatibility: a diminishing barrier to successful kidney transplantation? Expert Review of Clinical Immunology. 2010;6:893–900.
324. Sullivan KM. Immunomodulation in allogeneic marrow transplantation: use of intravenous immune globulin to suppress acute graft-versus-host disease. Clinical and Experimental Immunology. 1996;104(Suppl. 1):43–48.
325. Ichihara H, Nakamae H, Hirose A, et al. Immunoglobulin prophylaxis against cytomegalovirus infection in patients at high risk of infection following allogeneic hematopoietic cell transplantation. Transplantation Proceedings. 2011;43:3927–3932.
326. Planitzer CB, Saemann MD, Gajek H, et al. Cytomegalovirus neutralization by hyperimmune and standard intravenous immunoglobulin preparations. Transplantation. 2011;92:267–270.
327. Czer LS, Ruzza A, Vespignani R, et al. Prophylaxis of cytomegalovirus disease in mismatched patients after heart transplantation using combined antiviral and immunoglobulin therapy. Transplantation Proceedings. 2011;43:1887–1892.
328. Hwang S, Yu YD, Park GC, et al. Safety of ultra-rapid intravenous infusion of hepatitis B immunoglobulin in liver transplant recipients. Transplantation Proceedings. 2011;43:1780–1782.
329. Seite JF, Shoenfeld Y, Youinou P, et al. What is the contents of the magic draft IVIg? Autoimmunity Reviews. 2008;7:435–439.
330. Kotlan B, Stroncek DF, Marincola FM. Intravenous immunoglobulin-based immunotherapy: an arsenal of possibilities for patients and science. Immunotherapy. 2009;1:995–1015.
331. Siberil S, Elluru S, Negi VS, et al. Intravenous immunoglobulin in autoimmune and inflammatory diseases: more than mere transfer of antibodies. Transfusion and Apheresis Science. 2007;37:103–107.
332. Sapir T, Shoenfeld Y. Facing the enigma of immunomodulatory effects of intravenous immunoglobulin. Clinical Reviews in Allergy and Immunology. 2005;29:185–199.
333. Durandy A, Kaveri SV, Kuijpers TW, et al. Intravenous immunoglobulins–understanding properties and mechanisms. Clinical and Experimental Immunology. 2009;158(Suppl. 1):2–13.
334. Samuelsson A, Towers TL, Ravetch JV. Anti-inflammatory activity of IVIG mediated through the inhibitory Fc receptor. Science. 2001;291:484–486.
335. Siragam V, Crow AR, Brinc D, et al. Intravenous immunoglobulin ameliorates ITP via activating Fc gamma receptors on dendritic cells. Nature Medicine. 2006;12:688–692.
336. Augener W, Friedmann B, Brittinger G. Are aggregates of IgG the effective part of high-dose immunoglobulin therapy in adult idiopathic thrombocytopenic purpura (ITP)? Blut. 1985;50:249–252.
337. Teeling JL, Jansen-Hendriks T, Kuijpers TW, et al. Therapeutic efficacy of intravenous immunoglobulin preparations depends on the immunoglobulin G dimers: studies in experimental immune thrombocytopenia. Blood. 2001;98:1095–1099.
338. Desai DD, Harbers SO, Flores M, et al. Fc gamma receptor IIB on dendritic cells enforces peripheral tolerance by inhibiting effector T cell responses. Journal of Immunology. 2007;178:6217–6226.
339. Wenink MH, Santegoets KC, Roelofs MF, et al. The inhibitory Fc gamma IIb receptor dampens TLR4-mediated immune responses and is selectively up-regulated on dendritic cells from rheumatoid arthritis patients with quiescent disease. Journal of Immunology. 2009;183:4509–4520.
340. Flores M, Desai DD, Downie M, et al. Dominant expression of the inhibitory FcgammaRIIB prevents antigen presentation by murine plasmacytoid dendritic cells. Journal of Immunology. 2009;183:7129–7139.
341. Venkatesh J, Kawabata D, Kim S, et al. Selective regulation of autoreactive B cells by FcgammaRIIB. Journal of Autoimmunity. 2009;32:149–157.
342. Mihaylova N, Voynova E, Tchorbanov A, et al. Simultaneous engagement of FcgammaIIb and CD22 inhibitory receptors silences targeted B cells and suppresses autoimmune disease activity. Molecular Immunology. 2009;47:123–130.
343. Roopenian DC, Akilesh S. FcRn: the neonatal Fc receptor comes of age. Nature Reviews. Immunology. 2007;7:715–725.
344. Akilesh S, Petkova S, Sproule TJ, et al. The MHC class I-like Fc receptor promotes humorally mediated autoimmune disease. Journal of Clinical Investigation. 2004;113:1328–1333.
345. Thomson CW, Teft WA, Chen W, et al. FcR gamma presence in TCR complex of double-negative T cells is critical for their regulatory function. Journal of Immunology. 2006;177:2250–2257.
346. Lynch RG. Regulatory roles for FcgammaRIII (CD16) and FcgammaRII (CD32) in the development of T- and B-lineage lymphoid cells. Journal of Leukocyte Biology. 2000;67:279–284.
347. Kahwaji J, Sinha A, Toyoda M, et al. Infectious complications in kidney-transplant recipients desensitized with rituximab and intravenous immu-

第 18 章
未来的免疫调控通路

Allison B. Webber, Flavio Vincenti

引言

基于钙调磷酸酶抑制剂(CNI)的免疫抑制方案,虽然可降低移植后1年急性排斥反应,提高移植物存活率,但对1年后无此作用。自从1995年,长期的移植肾存活率已经保持不变[1]。并且,CNI伴有多系统副反应,包括肾毒性、代谢紊乱、高血压、高脂血症和葡萄糖耐受不良。CNI的代谢紊乱可导致心血管疾病明显增加,心血管疾病是非移植物失功死亡的主要死因[2-6]。此外,虽然CNI可有效抑制T细胞介导的急性排斥反应,但是其对慢性抗体排斥反应的作用较小,尤其是应用最小量方案时,这被认为对晚期移植物失功起到重要作用[7-9]。这表明,同种异体抗体及慢性体液排斥反应在晚期移植物失功中的显著作用,已经引发学者对B细胞新型治疗靶点的探索,包括应用CD40抗体阻断CD40-CD154共刺激通路,以及B细胞活化因子(BAFF)和增殖诱导配体(APRIL),这两个肿瘤坏死因子家族配体作为抗凋亡因子,对于B细胞系的成熟具有重要作用[10]。但是,T细胞依旧被认为是移植物排斥反应的中心。具有里程碑意义的研究确认,通过T细胞受体在MHC的背景下与抗原交互作用发出的信号1,对引发足量的T细胞反应是不够的,这引发了对共刺激分子的强烈兴趣。共刺激信号目前被认为可引发信号2,该信号可驱动活化T细胞的生存、扩增和分化[11,12]。正在积极探索的作为移植治疗靶点的最佳共刺激通路目前包括CD28/B7和CD40/CD154通路[13,14]。LFA-1/ICAM和CD2/LFA-3通路也在移植免疫中引发了研究兴趣。特异性地表达并针对这些通路的单克隆抗体和融合蛋白有望与CNI方案具有类似的抗排斥反应效果,并具有较少的副反应。但是,共刺激通路的复杂性,包括抑制T细胞活化的负性共刺激信号(例如,CTLA-4)的存在,以及这些分子在免疫活化的不同时间点和不同细胞亚群的变异表达,使应用临床试剂的试验颇具挑战[15]。最终,包括托法替尼、JAK激酶2/3抑制剂等小分子已经在动物模型中表现出可增加移植物存活,Ⅱa和Ⅱb期临床试验提示类似的结果,虽然具有更多的免疫抑制相关并发症,包括感染和移植后淋巴组织增生性疾病[16,17]。

本章主要论叙目前正在研究的移植通路,包括细胞内通路以及B细胞和T细胞表面受体、配体,将重点论述具有临床应用前景的免疫机制和新型靶点。移植治疗的终极目标是达到对移植物完全的免疫耐受,并且对其他抗原具有完整的免疫力。本章将论述意在达到此目标的治疗方案,可辅以第17章临床常用通路的描述。

移植中的共刺激通路

共刺激通路一直被认为是控制适应性免疫反应的重要靶点。虽然最近贝拉西普的批准预示着联合刺激通路治疗排斥反应的开端,但人们普遍认为,它们的真正前景才刚刚开始实现,而且贝拉西普的使用还将进一步完善,并随之出现许多其他化合物。本节以贝拉西普的开发为出发点,概述了在移植中可能探索的其他共刺激途径。

CD28/CTLA-4/B7 通路

T细胞在适应性免疫的启动和调解中扮演重要角色,需要两种协同信号以激活[18]。信号1通过T细胞受体与MHC和抗原递呈细胞上的抗原肽复合物交互作用而传递。信号2(共刺激通路)由T细胞表面受体与APC表面的配体相互作用而传递。当缺乏伴随信号2时,原始T细胞变得无能,妨碍了效应$CD4^+$ T细胞亚群的发生和活化毒性T细胞(CD8 T细胞)的增殖。最佳的正向通路是CD28/B7通路[13]。CD28是同聚二聚体的跨膜蛋白,表达于所有的原始$CD4^+$和$CD8^+$细胞[19],并具有两个已知配体，B7–1(CD80)和 B7–2(CD86)，前者是诱导性表达，后者表达于 APC 表面[19]。在缺乏 TCR 刺激时，CD28 与 B7 配体结合导致 T 细胞增殖，生成细胞因子(IL–2 和 IFN–γ)，增强 T 细胞生存(图 18.1)[13,14]。有趣的是，作为共刺激信号的一个复杂例子，活化 T 细胞上调毒性 T 细胞相关抗原 4(CTLA–4)的表达，该分子在结构上类似 CD28，但是与 B7–1、B7–2 的结合力更强，CTLA–4 结合提供了负性共刺激信号，下调 T 细胞反应，并形成负反馈调节。CTLA–4 对于 FoxP3⁺调节 T 细胞的功能具有重要作用，该细胞有助于促进免疫耐受[20,21]。

针对 CD28/CTLA–4/B7 通路，多种的生物制剂已被研发，最引人瞩目的是重组融合蛋白 CTLA–4–Ig(阿巴西普)，它含有 CTLA–4 的胞外域和 IgG1 的 Tc 部分。CTLA–4–Ig 的发生基于 CTLA–4 对 B7–1 和 B7–2 的高黏附性，以及其可结合于 B7–1 和 B7–2 而不是 CD28，因此阻断了正向共刺激通路[22]。虽然在啮齿类移植模型中，CTLA–4–Ig 延长了移植物存活期，但是该现象并未在非人灵长类中观察到[23,24]。该结果揭示 CTLA–4–Ig 对 B7–1(CD80)的抑制要强于对 B7–2(CD86)的抑制，它对 CD28/B7 通路的抑制对移植并未达到最优状态[22,25,26]。因此，贝拉西普(旧名 LEA29Y)是第二代 CTLA–4–Ig 融合蛋白（在结合位点有两个氨基酸替换)，它对 B7–2 有更强的结合力，在非人灵长类中与吗替麦考酚酯和激素合用可以延长移植肾生存期（图 18.2)[27]。此外，贝拉西普还可抑制抗供体抗体的产生[27]。

一项旨在研究贝拉西普对环孢素在预防排斥反应中非劣效性的多中心二期临床试验（应用两种剂量方案)的结果表明，相对于环孢素 A，两种贝拉西普剂量组在移植 1 年后，排斥反应率相当，肾小球滤过率更高，慢性移植物肾病更少[28]。基于这些可喜结果，研究者设计了两项三期临床试验，“基于贝拉西普的免疫抑制方案与环孢素在肾移植受体中的比较”(BENEFIT)和“超标准供体肾移植中贝拉西普与环孢素的比较”(BENEFIT–EXT)，研究在活体或尸体肾移植及超标准尸体肾移植的急性排斥反应率、GFR、受体及移植物 1 年存活率中，贝拉西普相对于环孢素是否等效或具有

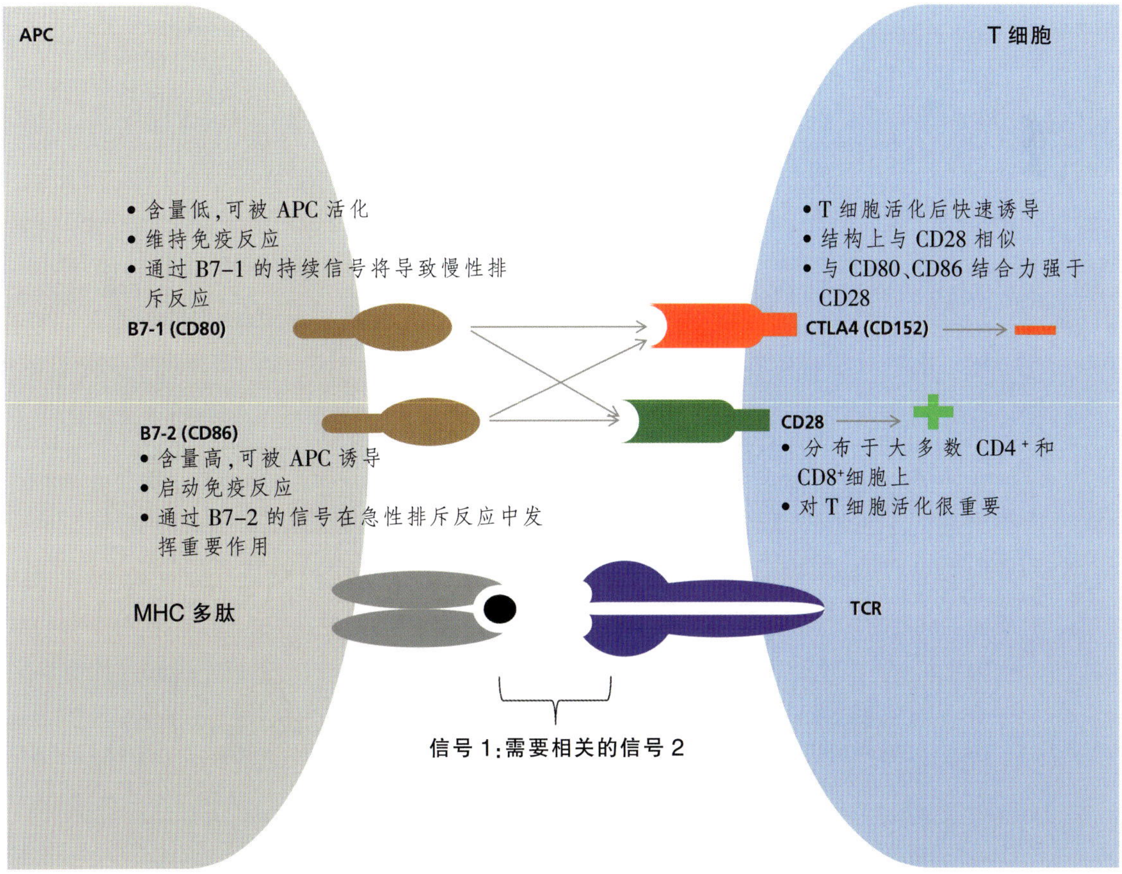

图 18.1 B7–1/2 和 CD28 信号通路在 T 细胞活化中起重要作用。此图显示了配体 B7–1 和 B7–2 与受体 CD28 和 CTLA4 之间的关系。注意，在共刺激信号相关之前，T 细胞受体(TCR)和 MHC(信号 1)之间的结合是必需的。APC，抗原呈递细胞。

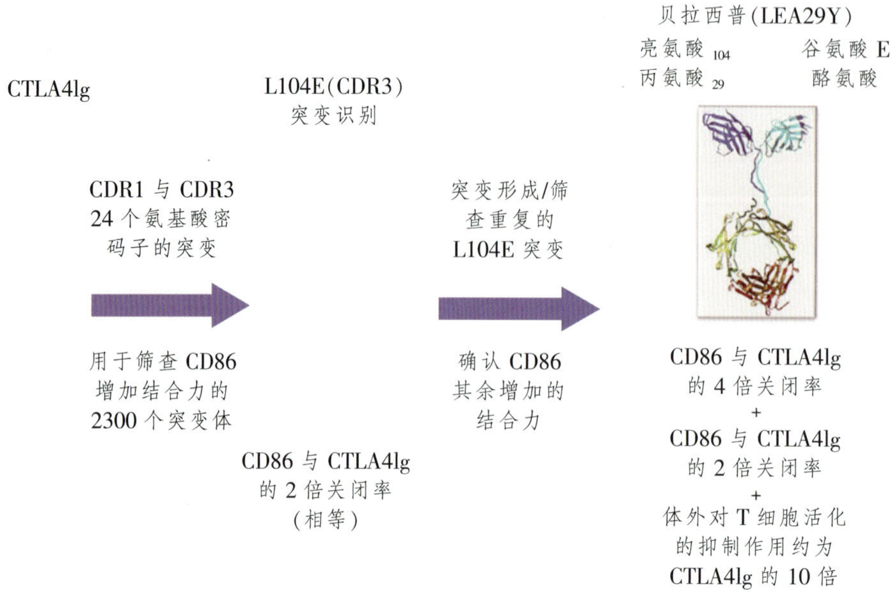

图 18.2 贝拉西普(LEA29Y)移植的合理设计。

优势。图 18.3 展示了两项研究中的治疗方案。BENEFIT 实验结果表明,相对于环孢素,贝拉西普高剂量组(MI)和低剂量组(LI)具有类似的受体及移植物存活率(MI组为 95%;LI 组为 97%;CsA 组为 93%)[29]。贝拉西普组 1 年后肾功能均优于环孢素组[平均 GFR MI组为 65mL/(min·1.73m²);LI 组为 63.4mL/(min·1.73m²);CsA 组为 50.4mL/(min·1.73m²),$P<0.0001$,MI 组和 LI 组对 CsA 组],随访 3 年,eGFR 组间差异继续增大。

相对于环孢素,贝拉西普组 1 年活组织检查证实为慢性移植物肾病的发生率小于环孢素组(MI 组为 18%;LI 组为 24%;CSA 组为 32%)。并且,心血管预后,包括血压、血脂,贝拉西普组均优于环孢素组(MI 组为 133/79,与 CsA 组比较:P=0.001;LI 组为 131/79,与 CsA 组比较:P=0.0273;CsA 组为 139/82)。移植后新发糖尿病(NODAT)发生率 3 组间无统计学差异。

但是,在贝拉西普组,急性排斥反应发生率(MI 组为 22%;LI 组为 17%;CsA 组为 7%)和 Banff ⅡB 级排斥反应发生率高于环孢素组。而且,安全终点评估,包括恶性肿瘤和泌尿系统、CMV 和 BKV 等感染在 3 组间无明显差异。重要的是,1 年 PTLD 在 3 组间发生例数分别是高剂量贝拉西普组 1 例,低剂量贝拉西普组 2 例,环孢素组 1 例。但是,1 年后,在高剂量贝拉西普组新出现 2

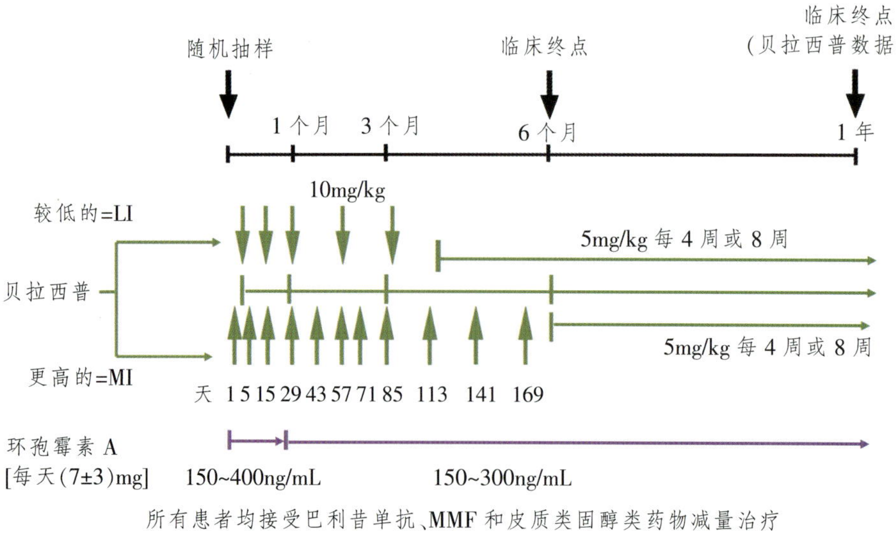

图 18.3 BENEFIT 和 BENEFIT-EXT 试验中的免疫抑制方案。

例中枢神经系统 PTLD。发生 PTLD 的受体发生血清学阴性的 EBV 感染的概率下降。在 BENEFIT-EXT 试验中，贝拉西普组 PTLD 发生率也增高(12 个月时：MI 组 1 例，LI 组 2 例，CsA 组 0；12 个月后：MI 组 2 例，LI 组 3 例，CsA 组 0)。3/5 EBV IgG 阴性[30]。另外，BENEFIT-EXT 试验的发现与 BENEFIT 试验类似，除了 3 组间类似的排斥反应发生率（MI 组为 17.9%；LI 组为 17.7%；CsA 组为 14.1%)，类似的慢性移植物肾病发生率(MI 组为 45%；LI 组为 46%；CsA 组为 52%）和环孢素组 1 年移植术后新发糖尿病发生率增加（MI 组为 2%；LI 组为 7%；CsA 组为 11%；P=0.0308，MI 组对 CsA 组)。低剂量贝拉西普具有较好的安全性，是 FDA 与 2011 年 6 月批准的用于 EBV 阳性受体肾移植的抗排斥治疗

贝拉西普治疗后组织学的严重性和排斥反应的增加表明共刺激通路阻断的复杂性。解释该现象的几项假说包括，贝拉西普在阻断 APC 上的 B7-1 和 B7-2 时也抑制了 CTLA-4 的结合，CTLA-4 是已知的负性共刺激信号，也是影响 FOXP3$^+$调节 T 细胞功能的重要分子之一[21,31]。并且，记忆 T 细胞是移植物免疫耐受的主要障碍，其对 CD28/B7-1/B7-2 的依赖较少，因此，被认为是对共刺激通路阻断抵抗的排斥反应的关键介质[32-35]。

一种合乎逻辑的方法是开发一种专门针对 CD28 的生物制剂。理论上，这将允许更多 CTLA-4/B7-1/B7-2 连接，并因此促进同种异体移植物耐受。但是几次人源化抗 CD28 单克隆抗体的尝试均以失败告终[36,37]。一项研究调查了一种超激动剂，TGN1412，它在临床前研究中可促进 T 调节细胞的扩增，导致 6 名志愿者出现细胞因子风暴和多器官衰竭[37]。然而，一种名为 Sc28AT 的嵌合人类/灵长类单价融合蛋白，与 B7-1 和 B72 竞争结合于 CD28，缺乏超激动剂活性，已经在非人类灵长类动物中进行了研究。在这项研究中，他们发现 Sc28AT 单药治疗显著延长了移植肾的存活时间，同时 Sc28AT 联合他克莫司治疗进一步延长了移植肾的存活时间[38]。此外，应用 Sc28AT 后，外周血 CD4$^+$调节 T 细胞数量增加，在移植肾活检中可见大量 FoxP3$^+$ CTLA-4$^+$调节 T 细胞以及少量 CD20$^+$ B 细胞，并且炎性因子表达下降[38]。在移植人群中，Sc28AT 或相关蛋白的临床研究很可能即将开始。

CD40/CD40L(CD154)通路

移植中另一条引起人们兴趣的共刺激通路是 CD40/CD40L(CD154)通路。CD40 在包括 B 细胞和树突细胞(DC)在内的 APC 上具有结构性表达，在炎症环境中，其在内皮细胞和成纤维细胞表达上调。此外，其自身的表达在激活后上调[39-41]。CD154 是 CD40 唯一的配体，在活化的 T 细胞、NK 细胞、嗜酸性粒细胞和血小板上表达[42]。CD40 与 CD154 结合促进树突细胞的活化和成熟，激活 B 细胞，促进免疫球蛋白类别转换。此外，CD40 下游信号通路增强 DC 细胞表面 MHC 复合物和共刺激分子(即 CD80 和 CD86)的表达，促进 TNF 和 IL-12 等炎性细胞因子的分泌(图 18.4)[41,43]。

CD40 的配体 CD154 是单克隆抗体抑制 CD40-CD154 通路的第一个靶点。靶向配体往往比靶向受体更安全，因为结合受体有可能促进激动信号。此外，与 CD40 相比，CD154 的表达更为有限。针对 CD154 单克隆抗体的早期试验在小鼠和非人类灵长类动物模型中的结果是鼓舞人心的，主要用于与其他疗法联合使用，包括 CTLA-4-Ig、供体特异性输血和西罗莫司[23,44-47]。在第一阶段两项应用人源化抗 CD154 单克隆抗体(Hu5C8)治疗系统性红斑狼疮及肾移植患者，以及稍后的在非人灵长类的研究中，血栓栓塞率高的出人意料，目前认为可能与表达于血小板上的 CD154 以及 CD154 对血凝块稳定性的作用有关[48,49]。Hu5C8 和其他抗 CD154 抗体的进一步研发已被暂停。但是，如果能改变抗 CD154 单克隆抗体的 Fc 片段以成功阻断其黏附于血小板上，则临床试验将可能重启。在此过渡期，阻断该通路的兴趣点已经转移到研发抗 CD40 单克隆抗体上。一种嵌合的抗 CD40 单克隆抗体(Chi220)与贝拉西普联用可延长非人灵长类胰岛移植物的存活期。在另一项非人灵长类模型中，与抗 CD86 单克隆抗体联用可延长移植肾存活期[23,45,50,51]。其他在研的抗 CD40 抗体中，包括目前在利妥昔单抗耐药的淋巴瘤患者中研究的 OM11-62MF(诺华制药，瑞士巴塞尔)、最近因志愿者招募不足而停止试验的用于银屑病性关节炎的 PG102(PanGenetics，瑞士乌得勒支)和目前唯一在移植受体中试验的人抗体 ASKP1240(安斯泰来制药)。一项在健康志愿者中进行的Ⅰa 期临床试验安全结束后，安斯泰来制药已经完成了一项在再次肾移植受体中研究 ASKP1240 药代动力学、药效学安全性和耐受性的Ⅰb 期全美多中心随机双盲安慰剂平行对照的临床研究(http://clinicaltrials.gov/ct2/show/NCT01279538)[52]。

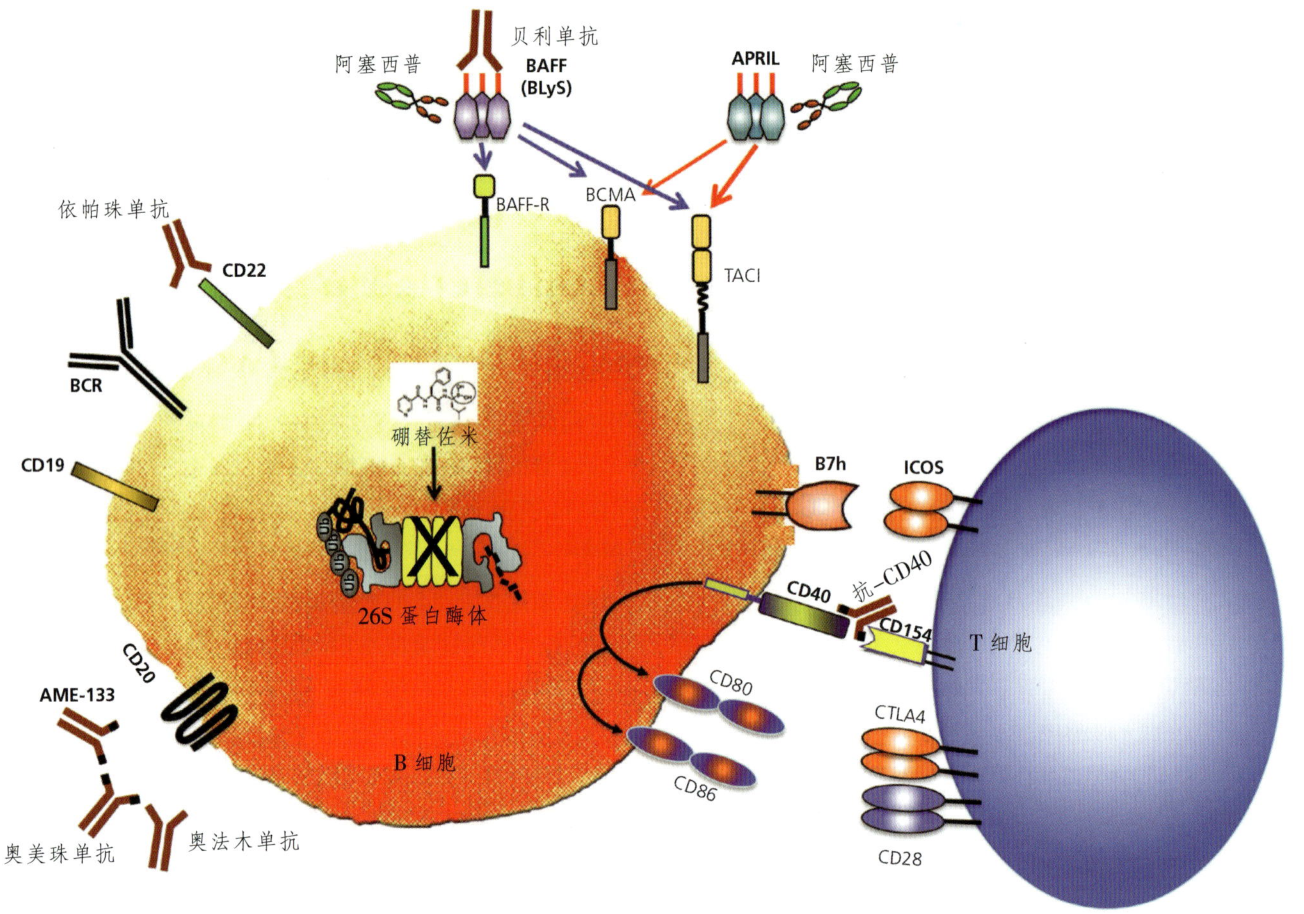

图 18.4 CD40-CD40L(CD154)通路。(Reproduced from[52] Webber A, Hirose R, Vincenti F. Novel strategies in immunosuppression:issues in perspective. Transplantation 2011; 91:1057 - 1064, with permission from Wolters Kluwer Health.)

记忆 T 细胞和 Ox40-Ox40L/LFA-3/CD2 通路

联合阻断 CD28/B7 和 CD40/CD154 通路以尝试在移植试验模型中促进移植物免疫耐受、延长移植物存活期已经取得成功[23,45]。但是,在移植排斥反应时,该联合用药并非总是有效[53,54],一种被称为"共刺激通路阻断剂耐药的排斥反应"的新现象出现,效应记忆 T 细胞被认为是主要元凶。效应记忆 T 细胞对 CD28 共刺激通路依赖少[55,56],甚至在共刺激通路阻断时仍可激活,被认为是抑制免疫耐受的一项障碍[57-59]。虽然 CNI 可有效抑制 CD8+记忆 T 细胞的增殖及其功能,但是 CNI 相关的毒性已经促使研究者探索新的药物[60]。

OX40(CD134)表达于活化的 T 细胞上,当其与表达于树突细胞、B 细胞、活化的内皮细胞、巨噬细胞上的配体 OX40L 结合时,可促进效应 T 细胞活化,以及通过 B 细胞增殖促进体液免疫反应[61,62]。相反,OX40/OX40L 在调节 T 细胞上结合后成为抑制信号(负性共刺激),并导致 FoxP3 下调,进而使抑制性调节 T 细胞功能丧失[63]。但是,最重要的也许是 OX40/OX40L 在 CD4+记忆 T 细胞增殖上的作用。OX40/OX40L 交互作用对于产生强效的 CD4+记忆 T 细胞是必需的[64,65]。

在研究皮肤移植的 CD28/CD154 双敲除小鼠模型中,主要通过 OX40 共刺激通路发生了严重的排斥反应[34]。在该研究中,联用 mCTLA-4-Ig 和抗 CD154 抗体或者单用抗 OX40L 抗体均无法阻止野生型小鼠的排斥反应,但是联用 mCTLA-4-Ig、抗 CD154 抗体和抗 OX40L 抗体,可维持皮肤移植物长期存活[34]。类似的,在大鼠心脏移植模型中,联用 mCTLA-4-Ig 和抗 OX40L 抗体可实现心脏移植物长期存活。因此,OX40/OX40L 通路成为未来实体器官移植免疫抗排斥的理想靶点。

就像 OX40-OX40L 共刺激通路对于 CD4+记忆 T 细胞的增殖和生成是必需的,CD2-LFA-3 通路对于 CD8+效应 T 细胞的功能也是必需的。CD2 是存在于活化的记忆 T 细胞表明蛋白，当它结合于其配体 LFA-3(CD58)时，可作为黏附分子和共刺激分子。阿法西普(人 LFA-3-IgG1 融合蛋白)是 FDA 批准用于银屑病的免疫调节治疗的融合蛋白。有趣的是，银屑病斑块以效应记忆 T 细胞的浸润为主，阿法西普可降低循环中和银屑病斑块中的效应记忆 T 细胞数量[68,69]。针对 BENEFIT 实验中应用贝拉西普治疗导致急性排斥反应增加的现象，一项应用流式细胞术旨在更好地探究共刺激通路阻断剂耐药的排斥反应中效应记忆 T 细胞的试验已经开始，该实验发现，与其他记忆 T 细胞亚群相比，效应记忆 T 细胞表达大多数的 CD2[70]，并且，同种异体反应的 $CD8^{+}CD2^{hi}$ $CD28^{-}$ T 细胞产生大多数细胞因子和所有 T 细胞亚群的细胞毒分子(IFN-γ，TNF 和 IL-2 颗粒酶 B，CD107a)，而且这些细胞可以耐受贝拉西普。所以，他们推测，这些细胞可能与 BENEFIT 试验中的高排斥反应率相关[29]。在体外实验中加入阿法西普，可抑制贝拉西普耐药的对同种异体抗原应答的 $CD8^{+}$ T 细胞[70]。同一团队前期已经证实，当联用 CTLA-4-Ig(阿巴西普)与西罗莫司，阿法西普可明显延长非人灵长类移植肾的存活期[71]。

比较阿法西普起始静脉注射然后皮下注射 3 个月方案与他克莫司为基础的免疫抑制方案的两项试验已经在美国和欧洲进行[72,73]。相对于他克莫司和吗替麦考酚酯，阿法西普组具有类似或更高的排斥率[72,73]。但是，正如在银屑病研究中显示的，循环中的记忆 T 细胞被耗尽，这种方法是不安全的。安斯泰来公司已经决定终止用于肾移植的阿法西普的研发。虽然联用 CTLA-4-Ig 和阿法西普具有前景，但是前期证实其可延长非人灵长类中移植物存活期，并耗尽效应记忆 T 细胞[71]，所以该临床试验不可能开展下去。

LFA-1/ICAM 通路

白细胞功能相关抗原-1(LFA-1)是一种 β 整合蛋白异二聚体，由一条唯一的 α 链(CD11a)和一条常见的 β 链(CD18)组成[74]。LFA-1 既是直接的共刺激分子[75]，也是稳定 T 细胞受体与 MHC 复合物免疫接口的主要部分。此外，它是淋巴细胞迁徙的重要细胞黏附分子，主要与细胞内的黏附分子-1(ICAM-1)相互作用[74,75]。它表达于 T 细胞、B 细胞上，类似 CD2，其在记忆 T 细胞上高表达[77,78]。

在肾移植中应用单克隆抗体阻断 LFA-1/ICAM 通路的多项试验已经开始[79-83]。依法利珠单抗是一种人抗 LFA-1 单克隆抗体，它已被 FDA 批准用于治疗银屑病[84-86]。依法利珠单抗用于肾移植的Ⅰ/Ⅱ期非盲多中心试验入组 38 例患者，分为低剂量组(0.5mg/kg)和高剂量组(2mg/kg)每周皮下注射，同时应用全量环孢素、吗替麦考酚酯和类固醇，或者半量环孢素、西罗莫司和泼尼松维持治疗[83]。虽然受体及移植物在术后 6 月的生存率很高，即使应用 2mg/kg 依法利珠单抗和全量环孢素，仍有 8%受体患有 PTLD[83]。患有Ⅰ型糖尿病的 8 例患者实施了胰岛细胞移植，并接受抗胸腺细胞球蛋白的免疫诱导，然后联用 0.5mg/kg 依法利珠单抗和西罗莫司或吗替麦考酚酯维持治疗。所有患者可实现胰岛素独立，且没有依法利珠单抗相关的副反应报道，有趣的是，循环中 $CD4^{+}$ $FoxP3^{+}$调节 T 细胞明显增加[87]。类似的，另一项依法利珠单抗用于糖尿病患者胰岛细胞移植的研究表明，单次胰岛细胞输注后，所有应用依法利珠单抗方案的患者实现胰岛素独立。在 2009 年 4 月，依法利珠单抗因为银屑病患者中有关进行性多灶性白质脑病(PML)的安全问题，自愿从美国市场退出(www.fda.gov/Safety/MedWatch/default.htm)。然而，考虑到近期对共刺激阻断耐药的排斥反应兴趣高涨，一项有效利用已知效应记忆 T 细胞上表达 LFA-1 增加的研究表明，一种小鼠抗人 CD11a 单克隆抗体 TS-1/22 当与巴利昔单抗、西罗莫司或贝拉西普联用时，可延长非人灵长类胰岛移植物的存活期[89]。未来的移植临床研究将可能探究联用生物制剂的效果，以活化原始 T 细胞的共刺激通路为靶点(即贝拉西普、抗 CD40 抗体)，还有对记忆 T 细胞增殖、活化有重大意义的通路(即阿法西普、抗 LFA-1 抗体、抗 OX40 抗体)，以及其他对于同种异体免疫具有重要意义的通路，包括补体和 B 细胞增殖通路。在一项小鼠心脏移植模型研究中，联用 CTLA-4-Ig 和补体 C5 的单克隆抗体(针对供体和受体)可明显延长移植物存活期。这些联用显示了移植试验中的巨大潜力[34,70,71,90,91]，但是在人体模型中，可能因为过度免疫抑制而受到限制。

未来 B 细胞及抗体介导损伤的治疗靶点

近期的数据表明，慢性抗供体抗体介导的损伤也许是导致晚期移植物失功的主要病理机制，针对 B 细胞和浆细胞的治疗已经在积极探索中[7,8,92,93]。目前的脱敏治疗方案以及针对急慢性抗体介导的排斥反应的治疗，包括血浆置换、静脉用免疫球蛋白、嵌合的抗 CD20 单克隆抗体和利妥昔单抗[94–98]。最新的成功治疗 AMR 及脱敏方法包括硼替佐米和依库丽单抗。硼替佐米是一种蛋白酶体抑制剂，以代谢活跃、分裂快速的细胞为靶点，通过选择性地抑制 26s 蛋白酶体和转录活化因子核因子 κB 而诱导细胞凋亡。虽然因为具有神经毒性而受到限制，但是 FDA 已经批准其用于治疗浆细胞恶病质，它以移植中的正常浆细胞为靶点，可减少供体特异性抗体，在一些个案中可抑制 AMR[99–104]。依库丽单抗是一种 FDA 批准用于补体相关性疾病(包括阵发性睡眠性血红蛋白尿和非典型溶血尿毒综合征，两者均发生于移植后，且易反复发作)[105–108]的人抗 C5 抗体[109]，可降低在脱敏方案中 AMR 和移植肾小球病的发生率[110]，提高移植后 AMR 的治疗效果。以补体瀑布为靶点用于抑制补体依赖的同种异体抗体介导的损伤的更多药物将可能在未来几年逐步面世。但是，需要更严格的临床试验来更好地定义硼替佐米和依库丽单抗的有效性和安全性。

注意到 B 细胞在多个层面参与同种异体免疫反应是很重要的。它们很明显是抗体介导损伤的主要部分，但是它们也是有效的抗原递呈细胞[111]，因此，对于 T 细胞活化是很重要的。因此，以 B 细胞本身为靶点的药物可能成为促使更持久的移植物耐受的有价值的治疗方法(图 18.5)。新的在生物制药流水线上的 B 细胞消耗抗体包括抗 CD20 单克隆抗体 atumumab，奥瑞珠单抗(ocrelizumab)，维妥珠单抗，以及正在进行Ⅱb 期临床试验用于治疗系统性红斑狼疮的 B 细胞消耗抗 CD22 抗体依帕珠单抗[112,113]。贝利木单抗和阿塞西普是主要在自身免疫疾病和血液系统恶性肿瘤治疗中研究的具有唯一靶点的新型 B 细胞疗法药物。贝利木单抗是完

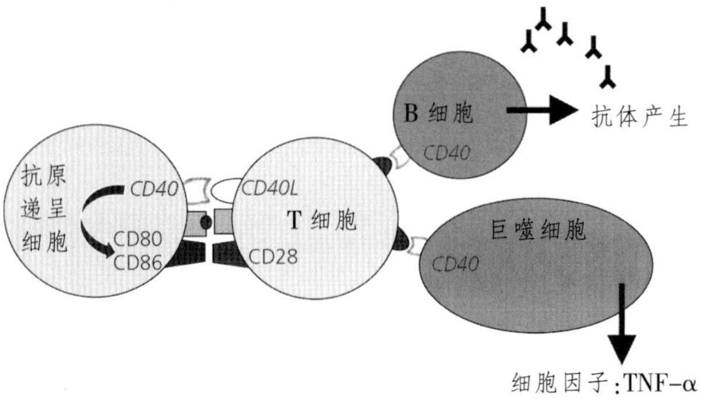

图 18.5 新的 B 细胞靶点。

全人单克隆抗体，与可溶性 B 细胞激活物(BLy，又称作 B 细胞活化因子 BAFF)结合并抑制其活性。BLy 是肿瘤坏死因子家族配体，当其与 BAFF 受体、B 细胞成熟蛋白(BCMA)、跨膜激活物、钙调节物以及亲环蛋白配体交互器结合时，可充当 B 细胞生存因子[10]。贝利木单抗可有效治疗系统性红斑狼疮，最近 FDA 已批准系统性红斑狼疮作为贝利木单抗的适应证[113–115]。宾夕法尼亚大学正在一项一年Ⅱ期研究中探究贝利木单抗作为减敏剂用于高度敏感的肾移植受体(www.clinicaltrials.gov)。

阿塞西普是一种由 TACI 细胞外域组成的融合蛋白，可与人 IgG1 的恒定区结合。当与增殖诱导配体(APRIL) 结合后，可与其靶点 BCMA 和 TACI 相互作用，因此，可阻碍 B 细胞活化和增殖。重要的是，APRIL 对于 B 细胞分化晚期和浆细胞生存是必须的[10]。一项阿塞西普联合吗替麦考酚酯用于狼疮肾患者的Ⅱ期研究因为感染并发症的增加而早早停止[113,116]。系统性红斑狼疮的进一步研究还在继续。目前，还没有探究阿塞西普用于移植的临床试验，但是考虑到其降低浆细胞和免疫球蛋白的潜力，其用于脱敏和抗体介导的排斥反应的前景美好。

IL–6

细胞因子 IL–6，既往被认为是急性期炎性反应的调节器，正逐渐成为重要的 TH17 细胞的促进剂和调节性 T 细胞的抑制剂[117]。IL–6 对自身免疫性疾病的影响与托珠单抗的关系已经确立，托珠单抗是第一个人抗 IL–6 抗体，已被批准用于类风湿关节炎。百时美施贵宝公司和再生元公司正在研究针对 IL–6 另外两个生物制剂。在试验中，与共刺激通路阻断剂联用时，抗 IL–6 治疗的效果最显著[118]。目前，在西达赛奈医学中心，一项托珠单抗作为脱敏药物提高移植存活率的单中心试验正在进行(NCT01594424)，在加州大学洛杉矶分校，托珠单抗治疗炎症和临界性排斥反应的试验也在进行中。如果这些试验成功，制药产业可能考虑将其用于器官移植领域。

小分子

JAK3/蛋白激酶 C

利用常见 γ 链的细胞因子受体(例如，T 细胞，B 细

胞受体 IL-2、4、7、9、15 和 21 等)均需要细胞质内酪氨酸激酶 JAK3 作信号通路。通过 JAK3 的细胞因子信号对于淋巴细胞活化和分化是十分重要的，是 T 细胞活化的第 3 个也是最后一个信号（前两个是 MHC-TCR 信号和共刺激信号)[119,120]。事实上,在淋巴细胞生物学 JAK3 具有潜在的作用，常见 γ 链和或 JAK3 的突变，会导致严重的重症综合性免疫缺陷表型[121]。JAK3 的表达主要受限于淋巴细胞和自然杀伤细胞，因此它是同种异体免疫反应的重要组分，也是防止同种异体排斥反应的潜在靶点。JAK3 的小分子抑制剂托法替尼(旧称 CP-690,550)对人自身免疫疾病具有显著疗效[123,124],因其在保护 $CD4^+$ $FOXP3^+$调节 T 细胞抑制性活动时,可选择性抑制效应 T 细胞的功能,所以托法替尼成为免疫抑制剂之一[125]。

在小鼠和非人灵长类器官移植模型成功应用托法替尼后[126-129],一项 JAK3 抑制剂用于肾移植受体的 I 期临床试验正在开展[130]。在这项剂量递增的研究中,28 例稳定的肾移植受体至少 12 个月联合应用不同剂量的托法替尼和吗替麦考酚酯,5~30mg tid 是可接受的安全性和耐受性的范围。在一项Ⅱa 期多中心、随机、开放标签试验中,比较了托法替尼两种剂量(15mg 对 30mg,口服,bid)与他克莫司在肾移植受体的作用,受体由抗 IL-2 受体抗体诱导,由 MPA 和类固醇维持,研究发现在术后 6 个月,15mg 托法替尼组(CP15)活检证实的急性排斥反应(BPAR)发生率为 5.3%,在 30mg 托法替尼组(CP30)是 21.1%,在他克莫司组是 4.8%。术后 6 个月和 12 个月估计肾小球滤过率在 3 组间类似，但是相对于他克莫司组,CP30 组 BK 病毒肾病（20%）和巨细胞病毒病(21.1%)发生率稍高。按照代谢指标，NODAT 发生率无差异。但是,血脂异常在托法替尼两组中更常见。所有的胆固醇指标在 CP15 组增加 34%，CP30 组增加 44%[16]。

一项Ⅱb 期临床试验的数据已经公布[131],在该试验中,322 名肾移植受体随机分为 3 组:两个托法替尼组(CP)和环孢素组,在托法替尼组 1 中先口服托法替尼 15mg bid 半年后减量为 10mg bid,组 2 口服托法替尼 15mg bid 3 个月后减量为 10mg bid[132,133]。所有受体接受抗 IL-2 受体抗体诱导免疫抑制，依靠吗替麦考酚酯和类固醇维持免疫抑制。两组托法替尼组在术后 6 个月和 12 个月的活检急性排斥反应发生率均表现出非劣效性。在术后 12 个月的估算肾小球滤过率统计学上明显升高(64.6mL/min CP1,64.7mL/min CP2,53.9mL/min 环孢素)。与环孢素组相比，两组托法替尼组 NODAT 发生率均下降,但是,免疫抑制剂相关并发症,包括感染和恶性肿瘤在托法替尼组均高于环孢素组。令人惊讶的是,托法替尼组 5 例患者出现 PTLD,而在环孢素组无 PTLD[132,133]。因此,托法替尼在移植中的作用仅局限于找到其不引起过度免疫抑制导致副反应而可抑制移植排斥反应的最佳剂量。

蛋白激酶 C

最后，蛋白激酶 C 亚型 PKCθ 和 PKCα 的小分子靶向药物 sotrastaurin，是针对非依赖钙调磷酸酶通路免疫抑制剂的另一例子。蛋白激酶 C 是淋巴细胞中抗原受体信号转导通路的中心,PKCθ 和 PKCα 分别是 IL-2 和 IFN-γ 产物的关键亚类。在啮齿类和非人灵长类模型中证实 sotrastaurin 可延长移植肾存活期[134],并且在一项银屑病的概念验证试验中 sotrastaurin 的实用性和安全性得到证实后[135-138],一项肾移植Ⅱ期临床试验研究了 sotrastaurin 口服制剂的安全性和有效性[139]。在该研究中,216 例患者随机分为 3 组,sotrastaurin 200mg bid + 他克莫司标准剂量(SET),sotrastaurin 200mg bid+减量的他克莫司(RET),他克莫司+MPA(对照组)[140]。在肾移植术后 3 个月,符合转换标准的 Sotrastaurin 受体将转为无 CNI 方案。所有患者接受 IL-2 受体抗体诱导免疫抑制,使用类固醇维持免疫抑制[140]。在 sotrastaurin 组,CNI 撤药前,主要疗效终点(包括 BPAR、移植物失功和死亡)在 3 组间相同,但是,在研究结束时(在 sotrastaurin 组 CNI 撤药后),对照组中 7.8%的患者到达主要疗效终点,但是 sotrastaurin+SET 和 sotrastaurin+RET 组分别有 44.8%和 34.1%的患者到达主要疗效终点。相反,胃肠道、心脏和感染等并发症发生率在 3 组间相等[140]。

一项最近的肾移植随机试验中，患者被随机分入他克莫司组和 sotrastaurin 组(300mg bid),试验结果也类似。也就是说,尽管 sotrastaurin 组术后 3 个月的估算肾小球滤过率有所提高(59mL/min 对 49.5mL/min),但是在统计学上 sotrastaurin 组到达主要效应终点多于对照组(25.7%对 2%),所以该试验被早期终止了,但是两组间的副反应类似[141]。

总结

H. U. Meier-Kriesche 和 B. Kaplan 撰写的社论题目是探索无 CNI 免疫抑制方案:没有免费的午餐,形象地比喻了研究新的移植药物靶点所遭遇的挫折[142]。虽然 JAK3 抑制剂在抑制移植物排斥反应方面与 CNI 类药物效果类似，但是也付出了更多副反应的代价。相反,PKC 抑制剂具有类似的感染和肿瘤发生率,但却无法提供类似的治疗效果，包括活检证实的急性排斥反应和移植物存活率。针对共刺激通路的药物对固有免疫反应具有明显的抑制效果，但是不太适合控制适应性免疫反应，这导致一种依赖受体既往免疫状态的有效性与副反应共存的现象。尽管如此,器官移植与探索无 CNI 免疫抑制方案的梦想还在继续。联用新型生物制剂,优化小分子的治疗窗或者某些药物的联用,最终能否在保证针对其他抗原具有完整免疫的同时，提供针对移植物的强效免疫抑制,还有待阐明。

(焦守斐 译 荀晓冬 李照 校)

参考文献

1. Meier-Kriesche HU, Schold JD, Srinivas TR, et al. Lack of improvement in renal allograft survival despite a marked decrease in acute rejection rates over the most recent era. American Journal of Transplantation. 2004;4:378-383.
2. Curtis JJ. Hypertension following kidney transplantation. American Journal of Kidney Diseases. 1994;23:471-475.
3. Curtis JJ. Hypertensinogenic mechanism of the calcineurin inhibitors. Current Hypertension Reports 2002;4:377-380.
4. Kobashigawa JA, Kasiske BL. Hyperlipidemia in solid organ transplantation. Transplantation. 1997;63:331-338.
5. Luke RG. Mechanism of cyclosporine-induced hypertension. American Journal of Hypertension. 1991;4:468-471.
6. Nankivell BJ, Borrows RJ, Fung CL, et al. The natural history of chronic allograft nephropathy. New England Journal of Medicine. 2003;349:2326-2333.
7. Gaston RS, Cecka JM, Kasiske BL, et al. Evidence for antibody-mediated injury as a major determinant of late kidney allograft failure. Transplantation. 2010;90:68-74.
8. Gourishankar S, Leduc R, Connett J, et al. Pathological and clinical characterization of the 'troubled transplant': data from the DeKAF study. American Journal of Transplantation. 2010;10:324-330.
9. Matas AJ, Leduc R, Rush D, et al. Histopathologic clusters differentiate subgroups within the nonspecific diagnoses of CAN or CR: preliminary data from the DeKAF study. American Journal of Transplantation. 2010;10:315-323.
10. Bossen C, Schneider P. BAFF, APRIL and their receptors: structure, function and signaling. Seminars in Immunology. 2006;18:263-275.
11. Lafferty KJ, Cunningham AJ. A new analysis of allogeneic interactions. Australian Journal of Experimental Biology and Medical Science. 1975;53:27-42.
12. Sayegh MH, Turka LA. The role of T-cell costimulatory activation pathways in transplant rejection. New England Journal of Medicine. 1998;338:1813-1821.
13. Li XC, Rothstein DM, Sayegh MH. Costimulatory pathways in transplantation: challenges and new developments. Immunological Reviews. 2009;229:271-293.
14. Pilat N, Sayegh MH, Wekerle T. Costimulatory pathways in transplantation. Seminars in Immunology. 2011;23:293-303.
15. Vincenti F, Kirk AD. What's next in the pipeline. American Journal of Transplantation. 2008;8:1972-1981.
16. Busque S, Leventhal J, Brennan DC, et al. Calcineurin-inhibitor-free immunosuppression based on the JAK inhibitor CP-690,550: a pilot study in de novo kidney allograft recipients. American Journal of Transplantation. 2009;9:1936-1945.
17. Vincenti F, Silva HT, Busque S. A phase 2B study of CNI-free immunosuppression with the JAK inhibitor CP-690,550 in de novo kidney transplant patients: 6-month interim analysis. American Journal of Transplantation. 2010;10:211.
18. Bretscher PA. A two-step, two-signal model for the primary activation of precursor helper T cells. Proceedings of the National Academy of Sciences of the United States of America. 1999;96:185-190.
19. Lenschow DJ, Walunas TL, Bluestone JA. CD28/B7 system of T cell costimulation. Annual Review of Immunology. 1996;14:233-258.
20. Sakaguchi S, Ono M, Setoguchi R, et al. Foxp3+ CD25+ CD4+ natural regulatory T cells in dominant self-tolerance and autoimmune disease. Immunological Reviews. 2006;212:8-27.
21. Wing K, Onishi Y, Prieto-Martin P, et al. CTLA-4 control over Foxp3+ regulatory T cell function. Science. 2008;322:271-275.
22. Linsley PS, Greene JL, Brady W, et al. Human B7-1 (CD80) and B7-2 (CD86) bind with similar avidities but distinct kinetics to CD28 and CTLA-4 receptors. Immunity. 1994;1:793-801.
23. Kirk AD, Harlan DM, Armstrong NN, et al. CTLA4-Ig and anti-CD40 ligand prevent renal allograft rejection in primates. Proceedings of the National Academy of Sciences of the United States of America. 1997;94:8789-8794.
24. Levisetti MG, Padrid PA, Szot GL, et al. Immunosuppressive effects of human CTLA4Ig in a non-human primate model of allogeneic pancreatic islet transplantation. Journal of Immunology. 1997;159:5187-5191.
25. Ronchese F, Hausmann B, Hubele S, et al. Mice transgenic for a soluble form of murine CTLA-4 show enhanced expansion of antigen-specific CD4+ T cells and defective antibody production in vivo. Journal of Experimental Medicine. 1994;179:809-817.
26. Sayegh MH, Akalin E, Hancock WW, et al. CD28-B7 blockade after alloantigenic challenge in vivo inhibits Th1 cytokines but spares Th2. Journal of Experimental Medicine. 1995;181:1869-1874.
27. Larsen CP, Pearson TC, Adams AB, et al. Rational development of LEA29Y (belatacept), a high-affinity variant of CTLA4-Ig with potent immunosuppressive properties. American Journal of Transplantation. 2005;5:443-453.
28. Vincenti F, Larsen C, Durrbach A, et al. Costimulation blockade with belatacept in renal transplantation. New England Journal of Medicine. 2005;353:770-781.
29. Vincenti F, Charpentier B, Vanrenterghem Y, et al. A phase III study of belatacept-based immunosuppression regimens versus cyclosporine in renal transplant recipients (BENEFIT study). American Journal of Transplantation. 2010;10:535-546.
30. Durrbach A, Pestana JM, Pearson T, et al. A phase III study of belatacept versus cyclosporine in kidney transplants from extended criteria donors (BENEFIT-EXT study). American Journal of Transplantation. 2010;10:547-557.
31. Friedline RH, Brown DS, Nguyen H, et al. CD4+ regulatory T cells require CTLA-4 for the maintenance of systemic tolerance. Journal of Experimental Medicine. 2009;206:421-434.
32. Larsen CP, Knechtle SJ, Adams A, et al. A new look at blockade of T-cell costimulation: a therapeutic strategy for long-term maintenance immunosuppression. American Journal of Transplantation. 2006;6:876-883.
33. Valujskikh A, Pantenburg B, Heeger PS. Primed allospecific T cells prevent the effects of costimulatory blockade on prolonged cardiac allograft survival in mice. American Journal of Transplantation. 2002;2:501-509.
34. Demirci G, Amanullah F, Kewalaramani R, et al. Critical role of OX40 in CD28 and CD154-independent rejection. Journal of Immunology. 2004;172:1691-1698.
35. Hamann D, Baars PA, Rep MH, et al. Phenotypic and functional separation of memory and effector human CD8+ T cells. Journal of Experimental Medicine. 1997;186:1407-1418.
36. Shiao SL, McNiff JM, Masunaga T, et al. Immunomodulatory properties of FK734, a humanized anti-CD28 monoclonal antibody with agonistic and antagonistic activities. Transplantation. 2007;83:304-313.
37. Suntharalingam G, Perry MR, Ward S, et al. Cytokine storm in a phase 1 trial of the anti-CD28 monoclonal antibody TGN1412. New England Journal of Medicine. 2006;355:1018-1028.
38. Poirier N, Azimzadeh AM, Zhang T, et al. Inducing CTLA-4-dependent immune regulation by selective CD28 blockade promotes regulatory T cells in organ transplantation. Science Translational Medicine 2010;2:17ra0.
39. Larsen CP, Pearson TC. The CD40 pathway in allograft rejection, acceptance, and tolerance. Current Opinion in Immunology. 1997;9:641-647.
40. van Kooten C, Banchereau J. Functions of CD40 on B cells, dendritic cells and other cells. Current Opinion in Immunology. 1997;9:330-337.
41. Ford ML, Larsen CP. Translating costimulation blockade to the clinic: lessons learned from three pathways. Immunological Reviews. 2009;229:294-306.

42. Grewal IS, Flavell RA. CD40 and CD154 in cell-mediated immunity. Annual Review of Immunology. 1998;16:111–135.
43. Yang Y, Wilson JM. CD40 ligand-dependent T cell activation: requirement of B7-CD28 signaling through CD40. Science. 1996;273:1862–1864.
44. Kirk AD, Burkly LC, Batty DS, et al. Treatment with humanized monoclonal antibody against CD154 prevents acute renal allograft rejection in nonhuman primates. Nature Medicine. 1999;5:686–693.
45. Larsen CP, Elwood ET, Alexander DZ, et al. Long-term acceptance of skin and cardiac allografts after blocking CD40 and CD28 pathways. Nature. 1996; 381:434–438.
46. Xu H, Montgomery SP, Preston EH, et al. Studies investigating pretransplant donor-specific blood transfusion, rapamycin, and the CD154-specific antibody IDEC-131 in a nonhuman primate model of skin allotransplantation. Journal of Immunology. 2003;170:2776–2782.
47. Elster EA, Xu H, Tadaki DK, et al. Treatment with the humanized CD154-specific monoclonal antibody, hu5C8, prevents acute rejection of primary skin allografts in nonhuman primates. Transplantation. 2001;72:1473–1478.
48. Kawai T, Andrews D, Colvin RB, et al. Thromboembolic complications after treatment with monoclonal antibody against CD40 ligand. Nature Medicine. 2000;6:114.
49. Sidiropoulos PI, Boumpas DT. Lessons learned from anti-CD40L treatment in systemic lupus erythematosus patients. Lupus. 2004;13:391–397.
50. Adams AB, Shirasugi N, Jones TR, et al. Development of a chimeric anti-CD40 monoclonal antibody that synergizes with LEA29Y to prolong islet allograft survival. Journal of Immunology. 2005;174:542–550.
51. Haanstra KG, Ringers J, Sick EA, et al. Prevention of kidney allograft rejection using anti-CD40 and anti-CD86 in primates. Transplantation. 2003;75:637–643.
52. Webber A, Hirose R, Vincenti F. Novel strategies in immunosuppression: issues in perspective. Transplantation. 2011;91:1057–1064.
53. Li XC, Strom TB, Blocking T. cell costimulation in transplantation: opportunities and challenges. Transfusion. 2000;40:139–142.
54. Williams MA, Trambley J, Ha J, et al. Genetic characterization of strain differences in the ability to mediate CD40/CD28-independent rejection of skin allografts. Journal of Immunology. 2000;165:6849–6857.
55. London CA, Lodge MP, Abbas AK. Functional responses and costimulator dependence of memory CD4+ T cells. Journal of Immunology. 2000;164: 265–272.
56. Slifka MK, Whitton JL. Activated and memory CD8+ T cells can be distinguished by their cytokine profiles and phenotypic markers. Journal of Immunology. 2000;164:208–216.
57. Koehn B, Gangappa S, Miller JD, et al. Patients, pathogens, and protective immunity: the relevance of virus-induced alloreactivity in transplantation. Journal of Immunology. 2006;176:2691–2696.
58. Adams AB, Williams MA, Jones TR, et al. Heterologous immunity provides a potent barrier to transplantation tolerance. Journal of Clinical Investigation. 2003;111:1887–1895.
59. Heeger PS, Greenspan NS, Kuhlenschmidt S, et al. Pretransplant frequency of donor-specific, IFN-gamma-producing lymphocytes is a manifestation of immunologic memory and correlates with the risk of posttransplant rejection episodes. Journal of Immunology. 1999;163:2267–2275.
60. Jones DL, Sacks SH, Wong W. Controlling the generation and function of human CD8+ memory T cells in vitro with immunosuppressants. Transplantation. 2006;82:1352–1361.
61. Rogers PR, Song J, Gramaglia I, et al. OX40 promotes Bcl-xL and Bcl-2 expression and is essential for long-term survival of CD4 T cells. Immunity. 2001;15: 445–455.
62. Stuber E, Strober W. The T cell-B cell interaction via OX40-OX40L is necessary for the T cell-dependent humoral immune response. Journal of Experimental Medicine. 1996;183:979–989.
63. Vu MD, Xiao X, Gao W, et al. OX40 costimulation turns off Foxp3+ Tregs. Blood. 2007;110:2501–2510.
64. Dawicki W, Bertram EM, Sharpe AH, et al. 4-1BB and OX40 act independently to facilitate robust CD8 and CD4 recall responses. Journal of Immunology. 2004;173:5944–5951.
65. Sugamura K, Ishii N, Weinberg AD. Therapeutic targeting of the effector T-cell costimulatory molecule OX40. Nature Reviews. Immunology. 2004;4:420–431.
66. Yuan X, Salama AD, Dong V, et al. The role of the CD134-CD134 ligand costimulatory pathway in alloimmune responses in vivo. Journal of Immunology. 2003;170:2949–2955.
67. Ellis CN, Krueger GG. Treatment of chronic plaque psoriasis by selective targeting of memory effector T lymphocytes. New England Journal of Medicine. 2001;345:248–255.
68. Chamian F, Lin SL, Lee E, et al. Alefacept (anti-CD2) causes a selective reduction in circulating effector memory T cells (Tem) and relative preservation of central memory T cells (Tcm) in psoriasis. Journal of Translational Medicine. 2007;5:27.
69. Chamian F, Lowes MA, Lin SL, et al. Alefacept reduces infiltrating T cells, activated dendritic cells, and inflammatory genes in psoriasis vulgaris. Proceedings of the National Academy of Sciences of the United States of America. 2005;102:2075–2080.
70. Lo DJ, Weaver TA, Stempora L, et al. Selective targeting of human alloresponsive CD8+ effector memory T cells based on CD2 expression. American Journal of Transplantation. 2011;11:22–33.
71. Weaver TA, Charafeddine AH, Agarwal A, et al. Alefacept promotes costimulation blockade based allograft survival in nonhuman primates. Nature Medicine. 2009;15:746–749.
72. Bromberg J, Cibrik D, Steinberg S, et al. Phase 2 study to assess the safety and efficacy of alefacept (ALEF) in de novo kidney transplant recipients. American Journal of Transplantation. 2011;11 (Suppl.s2):190.
73. Rostaing L, Mourad M, Charpentier B, et al. Efficacy and safety of alefacept in combination with tacrolimus, mycophenolate mofetil and steroids in de novo kidney transplantation. American Journal of Transplantation. 2011;11:98.
74. Nicolls MR, Gill RG. LFA-1 (CD11a) as a therapeutic target. American Journal of Transplantation. 2006;6:27–36.
75. Van Seventer GA, Shimizu Y, Horgan KJ, et al. The LFA-1 ligand ICAM-1 provides an important costimulatory signal for T cell receptor-mediated activation of resting T cells. Journal of Immunology. 1990;144:4579–4586.
76. Pribila JT, Quale AC, Mueller KL, et al. Integrins and T cell-mediated immunity. Annual Review of Immunology. 2004;22:157–180.
77. Sanders ME, Makgoba MW, Sharrow SO, et al. Human memory T lymphocytes express increased levels of three cell adhesion molecules (LFA-3, CD2, and LFA-1) and three other molecules (UCHL1, CDw29, and Pgp-1) and have enhanced IFN-gamma production. Journal of Immunology. 1988;140: 1401–1407.
78. Lee WT, Vitetta ES. The differential expression of homing and adhesion molecules on virgin and memory T cells in the mouse. Cellular Immunology. 1991;132:215–222.
79. Hourmant M, Bedrossian J, Durand D, et al. A randomized multicenter trial comparing leukocyte function-associated antigen-1 monoclonal antibody with rabbit antithymocyte globulin as induction treatment in first kidney transplantations. Transplantation. 1996;62:1565–1570.
80. Hourmant M, Le Mauff B, Le Meur Y, et al. Administration of an anti-CD11a monoclonal antibody in recipients of kidney transplantation. A pilot study. Transplantation. 1994;58:377–380.
81. Le Mauff B, Hourmant M, Rougier JP, et al. Effect of anti-LFA1 (CD11a) monoclonal antibodies in acute rejection in human kidney transplantation. Transplantation. 1991;52:291–296.
82. Le Mauff B, Le Meur Y, Hourmant M, et al. A dose-searching trial of an anti-LFA1 monoclonal antibody in first kidney transplant recipients. Kidney International. Supplement. 1996;53:S44–S50.
83. Vincenti F, Mendez R, Pescovitz M, et al. A phase I/II randomized open-label multicenter trial of efalizumab, a humanized anti-CD11a, anti-LFA-1 in renal transplantation. American Journal of Transplantation. 2007;7:1770–1777.
84. Joshi A, Bauer R, Kuebler P, et al. An overview of the pharmacokinetics and pharmacodynamics of efalizumab: a monoclonal antibody approved for use in psoriasis. Journal of Clinical Pharmacology. 2006;46:10–20.
85. Lebwohl M, Tyring SK, Hamilton TK, et al. A novel targeted T-cell modulator, efalizumab, for plaque psoriasis. New England Journal of Medicine. 2003; 349:2004–2013.
86. Leonardi CL, Papp KA, Gordon KB, et al. Extended efalizumab therapy improves chronic plaque psoriasis: results from a randomized phase III trial. Journal of the American Academy of Dermatology. 2005;52:425–433.
87. Posselt AM, Bellin MD, Tavakol M, et al. Islet transplantation in type 1 diabetics using an immunosuppressive protocol based on the anti-LFA-1 antibody efalizumab. American Journal of Transplantation. 2010;10:1870–1880.
88. Turgeon NA, Avila JG, Cano JA, et al. Experience with a novel efalizumab-based immunosuppressive regimen to facilitate single donor islet cell transplantation. American Journal of Transplantation. 2010;10:2082–2091.
89. Badell IR, Russell MC, Thompson PW, et al. LFA-1-specific therapy prolongs allograft survival in rhesus macaques. Journal of Clinical Investigation. 2010;120:4520–4531.
90. Raedler H, Vieyra MB, Leisman S, et al. Anti-complement component C5 mAb synergizes with CTLA4Ig to inhibit alloreactive T cells and prolong cardiac allograft survival in mice. American Journal of Transplantation. 2011;11: 1397–1406.
91. Metzler B, Gfeller P, Bigaud M, et al. Combinations of anti-LFA-1, everolimus, anti-CD40 ligand, and allogeneic bone marrow induce central transplantation tolerance through hemopoietic chimerism, including protection from chronic heart allograft rejection. Journal of Immunology. 2004;173:7025–7036.
92. Everly MJ, Everly JJ, Arend LJ, et al. Reducing de novo donor-specific antibody levels during acute rejection diminishes renal allograft loss. American Journal of Transplantation. 2009;9:1063–1071.

93. Hidalgo LG, Campbell PM, Sis B, et al. De novo donor-specific antibody at the time of kidney transplant biopsy associates with microvascular pathology and late graft failure. American Journal of Transplantation. 2009;9:2532–2541.
94. Becker YT, Becker BN, Pirsch JD, et al. Rituximab as treatment for refractory kidney transplant rejection. American Journal of Transplantation. 2004;4: 996–1001.
95. Stegall MD, Gloor J, Winters JL, et al. A comparison of plasmapheresis versus high-dose IVIG desensitization in renal allograft recipients with high levels of donor specific alloantibody. American Journal of Transplantation. 2006;6: 346–351.
96. Vo AA, Lukovsky M, Toyoda M, et al. Rituximab and intravenous immune globulin for desensitization during renal transplantation. New England Journal of Medicine. 2008;359:242–251.
97. Alausa M, Almagro U, Siddiqi N, et al. Refractory acute kidney transplant rejection with CD20 graft infiltrates and successful therapy with rituximab. Clinical Transplantation. 2005;19:137–140.
98. Faguer S, Kamar N, Guilbeaud-Frugier C, et al. Rituximab therapy for acute humoral rejection after kidney transplantation. Transplantation. 2007;83: 1277–1280.
99. Everly JJ, Walsh RC, Alloway RR, et al. Proteasome inhibition for antibody-mediated rejection. Current Opinion in Organ Transplantation 2009;14: 662–666.
100. Lonze BE, Dagher NN, Simpkins CE, et al. Eculizumab, bortezomib and kidney paired donation facilitate transplantation of a highly sensitized patient without vascular access. American Journal of Transplantation. 2010;10:2154–2160.
101. Perry DK, Burns JM, Pollinger HS, et al. Proteasome inhibition causes apoptosis of normal human plasma cells preventing alloantibody production. American Journal of Transplantation. 2009;9:201–209.
102. Sberro-Soussan R, Zuber J, Suberbielle-Boissel C, et al. Bortezomib as the sole post-renal transplantation desensitization agent does not decrease donor-specific anti-HLA antibodies. American Journal of Transplantation. 2010;10:681–686.
103. Wahrmann M, Haidinger M, Kormoczi GF, et al. Effect of the proteasome inhibitor bortezomib on humoral immunity in two presensitized renal transplant candidates. Transplantation. 2010;89:1385–1390.
104. Walsh RC, Everly JJ, Brailey P, et al. Proteasome inhibitor-based primary therapy for antibody-mediated renal allograft rejection. Transplantation. 2010;89: 277–284.
105. Chandran S, Baxter-Lowe L, Olson JL, et al. Eculizumab for the treatment of de novo thrombotic microangiopathy post simultaneous pancreas-kidney transplantation–a case report. Transplantation Proceedings. 2011;43:2097–2101.
106. Chatelet V, Fremeaux-Bacchi V, Lobbedez T, et al. Safety and long-term efficacy of eculizumab in a renal transplant patient with recurrent atypical hemolytic-uremic syndrome. American Journal of Transplantation. 2009;9:2644–2645.
107. Davin JC, Gracchi V, Bouts A, et al. Maintenance of kidney function following treatment with eculizumab and discontinuation of plasma exchange after a third kidney transplant for atypical hemolytic uremic syndrome associated with a CFH mutation. American Journal of Kidney Diseases. 2010;55:708–711.
108. Wilson CH, Brown AL, White SA, et al. Successful treatment of de novo post-transplant thrombotic microangiopathy with eculizumab. Transplantation. 2011;92:e42–e43.
109. Stegall MD, Diwan T, Raghavaiah S, et al. Terminal complement inhibition decreases antibody-mediated rejection in sensitized renal transplant recipients. American Journal of Transplantation. 2011;11:2405–2413.
110. Lonze BE. Complement inhibitors for treatment of antibody-mediated renal allograft injury. American Journal of Transplantation. 2010;10:564.
111. Zarkhin V, Li L, Sarwal M. To B or not to B?" B-cells and graft rejection. Transplantation. 2008;85:1705–1714.
112. Vincenti F, Cohen SD, Appel G. Novel B cell therapeutic targets in transplantation and immune-mediated glomerular diseases. Clinical Journal of the American Society of Nephrology 2010;5:142–151.
113. Yildirim-Toruner C, Diamond B. Current and novel therapeutics in the treatment of systemic lupus erythematosus. Journal of Allergy and Clinical Immunology. 2011;127:303–312; quiz 13-4.
114. Jacobi AM, Huang W, Wang T, et al. Effect of long-term belimumab treatment on B cells in systemic lupus erythematosus: extension of a phase II, double-blind, placebo-controlled, dose-ranging study. Arthritis and Rheumatism. 2010;62:201–210.
115. Wallace DJ, Stohl W, Furie RA, et al. A phase II, randomized, double-blind, placebo-controlled, dose-ranging study of belimumab in patients with active systemic lupus erythematosus. Arthritis and Rheumatism. 2009;61:1168–1178.
116. Clinical Trials. The efficacy and safety of atacicept in combination with mycophenolate mofetil used to treat lupus nephritis. Available at: http://www.clinicaltrials.gov/ct2/show/record/NCT00573157 (accessed January 2014).
117. Jones SA, Cheler J, Rose-John S. Therapeutic strategies for the clinical blockade of IL-6/gp130 signaling. Journal of Clinical Investigation. 2011;121(9): 3375–3383.
118. Zhao X, Boenisch O, Yeung M, et al. Critical role of proinflammatory cytokine IL-6 in allograft rejection and tolerance. American Journal of Transplantation. 2012;(1): 90–101.
119. Darnell JE Jr, Kerr IM, Stark GR. Jak-STAT pathways and transcriptional activation in response to IFNs and other extracellular signaling proteins. Science. 1994;264:1415–1421.
120. Podder H, Kahan BD. Janus kinase 3: a novel target for selective transplant immunosupression. Expert Opinion on Therapeutic Targets. 2004;8:613–629.
121. Buckley RH. The multiple causes of human SCID. Journal of Clinical Investigation. 2004;114:1409–1411.
122. Changelian PS, Flanagan ME, Ball DJ, et al. Prevention of organ allograft rejection by a specific Janus kinase 3 inhibitor. Science. 2003;302:875–878.
123. Riese RJ, Krishnaswami S, Kremer J. Inhibition of JAK kinases in patients with rheumatoid arthritis: scientific rationale and clinical outcomes. Best Practice and Research. Clinical Rheumatology. 2010;24:513–526.
124. Kaminska B, Swiatek-Machado K. Targeting signaling pathways with small molecules to treat autoimmune disorders. Expert Review of Clinical Immunology 2008;4:93–112.
125. Sewgobind VD, Quaedackers ME, van der Laan LJ, et al. The Jak inhibitor CP-690,550 preserves the function of CD4CD25FoxP3 regulatory T cells and inhibits effector T cells. American Journal of Transplantation. 2010;10: 1785–1795.
126. Borie DC, Changelian PS, Larson MJ, et al. Immunosuppression by the JAK3 inhibitor CP-690,550 delays rejection and significantly prolongs kidney allograft survival in nonhuman primates. Transplantation. 2005;79:791–801.
127. Borie DC, Larson MJ, Flores MG, et al. Combined use of the JAK3 inhibitor CP-690,550 with mycophenolate mofetil to prevent kidney allograft rejection in nonhuman primates. Transplantation. 2005;80:1756–1764.
128. Kudlacz E, Perry B, Sawyer P, et al. The novel JAK-3 inhibitor CP-690550 is a potent immunosuppressive agent in various murine models. American Journal of Transplantation. 2004;4:51–57.
129. Paniagua R, Si MS, Flores MG, et al. Effects of JAK3 inhibition with CP-690,550 on immune cell populations and their functions in nonhuman primate recipients of kidney allografts. Transplantation. 2005;80:1283–1292.
130. van Gurp E, Weimar W, Gaston R, et al. Phase 1 dose-escalation study of CP-690 550 in stable renal allograft recipients: preliminary findings of safety, tolerability, effects on lymphocyte subsets and pharmacokinetics. American Journal of Transplantation. 2008;8:1711–1718.
131. Vincenti F, Tedesco Silva H, Busque S, et al. Randomized phase 2b trial of tofacitinib (CP-690,550) in de novo kidney transplant patients: efficacy, renal function and safety at 1 year. American Journal of Transplantation. 2012; 12:2446–2456.
132. Silva H, Vinceti F, O'Connell P, et al. Renal-sparing effects of CP-690,550 in de novo kidney transplant patients in a phase 2b study. American Journal of Transplantation. 2011;11:98.
133. Vincenti F, Silva H, Busque S, et al. Efficacy and safety of CP-690,550-MPA combination regimens in de novo kidney transplant patients: 12-month final results of a phase 2b study. American Journal of Transplantation. 2011;11:30.
134. Spitaler M, Cantrell DA. Protein kinase C and beyond. Nature Immunology. 2004;5:785–790.
135. Wagner J, Evenou J-P, Zenke G, et al. The first-in-class oral protein kinase C (PKC) inhibitor NVP-AEB071 (AEB) prolongs renal allograft survival in non-human primates (NHP) and suppresses lymphocyte proliferation at safe exposures in human proof-of-concept studies. Transplantation. 2006;82:86.
136. Bruns C, Pally C, Beerli C, et al. NVP-AEB071 (AEB), a novel oral inhibitor of early T-cekll activation, prolongs rat cardiac allograft survival when used alone and in combination with cyclosporine, everolimus or FTY720. Transplantation. 2006;82:316.
137. Bigaud M, Wieczorek G, Riesen S, et al. NVP-AEB071 (AEB), a novel oral inhibitor of early T-cell activation, prolongs the survival of non-human primate (NHP) kidney allografts when used as monotherapy or at non-effective doses combined with a non-effective dose of cyclosporine (CsA). Transplantation. 2006;82:250.
138. Bigaud M, Wieczorek G, Preussing E, et al. NVP-AEB071 (AEB), the novel oral inhibitor of protein kinase C (PKC) and early T-cell activation, prolongs non-human primates (NHP) kidney allograft survival when combined with everolims (RAD), ERL080 (ERL) or FTY720 (FTY) without calcineurin inhibitor (CNI). Transplantation. 2006;82:251–252.
139. Skvara H, Dawid M, Kleyn E, et al. The PKC inhibitor AEB071 may be a therapeutic option for psoriasis. Journal of Clinical Investigation. 2008;118: 3151–3159.
140. Budde K, Sommerer C, Becker T, et al. Sotrastaurin, a novel small molecule inhibiting protein kinase C: first clinical results in renal-transplant recipients. American Journal of Transplantation. 2010;10:571–581.
141. Friman S, Arns W, Nashan B, et al. Sotrastaurin, a novel small molecule inhibiting protein-kinase C: randomized phase II study in renal transplant recipients. American Journal of Transplantation. 2011;11:1444–1455.
142. Meier-Kriesche HU, Kaplan B. The search for CNI-free immunosuppression: no free lunch. American Journal of Transplantation. 2011;11:1355–1356.

第 3 篇

器官获取

器官获取和分配

第 19 章 器官获取与分配的管理

Jennifer M. Porter, Lori E. Brigham, Susan Gunderson

引言

符合伦理并且实施成功的器官移植诚然是十分冗杂的，它需要耗费我们最专业的医护人员的大量精力去鉴别潜在供体，去得到捐献的许可，去判断供者是否适宜，去协调所有器官的复苏及分配，以及去维持移植过程中的花费等。在过去，这些工作都由仅有的几个成熟的移植中心中的专业医师来完成，但在最近的 40 年中，这些工作越来越多地被写入联邦和州的法律之中，并指定由专门的器官获取组织（OPO）来完成。本章探讨了 OPO 在器官复苏和分配工作中所扮演的角色——它是如何在法律法规的框架内组织和运作，以及将其整合到临床移植的工作中去。本章初步勾勒出 OPO 的结构基础，以及联邦和州的法律法规如何管理 OPO 的器官获取和分配行为。并让读者领会整个过程，注意到那些能影响器官移植成败的重要因素及其相互作用。

本章重点讨论的是美国模式，如此做的原因并不是否定其他模式，而是为了提供一种借鉴去系统地研究 OPO 的众多职责。作者已经意识到，美国模式虽十分重要，但并不是唯一的管理器官获取和分配的方法。本章的最后将简要讨论其他国家的组织形式，他们大多借鉴了西班牙模式，并在很多国家使用。

OPO 是什么？

在美国，OPO 在器官分配过程发挥了举足轻重的作用，它使得可移植人体器官这个宝贵而稀缺的资源能够合理地分配给那些在名单上苦苦等待器官移植的患者[1]。它是由政府指定的实体机构，其责任在于促进器官捐献事业的发展，鉴别潜在的器官捐献者，负责器官的复苏以及将可用的器官分配给需要器官移植的患者。OPO 是全国器官移植事件的管理者。

美国在 1984 年通过器官移植法案（NOTA），并以此法律为基础成立了 OPO[2]。该法案为 OPO 建立了一个全国的管理体系，用以复苏和分配已逝捐献者的器官。如今的 OPO 及其管理体系本质上与当初成立的组织基本一致。在第 128 章我们会对国家组织机构和移植活动的监管进行额外讨论。

每一个 OPO 负责专门的地理区域，即“捐献服务区”（DSA）。DSA 并不是统一而平均的，单一 DSA 的辖区地理面积可以从 3600 平方英里到 866 000 平方英里，辖区人口数量可以从 130 万到 1910 万人，辖区人群也是多样性的，包含了不同民族、不同种族、城市人口、郊区人口、农村人口等，辖区内的医院数量也从 1 家到 220 家急诊医院不等。全国划分为 58 个 DSA，由 58 个 OPO 分管，其中有 7 个 OPO 是由医院或者大学管理，其他都由独立的实体组织管理。众多的 OPO 是国家器官复苏和分配系统的基本组成单位，并由器官获取与移植网络协调。

NOTA 提出了 2 种联邦政府资金的来源途径：①在社会保障法（SSA）的规定下，医疗报销是肾脏获取的主要资金来源，②卫生资源和服务管理局（HRSA）对 OPO 的资助[3]。参与医疗报销系统需要 OPO 提供成本明细报告，它是医疗保险回顾性审核和调整的基础。此外，医疗保险还规定了 OPO 向移植医院提供一个肾脏所收取的金额[4]。

OPO 需要为它所提供的所有器官收取费用。移植中心所提供的器官获取费（OAC）也是 OPO 最大的单种经费来源。每个OPO根据自己的花费制订OAC,它包括获取费用(包括住院费、医疗费、实验室检验费、运输费以及其他医疗费用)和临床人员,信息技术,管理费用,以及在社区/公共场所举行的教育活动花费和对医院和医疗专业人员培训费用。

许多OPO在他们的辖区内也提供组织捐献的服务,包括角膜组织。对于这些人体组织的捐献流程,OPO也必须遵守食品和药物管理局(FDA)的规定,除了那些已经获得医疗保险和医疗补助服务中心(CMS)认证的中心所获取的人体组织。

NOTA和SSA把OPO直接处于卫生和人类服务部(HHS)部长的监管之下[5]。它们按照HHS、CMS的规章运行,也同时符合OPTN的政策和程序[6]。OPTN本身也处于HHS的卫生资源和服务管理局(HRSA)[7]的监管之下。OPO同时受到联邦和州的法律约束。

国家法律框架

从1967年世界上第一个成功实施的心脏移植开始,到1984年NOTA的发布,器官移植逐渐成为一种有效的主流医学治疗手段。在1978年,这门技术被联邦政府认可,并通过医疗保险报销终末期肾病患者的移植费用。社会对所有类型的可移植器官的需求迅速增长。于是,到目前为止,可供移植器官的数量大大超过了身患绝症等待器官移植的患者数量。

移植作为一种被认可的治疗手段,其在科学和医学上的进步都有不断完善的国家法律做保障。美国各州法律委员会全国会议(NCCUSL)[8]提出两部法案:1968年的国家解剖捐献法案(AGA)和1981年的国家死亡判定法案。这些国家法案的提出为器官移植作为一种医学治疗手段获得更大的应用性提供了法律保障。[NCCUSL(现在称为全国法律委员会)是国家支持的一个非营利的实体机构。通过一个广泛的合作过程中,它建议统一的法律对国家是十分重要的,依据法律是国家的责任。它称自己提供了“清晰和稳定的国家立法领域。”]这些国家法律是今天那些OPO和众多移植领域所依靠的基础。

国家死亡判定法(UDDA)

UDDA是NCCUSL在1981年发布。它提出一种新的医学和科学共识,除了传统的循环停止死亡判定标准外,可根据神经系统的损伤程度作为死亡判定标准(脑死亡)(在第21章和第22章分别讨论)。这种观点在普通法律中并没有先例,并且因为没有这种先例,对器官移植的复苏和移植造成了很大障碍。UDDA建议国家立法承认以神经系统功能停止作为死亡的判定标准。共有38个州采用了UDDA,但所有州都开始立法承认神经系统功能作为死亡判定标准。由于这一新法律的明确,那些已经符合神经系统死亡标准的供体立刻成为合法的捐献器官来源。

1968年国家解剖捐献法案及其接替法案

AGA于1968年推出,用来确定在新兴的移植科学中那些常规法律尚不明确的规定。AGA很快地被全国50个州及哥伦比亚特区所接受。

它在历史上第一次明确了捐献、接受、使用从供体捐献的解剖器官的权利。AGA承认明确死亡的个人或其家属有权利捐献器官、眼球和其他组织用于移植、治疗、研究或者教育。它同时明确了一些规定,关于谁可以行使器官的复苏、分配以及使用的权利。它从法律角度认可那些符合AGA规定进行器官捐献的工作,从而减少了社会对于发展中的器官捐献和移植过程参与者的过分关注[11]。

NCCUSL强调了AGA在鼓励人们捐献以及建立国家器官捐献与移植法律的重要性。它指出:“目前的普通法律及法律蓝图仍然是混乱的、多样的以及不足的……这部法律将为新兴的现代医学提供一个有效以及统一的国家法律环境”[12]。

由于新的联邦法律的推行、旧版本AGA遗留的不确定因素以及不断发展的移植科学,AGA分别于1987年及2006年进行了2次重大的修订。遵循联邦法律的1987版,明确规定:“为获取利益而进行的捐献器官买卖、获取、转让或者参与转让……以及任何参与器官捐献的行为(第10节)”是不合法的,并指出“获取利益”并不包括器官的去除、处理、保存、质控、储存运输、移植等这些“合理的花费”。国家捐献法案修订版(RUAGA),由NCCUSL于2006年发布,第一次将联邦和州法律进行统一。它也恢复了国家的法律统一,这是最早的AGA一直追求的,国家(以及NCCUSL)无法在不断发展的医学进步下维持联邦法律的不断更新。

RUAGA扩展以及简化了个人捐献器官的方法,它包括了目前所有的最有效的鼓励捐献的方法。例如,公民在驾驶证上登记,并在器官捐献处注册,通过健康管理机构或其他指定机构注明遗嘱或明确的捐献意愿。这就明确了谁有优先器官捐献的意愿。AGA认可个体器官捐献的权利;然而,OPO、医院、家庭、医生及其他医疗专业人员和整个社会常常接受失去亲人的家庭成员的意愿,这往往与死者的决定相符。RUAGA十分正视这个问题。如果一个人做出决定捐献或拒绝捐献,RUAGA禁止其他人改变这个决定[13]。这条规定适用于任何人,然而,OPO作为器官捐献过程中的一线角色,有责任去尊重捐献者的决定并保证其他人也是如此。RUAGA现在是46个州的法律,即使不是,法律同样要求尊重死者的决定。

为了响应当时的器官捐献和移植,AGA的1968年版本和1987年修订版本都允许医院、外科医生、医师接受捐献的器官或组织用来移植或者治疗。然而,2006年的RUAGA准许器官捐献给指定的单位进行移植和治疗,这个单位可以是移植的受体或眼球、其他组织指定保存机构。所有其他移植或治疗捐献必须捐献给合法的获取组织(即眼球、组织、器官)。用于研究和教育的捐献也必须捐献给指定机构[14]。

RUAGA还列出了OPO权利和义务的清单。当医院将潜在捐献者提交给OPO时(根据联邦法律的要求),OPO必须对机动车辆记录部门和捐助者登记处进行合理搜索,以查看被推荐个人是否注册为捐献者,并且必须合理合法的去匹配接受器官捐献的人。它授权OPO进行任何合理必要的检查,包括检查所有医疗和牙科记录,以确定可能是捐献器官的医疗适用性,并进一步规定,在进行该检查时,“采取必要的措施以确保该器官的医疗适用性不会改变,除非医院或器官分配组织知道该器官接受者其他的意图。”在捐献人去世后,RUAGA授权OPO进行任何必要的合理检查,以确保捐献器官为最初的目的而使用[15]。

当患者在医院中死亡时,州法律来判定患者是否已经死亡,以及此患者是否有合法的权利去完成器官捐献以用于医疗服务。

联邦法律框架

在1984年的NOTA之前,美国没有对器官捐献和分配工作进行有组织或连续的国家政策。该政策以特别的方式制订,是根据当地和区域情况以及当时的事件以特别方式制订的。而国家法律政策正是在这样不断的发展过程中产生的。器官获取机构(OPA)是在20世纪60年代开始成立,并且其功能是旨在扩大移植的应用性使得移植数目可以自然增长。到1984年,已经有接近90家OPA机构在美国运营。其中50家医院和40家独立的合法机构共同服务于多家医院和地区[16]。

在NOTA通过之前会举行国会听证会和公众讨论会,会议内容集中在持续性和不断增长的器官供应与现有流程无法解决所导致日益扩大的差距问题。而国家官方的回复会被视为解决问题答案的必要一部分,NOTA设法通过建立一个国家系统来解决鼓励捐献的这一资源短缺问题,并确保获取的器官得到公平分配和使用[17]。于是NOTA建立了美国器官复苏,分配和使用的一个基本制度框架;它创建了一个器官移植专责小组,负责对美国器官捐献和移植进行广泛的调查,并就如何改进该系统提出建议(见第137章)。

由NOTA创建的机构和系统

禁止出售器官

该法案宣布所有“故意获取,接受或以其他方式转让任何人体器官”为非法行为[18]。它还规定:“有价值的收费”并不包括与“人体器官捐献过程中的摘取、运输、植入、加工、保存、质量控制和储存或者是人员的行程、住宿和工资损失”所造成的所谓的由人体器官的捐献者与捐献有关“合理付费”。

OPO机构的创建

该法案组织了一个全国性的OPO网络来覆盖了之前90个OPA所具有的职能。NOTA又规定了这些OPO的结构、治理和职责。同时它还要求OPO设立一个咨询委员会,就常规委员会提出的有关器官获取和分配的所有事项提出建议。为了确保这一建议的独立性,NOTA规定,该咨询机构的成员应可以代表对器官复苏和获取感兴趣的所有各方,比如相关移植医院和外科医生、公众、捐献家庭、医院管理人员、眼睛和组织库,以及具有神经学和组织相容性的相关技术知识和经验的个人。

NOTA要求OPO成为新形成的OPTN的成员,该实体的成立是为了可以在国家一级协调OPO和制订需要移植的人的国家名单库而设立的。下面会更充分地讨论介绍 OPTN 的作用。

NOTA 和随后的修订建立了一个机制，强制与捐献过程中的所有其他参与者合作，例如，与捐献医院、移植医院以及组织和眼库，虽然它把如何解决合作中的问题留给了相关各方。这些要求以扩展形式纳入由 CMS 管理的联邦法规[19]。

OPTN 机构的创建

OPTN 的建立是为了：开发和维护一个计算机化的器官移植等待名单，现在称为 UNET；促进器官匹配和放置；制订基于共识的政策和程序来管理器官复苏，分配和运输的相关问题；收集和管理关于器官移植过程的科学数据；向政府和其他人提供数据，包括移植受者的科学登记数据（SRTR：有关此注册数据的更多详细信息，请参见第 133 章）；用于努力改善实体器官分配和移植；并提供关于捐献和移植的专业性和公共教育，OPTN 的活动和捐献的关键需要的内容[20]（见第 137 章）。

OPTN 是由一个私营但非营利性联合机构共享网络（UNOS）运营。UNOS 代表 OPTN 运作和维护 UNET。UNET 是用于接收捐献者和受体信息并促进器官分配和分布的计算机系统。移植医院负责将数据放在 UNET 等待名单程序中，并保存当前需要移植的患者的姓名和相关医疗信息。UNET 包含不同器官系统的下的不同列表。OPO 使用 UNET 的 DonorNet 模块为捐助者输入类似信息。然后，他们使用此程序将捐献者与 UNET 等待列表程序中列出的可能的相关匹配人进行匹配。

OPO 要求必须是 OPTN 的成员。OPTN 要求其成员遵守其相关政策和程序[21]。HHS 要求 OPO 遵守 OPTN 的“规则和要求”。OPTN 声明，HHS 应该具有法律效力[22]。与 CMS 一样，OPTN 也要衡量 OPO 功能的有效性。

SRTR 机构的创建

SRTR 由 NOTA 建立，作为在美国执行的所有器官移植的准确信息的存储库[23]。OPO 和其他组织需要定期向其提交指定的信息[24]。在数据表中收集的数据支持对美国实体器官移植状态的持续评估。

SRTR 还使用累积数据设计和实施科学数据研究，以更好地了解美国捐献和移植系统的性能。它还向相关移植团体传播其信息和分析（包括移植项目、OPO、决策者、移植专业人员、移植受益人、器官捐献者和捐助者家庭以及公众）。它还使合格的研究人员获得数据以帮助他们独立努力研究实体器官移植的各个方面的数据。

美国器官移植系统通过 OPO、移植团队团体、SRTR 和 OPTN 之间的合作努力采用基于证据政策的分配制度。政策制订是 OPTN 的责任；然而，SRTR 通过执行数据分析，为决策者提供做出明智决策所需的信息，发挥了重要作用。

SRTR 由明尼阿波利斯医学研究基金会的慢性疾病研究组为 HHS 所用[25]。

NOTA 要求 OPO 要有效

自国家制度建立开始以来，一个目标保持不变：那就是缩小可用器官与等待移植的人们之间的差距。1984 年，NOTA 希望捐献和移植过程的参与者共同努力将不断努力改善他们的表现。那段时间之后法律的变化均旨在加强这个初始和永久相关的想法。

2000 年的器官获取组织认证法，P.L. 106-505[26]，需要 CMS 制订一个应用标准来衡量 OPO 性能。该法案旨在纠正使用中的性能测量所产生的不确定性。2006 年，CMS 针对该立法颁布了新的绩效衡量标准[27]。这些政策规定 OPO（不包括非连续性国家地区）必须满足以下 3 项结果措施，以保持其作为 OPO 的认证[27]：

- 合格捐助者的捐献率作为符合资格的死亡率的百分比必须不超过合格捐助者的平均国家捐献率的 1.5 个标准差，在 OPO 重新认证周期的 4 年内的平均值。通过对心脏死亡后的每个捐献和对于 70 岁以上的每个捐献增加 1 来调整个体 OPO 的捐献率比率的分子和分母。
- 观察到的捐献率不显著低于用于再认证目的的 36 个月的数据中的 18 个月或更多月的预期率。
- 以下 3 个数量测量中的至少 2 个在重新认证周期的 4 年内平均值不超过国家平均值 1 个标准差：

1.每个标准供体包括用于胰岛细胞移植的胰腺移植的器官数量；

2.每个扩增的标准供体移植的器官数，包括用于胰岛细胞移植的胰腺；

3.用于每个供体的研究的器官的数量，包括用于胰岛细胞研究的胰腺。

未能满足所有结果的会导致自动取消认证。在OPO的数据团队内,这些结果被指责为未能提供任何有用的考察OPO性能的效果。OPO要求CMS修订法规。2013年7月,CMS发表对OPO的关注,并提出了几项监管修订要求[28]。特别是CMS规定,如果OPO能满足两个结果测量,而不是三个结果测量,就将保留其认证。OPO一直关注在规则制订程序期间他们的监管措施的有效性和效用,拟议规则于2013年12月最终定稿[29]。

CMS的性能评估

2014年1月,2006年修订的条例要求符合3个指标中的两个是衡量OPO性能的标准。OPO需要遵守该规定,以便通过CMS认证来使得OPO运行。

CMS设想,OPO如果不能满足这些指标,OPO将失去其作为OPO资格的认证。一旦OPO被取消认证,则其DSA可以由向CMS提交申请,并批准满足条件的任何其他实体接管OPO[30]。

如上所述,法律还要求OPO遵守OPTN的政策和程序以及规则和要求。OPTN会使用不同的方法来确定OPO是否在其工作中有效。

OPTN的性能评估

OPTN使用由SRTR开发的一套性能方法,使用一组基于在数据表中收集的实际捐献者信息为统计模型。这些模型考虑了可以不受OPO控制的各种特征,以试图调整每个OPO管理的捐献方类型的差异。对6个器官中的每一个使用单独的风险调整模型:心脏、肠、肾、肝、肺和胰腺。该模型基于从其中复苏至少一个器官用于移植目的(非必要性移植)和"产量"定义为最终移植的器官。为肾、肺、心脏、肝脏、胰腺和肠提供预期的产量。对于心脏、肝脏、胰腺、肺和肠,预期产量将在0~1范围内。例如,如果预期肝脏产量为0.7,人们将期望相似的供体在10次中产生移植的肝脏次数为7次。肺产量被建模型为产生至少一个肺用于移植的概率;因此,预期的肺预期产量范围从0~1而不是0~2。对于肾脏,预期产量将在0~2的范围内。然后将总的预期器官产量计算为器官特异性预期产量的和, 范围为0~7。在器官特异性基础上,模型预测根据具有类似特征的捐献者的国家经验, 来判断预计将有多少器官被回收和移植。

2012年7月,OPTN采用SRTR的预期产量方法来监测OPO的性能。性能要求载于OPTN章程,附录B(器官获取组织的会员要求),在B.2节[31]。本节还规定,OPTN成员和专业标准委员会 (MPSC) 将评估所有OPO, 以确定观察到的和预期的器官产量的差异是否可以由DSA或OPO的某一独特方面解释。

MPSC需要审查观察到的器官产量低于预期水平指定值的所有OPO。公式中的相关参数的绝对值对于不同的器官可以是不同的。因为根据OPTN理事会的同意,预计这些数值将定期审查和修改。

用于鉴定所有器官以及每种器官类型的低于预期器官产量的初始标准是:

- >每10个供体观察到的器官少于预期产量 (每100个供体观察到 – 每100个供体预期≤–10)。
- 观察到的预期率和期待值的比率<0.90。
- 双侧P值<0.05。

当OPO满足所有3个标准时会引发MPSC审查。如果OPO的器官产量率不能由所讨论的OPO或DSA的供体组合或某些其他特殊的临床方面来解释,则OPO成员需要与MPSC合作来实施功能的改善计划。如果不能按照这个流程做是违反OPTN义务的。

器官捐献和移植过程中的参与者都是自愿努力,在正式法律和监管框架之外,通过找到"最佳做法"来提高绩效,并通过更准确地有效的方法来反映OPO努力的有效性。这些努力中最深远和潜在的变革是器官捐献突破协作(ODBC或协作)。

ODBC

ODBC于2003年成立,作为HHS秘书在HRSA卫生保健系统局(HSB),移植部门(DoT)下开展的一项活动。其目的是大大增加可移植器官的可用性,并提供器官复苏和放置的最佳做法。HRSA与医疗改进研究所(IHI)、质量现实检查公司(QRC)、OPO团队以及他们的医院和移植中心合作伙伴一起合作,旨在从全国各地创造变革,能使器官捐献系统得到突破性转变。

该工作的初始重点是在国家范围内旨在提高器官捐献转换率(转换率是在医院发生的实际捐献数量与合格捐助者数量的比率),使医院每年有超过8名合格捐献者。所使用的方法是建立一个改进模版,采用国际认可的高效的IHI使用的性能改进方法。

在 ODBC 在 2003—2005 年进行的前两个周期，HRSA 和专家教师，包括来自全国各地高绩效组织的医疗保健专业人员，帮助每个参与组织尝试实现 HRSA 设定的目标：

- 及时通知 OPO 所有死亡或即将发生的死亡；
- 将参与医院的捐献授权率提高 30%；
- 增加供体转化率到 75%或者更高；
- 通知 OPO 所有未决决定，以便撤回不可生存条件患者的机械支持；
- 将经过培训、有效的捐献咨询小组来接受器官捐献咨询的成员数量增加到 100%；
- 90 分钟内回复所有死亡通知。

ODBC 的目标是确定最佳实践方案，并根据那些可以确定的做法来创建系统，在每个全国范围内的 DSA，准确和及时完成的捐献者转介、筛选、同意、器官复苏和安置。

2006 年，在 ODBC 的第 4 个周期，HRSA 引入了“每个捐献者移植的器官”(OTPD)作为评估 OPO 的另一种方式，包括移植程序和捐献医院的表现。OTPD 是移植的所有器官的数量与实际器官供体数量的比率。HRSA 建立的目标是实现每个供体移植超过 3.75 个器官的平均 OTPD 率。

2007 年，ODBC 将其国家学习战略推向区域层面，为正在进行的改进工作提供一个本地的、更便于访问的平台，并补充在正在进行的国家学习会议。目的是维持跨 DSA 学习机会，以追求国家绩效目标；使更多的 OPO、医院和移植中心代表能够获得跨 DSA 学习机会；并创造地方和区域 ODBC 领导机会，以增强个人的专业发展。这项战略慢慢证实它只是最低限度的成功，并作为一个主要焦点在 2012 年停止。其中每个 DSA 中所有合作伙伴提供的更广泛的方法似乎是实施最佳实践和评估结果的最有效手段。

HRSA 为每个 DSA 建立的成果目标是：

- 75%转换率；
- 10%在循环死亡(DCD)供体后捐献的所有供体；
- 3.75 OTPD；
- 移植的死亡供体器官的体积增加 20%。

ODBC 在器官捐献和移植取得了突破性增加。为了确保这一进展继续下去，ODBC 的工作已经在“捐献和移植实践社区(DTCP)”中制度化，它是一个包括在全国捐献和移植过程中涉及的所有各种学科和专业人员的分组。DTCP 由器官捐献和移植联盟(“联盟”)组织和协调，由 HRSA 拨款提供资金。联盟是一个在 2006 年成立的 501(c)(3)非营利，独立组织，目的是确保国家继续致力于增加器官的可用性和消除移植等待者死亡的机构。联盟提供了一个永久的结构，以寻求用文化和制度来影响器官捐献和移植的组织和个人中的持久文化变革。联盟通过继续开展具体活动，重点是满足和实现国家机构捐献和移植目标，这些的确立是由 HRSA 建立。联盟与 HRSA 合作、监督和组织会议，提供专题工作组和 DCTP 的学习机会。DTCP 和 OBDC 的经验表明，每年移植的 35 000 个器官的目标实现只有通过创建一个可以学习并有系统地参与监测，评估和改善自身表现的捐献和移植系统[32]。

系统如何工作？通过再分配实现逐步恢复

这一部分的总体主题是，当所有参与者，无论是个人(医生、护士、医院行政人员和管理人员以及 OPO 工作人员)或机构，所有参与者，了解器官捐献的重要性，把器官捐献和复苏作为一个使命，看作是它自己的权利，而不只是一个事后的想法，知道他们在这个过程中的角色，并合作完成共同的任务时会得到最大的发挥。在每一步，所有有关各方之间的合作以及及时的沟通和协调至关重要。关于有效捐献方法的更详细讨论，见文献[33,34]。

器官捐献和复苏过程仅适用于在医院发生的死亡。2010 年，美国有 246 万人死亡[35,36]。在每年死亡的人中，大约 30%(或 738 000)在医院死亡。最可能适合捐献的死亡是发生在医院急诊科(ED)或重症监护病房(ICU)的死亡。死亡捐献已经成为捐献器官的重要来源。OPTN 已经采纳了一些适用于这种捐献的政策和程序[35]，但这里描述的系统仅处理死亡后的捐献。

告知 OPO 所有死亡或即将发生的死亡

法律要求医院和 OPO 确保每个家庭都知道其器官捐献的权利[37]，并且为了确保这一权利不受损害，他们需要有一个协议，通知 OPO 每一个死亡或可能发生的在医院死亡情况。OPO 需要与医院和医院选择的相关眼库和组织库合作，以确保组织库和眼库及时收到可能的供体[38]。医院可以选择对组织和眼库单独进行转诊。然而,最常见的情况是,医院只向 OPO 或 OPO 的转诊呼叫中心发出一次呼叫。然后 OPO 与眼库和组织库协调,或在其他特殊情况下,根据与医院或与组织和眼库的协议执行组织恢复。这些监管他们有义务寻求确保可以达到的恢复眼球和组织的最大数量,以及器官的最大数量。他们还力求确保对成员采取协调一致的方法,使成员不受不同组织多次捐献请求的困扰。

自从通过 UDDA 和其他州法律识别脑死亡以来,大多数捐献者在停止神经功能——所谓的 DND 供体后捐献。最近,医学科学的进步引发了对 DCD(也称为循环死亡)的再次注意。所有 OPO 都需要有关于 DCD 恢复的政策,无论它是否需要执行它们[39]。如果 OPO 执行 DCD 恢复,OPO 与医院的协议就需要解决 DCD 恢复问题,尽管法律不要求医院进行此类恢复[40]。

具有严重的、不可恢复的神经损伤但没有临床进展发展成为神经系统死亡的患者是 DCD 捐献的候选者。撤销维持生命治疗的决定将通过预先医院医疗指示或法律代理人认定。当停止医疗干预(呼吸机),并且循环和呼吸功能停止时,然后在限定的心搏停止、心室纤维性颤动或无脉性电活动的时期之后,宣布患者死亡。为了成为活的器官供体,在移除呼吸机之后,患者必须在有限的时间内宣告死亡。时间限制可能因 OPO 协议而有所不同,但一般都在 60~90 分钟的时间内。然后快速进行器官的获取以确保器官活力。

转诊呼叫的临床触发标准

OPO 和医院会制订预先同意触发转诊呼叫的临床标准。但目前没有单一的标准临床触发标准供所有 OPO 和医院使用。特定触发的使用可以取决于 OPO 和相关医院的偏好和能力,例如,一些医院不执行 DCD 恢复。表 19.1 显示了一个 OPO 在其 DSA 中使用的临床触发器的说明情况。

一般来说,死亡发生后> 1 小时的转诊是不及时的。及早通知即将发生的死亡是最好的做法。临床触发定义何时将死亡为“即将发生”的死亡。他们打算在 OPO 被通知之前,医院不会移除呼吸机支持或做出任何排除捐献可能性的治疗决定。这将有助于确保 OPO 有足够的机会履行其法定责任,识别潜在的捐献者,并确保每个成员都知道捐献的选择。

表 19.1 医院面对即将死亡的临床患者时,应通知华盛顿地区移植组织(WRTC)

医院应通知 WRTC 以下内容:
1.每例符合以下一项或多项标准的患者:
• 格拉斯哥昏迷评分为 5 分或更低,且无持续镇静
• 正在考虑或进行脑死亡测试
• 接受治疗的患者不进行复苏(DNR)或家属确认临终关怀治疗
• 放弃生命支持治疗
• 家属主动提出有关捐献的想法
注意:这些标准是对非通气患者死亡所需通知的补充
2.上报每例患者死亡,并在死亡后 1 小时内上报

Reproduced with permission of WRTC.

捐助方识别和评估

OPO 24×7 小时开放,接收这些转诊需求电话,并开始识别潜在捐献者。图 19.1 和图 19.2 说明了关于 DND 和 DCD 捐献者的捐献者识别,恢复和分配时间表,其通过对在医院死亡的每个个人的死亡或即将死亡的转诊呼叫而发起。在接到呼叫时,OPO 具有审查患者的医疗记录的法定权利,并且在这一点上,OPO 开始执行其初始筛选以确定潜在捐献者的医疗适用性的权利。初步筛选可以通过电话或医院现场的 OPO 工作人员进行。

OPO 还进行检查(DMV)记录和捐献者登记处信息以确定患者是否做出解剖意愿。

成员在决定解剖意愿和获得授权方面的角色

如果患者在 DMV 或捐献者登记处作为捐献者注册(或已经做出任何其他的意愿文件),则不需要其他许可来使捐献有效,并且 OPO、医院、医生和捐献者家庭需要坚持患者的决定。如果患者不是捐献者,联邦法律要求每个家庭都有选择捐献或拒绝的权利。OPO 负责找到合法的决策者,通常是患者的亲属,必须向其提出捐献请求。家庭成员无论是授权还是通知家庭患者自己的决定,只有在 OPO 和医院工作人员协商后才可进行,并由接受过培训的工作人员进行。联邦法律要求对潜在捐助者家庭的情况,观点和信念酌情决定,并小心敏感地做出决定。联邦法律还详细说明了需要向家庭提供的信息[41]。

根据研究和经验，一直以来的做法是，在收到患者的终末预后并有时间接受患者的终末预后后，向家庭提供有关捐献的信息。最近，这个做法已经开始重新审查。新证据表明，当请求纳入尊重家庭成员悲伤的临终关怀过程中，并且与他们进行公开，与死亡情况和适当的沟通时，家庭更有可能对捐献请求做出积极回应并做出临终护理选择[42]。DCD 供体作为可用器官来源的新发现，其增加了在复苏之后继续进行的以整体方式解决临终护理的重要性的提议（图 19.1 和图 19.2）。

DCD 回收时间是非常敏感的，并且需要对供体实施一些预先复苏治疗以促进捐献。无论患者做出捐献决定还是放弃该决定，任何预先治疗需要在宣布死亡之前得到家庭的确认[43]。OPO 和医院正在研究如何最好地使这种方法，使家庭不会失去捐献的选择，不让直到器官的生存能力受损，移植捐献不再是一个选择。

死亡声明

患者的医生根据州法律宣布死亡。OPO 会确认死亡声明符合法律的要求。为了保护捐献过程的完整性并减轻捐献者及其家属的关注，即器官一旦需要终止生命决策，州和联邦法律禁止患者的医生和确定患者死亡的医生参与复苏或移植过程。一旦宣布死亡或家庭同意，如在上文讨论的 DCD 复苏的情况下，OPO 进行必要的剩余测试和检查以确定潜在供体在医学上是否适合作为供体。联邦法规和 OPTN 政策和程序规定了必要的测试内容，谁必须执行测试和在什么时间测试的框架，以及必须收集的潜在捐献者的信息，例如，医学病史和行为史（风险评估）。OPO 负责捐献者的评估和管理[44]。

器官分配

来自已故捐献者的所有器官都需要通过 NOTA 创建的国家系统进行回收和分发。所有需要移植的患者必须在国家候补名单上列出。除了 RUAGA 允许的捐献者指定特定个人接受捐献的罕见个例，并且指定的个人是匹配，否则任何患者都不能在该过程之外接收已故捐献器官。

当 OPO 确定个人在医疗上适合作为捐献者并且确认捐献授权时，OPO 在 OPTN 的国家器官分配计划

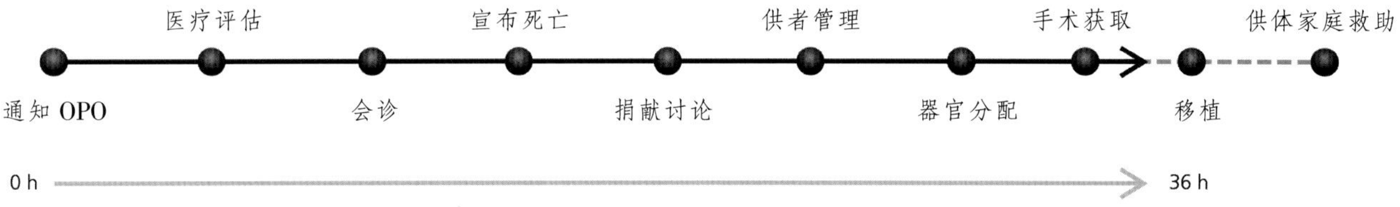

通知 OPO	➤	30~45 分钟告知相关信息；OPO 到达医院 1~1.5 小时
医疗评估	➤	30 分钟根据标准评估以确定捐献适用性
会诊	➤	5 分钟（可能需要 15 分钟到 1.5 小时完成所有会诊）
宣布死亡	➤	4~24 小时进行脑死亡测定（如果未明确诊断为脑死亡并且需要进行其他检查，则可能需要几个小时）
捐献讨论	➤	与家属/LNOK 进行 1~3 小时的讨论（包括与家属/LNOK 进行 1~2 小时的讨论以回顾既往的就诊史/社会史）
供体管理	➤	血清学检查和初步组织分型结果为 8~10 小时；等待 2~12 小时的特殊程序（超声心动图、支气管镜检查和特殊实验室等）
器官分配	➤	5 小时（肝、肾）和 24 小时（胸腔）用于器官分配给主要接受者和所需的后备接受者
手术获取	➤	外科手术器官获取 4~8 小时（手术延迟可能会增加 ICU 时间）
供体家庭救助	➤	两年计划，包括悲伤研讨会，丧偶支持小组，捐助者家庭务虚会，年度捐助者家庭聚会，促进捐助者家庭与受体之间的交流

图 19.1 所有医院的患者死亡或即将死亡时确认不抢救（DND）患者的供体识别、器官复苏和分配过程的最佳时间表。华盛顿地区移植组织（WRTC）使用的时间表。（Reproduced with permission of WRTC.）OPO，器官获取组织；LNOK，合法近亲；ICU，重症监护病房。

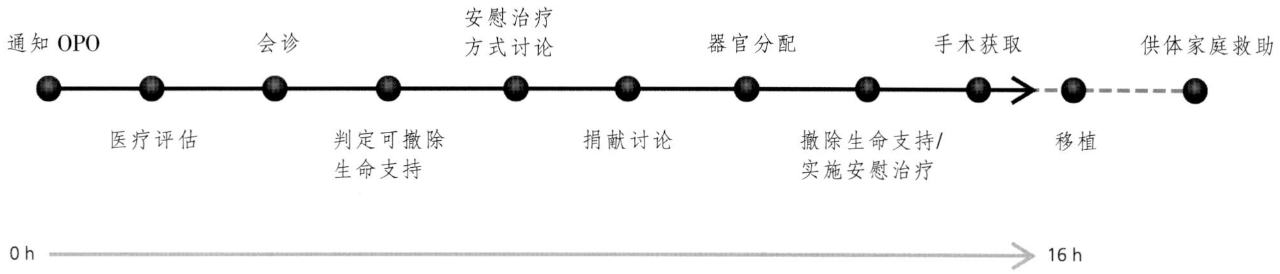

通知 OPO	➢ 30~45 分钟告知相关信息;OPO 到达医院 1~1.5 小时
医疗评估	➢ 30 分钟根据标准评估以确定捐献适用性
会诊	➢ 5 分钟(可能需要 15 分钟到 1.5 小时完成所有会诊)
捐献讨论	➢ 与家人/LNOK 进行 1~3 小时的讨论(包括与家人/LNOK 进行 1~2 小时的讨论以回顾既往的就诊史/社会史)
器官分配	➢ 2~12 小时用于器官分配给主要接受者和所需的后备接受者
手术获取	➢ 外科手术器官获取 2~4 小时(手术延迟可能会增加 ICU 时间)
供体家庭救助	➢ 两年计划,包括悲伤研讨会,丧偶支持小组,捐助者家庭务虚会,年度捐助者家庭聚会,促进捐助者家庭与受体之间的交流

图 19.2 所有医院的患者死亡或即将死亡时,启动循环死亡(DCD)患者的供体识别,器官复苏和分配过程的最佳捐献时间表。华盛顿地区移植社区(WRTC)使用的时间表。(Reproduced with permission of WRTC.)OPO,器官获取组织;LNOK,合法近亲;ICU,重症监护病房。

DonorNet 中输入捐献者的信息,包括血型和组织类型,因此,可以运行适合于特定器官的计算机算法来识别潜在的接受者[45]。计算机匹配运行根据可用的器官和基于由特定移植中心提供的筛选标准,按排序顺序产生潜在接受者的列表。然后,OPO 向移植中心或列出潜在接受者的中心提供可用的器官。移植中心有 1 小时接受或表示对器官的兴趣。OPO 主要负责提供器官;然而,移植中心在任何特定情况下决定是否将所提供的器官移植到患者中具有最终选择。OPTN 鼓励 OPO 提供后续服务,以确保避免可能的器官流失。

获取

OPO 负责协调获取,包括与捐献医院安排进入手术室和必要的工作人员支持,安排获取小组,并随后安排包装和安排将器官运送到其预期的目的地。器官获取可由任何有资格执行器官复苏的医生或技术人员执行。OPO 需要保持所有医生或其他从业者在 OPO 的 DSA 中定期获取器官的记录。还需要确保任何在其捐助医院进行康复的人员,包括来自 DSA 外的康复团队的成员,都得到合格和培训。OPO 医疗主任,需要是一名医生,负责实施 OPO 关于捐献者评估和管理以及器官获取和放置的协议。医疗主任也有法律规定要求其负责监管潜在捐献者的临床管理,以及在外科医生不能使用时协助管理捐献病例[46]。

数据保存

OPO 还负责获取和保持其 DSA 中恢复活动的记录,包括获取 DSA 恢复小组关于这些小组收回的器官的记录。OPO 保存的记录由 OPTN(如上所述)用于 OPO 评估,SRTR 用于研究目的。

质量保证义务

1984 年,NOTA 要求 OPO 每年评估其自身获得所有器官的有效性。从那时起,为了应对已故捐献器官的长期缺乏,这些要求变得更加具体。CMS 法规要求 OPO 具有正式的"数据驱动"质量评估和绩效改进计划。该计划必须涵盖 OPO 活动的所有领域,OPO 必须采取行动并监测任何已识别的缺陷问题。至少每月一次,OPO 必须在接受转诊的医院进行死亡记录审查,以识别错过的或操作不当的捐献可能性。CMS 还要求 OPO 制订书面政策和程序,以识别和纠正在其工作过程中发生的任何不良事件[47]。

器官获取组织协会(AOPO)已经开发了一个共同评审的认证计划,要求认证的 OPO 实施组织和道德标准,在许多方面比 CMS 要求更详细和严格。全国 58 个 OPO 中有 53 个由 AOPO 认证,另外 3 个正在获得认证。AOPO 每 3 年进行一次认证评审。OPO 是否满足 AOPO 和 CMS 质量标准的能力是这些审查的主要焦点。

这些计划提供了 OPO 可以获得对其自身操作的详细了解的手段,这是所需的自我改进努力的必要前提,这些努力标志着美国努力缩小移植所需器官和可用器官之间的差距。

除了这些明确的质量保证活动外,OPO 还要接受 CMS 和 OPTN 作为其监督责任的一部分进行的定期审计。来自 OPTN / UNOS 的调查小组对每个成员 OPO 进行持续和定期审查和评估, 以测定他们是否遵守 OPTN 规则和政策。OPTN 每 3 年对 OPO 进行一次调查。如果有证据显示 OPO 可能不符合这些规定,OPTN 也将对 OPO 进行特别审查,或者可能以危及患者安全的方式采取措施。

国际器官捐献模式

所有捐献活动都在某种形式的国家授权下进行捐献和移植。一个坚实的法律框架,提供捐献的权力,定义组织结构,制订机构分配政策,并规定融资模式对捐献和移植至关重要。

器官捐献职能的组织结构和人员配置在全球各不相同,每个国家对其独特性的挑战、资源、政治和法律框架都有不同反应。虽然没有被接受的统一的国际模式, 欧洲的大多数捐献系统一般遵循独立的基于 OPO 的美国模式或经常参考的西班牙模式[48]。

OPO 作为独立的非营利性公司组织起来, 服务于一个确定的地理区域, 在捐献医院或移植中心之外运作。相比之下,西班牙模式则是利用位于捐献医院内的器官获取人员进行(图 19.3)。被称为“移植获取管理(TPM)协调员”,工作人员是医院员工,他们对器官获取进行兼职。大多数移植协调员是 ICU 医生或麻醉师,负责识别和评估捐献者,捐助者管理和家庭授权。护士也担任这个角色。每个医院都有专门的工作人员,移植协调员通常不会去本国机构以外的捐献医院。通过处理医生和移植专业人员的双重角色, 对潜在捐献患者

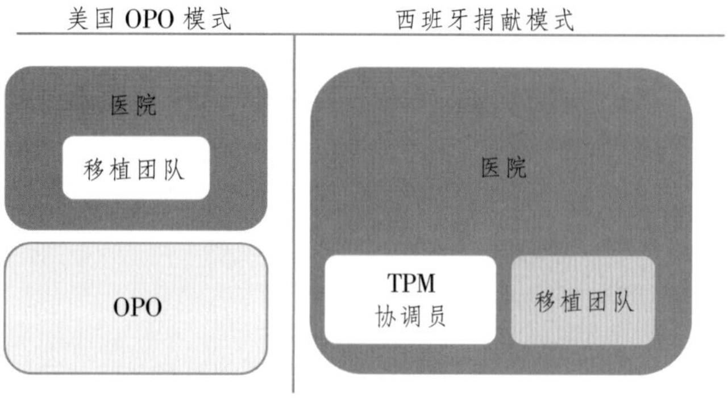

图 19.3 美国和西班牙模式之间的对比。西班牙聘用了位于捐献医院内的器官获取人员。(Reproduced from Vidal MM, et al. Transplant Coordination Manual, 2001; Transplant Procurement Management-TPM: A transplant coordination model to procure donors for transplantation, by permission of TPM-Les Heures, Universitat de Barcelona.)OPO,器官获取组织;TPM,移植获取管理。

的现场熟悉情况可以使得他们密切监测潜在的捐献,但他们需要清楚地分清自己的职责。

虽然 OPO 在许多情况下使用了内部捐献协调员,但这与西班牙移植协调员模式有很大不同。OPO 内部协调员由 OPO 雇用,并且没有担任患者护理和捐献的共同责任。专业方面也有着不同,大多数 OPO 协调员在护理、呼吸治疗或相关领域都具有临床背景。相比之下,在西班牙和其他几个欧洲国家,他们主要使用医师模型。

许多国家采用了美国和西班牙模式的关键组成部分,包括利用医院的兼职移植协调员。一些国家,如德国,建立了一个国家机关获取系统,即以集中监督和相对独立/区域机关获取小组的 OPO 结构为基础的 DSO。随着时间的推移,随着德国 DSO 的发展,例如,引入了一个试验性的基于医院的捐献者计划[49]。

器官分配和分布的职责也因国家而异。Eurotransplant,一个非营利组织,负责七个欧洲国家的器官分配和分布。其他国家如瑞士在 OPO 活动之外设有集中的机构共享办公室[50];在某些特殊情况下,地方器官获取小组也可以负责确定器官分配。除了 Eurotransplant 中心之外,其他地区器官分配政策比 UNOS / OPTN 采用的机制复杂得多。

虽然在欧洲捐献计划的结构、权威和操作范围有重大差异, 但所有计划仍然专注于提供移植器官的共同目标。要使得获取组织越来越专业化和国际化,他们的最佳做法的经验分享将导致全球捐款的改善。

总结

美国器官获取和分配系统在全国范围内运行，目的是最好和最公平地使用稀缺资源，捐献已故器官。该系统的诞生是由于可移植捐献器官的缺乏，并且继续受到持续稀缺的驱动而改善。

OPO 是美国最主要的公共捐献机构。他们负责在其地理服务区内负责教育公众进行器官捐献；说服市民使用正规途径和捐献登记成为器官捐献者；并与所有在医院死亡的潜在捐助者的家庭互动，必要时获得家庭授权捐献，如果没有捐献，向他们提供资料。捐献无论如何要向他们提供亲属丧亡的支持。

在医院环境中，OPO 负责确定潜在捐献者是否在医疗上适合捐献。它管理已故捐献者，直到复苏，并安排器官复苏的所有方面，包括协调和监督执行从已故捐献者移除器官的实际工作的医疗团队的安排。它通过 UNET 定位潜在的接受者，将提议扩展到已经列出潜在接受者的移植中心，并且在接受提议后，安排转移到相关的移植中心。

OPO 由 CMS 和 OPTN 监管，并接受审计检查，以审查其操作的所有方面，并且其在确定捐献者和复苏器官方面的表现也会受到衡量和频繁审查。大多数 OPO 也通过 AOPO 认证，并符合其标准和审核要求。OPO 对其绩效负责，并提出确定和实施改进措施。

在 1984 年推动 NOTA 通过的可用器官数量和移植所需数量之间的差距尚未结束。在任何给定的 DSA 中可用的器官数量受人口大小和位置（例如，农村、城市或郊区）以及其他人口特征（例如，年龄、种族、民族、宗教和公共卫生问题的发生率）的函数影响（HIV、高血压、糖尿病、心脏病）。器官捐献和移植团队及其监管机构已集中大量时间和努力来确定和理解捐献的社会障碍，以及社会本身内部存在的器官捐献和移植的文化和结构障碍。如果这些因素在 OPO 和医院的控制范围内，他们可以通过参与捐献和移植过程的所有机构和个人之间更密切的合作和协调来解决这些问题。该系统的最终有效性取决于所有各方、医院、医生、护士、管理人员及其 OPO 同事，他们之间的长期合作的效果使器官捐献成为重要的社会优先事项。

（张云凯 译 李照 校）

参考文献

1. United States Department of Health and Human Services, Centers for Medicare and Medicaid Services. Conditions for Coverage for Organ Procurement Organizations. Federal Register. 2006;71:30982.
2. National Organ Transplant Act (NOTA), PL 98-507, 98 Stat. 2339–2348 (Oct. 19, 1984), 42 USC §273 et seq. as amended.
3. NOTA §371, 42 USC §273, and 42 USC §1320b-8 (b) (1).
4. 42 CFR §413.200 (c)–(e).
5. Requirements for Certification and Designation and Conditions for Coverage of Organ Procurement Organizations, 42 CFR §486.301 et seq.
6. 42 CFR §121.10.
7. 42 CFR Subchapter K, Part 121.
8. http://www.uniformlaws.org/Default.aspx. [accessed February 18, 2013].
9. NCCUSL. Uniform Determination of Death Act of 1981. Available from: http://www.uniformlaws.org/Act.aspx?title=Determination%20of%20Death%20Act [accessed February 18, 2013].
10. NCCUSL. Revised Uniform Anatomical Gift Act of 2006. Available from: http://www.uniformlaws.org/shared/docs/anatomical_gift/uaga_final_aug09.pdf [accessed February 18, 2013].
11. Uniform Anatomical Gift Act [1968]. Available from: http://www2.sunysuffolk.edu/pecorip/scccweb/etexts/deathanddying_text/uaga.htm.
12. NCCUSL. Uniform Anatomical Gift Act of 1968, Comments.
13. RUAGA, Section 8.
14. RUAGA. Section 11.
15. RUAGA. Section 14.
16. Prottas J. Structure and effectiveness of the US organ procurement system. Inquiry. 1985;32:365, at 366.
17. Mintz B. Analyzing the OPTN Under the State Action Doctrine – Can UNOS's Organ Allocation Criteria Survive Strict Scrutiny. Columbia Journal of Law and Social Problems. 1995;28:339, 339–341.
18. NOTA, Section 301, 42 USC §274e.
19. 42 CFR §486.301 et seq.
20. 42 USC § 274.
21. OPTN. Charter, and policies and procedures. Available from: http://optn.transplant.hrsa.gov/policiesAndBylaws/nota.asp [accessed February 18, 2013].
22. 42 CFR §121.4.
23. NOTA, Section 373, 42 USC §274 a.
24. 42 CFR §486.328.
25. http://www.srtr.org/role.aspx.
26. 42 USC §273 (b) (1).
27. 42 CFR §486.318 (a). See 42 CFR § 486.318 (b) for the requirements applicable to non-contiguous jurisdictions.
28. 78 Federal Register 43671 (July 19, 2013).
29. 78 Federal Register 75141 (December 10, 2013).
30. 42 CFR §§486.312–486.316 for CMS's decertification and recertification and competition process.
31. OPTN. Policy Management/OPTN Bylaws. Available from: http://optn.transplant.hrsa.gov/policiesAndBylaws/bylaws.asp [accessed February 18, 2013].
32. History of the Organ Donation Breakthrough Collaborative process based on information provided by the Organ Donation and Transplantation Alliance [February 2013]. Available from: http://www.organdonationalliance.org/about-the-alliance/history/.
33. Institute of Medicine Committee on Increasing Rates of Organ Donation. Organ donation: Opportunities for action. Washington, DC: National Academies Press, 2006: Chapters 4–6.
34. Smith S. Organ and tissue donation and recovery. Organ Transplant. Medscape, 2003. Available from: http://www.medscape.com/viewarticle/451208?pa=ZOnDzCOxXY2sxAYlMpy0OLMWWK0ErkvO01TWeYQYcsOZpOguDYBcbtUYqxbz1F39s7CF3wx2Tu1U792SxywYLg%3D%3D [accessed February 18, 2010].
35. OPTN Policies 12 and 13. Available from: http://optn.transplant.hrsa.gov/policiesAndBylaws/policies.asp] [accessed February 18, 2013].
36. Centers for Disease Control and Prevention, Deaths and Mortality 2010. Available from: http://www.cdc.gov/nchs/fastats/deaths.htm [accessed February 18, 2013].
37. 42 USC §1320b-8 (a) (1), and 42 CFR §482.45.
38. 42 CFR §486.322 (c).
39. 42 CFR §486.324.
40. 42 CFR §486.344.

41. 42 CFR §486.342.
42. Institute of Medicine Committee, Committee on. Increasing Rates of Organ Donation. Organ donation: opportunities for action. Washington, DC: National Academies Press, 2006, 97. Available from: http://www.iom.edu/Reports/2006/Organ-Donation-Opportunities-for-Action.aspx.
43. Institute of Medicine, Committee on Non-Heart beating Transplantation II. Non-heart-beating organ transplantation: Practice and protocols. Washington, DC: National Academies Press, 2000.
44. 42 CFR §§486.344 and 486.346. See also, OPTN. Policy 2. Minimum Standards for an Organ Procurement Organization [rev. 9/1/2012]. Available from: http://optn.transplant.hrsa.gov/policiesAndBylaws/policies.asp [accessed February 18, 2013].
45. OPTN. Policy 3.2. Organ Distribution: UNOS Patient Waiting List [rev. 2/1/2013]. Available from: http://optn.transplant.hrsa.gov/policiesAndBylaws/policies.asp [accessed February 18, 2013]
46. 42 CFR §486.328(d).
47. 42 CFR §486.348.
48. Matesanz R. Factors influencing the adaptation of the Spanish Model of organ donation. Transplantation International. 2003;16:736–741.
49. Deutsche Stiftung Organtransplantation. 2011 Annual Report. Available from: http://www.dso.de/uploads/tx_dsodl/dso_jb2011_e_www.pdf.
50. Swisstransplant. http://www.swisstransplant.org/l4/.

第 20 章
死亡供体管理

John Fung, Koji Hashimoto, Bijan Eghtesad, Daniel J. Lebovitz, Melissa Watson

引言

器官移植仍然是越来越多患有重要器官功能衰竭的患者的唯一挽救生命的选择。移植技术的发展以及移植后并发症的预防和管理使得移植器官接受者的发病率和死亡率显著降低。器官移植的适应证也由此逐渐扩大。但这又导致对移植器官的需求增加,导致等待挽救生命的器官的患者数量增加。

器官捐献的发生既可以来自活体捐献者的自愿捐献,也可以在捐献者被宣布死亡时发生,即死亡后的器官捐献。第 23 章和第 24 章分别讨论了肾脏和肝脏移植的活体捐献。在可能发生死亡器官捐献的情况下,供体死亡时必须尽量保证可移植器官不会受到严重伤害。器官捐献者的死亡判定必须通过神经系统死亡捐献(DNC;以前称为"脑死亡捐献者")、循环衰竭死亡后捐献[DCDD;以前称为心死亡后捐献(DCD)]或心脏停跳捐献者(NHBD)。有关 DCDD 捐献的其他细节可以参见第 22 章。

DNC 是美国大多数地区和欧洲使用的捐献标准,并且每年为移植提供大量的潜在器官库。DCD 约占美国每年死亡捐献的 12%,每个捐献者捐献的器官也较少。根据器官获取和移植系统(OPTN)的最新数据,移植需求远未得到满足。截至 2010 年底,有超过 12 万例等待器官移植的患者,只有 22 000 例患者接受了移植手术,11 000 例患者在等待中死亡或病情加重而无法移植[1]。因此,需要器官移植的患者数量稳步增加,但可用于移植的器官数量增加缓慢,可用器官数量与需求之间的不平衡继续扩大。

在过去的 10 年中,美国努力让更多的国民意识到器官捐献的迫切需求,使得器官捐献的数量增加,器官捐献者的数量从每年约 5000 个增加到每年约 8000 个;然而,在过去的 5 年中,这已经趋于稳定。此外,我们尝试增加每个供体的器官利用也没有显著改变可供移植器官的数量,其保持在每个供体约 3 个器官。这是由于器官衰竭风险较高的捐献者增多,例如老年、糖尿病、超重、高血压和其他导致捐献者死亡的情况。因此,我们面临的主要问题是如何提高每个供体可获取并能够成功移植的器官数量,并改善器官移植后的器官功能来使每个受体获益。

关于器官捐献者的医疗管理几乎没有什么共识,通常是"最佳实践"方法、小型观察性研究或回顾性研究。在大多数情况下,捐献者管理由捐献者所在地区的器官获取组织(OPO)来负责。最近 OPO 的一个趋势是让重症监护医生协助管理死者捐献者,这可能是他们面临的一些最具挑战性的问题。这种做法取得了一些成功[2]。

已故器官捐献者的重症监护管理最简单的可分为两个阶段:一个是在宣布死亡之前,前 OPO 管理;以及在宣告死亡发生后(OPO 管理)。然而,实际操作起来要更加复杂,因为这是一个连续统一的整体过程,所有这些都符合重症监护治疗原则。最初,重症监护病房(ICU)患者的治疗包括维持心输出量和维持氧气输送,这对于抵抗疾病、提高患者生存率至关重要。此外,如果患者不幸病情加重并满足脑死亡的神经学标准,那么这种血流动力学支持增加了成功捐献器官的可能性,使得患者继续成为潜在器官捐献者。

及时识别有可能成为潜在供体的 ICU 患者,以及随后对其心肺系统的持续支持,对于减少器官功能损害至关重要。在 ICU 管理团队对重症患者的治疗期间,当治疗无效的可能性增大时,必须明确患者对身后事的意愿。在即将进展为脑死亡的情况下,应确定其有关器官捐献的意图——在本人同意的情况下,可通过器官捐献登记处或通过其他法律文件了解。如果缺少此信息，应明确捐献者其家庭成员的意愿，并与其接触。家庭拒绝捐献仍然是器官捐献的重大障碍。研究表明，通过ICU团队与家庭之间的适当互动，可以最大限度地减少这种情况，从而促进患者在ICU住院期间与家人的理解和沟通。

通过神经学标准正确识别和及时宣告死亡也是至关重要的。通过神经学标准延迟诊断或否认死亡是使器官捐献处于危险之中的另一个问题。然而，教育医疗专业人员关于临床特征和脑死亡的诊断可以有效解决这一点。

即使在诊断出DNC之后，尽管实施了OPO管理协议，但仍可能发生潜在供体的丢失。不幸的是，器官捐献者在临床表现出的这种特殊性，这些患者的治疗对于医疗专业人员来说是很具有挑战性的。DNC可以引发与血流动力学不稳定和终末器官损伤相关的许多生理变化。在DNC发展后，由于临床恶化，高达25%的潜在捐献者丧失[3]。因此，对潜在捐献者的适当管理对于预防器官损伤和损失至关重要[4,5]。随着对DNC生理学的理解和通过适当的重症监护管理策略减轻潜在的生理变化，可以实现可移植器官数量的显著增加以及接受者移植后器官功能的改善[6]。生理变化始于脑疝过程，如不及时治疗，可能导致快速恶化和心血管衰竭[7]。这些变化与激素的严重失调、大量细胞因子释放和许多电解质异常有关，这可能通过一些管理干预减弱、缓和甚至逆转。DNC后管理已经有了重大进展来维持或改善器官功能，并成功地增加了需要移植的人的供体数量[3,6,8]。

从这个意义上讲，一种标准化的方法侧重于多器官复苏，维持或改善氧气输送(DO_2)到可移植器官，将是指导全面进行整体捐献者管理的有用工具。这种理念需要采取积极的方式对捐献者进行干预，从脑死亡宣告到手术室，完成器官获取和保存的整个过程。

脑死亡的诊断

脑死亡诊断的神经学标准

通过神经学标准宣告死亡是在神经系统破坏性损伤后进行的临床诊断，通过连续神经系统检查证实的昏迷状态，显示由脑和脑干活动介导的所有反射活动的持续丧失[9,10]。脑死亡进展的最后一个事件是灾难性颅内压(ICP)升高的发展，导致由缺血、梗死、出血或脑疝引起的脑干功能丧失。已知多种脑病理学可起ICP升高。在脑死亡演变的早期过程中，幕上病变或进行性脑水肿的快速扩张导致上脑功能丧失，通常导致意识丧失。脑损伤的进一步发展导致幕下脑疝与幕下室压迫。

脑死亡被定义为一种临床病症，根据发布于1981年[11]和最近更新[12]的指南所述，其特征在于整个大脑功能完全和不可逆的丧失，包括大脑皮层和脑干。脑死亡是一种临床诊断，如果可以确定病因，消除可逆的昏迷原因，并进行包括呼吸暂停测试在内的完整神经系统检查，则可以在没有确认测试的情况下诊断。诊断需要证明皮质和脑干活动的缺失以及这种状态的不可逆性。在神经系统检查中，脑死亡的诊断需要记录昏迷或无反应、脑干反射丧失和呼吸暂停。在开始DNC测试之前，有必要排除可能混淆临床评估的可逆性医疗条件，包括：

- 电解质、酸碱和内分泌功能严重失衡；
- 药物中毒和中毒；
- 使用镇静剂或神经肌肉阻滞剂；
- 低血压[可抑制脑电图(EEG)活动]；
- 体温过低(核心温度<36℃，儿童需要>35℃)。

一旦确认不存在这些排除项，就用脑神经检查进行脑干反射测试。在DNC中，患者表现出瞳孔居中固定或瞳孔散大，没有对光反射，没有角膜反射，没有头眼反射(娃娃眼现象)，没有眼前庭反射(眼睛对冷刺激的强直性偏离)，没有呕吐反射或气管吸痰咳嗽反应，并且没有接受刺激后面部肌肉运动(由外周刺激引起的脊髓介导反射)[12]。一旦确认不存在脑干反射，则进行呼吸暂停测试以验证脑干功能的丧失。在进行呼吸暂停测试之前必须满足某些条件，以避免在测试期间可能发生的心律失常和全身性低血压。这些是进行呼吸暂停测试的先决条件：

- 正常血压；
- 正常体温；
- 血容量正常；
- 没有呼吸暂停；
- 没有低氧血症。

呼吸暂停测试或高碳酸血症测试的流程如表20.1所示。达到以下标准仍没有任何恢复呼吸的迹象，则确认呼吸暂停测试为没有反应：$PaCO_2$> 60mmHg；或高于

表 20.1 呼吸暂停测试

1.保持氧合 100%氧气 10~15 分钟，SaO_2> 95%
2.在开始呼吸暂停测试之前，降低呼吸机速率以保持正常的 PCO_2(40~45 范围)： • 如果患者患有慢性 CO_2 潴留，那么在开始呼吸暂停测试之前，应保持 pH 值为 7.35~7.40
3.获得初始动脉血气(ABG)
4.断开呼吸机－用鼻导管或其他导管供养，O_2 流量为 4~6L • 将患者留在机械呼吸机上可能导致自动循环通气，这可能与患者的自主呼吸相混淆
5.取下所有加温毯或其他器材，以便观察胸部上升，并监测自主呼吸运动的任何迹象
6.只要患者保持血流动力学稳定(血压或心率降低<20%)，O_2 饱和度仍> 90%，继续监测。在 10 分钟时，复查血气，并与呼吸暂停测试之前抽取的血气对比。如果在任何时候都不符合这些标准，请立即抽取 ABG 并与呼吸暂停测试之前抽取的血气对比
7.如果 $PaCO_2$ 分压上升到> 60，并且在没有自主呼吸的情况下超过基线>20，则认为是失败的高碳酸血症测试，并且与神经学标准(DNC)宣布死亡一致
8.如果 $PaCO_2$ 未能上升并且患者在脱离呼吸机时血流动力学稳定，则可以重复测试。应重新获得基线 ABG，重复测试更长一段时间，至少 12 分钟，并重复 ABG。(如果患者血流动力学稳定，则重复步骤 6~8，可以设定 12 分钟或更长时间)。如果测试不确定且由于患者不稳定而无法完成，则应进行辅助测试以帮助确定 DNC

基线 20mmHg 的慢性 CO_2 潴留。因为呼吸暂停测试可以引起进一步的临床恶化，例如低血压、严重的心律失常和 ICP 升高，所以应为脑死亡临床评估中进行的最后一项。当呼吸暂停测试无法确定或无法安全进行时，应考虑辅助测试[9,12]。

在脑死亡的临床测定中，系列观察进一步证实了脑损伤的不可逆性。建议重复评估脑死亡的基础发现。大多数专家建议初始间隔为 6 小时并重复临床观察以确定成年人脑死亡。

婴儿和儿童脑死亡宣告的特殊考虑

确定婴儿和儿童脑死亡的指南最初发表于 1987 年[13]，最近也有相关的更新[14]。在此更新中，已经对先前关于儿科 DNC 确定的建议进行了一些重大改变。

临床检查与检查期间的观察等待仍然是诊断的基石；然而，患者年龄范围已经改变[14]。

1.对于超过 37 周龄的胎儿至 30 天的婴儿，如果他们出生大于 24 小时并且在接受心肺复苏后超过 24 小时，则可以评估 DNC。对于这个年龄段，建议由两名独立的医生进行两次完整的神经系统检查，至少间隔 24 小时，并且在宣布死亡之前需要与 DNC 一致。

2.对于 31 天至 18 岁的儿科患者，时间间隔减少至 12 小时，但其他规定不变。

3.在无法完成全面检查或为减少等待期的情况下使用确认检测。

用于确定脑死亡的辅助测试

在大多数情况下，脑死亡的辅助检测并不是强制性的，但对于无法可靠评估临床检测特定成分结果的患者来说，有必要宣布脑死亡(表 20.2)。选择测试取决于执行脑死亡诊断的医生的酌处权。神经生理学技术和神经诊断测试是验证测试的黄金标准。

脑血管造影

选择性血管造影术是由神经放射学家进行的神经诊断测试。与脑死亡一致的血管造影发现，在颈动脉分叉或 Willis 环的入口上方没有脑血流，其中外部颈动脉循环是可以接受的。从技术角度来看，造影剂应在高压下注入前后循环。然而，脑灌注的存在并不意味着脑死亡没有发生[10]。

脑电图

脑电图可用于确定脑死亡。在脑死亡患者中，脑电图应显示在 30 分钟内对强烈的躯体感觉或视听刺激缺乏反应[9,15]。值得注意的是，脑电图结果受高巴比妥剂量的影响[16]。

经颅多普勒超声检查

经颅多普勒超声检查可能显示血流异常，如：无舒张期或反流；仅收缩期血流或舒张期反流；早期收缩期

表 20.2 需要确认性测试以确定脑死亡的临床情况

病因不明确的昏迷 • 不完整的脑干反射测试 • 不完整的呼吸暂停测试 • 有毒药物水平 • 年龄<1 岁的患儿 • 机构政策要求

的小收缩期峰值。血流速度可能受到$PaCO_2$、血细胞比容和心输出量的显著变化的影响[17]。完全没有血流可能不是一个可靠的发现，因为声纳的经颅窗口不足。10%的患者可能没有暂时的检查窗口。

脑闪烁显像

脑闪烁显像(锝核医学扫描)是另一种确定脑死亡的方法。在脑死亡中,脑闪烁显像显示没有摄取放射性同位素（空心现象)。同位素应在重建后30分钟内注入,并在几个时间点获得静态图像,分别为:立即,30~60分钟后,2小时。

体感和脑干听觉诱发电位

这可以在床边用便携式仪器进行，该仪器提供正中神经的双侧刺激。在脑死亡患者中,没有观察到对躯体感觉和脑干听觉诱发电位测试的反应。两种类型的测试都不如其他确认测试敏感。

脑死亡的生理学

严重的脑损伤或疾病会引起脑部的原发性损伤,导致继发性脑缺血。随着这种灾难性损伤进展为脑死亡,一系列广泛的、渐进的和不可逆的变化被激活,导致各种生理变化,包括交感神经和副交感神经反应、垂体–下丘脑功能障碍、促炎细胞因子释放和凝血功能异常。这些变化已被证明会导致各种并发症,可能危及重要的器官功能(图20.1)。并非所有这些变化都见于每个潜在的供体，但并发症的发生率和严重程度取决于脑死亡的病因和时间过程。脑死亡发生后,并发症的风险随着时间的推移而增加。这些并发症直接和间接地与重要器官功能的显著改变相关。

与大脑解剖相关的生理变化

脑死亡的发展伴随着可预测的体轴反射的脑结构锥形(表20.3)。当累及大脑时,发生迷走神经激活,导致心血管系统的抑制。这通常与下丘脑和脑下垂体的

表20.3 进行性脑脊髓缺血

脑结构受损	生理相关变化
大脑	↓心率,↓心输出量,↓血压
脑桥	↓心率,↑血压,呼吸紊乱
髓质	↑心率,↑血压,体温调节受损
脊髓	↓心率,↓心输出量,↓血压

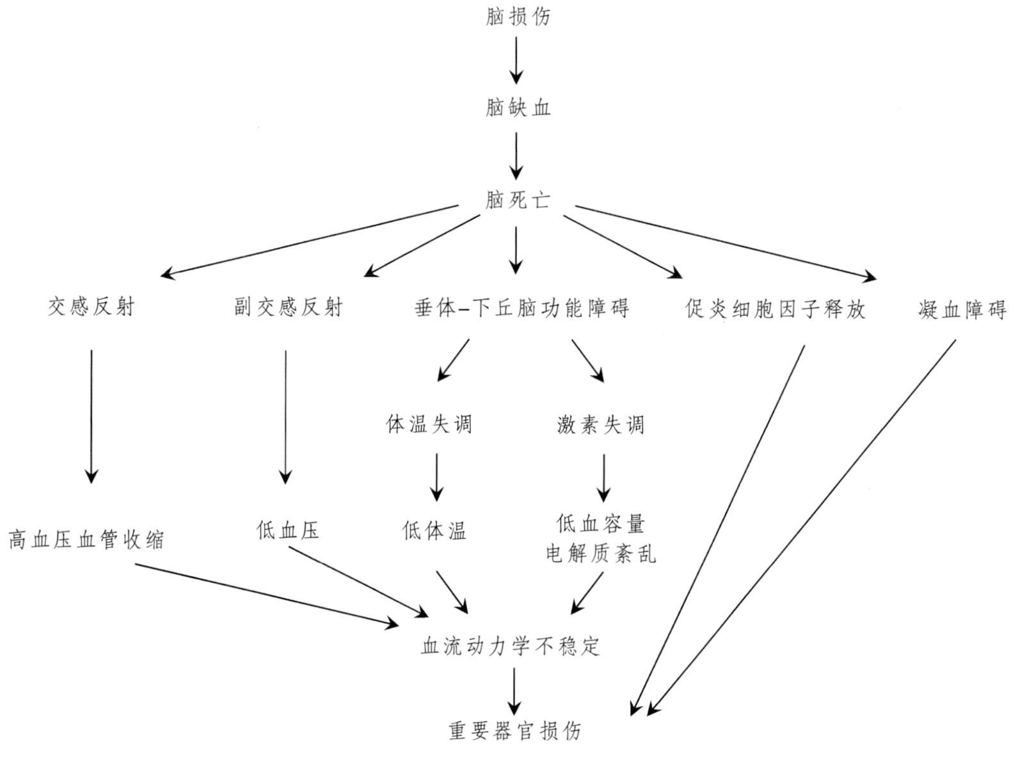

图20.1 脑死亡引起器官损伤的途径。

破坏同时发生，导致随后的温度和激素失调。脑桥缺血与库欣反射有关，导致混合性迷走神经和交感神经失控[18]。髓质缺血发生在脑干死亡的早期阶段，其特征是交感神经或自主神经风暴[19]。迷走神经和心脏运动核的局部缺血导致无对抗的儿茶酚胺激增。这导致强烈的全身和冠状动脉血管收缩、心动过速、高血压和 ICP 的进一步升高。这种过度交感神经状态可导致全身器官和组织缺血。升高的全身血管阻力（SVR）和肺血管阻力（PVR）导致肺毛细血管床压力增加和内皮损伤。下髓质呼吸中枢的缺血导致呼吸暂停。当脑干缺血完全发展时，可发生脊髓交感神经通路的逐渐丧失和全交感神经去神经支配。交感神经血管张力的全面丧失和 SVR 的显著降低导致心血管衰竭[20]。由于垂体缺血引起的交感神经激活和血管加压素缺乏的丧失，大多数潜在的供体不能维持血流动力学稳定性[4]。此外，垂体和下丘脑调节系统的缺血可以诱导各种稳态控制机制的丧失。

心血管改变

脑死亡与导致心血管不稳定和广泛器官损伤的复杂生理变化有关[4,5]。如前所述，脑死亡后的血流动力学不稳定性发生在两个连续阶段。第一阶段由儿茶酚胺储存动员的生理后遗症引起。在一项动物研究中，脑干死亡导致循环多巴胺、肾上腺素和去甲肾上腺素水平显著升高，分别为 800%、700%和 100%[21]。脑死亡的捐献者也出现类似的现象[22]。这种交感风暴引起强烈的血管收缩，导致严重的高血压和心动过速。虽然这会导致心肌需氧量的二次增加，但心肌氧供应没有增加，因为儿茶酚胺风暴也会引起冠状动脉血管收缩。这种供氧和供应的不平衡可能会导致早期心脏功能障碍，并可能导致脑死亡供体心肌的直接损伤[23]。脑死亡心肌损伤的特征是肌细胞溶解、心内膜下出血、水肿和间质炎症改变[19]。收缩带坏死是心肌损伤的常见病理变化之一，在脑死亡后的 90%患者中可观察到[24]。儿茶酚胺风暴可引起细胞内钙的显著增加，导致三磷酸腺苷（ATP）产生受损和自由基形成增加，这引起进一步的组织损伤。全身血管阻力的显著增加会增加后负荷并导致潜在供体的急性心力衰竭。由于静水压升高和毛细血管通透性增加，可能会出现急性肺水肿[25-27]。

交感神经失控的初始阶段之后是自主塌陷，伴有交感神经张力的丧失及与儿茶酚胺储存耗竭相关的全身血管阻力的显著降低，而不是心脏损伤。临床上，其特征是严重的低血压和心动过缓[3,18]。不受控制的血管舒张加速了热量损失和体温过低。由于血管容量和液体体积变化的增加、血管张力的丧失导致显著的功能性血容量不足。急性心电图异常在脑死亡中很常见，包括心房和室性心律失常、传导异常以及 ST 段的变化进一步损害血流动力学状态。

利尿剂和甘露醇等脑水肿的积极治疗会导致体积进一步减少并加剧血流动力学不稳定。尿崩症引起的不可治疗的液体流失也导致血流动力学不稳定。尿崩症引起的体积减少可超过 2L/h，导致全身水分迅速耗尽。密切监测尿量对于评估潜在捐献者的血流动力学至关重要。

肺部变化

严重脑损伤后肺功能障碍很常见[28]。随后的脑死亡常因肺炎、误吸和神经源性肺水肿而并发。在创伤患者中，肺挫伤和气胸常见，并且导致严重的呼吸功能障碍。与脑死亡有关的儿茶酚胺释放也会导致肺部细胞直接损伤[5]。严重的血管收缩导致肺毛细血管床中的压力增加和内皮损伤。炎症反应直接导致肺毛细血管通透性增加。液体复苏后的容量过载会增加肺水肿的风险。接受输血的患者也有移植相关急性肺损伤（TRALI）的风险。这些变化使成功的器官获取具有挑战性，并对移植结果产生负面影响[4,29]。

内分泌变化

随着脑死亡的发生，内分泌会发生许多变化，并可能导致代谢和血流动力学不稳定[27]。脑死亡破坏了下丘脑-垂体轴，导致血清激素耗竭。下丘脑和垂体系统的功能障碍导致体温调节的丧失，导致体温过高或体温过低。垂体后叶功能通常会丧失，导致高达 90%的脑死亡器官供体血管加压素水平低或检测不到[21,30]。这通常引起中枢性尿崩症，临床上以多尿为特征，导致严重的血容量不足、高渗性和高钠血症。

随着垂体前叶功能障碍，TSH、三碘甲状腺素（T3）、甲状腺素（T4）、促肾上腺皮质激素（ACTH）和生长激素（GH）通常被耗尽。随之而来的甲状腺功能减退和肾上腺功能不全可能导致线粒体丧失再生 ATP 的能力，导致功能性器官不稳定[31]。因此，降低的甲状腺激素水平可能导致一些供体的心脏功能和一般器官灌注的恶化。由于甲状腺刺激素(TSH)分泌受损以及从T4到T3的外周转换,脑死亡的游离T3迅速下降[31]。缺乏T3导致无氧代谢和酸中毒的转变。

脑死亡后皮质醇水平显著降低，导致应激反应受损。与T3耗竭协同作用下,这种变化可能对心血管系统产生负面影响。皮质醇水平的降低可能与垂体前叶腺中促肾上腺皮质激素(ACTH)的释放减少有关[21]。外源性皮质类固醇有助于器官功能的稳定。

高血糖是一种常见的内分泌失调。细胞内葡萄糖浓度降低是常见的,并且导致细胞能量缺乏,这不利于有氧代谢并诱导酸中毒。类固醇给药和儿茶酚胺水平升高可能进一步对高血糖症产生不利影响。通常需要大剂量胰岛素输注以防止高渗状态、严重的渗透性利尿和严重的血容量不足的发展。

炎症反应

脑死亡与各种全身炎症反应有关。炎性细胞因子水平升高与器官移植后的不良预后相关[32-35]。这种反应与免疫、凝血和补体系统的激活相互关联[36,37]。已知脑死亡引发各种细胞因子的产生，例如，肿瘤坏死因子(TNF)、白细胞介素(IL)-1和IL-6。脑死亡中细胞因子产生的机制尚不完全清楚,但报道了几种途径。已知缺血性脑组织将炎性细胞因子释放到体循环中[38]。脑死亡引发炎症状态，其可上调受损内皮细胞上的黏附分子表达，导致受体T淋巴细胞和巨噬细胞的黏附以及器官移植后移植物再灌注后炎性细胞因子的进一步释放[35]。通过与脑死亡相关的生理变化维持或扩大炎症反应[34,39]。这会影响所有重要器官,并且与供体中显著的器官损伤相关，并且随后的功能不良和接受者中移植物丢失的风险增加，其中促炎细胞因子水平升高和靶器官中受体的上调。

凝血功能障碍

凝血异常通常见于脑死亡。由于病理生理变化,脑死亡与弥散性血管内凝血(DIC)风险增加有关[40]。病因有两个主要原因:第一,从受损脑组织释放促凝血酶原激酶、纤维蛋白原和组织纤溶酶原;第二,由于大量液体复苏导致的循环凝血因子的稀释[3,41]。由于体温过低加剧了凝血功能障碍,因此,改善方法包括使用温热的静脉输液、加热毯和加热吸入的气体,以维持正常的体温核心温度。供体中DIC是否会损害供体器官活力一直存在争议。理论上,由于纤维蛋白和微血栓在移植器官中的沉积,DIC可能对移植物质量产生不利影响,并且许多移植中心认为微血栓的存在是器官捐献的相对禁忌证。然而,其他研究表明,这些供体的胸部和腹部器官都可以移植而不会影响受体结果[21,42,43]。

器官捐献管理

在诊断脑死亡之前，所有医疗工作都是针对严重受伤的患者，保持足够的心输出量以支持所有重要功能，包括保留潜在的残余脑功能和改善任何可逆性损伤。一旦确定了治疗无效并且神经学标准即将宣布死亡，则将治疗的重点转向维持和优化器官功能以允许器官捐献的机会。

一旦确认死亡宣告并确认器官捐献的同意，应避免不必要的延误，因为器官功能障碍的风险会逐渐增加。如果与脑死亡相关的生理变化未得到治疗或治疗不足，供体可能会在相对较短的时间内恶化并发生心脏骤停。及时了解捐献者管理和协调的重要性。器官获取必须在组织与个人协同共享下进行。捐献者管理需要OPO和临床护理团队之间的多学科协作方法。应在ICU环境中监测器官捐献者,以提供必须的监测治疗。密切的血流动力学监测和积极的复苏对于优化器官质量和最大限度地恢复移植器官的潜力至关重要[6]。标准化供体管理的应用显著增加了移植器官的数量而不影响移植后的结果[6,44]。

改善和维持供体的稳定增加了器官功能改善的机会,从而提高了器官捐献的成功率。在宣布DNC时,似乎无法使用的器官可以通过积极的供体管理进行功能改善,从而可以移植。虽然在过去,从宣告脑死亡到移植器官复苏的持续时间被视为影响移植器官的不利因素[45];最近的证据表明,良好的供体管理时期可以减少这种影响,并且实际上可以改善结果[46,47]。相反,未能维持供体稳定性与供体丢失率较高、移植器官较少和移植后器官功能受损有关。

UNOS供体管理标准

自移植早期以来，就知道不可逆的生理病理改变可导致潜在器官供体的功能恶化和心脏停搏。因此,制订了标准的重症监护方案，旨在保证更好的移植器官质量。然而,高达25%的潜在捐献者对其重要器官缺乏足够的灌注,使其不适合捐献[7]。

除了强化医疗护理外,OPO 人员还必须获得或确认器官捐献者或其家庭的同意,并为捐献者家庭提供情感支持。为应对这些挑战,UNOS 制订了旨在加强供体管理的准则[48]。该指南“供体管理标准”促进了供体的优质管理,并已被广泛使用,证实其对增加可用于移植的器官数量具有有益作用[6]。该标准旨在提供评估供体器官(包括心脏、肺、肝、肾和胰腺)功能状态所必需的信息,并确定改善和优化每个器官功能所需的管理步骤。这也促进了专业医务人员之间在器官供体护理方面的沟通。

管理标准的内涵

管理标准有 5 个不同但部分重叠的阶段。每个阶段都有可供专业医务人员照顾器官捐献者的小节,作为进行全面评估和管理的指南。

第一阶段(推荐)

当患有严重脑损伤的患者被确定为潜在的器官捐献者时,重症监护人员应启动该关键途径。这个初始步骤确定了医院与当地 OPO 之间的联系,并在潜在的器官捐献者脑死亡之前启动转诊。除非启动此步骤,否则器官捐献的可能性将减少。在这个阶段,器官获取协调员(OPC)对潜在的供体进行快速评估,以确定器官捐献的可行性。

第二阶段(脑死亡宣告和获得同意)

一旦潜在供体被确认为脑死亡,患者对器官捐献的选择将通过全州/地方捐献者登记处(通常通过机动车登记处或驾驶执照)进行评估,并且该家庭将获得此信息。如果没有首先得到本人的同意证件,则向家人询问器官捐献的意向。如果患者不在捐献者登记处,与其家人过早接触或由无经验的协调员负责协调,他们可能会因为无法接受而选择拒绝捐献。因此,只有在他们有足够的时间了解亲人的死亡之后,才应给予家庭捐献的选择[49,50]。如果家庭拒绝捐献,该途径将在此阶段终止,并应开始死后护理。如果患者是本人同意捐献,登记处或家庭同意捐献,则供体管理应优先开始实施。本人的同意意见优先于家庭其他成员的拒绝意见,在美国的许多州和 OPO 组织会选择捐献。

第三阶段(供体评估)

在通过捐献登记处获得或确认器官捐献的同意意见后,启动供体评估和管理协议。OPC 获得所有必要的历史记录和诊断测试的结果。死亡原因、脑死亡发生前的住院时间、估计或见证的停机时间(心肺骤停持续时间)、心肺复苏持续时间、胸部或腹部创伤以及生命体征是至关重要的信息。需要获得既往病史,包括高血压病史、糖尿病、冠状动脉疾病、肺病、肝病、肾病、恶性肿瘤、感染和血栓病史。如果有旧的医疗文书或供体的初级保健医生,可以收集更多有用的信息。外科手术史对器官获取外科医生非常重要。还应获得吸烟和酗酒的历史。如果供体有被监禁的历史、使用静脉注射药物或有多个性伴侣,则可能认为潜在的供体是传播人类免疫缺陷病毒(HIV)和肝炎病毒的高风险人群。彻底的身体检查对于排除可能影响捐献过程的发现也很重要,包括纹身、针迹痕迹或可疑病变或肿块的存在。实验室测试包括全血细胞计数、血清化学成分,包括肝功能测试(LFT)、动脉血气、凝血概况、传染病血清学测试和交叉匹配的组织分型。用于细菌和真菌的血液、尿液和痰培养物被送到实验室以筛查感染。除胸部 X 线片、心电图(ECG)、超声心动图和动脉血气外,需要通过胸部移植小组确定心导管检查和支气管镜检查的必要性。及时完成这些测试对于促进快速器官获取、移植和康复非常重要。

第四阶段(供体管理)

在评估供体的同时,还需要开始最佳管理以实现血流动力学稳定性,充分的氧合作用以及最佳的液体和电解质平衡。动脉导管和中心静脉导管的放置对于积极的呼吸和血流动力学监测是必要的,并且帮助改善供体的心肺状态。偶尔,微创血流动力学监测或肺动脉导管也被认为是有帮助的。这一治疗阶段的持续时间将取决于进入该阶段的供体的状态、供体的稳定性,以及对每个供体中认为可行移植的潜在器官的情况。目前的趋势是供体管理时间为 48~72 小时,以使移植前器官功能尽可能地改善。

第五阶段(器官复苏)

在确定了潜在的受体之后,将供体转移到获取器官的手术室。临床管理重点从供体管理转移到器官保存。所有器官康复团队应在获取程序之前尽可能解决可能存在的问题。

水晶城会议

联邦政府对器官捐献危机的认识促成了 2001 年 3 月在美国弗吉尼亚州水晶城召开的一次共识会议,

以制订初步可被大家接受的指导方针，以改善死者捐献者器官的恢复和移植。建立了5个工作组,重点是最大限度地利用心脏、肺、肝脏和肾脏,并增加使用具有恶性肿瘤史或丙型肝炎或乙型肝炎病毒阳性血清学检测的已故供体的器官。在这次会议上,多学科小组概述了一些管理方案,并给出了治疗建议,以提高上述高风险供体的个人器官或器官的效用。

心脏工作组提出了改善潜在心脏捐献者评估和利用的建议[41,51]。根据其建议,新的供体管理方式被纳入UNOS管理标准(表20.4)。在常规管理调整体积状态、酸碱平衡、氧合、贫血和正性肌力药物剂量后,进行超声心动图评估射血分数并排除结构异常。如果射血分数<45%,则启动激素复苏,旨在稳定和改善心脏功能:

- T3:4μg推注,然后连续输注3μg/h;
- 精氨酸加压素:1U推注，然后0.5~4.0U/h滴注(滴定至SVR为800~1200dyn·s/cm^5);
- 甲基强的松龙:15mg/kg推注(根据需要每24小时重复一次);
- 使用胰岛素滴注:以1U/h的最低速率,将血糖滴定至120~180mg/dL。

放置肺动脉导管以允许积极监测和管理心肺状态。这与激素复苏同时开始并持续至少2小时。每15分钟调整一次液体，正性肌力药和血管加压药应根据系列血流动力学测量，尽量减少α-激动剂的使用,并满足以下目标标准:平均动脉压> 60mmHg;中心静脉压4~12mmHg;肺毛细血管楔压8~12mmHg,SVR 800~1200dyn·s/cm^5 [5];心脏指数>2.4L/(min·m^2) [2];多巴胺或多巴酚丁胺10μg/(kg·min)。建议使用激素替代作为供体管理的一个组成部分[4,6,41,51]。激素替代物消除了与脑死亡相关的某些生理变化，导致心血管稳定和更好的器官灌注。这种效应使每个供体移植器官数量增加22.5%[6]。

表20.4 器官捐献者的关键管理标准(UNOS)

1.所有捐献者的早期超声心动图:
• 插入肺动脉导管以监测患者治疗情况[对于射血分数(EF)<45%的患者或大剂量正性肌力药物尤其重要]
2.流体和电解质:
• 维持 Na^+ <150mmol/L
• 维持 K^+> 4.0mmol/L
• 通过碳酸氢钠和轻度至中度过度通气(PCO_2 30~35mmHg)纠正酸中毒
3.通气条件:
• 维持潮气量10~15mL/kg
• 保持气道峰值压力<30mmHg
• 维持轻度呼吸性碱中毒(PCO_2 30~35mmHg)
4.激素复苏:
• 三碘甲状腺素
• 精氨酸
• 加压素
• 甲泼尼龙
• 胰岛素

体液和电解质管理

中枢性尿崩症的频繁发生存在特定的问题。如果患者因血浆钠和渗透压升高而出现不适当的利尿,则应考虑这一问题。尿崩症需要积极治疗,因其与器官捐献者的血流动力学不稳定密切相关[52]。可能需要低渗静脉液来恢复正常的钠水平，但面对未经治疗的尿崩症很少成功。因此,血容量、正常血容量和正常渗透压需要多重方法来纠正潜在的病理学改变(垂体衰竭)并用游离水代替体液缺乏。使用大量D5W可能导致血糖水平的二次升高,其也应用胰岛素治疗,优先选择胰岛素滴注。一些研究表明,高钠血症与移植后器官功能差相关[53],但实际上可能是整体供体管理不善的标志。然而,最近的一项研究表明,脑死亡供体中的高钠血症并不影响移植器官质量或移植器官存活[53]。

供体管理通常是复杂的，因为不同专业的优先级相互矛盾，这些胸腔和腹腔器官团队之间对供体内部的最佳体液平衡有不同的要求。通常,肺外科医生和胰腺移植外科医生更喜欢使静脉注射液最小化，以使肺和胰腺水肿最小化。通过限制液体量给药,使得这些器官的水肿或充血最小化。相比之下,心脏和肾脏的最佳体液管理截然相反。通过对供体进行积极扩容,可以很好地灌输肾脏,以保持尿量的快速增加,并可以优化心输出量。由于多个获取团队同时在器官管理和随后的多学科器官复苏中协调工作,因此,必须强调不同团队与OPO协调员之间沟通的重要性。

炎症反应

在肺和肝移植的随机研究中，向供体施用甲基强的松龙以试图减少炎症已被证明是有益的，并且通常在确认捐献计划后立即给予[54-56]。在最近对器官供体的观察评估中,较高的IL-6水平与接受者随后的器官结果恶化相关[36]。此外,同一组进行了最近的一项试验性研究,以探索使用血液吸附装置去除脑死亡供体中炎性细胞因子的可行性[57]。该装置能够适度降低血浆细胞因子水平;但是,没有足够临床移植结果的数据支撑。

凝血功能障碍

凝血功能障碍可能与供体病理学改变或受损脑组织中活化物质的释放有关。如果出现活动性出血,则需要进行治疗,并且在获取器官之前应考虑纠正明显异常的凝血状态。即时凝血测试,包括血栓弹力图,可能有助于治疗决策。必要时应考虑对ICU患者进行输血,除非TRALI发展。

器官复苏的术中管理

多器官捐献手术通常需要通过胸骨切开延长到腹部切开,即使不需要获取胸腔器官。与任何主要的体腔手术一样,有可能出现明显的失血和体温过低。在器官获取期间可能发生显著的心血管不稳定,即使血管活性药物输注可能正在进行中。围术期器官捐献者管理的目标是在器官复苏期间保持稳定,以允许有条不紊地移除复苏的器官。应进行手术安全检查。

应进行术中持续性加温,如果有任何延迟都会影响获取手术的进程。应加温静脉输液,如果需要,应立即提供血液和血液制品。由脊柱反射介导的心血管变化可能由于手术操作而被引发,并且可能需要用血管活性药物治疗。由于发生了脑干死亡,因此不需要麻醉。一些获取组织在获取期间使用可控制高血压的挥发性麻醉药物,因为它们可能对取出的器官具有有益的预处理效果,但没有证据证明这一点。协调药物给药是最重要的,特别是肝素。获取团队应熟练掌握腹腔和胸腔灌注技术。

评估供体的质量

由于对拯救生命的移植器官的巨大需求与器官捐献者数量有限之间的矛盾,大多数OPO在评估潜在器官捐献者时采用的一般前提是"每个器官每次评估"。目标是使得捐献器官的供体可以为移植外科医生及其患者提供所有可能移植的器官。不幸的是,并非所有希望在死亡时作为器官捐献者帮助他人的供体器官都是可捐献的。

OPO有责任审查每个潜在供体的现有信息,以评估每个潜在供体的质量,并确定每个特定供体的哪些器官可能是可移植的。OPO首先对潜在供体过去的医疗和社会经历进行彻底审查。供体质量的评估通常基于供体年龄、体重[特别是体重指数(BMI)]、一般病史、器官特定病史、吸烟史、注意恶性肿瘤、感染和高危行为,包括药物滥用[酒精或药物(静脉注射、吸入、口服等)]、多个性伴侣和监禁等。死因、住院时间、血流动力学状态(血压、心率、正性肌力支持)、肺功能、肝功能、尿量、葡萄糖水平和酸碱平衡在供体质量分析中也很重要。年龄增加、BMI较高、合并症史、缺血时间延长和血流动力学不稳定都已知会增加器官功能障碍和移植后存活率低的风险。

要知道,目前美国唯一的器官捐献绝对禁忌证是潜在供体的HIV诊断。这是目前的联邦法律,但正在根据南非最近发表的一篇文章进行重新评估,该文章显示HIV病毒阳性供体的器官可以成功捐献给HIV病毒阳性的受者[58]。捐献的其他潜在禁忌证是播散性恶性肿瘤、持续治疗癌症、未确定的脑膜脑炎病因和严重的多器官功能障碍。尽管如此,这些应根据具体情况进行评估,不应导致作为潜在供体的标准降低。

接下来,OPO将评估每个供体的死因情况,并再次评估其导致死亡的事件的潜在影响。一个考虑是缺氧时间以及是否进行心肺复苏(CPR),以及CPR的持续时间,直到自发循环恢复。同样重要的是,器官系统在严重损伤时间与神经学标准死亡宣告时之间的功能情况。任何呼吸、心血管、肾脏、肝脏和胰腺功能障碍都可能对器官的恢复和移植潜在产生负面影响。跟踪这些变量和评估ICU管理预期影响的一种机制是利用"供体管理目标(DMG)。"DMG是讨论出的一些参数,用于指导器官供体的管理。这些参数因程序/OPO/区域而异,但都基于针对心肺功能的正常生理终点,同时尽量减少额外支持(较少的正性肌力药),维持正常或接近正常的化学和pH值,并评估器官功能。满足更多DMG似乎与从供体中回收和移植的器官数量增加相关[59,60]。DMG的用法是为所有器官捐献者建立统一的目标DMG列表,以允许通过管理方法的变化以实现DMG中概述的生理参数,以及确定良好的管理结果。另一项建议是通过捐献者管理在不同时间评估DMG,并连续评估完成的DMG百分比。有证据表明,如果捐献者在OPO供体管理之前满足高水平的DMG,则每个捐献者移植更多器官的可能性将增加。在OPO参与之前,这可以用作OPO前管理策略的指南。应记录供体管理期间,DNC确定后以及移植器官复苏之前的问题的准确和详细说明,因为在此潜在供体管理期间可能发现许多潜在问题。

一旦收集和整理了所有信息,并解决了所有问题,这些信息将以电子方式提供给移植中心,以便评估和审查其中心通过OPTN计算机网络列出的合适受体。每个特定的中心都制订了自己独立的标准,通过该标准评估和确定受体的适合性。最终,移植外科医生和他们的患者必须根据接受者的状况和预期的供体器官质量的组合做出最终决定。供体器官质量评估中包括供体的潜在风险和预期的冷缺血时间,最终确定每个移植器官的可接受程度。从移植外科医生的角度评估器官的适用性可以参见第53章。

心脏

如前所述,影响捐献心脏潜在质量的因素很多。大多数移植计划的最大供体年龄标准为60~65岁，在这个年龄范围之外的非常适合的供体中都有一些例外。其他排除因素包括既往心脏病变、既往心脏手术,以及怀疑急性事件背后的原发性心脏病因，导致供体死亡(心肌梗死、原发性心律失常、心肌炎和心肌病等)。如果严重事件导致供体失去自发循环，那么没有灌注的时间是一个重要的问题,以及CPR的时间和自发循环恢复的时间。使用正性肌力药或血管加压药以及在捐献前护理和随后维持血流动力学稳定性所需的剂量可能会影响心脏移植的可能性。

我们之前讨论过脑死亡相关的生理变化；这些可能导致暂时性或永久性心脏功能障碍、心律失常和(或)心肌DO_2降低。评估心脏捐献的可能性取决于供体血流动力学崩溃后,通过儿茶酚胺风暴管理,并且直到可以建立具有正常SVR的正常生理心输出量(CO)/心脏指数(CI)。如果可以通过这些手段支持供体而不损害心脏功能，则可以重新评估心脏以确定成功移植的可能性。根据之前引用的数据,目前的做法是大多数OPO在所有潜在的心脏捐献者以及许多不是潜在心脏捐献者的供体中进行甲状腺替代治疗，以稳定血流动力学并允许减少或断绝正性肌力药物输注。关于T3或T4替换的决定,每个个体的剂量以及是否间歇或连续给药都是基于专家意见和当地实践。与器官供体管理的大多数方面一样,存在很少的随机数据。我们的局部实践是以10μg/h开始连续输注左旋甲状腺素（合成T4),并且只要能够容忍血流动力学效应而滴定至最大30μg/h，而没有副作用：最常见的是心动过速和高血压。此外,给予常规剂量的皮质类固醇并持续直至器官复苏。同样,客观数据是有限的,并且最佳实践在特定药物选择方面变化:即糖皮质激素和(或)盐皮质激素、使用的剂量和连续与间歇输注。

在评估心脏移植潜力时，通常的做法是在开始OPO管理时获得超声心动图;这种做法已经推迟到儿茶酚胺输注到最低限度,最好是完全停药后进行。除了评估足够的功能外,通常通过射血分数、心室壁厚度和运动动力学证明接近正常的功能。在较老的供体中,通常需要心脏导管插入以确定冠状动脉疾病是否使心脏不适合移植或者是否可以在冠状动脉旁路移植术后使用。

肺部动脉导管的使用已经明显下降，这是由于缺乏明显的益处，而且对插入和维持导管相关风险的认识以及大多数医院缺乏合格的人员和设备，即使其在ICU管理中一般都有。它已经被微创血流动力学监测器所取代，这些监测器在很大程度上利用脉冲轮廓来测量每搏输出量变化或脉压变化作为血流动力学状态的标志。一些OPO利用气管多普勒血流探针成功指导其供体管理。

肺脏

关于肺移植可行性的关键数据主要为最小机械呼吸机支持的PaO_2-FiO_2(P/F)比>300~350。与心脏一样，影响肺移植的因素包括年龄(<60岁)、病史、死亡原因、OPO前期供体管理以及OPO期间的管理。当致死性事件是创伤性或与CPR和呕吐有关时,我们应关注肺挫伤的程度、气胸的情况以及吸入胃内容物的可能性,所有这些都会影响肺移植的可能性。在有中度至重度哮喘、肺动脉高压或肺气肿史的供体中,肺移植不太可能。吸烟史超过20包/年或大麻使用很长一段时间也会减少肺部捐献的可能性。

由于长期机械通气需要,插管的持续时间和机械通气的程度以及气管造口管的放置是非移植的其他危险因素，因为它们引入感染和呼吸机引起损伤的可能性，例如，气压伤。在脑疝过程中释放的儿茶酚胺、激素和介质的综合反应可能导致肺组织的直接细胞损伤。经胸压力增加导致肺毛细血管床和内皮损伤，导致急性呼吸窘迫综合征(ARDS)事件，进一步导致肺功能障碍增加和持续的炎症级联反应。随着神经功能的停止、自主呼吸的丧失、咳嗽的丧失和自发运动的丧失，所有这些都导致黏液堵塞、肺不张和肺泡的损毁。另外，"神经源性肺水肿"发展，导致肺部进一步积水并进一步阻碍气体交换。此外，在血管塌陷阶段需要积极的液体复苏以支持血流动力学和肾功能，这将使肺水状况恶化。

早期胸部X线片检查有助于轻松识别肺部潜在问题，无须移动患者。开始胸部理疗(使用背心或床)和沙丁胺醇以增强黏膜纤毛清除有助于改善一些黏液堵塞。N-乙酰半胱氨酸也可以作为黏液溶解剂起作用。全身性皮质类固醇治疗的使用也已显示出改善肺功能，以及更好地评估和控制供体血容量状态以实现等容性状态。

机械呼吸机的肺部复苏策略包括圣安东尼奥肺移植(SALT)协议[61]、低潮气量(TV)、高呼气末正压(PEEP)复苏方法，以及使用倒置吸气的替代方法-呼气(I:E)压力比控制通气——BiVent或类似APRV的模式[62]。脑死亡的供体产生的CO_2很少，因此需要减少每分钟通气量，这种方法几乎没有什么缺点。供体管理的这两种策略都被证明可以增加成功复苏和随后肺部恢复和移植的可能性(Lebovitz等)。对于早期支气管镜检查，可以在大多数供体管理病例中进行论证，在过量黏液堵塞或吸入胃内容物以缓解阻塞并改善VQ匹配的情况下更应如此，从而改善P/F比。

虽然胸部X线检查是观察肺野的良好手段，但在早期OPO供体管理阶段，肺部CT扫描可能有助于评估既往没有肺气肿病史的吸烟者，以排除发生这种情况的可能。如果注意到肺气肿变化的证据，则肺不适合移植，并且可以使用较不积极的通气策略。

所有供体都需要被视为潜在的肺脏捐献者。解决上述众多问题是OPO管理阶段后期的最高优先级事项，因为它将管理目标的重点放在改善DO_2和肺动力学上，同时尽量减少气压伤和氧中毒的可能性。改善肺部和患者的液体状态。支持DO_2对于维持所有可移植器官的活力至关重要。如果P/F比率可以提高到350以上、峰值呼吸机压力低、PEEP为5cmH_2O、胸部X线片检查正常、OPO供体管理中肺部很少受到特殊管理，那么肺脏复苏和移植成功的可能性很高。

新的曙光即将出现，在复苏肺脏的过程，有些肺脏看起来似乎不能移植，但允许使用离体装置来修复和改善这些肺脏。已经使用该装置并且已发表的研究表明，这种办法可以回收、修复和移植一些边缘肺(即先前未用于移植的肺)[63]。美国食品和药物管理局(FDA)目前正在参与一些美国移植计划，以评估在美国使用的这些技术。

肝脏

肝脏是最能抵抗供体缺乏足够DO_2的器官之一。此外，供体的年龄不是移植后功能的一个因素。然而，当考虑肝脏移植潜力时，有许多独特的问题需要评估。捐献者的BMI是一个需要考虑的重要因素。体重指数>30的供体更有可能患有明显的脂肪肝，一些外科医生不会考虑进行移植。其他因素包括酒精摄入史——包括持续时间和数量。酒精滥用的病史导致肝脏纤维化和功能失调，不能移植。供体中存在或不存在病毒性肝炎对于供体肝脏质量的评估也是重要的。过去的乙型肝炎感染指标的存在或活跃的丙型肝炎血清学证据使得识别这种肝移植的受体更具质疑。如果不确定是否存在活动性感染或是否通过先前的免疫和其他因素解释，则可以进行额外的测试。因此，必须掌握必要的知识来解释血清学检测的结果，以便将这些肝脏移植给最合适的受体。如果肝脏移植可能性很小，对捐献者的肝脏进行床旁穿刺活检也是有帮助的。

供体中血清钠升高导致移植后这些肝脏结果不良的问题是有争议的，最近印第安纳州的一项研究似乎揭穿了这个神话[53]，但钠的升高实际上反映了供体的血容量状态不足，这可能是影响移植后肝功能的主要因素。

肾脏

到目前为止，肾脏是美国乃至全世界移植需求最高的器官。然而，年龄和其他常见的潜在医学疾病可能会限制他们作为供体捐献肾脏的可能性。

当患者在ICU接受高渗治疗、液体限制和血管收缩剂治疗致死性脑损伤时，为了降低颅内压并支持脑灌注压，结果可能是肾实质灌注不足。随着患者神经系统继续恶化，这些治疗会被进一步推动，从而加剧对其他重要器官的潜在伤害。一旦病情恶化并且患者被评估为DNC，则在同意捐献和OPO进程开始之前，初级治疗团队可以停止或不停止这些治疗。宣布DNC后，在捐献前和获取后的管理期间，肾脏发生恶化的急性肾小管坏死的风险很大。这是由于儿茶酚胺激增和随后的血流动力学崩溃发生时快速的体液移动和潜在供体的CO/CI变化。另外，下丘脑/垂体通路的丧失，导致尿崩症的发展，可能另外引起严重的血管内容量减低并加剧血流动力学不稳定性。

器官捐献者面临他们所遭受的院前事件（例如，创伤、低血压、摄入乙二醇等毒素）、医院事件（例如，败血症、肾毒性药物、如静脉肾盂造影染料或抗生素）或治疗方案引起的肾衰竭风险（例如，流体限制）。诸如挤压伤、药物过量（尤其是可卡因、海洛因、安非他明和PCP）、癫痫发作、严重缺氧和创伤等灾难性事件可导致横纹肌溶解，进而导致肌红蛋白沉积引起的肾损伤。DIC和微血栓形成会造成供体存在多器官系统衰竭的风险，肾脏同样面临这些风险。在心脏导管插入术等死者捐献者中需要静脉造影的程序可能会引起“造影剂肾病”。

因此，针对维持等血容量，增强尿量和提供保护免受毒性影响的积极辅助疗法是具有一些实用性的。在最近的一项研究中，在OPO管理阶段接受低剂量多巴胺的供体肾脏改善了受体移植后的肾功能[64]。

监测血清BUN、肌酸酐和每小时尿量，以最好地指示供体肾脏捐献的可能性。此外，肾活检和体外循环显示可改善移植后的肾功能，可以成为增加移植可行性和移植后功能恢复的有效手段。

胰腺和肠道

潜在供体中的胰腺和肠道都是极其脆弱的器官，潜在供体中的许多应激物可导致这些器官的不可移植性。它们特别容易受到自溶，其黏膜内层脱落和缺血、缺氧引起的损伤。

胰腺移植评估的最佳指标是正常的淀粉酶、脂肪酶和血红蛋白A1c。需要收集更多数据以确定是否存在有助于预测这些器官可能成功移植的指标。

传染病风险

移植中固有的是从供体到受体传播疾病的可能性。这可能是供体中预先存在的疾病或与当前医院疾病/损伤相关的急性治疗过程的结果。需要采取措施评估潜在的供体，在医院阶段对供体的治疗包括供体管理阶段以及移植受者的移植后治疗。关于供体衍生感染的详细讨论见第92章。

评估

根据当前UNOS政策2.2.4.1对供体的初步评估，要求对供体进行非血液稀释供体血清学检测，包括HIV 1和2、HepBsAg和HepBcAb、Hep C、巨细胞病毒（CMV）、Epstein-Barr病毒（EBV）、性病研究实验室（VDRL）或快速血浆反应素（RPR），以及血液、尿液和肺部捐献的急性细菌培养物、支气管镜检查/痰革兰染色和培养。如前所述，HIV阳性血清学检测目前在美国没有成为潜在供体的资格。这些筛选试验的其他阳性结果可能影响血清阳性供体特定器官的潜在移植或影响这些器官受体的移植后治疗。

核酸检测

捐献/移植专家最近就使用核酸测试系统（NAT）进行额外测试以筛选潜在捐献者的HIV、丙型肝炎和乙型肝炎病毒存在争议。这种新技术允许通过大量复制基因片段的过程检测少量DNA/RNA。NAT测试的优点是可以通过NAT测试缩短“窗口期”——个体感染与检测时间之间的时间段。

所有潜在供体的NAT测试的支持者（目前在血库工业中进行）表明，强制性NAT测试可以允许在血清学转换之前检测阳性个体，从而进一步降低意外传播的可能性。此外，对器官获取组织临床主任的调查表明，对丙型肝炎和HIV进行NAT检测可能会改善“高风险供体”器官利用[65]。

对于每种测试的病毒，“窗口期”的减少是不同的。对于HIV，标准血清学检测将在感染后17~22天给出阳性结果；增强的血清学（联合抗体-抗原）测试将此降低至7~16天，NAT将其降低至5~6天。对于乙型肝炎，标准血清学检测可在感染后35~44天内给出阳性结果；没有增强的测试可用，但NAT减少到20~22天。

最重要的是，丙型肝炎的平均窗口可以从标准血清学检测的约 70 天减少到血清学检测增强的 40~50 天，以及使用 NAT 时的 3~5 天[66-72]。

反对者仍然担心 NAT 对由于假阳性检测而导致的供体和移植器官丢失的潜在不利影响，已知这种情况是由于缺乏经验/不经常使用该测试，并且在移植前无法获得测试结果（测试地点的时间限制/血清到地点的旅行等）[73]。最近的一次专家共识会议得出结论："没有足够的证据建议使用现有的 NAT 平台对 HIV、HCV 和 HBV 的器官捐献者进行普遍前瞻性筛查。"进一步研究病毒筛查方式可以降低疾病传播风险而不会造成供体过多损失[74]。自这些建议公布以来，疾病控制和预防中心（CDC）已经分发并正在继续修订所有未来器官捐献者的生活和死亡测试指南。最近，关于其拟议修订指南的公众意见征询期引起了移植界的强烈抗议，并建议让所有各方进一步开会以平衡对立的观点。此修订可能会对将来对供体的测试产生影响。

供体的抗生素使用

在供体中使用抗生素取决于许多条件和情况，但应遵守标准的医学和手术指南。传统上，相对年轻的创伤受害者很少患有慢性病并且通常没有传染性风险，通常使用第一代头孢菌素来预防。然而，具有更复杂的医疗条件和潜在合并症的供体，或长期住院的供体，可能已获得抗生素耐药性细菌，包括耐甲氧西林金黄色葡萄球菌（MRSA），并有其他危险因素获得与重症患者的医院护理相关的感染。OPO 必须决定抗生素是否需要或有助于这些患者作为潜在供体的持续管理。具有已知特异性的抗生素应基于位点特异性培养物靶向，例如，脑脊液、呼吸道、泌尿道、血液或导管部位。在许多供体中，在 OPO 管理阶段使用广谱抗生素覆盖的方法反映了准备捐献的时间过短。一个问题是使用抗生素可能导致急性器官功能障碍并降低器官成功移植的可能性。最近的出版物评论了用哌拉西林-他唑巴坦治疗的重症患者急性肾功能不全/衰竭的可能性。另一个问题是，这种急性呼吸衰竭可能会因偶然使用万古霉素而恶化[75]。一般而言，除非有特定病菌需要更多毒性抗生素，否则建议使用扩大革兰阴性覆盖率的第四代头孢菌素。如果在供体管理过程中鉴定出革兰阳性球菌被认为是葡萄球菌属物种，则可以加入万古霉素并密切监测肾功能和万古霉素血药浓度。一旦获得敏感性，应立即转化为毒性较低的抗生素。

总结

可用于挽救生命的可移植器官严重短缺，并且死者捐献的数量在过去 5 年中保持不变。使捐献器官利用率提高的重任就落在了 DNC 期间的治疗团队（医生、护士、呼吸治疗师等）和 OPO 团队（协调员、床旁管理专业人员等）。潜在供体的管理标准有助于使管理有迹可循并使器官生理功能正常化，从而增加成功捐献和移植的可能性。

（张云凯 译　李照 校）

参考文献

1. http://optn.transplant.hrsa.gov/latestData/step2.asp. [accessed December 2011]
2. Singbartl K, Murugan R, Kaynar AM, et al. Intensivist-led management of brain-dead donors is associated with an increase in organ recovery for transplantation. American Journal of Transplantation. 2011;11(7):1517–1521.
3. Karcioğlu O, Ayrik C, Erbil B. The brain-dead patient or a flower in the vase? The emergency department approach to the preservation of the organ donor. European Journal of Emergency Medicine. 2003;10(1):52–57.
4. Dictus C, Vienenkoetter B, Esmaeilzadeh M, et al. Critical care management of potential organ donors: our current standard. Clinical Transplantation. 2009; 23(Suppl 21):2–9.
5. Smith M. Physiologic changes during brain stem death–lessons for management of the organ donor. Journal of Heart and Lung Transplantation. 2004;23(9 Suppl): S217–S222.
6. Rosendale JD, Chabalewski FL, McBride MA, et al. Increased transplanted organs from the use of a standardized donor management protocol. American Journal of Transplantation. 2002;2(8):761–768.
7. Mackersie R, Bronsther O, Shackford S. Organ procurement in patients with fatal head injuries. The fate of the potential donor. Annals of Surgery. 1991;213(2): 143–150.
8. Franklin GA, Santos AP, Smith JW, et al. Optimization of donor management goals yields increased organ use. American Surgeon. 2010;76(6):587–594.
9. Sullivan J, Seem DL, Chabalewski F. Determining brain death. Critical Care Nurse. 1999;19(2):37–46.
10. Henneman EA, Karras GE. Determining brain death in adults: a guideline for use in critical care. Critical Care Nurse. 2004;24(5):50–56.
11. Uniform determination of death act. Guidelines for the determination of death. Report of the medical consultants on the diagnosis of death to the President's Commission for the Study of Ethical Problems in Medicine and Biomedical and Behavioral Research. JAMA. 1981;246(19):2184–2186.
12. Wijdicks EFM, Varelas PN, Gronseth GS, et al. Evidence-based guideline update: determining brain death in adults. Neurology. 2010;74:1911–1918.
13. Task Force for the Determination of Brain Death in Children. Guidelines for the determination of brain death in children. Archives of Neurology. 1987;44: 587–588.
14. Nakagawa TA, Ashwal S, Mathuir M, Mysore M, the Society of Critical Care Medicine, Section of Critical Care and Section on Neurology of the American Academy of Pediatrics, and Child Neurology Society. Clinical report—Guidelines for the determination of brain death in infants and children: an update of the 1987 task force recommendations. Pediatrics. 2011;128:e720–e740.
15. Lovasik D. Brain death and organ donation. Critical Care Nursing Clinics of North America. 2000;12(4):531–538.
16. Arbour R. Continuous nervous system monitoring, EEG, the bispectral index, and neuromuscular transmission. AACN Clinical Issues. 2003;14(2):185–207.
17. Wijdicks EF. Determining brain death in adults. Neurology. 1995;45(5):

1003–1011.
18. Randell TT. Medical and legal considerations of brain death. Acta Anaesthesiologica Scandinavica. 2004;48(2):139–144.
19. Shivalkar B, Van Loon J, Wieland W, et al. Variable effects of explosive or gradual increase of intracranial pressure on myocardial structure and function. Circulation. 1993;87(1):230–239.
20. Pratschke J, Wilhelm MJ, Kusaka M, et al. Brain death and its influence on donor organ quality and outcome after transplantation. Transplantation. 1999;67(3): 343–348.
21. Chen EP, Bittner HB, Kendall SW, et al. Hormonal and hemodynamic changes in a validated animal model of brain death. Critical Care Medicine. 1996;24(8): 1352–1359.
22. Powner DJ, Hendrich A, Nyhuis A, et al. Changes in serum catecholamine levels in patients who are brain dead. Journal of Heart and Lung Transplantation. 1992;11(6):1046–1053.
23. Halejcio-Delophont P, Siaghy EM, Devaux Y, et al. Increase in myocardial interstitial adenosine and net lactate production in brain-dead pigs: an in vivo microdialysis study. Transplantation. 1998;66(10):1278–1284.
24. Baroldi G, Di Pasquale G, Silver MD, et al. Type and extent of myocardial injury related to brain damage and its significance in heart transplantation: a morphometric study. Journal of Heart and Lung Transplantation. 1997;16(10): 994–1000.
25. Bugge J. Brain death and its implications for management of the potential organ donor. Acta Anaesthesiologica Scandinavica. 2009;53:1239–1250.
26. Belzberg H, Shoemaker WC, Wo CC, et al. Hemodynamic and oxygen transport patterns after head trauma and brain death: implications for management of the organ donor. Journal of Trauma. 2007;63(5):1032–1042.
27. Novitzky D, Cooper DKC, Rosendale JD, et al. Hormonal therapy of the brain-dead organ donor: experimental and clinical studies. Transplantation. 2006;82(11): 1396–1401.
28. Bratton SL, Davis RL. Acute lung injury in isolated traumatic brain injury. Neurosurgery. 1997;40(4):707–712.
29. Avlonitis VS, Fisher AJ, Kirby UJA, et al. Pulmonary transplantation: the role of brain death in donor lung injury. Transplantation. 2003;75:1928–1933.
30. Howlett TA, Keogh AM, Perry L, et al. Anterior and posterior pituitary function in brain-stem-dead donors. A possible role for hormonal replacement therapy. Transplantation. 1989;47(5):828–834.
31. Novitzky D, Cooper DK, Morrell D, et al. Change from aerobic to anaerobic metabolism after brain death, and reversal following triiodothyronine therapy. Transplantation. 1988;45(1):32–36.
32. Birks EJ, Owen VJ, Burton PB, et al. Tumor necrosis factor-alpha is expressed in donor heart and predicts right ventricular failure after human heart transplantation. Circulation. 2000;102(3):326–331.
33. Nijboer WN, Schuurs TA, van der Hoeven JA, et al. Effect of brain death on gene expression and tissue activation in human donor kidneys. Transplantation. 2004;78(7):978–986.
34. Murugan R, Venkataraman R, Wahed AS, et al. Increased plasma interleukin-6 in donors is associated with lower recipient hospital-free survival after cadaveric organ transplantation. Critical Care Medicine. 2008;36(6):1810–1816.
35. de Vries DK, Lindeman JH, Ringers J, et al. Donor brain death predisposes human kidney grafts to a proinflammatory reaction after transplantation. American Journal of Transplantation. 2011;11(5):1064–1070.
36. Damman J, Daha MR, van Son WJ, et al. Crosstalk between complement and Toll-like receptor activation in relation to donor brain death and renal ischemia-reperfusion injury. American Journal of Transplantation. 2011;11(4):660–669.
37. Damman J, Hoeger S, Boneschansker L, et al. Targeting complement activation in brain-dead donors improves renal function after transplantation. Transplant Immunology. 2011;24(4):233–237.
38. Kostulas N, Pelidou SH, Kivisäkk P, et al. Increased IL-1beta, IL-8, and IL-17 mRNA expression in blood mononuclear cells observed in a prospective ischemic stroke study. Stroke; a Journal of Cerebral Circulation. 1999;30(10):2174–2179.
39. Ilmakunnas M, Höckerstedt K, Mäkisalo H, et al. Hepatic IL-8 release during graft procurement is associated with impaired graft function after human liver transplantation. Clinical Transplantation. 2010;24(1):29–35.
40. Hefty TR, Cotterell LW, Fraser SC, et al. Disseminated intravascular coagulation in cadaveric organ donors. Incidence and effect on renal transplantation. Transplantation. 1993;55(2):442–443.
41. Zaroff JG, Rosengard BR, Armstrong WF, et al. Consensus conference report: maximizing use of organs recovered from the cadaver donor: cardiac recommendations, March 28-29, 2001, Crystal City, Va. Circulation. 2002;106(7): 836–841.
42. Bennett WM, Hansen KS, Houghton DC, et al. Disseminated intravascular coagulation (DIC) in a kidney donor associated with transient recipient DIC. American Journal of Transplantation. 2005;5(2):412–414.
43. Valdivia M, Chamorro C, Romera MA, et al. Effect of posttraumatic donor's disseminated intravascular coagulation in intrathoracic organ donation and transplantation. Transplantation Proceedings. 2007;39(7):2427–2428.
44. Domínguez-Gil B, Delmonico FL, Shaheen FA, et al. The critical pathway for deceased donation: reportable uniformity in the approach to deceased donation. Transplant International. 2011;24(4):373–378.
45. Cantin B, Kwok BW, Chan MC, et al. The impact of brain death on survival after heart transplantation: time is of the essence. Transplantation. 2003;76(9): 1275–1279.
46. Inaba K, Branco BC, Lam L, et al. Organ donation and time to procurement: late is not too late. Journal of Trauma. 2010;68(6):1362–1366.
47. Nijboer WN, Moers C, Leuvenink HG, et al. How important is the duration of the brain death period for the outcome in kidney transplantation? Transplant International. 2011;24(1):14–20.
48. Holmquist M, Chabalewski F, Blount T, et al. A critical pathway: guiding care for organ donors. Critical Care Nurse. 1999;19(2):84–98.
49. Thompson TL, Robinson JD, Kenny RW. Family conversations about organ donation. Progress in Transplantation. 2004;14(1):49–55.
50. Chabalewski F, Norris MK. The gift of life: talking to families about organ and tissue donation. The American Journal of Nursing. 1994;94(6):28–33.
51. Rosengard BR, Feng S, Alfrey EJ, et al. Report of the Crystal City meeting to maximize the use of organs recovered from the cadaver donor. American Journal of Transplantation. 2002;2(8):701–711.
52. Wood KE, Becker BN, McCartney JG, et al. Care of the potential organ donor. New England Journal of Medicine. 2004;351(26):2730–2739.
53. Magnus RS, Fridell JA, Vianna RM, et al. Severe hypernatremia in deceased liver donors does not impact early transplant outcome. Transplantation. 2010;90: 438–443.
54. Venkateswaran RV, Patchell VB, Wilson IC, et al. Early donor management increases the retrieval rate of lungs for transplantation. Annals of Thoracic Surgery. 2008;85(1):278–286.
55. Venkateswaran RV, Steeds RP, Quinn DW, et al. The haemodynamic effects of adjunctive hormone therapy in potential heart donors: a prospective randomized double-blind factorially designed controlled trial. European Heart Journal. 2009;30:1771–1780.
56. Kotsch K, Ulrich F, Reutzel-Selke A, et al. Methylprednisolone therapy in deceased donors reduces inflammation in the donor liver and improves outcome after liver transplantation: a prospective randomized controlled trial. Annals of Surgery. 2008;248(6):1042–1050.
57. Kellum JA, Venkataraman R, Powner D, et al. Feasibility study of cytokine removal by hemoadsorption in brain-dead humans. Critical Care Medicine. 2008; 36(1):268–272.
58. Muller E, Khan D, Mendelson M. Renal transplantation between HIV-positive donors and recipients. New England Journal of Medicine. 2010;363:2336–2337.
59. Hagen M, McClean D, Falcon C, et al. Attaining specific donor management goals increases number of organs transplanted per donor: a quality improvement project. Progress in Transplantation. 2009;19:227–231.
60. Malinoski DJ, Daly MC, Patel MS, et al. Achieving donor management goals before deceased donor procurement is associated with more organs transplanted per donor. Journal of Trauma. 2011;71:990–996.
61. Angel LF, Levine DJ, Restrepo MI, et al. Impact of a lung transplantation donor-management protocol on lung donation and recipient outcomes. American Journal of Respiratory and Critical Care Medicine. 2006;174:710–716.
62. Hanna K, Ceder CW, Weinberger JB, et al. Airway pressure release ventilation and successful lung donation. Archives of Surgery. 2011;146:325–328.
63. Cypel M, Yeung JC, Liu M, et al. Normothermic ex vivo lung perfusion in clinical lung transplantation. New England Journal of Medicine. 2011;364:1431–1440.
64. Schunuelle P, Gottmann U, Hoeger S, et al. Effect of donor pretreatment with dopamine on graft function after kidney transplantation. A randomized controlled trial. JAMA. 2009;302:1067–1075.
65. Kucirka LM, Alexander C, Namuyinga R, et al. Viral nucleic acid testing and OPO-level disposition of high risk donor organs. American Journal of Transplantation. 2009;9:620–628.
66. Busch MP, Michael P, Glynn SA, et al. A new strategy for estimating risks of transfusion-transmitted viral infections based on rates of detection of recently infected donors. Transfusion. 2005;45:254–264.
67. Fiebig EW, Wright DJ, Rawal BD, et al. Dynamics of HIV viremia and antibody seroconversion in plasma donors: implications for diagnosis and staging of primary HIV infection. AIDS. 2003;17:1871–1879.
68. Owens SM, Yang C, Spira T, et al. Alternative algorithms for HIV infection diagnosis using tests that are licensed in the US. Journal of Clinical Microbiology. 2008;46:1588–1595.
69. Assal A, Barlet V, Deschaseaux M, et al. Sensitivity of two Hep B virus, Hep C virus, and HIV nucleic acid test systems relative to hep B surface Ag, anti-HCV,

anti HIV, and p24/anti-HIV combination assays in seroconversion panels. Transfusion. 2009;49:301–310.

70. Perry KR, Ramskill S, Eglin RP, et al. Improvement in the performance of HIV screening kits. Transfusion Medicine. 2008;18:228–240.

71. Marshall DA, Kleiman SH, Wong JB, et al. Cost-effectiveness of NAT screening of volunteer blood donations for hep B, hep C, and HIV in the US. Vox Sanguinis. 2004;86:28–40.

72. Kleinman SH, Busch MP. Assessing the impact of HBV NAT on window period reduction and residual risk. Journal of Clinical Virology. 2006;36(Suppl 1): S23–S29.

73. Shafer TJ, Schkade D, Schkade L, et al. Zero risk tolerance costs lives: loss of transplantable organs due to human immunodeficiency virus nucleic acid testing of potential donors. Progress in Transplantation. 2011;21(3):236–247.

74. Humar A, Morris M, Blumberg E, et al. Nucleic Acid Testing (NAT) of organ donors: is the 'Best' test the right test? a consensus conference report. American Journal of Transplantation. 2010;10:889–899.

75. Jensen JU, Hein L, Lundgren B, et al. Kidney failure related to broad-spectrum antibiotics in critically ill patients: secondary end point results from a 1200 patient randomized trial. BMJ (Clinical Research Edition). 2012;2:e000635.

第 21 章 脑死亡后器官获取技术

Rupert Oberhuber, Timm Heinbokel, Zain Khalpey, Sayeed Malek, Stefan G. Tullius

引言

迄今为止，脑死亡供体是用于移植的最大器官来源。在过去十年中，美国每年从脑死亡供体获取的器官数量逐年增加，到 2007 年达到峰值约 28 000 个器官。然而，从那时起，脑死亡供体的数量略有下降。与此同时，心死亡供体的捐献器官越来越多；目前，所有可用器官的 10%以上是在心死亡后从捐献者那里获得的[1,2]。

20 世纪 60 年代后期，哈佛医学院的委员会制订了脑死亡标准，其定义为由创伤、出血或梗死后广泛的和不可逆性中枢神经系统损伤引起的脑和脑干活动的不可逆转性损失[3]。定义脑死亡的临床标准包括昏迷、脑无反应、呼吸暂停、无脑干反射，以及这些表现持续 6~24 小时。虽然验证性测试不是强制性的，但相关的其他验证手段，如脑电图、经颅多普勒超声、体感和脑干听觉诱发电位、脑血流和磁共振成像可能有助于确诊。在确诊之前，必须排除镇静药物、体温过低、休克或可能抑制大脑功能的其他潜在可逆性疾病[4]。

脑死亡导致相当大的全身系统性变化，包括所谓的自主神经风暴、动脉低血压和高血压、凝血功能障碍和电解质平衡异常[5]。本章详细介绍了脑死亡供体器官获取的技术方法，特别关注脑死亡对这些技术的影响。器官获取是一种外科手术，有时会面临极端的意外发生，因此需要快速、精确地实施。对死者异常生理学的理解对于外科医生评估病例并与获取团队协调复苏器官非常重要。关于复苏前脑死亡供体管理的具体细节见第 20 章，第 22 章介绍了在心死亡后从非心脏跳动供体获取器官的具体技术。

脑死亡对心血管系统的深远影响

与脑死亡相关的颅内压的增高导致从大脑到脊髓的缺血（图 21.1）。这导致延髓的疝出，随后是迷走神经运动神经元缺血，最终导致全身性高血压和心动过速。外周缺血是交感神经过载导致血管阻力增加和随后的高血压的结果[6]。

尽管冠状动脉血流增加，心脏灌注仍然很差，导致整个心肌缺血和随后的结构变化，例如，间质出血、弥漫性散在的心内膜下坏死和单核细胞浸润。脑死亡后，“儿茶酚胺风暴”在结构上重塑心肌的方式类似于给予高剂量儿茶酚胺后观察到的变化[7,8]。

大型动物实验表明，心脏交感神经切除术可以限

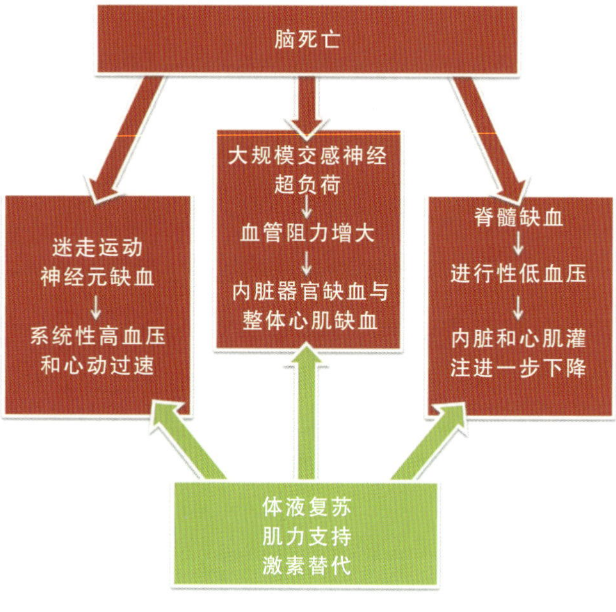

图 21.1　脑死亡后对心血管系统的影响和可能的治疗策略。

制局部儿茶酚胺的作用和脑死亡后的结构重塑。脑损伤的程度和颅内压水平通常与释放的儿茶酚胺的程度成正比[9]。

在最初的高血压后，外周血管阻力下降，脊髓缺血，并导致低血压发生。心脏和外周器官灌注不足是低血压、血管舒张、血容量不足、血管自动调节受损以及内皮依赖性血管舒张功能受损后微循环受损的综合效应[8,10]。

对供体心输出量、外周血管阻力和灌注压的适当管理决定了脑死亡供体器官的质量。液体复苏、正性肌力支持和激素替代通常用于维持供体稳定。脑死亡后的凝血功能障碍导致由游离血红蛋白引起的纤维蛋白沉积和器官损伤。预防这些事件的策略包括积极的补液、激素替代、凝血因子和尽早的器官获取。延迟获取来稳定供体是否有助于改善脑死亡的一些神经体液后果仍然存在争议[5](图 21.1)。

脑死亡导致内分泌发生变化(图 21.2)

脑死亡后的自主神经风暴导致血浆儿茶酚胺水平急剧增加。此外，脑死亡与所谓的垂体前叶和后垂体衰竭有关，导致下丘脑-垂体轴功能障碍。在动物模型中，脑死亡与血浆甲状腺激素、可的松和胰岛素水平显著下降有关。尽管一些临床报道描述了一些发现，但大多数作者认为脑死亡后可的松和胰岛素的水平正常[11,12]。

在存在不同程度的坏死、脑出血和垂体水肿的情况下，促甲状腺激素（TSH）、促肾上腺皮质激素(ACTH)和人生长激素(hGH)大多在正常范围内。然而，已经观察到甲状腺激素的浓度异常，并且 T4 的替代已被证明可以预防血流动力学和代谢改变[13,14]。

脑死亡后，几乎所有患者的垂体后叶功能均受损，导致尿崩症以及随后的血容量不足和电解质紊乱。缺乏血管加压素会加重外周血管扩张，这一点还会因与脑死亡相关的热调节受损而加重[15]。

脑死亡后供体器官的形态变化

脑死亡对器官形态和功能特性有着深远影响，不仅影响短期移植功能，还影响长期移植结果。脑死亡后的全身和局部炎症反应已被广泛探索。但值得注意的是，迄今为止，大多数研究都是描述性的，基本机制仍不清楚。

已经表明，颅内压的剧烈升高与促炎细胞因子(TNF-α、IFN-γ 和 IL-6)，趋化因子和细胞间黏附分子(ICAM、VCAM 和 LFA-1)的增加有关。脑死亡后，在肾脏和心脏中发现细胞浸润增加，可能增加供体器官的

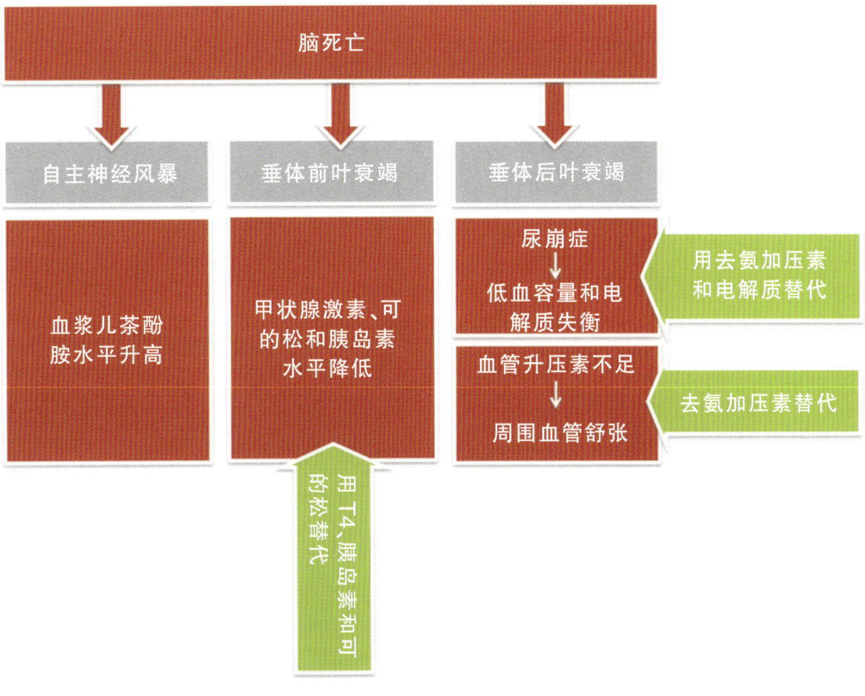

图 21.2 脑死亡的神经体液影响和治疗选择。

免疫原性，并导致强烈的同种免疫反应。假定的病理生理变化包括(图 21.3)：

1.脑死亡后，缺血性脑和脑干中炎性细胞因子的直接释放；

2.由于儿茶酚胺风暴导致的循环淋巴细胞和巨噬细胞的二次释放；

3.内皮细胞活化；

4.由于肠缺血导致的细菌移位[5,16]。

由于脑死亡后的交感风暴减少了冠状动脉灌注，导致的心脏结构变化与心脏缺血后观察到的结果吻合。此外，去甲肾上腺素从位于心外膜的交感神经末梢释放。局部和全身系统效应的结合导致氧气供应与消耗之间的不平衡。结果就是无氧代谢的发生并导致心肌内乳酸盐的积累。来自供体的心脏的形态学标志包括心内膜下坏死和瘀点出血、结蛋白和间质单核细胞浸润缺失。然而，即使在灌注良好的心脏中也会发生这些变化，并且胸交感神经切除术是有一定保护性的，儿茶酚胺的局部作用也似乎是至关重要的[17]。

在脑死亡与血流动力学失衡之后，肾脏灌注受到损害。灌注和炎症反应受损是脑死亡供体移植器官中肾脏损伤的主要原因。常见器官获取前脑死亡供体肾脏的组织形态学变化包括近端肾小管内层变性、内皮增生、周围神经炎、白细胞浸润和间质胶原沉积。此外，脑死亡导致肾脏活力的改变，因为脑死亡供体的肾脏中钠钾比率显著降低[18,19]。

有关脑死亡对肝脏影响的报道有限。肝脏似乎受脑死亡影响较小，可能与器官对灌注的相对抵抗力高有关。形态学特征包括中央和门静脉纤维化、弥漫性细胞坏死、脂肪变性和单核细胞浸润。临床上，供体用类固醇治疗已被证明可以减少肝脏中的促炎细胞因子，从而改善移植器官功能[6,20]。

肺部特别容易在脑死亡后受损，导致结构性损伤和肺水肿。儿茶酚胺的直接毒性作用、左心房压升高、全身性高血压、肺血管收缩和肺内皮损伤都最终导致肺毛细血管通透性增加。此外，液体复苏后的容量过载可能会增加肺水肿并危及气体交换的风险[21]。

心脏不停跳供体器官获取的技术考虑因素

供体的一般准备和定位

在获取程序之前，负责的外科医生需要验证供体的血型已经确定，并与受体血型的相容，供体的病史已经通过审查，并且脑死亡判定已经完成。

成功的器官复苏需要参与器官获取过程的所有手

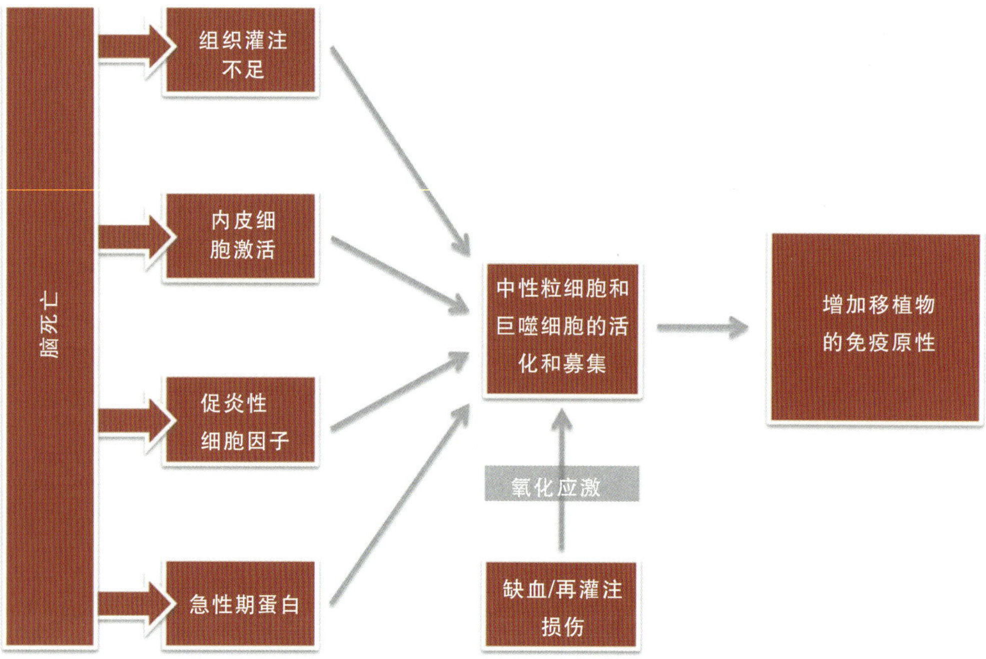

图 21.3 脑死亡后移植物免疫原性增加的病理生理学。

术团队之间的密切协调。主要的捐献外科医生应将获取小组介绍给手术室工作人员，并简要地与所有参与的小组一起审查程序的步骤，以便能够以同步和迅速的方式进行复苏。首先取出心胸器官(心脏和肺)，因为它们最容易受到 I/R 伤害，其次是小肠、肝脏、胰腺和肾脏。肝脏和胰腺可以整体取出，或者可以单独获取。供体仰卧位，双臂展开放置。手术部位备皮，并用无菌布帘覆盖供体。为了获得最佳视野，即使胸部器官不能被取出，也需要从胸骨上到耻骨做一长中线切口[22,23]。图 21.4 显示了暴露范围。电热止血应该用于所有步骤。适当的止血尤其重要，因为脑死亡与全身性外周血管扩张和凝血功能受损有关[24]。

在用胸骨锯进行正中胸骨切开术并且应用电热止血及骨蜡止血之后，插入自保持胸廓牵开器。在肝脏韧带和镰状韧带分离后，可以插入大型腹部牵开器。应切开心包左侧和右侧的隔膜以减轻张力。应彻底游离心包。随后，心包将被稳妥地固定。

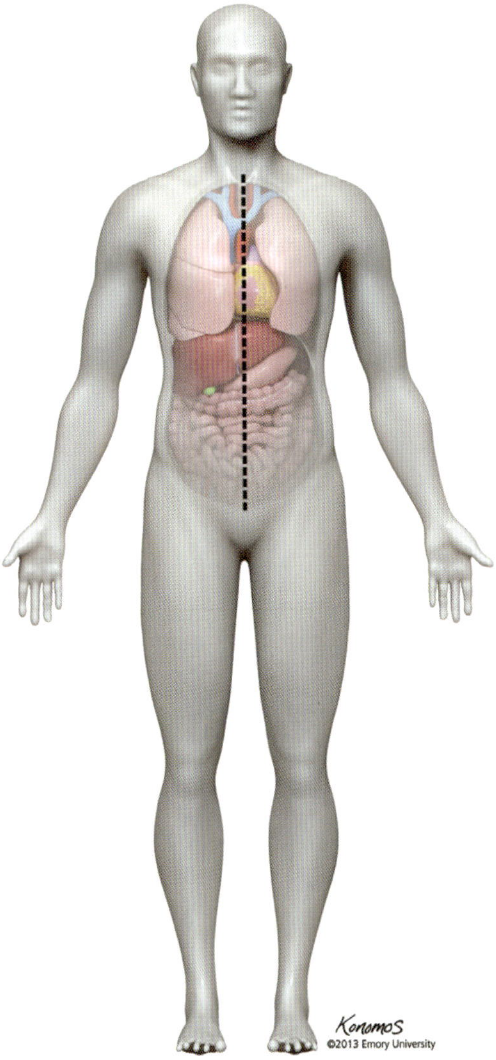

图 21.4 多脏器官获取手术的切口选择。

然后彻底检查所有腹部和胸部器官的明显病理改变。如果没有发现器官获取的潜在禁忌证，并且已确认 ABO 和组织相容性，则应告知受体中心移植程序可以启动[25]。

腹部器官

一般考虑

获取腹部器官有两种不同的技术。首先，“冷冻快速灌注技术”减少了手术时间，推荐用于血流动力学不稳定的供体以及从心死亡供体(DCD)获取器官时[26]。在这种方法中，腹主动脉被暴露并插管，无须进一步解剖，直到原位实现器官的核心冷却。目的是通过快速主动脉插管、放血和冷灌注来尽量减少器官缺血。在给予 30 000IU 肝素后，通过从剑突到耻骨进行中线切口来快速进入腹腔。放置牵开器，露出腹主动脉。将主动脉或髂总动脉和下腔静脉(IVC)插管并开始冲洗。为了快速冷却灌注，肝上腔静脉应从右心房游离出来。然后打开心包并将胸主动脉钳夹。碎冰块被填充在肝脏和肾脏周围，这可能需要进一步游离结肠以使肾脏充分冷却。在完成冷灌注后进行随后的解剖[26]。该程序有关的详细说明和讨论参见第 22 章。

其次，在标准的“维持体温解剖技术”中，在插管和灌注之前进行器官游离性解剖。一些证据表明，这种技术与血管痉挛引起的器官实质和血管损伤有关，可能导致较差的早期移植功能[27]。解剖后 30~60 分钟的复苏期可能能够逆转一部分这些不利影响。另一方面，冷冻解剖可能因更具挑战性的解剖结构而变得复杂。

供体手术有许多不同的方法。一些外科医生更喜欢使用快速技术进行所有获取。其他人使用不同程度的“冷”和“热”解剖。无论采用何种技术，都应精心进行多器官获取，以便能够在不受损害的情况下取出所有器官。供体手术的基本原则包括解剖胸部和腹部的大血管、分离主动脉以准备交叉钳夹、原位灌注和核心冷却，以及快速复苏以防止缺血。

准备步骤和插管

将回肠末端和盲肠与腹膜的附着处游离开，暴露腹膜后间隙。接下来，十二指肠通过 Kocher 切口游离，并且暴露肝下IVC和腹主动脉直至主动脉分叉和髂总动脉。此时,一些外科医生更喜欢在小肠系膜根部分离肠系膜上动脉(SMA),并在其周围放置血管环。这用于控制通过胰腺的主动脉血流量达到1~2L。肠系膜下动脉(IMA)可以在此阶段结扎并分开,注意不要损伤任何肾动脉[28]。在1%~3%的个体中,下肾动脉可以来自髂总动脉[29]。在这些病例中,髂总动脉必须向远端插管以确保附件远端肾动脉的灌注。为了确保血管重建成功,特别是在儿科或肝脏移植中,应保留IMA。对于严重的动脉硬化或远端主动脉动脉瘤,可以对胸主动脉进行插管以进行灌注。

通过断开并结扎圆韧带来游离肝脏。随后,游离镰状、左三角和肝胃韧带。在进行肝胃韧带的解剖之前,应探查源自胃左动脉发出的左肝动脉的存在。这种解剖变异存在于15%~23%的供体中,应谨慎保护[30]。

胆总管恰好位于十二指肠上方,并且可以在肝门后触及右肝动脉的存在。这种解剖变异在10%的供体中发现。接下来解剖肝十二指肠韧带,并且尽可能远离肝门并接近十二指肠,从外侧到内侧开始暴露胆总管。远端胆管用2-0丝线或Vicryl缝合线结扎并断开。

将胆囊管用3-0 Vicryl或Silk缝合线结扎离断之后,将胆囊从其胆囊床上移除,切开并用盐水冲洗胆管,直到来自断开的胆总管的内容物清除。该步骤防止冷藏期间胆管上皮细胞自溶[31]。

然后解剖腹主动脉以准备交叉夹闭。这是通过切开主动脉前筋膜,将食管向左推挤,以及分离右侧的膈肌纤维来完成的。腹主动脉被环绕起来,并在其周围放置止血带。

在插管前至少3分钟给予患者肝素(30 000IU或300IU/kg)。在等待胸部手术的同时,应用湿腹部纱布保护腹部器官。

将止血带绑在髂总动脉分叉处的水平,并行腹主动脉插管。然后抬起第二条带,切开腹主动脉,同时闭塞近端主动脉。插入灌注套管,助手将套管固定。套管尖端应位于肾动脉起点下方。现在可以放置用于门静脉冲洗的第二个插管[32]。

只要静脉切开处远离胰腺边缘,肠系膜上静脉(SMV)也可用于门静脉冲洗。或者,将肠系膜下静脉(IMV)在横结肠的肠系膜根部切开并分离,并插管以进行门静脉冲洗。应小心操作,注意不要将插管推得太深,以免损伤脾静脉。

外科医生应告知整个团队已完成初步解剖和插管,表明应做好冷灌注和器官切除的准备。

灌注

在外科医生横切下腔静脉或右心房并将腹部器官放血到腹部或右胸腔的同时,将腹主动脉用长而直的主动脉夹钳交叉钳夹。打开主动脉和门静脉插管以开始灌注,器官间填充雪泥和碎冰。应在灌注后立即使用冰和冷盐水局部冷却所有腹部器官。在腹膜后和小网膜囊中充满冷却液以允许充分冷却所有器官。

切除肝脏和胰腺

一旦从横断的IVC排出的流出物清亮,外科医生就开始移除腹部器官的过程。心包和膈肌双侧切开:左侧延伸至食管,右侧延伸至肝右叶、肾上腺和IVC后方。这导致肝脏回落至胸腔。始终保持肝脏被冰雪覆盖。图21.5详述了与肝脏和胰腺获取相关的解剖结构。

胃十二指肠动脉在十二指肠的上缘处,并且在近端发自肝总动脉。一旦确定了来自腹腔干动脉的肝总动脉,就可以结扎胃十二指肠动脉。在肝总动脉向近端解剖显露脾动脉,将其从腹腔干动脉的起始部离断。脾动脉不应切入胰腺组织,因为这可能会损伤背侧胰腺动脉分支。

沿着胃大弯解剖,游离胃短管直至膈肌食管裂孔。在幽门的远端将近端十二指肠闭合,并对钉线进行彻底消毒。在交叉钳夹之前,通过鼻胃管用抗真菌溶液冲洗胃和十二指肠。

如果排除了副肝动脉,则将左胃动脉游离并切断。然后将所有脾脏韧带离断并完全游离脾脏。Treitz韧带远端的近端空肠被闭合、离断和消毒;接下来,将脾结肠韧带分开,同时抬起胰腺尾部,将脾脏用作牵拉物。然后使用类似的方法解剖胰腺的背侧。

暴露小肠系膜的根部。然后可以单独结扎、缝合和游离SMA和SMV,注意保持肠系膜缝合线远离胰头和钩突,以避免损伤下胰十二指肠。

门静脉游离到冠状静脉水平,确保肝脏和胰腺均有足够的静脉长度。如果没有获取胰腺,则应在脾静脉汇合处分开门静脉。

然后在直视下切除SMA,确保识别肾动脉,肾动脉通常位于SMA原点的正下方。现在将肝下IVC游离到

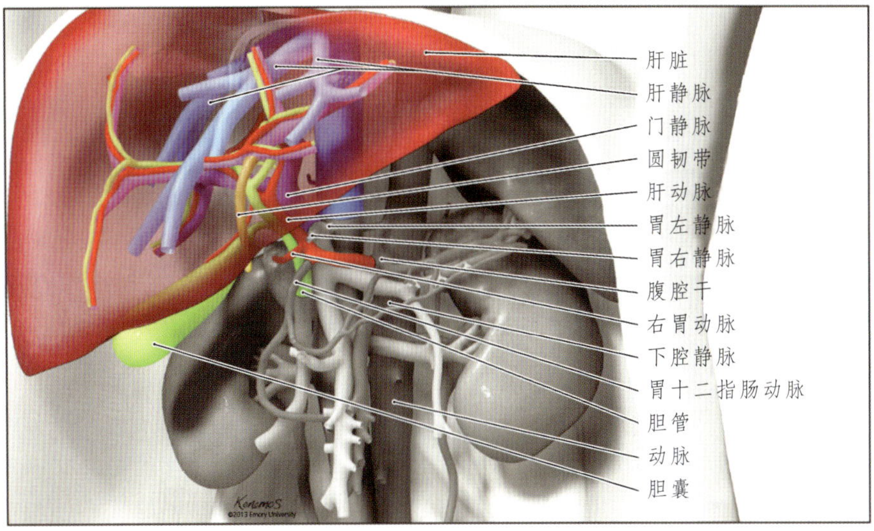

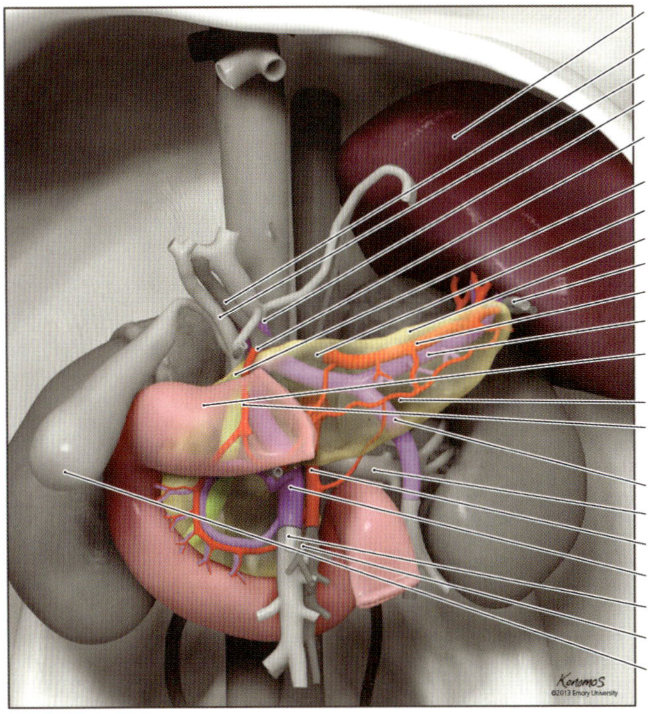

图 21.5 对于肝获取(A)和胰腺获取(B)重要的解剖关系。获取的解剖结构以彩色显示。

肾静脉上方。为了整体游离肝脏和胰腺,左右椎旁肌层(包括右肾上腺和左肾上腺)被分开。然后靠近近端主动脉和腹腔干切除 SMA。腹腔干周围的复杂神经组织可能会使这一步更复杂。如果存在变异的右肝动脉,则应将 SMA 游离至变异动脉的起点远端。在极少数情况下,副肝动脉会穿过胰腺的实质,在这种情况下,器官可能不能被移植[33]。

肾切除术

肾脏可以整体或单独切除。在移除肝脏和胰腺后,结肠和十二指肠被游离并向上收回到上腹部。仔细识别输尿管,留取足够的尿道周围组织以确保血液供应,并尽可能在远端离断。游离 IVC 直到髂总静脉分叉处上方,主动脉在主动脉插管水平处切断。然后通过切开椎前筋膜并使用锐性解剖将肾脏从侧面移动到内侧，并用 Gerota 的筋膜整体移除肾脏[25]。来自 5 岁以下供体的肾脏应始终采用完整的腹主动脉和下腔静脉进行整体获取。

肾脏获取的相关解剖关系如图 21.6 所示。

肾脏的离体准备

左肾静脉在 IVC 的水平离断，右肾保存完整的腔静脉。在成对的腰动脉之间切开主动脉，并且在从内部观察肾动脉的开口之后，分开主动脉的前部以便分离双侧肾脏。不应进行输尿管的进一步准备，因为这可能会影响输尿管的血液供应。通常在整个解剖过程中将止血钳放置在输尿管的尖端以便于识别。但是，输尿管应保持冷却，并且不要长时间暴露在保存液外。

获取髂动脉和静脉

在大多数情况下，髂动脉和静脉，常需与胰腺和（或）肝脏移植一起配合使用。应轻轻解剖髂骨分叉以避免牵引伤。髂内动脉的获取应包括二级分支。在严重动脉硬化的情况下，还应获取头臂动脉干。

小肠

在中线切开术后，应对小肠进行彻底检查，观察其是否有明显的病变，如充血和血肿、水肿、粘连、瘀点出血、血管发育不良或挫伤和腹膜炎的迹象。应评估小肠的活性。小肠被包裹在潮湿的腹部垫中。在获取时，通过鼻胃管输注抗生素（两性霉素 B /庆大霉素和多黏菌素 E）进行选择性肠道去污。

在游离右半结肠和 Kocher 切口后，腹主动脉和 IVC 得到充分暴露直至 SMA 水平（参见第 62 章，了解获取技术和肠道获取细节）。然后游离远端十二指肠和 Treitz 韧带。IMA 和 IMV 被游离暴露，并且显露 SMA 动脉弓。远端腹主动脉和远端 IVC 用两条 0–Vicryl 或 Silk 缝合线结扎。现在将大网膜分开，游离左侧结肠并确定结肠血管。肠道顺行减压是有争议的，并且已经被叫停[22]。

在靠近回盲瓣处用吻合器横切回肠末端，然后进行完整的结肠切除术。游离盲肠和右侧结肠，保留回肠动脉的回肠分支。进一步游离结肠中动脉、左结肠动脉和肠系膜下动脉。将乙状结肠闭合并横切以完全暴露肠系膜根部。在左侧向内侧内脏旋转（所谓的 Mattox 操作）之后，如前所述，游离胰腺尾部和脾脏。现在将近端空肠的肠系膜根部离断，并用距离 Treitz 韧带远 1~2 英寸（2.54~5.08cm）的吻合器分割空肠。SMA 和 SMV 通过于结肠中动脉和静脉水平的肠系膜根的横向解剖暴露[34]。关键是保留 SMA 门静脉轴。

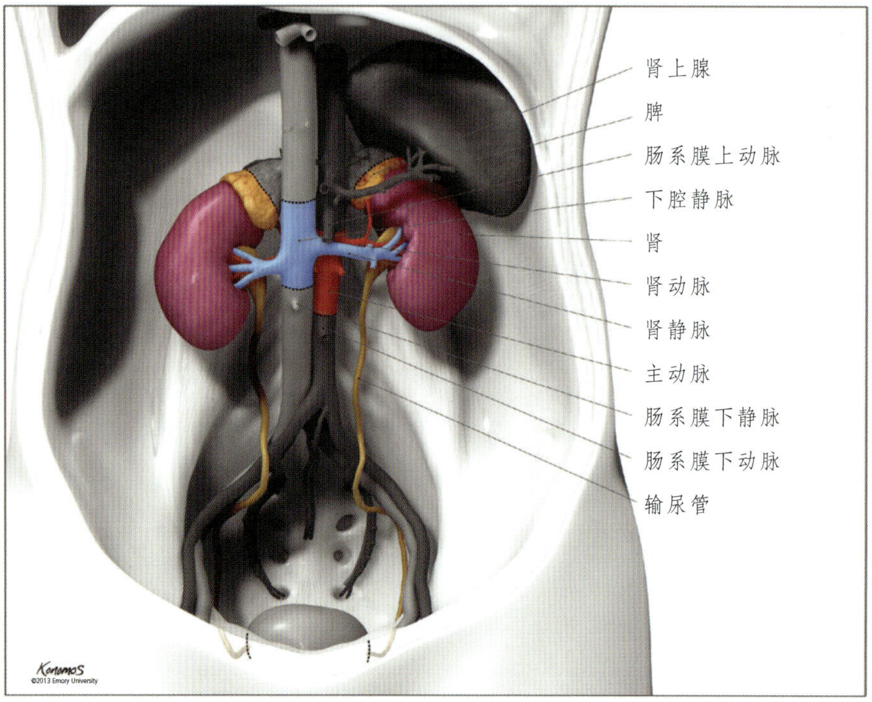

图 21.6 在左右肾脏的获取和准备中重要的解剖学细节。获取的解剖结构以彩色显示。

如果同时采集胰腺和小肠,则需密切注意SMA的早期分支。在这些情况下,应优先采用离体整体清除。胰十二指肠下动脉(IPA)起源于结肠中动脉起点附近,应与胰腺一起保存。由于在移除肝脏时牺牲了胰十二指肠上动脉(SPA),因此IPA的损伤将使胰腺的钩突部分血管供血不足。

在横切幽门远端的十二指肠之前,用缝合线标记肠系膜根的前侧。然后可以结扎左胃动脉并切断到脾脏的胃短血管。腹主动脉在膈肌远端结扎,肝素如前所述给药。腹主动脉交叉夹紧并开始灌注。小肠是灌注后第一个腹腔器官。之后结扎SMA和SMV的亚胰腺部分以防止血液回流到胰腺移植物中。

多器官获取

在腹腔内脏旋转后,胰腺和脾脏得到充分游离,左肝叶也游离至左肝静脉。打开小网膜囊,同时注意保护左肝动脉。将胃结肠韧带打开并暴露到远端食管。然后可以用闭合器横切贲门。接下来,腹膜主动脉游离到在膈肌下方水平,并在施用肝素后夹闭或结扎。开始如前所述的插管和灌注。然后可以整体去除腹部器官(肝脏、胰腺、小肠、胃和结肠)[35]。其他多器官获取和移植的有关细节可以参见第74章。

胸腔器官

一般准备

如前详述,沿中线切开胸廓后,打开心包并固定到皮肤。随后暴露升主动脉(直至主动脉弓)和肺动脉。

暴露上腔静脉(SVC)和IVC,并且在SVC头侧接近奇静脉处使用双重的丝线结扎。然后进行Sondergaard(Waterston)房间沟的解剖,以游离心脏和肺左心房袖口。在分离主动脉和肺动脉之后,将缝合线放置在升主动脉的前中部以插入灌注套管。然后,在肝素(30 000IU)输注至少3分钟后,可以将灌注套管插入升主动脉。使用类似的方法将插管置于远端主肺动脉中。

肺获取团队来决定是否在此时静脉内给予前列腺素。前列腺素E1是一种强有力的血管扩张剂,并且已在一些研究中显示可减少肺的缺血/再灌注损伤。向抗炎细胞因子的转变可能导致这种效应[36]。

相关解剖结构如图21.7所示。

然后在移除所有中心静脉线后将SVC结扎两次。与腹部团队协调,然后将升主动脉尽可能地向远侧交叉夹紧以增加移植组织的量。切开夹闭的IVC。如果仅切除心脏,则切开左肺上静脉或右肺上静脉;如果要获取心脏和肺部,则切开左心耳。如果要以逆行方式灌注肺,则切开肺动脉的主干。

在心脏空跳后开始灌洗保存过程。腹部灌注可以同时开始。在重力下通过肺动脉给予肺灌洗液,同时在80mmHg的压力下输注心脏停搏液。立即开始用冰水进行局部冷却。

通过小幅减少潮气量将冰盐水置于胸膜腔中,可以改善肺脏外部冷却。同理,向心包给予冷盐水溶液促进心脏冷却。呼吸停搏约需要5L冷Perfadex®肺保存液,而心脏停搏需要至少1L的冷晶体心脏停搏液。如果呼吸停搏和心跳停搏都需要的话,应在呼吸停搏期间持续输注心脏停搏液。在输注心脏停搏液期间必须持续监测主动脉根部压力和有无心室扩张。快速终止收缩和电活动终止是心脏停搏的标志。持续的电活动可能与未知的冠状动脉疾病或左心室肥大有关。在这种情况下,应使用更长时间的心脏停搏液灌注。在呼吸停搏期间,灌注液必须均匀地分布在两个肺部,并且应仔细监测左心房灌注液自由流动的逐渐减少过程。

在心脏停搏后,移除灌注套管并结扎缝合线。在SVC与升主动脉之间切开后心包以解剖隆突上方的气管。充分游离气管的前、外侧和内侧,以便在肺切除期间更快地找到气管。

切除心脏

游离IVC和SVC并切断。如果仅采集心脏,则肺静脉也在结扎线之间切断。如果要移除心脏和肺,则在左心房中形成横切口,在肺静脉周围留下足够大的左心房袖带。切口在左下肺静脉和冠状窦之间的中点处开始,向左心耳的基部和右侧的IVC的下缘延伸。然后将后心膜与后心包分开,可以从后纵隔游离左心房。

SVC和奇静脉在奇静脉上方和SVC结扎线的正下方横切。分开无名和左颈动脉。主动脉和肺动脉应尽可能在远端分开。然后可以移除心脏,并在离体后进行最终检查。其他细节和插图可以参见第58章。

肺切除

在获取程序开始之前,应进行支气管镜检查以明

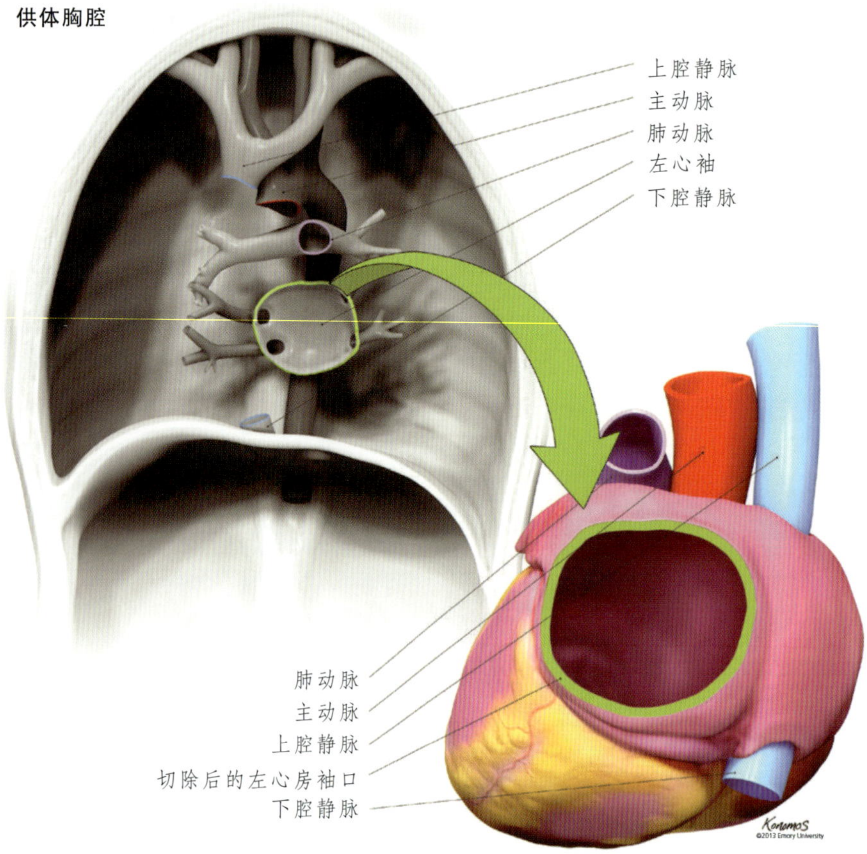

图 21.7 在(A)心脏(在获取肺之前)和(B)肺获取(在心脏已经获取之后)中重要的解剖关系。获取的解剖结构以彩色显示。(待续)

确肺部炎症、水肿、撕裂以及痰液的量和浓度。应留取痰液样品并进行支气管灌洗。此外,应进行动脉血气检查和胸部X线检查。

在胸骨切开术前应立即断开呼吸机，以避免在通气期间损伤肺部。

在沿中线胸骨切开后，无须烧灼止血直接进入胸膜腔,以防止肺部受伤。提起双肺,然后触诊肺部并彻底检查。我们关心的指标和病变包括尺寸和外观、粘连、肺不张、融合、漏气、肺大疱或水肿肿胀,以及其他任何病变。对于可能会影响移植进程或器官功能的异常应立即报告给受体的移植团队。其他细节和插图可以参见第70章。

将主肺动脉从升主动脉解剖出来,并将SVC与右肺动脉分开。置管后，取出所有中心静脉管并继续通气。结扎SVC并在膈肌正上方切开IVC。

打开左心耳以减压左心室。如果不获取心脏,则切开左心房。然后将升主动脉交叉夹闭并用心脏停搏液灌注。在排除左心室扩张后,可以开始肺灌注。此时应立即开始局部冷却，并使用吸引器去除灌注过程中的任何流出物。

在心脏和肺部停搏之后,两个插管被移除,断开呼吸机,将胸膜向两侧广泛张开。沿着肺门前方的膈神经移除前方心包。然后横向切除心包的后部。切断左侧的下肺韧带，暴露左肺并向右移动。靠近食管并向上解剖,将降主动脉在左锁骨下动脉的起点下方横断。对于右肺重复该步骤,其中解剖部位延伸至奇静脉的水平。

然后将远离气管的所有颈部血管断开。轻轻按摩两个肺并手动充气至30cmH_2O压力直至所有的肺不张组织完全扩张。然后将充气保持在中等通气水平,并且在移除气管导管后尽可能靠近头部切开闭合气管。离断所有剩余的纵隔黏连，堵塞双肺气管并从胸腔移除[37,38]。

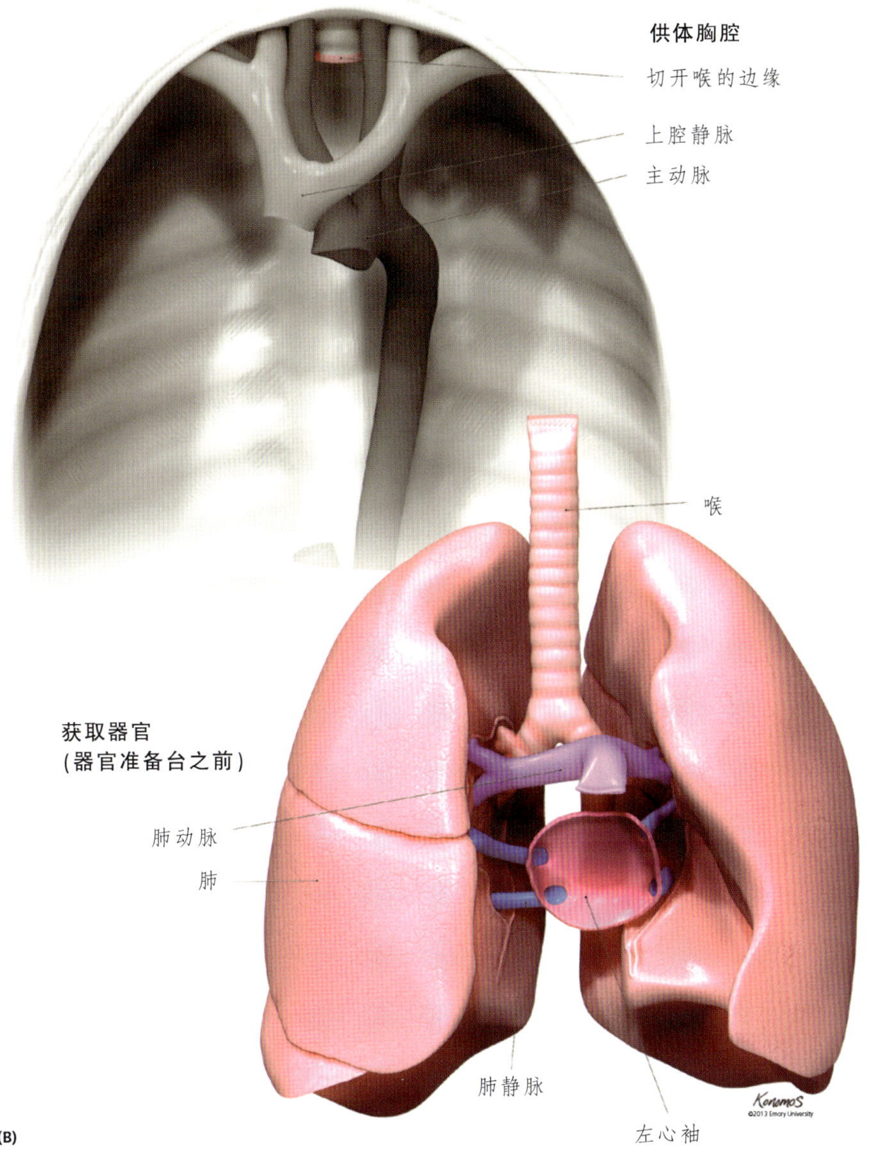

图 21.7(续)

肺部的离体准备

重新检查移出的双肺以除外所有前面提到的病变。将导尿管插入肺静脉逆行冲洗肺部，以便去除血栓栓塞物质，并确保保存液均匀分布到肺部。

应避免进一步解剖左支气管和右支气管以保护血管。只有当左肺和右肺分开移植时，两个支气管应该在隆突处用吻合器分开。

心脏和肺部整块清除

将胸膜和心包切除至肺门。然后将 SVC、IVC 和主动脉分开，尽可能多地留取心脏移植物的血管长度。

然后如前所述将气管切开闭合。为了整体切除心脏和肺部，应离断食管、主动脉、奇静脉和下肺动脉韧带上方的结缔组织[39]。

器官储存

从供体取出器官后，将器官置于无菌袋中，保持灌注溶液在 4℃下。将无菌袋放入装有无菌的冷冻林格乳酸盐或盐水的袋子中，并在这两个袋子外放置第三个空袋子，然后小心地将其标记并放入装有碎冰的保温运输箱中。肾脏、单肺和半肝分开存放，并且将明确的标签贴在第三个袋子上。将血管放入带有灌注溶液的单独袋中。将血液样本和脾脏段（或者，如果不存在，淋巴结）放入具有冷冻林格乳酸盐或盐水的盒子中。有关离体移植器官或捐供体的任何相关信息应核对并留置在运输箱中或附在运输箱上。然后应告知移植团队器官获取程序已完成。

获取后供体护理

在器官获取程序完成后，应除去供体内所有异物和液体，并仔细缝合所有伤口，并用伤口敷料覆盖。一定要注意，在我们充满敬意的转交尸体之前，尽量不要留下可见的痕迹。

总结

器官获取是一种要求十分严格的手术，术者通常在有时间压力和血流动力学不稳定的情况下进行手术。该手术通常在外科医生不熟悉的手术室中进行，在耗费精力的晚上进行，并且与之前没有合作过的其他外科同事一起进行。因此，该过程需要关于整个胸部和腹部解剖学的特殊知识以及对脑死亡的可预期后果的具体理解。手术前应有具体的手术计划，并在获取手术开始前解决潜在的风险。需知，供体获取是许多受体能够成功移植的第一步，也是向其他医院展示移植实力的机会。毫无疑问，它是器官移植领域中非常重要的一部分，并且确实是每个供体捐献移植成功的基础。

（张云凯 译 李照 校）

参考文献

1. http://optn.transplant.hrsa.gov/ar2009/. [accessed February 5, 2012]
2. Steinbrook R. Organ donation after cardiac death. New England Journal of Medicine. 2007;357(3):209–213.
3. A definition of irreversible coma. Report of the Ad Hoc Committee of the Harvard Medical School to Examine the Definition of Brain Death. JAMA. 1968;205(6):337–340.
4. Wijdicks EF. The diagnosis of brain death. New England Journal of Medicine. 2001;344(16):1215–1221.
5. Pratschke J, Neuhaus P, Tullius SG. What can be learned from brain-death models? Transplant International. 2005;18(1):15–21.
6. van Der Hoeven JA, Ter Horst GJ, Molema G, et al. Effects of brain death and hemodynamic status on function and immunologic activation of the potential donor liver in the rat. Annals of Surgery. 2000;232(6):804–813.
7. Galinanes M, Hearse DJ. Brain death-induced impairment of cardiac contractile performance can be reversed by explantation and may not preclude the use of hearts for transplantation. Circulation Research. 1992;71(5):1213–1219.
8. Szabo G, Buhmann V, Bahrle S, et al. Brain death impairs coronary endothelial function. Transplantation. 2002;73(11):1846–1848.
9. Mertes PM, Burtin P, Carteaux JP, et al. Brain death and myocardial injury: role of cardiac sympathetic innervation evaluated by in vivo interstitial microdialysis. Transplantation Proceedings. 1994;26(1):231–232.
10. Okamoto S, Corso CO, Kondo T, et al. Changes in hepatic microcirculation and histomorphology in brain-dead organ donors: an experimental study in rats. European Journal of Surgery. 1999;165(8):759–766.
11. Meyers CH, D'Amico TA, Peterseim DS, et al. Effects of triiodothyronine and vasopressin on cardiac function and myocardial blood flow after brain death. Journal of Heart and Lung Transplantation. 1993;12(1 Pt 1):68–79; discussion 80.
12. Wicomb WN, Cooper DK, Novitzky D. Impairment of renal slice function following brain death, with reversibility of injury by hormonal therapy. Transplantation. 1986;41(1):29–33.
13. Gramm HJ, Meinhold H, Bickel U, et al. Acute endocrine failure after brain death? Transplantation. 1992;54(5):851–857.
14. Taniguchi S, Kitamura S, Kawachi K, et al. Effects of hormonal supplements on the maintenance of cardiac function in potential donor patients after cerebral death. European Journal of Cardio-Thoracic Surgery. 1992;6(2):96–101; discussion 102.
15. Howlett TA, Keogh AM, Perry L, et al. Anterior and posterior pituitary function in brain-stem-dead donors. A possible role for hormonal replacement therapy. Transplantation. 1989;47(5):828–834.
16. Toyama H, Takada M, Suzuki Y, et al. Brain death-induced expression of ICAM-1 and VCAM-1 on rat hepatocytes. Hepato-Gastroenterology. 2003;50(54):1854–1856.
17. Wilhelm MJ, Pratschke J, Beato F, et al. Activation of the heart by donor brain death accelerates acute rejection after transplantation. Circulation. 2000;102(19):2426–2433.
18. Pratschke J, Wilhelm MJ, Kusaka M, et al. Accelerated rejection of renal allografts from brain-dead donors. Annals of Surgery. 2000;232(2):263–271.
19. Koo DD, Welsh KI, McLaren AJ, et al. Cadaver versus living donor kidneys: impact of donor factors on antigen induction before transplantation. Kidney International. 1999;56(4):1551–1559.
20. Jassem W, Koo DD, Cerundolo L, et al. Leukocyte infiltration and inflammatory antigen expression in cadaveric and living-donor livers before transplant. Transplantation. 2003;75(12):2001–2007.
21. Avlonitis VS, Fisher AJ, Kirby JA, et al. Pulmonary transplantation: the role of brain death in donor lung injury. Transplantation. 2003;75(12):1928–1933.
22. Wunderlich H, Brockmann JG, Voigt R, et al. DTG procurement guidelines in heart beating donors. Transplant International. 2011;24(7):733–757.
23. Abu-Elmagd K, Fung J, Bueno J, et al. Logistics and technique for procurement of intestinal, pancreatic, and hepatic grafts from the same donor. Annals of Surgery. 2000;232(5):680–687.
24. McKeown DW, Bonser RS, Kellum JA. Management of the heartbeating brain-dead organ donor. British Journal of Anaesthesia. 2012;108(Suppl 1):i96–i107.
25. Rosenthal JT, Shaw BW Jr, Hardesty RL, et al. Principles of multiple organ procurement from cadaver donors. Annals of Surgery. 1983;198(5):617–621.
26. Reich DJ, Mulligan DC, Abt PL, et al. ASTS recommended practice guidelines for controlled donation after cardiac death organ procurement and transplantation. American Journal of Transplantation. 2009;9(9):2004–2011.
27. Imagawa DK, Olthoff KM, Yersiz H, et al. Rapid en bloc technique for pancreas-liver procurement. Improved early liver function. Transplantation. 1996;61(11):1605–1609.
28. Starzl TE, Miller C, Broznick B, et al. An improved technique for multiple organ harvesting. Surgery, Gynecology and Obstetrics. 1987;165(4):343–348.
29. Kok NF, Dols LF, Hunink MG, et al. Complex vascular anatomy in live kidney donation: imaging and consequences for clinical outcome. Transplantation. 2008;85(12):1760–1765.
30. Hiatt JR, Gabbay J, Busuttil RW. Surgical anatomy of the hepatic arteries in 1000 cases. Annals of Surgery. 1994;220(1):50–52.
31. Moench C, Moench K, Lohse AW, et al. Prevention of ischemic-type biliary lesions by arterial back-table pressure perfusion. Liver Transplantation. 2003;9(3):285–289.
32. de Ville de Goyet J, Hausleithner V, Malaise J, et al. Liver procurement without in situ portal perfusion. A safe procedure for more flexible multiple organ harvesting. Transplantation. 1994;57(9):1328–1332.
33. Sollinger HW, Vernon WB, D'Alessandro AM, et al. Combined liver and pancreas procurement with Belzer-UW solution. Surgery. 1989;106(4):685–690; discussion 90–91.
34. Sindhi R, Fox IJ, Heffron T, et al. Procurement and preparation of human isolated small intestinal grafts for transplantation. Transplantation. 1995;60(8):771–773.
35. Nakazato PZ, Concepcion W, Bry W, et al. Total abdominal evisceration: an en bloc technique for abdominal organ harvesting. Surgery. 1992;111(1):37–47.

36. de Perrot M, Fischer S, Liu M, et al. Prostaglandin E1 protects lung transplants from ischemia-reperfusion injury: a shift from pro- to anti-inflammatory cytokines. Transplantation. 2001;72(9):1505–1512.
37. Zenati M, Dowling RD, Armitage JM, et al. Organ procurement for pulmonary transplantation. Annals of Thoracic Surgery. 1989;48(6):882–886.
38. Brodman RF, Goldsmith J, Veith FJ, et al. A technique for donor lung procurement and preservation for transplantation after completion of cardiac donation. Surgery, Gynecology and Obstetrics. 1988;166(4):363–366.
39. Hinkamp TJ, Montoya A, Bakhos M, et al. Heart and lung grafts harvested en bloc: operative technique, utilization, and results. Annals of Thoracic Surgery. 1993; 56(6):1381–1385.

第 22 章 心脏死亡后器官获取技术

Chandrasekar Santhanakrishnan, Anthony M. D'Alessandro

引言

在 1968 年通过脑死亡标准之前，大多数器官捐献的病例主要是无心脏跳动供体类型[1]。脑死亡作为死亡的标准在很大程度上是由哈佛大学专题委员会努力推动的，而且目前已经普遍接受这一原则，其中西方国家的大多数器官捐献是来自脑死亡供体或活体供体。在这两种情况下，器官获取、组织灌注同时持续进行。在 20 世纪 90 年代初，由于器官持续短缺和不断增长的等待名单死亡，人们对心脏死亡后捐献(DCD)产生新的兴趣，即从心肺停止的死亡个体中去除器官，并伴有进行性热缺血。本章将讨论 DCD 捐献者器官的获取技术。从脑死亡供体或活体肾脏或肝脏供体的器官获取的具体技术，可分别参阅第 21、23 和 24 章。

定义

DCD 供体是遭受毁灭性和不可逆性神经性损伤但不符合脑死亡标准的患者；或其死亡情况妨碍正式的脑死亡申报。死亡由心肺功能丧失决定，并按照 Maastricht 标准分类[2]：

第 1 类 – 到达医院时死亡；

第 2 类 – 复苏后死亡；

第 3 类 – 计划撤除生命支持后的死亡；

第 4 类 – 心脏骤停而脑死亡。

DCD 可以分为两类：可控和不可控。在不可控制的情况下，患者通常在到达医院之前已经心肺停止，进行或没有进行心肺复苏干预。在选定的中心，并在既定协议的指导下，一些已宣布心肺呼吸标准死亡的患者被置于心肺支持通路以维持一定程度的灌注到器官，通常不包括脑血管再灌注[3]。在可控情况下，患者在重症监护室(ICU)或手术室(OR)中进行生命支持撤除。死亡是由目睹心肺停止而宣告的，此后进行器官获取。我们的经验主要来自可控环境。然而，获取的技术细节在这两种情况下是相似的，包括器官获取的手段，灌注保鲜溶液和冰冻。

结论

DCD 捐献中的关键问题是由于心脏功能障碍，在获取、快速灌注和冷却过程中影响器官的热缺血。这影响器官的活性程度和移植后功能。然而，有越来越多的证据表明，脑死亡可能对器官的质量存在有害影响(见第 21 章)。从 DCD 供体中获取的器官可能不会遭受这种相同的炎症级联反应[4]。关于 DCD 供体器官相对于其他类别的供体器官的结果更完整的讨论可见第 65 章。

DCD 肾脏的结果比肝脏更令人鼓舞。Weber 等的研究已经表明，尽管 DCD 肾中早期移植肾功能障碍的比率较高，但移植肾和患者长期存活相当于脑死亡供体来源的肾脏[5]。DCD 供体的移植存活率在 10 年时为 78%；相比之下，脑死亡供体来源的肾为 76%。

Rudich 等的另一项研究在 1993 年和 2000 年之间，美国的 708 例 DCD 器官受者与 97 990 例脑死亡受者相比较[6]。与接受来自脑死亡供体器官的受体(23.3%)相比，DCD 肾受体具有更高的延迟肾功能恢复率(42.4%)。然而，同种异体移植存活率在 6 年结束时是相似的(DCD 为 73.2%，脑死亡为 72.5%)。

来自 DCD 供体的肝移植的结果比对于肾移植的结果差。尽管如此，DCD 捐献者在缩小移植肝脏供求之间差距方面发挥了重要作用，特别是当个体化风险–利益评估被特别考虑并被认为是有利时。Abt 等审查了从联合国索马里数据库获得的结果[7]。他们比较了从

144 个 DCD 供体采集的肝脏和 26 856 个脑死亡供体的肝脏。DCD 组的 1 年移植存活率较低(80%对 85%)。与脑死亡组相比,DCD 接受者具有更高的再移植率(14%对 8%)。

Foley 等也报道了从 DCD 供体获得的肝脏中血管和胆汁相关并发症的更高的发生率[8]。DCD 组在 1 年结束时的胆管狭窄率较高(33%对 10%)。然而,两组的肝动脉血栓形成和原发性无功能的发生率相同。这项研究还发现,与脑死亡组相比,DCD 组的移植物和患者存活率更差。DCD 组的亚组分析显示,与 40 岁以上的供体相比,40 岁以下的 DCD 供体具有更好的结果。来自 DCD 供体 40 岁以下的肝脏的 3 年移植肝存活率比来自超过 40 岁的 DCD 供体组(65%对 45%)的肝脏更好,尽管这不是统计学显著的。对于 3 年的患者存活率也是如此。

使用 DCD 供体的胰腺移植的结果是可接受的,尽管可能经受显著的选择偏倚。Qureshi 等比较了 2008 年和 2011 年之间, 在英国接受 DCD 供体的胰腺和那些从脑死亡供体接受胰腺的患者[9]。他们注意到,各组之间 1 年时移植物血栓形成率或血红蛋白 A1c 水平没有差异。胰移植存活率也没有显著差异。

由 Bellingham 等做的更大的研究在威斯康星大学也有类似的结果[10]。他们比较了 1993 年至 2008 年的患者。在 DCD 与脑死亡组之间,1 年、3 年和 10 年的胰腺移植物和患者存活率是相似的。此外,围术期并发症如组间血栓形成、胰漏和脓肿形成没有差异。

术前阶段

潜在捐献者在转诊到器官获取组织（OPO）后确定。这些患者具有毁灭性脑损伤,但没有达到脑死亡标准。这样的患者已被确定没有明显的机会康复。必须明确,移植团队不参与这些医疗决定。此外,作为 DCD 的潜在候选者的患者,在他/她心脏骤停后宣布死亡之前不是合法死亡或捐献者。

威斯康星大学 DCD 模型

成功的 DCD 恢复的关键是能够预测临床死亡是否会在支持撤除的 2 小时内发生。威斯康星大学已经开发了一种标准来评估潜在的 DCD 供体,并预测患者是否将在设定的时间内死亡, 从而使他/她成为 DCD 供体(表 22.1)[11]。基于以下内容计算得分:患者年龄、体重指数(BMI)、氧气饱和度、插管方法、自主呼吸水平和按压需求。如果得分较高,则患者在撤回支持后在适当的时间段内死亡的可能性较高。同样存在其他模型,但是模型之间的预期比较没有验证一个或另一个明显优越。

表 22.1　威斯康星大学标准,用于在撤回生命支持后预测心搏停止(死亡后捐献的评估工具)

标准	分值	患者评分
10 分钟后自发呼吸		
频率> 12	1	
频率<12	3	
TV> 200mL	1	
TV<200mL	3	
NIF> 20	1	
NIF <20	3	
无自发呼吸	9	
体重指数		
25	1	
25~29	2	
> 30	3	
减压器		
没有升压药	1	
单升压药	2	
多种升压药	3	
患者年龄		
0~30 岁	1	
31~50 岁	2	
>51 岁	3	
气管插管		
气管导管	3	
气管切开术	1	
10 分钟后充氧		
氧气饱和度> 90%	1	
氧气饱和度 80%~89%	2	
氧气饱和度<79%	3	
最终评分		
拔管日期拔管时间		
呼气日期呼气时间		
总时间		
TV=潮气量;NIF =负吸气力		
患者评分		
8~12 分:拔管后继续呼吸的高风险;		
13~18 分:拔管后继续呼吸的中度风险;		
19~24 分:拔管后继续呼吸的风险低。		

Reproduced from Lewis et al. [11], with permission from NATCO.

知情同意

器官捐献只有在家庭与原始治疗团队协商后决定撤除支持时才讨论。一旦患者被视为捐献者,就会从最近的亲属或其法定代理人那里获得详细的同意书。可以获得在死亡之前进行的程序的意见,例如,股动脉和静脉导管的放置,以及施用诸如肝素、酚妥拉明、两性霉素 B、微晶体、维生素 E 和泼尼松(Anderson M,个人交流)。

家人还保证,器官捐献不会发生,直到患者已经死亡并且由正在照顾患者并且独立于移植团队的医生宣布死亡。家人还被告知患者不能在设定的时间内(通常为 2 小时)死亡的可能性,并且这将阻止患者成为器官供体。如果发生这种情况,患者将被带回 ICU,在那里他/她将在没有器官捐献的情况下死亡。在实践中,根据具体的 OPO 方案,供体的血流动力学状态以及供体是否是潜在的肝脏供体等因素,在实践中可能存在变化。重要的是,这些局部变化对于维持 DCD 过程的完整性至关重要。因此,获取小组的成员必须认识和尊重现行环境下有关获取的具体指导方针。

生前药物管理

如上所述,OPO 可以在撤回支持之前从患者家属获得使用特殊药物的同意。这些药物可以使缺血/再灌注损伤最小化,并且具有在植入后改善器官功能的潜力。有一些证据表明,生前治疗可能对血管内皮有保护作用,因此对移植器官有益[12]。

在撤回支持之前使用肝素以降低捐献器官血栓的风险。肝素可能加速死亡的理论,缺乏证据。酚乙胺可以在获取之前输注以预防血管痉挛并促进适当的器官灌注。此药剂可能导致血压暂时下降;然而,这不认为促进心脏死亡。无论如何,最重要的原则是,移植小组不能干预死亡的进展,在这方面的怀疑应该解决,以消除家庭或捐献者护理团队的参与成员的任何关注。

手术技术

DCD 复苏的目标是快速获取器官以最小化热缺血损伤,确保器官不受损伤并且可用于移植的技术。外科恢复团队和捐献医院或团队之间的沟通是至关重要的。

在文献中已经描述了快速获取的不同方法。我们将描述在威斯康星大学使用的复苏方法[13]。

在手术室中的 DCD 复苏是优选的。这最小化在将患者运送到手术室时丢失的时间,并且在宣布死亡之后准备患者器官复苏。在撤除支持之前和之后,患者的家庭成员有机会与捐献者在一起。

促使从患者撤除生命支持的所有操作完全由负责照顾患者的医生来判断执行。外科手术复苏组不参与这些决定。如前所述,在撤除支持之前,并且在来自家庭和护理团队的同意的情况下,我们使用 30 000 IU 的肝素,10~20mg 的酚妥拉明和 12.5~25g 的甘露醇。相关药物管理,股动脉/静脉截取和撤回之前可能的插管将从家属授权。镇静剂、局部麻醉剂或麻醉剂由原始治疗小组自行决定使用,但不应由移植小组管理,或以促进心肺死亡的目的给予。

一旦患者被带到 OR,他/她就准备好,并从下颌到大腿近端披上手术巾。我们暴露股动脉和静脉,并在撤除生命支持之前插管(图 22.1)。这种手术使用局部麻

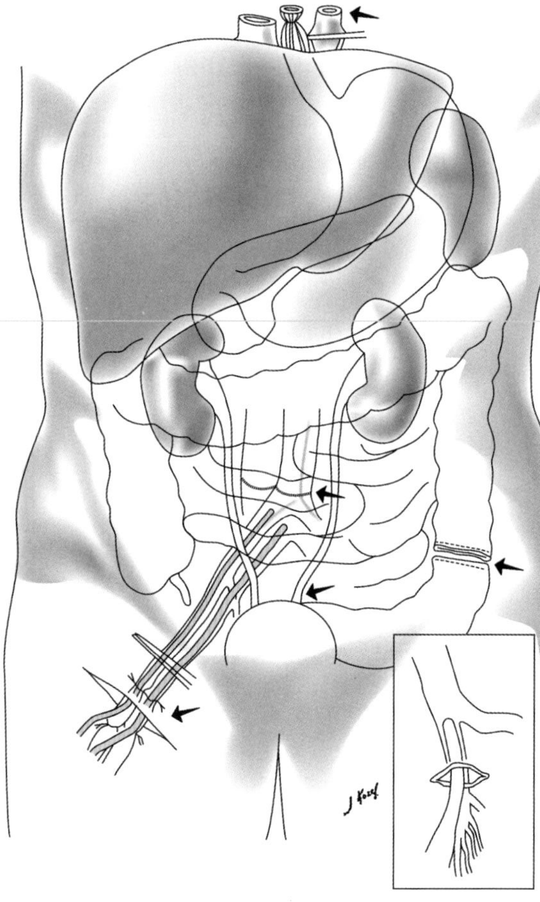

图 22.1 快速整体切除所有腹内器官的技术。箭头指示主要步骤,灌洗置管由离体肠系膜上/门静脉灌洗。(Redrawn from D'Alessandro et al.[13], with permission from Wolters Kluwer Health.)

醉进行。在此期间，重要的是认识到潜在的 DCD 供体是仍然存活的患者。18~20F 插管保持准备用于插管，这通常在患者宣告死亡并且强制 5 分钟等待时间过去之后进行。冷藏的保存溶液也保持准备好，管道打开，用于快速输注。

一旦执行如上所述的生前预干预，手术获取的成员离开 OR。OPO 的成员通常在退出过程中出现在手术室中。他/她记录在撤回支持后每分钟的血流动力学测量，以及死亡的确诊时间，5 分钟的等待时间，获取复苏开始时的时间和器官冲洗的时间。这些数据对于移植团队决定器官是否可用于移植是至关重要的。

患者的主要治疗团队撤除支持。该团队监测患者并记录心肺功能停止的时间。一旦捐献者被医生宣布死亡，我们在开始获取和灌注保存液之前等待另外 5 分钟。5 分钟的等待期是根据 1997 年出版的医学研究所指南[14]。确保不可逆转死亡的等待期问题一直在辩论。等待期是确保在心肺停止发生后没有自动复苏。DeVita 等审查了 1912—1970 年 108 例患者死亡而他们的生命体征受到监测的病例报告[15]。他们没有发现任何自动复苏的证据，在 65 秒后出现心肺停止。因此，重症监护医学学会认可了 2 分钟的等待期[16]。因此，这方面的辩论仍在继续。由于没有证据表明额外的 3 分钟改变结果，但更长的等待时间仍需谨慎。

在等待时间过去之后，外科手术获取复苏组返回到 OR。用预选的套管插入股动脉。将插管插入到大约耳廓交叉点。开始用冷保存溶液快速冲洗。同时，进行中间胸骨切开术，并且腹部从剑突到耻骨联合处急剧打开。打开心包并切开右心房。这用作冲洗溶液的流出口。股骨静脉也可以在胸部和腹部打开时切开作为通气孔。然后识别并夹紧胸主动脉。这确保腹部器官获得大部分冷冲洗。输注 2~3L 的保存溶液。腹部需充满冰块。

一旦冲洗完成并且流出物澄清，开始进行整体腹部器官的复苏。使用 GIA 缝合器分割食管。在胸主动脉上放置大夹子；这是一个有用的回缩工具。解剖开始于右心房的水平，所有腹膜后组织与隔膜一起快速分开。注意保持在椎体前方、主动脉和腔静脉后方。这个解剖平面一直延伸到主动脉分叉处。

然后将器官置于其解剖位置。左结肠和右结肠的侧向组织被游离。输尿管被识别并分开至膀胱。解剖进行到正好在主动脉分叉之上的水平。止血器放置在输尿管使它们容易识别。远端主动脉和静脉游离到分叉处。然后使用 GIA 缝合器分割乙状结肠。任何剩余的腹膜后组织被分开。然后整体取出腹部内脏，并放置在带有冰的大盆中。该程序的这一部分的通常操作时间小于 15~20 分钟。

一旦器官已被整体取出，肠系膜下静脉或肠系膜上静脉的分支被鉴定和插管。将 1L 保存溶液通过入口灌注。胆总管也被识别并分开接近十二指肠。胆道系统用 50mL 保存溶液冲洗。胆囊也被打开并且其内容物被排空，也用冰生理盐水冲洗。

主动脉的后壁纵向打开。明确腹腔干、肠系膜上动脉(SMA)和肾动脉孔。腹腔和 SMA 各自用 500mL 保存溶液冲洗。右肾动脉和左肾动脉也用 500mL 保存溶液冲洗。然后将整个器官储存在 4℃的保存溶液中，并转移到移植中心的离体器官准备台进一步修整。作为替代，器官可以在供体手术室中分开以运送到多个移植中心。

在完成供体操作之前，获得髂静脉和动脉用于可能的血管重建。保存溶液的选择仍然是有争论的问题，以及在获取之后对器官，特别是肾脏的静脉灌注与脉冲灌注的选择。这些要点的进一步讨论可以参见第 25 章和第 26 章。

Casavilla 等从匹兹堡中心已经描述了一种“超快速”技术(图 22.2 和图 22.3)[17]。在该技术中，腹部从剑突到耻骨联合开放。远端主动脉被识别并插管。开始用

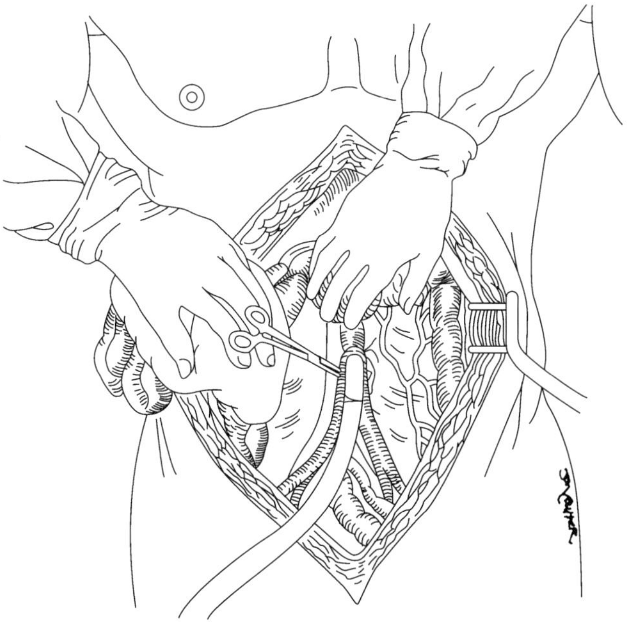

图 22.2　超快速技术。中线腹部切口和主动脉插管可立即冷保存溶液灌注。(Redrawn from Casavilla et al.[17], with permission from Wolters Kluwer Health.)

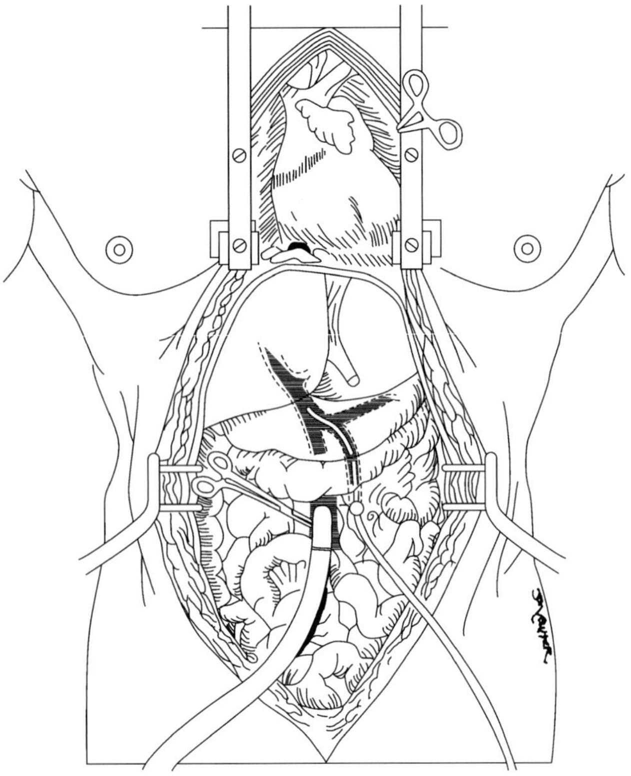

图 22.3 肠系膜下静脉的插管以低温灌注门静脉系统。(Redrawn from Casavilla et al. [17], with permission from Wolters Kluwer Health.)

冷保存溶液灌注器官。然后通过中间胸骨切开术打开胸部。然后将胸主动脉交叉夹紧,并打开腔静脉通气。然后将肠系膜下静脉插管以灌注门静脉系统。一旦器官被充分冲洗和冷却,就进行肝切除术。这之后是整体肾切除术。

Reich 描述了与上述"超快速"技术类似的恢复过程[18]。他详细描述了如何在冷的原位进行肝切除术,并且降低损伤右肝动脉的风险,防止花费时间获取胰腺。在这种情况下,肝脏与胰腺头部一起获得。作者建议,另一种方法是整体获得肝脏和胰腺。一旦去除肝脏,然后进行双侧肾切除术。

总结

等待名单上的患者数目与可供移植的器官数目之间的差距并没有减少。事实上,人们可能会认为,需求正在增加,供应仍然落后。DCD 供体提供可接受的器官来源并增加可用于移植的器官的数目。结果表明,来自 DCD 供体的肾脏和胰腺在适当选择的情况下长期预后良好。来自 DCD 供体的肝脏的结果显示较高的并发症发生率,但是当适当评估接受者的个体风险-收益平衡时,其在患者存活和移植物存活方面是可接受的。

DCD 获取的操作策略与脑死亡供体的有些不同。重点是一旦患者宣告死亡,安全,迅速而有效地获取复苏,而不对所获取的器官造成伤害。上述技术应该作为实现这一点的指南。

致谢

我们要感谢 Janet Fox 帮助本章的研究。此外,我们要感谢 UW OPO 提供关于 DCD 复苏/协议的文档。

(张云凯 译　李照 校)

参考文献

1. A definition of irreversible coma: report of the Ad Hoc Committee of the Harvard Medical School to Examine the Definition of Brain Death. JAMA 1968;205:337–340.
2. Koostra G, Daemen JH, Oomen AP. Categories of non-heart beating donors. Transplantation Proceedings. 1995;27:2893–2894.
3. Alvarez J, del Barrio R, Arias J, et al. Non-heart-beating donors from the streets: an increasing donor pool source. Transplantation. 2000;70:314–317.
4. Pratschke J, Willhelm MJ, Kusaka M, et al. Brain death and its influence on donor organ quality and outcome after transplantation. Transplantation. 1999;67:343.
5. Weber M, Dindo D, Demartines M, et al. Kidney transplantation from donors without a heartbeat. New England Journal of Medicine. 2002;347:248–255.
6. Rudich SM, Kaplan B, Magee JC, et al. Renal transplantations performed using non-heart-beating organ donors: going back to the future. Transplantation. 2002;74:1715–1720.
7. Abt PL, Crawford MD, Desai NM, et al. Liver transplantation from controlled and uncontrolled non-heart-beating donors: an increased incidence of biliary complications. Transplantation. 2003;75:1659–1663.
8. Foley DP, Fernandez LA, Leverson G, et al. Donation after cardiac death: the University of Wisconsin experience with liver transplantation. Annals of Surgery. 2005;242:724–731.
9. Qureshi MS, Callaghan CJ, Bradley JA, et al. Outcomes of simultaneous pancreas-kidney transplantation from brain-dead and controlled circulatory death donors. British Journal of Surgery. 2012;99:831–838.
10. Bellingham J, Santhanakrishnan C, Neidlinger N, et al. Donation after cardiac death: a 29 year experience. Surgery. 2011;150(4):692–702.
11. Lewis J, Peltier J, Nelson H, et al. Development of the University of Wisconsin donation after cardiac death tool. Progress in Transplantation. 2003;13:265–273.
12. Polyak MM, Arrington BO, Kapur S, et al. Donor treatment with phentolamine mesylate improves machine preservation dynamics and early renal allograft function. Transplantation. 2000;69:184–186.
13. D'Alessandro AM, Hoffmann RM, Knetchle SJ, et al. Successful extrarenal transplantation from non-heart-beating donors. Transplantation. 1995;59:977–982.
14. Institute of Medicine, National Academy of Sciences. Non-Heart-Beating Organ Transplantation: Medical and Ethical Issues in Procurement. Washington, DC: National Academy Press; 1997.
15. DeVita MA, Snyder JV, Arnold RM, et al. Observations of withdrawal of life-sustaining treatment from patients who became non-heart-beating organ donors. Critical Care Medicine. 2000;28:1709–1712.
16. Ethics Committee, American College of Critical Care Medicine; Society of Critical Care Medicine. Recommendations for non heart beating donation. A position paper by the Ethics Committee, American College of Critical Care Medicine, Society of Critical Care Medicine. Critical Care Medicine. 2001;29:1826–1831.
17. Casavilla A, Ramirez C, Shapiro R, et al. Experience with liver and kidney allografts from non-heart-beating donors. Transplantation. 1995;59:197–203.
18. Reich DJ. Non-heart-beating donor organ procurement. In: Humar A, Matas AJ, Payne WD, editors. Atlas of Organ Transplantation. London, UK: Springer; 2006: 23–33.

第 23 章
活体供肾获取技术

Andrew B. Adams, Ashtar Chami, Kenneth A. Newell

引言

活体供肾移植现在被广泛认可是对肾衰竭患者的最有效的治疗方法。与透析相比，它提供良好的器官功能和较高的生活质量。与已故供体移植相比，它降低可移植肾延迟功能恢复的风险，提高远期移植预后，降低排斥和增加移植手术的灵活性。然而，由于活体供体移植可能危害一个健康的人，因此，自从 1954 年提出这种方式以来，活体肾移植的使用指征仍然是一直争论的问题。推动更多地使用活体供肾的因素很多，包括逐渐减少的死亡器官捐献和越来越多的终末期肾病患者，社会对潜在死亡供体捐献的敏感程度，以及受体疾病的进行性恶化。逐渐老龄化的人口和逐渐加重的疾病形成鲜明的对比，使得大家更关心疾病的风险，尤其考虑到远期肾功能的时候。因此，适当的患者选择和手术技术在活体肾移植的进行中是至关重要的，为合适的受体提供优质器官，同时通过主要手术操作保证供体的安全，但要保证供体并没有获得利益。本章将讨论活体供体肾移植的进展，评估受体的选择，供体肾切除术的相关技术方面，以及可能影响其结果的因素。关于活体捐献伦理方面的深入讨论可以参见第 138 章。

活体肾移植的历史与现状

1954 年 12 月 23 日，一个由 Joseph Murray 博士领导的团队将当时 23 岁的 Ronald Herrick 的一个肾脏移植到他同一个孪生兄弟 Richard。这次手术的成功是肾移植和活体器官捐献发展的分水岭。Ronald Herrick 神圣的礼物给了他兄弟 8 年的高质量生活；在慢性透析出现之前，这是超出终末期肾病的患者预期的事件。Ronald Herrick 在他 79 岁去世，他的生活富裕且完美[1]。

从这个里程碑事件开始，肾移植和活体器官捐献在数量和成功率稳步增长。自 1998 年以来，美国共有 112 012 例活体肾脏供体[2]。在这段时间内，活体肾供体移植的数量从大约 2000 稳定地增加到平均每年>6000。虽然促进这种增长的因素仍然不确定，但是公众认为对于活体供体肾移植，新手术技术和不断变化的捐献者人口增长似乎很重要。肾移植对透析的终末期肾病(ESRD)患者能显著提高生存质量，以及来自活体供体的肾的短期和长期存活率远远大于死亡捐献者，这极大地促进了活体肾移植的进展(第 103 章深入讨论远期肾移植结果)。肾移植逐年增加的等待期(从 1999—2000 年列出的未感染 1276 天到 2003—2004 年列出的 1382 天)使得 ESRD 患者及其亲属和朋友考虑将活体捐献作为移植的方案来替代死亡捐献者的器官。在此期间，还报道了在透析之前的肾移植(预先移植)与远期移植肾的存活率相关[3]。对于大多数肾衰竭的患者，活体供体肾移植代表进行预先移植的唯一机会。在活体肾脏供体中引入微创手术进行肾切除术，虽然没有显著改变外科手术的风险，但已证明能减少手术后疼痛并加快供体的恢复，因此几乎肯定地导致活体肾捐献者的增多。这对于与受体不相关的供体的数目增加而言可能是特别有利的。在这种情况下，应该注意到，活体肾捐献的增长与捐献者的人口统计变化有关。这方面最引人注目的变化是在 1998—2008 年期间观察到的不相关捐献者以及配偶/亲友捐献者的增加[2,4]。这种增加已被相关活体肾捐献者的匹配度下降而抵消一部分。同时还发现活体肾供体的年龄逐渐增加的趋势。

尽管活体肾脏捐献有这些积极趋势，但是在 2004 年达到峰值 6647 之后，活体捐献者的数量逐年年下降到2008年的5968例。在2009年和2010年再次增加(分别为6387和6278)后,活体捐献者再次下降到2011年的5770例。由于对20世纪90年代和21世纪早期活体捐献者数量增加的因素了解不足,因此造成活体肾捐献者数量减少的因素也难以估计。一些人推测,这可能与在这段时间内美国经济的下降以及随之而来的潜在捐献者与活体肾捐献相关的成本支付能力有关。其他人已经推论,ESRD人群的年龄增长可能与有限数量的潜在活体捐献有关。与儿童活体供体移植率显著降低有关的一种因素是"共享35原则"。这项计划将35岁以下死亡器官捐献者的肾脏优先移植给小于18岁的患者,除非是HLA零匹配,用以挽救生命,非肾脏移植器官或受体为高度致敏人群。虽然共享35原则的目的是减少儿童肾脏移植的等待时间,但它导致减少儿童活体供体肾移植数量的意想不到的后果。最后,活体肾移植的实践中的地理和流程特异性差异可能影响活肾捐献的可用性。一般来说,活体供肾移植在新英格兰和美国中北部最高,在东南部最低[4]。最后,据报道,医学上复杂的活体肾捐献者的评估变数众多,其中最大的影响的是复杂活体供体[定义为具有较低的肾小球滤过率(GFR)供体、肥胖或高血压的供体等][6]。极为相似的是,最终愿意接受技术上或手术上复杂的捐献者也有类似的差异。潜在医学和外科手术复杂的捐献者是一个有争议的领域,值得仔细研究。然而,更多地传播理念和关于活体肾捐献的医学和外科原则更好的认识有助于增加ESRD的患者对活体供体肾移植的需求。目前正在实施和考虑其他一些促进活体供肾移植的倡议。所有潜在活体供体中,约1/3是ABO不相容的。这与高敏受者相结合导致许多接受者与医学上合适的供体不能使用标准方法进行活体供体肾移植。两个用来增加高敏感受体接受活体供体肾移植机会的策略是脱敏和匹配的供体交换流程[6]。促进这些方法的多种关键性进展包括引入用于检测抗HLA抗体的固相测定(参见第36章),以及使用蛋白酶体抑制剂硼替佐米或依库珠单抗(eculizumab)的抗体更有效地治疗抗体靶向补体蛋白C5介导的排斥反应(在第99章中更深入地讨论)[7]。脱敏最常应用于活体献血的过程,并直接解决对血型抗原或HLA分子特异的预先存在的抗体。两种最常见的脱敏方案利用单独的高剂量静脉内免疫球蛋白G(IVIG)或与血浆置换组合的低剂量IVIG。已将利妥昔单抗(一种抗CD20单克隆抗体)加入这些方案中的每一个中,以尝试耗尽负责产生供体指导的抗体的B细胞,从而增加每种治疗的有效性。现在有许多研究证明使用任一种方法的脱敏导致可接受的短期患者和移植物存活。然而,观察到的急性细胞和抗体介导的排斥的速率高于在没有供体指导的体液免疫的证据的受者中观察到的速率。此外,最新的数据表明,脱敏后的长期结果可能会低于在没有预先存在的供体适应性免疫的个体之间的移植中观察到的结果。

如第27章所详述,另一种方法,肾配对捐献(KPD),通过在最初预期的,免疫不相容的配对之间交换供体肾脏,从而避免与免疫记忆相关的有害作用,使得从免疫相容供体捐献给不同的受体[8,9]。不相容的供体和受体对之间的交换被运作以确保具有不相容的供体的每个受体接受免疫学上更合适的肾,避免负面的交叉匹配。使得受体的医疗管理更容易,并且几乎可靠地改善移植物功能和长期存活时间,但是KPD的实施在算法上和组织上是复杂的。虽然个别计划已取得了显著的成功[10],但为了优化KPD而需要大量不相容的配对,便产生了创建区域和国家KPD计划,例如国家肾脏登记处,配对捐献联盟和试验性KPD计划由器官获取和移植网络(OPTN)操作,由联合国器官共享网络(UNOS)管理。利他主义的非定向活体捐献者引入KPD计划允许创建超过30个供体-受体对的移植链。KPD发现,基于大KPD程序的数学建模表明高敏受体和O受体与A捐献将相对弱势。随着KPD的经验的增加,越来越明显的是,没有一种方法对于所有患者组是最佳的。由于排斥的风险已显示与供体特异性抗体(DSA)的强度相关,脱敏提供了及时移植的潜力,具有相对弱的DSA的受体具有良好的预后。对于不是广泛致敏但具有强DSA的接受者,KPD可提供接受活的供体肾的现实选择,而不增加免疫介导损伤的风险。对于既广泛致敏又具有许多高强度抗HLA抗体的那些患者,使用KPD鉴定已知DSA方面的最佳潜在供体的混合方法连同脱敏以使由低强度DSA引起的风险最小化可能提供最好的方法。

正在考虑的另一项倡议是某种形式的捐献者补偿,旨在至少部分抵消与活体肾捐献有关的财务支出和健康风险。调查结果表明捐献者肾脏捐献对其健康情况和财务状况有着负面影响,这些问题是活体肾捐献的重要障碍,并支持仔细考虑对活器官捐献者的有限补偿。然而,1984年的"国家器官移植法"(NOTA,见

第 19 章)认为取消对活体捐献者的任何形式的补偿。NOTA 使得购买或销售器官是非法的,并进一步规定,任何人故意获取, 接收或以其他方式转移任何人类器官,用于人类移植中是不合法的。活体肾捐献者在行程,工资损失和潜在的未来医疗风险和费用方面招致重大的个人开支,导致一些人建议为供体健康和财产提供有限的补偿,以及少量现金抵消间接与肾脏捐献有关的费用[11,12]。值得注意的是,尽管阿姆斯特丹共识会议明确表示反对补偿活体捐助者,但它确实要求向活体捐助者提供终身健康保险,这是一种补偿形式[13]。在所有主要工业化国家中,只有美国没有达到这一预期。因此,尽管法律,伦理和情感问题仍然存在,但越来越多的团体表示支持考虑有限和受监管的补偿制度,以抵消活体肾脏供体所承担的财务成本和风险。

活体肾捐献者的评估、选择和捐献后随访

对潜在活体供体的评价最开始要为获得基本医学信息以确定潜在捐献者的一般健康状态的谈话,并开始教育他/她关于与活体肾捐献相关的潜在风险(包括手术和长期)。必须强调,获得"知情同意"的过程不是一个孤立的事件,而是一种在整个评估和捐献过程中继续演变的对话。与这种方法一致,获得知情同意不是活体捐献者团队的任何单个成员的责任,而是需要多个团队成员的参与和告知的过程,包括但不限于肾科医生,外科医生,活体捐献者支持者,社会工作者和心理健康专家。知情同意对话中一个重要组成部分是明确潜在捐助者理解捐献过程完全是自愿的,他/她可以在任何时候终止该过程,而不受具体医疗原因的影响。在这种情况下,移植小组通常通过指出潜在捐献者不是肾脏捐献的合适候选人,而不是通知受体捐献者已经改变他/她的意见,反而来承担责任。除了向潜在的肾捐献者提供与由肾造成的可能的外科手术和长期的医疗风险有关的信息之外,还必须通知评估活体肾捐献的个体关于评估过程本身的风险。对于那些不密切参与活体肾脏捐献过程的人,评估过程的风险可能不是直观显而易见的。然而,除了评价医疗过程的潜在风险,例如用于腹部成像的造影剂的过敏反应,在评价过程中获得的信息本身可能是有害的或不想要的。甚至包括发现潜在捐献者未知的可能影响他/她就业、未来获得医疗保险、感染或恶性肿瘤的发生。在某些情况下,这些情况可能要求向卫生机构通报。这些发现也可能对潜在捐献者产生重大的财务影响。或者,在这些病症可能更易于治疗的时候对这些病症的早期诊断可被视为有益于潜在供体。评估过程的另一个潜在有害的后果与 HLA 分型的结果相关,可以证明有些家庭关系是不正确的[14]。由于这些原因,在活体供体肾移植中的评估过程和外科手术过程中要获得供体的单独同意。为了使捐献者和接受者确定活肾捐献和移植的潜在风险和益处的平衡,重要的是向他们提供国家结果数据和个体移植中心的数据。尽可能对可以提前改善这些数据预测的结果影响因素进行讨论。

评估过程的具体目标是审查潜在捐献者的医疗和心理社会健康的所有方面,以确定可能增加肾脏捐献风险的任何情况。UNOS 和 OPTN 的规则规定,精神病医生,心理学家或有移植经验的社会工作者必须完成心理社会评估。活体肾捐献者的心理社会评估侧重于确定个体是否有足够的社会支持系统和财政资源安全地进行活体肾捐献,以及评估捐献者的精神疾病和行为障碍。影响此评估的信息包括确定患者的就业和保险状况,以及与其配偶,家人和亲密朋友的人际关系的状态。心理社会评估还评估患者理解活体肾捐献的潜在短期和长期后果及其作出独立,知情决定的能力。心理社会评价的最后一个组成部分是评估当前或过去的药物使用或药物滥用。

医学检查的核心部分包括既往史和身体检查,特别关注肾脏疾病的家族史,实验室检验包括确定与预期接受者的免疫相容性和存在的传染病,腹部成像以明确肾脏解剖结构和年龄相符的健康筛查结果[15]。医学评估通常实施以便于早期检测可能排除活体肾捐献的医学状况,从而使评估的成本以及评估不合适的供体所花费的时间最小化,从而允许新供体被鉴定和更快地评价。标准活体肾供体评价的组分列于表 23.1 中。

医学评价通常从确定供体是否具有影响捐献的相关病史开始,包括肾脏疾病(包括蛋白尿、肾结石、频繁尿路感染或慢性使用肾毒性药物, 例如非甾体抗炎药),心血管或脑血管疾病,高血压(包括子痫或先兆子痫),糖尿病(包括妊娠糖尿病),自身免疫疾病,慢性感染或出血/血栓性/栓塞性疾病。没有器官捐献的明显禁忌证的供体测试评估它们与预期受体的免疫相容性。

表 23.1 标准的活体肾脏捐献者评估内容

在前往移植中心之前可能要进行的研究
1.初试
2.供体完成一份详细的健康调查表
3.为供体提供知情同意书,将其评估为潜在的活体肾脏供体
4.供体 ABO 分型
5.进行交叉匹配
6.此时可以进行供体的 HLA 分型
7. 24 小时尿液收集,以评估肾功能及蛋白尿情况
8.至少提供 3 次随机血压
9.由既往病史评估的其他测试:
(1)24 小时血压监测
(2)2 小时口服葡萄糖耐量测试±糖化血红蛋白
(3)有肾结石病史供体的代谢情况
在访问移植中心期间进行的研究
10.移植肾病学家和外科医生的详细病史和身体检查,包括至少测量 3 次完整的生命体征
11.独立的活体供体发起者和心理健康专家的详细访谈
12.实验室研究包括:
(1)全血细胞计数与血小板计数和差异
(2)电解质
(3)全面的代谢检查,包括空腹血糖和转氨酶测定
(4)空腹血脂
(5)凝血研究,包括凝血酶原时间(PT)、国际标准化比率(INR)和部分凝血活酶时间(PTT)
(6)尿液分析
(7)妊娠测试(如有需要)
(8)前列腺特异性抗原(根据供体年龄和家族史的建议)
(9)HIV 病毒、乙型和丙型肝炎血清学
(10)快速血浆反应素(RPR)
(11)结核病检测-结核病皮肤检测或量化-结核病金标准
(12)对来自流行地区供体的类线虫、克鲁斯锥虫和西尼罗河病毒进行检测
(13)心电图(ECG)
(14)胸部 X 线摄影
(15)使用 CTA 或 MRA 进行腹部成像
(16)所指示的超声心动图和心脏压力测试
(17)肺功能检查和胸部 CT 扫描显示
活体供体评估委员会将审查其他研究
13.适合年龄的癌症筛查结果
(1)妇科检查并宫颈涂片
(2)结肠镜检查
(3)乳腺钼靶 X 线摄影

这包括确定供体的 ABO 基团(与受体的比较),交叉匹配以确定是否存在供体指导的抗 HLA 抗体的存在和数量(如果存在),并且设置一些 HLA 分型。HLA 分型在评估过程早期对于多个潜在供体的设置中最常见;其可以使单个供体评估的过程快速结束,以降低在被确定为不合格肾供体的个体费用。在该阶段,可以提供希望进行的不相容的供体-受体配对,选择配对的供体交换程序,脱敏这两种方法的组合作为识别其他供体或等待已故供体捐献的肾脏替代方案。然后,相容的供体可以进行 24 小时尿液收集,以评估肾功能(肌酐清除率)和蛋白尿。病史可以规定特定的研究,例如在糖尿病风险增加的个体中口服葡萄糖耐量或糖化血红蛋白(HbA1c),在高血压风险增加的那些人的 24 小时血压研究,以及尿液收集以评估具有肾结石病史的个体中结石形成的风险。常规实验室研究,包括全血细胞计数,综合代谢分布,脂质分布,尿分析,凝血研究,肝炎和 HIV 血清学,梅毒的快速血浆反应试验(RPR)和结核病检测(TB 皮肤试验或还可以在此时获得干扰素-γ释放测定(例如,Quaniferon®-TB Gold)和尿培养物。对来自流行病地区的潜在供体,要对粪便检测,以及克氏锥虫和西尼罗病毒的另外的测试(参见第 92 章,用于额外考虑供体来源的感染)。潜在捐献者还应在随机时间提供一系列血压值。

其测试结果与活体肾献血相符的个体然后可以存在于移植中心以进行进一步的诊断研究和成像,其至少包括心电图(ECG),胸部 X 线,腹部成像和任何以前所述的实验室测试。50 岁以上或 40 岁以上具有冠状动脉疾病风险因素的个体,例如使用烟草历史,由单一药剂控制的高血压,异常 ECG 或早期冠状动脉疾病的家族史要进行心脏压力测试。发现有杂音的潜在捐献者应进行超声心动图检查。有晕厥,眩晕或心悸病史的捐献者应该接受超声心动图和动态心电图监测。具有持续吸烟史或胸部 X 线异常的潜在供者可能需要肺功能测试或胸部计算机断层扫描(CT)进行进一步评估。基于他们的性别,年龄和家族史,潜在的供者也应该根据美国癌症协会的建议进行宫颈癌,乳腺癌,前列腺癌,结肠癌和皮肤癌的筛查。

腹部成像是潜在活体肾捐献者评估的关键组成部分。它通常在评估过程后期进行,以最小化成本并避免由于其他原因的不能捐献的潜在捐献者暴露于辐射和造影剂的危害之中。这种方法的一个例外可以是早期使用超声波来筛选具有多囊肾病家族史的潜在供体,以排除那些具有明显肾囊肿的患者进行进一步评估。所使用的成像模式的选择随着新技术的引入和对现有腹部成像方法的改进而发展。血管造影术一直是评估活体供体的成像的主要手段,但由于其固有的风险和检测涉及除肾脏之外的器官,可能影响肾捐献的进行,现在很少使用。计算机断层扫描血管造影术(CTA)和磁共振血管造影术(MRA)各自广泛用于对潜在活供体的腹部器官成像。两者以高精确度限定肾脏的血管解剖结构,并且类似地有效地用于评估其他腹部器官和组织以用于解剖和病理大体,其可评估个体是否适合作为活体肾捐献者。CTA 具有将潜在的供体暴露于可能在易感个体中引起过敏反应的电离辐射和碘化造影剂的缺点。通过改进减少辐射暴露的扫描方案以及引入更安全的造影剂,在某种程度上改善了这些问题。CTA 与 MRA 相比的一个优点是其检测由 MRA 不可见的小到中等大小的肾和输尿管结石的能力。除了避免暴露于辐射和碘化造影剂,演变的 MRA 方案可以评估肾脏灌注和功能的定量。考虑到 CTA 和 MRA 的当前能力,用于对潜在活肾捐献者成像的两种方式之间的选择可能取决于个体考虑,包括可用设备和必要的解释专门知识。使用诸如 ^{99m}Tc-DTPA 或 ^{99m}Tc-标记的 MAG3 的放射性同位素肾造影还可以用来评估肾脏灌注和功能。随着横断面成像模式的能力已经改善,核医学图谱较少使用,但是仍然可以在显著体积差异的设置中提供有用的信息,这可能暗示右肾和左肾的功能有差异。

由多学科评估委员会审查活体肾脏供体评估结果是评价过程的关键组成部分。该评估小组的组成因机构而异,但通常应包括肾脏科医生,外科医生,活体捐献者协调员,独立的活体捐献者,社会工作者和(或)具有肾移植和捐献知识的精神健康专家组成。该组的成员应该独立于评估潜在肾移植受者的团队,以客观地评估对捐献者的风险,而不会由于考虑对受体的潜在益处而产生偏见。虽然标准因计划而有所不同,但活体捐献的普遍接受的排除标准如表 23.2 所示。委员会审议期间特别关注的领域如下所述[16]。

供体年龄

2007 年报告的调查结果显示,有接受老年人作为活体肾捐献者的趋势[15]。在美国调查的 132 个中心中,大约 21%的中心排除了 65 岁以上的活体捐献者候选人,而 60%的中心没有设定年龄上限。同时,移植计划更加仔细地审查年轻捐献者。18 岁以下的年龄被认为是几乎所有项目的活体肾脏捐献的禁忌,18 岁以上的捐献者被更详细地评估,特别是在他们的成熟度和捐献动机方面。这种更谨慎的方法是由于其相对较长的预期存活期,对肾功能随年龄增长而下降的速度的担心,以及有义务确定其自主决定捐献。活体捐献倡导者的作用是这一进程的核心。

高血压

虽然高血压以前被认为是活体肾捐献的绝对禁忌证,但是目前正在越来越多地考虑和评估那些可能具有高血压发展的危险因素,或者甚至可以被诊断为轻度,良好治疗的高血压的潜在供体。研究表明,基于 24 小时动态血压监测研究,基于在临床中进行的血压测量,被分类为高血压的个体的一定概率发现是正常血压[17]。为了分类活体候选供体,平均血压>135/85mmHg 被认为是高血压的诊断。对于明确诊断为患有高血压的那些人,越来越多的方案现在认为个体利用相对低剂量的单一抗高血压药(或更少地两种药剂),实现良好的血压控制,假设不存在末端器官损伤例如左心室肥大,

表 23.2 活体肾脏捐献的潜在禁忌证

年龄<18 岁或患有精神疾病,供体评估潜在风险或做出自主决定的能力不足

- 患有糖尿病或糖耐量减低
- 高血压
  - 需要多种药物或高剂量的单一药物进行控制
  - 有终末器官损伤的证据
  - 在肾脏损害高风险的人群中
- 当前或已治疗但有重大复发风险的癌症,但不包括已充分治疗的非色素性皮肤癌
- 传染病,如 HIV 病毒、乙型肝炎、丙型肝炎、西尼罗河病毒和美洲锥虫病
- 肾病的证据,包括肌酐清除率降低、蛋白尿或血尿
- 遗传性肾病风险
- 代谢异常的多发或复发性肾结石,易导致肾结石复发
- 肾脏异常,包括肾脏大小显著异常或肾脏脉管系统异常,使受体或供体增加手术并发症
- 冠状动脉或外周血管疾病
- 重大瓣膜性心脏病
- 自身免疫性疾病,例如,类风湿关节炎、克罗恩病或溃疡性结肠炎
- 慢性肺病
- 病态肥胖或病态肥胖伴合并症
- 重大血栓或出血事件的病史
- 没有完成戒断计划的药物滥用史

视网膜病变或蛋白尿可作为活体捐献的候选供体。具有心血管疾病风险因子的高血压个体,例如高胆固醇血症,肥胖,吸烟和冠状动脉疾病的高危家族史,也将被排除在活体捐献之外。接受具有良好控制的高血压的个体作为活体肾捐献者是基于以下报道:短期至中期随访提示具有轻度至中度原发性高血压和正常肾功能的活体供体与非高血压供体相比并没有增加对血压,蛋白尿或肾功能不利的影响[18,19]。具有轻度,良好控制的高血压的潜在供体的排除标准包括相对年轻的供体(年龄<45~50 岁),非裔美国人供体,以及捐献给更远相关/非相关受体的供体,假设他们将得到较少的心理/情感安慰。具有预先存在的高血压的那些符合活体肾脏捐献的选择标准的捐献者应当被告知迄今为止的高血压捐献者的短期随访相关的安全数据,并且被鼓励适当改变生活方式,包括坚持适当的饮食,从事适度的运动,以及承诺日常的定期医疗保健。

糖尿病

过度糖尿病,由美国糖尿病协会定义为>126mg/dL的空腹血浆葡萄糖,在 75g 口服葡萄糖刺激后 2 小时血浆葡萄糖水平为>200mg/dL,或 HbA1c>6.5,是活体肾捐献的禁忌证。类似的,葡萄糖耐量降低也是大多数中心的捐献禁忌,因为其与将来发展成糖尿病的风险增加相关。受损的葡萄糖耐量定义为空腹血浆葡萄糖在100~126mg/dL 之间,2 小时口服葡萄糖耐量试验中的葡萄糖在 140~200mg/dL 之间,或 HbA1c 在 5.7~6.5 之间。虽然正常空腹血糖值足以排除大多数供者的糖尿病和葡萄糖耐量受损,但具有过去葡萄糖耐量受损病史,妊娠糖尿病,出生体重>9lb(约 4kg)的儿童个体,糖尿病,非裔美国人和体质量指数(BMI)>27kg/m^2 的个体的所有亲属都应进行 2 小时口服葡萄糖耐量试验,以更准确地评估其未来的糖尿病风险。除了葡萄糖耐量测试,其 HbA1c 的测量可以在评估具有不符合糖尿病或葡萄糖耐量降低的诊断标准的糖尿病风险因子的潜在供体中提供有用的信息。此外,具有代谢综合征的多种危险因素的个体,包括高血压,>150mg/dL 的甘油三酯水平,对于男性<40mg/dL 和女性<50mg/dL 的高密度脂蛋白水平,也应筛选葡萄糖耐受不良。具有发生糖尿病风险但不满足葡萄糖耐量降低标准的个体可以在给予适当理解未来风险和与生活方式改变的需要相关的咨询的情况下进行捐献。减肥可以显著改善葡萄糖体内平衡和代谢参数,但是必须仔细评估对于供体保持健康的生活方式的能力。

肥胖

一些证据表明肥胖和病态肥胖活体捐献者肾捐献后肾功能障碍的风险增加[20]。他们肯定更容易患蛋白尿,高血压和高胆固醇血症;每个都增加了他们的心血管疾病的终生风险。事实上,不管肾捐献,肥胖个体相对于具有正常体重的那些个体具有较低的存活率。虽然有争论,但考虑到这些风险,许多方案对活体捐献者的 BMI 施加了上限。在施加限制的中心中最广泛使用的值是 BMI 为 35kg/m^2,也有少数中心将生活捐献候选者限制于 BMI<30kg/m^2 的个体。一种中间方法是允许 BMI 高达 35kg/m^2 的个体在没有与肥胖有关的其他病症的情况下进行捐献,而具有边界性高血压,临界葡萄糖耐受不良,高胆固醇血症和正在吸食香烟的那些患者需要达到≤30kg/m^2 的 BMI。

捐献者潜在肾病的评估

肾功能可能是评估肾脏健康和肾病的最佳单一预测因子。测定个体的肌酐清除率(CrCl)是最广泛使用的肾功能测量。使用公式估计 CrCl 可以提供一些见解,帮助决定对哪些潜在的活体肾捐献者进行评估,但不足以准确地用作评估预期活体肾捐献者的肾功能的唯一手段。当使用公式时,优选 CKD-epi 公式,因为与 Cockrault-Gault 公式的 MDRD 相比,它提供了在正常范围内 CrCl 的更精确的估计。24 小时尿液收集是最广泛使用的方法来测量预期捐献肾脏供体的 CrCl。然而,这种相对简单的测试受到许多影响,包括过多或过少收集,使其结果有偏差并非 100%可靠。另一种方法是使用放射性同位素或碘化示踪剂直接测量 CrCl。虽然概念上更准确,因为测试是直接监测,许多中心由于其逻辑复杂性而不使用这种方法。不管用何种方法测量潜在供体的肾功能水平,必须选择 CrCl 的阈值。历史上,许多程序选择 80mL/min 的值作为阈值。随着慢性肾脏疾病(CKD)阶段的定义,许多程序采用 90mL/min 的阈值,其定义为Ⅱ期 CKD。无论选择什么值,肾功能的测量应该通过表示为每 1.73/m^2 的值对供体大小进行归一化。越来越常见的方法是将可接受的阈值定义为在潜在捐献者的年龄和性别的正常值的 2 个标准偏差内,进而再考虑这些变量对肾功能的影响。

显著的蛋白尿和血尿是严重的潜在肾小球病理学和肾病的指标。蛋白尿可通过测定 24 小时尿液收集物中存在的蛋白质的量或通过测量点尿样品中的白蛋白与肌酐比值来定量。通常认为>250~300mg/24h 或>30mg/g 的值指示可能存在的重要的潜在病变，并且将排除在没有已知的良性原因例如姿势性蛋白尿的情况下的捐献。基于 24 小时尿液导致升高的蛋白尿测量的原因包括在收集期之前的大量运动和过多收集，其可以基于排泄的肌酐估算(女性为 15~20mg/kg，男性为 20~25mg/kg)。像蛋白尿一样，血尿可以指示严重的潜在肾病。微血尿的定义通过移植程序稍微改变，但通常定义为每个高倍视野中 5 个或更多个红细胞(RBC)。评估血尿的第一步是获得准确的病史。在月经的女性或已经剧烈运动的男性或女性中，可以在没有其他混杂事件的情况下再次收集尿样复测。通过获得腹部和骨盆的尿培养和 CT 扫描，可以排除尿路感染和肾结石作为微血肿的原因。如果这些诊断研究未能揭示血尿的原因并且它仍然存在，则应该完善尿细胞学和膀胱镜检查。如果这些研究不明确病因，对肾捐献仍然感兴趣的个体应进行肾活检以排除固有肾病形成的。在没有记录的良性原因例如轻度严重的薄基底膜疾病的情况下，应该进一步商榷有持续性血尿的潜在供对活体肾捐献的进行。

筛查遗传性肾病

对于具有显著肾病家族史的潜在活供体，除了腹部成像研究之外，遗传测试和肾活检可能是必要的，以评估其未来发展肾病的风险。具有显著遗传因素的肾病的实例包括成人多囊肾病(ADPKD)、系统性红斑狼疮(SLE)、薄基底膜疾病(TBM)、Alport 综合征和 IgA 肾病。ADPKD 是美国肾衰竭的第四大主要原因，并且是最常见的遗传性肾病。与 ADPKD 相关的基因座包括染色体 16(PKD1 基因座，85%的患者)和染色体 4(PKD2 基因座，15%的患者)上的突变。具有 PKD2 突变的患者可以在生命后期存在。通过高分辨率横断面腹部成像确定的不具有肾囊肿的 30 岁或更大的个体可以被认为没有发展 ADPKD 的风险。年龄<30 岁的潜在捐献者需要进行基因检测，以确定他们是否在未来有 ADPKD 的风险。SLE 可发生在约 12%或更多具有受影响的一级亲属的个体中。受 SLE 影响的家族成员的活体供体的评价应包括检测抗核抗体，抗磷脂抗体的存在和补体水平的测量。基于这些结果，认为有发展成为 SLE 风险的人应该排除捐献。存在血尿的家族性肾病包括 TBM 疾病、Alport 综合征和 IgA 肾病。TBM 通常具有常染色体显性遗传模式。受影响个体的一级亲属应筛选血尿以及高钙尿和高尿酸尿。在肾活检时没有严重薄基底膜的个体，没有蛋白尿或高血压，并且没有同时的 IgA 肾病或 Alport 综合征可以进行肾脏捐献，尽管潜在捐献者长期肾病的风险是肯定未知的。Alport 综合征具有不同的遗传模式，大多数是 X 连锁。Alport 综合征的组成包括感觉神经性听力损失，眼部发现例如小红细胞，白内障和视网膜病变，血尿和高血压。男性 20 岁或以上发现没有任何这些条件可以进行捐献。具有正常尿结果的受影响个体的女性兄弟姐妹也可以进行捐献。

肾结石

最近的一项调查结果表明，77%的移植应答机构允许有肾结石史的个体考虑用于活体肾捐献[21]。具有记录的肾结石的历史的患者应当进行代谢评估，以确定是否存在代谢状况，例如高钙尿症，低枸橼酸尿症，高尿酸血症，高草酸尿症或代谢性酸中毒，使得他们将来结石形成的风险增加。大多数排除潜在捐献者是因为肾脏的代谢原因不能纠正和那些多发结石或在年轻时即形成肾结石，因为这些个人有增加的复发的风险。活体肾脏捐献过程的最后一部分是试图确保活体捐献者被告知维持健康生活方式的必要性。这个讨论应该包括健康的饮食，适度的运动和日常的适当的医疗保健。至少，这应该包括常规测量血压和实验室检验，包括血清肌酐、尿常规、空腹血糖和空腹血脂。

手术技术

活体器官捐献是一种外科医生极少开展的手术，因为它本身不仅仅改善受体的身体状况，更重要的是，它将他/她的健康置于另一个人可能受到危害的风险中。虽然捐献者评估过程产生了有形和无形的利益，但与捐献有关的风险与大多数与手术相关。考虑到医学的原则是“primum non nocere”，即“首要是不能伤害”，外科医生特别需要理解并最终优化所使用的手术技术。

如上所述，活体捐献的评价过程可能相当复杂。虽然医学和心理社会指标是非常重要的，并且可能有助于长期预后，但捐献者是否适合手术和解剖变异，在手术术前评估中是至关重要的。

虽然先前已经讨论了包括需要额外测试的特殊人群的深入医学评估，同样也存在解剖学评估因素，并且不管所采用何种外科技术。在此期间必须完成术前腹部成像。具体采用CT或磁共振成像，主要由所在机构的专业考虑决定。我们喜欢用三维重建的CT成像，其给出了动脉和静脉解剖的极好描述(图23.1)。

虽然大多数早期微创供者肾切除术的经验认为供体存在血管变异，如多个肾动脉或环静脉肾静脉是捐献的禁忌证，但在当前不是这样的。目前，大多数中心将进行有两个甚至三个肾动脉，或者有复杂的静脉变异的活体肾切除术[22]。术前成像，包括CT和MRI，已被证明能够准确预测最终的术中发现，并为捐献外科医生提供关

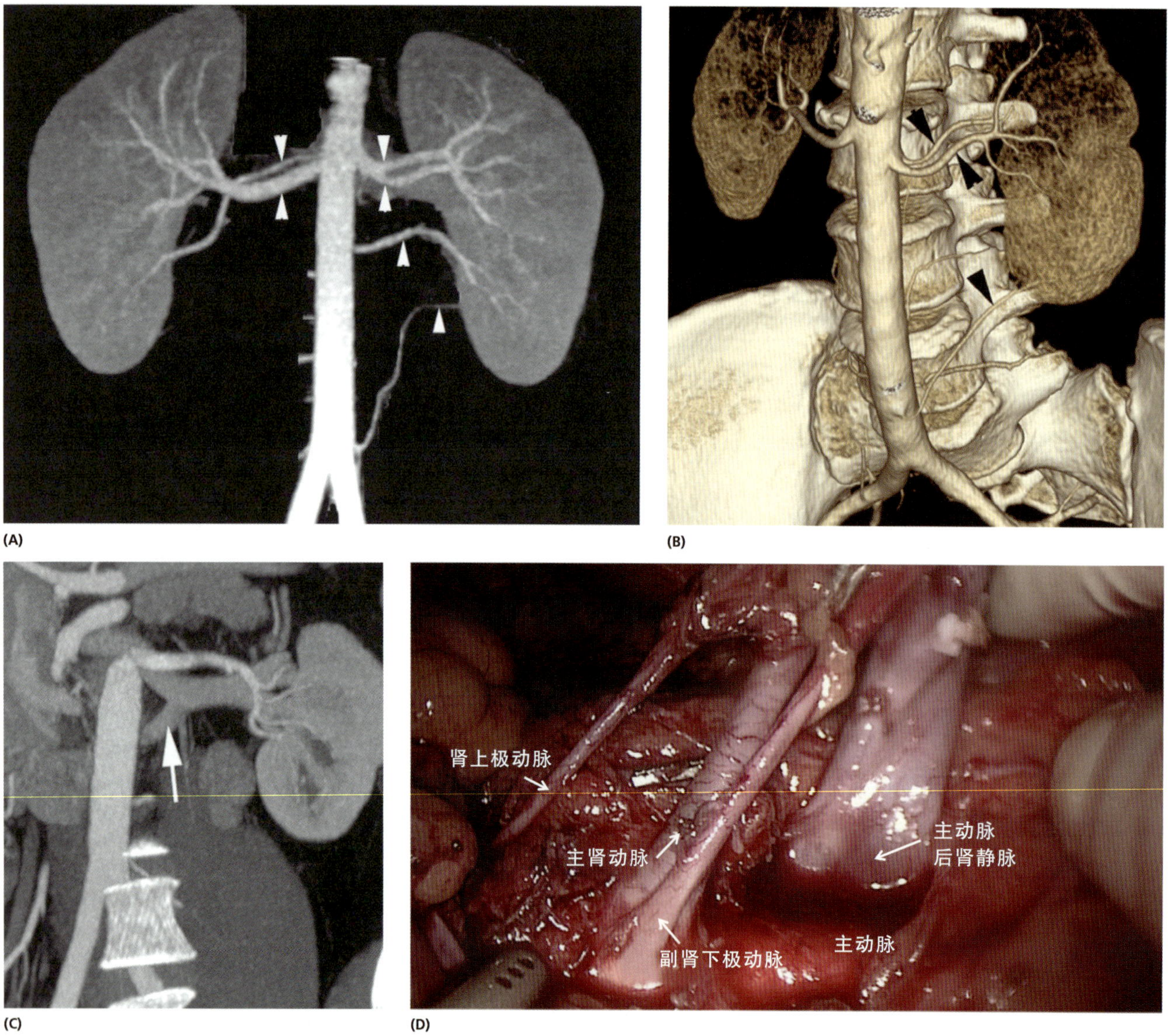

图23.1 腹部CT扫描重建表明解剖结构异常。(A)潜在供体的肾动脉解剖结构，其中有两条右肾动脉和四条左肾动脉(每个箭头表示一条独立的动脉)。值得注意的是，较小的右肾动脉起源于头侧主肾动脉，但供应肾脏的下极。左侧有一条小的下极肾动脉，出现在主动脉分叉处。这种动脉解剖结构可能会增加使用右肾或左肾的手术相关并发症的风险。(B)具有三条左肾动脉的供体，包括一条小动脉，该小动脉供应起源于主动脉分叉附近的下极(每个箭头表示一条独立的动脉)。值得注意的是，右肾动脉只有一条，因此右肾可能更适合捐献和移植。(C)具有环绕主动脉的左肾静脉供体重建CT(箭头标记了环主动脉肾静脉后方的主动脉部分)。(D)术中暴露的三条肾动脉和主动脉后方肾静脉的照片。尽管对于外科医生来说，在手术前了解这种异常的解剖结构很重要，但这一发现不会显著增加手术技术并发症的风险或影响使用哪种肾脏的选择。

键信息[23]。除了提供清晰的动脉和静脉解剖结构之外，术前成像也可以很好地评估肾实质，以及在排泄期间中的延迟序列评估收集系统和输尿管的情况。最后，但最重要的是，腹部成像可以评估外科医生任何可能导致捐献禁忌的腹腔内病变。

一旦已经确定有没有医疗，心理，或解剖禁忌，外科医生可以用敲定个性化的手术方案。活供体肾切除术的技术随着中心的不同而不同，并且随着时间的推移以及引入了更新的策略，较前有很大改变。我们将讨论传统的“开放式”的操作技术以及更近的微创方法，如何安全地取出供肾并且不危害患者安全或供体器官质量。

开放式供肾切除术

当 Ronald Herrick 在 50 多年前捐献他的肾脏给他的孪生兄弟时，Joseph Murray 和他的手术团队通过“开放”供体肾切除术获得肾脏。类似于当时其他的传统手术，没有想到创伤最小化的问题。开放式供体肾切除术是从移植供体安全获得肾脏公认的术式。患者抬高并暴露右侧或左侧腹部（取决于要去除哪个肾）。切口开始于第 12 肋的尖端，并沿脐的方向弯曲向前，直到到达腹直肌鞘的外侧边界。然后外科医生继续分离腹壁的肌肉层–腹外斜肌、腹内斜肌及腹横肌。如果需要，背阔肌也需向后牵拉离断。偶尔，可能需要移除第 12 肋的一部分以进行暴露。深达肌肉层，腹膜被识别并推动到中间以暴露腹膜后空间。输尿管从肾的下极发出并沿腰肌的前表面流动。游离过程中需保存大量的输尿管周围组织，以确保充足的血液供应。可以使血管环或游离带环绕固定输尿管以缓和收缩。然后切开 Gerota 筋膜，并将肾脏与周围的肾周围脂肪分离。然后分离出肾静脉，并向下腔静脉（IVC）内侧移动。当获取左肾时，静脉游离放到它穿过主动脉的区域。肾上腺静脉必须在上方分开，而性腺静脉和一个或多个腰静脉必须在下方识别清楚。较短的右肾静脉通常不具有任何连接分支，并且需要被游离到其进入 IVC 的区域。肾动脉在抬起肾脏并向前反折之后，在骨骼化其来自主动脉的近端。如果外科医生愿意的话，可以在此时给予一定剂量的肝素。然后将输尿管向远端结扎并横切。将肾动脉和肾静脉夹闭并分开，留下供体血管的足够的袖口以允许充分的吻合。将供体肾从场上移除并交给等待的受体外科医生。利用供体肾动脉进行冷灌注液冲洗器官并准备植入。然后用可吸收缝线将伤口分层闭合，并且等待患者麻醉苏醒并返回到恢复室。

对供体的早期术后护理与行腹内手术的其他人非常相似。密切监测生命体征，电解质，以及尿量。疼痛和其他术后症状，如恶心，应适当解决。应仔细观察捐献者是否有任何潜在的手术并发症，包括术后出血，肠损伤或伤口感染。应鼓励他们尽早行动，以尽量减少肺部并发症或深静脉血栓形成的风险。通常住院时间为 3~5 天，如果不需要剧烈的身体活动，则在 4 周内恢复就业。

与其他传统手术非常相似，开放性供者肾切除术与较新的微创技术相比，具有更长的住院时间，延长的术后疼痛，较差的美容术以及较慢的康复期[24]。在过去的 20 年中，在整个外科手术领域中，包括移植领域，都在大力开展微创技术。微创手术甚至已经取代了开放性胆囊切除术或传统阑尾切除术，在当前时代，开放性供者肾切除术是一种主要被归为教科书并且仅为特殊情况保留的术式。

腹腔镜供肾切除术

虽然腹腔镜检查已经用于简单的妇科手术多年，但直到计算机芯片彩色照相机的发展，腹腔镜检查的指征扩大到更复杂的手术。20 世纪 90 年代初，开始了腹腔镜胆囊切除术和阑尾切除术的为代表的简单手术腹腔镜时代。随着这些手术的最终成功和接受，腹腔镜手术的适应证扩大到包括实体器官。第一次腹腔镜肾切除术于 1991 年实施[25]。随后的研究表明，与开放性供体肾切除术相比，用于肾切除术的微创技术有着较少的术后疼痛，较短的住院时间和减少的恢复期。在短时间内，腹腔镜供体肾切除术被大家深入研究。首先在大型动物模型中试验，在 1995 年由 Ratner 等人详细地描述了人体手术的初步经验[26]。从那时起，手术技术上出现了几种变化。这些包括手辅助腹腔，完全腹腔镜，腹膜后腔镜，手辅助腹膜后腔镜，机器人辅助腹腔镜和腹腔镜单部位供体肾切除术。虽然有多种微创供体肾切除术，完全腹腔镜和手辅助腹腔镜方法是目前最广泛使用的。最终，所选择的技术取决于个体患者和外科医生的专业知识和偏好。我们将详细描述左侧肾的手辅助腹腔镜方法，因为这是我们在我们自己的机构中喜欢的。

手辅助腹腔镜供体肾切除术

患者被置于改良的侧卧位，确保采取适当的预防措施以避免与神经牵引或皮肤压力相关的医源性损伤(图 23.2)。一侧置于直立位置；这通常是左侧，因为大多数捐献者经历左侧供体肾切除术。术区表面被弯曲以扩大肋缘和髂嵴之间的面积。如果这样获取，肾脏靠垫可以垫高这一点。患者根据需要用固定袋和胶带或其他方法固定在适当位置。然后可以根据程序要求安全地旋转体位。脐下方进行 7cm 中线切口。插入凝胶口或类似的手部装置并建立气腹。然后用手将额外的端口插入腹部。对于左肾切除术，我们通常在直视下放置 3 个额外的端口：在髂嵴和肋缘之间中间的腋前线上的 12mm 端口(解剖端口)，一个 5mm 的端口(用于缩回的辅助端口)，位于中线旁边肋缘下方 2~3 个手指宽度；和一个额外的 12mm 端口(摄像头端口)位于脐侧上方。对于右侧手术需要类似的套管针，并且通常可以为肝牵开器放置另外的 5mm 的端口。

对于左侧手术，可使用超声刀从游离降结肠和乙状结肠。如果必要，脾曲部也可以游离，并且偶尔可能需要游离脾的隔膜韧带以允许脾向前和向内移动。游离结肠的内侧以暴露包围在 Gerota 筋膜中的肾脏。然后小心地游离在横结肠和后腹膜之间的自然平面。大部分的解剖可以通过分离直接完成，特别注意避免内疝的发生。一旦结肠和横结肠充分游离，就确定性腺静脉和输尿管的解剖结构。在确认结构确实是性腺静脉之后，将来自静脉前表面的组织从骨盆解剖到性腺静脉下边缘进入左肾静脉的水平。这种解剖操作向头端继续，以暴露肾静脉。在该解剖过程中明确输尿管的位置，并且将伴随输尿管的性腺静脉作为标记侧向游离，以确保收获足够的输尿管周围组织包裹。有时候，性腺静脉可以用于收缩，因为肾静脉被游离和周向解剖，但是必须小心不要使其从肾静脉上的起源偏离。最终，通常更容易分开性腺静脉，靠近与肾静脉的汇合处，允许后腰椎分支的更大的可视化，其必须被夹住和离断(图 23.3)。当肾静脉暴露时，肾上腺静脉将出现在上方，并且需要与夹子结扎并离断(图 23.4)。然后将肾静脉向内移动以确保足够的长度，通常到其通过主动脉前面的点是足够的。肾动脉位于肾静脉的后面，并且可以通过用钝的抓钳提起肾的下极或通过内侧旋转肾并且从后面接近血管而暴露。为了完全暴露肾动脉，周围的神经节组

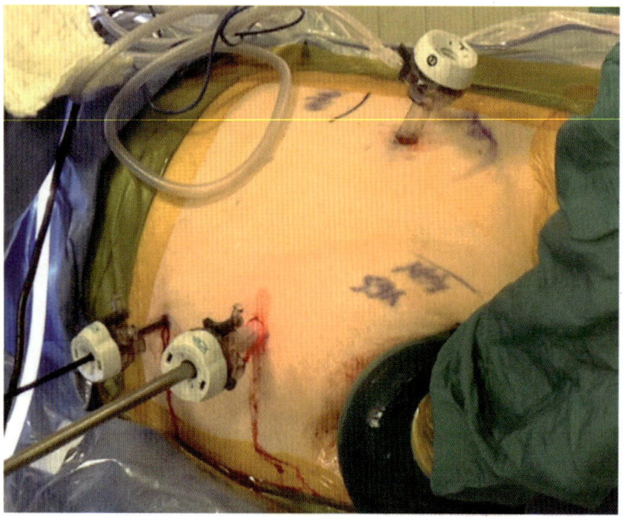

图 23.2 左侧手辅助腹腔镜供体肾切除术的典型定位和套管(Trocar)位置。将患者置于改良的侧卧位，确保采取适当的预防措施用以避免与神经牵引或皮肤受压有关的医源性伤害。

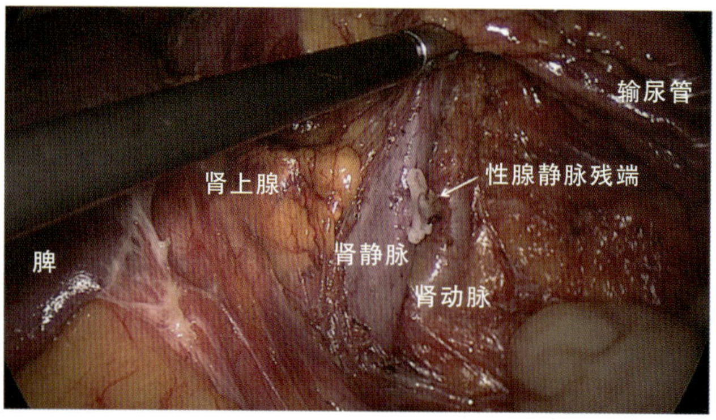

图 23.3 手术图片说明了性腺静脉(现已离断)、肾静脉、输尿管和肾动脉之间的关系。

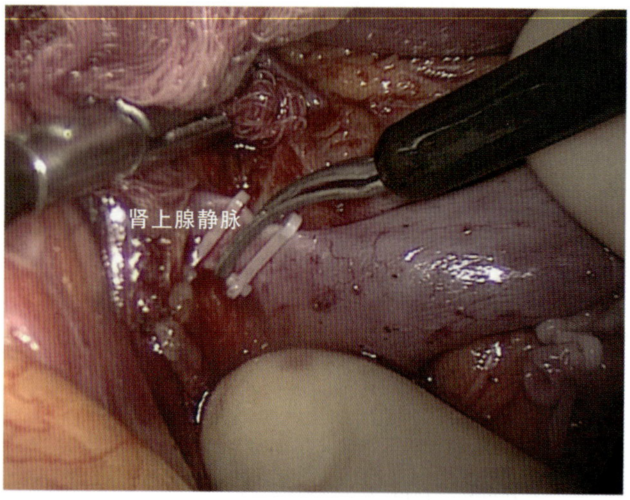

图 23.4 肾静脉与肾上腺静脉的夹闭离断。

织必须小心地分开到动脉与主动脉相交的水平（图 23.5）。在这一点上，在定义血管解剖结构的情况下，从其附件游离肾脏是有帮助的。

现在输尿管/性腺静脉复合体已经在纵向游离完毕，需要彻底离断。找到输尿管远端，一般在骨盆入口附近，穿过左髂动脉。然后可以轻轻地抓住输尿管，与性腺内静脉一起，包括周围的脂肪和结缔组织。然后用超声刀一起分成头尾方向，沿着腰肌的顶部朝向肾的下极移动。解剖的平面要沿着肾脏的侧表面，游离 Gerota 筋膜以暴露肾脏。然后分离后部附件，将肾从其外膜释放并朝向上部移动。为了分开肾上极附件，需要抓住肾并将其向下拉并且从一侧到另一侧旋转。最后的解剖平面沿着肾静脉的上边缘在肾上腺静脉和肾上极之间进行。该区域中的血管组织在夹闭之后离断，并且使用超声刀游离肾脏上极的所有结构。

然后肾脏从上部到下部并沿着其横向方向完全离断。应注意不要损伤肾脏的输尿管和下极之间的三角形组织，可能危及输尿管的血流。类似的，如果存在的话，也应保护供应肾脏下极的任何附属肾动脉，因为它也负责供应输尿管的血流（图 23.6）。随着肾脏完全游离，所有的血管结构显露，应该开始离断。在施用一定剂量的肝素后，我们首先将输尿管远端分开，穿过髂动脉；夹子夹闭输尿管的远侧。性腺静脉结扎并向远端游离。然后肾被外科医生抓住并提起，或者由助手侧向地牵拉以便显露动脉和静脉。缩回静脉头端提供了良好的视野暴露肾动脉。或者，肾脏可以向内旋转以从后面暴露肾动脉的起点。然后使用腹腔镜血管吻合器分割动脉。当缝合器被移除并重新装载时，如果需要，肾脏可以横向旋转，并且助手抓住并拉伸静脉。然后，当缝合器穿过主动脉时，静脉可以用缝合器离断，并确保足够的长度（图 23.7）。然后通过手术口取出肾并转移到处置台开始灌注。然后仔细检查止血，特别是在肾动脉残端的缝线处以及肾静脉分开的缝线的位置（图 23.8）。最后，检查分开的输尿管和性腺静脉残端（图 23.9）。在所有较大位置的筋膜缺损用可吸收缝合线缝合，如下中线切口。

术中/术后管理

类似于任何外科手术，活体供体的麻醉管理是至关重要的，并且需要麻醉师和外科医生之间的有效沟通。像任何腹腔镜手术一样，患者必须保持完全肌松以提供

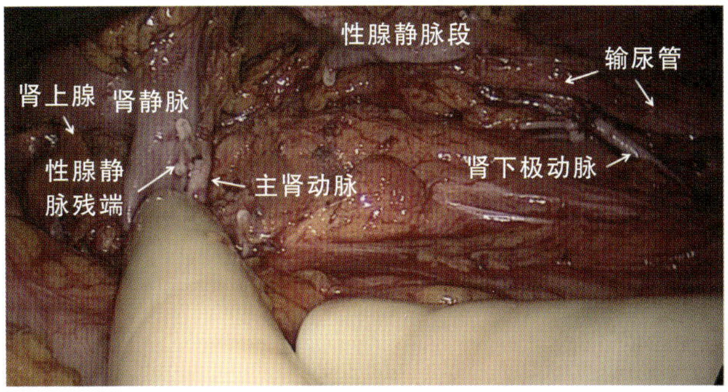

图 23.6 使用手助腹腔镜技术获取的供体肾脏。性腺静脉在其近端起源于肾静脉处和远端靠近骨盆入口处被离断。游离的部分是输尿管和输尿管周围组织。解剖时应注意保留任何辅助血管，例如下极动脉，如下图所示。

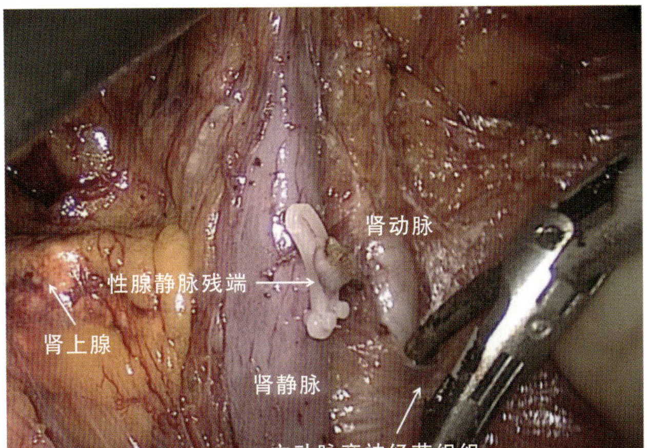

图 23.5 肾动脉与肾静脉的解剖关系。肾动脉位于肾静脉的后方。为了完全暴露肾动脉，必须将周围神经节组织游离到动脉与主动脉相接的水平。

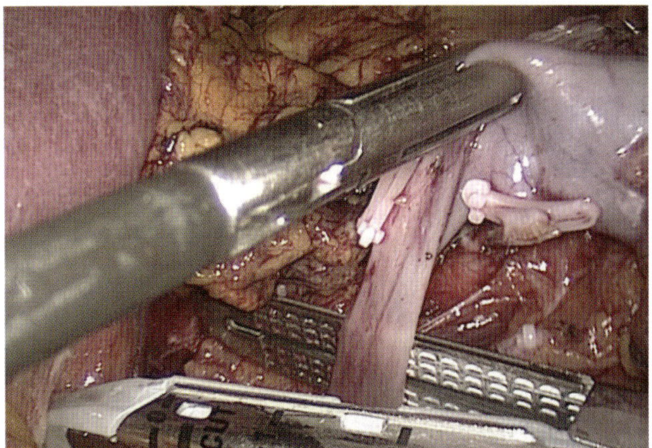

图 23.7 使用血管切割闭合器分割肾静脉。肾静脉可能会缩回，所以在横跨主动脉上方处时使用切割闭合器将静脉分开，以确保在接受者中有足够的长度进行重建。

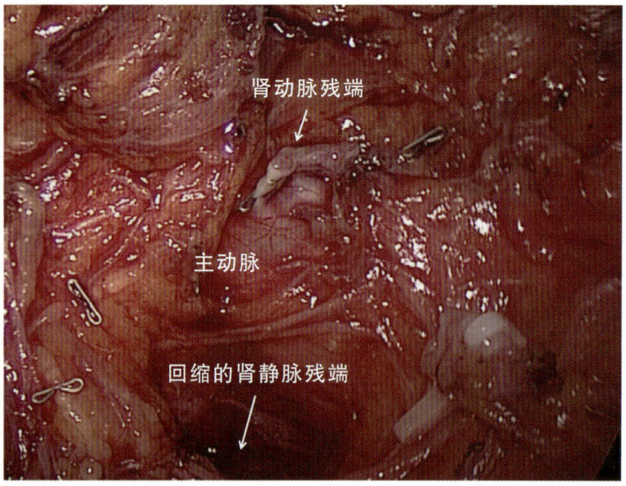

图 23.8 检查肾动脉残端和缩回的左肾静脉闭合处。

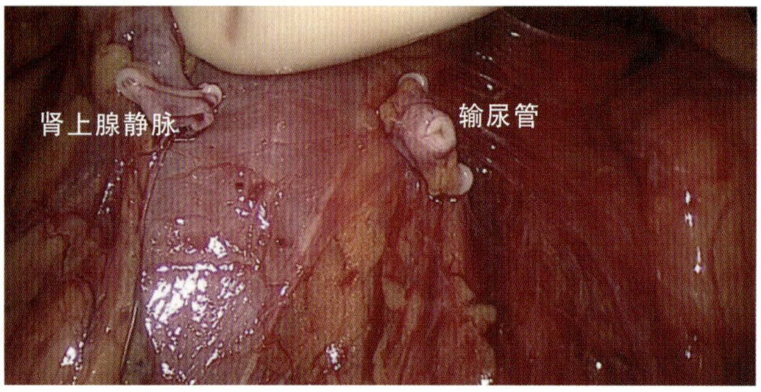

图 23.9 检查输尿管和性腺静脉断端是否有出血迹象。

足够的操作空间。这在肾血管即将被横切并且肾脏被提取的时期是特别重要的。我们发现在这个事件之前直接与麻醉团队沟通以确保肾脏的获取术中平稳。过去,我们常常在外植体之前用一剂量的呋塞米处理供体,以确保受体中的"充分利尿"。随后是重复剂量的呋塞米,并在灌注时间附近向接受者另外施用甘露醇。我们已经终止了这种做法,并选择保持捐献者血容量,滴定流体到足够的尿量,而不是单纯的利尿。

大多数进行腹腔镜肾切除术的供者在手术后保留在医院2~3天。在捐献后的前2个星期,他们逐渐恢复到正常的日常活动。在2周时,大多数供体能够耐受轻度运动。我们建议他们等待4~6周,然后重新开始任何剧烈的活动或重型举重。我们赞成使用静脉内酮咯酸以最小化术后疼痛,从而减少肠梗阻和恶心。

腹腔镜技术的影响

与普通外科手术中的其他腹腔镜技术非常相似,移除供体肾的微创技术在大多数移植中心很快获得了青睐。今天,腹腔镜供体肾切除术被认为是几乎普遍的手术标准。几项研究表明,腹腔镜供者的疼痛减轻,手术后麻醉剂使用减少,并且享受更短的住院时间和更快的恢复到完全的活动和工作[24,27-31]。与开放供体手术相比,腹腔镜供体的短期随访未能发现任何并发症增加的风险。然而,长期结局仍然未知,有待进一步研究。

与常规腹腔镜检查相比,手辅助技术的优点包括触觉反馈、控制出血的能力和触摸安全边缘,有利于更好地暴露和解剖结构,以及快速去除肾,导致较短的热缺血时间[32-35]。这些优势在有些中心特别有吸引力。大多数研究描述手辅助腹腔镜供体肾切除术的结论是:关于手术时间和失血,手辅助技术优于完全腹腔镜技术[34,36-41]。此外,一项荟萃分析表明,使用手辅助技术,中转开腹的风险较小[42]。

手辅助技术的缺点包括所需略大的切口,可以帮助游离和取出肾脏。纯腹腔镜技术可以将切口位置降低,可以更好地隐藏并且具有更小的切口尺寸,并使用标本袋递送肾脏。有一些理论提示,较低、较小的切口可能导致术后疼痛减少,但没有研究支持这一点。

其他技术

在美国和欧洲的许多中心,已经开始介绍并采用了各种其他技术。更常见的描述之一是腹膜后入路方法,其可以在有或没有手辅助的情况下进行。腹膜后镜下方法具有优于标准腹膜腹腔镜技术的优点,因为腹膜保持完整,具有较低的内脏损伤的理论风险和可能的较低的肠梗阻率。在几项小型研究中,手辅助腹膜镜下手术时间比标准腹腔镜供者肾切除术明显缩短[43-45]。总体而言,其他临床结果相似,这可能反映患者选择或外科医生对手术的熟悉程度。目前,腹膜后途径没有得到广泛的应用。

最近,各种外科专家在其手术中使用机器人辅助。有几个报告早期使用机器人辅助供体肾切除术,我们预计这将是一种越来越常见的技术[46-48]。机器人辅助技术的理论优点包括由操作臂的360°角接近腕部的移动自由度增加,导致更大的灵活性和可操作性。另一个优点是由于内置的稳定系统而造成的无震动操作的好处。减少疲劳和手术技术相关的外科医生的伤害也是机器人辅助方法的潜在优势。机器人技术的一个显著缺点是所需的金融投资以及与设备相关的学习曲线。

最后,微创手术的最新进展集中在单次切口单孔腹腔镜手术(SILS)和自然经口腔肠道内镜手术(NOTES)。有几项研究在讨论腹腔镜供体肾切除术的效用[49-51]。如预期的,总切口长度较少,接受单孔手术的接受者有着更快的恢复时间。这些研究还指出,此类手术需要更长的手术时间和更高的技术[52-53]。这些研究的样本量有限,影响了我们任何具体结论的权威性。目前有一项由康奈尔大学赞助的随机、前瞻性临床试验,评估常规腹腔镜供体肾切除术与单孔腹腔镜供体肾切除术的对比。试验中的评估内容包括手术时间、疼痛评分、镇痛要求、住院时间、手术瘢痕满意度,以及移植肾的功能和存活。有兴趣的可以关注这些技术之间是否有任何显著差异。未来的技术将使用独特的方法,如自然通道手术或NOTES技术。第一例供体肾切除术中的自然通道手术是在腹腔镜下获得的右侧肾切除术,但是不是通过标准切口提取肾脏,外科医生选择在先前经过子宫切除术的女性中通过阴道将其移除[54]。有趣的是,另一组研究描述了机器人辅助经阴道提取供体肾[55]。在两个报道中,捐献者没有接受任何术后麻醉静脉镇痛,并在24小时后出院回家。

活体供肾手术的未来可能包括这些技术的一些更替。但是,我们必须确保,无论采用哪种技术,对于那些选择不为自己的利益,而是为了改善他人而进行捐献的人,它必须保证捐献者的绝对安全。

活体肾捐献者术后的预后

与具有可接受的主要并发症和死亡率的大多数类型的外科手术不同,活体肾供体没有从外科手术得到任何益处,这导致对于肾脏捐献手术过程本身或手术过程相关的主要发病率和死亡率的推行零容忍策略。虽然在实践中不可能实现,但是这种心态可能反映了移植社群内的适当关注,即潜在的活体供体被保护免于过大的风险。被授权的调查者将捐献者死亡和与捐献过程相关的急性并发症(定义为捐献6周内或捐献者从外科手术护理中出院之前发生的死亡和急性并发症)上报到OPTN。手术相关供体死亡的风险估计约为1/3000。有报告显示,在1999年10月至2008年12月期间进行的51 153例活体肾脏供体手术中,有14例明确死亡[56]。在此期间,另有39名捐献者在捐献1年内死亡,其中所识别的原因反映了普通人群中常见的病症,例如,癌症、意外、脑血管和心血管疾病、杀人和自杀。有一些证据表明,活体肾捐献的手术和早期术后风险正在下降。OPTN数据表明,在2005—2009年之间进行的活供体肾切除术的手术后30天内只有3例死亡[2]。在此期间,捐献1年内因任何原因发生的活体捐献者死亡率为0.03%~0.08%。关于活体肾捐献的急性并发症,最常见的情况是需要输血的出血,其发生在约2%的供体中,需要再次手术的约为1/100。除了出血外,最常见的需要再次手术的并发症包括切口疝和肠梗阻。据报道,约1%的活肾捐献者发生这种情况。由于大多数供体肾脏切除术是通过腹腔镜进行的,转换为开放性手术被认为是并发症,并且据报道在2009年进行的所有腹腔镜供体肾脏切除术中的<1%。在当前时代,再入院率也低,其中约1%的活供体需要重新入院主要与腹内疾病有关,如腹痛、便秘、肠梗阻、恶心或呕吐。其他较不常见的报道,再入院原因包括深静脉血栓形成、肺栓塞、乳糜性腹水、胰腺炎或腹腔内感染。值得注意的是,没有证据表明,手术方法的选择影响供体中并发症的发生率或移植肾的功能。

与通常由于政策规定的统一要求而研究相关的风险相反,活体肾捐献的长期预后并没有被彻底研究。这部分是由于以下观点:活体捐献者在捐献之前是健康的,并且在从外科手术恢复之后返回到健康的生活方式;实际问题还妨碍了长期追踪肾脏供者健康的努力,许多捐献者与进行手术的移植中心相距较远,使得很难在肾脏捐献后返回移植中心进行常规健康评估。第二,大部分活体捐献者没有健康保险。由于没有预留资金用于支付前生活捐助者的长期医疗费用(包括日常医疗保健),因此捐助者和移植中心在进行全面,长期的后续行动方面存在重大财政问题。最后,活体肾捐献者常认为自己是健康的,他们的医生也是如此,并且没有看到肾脏捐献后用于常规健康评估的价值。自1996年以来,只记录了280个活体肾捐献者需要肾移植。鉴于他们以前的活体捐献者身份,这些个人具有移植优先权。在分配的时候,他们被授予4个额外的点,将其排在绝大多数的受者之前,但排除零HLA不匹配的受体和肾外器官的受体。虽然监测活肾捐献者的长期健康的障碍是巨大的,但是社会和移植社群有责任收集和传播关于活体肾捐献的长期预后的信息,这是一个迅速增长的共识。研究肾活体肾捐献的长期预后的必要性在21世纪由于活体肾捐献者不断变化的人口数目和日益增加的医疗复杂性而变得更加迫切。如所讨论的，活体肾捐献者比过去更年长，更具有种族多样性，并且与其受体关系不太密切。越来越多的活体捐献者也具有健康状况，例如，高血压、肥胖、脂质和葡萄糖体内平衡异常，每一种都增加了心血管和肾脏疾病的风险[56]。

尽管担心现有数据不足以告知潜在的活肾捐献者有关相关风险，但许多研究确实提供了有用的信息。对62名在第二次世界大战期间进行单侧肾切除术以进行创伤治疗的退伍军人的研究未能揭示相对于未经历肾切除术的同龄军人的死亡率或高血压的增加[57]。作者将死亡患者的肾脏疾病或活体内的功能障碍归因于肾脏切除术意外的原因，在45年的随访期，年轻男性的单肾切除术几乎没有严重的不良后遗症。肾脏捐献对捐献者的长期健康的影响的最早研究之一是检查57名捐献者，然后至少在捐献后20年[58]。与65名兄弟姐妹相比，血清肌酐、尿素氮和氮、肌酐清除率、平均血压或高血压或蛋白尿治疗的频率没有差异。随后对来自同一机构的大量肾捐献者的研究证实了活体肾捐献的相对安全性[59]。在第二项研究中，作者确定了3698名在1963—2007年期间捐献肾脏的个体的ESRD的生命状态和风险。他们还在2003—2007年间捐献的255名患者中进行了肾功能、肾损伤、高血压、一般健康状况和生活质量的特定测量。他们的结果表明，活体供体的存活与对照相当，符合年龄、性别、种族和民族的平均情况。类似的，与一般群体相比，供体的ESRD的风险没有显著差异。活体肾脏供者的生活质量和一般健康状况与从国家健康和营养调查（NHANES）获得的个体相比，与重要变量匹配的个体没有区别。基于这些发现，作者得出结论，活肾捐献者中显著的健康问题的发展与在一般人群中观察到的相似。虽然令人放心，但不确定这些研究结果在多大程度上是对高加索人捐献者的研究，其中许多人在20世纪70年代和80年代捐献，可以推广到今天更具种族和族裔多样性的捐献者，增加肥胖的流行及其相关的健康问题。为了解决不断变化的捐助者人口统计学和个人在美国的一般健康状况的影响，最近，第二组比较了在1994—2009年之间接受肾切除术的80 347名活体捐献者的国家登记数据，与在NHANES Ⅲ中的9364名参与者对比，其中排除了肾捐献禁忌证的患者[60]。虽然随访的持续时间较短（仅6年多），活体捐献者的死亡率与NHANES Ⅲ中年龄、性别和种族匹配的参与者没有不同。最近的第三份报告直接比较了活体捐献后种族对健康的影响[61]。该组检查了1987—2007年期间为肾脏供者的4650例个体的医疗记录，并在2000—2007年某时间由单一公司投保。这些活体肾脏供体的健康状况与NHANES的参与者进行比较。该分析表明，相对于白人肾供体，在黑人和西班牙活体肾供体中发生高血压、糖尿病或CKD的风险增加。然而，相对于来自NHANES的人口统计学匹配的对照个体，这些风险没有增加，表明种族和种族影响高血压、糖尿病和CKD的风险，但是活体肾捐献不进一步影响这些差异风险。ESRD，虽然在肾活体捐献后罕见，在非裔美国人更常见的发现值得进一步研究。一个可能的促成因素是最近描述编码APOL1的基因中的两个突变。这些突变称为G1和G2是相当常见的，发生在几乎1/3的所有非裔美国人，没有已知的肾病和2/3有肾脏疾病的人群。虽然存在单一风险的等位基因，G1或G2，赋予对抗“睡眠病”的锥虫病寄生虫的保护，两个拷贝的风险等位基因使ESRD的风险增加了一倍以上。这使得一些人实施了对非裔美国人潜在肾供体的APOL1的风险等位基因的存在的筛选[62]。虽然这是相对经济的，在没有关于这些突变对活肾供体的影响的数据情况下，它可能有助于进一步使非裔美国人在获得活体供体肾移植方面的尊重。

当结合在一起时，这些和其他研究提供了一些保证，活体肾脏捐献从操作风险的角度和单个肾的长期预后表明并没有禁忌。然而，到目前为止，所进行的几乎所有研究都缺乏真正反映活体肾脏供体的极好的健康状况的对照群体。与对活体肾脏供体候选者进行的彻底测试相反，大多数不必要的研究已经使用，基于目前已知的医疗条件或最少对少数患者的有限测试将自身鉴定为健康的对照组。尝试通过使用批准的活体肾捐献者解决这个问题，由于一个原因或另一个没有接受活体供体肾切除术被证明是困难的，因为许多这些医疗上合适的捐献者最终没有完成捐献，对参与长期研究没有兴趣。活体肾脏捐献的远期风险的研究由于偶尔发生严重的捐献相关不良事件及其在远离捐献的时间点的可能发生而更加复杂。这些观察对研究设计要求，为了提供信息，一项研究需要长时间跟踪大量活体捐献者。这具有明显的财务影响，因为目前存在有限的资金选择以抵消这种额外努力的成本。为了解决这些限制和关注，国家卫生研究院赞助了两项关于活体捐献结果的研究。ALTOLD（评估生活肾脏捐献的长期结果）是一项多中心，3年的研究，200名活肾捐献者和200个匹配的对照，用于肾、心血管、骨和电解质疾病的发展。这项研究是有限的，因为它不是设计用于检测罕见但严重的不良事件或那些发生在术后 3 年以上的并发症。RELIVE（肾和肺活体捐献者评估）是一项研究，旨在检查国家数据库，以确定之前 8951 例活体捐助者的 ESRD 的生命状况。这个大群体的子集将被选择进行额外的测试，以确定肾功能障碍、心血管疾病和生活质量的变化的发生率。目前正在进行一些其他的多中心联邦资助的研究，包括肾脏供体结果队列（KDOC）研究（ClinicalTrials.gov 标识符 NCT01427452），成为肾脏供体研究的长期影响（ClinicalTrials.gov 标识符 NCT00936078）和活肾脏捐献研究–横向和历史队列研究（ClinicalTrials.gov 标识符 NCT00951977）。尽管这些研究听取了移植专业人员、患者、资助组织的代表和联邦政府的广泛意见，这些研究的关键是告知潜在捐献者关于活体捐献的风险[63]，不可能最佳设计的研究将进行，直到得到适当的财政支持，以抵消参与长期研究的不利因素，因为没有明显的医疗资助。

总结

过去二十年来，活体肾捐献和移植发生了巨大变化。技术创新如腹腔镜供体肾切除术、机器人供体肾切除术和单孔腹腔镜肾切除术为捐献者提供更少术后疼痛和更快恢复的。有效脱敏接受者以及配对的供体交换程序的方案正在将活体供体肾移植的益处扩展到越来越多的致敏受体。捐助者人口的变化加上移植中心愿意考虑更多的医学和手术复杂的个人活体肾捐献的意愿，也导致过去 20 年活体肾捐献的近 3 倍增长。虽然现有数据表明，活体肾捐献具有可接受的短期和长期风险，但活体肾捐献进一步研究的设计和实施，来准确监测活体肾脏供体的长期预后，以充分告知未来捐献者相关风险。

（张云凯 译 李照 校）

参考文献

1. Murray JE. Ronald Lee Herrick Memorial: June 15, 1931-December 27, 2010. American Journal of Transplantation. 2011;11:419.
2. OPTN/SRTR 2010 Annual Data Report. Rockville, MD: Department of Health and Human Services, Health Resources and Services Administration, Healthcare Systems Bureau; 2011.
3. Meier-Kriesche HU, Kaplan B. Waiting time on dialysis as the strongest modifiable risk factor for renal transplant outcomes: a paired donor kidney analysis. Transplantation. 2002;74:1377–1381.
4. Axelrod DA, Millman D, Abecassis MM. US Health Care Reform and Transplantation, Part II: impact on the public sector and novel health care delivery systems. American Journal of Transplantation. 2010;10:2203–2207.
5. Reese PP, Feldman HI, McBride MA, et al. Substantial variation in the acceptance of medically complex live kidney donors across US renal transplant centers. American Journal of Transplantation. 2008;8:2062–2070.
6. Montgomery RA, Lonze BE, Jackson AM. Using donor exchange paradigms with desensitization to enhance transplant rates among highly sensitized patients. Current Opinion in Organ Transplantation. 2011;16:439–443.
7. Gloor J, Stegall MD. Sensitized renal transplant recipients: current protocols and future directions. Nature Reviews Nephrology. 2010;6:297–306.
8. Wallis CB, Samy KP, Roth AE, et al. Kidney paired donation. Nephrology, Dialysis, Transplantation. 2011;26:2091–2099.
9. Gentry SE, Montgomery RA, Segev DL. Kidney paired donation: fundamentals, limitations, and expansions. American Journal of Kidney Diseases. 2011;57:144–151.
10. Bingaman AW, Wright FH Jr, Kapturczak M, et al. Single-center kidney paired donation: the Methodist San Antonio experience. American Journal of Transplantation. 2012;12:2125–2132.
11. Gaston RS, Danovitch GM, Epstein RA, et al. Limiting financial disincentives in live organ donation: a rational solution to the kidney shortage. American Journal of Transplantation. 2006;6:2548–2555.
12. Matas AJ, Satel S, Munn S, et al. Incentives for organ donation: proposed standards for an internationally acceptable system. American Journal of Transplantation. 2012;12:306–312.
13. Delmonico F. Council of the Transplantation Society. A report of the Amsterdam forum on the care of the live kidney donor: data and medical guidelines. Transplantation. 2005;79(6 Suppl):S53–S66.
14. Young A, Kim SJ, Gibney EM, et al. Donor Nephrectomy Outcomes Research (DONOR) Network. Discovering misattributed paternity in living kidney donation: prevalence, preference, and practice. Transplantation. 2009;87(10):1429–1435.
15. Mandelbrot DA, Pavlakis M, Danovitch GM, et al. The medical evaluation of living kidney donors: a survey of US transplant centers. American Journal of Transplantation. 2007;7:2333–2343.
16. Taliercio JJ, Nurko S, Poggio ED. Living donor kidney transplantation: an update on evaluation and medical implications of donation. Minerva Urologica e Nefrologica. 2011;63:73–87.
17. Ommen ES, Schroppel B, Kim JY, et al. Routine use of ambulatory blood pressure monitoring in potential living kidney donors. Current Opinion in Organ Transplantation. 2007;2:1030–1036.
18. Textor S, Taler S. Expanding criteria for living kidney donors: what are the limits? Transplantation Reviews. 2008;22:187–191.
19. Ierino F, Boudville N, Kanellis J. The CARI guidelines. Donors at risk: hypertension. Nephrology. 2010;15(Suppl 1):S114–S120.
20. Nogueira JM, Weir MR, Jacobs S, et al. A study of renal outcomes in obese living kidney donors. Transplantation. 2010;90:993–999.
21. Ennis J, Kocherginsky M, Schumm LP, et al. Trends in kidney donation among kidney stone formers: a survey of US transplant centers. American Journal of Nephrology. 2009;30:12–18.
22. Saidi R, Kawai T, Kennealey P, et al. Living donor kidney transplantation with multiple arteries: recent increase in modern era of laparoscopic donor nephrectomy. Archives of Surgery. 2009;144:472–475.
23. Kawamoto S, Montgomery RA, Lawler LP, et al. Multidetector CT angiography for preoperative evaluation of living laparoscopic kidney donors. AJR. American Journal of Roentgenology. 2003;180:1633–1638.
24. Ratner LE, Kavoussi LR, Schulam PG, et al. Comparison of laparoscopic live donor nephrectomy versus the standard open approach. Transplantation Proceedings. 1997;29:138–139.
25. Clayman RV, Kavoussi LR, Soper NJ, et al. Laparoscopic nephrectomy. New England Journal of Medicine. 1991;324:1370–1371.
26. Ratner LE, Ciseck LJ, Moore RG, et al. Laparoscopic live donor nephrectomy. Transplantation. 1995;60:1047–1049.
27. Ratner LE, Kavoussi LR, Sroka M, et al. Laparoscopic assisted live donor nephrectomy–a comparison with the open approach. Transplantation. 1997;63:229–233.
28. Schulam PG, Kavoussi LR, Cheriff AD, et al. Laparoscopic live donor nephrectomy: the initial 3 cases. Journal of Urology. 1996;155:1857–1859.
29. Nanidis TG, Antcliffe D, Kokkinos C, et al. Laparoscopic versus open live donor nephrectomy in renal transplantation: a meta-analysis. Annals of Surgery. 2008;247:58–70.
30. Wolf JS Jr, Marcovich R, Merion RM, et al. Prospective, case matched comparison of hand assisted laparoscopic and open surgical live donor nephrectomy. Journal of Urology. 2000;163:1650–1653.
31. Wolf JS Jr, Merion RM, Leichtman AB, et al. Randomized controlled trial of hand-assisted laparoscopic versus open surgical live donor nephrectomy. Transplantation. 2001;72:284–290.

32. Slakey DP, Wood JC, Hender D, et al. Laparoscopic living donor nephrectomy: advantages of the hand-assisted method. Transplantation. 1999;68:581–583.
33. Minnee RC, Bemelman F, Kox C, et al. Comparison of hand-assisted laparoscopic and open donor nephrectomy in living donors. International Journal of Urology. 2008;15:206–209.
34. Dols LF, Kok NF, Ijzermans JN. Live donor nephrectomy: a review of evidence for surgical techniques. Transplant International. 2010;23:121–130.
35. Wolf JS Jr, Tchetgen MB, Merion RM. Hand-assisted laparoscopic live donor nephrectomy. Urology. 1998;52:885–887.
36. Ruiz-Deya G, Cheng S, Palmer E, et al. Open donor, laparoscopic donor and hand assisted laparoscopic donor nephrectomy: a comparison of outcomes. Journal of Urology. 2001;166:1270–1273; discussion 3–4.
37. El-Galley R, Hood N, Young CJ, et al. Donor nephrectomy: a comparison of techniques and results of open, hand assisted and full laparoscopic nephrectomy. Journal of Urology. 2004;171:40–43.
38. Lindstrom P, Haggman M, Wadstrom J. Hand-assisted laparoscopic surgery (HALS) for live donor nephrectomy is more time- and cost-effective than standard laparoscopic nephrectomy. Surgical Endoscopy. 2002;16:422–425.
39. Velidedeoglu E, Williams N, Brayman KL, et al. Comparison of open, laparoscopic, and hand-assisted approaches to live-donor nephrectomy. Transplantation. 2002;74:169–172.
40. Mateo RB, Sher L, Jabbour N, et al. Comparison of outcomes in noncomplicated and in higher-risk donors after standard versus hand-assisted laparoscopic nephrectomy. American Surgeon. 2003;69:771–778.
41. Kokkinos C, Nanidis T, Antcliffe D, et al. Comparison of laparoscopic versus hand-assisted live donor nephrectomy. Transplantation. 2007;83:41–47.
42. Silberstein J, Parsons JK. Hand-assisted and total laparoscopic nephrectomy: a comparison. JSLS: Journal of the Society of Laparoendoscopic Surgeons. 2009;13:36–43.
43. Sundqvist P, Feuk U, Haggman M, et al. Hand-assisted retroperitoneoscopic live donor nephrectomy in comparison to open and laparoscopic procedures: a prospective study on donor morbidity and kidney function. Transplantation. 2004;78:147–153.
44. Gjertsen H, Sandberg AK, Wadstrom J, et al. Introduction of hand-assisted retroperitoneoscopic living donor nephrectomy at Karolinska University Hospital Huddinge. Transplantation Proceedings. 2006;38:2644–2645.
45. Wadstrom J, Lindstrom P, Engstrom BM. Hand-assisted retroperitoneoscopic living donor nephrectomy superior to laparoscopic nephrectomy. Transplantation Proceedings. 2003;35:782–783.
46. Horgan S, Vanuno D, Sileri P, et al. Robotic-assisted laparoscopic donor nephrectomy for kidney transplantation. Transplantation. 2002;73:1474–1479.
47. Gorodner V, Horgan S, Galvani C, et al. Routine left robotic-assisted laparoscopic donor nephrectomy is safe and effective regardless of the presence of vascular anomalies. Transplant International. 2006;19:636–640.
48. Renoult E, Hubert J, Ladriere M, et al. Robot-assisted laparoscopic and open live-donor nephrectomy: a comparison of donor morbidity and early renal allograft outcomes. Nephrology, Dialysis, Transplantation. 2006;21:472–477.
49. Cannon RM, Eng M, Marvin MR, et al. Laparoscopic living kidney donation at a single center: an examination of donor outcomes with increasing experience. American Surgeon. 2011;77:911–915.
50. Wang GJ, Afaneh C, Aull M, et al. Laparoendoscopic single site live donor nephrectomy: single institution report of initial 100 cases. Journal of Urology. 2011;186:2333–2337.
51. Gimenez E, Leeser DB, Wysock JS, et al. Laparoendoscopic single site live donor nephrectomy: initial experience. Journal of Urology. 2010;184:2049–2053.
52. Afaneh C, Sheth S, Aull MJ, et al. Laparoendoscopic single-site nephrectomy in obese living renal donors. Journal of Endourology. 2012;26:140–146.
53. Afaneh C, Aull MJ, Gimenez E, et al. Comparison of laparoendoscopic single-site donor nephrectomy and conventional laparoscopic donor nephrectomy: donor and recipient outcomes. Urology. 2011;78:1332–1337.
54. Allaf ME, Singer A, Shen W, et al. Laparoscopic live donor nephrectomy with vaginal extraction: initial report. American Journal of Transplantation. 2010;10:1473–1477.
55. Pietrabissa A, Abelli M, Spinillo A, et al. Robotic-assisted laparoscopic donor nephrectomy with transvaginal extraction of the kidney. American Journal of Transplantation. 2010;10:2708–2711.
56. Davis CL, Cooper M. The state of U.S. living kidney donors. Current Opinion in Organ Transplantation. 2010;5:1873–1880.
57. Narkun-Burgess DM, Nolan CR, Norman JE, et al. Forty-five year follow-up after uninephrectomy. Kidney International. 1993;43:1110–1115.
58. Najarian JS, Chavers BM, McHugh LE, et al. 20 years or more of follow-up of living kidney donors. Lancet. 1992;340:807–810.
59. Ibrahim HN, Foley R, Tan L, et al. Long-term consequences of kidney donation. New England Journal of Medicine. 2009;360:459–469.
60. Segev DL, Muzaale AD, Caffo BS, et al. Perioperative mortality and long-term survival following live kidney donation. JAMA. 2010;303:959–966.
61. Lentine KL, Schnitzler MA, Xiao H, et al. Racial variation in medical outcomes among living kidney donors. New England Journal of Medicine. 2010;363:724–732.
62. Cohen DM, Mittalhenkle A, Scott DL, et al. African American living-kidney donors should be screened for APOL1 risk alleles. Transplantation. 2011;92:722–725.
63. Leichtman A, Abecassis M, Barr M, et al. Living kidney donor follow-up: state-of-the-art and future directions, conference summary and recommendations. American Journal of Transplantation. 2011;11:2561–2568.

第24章 活体供肝获取技术

Koji Hashimoto, Cristiano Quintini, Charles M. Miller

引言

面对愈发严重的器官捐献短缺，负责治疗终末期肝病患者的外科医生不得不由标准的脑死亡捐献扩大捐献指征。来自活体的部分移植器官是一个重要的器官来源。活体供肝移植(LDLT)的目的是为受体恢复部分肝功能的肝移植，并且留下足够的残余肝块以维持供体的健康与正常肝功能。然而,LDLT 的实际应用在一定程度上违背"primum non nocere"的伦理原则,即首要是不能伤害。活体器官捐献是医学中唯一的例外,为健康的、没有经历疾病的人实行的外科手术。在充分认识到这一问题的情况下,LDLT 的最初时代仅涉及成人向小儿科受者捐献一小部分肝脏。

在 1988 年，第一例手术是一位母亲为她的孩子捐献。由于严重的溶血和肾衰竭,患者在移植后 6 天死亡[1]。第一次成功的 LDLT 是 1989 年在澳大利亚为一例儿童患者进行的,为其移植了成人的肝左外叶[2]。左外叶切除术仅移除供体肝脏体积的 20%~25%,成人都能较好的耐受。成人-儿童 LDLT 获得广泛接受,因为该手术对于供体相对安全并且对儿童患者十分有效。

随着这一领域的成功,LDLT 的适应证慢慢地扩大到成年受体。Makuuchi 在 1993 年完成了第一例成功的成人 LDLT,使用的是肝左叶作为移植物[3]。不幸的是,成人-成人 LDLT 的早期病例经验并没有获得与在儿童接受者中同样令人满意的结果。受体所需的肝脏体积的理论值和实际值直接影响最终的效果。为了克服这个限制,外科医生开始使用更大的肝右叶。在 1996 年,第一个使用肝右叶移植的成人-成人 LDLT 在香港进行[4],然后这种技术迅速成为成人-成人 LDLT 中最常见的做法[5]。

使用肝右叶移植的成功使得东方和西方国家 LDLT 快速增加。虽然这使受体疾病预后有着明显改善，但是其也伴随着捐献者的发病率和死亡率的明显增加[6-9]。目前已有共识,捐献右叶与左叶移植物相比,供体发病率和死亡率的风险明显增加[10]。在 2002 年,随着广为人知捐献者死亡发生以及已故患者为终末期肝病(MELD)捐献程序的完善,成人-成人 LDLT 的需求和普及性在美国和欧洲急剧减少。相比之下,缺乏发达的已故捐献系统的东方国家对 LDLT 的需求持续上升。在 2010 年,LDLT 仅占美国进行的肝移植的 4.5%[11],但其在亚洲比例大于 90%。

因此直至今日，尽管 LDLT 在儿童中仍然安全有效,但成人-成人 LDLT 的应用仍然存在争议,特别是在世界上有成熟器官捐献系统的部分地区,LDLT 在成人中的应用仅是相对的。虽然世界上仍有几个中心,大多在亚洲,仍然利用 LDLT 用于高 MELD 评分的危重患者,但在西方,它通常保留用于低至中等 MELD 评分的患者[12-13]。在美国,肝右叶成人-成人 LDLT 在意向治疗分析中比那些必须等待死亡捐献者的患者显示出显著的生存优势[14-15]。即使在 MELD 评分<15 分的那些患者中,这种优势仍然持续,这是通常不会从死亡的供体肝移植受益的患者[16]。因此,随着最大限度地提高捐献者安全的新技术的发展,LDLT 的实行有可能被再次关注。

在本章中，我们将开始回顾 LDLT 中的捐献者评估和移植物的选择。活体供体的手术方面,肝切除术将被回顾,包括常规开放手术以及腹腔镜供体肝切除术。最后，我们将概述围术期供体管理和供体并发症。LDLT 受体程序的具体细节在第 57 章的附录中将会介绍。在死亡后捐献的供体肝脏的获取和心死亡后的捐献的技术方面可分别参阅第 21 章和第 22 章。

捐献者评估

捐献者的安全至关重要,这条原则没有例外。为了防止不必要的发病率,对潜在捐献者进行警惕性评估至关重要。理想情况下,捐献者的评估应由指定的捐献者宣传小组进行,该小组独立评估捐献者的候选资格,以避免利益冲突[17]。捐献者评估的目的是评估捐献者在医学、手术、情绪、心理和经济方面都适合做活体捐献。同样重要的是,还必须识别可能增加捐献者风险,以及可能危及捐献者或受体恢复的解剖变异。各种标准可能使潜在捐献者不适合活体捐献(表 24.1)。

捐献者必须充分知情同意。必须进行彻底的评估以确保没有胁迫。捐献者必须自愿做出决定,而不需要从捐献中获得任何直接或间接的经济利益。在评估期间,捐献者接受有关手术风险的教育。这包括讨论医学文献中报告的发病率和死亡率,以及将执行手术的医疗中心的发病率和死亡率结果[18]。在潜在捐献者的心理社会评价中需要尤其注意。在这个过程中,精神科医生和社会工作者在其个人行为基础上进行彻底的评估。重大的精神和情绪障碍是捐献的禁忌证。尽管在活体捐献者中矛盾是常见的,但是他们中的大多数可以在评估小组的支持下通过评价过程和捐献手术[19]。捐献者有权在手术前撤回他/她捐献意愿。读者可参考第 138 章对活体捐献的伦理进行更广泛的讨论。

表 24.1 活体肝脏捐献的相对禁忌

• 年龄<18 岁或> 55 岁(如果受体需要左外叶,则年龄>60 岁)
• 由于精神疾病而无法征得知情同意
• 病态肥胖
• 一般身体条件较差(例如,高血压、糖尿病)
• 凝血功能障碍的病史(例如,V 因子 Leiden 病)
• 出血病史
• 明显的心脏病史(冠状动脉疾病、瓣膜疾病)
• 周围血管疾病
• 慢性肺疾病
• 恶性肿瘤的近期病史,有远期复发风险(例如,乳腺癌)
• 黑色素瘤病史
• 活动感染
• 反复感染史
• 包括肝炎在内的肝脏疾病史
• 脂肪肝
• 无症状的 ZZ α-1 抗胰蛋白酶基因型
• 供体/受体肝脏大小不匹配(供体<受体)
• 供体未来的肝残留量<30%(通常将 35%作为安全裕度)
• 血管或胆管变异不适用于活体捐献

评估的第一步是从彻底的病史和体格检查开始。一般来说,潜在捐献者应该是完全健康的,在 18~55 岁之间。当接受者需要左外叶时,可以考虑直到 60 岁的捐献者。供体和受体应是血型相同或相容的。ABO 不相容的血型可以在死亡捐献极为稀缺的极端情况下被接受。优先选择与受体的有明确亲属关系的供体;然而,身体和精神健康的志愿者有时也可以作为神圣的捐献者。供体不能具有明显的疾病。然而,如果它们在医学上受到良好控制,例如,轻度高血压被认为是可接受的。在女性捐献者中,口服避孕药必须停药。高凝状态的既往史是捐献的禁忌证,由于其导致致命的血栓栓塞事件的风险较高。大量的吸烟者和饮酒者不应作为捐献者。如果潜在捐献者的体质量指数(BMI)>30kg/m^2,应进行肝活检,以排除脂肪肝的存在,这可能负面影响捐献者的安全性和受体的预后。

评估的下一步包括广泛的实验室分析和血清学测试。供体应具有正常的肝功能。系统性筛查凝血功能对于判别潜在的血栓形成风险很重要[20]。脂质谱也很重要;高脂血症与脂肪肝疾病之间有密切的关系[21]。

如果捐献者被认为是从医学和心理社会角度来看是一个好的候选人,那么下一步是评估解剖和外科方面。在解剖学的评估过程中,应该避免有创性检查。在 LDLT 的早期,常规地用血管造影术和内镜逆行胆管造影术评估供体。然而,这些有创性检查具有某些风险,这些风险不能作为对健康供体的常规评价的一部分。最近在使用多相计算机断层扫描(CT)扫描的肝脏三维重建已经能够精确的显示重要血管结构,非有创性绘图,允许对移植器官进行获取前的术前模拟(图 24.1a)。这使外科医生不仅可以直接看到详细的肝解剖,而且估计移植和残余肝体积(图 24.1b)。胆管成像可以用 MR 胆管造影术或 CT 胆管造影术来执行,以排除危及捐献者的显著解剖变异(参见下面的解剖变异)。在评估过程结束时,只有 30%~40%的有意愿的捐献者将被认为是活体捐献的良好供体。

移植器官的选择

为了理解在 LDLT 中使用的移植肝脏器官的类

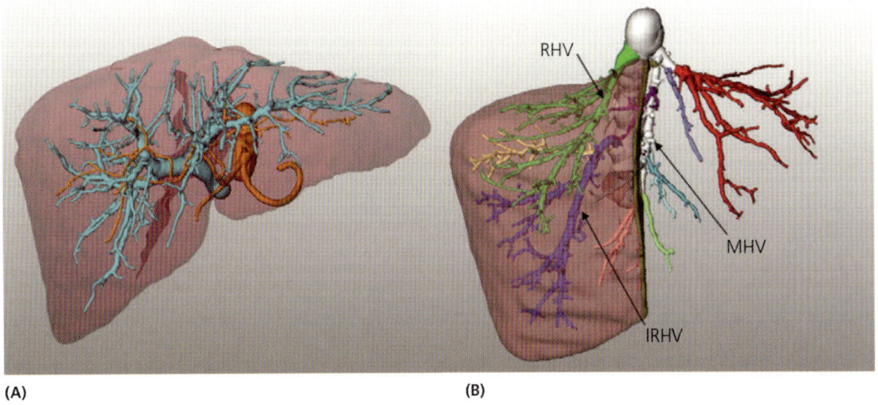

图 24.1　使用 CT 扫描对(A)肝动脉和门静脉进行三维重建，并(B)估计无肝中静脉的肝右叶移植物。RHV，右肝静脉；MHV，肝中静脉；IRHV，右肝下静脉。

型，有两个概念十分重要：剩余肝体积(FLR)和移植肝-受体体重比(GRWR)。FLR 是在捐献后估计保留的供体肝脏的比例。FLR 为 30%~35%被认为是安全和可接受的下限。在该下限下，捐献具有更高的术后肝功能衰竭发生的风险[22]。GRWR 是供体移植肝重量和受体体重之间的比率。成人-成人 LDLT 中移植肝可接受性的下限被认为是 0.6%~0.8%，其相当于受者标准肝体积的 30%~40%。然而，为应对某些特定的复杂情况，许多中心倾向于至少 1%的 GRWR 以给予受体安全余量。低于 0.6%~0.8%的 GRWR 增加了移植肝发生功能障碍的概率，称为小肝综合征(SFSS)。理想的移植肝是留下 FLR> 35%的供体并且同时提供相对于受体的足够的肝脏质量的移植物。

LDLT 中通常使用的移植肝主要有三种类型(图 24.2)：左外叶(2~3 段)，肝左叶与肝中静脉(1~4 段)，

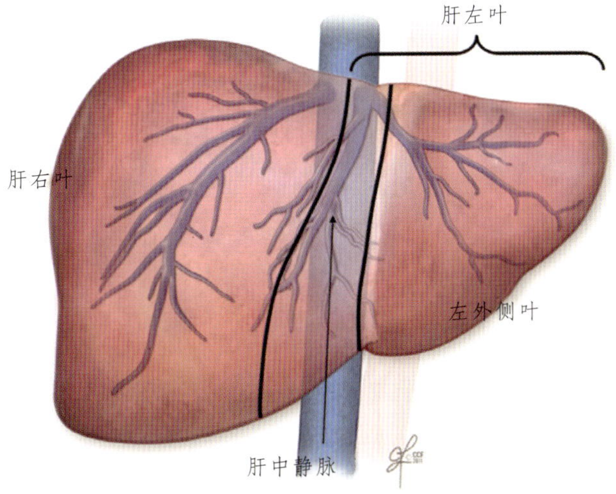

图 24.2　活体供体肝移植中常用的移植类型。

和无中肝静脉的肝右叶(5~8 段)。肝左外叶作为最小的常规移植肝，其通常占供体总肝体积的 20%~25%。这种移植肝通常捐献给儿童接受者。肝左叶占总肝脏体积的 30%~40%，通常提供给青少年或小体重成人。最后，肝右叶占总肝体积的 60%~70%，留给其余的成年受体。这是最大的移植肝，并在成人受体中有着最好的预后。然而，它同样导致捐献者发生最高的发病率和死亡率[10]。肝左叶通常具有单个静脉出口(左和中肝静脉的共同通道)，门静脉的单个左分支和单个左肝管。然而，肝左叶移植通常需要肝动脉的两个吻合[23]。相比之下，肝右叶移植物通常具有单个右肝动脉，但通常需要多个和复杂的静脉血管和胆管的重建[24]。

移植肝选择通依据由 3 个重要因素：肝解剖，供体-受体大小匹配和受体肝病的严重程度。在供体肝脏是否能够向受体提供足够的肝功能的决定因素中，最重要的是评估移植肝的功能储备。该评估被称为“移植肝功能性体积”，其是通过受体病情的严重程度、门静脉高压的严重程度和移植肝流出道可能受损的程度而制订的实际移植物肝体积的计算公式。较大的移植肝(肝右叶)更能提供足够的肝脏质量以满足受体的代谢需求，并且耐受成人肝硬化中常见的高动力内脏血流。然而，肝右叶通常需要复杂的静脉重建以确保最佳移植肝流出道。在使用肝左叶移植时，实际的移植物大小可能不总是超过 GRWR 的 0.8%或标准肝体积阈值的 40%。在这些病例中，肝左叶移植物具有优良的静脉流出道，如果受体的门静脉高压得到控制，也可提供足够的功能性肝脏体积。如果小的肝左叶移植用于高

MELD评分或严重的门静脉高压的患者，移植肝功能衰竭的风险非常高。

多个中心常规使用包括中肝静脉的扩大肝右叶移植[25]。这种移植肝为受体提供更大的肝脏质量和更好的静脉回流，但是与其他移植物肝种类相比，供体的安全性引起了关注。肝右后叶(6~7段)移植已经在一些罕见的情况下使用。这种移植肝需要复杂的外科技术，并且仅用于供体具有不成比例地小的肝左叶和罕见的门静脉解剖变异[26-27]。单节段移植肝仅用于小婴儿(体重<10kg)，以防止过大性移植肝功能衰竭[28-29]。一般来说，当肝左外叶对于这样的小婴儿来说太大时，外侧和尾部部分被去除以减小移植肝体积。这三种移植肝在技术上更具挑战性，但可以在经验丰富的中心也可以有良好的预后。

解剖变异

肝动脉

肝动脉重建仍然是LDLT中最重要和最具挑战性的步骤之一。肝动脉解剖的术前评价在供体和受体中是必须的。在活体肝脏供体中通常遇到动脉变异(约50%)。鉴别中肝动脉(A4)的起源很重要。当A4从右肝动脉产生时，肝左叶移植具有需要重建的两个分离的肝动脉。如果有肝内动脉侧支，可以牺牲较小的分支[30]。然而，通过重建两个分支可以减少胆道并发症的风险[23]。2段和3段各自的分支血管吻合直径较小(1~2mm)，增加左侧移植肝血栓形成的风险。

门静脉

需要多个血管吻合或导致捐献禁忌的门静脉的解剖变异比肝动脉或肝静脉的解剖变异发生的少[31]。一般人群中门静脉变异在占20%，三支分化是最常见的变异[32]。右前支可以从左门静脉产生。不过，该分支可以在肝门区域中鉴定，并且尽管其增加了手术复杂性但不是绝对禁忌证，它需要在肝右叶LDLT中重建两个单独的分支。当肝右叶的分支从左门静脉的脐部出现时，该门静脉分支的起点可能难以解剖和重建。

肝静脉

确保完美的静脉流出道是肝部分移植的关键，因为静脉回流是移植肝功能以及有效移植肝体积的非常重要的决定因素[5]。肝静脉解剖的预习能够术前明确最佳静脉重建的手术方案。由于左肝静脉对左叶几乎总是(92%)占优势，保留左肝中叶和中肝静脉的标准肝左叶移植通常能保证有效的流出道[33]。相比之下，在肝右叶移植中，右肝静脉和中肝静脉的各种解剖变异时常需要苛刻的重建技术[34]。现代三维CT技术可以提供对潜在拥塞段的精确估计。一般情况下，肝右前叶(5和8段)主要由肝中静脉回流。在不伴肝中静脉的供体肝右叶切除术中，5和8段静脉(V5和V8)的结扎可导致严重的静脉淤血。这导致两个问题：①拥塞区域不能完全发挥作用，降低功能性移植肝体积；②门静脉右前支变为流出道从而导致肝右后叶的门静脉高灌注。这种组合可引起严重的移植肝功能障碍和SFSS。当在成像时移植物充血导致肝体积明显变化时，应重建肝中静脉的主要分支。

20%~40%的供体中存在明显的肝右下静脉(直径>5mm)[35-36]。在这种情况下，应保留静脉以便随后在受体中重建。直径<4mm的肝右下静脉也可能是显著并且独立的负责6段的静脉回流。因此，值得临时阻断静脉以评估在相应的节段是否变得淤血拥塞[22]。当估计的拥塞面积最小，门静脉高压最低，或者GRWR较大时，没有复杂静脉重建的标准肝右叶移植足够了。相反，当预期较大体积的移植肝淤血时，强烈建议重建肝右下静脉。

胆管

胆管并发症是最常见的手术并发症，供体的胆管并发症发生率为25%[8,37,38]，受体的并发症发生率为40%[5,12,39]。异常或非标准胆管解剖成为成LDLT中的重大技术挑战。当存在多个胆管并且胆管口径非常小时，手术挑战更大。MR或CT胆管造影术可用于术前评估胆管解剖[40]，但术中胆管造影术仍然重要，以排除术前成像未显示的解剖变异。

相对于主右肝管的存在，胆道解剖学可分为两大类[41,42]。主右肝管的存在使得供体适合于肝左叶切除术或肝右叶切除术，留下将被重建的单个肝管。在没有主右肝管的情况下，前支和后支独立于左肝管和(或)肝总管。左支、右前和右后分支(12%)的分支包括在此变异中。在没有主右肝管的情况下，在肝右叶移植中需要显露出两个独立的肝管，需要复杂的胆管重建。肝左叶移植物几乎总是只有单个管道[24]。用于肝左外叶移植的胆管横切平面在肝圆韧带裂中，并且可以在左肝管的分叉的远侧到肝段胆管中。

应特别注意排除胆管解剖学的特殊变异。例如，最好是在胆囊切除术之前明确并术中分离由胆囊管分出的右肝管，该变异占 2%~3%[43]。左肝管（1%~2%）或右肝管（2%）变异也可导致供体肝切除术不能进行。

外科技术：常规开放手术

肝左外叶移植（图 24.3a）

通过上腹正中切口进行剖腹手术，是否向右延伸都可。镰状韧带是肝上、下腔静脉的分界点。在简要探查腹部器官后，游离左三角和冠状韧带。游离肝胃韧带以打开小网膜囊，但如果肝左动脉起源于胃左动脉，则必须保留。解剖肝左静脉的基部，目前不用挂线环绕。

外科海绵放置在肝右叶后面，以便游离肝脏内侧。没有必要通过手术游离肝右叶。在肝门，左肝动脉被游离显露。门静脉左支在左肝动脉后方找到确定。这都是无创性解剖。门静脉的尾状叶分支被结扎离断以游离整个门静脉左支。左肝管绕带并游离到脐裂的水平。采用缝扎控制小动脉出血。

在镰状韧带右侧 0.5cm 处用电刀标记横断线。肝实质的横切可以通过多种方法[例如，超声外科抽吸刀（CUSA）、夹钳破碎技术、水射流、双极电凝等]；该选择取决于操作者的经验和信任度，但应以最小化失血和最大化解剖精度为目标。肝实质分割直到达到肝左静脉。通过离断肝静脉韧带的头端，进入肝左静脉变得更容易。

静脉内给予 3000U 肝素后，左肝动脉结扎并离断。门静脉左支也被结扎和离断。用血管夹夹闭左肝静脉–中肝静脉连接，并离断左肝静脉。将移植肝立即移至后台并用冷保存溶液冲洗。当移植肝团队灌注移植物时，供体肝静脉的残端用丝线缝合。

肝左叶移植（图 24.3b）

向右侧延伸的上腹中线切口暴露最佳。通常不需要向左侧延伸。肝左叶的游离同肝左外叶切除术中相同。镰状韧带组织应保留在肝脏一侧，以便它可以用于将移植肝固定到受体的腹壁，以防止移植物错位到右膈下空间。尾状叶悬吊，通过分开腹膜后暴露肝后下腔静脉。

行胆囊切除术并且将胆囊管插管行胆管造影术。必须特别注意排除在术前影像学检查中未发现的解剖

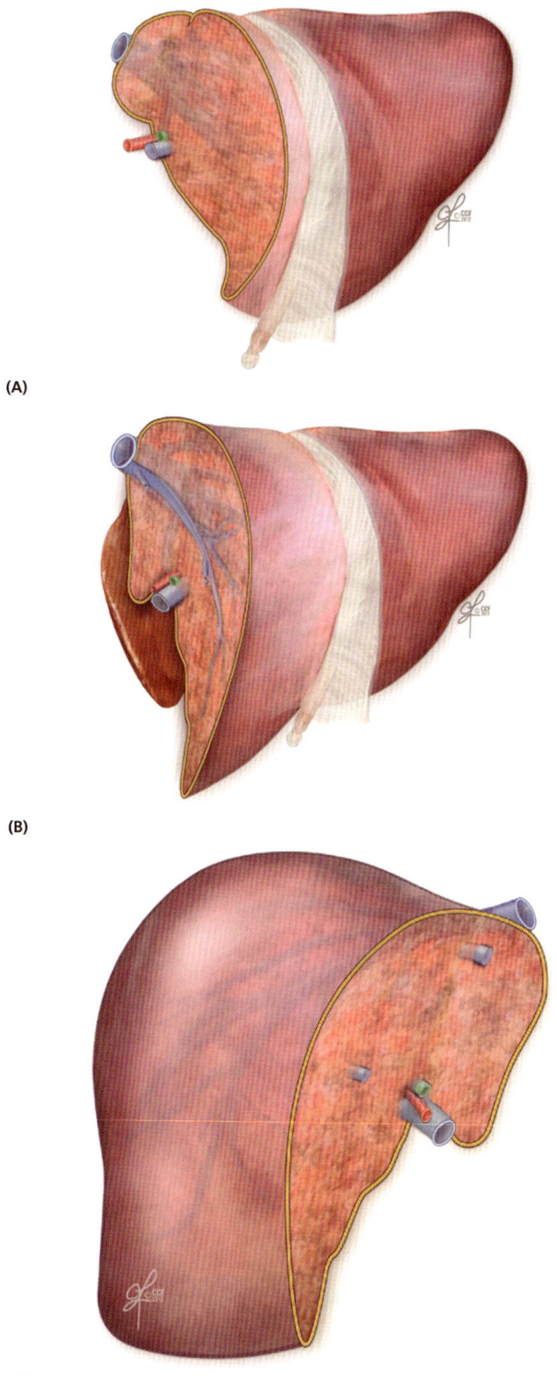

图 24.3 （A）左外叶移植，（B）左叶移植和（C）右叶移植。

变异。

在肝门离断期间，必须避免损伤右肝的解剖结构。左肝动脉显露至分叉的水平并离断。如果肝4段肝动脉起自右侧肝动脉，则动脉解剖延伸到分叉的右侧。然后在左肝动脉后显露门静脉左支并离断。努力保持一个小尾状血管分支，以确保其血液供应。

在肝门板内显露左肝管。将标记夹放置在左右肝管的分叉处左侧约0.5cm处，并再次胆管造影。如果右后肝管起源于左肝管，则最终的离断点必须在该管的左边。然后横切肝管和整个肝门板。

尾状叶与腔静脉之间的肝短静脉可结扎离断或用离断装置如Ligasure或harmonic夹横切。通常有一个主要的尾状静脉> 5mm，它可以与下腔静脉分支一起保留，以便它可以再次手术重建，以防止尾状叶的静脉充血[44]。

将左肝静脉和中肝静脉的汇合部在腔静脉入口处解剖至其基部。这需要结扎和横断左膈静脉，仔细离断从膈肌发出的穿通支。绕肝带从中肝静脉和右肝静脉之间的沟槽通过，并且在肝门结构后面通过，以将肝实质与腔静脉和肝门结构隔离。这样使肝脏悬吊，可以帮助暴露，减少失血，并指导肝实质横断的方向[45]。

进行术中超声以明确中肝静脉的解剖结构。中肝静脉支流的位置也得到证实。因为根据肝中静脉和胆囊窝的解剖学确定横断线，所以不需要通过临时的半肝血流阻断来确认分界线。该线在中肝静脉的右侧电刀标记，其来自胆囊窝，并沿着胆囊窝左侧肝脏的下表面向下到达胆管横切点。外科医生选择信任的技术和工具进行肝实质横断。一旦确定了中肝静脉，实质横断线最好在肝中静脉右侧1~2mm处，在解剖面和静脉之间有薄薄的肝实质。这可以防止中肝静脉的小分支的出血。在实质横断的最后部分，圆韧带的两端被轻轻拉动以产生向上牵引。然后完成横切并完全止血。给予肝素后，将左肝动脉和门静脉左支一起横切。随后，使用缝合装置缝合左肝静脉和中肝静脉的基部，并且在移植肝侧上横切静脉。立即取出肝移植物并用冷保存溶液冲洗。

在左肝管的残端突出之后，通过胆囊管行最终胆管造影以确保剩余胆管的完整性。

后台肝左叶移植物通常需要静脉成形术以优化静脉流出。将左肝静脉和中肝静脉之间的隔膜垂直切下并取出。内膜的缺损用单丝缝合闭合。这种技术还有助于扩大静脉孔的直径[46]。

肝右叶移植(图24.3c)

向右侧延伸的上腹中线切口。将圆韧带游离切断，然后将镰状韧带一直游离至肝上下腔静脉。在探查腹部脏器后，分割右三角韧带和冠状韧带。左叶不应游离，因为不必要的游离增加了残余肝脏错位的风险，并可能导致供者的术后肝功能不全。右叶在内侧旋转以完全游离，直到肝后下腔静脉出现。

行胆囊切除术，然后通过胆囊管行胆管造影。肝门解剖开始于肝门的右侧。这可以进行肝动脉分叉的解剖，而不接触肝动脉，以确保对普通肝管的血液供应不受干扰[47]。切除右肝动脉。然后解剖门静脉右支。尾状叶分支结扎并游离，保证足够的长度以确保当移除右肝时可放置血管夹。右肝管环绕肝门板。胆管造影定位后，在肝管和肝门板从分叉处横切0.5cm。

然后注意回到下腔静脉解剖。小心地游离下腔静脉韧带。肝短静脉在下腔静脉的右侧离断。中肝静脉和右肝静脉之间的沟槽被显露。分离右肝静脉，并使绕肝带通过该沟槽用于肝脏悬挂操作(图24.4a)[48]。绕肝带的尾端通过肝门结构后面，以隔离肝实质与腔静脉和肝门结构(图24.4b)。

同切除肝左叶一样确定切除线。肝实质切除以与肝左叶切除术相同的方式进行(见上文)。唯一的区别是，需要保留从右前叶进入肝中静脉的V5和V8(参见上面的解剖变异)。这些静脉被结扎在剩余的一侧，并被夹闭在右叶一侧。

在横断完成并完全止血后，给予静脉内肝素。然后右肝动脉和门静脉右支分别结扎离断。然后将右肝静脉沿着下腔静脉的边缘垂直缝合，并在移植肝侧充分游离。立即取出移植肝并用冷保存溶液冲洗。右肝管的残端用单丝缝合线穿过。通过胆囊管进行最终胆管造影以确认残余胆管的完整性。

在后台上，如果需要，重建V5和V8。该技术提供了与具有中间肝静脉的扩大肝右叶移植相当的功能性肝脏质量。血管移植物对于重建V5和V8是必需的。未使用的新鲜髂动脉和静脉移植物在死者供肝移植中是血管移植物的良好来源。可以使用自体移植物，例如，受体天然肝脏的肝内门静脉、肠系膜下静脉、性腺静脉和再通的脐静脉，其具有良好的开放性[49]。如果这

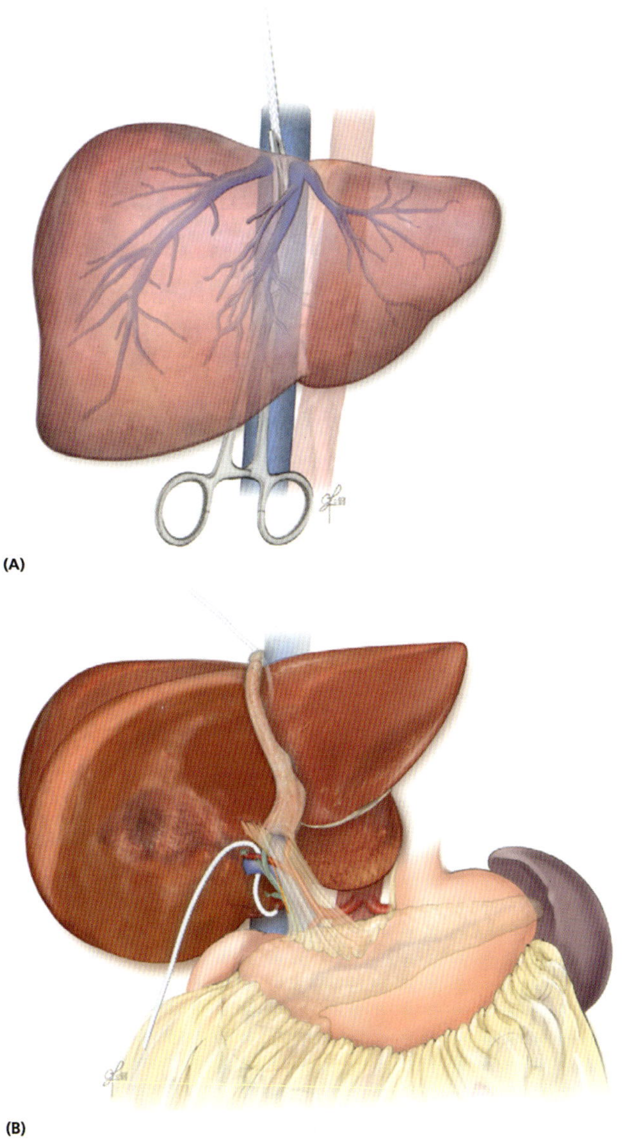

图 24.4　肝悬吊术以利于肝实质离断。

些不可用,来自尸体供体的冷冻保存的血管移植物是另一种选择[50]。已经报道了使用膨胀聚四氟乙烯(ePTFE)移植物用于 V5 和 V8 重建的有着良好的效果[51]。在那些情况中,ePTFE 移植物的通畅性在 1 个月时为 80%,在 4 个月时为 40%。早期阻塞 ePTFE 移植物的受试者在前段具有明显的充血,但是具有晚期阻塞的受试者是无症状的。患者和移植物存活率与扩大肝右叶移植(具有中肝静脉)的那些一样好。只要实现早期通畅,晚期静脉移植阻塞似乎对前段充血或生存没有影响。因为人工血管移植物的可用性没有限制,它们可能是右前叶引流的有效替代物。

腹腔镜供肝切除术

微创技术已经成功应用于活体供体肾脏获取,并且它们的优势使得该方式对许多潜在供体更具吸引力。一般来说,微创手术有更好的疼痛控制,具有更短的住院时间、更快的功能恢复,改善的美观和降低手术并发症的风险。事实上,自从引入腹腔镜供体肾脏切除术[52]以来,腹腔镜手术(见第 23 章)的好处已经被广泛认为,这种技术已迅速成为全世界活体供体肾移植的标准[53,54]。它已被证明是相对安全的,虽然有报道偶发性供体死亡由于错误夹闭肾动脉[55]。在尝试遵循微创肾脏获取的脚步,一些中心开始执行腹腔镜辅助活体供体肝切除术这些技术包括腹腔镜手术和手辅助腹腔镜手术。

关于腹腔镜肝脏手术,许多报告已经提出其用于切除良性和恶性肝肿瘤的安全性和可行性。随着腹腔镜肝脏手术的发展,其用于活体供肝切除术的应用已经提出,并且在法国首次尝试左外叶切除术[56]。本报道之后是一系列成功的 16 名捐献者[57]。最近,一个韩国团队报告了 11 名捐献者进行腹腔镜左外叶切除术;与常规开放性肝切除术相比,他们实现了较短的住院时间和较早的恢复饮食,无手术并发症[58]。

第一次腹腔镜辅助供体肝右叶切除术于 2006 年从西北大学报告[59]。4 名捐献者成功进行腹腔镜辅助程序,没有并发症。另一个韩国团队报道了 9 例腹腔镜肝右叶供肝肝切除术,其中唯一主要的手术并发症是 1 例患者的腹腔内脓肿[60]。此外,一个日本团队报道了 13 个成功的腹腔镜半肝脏获取,包括 3 个肝右叶切除术,他们使用无气腹壁提升技术,而不是气腹,以降低空气栓塞的风险[61]。

关于外科技术,很少进行纯腹腔镜供体肝切除术。相反,通常使用"混合"技术。这种技术包括肝辅助腹腔镜游离,随后是开放技术进行肝门解剖,实质横断和移植肝探查。除了小切口,该技术需要 10~12cm 长的上腹中线切口用于手动端口和移植物提取。通过避免肋下切口,混合技术可以减少供体的疼痛和发病率,并缩短恢复时间。

尽管最近有这些技术的报道,对活体供体的外科应对似乎取决于去除的肝脏体积。此外,仍然担心如果发生,通过小切口快速控制出血的能力。因此,似乎这种方法的常规应用仍有争议。在腹腔镜手术和常规供肝肝切除术的广泛经验的组合是成功应用这种方法的关键。需要进一步仔细的评估和讨论才能达成普遍的共识[62,63]。

围术期供体管理

在手术前一天,移植小组举行会议,通过一个最终清单,以确保评估已彻底完成。在麻醉诱导之前应该常规地进行试运行,以确保整个团队完全准备好并且所有设备都可用。如果在任一次会议上发现缺陷,应进行进一步评价,程序推迟或中止。

活体肝捐献者应该在术后24小时接受重症监护治疗。对生命体征的密切监测至关重要,并且应定期检查实验室数据。移植小组进行全面评估后,允许捐献者转入常规移植护理楼,医务人员熟悉肝脏切除术和肝移植患者的护理。这些团队应该熟悉与供体手术相关的常见并发症,例如,腹内出血、伤口感染、急性肾衰竭、胃膨胀,电解质紊乱和深静脉血栓形成。重症监护室和常规护理床都应该有适当的监测,以在这些并发症造成严重问题之前检测这些并发症。具有生命体征和实验室数据意外变化的捐献者需要立即评估。

由移植外科医生领导的多学科小组每天查房和评估捐献者,直到出院。疼痛管理是一个需要解决的主要问题。硬膜外麻醉可以提供良好的疼痛管理,但是存在并发症的风险,例如继发于血肿的急性脊髓压迫[64-66]和已报道的截瘫的病例。代替硬膜外镇痛,静脉内患者控制的镇痛是术后早期的一种选择。一些中心,包括我们自己,更喜欢使用短效的麻醉剂(24h),序列应用酮咯酸(Toradol)。由于长期使用麻醉剂会增加并发症的风险,因此强烈建议尽早切换到非麻醉药。

移植外科医生应该进行门诊随访,以检查伤口愈合,感染迹象和肝功能恢复。身体检查和实验室数据的任何异常应进一步评估。应至少监测肝功能测试,直到它们正常化。供体应该进行某种成像研究以确认充分的肝再生并排除任何手术并发症,包括胆汁泄漏、胆管狭窄、血栓形成和腹腔积液。没有临床症状,成像研究不需要重复。

关于活体捐献者的全面和准确的后续数据对于确保其安全至关重要。目前,联合国机构共享网络(UNOS)要求移植中心在捐献后至少2年内提交关于每个活体捐献者状态的信息[67]。随访方案可能因程序而异,但大多数中心每年继续跟踪捐献者,除外他们有任何并发症。

供体并发症

尽管捐献者的安全至关重要,但在世界范围内报道了一定的发病率和死亡率。尽管系统地利用肝右叶移植允许成人-成人LDLT的快速增长,并且在接受者中具有良好的结果,但是很快变得清楚的是,与肝左叶供体相比,右叶供体的发病率和死亡率远远更高。肝左外叶、肝左叶和肝右叶捐献后的供体并发症发生率约为15%、25%和35%~40%[8,9,37,68,69]。肝左叶的供体死亡率为0.1%,肝右叶捐献的死亡率为0.5%[10]。左叶和右叶捐献之间的发病率和死亡率的差异可以归因于两个因素:①肝左叶切除后留下较大的功能性肝残余物和②肝右叶切除术后常见的多发性胆汁漏。不应忽略单个胆管的优点,因为右叶受体的发病率通常由与多个胆管相关的并发症引起。

根据Clavien分级报告这些并发症很重要,根据严重程度的5个级别对其进行划分(表24.2)[70]。尽管如此,报告的并发症在不同的程序之间差异很大,可能是由于不同的经验或报告方法。

胆道并发症是在活体肝脏供体中最常见的并发症。伤口感染是第二常见的并发症。血管并发症较不常

表24.2 根据Clavien评分对并发症进行分级

1级	不需要药理治疗或外科手术,内镜和放射学干预而偏离正常术后过程的任何情况。允许的治疗方案是止吐药、退热药、止痛药、利尿药、电解质和物理疗法等药物。这个等级还包括在床边打开的伤口感染
2级	需要进行除1级并发症以外的药物治疗的并发症。还包括输血和全胃肠外营养
3级	需要手术、内镜或放射学干预的并发症
3a级	不在全身麻醉下进行干预
3b级	全身麻醉下的干预
4级	危及生命的并发症(包括中枢神经系统并发症)需要重症病房
4a级	单器官功能障碍(包括透析)
4b级	多器官功能障碍
5级	患者死亡

Reproduced from Dindo et al. [70], with permission from Wolters Kluwer Health.

见，但伴有显著的发病率和死亡率。胃滞留是罕见的(3%)，但严重危及左叶供体的生活质量[9]。已经报道了与麻醉和术后恢复相关的并发症(深静脉血栓形成、肺栓塞等)。在考虑 LDLT 和知情同意过程中，这些风险必须与捐献者及其家属详细讨论。一些捐献者需要在捐献后的早期或晚期的社会和心理支持[71,72]。社会工作者和精神病医生在支持和治疗他们方面发挥重要作用。在有重大问题的捐献者中可能需要考虑医疗服务。对于以上这些问题，移植团队和捐献者的初级保健医生之间的密切沟通也很重要。

总结

活体供肝移植已发展成为终末期肝病患者可行的选择，尽管在伦理上和技术上有些复杂。推动其成功实施的主要因素是适当的供体选择和对程序的解剖细节的高度注意。仔细考虑肝切除术对捐献者的影响以及术前必须明确手术对受体的必要性，并在术中进行持续评估。理想的移植肝同时为供体提供超过 35%的残余肝体积和受体具有> 0.8%的移植肝-受体重量比。一般来说，活体捐献仍然是开放手术为主，腹腔镜方法也正在探讨当中。多学科团队的围术期管理是重要的，LDLT 的实践应限于专门的，经过适当培训和资源充足的团队。其在短期内的执行将取决于这些小组的可用性和已故捐献机构的短缺。

(张云凯 译　李照 校)

参考文献

1. Raia S, Nery JR, Mies S. Liver transplantation from live donors. Lancet. 1989;2:497.
2. Strong RW, Lynch SV, Ong TH, et al. Successful liver transplantation from a living donor to her son. New England Journal of Medicine. 1990;322:1505–1507.
3. Hashikura Y, Makuuchi M, Kawasaki S, et al. Successful living-related partial liver transplantation to an adult patient. Lancet. 1994;343:1233–1234.
4. Lo CM, Fan ST, Liu CL, et al. Adult-to-adult living donor liver transplantation using extended right lobe grafts. Annals of Surgery. 1997;226:261–269.
5. Miller CM, Gondolesi GE, Florman S, et al. One hundred nine living donor liver transplants in adults and children: a single-center experience. Annals of Surgery. 2001;234:301–311.
6. Hwang S, Lee SG, Lee YJ, et al. Lessons learned from 1,000 living donor liver transplantations in a single center: how to make living donations safe. Liver Transplantation. 2006;12:920–927.
7. Yi NJ, Suh KS, Cho JY, et al. Three-quarters of right liver donors experienced postoperative complications. Liver Transplantation. 2007;13:797–806.
8. Ghobrial RM, Freise CE, Trotter JF, et al.; A2ALL Study Group. Donor morbidity after living donation for liver transplantation. Gastroenterology. 2008;135:468–476.
9. Taketomi A, Kayashima H, Soejima Y, et al. Donor risk in adult-to-adult living donor liver transplantation: impact of left lobe graft. Transplantation. 2009;87:445–450.
10. Barr ML, Belghiti J, Villamil FG, et al. A report of the Vancouver Forum on the care of the live organ donor: lung, liver, pancreas, and intestine data and medical guidelines. Transplantation. 2006;81:1373–1385.
11. Health Resources and Services Administration/Organ Procurement and Transplantation Network. HRSA/OPTN: Transplants by donor type. [cited December 3, 2011]; Available from: http://optn.transplant.hrsa.gov/latestData/rptData.asp.
12. Morioka D, Egawa H, Kasahara M, et al. Outcomes of adult-to-adult living donor liver transplantation: a single institution's experience with 335 consecutive cases. Annals of Surgery. 2007;245:315–325.
13. Selzner M, Kashfi A, Cattral MS, et al. Live donor liver transplantation in high MELD score recipients. Annals of Surgery. 2010;251:153–157.
14. Berg CL, Gillespie BW, Merion RM, et al.; A2ALL Study Group. Improvement in survival associated with adult-to-adult living donor liver transplantation. Gastroenterology. 2007;133:1806–1813.
15. Berg CL, Merion RM, Shearon TH, et al. Liver transplant recipient survival benefit with living donation in the model for endstage liver disease allocation era. Hepatology. 2011;54:1313–1321.
16. Merion RM, Schaubel DE, Dykstra DM, et al. The survival benefit of liver transplantation. American Journal of Transplantation. 2005;5:307–313.
17. Rudow DL. The living donor advocate: a team approach to educate, evaluate, and manage donors across the continuum. Progress in Transplantation. 2009;19:64–70.
18. Pruett TL, Tibell A, Alabdulkareem A, et al. The ethics statement of the Vancouver Forum on the live lung, liver, pancreas, and intestine donor. Transplantation. 2006;81:1386–1387.
19. Ann Simpson M, Kendrick J, Verbesey JE, et al. Ambivalence in living liver donors. Liver Transplantation. 2011;17:1226–1233.
20. Durand F, Ettorre GM, Douard R, et al. Donor safety in living related liver transplantation: underestimation of the risks for deep vein thrombosis and pulmonary embolism. Liver Transplantation. 2002;8:118–120.
21. Lee JY, Kim KM, Lee SG, et al. Prevalence and risk factors of non-alcoholic fatty liver disease in potential living liver donors in Korea: a review of 589 consecutive liver biopsies in a single center. Journal of Hepatology. 2007;47:239–244.
22. Fan ST. Live donor liver transplantation in adults. Transplantation. 2006;82:723–732.
23. Uchiyama H, Harada N, Sanefuji K, et al. Dual hepatic artery reconstruction in living donor liver transplantation using a left hepatic graft with 2 hepatic arterial stumps. Surgery. 2010;147:878–886.
24. Florman S, Miller CM. Live donor liver transplantation. Liver Transplantation. 2006;12:499–510.
25. Chan SC, Fan ST, Lo CM, et al. A decade of right liver adult-to-adult living donor liver transplantation: the recipient mid-term outcomes. Annals of Surgery. 2008;248:411–419.
26. Kokudo N, Sugawara Y, Imamura H, et al. Tailoring the type of donor hepatectomy for adult living donor liver transplantation. American Journal of Transplantation. 2005;5:1694–1703.
27. Tanimoto Y, Tashiro H, Itamoto T, et al. Hepatic venous outflow obstruction after right lateral sector living-donor liver transplantation, treated by insertion of an expandable metallic stent. Journal of Hepato-Biliary-Pancreatic Surgery. 2008;15:228–231.
28. Enne M, Pacheco-Moreira L, Balbi E, et al. Liver transplantation with monosegments. Technical aspects and outcome: a meta-analysis. Liver Transplantation. 2005;11:564–569.
29. Ogawa K, Kasahara M, Sakamoto S, et al. Living donor liver transplantation with reduced monosegments for neonates and small infants. Transplantation. 2007;83:1337–1340.
30. Ikegami T, Kawasaki S, Matsunami H, et al. Should all hepatic arterial branches be reconstructed in living-related liver transplantation? Surgery. 1996;119:431–436.
31. Nakamura T, Tanaka K, Kiuchi T, et al. Anatomical variations and surgical strategies in right lobe living donor liver transplantation: lessons from 120 cases. Transplantation. 2002;73:1896–1903.
32. Couinaud C. Liver anatomy: portal (and suprahepatic) or biliary segmentation. Digestive Surgery. 1999;16:459–467.
33. Radtke A, Sotiropoulos GC, Sgourakis G, et al. Hepatic venous drainage: how much can we learn from imaging studies? Anatomic-functional classification derived from three-dimensional computed tomography reconstructions. Transplantation. 2010;89:1518–1525.
34. Neumann JO, Thorn M, Fischer L, et al. Branching patterns and drainage territories of the middle hepatic vein in computer-simulated right living-donor hepatectomies. American Journal of Transplantation. 2006;6:1407–1415.
35. Uchida K, Taniguchi M, Shimamura T, et al. Three-dimensional computed tomography scan analysis of hepatic vasculatures in the donor liver for living donor liver transplantation. Liver Transplantation. 2010;16:1062–1068.
36. Hwang S, Ha TY, Ahn CS, et al. Reconstruction of inferior right hepatic veins in

living donor liver transplantation using right liver grafts. Liver Transplantation. 2012;18:238–247.
37. Azoulay D, Bhangui P, Andreani P, et al. Short- and long-term donor morbidity in right lobe living donor liver transplantation: 91 consecutive cases in a European Center. American Journal of Transplantation. 2011;11:101–110.
38. Hashikura Y, Ichida T, Umeshita K, et al. Japanese Liver Transplantation Society. Donor complications associated with living donor liver transplantation in Japan. Transplantation. 2009;88:110–114.
39. Chok KS, Chan SC, Cheung TT, et al. Bile duct anastomotic stricture after adult-to-adult right lobe living donor liver transplantation. Liver Transplantation. 2011;17:47–52.
40. Basaran C, Agildere AM, Donmez FY, et al. MR cholangiopancreatography with T2-weighted prospective acquisition correction turbo spin-echo sequence of the biliary anatomy of potential living liver transplant donors. AJR. American Journal of Roentgenology. 2008;190:1527–1533.
41. Kawarada Y, Das BC, Taoka H. Anatomy of the hepatic hilar area: the plate system. Journal of Hepato-Biliary-Pancreatic Surgery. 2000;7:580–586.
42. Ohkubo M, Nagino M, Kamiya J, et al. Surgical anatomy of the bile ducts at the hepatic hilum as applied to living donor liver transplantation. Annals of Surgery. 2004;239:82–86.
43. Kullman E, Borch K, Lindström E, et al. Value of routine intraoperative cholangiography in detecting aberrant bile ducts and bile duct injuries during laparoscopic cholecystectomy. British Journal of Surgery. 1996;83:171–175.
44. Yamazaki S, Takayama T, Makuuchi M. The technical advance and impact of caudate lobe venous reconstruction in left liver: additional safety for living-related donor liver transplantation. Transplant International. 2010;23: 345–349.
45. Ogata S, Belghiti J, Varma D, et al. Two hundred liver hanging maneuvers for major hepatectomy: a single-center experience. Annals of Surgery. 2007;245: 31–35.
46. Suehiro T, Shimada M, Kishikawa K, et al. Impact of graft hepatic vein inferior vena cava reconstruction with graft venoplasty and inferior vena cava cavoplasty in living donor adult liver transplantation using a left lobe graft. Transplantation. 2005;80:964–968.
47. Kokudo N, Sugawara Y, Imamura H, et al. Sling suspension of the liver in donor operation: a gradual tape-repositioning technique. Transplantation. 2003;76: 803–807.
48. Taketomi A, Morita K, Toshima T, et al. Living donor hepatectomies with procedures to prevent biliary complications. Journal of the American College of Surgeons. 2010;211:456–464.
49. Ikegami T, Soejima Y, Taketomi A, et al. Explanted portal vein grafts for middle hepatic vein tributaries in living-donor liver transplantation. Transplantation. 2007;84:836–841.
50. Sugawara Y, Makuuchi M, Akamatsu N, et al. Refinement of venous reconstruction using cryopreserved veins in right liver grafts. Liver Transplantation. 2004; 10:541–547.
51. Yi NJ, Suh KS, Lee HW, et al. An artificial vascular graft is a useful interpositional material for drainage of the right anterior section in living donor liver transplantation. Liver Transplantation. 2007;13:1159–1167.
52. Ratner LE, Ciseck LJ, Moore RG, et al. Laparoscopic live donor nephrectomy. Transplantation. 1995;60:1047–1049.
53. Sasaki TM, Finelli F, Bugarin E, et al. Is laparoscopic donor nephrectomy the new criterion standard? Archives of Surgery. 2000;135:943–947.
54. Nanidis TG, Antcliffe D, Kokkinos C, et al. Laparoscopic versus open live donor nephrectomy in renal transplantation: a meta-analysis. Annals of Surgery. 2008;247:58–70.
55. Friedman AL, Peters TG, Jones KW, et al. Fatal and nonfatal hemorrhagic complications of living kidney donation. Annals of Surgery. 2006;243: 126–130.
56. Cherqui D, Soubrane O, Husson E, et al. Laparoscopic living donor hepatectomy for liver transplantation in children. Lancet. 2002;359:392–396.
57. Soubrane O, Cherqui D, Scatton O, et al. Laparoscopic left lateral sectionectomy in living donors: safety and reproducibility of the technique in a single center. Annals of Surgery. 2006;244:815–820.
58. Kim KH, Jung DH, Park KM, et al. Comparison of open and laparoscopic live donor left lateral sectionectomy. British Journal of Surgery. 2011;98: 1302–1308.
59. Koffron AJ, Kung R, Baker T, et al. Laparoscopic-assisted right lobe donor hepatectomy. American Journal of Transplantation. 2006;6:2522–2525.
60. Suh KS, Yi NJ, Kim T, et al. Laparoscopy-assisted donor right hepatectomy using a hand port system preserving the middle hepatic vein branches. World Journal of Surgery. 2009;33:526–533.
61. Kurosaki I, Yamamoto S, Kitami C, et al. Video-assisted living donor hemihepatectomy through a 12-cm incision for adult-to-adult liver transplantation. Surgery. 2006;139:695–703.
62. Baker TB, Jay CL, Ladner DP, et al. Laparoscopy-assisted and open living donor right hepatectomy: a comparative study of outcomes. Surgery. 2009;146: 817–823.
63. Thenappan A, Jha RC, Fishbein T, et al. Liver allograft outcomes after laparoscopic-assisted and minimal access live donor hepatectomy for transplantation. American Journal of Surgery. 2011;201:450–455.
64. Ozkardesler S, Ozzeybek D, Alaygut E, et al. Anesthesia-related complications in living liver donors: the experience from one center and the reporting of one death. American Journal of Transplantation. 2008;8:2106–2110.
65. Hwang GS, McCluskey SA. Anesthesia and outcome after partial hepatectomy for adult-to-adult donor transplantation. Current Opinion in Organ Transplantation. 2010;15:377–382.
66. Clarke H, Chandy T, Srinivas C, et al. Epidural analgesia provides better pain management after live liver donation: a retrospective study. Liver Transplantation. 2011;17:315–323.
67. Health Resources and Services Administration/Organ Procurement and Transplantation Network. HRSA/OPTN: Proposed guidance for the medical evaluation of living liver donors. 2009. [cited December 3, 2011]; Available from: http://optn.transplant.hrsa.gov/PublicComment/pubcommentPropSub_247.pdf.
68. Humar A, Carolan E, Ibrahim H, et al. A comparison of surgical outcomes and quality of life surveys in right lobe vs. left lateral segment liver donors. American Journal of Transplantation. 2005;5:805–809.
69. Iida T, Ogura Y, Oike F, et al. Surgery-related morbidity in living donors for liver transplantation. Transplantation. 2010;89:1276–1282.
70. Dindo D, Demartines N, Clavien P-A. Classification of surgical complications: a new proposal with evaluation in a cohort of 6336 patients and results of a survey. Annals of Surgery. 2004;240(2):205–213.
71. Walter M, Papachristou C, Pascher A, et al. Impaired psychosocial outcome of donors after living donor liver transplantation: a qualitative case study. Clinical Transplantation. 2006;20:410–415.
72. Trotter JF, Hill-Callahan MM, Gillespie BW, et al. A2ALL Study Group. Severe psychiatric problems in right hepatic lobe donors for living donor liver transplantation. Transplantation. 2007;83:1506–1508.

第 25 章 腹部器官的保存和复苏

Henri G.D. Leuvenink，Rutger J. Ploeg

引言

现代器官移植，尤其是死亡捐献器官的移植，需要依赖一些科学的方法保持移植器官的活性，直到最终被移植后血管得到重建。的确，保存的质量是影响移植后器官功能的主要因素，因为有了科学的方法能够保存器官渡过重要的时期，所以几乎所有有关器官分配的创新都成为可能，本章会介绍一些现已出现的，在器官保存中非常重要的新概念，并强调一些临床数据来支持腹部器官保存和运输中的一些首选方法。它对第26章进行了补充，第26章讲述了适用于胸部器官的特有的类似的概念。这两章都介绍了关于器官复苏的新兴概念：用来改善离体器官的质量与功能的一些方法和操作。的确，这个概念代表着未来的发展，在这个未来的发展中，器官不仅仅被期望能被保存住原有的功能状态，而是达到另一状态，那就是器官可以随着时间而改善，而且通过离体操作使其更加适合器官移植。

影响现代器官保存发展的因素

在临床器官移植的早期，供受体是限制在同一家医院，大多数手术是在相邻的手术室进行的，这就允许器官的直接转移，便于移植。因此，除了血液灌注外，不需要其他的保存方法。随着移植项目发展成国家甚至是国际项目后，保存时间延长使器官移植从供体移植到HLA相匹配的受体身上变得更容易，减少由于排斥造成的移植失败的概率。在这一时期，适当的保存是必需的，它保证了一个有功能的、能够维持生命的器官在移植中被植入。因此，一个简单方法被采用使供体的移植器官顺利过渡到需要移植的患者身上，用冰块快速冷却和保存器官。然而，这种低温、低氧的保存方法会不可避免地带来一些有害的副作用，现在的保存方法已经被设计去抵消这些组织损伤的机制。另外，在过去的十年里，捐献器官的种类和质量都得到了显著的改善，在一些年龄较大、动力学不稳定的患者中，甚至在一些心脏停搏的患者中，移植器官都能得到显著的改善。

在保存期间维持器官的活性是器官移植成功的重要的先决条件。目前，大部分移植中心都是使用静态的低温保存器官。然而这种保存方法得到发展的年代，主要是以年轻的或者高质量的供体器官的可用性为特征的[1]。因为终末期器官衰竭需要器官移植的患者数量与来自脑死亡患者捐赠的高质量可用的器官数量之间差距与日俱增，使得很多移植协会被迫去接受仅供选择的可移植的器官。而对于肾移植，许多国家的现有的捐赠程序已经在一定程度上缩小了这种差距。而对于其他器官，这种的模式的捐赠要么不可能，要么会给捐赠者带来重大的风险。

考虑到高质量的供体的低利用率和可移植器官的持续的需求，接受移植的标准条件不断在扩充延伸。这些扩大标准供体器官(ECD;扩大标准供体将在第53章详细介绍)，相比于标准条件下脑死亡后捐赠的器官移植，平均受体生存率，移植物的存活和器官的功能都要差一些。如果预计校准后的移植器官衰竭的相对风险≥1.70，一个脑死亡后捐献的肾脏就被认为是一个扩大标准后的供体器官。扩大标准后捐赠肾脏的供体特征包括：年龄>60岁，或者年龄在50~59岁之间并符合以下条件中的两条：脑血管意外导致的死亡、已存在的高血压病、终端血清肌酐>1.5mg/dL。扩大标准供体的肝脏的特征：年龄>60岁、冷藏时间>12h、组织学上的脂肪肝、使用过血管活性药物。

在肾脏移植中，由于这类捐赠器官的使用的增加，导致移植器官延迟衰竭发生率从20世纪80年代末的15%增长到最近器官供应移植网络报道的25%。移植器官延迟衰竭已证明会给移植器官的存活产生负面影响，会产生1.7倍的相对风险。相对于标准条件下的捐赠器官1年后的生存率下降15%。

为了进一步增加器官捐献库，特别是最近几年，心脏死亡患者的捐献器官的使用也在增加。心脏死亡患者捐赠人是依据《马斯特里赫特标准》分类的。然而在大部分国家，仅仅符合马斯特里赫特标准的第3类捐献者或者可控的循环系统衰竭的捐献者是可以使用的。一些国家出台了不可控心脏死亡患者(第1类和第2类)的概念。可控循环系统衰竭捐献者是指那些有着广泛不可逆脑损伤的患者，进一步治疗无任何意义，但是，又没有达到脑死亡的标准。撤去通气支持后，患者会因为心脏骤停、循环停止而去世。经历一段“无感觉”的时间，器官能够被挽救并保存。

不可控的捐献者并没有经历脑损伤，而是死于原发性心脏骤停后的不成功复苏。无论是可控还是不可控的情况，热缺血时间的存在都会给潜在的移植器官带来损伤。

心脏死亡捐献者的肾脏有很高的原发性无功能的风险，并且会经历移植器官的延迟衰竭。更有趣的是，相比于那些来自脑死亡捐献的肾脏，尽管移植后发生功能衰竭的可能性较高，但是长期移植器官存活却是基本一样或者仅仅稍低一些。这有可能是选择性偏差。

由于较差的移植效果和频发的胆管并发症，心脏死亡捐献者器官的使用在肝脏移植中要比肾脏移植中更少被接受。会导致再次肝移植。然而，在一些移植中心，脑死亡捐献者和心脏死亡捐献者的肝移植有着相等的效果，这表明拥有好的捐献者管理和适当保存技术，这些捐赠者将会成为一个好的资源，减少等待移植患者的死亡率。

低温保存的原则

在循环停止后，组织代谢会持续一段时间；然而氧气和营养的缺乏很快会导致肾脏细胞主要的代谢障碍。因此，在器官保存期间，抑制代谢是保持器官活性所必需的。

与化学反应相似，生物系统中代谢率的减低依靠温度的下降。Q10温度系数被用来衡量温度每减低10℃生物或化学系统代谢率改变[2]。把这个应用到器官保存中，这就意味着把器官的中心体温降低到4℃，将会使细胞的代谢降低到原有的10%。并且会降低生物酶的活性(图25.1)。Calne等科学家表明：用冰水对肾脏进行简单低温保存可以保存肾脏的功能达12h[3]。针对低温保存中有害途径的保存措施的发展使得器官的保存时间变得更长，并且保存质量等到改善[4]。尽管有了低温保存有益的概念，但是因此产生的副作用仍然在发生(图25.2)，这些副作用仅有部分能被现有的保存方法抵消。

能量和酸中毒

器官保存期间组织缺氧会使细胞内的ATP水平快速下降。甚至温度降至0~4℃时，细胞内ATP的数量也在快速被消耗，细胞进而进行无氧代谢去支持细胞活动。这就会导致ATP更少的生成，而且会生成更多的乳酸，导致酸中毒[5,6]。在缺血损伤中，酸中毒起作用的程度和pH值相关。严重的酸中毒会激活磷脂酶和蛋白酶，造成溶酶体的损伤，最终导致细胞死亡。然而轻度的酸中毒(pH值6.9~7.0)证实有保护作用，通过抑制糖酵解的限速酶-磷酸果糖激酶[7,8]。因此，适当的控制pH值是保存液的一个重要功能。

细胞肿胀

在器官保存期间能观察到的细胞结构的变化就是细胞肿胀和突出袋的形成。这些改变的根本机制是

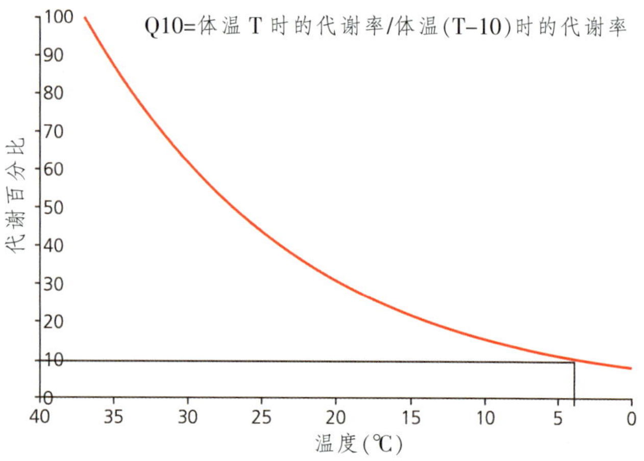

图25.1 温度和代谢活性的关系。

Na^+/K^+–ATP 泵的活性受损。钠排泄减少，钠离子在细胞质蛋白负电荷的吸引下被动进入细胞。这就形成了细胞内的高渗环境，随之水分就进入细胞内。为了重建被打乱的唐南平衡防止细胞肿胀，用非渗透物质和胶体来保存器官。

有效的非渗透物质是糖类和非糖类的阴离子。分子的大小决定细胞外的非渗透物质在器官保存的成功[10-12]。分子越大越成功。像淀粉等胶体是能够聚集在血管间隙的大分子。

活性氧

在器官缺血及缺血后再灌注的过程中，很多过程都可以产生活性氧[13]。大量的研究发现，活性氧是靠黄嘌呤氧化酶生成的，同时又能产生过氧化氢和超氧阴离子[14]。随之，在铁的催化下，过氧化氢减少生成氢氧自由基。在再灌注和缺血再灌注期间，活性氧会快速地与其他分子反应，造成磷脂、核苷酸和蛋白质的严重损伤[15,16]。另外，相比于啮齿动物，黄嘌呤氧化酶在肾移植中会有着较小的重要性，因为黄嘌呤氧化酶在人类细胞中并不丰富，其他的几个活性氧的产生源是重要的[17]。再灌注后白细胞浸润导致大部分过氧化物的生成(即著名的呼吸爆发)。

因为再灌注后呼吸链的部分减少，导致线粒体功能障碍，大量的活性氧的生成。活性氧的生成已经被认为是在组织再灌注期造成了细胞损伤，而不是在低温保存期[15,16]。然而一些报道表明，氧自由基是在组织再灌注期和低温保存期都会产生的[18]。

钙

正常环境下，细胞内和细胞外液中有着不同浓度的钙离子。这个不同是靠几个 ATP 依赖的钙离子的主动运输保持的，包括钙离子 ATP 酶和钠钙交换器[19]。在低温保存期，细胞 ATP 的下降导致细胞内钙离子增加。在低温期，钙离子的蓄积将会激活一些依赖钙离子的反应，例如，钙蛋白酶的激活和蛋白激酶 C 的信号传递。钙蛋白酶的激活会通过破坏细胞骨架蛋白造成细胞结构的丧失[20]。钙蛋白酶的活性被证实在低温状态下的肝细胞中也会增加，复温时进一步增加[21]。

酶

在器官保存期，细胞内的蛋白酶降解蛋白质，很可能是因为缺氧。而且基质金属蛋白酶在低温期被激活，导致内皮细胞和基质分离。研究发现，这种现象在低温保存的肝细胞中更明显，同样也会出现在肾脏保存中[22,23]。为了通过阻滞基质金属蛋白酶(特别是基质金属蛋白酶 2 和 9)，来减少这种有害的反应，威斯康星大学研究证实添加胶体和羟乙基淀粉的方法起到了关键的作用[23]。

另一个在低温保存时被激活的蛋白酶家族是与细胞凋亡相关的胱门蛋白酶[24-26]。在长期的器官保存中，游离的铁离子从细胞色素 P450 释放出来[27]。游离铁的释放结合过氧化氢，导致活性氧的大量生成[28,29]。近来，细胞的自噬作用被假设为随着低温缺血时间的增加导致损伤增加的一个可能的机制。尽管大部分的研究[30,31]来自肝脏的研究，但是临床前期的工作表明，自噬在肾脏中一样重要[32]。关于这方面，Minor 等科学家[33,34]也假设内质网的应激可能与缺血损伤有关。佩拉尔塔和布伦纳随后证实了这一假设[35]。

综上所述，在低温保存期，细胞内稳定不再保持不变。主要的紊乱是电解质的变化、pH 值的变化、细胞内酶和蛋白以及细胞内水分的增加，因此，器官保存液的组成成分用来抵消这些变化。

低温保存

随着肾脏移植程序的建立，对器官保存的需求更加明显。Belzer 和他的团队认为，在整个器官保存过程中，持续低温保存肾脏是最自然的方式，并且表明结果很好。由于静水压和抵抗水分进入组织间隙和细胞的机制缺乏，组织水肿是一个严重的问题。通过使用包括胶体试剂在内的液体来抵消产生的水肿。为了这个目的，人血白蛋白和冷沉淀蛋白被使用。贝尔泽和索斯纳德随后发明了一种合成的机器灌注液体，最终为 UW 的低温保存液提供了主要成分。程序的复杂性使研究者开始寻找可以替代的简单的方法。很多保存液被尝试，复杂性和疗效各不相同。随着保存液的不断发展，尽管近来随着心脏死亡和脑死亡捐献器官的使用，低温机器灌注再次激起研究者的兴趣，但是大部分移植中心现在把低温保存作为最主要的保存方法。

临床低温保存液的成分

大量的保存液被评估用于肾脏的静态低温保

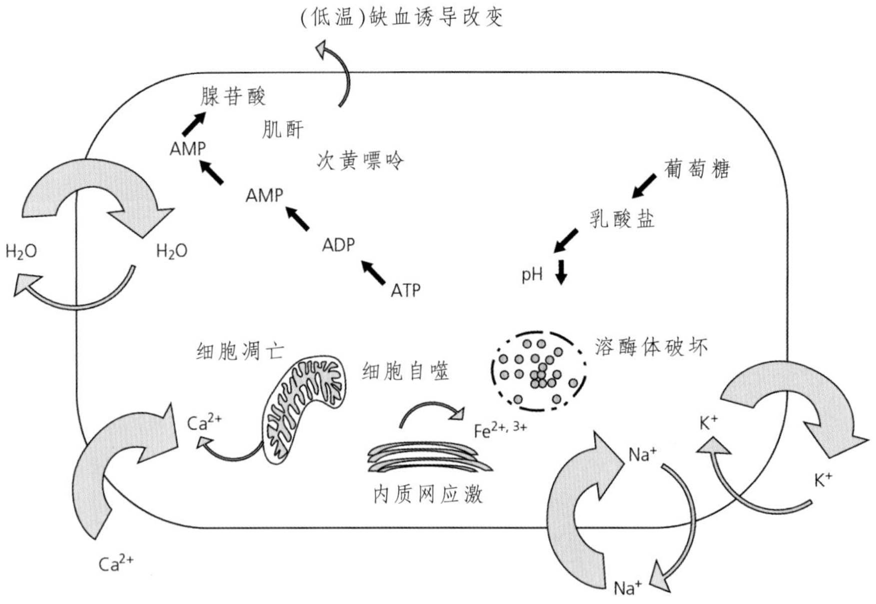

图 25.2 低温缺血的副作用:ATP 的分解,酸中毒,溶酶体酶的释放,内质网应激,钠离子和钙离子大量流入细胞,随后细胞肿胀。

表 25.1 保存液的成分

		EC	UW	HTK	HOC	Celsior	IGL-1
缓冲液(mM)	磷酸氢二钾	15	-	-	-	-	-
	磷酸二氢钾	43	25	-	-	-	25
	碳酸氢钠	10	-	-	10	-	-
	组氨酸	-	-	198	-	30	-
非渗透性溶质(mM)	葡萄糖	195	-	-	-	-	-
	乳酸醛酸盐	-	100	-	-	80	100
	柠檬酸盐	-	-	-	80	-	-
	甘露醇	-	-	38	185	60	-
	棉籽糖	-	30	-	-	-	30
电解质(mM)	氯离子	15	20	32	-	42	20
	钙离子	-	-	0.0015	-	0.25	-
	镁离子	-	5	4	40	13	5
	钾离子	115	120	9	84	15	25
	钠离子	10	30	15	84	100	120
活性氧清除剂(mM)	别嘌呤醇	-	1	-	-	-	1
	谷胱甘肽	-	3	-	-	3	3
	色氨酸	-	-	2	-	-	-
营养素(mM)	腺苷酸	-	5	-	-	-	5
	谷氨酸	-	-	-	-	20	-
	酮戊二酸	-	-	1	-	-	-
胶体(mM)	羟乙基淀粉	-	0.25	-	-	-	-
	聚乙二醇	-	-	-	-	-	0.03
渗透压(mM)		406	320	310	400	255	320

存[36]。其化学成分分析各不相同(表 25.1)。国际上临床实践中最重要的一些保存液的成分描述如下。

欧洲柯林液(EC)

第一个静态低温保存液是柯林在 20 世纪 60 年代末研制的[37,38]。欧洲器官移植基金会在 1976 年进行了小的调整,去除镁离子,形成了 EC 液。在 UW 保存液被研制前,EC 液是那个年代最常用的保存液。

EC 液是一个简单的类似细胞内液体的保存液。磷酸盐被用来调节 pH 值,葡萄糖用作渗透剂。由于葡糖糖能够透过细胞膜,柯林液提供了生成 ATP 需要的原料,以及无氧环境需要的乳酸盐,几小时后它抵制非渗透剂的功效就下降了[39,40]。大部分的移植中心现在都开始使用 UW 保存液。

威斯康星大学保存液(UW)

在 20 世纪 80 年代,通过 Belzer 和 Southard 长期系统的研究最后研制出了 UW 液,并在 1987 年提供了临床医学导论。代谢上,惰性底物和乳糖醛酸棉籽糖作为渗透剂(表 25.1)。羟乙基淀粉作为胶体液。胶体液起初被加入低温机器灌注保存液中,利用静水压防止组织水肿。Belzer 和 Southard 最初想研制出一种可以同时用于冷藏和低温机器灌注的保存液,所以在 UW 液中使用非渗透性羟乙基淀粉。作为一种胶体液,羟乙基淀粉在 UW 液的可行性受到了广泛的质疑。羟乙基淀粉可以防止组织间隙水肿并且对基质金属蛋白酶有益处。但是增加了黏性[41,42]。分析羟乙基淀粉对红细胞的影响,几个研究者发现:当使用大分子物质羟乙基淀粉时,红细胞的聚集会增加[41,42]。这个效应能从一定程度上解释血液的较低的流速,以及当 UW 液被使用时器官的不均匀灌注[43]。在 UW 液中,别嘌呤醇和谷胱甘肽的混合物被用来预防活性氧的生成。别嘌呤醇抑制黄嘌呤氧化酶,改善肾脏的保存,同时肝脏和胰腺的保存液几乎不受影响。

谷胱甘肽是一个三肽,具有捕获功能的游离自由基。这个重要的抗氧化物被氧化成谷胱甘肽二硫化物。实验研究表明, 谷胱甘肽在肾小管损伤的模型中和分离灌注肝脏有着很大的重要性。缺乏谷胱甘肽,ATP 的生成会更少,更多的乳酸脱氢酶被释放[46,48]。后来的研究证实了谷胱甘肽在肾移植后也有益处。而且谷胱甘肽在长期的肝脏保存中特别重要。

迄今为止,UW 保存液被认为是金标准的保存液,适用于肾脏、肝脏、胰腺和小肠[39,47–53]。

组氨酸-色氨酸-酮戊二酸保存液

组氨酸-色氨酸-酮戊二酸保存液最初是 20 世纪 70 年代布雷特施奈德在心脏手术中用作心脏停搏液[54,55]。基本设计是一个有效的缓冲剂:组氨酸联合两种氨基酸(表 25.1)。在 kyunerine 途径中,色氨酸通过其的氧化代谢作用充当膜稳定剂和抗氧化剂, 比如 5 羟基色氨酸。同时酮戊二酸作为器官保存中无氧代谢的底物。色氨酸通过拮抗活性氧介导的损伤保护器官。甘露醇是比葡萄糖分子大一些的单糖。但是它不像葡萄糖,不能被代谢也不能轻易通过细胞膜。而且,它被添加保存液也是因为它可以起到游离自由基清道夫的作用。在一个鼠的肝细胞的实验中,检测到大量的活性氧介导的损伤的标记物巴比妥酸反应物质。在器官保存的 24h 后,相比于保存肝细胞的 UW 液,巴比妥酸反应物质在组氨酸-色氨酸-酮戊二酸保存液明显的升高,表明由于谷胱甘肽和别嘌呤的联合,UW 液有更好的抗氧化的能力。

组氨酸-色氨酸-酮戊二酸保存液有很低的黏性,实现了器官的平衡灌注。在低流量保存液灌注器官时,高容量的保存液需要洗涤。

高渗的柠檬酸保存液

高渗的柠檬酸保存液(也是著名的马歇尔保存液)最初是在英国和澳大利亚用于肾脏的移植中。高渗的柠檬酸保存液是柠檬酸/碳酸氢钠的缓冲液,甘露醇作为非渗透剂。由于它的成分是高渗的,高渗的柠檬酸保存液防止水分进入细胞, 而且已经证实在实验中的肾脏保存中也有效。

CS 保存液

CS 保存液最初是在 20 世纪 90 年代研制的用于保存心脏,它和 UW 液的成分相似,因此,被证实可以用于肾脏、肝脏、胰腺的器官保存。但是不像 UW 保存液,它的钠浓度很高,钾浓度很低,而且黏性相对较低。同样并不包含羟乙基淀粉。像 UW 保存液的原理一样,它含有惰性渗透剂,有着 HTK 保存液一样强的缓冲能力。而且,CS 保存液含有乳酸醛酸盐和甘露醇非渗透剂,并以减量的谷胱甘肽作为抗氧化剂。

IGL-1 保存液

羟乙基淀粉的争论起始于一次寻找其他的胶体液,比如右旋糖酐、聚乙二醇。高黏性和羟乙基淀粉有关,而且在动物实验模型和试管中它更容易造成红细胞聚集,所以研究者寻找可以替代的成分,例如,聚乙二醇。聚乙二醇是一种中性、水溶性的,无毒的聚合物。尽管从化学的角度,它不是真正的胶体液,但是它像胶体液一样能结合水。另外,聚乙二醇能够结合细胞膜,形成一层结合水的结构。它通过干扰免疫系统细胞识别移植物为外源物质的过程,起到一种免疫保护。聚乙二醇抑制了再灌注诱导的炎性反应。这对移植效果有长期的益处,尤其通过干扰危险信号分子的产生。几篇研究报道:无论在实验中还是在临床中,证实了聚乙二醇对肝脏、肾脏、胰腺、小肠和心脏保存的有效性。

低温保存的临床使用

很难回答使用低温保存时哪种保存液最好。保存液的可行性、成本及本身颜色是个重要事情。甚至在肾脏移植方面,仅有限数量的高质量随机对照试验已经被施行。

下面部分就介绍不同器官的保存方法。

肾脏保存

现在,不考虑供体类型,静态低温保存是最流行的保存方法。除了美国有大约20%来自死亡供体的肾脏被灌注保存,大部分国家的首选低温保存。虽然保存解决方案几乎完全是用CS的机械灌注法,但泵灌注的变化更多。HTK和UW解决方案最常用。从20世纪90年代早期,UW保存液成为肾脏保存的金标准。在欧洲取代了EC液成为首选的保存液。一个关于EC液和UW保存液对比的随机对照试验造就了这个结果,而且试验表明移植肾功能延迟恢复在UW液保存中发生概率较低(23%对33%)。而且器官1年生存率UW保存液组较高[63,88]。同样在欧洲移植范围内,另一随机对照试验发现HTK保存液在减少移植肾脏功能延迟恢复方面优于EC保存液,但是缺少移植器官生存率的影响。在同一研究中发现,HTK和UW液没有明显区别。然而数据分析表明,UW保存液有着更低的器官无功能发生率和较低的移植器官无功能的风险,尤其在保存时间>18h时。

一项多中心的前瞻性随机试验将UW保存液和HTK保存液在肾脏保存中的作用进行对比发现:从移植肾功能延迟恢复的发生率看,两种保存液有着相同的作用(33%对33%)[49,74]。然而,对于用HTK保存液进行长时间低温保存(>24h)。几乎没有数据是可用的。一个单中心的研究报道:当低温缺血的时间>24h时,HTK保存的移植肾功能延迟恢复的发生率明显比UW高(50%对24%)。在最近的一篇研究中相反的结论被报道:相比于UW保存液,HTK保存液有着更高的移植肾功能延迟恢复发生率(56%对16%)[87,90]。由于每个研究对移植肾功能延迟恢复定义不同,直接比较这些争议的结论是不可能。其他被测试和UW保存液比较的是CS保存液和IGL-1保存液,他们被认为是和UW保存液相似。一些相对较小的研究发现:在移植肾功能延迟恢复和移植肾的存活率方面,CS保存液并不逊于UW保存液。在一些小的队列研究中,IGL-1和UW保存液在移植肾功能延迟恢复和移植肾脏存活率方面没有差别。然而,在IGL-1保存的肾脏,术后血肌酐较低,可能和其中的聚乙二醇相关。

最近英国关于临床实践中的器官保存液的系统分析表明:HOC保存液和UW保存液相比,或者HOC保存液和CS保存液相比,在器官移植的效果上没有很大的区别。尽管Kay等在最近的一次实验移植操作中发现:用HOC保存的肾脏相比UW保存液保存的水肿更重[93]。

随着来自脑死亡和心脏死亡捐献者的边缘肾脏的更多的使用,再次燃起了低温机器灌注的兴趣。来自器官共享联合网络的回顾性资料表明:它在减少移植肾功能延迟恢复方面会产生有益的影响。来自Wight等的一个很大的meta分析得到结论:低温机器灌注会减少20%的移植功能延迟恢复发生率。来自美国的回顾性资料也表明:低温机器灌注可以改善移植肾功能延迟恢复的发生率及移植存活率[75]。尽管来自欧洲器官移植范围内的最新机器灌注实验的A级证据仅表明低温机器灌注对标准捐献者、扩大标准捐献者、心脏死亡的捐献者的器官有益,但是移植肾功能延迟恢复发生率也较低,而且1年和3年存活率也更好[76,77]。有趣的是,移植肾功能延迟恢复对移植存活的影响在机器灌注肾脏中更小一些。Treckman等进行的机器灌注延伸试验表明，扩大标准捐献者捐献的肾脏经过机器灌注后,降低了移植肾功能延迟衰竭发生的风险,改善 1 年移植肾脏存活率和功能。

Jochmans 等关注于心脏死亡捐献者(《马斯特里赫特标准》分类的第 3 类)并且证明低温机器灌注能够降低移植肾脏功能延迟恢复的发生的风险以及肾脏移植后早期有着更好的器官功能直至移植后 1 个月。移植肾脏功能延迟恢复发生率从 70%降到 54%，并且移植存活率是相同的[80]。相比这个研究,英国 Watson 等在另一篇研究中并不能体现机器灌注在心脏死亡的捐献者捐献的肾脏有任何的影响[94]。这种在英国和欧洲移植肾脏出现的差异，一个可能的解释就是在英国研究的移植肾脏在灌注之前会经历低温保存。在英国的研究中，手臂的移植有着相似的功能延迟恢复发生率(56%对 58%)。这个概率和在欧洲移植试验中的相似。在 Hosgood 等的一篇研究中表示:直接进行灌注保存的肾脏的排斥反应随着功能的恢复会减小,而经过几小时低温保存的肾脏移植后排斥反应会随着器官功能的恢复而增加[95]。肾脏排斥和移植肾脏功能延迟恢复之间的关系被很多进行灌注保存肾脏的移植中心注意到,常以此为理由放弃要移植的肾脏。在机器灌注试验中,研究者忽视了肾脏排斥,肾脏排斥和移植肾脏功能延迟恢复之间的关系被确认有着很高的优势比。然而,预测值是低的,因此,作者得出结论:肾脏排斥反应作为一个单独的质量评估工具不能充分准确地预测移植后的效果[96,97]。

机器灌注另一个潜在的有趣的应用是一些用来选择和预测移植效果的灌注生物标记物的使用。最常使用和检测的生物标记物是谷胱甘肽硫转移酶，一种定位在肾小管的酶。它参与废物的早期排泄,被排到尿液中[97]。全部的谷胱甘肽硫转移酶已证实能准确地反映肾小管的损伤，而且与热缺血时间相关[98,99]。与移植肾脏功能延迟恢复有关。后来研究发现,氨基葡萄糖苷酶和心脏型脂肪酸结合蛋白都能独立成为移植肾功能延迟恢复的预测因子，但是不能预测原发性的移植物肾脏无功能和移植存活。其他潜在的生物标记物,如乳酸脱氢酶、谷草转氨酶和丙氨酸氨基肽酶都不具独立的预测的能力。灌注液的生物标记物浓度与低温保存时间无关,与灌注时的肾血管阻力无关。

肝脏保存

同肾脏保存一样,低温保存是最受欢迎的肝脏保存方法。使用的保存液也和保存肾脏使用的保存液一样。尽管 HTK 保存液和 CS 保存液的使用也在增加，但是在很长一段时间内,UW 保存液仍然被很多移植中心使用[100]。研究表明,UW 保存液和 HTK 或马歇尔保存液有着一样的保存能力,甚至有更长的保存周期[101-103]。移植存活和肾功能的即时恢复都得到了改善,所以 UW 保存液很快成为保存液的最佳选择。在肝脏移植中,没有高质量的研究可以用来比较各种保存液,很多已经发表的文献往往研究的病例<100,所以很可能证据不充分。尽管一些研究表明 HTK 保存液在胆管冲洗和胆管并发症的预防上更有效[53,104-108],但是大部分的研究表明两种保存液有着相似的效果。来自器官共享联合网络的数据回顾分析和一些最近的单中心研究报告表明,HTK 保存液会有一个高的移植肾失功的风险,尤其是低温缺血时间超过 8 小时和心脏死亡者捐献的器官。

UW 保存液在保存胆管系统上有较低的效果,很可能跟 UW 保存液中高钾成分有关,高钾离子浓度造成了血管痉挛。或者,可能和胶体的类型有关。羟乙基淀粉被证实能导致红细胞聚集达 5μm^2,这已经足够大,堵塞小的毛细血管。在 IGI-1 保存液中,钾离子的浓度较低,聚乙二醇代替了羟乙基淀粉。然而在法国的一个对照试验中,尽管没有胆汁流量和胆汁成分方面的报道,但是却发现了和护理标准类似的结果。

比较 CS 保存液和 UW 保存液发现,无论是无功能的发生率还是 1 年和 3 年的存活率上没有区别[48,64,70,91,110]。最近,Garcia-Gil 等报道再灌注后综合征的发生率从 UW 保存液组的 21.6%降低至 CS 保存液组的 5.9%。再灌注后综合征的定义是在移植物再灌注的第一个 5 分钟内,平均动脉压减少大于基线值的 30%以上超过 1 分钟。在同一篇文献中,在 5 年移植存活率方面没有区别,同样在这篇文献中,HTK 和 CS 保存液被进行比较,也显示了相同的结果[40]。

随着机器灌注肾脏的发展,也激起了研究者对机器灌注肝脏的兴趣。Monbaliu 等总结到,肝脏的灌注比肾脏的灌注更复杂。像肝脏血流和门静脉血流的竞争、胆管系统独立的供血动脉、肝窦内皮细胞的以及肝脏的高代谢率都使肝脏的灌注问题复杂化[112-115]。几组科学家依靠Starzl、Belzer和Bretschneider三人在20世纪60年代提供的遗产作为资金,正在研究适用于肝脏灌注的新的概念。能够显示在临床前期的研究中机器灌注疗效的新系统也即将进入临床领域。第一个也是最近仅有的已出版的使用低温肝脏保存临床研究由Guarera等完成,是在20例患者中用自制的机器灌注装置完成;结果是鼓舞人心的。血浆中损伤标记物的峰值在低温机器灌注保存的肝脏中更低。早期的同种异体移植的功能障碍发生率也从低温保存肝脏的25%降到了低温机器灌注保存肝脏的5%(P=0.08)[116]。

然而,还需要更大的研究去体现低温保存肝脏的优势,特别是在扩大标准捐献者和心脏死亡捐献者捐献的肝脏。剩下的问题就是灌注流速和灌注压、氧化作用的速度、单血管还是双血管以及灌注液的成分可能存在更多的争论。灌注温度也在调查研究中。

胰腺保存

胰腺的保存分为两个部分,即整个胰腺的保存和胰岛细胞的保存。在临床实践中,当一个胰腺被认为不适合进行整个胰腺移植时,会把胰腺进行胰岛分离(胰岛的产生和保存的细节会在第61章详细阐述)。无论是整个胰腺的移植还是胰岛细胞的移植,静态低温保存都是主要的保存方法。整个胰腺的保存几乎仅用UW保存进行保存,因为它是由Southard和Belzer研制的,在应用于其他的器官保存之前被证实是一个成功的保存液[117]。最近,一篇报道表明,其他保存液代替UW保存液也是有效的。

关于HTK和UW保存液的比较的文献大部分都是恢复性的和(或)单中心的研究。仅仅一些比较大的由Schneeberger等进行的随机对照研究表明,在移植存活率和移植功能方面两者有着同样的效果[118]。来自一个数量达4392个胰腺移植的注册中心的数据分析表明,HTK保存液的使用是移植器官无功能的一个独立的风险因子(风险比1.30;P=0.017),特别是低温缺血时间大于12小时(风险比1.42;P=0.017)。一些作者也报道移植后胰腺炎的高发生率可能是由于HTK保存液的大量使用造成了水肿。

第一个比较UW保存液和CS保存液在临床上胰腺移植中作用的前瞻性随机对照试验(n=50)表明,CS保存液和UW保存液在胰腺保存中有着相同的安全性。一个来自巴西的小一些,仅有30例胰腺移植的随机对照试验中没有发现两种保存液的区别。来自意大利的一篇回顾性分析表明,EC保存液在外科并发症发生率上可以比得上UW保存液[121]。另一个关于UW保存液(n=28)和CS保存液(n=44)用于胰腺移植的研究表明:2年受体存活率、2年移植存活率、胰漏发生率以及临床移植胰腺炎发生率上两组是相同的[67]。

针对独立的胰岛胰腺组织的保存大部分都使用UW保存液,尽管其他的方法和保存液也是可行。Kaddis等在2010年进行的meta分析显示用UW保存液保存胰腺能改善移植效果[122]。同样的,来自日内瓦的一篇报道回顾性地分析了376个分别用IGL-1保存液(n=95)、UW保存液(n=204)或低温(n=77)保存的从胰腺上分离的胰岛组织。表明在胰岛组织的移植功能上没有区别[124]。

低温机器灌注保存胰腺的报道仅限于Leeser等发表的。4个来自死亡捐献者的胰腺被获得,用低温机器灌注和用UW保存低温保存相比较。这个初步研究表明,低流速的动脉机器灌注保存长时间的低温缺血的胰腺也能收到好的效果,好的器官活性和功能,利用猪进行的实验性研究也表明,用机器灌注可以改善器官保存和改善移植后的效果。

两种层次的保存方法几乎仅存在于胰腺的保存中。在这两层次的保存方法中,胰腺在保存期间会直接被氟碳化合物氧化,这就可以使组织中保持一个高的ATP水平。这被认为是由于细胞完整性保持以及实质细胞和非实质细胞的保留[20,59,126,127]造成的。尽管最近有两篇大规模的研究表明,双层次保存方法在人类胰岛组织保存和移植中无有益的影响,但是大部分研究报道都证实了双层次的保存方法的有益影响[126,128]。

小肠保存

移植小肠的保存方法是足够的但大部分可能不是最佳的[129]。小肠的保存是困难的,因为小肠黏膜对缺血极其敏感[130]。肠道屏障功能障碍导致了移植后的细菌迁移[131]。为了防止这种移植后的并发症,低温缺血时间必须控制到最小。

与腹部其他器官一样,UW保存液是小肠保存最常用的[132]。仅有一篇回顾性分析比较UW保存液和HTK保存液的报道发现,两者在移植小肠功能和急性排斥反应方面没有区别[133]。Roover等进行的人小肠的实验研究表明，UW 保存液和 CS 保存液在保存小肠的能力方面是一样的。

比较不同保存液的实验模型表明：添加营养素在空腔脏器的保存上有着潜在的改善[68,135]。而且，氧气的添加也被证实是有益的。

复苏指南

心脏死亡捐献者的原位灌注

考虑到马斯特里赫特Ⅰ类和Ⅱ类心脏死亡捐献者器官可用性，来自这些资源的器官的使用将会减少等待移植患者的数量。2006 年，美国医学研究所建议移植协会努力增加捐献器官数量，尤其来自马斯特里赫特Ⅱ类的心脏死亡捐献者的器官。估计这个群体每年能增加 22 000 个移植资源。然而，由于不知缺血损伤的程度，器官质量的评估很困难，而且功能不良的风险也相当大。尤其在西班牙，每一百万名居民就有一名器官捐献者，是全世界最高的。来自心脏死亡捐献者的器官被广泛使用。使用严格选择标准，西班牙马德里的一个移植中心对来自马斯特里赫特Ⅰ类和Ⅱ类心脏死亡捐献者捐献的肾脏成功进行了移植[144,146]。对于合适的不可逆性心脏骤停的捐献者，在股动脉和股静脉放入导管，通过体外膜肺氧和保持器官的活性。体外膜肺氧和系统被广泛地用于支持重症监护室里心肺衰竭的患者。在确定器官捐献的情况下，马上用双球囊膨胀堵塞膈肌以上的血管，防止再循环通过大脑和心脏。这就使得在心脏停搏后温氧和血持续的在腹部器官循环。

这个方法被证实有效。在 1 年和 5 年存活率方面，比得上同一时期同一移植机构的脑死亡捐献肾脏移植的效果[146]。Ⅱ类肾脏经历不同时间段的热缺血时间，长者能达到 2 小时。因接受肾脏移植后的废弃率高达 33%。甚至在接受移植后，移植肾功能延迟恢复率（60%~80%）和无功能的（6%）的大量存在[144,145]。在西班牙巴塞罗那，一小系列的Ⅱ类和Ⅳ类捐献者的研究表明，常温的体外膜肺氧和低体温体外膜肺氧和用 EC 保存液相比，常温体外膜肺氧和移植肾功能延迟恢复和无功能发生率明显较低[147]。在法国巴黎进行了一系列马斯特里赫特Ⅰ类和Ⅱ类心脏死亡捐献者捐献的肾脏移植，这些肾脏的热缺血时间达 150 分钟，结果表明有着较高的废弃率（43%）和移植肾功能延迟恢复率（92%），但是有着较低的无功能率（2%）[148]。6 个月的移植存活率是 89%。相比较其他组，常温体外膜肺氧和有着较低的移植肾功能延迟恢复率，与原位灌注组相比有着较低的无功能发生率。

虽然体外膜肺氧和还没有广泛地用于可控的心脏死亡捐献者的捐献器官的保存，但是可以用于不可控心脏死亡捐献者捐献的器官保存。体外膜肺氧和提供了一种可能的方法，通过逆转撤去生命支持治疗的可控心脏死亡捐献者出现的酸中毒和低静脉氧和水平。随着 ICU 决定撤去治疗后，会询问家属是否愿意捐献器官。如果愿意，就会插入股动脉和静脉导管，然后撤去生命支持治疗。在心脏停搏 5 分钟后，动脉堵塞球囊被膨胀，紧接着体外膜肺氧和就开始了。来自美国密歇根州的一系列案例研究表明，对于马斯特里赫特Ⅲ类心脏死亡捐献者捐献的器官，这个方法有较低的移植肾脏功能延迟恢复率（8%）和无功能率（0%）[149]。

另一组来自美国北卡罗来纳州的研究者对可控心脏死亡捐献者捐献的肾脏在经过低于常温（22℃）的体外膜肺氧和后进行了移植[150]。在这个研究中有着较高的移植肾功能延迟恢复率（57%）。而且 1 年移植存活率是 87%。来自台湾台北的一系列案例表明，体外膜肺氧和对于来自马斯特里赫特Ⅰ类、Ⅱ类和Ⅳ类心脏死亡捐献者捐献的肾脏能产生极好的 5 年移植存活率，大约达 88%[151]。这个存活率赶得上同一时期同一机构进行的活体捐献的肾脏移植（89%）和脑死亡捐献肾脏的移植（83%）。

对于肝脏，体外膜肺氧和的方法仅使用于不可控的捐献者的器官保存。Fondevila 等和巴塞罗那组报道了第一次用体外膜肺氧和方法保存不可控心脏死亡捐献者肝脏保存的病例对照研究[152]。这个组选择严格标准接受和移植器官，导致 40 个捐赠器官仅有 10 个进行了移植。如果肝脏宏观上有脂肪肝或转氨酶升高或低灌注，就会被拒绝。长期热缺血时间的捐献器官也被排除在外。在进行了平均 23 个月的随访后发现，患者和移植器官的存活率比得上同一机构脑死亡捐献者捐献的肝脏移植。

来自西班牙的另一个病例对照研究分析了不可控心脏死亡捐献者的肝脏的同种异体移植[113,153]。Jimenez-Galanes 等和马德里组采用了严格的标准进行选择可接受的器官：捐献者的年龄必须小于 50 岁，心脏停搏时间小于 15 分钟，热缺血时间小于 50 分钟，能接受的最大的体外膜肺氧和时间是270分钟。来自43个潜在的器官捐献者的20个器官进行了同种异体移植。1年移植存活率是80%,比得上同一移植中心的脑死亡捐献的器官移植。无功能率也比得上这个系列(10%对5%)。然而,对于不可控心脏死亡捐献的肝脏移植者的再次肝移植率较高(15%对5%),因为有着峰值的谷丙转氨酶和谷草转氨酶水平。

不同温度的含氧机器灌注

在肾脏保存方面,未来的方法将旨于修复已损伤的肝脏,通过提供一定的机制支持代谢、排除代谢废物,抵消缺血再灌注损伤带来的不利影响。新的保存液将适用于在常温、低于常温的静态保存。这个已经在动物实验中被证实。AQIX,一种无磷酸盐缓冲剂的保存液已经用于猪的实验模型短期的低于常温的静态保存[154]。随着新的保存液的发展,静态低温保存的疗效也是有可能得到改善的。Polysol,一种低黏性的保存液,已经在猪的自体移植模型中被测试,结果显示相比UW保存液有着良好的肾脏血流和组织氧和作用[155]。相比HTK保存液,有着更好的肌酐清除率。

在器官保存期间,给移植器官进行氧气的输送已经成为很多研究的焦点。不仅有含氧全血的输送,在动物和试验研究中,各种方法被证实是有前景的。通过肾脏的脉管系统直接进行气态氧的充氧治疗被测试为肾脏缺氧损伤的一个挽救治疗。过滤的湿润的气态氧通过深静脉进入,通过微血管针形成的细小的针孔逸出。在动物研究中,相比低温静态保存和单独的灌注保存,随着氧气的冲入,自体肾脏移植后有着更高的肌酐清除率[157,158]。格罗宁根和普瓦捷的研究者们合作在低温机器灌注期间进行了含氧灌注的方法保存肾脏,这种方法也在心脏死亡的动物模型中和自体肾脏移植中进行试验[159,160]。联合机器灌注进行膜氧和保存器官被证实可以提高ATP的生成,甚至是在热缺血30分钟后[161]。机器灌注的氧化作用使用100%浓度的氧来实现较高的氧分压,这也成为机器灌注的一个辅助手段。而且这种方法被证实可以修复事先进行18h静态低温保存的肾脏[162]。进行了再灌注之后,肾脏进行了含氧再灌注后表现出改善的排尿和肌酐清除率。氧气也能通过溶氧载体进行运输。呼吸色素Hemarina-M101,一个来自海洋无脊椎动物的大分子血红蛋白,在静态低温保存的动物研究中,被用作标准保存液的补充[163]。随着保存器官的移植,Hemarina-M101能够改善保存细胞的代谢活性,增加ATP的水平,改善肌酐清除率,减少器官的纤维化[163]。

接下来最重要的步骤就是似乎就是常温保存联合持续的或动脉灌注移除代谢产物,保持血管环境的稳定。合成的保存液可能用于常温的灌注。Lifor,一种联合非蛋白溶氧载体的保存液,已经过测试用于短期的原位常温灌注[164]和猪模型中的低体温肾脏灌注[165]。Lifor被证实,与UW保存液相比,可以更好地保持肾脏的功能[164],减少排斥反应[165]。一种血红蛋白补充液体能够复苏经历2小时热缺血时间的肾脏。提供维持生命的功能[166]。另一个选择就是使用自己的血液,在一个动物实验中,用肝素化的全血进行常温灌注被证实能够保存肾脏的功能达6小时,即使是经历了40分钟的热缺血时间[167]。

在低温保存的开始和结束阶段给予常温和含氧灌注可能是有益的。理论上,这将会在保存的初期提供一定程度的缺血预处理,或者允许细胞保护机制帮助器官恢复。在静态低温保存16小时后进行自体血常温灌注2小时,就可以改善肾脏血流到静态保存2小时的血流水平[168]。这个技术最少相当于低温机器灌注18小时。体外常温灌注最近试验用于人体肾脏的移植中[169]。第一个刊登的案例是来自扩大标准供体的肾脏。在莱斯特移植中心接受前被6个英国移植中心拒绝。一个肾脏在移植前经过含氧血浆游离血红蛋白的保存液常温保存了35分钟。同时另一个肾脏单独进行静态低温保存。两个肾脏在第一周后的常规活检中都可以看到急性肾小管坏死和排斥反应。然而,经过灌注的肾脏的受体有了基本的功能,而静态低温保存的肾脏的受体需要长达4周的透析。莱斯特移植中心已经使用这种方法对16例移植器官进行了植入前的常温再循环,目前为止都有理想的结果[170]。

预防缺血再灌注损伤的一个方法就是“免疫伪装”,通过选定的聚合物和同种异体移植物细胞膜相互作用减少免疫细胞对移植物的侵袭。IGL-1保存液的聚乙二醇成分就是这样一种聚合物。动物研究已表明相比于IGL-1保存液或UW保存液,含有聚乙二醇的血浆有更好的保存效果,更少的免疫细胞浸润和改善的移植存活率[171]。

对于之前不能移植的肝脏低温机器灌注作为一种再复苏的方法现在已经进入临床前期的试验。Guarera 等用动脉灌注的方法保存了 10 个被废弃的人体肝脏达 10 小时,来测试这个技术的可行性[114]。同时在这个研究中,同样的方法保存了模拟心脏死亡捐献者的猪的肝脏,3 个经过低温机器灌注的肝脏完成了移植。所有的受体都表现出最初的移植功能,伴有血清酶下降[116]。Vekemans 等也在缺血再灌注的试验模型中测试低温机器灌注对废弃人体肝脏的挽救[172]。在静态低温保存一段时间后进行低温机器灌注 4 小时,并和单独的静态低温保存相比较。在低温保存后用血进行常温再灌注期间,低温机器灌注与谷草转氨酶和乳酸脱氢酶的释放减少有关,也与丝裂原活化蛋白激酶的降低有关。从两种保存方式的肝脏活检病理学检查发现两者是一样的。

低温机器灌注有作为心脏死亡捐献肝脏的再复苏治疗的能力,可能会进一步发展,在灌注期间进行含氧灌注(低温含氧灌注)。这个已经在心脏死亡捐献动物模型中进行了测试。在静态低温保存期的最后使用低温含氧灌注对器官进行预处理[115,173]。用含氧灌注预处理相比单纯的静态低温保存会减少细胞损伤,减少细胞坏死和脂肪氧化、增加细胞的 ATP 和胆汁流量。尽管实验动物无论是否经过低温含氧灌注都没有存活超过 18 小时的。但是经过低温含氧灌注保存的肝脏有着改善的移植存活率[173]。含氧机器灌注的使用进一步被测试,在常温和低体温的情况下使用含血的液体灌注[115]。在这种方法下低温含氧灌注也能逆转这些肝脏出现的微观和宏观的损伤,再灌注后谷草转氨酶释放减少,胆汁流量增加,减少了血清中的乳酸并且改善受体的存活[115]。在这个研究中,如果肝脏经历 120 分钟的热缺血,所有的实验动物都会在 24 小时内死亡[115]。

肝脏保存的未来发展将不得不处理移植互补名单的患者,通过让之前不能移植肝脏成为可行的。推测:添加氧气的保存方式通过保持代谢能让其成为可能。同样的对于肾脏,不同方法被试验增加离体肾脏的氧浓度。Minor 等已经在猪的移植模型中进行了气态氧的充入。在静态低温保存 10 小时后,在植入之前氧气泡会进入腔静脉达 2 小时[174]。肝脏接受氧气充入会极大地改善第一周的移植器官的存活率达 83%(在可控组是 0%)。尸检的组织学研究显示了在这个研究组保存肝脏的结构。血清的肝酶和凝血参数也都在正常范围内。充入气态氧气的后处理也在一小系列的人体肝脏中被测验,否则这些肝脏会因为之前的热缺血损伤而被拒绝[175]。这种复苏方法实现了 5 个肝脏的移植,并且所有的患者存活了下来,2 年随访都健康,没有进行再次移植的。氧气充入后细胞内的 ATP 显著增加。

作为实验模型中经历了长达 18 小时的静态低温保存的器官的复苏治疗,氧气充入也显示了良好的结果,降低了血清肝酶、乳酸脱氢酶和肿瘤坏死因子-α,并且增加了胆汁的产生量[162]。第一个氧气充入再复苏的随机对照试验最近正在招募[176]。与充氧的低温机器灌注相比,氧气充入在心脏死亡的动物模型中,在肝酶释放和胆汁的产生方面都更满意[177]。为了进一步适应低温机器灌注,使用高压氧舱泵入,增加组织的氧分压。在一个小系列的试验中,这个技术已经表明可以在再灌注后增加细胞 ATP 量和胆汁的产量,减少谷丙转氨酶的释放[178]。双层次方法,这个最初研究用于胰腺保存的方法(见上文),也在肝脏保存中进行了测试。持续的氧气充入直接联合保存液(典型的 HTK 和 UW 保存液)。在肝脏试验研究中,这种方法改善细胞 ATP 的水平,但是细胞形态学上并没有改善。

常温灌注

常温机器灌注提供了一个直观的、可能更好地替代低温机器灌注的方法。但是有相关的复杂性和技术挑战。为持续代谢的生理环境提供必需品实现了功能的评估和离体器官的复苏。Schön 和柏林研究组证实在移植前肝脏进行离体常温灌注 4 小时是安全的[180]。相比于静态低温保存,这个技术在热缺血一段时间以后似乎也能增加有益的影响。弗兰德和牛津的研究组接着这个研究报道猪的肝脏用含氧的灌注液进行常温机器灌注能保存长达 72 小时[181]。这些实验模型的进一步研究就是测验在再灌注期间肝脏的合成功能。然后这个研究组把用 UW 保存液静态低温保存和用含氧灌注液进行常温机器灌注相比较。常温机器灌注可以增加胆汁量和葡萄糖的产生、半乳糖的清除率,并且会减少肝酶的释放和组织学上的损伤[182]。同一组的研究者用心脏死亡捐献者的肝脏保存模型(60 分钟的热缺血时间)来证实常温机器灌注能够复苏功能,相比之下,静态低温保存没有表现出可行性的证据,无胆汁产生或废物利用[183]。在动物移植实验中，模仿心脏死亡捐献者和脑死亡捐献者，常温机器灌注显示出能够减少肝酶释放、增加患者存活率和改善肝脏组织学形态的能力。只要保存的时间够长(20小时)，这个有益影响是一致的[184]。最近，牛津研究团队、国王大学和伯明翰紧密合作，已经完成了第一个人体的初步研究：应用新的设备保存了包括脑死亡捐献者、心脏死亡捐献者和扩大标准供体的20个肝脏。第一个结果就非常鼓舞人心(个人信息)。巴塞罗那研究组和格罗宁根研究组已经完成了在经历了长热缺血时间(90分钟)的不可控心脏死亡捐献者的动物模型中运用常温机器灌注的实验。在这个研究中，在体外膜肺氧和后进行常温机器灌注，表现出能进一步改善经过静态低温保存后进行体外膜肺氧和的结果[185]。能看到肝功能的改善，肝脏宏观的和组织学上的改善[185]。Tolboom等对长时间热缺血(60分钟)的动物移植研究表明，肝脏的缺血损伤经过常温机器灌注能够获得一个很好的4周存活率(92%)，这个存活率比得上经静态低温保存或常温机器灌注的可控捐献者健康肝脏移植的存活率[186]。接受单独经静态低温保存的缺血损伤的肝脏的动物几乎全在移植后的12小时内死亡。一样是在经历60分钟的热缺血后，研究者们开始转向研究低体温的机器灌注[187]。20℃和30℃的机器灌注都能恢复缺血肝脏损伤，并且所有动物的生存期都超过1个月[187]。脂肪变的肝脏对缺血再灌注损伤尤其敏感，考虑到捐献资源的比例逐渐增加，这些器官的保存和再复苏变得越来越重要。在这些肝脏中，常温机器灌注有减轻明显肝损伤的水平，但是静态低温保存却不能[188]。

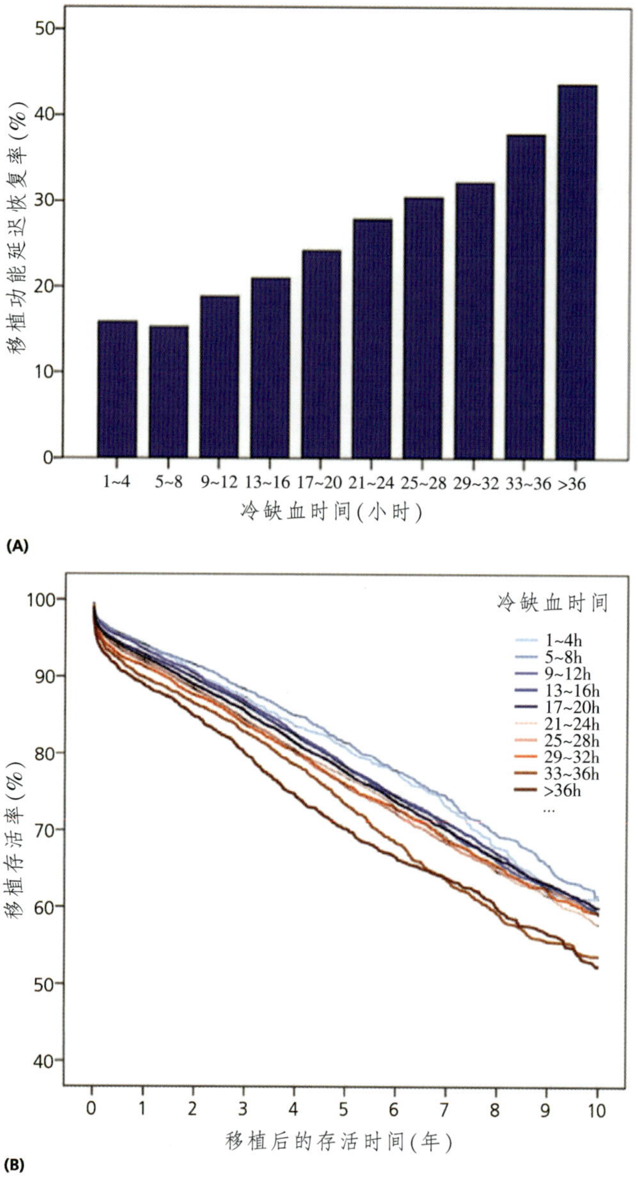

图 25.3 冷缺血时间对于移植功能延迟恢复率(A)和移植存活率的影响(B)。

冬眠策略

器官保存期间，在获得器官后会被冷却到4℃来防止损伤。然而，死亡捐献者的器官并不能无限地保持在4℃。在肾脏移植中，移植肾功能延迟恢复风险随着冷缺血的时间增加而增加[189]。冷缺血每增加6小时，移植肾功能延迟恢复率就增加23%，长时间的低温缺血时间与移植存活率负相关(图25.3)。

在人类肾脏移植的低温保存期间，肾小管细胞是凋亡的[32]。在植入时的热缺血再灌注期间，细胞凋亡和细胞坏死都会发生[18,190]。大量的研究者已经表明，冬眠代表器官保存和移植的一个自然的模型[191-193]，冬眠可以被视为等同于4℃的捐赠肾脏，然而，唤醒就相当于在器官植入时发生的热再灌注。哺乳动物每个冬天的冬眠都经历着核心体温的最大的降低。在冬眠期间，北极圈的冬眠动物的核心体温几天内就可以从38℃降低至零下3℃，温带的冬眠动物也可以降至2%~10℃[194]，冬眠动物经历着生理的改变，心跳从夏天的每分钟200~300次降到3~5次，它们的呼吸从每分钟100~200次降至每分钟4~6次[194]。有趣的是，在冬眠时期，动物对缺血再灌注损伤更加不敏感，这可能与免疫系统活性的减低有关[195,196]。Blackstone等在老鼠的研究中发现硫化氢诱导了类似冬眠的状态，被视为生命的暂停[197]，于是产生了一个想法：硫化氢可能在缺血再灌注损伤中起到保护作用[198,199]。无毒剂量的硫化氢气态的应用使这些保存的器官发生了类似在自然冬眠中观察到的生理改变[197,200]。在实验模型中，发现硫化氢的应用使肾脏和肝脏的缺血再灌注损伤降低[201]。然而，冬眠策略转变应用到临床中是复杂的，因为猪的实验并不能表现出明确的保护性[202,203]。

总结

20 世纪 60 年代，器官保存方法建立经过了一段创新和活跃的时间后，器官移植这个重要领域的进一步发展几乎沉寂，直到 20 世纪 80 年代晚期。移植中心明确地倾向于用保存液对器官进行低温保存。使用标准供体捐献的器官，单独的静态低温保存足够使其保存复苏，获得足够的功能。由于供体类型的改变，包括年老和高风险的供体的使用，目前的挑战已经驱使再灌注和保存进入一个令人兴奋的新的策略的发展和研究时期。持续低温机器灌注、原位常温再灌注以及使用小型设备联合生化方法的离体器官再复苏的使用，证明我们正在进入一个发展的新时期。先前的目标是为了在供体与受体之间搭建一个桥梁，使其仅有最小的损伤和功能的丧失，现在已经发展到在保存和运输的期间改善器官功能的概念，由于更多复杂的技术被应用于减少损伤和启动修复成为可能，这可能会被实现。为了去解决临床上在保存方面的问题，最近欧洲委员会支持建立了欧洲器官保存联盟，专注于用新的技术和含氧低体温或持续常温灌注的方法保存肝脏和肾脏的 3 个临床试验。器官保存在减少器官缺乏和缩小器官废弃上仍旧很关键，同时使之前不能移植的器官能够被移植。

致谢

本文在某种程度上得到了美国健康资源和服务管理局的支持，合约编号 234-2005-370011C。文章内容有作者单独负责，并不一定反映美国健康资源和服务管理局的观点和政策；同样的，商业名称、商业产品或组织的提及并不代表美国政府认可。

作者非常感谢 C. Moers 博士提供图 25.3 的数据。

（张长坤 译 李照 校）

参考文献

1. Belzer FO, Southard JH. The future of kidney preservation. Transplantation. 1980;30(3):161–165.
2. Storey KB. Out cold: biochemical regulation of mammalian hibernation – a mini-review. Gerontology. 2010;56(2):220–230.
3. Calne RY, Pegg DE, Brown FL. Renal preservation by ice cooling. An experimental study relating to kidney transplantation from cadavers. British Medical Journal. 1963;2(5358):651–655.
4. McAnullty JF, Reid TW, Waller KR, et al. Successful six-day kidney preservation using trophic factor supplemented media and simple cold storage. American Journal of Transplantation. 2002;2:712–718.
5. Marshall VC. Preservation by simple hypothermia. In: Collins G, Dubernard JM, Land W, et al., editors. Kidney Transplantation. Dordrecht/Boston/London: Kluwer Academic; 1997: 115–129.
6. Grace P. Ischaemia-Reperfusion Injury. Oxford: Blackwell Science; 1999.
7. Bonventre JV, Cheung JY. Effects of metabolic acidosis on viability of cells exposed to anoxia. American Journal of Physiology. 1985;249(1):C149–C159.
8. Hochachka PW, Mommsen TP. Protons and anaerobiosis. Science. 1983;219:1391–1397.
9. Jamieson NV, Sundberg R, Lindell S, et al. Preservation of the canine liver for 24-48 hours using simple cold storage with UW solution. Transplantation. 1988;46(4):517–522.
10. Hart NA, Leuvenink HGD, Ploeg RJ. New solutions in organ preservation. Transplantation Reviews. 2002;16:131–141.
11. Sumimoto R, Jamieson NV, Kamada N. Examination of the role of the impermeants lactobionate and raffinose in a modified UW solution. Transplantation. 1990;50(4):573–576.
12. Wahlberg JA, Love R, Landegard L, et al. 72-hour preservation of the canine pancreas. Transplantation. 1987;43:5–8.
13. McCord JM. Oxygen-derived free radicals in postischemic tissue injury. New England Journal of Medicine. 1985;312(3):159–163.
14. Kuppusamy P, Zweier JL. Characterization of free radical generation by xanthine oxidase. Evidence for hydroxyl radical generation. Journal of Biological Chemistry. 1989;264:9880–9884.
15. Byrne AT, Johnson AH. Lipid peroxidation. In: Grace P, Mathie R, editors. Ischaemia-Reperfusion Injury. Oxford: Blackwell Science; 1999: 148–156.
16. Kosieradzki M, Kuczynska J, Piwowarska J, et al. Prognostic significance of free radicals: mediated injury occurring in the kidney donor. Transplantation. 2003;75:1221–1227.
17. Simmonds HA, Goday A, Morris GS. Superoxide radicals, immunodeficiency and xanthine-oxidase activity- man is not a mouse. Clinical Science. 1985;68:561–565.
18. Salahudeen AK, Haider N, May W. Cold ischemia and the reduced long-term survival of cadaveric renal allografts. Kidney International. 2004;65:713–718.
19. Bernardi P. Mitochondrial transport of cations: channels, exchangers, and permeability transition. Physiological Reviews. 1999;79:1127–1155.
20. Goll DE, Thompson VF, Li H, et al. The calpain system. Physiological Reviews. 2003;83:731–801.
21. Kohli V, Gao W, Camargo CA, et al. Calpain is a mediator of preservation-reperfusion injury in rat liver transplantation. Proceedings of the National Academy of Sciences of the United States of America. 1997;94:9354–9359.
22. Topp SA, Upadhya GA, Strasberg SM. Cold preservation of isolated sinusoidal endothelial cells in MMP 9 knockout mice: effect on morphology and platelet adhesion. Liver Transplantation. 2004;10:1041–1048.
23. Upadhya GA, Strasberg SM. Glutathione, lactobionate, and histidine: cryptic inhibitors of matrix metalloproteinases contained in University of Wisconsin and Histidine/Tryptophan/Ketoglutarate liver preservation solutions. Hepatology. 2000;31:1115–1122.
24. Castaneda MP, Swiatecka-Urban A, Mitsnefes MM, et al. Activation of mitochondrial apoptotic pathways in human renal allografts after ischemia-reperfusion injury. Transplantation. 2003;76:50–54.
25. Duval M, Plin C, Elimadi A, et al. Implication of mitochondrial dysfunction and cell death in cold preservation- warm reperfusion-induced hepatocyte injury. Canadian Journal of Physiology and Pharmacology. 2006;84:547–554.
26. Oberbauer R, Rohrmoser M, Regele H, et al. Apoptosis of tubular epithelial cells in donor kidney biopsies predicts early renal allograft function. Journal of the American Society of Nephrology. 1999;10(9):2006–2013.
27. Huang H, Salahudeen AK. Cold induces catalytic iron release of cytochrome P-450 origin: a critical step in cold storage-induced renal injury. American Journal of Transplantation. 2002;2(7):631–639.

28. Rauen U, Petrat F, Li T, et al. Hypothermia injury/cold-induced apoptosis-evidence of an increase in chelatable iron causing oxidative injury in spite of low 02-H202 formation. FASEB Journal. 2000;14(13):1953–1964.
29. Wyllie S, Seu P, Gao FQ, et al. Deregulation of iron homeostasis and cold-preservation injury to rat liver stored in University of Wisconsin solution. Liver Transplantation. 2003;9(4):401–410.
30. Lu Z, Dono K, Gotoh K, et al. Participation of autophagy in the degeneration process of rat hepatocytes after transplantation following prolonged cold preservation. Archives of Histology and Cytology. 2005;68(1):71–80.
31. Gotoh K, Lu Z, Morita M, et al. Participation of autophagy in the initiation of graft dysfunction after rat liver transplantation. Autophagy. 2009;5(3): 351–360.
32. Turkmen K, Martin J, Akcay A, et al. Apoptosis and autophagy in cold preservation ischemia. Transplantation. 2011;91(11):1192–1197.
33. Manekeller S, Schuppius A, Stegemann J, et al. Role of perfusion medium, oxygen and rheology for endoplasmic reticulum stress-induced cell death after hypothermic machine preservation of the liver. Transplant International. 2008; 21(2):169–177.
34. Minor T, Manekeller S, Sioutis M, et al. Endoplasmic and vascular surface activation during organ preservation: refining upon the benefits of machine perfusion. American Journal of Transplantation. 2006;6(6):1355–1366.
35. Peralta C, Brenner C. Endoplasmic reticulum stress inhibition enhances liver tolerance to ischemia/reperfusion. Current Medicinal Chemistry. 2011;18(13): 2016–2024.
36. O'Callaghan JM, Knight SR, Morgan RD, et al. Preservation solutions for static cold storage of kidney allografts: a systematic review and meta-analysis. American Journal of Transplantation. 2012;12(4):896–906.
37. Collins GM, Bravo-Shugarman M, Terasaki P. Kidney preservation for transportation. Initial perfusion and 30 hours' ice storage. Lancet. 1969;294(7632): 1219–1222.
38. Ross H, Marshall VC, Escott ML. 72-hour canine kidney preservation using a new perfusate. Transplantation. 1976;21:498.
39. Mühlbacher F, Langer F, Mittermayer C. Preservation solutions for transplantation. Transplantation Proceedings. 1999;31(5):2069–2070.
40. Garcia-Gil FA, Serrano MT, Fuentes-Broto L, et al. Celsior versus University of Wisconsin preserving solutions for liver transplantation: postreperfusion syndrome and outcome of a 5-year prospective randomized controlled study. World Journal of Surgery. 2011;35(7):1598–1607.
41. Morariu AM, van der Plaats A, van Oeveren W, et al. Hyperaggregating effect of hydroxyethyl starch components and University of Wisconsin solution on human red blood cells: a risk of impaired graft perfusion in organ procurement? Transplantation. 2003;76(1):37–43.
42. van der Plaats A, t Hart NA, Morariu AM, et al. Effect of University of Wisconsin organ-preservation solution on haemorheology. Transplant International. 2004;17(5):227–233.
43. t Hart NA, Van Der Plaats A, Leuvenink HGD, et al. Initial blood washout during organ procurement determines liver injury and function after preservation and reperfusion. American Journal of Transplantation. 2004;4(11): 1836–1844.
44. Jamieson NV, Lindell S, Sundberg R, et al. An analysis of the components in UW solution using the isolated perfused rabbit liver. Transplantation. 1988;46: 512–516.
45. Biguzas M, Jablonski P, Thomas AC, et al. Evaluation of UW solution in a rat kidney preservation model. II. The effect of pharmacological additives. Transplantation. 1990;49:1051–1055.
46. Boudjema K, van Gulik T, Lindell SL, et al. Effect of oxidized and reduced glutathione in liver preservation. Transplantation. 1990;50:948–951.
47. Boggi U, Vistoli F, Del Chiaro M, et al. Pancreas preservation with University of Wisconsin and Celsior solutions: a single-centre, prospective, randomized study. Transplantation. 2004;77(8):1186–1190.
48. Cavallari A, Cillo U, Nardo B, et al. A multicenterpilot prospective study comparing Celsior and University of Wisconsin preserving solutions for use in liver transplantation. Liver Transplantation. 2003;9(8):814–821.
49. De Boer J, De Meester J, Smits JMA, et al. Eurotransplant randomized multicenter kidney graft preservation study comparing HTK with UW and Euro-Collins. Transplant International. 1999;12(6):447–453.
50. Fridell JA, Agarwal A, Milgrom ML, et al. Comparison of histidine-tryptophan-ketoglutarate solution and University of Wisconsin solution for organ preservation in clinical pancreas transplantation. Transplantation. 2004;77(8): 1304–1306.
51. Fridell JA, Mangus RS, Powelson JA. Histidine-tryptophan-ketoglutarate for pancreas allograft preservation: the Indiana University experience. American Journal of Transplantation. 2010;10(5):1284–1289.
52. Janssen H, Janssen PH, Broelsch CE. Celsior solution compared with University of Wisconsin solution (UW) and histidine-tryptophan-ketoglutarate solution (HTK) in the protection of human hepatocytes against ischemia-reperfusion injury. Transplant International. 2003;16:515–522.
53. Erhard J, Lange R, Scherer R, et al. Comparison of histidine-tryptophan-ketoglutarate (HTK) solution versus University of Wisconsin (UW) solution for organ preservation in human liver transplantation. Transplant International. 1994;7:177–181.
54. Bretschneider HJ. Myocardial protection. Thoracic and Cardiovascular Surgeon. 1980;28:295–302, 295.
55. Ben Mosbah I, Roselló-Catafau J, Franco-Gou R, et al. Preservation of steatotic livers in IGL-1 solution. Liver Transplantation. 2006;12(8):1215–1223.
56. Christen S, Peterhans E, Stocker R. Antioxidant activities of some tryptophan metabolites: possible implication for inflammatory diseases. Proceedings of the National Academy of Sciences of the United States of America. 1990;87: 2506–2510.
57. Feksa LR, Latini A, Rech VC, et al. Promotion of oxidative stress by l-tryptophan in cerebral cortex of rats. Neurochemistry International. 2006;49(1):87–93, 87.
58. Maathuis MH, Leuvenink HG, Ploeg RJ. Perspectives in organ preservation. Transplantation. 2007;83(10):1289–1298.
59. Rauen U, Reuters I, Fuchs A, et al. Oxygen free radical mediated injury to cultured rat hepatocytes during cold incubation in preservation solutions. Hepatology. 1997;26:351–357.
60. Marshall VC. Renal preservation. In: Morris PJ, editor. Kidney Transplantation: Principles and Practice. Philadelphia, PA: Saunders; 2001: 113–134.
61. Nicholson ML, Metcalfe MS, White SA, et al. A comparison of the results of renal transplantation from non-heart-beating, conventional cadaveric, and living donors. Kidney International. 2000;58(6):2585–2591.
62. Ahmad N, Hostert L, Pratt JR, et al. A pathophysiologic study of the kidney tubule to optimize organ preservation solutions. Kidney International. 2004; 66(1):77–90.
63. Roskott AM, Nieuwenhuijs VB, Dijkstra G, et al. Small bowel preservation for intestinal transplantation: a review. Transplant International. 2011;24(2): 107–131.
64. Lopez-Andujar R, Deusa S, Montalva E, et al. Comparative prospective study of two liver graft preservation solutions: University of Wisconsin and Celsior. Liver Transplantation. 2009;15(12):1709–1717.
65. Nicoluzzi J, Macri M, Fukushima J, et al. Celsior versus Wisconsin solution in pancreas transplantation. Transplantation Proceedings. 2008;40(10): 3305–3307.
66. Nunes P, Mota A, Figueiredo A, et al. Efficacy of renal preservation: comparative study of Celsior and University of Wisconsin solutions. Transplantation Proceedings. 2007;39(8):2478–2479.
67. Manrique A, Jimenez C, Herrero ML, et al. Pancreas preservation with the University of Wisconsin versus Celsior solutions. Transplantation Proceedings. 2006;38(8):2582–2584.
68. Wei L, Hata K, Doorschodt B, et al. Experimental small bowel preservation using Polysol: a new alternative to University of Wisconsin solution, Celsior and histidine-tryptophan-ketoglutarate solution? World Journal of Gastroenterology. 2007;13(27):3684–3691.
69. Montalti R, Nardo B, Capocasale E, et al. Kidney transplantation from elderly donors: a prospective randomized study comparing Celsior and UW solutions. Transplantation Proceedings. 2005;37(6):2454–2455.
70. Pedotti P, Cardillo M, Rigotti P, et al. A comparative prospective study of two available solutions for kidney and liver preservation. Transplantation. 2004; 77(10):1540–1545.
71. Candinas D, Largiader F, Binswanger U, et al. A novel dextran 40-based preservation solution. Transplant International. 1996;9(1):32–37.
72. Ben Mosbah I, Saidane D, Peralta C, et al. Efficacy of polyethylene glycols in University of Wisconsin preservation solutions: a study of isolated perfused rat liver. Transplantation Proceedings. 2005;37(9):3948–3950.
73. Nyberg SL, Baskin-Bey ES, Kremers W, et al. Improving the prediction of donor kidney quality: deceased donor score and resistive indices. Transplantation. 2005;80(7):925–929.
74. Bessems M, Doorschodt BM, Hooijschuur O, et al. Optimization of a new preservation solution for machine perfusion of the liver: which is the preferred colloid? Transplantation Proceedings. 2005;37(1):329–331.
75. Wight JP, Chilcott JB, Holmes MW, et al. Pulsatile machine perfusion vs. cold storage of kidneys for transplantation: a rapid and systematic review. Clinical Transplantation. 2003;17:293–307.
76. Moers C, Smits JM, Maathuis MHJ, et al. Machine perfusion or cold storage in deceased-donor kidney transplantation. New England Journal of Medicine. 2009;360(1):7–19.
77. Moers C, Pirenne J, Paul A, et al. Machine perfusion or cold storage in deceased-donor kidney transplantation. New England Journal of Medicine. 2012; 366(8):770–771.
78. Treckmann J, Moers C, Smits J, et al. Machine perfusion versus cold storage for

preservation of kidneys from expanded criteria donors after brain death. Transplant International. 2011;24(6):548–554.
79. Eugene M. Polyethylene glycols and immunocamouflage of the cells tissues and organs for transplantation. Cellular and Molecular Biology (Noisy-Le-Grand, France). 2004;50(3):209–215.
80. Jochmans I, Moers C, Smits JM, et al. Machine perfusion versus cold storage for the preservation of kidneys donated after cardiac death: a multicenter, randomized, controlled trial. Annals of Surgery. 2010;252(5):756–762.
81. Dondero F, Paugam-Burtz C, Danjou F, et al. A randomized study comparing IGL-1 to the University of Wisconsin preservation solution in liver transplantation. Annals of Transplantation: Quarterly of the Polish Transplantation Society. 2010;15(4):7–14.
82. Ben Abdennebi H, Elrassi Z, Scoazec J, et al. Evaluation of IGL-1 preservation solution using an orthotopic liver transplantation model. World Journal of Gastroenterology. 2006;12(33):5326–5330.
83. Badet L, Petruzzo P, Lefrancois N, et al. Kidney preservation with IGL-1 solution: a preliminary report. Transplantation Proceedings. 2005;37(1):308–311.
84. Codas R, Petruzzo P, Morelon E, et al. IGL-1 solution in kidney transplantation: first multi-center study. Clinical Transplantation. 2009;23(3):337–342.
85. Zheng TL, Lanza RP, Soon-Shiong P. Prolonged pancreas preservation using a simplified UW solution containing polyethylene glycol. Transplantation. 1991;51(1):63–66.
86. Itasaka H, Burns W, Wicomb WN, et al. Modification of rejection by polyethylene glycol in small bowel transplantation. Transplantation. 1994;57:645–648.
87. Wicomb WN, Hill JD, Avery J, et al. Optimal cardioplegia and 24-hour storage with simplified UW solution containing polyethylene glycol. Transplantation. 1990;49:261–264.
88. Ploeg RJ, van Bockel JH, Langendijk PT, et al. Effect of preservation solution on results of cadaveric kidney transplantation. The European Multicentre Study Group. Lancet. 1992;340(8812):129–137.
89. Roels L, Coosemans W, Donck J, et al. Inferior outcome of cadaveric kidneys preserved for more than 24 hr in histidine-tryptophan-ketoglutarate solution. Leuven Collaborative Group for Transplantation. Transplantation. 1998; 66(12):1660–1664.
90. Agarwal A, Powelson JA, Goggins WC, et al. Organ preservation with histidine-tryptophan ketogluatarate solution in clinical pancreas transplantation: an update of the Indiana university experience. Transplantation Proceedings. 2008;40(2): 498–501.
91. Nardo B, Bertelli R, Montalti R, et al. Preliminary results of a clinical randomized study comparing Celsior and HTK solutions in liver preservation for transplantation. Transplantation Proceedings. 2005;37(1):320–322.
92. Bond M, Pitt M, Akoh J, et al. The effectiveness and cost-effectiveness of methods of storing donated kidneys from deceased donors: a systematic review and economic model. Health Technology Assessment. 2009;13(38):iii–iv, xi–xiv, 1–156.
93. Kay MD, Hosgood SA, Bagul A, et al. Comparison of preservation solutions in an experimental model of organ cooling in kidney transplantation. British Journal of Surgery. 2009;96(10):1215–1221.
94. Watson CJE, Wells AC, Roberts RJ, et al. Cold machine perfusion versus static cold storage of kidneys donated after cardiac death: a UK multicenter randomized controlled trial. American Journal of Transplantation. 2010;10(9):1991–1999.
95. Hosgood SA, Mohamed IH, Bagul A, et al. Hypothermic machine perfusion after static cold storage does not improve the preservation condition in an experimental porcine kidney model. British Journal of Surgery. 2011;98:943–950.
96. Jochmans I, Moers C, Smits J, et al. The prognostic value of renal resistance during hypothermic machine perfusion of deceased donor kidneys. American Journal of Transplantation. 2011;11(10):2214–2220, 2214.
97. Moers C, Varnav OC, van Heurn E, et al. The value of machine perfusion perfusate biomarkers for predicting kidney transplant outcome. Transplantation. 2010;90(9):966–973.
98. van der Vliet JA, Kievit JK, Héné RJ, et al. Preservation of non-heart-beating donor kidneys: a clinical prospective randomised case-control study of machine perfusion versus cold storage. Transplantation Proceedings. 2001; 33(1–2):847.
99. Daemen JH, Heineman E, Kootstra G. Viability assessment of non-heart-beating donor kidneys during machine preservation. Transplantation Proceedings. 1995;27(5):2906–2907; discussion 2907–8.
100. Stewart ZA, Cameron AM, Singer AL, et al. Histidine-Tryptophan-Ketoglutarate (HTK) is associated with reduced graft survival in deceased donor livers, especially those donated after cardiac death. American Journal of Transplantation. 2009;9:286–293.
101. Badger IL, Michell ID, Buist LJ, et al. Human hepatic preservation using Marshall's solution and University of Wisconsin solution in a controlled, prospective trial. Transplantation Proceedings. 1990;22(5):2183–2184.
102. Kalayoglu M, Sollinger HW, Stratta RJ, et al. Extended preservation of the liver for clinical transplantation. Lancet. 1988;1(8586):617–619.
103. Todo S, Nery J, Yanaga K, et al. Extended preservation of human liver grafts with UW solution. JAMA. 1989;261(5):711–714.
104. Avolio AW, Agnes S, Nure E, et al. Comparative evaluation of two perfusion solutions for liver preservation and transplantation. Transplantation Proceedings. 2006;38(4):1066–1067.
105. Mangus RS, Fridell JA, Vianna RM, et al. Comparison of histidine-tryptophan-ketoglutarate solution and University of Wisconsin solution in extended criteria liver donors. Liver Transplantation. 2008;14(3):365–373.
106. Mangus RS, Tector AJ, Agarwal A, et al. Comparison of histidine-tryptophan-ketoglutarate solution (HTK) and University of Wisconsin solution (UW) in adult liver transplantation. Liver Transplantation. 2006;12(2):226–230.
107. Meine MH, Zanotelli ML, Neumann J, et al. Randomized clinical assay for hepatic grafts preservation with University of Wisconsin or histidine-tryptophan-ketoglutarate solutions in liver transplantation. Transplantation Proceedings. 2006; 38(6):1872–1875.
108. Pokorny H, Rasoul-Rockenschaub S, Langer F, et al. Histidine-tryptophan-ketoglutarate solution for organ preservation in human liver transplantation – A prospective multi-centre observation study. Transplant International. 2004; 17(5):256–260.
109. Stewart ZA, Cameron AM, Singer AL, et al. Histidine-tryptophan-ketoglutarate (HTK) is associated with reduced graft survival in pancreas transplantation. American Journal of Transplantation. 2009;9(1):217–221.
110. Lama C, Rafecas A, Figueras J, et al. Comparative study of Celsior and Belzer solutions for hepatic graft preservation: preliminary results. Transplantation Proceedings. 2002;34(1):54–55.
111. Monbaliu D, Brassil J. Machine perfusion of the liver: past, present and future. Current Opinion in Organ Transplantation. 2010;15(2):160–166.
112. Fondevila C, Hessheimer AJ, Maathuis MH, et al. Hypothermic oxygenated machine perfusion in porcine donation after circulatory determination of death liver transplant. Transplantation. 2012;94(1):22–29.
113. van der Plaats A, Maathuis MH, 'T Hart NA, et al. The Groningen hypothermic liver perfusion pump: functional evaluation of a new machine perfusion system. Annals of Biomedical Engineering. 2006;34(12):1924–1934.
114. Guarrera JV, Estevez J, Boykin J, et al. Hypothermic machine perfusion of liver allografts for transplantation: technical development in human discard and miniature swine models. Transplantation Proceedings. 2005;37:323–325.
115. Dutkowski P, Furrer K, Tian Y, et al. Novel short-term hypothermic oxygenated perfusion (HOPE) system prevents injury in rat liver graft from non-heart beating donor. Annals of Surgery. 2006;244(6):968–976; discussion 976–7.
116. Guarrera JV, Henry SD, Samstein B, et al. Hypothermic machine preservation in human liver transplantation: the first clinical series. American Journal of Transplantation. 2010;10(2):372–381.
117. Wahlberg JA, Southard JH, Belzer FO. Development of a cold storage solution for pancreas preservation. Cryobiology. 1986;23:477–482.
118. Schneeberger S, Biebl M, Steurer W, et al. A prospective randomized multicenter trial comparing histidine-tryptophan-ketoglutarate versus University of Wisconsin perfusion solution in clinical pancreas transplantation. Transplant International. 2009;22(2):217–224.
119. Potdar S, Malek S, Eghtesad B, et al. Initial experience using histidine-tryptophan-ketoglutarate solution in clinical pancreas transplantation. Clinical Transplantation. 2004;18(6):661–665.
120. Becker T, Ringe B, Nyibata M, et al. Pancreas transplantation with histidine-tryptophan-ketoglutarate (HTK) solution and University of Wisconsin (UW) solution: is there a difference? Journal of the Pancreas. 2007;8(3):304–311.
121. Boggi U, Coletti L, Vistoli F, et al. Pancreas preservation with University of Wisconsin and Celsior solutions. Transplantation Proceedings. 2004;36(3):563–565.
122. Kaddis JS, Danobeitia JS, Niland JC, et al. Multicenter analysis of novel and established variables associated with successful human islet isolation outcomes. American Journal of Transplantation. 2010;10(3):646–656.
123. Paushter DH, Qi M, Danielson KK, et al. Histidine-tryptophan-ketoglutarate and University of Wisconsin solution demonstrate equal effectiveness in the preservation of human pancreata intended for islet isolation: a large-scale, single-center experience. Cell Transplantation. 2013;22(7):1113–1121.
124. Niclauss N, Wojtusciszyn A, Morel P, et al. Comparative impact on islet isolation and transplant outcome of the preservation solutions Institut Georges Lopez-1, University of Wisconsin, and Celsior. Transplantation. 2012;93(7):703–708.
125. Taylor MJ, Baicu S, Greene E, et al. Islet isolation from juvenile porcine pancreas after 24-h hypothermic machine perfusion preservation. Cell Transplantation. 2010;19(5):613–628.
126. Papas KK, Hering BJ, Guenther L, et al. Pancreas oxygenation is limited during preservation with the two-layer method.[Erratum appears in Transplant Proc. 2006 May;38(4):1205 Note: Gunther, L [corrected to Guenther, L]]. Transplantation Proceedings. 2005;37(8):3501–3504.
127. Matsumoto S, Kuroda Y. Perfluorocarbon for organ preservation before trans-

plantation. Transplantation. 2002;74(12):1804–1809.
128. Qin H, Matsumoto S, Klintmalm GB, et al. A meta-analysis for comparison of the two-layer and university of Wisconsin pancreas preservation methods in islet transplantation. Cell Transplantation. 2011;20(7):1127–1137.
129. Roskott AMC, Nieuwenhuijs VB, Dijkstra G, et al. Small bowel preservation for intestinal transplantation: a review. Transplant International. 2011;24(2): 107–131.
130. Park PO, Haglund U, Bulkley GB, et al. The sequence of development of intestinal tissue injury after strangulation ischemia and reperfusion. Surgery. 1990;107(5):574–580.
131. Cicalese L, Sileri P, Green M, et al. Bacterial translocation in clinical intestinal transplantation. Transplantation. 2001;71(10):1414–1417.
132. Abu-Elmagd K, Reyes J, Bond G, et al. Clinical intestinal transplantation: a decade of experience at a single center. Annals of Surgery. 2001;234(3):404–416; discussion 416–7.
133. Mangus RS, Tector AJ, Fridell JA, et al. Comparison of histidine-tryptophan-ketoglutarate solution and University of Wisconsin solution in intestinal and multivisceral transplantation. Transplantation. 2008;86(2):298–302.
134. de Roover A, de Leval L, Gilmaire J, et al. A new model for human intestinal preservation: comparison of University of Wisconsin and Celsior preservation solutions. Transplantation Proceedings. 2004;36(2):270–272.
135. Fujimoto Y, Olson DW, Madsen KL, et al. Defining the role of a tailored luminal solution for small bowel preservation. American Journal of Transplantation. 2002;2(3):229–236.
136. Olson DW, Jijon H, Madsen KL, et al. Human small bowel storage: the role for luminal preservation solutions. Transplantation. 2003;76(4):709–714.
137. Oltean M, Joshi M, Herlenius G, et al. Improved intestinal preservation using an intraluminal macromolecular solution: evidence from a rat model. Transplantation. 2010;89(3):285–290.
138. Leuvenink HGD, van Dijk A, Freund RL, et al. Luminal preservation of rat small intestine with University of Wisconsin or Celsior solution. Transplantation Proceedings. 2005;37(1):445–447.
139. Tsujimura T, Salehi P, Walker J, et al. Ameliorating small bowel injury using a cavitary two-layer preservation method with perfluorocarbon and a nutrient-rich solution. American Journal of Transplantation. 2004;4(9):1421–1428.
140. Zhu JZJ, Castillo EG, Salehi P, et al. A novel technique of hypothermic luminal perfusion for small bowel preservation. Transplantation. 2003;76(1):71–76.
141. Guimaraes FAG, Taha MO, Simoes MJ, et al. Use of hyperbaric oxygenation in small bowel preservation for transplant. Transplantation Proceedings. 2006; 38(6):1796–1799.
142. Domínguez-Gil B, Haase-Kromwijk B, Van Leiden H, et al. Current situation of donation after circulatory death in European countries. Transplant International. 2011;24(7):676–686.
143. Hoogland ER, Snoeijs MG, Winkens B, et al. Kidney transplantation from donors after cardiac death: uncontrolled versus controlled donation. American Journal of Transplantation. 2011;11(7):1427–1434.
144. Alvarez J, del Barrio MR, Arias J, et al. Five years of experience with non-heart-beating donors coming from the streets. Transplantation Proceedings. 2002;34(7):2589–2590.
145. Alvarez J, del Barrio R, Arias J, et al. Non-heart-beating donors from the streets: an increasing donor pool source. Transplantation. 2000;70(2):314–317.
146. Sanchez-Fructuoso AI, Prats D, Torrente J, et al. Renal transplantation from non-heart beating donors: a promising alternative to enlarge the donor pool. Journal of the American Society of Nephrology. 2000;11(2):350–358.
147. Valero R, Cabrer C, Oppenheimer F, et al. Normothermic recirculation reduces primary graft dysfunction of kidneys obtained from non-heart-beating donors. Transplant International. 2000;13(4):303–310.
148. Fieux F, Losser M, Bourgeois E, et al. Kidney retrieval after sudden out of hospital refractory cardiac arrest: a cohort of uncontrolled non heart beating donors. Critical Care. 2009;13(4):R141.
149. Magliocca JF, Magee JC, Rowe SA, et al. Extracorporeal support for organ donation after cardiac death effectively expands the donor pool. Journal of Trauma. 2005;58(6):1095–1101; discussion 1101–2.
150. Farney AC, Singh RP, Hines MH, et al. Experience in renal and extrarenal transplantation with donation after cardiac death donors with selective use of extracorporeal support. Journal of the American College of Surgeons. 2008; 206(5):1028–1037; discussion 1037.
151. Lee C, Tsai M, Ko W, et al. Expanding the donor pool: use of renal transplants from non-heart-beating donors supported with extracorporeal membrane oxygenation. Clinical Transplantation. 2005;19(3):383–390.
152. Fondevila C, Hessheimer AJ, Ruiz A, et al. Liver transplant using donors after unexpected cardiac death: novel preservation protocol and acceptance criteria. American Journal of Transplantation. 2007;7(7):1849–1855.
153. Jimenez-Galanes S, Meneu-Diaz MJC, Elola-Olaso AM, et al. Liver transplantation using uncontrolled non-heart-beating donors under normothermic extracorporeal membrane oxygenation. Liver Transplantation. 2009;15(9):1110–1118.
154. Kay MD, Hosgood SA, Harper SJF, et al. Static normothermic preservation of renal allografts using a novel nonphosphate buffered preservation solution. Transplant International. 2007;20(1):88–92.
155. Schreinemachers MJM, Doorschodt BM, Florquin S, et al. Improved preservation and microcirculation with POLYSOL after transplantation in a porcine kidney autotransplantation model. Nephrology, Dialysis, Transplantation. 2009;24(3): 816–824.
156. Schreinemachers MCJM, Doorschodt BM, Florquin S, et al. Improved renal function of warm ischemically damaged kidneys using Polysol. Transplantation Proceedings. 2009;41(1):32–35.
157. Treckmann JW, Paul A, Saad S, et al. Primary organ function of warm ischaemically damaged porcine kidneys after retrograde oxygen persufflation. Nephrology, Dialysis, Transplantation. 2006;21(7):1803–1808.
158. Treckmann J, Nagelschmidt M, Minor T, et al. Function and quality of kidneys after cold storage, machine perfusion, or retrograde oxygen persufflation: results from a porcine autotransplantation model. Cryobiology. 2009;59(1): 19–23.
159. Manekeller S, Leuvenink H, Sitzia M, et al. Oxygenated machine perfusion preservation of predamaged kidneys with HTK and Belzer machine perfusion solution: an experimental study in pigs. Transplantation Proceedings. 2005; 37(8):3274–3275.
160. Maathuis MJ, Manekeller S, van der Plaats A, et al. Improved kidney graft function after preservation using a novel hypothermic machine perfusion device. Annals of Surgery. 2007;246(6):982–988; discussion 989–91.
161. Buchs J, Lazeyras F, Ruttimann R, et al. Oxygenated hypothermic pulsatile perfusion versus cold static storage for kidneys from non heart-beating donors tested by in-line ATP resynthesis to establish a strategy of preservation. Perfusion. 2011;26(2):159–165.
162. Koetting M, Kaiser G, Paul A, et al. Hypothermic reconditioning by gaseous oxygen improves survival after transplantation of marginally preserved livers in the pig. Langenbeck's Archives of Surgery. 2011;396(4):578–579.
163. Thuillier R, Dutheil D, Trieu MTN, et al. Supplementation with a new therapeutic oxygen carrier reduces chronic fibrosis and organ dysfunction in kidney static preservation. American Journal of Transplantation. 2011;11(9):1845–1860.
164. Regner KR, Nilakantan V, Ryan RP, et al. Protective effect of Lifor solution in experimental renal ischemia-reperfusion injury. Journal of Surgical Research. 2010;164(2):e291–e297.
165. Gage F, Leeser DB, Porterfield NK, et al. Room temperature pulsatile perfusion of renal allografts with Lifor compared with hypothermic machine pump solution. Transplantation Proceedings. 2009;41(9):3571–3574.
166. Brasile L, Green E, Haisch C. Warm ex vivo perfusion prevents reperfusion injury in warm ischemically damaged kidneys. Transplantation Proceedings. 1997;29(8): 3422–3423.
167. Harper S, Hosgood S, Kay M, et al. Leucocyte depletion improves renal function during reperfusion using an experimental isolated haemoperfused organ preservation system. British Journal of Surgery. 2006;93(5):623–629.
168. Bagul A, Hosgood SA, Kaushik M, et al. Experimental renal preservation by normothermic resuscitation perfusion with autologous blood. British Journal of Surgery. 2008;95(1):111–118.
169. Hosgood SA, Nicholson ML. First in man renal transplantation after ex vivo normothermic perfusion. Transplantation. 2011;92(7):735–738.
170. The first clinical series of normothermic perfusion in marginal donor kidney transplantation. 15th Annual Congress of the British Transplantation Society; 2012.
171. Thuillier R, Giraud S, Favreau F, et al. Improving long-term outcome in allograft transplantation: role of ionic composition and polyethylene glycol. Transplantation. 2011;91(6):605–614.
172. Vekemans K, Van Pelt J, Komuta M, et al. Attempt to rescue discarded human liver grafts by end ischemic hypothermic oxygenated machine perfusion. Transplantation Proceedings. 2011;43(9):3455–3459.
173. de Rougemont O, Breitenstein S, Leskosek B, et al. One hour hypothermic oxygenated perfusion (HOPE) protects nonviable liver allografts donated after cardiac death. Annals of Surgery. 2009;250(5):674–683.
174. Minor T, Koetting M, Kaiser G, et al. Hypothermic reconditioning by gaseous oxygen improves survival after liver transplantation in the pig. American Journal of Transplantation. 2011;11(12):2627–2634.
175. Treckmann J, Minor T, Saad S, et al. Retrograde oxygen persufflation preservation of human livers: a pilot study. Liver Transplantation. 2008;14(3): 358–364.
176. Minor T, Putter C, Gallinat A, et al. Oxygen persufflation as adjunct in liver preservation (OPAL): study protocol for a randomized controlled trial. Trials. 2011;12(1):234–234.
177. Stegemann J, Hirner A, Rauen U, et al. Gaseous oxygen persufflation or oxygenated machine perfusion with Custodiol-N for long-term preservation of ischemic

rat livers? Cryobiology. 2009;58(1):45–51.
178. Ijichi H, Taketomi A, Soejima Y, et al. Effect of hyperbaric oxygen on cold storage of the liver in rats. Liver International. 2006;26(2):248–253.
179. Odaira M, Aoki T, Miyamoto Y, et al. Cold preservation of the liver with oxygenation by a two-layer method. Journal of Surgical Research. 2009; 152(2):209–217.
180. Schön MR, Kollmar O, Wolf S, et al. Liver transplantation after organ preservation with normothermic extracorporeal perfusion. Annals of Surgery. 2001;233(1):114–123.
181. Butler AJ, Rees MA, Wight DGD, et al. Successful extracorporeal porcine liver perfusion for 72 hr. Transplantation. 2002;73(8):1212–1218.
182. Imber CJ, St Peter SD, Lopez de Cenarruzabeitia I, et al. Advantages of normothermic perfusion over cold storage in liver preservation. Transplantation. 2002;73(5):701–709.
183. St Peter SD, Imber CJ, Lopez I, et al. Extended preservation of non-heart-beating donor livers with normothermic machine perfusion. British Journal of Surgery. 2002;89(5):609–616.
184. Brockmann J, Reddy S, Coussios C, et al. Normothermic perfusion: a new paradigm for organ preservation. Annals of Surgery. 2009;250(1):1–6.
185. Fondevila C, Hessheimer AJ, Maathuis MJ, et al. Superior preservation of DCD livers with continuous normothermic perfusion. Annals of Surgery. 2011;254(6): 1000–1007.
186. Tolboom H, Pouw RE, Izamis M, et al. Recovery of warm ischemic rat liver grafts by normothermic extracorporeal perfusion. Transplantation. 2009;87(2): 170–177.
187. Tolboom H, Izamis M, Sharma N, et al. Subnormothermic machine perfusion at both 20°C and 30°C recovers ischemic rat livers for successful transplantation. Journal of Surgical Research. 2012;175(1):149–156.
188. Jamieson RW, Zilvetti M, Roy D, et al. Hepatic steatosis and normothermic perfusion-preliminary experiments in a porcine model. Transplantation. 2011;92(3):289–295.
189. Requiao-Moura LR, Durao Mde S, Tonato EJ, et al. Effects of ischemia and reperfusion injury on long-term graft function. Transplantation Proceedings. 2011;43(1):70–73.
190. Salahudeen AK. Cold ischemic injury of transplanted kidneys: new insights from experimental studies. American Journal of Physiology. 2004;287:F181–F187, F187.
191. Green C. Mammalian hibernation: lessons for organ preparation? Cryo Letters. 2000;21(2):91–98.
192. Zancanaro C, Malatesta M, Mannello F, et al. The kidney during hibernation and arousal from hibernation. A natural model of organ preservation during cold ischaemia and reperfusion. Nephrology, Dialysis, Transplantation. 1999;14(8): 1982–1990.
193. Bouma HR, Verhaag EM, Otis JP, et al. Induction of torpor: mimicking natural metabolic suppression for biomedical applications. Journal of Cellular Physiology. 2012;227(4):1285–1290.
194. Carey HV, Andrews MT, Martin SL. Mammalian hibernation: cellular and molecular responses to depressed metabolism and low temperature. Physiological Reviews. 2003;83(4):1153–1181.
195. Bouma HR, Henning RH, Kroese FG, et al. Hibernation is associated with depression of T-cell independent humoral immune responses in the 13-lined ground squirrel. Developmental and Comparative Immunology. 2012;39(3):154–160.
196. Bouma HR, Kroese FG, Kok JW, et al. Low body temperature governs the decline of circulating lymphocytes during hibernation through sphingosine-1-phosphate. Proceedings of the National Academy of Sciences of the United States of America. 2011;108(5):2052–2057.
197. Blackstone E, Morrison M, Roth MB. H2S induces a suspended animation-like state in mice. Science. 2005;308(5721):518.
198. Szabo C. Hydrogen sulphide and its therapeutic potential. Nature Reviews Drug Discovery. 2007;6(11):917–935.
199. Wagner F, Asfar P, Calzia E, et al. Bench-to-bedside review: hydrogen sulfide–the third gaseous transmitter: applications for critical care. Critical Care. 2009;13(3):213.
200. Bos EM, Leuvenink HG, Snijder PM, et al. Hydrogen sulfide-induced hypometabolism prevents renal ischemia/reperfusion injury. Journal of the American Society of Nephrology. 2009;20(9):1901–1905.
201. Bos EM, Snijder PM, Jekel H, et al. Beneficial effects of gaseous hydrogen sulfide in hepatic ischemia/reperfusion injury. Transplant International. 2012;25(8): 897–908.
202. Li J, Zhang G, Cai S, et al. Effect of inhaled hydrogen sulfide on metabolic responses in anesthetized, paralyzed, and mechanically ventilated piglets. Pediatric Critical Care Medicine: A Journal of the Society of Critical Care Medicine and the World Federation of Pediatric Intensive and Critical Care Societies. 2008;9(1):110–112.
203. Simon F, Giudici R, Duy CN, et al. Hemodynamic and metabolic effects of hydrogen sulfide during porcine ischemia/reperfusion injury. Shock. 2008; 30(4):359–364.

第 26 章
胸部器官的保存和复苏

Jonathan C. Yeung, Marcelo Cypel, John M. Craig, Shaf Keshavjee

引言

从 1983 年肺移植首次成功开始，肺保存已经取得了重大进展。肺保存起始于 20 世纪 80 年代，供、受体术间必须相邻，经历了静态冷浸式转运，发展当今的临床标准：低温灌注保存（低温、供氧、静态保存）。然而，供肺离体，在非自然状态时，完美的保存策略仍在研究。以前认为，供肺保存的中心原则是在器官被成功植入受体之前"延缓死亡"，如今，形成了器官保存过程中"保持存活"的概念，新的技术方法和保存策略也在朝着这个方向发展。这超越了器官保存，开启了"器官的个体化用药"时代，在这个时代，供肺的靶向诊疗应运而生。本章回顾目前的肺保存策略，并讨论未来可能出现的供肺保存和复苏方法。

通常认为供肺保存是器官位于捐献者体外的这段时间，实际上，保存策略贯穿于确认器官捐献直至器官移植后期的整个过程。本章连接着第 21、22 章和第 58、59 章，其内容涉及死亡供体或心脏死亡供体的器官获取和胸腔脏器移植程序。在器官获取和局部缺血之前，有效的供者处理措施可帮助器官复苏，增加脑死亡到器官获取期间的肺部供氧，可增加肺和心脏的复苏成功率[1-3]。

肺保存

供肺获取前阶段

在获取器官前，尤其是在脑死亡状态下，要特别注意维持容量状态，有助于避免神经源性肺水肿加重、容量超负荷性肺水肿的发生[4]。因此，必须监测中心静脉压，并控制在 4~10mmHg[5]。当怀疑左心功能不全时，同时需要以肺动脉导管监测肺动脉楔压。由于肺功能不全和去甲肾上腺素及肾上腺素相关，如有必要，升压药首选多巴胺[<10μg/(kg·min)]，其次可选用垂体加压素(<2.4U/h)[6]。另外，如果存在尿崩症，可以垂体加压素升高血压[7,8]，不仅有促血管收缩作用[9-11]，还有抗利尿作用。当有肺动脉导管时，体循环阻力应控制在 800~1200dyn·s/cm^5[12]。

避免气压伤是供肺保护的另一个原则。一般来说，供者的保护性通气策略和 ARDS 的治疗方案类似（潮气量 6~8mL/kg，PEEP 为 5cmH_2O，吸氧浓度<0.5）[13]。近期，Mascia 等完成的一项 RCT 研究表明，以潮气量 6~8mL/kg、PEEP 为 8~10cmH_2O 条件的机械通气在供肺中的应用有所增加[14]。供肺比较容易发生肺不张和肺炎，经常膨肺并进行吸痰是非常重要的，因此，规律肺复张预防肺不张、纤维支气管镜消除痰栓和肺泡盥洗应常规进行。胸片可用来观察肺部浸润影的改变，持续监测肺水肿的进展[1,6,12]。

即使是在脑死亡后数小时，应用甲强龙(15mg/kg)也有助于改善肺功能和提高移植后疗效[3,15]，但是，是因其抗炎作用还是脑死亡后 ACTH 缺乏时类固醇的替代作用目前尚无定论。其他激素替代治疗（如三碘甲状腺胺酸或左甲状腺素）的疗效，也有文献报道，但是在肺移植中没有明确获益[3]。现已证实，β_2-拟肾上腺素药的应用可加速离体肺（人和小鼠）肺泡液的清除[16]，为一项随机对照试验奠定了基础，其纳入了 500 例供肺[17]，通过对比沙丁胺醇喷雾剂和安慰剂，研究 β 受体激动剂对供肺氧合功能的影响。有趣的是，高剂量吸入沙丁胺醇组，并未改善供肺的氧合，也没有增加供肺利用率，因此暂不推荐常规使用 β_2-拟肾上腺素药[18]。

Angel 等进行的回顾性研究指出，对于质量较差的供体，供者的标准化治疗方案可以影响其复苏[2]。该方案实施的 4 年内，254 例供体初次评估时质量较差，其中有 135 例在标准化治疗结束时质量达到了理想状态，最后，初期认为质量较差的供体中，有 21%进行了肺移植。在标准化供者治疗方案实施之前，最初被认为质量较差的供体，利用率仅有 10%。Gabbay 等以提高氧合指数（PaO_2/FiO_2，P/F）为供者治疗策略[1]，140 例移植中，原来被拒绝使用的 20 例供肺，在肺移植后 30 天和 3 年的生存并没有受到影响。报道中还有一些其他的提高移植后疗效的供者治疗方案[3,19,20]。

供肺获取阶段

在当今的肺移植程序中，供者进行手术时才知道供体是否可用。一旦确定供体可用，将切取供肺，供肺的离体阶段也就开始了。通常情况下，供肺获取手术开始于评估供肺可用时，因此，减少供肺离体时的损伤非常重要。

在器官获取时，为了能更好地获取供肺，要采取很多措施[21]。在器官获取前阶段，为了避免出现气压伤，应用的肺通气策略类似于 ARDS 的治疗方案；在获取时，要全身肝素化（300U/kg）进行抗凝，以降低血管内凝血的风险；一旦完成供肺评估，立即经肺动脉给予前列腺素 E1（PGE1）以扩张肺血管并降低肺血管阻力（PVR），可促进随后进行的肺动脉灌洗，PGE1 还可以降低促炎性细胞因子对刺激的反应，或许可以减少原发性移植器官无功能（PGD）的发生[22]。PGE1 应用后，肺血管扩张，全身血压会继发性下降，此时即可开始对供体进行主动脉阻断，心脏停搏后，即可开始供肺获取[23]。通过肺血管灌注低温灌注液使供肺降温，并替换出供肺血管内血液，进一步减少可能存在的血凝块，并清除炎性细胞和免疫细胞。依据早期肺移植的经验，与其他器官应用细胞内液型溶液相反，应用细胞外液型溶液更有利于肺保存[24]。细胞内液型溶液可以导致肺血管收缩，影响肺血管灌注。右旋糖酐 40 是肺组织灌注液中的重要成分，有两方面作用：提高血管内的胶体渗透压以维持血管内压；减少红细胞、中性粒细胞和血小板的聚集。这可以帮助再灌注时维持毛细血管的通畅性，尤其是支气管的微循环中，可能起到减少支气管毛细血管网并发症的作用。葡萄糖是肺组织灌注液中的另一种重要成分。由于肺组织中储存有氧气，多出现缺血不缺氧的特殊情况，葡萄糖可维持肺保存阶段的有氧代谢。多个回顾性分析已经证实了低钾右旋糖酐 40 葡萄糖溶液优于细胞内液型溶液[25–29]。

灌注液要先经肺动脉进行顺行性灌注，再经每个肺静脉主干进行逆行性灌注。这种逆行灌注不仅可以帮助清除肺动脉中的栓子，并通过支气管的肺分流帮助灌注支气管血管[30]，可能还可以增加受低氧影响使肺动脉血管收缩区域的肺灌注[31]。顺行灌注时的灌注液用量约为 50~60mL/kg，逆行灌注为 1L。理想的灌注压不能太高，否则易导致肺血管损伤，也不能太低而出现灌注不充分。实际上，灌注液可以用 30cmH_2O 的压力依靠重力进行灌注。灌注完成后，移除供肺，并以 50%的氧浓度、20cmH_2O 的气道压进行膨肺，然后在冰中进行保存。膨肺有两个目的：首先，可以为肺组织的有氧代谢提供氧气；其次，可以维持肺泡结构并保存肺泡表面活性物质。因此，Van Raemdonck 等证实即使是用氮气膨肺也比出现肺不张好[32]。20cmH_2O 的气道压是理想条件。如果供肺进行空运，由于飞行时的低气压，尚需避免供肺过度膨胀，运输过程中，如果没有加压舱，供肺内气体膨胀后可能会导致气压伤。

直至今天，一旦供肺离体，通过降低温度来降低其代谢率依然是供肺保存的基本策略。Kayano 等在小鼠模型上证实肺保存的最佳温度大约为 10℃[33,34]，但是，为了简化运输管理，用冰降温至 4℃是最常用的方法。一旦器官离体，通常情况下要尽快开始器官移植手术。据报道，冷缺血时间超过 8 小时，将会增加 PGR 发生率和 30 天内死亡率[35]。也有冷缺血时间达到 10~12 小时移植成功的报道，但是这种选择仅限于供者和受者很少有其他危险因素的情况。

移植阶段

供肺获取的整个过程中，要小心避免热缺血，但是在供肺植入阶段，这是不可避免的。Date 等指出供肺植入过程中，其温度明显上升，供肺周围应用冰层降温可以延缓其发生[36]。尽管 Stammberger 等指出在模型猪肺移植中，2 小时的热缺血对移植后结果没有影响，移植肺没有出现损伤，但随访时间较短[37]。在供肺植入时应用冰层降温可能有好处，且不影响操作，因此我们应该常规使用。

再灌注可能使新肺出现损伤，是肺移植中的重要环节，需要重点关注。新肺植入后，历时 10min 缓慢打开肺动脉阻断带逐渐再灌注可以改善移植后情况[38]。有些学者主张在打开阻断带前以特制灌注液进行肺灌注，但是在大多数移植中心，这不是常规方法[39]。一旦开始再灌注,要同时开始进行低氧浓度(通常是21%)的肺通气,从而避免氧气相关的肺损伤。对于通过心肺转流术进行移植的患者,在新肺植入时,用10~15mmHg的脉冲性压力对准备好的新肺进行预灌注非常重要。Vienna团队对这种渐进性的、保护性的再灌注策略进行了延伸:Aigner等认为对于所有患者,肺移植过程中,当血流动力学或呼吸支持不稳定时,应用膜肺(ECMO)支持优于体外转流术[40],术中应用ECMO支持的130例患者中,51例患者在整个围手术期都应用了ECMO,使肺动脉再灌注逐渐增加的时间延长到了数小时甚至数天而不是几分钟。

移植后

再灌注之后,为了改善肺和支气管微循环,我们要常规静脉应用肝素(100U/h)和右旋糖苷40(10%的右旋糖酐40 500mL/24h)7天[41,42]。

在心脏死亡供者中

在国际上,文献报道,使用可控的心脏死亡后捐献(DCD)的供肺可以和传统肺移植达到相当的效果,并可以促进肺移植的发展。但是DCD供肺延长了心脏停跳到肺冷却之间热缺血时间,其应用给肺保存带来了新的挑战[43-48]。幸运的是,供肺对这种额外的热缺血表现出了较好的耐受性,或许和供肺代谢率低但肺内氧气充足相关[49,50]。实际上,Miyoshi等通过模型猪证实肺泡内的氧气非常重要,试验中,肺换气不足比循环停滞导致的移植后结果更差。临床上认为热缺血时间小于1h的供肺是可以用来做移植的[49,52-55]。通常情况下,这1个小时足够在DCD过程完成器官获取。然而,为了更好地保存DCD器官,Lund团队重新引入了原地局部降温的方法[56],胸腔内置管2根以灌注低温右旋糖苷40可以使供肺温度降至18℃。在动物模型和病例报告中,局部降温法可以使DCD供肺的热缺血时间从原来的1小时延长至6h。但是,实际上该策略最实用于不可控的DCD供肺保存。

在脑死亡供体捐献中,在循环停滞和脏器灌注降温之前要进行全身肝素化,但是在DCD中,由于涉及伦理问题,不能全部进行肝素化,因为其目的是获取器官,不能发生在供者死亡之前。为了解决该问题,大多数DCD器官获取协议中,都是在心脏停跳之后通过肺动脉注射进行肝素化。Okazaki等在犬肺移植模型上证实该方案是有效可行的[57]。临床数据也证实,两种肝素化方案中移植后的结果没有差异[58]。逆行性灌注在DCD供肺中对于清除血栓或栓子仍然是非常重要的措施。

常温下肺保存

当今临床上肺保存的基本观念是通过低温降低其代谢率,该方法较为理想,对供肺较好,被广泛接受。随着如今器官捐献的短缺,多数项目使用的超标准器官数量在逐步增加,肺功能不能达到理想状态。理想状态下,供肺在植入受者之前的离体时期,应该完成进一步评估和复苏。由于低温保存降低代谢率,影响供肺评估和复苏,为了实现该目的,需要使供体保存达到常温或接近常温。一种方法是离体肺灌注(EVLP,图26.1),模拟供肺在体内的通气和灌注条件。为了获取供肺时完成评估和保存,Carrel和Jirsch分别于1938年和1970年提出了该方案,并在不能维持血气屏障的供肺中进行了尝试,结果在离体肺灌注的过程中供肺出现了肺水肿和PVR增加[59,60]。

为了更客观地评估DCD供肺,Steen等在瑞典德隆市建立了可以快速评估离体肺功能的体外灌注系统[61]。他们应用了含有最佳胶体渗透压的缓冲式细胞外液型肺灌注液(Steen灌注液),这种灌注液既可以在灌注时帮助维持血管内压,也可以为供肺代谢提供营养,其组成成分和现在临床上应用的LPDG保存液很相似,以人血白蛋白为主要添加成分,人血白蛋白可以维持血管内较高胶体渗透压,能减少灌注时肺水肿的发生。Steen等在灌注液循环时混入了红细胞,并在大型动物模型对供肺进行了灌注和评估,长达1小时,没有出现肺水肿,移植效果也较好[61]。继其动物实验后,2007年,Steen首次报道了1例不符合条件的供肺在经历短暂EVLP后成功完成肺移植的案例[62]。后来,Steen团队有报道了6例不合格的供肺的短期灌注评估[63]。

Steen研究的最终目标是用EVLP作为供肺评估方法,使灌注次数减少。为了使EVLP应用于供肺保存、评估和功能修复,还需要投入更多的时间。Erasmus等第一次尝试把EVLP延长至6h,但是由于供肺在结束时出现PVR和气道压升高,不得不再一次考虑循环相关损伤[64]。我们将成功的长期(12h) EVLP定义为常温下进行通气,并应用非细胞型灌注的肺保护策略[65]。

为了达到稳定的12h灌注,采用了一些关键性供

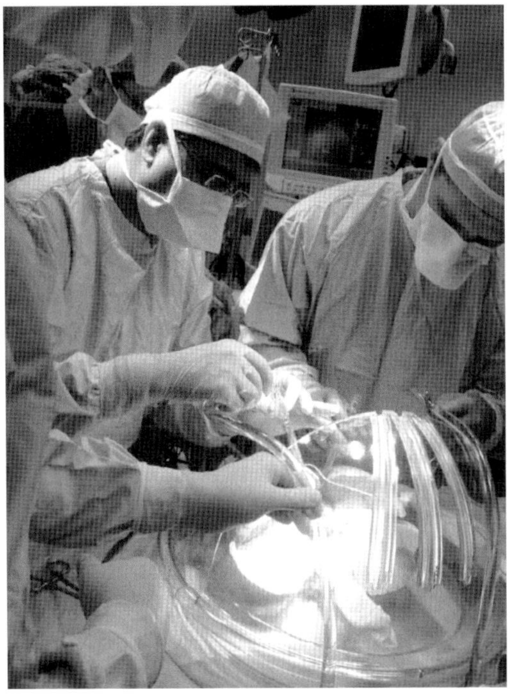
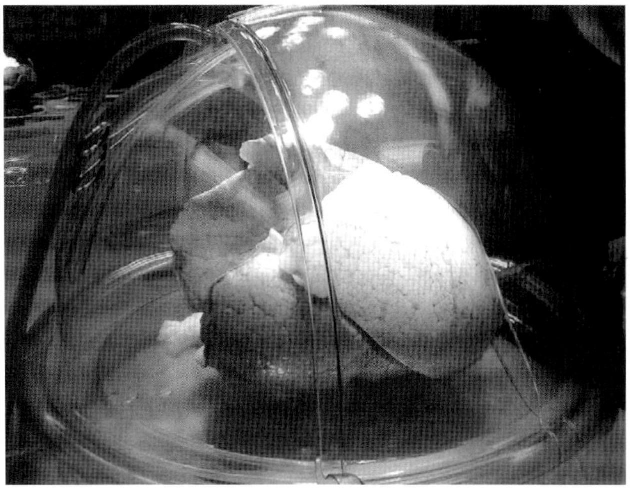

(A) (B)

图 26.1 体外肺灌注。(A)供肺正在被放入 EVLP 装置中，能够对供肺熟练完成包括支气管镜灌洗在内的操作，是 EVLP 和低温保存的重大优势；(B)供肺在 EVLP 装置中复苏，保存过程中可同时完成通气和灌注。

肺保护措施。首先应用了非细胞型灌注[65]。我们假设通过通气给肺供氧气，而不是通过血流，Egan 团队也支持该观念，他们在常温下为供肺只提供常温空气的肺通气，可以使细胞存活 24h[66,67]。此外，非细胞型灌注在临床应用中操作方便，还可以避免红细胞在灌注液微环境中寿命的限制。其次，肺灌注的最大流量要限制到心输出量的 40%而不是 100%。这种低流量可以减少因灌注导致的肺水肿，即使是对于供肺的流量依赖性区域，其 EVLP 供肺的组织学和移植后功能也是正常的。另外，我们发现左心房压力控制在 3~5mmHg 对于长期灌注至关重要。这种较低的左心房正压可以维持气道压升高和灌注流量降低时毛细血管和后毛细血管微静脉的开放，并避免微血管塌闭[68]。如果失去了左心房正压，会导致肺泡结构不稳定和肺顺应性下降[69]。最后，我们要重视离心泵的应用。通气时，膨胀的肺泡会压迫其周围血管，导致每次呼吸时 PVR 都会增加。离心泵的作用就是通过增加其后负荷来增加循环和流量。因此，在增加阻力时，泵会减少而不是促进灌注液通过，但是有可能诱发肺损伤或肺水肿。灌注的过程中，通过膜式氧和器清除氧气并提供二氧化碳来模拟细胞代谢。通过测量灌注液中的氧分压，以清除氧气进行肺功能评估；通过增加二氧化碳来帮助维持灌注液的 pH 值。这种可重复的安全的 12h 常温体外灌注方法已经在猪肺和人肺中取得了成功，这种 EVLP 方法已经用于冷缺血时间过长引起的缺血性损伤的治疗[65,70,71]。

体外供肺评估

目前，肺评估的临床过程非常依赖术中判断。但是一些评估要在器官获取前进行，比如胸部 X 线片和 ICU 纤维支气管镜，这些评估结果决定着器官是否可用。肺损伤可能已经发生，但是尚未表现出肺水肿，无意中，较低的氧合指数持续应用着。此外，由于血压不稳定，肺实质灌注不足而表现出的低 PaO_2 并不准确[72]，器官获取过程中捐献者的这种生理变化或许不适于进行全面准确的肺功能评估。作为 EVLP 过程中肺水肿进展的代表，肺损伤主要表现为肺顺应性和气道压的变化，比灌注液中氧分压的变化更早出现。因此，EVLP 过程中，要密切监测这些指标，用一段至少几个小时的时间来动态监测肺顺应性和气道压。为了减少肺移植过程中可能发生的肺不张，其基线时间点应该是在肺灌注复温和重新膨肺 1 小时后。所有随后测量的生理学指标(顺应性、气道压、PVR、灌注液氧分压)都要与这个时间点的相比较。肺功能评估通常需要寻找一个正常值或者截点，但是肺顺应性和气道压都是基于部分肺容量的测量结果,其测量值会有明显的下降。由于这些原因，测量值的变化趋势就比其绝对值本身更加重要,比如:肺顺应性的初始值是 80mL/cmH_2O,但是 4 小时后为 40mL/cmH_2O,比起初始值和 4 小时后测量值同为 40mL/cmH_2O 更有价值。当应用非细胞型灌注液对离体肺进行灌注时,需要理解其对氧分压影响的解释。因为氧分压-氧气容量曲线在此时是线性的,不同氧分压的灌注液混合在一起时,就像发生了肺分流,会导致更高的总体氧分压[72]。

关于 Cypel 等所提的 EVLP 和上边描述的评估方法,Toronto 肺移植项目开展了一项临床试验,用 EVLP 对高危供肺进行评估并决定其是否可用[73]。起初供肺是不符合标准的,但是经过 EVLP 评估,其 PVR、动态肺顺应性、吸气峰压是稳定的或者有所提高,吸入氧分压超过 350mmHg 时进行肺移植,其移植后结局和其他同期进行的移植并没有差异。

EVLP 的商业获取平台在不断发展,如 XVIVO 灌注的 XPS 系统、Vivoline 医药的 LS1、Transmedics 的 OCS 肺,这三者中,XPS 系统最有可能实现多伦多方案,不同之处在于添加了很多监控来帮助器官评估。LS1 系统和 Steen 等的肺功能评估系统最相似,与多伦多方案的不同之处在于其用的是滚筒泵、心房开放、以血液为基础的细胞型灌注液，英国正在用该装置进行临床试验。OCS 供肺装置被称作是可移动的供肺保存系统,其提供了一种被 Transmedics 称作是“保存模式”的供肺保存策略,其灌注液被循环进行的混合气体(12% O_2、2.5% CO_2、82.5% N_2)所替代。这样使需要的气体体积最小化了,使装置的运输更加方便,但是对供肺功能评估是不利的。剩下的“持续性监测”模型是更加方便的灌注措施,直接用空气进行通气,以静脉向肺动脉灌注来进行供肺评估。但是,持续性监测模型和供肺利用去氧灌注液进行氧和的 Toronto 和 Lund 方案相似,可自动测量，使预置在静脉内灌注液中氧饱和达到 73%、动脉中灌注液氧饱和度达到 93%,且不进一步去氧化所需的时间，该模型与 Toronto 方案不动之处也是应用了心房开放、滚筒泵、风箱而非呼吸机、以血液为基础的细胞型灌注液。OCS 供肺保存的报告仅限于个案报道,但是现在这是一个国际 INSPIRE 试验项目[75,76]。冷缺血对供肺不利这个假设,促进了像 OCS 供肺系统这样的移动性常温灌注措施的发展。有限的冷缺血是否真的对供肺不利仍然需要证明,尤其是 30 多的临床经验中,短期冷缺血作为唯一供肺保存方法也取得了较好疗效。即使是从器官获取到器官植入过程中应用常温保存,一些冷缺血的情况也难以避免。在供体循环阻断是需要用冷灌注和局部降温,在肺移植过程中也需要以植入前降温来保护供肺并使热缺血损伤最小化。实验及临床数据说明移动性连续性常温灌注优于短期间断冷缺血保存,但是,鉴于其运作带来的挑战性和增减的经济负担,为了标准器官或者超标准器官的应用,常温灌注评估和治疗方案需要证实其方便实用性。

不单是为了使冷缺血损伤最小化，以常温器官保存进行替代还为减少复苏导致的供肺损伤带来了很大希望。鉴于供肺损伤可能存在很多机制,如脑死亡、肺挫伤、吸气伤、肺感染、水肿和肺不张等,假设每种损伤都可以通过体外治疗来修复,供肺肯定会大量增加。但就要求灌注不单是为了评估,更为了修复。多数供肺可以通过 2~4h 的灌注进行评估,但进行可能需要的治疗性修复则要维持更长时间的稳定的无创性灌注。多伦多肺移植项目的 HELP 研究中，通过灌注原本不合格的供肺 23 例,使 20 例成功恢复,并进行了肺移植,其短期和中期生存也没有差异。随着通过 EVLP 来改善结果的临床经验不断积累，目前已经超过 50 例肺移植,这个数量会不断增加[77]。

其他用 EVLP 进行供肺修复的早期研究也有报道,但多数还只是一种抽象的形式。每项研究都是为了解决供肺损伤的一个方面，这样广度的探索最终会涌现出针对某一种供肺损伤的一大批体外供肺治疗方法。由于器官获取前脑死亡的生理性变化及 ECU 中的液体治疗,肺水肿是一种常见的供肺损伤。与正常机体内不同，肺灌注过程中应用特布他林可以加速肺泡液的清除[78]。另一种常见的机制是吸气性肺损伤,Inci 等曾试图通过酸性吸入来增加猪肺模型的损伤[79]。在EVLP 过程中,应用表面活性剂进行供肺灌洗,可以成功地提高供肺功能。鉴于许多供肺因为肺炎或者感染而被拒绝使用,EVLP 开始时可使用大剂量的抗生素。Newcastle 和 Toronto 团队的数据都显示,EVLP 中抗生素治疗后供肺感染的压力有减小的可能性。

基于 EVLP 的基因和细胞治疗也已经开始了探

素。应用腺病毒载体对离体肺进行基因治疗是有效的，并且由于载体相关炎症的减少，格外引人关注。此外，由于应用方便，该措施很容易与临床肺移植相结合[82]。对于不合格的供肺进行基于 EVLP 的 IL-10 基因治疗可以改善供肺功能，并可以使炎症相关生物标记物减少，预示着 IL-10 基因治疗可能会促进供肺再灌注时的恢复[71]。Lee 等提出，EVLP 过程中向供肺输注骨髓间充质干细胞，可以在内毒素引起肺损伤后使内皮细胞屏障的渗透性和肺泡液平衡恢复[83]。

心脏保存方法

缺血耐受时间是限制供体多少的一个主要因素。目前，最常用的心脏保存方法是 4℃含钾晶体液顺行性灌注，在冰中保存进行运输，4h 内开始再灌注。如何能够延长缺血耐受时间已经成为研究的焦点。改进保存液是减少缺血性损伤的新方法，以常温不停跳方法也正在进行试验。

心脏保存的早期实践中应用的是腹腔器官移植所使用的保存液，如 UW 液和 Erro-Collins 液，其电解质成分都与细胞内液相似，为低钠高钾型，另外，还加入一些非渗透性物质，以减轻细胞水肿。现已证实，对于心脏外科，用于心脏移植的器官保存液不仅要保护心肌细胞，还要保护血管内皮细胞。灌注液中的高钾状态可以损伤心脏血管内皮细胞，容易发生慢性移植物血管病变[84-87]。为了解决该问题，开发了新的器官保存液，HTK（Histidine-Tryptophan-Ketoglutarate）液和 Celsior 液，加入了能量物质，且为低钾型，更像是细胞外液。一些学者支持应用以血液为基础有心脏停搏作用的溶液，这需要从供者获取足够的血液，常使人难以接受。但是，文献报道，这种方案能够在器官保存过程中很好地保护血管内皮细胞，且不妨碍其他器官的获取[88]。一些比较性研究评估了各种保存液的优劣，表明能有效保护心肌的证据是非常重要的，还研究了一些新型的器官保存液添加成分，如帮助零下温度保存的抗冻蛋白[89]、加强保护血管内皮细胞的内皮素拮抗剂[90]、减轻缺血再灌注损伤的抗氧化剂[91]和最大程度使血管平滑肌舒张[92]、缺血心肌收缩及线粒体储存能量的试剂[93]。但是多数添加成分尚不能达到临床应用水平，但是改进器官保存液很有可能在某一天改善移植器官的功能或者延长缺血耐受时间。

常温下心脏灌注

应用持续性含氧灌注可能会改善心脏保存并提高心室功能[93]。其可以维持心脏不断进行有氧代谢，并清除缺血性代谢产物，如乳酸和腺苷酸[94]，从而很少产生自由基[95,96]。由于心肌细胞更耐受高温而不是低温，常温保存应该能防止温度造成的损伤[97]。结合了这两种策略的常温性机械灌注后心肌复苏和心肌功能要优于长达 4h 的静态冷保存[98]。应用常温不停跳灌注并运送供心是否可行在美国正进行Ⅱ期试验[99]。

小结

自临床心、肺移植开展以来，移植相关的临床和科研工作者一直试图在供体器官保存和运输过程中减少损伤和延长安全保存时间。伴随着世界范围内对终末期肺病的关注和肺移植的成熟，低温膨胀式和 Perfadex® 灌注式肺保存的改进已经达到顶峰。但心脏移植仍面临着很多限制。当今，肺保存的工作重心已经从减缓供肺死亡发展到促进供肺植入前复苏和修复，常温下 EVLP 供肺保存方法应运而生。EVLP 不仅在肺保存时十分有效，其在促进供肺复苏和修复方面也存在巨大潜力。器官移植过程中有效控制保存温度非常重要，如器官获取和植入时控制性降温，复苏和修复则在常温下进行(图 26.2)。体外进行供肺损伤的复苏和修复充满希望，是未来研究的重要方向。体外供体器官治疗措施可包含从药物治疗到基因及细胞治疗，将来有可能实现供体器官的个体化治疗。供肺损伤的个体化或靶向修复最终可能会使每一个潜在的供体都实现临床可用。

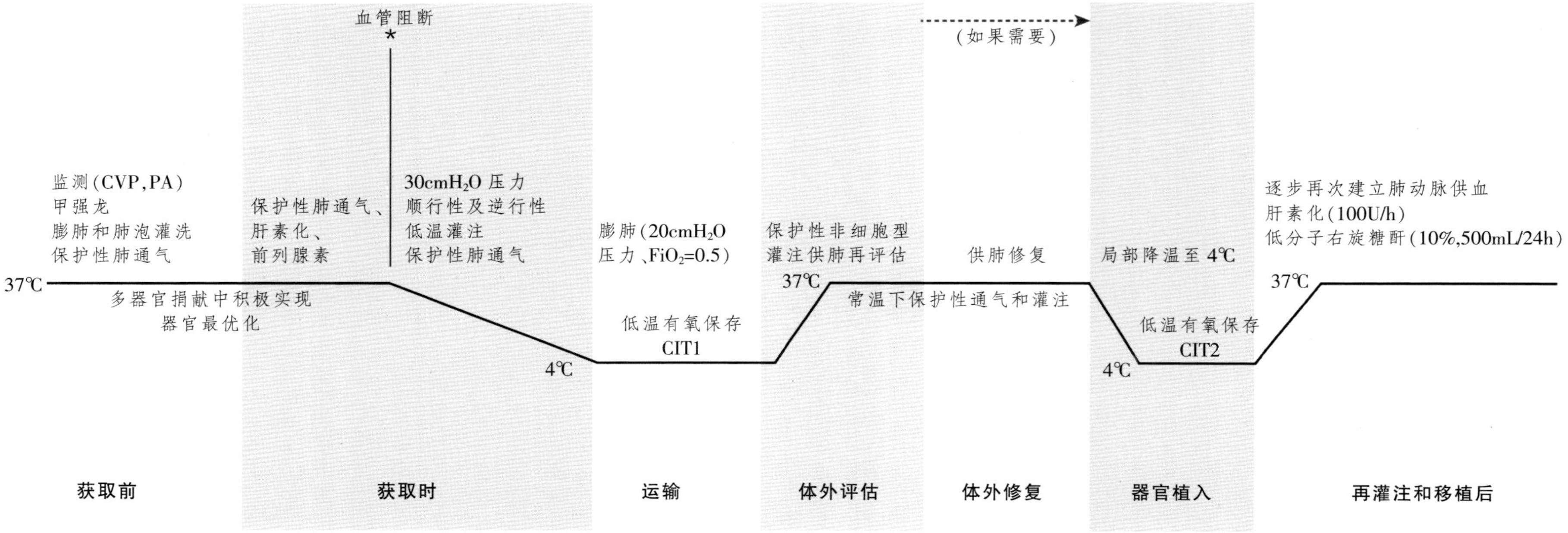

图 26.2 同期肺保存的轨道图。多器官捐献时,肺保存始于供者体内,经历低温有氧和常温有氧的体外保存期,结束于受者体内的再灌注;在每一步都有肺损伤的可能和进行预防及肺功能修复的机会;低温静态保存和常温积极治疗必须以温度变化为手段;必须监测 CVP、PA。

(张龙辉 译 张长坤 李照 校)

参考文献

1. Gabbay E, Williams TJ, Griffiths AP, et al. Maximizing the utilization of donor organs offered for lung transplantation. American Journal of Respiratory and Critical Care Medicine. 1999;160(1):265–271.
2. Angel LF, Levine DJ, Restrepo MI, et al. Impact of a lung transplantation donor-management protocol on lung donation and recipient outcomes. American Journal of Respiratory and Critical Care Medicine. 2006;174(6):710–716.
3. Venkateswaran RV, Patchell VB, Wilson IC, et al. Early donor management increases the retrieval rate of lungs for transplantation. Annals of Thoracic Surgery. 2008;85(1):278–286, discussion 86.
4. Novitzky D. Detrimental effects of brain death on the potential organ donor. Transplantation Proceedings. 1997;29(8):3770–3772.
5. Pennefather SH, Bullock RE, Dark JH. The effect of fluid therapy on alveolar arterial oxygen gradient in brain-dead organ donors. Transplantation. 1993; 56(6):1418–1422.
6. Shemie SD, Ross H, Pagliarello J, et al. Organ donor management in Canada: recommendations of the forum on medical management to optimize donor organ potential. CMAJ: Canadian Medical Association Journal. 2006;174(6):S13–S32.
7. Schnuelle P, Berger S, de Boer J, et al. Effects of catecholamine application to brain-dead donors on graft survival in solid organ transplantation. Transplantation. 2001;72(3):455–463.
8. Mukadam ME, Harrington DK, Wilson IC, et al. Does donor catecholamine administration affect early lung function after transplantation? Journal of Thoracic and Cardiovascular Surgery. 2005;130(3):926–927.
9. Rostron AJ, Avlonitis VS, Cork DM, et al. Hemodynamic resuscitation with arginine vasopressin reduces lung injury after brain death in the transplant donor. Transplantation. 2008;85(4):597–606.
10. Pennefather SH, Bullock RE, Mantle D, et al. Use of low dose arginine vasopressin to support brain-dead organ donors. Transplantation. 1995;59(1):58–62.
11. Debaveye YA, Van den Berghe GH. Is there still a place for dopamine in the modern intensive care unit? Anesthesia and Analgesia. 2004;98(2):461–468.
12. de Perrot M, Weder W, Patterson GA, et al. Strategies to increase limited donor resources. European Respiratory Journal. 2004;23(3):477–482.
13. The Acute Respiratory Distress Syndrome Network. Ventilation with lower tidal volumes as compared with traditional tidal volumes for acute lung injury and the acute respiratory distress syndrome. New England Journal of Medicine. 2000;342(18):1301–1308.
14. Mascia L, Pasero D, Slutsky AS, et al. Effect of a lung protective strategy for organ donors on eligibility and availability of lungs for transplantation: a randomized controlled trial. JAMA. 2010;304(23):2620–2627.
15. Follette DM, Rudich SM, Babcock WD. Improved oxygenation and increased lung donor recovery with high-dose steroid administration after brain death. Journal of Heart and Lung Transplantation. 1998;17(4):423–429.
16. Sakuma T, Folkesson HG, Suzuki S, et al. Beta-adrenergic agonist stimulated alveolar fluid clearance in ex vivo human and rat lungs. American Journal of Respiratory and Critical Care Medicine. 1997;155(2):506–512.
17. Ware LB, Koyama T, Billheimer D, et al. Advancing donor management research: design and implementation of a large, randomized, placebo-controlled trial. Annals of Intensive Care. 2011;1(1):20.
18. Ware LB, Landeck M, Koyama T, et al. A randomized trial of nebulized albuterol to enhance resolution of pulmonary edema in 506 brain dead organ donors. Journal of Heart and Lung Transplantation. 2012;31(4 Suppl):S116.
19. Straznicka M, Follette DM, Eisner MD, et al. Aggressive management of lung donors classified as unacceptable: excellent recipient survival one year after transplantation. Journal of Thoracic and Cardiovascular Surgery. 2002;124(2): 250–258.
20. Rosendale JD, Chabalewski FL, McBride MA, et al. Increased transplanted organs from the use of a standardized donor management protocol. American Journal of Transplantation. 2002;2(8):761–768.
21. Boasquevisque CH, Yildirim E, Waddel TK, et al. Surgical techniques: lung transplant and lung volume reduction. Proceedings of the American Thoracic Society. 2009;6(1):66–78.
22. de Perrot M, Fischer S, Liu M, et al. Prostaglandin E1 protects lung transplants from ischemia-reperfusion injury: a shift from pro- to anti-inflammatory cytokines. Transplantation. 2001;72(9):1505–1512.
23. Keshavjee SH, Yamazaki F, Cardoso PF, et al. A method for safe twelve-hour pulmonary preservation. Journal of Thoracic and Cardiovascular Surgery. 1989;98(4):529–534.
24. Keshavjee SH, Yamazaki F, Yokomise H, et al. The role of dextran 40 and potassium in extended hypothermic lung preservation for transplantation. Journal of Thoracic and Cardiovascular Surgery. 1992;103(2):314–325.
25. Struber M, Wilhelmi M, Harringer W, et al. Flush perfusion with low potassium dextran solution improves early graft function in clinical lung transplantation. European Journal of Cardio-Thoracic Surgery. 2001;19(2):190–194.
26. Muller C, Furst H, Reichenspurner H, et al. Lung procurement by low-potassium dextran and the effect on preservation injury. Munich Lung Transplant Group. Transplantation. 1999;68(8):1139–1143.
27. Oto T, Griffiths AP, Rosenfeldt F, et al. Early outcomes comparing Perfadex, euro-collins, and Papworth solutions in lung transplantation. Annals of Thoracic Surgery. 2006;82(5):1842–1848.
28. Rabanal JM, Ibanez AM, Mons R, et al. Influence of preservation solution on early lung function (Euro-Collins vs Perfadex). Transplantation Proceedings. 2003;35(5):1938–1939.
29. Ganesh JS, Rogers CA, Banner NR, et al. Does the method of lung preservation influence outcome after transplantation? An analysis of 681 consecutive procedures. Journal of Thoracic and Cardiovascular Surgery. 2007;134(5):1313–1321.
30. Varela A, Cordoba M, Serrano-Fiz S, et al. Early lung allograft function after retrograde and antegrade preservation. Journal of Thoracic and Cardiovascular Surgery. 1997;114(6):1119–1120.
31. Van De Wauwer C, Neyrinck AP, Geudens N, et al. Retrograde flush following warm ischemia in the non-heart-beating donor results in superior graft performance at reperfusion. Journal of Surgical Research. 2009;154(1):118–125.
32. Van Raemdonck DE, Jannis NC, Rega FR, et al. Extended preservation of ischemic pulmonary graft by postmortem alveolar expansion. Annals of Thoracic Surgery. 1997;64(3):801–808.
33. Kayano K, Toda K, Naka Y, et al. Identification of optimal conditions for lung graft storage with Euro-Collins solution by use of a rat orthotopic lung transplant model. Circulation. 1999;100(19 Suppl):II257–II261.
34. Wang LS, Nakamoto K, Hsieh CM, et al. Influence of temperature of flushing solution on lung preservation. Annals of Thoracic Surgery. 1993;55(3):711–715.
35. Lee JC, Christie JD. Primary graft dysfunction. Proceedings of the American Thoracic Society. 2009;6(1):39–46.
36. Date H, Matsumura A, Manchester JK, et al. Evaluation of lung metabolism during successful twenty-four-hour canine lung preservation. Journal of Thoracic and Cardiovascular Surgery. 1993;105(3):480–491.
37. Stammberger U, Schmid RA, Hillinger S, et al. Effect of a short period of warm ischemia after cold preservation on reperfusion injury in lung allotransplantation. European Journal of Cardio-Thoracic Surgery. 1998;13(4):442–447, discussion 7–8.
38. Pierre AF, DeCampos KN, Liu M, et al. Rapid reperfusion causes stress failure in ischemic rat lungs. Journal of Thoracic and Cardiovascular Surgery. 1998; 116(6):932–942.
39. Lick SD, Brown PS Jr, Kurusz M, et al. Technique of controlled reperfusion of the transplanted lung in humans. Annals of Thoracic Surgery. 2000;69(3):910–912.
40. Aigner C, Wisser W, Taghavi S, et al. Institutional experience with extracorporeal membrane oxygenation in lung transplantation. European Journal of Cardiothoracic Surgery 2007;31:468–474.
41. de Perrot M, Chaparro C, McRae K, et al. Twenty-year experience of lung transplantation at a single center: influence of recipient diagnosis on long-term survival. Journal of Thoracic and Cardiovascular Surgery. 2004;127(5):1493–1501.
42. Sekine Y, Fischer S, de Perrot M, et al. Bilateral lung transplantation using a donor with a tracheal right upper lobe bronchus. Annals of Thoracic Surgery. 2002;73(1):308–310.
43. Kootstra G, Daemen JH, Oomen AP. Categories of non-heart-beating donors. Transplantation Proceedings. 1995;27(5):2893–2894.
44. De Oliveira NC, Osaki S, Maloney JD, et al. Lung transplantation with donation after cardiac death donors: long-term follow-up in a single center. Journal of Thoracic and Cardiovascular Surgery. 2010;139(5):1306–1315.
45. Mason DP, Brown CR, Murthy SC, et al. Growing single-center experience with lung transplantation using donation after cardiac death. Annals of Thoracic Surgery. 2012;58(5):526–529.
46. Zych B, Popov AF, Amrani M, et al. Lungs from donation after circulatory death donors: an alternative source to brain-dead donors? Midterm results at a single institution. European Journal of Cardio-Thoracic Surgery. 2012;42(3): 542–549.
47. Cypel M, Sato M, Yildirim E, et al. Initial experience with lung donation after cardiocirculatory death in Canada. Journal of Heart and Lung Transplantation. 2009;28(8):753–758.
48. Van De Wauwer C, Verschuuren EA, van der Bij W, et al. The use of non-heart-beating lung donors category III can increase the donor pool. European Journal of Cardio-Thoracic Surgery. 2011;39(6):e175–e180, discussion e80.
49. Egan TM, Lambert CJ Jr, Reddick R, et al. A strategy to increase the donor pool: use of cadaver lungs for transplantation. Annals of Thoracic Surgery. 1991;52(5):1113–1120, discussion 20–21.
50. Van Raemdonck DE, Jannis NC, De Leyn PR, et al. Warm ischemic tolerance in collapsed pulmonary grafts is limited to 1 hour. Annals of Surgery. 1998; 228(6):788–796.
51. Miyoshi K, Oto T, Otani S, et al. Effect of donor pre-mortem hypoxia and hypotension on graft function and start of warm ischemia in donation after cardiac

death lung transplantation. Journal of Heart and Lung Transplantation. 2011; 30(4):445–451.
52. Steen S, Sjoberg T, Pierre L, et al. Transplantation of lungs from a non-heart-beating donor. Lancet. 2001;357(9259):825–829.
53. Van Raemdonck DE, Rega FR, Neyrinck AP, et al. Non-heart-beating donors. Seminars in Thoracic and Cardiovascular Surgery. 2004;16(4):309–321.
54. Rega FR, Jannis NC, Verleden GM, et al. Should we ventilate or cool the pulmonary graft inside the non-heart-beating donor? Journal of Heart and Lung Transplantation. 2003;22(11):1226–1233.
55. Rega FR, Neyrinck AP, Verleden GM, et al. How long can we preserve the pulmonary graft inside the nonheart-beating donor? Annals of Thoracic Surgery. 2004;77(2):438–444, discussion 44.
56. Steen S, Ingemansson R, Budrikis A, et al. Successful transplantation of lungs topically cooled in the non-heart-beating donor for 6 hours. Annals of Thoracic Surgery. 1997;63(2):345–351.
57. Okazaki M, Date H, Inokawa H, et al. Optimal time for post-mortem heparinization in canine lung transplantation with non-heart-beating donors. Journal of Heart and Lung Transplantation. 2006;25(4):454–460.
58. Iyer A, Harkess M, Havryk A, et al. Non heparinisation does not impair outcome of lung transplantation from maastricht category III donation after circulatory death (DCD) donors. Journal of Heart and Lung Transplantation. 2012;31(4 Suppl):S98.
59. Carrel A, Lindbergh CA. The culture of whole organs. Science. 1935; 81(2112):621–623.
60. Jirsch DW, Fisk RL. Couves cm. Ex vivo evaluation of stored lungs. Annals of Thoracic Surgery. 1970;10(2):163–168.
61. Steen S, Liao Q, Wierup PN, et al. Transplantation of lungs from non-heart-beating donors after functional assessment ex vivo. Annals of Thoracic Surgery. 2003;76(1):244–252, discussion 52.
62. Steen S, Ingemansson R, Eriksson L, et al. First human transplantation of a nonacceptable donor lung after reconditioning ex vivo. Annals of Thoracic Surgery. 2007;83(6):2191–2194.
63. Ingemansson R, Eyjolfsson A, Mared L, et al. Clinical transplantation of initially rejected donor lungs after reconditioning ex vivo. Annals of Thoracic Surgery. 2009;87(1):255–260.
64. Erasmus ME, Fernhout MH, Elstrodt JM, et al. Normothermic ex vivo lung perfusion of non-heart-beating donor lungs in pigs: from pretransplant function analysis towards a 6-h machine preservation. Transplant International. 2006; 19(7):589–593.
65. Cypel M, Yeung JC, Hirayama S, et al. Technique for prolonged normothermic ex vivo lung perfusion. Journal of Heart and Lung Transplantation. 2008; 27(12):1319–1325.
66. D'Armini AM, Roberts CS, Griffith PK, et al. When does the lung die? I. Histochemical evidence of pulmonary viability after "death". Journal of Heart and Lung Transplantation. 1994;13(5):741–747.
67. Alessandrini F, D'Armini AM, Roberts CS, et al. When does the lung die? II. Ultrastructural evidence of pulmonary viability after "death". Journal of Heart and Lung Transplantation. 1994;13(5):748–757.
68. Petak F, Habre W, Hantos Z, et al. Effects of pulmonary vascular pressures and flow on airway and parenchymal mechanics in isolated rat lungs. Journal of Applied Physiology. 2002;92:169–178.
69. Broccard AF, Vannay C, Feihl F, et al. Impact of low pulmonary vascular pressure on ventilator-induced lung injury. Critical Care Medicine. 2002;30(10): 2183–2190.
70. Cypel M, Rubacha M, Yeung J, et al. Normothermic ex vivo perfusion prevents lung injury compared to extended cold preservation for transplantation. American Journal of Transplantation. 2009;9(10):2262–2269.
71. Cypel M, Liu M, Rubacha M, et al. Functional repair of human donor lungs by IL-10 gene therapy. Science Translation Medicine. 2009;1(4):4ra9.
72. Yeung JC, Cypel M, Machuca TN, et al. Physiologic assessment of the ex vivo donor lung for transplantation. Journal of Heart and Lung Transplantation. 2012;31(10):1120–6. doi: 10.1016/j.healun.2012.08.016.
73. Cypel M, Yeung JC, Liu M, et al. Normothermic ex vivo lung perfusion in clinical lung transplantation. New England Journal of Medicine. 2011;364(15): 1431–1440.
74. Wallinder A, Ricksten SE, Hansson C, et al. Ex-vivo perfusion and transplantation of initially rejected donor lungs. Journal of Heart and Lung Transplantation. 2012;31(4 Suppl):S98.
75. Warnecke G, Haverich A, Massard G, et al. The inspire international lung trial with the Organ Care System Technology (OCS™). Journal of Heart and Lung Transplantation. 2012;31(4 Suppl):S115.
76. Souilamas R, Souilamas JI Jr, Saueressig M, et al. Advanced normothermic ex vivo lung maintenance using the mobile organ care system. Journal of Heart and Lung Transplantation. 2011;30(7):847–848.
77. Cypel M, Yeung J, Machuca T, et al. Experience with the first 50 ex vivo lung perfusions in clinical transplantation. Journal of Thoracic and Cardiovascular Surgery. 2012.
78. Frank JA, Briot R, Lee JW, et al. Physiological and biochemical markers of alveolar epithelial barrier dysfunction in perfused human lungs. American Journal of Physiology. Lung Cellular and Molecular Physiology. 2007;293(1): L52–L59.
79. Inci I, Ampollini L, Arni S, et al. Ex vivo reconditioning of marginal donor lungs injured by acid aspiration. Journal of Heart and Lung Transplantation. 2008;27(11):1229–1236.
80. Karamanou DM, Perry J, Walden HR, et al. The effect of ex-vivo perfusion on the microbiological profile of the donor lung. Journal of Heart and Lung Transplantation. 2010;29(2 Suppl):S94.
81. Bonato R, Machuca TN, Cypel M, et al. Ex vivo treatment of infection in human donor lungs. Journal of Heart and Lung Transplantation. 2012;31(4 Suppl): S97–S98.
82. Yeung JC, Wagnetz D, Cypel M, et al. Ex vivo adenoviral vector gene delivery results in decreased vector-associated inflammation pre- and post-lung transplantation in the pig. Molecular Therapy: Journal of the American Society of Gene Therapy. 2012;20(6):1204–1211.
83. Lee JW, Fang X, Gupta N, et al. Allogeneic human mesenchymal stem cells for treatment of E. coli endotoxin-induced acute lung injury in the ex vivo perfused human lung. Proceedings of the National Academy of Sciences of the United States of America. 2009;106(38):16357–16362.
84. Drinkwater DC, Rudis E, Laks H, et al. University of Wisconsin solution versus Stanford cardioplegic solution and the development of cardiac allograft vasculopathy. Journal of Heart and Lung Transplantation. 1995;14:891–896.
85. Mankad PS, Chester AH, Yacoub MH. Role of potassium concentration in cardioplegic solutions in mediating endothelial damage. Annals of Thoracic Surgery. 1991;51:89–93.
86. Sellke FW, Shafique T, Schoen FJ, et al. Impaired endothelium-dependent coronary microvascular relaxation after cold potassium cardioplegia and reperfusion. Journal of Thoracic and Cardiovascular Surgery. 1993;105:52–58.
87. Pearl JM, Laks H, Drinkwater DC, et al. Loss of endothelium-dependent vasodilatation and nitric oxide release after myocardial protection with University of Wisconsin solution. Journal of Thoracic and Cardiovascular Surgery. 1994; 107:257–264.
88. Luciani GB, Forni A, Rigatelli G, et al. Myocardial protection in heart transplantation using blood cardioplegia: 12-year outcome of a prospective randomized trial. Journal of Heart and Lung Transplantation. 2011;30:29–36.
89. Amir G, Rubinsky B, Horowitz L, et al. Prolonged 24-hour subzero preservation of heterotopically transplanted rat hearts using antifreeze proteins derived from arctic fish. Annals of Thoracic Surgery. 2004;77:1648–1655.
90. Fedak PW, Rao V, Verma S, et al. Combined endothelial and myocardial protection by endothelin antagonism enhances transplant allograft preservation. Journal of Thoracic and Cardiovascular Surgery. 2005;129:407–415.
91. Martin J, Lutter G, Sarai K, et al. Investigations on the new free radical scavenger polynitroxyl-albumin to prevent ischemia and reperfusion injury after orthotopic heart transplantation in the pig model. European Journal of Cardio-Thoracic Surgery. 2001;19:321–325.
92. Yang Q, Zhang RZ, Yim AP, et al. Effect of 11,12-epoxyeicosatrienoic acid as an additive to St. Thomas' cardioplegia and University of Wisconsin solutions on endothelium-derived hyperpolarizing factor-mediated function in coronary microarteries: influence of temperature and time. Annals of Thoracic Surgery. 2003;76:1623–1630.
93. Yang L, Yu T. Prolonged donor heart preservation with pinacidil: the role of mitochondria and the mitochondrial adenosine triphosphate-sensitive potassium channel. Journal of Thoracic and Cardiovascular Surgery. 2010;139: 1057–1063.
94. Rosenbaum DH, Peltz M, DiMaio JM, et al. Perfusion preservation versus static preservation for cardiac transplantation: effects on myocardial function and metabolism. Journal of Heart and Lung Transplantation. 2008;27: 93–99.
95. Abd-Elfattah AS, Jessen ME, Lekven J, et al. Differential cardioprotection with selective inhibitors of adenosine metabolism and transport: role of purine release in ischemic and reperfusion injury. Molecular and Cellular Biochemistry. 1998;180:179–191.
96. Abd-Elfattah AS, Jessen ME, Lekven J, et al. Myocardial reperfusion injury. Role of myocardial hypoxanthine and xanthine in free radical-mediated reperfusion injury. Circulation. 1988;78:III224–III235.
97. Hendry PJ, Walley VM, Koshal A, et al. Are temperatures attained by donor hearts during transport too cold? Journal of Thoracic and Cardiovascular Surgery. 1989;98:517–522.
98. Ozeki T, Kwon MH, Gu J, et al. Heart preservation using continuous ex vivo perfusion improves viability and functional recovery. Circulation Journal. 2007;71:153–159.
99. http://www.transmedics.com/wt/page/PROCEED_II.

第 27 章 肾脏配对捐献网络

Adam W. Bingaman, Cathi L. Murphey

引言

世界范围内肾移植等待者持续快速增长。在美国，过去的 10 年间，尸体器官捐献的效率没有明显增长，但是等待者数量却翻了一番[1]。美国每年大约有 4500 人死于等待肾移植的过程中。活体肾脏捐献移植为等待者提供了避免长期等待即可获得供肾的机会[2],因此这些年其优势越发明显。的确,对于一些接受移植疗效较好,却不能长期等待获取器官的老年患者,活体捐献移植是其唯一出路。相较于尸体器官捐献,活体器官捐献还有其他好处,不仅可以获得更好的免疫学配型,移植肾近期及远期功能更佳[2,3],还可以让移植手术成为择期手术,让患者为手术做最充分的准备,而且还能在透析开始之前优先选择移植。

很多患者接受活体肾脏捐献移植手术的巨大障碍是与供体之间的免疫学配型,配型实验包括 ABO 血型配型和人类白细胞抗原(HLA)配型。据评估,在肾移植等待者中,至少有 6000 人与健康的志愿捐献者配型失败[4]。1986 年,Rapaport 首次提出了肾脏配对捐献(KPD),其目的是为了让配型失败的活体器官捐献者重获成功的机会[5]。其定义是配型失败的两对供者和受者互换捐赠人来建立成功的配型，配型失败的两对之间互换供者并双双配型成功的概念如图 27.1a 所示[6]。图 27.1b 所示则为三组之间互换,虽然更复杂,却为配型成功提供了更大的可能性。最近,如图 27.1c 所示,由非定向捐献开启的链状移植，促成了一个个来自非定向捐献供体的大量移植，而非定向捐献实际上可以捐给任意受者。纵然 KPD 的概念增加了活体器官捐献移植的选择而备受好评,但是还需要克服来自伦理、法律、免疫学及运筹方面的重重阻碍。本章涵盖了这些问题,并描述了当代配对互换项目是如何取得成功的。本章和第 28、37 章组成了患者接受肾移植手术及肾移植等待者管理的总则。

哪些受者最易从 KPD 获益?

Segev 等报道了计算机预测供-受体配型失败队列中不同亚组患者在 KPD 项目中的匹配率。对于哪些患者能从 KPD 中获益、获益原因是什么,该数据是重要的预测根据。该研究发现群体反应性抗体(PRA)<80% 的受体等待者,与大部分血型的配型成功率约为 50%,与更大规模的配型失败队列相比,其获益仅有小幅度的提高。不出所料,中度敏感的非 O 型血受体或者 O 型血供体匹配成功的等待时间较短,而 AB 型血供者的配对鲜有成功。对于 PRA>80%的亚组,无论哪种血型,配型成功率都受到队列大小的显著影响。高度敏化的 AB 型血的受体等待者或 O 型血供体更易配型成功。

该模拟证明 KPD 中配型成功存在两个主要障碍。首先,在 KPD 项目中,血型比例失衡严重,O 型血的受者多,而非 O 型血的供者多,当然在大样本配型失败队列中,如果 O 型供者配对失败,通常情况下与受者高度敏化有关。其次,队列中高度敏化的受者需要去配对稀缺 HLA 配型的供体，例如,HLA 多位点纯合型供体和敏化的受者更易配型成功,但是这种类型的 HLA 是稀有的。

KPD 的匹配法则

匹配软件系统旨在预测配型成功率,可以是一组、双向或三方参与的配对。统计建模证明,与双向互换相比，三方互换更能充分利用 O 型血供体并帮助高敏受者[6]。四组或更大规模参与的闭环式互换会使运筹更加

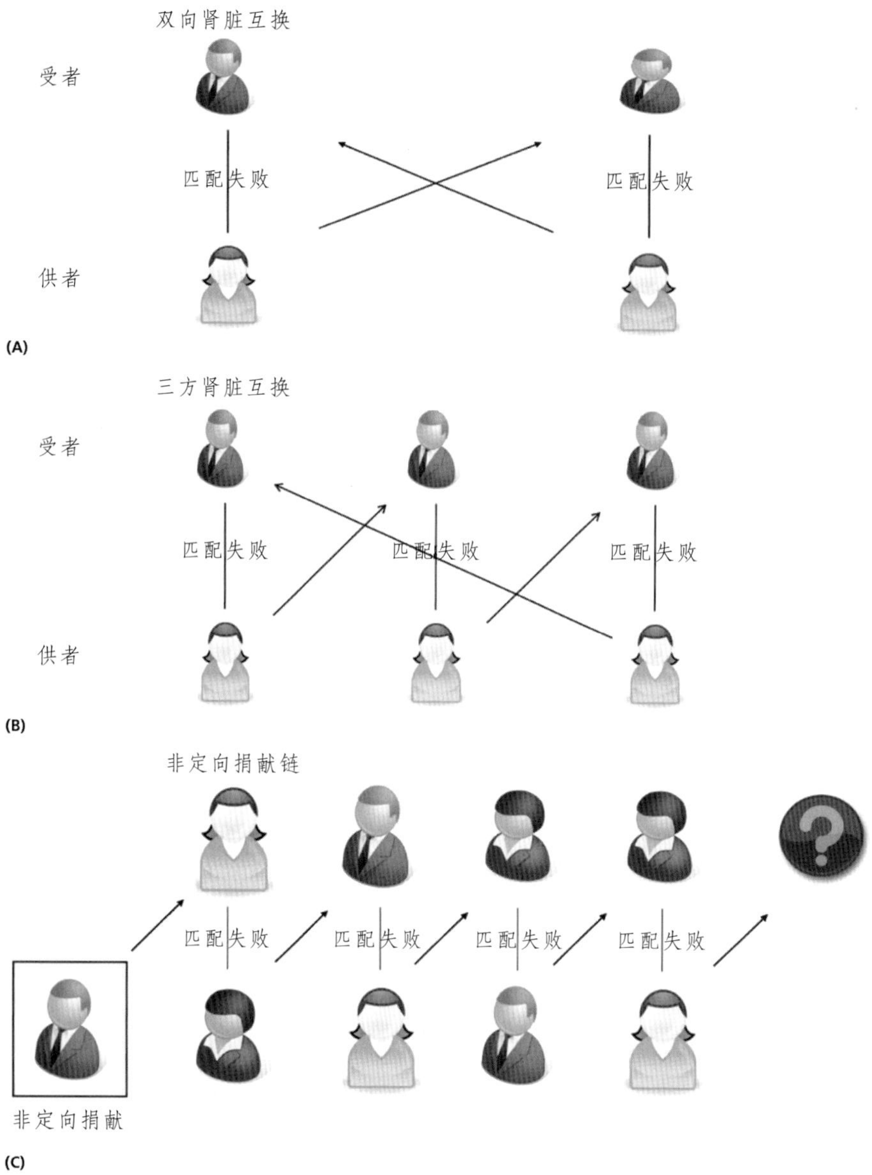

图 27.1 肾脏配对捐献移植的常见类型:(A)匹配失败的两组之间双向互换形成一个闭合环;(B)匹配失败的三组之间三方互换形成闭合环;(C)链式互换开始于非定向捐献,终止于捐给去世的供体等待者或者“桥式供者”开启另一个捐献连。

复杂,而获益甚少,因此不经常使用。采用非定向捐献(NDD)创立了一种非同时性、延展性、利他性的捐献链,可使大量患者受益。Rees 等于 2009 年 3 月首次对捐献链做了报道,其历时 8 个月,联合了 5 个州的 6 家移植中心,促成了 10 台移植手术[7]。随后出现了更大规模的捐献链,有跨地区的,也有单中心的报道,某中心的捐献连包含供者和受者各 23 例[8,9]。结束一个捐献连,有两种方式:①最后一位活体器官捐献者直接捐给去世的供体等待者;②运用“桥式捐献”开启了另外一个较晚的新捐献链。目前哪种方式的效能(移植数量)最高,还没有定论。Gentry 等的计算机模型指出,如果同时直接捐献给等待者,链长为 3 组时效能最高[10]。然而,Ashlagi 等应用无限链长的模型指出,虽然有浪费一个供体的风险,但“桥式捐献”有更高的效能[11,12]。显然,两种方法都需要更多的实践和数据,来证实哪种移植链终结途径能随着时间得推移产生最多的移植。

KPD 数据库、配型软件、固相抗体分析的应用

成功的 KPD 项目不仅需要大量的配型失败组,还需要精准的配型预测软件。所有的器官接受者和捐献

者都必须同意被纳入 KPD 数据库使数据库变得庞大。虽然不知道数据库促成配型成功效能最大化的临界值是多少,但是最少应不少于 100 组[13]。免疫学配型的早期教育和 KPD 项目中器官接受者和捐献者的选择性准入对 KPD 数据库的扩张是非常重要的两个方面,应鼓励纳入多对一的捐献以争取纳入更多的 O 型血和较好的 HLA 供者。很多 KPD 项目,尤其是跨地区或者国家项目,在捐献者纳入之前,全面评估必须进行,限制了那些没有足够时间和费用参加每次评估的捐献者。

纳入任何 KPD 项目,都需要录入一些基本信息,例如,接受者和捐献者的人口学信息,比如年龄、性别、血型和组织相容性信息。每组捐献者和接受者的 HLA 信息都必须被记录在案,并鉴定其不匹配性,这些数据将在更多 KPD 项目中应用。美国项目为零错配率做出了重要贡献。在大的 KPD 项目中,多数器官等待者都是敏化的,很难与捐献者匹配成功。因此,KPD 数据库中纳入的最具决定性的信息是依据敏感性 HLA 抗体鉴定实验被认为存在难结合抗原。这些实验是敏化的器官等待者配对成功的关键,对 KPD 项目的发展具有深远影响。因此,理解 KPD 之前,需要先了解 HLA 抗体鉴定实验(熟悉第 36 章和第 89 章)。

HLA 抗体鉴定的作用

免疫遗传学的高度发展,例如,基于 DNA 水平的 HLA 试验、固相抗体分析、流式细胞术交叉配型,使供受体匹配度的鉴定能力更加精确[14,15]。在美国,鉴定抗 HLA 抗体应用最广泛的技术是荧光磁珠被携带在个体 HLA 分子表面的固相分析。探测荧光即可作为探测抗体的标志。在供者确定之后,受者抗 HLA 抗体的鉴定被用在虚拟的交叉配型中去预测真实的交叉配型结果[16,17]。在 KPD 项目中,数据库中必须拥有所有敏化的器官等待者难结合抗原的抗体,配对程序才能排除有难结合抗原的供体。难结合抗原的准确匹配保证了交叉配型结果的准确性。相反,难结合抗原的过度匹配,尤其是对于高度敏化的等待者,会限制其移植的选择,可能失去一次成功配型的移植[18]。理想状态下,KPD 数据库中难结合抗原的匹配应该足够严格以筛除导致移植失败的阳性交叉配型,但是又不能严格到妨碍配对合适的移植[19,20]。实际上,抗 HLA 抗体鉴定的目的是促成更多成功的移植,而并非阻止可接受特殊抗体供者的等待者接受移植。该领域还有大量工作需要完成,其对 KPD 项目中高度敏化患者的移植将产生深远影响。此概念在美国称为"难结合抗原",而在欧洲移植协会使用的则是完全相反的系统,被称为"合适抗原"[21]。虽然在欧洲的方法不同,但是应用虚拟交叉配型来预测真实交叉配型的结果却是相同的。

全球 KPD 经验

KPD 影响着全球的活体器官捐献移植,世界范围内很多移植中心都采用这种策略来增加单中心、地区、甚至国家的移植量。

美国经验

在美国,尽管几十年前已经建立了活体器官移植的法律基础,1984 年国家器官移植法案的意向法律条款引起了大家对配对捐献的关注。规定"器官捐献中,任何人为了利益故意获取、接受或者转让任何人体器官都是违法的"[22](详见第 138 章活体器官捐献伦理学)。当然,不配对的供者把肾脏赠予不同的受者而从其他不匹配供者处获取匹配的肾脏,这样的肾脏交换方法同样是为了利益,是违法的。作为对器官移植团体和协会请求的回应,2007 年 10 月通过了 Charlie W. Norwood 活体器官捐献法案,并修订了国家器官移植法案,添加了"利益不包含人类器官配对捐献"的条例[23]。其他国家的 KPD 还面临着法律方面的阻碍,也限制了其在国际合作上的发展。

KPD 除了法律阻碍之外,还需要处理伦理问题。1997 年,来自芝加哥大学的 Ross 团队发出了关于 PKD 项目伦理学方面的讨论[24]。相继的,其他杂志也发表了配对捐献的伦理学基础[25,26]。生物医学伦理学有 4 条最高原则,活体器官捐献的理由是获益性、合法性、公平性、自愿性,通过配对捐献互换进行的非定向捐献没有违背或者改变这些原则[27]。然而对于强迫性的风险、隐匿性的维持的关注,使得配对捐献需要有深谋远虑,比如,配对失败可能使不情愿捐献感到恶意的欣慰,但是如果选择配对捐献,捐献过程中匹配失败将不再成为阻碍。因此,对纳入配对捐献的捐赠者采取额外的关照和举措来确保捐献是自愿的。当然,参与者有权在任何时候退出,因此,配对器官捐献移植手术需要有严谨的程序已确保器官接受者在移植开始之前其配对的捐献者不会捐出自己的器官。所以,在美国开展 KPD

的所有中心，同意和保障并重才能妥当处理这些特殊情况。

另外,在配对捐献过程中,如果涉及两对或更多,协议应保障每一对的隐私及各对之间的互不知情,需要涵盖临床查房、围术期全过程(术前、术中、术后监护)、家属等候室等方方面面。由于法律约束的存在、对生物医学伦理学指导原则的坚持和对这些特殊情况的关注,美国公众在很大程度上已经开始接受 KPD。

美国已经开展了单中心、多地区的 KPD 项目。2010 年,作为试点项目,启动了一个由各移植中心相互合作的国家项目[12,28,29]。美国自开展 KPD 以来,已经进行了 1000 多对 KPD 移植(图 27.2)[1,30,31]。Johns Hopkins 于 2000 年开展了首例单中心 KPD 移植，并于 2010 年 3 月报道了第 100 例。圣安东尼奥 Methodist 的 KPD 开始于 2008 年，到 2013 年 12 月，已经进行了 250 例[32]。这些单中心经验都是在 Inessa Kaplan 公司开发的电脑配对软件辅助下进行的。比较成功的跨地区项目有配对捐献联盟、新英格兰肾脏互换项目、配对捐献网、国家肾脏登记库[7,29,33,34]。每一个跨地区项目都有严格的共享准则、独特的匹配方法,其共享和成功的水平也存在差异。重要的是,KPD 移植受者的疗效和非 KPD 活体捐献具有可比性[35]。在美国,为了使 KPD 标准化并进行推广,2010 年美国器官分享网站开始在各移植中心逐步开展 KPD 的试点项目。

美国国家 KPD 项目操作指南在 2011 年进行了更新,陈述了器官分享细节[36]。在参与 KPD 项目之前,所有配对的参与者都要知情同意、接受全面评估并接受对移植和捐献审核。难结合抗原依据指南在当地中心使用固相单抗磁珠实验进行鉴别。配对算法采用基于要点加权系统的评分系统来排列匹配顺序（表 27.1）。所有的交叉配型实验都在受者所在当地移植中心进行，如果其反复确定交叉配型实验为阳性不能进行互换，移植中心需要转运其标本到参与项目的其他中心进行进一步分享。捐献的所有手术要同时进行,除非由于特殊原因需要改变顺序,在进行交换之前,各组供受者之间要保持距离,互不认识。多数情况下通过装运捐献的肾脏来避免转运供者或者使配对的供受者分开。

自 2011 年 12 月起,美国的 86 家移植中心参与了国家项目的器官分享,并完成了 10 例移植,而且随着近期加入的链状移植的加入，更多中心参与了器官分享,显著地扩展了这个项目。

韩国经验

世界上首例配对捐献移植是 1991 年韩国的两对 HLA 不匹配的器官接受者进行的双向交换。在韩国,死亡供体器官移植手术是被禁止的，但促进了活体捐献移植的发展。韩国接受不相关性活体捐献的标准要求 HLA-A/B 上的 4 个抗原中的 2 个相匹配或者至少 HLA-DR 上的一个抗原相匹配。韩国交换移植的原因包括血型不匹配、HLA 配型不符合标准或交叉配型不成功。交换移植的每对之间不需要保密。

韩国的一个移植中心报道了 1995 年至 2006 年间的 1090 例活体捐献肾移植,包括 692 例相关性活体捐献和 398 例不相关性活体捐献，不相关性活体捐献中有 129 例交换移植和 269 例非交换移植，接受交叉移植的患者中,84 例（65%）是因为血型不匹配,39 例(30%)不符合 HLA 配型标准,6 例(5%)则是交叉配型

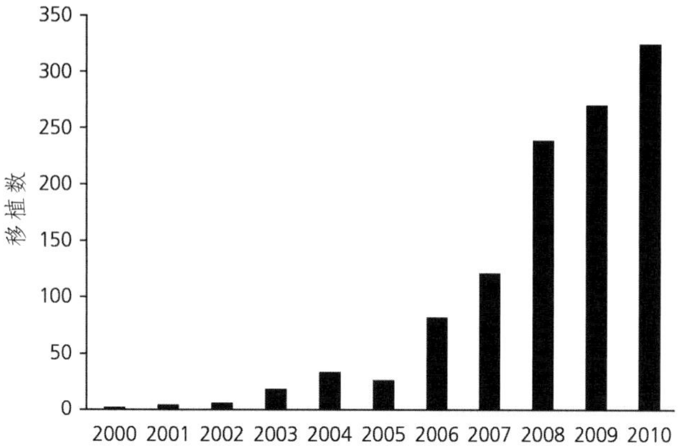

图 27.2 美国 2000—2010 年间肾脏配对移植的数量。

表 27.1 美国 KPD 项目评分表

配型特点	得分
等待者和潜在活体捐献者配型	200
等待者和潜在供体无抗原错配	200
等待者曾经捐献器官	150
PRA≥80%的高度敏化等待者	125
等待者≤18 岁	100
等待者和潜在供体在同一移植中心配型	75
等待者和潜在供体在同一器官分享区域	50
等待者和潜在供体在同一地区	25
等待者曾参加过配型但未进行移植	2
等待者存在单个或多个针对潜在供体的抗体	–5

PRA, 群体反应性抗体。

不成功。韩国没有报道交换或非交换移植中供体的敏化水平,但是有意思的是,交换移植组的二次移植的发生率显著低于非交换移植组。不相关性活体捐献中交换组和非交换组的移植成功率和患者生存资料之间没有差异。KPD 项目是活体捐献移植增加了 11.8%。韩国经验由大的单个移植中心而非国家项目提供,且由于近期更多非定向移植的应用,KPD 会持续增加。

罗马尼亚经验

罗马尼亚对死亡供体器官移植的限制也非常严格,因此对活体捐献器官移植有着强烈的推动作用。目前有两个肾移植项目,其中之一就是 2001 年开始的 KPD 项目。KPD 项目的纳入标准包括 ABO 血型不匹配、交叉配型失败、知情同意、亲属活体捐献。

2001 年 1 月至 2005 年 12 月,一共进行了 26 组配对捐献移植,包括 23 对双向互换、2 组三方互换和 1 组 4 对互换。双向或三方互换时,手术同时进行,而 4 对互换则是连续几天内完成。由于相互之间匿名是不必要也是不切实际的,术前他们已经相互熟识。无论 ABO 血型的比例、交叉配型不成功的移植,还是受体的敏化水平都没有相关报道。KPD 移受体的移植成功率为 98.2%,和定向活体器官捐献移植组的 97.7%相似,两组的急性排斥反应也没有明显的统计学差异。

罗纳尼亚经验来自其单个器官移植中心,因此,该中心的配对捐献水平是非常突出的。

荷兰经验

很明显,KPD 的成功和不匹配捐献的数量相关。基于此,2004 年,荷兰,一个 1600 万人口的国家,开展了一个非常成功的包含 7 个肾移植项目的国家项目,所有中心就一系列原则达成共识后,成立了荷兰移植基金,并运行了 KPD 分配系统。首先,所有的供者都要接受公共协议的评估,如果医学上具有可行性,每年每对可以被纳入系统 4 次。其次,计算机配对法则的运行要考虑一下情况:①成功配对量最大化;②血型配型完全相同;③高度敏化受者优先性;④短链优先性;⑤多中心分配。该项目认为,这种相对简单的算法没有考虑 HLA 配型、供者年龄、性别、器官大小等其他一些项目成功的重要因素。另外,患者配对的所有配型实验都是在国家 HLA 参考实验室进行,涉及交叉配型的标准性。最后,配对捐献手术同时进行,所有捐献者必须赶到受者所在的移植中心。配对法则最初只能进行双向互换,2005 年时加入了三方互换法则,长链互换法则则在 2007 年才开始使用。

2004 年 1 月到 2008 年 12 月间,登记了 312 对,其中 54%为 ABO 血型配型失败,另外 46%则是交叉配型不成功。对 169 对进行了鉴定,并成功开展了 131 组互换移植,是荷兰经验成为最成功的国家项目。

英国经验

英国在 2004 年建立了 KPD 项目的法律框架,由人体组织法案设立的人体组织局(HTA)规定所有的活体器官捐献移植。活体器官捐献经独立评估后推荐至 HTA 进行配对。至于 KPD,供体器官审批需要有三名 HTA 成员组成的专家组决定。KPD 的该批准方案较为恰当,英国器官移植也发展了配套的策略,其 23 家肾脏移植中心共同遵守。如果出现了 ABO 配型失败或交叉配型不成功,经过全面评估,审核批准后,则纳入 KPD 项目。鉴别潜在的双向或三方互换有成熟的运算法则,要依据以下 4 条标准进行匹配得分的计算:①供受者地理位置相近;②合适的抗体反应频率;③HLA-A、B 和 DR 配型失败;④双方供者年龄不同。每 3 个月进行一次配对,由参与的移植中心组织进行交叉配型实验。项目中各组配对者之间必须互不知情。要求同时进行供者手术并推荐装运供肾。最近,英国器官移植计划允许利他性的非定向捐献和链状捐献。

自 2007 年 4 月 KPD 项目在英国开始,到 2010 年 4 月,共进行了 64 组 KPD 移植,其效率略低于预期,但是随着应用非定向器官捐献的链状配对捐献的开展,将来的效率将明显提高。

澳大利亚经验

2007 年 10 月,位于西澳大利亚,佩斯的一个移植中心开始了 KPD 项目,其每年约进行 80 例活体捐献肾移植。项目开展后的 13 个月内,进行了 9 组 KPD 移植,包括 1 组双向互换,1 组三方互换,1 组非定向捐献者发起的双受者链,1 组非定向捐献发起的三受者链。5 位受者是敏化的,其中 3 位的 PRA 超过 70%。该 KPD 经验是西澳大利亚活体捐献器官移植增加了约 10%。西澳大利亚经验是其国家 KPD 项目(14 个器官移植中心开展活体捐献器官移植)的基础。为了保证匹配的公平性和各移植中心的平等性,国家器官匹配系统运用了基于荷兰分配法则的电脑软件。模仿西澳大利亚经验的国家经验估计可使活体器官捐献增加7%~10%,但是并没有相关数据的报道。

展望

应用匹配性配对

为了发展KPD,HLA配型失败的配对都建议纳入KPD项目。应用匹配性配对进行KPD移植被称为利他性非平衡配对肾脏互换(AUPKE)。Ratner等通过研究人们对于AUPKE的态度发现，很多配对者都倾向于这种方式,尤其是认为受者可能从中获益的情况下。如果匹配性捐献中供肾者较年轻,即存在可预测性的获益。有几个团队在KPD模拟系统中对匹配性捐献进行研究发现,获益显著。匹配性配对的加入增加了匹配非敏化受者的O型血供者,适度缓解了KPD项目中血型不平衡的问题。例如,一对非敏化的A型血受者及一个O型血供者可以和一对配对失败的O型血受者及年龄较小的A型血供者完成KPD移植(如图27.3a)。另外,稀有供体、受欢迎的HLA配型要应用于非常难配型的高度敏化的受者(如图27.3b)。将匹配性捐献纳入大型KPD项目计划使不匹配对的匹配成功率翻倍,这样对KPD项目的进一步发展会产生重大影响。伦理方面,由于KPD中匹配性配对的应用需要慎重考虑且可能限制其长远发展,需要进一步的讨论和研究。

KPD和脱敏结合

KPD和脱敏作为非匹配性配对移植中矛盾的双方,经常被关注,但是最近被关注确实因为其互补性。高度敏化的受者(PRA<90%)或者非O型血的中度敏化供者在KPD项目中配型成功都非常困难。理想状态下,这类受者适KPD和脱敏相结合。例如,对原始供体有高度活性抗体的受者可能和拥有低度活性抗体者互换供体以实现成功脱敏。该策略在加州大学洛杉矶分校约翰霍普金斯大学和圣安东尼奥的卫理公会医院被广泛应用,被认为是具有挑战性受者配对重要选择。该策略的结果未见报道,在推广之前,必须进行更加深入的研究。

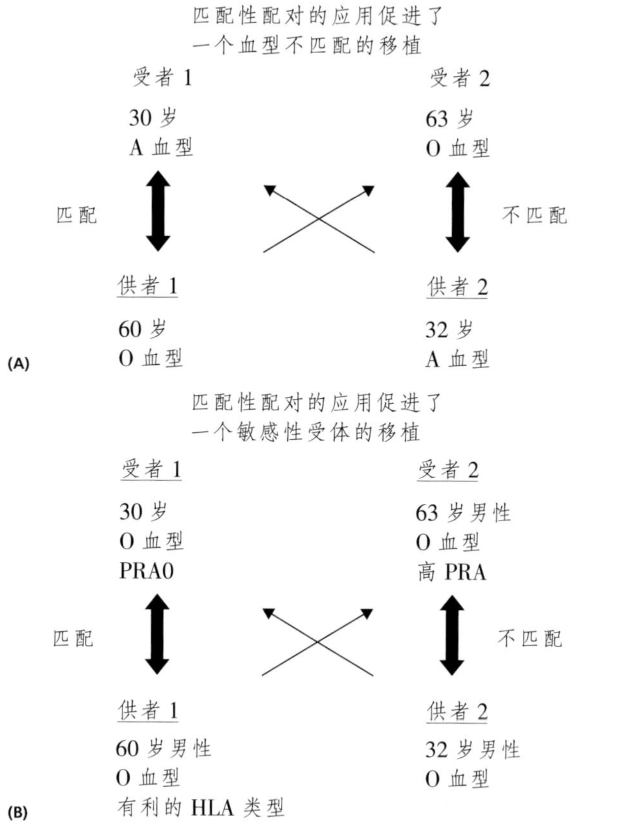

图27.3 匹配性配对的应用,以促进肾脏配对捐赠移植。(A)匹配性配对的应用促进血型不相容供受者的移植。(B)匹配性配对的应用促进敏感受体与交叉匹配不相容供体的移植。PRA,反应性抗体。

国际化

过去10年间,KPD项目的国家化使上千例患者在活体捐献肾移植中受益,否则需要等待多年进行尸体器官捐献肾移植。重要的是每例KPD移植的实施都是移植等待者名单中至少减少1人,是其他没有捐献者的等待者能够更快的接受移植。目前,已经跨越了很多伦理的、法律的、运筹上的障碍在欧洲、亚洲、澳大利亚、北美都建立了成功的KPD项目。多个研究报道认为长途装运活体捐献供肾和严重的功能延迟及不佳效果没有相关性。预计将来会出现国际间合作,建立更大范围的互助信息登记,使世界范围内的高度敏化患者受益。

小结

KPD被认为是死亡供肾捐献短缺潜在的解决办

法，也是延长死亡供体等待名单中患者等待时间的关键。无论如何，近来KPD项目的伦理学已经较健全，阻碍其广泛开展的运筹障碍也已经得到妥善处理。这些项目方兴未艾，估计在未来十年内，其应用的增加很可能为等待移植的敏化患者提供最好的选择。

（张龙辉 译 张长坤 李照 校）

参考文献

1. UNOS. Organ Procurement and Transplantation Network Data. Available from: http://www.unos.org.
2. Andreoni KA, Brayman KL, Guidinger MK, et al. Kidney and pancreas transplantation in the United States, 1996-2005. American Journal of Transplantation. 2007;7(5 Pt 2):1359-1375.
3. Kaneku HK, Terasaki PI. Thirty year trend in kidney transplants: UCLA and UNOS Renal Transplant Registry. Clinical Transplants. 2006:1-27.
4. Segev DL, Gentry SE, Warren DS, et al. Kidney paired donation and optimizing the use of live donor organs. JAMA. 2005;293(15):1883-1890.
5. Rapaport FT. The case for a living emotionally related international kidney donor exchange registry. Transplantation Proceedings. 1986;18(3 Suppl 2):5-9.
6. Saidman SL, Roth AE, Sonmez T, et al. Increasing the opportunity of live kidney donation by matching for two- and three-way exchanges. Transplantation. 2006; 81(5):773-782.
7. Rees MA, Kopke JE, Pelletier RP, et al. A nonsimultaneous, extended, altruistic-donor chain. New England Journal of Medicine. 2009;360(11):1096-1101.
8. Kidney transplant team continues to make history. 2012. Available from: http://www.texastransplantphysicians.com.
9. Bingaman A, Kapturczak M, Murphey C, et al. Kidney paired donation: a single center approach to increase living donor transplantation. Clinical Transplants. 2010:345-352.
10. Gentry SE, Montgomery RA, Swihart BJ, et al. The roles of dominos and nonsimultaneous chains in kidney paired donation. American Journal of Transplantation. 2009;9(6):1330-1336.
11. Ashlagi I, Gilchrist DS, Roth AE, et al. Nonsimultaneous chains and dominos in kidney- paired donation-revisited. American Journal of Transplantation. 2011; 11(5):984-994.
12. Gentry SE, Segev DL, Montgomery RA. Working together toward a national kidney paired donation program. American Journal of Transplantation. 2008; 8(2):464.
13. Bingaman AW, Wright FH, Murphey CL. Kidney paired donation in live-donor kidney transplantation. New England Journal of Medicine. 2010;363(11): 1091-1092.
14. Murphey CL, Forsthuber TG. Trends in HLA antibody screening and identification and their role in transplantation. Expert Review of Clinical Immunology. 2008;4(3):391-399.
15. Eckels DD. Solid phase testing in the HLA laboratory: implications for organ allocation. International Journal of Immunogenetics. 2008;35(4-5):265-274.
16. Bray RA, Nolen JD, Larsen C, et al. Transplanting the highly sensitized patient: the Emory algorithm. American Journal of Transplantation. 2006;6(10): 2307-2315.
17. Bingaman AW, Murphey CL, Palma-Vargas J, et al. A virtual crossmatch protocol significantly increases access of highly sensitized patients to deceased donor kidney transplantation. Transplantation. 2008;86(12):1864-1868.
18. Claas FH. HLA antibody testing: a tool to facilitate not to prevent organ transplantation. International Journal of Immunogenetics. 2008;35(4-5):275-277.
19. Ferrari P, Fidler S, Wright J, et al. Virtual crossmatch approach to maximize matching in paired kidney donation. American Journal of Transplantation. 2011;11(2):272-278.
20. Bingaman AW, Bray RA, Gebel HM, et al. Paired kidney donation: a (virtual) balancing act. American Journal of Transplantation. 2011;11(2):194-195.
21. Mayer G, Persijn GG. Eurotransplant kidney allocation system (ETKAS): rationale and implementation. Nephrology, Dialysis, Transplantation. 2006;21(1):2-3.
22. National Organ Transplant Act: Public Law 98-507. United States Statutes at Large. 1984;98:2339-2348.
23. Public law 110-144—DEC. 21, 2007 121 STAT. 1813. 2007. Available from: http://www.gpo.gov/fdsys/pkg/PLAW-110publ144/html/PLAW-110publ144.htm.
24. Ross LF, Rubin DT, Siegler M, et al. Ethics of a paired-kidney-exchange program. New England Journal of Medicine. 1997;336(24):1752-1755.
25. Woodle ES, Daller JA, Aeder M, et al. Ethical considerations for participation of nondirected living donors in kidney exchange programs. American Journal of Transplantation. 2010;10(6):1460-1467.
26. Patel SR, Chadha P, Papalois V. Expanding the live kidney donor pool: ethical considerations regarding altruistic donors, paired and pooled programs. Experimental and Clinical Transplantation. 2011;9(3):181-186.
27. Ghods AJ. Ethical issues and living unrelated donor kidney transplantation. Iranian Journal of Kidney Diseases. 2009;3(4):183-191.
28. Blumberg JM, Gritsch H, Veale JL. Kidney paired donation: advancements and future directions. Current Opinion in Organ Transplant. 2011;16(4):380-384.
29. Veale J, Hil G. The National Kidney Registry: transplant chains-beyond paired kidney donation. Clinical Transplants. 2009:253-264.
30. Wallis CB, Samy KP, Roth AE, et al. Kidney paired donation. Nephrology, Dialysis, Transplantation.2011;26(7):2091-2099.
31. Segev DL, Kucirka LM, Gentry SE, et al. Utilization and outcomes of kidney paired donation in the United States. Transplantation. 2008;86(4):502-510.
32. Kaplan I, Houp JA, Montgomery RA, et al. A computer match program for paired and unconventional kidney exchanges. American Journal of Transplantation. 2005;5(9):2306-2308.
33. Hanto RL, Reitsma W, Delmonico FL. The development of a successful multiregional kidney paired donation program. Transplantation. 2008;86(12): 1744-1748.
34. Veale J, Hill G. National Kidney Registry: 213 transplants in three years. Clinical Transplants 2010:333-344.
35. Montgomery RA, Zachary AA, Ratner LE, et al. Clinical results from transplanting incompatible live kidney donor/recipient pairs using kidney paired donation. JAMA. 2005;294(13):1655-1663.
36. OPTN Kidney Paired Donation Pilot Program: A transplant option for patients with an incompatible living donor.From UNOS. 2011. Available from: http://optn.transplant.hrsa.gov/resources/KPDPP.asp.
37. Kwak JY, Kwon OJ, Lee KS, et al. Exchange-donor program in renal transplantation: a single-center experience. Transplantation Proceedings. 1999;31(1-2): 344-345.
38. Park K, Moon JI, Kim SI, et al. Exchange-donor program in kidney transplantation. Transplantation Proceedings. 1999;31(1-2):356-357.
39. Huh KH, Kim MS, Ju MK, et al. Exchange living-donor kidney transplantation: merits and limitations. Transplantation. 2008;86(3):430-435.
40. Lee YJ, Lee SU, Chung SY, et al. Clinical outcomes of multicenter domino kidney paired donation. American Journal of Transplantation. 2009;9(10):2424-2428.
41. Huh KH, Kim HJ, Jeon KO, et al. Exchange-donor renal transplantation. Clinical Transplants. 2009:231-234.
42. Lucan M. Five years of single-center experience with paired kidney exchange transplantation. Transplantation Proceedings. 2007;39(5):1371-1375.
43. de Klerk M, Haase-Kromwijk BJ, Claas FH, et al. Living donor kidney exchange for both ABO-incompatible and crossmatch positive donor-recipient combinations. Transplantation Proceedings. 2006;38(9):2793-2795.
44. de Klerk M, Haase-Kromwijk BJ, Witvliet M, et al. [Favourable results of the first 2 years of the Dutch paired, living donor, kidney exchange programme]. Nederlands Tijdschrift Voor Geneeskunde. 2007;151(2):130-133.
45. de Klerk M, Keizer KM, Claas FH, et al. The Dutch national living donor kidney exchange program. American Journal of Transplantation. 2005;5(9): 2302-2305.
46. de Klerk M, Witvliet MD, Haase-Kromwijk BJ, et al. Hurdles, barriers, and successes of a national living donor kidney exchange program. Transplantation. 2008;86(12):1749-1753.
47. de Klerk M, Witvliet MD, Haase-Kromwijk BJ, et al. A highly efficient living donor kidney exchange program for both blood type and crossmatch incompatible donor-recipient combinations. Transplantation. 2006;82(12):1616-1620.
48. de Klerk M, Witvliet MD, Haase-Kromwijk BJ, et al. A flexible national living donor kidney exchange program taking advantage of a central histocompatibility laboratory: the Dutch model. Clinical Transplants. 2008:69-73.
49. Ferrari P, Woodroffe C, Christiansen FT. Paired kidney donations to expand the living donor pool: the Western Australian experience. Medical Journal of Australia. 2009;190(12):700-703.
50. Johnson RJ, Allen JE, Fuggle SV, et al. Early experience of paired living kidney donation in the United kingdom. Transplantation. 2008;86(12):1672-1677.
51. Ferrari P, de Klerk M. Paired kidney donations to expand the living donor pool. Journal of Nephrology. 2009;22(6):699-707.
52. Ross LF, Woodle ES. Ethical issues in increasing living kidney donations by expanding kidney paired exchange programs. Transplantation. 2000;69(8): 1539-1543.
53. Ratner LE, Rana A, Ratner ER, et al. The altruistic unbalanced paired kidney exchange: proof of concept and survey of potential donor and recipient attitudes. Transplantation. 2010;89(1):15-22.
54. Ratner LE, Ratner ER, Kelly J, et al. Altruistic unbalanced paired kidney exchange

at Columbia University/New York-Presbyterian hospital: rationale and practical considerations. Clinical Transplants. 2008:107-112.
55. Gentry SE, Segev DL, Simmerling M, et al. Expanding kidney paired donation through participation by compatible pairs. American Journal of Transplantation. 2007;7(10):2361-2370.
56. Roth AE, Sonmez T, Unver MU. Kidney paired donation with compatible pairs. American Journal of Transplantation. 2008;8(2):463.
57. Warren DS, Montgomery RA. Incompatible kidney transplantation: lessons from a decade of desensitization and paired kidney exchange. Immunologic Research. 2010;47(1-3):257-264.
58. Montgomery RA. Renal transplantation across HLA and ABO antibody barriers: integrating paired donation into desensitization protocols. American Journal of Transplantation. 2010;10(3):449-457.
59. Segev DL, Veale JL, Berger JC, et al. Transporting live donor kidneys for kidney paired donation: initial national results. American Journal of Transplantation. 2011;11(2):356-360.
60. Waki K, Terasaki PI. Paired kidney donation by shipment of living donor kidneys. Clinical Transplantation. 2007;21(2):186-191.
61. Connolly JS, Terasaki PI, Veale JL. Kidney paired donation-the next step. New England Journal of Medicine. 2011;365(9):868-869.

第 4 篇

移植患者的术前管理

第 28 章 肾移植的患者选择和适应证

Jeremy Goodman, Robert S. Gaston

引言

虽然实质脏器移植起源于同基因及同种异体肾移植,但现代肾移植的发展依然迅速,原因如下:第一,肾脏是成对器官,首例肾移植来源于活体供者,在随后的50年内,活体供者仍然为最主要的器官来源。第二,现在对于不可逆的肾衰竭有维持透析等治疗方法(在发达国家,维持透析应用广泛且效果良好)。一些其他器官移植的急性并发症并不常见于肾移植。虽然实质脏器移植的供体供不应求,但是长期透析的广泛使用使得患者不急于行移植手术。因此,肾脏替代治疗这章需要讨论肾移植的适应证、禁忌证和患者选择,这与其他器官移植有显著区别。本章将会总结肾移植的常见适应证。第37章将详细讨论移植患者等待名单的管理,并对本章内容进行补充说明。

表 28.1 美国的慢性肾病

(a)根据肾小球滤过率的 CKD 分期[1,96]

分期	描述	eGFR[mL/(min·1.73m²)]	普遍度(% US,成人,大于20岁)
1	有肾脏损伤的证据,但GFR正常(蛋白尿,血尿)	>90	5.7
2	轻度	60~89	5.4
3	中度	30~59	5.4
4	重度	15~29	0.4
5	肾衰竭(终末期肾病)	<15	

(b)终末期肾病的常见病因,2009年的不同病因的发病比例[2]

终末期肾病病因	不同病因的发病比例(%)
糖尿病肾病	44
高血压	28
肾小球肾炎	7
囊性肾病	2
其他原因	19

肾移植作为肾替代治疗的一种方法

晚期肾病是慢性肾病的终末表现(表28.1)[1]。随着年龄增长,慢性肾病的风险显著增加,大多数患者因为并发症而死亡,不能进展到第三期。基本上,在美国,每年大约有120 000例晚期肾病[2]。之前,几乎所有的患者均有致命性结局,直到1960年开始有了肾透析和肾移植。最初,透析是唯一的姑息疗法,予急性肾衰竭患者支持治疗直到康复或者不可逆疾病的移植治疗中的过度治疗。然而,因为不佳的移植效果和有限的肾移植供体,在1970年代,肾透析成为更普遍的治疗[3]。在1972年,美国社会保障机构将这个治疗措施列入治疗标准,联邦法律制定了晚期肾病的治疗方案,直到今天,仍然是美国唯一的关于器官的法律[4]。考虑到治疗有利于提高生活质量,移植治疗的供者有一定的适应证(年轻人和健康人是最好的候选者)和严格的患者筛选标准,通过这些筛选可以最大限度地获利并降低免疫反应的危害。在许多多学科选拔委员会选择通过透析治疗,移植治疗或者都不通过[5]。选拔的标准不仅包括健康状况,还有年龄、康复的概率,还有个人的社会价值[6]。在20世纪80年代,因为选拔的过程困难重重,这导致了这些委员会的废止,但是进行多学科评估“能否移植”在许多移植中心仍继续存在[7]。

在1980年到1990年,一些主要的研究改变了移植治疗的患者筛选标准。在1983年,环孢素的使用使得现代的有效免疫抑制能预防免疫排斥,皮质类固醇的用药剂量显著减少,控制并发症的发生,所有病例的疗效提高,特别是那些接受死亡供体的肾移植患者[8]。对移植供者和接受者来说,HLA 匹配要求更低意味着移植治疗能适用于更广泛的患者人群[9]。提前进行抗菌疗法,特别是抗真菌和抗病毒治疗,能使那些强壮或者不那么强壮的患者在早期不发生感染,使治疗更有效[10]。无独有偶,一个新兴的适用于晚期医疗保障治疗数据库的数据模型能够提供不同肾脏替代治疗的疗效[11]。不考虑年龄、种族,或者原有疾病,更不用说尝试与定义一个人的社会价值是无用的,肾脏移植比其他的替代治疗提供了更多的利处:存活时间比透析增加一倍。在一项关于分配死亡供体的研究中,移植后存活时间的概念被提出(LYFT)。LYFT 的概念是根据 USRDS 数据库提出的,统计透析患者的寿命,统计进行肾移植的类似患者的寿命,用后者减去前者[12]。无论年龄、性别、种族、原发肾脏疾病、血糖状态、地区和保险种类,接受死亡供体肾移植的患者(可能比活体移植更有优势),大幅度提升了终末期肾病患者的寿命。顺利的肾移植可能在余生中节省 330 000 美元(根据 2011 年的美元汇率,其中包括了质量调整寿命年)[13]。由于肾移植减少花费并且提高生活质量,需对每一名终末期肾病的患者进行肾移植评估。最近的研究表明,政策在不同的医疗中心中差异较大[14]。

目前,终末期肾病肾移植的指征比较宽泛,患者选择的重点主要在明确有无禁忌证。对于慢性肾病(CKD)患者的移植评估主要由移植中心的肾脏病专家进行。理想状态下,评估的同时应该进行透析治疗。CKD4 患者(肾小球滤过率为 20~29mL/min)可选择肾移植为首选治疗方案[15]。

移植指南可为每一例患者提供最佳方案。部分患者可以完成相关伦理审核,以亲属肾脏作为供体(等待的患者共有 100 000 人/年,只有大概 10 000 肾脏/年)[16]。然而,即便是有了供者,20%的患者可能从移植中获益。那些有望通过移植显著延长寿命的患者,却只能长时间行透析治疗,等待名单上的患者可能是供体的 10 倍[17]。解决方案主要是获得更多的肾源。

选择供体

如上所述,肾移植,或者在某种程度上说所有实体器官的移植,都归功于活体供者。首次成功的移植是在一对双胞胎之间实施的,因此彼此间没有太大的组织相容性差异[18]。随后,由于能够有效地抑制免疫排斥反应,大部分成功的同种异体移植都来自活体供者[19]。目前,从活体供者上得到肾脏器官的益处包括肾功能更好以及长期的器官生存率(目前 61%,10 年前 45%)[16]。另外,活体器官移植可以自行选择手术时间和有效地减少其他风险,如围术期心血管事件、移植物功能恢复延迟和急性免疫排斥反应。全国平均等待一个死亡供者器官的时间超过 3 年(在部分地区甚至更久),因此,活体供者最大的优势就是避免长时间地等待来源供体,以及等待过程伴随而来的透析的各种并发症。对于大部分受体患者来讲,活体器官移植能够提供及时的医疗干预和最大可能的成功,也同时使得供者在很多情况下能有选择的自主权。

肾移植最佳的时机

尽管仍存在争议,但目前比较公认的观点是延长透析的时间会增加同种异体之间肾脏移植失败的风险[20,21]。Meier-Kriesche 等 2002 年的研究指出,不管是接受活体供者还是死亡供者的肾脏,透析对受体而言是一种重要的有影响性的风险,透析治疗时间长达 6 个月会降低移植物的长期生存率[22]。随后的研究结果显示,首先是患者生存率的减少,而不是免疫性的移植失败、年龄或是种族差异[23]。Schold 等最近的研究指出,透析时间的影响可以分解成考虑移植前和等待移植的时间[24]。按这样来区分,对结果的影响就归功于从开始透析到申请移植的时间,而开始申请移植到进行移植的时间对结果没有影响。对于研究的数据,研究者解释为透析并发症和受体的社会经济地位是延迟考虑移植和增加死亡风险的主要原因。

移植最佳的时机是在透析开始之前,这样可以避免透析带来的并发症、维持较好的器官功能状态及改善移植的结局[15]。但是,由于等待移植的患者数量庞大,类似预购买这样的形式最大的障碍就是可用的活体供者的数量,而事实上对于终末期肾病患者而言,在透析之前能成功移植的也就只有 2%[16]。普遍的现象是购买第三方和移植中心会要求进行活体器官移植的受体肾功能至少是在慢性肾病分期的第 4 期(eGFR≤20mL/min);目前美国纽约器官分享(UNOS)指南要求 eGFR≤20mL/min 来增加器官分配得分[25]。但是,并没有指征证明移植前 eGFR 会对移植后移植物的功能或生存率有任何影响；预购买的益处是可以完全避免透析和透析的并发症[26]。因此，移植的最佳时机是等候移植的受体 eGFR≤20mL/min、没有或仅有轻微尿毒症表现及在慢性透析开始之前。值得注意的是，要实现这样的目标就需要申请移植的时间足够早（eGFR 20~29mL/min），这样才能确保移植的时机最佳[27]。

移植的评估

移植的评估包括：

- 教育部分：未来移植受体学习包括移植风险、获益、提高成功移植的策略方法、寻找适合的潜在活体供者的方法。
- 医学检测：确定是否有需要治疗或延迟移植的并发症（表 28.2），同时提供适当的患者咨询的风险分层。
- 心理评估：以评估潜在的候选人和他/她的支持人理解和遵循治疗的能力（表 28.3）。
- 金融咨询：以确保获得足以维持成功移植的资源（包括医疗保险、医疗补助、私人保险、个人财务）[28]。

表 28.2　肾脏移植的术前评估

1.主诉和体格检查
2.诊断评估
(1)超声心动图
(2)胸部影像学
(3)结肠镜(年龄>50 岁)
(4)泌尿系超声
(5)女性:子宫涂片+乳房 X 线片
(6)心脏评估:见内文
(7)泌尿系评估(膀胱功能失调及反复泌尿系感染)
(8)血管评估:盆腔 CT 平扫(年龄>50 岁或透析时间>5 年)
3.实验室检查
(1)常规:常规细胞计数和血小板计数、代谢测定、凝血酶原时间、部分活化凝血酶原时间
(2)尿常规、尿培养
(3) 血清学检查:HIV、HBV (表面抗体和核心抗体)、HCV、CMV、CBV、水痘、快速血清反应素试验
(4)前列腺特异性抗原:男性>50 岁
(5)免疫学检测:ABO 血型、HLA 抗原决定簇、抗 HLA 抗体、供体的交叉配型

Adapted from Pham et al.[28] with permission from John Wiley & Sons.

表 28.3　肾移植患者的生理及经济评估

1.个人评估
(1)体力
(2)智力
(3)性能力
(4)应变能力
(5)物质依赖
(6)医学依从性
2.疾病评估
(1)ESRD 的影响和生理状态
(2)患者对移植选择及移植步骤的理解
3.教育:最高教育水平
4.工作:工作的时间及稳定程度
5.财产:在移植前和移植后的收入来源及其他资源的丰富度(保险)
6.支持机制:家庭和社会
7.环境:家庭、交通、旅行的需要

Adapted from Pham et al. [28] with permission from John Wiley & Sons.

在大多数医疗中心，转诊结果根据患者的病史分流；明显的禁忌证会排除进一步的测试。后续的评估过程通常涉及多学科团队之间合作，包括协调员、肾病专家、手术医生、心理健康专业专家，社会工作者和财务顾问。医学检查通常是简单的，包括对测试结果的解释，对于阳性的测试结果（表 28.2）往往需要再行额外的检查项目。

作为常见的慢性病，成功的移植往往伴随着显著的心理和社会经济问题。在早期，精神问题被认为是肾移植的禁忌证。现在，精神疾病，如果得到适当的治疗，很少会阻碍移植的进行[29]。相反，大多数移植中心会要求精神障碍得到充分的治疗，并在开始移植前得到一个较好的治疗结果[30]。一个潜在的移植候选人的初步评估必须包括认知功能水平[29]。知情同意包括对与透析相关的移植风险和受益的理解。移植后，要有足够的认知能力，充分理解和遵循复杂的免疫抑制方案。有时，终末期肾病和一些严重的营养性疾病一样（如贫血、维生素缺乏等）可以损害认知，需要及时诊断和治疗。对于一些终末期肾病患者，认知功能障碍甚至可能会改善移植后尿毒症状态，因为这部分患者往往有明确的解决方案。有些情况下，即使是严重的患者，不可逆的认知功能障碍也可能会从移植中受益，因为认知障碍给他们带来更用心的照料人[31,32]。

一些非医疗因素（如社会经济地位、种族、教育成就、离移植中心的距离)对移植的实行以及随后患者的结果都有影响[33-35]。在美国,因其复杂和混乱的医疗融资体系,社会经济评估是大多数移植前的重要评估内容[36]。通常情况下,这项任务是由熟悉移植后各种要求的社会工作者执行,他们能够提供关于每个候选人的差异和移植后能带来的资源的咨询。后者包括保险覆盖面,去到和离开移植中心的能力,目前的就业,以及未来就业前景。对于终末期肾病患者,移植改变了他们获得社会经济资源的能力,并且使他们远离了慢性透析的过程。移植后的保险条款经常发生变化,患者可能会失去伤残津贴。移植前的社会经济评估简化了移植后事件的应对。

大多数终末期肾病患者在等待移植过程是由肾脏病学专家而非移植中心负责治疗[27,37]。随着等待移植时间的延长,新的医疗和心理-社会的挑战可能会出现[38]。确保出现的问题及时解决是医生的责任,而发生的任何改变移植中心需要被告知。同样,候选人和移植中心之间的接触日益规范,许多移植中心会每年对候选人重新作出评估。在医学中的地位、认知功能、保险覆盖或社会支持系统在决定是否进行器官移植时是至关重要的。

肾移植的禁忌证

任何关于肾移植禁忌证的讨论必须从两个方面来考虑。第一,禁忌证随时间改变,不管是由于护理标准的改变还是具体减轻其潜在风险的方法的改变[39]。在20世纪70年代,禁忌证包括糖尿病、年龄>55岁、胃肠道出血史等。前两者由于移植手术实践增多,第三个因素由于有效的药物治疗(H受体阻滞剂等)而不再成为禁忌。其次,不同的移植中心关于不同禁忌如何解释和如何对待看法不一,总的来说有限的预期移植后生存时间会阻碍移植;然而,因为基本上所有的情况与透析相比都会延长寿命,如果缺少一个特定的禁忌证,要以此来阻碍移植是一件比较困难的事情[40]。因此,大部分中心会评估医疗,心理和社会经济等来寻找是否有禁忌证;如果没有发现,被评估患者会被认为是可以接受的候选人[28]。

2014年的绝对禁忌证列表相对较短(表28.4),尤其是与前几十年相比。这些条件通常会对同种异体肾移植造成重要阻碍:一个开放的、膈下的血管手术和长期免疫抑制剂的使用。手术本身需要合适的血管解剖和足够的尿液流出。虽然后者很少是一个问题(手术重建的尿路,如有必要,也能够提供足够的尿液流出),而前者往往带来问题。标准手术入路涉及髂循环,CKD和透析时间的延长会造成转移性钙化,而因外周血管钙化不能吻合是常见的问题。同样,移植常见的构建足够循环的方法(主动脉-双股动脉旁路术)也是个问题。然而,在一些罕见的情况下,创造性的外科医生可以选择进行动脉内膜切除术或寻找可替代位置。对于主髂动脉支架植入术(这是越来越受欢迎),对支架远端放置位置的详细知识是很必要的。由于等待和透析时间的增加,盆腔静脉异常的情况可能变得更为重要。对于有大腿动静脉移植或长期股动脉导管失败史的候选人,应该评估他们的髂静脉和下腔静脉,以确保通畅的静脉流出。

表28.4 伯明翰亚拉巴马州大学的肾移植禁忌证

1.异常的血管解剖:
(1)主动脉双侧股动脉分流术或者主动脉支架延伸到两侧髂外动脉
(2)髂血管的周围血管钙化
(3)髂静脉血栓形成和下腔静脉血栓形成
2.晚期的心脏疾病:
(1)左心室射血分数≤20%的缺血性心肌病
(2)需要长期的家庭氧疗
3.2年内曾诊断为恶性肿瘤,包括皮肤黑色素瘤和小肾细胞癌<(2cm)
4.肥胖:体重指数≥40kg/m^2
5.活动性感染:(例如,肺结核、真菌性疾病骨髓炎)
6.活动性酗酒或药物滥用(包括吸烟)
7.生活状态:养老院

心脏功能测试是对大多数移植候选人进行评估的一部分(见下文)。严重的心脏和(或)肺部疾病作为手术禁忌证,会显著增加围术期风险,即使手术成功,也会影响术后的寿命。

依从性

在当今时代,术后遵循免疫抑制剂的使用是移植成功的关键。无法可靠地服用处方药物(无论何种原因)都必须被视为移植禁忌。由于药物滥用和不依从医疗治疗之间存在联系,滥用药物或酗酒也成为移植的绝对禁忌证[28]。即使没有药物滥用的情况,不遵医嘱史也可以被认为是一个相对禁忌，但不同移植中心对此的看法不同[41]。由于移植中心对于潜在候选人的了解是有限的，相关文件和后续透析单位或医生在评估和监测上也起了重要作用。这个问题尤其和青少年候选人有关，将会在第 120 章中深入探讨。

感染和恶性肿瘤

长期免疫抑制会损害受体有效地处理感染和恶性肿瘤的能力，这是移植两个主要的并发症。其次，长期的传统是完全消除移植前的感染，而现在，有效的抗菌药物的可得性已经使得标准改成在一定程度上控制而不是消灭。大多数移植中心推迟感染侵袭性细菌，真菌或分枝杆菌患者的移植，直到完成了有效的治疗。一些病毒感染的方法[特别是丙型肝炎（HCV）、乙型肝炎（HBV）和人类免疫缺陷病毒（HIV）]发生了巨大变化（见下文）。对于丙型肝炎病毒，患者即使在病毒存在的情况下进行移植，生存时间也超过透析，这使得移植（在晚期肝病或肝硬化的情况下）成为首选的治疗[42]。而对 HBV 和 HIV，尽管需要持续进行免疫抑制治疗，有效的抗病毒治疗仍可以控制病毒的复制[43,44]。

肿瘤也有类似的挑战。人群中非黑色素瘤很常见；尽管长期的免疫抑制可能会增加这种疾病的发病率和严重程度，但是很少危及生命，所以肺黑色素瘤不是移植的禁忌证。然而，由于免疫抑制治疗会促进肿瘤的生长，其他固体和造血恶性肿瘤仍是移植的禁忌[45-48]。对于有活动性肿瘤的潜在候选人而言，应避免移植[28]。传统上，经过适当的治疗后，肿瘤会进入一个“等待期”，它的时间长短因肿瘤的特点和复发风险而不同，此期可以实行移植（表 28.5）[29]。再次，随着对肿瘤生物学行为的认识深入和意识到移植的生存获益超过透析，有一些专门对于肿瘤“等待期”时间长短的评估。因此，以前可以接受的等待期为 5~10 年，现在被认为是不合适的，特别是给予更短的预期寿命与维持透析。在某种情况下，如果清楚认识到一些肿瘤尽管有等待期，也会出现肿瘤复发，那么此时知情同意是必不可少的。

患者自主选择的问题

在评估过程中如果患者出现担忧，尽管不会影响移植，但移植前仍需要额外的测试，治疗和（或）后续随访。这些“相对禁忌证”很少会被接受和适当的干预，因为目前的治疗方法和理解会随着时间而改变。它们本质上可以是医疗上的或心理社会层面的，虽然可能会影响到移植的成功，但是这些问题本身并不阻碍手术的进程或长期的免疫抑制治疗。例如，20 年前（和一些欧洲国家最近）年龄（>55 岁，或 60 岁，或 65 岁，或 70 岁）被认为是肾移植的禁忌证[49]。目前，已有的数据显示患者从移植中得到生存获益的最高年龄是 80 岁，但是对于年龄更大的患者，如果可以考虑的话，年龄也最多是一个相对禁忌证，因为对他们而言生命的质量比长短重要[17]。

表 28.5　恶性肿瘤与移植等待时间的关系。有恶性肿瘤病史的患者，需要评估其恶性肿瘤性质

如果评估为急需治疗者，不需要等待	
偶发的肾细胞癌	
膀胱原位癌	
子宫颈原位癌	
非黑色素皮肤癌	
等待时间至少 2 年	
大多数恶性肿瘤（包括肾母细胞瘤、膀胱癌、子宫癌）	
等待时间超过 2 年	
黑色素瘤	5 年
肾细胞癌	如果<5cm，2 年
	如果≥5cm，5 年
乳腺癌	2~5 年
淋巴瘤	2~5 年
结肠癌	2~5 年

Adapted from Pham et al. [28] with permission from John Wiley & Sons.

原有肾脏的肾小球疾病

移植后肾小球疾病复发是移植失败的常见原因，但复发性疾病的风险很少会是评估移植的决定性问题。过去，原发性局灶性肾小球硬化症被认为复发的频率很高，所以对于移植也是消极的态度[50-52]。目前的数据表明，复发率可能比以前认为的要低，因为疾病复发往往与临床管理也有关系。复发可能性最高的肾小球疾病是原发性局灶性肾小球硬化，年轻的白种人患者第一次移植复发的风险高达 50%，甚至高于那些接受移植后发生复发性疾病，再次进行移植的患者（表 28.6）。然而，移植与透析相比的好处是如此之大，复发的风险对候选人甚至是活体供者的影响是很轻微的。而狼疮性肾炎的复发是非常罕见的，大多数移植中心为了确保疾病的活动性很低，往往在移植前需要小剂

表 28.6 原发性肾病患者肾移植的治疗

原发性肾病	复发率	治疗
原发性局灶性肾小球肾炎	达 50%	在因为疾病复发导致移植肾失功的患者中,复发率可达 80%,这可能影响再次移植的选择
抗肾小球基底膜肾病	低	血清中的抗肾小球基底膜抗体可能增加危险度
韦格纳肉芽肿病	17%	ANCA 阳性和复发风险无关
IgA 肾病	20%~60%	组织学复发常见,但移植物失功罕见
HUS/TTP	达 75%	H 突变提示预后较差

Data from Golgert et al. [52].

量免疫抑制治疗;此外,抗心磷脂抗体的存在(狼疮抗凝物)可能需要预防性抗凝治疗。

多囊肾疾病

在移植前或是移植过程中, 需要考虑患者的多囊性肾病(PKD)。大多数多囊肾患者不需要切除肾脏,而有些患者切除肾脏可能会从中获益。体积较大的多囊肾,如果伸入骨盆,可能会阻碍移植物的植入;体格检查和腹部计算机断层扫描(CT)可以对肾脏的良恶性做出适当的评估。有明显症状或并发症的患者,包括顽固性疼痛、早期饱腹感、反复尿路感染和反复血尿,也应考虑行肾切除术。虽然传统上是在移植前进行,越来越多的成功经验指出, 肾脏切除术和肾脏移植可以同时进行[53]。

围术期并发症

一般来说,大多数医生都不愿意对蛋白质丢失甚至是严重低白蛋白血症的患者进行肾移植手术,因为这会增加围术期并发症的风险。对于有严重 CKD 的患者,使用药物(如血管紧张素转换酶抑制剂或非甾体抗炎药)通常可以控制尿道损失以逆转蛋白的丢失。

心血管疾病

与 CKD 相关的心血管负担是巨大的,并导致了一半以上的患者死亡[2]。尽管移植比透析更能降低心血管死亡的风险,与普通人相比,风险仍然很高[55,56]。普遍认为,传统的冠心病危险因素(如 Framingham 研究中建立的)与移植后的风险因素无关[57]。与移植后糖尿病、冠脉事件的发生和肾功能相比,移植前高血压、血脂异常、吸烟是相对较小的危险因素[58]。对于患者选择方面,筛选心血管疾病并在可能的情况下予以治疗,是评估过程中的重要组成部分,目的是解决两个主要问题[59]。首先是确定个人风险与移植手术本身的关系,有 5%患者本身会在围术期出现心肌梗死。二是评估移植成功后受体的寿命; 大部分情况下会考虑最大化利用从死者或活体供者得到的肾脏, 而移植给有高早期死亡率的患有不可逆性心功能不全的患者, 会被认为没有充分利用稀缺资源。不幸的是,对此并没有统一的适用标准[60]。事实上,最近的一个发人深省的文章指出,无症状患者常规筛查潜在的不利影响 (不必要的延迟移植的风险、造影剂肾病、抗血小板药物引起的术中出血、心理负担、动脉造影和血运重建的发病率和死亡率,低效利用医疗资源)抵消了其潜在的好处[61]。

界定进行筛选的人群(完整的病史和体格检查,心电图和胸部影像学)是第一个重大的挑战。毫无疑问有症状的患者(胸痛、呼吸困难、运动能力有限等)应进行检查。然而对于严重 CKD 患者而言,即使没有任何临床症状,心血管疾病的发病率仍很高,对于这部分患者该如何处理仍存在争议[61,62]。在极端的情况下,肾脏疾病预后质量倡议(KDOQI)指南指出,所有的候选人应该接受非侵入性的检测。美国心脏病学会(ACA)/美国心脏协会(AHA)建议应该针对危险因素对功能状态的影响选择测试内容[63,64]。指南所提及的指标需要更多的肾脏相关指标验证(图 28.1)[29,65]。最近的调查显示,大多数中心运用一些基于社会基础的版本,包括年龄、功能状态和按每个患者危险因素决定的检测水平。在最近一次对医疗数据的分析,认为有高缺血性心脏病(IHD)风险的患者(定义为糖尿病,以往缺血性心脏病,或>2 个心脏危险因素),移植后 3 年内发生急性心肌梗死的风险为 10%,其他患者的为 3%[58]。低 IHD 风险的患者,比高风险者组(20%对 65%)更可能没有进行心脏评估而行移植手术。急性心肌梗死的风险更可能与 IHD 有关,不管患者是否接受筛查,说明对风险因素的影响不仅有结果也是检查的做法(图 28.2)[59,66]。

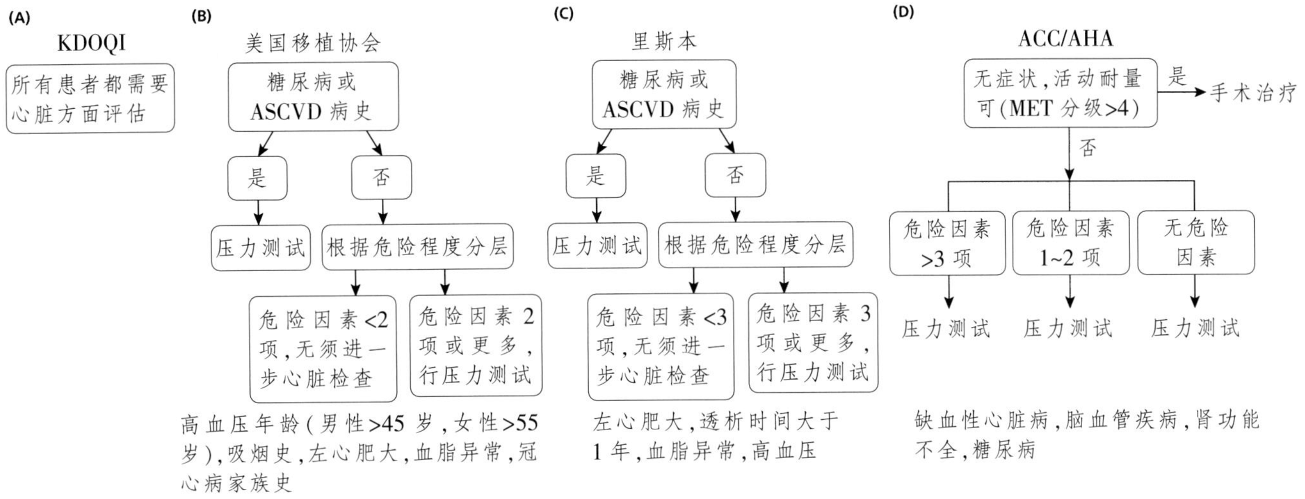

图 28.1 四项心脏风险评估的指南(A)肾脏病预后质量指南(K/DOQI);(B)美国移植协会;(C)肾移植接受者的里斯本会议(里斯本);(D) 美国心脏病学会/美国心脏协会;ASCVD 冠心病;MET: 代谢平衡。(Source: Friedman et al.[62]. Reproduced with permission from the American Society of Nephrology.)

对于此类患者仍然缺乏高级别的证据。

心脏检查对于移植前的患者是必须的,选择合适的检查十分重要。因为非侵入性检查的预测价值在 CKD 的患者中要比正常的患者更低。早期研究认为需要行血管造影检查。随着非侵入性检查的进展,血管造影主要用于冠心病或者有高危因素的患者。一项针对肾移植的研究先行非侵入性检查再行血管造影,结果显示二者差异较大,血管造影提示 40%的压力测试阴性的患者有冠脉病变[67,68]。有两项观察研究同样重要,其一是来自于梅奥诊所,还没被广泛认可,该研究提示与非侵入性试验相比,肌钙蛋白 T 是死亡率的更良好预测因子(可提示亚临床的缺血)[69]。第二项试验提示左心功能是独立于其他检查的,是等待期死亡率的最佳预测因子[70]。

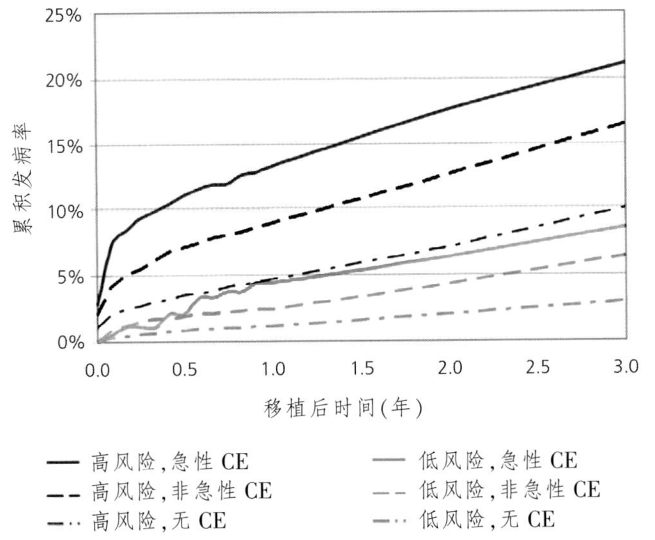

图 28.2 观察到的移植后急性心肌梗死发生率,根据临床缺血性心脏病 (IHD) 风险小组和移植前心脏评估状态的资料。(Source: Lentine et al.[59]. Reproduced with permission from the American Society of Nephrology)

非侵入性检查如表格 28.7 所示,通常,非特异性的非侵入性检查更为人所接受。专家意见认为,心脏检查推荐使用最有效和最可靠的检查。一项 META 分析建议,多巴酚丁胺刺激下的超声心动图可有效检查狭

表 28.7 对于接受肾移植患者的非侵入性心脏相关检查(Data from Friedman et al.[62])

应激状态下的超声心动图(运动或药物刺激,例如多巴酚丁胺刺激下的超声心动图)(DSE)
心肌灌注扫描(运动或药物刺激)
应激状态下的心电图(EST)
电子束 CT
超声心动图
运动下心室造影
数字减影荧光摄像(DSF)
静息状态下心电图
颈动脉内膜增厚(CIMT)
心肺功能测定
冠脉 CTA
MRA
心脏 MRI

窄程度大于50%的冠脉狭窄[71]。

如非侵入性检查阳性，需要冠脉造影检查，可能仍需要进一步血管重建治疗。根据数十年前的小样本临床研究，在ESRD的患者中，血管重建治疗比药物治疗更为重要[60,72]。针对普通人群的大样本研究提示，现代药物治疗(阿司匹林、他汀类药物、β受体阻断剂、血管活性药物抑制剂等)的效果几乎和血管重建治疗相同，除了三支病变(或等效)[73,74]。最近针对CKD患者的临床研究提示，CKD患者对于药物治疗的反应差于普通患者[75]。

糖尿病患者移植后的心血管发病率危险性较高[56,76]。非侵入性检查提示阳性结果提示可能需要心脏导管检查，这是糖尿病患者肾移植唯一的冠脉诊断性试验。

那些心脏检查的阳性结果足以停止肾移植手术。同样的，这是一个进展中的问题。目前，在大部分的中心中，心脏缺血但不能行血管重建治疗的患者无法进行肾移植。同样的，血管重建后的左心输出量不足(射血分数<20%~25%)同样是肾移植的禁忌证。不伴有冠心病的左心功能损伤患者可以进行心脏移植手术，很多研究中，此类患者在肾移植后肾功能有良好恢复。肺动脉高压常见于透析的患者，并且随着透析时间的延长而加重。最近研究提示，右心收缩压力(RVSP≥50mmHg)是移植的相对禁忌证。最后，严重的瓣膜疾病(严重的主动脉瓣狭窄，有症状的二尖瓣狭窄)应该先于肾移植手术治疗。

体重

严重的低体重和超体重是等待期和移植后患者死亡的高危因素。肥胖应该被重点评估[79]。即便是在1970年，肥胖是移植的禁忌证，在大多数中心中，现在还是禁忌证[80]。变化的是，肥胖在普通人群和ESRD人群中的普遍程度。肥胖增加了CKD的风险。最近的国际健康和营养调查数据提示，35%的美国人肥胖或病理性肥胖[BMI≥30kg/m^2]，但是RRT的BMI可能增加。大概超过20%的肾移植患者BMI>30kg/m^2[81]。

证据提示，BMI增高可能导致移植物失功能及死亡率风险增加。BMI≥36kg/m^{2}的风险最高，同时移植功能恢复减慢、急性排斥反应、伤口感染和冠脉事件的风险增加[82-84]。尽管如此，即便BMI≥36kg/m^2，甚至≥40kg/m^{2}肾移植后死亡率和并发症发生率仍低于透析患者[81]。因此，部分中心仍会对部分肥胖的患者进行肾移植手术。然而，大部分的中心会要求患者减重直至BMI<36~38kg/m^2，但是有部分研究提示术前减重不能给肾移植的患者带来获益[79]。对于病态肥胖的患者，肥胖手术可能带来获益，尽管ESRD患者肥胖手术的获益与风险尚未明确。

年龄

老年是移植的相对禁忌证。如上所述，无论年龄如何，肾移植都比透析治疗能有更大的生存获益。在等待手术的过程中，并发症的风险随着年龄和透析时间的增加而增加。根据美国供体扩展标准(ECD)，在部分欧洲国家，年老的供体会供给年老的患者[85,86]。符合ECD标准的年龄>65岁的肾移植患者，5年移植器官存活率为55%，不符合ECD的接受死亡供体的患者，5年移植器官存活率为64%，提示此类患者存在少量风险。然而，此类方法受到供体数量的限制，等待ECD肾脏的患者数目为35 000/年，能提供的肾脏1500/年[16]。同时，年龄>65岁的患者，如果接受活体肾脏，移植器官5年生存率为77%。考虑到ECD和非ECD患者的等待时间长度，部分患者仅对年龄>70岁实行活体移植。

HIV感染

考虑HIV感染患者有免疫抑制和不能耐受肾移植手术，HIV感染是肾移植的禁忌证[87]，目前，HIV是可控的慢性疾病，抗病毒药物可大幅延长HIV患者的生存期。因为HIV可能导致慢性肾衰竭，伴有HIV感染ESRD患者数目正在增加。尽管免疫抑制的治疗难度较大，药物间相互作用常见，伴有HIV感染ESRD患者行肾移植后的预后要优于长期透析的患者，现在不少中心可对HIV患者进行肾移植。

乙型病毒性肝炎和丙型病毒性肝炎

近年来，对于肾移植患者的肝炎状态评估的要求已经越来越低了，尽管HBV越来越少见，但HCV逐渐流行。肝脏纤维化或肝硬化的患者皆应避免肾移植，除非同时进行肾移植及肝移植。指南认为，需对肝炎或者进行肝脏穿刺活检[42]，此可明确患者是否存在进展期的肝脏纤维化或肝硬化，及进一步诊疗方案。

肝脏穿刺活检并不常见，原因如下。其一，可能影响肾移植的肝硬化一般程度较重，可以通过影像学、体格检查和实验室检查明确诊断。如果上述方法无效，可行终末期肝病评分(MELD)，此类患者可能评分较低，不适合进行肾移植。其二,现在 HBV 的治疗已经标准化、有效和易于执行,能常规用于术后治疗,并且 HBV 感染状态与肾移植的预后无关[43]。伴有 HCV 的 CKD 患者的治疗效果较差,副作用较大,并且移植术后是抗 HCV 治疗的禁忌证。因此,抗 HCV 治疗不是肾移植患者的常规治疗。如果需要抗 HCV 治疗,需在肾移植之前进行[88]。最后,在其他状态下,伴有 HBV 或 HCV 的患者进行肾移植能获得比透析治疗更好的预后,并且没有证据说明肾移植会加重病毒感染,并且再次强调可对肝炎病毒感染的患者进行肾移植。一项在伯明翰大学的研究提示,肝炎病毒感染的患者需要检测病毒载量、转氨酶、合成功能、肝脏影像学,如果上述指标变化提示肝脏纤维化加重或肿瘤负荷增加,需要按照上述建议对患者进行诊治。

特殊关注

1 型糖尿病

40 年前,1 型糖尿病是肾移植及透析的禁忌证。如今,糖尿病是 ESDR 的常见病因,1 型糖尿病多见于青年患者,他们是能从肾移植中获益最大的群体[12]。原因不是此类患者移植后有非常良好的结局,而是可以免于透析相关性死亡。因此,目前肾移植是 1 型糖尿病所致肾衰竭的首选治疗,术前治疗可有一定程度的获益[15]。

评价 1 型糖尿病患者的一个重要方面是肾移植入路(同样见于第 32 章和第 41 章,该章讨论了不同类型胰腺移植的适应证和胰腺移植等待名单管理的相关内容)。在单独行肾移植的患者中,仍有很高的糖尿病肾病发生率,但是其同样有很高的远期移植物存活率,几乎大于 10 年[89]。活体供者至少比尸体供者有两点好处,移植物平均寿命更长 (10 年移植物存活率,51%对 36%),避免了长期的等待和透析[16]。同时性胰腺及肾脏移植(SPK)的预后良好,研究显示,成功的胰腺移植可以降低远期死亡率,避免微血管并发症。然而胰腺、肾脏联合移植的等待时间可能为 2~3 年或更长,其远期移植肾存活时间仅稍高于活体供者的肾移植(10 年移植物存活率,63%对 51%)。对于先行肾移植,二期胰腺移植(PAK)的患者,移植胰腺的存活率稍低于 SPK。然而,移植胰腺的存活率在近十年有显著提高,与 SPK 相比 5 年的移植物存活率为(55%对 72%)。

患者该如何从此三种方案中选择呢? 通常,1 型糖尿病的 ESRD 患者的主要风险为透析时长。因此允许有确定活体供体的患者尽早进行移植,对于患者本人或其他等待器官的患者来说可能是最好的选择。PAK 移植可在某些患者中成功开展,特别是需要胰腺移植来控制血糖的患者。胰腺移植通常在肾脏移植的 2 个月后进行。PAK 预后不良的危险因素包括:GFR<45mL/L,肾脏移植和胰腺移植的间隔大于 1 年,肾排斥反应病史和蛋白尿,进行胰腺移植之前需要考虑上述危险因素[91]。

对于没有活体供者的患者,SPK 可能是更好的选择。与单纯肾移植相比,SPK 预后更好且等待时间更短。部分 1 型糖尿病的患者可能拒绝活体供者,从而选择 SPK 以减少透析的时间,这是可以理解的。安排 SPK 患者的等待时间时,要考虑该患者选择的是尸体供体。

多器官功能衰竭的患者

肾衰竭的患者可能伴有另一器官功能衰竭。首先,肾功能不全可能合并心功能或肝功能衰竭,此类患者通常同时需要心脏移植或者肝脏移植。2009 年,共有 444 例联合移植(占全部死亡供体的 4%),其中 82%为联合肝脏和肾脏移植,10%为联合心脏和肾脏移植[16]。其次是 ESRD 的在心脏、肺脏、肝脏和小肠移植的患者。此类患者在等待名单中约占 1%,但是现在已占等待名单中的 3%,并且约占接受死亡供者的 2%[92]。

评估心肾移植或肝肾移植是非常困难的,因为重症患者中肾功能不全有时是可逆的。即便是需要透析的患者,心脏或肝脏移植后肾脏功能依然可以得到一定程度的恢复。然而,肾功能不全可能对肾移植有影响。肾移植的时机选择主要考虑肾功能不全的严重性和病程长短[93]。根据最近指南,肝肾联合移植的主要指征如下:

1.终末期肾病伴有肝硬化和有症状的门脉高压症,或肝静脉压力>10mmHg;

2.CKD<30mL/min,同时合并肝功能衰竭;

3. 伴有肌酐>2.0mg/dL 和透析大于 8 周的急性肾衰竭或肝肾综合征;

4.肝功能衰竭合并 CKD,活检证实大于 30%的肾小球硬化,或大于 30%的纤维化[94]。

对于终末期心脏疾病的患者,暂无评估肾功能不全程度的共识。然而，最近一项UNOS的数据分析提示：eGFRS≤30mL/min时，不进行移植的患者预后远差于移植的患者[95]。

数据显示，进行移植后在出现ESRD的患者，长期透析的预后要低于肾移植，这可能表明此类患者选择合适免疫抑制剂的挑战性。此类患者可能更加需要预防性治疗，等待移植患者的标准需要更进一步标准化以反映区分此类患者。

总结

肾移植仍然是终末期肾病的最佳治疗手段。透析治疗、病例选择、围术期处理等取得了长足进展。如果合并疾病可被诊断及治疗，肾移植可以取得更加的结果，患者可有更客观的期待和药物依从性，禁忌证可被发现及排除。由于供体有限，合适的患者选择仍是移植最困难的步骤之一，同时，肾衰竭的患者需要内科医生参与治疗。

（刘以俊 译 张大方 校）

参考文献

1. National Kidney Foundation. K/DOQI Clinical practice guidelines for chronic kidney disease: executive summary. New York, NY: National Kidney Foundation; 2002.
2. United States Renal Data System. 2011 Annual Data Report. Minneapolis, MN; 2011.
3. Rennie D. Home dialysis and the costs of uremia. New England Journal of Medicine. 1978;298(7):399–400.
4. Rettig R. Special treatment-the story of Medicare's ESRD entitlement. New England Journal of Medicine. 2011;365:596–598.
5. Alexander S. They decide who lives, who dies: medical miracle puts a moral burden on a small committee. Life Magazine. 1962;53(19):102–104, 106, 108, 110, 115, 117, 118, 123, 124.
6. Rennie D, Rettig RA, Wing AJ. Limited resources and the treatment of end-stage renal failure in Britain and the United States. Quarterly Journal of Medicine. 1985;56(219):321–326.
7. Health Resources and Services Administration. HRSA transplant center growth and management collaborative: best practices final report. Washington, DC: U.S. Department of Health and Human Services; 2007.
8. Meier-Kriesche HU, Li S, Gruessner RW, et al. Immunosuppression: evolution in practice and trends, 1994–2004. American Journal of Transplantation. 2006;6(5 Pt 2):1111–1131.
9. Terasaki PI, Cecka JM, Gjertson DW, et al. High survival rates of kidney transplants from spousal and living unrelated donors. New England Journal of Medicine. 1995;333(6):333–336.
10. Fishman JA. Infection in solid-organ transplant recipients. New England Journal of Medicine. 2007;357:2601–2614.
11. Wolfe RA, Ashby VB, Milford EL, et al. Comparison of mortality in all patients on dialysis, patients on dialysis awaiting transplantation, and recipients of a first cadaveric transplant. New England Journal of Medicine. 1999;341(23):1725–1730.
12. Wolfe RA, McCullough KP, Schaubel DE, et al. Calculating life years from transplant (LYFT): methods for kidney and kidney-pancreas candidates. American Journal of Transplantation. 2008;8(4 Pt 2):997–1011.
13. Matas AJ, Schnitzler M. Payment for living donor (vendor) kidneys: a cost-effectiveness analysis. American Journal of Transplantation. 2004;4(2):216–221.
14. Kucirka LM, Grams ME, Balhara KS, et al. Disparities in provision of transplant information affect access to kidney transplantation. American Journal of Transplantation. 2012;12:351–357.
15. Abecassis M, Bartlett ST, Collins AJ, et al. Kidney transplantation as primary therapy for end-stage renal disease: a National Kidney Foundation/Kidney Disease Outcomes Quality Initiative (NKF/KDOQI) conference. Clinical Journal of the American Society of Nephrology. 2008;3:471–480.
16. Scientific Registry of Transplant Recipients. SRTR annual data report. 2011 [cited 2011 December 29, 2011]; Available from: http://www.srtr.org.
17. Schold JD, Srinivas TR, Kayler LK, et al. The overlapping risk profile between dialysis patients listed and not listed for renal transplantation. American Journal of Transplantation. 2008;8(1):58–68.
18. Murray JE, Merrill JP, Harrison JH. Renal homotransplantation in identical twins. Surgical Forum. 1955;6:432–436.
19. Murray JE, Merrill JP, Harrison JH, et al. Prolonged survival of human-kidney homografts by immunosuppressive drug therapy. New England Journal of Medicine. 1963;268:1315–1323.
20. Keith DS. Pre-emptive deceased donor kidney transplant not associated with patient survival benefit in minority kidney transplant recipients. Clinical Transplantation. 2012;26:82–86.
21. Kessler M, Ladriere M, Giral M, et al. Does pre-emptive kidney transplantation with a deceased donor improve outcomes? Results from a French transplant network. Transplant International. 2011;24(3):266–275.
22. Meier-Kriesche HU, Kaplan B. Waiting time on dialysis as the strongest modifiable risk factor for renal transplant outcomes: a paired donor kidney analysis. Transplantation. 2002;74(10):1377–1381.
23. Witczak BJ, Leivestad T, Line PD, et al. Experience from an active preemptive kidney transplantation program-809 cases revisited. Transplantation. 2009;88(5):672–677.
24. Schold JD, Sehgal AR, Srinivas TR, et al. Marked variation of the association of ESRD duration before and after wait listing on kidney transplant outcomes. American Journal of Transplantation. 2010;10(9):2008–2016.
25. United Network for Organ Sharing. OPTN/UNOS policy 3.5, 'Allocation of cadaveric kidneys'. 2005 [cited 2005 May 2, 2005]; Available from: http://optn.transplant.hrsa.gov/ContentDocuments/OPTN_Policies.pdf.
26. Akkina SK, Connaire JJ, Snyder JJ, et al. Earlier is not necessarily better in preemptive kidney transplantation. American Journal of Transplantation. 2008;8(10):2071–2076.
27. Gaston RS, Danovitch GM, Adams PL, et al. The report of a national conference on the wait list for kidney transplantation. American Journal of Transplantation. 2003;3(7):775–785.
28. Pham PT, Pham PA, Pham PC, et al. Evaluation of adult kidney transplant candidates. Seminars in Dialysis. 2010;23(6):595–605.
29. Kasiske BL, Cangro CB, Hariharan S, et al. The evaluation of renal transplantation candidates: clinical practice guidelines. American Journal of Transplantation. 2001;1(Suppl 2):3–95.
30. Ramos EL, Kasiske BL, Alexander SR, et al. The evaluation of candidates for renal transplantation. The current practice of U.S. transplant centers. Transplantation. 1994;57(4):490–497.
31. Dobbels F, De Geest S, Cleemput I, et al. Psychosocial and behavioral selection criteria for solid organ transplantation. Progress in Transplantation. 2001;11(2):121–130.
32. Benedetti E, Asolati M, Dunn T, et al. Kidney transplantation in recipients with mental retardation: clinical results in a single-center experience. American Journal of Kidney Diseases. 1998;31(3):509–512.
33. Alexander GC, Sehgal AR. Variation in access to kidney transplantation across dialysis facilities: using process of care measures for quality improvement. American Journal of Kidney Diseases. 2002;40(4):824–831.
34. Alexander GC, Sehgal AR. Why hemodialysis patients fail to complete the transplantation process. American Journal of Kidney Diseases. 2001;37(2):321–328.
35. Axelrod DA, Dzebisashvili N, Schnitzler MA, et al. The interplay of socioeconomic status, distance to center, and interdonor service area travel on kidney transplant access and outcomes. Clinical Journal of the American Society of Nephrology. 2010;5(12):2276–2288.
36. Gaston RS. Evolution of Medicare policy involving transplantation and immunosuppressive medications: past developments and future directions. In: Field MJ, Lawrence RL, Zwanziger L, editors. Extending Medicare Coverage for Preventive and Other Services. Washington, DC: National Academy Press; 2000: D23–D38.
37. Danovitch GM, Hariharan S, Pirsch JD, et al. Management of the waiting list for cadaveric kidney transplants: report of a survey and recommendations by the clinical practice guidelines Committee of the American Society of Transplantation. Journal of the American Society of Nephrology. 2002;13(2):528–535.
38. Kimmel PL. Psychosocial factors in dialysis patients. Kidney International. 2001;59:1599–1613.

39. Gaston RS, Deierhoi MH, Young CJ, et al. "High-risk" renal transplantation: evolving definitions at a single center. In: Cecka JM, Terasaki PI, editors. Clinical Transplants 2004. Los Angeles: UCLA Immunogenetics Laboratory; 2005: pp. 121-126.
40. Meier-Kriesche H-U, Schold JD, Gaston RS, et al. Kidneys from deceased donors: maximizing the value of a scarce resource. American Journal of Transplantation. 2005;5:1725-1730.
41. Prendergast MB, Gaston RS. Optimizing medication adherence: an ongoing opportunity to improve outcomes after kidney transplantation. Clinical Journal of the American Society of Nephrology. 2010;5(7):1305-1311.
42. Roth D, Gaynor JJ, Reddy KR, et al. Effect of kidney transplantation on outcomes among patients with hepatitis C. Clinical Journal of the American Society of Nephrology. 2011;22(6):1152-1160.
43. Reddy PN, Sampaio MS, Kuo HT, et al. Impact of pre-existing hepatitis B infection on the outcomes of kidney transplant recipients in the United States. Clinical Journal of the American Society of Nephrology. 2011;6(6):1481-1487.
44. Stock PG, Barin B, Murphy B, et al. Outcomes of kidney transplantation in HIV-infected recipients. New England Journal of Medicine. 2010;363(21):2004-2014.
45. Miao Y, Everly JJ, Gross TG, et al. De novo cancers arising in organ transplant recipients are associated with adverse outcomes compared with the general population. Transplantation. 2009;87(9):1347-1359.
46. Buell JF, Gross TG, Woodle ES. Malignancy after transplantation. Transplantation. 2005;80(2 Suppl):S254-S264.
47. Vajdic CM, McDonald SP, McCredie MR, et al. Cancer incidence before and after kidney transplantation. JAMA. 2006;296(23):2823-2831.
48. Kasiske BL, Snyder JJ, Gilbertson DT, et al. Cancer after kidney transplantation in the United States. American Journal of Transplantation. 2004;4(6):905-913.
49. Jordan ML, Novick AC, Steinmuller D, et al. Renal transplantation in the older recipient. Journal of Urology. 1985;134:243-246.
50. Ponticelli C. Recurrence of focal segmental glomerular sclerosis (FSGS) after renal transplantation. Nephrology Dialysis Transplantation. 2010;25(1):25-31.
51. Ponticelli C, Glassock RJ. Posttransplant recurrence of primary glomerulonephritis. Clinical Journal of the American Society Nephrology. 2010;5(12):2363-2372.
52. Golgert WA, Appel GB, Hariharan S. Recurrent glomerulonephritis after renal transplantation: an unsolved problem. Clinical Journal of the American Society Nephrology. 2008;3(3):800-807.
53. Kramer A, Sausville J, Haririan A, et al. Simultaneous bilateral native nephrectomy and living donor renal transplantation are successful for polycystic kidney disease: the University of Maryland experience. Journal of Urology. 2009;181(2): 724-728.
54. Kujovich JL. Thrombophilia and thrombotic problems in renal transplant patients. Transplantation. 2004;77(7):959-964.
55. Meier-Kriesche HU, Schold JD, Srinivas TR, et al. Kidney transplantation halts cardiovascular disease progression in patients with end-stage renal disease. American Journal of Transplantation. 2004;4(10):1662-1668.
56. Jardine AG, Gaston RS, Fellstrom BC, et al. Prevention of cardiovascular disease in adult recipients of kidney transplants. Lancet. 2011;378(9800):1419-1427.
57. Kasiske BL, Chakkera HA, Roel J. Explained and unexplained ischemic heart disease risk after renal transplantation. Journal of the American Society of Nephrology. 2000;11(9):1735-1743.
58. Israni AK, Snyder JJ, Skeans MA, et al. Predicting coronary heart disease after kidney transplantation: Patient Outcomes in Renal Transplantation (PORT) study. American Journal of Transplantation. 2010;10(2):338-353.
59. Lentine KL, Schnitzler MA, Brennan DC, et al. Cardiac evaluation before kidney transplantation: a practice patterns analysis in Medicare-insured dialysis patients. Clinical Journal of the American Society Nephrology. 2008;3(4):1115-1124.
60. Pilmore H. Cardiac assessment for renal transplantation. American Journal of Transplantation. 2006;6(4):659-665.
61. Kasiske BL, Israni AK, Snyder JJ, et al. Design considerations and feasibility for a clinical trial to examine coronary screening before kidney transplantation (COST). American Journal of Kidney Diseases. 2011;57(6):908-916.
62. Friedman SE, Palac RT, Zlotnick DM, et al. A call to action: variability in guidelines for cardiac evaluation before renal transplantation. Clinical Journal of the American Society Nephrology. 2011;6:1185-1191.
63. Fleisher LA, Beckman JA, Brown KA, et al. ACC/AHA 2007 guidelines on perioperative cardiovascular evaluation and care for noncardiac surgery: executive summary: a report of the American College of Cardiology/American Heart Association task force on practice guidelines (writing committee to revise the 2002 guidelines on perioperative cardiovascular evaluation for noncardiac surgery): developed in collaboration with the American Society of Echocardiography, American Society of Nuclear Cardiology, Heart Rhythm Society, Society of Cardiovascular Anesthesiologists, Society for Cardiovascular Angiography and Interventions, Society for Vascular Medicine and Biology, and Society for Vascular Surgery. Circulation. 2007;116(17):1971-1996.
64. Kidney Disease Outcomes Quality Initiative. K/DOQI clinical practice guidelines for cardiovascular disease in dialysis patients. American Journal of Kidney Diseases. 2005;45:S1-S153.
65. Abbud-Filho M, Adams PL, Alberu J, et al. A report of the Lisbon conference on the care of the kidney transplant recipient. Transplantation. 2007;83(8 Suppl): S1-S22.
66. Lentine KL, Hurst FP, Jindal RM, et al. Cardiovascular risk assessment among potential kidney transplant candidates: approaches and controversies. American Journal of Kidney Diseases. 2009;55:152-157.
67. De Lima JJ, Sabbaga E, Vieira ML, et al. Coronary angiography is the best predictor of events in renal transplant candidates compared with noninvasive testing. Hypertension. 2003;42(3):263-268.
68. Kahn MR, Fallahi A, Kim MC, et al. Coronary artery disease in a large renal transplant population: implications for management. American Journal of Transplantation. 2011;11(12):2665-2674.
69. Hickson LJ, Cosio FG, El-Zoghby ZM, et al. Survival of patients on the kidney transplant wait list: relationship to cardiac troponin T. American Journal of Transplantation. 2008;8(11):2352-2359.
70. de Mattos AM, Siedlecki A, Gaston RS, et al. Systolic dysfunction portends increased mortality among those waiting for renal transplant. Journal of the American Society of Nephrology. 2008;19(6):1191-1196.
71. Wang LW, Fahim MA, Hayen A, et al. Cardiac testing for coronary artery disease in potential kidney transplant recipients. Cochrane Database of Systematic Reviews. 2011;(12):CD008691.
72. Manske CL, Wang Y, Rector T, et al. Coronary revascularisation in insulin-dependent diabetic patients with chronic renal failure. Lancet. 1992;340(8826): 998-1002.
73. McFalls EO, Ward HB, Moritz TE, et al. Coronary-artery revascularization before elective major vascular surgery. New England Journal of Medicine. 2004; 351(27):2795-2804.
74. Poldermans D, Schouten O, Vidakovic R, et al. A clinical randomized trial to evaluate the safety of a noninvasive approach in high-risk patients undergoing major vascular surgery: the DECREASE-V pilot study. Journal of the American College of Cardiology. 2007;49(17):1763-1769.
75. Bansal N, Hsu CY, Chandra M, et al. Potential role of differential medication use in explaining excess risk of cardiovascular events and death associated with chronic kidney disease: a cohort study. BMC Nephrology. 2011;12:44.
76. Welsh RC, Cockfield SM, Campbell P, et al. Cardiovascular assessment of diabetic end-stage renal disease patients before renal transplantation. Transplantation. 2011;91(2):213-218.
77. Issa N, Krowka MJ, Griffin MD, et al. Pulmonary hypertension is associated with reduced patient survival after kidney transplantation. Transplantation. 2008;86:1384-1388.
78. American College of Cardiology Foundation/American Heart Association Task Force on Practice Guidelines. 2009 ACCF/AHA focused update on perioperative beta blockade incorporated into the ACC/AHA 2007 Guidelines on perioperative cardiovascular evaluation and care for noncardiac surgery. Circulation. 2009;120:e169-e276.
79. Schold JD, Srinivas TR, Guerra G, et al. A "weight-listing" paradox for candidates of renal transplantation? American Journal of Transplantation. 2007;7(3): 550-559.
80. Segev DL, Simpkins CE, Thompson RE, et al. Obesity impacts access to kidney transplantation. Journal of the American Society of Nephrology. 2008;19: 249-255.
81. Glanton CW, Kao T-C, Cruess D, et al. Impact of renal transplantation on survival in end-stage renal disease patients with elevated body mass index. Kidney International. 2003;63:647-653.
82. Lynch RJ, Ranney DN, Shijie C, et al. Obesity, surgical site infection, and outcome following renal transplantation. Annals of Surgery. 2009;250:1014-1020.
83. Meier-Kriesche HU, Arndorfer JA, Kaplan B. The impact of body mass index on renal transplant outcomes: a significant independent risk factor for graft failure and patient death. Transplantation. 2002;73:70-74.
84. Lentine KL, Rocca-Rey LA, Bacchi G, et al. Obesity and cardiac risk after kidney transplantation: experience at one center and comprehensive literature review. Transplantation. 2008;86(2):303-312.
85. Sung RS, Guidinger MK, Leichtman AB, et al. Impact of the expanded criteria donor allocation system on candidates for and recipients of expanded criteria donor kidneys. Transplantation. 2007;84(9):1138-1144.
86. Moers C, Kornmann NS, Leuvenink HG, et al. The influence of deceased donor age and old-for-old allocation on kidney transplant outcome. Transplantation. 2009;88(4):542-552.
87. Spital A. Should all human immunodeficiency virus-infected patients with end-stage renal disease be excluded from transplantation? The views of U.S. transplant centers. Transplantation. 1998;65(9):1187-1191.
88. Roth D, Bloom R. Selection and management of hepatitis C virus-infected patients for the kidney transplant waiting list. Contributions to Nephrology. 2012;176: 66-76.
89. Mauer SM, Goetz FC, McHugh LE, et al. Long-term study of normal

kidneys transplanted into patients with type I diabetes. Diabetes. 1989;38(4): 516–523.
90. Gruessner AC, Sutherland DE, Gruessner RW. Long-term outcome after pancreas transplantation. Current Opinion in Organ Transplantation. 2012;17(1):100–105.
91. Wiseman AC. Pancreas transplant options for patients with type 1 diabetes and chronic kidney disease: simultaneous pancreas kidney or pancreas after kidney. Current Opinion in Organ Transplantation. 2012;17(1):80–86.
92. Srinivas TR, Stephany BR, Budev M, et al. An emerging population: kidney transplant candidates who are placed on the waiting list after liver, heart, and lung transplantation. Clinical Journal of the American Society Nephrology. 2010; 5(10):1881–1886.
93. Papafragkakis H, Martin P, Akalin E. Combined liver and kidney transplantation. Current Opinion in Organ Transplantation. 2010;15(3):263–268.
94. Eason JD, Gonwa TA, Davis CL, et al. Proceedings of consensus conference on Simultaneous Liver Kidney transplantation (SLK). American Journal of Transplantation. 2008;8(11):2243–2251.
95. Russo MJ, Rana A, Chen JM, et al. Pretransplantation patient characteristics and survival following combined heart and kidney transplantation: an analysis of the United Network for Organ Sharing Database. Archives of Surgery. 2009; 144(3):241–246.
96. Centers for Disease Control. Prevalence of Chronic Kidney Disease and Associated Risk Factors – United States, 1999–2004. Atlanta, GA: Centers for Disease Control, 2007.

第 29 章 肝移植的患者选择和适应证

Kimberly A. Brown，Marwan Kazimi

引言

肝移植患者的选择必须对移植的风险及获益进行整体的医疗评估。医疗小组在做出移植决定时要充分权衡移植给患者带来的好处与风险。这是极具挑战的任务，原因如下。第一，我们缺乏特殊疾病的个体预后数据。我们有疾病的一般资料，这些资料可以运用于有特定疾病的群体，但是对个体的患者却未必合适。第二，现存的数据还不足以弄清多种并发症共存时对患者的影响。例如，老年患者合并丙型肝炎、肾功能不全、糖尿病及冠心病病史。尽管我们可能有单个医疗问题的数据，但是它们之间的相互关系尚不明了。最后，我们选择患者时要充分理解个体的效益风险比。然而，移植供体是有限的。因此，我们对某个患者做出的选择可能影响着其他等待或急需移植的患者。

为了引起人们对供体不足问题的关注，2011 年 12 月 16 日，工作人员对器官移植供应网络(OPTN)的数据进行了评估，发现截至当日共有 16148 名患者等待肝移植，而接受肝移植的患者只有 4734 人。事实上，在过去的几年，每年肝移植的病例在逐年减少，已经从 2006 年的 6651 例减少到 2011 年 12 月的 4734 例，这一例数与 1999 年的例数相近。因此，在我们选择肝移植患者时，我们应该清楚，在美国需要肝移植的患者在增加，而供体的数量却在减少。事实上，这些问题已经成为管理领域在挑选移植患者时必须明白的问题。

本章涵盖了成人肝移植的一般适应证和条例。儿科特定的问题将在 114 章深入讨论。本章是第 38 章的指南，第 38 章将讨论肝移植前的患者管理。

肝移植适应证

总论

目前，器官共享联合网络认定肝移植的适应证包括 7 类共 72 种肝脏疾病[1]。一般而言，肝移植的益处首先体现在肝脏方面。事实上，许多其他威胁人类健康的疾病会在移植过程及后续的治疗中急剧恶化。当然也有例外，例如，肝肾综合征时的肾衰竭，无论如何，这一过程是可怕的并且对受者造成一定的损害。因此，我们需要回归到对移植益处及风险的基本评估。

肝移植的主要适应证和禁忌证已在表 29.1 中列出。一般而言，多数肝硬化及急性肝功能衰竭患者，在评估后若移植造成死亡的风险比不移植而死亡的风险低，那么就是合适的人选。对于这些患者，肝功能衰竭是主要的问题，而肝移植能够恢复肝脏功能并且避免因肝功能衰竭而死亡。在其他类别中，移植的适应证更多的与患者的生活方式或预防已有肝脏疾病的并发症相关。对于这些患者，治疗目的主要在于改善患者健康和减少未来的风险，而总体生存率较为次要。

在美国，早于当前分配系统的是终末期肝病模型分配系统，该系统主要根据肝功能不全的程度及患者等待移植的时间进行肝脏分配。为了更好地明白和阐述移植患者选择问题，1997 年美国移植医师协会和美国肝病研究协会联合举办了国家会议[2]。那时肝移植患者的 1 年生存率约为 90%。因此，该会议推荐将预期一年生存率≤90%的患者列入移植名单。失代偿性肝硬化(包括黄疸、脑病、静脉曲张出血和腹水)与一年生存率的相关性为 70%~75%[3]。Child A 级肝硬化患者的中

表29.1 成人肝移植的适应证和禁忌证

适应证
急性肝功能衰竭
• 病毒感染
• 用药
• 局部缺血
• 肝豆状核变性(Wilson病)
• 自身免疫性
• 先天性肝脏疾病
失代偿性肝硬化
• 乙肝或丙肝
• 酒精性
• 非酒精性脂肪肝炎
• 胆汁淤积性疾病(原发性胆汁性肝硬化、原发性硬化性胆管炎、继发性胆汁性肝硬化、胆管缺如)
• 自身免疫性
• 代谢性(α-1抗胰蛋白酶缺乏、血色沉着病、肝豆状核变性)
• 恶性肿瘤(肝癌、胆管癌)
• 病因不明的
肝脏疾病的系统并发症
• 肝肺综合征
良性肝脏疾病
• 多囊肝
• 慢性布加综合征
全身代谢疾病
• 原发性高草尿酸症
• 家族性淀粉样变性
• 鸟氨酸循环障碍
• 糖原贮积症
二次肝移植
• 原发性失功能
• 原发病复发及移植物功能失调
• 血管并发症
• 胆汁并发症
禁忌证
• 肝外癌灶
• 肝癌超出Milan或UCSF准则
• 放射性物质或酗酒
• 严重心肺疾病
• 社会或资金支持不足
• 难以控制的精神病
• 解剖异常以至外科重建困难
• 难以控制的HIV感染
• 不遵守医疗规范

位生存期为6.4年,而Child C级患者中位生存期只有2个月[4],有学者建议将Child-Pugh评分大于7分的患者列入移植名单。对于进展期肝病及失代偿的患者,移植造成死亡的风险要比不移植的风险大。

对于非进展性肝功能衰竭患者,是否移植则更多地取决于诸如进行性肝脏疾病(如肝癌)、肝脏异常带来的并发症(如遗传性草酸过多症、家族性淀粉样多神经病)以及改善健康(如布加综合征、多囊肝)过程中存在的风险。且不论适应证如何,移植小组在评估患者是否需要移植时, 应充分权衡移植带来的潜在利益及移植及恢复过程中的总体风险。

乙型病毒性肝炎

在肝移植的早些年,乙肝病毒感染是肝移植的相对禁忌证。这是主要是由于其复发的风险很高、存在严重纤维瘀胆性肝炎的风险及移植后死亡率增高[5,6]。在1993年,欧洲人发表了一篇里程碑性的文章,该文章认为在移植时病毒停止复制或长期的HBV免疫预防能够降低HBV感染复发的风险,并能够降低死亡率[7]。

台湾一项大规模的研究表明,与对照组相比,拉米夫定能够显著地减缓乙肝患者的疾病发展过程(不用药和用药32个月分别为7.8%和17.7%)[8]。对于肝功能失代偿及HBV复制的患者,服用拉米夫定或阿德福韦酯都能够改善肝功能和缓解肝功能衰竭[9-12]。长期服用拉米夫定治疗的主要问题是耐药率较高(5年耐药率为70%)[13] 以及病毒反弹导致的谷丙转氨酶升高和肝功能进一步失代偿的风险[14]。恩替卡韦和替诺福韦是更为有效的核苷酸类似物,并且已经被美国FDA批准用于乙肝的治疗。Shim等将恩替卡韦用于70例HBV感染导致的失代偿性肝病患者[15]。他们发现在这些患者中, 恩替卡韦抑制病毒复制和清除e抗原的效果与在代偿肝病患者中的效果相当,并且恩替卡韦能够改善失代偿性肝病患者的肝脏储备。在此研究过程中没有发生耐药或病毒的反弹。基于这些研究,三个协会共同推荐在失代偿性肝硬化患者中,无论HBV DNA的水平如何都应该进行抗病毒治疗[16-18]。

可以肯定的是,口服抗病毒药物能够有效地减少乙肝及肝硬化患者进行肝移植的比例。事实上,自1990年以来,乙肝患者接受肝移植的比例从5.7%下降到1.5%。终末期肝病患者肝移植例数在下降而HBV

感染引起的肝癌患者移植例数在增加[19]。乙肝患者肝移植后的 5 年生存率已经由 1987 年到 1991 年之间的 53%上升到目前的 85%~94%[20,21]。

与早些年不同的是,乙型肝炎引起的肝脏失代偿或肝癌是肝移植的明确适应证。这些患者移植前后的管理将在第 38、78 和 82 章讨论。

丙型病毒性肝炎

丙型肝炎在 1945 年至 1965 年出生的人群中患病率最高[22]。由于丙肝自然进程缓慢,一些学者认为丙肝的慢性并发症带来的负担,包括肝移植需求的负担,会在未来数年继续增加[23]。早期研究表明,丙肝患者进行原位肝移植后,患者及移植物的存活时间与因其他慢性肝脏疾病而进行原位肝移植的时间相近。这些单中心的报道往往受到病例数和随访时间较短的限制。最近,一些注册分析报道,有 HCV 感染患者的移植物及患者存活时间减少。据 Forman 等在 UNOS 数据库报道[24],7459 例 HCV 阳性患者接受肝移植后,3 年生存率为 78%,而 20 743 例 HCV 阴性患者接受肝移植后的生存率为 82%(P=0.0001)。同样,与 HCV 阴性的患者相比,HCV 阳性患者在接受原位肝移植后,移植物的 3 年和 5 年的存活时间明显缩短。

早期研究表明,10%~15%的患者在原位肝移植后 5 年内会发展为肝硬化。而这一数据在后来的研究中上升为 40%,因此许多人提出 HCV 对移植受者的损害在逐渐增加。有人认为,HCV 感染患者移植后效果变差的原因为肝穿刺的常规使用、强效免疫抑制剂的使用、类固醇药物撤药太快及供者年龄增加[24]。Berenguer 等也发现,HCV 感染患者移植后移植物的存活时间变短,而 HCV 阴性的患者移植物存活时间都较长[25]。这些数据表明,我们行为的改变可能对 HCV 的复发和进展产生负面影响。

尽管 HCV 对肝移植后患者的发病率和死亡率都有负面影响,但是一旦患者进展到肝功能失代偿,肝移植仍然是最好的选择。

酒精性肝病

对于因酗酒而导致的晚期肝硬化和肝功能失代偿,肝移植是延长患者生存时间最好的选择。在美国,酒精性肝病是肝移植的第二大适应证[1]。戒酒后,酒精性肝病患者肝移植后 1~7 年的生存率与因其他疾病而进行移植患者的生存率相当[26,27]。酒精性肝病患者的总体适应证与其他肝脏疾病相同。不同的是,这些患者复发的风险主要取决于患者本身。

尽管有着严格的筛选原则,但是酒精性肝病患者移植后的复发率不尽相同,部分原因可能是由于对"喝一点"及"酗酒"的定义不同[28-30]。一个前瞻性研究发现,移植后 1 年内再度饮酒的患者占 22%[30],5 年内再度饮酒患者的比例为 42%,其中 26%的患者饮酒量超过警戒值。

因此,评估酒精性肝病患者预后应关注患者再饮酒的风险。一些潜在的预测因素正在被研究,包括家族史、社会支持度、相关精神疾病、治疗前旧习复燃及滥用非酒精物质。研究结果不尽相同,这使得很难用这些预测因素作为选择移植患者的绝对指标。2008 年的一项大样本的 Meta 分析结果表明,较差的社会支持体系、酗酒家族史及移植前戒酒≤6 个月是旧习复燃的重要预测因素[31]。鉴于认识水平的局限及患者不进行移植造成的严重后果,许多中心已经采用是否达到标准的戒酒时间(6 个月及以上)作为主要的选择患者的要素。

代谢综合征

在美国,代谢综合征的发病率逐渐升高。尽管非酒精性脂肪性肝病(NAFLD)的发病率及其引起肝硬化的概率尚不明了,但 NAFLD 已经逐渐成为肝移植的第三大适应证。目前在美国[1],男性肥胖率约为 28.7%,女性肥胖率约为 34.1%,其中重度肥胖(BMI 40~50kg/m^2)[32,33]的人数在逐渐增加。这一趋势可以从逐渐增加的 NAFLD 和非酒精性脂肪性肝病(NASH)患者数看出,然而,这些患者发展为肝硬化和肝功能失代偿的概率尚不清楚。基于 UNOS 数据库的一篇综述表明,1988 年至 1996 年,肝移植受者中 BMI>30kg/m^2 的患者占 16.8%,BMI>35kg/m^2 的患者占 5.3%,BMI>40kg/m^2 的患者占 2.1%[34]。从 2001 年至 2004 年,32.5%的移植受者患有肥胖症,其中 8.4%的患者重度肥胖,3.2%的患者为病态肥胖[35]。

Charlton 等[36]综合分析了移植受者科学注册系统(SRTR)的数据,他们发现原发或继发的需要肝移植的 NASH 患者逐渐增多(从 2001 年的 1.2%上升至 2009年的 9.7%)。此外,一些研究者认为,由于肝硬化过程中并非一定伴有脂肪变,因此真正的适合肝移植的 NASH

患者人数可能被低估了。在移植前被诊断为微小肝硬化的患者在表型上与NASH引起肝硬化的患者相似，这使得对这类患者的分类结果受到质疑[37,38]。

在选择代谢综合征或肥胖患者作为移植受者时，医师既要考虑复发的风险，也要考虑对患者及移植物的影响。NASH对移植后复发患者做了详细记录[39,40]。然而，在分析了SRTR数据后，Charlton等发现，原发或继发的NASH患者与有其他疾病而需要移植的患者相比，移植后患者和移植物的3年存活率相近。有研究者报道，复发的NASH相关的肝硬化和移植物失活的发生率为2.5%~5%，这也与其他疾病的发生率相近[41,42]。

对于BMI为30~35kg/m^{2}的NAFLD患者，短期(30天)的死亡率可能会增加，而长期(1~3年)死亡率与非NAFLD患者相近[43]。病态患者(BMI>35kg/m^2)的1年和2年死亡率及原发性功能丧失的情况比其他患者更糟糕[44]。一篇基于器官共享网络(UNOS)1987—2007年间的数据的综述表明，严重肥胖(BMI>340kg/m^2)的患者因感染性并发症及癌症而至死亡的例数比对照组患者多(P=0.02)。对3例不同时期肝移植患者进行多因素分析发现，重度低体重(BMI<18.5kg/m^2)或重度肥胖(BMI>40kg/m^2)是死亡重要的预测因素[45]。此外，许多肥胖患者常伴有糖尿病，这对严重影响了肝移植患者生存[46]。一项病例对照研究发现，糖尿病患者移植后5年内的死亡率比非糖尿病患者高40%[47]。

对于代谢综合征或肥胖患者，在选择移植受者时，既要考虑疾病复发对移植物的影响，也要考虑相关的副发病变对患者生存的影响。

自身免疫性肝脏疾病

原发性胆汁性肝硬化

最近，有学者对原发性胆汁性肝硬化(PBC)患者进行肝移植的情况做了调查。他们发现，从1995年到2007年，尽管肝移植的总体例数在增多，但是因PBC而接受肝移植的患者数量每年减少5.4例[48]。PBC患者是否进行肝移植仍然取决于患者是否出现肝功能失代偿的临床症状。在10年内，PBC患者中肝功能失代偿者占26%[49]。难治性的瘙痒或虚弱可能是由胆汁淤积引起的[50]。瘙痒通常用熊去氧胆酸治疗，但是有些研究表明其并不能明显缓解瘙痒症状[51]。对于药物治疗无法缓解的患者，移植可能是提高生活质量的唯一途径。而且，PBC患者中慢性疲劳者占80%[52]。尽管对于一些无明显肝功能失代偿的患者，移植的目的在于改善生活状态(如改善疲劳)，但是必须明白的是疲劳并不会在肝移植后持续改善[53]。

当患者移植后1年的生存率比仅用药物治疗的1年生存率高时才会将其作为理想的移植候选人。在所有进行肝移植的人群中，因胆汁淤积性肝病而进行肝移植的患者效果最好[1]。对大多数患者，当其Child评分达到C级或MELD评分≥15分时移植的益处最大。血清胆红素是预测PBC患者移植后预后的指标，一些学者将血清胆红素≥5.9mg/dL作为肝移植的绝对指征[54]。还有一些学者通过综合考虑多种因素来评估PBC患者是否需要进行肝移植，这些因素包括胆红素、白蛋白、凝血酶原时间、年龄、有无水肿及是否使用利尿剂(即Mayo风险评分)。移植中心可能会选择一个或多个评估方法来甄别患者能否从移植中获益。

尽管PBC患者在移植后复发率接近1/4，但是患者及移植物的存活时间在肝移植群体中效果突出[1]。

原发性硬化性胆管炎

原发性硬化性胆管炎(PSC)多见于50岁以下的男性。尽管PSC的进程较为缓慢，但是当患者发展为肝失代偿或有胆管狭窄并发症时，应考虑肝移植。与PBC的Mayo风险评分相似，对PSC患者进行评估的目的是选择合适的手术时机[56]。PSC的Mayo风险评分主要包括年龄、血清胆红素、血清白蛋白和曲张静脉出血史等方面[56]。MELD评分体系不像Mayo评分体系那样对PBC和PSC区别评分，但MELD评分体系确实能有效评估各种病因的患者[57]。

PSC特有的症状是胆管狭窄，这可能带来其他的并发症，如黄疸加重、阻塞和感染。另外，患者发展为胆管癌的风险增加(见下文)[58]。患者胆管炎复发时需要使用抗生素或住院治疗，这种情况常出现于MELD<15分的患者。对于这些患者，最好由区域审查委员会讨论决定，因为这些患者有败血症和胆管炎引起的并发症的风险。这类患者可能会有瘙痒症状，但是仅有瘙痒症状的患者是否需要移植需要谨慎考虑。

尽管PSC患者移植后复发率达10%~25%，但是其移植效果与PBC患者的移植效果相当[1,59,60]。

自身免疫性肝炎

自身免疫性肝炎患者移植的适应证是出现肝功能失代偿。大部分自身免疫性肝炎患者在移植前要接受免疫抑制治疗。因此,在评估移植风险时必须仔细审查移植前药物治疗的情况。类固醇类药物的使用可能会引起代谢综合征,因此,应该将其作为移植前整体评估的一部分(见评估部分)。

自身免疫性肝炎患者移植后复发率约为 23%[61],复发后可能因肝功能失代偿而需要再次移植[62]。与其他免疫性疾病相似,尽管自身免疫性肝炎移植后可能会复发,但其疗效也非常显著[1,61]。

遗传性肝病

无论是儿童还是成年人,α-1 抗胰蛋白酶缺乏都可能导致肝硬化[63]。出现 PiZZ 表型的患者中约 15%会发展肝脏疾病,并且这些患者发展为肝癌的风险增加[64]。α-1 抗胰蛋白酶缺乏导致的肝脏疾病尚无有效治疗措施,肝移植是唯一的治疗途径。由于 α-1 抗胰蛋白酶缺乏也累积到肺,所以这类患者在肝移植前要充分评估肺功能。α-1 抗胰蛋白酶缺乏患者肝移植后效果显著,1 年和 3 年的生存率分别为 88%和 84%[65]。

尽管血色沉着病的基因频率为 1/200,但是需要进行肝移植的患者很罕见[66]。对于这类患者,早期检测和铁缺乏检测能延缓或阻止肝脏疾病引起的并发症[67]。血色沉着病伴有肝硬化的患者发展为肝癌的风险增加[68]。对于肝硬化和肝功能失代偿的患者,肝移植仍然是唯一治疗方法。然而,有学者报道血色沉着病患者肝移植后生存率下降[69,70]。这些患者常发生心血管并发症、感染及肝癌复发,这反映出铁沉着发生在肝脏以外的器官[70]。对于这类患者,肝移植前应该进行充分的心血管评估及铁缺失检测[71]。

威尔逊病移植的适应证是出现肝硬化和肝功能失代偿或出现急性肝功能衰竭。部分患者可运用口服或注射针对铜确实的药物治疗而得到长期缓解[72]。对于由威尔逊病引起的肝功能失代偿或急性肝功能衰竭,肝移植是最好的选择[73]。肝移植后,除了严重的神经系统疾病,多数代谢相关症状会得到改善,这类患者的生存率也较好[74]。

恶性肿瘤

肝癌

1982 年,在华盛顿举办的美国国立卫生研究院发展大会上,肝移植被确定为终末期肝病和肝脏恶性肿瘤的治疗方法。25 年后,原位肝移植成为终末期肝病和肝癌的标准治疗方法。对于肝硬化和肝癌的患者,肝移植既能恢复肝功能,又能完整地切除肿瘤。然而,早期的原位肝移植生存率低且复发率高。如今,移植患者的选择标准得到重新定义,移植的疗效也得到显著的提高[75]。

米兰标准是由 Mazzaferro 等在 1996 年的研究会上制订的[76]。米兰标准综合评估了因终末期肝病和肝癌而接受肝移植患者的放射学及病理学结果。据报道,单个肿瘤≤5cm,或不超过 3 个肿瘤,每个肿瘤不超过 3cm 的肝癌患者,肝移植后总体生存率和无病生存率分别为 85%和 92%,4 年内肝癌总体复发率为 8%。超出米兰标准的患者总体生存率为 50%,并且只有 59%的存活患者无肿瘤复发。目前,UNOS 和美国国家老年医疗保险将米兰标准作为选择原位肝移植患者的指南,各个地区也不尽相同。

在过去的十几年中,多项研究挑战了米兰标准。这些研究报道,进展期肝癌在移植后也能得到较好的效果。Yao 等发现肝癌患者移植后 5 年生存率为 70.2%,这一研究补充了美国加州大学(UCSF)标准[77],该标准基于移植物病理学,将单个肿瘤直径≤6.5cm,或 3 个肿瘤最大直径≤4.5cm 和累积肿瘤直径之和≤8cm 纳入肝移植适应证。

巴塞罗那临床肝脏中心(BCLC)已经建立了肝癌原位肝移植的治疗体系,该体系基于肿瘤分级、肝功能、全身状态及肿瘤相关症状[78]。BCLC 体系强调对丢失率及意向治疗的分析,同时它也延伸了移植标准,即单个肿瘤<7cm;有 3 个以内肿瘤,每个<5cm;5 个以内肿瘤,每个<3cm;或传统米兰标准级别较低但在移植前运用辅助治疗的患者都是肝移植的适应证。通过也能用这一标准,巴塞罗那中心治疗的患者的移植后 5 年生存率已经超过 50%,而姑息治疗的 5 年生存率为 20%。

随后的研究也支持 UCSF 和 BCLC 标准,基于这些研究 Mazzaferro 等提出了决策分析模型[76]。该模型遵从的理论是：肿瘤直径越大和（或）肿瘤个数增多，那么肝癌复发的风险越大。尽管这一模型没有被广泛接受，移植医师和外科医师都默认肿瘤大小和肿瘤数目与肿瘤的复发有关，而且选择移植患者的重要参考。

胆管癌

如今，肝门部胆管癌（CCA）尚无有效治疗方法。虽然CCA的患病率不高，但是其死亡率却与胰腺癌相当。外科切除是目前延长生存期的唯一途径，但是只有20%的患者能进行手术[79]。大多数患者被诊断为CCA后都会感到绝望。

手术切除是唯一有希望治愈胆管癌的方法，但是影响患者长期生存的主要因素是能否做到切缘肿瘤为阴性。手术切缘是否有肿瘤细胞室预测复发和预后的重要指标[80]。理论上，通过完整的肝脏切除和原位肝移植能够提高达到切缘阴性的可能性。对于孤立的肝门部胆管癌，原位肝移植效果非常好。梅奥诊所也证实，原位肝移植结合严格筛选患者、放射治疗和化疗增敏能够使CCA患者获得长期生存[81]。运用这一治疗原则，患者的1年、3年和5年的生存率分别为92%、82%和82%。

肝门部胆管癌患者在考虑肝移植时应该充分评估潜在的肝外疾病，包括淋巴结扩散。CT对检测肝内胆管肿瘤、胆管阻塞情况及肝脏是否萎缩敏感性较高。此外，CT还能够鉴别相关淋巴结有无转移，在判断能够手术时，增强CT能提供比MRI更多信息。CT和MRI在肿瘤强化和胆管扩张的诊断上效果相当，但CT能够更好地评估是否存在肿瘤血管或邻近器官侵犯。

许多患者在术前存在腹膜种植和局部淋巴结转移，这是无法通过影像学发现的。运用超声内镜可能对判断肿瘤的边界和探查淋巴结，尤其是远处的淋巴结是否受到侵犯有帮助。另外，在剖腹探查之前的诊断性腹腔镜检查可以帮助明确诊断[83]。有研究分析了腹腔镜检查在肝胆管及胰腺肿瘤的作用，发现腹腔镜检查在30%的病例中能发现未知的转移灶[84]。此外，腹腔镜检查为术中肝脏超声提供机会，这有利于判断是否存在肝内转移。然而，最终能否进行肝脏切除或肝移植取决于全面的腹部探查。

胆管癌患者是否需要肝移植尚有争议，因为胆管癌移植后复发率很高，多家医疗中心也因此放弃将胆管癌作为肝移植的适应证。最近一项对207例接受肝移植的胆管癌患者的研究报道，移植后胆管癌患者1年、2年和5年的生存率分别为72%、48%和23%，但是有大于50%的患者在术后2年内复发[85]。另一项研究报道，移植后CCA患者的3年生存率为30%，并且肿瘤较小和单个肿瘤的患者预后较好[86]。

基于这些数据，胆管癌患者是否选择肝移植进行治疗仍然值得商榷。随之辅助治疗及新辅助治疗的发展，肝移植治疗胆管癌的效果可能会逐渐变好。De-Vreede等的研究能支持这一推断。他们严格选择一期和二期胆管癌患者，在肝移植前接受新辅助体外照射治疗、系统的5-FU治疗及近距离放射治疗。这项研究中，11例接受移植的患者中有7例生存时间大于36个月，有8例患者在随访的44个月内无肿瘤复发。另一项相似的研究选择Ⅰ~Ⅲa的肝门部胆管癌患者进行新辅助放化疗，其中位随访时间（7.5年）的生存率为45%（11例患者5例存活）[87]，但是有2例患者因肿瘤复发而死亡。这些研究表明早期的胆管癌患者或许是肝移植的适应证。

良性肝脏疾病

并非所有的肝移植患者都有肝功能异常。对于良性肝脏疾病（既非恶性肿瘤也非慢性疾病）的患者，是否需要肝移植取决于移植能否改善患者的症状。

布加综合征（BCS）是由肝静脉流出道阻塞造成的，这导致小叶中心淤血、坏死和纤维化，严重的还会导致肝硬化[88]。这类患者是否需要肝移植由肝脏损害及肝功能异常的程度决定。急性BCS患者可能会有严重的肝细胞坏死而使得肝功能无法恢复正常。另外，慢性流出道梗阻可能导致纤维化和肝硬化，这类患者在肝功能不全时应考虑肝移植[89]。移植后仍有潜在的血栓形成的可能，因此必须长期使用抗凝药物。在美国，骨髓外增殖异常是BCS的常见原因[90]。筛选BCS患者作为移植对象时必须考虑患者能否长期使用抗凝药物[91]。BCS患者与非BCS患者在接受原位肝移植后，移植物和患者的1年、3年及5年的生存率相近[92]。因此，当BCS患者在进行药物、手术及放射治疗后，若效果不佳或出现肝功能失代偿，则应该考虑肝移植。

目前，肝移植也是治愈多囊肝（PCD）的唯一选择。这类患者肝移植的适应证主要取决于其症状[93]。当患者出现疼痛、营养低下、呼吸困难、疲乏或反复囊腔感染时，可通过肝移植改善生活质量[94]。PCD患者移植后预后极好,5 年生存率接近 92%。肝移植、肾移植同时实施时应考虑肝脏囊肿大小带来的全身症状。并非所有考虑肾移植的患者都会累积到肝脏,只有一小部分患者因肝脏受累带来症状而需要肾移植和肝移植同时进行[95]。

急性肝功能衰竭

在无其他肝脏疾病状态下发生的肝功能失代偿伴有意识改变(肝性脑病)和凝血功能障碍称为急性肝功能衰竭(ALF)。从发病到发展为肝性脑病的时间小于 8 周则成为暴发性肝功能衰竭(FHF),在 8 周到 26 周之间发展为肝性脑病者则称为亚急性暴发性肝功能衰竭(也称为迟发型肝功能衰竭)[96]。上述临床表现均称为急性肝功能衰竭。ALF 患者会出现多种致命的症状,如脑水肿、血流动力学不稳定、肾衰竭、重度代谢失衡、对真菌和细菌敏感性增加以及凝血功能障碍。

ALF 少见但不罕见,在美国,每年大约有 2000 例,其死亡率接近 80%。因 ALF 接受肝移植的患者占美国肝移植总数的 6%[97]。多数患者会出现大范围的肝细胞坏死,而肝功能衰竭但不伴有肝细胞坏死是妊娠期脂肪肝和 Reye 综合征的典型表现,这表明肝细胞坏死并不是 ALF 的必要特征。无论发病原因如何,典型的病理特征是肝小叶广泛坏死。

早期研究报道,在美国,病毒性肝炎是引起 ALF 最常见的病因,但是最近的研究表明,对乙酰氨基酚过量和特殊的药物反应已经成为引起 ALF 的最常见病因[96]。恶性肿瘤并不是 ALF 的常见病因,影像学检查对 ALF 的诊断意义不大,但肝组织活检有利于诊断。其他较少见的引起 FHF 病因包括:药物反应(如抗生素和抗病毒药物)、自身免疫性肝炎、妊娠相关疾病(如急性妊娠期脂肪肝)、HELLP 综合征(溶血、肝酶升高和血小板降低)、BCS、威尔逊病和毒性物质的吸收(如蜡样芽孢杆菌毒素和鹅膏蕈毒素)。

肝移植已经成为拯救生命、提高生存率的重要手段。尽管部分 ALF 患者可能自行恢复,但是对于亚急性暴发性肝功能衰竭患者, 如不进行肝移植, 死亡率为 100%[96]。外科技术的提高、免疫抑制剂的使用以及综合治疗的改善使得患者在肝移植后的 1 年、5 年和 10 年生存率分别约为 65%、59%和 54%[1]。ALF 患者存活时间超过 3 个月后,其生存曲线与肝硬化患者移植后的生存曲线相近[97]。选择合适合适的 FHF 患者,判断患者仅在药物治疗情况下能否存活仍然是在判断 FHF 患者是否需要肝移植过程中最棘手的问题。细致的筛选原则、积极的支持治疗和术前治疗有希望提高患者的预后。在第 47 章中将阐述新的肝辅助设备在 ALF 治疗中的应用。

移植物失活

肝移植的患者可能由于技术原因、移植物功能丧失及疾病复发造成移植物的失活而引起肝功能失代偿。这部分患者大约占美国肝移植总数的 10%。再次移植时应考虑到患者及移植物的存活时间比首次移植缩短[1]。丙型肝炎复发和严重的自身免疫性疾病可能是这类患者在再次移植时额外的危险因素[98]。血清胆红素升高、肌酸酐升高、Child-Pugh 评分≥10 分或 MELD 评分>25 分都是预后差的因素[99,100]。

评估

肝移植的评估过程是权衡死亡风险与移植获益的过程。这能保证移植受者能从移植中获得最大益处。评估时应考虑以下内容:是否缺乏基础疾病的替代治疗、移植后期望的生存期与当前报道的生存期相当或是更长以及可以接受的疾病复发率[101]。多学科移植小组在进行移植评估时必须充分评估患者的肝脏疾病、总体医疗和心理健康、感染风险、社会支持及资金支持。评估内容见表 29.2。

在评估过程中要回答 3 个简单的问题:

1.肝脏疾病是否恶化到需要肝移植的地步? 换句话说,在无肝脏疾病的替代治疗时,肝移植的益处是否大于其风险?移植评估的过程是移植造成死亡的总体风险与药物治疗和对症治疗存在的风险之间的博弈。

2.患者是否适合移植?移植协会指出,在决定患者是否适合做肝移植时,要考虑到患者医疗和社会健康的多方面因素。患者有并发症时,死亡风险增加,移植的益处减少。若患者缺乏社会或资金支持,或不能够遵从医嘱,那么移植的成功率就会降低。这些问题会影响总体风险与效益的评估。

3.在移植小组确定移植为治疗疾病的最好途径时,患者及其家属是否愿意接受移植存在的风险? 患者可以拒绝医师肝移植的建议,但是在医师决定移植的风险大于益处时,患者则无权要求进行移植。

评估过程需要肝脏病学及外科学的移植专家进行

会诊，共同对并发症及社会心理做出评估(见表29.2)。患者接受一系列的检查主要是为了发现影响预后的并发症。要将保险和处方的覆盖范围告知患者及其看护人。最后，有必要要求患者及其家属参加家庭会议，通过会议明确患者的社会支持及资源，也能够进一步地了解患者及其家属对移植的需求。

心肺评估

在过去的20年中，肝移植的效果逐渐提升[102]，移植医师也越来越愿意接受风险较高的患者，这也反映出对肝移植受者的麻醉、手术及综合护理方面的进步。早期的绝对禁忌证如严重的心血管和肺部疾病已经成为相对禁忌证。移植中心已经建立了系统的术前心肺疾病的评估标准，目的在于最大可能地争取移植机会和降低风险。

肝移植前的评估主要分为两个方面：①个人评价和围术期并发症风险的评价；②评估远期疗效及潜在的肝外症状，以建立真实的风险效益比。对于潜在的活体肝脏的受者，还需要评估的是与受者生活质量相关的捐赠手术的风险，并且需要合理评估尸体肝移植的时间。肝移植本身的风险和供体短缺的现状使得移植医师必须选择能从肝移植中获益的患者进行手术。

心脏评估

当今的肝移植受者比20年前或30年前的受者年龄大，伴随疾病也较多。早期对肝移植受者的研究发现终末期肝病的患者很少伴有冠心病(CAD)。然而，最近的研究证实，与其他接受外科手术的患者相比，肝移植受者中冠心病的发病率并不低[103,104]。一些证据表明肝硬化引起的特异性心肌病可能会导致严重的心血管事件[105]。

据估计在肝移植期间，心血管事件的发生率为25%~70%[106,107]，心血管事件的发生将严重影响患者及移植物的存活时间。心血管疾病是除了肿瘤复发和新发肿瘤之外的导致肝移植患者远期死亡的最主要原因[108]。因此，肝移植患者术前的心脏评估已经引起重视，并且变得越来越重要，因为其对术后的疗效有着重要的影响。心脏评估的过程很复杂，并且不同中心评价方式也有差异。

与其他移植手术或腹部手术相比，肝移植能导致严重的血流动力学改变，从而诱发冠心病。尽管与之前的研究相比，心脏病的发病率和死亡率在升高，但是由于在患者筛选、冠心病的管理机移植患者围术期管理

表29.2 评估

医疗/外科
会诊
• 肝脏病学
• 移植外科
实验室
• 完善的血细胞计数，包括血小板
• 生化检查包括电解质、血尿素氮、肌酐及肝功能
• 凝血酶原时间(PT)、活化部分凝血酶原时间(PTT)、国际标准比值(INR)
• 肿瘤标志物甲胎蛋白(AFP)和癌胚抗原(CEA)，必要时检查CA19-9
• 抗人免疫缺陷病毒(HIV)/HIV2
• 性病实验室检查
• 血清学检查包括抗HCV抗体、HBsAg、抗-HBc抗体、抗HBs抗体、抗HAV IgG抗体、抗HSV IgG抗体、抗CMV IgG抗体、抗EB病毒核心抗原IgG抗体，抗弓形虫IgG抗体、抗带状疱疹IgG抗体
• 男性需检查前列腺抗原(PSA)
• 铁、总铁结合力(TIBC)和血清铁蛋白
• 抗核抗体(ANA)、抗线粒体抗体(AMA)抗平滑肌抗体(ASMA)
• 血清蛋白电泳(SPEP)
• 血浆铜蓝蛋白
• α-1抗胰蛋白酶
影像学
• 肝脏多普勒超声
• 肝脏CT或MRI
• 正、侧位胸片
心肺检查
• 心内科会诊
• 多巴酚丁胺超声心动图或其他非侵入性的心脏压力检查
• 动脉血气
• 心电图
• 部分患者肺部会诊
其他检查
• 女性乳腺X线片
• 结核菌素试验(PDD)
• 结肠镜(50岁以上的患者结肠癌风险增加)
• 肺功能检查(有吸烟史患者、有症状患者或存在肺部疾病风险的患者)
• 骨密度检查
• 部分行冠状动脉造影检查
心理评估
• 社会工作者评估
• 药物依赖评估(有药物滥用史)
• 心理筛查与评估
资金
• 确定移植及药物费用与患者的承受能力

方面的进步,其仍然比无冠心病的患者高。

肝移植受者最佳的筛查策略仍然是讨论的焦点,因为各个中心的非侵入性检查结果及算法各不相同。术前检查必须包括心血管病史检查,以发现存在的症状和危险因素。终末期肝患者群的冠心病症状可能并不典型,例如胸痛和呼吸短促可由运动诱发。因此,几乎所有的终末期肝病患者伴发冠心病时症状都不典型,因而有必要检查潜在的心脏疾病。

美国心脏病协会建议非心脏病手术也要进行围术期的心脏评估,这已经运用到肝移植前的评估体系中了[109]。非侵入性压力检查通常是移植前检查的第一步(各个机构有一定差异)。不幸的是,之前关于终末期肝病患者心脏病危险因素的研究已经失败,也没有形成最佳危险分层的策略[110]。一项研究对 45 岁以上无冠心病症状的肝移植受者进行了回顾性分析,冠状动脉造影结果表明 26%的受者存在中到重度的冠心病[111]。非酒精性脂肪性肝炎能是冠心病的独立危险因素[112]。

移植受者最常用的筛查冠心病的检查是多巴酚丁胺压力超声心动图(DSE)和心肌灌注闪烁显像(MPS)。若检查结果为阳性,则需进行冠状动脉造影检查,有些中心使用心脏 CT 或磁共振血管造影(MRA)来评估冠心病[109]。在普通人群中,DSE 和 MPS 能较好地发现冠心病,但是在终末期肝病患者中其敏感性和特异性分别为 12%~100%和 57%~100%[101]。在多数肝移植中心会选择 DSE 检查,因为 DSE 的敏感性比 MPS 高,而且能够提供左心室及瓣膜功能的整体情况。在所有的筛查方法中,必须关注某些特殊的人群,如频繁使用 β 受体阻滞剂的肝硬化患者及使用血管扩张药物的患者,这可能影响其对变时性药物如多巴酚丁胺或扩张药物如腺苷或双嘧达莫的反应[113,114]。

最近,心脏 CT 在检出和量化冠状动脉钙化方面的进步已经提高了心血管病在普通人群中的检出检出率。McAvoy 等最近的一项研究发现,在肝移植患者中,冠状动脉钙化与许多已知的心血管病的危险因素有强烈的相关性[115]。尽管使用钙化评级作为肝移植中预测心血管事件的依据需要进一步的评估,但其在其他外科手术中确实有一定的用武之地。

不同中心对患有阻塞性冠心病的移植受者的处理方法不尽相同。肝移植必须要推迟到血管重建或经皮冠状动脉介入治疗后,或者用合适的药物如 β 受体阻滞剂进行治疗[116,117]。然而,等待血管重建的过程是否会影响肝移植的时机尚不可知。在普通人群中,当无局部缺血或症状时,预防血管再生的药物并不优于传统的药物治疗[118]。另一方面,肝移植患者这一特殊群体具有的特征常常会掩盖了心脏疾病,而且移植手术本身带来的压力可能会影响 DSE 和 MPS 的结果。因此,要全面分析患者本身和总体的身体状况、副发病变及各种检查得到的结果。

肺部评估

肝移植受者的心脏检查得到了更多的重视,但已有的肺部疾病同样会增加围术期的风险。吸烟或其他病因引起的慢性阻塞性肺疾病(COPD)和肺气肿、原发性或门脉性肺动脉高压、肝肺综合征或肝性胸水都可能发生于肝硬化患者,这些无疑会给围术期患者肺部的管理带来新的挑战。肝移植时,确立诊断和判断潜在的肺部疾病同样重要。本部分将讨论终末期肝病患者最常见的影响移植的肺部问题。

COPD 在肝硬化患者中较常见,其在移植受者中的发病率为 18%[119,120]。尽管无统一的数据,但是 COPD 无疑会影响肝移植患者的长期生存[121]。当移植患者伴有 COPD 时,术后特护病房和院内住院时长、通气设备依赖、出院后康复及感染风险都会受到影响。另外,肝移植后再次吸烟可能会增加新发肝癌的风险[122]。

COPD 常用第 1 秒用力呼气容积(FEV_1)进行分级。BODE(体质指数、气道阻塞、呼吸困难和运动能力)指数是多方面的分级体系,该体系比单独的肺功能检查在预测各种原因及 COPD 引起的气道原因导致死亡风险上有更大的优势[123,124]。准确的气道评估,包括徒步实验,应该在伴有 COPD 的肝移植患者中强制实施。

肝硬化患者常有腹水和胸水,这会影响氧合和通气。肝性胸腔积液的定义是肝硬化患者无原发性心肺疾病而发生胸腔积液[125]。5%~12%的腹水患者伴有肝性胸腔积液。腹水会导致腹内压增高,隔膜升高,并引起肺容积和胸廓顺应性降低。终末期肝病患者的胸腔积液可能会因低蛋白血症和奇静脉压力增高而加重[126]。

胸腔积液形成的原因是由于腹水通过隔膜缺陷直接进入胸膜腔。当腹腔积液在胸膜腔积聚超过了胸膜的吸收能力就会形成肝性胸水。右侧胸腔较常出现不明原因的胸腔积液。有趣的是,在无临床可检测出的腹水患者中,有 20%的患者出现肝性腹水[126]。

对于有肝性胸水的肝移植受者,需进行胸部 X 线和胸部CT扫描来排除原发的引起胸腔积液的肺部疾病。重要的是判断有无纵隔淋巴结肿大以区别恶性胸水。检查包括诊断性胸腔穿刺,若为蛋白水平较低、细胞计数较少则为无菌渗出液。还应该评估培养物、真菌和革兰染色以及耐酸杆菌染色,并进行细胞学检查以排除恶性肿瘤。必须排除感染和恶性肿瘤,这可能需要胸腔镜进行胸膜活检。最后,腹水患者也应进行诊断性穿刺[127]。

肝肺综合征是指慢性肝脏疾病伴有呼吸困难、低氧和肺分流增加等症状。一些报道提出了解决肝移植后肝肺综合征的方法[128]。因此,尽管在肝移植前诊断和治疗肝肺综合征很重要,但不应将其作为肝移植的禁忌证。

肝硬化患者可能会有肺动脉高压,由于缺乏症状,可能在移植评估时才被诊断出来。肺动脉压增高的肝硬化患者死亡率比肺动脉正常的患者死亡率高。此外,肺动脉压高的患者围术期的死亡率增高,并且被认为是移植的禁忌证[129,130]。对静脉注射前列腺素敏感的患者可考虑进行肝移植[131],因为其肺动脉压力在移植后可能会恢复正常[132]。

心理评估

肝移植患者除了需要全面的临床评估以确定相关风险及移植的益处,还需要全面的心理评估。然而,对于移植前心理和社会筛查,基于证据的指南相对较少[133,134]。在多数移植中心是由精神科医生和社会工作者进行正式的心理评估,观察患者在移植前期对药物和医嘱的依从性与肝移植后1年预后有很强的相关性[135]。神经质和有限的社会支持可能会对肝移植产生负面影响,而积极的应对技能可能会使情况有所改善[136]。

对于有酗酒史的患者,“6个月”原则已经成为评估肝移植的标准方法[137]。一项Meta分析将戒酒6个月作为移植前预测移植后酒精复饮的三个因素之一[138],尽管目前戒酒的时间还有争议[139]。评估的目的是判断患者移植后保持戒酒状态的可能性。这需要成瘾疾病专家进行评估[140]。

应该对患者进行抑郁症的筛查,有抑郁症病史的患者应该由精神科医生进一步评估。心理健康问题在晚期肝病患者中较常见[141],而且抑郁症可能影响移植后精神病的患病率和依从性[142,143]。如果认为患者精神状态稳定,不影响恢复,则可进行肝移植。在等待期间或移植后,对精神病患者的随访建议应因患者而异。

尽管多数中心认为,持续使用成瘾的药物是肝移植的禁忌证[144],但是最近的研究发现56%的回应者接受肝移植患者持续使用美沙酮[145]。然而,该研究也发现32%的回应者认为在移植前应该终止美沙酮的使用。一些研究发现使用美沙酮替代药物的患者能成功地进行肝移植,且其预后与使用美沙酮的患者预后相似[146]。因此,各个中心有必要建立对药物成瘾患者进行移植的筛选原则。

感染性疾病的评估

对肝移植受者移植前感染性疾病的评估包括免疫病史、腹膜炎和胆管炎病史及旅游史。

推荐的检查包括肺结核、肝炎和曾经接触某种病毒或其他病原体(见表29.2)。这使得在移植前可以使用适当的疫苗,或者对有感染风险的患者采取一定的预防策略。

Schaffner概述了筛选肝移植受者的4个重要目标[147]:

1.确定移植受者对因移植而获得的一般病原体的免疫能力。

2.允许将来自感染了某种病原体的供体的器官分配给已经是病原体携带者的受体。

3.识别和治疗免疫抑制剂治疗后引起的感染。

4.避免为移植后预后较差的患者行移植手术。

建议通过实验室检查指导移植前后的筛选和感染的预防。

急性肝功能衰竭患者的选择

目前,对FHF患者进行肝移植的筛选原则尚无统一标准。急性肝功能衰竭患者与因慢性疾病而需要肝移植的患者的检查类似。最常用的标准是伦敦国王学院医院建立的,该标准基于对1973年至1985年间588例药物治疗的患者可能预后因素的回顾性、多因素分析[148](见表29.3)。其他中心已经注意到,尽管这一标准的实现对自发生存的预后不良,但若缺乏这一标准,可能会有更差的结果[149,150]。

最近的分析旨在考虑未纳入国王学院标准的其他因素是否与预后有关[150]。几项研究研究对白细胞计数、高血钾和乳酸盐水平进行了分析[151]。不幸的是,许多危险因素出现在临床晚期,只有在进行肝移植后才会好转,因此,这些因素就失去了其在决定肝移植时机及筛选移植受者中的作用。

肝移植已经成为拯救生命,提高生存率的重要手

表 29.3　急性肝功能衰竭的国王学院标准

对乙酰氨基酚过量
动脉血 pH 值<7.3 或满足以下三项：
• 凝血酶原时间>100s
• 肌酸酐>300μmol/L
• 3 期或 4 期肝性脑病
非对乙酰氨基酚过量
凝血酶原时间>100s 或国际标准比率 (INR)>6.7 或以下三项中任何一项
• 无直接原因（无甲型肝炎、乙型肝炎、氟烷性肝炎及药物性肝炎）
• 肝性脑病前出现黄疸>7 天
• 年龄<10 岁或>40 岁
• 凝血酶原时间>50s 或 INR>4
• 血清胆红素>300μmol/L

段。外科技术的进步、免疫抑制剂的使用及综合照护已经使得移植后患者的 1 年、5 年和 10 年生存率分别达到 65%、59%和 54%[1]。存活时间超过 3 个月后，患者的生存率与肝硬化而抑制的患者的生存率相当。选择合适的 FHF 患者，决定哪些患者仅在药物治疗就能下能好转，这仍然是目前较为棘手的问题。进一步地弄清筛选标准、重症监护支持和围手术期的护理的提高可能会提高患者的临床预后。

肝癌患者的选择

迄今为止，对肝移植中肝癌患者的最大的前瞻性单机构的研究来自加利福尼亚大学洛杉矶分校，该研究证实患者预后差的因素包括肿瘤数目、淋巴血管侵犯及肿瘤分化差。这些发现确认了之前的一系列研究，也强调了肿瘤的生物学特征而不是大小或数量决定了肝癌患者进行肝移植的预后[152]。因此，有些研究者认为术前的影像学检查是有好处的，经导管动脉消融(TACE)或射频消融(RFA)拥有更好的价值。要阐述这一理论还需要更多的研究，尤其在移植前评估肿瘤生物学行为的最好方法方面，是血清学还是影像学检查。

长期的供体短缺和肝癌生长引起的移植受者的高丢失率，使得移植受者的选择成为治疗晚期肝癌的决定因素，并且，移植前的辅助治疗也成为重要的组成部分。在等待供体期间的，控制肿瘤的生长益处良多，包括避免移植前死亡、降低移植后肝癌复发率和提高这类患者的总体生存率。

尽管单一治疗能减缓肝癌生长，但是综合治疗更能促进肿瘤的坏死，因而，移植后的复发率会降低。许多中心，尤其是加州大学旧金山分校，通过非控制性实验已经发现综合治疗能使患者在等待移植时的丢失率降低，提高生存率，及降低复发率[77]。同时，Freeman 等通过对 1997 年至 2006 年间 SRTR 数据库中的病例做了回顾性的研究[153]，他们也得到了相似的结论。他们注意到，在等待期间进行肝癌切除或局部消融的移植等待者移植后 3 年的生存率有所提高。

基于这些发现，来自加州大学洛杉矶分校的 Duffy 等提出，术前肿瘤的分期最好在进行肝移植的 6 个月内通过 CT 或 MRI 扫描进行，或者通过肝组织活检对病理分级进行评估，及判断有无血管、淋巴管的转移[154]。由于对于肝硬化患者，肝组织活检确实存在取样错误、出血及肿瘤扩散等风险，有些医师认为只有当肿瘤直径≥3cm 时，或肿瘤对局部治疗不敏感是才考虑使用肝组织活检。

建立筛选委员会

一旦患者完成了内科、外科及心理/经济评估，那么筛选委员会就可以对其移植过程进行讨论。委员会一般由代表肝脏病学及外科学、移植护理、精神病学、药物依赖、经济支持、饮食及社会工作等领域的专家组成。在评估患者过程中，有些问题可能需要进一步的协商或考查。讨论过程能使得委员会在评估过程中获得完整的数据，如决定相关风险、利益，并且为最终决定移植受者提供建议。

总结

当肝移植给患者带来的总体好处大于风险时才会考虑肝移植。在评估过程中应当考虑总体内科和外科风险、心理支持和经济支持。移植小组应该共同合作做出移植的决定，并综合考虑患者各个方面的检查。对于进行性肝功能衰竭的患者，是否移植可能会受到疾病的预后及并发症的死亡风险影响。对于肝癌患者，移植的好处可能在于减少肿瘤的复发。对于其他类型的患者，肝移植的总体需求/好处或许在于提高生活质量。无论适应证如何，移植小组对每个患者的评估过程就是在权衡移植给患者带来的总体风险和潜在利益。

（王亚洲　译　张大方　校）

参考文献

1. Health Resources and Services. Administration/Organ Procurement and Transplantation Network. [accessed December 16, 2011]; Available from: http://optn.transplant.hrsa.gov/latestData.
2. Lucey MR, Brown KA, Everson GT, et al. Minimal criteria for placement of adults on the liver transplant waiting list: a report of a national conference organized by the American Society of Transplant Physicians and the American Association for the Study of liver Diseases. Liver Transplantation and Surgery. 1997;3(6): 628–637.
3. D'Amico G, Garcia-Tsao G, Pagliaro L. Natural history and prognostic indicators of survival in cirrhosis: a systematic review of 118 studies. Journal of Hepatology. 2006;44:217–231.
4. Christensen E, Schlichting P, Fauerholdt L, et al. Prognostic value of Child-Turcotte criteria in medially treated cirrhosis. Hepatology. 1984;4(3): 430–435.
5. Lake JR, Wright TL. Liver transplantation for patients with hepatitis B: what have we learned from our results? Hepatology. 1991;13:769–9.
6. Todo S, Demetris AJ, Van Thiel D, et al. Orthotropic liver transplantation for patients with hepatitis B virus-related liver disease. Hepatology. 1991;13: 619–626.
7. Samuel D, Muller R, Alexander G, et al. Liver transplantation in European patients with the hepatitis B surface antigen. New England Journal of Medicine. 1993;329:1842–1847.
8. Liaw YF, Sung JJ, Chow WC, et al. Lamivudine for patients with chronic hepatitis B and advanced liver disease. New England Journal of Medicine. 2004; 351:1521–1531.
9. Kapoor D, Guptan RC, Wakil SM, et al. Beneficial effects of lamivudine in hepatitis B virus-related decompensated cirrhosis. Journal of Hepatology. 2000; 33:308–312.
10. Yao FY, Terrault NA, Freise C, et al. Lamivudine treatment is beneficial in patients with severely decompensated cirrhosis and actively replicating hepatitis B infection awaiting liver transplantation: a comparative study using a matched, untreated cohort. Hepatology. 2001;34:411–416.
11. Villeneuve JP, Condreay LD, Willems B, et al. Lamivudine treatment for decompensated cirrhosis resulting from chronic hepatitis B. Hepatology. 2000;31: 207–210.
12. Schiff E, Lai CL, Hadziyannis S, et al. Adefovir dipivoxil for wait-listed and post-liver transplantation patients with lamivudine-resistant hepatitis B: final long-term results. Liver Transplantation. 2007;13:349–360.
13. Lok AS, Lai CL, Leung N, et al. Long-term safety of lamivudine treatment in patients with chronic hepatitis B. Gastroenterology. 2003;125:1714–1722.
14. Natsuizaka M, Hige S, Ono Y, et al. Long-term follow-up of chronic hepatitis B after the emergence of mutations in the hepatitis B virus polymerase region. Journal of Viral Hepatitis. 2005;12:154–159.
15. Shim JH, Lee HC, Kim KM, et al. Efficacy of entecavir in treatment-naïve patients with hepatitis B virus-related decompensated cirrhosis. Journal of Hepatology. 2010;52:176–182.
16. Keeffe EB, Dieterich DT, Han SH, et al. A treatment algorithm for the management of chronic hepatitis B virus infection in the United States: 2008 update. Clinical Gastroenterology and Hepatology. 2008;6:1315–1341.
17. Lok AS, McMahon BJ. Chronic hepatitis B. Hepatology. 2007;45:57–39.
18. European Association for the Study of the Liver. EASL clinical practice guidelines: management of chronic hepatitis B. Journal of Hepatology. 2009;50: 227–242.
19. Kim RW, Terrault NA, Pedersen RA, et al. Trends in waiting list registration for liver transplantation for viral hepatitis in the United States. Gastroenterology. 2009;137:1680–1686.
20. Kim WR, Poterucha JJ, Kremers WK, et al. Outcome of liver transplantation for hepatitis B in the United States. Liver Transplantation. 2004;10:968–974.
21. Bzowej N, Han S, Degertekin B, et al. Liver transplantation outcomes among Caucasians, Asian Americans, and African Americans with hepatitis B. Liver Transplantation. 2009;15(9):1010–1020.
22. Armstrong GL, Wasley A, Simard EP, et al. The prevalence of hepatitis C infection in the United States, 1999 through 2002. Annals of Internal Medicine. 2006;144: 705–714.
23. Davis G, Albright J, Cook S, et al. Projecting the future healthcare burden from hepatitis C in the United States. Hepatology. 1998;28:390A.
24. Forman L, Lewis JD, Berlin JA, et al. The association between hepatitis C infection and graft survival after liver transplantation. Gastroenterology. 2002;122: 889–896.
25. Berenguer M, Prieto M, Rayon JM, et al. Natural history of clinically compensated hepatitis C virus-related graft cirrhosis after liver transplantation. Hepatology. 2000;32:852–858.
26. Belle SH, Beringer KC, Detre KM, et al. Liver transplantation for alcoholic liver disease in the United States: 1988 to 1995. Liver Transplantation and Surgery. 1997;3:212–219.
27. Gedaly R, McHugh PP, Johnston TD, et al. Predictors of relapse to alcohol and illicit drugs after liver transplantation for alcoholic liver disease. Transplantation. 2008;86:1090–1095.
28. Gish RG, Lee AH, Keefe EB, et al. Liver transplantation for patients with alcoholism and end-stage liver disease. American Journal of Gastroenterology. 1993;88: 1337–1342.
29. Foster PF, Fabrega F, Karademir S, et al. Prediction of abstinence from ethanol in alcoholic recipients following liver transplantation. Hepatology. 1997;25: 1469–1477.
30. DiMartini A, Day N, Dew MA, et al. Alcohol consumption patterns and predictors of use following liver transplantation for alcoholic liver disease. Liver Transplantation. 2006;12:813–820.
31. Dew M, DiMartini AF, Steel J, et al. Meta-analysis of risk for relapse to substance use after transplantation of the liver or other solid organs. Liver Transplantation. 2008;14:159–172.
32. Ogden CL, Carroll MD, Curtin LR, et al. Prevalence of overweight and obesity in the United States, 1999–2004. JAMA. 2005;295:1549–1555.
33. Sturm R. Increases in clinically severe obesity in the United States, 1986–2000. Archives of Internal Medicine. 2003;163:2146–2148.
34. Nair S, Verma S, Thuluvath PJ, et al. Obesity and its effect on survival in patients undergoing orthotropic liver transplantation in the United States. Hepatology. 2002;35:105–109.
35. Pelletier SJ, Schaubel DE, Wei G, et al. Effect of body mass index on the survival benefit of liver transplantation. Liver Transplantation. 2007;13:1678–1683.
36. Charlton MR, Burns JM, Pedersen RA, et al. Frequency and outcomes of liver transplantation for non-alcoholic steatohepatitis in the United States. Gastroenterology. 2011;141:1249–1253.
37. Caldwell SH, Lee VD, Kleiner DE, et al. NASH and cryptogenic cirrhosis; a histological analysis. Annals of Hepatology. 2009;8:346–352.
38. Caldwell SH, Oelsner DH, Lezzoni JC, et al. Cryptogenic cirrhosis; clinical characterization and risk factors for underlying disease. Hepatology. 1999;29: 664–669.
39. Kim WR, Poterrucha JJ, Porayko MK, et al. Recurrence of nonalcoholic steatohepatitis following liver transplantation. Transplantation. 1996;62:1802–1805.
40. McCaughan GW. Recurrence of nonalcoholic steatohepatitis (NASH) post-liver transplantation. Liver Transplantation and Surgery. 1997;3:683.
41. Bhagat V, Mindikoglu AL, Nudo CG, et al. Outcomes of liver transplantation in patients with cirrhosis due to nonalcoholic steatohepatitis versus patients with cirrhosis due to alcoholic liver disease. Liver Transplantation. 2009;15: 1814–1820.
42. Malik SM, DeVera ME, Fontes P, et al. Outcome after liver transplantation for NASH cirrhosis. American Journal of Transplantation. 2009;9:782–793.
43. Barritt SA, Dellon ES, Kozlowski T, et al. Influence of non alcoholic fatty liver disease and associated co-morbidities on transplant outcomes. Liver Transplantation. 2009;15:968–977.
44. Nair S, Verma S, Thuluvath PJ. Obesity and its effect on survival in patients undergoing orthotropic liver transplantation in the United States. Hepatology. 2002;35:105–109.
45. Dick AA, Spitzer AL, Seifert CF, et al. Liver transplantation at the extremes of the body mass index. Liver Transplantation. 2009;15(8):968–977.
46. Shields PL, Tang H, Neuberger JM, et al. Poor outcome in patients with diabetes mellitus undergoing liver transplantation. Transplantation. 1999;68:530–535.
47. John PR, Thuluvath PJ. Outcome of liver transplantation in patients with diabetes mellitus; a case-control study. Hepatology. 2001;34:889–895.
48. Lee J, Belanger A, Doucette JT, et al. Transplantation trends in primary biliary cirrhosis. Clinical Gastroenterology and Hepatology. 2007;5:1313–1315.
49. Tinmouth J, Tomlinson G, Heathcote EJ, et al. Benefit of transplantation in primary biliary cirrhosis between 1985–1997. Transplantation. 2002;73:224–227.
50. Bergasa NV. The pruritus of chronic cholestasis. Gut. 2004;53:475–477.
51. Heathcoate EJ, Cauch-Dudek K, Walker V, et al. The Canadian multicenter trial double-blind randomized controlled trial of ursodeoxycholic acid in primary biliary cirrhosis in Ontario, Canada. Hepatology. 1990;12:98–105.
52. Huet PM, Deslauriers J, Tran A, et al. Impact of fatigue on the quality of life in patients with primary biliary cirrhosis. American Journal of Gastroenterology. 2000;95:760–767.
53. Gross CR, Malinchoc M, Kim WR, et al. Quality of life before and after liver transplantation for cholestatic liver disease. Hepatology. 1999;29:356–364.
54. Christensen E, Gunson B, Neuberger J. Optimal timing of liver transplantation

for patients with primary biliary cirrhosis, use of prognostic modeling. Journal of Hepatology. 1999;29:356–364.
55. Dickson ER, Grambsch PM, Fleming TR, et al. Prognosis in primary biliary cirrhosis: model for decision making. Hepatology. 1989;10:1–7.
56. Kim WR, Therneau TM, Wiesner RH, et al. A revised natural history model for primary sclerosing cholangitis. Mayo Clinic Proceedings. Mayo Clinic. 2000;75:688–694.
57. Said A, Williams J, Holden J, et al. Model for end stage liver disease score predicts mortality across a broad spectrum of liver disease. Journal of Hepatology. 2004; 40(6):897–903.
58. Burak K, Anjulo P, Pasha TM, et al. Incidence and risk factors for cholangiocarcinoma in primary sclerosing cholangitis. American Journal of Gastroenterology. 2004;99(3):523–526.
59. Goss JA, Shackleton CR, Farmer DG, et al. Orthotropic liver transplantation for primary sclerosing cholantitis: a 12-year single center experience. Annals of Surgery. 1997;225(5):472–483.
60. Duclos-Vallee JC, Segagh M. Recurrence of autoimmune disease, primary sclerosing cholangitis, primary biliary cirrhosis, and autoimmune hepatitis after liver transplantation. Liver Transplantation. 2009;15:S25–S34.
61. Gautam M, Cheruvattath R, Balan V, et al. Recurrence of autoimmune liver disease after liver transplantation; a systematic review. Liver Transplantation. 2006;12:1813–1824.
62. Reich DJ, Fiel I, Guarrera JV, et al. Liver transplantation for autoimmune hepatitis. Hepatology. 2000;32:693–700.
63. Vennarecci G, Gunson BK, Ismail T, et al. Transplantation for end stage liver disease related to alph-1-antitrypsin. Transplantation. 1996;6:1488–1495.
64. Elzouki AN, Erillsson S. Risk of hepatobiliary disease in adults with severe alpha-1-antitrypsin deficiency (PiZZ); is chronic viral hepatitis B or C an additional risk factor for cirrhosis and hepatocellular carcinoma? European Journal of Gastroenterology and Hepatology. 1996;8:989–994.
65. Roberts MS, Angus DC, Bryce CL, et al. Survival after liver transplantation in the United States; a disease-specific analysis of the UNOS database. Liver Transplantation. 2004;10:886–897.
66. Mainous AG, Gill JM, Pearson WS, et al. Should we screen for hemochromatosis? An examination of evidence of downstream effects on morbidity and mortality. Archives of Internal Medicine. 2002;162:1769–1774.
67. Niederau C, Fischer R, Sonnenberg A, et al. Survival and causes of death in cirrhotic and non-cirrhotic patients with primary hemochromatosis. New England Journal of Medicine. 1985;313:1256–1262.
68. Kowdley KV, Hassanein T, Kaur S, et al. Primary liver cancer and survival in patients undergoing liver transplantation for hemochromatosis. Liver Transplantation and Surgery. 1995;1:237–241.
69. Brandhagen DJ, Alvarez W, Therneau TM, et al. Iron overload in cirrhosis-HFE phenotypes and outcome after liver transplantation. Hepatology. 2000;31: 456–460.
70. Crawford DH, Fletcher LM, Hubscher SG, et al. Patient and graft survival after liver transplantation for hereditary hemochromatosis; implications for pathogenesis. Hepatology. 2004;39:1655–1662.
71. Murray KF, Carithers RL. AASLD practice guidelines: evaluation of the patients for liver transplantation. Hepatology. 2005;41:1–26.
72. Schilsky MI, Scheinberg IH, Sternlieb I, et al. Prognosis of Wilsonian chronic active hepatitis. Gastroenterology. 1991;100:762–767.
73. Guarino M, Stracciari A, D'Alessandro R, et al. No neurological improvement after liver transplantation for Wilson's disease. Acta Neurologica Scandinavica. 1995;92:405–408.
74. Bellary S, Hassanein T, Van-Thiel DH, et al. Liver transplantation for Wilson's disease. Journal of Hepatology. 1995;23:373–381.
75. Llovet JM, Schwartz M, Mazzaferro V, et al. Resection and liver transplantation for hepatocellular carcinoma. Seminars in Liver Disease. 2005;25:181–200.
76. Mazzaferro V, Regalia E, Doci R, et al. Liver Transplantation for the treatment of small hepatocellular carcinomas in patients with cirrhosis. New England Journal of Medicine. 1996;334:693–699.
77. Yao FY, Kinkhabwala M, LaBerge JM, et al. The impact of pre-operative loco regional therapy on outcome after liver transplantation for hepatocellular carcinoma. American Journal of Transplantation. 2005;5(4 Pt 1):795–804.
78. Llovet JM, Fuster J, Bruix J, et al. The Barcelona approach: diagnosis, staging, and treatment of hepatocellular carcinoma. Liver Transplantation. 2004; 10(2 Suppl 1):S115–S120.
79. Freeman RB Jr, Steffick DE, Guidinger MK, et al. Liver and intestine transplantation in the United States, 1997–2006. American Journal of Transplantation. 2008;8(4 Pt 2):958–976.
80. Nagorney DM, Donohue JH, Farnell MB, et al. Outcomes after curative resections of cholangiocarcinoma. Archives of Surgery. 1993;128:871–877; discussion 877–879.
81. De Vreede I, Steers JL, Burch PA, et al. Prolonged disease-free survival after orthotropic liver transplantation plus adjuvant chemoirradiation for cholangiocarcinoma. Liver Transplantation. 2000;6:309–16.
82. Valls C, Guma A, Puig I, et al. Intrahepatic peripheral cholangiocarcinoma: CT evaluation. Abdominal Imaging. 2000;25:490–496.
83. Corvera CU, Weber SM, Jarnagin WR, et al. Role of laparoscopy in the evaluation of biliary tract cancer. Surgical Oncology Clinics of North America. 2002;11:877–891.
84. Callery MP, Strasberg SM, Doherty GM, et al. Staging laparoscopy with laparoscopic ultrasonography: optimizing respectability in hepatobiliary and pancreatic malignancy. Journal of the American College of Surgeons. 1997;185:33–39.
85. Meyer CG, Penn I, James L, et al. Liver transplantation for cholangiocarcinoma: results in 207 patients. Transplantation. 2000;69:1633–1637.
86. Shimoda M, Farmer DG, Colquhoun SD, et al. Liver transplantation for cholangiocellular carcinoma: analysis of a single-center experience and review of the literature. Liver Transplantation. 2001;7:1023–1033.
87. Sudan D, DeRoover A, Chinnakotla S, et al. Radiochemotherapy and transplantation allow long-term survival for non-respectable hilar cholangiocarcinoma. American Journal of Transplantation. 2002;2:774–779.
88. Tanaka M, Wanless IR. Pathology of the liver in Budd-Chiari syndrome: portal vein thrombosis and the histogenesis of veno-centric cirrhosis, veno-portal cirrhosis, and large regenerative nodules. Hepatology. 1998;27:488.
89. Klein AS, Molmenti EP. Surgical treatment of Budd-Chiari syndrome. Liver Transplantation. 2003;9:891.
90. Cruz E, Ascher NL, Roberts JP, et al. High incidence of recurrence and hematologic events following liver transplantation for Budd-Chiari syndrome. Clinical Transplantation. 2005;19:501.
91. Srinivasan P, Rela M, Prachalias A, et al. Liver transplantation for Budd-Chiari syndrome. Transplantation. 2002;73:973.
92. Melear JM, Goldstein RM, Levy MF, et al. Hematologic aspects of liver transplantation for Budd-Chiari. Transplantation. 2002;7:1090–1095.
93. Drenth J, Chrispijn M, Nagorney D, et al. Medical and surgical treatment options for polycystic liver disease. Hepatology. 2010;52:2223–2230.
94. Stickel F, Inderbitzin D, Candinas D, et al. Role of nutrition in liver transplantation for end-stage chronic liver disease. Nutrition Reviews. 2008;66:47–54.
95. Teperman L. Systematic review; the pathophysiology and management of polycystic liver disease. Alimentary Pharmacology and Therapeutics. 2011;34(7): 702–713.
96. Lee WM. Acute liver failure. New England Journal of Medicine. 1993;329: 1862–1872.
97. US Scientific Registry (UNOS). Richmond (VA); United Network for Organ Sharing. [Accessed January 12, 2012]; Available from: http://www.unos.org.
98. Yoo HY, Maheshwari A, Thuluvath PJ, et al. Re-transplantation of the liver: primary graft non-function and hepatitis C virus are associated with worse outcome. Liver Transplantation. 2003;9:897–904.
99. Biggins SW, Beldecos A, Rabkin JM, et al. Re-transplantation for hepatic allow graft failure; prognostic modeling and ethical considerations. Liver Transplantation. 2002;8:313–322.
100. Azoulay D, Linhares MM, Huguet E, et al. Decision for re-transplantation of the liver: an experience and cost based analysis. Annals of Surgery. 2002;236: 713–721.
101. Larson AM. Adult liver transplantation in the USA. Current Opinion in Gastroenterology. 2011;7:240–247.
102. Xia VW, Taniguchi M, Steadman TH, et al. The changing face of patients presenting for liver transplantation. Current Opinion Organ Transplantation. 2008;3: 280–284.
103. Johnston SD, Morris JK, Cramb R, et al. Cardiovascular morbidity and mortality after orthotropic liver transplantation. Transplantation. 2002;6:901–906.
104. Guckelberger O, Byram A, Klupp J, et al. Coronary event rates in liver transplant recipients reflect the increased prevalence of cardiovascular risk factors. Transplant International. 2005;8:967–974.
105. Wong F. Cirrhotic cardiomyopathy. Hepatology International . 2009;1:294–304.
106. Pruthi J, Medkiff KA, Esrason KT, et al. Analysis of causes of death of liver transplant patients who survived more than three years. Liver Transplantation. 2001;9:811–815.
107. Dec GW, Kondo N, Farrell ML, et al. Cardiovascular complications following liver transplantation. Clinical Transplantation. 1995;6:463–471.
108. Appleton CP, Hurst RT, Lee KS, et al. Long-term cardiovascular risk in the orthotropic liver transplant population. Liver Transplantation. 2006;3:352–355.
109. Fleisher LA, Beckman JA, Brown KA, et al. ACC/AHA 2007 guidelines on perioperative cardiovascular evaluation and care for non-cardiac surgery. Journal of the American College of Cardiology. 2007;17:1707–1732.
110. Lester SJ, Hurst RT. Liver transplantation: do you have the heart for it? Liver Transplantation. 2006;4:520–522.

111. Tiukinhoy-Laing SD, Rossi JS, Bayram M, et al. Cardiac hemodynamic and coronary angiographic characteristics of patients being evaluated for liver transplantation. American Journal of Cardiology. 2006;2:178–181.
112. Targher G, Arcaro G. Non-alcoholic fatty liver disease and increased risk of cardiovascular disease. Atherosclerosis. 2007;2:235–240.
113. Ehtisham J, Altieri M, Salame E, et al. Coronary artery disease in orthotropic liver transplantation: pre-transplant assessment and management. Liver Transplantation. 2010;5:550–557.
114. Williams K, Lewis JF, Davis G, et al. Dobutamine stress echocardiography in patients undergoing liver transplant evaluation. Transplantation. 2000;11:2354–2356.
115. McAvoy NC, Kochar N, McKillop G, et al. Prevalence of coronary artery calcification in patients undergoing assessment for orthotropic liver transplantation. Liver Transplantation. 2008;12:1725–1731.
116. Safadi A, Homsi M, Maksoum W, et al. Perioperative risk predictors of cardiac outcomes in patients undergoing liver transplantation surgery. Circulation. 2009;13:1189–1194.
117. Rybak D, Fallon MB, Krowka MJ, et al. Risk factors and impact of COPD in candidates for liver transplantation. Liver Transplantation. 2008;9:1357–1365.
118. Ehlers SL, Rodrigue JR, Widows MR, et al. Tobacco use before and after liver transplantation: a single center survey and implications for clinical practice and research. Liver Transplantation. 2004;3:412–417.
119. Murray CJ, Lopez AD. Global mortality, disability, and the contribution of risk factors: Global Burden of Disease Study. Lancet. 1997;9063:1436–1442.
120. Van der Heide F, Dijkstra G, Porte RJ, et al. Smoking behavior in liver transplant recipients. Liver Transplantation. 2009;6:648–655.
121. Pauwels Ram Buist AS, Ma P Jenkins CR, Hurd SS, et al. Global strategy for the diagnosis, management, and prevention of COPD. Respiratory Care. 2001;8: 798–825.
122. Celli BR, Cote CG, Marin JM, et al. The body-mass index, airflow obstruction, dyspnea, and exercise capacity index in COPD. New England Journal of Medicine. 2004;10:1005–1012.
123. Lazardis KN, Frank JW, Krowka MJ, et al. Hepatic hydrothorax: pathogenesis, diagnosis, and management. American Journal of Medicine. 1999;10:262–267.
124. Strauss RM, Boyer TD. Hepatic hydrothorax. Seminars in Liver Disease. 1997;17:227–232.
125. Krowka MT, Cortese DA. Pulmonary aspects of chronic liver disease and liver transplantation. Mayo Clinic Proceedings. 1985;60:407–418.
126. Lazaridis KN, Frank JW, Krowka MJ, et al. Hepatic hydrothorax: pathogenesis, diagnosis, and management. American Journal of Medicine. 1999;107(3): 262–267.
127. Krowka MJ, Wiseman GA, Burnett OL, et al. Hepatopulmonary syndrome: a prospective study of relationships between severity of liver disease, PaO_2, response to 100% oxygen, and brain uptake after (99m) Tc MAA lung scanning. Chest. 2000;118:615–624.
128. Stoller JK, Lange PA, Westveer MK, et al. Prevalence and reversibility of hepatopulmonary syndrome after liver transplantation. The Cleveland Clinic experience. Western Journal of Medicine. 1995;163(2):133–138.
129. Krowka MJ, Plevak DJ, Findlay JY, et al. Pulmonary hemodynamics and perioperative cardiopulmonary-related mortality in patients undergoing liver transplantation. Liver Transplantation. 2000;6:443–450.
130. Starkel P, Vera A, Gunson B, et al. Outcome of liver transplantation for patients with portopulmonary hypertension. Liver Transplantation. 2002;8:382–388.
131. Plotkin J, Kuo PC, Rubin LJ, et al. Successful use of chronic epoprostenol as a bridge to liver transplantation in severe portopulmonary hypertension. Transplantation. 1998;65:457–459.
132. Koneru B. Resolution of pulmonary hypertension of cirrhosis after liver transplantation. Transplantation. 1994;58:1133–1135.
133. Olbrisch ME, Benedict SM, Haller DL, et al. Psychosocial assessment of organ transplant candidates. Current status of methodological and philosophical issues. Psychosomatics. 1995;36:236–241.
134. Dobbels F, De Geest S, Cleemput I. Psychosocial and behavioral selection criteria for solid organ transplantation. Progress in Transplantation. 2001;11:121–126.
135. Dobbels F, Vanhaecke J, Dupont L, et al. Pre-transplant predictors of post-transplant adherence and clinical outcome: an evidence base for pre-transplant psychosocial screening. Transplantation. 2009;87(10):1497–1504.
136. Telles-Correia D, Barbosa A, Mega I, et al. Psychiatric and psychosocial predictors of medical outcome after liver transplantation: a prospective, single-center study. Transplantation Proceedings. 2011;43:155–157.
137. Everhart JE, Beresford TP. Liver transplantation for alcoholic liver disease: a survey of transplantation programs in the United States. Liver Transplantation and Surgery. 1997;3:220–226.
138. Dew MA, DiMartini AF, Steel J, et al. Meta-analysis of risk for relapse to substance use after transplantation of the liver or other solid organs. Liver Transplantation. 2008;14:159–172.
139. Beresford TP. Psychiatric assessment of alcoholic candidate for liver transplantation. In: Lucey MR, editor. Liver Transplantation and the Alcoholic Patient: Medical, Surgical and Psychosocial issues. Cambridge, UK: Cambridge University Press; 1994: 29–49.
140. Murray KF, Carithers RL. AASLD practice guidelines: evaluation of the patients for liver transplantation. Hepatology. 2005;41:1407–1432.
141. Guimaro MS, Lacerda SS, Karem CH, et al. Psychosocial profile of patients on the liver transplant list. Transplantation Proceedings. 2008;40:782–784.
142. Rogal SS, Landsittel D, Surman O, et al. Pre-transplant depression, antidepressant use, and outcomes of orthotropic liver transplantation. Liver Transplantation. 2011;17:251–260.
143. Levenson JL, Olbrisch ME. Psychosocial evaluation of organ transplant candidates; a comparative survey of process, criteria, and outcomes in heart, liver, and kidney transplantation. Psychosomatics. 1993;34:314–323.
144. Koch M, Banys P. Liver transplantation and opioid dependence. JAMA. 2001;285(8):1056–1058.
145. Kanchana TP, Kaul V, Manzarbietia C, et al. Liver transplantation for patients on methadone maintenance. Liver Transplantation. 2002;8(9):778–772.
146. Weinrieb RM, Barnett R, Lynch KG, et al. A matched comparison study of medical and psychiatric complications and anesthesia and analgesia requirements in methadone-maintained liver transplant recipients. Liver Transplantation. 2004;10(1):97–106.
147. Schaffner A. Pretransplant evaluation of infections of donors and recipients of solid organs. Clinical Infectious Diseases. 2001;33(Suppl 1):S9–S14.
148. O'Grady JG, Alexander GJM, Hayllar KM. Early indicators of prognosis in fulminant hepatic failure. Gastroenterology. 1989;97:439–445.
149. Shakil AO, Kramer D, Mazariegos GV. Etiology and outcome for 295 patients with acute liver failure in the United States. Liver Transplantation and Surgery. 1999;5:29–34.
150. Anand AC, Nightingale P, Neuberger JM. Early indicators of prognosis in fulminant hepatic failure: an assessment of the King's criteria. Journal of Hepatology. 1997;26:62–68.
151. Bernal W, Donaldson N, Wyncoll D. Blood lactate as an early predictor of outcome in paracetamol-induces acute liver failure: a cohort study. Lancet. 2002;359:558–563.
152. Schmidt C, Marsh JW. Molecular signature for HCC: role in predicting outcomes after liver transplant and selection for potential adjuvant treatment. Current Opinion Organ Transplantation. 2002;15:277–282.
153. Freeman RB, Steffick DE. Liver and intestine transplantation in the United States, 1997–2006. American Journal of Transplantation. 2008;8(4 Pt 2):958–976.
154. Duffy JP, Vardanian A, Benjamin E. Liver transplantation criteria for hepatocellular carcinoma should be expanded. Annals of Surgery. 2007;246:502–511.

第 30 章 心脏移植的患者选择和适应证

Andrew L. Smith，Daniel B. Sims

引言

美国每年实施心脏移植的患者有 2300 名，其中约 1950 名是 18 岁以上的成年人。尽管放宽了捐助者的标准，但是心脏移植手术量十年来不曾变化。据统计，全世界每年实施 5000 例心脏移植[1]。心力衰竭的发病率增加，导致登记等待移植的患者数量远大于心脏移植手术的实施量。此外，现在左心室辅助装置(LVAD)植入和心脏移植一样频繁。LVAD 是没有在移植名单上或者没有合适供体的患者在心脏移植前的一个过渡[2]。幸运的是，对于日益增长的心力衰竭患者，近年来相应的治疗措施也随之有所改善，部分严重的心肌功能障碍患者的预后得到改善。

心脏移植的一般适应证(表 30.1)在过去的几十年中一直没有变化。然而许多其他治疗方法的加入已经改变了对于难治性心力衰竭的定义[3]。神经内分泌药物的调节作用、植入心脏除颤器减少心脏猝死、再同步设备改善了宽 QRS 波患者的心肌收缩[4]。因此，心脏移植的风险评估也随之改变，器官可用性也随之下降。本章将重点讨论心脏移植患者的选择与分配政策的变化，这将对接受心脏移植的患者的选择上产生重大影响。本章是对第 39 章的一个补充，涵盖了等待心脏移植候患者的管理，第 44 章、第 48 章和第 49 章也做了补充，分别介绍了心力衰竭的患者的重症监护病房管理以及心室辅助装置和人工心脏的出现。

表 30.1 心脏移植的一般适应证

常见适应证
• 严重的收缩功能障碍，治疗无法改善晚期症状，客观证据支持小于 1 年的生存率
不常见适应证
• 复杂先天性心脏病伴严重症状，不适合姑息或矫正手术
• 限制性或肥厚性心肌病伴严重心力衰竭，难治疗
• 持续的危及生命的难治性室性心律失常
• 严重、致使缺血，不适合血运重建

心力衰竭:症状及进展性综合征

心力衰竭是一种常见的慢性疾病，在美国超过 600 万的患者经历着心力衰竭。纽约心脏协会(NYHA)症状分级长期以来被用于心力衰竭的分类，从无症状或轻度症状（Ⅰ~Ⅱ级）到有明显或严重受限制的症状(Ⅲ~Ⅳ级)。针对液体淤滞的治疗往往可以改善症状，但随着时间的推移可能变得难治。因此，对疾病的进展状态进行分期，对于判断患者预后有重要的影响。难治性终末期心力衰竭被定为 D 期[5]。虽然对心力衰竭的评估存在差异，但在美国有多达 15 万心力衰竭的患者可能已经进入 D 期。其中 75%的患者年龄在 65 岁以上，并且伴有相关并发症，包括糖尿病、慢性肾脏病和外周血管疾病。然而，如果存在合适的供体，成千上万的 D 期患者将通过心脏移植延长生命。由于供体心脏的需求和可用性不匹配，心脏移植的过程不仅基于个体的结果，也基于分配稀有资源的伦理问题。

心脏移植候补名单的结果

近年来，心脏移植的结果有所改善，1 年生存率为 88%~90%，而在 20 世纪 90 年代为 80%(图 30.1)。5 年生存率约为 75%。对于存活 1 年的成年患者，1/2 预期可以生活 14 年，接近 1/3 可以生活 20 年[1]。根据器官共享联合网络(UNOS)，在 2008 年等待心脏移植的成年患者中，60%在 12 个月内接受了移植，25%仍在等待，10%死亡，5%因改善或恶化的原因被移除。到 36 个月时，70%接受移植，8%等待，12%死亡，10%被移

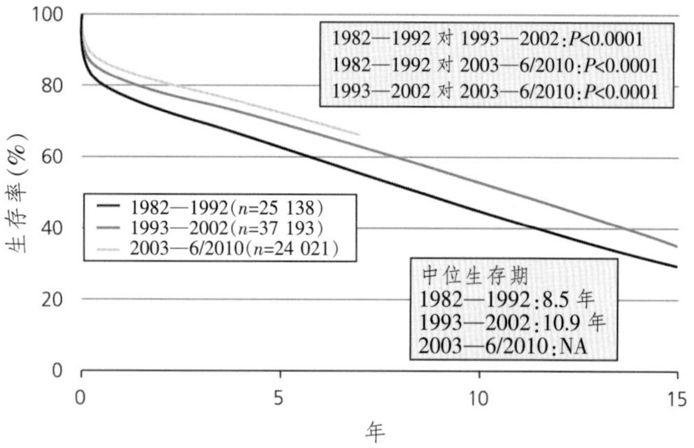

图 30.1　成人心脏移植生存率。NA,不可用。(Data from the ISHLT https://www.ishlt.org/registries.)

除。近年来,每年约有 3400 名候选人被列入名单[6]。

值得注意的是,77%的心脏移植中心每年进行的移植少于 20 例。较大规模的中心,每年实施超过 20 例心脏移植,完成总移植的 52%(图 30.2)[1]。

左心室辅助装置:改变 D 期心力衰竭治疗的前景

正如第 48 章中深入讨论的,机械循环辅助装置已经可用多年,包括 LVAD、右心室辅助装置(RVAD)或双心室辅助装置(BiVAD)来负责危重患者心脏移植的过渡阶段。连续流动 LVAD 的普及极大推动了心力衰竭预后的改善(图 30.3)。这些泵比前一代装置更小且更可靠,并且有助于改善治疗结果,不仅对于等待移植的患者,而且对于作为永久性或“目的地”治疗的患者,都改善了患者预后。在植入 LVAD 后,患者可在 2 周内出院,并且在前 2 个月内具有良好的活动状态。机械辅

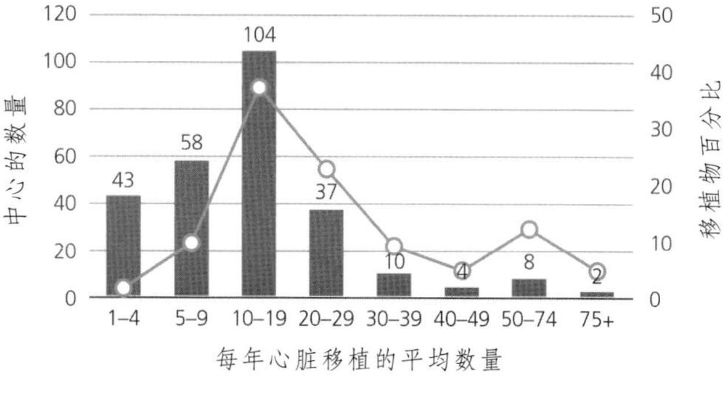

图 30.2　2006 年 1 月—2011 年 6 月期间执行指定数量的移植中心(柱状)和这些中心做的移植物总数的百分比(线状)。(Data from https://www.ishlt.org/registries.)

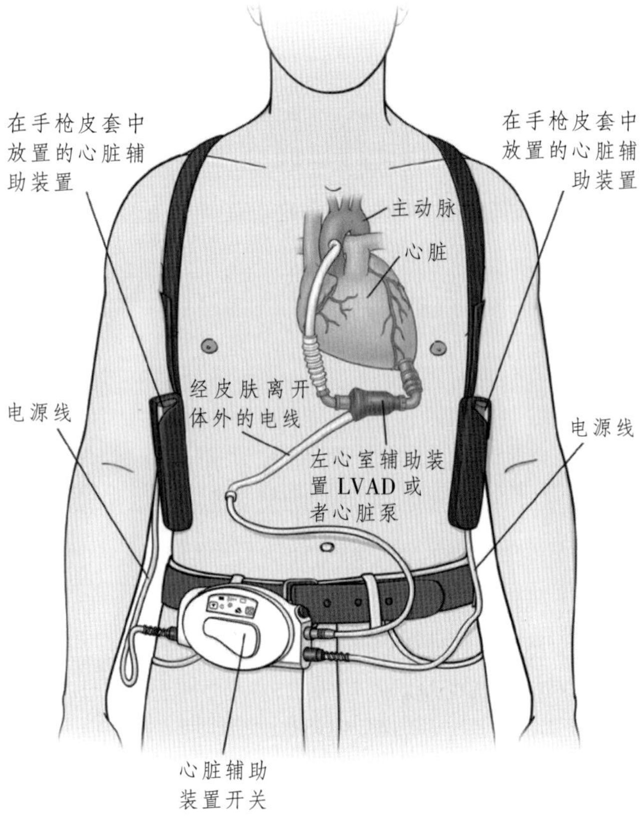

图 30.3　Thoratec HeartMate Ⅱ 左心室辅助装置(LVAD)。血液从左心室流经叶轮泵进入主动脉。(Reprinted with the permission of Thoratec Corporation)

助循环支持机构间登记处 (Intermacs) 报告, 在美国 2009 年约 1000 个接受移植的患者和 2011 年 1800 个接受移植的患者,这已经接近心脏移植的数量[2]。这些植入物的适应证是连续性肌力支持退化的患者作为移植候选人的过渡阶段,即潜在的禁忌证被解决;或作为长期治疗目标(DT)。2011 年,23%的植入物为 BTT,37%为 BTC,38%为 DT[7]。因 BTT 而使用 LVAD 显著增加,2010 年约 1/3 的移植患者得到了这些装置的支持(图 30.4)。

LVAD 技术的改进提高了严重心力衰竭患者的生存率。目前,连续流动 LVAD 支持的患者的 1 年生存率约 75%,2 年生存率 62%。LVAD 的临床结果与植入时疾病的严重程度密切相关。心源性休克患者的临床结果较差。如果排除这些患者以及具有严重并发症的患者,2 年生存率约 80%,这与心脏移植类似[7]。长期数据有限。

尽管 LVAD 技术有所提高,但感染、血栓形成和出血等问题仍然存在。目前,超过 25%的植入 LVAD 的患

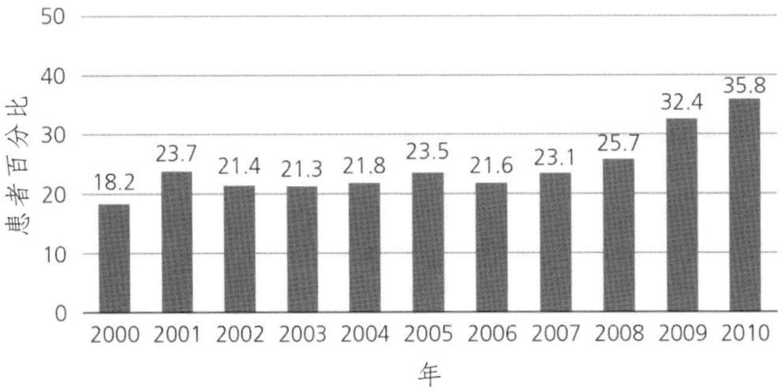

图 30.4 使用左心室辅助装置、右心室辅助装置或全人工心脏过渡到移植的患者百分比。(Data from the ISHLT https://www.ishlt.org/registries)。

者使用抗生素治疗细菌感染,最常见的是连接电池和控制器的传动系统所在的皮肤[8]。患者需要使用华法林进行长期抗凝治疗。设备形成的血栓可能导致中风或设备故障,这种情况可能需要更换泵。这些患者长期抗凝和凝血因子缺乏可能导致动静脉畸形,从而引发消化道出血,临床出血发生在高达 20%的患者中[9]。基于这些影响长期结果的并发症,心脏移植仍然是优于永久性 LVAD 治疗的治疗方法。

LVAD 越来越多地被用于过渡不稳定患者进行移植。即使手术复杂性增加,但总体结果与非装置患者相当。除了提到的潜在并发症之外,LVAD 过渡性治疗还有其他缺点。LVAD 患者有发展同种异体抗体的风险,由升高的群体反应性抗体(PRA)百分比表示(将在第 89 章深入讨论)。这对找到合适供体的可能性有影响。PRA 升高可能是由于手术或胃肠道出血而采取的输血;然而,没有输血的患者在植入术后 PRA 升高。自体与来自 LVAD 的物质相互作用导致的免疫系统激活可能参与了这一过程,尽管并不是所有 LVAD 抗体中都可以检测到 HLA 抗体[10]。一些心脏移植的候选人使用 LVAD 出现并发症的风险较高。这些候选人包括严重右心室衰竭、非扩张型心肌病、多次胸骨切开术或机械瓣膜置换术,特别是主动脉瓣置换的患者。因此,应首先对患者进行移植评估,如果是候选人,应评估使用 LVAD 发生恶性事件的风险。未接受移植的患者应评估对 DT 的适合性。

美国的心脏分配

美国捐赠器官的分配由 UNOS 政策决定[10]。由移植医生、护士协调员、移植医院代表、器官获取组织(OPO)代表和患者代表组成的胸部器官移植委员会制定和监测心肺分配政策。区域审查委员会提供额外的监督,包括额外审查高优先级的请求。心脏分配由三个优先级状态组成,旨在向更危重的候选者提供心脏(表 30.2)。

如表所示,最高优先级(1A)的候选人可能在移植中心医院病情恶化,或者在 30 天规则下出现 LVAD 或严重并发症,如血栓形成、感染或机械故障。使用 LVAD 但达不到以上标准的则为 1B,需要长期心脏支持患者也是 1B。不符合这些标准的门诊患者是状态 2,并且不适合立即被移植的患者可以暂时失活至状态 7。等待时间在同一水平时才有意义。例如,列出 1A 为 1 天的患者将优先于 1B 为 3 个月或状态 2 为 3 年的患者。关于 ABO 血型,O 型血心脏优先给予 O 型血或 B 型血受者,A 型血心脏优先给予 A 型血或 AB 型血受者,B 型血心脏优先给予 B 型血或 AB 型血受者。

在 2006 年,如果一个 1A 或 1B 患者在当地移植中心和供者心脏不匹配,那么会优先给方圆 500 英里(1 英里≈1.61km)范围内的医院的 1A 或 1B 患者,而不给当地医院的 2 级候选人。这种地理设计旨在降低等待名单中患者的死亡率,同时保证器官缺血时间<4 小

表 30.2 UNOS 中心脏移植优先的状态

状态 1A——允许进入移植医院和以下情况之一:
• 血流动力学监测和连续输注大剂量或多剂量强心药
• 机械循环支持主动脉内球囊泵、体外膜氧合器(ECMO)或全人工心脏
• 机械通气机
状态 1A——不需要住院:
• 左心室辅助装置(LVAD)和(或)右心室辅助装置(RVAD)可能为 1A,计划在 30 天内的任何时间点住院治疗
• 对于 LVAD 或 RVAD,客观证据显示明显器械相关并发症或危及生命的室性心律失常
状态 1B:
• 连续输注肌力
• LVAD 或 RVAD
状态 2:
• 所有不符合 1A 或 1B 标准的候选人

根据器官获取和移植网络(OPTN)的指导方针,组织分配:胸腔器官分配。美国卫生和公共服务部,美国健康资源和服务管理局,美国医疗保健系统,美国移植部门。Available at:http://optn.transplant.hrsa.gov/Policiesand-Bylaws2/policies/pdfs/policy_9.pdf. (2013 年 1 月 15 日访问)

时,以使移植成功率不会下降(表30.3)[11]。结果,移植状态2的患者接受的心脏显著减少，但对整体移植结果没有不利影响[12]。

在2011年，只有6%的心脏移植是状态2,62%的是状态1A和32%的是状态1B(表30.4)。目前,植入式心脏除颤器治疗(ICD)和猝死的减少,使得等待名单上状态2的患者的与接受心脏移植的状态2的患者1年生存率类似。这一事实,以及患者被列为状态2的可能性较低，导致一些人质疑是否需要列出此类患者[12,13]。然而,很大一部分的状态2患者将在短时间内恶化,为此,有人倡导当前的候补名单制度[14]。在移植的等待时间和等待移植的状态2的患者的数量方面存在区域变异性。等待时间也受个体体型、ABO血型和同种异体敏化的影响。在一些地区,O型血、体型大的男性期望基于1A等待时间接受移植可能是合理的。将患者列为状态2在接受心脏移植时不会受到影响。

很明显,器官的可用性限制了从心脏移植受益的患者的数量。活到心脏移植的那一天对患者和其家庭都是一个挑战。患有心力衰竭的患者在医院经常需要延长住院时间,可能还需要在家里注射强心剂,并且超过1/3的患者可能需要主动脉内球囊泵或LVAD作为BTT。接受LVAD置入的患者将有一段恢复期,随后是不确定的等待期,通常因为发生了严重并发症,被确定为最高优先级来获得移植机会。移植中心会告知患者他们在等待接受移植过程中的艰难,尽管等待移植患者的个体不确定性使得确定每个患者的未来都变得十分困难。

移植患者名单是由多学科委员会决定的，期望那些列出的患者将最终通过移植得到良好的结果。我们需要一个有利的结果来确保有限的器官被充分利用，

表30.3　优先分配

- 本地:状态1A,然后是1B
- A区(500英里内):状态1A,然后1B
- 本地:状态2

表30.4　心脏移植的百分比(按状态)

年份	状态1A	状态1B	状态2
2005	40	34	26
2011	62	32	6

基于器官获取和移植网络(OPTN)数据。Available at http://optn.transplant.hrsa.gov/latestData/rptData.asp.(2013年1月15日访问)

以减少患者的痛苦，并在严格审查的监管环境中保护移植计划的可持续发展。因此,选择进行心脏移植的受体时,不仅仅要考虑是否可能延长患者的生存时间。由于适于移植的器官的差异，心脏移植程序具有比肾脏和肝脏移植程序更严格的排除标准。

纳入心脏移植名单的患者选择标准

对于心脏移植的患者的评估可能是对医院中病情不稳定患者的紧急评估,或者是对门诊患者的综合评估,包括对治疗的适应能力,治疗是否有效,以及是否坚持评估。

在把一个患者列入心脏移植名单之前，需要考虑以下问题：

1.患者是否有难治性终末期心脏病？这包括对所有合理治疗方案的回顾,包括医学治疗的优化。

2.患者是否有影响移植后的生存率和生活质量的并发症？

3.是否有足够的支持机制来保证成功的结果？

4.患者是否明白自己有度过等待期、移植期和其余生的义务？

5.根据患者的期望和愿望,患者是否自主决定接受移植？

终末期心脏病的定义

超过95%的患者进行心脏移植是因为心肌或“泵”的衰竭,并且常常是慢性心力衰竭。在不存在严重心肌衰竭的情况下,难治性心绞痛或危及生命的心律失常的移植极为少见。根据国际心肺移植协会(ISHLT)报告,在过去5年中,非缺血性扩张型心肌病占54%,缺血性心肌病占37%。先天性心脏病、瓣膜性心脏病和再移植各占移植总数的3%[1]。

由于20世纪80年代心脏移植项目的发展，促进了晚期心力衰竭和心脏移植的心脏病学分支学科认证的发展。随着转诊和等待时间的增加,建立了心力衰竭诊所,以照顾晚期慢性病患者人群。这些中心的心脏病学家在一个多学科团队中工作，以评估和长期管理严重左心室功能障碍的患者。之前被诊断为难治性心力衰竭症状的患者通过这些治疗方案,病情得到了改善。

从那时起,许多研究慢性心力衰竭的大型临床试验已经为收缩性心力衰竭患者制定了适当的治疗方案[4]。

最佳药物治疗组合为 ACEI、β-受体阻滞剂、醛固酮拮抗剂的使用和调整剂量的袢利尿剂以保持适当的状态。非裔美藉患者额外增加肼屈嗪/硝酸盐后会获益。一部分经过筛选的宽 QRS 持续时间的患者将从心脏再同步治疗(CRT)中获益。β-受体阻滞剂和 CRT 治疗都被证明可改善心肌结构和功能,并可逆转心脏扩张。左心室射血分数(LVEF)<35%的患者可能从 ICD 治疗中获益。指南已经推荐将难治性心力衰竭的患者转诊到多学科疾病管理团队[5]。心力衰竭疾病管理的组成部分[15]列于表 30.5。这些可以改善心力衰竭患者的生活,并且可以影响移植的需要。

最重要的是我们需要认识到,患者由于心力衰竭的症状而寻求医疗帮助时,多种疾病状态同时存在可能是他/她出现症状的根本原因所在。在一些情况下,对这些根本原因的治疗可导致收缩功能障碍的逆转。在列表的一端是有症状的患者,其由于心动过速介导心肌病,LVEF 为 15%。在心房或心室的电极的导管因电极消融造成的心动过速可能是治愈的[16]。此外,某些扩张型心肌病和左束支传导阻滞的患者可能是双心室起搏系统 CRT 治疗的"超级反应者"[17]。在不可逆转的末端是患有远端大片心肌梗死的患者,已经发展为难治性低血压、心动过速和利尿剂抵抗。介于两者之间的是慢性严重左心室功能障碍的患者,其可能 β-受体阻滞剂使用剂量不足,并且有未充分治疗的高血压,由于药物和饮食依从性问题而导致的慢性体液超负荷、未经治疗的阻塞性睡眠呼吸暂停或房颤控制不良,某些处于 NYHA Ⅳ级的慢性疾病状态/共病的患者经过合适的治疗,能会出现症状缓解或无症状生存。

需要评估确定移植

住院患者

大多数心脏移植评估可以在门诊进行,然而,某些患者可能需要转到移植中心进行紧急评估。疑似暴发性心肌炎的心源性休克的患者可能需要机械支持和移植评估,特别是通过活检被确定为巨细胞性心肌炎的患者[18]。包括因急性心肌梗死行冠状动脉介入术,或具有难治性室性心律失常所致血流动力学不稳定的患者。对于慢性心力衰竭的患者,如果不能停止心肌辅助支持,心功能或肝功能进行性恶化或复发性心律失常,应该迅速将其转移到移植中心。

表 30.5 心力衰竭疾病管理的组成部分

- 个性化教育和咨询
- 促进自我保健,包括体重监测和利尿调节
- 促进遵守的策略
- 优化治疗
- 主动干预症状变化
- 社会和经济方面的支持
- 需要时访问供应者

慢性心力衰竭患者的治疗

大多数严重左心室功能障碍的患者都会接受较为复杂的医疗方案,并且通常具有防止心源性猝死的 ICD。他们的慢性治疗管理通常由当地心脏病门诊负责。这些患者多数都具有很好的生活质量,偶尔症状加剧可通过药物剂量调整和生活方式的干预来管理。确定需要进一步治疗来控制预后下滑的时间点是一个难题。

移植评估的合适时机说的是,患者可能需要时间来满足候选名单的要求,以及参与关于高级治疗的共同决策[19]。尽管移植检测结果可能很快获得,但许多患者需要进一步评估,包括通过结肠镜检查进行常规健康评估或对糖尿病等合并症进行专门检查。此外,具有多种并发症或社会心理问题的患者可能需要在中心随访一段时间以证明他们能够承受复杂的治疗计划。相反,对患者过早的评价可能导致过度的检查和费用。此外,不适当的早期移植评估可能会给我们目前的医疗保险和监管系统带来压力。一旦移植评估阶段开始,将有许多人参与,并且需要沟通所需的文件。因此,在评估阶段开始之前,通常心力衰竭心脏病专家会先在晚期心力衰竭门诊中对患者进行问诊。

心力衰竭的临床过程是相当多变的,使得在临床实践中对患者做出预后变得困难。然而,临床医生应该注意到某些预警迹象表明患者的预后已经恶化,并且需要考虑进一步的治疗。欧洲心脏病学会已经确定晚期慢性心力衰竭的标准,引导临床医生参考移植或 LVAD。所有列出的标准应该在实施或尝试最佳治疗后出现(表 30.6)[20]。

其余的独立危险因素应该特别注意,包括非自愿减肥,症状性低血压导致的 ACEI 或 β-受体阻滞剂不耐受和心肾综合征的先兆[23]。

患者最好在门诊进行客观的评估。在门诊患者中,

表 30.6 欧洲心脏病学会关于晚期慢性心力衰竭的标准

1.中度至重度的呼吸困难症状和(或)休息时疲劳的症状,或最小消耗(NYHA 功能Ⅲ或Ⅳ级)
2.液体淤滞和(或)心输出量减少
3.证明严重心脏功能障碍的客观证据,至少为以下之一:
(a)左心室射血分数<30%
(b)多普勒超声假性正常或限制性二尖瓣流入模式
(c)左心室和(或)右心室充盈压力高
(d)B 型利尿钠肽升高
4.功能状态严重受损,无法锻炼、6 分钟步行距离<300m,或吸氧峰值<12~14mL/(g·min)
5.过去 6 个月内至少有一次住院史
6.药物治疗无效

心肺运动测试可以量化功能限制,确定该限制是否主要与心力衰竭相关,并且以后为患者提供重要的预后信息。峰值氧耗量(峰值 VO_2),假设充分的努力并达到无氧阈值,有助于将患者分为风险类别。之前已经将峰值 VO_2<14mL/(kg·min)用作心脏移植的指征[24]。然而,对β-受体阻滞剂、ICD 和再同步装置的研究已经导致较低的临界点<10~12mL/(kg·min)[25,26]。临床稳定和峰值 VO_2 结果良好的患者可以保证至少有 1 年的良好预后。

已经有超过 100 例患者统计研究显示人口学、临床和实验室变量与心力衰竭相关,包括缺血性病变、静息心率、QRS 波群延长、低血压、血清钠、尿酸、血红蛋白、脑钠肽(BNP)水平、射血分数和左心室大小等。多变量风险评分已被用来评估心力衰竭的门诊患者的预后。

20 种可变量的西雅图心力衰竭模型(SHFM)已经在大量的心力衰竭患者中得到验证,以提供 1~5 年的生存率和平均寿命的估计值(http://depts.wahington.edu/shfm/)。它往往低估非常晚期阶段的风险[27]。心力衰竭生存评分(HFSS)专门用于移植选择,但是它出现在β-受体阻滞剂使用和 ICD 治疗之前。它可能会增加确定那些可以安全推迟移植的低风险患者的价值[28]。这些分数不能单独用于确定移植候选者资格,但它们确实帮助临床医生来确定哪些患者可能需要正式评估。一些中心将这些信息包括在决定列入或拒绝列入名单的决定中[25]。

心脏移植评价阶段

在晚期心力衰竭门诊进行彻底评估后,被评估需要心脏移植而且没有心脏移植绝对禁忌证的患者有机会进入移植评估阶段。这项工作由多学科团队完成,包括与移植护士协调员、社会工作者、营养学家、心理健康专家和财务协调员的会面,以及药剂师的药物审查。此外,还需要进行多种测试以进一步评估移植的必要性、移植的禁忌证和供体器官相容性[ABO 型和群体反应性抗体(PRA)]。在本中心进行的测试和结果在表 30.7 中给出。

在美国,心脏移植的标准是由当地移植项目组确定的,通常通过满足标准的多学科选择委员会来确定。每个心脏移植程序基于经验和登记结果确定绝对和相对禁忌证,是根据有限的随机临床试验数据得出的。已发表的临床指南提供了通用的方法[26,29]。禁忌证是基于手术风险以及对寿命、生活质量和移植后免疫抑制治疗可能干扰或加重的潜在的程度。

绝对和相对禁忌证见表 30.8。相对禁忌证列出的是那些可以被修改的,可以基于程度确定,或者可以被认为在一些但不是所有程序都可接受的情况。

有助于考虑潜在禁忌证和心力衰竭疾病状态之间的关系:

表 30.7 心脏移植评估

• 当有指征时,右心导管插管时进行血管扩张剂激发实验
• 心肺运动测试(CPX)——可以在门诊基础上进行预评估
• 心电图(ECG)
• 超声心动图
• 支气管扩张剂和一氧化碳扩散能力(DLCO)的肺功能检查(有尼古丁使用史,哮喘或胺碘酮治疗史的患者)
• 与心理健康社会工作者、社会工作者、财务协调员和营养学家协商。通知药剂师进行图表审阅;可根据需要进一步咨询
• 血液学特征差异、血小板计数、PT 和 PTT、综合代谢状况、TSH、PSA(如果男性患者>50 岁)、脂质分布、Mg
• HIV、乙型和丙型肝炎的血清学检测
• CMV、EBV,弓形虫(移植后影响)
• PRA 抗体筛查
• 尼古丁尿液测试
• 血型测定和筛查×2
• 24 小时尿液收集以清除肌酐和蛋白质
• PPD 皮肤试验、肺炎疫苗(如果没有接种)、乙型肝炎疫苗
• 附加诊断或咨询

PT,凝血酶原时间;PTT,部分凝血活酶时间;TSH,促甲状腺激素;PSA,前列腺特异性抗原;CMV,巨细胞病毒;EBV,爱波斯坦-巴尔病毒;PPD,纯化蛋白衍生物。

表 30.8　心脏移植禁忌证

绝对禁忌证：
• 严重、不可逆的肺动脉高压
• 活跃的恶性肿瘤
• 预后不良的全身性疾病
• 严重阻塞性肺病
相对禁忌证：
• 高龄(>70 岁)
• 不受控制的感染
• 活动性消化性溃疡病
• 控制不良或终末器官损伤的糖尿病(神经病，肾病或增殖性视网膜病变)
• 严重肥胖
• 恶病质
• 严重的外周血管疾病
• 严重脑血管病
• 肾小球滤过率降低的固有性肾脏疾病(eGFR)<40mL/(min·1.73m^2)
• 肝功能异常胆红素>2.5mg/dL 或转氨酶是正常值的 3 倍
• 肝硬化
• 慢性病毒感染(乙型肝炎、丙型肝炎、HIV)
• 淀粉样变性
• 活跃的系统性红斑狼疮
• 多系统参与的活动性结节
• 近期肺梗死(由于免疫抑制的脓肿风险)
• 中风或肌营养不良导致的功能状态不佳
• 吞咽或呕吐障碍
• 控制不良的高血压
• 频繁或近期滥用药物(烟草、酒精、非法药物)
• 不稳定的精神疾病
• 近期不遵守治疗
• 缺乏社会支持结构
• 严格遵守药物的社会心理或经济障碍
• 移植中心随访沟通不足

1.一些情况可能是由于慢性或急性低输出性心力衰竭、心脏内压升高、组织充血、激活的神经激素或在医院治疗期间并发症导致的容量过载。随着心力衰竭的治疗，这些情况可能是可逆的。

2.其他禁忌证可能导致心脏衰竭的病因，如果不去改变，可能导致移植后发生持续的健康问题。

3.免疫抑制治疗可使一些禁忌证恶化。

肺血管阻力

继发性肺动脉高压发生在大多数患有心力衰竭的患者中，并且如果不可逆，在移植时可导致急性右心室衰竭。心脏移植后早期死亡的 20%是由于右心室衰竭[30]。供体心脏通常会因为脑死亡以及获得和植入产生的缺血时间导致功能异常。在这种情况下，因为右心室无法将足够的血量泵送到左侧，高肺血管阻力(PVR)可能导致循环休克。ISHLT 登记表一直展示 PVR 和移植后死亡率之间的线性关系[1]。常见的排除标准包括 PVR>6 Wood 单位或跨肺梯度>15。然而，肺动脉压迫通常可以通过肺血管舒张疗法迅速得到改善；如果未能在患者身上看到即刻的反应，不应该将患者永久排除在考虑范围之外。米力农、多巴酚丁胺或前列腺素 E 1 的慢性输注可以改善肺血流动力学。慢性西地那非或波生坦治疗似乎也是安全的，并已成功地运用于移植中[30,31]。以前固定的肺动脉高压的可逆性已经在慢性 LVAD 辅助下得到证实，这种治疗方法可以减少左心房压力并减少心输出量[32]。使用这些疗法，似乎大多数最初被认为因肺阻力而不能接受移植的患者最终不会因为这个原因而被排除。一旦列入移植名单，应考虑每 6~12 个月进行一次右心导管插入术，以排除原发性肺动脉高压的发生。

恶性肿瘤

除了某些皮肤癌之外，由于免疫抑制对肿瘤生长速度和存活时间的影响，所以活动性恶性肿瘤是移植的禁忌证。此外，难以同时使用化疗和移植免疫抑制药物。对于病情缓解的候选者，肿瘤会诊旨在确定复发或第二恶性肿瘤的风险，以确定是否需要特定的无肿瘤等待周期来评估预后。我们的中心将考虑复发率<10%的患者。

因化疗导致的心脏病患者数量正在增加[33]。蒽环类药物改善了乳腺癌、淋巴瘤、肉瘤和白血病患者的生存率。较新的药剂，包括曲妥珠单抗和酪氨酸激酶抑制剂，已经被证实参与了心脏毒性和化疗诱导的心肌病(CCMP)的发展。2/3 进行 CCMP 心脏移植的患者是女性，有趣的是，大约 75%的心脏移植受体是男性。癌症复发率一直较低。与扩张型心肌病患者相比，感染和皮肤癌的发生率更高，但是相对于生存率来说，排斥发生率较低。需要 LVAD 治疗的 CCMP 患者可能具有更高的右心室衰竭的风险，并且更有可能需要右心室辅助装置支持[34]。

有纵隔放射史的心脏移植患者因纵隔瘢痕所致的

手术出血和术后肺部并发症发生率较高。这部分患者移植的安全性和功效已引起关注。有纵隔放射的患者通常有心脏手术史,也增加了上述风险。此外,这些患者的恶性肿瘤复发率似乎更高[35,36]。

年龄

心脏移植患者的中位年龄为54岁;超过25%的受者年龄超过60岁,而只有2%的年龄大于70岁[1]。年龄较大的心脏移植患者更可能患有并发症，并且更容易出现免疫抑制性并发症,例如肾功能障碍、骨质疏松、类固醇诱导糖尿病和恶性肿瘤。老年受者不太可能有排斥反应,可能需要较少的强化免疫抑制[37]。2006年的ISHLT更新指出,如果患者年龄≤70岁,就应该慎重考虑移植[26]。中心一般基于生理参数做出决定,65岁以上的患者有更严格的标准[38,39]。捐赠者心脏日益稀缺造成了伦理困境:为老年人提供有限的资源可能会阻止年轻的患者接受移植。因此,一些中心使用边缘供体心脏创建了替代名单,尽管LVAD的改善结果可能是首选[40]。

糖尿病

约25%收缩性心力衰竭的门诊患者和约40%的住院患者患有糖尿病[41]。近年来,25%的心脏移植患者有糖尿病[1]。许多中心认为终末器官的损伤,包括肾病、神经病变或增生性视网膜病变,作为排除标准。自主神经功能障碍的患者被认为具有较高的并发症风险[26]。最近的注册数据发现,糖尿病对5年生存率的影响不大[1]。这可能反映了选择风险较低的患者以及手术期间改善的血糖管理。用类固醇和他克莫司（特别是非洲裔美国人)的免疫抑制可能导致移植后糖尿病的发生或恶化。接近40%的患者在移植后的前5年内患有糖尿病[1]。

肥胖

体重指数(BMI)>30kg/m^{2}或理想体重百分比(PIBW)>140%与心脏移植后的不良预后相关。肥胖患者心脏在手术后并发症增加,包括感染、静脉血栓栓塞和肺部并发症。在心脏和其他实体器官移植受者的排斥反应也有所增加[42,43]。体重增加在所有心脏移植受者中都很常见,并且肥胖可以通过类固醇免疫抑制恶化,特别是在第一年。近40%的心脏受者在移植后5年内BMI>30kg/m^2。许多中心在移植前需要减重至理想体重的140%以内。具有严重损害的患者可以在减肥的同时进行LVAD植入以维持生命。这可以成功;然而,对于严重肥胖的患者,在LVAD置入后很难达到或维持体重减轻,并且这些患者长期处于LVAD支持的状态[44,45]。

肾功能障碍

心脏移植后的肾功能障碍是多因素的，并且与长期结果密切相关。超过16%的患者在5年内肌酐>2.5mg/dL，这种程度功能障碍的患者比正常患者死亡的风险高出4倍[46,47]。预测哪些患者将在移植后具有严重的肾脏疾病是很重要的。肾功能障碍在晚期心力衰竭的患者中是常见的，并且通常可通过血流动力学的改善而变得可逆。然而,引起心脏病(包括高血压、糖尿病和动脉粥样硬化）的病症也是内源性肾病的主要危险因素。此外,心力衰竭可通过慢性神经激素激活以及慢性灌注不足引起肾脏永久性纤维化。肾功能应通过估计肾小球滤过率(eGFR)或肌酐清除率评估,最好是在患者状态稳定时进行。肾脏超声应该在那些具有异常结果的患者中进行。严重的回声或双侧肾脏萎缩的存在表示严重的内源性疾病。然而,明显灌注不足的肾脏可能在超声上显示异常。在这些患者中,肾活检以确定病因以及评估纤维化的严重性可能有助于候选人选择[48]。一些中心列出不可逆的肾功能障碍,肌酐清除率<40mL/min作为禁忌证,但实践各不相同。我们的中心没有肌酐清除率的绝对界限，但决定是基于功能障碍、活检结果和其他并发症考虑。联合心脏和肾脏移植可以在某些选定患者中进行,效果良好。

淀粉样变性

淀粉样变性是由错误折叠的不溶性蛋白质在组织中沉积引起的临床疾病。淀粉样变性有许多不同的类型,有两种关于心脏移植的常见类型值得讨论。在轻链(AL)淀粉样变性中,蛋白质由骨髓浆细胞的克隆群产生。在几个月的时间内许多器官浸润是常见的，多达50%的患者可能有心脏受累的迹象。只有5%的患者患有与心脏无关的疾病[49]。淀粉样蛋白最初影响间质,并且随着进展导致心肌坏死。临床上,心肌肥厚限制心脏收缩,最终导致射血分数下降。收缩功能障碍的常规疗法包括ACEI和β-受体阻滞剂,通常没有帮助,并且耐受性差。应避免使用地高辛。文献报道了不到100例AL淀粉样变性的患者接受了心脏移植，并随访了5年。近年来,患者心外受累已经被严密监控,并且在移植后进行化疗，有时会进行造血干细胞移植。尽管如此，这部分患者5年生存率明显低于没有AL淀粉样蛋白的患者，并且在其他器官中经常发现疾病进展[50,51]。许多中心不会考虑在AL淀粉样蛋白患者中进行移植。不幸的是，心脏性淀粉样变性通常发生在以前健康的患者中，使这成为一种情感障碍的疾病。

甲状腺素运载蛋白(TTR)淀粉样蛋白也常浸润心脏。与AL淀粉样蛋白不同，它是缓慢进展的，但可导致晚期心力衰竭。家族遗传形式的TTR淀粉样蛋白是由于在肝脏中产生的突变的TTR。肝移植是没有显著心脏受累患者的潜在选择，并且已经有约26例心脏-肝移植用于严重的心脏病。新型小分子药物可以控制疾病，使得最终不需要肝移植[52]。散发型TTR是另一种形式，肝脏不受影响。TTR淀粉样蛋白的患者似乎比患有AL淀粉样蛋白的患者有更好的预后，这与较慢的进展过程相关。但是，数据有限。

所有限制性生理学的淀粉样蛋白类型的病因依然存在，使得管理等待名单上的患者变得困难；大家担心新的心脏将再次受累或心脏外受累将会减少患者生存时间。

慢性病毒感染

十多年前的研究显示，移植前乙型肝炎表面抗原阳性的患者肝脏并发症的发生有显著性差异，但对生存率没有明显的影响[53]。在当前时代，对于乙型肝炎的抗病毒治疗耐受性良好，肝脏并发症似乎可以用拉米夫定治疗进行控制。一些患者出现了耐药性，需要替代的抗病毒药物[54-56]。丙型肝炎因为一些原因引起人们的重视。抗病毒治疗的耐受性差得多。此外，一项大型回顾性研究显示，移植后丙型肝炎病毒阳性患者的生存率降低。值得注意的是，丙型肝炎患者的5年，10年和15年生存率分别为73%、47%和25%，而与之相对应的非丙型肝炎患者为77%、67%和47%，表明患有丙型肝炎的患者受到显著影响[57]。

传统上，人类免疫缺陷病毒(HIV)感染被认为是实体器官移植的禁忌证。高效抗逆转录病毒治疗(HAART)的使用显著改善了HIV患者的预后，并且在肾脏和肝脏群体中进行了移植[58]。在肾移植中，一项针对150名仔细选择的患者的非随机试验显示在1年和3年的移植存活率是可接受的，尽管低于整体肾移植结果[59]。由于蛋白酶抑制剂和钙调磷酸酶抑制剂之间的药物相互作用，这些患者的免疫抑制治疗非常复杂。在这些患者中排斥反应率出乎意料地高。已有关于HIV患者的心脏移植的独立报告表明短期预后良好，但是经验似乎限于文献中少于15例报告病例的几个中心[58,60]。因为HAART可导致冠状动脉粥样硬化，所以在该类患者中心脏病的发病率可能增加。

社会心理因素

虽然在移植的结果方面，医学因素已经被更好地定义和更为深入的评估，但社会心理因素被认为在排斥反应、移植功能、感染和存活的关系中非常重要[61]。移植后的成功取决于支付药费的能力，每月基本会超过1000美元，并且可能涉及20%的共同支付(即医疗保险接受者)，以及遵循复杂的药物计划和服用治疗免疫抑制副作用的药物[62]。对于排斥和感染的早期干预取决于患者和护理者对状态变化的认识，以及适当地运送到医疗中心以进行紧急或常规后续护理。抑郁症、社会孤立、既往的不入依从史和药物滥用都与不良预后相关[61]。患者在心脏移植之前和之后经历的严重身体损伤可能导致暂时性精神损伤；因此，许多心脏移植程序需要固定的心理辅导人员。已婚患者似乎有更好的结果[63]。

选择委员会包括社会工作者、心理健康专家和其他团队成员，以确定患者是否具有管理疾病的能力、适当的支持系统、心理稳定性和适当的生活方式以确保成功。迄今为止，评估尚未在各个项目中实现标准化，但正在尝试制定标准来识别可能具有过度风险的患者，从而为接受者选择建立标准化标准[64]。

复杂先天性心脏病和心脏移植结果

复杂先天性心脏病患者是一个独特的群体。儿科心脏手术的成功使得先天性心脏病患者能够活到成年。不幸的是，衰弱性心力衰竭会逐渐恶化。因先天性心脏病而移植的患者由于再次手术的并发症和侧支循环出血而具有较差的短期预后。与单心室生理学移植的患者似乎比双心室生理学的患者有更高的风险[65]。慢性肝淤血可能是其中原因。尽管1年死亡率较高，但10年生存率与没有先天性疾病的患者相同[66]。

潜在候选人的评估

潜在的心脏移植受者的风险分层包括多方面的考

虑，包括心力衰竭的病因、既往的手术或治疗（即放射）、伴随的慢性疾病，以及导致多器官损害的患者敏锐度。精神稳定、康复潜力和社会支持是很重要的，但更难以量化。每个候选人克服移植前的困难或手术期并发症的能力应该在委员会以及与患者和家人进行讨论和评估。有几种可能降低生存率的特征的患者需要仔细考虑。正在尝试制定风险分层评分，以确定1年生存率差的患者是否具有不可接受的高风险[67]。

决定移植清单

我们的计划中心脏移植评估的方法在图30.5中进行了回顾。在晚期心力衰竭治疗委员会进行评估后，以确定移植和(或)LVAD治疗的候选资格。委员会使用由我们制定的排除标准，并尝试一致地应用这些标准。我们的标准由委员会定期审查和修改。坚持治疗的潜在问题很受关注，我们会议上的大部分讨论涉及这些问题。被排除在移植之外的患者将会得到口头和书面通知，他们可以在另一个中心寻求意见。

中心的标准各不相同，可能需要根据中心的结果调整这些标准。在美国，通过美国移植受者科学委员会(SRTR)公开报告详细的特定方案和数据。报告每6个月更新一次，包括等待名单死亡率、移植率和生存率，根据观察结果和预期结果进行调整。监管机构、保险提供商、医疗专业人员和患者可以轻易地在互联网上访问这些信息。如果中心的结果大大偏离预期，那么中心可能会失去认证。事实上，不仅用移植方案来评估患者，而且美国的项目正在通过公开报告进行高度评估。

心脏移植计划与肾脏和肝脏计划相比，体积较小，因此需要进行风险限制，以确保有利的结果，不仅要确保器官的最佳使用，而且从实践的角度来维持该计划的存在。有人认为，在不断变化的环境中，SRTR充分调

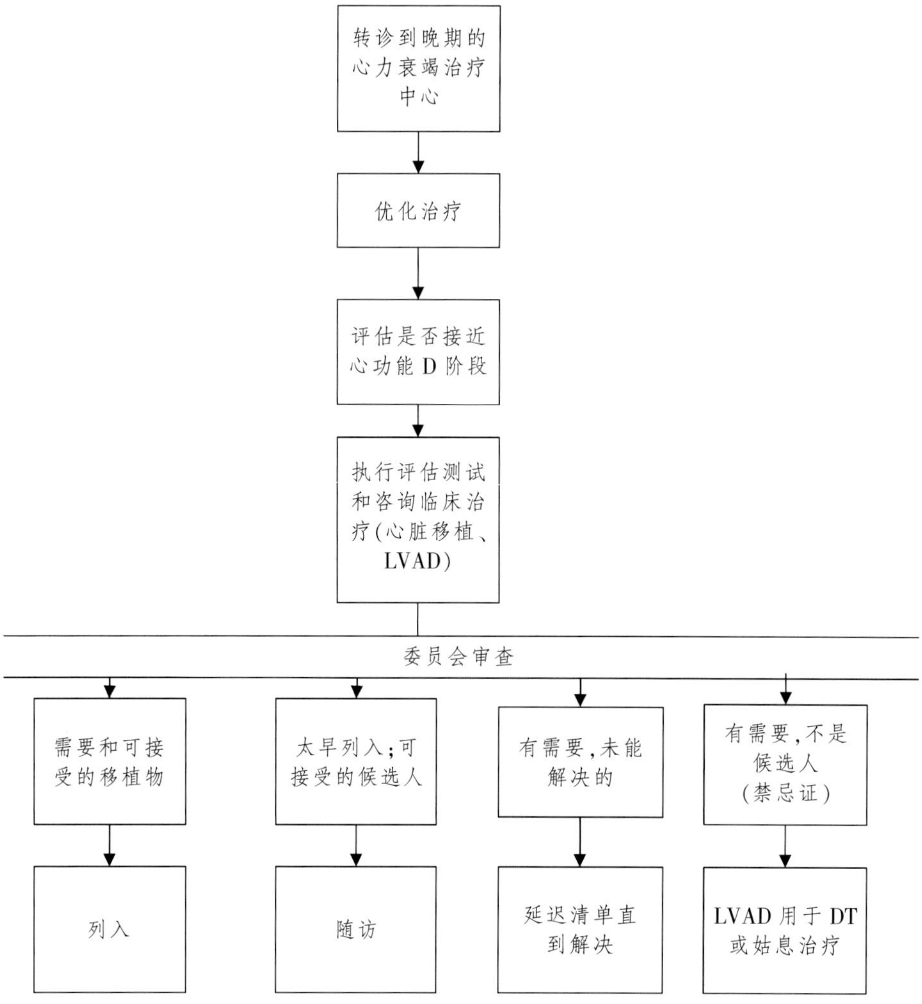

图30.5 心脏移植方法。

整风险的结果是具有挑战性的。一份与所有实体器官移植相关的共识报告指出,不适当的风险调整可能会导致避免对合适的但手术风险更高的患者进行移植[68]。许多移植禁忌证是相对的,而且它们还是动态的,随着并发症的药物治疗改善以及免疫抑制剂的应用的改变。鉴于相对缺乏随机临床数据,移植计划通常逐渐地小心测试障碍,而不是突然改变许多标准。

晚期心力衰竭的决策

晚期心力衰竭治疗委员会在移植中心为每位患者提供合适的治疗方案。这些选项同时被患者和家人所回顾,认识到心脏移植和 LVAD 治疗是可以提高寿命和生活质量的疾病交换疗法,但是需要适应移植存活的负担以及长期维持所需的治疗[69,70]。理想情况下,所有患者都应接受姑息治疗和支持性的护理咨询,以帮助他们及其家减轻疾病负担。这种护理包括考虑患者和家庭的生理、心理、精神和社会需求。一些患者可能不是心力衰竭进展的候选对象,或者可能不接受最大化的治疗。对于晚期心力衰竭小组来说,重要的是继续提供超出委员会决定和患者决定的护理。

总结

心脏移植对于终末期心力衰竭是一种有效的治疗方案,但其实施仍然严重受限于捐赠者心脏的短缺。这种有限的供体可用性和心力衰竭的日益普遍导致需要心脏移植的人和将接受移植的人之间的差距扩大。因此,心脏移植候选者比其他器官的候选者更具限制性,候选者的考虑不仅需要确定患者对手术的适应性,而且涉及替代性治疗的实用性考虑。幸运的是,心力衰竭的治疗正在改善,这可以减少或延长移植的时间。此外,慢性 LVAD 技术的改进已具有更好的效果,以桥接患者移植和提高非移植候选患者的生存率。基于疾病严重程度的心脏分配策略使得未进行连续肌力支持治疗或 LVAD 治疗的患者分配到心脏的情况较为少见。因此,对优势系统的理解很重要,不仅在管理患者的疾病,而且在管理他/她的期望方面。总而言之,在特定条件下需要心脏移植的患者及时地并且在有利于从过程中恢复的条件下被递送到候选名单,这样选择候选人的方式才是最佳的。

(谢文勇 译 张大方 校)

参考文献

1. Stehlik J, Edwards LB, Kucheryavaya AY, et al. The registry of the International Society for Heart and Lung Transplantation: 29th official adult heart transplant report–2012. Journal of Heart and Lung Transplantation. 2012;31:1052–1064.
2. Kirklin JK, Naftel DC, Kormos RL, et al. The fourth INTERMACS Annual Report: 4,000 implants and counting. Journal of Heart and Lung Transplantation. 2012;31:117–126.
3. Jessup M, Abraham WT, Casey DE, et al. 2009 focused update: ACCF/AHA Guidelines for the Diagnosis and Management of Heart Failure in Adults: a report of the American College of Cardiology Foundation/American Heart Association Task Force on Practice Guidelines: developed in collaboration with the International Society for Heart and Lung Transplantation. Circulation. 2009;119:1977–2016.
4. McMurray JJ. Clinical practice. Systolic heart failure. New England Journal of Medicine. 2010;362:228–238.
5. Hunt SA, Abraham WT, Chin MH, et al. ACC/AHA 2005 guideline update for the diagnosis and management of chronic heart failure in the adult: summary article: a report of the American College of Cardiology/American Heart Association Task Force on Practice Guidelines (Writing Committee to update the 2001 Guidelines for the Evaluation and Management of Heart Failure). Circulation. 2005;112: 1825–1852.
6. Organ Procurement and Transplantation Network (OPTN) and Scientific Registry of Transplant Recipients (SRTR). OPTN / SRTR 2011 Annual Report. Heart Rockville, MD, Department of Health and Human Services, Health Resources and Services Administration, Healthcare Systems Bureau, Division of Transplantation, 119–146, 2011 Available from: http://srtr.transplant.hrsa.gov/annual_reports/2011/pdf/05_heart_12.pdf.
7. Kirklin JK, Naftel DC, Pagani FD, et al. Long-term mechanical circulatory support (destination therapy): on track to compete with heart transplantation? Journal of Thoracic and Cardiovascular Surgery. 2012;144:584–603.
8. Goldstein DJ, Naftel D, Holman W, et al. Continuous-flow devices and percutaneous site infections: clinical outcomes. Journal of Heart and Lung Transplantation. 2012;31:1151–1157.
9. Demirozu ZT, Radovancevic R, Hochman LF, et al. Arteriovenous malformation and gastrointestinal bleeding in patients with the HeartMate II left ventricular assist device. Journal of Heart and Lung Transplantation. 2011;30:849–853.
10. Urban M, Gazdic T, Slimackova E, et al. Alloimmunosensitization in left ventricular assist device recipients and impact on posttransplantation outcome. ASAIO Journal. 2012;58:554–561.
11. Colvin-Adams M, Valapour M, Hertz M, et al. Lung and heart allocation in the United States. American Journal of Transplantation. 2012;12:3213–3234.
12. Vega JD. The change in heart allocation policy in the United States: is it working as designed? Journal of Heart and Lung Transplantation. 2010;29:255–256.
13. Young JB. Heart failure's near dead and dying: reconsidering our heart transplant wait list scheme. Journal of the American College of Cardiology. 2007;50: 1291–1293.
14. Dardas TF, Cowger J, Koelling TM, et al. The effectiveness of united network of organ sharing status 2 transplantation in the modern era. Journal of Heart and Lung Transplantation. 2011;30:1169–1174.
15. Hauptman PJ, Rich MW, Heidenreich PA, et al. The heart failure clinic: a consensus statement of the heart failure society of America. Journal of Cardiac Failure. 2008;14:801–815.
16. Umana E, Solares CA, Alpert MA. Tachycardia-induced cardiomyopathy. American Journal of Medicine. 2003;114:51–55.
17. Hsu JC, Solomon SD, Bourgoun M, et al. Predictors of super-response to cardiac resynchronization therapy and associated improvement in clinical outcome: the MADIT-CRT (multicenter automatic defibrillator implantation trial with cardiac resynchronization therapy) study. Journal of the American College of Cardiology. 2012;59:2366–2373.
18. Shabetai LT. Idiopathic giant-cell myocarditis–natural history and treatment. Multicenter Giant Cell Myocarditis Study Group Investigators. New England Journal of Medicine. 1997;336:1860–1866.
19. Allen LA, Stevenson LW, Grady KL, et al. Decision making in advanced heart failure: a scientific statement from the American Heart Association. Circulation. 2012;125:1928–1952.
20. Metra M, Ponikowski P, Dickstein K, et al. Advanced chronic heart failure: a position statement from the Study Group on Advanced Heart Failure of the Heart Failure Association of the European Society of Cardiology. European Journal of Heart Failure. 2007;9:684–694.
21. Clark AL, Anker SD. Body mass, chronic heart failure, surgery and survival. Journal of Heart and Lung Transplantation. 2010;29:261–264.
22. Kittleson M, Hurwitz S, Shah MR, et al. Development of circulating-renal limitations to angiotensin-converting enzyme inhibitors identifies patients with severe

heart failure and early mortality. Journal of the American College of Cardiology. 2003;41:2029–2035.
23. Cole RT, Masoumi A, Triposkiadis F, et al. Renal dysfunction in heart failure. Medical Clinics of North America. 2012;96:955–974.
24. Mancini DM, Eisen H, Kussmaul W, et al. Value of peak exercise oxygen consumption for optimal timing of cardiac transplantation in ambulatory patients with heart failure. Circulation. 1991;83:778–786.
25. Mancini D, Leitz K. Selection of cardiac transplantation candidates in 2010. Circulation. 2010;122:173–183.
26. Mehra MR, Kobashigawa J, Starling R, et al. Listing criteria for heart transplantation: International Society for Heart and Lung Transplantation guidelines for the care of cardiac transplant candidates - 2006. Journal of Heart and Lung Transplantation. 2006;25:1024–1042.
27. Kalogeropoulos AP, Georgiopoulou VV, Giamouzis G, et al. Utility of the Seattle Heart Failure Model in patients with advanced heart failure. Journal of the American College of Cardiology. 2009;53:334–342.
28. Goda A, Williams P, Mancini D, et al. Selecting patients for heart transplantation: comparison of the Heart Failure Survival Score (HFSS) and the Seattle Heart Failure Model (SHFM). Journal of Heart and Lung Transplantation. 2011;30:1236–1243.
29. Banner NR, Bonser RS, Clark AL, et al. UK guidelines for referral and assessment of adults for heart transplantation. Heart. 2011;97:1520–1527.
30. Pons J, Leblanc MH, Bernier M, et al. Effects of chronic sildenafil use on pulmonary hemodynamics and clinical outcomes in heart transplantation. Journal of Heart and Lung Transplantation. 2012;31:1281–1287.
31. Perez-Villa F, Farrero M, Sionis A, et al. Therapy with sildenafil or bosentan decreases pulmonary vascular resistance in patients ineligible for heart transplantation because of severe pulmonary hypertension. Journal of Heart and Lung Transplantation. 2010;29:817–818.
32. Beyersdorf F, Schlensak C, Berchtold-Herz M, et al. Regression of "fixed" pulmonary vascular resistance in heart transplant candidates after unloading with ventricular assist devices. Journal of Thoracic and Cardiovascular Surgery. 2010;140:747–749.
33. Eschenhagen T, Force T, Ewer MS, et al. Cardiovascular side effects of cancer therapies: a position statement from the Heart Failure Association of the European Society of Cardiology. European Journal of Heart Failure. 2011;13:1–10.
34. Oliveira GH, Hardaway BW, Kucheryavaya AY, et al. Characteristics and survival of patients with chemotherapy-induced cardiomyopathy undergoing heart transplantation. Journal of Heart and Lung Transplantation. 2012;31:805–810.
35. Uriel N, Vainrib A, Jorde UP, et al. Mediastinal radiation and adverse outcomes after heart transplantation. Journal of Heart and Lung Transplantation. 2010;29:378–381.
36. Nohria A. Should we avoid heart transplantation in cardiomyopathy due to radiotherapy/chemotherapy or amyloidosis? The devil is in the details. Journal of Heart and Lung Transplantation. 2012;31:1253–1256.
37. George JF, Pamboukian SV, Tallaj JA, et al. Balancing rejection and infection with respect to age, race, and gender: clues acquired from 17 years of cardiac transplantation data. Journal of Heart and Lung Transplantation. 2010;29:966–972.
38. Hunt SA. Heart transplant recipient selection issues: limited assets, infinite possibilities. Journal of Heart and Lung Transplantation. 2012;31:675–676.
39. Goldstein DJ, Bello R, Shin JJ, et al. Outcomes of cardiac transplantation in septuagenarians. Journal of Heart and Lung Transplantation. 2012;31:679–685.
40. Daneshmand MA, Rajagopal K, Lima B, et al. Left ventricular assist device destination therapy versus extended criteria cardiac transplant. Annals of Thoracic Surgery. 2010;89:1205–1209.
41. Adams KF Jr, Fonarow GC, Emerman CL, et al. Characteristics and outcomes of patients hospitalized for heart failure in the United States: rationale, design, and preliminary observations from the first 100,000 cases in the Acute Decompensated Heart Failure National Registry (ADHERE). American Heart Journal. 2005;149:209–216.
42. Grady KL, Naftel D, Pamboukian SV, et al. Post-operative obesity and cachexia are risk factors for morbidity and mortality after heart transplant: multi-institutional study of post-operative weight change. Journal of Heart and Lung Transplantation. 2005;24:1424–1430.
43. Gore JL, Pham PT, Danovitch GM, et al. Obesity and outcome following renal transplantation. American Journal of Transplantation. 2006;6:357–363.
44. Emani S, Brewer RJ, John R, et al. Patients with low compared with high body mass index gain more weight after implantation of a continuous-flow left ventricular assist device. Journal of Heart and Lung Transplantation. 2013;32:31–35.
45. Dhesi P, Simsir SA, Daneshvar D, et al. Left ventricular assist device as 'bridge to weight loss' prior to transplantation in obese patients with advanced heart failure. Annals of Transplantation. 2011;16:5–13.
46. Ojo AO, Held PJ, Port FK, et al. Chronic renal failure after transplantation of a nonrenal organ. New England Journal of Medicine. 2003;349:931–940.
47. Rogers JG. Editorial commentary: renal failure after cardiac transplantation: of bravery, wisdom and honesty. Journal of Heart and Lung Transplantation. 2012;31:231–232.
48. Labban B, Arora N, Restaino S, et al. The role of kidney biopsy in heart transplant candidates with kidney disease. Transplantation. 2010;89:887–893.
49. Desai HV, Aronow WS, Peterson SJ, et al. Cardiac amyloidosis: approaches to diagnosis and management. Cardiology in Review. 2010;18:1–11.
50. Bradshaw SH, Veinot JP. Cardiac amyloidosis: what are the indications for transplant? Current Opinion in Cardiology. 2012;27:143–147.
51. Varr BC, Liedtke M, Arai S, et al. Heart transplantation and cardiac amyloidosis: approach to screening and novel management strategies. Journal of Heart and Lung Transplantation. 2012;31:325–331.
52. Ruberg FL, Berk JL. Transthyretin (TTR) cardiac amyloidosis. Circulation. 2012;126:1286–1300.
53. Hosenpud JD, Pamidi SR, Fiol BS, et al. Outcomes in patients who are hepatitis B surface antigen-positive before transplantation: an analysis and study using the joint ISHLT/UNOS thoracic registry. Journal of Heart and Lung Transplantation. 2000;19:781–785.
54. Chen YC, Chuang MK, Chou NK, et al. Twenty-four year single-center experience of hepatitis B virus infection in heart transplantation. Transplantation Proceedings. 2012;44:910–912.
55. Zampino R, Marrone A, Ragone E, et al. Heart transplantation in patients with chronic hepatitis B: clinical evolution, molecular analysis, and effect of treatment. Transplantation. 2005;80:1340–1343.
56. Potthoff A, Tillmann HL, Bara C, et al. Improved outcome of chronic hepatitis B after heart transplantation by long-term antiviral therapy. Journal of Viral Hepatitis. 2006;13:734–741.
57. Lee I, Localio R, Brensinger CM, et al. Decreased post-transplant survival among heart transplant recipients with pre-transplant hepatitis C virus positivity. Journal of Heart and Lung Transplantation. 2011;30:1266–1274.
58. Grossi PA. Update in HIV infection in organ transplantation. Current Opinion in Organ Transplantation. 2012;17:586–593.
59. Stock PG, Barin B, Murphy B, et al. Outcomes of kidney transplantation in HIV-infected recipients. New England Journal of Medicine. 2010;363:2004–2014.
60. Sims DB, Uriel N, González-Costello J, et al. Human immunodeficiency virus infection and left ventricular assist devices: a case series. Journal of Heart and Lung Transplantation. 2011;30:1060–1064.
61. Kop WJ. Role of psychological factors in the clinical course of heart transplant patients. Journal of Heart and Lung Transplantation. 2010;29:257–260.
62. Allen JG, Weiss ES, Arnaoutakis GJ, et al. Insurance and education predict long-term survival after orthotopic heart transplantation in the United States. Journal of Heart and Lung Transplantation. 2012;31:52–60.
63. Tam V, Arnaoutakis GJ, George TJ, et al. Marital status improves survival after orthotopic heart transplantation. Journal of Heart and Lung Transplantation. 2011;30:1389–1394.
64. Maldonado JR, Dubois HC, David EE, et al. The Stanford Integrated Psychosocial Assessment for Transplantation (SIPAT): a new tool for the psychosocial evaluation of pre-transplant candidates. Psychosomatics. 2012;53:123–132.
65. Karamlou T, Diggs BS, Welke K, et al. Impact of single-ventricle physiology on death after heart transplantation in adults with congenital heart disease. Annals of Thoracic Surgery. 2012;94:1281–1287.
66. Davies RR, Russo MJ, Yang J, et al. Listing and transplanting adults with congenital heart disease. Circulation. 2011;123:759–767.
67. Hong KN, Iribarne A, Worku B, et al. Who is the high-risk recipient? Predicting mortality after heart transplant using pretransplant donor and recipient risk factors. Annals of Thoracic Surgery. 2011;92:520–527.
68. Kasiske BL, McBride MA, Cornell DL, et al. Report of a consensus conference on transplant program quality and surveillance. American Journal of Transplantation. 2012;12:1988–1996.
69. Allen LA, Stevenson LW, Grady KL, et al. Decision making in advanced heart failure: a scientific statement from the American Heart Association. Circulation. 2012;125:1928–1952.
70. Schwarz ER, Philip KJ, Simsir SA, et al. Maximal care considerations when treating patients with end-stage heart failure: ethical and procedural quandaries in management of the very sick. Journal of Religion and Health. 2011;50:872–879.

第 31 章 肺移植的患者选择和适应证

Julia B. Becker, Edward R. Garrity Jr

引言

肺移植主要用于治疗终末期肺病，如 COPD、特发性肺纤维化(IPF)、囊性纤维化(CF)等。为了获得生存获益，移植的转诊应考虑到任何特定情况的预后。移植前需仔细评估患者情况，这对移植后的生存有重要影响。本章将详细讨论肺移植的适应证和禁忌证。我们回顾了推荐的肺移植标准及近期的关于患者选择的相关文献。本章及第 40 章将讨论肺移植患者的评分及等待名单管理。

适应证

2012 年国际心肺移植学会（ISHLT）发布了第 29 次肺及心肺联合移植登记报告。肺移植逐渐成为一种常见手术，2010 年施行 3519 例。移植比例的增长表现为两个方面[1,2]，COPD 和特发性肺纤维化(IPF)是肺移植的主要适应证。其中 IPF 的比例由 2000 年的 16%增长到 2010 年的 28.3%(表 31.1)[1]。

2006 年，ISHLT 发布了肺移植的患者选择指南[3]。

与其他实体器官移植相比，肺移植更容易出现慢性排斥反应及高死亡率，再加上供体紧缺，肺移植应该仅限于那些预期有生存益处的患者。根据近期文献，总体中位生存时间为 5.5 年，生存时间超过 1 年的患者，总体中位生存时间为 7.7 年[1]。因此适合肺移植的患者应为最大药物剂量仍无法控制的终末期肺病患者，并且具有明显症状或 50%预期生存时间<2~3 年。ISHLT 采用纽约心脏病协会(NYHA)的分级来评价患者肺功能，Ⅲ期(少量活动后有症状)和Ⅳ期(休息时仍出现症状)为肺移植的适应证[3]。此外，接受肺移植的患者需处于一个相对较好的身体状态。

禁忌证

绝对禁忌证

2006 年的 ISHLT 指南中包括了肺移植的绝对禁忌证(表 31.2)，其中某些禁忌证已经有所改动。

恶性肿瘤

总体来讲，恶性肿瘤是肺移植的绝对禁忌证，其中某些类型的恶性肿瘤可作为相对适应证。原位腺癌及微浸润腺癌在最近的分类中取代了支气管肺泡癌[4]。双侧或多发的此类型肿瘤行肺移植术后，未见短期复发[5,6]。然而，多项关于进展期微浸润腺癌肺移植的研究提示较高的复发率[7,8]。

意外发现，终末期肺病及Ⅰ期非小细胞肺癌(NSCLC)行肺移植后常有良好疗效。ISHLT 肺移植中心报告了 43 例因其他适应证行肺移植时意外发现原发性肺癌的患者，其中Ⅰ期肺癌及微浸润腺癌具有低复发率及低转移率。Ⅱ~Ⅲ期的 NSCLC 则具有高复发率及高死亡率[9]。克利夫兰中心报道了 1991—2000 年 214 例肺移植的患者，其中 2%(4 例)意外发现了肺癌，其中 3 例为Ⅰ期患者，无证据表明复发或远期生存受影响。值得注意的是，此研究的年代尚未普及常规 CT 检查，根据当前诊疗指南，部分患者可能不适合行肺移植治疗[10]。

明显的胸壁及脊柱畸形

由于手术难度及术后需机械通气和肺部清洁，明显畸形的患者少有行肺移植。有文献报道了因严重脊柱侧弯或胸壁畸形而行肺移植的患者[11-13]，其中至少 1 例患者因脊柱侧弯而气道梗阻复发，需要反复气管镜

表 31.1 成人肺移植的适应证(1995 年 1 月—2000 年 6 月[1])

诊断	单肺(n=13 721)数量(%)	双肺(n=20 831)数量(%)	总共(n=34 102)数量(%)
慢性阻塞性肺疾病/肺气肿	6048(45.6)	5549(26.6)	11 587(34.0)
肺纤维化			
特发性	4420(33.4)	3495(16.8)	7925(23.2)
其他	498(3.8)	659(3.2)	1157(3.4)
囊性纤维化	219(1.7)	5469(26.3)	5688(16.7)
α1-抗胰蛋白酶缺乏	741(5.6)	1332(6.4)	2073(6.1)
肺动脉高压	82(0.6)	982(4.7)	1064(3.1)
支气管扩张	54(0.4)	891(4.3)	945(2.8)
结节病	251(1.9)	614(2.9)	865(2.5)
闭塞性细支气管炎	91(0.7)	260(1.2)	351(1.0)
再次移植			
闭塞性细支气管炎	259(2.0)	254(1.2)	513(1.5)
非闭塞性细支气管炎	166(1.3)	191(0.9)	357(1.0)
结缔组织疾病	140(1.1)	281(1.3)	421(1.2)
淋巴管平滑肌瘤病	122(0.9)	241(1.2)	363(1.1)
先天性心脏病	45(0.3)	248(1.2)	293(0.9)
肿瘤	6(0.0)	28(0.1)	34(0.1)
其他	119(0.9)	347(1.7)	466(1.4)

表 31.2 肺移植的绝对禁忌证

1. 2 年内曾患有恶性肿瘤，除了皮肤鳞状细胞癌及基底细胞癌。总体上,5 年生存率较低
2.重要脏器(心脏、肝脏、肾脏)的不可逆功能障碍。患有冠心病,但未行经皮冠状动脉介入治疗或搭桥手术,或者显著的左心室功能障碍,是肺移植的禁忌证,但是心肺联合移植可用于进行过严格选择的患者
3.不可治愈的慢性肺外感染,包括慢性活动性乙、丙型肝炎病毒感染和人类免疫缺陷病毒(HIV)感染
4.严重的胸壁畸形
5.无法遵嘱进行诊疗及随访
6.无法治愈的精神及心理疾病,从而导致无法配合治疗
7.缺乏持续和可依靠的社会支持系统
8.目前或既往 6 个月内有物质成瘾(酒精、烟草、毒品)

检查及介入治疗[14]。如需进行肺移植,需根据胸腔大小来决定手术入路和供体选择[13]。

不可治愈的慢性肺外感染

近 30 年来，对于 HIV 的研究进展改善了 HIV 患者的预后。有报道,1 例合并 HBV 及 HIV 感染的患者因囊性纤维化行肺移植手术，术后两年肺功能良好及无异常并发症[15]。有文献回顾 170 例 HCV 血清反应阳性的肺移植患者,发现生存率无统计学差异,但是大部分患者的 HCV RNA 阴性[16]。克利夫兰诊所的一小组丙型肝病毒阳性的肺移植受者没有肝硬化的迹象表明死亡率没有增加[17]。

重要脏器的不可逆功能障碍

总体上，进展期重要脏器功能障碍是肺移植的禁忌证。但是可考虑器官联合移植。根据器官获取和移植网络(OPTN)的 2011 年 11 月 25 日数据,美国自 1988 年来共有 17 例肺肾联合移植、44 例肝肺联合移植、2 例心肺肾的联合移植、2 例胰腺肺的联合移植、1 例肝胰腺肺的联合移植。

透析患者行肺移植会增加 1 年死亡率[1,2,18],但研究数据有限。

联合移植方面的最主要经验来自肝肺联合移植，特别是肝硬化合并肺囊性纤维化、门脉性肺动脉高压或肝硬化合并肝肺综合征。有效数据显示,其生存率和单器官移植无显著差异[19-26]。

依从性和成瘾

仔细评估社会支持的力度是很重要的，有经验的移植相关心理学家及社会工作者的支持同样重要。一个可用的工具是移植评估量表，此表用于器官移植及骨髓移植前的患者[27]。

不遵守移植后免疫抑制、生活方式的改变及药物治疗在移植的患者中十分常见，约 50%的患者可出现上述问题，包括独自居住的患者[28]。移植前不遵医嘱与晚期急性排斥反应有关[29]。对于移植术后需要服用抗排斥药物 1 年的患者，术前不遵医嘱地服用药物、较低的社会支持、较低的责任感、较高的教育程度是不遵医嘱的行为的预测因素[29]。肺移植患者遵医嘱的比例在不同的研究中有较大差别，主要是因为不同研究对遵医嘱的定义不同[30,31]。与其他器官移植相比，肺移植的不遵医嘱可能性更高，因为肺移植术后需要更多的药物治疗[30]。

终末期肺病的患者多有吸烟史，所以应该强调戒烟。一项研究表明移植术后戒烟率达 100%[32]。然而与尿可铁宁检测相比，自我评价量表可能低估了吸烟率[33]。肺移植患者自称已戒烟从心理上是可以理解的。我们建议对再吸烟可能性大的患者进行生物学检测。

相对禁忌证

对于肺移植的相对禁忌证，存在更多的争论。

年龄

尽管 2006 年的 ISHLT 不建议对 65 岁以上的患者进行肺移植[3]，但这是有争议的。登记数据显示老年患者的肺移植手术不断增加，2000 年年龄≥66 岁的肺移植手术共 28 台(1.6%)。尽管老年患者移植的死亡率更高，但在 2011 年的上半年，共有 13.5%的肺移植手术患者≥66 岁[1]。目前仍无法得出应限制的肺移植的精确年龄，因为不同研究对老年的定义不一。一项多伦多的配对队列研究将 42 例 60 岁以上的患者与 60 岁以下的患者进行对比，老年组的 1 年、2 年、3 年、4 年、5 年生存率显著低于对照组。首要原因是移植早期感染风险更高，其次是恶性肿瘤风险增加[34]。另一项研究纳入了 1999—2006 年 UNOS 数据库 8000 多例患者，结果显示>60 岁的患者 1~2 年的死亡风险增加 37%，但是短期死亡率(30 天及 60 天)和<60 岁的患者无差异。在>60 岁的患者中，>70 岁的人群与<70 岁相比短期死亡率更高。与其他研究不同的是，此研究认为年龄是防止感染和排斥反应的保护因素[35]。最新的 ISHLT 报告显示，年龄>65 岁的患者的中位生存时间比 35~49 岁的患者更短(3.6 年对 6.5 年)，与年龄<65 岁的患者相比，其长期生存率更低(5 年生存率 39%对 51%~56%)[1]。

在其他纳入标准严格的研究中，结果显示高龄组和对照组的术后死亡率相当[36-38]。指南通过 BMI 等来选择高龄患者，但忽视了冠心病、外周血管及脑血管疾病和肾功能不全或衰竭[38]。一项大型研究纳入了 2006 年 1 月至 2008 年 5 月的患者，分为 60 岁以下、60~65 岁、65 岁以上 3 组，结果显示生存率并无统计学差异，但是高龄组并发症的发生率更高，且恶性疾病及药物毒性更常见，而排斥反应多见于 60~65 岁年龄组的患者[39]。

有研究提示，单肺移植可能更适用于老年患者，部分移植中心对移植患者仅行单肺移植手术。Meyer 等回顾分析了 2260 例患者，其中 1835 例接受单肺移植，425 例接受双肺移植，结果显示 60 岁之前行双肺移植有生存优势，60 岁之后行单肺移植生存优势更佳[40]。一项关于肺纤维化的类似研究表明双肺移植并没有比单肺移植更具有优势[41]。然而，也有研究得出相反结论。有研究表明，在 60 岁以上的患者中，双肺移植和单肺移植的术后 30 天 [42]、1 年、2 年、5 年的生存率无统计学差异[43]。一项基于 UNOS 数据的研究表明，60 岁以上的患者行双肺和单肺移植的死亡率无统计学差异[44]。

营养状态

慢性肺病患者的营养状态时有异常。在一项研究中，仅有 1/2 的患者营养状态正常，剩余患者或是体重过低，或是超重[45]。ISHLT 指南不建议对 BMI≥30kg/m^2 的患者进行移植手术，但是没有对体重过低患者做相关建议[3]。

BMI 和死亡率的关系是相当密切的，建议将 BMI 作为移植禁忌证的相关指标。多伦多的研究同样发现超重会产生类似结果[46-48]。一项西班牙的研究纳入了 256 例移植后的患者，其中 38 例为肥胖，肥胖组和对照组的死亡率无统计学差异，但肥胖组有死亡率更高及机械通气时间更长的倾向[49]。超重和肥胖也与移植后肺功能丧失有关[50]。

体重过低是死亡的一个高危因素[51]，最近一项大型回顾性研究将肺移植的患者根据 BMI 分为：低体重(BMI<18.5kg/m^2)、正常体重(BMI 18.5~24.9kg/m^2)、超重

(BMI 25~29.9kg/m^2)、肥胖(BMI>30kg/m^2)。Lederer等在UNOS中回顾了5978例患者，其中包括囊性纤维病、COPD、弥漫性肺实质病变患者，以此评估BMI对肺移植的影响。异常的BMI会导致1年、5年生存率降低。低体重患者的HR为1.15~1.16，超重患者的HR为1.14~1.17，肥胖患者的HR为1.2~1.25[52]。Allen等的研究从UNOS中纳入1998—2008年的11 411例肺移植患者，并根据BMI进行分类，结果显示BMI过高或过低都会导致死亡率增加，有统计学意义，并不显著。多因素分析提示，超重患者的OR值是1.06，肥胖患者的OR值为1.16，低体重患者的OR值为1.14。超重或肥胖患者死亡率的增加主要表现为短期死亡率(1年内)，但低体重患者主要是长期死亡率增加(1年后)[53]。

其他未导致器官终末期病变的疾病

冠状动脉疾病

一项巴西的单因素分析提示，潜在的冠状动脉疾病(CAD)可导致肺移植手术死亡率增加[54]。对潜在的CAD可能需要术前干预。最近UCLA报道了一项10年的研究，该研究对27例左心射血分数良好的单处冠脉病变的患者在肺移植前进行了冠脉血管重建研究，结果是试验组的死亡率和死亡原因与对照组无差别[55]。其他研究也得出类似结论[56,57]。值得注意的是，所有的患者皆为单处冠脉病变且心功能良好。

糖尿病

在肺移植的患者中(特别是CF患者)，糖尿病是一种常见的合并症。Plantier等[58]发现糖尿病是肺移植患者术后全因死亡及因心血管事件死亡的独立高危因素，但是该研究中糖尿病患者的病例数较少。一项纳入25例患者的回顾性研究表明，合并糖尿病的CF患者，肺移植后的并发症发生率及死亡率更高[59]。但有趣的是，大型临床研究提示合并糖尿病对CF患者的肺移植无影响，糖尿病前期的CF患者肺移植后的1年生存率更高[60]。Bradbury等[59]认为术后血糖控制不良与移植后再入院有关，但是，目前暂无关于术后血糖控制作用的系统性研究。我们建议术前应仔细选择血糖控制良好的患者，将强化控制血糖作为肺移植手术术前管理的专家共识。

胃食管反流疾病

胃反流性疾病已经被认为是导致同种异体器官移植后器官功能丧失的原因之一，其会导致阻塞性细支气管炎和急性排斥反应[61,62]，此外还会降低FEV_1和短期生存率[63]。胃食管反流疾病在肺移植患者中发病率高，并且可能无症状，需要侵入性检查[64-66]。肺移植手术后病情可能恶化[67]，其可能与医源性胃瘫有关[68]。

治疗上可能需要外科手术。质子泵抑制剂可以减少胃酸分泌，但是不可治疗非酸性反流和预防胃内容物误吸[69]。胃底折叠术可能导致阻塞性细支气管肺炎发生率的增加[70]。移植前患者可成功实施腹腔镜下胃底折叠术[71]，并且可对移植前和移植后患者的肺功能无显著影响[72,73]。

因此，建议对移植前的患者进行食管反流相关的侵入性检查，症状明显的难治性食管反流疾病应当作为肺移植的相对禁忌证。

危急或不稳定的情况

机械通气、人工肺替代、住院时间长都可增加肺移植患者的1年死亡率。根据ISHLT的数据，紧急移植可导致死亡率的增加[1,2]。欧洲的研究表明，与传统移植相比，紧急移植的生存率更低[74]。对于危重患者(机械通气、人工肺替代)的肺移植才刚刚起步。

在移植时需要机械通气与早期死亡率增加有关。2011年的ISHLT报告指出，1996—2009年390例移植前需要机械通气的患者的1年死亡率是COPD患者的1.57倍。根据美国和欧洲的经验，需要机械通气和体外膜肺氧合(ECMO)的患者1年生存率显著低于常规肺移植患者[75-77]，但与不移植相比可有生存获益[75,76]。根据UNOS数据，一项主要纳入年轻的肺纤维化患者的研究表示，需要机械通气的患者的1个月、6个月、12个月和24个月的生存率分别为83%、67%、62%和57%。需要ECMO的患者1个月、6个月、12个月和24个月的生存率分别为72%、53%、50%和45%。常规肺移植患者的1个月、6个月、12个月和24个月的生存率分别为93%、85%、79%和70%[75]。小样本研究的结果多样[78-81]。目前的经验建议，对需要机械通气的患者进行肺移植时，需注意限制已有单器官功能衰竭、无气道菌群定植和有能力进行物理和康复治疗的患者[82,83]。

单中心的研究提示，ECMO的患者进行肺移植后围术期死亡率及短期死亡率更高，但是中期生存率可接受，3个月生存率甚至可与常规移植相当[84]。其他小规模研究发现静脉分流设备[85,86]或者二氧化碳清除设备(不会导致低氧血症)[87]可成功用于肺移植的过渡期。

可移动的设备及物理治疗可在早期用于肺移植成为可能[88-92]。有趣的是，仅行 ECMO 的患者比需要机械通气的患者有更好的生存获益[93-95]。但是现在尚无关于使用 ECMO 方法和时机的指南。人工肺替代和机械通气将在第 50 章中详细讲述。

高度耐药性或致病性细菌、真菌或分歧杆菌定植

现症感染是移植的禁忌证，因为使用免疫抑制后可能引起脓毒血症而导致死亡。伴有化脓的肺部疾病(囊性纤维化或不伴有囊性纤维化的支气管扩张)，可能有耐药细菌的定植。暂无关于非囊性纤维化患者行肺移植的危险因素的研究。囊性纤维化患者的气道细菌定植将在疾病相关章节中描述。

严重的或者有症状的骨质疏松

肺移植的患者多有骨质疏松和骨量减少[96-98]。双膦酸盐和阻抗训练可用于肺移植患者的预防性治疗[99,100]。但是，移植前疾病处于进展期的患者容易出现严重并发症，因为骨质疏松常会在移植后加重[98,101,102]。移植后使用类固醇激素可能增加严重或有症状的骨质疏松患者的术后并发症发生率。

其他

既往胸科手术

既往胸科手术，特别是涉及胸膜的手术，与肺移植围术期出血增加有关，但不会导致死亡率增加[103-105]，并且不应作为移植的禁忌证。然而，胸膜粘连会提高对手术技巧的要求[106]。

需根据不同的手术情况调整手术方式，既往行肺切除、心脏移植、单侧胸膜粘连等情况可能增加手术风险[107-109]。

阻塞性肺疾病

慢性阻塞性肺疾病

慢性阻塞性肺疾病(COPD)是肺移植最常见的指征[1,18]。COPD 表现多样，预后差别大，因此增加了选择合适移植患者的难度。

生存获益

结合 COPD 预后的明显差别，COPD 患者肺移植的生存获益无明显差别。根据早期的经验，那时尚未实行现在的器官分配制度，肺气肿患者的等待期生存率最高[110]。Thabut 等创立了一套统计学模型，分析了 8182 例等待肺移植的患者，50.1%的单肺移植和 63.7%的双肺移植患者可有生存获益，但这一模型尚未得到进一步的验证[111]，Charman 等的研究同样发现肺移植可提高 COPD 患者的生存获益[112]。

预后

最近的大型临床研究提示 COPD 的预后具有较大的异质性。一项纳入 2163 例 COPD 患者的回顾性研究提示，COPD 患者 3 年 FEV_1 下降程度的比例差别较大，38%的患者 FEV_1 下降>40mL/y，31%的患者 FEV_1 下降 21~40mL/y，23%的患者变化为从减少 20mL/y 到增加 20mL/y，8%的患者增加>20mL/y。重度 COPD 患者的下降幅度小于轻度 COPD 患者的下降幅度[113]。FEV_1、肺过度充气、体重减轻至 BMI 过低、贫血、活动耐量、呼吸困难、健康相关的生活质量和活跃程度、需要氧疗、肺气肿的加重可以作为预测 COPD 患者肺移植术后死亡率的指标[114-117]。

FEV_1

在早期的研究中，Burrows 等使用 FEV_1 来预测 COPD 的预后，该研究纳入 200 例患者，随访 7 年，总体死亡率为 58%。FEV_1<0.75L 的患者预后显著差于 FEV_1 为 0.75~1.24L 的患者，预后最好的是 FEV_1>1.24L 的患者。研究提示 FEV_1 每年下降 56mL，但是个体差异较大[118]。

一项观察性研究纳入了无低氧血症的 COPD 患者，随访 3 年，发现支气管扩张后的 FEV_1 与肺移植后的死亡率有关[119]。

恶化

入院后 COPD 急性加重可导致术后 1 年死亡率的上升，根据不同文献报道，1 年死亡率为 22%~59%，当二氧化碳分压>50mmHg 时，死亡率可达 49%[120]，进入 ICU 的可能性为 59%[120-123]。一项研究纳入了 304 例 COPD 患者，随访时间为 5 年，研究了反复急性加重和死亡率的关系。与无急性加重的 COPD 患者相比，加重 3~4 次/年的患者死亡的 HR 为 4.13，加重 1~2 次/年的患者

死亡的 HR 为 2.0。独立危险因素是肺功能和年龄[115]。最近，一项大样本的研究提示，无论总共的加重次数及基础肺功能如何，每一次加重都可导致死亡率的增加[124]。

肺动脉高压

舒张期肺动脉压力与肺气肿患者肺移植后死亡率有关[125]。

BODE 指数

Celli 等于 2004 年发表了一个具有里程碑意义 COPD 严重程度的预后评分，即 BODE 指数。BODE 是指 BMI(B)、气流阻塞的程度(O)、呼吸困难程度(D)和运动能力(E)，并通过 6 分钟步行试验(6MWT)来测定。BODE 评分高的患者死亡率更高(表 31.3)。与 FEV_1 的预测结果基本相符合[126]。

通过 BODE 指数来推测移植的作用是有限的，因为该指标主要在老年或男性群体中得到验证[126]。然而，Lahzami 研究发现 BODE 指数≥7 提示患者可从肺移植中获益[127]。更进一步的观察性研究或单中心研究均提示 BODE 指数对预后有帮助。Martinez 等回顾了 609 例重度肺气肿的患者(FEV_1≤45%，残气量≥150%)，发现标准化 BODE 指数越高死亡率越高[117]。进一步研究发现标准化 BODE 指数在 6 个月、12 个月、24 个月的变化可以预测死亡率[128]。一项前瞻性研究纳入了 1997—2008 年美国和西班牙的 751 例患者，长期以至少 3 种方法监测 BODE 评分和 FEV_1，结果显示，BODE 评分增加但 FEV_1 正常的病例(n=69)死亡率更高[129]。

结合 VO_{2max} 的心肺运动功能测定(CPET)的标准化 BODE 并不能增加预测的准确性[130]。一例急性加重的 COPD 患者的 6 分钟步行试验结果同样良好，可以简化评分[131]。需要强调的是，尽管 BODE 评分等可以被推荐为移植的评价标准，但并不适用于肺移植供体分配。

表 31.3 BODE 指数的分值

变量	分数			
	0	1	2	3
BMI(kg/m²)	>21	≤21		
FEV_1(%预测值)	≥65	50~64	36~49	≤35
MMRC(scal)	0~1	2	3	4
6MWT(m)	≥350	250~349	150~249	≤149

From Celli et al.[126] Copyright © 2004 Massachusetts Medical Society. Reprinted with permission from the Massachusetts Medical Society.

同时也有其他的评分运用于临床，如 HADO 评分(健康状态、活动能力、呼吸困难程度、梗阻)[132]和 CART(分类树及回归树)，后者利用年龄、FEV_1、呼吸困难程度、活动能力、一般健康情况、2 年内住院情况进行分析[133]。目前尚未取代 BODE 的评分，也没有常规用于肺移植的评估。

肺减容术

肺减容术可被看作是适合行肺移植术患者的一种替代方式或是桥梁。它已被运用于改善异质性肺气肿患者的过度充气，并且已被证明可以改善阻塞性通气障碍、气潴留、氧合及运动耐量等生理学参数[134]。一组随机对照试验显示，肺减容术可以改善有上肺叶明显病变及较差运动能力的患者的死亡率[135]。经手术治疗的患者其修正 BODE 评分有所改善，而该评分与死亡率相关[128]。成功的肺减容术延长了患者肺移植前的时间，并且不会影响肺移植后的发病率和死亡率[136-140]。对于肺减容术失败的这部分患者，其本身就代表有较高风险需行肺移植术[139,140]。一项报道显示，31 例在肺移植等待名单中的患者，有 24 例在行肺减容术后被从名单中移除了[136]。FEV_1<20%、一氧化碳弥散量(DLCO)<20%或均质肺气肿的患者行肺减容术有较高的死亡风险，因而不适宜行该手术。

手术选择

慢性阻塞性肺疾病(COPD)患者可行单侧或双侧肺移植，后者更获得青睐。国际心肺移植协会/器官共享联合网络(ISHLT/UNOS)的一项 1991—1997 年的研究共纳入了 2260 例行肺移植术的 COPD 患者（其中 1835 例行单侧肺移植术，425 例行双侧肺移植术)，该项研究结果显示年龄<60 岁的患者行双侧肺移植术有更高的生存率；年龄>60 岁行单侧肺移植死亡率更高[40]。华盛顿大学 2002 年发表的一项研究纳入了 1998—2000 年 306 例肺气肿患者，结果发现慢性阻塞性肺疾病和 α1-抗胰蛋白酶缺失患者行双侧肺移植术的 5 年生存率更高，而早期住院期间生存率及 5 年生存率在两种疾病之间并没有区别[142]。

移植指南

基于上述信息，ISHLT 建议 BODE 评分>5 分的患者可考虑行肺移植术，而 BODE 评分为 7~10 分或是满足以下至少一项者：有与急性高碳酸血症相关的住院史、肺动脉高压和（或）肺心病、FEV_1<20%或 DLCO<20%或均质肺气肿，应行肺移植术。

α1-抗胰蛋白酶缺失

肺气肿与α1-抗胰蛋白酶缺失（AATD）有关，AATD 是一种常染色体显性遗传病，是需行肺移植术的第 4 大常见疾病，占 ISHLT 注册的移植患者的 7%[18]。它是导致阻塞性肺疾病的一种因素[143]，会加速年轻患者的肺部疾病的进展[144]，特别是对于有吸烟史的患者[145]。最普遍也是最严重的情况是 ZZ 等位基因同时缺失，临床表现为肺气肿和（或）终末期的肝脏疾病[143]。美国[146]和丹麦[147]的注册库资料显示 AATD 患者死亡率和肺气肿相关，不管患者吸烟与否[148,149]。移植的标准与非 AATD 性肺气肿一样，以 FEV_1 作为选择的标准之一。AATD 的死亡率和 FEV_1 相关，FEV_1 在最低百分位点（<35%~37.5%预测值）的这部分患者的死亡率最高[145,150,151]。此外，DLCO 和 CT 扫描的得分与呼吸性死亡相关[150,151]。所有患者均应考虑酶替治疗，因为它可以延缓 FEV_1 的衰减和改善总体死亡率[145]。

弥散性肺实质疾病

弥散性肺实质疾病是肺移植常见的指征。特发性肺纤维化（IPF）是目前肺移植的第二常见指征，并且在肺移植中所占的比例逐渐递增。而对于其他弥散性肺实质疾病，如淋巴管平滑肌瘤病、结节病、胶原血管病相关的间质性肺疾病（ILDS），也常需要行肺移植术[2,18]。

特发性肺纤维化和纤维化非特异性间质性肺炎

预后

美国胸科学会发布了最新的关于特发性间质性肺炎的组织学分类[152]。与其他类型相比，病理学表现为普通型间质性肺炎（UIP）的特发性肺纤维化（IPF）的预后更差，因而当考虑患者需行肺移植时应当做出正确的诊断。脱屑性间质性肺炎（DIP）和呼吸性毛细支气管性间质性肺炎（RBILD）的 5 年生存率为 80%，纤维化非特异性间质性肺炎（NSIP）的生存率为 70%，而普通型间质性肺炎（UIP）的 5 年生存率仅有 20%[153]。相似的，一项对于 315 例弥散性肺实质疾病患者的回顾性研究显示，IPF 的生存率（2 年生存率为 48.4%，5 年生存率为 35.4%）比其他疾病（2 年生存率为 74.9%~100%，5 年生存率为 69.5%~91.6%）更低[154]。一些针对 IPF 行移植术的生存效益的评估已经被建立[112,155,156]。

列入移植名单和移植的时机需要考虑患者的预后，目的是识别短期内有高死亡风险的患者被列入名单，而暂缓对预期疾病进展可能缓慢的患者的移植。这种评估对于 IPF 患者更具挑战性，因为疾病进展快速且很难预测患者情况的恶化[157]。一项观察性研究发现，有轻微至中等程度的 IPF 患者，可以急性、突发或是亚急性恶化伴呼吸困难进行性加重而后逐渐衰减以至死亡[158]。起初认为 IPF 生存时间的中位数是 2~3 年，然而，逐渐地认识发现临床进展大相径庭，一些患者可以有更长的生存期[157]。最近的注册数据显示，轻微程度患者的中位生存时间是 55.6 个月，而用力肺活量（FVC）低的严重程度的患者的中位生存时间是 27.4 个月[156]。2006 年 ISHLT 关于间质性肺疾病转诊的参考指南包括有组织学或影像学证据而与肺活量无关的普通型间质性肺炎（UIP），以及有组织学证据的纤维性非特异性间质性肺炎（NSIP）[3]。组织学同时诊断为 UIP 和 NSIP（有活组织切片证据）的患者的预后与单独为 UIP 的患者的预后相似，同样需要考虑行肺移植术[159]。

预后

肺功能

反映肺功能的不同参数均与生存情况有关。基线肺活量的评估与死亡率有关，尽管在不同的研究中具体增加相关风险的数值不同：≤60%预测值[160]，而用力肺活量的切断点为 60%~83%[161]。最近，Nathan 等注意到，以用力肺活量为划分（轻度≥70%，中等程度 55%~69%，重度<55%），中位生存期分别为 55.6 个月、38.7 个月及 27.4 个月[156]。Latsi 等发现短期死亡率（2 年）高的患者，其基线用力肺活量更低（62.0%对 78.7%）[162]。

用力肺活量的纵向改变在多项研究中均显示为与死亡率的增加有关[163-167]，甚至横向变化（6 个月内 5%~10%的改变）也比稳定的患者有更高的死亡率[164]。

DLCO

DLCO 也与生存率相关，尽管像 FVC 一样，具体数值在不同研究中不尽相同（30%~45%）。有研究表示，

DLCO<50%预测值的逐渐减小伴随着死亡率的逐渐增高，而DLCO<20%预测值的患者预后最差[156,161,162,168,169]。梅奥诊所针对487例IPF患者的一项研究显示，DLCO每10%的减少伴随着相对风险1.4的增加[166]。Mogulkoc等经过多因素分析也发现DLCO和生存率相关，并且DLCO每减少1%相对死亡风险增加4%[169]。纵向分析显示，DLCO 1年减少>20%和死亡率相关[167]，尽管更低水平的改变没有发现统计学意义[164,170]。

肺泡-动脉血氧梯度(A-a梯度)

关于肺泡-动脉血氧梯度与死亡率是否相关，不同的研究则有不同的结果[165,170]。

肺动脉高压

肺动脉高压[160,168,171]，或是合并有肺纤维化和肺气肿[172]与IPF的预后差相关，平均肺动脉压力升高超过17mmHg伴随着5年生存率的下降。

运动耐量

6分钟步行试验(6MWT)可以提供一些反映疾病预后的信息。一项纳入了822例患者的纵向比较显示，6MWT距离减少超过50m，死亡风险增加4倍，距离减少26~50m，死亡风险增加3倍[173]。另一项前瞻性研究也发现风险增加3倍，距离减少29~34m[174]。以色列的一份正在等待肺移植的患者资料显示，6MWT的步行距离和死亡风险相关[175]。

相似的，6MWT后不正常的心率恢复的时间（1~2分钟）、血氧饱和度的改变、爬山或是6MWT时的最低血氧饱和度也与较差的预后相关，并且或许也与肺高压相关[176-178]。

影像学

研究发现，高分辨率CT(HRCT)的特征可预测死亡率[169,179,180]。纤维化的程度和死亡风险的增加相关，而有更多纤维化的患者更可能有低的DLCO和FVC，以及肺泡-动脉血氧梯度的增加[180]。HRCT纤维化得分每增加一个单位，则死亡风险增加106%[169]。

机械通气

因为急性呼吸衰竭而需要机械通气的IPF患者，其死亡率极高。传统上，需要机械通气的患者将不再被考虑行移植手术[161]。一项针对34例伴呼吸衰竭的IPF患者的回顾性调查显示，15例使用有创机械通气的患者有100%的院内死亡率；19例使用无创机械通气的患者有74%的死亡率。存活的5例患者中，有4例在回访的6个月内死亡[181]。

移植指南

基于上述大部分信息，2006年ISHLT指南建议UIP或是纤维化NSIP患者均应申请肺移植，而组织学或是影像学支持的UIP伴DLCO<39%预测值、FVC 6个月下降≥10%、6MWT期间血氧饱和度<88%或HRCT呈蜂窝状，则需行移植术。对于NSIP患者，如果DLCO<35%、FVC下降≥10%或是6个月DLCO下降>15%，则推荐行移植术[3]。

即使有关于预后的临界值的变化范围，但确切的生理学指标也可能存在争议。例如，Flaherty等建议FVC或总肺活量≤65%预测值以及DLCO≤45%预测值的患者应被列入肺移植名单[161]。一些主观的指标，如进行性呼吸困难和咳嗽与死亡率相关，但并未被列入指南中[165,177,182]。因此，在做出决策时应全面地评估患者的临床进程和并发症。

单侧和双侧肺移植

多项研究发现双侧肺移植比单侧肺移植的生存率更高，尽管最初手术的挑战性更大(手术时间更长、手术复杂性更高)。1987—2008年UNOS的数据库资料显示，年轻组患者的1年生存率双侧肺移植优于单侧[183]。而UNOS 2005—2007年的数据库资料显示，肺分配指数(见第40章)高的患者，1年生存率也是双侧优于单侧[184]。另一项针对IPF患者的评估发现，行双侧肺移植患者移植后6MWT和FEV_1更佳，同时1年生存率、总体生存率和没有闭塞性细支气管炎综合征的生存率更高，尽管行双侧肺移植患者的术前平均肺动脉压力更高[185]。其他评估显示，IPF患者比其他诊断的患者的总体30天和1年生存率更差，而单侧与双侧比较则没有统计学差异[41,186]。

其他弥散性肺实质性疾病

结缔组织疾病和相关的肺部疾病

行移植术的肺纤维化相关的结缔组织疾病患者仅占肺移植患者总数的0.8%[18]，部分原因是患者因伴有系统性疾病而导致手术的复杂化，与此同时，患者的预后较IPF患者好[187]。弥散性肺实质疾病和多发的结缔组织疾病有关，包括系统性硬化、多肌炎和皮肌炎、风湿性关节炎、混合性结缔组织疾病、系统性红斑狼疮和干燥综合征[161]。由于临床经验有限,暂未有关于考虑移植和实行移植最佳时机的推荐。

系统性硬化

肺部病变几乎存在于所有系统性硬化患者，但仅有少数患者存在进行性恶化[188]。已有不少成功进行肺移植的案例[189-192],一项单中心的对于 14 例系统性硬化患者行肺移植的研究显示，尽管术后急性排斥发生的概率比 IPF 移植患者更高，但是总体 1 年生存率并无差异[189]。和硬皮病相关的系统性疾病会影响移植,包括皮肤溃疡、慢性肾脏疾病和食管运动障碍[193]。对于硬皮病考虑行肺移植的患者，应有进行性恶化的肺部病变和最小化的系统性疾病。

特发性炎性肌病(ILD)

多肌炎、皮肌炎、临床无肌病性皮肌炎和抗合成酶综合征在 35%~40%的患者中与 ILD 相关,其中一些伴随有进展性呼吸衰弱[194]。相关的肌肉衰弱可能是不支持移植的指征[161],因为它会延缓术后修复和降低肺清除率。有进展性肺部疾病的患者需行多项肺功能测试后才能考虑移植，并且如伴有系统性疾病应是非活动性的。

风湿性关节炎、混合性结缔组织疾病、系统性红斑狼疮和干燥综合征

ILD 在风湿性关节炎中发生的概率各异，在 1%~4%的患者中伴有衰弱的肺部疾病;严重的炎症性关节炎是这部分患者进行肺移植的最大禁忌证[161]。在风湿性关节炎中,HRCT 和活体组织学检查发现的 UIP 比其他结缔组织疾病相关的 ILD 更为常见,相对来说预后也更差[195]。胸膜性疾病在系统性红斑狼疮中很普遍,但是明显的肺纤维化进展很罕见,并且这种疾病本身进展很缓慢;一项对于 14 例间质性疾病和狼疮患者的研究显示,仅有 2 例患者最终死于进展性的肺部疾病[196,197]。另一项对于 144 例混合性结缔组织病(MTCD)患者的研究显示,其中 96 例(66.6%)有急性 ILD,大部分在治疗后得到缓解,尽管 13 例患者 HRCT 上仍有一些纤维化的表现,其中 1 例呈蜂窝状影像[198]。MTCD 患者的食管扩张与 ILD 有关[199],提示这可能是移植的禁忌证。最后,ILD 使干燥综合征患者的疾病进展更加复杂化，在一项研究中影响了 20 例患者中的 9 例[200]。

移植的方法和其他结缔组织疾病相似，有进展性肺部疾病和微小系统性疾病的患者应转诊至移植中心。

结节病(肉状瘤病)

结节病是一种多系统疾病，可以导致其他器官的损伤(如心脏和肝脏),而这会妨碍移植的顺利进行。这种疾病目前占所有肺移植的 2.6%[18]。患有晚期肺结节病的患者在等待移植过程中有很高的死亡率。美国宾夕法尼亚大学医疗中心的 43 例结节病患者在等待肺移植的过程中,其中 23 例(53%)在移植前死亡。所有等候的患者 3 年生存率是 31%,而 12 例移植患者的 3 年生存率为 50%[201]。等待生存率与 IPF 类似,尽管结节病患者要担负更大的肺高压[202]。

预后

肺高压是影响结节病最重要的危险因素[203]。多因素分析显示,右心房压力(RAP)≥15mmHg 是导致死亡的独立危险因素[201]。1995—2000 年的一项针对美国 405 例等候移植的结节病患者的研究显示，死亡的风险和肺动脉压力的增加、供氧需求增加及非裔美国人种相关[204]。

移植指南

基于上述发现,2006 年 ISHLT 指南建议：对于结节病患者,若 NYHA 心功能评分Ⅲ级或Ⅳ级,应考虑行移植术;若 NYHA 心功能评分Ⅲ级或Ⅳ级,且伴休息时低氧血症、肺高压或右肺动脉压力>15mmHg,则应行肺移植术[3]。

淋巴管平滑肌瘤病

基于目前 ISHLT 报道，淋巴管平滑肌瘤病(LAM)占肺移植患者的 1.1%[18]，是一种被认为仅发生在育龄妇女的罕见疾病。并且,其在发病的 10 年内迅速致命[205,206]。随着对该疾病意识的提高、对该疾病的筛查及对该罕见疾病数据库的建立[207],我们发现患者群包括更年老的妇女，并且部分 LAM 患者疾病进展缓慢,10 年生存率可高达 91%[208-211]。LAM 注册数据库纳入了 1998—2001 年的 LAM 患者,发现 1/3 的患者已经接受或正在等候肺移植[212]。

移植考虑

虽然移植后的生存率可与其他疾病相当，但是术后有一些特异性的并发症，如经常发生的气胸、乳糜胸，可能需要进行辅助通气，并且如果已有胸膜手术

史,手术过程中出血的概率会增加[104,213-215]。LAM的移植也很少因反复发作而复杂化[214-216]。因此,这些风险必须在移植评估过程中充分传达给患者。

预后

最大氧耗的减少和以FEV_1及DLCO评估的疾病严重性一致。一项研究显示已接受移植的患者,其平均VO_{2max}预测值为41.7%[217]。疾病进展通常由FEV_1和(或)DLCO的减少来定义,两者均和CT扫描的影像学结果及组织学评分相关[218,219]。

移植指南

FEV_1和DLCO的减少范围是很广的。对于快速进展的LAM患者,其FEV_1每年可减少0~285mL[218],平均减少110mL/y[208]。而在治疗上,仅有西罗莫司已被证明可有效减缓肺功能的下降[220];而对疾病进展至肺移植的影响仍待观察。

肺功能和功能肺活量仍是评估患者是否需要移植的最佳方法。2006年ISHLT指南建议:若患者的NYHA心功能评分Ⅲ级或Ⅳ级,应考虑行移植术;如果肺功能严重受损,并且休息时出现运动耐力不足或低氧血症,则应行肺移植术[3]。如果一系列肺功能的测量均显示肺功能的快速下降,不管治疗与否,应尽早考虑行移植术。

肺朗格汉斯细胞组织细胞增生症(嗜酸性肉芽肿)

移植

肺朗格汉斯细胞组织细胞增生症(PLCH)是肺移植中的一种罕见疾病,提示许多PLCH患者的疾病趋于稳定或消退[221]。

法国的一项针对39例PLCH患者的回顾性调查显示,PLCH的1年生存率为76.9%,2年生存率为63.6%,5年生存率为57.2%,10年生存率为53.7%[222]。中位生存率在两项回顾性调查中相似,分别为12.5年和13年[223,224]。疾病终末期通常和严重肺高压有关,而与肺功能损伤的程度无关,同时疾病可以直接导致肺血管病变[221,222,225-227]。肺高压在肺移植的患者中几乎无处不在[222]。

移植时机

和LAM一样,肺功能和功能肺活量是评估患者是否需要移植的方法,因为这种罕见疾病并没有任何精确的预测手段。等待移植过程中需要注意患者肺高压的恶化程度。2006年ISHLT指南建议,NYHA心功能评分Ⅲ级或Ⅳ级的患者需考虑行移植术,而伴有严重肺功能损伤以及在休息时出现运动耐力不足或是低氧血症的患者,则需行肺移植术[3]。

囊性纤维化和导致支气管扩张的其他因素

囊性纤维化(CF)是肺移植的重要指征,占1995—2010年期间肺移植数的16%[2]。与行肺移植的其他诊断相比,CF是一种多系统疾病且患者更为年轻。CF患者接受肺移植术后能显著改善生存率[110,112,228,229]。一些分析显示,其是所有移植诊断中获益最大的[228,229]。

除CF外,引起支气管扩张的因素有很多,包括先天性的、自身免疫疾病或是肿瘤引起的、与感染有关的,或是免疫缺陷相关的因素[230]。对于这些不同因素引起的支气管扩张的移植处理,与CF类似[3]。

移植指南

2006年ISHLT指南建议:如果患者FEV_1<30%或FEV_1快速下降,尤其是年轻女性患者、病情恶化需要住ICU的患者、恶化频率增加需要使用抗生素的患者、顽固性或经常发作的气胸的患者,或者栓塞不能控制的反复咯血的患者,需要考虑行移植术[3]。若患者存在氧依赖性呼吸衰竭、高碳酸血症或是肺高压,则需行肺移植术[3]。

预后

近几年,CF的预后在逐渐改善。根据囊性纤维化基金会截至2010年度的注册数据显示,CF中位生存率已从1986年的27岁增加到了2010年的38.3岁。呼吸衰竭仍是导致CF死亡的最普遍因素[231]。与生存率相关的指标有FEV_1、年龄、性别、肺部血流动力学、供氧需求、高碳酸血症以及恶化的频率,这些指标均被纳入2006年的ISHLT移植指南[3]。其他可能增加死亡率的因素包括糖尿病、6MWT和营养状态[232-235]。

FEV_1

FEV_1的传统移植参考值FEV_1<30%预测值来自Kerem等早在1992年的研究。1977—1989年的一项纳入673例患者的回顾性研究显示,FEV_1<30%预测值、

PaO_2<55mmHg 及 $PaCO_2$>50mmHg 的患者 2 年死亡率高达 50%[236]。死亡率数据提示需要适当的移植时机来达到生存获益。在等待移植的过程中 FEV_1 逐渐恶化也与死亡相关。一项研究显示,与成功进行移植的患者的 FEV_1 相比(21%预测值),等待移植过程中死亡患者的 FEV_1 更低(15%预测值),6MWT 的距离也更低[237]。FEV_1%预测值已被纳入多个模型来预测 CF 的生存率[233,238,239]。

由于 CF 的生存率有所改善，近年来的研究认为 FEV_1 30%的临界值已经不足以作为评估移植的单独临界值。Augarten 等通过对 40 例 FEV_1<30%预测值的患者的评估,发现即使未行肺移植术的患者,也存在生存率的改善[240]。

Kerem 等提出 CF 的 2 年死亡率为 50%，这个值并没有根据后期对肺功能严重下降的患者的随访而不断更新,提示 CF 治疗的改革已经使生存率有所提升。明尼苏达大学对 61 例 FEV_1<30%预测值的患者进行回顾性调查，结果发现 FEV_1<30%预测值的 49 例已故患者中，在死亡的 2 年内 FEV_1 才达到临界值的只有 1/3。剩下的患者在 2~14 年间 FEV_1 一直持续<30%。生存分析指出 FEV_1<30%预测值的患者中位生存时间为 3.9 年[241]。另一项对于 178 例 FEV_1<30%预测值的研究则显示中位生存时间为 4.6 年,其中移植前时代(1986—1990 年)25%患者的生存时间>9 年[242]。在英国,George 等开展了一项单中心研究,随访 1990—2003 年 FEV_1<30%预测值的 276 例患者直到 2007 年，发现中位生存时间从 1990 年的 1.2 年增加到了 2003 年的 5.3 年。而最长的中位生存时间是 1994—1997 年,与英国成功提取 DNA 酶以及队列研究营养状态的改善时间一致[243]。

FEV_1 衰减的比例是预测死亡率和移植时机的有用指标[244]。对于生存时间短于中位生存时间的患者，FEV_1 衰减的比例更高(每年 1.8%预测值)。相反,长于中位生存时间的患者,FEV_1 衰减的比例较低（每年 0.73%预测值),提示 FEV_1 衰减的比例是预测死亡有意义的指标。总的来说,FEV_1 每衰减 1%预测值(每年),相对死亡风险增加 1.3 倍[241]。Augarten 等也发现,FEV_1 衰减的比例是导致死亡的独立危险因素[240]。

性别

许多研究均显示，女性和死亡风险的增加相关[231,233,236,245-248],尽管少数研究并没有发现两者之间的联系[240,241,249]。性别差异的具体影响机制仍未知。

年龄

年龄小也与死亡率增加有关。年龄<18 岁的患者生存时间更短[235,236,241]。Kerem 等发现,年龄<18 岁的患者相关死亡风险增加 2.0 倍[236]。

恶化频率

病情的急性恶化与较差的预后相关，而次数的多少与死亡率相关[248,250]。同时,需要 ICU 干预的严重程度恶化的患者预后更差[235,251]。

肺血流动力学

肺高压和死亡相关，因此已被纳入到移植参考标准中。在等待肺移植过程中死亡的患者更可能有严重程度的肺高压,表现在更高的肺动脉阻力、$PaCO_2$ 和全身血管阻力[252]。一项仅有 27 例患者的研究也发现,肺高压的严重程度和死亡相关[248]。另一项针对 Barnes Jewish 医院等候肺移植的 146 例 CF 患者的研究则发现，较高的肺动脉压力是等待移植过程中死亡的独立危险因素[232]。

预测模型

2001 年建立了一个以 CF 5 年生存与否为因变量的预测模型。该模型的数据来源是囊性纤维化基金会注册的患者数据库,自变量纳入了年龄、FEV_1、性别、年龄体重 Z 评分、胰腺分泌功能、糖尿病、金黄色葡萄球菌感染、洋葱伯克霍尔德菌属感染以及每年急性肺部恶化的次数[233]。同一学者还发现,运用该模型来识别 5 年生存率<30%的患者，会发现患者能从肺移植中获益,而仅用 FEV_1<30%预测值的单一指标不能确切得出移植能改善生存率的结果。但是,该模型运用在 5 年生存率更高组别的群体却得出肺移植不能带来生存获益的结果[253]。尽管如此,该模型未被纳入移植参考指南中。

感染风险

气道微生物的定植和感染是 CF 患者长期存在的问题。基于这个原因,几乎所有 CF 患者行肺移植术都采用双侧。

均应评估每例患者体内微生物环境对死亡率和移植风险的影响。Liou 等的预测模型发现,洋葱伯克霍尔德菌属感染和死亡相关,OR 值为 4.12[233]。相似的研究发现，洋葱伯克霍尔德菌属感染也与移植后感染引起的死亡风险增加有关[254,255],并且很多单位将该病菌的感染作为移植的禁忌证。近来的研究均表明与死亡风险增加有关的感染尤其特指洋葱伯克霍尔德菌属的感染[255-257]。一项75例移植患者的研究结果显示，该菌属感染和随后生存率的下降有关，而非该菌属感染未能得出相似的结果[256]。

其他非洋葱伯克霍尔德菌属的微生物定植并未发现对CF有严重的影响。Liou等的预测模型发现金黄色葡萄球菌的定植能带来生存获益[233]。一项单中心研究显示，除洋葱伯克霍尔德菌属外全耐药的患者与其他患者相比，生存率会有所下降，尽管下降后的生存率仍不比UNOS数据库CF患者的生存率低。该项研究的定植菌属包括假单胞菌、寡养单胞菌和无色杆菌[258]。

肝脏疾病

严重的肝脏疾病在CF患者中很普遍，如肝硬化。27%~35%的患者有肝脏受累，大部分是局部胆汁性肝硬化，少部分患者进展到多胆管肝硬化并出现终末期肝脏疾病并发症[259]。肝脏疾病是死亡或肺移植的独立危险因素[260]。对于伴有肝脏疾病的CF患者，成功的肺移植保护了肝脏的合成功能而对患者预后没有不良影响[261,262]。对于同时有终末期肝脏疾病和肺部疾病的患者可考虑采用肺肝联合移植。

危重病和机械通气

一些研究报道了需行机械通气的CF成功进行肺移植的案例[78-80]。然而，移植应仅限于没有全身性感染，仅有单个器官衰竭且术后能够参与物理治疗的患者[263]。

肺动脉高压

肺动脉高压可由多种因素造成[264]，并且长期以来一直是肺移植的指征。特发性肺动脉高压（IPAH）是肺动脉高压最常见的一种，自1995年起占肺移植数的3.1%[1]。IPAH患者的短期死亡率很高，但相对其他移植患者而言长期生存率较高，仅次于CF移植患者[1,2]。近年来由于治疗的进展，IPAH患者的预后有所改善，行移植术的比例也有所下降。

预后

在治疗以前，肺动脉高压患者的预后很差。一组57例未接受移植的肺高压患者3年生存率为35%[265]。NIH注册数据显示的中位生存期是2.8年，并且平均肺动脉压力（≥85mmHg对≤55mmHg）、平均右心房压力（<10mmHg对≥20mmHg）和平均心指数[<2L/(min·m^2)对≥4L/(min·m^2)]均会对生存率造成负面的影响[266]。随后的研究显示右心衰竭和右心房压力≥12mmHg和较差的生存率相关[267]。

长期输注前列环素可以降低死亡率[266,268,269]，并且导致考虑移植的患者减少。治疗无反应是死亡和考虑移植的预测因素。NYHA心功能评分Ⅳ级患者的预后比Ⅲ级患者差，且患者无心功能改善或肺阻力下降30%死亡率更高[267]。

6MWT与死亡率相关，6MWT距离<332m患者的生存率下降[270]。运用促红细胞生成素的随机对照试验显示，死亡的患者同时6MWT距离更短[268]。

移植参考

基于上述预后数据，ISHLT建议：若NYHA心功能评分Ⅲ级或Ⅳ级，或是伴病情快速进展的患者，均应考虑行移植术，而治疗后仍为NYHA心功能评分Ⅲ级或Ⅳ级、6MWT<350m或是逐渐减少、前列环素治疗无效、心指数<2L/(min·m^2)或右心房压力>15mmHg的患者应行移植术[3]。

尽管药物治疗是有效的，但接受肺移植术患者的生存率比处于疾病严重状态的患者高[271]，尽管最近实施的肺分配评分（见第40章）并没有使等待移植患者的死亡率有所改善[272]。另外还有一些评估方法对于识别病程逐渐恶化的患者进行手术治疗的时机具有重要的意义[273]。

总结

肺移植仍然是一个复杂的手术，如果实施成功，患者将能从中持续受益。虽然很多终末期肺病都可以考虑移植（常见有COPD、IPF和CF），但彻底评估患者的并发症、解剖因素和社会状况尤为重要。旨在优化患者的移植条件和适用性，以获得最佳治疗结果，转诊医生和移植机构之间的良好合作也十分必要。

致谢

本书受到健康资源和服务管理合同234-2005-37011C的资助。内容仅由作者负责，并不一定反映卫生与公众部门的观点和政策，提及的商标、商业产品或组织并不意味着得到美国政府的认可。

（刘以俊 译　张大方 校）

参考文献

1. Christie JD, et al. The Registry of the International Society for Heart and Lung Transplantation: 29th adult lung and heart-lung transplant report-2012. Journal of Heart and Lung Transplantation. 2012;31(10):1073–1086.
2. Christie JD, et al. The Registry of the International Society for Heart and Lung Transplantation: twenty-eighth adult lung and heart-lung transplant report–2011. Journal of Heart and Lung Transplantation. 2011;30(10):1104–1122.
3. Orens JB, et al. International guidelines for the selection of lung transplant candidates: 2006 update–a consensus report from the Pulmonary Scientific Council of the International Society for Heart and Lung Transplantation. Journal of Heart and Lung Transplantation. 2006;25(7):745–755.
4. Travis WD, et al. International Association for the Study of Lung Cancer/American Thoracic Society/European Respiratory Society International multidisciplinary classification of lung adenocarcinoma. Journal of Thoracic Oncology. 2011;6(2):244–285.
5. Etienne B, et al. Successful double-lung transplantation for bronchioalveolar carcinoma. Chest. 1997;112(5):1423–1424.
6. Wang Y, Chen J. [Lung transplantation for lung carcinoma: a case report and literature review]. Zhongguo Fei Ai Za Zhi. 2011;14(7):633–636.
7. Zorn GL Jr, et al. Pulmonary transplantation for advanced bronchioloalveolar carcinoma. Journal of Thoracic and Cardiovascular Surgery. 2003;125(1):45–48.
8. de Perrot M, et al. Role of lung transplantation in the treatment of bronchogenic carcinomas for patients with end-stage pulmonary disease. Journal of Clinical Oncology. 2004;22(21):4351–4356.
9. de Perrot M, et al. Management of lung transplant recipients with bronchogenic carcinoma in the native lung. Journal of Heart and Lung Transplantation. 2003;22(1):87–89.
10. Abrahams NA, et al. Incidence of primary neoplasms in explanted lungs: long-term follow-up from 214 lung transplant patients. Transplantation Proceedings. 2004;36(9):2808–2811.
11. Su JW, et al. Successful double lung transplantation in 2 patients with severe scoliosis. Journal of Heart and Lung Transplantation. 2008;27(11):1262–1264.
12. Fukahara K, et al. Successful heart-lung transplantation in a patient with kyphoscoliosis. Journal of Heart and Lung Transplantation. 2003;22(4):468–473.
13. Piotrowski JA, et al. Single-lung transplantation in a patient with cystic fibrosis and an asymmetric thorax. Annals of Thoracic Surgery. 1997;64(5):1456–1458, discussion 1458–1459.
14. Garcha PS, et al. Clinical course after successful double lung transplantation in a patient with severe scoliosis. Journal of Heart and Lung Transplantation. 2011;30(2):234–235.
15. Bertani A, et al. Successful lung transplantation in an HIV- and HBV-positive patient with cystic fibrosis. American Journal of Transplantation. 2009;9(9):2190–2196.
16. Fong TL, et al. Outcomes after lung transplantation and practices of lung transplant programs in the United States regarding hepatitis C seropositive recipients. Transplantation. 2011;91(11):1293–1296.
17. Sahi H, et al. Outcomes after lung transplantation in patients with chronic hepatitis C virus infection. Journal of Heart and Lung Transplantation. 2007;26(5):466–471.
18. Christie JD, et al. The Registry of the International Society for Heart and Lung Transplantation: twenty-seventh official adult lung and heart-lung transplant report–2010. Journal of Heart and Lung Transplantation. 2010;29(10):1104–1118.
19. Barshes NR, et al. Combined lung and liver transplantation: the United States experience. Transplantation. 2005;80(9):1161–1167.
20. Corno V, et al. Combined double lung-liver transplantation for cystic fibrosis without cardio-pulmonary by-pass. American Journal of Transplantation. 2007;7(10):2433–2438.
21. Couetil JP, et al. Combined lung and liver transplantation in patients with cystic fibrosis. A 4 1/2-year experience. Journal of Thoracic and Cardiovascular Surgery. 1995;110(5):1415–1422, discussion 1422–1423.
22. Couetil JP, et al. Combined heart-lung-liver, double lung-liver, and isolated liver transplantation for cystic fibrosis in children. Transplant International. 1997;10(1):33–39.
23. Dennis CM, et al. Heart-lung-liver transplantation. Journal of Heart and Lung Transplantation. 1996;15(5):536–538.
24. Gandhi SK, et al. Case report of combined pediatric heart-lung-liver transplantation. Transplantation. 2002;73(12):1968–1969.
25. Praseedom RK, et al. Combined transplantation of the heart, lung, and liver. Lancet. 2001;358(9284):812–813.
26. Wise PE, et al. Heart-lung-liver transplant for cystic fibrosis. Transplantation Proceedings. 2001;33(7–8):3568–3571.
27. Erim Y, et al. Psychosomatic evaluation of patients awaiting lung transplantation. Transplantation Proceedings. 2009;41(6):2595–2598.
28. Germani G, et al. Nonadherent behaviors after solid organ transplantation. Transplantation Proceedings. 2011;43(1):318–323.
29. Dobbels F, et al. Pretransplant predictors of posttransplant adherence and clinical outcome: an evidence base for pretransplant psychosocial screening. Transplantation. 2009;87(10):1497–1504.
30. De Bleser L, et al. The spectrum of nonadherence with medication in heart, liver, and lung transplant patients assessed in various ways. Transplant International. 2011;24(9):882–891.
31. Bosma OH, et al. Adherence to immunosuppression in adult lung transplant recipients: prevalence and risk factors. Journal of Heart and Lung Transplantation. 2011;30(11):1275–1280.
32. Evon DM, et al. Tobacco and alcohol use in lung transplant candidates and recipients. Clinical Transplantation. 2005;19(2):207–214.
33. Gorber SC, et al. The accuracy of self-reported smoking: a systematic review of the relationship between self-reported and cotinine-assessed smoking status. Nicotine and Tobacco Research. 2009;11(1):12–24.
34. Gutierrez C, et al. The effect of recipient's age on lung transplant outcome. American Journal of Transplantation. 2007;7(5):1271–1277.
35. Weiss ES, et al. Lung allocation score predicts survival in lung transplantation patients with pulmonary fibrosis. Annals of Thoracic Surgery. 2009;88(6):1757–1764.
36. Smith PW, et al. Lung transplantation in patients 60 years and older: results, complications, and outcomes. Annals of Thoracic Surgery. 2006;82(5):1835–1841, discussion 1841.
37. Machuca TN, et al. Lung transplantation for patients older than 65 years: is it a feasible option? Transplantation Proceedings. 2011;43(1):233–235.
38. Mahidhara R, et al. Lung transplantation in older patients? Journal of Thoracic and Cardiovascular Surgery. 2008;135(2):412–420.
39. Vadnerkar A, et al. Age-specific complications among lung transplant recipients 60 years and older. Journal of Heart and Lung Transplantation. 2011;30(3):273–281.
40. Meyer DM, et al. Single vs bilateral, sequential lung transplantation for end-stage emphysema: influence of recipient age on survival and secondary end-points. Journal of Heart and Lung Transplantation. 2001;20(9):935–941.
41. Meyer DM, et al. Impact of recipient age and procedure type on survival after lung transplantation for pulmonary fibrosis. Annals of Thoracic Surgery. 2005;79(3):950–957, discussion 957–958.
42. Minambres E, et al. Early outcome after single vs bilateral lung transplantation in older recipients. Transplantation Proceedings. 2008;40(9):3088–3089.
43. Palmer SM, et al. Successful bilateral lung transplant outcomes in recipients 61 years of age and older. Transplantation. 2006;81(6):862–865.
44. Nwakanma LU, et al. Impact of bilateral versus single lung transplantation on survival in recipients 60 years of age and older: analysis of United Network for Organ Sharing database. Journal of Thoracic and Cardiovascular Surgery. 2007;133(2):541–547.
45. Souza SM, et al. Nutritional profile of lung transplant candidates. Jornal Brasileiro de Pneumologia: Publicacao Oficial da Sociedade Brasileira de Pneumologia e Tisilogia. 2009;35(3):242–247.
46. Kanasky WF Jr, et al. Impact of body weight on long-term survival after lung transplantation. Chest. 2002;121(2):401–406.
47. Culver DA, et al. Discordant utility of ideal body weight and body mass index as predictors of mortality in lung transplant recipients. Journal of Heart and Lung Transplantation. 2005;24(2):137–144.
48. Madill J, et al. Nutritional assessment of the lung transplant patient: body mass index as a predictor of 90-day mortality following transplantation. Journal of Heart and Lung Transplantation. 2001;20(3):288–296.
49. de la Torre MM, et al. Influence of body mass index in the postoperative evolution after lung transplantation. Transplantation Proceedings. 2010;42(8):3026–3028.
50. Lederer DJ, et al. Obesity and primary graft dysfunction after lung transplantation: the LTOG obesity study. American Journal of Respiratory and Critical Care Medicine. 2011;184(9):1055–1061.
51. Plochl W, et al. Nutritional status, ICU duration and ICU mortality in lung transplant recipients. Intensive Care Medicine. 1996;22(11):1179–1185.
52. Lederer DJ, et al. Obesity and underweight are associated with an increased risk of death after lung transplantation. American Journal of Respiratory and Critical

Care Medicine. 2009;180(9):887–895.
53. Allen JG, et al. The impact of recipient body mass index on survival after lung transplantation. Journal of Heart and Lung Transplantation. 2010; 29(9):1026–1033.
54. Machuca TN, et al. Prognostic factors in lung transplantation: the Santa Casa de Porto Alegre experience. Transplantation. 2011;91(11):1297–1303.
55. Sherman W, et al. Lung transplantation and coronary artery disease. Annals of Thoracic Surgery. 2011;92(1):303–308.
56. Parekh K, et al. Outcome of lung transplantation for patients requiring concomitant cardiac surgery. Journal of Thoracic and Cardiovascular Surgery. 2005;130(3):859–863.
57. Patel VS, et al. Clinical outcome after coronary artery revascularization and lung transplantation. Annals of Thoracic Surgery. 2003;75(2):372–377, discussion 377.
58. Plantier L, et al. Impact of previous cardiovascular disease on the outcome of lung transplantation. Journal of Heart and Lung Transplantation. 2010; 29(11):1270–1276.
59. Bradbury RA, et al. Prior diabetes mellitus is associated with increased morbidity in cystic fibrosis patients undergoing bilateral lung transplantation: an 'orphan' area? A retrospective case-control study. Internal Medicine Journal. 2009; 39(6):384–388.
60. Hofer M, et al. Diabetes mellitus and survival in cystic fibrosis patients after lung transplantation. Journal of Cystic Fibrosis. 2012;11(2):131–136.
61. Palmer SM, et al. Gastroesophageal reflux as a reversible cause of allograft dysfunction after lung transplantation. Chest. 2000;118(4):1214–1217.
62. Shah N, et al. Gastroesophageal reflux disease is associated with an increased rate of acute rejection in lung transplant allografts. Transplantation Proceedings. 2010;42(7):2702–2706.
63. Murthy SC, et al. Pretransplant gastroesophageal reflux compromises early outcomes after lung transplantation. Journal of Thoracic and Cardiovascular Surgery. 2011;142(1):47–52.e3.
64. Reid KR, et al. Importance of chronic aspiration in recipients of heart-lung transplants. Lancet. 1990;336(8709):206–208.
65. Sweet MP, et al. The prevalence of distal and proximal gastroesophageal reflux in patients awaiting lung transplantation. Annals of Surgery. 2006;244(4): 491–497.
66. Fortunato GA, et al. Prevalence of gastroesophageal reflux in lung transplant candidates with advanced lung disease. Jornal Brasileiro de Pneumologia: Publicacao Oficial da Sociedade Brasileira de Pneumologia e Tisilogia. 2008; 34(10):772–778.
67. Young LR, et al. Lung transplantation exacerbates gastroesophageal reflux disease. Chest. 2003;124(5):1689–1693.
68. D'Ovidio F, Keshavjee S. Gastroesophageal reflux and lung transplantation. Diseases of the Esophagus. 2006;19(5):315–320.
69. Blondeau K, et al. Gastro-oesophageal reflux and gastric aspiration in lung transplant patients with or without chronic rejection. European Respiratory Journal. 2008;31(4):707–713.
70. Davis RD Jr, et al. Improved lung allograft function after fundoplication in patients with gastroesophageal reflux disease undergoing lung transplantation. Journal of Thoracic and Cardiovascular Surgery. 2003;125(3):533–542.
71. Gasper WJ, et al. Antireflux surgery for patients with end-stage lung disease before and after lung transplantation. Surgical Endoscopy. 2008;22(2):495–500.
72. Hoppo T, et al. Antireflux surgery preserves lung function in patients with gastroesophageal reflux disease and end-stage lung disease before and after lung transplantation. Archives of Surgery. 2011;146(9):1041–1047.
73. Hartwig MG, Appel JZ, Davis RD. Antireflux surgery in the setting of lung transplantation: strategies for treating gastroesophageal reflux disease in a high-risk population. Thoracic Surgery Clinics. 2005;15(3):417–427.
74. Boussaud V, et al. One-year experience with high-emergency lung transplantation in France. Transplantation. 2012;93(10):1058–1063.
75. Mason DP, et al. Should lung transplantation be performed for patients on mechanical respiratory support? The US experience. Journal of Thoracic and Cardiovascular Surgery. 2010;139(3):765–773.e1.
76. Gottlieb J, et al. Outcome of critically ill lung transplant candidates on invasive respiratory support. Intensive Care Medicine. 2012;38(6):968–975.
77. Algar FJ, et al. Lung transplantation in patients under mechanical ventilation. Transplantation Proceedings. 2003;35(2):737–738.
78. Flume PA, et al. Lung transplantation for mechanically ventilated patients. Journal of Heart and Lung Transplantation. 1994;13(1 Pt 1):15–21, discussion 22–23.
79. Massard G, et al. Double-lung transplantation in mechanically ventilated patients with cystic fibrosis. Annals of Thoracic Surgery. 1993;55(5):1087–1091, discussion 1091–1092.
80. Bartz RR, et al. Pre-transplant mechanical ventilation and outcome in patients with cystic fibrosis. Journal of Heart and Lung Transplantation. 2003;22(4): 433–438.
81. Elizur A, et al. Pre-transplant mechanical ventilation increases short-term morbidity and mortality in pediatric patients with cystic fibrosis. Journal of Heart and Lung Transplantation. 2007;26(2):127–131.
82. Vermeijden JW, et al. Lung transplantation for ventilator-dependent respiratory failure. Journal of Heart and Lung Transplantation. 2009;28(4):347–351.
83. Baz MA, et al. Lung transplantation after long-term mechanical ventilation : results and 1-year follow-up. Chest. 2001;119(1):224–227.
84. Bermudez CA, Rocha RV, Toyoda Y, et al. Extracorporeal membrane oxygenation as a bridge to lung transplant: midterm outcomes. Annals of Thoracic Surgery. 2011; 92(4):1226–1231; discussion 1231–1232.
85. Fischer S, et al. Bridge to lung transplantation with the extracorporeal membrane ventilator Novalung in the veno-venous mode: the initial Hannover experience. ASAIO Journal. 2007;53(2):168–170.
86. Fischer S, et al. Bridge to lung transplantation with the novel pumpless interventional lung assist device NovaLung. Journal of Thoracic and Cardiovascular Surgery. 2006;131(3):719–723.
87. Ricci D, et al. The use of CO2 removal devices in patients awaiting lung transplantation: an initial experience. Transplantation Proceedings. 2010;42(4): 1255–1258.
88. Garcia JP, et al. Ambulatory extracorporeal membrane oxygenation: a new approach for bridge-to-lung transplantation. Journal of Thoracic and Cardiovascular Surgery. 2010;139(6):e137–e139.
89. Turner DA, et al. Active rehabilitation and physical therapy during extracorporeal membrane oxygenation while awaiting lung transplantation: a practical approach. Critical Care Medicine. 2011;39(12):2593–2598.
90. Reeb J, et al. Double lumen bi-cava cannula for veno-venous extracorporeal membrane oxygenation as bridge to lung transplantation in non-intubated patient. Interactive Cardiovascular and Thoracic Surgery. 2012;14(11): 125–127.
91. Hayes D Jr, et al. Ambulatory venovenous extracorporeal respiratory support as a bridge for cystic fibrosis patients to emergent lung transplantation. Journal of Cystic Fibrosis. 2012;11(1):40–50.
92. Hammainen P, et al. Usefulness of extracorporeal membrane oxygenation as a bridge to lung transplantation: a descriptive study. Journal of Heart and Lung Transplantation. 2011;30(1):103–107.
93. Nosotti M, et al. Bridge to lung transplantation by venovenous extracorporeal membrane oxygenation: a lesson learned on the first four cases. Transplantation Proceedings. 2010;42(4):1259–1261.
94. Nosotti M, et al. Extracorporeal membrane oxygenation with spontaneous breathing as a bridge to lung transplantation. Interactive Cardiovascular and Thoracic Surgery. 2013;16(1):55–59.
95. Fuehner T, et al. Extracorporeal membrane oxygenation in awake patients as bridge to lung transplantation. American Journal of Respiratory and Critical Care Medicine. 2012;185(7):763–768.
96. Lakey WC, et al. Osteoporosis in lung transplant candidates compared to matched healthy controls. Clinical Transplantation. 2011;25(3):426–435.
97. Jastrzebski D, et al. Osteoporosis in patients referred for lung transplantation. European Journal of Medical Research. 2010;15(Suppl 2):68–71.
98. Spira A, et al. Osteoporosis and lung transplantation: a prospective study. Chest. 2000;117(2):476–481.
99. Braith RW, et al. Comparison of alendronate vs alendronate plus mechanical loading as prophylaxis for osteoporosis in lung transplant recipients: a pilot study. Journal of Heart and Lung Transplantation. 2007;26(2):132–137.
100. Mitchell MJ, et al. Resistance training prevents vertebral osteoporosis in lung transplant recipients. Transplantation. 2003;76(3):557–562.
101. Seijas R, et al. Bilateral pathological hip fractures in a patient with a bipulmonary transplant: a case report. Journal of Orthopaedic Surgery (Hong Kong). 2009;17(2):240–242.
102. Aris RM, et al. Severe osteoporosis before and after lung transplantation. Chest. 1996;109(5):1176–1183.
103. Detterbeck FC, Egan TM, Mill MR. Lung transplantation after previous thoracic surgical procedures. Annals of Thoracic Surgery. 1995;60(1):139–143.
104. Almoosa KF, et al. Management of pneumothorax in lymphangioleiomyomatosis: effects on recurrence and lung transplantation complications. Chest. 2006; 129(5):1274–1281.
105. Koulouri S, et al. Previous thoracic surgery does not increase peri-operative mortality in pediatric heart-lung transplant recipients. Journal of Heart and Lung Transplantation. 2004;23(11):1228–1230.
106. Rolla M, et al. Lung transplantation for cystic fibrosis after thoracic surgical procedures. Transplantation Proceedings. 2011;43(4):1162–1163.
107. Le Pimpec-Barthes F, et al. Single-lung transplantation in patients with previous contralateral pneumonectomy: technical aspects and results. European Journal of Cardio-Thoracic Surgery. 2009;36(5):927–932.
108. Diethrich EB, et al. Postoperative complications necessitating right lower lobec-

tomy in a heart-lung transplant recipient with previous sternotomy. Journal of Thoracic and Cardiovascular Surgery. 1987;94(3):389–392.
109. Kawaguchi A, et al. Heart and unilateral lung transplantation in patients with end-stage cardiopulmonary disease and previous thoracic operations. Journal of Thoracic and Cardiovascular Surgery. 1989;98(3):343–349.
110. De Meester J, et al. Listing for lung transplantation: life expectancy and transplant effect, stratified by type of end-stage lung disease, the Eurotransplant experience. Journal of Heart and Lung Transplantation. 2001;20(5):518–524.
111. Thabut G, et al. Determinants of the survival benefit of lung transplantation in patients with chronic obstructive pulmonary disease. American Journal of Respiratory and Critical Care Medicine. 2008;177(10):1156–1163.
112. Charman SC, et al. Assessment of survival benefit after lung transplantation by patient diagnosis. Journal of Heart and Lung Transplantation. 2002;21(2): 226–232.
113. Vestbo J, et al. Changes in forced expiratory volume in 1 second over time in COPD. New England Journal of Medicine. 2011;365(13):1184–1192.
114. Celli BR, et al. Predictors of Survival in COPD: more than just the FEV1. Respiratory Medicine. 2008;102(Suppl 1):S27–S35.
115. Soler-Cataluna JJ, et al. Severe acute exacerbations and mortality in patients with chronic obstructive pulmonary disease. Thorax. 2005;60(11):925–931.
116. Celli BR. Predictors of mortality in COPD. Respiratory Medicine. 2010;104(6): 773–779.
117. Martinez FJ, et al. Predictors of mortality in patients with emphysema and severe airflow obstruction. American Journal of Respiratory and Critical Care Medicine. 2006;173(12):1326–1334.
118. Burrows B, Earle RH. Course and prognosis of chronic obstructive lung disease. A prospective study of 200 patients. New England Journal of Medicine. 1969;280(8):397–404.
119. Anthonisen NR, Wright EC, Hodgkin JE. Prognosis in chronic obstructive pulmonary disease. American Review of Respiratory Disease. 1986;133(1):14–20.
120. Connors AF Jr, et al. Outcomes following acute exacerbation of severe chronic obstructive lung disease. The SUPPORT investigators (Study to Understand Prognoses and Preferences for Outcomes and Risks of Treatments). American Journal of Respiratory and Critical Care Medicine. 1996;154(4 Pt 1):959–967.
121. Seneff MG, et al. Hospital and 1-year survival of patients admitted to intensive care units with acute exacerbation of chronic obstructive pulmonary disease. JAMA. 1995;274(23):1852–1857.
122. Groenewegen KH, Schols AM, Wouters EF. Mortality and mortality-related factors after hospitalization for acute exacerbation of COPD. Chest. 2003;124(2):459–467.
123. Almagro P, et al. Mortality after hospitalization for COPD. Chest. 2002; 121(5):1441–1448.
124. Garcia-Aymerich J, et al. Lung function impairment, COPD hospitalisations and subsequent mortality. Thorax. 2011;66(7):585–590.
125. Egan TM, et al. Predictors of death on the UNOS lung transplant waiting list: results of a multivariate analysis. Journal of Heart and Lung Transplantation. 2001;20(2):242.
126. Celli BR, et al. The body-mass index, airflow obstruction, dyspnea, and exercise capacity index in chronic obstructive pulmonary disease. New England Journal of Medicine. 2004;350(10):1005–1012.
127. Lahzami S, et al. Survival impact of lung transplantation for COPD. European Respiratory Journal. 2010;36(1):74–80.
128. Martinez FJ, et al. Longitudinal change in the BODE index predicts mortality in severe emphysema. American Journal of Respiratory and Critical Care Medicine. 2008;178(5):491–499.
129. Casanova C, et al. The progression of chronic obstructive pulmonary disease is heterogeneous: the experience of the BODE cohort. American Journal of Respiratory and Critical Care Medicine. 2011;184(9):1015–121.
130. Cote CG, et al. The modified BODE index: validation with mortality in COPD. European Respiratory Journal. 2008;32(5):1269–1274.
131. Soler-Cataluna JJ, et al. Severe exacerbations and BODE index: two independent risk factors for death in male COPD patients. Respiratory Medicine. 2009; 103(5):692–699.
132. Esteban C, et al. BODE-Index vs HADO-score in chronic obstructive pulmonary disease: which one to use in general practice? BMC Medicine. 2010;8:28.
133. Esteban C, et al. Development of a decision tree to assess the severity and prognosis of stable COPD. European Respiratory Journal. 2011;38(6): 1294–1300.
134. Cooper JD, et al. Results of 150 consecutive bilateral lung volume reduction procedures in patients with severe emphysema. Journal of Thoracic and Cardiovascular Surgery. 1996;112(5):1319–1329, discussion 1329–1330.
135. Fishman A, et al. A randomized trial comparing lung-volume-reduction surgery with medical therapy for severe emphysema. New England Journal of Medicine. 2003;348(21):2059–2073.
136. Bavaria JE, et al. Effect of volume reduction on lung transplant timing and selection for chronic obstructive pulmonary disease. Journal of Thoracic and Cardiovascular Surgery. 1998;115(1):9–17, discussion 17–18.
137. Burns KE, et al. Outcomes of lung volume reduction surgery followed by lung transplantation: a matched cohort study. Annals of Thoracic Surgery. 2002;73(5):1587–1593.
138. Meyers BF, et al. Outcome of bilateral lung volume reduction in patients with emphysema potentially eligible for lung transplantation. Journal of Thoracic and Cardiovascular Surgery. 2001;122(1):10–17.
139. Senbaklavaci O, et al. Successful lung volume reduction surgery brings patients into better condition for later lung transplantation. European Journal of Cardio-Thoracic Surgery. 2002;22(3):363–367.
140. Wisser W, et al. Lung transplantation following lung volume reduction surgery. Journal of Heart and Lung Transplantation. 2000;19(5):480–487.
141. National Emphysema Treatment Trial Research Group. Patients at high risk of death after lung-volume-reduction surgery. New England Journal of Medicine. 2001;345(15):1075–1083.
142. Cassivi SD, et al. Thirteen-year experience in lung transplantation for emphysema. Annals of Thoracic Surgery. 2002;74(5):1663–1669, discussion 1669–1670.
143. Stoller JK, Aboussouan LS. Alpha1-antitrypsin deficiency. Lancet. 2005; 365(9478):2225–2236.
144. Browne RJ, Mannino DM, Khoury MJ. Alpha 1-antitrypsin deficiency deaths in the United States from 1979-1991. An analysis using multiple-cause mortality data. Chest. 1996;110(1):78–83.
145. Survival and FEV1 decline in individuals with severe deficiency of alpha1-antitrypsin. The Alpha-1-Antitrypsin Deficiency Registry Study Group. American Journal of Respiratory and Critical Care Medicine. 1998;158(1):49–59.
146. McElvaney NG, et al. Baseline characteristics of enrollees in the National Heart, Lung and Blood Institute Registry of alpha 1-antitrypsin deficiency. Alpha 1-Antitrypsin Deficiency Registry Study Group. Chest. 1997;111(2):394–403.
147. Seersholm N, Kok-Jensen A, Dirksen A. Survival of patients with severe alpha 1-antitrypsin deficiency with special reference to non-index cases. Thorax. 1994;49(7):695–698.
148. Stoller JK, et al. Mortality in individuals with severe deficiency of alpha1-antitrypsin: findings from the National Heart, Lung, and Blood Institute Registry. Chest. 2005;127(4):1196–1204.
149. Seersholm N, Kok-Jensen A. Clinical features and prognosis of life time non-smokers with severe alpha 1-antitrypsin deficiency. Thorax. 1998;53(4): 265–268.
150. Dawkins P, et al. Mortality in alpha-1-antitrypsin deficiency in the United Kingdom. Respiratory Medicine. 2009;103(10):1540–1547.
151. Dawkins PA, et al. Predictors of mortality in alpha1-antitrypsin deficiency. Thorax. 2003;58(12):1020–1026.
152. American Thoracic Society, European Respiratory Society. American Thoracic Society/European Respiratory Society international multidisciplinary consensus classification of the idiopathic interstitial pneumonias. This joint statement of the American Thoracic Society (ATS), and the European Respiratory Society (ERS) was adopted by the ATS board of directors, June 2001 and by the ERS Executive Committee, June 2001. American Journal of Respiratory and Critical Care Medicine. 2002;165(2):277–304.
153. Bjoraker JA, et al. Prognostic significance of histopathologic subsets in idiopathic pulmonary fibrosis. American Journal of Respiratory and Critical Care Medicine. 1998;157(1):199–203.
154. Thomeer MJ, et al. Interstitial lung diseases: characteristics at diagnosis and mortality risk assessment. Respiratory Medicine. 2004;98(6):567–573.
155. Thabut G, et al. Survival benefit of lung transplantation for patients with idiopathic pulmonary fibrosis. Journal of Thoracic and Cardiovascular Surgery. 2003;126(2):469–475.
156. Nathan SD, et al. Long-term course and prognosis of idiopathic pulmonary fibrosis in the new millennium. Chest. 2011;140(1):221–229.
157. Raghu G, et al. An official ATS/ERS/JRS/ALAT statement: idiopathic pulmonary fibrosis: evidence-based guidelines for diagnosis and management. American Journal of Respiratory and Critical Care Medicine. 2011;183(6):788–824.
158. Martinez FJ, et al. The clinical course of patients with idiopathic pulmonary fibrosis. Annals of Internal Medicine. 2005;142(12 Pt 1):963–967.
159. Monaghan H, et al. Prognostic implications of histologic patterns in multiple surgical lung biopsies from patients with idiopathic interstitial pneumonias. Chest. 2004;125(2):522–526.
160. Jezek V, et al. The prognostic significance of functional tests in cryptogenic fibrosing alveolitis. Bulletin Europeen de Physiopathologie Respiratoire. 1980;16(6): 711–720.
161. Flaherty KR, et al. Timing of lung transplantation for patients with fibrotic lung diseases. Seminars in Respiratory and Critical Care Medicine. 2001;22(5): 517–532.
162. Latsi PI, et al. Fibrotic idiopathic interstitial pneumonia: the prognostic value of

longitudinal functional trends. American Journal of Respiratory and Critical Care Medicine. 2003;168(5):531-537.
163. Taniguchi H, et al. The clinical significance of 5% change in vital capacity in patients with idiopathic pulmonary fibrosis: extended analysis of the pirfenidone trial. Respiratory Research. 2011;12:93.
164. Zappala CJ, et al. Marginal decline in forced vital capacity is associated with a poor outcome in idiopathic pulmonary fibrosis. European Respiratory Journal. 2010;35(4):830-836.
165. Collard HR, et al. Changes in clinical and physiologic variables predict survival in idiopathic pulmonary fibrosis. American Journal of Respiratory and Critical Care Medicine. 2003;168(5):538-542.
166. Douglas WW, Ryu JH, Schroeder DR. Idiopathic pulmonary fibrosis: impact of oxygen and colchicine, prednisone, or no therapy on survival. American Journal of Respiratory and Critical Care Medicine. 2000;161(4 Pt 1):1172-1178.
167. Hanson D, et al. Changes in pulmonary function test results after 1 year of therapy as predictors of survival in patients with idiopathic pulmonary fibrosis. Chest. 1995;108(2):305-310.
168. Hamada K, et al. Significance of pulmonary arterial pressure and diffusion capacity of the lung as prognosticator in patients with idiopathic pulmonary fibrosis. Chest. 2007;131(3):650-656.
169. Mogulkoc N, et al. Pulmonary function in idiopathic pulmonary fibrosis and referral for lung transplantation. American Journal of Respiratory and Critical Care Medicine. 2001;164(1):103-108.
170. King TE Jr, et al. Analyses of efficacy end points in a controlled trial of interferon-gamma1b for idiopathic pulmonary fibrosis. Chest. 2005;127(1):171-177.
171. Nadrous HF, et al. The impact of pulmonary hypertension on survival in patients with idiopathic pulmonary fibrosis. Chest. 2005;128(6 Suppl):616S-617S.
172. Mejia M, et al. Idiopathic pulmonary fibrosis and emphysema: decreased survival associated with severe pulmonary arterial hypertension. Chest. 2009;136(1): 10-15.
173. du Bois RM, et al. Six-minute-walk test in idiopathic pulmonary fibrosis: test validation and minimal clinically important difference. American Journal of Respiratory and Critical Care Medicine. 2011;183(9):1231-1237.
174. Holland AE, et al. Small changes in six-minute walk distance are important in diffuse parenchymal lung disease. Respiratory Medicine. 2009;103(10): 1430-1435.
175. Shitrit D, et al. Risk factors for death while awaiting lung transplantation in Israeli patients: 1997-2006. European Journal of Cardio-Thoracic Surgery. 2008;34(2): 444-448.
176. Swigris JJ, et al. Heart rate recovery after 6-min walk test predicts survival in patients with idiopathic pulmonary fibrosis. Chest. 2009;136(3):841-848.
177. Nishiyama O, et al. A simple assessment of dyspnoea as a prognostic indicator in idiopathic pulmonary fibrosis. European Respiratory Journal. 2010;36(5): 1067-1072.
178. Shitrit D, et al. The 15-step oximetry test: a reliable tool to identify candidates for lung transplantation among patients with idiopathic pulmonary fibrosis. Journal of Heart and Lung Transplantation. 2009;28(4):328-333.
179. Wells AU, et al. Serial CT in fibrosing alveolitis: prognostic significance of the initial pattern. AJR. American Journal of Roentgenology. 1993;161(6): 1159-1165.
180. Lynch DA, et al. High-resolution computed tomography in idiopathic pulmonary fibrosis: diagnosis and prognosis. American Journal of Respiratory and Critical Care Medicine. 2005;172(4):488-493.
181. Mollica C, et al. Mechanical ventilation in patients with end-stage idiopathic pulmonary fibrosis. Respiration; International Review of Thoracic Diseases. 2010;79(3):209-215.
182. Ryerson CJ, et al. Cough predicts prognosis in idiopathic pulmonary fibrosis. Respirology. 2011;16(6):969-975.
183. Force SD, et al. Bilateral lung transplantation offers better long-term survival, compared with single-lung transplantation, for younger patients with idiopathic pulmonary fibrosis. Annals of Thoracic Surgery. 2011;91(1):244-249.
184. Weiss ES, et al. Survival after single versus bilateral lung transplantation for high-risk patients with pulmonary fibrosis. Annals of Thoracic Surgery. 2009; 88(5):1616-1625, discussion 1625-1626.
185. Neurohr C, et al. Potential functional and survival benefit of double over single lung transplantation for selected patients with idiopathic pulmonary fibrosis. Transplant International. 2010;23(9):887-896.
186. Algar FJ, et al. Results of lung transplantation in idiopathic pulmonary fibrosis patients. Transplantation Proceedings. 2010;42(8):3211-3213.
187. Navaratnam V, et al. Does the presence of connective tissue disease modify survival in patients with pulmonary fibrosis? Respiratory Medicine. 2011; 105(12):1925-1930.
188. Greenwald GI, et al. Longitudinal changes in lung function and respiratory symptoms in progressive systemic sclerosis. Prospective study. American Journal of Medicine. 1987;83(1):83-92.
189. Saggar R, et al. Systemic sclerosis and bilateral lung transplantation: a single centre experience. European Respiratory Journal. 2010;36(4):893-900.
190. Schachna L, et al. Lung transplantation in scleroderma compared with idiopathic pulmonary fibrosis and idiopathic pulmonary arterial hypertension. Arthritis and Rheumatism. 2006;54(12):3954-3961.
191. Massad MG, et al. Outcomes of lung transplantation in patients with scleroderma. World Journal of Surgery. 2005;29(11):1510-1515.
192. Shitrit D, et al. Lung transplantation in patients with scleroderma: case series, review of the literature, and criteria for transplantation. Clinical Transplantation. 2009;23(2):178-183.
193. Rosas V, et al. Lung transplantation and systemic sclerosis. Annals of Transplantation: Quarterly of the Polish Transplantation Society. 2000;5(3):38-43.
194. Connors GR, et al. Interstitial lung disease associated with the idiopathic inflammatory myopathies: what progress has been made in the past 35 years? Chest. 2010;138(6):1464-1474.
195. Kim EJ, Collard HR, King TE Jr. Rheumatoid arthritis-associated interstitial lung disease: the relevance of histopathologic and radiographic pattern. Chest. 2009;136(5):1397-1405.
196. Weinrib L, Sharma OP, Quismorio FP Jr. A long-term study of interstitial lung disease in systemic lupus erythematosus. Seminars in Arthritis and Rheumatism. 1990;20(1):48-56.
197. Cheema GS, Quismorio FP Jr. Interstitial lung disease in systemic lupus erythematosus. Current Opinion in Pulmonary Medicine. 2000;6(5):424-429.
198. Bodolay E, et al. Evaluation of interstitial lung disease in mixed connective tissue disease (MCTD). Rheumatology. 2005;44(5):656-661.
199. Fagundes MN, et al. Esophageal involvement and interstitial lung disease in mixed connective tissue disease. Respiratory Medicine. 2009;103(6):854-860.
200. Deheinzelin D, et al. Interstitial lung disease in primary Sjogren's syndrome. Clinical-pathological evaluation and response to treatment. American Journal of Respiratory and Critical Care Medicine. 1996;154(3 Pt 1):794-799.
201. Arcasoy SM, et al. Characteristics and outcomes of patients with sarcoidosis listed for lung transplantation. Chest. 2001;120(3):873-880.
202. Shorr AF, Davies DB, Nathan SD. Outcomes for patients with sarcoidosis awaiting lung transplantation. Chest. 2002;122(1):233-238.
203. Shorr AF, et al. Pulmonary hypertension in advanced sarcoidosis: epidemiology and clinical characteristics. European Respiratory Journal. 2005;25(5):783-788.
204. Shorr AF, Davies DB, Nathan SD. Predicting mortality in patients with sarcoidosis awaiting lung transplantation. Chest. 2003;124(3):922-928.
205. Corrin B, Liebow AA, Friedman PJ. Pulmonary lymphangiomyomatosis. A review. American Journal of Pathology. 1975;79(2):348-382.
206. Silverstein EF, et al. Pulmonary lymphangiomyomatosis. American Journal of Roentgenology, Radium Therapy, and Nuclear Medicine. 1974;120(4):832-850.
207. Peavy H, et al. A National Heart, Lung, and Blood Institute history and perspective on lymphangioleiomyomatosis. Lymphatic Research and Biology. 2010; 8(1):5-8.
208. Cohen MM, Pollock-BarZiv S, Johnson SR. Emerging clinical picture of lymphangioleiomyomatosis. Thorax. 2005;60(10):875-879.
209. Johnson SR, Tattersfield AE. Clinical experience of lymphangioleiomyomatosis in the UK. Thorax. 2000;55(12):1052-1057.
210. Taylor JR, et al. Lymphangioleiomyomatosis. Clinical course in 32 patients. New England Journal of Medicine. 1990;323(18):1254-1260.
211. Urban T, et al. Pulmonary lymphangioleiomyomatosis. A study of 69 patients. Groupe d'Etudes et de Recherche sur les Maladies "Orphelines" Pulmonaires (GERM"O"P). Medicine (Baltimore). 1999;78(5):321-337.
212. Maurer JR, et al. Lung transplantation in the management of patients with lymphangioleiomyomatosis: baseline data from the NHLBI LAM Registry. Journal of Heart and Lung Transplantation. 2007;26(12):1293-1299.
213. Boehler A. Lung transplantation for cystic lung diseases: lymphangioleiomyomatosis, histiocytosis x, and sarcoidosis. Seminars in Respiratory and Critical Care Medicine. 2001;22(5):509-516.
214. Boehler A, et al. Lung transplantation for lymphangioleiomyomatosis. New England Journal of Medicine. 1996;335(17):1275-1280.
215. Pechet TT, et al. Lung transplantation for lymphangioleiomyomatosis. Journal of Heart and Lung Transplantation. 2004;23(3):301-308.
216. Bittmann I, et al. Lymphangioleiomyomatosis: recurrence after single lung transplantation. Human Pathology. 1997;28(12):1420-1423.
217. Taveira-DaSilva AM, et al. Maximal oxygen uptake and severity of disease in lymphangioleiomyomatosis. American Journal of Respiratory and Critical Care Medicine. 2003;168(12):1427-1431.
218. Taveira-DaSilva AM, Pacheco-Rodriguez G, Moss J. The natural history of lymphangioleiomyomatosis: markers of severity, rate of progression and prognosis. Lymphatic Research and Biology. 2010;8(1):9-19.
219. Yao J, et al. Computer-aided grading of lymphangioleiomyomatosis (LAM) using HRCT. Proceedings of the IAPR International Conference Pattern Recognition.

2008;2008 (8-11 Dec. 2008):1-4.
220. McCormack FX, et al. Efficacy and safety of sirolimus in lymphangioleiomyomatosis. New England Journal of Medicine. 2011;364(17):1595-1606.
221. Sundar KM, et al. Pulmonary Langerhans cell histiocytosis: emerging concepts in pathobiology, radiology, and clinical evolution of disease. Chest. 2003; 123(5):1673-1683.
222. Dauriat G, et al. Lung transplantation for pulmonary Langerhans' cell histiocytosis: a multicenter analysis. Transplantation. 2006;81(5):746-750.
223. Delobbe A, et al. Determinants of survival in pulmonary Langerhans' cell granulomatosis (histiocytosis X). Groupe d'Etude en Pathologie Interstitielle de la Societe de Pathologie Thoracique du Nord. European Respiratory Journal. 1996;9(10):2002-2006.
224. Vassallo R, et al. Clinical outcomes of pulmonary Langerhans'-cell histiocytosis in adults. New England Journal of Medicine. 2002;346(7):484-490.
225. Fartoukh M, et al. Severe pulmonary hypertension in histiocytosis X. American Journal of Respiratory and Critical Care Medicine. 2000;161(1):216-223.
226. Harari S, et al. Advanced pulmonary histiocytosis X is associated with severe pulmonary hypertension. Chest. 1997;111(4):1142-1144.
227. Kiakouama L, et al. Severe pulmonary hypertension in histiocytosis X: long-term improvement with bosentan. European Respiratory Journal. 2010;36(1): 202-204.
228. Hosenpud JD, et al. Effect of diagnosis on survival benefit of lung transplantation for end-stage lung disease. Lancet. 1998;351(9095):24-27.
229. Titman A, et al. Disease-specific survival benefit of lung transplantation in adults: a national cohort study. American Journal of Transplantation. 2009;9(7): 1640-1649.
230. Goeminne P, Dupont L. Non-cystic fibrosis bronchiectasis: diagnosis and management in 21st century. Postgraduate Medical Journal. 2010;86(1018):493-501.
231. Nick JA, et al. Effects of gender and age at diagnosis on disease progression in long-term survivors of cystic fibrosis. American Journal of Respiratory and Critical Care Medicine. 2010;182(5):614-626.
232. Vizza CD, et al. Outcome of patients with cystic fibrosis awaiting lung transplantation. American Journal of Respiratory and Critical Care Medicine. 2000;162(3 Pt 1):819-825.
233. Liou TG, et al. Predictive 5-year survivorship model of cystic fibrosis. American Journal of Epidemiology. 2001;153(4):345-352.
234. Sharma R, et al. Wasting as an independent predictor of mortality in patients with cystic fibrosis. Thorax. 2001;56(10):746-750.
235. Weiss ES, et al. Lung transplantation in older patients with cystic fibrosis: analysis of UNOS data. Journal of Heart and Lung Transplantation. 2009;28(2): 135-140.
236. Kerem E, et al. Prediction of mortality in patients with cystic fibrosis. New England Journal of Medicine. 1992;326(18):1187-1191.
237. Ciriaco P, et al. Analysis of cystic fibrosis referrals for lung transplantation. Chest. 1995;107(5):1323-1327.
238. Hayllar KM, et al. A prognostic model for the prediction of survival in cystic fibrosis. Thorax. 1997;52(4):313-317.
239. Buzzetti R, et al. Validation of a predictive survival model in Italian patients with cystic fibrosis. Journal of Cystic Fibrosis. 2011;11(1):24-29.
240. Augarten A, et al. Prediction of mortality and timing of referral for lung transplantation in cystic fibrosis patients. Pediatric Transplantation. 2001;5(5): 339-342.
241. Milla CE, Warwick WJ. Risk of death in cystic fibrosis patients with severely compromised lung function. Chest. 1998;113(5):1230-1234.
242. Doershuk CF, Stern RC. Timing of referral for lung transplantation for cystic fibrosis: overemphasis on FEV1 may adversely affect overall survival. Chest. 1999;115(3):782-787.
243. George PM, et al. Improved survival at low lung function in cystic fibrosis: cohort study from 1990 to 2007. BMJ (Clinical Research Edition). 2011;342: d1008.
244. Rosenbluth DB, et al. Lung function decline in cystic fibrosis patients and timing for lung transplantation referral. Chest. 2004;126(2):412-419.
245. Rosenstein BJ, Zeitlin PL. Prognosis in cystic fibrosis. Current Opinion in Pulmonary Medicine. 1995;1(6):444-449.
246. Rosenfeld M, et al. Gender gap in cystic fibrosis mortality. American Journal of Epidemiology. 1997;145(9):794-803.
247. Konstan MW, et al. Risk factors for rate of decline in forced expiratory volume in one second in children and adolescents with cystic fibrosis. Journal of Pediatrics. 2007;151(2):134-139, 139 e1.
248. Baghaie N, et al. Determination of mortality from cystic fibrosis. Pneumologia (Bucharest, Romania). 2010;59(3):170-173.
249. Verma N, Bush A, Buchdahl R. Is there still a gender gap in cystic fibrosis? Chest. 2005;128(4):2824-2834.
250. de Boer K, et al. Exacerbation frequency and clinical outcomes in adult patients with cystic fibrosis. Thorax. 2011;66(8):680-685.
251. Ellaffi M, et al. One-year outcome after severe pulmonary exacerbation in adults with cystic fibrosis. American Journal of Respiratory and Critical Care Medicine. 2005;171(2):158-164.
252. Venuta F, et al. Pulmonary hemodynamics contribute to indicate priority for lung transplantation in patients with cystic fibrosis. Journal of Thoracic and Cardiovascular Surgery. 2000;119(4 Pt 1):682-689.
253. Liou TG, et al. Survival effect of lung transplantation among patients with cystic fibrosis. JAMA. 2001;286(21):2683-2689.
254. Chaparro C, et al. Infection with Burkholderia cepacia in cystic fibrosis: outcome following lung transplantation. American Journal of Respiratory and Critical Care Medicine. 2001;163(1):43-48.
255. Aris RM, et al. Lung transplantation for cystic fibrosis patients with Burkholderia cepacia complex. Survival linked to genomovar type. American Journal of Respiratory and Critical Care Medicine. 2001;164(11):2102-2106.
256. Alexander BD, et al. Survival after lung transplantation of cystic fibrosis patients infected with Burkholderia cepacia complex. American Journal of Transplantation. 2008;8(5):1025-1030.
257. De Soyza A, et al. Lung transplantation for patients with cystic fibrosis and Burkholderia cepacia complex infection: a single-center experience. Journal of Heart and Lung Transplantation. 2010;29(12):1395-1404.
258. Hadjiliadis D, et al. Survival of lung transplant patients with cystic fibrosis harboring panresistant bacteria other than Burkholderia cepacia, compared with patients harboring sensitive bacteria. Journal of Heart and Lung Transplantation. 2007;26(8):834-838.
259. Debray D, et al. Best practice guidance for the diagnosis and management of cystic fibrosis-associated liver disease. Journal of Cystic Fibrosis. 2011;10(Suppl 2):S29-S36.
260. Chryssostalis A, et al. Liver disease in adult patients with cystic fibrosis: a frequent and independent prognostic factor associated with death or lung transplantation. Journal of Hepatology. 2011;55(6):1377-1382.
261. Klima LD, et al. Successful lung transplantation in spite of cystic fibrosis-associated liver disease: a case series. Journal of Heart and Lung Transplantation. 1997;16(9):934-938.
262. Nash EF, et al. Outcomes of patients with cystic fibrosis undergoing lung transplantation with and without cystic fibrosis-associated liver cirrhosis. Clinical Transplantation. 2011;26(1):34-41.
263. Orens JB, et al. Thoracic organ transplantation in the United States, 1995-2004. American Journal of Transplantation. 2006;6(5 Pt 2):1188-1197.
264. Simonneau G, et al. Updated clinical classification of pulmonary hypertension. Journal of the American College of Cardiology. 2009;54(1 Suppl):S43-S54.
265. Hopkins WE, et al. Comparison of the hemodynamics and survival of adults with severe primary pulmonary hypertension or Eisenmenger syndrome. Journal of Heart and Lung Transplantation. 1996;15(1 Pt 1):100-105.
266. D'Alonzo GE, et al. Survival in patients with primary pulmonary hypertension. Results from a national prospective registry. Annals of Internal Medicine. 1991;115(5):343-349.
267. Sitbon O, et al. Long-term intravenous epoprostenol infusion in primary pulmonary hypertension: prognostic factors and survival. Journal of the American College of Cardiology. 2002;40(4):780-788.
268. Barst RJ, et al. A comparison of continuous intravenous epoprostenol (prostacyclin) with conventional therapy for primary pulmonary hypertension. The Primary Pulmonary Hypertension Study Group. New England Journal of Medicine. 1996;334(5):296-302.
269. McLaughlin VV, Shillington A, Rich S. Survival in primary pulmonary hypertension: the impact of epoprostenol therapy. Circulation. 2002;106(12): 1477-1482.
270. Miyamoto S, et al. Clinical correlates and prognostic significance of six-minute walk test in patients with primary pulmonary hypertension. Comparison with cardiopulmonary exercise testing. American Journal of Respiratory and Critical Care Medicine. 2000;161(2 Pt 1):487-492.
271. Dandel M, et al. Survival of patients with idiopathic pulmonary arterial hypertension after listing for transplantation: impact of iloprost and bosentan treatment. Journal of Heart and Lung Transplantation. 2007;26(9):898-906.
272. Chen H, et al. Impact of the lung allocation score on lung transplantation for pulmonary arterial hypertension. American Journal of Respiratory and Critical Care Medicine. 2009;180(5):468-474.
273. Nickel N, et al. The prognostic impact of follow-up assessments in patients with idiopathic pulmonary arterial hypertension. European Respiratory Journal. 2011;39(3):589-596.

第32章 胰腺和胰岛移植的患者选择和适应证

Alexandra Turner, Nicole A. Turgeon

引言

1 型糖尿病(T1DM)是一种不能规律控制自身血糖的疾病,主要原因是自身免疫破坏了胰腺 β 细胞。胰腺组织中含有 1%~2%的 β 细胞。在美国,患有 1 型糖尿病的患者超过 100 万。1 型糖尿病是一种能够导致肾病、神经系统疾病、胃病、心血管疾病、周围血管疾病以及视网膜病变的多系统疾病[1,2]。在过去,1 型糖尿病患者在 20 年的病情发展中,有 1/5 的患者死亡,1/4 的患者发展为终末期肾病。强化胰岛素治疗时代的到来改善了 1 型糖尿病的预后,强化胰岛素治疗最初发表在 1993 年的糖尿病控制和并发症试验上,它是一篇具有里程碑意义的论文[3]。现在 1 型糖尿病的长期生存率已经有显著的提高,而且终末期肾病的发生率也趋于平稳。和传统的治疗方法相比,加强血糖的控制延缓了糖尿病肾病、视网膜病变以及神经系统病变的发生和进展[3]。多项纵向研究表明,在严重的糖尿病并发症的治疗上强化胰岛素治疗 1 型糖尿病患者相比于传统治疗有显著提高,其中肾病的发病率对比传统的队列研究是 9%比 25%,视网膜病变的发病率从 47%改善到 21%,终末期肾病的发病率从 2%改善到 1%[4,5]。但是,强化胰岛素治疗方案更容易导致低血糖事件的发生,是传统治疗方案的 3 倍[3]。尽管强化胰岛素治疗有其优点,但是它却没有完全消除糖尿病的继发并发症。此外,患者每天都要测血糖和注射胰岛素,并且还要遵守严格的饮食,所有的这些都将会对生活质量和医疗保健费用有负面的影响。

实体器官胰腺移植是治疗 1 型糖尿病的外科方法。患者进行胰腺移植最大的好处就是提高生活质量,患者不用太多关注血糖管理[6,7]。目前治疗 1 型糖尿病和终末期肾病的"金标准"就是联合胰肾移植(SPK),这将同时使糖化血红蛋白恢复正常以及消除无意识的低血糖发生。联合胰肾移植(SPK)在实体胰腺移植中最常见,据统计占 2007 年美国胰腺移植的 65%,而且还是最耐用持久的移植器官,目前具有 12~16 年的移植中位生存时间。

肾移植术后胰腺移植是治疗已经接受死亡供体或活体供体肾移植并患有 1 型糖尿病患者的另一种选择。对于无法药物控制无意识低血糖发生以及不稳定的血糖管理但保存肾功能的患者,单纯的胰腺移植和胰岛细胞移植也是一种选择。胰岛移植是一种微创技术,它可以清除腺体的外分泌部分。胰岛移植比胰腺移植有更少的围术期并发症[8]。本章将讲述一些因素,其关于选择能从胰腺和胰岛移植中获益的患者,并将这些患者从可以靠药物管理其疾病受益的患者中区别开来。本章还会讲述影响与糖尿病肾病患者胰腺移植相关的肾移植时机的相关因素。本章将补充第 41 章所讲述的关于等待胰腺移植患者候补名单的管理。

历史

第一次胰腺移植于 1966 年明尼苏达大学进行,同时将导管结扎的部分胰腺和来自死者供体的肾脏一起移植(表 32.1)。该患者体内独立的胰岛素保留 6 天,但是由于导管的结扎导致了多种并发症[9]。当时胰腺移植的主要目的是阻止糖尿病肾病在肾移植术后复发。胰腺移植的成功主要与先进的外科技术和免疫抑制的管理有关。在胰腺移植的发展中操作胰管是主要的外科挑战。1967 年第二例联合胰肾移植通过十二指肠皮肤瘘管引流外分泌物。在被移植排斥前该移植保持 2 个月的器官功能[9]。随后的变化包括用丙烯酸酯胶和氯丁橡胶的导管阻塞,导致胰腺炎和外分泌纤维化[10,11],以及导管引流液引流到腹膜,导致化学性腹膜炎[12]。1973

表 32.1 胰腺移植的进展。主要的挑战是胰管的管理。随着技术和免疫抑制的改善,肠道引流是当今最常用的技术

时间(年)	发展	结果	机构
1966	第一次胰腺移植节段腺管结扎	6 天内独立分泌胰岛素,因为胰腺炎失败	明尼苏达大学
1967	导管通过十二指肠皮肤瘘引流	2 个月后出现排斥反应	明尼苏达大学
1973	导管通过输尿管引流	输尿管结石、酸中毒、排尿困难	艾尔伯特爱因斯坦医学院/蒙特菲奥雷医疗中心
1977	通过丙烯酸酯胶导管堵塞	胰腺炎、外分泌腺体纤维化	悉尼大学/威斯康星大学
1979	导管通过腹膜引流	化学性腹膜炎	迈阿密大学
1983	导管通过膀胱引流	膀胱尿结石、酸中毒、排尿困难;更容易管理的渗漏和检测的排斥	威斯康星大学
1996	导管通过肠道引流(侧面近端空肠)	生理通道,很难管理渗漏	斯德哥尔摩,卡罗林斯卡学院

年描述了可接受的输尿管引流[13],进行改进之后通过胰腺膀胱造口引流到膀胱[14]。后来又改进为十二指肠胆囊造口吻合术[15]。用 Roux-en-Y 的一个分支做肠道引流被同时描述[16]。

早期尝试的全胰腺移植导致很高的死亡率和并发症发生率,并且具有很少的独立胰岛素。1980 年,国际胰腺移植登记处(IPTR)报道 1 年移植存活率为 21%,1 年死亡率为 39%[17]。20 世纪 70 年代至 90 年代在外科技术、器官保存和免疫抑制方面取得了显著进步,结果得到显著改善。随着环孢菌素的出现以及十二指肠胆囊造口吻合技术的进步,Sollinger 在 1983 年报道胰腺移植 1 年生存率为 80%[18]。在下一个 10 年里,胰腺移植主要应用这种方法,因为膀胱引流有很好管理吻合口漏的优点(通过 Foley 导尿管),而且能很容易测出移植排斥反应(通过尿液中淀粉酶的下降)。但是术后泌尿系统并发症发生率为 15%~30%,因此有必要转换成肠道引流。由于在膀胱引流中胰腺外分泌物的减少导致脱水和代谢性酸中毒[19]。在 20 世纪 90 年代,随着手术技术的提高,越来越多的有效免疫抑制药,比如他克莫司出现,肠道引流成为最主要的技术。国际胰腺移植登记处(IPTR)报道从 2003 年开始有超过 80%的胰腺移植采用肠道引流[18]。有几项研究表明,两种引流方法在移植生存率和手术并发症的发病率上相当[20-24]。其他关于胰腺移植过程历史的讨论可以见第 60 章。

患者选择

对于选择候选者以及候补名单的标准,每个移植中心都不一样。对于联合胰肾移植(SPK),缺乏内源性胰岛素和肾小球滤过率(GFR)<40mL/(min·1.73m^2)是入选的绝对要求。年龄、胰岛素需求、体重指数(BMI)、心血管状态、外周血管疾病和吸烟状态也是重要的考虑因素。术后前 90 天内胰腺移植与单纯肾移植相比,绝对死亡率高 2%[25]。胰腺移植和肾移植的绝对死亡率在术后 12~24 个月是相当的。与剩下等待移植的名单相比,相对死亡的风险在移植后的前 90 天内相似地增加,而死亡风险比等待名单上的患者死亡风险更高。Gruessner 等比较了 1995—2003 年器官共享联合网络(UNOS)/IPTR 数据库的移植患者的等待患者死亡率[26]。移植后的前 90 天,SPK 的死亡率为 1.95%,PAK 的死亡率为 4.64%(P<0.0001)。90 天后死亡率危险比<1。患者最有可能在术后早期通过功能性移植而死于心血管或脑血管疾病。死亡率独立地与 45 岁以上的受体年龄和移植前透析相关。

总之,为了从胰腺移植获得益处,患者必须在手术中存活,因为术后早期死亡率显著高于肾脏移植。因此,选择胰腺受体的相对适应性以试图优化生存效益。

联合胰肾移植

目前联合胰肾移植(SPK)是治疗 T1DM 和 ESRD 患者的"黄金标准"。对胰腺移植患者最直接的益处是改善生活质量:免于胰岛素注射、频繁的血糖监测和透析[6,7]。虽然胰腺移植已经显示可减轻糖尿病肾病、视网膜病变和心血管病变的发展,但是与单独的肾移植相比,其是否可转化为患者的生存利益还不清楚[27]。最近的研究在联合胰肾移植(SPK)患者中的生存获益有不同看法,一些研究显示与仅进行活供体肾移植相比功

能性肾移植在10年后更受益[28-30],其他研究显示与联合胰肾移植(SPK)相比,活体供肾移植患者10年并没有明显生存获益[31-34]。联合胰肾移植(SPK)接受者与死亡供体肾移植受体相比显著改善了移植物和患者的存活。然而,Rayhill等在1986—1996年间在单个中心的600例患者中检查了联合胰肾移植(SPK)术后患者存活、活体相关和不相关肾移植(LRT)的患者存活,以及死亡供体肾移植(DDK)的患者存活。SPK和LRT患者的10年生存率是相似的,分别为75%和80%。死亡供体移植的受者具有更差的10年患者存活率,为62%($P<0.01$)。此外,联合胰肾移植(SPK)和活体相关供体(LRD)组之间的肾脏同种异体移植存活率在10年时相似,并且与死亡供体肾移植(DDK)的受体相比,在这些组中更高[34]。对1988—1997年在胰腺移植等待名单中登记的13 000例T1DM患者的登记分析证实了这些发现。对于调整后的10年生存率,SPK接受者为67%,LRD接受者为65%,DDK接受者为46%($P=0.05$)[33]。

联合胰肾移植(SPK)和活体供体肾移植后10年的等效生存可能反映了用于胰腺移植的高质量器官选择;供体通常年轻,具有低BMI(<35kg/m^2),并且在捐献之前没有心血管疾病或血流动力学不稳定性。供体胰腺和同时移植的肾脏的最小化器官保存时间也有助于改善这一群体的长期存活率[35-37]。这些因素已被证明与胰腺移植物血栓形成的发生率较低和移植物存活率改善相关[36]。联合胰肾移植(SPK)的受者通常也较年轻,并且比仅肾移植的受者具有更好的健康状况,进一步对SPK、DDK和LRT的受者之间进行了比较。最近的研究检查了应用来自相同供体器官的SPK和DDK之间的受者结果,以消除两组之间的供体特异性变量。在移植后9年内,经调整的肾同种异体移植物和患者存活率没有差异[38]。尽管如此,联合胰肾移植(SPK)的器官质量可能更接近于来自活的供体而不是死亡的供体的肾移植[37,39]。

然而,在移植后10年以上,联合胰肾移植(SPK)与活体相关和不相关肾移植(LRT)相比,具有生存获益。这归因于少数心血管死亡,反映了正常血糖的长期系统影响。Morath等检查了11 000例联合胰肾移植(SPK)、活体相关供体(LRD)和死亡供体肾移植体(DDK)患者,并报告于1984—2000年的协作移植研究(CTS)。所有患者均为45岁以下的终末期肾病(ESRD)的T1DM患者。在1984—1990年间移植的那些患者中,功能性肾同种异体移植物移植后10年,联合胰肾移植(SPK)与活体相关供体(LRD)患者的18年患者生存率显著改善。联合胰肾移植(SPK)受者18年的患者存活率为74%,活体相关和不相关肾移植后为60%,死亡供体肾移植(DDK)后为40%($P\leq0.001$)。联合胰肾移植(SPK)患者在移植后10年时具有功能性胰腺,与没有功能性胰腺的患者(80%对50%;$P<0.0001$)比较时,显著改善了长期存活。Cox回归分析证实联合胰肾移植(SPK)存活优于活体相关和不相关肾移植(LRT),其中考虑植入前心脏风险(HR:0.55;$P=0.0005$)。多变量分析证实联合胰肾移植(SPK)的受者,相对活体相关和不相关肾移植(LRT)(RR:0.56;$P=0.007$)和死亡供体肾移植体(DDK)(RR:0.77;$P=0.049$)的受者,其心血管死亡风险显著降低。与移植后10年功能性肾脏移植患者的活体相关和不相关肾移植或死亡供体肾移植体(DDK)相比,联合胰肾移植(SPK)后的长期患者存活率更高,并且在该组中,功能性胰腺的患者具有比没有功能性胰腺的患者存活得更好。在没有胰腺移植的患者中,死亡更常见于心血管疾病,这可能反映长期血糖正常对心血管的显著积极影响[28]。

总之,联合胰肾移植(SPK)是治疗T1DM和终末期肾病患者的金标准。与接受单纯肾移植的患者相比,联合胰肾移植(SPK)后最直接的有益效果是生活质量的改善。有证据表明联合胰肾移植(SPK)可减少糖尿病肾病、视网膜病变和心血管疾病的发展。与单独的活体相关肾移植后的T1DM相比,SPK受者在10年后具有功能性胰腺和肾同种异体移植物的生存益处是明显的。SPK受者比LRT受者的心血管事件少,反映了血糖正常的长期系统性影响[28]。

肾移植后胰腺移植

对于已经接受活体供体或死亡供体肾移植的终末期肾病的T1DM患者可考虑为肾移植后胰腺移植(PAK)。即使等待SPK的患者具有很高的死亡率(4年内46%)以及证明肾移植有利于T1DM患者[40],对于长时间等待SPK的患者或者有很好的肾移植活体供体配型的患者,追求单纯肾移植比胰腺移植更可行。

从历史的观点来说PAK很具有争议。肾脏移植与透析相比更具有生存优势。危害一个有功能的肾同种异体移植对于一个没有明确生存获益的胰腺移植可能并不太好[40,41]。早期的研究表明了相反的结果,一项研究表明 PAK 的长期不利生存(和单纯肾移植相比),另一项研究表明同种异体胰腺移植 4 年后将有利于生存获益[26,42]。随着外科技术的提高以及免疫抑制剂的发展,最近的文献报道表明活体供体肾移植后胰腺移植患者的生存以及移植术后 10 年肾小球滤过率比单纯的活体供体肾移植有所增加或者相当[43,44]。

PAK 比 SPK 表现出更差的肾小球滤过率[45]。结果,明确最能获益的患者群体是调查的主要目的。尤其是,肾小球滤过率的降低考虑是增加免疫抑制剂和大剂量的肾毒性钙调磷酸酶抑制剂联合的结果,以及是肾移植手术本身的影响和免疫因子,例如能增加排斥发作的同种异性抗原[44]。一个关于 126 例 PAK 患者术后 3 年的分析表明,肾移植损伤的危险因素包括 PAK 术前肾小球滤过率<45mL/(min·1.73m^2)、PAK 术前发生急性排斥、PAK 术前出现蛋白尿,以及肾移植术后胰腺移植间隔期>1 年[46]。一项纳入了 2776 例患者的研究认为,在控制了选择偏差之后,PAK 和年轻 T1DM 肾移植患者相比具有更高的总体肾移植生存率。通过肾小球滤过率的分层次 PAK 相关的同种异体肾移植生存,提高了 10 年同种异体移植生存,记录下的移植前肾小球滤过率为 40~49mL/(min·1.73m^2)、50~59mL/(min·1.73m^2)以及 60~69mL/(min·1.73m^2)。移植前肾小球滤过率为 30~39mL/(min·1.73m^2),与通过单纯肾移植并没有关联性,尽管这些患者的 10 年移植生存率依然是 69%。胰腺同种异体移植的失败是肾同种异体移植失败的重要危险因素。该研究发现 PAK 时机与肾移植失败没有关系[47]。

总之,PAK 和提高长期患者生存率和提高肾移植生存率 [移植前受者的肾小球滤过率>40mL/(min·1.73m^2)]有相关性。术前发生肾脏排斥反应的患者,以及具有高免疫学风险或者边缘性肾同种异体移植功能的患者可能不会从 PAK 中获益。就像其他形式的胰腺移植一样,患者必须足够适合才能从手术中获益[48]。

联合胰肾移植(SPK)与肾移植后胰腺移植(PAK)的比较

虽然 PAK 的预后有所改善,但 SPK 的胰腺移植物中位存活率仍然较高。SPK 移植物的中位生存期为 12~16 年,PAK 为 7 年[49]。PAK 的移植物存活率降低与免疫移植物损失率的增加有关,推测是单独的抗原刺激或难以监测胰腺同种异体移植物的急性排斥反应所致[25]。2004—2008 年,在所有美国和国际胰腺移植物的注册表分析中,PAK 的 3 年免疫性胰腺移植物损失率为 14%,SPK 为 5%[25]。在 2000—2007 年的器官获取和移植网络(OPTN)/UNOS 数据库中,对 T1DM 患者中 SPK 与 PALK 的比较证实了这些发现。死亡检测胰腺同种异体移植物与 SPK 对 PALK 显著独立相关;SPK 的 5 年生存率为 80%,PALK 的 5 年生存率为 64%($P<0.01$)。胰腺移植后 5 年两组患者总体生存率相似。值得注意的是,与 SPK 相比,PALK 移植后 1 年的排斥反应明显高于 SPK(16.88%对 10.97%;$P<0.01$)[50]。

患者接受 SPK 与 PALK 最终取决于 SPK 的等待时间。同样的,SPK 是需要肾移植的 T1DM 患者的金标准。等待名单上的时间长度必须与透析时间和活体捐献者的可用性相平衡。SPK 等待时间因血型和区域而异。根据"移植受者科学注册(SRTR)"数据库,2007 年,美国 SPK 移植的中位时间分别为:O、A、B 和 AB 血型分别对应 498 天、341 天、337 天和 165 天[48]。更长的等待时间与 SPK 的患者死亡率升高相关,1995—2003 年对 12 478 例 SPK 患者登记分析,报告显示候诊名单中患者的 4 年后死亡率为 46%(图 32.1)。PAK 列出的患者在相同时间内死亡率高达 18%,突显了 ESRD 对患者死亡率的潜在影响[26]。因此,进行 SPK 对 PALK 的决定应该由个人/中心进行。等待长时间 SPK 的透析患者,应该进行活体供体肾移植(如果有的话),而透析前患者应该进行 SPK(图 32.2)[48]。

单独胰腺移植和胰岛细胞移植的适应证

单独的胰腺移植(PTA)占美国全部胰腺移植的 10%。胰岛移植(IT)当前是实验性的,仅在研究协议下可用。PTA 和胰岛细胞移植的适应证是相似的,并且包括频繁的急性和虚弱的代谢并发症,例如低血糖症、高血糖症和酮症酸中毒;对外源胰岛素治疗无效是一种临床挑战;并且外源性胰岛素缓解了对这些并发症治疗失败[8]。用 PTA 或 IT 解决这些并发症的好处应该超过与终身免疫抑制相关的风险,如严重的感染和癌症。候选人包括具有肾功能保护且能够承受 CNI 的肾

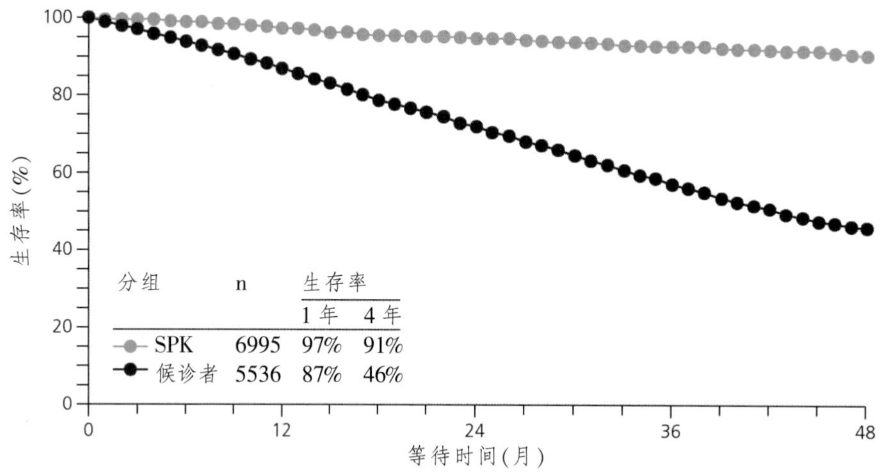

图 32.1 进行联合胰肾移植(SPK)后患者的4年生存率与其他候诊者的比较。更长的等待时间与SPK列出的患者死亡率增加有关,在对1995—2003年间列出的12 478例SPK患者的登记分析中,在等待名单上报告了4年后46%的死亡率。Reproduced from White et al.[39] with permission from Elsevier. Copyright ⓒ 2009, Elsevier.

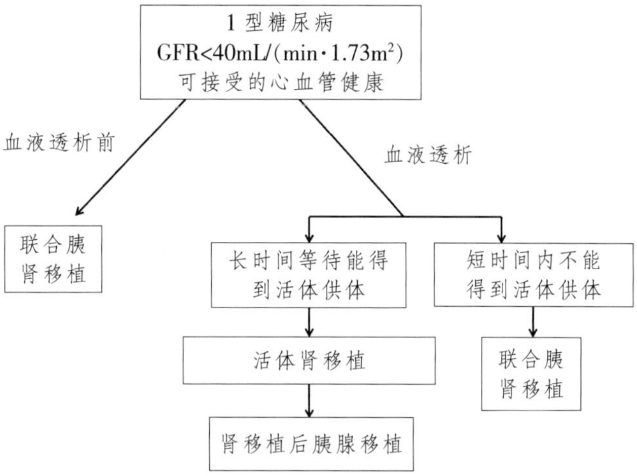

图 32.2 联合胰肾移植(SPK)与肾移植后的胰腺移植(PAK)的选择。SPK是治疗需要肾脏移植的1型糖尿病患者的首选手术方法。鉴于在SPK等候名单上较高的死亡率(图32.1),候诊时间必须与候选人的肾脏活体供体移植平衡。透析患者面临长时间的SPK等待,应该继续进行活体供体肾移植(如果有的话),然后选择PAK移植。透析患者具有短时间的SPK等待时,应该被列为SPK。透析前的患者应该被列为SPK。Date from [26,48].

毒性作用的患者:GFR>80mL/(min·1.73m²)和(或)血清肌酐<1.5mg/dL(移植前)(图32.3)。如果满足这些标准,受者不太可能发生需要透析或未来肾移植的肾衰竭[51]。在PTA 5年后,两个大型单中心系列报道肾衰竭的总体发生率为10%~15%[51,52]。选择PTA的患者必须足够合适,以考虑其相关的发病率和死亡率。IT与显著减少手术并发症和死亡率有关,将在下文详细讨论。第61章涵盖了IT的程序方面。

单独的胰腺移植

患有T1DM的患者经历代谢并发症,如血糖不稳定、频发低血糖和低血糖无意识的发生,严重损害了生活质量。另外,低血糖无意识也有致命的可能[2,53],频发低血糖对儿童和成人产生不利影响[2]。对于T1DM患者,考虑PTA。与SPK或PAK相比,PTA耐受性差,移植半衰期为5年[49]。

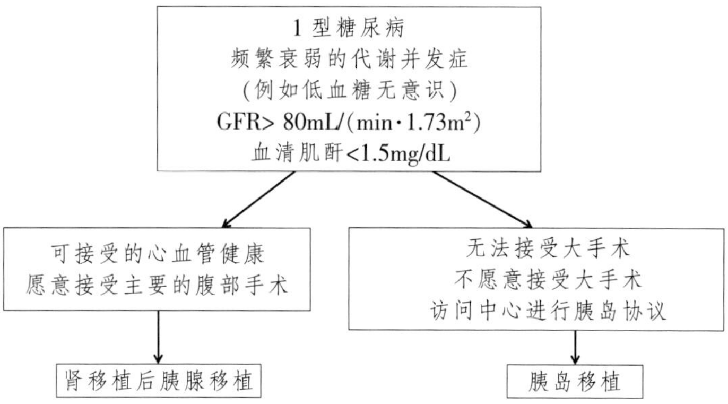

图 32.3 胰腺移植(PTA)与胰岛移植的算法。PTA和胰岛移植被认为是1型糖尿病患者潜在致命的代谢并发症,如低血糖无意识。患者必须保留足够的肾脏功能以能够抵抗钙调磷酸酶抑制剂的肾毒性作用,这是移植后免疫抑制的主要因素。愿意和能够进行主要腹部手术的患者,应该进行PTA,因为这是实现胰岛素独立的最持久方式。胰岛移植目前是实验性的,仅在几个移植中心提供。对于不符合条件或者不希望做主要腹部手术的患者,这是一种选择。

文献中讨论了 PTA 的理论依据,缺乏与低血糖意识障碍有关的死亡率数据的直接结果。选择应用 PTA 的患者没有肾衰竭,因此不应该认为具有立即危及生命的状况,很难将候诊死亡率作为结果测量。Venstrom 等分析了 1995 年—2000 年 672 例的 PTA 患者候选人,发现相对于那些候诊者,PTA 后的相对死亡风险更高(RR:1.57;P=0.06)[42]。Gruessner 等分析了相同的患者,但排除了多个移植中心列表的患者,使得每例患者只统计一次。另外,他们也统计了从等候名单中被移除以接受 KTA 的患者。经过这些调整,PTA 后死亡率的总体风险比为 0.66(P=0.12),是有利于移植的趋势。重要的是,第 366 天后的风险比为 0.15(P<0.0001)[26]。因此,随机选择的一组患者,其生存期至少等同于候选者,并且对于具有功能性胰腺同种异体移植物的患者,其生存期>1 年,并且受者的存活率得到改善。PTA 的死亡率优势不如 SPK 和 PAK 受者,而且应该为经历衰弱性代谢并发症的患者保存这一程序[26]。

选择 PTA 的患者必须具有足够的肾功能,以抵御 CNI 的肾毒性作用,这是胰腺移植后免疫抑制的主要作用。一项针对 131 例患者的单中心评估报告显示,PTA 是移植后肾衰竭的独立危险因素。移植后 4 年平均 GFR 降低 33mL/(min·1.73m^2)(P<0.0001)[52]。10%的发生肾功能不全的患者需要透析。在 GFR≥40mL/(min·1.73m^2)的患者中,多变量分析的唯一重要危险因素是 BMI;70%的 BMI>30kg/m^2 的患者在移植后 GFR 下降>40mL/(min·1.73m^2)[52]。

报道的最大的 PTA 患者系列来自明尼苏达大学(n=513),并证实接受他克莫司治疗的患者(n=239)中有 12%发生肾功能衰竭。作者通过多变量分析发现肌酐>1.5mg/dL,年龄<30 岁,是移植后肾功能衰竭的重要危险因素(P<0.0001 和 P<0.07)。在接受两次或更多次排斥反应的患者中发现肾衰竭的趋势,并得出结论,随着年轻患者出现更多的治疗排斥反应,其肾功能衰竭的风险更高[51]。

尽管肾衰竭是 PTA 的风险因素,但有证据表明胰腺移植提供的长期代谢控制对糖尿病肾病有益。已经证明,单独的胰腺移植可以改善 10 年正常血糖后与肾病相关的糖尿病病变[54]。Fioretto 等对 8 例移植前患者进行了组织活检,其处于移植后 5 年和 10 年间隔,发现移植后 10 年肾小球和肾小管基底膜厚度有统计学显著的降低(P<0.0001)。移植前和移植后 GFR 没有改善,虽然有尿白蛋白排泄减少的趋势[54]。类似地,Coppelli 等记录了 6 例 PTA 患者肾脏综合征消失(随访 36 个月),并且肌酐清除率没有显著变化[55]。

总之,推荐 PTA 作为伴有代谢不良引起低质量的生活或致命的并发症的 T1DM 患者的一种选择方式。选择 PTA 的患者应具有良好的肾功能,肌酐<1.5mg/dL,GFR>80mL/(min·1.73m^2)以预测 CNI 暴露后不会发生肾功能衰竭的患者[51]。肾衰竭的其他危险因素包括 BMI>30kg/m^2 和年龄<30 岁,在选择手术患者时应考虑[51,52]。患者也应该具有良好的心血管健康,以优化其围术期结果。

胰岛细胞移植

强化胰岛素治疗显著改善继发性糖尿病并发症的发生率和进展,代价是严重低血糖频繁发作。在过去 10 年中,IT 是获得血糖控制的非生物学方法,并且已经显示在选定的 T1DM 患者中实现胰岛素的独立性。

IT 代表 PTA 的微创替代方法。两个方法的适应证是相同的,即具有低血糖无意识和(或)极度代谢不适的 T1DM 患者,并对生活质量产生不利影响[8]。IT 目前是实验性的,在全球不到十几个中心进行[56]。

第一次成功的同种异体胰岛细胞移植在 1990 年密苏里州圣路易斯的华盛顿大学进行;在移植后持续分泌有效的胰岛素 25 天[57]。然而,难以解释 IT 后长期胰岛素独立性,直到 2000 年描述埃德蒙顿议定书的里程碑式出版物的出现[58]。埃德蒙顿议定书包括胰岛加工的精制技术、输入的胰岛数量以及类固醇免疫抑制方案,包括他克莫司、西罗莫司和达利珠单抗。所有 7 名接受 IT 治疗的患者均在移植后 1 年无胰岛素治疗[58]。埃德蒙顿议定书在其他中心可重现。在 3 个中心,1 年的胰岛素独立率为 90%[59]。第一次使用埃德蒙顿方案的多中心试验发生在 2006 年[60]。在 36例参加试验的患者中,44%患者的胰岛素独立性为 1 年,13%的患者为胰岛素依赖性 2 年。结果各不相同,因为最熟悉 IT 的中心能够取得最佳效果:1 年内有 67%的患者胰岛素独立。移植后 1 年,28%的患者完成移植物丢失,定义为 C-肽降至<0.3ng/mL(C-肽由胰岛产生,在数量上等于同于胰岛素,并且与胰岛素水平相比,其是内源性胰岛素生产的更可靠指标)。剩余的 28%的患者具有部分移植功能(C-肽>0.3ng/mL,并且需要足够的外源胰岛素来控制血糖)。具有部分移植功能的患者改善了的血糖的控制和预防严重的低血糖发作,然而,伴有移植前 HbA1c、胰岛素需求和空腹血糖中的降低。作者认为,虽然长期胰岛素非依赖性很难实现,但 IT 对大多数具有部分移植物功能的患者提供了有益的代谢效果[60]。

与 PTA 相比,尽管 IT 具有显著降低的发病率和死亡率,但结果却显著低于整体器官移植。移植后 5 年,10%的原始埃德蒙顿胰岛受试者仍然胰岛素独立,而 PTA 受试者的概率为 50%[49,51,61]。尽管很少患者仍然保持胰岛素独立性,但 80%的 C-肽阳性并改善血糖控制,而无降低血糖无意识[61]。在 1999—2007 年间向国际胰岛移植登记处(CITR)报告的所有异体移植物中,23%的 IT 受试者在移植后 3 年仍保持胰岛素独立性,29%为胰岛素依赖性,并具有阳性 C-肽水平,明显改善血糖控制和低血糖无意识。报告给 CITR 的大多数患者接受了来自多个捐助者的胰岛[62]。

如同 PTA,IT 涉及的风险与利益之比必须以个体患者为基础来确定。已经证明,随着一些残留移植物功能的存在,IT 可以改善严重低血糖和低血糖无意识的症状[63,64]。具有功能性胰岛移植的患者被报告由于担心低血糖,生活质量得到改善[65-67]。这些益处必须平衡终身免疫抑制的风险。埃德蒙顿方案中使用的原始免疫抑制药物(他克莫司和西罗莫司)可能会产生有害影响。已知他克莫司对肾功能有不良影响[68],并且均显示两种药物对胰岛素敏感性和胰岛血管形成有不良影响[69,70]。在参与原始埃德蒙顿试验的患者中证实了胰岛移植后 GFR 逐渐下降:GFR 每月下降 0.39mL/(min·1.73m^2)[71]。埃德蒙顿议定书随后的多中心试验也注意到 GFR 降低:每月 GFR 平均下降 0.45mL/(min·1.73m^2)[60]。

然而,与接受强化疗法的 T1DM 患者相比,Warnock 等发现 GFR 的下降没有显著差异。这项研究对维持他克莫司或西罗莫司的 IT 受者与进行药物治疗的 T1DM 患者进行比较(平均随访 3 年)[72]。另外,与对照组相比,在 IT 受者中,HbA1c 和视网膜病变进展有了改善[72]。然而,仍然认识到 IT 的好处并没有被免疫抑制的风险所抵消[73]。随后,单中心研究对来自单一供体的 IT 成功地采用了无 CNI 或 CNI 最小化方案,以尽量减少风险[74,75]。

最近的一些研究已经证明 IT 对糖尿病微血管/大血管病变、心血管功能、肾脏同种异体移植物存活率的有益作用,并且已经免疫抑制[76-78]。Fiorina 等发现,与接受 KTA 的患者相比,在 IT 6 年后肾脏同种异体移植物存活率有所改善[78]。Gerber 等报道 SPK 后 5 年患者和同时接受了肾移植和 IT 的患者的可观的血糖控制[79]。

迄今为止,大多数 IT 需要多个供体以获得足够的胰岛,从而实现胰岛素独立,潜在地使患者处于 HLA 敏化的危险之中[62]。Campbell 等报告,34%的患者在 IT 失败后发展了新生抗 HLA 抗体,其中大多数患者已经从两个供体接收了胰岛。接受免疫抑制的受试者中,有 70%具有> 50%的群体反应性抗体(PRA)。这种敏感度会使随后的肾脏或胰腺移植更加困难。作者承认 HLA 与胰岛受试者匹配是不可行的,因为捐赠者极其有限。来自单个供体的移植胰岛将减少 HLA 错配的数量,但是如果存在来自单个供体的许多不匹配表位,则仍然可以存在很大的敏感性[80]。与埃德蒙顿方案治疗对照组相比较,最近使用基于生物制剂 efaluzimab(抗 LFA-1)和 abatacept(CTLA4-Ig)的替代性免疫抑制的试验没有显示同种致敏作用[75]。新的免疫抑制方案以及在移植时列出的不可接受的 HLA 抗原的能力可能有利于该 HLA 群体中抗 HLA 抗体的发展。

总之,IT 是实验性的,并且最好在经验丰富的临床研究中心进行。虽然长期的胰岛素独立性很难达到,但大多数移植后 5 年的患者至少具有局部移植功能,可以防止极端低血糖或降血糖意识,这是移植的主要指征[61]。

对于 T1DM 经历低血糖无意识者,以及衰弱性代谢并发症者,PTA 仍然是治疗的"金标准"。选择 PTA 的患者必须具有良好的肾功能,并且应该足够健康以进行手术。像 PTA 候选人一样,IT 候选人也应该具有良好的肾功能,从而能够抵御 CNI 的肾脏毒性作用。虽然 IT 仍然是一种实验性治疗,但对于不符合或不选择主要腹部手术的患者,IT 是 PTA 的替代方案。对于两种手术的风险和收益,应以患者具体情况为基础进行权衡。

总结

所有形式的胰腺移植对于具有进行性继发并发症且具有生理能力的 T1DM 患者来说仍然是合理的,其效果随着时间也在提高,但仍然与不显著的发病率相关,因此不应仅仅视为消除对外源性胰岛素需要的手段。IT 远不如全器官胰腺移植成功,但并发症较少。因此，IT 仍然是严重低血糖无意识患者的主要研究替代方案。两者都是由于合适的供体器官相对短缺而被接受的。因此，对于最有可能受益的患者，应仔细考虑和保留该资源的配置。

（谢文勇 译 张大方 校）

参考文献

1. Cowie CC, et al. Full accounting of diabetes and pre-diabetes in the U.S. population in 1988–1994 and 2005–2006. Diabetes Care. 2009;32(2):287–294.
2. Daneman D. Type 1 diabetes. Lancet. 2006;367(9513):847–858.
3. The Diabetes Control and Complications Trial Research Group, United States National Institute of Diabetes and Digestive and Kidney Diseases (NIDDK). The effect of intensive treatment of diabetes on the development and progression of long-term complications in insulin-dependent diabetes mellitus. New England Journal of Medicine. 1993;329(14):977–986.
4. Nathan DM, et al. Modern-day clinical course of type 1 diabetes mellitus after 30 years' duration: the diabetes control and complications trial/epidemiology of diabetes interventions and complications and Pittsburgh epidemiology of diabetes complications experience (1983–2005). Archives of Internal Medicine. 2009;169(14):1307–1316.
5. de Boer IH, et al. Intensive diabetes therapy and glomerular filtration rate in type 1 diabetes. New England Journal of Medicine. 2011;365(25):2366–2376.
6. Gross CR, et al. Impact of transplantation on quality of life in patients with diabetes and renal dysfunction. Transplantation. 2000;70(12):1736–1746.
7. Sutherland DE, et al. Lessons learned from more than 1,000 pancreas transplants at a single institution. Annals of Surgery. 2001;233(4):463–501.
8. Robertson P, et al. Pancreas transplantation in type 1 diabetes. Diabetes Care. 2004;27(Suppl 1):S105.
9. Kelly WD, et al. Allotransplantation of the pancreas and duodenum along with the kidney in diabetic nephropathy. Surgery. 1967;61(6):827–837.
10. Little JM, Lauer C, Hogg J. Pancreatic duct obstruction with an acrylate glue: a new method for producing pancreatic exocrine atrophy. Surgery. 1977;81(3):243–249.
11. Dubernard JM, et al. A new method of preparation of segmental pancreatic grafts for transplantation: trials in dogs and in man. Surgery. 1978;84(5):633–639.
12. Sutherland DE, et al. Segmental pancreas transplantation from living related and cadaver donors: a clinical experience. Surgery. 1981;90(2):159–169.
13. Gliedman ML, et al. Clinical segmental pancreatic transplantation with ureter-pancreatic duct anastomosis for exocrine drainage. Surgery. 1973;74(2):171–180.
14. Cook K, et al. Pancreaticocystostomy: an alternative method for exocrine drainage of segmental pancreatic allografts. Transplantation. 1983;35(6):634–636.
15. Nghiem DD, Schulak JA, Corry RJ. Duodenopancreatectomy for transplantation. Archives of Surgery. 1987;122(10):1201–1206.
16. Tyden G, et al. Improved results with a simplified technique for pancreaticoduodenal transplantation with enteric exocrine drainage. Clinical Transplantation. 1996;10(3):306–309.
17. Sutherland DE. International human pancreas and islet transplant registry. Transplantation Proceedings. 1980;12(4 Suppl 2):229–236.
18. Lam VW, et al. Evolution of pancreas transplant surgery. ANZ Journal of Surgery. 2010;80(6):411–418.
19. Odorico JS, Sollinger HW. Technical and immunosuppressive advances in transplantation for insulin-dependent diabetes mellitus. World Journal of Surgery. 2002;26(2):194–211.
20. Kaufman DB, et al. Simultaneous pancreas-kidney transplantation in the mycophenolate mofetil/tacrolimus era: evolution from induction therapy with bladder drainage to noninduction therapy with enteric drainage. Surgery. 2000;128(4):726–737.
21. Bloom RD, et al. Long-term pancreas allograft outcome in simultaneous pancreas-kidney transplantation: a comparison of enteric and bladder drainage. Transplantation. 1997;64(12):1689–1695.
22. Kuo PC, et al. Simultaneous pancreas/kidney transplantation–a comparison of enteric and bladder drainage of exocrine pancreatic secretions. Transplantation. 1997;63(2):238–243.
23. Pearson TC, et al. Drainage of the exocrine pancreas in clinical transplantation: comparison of bladder versus enteric drainage in a consecutive series. Clinical Transplantation. 1997;11(3):201–205.
24. Stratta RJ, et al. Portal-enteric pancreas transplantation at the University of Tennessee, Memphis. Clinical Transplants. 2000;217–237.
25. Gruessner AC, Sutherland DE, Gruessner RW. Pancreas transplantation in the United States: a review. Current Opinion in Organ Transplantation. 2010;15(1):93–101.
26. Gruessner RW, Sutherland DE, Gruessner AC. Mortality assessment for pancreas transplants. American Journal of Transplantation. 2004;4(12):2018–2026.
27. Gremizzi C, et al. Impact of pancreas transplantation on type 1 diabetes-related complications. Current Opinion in Organ Transplantation. 2010;15(1):119–123.
28. Morath C, et al. Metabolic control improves long-term renal allograft and patient survival in type 1 diabetes. Journal of the American Society of Nephrology: JASN. 2008;19(8):1557–1563.
29. Morath C, et al. Transplantation of the type 1 diabetic patient: the long-term benefit of a functioning pancreas allograft. Clinical Journal of the American Society of Nephrology. 2010;5(3):549–552.
30. Young BY, et al. Living donor kidney versus simultaneous pancreas-kidney transplant in type I diabetics: an analysis of the OPTN/UNOS database. Clinical Journal of the American Society of Nephrology: CJASN. 2009;4(4):845–852.
31. Reddy KS, et al. Long-term survival following simultaneous kidney-pancreas transplantation versus kidney transplantation alone in patients with type 1 diabetes mellitus and renal failure. American Journal of Kidney Diseases. 2003;41(2):464–470.
32. Weiss AS, Smits G, Wiseman AC. Simultaneous pancreas-kidney versus deceased donor kidney transplant: can a fair comparison be made? Transplantation. 2009;87(9):1402–1410.
33. Ojo AO, et al. The impact of simultaneous pancreas-kidney transplantation on long-term patient survival. Transplantation. 2001;71(1):82–90.
34. Rayhill SC, et al. Simultaneous pancreas-kidney transplantation and living related donor renal transplantation in patients with diabetes: is there a difference in survival? Annals of Surgery. 2000;231(3):417–423.
35. Troppmann C, et al. Vascular graft thrombosis after pancreatic transplantation: univariate and multivariate operative and nonoperative risk factor analysis. Journal of the American College of Surgeons. 1996;182(4):285–316.
36. Troppmann C. Complications after pancreas transplantation. Current Opinion in Organ Transplantation. 2010;15(1):112–118.
37. Stegall MD, et al. The rationale for the new deceased donor pancreas allocation schema. Transplantation. 2007;83(9):1156–1161.
38. Waki K, Terasaki PI. Kidney graft and patient survival with and without a simultaneous pancreas utilizing contralateral kidneys from the same donor. Diabetes Care. 2006;29(7):1670–1672.
39. White SA, Shaw JA, Sutherland DE. Pancreas transplantation. Lancet. 2009;373(9677):1808–1817.
40. Wolfe RA, et al. Comparison of mortality in all patients on dialysis, patients on dialysis awaiting transplantation, and recipients of a first cadaveric transplant. New England Journal of Medicine. 1999;341(23):1725–1730.
41. Gaston RS, et al. Transplantation in the diabetic patient with advanced chronic kidney disease: a task force report. American Journal of Kidney Diseases. 2004;44(3):529–542.
42. Venstrom JM, et al. Survival after pancreas transplantation in patients with diabetes and preserved kidney function. JAMA. 2003;290(21):2817–2823.
43. Kleinclauss F, et al. Pancreas after living donor kidney transplants in diabetic patients: impact on long-term kidney graft function. Clinical Transplantation. 2009;23(4):437–446.
44. Sampaio MS, et al. Transplantation with pancreas after living donor kidney vs. living donor kidney alone in type 1 diabetes mellitus recipients. Clinical Transplantation. 2010;24(6):812–820.
45. Larson TS, et al. Pancreas-after-kidney transplantation: an increasingly attractive alternative to simultaneous pancreas-kidney transplantation. Transplantation. 2004;77(6):838–843.
46. Pavlakis M, et al. Renal allograft failure predictors after PAK transplantation: results from the New England Collaborative Association of Pancreas Programs. Transplantation. 2010;89(11):1347–1353.
47. Browne S, et al. The impact of pancreas transplantation on kidney allograft survival. American Journal of Transplantation. 2011;11(9):1951–1958.
48. Wiseman AC. Pancreas transplant options for patients with type 1 diabetes mellitus and chronic kidney disease: simultaneous pancreas kidney or pancreas after kidney? Current Opinion in Organ Transplantation. 2012;17(1):80–86.
49. Lodhi SA, Lamb KE, Meier-Kriesche HU. Solid organ allograft survival improvement in the United States: the long-term does not mirror the dramatic short-term success. American Journal of Transplantation. 2011;11(6):1226–1235.
50. Poommipanit N, et al. Pancreas after living donor kidney versus simultaneous pancreas-kidney transplant: an analysis of the organ procurement transplant network/united network of organ sharing database. Transplantation. 2010;89(12):1496–1503.
51. Gruessner RW, et al. Over 500 solitary pancreas transplants in nonuremic patients with brittle diabetes mellitus. Transplantation. 2008;85(1):42–47.

52. Scalea JR, et al. Pancreas transplant alone as an independent risk factor for the development of renal failure: a retrospective study. Transplantation. 2008;86(12): 1789–1794.
53. Gale EA. Type 1 diabetes in the young: the harvest of sorrow goes on. Diabetologia. 2005;48(8):1435–1438.
54. Fioretto P, et al. Reversal of lesions of diabetic nephropathy after pancreas transplantation. New England Journal of Medicine. 1998;339(2):69–75.
55. Coppelli A, et al. Disappearance of nephrotic syndrome in type 1 diabetic patients following pancreas transplant alone. Transplantation. 2006;81(7):1067–1068.
56. Vardanyan M, et al. Pancreas vs. islet transplantation: a call on the future. Current Opinion in Organ Transplantation. 2010;15(1):124–130.
57. Scharp DW, et al. Insulin independence after islet transplantation into type I diabetic patient. Diabetes. 1990;39(4):515–518.
58. Shapiro AM, et al. Islet transplantation in seven patients with type 1 diabetes mellitus using a glucocorticoid-free immunosuppressive regimen. New England Journal of Medicine. 2000;343(4):230–238.
59. Shapiro AM, Ricordi C, Hering B. Edmonton's islet success has indeed been replicated elsewhere. Lancet. 2003;362(9391):1242.
60. Shapiro AM, et al. International trial of the Edmonton protocol for islet transplantation. New England Journal of Medicine. 2006;355(13):1318–1330.
61. Ryan EA, et al. Five-year follow-up after clinical islet transplantation. Diabetes. 2005;54(7):2060–2069.
62. Alejandro R, et al. Update from the Collaborative Islet Transplant Registry. Transplantation. 2008;86(12):1783–1788.
63. Faradji RN, et al. Simple measures to monitor beta-cell mass and assess islet graft dysfunction. American Journal of Transplantation. 2007;7(2):303–308.
64. Pileggi A, et al. Twenty years of clinical islet transplantation at the Diabetes Research Institute–University of Miami. Clinical Transplants. 2004;177–204.
65. Toso C, et al. Quality of life after islet transplant: impact of the number of islet infusions and metabolic outcome. Transplantation. 2007;84(5):664–666.
66. Poggioli R, et al. Quality of life after islet transplantation. American Journal of Transplantation. 2006;6(2):371–378.
67. Tharavanij T, et al. Improved long-term health-related quality of life after islet transplantation. Transplantation. 2008;86(9):1161–1167.
68. Ojo AO, et al. Chronic renal failure after transplantation of a nonrenal organ. New England Journal of Medicine. 2003;349(10):931–940.
69. Johnston O, et al. Sirolimus is associated with new-onset diabetes in kidney transplant recipients. Journal of the American Society of Nephrology. 2008;19(7): 1411–1418.
70. Cantaluppi V, et al. Antiangiogenic and immunomodulatory effects of rapamycin on islet endothelium: relevance for islet transplantation. American Journal of Transplantation. 2006;6(11):2601–2611.
71. Senior PA, et al. Changes in renal function after clinical islet transplantation: four-year observational study. American Journal of Transplantation. 2007;7(1):91–98.
72. Warnock GL, et al. A multi-year analysis of islet transplantation compared with intensive medical therapy on progression of complications in type 1 diabetes. Transplantation. 2008;86(12):1762–1766.
73. Khan MH, Harlan DM. Counterpoint: clinical islet transplantation: not ready for prime time. Diabetes Care. 2009;32(8):1570–1574.
74. Hering BJ, et al. Single-donor, marginal-dose islet transplantation in patients with type 1 diabetes. JAMA 2005;293(7):830–835.
75. Turgeon NA, et al. Experience with a novel efalizumab-based immunosuppressive regimen to facilitate single donor islet cell transplantation. American Journal of Transplantation. 2010;10(9):2082–2091.
76. Fiorina P, et al. Long-term beneficial effect of islet transplantation on diabetic macro-/microangiopathy in type 1 diabetic kidney-transplanted patients. Diabetes Care. 2003;26(4):1129–1136.
77. Fiorina P, et al. Islet transplantation is associated with an improvement of cardiovascular function in type 1 diabetic kidney transplant patients. Diabetes Care. 2005;28(6):1358–1365.
78. Fiorina P, et al. Natural history of kidney graft survival, hypertrophy, and vascular function in end-stage renal disease type 1 diabetic kidney-transplanted patients: beneficial impact of pancreas and successful islet cotransplantation. Diabetes Care. 2005;28(6):1303–1310.
79. Gerber PA, et al. Simultaneous islet-kidney vs pancreas-kidney transplantation in type 1 diabetes mellitus: a 5 year single centre follow-up. Diabetologia. 2008; 51(1):110–119.
80. Campbell PM, et al. High risk of sensitization after failed islet transplantation. American Journal of Transplantation. 2007;7(10):2311–2317.

第 33 章
小肠和多脏器器官移植的患者选择和适应证

Douglas G. Farmer, Robert S. Venick

引言

在过去的 20 年间,小肠移植和多脏器联合移植已经从实验性操作发展成为世界上多个移植中心的常规手术。这一领域向前发展的重要一步是对其移植指征的首次阐述[1]。由此开始,已有多篇文章来论述移植指征[2-6]。然而,尽管患者选择是否影响手术成功及预后仍存在争议,这些年来移植指征几乎没有变化。在本章中,我们将介绍小肠移植的指征,包括单纯小肠移植以及多脏器联合移植。本章内容对于理解第 42、62 和 63 章等内容大有裨益,因为这几章介绍了等待小肠移植患者的管理及移植手术过程。

小肠衰竭

不可逆小肠衰竭是大多数小肠移植手术的基础,也是在应用多脏器联合移植治疗严重复杂疾病时,把小肠纳入移植物的重要原因。小肠衰竭是指一个人无法通过胃肠道获取维持机体所需的水、电解质、能量、各类营养素[7]。临床工作中,小肠衰竭是指肠外营养需要持续 60~90 天,可致儿童无法正常生长发育。类似其他实质器官衰竭,肠衰竭病因可分为可逆因素及不可逆因素。常见的病因为黏膜功能紊乱、肠道动力紊乱、手术损伤或先天性畸形等。手术损伤通常是指短肠综合征。

可逆性小肠衰竭患者不应考虑进行小肠移植或者包含肠道的多脏器联合移植。相反,不可逆性小肠衰竭患者可以考虑。表 33.1 显示了判断肠衰竭恢复潜力的预后因素[8-10]。需要注意的是,这些因素主要应用于手术因素导致的肠衰竭的预后判断。

表 33.1 影响肠衰竭的预后因素

• 年龄
• 肠衰竭持续时间
• 残余小肠长度
• 残余小肠的解剖部位
• 回盲瓣是否存在
• 残余结肠长度
• 肠造口是否存在
• 基础肠病是否存在

肠适应是指受损的肠道恢复所有的功能和节律的过程,包括肠绒毛的延长、腺窝的加深、胃肠道蠕动的减少、肠道的扩张及延长等。这一过程是依赖于能量的,需要充足的能量和营养物质供应。这一过程可能持续数月至数年。因此,此类患者需要肠外营养。

显然,年轻的患者拥有更好的适应潜能。大多数的研究认为适应过程的最大化发生在肠道衰竭后的 24~36 个月,也有研究报道了晚期适应。残余小肠的长度和解剖部位对于适应是至关重要的。残余肠道越长,适应潜能越高。回肠比空肠有更好的适应潜能。回盲瓣影响肠适应的原因仍存有争议。一些学者认为回盲瓣会有良好的预后是由于回盲瓣不可避免地带有部分回肠。同理,回盲瓣的存在也意味着部分结肠的存在。另外一些学者认为原因在于回盲瓣可阻止结肠内容物反流和防止细菌过度生长。总而言之,有回盲瓣的患者有更好的预后。结肠对于适应也很重要。在这些病例中,结肠不仅可以吸收过多的液体,而且可以通过肠道细菌的作用吸收一些能量。因此,通过手术重建肠道的完整性对于适应的发生非常重要。除此之外,残余肠道的健康程度及功能也很关键。如果残余肠道存在缺血损伤或者活动性疾病,如炎症性肠病,则会影响适应过程,此时不需考虑以上介绍的其他因素。

肠外营养相关并发症

一般说来，仅仅不可逆性小肠衰竭不是小肠移植的绝对适应证,对于此类患者,术者不应在行多脏器联合移植时考虑添加小肠移植。小肠移植适用于永久肠衰竭并且长期全肠外营养有死亡风险的患者。因为在多数情况下，在家进行不复杂的全肠外营养的永久肠衰竭的患者的预后，可以相当于甚至优于肠道移植术后的患者[11]。例外情况确实存在,下面一一介绍。

如果不可逆性小肠衰竭的患者出现主要的肠外营养并发症,则需考虑进行小肠移植。在这些病例中,与进行长期复杂的全肠外营养的患者相比，移植患者的预后更好。

最令人关注的全肠外营养的并发症是肝脏损伤,包括全肠外营养胆汁淤积、肠外营养相关肝损伤(PNALD)、肠衰竭相关肝损害(IFALD)等。此类疾病仍然是此类患者死亡的主要原因。该类肝病的确切病因仍不清楚,但有几个理论来解释,比如肠道缺乏胆汁分泌的刺激,肠外营养成分的缺失等;这里不详细讨论[12]。IFALD 的风险因素包括:早产,低出生体重,肠内营养的缺乏,中心静脉导管感染,小肠细菌过度增殖,肠外营养包含过多的碳水化合物、蛋白或者脂肪等。儿童的 IFALD 可表现为胆汁淤积性肝损伤,进一步可发展为胆汁淤积性肝硬化。成人的 IFALD 更多地表现为脂肪变性肝损伤,伴或不伴炎症性肝病。它可归于非酒精性脂肪肝(NASH)。肝损害一旦发生,其逆转十分困难,将逐步进展为终末期肝病。

一般说来，不可逆性小肠衰竭合并肝病是小肠移植的主要指征。一些组织主张在肝病的初期进行小肠移植以避免肝损伤进展为终末期肝病。这是一个合理的做法，它避免了该类患者以后进入漫长的死亡率更高的肝移植等待名单。然而,随着对早期 IFALD 的新的防治策略的出现,这种做法的合理性需要重新讨论。当然,一旦肝病进展为肝硬化,则需要进行肝肠联合移植或者多脏器联合移植。因为当 IFALD 的患者进入肝硬化失代偿期,将很快死亡。

另一个小肠移植的常见指征与中心静脉相关。主要中心静脉发生梗阻或者发生血栓的患者需要考虑进行移植手术，特别是两个以上中心静脉甚至腔静脉受累时。现在有一些介入放射的技术可对慢性或者狭窄的中心静脉进行扩张、支架和溶栓等治疗[13],然而这些技术不应作为该类患者的一种有效的长期治疗方法，而应作为保证移植手术安全的围术期管理手段。

另外一种中心静脉相关的并发症是血行感染(BSI),此类患者推荐进行小肠移植。血行感染在全肠外营养的患者中十分常见，最好的报道是每年仅发生 0.5 次[14]。大量的患者有更高的血行感染发生率,此类患者常常因此而拔除中心静脉置管。血行感染高发生率是小肠移植的指征。除此之外,耐药菌或者真菌血行感染,转移性感染灶,比如心内膜炎、脓肿,全身炎症反应需要重症监护和(或)机械通气,也是小肠移植的指征。表 33.2 总结了常见的移植手术指征,以及与最近文献报道的上文提到的共病的关系。

没有达到经典标准的其他指征

不可切除的硬纤维瘤或者胃肠道间质瘤

低度恶性肿瘤或者有潜在发展为低度恶性肿瘤的疾病可以是小肠移植的指征。根据肿瘤侵犯的程度,如果需要切除的范围较大，则会需要进行多脏器联合移植[15]。一些疾病通过常规手术方法是无法切除的,此类疾病通常是硬纤维瘤样肿瘤或者胃肠道间质瘤等侵及肠系膜根部的肿瘤。家族性腺瘤性息肉病(Gardner 综合征)也是小肠移植的指征[16]。肿瘤完整切除、阴性切缘是必须的,常用多脏器联合移植来替代切除的器官。然而,新的技术,比如体外肿瘤切除联合自体器官移植,正在应用于此类患者,从而改变了移植手术的指征[17]。

门-脾-肠系膜静脉血栓

对于门静脉、肠系膜、合并或者不合并脾静脉血栓的患者，标准的疗法是内镜和药物治疗后进行外科分流术。然而,一些患者由于基础肝病,需要进行移植手术。对大多数病例,标准疗法是单纯肝脏移植联合门静脉取栓、使用静脉导管或门体分流[18]。然而,还有一小部分患者，仅进行单纯的肝脏移植是没有办法打通静脉的。这些患者应该考虑进行多脏器联合移植。以上经验仅限在专门的移植中心,每年只有少量的病例[19]。

表 33.2　小肠移植的手术指征

作者	不可逆 IF	肝病	BSI	血管通路	其他表现	备注
Kaufman 等[1]	有	有	有(转移性感染灶;SIRS;Tx 耐药)	有(2/4 婴儿;3/6 儿童)	严重的 SGS、胃结肠不连续,先天性肠黏膜功能障碍,无法控制的水电解质平衡紊乱,慢性疼痛	无
AGA 综述[2]	有	有	有 (2 年 SIRS 2/2 菌血症;1 年 SIRS 2/2 真菌感染)	有(2/6 成人)	频繁的严重脱水	无
CMS[3]	有	有	有 (2 年 SIRS 2/2 菌血症;1 年 SIRS 2/2 真菌感染)	有(2/6 成人)	频繁的严重脱水	无
Pironi 等[4]	有	有	有(>1/1000 天;转移性感染灶)	有(2/4 婴儿;3/6 儿童/成人)	严重的 SGS、胃结肠不连续,先天性肠黏膜功能障碍,肿瘤所致大范围切除,肠系膜血管缺血 2/2 血栓形成	生活质量差
Avitzur & Grant[5]	有	有	有 (2 年 SIRS 2/2 菌血症;1 年 SIRS 2/2 真菌感染;1 年休克;1 年 ARDS)	有(2/6 所有)	严重的 SGS、胃结肠不连续,频繁的严重脱水先天性肠黏膜功能障碍,肿瘤所致大范围切除	生活质量差

IF,肠衰竭;BSI,血流感染;Tx,治疗;ARDS,急性呼吸窘迫综合征;SGS,短肠综合征;SIRS,全身炎症反应综合征。

无法吻合的胃肠道或者短肠综合征

无法吻合的胃肠道多发生于中肠的缺失，使得无法进行前肠和后肠的外科吻合，这些患者通常有十二指肠盲端,里面有引流管引流前肠的分泌物。短肠综合征的患者则只有不到 10cm 的小肠与结肠相连接。在这两种情况中,预后较差,肠外营养的并发症频繁发生。另外,这些患者还会频繁发生脱水、电解质紊乱,给临床管理带来挑战。该类患者应更积极地进行移植手术以期更好的预后[20]。

移植指征的展望

一直以来被广泛接受的小肠移植指征已被新的预防性的治疗手段所挑战。特别是静脉脂类的减少和 ω-3 脂类的使用,减少了 IFALD 的发生,因此改变了肠衰竭管理的现状。脂类减少技术[≤1g/(kg·d)]已经成为 IFALD 患者的一种相对常见的预防和治疗手段。在一些小样本单中心研究中，这种治疗手段成功地改善了胆汁淤积,给外科医生提供了继续肠道适应的机会[21]。最近,ω-3 脂肪酸(O3FA)乳剂在欧美、亚洲越来越常见,并且在美国已基于研究并投入使用,它可以预防和逆转大多数 IFALD 儿童的胆汁淤积[22,23,24]。O3FA 溶液缺乏甾醇,含有更多的维生素 E,建议用量为 1g/(kg·d)。新的乳剂含有豆油、中链脂肪酸、橄榄油和鱼油,被宣称有更好的生理平衡,在预防 IFALD 方面更加有效[25]。虽然新的脂质疗法更加安全,有效地改善了胆汁淤积,但是其长期有效性在无法脱离肠外营养的高危肠衰竭患者中仍不清楚。

总结

小肠移植和多脏器联合移植在过去的 20 多年里取得了重大进展,已经成为肠衰竭患者、需要切除肠道以治疗局部进展肿瘤的患者的治疗范式。随着经验的丰富,移植手术的指征会逐步明晰。现有指征的发展需要等待新的研究进展。在管理肠衰竭患者方面的新的进展，将会影响小肠移植和多脏器联合移植的手术指征。未来的发展,我们拭目以待。

(李照　译　朱继业　校)

参考文献

1. Kaufman SS, Atkinson JB, Bianchi A, et al. American Society of Transplantation. Indications for pediatric intestinal transplantation: a position paper of the American Society of Transplantation. Pediatric Transplantation. 2001;5(2):80–87.
2. Buchman AL, Scolapio J, Fryer J. AGA technical review on short bowel syndrome and intestinal transplantation. Gastroenterology. 2003;124(4):1111–1134.
3. National Coverage Determination for intestinal and multivisceral transplantation (260.5). Available from: www.cms.gov.
4. Pironi L, Spinucci G, Paganelli F, et al. Italian guidelines for intestinal transplantation: potential candidates among the adult patients managed by a medical referral center for chronic intestinal failure. Transplantation Proceedings. 2004;36(3): 659–661.
5. Avitzur Y, Grant D. Intestine transplantation in children: update 2010. Pediatric Clinics of North America. 2010;57(2):415–431.
6. Pironi L, Hébuterne X, Van Gossum A, et al. Candidates for intestinal transplantation: a multicenter survey in Europe. American Journal of Gastroenterology. 2006;101(7):1633–1643.
7. Jeejeebhoy KN. The etiology and mechanism of intestinal failure. In: Matarese L, Steiger E, Seidner DL, editors. Intestinal Failure and Rehabilitation: A Clinical Guide. New York, NY: CRC Press; 2005: p26.
8. Beath S, Pironi L, Gabe S, et al. Collaborative strategies to reduce mortality and morbidity in patients with chronic intestinal failure including those who are referred for small bowel transplantation. Transplantation. 2008;85:1378–1384.
9. Pironi L, Joly F, Forbes A, et al. Home artificial nutrition & chronic intestinal failure working group of the European Society for Clinical Nutrition and Metabolism (ESPEN). Long-term follow-up of patients on home parenteral nutrition in Europe: implications for intestinal transplantation. Gut. 2011;60(1):17–25.
10. Quirós-Tejeira RE, Ament ME, Reyen L, et al. Long-term parenteral nutritional support and intestinal adaptation in children with short bowel syndrome: a 25-year experience. Journal of Pediatrics. 2004;145(2):157–163.
11. Lloyd DA, Vega R, Bassett P, et al. Survival and dependence on home parenteral nutrition: experience over a 25-year period in a UK referral centre. Alimentary Pharmacology and Therapeutics. 2006;24(8):1231–1240.
12. Kelly DA. Preventing parenteral nutrition liver disease. Early Human Development. 2010;86:683–687.
13. Warren P, Burke C. Endovascular management of chronic upper extremity deep vein thrombosis and superior vena cava syndrome. Seminars in Interventional Radiology. 2011;28(1):32–38.
14. Colomb V, Dabbas-Tyan M, Taupin P, et al. Long-term outcome of children receiving home parenteral nutrition: a 20-year single-center experience in 302 patients. Journal of Pediatric Gastroenterology and Nutrition. 2007;44(3):347–353.
15. Moon JI, Selvaggi G, Nishida S, et al. Intestinal transplantation for the treatment of neoplastic disease. Journal of Surgical Oncology. 2005;92(4):284–291.
16. Cruz RJ Jr, Costa G, Bond GJ, et al. Modified multivisceral transplantation with spleen-preserving pancreaticoduodenectomy for patients with familial adenomatous polyposis "Gardner's Syndrome". Transplantation. 2011;91(12):1417–1423.
17. Kato T, Lobritto SJ, Tzakis A, et al. Multivisceral ex vivo surgery for tumors involving celiac and superior mesenteric arteries. American Journal of Transplantation. 2012;12(5):1323–1328.
18. Stieber AC, Zetti G, Todo S, et al. The spectrum of portal vein thrombosis in liver transplantation. Annals of Surgery. 1991;213(3):199–206.
19. Vianna R, Giovanardi RO, Fridell JA, et al. Multivisceral transplantation for diffuse portomesenteric thrombosis in a patient with life-threatening esophagogastroduodenal bleeding. Transplantation. 2005;80(4):534–535.
20. Fishbein T, Schiano T, Jaffe D, et al. Isolated intestinal transplantation in adults with nonreconstructible GI tracts. Transplantation Proceedings. 2000;32(6): 1231–1232.
21. Colomb V, Jobert-Giraud A, Lacaille F, et al. Role of lipid emulsions in cholestasis associated with long-term parenteral nutrition in children. Journal of Parenteral and Enteral Nutrition. 2000;24(6):345–350.
22. Puder M, Valim C, Meisel JA, et al. Parenteral fish oil improves outcomes in patients with parenteral nutrition-associated liver injury. Annals of Surgery. 2009;250(3):395–402.
23. Diamond IR, Sterescu A, Pencharz PB, et al. Changing the paradigm: omegaven for the treatment of liver failure in pediatric short bowel syndrome. Journal of Pediatric Gastroenterology and Nutrition. 2009;48(2):209–215.
24. Calkins K, Dunn J, Shaw S, et al. Pediatric intestinal failure - associated liver disease is reversed with 6 months of intravenous fishoil. Journal of Parenteral and Enteral Nutrition. 2013: epub ahead of print.
25. Goulet O, Antébi H, Wolf C, et al. A new intravenous fat emulsion containing soybean oil, medium-chain triglycerides, olive oil, and fish oil: a single-center, double-blind randomized study on efficacy and safety in pediatric patients receiving home parenteral nutrition. Journal of Parenteral and Enteral Nutrition. 2010;34(5):485–95.

第34章 初期保健医师在腹部器官移植患者转诊和诊治中的角色

Peggy B. Hasley, Kristine S. Schonder, Ron Shapiro

引言

截至2007年底,183 222位接受了功能性实体器官移植的患者被器官获取和移植网络(OPTN)记录在案[1]。在美国,每年有27 000名患者接受器官移植。除外单独胰腺移植、胰肾联合移植和小肠移植,在其他所有类型的实体器官移植中,患者的存活率都得到了改善。大多数器官移植受体的5年生存率都高于70%[1]。在目前移植技术取得巨大成功的条件下,预计越来越多的患者会活着离开医院,并最终回到自己的初期保健医师那里获取后续的治疗。

随着越来越多的移植受体在手术后的最初几个月存活下来,由于接受了免疫抑制治疗,他们被认为更有可能患上以下慢性疾病:高血压、糖尿病、高脂血症、肥胖、心脑血管疾病、慢性肾病和骨质疏松症。而初期保健医师专注于慢性病的一级和二级预防,因此其非常适合为移植后患者提供医疗服务。在美国多个肝脏移植中心的一项调查显示,有40%的移植中心表示初期保健医师应该是移植后1年内的主要医疗服务提供者。另外40%的移植中心采用专科医师和初期保健医师的组合来管理其移植接受者[2]。初期保健医师应做好管理移植患者初期保健的准备。

本章的目的是协助初期保健医师管理腹部器官移植后发生的慢性疾病,同时通过筛查、免疫治疗、避孕等方面为特定疾病的预防提供建议。一个涵盖相似主题的有关胸部器官移植的章节将在第35章呈现。

医疗协作

初期保健医师、专科医师和外科医师三者之间的医疗协作对于优化移植患者的预后至关重要,还能尽可能减少各种重复检查,同时避免很多错误。一项关于初期保健医师和专科医师之间医疗协作的荟萃分析报告显示,执业医师之间的有效互动能改善患者在心理健康和糖尿病治疗上的预后[3]。虽然医疗协作已被证实有效,但协作的最优策略还有待开发。虽然采用卫生信息技术系统和绩效报告制度是现行初期保健实践的行之有效的组成部分,但改善执业医师之间沟通的方法尚不成熟[4]。在移植肝脏病学家中的一项调查显示[5],超过60%肝脏病学家表示,移植后的慢性疾病应该由初期保健医师进行管理。然而,少于40%的肝脏病学家对初期保健医师在其患者治疗中的参与程度表示满意。虽然70%的被调查者表示,他们与初期保健医师保持着适当的沟通,但多数受访者都不满意初期保健医师给他们的反馈。最终,移植肝脏病学家认为他们的患者在移植后,慢性疾病方面并没有接受到足够的控制。

用于移植受者的一个协作治疗模式可能把初期保健医师包含在移植团队之内,以帮助优化移植后治疗。其他模式可能包括共享电子病历、基于电子邮件的复杂医疗决策信息传递或跨学科团队成员之间的交流。

在电子病历得到发展之前,初期保健医师使用电话与专科医师沟通。在通话过程中,被咨询的相关背景信息和问题可以得到交流。开始使用电子病历系统之后,首先进行电话沟通的做法被取消。在移植患者术后慢性疾病的共同管理方面，专科教授人力资源委员会为初期保健医师和专科医师的沟通交流制定了一些准则[6]。在这些准则中有以下建议：

1.初期保健医师应该发送一份原始记录，其中包括咨询的原因、咨询的问题和已收集到的背景资料。

2.初期保健医师应在患者转诊后发送一份临床记录副本。

3.专科医师应考虑使用“特定疾病模板”以与初期保健医师做指南和建议上的交流。

其他移植前的治疗包括建立包括高级护士在内的多学科诊疗团队[7]和使用远程医疗以对位于农村的患者提供移植前保健[8]。

移植前初期保健医师，在患者移植后的长期预后方面扮演了重要角色。建立公开的同专科医师进行沟通的渠道、恰当转诊的时机、对可控危险因素的识别和处理、与患者一起改善治疗计划以提高患者的依从性，是移植前保健的重要目标。

专科医师的转诊时机选择

通过参照其他慢性疾病指南要求的治疗目标，初期保健医师可以优化移植后预后、降低死亡率和发病率。在一项包含5978例合并严重肺部疾病成人患者的队列研究中，cox模型被用来确定移植前体重指数(BMI)和移植后死亡风险的关联。这项研究表明，在4.2年的平均随访时间过后，低体重和超重患者的死亡率比正常体重的移植接受者高出15%[9]。其他慢性疾病，包括移植前慢性肾病(CKD)，已被证明会增加移植后其他疾病的发病率[10,11]。

对大多数慢性疾病来说，有关转诊到专科医师处适当时机的研究尚不成熟，但慢性肾病除外。初期保健医师和专科医师协作组已经制定了关于心血管疾病、糖尿病、慢性肾病、哮喘和慢性阻塞性肺疾病、骨关节炎和风湿性多肌痛、肠易激综合征和炎症性肠疾病的共同管理初步准则[6]。作者认为这是一个需要更多研究来指导初期保健医师和专科医师明确自身和共同角色的领域。

对于慢性肾病患者，已显示延迟转诊至专科医师会导致发病率、死亡率和医疗成本的增加[12-16]。Cass等已表明被转诊至亚专科医师处的处于3个月初始肾脏替代治疗内的慢性肾病患者是不太可能进入等待移植名单，并且在该治疗结束后2年内不太可能接受移植。作者推测，这种无法获得移植的原因是患者在初始肾脏替代治疗开始时病情更重，并且没有足够的时间通过移植前评估，以使患者绕过透析直接接受移植[13]。初期保健医师可以在需要依赖性肾保健之前通过咨询肾脏病学家使患者获取更恰当的治疗。

改善依从性

药物依从性和积极的自我保健是获得移植后成功的关键因素。几项研究已经表明，即使是免疫抑制药物依从程度上的微小偏差也与移植物排斥相关。此外，药物依从性差的患者临床无病生存期较短[17-19]。在一项关于移植后免疫抑制药物依从性的研究中，Dew等显示患者所接受的保健服务质量是依从性的一个重要决定因素[20]。初期保健医师通常在移植前和患者建立了一个长期的关系。因此，初期保健医师非常适合发现患者可能存在缺乏依从性的危险信号并使用一定策略协助其患者提高对医疗方案的依从性。已被证明具有降低依从性的患者因素包括男性、较低的自我效能、焦虑和抑郁、人格障碍、神经认知障碍和缺乏社会支持。可预测移植后缺乏依从性的患者移植前的行为，包括移植前不规范服药、酗酒和不服从生命体征监测[21,22]。初期保健医师可以协助移植前依从性评估，可以告诫患者药物和生活方式依从性的重要性，以此为手段从而改善移植前后生存质量和获得移植的可能性。初期保健医师可以通过诊治焦虑和抑郁，提供药丸收纳盒，采用指南支持的方法干预烟草使用、酒精滥用和依赖，并安排更好的社会支持系统，以提高移植后的结果。Bell等开发了很多由青少年过渡到成人保健之前需要达成的目标，可以应用到移植前患者，从而提高移植后的依从性[23](表34.1)。

移植后慢性疾病

高血压

心血管疾病是移植受者死亡的最常见原因[24,25]。高血压病，在国家联合委员会有关预防、诊断、评估和治疗高血压第八版中的定义为收缩压>140mmHg和舒张压>90mmHg，或者需要降压治疗[26]。在移植受者中，供

表 34.1　建议患者在移植准备阶段达到的目标

- 了解并能描述其器官衰竭的根本原因以及移植的必要性
- 拥有一个简洁、便携、随时可获取的自身医疗信息概要
- 意识到移植的远期和短期并发症对其整体健康状况及其生活其他方面的影响(例如预防感染、癌症监测)
- 理解其疾病对性和生殖健康的影响,包括:
  - 怀孕对自身幸福的影响
  - 药物对生育能力的影响
  - 药物所具备的任何潜在的致畸性
  - 遗传咨询的作用, 以及在后代中再出现和他目前状况相关的这种疾病的遗传风险
  - 自身对性传播疾病的易感性增加
- 表现出对自身医疗保健负有责任感:
  - 知道移植及辅助药物的名称(和形状/颜色)、适应证和剂量(或钱包/手袋里携带以上信息)
  - 请求自己处方的补充和更新
  - 如果不是由他们的药剂师完成,应准备自己的药物剂量盒
  - 将其医疗保健需求独立地传达给其提供者
  - 知道何时以及如何寻求紧急医疗服务,包括急救电话号码
  - 能够制作、保存并遵循一个含有健康服务预约信息的日历
  - 了解他们的医疗保险覆盖范围和资格要求
- 大多数时候能独立照顾自己的能力

Adapted from Bell et al.[23] with permission from John Wiley and Sons [192].

者因素、宿主因素和免疫抑制剂共同促进了高血压病的发展[27,28]。增加高血压患病风险的宿主因素包括移植前高血压、高体重指数、慢性肾病,以及移植后甲亢。可导致高血压病的供者因素包括高龄、男性和高血压病[29-31]。目前还没有大型前瞻性研究得出移植受者血压控制的适当目标,但最近的指南指出,肝、肾移植受者的目标血压应<130/80mmHg[32,33]。

对移植受者的高血压病的诊断富有挑战性。通过对在办公室的血压读数与上班前和下班后的血压读数进行比较,可以发现其中存在一个典型的白领高血压效应[34,35]。血压的自我测量值在移植受者中显著增高[36]。一项针对 200 例肾移植受者的研究表明,连续 24 小时动态血压监测在诊断高血压时具备非常高的灵敏度。在这个群体中发现的夜间高血压为非杓型[37]。

一般群体中的高血压的传统治疗包括减肥、低钠饮食和规律锻炼。很少有数据表明这些干预措施对移植受者有效。当尿钠排泄被用作衡量肾移植受者群体膳食中盐摄入量时, 并未发现钠排泄和血压之间存在关联[38]。然而,对于合并高血压的肾移植受者,指南仍推荐每日钠摄入量<2.4g、保持正常体重和规律锻炼[39]。

几类抗高血压药,包括钙通道阻滞剂、血管紧张素转换酶(ACE)抑制剂、血管紧张素受体阻滞剂、β-受体阻滞剂和利尿剂已被证明对移植受者有效。一项比较硝苯地平与赖诺普利疗效大型的前瞻性试验证实硝苯地平组中移植肾功能更好[52]。针对肝移植受者的一项回顾性研究发现,与服用他克莫司的患者相比,服用环孢素的患者中高血压的发生率并不会更高[53]。然而,移植后钙调磷酸酶抑制剂(CNIS)剂量的仔细削减与血压控制的改善有关[54]。

通常移植患者的高血压很难控制[55,56],经常需要同时服用两种或三种药物。更好的控制已经显示能减少肾移植群体的并发症发病率和心血管疾病死亡率[57]。通过加入二氢吡啶类钙通道阻滞剂可以提高钙调磷酸酶抑制剂水平,因此,这些阻滞剂经常得到应用,这样可以减少价格昂贵的钙调磷酸酶抑制剂的使用剂量。另外,需要特别考虑的是在移植群体中,钙调磷酸酶抑制剂(特别是他克莫司)可能会导致高血钾。因此,若使用血管紧张素转换酶抑制剂、血管紧张素受体阻滞剂或保钾利尿剂,用药过程中需密切监测血钾水平。预期利尿剂会抵消 CNIS 和泼尼松的钠和流体保持效果。患者并发心肌梗死、蛋白尿和痛风,β-受体阻滞剂、ACE 抑制剂和缬沙坦应当分别作为这些疾病的临床用药。

高脂血症

高脂血症在实体器官移植术后比较常见。移植术后 1 年 66%的肝移植受者和 60%的肾移植受者存在血脂异常[58-66]。在移植群体中高脂血症的原因是多因素的,包括移植后肥胖、糖尿病,以及甲状腺功能减退。此外, 抗高血压药和免疫抑制剂的选择也已显示可以影响血脂水平[62,64-66]。

针对肝肾移植患者的血脂控制目标指南已经发布[67,68]。国家肾脏基金会的肾病预后质量倡议建议将肾移植的患者安置在美国国家胆固醇教育小组(NCEP)第三成人治疗组(ATP)的心脏等风险组[67]。因此,低密度脂蛋白(LDL)胆固醇的控制目标设定为<100mg/dL,当该值> 130mg/dL 时应开始药物治疗 (>100mg/dL 时应考虑给予药物治疗)。两个大型随机对照试验(RCT)已显示当移植受者的高脂血症得到治疗后成功降低了心血管相关的疾病发病率和整体的死亡率[69,70]。

高脂血症的一般治疗应注重减肥、饮食调整和鼓

励锻炼。每日摄入低于总能量25%的脂质,低于总能量10%的饱和脂肪,并且胆固醇摄入量每天低于500mg,这样的饮食可以显著降低肾移植受者的低密度脂蛋白胆固醇,但还没有低到足以达到<100mg/dL的低密度脂蛋白的目标。美国第3阶段饮食被证明可减少肾移植群体的脂质水平[72]。虽然没有研究显示体育锻炼能有效地改善脂质状态并降低移植群体死亡率,并且移植后的体育锻炼水平又通常较低[73],但已有研究表明移植受者仍旧可以耐受各种运动项目并且可以达到和非移植群体同样高的运动强度[74]。如果通过饮食和锻炼无法完全达到低密度脂蛋白目标值,初期保健医师应同移植医师共同考虑调整免疫抑制治疗方案是否可行。减少暴露于环孢素和皮质类固醇的免疫抑制治疗方案已被证实可以改善血脂异常[75-78]。

对于通过饮食和锻炼还不能达到低密度脂蛋白胆固醇控制目标的患者,建议使用药物治疗。各种降脂药物,包括他汀类药物、胆汁酸树脂、胆固醇吸收抑制剂、贝特类、烟酸和ω-3脂肪酸等已在移植群体中得到研究[69,70,72-107]。

他汀类被认为是移植受者的一线治疗药物[67]。氟伐他汀和普伐他汀不是由CYP450 3A4系统代谢,因此不太可能影响钙调磷酸酶抑制剂的水平。初期保健医师应当知道患者患上他汀类药物相关肌病的危险性会增加,并应在开始治疗或剂量调整后的4~6周检查肌磷酸激酶(CPK)和转氨酶的水平。对于通过3A4途径代谢的他汀类,如辛伐他汀和阿托伐他汀,应从较低的剂量开始使用,并应频繁检查钙调磷酸酶抑制剂水平。

通常胆汁酸结合树脂的耐受性没有他汀类好[84],但可以考虑应用于对他汀类药物有严重副作用的患者。这类药物的用处经常在移植受者群体中引起争议,因为其对免疫抑制剂吸收的影响还存在分歧[108,109]。

只有一种称为依泽替米贝的胆固醇吸收抑制剂已在移植受者中得到研究。依泽替米贝与他汀类药物的联合应用已显示可引起脂质更安全地降低[99-103]。然而,暂无长期的研究证明其在减少心血管疾病患病率和死亡率方面有显著益处。

贝特类药物用于治疗移植受者高脂血症应受到限制。只有几项较小的研究已显示出该类药物的效果,但是其并存的药物相关性肌病风险依然受到关注[110]。贝特类药物应限制适用于不耐受他汀类药物治疗并伴有甘油三酯严重升高的患者。

烟酸尚未在移植群体中得到大量研究,可能是因为其已知的损害胃肠道、肾和肝功能,以及潮红的副作用。最新的一项研究中报告,烟酸对于改善脂质谱是安全和有效的[91]。

ω-3脂肪酸已显示可替代贝特类药物治疗严重的高甘油三酯血症。有关ω-3脂肪酸在肾移植患者中应用的一项荟萃分析显示,甘油三酯有显著降低,同时不伴随肾小球滤过率(GFR)、移植物存活率、排斥反应的任何变化[107]。

糖尿病

在2005年,移植后新发糖尿病(NODAT)被定义为空腹血糖≥126mg/dL(7.0mmol/L)。而空腹血糖为110~125mg/dL(6.1~6.9mmol/L)的患者被定义为糖耐量减低,空腹血糖<110mg/dL(6.1mmol/L)被定义为血糖正常。这些定义都是基于世界卫生组织制定的糖尿病诊断标准[111]。自从这些定义被公布以后,美国糖尿病协会就已经调整了糖耐受减低定义的区间为空腹血糖100~125mg/dL(5.6~6.9mmol/L)[112]。在一项文献的系统评价中,Montori等表明在实体器官移植患者中,移植后新发糖尿病的发病率为2%~50%[113]。最新的一项来自美国的单中心研究表明,74%的肾移植受者患有移植后新发糖尿病[114]。这些研究均完成于美国糖尿病协会批准的最新糖尿病诊断标准公布之前,预期这会增加移植受者被诊断为糖尿病患者的比例。

对于肾移植和肝移植受者来说,其发展成糖尿病的危险因素相似。糖尿病的不可控危险因素包括年龄、非白种人、男性、糖尿病家族史、丙型肝炎和多囊肾。可控危险因素包括移植前体重、类固醇的使用、钙调磷酸酶抑制剂(尤其是他克莫司)和移植前糖耐量减低的程度[115-122]。

为了诊断移植后新发糖尿病,最新发布的指南建议移植后4周应每周检测一次空腹血糖,之后在移植后的3个月、6个月、12个月分别检测一次,此后每年都应检测一次[123]。糖化血红蛋白A1cs(HbA1cs)不应该在移植后立即进行检测,因为许多移植受者都接受了大量红细胞输血,因此会改变检测结果。然而,一旦患者被诊断为移植后新发糖尿病,HbA1cs应常规检测[123]。

很少有研究涉及移植群体糖尿病治疗的有效性和安全性。针对肾移植受者的共识会议指南也已发布[123,124]。Reynolds等已经提出了一个针对移植后新发糖尿病管理的简化算法。对于空腹血糖> 250mg/dL 的患者来说,初始治疗应包括饮食治疗、运动疗法和胰岛素治疗。为了改善血糖控制和减少组织的胰岛素抵抗,建议加用二甲双胍、噻唑烷二酮类或普兰林肽。对于确诊时空腹血糖< 250mg/dL 的患者,一线治疗应是饮食治疗、运动疗法和二甲双胍。如果 3 个月后的 HbA1c>7%,应开始加用噻唑烷二酮类、艾塞那肽或西他列汀。如果治疗 3 个月后 HbA1c 仍> 8%,则建议加用胰岛素。如果 HbA1c 为 7%~8%,那么噻唑烷二酮类、艾塞那肽或西他列汀中任何其一都可被认为可以替代胰岛素[125]。最新数据表明噻唑烷二酮类与心力衰竭之间存在关联,使得这类药物并不是移植受者的一个理想选择[126]。

骨质疏松

在患有终末期实质器官疾病的群体中,肝衰竭患者有 31%患有骨质疏松症,而在肾衰竭患者中这一数字是 24%[127]。接受移植后,患者暴露于各种免疫抑制剂,包括类固醇、西罗莫司、环孢素、麦考酚酯之中增加了骨密度降低的可能性[128-130]。已显示在移植后的最初几年里,肾移植患者的骨密度会进一步下降[131]。除了免疫抑制之外,合并的糖尿病[132]、体重下降和移植后肌酐增高[130]已被证明能增加这个群体患上骨质疏松症的风险。已有一项研究表明,双能 X 线骨密度测试低 T 值和脊椎骨折之间存在关联[133]。在这项研究中,Cox 回归分析显示,合并骨质疏松症的患者骨折的风险增加了 3.5 倍(95% CI:1.8~6.4),而在骨量减少的患者中增加了 2.7 倍(95% CI:1.6~4.6)[133]。一项包含 33 479 例肾移植受者的回顾性调查揭示了调整后的骨折发病比为 4.59(95% CI:3.29~6.31)。对于住院的髋部骨折患者,这一群体的死亡风险比为 1.60(95% CI:1.13~2.26)[134]。由于在移植后第 1 年内骨质流失进展迅速,移植后应尽早进行骨密度检测,对于满足骨量减少标准的患者应尽早进行预防。

虽然还没有针对移植患者骨质疏松症治疗的研究提出其可降低骨折发生率,但几种治疗方法已显示出其能减缓移植后骨密度的降低。一项针对 57 例肾胰联合移植受者的研究展示了在 4 年的随访期内腰椎和股骨颈的 T 值增加[129]。该研究的成功归因于在该群体中使用了激素节制免疫抑制疗法和积极的治疗方案[129]。其他被证明对骨密度有益处的疗法包括使用维生素 D[135]和降钙素[136]。一项针对双膦酸盐治疗 180 例肾移植受者共 5 个随机对照试验的荟萃分析表明,该治疗方法使移植后 6~12 个月内骨密度跌幅减小。在该群体中未发现双膦酸盐治疗有任何严重的副作用[137]。

Palmer 等针对肾移植患者进行了一项包括 24 个随机对照试验(共 1299 例)的荟萃分析,结果显示双膦酸盐、维生素 D、降钙素能有效地改善髋关节骨密度。但这些干预措施都没有使骨折减少[138]。

一项针对移植群体的基于现有指南的用于检测、治疗、监测骨质疏松症的协定改善了肾脏和胰腺移植患者中骨质疏松症的筛查和预防措施[139]。

除了类固醇激素剂量最小化,应鼓励移植受者通过定期负重运动、戒烟、戒酒来预防骨质疏松症。建议保持适量的钙摄入(男性为 1000mg/d,绝经前妇女为 1200mg/d,绝经后妇女为 1500mg/d)和维生素 D 摄入(400~1000IU/d)。然而,最近的一项针对非移植群体的研究表明,补充钙和维生素 D 和心血管疾病死亡率之间可能存在关联,这可能会导致以上建议被修改[140]。对于 T 值<-2.5 的患者应考虑双膦酸盐治疗。使用双膦酸盐预防骨质疏松应个体化,因为目前并没有任何证据证明其能防止骨折发生。目前暂无相关研究表明,微量元素锶、选择性雌激素受体调节剂、周期性甲状旁腺激素、核因子 κ B 受体活化因子配体抑制剂(狄诺塞麦)在移植群体中应用的有效性或安全性。

生育和避孕

现已证明,对于接受肾脏和肝脏移植的妇女来说,移植前已存在的正常月经功能受损可在移植后得到解决[141,142]。在男性中同样也有移植后恢复正常生育能力的报道[143-145]。和没有接受西罗莫司治疗的患者相比,在移植后接受西罗莫司免疫抑制治疗的男性肾移植受者会出现精子总数的显著减少,活性精子的比例下降,妊娠概率降低[146]。

目前国家移植登记数据库报告,在 919 例移植受者中,已有 1418 例妊娠和 1451 个活产,包括双胞胎和三胞胎[147]。由于生育能力的恢复,初期保健医师应在移植前后给患者提供关于避孕的咨询服务。

已有研究报道了在移植群体中激素组合避孕的效果[148-150]。针对肾移植受者的一项研究表明,在肾移植群体中宫内节育器的有效性已降低[151]。迄今没有研究报道过单纯孕激素口服避孕、长效醋酸甲羟孕酮、屏障避孕和紧急避孕在该群体中的有效性。大多数专家认为屏障避孕是移植群体最安全的避孕方式。

以下问题在移植群体中受到特别关注。口服避孕药组合已被证明能够抑制细胞色素 P450 3A4 通路[152],因此可以导致钙调磷酸酶抑制剂水平的升高。它们也可引起减少类固醇激素比如泼尼松龙的清除[153],从而增加了类固醇激素相关副作用发生的风险。长期服用钙调磷酸酶抑制剂的患者患上动脉粥样硬化的风险持续增加。因此,任何已知患有心脑血管疾病的移植患者是口服避孕药的绝对禁忌证。患有高血压、糖尿病或高脂血症是其相对禁忌证。而对于使用该试剂,首先需考虑在使用该药时移植受者患上骨质疏松症的风险增加。除了担忧有效性,宫内节育器也带来与免疫抑制治疗后感染风险增加相关的一系列问题。

表 34.2 在移植受者中禁忌和安全的疫苗

禁忌的活病毒疫苗	安全的病毒灭活疫苗
• 水痘	• 人乳头瘤病毒
• 带状疱疹	• 甲型肝炎
• 鼻内减毒流感病毒	• 乙型肝炎
• 麻疹、腮腺炎、风疹	• 流感(注射形式)
• 口服脊髓灰质炎病毒	• 白喉类毒素
• 口服活减毒伤寒杆菌	• 破伤风类毒素
• 卡介苗(BCG)	• 百日咳
• 黄热病	• B型流感嗜血杆菌(HIb)
	• 灭活脊髓灰质炎
	• 肺炎球菌
	• 脑膜炎球菌
	• 狂犬病
	• 伤寒
	• 日本脑炎病毒

免疫接种

用于移植受者的强效免疫抑制剂已成为各种合适免疫治疗方案青睐的对象。虽然灭活病毒的和毒素源性的疫苗在移植受者中使用是安全的，但是许多移植受者(高达 89%)没有充分了解疫苗接种[155]。灭活病毒疫苗接种后产生的抗体反应已被证明可以预防流感病毒[156-159]、肺炎球菌[160,161]和乙肝病毒[162,163]。当移植患者接受了甲型肝炎免疫接种之后，甲型肝炎病毒的滴度出现明显下降[164]。

由于在移植群体中免疫接种后抗体反应的快速消退,针对强化免疫接种效果的研究正在进行中。一个强化的流感病毒免疫接种策略已显示可以在肝移植患者中增加治疗性抗体滴度[165]。

初期保健医师应建议患者在移植前更新所有免疫接种史，并应告知患者 2 周内避免接触接种过活病毒疫苗的家庭成员。虽然初步研究表明,麻疹、腮腺炎、风疹和水痘的活病毒疫苗对经过选择的儿童肝移植受者是安全的[166],但初期保健医师仍应继续告知成人移植受者避免接种活病毒疫苗。表 34.2 显示了哪些疫苗对移植受者来说是安全的和哪些是禁忌的。

移植受者的吸烟问题

疾病预防控制中心(CDC)报告说,吸烟者占美国总人口的 25.5%。因此,在移植受者中烟草使用很普遍这一点并不奇怪。已有研究证明,吸烟已成为肝移植、肾移植、肾脏-胰腺联合移植受者并发症发生率和死亡率增高的独立危险因素。在肝移植受者中,吸烟已被证明会增加死亡率[167]、恶性肿瘤发生率[168,169]、胆道并发症发生率[170],以及移植后的住院时间和医疗资源消耗[171]。也显示有吸烟史的肾移植受者生存时间更短[172-174],移植失败[173,175]、常见心血管疾病、恶性肿瘤[173]发生的风险更高。

Nogueria 等在一项包含 997 例活体肾移植受者的回顾性研究中表明,和从不吸烟者相比,有吸烟史的患者死亡风险更高(HR:1.47;95% CI:1.08~1.99;P=0.01)[172],甚至那些在接受移植前从未主动吸烟的被动吸烟者也表现出死亡风险增高。Kasiske 等用图表的形式回顾性研究了 1228 例肾移植受者,结果发现烟草对死亡率的影响有剂量依赖效应，如果移植受者在移植前已经戒烟 5 年以上,死亡率会降低[173]。在肾脏-胰腺联合移植的患者中，也已显示吸烟会导致大血管病变的进展和 1 型糖尿病死亡率的增加[176]。

Banas 等报告说,很大一部分肾移植患者(27.6%)都是能够戒烟的[177]。DiMartini 等在一项队列研究中发现，因酒精性肝病而接受了肝移植的患者在移植后 3 个月,50%的患者又开始了吸烟[178]。

尽管烟草对移植受者有不利影响，但目前还没有关于戒烟评估与咨询以及药物干预的有效性数据。在一般群体中已被证明的成功有效的戒烟方法，如动机性访谈、尼古丁替代疗法和安非他酮可以考虑用于移植群体。虽然瓦伦尼克林可用于一般群体，但在移植群体中应该慎用，因为使用该药物会增加发生药物相关性焦虑和抑郁的风险[179,180]。目前针对肾移植受者治疗的指南指出："建议采取积极措施控烟"[181]。

癌症筛查

免疫抑制治疗通过削弱肿瘤免疫监视作用增加了恶性肿瘤发生风险，同时也增加了肿瘤促进的病毒感染风险，可能和免疫抑制剂的直接致癌作用有关。其结果是，移植受者的患癌风险是一般群体的 3~4 倍[182]。标准化发病率的定义为实际肿瘤发生例数与预期肿瘤发生例数的比值，而在非霍奇金淋巴瘤、子宫颈癌、外阴癌、肾癌、甲状腺癌、卡波西肉瘤和非黑色素瘤性皮肤癌中这一比值在不断增加[183]。移植群体中肿瘤发生的独立危险因素包括持续免疫抑制的持续时间和强度[184]、丙型肝炎病毒感染、吸烟、酗酒、日光照射[185]、男性和年龄超过 45 岁[184]。

尽管恶性肿瘤是移植后死亡率升高最常见的原因之一[186,187]，但移植受者往往并不知晓这种升高的风险[188]。在一项包括 338 例移植受者的独立调查中，Kauffman 等表明，35.5%的受访者对癌前征兆知晓程度为"无"或者"不多"。不到一半的受访者了解"很多"或"全部"的有关癌症的重要危险因素。只有 30.3%的受访者表示，他们已经学会了"足够的"关于预防癌症的知识。因此，在一项电话调查了 60 例肝移植受者的移植学术项目中，每年只有 40%的患者进行了皮肤或口腔癌的筛查，这并不奇怪。38%的女性进行了乳腺癌筛查，而在过去的 2 年里有 11%的女性曾接受了宫颈癌筛查[189]。

初期保健医师应当了解到这种风险在自己所管理的移植受者中正在增加，并遵循由美国疾病预防工作组、加拿大医学会、美国癌症学会颁布的癌症预防和监测指南[190-192]。虽然这些出版物并不包括移植群体的筛查指南，但是最近的指南已经包括了肝[68]、肾移植[39]受者的癌症筛查。除此之外，初期保健医师应在移植前明确告知患者移植后患上恶性肿瘤的风险会增加，并告知患者在移植前需要采取多种措施预防癌症，比如戒烟戒酒、预防肥胖、每日健康饮食、使用 SPF 值 30 以上的防晒霜和接种人乳头瘤病毒疫苗，这一点非常重要。

药物相互作用

药物相互作用通常见于有关免疫抑制药物的报道，表现为药代动力学或药效动力学的相互作用。药代动力学相互作用发生于药物的吸收、代谢、分布和清除，并可能导致药物浓度的增加或减少。药效动力学相互作用由两种药物毒性叠加引起。表 34.3 总结了服用免疫抑制剂患者的药物相互作用。

钙调磷酸酶抑制剂、环孢素和他克莫司是细胞色素 P450 3A4 酶系的底物，这一酶系同时也是许多药物代谢的一个共同途径。其结果是，许多药代动力学的药物相互作用报告都与钙调磷酸酶抑制剂有关。细胞增殖信号抑制剂(PSI)西罗莫司和依维莫司也是该酶系的底物。虽然关于细胞增殖信号抑制剂的药物相互作用少有报道，但是这主要是因为该类药物远不如钙调磷酸酶抑制剂应用得广泛。有人预计，与钙调磷酸酶抑制剂相互作用的药物也将以同样的方式改变细胞增殖信号抑制剂水平。抑制细胞色素 P450 3A4 酶系活性的药物会降低钙调磷酸酶抑制剂和细胞增殖信号抑制剂的代谢，从而提高了免疫抑制剂的血清浓度。这些相互作用通常由细胞色素 P450 酶系的竞争性抑制介导，因此免疫抑制剂的血清浓度将有望在使用相互作用药物后 24 小时内立即增加。如果已知相互作用的程度，那么明智的做法是在相互作用药物开始使用后相应地减少免疫抑制剂的用量。相应地，诱导细胞色素 P450 酶系活性的药物将会增加钙调磷酸酶抑制剂和细胞增殖信号抑制剂的代谢，从而降低免疫抑制剂的血药浓度。和抑制细胞色素 P450 酶系活性的过程不同，诱导其活性增强通常需要几天时间使酶合成上调。因此，免疫抑制剂血清浓度不会像预期的那样在几天内一直降低，也不会在应用相互作用药物后的约一个星期的时间内达到稳态最低点。当开始应用已知可诱导细胞色素 P450 酶系活性增强的药物之后，最好通过更频繁地监测免疫抑制剂血清浓度来管理药物相互作用，并在血清浓度开始下降时及时调整用药剂量。

应尽可能避免使用可激活免疫系统的西药和中草药，以防止发生潜在的排斥反应。已知的可激活免疫系统的中草药包括但不限于：紫锥花、苜蓿、黑升麻。

表34.3 常用药物与免疫抑制剂的相互作用

药物	相互作用	注释
钙调磷酸酶抑制剂(CNI):环孢菌素(CSA);他克莫司(TAC)		
唑类抗真菌剂:	增加CNI浓度:	降低CNI剂量并每周监测两次
氟康唑	增加30%~40%	
伊曲康唑	增加50%	
酮康唑	增加高达80%	
泊沙康唑	CSA增加25%;TAC增加66%	
伏立康唑	增加40%~50%	
二氢吡啶类钙通道阻滞剂:	增加CNI浓度:	每周监测一次或两次CNI水平
地尔硫䓬	增加25%~50%	
维拉帕米	增加≤25%	
大环内酯抗生素:	增加CNI浓度:	阿奇霉素是最好的替代方案,相互作用的潜力较小
克拉霉素	增加25%~50%	
红霉素	增加50%	
其他抗菌药物:		
两性霉素B	肾毒性增加	如果可能,使用脂质产品或替代性抗真菌药
氨基糖苷类	肾毒性增加	如果可能,使用替代性抗菌药物
阿尼芬净	阿尼芬净浓度增加(仅CSA)	无需剂量调整
卡泊芬净	卡泊芬净浓度增加	避免与CSA合用;与TAC合用时监测肝功能
利福布汀	CNI浓度降低	每周监测一次或两次CNI水平
利福平	CNI浓度降低	每周监测一次或两次CNI水平
HMG Co-A还原酶抑制剂(他汀类):	增加他汀类药物浓度(CSA> TAC)	以较低剂量开始用药,缓慢增加剂量,密切监测
阿托伐他汀		横纹肌溶解
氟伐他汀		避免将CSA、TAC与洛伐他汀合用
洛伐他汀		氟伐他汀和普伐他汀可能具有较少的相互作用潜力
普伐他汀		避免CSA与辛伐他汀合用
瑞舒伐他汀		
辛伐他汀		
胆汁酸树脂:	减少CNI吸收	CNI与胆汁酸树脂用药间隔4小时
消胆胺		
考来维仑		
考来替泊		
选择性5-羟色胺再摄取抑制剂:	增加CNI浓度:	如果可能,使用替代的选择性5-羟色胺再摄取抑制剂或抗抑郁药
氟伏沙明	仅在高剂量下增加浓度	
氟西汀		
帕罗西汀		
其他抗抑郁药:		
奈法唑酮	增加CNI浓度	避免合用,使用替代性抗抑郁药
圣约翰草	增加CNI浓度	避免合用,与CSA合用有排斥报道
抗惊厥药:	CNI浓度降低	每周监测一次或两次CNI水平
卡马西平		尽可能使用替代药物(例如用于神经病变的药物)
苯巴比妥		
苯妥英钠		
蛋白酶抑制剂:	增加CNI浓度(基于利托那韦的方案>100%)	对于基于利托那韦的方案:使用单次低剂量CNI(CSA 25mg或TAC 0.5mg),并在再次检测前每日监测CNI水平;CNI通常每周单次给药
安普那韦		

(待续)

表 34.3(续)

药物	相互作用	注释
阿扎那韦		福沙那韦的效果较差;阿扎那韦和替拉那韦的剂量未知(可能每天两次使用较低的 CNI 剂量,并监测 CNI 水平)
福沙那韦		
印地那韦		
洛匹那韦		
奈非那韦		
利托那韦		
沙奎那韦		
替拉那韦		
非核苷类逆转录酶抑制剂:	改变 CNI 浓度:	监测 CNI 水平并相应调整剂量
拉韦啶	增加 CNI 浓度	
依法韦仑	CNI 浓度降低	
依曲韦林	增加 CNI 浓度	
奈韦拉平	CNI 浓度降低	
抑酸药	减少 TAC 吸收(仅仅)	给药时间与 TAC 间隔 2 小时以上
其他药物		
西咪替丁	CNI 浓度增加	使用替代的 H_2 受体阻滞剂
霉酚酸酯(MMF);霉酚酸(MPA)		
抑酸药	减少 MMF/MPA 吸收	给药时间与 MMF/MAP 间隔 2 小时以上
抗病毒药物:	增加骨髓抑制:	监测全血细胞计数(CBC)以发现骨髓抑制的证据
阿昔洛韦	肾衰竭	相应减少 MMF/MPA 剂量
更昔洛韦	增加 MPA 浓度	相应降低抗病毒药剂量
伐昔洛韦	增加抗病毒药浓度	
缬更昔洛韦		
胆汁酸树脂:	减少 MMF/MPA 吸收	MMF/MPA 与胆汁酸树脂用药间隔 4 小时
消胆胺		
考来维仑		
考来替泊		
质子泵抑制剂:	减少 MMF/MPA 吸收	使用 H_2 受体阻滞剂或增加 MMF/MPA 剂量
兰索拉唑		
奥美拉唑		
泮托拉唑		
雷贝拉唑		
硫唑嘌呤		
胆汁酸树脂:	减少硫唑嘌呤吸收	硫唑嘌呤与胆汁酸树脂用药间隔 4 小时
消胆胺		
考来维仑		
考来替泊		
黄嘌呤氧化酶抑制剂:	增加硫唑嘌呤浓度	将硫唑嘌呤的剂量减少 50%~75%
别嘌呤醇		
非布索坦		
刺激增殖抑制剂;西罗莫司;依维莫司		
与钙调磷酸酶抑制剂相同的相互作用		

表 34.4 移植患者初期保健建议总结

医疗协作	初期保健医师和专家应确保他们与移植患者密切合作；在专家和全科医生之间建立劳动分工将优化医疗服务并减少裁员
转诊时机	慢性肾脏疾病(CKD)患者的早期转诊增加了提前移植的可能性并可以减少并发症率、死亡率和治疗成本
优化依从性	初期保健医师应通过诊断和治疗抑郁、焦虑和药物滥用来改善依从性
高血压	• 对于肝肾移植受者和所有合并慢性肾脏疾病或其他等同心脏风险的移植受者，血压控制目标<130mmHg/<80mmHg • 所有类型的降压药已显示在移植群体中有效
高脂血症	• 肾移植受者的目标低密度脂蛋白(LDL)<100 mg / dL • 不被细胞色素 P450 3A4 酶系代谢的 HMG-CoA 还原酶抑制剂应被视为一线药物治疗高脂血症(氟伐他汀、普伐他汀) • 服用钙调磷酸酶抑制剂(CNI)的移植受者患上他汀类药物相关性肌病的风险增加，因此应在随访期间检查磷酸肌酸激酶(CPK)和转氨酶水平
糖尿病	• 移植受者应在移植后仔细筛查新发糖尿病 • 美国糖尿病协会的建议应适用于移植人群
骨质疏松症	• 移植受者发生骨质疏松症的风险增加 • 维生素 D 补充剂、降钙素和双膦酸盐已被证明可以在一定时期内减少骨密度的下降
生育和避孕	• 育龄妇女应该在移植后被告知需要避孕 • 在移植群体中，屏障避孕法被认为是最安全的避孕方式 • 激素组合避孕法已显示在该群体中有效，但可能导致钙调磷酸酶抑制剂(CNI)水平的升高
免疫接种(见表 34.2)	• 灭活病毒和毒素疫苗在移植受体中是安全的 • 移植受者应避免接种活病毒疫苗，同时 2 周内避免接触接种过活病毒疫苗的家庭成员
吸烟	• 建议采取积极措施，包括激励性访谈和尼古丁替代治疗
癌症筛查	• 与普通人群相比，移植受者发生癌症的风险增加 3~4 倍 • 初期保健医师应遵循为肝肾移植受者发布的癌症筛查指南

总结

初期保健医师有机会显著改善实体器官移植后免疫抑制治疗所带来的慢性疾病负担。表 34.4 提供了关于初级保健移植受体的总结性建议。

（李仕进 译　向骁 朱继业 校）

参考文献

1. U.S. Department of Health and Human Services HRaSA, Healthcare Systems Bureau, Division of Transplantation. 2009 Annual Report of the U.S. Organ Procurement and Transplantation Network and the Scientific Registry of Transplant Recipients: Transplant Data 1999–2008.2009.
2. McCashland TM. Post transplantation care: role of the primary care physician versus transplant center. Liver Transplantation. 2001;11B:s2–s12.
3. Foy R, Hempel S, Rubenstein L, et al. Meta-analysis: effect of interactive communication between collaborating primary care physicians and specialists. Annals of Internal Medicine. 2010;152(4):247–258.
4. Fisher ES. Building a medical neighborhood for the medical home. New England Journal of Medicine. 2008;359(12):1202–1205.
5. Heller JC, Prochazka AV, Everson GT, et al. Long-term management after liver transplantation: primary care physician versus hepatologist. Liver Transplantation. 2009;15(10):1330–1335.
6. Linzer M, Myerburg RJ, Kutner JS, et al. Exploring the generalist-subspecialist interface in internal medicine. American Journal of Medicine. 2006;119:528–537.
7. McNatt GE, Easom A. The role of the advanced practice nurse in the care of organ transplant recipients. Advances in Renal Replacement Therapy. 2000;7(2):172–176.
8. Hilty DM, Nesbitt TS, Canning RD, et al. Telepsychiatry for the management of a liver transplantation candidate in the primary care setting. General Hospital Psychiatry. 2000;22:122–136.
9. Lederer DJ, Wilt JS, D'Ovidio F, et al. Obesity and underweight are associated with an increased risk of death after lung transplantation. American Journal of Respiratory and Critical Care Medicine. 2009;180(9):887–895.
10. Lee CK, Christensen LL, Magee JC, et al. Pre-transplant risk factors for chronic renal dysfunction after pediatric heart transplantation: a 10 year national cohort study. Journal of Heart and Lung Transplantation. 2007;26(5):458–465.
11. Vossler MR, Ni H, Toy W, et al. Pre-operative renal function predicts development of chronic renal insufficiency after orthotopic heart transplantation. Journal of Heart and Lung Transplantation. 2002;21:651–657.
12. Levin A. Consequences of late referral on patient outcomes. Nephrology, Dialysis, Transplantation. 2000;15(3):8–13.
13. Cass A, Cunningham J, Snelling P, et al. Late referral to a nephrologist reduces access to renal transplantation. American Journal of Kidney Diseases. 2003;42(5):1043–1049.
14. Chan MR, Dall AT, Fletcher KE, et al. Outcomes in patients with chronic kidney disease referred late to nephrologists: a meta-analysis. American Journal of Medicine. 2007;120(12):1063–1070.
15. Chen SC, Chang JM, Chou MC, et al. Slowing renal function decline in chronic kidney disease patients after nephrology referral. Nephrology. 2008;

13(8):730–736.
16. Roubicek C, Brunet P, Huiart L, et al. Timing of nephrology referral: influence on mortality and morbidity. American Journal of Kidney Diseases. 2000; 36(1):35–41.
17. Didlake RH, Dreyfus K, Kerman RH, et al. Patient non-adherence: a major cause of late graft failure in cyclosporine-treated renal transplants. Transplantation Proceedings. 1988;20(Suppl 3):63–69.
18. Michelon TF, Piovesa F, Pozza R, et al. Non-adherence as cause of renal graft loss. Transplantation Proceedings. 2002;34:2768–2770.
19. Vlaminck H, Maes B, Evers G. Prospective study on late consequences of subclinical non-adherence with immunosuppressive therapy in renal transplant patients. American Journal of Transplantation. 2004;4:1509–1513.
20. Dew MA, DiMartini AF, De Vito Dabbs A. Adherence to the medical regimen during the first two years after lung transplantation. Transplantation. 2008;85: 193–202.
21. Denhaerynck K, Steiger J, Bock A, et al. Prevalence and risk factors of non-adherence with immunosuppressive medication in kidney transplant patients. American Journal of Transplantation. 2007;7(1):108–116.
22. Dobbels F, Verleden G, Dupont L, et al. To transplant or not? The importance of psychosocial and behavioural factors before lung transplantation. Chronic Respiratory Disease. 2006;3(1):39–47.
23. Bell LE, Bartosh SM, Davis CL, et al. Adolescent transition to adult care in solid organ transplantation: a consensus conference report. American Journal of Transplantation. 2008;8(11):2234.
24. Kasiske BL, Epidemiology of cardiovascular disease after renal transplantation. Transplantation. 2001;72:55–58.
25. Pruthi J, Medkiff KA, Esrason KT, et al. Analysis of causes of death in liver transplant recipients who survived more than 3 years. Liver Transplantation. 2001;7:811–815.
26. James PA, Oparil S, Carter BL, et al. 2014 Evidence-based guideline for the management of high blood pressure in adults. Report from the panel members appointed to the eighth joint national committee (JNC 8). Journal of American Medical Association. 2014;311(5):507–520.
27. Canzanello VJ, Textar SC, Taler SJ, et al. Late hypertension after liver transplant: a comparison of cyclosporine and tacrolimus (FK 506). Liver Transplantation and Surgery. 1998;4:328–334.
28. Moss NG, Powell SL, Falk RJ. Intravenous cyclosporine activates afferent and efferent renal nerves and causes sodium retention in innervated kidneys in rats. Proceedings of the National Academy of Sciences. 1985;85:8222–8226.
29. Mangray M, Vella J. Hypertension after kidney transplant. American Journal of Kidney Diseases. 2011;57(2):331–341.
30. Prassad GVR, Ruzicka M, Burns KD, et al. Hypertension in dialysis and kidney transplant patients. Canadian Journal of Cardiology. 2009;25(5): 309–314.
31. Rubin M. Hypertension following kidney transplantation. Advances in Chronic Kidney Disease. 2011;18(1):17–22.
32. Mells G. Reducing the risks of cardiovascular disease in liver allograft recipients. Transplantation. 2007;83:1141–1150.
33. Kidney Disease: Improving Global Outcomes (KDIGO) Transplant Work Group. KDIGO clinical practice guideline for the care of kidney transplant recipients. American Journal of Transplantation. 2009;9(Suppl 3):S1–S157.
34. Beltran S, Crespo J, Kanter J, et al. Ambulatory blood pressure monitoring in renal transplant patients: should it be routinely performed? Transplantation Proceedings. 2010;42(8):2868–2870.
35. Prasad GV, Nash MM, Zaltzman JS. A prospective study of the physician effect on blood pressure in renal-transplant recipients. Nephrology, Dialysis, Transplantation. 2003;18(5):996–1000.
36. Stenehjem AE, Gudmundsdottir H, Os I. Office blood pressure measurements overestimate blood pressure control in renal transplant patients. Blood Pressure Monitoring. 2006;11(3):125–133.
37. Haydar AA, Covic A, Jayawardene S, et al. Insights from ambulatory blood pressure monitoring: diagnosis of hypertension and diurnal blood pressure in renal transplant recipients. Transplantation. 2004;77(6):849–853.
38. Prasad GV, Huang M, Nash MM, et al. Role of dietary salt intake in posttransplant hypertension with tacrolimus-based immunosuppression. Transplantation Proceedings. 2005;37(4):1896–1897.
39. K/DOQI. Clinical practice guidelines on hypertension and anti hypertensive agents in chronic kidney disease. American Journal of Kidney Diseases. 2004;43(5):S14–S290.
40. Galioto A, Semplicini A, Zanus G, et al. Nifedipine versus carvedilol in the treatment of de novo arterial hypertension after liver transplant: results of a controlled clinical trial. Liver Transplantation. 2008;14:1020–1028.
41. Hausberg M, Barenbrock M, Hohage H, et al. ACE inhibitor versus beta-blocker for the treatment of hypertension in renal allograft recipients. Hypertension. 1999;33:862–868.
42. Hernandez D, Lacalzada J, Salido E, et al. Regression of left ventricular hypertrophy by lisinopril after renal transplantation: role of ACE gene polymorphism. Kidney International. 2000;58:889–897.
43. Hiremath S, Fergusson D, Doucette S, et al. Renin angiotensin system blockade in kidney transplantation. American Journal of Transplantation. 2007;7(10): 2350–2360.
44. Ladefoged SD, Andersen CB. Calcium channel blockers in kidney transplantation. Clinical Transplantation. 1994;8(2 Pt 1):128–133.
45. Madsen JK, Sorensen SS, Hansen HE, et al. The effect of felodipine on renal function and blood pressure in cyclosporine-treated renal transplant recipients during the first three months after transplantation. Nephrology, Dialysis, Transplantation. 1998;13:2327–2334.
46. Midtvedt K, Ihlen H, Hartmann A, et al. Reduction of left ventricular mass by lisinopril and nifedipine in hypertensive renal transplant recipients: a prospective randomized double-blind study. Transplantation. 2001;72:107–111.
47. Mourad G, Ribstein J, Mimran A. Converting-enzyme inhibitor versus calcium antagonist in cyclosporine-treated renal transplants. Kidney International. 1993;43:419–425.
48. Rahn KH, Barenbrock M, Fritschka E, et al. Effect of nitrendipine on renal function in renal transplant patients treated with cyclosporine: a randomized trial. Lancet. 1999;354:1415–1420.
49. Tylicki L, Biedunkiewicz B, Chamienia A, et al. Randomized placebo controlled study on the effects of losartan and carvedilol on albuminuria in transplant recipients. Transplantation. 2006;18:52–56.
50. Van den Dorpel MA, Zietse R, Ijzermans JN, et al. Prophylactic isradipine treatment after kidney transplantation: a prospective double-blind placebo-controlled randomized trial. Transplant International. 1994;7(Suppl 1):270–274.
51. van Riemsdijk IC, Mulder PG, de Fijter JW, et al. Addition of isradipine (lomir) results in a better renal function after kidney transplantation: a double-blind randomized, placebo-controlled, multi-center study. Transplantation. 2000;70: 122–126.
52. Midtvedt K, Hartmann A, Foss A, et al. Sustained improvement of renal graft function for two years in hypertensive renal transplant recipients treated with nifedipine as compared to lisinopril. Transplantation. 2001;72(11):1787–1792.
53. Rossetto A, Bitetto D, Bresadola V, et al. Cardiovascular risk factors and immunosuppressive regimen after liver transplantation. Transplantation Proceedings. 2010;42(7):2576–2578.
54. Liefeldt L, Budde K. Risk factors for cardiovascular disease in renal transplant recipients and strategies to minimize risk. Transplant International. 2010;23(12): 1191–1204.
55. Malyszko J, Malyszko JS, Bachorzewska-Gajewska H, et al. Inadequate blood pressure control in most kidney transplant recipients and patients with coronary artery disease with and without complications. Transplantation Proceedings. 2009;41(8):3069–3072.
56. Przybylowski P, Malyszko J, Malyszko JS, et al. Blood pressure control in orthotopic heart transplant and kidney allograft recipients is far from satisfactory. Transplantation Proceedings. 2010;42(10):4263–4266.
57. Opelz G, Dohler B. Improved long-term outcomes after renal transplantation associated with blood pressure control. American Journal of Transplantation. 2005;5(11):2725–2731.
58. Aakhus S, Dahl K, Wideroe T. Hyperlipidemia in renal transplant recipients. Journal of Internal Medicine. 1996;239:407–415.
59. Brown JH, Murphy BG, Douglas AF, et al. Influence of immunosuppressive therapy on lipoprotein (A) and other lipoproteins following renal transplantation. Nephron. 1997;75:277–282.
60. Gisbert C, Prieto M, Berenguer M, et al. Hyperlipidemia in liver transplant recipients: prevalence and risk factors. Liver Transplantation and Surgery. 1997;3(4):416–422.
61. Gonyea JE, Anderson CF. Weight change and serum lipoproteins in recipients of renal allografts. Mayo Clinic Proceedings. 1992;67:653–657.
62. McDiarmid SV, Gornbein JA, Fortunat M, et al. Serum lipid abnormalities in pediatric liver transplant patients. Transplantation. 1992;53:109–115.
63. Moore R, Thomas D, Morgan E, et al. Abnormal lipid and lipoprotein profiles following renal transplantation. Transplantation Proceedings. 1993;25: 1060–1061.
64. Munoz SJ. Hyperlipidemia and other coronary risk factors after orthotopic liver transplantation: pathogenesis, diagnosis and management. Liver Transplantation and Surgery. 1995;5(Suppl 1):29–38.
65. Munoz SJ, Deems RO, Mortiz MJ. Hyperlipidemia and obesity after liver transplantation. Transplantation Proceedings. 1991;23(1 Pt 2):1480–1483.
66. Stegall MD, Everson G, Schroter G, et al. Metabolic complications after liver transplant: diabetes, hypercholesterolemia, hypertension and obesity. Transplantation. 1995;60:1057–1060.
67. Kasiske BL, Cosio FG, Beto J, et al. Clinical practice guidelines for managing

dyslipidemias in kidney transplant patients: a report from the managing dyslipidemias in chronic kidney disease work group of the National Kidney Foundation kidney diseases outcomes quality initiative. American Journal of Transplantation. 2004;4(Suppl 7):13–53.
68. McGuire BM, Rosenthal P, Brown CC, et al. Long-term management of the liver transplant patient: recommendations for the primary care doctor. American Journal of Transplantation. 2009;9:1988–2003.
69. Kasiske BL, Tortorice KL, Heim-Duthoy KL, et al. Lovastatin treatment of hypercholesterolemia in renal transplant recipients. Transplantation. 1990;49:95–100.
70. Wenke K, Meiser B, Thiery J, et al. Simvastatin initiated early after heart transplantation. Circulation. 2003;107:93–97.
71. Zaffari D, Losekann A, Santos AF, et al. Effectiveness of diet in hyperlipidemia in renal transplant patients. Transplantation Proceedings. 2004;36:889–890.
72. Sapan M, Ozben B, Yakupoglu G, et al. Effects of diet and gemfibrozil on posttransplant hyperlipidemia in renal transplant Recipients. Journal of Investigative Medicine. 2009;57(2):456–459.
73. Evangelista LS, Dracup K, Doering L, et al. Physical activity patterns in heart transplant women. Journal of Cardiovascular Nursing. 2005;20(5):334–339.
74. Painter P. Exercise following organ transplantation: a critical part of the routine post transplant care. Annals of Transplantation: Quarterly of the Polish Transplantation Society. 2005;10(4):28–30.
75. Perrea DN, Moulakakis KG, Poulakou MV, et al. Correlation between lipid abnormalities and immunosuppressive therapy in renal transplant recipients with stable renal function. International Urology and Nephrology. 2008;40(2):521–527.
76. Roy A, Kneteman N, Lilly L, et al. Tacrolimus as intervention in the treatment of hyperlipidemia after liver transplant. Transplantation. 2006;82(4):494–500.
77. Kniepeiss D, Iberer F, Shcaffellner S, et al. Dyslipidemia during sirolimus therapy in patients after liver transplantation. Clinical Transplantation. 2004;18(6):642–646.
78. Moore R, Hernandez D, Valantine H. Calcineurin inhibitors and post-transplant hyperlipidaemias. Drug Safety. 2001;24(10):755–766.
79. Gomez G, Alvarez ML, Errasti F, et al. Fluvastatin in the treatment of hypercholesterolemia in renal transplantation. Transplantation Proceedings. 1999;31:2326–2327.
80. Alvarez ML, Errasti P, Gomez G, et al. Effect of atorvastatin on the treatment of hypercholesterolemia after renal transplantation. Transplantation Proceedings. 1999;31:2328–2329.
81. Yoshimura N, Oka T, Okamoto M, et al. The effects of pravastatin on hyperlipidemia in renal transplant recipients. Transplantation. 1992;53:94–99.
82. Imagawa DK, Dawson S, Holt CD, et al. Hyperlipidemia after liver transplantation: natural history and treatment with the hydroxylmethlglutaryl-coenzyme a reductase inhibitor pravastatin. Transplantation. 1996;62:934–942.
83. Imamura R, Ichimaru N, Moriyama T, et al. Long term efficacy of simvastatin in renal transplant recipients treated with cyclosporine or tacrolimus. Clinical Transplantation. 2005;19:616–621.
84. Pfugfelder PW, Huff M, Oskalns R, et al. Cholesterol-lowering therapy after heart transplantation: a 12-month randomized trial. Journal of Heart and Lung Transplantation. 1996;15:539–540.
85. Zachoval R, Gerbes AL, Schwandt P, et al. Short-term effects of statin therapy in patients with hyperlipoproteinemia after liver transplantation: results of a randomized crossover trial. Journal of Hepatology. 2001;35:86–91.
86. Renders L, Mayer-Kadner I, Koch C, et al. Efficacy and drug interactions of the new HMG-CoA reductase inhibitors cerivastatin and atorvastatin in CsA-treated renal transplant recipients. Nephrology, Dialysis, Transplantation. 2001;16:141–146.
87. Santos AF, Keitel E, Bittar AE, et al. Safety and efficacy of simvastatin for hyperlipidemia in renal transplant recipients: a double-blind randomized, placebo-controlled study. Transplantation Proceedings. 2001;30:2054–2057.
88. Lepre F, Rigby R, Hawley C, et al. A double-blind placebo controlled trial of simvastatin for the treatment of dyslipidaemia in renal allograft recipients. Clinical Transplantation. 1999;13:520–525.
89. Melchor JL, Gracida C. Treatment of hypercholesterolemia with fluvastatin in kidney transplant patients. Transplantation Proceedings. 1998;30:2054–2057.
90. Castro R, Queiros J, Fonseca I, et al. Therapy of post renal transplantation hyperlipidaemia: comparative study with simvastatin and fish oil. Nephrology, Dialysis, Transplantation. 1997;12:2140–2143.
91. Lal SM, Hewett JE, Petroski GF, et al. Effects of nicotinic acid and lovastatin in renal transplant patients: a prospective randomized, open-labeled crossover trial. American Journal of Kidney Diseases. 1995;25:616–622.
92. Hanes DS, Nicholson PG, Raval DD, et al. A crossover comparison of the efficacy and safety of lovastatin and gemfibrozil in the treatment of hyperlipidemic organ transplant recipients. American Journal of Therapeutics. 1997;4(2-3):85–91.
93. Kobashigawa JA, Katznelson S, Laks H, et al. Effect of pravastatin on outcomes after cardiac transplantation. New England Journal of Medicine. 1995;333:621–627.
94. Holdaas H, Fellstrom P, Jardine AG, et al. Assessment of LEscol in Renal Transplantation (ALERT) Study Investigators. Effect of fluvastatin on cardiac outcomes in renal transplant recipients: a multi-center randomized placebo-controlled trial. Lancet. 2003;361(9374):2024–2031.
95. Buchanan C, Smith L, Corbett J, et al. A retrospective analysis of ezetimibe treatment in renal transplant recipients. American Journal of Transplantation. 2006;6:770–774.
96. Taylor PJ, Kubler PA, Lynch SV, et al. Effect of atorvastatin on cyclosporine pharmocokinetics in liver transplant recipients. Annals of Pharmacotherapy. 2004;38(2):205–208.
97. Samman A, Imai C, Straatman L, et al. Safety and efficacy of rosuvastatin therapy for the prevention of hyperlipidemia in adult cardiac transplant recipients. Journal of Heart and Lung Transplantation. 2005;24(8):1008–1013.
98. Tokumoto T, Tanabe K, Ishida H, et al. Impact of fluvastatin on hyperlipidemia after renal transplantation. Transplantation Proceedings. 2004;36(7):2141–2144.
99. Langone AJ, Chuang P. Ezetimibe in renal transplant patients with hyperlipidemia resistant to HMG-CoA reductase inhibitors. Transplantation. 2006;81(5):804–807.
100. Chuang P, Langone AJ. Ezetimibe reduces Low-Density Lipoprotein Cholesterol (LDL-C) in renal transplant patients resistant to HMG-CoA reductase inhibitors. American Journal of Therapeutics. 2007;14(5):438–441.
101. Rodriguez-Ferrero ML, Anaya F. Ezetimibe in the treatment of uncontrolled hyperlipidemia in kidney transplant patients. Transplantation Proceedings. 2008;40(10):3492–3495.
102. Lopez V, Gutierrez C, Gutierrez E, et al. Treatment with ezetimibe in kidney transplant recipients with uncontrolled dyslipidemia. Transplantation Proceedings. 2008;40(9):2925–2926.
103. Savvidaki E, Koukoulaki M, Benou A, et al. Ezetimbe is effective in the treatment of persistent hyperlipidemia of renal allograft recipients. Clinical Nephrology. 2011;75(2):107–112.
104. Shaw SM, Chaggar P, Ritchie J, et al. The efficacy and tolerability of ezetimibe in cardiac transplant recipients taking cyclosporin. Transplantation. 2009;87(5):771–775.
105. Moro J, Almenar L, Martinez-Dolz L, et al. Ezetimibe in heart transplantation: initial experience. Transplantation Proceedings. 2007;39(7):2389–2392.
106. Kohnle M, Pietruck F, Kribben A, et al. Ezetimibe for the treatment of uncontrolled hypercholesterolemia in patients with high-dose statin therapy after renal transplantation. American Journal of Transplantation. 2006;6(1):205–208.
107. Tatsioni A, Chung M, Sun Y, et al. Effects of fish oil supplementation on kidney transplantation: a systematic review and meta-analysis of randomized, controlled trials. Journal of the American Society of Nephrology. 2005;16(8):2462–2470.
108. Kasiske BL. Clinical practice guidelines for managing dyslipidemias in kidney transplant patients. American Journal of Transplantation. 2003;5(6):1576.
109. Jensen RA, Lal SM, Diaz-Arias A, et al. Does cholestyramine interfere with cyclosporine absorption? A prospective study in renal transplant patients. American Society for Artificial Internal Organs Journal. 1995;41(3):M704–M706.
110. Vergoulas G, Miserlis G, Solonaki F, et al. Combined treatment of hypercholesterolemia of renal transplant allograft recipients with fluvastatin and gemfibrozil. Transplant International. 2000;13(Suppl 1):S64–S67.
111. Alberti KG, Zimmet PZ. Definition diagnosis and classification of diabetes mellitus and its complications. Part 1: diagnosis and classification of diabetes mellitus provision report of a WHO consultation. Diabetic Medicine. 1998;15:539.
112. American Diabetes Association. Standards of medical care in diabetes. Diabetes Care. 2011;34(Suppl 1):S11–S62.
113. Montori VM, Basu A, Erwin PJ, et al. Posttransplantation diabetes: a systematic review of the literature. Diabetes Care. 2002;25(3):583–592.
114. Kiberd M, Panek R, Kiberd BA. New onset diabetes mellitus post-kidney transplantation. Clinical Transplantation. 2006;20(5):634–639.
115. Saab S, Shapner A, Zhao Y, et al. Prevalence and risk factors for diabetes mellitus in moderate term survivors of liver transplantation. American Journal of Transplantation. 2006;6(8):1890–1895.
116. Salvadori M, Bertoni E, Rosati A, et al. Post-transplant diabetes mellitus. Journal of Nephrology. 2003;16(5):626–634.
117. Nieuwenhuis MG, Kirkels JH. Predictability and other aspects of post-transplant diabetes mellitus in heart transplant recipients. Journal of Heart and Lung Transplantation. 2001;20(7):703–708.
118. Razeghi E, Heydarian P, Amerian M, et al. The risk factors for diabetes mellitus after kidney transplantation. Saudi Journal of Kidney Diseases and Transplantation. 2010;21(6):1038–1043.
119. Duclos A, Flechner LM, Faiman C, et al. Post-transplant diabetes mellitus: risk reduction strategies in the elderly. Drugs and Aging. 2006;23(10):781–793.
120. Joss N, Staatz CE, Thomson AH, et al. Predictors of new onset diabetes after renal

transplantation. Clinical Transplantation. 2007;21(1):136–143.
121. Mora PF. New-onset diabetes after renal transplantation. Journal of Investigative Medicine. 2010;58(6):755–763.
122. Kahn J, Rehak P, Schweiger M, et al. The impact of overweight on the development of diabetes after heart transplantation. Clinical Transplantation. 2006;20(1):62–66.
123. Wilkinson A, Davidson J, Dotta F, et al. Guidelines for the treatment and management of new-onset diabetes after transplantation. Transplantation. 2005;19(3): 291–298.
124. Davidson J, Wilkinson A, Dantal J, et al. New-onset diabetes after transplantation: 2003 international consensus guidelines. proceedings of an international expert panel meeting. Transplantation. 2003;75(10):SS3–SS24.
125. Reynolds LR, Tannock L. Management of new-onset diabetes mellitus after transplantation. Postgraduate Medicine. 2008;120(2):60–66.
126. Nesto RW, Bell D, Bonow RO, et al. Thiazolidinedione use, fluid retention, and congestive heart failure: a consensus statement from the American Heart Association and American Diabetes Association. Circulation. 2003;108: 2941–2948.
127. Dolgos S, Hartmann A, Isaksen GA, et al. Osteoporosis is a prevalent finding in patients with solid organ failure awaiting transplantation – a population based study. Clinical Transplantation. 2010;24(5):E145–E152.
128. Sessa A, Esposito A, Lavicoli GD, et al. Immunosuppressive agents and bone disease in renal transplant patients with hypercalcemia. Transplantation Proceedings. 2010;42(4):1148–1155.
129. Pereira S, Pedroso S, Martins L, et al. Bone mineral density after simultaneous kidney-pancreas transplantation: four years follow-up of 57 recipients. Transplantation Proceedings. 2010;42(2):555–557.
130. Ahmadpoor P, Reisi S, Makhdoomi K, et al. Osteoporosis and related risk factors in renal transplant recipients. Transplantation Proceedings. 2009; 41(7):2820–2822.
131. Bayat N, Einollahi B, Pourfarzian V, et al. Bone mineral density changes within 11 months of renal transplantation in Iranian patients. Transplantation Proceedings. 2007;39(4):1039–1043.
132. Rakel A, Sheehy O, Rahme E, et al. Does diabetes increase the risk for fractures after solid organ transplantation? A nested case-control study. Journal of Bone and Mineral Research. 2007;22(12):1878–1884.
133. Akaberi S, Simonsen O, Lindergard B, et al. Can DEXA predict fractures in renal transplant patients? American Journal of Transplantation. 2008;8(12): 2647–2651.
134. Abbott K, Oglesby R, Hypolite I, et al. Hospitalizations for fractures after renal transplantation in the United States. Annals of Epidemiology. 2001;11(7): 450–457.
135. Sikgenc MM, Paydas S, Balal M, et al. Bone disease in renal transplantation and pleotropic effects of vitamin D therapy. Transplantation Proceedings. 2010;42(7): 2518–2526.
136. Wang HH, Chang PC, Chu SH, et al. Osteoporosis after kidney transplantation: preliminary report from a single center. Transplantation Proceedings. 2008;40(7): 2412–2413.
137. Mitterbauer C, Schwarz C, Haas M, et al. Effects of bisphosphonates on bone loss in the first year after renal transplantation - a meta-analysis of randomized controlled trials. Nephrology, Dialysis, Transplantation. 2006;21(8):2275–2281.
138. Mainra R, Elder G. Review article: managing bone complications after kidney transplantation. Nephrology. 2009;14:437–442.
139. Taber D, Ashcraft EA, Baillie GM, et al. Use of bone health protocol to identify and prevent bone disease in kidney and pancreas transplant recipients. Annals of Pharmacotherapy. 2007;41:944–950.
140. Bolland M, Grey A, Avenell A, et al. Calcium supplements with or without vitamin D and risk of cardiovascular events: reanalysis of the women's health initiative limited access dataset and meta-analysis. British Medical Journal (Clinical Research Edition). 2011;342:2040.
141. Riley CA. Contraception and pregnancy after liver transplantation. Liver Transplantation. 2001;7(11 Suppl 1):S74–S76.
142. de Koning ND, Haagsma EB. Normalization of menstrual pattern after liver transplantation: consequences for contraception. Digestion. 1990;46(4): 239–241.
143. Xu LG, Wang HW, Jin LM, et al. Marital status and fertility of 185 male renal transplant recipients in China. Journal of Andrology. 2008;29(6):618–621.
144. De Celis R, Pedron-Nuevo N. Male fertility of kidney transplant patients with one to ten years of evolution using a conventional immunosuppressive regimen. Archives of Andrology. 1990;42(1):9–20.
145. Haberman J, Karwa G, Greenstein SM, et al. Male fertility in cyclosporine-treated renal transplant patients. Journal of Urology. 1991;145(2):294–296.
146. Zuber J, Anglicheau D, Elie C, et al. Sirolimus may reduce fertility in male renal transplant recipients. American Journal of Transplantation. 2008;8(7): 1471–1479.
147. Armenti VT, Radomski JS, Moritz MJ, et al. Report from the National Transplantation Pregnancy Registry (NTPR): Outcomes of pregnancy after transplantion. In: Cecka JM, Terasaki PI, editors. Clinical Transplants 2004. Los Angeles: UCLA Immunogenetics Center, 2004: 103–114.
148. Jabiry-Zieniewicz Z, Bobrowska K, Kaminski P, et al. Low-dose hormonal contraception after liver transplantation. Transplantation Proceedings. 2007;39(5): 1530–1532.
149. Pietrzak B, Bobrowska K, Jibiry-Zieniewicz Z, et al. Oral and transdermal hormonal contraception in women after kidney transplantation. Transplantation Proceedings. 2007;39(9):2759–2762.
150. Dourakis SP, Tolis G. Sex hormonal preparations and the liver. European Journal of Contraception and Reproductive Health Care. 1998;3:7–16.
151. Zerner J, Doil KL, Drewry J, et al. Intrauterine contraceptive device failure in renal transplant patients. Journal of Reproductive Medicine. 1981;26:99–102.
152. Bush WW. Overview of transplantation immunology and the pharmacotherapy of adult solid organ transplant recipients: focus on immunosuppression. American Association of Critical-Care Nurses Clinical Issues. 1999;10:253–269.
153. Gustavson LE, Legler UF, Benet LZ. Impairment of prednisolone disposition in women taking oral contraceptives or conjugated estrogens. Journal of Clinical Endocrinology and Metabolism. 1986;62:234–237.
154. Scholes D, LaCroix AZ, Ichikawa LE. Injectable hormone contraception and bone density: results from a prospective study. Epidemiology. 2002;13:581–587.
155. Chesi C, Gunther M, Huzly D, et al. Immunization of liver and renal transplant recipients: a seroepidemiological and sociodemographic survey. Transplant Infectious Disease. 2009;11(6):507–512.
156. Dopp JM, Wigert NA, Moran JJ, et al. Effect of annual influenza immunization on antibody response in lung transplant patients. Progress in Transplantation. 2009;19(2):153–159.
157. Sanchez-Fructuoso AI, Pratts D, Narajo P, et al. Influenza virus immunization effectivity in kidney transplant patients subjected to two different triple-drug therapy immunosuppression protocols: mycophenolate versus azathioprine. Transplantation. 2000;69(3):436–439.
158. Huang KL, Armstrong JA, Ho M, et al. Antibody response after influenza immunization in renal transplant patients receiving cyclosporin A or azathiprine. Infection and Immunity. 1983;40(1):421–424.
159. Keshtkar-Jahromi M, Argani H, Rhnavardi M, et al. Antibody response to influenza immunization in kidney transplant recipients receiving either azathioprine or mycophenolate: a controlled trial. American Journal of Nephrology. 2008;28(4):654–660.
160. Bortoluss R, Marrie TJ, Cunningham J, et al. Serum antibody and opsonic responses after immunization with pneumococcal vaccine in kidney transplant recipients and controls. Infection and Immunity. 1981;34(1):20–25.
161. Kazancioglu R, Sever MS, Yuksel-Onel D, et al. Immunization of renal transplant recipients with pneumococcal polysaccharide vaccine. Clinical Transplantation. 2000;14(1):61–65.
162. Bienzle U, Gunther M, Neuhaus R, et al. Immunization with an adjuvant hepatitis B vaccine after liver transplantation for hepatitis B-relate disease. Hepatology. 2003;38(4):811–819.
163. Gunther M, Neuhaus R, Bauer T, et al. Immunization with an adjuvant hepatitis B vaccine in liver transplant recipients: antibody decline and booster vaccination with conventional vaccine. Liver Transplantation. 2006;12(2):316–319.
164. Gunther M, Stark K, Neuhaus R, et al. Rapid decline of antibodies after hepatitis A immunization in liver and renal transplant recipients. Transplantation. 2001;71(3):477–479.
165. Soesman NMR, Rimmelzwaan GF, Nieunkoop NJ, et al. Efficacy of influenza vaccination in adult liver transplant recipients. Journal of Medical Virology. 2006;61:83–93.
166. Khan S, Erlichman J, Rand EB. Live virus immunization after orthotopic liver transplantation. Pediatric Transplantation. 2006;10(1):78–82.
167. Leithead JA, Ferguson JW, Hayes PC. Smoking-related morbidity and mortality following liver transplantation. Liver Transplantation. 2008;14(8):1159–1164.
168. van der Heide F, Dijkstra G, Porte RJ, et al. Smoking behavior in liver transplant recipients. Liver Transplantation. 2009;15(6):648–655.
169. Herrero JI, Pardo F, D'Avola D, et al. Risk factors of lung, head and neck, esophageal, and kidney and urinary tract carcinomas after liver transplantation: the effect of smoking withdrawal. Liver Transplantation. 2011;17:402–408.
170. Mathur A, Ranney D, Patel S, et al. The effect of smoking on biliary complications following liver transplantation. European Society for Organ Transplantation. 2010;24:58–66.
171. McConathy K, Turner V, Johnston T, et al. Analysis of smoking in patients referred for liver transplantation and its adverse impact of short-term outcomes. Journal of the Kentucky Medical Association. 2007;105(6):261–266.
172. Nogueira JM, Haririan A, Jacobs SC, et al. Cigarette smoking, kidney function, and mortality after live donor kidney transplant. American Journal of Kidney Diseases. 2010;55(5):907–915.

173. Kasiske BL, Klinger D. Cigarette smoking in renal transplant recipients. Journal of the American Society of Nephrology. 2000;11:753–759.
174. Cosio FG, Falkenhain ME, Pesavento TE, et al. Patient survival after renal transplantation: II. The impact of smoking. Clinical Transplantation. 1999;13(4): 336–341.
175. Gombos P, Langer RM, Korbely R, et al. Smoking following renal transplantation in Hungary and its possible deleterious effect on renal graft function. Transplantation Proceedings. 2010;42:2357–2359.
176. Biesenbach G, Biesenbach P, Bodlaj G, et al. Impact of smoking on progression of vascular diseases and patient survival in type-1 diabetic patients after simultaneous kidney-pancreas transplantation in a single centre. Transplant International. 2008;21(4):357–363.
177. Banas MC, Banas B, Wolf J, et al. Smoking behavior of patients before and after renal transplantation. Nephrology, Dialysis, Transplantation. 2008;23(4): 1442–1446.
178. DiMartini A, Lubna J, Russell S, et al. Tobacco use following liver transplantation for alcoholic liver disease: an underestimated problem. Liver Transplantation. 2005;11:679–683.
179. McClure JB, Swan GE, Jack L, et al. Mood, side-effects and smoking outcomes among persons with and without probable lifetime depression taking varenicline. Journal of General Internal Medicine. 2009;24(5):563–569.
180. McIntyre RS. Varenicline and suicidality: a new era in medication safety surveillance. Expert Opinion on Drug Safety. 2008;7(5):511–514.
181. EBPG Expert Group on Renal Transplantation. European best practice guidelines for renal transplantation. Section IV: long-term management of the transplant recipients. IV.5.6 cardiovascular risks. Smoking. Nephrology, Dialysis, Transplantation. 2002;17(Suppl 4):29.
182. Kinlen LJ. Incidence of cancer in rheumatoid arthritis and other disorders after immunosuppressive treatment. American Journal of Medicine. 1985;78(Suppl 1A):44–49.
183. Gutierrez-Dalmau A, Campistol JM. Immunosuppressive therapy and malignancy in organ transplant recipients a systematic review. Drugs. 2007;67(8): 1167–1198.
184. Einollahi B, Nemati E, Lessan-Pezeshki M, et al. Skin cancer after renal transplantation: results of a multicenter study in Iran. Annals of Transplantation. 2010;15(3):44–50.
185. Chak E, Saab S. Risk factors and incidence of de novo malignancy in liver transplant recipients: a systematic review. Liver International. 2010;30(9): 1247–1258.
186. Gallo P, Agozzino L, Angelini A, et al. Causes of late failure after heart transplantation: a ten year survey. Journal of Heart and Lung Transplantation. 1997;16:1113.
187. Jain AB, Yee LD, Nalesnik MA, et al. Comparative incidence of de novo nonlymphoid malignancies after liver transplantation under tacrolimus using surveillance epidemiologic end result data. Transplantation. 1998;66:1193.
188. Kauffman HM, Woodle ES, Cole EH, et al. Transplant recipient's knowledge of posttransplant malignancy risk: implication for education programs. Transplantation. 2008;85(7):928–933.
189. Zeldin GA, Maygers J, Klein A, et al. Vaccination, screening for malignancy and health maintenance of the liver transplant recipient. Journal of Clinical Gastroenterology. 2001;32(2):148–150.
190. Ringash J, the Canadian Task Force on Preventive Health Care. Preventive Health Care, 2001 update: screening mammography among women aged 40–49 years at average risk of breast cancer. Canadian Medical Association Journal. 2001;164: 469–476.
191. U.S. Preventive Services Task Force. The Guide to Clinical Preventive Services 2006: Recommendations of the United States Preventive Services Task Force. Alexandria, VA: International Medical Publishing Inc; 2006.
192. Smith RA, Brooks D, Cokkinides V, et al. Cancer screening in the United States, 2013: A review of current American Cancer Society Guidelines, current issues in cancer screening, and new guidance on cervical cancer screening and lung cancer screening. CA: A Cancer Journal for Clinicians. 2013;63:87–105.

第 35 章 初期保健医师在胸部器官移植患者转诊和诊治中的角色

Remzi Bag, Arvind Bhimaraj, Sireesha Garikipati

引言

自从 1967 年 Christiaan Barnard 成功实施了首例心脏移植和 1981 年 Bruce Reitz 和 Norman Shumway 又成功进行了心肺联合移植术以后，胸部器官移植领域在患者选择、手术技术、重症监护管理、免疫抑制、长期筛查和随访等方面取得了多项重大进展。虽然没有关于需要肺移植的肺衰竭患病率的数据，但 10%的心力衰竭患者可能处于晚期(ACC/AHA D 期)[1]。对于接受了最佳治疗和其他手术干预之后症状无明显好转的患者,移植已经成为越来越可行的选择。截至 2011 年底,国际心肺移植学会(ISHLT)已收到约 10 万例心脏、38 000 例肺和 4200 例心肺联合移植的报告[2]。虽然每年在美国进行的肺移植数量正在逐渐增加，但心脏移植的数量在过去 10 年间一直存在波动[3],在 2009 年有 1670 例成年患者接受了肺移植,1853 例接受了心脏移植[4]。随着这些年来生存率的提高,2009 年存活的心脏或肺移植患者的数量分别逐渐增加到 20 369 人和 7425 人[4]。因此,当前有更多的患者接受了移植评估,并由移植中心和非移植医生共同管理,同时等待可用的器官,数量比以往任何一年都多。随着移植后患者寿命延长,预计他们将会患上新的慢性疾病,其中一些与其原始疾病相关,另一些为免疫抑制治疗的后遗症。此外,在接受移植多年以后,特别是稳定的患者对免疫排斥的警惕性降低了,也不再定期随访,可能会因为与移植无关的一般医疗问题而再次就诊于他们的初期保健医师(PCP)。因此,需要移植和非移植医生之间保持合作,在及时转诊、评估、移植时机、最优化处理合并症、移植前准备等方面为移植候选人提供全面的医疗服务，并应在移植前和新出现合并症的长期治疗和管理中提供一样的服务。初期保健医师可以处理胸部器官移植患者出现的最常见的合并症,包括高血压、糖尿病、血脂异常、骨质疏松症和感染,并帮助患者保持健康的生活方式、合理饮食和适当运动,并可作为一线医师筛查恶性肿瘤(表 35.1)。

表 35.1 非移植医疗保健医师主要服务领域

移植前阶段

- 确定移植候选人
- 及时转诊
- 优化慢性呼吸或心力衰竭的治疗
  - 药物治疗
  - 肺或心脏康复
  - 依从性
- 治疗先前已存在的合并症
  - 高血压
  - 糖尿病
  - 血脂异常
  - 骨质疏松症/骨质减少
  - 情绪障碍(焦虑、抑郁)
- 通过限制血制品的输注来避免致敏
- 健康维护
  - 预防性治疗和适龄癌症筛查
  - 药物使用咨询
  - 运动、心脏或肺部康复
  - 体重优化
  - 免疫接种

移植后阶段

- 对排斥和感染的高怀疑指数
- 避免药物相互作用
- 联系移植中心,如表 35.2 所示
- 治疗先前已存在的和新出现的合并症(如上)
- 健康维护(如上)
- 依从性

本章的目的是帮助初期保健医师管理胸部移植后发生的慢性疾病，以及在筛查、疫苗接种、性和生殖健康以及健康维护等方面为特定疾病预防提供建议。第34章是一个涵盖相似主题的有关腹部器官移植的章节。

医疗协作

虽然认识到专家和社区医生之间的合作可以改善患者预后[5]，并通过信息共享消除错误，但心脏、肺移植医疗协作的标准尚未建立。移植团队和全科医生之间的沟通是改善移植受者治疗的基本特征。医疗提供者沟通不力可能损害患者安全，降低患者满意度，并增加医疗经济负担。直接语音或书面交流已经成为了信息交换的主要方式，同时也具有公认的限制性。今后，卫生信息系统更广泛地被利用有望使各专业之间更好地沟通和配合，从而改善医疗协作。初步咨询请求应包括收集背景资料和需要回答的问题。即使在状态没有变化或变化很小的情况下，临床记录副本也应该及时地在医疗提供者之间共享[6]。一般来说，考虑到他们与患者在距离上的邻近和关系上的亲近，非移植医生可以最好地实现对健康维护、预防性治疗和常见慢性合并症的持续管理[6]。全科医生办公室专门为这些服务提供适当的设施、电子提醒、支持人员和适当的患者教育材料。

心脏和(或)肺移植患者的医疗服务是独特的，因为存在急性或慢性排斥的可能；免疫抑制及其相关的毒性、感染和恶性肿瘤的风险；抗排斥药物的使用改变了初诊体征和症状；以及抗排斥药物带来的毒性和药物相互作用。此外，存在同种异体移植物特有的问题，例如心脏移植受者的无痛性心肌缺血，肺移植受者的气道狭窄以及自体肺的过度膨胀。因为管理事项的独特性，美国移植学会建议将移植受者临床状况的重大变化及时传达给移植中心(表35.2)[7]。这样的沟通对于等待名单上的患者也很重要，这些患者通常在经过指导后将临床上的各种变化直接报告并咨询移植团队。根据器官获取和移植网络(OPTN)数据，每天约有700~800名患者在心脏或肺部移植的等待名单上[8]。不断恶化的需要正性肌力药物支持的心力衰竭可能潜在地需要更多的干预，因此可以在等待名单上获得升位。在肺移植候选者中，肺功能储备的变化，伴随氧需求不断增加的氧合状况的恶化、需要持续机械通气、肺动脉高压、肺活量的变化、肌酐或动脉血气等信息应当被传送到移植中心，因为它们影响器官分配的顺序。住院和疾病，比如感染、肺栓塞和中风，也应通知器官分配中心，以使移植候选人位置发生变化。

表35.2 非移植医师联系移植中心的指征

一般情况
• 住院
• 药物改变(添加或删除)
• 低血压或无法解释的收缩压较基线下降20mmHg
• 静息心率较基线增加>10bpm
• 发烧≥101°F(1℃=33.8°F)或任何无法解释的发烧≥100.5°F(≥48小时)
• 1周内体重增加≥2磅(1磅≈0.45kg)
• 不明原因的体重减轻>5磅
• 选择手术
心肺
• 呼吸急促
• 肺炎
• 肺移植患者的任何呼吸道感染
• 肺移植患者 FEV_1 降低>10%
• 晕厥
• 肌肉骨骼以外的胸痛
• 心肌梗死、心律失常、射血分数变化
胃肠道
• 便秘或胀气以外的腹痛
• 恶心、呕吐或腹泻
• 重大腹部疾病
神经
• 脑血管事件
• 癫痫发作
• 精神状态改变
其他
• 新发肾衰竭
• 恶性肿瘤
• 不耐受口服药物
• 不依从

Modified from the American Society of Transplantation guidelines[7].

移植前期

早期发现和转诊患有终末期心脏或肺部疾病的患者使其接受更好的治疗是治疗慢性心脏或呼吸衰竭的重要一步，在第30章和第31章中有详细讨论。移植问题应在患者健康状况出现恶化的早期就得到讨论，而不是在患者需要把移植作为一个紧急的个人选择而去面对的时候。及时转诊要求彻底的评估、发现和缓解先前未知的合并症、改善营养和功能状况,以及患者及其家人做好面对移植所带来的改变人生的一系列事件的准备。虽然在2005年美国引入肺脏分配评分系统之后，患者从名单登记到接受移植的平均等待时间已经大大改善,但是一些亚组的等待时间,例如带有人类白细胞抗原(HLA)抗体的患者,其等待时间可长达2年。特定疾病候选人的移植选择通常遵循已公布的国际指南,这在第30章和第31章中已详细谈到[9-13]。

优化医疗

随着重症监护和免疫抑制的进展,正如第79章和第106章所述,在过去10年里胸部器官移植后的短期和长期生存率都有所改善。然而,胸部器官移植的收益逊于肝脏或肾脏移植。努力在身体、医疗、情绪和心理上使患者处于最佳状态并使其为手术做好充分准备,可以降低并发症的风险并改善预后。

肺和心脏康复

慢性呼吸或心力衰竭患者的运动能力降低。功能障碍由有氧代谢能力和最大氧耗降低所致，并且与呼吸困难、肌肉力量、肺功能或中枢和外周循环异常相关。骨骼肌功能障碍在慢性阻塞性肺疾病(COPD)和充血性心力衰竭(CHF)中均有详细记录,但也存在于其他形式的慢性呼吸衰竭中[14-17]。

有氧代谢能力(心肺运动试验中的最大耗氧量,6分钟步行试验,功能类临床分期等)的测定是慢性心脏和呼吸衰竭患者的重要预后因素。较低的运动能力与患有这些疾病的患者的较低存活率相关。因此,它可能对移植患者的生存有更大的影响[18-23]。

肺和心脏移植是具有围术期并发症和死亡重大风险的主要外科手术。虽然缺乏肺移植前肺康复益处的随机对照试验,但保留有最大运动耐力和进行术后康复的患者在胸部手术后有更快的恢复和更好的效果。体育训练对于改善慢性阻塞性肺疾病、间质性肺病、囊性纤维化、肺动脉高压和心力衰竭者的肺功能、呼吸困难和健康相关生活质量是安全和有效的[24-29]。一项大型队列研究表明,运动训练与慢性心力衰竭患者住院率、全因死亡率和心血管疾病相关死亡率的显著降低有关[30]。

术前肺部或心脏康复可以识别依从性不好的、太虚弱的或缺乏足够社会支持的患者，因此可判断谁是贫困的或次优移植候选人[31]。

尽管对运动训练在运动不耐受的改变中的作用的验证越来越多,但是其常规治疗实践仍然存在挑战,包括接受、有限的保险覆盖、定制运动程序以最好地满足亚组患者的需要，以及改善短期和长期的对运动训练和积极锻炼生活方式的依从性[32]。在诊断确立时和移植成功以后，就应鼓励患者咨询医生获取以心脏或肺康复和日常锻炼计划为形式的运动训练内容，以作为慢性心脏或呼吸衰竭患者管理的辅助干预措施。

优化体重和营养状况

移植前营养状况根据潜在的肺部疾病而变化,并且可能导致低体重、超重或肥胖。患有晚期肺病或心脏病的个体营养不良的原因是多因素的,包括饮食摄入减少、能量消耗增加、炎症细胞因子的释放、吸收不良和频繁住院。体重指数(BMI)通常用于分类体重不足(BMI<18.5kg/m^2)、超重(BMI 25~29.9kg/m^2)、肥胖(BMI≥30kg/m^2)和极度肥胖(BMI≥40kg/m^2)。肥胖是一种世界性流行病,在最近几十年越来越普遍。2007—2008年国家健康和营养调查(NHANES)的结果表明,估计73.9%的美国成年人的BMI≥25kg/m^2,34.2%超重,33.8%肥胖,5.7%极度肥胖[33]。

肥胖在国际指南中被列为选择肺移植候选者的相对禁忌证[13]。器官共享联合网络(UNOS)数据显示,在美国，超过15%的肺移植在肥胖患者身上实施。假设73.9%的美国成年人超重或肥胖,这一比例很可能会上升。超重和肥胖患者被认为有患上相关合并症的风险,例如高血压、血脂异常、2型糖尿病、冠心病、中风、恶性肿瘤和其他疾病，因此围术期和长期的死亡率和合并症发病率更高。此外,肥胖是一个独立的危险因素,它使原发性移植物功能障碍的风险增加2倍，排在移植中心调整、诊断、体外循环和移植手术之后[34]。单中心回顾性研究表明，肥胖个体的死亡风险比非肥胖个体的死亡风险高3倍以上[35,36]。在大型回顾性多机构数据分析中,肺移植后肥胖患者死亡风险增加15%,低体重(BMI <18.5kg/m^2)患者增加14%[37]。在另一项有关美国的一群患有慢性阻塞性肺疾病、囊性纤维化和弥漫性实质性肺病(肺移植最常见的3个诊断组)患者的回顾性分析中，对于任何处于正常BMI之外的患者,术后1年和5年的校正死亡率都明显升高，与正常体重

受者相比，超重、肥胖和低体重患者术后1年死亡率分别增加了27%、40%和34%[38]。增加的死亡风险由超重和肥胖患者中的原发性移植物功能障碍、呼吸衰竭、感染、心脏病和癌症介导。低体重患者的死亡可归因于感染、膈肌无力、与营养状况不良相关的呼吸衰竭和慢性同种异体移植物功能障碍[34,37,38]。在等候移植时，营养缺乏和低体重也是死亡的危险因素[39,40]。

强有力的证据表明体重减轻降低了移植的并发症和死亡率[41]。由于大多数肺移植受者在正常BMI范围之外，因此存在改善生存受益的绝好机会。应鼓励初期保健提供者遵循现有指南，通过适当的戒断和避免摄入糖皮质激素、营养咨询和膳食改良(包括低体重患者的肠内营养支持)、改变运动和生活方式，来优化移植候选人的营养状况，并对特殊选定的患者采取手术或其他治疗方法[42,43]。安非他酮和高剂量(60mg/d)的选择性5-羟色胺再摄取抑制剂(SSRI)氟西汀具有食欲抑制和情绪改变的属性。在大型公开对照试验中，外科减肥手术后的早期死亡率为1%或更低。在肺移植候选人的病例报道中，减肥手术不仅帮助实现了持续的体重减轻，而且导致了合并症的减少[44,45]。

与正常体重受者相比，超重和肥胖肺移植受者具有较低的去脂肪体重、较低的体育活动水平和静息能量消耗。此外，体重的显著增加发生在肺移植后第一年，由于异常BMI而导致晚期死亡风险增加[38,46,47]。因此，肺移植受者应该继续关注他们的饮食摄入，并参与肺移植后的肺康复和运动计划，以防止发展为超重或肥胖。

对于心脏移植候选者，BMI是等待移植时生存和移植预后的重要预测因素，包括围术期合并症发病率、移植后心血管并发症、远期并发症和死亡率[48]。国际心脏和肺移植协会的指南建议候选人在被列为心脏移植等待者之前应达到BMI<30kg/m^2(或与理想体重的百分比<140%)[12]。肥胖个体在原位心脏移植(OHT)的人口统计学中代表性不足，对器官的等待时间明显更长，并且在等待名单上不太可能接受原位心脏移植。此外，心脏移植前和(或)其在心脏移植后早期出现的代谢综合征可负面影响远期预后[49]。对器官共享联合网络数据库中19 593名原位心脏移植受者的分析发现，BMI为18.5~34.9kg/m^{2}时对死亡率、围术期合并症发病率、移植后心血管并发症和移植的远期并发症没有显著影响[50]。因此，移植前代谢综合征或BMI>30~34.9kg/m^{2}的肥胖的存在不一定是心脏移植的禁忌证。相反，这类患者需要密切监测和替代治疗方案。然而，BMI和移植预后之间的关系是U型的极端，比如，低体重(BMI<18.5kg/m^2)和肥胖(BMI>35kg/m^2)患者的预后更差。在低体重患者中，生存率下降是由于移植后第一年合并症发病率过高，而对于BMI>35kg/m^{2}的患者，其生存率下降似乎是由于术后一年以后死亡率开始增加[50]。因此，由于关注到术后和远期生存率的下降，许多中心以BMI>35kg/m^{2}作为原位心脏移植的禁忌证。因为营养状况是潜在可控的危险因素，所以设计用于改善终末期心力衰竭患者营养状况的策略可延长移植前存活时间并减少移植后期的短期风险，从而扩大移植的益处[51-54]。

优化依从性

移植患者的治疗方案由以下几方面组成：终身药物治疗(包括免疫抑制剂)，监测排斥、感染以及其他并发症的症状和体征，避免心血管疾病和癌症的危险因素(即饮食和运动处方、戒烟)，避免滥用/依赖酒精或非法药物，以及参加定期的临床检查和治疗药物监测[55]。不依从治疗方案的现象广泛存在，在心脏或肺移植中这一比例为7.5%~37%[55-61]。

尽管心理因素和治疗依从性对移植预后的重要性不言而喻(并且在第120章中有特别描述)，但目前没有对心脏或肺移植候选者进行心理评估的标准方法[62-64]。不依从在青少年和伴有焦虑和抑郁、人格障碍和神经认知障碍的患者中更常见。在独居、失业或缺乏社会支持的患者中更加糟糕[65]。胸部器官移植候选人在等待移植时经历着相当严重的精神困扰，而且研究已发现移植前和移植后的心理功能状态可预测移植后的生活质量、治疗依从性和预后[66]。由于他们渴望被移植团队接受，因此一些患者可能会出于自我保护而不会与移植中心专业人士分享他们的担忧[66]。此时，如果你去请教与患者建立长期关系的医生，会发现他们有特别的资格识别哪些患者不依从或哪些能从依从性强化干预中获益。没有单一的干预措施被证明在增加器官移植中药物依从性方面是优越的，但是包括以患者为中心的认知、教育、行为咨询和心理干预在内的干预措施的组合可能是长期有效的[67,68]。初期保健医师也有助于提高生活方式干预(运动、烟草、酒精和药物使用)的依从性，诊断和治疗焦虑和抑郁，以及为他们的患者提供社会支持。

避免输注血制品

移植受者血清中抗 HLA 抗体的存在或“体液免疫致敏”与急性排斥频率增加和存活率降低有关。未被致敏并被列入等待移植名单的患者可能由于各种原因而致敏，其中通过输注血制品而暴露于外部抗原是重要的潜在可避免的病因。不到万不得已不要输血，只有当输注任何血制品的益处超过移植候选人致敏风险时才能进行输血。

移植后期

在治疗胸部器官移植受者时要考虑的重要原则为：已改变的免疫系统、去神经移植物（心脏或肺）和高度潜在的药物间相互作用。

同种异体移植排斥

在移植后最初几周之后的排斥可分为急性细胞排斥（T 细胞介导）、急性体液排斥（抗体，因此为 B 细胞介导）和慢性排斥。肺部的急性排斥表现为急性血管排斥或气道炎症。慢性排斥主要是针对心脏的冠状动脉同种异体移植物血管病变和针对肺移植物的慢性气道排斥（闭塞性细支气管炎）。慢性血管排斥在肺中很少被识别，因为它需要开放式肺活检。排斥的复杂性和争议超出了本章的范围，将在第 71 和 72 章讨论。用于检测、定义和治疗各种排斥的技术在各中心之间存在显著差异。

虽然急性细胞排斥在心脏移植后的前 6 个月至 1 年中最常见，而在超过 3 年的移植患者中其对死亡率的贡献显著下降，但是原发性移植物衰竭（未检测到排斥的心功能丧失）占移植后 1 年以上死亡患者的 15%~20%[3]。不考虑原因，心脏移植物功能的任何损害将改变临床预后。因此，高度怀疑和早期识别排斥或移植物衰竭对于使用更高水平的免疫抑制进行干预非常重要。大多数中心经常在移植后第 1 年进行心内膜活检监测。外周血单核细胞（Allomap®）的基因表达谱也可以用作非侵入性监视工具。在任一策略中，监测仅表示为横截面取样，并且不能可靠地预测带有显著残留排斥风险的未来何时发作。医疗保健提供者需要警惕非典型和微妙的心力衰竭征象可能是移植物功能障碍的表现。由于心脏去神经，患者可能没有由于缺血或左心室高充盈压而造成的胸部不适。一些非典型的表现包括全身不适、早饱、恶心和由于肠道充血引起的呕吐。

与其他常见的实体器官移植相比，排斥反应在肺移植受者中更常见。约 35%的肺移植受者在移植后的第 1 年接受了同种异体移植排斥反应治疗[2]。第 1 年后，急性排斥的风险显著降低，但并不会从此消除。成人肺移植受者的总体中位生存期为 5.5 年，死因主要为慢性排斥，其发生率在移植后的最初几个月后开始增加，移植后 5 年可达到 50%[2]。排斥发作可以是无症状的或表现为呼吸困难、咳嗽、咳痰、发热、缺氧、湿啰音、喘息或干啰音。X 线片异常（如果存在）是非特异性的。肺功能测定可能会显示 1 秒用力呼气量（FEV_1）和用力肺活量（FVC）在高达 60%的排斥发作中减少[69]，但是不能区分排斥和引起同种异体移植物功能障碍的其他原因，例如感染、气道并发症（特别是狭窄）或胸腔积液。使用家用肺功能检测的中心确认了正式肺功能测定中任何> 10%下降。由于临床表现，实验室和放射学检查结果是非特异性的，并且不能区分移植物功能障碍的各种病因，包括感染、排斥、恶性肿瘤和气道狭窄等，所以鼓励非移植医生与移植中心讨论这些发现并安排明确的诊断性研究。

心脏同种异体移植物血管病变（CAV）涉及冠状动脉血管系统的整个范围，并且其特征在于由于平滑肌细胞增殖和细胞外基质沉积并伴有不同程度炎性细胞浸润的内膜增厚。钙化和动脉粥样硬化形成并不常见[70]。在移植后 10 年受到 CAV 导致的远期并发症和死亡影响的受者>50%，10%的患者在诊断后 1 年内死亡。冠状动脉造影常用于筛查 CAV。血管内冠状动脉超声（IVUS）更敏感，但没有得到普遍应用。计算机断层扫描（CT）血管造影也正在成为识别血管病变和移植物功能障碍的新技术[71,72]。多巴胺应激超声心动图不仅能检测显著的 CAV，而且是一个良好的预测死亡的标志物[73]。

尽管免疫机制在心脏同种异体移植物血管病变（CAV）的发病机理中起主要作用，但许多代谢危险因素，包括胰岛素抵抗和高胆固醇血症均有助于 CAV 的发生和进展[74-76]。在最近使用血管内冠状动脉超声定义的 CAV 的研究中，患有代谢综合征患者的 CAV 发生率增加了 8 倍[77]。冠状动脉粥样硬化的典型危险因素，如年龄和高血压，并不与 CAV 密切相关[77-80]。目前对任何代谢危险因素的治疗目标没有达成共识。然而，对于心脏移植受者来说,应该像非移植个体一样,将控制血压、脂质水平、体重优化和戒烟列为目标。非移植医生在控制这些风险因素和可能减少 CAV 负担方面发挥了至关重要的作用。

一旦心脏同种异体移植物血管病变(CAV)发生,暂无有效的疗法影响其预后。一些小型研究表明,钙通道阻滞剂和血管紧张素转换酶(ACE)抑制剂对 CAV 的发展有保护作用[81,82]。如这些小型研究所示,增殖抑制剂西罗莫司和依维莫司能降低进展速率,并可能降低死亡率,但这些药物的副作用特征阻碍了其广泛使用。所有心脏移植受者都应该给予他汀类药物,而不考虑他们的胆固醇分布,因为这些药物延迟了 CAV 的发病和进展[83,84]。除了降脂,这类药物抑制了抗原在内皮细胞、单核细胞和巨噬细胞上的诱导[85]。术后早期应用已被证明是有益的,同时影响死亡率和排斥[86]。与钙调磷酸酶抑制剂(CNI)和 mTOR 抑制剂的相互作用可导致发生肌病和横纹肌溶解的风险增高。因此,由于其最小的药物相互作用,推荐使用普伐他汀和氟伐他汀。接受这些免疫抑制剂的患者的每日最大允许剂量为 80mg。通过密切的临床和肌酶监测,阿托伐他汀可以考虑用于中重度高胆固醇血症,尽管部分会通过细胞色素 P450 系统代谢。

感染

由于强烈的免疫抑制,胸部移植受体处于各种感染的高风险中,特别是在前 12 个月和在用于治疗排斥发作所增加时间中。肺移植受者感染的其他诱因包括由于去神经支配引起的咳嗽反射的丧失,无效的黏膜纤毛清除,以及术后由于缺乏支气管动脉血管化和无效淋巴引流所引起的细胞死亡而导致黏膜屏障缺失。此外,被移植的下呼吸道系统对环境保持开放,持续暴露于各种刺激物和微生物。第 94 章专门讨论了长期移植受者的感染问题。

为了避免感染,移植患者接受了关于改变生活方式的广泛教育,如第 94 章所述[87]。预防性抗菌方案因胸腔器官移植中心而异,通常包括用于肺囊虫、弓形虫、念珠菌感染和巨细胞病毒(CMV)的药物。一些肺移植方案还会药物预防曲霉菌种。感染性心内膜炎在原位心脏移植中并不常见,但有高达 80%的死亡风险。因此,在牙科手术中药物预防是一个合理的选择[88,89]。

由于免疫抑制剂诱导的固有和获得性免疫的变化,移植受者可能不会总是出现感染的典型体征和症状。模糊和普通的不适和疲劳的症状可能表明存在显著的菌血症和败血症,即使缺乏全身性炎症反应综合征。此外,非感染性发热,例如在胸部器官移植受者中很常见。否则,非典型的罕见的细菌、分枝杆菌、真菌和病毒生物体将可能在免疫抑制的胸部器官移植受者中引起严重的感染。流行病学暴露(医院、社区、捐赠者或受体来源的感染)、旅行和宠物史可以为最可能的病因提供线索。

移植患者的感染时间线(不限于胸部移植)可分为移植后第 1 个月;1~6 个月;6 个月以后[90]。1~6 个月是免疫调节病毒(巨细胞病毒、EB 病毒、人类疱疹病毒 6 型以及乙型、丙型肝炎病毒)引起临床疾病的时期,并且与更高的免疫抑制剂水平组合可以导致机会性感染,例如单核细胞增多性李斯特菌、烟曲霉菌和肺囊虫,即使没有受到很强的暴露。6 个月以后,大多保留了移植物功能的患者主要面临社区获得性呼吸道感染,包括病毒(流感、副流感和呼吸道合胞病毒),而那些发生了移植物功能障碍和(或)排斥的患者因长期维持在较高剂量的免疫抑制剂当中,因此具有更高的机会性感染风险,例如肺囊虫、单核细胞增多性李斯特菌、新型隐球菌和星状诺卡菌。

早期术后筛查、预防和先发制人治疗方案降低了感染的发生率。虽然这些策略改变了时间线,但也导致出现了由抗生素耐药病原体引起的感染。早期和特异性的微生物学诊断对于指导治疗和最小化非必需药物治疗至关重要[91]。通常需要有创性诊断措施来获取准确和及时的诊断。对感染和排斥的诊断需要时刻保持一个临床怀疑状态,因为很多症状和体征都是非特异性的。鼓励非移植医生在怀疑感染或排斥发生时联系移植中心,以协调诊断研究以及适当和及时的治疗,特别是免疫抑制最强烈的时期,以避免移植后第 1 年的高排斥风险。

高血压

高血压在心脏或肺移植后很常见,发生于 50%~90%的受者[2,92]。患者通常有一个异常的昼夜血压分布,伴有夜间和舒张期高血压,使得自我监测在发现和治疗高血压至目标血压方面至关重要[93,94]。典型的移植前危险因素,如高 BMI、慢性肾脏疾病和甲状腺功能亢进均促进移植后高血压的发生。此外,动脉硬化[95]、钙调磷酸酶抑制剂(全身血管收缩、肾血管收缩和高交感兴奋状态、前列腺素与血栓素和内皮素之间存在失衡)[96,97]、异常压力感受器[98]和盐敏感性[99]被认为参与了移植后高血压的发展。在使用他克莫司和环孢霉素治疗的患者中,高血压和肾功能不全的发生率相当[100]。高血压以及其他危险因素被怀疑促进了心脏移植受者同种异体移植物血管病变(CAV)的发生和恶化[80]。

高血压评估、治疗目标和生活方式改变（包括减肥、避免钠盐摄入和坚持锻炼)与一般人群相似[101]。当选择某种抗高血压药物时，应综合考虑并发症和药物相互作用。钙通道阻滞剂可能具有抗钙调磷酸酶抑制剂(CNI)所介导的高血压的生理优势。地尔硫草与 CNI 具有显著的相互作用(增加血清水平),而氨氯地平没有,因此其可以作为安全的第一选择,其次是血管紧张素转换酶抑制剂(ACEI)或血管紧张素受体阻断剂(ARB)。如果合并蛋白尿或糖尿病,优选 ACEI 或ARB,同时需要密切监测血钾和肾功能[102]。若同时使用了硫唑嘌呤,ACEI 可能引起骨髓抑制,应该避免使用。利尿剂有助于减少循环负荷过重。地尔硫草也能延缓心脏移植受者中同种异体移植物血管病变(CAV)的进展。β-受体阻滞剂应用于肺移植受者是安全的，但在原位心脏移植患者(OHT)中应避免使用,特别是在术后早期,因为去神经支配的心脏更容易发生心动过缓。

糖尿病

在国际心肺移植协会的登记中,对于肺移植受者,其术后 1 年和 5 年的糖尿病患病率分别为 26.2%和 39.6%,这一数字在心脏移植受者中分别为 28%和 40%[2,103]。而在囊肿性纤维化患者中有高达 65%的发病率[104]。在器官共享联合网络(UNOS)数据库中,肺移植后的新发糖尿病在 2 年的中位随访期间占 2991 例肺移植受者的 33.4%[105]。约占总受者 1/5 的已经患有糖尿病的受者可能由于激素和钙调磷酸酶抑制剂(CNI)的使用而使糖尿病恶化。糖皮质激素诱导胰岛素抵抗、刺激脂肪分解和增加肝脏葡萄糖产出，而 CNI 通过与转录因子的相互作用和改变线粒体功能而抑制胰岛素分泌[106,107]。

尽管移植后糖尿病(DM)被认为是心血管事件、感染和移植物衰竭的独立危险因素，但是肺移植后糖尿病的影响尚未得到充分研究，因其对预后的影响还存在争议[104,108,109]。类固醇激素、钙调磷酸酶抑制剂(特别是他克莫司)的使用,体重增加与随之而来的胰岛素抵抗，术后应激和感染均增加了患上糖尿病的风险或对糖尿病的控制造成了挑战[100,110,111]。移植后新发糖尿病的其他危险因素包括男性、受体年龄>50 岁、非洲裔美国人和囊性纤维化[105]。

其诊断标准与非移植患者类似，除了糖化血红蛋白 A1c(HbA1c)结果不应当在移植后即刻使用,因为已输注的大量红细胞可以改变其结果。关于移植后新发糖尿病的国际共识指南建议术后第 1 个月每周监测 1 空腹血糖,然后改为每 3 个月 1 次,持续 1 年,之后改为每年监测 1 次。还建议对空腹血糖调节受损的患者进行葡萄糖耐量试验,以增加诊断率[112]。

移植后糖尿病的管理与非移植患者的管理相似,同时需要考虑药物的毒性或相互作用。在正常或有足够肾功能、肝功能和心功能的患者中,可以在使用胰岛素治疗前尝试大多数可用的药物种类（包括胰岛素增敏剂、促胰岛素促分泌剂和肠降糖素)。药剂的选择应该针对患者进行个体化定制。可以考虑使用 2 种或 3 种降糖药的组合。然而,当使用二甲双胍时,具有不稳定肾小球滤过率的患者发生乳酸性酸中毒的风险可能会增加。当使用大剂量糖皮质激素用于诱导免疫抑制或治疗急性排斥时，可能需要临时的胰岛素治疗以控制血糖。胰岛素治疗可以采用睡前单次注射中效或长效胰岛素的形式。可以用较低的胰岛素剂量加上口服降糖药来实现更好的血糖控制。如果初始治疗无法达到理想的控制水平,则需要采用更积极的方法,比如胰岛素泵[112]。出院后,建议在第 1 年内密切监测血糖。

长期血糖控制不佳可能需要将他克莫司改为环孢素。一些移植中心试图最小化糖皮质激素的使用。糖皮质激素剂量减少需要权衡排斥的风险，因此只能由移植中心在选定的患者中进行。建议改变生活方式,比如运动和体重优化，采用减少饱和脂肪和胆固醇摄入的心脏健康饮食,增加复合碳水化合物和纤维素摄入。除了高血糖,需要改善对并发症和合并症,如血脂异常和高血压的适当监测[113]。应像对待一般群体那样,每年对糖尿病并发症进行筛查。

血脂异常

肺移植受者中高脂血症的 1 年和 5 年患病率分别为 24.7%和 57.5%[2]。尽管普遍使用他汀类药物,约 66%的原位心脏移植受者具有至少一种血脂异常[114]。危险因素包括个人或家族史、不活动、不良饮食习惯、肥胖、甲状腺功能减退、糖尿病和免疫抑制药物，包括糖皮质激素、西罗莫司和钙调磷酸酶抑制剂(CNI)。在一项关于212名心脏移植受者的研究中，高龄、使用依维莫司、缺乏他汀类和(或)他克莫司使用与低密度脂蛋白(LDL)水平增加相关，而在一项多变量分析中，男性、移植前确诊冠心病和较低的射血分数与高密度脂蛋白(HDL)低水平有关[114]。只有较高的BMI与高甘油三酯水平相关。血脂异常和特定脂质参数与同种异体移植物血管病变(CAV)或死亡率的关系尚未得到证实，但在更大型的研究中，已显示高血脂与动脉粥样硬化发展存在关联[115,116]。最佳脂质水平控制目标暂时未知。在没有针对肺或心脏移植受者的具体指南的情况下，可以使用肾移植受者指南和国家胆固醇教育计划(NCEP)最近更新的建议(LDL胆固醇目标<100mg/dL)[117,118]。在经历3个月由饮食调节和运动组成的生活方式的干预后，若LDL>130mg/dL(至少>100mg/dL)，应开始药物治疗。高胆固醇血症的初始治疗药物应选择他汀类[119,120]。他汀类药物通过预防急性和慢性排斥改善了肺同种异体移植物的功能和存活[121]，并延迟心脏移植受者中同种异体移植物血管病变(CAV)的发生，也延缓了其进展[83,84]。如果效果不佳，可以将依折麦布加入他汀类药物[122,123]。虽然他汀类药物的副作用并不常见，但需要仔细监测这些情况，包括糖尿病、记忆丧失、精神错乱、肌肉无力，以及肌病和横纹肌溶解相关性疼痛。在他汀类药物中，当与钙调磷酸酶抑制剂(CNI)联合使用时，氟伐他汀和普伐他汀具有较低的横纹肌溶解风险。非移植医生应该意识到使用他汀类和钙调磷酸酶抑制剂(CNI)的药物组合会增加横纹肌溶解的风险。肌酶，如肌酸磷酸激酶和醛缩酶应在治疗开始后或剂量变化后跟踪监测。其他潜在的治疗药物包括吉非罗齐、烟酸和高剂量的鱼油补充剂[124,125]。贝特类与他汀类药物合用需要谨慎和密切随访，并限用于甘油三酯严重升高的患者。一些小型研究表明，在应用mTOR抑制剂的患者中，使用ω-3脂肪酸对降低甘油三酯很有益[125]。胆汁酸结合树脂可能减少免疫抑制药物的吸收，特别是与脂质结合的免疫抑制剂[118]。因此，应谨慎地避免在CNI给药前1小时至给药后4小时使用胆汁酸螯合剂，并应监测治疗药物水平。

骨健康

由于存在诸如吸烟、不活动、维生素D缺乏、低BMI和既往使用过糖皮质激素的危险因素，据报道肺移植候选人的骨质疏松症患病率高达61%[126,127]。其他危险因素，如吸收不良和高分解代谢状态使得囊肿性纤维化患者的骨密度(BMD)比那些由其他原因导致的终末期慢性呼吸衰竭患者更低[128-130]。在超过1/2的患有重度慢性心力衰竭的移植前患者中可以观察到骨质减少或骨质疏松症[131]。由于骨质减少和骨质疏松症的高患病率，维生素D水平和骨密度检查应当常规地包括在肺或心脏移植候选人的评估中。转诊医生和移植中心应该在移植前主动开始治疗骨密度异常和维生素D缺乏。由于使用了高剂量的糖皮质激素和免疫抑制治疗，在心脏或肺移植后第1年，腰椎和股骨颈的骨密度会显著降低[132-136]。有报道称，在肺移植后的第1年，非创伤性骨折率为18%~38%，骨密度损失了4%~12%[130,135-137]。在遭受骨质流失和(或)骨折的患者中，标志骨重吸收的生化标记物有显著增高[135]。

为防治骨质减少和骨质疏松，应鼓励体育活动，包括定期负重训练，鼓励戒烟戒酒[138-141]。所有患者都应按照建议量每日摄入钙1000~1500mg和维生素D 400~800 IU。任何维生素D缺乏都应予以治疗，以保持血清25-OH维生素D水平高于30ng/mL。维生素D和钙的替代治疗剂量并不能可靠地预防移植后临床上显著的骨丢失[134-136]。已显示骨化三醇在肺或心脏移植后第1年能降低骨丢失率，但还需要密切监测血钙和尿钙[142,143]。已显示降钙素在移植后预防早期骨丢失方面没有益处，因此不应使用[144,145]。

心脏和肺移植受者的随机和非随机对照试验和国际心肺移植协会指南指出，预防移植后早期骨吸收和快速骨丢失的最有效的选择是双膦酸盐[146-150]。静脉注射(帕米膦酸盐、唑来膦酸、伊班膦酸盐)和口服(阿仑膦酸盐、利塞膦酸盐)制剂均适用。双膦酸盐稍微增加了非典型性股骨骨折的风险。目前尚不清楚口服双膦酸盐治疗是否与增加的食管癌风险相关。双膦酸盐应该在早晨醒来后即刻用一整杯纯净水服用。患者在服药后应保持直立至少30~60分钟。重组人甲状旁腺激素（特立帕肽）对治疗糖皮质激素诱导的骨质疏松有效，但没有显示在肾移植后早期可以改善骨密度[151,152]。由于成本的原因，应将其保留给那些严重的骨质疏松或食管功能障碍(狭窄、贲门失弛缓症、硬皮病食管等)或不耐受双膦酸盐的患者。

对于随访，应在移植后1年使用双能X线吸收仪或等效扫描设备对所有成年移植患者进行股骨近端和腰椎骨密度的评估，若患者长期服用糖皮质激素，则此后每年都需评估一次[149]。根据是否存在骨量减少或骨密度是否正常，随访测试时间可为 2~3 年。

心理问题

移植专业人士通常对接受了胸部器官移植患者的心理应激认识不够[153]。意大利的一项研究表明，41%的心脏移植患者被发现患有重度抑郁症，而 12%患有移植相关创伤后应激障碍[154]。人格障碍、应对策略功能障碍、并发症和免疫抑制药物的副作用、压力事件、工作表现受限、性功能障碍和缺乏心理社会支持均促进了抑郁症的发生[155]。包括慢性排斥的并发症的发生可导致与抑郁症状急剧增加相关的功能状态下降。心理疾病对受者应对新器官的能力造成负面影响，并可能导致生活质量下降、期望落空和不依从康复和药物治疗。针对抑郁和焦虑的有效和可靠的心理治疗或精神药物干预可以改善依从性和健康相关的生活质量。选择性 5-羟色胺再摄取抑制剂(SSRI)对抑郁症、惊恐障碍和创伤后应激障碍的治疗既有效又具有良好的耐受性，并且代替三环类抗抑郁药而成为一线干预药物。其中，西酞普兰和依他普仑似乎具有最小的药物间相互作用风险[156]。当存在肾脏或肝脏损伤时，需要调整剂量。虽然苯二氮䓬类药物通常用于治疗与抑郁症状相关的焦虑和失眠，但建议在肺移植候选者和受者中谨慎使用这些药物，因为其具有药物依赖、上呼吸道肌张力降低和对高碳酸血症反应迟钝的风险[157]。米氮平对焦虑症和伴有厌食和失眠的抑郁症有效。其他疗法和人际关系、社群、家庭、支持或认知心理治疗可能有助于受者在心理上适应移植状态[62,155]。已发现一个高强度运动计划能够改善心脏移植受者的运动能力、健康自评、焦虑和抑郁[158]。

不鼓励自行使用圣约翰草治疗抑郁症，因为它存在严重的问题，包括毒性，被重金属、微生物和农药污染，掺假和药物间相互作用导致环孢素水平降低[155]。

在胸部移植候选人或受者中出现的抑郁通常被认为是对身体疾病的正常、可理解和可预测的反应，并且仍未被诊断和治疗[159]。此外，这类人群中的抑郁症状可能更难以被检测，因为可能存在诸如易激惹、认知障碍、挫败感、头痛、胃肠道不适、疲劳、睡眠问题、食欲下降或模糊性躯体疼痛等非典型特征[160]。非移植初期保健提供者可以通过对心理应激因素保持警惕，并利用标准仪器筛查识别相关的疾病和参考以上讨论的附加说明以治疗常见的情绪障碍，从而对移植患者的健康和生存做出显著贡献。对于严重的病例，可能需要转诊到专攻移植相关精神障碍的精神科医生处进行治疗和监测。

重返工作、娱乐和生活

移植患者在移植后很快就会看到并感知到其自我，并且很多患者希望回到其移植前的健康生活方式。在美国和其他国家，随访 1~12 年发现，移植后就业率为 22%~86%，变化较大。当使用广义的就业一词时，包括任何有酬工作或返校，都会发现这一比率更高[161-165]。许多患者面临着维持正常生计的问题，因为雇主担心体内有移植器官的雇员会有更高的健康保险负担和更多的病假。尽管这些患者重新融入社会的任务十分复杂，但应鼓励他们积极和富有成效地实现更好的身心成果。唯一需要强制限制的是避免从事可能暴露于感染的活动。应避免使感染风险升高的娱乐活动。公共泳池是感染的来源，因此应该避免，特别是当人多拥挤时。应避免在活动(烹饪或打猎)期间食用和处理生肉。

没有具体研究提出对心脏或肺移植患者进行驾驶和操作车辆的限制。心脏移植受者中晕厥的发生率为 3%~10%，与该症状发生相关的限制是适用的。每个州的法律都不尽相同，但大多数都要求在重新驾驶车辆之前需要 6 个月的无晕厥发作期。应尽一切努力识别和纠正导致晕厥的原因。症状性心动过缓的患者应该保证放置永久性心脏起搏器。窦房结功能障碍的发生率正在下降，因为许多中心采用了双心室手术技术，而不是旧式心脏移植中双心房方法[166]。虽然一项小型研究报告了心源性猝死的发生率为 18%，但由于缺乏尸体解剖研究，该病的真实发生率仍然未知[167]。

性和生殖健康

大多数患者在经历心脏或肺移植后所拥有的正常生育能力带来了复杂的医疗、社会心理和伦理问题。这一复杂问题将在第 97 章进行深入讨论。众多的不确定性仍然存在，包括怀孕对移植物和患者本身的风险，以及对胎儿的远期风险[168]。国家移植妊娠登记处(NTPR)在女性移植受者中获得了 2000 例妊娠结局的经验：怀孕的女性肾脏受者中 71%~76%顺利分娩，对于其他器官，活产率为 50%~86%[169]。新生儿出生缺陷的发生率似乎与一般人群相似，但对于接受了霉酚酸酯治疗的受者，其胎儿有23%的出生缺陷发生率[169,170]。对移植受者后代的长期随访再次验证了这一说法[169]。美国移植生殖问题共识会议建议在提供妊娠时机建议时应考虑各种个体因素，包括急性排斥和感染的风险，具有潜在毒性和致畸性药物的使用，以及移植物功能是否充足[168]。尽管这些患者存在发生母体、胎儿和新生儿并发症（包括高血压、先兆子痫、感染、早产和低出生体重）的风险，但在心脏或肺移植后仍有成功的妊娠结局[171]。有怀孕计划的心脏移植受者需要在过去半年内通过血管造影来给移植物做一个基线评估，以记录未发生同种异体移植物血管病变（CAV）和具备完整的移植物功能。在肺移植受者中，肺功能基线测定应有稳定的结果。在具备完整移植物功能的条件下，心脏移植患者怀孕后产生的生理变化通常都能良好耐受。

虽然有关肺移植后怀孕的信息很有限，但在怀孕期间和怀孕后同种异体移植物排斥的风险是显著的。在患有囊肿性纤维化的肺移植受者中妊娠是可行的，但仍应被视为一个危险的举动，因为有超过半数的受者在分娩后发生急性排斥的风险增高，另外所有受者在分娩后发生进展型同种异体移植物功能不全的风险也会增高[172]。

随着各种尚未确立妊娠安全性的新药的出现，尚不清楚如何最好地修改免疫抑制剂或治疗妊娠期间发生的免疫排斥。为了最小化移植物排斥的风险，应在整个怀孕期间保持一个合适的免疫抑制水平并密切监测，并谨记在产后会出现由体液改变和肾小球功能变化带来的药物浓度波动。随着最近辅助生殖技术的发展，控制性超排卵和代孕可能对希望有一个继承自己遗传基因的后代的胸部器官移植患者来说是一种更安全的选择[173,174]。

遗传咨询对于患有遗传性疾病的患者至关重要，包括作为其移植主要病因的先天性心脏病、家族性心肌病、遗传性肺动脉高压、囊肿性纤维化、家族性肺纤维化和α1-抗胰蛋白酶缺乏症。对于因围生期心肌病而进行心脏移植的妇女，由于存在高复发风险，应避免怀孕。

对于心脏移植后受孕的时间，一直存在争议。多数建议等待2年再怀孕。患者需要被告知胸部器官移植受者相对有限的远期存活率和怀孕对远期预后的影响会使其难以抚养子女长大成人。

可用的避孕选择与非移植患者相似。因为害怕感染，大部分患者都避免使用宫内节育器。提前做好屏障措施，成人中自己或配偶绝育，以及青少年的激素避孕法均是有效的选择。醋酸去甲羟孕酮每3个月肌内注射是有效的，但与骨密度降低有关。联合口服避孕药可引起类固醇激素清除率降低和抑制细胞色素P450 3A4通路，导致钙调神经磷酸激酶抑制剂（CNI）水平升高。如果考虑激素组合避孕，很有必要彻底筛查高凝状态和监测免疫抑制剂药物水平。激素避孕法不应用于患有显著高血压、血管病变、肝脏疾病和雌激素敏感性癌症的患者。

感染的风险是显著的，在常规阴道检查中需要采取严苛的无菌预防措施。疑似感染需要在等待培养结果时及时治疗。在分娩时也建议常规应用抗生素预防感染。具有多个性伴侣的个体应该接受安全性行为建议，并筛查性传播疾病。

虽然例数很少，但可用的数据表明心脏移植受者的亲子关系可能是安全的[175]。勃起和性功能障碍在心脏移植后比较常见，影响了感知方面的生活质量[176,177]。在开始治疗之前需要解决特定的心理原因。磷酸二酯酶抑制剂作为一线治疗药物是安全的[178]。使用mTOR抑制剂西罗莫司和依维莫司治疗会引起睾酮水平的降低，并破坏精子，降低其计数和活性[179]。

免疫接种

疫苗可预防的疾病发病率很高，在美国每年约有45 000个成年人死于这些疾病，大多数死于流感。建议初期保健医师和患者在移植前按照国家指南完成所有常规疫苗接种。一项关于儿童肺移植项目的调查显示，初期保健医师在移植前（69%）提供疫苗更常见，相对于移植后（38%）来说[180]。免疫接种计划会定期更新[181,182]。美国疾病控制和预防中心（CDC）国家免疫和呼吸疾病中心网站提供了可直接获取的疫苗接种建议和与其他疫苗接种相关网站的链接（http://www.cdc.gov/vaccines）。

一般认为实体器官移植受者的免疫活性已被改变，故不应使用减毒活疫苗。使用大剂量类固醇激素［相当于给予泼尼松≥2mg/kg（体重）或≥20mg/d，给药≥14天］或免疫抑制药物的移植前患者也应避免使用减毒活疫苗，包括鼻内减毒活流感病毒、水痘、带状疱疹、麻疹、腮腺炎和风疹[183]。由于没有前述最后5种病毒疫苗的替代物，因此特别重要的一点是，针对这些病毒的疫苗系列应像指示的那样在移植前接种完毕。建议患者至少 2 周内避免接触接受过减毒活疫苗接种的家庭成员。

CDC 认为心脏或肺移植候选人或受者发生医疗事件的风险很高，并建议他们定期接受流感和肺炎球菌疫苗接种。

癌症筛查

恶性肿瘤是心脏和肺移植存活者晚期死亡的主要原因[184]。这一主题将在第 95 章进行讨论。除了一般人群中常见的危险因素(如接触烟草和酒精、年龄、遗传)，免疫抑制诱导的癌症免疫监视削弱和更高致癌性病毒感染风险均促进了发病率的上升[185]。免疫抑制的同种异体移植物受者的器官发生肿瘤的风险增加了 3~4 倍,但发生某些癌症的风险增加了几百倍[186]。除了乳腺癌和前列腺癌，在普通人群中能看到的大多数常见恶性肿瘤的发病率都会增加[187]。此外,一些相对罕见的肿瘤出现的频率更高，包括移植后淋巴瘤和淋巴增殖性疾病(PTLD)、卡波西肉瘤(KS)、肾癌、子宫颈原位癌、肝胆恶性肿瘤、肛门癌和各种肉瘤。

心脏或肺移植后肺癌的发生率增加[188-191]。在单肺移植受者中,其发生在自体肺,特别多见于患有原发性慢性阻塞性肺疾病(COPD)或特发性肺纤维化和有吸烟史的患者。这类癌症被诊断时通常已到晚期,预后很差[192]。建议尽力加强筛查,因为积极的管理和治疗可能对更早期疾病有利[188]。囊肿性纤维化患者的结肠癌发病率显著(5.7%),多发生于移植后 246 天至 9.3 年[193]。结肠镜筛查可以识别患有结肠癌前病变的患者并防止其发展成结肠恶性肿瘤。

皮肤癌,特别是鳞状细胞癌和基底细胞癌,是器官移植受者中最常见的恶性肿瘤。其他皮肤癌类型,包括黑色素瘤、梅克尔细胞癌和卡波西肉瘤,也比非移植人群更常见。伏立康唑是一种经常用于肺移植的唑类抗真菌剂,由于其能诱导光敏性,因此增加了移植后患上皮肤癌的风险[194]。

实体器官移植后发生的大多数恶性淋巴细胞增殖性紊乱属于 B 细胞起源的移植后淋巴细胞增殖性疾病(PTLD)[195]。预防措施包括将免疫抑制降低至与保持移植物功能相适应的最低水平，并采取预防措施以防止某些病毒感染。

使用 mTOR 抑制剂西罗莫司和依维莫司来维持免疫抑制可显著降低发生各种移植后新发恶性肿瘤和非皮肤实体恶性肿瘤的风险[196]。

关于胸部器官移植受者的癌症筛查和预防还没有得到彻底研究。在一项针对心脏移植受者的单中心观察性研究中,对胸部、腹部和骨盆进行计算机断层扫描(CT)并无作用[197]。对于胸部移植受者的筛查和癌症监测,初期保健医师可以遵循美国移植学会、美国预防服务工作组和美国癌症协会当前公布的指南进行肾移植患者的癌症筛查[198,199]。其他预防措施包括适当的抗病毒预防和疫苗接种,患者行为教育和修正(戒烟戒酒、健康饮食等),经常使用防晒霜,每月自我检查和每年的皮肤病检查[200-202]。

准备外科手术

在谨慎对待某些方面治疗的前提下，胸部器官移植受者可以安全地进行手术。服用西罗莫司和依维莫司的个体可能出现伤口愈合能力受损。为了重大手术而停用这些药物的风险和益处应得到讨论。在重大手术期间，大量糖皮质激素暴露需要冒着肾上腺功能不全的风险使用应激剂量的类固醇激素。当患者口服摄入量为零时，应与移植医生协商将钙调磷酸酶抑制剂(CNI)和细胞周期抑制剂转化为静脉内或舌下制剂,同时治疗药物水平必须加以监测。虽然白细胞减少可能减少致敏,但最好避免不必要的血制品输注。对未行巨细胞病毒免疫接种的患者，应输注巨细胞病毒(CMV)阴性的血制品。

药物相互作用

通常用于移植医学的免疫抑制剂包括糖皮质激素、钙调磷酸酶抑制剂(环孢素、他克莫司)、mTOR 抑制剂(西罗莫司、依维莫司)和抗代谢物细胞周期阻滞剂[硫唑嘌呤和霉酚酸酯(MMF)或衍生物]。这些药物会在第 98 章中深入讨论，它们具有狭窄的治疗指数,剂量或浓度相对较小的变化将导致严重的治疗失败或药物不良反应。这些后果可能是持续的,不可逆的,慢性可逆的或危及生命的,并可能导致住院,持续或显著的残疾,移植物损失或丧失工作能力甚至死亡[203]。因此需常规对 mTOR 抑制剂和 CNI 进行治疗药物监测。靶血清水平根据移植时间和个体患者排斥负荷而变化。CNI 和 mTOR 抑制剂通过细胞色素 P450 系统代谢并且与许多其他常用药物有显著的相互作用，从而导致亚治疗或毒性水平(表 35.3)。开始或停止使用这些药物治

表 35.3 细胞色素 P450 系统相关的重要药物相互作用

诱导剂(排斥风险)	抑制剂(中毒风险)
卡马西平	胺碘酮
奈夫西林	唑类抗真菌剂:
苯妥英钠	氟康唑
苯巴比妥	伊曲康唑
吡格列酮	酮康唑
利福布汀	泊沙康唑
利福平	伏立康唑
曲格列酮	钙通道阻滞剂:
圣约翰草	地尔硫䓬
	尼卡地平
	维拉帕米
	西咪替丁
	环丙沙星
	大环内酯类:
	克拉霉素
	红霉素
	糖皮质激素
	印地那韦
	葡萄柚汁

疗需要查看文献并与移植中心协调,同时要频繁(有时每天)进行治疗药物监测。制药商已明令禁止西罗莫司和唑类抗真菌剂的共同给药。然而,当伏立康唑和泊沙康唑的剂量分别预先降低 90%和 33%~50%时,两种病例组并没有发现临床上显著的毒性和稳定的谷浓度[204,205]。

与硫唑嘌呤同时使用以下药物可能导致严重的骨髓抑制和血细胞减少:别嘌呤醇、卡托普利和其他血管紧张素转换酶抑制剂(ACEI)[206,207]。同时使用霉酚酸酯(MMF)和质子泵抑制剂可能导致对 MMF 活性代谢产物的暴露减少,从而导致排斥风险增加。

免疫抑制药物的所有变化只应由移植中心决定[7]。如果要添加或删除任何其他药物,应查询文献和药物相互作用表。如果发生药物的任何改变,包括以仿制药替代,应通知移植中心,以便可以实现高度紧密的治疗药物监测,直至达到药物的稳定水平。

总结

胸部器官移植已经成为医疗中越来越常见的组成部分,同时其愈发改善的存活率已使成千上万的患者能够回归社区安居乐业,但这一部分患者还需要得到医疗专业人员的重点关注。一般来说,长期存活的移植受者所面临的问题与普通人群相似,尽管它们的临床表现会被免疫抑制药物改变。现实仍需要移植医生和非移植医生之间的紧密合作,以为移植候选人在及时转诊、评估、最大化治疗合并症和移植前准备方面提供优质医疗服务,同时为移植受者在常见合并症,免疫接种,恶性肿瘤筛查和健康生活方式咨询方面提供管理服务。在这个过程中最重要的一个因素是初期保健医师和移植团队之间的持续沟通。

(李仕进 译 向骁 朱继业 校)

参考文献

1. Lietz K, Long JW, Kfoury AG, et al. Outcomes of left ventricular assist device implantation as destination therapy in the post-REMATCH era: implications for patient selection. Circulation. 2007;116(5):497–505.
2. Christie JD, Edwards LB, Kucheryavaya AY, et al. The registry of the International Society for Heart and Lung Transplantation: twenty-eighth adult lung and heart-lung transplant report–2011. Journal of Heart and Lung Transplantation. 2011;30(10):1104–1122.
3. Stehlik J, Edwards LB, Kucheryavaya AY, et al. The registry of the International Society for Heart and Lung Transplantation: twenty-eighth adult heart transplant report–2011. Journal of Heart and Lung Transplantation. 2011;30(10):1078–1094.
4. Scientific Registry of Transplant Recipients. 2011 [cited 2011 December 25, 2011]; Available from: http://www.srtr.org/.
5. Indridason OS, Coffman CJ, Oddone EZ. Is specialty care associated with improved survival of patients with congestive heart failure? American Heart Journal. 2003;145(2):300–309.
6. Linzer M, Myerburg RJ, Kutner JS, et al. Exploring the generalist-subspecialist interface in internal medicine. American Journal of Medicine. 2006;119(6):528–537.
7. American Society of Transplantation. AST guidelines for non-transplant physicians caring for heart and/or lung transplant recipients. Available from: http://www.a-s-t.org/content/non-transplant-physicians.
8. Organ Procurement and Transplantation Network (OPTN) and Scientific Registry of Transplant Recipients (SRTR). OPTN/SRTR 2010 annual data report. Department of Health and Human Services, Health Resources and Services Administration, Healthcare Systems Bureau, Division of Transplantation 2011. 2012 [cited 2012 January 01, 2012]; Available from: http://www.srtr.org/annual_reports/2010/default.htm.
9. Banner NR, Bonser RS, Clark AL, et al. UK guidelines for referral and assessment of adults for heart transplantation. Heart. 2011;97(18):1520–1527.
10. Costanzo MR, Augustine S, Bourge R, et al. Selection and treatment of candidates for heart transplantation. A statement for health professionals from the committee on heart failure and cardiac transplantation of the council on clinical cardiology, American Heart Association. Circulation. 1995;92(12):3593–3612.
11. Mancini D, Lietz K. Selection of cardiac transplantation candidates in 2010. Circulation. 2010;122(2):173–183.
12. Mehra MR, Kobashigawa J, Starling R, et al. Listing criteria for heart transplantation: International Society for Heart and Lung Transplantation guidelines for the care of cardiac transplant candidates–2006. Journal of Heart and Lung Transplantation. 2006;25(9):1024–1042.
13. Orens JB, Estenne M, Arcasoy S, et al. International guidelines for the selection of lung transplant candidates: 2006 update–a consensus report from the Pulmonary Scientific Council of the International Society for Heart and Lung Transplantation. Journal of Heart and Lung Transplantation. 2006;25(7):745–755.
14. Conraads VM, Van Craenenbroeck EM, De Maeyer C, et al. Unraveling new mechanisms of exercise intolerance in chronic heart failure. Role of exercise training. Heart Failure Reviews. 2013;18(11):65–77.
15. Carrai R, Scano G, Gigliotti F, et al. Prevalence of limb muscle dysfunction in patients with chronic obstructive pulmonary disease admitted to a pulmonary

rehabilitation centre. Clinical Neurophysiology. 2012;123(11):1547–1553.
16. Sahlberg ME, Svantesson U, Thomas EM, et al. Muscular strength and function in patients with cystic fibrosis. Chest. 2005;127(5):1587–1592.
17. Nishiyama O, Taniguchi H, Kondoh Y, et al. Quadriceps weakness is related to exercise capacity in idiopathic pulmonary fibrosis. Chest. 2005;127(6): 2028–2033.
18. Keteyian SJ, Pina IL, Hibner BA, et al. Clinical role of exercise training in the management of patients with chronic heart failure. Journal of Cardiopulmonary Rehabilitation and Prevention. 2010;30(2):67–76.
19. Cote CG, Pinto-Plata V, Kasprzyk K, et al. The 6-min walk distance, peak oxygen uptake, and mortality in COPD. Chest. 2007;132(6):1778–1785.
20. Horwich TB, Broderick S, Chen L, et al. Relation among body mass index, exercise training, and outcomes in chronic systolic heart failure. American Journal of Cardiology. 2011;108(12):1754–1759.
21. Lederer DJ, Arcasoy SM, Wilt JS, et al. Six-minute-walk distance predicts waiting list survival in idiopathic pulmonary fibrosis. American Journal of Respiratory and Critical Care Medicine. 2006;174(6):659–664.
22. Wensel R, Opitz CF, Anker SD, et al. Assessment of survival in patients with primary pulmonary hypertension: importance of cardiopulmonary exercise testing. Circulation. 2002;106(3):319–324.
23. Martinu T, Babyak MA, O'Connell CF, et al. Baseline 6-min walk distance predicts survival in lung transplant candidates. American Journal of Transplantation. 2008;8(7):1498–1505.
24. Ferreira A, Garvey C, Connors GL, et al. Pulmonary rehabilitation in interstitial lung disease: benefits and predictors of response. Chest. 2009;135(2):442–447.
25. Holland A, Hill C. Physical training for interstitial lung disease. Cochrane Database of Systematic Reviews (Online). 2008;(4):CD006322.
26. Puhan M, Scharplatz M, Troosters T, et al. Pulmonary rehabilitation following exacerbations of chronic obstructive pulmonary disease. UIN–Cochrane Database Systematic Reviews. 2011;(10):CD005305, PMID: 21975749.
27. Ries AL, Bauldoff GS, Carlin BW, et al. Pulmonary rehabilitation: joint ACCP/AACVPR evidence-based clinical practice guidelines. Chest. 2007;131(5 Suppl): 4S–42S.
28. Mereles D, Ehlken N, Kreuscher S, et al. Exercise and respiratory training improve exercise capacity and quality of life in patients with severe chronic pulmonary hypertension. Circulation. 2006;114(14):1482–1489.
29. Karapolat H, Yagdi T, Zoghi M, et al. Does pretransplantation etiology have any effect on exercise results in heart transplant patients? Transplantation Proceedings. 2010;42(5):1779–1783.
30. O'Connor CM, Whellan DJ, Lee KL, et al. Efficacy and safety of exercise training in patients with chronic heart failure: HF-ACTION randomized controlled trial. JAMA. 2009;301(14):1439–1450.
31. Rochester CL. Pulmonary rehabilitation for patients who undergo lung-volume-reduction surgery or lung transplantation. Respiratory Care. 2008;53(9): 1196–1202.
32. Downing J, Balady GJ. The role of exercise training in heart failure. Journal of the American College of Cardiology. 2011;58(6):561–569.
33. Flegal KM, Carroll MD, Ogden CL, et al. Prevalence and trends in obesity among US adults, 1999–2008. JAMA. 2010;303(3):235–241.
34. Lederer DJ, Kawut SM, Wickersham N, et al. Obesity and primary graft dysfunction after lung transplantation: the lung transplant outcomes group obesity study. American Journal of Respiratory and Critical Care Medicine. 2011;184(9): 1055–1061.
35. Gonzalez-Castro A, Llorca J, Suberviola B, et al. Influence of nutritional status in lung transplant recipients. Transplantation Proceedings. 2006;38(8): 2539–2540.
36. Kanasky WF Jr, Anton SD, Rodrigue JR, et al. Impact of body weight on long-term survival after lung transplantation. Chest. 2002;121(2):401–406.
37. Allen JG, Arnaoutakis GJ, Weiss ES, et al. The impact of recipient body mass index on survival after lung transplantation. Journal of Heart and Lung Transplantation. 2010;29(9):1026–1033.
38. Lederer DJ, Wilt JS, D'Ovidio F, et al. Obesity and underweight are associated with an increased risk of death after lung transplantation. American Journal of Respiratory and Critical Care Medicine. 2009;180(9):887–895.
39. Schwebel C, Pin I, Barnoud D, et al. Prevalence and consequences of nutritional depletion in lung transplant candidates. European Respiratory Journal. 2000; 16(6):1050–1055.
40. Snell GI, Bennetts K, Bartolo J, et al. Body mass index as a predictor of survival in adults with cystic fibrosis referred for lung transplantation. Journal of Heart and Lung Transplantation. 1998;17(11):1097–1103.
41. Pontiroli AE, Morabito A. Long-term prevention of mortality in morbid obesity through bariatric surgery. A systematic review and meta-analysis of trials performed with gastric banding and gastric bypass. Annals of Surgery. 2011; 253(3):484–487.
42. Clinical guidelines on the identification, evaluation, and treatment of overweight and obesity in adults–the evidence report. National Institutes of Health. Obesity Research. 1998;(6 Suppl 2):51S–209S.
43. Snow V, Barry P, Fitterman N, et al. Pharmacologic and surgical management of obesity in primary care: a clinical practice guideline from the American College of Physicians. Annals of Internal Medicine. 2005;142(7):525–531.
44. Martin MJ, Bennett S. Pretransplant bariatric surgery: a new indication? Surgery for Obesity and Related Diseases. 2007;3(6):648–651.
45. Takata MC, Campos GM, Ciovica R, et al. Laparoscopic bariatric surgery improves candidacy in morbidly obese patients awaiting transplantation. Surgery for Obesity and Related Diseases. 2008;4(2):159–164, discussion 64–65.
46. Bossenbroek L, den Ouden ME, de Greef MH, et al. Determinants of overweight and obesity in lung transplant recipients. Respiration; International Review of Thoracic Diseases. 2011;82(1):28–35.
47. Singer LG, Brazelton TR, Doyle RL, et al. Weight gain after lung transplantation. Journal of Heart and Lung Transplantation. 2003;22(8):894–902.
48. Weiss ES, Allen JG, Russell SD, et al. Impact of recipient body mass index on organ allocation and mortality in orthotopic heart transplantation. Journal of Heart and Lung Transplantation. 2009;28(11):1150–1157.
49. Sanchez-Lazaro IJ, Sanchez-Gomez JM, Almenar-Bonet L, et al. Long-term prognostic implications of metabolic syndrome in heart transplant recipients. Transplantation Proceedings. 2011;43(6):2257–2259.
50. Russo MJ, Hong KN, Davies RR, et al. The effect of body mass index on survival following heart transplantation: do outcomes support consensus guidelines? Annals of Surgery. 2010;251(1):144–152.
51. Clark AL, Chyu J, Horwich TB. The obesity paradox in men versus women with systolic heart failure. American Journal of Cardiology. 2012;110(1):77–82.
52. Clark AL, Fonarow GC, Horwich TB. Waist circumference, body mass index, and survival in systolic heart failure: the obesity paradox revisited. Journal of Cardiac Failure. 2011;17(5):374–380.
53. Amarelli C, Buonocore M, Romano G, et al. Nutritional issues in heart transplant candidates and recipients. Frontiers in Bioscience. 2012;4:662–668.
54. Guida B, Perrino NR, Laccetti R, et al. Role of dietary intervention and nutritional follow-up in heart transplant recipients. Clinical Transplantation. 2009;23(1): 101–107.
55. De Geest S, Dobbels F, Fluri C, et al. Adherence to the therapeutic regimen in heart, lung, and heart-lung transplant recipients. Journal of Cardiovascular Nursing. 2005;20(5 Suppl):S88–S98.
56. Bosma OH, Vermeulen KM, Verschuuren EA, et al. Adherence to immunosuppression in adult lung transplant recipients: prevalence and risk factors. Journal of Heart and Lung Transplantation. 2011;30(11):1275–1280.
57. Dew MA, Roth LH, Thompson ME, et al. Medical compliance and its predictors in the first year after heart transplantation. Journal of Heart and Lung Transplantation. 1996;15(6):631–645.
58. Matthees BJ, Anantachoti P, Kreitzer MJ, et al. Use of complementary therapies, adherence, and quality of life in lung transplant recipients. Heart and Lung: The Journal of Critical Care. 2001;30(4):258–268.
59. McAllister S, Buckner EB, White-Williams C. Medication adherence after heart transplantation: adolescents and their issues. Progress in Transplantation. 2006;16(4):317–323.
60. Teichman BJ, Burker EJ, Weiner M, et al. Factors associated with adherence to treatment regimens after lung transplantation. Progress in Transplantation. 2000;10(2):113–121.
61. Shapiro PA, Williams D, Gelman I, et al. Compliance complications in cardiac patients. American Journal of Psychiatry. 1997;154(11):1627–1628.
62. Craven JL, Bright J, Dear CL. Psychiatric, psychosocial, and rehabilitative aspects of lung transplantation. Clinics in Chest Medicine. 1990;11(2):247–257.
63. Dobbels F, Verleden G, Dupont L, et al. To transplant or not? The importance of psychosocial and behavioural factors before lung transplantation. Chronic Respiratory Disease. 2006;3(1):39–47.
64. Spaderna H, Smits JM, Rahmel AO, et al. Psychosocial and behavioural factors in heart transplant candidates–an overview. Transplant International: Official Journal of the European Society for Organ Transplantation. 2007;20(11): 909–920.
65. Germani G, Lazzaro S, Gnoato F, et al. Nonadherent behaviors after solid organ transplantation. Transplantation Proceedings. 2011;43(1):318–323.
66. Barbour KA, Blumenthal JA, Palmer SM. Psychosocial issues in the assessment and management of patients undergoing lung transplantation. Chest. 2006; 129(5):1367–1374.
67. De Bleser L, Matteson M, Dobbels F, et al. Interventions to improve medication-adherence after transplantation: a systematic review. Transplant International: Official Journal of the European Society for Organ Transplantation. 2009; 22(8):780–797.
68. O'Grady JG, Asderakis A, Bradley R, et al. Multidisciplinary insights into optimizing adherence after solid organ transplantation. Transplantation. 2010; 89(5):627–632.

69. Van Muylem A, Melot C, Antoine M, et al. Role of pulmonary function in the detection of allograft dysfunction after heart-lung transplantation. Thorax. 1997;52(7):643–647.
70. Mitchell RN. Graft vascular disease: immune response meets the vessel wall. Annual Review Pathology. 2009;4:19–47.
71. Gregory SA, Ferencik M, Achenbach S, et al. Comparison of sixty-four-slice multidetector computed tomographic coronary angiography to coronary angiography with intravascular ultrasound for the detection of transplant vasculopathy. American Journal of Cardiology. 2006;98(7):877–884.
72. Pichler P, Loewe C, Roedler S, et al. Detection of high-grade stenoses with multislice computed tomography in heart transplant patients. Journal of Heart and Lung Transplantation. 2008;27(3):310–316.
73. Dipchand AI, Bharat W, Manlhiot C, et al. A prospective study of dobutamine stress echocardiography for the assessment of cardiac allograft vasculopathy in pediatric heart transplant recipients. Pediatric Transplantation. 2008;12(5):570–576.
74. Kato T, Chan MC, Gao SZ, et al. Glucose intolerance, as reflected by hemoglobin A1c level, is associated with the incidence and severity of transplant coronary artery disease. Journal of the American College of Cardiology. 2004;43(6):1034–1041.
75. Eich D, Thompson JA, Ko DJ, et al. Hypercholesterolemia in long-term survivors of heart transplantation: an early marker of accelerated coronary artery disease. Journal of Heart and Lung Transplantation. 1991;10(1 Pt 1):45–49.
76. Kapadia SR, Nissen SE, Ziada KM, et al. Impact of lipid abnormalities in development and progression of transplant coronary disease: a serial intravascular ultrasound study. Journal of the American College of Cardiology. 2001;38(1):206–213.
77. Sanchez-Gomez JM, Martinez-Dolz L, Sanchez-Lazaro I, et al. Influence of metabolic syndrome on development of cardiac allograft vasculopathy in the transplanted heart. Transplantation. 2012;93(1):106–111.
78. Bogot NR, Durst R, Shaham D, et al. Cardiac CT of the transplanted heart: indications, technique, appearance, and complications. Radiographics. 2007;27(5):1297–1309.
79. Braga JR, Santos IS, McDonald M, et al. Factors associated with the development of cardiac allograft vasculopathy–a systematic review of observational studies. Clinical Transplantation. 2012;26(2):E111–E124.
80. Radovancevic B, Poindexter S, Birovljev S, et al. Risk factors for development of accelerated coronary artery disease in cardiac transplant recipients. European Journal of Cardio-Thoracic Surgery. 1990;4(6):309–312, discussion 13.
81. Schroeder JS, Gao SZ, Alderman EL, et al. A preliminary study of diltiazem in the prevention of coronary artery disease in heart-transplant recipients. New England Journal of Medicine. 1993;328(3):164–170.
82. Mehra MR, Ventura HO, Smart FW, et al. An intravascular ultrasound study of the influence of angiotensin-converting enzyme inhibitors and calcium entry blockers on the development of cardiac allograft vasculopathy. American Journal of Cardiology. 1995;75(12):853–854.
83. Wenke K, Meiser B, Thiery J, et al. Simvastatin reduces graft vessel disease and mortality after heart transplantation: a four-year randomized trial. Circulation. 1997;96(5):1398–1402.
84. Kobashigawa JA, Katznelson S, Laks H, et al. Effect of pravastatin on outcomes after cardiac transplantation. New England Journal of Medicine. 1995;333(10):621–627.
85. Kwak B, Mulhaupt F, Myit S, et al. Statins as a newly recognized type of immunomodulator. Nature Medicine. 2000;6(12):1399–1402.
86. Wang SS. Treatment and prophylaxis of cardiac allograft vasculopathy. Transplantation Proceedings. 2008;40(8):2609–2610.
87. Strategies for safe living following solid organ transplantation. American Journal of Transplantation. 2004;4(Suppl 10):156–159.
88. Sherman-Weber S, Axelrod P, Suh B, et al. Infective endocarditis following orthotopic heart transplantation: 10 cases and a review of the literature. Transplant Infectious Disease. 2004;6(4):165–170.
89. Wilson W, Taubert KA, Gewitz M, et al. Prevention of infective endocarditis: guidelines from the American Heart Association: a guideline from the American Heart Association Rheumatic Fever, Endocarditis and Kawasaki Disease Committee, Council on Cardiovascular Disease in the Young, and the Council on Clinical Cardiology, Council on Cardiovascular Surgery and Anesthesia, and the Quality of Care and Outcomes Research Interdisciplinary Working Group. Journal of the American Dental Association. 2007;138(6):739–745, 47–60.
90. Introduction to the guidelines. American Journal of Transplantation. 2004;4(Suppl 10):6–9.
91. Fishman JA. Infection in solid-organ transplant recipients. New England Journal of Medicine. 2007;357(25):2601–2614.
92. Lindenfeld J, Page RL 2nd, Zolty R, et al. Drug therapy in the heart transplant recipient: part III: common medical problems. Circulation. 2005;111(1):113–117.
93. Walker AH, Locke TJ, Braidley PC, et al. The importance of 24 hour ambulatory blood pressure monitoring after thoracic organ transplantation. Journal of Heart and Lung Transplantation. 2005;24(11):1770–1773.
94. Vandergheynst A, Van de Borne P, Melot C, et al. High prevalence of nocturnal arterial hypertension and non-dipping in lung transplant recipients. Acta Cardiologica. 2010;65(4):395–400.
95. Klinge A, Allen J, Murray A, et al. Increased pulse wave velocity and blood pressure in children who have undergone cardiac transplantation. Journal of Heart and Lung Transplantation. 2009;28(1):21–25.
96. Kaye D, Thompson J, Jennings G, et al. Cyclosporine therapy after cardiac transplantation causes hypertension and renal vasoconstriction without sympathetic activation. Circulation. 1993;88(3):1101–1109.
97. Porter GA, Bennett WM, Sheps SG. Cyclosporine-associated hypertension. National high blood pressure education program. Archives of Internal Medicine. 1990;150(2):280–283.
98. Dalla Pozza R, Kleinmann A, Bechtold S, et al. Hypertension in heart and heart-lung transplanted children: does impaired baroreceptor function play a role? Transplantation. 2006;81(1):71–75.
99. Braith RW, Mills RM Jr, Wilcox CS, et al. Breakdown of blood pressure and body fluid homeostasis in heart transplant recipients. Journal of the American College of Cardiology. 1996;27(2):375–383.
100. Fan Y, Xiao YB, Weng YG. Tacrolimus versus cyclosporine for adult lung transplant recipients: a meta-analysis. Transplantation Proceedings. 2009;41(5):1821–1824.
101. Chobanian AV, Bakris GL, Black HR, et al. Seventh report of the Joint National Committee on Prevention, Detection, Evaluation, and Treatment of High Blood Pressure. Hypertension. 2003;42(6):1206–1252.
102. Morath C, Schmied B, Mehrabi A, et al. Angiotensin-converting enzyme inhibitors and angiotensin II type 1 receptor blockers after renal transplantation. Clinical Transplantation. 2009;23(Suppl 21):33–36.
103. Stehlik J, Edwards LB, Kucheryavaya AY, et al. The Registry of the International Society for Heart and Lung Transplantation: twenty-eighth Adult Heart Transplant Report–2011. Journal of Heart and Lung Transplantation. 2011;30(10):1078–1094.
104. Hofer M, Schmid C, Benden C, et al. Diabetes mellitus and survival in cystic fibrosis patients after lung transplantation. Journal of Cystic Fibrosis. 2012;11(2):131–136.
105. Ye X, Kuo HT, Sampaio MS, et al. Risk factors for development of new-onset diabetes mellitus after transplant in adult lung transplant recipients. Clinical Transplantation. 2011;25(6):885–891.
106. Heit JJ, Apelqvist AA, Gu X, et al. Calcineurin/NFAT signalling regulates pancreatic beta-cell growth and function. Nature. 2006;443(7109):345–349.
107. Rostambeigi N, Lanza IR, Dzeja PP, et al. Unique cellular and mitochondrial defects mediate FK506-induced islet beta-cell dysfunction. Transplantation. 2011;91(6):615–623.
108. Bradbury RA, Shirkhedkar D, Glanville AR, et al. Prior diabetes mellitus is associated with increased morbidity in cystic fibrosis patients undergoing bilateral lung transplantation: an 'orphan' area? A retrospective case-control study. Internal Medicine Journal. 2009;39(6):384–388.
109. Hadjiliadis D, Madill J, Chaparro C, et al. Incidence and prevalence of diabetes mellitus in patients with cystic fibrosis undergoing lung transplantation before and after lung transplantation. Clinical Transplantation. 2005;19(6):773–778.
110. Prokai A, Fekete A, Pasti K, et al. The importance of different immunosuppressive regimens in the development of posttransplant diabetes mellitus. Pediatric Diabetes. 2012;13(1):81–91.
111. Grimm M, Rinaldi M, Yonan NA, et al. Superior prevention of acute rejection by tacrolimus vs. cyclosporine in heart transplant recipients–a large European trial. American Journal of Transplantation. 2006;6(6):1387–1397.
112. Wilkinson A, Davidson J, Dotta F, et al. Guidelines for the treatment and management of new-onset diabetes after transplantation. Clinical Transplantation. 2005;19(3):291–298.
113. Lane JT, Dagogo-Jack S. Approach to the patient with new-onset diabetes after transplant (NODAT). Journal of Clinical Endocrinology and Metabolism. 2011;96(11):3289–3297.
114. Zakliczynski M, Boguslawska J, Wojniak E, et al. In the era of the universal use of statins dyslipidemia's are still common in heart transplant recipients: a cross-sectional study. Transplantation Proceedings. 2011;43(8):3071–3073.
115. Hess ML, Hastillo A, Mohanakumar T, et al. Accelerated atherosclerosis in cardiac transplantation: role of cytotoxic B-cell antibodies and hyperlipidemia. Circulation. 1983;68(3 Pt 2):II94–II101.
116. Gao SZ, Schroeder JS, Alderman EL, et al. Clinical and laboratory correlates of accelerated coronary artery disease in the cardiac transplant patient. Circulation. 1987;76(5 Pt 2):V56–V61.

117. Third Report of the National Cholesterol Education Program (NCEP). Expert Panel on Detection, Evaluation, and Treatment of High Blood Cholesterol in Adults (Adult Treatment Panel III) final report. Circulation. 2002;106(25): 3143–3421.
118. Kasiske B, Cosio FG, Beto J, et al. Clinical practice guidelines for managing dyslipidemias in kidney transplant patients: a report from the Managing Dyslipidemias in Chronic Kidney Disease Work Group of the National Kidney Foundation Kidney Disease Outcomes Quality Initiative. American Journal of Transplantation. 2004;4(Suppl 7):13–53.
119. Moreso F, Calvo N, Pascual J, et al. Early statin use is an independent predictor of long-term graft survival. NDT Plus. 2010;3(Suppl 2):ii26–ii31.
120. Navaneethan SD, Perkovic V, Johnson DW, et al. HMG CoA reductase inhibitors (statins) for kidney transplant recipients. Cochrane Database of Systematic Reviews (Online). 2009;(2):CD005019.
121. Johnson BA, Iacono AT, Zeevi A, et al. Statin use is associated with improved function and survival of lung allografts. American Journal of Respiratory and Critical Care Medicine. 2003;167(9):1271–1278.
122. Niemczyk M, Paczek L. Ezetimibe in sirolimus-associated hyperlipidemia: to add or not to add to statins? Annals of Transplantation: Quarterly of the Polish Transplantation Society. 2011;16(3):132–134.
123. Yoon HE, Song JC, Hyoung BJ, et al. The efficacy and safety of ezetimibe and low-dose simvastatin as a primary treatment for dyslipidemia in renal transplant recipients. Korean Journal of Internal Medicine. 2009;24(3):233–237.
124. Broeders N, Knoop C, Antoine M, et al. Fibrate-induced increase in blood urea and creatinine: is gemfibrozil the only innocuous agent? Nephrology, Dialysis, Transplantation. 2000;15(12):1993–1999.
125. Celik S, Doesch A, Erbel C, et al. Beneficial effect of omega-3 fatty acids on sirolimus- or everolimus-induced hypertriglyceridemia in heart transplant recipients. Transplantation. 2008;86(2):245–250.
126. Tschopp O, Boehler A, Speich R, et al. Osteoporosis before lung transplantation: association with low body mass index, but not with underlying disease. American Journal of Transplantation. 2002;2(2):167–172.
127. Caplan-Shaw CE, Arcasoy SM, Shane E, et al. Osteoporosis in diffuse parenchymal lung disease. Chest. 2006;129(1):140–146.
128. Grey AB, Ames RW, Matthews RD, et al. Bone mineral density and body composition in adult patients with cystic fibrosis. Thorax. 1993;48(6):589–593.
129. Stephenson A, Jamal S, Dowdell T, et al. Prevalence of vertebral fractures in adults with cystic fibrosis and their relationship to bone mineral density. Chest. 2006;130(2):539–544.
130. Aris RM, Neuringer IP, Weiner MA, et al. Severe osteoporosis before and after lung transplantation. Chest. 1996;109(5):1176–1183.
131. Shane E, Mancini D, Aaronson K, et al. Bone mass, vitamin D deficiency, and hyperparathyroidism in congestive heart failure. American Journal of Medicine. 1997;103(3):197–207.
132. Shane E, Rivas M, McMahon DJ, et al. Bone loss and turnover after cardiac transplantation. Journal of Clinical Endocrinology and Metabolism. 1997; 82(5):1497–1506.
133. Sambrook PN, Kelly PJ, Fontana D, et al. Mechanisms of rapid bone loss following cardiac transplantation. Osteoporosis International. 1994;4(5):273–276.
134. Ferrari SL, Nicod LP, Hamacher J, et al. Osteoporosis in patients undergoing lung transplantation. European Respiratory Journal. 1996;9(11):2378–2382.
135. Shane E, Papadopoulos A, Staron RB, et al. Bone loss and fracture after lung transplantation. Transplantation. 1999;68(2):220–227.
136. Spira A, Gutierrez C, Chaparro C, et al. Osteoporosis and lung transplantation: a prospective study. Chest. 2000;117(2):476–481.
137. Dodd VA, Staron RB, Papadopoulos A, et al. Bone densitometry should be included in the evaluation of candidates for lung transplantation. Journal of Transplant Coordination. 1999;9(2):119–123.
138. Braith RW, Magyari PM, Fulton MN, et al. Resistance exercise training and alendronate reverse glucocorticoid-induced osteoporosis in heart transplant recipients. Journal of Heart and Lung Transplantation. 2003;22(10):1082–1090.
139. Braith RW, Magyari PM, Fulton MN, et al. Comparison of calcitonin versus calcitonin + resistance exercise as prophylaxis for osteoporosis in heart transplant recipients. Transplantation. 2006;81(8):1191–1195.
140. Braith RW, Mills RM, Welsch MA, et al. Resistance exercise training restores bone mineral density in heart transplant recipients. Journal of the American College of Cardiology. 1996;28(6):1471–1477.
141. Mitchell MJ, Baz MA, Fulton MN, et al. Resistance training prevents vertebral osteoporosis in lung transplant recipients. Transplantation. 2003;76(3):557–562.
142. Sambrook P, Henderson NK, Keogh A, et al. Effect of calcitriol on bone loss after cardiac or lung transplantation. Journal of Bone and Mineral Research. 2000;15(9):1818–1824.
143. Shane E, Addesso V, Namerow PB, et al. Alendronate versus calcitriol for the prevention of bone loss after cardiac transplantation. New England Journal of Medicine. 2004;350(8):767–776.
144. Cremer J, Struber M, Wagenbreth I, et al. Progression of steroid-associated osteoporosis after heart transplantation. Annals of Thoracic Surgery. 1999;67(1): 130–133.
145. Garcia-Delgado I, Prieto S, Gil-Fraguas L, et al. Calcitonin, etidronate, and calcidiol treatment in bone loss after cardiac transplantation. Calcified Tissue International. 1997;60(2):155–159.
146. Aris RM, Lester GE, Renner JB, et al. Efficacy of pamidronate for osteoporosis in patients with cystic fibrosis following lung transplantation. American Journal of Respiratory and Critical Care Medicine. 2000;162(3 Pt 1):941–946.
147. Henderson K, Eisman J, Keogh A, et al. Protective effect of short-term calcitriol or cyclical etidronate on bone loss after cardiac or lung transplantation. Journal of Bone and Mineral Research. 2001;16(3):565–571.
148. Trombetti A, Gerbase MW, Spiliopoulos A, et al. Bone mineral density in lung-transplant recipients before and after graft: prevention of lumbar spine post-transplantation-accelerated bone loss by pamidronate. Journal of Heart and Lung Transplantation. 2000;19(8):736–743.
149. Costanzo MR, Dipchand A, Starling R, et al. The International Society of Heart and Lung Transplantation Guidelines for the care of heart transplant recipients. Journal of Heart and Lung Transplantation. 2010;29(8):914–956.
150. Krieg MA, Seydoux C, Sandini L, et al. Intravenous pamidronate as treatment for osteoporosis after heart transplantation: a prospective study. Osteoporosis International. 2001;12(2):112–116.
151. Saag KG, Shane E, Boonen S, et al. Teriparatide or alendronate in glucocorticoid-induced osteoporosis. New England Journal of Medicine. 2007;357(20): 2028–2039.
152. Cejka D, Benesch T, Krestan C, et al. Effect of teriparatide on early bone loss after kidney transplantation. American Journal of Transplantation. 2008;8(9): 1864–1870.
153. Cupples S, Dew MA, Grady KL, et al. Report of the Psychosocial Outcomes Workgroup of the Nursing and Social Sciences Council of the International Society for Heart and Lung Transplantation: present status of research on psychosocial outcomes in cardiothoracic transplantation: review and recommendations for the field. Journal of Heart and Lung Transplantation. 2006;25(6): 716–725.
154. Favaro A, Gerosa G, Caforio AL, et al. Posttraumatic stress disorder and depression in heart transplantation recipients: the relationship with outcome and adherence to medical treatment. General Hospital Psychiatry. 2011;33(1):1–7.
155. Fusar-Poli P, Lazzaretti M, Ceruti M, et al. Depression after lung transplantation: causes and treatment. Lung. 2007;185(2):55–65.
156. Crone CC, Gabriel GM. Treatment of anxiety and depression in transplant patients: pharmacokinetic considerations. Clinical Pharmacokinetics. 2004; 43(6):361–394.
157. George CF. Perspectives on the management of insomnia in patients with chronic respiratory disorders. Sleep. 2000;23(Suppl 1):S31–S35, discussion S6–S8.
158. Christensen SB, Dall CH, Prescott E, et al. A high-intensity exercise program improves exercise capacity, self-perceived health, anxiety and depression in heart transplant recipients: a randomized, controlled trial. Journal of Heart and Lung Transplantation. 2012, 31(1):106–107.
159. Fusar-Poli P, Martinelli V, Klersy C, et al. Depression and quality of life in patients living 10 to 18 years beyond heart transplantation. Journal of Heart and Lung Transplantation. 2005;24(12):2269–2278.
160. De Vito Dabbs A, Dew MA, Stilley CS, et al. Psychosocial vulnerability, physical symptoms and physical impairment after lung and heart-lung transplantation. Journal of Heart and Lung Transplantation. 2003;22(11):1268–1275.
161. White-Williams C, Jalowiec A, Grady K. Who returns to work after heart transplantation? Journal of Heart and Lung Transplantation. 2005;24(12):2255–2261.
162. Paris W, White-Williams C. Social adaptation after cardiothoracic transplantation: a review of the literature. Journal of Cardiovascular Nursing. 2005;20(5 Suppl):S67–S73.
163. Petrucci L, Ricotti S, Michelini I, et al. Return to work after thoracic organ transplantation in a clinically-stable population. European Journal of Heart Failure. 2007;9(11):1112–1119.
164. Paris W, Diercks M, Bright J, et al. Return to work after lung transplantation. Journal of Heart and Lung Transplantation. 1998;17(4):430–436.
165. Cicutto L, Braidy C, Moloney S, et al. Factors affecting attainment of paid employment after lung transplantation. Journal of Heart and Lung Transplantation. 2004;23(4):481–486.
166. Meyer SR, Modry DL, Bainey K, et al. Declining need for permanent pacemaker insertion with the bicaval technique of orthotopic heart transplantation. Canadian Journal of Cardiology. 2005;21(2):159–163.
167. Alexander RT, Steenbergen C. Cause of death and sudden cardiac death after heart transplantation. An autopsy study. American Journal of Clinical Pathology. 2003;119(5):740–748.
168. McKay DB, Josephson MA, Armenti VT, et al. Reproduction and transplantation: report on the AST consensus conference on reproductive issues and transplanta-

tion. American Journal of Transplantation. 2005;5(7):1592–1599.
169. Coscia LA, Constantinescu S, Moritz MJ, et al. Report from the National Transplantation Pregnancy Registry (NTPR): outcomes of pregnancy after transplantation. Clinical Transplants. 2010:65–85.
170. Miniero R, Tardivo I, Centofanti P, et al. Pregnancy in heart transplant recipients. Journal of Heart and Lung Transplantation. 2004;23(7):898–901.
171. Wu DW, Wilt J, Restaino S. Pregnancy after thoracic organ transplantation. Seminars in Perinatology. 2007;31(6):354–362.
172. Gyi KM, Hodson ME, Yacoub MY. Pregnancy in cystic fibrosis lung transplant recipients: case series and review. Journal of Cystic Fibrosis. 2006;5(3):171–175.
173. Huang JQ, Shahine LK, Gupta N, et al. Controlled ovarian hyperstimulation and gestational surrogacy in a patient with lung transplant: a case report. Journal of Reproductive Medicine. 2010;55(11–12):509–510.
174. Douglas NC, Shah M, Sauer MV. Fertility and reproductive disorders in female solid organ transplant recipients. Seminars in Perinatology. 2007;31(6):332–338.
175. Wagoner LE, Taylor DO, Price GD Sr, et al. Paternity by cardiac transplant recipients. Transplantation. 1994;57(9):1337–1340.
176. Mulligan T, Sheehan H, Hanrahan J. Sexual function after heart transplantation. Journal of Heart and Lung Transplantation. 1991;10(1 Pt 1):125–128.
177. Phan A, Ishak WW, Shen BJ, et al. Persistent sexual dysfunction impairs quality of life after cardiac transplantation. Journal of Sexual Medicine. 2010;7(8):2765–2773.
178. Schofield RS, Edwards DG, Schuler BT, et al. Vascular effects of sildenafil in hypertensive cardiac transplant recipients. American Journal of Hypertension. 2003;16(10):874–877.
179. Huyghe E, Zairi A, Nohra J, et al. Gonadal impact of target of rapamycin inhibitors (sirolimus and everolimus) in male patients: an overview. Transplant International. 2007;20(4):305–311.
180. Benden C, Danziger-Isakov LA, Astor T, et al. Variability in immunization guidelines in children before and after lung transplantation. Pediatric Transplantation. 2007;11(8):882–887.
181. Recommended adult immunization schedule: United States, 2012. Annals of Internal Medicine. 2012;156(3):211–217.
182. Kumar D, Morris MI, Kotton CN, et al. Guidance on novel influenza A/H1N1 in solid organ transplant recipients. American Journal of Transplantation. 2010;10(1):18–25.
183. General recommendations on immunization–recommendations of the Advisory Committee on Immunization Practices (ACIP). MMWR Recommendations and Reports. 2011;60(2):1–64.
184. Gallo P, Agozzino L, Angelini A, et al. Causes of late failure after heart transplantation: a ten-year survey. Journal of Heart and Lung Transplantation. 1997;16(11):1113–1121.
185. Gutierrez-Dalmau A, Campistol JM. Immunosuppressive therapy and malignancy in organ transplant recipients: a systematic review. Drugs. 2007;67(8):1167–1198.
186. Penn I. Post-transplant malignancy: the role of immunosuppression. Drug Safety. 2000;23(2):101–113.
187. Engels EA, Pfeiffer RM, Fraumeni JF Jr, et al. Spectrum of cancer risk among US solid organ transplant recipients. JAMA. 2011;306(17):1891–1901.
188. Raviv Y, Shitrit D, Amital A, et al. Lung cancer in lung transplant recipients: experience of a tertiary hospital and literature review. Lung Cancer. 2011;74(2):280–283.
189. Bruschi G, Conforti S, Torre M, et al. Long-term results of lung cancer after heart transplantation: single center 20-year experience. Lung Cancer. 2009;63(1):146–150.
190. Bellil Y, Edelman MJ. Bronchogenic carcinoma in solid organ transplant recipients. Current Treatment Options in Oncology. 2006;7(1):77–81.
191. Anyanwu AC, Townsend ER, Banner NR, et al. Primary lung carcinoma after heart or lung transplantation: management and outcome. Journal of Thoracic & Cardiovascular Surgery. 2002;124(6):1190–1197.
192. Minai OA, Shah S, Mazzone P, et al. Bronchogenic carcinoma after lung transplantation: characteristics and outcomes. Journal of Thoracic Oncology. 2008;3(12):1404–1409.
193. Meyer KC, Francois ML, Thomas HK, et al. Colon cancer in lung transplant recipients with CF: increased risk and results of screening. Journal of Cystic Fibrosis. 2011;10(5):366–369.
194. Zwald FO, Brown M. Skin cancer in solid organ transplant recipients: advances in therapy and management: part I. Epidemiology of skin cancer in solid organ transplant recipients. Journal of the American Academy of Dermatology. 2011;65(2):253–261.
195. Preiksaitis JK. Epstein-Barr virus infection and malignancy in solid organ transplant recipients: strategies for prevention and treatment. Transplant Infectious Disease. 2001;3(2):56–59.
196. Kauffman HM, Cherikh WS, Cheng Y, et al. Maintenance immunosuppression with target-of-rapamycin inhibitors is associated with a reduced incidence of de novo malignancies. Transplantation. 2005;80(7):883–889.
197. Dasari TW, Pavlovic-Surjancev B, Dusek L, et al. Utility of screening computed tomography of chest, abdomen and pelvis in patients after heart transplantation. European Journal of Radiology. 2011;80(3):e381–e384.
198. American Cancer Society Guidelines for the early detection of cancer. 2012. Available from: http://www.cancer.org/Healthy/FindCancerEarly/CancerScreeningGuidelines/american-cancer-society-guidelines-for-the-early-detection-of-cancer.
199. Kasiske BL, Vazquez MA, Harmon WE, et al. Recommendations for the outpatient surveillance of renal transplant recipients. Journal of the American Society of Nephrology. 2000;11(Suppl 15):S1–S86.
200. Wu C, Shapiro R. Post-transplant malignancy: reducing the risk in kidney transplant recipients. Expert Opinion on Pharmacotherapy. 2011;12(11):1719–1729.
201. Ulrich C, Jurgensen JS, Degen A, et al. Prevention of non-melanoma skin cancer in organ transplant patients by regular use of a sunscreen: a 24 months, prospective, case-control study. British Journal of Dermatology. 2009;161(Suppl 3):78–84.
202. Reichrath J, Nurnberg B. Solar UV-radiation, vitamin D and skin cancer surveillance in organ transplant recipients (OTRs). Advances in Experimental Medicine and Biology. 2008;624:203–214.
203. Uber PA, Ross HJ, Zuckermann AO, et al. Generic drug immunosuppression in thoracic transplantation: an ISHLT educational advisory. Journal of Heart and Lung Transplantation. 2009;28(7):655–660.
204. Kubiak DW, Koo S, Hammond SP, et al. Safety of posaconazole and sirolimus coadministration in allogeneic hematopoietic stem-cell transplants. Biology of Blood and Marrow Transplantation. 2012;18(9):1462–1465.
205. Marty FM, Lowry CM, Cutler CS, et al. Voriconazole and sirolimus coadministration after allogeneic hematopoietic stem cell transplantation. Biology of Blood and Marrow Transplantation. 2006;12(5):552–559.
206. Gossmann J, Kachel HG, Schoeppe W, et al. Anemia in renal transplant recipients caused by concomitant therapy with azathioprine and angiotensin-converting enzyme inhibitors. Transplantation. 1993;56(3):585–589.
207. Kuriyama R, Kogure H, Itoh S, et al. Angiotensin converting enzyme inhibitor induced anemia in a kidney transplant recipient. Transplantation Proceedings. 1996;28(3):1635.

第 36 章 同种抗体、致敏性和虚拟交叉配型

Howard M. Gebel, Robert A. Bray

引言

在 1969 年,Patel 和 Terasaki 报道称, 移植前受体血清和供体淋巴细胞之间的阳性交叉反应与超急性肾脏同种异体移植排斥的高风险相关(见第 3 章)[1]。随后指出, 当阳性交叉匹配是由于预先存在针对供体 HLA 抗原的抗体时,特别是当这些抗体联合补体时,排斥风险最强。移植前存在的针对供体 HLA 的抗体和同种异体移植物排斥之间的关联较为紧密, 以致于 Patel 和 Terasaki 默认,在移植前不进行交叉匹配的情况下给患者移植是不正当行为。这种情况意味着支持移植程序的组织相容性实验室需要全天候运行, 以随时执行预期的淋巴细胞交叉匹配。该模式不复杂:能够容易地避免具有表达一种或多种相应 HLA 抗原的供体器官和具有相应 HLA 抗体(即致敏受体)的患者匹配移植。早期研究[2,3]表明,通过对患者血清的详细预筛选来鉴定 HLA 抗体, 可以预测在进行物理交叉匹配之前要避免的 HLA 抗原。今天被称为虚拟交叉匹配(vXM),这一概念的出现在当时是完全合理的,但其实用性受到当时技术局限性的严重阻碍。此外,认为所有的阳性反应都是临床相关的 HLA 抗体的结果,并且所有的阴性反应都能确保长期的移植物存活的设想都不是正确的。在某种程度上,这是因为用于鉴定 HLA 抗体和进行交叉匹配的早期测定既不充分, 也不足以识别所有相关的 HLA 抗体[4]。因此,虽然避免针对供体 HLA 的抗体在概念上是吸引人的, 但是目前的方法还达不到预期目标。除了这些严重的问题之外,用于分配 HLA 抗原的血清学 HLA 分型测定常常是主观和不完善的,这意味着 HLA 抗原并不总是被正确或完全识别。

近年来,随着使用纯化的 HLA 抗原(Ⅰ类或Ⅱ类)的固相测试平台技术的发展, 允许以前所未有的特异性和灵敏度来对 HLA 抗体进行鉴定[5,6]。类似地,分子分型方法的实现使得精细分辨 HLA 抗原和单个等位基因的表征/定义[7,8]成为现实。总而言之,这些发展使得目前可以客观地鉴定由潜在的器官供体表达的 HLA 抗原以及精确评估敏感受体血清中存在的 HLA 抗体。虚拟交叉匹配的概念已经准备好从理论转向实践。本章将总结现代移植组织相容性检测中使用的基本测定方法的发展及其在临床上合理应用的原则。本章还补充了第 6 章抗体介导的排斥的基本机制, 第 4 章组织相容性分子的结构和功能,第 89 章详细介绍了抗体检测作为术后生物标志物的用途的内容。

测定

血清抗体检测

最初,前瞻性地使用补体依赖性细胞毒性(CDC)测定法来确定等待移植的患者是否对 HLA 抗原敏感[9-12]。简而言之, 来自至少 30 个供体的 HLA 型细胞与患者血清和补体一起孵育。解释靶细胞死亡意味着小组成员表达至少一种患者血清相应抗体的 HLA 抗原。这个测试蕴含着双重的逻辑。首先,它向患者提供了有价值的信息,即他/她与随机供体相互兼容(因此可移植)的可能性。第二,可以定义 HLA 特异性,然后可以将其用于预测与特定供体的相容性。在其最简单的形式中,与患者血清反应的受测群体细胞的百分比被认为对应于他/她的致敏程度。例如,如果 30 个受测群体细胞中的 10 个与来自患者的血清反应, 则该患者被认为具有

33%的群体反应性抗体(PRA)活性。然后,该患者将被告知他/她将与每3名随机捐赠者中的2名交叉匹配。然而,这种解释的有效性取决于受试细胞组中HLA抗原的频率是否反映了供体群体中抗原的频率。最初,使用随机选择的健康志愿者供体或基于其HLA表型在移植中心组装细胞组。随后,冷冻细胞板从几个供应商处商购获得。不幸的是,缺乏选择捐助者作为小组成员的标准方法。因此,小组成员的HLA表型组成不一定反映了死亡供体群体中HLA抗原的频率。因此,如果上述血清样品含有针对HLA-A*01的抗体, 并且在3种不同的细胞板上进行测试,其中没有、一半或全部靶细胞表达HLA-A*01,则PRA将分别被正确解释为0、50%和100%。哪些结果最准确地反映HLA-A*01在成为器官捐赠者的个体中的分布?实际上,美国供体人群HLA-A*01的频率为23%[13], 这意味着上述实例中的PRA值都不正确。

使用由随机HLA表型组成的受测细胞群体产生的PRA值的另一个意义重大的疑问是当所有抗体都未被鉴定时其对死亡供体肾脏分配的影响。众所周知,与非致敏性患者相比,高度致敏性患者(目前定义为PRA≥80%的患者)更难以寻找到可相容的供体[14]。在美国,根据积分制决定肾移植的顺序。患者累积的分数越多,他们在由联合国器官分享网络(UNOS)管理的等待名单上排名越靠前[15]。当患者的分数足够将他/她列入等待名单的顶部时,他/她将有机会与血型相容的捐助者进行交叉匹配。积分的高低决定着受者与预期供体HLA-DR的匹配程度 (两个HLA-DRB1*匹配得2分,一个HLA-DRB1*匹配得1分)和等待时间(每等待1年得1分)。为了减少高度致敏性和非致敏性患者之间的移植差异,UNOS向高度致敏性(PRA≥80%)患者提供了4个附加分。目前有近10万名患者正在等待死亡供体肾脏[16],积分制被认为是死亡供体肾脏分配的公平方法。高度致敏性患者在等待时间方面也累积了一定分值(毕竟难以匹配),并且还有4个PRA额外加分:这类患者常常位列榜首。但是,在列表的顶部并不能保证患者能够尽快进行移植。患者仍然必须与他/她的捐助者交叉匹配。历史上,原始交叉匹配是作为分诊分步进行的, 过滤掉具有阳性交叉匹配的患者,并允许阴性交叉匹配的患者移动到下一个(或"最终")阶段,也就是来自患者与来自预期供体的细胞进行交叉匹配。这种所谓的"最终交叉匹配"必须是兼容的(即,阴性的),才能让患者进行移植。

直到最近, 与高度致敏性患者的血清交叉匹配常常是阳性的[17]。至少部分原因是使用HLA型细胞板不能完全分配不可接受的抗原[18]。例如,在表36.1中,与患者血清反应的所有细胞都表达HLA-A*02抗原,而没有任何非反应性细胞表达HLA-A*02。该反应模式表明患者具有针对HLA-A*02抗原的单一HLA抗体。因此,只有HLA-A*02被认为是患者不可接受的抗原。具有所有其他HLA抗原的供体将被认为与患者暂时相容(即vXM阴性)。然而,仔细检查表36.1发现,表达HLA-B*44的所有细胞也表达HLA-A*02。如果患者还具有HLA-B*44的抗体, 则其检测将被HLA-A*02抗体掩蔽。在这个例子中,如果HLA-A*02被认为是唯一不可接受的HLA抗原, 则表达HLA-B*44 (但不是HLA-A*02)的供体将被认为是可接受的;不过,意想不

表36.1 这两个表格代表了一个HLA类型(仅限Ⅰ类)的细胞板。在此示例中,有24种类型的板成员正在使用患者血清进行测试。这24个细胞中有12个细胞(深色阴影)与患者血清反应,对应的群体反应性抗体(PRA)活性为50%。所有12个细胞均表达HLA-A2,这意味着抗体特异性针对该抗原。但是请注意,有4个HLA-A2阳性细胞也表达HLA-B44。由于HLA-B44只伴随HLA-A2表达,因此有可能存在针对HLA-B44的第二抗体

A		B		C	
2	11	35	75	8	7
2	23	53	81	4	6
2	24	7	44	5	8
2	24	35	37	4	6
2	24	44	35	4	6
2	24	35	50	2	6
2	26	39	46	1	7
2	29	44	62	4	5
2	29	7	44	2	9
2	30	45	56	1	7
2	31	35	47	4	6
2	32	27	63	2	5

A		B		C	
1	3	35	63	4	7
1	11	37	52	4	6
1	25	35	52	5	7
1	26	27	57	2	6
1	26	38	73	2	8
1	32	42	50	5	6
1	33	8	62	7	10
1	34	35	57	6	7
1	66	50	58	4	7
1	74	8	72	2	7
1	11	13	55	1	7
1	11	13	46	1	6

到的是，最后的交叉匹配是阳性的。除了由于掩蔽抗体而导致的不完全鉴定之外，细胞组不能够确定广泛致敏(即≥80%PRA)患者中整个抗体谱系的理想测试目标。因此，他们的血清通常与任何与血型相容的供体交叉匹配。如果交叉匹配是阳性的，那么供体被认为与该患者不相容。更为复杂的是进行交叉匹配的敏感性[19]。当首次实施时，使用补体依赖性细胞毒性(CDC)测定进行交叉匹配的目的是鉴定与临床结果相关的抗体。然而，很快发现，没有 CDC-可检测抗体的患者仍然经历早期抗体介导的移植物排斥/移植物损失。这促使了对测定的修改，包括延长的孵育、额外的洗涤和用抗人球蛋白(AHG)试剂的增强[10]，后者最终成为多年的实验室金标准(表 36.1)。然而，即使使用这种增强技术来鉴定抗体，仍然有一组患者经历由于供体导向的抗体而引起的早期排斥反应或移植物丢失。此外，细胞毒性测试通常仅鉴定Ⅰ类 HLA 抗体。随着器官移植领域的成熟，显而易见的是，在移植前，还要确定患者是否具有针对Ⅱ类特异性的抗体(例如 HLA-DR、HLA-DQ)[20]。

流式细胞术交叉配型(FCXM)的发展和运用为移植界提供了一种极为灵敏的新测定法，该方法可以同时评估 T 淋巴细胞和 B 淋巴细胞，这意味着目前可以使用一种测定法来观察靶细胞(B 细胞)表达Ⅱ类组织相容性抗原。当时，公开的数据表明Ⅱ类 HLA 抗体的临床意义很小，只要 T 细胞交叉配型为阴性，大多数移植中心就开始进行移植。但是，这些早期研究的可靠性值得怀疑，因为它们通常仅仅基于必须与 T 细胞物理分离的少量 B 细胞。此外，未能识别出 B 细胞像 T 细胞一样表达的Ⅰ类抗原。多项研究表明，针对供体Ⅰ类抗原的低滴度抗体导致的 T 细胞阴性、B 细胞阳性交叉配型与早期移植物丢失有关（移植物 1 年存活率为 50%~67%；综述于[19]）。

FCXM 的另一个特点是，它能识别供者体内未与补体结合的抗体。这种抗体对临床的影响，尽管值得怀疑，但其真正的意义可能并不像人们预测那样。尽管仅通过流式细胞术检测到的抗体确实与排斥反应和移植物丢失的增加有关[21-23]。然而，其他研究指出与细胞毒性交叉配型相比，FCXM 并没有带来更多益处[24]。尽管明显矛盾，但对这些差异的一种解释是某些阳性 FCXM 不是由于 HLA 抗体引起的。自身抗体、免疫复合物的非特异性结合(常见于自身免疫性疾病，如系统性红斑狼疮）和/或 IgG 分子与淋巴细胞上表达的 Fc 受体的 Fc 结合可能导致明显的假阳性交叉配型[25,26]。B 细胞特别容易受到这些非特异性结合问题的影响。一项研究提出，高达 75%的 B 细胞阳性交叉配型反应是由于非 HLA 抗体引起的，因此与临床无关[27]。但是，该研究还表明，当阳性 B 细胞交叉配型反应归因于 HLA 抗体(特别是Ⅱ类抗体)时，移植物存活率显著降低。这项研究强调了使用 B 细胞作为靶标的隐患，以及当 B 细胞交叉配型意外呈阳性时需要考虑其他解释的必要。

注意点

在 20 世纪 90 年代初，分子生物学的进展(特别是聚合酶链式反应的发展)使得能够进行基于 DNA 的 HLA 抗原测试。到 20 世纪 90 年代中期，引入多重微粒技术和基于细胞计数的仪器可以对 HLA 抗体进行详细的评估，并准确测定个体的 HLA 类型。目前，基于多重荧光的固相测定技术是临床 HLA 实验室中最常用的平台。该技术有能力同时区分和分析多达 100 个独特的涂层微粒[4,28](可参阅后续相关章节)。通过记录患者血清是否具有供体反应性 HLA 抗体，现在可以更可靠地解释淋巴细胞交叉配型(阳性或阴性)。事实上，使用固相数据，可以将阳性淋巴细胞交叉匹配分为临床

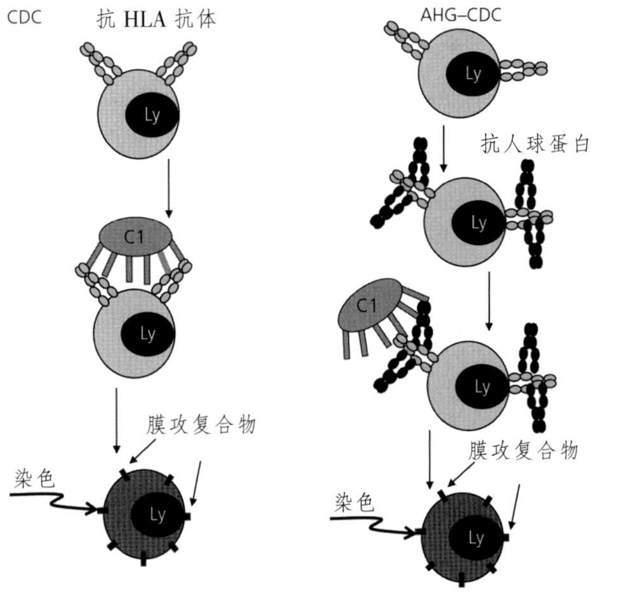

图 36.1　补体依赖性和抗人球蛋白增强的补体依赖性细胞毒性试验检测 HLA 抗体。将供体淋巴细胞与患者血清和补体(CDC 测定)或患者血清、抗人球蛋白和补体(AHG-CDC)一起孵育。抗体本身或用 AHG 增强激活补体，最终可通过摄取重要染料来检测淋巴细胞膜的损伤。Ly，淋巴细胞；CDC，补体依赖性细胞毒性试验。

无关性与相关性，如果相关，阳性交叉匹配可被解释为排斥反应的危险因素或肾移植的明确禁忌证[19]。因此，与 20 世纪 80 年代早期作为免疫抑制剂的钙调神经磷酸酶抑制剂引入移植医学的方式类似，多重微粒技术彻底改变了临床组织相容性检测。

固相测试的变革

由于 T 淋巴细胞和 B 淋巴细胞除了 HLA 之外还表达许多膜蛋白，因此使用膜依赖性测定法特异性分配 HLA 抗体十分困难。使用不含其他所有细胞膜组分的纯化 HLA 蛋白的固相测定方法的研发有助于使抗体识别更可控。固相测试的第一步是使用从血小板分离的亲和纯化 HLA Ⅰ类抗原作为靶抗原的酶联免疫吸附测定(ELISA)来检测患者血清中的 HLA Ⅰ类抗体[29]。虽然这种方法将 HLA 与非 HLA 抗体区分开，但是阳性血清的特异性不易识别。虽然 ELISA 是膜依赖性测定的改进，但它们是复杂的，其敏感性低于基于流式细胞术的方法。此外，即使在实施 ELISA 以鉴定Ⅱ类 HLA 抗原的抗体后，也需要进行单独的检测来区分Ⅰ类与Ⅱ类抗体。

HLA 抗体测试的下一个突破是 Pei 等描述的一种方法，其中将从 EB 病毒(EBV)转化的细胞系中分离的纯化的 HLA Ⅰ类和Ⅱ类蛋白连接到微粒上并通过流式细胞术进行分析[5]。与 ELISA 相反，FlowPRA® 允许在标准流式细胞仪上同时鉴定 HLA Ⅰ类和Ⅱ类抗原的抗体。抗体固相分析的其他优点包括数据的客观和半定量分析，无需活的靶细胞，以及持续一致且可再生的 HLA 抗原包被的微粒。自从成立以来，基于微粒的测定方法已经经历了若干种不同的配置。FlowPRA®是确定 HLA 抗体是否存在的简单、直接的检测方法。简而言之，它包含了 60 个单独的微粒，30 个包被有Ⅰ类抗原，另外 30 个包被有Ⅱ类抗原(图 36.2A)。混合物中的每单个微粒用来自单个 EBV 转化的细胞系的不同Ⅰ类(A、B、C)或Ⅱ类(DR、DQ、DP)表型包被。基于两个参数，尺寸和荧光，可以从Ⅱ类包被的微粒中鉴别出Ⅰ类包被颗粒。与Ⅱ类包被微粒相比，Ⅰ类表型包被微粒

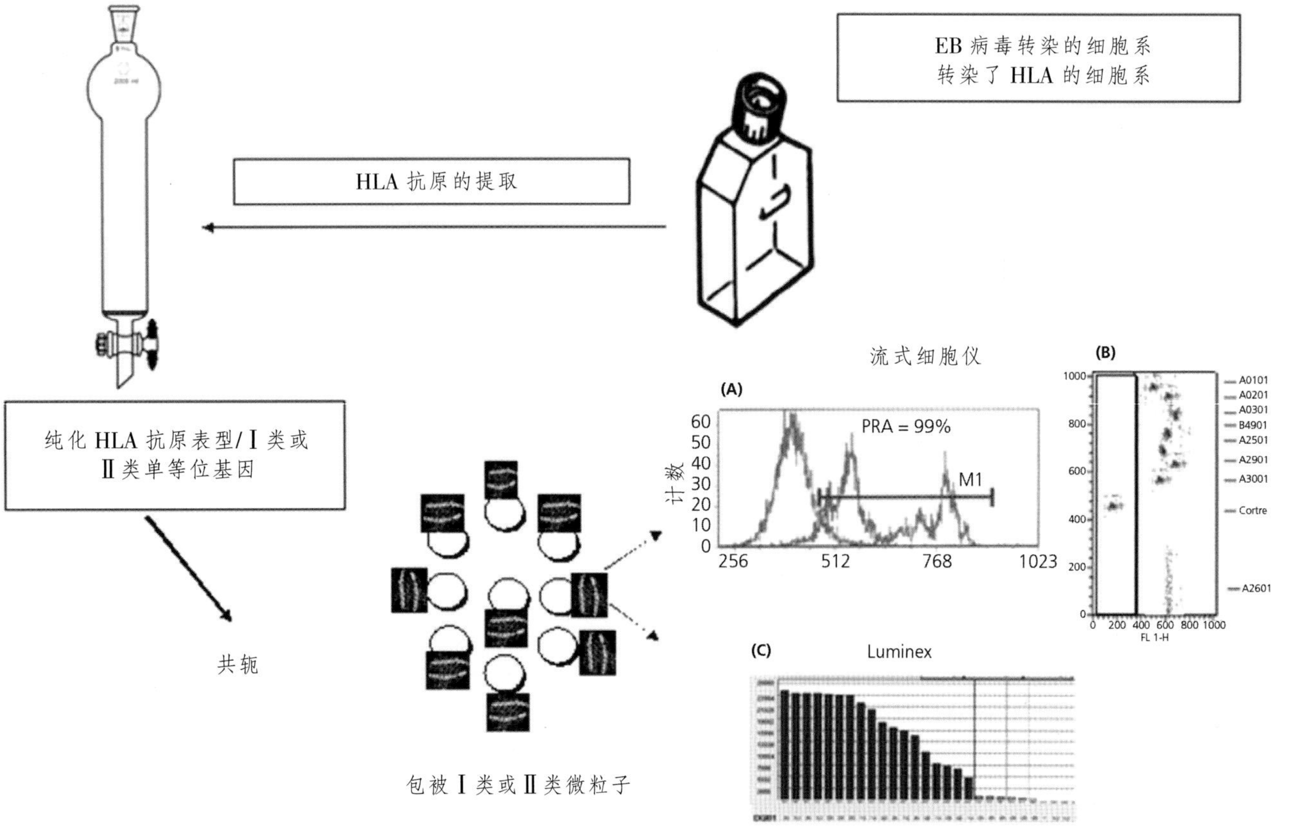

图 36.2 从细胞系中提取和纯化 HLA Ⅰ类和Ⅱ类抗原(整个表型或单个等位基因簇)并包被在微粒上。将单个微粒(n=30)组合以产生在流式细胞仪上可分析的 HLA 抗原筛选池(A)。根据磁珠反应性百分比计算群体反应性抗体(PRA)的百分比。或者，通过流式细胞仪(B)或 Luminex(C)测定个体微粒以评估抗体特异性。磁珠反应性百分比允许计算 PRA 的百分比。

更大且无荧光，而Ⅱ类表型包被微粒体积较小并且内部呈现红色荧光染料染色。当与背景对照相比,用荧光的抗人 IgG 染色时显示出增强的荧光磁珠被认为是阳性的。阳性反应强度由微粒的数量和荧光强度决定。由于单个Ⅰ类或Ⅱ类微粒代表事件总数的 30%(约 3%)，每个阳性反应必须表现出明显高于阴性对照的荧光峰,并且要考虑至少还有总数 3%的门控事件。

尽管 FlowPRA®识别 HLA 抗体与基于细胞的测定方法和 ELISA 相比更为敏感和特异，但是该测定方法不能确定所针对的 HLA 特异性,基于此原因开展了另一项测试,即基于流式的特异性检测。在该测定中,从 EBV 细胞系分离的 HLA 表型簇(Ⅰ类或Ⅱ类)如同对 FlowPRA®筛选试验所述一样连接到个体化的珠群上。然而，每个单独的微粒在内部用特定量的红色荧光染料进行染色。可以在单个荧光轴上单独识别多达 11 个不同的磁珠,并使用这样一组靶标,可以评估单个抗体特异性(图 36.2B)[6]。

虽然 FlowPRA®为识别 HLA 抗体特异性开辟出一条道路,但目前仍有两个绊脚石：

1. HLA 受体复合物的广泛多态性阻碍了目标阵列的设计；

2.一次只可以测试 11 个磁珠(这降低了技术效率)。

另一种基于流式细胞术的仪器(Luminex)的出现在鉴定 HLA 抗体上是一种改进,因为该方法允许同时评估多达 100 个单个微粒(所谓的多重测定)[28]。每个微粒具有独特的荧光标记序列，其通过在微粒上掺入具有不同量的两个荧光标签而得到。对于每个荧光标签,有 10 个不同的色度,意味着可以建立一个 10×10 的矩阵,从而产生一组 100 个唯一可识别的微粒。荧光的读取或“报告”分子是可以在基质中的每个磁珠上测量到的不同的颜色而定。然后,每个微粒与另一个不同的 HLA 抗原或核苷酸序列缀合,允许阳性免疫测定结果与独特的 HLA 特异性自动相关(图 36.2C)。在理论上,这种测定体系可以包含第三和第四组染料,那么同时检测 1000 或 10 000 个分析物将成为可能。增加测试分析物数量的另一种方法是使用一组与原始组大小不同的微粒。可以同时分析的分析物越多,测试的效率就越高。

等待移植的患者中有相当一部分具有这样广泛活性的 HLA 抗体,这些抗体与所有 HLA 抗原包被的微粒的反应都是阳性的[30]。然而,实际上患者身上并不存在这种 100%的 PRA,而是具有多种抗体,且只与几种常见的 HLA 发生特异性反应[31,32]。随着重组技术的应用,单个 HLA 蛋白可以纯化并附着于微粒。然后使用这些所谓的单抗原珠面板来清楚地描绘抗体反应性。

在新技术的应用使抗体检测和鉴定方法改进的同时对 HLA 抗原分型的水平也在不断提高。在过去 20 年中,HLA 抗原的分型从血清学转变为基于分子的分型方法,可以仅靠单个氨基酸的不同而检测出两种不同抗原(例如 HLA-B*44:02 对 HLA-B*44:03)[33]。虽然血清学分型鉴别了有限数量的 HLA 特异性,但基于分子的方法可以识别所有 HLA 等位基因。只要知道包被在微粒上的独特的等位基因，很快就能发现患者具有产生等位基因特异性抗体的能力，即与抗原家族的某个等位基因反应的抗体。实际上,等位基因抗体并不罕见,这一认识开始强调了在等位基因而不是抗原水平上对供体分型的可能性,至少对于那些可供选择等位基因的频率足够高并且已鉴定出等位基因抗体的那些抗原。显然，如果捐献者没有进行全面的分子分型,则 vXM 是不可能的。显然血清学 HLA 分型的时代已经过去了。而第 3 章综述了基于分子的 HLA 分型技术[34]。

虚拟交叉匹配的临床应用

虽然虚拟交叉匹配的概念已经有近 30 年历史[2],但在 2006 年之前,这项程序在临床上并没有得到合理的应用。随后,使用固相抗体测定来确定 HLAⅠ类和Ⅱ类抗体体现出准确性和敏感性,埃默里大学和杜克大学发表了他们使用虚拟交叉匹配的成功经验,以预测接受死亡供体肾脏和肺移植的高度致敏性患者之间的相容性[35,36]。随后,一项国家研究测试了虚拟交配的能力，预测了 UNOS 候选人高度致敏性患者的阳性交叉匹配,并报告了超过 90%的预测值[37]。然而,在这项研究中,预测阴性交叉配型反应的能力欠佳(约 50%)。随后的研究表明，至少部分无法预测阴性交叉匹配是因为关于这些高度致敏性患者所具有的所有抗体的信息不完全,特别是针对 HLA-C、HLA-DQ 和 HLA-DP 抗原的抗体[38]。尽管这些抗体可能已经被鉴定,但是它们不是常规地被列为不可接受的，部分原因是因为 UNOS 只要求对死亡供体器官进行 HLA-A、HLA-B 和 HLA-DRB1 位点的抗原测试和报告,暗示其他 HLA 位点的抗体在临床上是不相关的。这不再是 UNOS 的工作模式。目前已经发表了几项研究，证明当具有相应抗原的器官移植于那些相应抗体的患者时，HLA-C、HLA-DQB1 和 HLA-DPB1 的抗体与排斥反应和移植物丢失发生相关[39-42]。2011 年 6 月，UNOS 要求为 HLA-A、HLA-B、HLA-C、HLA-DRB1 和 HLA-DQB1 位点报告 HLA 分子分型数据。目前，HLA-DPB1 或 HLA-DQα 抗原不需要强制分型，即使潜在受体群体中这些抗体的频率正在上升。如果这些位点的分型最终成为强制性的，也并不奇怪。

自从这些早期报告以来，vXM 已经被广泛接受，不仅对于死亡捐助者[43,44]，而且对于活着的捐助者也是如此，特别是那些参与配对的捐献者[45]。对于胸部器官移植，vXM 减少了候诊者的死亡人数，允许器官从 500 英里(1 英里≈1.61km)外的中心引进，这在以前是不可能的，因为没有足够的时间进行预期的物理交叉匹配[46]。vXM 已经有效地消除了在美国几乎所有实验室中对昂贵和耗时的初步交叉配型程序。在欧洲，Claas 等通过可接受的不匹配的国际方案，大大增加了移植到高度致敏性患者身上的死亡供体肾脏数量[47]。英国还将全国范围的广泛致敏性患者优先考虑用于基于 vXM 的移植[48]。2014 年底，UNOS 将实施一项分配计划，旨在扩大对高度致敏性患者接受移植的指征。具体来说，对于 98%、99%和 100%的 cPRA 患者，将分别以地方、区域和国家为单位强制性地分配器官。

使用固相 HLA 抗体检测测定法可以将患者至少分为 3 类：

1.无 HLA 抗体；

2.具有无供体特异性的 HLA 抗体；

3.具有供体特异性的 HLA 抗体(DSA)。

预计第一类患者交叉匹配的结果为阴性。事实上，如果这类患者的物理交叉匹配是阳性的，那么通常不被认为是移植的禁忌证。第二类患者也是 vXM 阴性。当移植时，这些患者由抗体介导的排斥反应/移植物丢失的风险很低，并且具有令人满意的长期移植物存活率[35,49-51]。对于第三类患者，vXM 将为阳性。重要的是要认识到，对于具有抗体的患者，相同的抗体对于一些供体可能不具有 DSA，而 vXM 将为阴性，但对于其他供体，可能存在一种或多种供体特异诱导抗体，并且 vXM 将是阳性(图 36.3)。最近的数据表明，DSA 患者的物理交叉匹配并不总是阳性的[52-54]，这种现象产生一个疑问，在进行移植时决定因素应该是什么：DSA 还是阳性交叉匹配？

模式转变

如上所述，HLA 型体系(细胞或微粒)的组成可以容易地影响致敏性患者是否达到额外 4 分的 80%阈值。直到最近，对于报告的 PRA≥80%的患者，即使仅鉴定出一种不可接受的抗原[55]，也获得了 4 分。这种方

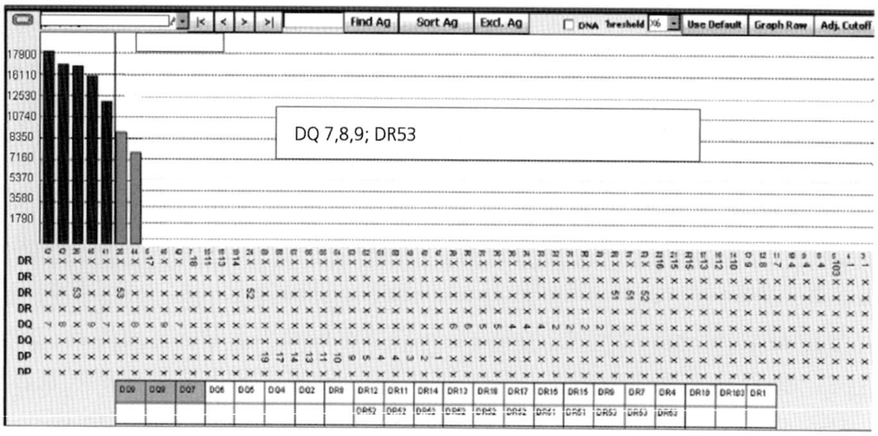

潜在的供体：
DRB1*04, DRB1*07; DRB4*PRESENT, -;
DQB1*02, DQB*03:02 (8)

潜在的供体：
DRB1*15, DRB1*16; DRB5*PRESENT, -;
DQB1*05, DQB1*06

图 36.3 直方图中的血清具有 HLA-DQB1*03:01、03:02 和 03:03(DQ7、DQ8 和 DQ9)以及 DRB4*(DR53)的抗体。对应于这些抗体的抗原将被列为“不可接受的”抗原。左侧的供体将被认为是不可接受的，因为抗体将被认为是供体特异性抗体(DSA)，并且虚拟交叉匹配是阳性的。相比之下，对于右侧的供体，存在相同的抗体，但它们不是 DSA，与这个供体的虚拟交叉是阴性的。

法不是特别有效，因为已经等待多时的广泛致敏性患者接受了 4 分额外加分后常规地出现在每个血型相容供体的每次匹配运行的前列。在这些广泛致敏性的患者中，阳性的最终交叉匹配是常见的[17]，并且正在以远低于其等待移植率的比例被移植。对这个现象的认识促使了国家器官分配体系的一些变化。2009 年 10 月，UNOS 实施了一项新政策，规定当且仅当患者的不可接受的 HLA 抗原百分比≥80%时，才能获得 4 个额外加分。对 HLA 抗原频率的评估是根据 UNOS 数据库中>12 000 名 HLA 型死亡供体确定的。根据这些新规则，PRA 是可以被计算的，而不是被分配的。获得 4 个额外加分的患者不会被视为表达一种或多种被列为不可接受的 HLA 抗原的捐献者的接受者。新的 cPRA 政策旨在确定报告患者致敏性时的问责制和统一性，并通过消除不兼容的供肾来提高肾脏分配的效率，从而减少已达到等待名单的前列患者的阳性的交叉配型反应的数量。实际上，由 cPRA 确定的列表前列的高度致敏性患者将更有可能与其供体相容[17]。简单来说，排名前列的患者之间的阳性交叉数量预计将大幅度减少。这种政策变化从根本上改变了肾脏移植候选人在等待列表上的排序方式。随后对国家数据的审查表明，在新的 cPRA 政策实施后 2 年内，因为患者与潜在供者产生阳性交叉匹配而配型失败的数量比新政策实施前减少了至少 90%以上[56]。此外，高度致敏性患者似乎特别受益于 cPRA 政策，基于观察到在 cPRA 政策实施前后 cPRA ≥80% 的患者百分比增加（分别为 7.2% 和 15.8%）。这些数据与以下宗旨相一致：即使在国家层面，在等待列表上（并将信息保持在最新的 UNOS 数据库上），对于高度致敏性候选人中仔细鉴定不可接受的 HLA 抗原也增加了这些患者将会与筛选出的供者产生阴性交叉匹配的概率。

HLA 抗原何时被认为是不可接受的？

作为一个整体，与没有 DSA 的患者相比，针对供体 HLA 抗原移植 DSA 的患者具有更高的抗体介导的移植物损伤风险[57]。是否有阈值水平低于 DSA 没有临床意义？目前最常见的固相抗体检测系统使用 Luminex 技术，其基于免疫荧光反应性，其定义为任意单位的平均荧光强度（MFI）。MFI 值越高，荧光信号越强，表明抗体结合量越大。MFI 数值范围为 0~20 000，一般情况下（但不是普遍的），MFI 值为 300~2000 被认为是弱的，2000~5000 为中等偏弱，5000~10 000 为中等偏强，>10 000 为强大。将抗原考虑为不可接受的实际阈值是中心对中心的决定，并基于每个中心的理念和风险规避。中等到强的抗体通常导致阳性流式（并且通常是细胞毒性的）交叉匹配，而与弱到中等偏弱强度抗体的流式细胞术交叉匹配可以是阳性或阴性。后一种类型的抗体是当前移植领域面临的挑战。如果交叉匹配是阴性的，DSA 是否在临床上无关？显而易见，如果将不能接受的抗体的阈值设置得太低，则会有患者失去接受能够与之相容的器官进行移植的机会[58]。相反，如果阈值设置得太高，患者可能会经历抗体介导的排斥反应，从而降低同种异体移植物的功能寿命[59]。文献分为两组，一些研究组报告，仅通过固相检测的抗体对移植结果没有影响，而其他组则报告，这种抗体（就算强度很弱）确实与抗体介导的排斥反应和移植物损失的风险增加有关。

在微粒上检测到的 DSA 和在细胞上检测到的差异可能是技术和生物变量的组合。例如，在微粒上检测到的 HLA 抗体是针对某种给定等位基因的特异性抗原，例如，HLA-B*44:02 及靶细胞可能表达 HLA-B*44:03。即使在 44:02 和 44:03 之间只有一个氨基酸的差异，这足以使 B*44:02 抗体与 B*44:02 细胞产生阳性交叉匹配，而不与表达 B*44:03 的细胞产生阳性反应。另一个解释是供体细胞在病毒感染后或在某些药物的作用下使 HLA 的表达减少了[60,61]。其他可能性包括锚定于微粒的抗体与锚定于细胞的抗体的活性不同，亦或是微粒上的 HLA 抗原/表位发生了降解或隐蔽，而细胞上的并未发生。来自一些患者（甚至没有已知致敏事件的患者）的血清与变性的非天然 HLA 抗原结合（因此结合到微粒而不是淋巴细胞）。这些抗体的作用和刺激它们产生的原因是未知的。在最近的研究中，一名心肺移植患者和两名肾脏移植患者显示了对变性抗原的抗体，移植了表达相关天然抗原的供体器官[52,62]。一名患者（肾移植的接受者）在移植后 5 年没有出现排斥反应。而另外两名患者在移植后只有 4 个月和 1 年，也没有出现任何排斥的迹象。还存在有些患者似乎没有 HLA 抗体而呈现阳性交叉匹配的实例。最合乎逻辑的解释是这些交叉匹配是由于非 HLA 抗体引起的。但是，并不总是如此。一个简单的例子是，存在于供体上的 HLA Ⅰ/Ⅱ型抗原的谱系在用于筛选/鉴定 HLA 抗体的微粒上不完全表达。与微粒相比，另一种解释是靶细胞上的 HLA 抗原密度更高。如果供者表达两种或多种抗原，而接受者具有低水平抗体(低于阈值水平为阳性)，则交叉匹配可能是出乎意料地呈现阳性。随着抗原表达的增加，可以在细胞表面上沉积更多的抗体，从而产生更高的荧光信号。此外，针对单个表位的抗体可以分布在所有表达该表位的多个微粒上(例如，Bw4 的抗体将存在于约 60%的靶组织)，并且抗体可以在多个磁珠上稀释，没有磁珠显示 MFI 值高于阈值。总的来说，这些数据表明，单独的临界值可能不是将抗体确定为阳性的适当方法。必须考虑到其他几个因素的存在，包括患者的致敏史和(或)低于阈值的 MFI 值(但不是阴性)的磁珠是否具有抗体特异性的模式。否则，假阳性和假阴性结果并不罕见，并且导致 vXM 和物理交叉匹配之间的不一致结果。Tambur 等的研究表明约 10%的患者出现不一致的情况[38]。

总结

组织相容性的领域不断发展。在过去 20 年中，HLA 分型已经从血清学为主转变为分子技术为主，HLA 抗体检测/分析已经从基于细胞的方法转变为依赖于固相基质的检测方法。这些进展引起了美国器官分配制度的重大变化，从而使虚拟交叉匹配成为现实。使用敏感固相测定法鉴定不可接受的抗原可有效地用于分类致敏受体，使得时间或资源不会浪费在与其预期供体不相容的个体。缺血时间减少，高度致敏性患者比过去有更多机会接受移植。筛选 HLA 抗体将决定患者是否可以直接进行移植(例如，没有 HLA 抗体)或需要进一步研究来鉴定Ⅰ类和Ⅱ类抗体。如果后者可以鉴定出不可接受的抗原并进入国家计算机系统，使得拥有一种或多种不可接受的抗原的供体不被考虑用于分配给相应的受体(图 36.4)。显然，vXM 的应用

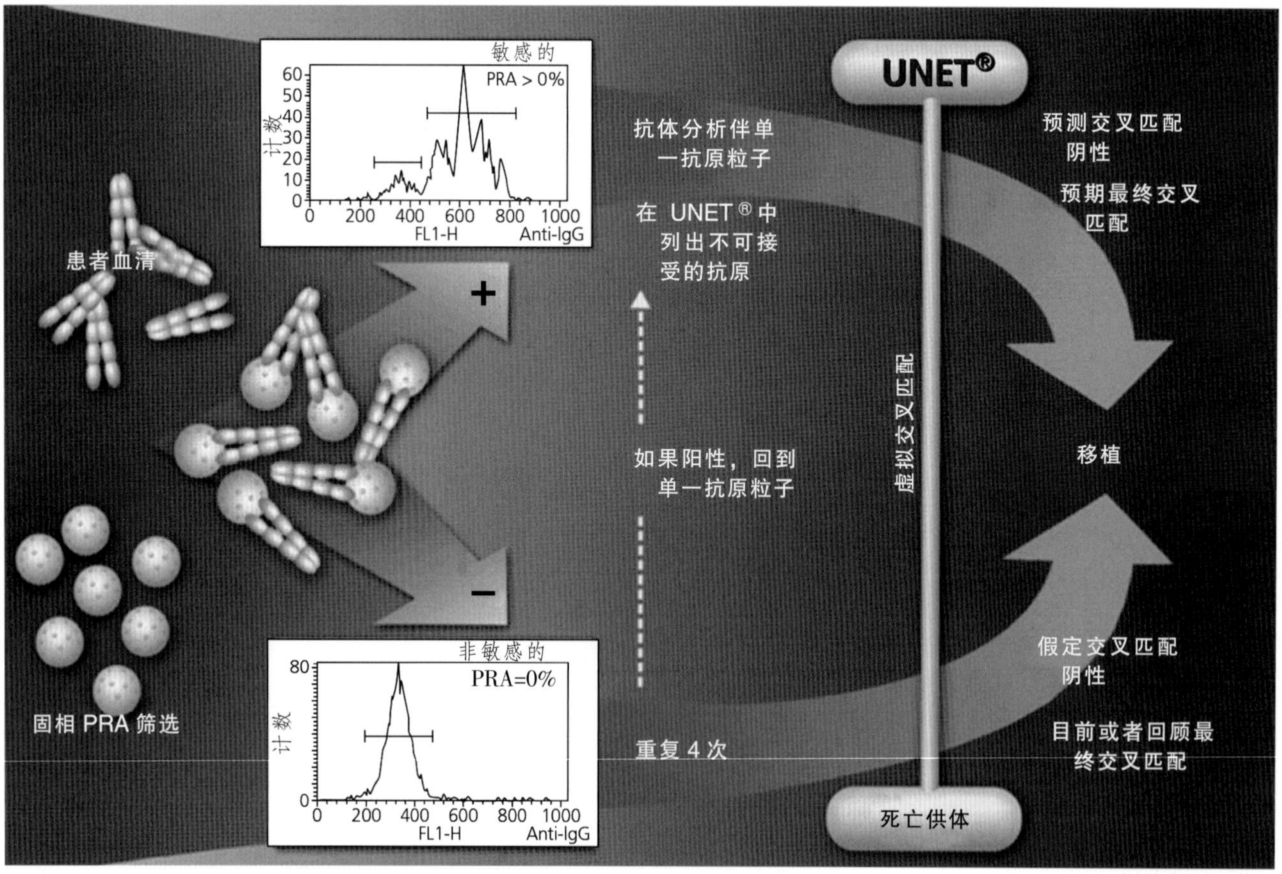

图 36.4 虚拟交叉匹配(vXM)算法。对来自潜在移植受者的血清进行筛选，以鉴定是否存在 HLA Ⅰ类和Ⅱ类抗体。血清Ⅰ类和Ⅱ类抗体阴性的患者可以直接进行移植，并可追溯进行物理交叉匹配。如果Ⅰ类和(或)Ⅱ类抗体血清阳性，则用 HLA 抗原包被的微粒进行详细的抗体特异性分析。在 UNOS 数据库，能够被对应的鉴定抗体识别的特异性 HLA 抗原被列为“不可接受的”抗原。当供体器官可用于这些患者时，其不可接受的抗原用于区分不相容组合。只有 vXM 为阴性的组合才会进行最终的交叉匹配和移植(如果为阴性)。

在识别兼容的供体-受体对方面发挥了重要作用。

不幸的是,vXM 并不完美。此时更有争议的话题之一是如何界定不可接受的抗原。对于任何给定患者的阈值是否设置得太高或太低?目前的难点是将可接受的 DSA 与不可接受的 DSA 区分开来。即使移植前抗体是同种异体移植结果的唯一危险因素,也需要更多简单的抗体水平定量方法来确定其长期结果。可能需要评估诸如记忆 B 细胞和浆细胞的数量和特异性、抗体亲和力、补体结合属性、抗体滴度和抗体类型等因素。目前,对于 DSA 移植前具有相同特异性和明显强度的患者,没有常规检查可以可靠地区分哪些患者预后较好,哪些患者预后较差。是否继续移植是一项依赖各中心自行决定的伦理问题[63]。在一个移植中心可接受移植的患者,在另一个中心可能判定为不能进行移植。目前已经认识到非 HLA 同种异体抗体(例如抗内皮细胞抗体)是移植存活的危险因素,并且对这种抗体的监测正在增加。最终,这种抗体及其相应的抗原将被并入未来的 vXM 中。现在可用于检测和鉴定 HLA 抗体的工具虽然不完美,但代表了目前技术发展的前沿。随着这项技术的发展,我们将其应用于患者身上使其获益的能力也随之变强。

(胡士华 译 李勇剑 朱继业 校)

参考文献

1. Patel R, Terasaki PI. Significance of the positive crossmatch test in kidney transplantation. New England Journal of Medicine. 1969;280:735–739.
2. Delmonico FL, Fuller A, Cosimi AB, et al. New approaches to donor crossmatching and successful transplantation of highly sensitized patients. Transplantation. 1983;36:629–633.
3. Oldfather JW, Anderson CB, Phelan DL, et al. Prediction of crossmatch outcome in highly sensitized dialysis patients based on the identification of serum HLA antibodies. Transplantation. 1986;42:267–270.
4. Gebel HM, Bray RA. The evolution and clinical impact of Human Leukocyte Antigen technology. Current Opinion in Nephrology and Hypertension. 2010; 19:598–602.
5. Pei R, Wang G, Tarsitani C, et al. Simultaneous HLA Class I and Class II antibodies screening with flow cytometry. Human Immunology. 1998;5:313–322.
6. Pei R, Lee J-H, Shih N-J, et al. Single human leukocyte antigen flow cytometry beads for accurate identification of human leukocyte antibody specificities. Transplantation. 2003;75:43–49.
7. Welsh K, Bunce M. Molecular typing for the MHC with PCR-SSP. Reviews in Immunogenetics. 1999;1:157–176.
8. Tiercy JM, Jeannet M, Mach B. A new approach for the analysis of HLA class II polymorphism: 'HLA oligotyping'. Blood Reviews. 1990;4:9–15.
9. Amos DB, Bashir H, Boyle W, et al. A simple microcytotoxicity test. Transplantation. 1989;7:220–223.
10. Johnson AH, Rossen RD, Butler WT. Detection of alloantibodies using a sensitive antiglobulin microcytotoxicity test: identification of low levels of preformed antibodies in accelerated allograft rejection. Tissue Antigens. 1972; 2:215–226.
11. Cross DE, Whittier FC, Weaver P, et al. A comparison of the antiglobulin versus extended incubation time crossmatch: results in 223 renal transplants. Transplantation Proceedings. 1977;9:1803–1806.
12. Fuller TC, Cosimi AB, Russell PS. Use of an antiglobulin-ATG reagent for detection of low levels of alloantibody-improvement of allograft survival in presensitized recipients. Transplantation Proceedings. 1978;10:463–466.
13. Gonzalez-Galarza FF, Christmas S, Middleton D, et al. Allele frequency net: a database and online repository for immune gene frequencies in worldwide populations. Nucleic Acid Research. 2011;39:D913–D919.
14. Gebel HM, Bray RA. Approaches for transplanting the sensitized patient: biology versus pharmacology. Nephrology, Dialysis, Transplantation. 2008;23: 2454–2457.
15. UNOS Rationale for Objectives of Equitable Organ Allocation. Richmond, VA: United Network for Organ Sharing; 1994; Available from: http://www.unos.org/resources/bioethics.asp?index=8.
16. OTPN/SRTR Annual Report. 2010; Available from: http://www.srtr.org/annual_reports/2010/.
17. Cecka JM. Calculated PRA (CPRA): the new measure of sensitization for transplant candidates. American Journal of Transplantation. 2010;10:26–29.
18. Bray RA, Tarsitani C, Gebel HM, et al. Clinical cytometry and progress in HLA antibody detection. Methods in Cell Biology. 2011;103:285–310.
19. Gebel HM, Bray RA, Nickerson PW. Pretransplant assessment of donor reactive, HLA specific antibodies in renal transplantation: contraindication vs risk. American Journal of Transplantation. 2003;3:1488–1500.
20. Pollinger HS, Stegall MD, Gloor JM, et al. Kidney transplantation in patients with antibodies against donor HLA class II. American Journal of Transplantation. 2007;7:857–863.
21. Mahoney RJ, Ault KA, Given SR, et al. The flow cytometric crossmatch and early renal transplantation. Transplantation. 1990;49:527–535.
22. Ogura K, Terasaki PI, Johnson C, et al. The significance of a positive flow cytometric crossmatch in primary renal transplantation. Transplantation. 1993;56: 294–298.
23. Bryan CF, Baier KA, Nelson PW, et al. Long-term graft survival is improved in cadaveric renal retransplantation by flow cytometric crossmatching. Transplantation. 1998;66:1827–1832.
24. Kerman RH, Susskind B, Buyse I, et al. Flow cytometry-detected IgG is not a contraindication to renal transplantation: IgM may be beneficial to outcome. Transplantation. 1999;68:1855–1858.
25. Ettenger RB, Jordan SC, Fine RN. Cadaver renal transplant outcome in recipients with autolymphocytotoxic antibodies. Transplantation. 1983;35:429–431.
26. Vaidya S, Cooper TY, Avandsalehi J, et al. Improved flow cytometric detection of HLA alloantibodies using pronase. Transplantation. 2001;72:422–428.
27. Le Bas-Bernardet S, Hourmant M, Valentin N, et al. Identification of the antibodies involved in B cell crossmatch positivity in renal transplantation. Transplantation. 2003;75:477–482.
28. Cesbron-Gautier A, Simon P, Achard L, et al. Luminex technology for HLA typing by PCR-SSO and identification of HLA antibody specificities. Annales de Biologie Clinique. 2004;62:93–98.
29. Kao KJ, Scornik JC, Small SJ. Enzyme-linked immunoassay for anti-HLA antibodies–an alternative to panel studies by lymphocytotoxicity. Transplantation. 1993;55:192–196.
30. Bray RA, Nickerson PW, Kerman RH, et al. Evolution of HLA antibody detection: technology emulating biology. Immunologic Research. 2004;29:41–54.
31. Claas FH, van Leeuwen A, van Rood JJ. Hyperimmunized patients do not need to wait for an HLA identical donor. Tissue Antigens. 1989;34:23–29.
32. Rodey GE, Neylan JF, Whelchel JD, et al. Epitope specificity of HLA class I alloantibodies. I. Frequency analysis of antibodies to private versus public specificities in potential transplant recipients. Human Immunology. 1994;39: 272–280.
33. Fleischhauer K, Kernan NA, Dupont B, et al. The two major subtypes of HLA-B44 differ for a single amino acid in codon 156. Tissue Antigens. 1991;37:133–137.
34. Phelan DL, Mickelson EM, Noreen HS, et al. ASHI Laboratory Manual. 4th ed. Mt. Laurel, NJ: American Society for Histocompatibility and Immunogenetics; 2001.
35. Bray RA, Nolen JD, Larsen C, et al. Transplanting the highly sensitized patient: The Emory algorithm. American Journal of Transplantation. 2006;6:2307–2315.
36. Appel JZ 3rd, Hartwig MG, Cantu E 3rd, et al. Role of flow cytometry to define unacceptable HLA antigens in lung transplant recipients with HLA-specific antibodies. Transplantation. 2006;81:1049–1057.
37. Nikaein A, Cherikh W, Nelson K, et al. Organ procurement and transplantation network/united network for organ sharing histocompatibility committee collaborative study to evaluate prediction of crossmatch results in highly sensitized patients. Transplantation. 2009;87:557–562.
38. Tambur AR, Ramon DS, Kaufman DB, et al. Perception versus reality?: virtual crossmatch-how to overcome some of the technical and logistic limitations. American Journal of Transplantation. 2009;9:1886–1893.
39. Bachelet T, Couzi L, Guidicelli G, et al. Anti-Cw donor-specific alloantibodies can

lead to positive flow cytometry crossmatch and irreversible acute antibody-mediated rejection. American Journal of Transplantation. 2011;11:1543–1544.
40. Goral S, Prak EL, Kearns J, et al. Preformed donor-directed anti-HLA-DP antibodies may be an impediment to successful kidney transplantation. Nephrology, Dialysis, Transplantation. 2008;23(1):390–392.
41. Thaunat O, Hanf W, Dubois V, et al. Chronic humoral rejection mediated by anti-HLA-DP alloantibodies: insights into the role of epitope sharing in donor-specific and non-donor specific alloantibodies generation. Transplant Immunology. 2009;20:209–211.
42. Iniotaki-Theodoraki AG, Boletis JN, Trigas G, et al. Humoral immune reactivity against human leukocyte antigen (HLA)-DQ graft molecules in the early post-transplantation period. Transplantation. 2003;75:1601–1607.
43. Bingaman AW, Murphey CL, Palma-Vargas J, et al. A virtual crossmatch protocol significantly increases access of highly sensitized patients to deceased donor kidney transplantation. Transplantation. 2008;86:1864–1868.
44. Stehlik J, Islam N, Hurst D, et al. Utility of virtual crossmatch in sensitized patients awaiting heart transplantation. Journal of Heart and Lung Transplantation. 2009;28:1129–1133.
45. Ferrari P, Fidler S, Wright J, et al. Virtual crossmatch approach to maximize matching in paired kidney donation. American Journal of Transplantation. 2011;11: 272–278.
46. Zangwill S, Ellis T, Stendahl G, et al. Practical application of the virtual crossmatch. Pediatric Transplantation. 2007;11:650–654.
47. Claas FH, Rahmel A, Doxiadis II. Enhanced kidney allocation to highly sensitized patients by the acceptable mismatch program. Transplantation. 2009;88:447–452.
48. Taylor CJ, Kosmoliaptis V, Summers DM, et al. Back to the future: application of contemporary technology to long-standing questions about the clinical relevance of human leukocyte antigen specific alloantibodies in renal transplantation. Human Immunology. 2009;70:563–568.
49. Bielmann D, Honger G, Lutz D, et al. Pretransplant risk assessment in renal allograft recipients using virtual crossmatching. American Journal of Transplantation. 2007;7:626–632.
50. Amico P, Honger G, Mayr M, et al. Clinical relevance of pretransplant donor-specific HLA antibodies detected by single-antigen flow beads. Transplantation. 2009;87:1681–1688.
51. Issa N, Cosio FG, Gloor JM, et al. Transplant glomerulopathy: risk and prognosis related to anti-human leukocyte antigen class II antibody levels. Transplantation. 2008;86(5):681–685.
52. Pereira S, Perkins S, Lee JH, et al. Donor-specific antibody against denatured HLA-A1: clinically nonsignificant? Human Immunology. 2011;72:492–498.
53. Patel AM, Pancoska C, Mulgaonkar S, et al. Renal transplantation in patients with pre-transplant donor-specific antibodies and negative flow cytometry crossmatches. American Journal of Transplantation. 2007;7:2371–2377.
54. Couzi L, Araujo C, Guidicelli G, et al. Interpretation of positive flow cytometric crossmatch in the era of the single-antigen bead assay. Transplantation. 2011;91: 527–535.
55. OPTN/UNOS Histocompatibility Committee. Interim report: Implementation of policy 3.5.11.3 calculate panel reactive antibody (CPRA). Richmond, VA: United Network for Organ Sharing, 2007; Available from: http://optn.transplant.hrsa.gov/CommitteeReports/interim_main_HistoCommittee_9_25_2007_15_51.pdf.
56. Cecka JM, Kucheryavaya AY, Reinsmoen NL, et al. Calculated PRA: initial results show benefits for sensitized patients and a reduction in positive crossmatches. American Journal of Transplantation. 2011;11:719–724.
57. Montgomery RA. Renal transplantation across HLA and ABO antibody barriers: integrating paired donation into desensitization protocols. American Journal of Transplantation. 2010;10:449–457.
58. Lefaucheur C, Antoine C, Suberbielle C, et al. Mastering the risk of HLA antibodies in kidney transplantation: an algorithm based on pretransplant single-antigen flow bead techniques. American Journal of Transplantation. 2011;11:1592–1598.
59. Lefaucheur C, Loupy A, Hill GS, et al. Preexisting donor-specific HLA antibodies predict outcome in kidney transplantation. Journal of the American Society of Nephrology. 2010;21:1398–1406.
60. Lin A, Xu H, Yan W. Modulation of HLA expression in human cytomegalovirus immune evasion. Cellular and Molecular Immunology. 2007;4:91–98.
61. Kuipers K, Biesta P, Groothuis T, et al. Statins affect cell-surface expression of major histocompatibility complex II molecules by disrupting cholesterol containing microdomains. Human Immunology. 2005;66:653–665.
62. Jacob EK, De Goey SR, Gandhi MJ. Positive virtual crossmatch with negative flow crossmatch results in two cases. Transplant Immunology. 2011;25:77–81.
63. Gebel HM, Moussa O, Eckels DD, et al. Donor-reactive HLA antibodies in renal allograft recipients: considerations, complications, and conundrums. Human Immunology. 2009;70:610–617.

第 37 章 肾移植等待名单管理

Phuong-Thu T. Pham, Phuong-Chi T. Pham, Gabriel M. Danovitch

引言

死亡供肾的数量仍然远低于需求的增长，导致移植等待名单的患者数量持续增加、等待时间延长、等待名单死亡人数增加。器官获取和移植网络/器官共享联合网络（OPTN/UNOS）数据库显示，在过去 10 年，每年有 22 000~34 000 的肾移植候选者被列入等待名单。在同一时期，每年有 4300~6700 的患者因死亡或医疗条件发生改变不适于移植而从等待名单移除。目前，估计有 1/2 等待名单中的死亡患者为“非活跃状态”名单的患者。因此，管理等待名单患者已经成为移植中心面临的最大问题。本章讨论 OPTN/UNOS 提出的等待名单状态分类、移植肾等待时间的影响因素、活跃等待名单中成人肾移植候选者管理指南以及存在医疗或社会心理问题患者的管理指南，是对论述肾移植适应证的第 28 章的补充。

器官共享联合网络（UNOS）等待名单状态

死亡供者等待名单的肾移植候选者会被列为状态 1 或状态 7 这两种状态之一。当患者的医学和社会心理状态被认为适合移植时会被列入状态 1。与此相反，状态 7 代表暂停状态，处于这一状态的患者由于并发症而暂时无法获得器官分配。OPTN/UNOS 的政策规定患者医学状态的改变需要向 OPTN 报告。以前，注册者被置于暂停状态 1 个月后其等待时间将停止增长，只有当医学并发症得以解决并报告给 OPTN 后才能重新开始等待时间。然而，这一政策被认为妨碍移植中心向 OPTN 准确报告注册者的状态，导致获得器官延迟。2003 年 11 月，实施了一项重要改变，由于任何紧急事件被置于状态 7 的候选者的等待时间继续自然增长，以此来减少准确报告导致的妨碍。

患者可能因为多种医学或社会心理原因而被置于状态 7。医学因素包括：其他疾病或住院、无瘤等待时间、减肥以获得可接受的体重指数、心脏或神经康复。社会心理因素包括：医学不依从、频繁的药物滥用或精神疾病、缺乏社会心理支持。等待名单中的患者会因临时事件从状态 1 调至状态 7，反之亦然。然而，那些发生了诸如转移癌、严重冠状动脉疾病、严重的卒中等不可逆并发症而禁忌实施移植的患者，将从等待名单移除。UNOS 列入和移除程序的算法列于图 37.1。

等待名单上移植候选者的等待时间

死亡供肾的等待时间存在很大差异，主要是基于以下因素：ABO 血型、种族背景、致敏作用（群体反应性抗体），以及美国的不同器官获取组织（OPO）区域。其他因素包括：接受扩大标准供肾（ECD）或当单一扩大标准肾脏被认为不适合时使用双扩大标准供肾，循环死亡供体（DCD）肾脏，公共卫生服务部（PHS）高危供体肾脏或有慢性丙型肝炎感染记录的丙型肝炎病毒（HCV）供体肾脏。

了解可能影响等待时间的主要因素后，临床医生和移植协调员制定临床计划以确保等待名单顶端的候选者确实适于移植，尽量避免最后一分钟取消的情况，避免未达到最优风险管理的候选者被不适当地进行了移植。

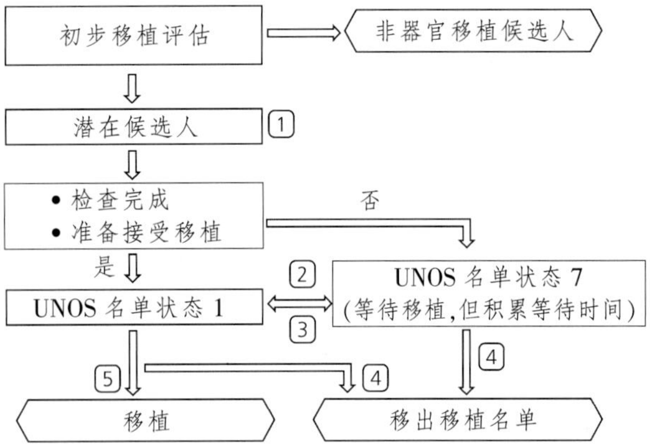

图 37.1 器官共享联合网络(UNOS)关于列入移植名单和移出移植名单的流程算法。

1.讨论项目(见文本):活体肾捐献、ECD、ECD 肾脏双重移植、DCD、PHS 高风险、来自丙型肝炎捐赠者的肾脏。

2.新的医疗和(或)心理问题(状态 1→状态 7)。

3.检查完成。所有问题解决(状态 7→状态 1)。

4.不可逆转的并发症发生导致不适合移植。

5.持续健康维护和筛查(见文本)。

UNOS,器官共享联合网络;ECD,扩大标准供体;DCD,循环死亡供体;PHS, 公共卫生服务。

患者内在因素对等待时间的影响

ABO 血型

OPTN/UNOS 数据库显示,1999—2004 年等待名单中注册者的 Kaplan-Meier 中位等待时间在不同血型存在区别,O 型为 1763~1852 天,A 型为 1085~1208 天,B 型为 1967~2033 天,AB 型为 597~855 天[1]。因此,O 型和 B 型患者等待时间最长。

种族背景

在美国,列入等待名单中的白种人和非洲裔美国人的比例在过去 10 年没有发生改变。非洲裔美国人大约占等待名单中注册者的 35%,这一比例与他们的慢性透析人群相似,大约是普通人群的 3 倍[2]。新加入的非洲裔美国人的比例低于等待名单中已经存在的比例(30%对 35%),提示他们移植率较低。与此相反,新列入的白种人的比例高于已经存在于等待名单中的比例(64%对 53%),反映出他们的移植率较高[2]。西班牙裔和拉丁裔在等待名单和新注册者中占 17%~18%[2]。一项针对 1995—2006 开始维持透析的非老年患者(18~64 岁)的研究也证实,非白人患者较白人患者死亡供肾肾移植率较低[3]。美国印第安人、阿拉斯加原住民和黑人中死亡供肾肾移植率的降低反映了等待名单比例和等待名单患者移植率的降低。然而,亚裔、太平洋岛民和西班牙裔进入等待名单的人等待时间更长。

OPTN/UNOS 数据库显示,1999—2004 年进入等待名单的白人注册者的 Kaplan-Meier 中位等待时间较黑人、西班牙裔、亚裔和非西班牙裔短 30%~35%,较美国印第安人短 15%。在所有种族中,太平洋岛民的等待时间最长[1]。

不同种族等待时间和移植率的差异被认为与多种因素有关,包括器官移植和器官捐献的个人和文化信仰,HLA 错配的频率,社会经济状态和教育水平,因 ABO 血型和地理位置导致进入移植的变异性等。

高度致敏移植候选者

在美国,约 40%的等待名单中的移植候选者存在高水平的抗-HLA 抗体,也称为高群体反应性抗体(PRA)。通常认为,高 PRA 水平是由于既往暴露于非己 HLA 抗原(例如妊娠、输血或既往失败的移植)所致。高 PRA 候选者获得交叉匹配相容的等待时间会明显延长。OPTN/UNOS 数据库显示,在 2001—2002 年,移植候选者 PRA 水平为 0~9%、10%~79%和≥80%的 Kaplan-Meier 中位等待时间分别为 1329 天(约 3.6 年)、1920 天(约 5.3 年)和 3649 天(约 9.9 年)[1]。在过去 5 年,各种降敏措施(第 68 章深入讨论)被开发出来用于高敏患者以便成功移植,包括静脉注射免疫球蛋白、血浆置换或免疫吸附、利妥昔单抗(一种 CD-20 单克隆抗体)。最近,硼替佐米(一种蛋白酶抑制剂)和依库丽单抗(一种抗补体 C5 单克隆抗体)被用于多种降敏程序。目前,一些中心为处于死亡供者等待名单顶端的明显致敏患者提供降敏治疗。在洛杉矶加利福尼亚大学,基于透析开始日期识别出每种血型的前 30 例候选者。高致敏患者进入匹配程序后,临床会监测到并给予参加降敏治疗的机会。通常,在同一时间每种血型(AB 型除外)会有一名患者被给予降敏治疗。

患者居住地对等待时间的影响

美国分为 11 个 OPO 区域。不同 OPO 区域的等待时间差别巨大[4]。这导致一些预期接受移植的候选者寻求进入不同 OPO 代理处的多个移植中心的等待名单,以便增加他们获得移植的可能性。

UNOS 注册数据显示，多重登记增加 88%的肾移植概率，减少等待时间约 50%(在 1995 年 1 月 7 日至 2000 年 6 月 30 日登记的候选者中，单一登记和多重登记的中位等待时间分别为 156 周和 83 周)[5]。显而易见,多重注册几乎使得所有人口统计学、生物学和社会经济学亚群提高移植率，包括那些已知的明显不容易实现移植的患者,例如非洲裔美国人、女性以及 O 型和 B 型血患者。多重注册似乎不能使健康维护组织覆盖的患者获益。这提示多重注册趋于减少不同 OPO 之间等待时间的差距,因为第二个注册的 OPO 通常比首个 OPO 等待时间更短。尽管如此,需要注意的是,当在等待时间长的中心等待移植的患者在等待时间短的中心多重注册后可能会获益，但是如果在等待患者很多的中心再次注册却是昂贵且无效的[6]。

减少等待时间的特殊选项

候选者罹患慢性丙型肝炎

同意接受丙肝供体肾脏的等待名单中丙肝抗体阳性移植候选者的人数普遍较少（作者所在中心在写作本文时的数量<20）。丙肝死亡供体肾脏的等待时间相对较短(我们中心目前为 2~3 年)。因此,应该密切随访同意接受丙肝供肾的患者，确保他们在医学和社会心理方面随时做好移植准备。

公共卫生服务部高危供体肾脏

公共卫生服务部实行了定义供者存在传播病毒性疾病(包括人免疫缺陷病毒 HIV、丙型肝炎)高度风险的标准。在捐献 1 年之内的危险因素包括：

1.男性同性恋接触。

2.非医疗静脉注射、肌肉注射或皮下注射药物。

3.以金钱或毒品为目的的乱交。

4.在 12 个月内与上述 1~3 描述的人有性接触,或是与明确的或可疑的 HIV 感染者有经皮肤接种、经开放伤口、不完整皮肤或黏膜接触。

5.明确或可疑罹患性传播疾病者。

6.被惩教系统收容者。

7.由于拒绝检测、血液样本不足(例如血液稀释导致假阴性结果)或其他原因不能检测 HIV 感染者。

8.不论附加检测结果如何,需要重复 HIV_1 或 HIV_2 抗体反应性筛查实验者。

9 病史、体检、医疗记录或活检报告显示其他 HIV 感染证据或高危行为(例如诊断 AIDS、无法解释的体重减轻、夜间盗汗、皮肤或黏膜典型的卡波西肉瘤病变、无法解释的持续淋巴结肿大>1 个月、无法解释的体温>38.6℃超过 10 天、无法解释的持续咳嗽和呼吸急促、机会性感染、无法解释的持续腹泻、注射瘢痕或其他静脉滥用药物的体征)者。

公共卫生服务部高危供肾传播病毒性疾病的风险尚不明确,但其范围是 1/10 000~1/300。尽管如此,对于预期等待时间延长或透析穿刺部位耗尽病例应用此类供肾进行移植较保持透析存在更好的生存获益。需要注意的是，卫生服务部定义的高危供肾没有包括供体器官向受者传播未发现的恶性肿瘤的风险。完整的公共卫生服务部指南网址如下 http://www.publichealthreports.org/issuecontents.cfm?Volume=128&Issue=4。

扩大标准供肾

目前，许多年老的移植候选者在等待标准死亡供体肾脏的过程中死亡。而且,移植前等待时间显著增加死亡导致的移植物丢失和移植后患者死亡风险[7]。我们中心现在向所有 50 岁以上的候选者建议扩大标准供肾(ECD)项目。ECD 肾脏由供者特征定义,与对照组相比,移植物失败的风险增加 70%,对照组为 10~39 岁的无高血压病供者，死亡原因不是脑血管病并且末次肌酐≤1.5 mg/dL。增加移植物失败概率的供者因素包括：年龄≥60 岁,或者年龄介于 50~59 岁,合并至少两个共患因素。所谓的共患因素包括：死亡原因为脑血管病、高血压,和(或)末次肌酐>1.5mg/dL(表 37.1)。患者应被告知 ECD 肾脏候选者会被同时列入标准供肾和 ECD 供肾等待名单中。在经过挑选的患者中,双 ECD 供肾移植给高龄患者,可以获得良好的短期和中期效果。对 OPTN/UNOS 数据库中 625 例双肾移植(DKT)和 7686 例单 ECD 肾移植的研究证实,两组移植受者的 3 年总体移植物存活率是相似的(分别为 79.8%和 78.3%)[8]。有人认为,DKT 的优势在于拥有更多有活力的肾单位。

心脏死亡供肾

扩大死亡供者器官供给的一个途径是应用心脏死亡供者(DCD)的器官。DCD 肾脏明显受到不同程度热缺血损伤的影响，应用后不可避免地会增加移植物功

表 37.1 确定扩大标准供体的因素(UNOS 定义)

供体状态	供体年龄分类(岁)	
	50~59	≥60
CVA+HTN+肌酐>1.5mg/dL	X	X
CVA+HTN	X	X
CVA+肌酐>1.5mg/dL	X	X
HTN+肌酐>1.5mg/dL	X	X
CVA		X
HTN		X
肌酐 >1.5mg/dL		X
以上都不是		X

X,扩大标准供体;CVA,脑血管意外为死亡原因;HTN,任何时期的高血压病史。

Adapetd from UNOS.

能恢复延迟(DGF)和原发无功能。美国肾脏资料系统数据库证实,DCD 肾移植受者 DGF 的发生率约是有心跳供肾移植受者的两倍(分别为 42.3%和 23.3%)。尽管如此,DCD 供肾移植和有心跳死亡供者供肾移植随访 6 年后的移植物存活率相似(分别为 73.2%和 72.5%,*P*=NS)[9]。有趣的是,DCD 肾移植受者比有心跳供体肾移植受者的 6 年存活率有更好的趋势(分别为 80.9%和 77.8%,*P*=NS)。DCD 供肾肾移植受者移植物丢失的重要危险因素包括:再次移植、DGF、供者年龄大于 35 岁、头外伤为初期损伤的原因。为了优化 DCD 肾脏的应用,大量中心使用了机械灌注参数和生存能力测试来评估肾损伤的程度和预测移植物功能。在作者所在的机构,DCD 肾脏提供给事先识别好的并经过知情同意的等待名单中的候选者。

在最初评估和随访过程中,应和潜在的移植候选者详细讨论是否选择 HCV、ECD、双 ECD 供肾肾移植、DCD 和 PHS 高危死亡供肾。这些选择在第 21、22 和 53 章被特别讨论。活体供肾也应被讨论(关于活体移植的处理和伦理问题分别在第 23 章和第 138 章进行深入讨论)。

发展新的肾脏分配系统:透析时间

2002 年 3 月在费城召开的肾移植等待名单国家会议上,来自 9 个美国机构的代表组成的专家组建议,移植等待时间应该从开始维持透析算起,而不是从完成移植评估开始[10]。这一建议旨在消除早进入等待名单患者的优势,给所有适合移植的候选者提供公平的获得移植的机会,特别是少数民族和经济弱势群体患者。一项评估肾移植患者移植等待时间从首次透析开始或达到肾衰竭医疗定义标准的影响的初步研究于 2003 年 11 月首次被 OPTN/UNOS 指导委员会批准。

来自两个 OPO(CAOP 和 MIOP)的早期报告采用了透析等待时间分配系统,证实在政策实施的 18 个月,平均透析时间有增加趋势,而接受死亡供肾移植受者在等待名单的平均等待时间有减少趋势。表面上矛盾的移植前透析时间增加和等待时间缩短反映出很多移植患者来自大量长期依赖透析延迟转介到移植中心的患者。而在没有执行这一政策的 OPO 没有观察到这一趋势[11]。CAOP 在政策改变前(2004 年 4 月 28 日前)后(2004 年 4 月 29 日后)的 18 个月中,死亡供肾移植受者的平均透析时间分别为 3.9 年和 4.8 年。相反,政策改变后可看到等待名单中时间减少(政策改变后为 2.3 年,政策改变前为 2.7 年)。CAOP 和 MIOP 的透析时间增加和等待名单中时间减少在所有种族中是一致的(MIOP 的西班牙裔和亚裔除外)。有些州观察到非洲裔美国人的移植率有轻度增加。有人推测,这种效果在等待时间存在差异的区域还不明显,需要更长期的随访。总体来说,所有种族的等待时间都有降低。

基于初步报告,OPTN 肾移植委员会近期建议透析时间应纳入国家分配政策。透析等待时间和估计肾小球滤过率 (eGFR)<20 cc/min 将于 2014 年的国家分配运算法则中实施。

维护和监测等待名单中的患者

分配政策要求所有等待名单中状态为 1 的患者做好随时移植的准备。但是缺乏维护和监测等待名单中活跃患者的指南。患者的健康状态,特别是心血管状态可能随着透析时间的延长而恶化。接下来的部分讨论等待名单中患者的管理指南,包括随访频率、血清储存用于移植前交叉配型,以及总体健康维护。总体健康维护包括心血管和心瓣膜疾病、恶性肿瘤以及感染性疾病筛查。需要指出的是,不同移植中心在实践中的差别很大。

随访频率

随着等待名单中患者数量的不断增加,以及器官供给和需求的扩大,定期或每年对所有等待移植的候选者进行随访变得不切实际,特别是在大的移植中心,其等待患者数量通常超过 1500 人/年。因此,为更新患者数据而制订运算法则仍然是移植医师、协调员和社会工作者面临的挑战,特别是在等待时间常规超过 6~7 年的区域。

在洛杉矶加利福尼亚大学,在过去 5 年,每年有超过 1500~2000 名患者在等待名单中。目前我们每年对每种 ABO 血型的前 30 名患者和身份信息进入匹配程序的患者进行随访,再评估其总体健康状态和人口学问题。在美国,配型由中央计算机网络来完成,死亡供者的医学信息与移植候选者进行匹配。这一匹配过程自动为每个器官产生一个适合的候选者排名表,依据的因素包括供者和移植候选者的组织配型、ABO 血型、PRA 水平、在等待名单中的时间、儿童候选者以及潜在的受者和供者的地域距离。

移植前交叉配型的血清的储存

当从等待移植患者采集的血清在预定的间隔并且可以被 HLA 实验室获得时,即可完成最后的交叉配型而不需要从患者获取新鲜标本。在作者所在的机构,前 25%的非致敏移植候选者每个季度采集一次血清,其余非致敏患者每半年采集一次。对于高度致敏候选者,每个月需要进行筛查检查。在供体 HLA 分型检查时通过适当的方式对供者细胞进行检测以完成初步的交叉配型。

健康维护

心血管和瓣膜性心脏病

心血管筛查

由于终末期肾病患者中无临床症状冠心病的患病率很高,大多数移植中心将心血管筛查作为移植前评估的一项基本内容。而且,心血管疾病是肾移植后死亡的首要原因。移植后 30 天内发生功能性移植物死亡的肾移植受者约 1/2 是由于缺血性心脏病。详细的心血管病史不仅有助于预测手术风险,而且能够帮助移植后的心脏管理,提高短期和长期的心脏预后。然而,用于预防围术期心脏事件的移植前评估和管理冠状动脉疾病的最佳策略仍存在争议。另外,在选择哪些候选者重复检查以及在长时间等待期间如何确定检查频率等方面尚未达成一致。美国移植协会建议对高危肾移植候选者进行心脏负荷检查,高危患者定义为:患者合并糖尿病、既往缺血性心脏病史、心电图异常或者年龄≥50 岁。只有心脏负荷试验阳性的患者才应考虑冠状动脉造影[12]。但是多年以来,这一策略受到质疑,因为现在认识到,与普通人群相比,肾移植患者非侵袭性检查的敏感性和特异性降低。在普通人群,心肌灌注检查的异常与冠状动脉心脏病的出现相一致,平均灵敏度和特异度分别为 88%和 74%[13],而在终末期肾病患者,有报道显示灵敏度和特异度的范围分别为 37%~90%和 40%~90%[14]。大量移植中心建议对高危患者直接行冠状动脉造影检查。

作者对于等待名单中患者的初次心脏评估和后续心脏监测的建议分别列在图 37.2 和表 37.2。作者建议的指南部分基于 Lee 心脏风险评估模型[15],2007 年美国心脏病学会(ACC)和美国心脏病协会(AHA)外科风险分层[16],国家胆固醇教育项目专家组的成人高胆固醇血症发现、评估和治疗指南[17],以及 K/DOQI 透析患者心血管疾病临床实践指南[18]。对于肾移植候选者心脏风险的详细讨论超出了本章的范围,感兴趣的读者可以参考 Pham 等的文章[19]。

瓣膜性心脏病

终末期肾病维持透析的患者常常由于继发性甲状旁腺功能亢进、钙-磷酸产物升高、高钙血症和高磷酸盐血症而发生瓣膜性心脏病。其他危险因素包括高血压、糖尿病、高脂血症、左心室肥大、尿毒症环境和贫血等[20]。最常见的异常包括瓣膜和环增厚、任何心瓣膜钙化导致的反流和狭窄。主动脉瓣和二尖瓣增厚或狭窄的发生率分别为 55%~69%和 40%~60%[20]。以往认为瓣膜硬化没有临床意义,但是目前认识到瓣膜硬化是瓣膜进行性狭窄和心血管死亡的一个潜在原因。二尖瓣环钙化发生于 10%~50%的患者,主动脉瓣钙化在透析患者中的发生率为 25%~55%。三尖瓣和肺动脉瓣钙化较为罕见[20]。目前,K/DOQI 对透析患者心瓣膜疾病的临床实践指南[18]推荐根据 ACC/AHA 的指南评估透析患者瓣膜性心脏病的出现。对透析患者瓣膜性心脏病的随访也依据普通人群的指南,主动脉瓣狭窄的随访频率除外(下面会进一步讨论)[18]。

存在心脏瓣膜疾病的患者的最佳随访频率尚无明确定义,但大多数医生建议无症状患者应每年进行病史和体格检查。另外,ACC/AHA 指南推荐无症状重度主动脉瓣狭窄患者每年检查心脏超声,中度主动脉瓣狭窄患者每 1~2 年检查心脏超声,轻度主动脉瓣狭窄

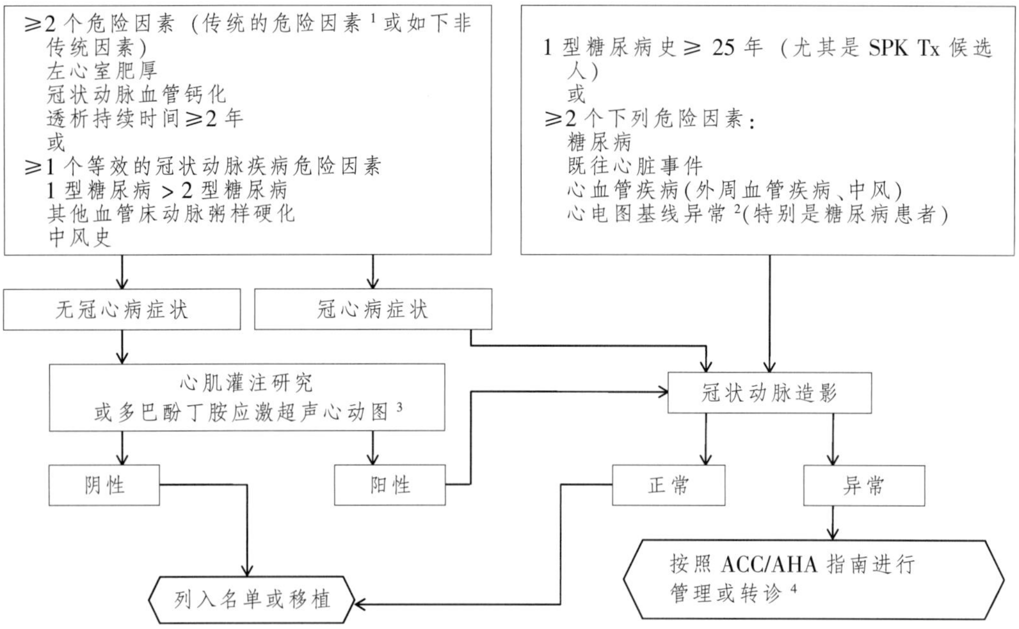

图 37.2　移植前心脏评估的推荐流程。(Reproduced from Pham et al. [19] with permission from John Wiley and Sons Ltd.)

1 参考表 37.2 脚注。

2 心电图结果提示陈旧性心肌梗死，ST-T 波改变。

3 根据中心具体情况。

4 如果可能，应在列入移植名单或移植前进行 PCI 或 CABG 和心脏病康复治疗。

SPK，胰肾联合移植；Tx，移植；ACC/AHA，美国心脏病学会/美国心脏病协会；PCI，经皮冠状动脉介入治疗；CABG，冠状动脉旁路移植术。

患者每 3~5 年检查一次心脏超声（Ⅰ级）。然而，等待名单中的无症状的中度或更严重的主动脉瓣狭窄（或者任何存在主动脉瓣置换的透析患者）的移植候选者应每年进行心脏超声检查。有人认为透析患者主动脉瓣狭窄的进展速度比普通人群更快。任何临床症状发生变化的患者也应进行心脏超声检查（Ⅰ级）。无症状患者如果由于静态的生活方式而导致临床状态可疑，应考虑进行运动试验以诱发症状并评估血流动力学应答（Ⅱb 级）[21]。类似的指南通常被推荐用于等待名单中的透析患者。需要注意的是，K/DOQI 临床实践指南推荐在试验前优化患者的干重[18]。对于其他瓣膜性心脏病没有特殊建议。

恶性肿瘤筛查

对接受透析或移植治疗的终末期肾病患者和艾滋病患者的研究显示，肿瘤可以分为终末期肾病相关的肿瘤、免疫缺陷相关的肿瘤、与免疫缺陷无关的肿瘤以及不确定状态（表 37.3）[22]。终末期肾病相关的肿瘤包括肾、尿路、甲状腺肿瘤和多发性骨髓瘤。虽然关于等待名单中肾移植候选者恶性肿瘤筛查的类型和频率尚未达成共识，但是所有患者都应坚持标准的适龄的肿瘤监测。推荐的肿瘤筛查指南列在表 37.4。另外，成人肾移植候选者的恶性肿瘤筛查应聚焦于肾和尿路，而透析依赖的终末期肾病患者更是如此（下文进一步讨论）。年龄大于 60 岁的患者都应进行血清免疫固定电泳检查。慢性乙型肝炎和丙型肝炎病毒感染患者应筛查肝癌。虽然观察到透析患者比普通人群甲状腺癌的发生率增加，但是甲状腺超声不是移植前筛查的常规项目。虽然没有研究证实或反对，但仍建议透析患者有理由常规进行甲状腺超声检查[23]。因此，肾移植候选者是否进行甲状腺癌筛查应由临床医生决定。

获得性囊性肾病和肾细胞癌筛查

获得性囊性肾病（ACKD）定义为没有遗传性囊性疾病病因的患者每侧肾脏存在多于 3~5 个肉眼可见的囊肿。文献报道，与普通人群相比，ACKD 患者囊肿恶变的发生率<1%~7%，肾细胞癌（RCC）的发生风险高达 40 倍。RCC 约占尿毒症患者肾细胞肿瘤的 80%，约 85%的患者是无症状的[23]。已提出的危险因素包括：男

表 37.2 针对等待名单中的候选人建议进行的心脏监测

无已知 CAD 或初始评价阴性	
(a)糖尿病终末期肾病	每年
(b)无糖尿病+下列任何：	每 2 年
≥2 个传统[1]或非传统[2]危险因素	
或≥1 个等效的 CAD 危险因素[3]	
(c)"更低风险"[4]	每 3 年
已知 CAD	
根据 ACC/AHA 治疗指南进行治疗管理	每年
之前成功进行了 PCI 术	每年
成功的 CABG 手术史	CABG 术后 3 年，之后每年
无症状的主动脉瓣狭窄[5]	
轻度	超声心动图每 3~5 年
中等[6]	超声心动图每年

[1] 传统危险因素：男性年龄>45 岁和女性年龄>55 岁、糖尿病、高血压、血脂异常、肥胖、心绞痛病史、充血性心力衰竭、既往心脏事件、吸烟、家族史。

[2] 非传统危险因素：左心室肥大(LVH)、冠状动脉血管钙化、透析持续时间≥2 年。

[3] 等效的 CAD 危险因素：1 型糖尿病>2 型糖尿病、其他血管床动脉粥样硬化、中风史。

[4] 更低风险：不满足上述的(a)或(b)标准。

[5] 每年临床评估。

[6] 建议心脏病咨询。

CAD，冠状动脉疾病；PCI，经皮冠状动脉介入治疗；CABG，冠状动脉旁路移植术；ACC，美国心脏病学会；AHA，美国心脏学协会。

表 37.3 终末期肾病人群癌症的分类

ESKD 相关
- 肾脏
- 尿道
- 甲状腺
- 骨髓瘤

免疫缺乏相关
- 霍奇金淋巴瘤
- 非霍奇金淋巴瘤
- 白血病
- 皮肤黑色素瘤
- 卡波西肉瘤
- 癌：
  - 唇
  - 口、舌、扁桃体、口咽
  - 食管
  - 胃
  - 肛门
  - 肝
  - 喉
  - 肺
  - 宫颈、子宫、阴道、外阴
  - 阴茎
  - 眼(仅鳞状细胞癌)

与免疫缺乏不相关
- 直肠
- 乳腺
- 卵巢
- 前列腺

状况不确定
- 所有其他癌

Data from Steward et al.[22]

性(男女比例为 7:1)、非洲裔美国人、透析持续时间、严重 ACKD 伴明显的器官增大[23]。

对于等待名单中患者进行肾肿瘤筛查的频率尚未达成一致。然而，所有适合移植的候选者都应进行基线肾脏超声检查。筛查频率应该依据为透析患者制定的指南。如果在最初筛查时没有 ACKD 的证据，超声可以每年或每两年复查一次[23]。已经持续透析 3~5 年的患者应每年筛查[24]。良性囊肿(Bosniak Ⅰ和Ⅱ)需要每 6 个月或 12 个月复查超声，病变进展者应进一步行增强计算机断层扫描(CT)或磁共振成像(MRI)检查。存在中度复杂囊肿(Bosniak ⅡF)的患者应每 3 个月复查超声，每 12 个月做一次增强 CT 或 MRI。如果出现不确定的囊性肿块(Bosniak Ⅲ)或明显恶性的囊性肿块(Bosniak Ⅳ)，则必须进一步应用增强 CT 或 MRI 进行评估并向泌尿科转诊[23]。RCC 患者需要的移植前无瘤等待时间取决于肿瘤分期及病变范围(见第 28 章)。已提出的针对 ACKD 和肾肿瘤的筛查方案列于图 37.3。

需要注意的是，原有肾脏囊肿(NRC)和透析持续时间也被认为是移植后 RCC 的危险因素[25]。在一项包含 1036 例肾移植受者的单中心研究中，常规应用超声对原有肾脏和移植肾脏进行筛查(首次检查在术后 1个月内，无囊肿者每 5 年一次，有囊肿者每 2 年一次)，10 例无症状的肾移植受者被诊断为 RCC，中位移植后时间为 5.8 年。根据是否存在 NRC 和时间，移植受者分为无 NRC 组(No-NRC，n=392)，新发 NRC 组(New-NRC，n=166)，移植前已存在 NRC 组(Pre-NRC，n=274)和时间不确定 NRC 组(TI-NRC，n=204)。在研究期间，移植前已

表 37.4 针对等待名单中移植候选人的癌症监测的预防性保健建议

筛查对象	开始年龄(岁)	早期检测和预防保健	筛查频率
结肠直肠癌	平均风险:50	早期检测与预防(首选)	结肠镜:每 10 年,或每 5 年可屈性乙状结肠镜检查,或每 5 年 CT 结肠成像
		只进行早期检测	每年查粪便潜血,或每年进行粪便免疫化学试验
	风险增加:40	结肠镜	每 5 年,如果一级亲属在 60 岁前患结直肠癌
			@年龄小于最年轻的诊断患有结直肠癌的家庭成员 10 岁
			每 10 年,如果亲属在 60 岁时诊断为结肠癌
			如果两位或以上的一级亲属患有结直肠癌,应考虑转诊到医学遗传学科室
女性			
乳腺癌	50~75	乳腺检查和乳腺 X 线筛查	每 1 或 2 年
	40~49	乳腺检查和乳腺 X 线筛查	每 1 或 2 年(目前对该年龄组无支持或反对证据)
	30 岁以前 (如果患者母亲或姐妹患有乳腺癌)		
宫颈癌[1]	性交发生后 3 年或 21岁,以先到者为准	巴氏涂片和盆腔检查	每年进行常规细胞学检查
			每 2 年进行液基细胞学检查
男性			
前列腺癌[2]	50	PSA 检测(伴或不伴直肠指检)	每年,如果 PSA>2.5ng/mL
	40~45[3]	PSA 检测(伴或不伴直肠指检)	每 2 年,如果 PSA<2.5ng/mL

[1] 对于年龄>30 岁的患者,若无高危因素且连续 3 次涂片结果正常,每 2 年进行检查。
[2] 美国癌症协会推荐。
[3] 非洲裔美国人,有亲属在 65 岁前患前列腺癌,或携带 *BRCA1* 和(或)*BRCA2* 突变的男性。
PSA,前列腺特异性抗原。

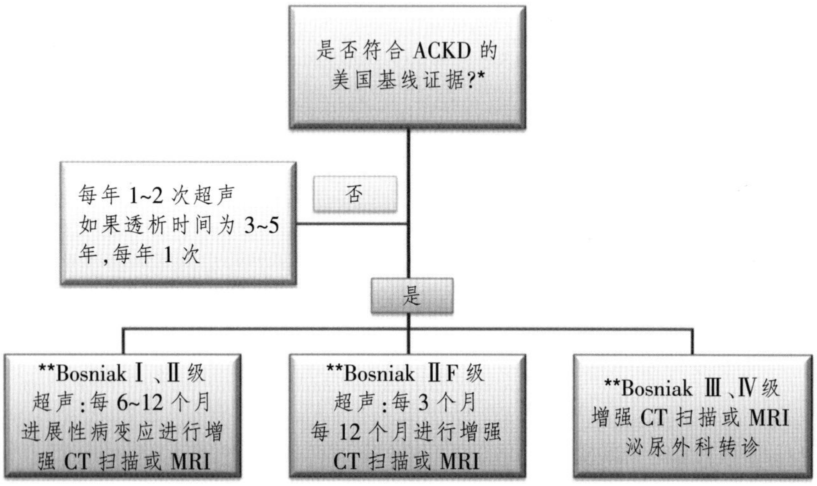

图 37.3 对获得性肾囊肿(ACKD)和肾脏肿瘤患者推荐的筛查流程。
*ACKD:每个肾脏>3~5 个囊肿。
**Bosniak Ⅰ、Ⅱ级,良性囊肿;Bosniak ⅡF 级,中度复杂囊肿;Bosniak Ⅲ级,不能定性的囊性肿物;Bosniak Ⅳ级,明确的恶性肿瘤。

存在 NRC 组和时间不确定 NRC 组发生了 10 例 RCC,无 NRC 组和新发 NRC 组没有出现 RCC。移植前已存在 NRC 组和时间不确定 NRC 组的透析持续时间长于无 NRC 组和新发 NRC 组[(6.7±3.9)年和(3.3±3.2)年对(2.7±3.1)年和(2.6±2.4)年]。这一研究结果显示,NRC 和增加的透析持续时间是移植后 RCC 的危险因素[25]。

感染性疾病筛查

虽然不同移植中心的工作有一定差别，但通常接受的标准筛查内容包括肝炎血清学检查（乙肝表面抗原，乙肝核心抗体 IgM 和 IgG，乙肝表面抗体，丙肝抗体）、HIV_1 和 HIV_2 抗体、巨细胞病毒 IgG 抗体、快速血浆反应素试验(RPR)或梅毒螺旋体颗粒凝集试验(TP-PA)、EB 病毒抗体组合(EBV)、单纯疱疹病毒(HSV)和水痘-带状疱疹病毒 (VZV)IgG 抗体、PPD 皮肤试验或 QuantiFERON TB Gold 试验。近些年，传统的 PPD 皮肤试验逐渐被 QuantiFERON TB Gold 试验取代。后者在接种过卡介苗的患者中有助于区分 PPD 试验中的卡介苗接种反应和 TB 反应。所有预期接受移植的患者在初始评估时都要完成检测。基于流行病学风险和暴露历史的特殊血清学试验包括球孢子菌 IgM 和 IgG 抗体、组织胞浆菌免疫扩散抗体或尿抗原、人 T 细胞淋巴病毒(HTLV-Ⅰ/Ⅱ)抗体，类圆线虫抗体和锥形虫抗体[26]。

等待移植过程中是否需要重复肝炎和 HIV 血清学检查通常取决于肾病专家的判定。2002 年在费城召开了管理等待名单中患者的国家共识会议，专家组制定了等待名单中患者定期监测特定感染性疾病的指南(表 37.5)[27]。

表 37.5 等待名单中移植候选人的传染病监测

人类免疫缺陷病毒(HIV)	高危人群应进行年度筛查
丙型肝炎病毒(HCV)	ELISA 阴性的患者应进行年度筛查 转氨酶水平异常的 ELISA 阴性患者应考虑进行 PCR 检测 HCV 阳性的患者需要持续治疗，高等级组织学病变可能导致移植终止
乙型肝炎病毒(HBV)	之前未暴露过的患者应进行免疫接种，同时每年检测抗体水平，如有需要应进行强化注射
结核 *	PPD 阳性的患者应接受标准的化学预防治疗，并应每年进行胸部 X 线检查
类圆线虫	流行地区应进行年度筛查
EB 病毒、弓形虫、巨细胞病毒、单纯疱疹病毒	无特殊情况应进行年度检查

* 近年来，PPD 皮肤试验已经逐渐被 QuantiFERON TB Gold 检验代替。后者可区分卡介苗接种患者 PPD 试验结果中卡介苗接种的反应结果和 TB 的反应结果。

名单状态知晓

一项应用透析患者移植问卷(DPTQ)进行的单中心调查研究发现，>50%(34 人中的 18 人）的正在进行移植前检查的患者不知道他们准确的名单状态[28]。这些患者中，88.9%(18 人中的 16 人)的患者错误地认为他们已经进入等待名单，11%的患者不清楚他们的名单状态。在 32 个等待名单中的患者中，81.3%的患者准确地知道他们在等待名单中，6.2%的患者错误地认为他们尚未进入等待名单，12.5%的患者不确定。所有等待名单中不清楚等待状态的患者都是状态 7 的患者，这些患者需要进一步检查或是患有并发症。将近 2/3 的受调查者完成了高中教育，11%的受调查者完成了某种程度的大学教育。虽然这一研究对象主要为非洲裔美国人(82.8%)并且结果尚未在其他种族背景得到验证，对等待状态缺乏意识大多发生于高中毕业生的结果显示在移植团队、患者以及转诊肾病内科医生之间缺乏交流。有人建议应用 DPTQ 收集自我报告数据并将其与 UNOS 等待名单数据库进行比较是对可纠正的问题的快速且不昂贵的筛查办法。

在作者所在的中心，所有等待名单中的移植候选者每年都会通过邮件被告知他们的 UNOS 等待名单状态。患者被建议在人口学或健康状态发生改变时要通知他们的移植协调员(或者移植团队其他成员)，这些状态包括：迁居、转诊至其他透析中心、联系方式改变、并发症或住院。我们的政策还包括每个季度将所有等待名单中移植候选者及其当前状态发给相应的透析单位的社会工作者。

管理死亡供体等待名单：国家调查

在美国，一项包含 192 个 UNOS 认证的中心的国家调查显示，71%的中心支持对所有等待名单中的患者进行常规随访监测，监测可以通过有计划的访视或是中心发起的电话联系进行[27]。随访频率和贯彻标准癌症预防筛查(乳腺、宫颈和结肠)在一定程度上受移植中心规模的影响。与大的移植中心相比，小的移植中心更能够遵守标准癌症筛查建议(<500 名患者的中心占 72%，>500 名患者的中心占 54%；$P<0.05$)。80%的中

心要求定期进行肝炎病毒血清学检查,52%的中心要求进一步检查其他感染性疾病。79%的中心要求规律监测前列腺特异性抗原。无症状心脏高风险候选者定义为存在已确定的CAD、糖尿病、高龄或肥胖,需要每年进行心脏筛查。大多数中心采取无创心脏检查,超过50%的移植中心具有指定的心脏病医生或心脏病医生团队。

虽然定期的随访和持续更新患者的医学、社会心理学和人口学资料给移植中心增加了大量的负担,但是如果缺乏这些监测会增加患者由于人口学变化而下落不明的可能性,增加由于意外的或是未曾发现的新的医疗问题导致的移植手术取消的概率,如果这些问题被忽视会导致围术期并发症发生率和死亡率的增加。与大的中心相比,小的中心的患者因为意外的医学问题而被送回家的频率更低。这种事件在61%的移植中心受影响的预期的受者不到2%(80%为小的中心;与大的中心相比 $P<0.001$)。7个中心表明超过10%的患者因为未认识到的或未预见到的医学问题而被送回家。

随着进入死亡供体等待名单中的人数日益增多,特别是老年候选者越来越多,移植中心管理移植候选者的难度逐渐增加。在漫长的等待过程中,患者的健康状况和功能状态可能会恶化,也可能出现新的医学或社会心理问题。这些变化可能会使患者不适于进行移植,或者需要进一步诊断性检查或管理。由于没有针对每个移植中心该如何处理这些问题的具体建议,这里把通用的指南列于表37.6。

等待名单移除

由于死亡、移植、发生了无法逆转的移植禁忌证或是其他任何原因而从等待名单移除时,应在24小时内报告至OPTN。

今后的研究

下述问题需要进一步研究:

- 心脏事件高危风险的定义需要仔细研究并在前瞻性研究中验证,避免重复试验增加成本和不便[28]。
- 应设计和实施前瞻性研究评估非侵袭性心脏检查在等待名单中患者中的作用,确定重复检查的最理想的和最低的需求[28]。

表37.6 等待名单中移植候选人管理的一般原则

1.每个移植中心应承担以下职责:
(a)建立一个结构良好的系统以保持其与等待名单中患者的持续接触
(b)建立与肾脏内科医生和透析人员的通畅沟通[28]
(c)明确对患者、他们的肾脏内科医生以及透析人员的期望。(例如,任何医疗或心理问题应被及时通报给移植项目组,确保患者的血液样本在预定的时间内被发送到HLA实验室。这将允许HLA实验室在获得可用肾源时无需患者新鲜样本即可进行最终的交叉配型)
(d)密切监测心脏事件高危患者。一种用于等待名单患者持续心脏监测的推荐算法见表37.2[19]
(e)如果可行的话,应指定专家协助等待名单患者的护理计划
(f)建立将患者移入或移出等待名单的标准,以防止肾脏被分配给在医学上不适宜接受移植的患者
(g)进行定期的多学科团队会议,积极解决患者的医疗、手术以及与患者移植候选人资格相关的社会心理问题。根据团队的共识意见,患者被分为下列几种状态:列入名单;维持;延期;移除名单;移植启动
(h)根据"匹配"结果在ABO每个血型组确定前10~20位移植候选人,重新评估他们的整体健康状况和人口问题,以确保他们随时准备移植
(i)建立一个系统,每年告知名单中候选人的UNOS等待状态(或由单独的移植项目建立,定期提醒)
2.移植前的其他方面也应当加以考虑:
(a)成本的影响,对于重复患者评估和心脏检查的医疗、护理和管理要求应引起政府机构、第三方保险公司和医院管理部门的重视[28]
(b)应密切关注等待名单中移植候选人的健康状况,特别是应谨慎对待其心脏风险,以优化移植相对于透析的最终获益和存活优势[28]
(c)关于扩大标准供体(ECD),ECD肾脏双侧移植,以及公共卫生服务高风险下死亡的供体肾脏的选项,应在初始评估时与患者进行讨论,且这些选项应在随访期间重新申明,以促进这些器官能够被及时而妥当地分配给事先同意的患者
(d)对于心脏风险较高的患者和等待进行胰腺移植的患者,应考虑提高随访频率

• 随机对照研究，比较常规筛查与非常规筛查对主要不良心脏事件的影响[29]。

总结

等待名单管理是一个积极的过程，在透析单位、患者、移植协调员和移植中心之间不间断地进行交流。大多数移植中心尝试每年访视一次移植候选者。但是随着进入等待名单中患者数量的日益增加，对所有移植候选者进行定期或是每年的随访变得不现实。了解可能影响等待时间的因素可以让临床医生和移植协调员制定切实可行的步骤，确保等待名单顶部的患者随时适于移植。在洛杉矶加利福尼亚大学，我们每年对各个 ABO 血型排名前 30 的患者和个人信息出现在配型程序中的患者进行随访，对他们的总体健康情况和人口学情况进行再次评估。在访视时，也会回顾常规健康维护状态和与年龄、性别相适应的癌症筛查，癌症筛查内容包括前列腺特异性抗原、乳腺 X 线、宫颈涂片和结肠镜。虽然各移植中心之间对等待名单中患者进行心脏监测的建议差别很大，但是大多数中心都支持对合并糖尿病的移植候选者每年进行心脏筛查。

除了再次评估患者的医学和社会心理状况，活体供体的可获得性应再次被提及。目前，为最大化利用活体供肾，我们实施了一项评估交叉配型阳性和 ABO 不相容供受体的方案。患者被建议选择活体供体，包括配对交叉移植，通过脱敏方案的阳性交叉配型和 ABO 不相容移植，ABO 不相容交叉配型阳性的患者通过活体供肾交换移植。对于老年移植候选者，应告知其 ECD 肾移植的优点和缺点。

最后，患者的初始肾病专家和移植中心的有效沟通是非常重要的，可以使患者在可以获得死亡供肾时处于最理想的医学健康状态。虽然不同移植中心的实践指南有所差别，但是等待名单管理也需要适应变化的肾脏分配系统。将透析等待时间和 eGFR≤20cc/min 纳入分配系统使得移植中心更好地预测在一定的时间内哪个候选者最可能分配到器官。因此，移植中心应确保每个血型未致敏的患者中等待时间最长者随时在医学和社会心理方面适于移植。

（高鹏骥 译　高鹏骥 校）

参考文献

1. OPTN/UNOS Database as of August 26, 2011. Available from: http://www.unos.org.
2. Danovitch GM. The Kidney Transplant Waiting List. UptoDate. 2011. Available from: http://www.uptodate.com.
3. Hall YN, Choi AI, Xu P, et al. Racial ethnic differences in rates and determinants of deceased donor kidney transplantation. Journal of the American Society of Nephrology. 2011;22:743–751.
4. Adams PL, Graham WK, Gunderson S. Kidney allocation: role of UNOS and OPOs. In: McKay DB, Steinberg SM, editors. Kidney Transplantation: A Guide to the Care of Kidney Transplant Recipients, 1st ed. New York: Springer; 2010: 57–72.
5. Merion RM, Guidinger MK, Newmann JM, et al. Prevalence and outcomes of multiple-listing for cadaveric kidney and liver transplantation. American Journal of Transplantation. 2004;4:94–100.
6. Kumar V, Julian BA, Deierhoi MH, et al. Secondary listing for deceased-donor kidney transplantation does not increase likelihood of engraftment at a large transplant center. American Journal of Transplantation. 2009;9:1671–1673.
7. Meier-Kriesche HU, Port FK, Ojo AO, et al. Effect of waiting time on renal transplant outcome. Kidney International. 2000;58(3):1311–1317.
8. Gill J, Cho YW, Danovitch GM, et al. Outcomes of dual kidney transplantation in the United States: an analysis of the OPTN/UNOS database. Transplantation. 2008;85(1):62–68.
9. Rudich SM, Kaplan B, Magee JC, et al. Renal transplantations performed using non-heart-beating organ donors: going back to the future? Transplantation. 2002;74:1715–1720.
10. Gaston RS, Danovitch GM, Adams PL, et al. The report of a national conference on the wait list for kidney transplantation. American Journal of Transplantation. 2003;3:775–785.
11. Analysis for the OPTN Minority Affairs Committee Meeting on 03/11/2008. Data prepared by the Scientific Registry of Transplant Recipients.
12. Kasiske BL, Cangro CB, Hariharan S, et al. The evaluation of the renal transplant candidates: clinical practice guidelines. American Journal of Transplantation. 2001;1(Suppl 1):5–95.
13. Klocke FJ, Baird MG, Lorell BH, et al. ACC/AHA/ASNC guidelines for the clinical use of cardiac radionuclide imaging -executive summary: a report of the American College of Cardiology/American Heart Association Task Force on Practice Guidelines (ACC/AHA/ASNC Committee to Revise the 1995 Guidelines for the Clinical Use of Cardiac Radionuclide Imaging). Journal of the American College of Cardiology. 2003;42:1318–1333.
14. Lentine KL, Hurst FP, Jindal RM, et al. Cardiovascular risk assessment among potential kidney transplant candidates: approaches and controversies. American Journal of Kidney Diseases 2009;55(1):152–167.
15. Lee TH, Marcantonio ER, Mangione CM, et al. Derivation and prospective validation of a simple index for prediction of cardiac risk of major noncardiac surgery. Circulation. 1999;100:1043–1049.
16. Fleisher LA, Beckman JA, Brown KA, et al. ACC/AHA 2007 guidelines on perioperative cardiovascular evaluation and care for noncardiac surgery. A report of the American College of Cardiology/American Heart Association Task Force on Practice Guidelines (writing committee to revise the 2002 Guidelines on Perioperative Cardiovascular Evaluation for Noncardiac Surgery). Journal of the American College of Cardiology. 2007;50:e159–e241.
17. Benitez RM, Conolly HM, Freeman RV, et al. Coronary artery disease: Risk factors for coronary artery disease. In: Otto CM, Weitz HH, editors. Cardiovascular Medicine. Medical Knowledge Self-Assessment Program 15; 2009: 10–12.
18. K/DOQI Work Group. K/DOQI clinical practice guidelines for cardiovascular disease in dialysis patients. American Journal of Kidney Diseases. 2005;45(4 Suppl 3):S1–S153.
19. Pham PT, Pham PA, Pham PC, et al. Evaluation of adult kidney transplant candidate. Seminars in Nephrology. 2010;23(6):595–605.
20. Cunningham R. Valvular heart disease in patients with end-stage renal disease. 2011 UpToDate. Available from: http://www.uptodate.com.
21. Bonow RO, Carabello BA, Chatterjee K, et al. ACC/AHA 2006 guidelines for the management of patients with valvular heart disease. A report of the American College of Cardiology/American Heart Association Task Force on Practice Guidelines. Journal of the American College of Cardiology. 2006;48(3):e1–e148.
22. Steward JH, Vajdic CM, van Leewen MT, et al. The pattern of excess cancer in dialysis and transplantation. Nephrology, Dialysis, Transplantation. 2008;24: 3225–3231.
23. Eitner F. Acquired cystic kidney disease and malignant neoplasms. In: Floege J, Johnson RJ, Feehally J, editors. Comprehensive Clinical Nephrology, 4th ed. St. Louis, MO: Elsevier Saunders; 2010: 1010–1015.
24. Chapman AB Acquired cystic disease of the kidney in adults. Upto Date. 2011;

Available from: http://www.uptodate.com.

25. Goh A, Vathsala A. Native renal cysts and dialysis duration are risk factors for renal cell carcinoma in renal transplant recipients. American Journal of Transplantation. 2010;10:1–7.
26. Pegues DA, Kubak BM, Maree CL, et al. Infections in kidney transplantation. In: Danovitch GM, editor. Handbook of Kidney Transplantation, 5th ed. Philadelphia, PA: Lippincott Williams & Wilkins; 2010: 251–279.
27. Danovitch GM, Hariharan S, Prirsch JD, et al. Management of the waiting list for cadaveric kidney transplants: report of a survey and recommendations by the Clinical Practice Guidelines Committee of the American Society of Transplantation. Journal of the American Society of Nephrology. 2002;13:528–535.
28. Gillespie A, Hammer H, Lee J, et al. Lack of listing status awareness: results of a single-center survey of hemodialysis patients. American Journal of Transplantation. 2011;11:1522–1526.
29. Kasiske BL, Israni AK, Snyder JJ, et al. Design considerations and feasibility for a clinical trial to examine coronary screening before kidney transplantation (COST). American Journal of Kidney Diseases. 2011;57(6):908–916.

第 38 章
肝移植等待名单管理

John G. O’Grady

引言

列入肝移植等待名单的患者直到移植前都需要积极的诊疗。等待名单上的患者大致可以分为四类:慢性肝病、肝细胞癌、急性肝衰竭和其他疾病。大多数患者有慢性肝病和一些肝衰竭的并发症，这些是肝移植的指征。肝细胞癌(HCC)在其全病程中可以并发肝硬化,从完全代偿性疾病到一定程度肝衰竭，各个阶段都有必要行肝移植。这对等待移植期间如何管理疾病的恶性组成有重要启示。移植的其他指征与肝硬化的严重程度无关。例如,比起肝硬化的严重程度,肝肺综合征(HPS)和门静脉高压的严重程度更相关。急性肝衰竭由急诊移植负责诊疗,等待时间数以天计,这个时期正处于临床强化活动期。

有时,列入等待名单的患者病情恢复到一定程度,有可能被从名单上移除（如果最小列表标准适用),或因未达到终末期肝病评分模型(MELD)的标准而不能被分配器官。这种情况最常见于潜在病因为酒精性或病毒性肝炎,因戒酒或抗病毒治疗有所缓解的患者。然而,更典型的临床情况是恶化,因死亡、病情过重,或肿瘤生长超过移植标准,20%~30%列入等待名单的慢性肝病患者不能接受移植。这些不能维持患者处于适合移植情况的例子说明，移植等待名单管理面临着巨大挑战。类似地,一部分急性肝衰竭患者,有可能病情恶化到一定程度以至于不能接受移植，或未移植而存活下来。

本章肝病管理的重点不是回顾治疗方案和选择,而是对于即将进行肝移植的患者，如何改善和应用标准的护理方法。本章与第 29 章(介绍肝移植的适应证)和第 43 章(详述肝衰竭患者的重症监护管理)互为补充。

等待名单

在美国,等待-移植的比例大约是 2.5:1,英国大约是 1.5:1。最完整的关于等待名单组成的数据来源于美国。移植受者科学注册系统(SRTR)1997—2006 年数据显示,这段期间内有 12 000 位登记者,其中 72%年龄超过 50 岁,72%为白种人,61%为男性[1]。除了 3%的登记者,其他人都在等待他们的第一次移植。血型分布为 50%O 型,38%A 型,11%B 型和 2%AB 型。2006 年底,64%的人等待时间> 1 年,47%> 2 年,移植的中位时间是 306 天。死亡率稳步下降,根据种族不同,变化范围为 9%~14%。不同临床情况的死亡率见表 38.1。终末期肝病评分>30 的患者，几乎 1/2 可以在 30 天内进行移植,而 1/5 则在这段期间内死亡。一些地区等待名单的死亡率已经下降,尤其是在西班牙和法国,实现了死亡率低于 5%。

表 38.1　不同临床情况下的死亡率——SRTR 数据 2006 年

临床情况	死亡率
总体	11.7%
MELD 评分 6~10	3.4%
MELD 评分 21~30	6.5%
MELD 评分>30	36.7%
急性肝衰竭	18.7%
代谢障碍	14.3%
恶性疾病	12.3%
硬化(胆汁郁积症除外)	10.9%
胆汁郁积症	7.7%
肝细胞癌除外	11%
其他情况	15.0%

影响等待时间的因素

患者等待移植的时间长短取决于一系列因素(表38.2)。以MELD为基础的和相关的分配系统推广这样的原则:病情最重的患者优先考虑移植,与其列入等待名单的时间长短无关。在美国系统中,等待时间的唯一作用是对于具有相同MELD评分的患者进行决断。然而,约25%的等待移植的患者会具有低且稳定的MELD评分,包括肝细胞癌或其他适应证的患者(例如肝肺综合征、家族性淀粉样多神经病),如果他们要接受移植,还需要额外给予积分。有很多方法解决这个问题,其中一个比较复杂的是法国个性化系统,增加了有关13种临床情况的积分[2]。等待时间也受到器官供体–受体匹配程度的影响。这可以通过正式的捐赠者风险指数(DRI)评价,或仅是达到避免不利配对的目的,如一个老人的脂肪变供肝供给一个丙型肝炎病毒(HCV)相关疾病的患者。

表38.2　影响等待时间和器官分配的因素

因素	注释
主要决定因素	
原始MELD评分	广泛使用的决定因素
调整MELD评分	补偿不能由原始MELD评分反映需求的患者
列入等待名单的时间	在英国和欧洲一些地区是重要因素
次要决定因素	
血型	O型血患者倾向于等待更长时间,对其他血型作用随种族而异
捐赠者风险指数(DRI)	目标是寻找合适的匹配以得到更好的结果
脂肪变性的程度	和DRI概念相同
体型	体型娇小的成年人与儿童竞争的问题
捐赠者年龄	可能影响丙肝患者的器官分配,虽然实践倾向于反映降低疾病复发的期望
病毒感染史	有HBV、HCV或HIV病毒感染的证据,可能要与有相同感染的患者匹配
很少或没有影响	
组织相容性	很少用于肝脏分配
捐赠者年龄	不存在影响疾病复发的证据

肝硬化和相关并发症

常规监测

临床和实验室监测的频率可以反映肝脏疾病的严重程度、相对稳定性或患者的其他情况。每隔1~2个月的门诊监测对于这个人群是相当平常的。基于MELD的器官分配系统或相关系统可能会要求实验室更新结果的频率。监测的目的是记录肝脏疾病严重程度的变化情况、电解质情况和需要治疗的肾功能情况。

肝硬化患者的常规监测为门静脉高压和HCC。监测内容的细节可能因机构或国家而异,但是这些应在患者列入等待名单后持续进行。每隔4~6个月进行肝脏超声检查,可以解决监测的两个部分,因为超声通常是HCC的筛查项目(经常与甲胎蛋白结合),同时可以评估门静脉的通畅性。早期HCC也许能通过超声检测到,进行分期则需要依赖其他手段,通常使用计算机断层摄影(CT)和(或)磁共振成像(MRI)。这些HCC中的一小部分超过了移植标准,则这些患者应从等待名单移除。更典型的是,新诊断HCC考虑桥接治疗的患者,仍列于等待名单上。

门静脉血栓的发展与移植手术医生相关,非常广泛的血栓形成可能改变患者进行肝移植的适用性。虽然抗凝不是门静脉血栓形成并发肝硬化的标准措施,其作用需要在等待移植的患者中进行评估。考虑到血栓可能增加手术的复杂性,预防血栓扩大需要考虑出血风险。新形成的门静脉血栓可以导致门静脉压力的突然增加,显著增大静脉曲张破裂出血的风险。因此,食管和胃底静脉曲张的内镜评估是需要的。

腹水

顽固性腹水可以是肝移植的主要指征,并且在这种情况下,几乎没有其他治疗可以选择。这种情况下的重点是限制可能影响移植的治疗相关的副作用。利尿剂可引起或加重低钠血症和肾功能损害。一致认为肾功能与移植后的结果相关,最大程度降低对肾功能的不良影响是合理的。由于这两个原因,利尿剂的选择应该以安全性为首要考虑因素而不是功效,特别是当患者接近于有机会被分配器官的时间。在基于MELD的分配系统中,肌酐升高可能需要减少或停止利尿剂使用,以免在器官分配方面获得优势。定期或程序性穿刺可能是顽固性腹水患者的唯一选择,而每次穿刺都有出血或感染的风险。

在其他情况下,腹水可能会发展或恶化,而成为优先肝移植的指征。初始诊疗方法是沿着标准线,遵守注意事项(表 38.3),包括限制盐、限制液体摄入在 800~1500mL/d、利尿剂和穿刺。管理腹水的常规方案可以扩展到在合成功能良好和无肝性脑病病史的患者中,应用经静脉肝内门体分流术(TIPS)。然而,这种情况的患者更有可能已列入移植等待名单,而不适合接受 TIPS。在没有 HCC 的情况下,由于 TIPS 可能不利于移植和 TIPS 错位的可能性,限制了这种治疗方案的吸引力。

自发性细菌性腹膜炎(SBP)是等待肝移植患者的一种严重的并发症。抗生素预防 SBP,通常用喹诺酮(如诺氟沙星 400mg/d),可以常规用于有腹水的患者,或既往有 SBP 发作的风险增加的患者,或腹水中白蛋白水平非常低的患者。使用上述治疗时,应考虑对移植等待名单上的所有患者均预防性用药。反复发作 SBP 的患者可并发肠襻粘连,后期常呈茧形。茧腹症增加了移植手术的复杂性,并有可能引起移植后营养不良。

低钠血症

约 30%的肝硬化患者会发生低钠血症,通常与利尿剂使用相关,调整这些药物的使用可能会改善低钠血症。低钠血症也可以独立发生,这种情况更难以纠正,而且提示预后不良。因此,一些评分系统中包括血钠水平,如 MELD-Na 和英国终末期肝病(UKELD)。限制液体摄入是目前唯一可行的诊疗自发性低钠血症的方法。如果当分配到器官时,血钠低于 125mEq/L,需要在移植前进行超滤纠正,因为围手术期发生的血钠水平的快速波动,可导致脑桥中央髓鞘溶解症。

肝肾综合征

对于等待肝移植患者,肝肾综合征(HRS)是肝硬化最关键的并发症,住院患者中高达 25%,重症监护患者中达 40%~60%[2]。1 型肾功能快速进行性恶化,并在几个星期内演变(表 38.4)。2 型症状不明显,病情较轻。相比 2 型 HRS,1 型与晚期肝病更相关,常见于严重的门静脉高压患者。1 型和 2 型 HRS 均与固有肾脏疾病无关,相对更常见于肝硬化患者。基于 MELD 的器官分配系统不可避免地增加了存在肾功能障碍的肝移植患者的积分。

HRS 的治疗方案包括血浆扩容、血管活性药物和肝移植。在欧洲,特利加压素是首选的血管收缩药,而美国更常用米多君或肾上腺素。白蛋白和特利加压素联合应用被认为是 1 型 HRS 的一线治疗,在高达 50%的病例中有显效[3,4]。敏感性高的患者表现为早期疾病和平均动脉压持续升高,虽然后者不一定改善肾功能[5]。这种治疗的价值体现在移植的桥接治疗,而不是直接改善生存率。肾功能正常或接近正常的患者移植后在肾脏支持的需求方面、住院时间和生存率方面均有明显的获益[2]。支持 2 型 HRS 患者使用这种方案的证据较少。基本上,这些患者和急性肾小管坏死致肾衰的患者,可能等待肝移植期间均需要肾脏替代治疗。

基于 MELD 的分配系统的一个意外结果是同时需要肝移植和肾移植的患者数量急剧增加。肝移植时伴有肾衰的患者可以同时接受肝、肾移植,但是一些患者的肾功能在肝移植成功后可以得到恢复,包括至少 30%接受联合移植的患者。针对联合移植的患者选择的指南正在改进,但尚未完全确定。相比急性肾小管坏死(ATN),HRS 患者的肾功能更有可能恢复。在一项研究中,移植后 90 天观察到 88%的 HRS 患者肾功能有改善,71%的 ATN 患者有改善[6]。移植前肾脏支持的持续时间也影响功能恢复的可能性。当透析的持续时间

表 38.3 腹水的管理

注意事项	注释
限制盐摄入	不要损害营养状态
限制液体摄入	优先保持血钠>130mmol/L
利尿剂	优先考虑安全性,而不是疗效
穿刺	白蛋白替代治疗可能也有益
经静脉肝内门体分流术(TIPS)	尽量避免
抗生素	考虑预防自发性细菌性腹膜炎

表 38.4 1 型和 2 型肝肾综合征的定义和特点

1 型
血肌酐 2 周内成倍增长,超过 2.5mg / dL
或
肌酐清除率减少至少 50%至<20 mL / min
晚期肝衰竭患者出现快速、进行性并且无法解释原因的肾衰竭
2 型
血肌酐 1.5~2.5mg / dL
比 1 型增长慢
通常肝功能良好,但有明显的门静脉高压

不超过4周可以观察到最好的结果[7]。这个标准等同于6~12周的联合治疗。这个讨论的实际意义是:是否需要肾活检对个体案例做出决定。肾脏组织学可以提供很好的预后信息，但这需要与活检后出血的风险进行平衡。

静脉曲张破裂出血

静脉曲张破裂出血是肝移植患者所面临的潜在不稳定事件中最急性的。虽然静脉曲张破裂出血后的总生存率显著提高，但肝移植等待患者的死亡风险仍在30%左右[8]。除非对药物不耐受,否则应该维持予普萘洛尔一线或二线预防,使脉搏保持在60次/分左右。这种情况下,低血压是主要的限制因素。没有数据支持在列入移植等待名单后改为内镜监测曲张静脉或内镜预防的方案。

静脉曲张破裂出血的诊疗应遵循标准的规程[9]。只要患者给予适当的晶体、胶体、血液和血液制品复苏后,内镜仍为一线治疗。血管活性药物,如特利加压素、生长抑素及其类似物,可以引起肝动脉收缩,但并不影响移植的成功率。TIPS用于抢救内镜和药物干预无效的患者。这种情况下,TIPS的风险效益比要优于顽固性腹水,对治疗无效和(或)有胃底静脉曲张破裂出血的患者抢救时应考虑TIPS。放置TIPS时应小心,避免将分流延伸到手术区域。多达66%的患者出现细菌感染合并静脉曲张破裂出血，因此可以短期预防性应用抗生素[2]。

有些情况下,患者被分配到器官时,其正在处理活动性静脉曲张破裂出血，这时需要决定进行移植是否合适。没有数据协助决定,需要根据临床经验。门静脉压力在移植过程的早期可以降低，如果有必要建立临时分流或者体外静脉 - 静脉旁路技术,将有助于控制出血。因此,出血本身不是移植的禁忌证。但是,经常出现出血可引起肝硬化的其他并发症，这时最好在手术前稳定患者的情况。败血症、吸出入性肺炎、血流动力学不稳定和代谢异常是这种情况下常见的并发症。

脑病

肝移植受体的状态对预防脑病的方法影响有限。治疗方法如乳果糖和利福昔明，标准应用于脑病的预防。但是,限制蛋白摄入以降低脑病的发病率可能与改善营养状态相冲突,因此蛋白摄入不应过度(<60g/d)。脑病急性发作的标准管理由三部分组成:静脉输液、抗生素和导泻。此外,应该要去除诱因。

重症脑病的患者通常需要机械通气，以保护气道和维持气体交换。这与肝移植有关,因为对于分配到器官时仍插管的患者,生存率会显著降低。然而,有理由相信这可能不适用于那些插管主要是为了度过一次脑病发作的患者。这些包括相对较短的插管时间,不存在使死亡率增加的并发症。肝移植成功后,脑病逆转非常迅速,术后不需要显著延长通气时间。相比之下,移植时多器官衰竭的脑病患者需要延长相关风险的支持时间。

营养

体重指数(BMI)对肝移植的结果有影响,因此营养可能是移植前相当关注的焦点。低BMI(<18kg/m^2)患者需要加强营养支持是最明显的证据，在严重的晚期肝病患者中,获益会低于摄入热量的预期值。营养支持的一般原则适用于这样的人群[11]。常规使用营养补充剂或鼻饲营养。

有关BMI升高的影响的证据仍不太清楚,一些研究发现BMI>(35~40)kg/m^{2}的患者有相似的结果,而其他研究则显示相互矛盾的数据。不考虑证据,许多肝移植项目经验性地推荐肥胖患者在等待移植时减轻体重。肥胖患者在增加运动方面的选择有限,因此限制热量摄入是其主要方法。

急性失代偿发作

上述讨论的并发症通常在急性失代偿发作期间共同存在。最近,慢性肝衰竭急性发作已被用于描述这种情况,但这个术语不被普遍接受,一些权威人士更愿意仍使用“慢性肝衰竭急性发作”,因为它保留了与肝硬化无关的含义。感染和静脉曲张破裂出血是引起多器官衰竭最常见的原因,这些又反过来引起脑病、血流动力学不稳定和肾功能障碍(图38.1)。这些患者通常在重症监护室中管理,并且很有可能插管。

这种情况下,有器官供应时,可能非常困难做出是否进行移植的决定。死亡率在40%,大多数发生在进入重症监护一周内[2]。另一方面,肝移植的1年生存率在这种情况下大约是60%，或比有慢性肝病的门诊患者低25%~30%[1]。需要判断患者的病情改善有多大的可能性,从而增加患者的最终生存机会。现有的预后模型

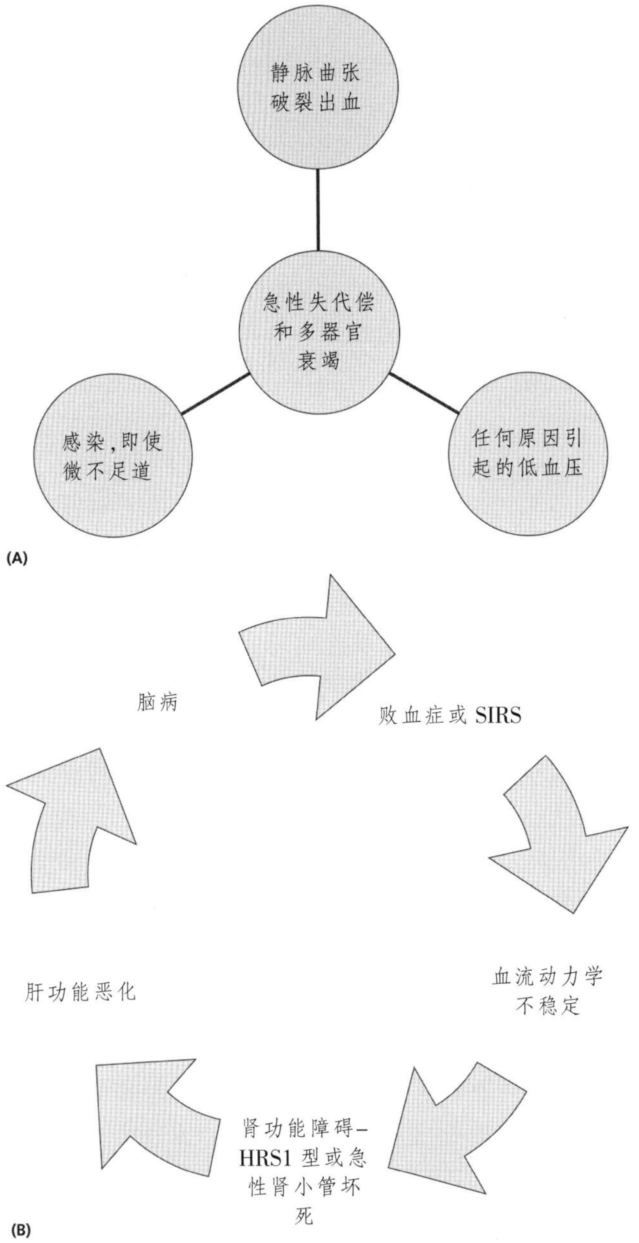

图 38.1 (A)慢性肝病的急性失代偿有三个主要诱因。(B)是一个并发症相互作用的恶性循环。SIRS，全身炎症反应综合征；HRS，肝肾综合征。

没有极大的精确度，最终的决定需要依赖共同的临床判断。MELD 评分<26，序贯器官衰竭估计(SOFA)评分<9，因静脉曲张破裂出血或脑病进入重症监护室的患者最有可能恢复[2]。供体器官的质量是做出决策的另一个因素。进行性恶化的患者越早获得可用的器官获益越大，而相对稳定的患者可能更愿意等待一个质量更好的器官。

抗病毒治疗

根据地理位置不同，在 25%~50%的病例中，慢性病毒性肝炎是肝移植的指征。在美国和欧洲，丙型肝炎病毒(HCV)占主导地位，而在亚洲更常见的是乙型肝炎病毒(HBV)。HCC 与两种病毒均相关，HCC 见于 1/3 的 HCV 病例。HBV 患者中合并 HCC 的比例更高，这是因为抗病毒治疗显著减少了终末期慢性肝病移植的需求。历史上，HBV 复发是一个主要问题，但现在已经可以在大多数病例中得到预防或管理。而 HCV 的复发仍然是一个主要问题，直至最近才开始形成对抗它的策略。

乙型肝炎

随着移植后乙型肝炎免疫球蛋白的应用，乙肝患者肝移植的效果显著改善。从开始就很明显，这种策略的成功取决于移植时血液中的低 HBV DNA 水平。可有效控制 HBV 复制的一系列抗病毒药物的发展，使大多数患者在选择肝移植时 HBV DNA 阴性。药物的选择受到控制病毒复制的速度和病毒的耐药现状的影响。当需要获得快速病毒学应答时，更倾向于使用拉米夫定和替诺福韦。维持抗病毒治疗的患者在等待移植时，应每隔 6 个月筛查耐药性。

丙型肝炎

与 HBV 一样，移植前清除病毒血症对患者也有潜在的益处。高达 70%的移植时 HCV RNA 阴性的患者可能不会复发。然而，只有少数感染 HCV 的等待移植患者可以达到 HCV RNA 阴性。聚乙二醇干扰素和利巴韦林的标准治疗方案，实际上只能用于完全代偿的肝硬化患者，因此只有一部分 HCC 患者可以选择这种方案。其余患者有一种替代方案，称为低剂量快速摄入方案(LADR)，这是一种滴定方法，如果治疗的耐受性良好，可以增加剂量[12]。抗病毒治疗主要关注肝功能的恶化情况，停止治疗后可能不会扭转并导致需要肝移植，甚至死亡的紧急事件发生。理论上，抗病毒治疗对血液系统的副作用可能会导致术中和术后出现问题，但实际上大多数可以得到有效诊疗。

移植前 HCV 的治疗取得相对迅速的进展是相当

乐观的。首先,两个新药的使用,特拉匹韦和博赛泼维,增加了对基于干扰素的抗病毒治疗的应答, 并缩短了治疗时间;第二,开始治疗后依据个体的HCV基因型、IL28b基因型和病毒动力学,使评估患者是否适合抗病毒治疗变得更加容易;第三,预期有一种药物组合将出现,允许无干扰素抑制病毒复制,模仿HBV的进展。但是,目前没有预期像预防HBV复发一样将免疫球蛋白用于HCV。

HIV 病毒感染

已经有感染人类免疫缺陷病毒(HIV)的患者进行肝移植的案例,但程序仍然是实验性的,并且只应用于高度选择的患者。典型的方案要求患者的病毒载量降到无法检测, 并且如果出现耐药可以有其他抗病毒药物选择。因此, 整个等待期间均需要密切监测这些参数。艾滋病界定疾病在免疫重建后通常是移植的禁忌证,如果列入等待名单后疾病进展,则应该重新评估移植的资格。在合理选择的案例中,肝移植的结果与一般人群相当,除了HCV患者,他们的3年移植生存率只有53%[13]。低BMI(<18kg/m^2)和肾功能受损已经确定与不良预后有关,有这些特征的患者不应进行移植。

肝脏支持装置

支持衰竭肝脏的策略与等待肝移植的患者有特殊的相关性。肝脏支持装置不能提高生存率,但一些研究的证据表明,预期这些装置可以起到移植的桥接作用。这些装置将在第47章深入讨论,根据它们是否含有细胞组分,可以分为非生物和生物的。细胞组分包括正常的人肝细胞,来自人肿瘤细胞系或猪的肝细胞。还有一些方法是混合性的,它们结合了非生物和生物装置。解毒是所有人工装置的一个目的, 一系列非生物装置已经发展到可以清除水溶性和(或)蛋白结合性的毒素。只有生物装置有可能进行蛋白质合成,包括猪肝细胞、来自肿瘤细胞系或不适合肝移植的器官的人肝细胞。

白蛋白透析是最广泛应用的装置。血液或血清与白蛋白接触,使蛋白结合毒素转移。分子吸附再循环系统(MARS)既是原型,也是这些装置里最广泛使用的。一份早期报告显示, 它对重度黄疸伴肾功能不全患者有明显的改善,随后的系统综述显示,慢性肝衰竭急性发作患者的死亡率降低33%, 但对移植患者的桥接治疗无显著效果。两项随机对照试验不能证明MARS或超过标准护理的Prometheus可以提高生存率[14,15]。尽管对此有巨大热情,但白蛋白透析并没有被广泛使用。列入移植等待名单的患者使用生物系统的经验甚至更有限。最近一次包括62名患者的试验也不能证明使用体外肝脏辅助装置(ELAD)可以提高生存率或移植成活率[16]。

肝细胞癌

大多数肝移植项目对列入等待名单的患者有严格的标准,标准基于肿瘤的体积(用结节的数量和大小定义),并且要求直到移植时都符合这些标准。最原始和最广泛使用的标准是米兰标准,允许一个孤立结节占位直径≤5cm, 或多发占位≤3个且直径均≤3cm。许多其他标准较少受到占位边界易变的限制,包括加州大学旧金山分校(UCSF)标准和7s规则。HCC的生物学行为变化很大,开始时难以预测,对治疗干预的反应也是如此。列入等待名单的这些患者的诊疗复杂,且强度高,需要动态研究程序化,再分期和治疗选择的再评估。

终末期肝病或有任何失代偿症状的患者不适合局部治疗, 依赖这些生物学特性也能使其保持在移植标准内。每隔2~3个月进行一次CT和(或)MRI影像学检查, 以评估肿瘤体积, 确认没有血管侵犯和肝外疾病。绝对和相对的甲胎蛋白水平也用于评估。另一方面,完全代偿期肝硬化患者可能适合用局部治疗,如动脉化疗栓塞(TACE),消融技术或两者结合。局部治疗也推荐用于肿瘤直径>2cm,预计等待时间超过6个月的患者[17,18]。TACE是最常用的主要治疗,尽管有一些证据表明,射频消融(RFA)可能杀死肿瘤细胞的效果更好[19]。迄今还没有数据表明抗血管生成药物更优于移植。

对局部治疗的反应是评估患者的重要部分。有一个良好的初始反应,随后3~9个月内进行肝移植被认为是最好的情况。高达25%的患者尽管接受了局部治疗,但病情仍进展而从等待名单中移除。一些人认为这是由于治疗失败,其他人认为这是肿瘤生物学和患者选择相互作用的结果。同样,未列入等待名单的患者,病情好转符合标准后,越来越被认为适合进行肝移植[20,21]。在这样的患者中已经取得了良好的结果, 移植后4年生存率为92%,相同时间总的介入治疗生存率为69%[21]。

急性肝衰竭

列入移植名单的患者,或者是符合该标准,即预后模型提示不良预后,或者是被评估为病情很有可能恶化到需要移植的阶段。前者的预后模型特异性更高,后者的评估敏感性更高。患者的病情可能恶化或改善,因此需要经常评估肝移植的需求和适合性。一系列数据显示,总人群中有 6%~18%从等待名单中移除或在获得器官前死亡。在这个过程中,当有器官可用时,可做出器官移植的最终决定。

大多数等待急诊肝移植的患者会住进重症监护,并因严重脑病而需要机械通气。一些亚急性肝衰竭和轻度脑病的患者可能例外。急性肝衰竭的管理很复杂,因为几乎每个生理系统都有可能衰竭[22]。针对这些患者的诊疗具体方案是有效的,这里将不再详细回顾。然而,许多诊疗需要根据患者等待移植时的情况进行改进。其中最重要的是颅内压的侵入性监测,这是有争议的,因为缺少其影响生存和相关风险的证据,特别是颅内出血。但是当为了安全桥接治疗时,其使用被高度支持。

另一个有争议的领域是在没有症状的情况下用新鲜冷冻血浆纠正凝血障碍。反对这种做法是基于这样的论点:它没有明显的临床获益,而且破坏了进行中的预后评估。在列入等待名单的情况下,临床获益表现在手术准备方面,而且大部分案例的预后已经被评估为较差。通常重组Ⅶ因子不用于急性肝衰竭患者,也应避免其在等待移植的患者中使用,因为这可能增加血栓形成事件的风险,从而导致移植后出现严重的后果,如肝动脉血栓形成。

未治疗的败血症是另一个可以导致移植不成功的并发症,一旦患者列入等待名单,预防性应用抗菌药物(包括抗细菌和抗真菌)是合理的,而且这对于较早开始肾替代治疗的患者,可以在开始手术时将代谢紊乱降到最低。

识别那些病情太重以致不能从移植受益的患者,或是从等待名单中移除那些病情严重到移植无效的患者,是很困难的,但这对于尽量减少宝贵资源的消耗是很重要的。

两项大型研究已经确定了一些提示肝移植预后不良的指标,但其临床效用在这些情况下有限(表 38.5)[23,24]。年龄在两项研究中均被确定为不良预后的指标,临界值分别是 45 岁和 50 岁。其他临床因素呈弱相关,尽管美国的研究显示,死亡率随着不良预后指标的积累而增加[23](图 38.2)。但是,4 项标准里符合 3 项的生存率是 57%;只有 2%的患者符合全部 4 项标准,其生存率为 42%。英国的研究重点强调供体器官质量的重要性[24],并且这是针对改善结果的决策过程中,能够被操纵的一部分。

历史上,曾担忧移植手术成功后会出现不可逆的脑损伤,但最近几年这种担忧已经明显减少。在美国,只有 13%的肝移植后死亡被认为是神经系统的原因[23]。然而,有瞳孔固定散大或其他脑干疝证据的患者是肝移植的禁忌证。已经证明颅内压和脑灌注压在确定这个问题时是不可靠的。血管收缩剂的使用,不能控制的败血症和严重的呼吸衰竭是不确切的移植禁忌证。这些禁忌证与年龄易感性有关,年轻的患者复原力强,肝移植后也更有可能扭转这些并发症。

表 38.5 影响急性肝衰竭患者移植预后的因素

	风险比(HR)
美国	
BMI>29kg/m²	1.5
血肌酐>2mg/dL	1.4
年龄>50 岁	1.4
机械通气	1.4
英国	
年龄>45 岁	3.0
列入名单时正在使用血管收缩剂	2.2
高风险供体	2.4
时代因素	1.9

Data from [23] and [24].

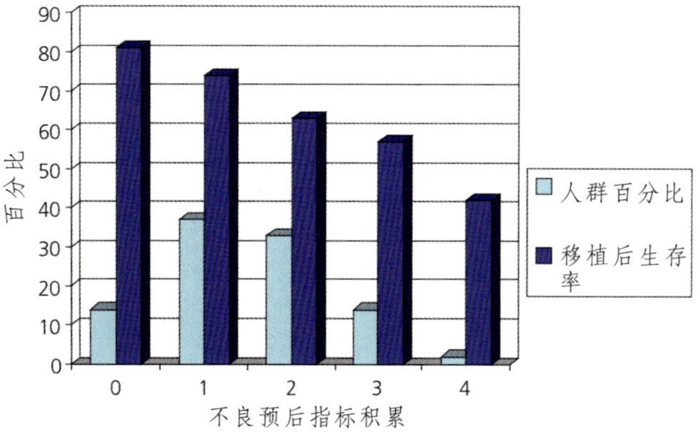

图 38.2 死亡率随着不良预后指标的积累而增加。危险因素的人群分布如图。

酒精和吸烟筛查

酒精性肝病是肝移植患者面临的第二大病因。虽然不同项目酒精政策不同,但普遍都期望等待移植的患者能终身戒酒。等待移植的时间为评估这一承诺提供了机会。如何评估承诺有很大的变异性。有一种严格的方法是利用书面合同,随机进行呼吸、血液或尿液的酒精筛查。定期与支持禁酒的项目互动也可能是必要条件,如戒酒互助会,虽然这可能不适用于不酗酒的酒精性肝病患者。另一个极端是基于信任的系统,当出现临床事件或实验室检查结果怀疑活跃饮酒时,才进行酒精筛查。

如前所述,患者戒酒后,肝功能通常有所改善。列入肝移植等待名单时, 假设大部分或全部的改善能力都很明显,随着等待时间的延长,一组少但值得注意的患者继续改善直到戒酒 18~24 个月。器官分配系统如 MELD,这些患者可以继续列入名单中,但优先级会较低。但是,器官分配系统需要有主动将这些患者从等待名单中移除的决定,而不是结合最低列入标准与等待时间。

关于持续吸烟的政策甚至更不统一。当患者列入等待名单时,他们可能会被建议戒烟,这有助于改善移植时的呼吸功能,减少长期心血管和恶性事件的风险。此政策的监测范围尚不明确。

总结

肝移植的等待时间普遍在增加, 特别是随着基于 MELD 的分配系统的应用, 因此等待移植的患者在分配到器官前会病情加重, 并且在列入名单到获得器官期间,死亡率在 5%~20%。肝硬化患者可能会稳定地恶化,或急剧出现危及生命的并发症。肝硬化患者最常见的问题包括腹水、静脉曲张破裂出血、脑病和肾功能不全,这些并发症都有可能引起多器官衰竭。其他问题与感染易感性和营养不良有关。

HCC 患者的治疗还需要抑制疾病进展, 以免超过移植的标准。这些管理方案需要适应等待肝移植患者的需要。"移植的桥接治疗"概念的建立是为了评估一些更复杂或更昂贵的治疗, 如肝脏支持装置——一个不同于其他生存获益标准的衡量。

(马慧云 译 高鹏骥 校)

参考文献

1. Freeman RB, Steffick DE, Guidinger MK, et al. Liver and intestine transplantation in the United States, 1997–2006. American Journal of Transplantation. 2008;8: 958–976.
2. Francoz C, Belghiti J, Castaing D, et al. Model of end-stage liver disease exceptions in the context of the French model for end-stage liver disease score-based liver allocation system. Liver Transplantation. 2011;17:1137–1151.
3. Gines P, Fernandez J, Durand F, et al. Management of critically-ill cirrhotic patient. Journal of Hepatology. 2012;56:S13–S24.
4. Gines P, Schrier RW. Renal failure in cirrhosis. New England Journal of Medicine. 2009;361:1279–1290.
5. Gluud LL, Christensen K, Krag A. Systematic review of randomized trials on vasoconstrictor drugs for hepatorenal syndrome. Hepatology. 2010;51: 576–584.
6. Boyer TD, Sanyal AJ, Garcia-Tsao G, et al. Predictors of response to terlipressin plus albumin in hepatorenal syndrome (HRS) type 1: relationship of serum creatinine to hemodynamics. Journal of Hepatology. 2011;55:315–321.
7. Nadim MK, Genyk YS, Tokin C, et al. Impact of the etiology of acute kidney injury on outcomes following liver transplantation: acute tubular necrosis versus hepatorenal syndrome. Liver Transplantation. 2012;18:539–548.
8. Ruiz R, Kunitake H, Wilkinson AH, et al. Long-term analysis of combined liver and kidney transplantation at a single center. Archives of Surgery. 2006;141: 735–741.
9. Carbonnel N, Pauwels A, Serfaty L, et al. Improved survival after variceal bleeding in patients with cirrhosis over the past two decades. Hepatology. 2004;40: 652–659.
10. De Franchis R. Revising consensus in portal hypertension: report of the Baveno V consensus workshop on methodology of diagnosis and therapy in portal hypertension. Journal of Hepatology. 2010;53:762–768.
11. McCullough AJ. Malnutrition in cirrhosis. In: Bacon BR, O'Grady JG, Di Bisceglie AM, et al., editors. Comprehensive Clinical Hepatology. Philadelphia, PA: Elsevier; 2006: 177–190.
12. Everson G. Should we treat patients with chronic hepatitis C on the waiting list? Journal of Hepatology. 2005;42:456–462.
13. Terrault N, Roland M, Schiano T, et al. Outcomes of liver transplantation in HCV-HIV coinfected recipients. Liver Transplantation. 2012;10:716–726.
14. Banares R, Nevens F, Larsen FS, et al. Extracorporeal liver support with the molecular absorbent recirculating system (MARS) in patients with acute-on-chronic liver failure. Journal of Hepatology. 2010;52:S459.
15. Rifai K, Kribben A, Gerken G, et al. Extracorporeal liver support by fractionated plasma separation and absorption (Prometheus) in patients with acute-on-chronic liver failure(HELIOS) study: a prospective randomized controlled multicenter study. Journal of Hepatology. 2010;52:S3.
16. Teperman L. A phase 2b study of safety and efficacy of a human cell-based biological liver support system (ELAD) in patients with acute-on-chronic hepatitis (AOCH) due either to acute alcoholic hepatitis or acute decompensation of cirrhosis. Liver Transplantation. 2012;18:S82.
17. Manjo PE, Lencioni R, Mornex F, et al. Is treatment of HCC on the waiting list necessary? Liver Transplantation. 2011;17:S98–S108.
18. Clavien PA, Lesurtel M, Bossuyt PMM, et al. Recommendations for liver transplantation for hepatocellular carcinoma: an international consensus conference report. Lancet Oncology. 2012;13:e11–e22.
19. Martin AP, Goldstein RM, Dempster J, et al. Radiofrequency ablation procedures in cirrhotic patients with hepatocellular carcinoma before liver transplantation – a clinical and histological examination. Clinical Transplantation. 2006;20:695–705.
20. Lesurtel M, Mullhaupt B, Pestalozzi BC, et al. Transarterial chemoembolization as a bridge to liver transplantation for hepatocellular carcinoma: an evidence-based analysis. American Journal of Transplantation. 2006;6:2644–2650.
21. Yao FY, Kerlan RK, Hirose R, et al. Excellent outcome of down-staging of hepatocellular carcinoma prior to liver transplantation: an intention-to-treat analysis. Hepatology. 2008;48:819–827.
22. Stravitz RT, Kramer DJ. Management of acute liver failure. Nature Reviews. Gastroenterology & Hepatology. 2009;6:542–553.
23. Barshes NR, Lee TC, Balkrishnan R, et al. Risk stratification of adult patients undergoing orthotopic liver transplantation for fulminant hepatic failure. Transplantation. 2006;81:195–201.
24. Bernal W, Cross TJS, Auzinger G, et al. Outcome after wait-listing for emergency liver transplantation in acute liver failure: a single centre experience. Journal of Hepatology. 2009;50:306–313.

第 39 章

心脏移植等待名单管理

Howard J. Eisen

引言

患者入选心脏移植名单是基于不良临床指征的数量、衰退的心功能及不良预后等指标。未能正确参照标准医疗、器械相关和(或)外科治疗也许会对心脏移植患者的远期生存率产生影响。从被列于心脏移植的候选名单开始，潜在的移植受者需要很细致地执行对各种治疗中一定会产生的临床状态变化，以及可能出现的影响移植名单上患者优先顺序的临床状态改变的监测。本章讲述等待心脏移植患者的常规诊疗。这章可作为讲述心脏移植指征的第 30 章的姊妹篇,同时也是对分别详述重症监护病房对心衰患者的诊疗、心室辅助装置患者及人工心脏的出现的第 44 章、第 48 章、第 49 章的补充。

列入心脏移植等待名单的晚期心衰患者的诊疗

口服制剂

已列入心脏移植名单上的患者应已接受过最优或者最大量可耐受量的口服药物治疗。这个治疗是在由美国大学心脏病学(ACC)、美国心脏协会(AHA)和美国心衰协会(HFSA)[1-3]所制订的指南指导下完成。这些治疗包括在临床实验中表现出对心衰患者生存有帮助的 β 受体阻滞剂[4-7],血管紧张素转换酶(ACE)抑制剂,或血管紧张素受体阻滞剂(患者不能耐受 ACE 抑制剂的情况下),醛固酮受体拮抗剂以及特别是在非裔美国人中常联合使用的血管舒张药物肼苯哒嗪及硝酸盐类[8-15]。肾素-血管紧张素-醛固酮系统阻滞剂将维持在由 ACC/AHA 和 HFSA 指定的指南所描述的目标剂量,或是根据能体现患者对药物耐受程度的系统血压、肾功能、血清钾及临床症状来判定的目标剂量。卡维地洛、长效美托洛尔或比索洛尔也维持在指南所指导的目标剂量或是根据血压判定耐受程度所显示的目标剂量。额外的一些常用以及需要在晚期心衰患者体内维持的口服药物，包括给有明显淤血症状患者的袢利尿剂及减轻痛苦的强心苷[16]。

装置

列入心脏移植名单的患者，依照他们的心衰症状分级,至少都是纽约心脏协会(NYHA)Ⅲ级以上的,并且他们被列入移植名单前都优先选择植入自动植入型心律转复除颤器(ICD)[17-19]。ICD 在患者被列入名单时以及每次到门诊办公室复查时，都需要核对以判断是否存在需要抗心动过速起搏或除颤的心律失常,以及这些心律失常出现的频率。审核 ICD 的情况将能提供关于除颤阈值、起搏阈值、导向功能和电池寿命的信息。这些 NYHAⅢ级的患者中尽管服用了最大剂量的药物治疗，仍然在心电图上出现 QRS 间期>120ms 的患者,应该连同 ICD 一起植入额外一个双心室起搏器，以提高运动耐量及提高有利于心室功能和生存的效果[20-22]。这些设备在门诊办公室复查时需要被审核，也是为了从根本上判断患者是否正在起搏以决定是否接受心脏再同步治疗。如果患者只花一小部分时间在心脏再同步治疗上,将导致运动耐量和心功能的减退,而且可能将其错误地解释成患者心衰的过程。同时需要投入精力于核实装有双心室起搏器的患者真正在接受心脏再同步化治疗，包括随着双心室起搏器功能优化后的房颤抑制或复律。

静脉注射

出现 NYHA Ⅳ 级心衰症状的患者尽管在接受最

大剂量药物治疗以及心脏再同步化治疗，视患者病情也应行右心导管术以评估心输出量、心指数、肺动脉和肺毛细血管楔压(PCWP)、跨肺动脉瓣压力阶差(TPG)以及肺血管阻力 (PVR)(见表39-1,TPG及PVR的公式计算)[23]。右心导管术的检查结果常用来指导下一步治疗，包括口服药物可能的进一步优化，对PCWP增高、提示容量负荷过度的患者加强利尿,以及开始使用静脉注射交感神经多巴酚丁胺或磷酸二酯酶3抑制剂药物进行强心的治疗。这些可用于短期的几天内增加口服心衰药物及利尿药以提高心输出量及心指数,或者对于被证明是依赖强心治疗以维持心输出量的患者也许可以尝试长期维持治疗。这通常取决于脱机强心治疗及血流动力学的再评估，包括重复的右心导管术所评估的心输出量。需要永久强心治疗以维持心输出量的患者将可以留置导管，如PICC或者静脉导管,以便于持续地把控强心治疗的进行。这些患者通常可以在家里等待接受移植,但是需要复查他们的ICD,因为强心治疗会导致心律失常并且可能导致室性心动过速或室颤。持续使用强心治疗与较低的一年生存率有密切关系，这个问题在正在接受药物治疗等待心脏移植的患者中需要被处理[24,25]。家庭护理支持则通常对在家接受静脉内强心治疗的患者提供帮助。口服心衰药物治疗通常是需要继续维持的，尽管若强心治疗引起了低血压,则口服药物剂量可能被缩减。

当检查右心导管术结果时，另一个需要处理的重要问题是是否存在肺动脉高压以及肺动脉高压的类型。患有晚期心衰的患者通常伴有WHO Ⅱ级的肺动脉高压[23]。这在移植评估的过程中就已经被评估过了，如果TPG或PVR被评估后 (TPG≥15mmHg;PVR>3.0伍德单位,肺动脉收缩压≥50mmHg),已证明可出现当维持体循环收缩期动脉压>85mmHg，给予静脉或者吸入肺血管扩张药物干预[即硝普酸、硝酸甘油、一氧化氮、前列环素(PGI2),奈西立肽],这些血流动力学参数可以被降低或者逆转。这是很重要的一点,以便阻止致命的移植后右心衰的发生。当没有或者仅存在最低限度的固有肺动脉高压时已经证明TPG和PVR是可逆的,这也为当时心脏移植减少TPG和PVR提供了药理学策略。不幸的是,持续的给量使晚期心衰患者患者负荷过多,这可能会导致内在肺动脉损害[23]。因此,重复右心导管检查通常是必要的，尤其对于之前TPG和PVR有升高的患者要确保肺动脉高压仍能被血管扩张剂逆转。

表39.1 肺血流动力计算公式

$\overline{PAP}$=(SPAP+2×DPAP)/3
TPG=$\overline{PAP}$−$\overline{PCWP}$
PVR=($\overline{PAP}$−$\overline{PCWP}$)/CP
$\overline{PAP}$,肺动脉压均值;SPAP,肺动脉收缩压;DPAP,肺动脉舒张压;$\overline{PCWP}$,肺毛细血管楔压均值;TPG,跨肺压;PVR,肺血管阻力;CO,心输出量。
正常值
PVR:1.0~1.5Wood单位(1 Wood单位=80dyns/cm^5)
TPG:8~12mmHg

Source:Mehra et al. [23] Reproduced with permission from Elsevier.

机械辅助循环

很多接受口服药物治疗和(或)利尿药的晚期心衰患者,仍将进展为血流动力学恶化。这些患者常常临床上出现心力衰竭恶化的症状,包括疲劳和腹痛、心律失常、血压过低和伴有四肢冰凉以及逆脉的低灌注迹象。心力衰竭恶化的实验室检查包括肌酐上升、血尿素氮、肝功试验和脑钠素，这也为血流动力学恶化提供了证据。对于这些患者,机械辅助循环成了移植的桥梁,要求要使终末器官功能正常化并改善心脏移植患者的生命质量并延长生存,在第48章中有深入阐述。理想状况下，机械辅助循环应该在终末器官功能严重恶化之前启用。美国食品药物管理局(FDA)批准最常用于移植桥梁装置的是心室辅助装置，连续流动式左心室辅助装置(LVAD)已经取代了早期的脉动流装置,因其一年生存率更高，具有更少的不良反应以及在随机临床试验中更好的耐久性[26,27]。美国食品药物管理局最近也批准将HeartWare HVAD仪器用于移植的桥梁而Jarvik VAD仪器仍处于临床试验研究中[28]。大部分晚期心衰的患者都需要机械辅助循环，单纯左心室辅助装置只能作为移植的桥梁。然而,在左心室辅助装置植入后出现右心室功能障碍也是一个常见的现象。几个评分系统已经发展为在左心室辅助装置植入之前预见出现右心室功能障碍可能性的系统[29,30]。如果出现了右心室功能障碍,系统通常在术中或术前显示出来。应对该情况的策略包括持续收缩药物支持，在更严重的情况下,诸如TCM右心室辅助支持会作为临时设备。如果一个患者在术前被认为右心室功能障碍出现的风险极高，严重到只能采取折中的办法就是单纯采用左心室辅助装置，备选方案是采用 PVAD 仪器或植入式心室辅助装置(IVAD)的两心室辅助支持，这两种都可以在家使用，或者采用 the SynCardia CardioWest 人工心脏，其有一个外部驱动器同样可以在家使用。之后的设备已经证明，将机械辅助循环作为重症患者移植的桥梁需要心室手术摘除，这与心室辅助装置相反[31]。

国际心肺移植学会(ISHLT)的数据显示，采用机械辅助循环的待心脏移植手术患者的比例在 2000—2010 年有所增加(图 39.1)。采用左心室辅助装置和右心室辅助装置(RVAD)的患者与其他组相比，结果更差。那些没有采用机械辅助循环的患者相比采用任何形式的机械辅助循环的患者，有着更高的移植后存活率(图 39.2)。

晚期心衰患者列入心脏移植等待名单

患者可通过当地器官获取组织(OPO)被列入心脏移植等待名单，他们的优先顺序取决于药物治疗的程度或他们接受的机械支持。该优先体制在表 39.2 中有说明，该体制是由联合器官共享网络(UNOS)和美国卫生及公共服务部的卫生资源和服务部门的器官获取和移植网络(OPTN)所明确的[32]。采用机械辅助循环的患

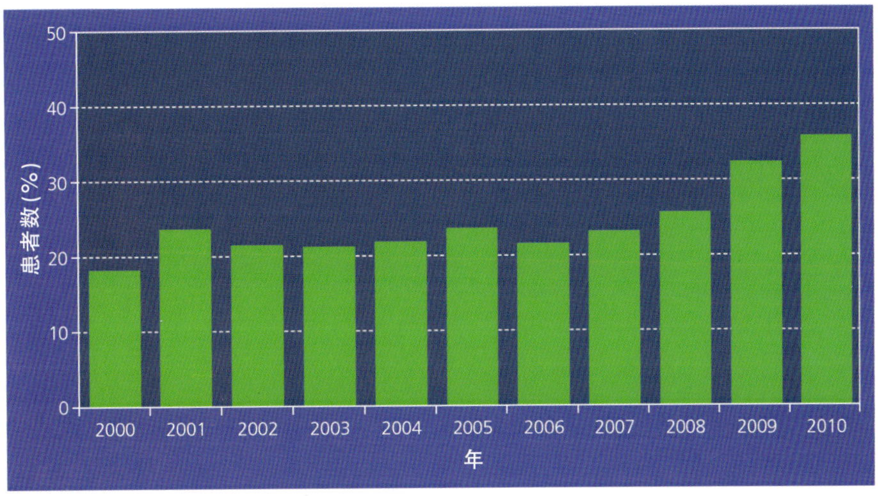

图 39.1　在心脏移植等待名单中需要机械辅助循环的成年患者比例有所增加。数据来源于国际心肺移植学会。

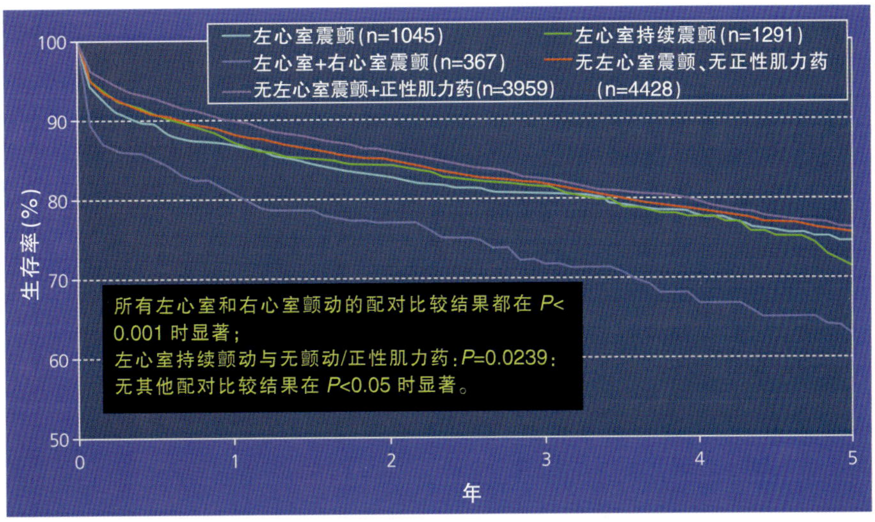

图 39.2　移植前机械辅助循环的效果和支持类型的移植后成活率。LVAD，左心室辅助装置，RVAD，右心室辅助装置。数据来源于国际心肺移植学会登记处。

者可能在术后任意30天内被列为1A状态。

这通常在患者术后恢复并能走动时完成，采用机械辅助循环的患者如果有跟主要设备相关的并发症的显而易见和明确的证据，也可能被列为1A状态，比如感染、设备机械故障、血栓栓塞或潜在的恶性心律失常[32]。其他所有采用机械辅助循环的患者会被列为1B状态。更多的患者可能列为1A状态，包括那些采用连续14天机械呼吸机支持并且后续每14天更新的患者（这些患者确实在移植后出现更糟糕的结果）；接受一次性大剂量的正性肌力药物或多种该类药物持续静脉输注的患者，要接受7天左心室充盈压的连续血流动力学监测，如果上述情况没有改变的话还有一次延长7天的选择权。最终，没有出现上述情况的患者可能被认作1A状态，如果他们有可以被器官共享联合网络区域审查委员会证明并认定的足够严重的紧急状况和临床情况。

所有没有出现上述情况，采用静脉收缩药物支持或机械辅助循环的患者被列为1B状态[52]。只采用口服药的患者被列为状态2，在名单上但由于种种情况目前还不能移植的患者被列为状态7和“未激活”。

器官分配

捐赠者的心脏根据器官获取和移植网络的政策分配并由联合器官共享网络执行。捐赠者心脏优先在当地分配并在当地器官获取组织界定的范围内根据移植者病情严重程度来分配。如果在规定的状态水平下有超过一个潜在心脏移植者，优先权给予等待时间最长的。如果当地鉴定没有合适的受者，捐赠者心脏将会根据地理距离从捐赠医院优先分配。该算法依照相继同心圆：从捐赠医院起到500英里（A区）（编者注：1英里约等于1600米），从捐赠医院起到500~1000英里（B区），从捐赠医院起到1000~1500英里（C区），从捐赠医院起到1500~2500英里（D区），从捐赠医院起超过2500英里（E区）[32]。

心脏移植等待名单中的致敏患者的诊疗

等待移植的晚期心力衰竭患者可能从若干来源发展出同种致敏作用，包括怀孕前、输入血制品前（包括

表39.2 成年心脏移植受体优先级别

1A状态

a i.装有左和（或）右心室辅助装置的机械辅助循环患者可能在设备移植后30天处于1A状态，只要患者被认定为在临床上已经做好心脏移植的准备（患者可能在家）

a ii.全人工心脏

a iii.主动脉内球囊反搏

a iv.体外膜式氧合法

对于满足a ii、a iii或a iv条件的患者必须在列表上的移植中心入院治疗。初步的1A状态有效期是14天，然后从列表上的初始日期开始每14天必须由患者的主治医生重新鉴定

b.装有机械辅助循环的记录在案患者，重大的设备相关并发症的客观证据指出，最常见的是设备机械故障、设备感染、血栓栓塞事件或设备血栓，或危及生命的心率不齐。患者有可能在家。初步的1A状态有效期是14天，然后从列表上的初始日期开始每14天必须由患者的主治医生重新鉴定

c.装有持续机械通气的患者。初步的1A状态有效期是14天，然后从列表上的初始日期开始每14天必须由患者的主治医生重新鉴定

d.接受一次性大剂量正性肌力药物（多巴酚丁胺或米力农）的持续静脉输注患者，或多种协同药物以及接受左心室充盈压的连续有创血液动力学监测患者。患者有可能在家。初步的1A状态有效期是14天，然后从列表上的初始日期开始每14天必须由患者的主治医生重新鉴定

例外：在移植候选名单上没有满足上述条件但其移植医生认为有足够的临床紧迫性，并且可以从移植中获得实质利益的患者。该请求的正当理由必须由其移植医生递交给区域审查委员会批准。该例外下的名单有效期是14天。随后的1A状态的扩展名单——例外名单必须由区域审查委员会事先批准。诸如1A状态名单若未经批准将被提交到胸器官移植委员会和会员与专业标准委员会

1A状态的正当理由表格应通过UNet提交初步名单或扩展名单。一旦1A状态时间期满，患者会自动降级到1B状态

1B状态

aa 左和（或）右心室辅助装置

bb 正性肌力药物的持续静脉输注

例外：在移植候选名单上没有满足上述条件但其移植医生认为有足够的临床紧迫性，并且可以从移植中获得实质利益的患者。该请求的正当理由必须由其移植医生递交给区域审查委员会批准。区域审查委员会的决定报告供胸器官移植委员会和会员与专业标准委员会的审查参考。

1B状态的正当理由表格应通过UNet提交初步名单或扩展名单

状态2

没有满足1A状态或1B状态条件的心脏移植受体（没有正性肌力药物、机械辅助循环或呼吸机支持）

（待续）

表 39.2 成年心脏移植受体优先级别(续)

状态 7 在心脏移植名单上但被定为暂时不适合移植的患者。这些患者保留他们之前累积的移植等待时间，但不产生新的时间并且不被提供捐赠者心脏。被定为无限期或永久不适合移植的患者将会被移出名单

Source: United Network for Organ Sharing/Organ Procurement and Transplant Network of the Health Resources and Service Administration [32]. Available at: http://optn.transplant.hrsa.gov/PoliciesandBylaws2/policies/pdfs/policy_9.pdf

血小板)、实体器官移植前或用于机械辅助循环的心室辅助装置的存在[33]。同种致敏作用向移植提出了挑战，它把受体置于危险之中，因为如果捐赠者心脏被移植到对那些心脏的内皮细胞表层的抗原有抗体特性的患者身上，就会导致抗体介导性排斥反应和移植失败。根据 ISHLT 的登记记录显示，致敏患者[群体反应性抗体(PRA)>10%]在移植后五年有更高的死亡率(表 39.3)。有时同种致敏非常强烈，已经致敏的患者会对抗移植器官，这导致移植医生和外科医生寻求不让已致敏患者获得潜在的器官。虚拟交叉匹配(见第 89 章)的运用有助于优化捐赠者可用性。然而，设法调节同种免疫反应以缩小同种致敏作用的程度，从而增加潜在捐赠者心脏适用于心脏移植列表中特殊潜在受体的数量这种做法是很诱人的，从而使大量降低同种致敏作用的脱敏治疗策略发展起来。该主题已在 68 章中作深入探讨。脱敏疗法常常在计算出的群体反应性抗体超过 10%时发起。这些疗法是针对 B 细胞抗体生成并且包括静脉注射免疫球蛋白(IVIG)、血浆除去法、霉酚酸酯、利妥昔单抗的治疗方法[34]。虽然静脉注射免疫球蛋白已经在临床研究中证明了疗效，但是并没有可用的确切信息，且没有在等待心脏移植的患者身上实施的临床试验[35]。一项回顾性研究显示血浆除去法、静脉注射免疫球蛋白、利妥昔单抗的结合将群体反应性抗体从 70.5%降低到 30.2%，并有移植后五年存活率和免于心脏移植物血管病变，与那些非致敏患者一样[34]。通常，这些治疗方法是无效的，最近，蛋白酶体抑制剂硼替佐米已经结合血浆除去法和利妥昔单抗，用于难以接受其他治疗方案的患者。包含 10 个患者的两个小型报告指出，硼替佐米对于降低使用其他方法不奏效的患者的群体反应性抗体也许有帮助[36,37]。不幸的是，没有脱敏疗法的前瞻性对照试验在心脏移植等待名单的患者身上尝试过，所以该治疗方法主要靠经验。

心脏移植候选患者的临床评估

因为晚期心衰是一个动态变化的疾病，所以心脏移植候选患者需要进行频繁的临床评估来决定他们在等候移植名单中的排位是否改变。举个例子，状态等级 2 的患者可能需要强心治疗措施，或者有严重血流动力学障碍者需要植入左心室辅助装置。这样他们就可能变成状态等级 1B。一个植入左心辅助装置的 1B 患者，可能由于威胁生命的设备感染以及血栓形成使状态等级上升至 1A。关于列入心脏移植名单后随访的推荐规范已被列入 2006 年国际心肺移植协会列表标准指南[23]。表 39.4 概述了心脏移植候选患者的门诊人次及手术安排。目前的门诊患者，包括大部分接受强心治疗或机械辅助循环治疗的行动便利的患者，应完善病史和查体，以及实验检查评估其肝肾功能及电解质水平。肾小球滤过率以肾病膳食改良试验公式计算，并且

表 39.3 升高的移植前群体反应性抗体(PRA)(>10%)是危险因素之一，因其增加了移植后五年死亡率(n=10 507)

可变因素	n	相对风险度	P 值	95%置信区间
孕前女性受体/男性捐赠者对男性受体/男性捐赠者	780	1.22	0.0286	1.02~1.45
PRA>10%	766	1.21	0.0066	1.06~1.40
感染的受体在移植前两周内需要静脉药物治疗	1161	1.18	0.0082	1.04~1.33
有糖尿病历史的受体	2177	1.14	0.0062	1.04~1.26
诊断:冠状动脉疾病对心肌病	4792	1.14	0.0063	1.04~1.25
移植前没有住院	5516	0.92	0.0475	0.84~1.00

PRA，群体反应性抗体

Data from the ISHLT registry.

每3个月评估一次[38,39]。右心置管应被应用于所有的患者，并且在6个月观测的基础上判定是否有跨肺动脉瓣压力阶差、肺血管阻力以及肺动脉收缩压的升高；如果目前发现这些现象，则在这些肺高压指标可逆的基础上，应使用之前提到的肺血管扩张药物治疗。除此之外，右心置管提供关于心输出量的信息可能引起过度的强心和机械辅助循环治疗。对于跨肺动脉瓣压力阶差及肺血管阻力或肺动脉收缩压已经升高的患者，这些评估可能需要更频繁地重复，并且应该执行在移植名单中表现出低心输出量症状和体征，或者那些尽管服用了药物治疗但仍出现进行性心衰的患者身上。装有植入式心脏复律除颤器或在进行心脏再同步化治疗的患者应该拥有他们的设备审查。装有左心室辅助装置或其他形式的机械辅助循环患者应每月去检查，并且他们的支持设备应做详细检查。群体反应性抗体>10%的患者或装有左心室辅助装置的患者应每1~2个月检查一次群体反应性抗体[23]。需要输血的患者应两周后测量群体反应性抗体，然后接下去6个月要每个月测量一次[23]。移植中心应该和当地器官获取组织联系来为特殊患者更新不可接受的抗原，基于最近的群体反应性抗体结果。由于等待移植超过一年的患者数量增加，超声心动图应每年进行一次。装有左心室辅助装置的患者如果出现了心律失常，也许需要更频繁的超声心动图。超声心动图在这些患者身上也很有用，以评定从装载左心室辅助装置进行心室排空。状态2的患者应进行心肺运动试验，以决定他们的功能等级是否提升到他们不再从心脏移植中获得好处的阶段[23]。

在医院等待移植的患者代表着应该进行更严格的审查的患者群体。这可能包括更频繁的有创血流动力学监测和左心室辅助装置功能评估。

总结

列入心脏移植名单中的晚期心衰患者应进行持续监测和最优化的心衰治疗。需要密切关注临床恶化情况，因为这有可能使更多积极的支持治疗，如正性肌力药物或机械循环支持成为必要的措施。终末期器官的功能变化也应密切监测，以根据情况进行最优化的治疗调整。治疗力度的变化应该反映在与患者的治疗及移植前预后判断相符合的移植候选名单排位变化中。左心室辅助装置感染或者功能紊乱将导致患者的联合器官共享网络情形上升至1A级。对群体反应性抗体上升>10%或者有进行性上升风险的群体反应性抗体需要进行纵向的评估，包括带有左心室辅助装置的患者及近期输血的患者。脱敏治疗在心脏移植候选患者中

表39.4 推荐计划表，用于跟进列入心脏移植候选名单的患者

病史和身体检查(包括体重，身高和体质指数计算)	每月一次，尤其是使用正性肌力药物或机械辅助循环的患者
PRA和流式细胞术>10%	每1~2个月
VAD	每1~2个月
输血后	输血后两周，然后连续6个月每月一次
实验室试验(CBC,CMP,BNP)	每月一次并要门诊就医
PT/INR	每月一次，或根据需要若为心房颤动、VAD或机械心脏瓣膜抗凝血
GFR评估(MDRD方法)	每3个月
右心导管术和肺血流动力学评估并根据需要使用血管舒张药	至少每6个月(根据临床需要可以更频繁)
VAD评估	每月一次，根据需要可以更频繁
ICD，双腔起搏器检查	每4个月，根据临床上需要可以更频繁
心肺压力测试	每年一次(状态2患者)
超声波心动图	每年一次，根据装有VAD的患者需要可以更频繁
ECG	每年一次

PRA，群体反应性抗体；VAD，心室辅助装置；CBC，全血计数；CMP，代谢功能全套试验；BNP，脑钠肽；PT/INR，凝血酶原时间/国际标准化比率；GFR，肾小球滤过率；MDRD，肾脏病膳食改良试验；ICD，植入式心脏复律除颤器；ECG，心电图。

Adapted from Mehra et al. [23] with permission from Elsevier.

的作用在前瞻性临床试用中尚未被很好地建立，未来可能在未能接受供体心脏的高群体反应性抗体患者中得到结论。

（王辉杭 译 高鹏骥 校）

参考文献

1. Hunt SA, Abraham WT, Chin MH, et al. 2009 focused update incorporated into the ACC/AHA 2005 Guidelines for the Diagnosis and Management of Heart Failure in adults a report of the American College of Cardiology Foundation/American Heart Association Task Force on Practice Guidelines developed in collaboration with the International Society for Heart and Lung Transplantation. Circulation. 2009;119:e391–e479. Journal of the American College of Cardiology. 2009;54:2464.
2. Heart Failure Society of America. HFSA 2010 comprehensive heart failure practice guidelines. Journal of Cardiac Failure. 2006;16:e73–e97.
3. Jessup M, Banner N, Brozena S, et al. Optimal pharmacologic and non-pharmacologic management of cardiac transplant candidates: approaches to be considered prior to transplant evaluation: International Society for Heart and Lung Transplantation guidelines for the care of cardiac transplant candidates–2006. Journal of Heart and Lung Transplantation. 2006;25:1003–1023.
4. Garg R, Yusuf S, for the Collaborative Group on ACE Inhibitor Trials. Overview of randomized trials of angiotensin-converting enzyme inhibitors on mortality and morbidity in patients with heart failure. JAMA. 1995;273:1450–1456.
5. The CONSENSUS Trial Study Group. Effects of enalapril on mortality in severe congestive heart failure. Results of the Cooperative North Scandinavian Enalapril Survival Study (CONSENSUS). New England Journal of Medicine. 1987;316:1429–1435.
6. Cohn JN, Johnson G, Ziesche S, et al. A comparison of enalapril with hydralazine-isosorbide dinitrate in the treatment of chronic congestive heart failure. New England Journal of Medicine. 1991;325:303–310.
7. The SOLVD Investigators. Effect of enalapril on survival in patients with reduced left ventricular ejection fractions and congestive heart failure. New England Journal of Medicine. 1991;325:293–302.
8. CIBIS-II Investigators and Committee. The Cardiac Insufficiency Bisoprolol Study II (CIBIS-II): a randomised trial. Lancet. 1999;353:9–13.
9. Hjalmarson A, Goldstein S, Fagerberg B, et al. for the MERIT-HF Study Group. Effects of controlled-release metoprolol on total mortality, hospitalizations, and well-being in patients with heart failure: the Metoprolol CR/XL Randomized Intervention Trial in congestive heart failure (MERIT-HF). JAMA. 2000;283:1295–1302.
10. Packer M, Bristow MR, Cohn JN, et al. for the U.S. Carvedilol Heart Failure Study Group. The effect of carvedilol on morbidity and mortality in patients with chronic heart failure. New England Journal of Medicine. 1996;334:1349–1355.
11. Packer M, Coats AJ, Fowler MB, et al. Effect of carvedilol on survival in severe chronic heart failure. New England Journal of Medicine. 2001;344:1651–1658.
12. Granger CB, McMurray JJ, Yusuf S, et al. Effects of candesartan in patients with chronic heart failure and reduced left-ventricular systolic function intolerant to angiotensin-converting-enzyme inhibitors: the CHARM-Alternative trial. Lancet. 2003;362:772–776.
13. Cohn JN, Tognoni G. A randomized trial of the angiotensin receptor blocker valsartan in chronic heart failure. New England Journal of Medicine. 2001; 345:1667–1675.
14. Taylor AL, Ziesche S, Yancy C, et al. Combination of isosorbide dinitrate and hydralazine in blacks with heart failure. New England Journal of Medicine. 2004;351:2049–2057.
15. Pitt B, Zannad F, Remme WJ, et al. for the Randomized Aldactone Evaluation Study Investigators. The effect of spironolactone on morbidity and mortality in patients with severe heart failure. New England Journal of Medicine. 1999;341:709–717.
16. The Digitalis Investigation Group. The effect of digoxin on mortality and morbidity in patients with heart failure. New England Journal of Medicine. 1997;336:525–533.
17. Gronda E, Bourge RC, Costanzo MR, et al. Heart rhythm considerations in heart transplant candidates and considerations for ventricular assist devices: International Society for Heart and Lung Transplantation guidelines for the care of cardiac transplant candidates–2006. Journal of Heart and Lung Transplantation. 2006;25:1043–1056.
18. Bardy GH, Lee KL, Mark DB, et al. Amiodarone or an implantable cardioverter-defibrillator for congestive heart failure. New England Journal of Medicine. 2005;352:225–237.
19. Moss AJ, Zareba W, Hall WJ, et al. Prophylactic implantation of a defibrillator in patients with myocardial infarction and reduced ejection fraction. New England Journal of Medicine. 2002;346:877–883.
20. Cleland JG, Daubert JC, Erdmann E, et al. The effect of cardiac resynchronization on morbidity and mortality in heart failure. New England Journal of Medicine. 2005;352:1539–1549.
21. Abraham WT, Fisher WG, Smith AL, et al. Cardiac resynchronization in chronic heart failure. New England Journal of Medicine. 2002;346:1845–1853.
22. Bristow MR, Saxon LA, Boehmer J, et al. Cardiac-resynchronization therapy with or without an implantable defibrillator in advance chronic heart failure. New England Journal of Medicine. 2004;350:2140–2150.
23. Mehra MR, Kobashigawa J, Starling R, et al. Listing criteria for heart transplantation: International Society for Heart and Lung Transplantation guidelines for the care of cardiac transplant candidates—2006. Journal of Heart and Lung Transplantation. 2006;25:1024–1042.
24. Rose EA, Gelijns AC, Moskowitz AJ, et al. Long-term mechanical left ventricular assistance for end-stage heart failure. New England Journal of Medicine. 2001; 345:1435–1443.
25. Stevenson LW. Clinical use of inotropic therapy for heart failure: looking backward or forward? Part II: chronic inotropic therapy. Circulation. 2003;108:492–497.
26. Miller LW, Pagani FD, Russell SD, et al. Use of a continuous-flow device in patients awaiting heart transplantation. New England Journal of Medicine. 2007; 357:885–896.
27. Slaughter MS, Rogers JG, Milano CA, et al. Advanced heart failure treated with continuous-flow left ventricular assist device. New England Journal of Medicine. 2009;361:2241–2251.
28. Aaronson K. Evaluation of the HeartWare Ventricular Assist System for the Treatment of Advanced Heart Failure (ADVANCE) LBCT I, Abstract 21723. Presented at: American Heart Association Scientific Sessions 2010; Nov.13-17; Chicago. Available from: http://www.scientificsessions-365.com/highlight.aspx?id=2270&p=202.
29. Matthews JC, Koelling TM, Pagani FD, et al. The right ventricular failure risk score a pre-operative tool for assessing the risk of right ventricular failure in left ventricular assist device candidates. Journal of the American College of Cardiology. 2008;51:2163–2172.
30. Fitzpatrick JR 3rd, Frederick JR, Hsu VM, et al. Risk score derived from pre-operative data analysis predicts the need for biventricular mechanical circulatory support. Journal of Heart and Lung Transplantation. 2008;27:1286–1292.
31. Copeland JG, Smith RG, Arabia FA, et al. Cardiac replacement with a total artificial heart as a bridge to transplantation. New England Journal of Medicine. 2004;351:859–867.
32. United Network for Organ Sharing/Organ Procurement and Transplant Network of the Health Resources and Service Administration. 3.7 Organ Distribution: Allocation of Thoracic Organs. 15 November 2011; Available from: http://optn.transplant.hrsa.gov/PoliciesandBylaws2/policies/pdfs/policy_9.pdf.
33. Velez M, Johnson MR. Management of allosensitized cardiac transplant candidates. Transplantation Reviews. 2009;23:235–247.
34. Kobashigawa JA, Patel JK, Kittleson MM, et al. The long-term outcome of treated sensitized patients who undergo heart transplantation. Clinical Transplantation. 2011;25:E61–E67.
35. Jordan SC, Toyoda M, Kahwaji J, et al. Clinical aspects of intravenous immunoglobulin use in solid organ transplant recipients. American Journal of Transplantation. 2011;11:196–202.
36. Patel J, Everly M, Chang D, et al. Reduction of alloantibodies via proteosome inhibition in cardiac transplantation. Journal of Heart and Lung Transplantation. 2011;30:1320–1326.
37. Weston M, Rolfe M, Haddad T, et al. Desensitization protocol using bortezomib for highly sensitized patients awaiting heart or lung transplants. Clinical Transplants. 2009:393–399.
38. Rule AD, Larson TS, Bergstralh EJ, et al. Using serum creatinine to estimate glomerular filtration rate: accuracy in good health and in chronic kidney disease. Annals of Internal Medicine. 2004;141:929–937.
39. Levey AS, Coresh J, Balk E, et al. National Kidney Foundation practice guidelines for chronic kidney disease: evaluation, classification, and stratification. Annals of Internal Medicine. 2003;139:137–147.

第 40 章 肺移植等待名单管理

E. Clinton Lawrence, David C. Neujahr

引言

自列入肺移植候选人名单之后，移植前等待时间通常需要几周到几个月不等，这段时间对于反映肺移植优先度和移植肺根据疾病严重程度以进行合理分配来说相对较短。因此,对肺移植的等待名单管理需要高度理解，并对移植肺的分配和需求以及出现终末肺衰竭状态的处理需要达成工作共识。本章将回顾当前肺移植分配评分系统(LAS),它将解决肺移植中心面临的实际问题,包括如何教育、开导、优化患者,确保他们能获取最大机会,成功地进行移植。本章还将讨论包括HLA 致敏、生理缺陷、患者依从性、受者大小尺寸在内的问题。本书第 31 章介绍了录入肺移植名单的明确指征,本章还将对其进行补充。

肺移植名单

美国方案

最近通过美国的器官共享网络(UNOS)回顾了选出肺移植个体和器官分配过程的历史[1]。1984—2005年可以被视为 LAS 评分系统之前的时代,当时移植器官仅分配给名单上等待时间最长的患者，除此之外也考虑到了受者-供体匹配性和 ABO 血型相容性等特殊问题。然而随着等待时间的延长,包括患有特发性肺间质纤维化(IPF)在内的很多患者在移植之前就已经死亡,其比例不可忽视。尽管 1995 年给予 IPF 患者减少额外90 天的等待时间,其肺移植死亡率仍然高得令人难以接受。考虑到当时分配系统存在的不平等性,以及一定程度上增加移植名单上的患者在移植后存活一年以上的可能性,美国器官移植工作组的建议被采纳,最终在2005 年采用了 LAS 评分系统[2,3]。

在目前的 LAS 评分时期,12 岁以上的肺移植候选人被归为四个诊断群组之一(表 40.1)。将各种人口统计学、生理学和疾病相关数据输入到一个计算公式[2]中,LAS 从 0~100 之间为患者评分,随着患者的状况变化做候诊名单上次序的修改。样本 LAS 评分计算器可供临床医生和患者使用(网址:http://optn.transplant.hrsa.gov/resources)。LAS 的明确目标是按轻重缓急进行器官分配，以获得等待患者的死亡率最小化和移植后生存比例最大化。重要的是在当前系统下,LAS 将等待列表死亡率加权为移植后存活概率的两倍。器官仍然在受者身高范围和 ABO 血型相容的基础上进行分配。首先在每个列表区域(本地、区域 A、区域 B 等)内由本地向可用器官 LAS 评分最高的患者提供供体肺。因此,肺首先提供给当地器官获取组织(OPO)的移植中心。

表 40.1 肺分配评分系统(LAS)诊断分组及主要临床诊断

A 组:阻塞性肺病
包括慢性阻塞性肺疾病(COPD);肺气肿;α-1 抗胰蛋白酶缺乏症;淋巴管肌瘤病(LAM);支气管扩张,包括原发性纤毛运动障碍;平均肺动脉(PA)压力≤30mmHg 的结节病
B 组:肺血管疾病
包括原发性肺动脉高压(PPH);艾森曼格综合征;其他特定的肺血管疾病,包括肺静脉阻塞性疾病、慢性肺血栓栓塞性疾病
C 组:囊性纤维化或免疫缺陷病障碍
囊性纤维化;常见变异型免疫缺陷病;低丙种球蛋白血症
D 组:限制性肺部疾病
特发性肺纤维化(IPF);肺纤维化(其他原因);平均肺动脉压力>30mmHg 的结节病;硬皮病/CREST;支气管肺泡癌(BAC);肺移植后闭塞性细支气管炎综合征(BOS);肺移植后的原发性移植物衰竭;嗜酸性肉芽肿

Reproduced from Egan et al. [2] with permission from John Wiley and Sons.

如果合适的受者不在本地，则肺由相应区域提供，每个区域(A、B 等)对应于距捐赠医院 500 海里半径的同心圆内。在每个列表中，肺首先提供给 ABO 血型相同的患者，然后是 ABO 相容的患者。自从实施 LAS 系统以来，很多 IPF 患者接受了肺移植[4]，等待时间和等待名单死亡率均有下降[1]。虽然在 LAS 系统下总的 1 年生存率没有改变，但有数据显示，LAS 评分较高的患者(较严重的患者)具有更高的发病率[5]、更高的成本[6]和也许日后较低的生存期[7,8]。

已经注意到，LAS 系统未能充分计算等待名单上特发性肺动脉高压(IPAH)患者死亡的可能性[9-11]。因此实施了一个申请机制，以提高选定患者的 LAS 评分；例如合并有 IPAH 的患者，当右心房压力>15mmHg 和心脏指数<1.8L/min/m² 时，可以申请提高其 LAS 到第 90 百分位。LAS 也进行了其他修改，例如增加 Pco_2 和胆红素的评估，随着数据的增多将来还会做进一步改进。考虑在区域分配之前仍然首先在本地 OPO 列表中提供肺，如果在本地列表上没有其他类似的患者，则受者仍然可以在相对短的时间段内接受肺移植。美国在移植的中位等待时间方面存在很大的异质性，这一点并不稀奇。在肺移植社区中，存在部分疾病比本地患者更严重的区域受者，他们已经提出建议，应比对心脏分配规则以修改肺移植的分配规则。目前，如何定位这种高度紧急的患者存在相当大的争议。

其他国家的方案

鉴于 LAS 系统为美国独有，其他国家对于器官的公平分配问题亦有自己的方法。例如，欧洲的七个国家(奥地利、比利时、克罗地亚、荷兰、卢森堡、德国和斯洛文尼亚)组成了欧洲移植(ET)地区。欧洲移植区的肺移植等待者被分为一般、紧急(U)或高度紧急(HU)，其中高度紧急患者通常在重症监护病房中并且通常需要辅助通气[12]。在这些亚组中，名单上的等待时间被列入考虑范围之内。在 Smits 等[12]的论文中，对使用 LAS 和 LAS+分组的患者进行了一项初步研究，发现 LAS 可以预测他们在危重疾病群组中的死亡率，表明某些版本的 LAS 可能在欧洲移植地区实施。在英国有 6 个地区可执行肺移植。肺移植捐赠者被首先分配到他们居住的固定区域，然后分配遵循轮转系统，将捐赠器官分配到列表中下一个区域。没有以医疗紧急程度为标准对受者进行排序的标准，虽然有建议提出应该这样做。

尽管加拿大与美国的平均人口肺移植率几乎相同，但在加拿大却没有类似的器官共享(UNOS)系统用于器官分配。2001 年起，加拿大就试图集中进行包括肺移植在内的器官分配，但到目前为止，大多数器官分配仍然驻留在省级水平。2008 年，加拿大血液服务处开始着手将捐献者分配集中的任务。2010 年建立了一个与生存有关的肾脏捐赠国家登记册[13]。其预期最终将制订用于捐赠者分配和接受者排序的标准化方案。在加拿大有 5 个集中式肺移植中心，最近这些中心的主任提出了一种用于捐赠者分配的算法，其首先推荐本地分配，然后是区域，然后是全国，类似于美国的算法。关于器官受者的排序，目前的加拿大系统仅将患者分类为状态 1 或状态 2。状态 1 患者被认为是稳定的，而状态 2 患者则需要紧急移植。如预期的一样，状态 2 接受者的等待时间中间值比状态 1 接受者短得多。

澳大利亚使用类似的分散式系统进行肺移植分配。澳大利亚 6 个州有 4 个移植中心。捐赠者首先被分配到本地移植中心，如果没有合适的接受者，他们被轮流提供给随后的其他州。该分配系统还通过 ABO 相容性以及大小匹配性对接受者进行优先级排序，然后基于接受者的疾病严重程度来进行分配。

值得强调的是，在加拿大和澳大利亚都采用供体-受体匹配的分散化管理过程，因此移植程序在接受者选择方面需要高度的考量。在采用 LAS 和 UNOS 的高度集中化管理的美国系统中，这种考量就无须过于谨慎了。

名单上患者的管理

教育

无论是在肺移植期间和列入名单后、移植之前等待期间，患者及其支持人员对移植过程的方方面面都进行充分了解是相当重要的。最近，美国医疗保险和医疗补助中心(CMS)已经使用一个长篇幅的教育文件来将这个过程程式化，患者必须在移植评估过程开始时已完成这个教育文件。该文件有八个核心方面内容：

1.评估过程；

2.手术程序；

3.替代治疗；

4.潜在医疗或心理社会风险；

5.国家和移植中心具体结局，取自最新的移植受者科学注册中心(SRTR)特定报告；

6.可能影响患者移植成功和健康的器官供体的危险因素；

7.患者拒绝移植的权利；

8.如果移植发生在非医疗保险批准的中心，则可能影响患者在医疗保险B部分支付其免疫抑制药物的能力。

很明显，关键的是潜在的移植候选人对肺移植的潜在益处和局限性有现实性的理解，并能够做出有关是否进行肺移植的知情决策。对于每个患者来说都很重要的是，应了解器官分配的过程是基于ABO血型、LAS评分系统、单一或双侧移植以及诸如对供体HLA抗原、受体巨细胞病毒(CMV)和乙型肝炎病毒(HBV)免疫状态等混杂因素。对于患者和其支持人员来说，了解移植后所需的药物及其副作用、药物相互作用和避免使用的药物(例如非甾体抗炎药)也是非常重要的。在移植围手术期期间，有必要制订家庭或其他个人支持计划。教育过程还强调了解治疗成本和移植后药物，并且还包含获得这种费用的资源和(或)制订处理经济负担的计划。非医疗因素确实会影响患者的结局，最近的一项研究报告表明，保险覆盖类型与肺移植后的长期结局相关[14]，医疗保险患者或医疗救助金患者的长期生存率低于私人保险患者。愿意与其移植护理人员合作，并遵循关于移植后护理和药物依从性的指示也是移植后成功结局的关键。最后，充分的社会支持对于处理移植过程中的心理压力和医疗问题至关重要[15]。

免疫

通过常规免疫预防某些特定感染通常在列入肺移植等待名单之前或同时完成。普遍认同的是针对肺炎链球菌的免疫接种（一个中心的回顾性研究发现只有62%的移植参照者先前进行过免疫接种[16]）；捐献者之前有HBV感染证据的话，受者免疫缺乏时应免疫接种预防[17]；每年接种流感疫苗，使用灭活疫苗而不是活疫苗。重要的是在移植前后，家庭成员每年也应接种灭活的疫苗免疫，因为免疫功能不全的移植受者可能对疫苗本身难以产生足够的抗体反应[18]。

肺康复

有许多令人信服的研究支持有组织性锻炼计划的重要性，为等待肺移植的患者优选通过肺康复计划[19-26]。事实上，在6分钟步行测试(6MWT)中行走的距离已经显示出在肺移植等待名单上的患者[27]、尤其是在IPF患者[28]中与存活率有着高度的相关性。因此，几乎所有肺移植项目都规定需要注册肺康复计划，一些项目甚至让患者搬迁到中心附近以参加他们的肺康复计划。在某些情况下，第三方支付财政紧缩和(或)缺乏可能需要替换为以家庭为基础的锻炼计划。无论肺康复计划如何实现，肺移植候补名单上的患者必须保持尽可能的活动度，并且需要监测他们对锻炼计划的参与度。

肺移植名单人员的医疗监测和治疗

虽然在LAS系统下从上市到移植的时间中位数已经减少到几个月[29,30]，但由于各种原因，相当多患者的等待时间会有一定延长。因此，有一个能随时间更新的患者LAS系统评分、检测新的医学或心理社会问题并确定患者是否一直满足肺移植标准的监测系统是十分重要的。患者和护理者应当了解到，LAS评分类似于用于对肝脏受体分级的终末期肝病模型(MELD)评分，是反映患者的医疗状态变化的动态评分。LAS中严重影响得分的几个因素是静息时的氧使用程度和6MWT距离。因此，必须将这些因素的任何变化均报告给移植中心，以便可以将最新的数值输入到分配系统中。LAS中的三个因素有效期为6个月；在6个月之后，需要新的测试来评估这三个因素。这三个因素分别为用力肺活量、6MWT和血清肌酐水平。肺移植计划的基础设施应确保这些临床数值保持最新。

待移植患者的临床监测和测试相对比较集中。用于确保移植持续适合的测试包括肺功能测试、动脉血气、血清肌酐和胆红素等常规实验室检测；囊性纤维化(CF)或支气管扩张的患者的痰培养；测试针对人白细胞抗原(HLA)的群体反应性抗体(PRA)；每6个月左右为可能患恶性病[慢性阻塞性肺病(COPD)/IPF]或真菌感染(囊性纤维化/结节病)风险的患者进行胸部CT成像；重复测量6MWT；肺动脉高压患者要重复进行经胸部超声心动图，如果肺动脉压力过高，可能需要重复进行右心导管插入术。根据UNOS的要求更新LAS系统最新数据。

鉴于严重营养不良和肥胖是移植后不良结果的风险因素[31]，在移植中心的门诊访问期间可询问关于体重增减的问题。在此期间还可以确认肺康复计划的参与文件、一般医疗合规以及患者心理社会支持和保险范围的任何变化。有风险因素的患者中可能随机筛选药物和(或)尼古丁滥用,若发现阳性则可能被从等候名单中移除。

患者在等待移植期间经历焦虑和(或)抑郁症状并不罕见,这些问题应该通过药物治疗和(或)转诊给精神病医生或心理学家来探讨和处理。抑郁与等待肺移植期间的死亡率升高有关[32]。一些移植程序需要在移植前将肺移植候选者移至其当地区域,这可能对患者和家庭造成额外的困难,可能导致进一步的抑郁风险。因此,计划中有制订距移植中心最短距离的中心政策,并且将这些政策在移植前早期传达是相当重要的。

列入等候名单上的患者在初始和随访期间,应评估其合并的临床问题如高血压和糖尿病并充分控制。骨质疏松症和维生素 D 缺乏在各种肺部疾病患者中很常见[33,34],因此移植患者出现骨密度降低时,应使用连续的骨密度扫描以及钙、维生素 D、双膦酸盐和(或)其他药物的治疗[35]。

肺移植计划还需要建立相应机制,以确保适合移植的潜在受者持续位于移植候补名单上。2011 年的美国,约有 500 名患者在未接受移植的情况下从候补名单中删除,其中约 300 名患者因健康达标或病情过重而不必接受移植。这些数据强调了移植适应性仍然是一个需要密切监测的持续性问题。没有明确指导如何进行这种监测的方针,但仍存在几条广泛的共识。例如,大多数人认为,具有高 LAS 评分(> 40)的重病患者应该比相对稳定的患者的监测更频繁。具有高 LAS 评分的患者,尤其是患者出现病情恶化时,监测频率应至少每月一次,稳定的 COPD 患者监测的时间间隔不应超过 3 个月。确保移植适用性的另一个策略是每周使用诸如打电话或电子邮件之类的方法维持与待移植患者的联系。第二条广泛共识是住院的等待列表上待移植患者需要加大审查与监测的力度,大多数美国中心有一个含蓄或明确的最小 6MWT,患者必须达到该标准才认定为适合移植,病情急性恶化的住院患者步行距离可能降至该标准以下,在这种情况下,可以接受入选标准以外的供体肺。

在何种程度上应向需要机械通气和(或)体外膜肺氧合(ECMO)的患者提供肺移植仍然是持续争议的话题。来自国际心脏和肺移植学会(ISHLT)的注册数据表明,机械通气患者的移植后 1 年存活率显著降低[4]。然而,病例系列研究已经证明移植在特殊选择个体中的可行性,其结果与历史病例对照相当[36-38]。这些病例存在一个共同点:大多数患者相对年轻且没有其他医疗共病,因此,如果将机械通气用作移植前的桥梁,应用于移植后存活的概率相对较高的患者可能为其中一项指导原则。尽管对于通气患者的移植存在一些不确定性,但是 ECMO 的经验更不甚清楚。这可能部分源于 ECMO 技术在过去几年中快速的发展,包括技术进步以及新的临床决策方法。关于前者,使用独立的小 ECMO 电路,其利用了新的双腔插管,需要的手动操作大大减少,可最终导致一种类型的 ECMO 模式,其可以在大群组患者中进行实际疗效的测试。关于后者,一些临床医生建议使用 ECMO 作为终末期肺衰竭患者的前期治疗,而不是将其作为最后的治疗手段。前期治疗应用 ECMO 的理论优点是其可允许肌肉调节和较低误吸风险的持续口服营养,从而当供体肺可用时优化受者。来自欧洲的几个小样本病例系列研究使用 ECMO 作为肺移植的桥梁,已经证明了这种方法的可行性,然而对大样本患者的长期随访研究仍然缺乏。

克服肺移植的障碍

有几个因素可能导致某些肺移植候选者比其他人等待供体肺的时间更长。在这种情况下,考虑在多个移植中心登记(“双重登记”)可能符合患者的最佳利益。一般来说,双重登记涉及在两个或更多个中心的肺移植列表上登记,其中每个中心在不同的本地器官获取组织(OPO)处是“本地的”。这样的列表可有效地让受者被认为是在多个列表上的本地受者,从而增加找到捐献者的概率。在进行双重登记之前,患者和所有涉及的中心必须提前决策好哪个中心将进行患者术后的护理。在大多数情况下,短期和长期的护理仍是移植中心的责任,因为患者的生存率只计入移植中心的统计数据。

限制个体患者及时接受供体器官的另一常见因素是存在针对预期供体的抗 HLA 抗体。这个因素限制了可接受的供体选择范围,因此延长了等待时间。防止这种致敏受体对肺同种异体移植物急性排斥的传统方法是使用受体血清和供体细胞进行预交叉匹配。然而,运输问题和时间限制使得这种方法在许多情况下不切实际,因此增加了等待名单上的时间。所幸这个问题已经通过使用“虚拟交叉匹配”来解决[39,40]。实质上,移植前测试将限定供体抗HLAI类和II类特异性抗体。在本地器官获取组织(OPO)的供体评价过程期间,先确定供体HLA抗原,使移植小组可确定潜在受者是否具有对供体HLA特异性的抗体,可以基于这些数据接受或拒绝供体肺。这种方法有许多注意事项,但虚拟交叉匹配确实提供了一种解决致敏患者长时间等待捐赠者的方法。

一种可以确定找到适当匹配的供体的有效工具是CPRA计算器,其将不可接受的抗原输入到计算机化算法中,然后针对这些不可接受的抗原运行先前超过12 000个患者等位基因的数据库,以计算出下一个器官没有任何不可接受的HLA抗原表位的可能值。然后,该数值可用于建议患者其将接受移植的机会,以及决定在哪些患者中必须进行某种类型的干预。例如,一些程序试图在移植时用血浆置换法和静脉注射免疫球蛋白G(IVIG)移除抗供体HLA抗体[41],或在移植前使用各种方法减少受体中的抗体产生,即脱敏疗法,这在本书第68章[42]中有所描述。然而,迄今为止这些方法均未得到充分研究,长期随访被认为是诊疗致敏化肺移植患者的公认方法。当移植前抗HLA抗体水平太高时,也可以考虑与其他移植中心“双重登记”。

肺移植候选人可能没有快速接受捐献的另一个原因是受者较小。在特定个体如体型较小的CF患者中,用于肺移植的活供体肺叶是可以选择的[43],尽管该技术的临床经验目前仅限于几个中心。或者,供体肺可能需要手术减小至适合接受者的大小。另外在预期受者大小/结构问题可能增加等待时间的情况下,双重登记可以增加患者接受捐献的机会。

患者在等待移植时可能会出现临床症状恶化。如果恶化是由多重感染发展而来,例如肺炎等,在感染得到充分控制之前患者可出现暂时性萎靡。如果临床恶化由基础疾病过程的进展引起,则LAS评分将增加,这使得患者可能因此接受捐献。然而,采取各种措施以稳定和(或)改善这些患者的状态,包括短期应用皮质类固醇、增加氧流量或改为面罩给氧或双水平式气道正压通气(BIPAP)给氧、通过经气管导管给氧乃至机械通气插管[44]。如上所述,具有严重通气功能衰竭的特定患者在移植完成前甚至可一直给予ECMO支持[45-47],该方法和其他人工辅助通气设备在本书第50章中进行了深入讨论。显然,这些危重患者在移植之前死亡率相对较高,移植后并发症和花费也相对高很多[5,6]。

自从实施LAS系统以来,等待时间和等待捐献者死亡率都在下降[1],部分原因是器官的可用性增加[4]。尽管如此,仍然没有足够数量合适的供体肺,仍有个体在等待肺移植期间死亡。有一种可增加供体肺移植数目的方法,是将不确定是否合格的移植肺进行常温体外肺灌注(EVLP;在第26章有深入讨论)[49]。在EVLP 4小时后,该种类型的肺移植成功的比例相当高且具有极好的短期结果。在美国,正在进行相关研究以获得食品和药物监督管理局(FDA)批准EVLP装置和其他相关材料在临床肺移植实践中实施。

从肺移植等待名单中移除

在以下情况下应将患者从肺移植等待名单中移除:

1.患者可能由于并发疾病、旅行或社会心理环境的变化而暂时处于失活状态,一旦这些问题得到解决会重新激活。

2.若已证实患者复发药物滥用,可能会将患者从名单上永久删除。

3.患者被认为已经进展到不再是合适的候选者的程度。例如脓毒性休克和多器官衰竭综合征等重度感染。

4.少数患者可能对同时进行的相关治疗有反应,并且被认定为可以不用移植治疗。

5.患者可能改变主意,决定放弃肺移植疗法。

6.当匹配的器官可用并且患者完成移植的相关程序后。这也是整个移植团队的目标,我们与患者和家人同乐。

总结

患有终末期肺衰竭的患者病情危重且呈进展性恶化,并且在肺移植的等待期间需要相对频繁的医疗监测。虽然最近引入的肺分配算法有助于将等待肺移植的患者进行标准化管理,但是在等待时间方面仍然存在与局部实践模式和器官供应相关的区域异质性。应尽可能合理安排等待合适移植器官的时间,应优化受者的心肺储备,通过疫苗接种和避免致敏事件为受者进行免疫方面的准备，还应合理教育受者进行康复训练和药物治疗。

（秋宇典 译 高鹏骥 校）

参考文献

1. Eberlein M, Garrity ER, Orens JB. Lung allocation in the United States. Clinics in Chest Medicine. 2011;32(2):213–222.
2. Egan TM, Murray S, Bustami RT, et al. Development of the new lung allocation system in the United States. American Journal of Transplantation. 2006;6(5 Pt 2):1212–1227.
3. Davis SQ, Garrity ER Jr. Organ allocation in lung transplant. Chest. 2007; 132(5):1646–1651.
4. Christie JD, Edwards LB, Kucheryavaya AY, et al. The Registry of the International Society for Heart and Lung Transplantation: twenty-eighth adult lung and heart-lung transplant report–2011. Journal of Heart and Lung Transplantation. 2011; 30(10):1104–1122.
5. Kozower BD, Meyers BF, Smith MA, et al. The impact of the lung allocation score on short-term transplantation outcomes: a multicenter study. Journal of Thoracic and Cardiovascular Surgery. 2008;135(1):166–171.
6. Arnaoutakis GJ, Allen JG, Merlo CA, et al. Impact of the lung allocation score on resource utilization after lung transplantation in the United States. Journal of Heart and Lung Transplantation. 2011;30(1):14–21.
7. Merlo CA, Weiss ES, Orens JB, et al. Impact of U.S. lung allocation score on survival after lung transplantation. Journal of Heart and Lung Transplantation. 2009;28(8):769–775.
8. Russo MJ, Iribarne A, Hong KN, et al. High lung allocation score is associated with increased morbidity and mortality following transplantation. Chest. 2010;137(3):651–657.
9. Benza RL, Miller DP, Frost A, et al. Analysis of the lung allocation score estimation of risk of death in patients with pulmonary arterial hypertension using data from the REVEAL Registry. Transplantation. 2010;90(3):298–305.
10. Chan KM. Idiopathic pulmonary arterial hypertension and equity of donor lung allocation in the era of the lung allocation score: are we there yet? American Journal of Respiratory and Critical Care Medicine. 2009;180(5):385–387.
11. Chen H, Shiboski SC, Golden JA, et al. Impact of the lung allocation score on lung transplantation for pulmonary arterial hypertension. American Journal of Respiratory and Critical Care Medicine. 2009;180(5):468–474.
12. Smits JM, Nossent GD, de Vries E, et al. Evaluation of the lung allocation score in highly urgent and urgent lung transplant candidates in Eurotransplant. Journal of Heart and Lung Transplantation. 2011;30(1):22–28.
13. Organ Registry Team. Organ and Tissue Donation and Transplantation (OTDT) Team. CANNT Journal. 2011;21(1):12–13.
14. Allen JG, Arnaoutakis GJ, Orens JB, et al. Insurance status is an independent predictor of long-term survival after lung transplantation in the United States. Journal of Heart and Lung Transplantation. 2011;30(1):45–53.
15. Phillips KM, Burker EJ, White HC. The roles of social support and psychological distress in lung transplant candidacy. Progress in Transplantation. 2011;21(3): 200–206.
16. Gasink LB, Wurcell AG, Kotloff RM, et al. Low prevalence of prior streptococcus pneumoniae vaccination among potential lung transplant candidates. Chest. 2006;130(1):218–221.
17. Hartwig MG, Patel V, Palmer SM, et al. Hepatitis B core antibody positive donors as a safe and effective therapeutic option to increase available organs for lung transplantation. Transplantation. 2005;80(3):320–325.
18. Agarwal N, Ollington K, Kaneshiro M, et al. Are immunosuppressive medications associated with decreased responses to routine immunizations? A systematic review. Vaccine. 2011;30(8):1413–1424.
19. Manzetti JD, Hoffman LA, Sereika SM, et al. Exercise, education, and quality of life in lung transplant candidates. Journal of Heart and Lung Transplantation. 1994;13(2):297–305.
20. Palmer SM, Tapson VF. Pulmonary rehabilitation in the surgical patient. Lung transplantation and lung volume reduction surgery. Respiratory Care Clinics of North America. 1998;4(1):71–83.
21. Van Der Woude BT, Kropmans TJ, Douma KW, et al. Peripheral muscle force and exercise capacity in lung transplant candidates. International Journal of Rehabilitation Research. 2002;25(4):351–355.
22. Mitchell MJ, Baz MA, Fulton MN, et al. Resistance training prevents vertebral osteoporosis in lung transplant recipients. Transplantation. 2003;76(3):557–562.
23. Ries AL. Pulmonary rehabilitation and COPD. Seminars in Respiratory and Critical Care Medicine. 2005;26(2):133–141.
24. Takaoka ST, Weinacker AB. The value of preoperative pulmonary rehabilitation. Thoracic Surgery Clinics. 2005;15(2):203–211.
25. Mathur S, Hornblower E, Levy RD. Exercise training before and after lung transplantation. Physician and Sports Medicine. 2009;37(3):78–87.
26. Turner DA, Cheifetz IM, Rehder KJ, et al. Active rehabilitation and physical therapy during extracorporeal membrane oxygenation while awaiting lung transplantation: a practical approach. Critical Care Medicine. 2011;39(12): 2593–2598.
27. Tuppin MP, Paratz JD, Chang AT, et al. Predictive utility of the 6-minute walk distance on survival in patients awaiting lung transplantation. Journal of Heart and Lung Transplantation. 2008;27(7):729–734.
28. Lederer DJ, Arcasoy SM, Wilt JS, et al. Six-minute-walk distance predicts waiting list survival in idiopathic pulmonary fibrosis. American Journal of Respiratory and Critical Care Medicine. 2006;174(6):659–664.
29. Iribarne A, Russo MJ, Davies RR, et al. Despite decreased wait-list times for lung transplantation, lung allocation scores continue to increase. Chest. 2009; 135(4):923–928.
30. Yusen RD, Shearon TH, Qian Y, et al. Lung transplantation in the United States, 1999-2008. American Journal of Transplantation. 2010;10(4 Pt 2): 1047–1068.
31. Allen JG, Arnaoutakis GJ, Weiss ES, et al. The impact of recipient body mass index on survival after lung transplantation. Journal of Heart and Lung Transplantation. 2010;29(9):1026–1033.
32. Evon DM, Burker EJ, Galanko JA, et al. Depressive symptoms and mortality in lung transplant. Clinical Transplantation. 2010;24(5):E201–E206.
33. Shane E, Silverberg SJ, Donovan D, et al. Osteoporosis in lung transplantation candidates with end-stage pulmonary disease. American Journal of Medicine. 1996;101(3):262–269.
34. Jastrzebski D, Lutogniewska W, Ochman M, et al. Osteoporosis in patients referred for lung transplantation. European Journal of Medical Research. 2010;15(Suppl 2):68–71.
35. Ebeling PR. Approach to the patient with transplantation-related bone loss. Journal of Clinical Endocrinology and Metabolism. 2009;94(5):1483–1490.
36. Baz MA, Palmer SM, Staples ED, et al. Lung transplantation after long-term mechanical ventilation : results and 1-year follow-up. Chest. 2001;119(1):224–227.
37. Vermeijden JW, Zijlstra JG, Erasmus ME, et al. Lung transplantation for ventilator-dependent respiratory failure. Journal of Heart and Lung Transplantation. 2009;28(4):347–351.
38. Massard G, Shennib H, Metras D, et al. Double-lung transplantation in mechanically ventilated patients with cystic fibrosis. Annals of Thoracic Surgery. 1993;55(5):1087–1091, discussion 91–92.
39. Appel JZ 3rd, Hartwig MG, Cantu E 3rd, et al. Role of flow cytometry to define unacceptable HLA antigens in lung transplant recipients with HLA-specific antibodies. Transplantation. 2006;81(7):1049–1057.
40. Murphey CL, Forsthuber TG. Trends in HLA antibody screening and identification and their role in transplantation. Expert Review of Clinical Immunology. 2008;4(3):391–399.
41. Robinson JA, Radvany RM, Mullen MG, et al. Plasmapheresis followed by intravenous immunoglobulin in presensitized patients awaiting thoracic organ transplantation. Therapeutic Apheresis. 1997;1(2):147–151.
42. Weston M, Rolfe M, Haddad T, et al. Desensitization protocol using bortezomib for highly sensitized patients awaiting heart or lung transplants. Clinical Transplants. 2009:393–399.
43. Date H. Update on living-donor lobar lung transplantation. Current Opinion in Organ Transplantation. 2011;16(5):453–457.
44. O'Brien G, Criner GJ. Mechanical ventilation as a bridge to lung transplantation. Journal of Heart and Lung Transplantation. 1999;18(3):255–265.
45. Broome M, Palmer K, Schersten H, et al. Prolonged extracorporeal membrane oxygenation and circulatory support as bridge to lung transplant. Annals of Thoracic Surgery. 2008;86(4):1357–1360.
46. Cypel M, Keshavjee S. Extracorporeal life support as a bridge to lung transplantation. Clinics in Chest Medicine. 2011;32(2):245–251.
47. Hammainen P, Schersten H, Lemstrom K, et al. Usefulness of extracorporeal membrane oxygenation as a bridge to lung transplantation: a descriptive study. Journal of Heart and Lung Transplantation. 2011;30(1):103–107.
48. Stern JB, Mal H, Groussard O, et al. Prognosis of patients with advanced idiopathic pulmonary fibrosis requiring mechanical ventilation for acute respiratory failure. Chest. 2001;120(1):213–219.
49. Cypel M, Yeung JC, Liu M, et al. Normothermic ex vivo lung perfusion in clinical lung transplantation. New England Journal of Medicine. 2011;364(15): 1431–1440.

第 41 章
胰腺和胰岛移植等待名单管理

Jon S. Odorico

引言

对于尿毒症性和非尿毒症性糖尿病患者而言，他们可供选择的胰腺和胰岛移植方案有很多。移植中心可为患者提供一种或多种方案，同时所有相关的移植方案也会列入讨论。对于尿毒症性糖尿病患者，胰腺-肾脏联合(SPK)移植和肾脏-胰腺序贯(PAK)移植都是首选方案，而如果移植中心可以提供胰岛移植，那么可供选择的方案还可包括胰岛-肾脏联合(SIK)移植或肾脏-胰岛序贯(IAK)移植，后者更为常见。对于非尿毒症性糖尿病患者，首选移植方案是胰腺单独移植(PTA)或胰岛单独移植(ITA)，后者仅限于已批准的临床试验。如果想要了解更多有关胰腺和胰岛移植方案选择的相关细节，可参考第 32 章，该章详述了患者选择和胰腺及胰岛移植的适应证。移植中心最终推荐的移植方案决定了患者的等待时间，反之，预期的等待时间也会影响移植方案的选择。因此，向患者推荐哪种移植方案受到多种因素的影响，包括在 SPK 或单独肾脏移植等待名单上的患者需要进行肾移植的预期等待时间；尿毒症糖尿病患者是正在透析还是透析前状态，或者是否肾功能正常；同种致敏状态；心血管状态；该移植中心的胰腺移植效果；对于其他胰腺移植方案的预期胰腺等待时间；胰岛移植方案是否为试验性；患者意愿。由于为代替患者丧失的 β 细胞功能而进行的移植方案是多种多样的，患者会归属在不同的等待名单上面。

糖尿病患者的等待名单并不是单一的列表，而经常包含着多个不同的列表。例如，在某些移植中心，尿毒症性糖尿病患者和非尿毒症性糖尿病患者位于同一个等待名单上，然而在其他移植中心，尿毒症性糖尿病患者被分配在一个单独的 SPK 等待名单上。单独胰腺移植的患者(PAK 和 PTA 方案)常常被安排在同一个等待名单上，但同时与 SPK 患者是分开的。对于尿毒症性患者，也可能被列在两个等待名单上(例如单独肾移植或 SPK)。因此，在评估过程中决定某一患者归属于哪个等待名单，是一个非常复杂烦琐的过程，而管理这些等待移植的患者无论其在哪个等待名单上，只要出现过一次，也同样复杂。

本章主要讨论等待移植的伴或不伴慢性肾脏病(CKD)的糖尿病患者的健康维护问题以及频变的医疗状态。在众多健康维持问题中，最重要的是心血管疾病评估和监测。本章还概述了影响移植等待时间的因素，以及预期等待时间如何影响胰腺移植的方案推荐。最后，由于美国胰腺移植系统将会在近几年发生变化，我们也会讨论当前体系的局限以及新的移植体系会如何提高移植效率和器官利用度。

移植等待名单中患者移植活跃状态的监测及维持

频发的医疗问题和总在变化的等待名单状态

1 型糖尿病患者(T1DM)如果进展到需要移植的程度通常会合并诸多医疗问题，因此密切关注和检查病情以达到合理的风险管理是很必要的。常见的移植前医疗问题包括冠状动脉疾病、外周血管疾病、视网膜病变、外周和自主神经病变、胃轻瘫、低血糖昏迷，或其他可以导致急症并可能导致移植延期的自身免疫性疾病。由于这些慢性医疗问题以及它们可能导致的急性疾病的存在，待移植名单上的患者常常被归为移植保留或移植不活跃状态。事实上，维持移植不活跃状态超过一年的患者并不罕见。略观美国器官共享联合网络

(UNOS)的胰腺移植等待名单,在任何时间,胰腺移植等待名单上都有接近 50%的患者处于移植不活跃状态[1]。比如,在 2009 年末,约 3500 名患者在所有类型的胰腺移植等待名单上,然而其中只有 1600 位患者被评估为移植活跃状态。在 2010 年末,在欧洲国家移植中心的胰腺移植等待名单上,有 40%的患者被评估为移植不活跃状态[2]。现在在美国,移植不活跃状态患者(即状态 7)仍能延长等待时间节点。

等待胰腺移植的糖尿病患者的医疗状态和等待状态是频繁变化的,这对移植中心来说是不小的挑战。挑战之一便是沟通问题。由于患者会随着急性疾病的出现和恢复而在移植不活跃和活跃状态之间变换,维持患者和临床医生之间沟通交流的透明性就变得十分重要。沟通的内容包括检索新的记录、反复评估患者状态、反复在多学科候选者选择会议中讨论和更新患者的 UNOS 注册状态。临床医生(或者称之为初级保健医生)与移植中心之间的交流是很重要的,而移植中心与患者之间关于患者状态的交流也同等重要。最近的一项关于透析患者的研究[3]表明,在进行移植前检查的患者中,有超过一半的人不清楚自己准确的在等待名单上的状态。完成透析的患者不清楚自己移植问卷的准确等待状态的患者中,有 89%的人误认为自己是在移植名单中的,11%的人则不确定自己目前的等待状态。在等待名单上的患者中,大多数人能准确地知道自己的等待状态,但有 6%的人误认为自己没有被列在名单上,12.5%的人则不确定。重要的是,所有不清楚自己等待状态的名单上的患者都被列为移植不活跃状态患者(即状态 7),这表明,他们或者已经出现了新发疾病,或者需要进一步的随访检查。尽管这项单中心研究主要涉及的是非洲裔美国人透析患者,并且研究的结果仍需要在其他种族和糖尿病群体中验证,研究结果中患者对自己等待状态知晓的大量缺乏,表明在移植项目、患者以及临床医生之间沟通效率的提高是十分重要的。因此,初始的等待名单状态以及后续的所有改变都应以书面文字方式及时地传达给患者。

许多患者的等待状态是持续变化的,这就需要等待名单管理的前期工作,当然,这些工作是需要更多的付出,但对于维持患者的可移植状态是十分重要的。在众多导致糖尿病患者被列为移植不活跃状态的情况中,常见的问题是:近期心脏事件或需要完成或更新的心脏试验、足部感染和(或)溃疡、截肢、血管疾病介入治疗、眼部手术、肺炎和透析导管相关性感染。患者通常是在较远地区由内分泌科医生、肾脏科医生、初级保健医师管理,因此有关患者医疗状态改变的沟通对移植中心来说并不总是很及时。然而,在器官提供时期避免出现未经控制的医疗问题是十分重要的。如果不能将患者列为保留(例如,移植不活跃状态),或者未能及时处理患者的疾病,又或者不能识别恶化中的医疗状态,这些都会导致在器官提供期间患者不能接受移植。如果患者存在持续进展的急性医疗情况但在等待名单上仍保持着移植活跃状态并接受器官移植,那么移植手术必须取消,因为这种情况会延长冷缺血时间;或者,如果移植手术进行,患者则被放置于一种不必要的或无法预见的风险之中。因此,尽管管理远程患者具有挑战性,移植中心也乐于主动沟通,以从患者及其临床医生处获得医疗状态信息的更新。结果就是,许多移植中心力求每年都再次评估患者,并经常和患者沟通一次,持续评估他们的医疗状态和移植的准备情况。然而,与明显人数较少的 SPK 或单独胰腺移植等待名单上的长时间等待患者相比,人数众多的肝脏或肾脏移植等待名单的再评估过程需要优先进行。事实上,胰腺移植等待名单上的患者变少,以及 SPK 移植受者经常与非糖尿病尿毒症患者在同一等待名单上,这些更加强调了为使胰腺移植效率和移植率最大化,优化患者的医疗状态十分重要。

影响等待时间的因素

移植医生常常被患者及其临床医生问到的问题是:胰腺移植的预期等待时间有多长?然而要回答这一问题,需要多种因素的考量,包括移植中心/地区以及敏感度。预期等待时间可以分为短(3~6 个月)、中(6 个月~2 年)或较长(>2 年)三种,而预期等待时间的长短会影响患者移植前期的临床管理以及移植方案的选择,所以对预期等待时间的考量通常是很慎重的。因此,明确影响等待时间的关键因素可以指导移植医生们评估移植时间并制订特定的健康维护和监控计划,以确保合适的移植受者的可移植状态,从而最大限度地减少临时取消移植的可能性。

等待时间在美国不同区域之间有着明显的不同,尤其是在 SPK 移植中,因此不能确保每次对等待时间的预测都是准确的。影响 SPK 移植等待时间的主要因素是患者与非糖尿病性尿毒症患者是否处于同一名单上。与非糖尿病性尿毒症患者的名单分开的SPK移植受者往往等待时间会相对较短。一项UNOS的分析[4]指出,等待名单单独列表的SPK移植受者与和肾移植联合列表的SPK移植受者相比,前者等待时间较短(所有的SPK移植受者对应的中位等待时间:177天对645天,非致敏的透析依赖SPK移植受者对应的中位等待时间:144天对486天)。在一个特定的移植中心或捐助服务区,预测等待时间比较容易一些,但仍会有变动,取决于移植受者的血型、种族、移植类型以及同种致敏程度。这些患者特异性因素将在后文更详细地阐述。

在美国,胰腺移植的等待时间在过去的10年中逐渐延长[1]。与1998年有将近60%的患者等待时间短于1年相比,现在仅有40%的患者在被列入等待名单上1年之内接受了移植。相似的,10年前只有1%~2%的人等待时间超过5年,但是现在有接近10%的患者等待时间超过5年。这种等待时间的逐渐延长与等待名单上移植不活跃患者数目的增多和再移植以及敏感患者的增多有关,后者因为难以找到合适的匹配,往往等待时间更长。在成人胰腺移植中,等待时间的延长与10年内美国明显下降的移植率有关[1]。所有的胰腺移植加起来,1998年的移植率是将近60%/100人-年,但在2009年已下降到低于40%/100人-年。这期间移植率的下降最明显的是PAK移植,从1998年的接近72%下降至2009年仅20%[1]。相反地,SPK移植率在这一时期仅略有下降,为60%~48%。

在美国,胰腺移植的预期等待时间是多久?名单上活跃的移植受者的中位等待时间在2005—2009年为:PTA移植等待7个月,SPK移植等待11.5个月,PAK移植等待12.8个月[1]。当然,在列入名单时被登记为移植名单不活跃者的等待时间明显长于移植活跃者。例如,不活跃的PTA移植患者中位等待时间约40个月,SPK移植患者约等待25个月,PAK移植患者等待超过60个月。记录在案的PAK移植患者的等待时间较长,部分原因可能是一些中心会在活体供肾移植时使PAK移植等待名单上的尿毒症性T1DM患者变成移植活跃状态,以便在同时可行死者供体胰腺移植,因此人为地延长了尿毒症性T1DM患者的等待时间。无论是哪种移植类型,美国的胰腺移植的中位时间都表现出明显的地理差异[1]。在三种胰腺移植类型中,美国PAK移植患者在移植3年后仍等待移植的可能性略高。例如,在移植后第3年年底,仍等待PTA、SPK和PAK移植的患者分别是20%、16.1%和24.9%。PAK移植等待时间的延长与美国2009年做PAK移植的中心较2004年减少有关。与之相反,在此期间,越来越多的中心在做PTA移植,而从事SPK移植的中心数量一直保持稳定。

不幸的是,在美国,胰腺移植的中位等待时间在过去10年有所增加[1],部分原因是由于供体提供的合适的胰腺移植物减少了。自2002年以来,每个供体的胰腺回收率和移植率持续下降,2002年回收率和移植率达到峰值,分别是0.3和0.24,到2009年已经是0.21和0.15。导致下降的原因很可能与供者年龄较大、肥胖和糖尿病患病的增加有关。与此同时,自1998以来,胰腺丢弃率在各年龄组都有所上升。尽管美国循环死亡后供者(DCD)的胰腺回收率升高,以及器官获取组织(OPO)在选择最合适胰腺移植物中做出的努力,整个美国的胰腺回收率和移植率(即利用率)仍然是高度可变的,并显著低于肾移植和肝移植。

等待移植患者的死亡率和新发的与移植适应证相悖的医疗问题影响着对其能否进行移植的评估。无论是什么类型的胰腺移植,因死亡或医疗原因将患者从等待名单上去除的总去除率往往是相似的[1]。在过去3年里,美国患者的去除率往往高达20%,这再次强调了经常监测和重复评估的重要性。因医疗问题被去除的患者中,PAK和PTA移植患者的去除率最高,而SPK移植等待名单的患者则最低。另一方面,SPK移植患者在任何类型的胰腺移植等待名单中死亡率最高,这是尿毒症和糖尿病相关死亡联合的结果。到第3年,有3.3%的PTA移植等待名单上的患者死亡,SPK移植等待患者中则有9.4%死亡,PAK移植等待患者死亡率为2.5%。由于等待SPK移植的尿毒症性T1DM患者死亡率相当高,再加上漫长的SPK移植等待时间,在美国,一些地区对于这些患者群体是采取SPK移植还是活体供者肾移植术后再加PAK移植的决策是十分慎重的(亦可见后面部分)。

ABO血型、致敏、再次移植及种族因素

等待时间的长短也取决于ABO血型、人白细胞抗原(HLA)致敏的程度和再次移植的状态(在第36章详述)[1]。在美国,O型和B型患者的等待时间几乎是A型和AB型患者的两倍(即2009年的中位等待时间分

别为约 20 个月和约 10 个月），在过去的 10 年里这种差距越来越大,但原因未知。

正如肾移植一样，移植受者的同种致敏是所有类型胰腺移植等待时间延长的危险因素。由于近几年再次移植受者的数量增加，等待名单上非致敏胰腺移植受者的比例有所下降[1]。此外,越来越多敏感的 HLA 抗体检测方法的使用,如 Luminex®单珠检测,可能是导致致敏患者的比率升高的原因。中度及高度致敏的患者[20%~79%群体反应抗体(cPRA)]的等待时间明显长于低致敏(<20% cPRA)或非致敏患者。对于高度致敏的尿毒症性糖尿病患者，临床医生应特别考虑几种可能的治疗方案。其中最好的选择是迅速纠正患者的 CKD 状态，从而降低患者在透析时的死亡率。关于方案的选择,其一是死亡供体的 SPK 移植,这种移植方式不需要等待名单脱敏，但预期的等待时间要长于平均等待时间。另一种选择是等待名单脱敏后行 SPK 移植术或死亡供体肾移植，但这一方式可能会需要大量的管理工作。第三种选择是如果 ABO 血型不合或交叉配血阳性的活体供者存在，可通过国家肾脏登记处或当地捐助者交换计划行活体供体肾单独移植。最后,无论哪种方案首先适用，都应将患者放在死亡供体 SPK 移植或肾脏单独移植的双重等待名单上，也可以建议考虑将患者放在不同捐赠服务地区的移植中心的多个等待名单上。一项关于 UNOS 肾脏移植等待名单的分析[5]显示,无论移植受者的人口学、生物学和社会经济学状态如何，位于多个等待名单上可以使其获得减少 50%的中位等待时间和相对较高的移植率。虽然在其他等待名单人数明显少的移植中心加入多个等待名单已被证明是有益的，但如果在其他中心也需要同样长的等待时间，这种加入多个等待名单的方法可能不会有明显的成效[6]。虽然目前还没有和胰腺移植相关的类似数据，但将这些数据在概念上推演到胰腺移植是很可能成立的。

尽管在过去黑人或非洲裔美国人作为移植受者需要更长的等待时间，目前在美国根据种族分层时的等待时间差别不大[1]。

慢性肾脏疾病和 1 型糖尿病患者的移植选择

对尿毒症性 T1DM 患者而言，胰腺移植和肾移植的选择方案有很多[7]。其中最主要的是 SPK 移植或活体供体肾移植后的死亡供体胰腺移植。虽然这些都不是唯一的选择，但在其他病情稳定并很少发生并发症的患者中，术后透析或单独接受死亡供体肾移植是不理想的结果,并且通常伴有更高的死亡率[8-10]。一个连续的 PAK 移植涉及两个手术和两个来自不同供体的器官，治疗过程中需要监测每一个供体器官的排斥反应，并且通常会出现很低的胰腺同种异体移植物存活率（3 年胰腺移植物存活率:PAK 移植是 68%,SPK 移植是 78%）[1]。然而,在 PAK 移植中,患者因为在短期接受了活体供体肾移植，因而能迅速逆转 CKD 病情,所以也能从 PAK 移植中潜在获益。另一方面,从相同供者处进行 SPK 移植可以通过一次手术和仅监测对一个供者的排斥反应让患者同时纠正肾脏疾病和糖尿病病情，从而使患者——与活体供体肾移植相比——拥有更高的胰腺移植物存活率与相似的肾脏存活率[7]。

应该推荐哪种移植方式给患者在很大程度上取决于在特定地区的 SPK 移植的预期等待时间。这样说的依据是什么呢？鉴于 CKD 糖尿病联合导致非常高的死亡率以及记录在案的肾移植对患者的强大生存获益，这些患者的等待名单死亡率很高，因此不能长时间等待肾移植。在美国和世界各地的一些移植中心,SPK 移植受者与许多非糖尿病 CKD 患者在同一名单上,因此等待时间是很长的，那么为了达到成功的肾移植的首要目的，活体供体肾移植是最好的选择。因此，如果 SPK 移植受者的预计等待时间很长（可能超过 1~2 年）,无论是移植中心的因素还是患者个人原因,活体供体肾单独移植可能是一个非常有益的选择。在其他情况下，预计 SPK 移植的等待时间短一些，那么 SPK 移植就优于 PAK 移植。上述建议的活体供体肾移植后 PAK 移植术的前提是这个患者有活体供体肾的选择，如果没有,那么 SPK 移植与单独死者供体肾移植相比，在改善患者长期生存和更好的生活质量方面，显然是一个更好的长期选择[9]。

值得一提的是，为了调节移植方式的相对获益还有一些其他的考虑。如果有 HLA 相合的活体供体肾脏可用,则活体供体肾移植和连续的 PAK 移植或许是一个好的选择,因为 HLA 相合肾脏移植的排斥反应率通常很低并能显著地延长寿命[11]。另一方面,如果糖尿病患者同时伴有低血糖意识受损和频繁低血糖发作,那么有可能会更积极地考虑早期胰腺移植和联合移植。高度致敏的尿毒症糖尿病患者的病例也值得考虑。通常情况下，如果缺乏肾移植的活体供体，这类患者将被列于 SPK 移植等待名单上，因为胰腺-肾脏联合移植与单独死亡供体肾移植相比患者收益更大。然而，由于高致敏患者只能接受一部分匹配良好供者的供体移植，同时只有一部分的供者(美国平均 15/100)能提供一个合适的胰腺移植物，这些患者可能要为了一次 SPK 移植等待很长时间。在这种情况下，与患者本人沟通将其既列于 SPK 等待名单上，同时也列于单独肾脏移植等待名单上，并当供者的胰腺不可移植时选择接受匹配良好的肾移植也是很有意义的。最后，对那些没有适合的活体供者的患者，他们可以在国家肾脏登记处通过其他途径获得活体供体肾脏。

监测频率

大多数移植中心至少每年一次或每两年一次重新评估等待名单上的移植受者。一项关于美国移植项目的调查表明，71%的移植中心会试图通过约定见面或电话联系的方式跟踪监测所有等待肾移植的受者[12]。及时更新患者的心脏情况、免疫性、精神性和感染性疾病以及恶性状态是至关重要的，这样可以避免在器官提供时不可移植状态的发生，或避免因忽视相关问题后进行移植而引起的围手术期发病率的升高。在威斯康星大学，我们的目标是重新评估在肾脏和胰腺移植等待名单上的所有发生显著医疗状况变化的、显著的体重增加的，或已经在等候名单上超过一年的患者。

移植中心通常每月收集血清进行交叉匹配和抗 HLA 抗体的检测。在威斯康星大学，我们每月收集 Luminex®抗 HLA 抗体检测的血液样本，并对致敏患者每个季度测试一次，对非致敏患者每半年测试一次，或者在任何潜在致敏事件，如输血制品、怀孕或移植后测试一次。

心脏筛查

在所有 CKD 患者中，合并有 T1DM 的患者有晚期缺血性心脏病和未识别的心血管疾病的风险最高。因此，至少在移植术前和移植术后需要经常进行心脏负荷试验。然而，仅仅依靠非侵入性心脏负荷试验的方法已经受到人们的质疑[13]。事实上，糖尿病性尿毒症患者的心脏高风险提示心脏病筛查需要积极进行。积极进行心血管疾病筛查的原则来源于以下观察数据：①患者具有心脏病的高患病率[14,15]；②心肌缺血和梗死通常不易被发现[16]和③心脏负荷试验有高的假阴性[13,17-19]。例如，Vandenberg 等在 47 例无症状糖尿病移植受者中应用了非侵入性测试（应力铊显像或运动核素心室造影）和冠状动脉造影，能检测到 75%或更大的冠状动脉狭窄的敏感度，在应力铊显像和运动核素心室造影中分别为 62%和 50%[13]。在另一项前瞻性研究中，多巴酚丁胺负荷超声心动图敏感度为 75%，特异度为 76%[17]。Selek 等的研究显示，无论是进行运动核负荷试验、药物负荷试验还是负荷超声心动图，需要移植评估的糖尿病尿毒症患者在社区进行心脏负荷试验的敏感度都为 27%~47%[19]。这些研究和临床证据都提示在将 SPK 或单独肾脏移植等待名单上的患者认定为移植活跃之前，对糖尿病患者需要经常进行冠状动脉造影以筛查心脏疾病和心肌代谢清除情况。以冠状动脉造影作为这群高危人群的心脏筛查金标准的优势还体现在，SPK 移植等待者常常死亡，尽管死亡前不久的核或跑步机负荷试验结果是阴性。同时，SPK 移植后最常见的死亡原因常与心血管疾病有关[9]。此外，SPK 移植患者移植后发生心肌缺血事件的情况是有明确发生率的，在某项研究中最高可达到 20%，尽管术前心脏负荷试验结果是阴性[17]。因此，在笔者所属的机构中，绝大多数移植评估中的糖尿病患者需要进行冠状动脉造影。

许多大型胰腺移植中心倾向于采用冠状动脉造影评估尿毒症透析前的 SPK 移植受者，而不管负荷试验的结果，尤其是年龄>45 岁，糖尿病病史>25 年，有吸烟史，或列入等待名单前存在心脏疾病的患者。移植中心希望通过采取这种方式干预围手术期心脏事件的发生。这种检查方式并不是对那些已经在透析的患者而言的，然而，在透析前患者中，冠状动脉造影可能会导致肾功能不全的进展，并有可能需要开始进行透析，这是一个临床难题。数据清楚地表明肾脏移植患者在透析前检查是可以获益的，并且可提高患者和肾脏移植物的存活率[20]。鉴于糖尿病患者透析死亡率高的事实，人们希望上述研究结果也可以推论到 1 型糖尿病患者和肾脏病患者中。因此，继续推荐早期肾脏疾病患者进行移植检查似乎是很重要的。鉴于出现肾衰竭的风险，移植中心往往在透析前患者中有选择地进行心脏置管或避免做冠状动脉造影。在这种情况下，患者可以在不做心室造影的前提下接受冠状动脉造影同时保护肾脏功能，或只保护肾脏功能而不检查冠状动脉，尤其是在患者肌酐水平较低的情况下。另外，仅心脏负荷试验阴性且冠状动脉造影推迟的患者可以被添加到 SPK 移植等待名单中,等待到透析开始为止。在患者 UNOS 等待名单上可以被登记为移植非活跃状态，这样可以增加等待时间,直到开始透析后进行冠状动脉造影检查,在此之后再认定为移植活跃状态。

如果冠状动脉造影显示病变> 75%，患者应该接受血管成形术和支架置入或冠状动脉旁路移植术。Manske 等研究了 26 位发现有 75%冠状动脉狭窄的无症状糖尿病患者，并将他们随机分为术前血管重建组和单独药物治疗组[18]。他们发现,单独药物治疗组的患者在移植后发生心脏事件的概率明显比接受介入治疗的患者要大。

综上所述，现有的对糖尿病尿毒症移植受者的心血管筛查数据表明，移植前积极的诊断和恰当的干预是十分有益的。

外周血管筛查

由于血流在影响同种异体移植物功能上是一个关键的决定因素,在评估胰腺和(或)肾脏移植的糖尿病患者时，明确髂血管病变范围和是否对称是极其重要的。相比于糖尿患者群中普遍存在的远端下肢疾病,存在或不存在髂血管病应作为关注的焦点。多年来,有许多不同的血管成像技术已被用于评估这些患者，但却很少有比物理诊断效果更好的。由于严重钙化的血管是不可压缩的，下肢的多普勒容积记录的不准确性众所周知,而下肢动脉造影不能完全评估双侧髂血管,这使得该检查也失去其诊断优势。腹部平片可观察髂血管系统中的血管钙化情况,但其灵敏度较低。下肢截肢患者,尤其是那些由骨髓炎导致的患者,一般不会有髂动脉病变,因此可不作为移植的排除因素。对于需要植入一个或多个同种异体移植物患者来说，最适合移植的血管状态是良好的股脉搏检查和(或)无静脉造影的腹部或骨盆的计算机断层扫描(CT)。移植等待期间的血管筛查的最佳频率尚未确定，但如果患者有暂时的双侧或严重的单侧病变的进展，可能需要再次评价患者作为 SPK 移植受者的资格。

其他

有些患者在特殊情况下可能适合或可能不适合从疾病预防控制中心(CDC)接受器官高危或丙型肝炎病毒患者的器官。当地移植和分配政策应该规定这些器官分配的条件和方法。当地等待名单机构应明确指明患者是否自愿接受 CDC 提供的高危或丙型肝炎病毒患者的胰腺，并且患者的选择随着时间的推移在等待过程中可能会发生改变。在笔者所在的机构,我们采取这样的政策:对于丙型肝炎病毒携带者的 SPK 移植受者，只考虑丙型肝炎病毒阳性的移植供者这种原则在肾脏移植中同样适用，即丙型肝炎病毒阳性供者的器官只能移植给丙型肝炎病毒携带者受体。关于 CDC 高危人群供者器官的分配，只有移植受者同意且只有供者的核酸检测(NAT)为阴性,移植才可以进行。重要的是,在对患者等待状态评估的同时,应该重新评估患者对于 CDC 高危和丙型肝炎病毒患者供者移植的意愿。

从等待名单中去除

死亡、移植和不可纠正的禁忌证的出现都是将患者从器官共享移植网络(OPTN)等候名单中去除的原因,且需要在移植中心知晓上述事件后的 24 小时内完成。

目前美国的胰腺移植物分配系统

在美国，胰腺移植物首先被分配给胰腺全器官移植受者,其次是胰岛移植受者[21]。胰腺是首先分配在当地的医院的供体服务区(DSA),然后分配在 11 个不同的 OPTN 区域,最后在全国范围内分配。高度致敏移植受者中的胰腺移植物分配为,无 HLA 不匹配患者优先于存在 HLA 不匹配者，存在 HLA 不匹配者优先于其他等待名单上的患者。在每个 DSA 中,致敏受者优先于其他受者。然后再根据等待时间长短对患者进行分层。

对于其他 DSA 的胰腺和 SPK 移植供者,移植中心可能要明确中心特定的标准以保证该器官不适合被移植。年龄<50 岁且身体质量指数(BMI)<30kg/m^2 的捐赠者的胰腺首先被用于胰腺移植，如果捐赠者的胰腺对所有的移植受者而言都不适合，则该捐赠者的胰腺将被用于胰岛移植或研究。年龄>50 岁或 BMI>32kg/m^2 的捐赠者的胰腺则首先被用于胰岛移植。制订本项政策的目的是要便于利用一般认为不适合全器官移植的胰腺,并提高胰岛移植受者的移植物分配率。

由于目前的胰腺分配政策只考虑胰腺全器官移植的分配,导致美国国内 UNOS 地区的政策不统一。在一些地区，“肾脏移植后胰腺移植”受者和SPK移植受者和许多非糖尿病肾移植受者位于同一等待名单上，而在其他地区，“胰腺移植后肾脏移植”受者和SPK移植受者以及肾移植受者分属于不同的等待名单上。因此，移植中心和地区产生了差异或例外，由此导致美国胰腺全器官移植分配政策的混乱和不一致。这些差异的结果之一是，胰腺利用、移植途径和移植等待时间的地理不平衡仍然十分明显。

此外，目前的系统对于等待胰腺移植患者，除了“被诊断为糖尿病或胰腺外分泌功能不全”之外，没有具体的糖尿病相关的评判标准，这可能反过来会导致越来越多的2型糖尿病和CKD患者接受SPK移植。最后，许多中心对胰腺全器官移植受者提供至少两个单独的等待名单：一个是SPK移植等待名单，一个是单独胰腺移植等待名单，然而这两个名单在两个群体中本可以简化为一个名单即可。

未来美国胰腺移植物分配展望

最近UNOS董事会表示，UNOS胰腺移植委员会制订了一个详细的提议，以期到2011年制订并实现一个更高效、统一的国家胰腺分配系统。提议的新分配制度的目标是通过将胰腺分配从肾脏分配中分离，使胰腺分配效率提高，以及最大限度地利用胰腺移植物并纠正胰腺移植途径和等待时间在地理上的不平衡[4]。

新提议的政策旨在：

1.将单独胰腺移植和SPK移植受者归为一个联合等待名单，同时允许联合等待名单上的受者在接受胰腺分配后仍能在单独肾脏匹配中获得单独肾移植，只要该患者符合特定的评判标准。

2.出台针对SPK移植受者的肾功能障碍和糖尿病相关的客观的医学评判标准，以延长等待时间。

3.将死亡供体胰腺和当前的肾脏分配系统中分离出来，以便胰腺移植受者能在肾脏移植前并优先于儿童及成人单独肾移植受者得到器官分配[4]。

为了使评判标准规范化和防止大量2型糖尿病患者和尿毒症患者被归为SPK移植，符合下列医疗评判标准的SPK移植受者将能够增加时间并接受移植[4,22]：

- SPK移植受者必须符合当前肾脏移植的评判标准。即他们必须符合在透析中或肾小球滤过率(GFR)≤20mL/min或肌酐清除率≤20mL/min。
- 关于糖尿病的资格标准，移植受者必须满足以下标准之一：①正在使用胰岛素或C肽≤2ng/mL；②正在使用胰岛素且C肽> 2ng/mL，且BMI达到最大允许阈值，为28~30kg/m^2。BMI的阈值可通过器官获取组织(OPO)负责人动态调整。
- 单独胰腺移植的等待名单标准仍与之前相同[4]。

有意为之的这些改变使所有胰腺移植受者都位于同一等待名单上，从而消除了胰腺分配的一部分复杂性，并建立了统一的全国性的系统。此外，所有类型的胰腺移植受者获得高质量器官的机会是均等的。重要的是，通过建模可以证明，在单独胰腺移植的病例中，该系统能在肾脏分配系统中保留高质量的肾脏移植物。此外，新分配模式中的“胰腺移植后的肾脏移植”与其他肾外器官的同种异体肾移植的分配是一致的。预计新分配模式将在2014年秋季实行，而实行之后SPK移植的总等待时间将会减少，并且胰腺移植的总利用率和胰腺移植率将会有所提高。

胰岛移植等待名单的注意事项

美国的胰岛移植仅由食品和药物管理局(FDA)和机构审查委员会(IRB)批准的临床试验中提供。因此，等待名单的管理在很大程度上取决于临床试验的设计方案或当地政策。胰岛胰腺移植的一个重要特征是，要达到不依赖外源性胰岛素的状态，往往需要不止一个胰腺的胰岛。普遍认同的看法是，在两个或两个以上的胰岛供体的胰岛输注间期进行短期干预是有益的。接受至少一次胰岛输注的移植受者通常优先进行第二次胰岛输注，并可以在等待名单上保持移植活跃状态。

总结

T1DM患者的等待名单管理受许多因素影响，包括并发症的显著进展（尤其是心血管疾病），β细胞替代方案的多样性，以及多种名单共存的可能。分配政策的不一致性进一步复杂化了名单管理过程。移植中心需要仔细地考虑对患者影响最大的因素，以便处理移植前出现的各种问题。定期检查是必需的，特别是筛查心血管疾病和无症状心肌缺血，以确保患者的健康状况在其获得死亡供体器官之前都维持良好状态。

致谢

笔者敬谢 Dixon Kaufman 博士和高级临床移植协调员 Mike Armbrust 对本书稿的审阅。

（林天雨 译 高鹏骥 校）

参考文献

1. OPTN and SRTR Annual Data Report 2010: pancreas. American Journal of Transplantation. 2012;12(Suppl 1):33–52.
2. Annual Report 2011, Eurotransplant International Foundation. 2012 [cited 2012 May 24, 2012]; Available from: http://www.eurotransplant.org.
3. Gillespie A, et al. Lack of listing status awareness: results of a single-center survey of hemodialysis patients. American Journal of Transplantation. 2011;11:1522–1526.
4. Organ Procurement Transplantation Network Pancreas Transplantation Committee. Proposal to develop an efficient, uniform pancreas allocation system. 2010 [cited 2010 May 24, 2012]; Available from: http://optn.transplant.hrsa.gov/PublicComment/pubcommentPropSub_259.pdf.
5. Merion RM, et al. Prevalence and outcomes of multiple-listing for cadaveric kidney and liver transplantation. American Journal of Transplantation. 2004;4:94–100.
6. Kumar V, Julian BA, Deierhoi MH, et al. Secondary listing for deceased-donor kidney transplantation does not increase likelihood of engraftment at a large transplant center. American Journal of Transplantation. 2009;9:1671–1673.
7. Wiseman AC. Pancreas transplant options for patients with type 1 diabetes mellitus and chronic kidney disease: simultaneous pancreas kidney or pancreas after kidney? Current Opinion in Organ Transplantation. 2012;17:80–86.
8. Becker BN, et al. Simultaneous pancreas-kidney transplantation reduces excess mortality in type 1 diabetic patients with end-stage renal disease. Kidney International. 2000;57:2129–2135.
9. Sollinger HW, Odorico JS, Becker YT, et al. One thousand simultaneous pancreas-kidney transplants at a single center with 22-year follow-up. Annals of Surgery. 2009;250:618–630.
10. Tyden G, et al. Improved survival in patients with insulin-dependent diabetes mellitus and end-stage diabetic nephropathy 10 years after combined pancreas and kidney transplantation. Transplantation. 1999;67:645–648.
11. Rayhill SC, et al. Simultaneous pancreas-kidney transplantation and living related donor renal transplantation in patients with diabetes: is there a difference in survival? Annals of Surgery. 2000;231:417–423.
12. Danovitch GM, et al. Management of the waiting list for cadaveric kidney transplants: report of a survey and recommendations by the Clinical Practice Guidelines Committee of the American Society of Transplantation. Journal of the American Society of Nephrology. 2002;13:528–535.
13. Vandenberg BF, et al. Evaluation of diabetic patients for renal and pancreas transplantation: noninvasive screening for coronary artery disease using radionuclide methods. Transplantation. 1996;62:1230–1235.
14. Haffner SM, Lehto S, Ronnemaa T, et al. Mortality from coronary heart disease in subjects with type 2 diabetes and in nondiabetic subjects with and without prior myocardial infarction. New England Journal of Medicine. 1998;339:229–234.
15. Stamler J, Vaccaro O, Neaton JD, et al. Diabetes, other risk factors, and 12-yr cardiovascular mortality for men screened in the multiple risk factor intervention trial. Diabetes Care. 1993;16:434–444.
16. Valensi P, Lorgis L, Cottin Y. Prevalence, incidence, predictive factors and prognosis of silent myocardial infarction: a review of the literature. Archives of Cardiovascular Diseases. 2011;104:178–188.
17. Herzog CA, et al. Dobutamine stress echocardiography for the detection of significant coronary artery disease in renal transplant candidates. American Journal of Kidney Diseases. 1999;33:1080–1090.
18. Manske CL, Wang Y, Rector T, et al. Coronary revascularisation in insulin-dependent diabetic patients with chronic renal failure. Lancet. 1992;340:998–1002.
19. Selek A, et al. Should diabetic patients undergoing transplant evaluation routinely have cardiac angiography? American Journal of Transplantation. 2011;11(Suppl 2):102.
20. Meier-Kriesche HU, et al. Effect of waiting time on renal transplant outcome. Kidney International. 2000;58:1311–1317.
21. OPTN and SRTR Annual Data Report 2010: allocation policies. American Journal of Transplantation. 2012;12(Suppl 1):135–142.
22. Kaufman DB, Sutherland DE. Simultaneous pancreas-kidney transplants are appropriate in insulin-treated candidates with uremia regardless of diabetes type. Clinical Journal of the American Society of Nephrology. 2011;6:957–959.

第 42 章
小肠及多脏器联合移植等待名单管理

Kareem M. Abu-Elmagd, Guilherme Costa

引言

在过去的 20 年中，随着小肠移植（不论是单独移植还是多脏器联合移植）可操作性的提升，联合器官共享网络（UNOS）等待名单中的等候者数目也在稳定上升[1,2]。因此，为了降低等候者的死亡率以及最有效地利用已捐献的器官，建立一个管理等候者的临床指南是至关重要的。

本章通过同种异体移植脏器的类型、现行 UNOS 管理条例、危险因素等方面来介绍器官移植等候者的临床管理。

同种异体移植脏器的类型

近年来，各种不同的同种异体移植脏器都有了明确的定义[1,3,4]。伴有小肠衰竭或复杂腹部病变的患者，可能需要小肠单独移植或小肠联合其他脏器和实质器官移植（图 42.1）。三种主要的移植脏器类型包括独立的小肠、小肠-肝脏联合、包括胃在内的伴或不伴肝脏的多脏器。有指征时，部分结肠肠段和（或）单个肾脏也会同独立小肠或其他多脏器进行联合移植。

脏器移植的指征在其他文献[5]及本书第 30 章均有详细的论述。简而言之，器官衰竭是移植替换的基础。包括胰腺在内的小肠-肝脏联合移植通常需要同种异体移植物保持其血管的完整性和连续性。在多脏器联合移植中，由于患者实质脏器和空腔脏器会发生大范围的血管功能紊乱，通常胰腺和胃也需要被替换。

现行 UNOS/OPTN 管理条例及分配政策

名单

经过全面的评估后，机构评选委员会决定患者的等候资格。在通过保险人的财务审批后，患者会根据

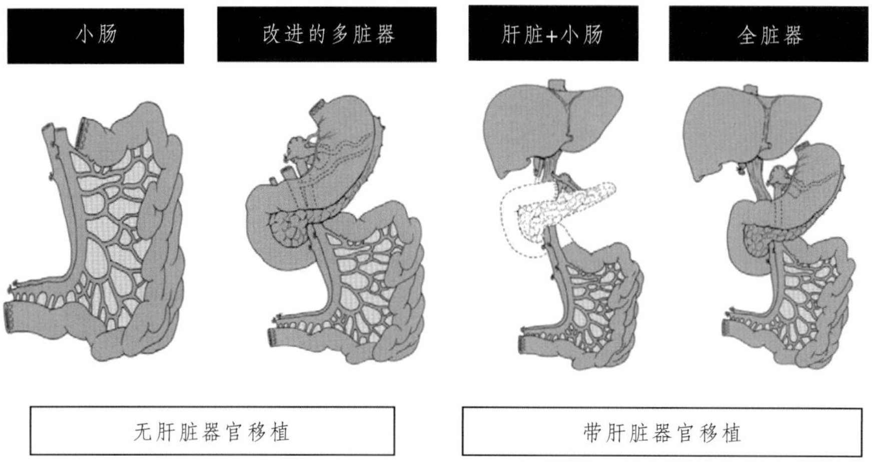

图 42.1 同种异体移植脏器的类型：小肠、小肠-肝脏联合、多脏器联合。胰十二指肠复合物（图中非阴影部分）是肝脏-小肠联合移植的可选部分。多器官移植必须包括完整的胃以及其他多脏器（改进的多脏器或全脏器）。当肾脏只能单独移植时，结肠、胰腺和肾脏也可以完整地加入到无肝移植物中。

UNOS 指南被列在名单上。一般来说,等待名单中没有指定哪个患者需要进行联合移植,同样地,每个器官也是单独被列出来的。从对腹腔和胸腔器官统筹管理的相似性角度来说,因为腹部区域的挛缩问题,尤其是对患有短肠综合征的患者而言,内脏移植等候者往往优先匹配给那些所需脏器更小的同血型患者。

脏器移植等候者在 UNOS 等待名单中的分层地位是根据所需移植物的类型来决定。需要无肝移植物的患者,当存在威胁生命的家庭肠外营养相关并发症,如静脉通路消失、进行性肝损害时,将在名单中被列为第一位,其他情况的患者将被列为第二位。

目前,肝脏-小肠联合或多脏器联合移植在 UNOS 等待名单上的优先次序是由儿科终末期肝病/终末期肝病模型(PELD/MELD)评分来指导的。然而,由于疾病的严重性以及患者的复杂性,肝脏-小肠联合移植的等候者是被 PELD/MELD 评分拒之在外的,无法被评估[6]。关于肝脏-小肠联合移植的分配政策及其对当前等候者死亡率的影响将在下文讨论。

目前单独列出构成联合内脏移植物的各种脏器和实体器官的现行方法存在着显著的缺陷,具有使临床、生物学、免疫学指标发生偏移的可能,尤其是当 UNOS 或移植受者科学注册系统(SRTR)的数据被用于包括结果测量的临床研究时。近期观察发现,一些接受联合脏器移植物的患者在 SRTR 的报告中是根据移植物中某一器官进行分类的,而忽视了小肠才是整个器官移植物的核心。另一种潜在缺陷是,在与胰腺移植相关的临床研究中,接受胰腺及其他器官联合移植的受者存在不同的免疫学和非免疫学差异[7,8]。

等候时间

名单中的等候时间是多种临床因素和立法因素作用的结果。最重要的因素包括移植物类型、在等待名单中的地位、器官获取组织(OPO)的地理位置以及捐献者位置的可及性,其他决定性因素包括接受者的年龄、体重、血型、腹腔容积。对于需要无肝移植物的患者,其血清巨细胞病毒(CMV)是否阳性,以及是否存在同种异体抗体,尤其是交叉配型阳性时产生的供体特异性抗体,都将作为决定等候时间的相关指标。

在当前器官供应移植网络(OPTN)的器官配置政策下,脏器移植物的类型是决定患者从列入名单到实行移植的等候时间的主要决定因素(图 42.2)。当前单独小肠移植物的需求量较少,该类移植物的等候时间大约在几天到 250 天[1]。如此宽泛的范围反映了不同移植中心采取了多种管理协议,包括终止 CMV 阳性供者对 CMV 阴性受者的移植以及交叉反应阳性的无肝脏器移植。其他重要的影响因素包括 OPO 对小肠的非最优化利用,冷缺血时间受限于供者的地理位置,包括低年龄、血流动力学稳定、无心肺骤停病史等在内的严格的供者选择标准。由于体重和体形的限制,儿童群体需要更长的等候时间[1]。

近些年来,那些需要改良的无肝多脏器移植的患者,他们的等候时间变得越来越长。移植物保留腹腔干以保证移植胃的血供,此项操作越来越难以得到全国肝脏移植外科医生的批准[9,10]。需要实施该手术的患者通常是弥漫性胃肠功能紊乱和严重的腹部病变的患者,尤其是具有严重的胃动力障碍、加德纳综合征和前胃切除术的患者。

根据最新的 SRTR 年度报告,不论是进行单独小肠移植还是肝脏-小肠联合移植,患者等候移植物的中位时间均是逐渐且优先减少的(图 42.2)。这一成就反映了 UNOS 分配政策的持续变化以及该领域的不断进展。这两个重要的演变对肝脏-小肠移植的等候者有一定的益处,而对无肝移植的等候者没有显著影响。尽管如此,每年移植等候的中位时间的显著变化,反映了转诊模式、肠道康复活动、UNOS/OPTN 分配政策的不断变化(表 42.1)。

等待名单死亡率

由于疾病的复杂性和严重性,在 UNOS 等待名单

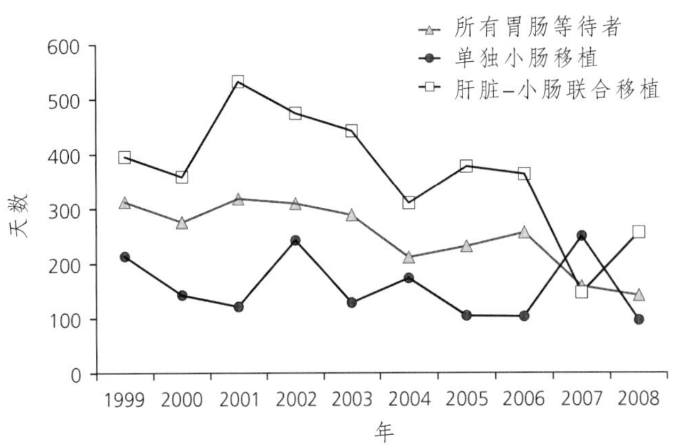

图 42.2 1999-2008 年 UNOS 登记注册的小肠移植中位等候时间。(Modified from Mazariegos et al. [1], with permission from John Wiley and Sons Ltd.)

上的内脏移植等候者有很高的死亡率[11-15]。根据UNOS数据库,与其他胸部和腹部器官的等候患者相比,这些患者具有更高的死亡率(图42.3)[1]。紧急转诊、等候者死亡以及早期移植后死亡率的预测因素在其他地方已有全面讨论[16-22]。简而言之,肝脏损伤程度、移植时住院治疗、肠道衰竭的因素和麻醉依赖性是不良预后的最重要危险因素。

最近在UNOS/OPTN分配政策中引入的一系列变化(表42.1)降低了肝脏-小肠等待名单中小儿等候者的死亡率,而成人的死亡率将持续明显高于单独肝脏移植的候选者(图42.4)[13]。因此,本章的主要作者于2009年6月联系了UNOS肝脏-小肠移植委员会,并提出了循证建议,进一步修订当前UNOS条例,以增加已故患者的器官对这些高危的肝脏-小肠等候者的可利用性。上述对当前SRTR数据的分析显示,肝脏-小肠等候者的死亡率为单独肝脏移植等候者的3倍(图42.5)。因此,UNOS/OPTN委员会确定了最终方案,允许MELD评分≥29的肝脏-小肠等候者能够在全国范围内获得已故捐赠者的器官[23]。

改善预后的努力

由于联合肝脏-小肠的供体十分有限,早期转诊越来越被重视,以此来避免患者发展到需要肝脏移植的阶段[16-19,24-27]。此外,利用创新的药物和外科模式恢复肠功能的多学科会诊的概念被引入,用此方法有可能避免移植的需要[28]。

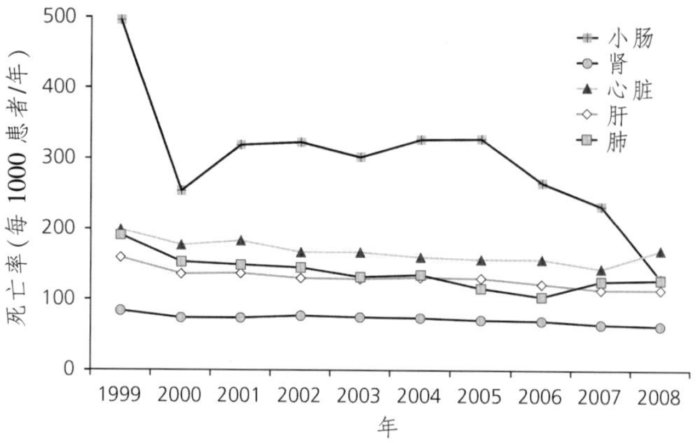

图 42.3 1999-2008年联合器官共享网络(UNOS)等待名单中患者的未调整千人死亡率。(Modified from Mazariegos et al. [1], with permission from John Wiley and Sons Ltd.)

可以想象,减少UNOS名单中等候者的等候时间,无论是无肝移植还是带肝移植的等候者,都可能降低他们的死亡率。对于无肝移植物,技术的创新、活体供体的利用以及已故供体库的审慎扩张等方式已经成功地应用[9,29-31],其优势在于开辟了从同一供体同时获取小肠和胰腺并将其移植到两个不同受体的方法[9]。我们

表 42.1 肝脏-小肠移植等候者OPTN政策的变化

描述	UNet℠ 应用时间
Ⅰ 对于肝脏-小肠联合移植的等候者,可以使用小肠名单来分配肝脏,除非该地区中有分类地位为第一地位的患者。在此阶段使用了不同的名单地位标准	1990年5月~2005年2月
Ⅱ 所有在两个等待名单上登记的肝脏-小肠联合移植的等候者,将自动获得相当于3个月死亡率风险为10%的MELD/PELD评分的增加	2005年3月
Ⅲ 3.9.3修改为"肝脏可以由当地OPO分配给当地、整个地区或全国的小肠等候者,基于小肠等待名单中的优先次序,除非当地、整个地区或国家中有1A或1B地位的肝脏等候者"	2007年6月
Ⅳ 小儿肝脏-小肠等候者获得另外23分的分数。成人仍然获得额外的10%	2007年6月
Ⅴ 小儿捐献的脏器优先提供给需要肝脏或肝脏-小肠移植的小儿患者	2007年6月
Ⅵ 政策修订后声明:在根据小肠匹配运行顺序将移植物提供给进行肝脏-小肠移植的潜在受者之前,肝脏必须根据国家提供的1A和1B地位按顺序分配给每个潜在的肝脏受者(包括所有MELD/PELD潜在受者)	N/A
Ⅶ 0~10岁儿童供者的肝脏优先提供给1A地位的0~11岁的肝脏和肝脏-小肠移植等候者,然后再提供给当地1A地位的成年等候者	2010年11月
Ⅷ 成人供体算法将被修改,使得当整个区域没有1A/1B地位的候选者或者当地没有MELD/PELD积分≥29分的候选者时,肝脏可以全国性地分配给肝脏-小肠移植等候者	2011年11月

UNetSM,由联合器官共享网络(UNOS)管理的一个集中式计算机网络,用于匹配已故捐赠者和潜在接受者之间的器官。
MELD/PELD,儿科终末期肝病/终末期肝病模型;OPO,器官获取组织。

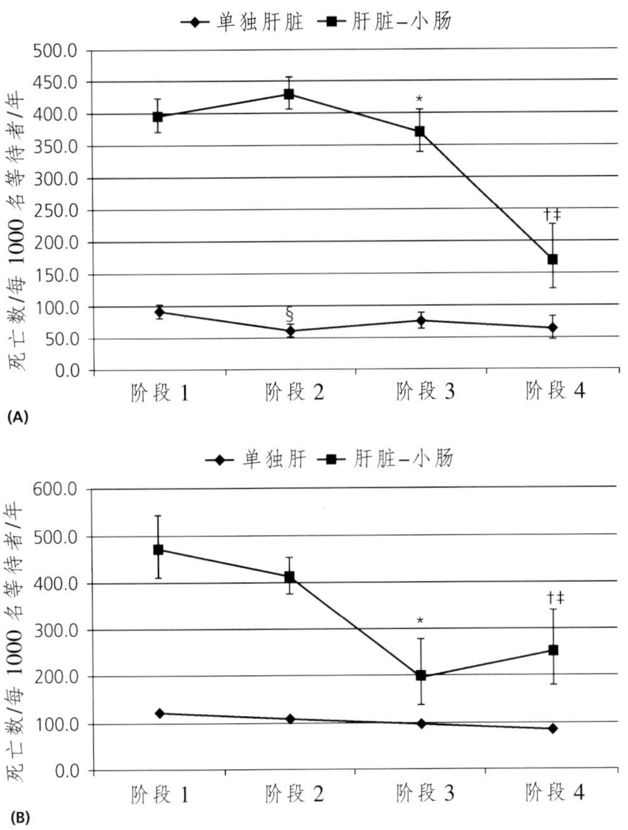

图 42.4 (A)MELD/PELD 的修订对成年候选者中肝脏–小肠移植及单独肝脏移植的死亡率的影响。与阶段 2 相比,*$P<0.05$;与阶段 1 和阶段 2 相比,†$P<0.05$;与阶段 3 相比,‡$P<0.01$;与阶段 1 相比,§$P<0.05$。I 条表示 95%置信区间。(Reproduced from Kaplan et al.[13],with permission from John Wiley and Sons Ltd.)(B)小儿候选者中肝脏–小肠移植及单独肝脏移植的死亡率对比。与阶段 1 和阶段 2 对比,*$P<0.001$;与阶段 2 对比,†$P<0.05$;与阶段 1 对比,‡$P<0.01$。I 条表示 95%置信区间。(Reproduced from Kaplan et al.[13],with permission from John Wiley and Sons Ltd.)

建议,仅针对没有遗传性疾病的同卵双胞胎,以及在法律不允许脑死亡个体捐献器官的的国家,方可采用来源于活体的节段性小肠移植。

对于带肝移植的等候者,UNOS 分配政策的不断演变有助于降低其死亡率,尤其是进行肝脏–小肠移植的小儿候选者。在实施器官分配的新算法(表 42.1)后,成年等候者也可以得到类似的预期结果。同时,在短肠综合征的患儿中利用单独肝脏移植来进行肠道恢复的方法已经被成功采用[32]。为数较少的 ABO 兼容的移植物也已被用于病情极度严重的候选者身上[27,33,34]。源于活体的节段性小肠和肝脏联合移植也被小心地引入,其预期的潜在风险也在相应地逐步上升[35]。

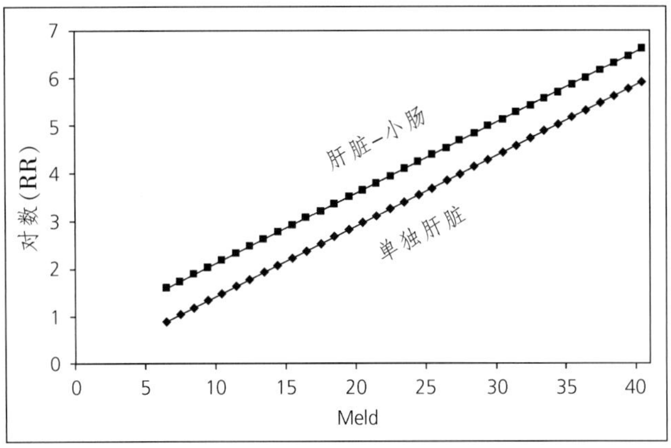

图 42.5 在器官供应移植网络(OPTN)等待名单中,肝脏–小肠移植与单独肝脏移植的等候者死亡率的相对危险度(RR)对数的比较。数据由移植受者科学注册系统(SRTR)提供,并提交给联合器官共享网络(UNOS)肝脏–小肠委员会。2011 年 11 月,UNOS/OPTN 委员会批准了表 42.1 中所列的修改建议。

法规遵从

与其他器官移植的政策相同,UNOS/OPTN 的分配政策必须被遵从。包括将候选者列入名单或从中移除时的告知,加入多个名单的权利,以及在名单中等候者地位的定期更新。严格实行这些规定,可以更好地实现患者的护理和器官的利用。

临床管理

患者

维持疗法

包括家庭肠外营养(HPN)治疗在内的肠道衰竭的管理,是患者护理的一大难点。应密切监测的危及生命的 HPN 并发症主要是脓毒血症、中心静脉血栓形成和肝衰竭。所有患者都应每周进行血培养,监测是否有血行感染。临床怀疑的中心静脉血栓形成应行多普勒超声和(或)中心静脉造影以进行影像学诊断。无肝移植的等候者也应密切监测肝损伤的进展,必要时行肝脏移植。与此相反,带肝移植的等候者应监测肝损伤是否改善,有些情况可以避免进行接下来的肝脏移植。近几年来我们已经观察到数个上述监测后改变移植方式的例子。

随访研究

对于大多数患者来说，每周进行定期的测试是必须的，应包括肾功能评估和综合代谢评估，用以监测和调整 HPN 的治疗。此外还需要进行肝酶评估、肝功能检查和血清微量营养素水平的测定。如我们最近的出版物所指出的，强烈建议患者每年评估骨骼健康程度，包括双能 X 线吸收测定（DXA）、血清激素和维生素 D 水平测定[36,37]。

与移植中心相距很远的患者应由初级护理或转诊医生密切跟踪。患者被强制要求与护理医生每周保持联系，且定期访问指定的移植中心。

肠道康复

尽管已列入移植等待名单上，等候者还是应该继续利用综合全面的药物和外科治疗手段来进行肠道康复。临床及营养数据提示肠道吸收功能明显改善的等候者，应逐步脱离 HPN 治疗，并列入暂缓等待名单中。同时，应审慎考虑对具有残余肝功能的患者进行自体手术重建以及对终末期肝衰竭的患者进行独立肝脏移植[32,38]。

静脉通路

留置中心静脉导管的管理是患者护理的一个重要组成部分。为了避免危及生命的并发症，以及在移植期间保持可靠的中心静脉通路用于液体复苏，必须进行导管置换，最好由经验丰富的介入放射学团队进行操作。对于中心静脉导管的正确放置和维护的详细讨论超出了本章的范畴。然而在实际操作中，由于存在隐源性导管相关感染的可能性，移植时严禁使用先前放置的中心静脉导管。

感染

伴有发热和（或）血培养阳性的等候者应当迅速进行中心导管置换以及抗菌治疗。在患有超短肠和假性梗阻综合征的患者中，复发性吸入性肺炎并不罕见。为了避免这种风险，需要采取有效的预防措施，利用影像学进行诊断以及有指征时积极治疗。对于患有进展性空腔脏器肌病/神经病变的等候者，复发性尿路感染也是常见的感染源，其可以通过无菌性导管插入和间歇性抗生素治疗来部分消除。

伴有复杂性腹部病变的患者，尤其是患有炎症性肠病和放射性肠炎的患者，必须谨慎留意发生腹腔内脓肿、穿孔和肠外瘘的可能。在这种情况下，患者应列入暂缓等待名单中，并优先考虑完成肠切除术和控制腹腔感染，尤其是那些具有残留肝功能的患者。

监测方案

等待名单上的所有等候者都应每年进行一次恶性肿瘤筛查，特别是先前患过癌症或有明显癌症家族史的高危患者。监测应包括女性乳房 X 线检查和宫颈涂片，有吸烟史患者的胸部影像学检查，以及包括加德纳综合征在内的肿瘤性疾病患者的胃肠内镜检查。对于患有包括 Jak-2 突变、心血管疾病或复发性肺栓塞病史在内的高凝状态疾病患者，也建议每年评估一次心肺功能。在等待内脏移植的过程中，我们在一些患者身上发现了新发的恶性肿瘤，例如黑素瘤和其他皮肤癌。同样地，进展的原发性心血管疾病以及可能影响移植的致命并发症也可能出现。

移植物

带肝或无肝内脏移植的适应证在其他文章有详细的描述[5,27]。必须注意的是，出于技术上和生理学上的考虑，胰腺通常与肝脏-小肠一同移植，或作为多脏器移植物的一部分进行完整的移植[5,7,9]。以胃作为主要器官的多脏器移植物应仅用于患有广泛胃肠道疾病的患者以及伴有肝衰竭和肝门静脉/脾静脉血栓形成的患者。多脏器移植物也常用于肝脏-小肠移植术后腹部情况不佳而需要再移植的患者[27]。

为了更好地进行患者护理以及最佳地利用已故者器官，必须定期评估所列器官进行移植的必要性。由于肝衰竭或肾衰竭的进展，特别是在具有边缘供肝、需要再移植的患者中，在最初的器官清单上再添加肝脏或肾脏并不罕见。根据最新的 SRTR/OPTN 报告，在小肠移植的等候者中，最常见的再添加移植器官是胰腺（20%），其次是肝脏（10%）和肾脏（4%）。在最初所列器官为小肠和肝脏的成年等候者中，有 58%的患者随后需要额外的器官，由于胰腺整体移植技术的提高，最常见的再添加器官是胰腺[39]。在最初所列器官为单独小肠以及小肠-胰腺的儿童等候者中，分别有 32%和 36%的患者随后需要再添加肝脏。此外，在最初所列器官为小肠和肝脏联合的儿童等候者中，有 27%随后需要再添加胰腺[1]。

在肠道吸收功能或其他腹部器官功能显著改善的等候者中，应当考虑从列表中剔除一个或多个所列器官。通过对家庭肠外营养配方的精细调整，例如使用 ω 脂肪酸，我们已经可以单独移植小肠而不再需要进行肝脏及胰腺的置换。在某些情况下，上述减少移植物的决策是在移植进行时决定的，保留下的移植物将按照等待名单中的优先次序用于其他等候者。

捐献者

由于肠道对缺血-再灌注损伤的高敏感性以及受体移植手术的复杂性，对于大多数等候者来说，仅应考虑来源于最佳捐献者的移植物。目前采用的捐赠者标准包括年轻（≤55 岁）、低身体质量指数（BMI≤$30kg/m^2$）、血流动力学稳定性、最小升压支持、没有或仅短时间心肺停搏。有利的生化标志物包括正常肝酶、低血清肌酐、正常的血清乳酸水平，以及没有弥漫性血管内凝血的证据。尽管器官十分短缺，特别是肝脏，对于边缘供体的利用尤其应该谨慎考虑[31]。同时也建议避免选用带有脂肪性肠系膜的小肠移植物。

对于所有脏器等候者，我们建议使用 ABO 血型相同的供体。根据目前交叉配型的有效性，最好避免将无肝移植物移植到表达多种供体特异性抗体的患者身上[8]。对于腹腔挛缩的患者，建议使用小体积的供体。此外，还建议对需要无肝移植的 CMV 阴性候选者使用 CMV 阴性供体。通过同步供体和受体的操作时间来缩短冷缺血时间同样重要。

总结及未来展望

为了持续改善移植前后患者的生存预后，对 UNOS 名单上脏器移植等候者的管理是十分有必要的。最为重要的是早期转诊、适当管理等待名单以及进一步完善目前的 UNOS/OPTN 分配政策。通过早期转诊，可以降低疾病的严重程度，减少中心静脉血栓形成的风险，以及降低肝脏置换的概率。通过对导管性/全身性败血症、中心静脉血栓形成和肝血管或实质失代偿的有效预防和积极治疗，可以进一步降低等待名单的死亡率。通过监测，可以早期诊断恶性疾病、心血管疾病及其他危及生命的疾病，并及时采取更好的治疗以改善预后。进一步完善 UNOS/OPTN 的分配制度将有助于更好地利用国家供体库，以缩短等候时间、改善等候者预后。

对于无肝移植物，为了减少患者等候时间，尤其是体内表达供体特异性抗体以及交叉配型阳性的等候者，有必要出台新的匹配政策以更好地进行 HLA 匹配。此外，未来需要转化性研究来识别、验证和改善捐献者的风险因素（表 42.2），以增加器官的可利用性。

对于带肝移植物的等候者，更广泛地获取 UNOS 死亡捐助者的国家供体库对于改善目前的结果至关重要。最近的小肠移植登记报告中观察到临床上移植例数越来越多[40]，上述类似的政策应该在全世界范围内采用。

表 42.2 影响脏器移植等待名单死亡率的危险因素

- 肝脏损害的程度（组织学和生物化学）[15-18,20,22]
- 住院治疗[19]
- 引起肠道衰竭的因素[16,20,22]
- 麻醉依赖[20,22]

（李博 译　高鹏骥 校）

参考文献

1. Mazariegos GV, Steffick DE, Horslen S, et al. Intestine transplantation in the United States 1999-2008. American Journal of Transplantation. 2010;10(2):1020-1034.
2. Berg CL, Steffick ED, Edwards EB, et al. Liver and intestine transplantation in the United States 1998-2007. American Journal of Transplantation. 2009;9(2):907-931.
3. Abu-Elmagd KM. Preservation of the native spleen, duodenum, and pancreas in patients with multivisceral transplantation: nomenclature, dispute of origin, and proof of premise. Transplantation. 2007;84(9):1208-1209.
4. Abu-Elmagd KM. The small bowel contained allografts: existing and proposed nomenclature. American Journal of Transplantation. 2010;11(1):184-185.
5. Abu-Elmagd K. Indications and patient selection. In: Langnas A, Goulet O, Quigley E, et al., editors. Intestinal Failure: Diagnosis, Management and Transplantation. Oxford: Blackwell Publishing; 2008: 245-253.
6. Freeman RB Jr, Wiesner RH, Harper A, et al. The new liver allocation system: moving toward evidence-based transplantation policy. Liver Transplantation. 2002;8:851-858.
7. Thai N, Abu-Elmagd K, Khan A, et al. Pancreatic transplantation under a regimen of campath-1H. In: Terasaki PL, Cecka JM, editors. Clinical Transplants 2004. Los Angeles, CA: UCLA Tissue Typing Laboratory; 2005: 205-214.
8. Abu-Elmagd K, Wu G, Costa G, et al. Preformed and de novo donor specific antibodies in visceral transplantation: long-term outcome with special reference to the liver. American Journal of Transplantation. 2012;12(11):3047-3060.
9. Abu-Elmagd KM, Fung JJ, Bueno J, et al. Logistics and technique for procurement of intestinal, pancreatic, and hepatic grafts from the same donor. Annals of Surgery. 2000;232(5):680-687.
10. Cruz RJ, Costa G, Bond GJ, et al. Modified liver-sparing multivisceral transplant with preserved native spleen, pancreas and duodenum: Technique and long-term outcome. Journal of Gastrointestinal Surgery. 2010;14(11):1709-1721.
11. Cherikh W, Kramer B, Baker TM, et al. Data provided to the OPTN/UNOS Pediatric Transplantation Committee. 2010. Available from: http://optn.transplant.hrsa.gov/CommitteeReports/board_main_PediatricTransplantationCommittee_6_24_2010_9_9.pdf.
12. Berg CL, Steffick DE, Edwards EB, et al. Liver and intestine transplantation in the United States 1998-2007. American Journal of Transplantation. 2009;9(4):907-931.
13. Kaplan J, Han L, Halgrimson W, et al. The impact of MELD/PELD revisions on

the mortality of liver-intestine transplantation candidates. American Journal of Transplantation. 2011;11:1896–1904.
14. Fryer JP, Pellar S, Ormond D, et al. Mortality in candidates waiting for combined liver-intestine transplants exceeds that for other candidates waiting for liver transplants. Liver Transplantation. 2003;9:748–753.
15. Chungfat N, Dixler I, Cohran V, et al. Impact of parenteral nutrition-associated liver disease on intestinal transplant waitlist dynamics. Journal of the American College of Surgeons. 2007;205(6):755–761.
16. Javid PJ, Malone FR, Bittner R, et al. The optimal timing of referral to an intestinal failure program: the relationship between hyperbilirubinemia and mortality. Journal of Pediatric Surgery. 2011;46:1052–1056.
17. Middleton SJ, Nishoda S, Tzakis A, et al. Cambridge-Miami score for intestinal transplantation preoperative risk assessment: initial development and validation. Transplantation Proceedings. 2010;42:19–21.
18. Grant D, Abu-Elmagd K, Reyes J, et al. 2003 Report of the intestine transplant registry: a new era has dawned. Annals of Surgery. 2005;241(4):607–613.
19. Beath S, Pironi L, Gabe S, et al. Collaborative strategies to reduce mortality and morbidity in patients with chronic intestinal failure including those who are referred for small bowel transplantation. Transplantation. 2008;85(10):1378–1384.
20. Reyes J, Mazariegos GV, Bond GJ, et al. Pediatric intestinal transplantation: historical notes, principles and controversies. Pediatric Transplantation. 2002;6:193–207.
21. Gondolesi GE, Almau HM. Intestinal transplantation outcomes. Mount Sinai Journal of Medicine. 2012;79:246–255.
22. Farmer DG, Venick RS, Colangelo J, et al. Pretransplant predictors of survival after intestinal transplantation: analysis of a single-center experience of more than 100 transplants. Transplantation. 2010;90(12):1574–1580.
23. United States of Department of Health and Human Services. HRSA/OPTN. 2012 [cited June 5, 2012]; Available from: http://optn.transplant.hrsa.gov/Shared ContentDocuments/ExecutiveSummary_1111.pdf.
24. Bueno J, Ohwada S, Kocoshis S, et al. Factors impacting the survival of children with intestinal failure referred for intestinal transplantation. Journal of Pediatric Surgery. 1999;34(1):27–33.
25. Abu-Elmagd K. Intestinal transplantation for short gut syndrome and gut failure: rewarding outcomes and current consensus. Gastroenterology. 2006;130(2):132–137.
26. Mazariegos GV, Superina R, Rudolph J, et al. Current status of pediatric intestinal failure, rehabilitation, and transplantation: summary of a colloquium. Transplantation. 2011;62(11):1173–1180.
27. Abu-Elmagd KM, Costa G, Bond GJ, et al. Five hundred intestinal and multivisceral transplantation at a single center: major advances with new challenges. Annals of Surgery. 2009;250(4):567–581.
28. Abu-Elmagd KM, Bond G, Matarese L, et al. Gut rehabilitation and intestinal transplantation. Therapy. 2005;2(6):853–864.
29. Gruessner RW, Sharp HL. Living-related intestinal transplantation: first report of a standardized surgical technique. Transplantation. 1997;64:1605–1607.
30. Pollard SG. Intestinal transplantation: living related. British Medical Journal. 1997;53(4):868–878.
31. Matsumoto CS, Kaufman SS, Cirlanda R, et al. Utilization of donors who have suffered cardiopulmonary arrest and resuscitation in intestinal transplantation. Transplantation. 2008;86(7):941–946.
32. Botha JF, Grant WJ, Torres C, et al. Isolated liver transplantation in infants with end-stage liver disease due to short bowel syndrome. Liver Transplantation. 2006;12(7):1062–1066.
33. Reyes J, Fishbein T, Bueno J, et al. Reduced-size orthotopic composite liver-intestinal allograft. Transplantation. 1998;66(4):489–492.
34. Bueno J, Abu-Elmagd K, Mazariegos G, et al. Composite liver-small bowel allografts with preservation of donor duodenum and hepatic biliary system in children. Journal of Pediatric Surgery. 2000;35(2):291–296.
35. Raofi V, Beatty E, Testa G, et al. Combined living-related segmental liver and bowel transplantation for megacystis-microcolon-intestinal hypoperistalsis syndrome. Journal of Pediatric Surgery. 2008;43:e9–e11.
36. Resnick J, Gupta N, Wagner J, et al. Skeletal integrity and visceral transplantation. American Journal of Transplantation. 2010;10(10):2331–2340.
37. Abu-Elmagd KM, Kosmach-Park B, Costa G, et al. Long-term survival, nutritional autonomy, and quality of life after intestinal and multivisceral transplantation. Annals of Surgery. 2012;256(3):494–508.
38. Thompson J, Sudan D. Intestinal lengthening for short bowel syndrome. Advances in Surgery. 2008;42:49–61.
39. Abu-Elmagd K, Reyes J, Todo S, et al. Clinical intestinal transplantation: new perspectives and immunologic considerations. Journal of the American College of Surgeons. 1998;186(5):512–527.
40. Intestinal Transplant Association. Intestinal Transplant Registry. 2012 [cited June 5, 2012]; Available from: http://intestinaltransplantassociation.com/?cat=9.

第 43 章 肝功能衰竭的重症监护

Jenny E. Han, Ram M. Subramanian

引言

在肝功能衰竭的诊断、治疗及管理过程中,快速区分急性肝功能衰竭(ALF)与慢加急性肝功能衰竭(A-CLF)非常重要。两种类型的肝功能衰竭均可引起多器官功能衰竭、脓毒症,甚至死亡。临床医生需要根据两者不同的病理生理学过程,对他们各自所导致的肝内及肝外的器官功能障碍进行监测及治疗。尤其是在肝性脑病发生过程中,ALF 可能会出现颅内高压甚至脑疝。晚期出现多器官功能障碍(包括心肺功能、肾功能、神经系统功能障碍)的重症患者,维持肝内、肝外内环境稳定对成功进行肝移植十分必要。

本章内容包括对 ALF 与 ACLF 患者多器官功能的监护处理。并对第 38 章中等待肝移植患者的处理内容进行补充,同时也会对第 47 章中肝功能衰竭处理中肝脏辅助装置的应用部分进行详细介绍。

急性肝功能衰竭

ALF 是指既往没有肝脏疾病的患者在出现肝功能不全症状的 8 周内出现肝性脑病的病理生理过程。ALF 脑病的一个特点是有进展为颅内压增高及脑疝的风险。肝性脑病的出现常伴有凝血障碍,而这两个因素的进展同时也提示肝功能的恶化,从而强调了进行肝移植的必要性。在美国每年约有 2000 例 ALF 患者[1]。其中有 15%的成人患者无法确定病因[2]。约有 45%的患者仅需对症支持治疗即可存活,约 25%的患者需要肝移植,30%的患者死亡(未进行肝移植手术)。ALF 的病因不同预后也不同(表 43.1)。其中以对乙酰氨基酚过量、甲型肝炎、缺血所致的 ALF 预后最好,60%仅给予对症支持治疗即可存活。药物性 ALF 和乙型肝炎所致的 ALF 预后差,仅有 25%的患者对症支持治疗后可以存活。

病理生理学

ALF 的病理生理学主要是大量肝细胞坏死。肝性脑病与凝血障碍的特征性临床表现分别继发于高血氨血症和凝血因子缺乏。根据从黄疸进展至脑病的时间将 ALF 分成三种类型:超急性 ALF(0~7 天),可能快速进展为致命性脑水肿,但是该类型预后最好;急性 ALF(8~28 天)或亚急性 ALF(5~12 周),脑水肿的发生概率较低,但预后差[3]。

诊断

对可疑 ALF 的患者,需要认真快速地评估肝功能衰竭的原因(表 43.1),并排除已存在慢性肝脏疾病。在对这些患者早期诊断和处理的过程中,应考虑进行移植评估,并确定影响肝移植的因素,例如,缺乏社会支持、并存的基础疾病、活动性肿瘤或感染。

可以进行一系列的检查来寻找 ALF 的潜在病因(见表 43.1),其中精神状态评估十分重要。实验室检查包括肝酶、凝血指标包括国际标准化比值(INR)、动脉血 pH 值、乳酸水平等。腹部 CT 或 MRI 检查对于排除慢性肝病非常有意义,常表现为慢性门脉高压,例如,肝硬化的外观表现、脾大、静脉曲张等。此外,影像学检查还可以帮助移植医生对患者的血管状态进行评估。如果患者状态不允许外出行 CT 或 MRI 检查,床旁超声检查也可以提供有价值的数据。肝组织活检在 ALF 患者中应用有限,但对于可疑淋巴瘤的患者或者无法确定病因的亚急性肝功能衰竭患者尚有一定价值。

由于起初稳定的 ALF 患者的临床及生化学指标

表 43.1 ALF 病因

药物性(对乙酰氨基酚最常见)	
处方药 抗生素 抗癫痫药 抗抑郁药 降脂药 降压药 化疗药 HIV 相关药物	大部分病例具有异质性，常发生于起始治疗的6个月内 损伤机制包括肝细胞坏死、胆汁淤积、混合型、脂肪变性、自身免疫、高敏过敏反应、磷脂质病、线粒体毒性、肝窦阻塞综合征 如怀疑为高敏反应，可应用类固醇激素
非处方镇痛药	
毒品	甲型肝炎
病毒(美国12%的病例为甲肝和乙肝病毒)	乙型肝炎(应用抗病毒药物治疗) 丁型肝炎(混合或重叠感染) 戊型肝炎(妊娠女性死亡率20%) 丙型肝炎(罕见) 单纯性疱疹(应用阿昔洛韦治疗) 水痘带状疱疹(应用阿昔洛韦治疗) 巨细胞病毒(应用抗病毒治疗) EB 病毒
毒素	毒鹅膏菌(蘑菇) 有机溶剂 中草药 细菌毒素(例如，蜡样芽孢杆菌)
威尔逊病	慢性疾病 可能出现溶血性贫血和肾衰竭 碱性磷酸酶降低 尿酸降低 如果不做移植死亡率100%
妊娠相关(胎儿娩出后好转)	妊娠期急性脂肪肝 HELLP 综合征
自身免疫性肝炎	类固醇治疗
恶性肿瘤	淋巴瘤 转移性疾病
缺血性肝病	休克 可卡因 急性动脉血栓形成/损伤
热休克	病史重要性
急性布加综合征	高凝状态
广泛肝切除术后	取决于肝脏切除部分所占百分比，及所剩肝脏组织的功能状态
不确定病因(15%~20%)	高达20%的病例可能是由于未确定的对乙酰氨基酚中毒 肝活组织检查不一定有帮助

Reproduced from Ford et al.[19], with permission from Elsevier. Copyright © 2010, Elsevier.

可能会快速恶化，建议早期将患者转移至肝移植中心。转运及接受的设备需根据患者的神经系统、心肺系统、肝脏、血液及肾脏状态决定。由于在转运过程中可能会出现进展性脑病，在转运之前可以选择气管插管进行气道保护。此外，进展性 ALF 患者存在多器官功能衰竭，治疗上需遵从多系统、目标导向的治疗策略。

处理

脑水肿和颅内高压

ALF 处理过程中一个重要的特点即为对脑水肿和颅内高压的评估及治疗。与 ACLF 不同的是，ALF 的高血氨症会引起星形胶质细胞肿胀进而引起脑水肿和颅内压升高(ICP)。20%~30%的 ALF 患者会出现颅内压升高[4]。连续神经系统评估有助于发现进行性加重的颅内高压，表现为脑病的恶化。利用 West Haven 标准对肝性脑病进行分级(表 43.2)对评估和记录神经系统检查以及 ICP 检测仪的置入时机很有意义。Ⅲ级和Ⅳ级肝性脑病伴有脑水肿需要紧急气管插管气道保护、ICP 监测和降低颅内压。需要注意的是，CT 或 MRI 对评估 ALF 的脑水肿及高颅压并不够敏感，因此影像学正常不能排除高颅压。

颅内压的监测和治疗

在不同的医疗机构 ICP 监测方法也不相同。目前尚没有关于 ALF 进行 ICP 监测的临床意义的随机研究。ICP 监测已在一些欧洲和美国的神经重症监护中应用，但鉴于可能存在由凝血功能障碍导致颅内出血的风险尚没有被广泛应用。晚期脑病需要进行气管插管和机械通气治疗，而镇静治疗会限制 ICP 监测的应用，因此，更精确客观的 ICP 监测设备可以帮助检测颅内高压还可以指导临床治疗、预后以及肝移植候选可能。脑实质监测可以平衡监测的准确性与安全性，是目前 ALF 患者最广泛的颅内压监测方法。

脑实质监测可以由受过培训的专业人员快速安全地实施。ALF 的凝血障碍可以用活化的凝血Ⅶa(40μg/kg)快速纠正，从而使手术相关的出血风险降至最低。ICP 升高被定义为 ICP>25mmHg 超过 10min。ICP 监测还可以帮助计算脑灌注压(CPP)，公式为 CPP 等于平均动脉压(MAP)减去颅内压(CPP=MAP−ICP)。药物治疗目标为 ICP<25mmHg，CPP>60mmHg。在 ICP 升高的情况下，如要达到最佳 CPP 可以使用血管活性药物(如去甲肾上腺素)提高 MAP。图 43.1 为 ICP 升高的药物治疗方法提供了一个算法[5]。

在开始药物治疗前，Ⅲ级或Ⅳ级脑病的患者应先进行气管插管气道保护。插管前预先给予气管内或静脉内利多卡因可以降低 ICP 升高的风险。如果出现癫痫发作应给予苯妥英钠治疗，但不推荐预防性应用苯妥英钠。对气管插管的患者,应持续给予镇痛镇静以预防因气管插管刺激所致的 ICP 骤增。

颅内压升高的药物治疗

甘露醇是 ALF 患者 ICP 升高的有效初始治疗药物,根据血清渗透压和肾功能(甘露醇经肾脏清除)调整用量。甘露醇通过增加血浆渗透压并利用渗透梯度将脑组织内的水分渗透至血管内。甘露醇通过降低脑水肿可以提高患者生存率[6]。如果患者血浆渗透压小于 320mOsm/L 并且无肾衰竭,给予 0.5~1g/kg 的负荷剂量可以有效改善 ICP 升高。高钠血症和高渗透压会激发肺水肿和高血容量,因此,对渗透压和电解质的密切监测十分必要。

除甘露醇外，高渗盐水也通过增加血浆渗透压来达到降低和维持 ICP 的目的,研究显示此种干预措施是有效的[7]。静脉给予 23%的高渗盐水(30mL q2h)使钠离子水平达 145~155mmol/L。此外,适当降低体温,使目标核心体温达到 32℃~34℃也可以有效降低 ICP,尤其在上述药物干预无效的情况下[8]。以作者经验,联合应用高渗盐水和低体温治疗可以有效降低 ALF 患者的颅内高压。对上述治疗无效的难治性颅内高压患者,可以考虑巴比妥昏迷疗法。在逐渐增加巴比妥用量时,需要持续监测脑电图(EEG),以确定出现了爆发性抑制。巴比妥昏迷的副作用之一是心肌抑制与低血压，这限制了该种方法的使用[9]。吲哚美辛作为脑血管收缩剂，静脉使用时因其快速降低 ICP 的作用而成为颅内高压治疗的最后一道防线[10]。需要注意的是,以上改善 ICP 和 CPP 的措施可以稳定患者的神经系统状态，进而为进行肝移植争取一定时间。如果在肝移植前已进行 ICP 监测，应该保留至移植术后 24~48 小时来帮助确定颅内压已降至正常水平。

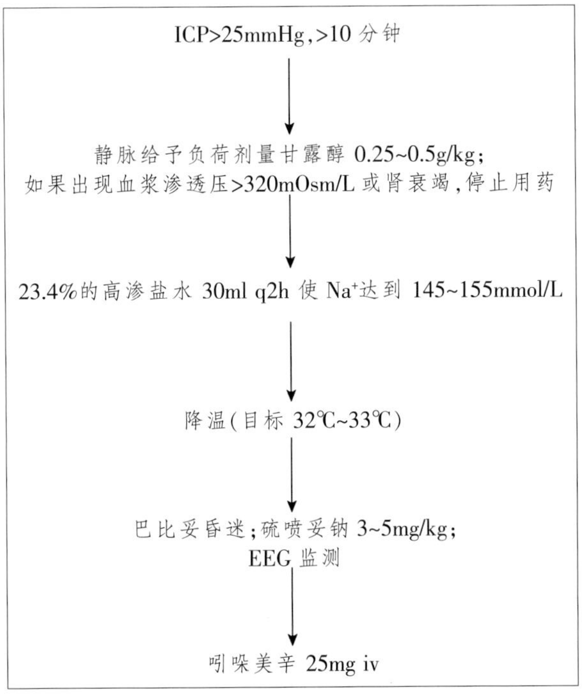

图 43.1 急性肝功能衰竭患者颅内压增高的处理流程。EEG,脑电图。(Reproduced from Ford et al. [19], with permission from Elsevier. Copyright © 2010, Elsevier.)

血流动力学异常

ALF 患者 PT/INR 延长可以证明存在凝血障碍。凝血因子(例如,Ⅴ因子和Ⅶ因子)和 INR 是判断肝功能恢复情况最敏感的生化指标,INR 可以作为肝功能恢复的指标，并且在没有活动性出血的情况下不应该用输注血制品来纠正。除促凝血因子的缺失外,肝脏合成的抗凝蛋白(例如,蛋白 C 和 S)也会下降。因此,INR 的升高不一定意味着活动性出血的风险也增加。如果患者需要进行侵入性操作或有活动性出血,可以应用重组凝血因子Ⅶ来纠正 INR,推荐使用最小剂量 40μg/kg 来短暂纠正凝血功能障碍，治疗时间窗为操作前 2 小时。重组凝血因子Ⅶ非常适用于 ALF 患者,它可以在患者进行侵入性操作时短暂的纠正凝血异常，保证操作安全，而在操作完成后迅速恢复至未纠正前的 INR 值,继续作为追踪肝功能的生化学指标。

ALF 患者经常出现血小板减少症。虽然患者血小板降低,但很少有明显的出血症状。由于 ALF 不会出现慢性门脉高压,静脉曲张出血的风险也很小。如果患者没有活动性出血的证据，当血小板>10 000/mm^3 时，不推荐常规输注血小板。如患者需要进行侵入性操作，建议使血小板>50 000/mm^3。

在纠正血流动力学紊乱过程中，需要警惕输血相关急性肺损伤(TRALI)。其中新鲜冰冻血浆(FFP)风险最大,血小板与压积红细胞(pRBC)也会导致 TRALI。TRALI 常发生于血制品输注后 6 小时内。

心肺异常

心血管

ALF进展过程中，全身炎性反应可以引起高动力循环和低外周血管阻力。ALF患者处于免疫抑制状态，有发生感染并发症的风险，会加重已存在的低血压状态。脓毒性休克常用血管活性药物包括去甲肾上腺素和小剂量的血管升压素。在存在心功能障碍的情况下，可以考虑应用多巴酚丁胺和米力农进行支持治疗。根据前文所述，在ICP升高时也可以用血管活性药物(例如，去甲肾上腺素)来升高血压以达到最佳CPP。

肺脏

出现晚期脑病的患者有必要进行气管插管气道保护，给予充分的镇痛(例如，芬太尼)和镇静(例如，丙泊酚和右美托咪定)治疗以保证人机协调。关于呼吸机模式选择目前尚无基于证据的指南推荐，容量控制模式与压力控制模式可供选择。感染或非感染因素均可导致ALF患者出现急性肺损伤。TRALI即是ALF患者最易出现的由非感染因素引起的急性肺损伤，是由输注血制品纠正凝血功能障碍与血小板减少引起的。至于预防措施，在ICU常规操作中可将床头抬高30°以降低呼吸机相关性肺炎，同时还可以降低ICP。至于呼吸机设置，降低胸膜腔内压可以促进静脉回流，从而改善ICP；因此，将潮气量设置为6~8mL/kg(理想千克体重)，并将PEEP设置为保证足够氧合的最低PEEP。

肾衰竭

AKI在ALF患者中亦很常见，但却很少被诊断。AKI的诊断检查应包括肾前性、肾性、肾后性病因。需要强调的是ALF患者出现的AKI并非一定是由于肝肾综合征(HRS)，因为HRS的病理生理学需要存在慢性门脉高压异常。ALF患者出现AKI常需要肾脏替代治疗，尤其当存在迅速恶化的乳酸酸中毒性代谢性酸中毒。一旦开始肾脏替代治疗，即使在血流动力学稳定的患者也应该选用持续血透模式，这是由于间断血液透析会导致血流动力学不稳定并增加ICP[12]。研究显示高通量的血液滤过可以降低血清乳酸水平、碱缺失及血管活性药物的使用[13]。

N-乙酰半胱氨酸治疗

在由对乙酰氨基酚或非对乙酰氨基酚导致的肝功能障碍治疗过程中，可以使用N-乙酰半胱氨酸(NAC)，尤其在静脉注射对乙酰氨基酚的12小时内。NAC增加谷胱甘肽的生成，其作为抗氧化剂可以减轻肝毒性，作用持续48~72小时[14]。对于非对乙酰氨基酚导致的肝功能衰竭，研究显示NAC可以改善终末器官氧输送及血流动力学稳定性[15]。因此，所有ALF患者均应接受NAC治疗。NAC可以口服或静脉给药，其副作用小耐受性良好。口服负荷剂量为140mg/kg，接下来每4小时给药70mg/kg；静脉给药剂量150mg/kg(溶于5%葡萄糖溶液)，接下来每4小时50mg/kg，继而每16小时100mg/kg[16]。当患者脑病及凝血功能好转(INR<1.5)，即肝功能好转后可暂停NAC治疗。

综上所述，ALF的治疗包括多器官系统紊乱，尤其注意肝性脑病和凝血功能障碍的治疗。多种预后预测模型证明，这两个因素对预测自发肝功能恢复或是否需要肝移植十分有效。

慢加急性肝功能衰竭

ACLF病理生理学包括慢性门脉高压导致的脏器及全身系统性紊乱。多器官系统紊乱可导致威胁生命的静脉曲张出血、休克、气体交换障碍及HRS导致的AKI。早期发现并预测需重症监护支持是重要的移植前干预措施。

门脉高压

肝硬化门脉高压是门脉回流障碍与门脉血流量增加的综合结果。门脉回流障碍原因包括器质性和功能性两方面因素。器质性病变是由于肝窦纤维化和再生结节压迫。功能性因素继发于肝内一氧化氮减少和肝内血管收缩。肝内一氧化氮的减少与肝外一氧化氮生成增加的矛盾导致内脏血管舒张和门脉血流增加。综上，门脉回流障碍与门脉血流量增加共同导致了门脉高压[17]。此外，内脏血管舒张导致心脏泵出的血液在内脏循环系统内的分流以及其他器官的有效灌注减少。上述内脏及循环系统异常即是移植前失代偿期肝硬化患者治疗方案的基础。ACLF患者循环系统障碍治疗的核心是使用内脏血管收缩剂来纠正内脏血管的舒张。

肝性脑病

肝性脑病是ACLF患者门脉高压的一个严重并发

症，神经精神系统表现可以从轻度认知障碍到严重昏迷。病理生理学上认为肝性脑病的发生是由于肝脏对胃肠道吸收毒素清除障碍，尤其是血氨。

导致肝性脑病的毒素种类是一个持续争论的问题，由于血氨对星形胶质细胞的影响，血氨升高一直被认为在肝性脑病的病理生理学过程中起着重要作用。星型胶质细胞在慢性肝病时呈现出阿尔茨海默病样的形态学被称为阿尔茨海默病Ⅱ型星型胶质细胞。慢性肝脏疾病时，过度升高的血氨改变了星型胶质细胞的神经元蛋白，导致谷氨酸盐转运异常，这可能是肝性脑病过程中神经递质异常的原因。其他研究显示羟色胺与 GABA 受体、锰以及儿茶酚胺通路在肝性脑病发病过程中也起到一定作用[18]。

患者的临床表现可以从轻度的睡眠觉醒周期改变到昏睡甚至进一步出现意识障碍（包括嗜睡和昏迷）。肝性脑病的 West Haven 分级标准根据患者意识状态、智力功能和行为水平分为Ⅰ~Ⅳ级（表 43.2）。查体时神经系统异常可表现为扑翼样震颤、腱反射的过度活跃和偏瘫。

肝性脑病的初始处理包括快速进行脑病分级，对于Ⅲ级和Ⅳ级脑病患者选择性进行气管插管气道保护。机械通气过程中仅需要最小剂量的镇静治疗。可选择的镇静药物包括丙泊酚和右美托咪定。由于苯二氮䓬类药物有加重肝性脑病的风险，因此不建议使用。影像学检查可以用来排除引起神志改变的其他原因，包括脑血管意外（CVA）、颅内出血或占位病变。需要确定肝性脑病的病因并尽快治疗。包括胃肠道出血、感染、电解质紊乱、脱水、近期经颈静脉门体静脉分流术（TIPS）手术、便秘、药物、镇静剂或进展期肝功能障碍。支持治疗包括静脉液体输注、纠正电解质紊乱及预防性治疗等。

与 ALF 相反，ACLF 患者肝性脑病过程中出现脑水肿及颅内高压的风险很小。因此，ICP 监测和渗透疗法不作为常规推荐。推测原因是 ACLF 的肝功能障碍进程缓慢，从而为肝外器官（例如肌肉）调节血氨水平提供了时间。因此，在急性损害导致高血氨状态时，中枢神经系统不会因为血氨升高而出现星形胶质细胞水肿。

表 43.2 West Haven 标准意识状态的半定量分级

1 级	认知的轻度缺乏、欣快或焦虑、注意力缩短、加法运算能力受损
2 级	冷漠或倦怠、对时间或地点轻度认知混乱、轻度的人格改变、行为不正常、减法运算能力受损
3 级	嗜睡，但对言语刺激有反应、定向障碍
4 级	昏迷，对语言或刺激没有反应

肝性脑病时，非可吸收性双糖（例如，乳果糖）是帮助清除血氨最主要的药物。这些药物可以减少肠道内氨的产生并促进氮的排泄。并且，当口服乳果糖到达盲肠后可以被肠道细菌代谢，降低肠道内 pH 值，从而促进涉氨细菌的生长，肠黏膜吸收氨减少。如果患者不能口服乳果糖，则需要置入鼻胃管进行肠内喂养或乳果糖灌肠。剂量需要根据排便情况调整，以每天排便 3 次为宜。抗生素如甲硝唑、利福昔明和万古霉素在治疗肝性脑病过程中同样有效，原因主要是由于清除了产脲酶菌。虽然这些药物可以降低血氨并改善精神症状，但需要注意的是，并无证据显示脑病分级与血氨水平有相关性。其他治疗方法，例如补锌及降低蛋白质的涉入等也在临床上使用，但没有充分的证据支持。除了上述降低血氨的治疗外，去除诱发因素同样重要，尤其是发现并治疗潜在的感染。

血流动力学紊乱

肝硬化时由于全身血管舒张导致外周血管阻力降低，为满足终末器官灌注，心输出量也会增加。这一病理生理过程与脓毒症类似，表现为低 MAP、脉压差增加、心率增快。在肝功能逐渐恶化或存在感染时，这一生理过程可能快速进展成脓毒性休克。去甲肾上腺素是最常用的血管活性药物，它作用于 α 受体和 β1 受体，从而增加血管张力改善心输出量。在去甲肾上腺素效果不佳时可以加用血管升压素。多巴胺由于其可以扩张内脏血管而加重门脉高压需慎用。液体复苏会加重腹水导致腹腔间隙综合征，并压迫下腔静脉（IVC）降低心脏前负荷而继发低血量性低血压[19]，因此需在密切监测下进行。

肺部并发症

肝肺综合征

肝肺综合征（HPS）以低氧血症为特点，定义为肝脏疾病过程中出现的肺泡-动脉氧分压差（A-a）增加和肺内血管扩张[20]。HPS 的发病率为 4%~29%，约有 20%

的 HPS 患者等待肝移植[21]。HPS 是由肺内血管扩张或肺内动静脉畸形引起的。实验模型显示肺内内皮素 B 受体的激活使一氧化氮水平增加，进而导致肺内血管病理性扩张。扩张的肺血管阻碍了氧气从肺泡弥散到毛细血管内的血红蛋白分子内，从而导致低氧血症。

临床表现包括呼吸急促、低氧、杵状指、发绀、仰卧呼吸(直立位时呼吸短促)以及直立位低氧(直立位时血氧下降)。低氧加重的原因是由于直立位时以肺基底部血管病理性扩张为主，血流多分布至基底部，使得 HPS 相关低氧血症加重。HPS 患者的胸部影像学表现多正常。因此，当患者出现低氧血症而影像学正常时需考虑 HPS。

诊断标准为吸空气情况下，PaO_2<70mmHg，肺泡–动脉氧分压差>20mmHg[22]，可以应用超声心动或肺灌注扫描寻找肺内分流的影像学证据。前者可以根据左右心情况评估右向左分流，生理盐水气泡经过外周静脉进入外周静脉，气泡延迟(3~6 个心动周期)进入左心提示肺内分流，因气泡需在病理性扩张的肺循环内穿过。但气泡延迟出现需与“早期出现气泡”对比，“早期出现气泡”可以在心内分流的情况下出现。在正常人肺血管床内可以用锝–99 标记的大颗粒聚合白蛋白进行追踪，但是在肺血管扩张的患者中，这种大分子白蛋白可以穿过肺血管而出现在肾脏和脑内。

氧疗可以作为支持治疗。对胸部影像学显示存在动静脉畸形的患者可以选择栓塞治疗。HPS 患者如果在吸空气情况下 PaO_2<60mmHg 则符合终末期肝病模型，肝移植对彻底纠正低氧血症是有效的。吸空气时 PaO_2<50mmHg 被定义为严重 HPS，研究显示此类患者围术期死亡率明显增高[23]，但最新研究显示严重 HPS 患者可以进行移植而不增加死亡率，因此不应作为肝移植的禁忌证[24]。

肺动脉高压

另外一个仅出现在肝硬化患者中的肺部病变为门脉性肺动脉高压（PPH），是肺动脉高压的一种。2%~10%的肝硬化患者有出现肺动脉高压的风险，涉及肝移植的患者中 16%伴有门脉高压[22]。PPH 的诊断标准包括平均肺动脉压(mPAP)≥25mmHg，外周血管阻力(PVR)≥120dynes.s/cm^5，肺毛细血管楔压(PCWP)≤15mmHg[22]。

尽管目前对门脉高压发病机制尚无明确的阐述，但肝脏对内毒素和细胞因子的清除率降低，导致这些因子进入肺循环，激活肺动脉血管内皮细胞增生，这一病理过程与门脉高压的发生相关。增生的肺动脉内皮细胞和平滑肌细胞引起肺血管收缩及肺动脉壁肥厚、管腔闭塞及肺血管丛重构，这也是肺动脉高压的主要特点[25]。重度 PPH 可引起肺心病和右心衰竭。中重度 PPH 定义为 mPAP≥35mmHg，aPVR≥250dynes.s/cm^5，此类患者肝移植后由于再灌注损伤导致急性右心衰竭死亡率>50%；因此，中重度 PPH 被列为肝移植禁忌证[23]。

典型症状包括活动后呼吸困难、心悸、胸痛、晕厥，并可能进展为右心衰竭。超声心动图是筛查肺动脉高压的有效无创检查。超声心动图提示肺动脉压>50mmHg，则需要置入右心导管获得更多数据。目前研究证明静脉输注前列环素可以降低 mPAP 水平，治疗 PPH 的效果可与肝移植相比拟[22]。其他治疗 PPH 的药物包括西地那非、磷酸二酯酶–5 抑制剂和内皮素受体拮抗剂(例如，波生坦)。与 HPS 相反，PPH 在肝移植后很难逆转；大部分患者在移植后短期内需要继续药物治疗。

肝性胸水

肝性胸水是腹水在胸膜腔积聚引起呼吸困难甚至呼吸衰竭。由于胸腔相对于腹腔而言为负压，因此腹水会通过横隔孔进入胸腔并在胸膜腔积聚，并以右侧最常见(见于 66%的胸腔积液患者)。治疗以利尿为主，如果出现急性呼吸困难，可行胸腔穿刺术。为避免出现低血容量甚至低血容量性休克建议使用细管径的引流管。对复发性肝性胸水，不建议施行胸膜固定术，因为持续积聚的液体可以隔断脏层胸膜和壁层胸膜。大剂量利尿剂和胸腔穿刺术对复发性肝性胸水效果不佳，TIPS 是有效的治疗措施。

胸腔积液多为漏出液。如胸水化验提示为渗出液则需要考虑伴发肺炎的可能。肝性胸水可出现感染并导致自发性细菌性胸膜炎（中性粒细胞数绝对升高>250/mm^3 或胸水培养阳性），治疗方法同自发性腹膜炎[26]。

呼吸衰竭

在 ICU 中，肝硬化患者由于意识状态障碍、急性肺损伤、脓毒症或多器官功能衰竭常需要呼吸机辅助呼吸。肝硬化患者由于肺内或肺外损伤，可能出现急性肺损伤或急性呼吸窘迫综合征[27]。对于出现急性肺损伤或急性呼吸衰竭[急性呼吸窘迫综合征(ARDS)]的肝硬化患者的最佳呼吸机条件选择尚无基于证据支持的指南,但目前推荐给予小潮气量(6mL/理想千克体重)[28]。此外,肝硬化患者常出现腹水、胸水、胸壁水肿,这些都会影响肺的机械活动,在机械通气过程中还会增加气压伤和容积伤。对于需要长期机械通气的肝性脑病患者,可以进行经皮气切或手术气管切开。

静脉曲张破裂出血

食管胃底静脉曲张破裂出血是肝硬化的严重并发症。门脉高压导致内脏血管扩张,从而使门脉血流增加。食管胃底静脉曲张是门脉回流受阻以及肝内阻力增加共同作用的结果。静脉曲张的严重程度与肝窦阻力直接相关,肝窦阻力可以通过肝静脉压力梯度(HVPG)测量,压力为 10~12mmHg。曲张的静脉具有破裂并引起消化道大出血的风险。

初始治疗包括建立静脉通路进行液体复苏及输血。密切的血流动力学监测十分必要,因为过度液体复苏会增加门脉压力并加重出血。在出现呕血或休克时,建议选择性气管插管保护气道并方便内镜检查。纠正贫血及凝血障碍同样重要,可以输注压缩红细胞、血小板、FFP改善血液系统异常。此外,预防性应用抗生素可以降低静脉曲张出血后细菌感染的风险,推荐选择喹诺酮类或头孢菌素类抗生素并持续应用 7 天。研究显示包含抗生素的初始治疗可以降低再出血及死亡率[30]。

建议尽早使用收缩内脏血管的药物治疗,例如奥曲肽(生长抑素类似物)或特利加压素。并应进行急诊内镜检查。食管静脉曲张出血时,内镜下结扎术可以有效止血。对于内镜止血困难的孤立性胃静脉曲张出血或食管静脉曲张出血,在等待 TIPS 手术期间可置入三腔两囊管暂时止血稳定循环。

肾功能障碍与肝肾综合征

肾衰竭是 ACLF 的一个常见并发症。肾功能障碍可以是由肾前、肾性或肾后性原因所致。肾损伤的病因检查包括尿液检查和超声影像学检查。ACLF 发生 AKI 的原因包括休克、肾毒性药物、既往肾脏疾病。HRS 是肝硬化患者一个独立的肾前性因素,并可增加死亡率。晚期门脉高压患者发生 HRS 的原因是内脏血管舒张导致肾脏动脉血液灌注下降,肾血管代偿性收缩,进一步导致肾小球滤过率(GFR)下降[31]。

HRS 分为两型。HRS-I 型为急进型表现为急性进展型肾衰竭,在 2 周内血清肌酐倍增达 2.5mg/L 以上,或肌酐清除率 24 小时下降 50%,降至 20mL/min 以下。HRS-Ⅱ型表现为肾功能障碍(血清肌酐 1.5~2.5mg/dL)无快速进展,通常伴有典型的难治性腹水。HRS 是一个排除性诊断,HRS 与肾前性氮质血症的区别在于它对晶体和胶体液复苏无反应[32]。联合治疗的目标为内脏和全身血管收缩,奥曲肽(生长抑素)和米多君(α-肾上腺素受体激动剂)是潜在的治疗方法。特利加压素是强效内脏血管收缩剂,并有证据显示其可以改善 HRS 患者的肾功能[33-35]。目前美国正在进行Ⅲ期临床试验,FDA 尚未批准上市。如果 HRS 患者肾功能障碍对药物治疗无反应,则需要开始肾脏替代治疗。对 HRS 患者尤其是肾脏替代治疗超过 6 周的患者需考虑肝脏和肾脏移植[36]。

腹水和自发性细菌性腹膜炎

腹水

腹水是由门脉高压和肾素血管紧张素系统紊乱所致,从而引起肾脏钠水吸收障碍。新发或加重的腹水患者评估急性肠系膜静脉血栓,尤其需评估门静脉和肝静脉血栓。对于保留肾功能的患者,可以应用螺内酯和呋塞米联合利尿治疗以减少腹水。但对于 ACLF 合并 AKI 患者,利尿治疗则为禁忌,可以选择大量放腹水(LVP)。如放出腹水大于 5L,则需同时输注白蛋白 5g/L 以预防循环障碍及低血压肾损伤。持续性腹水需要反复 LVP 时则需考虑 TIPS。

需要注意的是,张力性腹水可能导致腹腔内高压,并与腹腔间隔室综合征(ACS)相关。ACS 可以表现为低血压,这是由于下腔静脉受压迫而使得静脉回流障碍,也可因肾血管受压而出现少尿,并可因胸壁顺应性下降而使得气道峰压和平台压升高,内脏血管受压可引起肠系膜缺血。测量膀胱压可间接评估腹腔内压力,如>20mmHg 则为病理状态。ACS 的治疗包括大量放腹水和胃肠减压。

自发性细菌性腹膜炎

持续性腹水可发展为自发性细菌性腹膜炎(SBP)。据报道肝硬化 ACLF 合并 SBP 的患者超过 12%需要住院治疗；因此，肝硬化患者入院后需进行腹腔穿刺评估 SBP[32]。如腹水中中性粒细胞绝对值>250 个/mm³ 或腹水培养阳性则可诊断 SBP。治疗可选用三代头孢菌素(例如，头孢噻肟 2g q8h)。至于抗生素使用时间，RCT 研究显示 5 天与 10 天效果无显著差异[37]。需要注意，除了细菌性 SBP，真菌性 SBP 的发病率逐渐增加，因此如经验性抗生素治疗无效，需考虑真菌性 SBP 的可能性。

除了抗菌药物治疗，研究证明在诊断 SBP 6 小时内给予白蛋白 1.5g/kg 输注，在诊断后第 3 天给药 1g/kg 白蛋白输注与单独给药抗生素治疗相比，可以有效降低肾功能障碍的发生率和死亡率。

脓毒症

肝硬化患者具有发展为脓毒症、严重脓毒症及脓毒性休克的风险。据报道，肝硬化合并脓毒性休克患者死亡率高达 70%[39]。肝硬化患者出现细菌和真菌感染的机制尚不明确，有研究显示细胞因子缺乏和巨噬细胞调节异常可能起到一定作用。最常见的感染为 SBP 继发尿路感染、肺炎、菌血症及蜂窝织炎。50%~70%的患者培养阳性，且通常为 G−菌，尤其大肠埃希菌。G+球菌见于 30%~35%的患者。鉴于经验性抗菌药物应用的增加，院内真菌感染的发生率在逐渐增加。由于基线 MAP 和全身血管阻力的降低，感染可以引起血流动力学紊乱迅速加重出现脓毒性休克。此外，肝硬化合并脓毒性休克的患者肾上腺功能不全的发生率极高(51%~68%)，这可能是由于肾上腺灌注长期不足[40]。

肝硬化患者脓毒症和脓毒性休克的治疗与 ICU 内其他脓毒性休克患者的治疗方案相似；包括早期目标导向治疗包括液体复苏以保证组织器官灌注及血管活性药物支持，经验性广谱抗生素治疗，机械通气肺保护策略。

总结

肝功能衰竭患者的治疗需要基于系统的多器官支持治疗。ALF 与 ACLF 的病理生理学不同，需要给予不同的肝内及肝外处理方案。临床决策的制订需要团队合作，包括肝脏移植病学专家、外科医生和重症医学科医生的共同讨论治疗，在移植前稳定患者的生命体征。

(肖增丽 译 朱凤雪 校)

参考文献

1. Hoofnagle JH, Carithers RL Jr, Shapiro C, et al. Fulminant hepatic failure: summary of a workshop. Hepatology. 1995;21(1):240–252.
2. Lee WM, Squires RH Jr, Nyberg SL, et al. Acute liver failure: summary of a workshop. Hepatology (Baltimore, Md.). 2008;47(4):1401–1415.
3. O'Grady JG, Schalm SW, Williams R. Acute liver failure: redefining the syndromes. Lancet. 1993;342(8866):273–275.
4. Bernal W, Wendon J. Liver transplantation in adults with acute liver failure. Journal of Hepatology. 2004;40(2):192–197.
5. Rabinstein AA. Treatment of brain edema in acute liver failure. Current Treatment Options in Neurology. 2010;12(2):129–141.
6. Canalese J, Gimson AE, Davis C, et al. Controlled trial of dexamethasone and mannitol for the cerebral oedema of fulminant hepatic failure. Gut. 1982;23(7):625–629.
7. Murphy N, Auzinger G, Bernel W, et al. The effect of hypertonic sodium chloride on intracranial pressure in patients with acute liver failure. Hepatology. 2004;39(2):464–470.
8. Jalan R, Davies NA, Olde Damink SW. Hypothermia for the management of intracranial hypertension in acute liver failure. Metabolic Brain Disease. 2002;17(4):437–444.
9. Forbes A, Alexander GJ, O'Grady JG, et al. Thiopental infusion in the treatment of intracranial hypertension complicating fulminant hepatic failure. Hepatology. 1989;10(3):306–310.
10. Tofteng F, Larsen FS. The effect of indomethacin on intracranial pressure, cerebral perfusion and extracellular lactate and glutamate concentrations in patients with fulminant hepatic failure. Journal of Cerebral Blood Flow and Metabolism. 2004;24(7):798–804.
11. O'Grady JG, Alexander GJ, Hayllar KM, et al. Early indicators of prognosis in fulminant hepatic failure. Gastroenterology. 1989;97(2):439–445.
12. Davenport A. The management of renal failure in patients at risk of cerebral edema/hypoxia. New Horizons. 1995;3(4):717–724.
13. Davenport A. Dialysate and substitution fluids for patients treated by continuous forms of renal replacement therapy. Contributions to Nephrology. 2001;132:313–322.
14. Harrison PM, Wendon JA, Gimson AE, et al. Improvement by acetylcysteine of hemodynamics and oxygen transport in fulminant hepatic failure. New England Journal of Medicine. 1991;324(26):1852–1857.
15. Lee WM, Hynan LS, Rossaro L, et al. Intravenous N-acetylcysteine improves transplant-free survival in early stage non-acetaminophen acute liver failure. Gastroenterology. 2009;137(3):856–864, 64 e1.
16. Kociancic T, Reed MD. Acetaminophen intoxication and length of treatment: how long is long enough? Pharmacotherapy. 2003;23(8):1052–1059.
17. Garcia-Tsao G. Portal hypertension. Current Opinion in Gastroenterology. 2006;22(3):254–262.
18. Butterworth RF. Hepatic encephalopathy: a central neuroinflammatory disorder? Hepatology. 2011;53(4):1372–1376.
19. Ford RM, Sakaria SS, Subramanian RM. Critical care management of patients before liver transplantation. Transplantation Reviews. 2010;24(4):190–206.
20. Martinez GP, Barbera JA, Visa J, et al. Hepatopulmonary syndrome in candidates for liver transplantation. Journal of Hepatology. 2001;34(5):651–657.
21. Bozbas SS, Eyuboglu F. Evaluation of liver transplant candidates: a pulmonary perspective. Annals of Thoracic Medicine. 2011;6(3):109–114.
22. Krowka MJ, Mandell MS, Ramsay MA, et al. Hepatopulmonary syndrome and portopulmonary hypertension: a report of the multicenter liver transplant database. Liver Transplantation. 2004;10(2):174–182.
23. Sharma P, Rakela J. Management of pre-liver transplantation patient–part 2. Liver Transplantation. 2005;11(3):249–260.
24. Gupta S, Castel H, Rao RV, et al. Improved survival after liver transplantation in patients with hepatopulmonary syndrome. American Journal of Transplantation. 2010;10(2):354–363.
25. Hoeper MM, Krowka MJ, Strassburg CP. Portopulmonary hypertension and hepatopulmonary syndrome. Lancet. 2004;363(9419):1461–1468.
26. Kinasewitz GT, Keddissi JI. Hepatic hydrothorax. Current Opinion in Pulmonary Medicine. 2003;9(4):261–265.
27. TenHoor T, Mannino DM, Moss M. Risk factors for ARDS in the United States: analysis of the 1993 national mortality followback study. Chest. 2001;119(4):1179–1184.
28. Ventilation with lower tidal volumes as compared with traditional tidal volumes for acute lung injury and the acute respiratory distress syndrome. The Acute Respiratory Distress Syndrome Network. New England Journal of Medicine. 2000;342(18):1301–1308.
29. Garcia-Tsao G, Groszmann RJ, Fisher RL, et al. Portal pressure, presence of gas-

troesophageal varices and variceal bleeding. Hepatology. 1985;5(3):419–424.
30. Soares-Weiser K, Brezis M, Tur-Kaspa R, et al. Antibiotic prophylaxis for cirrhotic patients with gastrointestinal bleeding. Cochrane Database of Systematic Reviews. 2002;(2):CD002907.
31. Arroyo V, Gines P, Gerbes AL, et al. Definition and diagnostic criteria of refractory ascites and hepatorenal syndrome in cirrhosis. International Ascites Club. Hepatology. 1996;23(1):164–176.
32. Runyon BA. Management of adult patients with ascites due to cirrhosis: an update. Hepatology. 2009;49(6):2087–2107.
33. Sanyal AJ, Boyer T, Garcia-Tsao G, et al. A randomized, prospective, double-blind, placebo-controlled trial of terlipressin for type 1 hepatorenal syndrome. Gastroenterology. 2008;134(5):1360–1368.
34. Boyer T, Sanyal AJ, Garcia-Tsao G, et al. Predictors of response to terlipressin plus albumin in hepatorenal syndrome (HRS) type 1: Relationship of serium creatine to hemodynamics. Journal Hepatology. 2011;55(2):315–321.
35. Velez J, Nietert P. Therapeutic response to vasoconstriction in hepatorenal syndrome parallels increase in mean arterial pressure: A pooled analysis of clinical trials. American Journal Kidney Disease. 2011;58(6);928–938.
36. Chava SP, Singh B, Zaman MB, et al. Current indications for combined liver and kidney transplantation in adults. Transplantation Reviews. 2009;23(2):111–119.
37. Runyon BA, McHutchison JG, Antillon MR, et al. Short-course versus long-course antibiotic treatment of spontaneous bacterial peritonitis. A randomized controlled study of 100 patients. Gastroenterology. 1991;100(6):1737–1742.
38. Sort P, Navasa M, Arroyo V, et al. Effect of intravenous albumin on renal impairment and mortality in patients with cirrhosis and spontaneous bacterial peritonitis. New England Journal of Medicine. 1999;341(6):403–409.
39. Gustot T, Durand F, Lebrec D, et al. Severe sepsis in cirrhosis. Hepatology. 2009;50(6):2022–2033.
40. Tsai MH, Peng YS, Chen YC, et al. Adrenal insufficiency in patients with cirrhosis, severe sepsis and septic shock. Hepatology. 2006;43(4):673–681.

第 44 章

心力衰竭的重症监护

Josef Stehlik, Michael S. Kiernan, Deborah Budge, Maryl R. Johnson

引言

心血管疾病成为移植患者护理的重要问题。非心脏移植的适应证有很多,例如,高血压性肾小球硬化或胰岛素抵抗性糖尿病等,可以引起心肌缺血的疾病。此外,人口老龄化问题的逐渐加重,也增加了移植患者的心血管风险。脑死亡也会影响患者的心脏功能,并且心脏支持治疗也会进一步影响其他器官的功能。重度心力衰竭会引起严重的血流动力学紊乱从而影响其他重要器官的功能,使得这部分患者需要重症监护治疗。本章主要介绍重度心力衰竭患者的处理方法, 包括血管活性药物、主动脉内球囊反搏术以及机械通气等。本章对第39 章中等待心脏移植重症患者名单的处理问题做了补充说明, 并包含第 48 章中心室辅助装置的应用的相关问题。本章还介绍了由心脏功能继发的其他器官系统功能障碍的病理生理学机制和处理方法,例如,肺动脉高压、心肾综合征、肝功能衰竭。因此,本章内容同样适用于其他器官移植后出现心血管并发症的重症患者。

静脉用血管活性药物

重度心力衰竭患者可能会出现血流动力学紊乱,包括低血压、呼吸窘迫或进展性终末器官功能障碍等。在此类情况下,常需要血管活性药物来维持血流动力学稳定并保护终末器官功能。

根据患者血流动力学监测情况决定血管活性药物的种类及剂量,主要关注参数包括收缩压、容量状态、心输出量、体循环血管阻力。体格检查可以对这些参数做出很好的评估, 客观指标可以通过右心导管获得(Swanz-Ganz 导管)。对于危重症患者置入肺动脉导管的优势问题尚存在争议。随机对照研究显示常规置入肺动脉导管并不能降低死亡率或住院率[1–3]。当然在一些特定情况下,肺动脉导管仍有应用价值。例如,在重度心力衰竭患者,尤其是存在进展性终末器官功能障碍的患者,单纯体格检查不能准确评估患者血流动力学状态或基于临床评估的初始治疗未能达到预期效果[4–7]。通过右心导管获得的血流动力学参数可以指导临床医生选择合适的血管活性药物。

分类

正性肌力药

心输出量的显著降低是重症患者出现心力衰竭症状及终末器官功能障碍的主要原因。多巴酚丁胺和米力农是心力衰竭时增加心输出量最常见的两种正性肌力药。两者作用机制均是增加心肌和血管平滑肌细胞内的 cAMP 水平(图 44.1)[8–11]。在心肌细胞,cAMP 水平的增加可以促进 Ca^{2+}内流,从而增强心肌收缩性及变时效应。在血管内皮细胞,cAMP 水平的增加可以促进肌浆网钙摄取和血管舒张。

多巴酚丁胺为合成类儿茶酚胺药物,是 β_1 和 β_2 受体激动剂。与心肌 β_1 受体结合导致 cAMP 合成增加引起较强的正性肌力作用和较弱的变时作用[12]。与血管平滑肌细胞 α_1 和 β_2 受体结合的效应取决于多巴酚丁胺的剂量,小剂量[≤5μg/(kg·min)]应用时效应为轻度血管舒张,中等剂量[5~15μg/(kg·min)]应用外周血管阻力无明显改变,大剂量[>15μg/(kg·min)]应用时血管收缩作用占主导[13]。

米力农通过阻断磷酸二酯酶 3(PDE3),从而阻断 cAMP 降解为 AMP 来增加心肌和血管平滑肌内 cAMP 水平(图 44.1)[14]。米力农具有强效的心肌收缩作用并改善舒张功能[15–17]。全身及肺血管舒张作用强于多巴酚丁胺[18,19]。米力农通过肾脏代谢,因此肾功能不全患者

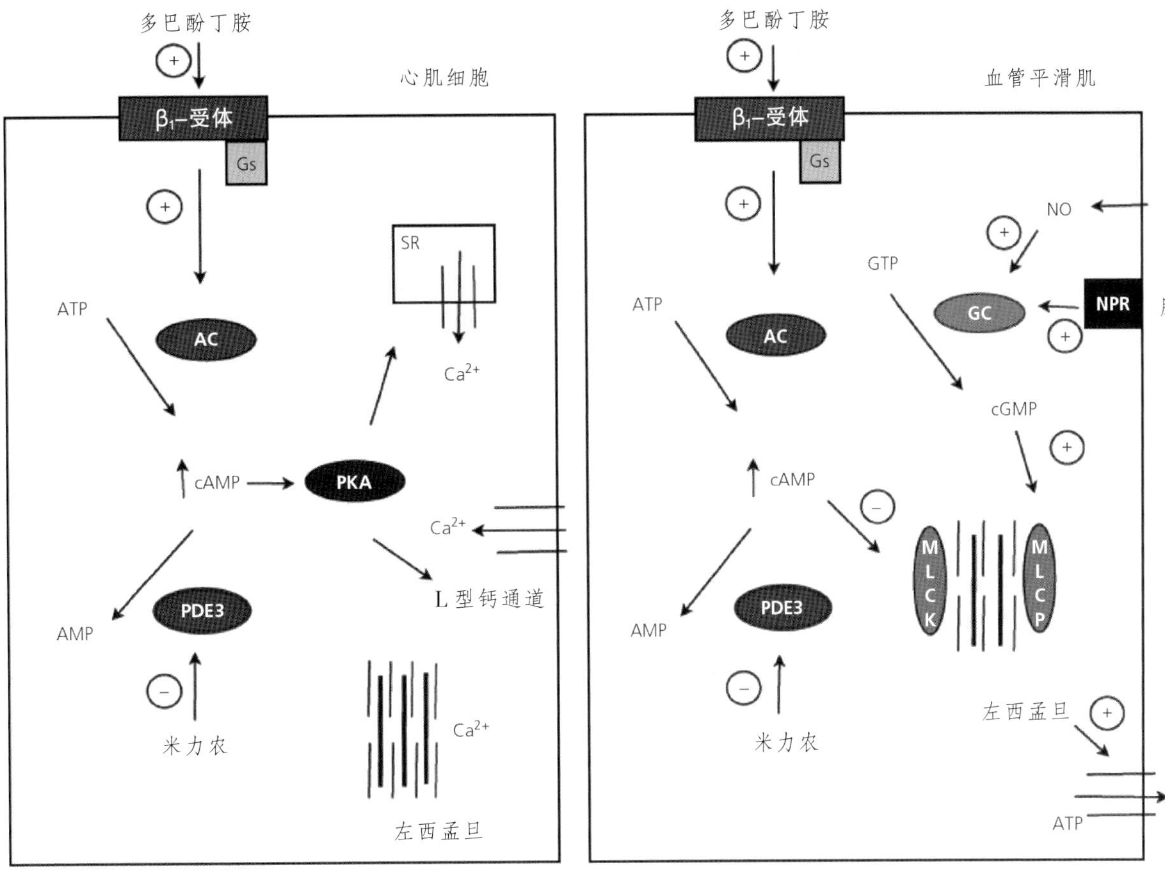

图 44.1　(A)β-激动剂(例如,多巴酚丁胺)通过 G 蛋白(Gs)激活腺苷酸环化酶(AC)增加环腺苷酸(cAMP)浓度。米力农通过阻断磷酸二酯酶 3(PDE3)以及 cAMP 的降解来增加 cAMP 水平。在心肌细胞,cAMP 激活蛋白激酶 A(PKA),导致 L 型钙通道的磷酸化促进 Ca^{2+}内流并增加肌浆网(SR)Ca^{2+}的释放,导致心肌收缩力增强。左西孟旦增加心肌肌丝对 Ca^{2+}敏感性。(B)在血管平滑肌,cAMP 阻断肌球蛋白轻链激酶(MLCK)导致平滑肌松弛。一氧化氮(NO)和钠尿肽(NPR)通过鸟苷酸环化酶(GC)增加环鸟苷酸(cGMP)浓度激活肌球蛋白轻链磷酸酶(MLCP)导致平滑肌松弛。左西孟旦激活 ATP 依赖的 K^+通道引起血管舒张。

应用时需酌情减量。

研究显示,多巴酚丁胺和米力农的临床预后相似,包括血流动力学效果和潜在致心律失常作用[20]。但在特定情况下,两者仍有各自的优势。多巴酚丁胺的血管舒张功能相对较弱,因此更适用于低血压的患者,尤其是收缩压≤85mmHg 的患者。由于一些患者对 β 肾上腺素受体反应迟钝或正在应用 β 受体阻滞剂,使得多巴酚丁胺治疗效果减弱[21]。由于米力农是通过非 β 肾上腺素通路起作用,所以这些因素不会影响米力农的作用。此外,由于米力农具有强效肺血管舒张作用可以降低右心室(RV)后负荷,因此,更适用于肺动脉高压和(或)右心功能障碍患者。长期使用多巴酚丁胺和米力农的死亡率无明显差异。急性期短期使用正性肌力药的使用可以改善血流动力学状态,长期使用多巴酚丁胺和米力农可以增加心肌氧耗并可能增加死亡率[22-27]。

钙增敏剂

钙增敏剂是一种新型正性肌力药,左西孟旦是目前研究最为广泛的一种。在心脏,左西孟旦与肌钙蛋白 C 结合,心肌肌丝对钙离子敏感性增加从而增加心肌收缩力。在血管平滑肌,左西孟旦可以使 ATP 依赖的钾通道开放,引起血管舒张从而降低心脏前后负荷[28,29]。研究显示,左西孟旦可以明显改善急性失代偿性心力衰竭的症状,但与持续应用多巴酚丁胺相比存活率无明显差异[30,31]。

其他拟交感药物

多巴胺是一种去甲肾上腺素前体,剂量不同其对心脏及血管的作用效果亦不同[32,33]。小剂量[1~3μg/(kg·min)]应用时肾脏和内脏动脉上多巴胺受体兴奋可以促进血管舒张并增加这些血管的血流。中等剂量[3~10μg/(kg·min)]应用时,多巴胺与 β_1 受体结合增加心肌收缩力和心率同时轻度增加外周血管阻力。大剂量[10~20μg/(kg·min)]应用时,外周血管 α_1 肾上腺素受体兴奋占主导地位,引起外周血管收缩、血压升高。

去甲肾上腺素是一种强效 α_1 受体激动剂,β 受体激动作用相对较弱。去甲肾上腺素可以引起强烈的血管收缩而心脏变力和变时效应相对较弱。在严重低血压患者中可以短期应用;然而,长期使用则与心肌毒性和心律失常直接相关。

肾上腺素作用于心脏和血管,是一种强效的 α 和 β 受体激动剂。小剂量应用时 β 受体激动占主导作用,大剂量应用时,则 α 受体激动占主导作用引起动脉和静脉血管收缩。肾上腺素常用于心脏移植前改善低心输出量状态。它在心力衰竭患者中应用较为局限,因其与心脏耗氧量增加明显相关,并会增加心脏后负荷以及心律失常发生率;建议在严重低血压时短期应用。

异丙肾上腺素是一种非选择性 β 受体激动剂,对 α 受体作用较弱。异丙肾上腺素有强力的变力和变时效应,常在心脏移植后即刻应用以维持较快的心率[34]。在除此之外的重度心力衰竭患者中的应用较为局限。

血管升压素

加压素通过激活血管平滑肌加压素 V1 受体。加压素可以引起外周血管收缩并增加血管平滑肌对儿茶酚胺的反应性[35]。加压素适用于由外周血管舒张导致严重低血压的心力衰竭患者。与其他血管加压药不同,加压素不会引起明显的心律失常。

静脉用血管扩张剂

慢性心力衰竭会引起交感神经系统活化及外周血管收缩,导致外周血管阻力、心脏后负荷增加、心输出量减少,心功能进一步恶化。在血压允许的情况下,静脉用血管舒张剂可以改善血流动力学状态。

硝普钠是一种作用于体循环及肺循环的强效动脉和静脉血管扩张剂。硝普钠代谢产生一氧化氮(NO)通过细胞内谷胱甘肽降低硝普盐浓度产生血管扩张作用。对于心输出量降低而不伴有低血压的患者,由于硝普盐不会增加心肌氧耗及心律失常的发生率,而优于强心药[36,37],但在伴有低血压的患者中应用受限。其他副作用则与其代谢产物相关。氰化物是硝普盐的代谢产物之一,会在肝功能障碍的患者体内积聚,但也有肝功能正常的患者出现氰化物中毒的报道。氰化物中毒的临床表现包括乳酸酸中毒、恶心、躁动、高铁血红蛋白血症。肾功能不全的患者可能出现硫氰酸盐(氰化物的一种代谢产物)中毒,表现为虚弱、震颤、恶心、反射亢进、昏迷罕见[38,39]。

硝酸盐产生 NO 的主要作用为静脉扩张,但在大剂量应用时也会出现动脉扩张。对利尿剂反应不佳的失代偿心力衰竭患者,尤其是右心衰竭患者,建议给予静脉用硝酸甘油。限制硝酸甘油使用的原因在于其易出现耐药性[40,41]。

奈西利肽是一种重组人 B 型利钠肽(BNP),减轻内源性 BNP 的作用。奈西利肽可以产生动脉及静脉血管扩张作用,并可以降低肺毛细血管楔压和右房压。研究显示,奈西利肽可以改善急性失代偿性心力衰竭患者的临床症状,但对死亡率没有明显改善[42-44]。在心脏移植时,奈西利肽可以用于对其他治疗无反应的重症患者[45]。奈西利肽的主要副作用为低血压。

临床应用

血管活性药物在心力衰竭患者中的应用一直存在争议。关于正性肌力药在重度心力衰竭患者中应用是否获益的研究尚不足够。但在无心脏移植打算的相对较轻的进展性心力衰竭患者中,无论短期还是长期使用正性肌力药均会增加患者的死亡率[24,46,47]。这些不良反应的机制主要与细胞内钙离子浓度增加和肌浆网内钙离子超载相关,进而引起心律失常和心肌重构[48,49]。对于急性失代偿性心力衰竭患者,指南不推荐常规使用这些血管活性药物,但在等待心脏移植的患者中可以长期应用强心药,或可以用于终末期患者的保守治疗[50]。

血管活性药物常作为急性心力衰竭恶化及等待心脏移植患者的初始治疗方案。药物的选择需要根据患者的血流动力学状态以及药物的属性。具有明显低血压的患者需要选择血管舒张作用较小的药物,例如,多巴胺、肾上腺素和去甲肾上腺素。关于几种具有血管加压作用药物对比的研究较少[51]。在低心输出量不伴有低血压的患者中,米力农或多巴酚丁胺为最常用的正性肌力药。与多巴酚丁胺相比,米力农的耐药率相对较低并且对肺血管的舒张作用更强;然而,由于缺乏有力的临床对照研究,目前认为这两种药物临床结局相似[52]。当联合使用时，多巴酚丁胺的 β 受体激动作用和米力农的 PDE3 阻滞作用可以使对单独应用效果欠佳的患者获益。

一旦血流动力学得到改善，需尽快改为口服治疗。然而在一些患者中，撤除静脉血管活性药物支持可能会进一步引起血流动力学不稳，加重心力衰竭并引起终末器官功能障碍[48]。排除其他因素后，认为这部分患者为强心药依赖型，在等待移植过程中可能需要持续的静脉强心药物支持。这一临床状态十分常见，根据国际心肺移植学会注册显示，2002—2010 年 27 387 例患者中，有 45%在移植期间使用正性肌力药物支持[53]。等待肝移植患者，如果在使用正性肌力药则需要严密观察。鉴于正性肌力药的致心律失常特性，应在患者出院前置入植入型心律转复除颤器[54-56]。如果等待移植的患者出现正性肌力药物依赖，提示患者心力衰竭处于进展阶段并与高死亡率相关[57]，一些器官分配系统使这些患者处于更高危状态。例如，在美国如果患者持续静脉使用单一高剂量正性肌力药 [多巴酚丁胺≥7.5μg/(kg·min)]，米力农≥0.5μg/(kg·min)，多巴胺≥7.5μg/(kg·min)，或肾上腺素≥0.02μg/(kg·min)或两种或两种以上正性肌力药，并有持续血流动力学监测，则属于最高危 1A 期。如果患者静脉使用持续正性肌力药，包括使用单一药物的患者以及门诊患者，则属于 1B 期[58]。

正性肌力药依赖患者，如果等待移植时间超出预期，或在使用正性肌力药物过程中出现进展性血流动力学恶化，则需要考虑机械支持治疗，例如，机械通气或人工心脏支持治疗。这部分内容详见第 48 章和第 49 章。

主动脉内球囊反搏

主动脉内球囊反搏(IABP)技术常用于对药物治疗效果不佳的心力衰竭患者。主动脉反搏的概念由 Moulopoulos 及其同事于 20 世纪 60 年代早期第一次提出[59]，并在 1968 年由 Kantrowitz 教授第一次应用于临床[60]。目前 IABP 的应用现状包括心源性休克支持治疗、高危冠状动脉介入治疗、难治性心绞痛的治疗、心肺转流术脱机过程支持[61,62]。IABP 仍是最常用的机械循环支持方式。

血流动力学作用

IABP 是经皮置入一个可充气的球囊，通常由股动脉至降主动脉。体外控制台在心脏循环间期通过膨胀和压缩球囊：心室舒张期球囊充气膨胀，而在心室收缩前放气。心脏舒张期球囊扩张大部分血流逆行向上升高主动脉根部压力，增加舒张压和冠状动脉血流，同时也增加舒张期其他器官的血流灌注。收缩期，球囊放气产生真空效应，降低心脏后负荷并增加心输出量。很多人相信对于左心室功能(LV)不全的患者，降低后负荷可以使患者最大程度获益[63,64]。Scheidt 等报道，对于心源性休克的患者，IABP 反搏的平均结果为收缩压降低 20%、舒张压升高 30%、心输出量升高 20%、肺毛细血管楔压(PCWP)降低 20%[65]。要得到最佳血流动力学结果，需保证 IABP 球囊的膨胀与收缩与心脏周期同步。技术进步有助于 IABP 控制系统自动调节球囊最佳膨胀与收缩时间。

临床应用

在过去 20 年间，IABP 已帮助约 7%的等待移植患者成功过渡到移植手术[53]。使用 IABP 成功过渡到移植的患者移植术后死亡率并不增加[53,66]。

IABP 最常用于 ST 段抬高型心梗(STEMI)导致的心源性休克患者。与正性肌力药和血管加压药相反，IABP 不会增加心肌缺血患者的氧耗。目前尚在对 IABP 的有效性进行进一步审查。一项对 9 个 STEMI 和心源性休克研究的 Meta 分析显示，在接受溶栓治疗的患者中 IABP 与 30 天死亡率降低相关，但在全部队列研究中未见明显获益(n=10 529)[67]。心肌梗死国家注册系统中的数据未显示 IABP 与直接经皮冠状动脉介入治疗患者降低相关，但在 IABP 使用率更高的医院显示IABP 可以使患者获益[68]。最近，一项多中心随机研究，纳入 600 例由急性心肌梗死患者导致的心源性休克计划行血管重建的患者，分为使用 IABP 组和不使用 IABP，研究结果未显示出两组患者 30 天死亡率存在差异[69]。由于缺乏明确的临床疗效数据，在这种临床情况下 IABP 技术可以使患者血流动力学获益，因此 STEMI 临床指南推荐在对药物治疗反应不佳的心源性休克患者可以使用 IABP[70]。IABP 可以用于血管重建术、其他机械循环辅助支持或心脏移植的过度治疗。

在非缺血性心肌病伴有心输出量降低及终末器官功能障碍的患者中，IABP 也有一定的应用价值。虽然 IABP 可以改善心肌氧供和氧耗比例，但此作用会被心肌储备功能和心肌收缩力所限制[71]。对没有冠心病和心肌缺血的患者，IABP 的优势会有所减少。在使用

IABP 的患者中，慢性心力衰竭、左心室射血分数<30%、纽约心脏协会心功能分级(NYHA)Ⅳ级和急性心肌梗死患者的存活率更低[72]。因此，在伴有严重休克、终末器官功能障碍、明显心律失常的心肌病患者，IABP会有一定益处，但同时也要制订应用其他机械支持治疗的计划。

IABP 与血管活性药物联合治疗可以用于降低等待心脏移植患者的肺动脉压。新型治疗还包括磷酸二酯酶-5(PDE5)抑制剂和左心室辅助装置，在后面还会提及这部分内容。

IABP 应用的禁忌证包括严重的外周血管疾病和重度主动脉瓣关闭不全。潜在并发症包括肢端缺血、出血、血管撕裂等血管事件，以及感染和休克。IABP 应用的主要限制为稳定性问题，使得 IABP 只能短期使用。如果通过左侧腋动脉置管则可以允许患者走动，但这种方法很少使用[73]。目前已经有更永久的心室辅助装置，因此对于有更多的机械辅助装置选择的患者，将 IABP 的使用限制在 1 周内似乎是合理的。

机械通气在移植候选人中的应用

进展性心力衰竭患者可能会伴有呼吸功能不全而需要机械通气治疗。机械通气治疗的目标包括改善气体交换、降低呼吸做功及降低心肌耗氧。机械通气患者心肺系统的相互作用很复杂[74,75]。接下来简要介绍心力衰竭患者机械通气的基本原理。

血流动力学作用

正常自主呼吸情况下，吸气时肺泡内压和胸膜内压降低，增加心脏血管静脉回流[76]。正压机械通气的应用增加了胸腔内压，由于改变了压力梯度，继而可以改变全身静脉回流及回心血量[77]，导致全身静脉回流减少和左心室后负荷降低。净效应为胸腔内血容量降低和心脏做功减少[75]。这些血流动力学改变理论上对心源性肺水肿患者是有益的。机械通气的额外好处得益于动脉氧合的改善和呼吸肌氧需的降低[78]。

机械通气在右心室功能的影响的研究相对较少，而在急性呼吸窘迫综合征(ARDS)患者中应用的研究较多。正压机械通气可以降低右心室前负荷。机械通气期间，高平台压和高呼气末正压(PEEP)会导致右心室后负荷的增加[79,80]。这些效应可以用于需要机械通气的右心室功能不全的患者。

临床应用

伴有急性呼吸功能不全的心力衰竭患者接受机械通气治疗的适应证为心源性肺水肿。在这种情况下，左心房压增加导致液体渗入到组织间隙和肺泡，并进一步引起肺实变和通气血流比例失调导致低氧血症、CO_2储留、增加呼吸做功。除利尿剂和血管扩张剂外，初始治疗可能还包括无创正压通气（NIPPV），NIPPV 已被证明可以改善氧合并降低心源性肺水肿患者有创机械通气的可能性[81-85]。以上治疗失败或患者出现血流动力学不稳定或呼吸肌疲劳时，可以进行气管插管与有创机械通气治疗。对于进展性心力衰竭患者，其他机械通气治疗的适应证包括心肌梗死的机械性并发症、顽固性心律失常、肺栓塞、多器官功能衰竭。这些情况下机械通气的益处包括改善组织的最大氧供、纠正酸碱失衡、降低心肌氧耗。

除了一些特殊的适应证，心脏移植患者如需要机械通气支持是死亡率增加的一个危险因素，但只有一小部分需要机械通气的患者被考虑进行心脏移植。2004—2009 年间 ISHLT 注册的 10 271 例心脏移植患者，只有<3%的患者在移植期间接受机械通气治疗。多变量分析校正其他临床危险因素后，机械通气与 1 年死亡率增加 60%相关[53]。因此，移植患者进行机械通气治疗应该慎重。如果进行机械通气治疗的首要原因是由心力衰竭加重或进展导致的血流动力学不稳定，那么应该考虑正性肌力药物支持或机械循环辅助支持以稳定循环、方便脱机、恢复器官功能。如果不是由血流动力学不稳定引起的呼吸衰竭，那么移植或永久机械循环支持治疗的预后较差。

终末期心力衰竭患者的肺脏

由左心室功能障碍导致的肺动脉高压被称为左心疾病相关性肺动脉高压，肺静脉或毛细血管后肺动脉高压[86]。严重的左心室收缩功能障碍患者有 60%伴有肺动脉高压，而在心脏舒张功能障碍的患者中发病率更高[87]，并与发病率和死亡率升高相关[88,89]。一项研究显示，心力衰竭和中重度肺动脉高压患者的死亡率是无肺动脉高压患者的 3 倍[90]。

>50%接受心脏移植评估的患者伴有肺血管阻力

增加[91,92]。跨肺压(TPG)>16mmHg 增加移植后右心衰竭的风险和死亡率[91-93]。使用血管扩张剂后肺血管阻力(PVR)>2.5WU 和（或)TPG>15mmHg 的患者移植后早期死亡率增加 3 倍,且移植后晚期预后不佳。如果患者的肺动脉高压(PVR<2.5WU)表现出明显的可逆性并且不伴有全身低血压表现，则此类移植患者的预后与基线 PVR<2.5WU 的患者相似[92]。

心肺疾病的病理生理学

由左心疾病引起的肺动脉高压的发病机制十分复杂(图 44.2)[94]。由心脏收缩[88,89]、心脏舒张[95]、或心脏瓣膜病[96]引起的左心压力升高会导致肺静脉压和平均肺动脉压被动升高。毛细血管后肺动脉高压患者有两种血流动力学表现形式[97]。第一种,被动的肺动脉高压,平均肺动脉压的升高是对 PCWP 升高的反应,TPG 轻度升高。毛细血管后肺动脉高压是对下游压力增加的一种代偿反应,以保证前向血流[97]。被动毛细血管后肺动脉高压患者 PCWP 降低会引起平均肺动脉压的降低[98]。左心室疾病相关肺动脉高压的第二种形式为反应性肺动脉血管收缩,是在被动肺动脉高压基础上出现的。肺静脉收缩导致 PVR 反应性增加的具体机制尚不明确。内皮细胞通过一氧化氮和内皮素通路在维持血管紧张性上起到核心作用[94]。在心力衰竭患者中,一氧化氮依赖的血管舒张作用受损[99],内皮素释放上调[94]。

心力衰竭患者肺血管反应的异常,一部分原因是内皮功能紊乱和这些通路的失衡[94]。在反应性肺动脉高压患者，即使在左心室充盈压下降后,TPG 和 PVR 仍处于较高水平。长期反应性肺动脉高压会引起肺血管床重塑[100]。肺泡和毛细血管基膜增厚[101,102]会降低毛细血管滤过和微血管通透性。最初血管重塑是为了阻止肺水肿的发展;然而,与心力衰竭时神经内分泌的级联反应相似,这些代偿性改变会导致肺顺应性降低、PVR 增加、气体弥散率降低及通气不足[101,102]。反应性肺动脉高压的可逆性可以用血管扩张剂试验。急性血流动力学试验后肺动脉压、TPG、PVR 下降不明显者被定义为“顽固性肺动脉高压”；但缺乏急性反应并不一定意味着永久性改变。一些患者虽然在急性试验后未显示出肺动脉压的下降，但经过适当的药物治疗数周或数月后肺循环血流动力学仍可逐渐改善[97]。最新研究显示，在由左心室疾病导致血流动力学异常的患者中，使用 LVAD 可以明显减轻心脏负担,并降低肺动脉压[103,104]。

一项研究显示,急性失代偿性心力衰竭住院患者中,有 51%患者出现被动性肺动脉高压,25%出现反应性肺动脉高压[105]。与被动性肺动脉高压相比,反应性肺动脉高压与死亡相关性更高(与正常肺动脉压患者对比,校正 HR 值:4.8 对 2.8,P=0.0001)[105]。

肺循环是右心后负荷的主要决定性因素,由心肺疾病导致的死亡与右心功能障碍密切相关[106-108]。右心衰竭引起心输出量和心肌收缩力降低,从而导致器官功能衰竭(见肾脏和肝脏部分)。右室壁薄可以适应静脉回流的增加并向低阻力的肺循环继续泵血[109]。右心后负荷增加导致右心扩张,增加氧消耗,降低心肌收缩力[110]。由于左右心室相互比邻,右心室扩张会导致室间隔矛盾运动,同时右心室充盈压增加也会传至左心室,并影响左心室充盈压[111-114]。此外,由容量负荷导致室壁张力增加同时心肌纤维长度也会增加,一旦超过 Frank-Starling 曲线的最佳长度，则会出现心室收缩力下降[115]。肺动脉压更依赖于右心功能。正常情况下,右心室收缩压可达到 40~50mmHg,但如果出现心室肥厚,则可产生更高的收缩压[94]。当右心室功能下降时,即使 PVR 显著升高,平均肺动脉压仍会下降[113]。

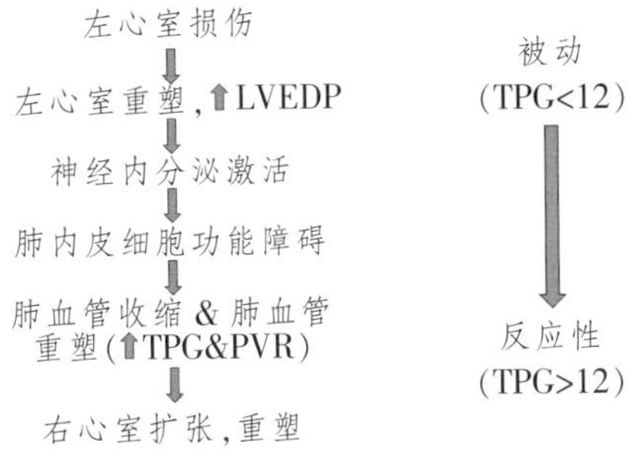

图 44.2 由左心室疾病引起的肺动脉高压的病理学改变。慢性心力衰竭导致神经内分泌调节异常,一氧化氮(NO)的血管扩张效应与内皮素(ET1)的血管收缩作用失衡。左心室(LV)收缩或舒张功能障碍,导致左心室舒张末期压力(LVEDP)增加,并被动传递至肺血管床,导致肺动脉压升高。初期跨肺压(TPG)低,肺动脉压与左心室压力成比例增加。内皮功能障碍可能会引起肺动脉血管反应性舒张及肺血管重塑，此时肺动脉压与左心室压力不成比例增加(TPG 增加)。肺动脉高压会导致右心室(RV)重塑并进一步引起右心室功能障碍。

肺动脉高压的诊断

超声心动图可以作为一种筛查手段,来评估右心室收缩压。超声心动可以发现左心室舒张异常包括左心房扩大、左心室肥厚、二尖瓣血流异常以及二尖瓣环组织多普勒信号异常[116,117]。但是,右心导管评估血流动力学仍是肺动脉高压的客观诊断标准[87,116]。右心导管可以检测心室充盈压、肺动脉压、PCWP及心输出量,通过这种方法还可以检测TPG和PVR。在存在肺动脉高压时,右心导管还可以帮助分析其是由毛细血管前还是毛细血管后原因所致。推荐使用肺血管扩张剂进行肺血管扩张试验来评估心脏移植患者肺动脉高压的可逆性。在肺动脉收缩压>50mmHg、TPG>15mmHG或PVR>3WU的患者,最常使用的血管扩张剂包括硝普钠、吸入性一氧化氮和前列环素,目标为肺动脉收缩压<40mmHg、TPG<15mmHG或PVR<3WU,且不伴有心输出量下降,并维持收缩压>85mmHg[118]。

肺动脉高压的治疗

治疗需针对引起疾病的直接原因及左心室充盈压[116]。治疗的总体目标为恢复右心室与肺动脉直接的生理关系以改善肺血流。一些药物(如利尿剂、硝酸盐、肼屈嗪、血管紧张素转换酶抑制剂、血管紧张素Ⅱ受体阻断剂、奈西立肽、米力农)和操作(心脏瓣膜手术、LVAD植入术)的干预也可以通过降低左心室充盈压来降低平均肺动脉压。此外,一些治疗的目标是改善右心室功能。接下来介绍具体治疗方法。

血管扩张剂

非选择性和选择性肺血管扩张剂都可以通过降低右心后负荷降低PVR和增加右心输出量。吸入性一氧化氮和前列环素是肺血管扩张剂,起效快并可以改善血流动力学效应[119-121]。由于在呼吸机循环中需要持续输送一氧化氮,因此,肺动脉高压在脱机过程中可能会复发[122]。对左心衰竭引起的肺动脉高压患者使用选择性肺血管扩张剂的研究结果并未显示出其对临床预后有益。而大型随机对照研究显示,前列环素与标准治疗相比会导致更高的死亡率[123]。内皮素拮抗剂波生坦片在慢性心力衰竭患者中也未显示出有利的影响,虽然并未对毛细血管后肺动脉高压患者做单独研究[124]。选择性肺血管扩张剂可能会增加右心输出量,并会导致急性肺水肿[119,125-127]。

硝普钠可以降低肺血管和全身血管阻力,使左心室后负荷降低,从而可以抵消由右心功能改善导致的左心室充盈量的增加。硝普钠被用作肺动脉高压可逆性的急性血流动力学检测用药,也可以作为急性失代偿性心力衰竭的短期治疗[128]。重组脑钠肽奈西立肽也可以降低毛细血管后肺动脉高压患者的肺动脉压和PVR[43,129];然而,尚未证明其有除了改善血流动力学以外的其他优势。

西地那非,PDE5抑制剂,是一种选择性肺血管扩张剂[130-132]。一些临床研究显示,西地那非可能改善血流动力学状态、运动耐量,以及由左心室功能下降导致的慢性心力衰竭患者的生活质量[133-135]。也有研究证明西地那非可以改善心脏舒张功能的测量结果[136]。西地那非通过抑制PDE3还可以产生类米力农效应,改善右心室功能[137]。然而,随机研究显示与安慰剂相比,西地那非不能改善舒张性心力衰竭患者的运动耐量[138]。有研究显示,西地那非在术后急性右心功能障碍患者中有一定作用[139,140]。由于没有足够的证据支持,PDE5抑制剂在毛细血管后肺动脉高压患者中常规使用尚未被推荐,但在心脏移植候补者中其常被用来降低肺动脉压[140-142]。

右心室功能障碍的治疗

目前尚缺乏对肺动脉高压导致的右心室功能障碍的有效治疗。治疗策略包括改善右心室前负荷和收缩功能,以及降低右心室后负荷[115]。首先,需要纠正引起PVR升高的可逆性因素,例如低氧血症。睡眠呼吸暂停在心力衰竭患者中很常见,而纠正睡眠呼吸暂停可以降低肺动脉压并改善右心室功能。正性肌力药可以改善右心室收缩性,例如,多巴酚丁胺和米力农(见本章前部分)。

右心衰竭时由于容量负荷过重会导致室间隔移位影响左心室充盈,并降低左心室容量[143-145]。在右心功能障碍患者中,不建议在无监测的情况下进行快速补液[115]。有创血流动力学监测目标是维持初始中心静脉压在10mmHg。

移植与机械支持

经药物治疗无效的终末期心力衰竭和肺动脉高压患者,可以考虑LVAD治疗[146]。经过LVAD治疗,可以通过改善左心室充盈压而逐渐降低PVR[103,104]。在严重右心衰竭患者中,在等待移植过程中,右心辅助装置(RVAD)可以与LVAD联合使用。对于全心衰竭患者,在等待确切的治疗前,可以先使用主动脉内球囊反搏和体外膜肺氧合[147,148]。接受机械通气治疗的患者需进行保护性肺通气策略以降低平台压,并避免右心功能障碍加重[149]。对于药物治疗和机械支持治疗效果不佳的顽固性肺动脉高压患者，可以考虑心肺联合移植[150]。

终末期心力衰竭患者的肾脏

心肾轴对调节水电解质平衡、血压及全身血液灌注十分重要。心肾综合征是指由心脏和肾脏的急性或慢性功能障碍引起其他器官的功能改变[151]。急性心力衰竭患者，缓解心脏充血的治疗过程中可能会加重肾功能的恶化。心力衰竭治疗的挑战在于避免肾小球滤过率(GFR)进一步恶化的同时缓解液体过负荷。

避免肾功能的进一步恶化十分重要，因为与左心室射血分数下降相比，GFR 的下降对死亡率的预测能力更强[152]，并且独立于心力衰竭症状的严重程度[153-159]。一项对>80 000 例心力衰竭患者的系统性评价显示，正常 GFR 患者的 1 年死亡率为 24%，GFR 轻度下降者为 38%，中重度下降者为 51%[160]。在心力衰竭治疗过程中，患者血肌酐升高也与预后不佳相关，包括住院时间延长、再住院率升高、院内及远期死亡率增加[157-159,161-167]。

心力衰竭合并血肌酐升高的患者，区分心肾综合征(由心力衰竭导致血流动力学紊乱所致)和潜在的原发的慢性肾病十分重要。鉴于许多心力衰竭患者同时存在两种情况，因此区分起来十分困难[168]。支持原发肾脏疾病的检测包括：严重蛋白尿(>1g/d)，尿沉渣检测(血尿、脓尿、细胞管型)和(或)影像学显示肾结构异常。

心肾综合征的病理生理学

心肾综合征是一种复杂的血管运动性肾病，有多种因素可以导致肾功能恶化[161,162,169,170]。了解病理生理学机制包括神经内分泌激活、肾灌注下降、肾静脉压增高、右心室功能障碍和全身感染。

神经内分泌激活

心力衰竭患者每搏量和心输出量降低，导致有效动脉血容量减少和动脉充盈不足，导致左心室、主动脉弓、颈动脉窦、肾小球旁器压力感受器上的机械性感受器触发减少。反过来，这会导致一系列神经内分泌通路的激活——交感神经传出增加，肾素-血管紧张素-醛固酮系统激活，抗利尿激素和内皮素-1 的释放，目的在于通过全身血管收缩和水钠潴留来恢复器官灌注[171-173]。随着时间延长，这些过程逐渐出现适应不良，并逆调节利钠肽、一氧化氮、前列环素和缓激肽的血管舒张和尿钠排泄通路[162,169,174]。钠尿肽受体下调，使得这些机制在肾脏的效应会有所衰减[172,175]，肾血管收缩、钠离子向远侧肾单位转运减少，进而引起水钠潴留[171,176,177]。

心力衰竭患者使用袢利尿剂可以促进钠向远曲小管传递，导致腺苷分泌增加[178]。血清腺苷水平增加，促进入球小动脉收缩和近曲小管钠重吸收[163,179]，导致 GFR 进一步降低，促进水钠潴留，并可能会降低利尿剂的反应性。

因此，心力衰竭患者神经内分泌激活导致血管收缩、增加心脏后负荷、降低心输出量和肾血流减少。

肾血流减少

心力衰竭加重期间肾功能的恶化常由心输出量减少和肾脏低灌注所导致，这种情况常出现在低血压或心源性休克患者中；然而，心输出量与肾功能之间的相关性并不是线性的[164,165]，只要心指数不低于 1.5L/(min·m^2)，肾脏自身调节机制仍可维持肾血流[166]。绝大部分心力衰竭合并肾功能不全的住院患者并不存在低血压或休克[153,180,181]，因此，心肾综合征的发病机制除了低心输出量还有其他更重要的因素。

静脉淤血

绝大多数急性心力衰竭患者会出现静脉淤血的症状和体征[153]。但即使没有外周水肿的表现，患者仍可能存在血容量和心脏充盈压的增加[167]。

腹水、内脏水肿、内脏循环充血会导致腹腔内压力增加，肾外血管被压缩，肾功能下降[181]。肾灌注压取决于平均动脉压与肾静脉压的差值[182]，静脉淤血的加重会阻碍肾脏的前向血流[183,184]，减少尿液产生和钠离子的排泄[185]。这是全身静脉淤血与 GFR 下降独立相关的原因[168,186,187]；也是心力衰竭恶化治疗过程中外周静脉压下降不足与肾功能下降(与心输出量下降相比)更加相关的原因[168]。在 ESCAPE 研究[1]中，右房压是与基线肾功能相关的唯一血流动力学变量[164]。

由于肾小囊的不可扩张性，间质水肿会进一步加重肾间质和肾静脉压(图 44.3)[182]。肾静脉压的增加会刺激局部交感神经激活，导致肾动脉血管收缩和 GFR 下降[188-190]。

右心功能

在急性心力衰竭恶化患者中，超声心动图证实存

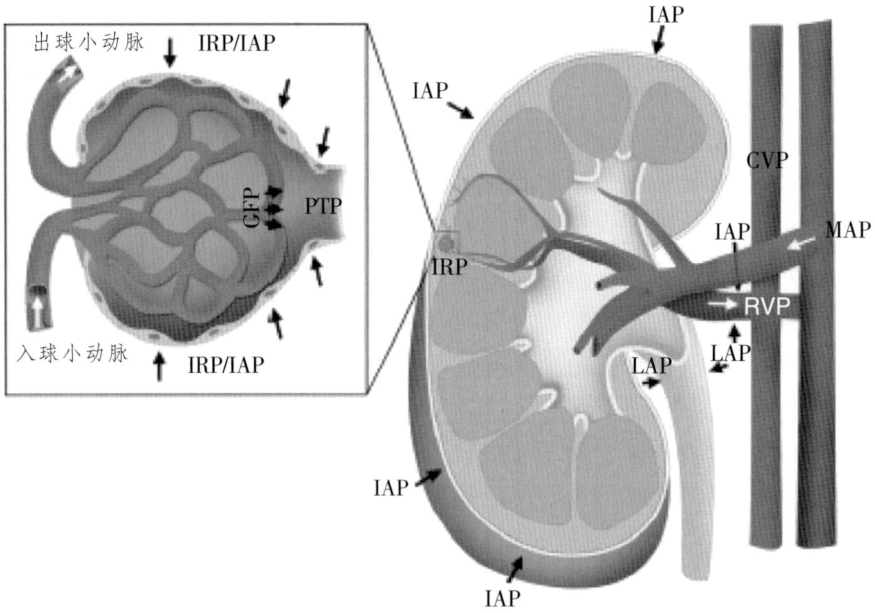

图 44.3 决定肾小球滤过率(GFR)的血流动力学因素。除肾单位数量和治疗外,GFR 还与多种血流动力学因素相关。促使血流从肾小球毛细血管向肾小囊腔流动的机械作用为滤过梯度(FG),相当于肾小球滤过压(GFP)- 近曲小管压力(PTP)。PTP 与肾间质压力(IRP)和腹内压(IAP)相关,而这两者都会因静脉淤血而升高。GFP 取决于肾血流[肾灌注压;平均动脉压(MAP)-肾静脉压(RVP)/肾血管阻力]。RVP 与中心静脉压(CVP)密切相关,因此,当存在静脉淤血时 CVP 会升高。GFP 则受入球小动脉和出球小动脉的收缩和舒张的调节。(Reproduced from Dupont et al.[182], with kind permission from Springer Science+Business Media.)

在右心功能障碍患者的肾功能损伤重于右心功能正常的患者[191]。右心功能障碍导致外周静脉压升高,进而会影响肾功能(如前述)。此外,由于心包的束缚,右心扩张会影响左心充盈,限制每搏输出量和心输出量[192]。通过以上两种机制,右心功能在心肾综合征的进展中起到重要作用。

炎症

心力衰竭可以导致内皮激活[193-195]。周向应力改变会作用于内皮细胞产生炎症介质,例如,内皮素-1、白细胞介素-6、肿瘤坏死因子-α[182,196-199]。氧化应激会进一步降低一氧化氮的生物利用度[182],会影响内皮一氧化氮介导的静脉张力,可能会导致心肾综合征[197]。

影响治疗效果的因素

血浆再充盈率

血浆再充盈是指在血容量降低时液体由血管外向血管内流动,例如使用利尿剂或超滤时。血浆再充盈率取决于血管内外的胶体渗透压和静水压差[200]。如血浆再充盈率过高,则会导致肾功能恶化和低血压。因此,使用利尿剂时,血清肌酐的下降并不意味着充血的减轻,相反,可能是由于血管内液体排出过多与血浆再充盈不匹配[201]。

利尿剂抵抗

利尿剂抵抗是指患者对同等剂量利尿剂的反应减弱[202]。利尿剂抵抗的机制有很多。药物生物利用度会因肠道灌注减少和内脏水肿而下降[203]。进展性心力衰竭还可能引起蛋白丢失和低白蛋白血症[204],降低血管内胶体渗透压,增加袢利尿剂的分布容量,减少其向近曲小管的转运[205]。肾功能障碍导致有机酸在体内积聚并抑制袢利尿剂的肾小管分泌[185]。即使在有足够的药物吸收和转运的情况下,利尿剂的药理作用仍会受到影响。肾功能障碍时会降低钠离子的滤过,限制利尿剂的反应。利尿剂对近端 $Na^+/K^+/Cl^-$转运体慢性阻滞作用,导致钠向远端小管转运增加,并最终引起肾小管细胞肥大[185],此外还存在"刹车效应",即钠输送增加导致远端肾小管重吸收反弹增加[206]。神经内分泌激活效应与利尿剂对肾脏的效应相互抵消;相反,心力衰竭时去甲肾上腺素水平下降则可以改善利尿剂的反应性[207]。

心肾综合征的治疗

由于缺乏增加 GFR 的特异性疗法，合并心肾综合征的心力衰竭患者的治疗目标是缓解体循环充血和恢复终末器官灌注。有效的血流动力学改变可以重建有效的肾动静脉压力梯度并改善 GFR[168]。通过利尿、超滤或穿刺术减少液体负荷可以降低腹腔内压力并改善肾功能[208]。

限制水钠吸收

虽然没有随机研究证实，但限盐治疗在避免淤血加重上十分重要[209]，建议钠盐摄入限制在<2g/d。并建议液体摄入<2L/d，尤其对低钠血症患者(<130mmol/L)或利尿剂抵抗患者[209]。

利尿剂

虽然尚缺乏其安全性和有效性的证据，利尿剂仍是治疗体循环充血的主要药物[209]。心力衰竭患者对袢利尿剂的反应常存在一种不可预测的剂量反应曲线，因此这些药物的剂量需要谨慎滴定以达到预期治疗效果(图 44.4)[210]。过度利尿会引起低血容量、低血压、心输出量降低及神经内分泌激活，导致肾功能进一步恶化，而更大剂量的利尿剂则与死亡率相关[211-213]。利尿剂抵抗患者，增加剂量可以提高患者对利尿剂的反应。在全天剂量相同情况下，持续静脉输注和间断负荷剂量给药效果相似[214]。加用噻嗪类利尿剂也可以改善利尿剂抵抗。噻嗪类利尿剂作用于远曲小管，与袢利尿剂具有协同作用。噻嗪类利尿剂与袢利尿剂联合使用可以克服长期使用袢利尿剂后出现的肾小管肥厚和快速钠重吸收[215]。

所有的利尿剂都可以改变血电解质浓度，并对心脏节律和神经肌肉活动有潜在影响作用。所有利尿治疗都需要密切监测电解质，尤其当袢利尿剂和噻嗪类利尿剂联合使用时。补钾治疗及使用保钾利尿剂可以平衡钾离子的丢失，目标是维持钾离子>4.0mmol/L，并维持镁离子水平在 0.75~1mmol/L。

超滤

对心力衰竭和容量超负荷的患者，如果对利尿剂反应不佳，可以考虑超滤治疗。尽管利尿剂使钠浓缩增加，但相对于血浆，尿液仍为低渗，例如，使用袢利尿剂后，平均尿钠浓度为 60mmol/L，而血浆钠浓度为 140mmol/L[210]。理论上，由于超滤使用的是等张液，因此其优势之一为可以去除更大量的钠离子；此外，通过控制液体清除率，超滤的另一个优势在于可以根据调节超滤量达到预计的血浆再充盈率。根据心力衰竭患者使用静脉–静脉超滤的经验，该治疗耐受性好，不会导致血流动力学恶化[216,217]。与静脉使用利尿剂相比，超滤会使体重下降更明显，并可以移除更多液体，但血肌酐水平改变相似[216,218]。如果液体移除率不能超过血浆再灌注率(12~14mL/min)，并可以避免肾素–血管紧张素–醛固酮系统的进一步激活[200]。

超滤是否可以帮助治疗心肾综合征尚明确。一些研究显示，通过超滤使体重减轻可以改善利尿剂的反应性，且与袢利尿剂相比充血的缓解也更明显[207,2018-220]。需要注意过度超滤会增加神经内分泌激活，降低肾灌注，并导致肾功能恶化[183]。随机研究显示，急性心力衰竭伴持续充血和肾功能恶化的住院患者，在 96 小时体重下降相似的情况下，与阶梯式药物治疗策略相比，超滤治疗的肾功能恶化和恶性事件比例更高[221]。目前，超滤适用于使用大剂量利尿剂仍无法维持负平衡的患者[209,222,223]。严重肾功能障碍患者可能需要血液

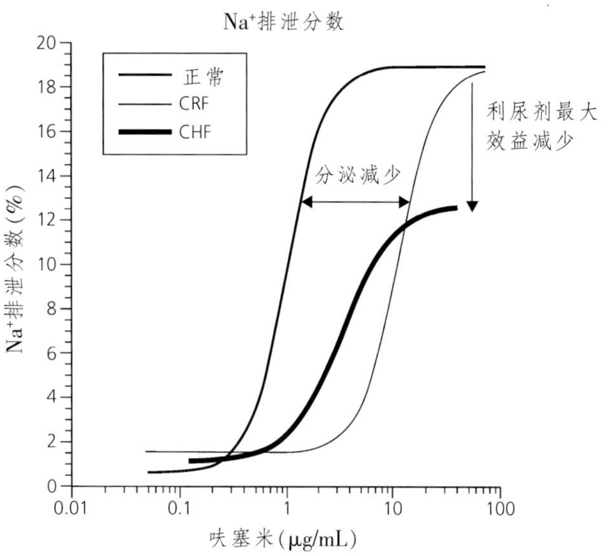

图 44.4 袢利尿剂的剂量反应曲线。Na+排泄分数(FENa+)可以评估袢利尿剂浓缩功能。与健康对照组相比，由于慢性肾衰竭(CRF)患者利尿剂排泄受到影响，使剂量反应曲线右移，当表示为 FENa+时，利尿剂最大效益会得到保留，但绝对 Na+排泄则会减少。慢性心力衰竭(CHF)患者的剂量反应曲线向右下移位，即使在用 FENa+表示时仍是这种情况，即利尿剂抵抗明显。(Reproduced from Ellison[210], with permission from S. Karger AG, Basel.)

滤过或血液透析，而非静脉-静脉超滤。在无法建立静脉通路、高凝状态或存在休克或低血压需要血管活性药物等情况下，也应该避免使用超滤治疗[183]。

血管活性药物治疗

目前尚没有关于血管活性药物治疗心肾综合征效果的证据。常用的血管活性药物包括硝酸甘油、硝普钠、奈西立肽和多巴酚丁胺，虽然这些药物可以改善心输出量，但在改善肾功能的作用上效果不一[224-227]。许多药物可以通过扩张动静脉来减轻心脏的前后负荷[228]。血管扩张剂通过增加肾血流，降低肾静脉压，可以改善肾功能。然而，根据某种药物对肾血管(入球和出球小动脉)的相对效应和血流动力学的影响，其最终对肾血流和GFR的净效应很难预测。血管扩张剂引起低血压的副作用可以抵消其对静脉压和心输出量的有效作用[229]。急性心力衰竭和肾功能障碍患者，与对照剂相比，小剂量奈西立肽[0.005μg/(kg·min)]联合利尿剂治疗不能加强其减轻充血或改善肾功能的作用[230]。虽然未证明肺动脉导管的常规使用可以改善预后，但它适用于使用临床评估无法确定应用血管活性药物患者的血容量状态和心脏充盈压[209]。

由于临床研究结果并不统一，因此，小剂量多巴胺对心力衰竭和心肾综合征患者肾功能恶化的预防作用尚不确定[231-233]。一项研究显示，小剂量多巴胺[5μg/(kg·min)]和小剂量呋塞米(5mg/h)联合使用的效果与大剂量呋塞米(20mg/h)静脉注射在缓解充血方面效果相当，可以减少肾功能障碍的发生，并维持钾离子平衡[234]。然而，一项对急性心力衰竭和肾功能障碍患者的研究显示，与对照剂相比，小剂量多巴胺[2μg/(kg·min)]不能加强其减轻充血或改善肾功能的作用[230]。我们需要并且正在进行更具权威性的研究。

急性心力衰竭患者静脉使用正性肌力药可以通过增加心输出量和降低心脏充盈压，从而改善临床症状和肾功能。但一系列临床研究却增加了对正性肌力药增加死亡率的担忧[27,235]。虽然米力农可以轻度改善肾功能，但这不等于其可以降低死亡率或再入住率[236]。因此，并不推荐在慢性心力衰竭患者中常规使用正性肌力药。在合并肾功能障碍的心脏移植候选者中，静脉使用正性肌力药可以稳定血流动力学状态，并帮助这部分患者过度至机械支持或移植。

移植和机械支持

对进展性心力衰竭和可逆性肾脏疾病患者，可以考虑心肾联合移植。根据来自器官共享联合网络(UNOS)的数据，在1995—2005年间，美国有1.4%(n=264)的心脏移植受者同时接受了肾脏移植[237]。虽然目前尚没有社会统一认可的指南对心肾联合移植受者做出说明，但肾小球滤过率估计值(eGFR)<33mL/min且预计无肾功能恢复可能的患者是此项治疗的合适候选人，与单独心脏移植相比预后更佳[237]。心肾移植受者的预期生存率与单独心脏移植受者相似[238]。但透析依赖患者如单独接受心脏移植则预后不佳。因此，终末期肾病被认为是心脏移植的禁忌证，除非同时考虑肾脏移植[238]。

进展性心力衰竭合并心肾综合征患者，机械循环支持通常可以改善肾功能[239,240]。但其他报道显示置入LVAD后肾功能的改善多数是暂时性的[241]。但对于即使改善了血流动力学也无法恢复肾功能的患者，则不建议置入LVAD，除非考虑进行心肾联合移植。

终末期心力衰竭患者的肝脏

“心肝”综合征由两种临床综合征组成。第一，缺血性肝炎或“休克肝”，与急性心力衰竭和心源性休克相关。第二，充血性肝病，与慢性心力衰竭的关系更加密切。但这两种综合征在临床上有很多重叠之处。且不同患者间有很大差异，例如，很多轻度心力衰竭患者即可出现肝功能检测(LFT)异常，而另一些重度心力衰竭患者并未发现肝功能障碍证据[242]，说明这种异质性并不确切。心力衰竭并发肝功能异常的患者，仍需要完善相关检查以除外原发性肝脏疾病可能，例如，感染性、自身免疫性以及胆源性肝病等。

缺血性肝炎

缺血性肝炎或“休克肝”的特点为血清转氨酶可逆性升高，至少大于正常值上限20倍，并需要除外其他原因[243,244]。缺血性肝炎最常见原因为心源性—急性心肌梗死所致心源性休克、慢性心力衰竭急性加重、心律失常及心脏压塞等[243]。低血容量所致缺血性肝炎相对少见。约有20%的心源性休克患者会出现急性缺血性肝炎[245]。

病理生理学

缺血性肝炎的病理生理学机制尚不明确。肝脏为双重血供器官。肝脏的血供 80%来自门静脉,20%来自肝动脉[244,246]。低血压时,代偿性神经内分泌和交感神经系统激活使心输出量重新分配,主要供应心脏和脑[244]。内脏血管收缩会减少门静脉血流;但肝脏可以通过增加氧摄取率来维持正常摄氧量[246]。这种代偿机制可以在一定程度上帮助肝脏抵抗缺血性损伤,也因此在其他类型休克时很少出现肝损伤[247,248]。此外,如既往未曾发生肝损伤,则缺血性损伤通常呈自限性和可逆性[246]。由于小叶中心区域对缺氧最为敏感[244],因此缺血性肝炎患者常伴小叶中心坏死[243,249]。最常见机制是由低血压和心输出量降低引起肝细胞缺氧导致肝脏低灌注[243],肝静脉瘀血也起到重要作用[243]。心输出量降低伴中心静脉升高的患者比单独低心输出量的患者更容易出现缺血性肝炎[245],而创伤引起的严重休克患者很少出现 LFT 异常[243]。因此认为被动充血使肝细胞更容易受到缺氧性损伤,因为中心静脉淤血会引起门脉高压,改变肝脏血流[243]。低血压可能会使已经异常的肝血流更加恶化。另一方面,如果肝细胞长期暴露于高血压则更易受到损伤。此外,慢性心力衰竭患者由于存在潜在的低灌注和低氧血症,肝细胞更容易受到慢性反复的损伤[243]。因此,缺血性肝炎患者的前向和后向血流可能都存在异常[242]。

治疗

支持治疗的目标为改善肝脏灌注和缓解肝脏充血。这些治疗如前所述,包括药物治疗(血管加压药、正性肌力药、血管扩张剂、利尿剂)和机械支持(IABP、心室辅助装置、超滤)。

慢性充血性肝病

充血性肝病的特点包括心力衰竭、FT 异常,并除外其他引起 LFT 异常的原因[250]。右心衰竭、限制性心肌病或缩窄性心包炎引起的充血都可以导致充血性肝病。LFT 患者常合并右心衰竭[249],右心衰竭患者体格检查常常出现肝大[251]。右心衰竭引起的 LFT 异常表现为胆汁淤积性而非肝源性[250,252]。坎地沙坦降低心力衰竭死亡率和发病率的评价研究(CHARM)的 2679 例患者中,13%总胆红素升高,14%碱性磷酸酶升高,18%血清白蛋白降低[252]。4%的患者直接胆红素,3%的患者谷丙转氨酶升高和 4%的患者谷草转氨酶升高[250,251]。容量负荷过重的患者的总胆红素相对更高[252]。三尖瓣反流的严重程度也与 LFT 异常相关,中重度三尖瓣反流患者的胆汁淤积性 LFT 明显增加[250]。总胆红素是心力衰竭患者死亡的强预测指标[204,252]。即使术前胆红素已升高,总胆红素仍是 LVAD 置入术后死亡率的预测指标[253,254]。

病理生理学

肝静脉后充血及三尖瓣关闭不全引起的搏动性损伤,可能会导致慢性心力衰竭患者的肝损伤[250]和肝细胞功能异常,并引起直接和间接胆红素升高[255]。组织病理学观察显示肝小叶中央区充血和淤血,也称为"槟榔肝"[250,255]。接下来可能会出现充血性肝纤维化,从胶原蛋白的轻度沉积到重度纤维化[246],这是静脉压增加、低氧血症和(或)肝细胞坏死共同作用的结果[256]。充血性肝纤维化可以进展为肝硬化。有趣的是,心源性肝硬化患者的肝合成功能可以被保留,而 LFT 无任何异常。心源性肝硬化的诊断标准为右心衰竭伴肝大和利尿剂无效的难治性腹水[246]。心源性肝硬化患者的腹水蛋白含量通常较高(>0.5g/dL),血清-腹水蛋白梯度>1g/dL,与门脉高压的异常表现相似[246,257]。

治疗

充血性肝病的治疗与慢性心力衰竭相似。血管扩张剂、利尿剂及限盐治疗可以用来缓解充血。难治性腹水可以采用穿刺术;然而,由于心源性肝硬化患者的合成功能正常,因此不需要补充白蛋白[246]。

正在进行心脏移植评估的患者,如果存在腹水则需进行肝脏影响血检查,例如,超声或 CT 检查,如果提示存在肝硬化,则还需完善肝穿刺活检。如果存在肝硬化,对于合适的患者则需考虑心脏-肝脏联合移植。存在肝硬化的患者不建议进行单独的心脏移植。由于心脏-肝脏联合移植并非常规手术,目前尚没有统一的公认指南,在 2005—2010 年间 ISHLT 注册的只有 51 项报道[53]。心脏-肝脏联合移植的 1 年和 3 年生存率分别为 80%和 70%,与单独心脏移植结果相似[258]。由于肝硬化不适合进行心脏移植的患者可以考虑机械支持治疗;置入 LVAD 常可改善肝功能的异常[239]。然而,LFT 升高与置入 LVAD 后右心支持需求增加相关[254]。

总结

心力衰竭在移植的很多方面都起着重要作用，既是心脏移植的直接原因又是合并疾病的结果。心力衰竭患者可以出现心脏以外的其他器官系统的不良表现，心力衰竭也是肝脏、肺脏和肾脏系统衰竭终末期的鉴别诊断之一。同样的，心脏循环支持和重症监护治疗仍是所有移植医生需要了解的重要知识。很多的心血管活性药物可以用来支持衰竭的心脏，此外，IABP到人工心脏支持治疗都可以帮助心力衰竭患者过渡。由于心力衰竭普遍存在，且治疗复杂，使得心脏病学和心胸外科手术成为甚至非心脏移植手术的重要部分。

（肖增丽 译 朱凤雪 校）

参考文献

1. Binanay C, Califf RM, Hasselblad V, et al. Evaluation study of congestive heart failure and pulmonary artery catheterization effectiveness: the ESCAPE trial. JAMA. 2005;294:1625-1633.
2. Shah MR, Hasselblad V, Stevenson LW, et al. Impact of the pulmonary artery catheter in critically ill patients: meta-analysis of randomized clinical trials. JAMA. 2005;294:1664-1670.
3. Harvey S, Harrison DA, Singer M, et al. Assessment of the clinical effectiveness of pulmonary artery catheters in management of patients in intensive care (PAC-Man): a randomised controlled trial. Lancet. 2005;366:472-477.
4. Nohria A, Lewis E, Stevenson LW. Medical management of advanced heart failure. JAMA. 2002;287:628-640.
5. Nieminen MS, Bohm M, Cowie MR, et al. Executive summary of the guidelines on the diagnosis and treatment of acute heart failure. The Task Force on Acute Heart Failure of the European Society of Cardiology. European Heart Journal. 2005;26:384-416.
6. Hunt SA, Abraham WT, Chin MH, et al. 2009 focused update incorporated into the ACC/AHA 2005 guidelines for the diagnosis and management of heart failure in adults. Circulation. 2009;119:e391-e479.
7. Stevenson LW. Are hemodynamic goals viable in tailoring heart failure therapy? Hemodynamic goals are relevant. Circulation. 2006;113:1020-1033.
8. Silver PJ, Harris AL, Canniff PC, et al. Phosphodiesterase isozyme inhibition, activation of the cAMP system, and positive inotropy mediated by milrinone in isolated guinea pig cardiac muscle. Journal of Cardiovascular Pharmacology. 1989;13:530-540.
9. Gillies M, Bellomo R, Doolan L, et al. Bench-to-bedside review: inotropic drug therapy after adult cardiac surgery: a systematic literature review. Critical Care. 2005;9:266-279.
10. Lowes BD, Simon MA, Tsvetkova TO, et al. Inotropes in the beta-blocker era. Clinical Cardiology. 2000;23:1-6.
11. Feldman MD, Copelas L, Gwathmey JK, et al. Deficient production of cyclic AMP: pharmacologic evidence of an important cause of contractile dysfunction in patients with end-stage heart failure. Circulation. 1987;75:331-339.
12. Sonnenblick EH, Frishman WH, LeJemtel TH. Dobutamine: a new synthetic cardioactive sympathetic amine. New England Journal of Medicine. 1979;300:17-22.
13. Ruffolo RR Jr. The pharmacology of dobutamine. American Journal of the Medical Sciences. 1987;294:244-248.
14. Movsesian M, Stehlik J, Vandeput F, et al. Phosphodiesterase inhibition in heart failure. Heart Failure Reviews. 2009;14:255-263.
15. Monrad ES, McKay RG, Baim DS, et al. Improvement in indexes of diastolic performance in patients with congestive heart failure treated with milrinone. Circulation. 1984;70:1030-1037.
16. Jaski BE, Fifer MA, Wright RF, et al. Positive inotropic and vasodilator actions of milrinone in patients with severe congestive heart failure. Dose-response relationships and comparison to nitroprusside. Journal of Clinical Investigation. 1985;75:643-649.
17. Anderson JL. Hemodynamic and clinical benefits with intravenous milrinone in severe chronic heart failure: results of a multicenter study in the United States. American Heart Journal. 1991;121:1956-1964.
18. Colucci WS, Wright RF, Jaski BE, et al. Milrinone and dobutamine in severe heart failure: differing hemodynamic effects and individual patient responsiveness. Circulation. 1986;73:175-183.
19. Monrad ES, Baim DS, Smith HS, et al. Milrinone, dobutamine, and nitroprusside: comparative effects on hemodynamics and myocardial energetics in patients with severe congestive heart failure. Circulation. 1986;73:168-174.
20. Aranda JM Jr, Schofield RS, Pauly DF, et al. Comparison of dobutamine versus milrinone therapy in hospitalized patients awaiting cardiac transplantation: a prospective, randomized trial. American Heart Journal. 2003;145:324-329.
21. Unverferth DV, Blanford M, Kates RE, et al. Tolerance to dobutamine after a 72 hour continuous infusion. American Journal of Medicine. 1980;69:262.
22. Hershberger RE, Nauman D, Walker TL, et al. Care processes and clinical outcomes of continuous outpatient support with inotropes (COSI) in patients with refractory endstage heart failure. Journal of Cardiac Failure. 2003;9:180-187.
23. Felker GM, Benza RL, Chandler AB, et al. Heart failure etiology and response to milrinone in decompensated heart failure: results from the OPTIME-CHF study. Journal of the American College of Cardiology. 2003;41:997-1003.
24. O'Connor CM, Gattis WA, Uretsky BF, et al. Continuous intravenous dobutamine is associated with an increased risk of death in patients with advanced heart failure: insights from the Flolan International Randomized Survival Trial (FIRST). American Heart Journal. 2000;138:78-86.
25. Ewy GA. Inotropic infusions for chronic congestive heart failure: medical miracles or misguided medicinals? Journal of the American College of Cardiology. 1999;33:572-575.
26. Dies F, Krell MJ, Whitlow P, et al. Intermittent dobutamine in ambulatory outpatients with chronic heart failure. Circulation. 1986;74:38.
27. Abraham WT, Adams KF, Fonarow GC, et al. In-hospital mortality in patients with acute decompensated heart failure requiring intravenous vasoactive medications. Journal of the American College of Cardiology. 2005;46:57-64.
28. Sorsa T, Pollesello P, Rosevear PR, et al. Stereoselective binding of levosimendan to cardiac troponin C causes Ca^{2+}-sensitization. European Journal of Pharmacology. 2004;486:1-8.
29. Kopustinskiene D, Pollesello P, Saris NE. Effect of levosimendan on cardiac mitochondrial ATP-dependent potassium channel. Biochemical Pharmacology. 2004;68:807-812.
30. De Luca L, Colucci WS, Nieminen MS, et al. Evidence-based use of levosimendan in different clinical settings. European Heart Journal. 2006;27:1908-1920.
31. Mebazaa A, Nieminen MS, Packer M, et al. Levosimendan vs dobutamine for patients with acute decompensated heart failure: the SURVIVE randomized trial. JAMA. 2007;297:1883-1891.
32. Murphy MB, Elliott WJ. Dopamine and dopamine receptor agonists in cardiovascular therapy. Critical Care Medicine. 1990;18:514-518.
33. Lollgen H, Drexler H. Use of inotropes in the critical care setting. Critical Care Medicine. 1990;18:S56-S60.
34. Stinson EB, Caves PK, Griepp RB, et al. Hemodynamic observations in the early period after human heart transplantation. Journal of Thoracic and Cardiovascular Surgery. 1975;69:264-270.
35. Holmes CL, Patel BM, Russell JA, et al. Physiology of vasopressin relevant to management of septic shock. Chest. 2001;120:989-1002.
36. Mullens W, Abrahams Z, Francis GS, et al. Sodium nitroprusside for advanced low-output heart failure. Journal of the American College of Cardiology. 2008;52:200-207.
37. Stevenson LW, Bellil D, Grover-McKay M, et al. Effects of afterload reduction (diuretics and vasodilators) on left ventricular volume and mitral regurgitation in severe congestive heart failure secondary to ischemic or idiopathic dilated cardiomyopathy. American Journal of Cardiology. 1987;60:654-658.
38. Tinker JH, Michenfelder JD. Sodium nitroprusside: pharmacology, toxicology and therapeutics. Anesthesiology. 1976;45:340-354.
39. Nessim SJ, Richardson RMA. Dialysis for thiocyanate intoxication: a case report and review of the literature. American Society for Artificial Internal Organs Journal. 2006;52:479-481.
40. Elkayam U, Kulick D, McIntosh N, et al. Incidence of early tolerance to hemodynamic effects of continuous infusion of nitroglycerin in patients with coronary artery disease and heart failure. Circulation. 1987;76:577-584.
41. Elkayam U. Tolerance to organic nitrates: evidence, mechanisms, clinical relevance, and strategies for prevention. Annals of Internal Medicine. 1991;114:667-677.
42. O'Connor CM, Starling RC, Hernandez PW, et al. Effect of nesiritide in patients with acute decompensated heart failure. New England Journal of Medicine.

2011;365:32–43.
43. Colucci WS, Elkayam U, Horton DP, et al. Intravenous nesiritide, a natriuretic peptide, in the treatment of decompensated congestive heart failure. Nesiritide study group. New England Journal of Medicine. 2000;343:246–253.
44. VMAC Investigators. Intravenous nesiritide vs nitroglycerin for treatment of decompensated congestive heart failure: a randomized controlled trial. JAMA. 2002;287:1531–1540.
45. Hill JA, Hsu K, Pauly DF, et al. Sustained use of nesiritide to aid in bridging to heart transplant. Clinical Cardiology. 2003;26:211–214.
46. Packer M, Carver JR, Rodeheffer RJ, et al. Effect of oral milrinone on mortality in severe chronic heart failure. New England Journal of Medicine. 1991;325: 1468–1475.
47. Felker GM, O'Connor CM. Inotropic therapy for heart failure: an evidence-based approach. American Heart Journal. 2001;142:393–401.
48. Stevenson LW. Clinical use of inotropic therapy for heart failure: looking backward or forward? Part II: chronic inotropic therapy. Circulation. 2003;108: 492–497.
49. Goldhaber JI, Hamilton MA. Role of inotropic agents in the treatment of heart failure. Circulation. 2010;121:1655–1660.
50. Hunt SA, et al. ACC/AHA 2005 guideline update for the diagnosis and management of chronic heart failure in the adult-summary article: a report of the American College of Cardiology/American Heart Association task force on practice guidelines. Circulation. 2005;112:1825–1852.
51. De Backer D, Biston P, Devriendt J, et al. Comparison of dopamine and norepinephrine in the treatment of shock. New England Journal of Medicine. 2010;362:779–789.
52. Mehra MR, Ventura HO, Kappor C, et al. Safety and clinical utility of long-term intravenous milrinone in advanced heart failure. American Journal of Cardiology. 1997;80:61–64.
53. Stehlik J, Edwards LB, Kucheryavaya AY, et al. The Registry of the International Society for Heart and Lung Transplantation: twenty-eighth adult heart transplant report—2011. Journal of Heart and Lung Transplantation. 2011;30:1078–1094.
54. Upadya S, Lee FA, Saldarriaga C, et al. Home continuous positive inotropic infusion as a bridge to cardiac transplantation in patients with end-stage heart failure. Journal of Heart and Lung Transplantation. 2004;23:466–472.
55. Brozena SC, Twomey C, Goldberg LR, et al. A prospective study of continuous intravenous milrinone therapy for status IB patients awaiting heart transplant at home. Journal of Heart and Lung Transplantation. 2004;23:1082–1086.
56. Gronda E, Bourge RC, Costanzo MR, et al. Heart rhythm considerations in heart transplant candidates and considerations for ventricular assist devices: International Society for Heart and Lung Transplantation guidelines for the care of cardiac transplant candidates—2006. Journal of Heart and Lung Transplantation. 2006;25:1043–1056.
57. Johnson MR, Meyer KH, Haft J, et al. Heart transplantation in the United States, 1999–2008. American Journal of Transplantation. 2010;10:1035–1046.
58. Organ Procurement and Transplantation Network. Policy 3.7. Organ distribution: allocation of thoracic organs. 2011 [cited 2011 November 23, 2011]; Available from: http://optn.transplant.hrsa.gov/policiesAndBylaws/policies.asp.
59. Moulopoulos SD, Topaz S, Kolff WJ. Diastolic balloon pumping (with carbon dioxide) in the aorta—a mechanical assistance to the failing circulation. American Heart Journal. 1962;63:669–675.
60. Kantrowitz A, Tjonneland S, Freed PS, et al. Initial clinical experience with intraaortic balloon pumping in cardiogenic shock. JAMA. 1968;203:113–118.
61. Santa-Cruz RA, Cohen MG, Ohman EM. Aortic counterpulsation: a review of the hemodynamic effects and indications for use. Catheterization and Cardiovascular Interventions. 2006;67:68–77.
62. Ferguson JJ 3rd, Cohen M, Freedman RJ Jr, et al. The current practice of intraaortic balloon counterpulsation: results from the Benchmark Registry. Journal of the American College of Cardiology. 2001;38:1456–1462.
63. Buckley MJ, Leinbach RC, Kaston JA, et al. Hemodynamic evaluation in intraaortic balloon pumping in man. Circulation. 1970;45(Suppl 2):130–134.
64. Rose EA, Marrin CAS, Bregman D, et al. Left ventricular mechanics of counterpulsation and left heart bypass, individually and in combination. Journal of Thoracic and Cardiovascular Surgery. 1979;77:127–137.
65. Scheidt S, Wilner G, Mueller H, et al. Intraaortic balloon counterpulsation in cardiogenic shock. New England Journal of Medicine. 1973;288:979–984.
66. Gjesdal O, Gude E, Arora S, et al. Intra-aortic balloon counterpulsation as a bridge to heart transplantation does not impair long-term survival. European Journal of Heart Failure. 2009;11:709–714.
67. Sjauw KD, Engstrom AE, Vis MM, et al. A systematic review and meta-analysis of intra-aortic balloon pump therapy in ST-elevation myocardial infarction: should we change the guidelines? European Heart Journal. 2008;30:459–468.
68. Chen EW, Canto JG, Parsons LS, et al. Relation between hospital intra-aortic balloon counterpulsation volume and mortality in acute myocardial infarction complicated by cardiogenic shock. Circulation. 2003;108:951–957.
69. Thiele H, Zeymer U, Neumann FJ, et al. Intraaortic balloon support for myocardial infarction with cardiogenic shock. New England Journal of Medicine. 2012;367: 1287–1296.
70. O'Gara PT, Kushner FG, Ascheim DD, et al. 2013 ACCF/AHA guideline for the management of ST-elevation myocardial infarction: a report of the American College of Cardiology Foundation/American Heart Association Task Force on Practice Guidelines. Journal of the American College of Cardiology. 2013;61: e78–140.
71. Naka Y, Chen JM, Rose EA. Assisted circulation in the treatment of heart failure. In: Zipes DP, Libby P, Bonow RO, et al., editors. Braunwald's Heart Disease. Philadelphia: Elsevier Saunders; 2005: 625.
72. Pi K, Block PC, Warner MG, et al. Major determinants of survival and nonsurvival of intraaortic balloon pumping. American Heart Journal. 1995;130: 849–853.
73. Cochran RP, Starkey TD, Panos AL, et al. Ambulatory intraaortic balloon pump use as bridge to heart transplant. Annals of Thoracic Surgery. 2002;74:746–752.
74. Pinsky MR. The hemodynamic consequences of mechanical ventilation: an evolving story. Intensive Care Medicine. 1997;23:493–503.
75. Steingrub JS, Tidswell M, Higgins TL. Hemodynamic consequences of heart-lung interactions. Journal of Intensive Care Medicine. 2003;18:92–99.
76. Wise RA, Robotham JL, Summer WR. Effects of spontaneous ventilation on the circulation. Lung. 1981;159:175–186.
77. Monnet X, Teboul JL, Richard C. Cardiopulmonary interactions in patients with heart failure. Current Opinion in Critical Care. 2007;13:6–11.
78. Lenique F, Habis M, Lofaso F, et al. Ventilatory and hemodynamic effects of continuous positive airway pressure in left heart failure. American Journal of Respiratory and Critical Care Medicine. 1997;155:500–505.
79. Bouferrache K, Vieillard-Baron A. Acute respiratory distress syndrome, mechanical ventilation, and right ventricular function. Current Opinion in Critical Care. 2011;17:30–35.
80. Fougeres E, Teboul JL, Richard C, et al. Hemodynamic impact of a positive end-expiratory pressure setting in acute respiratory distress syndrome: importance of the volume status. Critical Care Medicine. 2010;38:802–807.
81. Masip J, Betbese AJ, Paez J, et al. Non-invasive pressure support ventilation versus conventional oxygen therapy in acute cardiogenic pulmonary oedema: a randomised trial. Lancet. 2000;356:2126–2132.
82. Masip J, Roque M, Sanchez B, et al. Noninvasive ventilation in acute cardiogenic pulmonary edema: systematic review and meta-analysis. JAMA. 2005;294: 3124–3130.
83. Winck JC, Azevedo LF, Costa-Pereira A, et al. Efficacy and safety of non-invasive ventilation in the treatment of acute cardiogenic pulmonary edema- a systematic review and meta-analysis. Critical Care. 2006;10:69.
84. Weng CL, Zhao YT, Liu QH, et al. Meta-analysis: noninvasive ventilation in acute cardiogenic pulmonary edema. Annals of Internal Medicine. 2010;152:590–600.
85. Gray A, Goodacre S, Newby DE, et al. Noninvasive ventilation in acute cardiogenic pulmonary edema. New England Journal of Medicine. 2008;359:142–151.
86. Guazzi M, Arena R. Pulmonary hypertension with left-sided heart disease. Nature Reviews. Cardiology. 2010;7:648–659.
87. Hoeper MM, Barbera JA, Channick RN, et al. Diagnosis, assessment, and treatment of non-pulmonary arterial hypertension pulmonary hypertension. Journal of the American College of Cardiology. 2009;54:S85–S96.
88. Ghio S, Gavazzi A, Campana C, et al. Independent and additive prognostic value of right ventricular systolic function and pulmonary artery pressure in patients with chronic heart failure. Journal of the American College of Cardiology. 2001;37:183–188.
89. Grigioni F, Potena L, Galie N, et al. Prognostic implications of serial assessments of pulmonary hypertension in severe chronic heart failure. Journal of Heart and Lung Transplantation. 2006;25:1241–1246.
90. Abramson SV, Burke JF, Kelly JJ Jr, et al. Pulmonary hypertension predicts mortality and morbidity in patients with dilated cardiomyopathy. Annals of Internal Medicine. 1992;116:888–895.
91. Chang PP, Longenecker JC, Wang NY, et al. Mild vs severe pulmonary hypertension before heart transplantation: different effects on posttransplantation pulmonary hypertension and mortality. Journal of Heart and Lung Transplantation. 2005;24:998–1007.
92. Costard-Jackle A, Fowler MB. Influence of preoperative pulmonary artery pressure on mortality after heart transplantation: testing of potential reversibility of pulmonary hypertension with nitroprusside is useful in defining a high risk group. Journal of the American College of Cardiology. 1992; 19:48–54.
93. Butler J, Stankewicz MA, Wu J, et al. Pre-transplant reversible pulmonary hypertension predicts higher risk for mortality after cardiac transplantation. Journal of Heart and Lung Transplantation. 2005;24:170–177.

94. Moraes DL, Colucci WS, Givertz MM. Secondary pulmonary hypertension in chronic heart failure: the role of the endothelium in pathophysiology and management. Circulation. 2000;102:1718–1723.
95. Lam CS, Roger VL, Rodeheffer RJ, et al. Pulmonary hypertension in heart failure with preserved ejection fraction: a community-based study. Journal of the American College of Cardiology. 2009;53:1119–1126.
96. Enriquez-Sarano M, Rossi A, Seward JB, et al. Determinants of pulmonary hypertension in left ventricular dysfunction. Journal of the American College of Cardiology. 1997;29:153–159.
97. Rich S, Rabinovitch M. Diagnosis and treatment of secondary (non-category 1) pulmonary hypertension. Circulation. 2008;118:2190–2199.
98. Drazner MH, Hamilton MA, Fonarow G, et al. Relationship between right and left-sided filling pressures in 1000 patients with advanced heart failure. Journal of Heart and Lung Transplantation. 1999;18:1126–1132.
99. Kumar P, Francis GS, Tang WH. Phosphodiesterase 5 inhibition in heart failure: mechanisms and clinical implications. Nature Reviews. Cardiology. 2009;6:349–355.
100. Delgado JF, Conde E, Sanchez V, et al. Pulmonary vascular remodeling in pulmonary hypertension due to chronic heart failure. European Journal of Heart Failure. 2005;7:1011–1016.
101. Huang W, Kingsbury MP, Turner MA, et al. Capillary filtration is reduced in lungs adapted to chronic heart failure: morphological and haemodynamic correlates. Cardiovascular Research. 2001;49:207–217.
102. Kingsbury MP, Huang W, Donnelly JL, et al. Structural remodelling of lungs in chronic heart failure. Basic Research in Cardiology. 2003;98:295–303.
103. Salzberg SP, Lachat ML, von Harbou K, et al. Normalization of high pulmonary vascular resistance with LVAD support in heart transplantation candidates. European Journal of Cardio-Thoracic Surgery. 2005;27:222–225.
104. Tedford RJ, Hemnes AR, Russell SD, et al. PDE5A inhibitor treatment of persistent pulmonary hypertension after mechanical circulatory support. Circulation. Heart Failure. 2008;1:213–219.
105. Aronson D, Eitan A, Dragu R, et al. Relationship between reactive pulmonary hypertension and mortality in patients with acute decompensated heart failure. Circulation. Heart Failure. 2011;4:644–650.
106. Bangalore S, Yao SS, Chaudhry FA. Role of right ventricular wall motion abnormalities in risk stratification and prognosis of patients referred for stress echocardiography. Journal of the American College of Cardiology. 2007;50:1981–1989.
107. de Groote P, Millaire A, Foucher-Hossein C, et al. Right ventricular ejection fraction is an independent predictor of survival in patients with moderate heart failure. Journal of the American College of Cardiology. 1998;32:948–954.
108. Meyer P, Filippatos GS, Ahmed MI, et al. Effects of right ventricular ejection fraction on outcomes in chronic systolic heart failure. Circulation. 2010;121:252–258.
109. Sheehan F, Redington A. The right ventricle: anatomy, physiology and clinical imaging. Heart. 2008;94:1510–1515.
110. Sibbald WJ, Driedger AA. Right ventricular function in acute disease states: pathophysiologic considerations. Critical Care Medicine. 1983;11:339–345.
111. Bossone E, Bodini BD, Mazza A, et al. Pulmonary arterial hypertension: the key role of echocardiography. Chest. 2005;127:1836–1843.
112. Taylor RR, Covell JW, Sonnenblick EH, et al. Dependence of ventricular distensibility on filling of the opposite ventricle. American Journal of Physiology. 1967;213:711–718.
113. Greyson CR. Pathophysiology of right ventricular failure. Critical Care Medicine. 2008;36:S57–S65.
114. Louie EK, Rich S, Brundage BH. Doppler echocardiographic assessment of impaired left ventricular filling in patients with right ventricular pressure overload due to primary pulmonary hypertension. Journal of the American College of Cardiology. 1986;8:1298–1306.
115. Price LC, Wort SJ, Finney SJ, et al. Pulmonary vascular and right ventricular dysfunction in adult critical care: current and emerging options for management: a systematic literature review. Critical Care. 2010;14:R169.
116. Galie N, Hoeper MM, Humbert M, et al. Guidelines for the diagnosis and treatment of pulmonary hypertension: the Task Force for the Diagnosis and Treatment of Pulmonary Hypertension of the European Society of Cardiology (ESC) and the European Respiratory Society (ERS), endorsed by the International Society of Heart and Lung Transplantation (ISHLT). European Heart Journal. 2009;30:2493–2537.
117. Paulus WJ, Tschope C, Sanderson JE, et al. How to diagnose diastolic heart failure: a consensus statement on the diagnosis of heart failure with normal left ventricular ejection fraction by the Heart Failure and Echocardiography Associations of the European Society of Cardiology. European Heart Journal. 2007;28:2539–2550.
118. Mehra MR, Kobashigawa J, Starling R, et al. Listing criteria for heart transplantation: International Society for Heart and Lung Transplantation guidelines for the care of cardiac transplant candidates–2006. Journal of Heart and Lung Transplantation. 2006;25:1024–1042.
119. Loh E, Stamler JS, Hare JM, et al. Cardiovascular effects of inhaled nitric oxide in patients with left ventricular dysfunction. Circulation. 1994;90:2780–2785.
120. Fojon S, Fernandez-Gonzalez C, Sanchez-Andrade J, et al. Inhaled nitric oxide through a noninvasive ventilation device to assess reversibility of pulmonary hypertension in selecting recipients for heart transplant. Transplantation Proceedings. 2005;37:4028–4030.
121. Haraldsson A, Kieler-Jensen N, Nathorst-Westfelt U, et al. Comparison of inhaled nitric oxide and inhaled aerosolized prostacyclin in the evaluation of heart transplant candidates with elevated pulmonary vascular resistance. Chest. 1998;114:780–786.
122. Atz AM, Adatia I, Wessel DL. Rebound pulmonary hypertension after inhalation of nitric oxide. Annals of Thoracic Surgery. 1996;62:1759–1764.
123. Califf RM, Adams KF, McKenna WJ, et al. A randomized controlled trial of epoprostenol therapy for severe congestive heart failure: the Flolan International Randomized Survival Trial (FIRST). American Heart Journal. 1997;134:44–54.
124. Kalra PR, Moon JC, Coats AJ. Do results of the ENABLE (Endothelin Antagonist Bosentan for Lowering Cardiac Events in Heart Failure) study spell the end for non-selective endothelin antagonism in heart failure? International Journal of Cardiology. 2002;85:195–197.
125. Bocchi EA, Bacal F, Auler Junior JO, et al. Inhaled nitric oxide leading to pulmonary edema in stable severe heart failure. American Journal of Cardiology. 1994;74:70–72.
126. Palmer SM, Robinson LJ, Wang A, et al. Massive pulmonary edema and death after prostacyclin infusion in a patient with pulmonary veno-occlusive disease. Chest. 1998;113:237–240.
127. Preston IR, Klinger JR, Houtchens J, et al. Pulmonary edema caused by inhaled nitric oxide therapy in two patients with pulmonary hypertension associated with the CREST syndrome. Chest. 2002;121:656–659.
128. Mullens W, Abrahams Z, Francis GS, et al. Sodium nitroprusside for advanced low-output heart failure. Journal of the American College of Cardiology. 2008;52:200–207.
129. Michaels AD, Chatterjee K, De Marco T. Effects of intravenous nesiritide on pulmonary vascular hemodynamics in pulmonary hypertension. Journal of Cardiac Failure. 2005;11:425–431.
130. Alaeddini J, Uber PA, Park MH, et al. Efficacy and safety of sildenafil in the evaluation of pulmonary hypertension in severe heart failure. American Journal of Cardiology. 2004;94:1475–1477.
131. Melenovsky V, Al-Hiti H, Kazdova L, et al. Transpulmonary B-type natriuretic peptide uptake and cyclic guanosine monophosphate release in heart failure and pulmonary hypertension: the effects of sildenafil. Journal of the American College of Cardiology. 2009;54:595–600.
132. Botha P, Parry G, Dark JH, et al. Acute hemodynamic effects of intravenous sildenafil citrate in congestive heart failure: comparison of phosphodiesterase type-3 and -5 inhibition. Journal of Heart and Lung Transplantation. 2009;28:676–682.
133. Guazzi M, Samaja M, Arena R, et al. Long-term use of sildenafil in the therapeutic management of heart failure. Journal of the American College of Cardiology. 2007;50:2136–2144.
134. Lewis GD, Lachmann J, Camuso J, et al. Sildenafil improves exercise hemodynamics and oxygen uptake in patients with systolic heart failure. Circulation. 2007;115:59–66.
135. Lewis GD, Shah R, Shahzad K, et al. Sildenafil improves exercise capacity and quality of life in patients with systolic heart failure and secondary pulmonary hypertension. Circulation. 2007;116:1555–1562.
136. Guazzi M, Vicenzi M, Arena R, et al. PDE5 inhibition with sildenafil improves left ventricular diastolic function, cardiac geometry, and clinical status in patients with stable systolic heart failure: results of a 1-year, prospective, randomized, placebo-controlled study. Circulation. Heart Failure. 2011;4:8–17.
137. Michelakis E, Tymchak W, Lien D, et al. Oral sildenafil is an effective and specific pulmonary vasodilator in patients with pulmonary arterial hypertension: comparison with inhaled nitric oxide. Circulation. 2002;105:2398–2403.
138. Redfield MM, Chen HH, Borlaug BA, et al. Effect of phosphodiesterase-5 inhibition on exercise capacity and clinical status in heart failure with preserved ejection fraction. A randomized clinical trial. JAMA. 2013;309:1268–1277.
139. Guazzi M, Casali M, Berti F, et al. Endothelium-mediated modulation of ergoreflex and improvement in exercise ventilation by acute sildenafil in heart failure patients. Clinical Pharmacology and Therapeutics. 2008;83:336–341.
140. De Santo LS, Mastroianni C, Romano G, et al. Role of sildenafil in acute posttransplant right ventricular dysfunction: successful experience in 13 consecutive patients. Transplantation Proceedings. 2008;40:2015–2018.
141. Gomez-Moreno S, Lage E, Hernandez A, et al. Use of oral sildenafil in patients with irreversible pulmonary hypertension not eligible for heart transplantation.

Transplantation Proceedings. 2005;37:1550–1551.
142. Zakliczynski M, Maruszewski M, Pyka L, et al. Effectiveness and safety of treatment with sildenafil for secondary pulmonary hypertension in heart transplant candidates. Transplantation Proceedings. 2007;39:2856–2858.
143. Banerjee D, Haddad F, Zamanian RT, et al. Right ventricular failure: a novel era of targeted therapy. Current Heart Failure Reports. 2010;7:202–211.
144. Dell'Italia LJ, Starling MR, Blumhardt R, et al. Comparative effects of volume loading, dobutamine, and nitroprusside in patients with predominant right ventricular infarction. Circulation. 1985;72:1327–1335.
145. Gayat E, Mebazaa A. Pulmonary hypertension in critical care. Current Opinion in Critical Care. 2011;17:439–448.
146. Slaughter MS, Rogers JG, Milano CA, et al. Advanced heart failure treated with continuous-flow left ventricular assist device. New England Journal of Medicine. 2009;361:2241–2251.
147. Gregoric ID, Chandra D, Myers TJ, et al. Extracorporeal membrane oxygenation as a bridge to emergency heart-lung transplantation in a patient with idiopathic pulmonary arterial hypertension. Journal of Heart and Lung Transplantation. 2008;27:466–468.
148. Arafa OE, Geiran OR, Andersen K, et al. Intraaortic balloon pumping for predominantly right ventricular failure after heart transplantation. Annals of Thoracic Surgery. 2000;70:1587–1593.
149. Vieillard-Baron A, Schmitt JM, Augarde R, et al. Acute cor pulmonale in acute respiratory distress syndrome submitted to protective ventilation: incidence, clinical implications, and prognosis. Critical Care Medicine. 2001;29:1551–1555.
150. Christie JD, Edwards LB, Kucheryavaya AY, et al. The Registry of the International Society for Heart and Lung Transplantation: twenty-eighth adult lung and heart-lung transplant report–2011. Journal of Heart and Lung Transplantation. 2011;30:1104–1122.
151. Ronco C, Haapio M, House AA, et al. Cardiorenal syndrome. Journal of the American College of Cardiology. 2008;52:1527–1539.
152. Hillege HL, Girbes AR, de Kam PJ, et al. Renal function, neurohormonal activation, and survival in patients with chronic heart failure. Circulation. 2000; 102:203–210.
153. Adams KF Jr, Fonarow GC, Emerman CL, et al. Characteristics and outcomes of patients hospitalized for heart failure in the United States: rationale, design, and preliminary observations from the first 100,000 cases in the Acute Decompensated Heart Failure National Registry (ADHERE). American Heart Journal. 2005;149:209–216.
154. Bhatia RS, Tu JV, Lee DS, et al. Outcome of heart failure with preserved ejection fraction in a population-based study. New England Journal of Medicine. 2006;355:260–269.
155. Dries DL, Exner DV, Domanski MJ, et al. The prognostic implications of renal insufficiency in asymptomatic and symptomatic patients with left ventricular systolic dysfunction. Journal of the American College of Cardiology. 2000;35: 681–689.
156. Hillege HL, Nitsch D, Pfeffer MA, et al. Renal function as a predictor of outcome in a broad spectrum of patients with heart failure. Circulation. 2006;113: 671–678.
157. Owan TE, Hodge DO, Herges RM, et al. Secular trends in renal dysfunction and outcomes in hospitalized heart failure patients. Journal of Cardiac Failure. 2006;12:257–262.
158. Shlipak MG, Smith GL, Rathore SS, et al. Renal function, digoxin therapy, and heart failure outcomes: evidence from the digoxin intervention group trial. Journal of the American Society of Nephrology. 2004;15:2195–2203.
159. Yancy CW, Lopatin M, Stevenson LW, et al. Clinical presentation, management, and in-hospital outcomes of patients admitted with acute decompensated heart failure with preserved systolic function: a report from the Acute Decompensated Heart Failure National Registry (ADHERE) Database. Journal of the American College of Cardiology. 2006;47:76–84.
160. Smith GL, Lichtman JH, Bracken MB, et al. Renal impairment and outcomes in heart failure: systematic review and meta-analysis. Journal of the American College of Cardiology. 2006;47:1987–1996.
161. Bock JS, Gottlieb SS. Cardiorenal syndrome: new perspectives. Circulation. 2010;121:2592–2600.
162. Sarraf M, Masoumi A, Schrier RW. Cardiorenal syndrome in acute decompensated heart failure. Clinical Journal of the American Society of Nephrology. 2009;4:2013–2026.
163. Vallon V, Muhlbauer B, Osswald H. Adenosine and kidney function. Physiological Reviews. 2006;86:901–940.
164. Nohria A, Hasselblad V, Stebbins A, et al. Cardiorenal interactions: insights from the ESCAPE trial. Journal of the American College of Cardiology. 2008; 51:1268–1274.
165. Weinfeld MS, Chertow GM, Stevenson LW. Aggravated renal dysfunction during intensive therapy for advanced chronic heart failure. American Heart Journal. 1999;138:285–290.
166. Ljungman S, Laragh JH, Cody RJ. Role of the kidney in congestive heart failure. Relationship of cardiac index to kidney function. Drugs. 1990;39(Suppl 4):10–21, discussion 2–4.
167. Androne AS, Katz SD, Lund L, et al. Hemodilution is common in patients with advanced heart failure. Circulation. 2003;107:226–229.
168. Mullens W, Abrahams Z, Francis GS, et al. Importance of venous congestion for worsening of renal function in advanced decompensated heart failure. Journal of the American College of Cardiology. 2009;53:589–596.
169. Liang KV, Williams AW, Greene EL, et al. Acute decompensated heart failure and the cardiorenal syndrome. Critical Care Medicine. 2008;36:S75–S88.
170. Shamseddin MK, Parfrey PS. Mechanisms of the cardiorenal syndromes. Nature Reviews. Nephrology. 2009;5:641–649.
171. Schrier RW, Abraham WT. Hormones and hemodynamics in heart failure. New England Journal of Medicine. 1999;341:577–585.
172. Schrier RW. Body fluid volume regulation in health and disease: a unifying hypothesis. Annals of Internal Medicine. 1990;113:155–159.
173. Schrier RW, Berl T, Anderson RJ. Osmotic and nonosmotic control of vasopressin release. American Journal of Physiology. 1979;236:F321–F332.
174. Cadnapaphornchai MA, Gurevich AK, Weinberger HD, et al. Pathophysiology of sodium and water retention in heart failure. Cardiology. 2001;96:122–131.
175. Schrier RW. Role of diminished renal function in cardiovascular mortality: marker or pathogenetic factor? Journal of the American College of Cardiology. 2006;47:1–8.
176. Braunwald E, Plauth WH Jr, Morrow AG. A method for the detection and quantification of impaired sodium excretion. Results of an oral sodium tolerance test in normal subjects and in patients with heart disease. Circulation. 1965; 32:223–231.
177. Mokotoff R, Ross G, Leiter L. Renal plasma flow and sodium reabsorption and excretion in congestive heart failure. Journal of Clinical Investigation. 1948;27:1–9.
178. Funaya H, Kitakaze M, Node K, et al. Plasma adenosine levels increase in patients with chronic heart failure. Circulation. 1997;95:1363–1365.
179. Dohadwala MM, Givertz MM. Role of adenosine antagonism in the cardiorenal syndrome. Cardiovascular Therapeutics. 2008;26:276–286.
180. Fonarow GC, Adams KF Jr, Abraham WT, et al. Risk stratification for in-hospital mortality in acutely decompensated heart failure: classification and regression tree analysis. JAMA. 2005;293:572–580.
181. Mullens W, Abrahams Z, Skouri HN, et al. Elevated intra-abdominal pressure in acute decompensated heart failure: a potential contributor to worsening renal function? Journal of the American College of Cardiology. 2008;51: 300–306.
182. Dupont M, Mullens W, Tang WH. Impact of systemic venous congestion in heart failure. Current Heart Failure Reports. 2011;8:233–241.
183. Costanzo MR, Jessup M. Treatment of congestion in heart failure with diuretics and extracorporeal therapies: effects on symptoms, renal function, and prognosis. Heart Failure Reviews. 2012;17(2):313–324.
184. Merrill AJ. Edema and decreased renal blood flow in patients with chronic congestive heart failure: evidence of "Forward Failure" as the primary cause of edema. Journal of Clinical Investigation. 1946;25:389–400.
185. Swan SK. Diuretic strategies in patients with renal failure. Drugs. 1994;48: 380–385.
186. Damman K, van Deursen VM, Navis G, et al. Increased central venous pressure is associated with impaired renal function and mortality in a broad spectrum of patients with cardiovascular disease. Journal of the American College of Cardiology. 2009;53:582–588.
187. Firth JD, Raine AE, Ledingham JG. Raised venous pressure: a direct cause of renal sodium retention in oedema? Lancet. 1988;1:1033–1035.
188. Dilley JR, Corradi A, Arendshorst WJ. Glomerular ultrafiltration dynamics during increased renal venous pressure. American Journal of Physiology. 1983;244:F650–F658.
189. Haddy FJ, Scott J, Fleishman M, et al. Effect of change in renal venous pressure upon renal vascular resistance, urine and lymph flow rates. American Journal of Physiology. 1958;195:97–110.
190. Kostreva DR, Seagard JL, Castaner A, et al. Reflex effects of renal afferents on the heart and kidney. American Journal of Physiology. 1981;241: R286–R292.
191. Testani JM, Khera AV, St John Sutton MG, et al. Effect of right ventricular function and venous congestion on cardiorenal interactions during the treatment of decompensated heart failure. American Journal of Cardiology. 2010;105: 511–516.
192. Schrier RW, Bansal S. Pulmonary hypertension, right ventricular failure, and kidney: different from left ventricular failure? Clinical Journal of the American Society of Nephrology. 2008;3:1232–1237.
193. Colombo PC, Onat D, Sabbah HN. Acute heart failure as "acute endothelitis"–Interaction of fluid overload and endothelial dysfunction. European Journal of

Heart Failure. 2008;10:170–175.
194. Colombo PC, Banchs JE, Celaj S, et al. Endothelial cell activation in patients with decompensated heart failure. Circulation. 2005;111:58–62.
195. Gimbrone MA Jr, Nagel T, Topper JN. Biomechanical activation: an emerging paradigm in endothelial adhesion biology. Journal of Clinical Investigation. 1997;100:S61–S65.
196. Hasdai D, Holmes DR Jr, Garratt KN, et al. Mechanical pressure and stretch release endothelin-1 from human atherosclerotic coronary arteries in vivo. Circulation. 1997;95:357–362.
197. Ganda A, Onat D, Demmer RT, et al. Venous congestion and endothelial cell activation in acute decompensated heart failure. Current Heart Failure Reports. 2010;7:66–74.
198. Harrison DG, Widder J, Grumbach I, et al. Endothelial mechanotransduction, nitric oxide and vascular inflammation. Journal of Internal Medicine. 2006;259:351–363.
199. Wang BW, Chang H, Lin S, et al. Induction of matrix metalloproteinases-14 and -2 by cyclical mechanical stretch is mediated by tumor necrosis factor-alpha in cultured human umbilical vein endothelial cells. Cardiovascular Research. 2003;59:460–469.
200. Marenzi G, Lauri G, Grazi M, et al. Circulatory response to fluid overload removal by extracorporeal ultrafiltration in refractory congestive heart failure. Journal of the American College of Cardiology. 2001;38:963–968.
201. Boyle A, Sobotka PA. Redefining the therapeutic objective in decompensated heart failure: hemoconcentration as a surrogate for plasma refill rate. Journal of Cardiac Failure. 2006;12:247–249.
202. Krum H, Iyngkaran P. Lekawanvijit S. Pharmacologic management of the cardiorenal syndrome in heart failure. Current Heart Failure Reports. 2009;6: 105–111.
203. Sica DA. Pharmacotherapy in congestive heart failure: drug absorption in the management of congestive heart failure: loop diuretics. Congestive Heart Failure. 2003;9:287–292.
204. Batin P, Wickens M, McEntegart D, et al. The importance of abnormalities of liver function tests in predicting mortality in chronic heart failure. European Heart Journal. 1995;16:1613–1618.
205. Kramer BK, Schweda F, Riegger GA. Diuretic treatment and diuretic resistance in heart failure. American Journal of Medicine. 1999;106:90–96.
206. Almeshari K, Ahlstrom NG, Capraro FE, et al. A volume-independent component to postdiuretic sodium retention in humans. Journal of the American Society of Nephrology. 1993;3:1878–1883.
207. Cipolla CM, Grazi S, Rimondini A, et al. Changes in circulating norepinephrine with hemofiltration in advanced congestive heart failure. American Journal of Cardiology. 1990;66:987–994.
208. Mullens W, Abrahams Z, Francis GS, et al. Prompt reduction in intra-abdominal pressure following large-volume mechanical fluid removal improves renal insufficiency in refractory decompensated heart failure. Journal of Cardiac Failure. 2008;14:508–514.
209. Jessup M, Abraham WT, Casey DE, et al. 2009 focused update: ACCF/AHA Guidelines for the Diagnosis and Management of Heart Failure in Adults: a report of the American College of Cardiology Foundation/American Heart Association Task Force on Practice Guidelines: developed in collaboration with the International Society for Heart and Lung Transplantation. Circulation. 2009;119: 1977–2016.
210. Ellison DH. Diuretic therapy and resistance in congestive heart failure. Cardiology. 2001;96:132–143.
211. Wang DJ, Gottlieb SS. Diuretics: still the mainstay of treatment. Critical Care Medicine. 2008;36:S89–S94.
212. Wargo KA, Banta WM. A comprehensive review of the loop diuretics: should furosemide be first line? Annals of Pharmacotherapy. 2009;43: 1836–1847.
213. Levy WC, Mozaffarian D, Linker DT, et al. The Seattle heart failure model: prediction of survival in heart failure. Circulation. 2006;113:1424–1433.
214. Felker GM, Lee KL, Bull DA, et al. Diuretic strategies in patients with acute decompensated heart failure. New England Journal of Medicine. 2011;364: 797–805.
215. Boerrigter G, Burnett JC Jr. Cardiorenal syndrome in decompensated heart failure: prognostic and therapeutic implications. Current Heart Failure Reports. 2004;1:113–120.
216. Bart BA, Boyle A, Bank AJ, et al. Ultrafiltration versus usual care for hospitalized patients with heart failure: the relief for acutely fluid-overloaded patients with decompensated congestive heart failure (RAPID-CHF) trial. Journal of the American College of Cardiology. 2005;46:2043–2046.
217. Jaski BE, Ha J, Denys BG, et al. Peripherally inserted veno-venous ultrafiltration for rapid treatment of volume overloaded patients. Journal of Cardiac Failure. 2003;9:227–231.
218. Costanzo MR, Guglin ME, Saltzberg MT, et al. Ultrafiltration versus intravenous diuretics for patients hospitalized for acute decompensated heart failure. Journal of the American College of Cardiology. 2007;49:675–683.
219. Agostoni PG, Marenzi GC, Sganzerla P, et al. Lung-heart interaction as a substrate for the improvement in exercise capacity after body fluid volume depletion in moderate congestive heart failure. American Journal of Cardiology. 1995;76: 793–798.
220. Agostoni P, Marenzi G, Lauri G, et al. Sustained improvement in functional capacity after removal of body fluid with isolated ultrafiltration in chronic cardiac insufficiency: failure of furosemide to provide the same result. American Journal of Medicine. 1994;96:191–199.
221. Bart BB, Goldsmith SR, Lee KL, et al. Ultrafiltration in decompensated heart failure with cardiorenal syndrome. New England Journal of Medicine. 2012;367:2296–2304.
222. Dickstein K, Cohen-Solal A, Filippatos G, et al. ESC guidelines for the diagnosis and treatment of acute and chronic heart failure 2008: the Task Force for the Diagnosis and Treatment of Acute and Chronic Heart Failure 2008 of the European Society of Cardiology. Developed in collaboration with the Heart Failure Association of the ESC (HFA) and endorsed by the European Society of Intensive Care Medicine (ESICM). European Heart Journal. 2008; 29:2388–2442.
223. Howlett JG, McKelvie RS, Costigan J, et al. The 2010 Canadian Cardiovascular Society guidelines for the diagnosis and management of heart failure update: heart failure in ethnic minority populations, heart failure and pregnancy, disease management, and quality improvement/assurance programs. Canadian Journal of Cardiology. 2010;26:185–202.
224. Bayram M, De Luca L, Massie MB, et al. Reassessment of dobutamine, dopamine, and milrinone in the management of acute heart failure syndromes. American Journal of Cardiology. 2005;96:47G–58G.
225. Leier CV, Bambach D, Thompson MJ, et al. Central and regional hemodynamic effects of intravenous isosorbide dinitrate, nitroglycerin and nitroprusside in patients with congestive heart failure. American Journal of Cardiology. 1981; 48:1115–1123.
226. Leier CV, Heban PT, Huss P, et al. Comparative systemic and regional hemodynamic effects of dopamine and dobutamine in patients with cardiomyopathic heart failure. Circulation. 1978;58:466–475.
227. Wang DJ, Dowling TC, Meadows D, et al. Nesiritide does not improve renal function in patients with chronic heart failure and worsening serum creatinine. Circulation. 2004;110:1620–1625.
228. Publication Committee for the VMAC Investigators (Vasodilatation in the Management of Acute CHF). Intravenous nesiritide vs nitroglycerin for treatment of decompensated congestive heart failure: a randomized controlled trial. JAMA. 2002;287:1531–1540.
229. Riter HG, Redfield MM, Burnett JC, et al. Nonhypotensive low-dose nesiritide has differential renal effects compared with standard-dose nesiritide in patients with acute decompensated heart failure and renal dysfunction. Journal of the American College of Cardiology. 2006;47:2334–2335.
230. Chen HH, Anstrom KJ, Givertz MM, et al. Low-dose dopamine or low-dose nesiritide in acute heart failure with renal dysfunction. The ROSE acute heart failure randomized trial. JAMA. 2013;310:2533–2543.
231. Friedrich JO, Adhikari N, Herridge MS, et al. Meta-analysis: low-dose dopamine increases urine output but does not prevent renal dysfunction or death. Annals of Internal Medicine. 2005;142:510–524.
232. Bellomo R, Chapman M, Finfer S, et al. Low-dose dopamine in patients with early renal dysfunction: a placebo-controlled randomised trial. Australian and New Zealand Intensive Care Society (ANZICS) Clinical Trials Group. Lancet. 2000;356:2139–2143.
233. Kellum JA, Decker MJ. Use of dopamine in acute renal failure: a meta-analysis. Critical Care Medicine. 2001;29:1526–1531.
234. Giamouzis G, Butler J, Starling RC, et al. Impact of dopamine infusion on renal function in hospitalized heart failure patients: results of the Dopamine in Acute Decompensated Heart Failure (DAD-HF) trial. Journal of Cardiac Failure. 2010;16:922–930.
235. Cuffe MS, Califf RM, Adams KF Jr, et al. Short-term intravenous milrinone for acute exacerbation of chronic heart failure: a randomized controlled trial. JAMA. 2002;287:1541–1547.
236. Klein L, Massie BM, Leimberger JD, et al. Admission or changes in renal function during hospitalization for worsening heart failure predict postdischarge survival: results from the Outcomes of a Prospective Trial of Intravenous Milrinone for Exacerbations of Chronic Heart Failure (OPTIME-CHF). Circulation. Heart Failure. 2008;1:25–33.
237. Russo MJ, Rana A, Chen JM, et al. Pretransplantation patient characteristics and survival following combined heart and kidney transplantation: an analysis of the United Network for Organ Sharing Database. Archives of Surgery. 2009;144: 241–246.
238. Gill J, Shah T, Hristea I, et al. Outcomes of simultaneous heart-kidney transplant

in the US: a retrospective analysis using OPTN/UNOS data. American Journal of Transplantation. 2009;9:844–852.
239. Russell SD, Rogers JG, Milano CA, et al. Renal and hepatic function improve in advanced heart failure patients during continuous-flow support with the HeartMate II left ventricular assist device. Circulation. 2009;120:2352–2357.
240. Kirklin JK, Naftel DC, Kormos RL, et al. Quantifying the effect of cardiorenal syndrome on mortality after left ventricular assist device implant. Journal of Heart and Lung Transplantation. 2013;32:1205–1213.
241. Brisco MA, Kimmel SE, Coca SG, et al. Prevalence and prognostic importance of changes in renal function after mechanical circulatory support. Circulation. 2014;7:68–75.
242. Kubo SH, Walter BA, John DH, et al. Liver function abnormalities in chronic heart failure. Influence of systemic hemodynamics. Archives of Internal Medicine. 1987;147:1227–1230.
243. Seeto RK, Fenn B, Rockey DC. Ischemic hepatitis: clinical presentation and pathogenesis. American Journal of Medicine. 2000;109:109–113.
244. Wadia Y, Etheridge W, Smart F, et al. Pathophysiology of hepatic dysfunction and intrahepatic cholestasis in heart failure and after left ventricular assist device support. Journal of Heart and Lung Transplantation. 2005;24:361–370.
245. Henrion J, Descamps O, Luwaert R, et al. Hypoxic hepatitis in patients with cardiac failure: incidence in a coronary care unit and measurement of hepatic blood flow. Journal of Hepatology. 1994;21:696–703.
246. Naschitz JE, Slobodin G, Lewis RJ, et al. Heart diseases affecting the liver and liver diseases affecting the heart. American Heart Journal. 2000;140:111–120.
247. Henrion J, Colin L, Schmitz A, et al. Ischemic hepatitis in cirrhosis. Rare but lethal. Journal of Clinical Gastroenterology. 1993;16:35–39.
248. Irie H, Mori W. Fatal hepatic necrosis after shock. Acta Pathologica Japonica. 1986;36:363–374.
249. Killip T 3rd, Payne MA. High serum transaminase activity in heart disease. Circulatory failure and hepatic necrosis. Circulation. 1960;21:646–660.
250. Lau GT, Tan HC, Kritharides L. Type of liver dysfunction in heart failure and its relation to the severity of tricuspid regurgitation. American Journal of Cardiology. 2002;90:1405–1409.
251. Richman SM, Delman AJ, Grob D. Alterations in indices of liver function in congestive heart failure with particular reference to serum enzymes. American Journal of Medicine. 1961;30:211–225.
252. Allen LA, Felker GM, Pocock S, et al. Liver function abnormalities and outcome in patients with chronic heart failure: data from the Candesartan in Heart Failure: Assessment of Reduction in Mortality and Morbidity (CHARM) program. European Journal of Heart Failure. 2009;11:170–177.
253. Reinhartz O, Farrar DJ, Hershon JH, et al. Importance of preoperative liver function as a predictor of survival in patients supported with Thoratec ventricular assist devices as a bridge to transplantation. Journal of Thoracic and Cardiovascular Surgery. 1998;116:633–640.
254. Matthews JC, Koelling TM, Pagani FD, et al. The right ventricular failure risk score: a pre-operative tool for assessing the risk of right ventricular failure in left ventricular assist device candidates. Journal of the American College of Cardiology. 2008;51:2163–2172.
255. Giallourakis CC, Rosenberg PM, Friedman LS. The liver in heart failure. Clinics in Liver Disease. 2002;6:947–967, viii–ix.
256. Valla D. [Cirrhosis of vascular origin]. La Revue Du Praticien. 1991; 41:1170–1173.
257. Runyon BA, Montano AA, Akriviadis EA, et al. The serum-ascites albumin gradient is superior to the exudate-transudate concept in the differential diagnosis of ascites. Annals of Internal Medicine. 1992;117:215–220.
258. Porrett PM, Desai SS, Timmins KJ, et al. Combined orthotopic heart and liver transplantation: the need for exception status listing. Liver Transplantation. 2004;10:1539–1544.

第 45 章
肺功能衰竭的重症监护

John Adam Reich, Richard Eliot Fagley

引言

呼吸衰竭可以是急性、慢性或混合性,随病情进展至终末期呼吸功能衰竭时可能需要进行肺移植治疗。然而移植患者的最终结局不仅与治疗期间基础情况密切相关,高质量的护理对重症呼吸衰竭的患者也同样非常重要。实际上,其他器官移植的危重患者常继发呼吸功能衰竭,尤其是心脏和肝移植患者。本章将对急性和慢性呼吸衰竭的生理及病理生理进行回顾,并对改善肺功能的药物及非药物治疗进行讨论。简单介绍机械通气的应用,强调可以减轻肺脏或其他终末器官进一步损伤的通气策略。此外,本章将对可以从实体器官移植中获益的最常见肺疾病进行回顾性介绍。

呼吸系统的生理及病理生理

氧气及二氧化碳进行充分交换需要有以下几方面保证:吸入气体可传至肺泡,有效通气(V)和肺泡毛细血管的血流[灌注(Q)]。最理想的肺部情况是通气血流比值为 1(V/Q=1)[1]。有灌注但是通气不足(V/Q<1),称为分流。有通气但是灌注不足(V/Q>1),称为无效腔[1]。解剖无效腔(V_{Danat})是指存在于较大气道如气管、支气管及传导气道中不进行气体交换的气量[2]。肺泡无效腔(V_{Dalv})指存在于肺泡内未进行血气交换(Q=0)的气量,是潮气量(V_T)的一部分[2]。正常生理情况下,V_{Dalv} 很小,可以忽略不计,但如果发生肺部疾病,V_{Dalv} 可以快速增加[2]。解剖无效腔和肺泡无效腔共同构成了生理无效腔($V_{Dphysiol}$)[2]。生理无效腔的改变对患者有一定的意义。生理无效腔、解剖无效腔和肺泡无效腔的关系如下:

$$V_{Dphysiol}= V_{Danat}+ V_{Dalv}$$

正常人解剖无效腔和肺泡无效腔的总和占潮气量的 20%~30%[1]。当 $V_{Dphysiol}$ 达到 100%时,V/Q 近乎无穷大($V/Q=\infty$)。有些疾病如肺气肿,由于有效肺组织明显减少,使得无效腔增加。而有些疾病如肺栓塞或失血性休克,由于限制或改变了肺血流而造成无效腔增加。无效腔的增加最终可以造成高二氧化碳和低氧血症的发生。

假设每一个有灌注的肺泡和肺毛细血管都处于平衡关系,即动脉气体张力等于肺泡气体张力,在此前提下,可以计算无效腔量。生理无效腔量 Bohr 计算公式[2]:

$$V_{Dphysiol}/V_T = PaCO_2-PECO_2/PaCO_2$$

值得注意的是,公式中 $PECO_2$ 代表呼出气体 P_{CO_2},不同于二氧化碳监测中的呼吸末二氧化碳[1]。$PaCO_2$ 代表动脉血液中 CO_2 张力。

有灌注但通气不足称为分流(V/Q<1)。与无效腔相似,分流可以分为两种类型,真性分流(完全没有气体交换)和静脉血掺杂(仅部分通气进行气血交换)。在真性分流中,V/Q=0。例如,有些疾病导致气道阻塞而没有气体通过或者因通过肺毛细血管的血流过多造成分流,如急性呼吸窘迫综合征(ARDS)、肺炎、肝肺综合征和肺水肿。任何肺泡填充过程如果伴有缺氧性肺血管收缩,同样可以造成一定程度的分流发生。一旦发生分流,可能造成低氧血症伴 $PaCO_2$ 升高。分流情况越严重,患者对氧疗的反应越差。事实上,当分流比例超过 50%,PaO_2 的改变受 FiO_2 影响较小[3]。图 45.1 为 V/Q 改变的示意图,从分流(图 45.1b)到无效腔(图 45.1c)。理想 V/Q 比值为 1:1(图 45.1a)。

分流率可以通过以下公式进行计算,其中 CcO_2 代表终末端肺毛细血管内氧气含量,CaO_2 代表动脉血中氧气含量,CvO_2 代表肺混合静脉氧含量:

$$Qs/Qt=(CcO_2-CaO_2)/(CcO_2-CvO_2)$$

这个公式有些复杂。分母(CcO_2-CvO_2)代表全部肺血流,分子代表没有进行气体交换的血流。另一种说

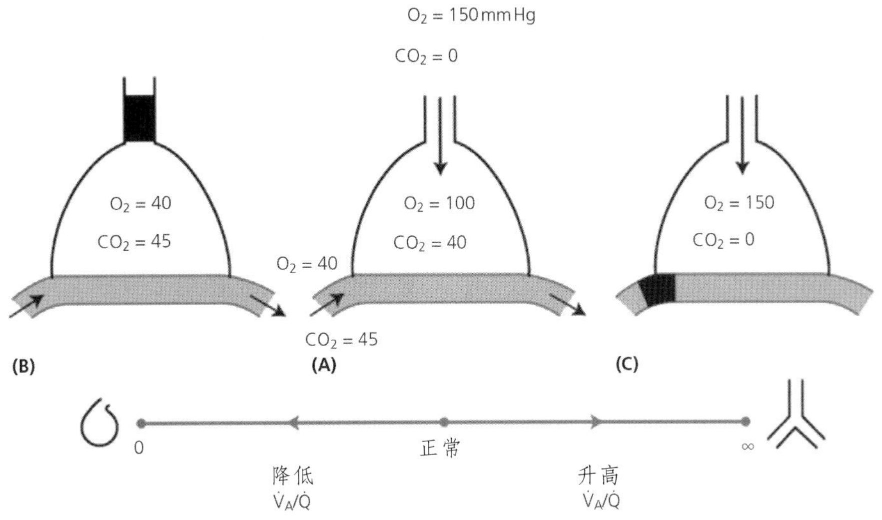

图 45.1　(A)理想 *V/Q* 比。(B)真性分流。(C)真性无效腔 *V/Q*=无穷大(Adapted From West JB. Respiratory Physiology: The Essentials, 9th ed. 2011. Reproduced by permission of Wolter Kluwer Health.)

法,分流量是对全身动脉血氧含量(CaO_2)、混合静脉氧含量(CvO_2)和肺毛细血管氧含量(CcO_2)的比较。但是由于临床上很难得到终末端肺毛细血管内血样，所以此公式在临床使用上有所限制。临床上常用 PaO_2/FiO_2 估算有肺部疾病患者如 ARDS 的分流率[4]。$PaO_2/FiO_2<200$ 通常预示分流率>20%(Qs/Qt)[4]。

临床上,若 *V/Q* 不正常,还可以通过计算肺泡(A)氧分压和动脉(a)氧分压差,即肺泡-动脉(A-a)氧分压差来估算。肺泡氧分压可通过以下公式计算：

$$PAO_2=PIO_2-(PaCO_2/RQ)$$

其中 PAO_2 代表肺泡内氧分压,PIO_2 代表吸入气体氧分压,$PaCO_2$ 代表动脉血二氧化碳分压,RQ 代表呼吸商,即相对气体交换率。在海平面,呼吸空气情况下的 A-a 梯度为 10mmHg。随着年龄的增长,A-a PO_2 会随之增加,这是因为小气道弹性降低导致肺泡塌陷,造成分流的增加，同时无效通气的肺容量增加,*V/Q* 亦会出现明显的差异性[5]。此外,随着 FiO_2 的增加,A-a PO_2 也会增加,可能是因为在原本低通气的肺组织,高浓度吸氧一定程度上可以缓解由低氧造成的肺血管收缩,虽灌注有所改善但通气并未得到改善。因此,增加肺泡氧分压可能会导致 *V/Q* 不匹配,继而增加分流率,加大 A-a 梯度[1]。

肺相关药理学

呼吸衰竭的治疗是通过纠正潜在的病理状态,改善肺功能和呼吸力学。最终目的是帮助患者改善症状、恢复正常生活状态。以下将对呼吸衰竭患者常用到的静脉及雾化药物的机制进行简单的介绍。

血管舒张药:氧气、一氧化氮及前列环素

氧疗是呼吸衰竭的一线治疗。如前所述,某种特定情况下,如患者存在较大的分流率时,氧疗对改善动脉血氧分压的作用是极其有限的。此外,如果患者血红蛋白数量及功能正常，增加动脉血氧分压并不能很好地改善血氧含量。详见以下公式：

$$CaO_2=(Hgb\times1.36\times SaO_2)+(0.0031\times PaO_2)$$

其中 CaO_2 代表氧含量,Hgb 代表血红蛋白浓度,单位为 g/dL,SaO_2 代表动脉血氧饱和度即动脉血中与氧气结合的血红蛋白的比例。

氧气可以减少缺氧性肺血管收缩(HPV),从而降低肺血管阻力。肺动脉高压患者可能从中获益,但在其他病例中可能会造成 A-a 梯度的增加或加重 *V/Q* 失调,如慢性阻塞性肺疾病(COPD)患者[6]。如果想避免终末器官损伤,必须要保证有充足的氧气供给。然而,在静息状态下，即使是伴有严重肺功能不全的患者(PaO_2 为 20~30mmHg),血乳酸水平也并没有提高[7],并且正常静息状态下,器官和组织的氧含量极低。因此,在对肺功能严重受损的患者的临床处理上，我们可能过分强调了提高氧输送的治疗[1]。

氧疗同样可能存在危害。氧中毒的机制可能是由于产生了氧自由基和其他活性氧物质造成细胞的炎性

损伤[8]。相对而言，新生儿发生氧中毒的风险更高，如早产儿视网膜病变[9]。因此，在进行氧疗时要尽可能地避免过度治疗。尽量控制 FiO_2<60%是合理的。

人体本身可以产生一氧化氮(NO)，而肺脏本身也存在大量可以产生 NO 的细胞，包括血管内皮细胞、上皮细胞、平滑肌细胞和炎性细胞[10]。在血管内皮，NO 可以提高环磷酸鸟苷(cGMP)水平，从而降低血管平滑肌中对钙离子的结合，导致血管舒张[10]。目前，认为吸入 NO(iNO)可能有一定的临床获益，因为吸入治疗可以直接作用于有通气的肺泡，从而大幅减少了 NO 造成的全身副反应。吸入 NO 可以选择性扩张肺血管，使更多的心排血量流向有充足通气的肺组织。iNO 可以明显改善绝大部分患者 *V/Q* 及氧和情况，但并不能降低 ARDS 患者的死亡率[11]。NO 的最大优势在于代谢快而且可选择性扩张肺血管[10]。因此，临床上常采用 iNO 治疗肺动脉高压和右心功能不全[10]。

前列环素由体内花生四烯酸代谢产生，它通过提高细胞内环磷酸腺苷(cAMP)水平，降低钙离子水平，从而使血管舒张[10]。前列环素可以静脉给药或雾化吸入。如果是静脉给药，则需要特殊的泵。而前列环素雾化不仅可以改善患者 *V/Q*，而且在价格上较 iNO 有明显优势，因此目前已普遍应用于难治性低氧血症患者。遗憾的是，至今还没有任何关于前列环素对 ARDS 患者临床意义的随机对照研究[12]。

支气管扩张剂：β_2 受体激动剂及抗胆碱能类药物

β_2 受体激动剂

β_2 受体激动剂可以通过静脉给药(肾上腺素、异丙肾上腺素)，但对于支气管痉挛、气道阻力增高患者，雾化给药可能更有效，并且可以减少药物的全身副反应。β_2 受体激动剂作用于 G 蛋白受体，提高 cAMP 水平，从而减少细胞内游离钙浓度，松弛平滑肌[13]。短效制剂(沙丁胺醇、左旋沙丁胺醇)可以用于急性支气管痉挛的治疗，而像福莫特罗、沙美特罗等长效制剂则常用于哮喘或 COPD 的长期治疗。现有研究表明，长效制剂可以明显减少哮喘患者发生急性加重并缓解其症状，但可能会使部分患者的死亡率增加，安全性有待进一步研究[14]。因此，治疗急性发作患者时，很多临床医生会停止使用长效制剂，单纯应用短效制剂。β 受体激动剂的副作用较多，其中心动过速最为常见。针对此问题，已研发出左旋沙丁胺醇并已上市，其药效与沙丁胺醇相似并且可以避免心动过速和快速心律失常等副作用发生。但哮喘缓患者的相关临床研究并不充足[15]。

抗胆碱能类药物

抗胆碱能药物用于治疗支气管扩张，常选用雾化剂型，而非静脉剂型。该类药物通过阻断支气管平滑肌毒蕈碱型受体(M_1、M_2 和 M_3)，松弛气道平滑肌。吸入型抗胆碱能药物异丙托溴铵和噻托溴铵均为季铵类化合物，异丙托溴铵为非选择性毒蕈碱拮抗剂，可阻滞三种亚型 M 受体。噻托溴铵在肺中也可以拮抗三种亚型 M 受体，但对 M_1 及 M_3 的作用半衰期更长，从而支气管扩张效果理论上会更强(M_2 型拮抗剂可以导致支气管收缩)[16]。由于雾化抗胆碱能药物为季铵类化合物，不易通过血脑屏障，很少发生抗胆碱能综合征[16]。目前，临床上将异丙托溴铵作为哮喘急性加重治疗的二线药物，而噻托溴铵仅用于 COPD 的慢性治疗[16]。

抗感染治疗：激素及白三烯抑制剂

激素

激素在呼吸功能衰竭患者中的应用存在很大的争议。无论感染还是非感染类疾病发生时，肺组织都会受到炎性反应的影响而受到损伤。而激素可以减轻人体的炎性反应，从而避免组织的进一步损伤。目前已证实，系统性应用激素可以使 COPD 和哮喘急性加重患者获益[17]。但还未证实，哮喘急性发作患者应用“双倍剂量”雾化激素可以有效减少预防性全身激素的用量[18]。此外，有大量研究探讨糖皮质激素在 ARDS 患者中的价值，但并未发现应用糖皮质激素可以明显改善死亡率[19]。

白三烯抑制剂

白三烯是花生四烯酸代谢产生的一种炎性介质，在肺部病变尤其是哮喘等疾病中起到关键作用。白三烯具有很强的诱导支气管收缩作用，白三烯的拮抗作用在运动诱导型哮喘和阿司匹林诱导型哮喘的治疗中效果显著。白三烯除了可以诱导支气管收缩，还可以调节肺毛细血管通透性、黏液产生及传导通路活性[20]。白三烯抑制剂在炎性介导肺病的长期治疗中有一定的优势,但并不适合在急性期使用。因此,常作为过敏性哮喘长期治疗的基础辅助用药。

磷酸二酯酶抑制剂

磷酸二酯酶(PDE)是环核苷酸的催化水解酶。PDE 共 11 种亚型,大多可以调节平滑肌收缩,而不同亚型的 PDE 在不同组织中的表达各有差异,因此我们希望研发出具有较强针对性的药物以达到确切的治疗效果[21]。茶碱是目前仍在使用的最原始的 PDE 抑制剂,尽管其磷酸二酯酶抑制作用很弱[21]。PDE3 抑制剂有很强的正性肌力作用,可作用于肺及全身血管平滑肌,造成血管舒张[21]。以米力农为例,其是一种 PDE3 抑制剂具有正性肌力作用及血管扩张作用,被用于终末期肺动脉高压伴右心衰竭的治疗。PDE5 抑制剂——西地那非因安全性高及疗效好,已经被广泛应用于终末期肺动脉高压的治疗[22]。在重症监护室(ICU),患者脱机时,可以尝试应用 PDE5 抑制剂辅助脱机或代替雾化前列环素、iNO 等肺血管扩张药。

黏膜纤毛类药物

近年来,以 N-乙酰半胱氨酸、愈创甘油醚、碘甘油为代表的一类药物,用于促进黏液分泌、改善黏液质量,从而提高气道自洁能力[23]。但有趣的是,目前几乎没有任何证据支持对重症患者应用此类药物。众所周知,N-乙酰半胱氨酸有很强的抗氧化特性,但目前一系列相关研究并没有证实其对死亡率有显著影响[24]。

呼吸衰竭患者的机械通气

机械通气的合理应用对重症呼吸衰竭患者的病情改善起到至关重要的作用。机械通气并非单纯对肺部进行治疗,而是通过提供合理的呼吸系统支持帮助患者满足通气需求,改善氧合以保证患者生存。在应用机械通气过程中,要避免参数设置不合理造成机械通气相关肺损伤,并且及时评估患者情况以尽早脱机。

本章重点介绍机械通气相关术语,这是临床医生在对呼吸衰竭患者进行管理过程中必须掌握的内容。为了较好地理解现代机械通气,我们将其分为三个变量:触发变量、限制变量、周期变量。触发变量是呼吸机计算机程序中的一个输入变量,用于控制患者每一次呼吸开始,触发模式由操作者选择,每个呼吸机都有一个触发预设值,但有时会根据临床需求来调节。例如,在触发模式下,可以选择流量触发即呼吸机感受到流量缺失达到预设流速(单位 L/min)或压力触发即呼吸机感受到气道压力下降达到某个数值以下预设压力(单位 cmH_2O)。限制变量是指呼吸机在送气过程中的通气目标,就像司机在旅行中尝试限制车速以达到最佳的旅行效果。限制变量通常为吸气压力或流速。而周期变量是用来决定每一次正压吸气的结束,可以是时间(单位 s)、容量(单位 mL)、流速(L/min)。

最常用的通气模式是辅助-控制通气(ACV)。在这种模式中,临床医生会预设呼吸频率。当患者没有自主呼吸时,呼吸机会按照预设频率进行正压通气。如果患者触发呼吸机送气,呼吸机会同步给予患者预设的潮气量进行辅助通气。但不论是控制通气,还是辅助通气限制变量和循环变量都是由临床医生预设的。由于在吸气过程中可以选择达到预设容量或预设压力,所以这种通气模式全程为容量辅助控制通气(ACV)或压力辅助控制通气(ACP)。总之,ACV 是容量限制、时间切换,ACP 是压力限制、时间切换。

同步间隙指令通气(SIMV)是一种改良版的辅助控制通气。SIMV 与辅助控制通气一样可以由容量控制或压力控制。在这种模式中,临床医生同样需要设定呼吸频率。如果患者自主呼吸很弱或者呼吸频率小于预设呼吸频率,那么就按照预设频率进行通气。如果患者呼吸频率高于预设频率,那么呼吸机会额外给予患者一定水平的压力支持。压力支持通气是压力限制流量切换。这种模式的设计使患者有更多的机会锻炼自身呼吸肌肉的力量。人们一直认为 SIMV 伴压力支持这种通气模式对困难脱机的重症呼吸衰竭患者脱机是有益处的,但回顾现有文献,并没有证据支持这种优势[25]。压力支持通气可以作为独立的模式使用,在这种模式中,呼吸频率及分钟通气量由患者决定。因此,后备通气是这种模式的一项非常重要的安全保障设置,避免患者低通气或窒息的发生。

压力调节容量控制通气(PRVC)是一种压力限制时间切换的通气模式,但需要设置目标潮气量。呼吸机的微处理器会评估每次通气是否达到预设潮气量,并反馈调节压力限制来达到预设容量目标。这是目前向“智能通气”模式发展的一个代表,也是临床医生必须掌握的一种模式。但应用 PRVC 模式同样存在危险。例如,如果患者有自发性气胸,并存在一定的张力,应用

PRVC模式时闭合环路通过反馈调节，呼吸机会不断增加送气压力以达到目标潮气量，直到超过到压力上限，这样会加重气胸，甚至造成爆发性心肺功能衰竭。这种“智能通气”需要设定相应的报警参数以避免不必要的危害发生，但临床医生必须对这些变量限制导致的呼吸系统顺应性和(或)潮气量变化做出准确判断，并做出相应处理。

气道压力释放通气(APRV)是一种新型通气模式，旨在维持相对较高的平均气道压(MawP)以改善氧合。APRV是时间触发、压力限制、时间切换的通气模式[26]。需要设置的参数包括高压(P_{high})、高压相时间(t_{high})、低压(P_{low})、低压相时间(t_{low})，通常此模式的初始设置为每分钟6~10个呼吸周期，P_{high}=30mmHg，t_{high}=5.2s，P_{low}=0mmHg，t_{low}=0.8s。在传统模式中，大部分肺泡都是较低肺容积时利用呼气末正压(PEEP)达到肺复张效果的，而APRV有所不同，t_{low}是决定肺复张的关键。由于t_{low}设置非常短，造成呼气不完全，从而导致内源性PPPE的产生。临床医生应用邻近闭合压力的内源性PEEP打开肺组织。APRV的另一大优势是可以避免不张肺组织通气时产生的剪切伤。在整个通气过程中允许患者自主呼吸，由于吸气阀及呼气阀都没有完全关闭，因此不会增加患者呼吸阻力，整体上提高了患者舒适度，改善人机同步性。例如，患者可以在P_{high}或P_{low}相上进行很小的呼吸运动，且保留自主呼吸可以改善V/Q匹配程度和血流动力学。相比传统通气，APRV通过延长肺部膨胀的时间，提高MawP，从而明显改善低氧血症患者的氧合。有研究证实，APRV相比压力支持通气，可以明显增加ARDS患者的有效通气肺容积[27]。但是对于需要延长呼气时间的阻塞性肺疾病患者，应用这种模式的风险相对较大。此外，应用此模式，临床医生不能很好地控制高压相产生的潮气量，理论上会有造成肺过度膨胀，产生容积伤的潜在风险。理论上，APRV不仅是一种通气模式，同时具有肺复张的效果，可以打开并维持肺泡开放，改善患者的通气并提高氧合。但现有临床研究并未证实患者可以从此种通气模式中获益[26]。

高频振荡通气(HFOV)常应用于肺依从性极差的ARDS患者。类似立体扬声器的振动器，HFOV利用震动活塞以很高的频率移动膈膜，达到3~10Hz，每分钟180~600次呼吸[28]。其中参数偏流是指引入新鲜气体的流量，可以达到40~60L/min，FiO_2为0.8~1[28]。呼气阀允许气体流通并维持在设定的平均气道压[29]。值得注意的是，HFOV的最大优势就是可以分别调节氧合和通气[28]。影响氧合的参数包括FiO_2、平均气道压和偏流量[28]，而影响通气的参数包括频率及振幅(力度)[28]。现有研究表明，相比传统通气，应用HFOV可能会改善急性肺损伤或ARDS患者30天的死亡率，但仍需更多更严谨的研究进行进一步验证[30]。

如前所述，对呼吸衰竭患者应用机械通气并不只是为了治疗肺部疾病。临床工作者应时刻评估患者是否具备脱机的条件。研究发现，如果没有较强的脱机意识，不能及时评估患者是否可以脱机，往往会造成患者脱机延迟。研究证明，镇静药物的每日中断可以明显减少机械通气时间[31]，联合应用呼吸控制实验、每日镇静中断及自主呼吸实验可以显著缩短患者住ICU时间及住院时间[32]。仅联合应用镇静中断和自主呼吸实验，同样可以缩短机械通气时间并减少机械通气相关并发症。

急性呼吸窘迫综合征

1967年报道了第一例ARDS。此后，ARDS逐步得到关注，很多相关临床研究得以开展。最初ADRS的死亡率超过60%，目前已下降至30%[33]。1994年发布的一项会议共识，对这种临床综合征的特点进行了概括：①急性起病；②PaO_2/FiO_2<200；③胸片显示浸润影；④肺毛细血管楔压(PCWP)<18mmHg[34]。ARDS主要是由肺泡毛细血管膜破坏所造成的。由于目前肺动脉导管的应用逐渐减少，可以用缺乏心源性肺水肿证据替代PCWP>18mmHg。

ARDS从病理上可以分为三个阶段(并不是所有患者都具有这三个阶段)：渗出期、增生期及纤维化期[35]。渗出期出现肺泡毛细血管膜的破坏，导致富含蛋白及中性粒细胞的液体进入肺泡。增生期是指透明膜的形成，发生在病程两周左右，最终导致纤维化形成。从第一阶段开始，由于肺泡弥漫性的损伤，导致功能性分流的产生，从而影响正常的气体交换，导致低氧血症的发生。如前所述，随着患者分流量增加，对氧疗的反应性会明显降低。此外，如果ARDS患者早期无效腔通气量明显增加则提示患者预后不佳[36]。

ARDS的病因有很多，可以是直接作用于肺部(即肺源性)的，如误吸、溺水、肺炎、吸入有毒物或肺部挫伤；也可以是间接作用于肺部(即非肺源性)的，如创伤但并未累及胸廓、脓毒症、血液输注、心肺转流[34]。总之，是肺泡毛细血管膜遭到破坏，肺部遭到炎性反应的进一步损坏。

临床上努力尝试应用药物治疗来改善 ARDS 的症状，但均未取得明显效果。例如，表面活性药物治疗，理论上由于 ARDS 患者表面活性物质缺乏，导致肺泡易于塌陷，额外提供可以降低肺泡表面张力。然而，在针对所有 ARDS 的患者研究中并未发现，应用表面活性物质可以改善死亡率，但部分荟萃分析发现其对误吸或肺炎导致的 ARDS 患者，可能有一定的益处[37]。iNO 虽然可以改善氧合，但不能降低死亡率[38]。同样激素也不能改善死亡率，但可以减少患者机械通气的时间[39]。

2000 年，急性呼吸综合征网络工作组(ARDSnet)进行了一项具有里程碑意义的研究，对比了传统潮气量通气(12mL/kg 理想体重)和小潮气量通气(6mL/kg 理想体重)对 ARDS 患者的影响。研究的设计是基于先前大量动物及临床实验，发现小潮气量的应用可以减少肺损伤的发生。此研究收录至大约 800 例患者时，小潮气量组死亡率从 39%降至 31%，因伦理规定提前终止了研究[40]。

ARDS 患者胸部 CT 可表现出不均质病变，通气好的肺组织及受损伤的肺组织共同存在[41]。如前所述，毛细血管通透性增加导致液体进入肺泡，从而造成顺应性的改变。当患者应用正压通气时，气体更容易流向健康的、顺应性好的肺泡，而这种不利的再分配会导致原本正常的肺泡由于通气过度造成抻拉并产生剪切力，进一步加重炎性反应及肺泡损伤。因此，小潮气量通气策略使患者受益，可能是因为减少了机械通气对健康肺组织造成的损伤。

存在 ARDS 时，肺部遭受炎症介质的不断刺激，加之应用机械通气很容易产生机械通气相关肺损伤(VALI)。例如，气压伤(高容量导致的损伤)、肺不张(低潮气量造成的损伤)和生物伤(肺外器官损伤)[41]。气压伤是由于大潮气量导致肺泡过度抻拉，造成肺泡毛细血管膜的损伤。临床上可以采用肺保护性通气策略，即小潮气量及维持平台压(代替肺泡压)小于 35cmH_2O[41]。但平台压并不能真正反映作用在肺泡上的压力，但可以间接反映非气体交换气道和通气回路阻力的函数关系[41]。肺不张使闭合肺容积大于功能残气量。每一次正压通气时，小的气体交换气道和塌陷肺泡会被打开，呼气时会再次陷闭，伴随着呼吸，反复地开放闭合，对肺泡产生剪切力，造成肺损伤[41]。合理地应用 PEEP 可以维持肺泡开放，避免大部分肺泡发生陷闭。在动物研究中，已证明此方法是有益的。但现有大规模关于高 PEEP 和低 PEEP 联合小潮气量通气的临床随机对照试验，并未发现两组在死亡率或其他研究终点上有明显差异[42]。因此，对于预防 VALI 的发生，小潮气量通气策略更为重要[42]。同时也推荐合理应用 PEEP 改善氧合，临床医生应根据临床情况具体调节。生物伤也是 ARDS 患者进行机械通气时可能出现的损伤，患者进行机械通气治疗时，会造成肺部释放一些炎症因子并随血流流向其他器官，进而导致多器官系统的衰竭[41]。此外，其他器官释放的炎症介质同样会造成肺组织的损伤。ARDSnet 的研究发现，在小潮气量通气组中，血清中白介素(IL)-6 明显降低[40]，即小潮气量可能减少由 IL-6 介导的肺损伤。

总之，ARDS 是一种临床综合征，病因病理表现多样，但最终临床结果相似。有很多药理学及机械通气干预相关的研究，但大部分都未得到其有益的结论。研究显示，仅少数 ARDS 患者真正死于不可逆的肺损伤，而大部分都是死于其他疾病，以脓毒症为主[43]。对 ARDS 患者的治疗原则是纠正基础疾病，给予患者最大的支持直至好转。应用小潮气量保护性通气策略，以最大限度减少 VALI 的发生。

慢性呼吸衰竭相关疾病

如前所述，大部分 ARDS 患者的死因并不是不可逆的肺部损伤。而对于慢性呼吸衰竭，其病程通常呈渐进性，间歇性感染或炎性诱导的急性发作都会加重病情。一旦发生威胁生命的呼吸衰竭，肺移植是终末期患者可以有质量生存的唯一治疗方法。

肺移植的对象一般病情重、进展快且移植后不易复发的患者。一项全球范围的肺移植调查显示，接受肺移植的疾病种类主要包括 COPD(31%)、特发性肺纤维化(21%)、肺囊性纤维化(16%)、α-1 抗胰蛋白酶缺乏(7%)[44]。下面简要介绍这几种疾病的病理特点及移植后的管理。其他相关治疗详见第 31 章。

慢性阻塞性肺疾病

COPD 给美国甚至全世界带来了极大的医疗负担[45]。预计到 2020 年，会成为世界第五大致死疾病[46]。COPD

患者可能合并慢性支气管炎及肺气肿，在进行肺功能监测时都存在一定程度的气流阻塞。慢性支气管炎是小气道病变，可造成呼气末气道阻塞。肺气肿与其相似,但会进一步造成肺实质的弹性组织减少,造成呼气功能受损。

COPD 的诊断包括两部分，即临床病史和肺功能检测。临床上,通常患者会同时存在慢性支气管炎和肺气肿,还有一些患者可能合并哮喘,会干扰诊断的准确性。肺功能监测中,β2 受体激动剂试验可以帮助判断气道阻塞的可逆性。COPD 患者按一秒用力呼气肺容积(FEV1)/用力肺活量(FVC)的比值情况,可以将病情分为轻、中、重、极重。按照疾病严重程度的不同,接受相应的治疗。对于轻度 COPD 患者,即 $FEV_1/FVC<0.70$ 且 $FEV_1>80\%$预计值,治疗方案主要是避免危险因素,适当接种流感疫苗,必要时使用短效支气管扩张剂。对于中度 COPD 患者,即 $FEV_1/FVC<0.70$ 且 $50\%<FEV_1<80\%$预计值，此时应加用长效支气管扩张剂并考虑进行肺康复治疗。当病情继续进展至重度 COPD 时，$FEV_1/FVC<0.70$ 且 $30\%<FEV_1<50\%$预计值，除上述治疗外,在急性加重期可考虑增加激素吸入治疗。最终发展至极重度时,$FEV_1/FVC<0.70$ 且 $FEV_1<30\%$预计值或 $FEV_1<0\%$合并慢性呼吸衰竭，则应考虑增加慢性长期氧疗及手术干预[47]。

由于同时存在呼气受限和弹性组织缺失,COPD 患者往往会存在很多并发症,如气胸、肺心病、肺大疱及肺炎[48]。

COPD 的发病机制并不明确,造成肺损伤的很多原因都可以造成 COPD,其中如吸烟等环境因素是导致肺部炎性改变的一大因素。通常,COPD 患者存在慢性支气管扩张导致杯状细胞增生，使大气道内黏液分泌增加[49]。但这类患者的气道阻塞并不发生在大气道,而发生在更小的气道,即直径在 2mm 以下的气道[49]。复杂的炎性机制因素目前尚未完全掌握，但可以确定的是，COPD 患者的细支气管肺组织中被大量的中性粒细胞浸润[50],而平滑肌的肥大可能是造成气道阻力增加的一个原因,同时存在肺组织的破坏,造成非正常的肺泡弹性回缩导致无效腔的增加。由于肺气肿或气流阻塞所造成的不良后果,患者病情及程度差异很大。除了肺弹性的改变,COPD 患者由于肺实质重建造成肺毛细血管血流减少,二氧化碳弥散能力降低[51]。

目前治疗包括戒烟、应用支气管扩张剂以及肺康复治疗。对于重症患者，可以加用吸入性激素治疗。"COPD 急性加重"可能会危及患者生命,称为症状性急性加重。因此,COPD 治疗的第一步就是避免急性加重。吸入性激素可以使 COPD 急性加重的发生率降低 20%[47]。研究证明，噻托溴铵可以改善 COPD 患者的生活质量，且与异丙托溴铵相比，前者可以使 COPD 急性加重的发生率降低 24%[52]。沙美特罗和氟替卡松联合治疗可以使 COPD 的发生率降低 25%。支气管扩张剂——短效和长效 β2 受体激动剂可以使 FEV_1 增加 100~150mL[48]。COPD 急性加重患者使用经验性抗生素治疗可以使治疗失败率降低 46%、院内死亡率降低 78%[53]。14 天以内的短期类固醇治疗可以使治疗失败率降低 46%[53]。氧疗可使氧饱和度>88%~90%[49]。对于存在低氧血症的 COPD 患者，长程氧疗可以改善生存率,24 小时全天氧疗的效果优于间断吸氧[54]。

COPD 急性加重患者使用呼吸机支持治疗的效果需要进一步讨论。COPD 急性加重期间,由于小气道气流受限,肺容量会增加[55]。充气过度限制了呼吸肌并增加呼吸做功。此外,由于在呼吸循环过程中不能完全将气体呼出,会引起呼吸性酸中毒,进一步影响换气[55]。随机对照研究的系统评价显示，对于 COPD 急性加重患者,与常规治疗相比,使用无创正压通气(NIPPV)会使死亡率降低 48%[55]，并使气管插管率降低 59%[55]。NIPPV 对于 COPD 急性加重和急性充血性心力衰竭患者有独特优势。而对其他患者人群,NIPPV 的优势尚未证实,甚至有时会延迟进行气管插管的时间。NIPPV 明显降低 COPD 和充血性心力衰竭(CHF)患者死亡率的原因可能是降低了气管插管率，从而减少了与其相关的危险因素,包括气道分泌物清除、镇痛镇静的使用及呼吸机相关性肺炎。

囊性纤维化

囊性纤维化(CF)是一种由囊性纤维化跨膜传导调节因子(CFTR)突变所致的常染色体遗传性疾病。这种疾病具有变异性,但主要表现为慢性感染、气道梗阻、胰腺外分泌不足以及胃肠道功能障碍[56]。此病常见于北欧人群,2%~5%高加索人群中携带 CF 基因突变[56]。CF 患者的肺上皮细胞功能障碍。CFTR 蛋白在氯离子转运过程中十分重要,而蛋白的缺陷会导致气道表面水分的耗竭[57],使得剩余的黏液更厚且与细胞黏附得更紧,从而导致气道梗阻,并成为感染病灶[56]。黏液纤毛更难清除这些黏液。由于慢性气道梗阻,患者更易感染致病菌。

CF 急性加重患者的治疗:①抗生素治疗以降低细菌负担;②清洁气道;③适当的营养支持[58]。常见的致病菌包括金黄色葡萄球菌和铜绿假单胞菌[56]。继发于 CF 急性加重的呼吸功能不全患者需要进行痰培养以发现细菌种类和药物敏感度。因为,CD 患者感染的致病菌常为多重耐药的 G−菌,例如,有 1/3 的患者培养结果为洋葱伯克霍尔德菌[59]。初始抗生素选择应该基于既往培养结果并包含两种抗假单胞菌的药物[58]。感染学专家可以指导治疗。目前对门诊患者普遍采用吸入性妥布霉素进行抑制性抗菌治疗,并降低 CF 急性加重的发生率[58]。研究显示,大环内酯类药物治疗(主要为阿奇霉素)可以改善肺功能,尤其对于假单胞菌感染患者[60],由于它没有抗假单胞菌活性,目前认为炎症和免疫调节可能是阿奇霉素改善肺功能的机制[60]。

通过物理引流辅助装置和吸入性化痰药来清理气道。体位引流法、人工叩背与振动等方法可以增加排痰量[61]。体位引流法、人工叩背、振动与运动联合治疗,可以达到增加 FEV_1 的效果[61]。治疗仪器包括振动床和排痰背心。在化痰治疗方面,重组人脱氧核糖核酸酶 I (rhDNaseI)是一种人工合成的生物制剂。CF 患者黏液的特性源于细胞外 DNA。每天吸入两次 rhDNase,与对照剂相比,可以使 CF 急性加重的发生率降低 37%[62]。使用高渗盐水喷雾来增加 CF 患者的黏液清除率,其机制为通过增加渗透压使水分流动,使黏液再水化,降低其黏度而促进排痰,但目前证据尚不足够[63]。

由于研究显示营养状态差和低体重指数(BMI)与不良预后相关,因此,保证患者的营养状态是 CF 治疗的重要组成部分[58]。虽然并未推荐特殊饮食,但鼓励进食高热量食物,并可以适当联合应用胰酶制剂[58]。低 BMI 甚至成为肺移植的一项障碍。

CF 患者呼吸系统的支持治疗与其他原因所致的呼吸衰竭相似。氧疗可以通过降低肺动脉高压和肺心病而使患者获益,但对 CF 患者的研究相对较少,并且多数数据来自 COPD 患者人群[58]。高碳酸血症患者短期使用无创通气治疗是否获益目前尚不明确[64]。CFTR 在其他组织也有表达,尤其是胃肠道系统,因此对其他器官系统的支持也非常重要。可以通过消化酶的补充来治疗胰腺功能不全。高血糖通常在 20~30 岁时出现[56]。由于经常暴露于氨基糖苷类抗生素,患者经常存在肾功能不全。除其他相关并发症以外,还可能发生肝硬化[56]。

特发性肺间质纤维化

特发性肺间质纤维化(IPF)常表现为无痰性干咳和劳力性呼吸困难,因而不易被发现。其临床特点为限制性肺疾病,顺应性下降与肺纤维化相关。IPF 的诊断主要靠肺部活检[65]。IPF 如果不能缓解则会致命。诊断后 5 年生存率为 20%~30%[66],疾病进展死亡率为 39%,死于心血管原因患者占 24%(主要为肺心病),死于支气管癌患者占 10%,死于肺栓塞患者占 7%[67]。

类固醇皮质激素为主要治疗药物,但并没有证据支持其作为单独治疗[68]。IPF 诊断后要立即将患者送至有治疗此类疾病经验的医院,并需要考虑肺移植。2005 年开始进行肺移植器官分配评分,目的是降低患者在等待移植过程中的死亡率,这明显增加了移植患者的数量[69]。此时,试验性治疗方案包括抗炎药物和支持治疗。目前有很多关于抗纤维化和抗炎药物的研究正在进行。

IPF 常伴有肺动脉高压,应该考虑置入右心导管,并根据监测结果实施治疗[70]。对于进展性 IPF 患者,应避免气管插管,除非可以立即进行相应治疗[71]。一项研究显示,IPF 合并急性呼吸衰竭的患者在进行气管插管机械通气后,只有 1 例患者存活,是由于在机械通气后 6 小时接受了肺移植治疗[71]。

肺动脉高压

肺动脉高压定义为右心导管监测结果显示平均动脉压≥25mmHg、肺动脉楔压<15mmHg[72]。世界卫生组织将肺动脉高压进行了分组(表 45.1)[73]。特发性肺动脉高压(IPAH)归于第一组。该疾病的进展机制尚不明确,但最近有证据指出是由于三层血管壁内的细胞生长及增殖[73]。呼吸困难为最常见的症状,超声心动图检查有一定帮助,联合右心导管监测结果共同做出诊断[73]。治疗包括支持治疗、适当锻炼、华法林抗凝、利尿及肺血管扩张剂治疗[73]。根据患者的功能状态分级使用肺血

表 45.1 世界卫生组织对肺动脉高压的分组

第1组	肺动脉高压
第1′组	肺静脉闭塞性疾病
第2组	左心疾病所致肺动脉高压
第3组	慢性肺疾病或低氧血症所致肺动脉高压
第4组	慢性血栓栓塞性肺疾病
第5组	病因不明的多种病因所致的肺动脉高压

管扩张剂[72]。根据指南,肺动脉高压患者使用血管扩张剂治疗可以延长生存时间,改善生活质量,并降低肺移植风险。

体外生命支持

对于出现呼吸衰竭的患者,在疾病晚期使用呼吸机辅助治疗也可能无法提供足够的氧合。在这种情况下,需要额外的支持治疗来为患者争取一定恢复时间或帮助患者过渡到肺移植[74]。最常用的肺部支持治疗为体外膜肺氧合(ECMO)(参见第50章)。ECMO分为两种类型:静脉-静脉(V-V)和静脉-动脉(V-A)。V-V ECMO通过中心静脉导管引出去氧血液,在体外进行氧合后再回输入中心静脉循环。相反,V-A ECMO主要进行心肺支持,与心脏手术过程中的心肺分流术相似。ECMO的获益及死亡率取决于患者的选择、潜在疾病的进展情况及ECMO实施中心的专业素质。既往的研究并未发现其在生存率上的优势。最近发表的研究显示,使用ECMO的严重ARDS患者的生存率高于单独使用机械通气而不使用ECMO的患者[75]。ECMO是否为提高生存率的必要治疗以及是否有必要将患者转至医疗质量更好的医院,这类问题还需进一步研究证实。

总结

肺脏是维持血流动力学的必要器官之一,它可以提供氧合、通气以及激素分泌。健康的呼吸系统具有强大的内在储备功能,因此可以承受单肺通气。然而,由于肺脏直接暴露于外界环境,因此极易受到误吸、吸入剂、雾化剂等影响,并易暴露于感染因素。当患者无法通过自身肺组织得到足够的氧合来维持生存时,机械通气可以维持组织氧合和通气。当患者病情加重时,需要使用ECMO来维持身体需求或帮助患者过渡到移植手术。

(肖增丽 译 朱凤雪 校)

参考文献

1. Marino PL. The ICU Book. 3rd ed. Philadelphia: Lippincott Williams and Wilkins; 2006.
2. Hlastala MP, Albert AJ. Physiology of Respiration, 2nd ed. Oxford: Oxford University Press; 2001.
3. D'Alonzo GE, Danzker DR. Respiratory failure, mechanisms of abnormal gas exchange, and oxygen delivery. Medical Clinics of North America. 1983;67(3):557–571.
4. Covelli HD, Nessan VJ, Tuttle WK. Oxygen derived variables in acute respiratory failure. Critical Care Medicine. 1983;11(8):646–649.
5. Janssens P, Pache JC, Nicod LP. Physiological changes in respiratory function associated with ageing. European Repiratory Journal. 1999;13:197–205.
6. Robinson TD, Freiberg DB, Regnis JA, et al. The role of hypoventilation and ventilation-perfusion redistribution in oxygen-induced hypercapnia during acute exacerbations of chronic obstructive pulmonary disease. American Journal of Respiratory and Critical Care Medicine. 2000;161:1524–1529.
7. Eldridge F. Blood lactate and pyruvate in pulmonary insufficiency. New England Journal of Medicine. 1966;274(16):878–883.
8. Jackson R. Pulmonary oxygen toxicity. Chest. 1985;88:900–905.
9. Kotecha S, Allen J. Oxygen therapy for infants with chronic lung disease. Archives of Disease in Childhood. 2000;87(3):234.
10. Siobal MS. Pulmonary vasodilators. Respiratory Care. 2007;52(7):885–889.
11. Taylor R, Zimmerman JL, Dellinger RP, et al. Low-dose inhaled nitric oxide in patients with acute lung injury. A randomized controlled trial. JAMA. 2004;291(13):1603–1609.
12. Puri N, Dellinger RP. Inhaled nitric oxide and inhaled prostacyclin in acute respiratory distress syndrome: what is the evidence. Critical Care Clinics. 2011;27(3):561–587.
13. Johnson M. Molecular mechanisms of B2-adrenergic receptor function, response, and regulation. Journal of Allergy and Clinical Immunology. 2005;117(1):18–24.
14. Walters EH, Gibson PG, Lasserson TJ, et al. Long-acting beta2-agonists for chronic asthma in adults and children where background therapy contains varied or no inhaled corticosteroid. Cochrane Database of Systemic Reviews. 2007;24(1):1385.
15. Lötvall J, Palmqvist M, Arvidsson P, et al. Levalbuterol and racemic albuterol: are there therapeutic differences? Journal of Allergy and Clinical Immunology. 2001;108(5):726–731.
16. Flynn RA, Glynn DA, Kennedy MP. Anticholinergic treatment in airways diseases. Advances in Therapy. 2009;26(10):908–919.
17. Walters JA, Gibson PG, Wood-Baker R, et al. Systemic corticosteroids for acute exacerbations of chronic obstructive pulmonary disease. Cochrane Database of Systematic Reviews. 2009;1:CD001288.
18. Quon BS, Fitzgerald JM, Lemiere C, et al. Increased versus stable doses of inhaled corticosteroids for exacerbations of chronic asthma in adults and children. Cochrane Database of Systematic Reviews. 2010;12:CD007524.
19. Peter JV, John P, Graham PL, et al. Corticosteroids in prevention and treatment of acute respiratory distress syndrome (ARDS) in adults: meta-analysis. British Medical Journal. 2008;3(336):1006–1009.
20. Hay DWP. Pharmacology of leukotriene receptor antagonists: more than inhibitors of bronchoconstriction. Chest. 1997;111:35S–45S.
21. Boswell-Smith V, Spina D, Page CP. Phosphodiesterase inhibitors. British Journal of Pharmacology. 2006;147:S252–S257.
22. He B, Zhang F, Li X, et al. Meta-analysis of randomized controlled trials on treatment of pulmonary arterial hypertension. Circulation Journal. 2009;74(7):1458–1464.
23. Bolser DC. Cough suppressant and pharmacologic protussive therapy: ACCP evidence-based clinical practice guidelines. Chest. 2006;129:238S–249S.
24. Adhikari N, Burns KE, Meade MO, et al. Pharmacologic therapies for adults with acute lung injury and acute respiratory distress syndrome (Review). Cochrane Database of Systematic Reviews. 2010;7:1–55.
25. Ortiz G, Frutos-Vivar F, Ferguson ND, et al. Outcomes of patients ventilated with synchronized intermittent mandatory ventilation with pressure support: a comparative propensity score study. Chest. 2009;137(6):1265–1277.
26. Myers TR, MacIntyre NR. Respiratory controversies in critical care setting. Does airway pressure release ventilation offer important new advantages in mechanical

ventilator support? Respiratory Care. 2007;52(4):452–460.
27. Yoshida T, Rinka H, Kaji A, et al. The impact of spontaneous ventilation on distribution of lung aeration in patients with acute respiratory distress syndrome: airway pressure release ventilation versus pressure support ventilation. Anesthesia and Analgesia. 2009;109(6):1892–1900.
28. Chan KP, Stewart TE, Mehta S. High-frequency oscillatory ventilation for adult patients with ARDS. Chest. 2007;131(6):1907–1916.
29. Slutsky AS, Brown R, Lehr J, et al. High-frequency ventilation: a promising new approach to mechanical ventilation. Medical Instrumentation. 1981;15(4): 229–233.
30. Sud S, Sud M, Friedrich JO, et al. High frequency oscillation in patients with acute lung injury and acute respiratory distress syndrome (ARDS): systemic review and meta-analysis. British Medical Journal. 2010;18(340):1–11.
31. Kress JP, Pohlman AS, O'Connor MF, et al. Daily interruption of sedative infusions in critically ill patients undergoing mechanical ventilation. New England Journal of Medicine. 2000;342(20):1471–1477.
32. Girard TD, Kress JP, Fuchs BD, et al. Efficacy and safety of a paired sedation and ventilator weaning protocol for mechanically ventilated patients in intensive care (Awakening and Breathing Controlled trial): a randomised controlled trial. Lancet. 2008;371:126–134.
33. Zambon M, Vincent JL. Mortality rates for patients with acute lung injury/ARDS have decreased over time. Chest. 2008;133(5):1120–1127.
34. Bernard GR, Artigas A, Brigham KL, et al. The American-European Consensus Conference on ARDS. Definitions, mechanisms, relevant outcomes, and clinical trial coordination. American Journal of Respiratory Critical Care Medicine. 1994;149(3):818–824.
35. Tomashefski J. Pulmonary pathology of adult respiratory distress syndrome. Clinics in Chest Medicine. 1990;11(4):593–619.
36. Nuckton TJ, Alonso JA, Kallet RH, et al. Pulmonary dead-space fraction as a risk factor for death in the acute respiratory distress syndrome. New England Journal of Medicine. 2002;346(17):1281–1286.
37. Taut FJ, Rippin G, et al. A search for subgroups of patients with ARDS who may benefit from surfactant replacement therapy: a pooled analysis of five studies with recombinant surfactant protein-C surfactant (Venticute). Chest. 2008;134(4): 724–732.
38. Dellinger RP, Zimmerman JL, et al. Effects of inhaled nitric oxide in patients with acute respiratory distress syndrome: results of randomized phase II trial. Inhaled Nitric Oxide in ARDS Study Group. Critical Care Medicine. 1998; 26(1):15–23.
39. Steinberg KP, Hudson LD, Goodman RB, et al. Efficacy and safety of corticosteroids for persistent acute respiratory distress syndrome. New England Journal of Medicine. 2006;354(16):1671–1684.
40. Ventilation with lower tidal volumes as compared with traditional tidal volumes for acute lung injury and the acute respiratory distress syndrome. The Acute Respiratory Distress Syndrome Network. New England Journal of Medicine. 2000;343(18):1301–1308.
41. Moloney ED, Griffiths MJ. Protective ventilation of patients with acute respiratory distress syndrome. British Journal of Anaesthesia. 2004;92(2):261–270.
42. Brower RG, Lanken PN, MacIntyre N, et al. Higher versus lower positive end-expiratory pressures in patients with the acute respiratory distress syndrome. New England Journal of Medicine. 2004;351(4):327–336.
43. Montgomery AB, Stager MA, Carrico CJ, et al. Causes of mortality in patients with adult respiratory distress syndrome. American Review of Repiratory Disease. 1985;132(3):485–489.
44. Christie JD, Edwards LB, Aurora P, et al. The Registry of the International Society for Heart and Lung Transplantation: twenty-sixth Official Adult Lung and Heart-Lung Transplantation Report-2009. Journal of Heart and Lung Transplantation. 2009;28(10):1031–1049.
45. Centers for Disease Control and Prevention (CDC). Deaths from chronic obstructive pulmonary disease–United States, 2000–2005. MMWR. Morbidity and Mortality Weekly Report, 2008; 57(45):1229–1232.
46. Murray CJ, Lopez AD. Alternative projections of mortality and disability by cause 1990–2020: Global Burden of Disease Study. Lancet. 1997;349(9063):1498–1504.
47. Rabe KF, Hurd S, Anzueto A, et al. Global strategy for the diagnosis, management, and prevention of chronic obstructive pulmonary disease: GOLD executive summary. American Journal of Respiratory and Critical Care Medicine. 2007;176(6):532–555.
48. Shapiro S, Reilly J, Rennard S. Chronic Bronchitis and Emphysema. In: Murray and Nadel's Textbook of Respiratory Medicine. Philadelphia, PA: Elsevier Saunders; 2010: 919–967.
49. Shapiro SD, Ingenito EP. The pathogenesis of chronic obstructive pulmonary disease: advances in the past 100 years. American Journal of Respiratory Cell and Molecular Biology. 2005;32(5):367–372.
50. Thompson AB, Daughton D, Robbins RA, et al. Intraluminal airway inflammation in chronic bronchitis. Characterization and correlation with clinical parameters. American Review of Repiratory Disease. 1989;140(6):1527–1537.
51. Terzano C, Conti V, Petroianni P, et al. Effects of postural variations on carbon monoxide diffusing capacity in healthy subjects and patients with chronic obstructive pulmonary disease. Respiration; International Review of Thoracic Diseases. 2009;77(1):51–57.
52. Vincken W, van Noord JA, Greefhorst AP, et al. Improved health outcomes in patients with COPD during 1 yr's treatment with tiotropium. European Respiratory Journal. 2002;19(2):209–216.
53. Quon BS, Gan WQ, Sin DD. Contemporary management of acute exacerbations of COPD: a systematic review and metaanalysis. Chest. 2008;133(3):756–766.
54. Nocturnal-Oxygen-Therapy-Trial-Group. Continuous or nocturnal oxygen therapy in hypoxemic chronic obstructive lung disease: a clinical trial. Annals of Internal Medicine. 1980;93(3):391–398.
55. Ram FS, Picot J, Lightowler J, et al. Non-invasive positive pressure ventilation for treatment of respiratory failure due to exacerbations of chronic obstructive pulmonary disease. Cochrane Database of Systematic Reviews. 2004;(3):CD004104, 1–73.
56. Boucher R, K. M, Yankaskas J. Cystic Fibrosis. In: Murray and Nadel's Textbook of Respiratory Medicine. 5th ed. Philadelphia, PA: Elsevier Saunders; 2010: 985–1084.
57. Mogayzel PJ Jr, Flume PA. Update in cystic fibrosis 2009. American Journal of Respiratory and Critical Care Medicine. 2010;181(6):539–544.
58. Yankaskas JR, Marshall BC, Sufian B, et al. Cystic fibrosis adult care: consensus conference report. Chest. 2004;125:1S–39S.
59. Burns JL, Emerson J, Stapp JR, et al. Microbiology of sputum from patients at cystic fibrosis centers in the United States. Clinical Infectious Diseases. 1998;27(1): 158–163.
60. Cai Y, Chai D, Wang R, et al. Effectiveness and safety of macrolides in cystic fibrosis patients: a meta-analysis and systemic review. Journal of Antimicrobial Chemotherapy. 2011;66:968–978.
61. Thomas J, Cook DJ, Brooks D. Chest physical therapy management of patients with cystic fibrosis. American Journal of Respiratory and Critical Care Medicine. 1995;151(3 Pt 1):846–850.
62. Fuchs HJ, Borowitz DS, et al. Effect of aerosolized recombinant human DNase on exacerbations of respiratory symptoms on pulmonary function in patients with cystic fibrosis. The Pulmozyme Study Group. New England Journal of Medicine. 1994;8(331):637–642.
63. Wallis C. Mucolytic therapy in cystic fibrosis. Journal of the Royal Society of Medicine. 2001;94(Suppl 40):17–24.
64. Fauroux B. Why, when and how to propose noninvasive ventilation in cystic fibrosis? Minerva Anesthesiologica. 2011;77(11):1108–1114.
65. Flaherty KR, King TJ Jr, Raghu G, et al. Idiopathic interstitial pneumonia: what is the effect of a multidisciplinary approach to diagnosis? American Journal of Respiratory and Critical Care Medicine. 2004;170(8):904–910.
66. Noble P. Idiopathic pulmonary fibrosis: natural history and prognosis. Clinics in Chest Medicine. 2006;27(1 Suppl 1):S11–S16.
67. Panos RJ, Mortenson RL, Niccoli SA, et al. Clinical deterioration in patients with idiopathic pulmonary fibrosis: causes and assessment. American Journal of Medicine. 1990;88(4):396–404.
68. Selman M, Morrison L, Noble P, et al. Infiltrative and Interstitial Lung Diseases. In: Murray and Nadel's Textbook of Respiratory Medicine. Philadelphia, PA: Elsevier Saunders; 2010: 1356–1397.
69. Kozower BD, Meyers BF, Smith MA, et al. The impact of the lung allocation score on short-term transplantation outcomes: a multicenter study. Journal of Thoracic and Cardiovascular Surgery. 2008;135(1):166–171.
70. Nathan SD, Noble PW, Tuder RM. Idiopathic pulmonary fibrosis and pulmonary hypertension: connecting the dots. American Journal of Respiratory and Critical Care Medicine. 2007;175(9):875–880.
71. Stern JB, Mal H, Groussard O, et al. Prognosis of patients with advanced idiopathic pulmonary fibrosis requiring mechanical ventilation for acute respiratory failure. Chest. 2001;120(1):213–219.
72. Badesch DB, Abman SH, Simonneau G, et al. Medical therapy for pulmonary arterial hypertension: updated ACCP evidence-based clinical practice guidelines. Chest. 2007;131(6):1917–1928.
73. Channick R, Lewis R. Pulmonary Hypertension. In: Murray and Nadel's Textbook of Respiratory Medicine. Philadelphia, PA: Elsevier Saunders; 2010:1224–1243.
74. Ota K. Advances in artificial lungs. Journal of Artificial Organs. 2010;13(1): 13–16.
75. Peek GJ, Mugford M, Tiruvoipati R, et al. Efficacy and economic assessment of conventional ventilatory support versus extracorporeal membrane oxygenation for severe adult respiratory failure (CESAR): a multicentre randomised controlled trial. Lancet. 2009;374:1351–1363.

人工器官和辅助设备

第 46 章
透析

Myriam Farah, John S. Gill

引言

当前肾移植离不开透析的使用。与其他维持生命的器官移植不同，在其他移植领域中，缺乏终末期器官衰竭可靠的、长期的替代物（例如，肝、肺）或者只是最近期才获得了可靠的替代物（心脏、小肠），肾移植出现的同时伴随着透析技术的改善。确实可以这样说，大部分肾移植的存在是由于肾移植可以缓解肾衰竭的急性后果，并且这样做使得移植团队可以参与移植物工作。同样地，肾移植的财务处理也受到与透析范围有关的政策（见第 140 章和第 143 章）的极大影响。同样，全面掌握肾移植内容需要适当了解透析操作，并且获得、维持透析通路的技术也是移植医生必备的技能。

本章将向读者介绍透析概况，分为以下三部分：回顾透析的应用及不同透析方法对肾移植预后影响的流行病学资料；透析技术概述及相关的体外循环疗法；肾移植和非肾移植受体应用透析的详细讨论。阅读本章可同时参考第 28 章和第 37 章，这两章介绍了移植受体选择、移植指征以及等待肾移植手术的患者的管理。

流行病学

透析对肾移植预后的影响

透析可清除部分代谢废物。尿毒症、血容量过多伴随其他代谢异常（如氮质血症、钙磷代谢异常）可加速病理状态的进展，包括动脉硬化性疾病、血管钙化和左室肥厚，从而导致透析患者死亡率升高。透析和医疗手段的进展改善了透析患者的生存，然而移植等待者的年死亡率仍为 3%~5%[1]。患者对于尿毒症的耐受是不同的，糖尿病及老年患者透析的死亡率最高。

移植前透析治疗的维持期越长，这与移植物的生存期下降有关，可能是因为透析时并发疾病的进展在移植后没有得到逆转[2]。这部分基于以下事实：有功能的异体移植物存活的患者常合并肾功能受损，可能会继续处于慢性肾病相关并发症的风险之中[3]。未行透析的初次移植患者移植术后预后最好[4]。初次移植患者的预后更好是由于初次移植与非初次移植受体不同，而不是相对较短的尿毒症暴露的不良影响造成的，这通过目前可获得的观察性研究无法解决。

初次移植的时机仍未有定论。在 1994—2000 年一项美国初次移植成人受体的研究中，移植时估计肾小球滤过率（GFR）小于或超过 15mL/min 对于预后没有影响[5]。在临床实践中，GFR<20mL/min 并且没有尿毒症症状及体征是考虑行初次肾移植的最重要指征。对于初次肾移植的患者，要严密观察肾功能受损速度、尿毒症症状及体征。对于初次肾移植的患者，如果出现体征或者生化指标异常且无法通过常规医疗手段进行控制，利用短期的透析来纠正尿毒症也许是必需的（表 46.1）。

透析死亡率对肾移植预后的影响

目前单中心研究缺乏鉴别移植预后差异的能力，

表 46.1　急诊透析指征

- 难以纠正的高钾血症
- 难以纠正的酸中毒
- 难治性肺水肿
- 尿毒症性心包炎或者心包积液
- 尿毒症性脑病

而注册病例分析研究中混杂因素较多，因此透析死亡率和肾移植预后的关系尚不清楚。腹膜透析(PD)可以自我管理,因而为需要弹性透析治疗时间表和(或)有旅游需求的患者所钟爱。相应地,相较于血液透析,腹膜透析的患者生活中更加积极向上，有更好的功能状态和更少的伴随疾病的负担。在注册病例的研究中,这些差异没有进行充分的阐释。与此观点相一致的发现是腹膜透析患者比血液透析患者有更大的可能性接受移植[6]。

在一项基于美国肾脏病数据系统(USRDS)数据的研究分析中发现,腹膜透析与血液透析的患者相比,移植物的长期存活或者死亡并没有差异，尽管腹膜透析患者死亡供体移植物失败的风险稍高并且存在统计学差异[6]。死亡供体移植物损失的长期风险主要由于移植后 3 个月内移植物有较高的失活风险。在腹膜透析的患者中,死亡供体移植物移植早期损失的风险较高,而移植物延迟功能恢复的概率较低（可能由于腹膜透析患者的自体肾有更好的残余功能)。腹膜透析患者移植物早期失败较多的原因尚不清楚。然而,在一组资料可用于分析移植物失败原因的病例研究中，移植物失败的患者有较高的移植物血栓形成概率[6,7]。急性排斥反应并无差异。其他研究也证实腹膜透析患者有更高的移植物血栓形成概率,在理论上也可以解释:由于抗凝蛋白透过腹膜透析膜而丢失，机体处于获得性高凝状态[7]。一项小样本回顾性单中心研究发现,预防性使用阿司匹林可降低肾血管血栓形成的发生[8]。然而,在向腹膜透析患者推荐任何干预方法之前，大样本对照研究是必需的。

目前的研究没有发现腹膜透析和血液透析患者存在急性排斥反应差异。对于移植物延迟功能恢复,先前的研究发现腹膜透析患者有更高的霉酚酸(MPA)清除率[9];然而,近期的研究却没有发现腹膜透析与血液透析患者之间的这种差异,并且保持 MPA 的剂量可能对于透析患者维持其治疗有效性是必需的。然而,霉酚酸葡萄糖苷(MPAG)确实在透析患者机体积聚,并可能导致胃肠不耐受[9,10]。

过去已有大量研究不断指出腹膜透析患者容易出现腹腔、血液、手术切口及置管位置的细菌感染;然而,相较于血液透析患者,感染风险是否更高尚不清楚[11,12]。

没有研究分析透析治疗(比如通过夜间血液透析、日常血液透析或者血液透析滤过增加代谢废物的清除)是否会缓解尿毒症对于移植预后的影响。

透析及相应的体外治疗

透析指征

急诊透析用于治疗尿毒症无法纠正的致命并发症(表 46.1)。急诊透析指征也适用于长期慢性透析患者、进展期慢性肾脏病患者尚未开始透析治疗以及急性肾损伤患者,亦包含移植物延迟功能恢复患者。

血液透析

过程

血液透析中，血液在包含透析膜的体外通路中流转,多余的水分和溶质被透析膜清除后流回患者体内[13]。血液和透析液在透析膜的两边相对流动。溶质渗透通过透析膜而被清除，而水分的清除则是利用透析膜两边的静水压差。常规血液透析中,渗透是溶质清除的主要形式;而在血液透析滤过中,溶质也可以经由对流清除。

透析环路

透析环路包括一个血管通路(将血液从患者体内导出)、透析通路(可以连接患者到体外循环通路)、透析机、透析液和透析膜(图 46.1)。现代透析机可以精确控制液体清除,并且可以不清除溶质而仅仅清除液体。需要使用抗凝剂以避免体外环路中血液凝固，通常使用肝素。

透析处方

透析处方包含治疗的频率和持续时间、血液和透析液的流速,透析膜的类型以及透析液的成分。可以增加透析治疗的频率和持续时间以提高代谢废物和液体的清除率,在长期血液透析的患者中可见临床获益[14-16]。在急诊透析中，透析治疗的频率和持续时间依赖于透析的指征。表 46.2 显示了常用的透析处方。

血管通路

长期血液透析患者的经典血管通路有动静脉造瘘(AVF)、动静脉移植物(AVG)及中心静脉导管(CVC)。CVC 是联通中心静脉循环的皮下通路（深静脉长期留

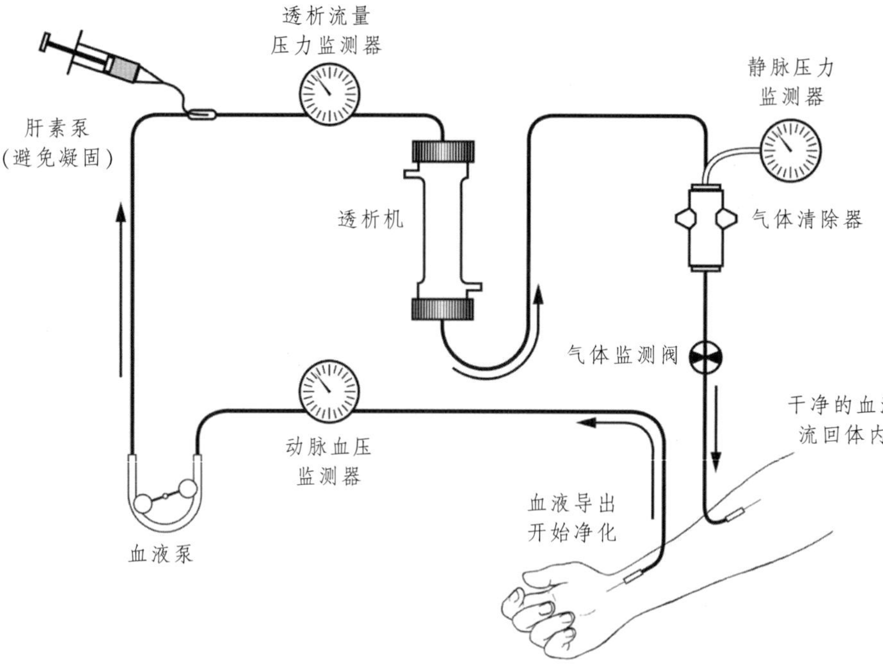

图 46.1 血液透析环路。透析环路包括一个血管通路可以将血液从患者体内导出、透析通路可以连接患者到体外循环通路、透析机(未显示)、透析液(未显示)和透析膜。血液和透析液(未显示)在透析膜的两边反向流动。通过分子渗透通过透析膜来实现溶质的清除,溶质则是向低渗透压的方向流动透过透析膜被清除。整个环路通常使用肝素避免血液凝固。(Reproduced from http://www.catalog.niddk.nih.gov/imagelibrary.)

表 46.2 血液透析处方

	经典处方	变动
透析膜	合成中空纤维;高流量;表面积 1.8m²	纤维素合成中空纤维;低流量;表面积 1.8~2.5m²
透析液		
钠(mEq/L)	138~140	130~155
钾(mEq/L)	2	0~4
碳酸氢盐(mEq/L)	35	28~40
钙(mmol/L)	1.25	1.25~1.75
镁(mmol/L)	0.75	0.5~1.0
葡萄糖和氯	标准	
透析液流速(mL/min)	500	300~800
血液流速(mL/min)	350	200~400
抗凝	肝素 500U,初始 500U/h,维持	肝素 500~1500U,初始 500~1500U/h,维持 其他替代治疗:不使用肝素,局部使用柠檬酸盐,局部使用肝素并用鱼精蛋白拮抗,达那肝素钠
持续时间(h)	4	2~8
透析频率(次数/周)	3	3~7
液体移除(L/每次治疗)	2L	0~5L
透析液温度(℃)	36.5	35~37

置导管)。

AVF 是动静脉的直接吻合,AVG 是使用合成材料来连接动静脉(图 46.2)。AVF 和 AVG 在使用前需要 4~8 周的成熟时间。透析时,穿刺针直接置入 AVF 或者 AVG 用于血液的导出和回流。CVC 是双腔导管,通常置入颈内静脉、锁骨下静脉或者股静脉(图 46.2)。CVC 置入后可以立即使用。不用时,CVC 需要使用抗凝药封管。

并发症

由于液体及溶质清除所致

透析失衡综合征是由于颅内水肿所致的神经症状和体征[17]。确切的病因尚不清楚,但是与快速液体、溶质清除相关。由于血钾、钙快速清除所致心律失常、血钠和钙快速改变所致癫痫、快速液体清除所致低血压则是其他常见的并发症[18]。

由于血液暴露于体外环路所致

尽管技术取得了很大的进步,血液流经体外通路仍然会有各种各样的问题,包括出血、血液凝固、血小板减少症、感染及空气栓塞。当血液接触透析膜时会导致细胞因子释放和补体激活。现代使用的透析膜多为生物相容材料,与以前的纤维素透析膜相比,减少了细胞因子的释放。然而,透析器反应仍然会发生。这种反

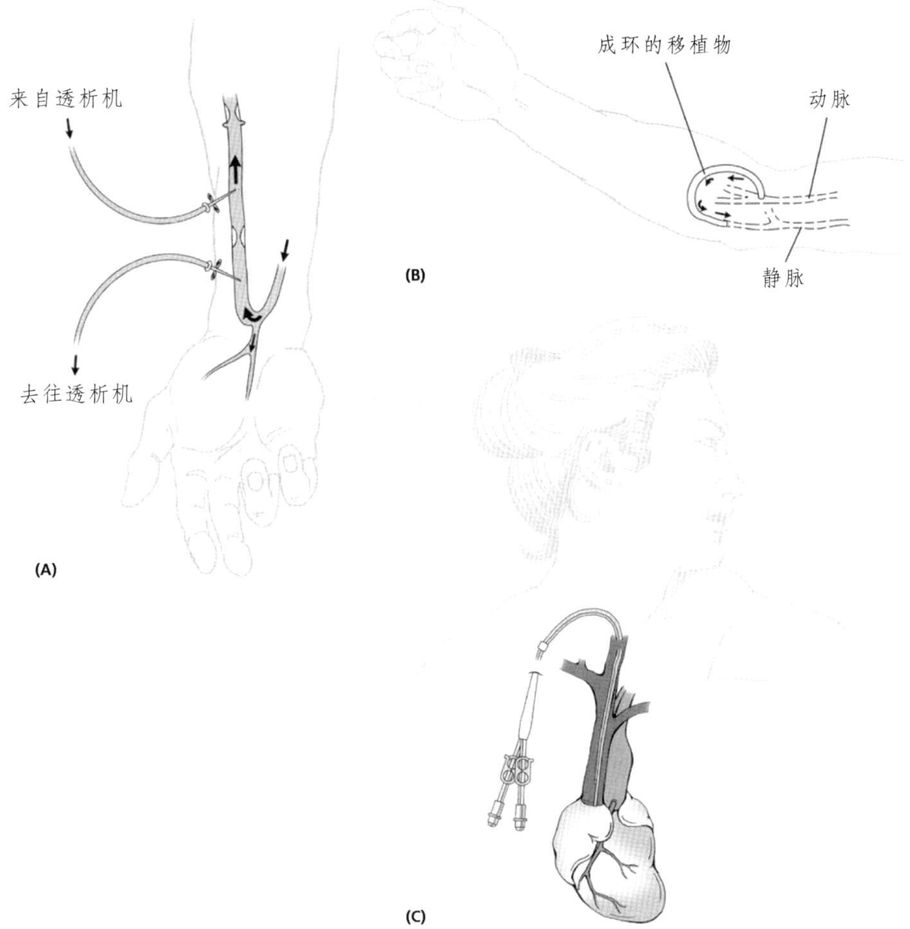

图 46.2 不同的透析血管通路。经典的血液透析通路有(A)动静脉造瘘(AVF)、(B)动静脉移植物(AVG)及(C)中心静脉导管(CVC)。CVC 是联通中心静脉循环的皮下通路(深静脉长期留置导管)。(Reproduced from http://www.catalog.niddk.nih.gov/imagelibrary.)

应可以是轻微的过敏反应,也可能是过敏性休克[19]。

透析液相关并发症

血液透析的患者暴露于大量的透析液。液体必须经过过滤、软化、升温、调整 pH、反向渗透纯化,并且有机溶质必须吸收后才能进入透析环路。患者可能暴露于矿物质污染物、化学污染物或者细菌内毒素才会出现感染或者溶血[20]。

血管通路相关并发症

AVF/AVG 最主要的并发症是感染、血栓形成和盗血综合征。感染可表现为炎症、败血症或外周播散(心内膜炎、骨髓炎)等局部症状。治疗包括检查(血液和局部引流液的培养)、抗感染治疗和偶尔的外科干预[21]。血栓形成可能由于狭窄或者局部、系统性的低血压导致的血流缓慢所致。应尽量避免在有 AVG、AVF 的肢体进行血压测量、放血、外周静脉导管穿刺置入。避免低血压和局部压迫也是十分重要的[22]。动脉血流经由 AVF/AVG 分流可能会导致远端肢体缺血(盗血综合征)。肢体缺血或者疼痛,尤其在透析时,通常提示盗血综合征。移植术前应评估盗血综合征的症状和体征来了解在移植术中是否需要手术干预以保护肢体功能[23]。

CVC 比 AVF/AVG 具有更高的感染概率。感染可以是局部的或者全身的。疑似感染时的检查和治疗与 AVF/AVG 感染类似。移除导管时要综合考虑患者血流动力学状态、微生物培养结果、治疗反应及是否同时存在透析导管或置管位置局部感染[24]。导管功能不良表现为透析时无法获得合适的血流速度和由于导管内环流的发生率增高导致的代谢废物清除率下降。导管功能不良的主要原因包括置管位置不佳、导管折曲、导管内纤维蛋白鞘形成。干预措施包括调整患者或者导管的位置、导管内溶栓治疗,甚至有时需要重新置管[25]。

中心静脉狭窄可以发生在所有类型的血管通路[26]。通常表现为上肢水肿;其他表现包括胸膜渗出、侧支循环的形成、穿刺困难以及上腔静脉综合征。

腹膜透析

过程

留置的腹膜透析导管用于向腹膜腔滴注和移除透析液。患者自身的腹膜被用作透析膜,使得分子和水分渗透进入透析液,随后被引流出体外。腹膜透析液包含渗透性分子,可以促使液体离开腹膜血管透过腹膜进入腹膜腔里的透析液中。通过重复灌注、引流这一过程,腹膜透析取得逐渐且持续的溶质和液体清除[27]。

患者经过训练可以日常在家中进行腹膜透析,或者手工进行[持续不卧床腹膜透析(CAPD)],或者使用循环机器[自动腹膜透析(APD)]。在没有进行交换时,腹膜腔可以是空置的("干腹"),也可以充满溶液("湿腹")。CAPD的患者通常使用右旋葡萄糖溶液在白天进行3~4次交换,夜晚间歇。APD的患者则在夜间进行几次交换,白天间歇。治疗的选择通常基于患者的偏好。通常不需要系统性抗凝治疗。

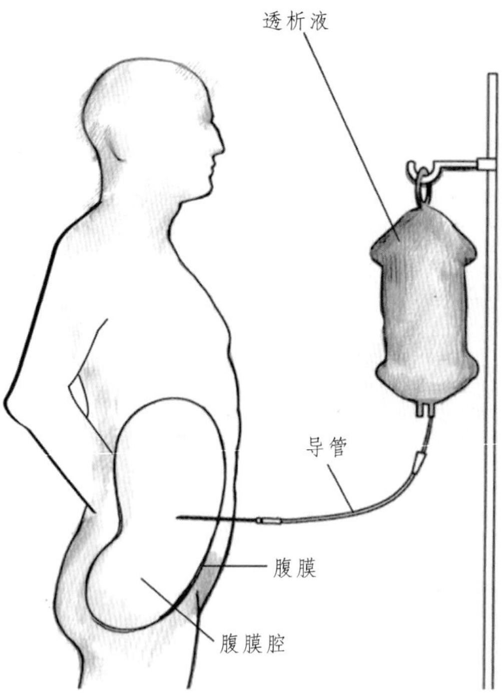

图46.3 腹膜透析过程。腹膜透析装置包括导管、透析液、连接管和转换装置。腹膜透析导管用于向腹膜腔滴注和移除透析液。患者自身的腹膜被用作透析膜,使得分子和水分渗透进入透析液,随后被引流出体外。(Reproduced from http://www.catalog.niddk.nih.gov/imagelibrary.)

装置

腹膜透析装置包括导管、透析液、连接管和转换装置(图46.3)。透析液已预先包装好,由无菌液体混合渗透性物质、电解质和缓冲液构成。渗透性物质的类型和浓度以及间歇的时间决定了液体量和交换中清除的溶质量。高渗透性的溶液清除更多的液体和溶质。最常使用的渗透性物质是右旋葡萄糖和艾考糊精,一种高分子葡萄糖多聚体。腹膜透析导管包含一个远端的腹内部分和皮下通道部分[28]。导管的变动包括导管腹内段远端的形状(直或者弯曲的)、植入腹壁的袖口数目(一个或者两个)以及皮下通道部分的设计式样(直或者永久弯曲的)。最常用的导管是双袖Tenckhoff导管(图46.4)。

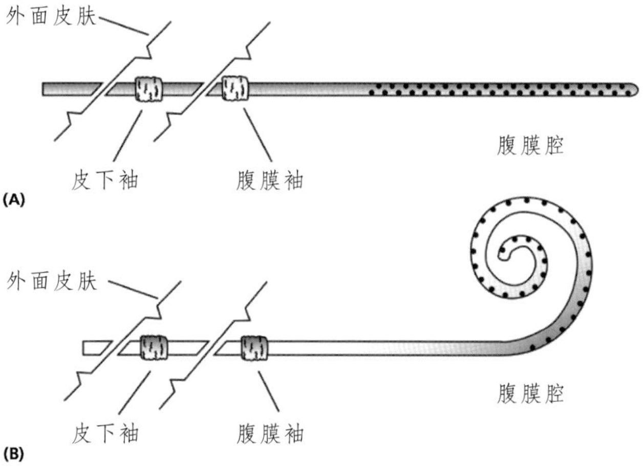

图46.4 双袖Tenckhoff导管,是最常使用的腹膜透析导管。腹膜透析导管包含一个远端进入腹腔的部分、一个中间植入腹壁的部分和一个皮下通道。(Reproduced from http://www.catalog.niddk.nih.gov/imagelibrary.)

处方

经典的腹膜透析处方及其变动可见表46.3。透析处方需要经常进行再评估,因为腹膜的交换功能和残余肾脏功能会随着时间而不断变化,导致液体和溶质的清除量发生改变[29]。腹膜炎也会引起腹膜交换功能的急性改变,需要改变腹膜透析处方。

并发症

感染

腹膜透析导管相关感染可以表现为出口感染、皮

表 46.3　腹膜透析处方

	经典处方	变动
交换频率	每天 3 次	每天 3~5 次(CAPD),每夜 3~5 次(CCPD)
每次交换容量(L)	2	1.0~2.5
腹膜透析液	1.5%右旋葡萄糖	0.5%,1.5%,2.5%,或者 4.25%右旋葡萄糖,或者碳酸氢盐,氨基酸
间歇抗凝	一夜,7.5%艾考糊精无	一夜干腹(无液体),如果 CCPD 则一白天肝素注射进入腹膜透析液
标准电解质构成	钠 130~137mEq/L 钾 0~2mEq/L 钙 1.25~1.75mmol/L 镁 0.5~1.5mmol/L 乳酸 35~40mEq/L	

CAPD,连续非卧床腹膜透析;CCPD,持续循环腹膜透析。

下通道感染或者腹膜炎。出口和皮下通道感染表现为局部炎症反应和(或)渗出。腹膜炎通常是由滴入或引流透析液时腹膜腔污染引起的。腹膜炎的诊断标准见表 46.4。与腹腔内疾病所致腹膜炎进行区分,需要回顾围术期的处置,并常常需要相应影像学检查的帮助。单独的、不复杂的出口感染可经由仔细的护理和抗感染治疗(局部或口服)治愈。如果出口感染进展或者合并腹膜炎、皮下通道感染,那么腹膜透析导管必须被移除[30]。通常应用腹腔内抗感染疗法来治疗腹膜炎,对于真菌、分枝杆菌、复杂细菌、难治性及复发性腹膜炎,拔除导管是必须的。

表 46.4　腹膜炎的诊断

可疑 PD 腹膜炎	确诊 PD 腹膜炎	怀疑继发性腹膜炎
至少满足以下 1 条: 腹膜刺激征 发热 透析液浑浊 血白细胞升高 另外: 透析液 WBC >100 个/mL 同时中性粒细胞 >50 个/mL	透析液阳性涂片或者培养	透析液培养阳性,发现多种致病菌 透析液粪样物质 透析液淀粉酶升高 透析液脂肪酶升高

PD,腹膜透析;WBC,白细胞计数。

机械并发症

腹膜透析导管留置于皮下通道和出口,可能使腹膜力量减弱,进而导致腹壁疝形成。管周渗漏表现为皮下肿胀、引流量减低或液体积聚于导管周围。部分患者腹壁或者会阴的水肿会进展,需要外科干预和(或)拔除腹膜透析导管[31]。单侧胸膜强积液提示存在腹膜腔和胸膜腔的交通。引流失败常常与便秘或导管相关问题有关,如导管移位、弯折、管腔被血栓阻塞或者被网膜压迫阻塞。腹膜透析导管的腹腔段很少引起腹腔器官的损伤而出现血性透析液。其他引起血腹的原因包括多囊肾囊破裂、排卵、子宫内膜异位症或者月经逆行。

腹膜透析液溶质相关并发症

传统的腹膜透析液使用乳酸进行缓冲,pH 值偏酸性,并且含有右旋葡萄糖。所有这些因素使得腹膜透析液部分生物不相容,从而随着时间延长导致腹膜功能丧失。基于右旋葡萄糖的透析液可以导致葡萄糖吸收引起代谢异常,包括高能量、高血糖症和血脂异常[27]。

持续肾脏替代疗法

持续肾脏替代疗法(CRRT)的主要形式是持续静脉-静脉血液透析(CVVHD)、持续静脉-静脉血液滤过(CVVH)和持续静脉-静脉血液透析滤过(CVVHDF)。增加血液滤过使得仅通过血液透析无法去除的大分子也可以被清除。

与常规血液透析相比,CRRT 使用更小的血液透析膜,血流及透析液的流速更低,因此透析的效率稍低[32]。透析效率通过 24 小时持续不断的透析得以弥补,从而全天溶质和液体的清除可以获得类似间断透析的效果。

技术

CRRT 环路的设置与常规血液透析类似,但也有一些值得注意的不同之处(表 46.5)。大多 CRRT 装置使用预包装的透析液和替换液。电解质和缓冲液已经设定好,在常规血液透析中无法进行改变。电解质和酸碱平衡紊乱的患者需要进行系统纠正。治疗中通常不会使用先前存在的 AVF/AVG,而倾向于使用透析导管。需要进行局部或者系统性抗凝。在大多数病情较重的患者中更倾向于使用局部柠檬酸盐抗凝。

优势、不足及指征

血流动力学不稳定的患者比起常规血液透析更加

表 46.5 CRRT 与常规间断血液透析(HD)的比较

	CRRT	间断 HD
每日持续时间(h)	24	4
血流速率(mL/min)	100~200	250~350
透析液速率(mL/min)	15~45	300~800
置换液速率(mL/min)	15~45	N/A
小时滤过速率(mL/min)	50~150	100~1500
透析膜面积	0.9~1.2m²	1.8~2.5m²
抗凝治疗	1.局部柠檬酸盐 2.肝素 3.不使用	1.肝素 2.Citrasate 透析液 3.达那肝素钠 4.普通盐水冲洗
透析液成分	确定的(几种可用的溶质)	可变动的
置换液成分	确定的(几种可用的溶质)	N/A

耐受 CRRT。CRRT 提供了虽然相对缓慢但持续的溶质和液体的清除，因此可以实时根据临床反应和液体状态进行调整。对于大多数患者而言,该技术使得使用血液制品、全肠外营养和用药变得更加容易,避免了容量负荷过多和电解质紊乱。

实际透析量常常远远少于 CRRT 要求的剂量。CRRT 常常被各种各样的原因打断，由于该技术透析相对缓慢,丢失的时间很难被弥补回来。尽管有抗凝方面的优势,CRRT 滤网的半衰期较短,每 48~72 小时需要更换滤网[33]。用局部柠檬酸盐抗凝来代替系统肝素抗凝,需要时时进行监测以免出现高钙血症、高钠血症和碱中毒。因此,CRRT 是一种昂贵的、耗费大量人力的透析方法[34]。

尽管存在诸多优点,CRRT 并没有改善危重患者的生存或者肾功能恢复情况[35]。尽管如此,该方法对于血流动力学不稳定的患者仍然是最可行的透析方法。CRRT 不应该用于需要快速液体或溶质清除的临床情况，包括摄取毒物的患者和危及生命的高钾血症等情况。

治疗性血浆置换

治疗性血浆置换(TPE)是一种体外治疗方法,用于清除血浆中大分子量的物质(如抗体、异常蛋白)或补充不足的血浆因子。

技术

血液中分离血浆可以通过离心分离或者膜过滤[36]。离心分离通常使用特殊的离心机。离心的好处包括可以通过使用双腔静脉导管从外周静脉循环中导出和回输血液,并且可以选择性地从血液中分离细胞(细胞净化)。这种低效率方法的劣势是治疗时间较长、血小板减少症发生率较高及使用柠檬酸盐抗凝存在相关并发症。与之相对比,膜过滤需要使用高透过性膜和一个标准的透析机器,并且需要置入双腔 CVC 来获得充足的血流速率。虽然可以使用柠檬酸盐抗凝,肝素仍然是最常用的抗凝剂。

当血浆被移除后，静脉内容量必须被补足以避免低血压的发生。置换所选用的液体依赖于 TPE 的指征[37]。新鲜冰冻血浆(FFP)替换正常血浆蛋白,避免凝血因子和免疫球蛋白的损耗。FFP 的劣势则包括血液转播疾病的风险、输血相关肺损伤、柠檬酸盐相关低钙血症和荨麻疹,以及罕见的过敏反应。只有需要进行血浆因子置换时才推荐 FFP，比如发生 HUS/TTP 或者有出血风险。白蛋白是大多数情况下置换液体的首选,因为它没有血液传播疾病的风险，并且过敏反应的风险较低。白蛋白结合的盐溶液当发生低渗透时可以考虑使用。在血浆置换中快速移除和输注含蛋白溶液可造成血管内压力分布不均,因此,即使很小的移除和输注液体量的不匹配也会对血压造成较大影响。相应地,输注的盐溶液的量应该控制在总置换容量的 20%~40%。

1 倍血浆容量进行置换可降低 65%的 IgG,1.5 倍血浆容量的置换则可使之降低 75%[38]。血浆置换容量的计算主要依靠患者体重及血细胞比容(hct),可以依据下面的简化公式进行估算：

血浆容量=0.07×体重(kg)×(1−hct)

治疗性血浆置换的量取决于治疗的指征、患者的耐受程度和临床治疗反应。血浆置换中移除大分子物质受限于每次治疗后血管外间隙的再分布(反弹)。一般而言,在达到预期抗体降低水平之前需要 3~5 次治疗(图 46.5)。表 46.6 显示了常用的血浆置换处方及相应的变动。

并发症

轻微过敏反应(如皮肤瘙痒、皮疹)发生率在 5%~10%。中等治疗反应如低血压或者心律失常(由于低钾血症或者低钙血症)的发生率大约为 5%,而严重过敏反应则<3%。该疗法相关死亡率很低(<0.05%)[39]。

当使用 FFP 进行 TPE 时并发症更加常见,包括过敏反应、严重支气管痉挛和输血相关肺损伤。在使用

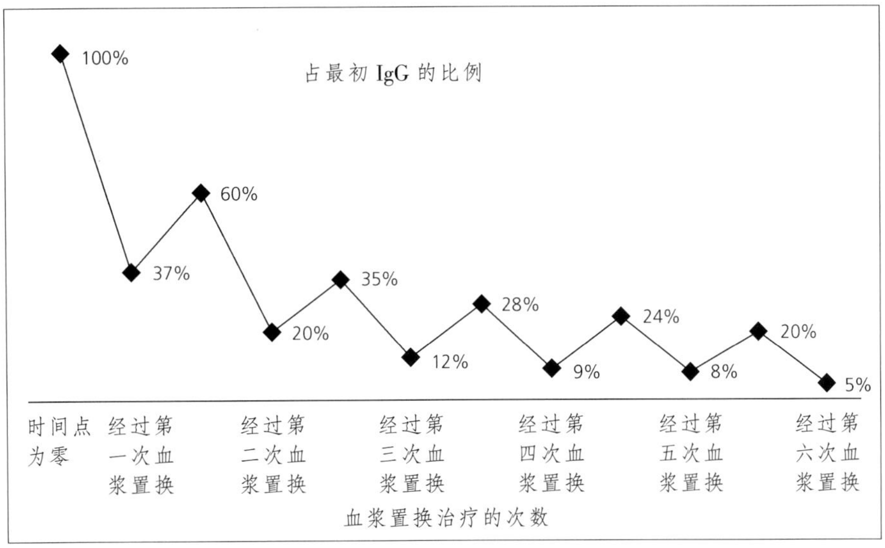

图 46.5 血浆置换治疗后血浆 IgG 水平的变化。一般而言,1 倍血浆容量进行置换可降低 65%的 IgG,血浆置换中移除大分子物质受限于每次治疗后血管外间隙的再分布(反弹)。在达到预期抗体降低水平之前需要 3~5 次治疗。

表 46.6 治疗性血浆置换处方

	经典处方	变动
模式	离心或者膜过滤	
置换容量	1 倍血浆容量	1~2 倍血浆容量
置换液	白蛋白加盐溶液(生理盐水或者格林液)	新鲜冰冻血浆
血浆清除速率(mL/min)	60	30~100
抗凝药物	柠檬酸盐(联合预防性补钙)	肝素
治疗策略	基于治疗指征及治疗反应的个体化治疗	

ACEI 类药物的患者中过敏反应也许更加常见。FFP 中使用的柠檬酸盐可以结合钙,从而降低离子钙而不影响总钙浓度,这可以导致许多症状,如感觉异常、肌肉痉挛、恶心、呕吐、QT 间期延长及心律不齐、低血压和手足抽搐。可以预防性地使用静脉补充钙(如血浆置换开始 15 分钟后,将 10mL 浓度为 10%的氯化钙溶液在超过 30 分钟的时间内输入)。柠檬酸盐也会引起碱血症,特别是并发肾功能衰竭的患者。容量相关并发症包括由于移除和置换液体容量不匹配引发的低血压和肺水肿。低血压和呼吸困难也可由于血液与体外循环通路接触导致的补体激活或者对消毒用的环氧乙烷敏感而引起。低钾血症导致的心律失常可在白蛋白置换中发生。钾离子通常会加入到白蛋白溶液中以避免低钾血症发生。移除凝血因子可导致出血倾向。在出血风险较高的患者中,应该考虑使用 FFP 作为置换液。移除免疫球蛋白和补体可导致感染风险升高,同时使用的免疫抑制药物可增大该风险。血浆置换可有效清除药物,因此,治疗药物应在血浆置换后再使用,并且增加对重要治疗药物浓度的监测可能是必要的。

肾移植及非肾移植受体的透析管理

肾移植等待者

移植前评估

肾移植等待者的初次评估可发生于移植前的几天到几年不等。表 46.7 列举了与移植联系最为密切的透析相关问题。

透析史

了解首次透析治疗的日期对于预测移植时间和制订移植计划是十分重要的。虽然死亡捐献者移植时机不能被准确地预测,了解 ABO 血型和群体反应性抗体(PRA)能够提供等待时间的合理评估。基于预期的等待时间和合并症病史,可以帮助决定移植等待者的管理策略,包括追踪性调查和重复临床或者手术评估[40-42]。

表 46.7 透析患者的移植前评估

透析史	初次透析治疗的日期及指征，更改治疗模式的原因
透析通路	血液透析通路、腹膜透析导管
透析充分程度	透析是否充分的临床评估和计量
残余肾脏功能	残余肾脏功能的评估及保护
药物治疗的干预	移植前、移植后

透析通路

充分了解目前血液透析和腹膜透析的位置、类型及健康状态。

血液透析患者长期使用中心静脉透析通路可导致中心静脉狭窄及瘢痕形成，使得移植时留置中心静脉导管变得困难。有频繁AVF/AVG血栓形成病史的患者需要进一步的评估。有复发性血管通路血栓形成的患者在移植时如何管理仍不清楚。血管通路狭窄是血栓形成最常见的原因，移植前并不需要特殊的处理。然而，在一些情况下，有必要进行血栓形成倾向的诊断检查以除外系统性凝血异常，这些异常可能导致移植物血栓形成。当抗凝治疗仅仅是为了维持血管通路而没有系统性凝血异常，在移植中和移植后不应该使用抗凝治疗。

在腹膜透析的患者中，应该充分了解先前腹膜透析导管相关的并发症及导管缺失的原因。因严重的腹膜感染合并间歇性肠梗阻或者腹腔积液而移除腹膜透析管，也许提示存在包裹性腹膜硬化症，这是一种不常见的疾病，可使得移植手术变得困难，术后可能导致肠梗阻的发生[43]。

透析充分程度

评估透析的充分程度需要评估尿毒症的症状和体征，并使用数学公式计算透析时代谢废物的清除率（表46.8）。有多种方法可估计血液透析或腹膜透析的代谢废物的清除率，但是这些方法不在本章论述范围内[44,45]。不充分的透析通常预示着透析环路或者透析膜存在问题，或者患者没有严格遵守透析处方。改善透析处方可帮助优化移植前患者的管理。

残余肾脏功能

了解残余肾脏功能和尿量对于移植术后立即评估移植物功能十分重要。由于血清肌酐水平与GFR非线性相关，GFR的微小改变将引起晚期肾脏病患者血肌酐水平的巨大改变。残余肾脏功能不应该仅仅通过血肌酐水平来监测。24小时尿量和肌酐清除率能更精确地评估残余肾脏功能。然而，由于患者收集尿液不方便，此检测方法的有效性受到限制并且容易出现误差。另外，肾小管分泌的肌酐可造成肾脏功能被高估。

有多种基于血清肌酐水平的公式可用来评估肾脏功能（表46.9）[46]。Cockcroft-Gault公式基于年龄、体重、身高和血清肌酐水平来评估肌酐清除率。在临床实践中，体重和身高有时会限制该公式的应用。来自于肾脏病膳食改变（MDRD）研究的公式不需要测量身高和体重，目前在临床中广泛应用。最初的6变量MDRD公式需要测量血白蛋白、血肌酐，不如4变量公式简单。MDRD公式还没有在病态肥胖患者及除了非裔美国人的少数民族人群中得到证实。在MDRD研究中，为了克服血肌酐测量相关的GFR偏倚，研究者推荐世界范围内使用同位素稀释浓度光谱法（IDMS）来作为肌酐测量的标准方法。一个新的因子“175”（不同于“186”）随后被推荐用于MDRD公式中肌酐试验。MDRD公式在肾功能基本正常的患者中符合性较差。在这种情况下，最近提出的慢性肾脏病流行病学协作（CKD-EPI）公式更加适用[47]。Cockcroft-Gault公式和MDRD公式均可用于监测终末期慢性肾脏病患者的肾脏功能，也包含先行移植手术等待者。

表 46.8 评估透析充分程度

	血液透析患者	腹膜透析患者
透析不充分的临床表现	难治性高血压、难治性充血性心力衰竭、进行性左室肥厚、难治性高磷血症、难以纠正的酸中毒、意识模糊、认知改变、恶心、呕吐、皮肤瘙痒不明原因的乏力	
透析不充分的数学指标	Kt/V<1.2（临床目标>1.4），URR<65%（临床目标>70%）	每周Kt/V<1.7，每日腹膜透析超滤量<750mL（或者如果残余肾无功能则小于250mL）

Kt/V，透析量，K是透析膜清除率（mL/min），t是透析治疗持续时间（min），V是尿素分布容积（mL）。URR，尿素降低比率。

表 46.9　评估肾脏功能的公式

名称	公式	变量
肌酐清除率(mL/min) 需要体表面积来调整	$GFR=[U_{Cr}\times V]/S_{Cr}$	U_{Cr}=尿肌酐浓度(umol/L) S_{Cr}=血清肌酐浓度(umol/L) V=24 小时尿量(L)
Cockcroft-Gault 需要体表面积来调整	$[(140-年龄)\times W(kg)/Cr\times 72]\times 0.85$(如果女性)	W=清瘦者的体重 Cr=血清肌酐浓度(mg/dL)
最初 6 变量 MDRD	$170\times S_{cr}^{0.999}\times 年龄^{0.176}\times BUN^{-0.170}\times Alb^{+0.318}\times 0.762$ (如果女性)×1.18(如果黑人)	S_{Cr}=血清肌酐水平(mg/dL) 年龄使用年来计数 BUN=血浆尿素氮浓度(mg/dL) Alb=血白蛋白浓度(g/dL)
改良 4 变量 MDRD	$186.3\times S_{Cr}^{-1.154}\times 年龄^{-0.203}\times 0.742$(如果女性)×1.21(如果黑人)	S_{Cr}=血清肌酐水平(mg/dL) 年龄使用年来计数
改良 4 变量 MDRD IDMS	$175\times S_{Cr}^{-1.154}\times 年龄^{-0.203}\times 0.742$(如果女性)×1.21(如果黑人)	S_{Cr}=血清肌酐水平(mg/dL) 年龄使用年来计数
CKD-EPI	$141\times \min(S_{Cr}/\kappa,1)^{\alpha}\times \max(S_{Cr}/\kappa,1)^{-1.209}\times 0.993^{(年龄)}\times 1.018$ (如果女性)×1.159(如果黑人)	S_{Cr}=血清肌酐水平(mg/dL) κ=女性为 0.7,男性为 0.9 α=女性为-0.329,男性为-0.411 min=S_{Cr}/κ 的最小值或 1 max=S_{Cr}/κ 的最大值或 1 年龄使用年来计数

残余肾脏功能是透析患者生存的重要预测指标[48]。医生应该尽量保护残余肾脏功能，特别是先行和腹膜透析患者。比如避免使用肾毒性药物、低血压及放射造影剂。当这些损害无法避免时，应邀请肾脏病专家会诊,以尽量采取预防性手段来缓解肾毒性。

用药管理

慢性透析患者的大多数药物在移植术后都不再使用。由于与免疫抑制药物的相互作用或者移植肾功能的建立，某些药物需要在移植术后进行剂量调整（表46.10)。药物剂量调整超出了本章的讨论范围,建议用药时与医院药剂专家进行沟通以保证患者安全。

表 46.10　围移植术期用药管理

通常停用的药物	继续使用的药物但需要进行剂量调整
磷结合剂(如碳酸钙、sevalemer、镧),华法林(如果只是用于维持血管通路)，血小板 P2Y12 受体抑制剂★(如氯吡格雷、噻氯匹定、普拉格雷),维生素 D 类似物(如 1-α 骨化三醇),利尿药,ACEI,他汀类	胰岛素和口服降糖药 抗痉挛药 阿司匹林 抗心律失常药物 抗抑郁药物 β 受体阻滞剂 可乐定

★依赖于指征。裸金属冠状动脉支架需要双重抗血小板治疗,需联合阿司匹林和血小板 P2Y12 受体抑制剂应用至少 1 个月,最好 6 个月;药物洗脱支架需要至少 6 个月,最好 12 个月。推荐咨询心脏病学专家。

围术期管理

急诊移植前透析

移植时很容易忽视透析相关的管理问题。移植前透析的绝对适应证见表 46.1。除了绝对适应证,透析通常基于最后一次透析治疗的时间、患者的临床评估或者由于捐献者的原因或者冷缺血时间造成的移植物延迟功能恢复。

移植前处方的优化

肝素通常在血液透析患者的处方中被停用，以减少移植术中出血的风险。血液透析前测量血钾浓度并且调整透析液中血钾浓度，可以减少术中高钾和低钾血症的风险。依据手术时机,高容量患者血液透析的时间可以延长至达到目标体重。移植前血液透析治疗,尤其是应用了生物不相容的透析膜，可能会激活炎症介质,但是这种担忧仍然仅存在于理论中。并且,生物相容透析膜的广泛应用更是减少了这种担忧。如果有条件,移植前的透析治疗应优先使用生物相容透析膜。

腹膜透析可一直持续到移植手术。如果需要快速纠正高容量负荷或者高钾血症,可以每30~90分钟进行一次快速腹膜透析,可以手动也可以使用循环机器[49]。在快速腹膜透析时,不应使用艾考糊精透析液。在术前,应清空腹膜腔内的透析液。

长时间或者频繁透析的患者,也包括进行夜间透析的患者,也许会有较低的围术期血压,然而此类患者移植物延迟功能的发生率并不高[50,51]。一些移植中心常规将夜间透析的患者在活体移植术前1周改为血液透析,以降低移植术后低血压的风险(私下交流自Chris Chan,Toronto General Hospital)。

透析通路的维护

围术期要优先考虑保护性措施来维护AVF/AVG[52]。在移植术前,CVC导管每次透析后均需行抗凝处理。腹膜透析导管可以移除,也可以在术后留在原位晚些时候移除。保留腹膜透析管的好处是移植术后如果需要可以经此进行透析,主要的不便则包括导管相关感染的风险、移植术后导管需要护理,以及之后需要额外的操作来移除导管[53]。保留还是移除腹膜透析管需要权衡移植术后透析的可能性和腹膜透析管相关感染的风险。腹膜炎发生的风险可以通过腹膜炎病史及移植术前对腹膜透析管出口的临床检查来进行衡量[54]。

术后管理

移植术后透析的时机

移植术后透析的绝对适应证见表46.1。对于移植术后生命体征不平稳的患者,最重要的是患者的安全。急诊透析可能会影响检查移植物失功的原因。

严重的术后高钾血症是医学急症,在准备紧急透析同时需要进行临时的医学处置。包括静脉注射碳酸氢盐、钙剂、胰岛素和葡萄糖。肛塞降钾树脂可能引起结肠扩张,甚至穿孔,在术后早期最好避免使用。

少尿或者无尿的患者通常处于容量高负荷状态。对血容量过多的耐受也受基础心肺功能状态的影响,包括既往充血性心力衰竭、心脏瓣膜病、慢性肺病、睡眠呼吸暂停和肥胖。对于这些患者,如果没有血流动力学不稳定,应适当限制容量复苏。对于尿量稀少的情况,在尿量恢复或者透析完成之前,避免拔管是明智的。通过常规血液透析或者单独的超滤可以进行紧急降低容量负荷。

术后应立即评估透析通路的功能完整性。造瘘应是通畅的,术中透析导管应妥善放置。在进行血液透析之前,需要临床试验检查造瘘及影像学检查确认中心静脉透析导管的位置。罕见情况下,可以通过透析通路灌注重要的药物,并且在没有透析适应证的情况下,必须确认透析导管的位置。对于腹膜透析导管的病例,在进行腹膜透析之前,需要与移植医生直接沟通以确认腹膜的完整性。

对于少尿的患者,需要了解移植前残余肾脏功能、尿量及透析的时机,以评估移植物的功能。需要回顾麻醉记录来确认输入的静脉溶液、血液制品的量及类型,是否发生低血压、心律失常,失血量及术中总尿量。回顾手术记录、与移植医生沟通对于了解任何供体相关或者手术相关的问题是十分重要的,这些也许会影响移植术后早期透析的决定及时机。

对移植物状态及术中情况的了解有帮于进行透析决策。特别是来自于扩大标准的死亡供体、延长的冷缺血或者热缺血时间以及进行了复杂血管吻合的移植均可提供重要的预后信息。了解另外一个肾脏是否出现移植物延迟功能也是十分有用的。

移植物延迟功能恢复的透析处置

除了透析的绝对适应证,在不同的移植单位透析的指征通常具有主观性且十分多样。因此,在移植术后第1周通过透析来定义移植物延迟功能恢复是有问题的,这也造成了临床回顾分析移植物延迟功能恢复的发生率及预后不一致。另外,一些研究发现移植物延迟功能恢复与移植物生存降低有关,通过是否需要行透析治疗来定义移植物延迟功能恢复会导致这样的认知,即透析对移植物是有害的。

实验和临床观察发现,人体血液暴露于生物不相容的透析膜可导致移植物延迟功能恢复的时间延长。20个世纪90年代末期,三项小的随机试验没有显示出使用生物相容性透析膜和生物不相容性透析膜对移植物延迟功能恢复影响的差异[55-57]。虽然这些研究没有充分的证据来回答这个问题,目前生物相容性透析膜的广泛使用已经使这类研究缺乏意义。

透析中的低血压会导致移植物灌注不足、移植物延迟功能恢复延长,甚至还会造成移植物血栓形成。在血液透析的患者中,频繁、延长的透析和低温透析能够预防透析低血压的发生[58]。同样,单独的超滤能够仅仅去除多余的液体。具备功能良好的腹膜透析管并且没有手术禁忌证的患者，在治疗移植物延迟功能恢复时可以使用腹膜透析，因为比起血液透析，腹膜透析出现低血压的风险更低。在血流动力学不稳定的患者中，推荐使用CRRT。

仔细评估容量状态，限制或者避免使用加重低血压的药物是十分重要的。特别是对于已经诊断为移植物延迟功能恢复的患者，使用淋巴细胞消耗抗体和血液透析是有益的。

移植术后管理

血液透析通路

成功的移植受体不再需要进行透析，为避免导管相关感染，移植术后几周将安排拔除透析导管。当透析导管在原位时，直到拔除之前，需每周评估透析位置的健康状态，并用抗凝药物进行冲洗、封管。

血液透析、动静脉瘘、移植物

少数患者会出现自发性的AVF/AVG关闭[59]。对于已经建立移植物功能的患者，何时行常规手术封闭功能良好的AVF/AVG尚未形成共识[60]。维持造瘘的好处包括保留将来透析的通道和避免手术。过去较少血管通路选择的患者更倾向于维持造瘘。缺点则是动静脉瘘对心脏功能有潜在的害处[61]。有研究发现存在基础心脏疾病的患者在建立动静脉瘘之后出现了心力衰竭[62]。

对于移植受体术后关闭造瘘的影响，有研究得出了不一致的结果。两项小的前瞻性观察性研究发现，关闭造瘘可以改善超声观测的心脏三维结构，然而这些改变何时能改善患者的预后仍不清楚，因此并不推荐常规术后关闭造瘘[63,64]。手术关闭造瘘的指征包括心脏血流动力学恶化、造瘘相关并发症(如感染、盗血综合征)及患者进行高危活动的安全考虑[60]。

腹膜透析通路

移除前应每周检查、冲洗腹膜透析通路以避免感染。移除腹膜透析通路的主要目的是减少感染和腹膜炎的发生风险[65]。

心脏移植等待者

等待移植的慢性透析患者

各种因素相互影响，包括心输出量减低、神经内分泌通路紊乱导致的水钠潴留以及药物的作用，使等待心脏移植并且依赖透析的患者清除多余的液体变得十分困难[66]。由于液体和溶质的快速交换，此类患者通常无法耐受常规血液透析。对于此类患者，通常需要增加透析的频率和(或)时间。腹膜透析也许更加理想，因为腹膜透析中液体、溶质的清除更加温和、更容易被耐受[67]。

不需要透析的失代偿心力衰竭患者

心力衰竭患者没有合并终末期肾病，但是对利尿药产生抵抗并且出现急性心力竭衰失代偿，外周血静脉-静脉超滤（UF）和缓慢持续的超滤便于液体的清除。在一项没有设置盲法的研究中，200例急性失代偿心力衰竭患者被随机分组进行超滤或者利尿药治疗。在最初的48小时内，体重减轻和呼吸困难改善没有显著差异。然而，超滤组在90天内有更高的体重下降和液体清除率，以及更低的再入院率。两者在肾功能和低钾血症的发生率方面没有差异。可能的机制是超滤组去除了等张的液体，而利尿药去除了低张的液体[68]。超滤是心力衰竭失代偿患者大剂量利尿药的重要替代疗法，特别是肾功能受损或者利尿药抵抗的患者。然而，在超滤常规用于终末期心力衰竭患者之前，仍然需要进一步的研究来证实。

需要透析的重症患者

对于心源性休克的患者，CRRT是首选的透析形式。当CRRT无法获得时，应改良常规血液透析环路和处方使其尽可能与CRRT类似。频繁(最好每天)和长时间(超过8h)的透析，并且保持血液及透析液的流速缓慢，可以使透析近似于CRRT。这项技术[缓慢、低效率透析(SLED)]也可以和CRRT一样被血流动力学不稳定的患者所耐受[69]。

需要机械辅助装置的患者

需要主动脉内球囊反搏、心室辅助装置进行心脏支持的患者，透析准备包括了解这些装置在体内的位置、经皮通路的位置和抗凝治疗的类型[70]。曾有报道指出持续静脉-静脉血液透析(CVVHD)系统和主动脉内球囊反搏(IABP)相互作用存在一定的危险[71]。CVVHD系统的滚压泵活动造成的电活动会被主动脉球囊所识别，从而产生加压和减压。电支持装置可以相互作用，在联合应用之前需充分检测它们的相容性。

需要体外膜肺氧合的患者

不可逆心源性休克的患者需要完全的心肺旁路支持，主要是动静脉体外膜肺氧合(VA-ECMO)[72]。在常规VA-ECMO中，大量的血液从股静脉中被抽出，流经氧气机和热交换器，在那里血红蛋白和氧气结合并释放二氧化碳，然后血液回流进入股动脉。流经ECMO环路的血流为4~5L/min。ECMO环路需要持续地抗凝，因而溶血和出血的风险较高。

心源性休克的ECMO支持患者经常并发急性肾功能损伤，需要进行肾脏替代疗法。这可以通过三种方法实现[73-75]。第一种方法是建立一个独立的血管透析环路，使CRRT环路与ECMO环路完全独立。这也许会受限于静脉通路的不足以及ECMO时系统的抗凝治疗。第二种方法是在氧气机后面增加血液透析膜。这种方法的缺点是不允许透析的参数调整独立于ECMO的参数。第三种方法是从ECMO环路中虹吸部分血液，让其流经CRRT透析环路，然后回流进入ECMO环路进行氧合。当地中心的医生应依据经验决定使用哪种方法。

术中透析

通过连接血液透析环路到心肺旁路泵(CBP)可以于术中施行血液透析。这可用于术中控制电解质(尤其是钾)和液体容量，从而避免术后急诊血液透析[76]。

心脏移植术后透析

心脏移植术后患者可以使用CRRT或者常规血液透析来进行透析。需要特别关注透析环路的抗凝和容量设定，这对于右心衰竭的患者十分重要。腹膜透析的患者移植术后可以继续进行腹膜透析，但需要管理好容量状态和通气参数。使用低容量的快速腹膜透析(每30~90min)需要避免容量负荷过多。

肝移植等待者

肝病患者并发肾功能不全，则死亡率较高[77]。第43章已进行过探讨，此类患者的管理充满挑战，经常需要对衰竭的肾脏进行支持治疗。透析只能用于急性肾功能损伤有望恢复肝衰竭患者，以及肝移植等待者或者正在进行评估肝移植的患者[78]。由于系统性血管扩张及短路导致系统性低血压、营养不良所致血浆渗透压减低及肝功能异常、凝血障碍、血小板减低导致出血风险增加等，透析变得十分困难[79]。肝脏清除血管扩张因子的能力降低，造成有效循环容量不足和水钠潴留。对于系统性低血压，血液透析很难去除腹水和外周水肿。

使用间断透析或者CRRT进行治疗是基于患者血流动力学稳定。CRRT理论上的优点是可逐渐纠正低钠血症，并且对颅内压力的影响较小[78]。CRRT环路中应避免使用局部柠檬酸盐抗凝剂，因为这会导致肝功能不全的患者柠檬酸盐中毒[33]。替代方法包括高流量CRRT而不使用抗凝治疗，以及局部肝素-鱼精蛋白抗凝。CRRT更适用于暴发性肝衰竭的患者，因为与常规血液透析相比，该疗法不会增加颅内压力[80]。

虽然能够获得部分小分子溶质及尿毒症毒物的清除，常规血液透析只能清除小分子溶质及尿毒症患者的部分毒性物质，大分子与蛋白结合的毒物无法清除，而在肝衰竭患者中，该类毒物大量积聚。对于严重肝功能不全的患者，增加大分子物质的清除率、改良血液透析的形式也许是有益的，但这需要更深入的研究来证实[81,82]。

对部分肝衰竭患者而言，腹膜透析也许是最可行的透析形式。相较于血液透析，腹膜透析的优势包括不需要使用抗凝治疗、更加缓和的液体清除、持续的溶质清除、引流腹水和含右旋葡萄糖的腹膜透析液。不足则是透析液中蛋白的丢失[83]。以前对于腹膜炎高发生率及患者中途退出的担心没有得到证实。

一些新的技术已经出现，可为肝肾衰竭患者提供支持帮助。包括膜系统或者吸附剂系统来提供透析、解毒治疗(如血液灌注、血液透析再吸收、血浆提取和选择性血浆滤过疗法)和基于细胞的疗法来复制肝脏的代谢功能。这些技术尚未经严格的试验证实，仍属试验性疗法。分子吸收再循环系统(MARS)通过白蛋白透析和CRRT来清除白蛋白结合毒素[84]。白蛋白透析液通过联合应用活性炭及阴离子交换树脂实现再生。MARS已经在少量肝肾综合征患者中试验性应用，并且与血液透析相比改善了这些患者的生存和血流动力学状态[85]。另外一些研究则发现对血管活性药物抵抗的肝肾综合征患者并没有获益[86]。一个类似但是相对简单的系统，单次白蛋白滤过透析(SPAD)使用常规血液透析环路，但是灌注白蛋白作为透析液。白蛋白通过透析环路,然后被清除。先前的研究比较了 SPAD 和 MARS,发现两者效用类似[87]。

在肝移植术中,切除病肝时下腔静脉和门静脉会被横断,这会降低静脉回流,心输出量会降低 40%~50%。门静脉吻合完成后,门静脉开放导致大量稀释的血液、钾离子及乳酸进入血液循环,引起低血压、高钾血症、代谢性酸中毒及凝血障碍(再灌注综合征)[88,89]。通常,移植术中会需要大量的血液及血浆。为了缓和这些因素的影响,术中透析(如 CRRT)已经在肝移植术中被采用。这特别适用于严重肾功能不全或者术前需要肾脏替代疗法的患者。这是部分中心术中采用 CRRT 的经验。然而,仍需研究明确术中 CRRT 的指征[89,90]。

总结

透析提供了有限但是可以耐受的代谢废物清除率,通过透析可以控制尿毒症、急性电解质紊乱和容量负荷过多所致的肾衰竭。有各种各样的透析方法和形式存在。这些方法适用于不同类型的肾衰竭,从急性肾衰竭患者等待肾功能恢复的短暂支持治疗,到等待肾移植或者无法行肾移植的患者的长期支持治疗,甚至到终末期的支持治疗。考虑到肾衰竭经常合并肝衰竭和心力衰竭,透析疗法是一种重要的支持疗法,不仅影响肾移植,还影响肝移植和心脏移植。透析疗法及各种各样的透析方法设备,仍然是每一名移植医生全部医疗设备的重要组成部分。

(刘晓 译 荀晓冬 朱继业 校)

参考文献

1. USRDS. Annual Data Report: Atlas of End Stage Renal Disease in the United States. National Institute of Health, National Institute of Diabetes and Digestive and Kidney Disease, 2010.
2. Meier-Kriesche HU, Port FK, Ojo AO, et al. Effect of waiting time on renal transplant outcome. Kidney International. 2000;58(3):1311–1317.
3. Gill JS, Pereira BJ. Chronic kidney disease and the transplant recipient. Blood Purification. 2003;21(1):137–142.
4. Kasiske BL, Snyder JJ, Matas AJ, et al. Preemptive kidney transplantation: the advantage and the advantaged. Journal of the American Society of Nephrology. 2002;13(5):1358–1364.
5. Ishani A, Ibrahim HN, Gilbertson D, Collins AJ. The impact of residual renal function on graft and patient survival rates in recipients of preemptive renal transplants. American Journal of Kidney Diseases. 2003;42(6):1275–1282.
6. Snyder JJ, Kasiske BL, Gilbertson DT, et al. A comparison of transplant outcomes in peritoneal and hemodialysis patients. Kidney International. 2002;62(4):1423–1430.
7. Ojo AO, Hanson JA, Wolfe RA, et al. Dialysis modality and the risk of allograft thrombosis in adult renal transplant recipients. Kidney International. 1999;55(5):1952–1960.
8. Robertson AJ, Nargund V, Gray DW, et al. Low dose aspirin as prophylaxis against renal-vein thrombosis in renal-transplant recipients. Nephrology, Dialysis, Transplantation. 2000;15(11):1865–1868.
9. Morgera S, Budde K, Lampe D, et al. Mycophenolate mofetil pharmacokinetics in renal transplant recipients on peritoneal dialysis. Transplant International. 1998;11(1):53–57.
10. MacPhee IA, Spreafico S, Bewick M, et al. Pharmacokinetics of mycophenolate mofetil in patients with end-stage renal failure. Kidney International. 2000;57(3):1164–1168.
11. Passalacqua JA, Wiland AM, Fink JC, et al. Increased incidence of postoperative infections associated with peritoneal dialysis in renal transplant recipients. Transplantation. 1999;68(4):535–540.
12. Vanholder R, Heering P, Loo AV, et al. Reduced incidence of acute renal graft failure in patients treated with peritoneal dialysis compared with hemodialysis. American Journal of Kidney Diseases. 1999;33(5):934–940.
13. Himmelfarb J, Ikizler TA. Hemodialysis. New England Journal of Medicine. 2010;363(19):1833–1845.
14. Chertow GM, Levin NW, Beck GJ, et al. In-center hemodialysis six times per week versus three times per week. New England Journal of Medicine. 2010;363(24):2287–2300.
15. Culleton BF, Walsh M, Klarenbach SW, et al. Effect of frequent nocturnal hemodialysis vs conventional hemodialysis on left ventricular mass and quality of life: a randomized controlled trial. JAMA 2007;298(11):1291–1299.
16. Rocco MV, Lockridge RS, Beck GJ, et al. The effects of frequent nocturnal home hemodialysis: the Frequent Hemodialysis Network Nocturnal Trial. Kidney International. 2011;80(10):1080–1091.
17. Lopez-Almaraz E, Correa-Rotter R. Dialysis disequilibrium syndrome and other treatment complications of extreme uremia: a rare occurrence yet not vanished. Hemodialysis International 2008;12(3):301–306.
18. Davenport A. Intradialytic complications during hemodialysis. Hemodialysis International. 2006;10(2):162–167.
19. Cheung AK. Biocompatibility of hemodialysis membranes. Journal of the American Society of Nephrology. 1990;1(2):150–161.
20. Hoenich NA, Levin R. The implications of water quality in hemodialysis. Seminars in Dialysis. 2003;16(6):492–497.
21. Jindal K, Chan CT, Deziel C, et al. Hemodialysis clinical practice guidelines for the Canadian Society of Nephrology. Journal of the American Society of Nephrology. 2006;17(3 Suppl 1):S1–S27.
22. Work J. Role of access surveillance and preemptive intervention. Seminars in Vascular Surgery. 2011;24(2):137–142.
23. Scali ST, Huber TS. Treatment strategies for access-related hand ischemia. Seminars in Vascular Surgery. 2011;24(2):128–136.
24. Mermel LA, Allon M, Bouza E, et al. Clinical practice guidelines for the diagnosis and management of intravascular catheter-related infection: 2009 Update by the Infectious Diseases Society of America. Clinical Infectious Diseases. 2009;49(1):1–45.
25. Chan MR. Hemodialysis central venous catheter dysfunction. Seminars in Dialysis. 2008;21(6):516–521.
26. Kundu S. Central venous disease in hemodialysis patients: prevalence, etiology and treatment. Journal of Vascular Access. 2010;11(1):1–7.
27. Teitelbaum I, Burkart J. Peritoneal dialysis. American Journal of Kidney Diseases. 2003;42(5):1082–1096.
28. Gokal R, Alexander S, Ash S, et al. Peritoneal catheters and exit-site practices toward optimum peritoneal access: 1998 update. (Official report from the International Society for Peritoneal Dialysis). Peritoneal Dialysis International. 1998;18(1):11–33.
29. Tzamaloukas AH, Raj DS, Onime A, et al. The prescription of peritoneal dialysis. Seminars in Dialysis. 2008;21(3):250–257.
30. Li PK, Szeto CC, Piraino B, et al. Peritoneal dialysis-related infections recommendations: 2010 update. Peritoneal Dialysis International. 2010;30(4):393–423.
31. Bernardini J. Peritoneal dialysis catheter complications. Peritoneal Dialysis International. 1996;16(Suppl 1):S468–S471.
32. O'Reilly P, Tolwani A. Renal replacement therapy III: IHD, CRRT, SLED. Critical Care Clinics. 2005;21(2):367–378.
33. Oudemans-van Straaten HM, Kellum JA, Bellomo R. Clinical review: anticoagulation for continuous renal replacement therapy–heparin or citrate? Critical Care. 2011;15(1):202.
34. Manns B, Doig CJ, Lee H, et al. Cost of acute renal failure requiring dialysis in the intensive care unit: clinical and resource implications of renal recovery. Critical Care Medicine. 2003;31(2):449–455.
35. Rabindranath K, Adams J, Macleod AM, et al. Intermittent versus continuous renal replacement therapy for acute renal failure in adults. Cochrane Database of Systematic Reviews. 2007;(3):CD003773.
36. Kaplan AA. Therapeutic plasma exchange: core curriculum 2008. American Journal of Kidney Diseases. 2008;52(6):1180–1196.

37. Okafor C, Ward DM, Mokrzycki MH, et al. Introduction and overview of therapeutic apheresis. Journal of Clinical Apheresis. 2010;25(5):240–249.
38. Ward DM. Conventional apheresis therapies: a review. Journal of Clinical Apheresis. 2011;26(5):230–238.
39. Mokrzycki MH, Balogun RA. Therapeutic apheresis: a review of complications and recommendations for prevention and management. Journal of Clinical Apheresis. 2011;26(5):243–248.
40. Gill JS, Rose C, Pereira BJ, et al. The importance of transitions between dialysis and transplantation in the care of end-stage renal disease patients. Kidney International. 2007;71(5):442–447.
41. Gill JS, Ma I, Landsberg D, et al. Cardiovascular events and investigation in patients who are awaiting cadaveric kidney transplantation. Journal of the American Society of Nephrology. 2005;16(3):808–816.
42. Pilmore H. Cardiac assessment for renal transplantation. American Journal of Transplantation. 2006;6(4):659–665.
43. Korte MR, Sampimon DE, Betjes MG, et al. Encapsulating peritoneal sclerosis: the state of affairs. Nature Reviews Nephrology. 2011;7(9):528–538.
44. Group HAW. Clinical practice guidelines for hemodialysis adequacy, update 2006. American Journal of Kidney Diseases. 2006;48(Suppl 1):S2–S90.
45. Group PDAW. Clinical practice guidelines for peritoneal adequacy, update 2006. American Journal of Kidney Diseases. 2006;48(Suppl 1):S91–S97.
46. Stevens LA, Padala S, Levey AS. Advances in glomerular filtration rate-estimating equations. Current Opinion in Nephrology and Hypertension. 2010;19(3): 298–307.
47. Stevens LA, Li S, Kurella Tamura M, et al. Comparison of the CKD Epidemiology Collaboration (CKD-EPI) and Modification of Diet in Renal Disease (MDRD) study equations: risk factors for and complications of CKD and mortality in the Kidney Early Evaluation Program (KEEP). American Journal of Kidney Diseases. 2011;57(3 Suppl 2):S9–S16.
48. Perl J, Bargman JM. The importance of residual kidney function for patients on dialysis: a critical review. American Journal of Kidney Diseases. 2009;53(6): 1068–1081.
49. Burdmann EA, Chakravarthi R. Peritoneal dialysis in acute kidney injury: lessons learned and applied. Seminars in Dialysis. 2011;24(2):149–156.
50. Pauly RP, Asad RA, Hanley JA, et al. Long-term clinical outcomes of nocturnal hemodialysis patients compared with conventional hemodialysis patients post-renal transplantation. Clinical Transplantation. 2009;23(1):47–55.
51. McCormick BB, Pierratos A, Fenton S, et al. Review of clinical outcomes in nocturnal haemodialysis patients after renal transplantation. Nephrology, Dialysis, Transplantation. 2004;19(3):714–719.
52. Chang TI, Paik J, Greene T, et al. Intradialytic hypotension and vascular access thrombosis. Journal of the American Society of Nephrology. 2011;22(8): 1526–1533.
53. Gokal R, Kost S. Peritoneal dialysis immediately post transplantation. Advances in Peritoneal Dialysis. 1999;15:112–115.
54. Bakir N, Surachno S, Sluiter WJ, et al. Peritonitis in peritoneal dialysis patients after renal transplantation. Nephrology, Dialysis, Transplantation. 1998;13(12): 3178–3183.
55. Valeri A, Radhakrishnan J, Ryan R, et al. Biocompatible dialysis membranes and acute renal failure: a study in post-operative acute tubular necrosis in cadaveric renal transplant recipients. Clinical Nephrology. 1996;46(6): 402–409.
56. Romão JE, Abensur H, de Castro MC, et al. Effect of dialyser biocompatibility on recovery from acute renal failure after cadaver renal transplantation. Nephrology, Dialysis, Transplantation. 1999;14(3):709–712.
57. Woo YM, Craig AM, King BB, et al. Biocompatible membranes do not promote graft recovery following cadaveric renal transplantation. Clinical Nephrology. 2002;57(1):38–44.
58. Davenport A. Using dialysis machine technology to reduce intradialytic hypotension. Hemodialysis International. 2011;15(Suppl 1):S37–S42.
59. De Lima JJ, Vieira ML, Molnar LJ, et al. Cardiac effects of persistent hemodialysis arteriovenous access in recipients of renal allograft. Cardiology. 1999;92(4): 236–239.
60. Manca O, Pisano GL, Carta P, et al. The management of hemodialysis arteriovenous fistulas in well functioning renal transplanted patients: many doubts, few certainties. Journal of Vascular Access. 2005;6(4):182–186.
61. Ferro CJ, Savage T, Pinder SJ, et al. Central aortic pressure augmentation in stable renal transplant recipients. Kidney International. 2002;62(1):166–171.
62. Stern AB, Klemmer PJ. High-output heart failure secondary to arteriovenous fistula. Hemodialysis International. 2011; Jan 12 [Epub ahead of print].
63. van Duijnhoven EC, Cheriex EC, Tordoir JH, et al. Effect of closure of the arteriovenous fistula on left ventricular dimensions in renal transplant patients. Nephrology, Dialysis, Transplantation. 2001;16(2):368–372.
64. Unger P, Wissing KM, de Pauw L, et al. Reduction of left ventricular diameter and mass after surgical arteriovenous fistula closure in renal transplant recipients. Transplantation. 2002;74(1):73–79.
65. McDonald MW, Sterioff S, Engen DE, et al. Renal transplantation in patients with indwelling continuous ambulatory peritoneal dialysis catheters. Journal of Urology. 1987;137(5):849–851.
66. House AA, Haapio M, Lassus J, et al. Therapeutic strategies for heart failure in cardiorenal syndromes. American Journal of Kidney Diseases. 2010;56(4): 759–773.
67. Cnossen N, Kooman JP, Konings CJ, et al. Peritoneal dialysis in patients with congestive heart failure. Nephrology, Dialysis, Transplantation. 2006;21(Suppl 2): ii63–ii66.
68. Costanzo MR, Guglin ME, Saltzberg MT, et al. Ultrafiltration versus intravenous diuretics for patients hospitalized for acute decompensated heart failure. Journal of the American College of Cardiology. 2007;49(6):675–683.
69. Fieghen HE, Friedrich JO, Burns KE, et al. The hemodynamic tolerability and feasibility of sustained low efficiency dialysis in the management of critically ill patients with acute kidney injury. BMC Nephrology. 2010;11:32.
70. Basra SS, Loyalka P, Kar B. Current status of percutaneous ventricular assist devices for cardiogenic shock. Current Opinion in Cardiology. 2011;26(6): 548–554.
71. Sakiewicz PG, Wright E, Robinson O, et al. Abnormal electrical stimulus of an intra-aortic balloon pump with concurrent support with continuous veno-venous hemodialysis. ASAIO Journal. 2000;46(1):142–145.
72. Westaby S, Anastasiadis K, Wieselthaler GM. Cardiogenic shock in ACS. Part 2: role of mechanical circulatory support. Nature Reviews Cardiology. 2012.
73. Yap HJ, Chen YC, Fang JT, et al. Combination of continuous renal replacement therapies (CRRT) and extracorporeal membrane oxygenation (ECMO) for advanced cardiac patients. Renal Failure. 2003;25(2):183–193.
74. Santiago MJ, Sánchez A, López-Herce J, et al. The use of continuous renal replacement therapy in series with extracorporeal membrane oxygenation. Kidney International. 2009;76(12):1289–1292.
75. Rubin S, Poncet A, Wynckel A. Baehrel B. How to perform a haemodialysis using the arterial and venous lines of an extracorporeal life support. European Journal of Cardio-Thoracic Surgery. 2010;37(4):967–968.
76. Ilson BE, Bland PS, Jorkasky DK, et al. Intraoperative versus routine hemodialysis in end-stage renal disease patients undergoing open-heart surgery. Nephron. 1992;61(2):170–175.
77. Wong LP, Blackley MP, Andreoni KA, et al. Survival of liver transplant candidates with acute renal failure receiving renal replacement therapy. Kidney International. 2005;68(1):362–370.
78. Wadei HM, Davis CL. Renal replacement therapy in the liver transplant candidate. Advances in Chronic Kidney Disease. 2009;16(4):250–255.
79. Oliver JA, Verna EC. Afferent mechanisms of sodium retention in cirrhosis and hepatorenal syndrome. Kidney International. 2010;77(8):669–680.
80. Gonwa TA, Wadei HM. The challenges of providing renal replacement therapy in decompensated liver cirrhosis. Blood Purification. 2012;33(1-3): 144–148.
81. Ozdemir FN, Tutal E, Sezer S, et al. Effect of supportive extracorporeal treatment in liver transplantation recipients and advanced liver failure patients. Hemodialysis International. 2006;10(Suppl 2):S28–S32.
82. Arata S, Tanaka K, Takayama K, et al. Treatment of hepatic encephalopathy by on-line hemodiafiltration: a case series study. BMC Emergency Medicine. 2010;10:10.
83. Chaudhary K, Khanna R. Renal replacement therapy in end-stage renal disease patients with chronic liver disease and ascites: role of peritoneal dialysis. Peritoneal Dialysis International. 2008;28(2):113–117.
84. Hassanein TI, Schade RR, Hepburn IS. Acute-on-chronic liver failure: extracorporeal liver assist devices. Current Opinion in Critical Care. 2011;17(2): 195–203.
85. Mitzner SR, Stange J, Klammt S, et al. Improvement of hepatorenal syndrome with extracorporeal albumin dialysis MARS: results of a prospective, randomized, controlled clinical trial. Liver Transplantation. 2000;6(3):277–286.
86. Wong F, Raina N, Richardson R. Molecular adsorbent recirculating system is ineffective in the management of type 1 hepatorenal syndrome in patients with cirrhosis with ascites who have failed vasoconstrictor treatment. Gut. 2010;59(3):381–386.
87. Kortgen A, Rauchfuss F, Götz M, et al. Albumin dialysis in liver failure: comparison of molecular adsorbent recirculating system and single pass albumin dialysis–a retrospective analysis. Therapeutic Apheresis and Dialysis. 2009;13(5):419–425.
88. Rettke SR, Janossy TA, Chantigian RC, et al. Hemodynamic and metabolic changes in hepatic transplantation. Mayo Clinic Proceedings. 1989;64(2): 232–240.
89. Sedra AH, Strum E. The role of intraoperative hemodialysis in liver transplant patients. Current Opinion Organ Transplantation. 2011;16(3):323–325.
90. Townsend DR, Bagshaw SM, Jacka MJ, et al. Intraoperative renal support during liver transplantation. Liver Transplantation. 2009;15(1):73–78.

第 47 章
人工肝、体内组织工程及器官打印

Igor M. Sauer, Nathanael Raschzok, Peter Neuhaus

引言

自 1963 年起，经过多年的发展，肝移植已经从一个试验性的治疗方法变成治疗致命性肝衰竭的标准治疗方法。然而，肝移植事业却逐渐受限于供肝的稀缺。为了改善合适供肝数目和等待移植患者数量的不匹配，人们在以下几方面进行了努力：优化器官分配、寻找死亡供肝的替代方法、发展支持或替代衰竭器官的体外方法。医生和基础研究者们迫切希望找到器官移植的替代方法和技术。为扩大捐献池，边缘器官获取和心脏死亡后捐献被广泛接受。然而，使用这些替代方法的器官和患者的生存率是降低的。肝脏支持装置是通过提供患者器官再生的环境（连接再生），或支持患者直到可以施行器官移植手术（连接移植）来改善预后的。在肝源性代谢紊乱的治疗中，肝脏细胞移植（LCT）是肝移植的替代治疗方案。LCT 在急性或慢性肝衰竭的治疗中可能是有用的。生物打印，或组织和器官样结构的逐层添加式生物制造，以及对供体器官的脱细胞所提供的脱细胞的、天然的三维支架，都是有希望改变组织工程学的新兴技术。本章总结了从体外肝脏支持、肝脏细胞移植、新兴的生物工程技术替代传统肝脏移植的最新进展。这些内容与第 38 章和第 43 章有关，这两章介绍了等待肝移植患者的照顾和肝衰竭患者的监护治疗。

体外肝脏支持

肝脏支持装置是通过提供器官再生的环境（连接再生），或支持患者直到可以施行器官移植手术（连接移植）来改善肝衰竭患者预后的。因此，肝脏支持装置应当具备肝脏的三大功能：解毒、合成和调节。

肝衰竭最严重的临床症状是由于衰竭的肝脏无法清除有害物质而使之蓄积。基于这一假说，清除脂溶性、白蛋白结合的物质，如胆红素、胆酸、氨基酸代谢产物、中链脂肪酸和细胞因子，应是对肝衰竭患者有益的。这一理论导致人工过滤和吸收装置的产生——人工肝脏支持装置。肝脏复杂的调节和合成功能仍然由肝细胞来完成，这使得人工肝脏支持系统的应用成为可能。

人工肝脏支持

人工肝脏支持系统用于支持替换肝脏的解毒功能。在 20 世纪 80 年代广泛应用的血浆置换在近年来重新成为一项治疗选择。Larsen 等的多中心研究发现，急性肝衰竭患者经过三次大量（10L）血浆置换治疗可以显著改善肝移植预后[1]。条件性的血液透析（HD）联合持续静脉-静脉血液滤过（CVVHDF）对于清除水溶性毒物是有效的。为了清除血液中白蛋白结合的疏水物质，需要额外的吸收底物来加强物质交换功能。大多数人工肝脏支持装置是基于联合吸附剂的分离膜装置，包括活性炭和阴离子、阳离子交换物。在人体血液中，白蛋白是最常见的毒物载体，因此白蛋白可能是一种理想的吸收底物。基于这一想法，白蛋白已经被加入改良血液透析系统中。来自德国罗斯托克的 Stange 和 Mitzner 发明了基于白蛋白透析的解毒系统——分子吸附再循环系统（MARS；Gambro，Stockholm，瑞典）[2]。白蛋白溶液在一个封闭的环路中循环，被一个高流量的血液透析过滤器与人体血液分隔开（图 47.1A）。白蛋白作为白蛋白结合毒物的吸收底物，并且可以在一个封闭的环路中通过阴离子交换和活性炭吸附而部分再生。单通道白蛋白透析（SPAD）是一种简单的透析方法，使用标准的肾脏交换疗法，没有额外的灌注泵装置，患者的血液流过一个装有高流量中空纤维的血液

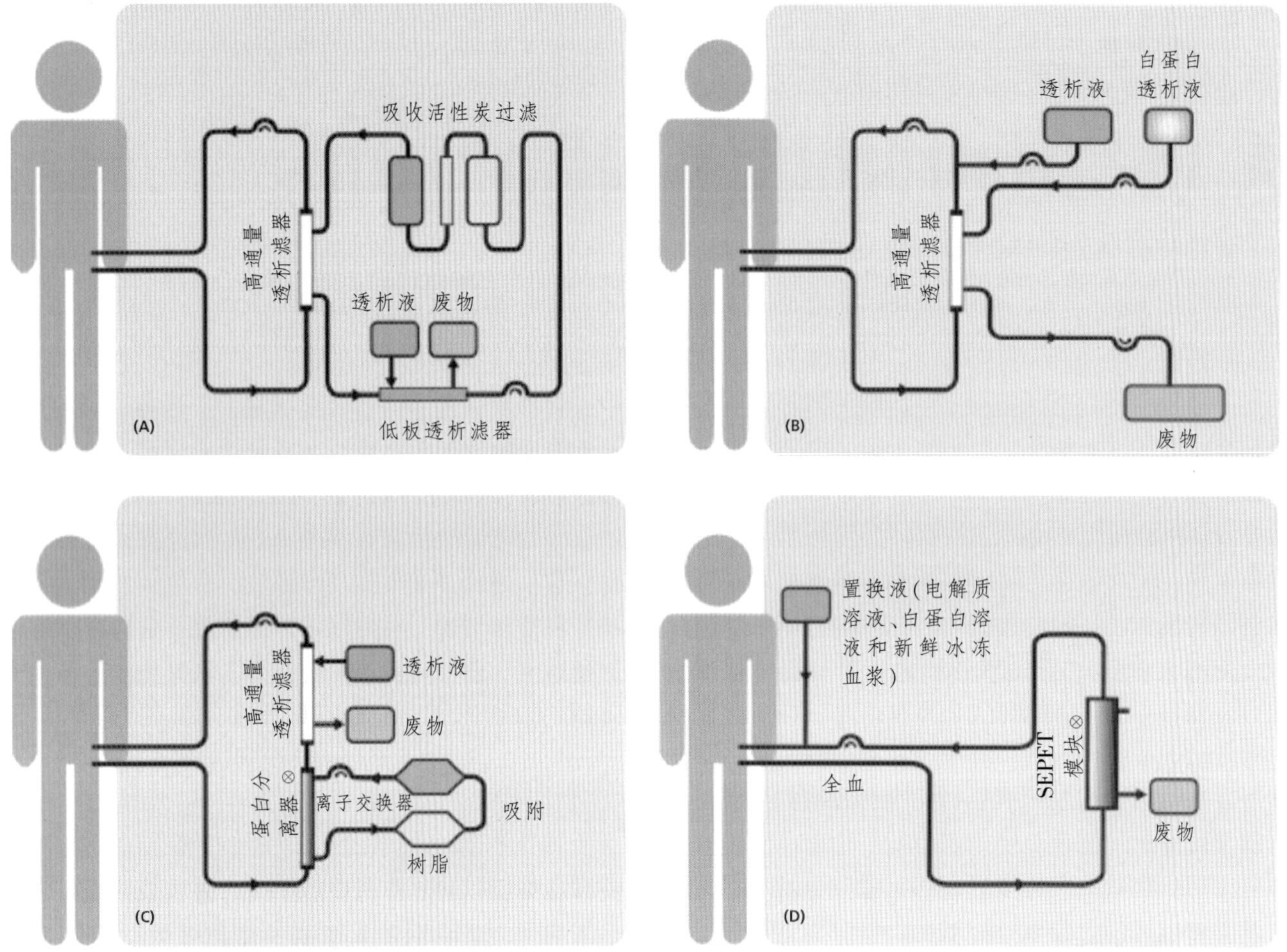

图 47.1 人工肝支持系统。(A)分子吸附再循环系统(MARS);(B)单通道白蛋白透析(SPAD);分级血浆分离与吸收(FPSA,Prometheus),和(D)选择性血浆滤过治疗(SEPET)。(Reproduced from Jörres A, Ronco C, Kellum JA. (2009) Management of acute kidney problems: Extracorporeal liver support, with kind permission of Springer Science +Business Media.)

透析环路。透析膜的另一面通过对流的白蛋白溶液来清洁,白蛋白溶液流过过滤器后被丢弃(图 47.1B)[3]。

下一步使用更大孔隙的透析膜来把特定分子量的血浆蛋白,包括结合有毒物质的白蛋白从血液中清理出去。分级血浆分离与吸收(FPSA;Prometheus,Fresenius Medical Care,Bad Homburg,德国)使得患者自身的白蛋白可以通过在次级环路中穿过两个吸收基质而再生(图 47.1C)。与 SPAD 和 MARS 相比,可透过白蛋白的聚砜膜被用来过滤患者的白蛋白,使之可以进入次级环路。在次级环路中,结合有毒物质的白蛋白被各种吸附剂净化。之后,在初级环路中进行常规高流量透析[4]。

Rozga 等发明了选择性血浆交换疗法(SEPET;Arbios Systems,Allendale,NJ,美国)。该方法尝试融合 SPAD 和 Prometheus 的优点(图 47.1D)。在 Prometheus 系统中,分级的血浆流经一个白蛋白通透的、基于分子量选择的透析膜。分子量<100kDa 的成分被去除,分子量>100kDa 的成分,包括免疫球蛋白、补体系统蛋白、大多数血液凝集因子和肝细胞再生刺激因子则保留在血液循环中。然而,同 SPAD 系统一样,该系统没有白蛋白再生功能。结合有毒物质的白蛋白被清除,而用电解质溶液、白蛋白溶液和新鲜冰冻血浆来进行置换[5]。

Ash 等所开发的 BioLogic-DT 系统将血液分离吸收与推拉式的基于附着剂的血液成分提取相结合,后者是基于纤维素透析器、以活性炭和阳离子交换剂的混悬液作为透析液。该系统被重新设计并改名为肝脏透析装置(HemoCleanse,Lafayette,IN,美国),但没有上市[6]。

生物人工肝脏支持

生物人工肝脏支持装置只能支持衰竭肝脏的解毒功能。由于肝脏不仅具有解毒功能,肝衰竭的临床症状更可能由衰退的调节功能(如酸碱状态、氨基酸)和更重要的合成功能(如白蛋白、葡萄糖、脂类、凝血因子及其他成分)引起。这些任务只能由肝脏细胞完成。

在20世纪60年代开始进行的体外肝脏灌注需要复杂的后勤工作。因为器官在用于治疗之前必须保证其新鲜状态,然后在无菌状态下接入患者的血液循环。所以为了应对此类问题,发明了几种不同的肝脏支持生物反应器,它可以用来在更适宜的状态下培育离体肝脏细胞,从而集成临床灌注系统。

Demetriou 等发明的肝脏辅助系统是基于$(5\sim7)\times10^9$冷藏保存的毛细血管间的猪肝细胞,类似于改良的透析灌流器。患者的血浆通过活性炭吸附器和氧气机,流经该灌流器[7]。

离体肝脏辅助装置(ELAD)是由 Sussman 等发明的。该装置使用大约200g一种来自人类肝母细胞瘤(C3A,从 HepG2 衍化而来)的细胞系。通过中空纤维膜将细胞与血浆分离开,一个活性炭吸附器和氧气机来提供解毒功能和细胞的氧气供应[8]。

Gerlach 等在20世纪80年代发明的一种生物反应装置被整合入模块化体外肝脏支持(MELS)系统。该生物反应装置包含两个亲水的聚醚砜膜束和一个用于氧合的疏水的多层中空纤维束[9]或人类肝脏细胞[10]。MELS 将 CVVHD 和 SPAD 与该生物反应装置整合在一起,分别用于清除水溶性和白蛋白结合的毒物。

学术医学中心人工生物肝脏(AMC-BAL)由 Chamuleau 等发明,不同于其他临床应用系统的一个主要方面是:在该系统中,患者的血浆与细胞直接接触,而不是通过膜将其与体外肝脏细胞分隔开。在圆柱状的装置中,一个非织造聚酯基质提供了巨大的表面,原始猪细胞可以接种其上并在纤维间形成聚合[11]。

评估

对于肝衰竭临床研究的设计十分困难。考虑到组织再生能力和预后,ALF 和慢性肝衰竭急性发作(AoCLF)是迥然不同的疾病。当发生 ALF 时,患者的肝脏支持治疗通常会在24~48h终止,因为该类患者将进行紧急肝脏移植。此外,缺乏敏感有效的临床终点[12]。

由于大多数临床研究是非盲法的,并且没有设置对照,因此目前缺乏随机对照试验和有足够说服力的研究。目前对于人工肝脏支持系统有较多的临床数据,而生物人工概念却没有。

一个关于体外肝脏支持系统应用于 ALF 和 AoCLF 治疗的 Cochrane 系统综述回顾了2002年9月之前的研究,认为这些系统对于死亡率没有显著影响,而对于 AoCLF 的患者似乎有生存获益[13]。最近,Stutchfield 等发表的系统综述纳入了一些 RCT 研究,探讨了体外肝脏支持装置对 ALF 和 AoCLF 生存的影响。也有系统综述总结分析了体外肝脏支持对于临床和生化指标的影响[14]。Stutchfield 等分析了74个临床研究(17个 RCT 研究,5个病例对照研究和52个队列研究)。8个 RCT 研究分析了体外肝脏支持在 ALF (3个研究,198名参与者)和 AoCLF(5个研究,157名参与者)中的效用。在6个研究中使用了人工肝脏支持装置(5个使用了 MARS,1个使用了 Biologic DT),2个研究评估了生物人工系统(ELAD 和 HepatAssist)。这些研究均没有报道在不良事件中,标准疗法与体外肝脏支持装置存在显著差异。也没有报道任何特殊的生物不相容事件。有趣的是,体外肝脏支持治疗显著改善了 ALF 患者的生存(风险比0.70,P=0.05)。而对于 AoCLF 患者,则没有显著生存获益(风险比0.87,P=0.37)。

一个欧洲多中心随机对照研究未纳入上述系统综述中。该研究将 Prometheus/FPSA 用于145例 AoCLF 患者的治疗。在该研究(HELIOS 研究)中,各组的总体生存率并没有显著不同。然而,两个预先确定使用 FPSA 治疗的亚组有明显的生存获益,这些患者有Ⅰ型肝肾综合征且 MELD 评分>30[4]。

与移植后移植肝效应的大规模临床研究相比,这些研究结果备受质疑。这些概念有没有充分评估?虽然概念正确,研究规模太小。大多数研究评估了人工肝脏支持系统,所有生物组件都必须具备吗?基于细胞的生物人工肝脏支持系统完成了包括解毒、调节、合成等复杂的肝脏功能,但仍然存在诸多共通的生物和物理的不足:大多数系统使用中空纤维膜,限制了患者血液和体外肝脏细胞的大规模交换。出于技术方面的原因,血浆对生物反应装置的灌注速率限定于100~300mL/min,远远低于正常生理状态下肝脏灌注血流1500mL/min。因此,生物反应装置的最大清除速率远低于人体肝脏的效率。另一个当前生物反应装置的不足是缺失功能性的胆汁分泌于特定腔室。处于三维培养条件下的肝脏细胞可以形成有功能的胆小管，但仍然不知道胆汁性混合物会在细胞内聚集到何种程度，也不知道这些是否会降低细胞活力[15]。然而，这些担忧可以通过添加特定的解毒组件来解决，如 MELS 中的 SPAD 或 ELAD 中的活性炭吸附装置。

最后，肝细胞重量似乎是受限的。通常，肝脏支持装置中的生物反应装置仅装载了 100~200g（一些装置甚至达到了 600g）肝脏组织细胞，这也许是不足的。在活体供体肝脏移植（LD-LTx）中，移植物的体积小于受体理想肝脏重量的 40%或更少，将无法满足受体的代谢需要，受体将处于移植物衰竭的风险中[16]。当在体外环路中时，尤其是考虑到血浆流速和物质交换的限制时，应提供更大量的细胞[17]。

所有生物人工支持系统的最主要限制仍然是细胞来源问题。广泛可及的细胞通常伴随着代谢不兼容、异种生物细胞感染的风险、转移瘤的风险及肝脏特定代谢功能低下（肿瘤细胞系）。原始人类肝脏细胞在临床应用中越来越受欢迎。无法使用的供体器官也许可以作为分离原始人类肝脏细胞的来源。然而，除了来源不足，由于组织分化、保存及分离过程等的影响，从这些器官获得的原始肝脏细胞，其代谢和再生能力受限。在我们能获得可靠的、安全的、高度代谢活性和容易扩展的人类细胞来源之前，生物人工肝脏支持系统获得重大突破是不可能的。

肝脏细胞移植

LCT 是肝移植的备选治疗方案，可用于肝脏相关的代谢紊乱和急性或慢性肝衰竭[18]。LCT 是将混悬液中的肝脏细胞进行灌注（图 47.2）。肝细胞来自供体肝脏、肝移植时不需要的或排斥的肝叶[19]。采用胶原酶灌注技术实现细胞分离，然后进行离心获得细胞纯化。分离后的肝细胞立即或冷藏保存再融化后进行移植。分离的肝细胞通过门静脉输注进入受体的肝脏或移植到其他部位，如脾脏或腹膜。经门脉灌注是目前最主要的细胞输注通道，肝脏将作为移植的肝细胞的基质。进入门脉的血管通路通常选择经皮或经颈静脉肝脏穿刺、肠系膜上静脉置管，新生儿也可以使用脐静脉。在门脉聚集的肝细胞将引起短暂的门脉高压及缺血再灌注损伤，黏附于活化的内皮细胞，移位并嫁接于肝板。在合适的条件下，如在再生刺激存在或具备生存优势时，供体肝细胞增殖并替代受体肝脏。在持续监测门脉压力的情况下，持续输注达到每千克体重 108 个细胞是安

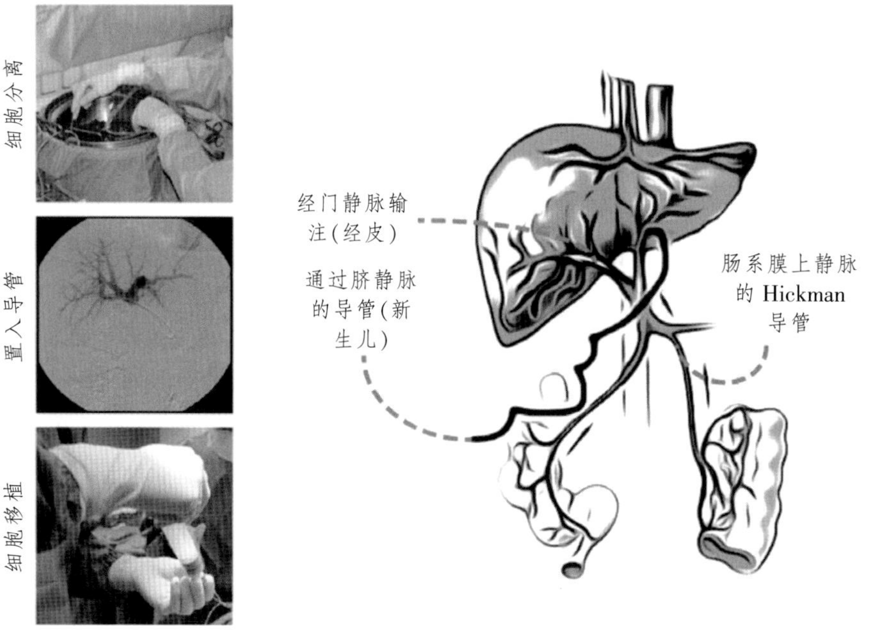

图 47.2 肝脏细胞移植。肝细胞移植是将混悬液中的肝脏细胞进行灌注。利用酶灌注技术可以将肝脏细胞从供体肝脏中分离出来。通过门脉将肝细胞输注到受体肝脏中。门脉血管通路通常选择经皮或经颈静脉肝穿刺、脐静脉置管或在肠系膜上静脉置入 Hickman 导管。

全的,并且可达到 5%受体肝脏细胞重量的置换[20]。

从概念上来说,与肝移植相比,细胞移植有如下优势:

(1)肝细胞可以低温处理,保存于细胞仓库,从而实现紧急或择期使用。

(2)细胞输注比整个器官移植的创伤小,可用于治疗病情危重或非常年轻不适合进行器官移植的患者。

(3)受体的肝脏留在原位,使得其功能有恢复的可能,这也意味着移植物功能衰竭不再是致命的。

(4)可以依据受体的需要调整细胞输注的剂量,在移植之前这些细胞可以从遗传方面进行优化或使用对比剂进行标注。

ALF 或代谢紊乱的动物模型的实验研究显示 LCT 改善了生存或生化异常。基于这些研究,临床 LCT 在过去的 10 年里取得了巨大进步。目前的综述列举了大约 13 个中心的超过 80 例临床人类肝脏细胞移植[21]。本部分将探讨临床中 LCT 用于治疗代谢性肝病、ALF 和慢性肝病的当前进展,并且指明其理论上和临床实践中的不足。

代谢性肝病的治疗

在所有指征中,目前 LCT 在治疗新生儿代谢性肝病中尤为有效。在特定基因缺失的病例中,表达该基因的供体肝细胞将补足缺失的功能,而无需替换整个器官。移植的细胞整合进入正常的受体肝脏中,改善肝脏缺失的特定功能,无需完成所有的肝脏功能。已有报道大约 35 个儿童和成人接受 LCT 用于治疗代谢性肝病,大多数研究在过去的几年里完成[21-24]。在所有病例中,LCT 经由门静脉输注完成,单次或多次输注,使用新鲜的或冷藏保存的肝细胞。作为第一次尝试使用肝细胞治疗代谢性肝病,Grossmann 等于 1994 年使用 LCT 治疗家族性高胆固醇血症[25]。他们分离的肝脏细胞来自 5 个成人切除的肝脏组织,在体外用表达 LDL 受体的逆转录病毒质粒进行转染,切除术后 3 天将这些细胞经门静脉输入,从而可以充分利用部分肝脏切除术后的增生刺激。研究者们发现大约 20% LDL 胆固醇水平降低,但移植后早期即出现转染基因的下降。现在,存在尿酸循环缺陷的患者是施行 LCT 的最常见人群[21]。在这些患者中,10 名儿童(年龄为 1 天~5 岁)患有氨甲酰基转移酶(OTC)缺陷症,在 LCT 术后出现血氨水平降低,并且可以在后期成功实施肝移植。2 名患有瓜氨酸血症和 1 名患有精氨酸琥珀酰酶缺陷的患者其代谢状态保持平稳。8 例使用肝细胞治疗 1 型家族性非溶血型黄疸的病例已被报道。经过门静脉输注 5%肝脏重量的肝细胞,胆红素水平降低了 30%~60%。然而对于大多数病例,几个月后仍需进行肝移植。其他使用 LCT 成功治疗的疾病包括糖原贮积病、雷夫叙姆综合征和Ⅶ因子缺乏。

总之,通过发表的病例可见 LCT 对于代谢性肝病的短暂治疗是安全、有效的。LCT 的相关并发症未被报道。然而,大多数病例的代谢性缺陷只能在短时间被纠正,提示可能由于移植不充分[26]或移植物排斥[27]造成移植细胞的活性降低。并且由于缺乏对照研究,使得这些发现的阐释尤为困难。

急性肝衰竭的治疗

在 D-半乳糖中毒的动物研究中,脾、门静脉或腹膜肝细胞移植可以缓解该病。基于该研究,LCT 被用于人类 ALF,作为等待自身肝功能恢复或肝移植[28,29]。Fisher 等回顾了 37 例使用肝细胞移植治疗的 ALF 患者[30]。在这些患者中,10 名儿童通过门静脉进行肝细胞输注。之后 3 名儿童成功进行了肝移植,2 名儿童肝功能恢复未进行肝移植。在 27 名成人中,肝细胞输注治疗后,4 人成功进行了肝移植,5 人自身肝功能恢复。在 13 名将肝细胞移植到脾的成人中,3 人成功进行了肝移植,1 人自身肝功能恢复。细胞输注相关并发症,如肝细胞肺栓子、脾和肠系膜静脉血栓形成,或由于介入肝脏通路造成的出血,可在严重 ALF 患者中出现[31,32]。LCT 使得 ALF 患者的血氨和血胆红素水平下降,肝性脑病有所缓解。但报道的发病率和死亡率仍然相对较高。这也许是由于通过门静脉和脾输注的细胞量不足,从而不足以挽救肝衰竭患者。由于治疗方法(如细胞量和输注方法位置)和使用肝细胞移植治疗的患者差异很大,同时缺失 RCT 研究,使得 LCT 有效性的评估无法进行。

慢性肝病的治疗

在慢性肝病的治疗中,LCT 可以利用肝细胞移植替代病肝的部分功能或使用移植的肝细胞重新注入病肝。发表的数据中有 20 名患有慢性肝病并进行肝脏细胞移植的患者的资料是可及的[21]。动物研究显示,扰乱的肝脏构造使得肝细胞植入变得困难,肝内门体分流会造成门静脉移植细胞的全身分布。因此在发表的大多数临床研究中选择脾脏作为移植位点[33]。

Mito 等最先使用肝细胞治疗肝硬化患者[34]。他们切除丙型病毒性肝炎患者的左外侧叶，分离并将自体肝细胞回输进入患者的脾脏。1 名患者获得了完全恢复,LCT 之后 11 个月可通过放射性同位素显像检测到肝细胞。然而,另外 9 名患者没有临床获益。在更进一步的研究中，分离自非硬化肝的异体肝脏细胞被用于移植。

虽然已经取得了一些临床进展,LCT 似乎仅在一些患有慢性肝病的患者中取得了一定疗效。这也许是由于在大多数研究中,只有少量的细胞被输入。肝硬化患者也许会从异位肝细胞移植中获益，但如果硬化的肝脏被留在原位，将无法处理并存的门脉高压症和肝细胞肝癌的发生风险[35]。

理论上和临床实践中的不足

在过去 10 年中,LCT 的安全性和可能性已经得到了证实,特别是用于治疗代谢性肝病。然而,在成功使用肝细胞移植治疗肝病之前仍然存在诸多问题和障碍。

肝细胞移植的细胞来源

同器官移植中供肝严重不足一样，用于获取肝细胞的供肝十分稀缺。为获得足够的细胞供给用于 LCT,可替代的来源,如无心跳供体的肝脏,可以用来分离肝脏细胞[36]。另外的细胞来源可以是干细胞或诱导的多能细胞[37,38]。尽管从该类细胞中获得肝样细胞的增殖结果令人振奋,许多人仍然对此存有安全性顾虑,特别是干细胞的致瘤潜力。

移植细胞的植入和存活

LCT 的另外一个重要方面是移植细胞未充分植入和移植肝细胞的长期生存问题。也许许多细胞没有存活足够长的时间以进入肝脏结构,动物实验显示,高达 80%的细胞在输入后 24~48h 内损失[39]。体外研究发现，类似胰岛移植，分离的肝细胞导致急性血液源性炎症反应,这也许是体内大量细胞损失的原因[40]。此外,由于先天免疫系统的存在,即使 OLT 之后使用了免疫抑制药物，肝细胞需要面对适应性免疫反应和非适应性免疫反应，如细胞凋亡或特异性的细胞介导的或体液免疫[41]。肝细胞植入也受限于细胞需要穿过并整合进入肝实质。在动物模型和使用肝细胞移植的肝脏中,组织病理学分析显示细胞陷于远端门静脉分支[26]。可能这些细胞在以后会失去代谢活性。在临床 LCT 中,目前有两种策略被用于增加肝脏细胞的植入：肝脏辐射和部分栓塞。在动物实验中,肝脏辐射可以抑制肝细胞增殖,扰乱肝窦内皮细胞,抑制枯否细胞的功能[42]。部分可逆的门静脉栓塞可以刺激肝脏的增生反应，对于移植细胞是有益的[43]。也许联合应用可逆门静脉栓塞和肝脏辐射能获得最好的效果。

追踪移植的肝细胞

遗憾的是,对于 LCT 术中、术后生理过程的了解很少。因为供体肝细胞分布和植入的研究受限于组织标本的检查。临床中应用的用于监测移植细胞的方法目前并不适用。放射性同位素标记的细胞用于一名患者来显示移植后肝细胞的生理分布[44]。然而,放射性同位素显像受限于放射性同位素半衰期较短和分辨率较低。磁共振成像(MRI)是目前临床中最主要的手段来实时、无创地监测细胞移植。MRI 在实性器官中提供较高的分辨率,并可以实现动态显像。细胞必须使用细胞内造影剂进行标记,从而可以被 MRI 识别。体外实验已经显示使用 MRI 造影剂标记人类肝脏细胞的可行性。动物实验则已经表明 MRI 在生理条件下追踪肝细胞的可行性[45,46]。然而,需要进行更多的研究来将其转变为临床可用的技术。

肝细胞的植入部位

肝细胞异位植入位置是必要的，特别是在治疗慢性肝病时[21]。临床研究多关注脾脏,但肝细胞的长期生存尚未确切阐释。脾脏的肝样变仍然是个谜。ALF 是需要的肝细胞量无法安全地移植入脾。并且,肝细胞暴露于脾脏的免疫环境中是不利的。肝细胞胶囊化是一种对肝细胞进行免疫保护的有潜力的方法，还可以同时进行异位植入。Mei 等发现使用藻酸钙微球进行肝细胞胶囊化,足够量的(50%肝脏重量)胶囊化的肝细胞可以植入腹膜腔,来挽救暴发性肝衰竭的动物[47]。需要进行更深入的研究来探讨和评估可用的肝外植入位点或基于组织工程的可进行体外肝脏细胞支持的构造[35]。

生物工程解决方案

由于供者器官的稀缺性以及肝外肝支持和 LCT 尚未解决的问题,我们需要寻求其他的解决方案。生物工程方法结合了体外和体内组织工程学，可能实现生物人工肝移植的终极目标。这部分将集中讨论目前有关生物工程肝的最激动人心的两个概念：器官打印和器官再细胞化。

器官打印:人体器官的生物制造

器官打印是进行完全从头开始的生物制造三维血管化的有功能的人体器官的技术。器官打印基于对有功能的三维组织进行逐层自动化生物制造[48]。其将不同来源的细胞以生理方式彼此相邻放置，以模拟完整模板器官中的细胞分布。自动化生物打印机是基于传统喷墨打印机的概念，它和生物反应器是器官生物制造线的必要组分(图 47.3A)[49]。

与其他用于肝脏的基于组织工程学的方法相比，如为异位肝种子细胞提供支架或肝细胞移植，器官打印有一些竞争性优势：它能够让几种类型的细胞同时精确地进行三维定位,像自然状态下一样理想;它能够使创造的组织具有高水平的细胞密度；它能够解决较厚组织结构中血管化的问题;它能够自动化,并且提供了可扩展至制造工程器官的方法[50]。

在基于组织工程学构建有功能的肝组织时,对脉管的生物制造以保证供血和胆汁排泄通常是限制性问题。器官打印能够解决这些问题,如使用逐层沉积技术[51]。如 Visconti 等所描述的,打印一片生物相容的水凝胶,将组织球嵌入水凝胶中[52]。组织球由细胞悬液

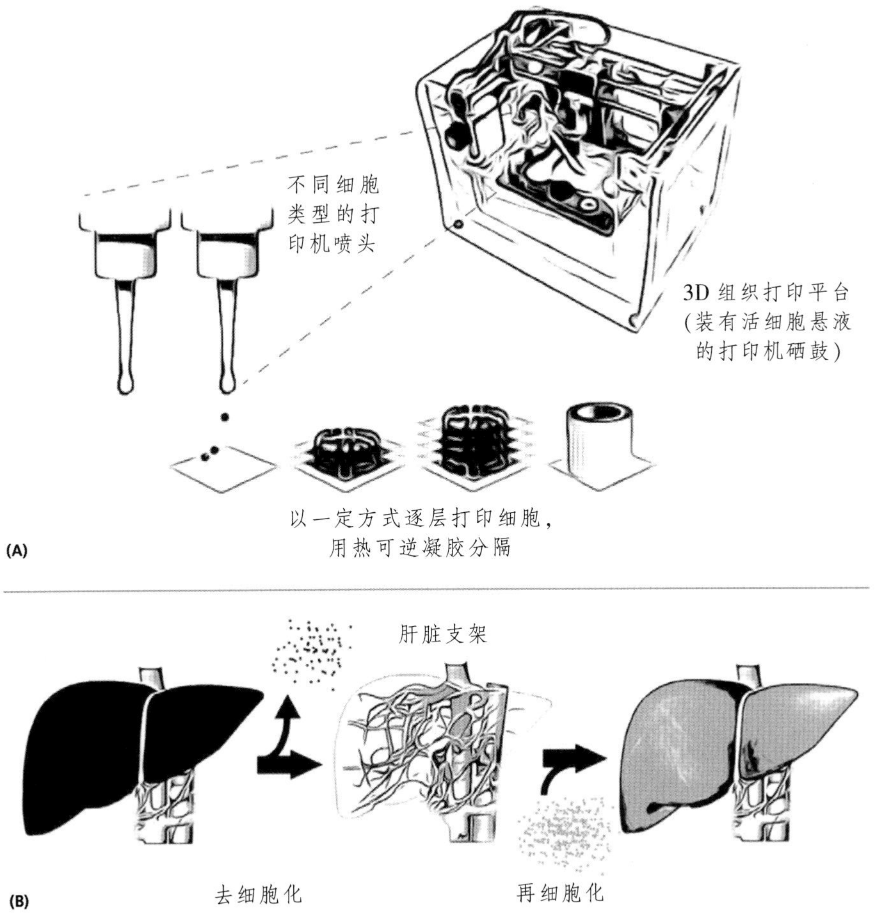

图 47.3 肝脏的生物工程解决方案。(A)器官打印是基于细胞或球体的三维打印。细胞以一定的方式逐层打印,由热可逆凝胶分开以形成管状结构。活细胞为基础的结构是由细胞打印及打印后的细胞融合形成。(Adapted from Mironov et al.[51])(B)肝脏的去细胞化和再细胞化。肝脏去细胞化是通过灌注去污剂以溶解细胞和细胞质成分。顺序用肝细胞和内皮细胞或前体细胞使去细胞化的肝脏支架再细胞化,从而获得有功能的肝组织。

制备而成,可以是同种类或不同种类的,可以包含单一细胞类型或混合几种细胞类型（如肝细胞与内皮细胞或胆管细胞）。根据预先确定的预期三维结构蓝图,如管状结构,进行水凝胶和组织球的逐层沉积。随着组织球之间的融合以及水凝胶的去除，数天后就能形成空心管。经过打印和打印后融合过程形成了活细胞为基础的结构,将其放入培养箱,就将形成最终的三维结构以及适当的生物机械特性。已有概念证明研究显示可以“构建”较厚的组织片以及直线型和有分支的管状结构[53]。

器官打印是一种高度创新和宏大的技术。到目前为止,只发表了几项成功的应用。例如,使用生物打印为基础的技术已成功得到骨移植物。Fedorovich 等使用器官打印技术制造了包含内皮前体细胞和多能基质细胞的多孔结构[54]。他们证明将这些移植物植入免疫缺陷小鼠的皮下之后,仍保留多种细胞结构。细胞分化使前体细胞沉积部位形成组织。此结构中的内皮前体细胞部位形成灌注的血管，打印的移植物中多能基质细胞部位则出现骨的形成。另一个成功应用生物打印技术的例子是 Xu 等证明自动化细胞打印系统可以用来打印癌细胞和正常成纤维细胞的三维共培养模型。生物打印能够对共培养细胞的打印进行高度的空间调控,有利于研究特定细胞之间的相互作用[55]。此外,生物打印可用于拟胚体形成，为得到可控的尺寸均一的拟胚体提供了有效的工具[56]。

关于肝器官打印的研究尚未发表。但这项技术很可能被用于制造血管和胆管，在这些结构的间隙中放入肝细胞和非实质肝细胞。根据报道的其他细胞和组织充满希望的结果,以及这项新兴技术的不断发展,可以想象，器官打印终将成功制造出适合手术移植的人的肝脏。

去细胞化器官的再细胞化

再细胞化是另一个近年迅速发展的新兴概念。再细胞化是从供肝去除所有细胞和抗原呈递组分，再将其他来源的细胞播种在这个肝脏支架里(图 47.3B)。去细胞化完美保存了整个器官的大血管骨架，包括天然微脉管系统的功能区域、细胞外基质以及三维结构,使得再细胞化器官的基质完美适合播种细胞[57]。由于无心跳供体的器官(以及可预知异种器官)可以用来去细胞化,这个概念有希望克服器官稀缺的问题[58]。再细胞化可以使用患者自己的细胞，可以是干细胞或使用诱导多能干细胞的技术，这就不再需要移植后终生进行免疫抑制。

已有其他组织的组织工程去细胞化的成功示范,包括膀胱、动脉和器官,一些团队已经开始研发肝脏去细胞化和再细胞化技术。Uygun 等最早报道制造出了可移植的再细胞化肝脏[59]。他们使用灌注 SDS 的方法对大鼠肝脏进行了全器官的去细胞化,SDS 是一种阴离子去污剂,能够溶解细胞和细胞质成分。在完全去细胞化之后，作者通过门静脉反复灌注肝细胞的方法重建肝实质，此外向肝脏灌注微脉管内皮细胞作为非实质组分。作为证明,他们将生物工程肝移植物连接到肾切除术后大鼠的肾动脉和肾静脉，对其进行在体灌注8h。对灌注后的器官进行组织学分析,结果显示肝细胞已经迁移到较大脉管周围并填充了脉管周围的肝实质，提示细胞跨过基质屏障迁移到了去细胞化的窦状腺间隙。内皮细胞能够形成肝细胞所围绕的脉管系统的内膜。移植后,肝细胞恢复了正常的形态和功能。

根据这些充满希望的结果，进一步的研究对肝脏去细胞化和再细胞化过程进行了优化。Baptista 等证明了小鼠、大鼠和成年猪的肝脏都能够成功地用人内皮细胞和人胎肝细胞再细胞化[60]。Soto-Gutierrez 等研发出一种肝脏全器官去细胞化的方法，只会造成很小的破坏[61]。使用该方法,他们能够保存肝脏天然的微脉管系统、胆汁引流系统和高达 50%的生长因子成分。Bao 等使用肝素对去细胞化的移植物进行改进，以避免血管内血栓形成[62]。通过这种内表面抗凝的改进之后,他们能够将播种细胞的数量增加，增加量相当于高达 10%的全肝当量。他们将再细胞化的移植物植入体内,使之与残余天然肝相串联,以门静脉对其进行灌注,结果显示肝功能有改善，并且 90%的肝切除术后大鼠生存时间延长超过了 72h。最后,Barakat 等将人胎肝细胞与胎星形细胞共培养后，将其移植到去细胞化的猪肝脏基质,制造出了人化的猪肝[63]。

这些前期研究结果非常吸引人，证明了制造再细胞化肝脏移植物的可行性。然而,再细胞化肝脏移植物用于临床仍需巨大的努力。去细胞化的方法需要进一步优化和标准化,这样才能有效地去除所有细胞成分,同时保留肝脏的微结构和细胞外基质。必须增加播种的细胞数，并且需要刺激播种的细胞使其填充去细胞化的基质。此外,需要进一步研究再细胞化移植物中的肝细胞能否保留它们的生理特性并形成有功能的组织。最后,需要动物实验来证明再细胞化的肝脏和天然肝脏移植物功能相似。尽管面临着这些挑战,很显然的是,这项技术如果最终取得成功,将会对临床肝移植产生广泛的影响,有希望克服肝移植所面临的器官稀缺问题。

总结

肝移植受到器官供应以及无法完全预测患者从ALF中恢复能力的限制。不同形式的肝脏支持装置已应用了数十年,其作为患者痊愈或是移植前的衔接治疗仍然是具有极大吸引力的概念。但这些装置的有效性有待证明,想要实现其概念上的潜质仍需对这些装置进行很多优化。能够取代肝脏各种各样功能的合适的人造产品以及生物人工混合装置中合适的肝细胞来源仍然是限制性因素。LCT是实体肝移植的替代治疗方法,尤其是治疗肝脏引起的代谢性疾病,治疗急性或慢性肝衰竭也可获益。由于替代供体器官移植的明确需求和其他已有技术的缺陷,许多新方法都正在开发测试,其中包括生物打印和将去细胞化的器官再细胞化,这些方法提供了肝细胞的新来源。

(刘晓 译 荀晓冬 朱继业 校)

参考文献

1. Kramer L, Kodras K. Detoxification as a treatment goal in hepatic failure. Liver International. 2011;31:1–4.
2. Mitzner SR. Extracorporeal liver support-albumin dialysis with the Molecular Adsorbent Recirculating System (MARS). Annals of Hepatology. 2011;10:21–28.
3. Sauer IM, Goetz M, Steffen I, et al. In vitro comparison of the molecular adsorbent recirculation system (MARS) and single-pass albumin dialysis (SPAD). Hepatology. 2004;39:1408–1144.
4. Rifai K. Fractionated plasma separation and adsorption: current practice and future options. Liver International. 2011;31:13–15.
5. Rozga J, Umehara Y, Trofimenko A, et al. A novel plasma filtration therapy for hepatic failure: preclinical studies. Therapeutic Apheresis and Dialysis. 2006;10:138–144.
6. Ash SR, Steczko J, Knab WR, et al. Push-pull sorbent-based pheresis and hemodiabsorption in the treatment of hepatic failure: preliminary results of a clinical trial with the BioLogic-DTPF System. Therapeutic Apheresis. 2000;4:218–228.
7. Demetriou AA, Brown RS Jr, Busuttil RW, et al. Prospective, randomized, multicenter, controlled trial of a bioartificial liver in treating acute liver failure. Annals of Surgery. 2004;239:660–670.
8. Sussman NL, Gislason GT, Conlin CA, et al. The Hepatix extracorporeal liver assist device: initial clinical experience. Artifical Organs. 1994;18:390–396.
9. Sauer IM, Kardassis D, Zeillinger K, et al. Clinical extracorporeal hybrid liver support-phase I study with primary porcine liver cells. Xenotransplantation. 2003;10:460–469.
10. Sauer IM, Zeilinger K, Pless G, et al. Extracorporeal liver support based on primary human liver cells and albumin dialysis-treatment of a patient with primary graft non-function. Journal of Hepatology. 2003;39:649–653.
11. van de Kerkhove MP, Di Florio E, Scuderi V, et al. Phase I clinical trial with the AMC-bioartificial liver. International Journal of Artificial Organs. 2002;25: 950–959.
12. O'Grady JG. Perspectives and future of artificial and bioartificial devices. In: Henne-Bruns D, Buttenschön K, Fuchs M, et al., editors. Artificial Liver Support—Proceedings of the Falk Symposium 145. Heidelberg: Springer Verlag; 2006: 72–75.
13. Liu JP, Gluud LL, Als-Nielsen B, et al. Artificial and bioartificial support systems for liver failure. Cochrane Database of Systematic Reviews. 2004;(1):CD003628.
14. Stutchfield BM, Simpson K, Wigmore SJ. Systematic review and meta-analysis of survival following extracorporeal liver support. British Journal of Surgery. 2011;98:623–631.
15. Chamuleau RA. Future of bioartificial liver support. World Journal of Gastrointestinal Surgery. 2009;1:21–25.
16. Lo CM, Fan ST, Liu CL, et al. Adult-to-adult living donor liver transplantation using extended right lobe grafts. Annals of Surgery. 1997;226:261–270.
17. Iwata H, Ueda Y. Pharmacokinetic considerations in development of a bioartificial liver. Clinical Pharmacokinetics. 2004;43:211–225.
18. Dhawan A, Puppi J, Hughes RD, et al. Human hepatocyte transplantation: current experience and future challenges. Nature Reviews. Gastroenterology & Hepatology. 2010;7:288–298.
19. Dhawan A, Strom SC, Sokal E, et al. Human hepatocyte transplantation. Methods in Molecular Biology. 2010;640:525–534.
20. Hughes RD, Mitry RR, Dhawan A. Current status of hepatocyte transplantation. Transplantation. 2012;93(4):342–347.
21. Fitzpatrick E, Mitry RR, Dhawan A. Human hepatocyte transplantation: state of the art. Journal of Internal Medicine. 2009;266:339–357.
22. Puppi J, Tan N, Mitry RR, et al. Hepatocyte transplantation followed by auxiliary liver transplantation–a novel treatment for ornithine transcarbamylase deficiency. American Journal of Transplantation. 2008;8:452–457.
23. Meyburg J, Das AM, Hoerster F, et al. One liver for four children: first clinical series of liver cell transplantation for severe neonatal urea cycle defects. Transplantation. 2009;87:636–641.
24. Legido-Quigley C, Cloarec O, Parker DA, et al. First example of hepatocyte transplantation to alleviate ornithine transcarbamylase deficiency, monitored by NMR-based metabonomics. Bioanalysis. 2009;1:1527–1535.
25. Grossman M, Raper SE, Kozarsky K, et al. Successful ex vivo gene therapy directed to liver in a patient with familial hypercholesterolaemia. Nature Genetics. 1994;6:335–341.
26. Quaglia A, Lehec SC, Hughes RD, et al. Liver after hepatocyte transplantation for liver-based metabolic disorders in children. Cell Transplantation. 2008;17: 1403–1414.
27. Allen KJ, Mifsud NA, Williamson R, et al. Cell-mediated rejection results in allograft loss after liver cell transplantation. Liver Transplantation. 2008;14:688–694.
28. Sutherland DE, Numata M, Matas AJ, et al. Hepatocellular transplantation in acute liver failure. Surgery. 1977;82:124–132.
29. Baumgartner D, LaPlante-O'Neill PM, Sutherland DE, et al. Effects of intrasplenic injection of hepatocytes, hepatocyte fragments and hepatocyte culture supernatants on D-galactosamine-induced liver failure in rats. European Surgical Research. 1983;15:129–135.
30. Fisher RA, Strom SC. Human hepatocyte transplantation: worldwide results. Transplantation. 2006;82:441–449.
31. Sterling RK, Fisher RA. Liver transplantation. Living donor, hepatocyte, and xenotransplantation. Clinics in Liver Disease. 2001;5:431–460, vii.
32. Bilir BM, Guinette D, Karrer F, et al. Hepatocyte transplantation in acute liver failure. Liver Transplantation. 2000;6:32–40.
33. Kasai S, Sawa M, Kondoh K, et al. Intrasplenic hepatocyte transplantation in mammals. Transplantation Proceedings. 1987;19:992–994.
34. Mito M, Kusano M, Kawaura Y. Hepatocyte transplantation in man. Transplantation Proceedings. 1992;24:3052–3053.
35. Soltys KA, Soto-Gutiérrez A, Nagaya M, et al. Barriers to the successful treatment of liver disease by hepatocyte transplantation. Journal of Hepatology. 2010;53: 769–774.
36. Hughes RD, Mitry RR, Dhawan A, et al. Isolation of hepatocytes from livers from non-heart-beating donors for cell transplantation. Liver Transplantation. 2006; 12:713–717.
37. Touboul T, Hannan NR, Corbineau S, et al. Generation of functional hepatocytes from human embryonic stem cells under chemically defined conditions that recapitulate liver development. Hepatology. 2010;51:1754–1765.
38. Espejel S, Roll GR, McLaughlin KJ, et al. Induced pluripotent stem cell-derived hepatocytes have the functional and proliferative capabilities needed for liver regeneration in mice. Journal of Clinical Investigation. 2010;120:3120–3126.
39. Rajvanshi P, Kerr A, Bhargava KK, et al. Studies of liver repopulation using the dipeptidyl peptidase IV-deficient rat and other rodent recipients: cell size and structure relationships regulate capacity for increased transplanted hepatocyte mass in the liver lobule. Hepatology. 1996;23:482–496.

40. Gustafson EK, Elgue G, Hughes RD, et al. The instant blood-mediated inflammatory reaction characterized in hepatocyte transplantation. Transplantation. 2011;91:632–638.
41. Han B, Lu Y, Meng B, et al. Cellular loss after allogenic hepatocyte transplantation. Transplantation. 2009;87:1–5.
42. Yamanouchi K, Zhou H, Roy-Chowdhury N, et al. Hepatic irradiation augments engraftment of donor cells following hepatocyte transplantation. Hepatology. 2009;49:258–267.
43. Dagher I, Nguyen TH, Groyer-Picard MT, et al. Efficient hepatocyte engraftment and long-term transgene expression after reversible portal embolization in nonhuman primates. Hepatology. 2009;49:950–959.
44. Bohnen NI, Charron M, Reyes J, et al. Use of indium-111-labeled hepatocytes to determine the biodistribution of transplanted hepatocytes through portal vein infusion. Clinical Nuclear Medicine. 2000;25:447–450.
45. Puppi J, Modo M. Use of magnetic resonance imaging contrast agents to detect transplanted liver cells. Topics in Magnetic Resonance Imaging. 2009;20:113–120.
46. Raschzok N, Teichgräber U, Billecke N, et al. Monitoring of liver cell transplantation in a preclinical swine model using magnetic resonance imaging. Cell Medicine. 2010;1:123–135.
47. Mei J, Sgroi A, Mai G, et al. Improved survival of fulminant liver failure by transplantation of microencapsulated cryopreserved porcine hepatocytes in mice. Cell Transplantation. 2009;18:101–110.
48. Jakab K, Norotte C, Marga F, et al. Tissue engineering by self-assembly and bioprinting of living cells. Biofabrication. 2010;2:022001.
49. Mironov V, Kasyanov V, Markwald RR. Organ printing: from bioprinter to organ biofabrication line. Current Opinion in Biotechnology. 2011;22:667–673.
50. Mironov V, Kasyanov V, Drake C, et al. Organ printing: promises and challenges. Regenerative Medicine. 2008;3:93–103.
51. Mironov V, Visconti RP, Kasyanov V, et al. Organ printing: tissue spheroids as building blocks. Biomaterials. 2009;30:2164–2174.
52. Visconti RP, Kasyanov V, Gentile C, et al. Towards organ printing: engineering an intra-organ branched vascular tree. Expert Opinion on Biological Therapy. 2010;10:409–420.
53. Jakab K, Norotte C, Damon B, et al. Tissue engineering by self-assembly of cells printed into topologically defined structures. Tissue Engineering. Part A. 2008;14:413–421.
54. Fedorovich NE, Wijnberg HM, Dhert WJ, et al. Distinct tissue formation by heterogeneous printing of osteo- and endothelial progenitor cells. Tissue Engineering. Part A. 2011;17:2113–2121.
55. Xu F, Celli J, Rizvi I, et al. A three-dimensional in vitro ovarian cancer coculture model using a high-throughput cell patterning platform. Biotechnology Journal. 2011;6:204–212.
56. Xu F, Sridharan B, Wang S, et al. Embryonic stem cell bioprinting for uniform and controlled size embryoid body formation. Biomicrofluidics. 2011;5:22207.
57. Badylak SF. The extracellular matrix as a biologic scaffold material. Biomaterials. 2007;28:3587–3593.
58. Fukumitsu K, Yagi H, Soto-Gutierrez A. Bioengineering in organ transplantation: targeting the liver. Transplantation Proceedings. 2011;43:2137–2138.
59. Uygun BE, Soto-Gutierrez A, Yagi H, et al. Organ reengineering through development of a transplantable recellularized liver graft using decellularized liver matrix. Nature Medicine. 2010;16:814–8120.
60. Baptista PM, Siddiqui MM, Lozier G, et al. The use of whole organ decellularization for the generation of a vascularized liver organoid. Hepatology. 2011;53:604–617.
61. Soto-Gutierrez A, Zhang L, Medberry C, et al. A whole-organ regenerative medicine approach for liver replacement. Tissue Engineering. Part C, Methods. 2011;17:677–686.
62. Bao J, Shi Y, Sun H, et al. Construction of a portal implantable functional tissue-engineered liver using perfusion-decellularized matrix and hepatocytes in rats. Cell Transplantation. 2011;20:753–766.
63. Barakat O, Abbasi S, Rodriguez G, et al. Use of Decellularized Porcine Liver for Engineering Humanized Liver Organ. Journal of Surgical Research. 2012;173(1):e11–25.

第 48 章
心室辅助装置

O.H. Frazier, Steven M. Parnis

引言

使用心室辅助装置(Ventricular Assist Devices,VAD)来治疗严重的心力衰竭以及作为心脏移植前的衔接治疗已经成为心血管临床医学中被普遍认可和常规的手段。心室辅助装置在心脏移植患者治疗中的普及和广泛使用使其成为心脏移植的必需品,事实上,通常将VAD装置和移植装置一起作为心力衰竭患者多学科治疗的一部分。本章将介绍VAD的起源、发展和现代使用,并且是第30章和第39章的姊妹章节,这两章分别讨论了心脏移植的术前评估和等待者名单管理。

历史

Gibbon最早开始针对血液循环的临时机械支持进行研究,其也是第一个成功将体外循环装置用于临床的人[1,2]。此外,Dodrill使用左心转流成功进行了二尖瓣修复术。然而,该技术被视为专用于二尖瓣手术,而非长期的左心室(Left Ventricular,LV)机械支持[3]。对首批使用体外循环的患者的观察显示,有时术后的长期支持有利于心脏的恢复。一旦心脏功能恢复,这些患者就可以成功地脱离体外循环装置。该发现显著推动了循环机械支持的发展。然而,当时使用的氧合器会导致血液系统损害,从而限制了体外循环中的心室恢复。因此,在那个年代,只有在患者自身肺脏可以作为氧合器使用、仅需要循环支持的情况下,使用VAD才能够使心脏恢复。

1961年,Dennis等[4]使用体外滚压泵直接辅助衰竭的左心室。通过大量的研究和详尽的解剖,他们能够通过右颈静脉,跨过房间隔将导管置入左心房。然后借由滚压泵通过股动脉将血液泵回。该跨房间隔的流入导管是盲法置入的,值得注意的是,在8名严重心肌梗死后心力衰竭的患者中,它成功支持了7名患者[4](Spencer和Dennis最早使用了该方法,形成了目前广泛使用的Tandem Heart的基础)。同样的,在1965年,Spencer等也成功地将滚压泵用于临时的循环支持,使心室得以恢复[5]。

DeBakey和Spencer同时报道了一例在长期部分体外循环支持后成功恢复的患者[5,6]。这项工作在心脏直视手术后高死亡率的年代逐渐发展。因此,此研究的最初目标是开发出能够临时支持心脏的泵,直到心肌功能恢复能够使泵移除。1963年,DeBakey医生领导的Baylor小组报道了第一例体内搏动性左心室辅助装置(Left Ventricular Assist Device,LVAD)的植入[7]。在装置支持期间,循环得以很好的维持,心肌也有好转的表现,但患者在此过程中的神经损伤未能恢复。1966年8月,DeBakey医生再次放置一例LVAD,这次是体外放置,患者是一名在双瓣膜置换术后无法脱离体外循环的37岁女性[6]。10天后,泵成功移除,这名患者存活了6年且心功能良好,最终不幸死于车祸。

关于短期LVAD的研究在20世纪60年代继续进行,但很快就被心脏移植的开展所超越:1967年,Barnard成功施行了第一例心脏移植[8]。然而,虽然心脏移植在手术和医学上获得了短期成功,其远期预后令人失望,使得该手术明显减少,短期和长期机械循环支持装置重新引起了大家的兴趣。1972年,在国立卫生研究院(National Institutes of Health,NIH)的支持下,由学术上资深的临床医生组成了委员会,他们在华盛顿会面并建议进一步发展长期植入式LVAD。由于在当时不考虑移植,开发这些装置的一个目标是长期的心脏支持(“替代治疗”)。然而,最初的植入式LVAD再次仅被用于心脏直视手术后无法脱离体外循环的患者恢复前的短期衔接治疗。当时,在John Norman医生的指导下，得克萨斯心脏研究所拥有最多的腹腔内LVAD的临床经验[9]。虽然这些LVAD的使用未能获得有意义的长期存活，这些装置成功提供了短期的循环支持，1978年第一次使用LVAD作为衔接治疗进行了移植[10]。

在上述开发临时腹腔内LVAD的同时，也有人在尝试开发长期的、完全植入性的LVAD。这项研究也由国立心肺血液研究所支持（National Heart, Lung, and Blood Institute, NHLBI）。1976年和1978年发布了需求建议书（Requests For Proposals, RFP），以求达到使终末期心力衰竭患者恢复至纽约心脏协会（New York Heart Association, NYHA）心功能Ⅰ级状态的最终目标。正如已提到的，这些只是左心室泵，希望通过长期的左心室卸载和临时的药物支持，右心室（Right Ventricle, RV）能够得以支持。

如前所述，心脏移植的出现是植入性LVAD应用于临床的重要促进因素。在使用环孢素之前，曾植入3种LVAD作为移植前的衔接治疗（表48.1）。遗憾的是，虽然机械支持作为移植前的衔接治疗是有效的，由于当时使用的预防移植排斥反应的药物引起极度的多种免疫抑制，从而导致感染，这些患者最终都死于严重的败血症。随着环孢素的问世，将这些泵作为移植前衔接治疗的方法再次得以应用。1984年，我们医院一例活动性葡萄球菌、链球菌和念珠菌败血症患者的存活证明了在使用新型免疫抑制药物的情况下，即使严重感染的患者也能够顺利进行心脏移植手术[11]。因此，人们认为接受LVAD支持的患者，使用环孢素免疫抑制治疗也有可能顺利进行心脏移植，从而使LVAD成为移植前衔接治疗的可行选择。在这个病例被报道后不久，Portner和Oyer描述了将Novacor LVAD用于移植前衔接的情况（图48.1）[12]。此外，Thermo Cardiosystems公司（TCI）的LVAD在NHLBI的支持下也得以开发，在1986年首次植入作为移植前的衔接治疗[13]。

表48.1 两阶段的心脏置换

患者	诊断	年	过程	持续时间
47岁男性	CAOD、LVA	1969	TAH	64h
		1969	异体移植	32h
21岁男性	SBE、MR、AR、石头心	1978	LVAD	5天
		1978	异体移植	14天
36岁男性	CAOD	1981	TAH	54h
		1981	异体移植	7天

CAOD，冠状动脉闭塞性疾病；LVA，左心室壁瘤；SBE，亚急性细菌性心内膜炎；MR，二尖瓣反流；AR，主动脉瓣反流；TAH，全人工心脏；LVAD，左心室辅助装置。

虽然移植前衔接治疗并非这项技术最初设想的作用，环孢素的引入使得应用机械辅助装置后能够顺利进行移植，再次引起了对长期植入性循环支持的兴趣[14]。因此，使用这些植入型泵作为移植前衔接治疗在20世纪80年代开始增加，在20世纪90年代该领域出现指数型增长[14]。

随着供体器官等待时间的增加，LVAD支持的持续时间也随之增加。最初只有限制性气动LVAD可供选择，使用了这种装置的移植候选人由NYHA Ⅳ级状态康复至NYHA Ⅰ级或Ⅱ级状态，但遗憾的是，他们被迫住院直至移植术后。LVAD技术在1991年有了显著进步，此时首例患者接受了非限制性、可穿戴式、植入性、电子动力的TCI LVAD治疗（图48.2）。这名患者最终在1993年出院，成为首例有植入性LVAD的出院患者[15]。除了使患者有了出院的自由，这些便携式装置也能够改善终末器官功能和运动耐力，使血流动力学正常化，提高生活质量[16-19]。

当时，两种主要的搏动性植入式泵分别是Novacor和TCI[19]。1994年，气动式的HeartMate（原名TCI LVAD）首获美国食品药品监督管理局（Food and Drug

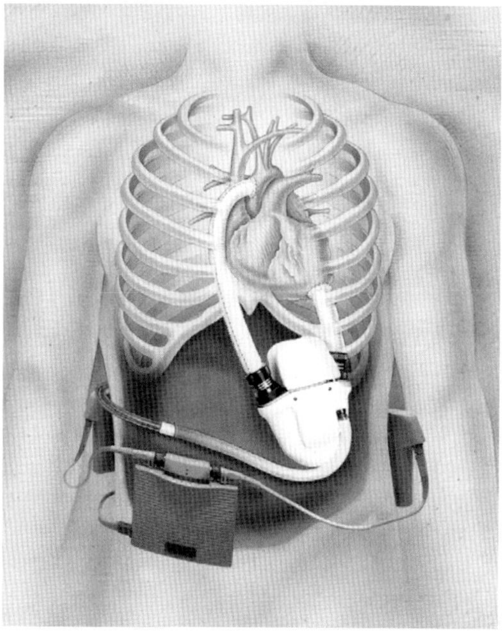

图48.1 Novacor电子动力的植入性左心室辅助装置。1984年，Oyer和Portner使用该装置首次成功进行了移植前衔接。

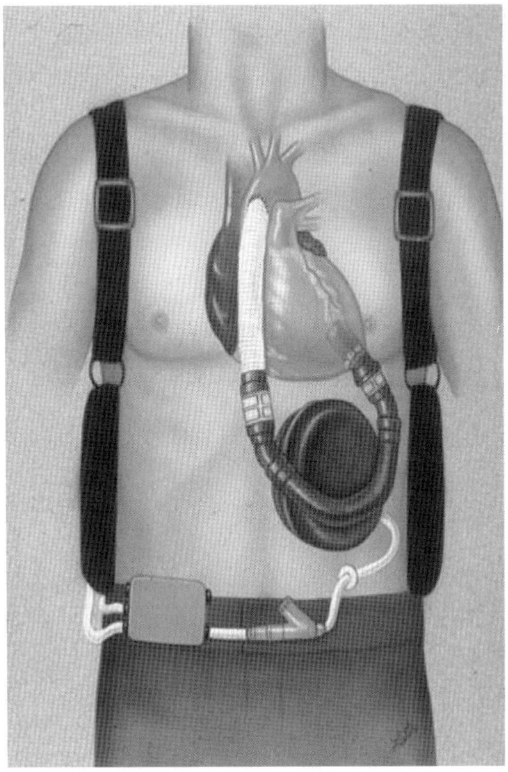

图 48.2　TCI HeartMate 左心室辅助装置(LVAD),首个允许患者出院的非限制性 LVAD。

Administration,FDA)的批准。1996 年,电子动力的 TCI 和 Novacor 植入型泵都获得了 FDA 的批准。

REMATCH 和替代治疗:起始的终点

自 20 世纪 70 年代发展这些技术作为移植替代方案的最初版本 RFP 发布以来,对于 NHLBI 非常重要的是用此目标来评估这些技术。因此,在 NHLBI 的支持下,启动了机械辅助治疗充血性心力衰竭试验的随机评价(Randomized Evaluation of Mechanical Assistance for the Treatment of Congestive Heart Failure Trial,REMATCH)。这项研究分析了非心脏移植候选者的患者使用长期 LVAD 的情况,将他们的预后与随机队列中药物治疗的患者相比较。这项研究显示,NYHA Ⅳ级症状的患者植入 LVAD 是一种可接受的治疗方案,这些患者使用 LVAD 可获得临床有意义的生存获益和生活质量的提高[20]。

这些可植入的搏动性装置作为挽救生命的技术用于经过选择的因心力衰竭而面临死亡的患者时发挥着重要作用。该装置作为移植前的衔接治疗用于这些患者非常有效。这些可植入的搏动性泵最主要的限制是尺寸和持久性。由于这些泵的尺寸很大,它们只适宜安装于正常体型的成年人。此外,由于移植的等待时间延长,这些泵的持久性就成了其最大的限制。这些泵所需要的弯曲的、非润滑的膜每 24h 会启动超过 100 000 次或每年至少启动 3800 万次,因此使其发挥 2 年功能是一个很高的目标。完成 2 年的目标是一项显著的成就。然而,超过这个时间段的成功使用还是受限的,为了达到这样的持久性通常还需要进行多次更换。因此,持久性的问题阻碍了搏动性泵进行有意义的长期心脏支持。因此,这项技术的主要用处只能是移植前衔接治疗。

旋转式血泵系统

自20 世纪 50 年代首次使用心肺机以来,对使用持续性流泵的兴趣一直存在。早在 1960 年,Saxton 等[21]就引入了将持续性流泵用于长期支持的概念。然而,当时这项技术在临床上仅用于制动患者的临时支持。由于工程学的限制以及这项技术的生理学障碍,当时并没有将旋转式血泵技术用于长期的心脏支持。

Richard Wampler 医生在 1986 年引入了血泵的概念,显示可植入的持续性流泵技术可以切实支持衰竭的心脏。为了探索该装置的潜力,资深学者(OHF)和 Wampler 医生进行了体内研究,他们使用植入性的阿基米德螺旋泵以超过 25 000rpm 的速度旋转,直接减轻了衰竭的心室负荷。这些研究显示该泵可以有效地工作,可以对抗生理压力泵到 4L,它快速的旋转不会引起溶血。1988 年首次成功将血泵应用于临床。与此同时,我们实验室也和 Robert Jarvik 合作,利用浸血轴承研发长期的可植入的阿基米德螺旋式持续性流泵。在上述研究开展之前,人们认为快速的旋转应用于血管内会造成溶血,并且通常认为无润滑式的浸血轴承无法长期植入血管系统。上述实验对于旋转式血泵作为临时或长期的心脏支持应用于临床必不可少。

与以前的容积式泵相比,旋转式血泵有几方面的优势。旋转式血泵较其前体小,因此可用于体型小的成人甚至儿童,这就使手术植入更简单,容许更合适的解剖位置。重要的是,由于流动是单向的,旋转式血泵不需要阀门,节省了一大笔费用。这种泵通常只有一个运转部件—叶轮或转子,使其机械寿命延长,并且动力传动系统较小。搏动性泵随着搏动产生负压,因此需要经皮动力传动系统作为孔口,这在持续性流泵中是不需要的,这就允许了透皮动力输送,从而完全避免了外部污染。而且，与以前的容积式泵相比，旋转式泵需要较少的动力就能够提供同水平的支持[22]。

20 世纪 90 年代末和 21 世纪初，欧洲和美国开始了旋转式血泵植入的临床使用。最初的泵使用浸血轴承的轴流阿基米德螺旋泵。MicroMed、Jarvik 和 HeartMate Ⅱ分别于 1998 年、1999 年和 2001 年被引入临床。所有这些泵的操作方法都是相似的，主要区别是是否有入口套管(Jarvik)及其长度、泵与心脏的解剖位置以及所用浸血轴承的类型。2000 年 6 月，Jarvik 泵成为第一个被用于替代治疗而非移植前衔接治疗的长期泵。这名患者由泵支持了 7.5 年。在他去世时，泵仍维持着良好的工作状态，只有轻微的轴承磨损(图 48.3)。

目前临床使用的持续性流泵

轴流泵

Heart Mate Ⅱ

HeartMate Ⅱ(图 48.4；Thoratec 公司，普莱森顿，加利福尼亚，美国)是一种植入性的轴流 LVAD，本质上是血泵原理的长期应用(图 48.5)。与此相关的研究开始于 20 世纪 80 年代，在 20 世纪 90 年代由匹兹堡大学 Bartley Griffith 所带领的研究团队进一步深入[23]。

这种电池供电的 LVAD 通过经皮导线与外部的控制器及电池相连。外部系统控制转速、监测系统功能并供电。血泵重 375g，直径 4cm，长 6cm。叶轮是该装置的唯一运转部件，由浸血轴承固定位置，由内嵌在泵壳的电磁马达所控制。叶轮转速为 6000~15 000rpm，能够产生高达 10L/min 的流量。虽然此系统无需体外循环即可植入，通常情况下，通过正中胸骨切开术并且患者置于体外循环时植入该系统[24]。该装置的流入导管通过心尖部的缝合环放在左心室腔内，或是通过左心室的膈肌面游离壁，这样导管可与室间隔保持平行。这种方法和我们目前用来植入 HeartWare LVAD 的方法相似(图 48.6)[25]。泵的流出部通过端-侧吻合的方式吻合在升主动脉。患者术后长期服用华法林以维持国际标准化比值(International Normalized Ratio，INR)在 1.5~3[26]。

2003 年在美国开始了临床试验[23,27]。到 21 世纪初，从植入 HeartMate Ⅱ的患者观察到了非常好的结果。2008 年，Thoratec 的 HeartMate Ⅱ轴流 LVAD 获得 FDA 的批准可用于心脏移植的衔接治疗，使得 HeartMate Ⅱ LVAD 的植入数量增加。获批后的一项前瞻性研究对 HeartMate Ⅱ的受者进行随访，发现接受 HeartMate Ⅱ VAD 的患者的生存率得到进一步提高，如果他们在病程早期就植入泵则尤其明显[28]。目前(2012 年 8 月)，有超过 11 000 名患者使用 HeartMate Ⅱ血泵作

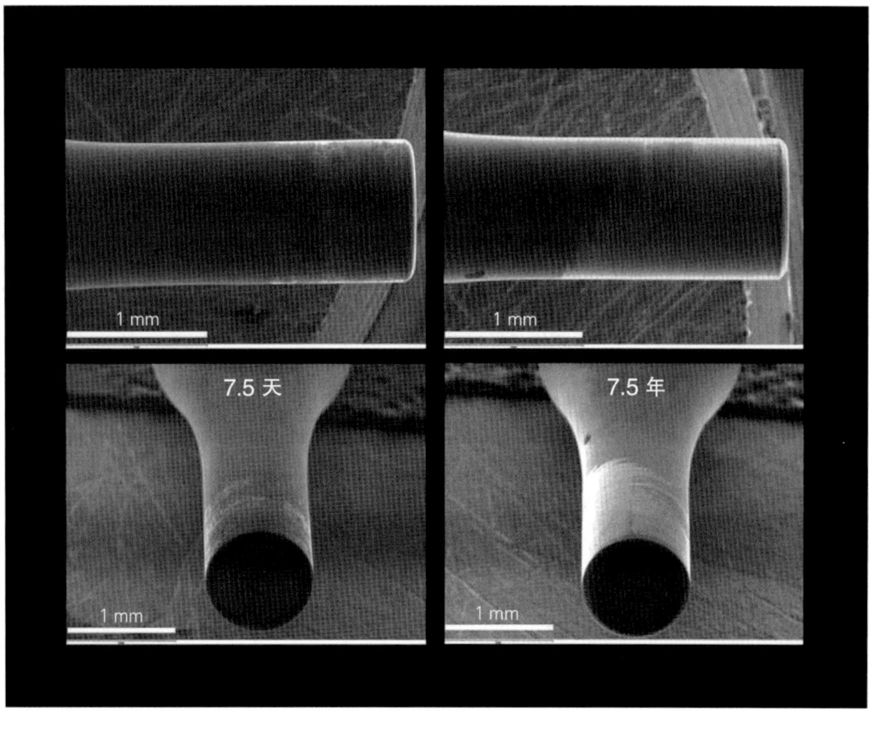

图 48.3 植入 7.5 年后，Jarvik 2000 只有轻微的轴承磨损。

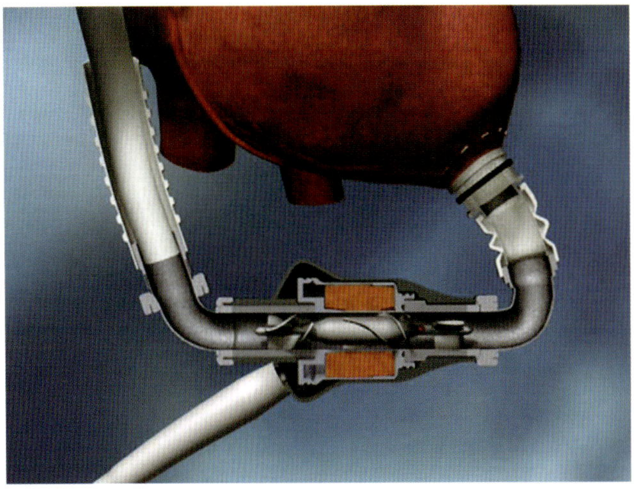

图 48.4 HeartMate Ⅱ,注意其浸血轴承。

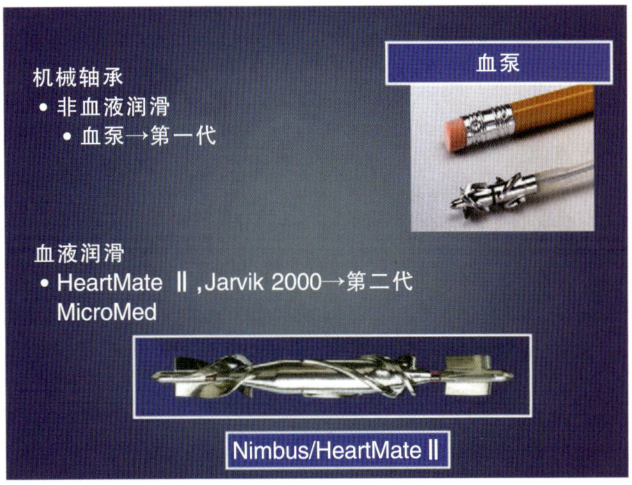

图 48.5 从血泵向 HeartMate Ⅱ 的演变。

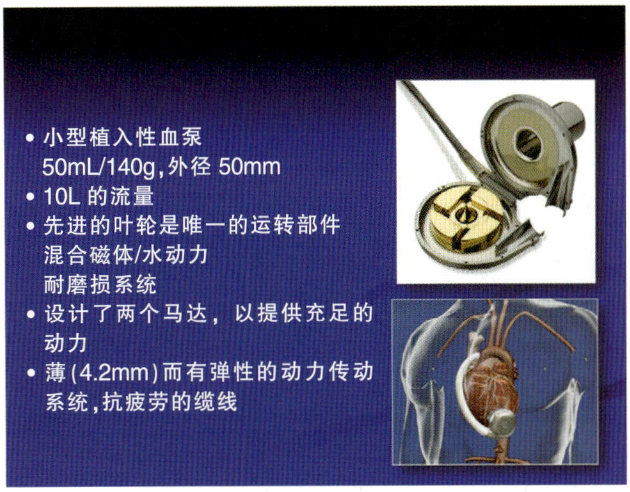

图 48.6 HeartWare 心室辅助系统。

为循环支持，意味着 HeartMate Ⅱ 是使用最广泛的植入性 LVAD。

Jarvik 2000

Jarvik 2000(Jarvik Heart 公司,纽约市,纽约州,美国)是小型的(直径 25mm,重 90g)植入性轴流 LVAD,也是在 NIH 的支持下于 20 世纪 90 年代到 21 世纪初研发出来的[29]。这种电池供电的 LVAD 通过穿出腹腔的小型经皮导联或耳后的基座与外部的控制器以及电池相连[30]。外部系统控制转速、监测系统功能以及供电。与其他轴流泵相同，叶轮是该装置的唯一运转部件,由浸血轴承固定位置。叶轮转速为 8000~12 000rpm。在生理压力下,此泵能够产生高达 7L/min 的流量[31]。为了解决可能出现的血液停滞问题,2005 年研发并应用了周期性速度控制器。该控制器每分钟将泵速降低至 7000rpm/6s。通过降低泵速,心室得以充盈并通过主动脉瓣射血。心室射血可以冲洗主动脉根部,从而预防血液停滞和血栓形成[32]。此外,通过开放主动脉瓣,可以预防主动脉瓣融合以及由此导致的主动脉瓣关闭不全和狭窄。

可以通过正中胸骨切开术植入 Jarvik 2000，泵的流出部吻合在升主动脉(图 48.7)。最初的设计是通过左胸切口植入[33]。这一技术避免了胸壁与泵接触界面造成的压力以及流出部的变形，避免了移植时反复胸骨切开。无论有无体外循环均可进行泵的植入[34,35]。该装置的独特之处在于整个血泵都可以放入左心室腔,因此无需腹膜前间隙的泵囊。没有了泵囊,感染的概率就会明显降低[36]。胸廓切开术植入的泵的流出部通过端-侧吻合的方式吻合在胸主动脉降部。华法林抗凝治疗要根据主动脉瓣的开放情况。另一种放入泵的方法是经左肋缘下切口通过心室的膈面放入。该方法尤其有利于曾接受过正中胸骨切开术的患者，通常无需体外循环就可放入装置[37]。如果使用周期性速度控制器,可以成功保持主动脉瓣开放(图 48.8),INR 应维持在 1.5~2.0。如果主动脉瓣开放极小,INR 的控制目标是 2.5~3.0[32]。Jarvik 2000 的临床试验开始于 2000 年 4 月。根据厂商的说法,目前 Jarvik 2000 在临床上已经应用于超过 360 名患者[33,34]。

InCor

InCor LVAD(Berlin Heart AG,柏林,德国)是植入

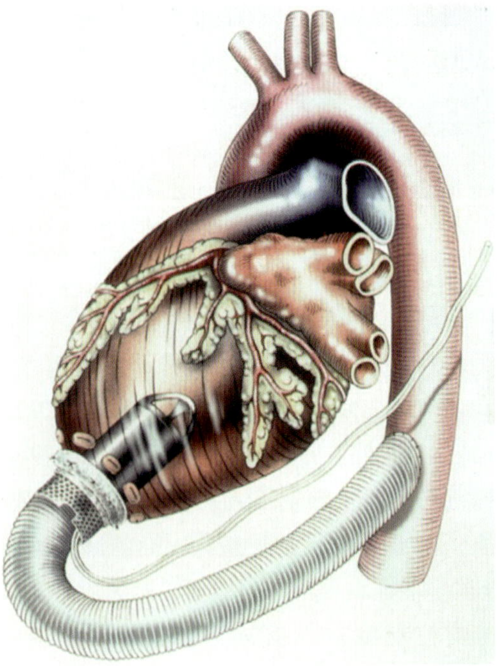

图 48.7 Jarvik 泵在心室内的放置。

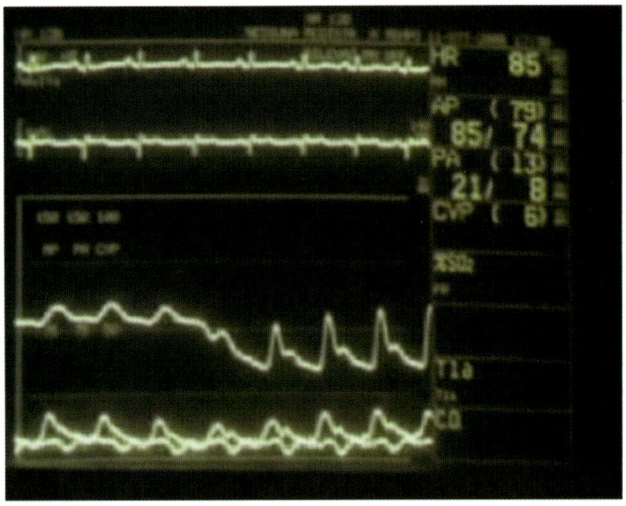

图 48.8 Jarvik 泵的周期性速度控制器保证了主动脉瓣的开放，是对该领域的重要贡献。

性的轴流 LVAD，其采用磁悬浮马达，主动轴向电磁轴承定位于马达的两端。泵重为 200g。此泵尺寸为(30×120)mm，置换容积为 80mL[38]。系统运行转速为 5000~10 000rpm，能够产生高达 7L/min 的血流[38]。一般情况下，患者在体外循环的情况下，经正中胸骨切开术植入此系统[39]。该装置的流入导管通过心尖部的缝合环放在左心室腔内。泵的硅胶流出导管通过端-侧吻合的方式吻合在升主动脉。将泵植入胸腔的心包腔内，沿着心脏的膈面放置。患者右侧的驱动电缆将泵连接于小型控制系统，后者调整和监测着整个系统。使用电池供电保证患者的活动性。InCor 接触血液的表面应覆盖 Carmeda®生物活性涂层，以降低血栓形成的风险。对于长期使用者，应进行抗凝治疗，维持 INR 在 2.8~3.2[40]。目前该系统已在全球范围内植入于超过 500 名患者[41]。

离心泵

在离心泵或径流泵中，血液垂直于泵的流出部分进入泵内，由叶轮加速，然后径向流出。虽然离心泵的直径略大于轴流泵，离心泵的整体几何结构设计符合解剖，很容易放入正常体型成年人的心包间隙。离心血泵比轴流血泵的转速低(1400~4000rpm)，无需固定叶片或定子维持泵流出部位的血流方向稳定性。

HeartWare HVAD

HeartWare HVAD(HeartWare International，迈阿密湖，佛罗里达州，美国)是植入心包腔的离心泵[42]。此泵包括一个宽幅叶片并内嵌磁石的旋转叶轮、一个内嵌磁石的中心柱和前后罩壳，各有一个密封的电动机定子。当泵启动时，叶轮开始旋转，由水动力轴承和磁石接触产生的被动磁悬浮支持。叶轮转速为 1800~4000rpm，能够产生高达 10L/min 的血流。HeartWare HVAD 重 145g，置换容积为 50mL。前罩壳包含一个综合流入导管，使得该装置能够放入左心室。

一般情况下，患者在体外循环的情况下，经正中胸骨切开术植入 HeartWare HVAD 系统。该装置的综合流入导管通过左心室膈面或心尖部的缝合环放在左心室腔内。膈面的放置方法使导管能够位于左心室的中间部分、朝向二尖瓣并平行于室间隔(图 48.9)[25]。泵的 10mm 流出部通过端-侧吻合的方式吻合在升主动脉。该泵放于心包腔内，无需腹膜前间隙的泵囊，降低了植入手术的级别。患者一侧薄而有弹性的驱动电缆连接于外部系统，后者包含可穿戴式控制器和电池，监测和控制着整个系统并为系统提供电力。长期使用则要求患者接受华法林抗凝治疗，以维持 INR 在 2.5~3[43]。目前已经植入了超过 1700 台 HeartWare HVAD。

EVAHEART

EVAHEART 系统(EVAHEART Medical USA 公司，匹兹堡，宾夕法尼亚州，美国)是植入性 LVAD，其将使用

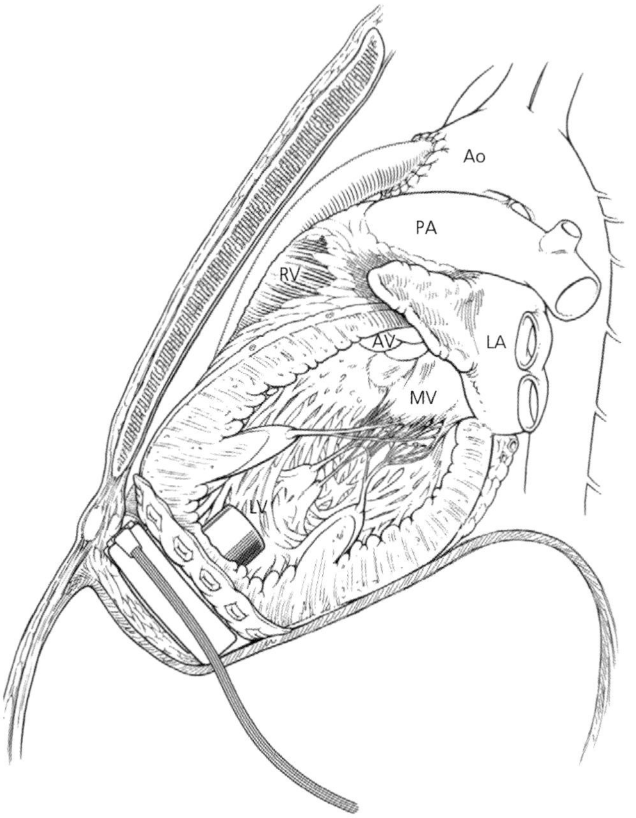

图 48.9　膈面放置流入导管可优化流入方向。LV，左心室；Ao，主动脉；PA，肺动脉；LA，左心房；AV，房室瓣；MV，二尖瓣。（Reproduced from Gregoric et al.[25], with permission from Elsevier. Copyright © 2011, Elsevier.）

离心血泵产生血流和压力与体外液体再循环系统相结合。该泵由开放式叶轮组成，叶轮安装在轴上，由重 420g 的马达驱动[44,45]。水动力轴承为旋转叶轮轴提供润滑和支持。来自体外再循环系统的液体由经皮通道泵入，发挥传热作用并防止血液蛋白的热变性。经皮动力传动系统将泵与控制器相连接。该泵可以对抗将近 90mmHg 的主动脉压力，产生高达 8L/min 的血流。EVAHEART 泵与血液接触的表面涂有 2-甲基丙烯酰氧乙基磷酰胆碱（MPC），这是一种模拟血管内膜的聚合物，提供了血液相容性表面。通过正中胸骨切开术植入 EVAHEART 血泵。16mm 的聚四氟乙烯流入和流出导管分别与左心室心尖部以及升主动脉相连接。评估 EVAHEART 的临床试验正在日本进行，近期也已在美国开始。

并发症

在过去十年里，我们处理并发症的能力已经有了进步。持续流动技术的使用给设备管理带来了深刻变化。临床上出现的旋转式血泵 LVAD 相关并发症与早期搏动性 LVAD 的并发症有很大程度的相似。然而，搏动性泵发生多数类别的不良事件的频率较高。

右心功能不全

LVAD 术前评估应包括右心室功能。慢性左心及肺动脉压力升高会导致右心室功能不全。机械辅助循环跨部门登记处（Interagency Registry for Mechanically Assisted Circulatory Support，INTERMACS）的数据显示，单纯 LVAD 支持足以支持绝大多数心力衰竭患者[46]。植入 LVAD 应可以进行临时的右心支持。大多数右心衰竭发生于手术过程中或术后早期，使用血液制品可使其加重。在植入手术过程中应进行右心室功能的评估。一旦 LVAD 启动，快速的左心室卸载会导致室间隔从右向左偏移，从而减少室间隔在右心室收缩过程中所发挥的作用，减少右向左的血流。对 LVAD 的适当调整可以帮助代偿右室功能不全并可以减少右室辅助的需求。近期，Kirklin 等的文章通过使用 INTERMACS 的数据显示，右室辅助会使死亡率增加 2 倍[47]。死亡率增加不仅和更多的血液丢失有关，也和右室辅助植入的延误有关。如果有需要，使用临时右室辅助不应被延误。

虽然最初研发植入性长期机械辅助装置是针对左心室的，现在的技术，尤其是 HeartWare 泵和在某些情况下的 Jarvik，可以应用于右心。2003 年进行了第一例右心室辅助装置（Right Ventricular Assist Device，RVAD）的植入，这是一名 Jarvik 的患者，在植入右心和左心 VAD 后不久就出现了严重的右心衰竭[48]。在此之后，有了用植入型泵进行长期右心支持的其他病例，其中，德国的中心数量最多[49]。衔接治疗取得了非常好的结果[49]。

感染

感染是管理 LVAD 受者中最大的挑战之一，仍然是 LVAD 受者最主要的死亡原因之一[50]。虽然泵和动力传动系统尺寸的减小以及经验的增加改善了使用持续流 LVAD 的预后[51]，感染和与之相关的败血症仍然是接受 LVAD 植入患者在等待心脏移植期间的主要并发症[52]。LVAD 相关的感染包括：动力传动系统出口部位的感染，有可能沿着动力传动系统，从出口部位蔓延至泵；泵囊的感染。感染相关的并发症也可能不在

LVAD本身的位置，如肺炎、胸骨伤口、泌尿系感染以及全身性感染。

消化道出血

自从长期LVAD支持开始，紧急手术后的消化道出血一直是患者管理过程中的一个挑战。气动式HeartMate和HeartMateXVE确实降低了出血的风险，因为该技术无需全身抗凝。Novacor泵需要全身抗凝，其消化道出血风险高达19%[53]。使用持续流技术就伴随着抗凝。并不是泵需要抗凝，因为泵内的流动是持续的，不存在Virchow三角的任何元素。然而，人们感觉抗凝是必须的，尤其是主动脉根部或泵入口底部周围可能会有血凝块形成。在使用LVAD的早期，人们观察到动静脉畸形处的消化道出血[54]。随着HeartMate Ⅱ泵的广泛使用，受此并发症所累的患者数量增加。这个问题被认为与使用持续性流泵引起的脉压降低有关。1958年，Heyde首先描述了严重主动脉瓣狭窄患者动静脉畸形处的出血[55]。其病因仍不清楚，但预计会有10%~15%的植入后患者出现。可以通过降低泵的转速以及尽量减少抗凝剂量解决这个问题，其中降低泵的转速可以使脉压升高。

总结

在美国，心血管相关死亡原因中心力衰竭占了34%[32,56]。由于急性心肌梗死患者的生存改善以及人群年龄的增长，心力衰竭将会持续增加成为美国一个主要的健康问题[57-60]。长期的机械性心脏支持已经成为管理等待心脏移植患者的重要且有效的工具。在过去5年中，已证实使用旋转式血泵支持可以改善等待心脏移植的严重心力衰竭患者的肾脏和肝脏功能[61]。随着更多的此类装置投入使用，临床研究提供了更强的证据支持此类装置的安全性，医学界和患者都更愿意在患者濒临死亡之前的病程早期植入此类装置。持久性延长、HeartMate Ⅱ相关的短期及长期死亡率降低减少了紧急心脏移植的需求[62]。

无法预测供者器官的等待时间，这主要是由于移植等待名单上患者数量的增加以及每年可用的供者心脏数量稳定，目前对VAD技术的使用远超过作为移植前衔接治疗的使用。VAD现在主要作为严重心力衰竭患者的长期支持，这些患者的最终目标是移植[46]。理想情况下，将来伴随更好的医疗条件和辅助疗法以及设计更合理的装置，心脏功能得以足够改善，支持的装置可以被移去[53]。

机械支持需求的增加反映了现代医疗在治疗各种循环系统疾病中的成功。如果在潜在过程就能发现并进行治疗，我们将能够攻克心脏疾病，在此之前，VAD将在恢复终末期心力衰竭患者的循环功能中持续扮演重要的角色，从而使这些患者过上完整和满意的生活。

（刘晓 译 苟晓冬 朱继业 校）

参考文献

1. Dennis C, Spreng DS Jr, Nelson GE, et al. Development of a pump-oxygenator to replace the heart and lungs; an apparatus applicable to human patients, and application to one case. Annals of Surgery. 1951;134:709–721.
2. Gibbon JH Jr. Application of a mechanical heart and lung apparatus to cardiac surgery. Minnesota Medicine. 1954;37:171–185.
3. Dodrill FD, Hill E, Gerisch RA. Temporary mechanical substitute for the left ventricle in man. Journal of the American Medical Association. 1952;150: 642–644.
4. Dennis C, Carlens E, Senning A, et al. Clinical use of a cannula for left heart bypass without thoracotomy: experimental protection against fibrillation by left heart bypass. Annals of Surgery. 1962;156:623–637.
5. Spencer FC, Eiseman B, Trinkle JK, et al. Assisted circulation for cardiac failure following intracardiac surgery with cardiopulmonary bypass. Journal of Thoracic and Cardiovascular Surgery. 1965;49:56–73.
6. DeBakey ME. Left ventricular bypass pump for cardiac assistance. Clinical experience. American Journal of Cardiology. 1971;27:3–11.
7. DeBakey ME, Liotta D, Hall CW. Left heart bypass using an implantable blood pump. In: Mechanical Devices to Assist the Failing Heart; Proceedings. Washington, D.C.: National Academy of Sciences-National Research Council; 1966: xiv: 287.
8. Barnard CN. The operation. A human cardiac transplant: an interim report of a successful operation performed at Groote Schuur Hospital, Cape Town. South African Medical Journal. 1967;41:1271–1274.
9. Norman JC, Duncan JM, Frazier OH, et al. Intracorporeal (abdominal) left ventricular assist devices or partial artificial hearts: a five-year clinical experience. Archives of Surgery. 1981;116:1441–1445.
10. Norman JC, Brook MI, Cooley DA, et al. Total support of the circulation of a patient with post-cardiotomy stone-heart syndrome by a partial artificial heart (ALVAD) for 5 days followed by heart and kidney transplantation. Lancet. 1978;1:1125–1127.
11. Frazier OH, Cooley DA, Okereke OU, et al. Cardiac transplantation in a patient with septicemia after prolonged intraaortic balloon pump support: implications for staged transplantation. Texas Heart Institute Journal. 1986;13:13–18.
12. Portner PM, Oyer PE, McGregor C. First human use of an electrically powered implantable ventricular assist system. Artificial Organs. 1985;9:36–41.
13. Frazier OH, Duncan JM, Radovancevic B, et al. Successful bridge to heart transplantation with a new left ventricular assist device. Journal of Heart and Lung Transplantation. 1992;11:530–537.
14. Frazier OH, Rose EA, Macmanus Q, et al. Multicenter clinical evaluation of the HeartMate 1000 IP left ventricular assist device. Annals of Thoracic Surgery. 1992;53:1080–1090.
15. Frazier OH. First use of an untethered, vented electric left ventricular assist device for long-term support. Circulation. 1994;89:2908–2914.
16. Catanese KA, Goldstein DJ, Williams DL, et al. Outpatient left ventricular assist device support: a destination rather than a bridge. Annals of Thoracic Surgery. 1996;62:646–652; discussion 53.
17. Frazier OH, Rose EA, McCarthy P, et al. Improved mortality and rehabilitation of transplant candidates treated with a long-term implantable left ventricular assist system. Annals of Surgery. 1995;222:327–336; discussion 36–38.
18. Moskowitz AJ, Weinberg AD, Oz MC, et al. Quality of life with an implanted left ventricular assist device. Annals of Thoracic Surgery. 1997;64:1764–1769.
19. Portner PM, Oyer PE, Pennington DG, et al. Implantable electrical left ventricular assist system: bridge to transplantation and the future. Annals of Thoracic Surgery.

1989;47:142–150.
20. Rose EA, Gelijns AC, Moskowitz AJ, et al. Long-term use of a left ventricular assist device for end-stage heart failure. New England Journal of Medicine. 2001;345: 1435–1443.
21. Saxton GA Jr, Andrews CB. An ideal heart pump with hydrodynamic characteristics analogous to the mammalian heart. Transactions – American Society for Artificial Internal Organs. 1960;6:288–291.
22. Slaughter MS, Rogers JG, Milano CA, et al. Advanced heart failure treated with continuous-flow left ventricular assist device. New England Journal of Medicine. 2009;361:2241–2251.
23. Griffith BP, Kormos RL, Borovetz HS, et al. HeartMate II left ventricular assist system: from concept to first clinical use. Annals of Thoracic Surgery. 2001;71:S116–S120; discussion S4–6.
24. Gregoric ID, La Francesca S, Myers T, et al. A less invasive approach to axial flow pump insertion. Journal of Heart and Lung Transplantation. 2008;27:423–426.
25. Gregoric ID, Cohn WE, Frazier OH. Diaphragmatic implantation of the HeartWare ventricular assist device. Journal of Heart and Lung Transplantation. 2011;30:467–470.
26. John R. Current axial-flow devices–the HeartMate II and Jarvik 2000 left ventricular assist devices. Seminars in Thoracic and Cardiovascular Surgery. 2008;20: 264–272.
27. Frazier OH, Delgado RM 3rd, Kar B, et al. First clinical use of the redesigned HeartMate II left ventricular assist system in the United States: a case report. Texas Heart Institute Journal. 2004;31:157–159.
28. Starling RC, Naka Y, Boyle AJ, et al. Results of the post-U.S. Food and Drug Administration-approval study with a continuous flow left ventricular assist device as a bridge to heart transplantation: a prospective study using the INTERMACS (Interagency Registry for Mechanically Assisted Circulatory Support). Journal of the American College of Cardiology. 2011;57:1890–1898.
29. Frazier OH, Myers TJ, Jarvik RK, et al. Research and development of an implantable, axial-flow left ventricular assist device: the Jarvik 2000 Heart. Annals of Thoracic Surgery. 2001;71:S125–S132; discussion S44–6.
30. Siegenthaler MP, Frazier OH, Beyersdorf F, et al. Mechanical reliability of the Jarvik 2000 Heart. Annals of Thoracic Surgery. 2006;81:1752–1758; discussion 8–9.
31. Parnis SM, Conger JL, Fuqua JM Jr, et al. Progress in the development of a transcutaneously powered axial flow blood pump ventricular assist system. ASAIO Journal. 1997;43:M576–M580.
32. Goldstein DJ, Zucker M, Pagani FD, et al. Rotary Ventricular Assist Devices. In: Frazier OH, Kirklin JK, editors. ISHLT Monograph Series, Vol. 1, Mechanical Circulatory Support. Addison, TX: The International Society for Heart & Lung Transplantation, 2006.
33. Sorensen EN, Pierson RN 3rd, Feller ED, et al. University of Maryland surgical experience with the Jarvik 2000 axial flow ventricular assist device. Annals of Thoracic Surgery. 2012;93:133–140.
34. Frazier OH. Implantation of the Jarvik 2000 left ventricular assist device without the use of cardiopulmonary bypass. Annals of Thoracic Surgery. 2003;75: 1028–1030.
35. Westaby S, Frazier OH, Pigott DW, et al. Implant technique for the Jarvik 2000 Heart. Annals of Thoracic Surgery. 2002;73:1337–1340.
36. Siegenthaler MP, Martin J, Pernice K, et al. The Jarvik 2000 is associated with less infections than the HeartMate left ventricular assist device. European Journal of Cardio-Thoracic Surgery. 2003;23:748–754; discussion 54–5.
37. Frazier OH, Gregoric ID, Cohn WE. Initial experience with non-thoracic, extraperitoneal, off-pump insertion of the Jarvik 2000 Heart in patients with previous median sternotomy. Journal of Heart and Lung Transplantation. 2006;25: 499–503.
38. Pagani FD. Continuous-flow rotary left ventricular assist devices with "3rd generation" design. Seminars in Thoracic and Cardiovascular Surgery. 2008;20: 255–263.
39. Attisani M, Centofanti P, La Torre M, et al. Safety and effectiveness of low dosing of double antiplatelet therapy during long-term left ventricular support with the INCOR system. Journal of Artificial Organs. 2010;13:202–206.
40. Schmid C, Tjan TD, Etz C, et al. First clinical experience with the Incor left ventricular assist device. Journal of Heart and Lung Transplantation. 2005;24: 1188–1194.
41. Timms D. A review of clinical ventricular assist devices. Medical Engineering and Physics. 2011;33:1041–1047.
42. Larose JA, Tamez D, Ashenuga M, et al. Design concepts and principle of operation of the HeartWare ventricular assist system. ASAIO Journal. 2010;56:285–289.
43. Wieselthaler GM, O'Driscoll G G, Jansz P, et al. Initial clinical experience with a novel left ventricular assist device with a magnetically levitated rotor in a multi-institutional trial. Journal of Heart and Lung Transplantation. 2010;29: 1218–1225.
44. Golding L, El-Banayosy A, Kormos RL, et al. Emerging left ventricular assist devices. In: Frazier OH, Kirklin JK, editors. ISHLT Monograph Series, Vol. 1, Mechanical Circulatory Support. Addison, TX: The International Society for Heart & Lung Transplantation; 2006: 205–217.
45. Takatani S, Matsuda H, Hanatani A, et al. Mechanical circulatory support devices (MCSD) in Japan: current status and future directions. Journal of Artificial Organs. 2005;8:13–27.
46. Kirklin JK, Naftel DC, Kormos RL, et al. Third INTERMACS Annual Report: the evolution of destination therapy in the United States. Journal of Heart and Lung Transplantation. 2011;30:115–123.
47. Kirklin JK, Naftel DC, Pagani FD, et al. Long-term mechanical circulatory support (destination therapy): on track to compete with heart transplantation? Journal of Thoracic and Cardiovascular Surgery. 2012;144:584–603; discussion 597–598.
48. Frazier OH, Myers TJ, Gregoric I. Biventricular assistance with the Jarvik FlowMaker: a case report. Journal of Thoracic and Cardiovascular Surgery. 2004; 128:625–626.
49. Krabatsch T, Potapov E, Stepanenko A, et al. Biventricular circulatory support with two miniaturized implantable assist devices. Circulation. 2011;124: S179–S186.
50. Kirklin JK, Naftel DC, Kormos RL, et al. Second INTERMACS annual report: more than 1,000 primary left ventricular assist device implants. Journal of Heart and Lung Transplantation. 2010;29:1–10.
51. Pagani FD, Miller LW, Russell SD, et al. Extended mechanical circulatory support with a continuous-flow rotary left ventricular assist device. Journal of the American College of Cardiology. 2009;54:312–321.
52. Miller LW, Pagani FD, Russell SD, et al. Use of a continuous-flow device in patients awaiting heart transplantation. New England Journal of Medicine. 2007;357: 885–896.
53. Frazier OH. Unforeseen consequences of therapy with continuous-flow pumps. Circulation. Heart Failure. 2010;3:647–649.
54. Letsou GV, Shah N, Gregoric ID, et al. Gastrointestinal bleeding from arteriovenous malformations in patients supported by the Jarvik 2000 axial-flow left ventricular assist device. Journal of Heart and Lung Transplantation. 2005;24: 105–109.
55. Heyde EC. Gastrointestinal bleeding in aortic stenosis [letter]. New England Journal of Medicine. 1958;259:196.
56. Roger VL, Go AS, Lloyd-Jones DM, et al. Heart disease and stroke statistics–2011 update: a report from the American Heart Association. Circulation. 2011;123: e18–e209.
57. Fonarow GC. Epidemiology and risk stratification in acute heart failure. American Heart Journal. 2008;155:200–207.
58. Gottlieb SS, Khatta M, Friedmann E, et al. The influence of age, gender, and race on the prevalence of depression in heart failure patients. Journal of the American College of Cardiology. 2004;43:1542–1549.
59. He J, Ogden LG, Bazzano LA, et al. Risk factors for congestive heart failure in US men and women: NHANES I epidemiologic follow-up study. Archives of Internal Medicine. 2001;161:996–1002.
60. Masoudi FA, Havranek EP, Smith G, et al. Gender, age, and heart failure with preserved left ventricular systolic function. Journal of the American College of Cardiology. 2003;41:217–223.
61. Russell SD, Rogers JG, Milano CA, et al. Renal and hepatic function improve in advanced heart failure patients during continuous-flow support with the HeartMate II left ventricular assist device. Circulation. 2009;120:2352–2357.
62. John R, Pagani FD, Naka Y, et al. Post-cardiac transplant survival after support with a continuous-flow left ventricular assist device: impact of duration of left ventricular assist device support and other variables. Journal of Thoracic and Cardiovascular Surgery. 2010;140:174–181.

第 49 章

人工心

Hannah Copeland, Jennifer Berumen, Richard G. Smith, Jack G. Copeland

引言

Syncardia CardioWest 的全人工心脏(TAH)是美国食品药品监督管理局(FDA)唯一批准的全人工心脏。TAH 被批准用于患有严重全心衰竭的潜在心脏受体。这些患者有时存在多系统器官衰竭，数小时到数天内存在死亡的风险。与左心室辅助装置相比,TAH 替代了两个心室。TAH 是第一个植入器官的替代疗法。它很可能代表了未来器官移植的新观点，即器官替代疗法可以实现，而不用担心免疫抑制的发生和供体器官的供应，而供体器官的供应基本主导着目前的器官移植实践过程。本章将介绍 TAH,它不仅独立于心室辅助装置(参见第 48 章),而且也与移植治疗模式相关。因此,本章补充了第 39 章和第 44 章的内容，这两章分别讨论了等待心脏移植患者的治疗和心力衰竭患者的重症监护。

历史

Akutsu 和 Kolff 早期进行了气动式 TAH 的研究，他们成功使犬存活了 90 分钟[1]。接下来的几年中,在牛中所进行的心脏移植的研究取得了令人鼓舞的结果，并于 1964 年,美国国会通过了国家心脏倡议,支持为人类研制 TAH。

1969 年,Denton Cooley 医生为患者植入了 Liotta 型 TAH,作为心脏移植前的过渡治疗,这位患者坚持了 64 小时后实施了心脏移植[2],但患者在移植术后 32 小时死于感染。1981 年,Cooley 医生为患者植入 Aktusu 型 TAH,患者直到移植前坚持了 53 小时[3],术后存活 8 天,也死于感染。同年,美国犹他大学的 DeVries、Kolff 和 Jarvik 获得 FDA 批准可植入 Jarvik-7 型 TAH 作为永久性心脏置换装置。他们的第一位患者 Barney Clark,于 1982 年接受了 Jarvik-7 型 TAH,治疗 112 天后死于一系列脑血栓栓塞并发症。TAH 促凝血的特性与由此产生的抗凝需求,迅速被认为是 TAH 能否成功的核心问题[4]。

1985 年 3 月,美国亚利桑那大学的 Jack Copeland 医生为救助一位急性心脏移植物功能衰竭的患者,为其植入了 Phoenix 型 TAH[5]。这名患者支撑了 12 小时后进行了再次移植，在第二次移植后 33 小时死于感染。使用未经 FDA 批准的装置是有争议的，但最终 FDA 做出了具有里程碑意义的裁决。自从 1985 年后，FDA 允许任何医生有一次机会使用未经 FDA 批准的装置,可以在“真正的紧急时刻”救助患者的生命。

随后在 1985 年 8 月 29 日,Copeland 和其团队将 Jarvik-7 型 TAH 植入到 Michael Drummond 体内[6],TAH 支持 9 天后,他成功地过渡到移植,并且在移植后存活超过 5 年。

Michael Drummond 移植前过渡的成功引起了随后 Jarvik-7 型 (100mL)TAH 及后来 Jarvik-7 型(70mL) TAH 的使用。1990 年，随着其他类型 TAH 植入的成功,FDA 认为生产 Jarvik-7 的 Symbion 公司不合规定，并停止了 Symbion 在美国行 TAH 植入的器械研究临床豁免(IDE)试验。从 1991 年开始,所有美国的心脏移植计划都暂停了。在巴黎 La Pitie 医院,Szfener 等发表报告称,基于抗凝及抗血小板的抗凝原则,连续 60 名接受 Jarcik-7 型的患者均未出现神经系统并发症[7]。对于强调血小板聚集和血栓弹力图研究的最初原则,许多项目从中获得了重要的内容。

经过启发,Jarvik-7 型 TAH 得到重新使用,这个装置于 1993 年更名为 CardioWest TAH，新的 IDE 研究在 5 个中心启动。研究的第一位患者于 1993 年 1 月在大学医疗中心(UMC)接受植入治疗。TAH 支持 186 天后她接受了移植手术,术后又存活 6 年。到 2002 年,总共研究了 81 名患者,历时 9 年的试验完成。后来,在同年,许多小型人工心脏公司因金融压力破产。面对金融压力,为“保存这项技术”,Symbion 公司得以重建并命名为 SynCardia 系统, 最后人工心脏也更名为 SynCardia TAH。IDE 研究表明,对于双心衰竭而等待心脏移植的非常严重的患者,SynCardia CardioWest TAH 能成功作为其移植前的过渡。FDA 将 2004 年提出的数据[6]作为 TAH 成为移植前过渡的唯一批准。4 年后,SynCardia TAH 被医疗保险基金认可, 从此便得到美国医疗保险和私人保险公司的赞助。

一共有超过 1000 个 SynCardia TAH 在 50 个医学中心被植入,美国和西欧各占一半。另有 39 个机构接受了培训并准备植入术的进行。现在小型驱动器可在院内和院外治疗,院外治疗需要有超过 25 年的患者治疗经验,大多经验都来自欧洲。这种装置在移植前用于过渡的时间最长可达 3.75 年。过去几年里,全世界每年都有 60~70 个 TAH 被使用。2012 年最初 2 个月内有超过 20 个 TAH 被使用。从 20 世纪 90 年代早期开始,TAH 使用的数量就稳定增加,过去 5 年内,其被快速接受并使用。

患者选择

心力衰竭患者是选择左心室辅助装置(LVAD)、双心室辅助装置(BiVAD),还是 TAH 植入物,还存在争议。有研究表明,TAH 植入的适应证包括不可逆的双心室衰竭、心脏切开术后的急性失代偿、急性心肌梗死后心源性休克、“石头心”、不可逆的心脏排斥、严重的移植物冠状动脉血管病变、不能使用 LVAD 或 BiVAD、左心室血栓致心力衰竭失代偿、获得性室间隔缺损、心源性休克或无反应性室性心律失常患者存在假体或本身功能不全的主动脉瓣。后面 6 种患者只适合 TAH 植入,而其他的患者可以使用 LVAD、BiVAD 或 TAH。如第 48 章中所述,LVAD 或 BiVAD 的适应证包括不伴有右心衰竭的左心室衰竭,以及潜在可逆的心力衰竭,如病毒性心肌炎,应避免行心脏移植。

关于 TAH 试验,FDA 注意到 CardioWest TAH 作为移植前的过渡能有 79%的存活率[8]。入选标准很严格且有选择性:

- 纽约心脏协会(NYHA)心功能分级为Ⅳ级;
- 体表面积为 1.7~2.5m^2;
- 血流动力学不稳定,指心脏指数<2.0L/(min·m^2),并满足以下 1 项:收缩压<90mmHg,或中心静脉压(CVP)>18mmHg;或满足以下 2 项:多巴胺每分钟以 10μg/kg 泵入,多巴酚丁胺每分钟以 10μg/kg 泵入,肾上腺素每分钟以 2μg/kg 泵入或血管加压药以最大剂量泵入,主动脉球囊反搏或体外循环。

这些标准便是新的国际机械辅助循环协会登记系统(INTERMACS)中的第 1 类,即撞伤和烧伤患者。2001 年,Copeland 等人发表一项回顾性研究, 对 CardioWest TAH、Novacor 和 Thoratec 作为移植前过渡的使用进行了比较[7]。研究表明,对于双心室衰竭、心源性休克、多系统器官衰竭或目前 INTERMACS 1 类(严重的心源性休克)或 2 类(心功能进行性下降)的患者,CardioWest TAH 是最好的选择[8]。

CardioWest TAH 旨在使那些对 LVAD、右心室辅助装置(RVAD)或 BiVAD 无效的患者受益,这些患者往往存在严重的多系统器官衰竭,如肾衰竭和(或)肝衰竭。在 2008 年公布的风险因素分析中, 已证明与 LVAD 装置(如 Novacor、HeartMate Ⅰ 或 Thoratec)并未增加 CardioWest TAH 的植入和生存风险[9]。同时控制左、右双心室的循环是 TAH 独有的。它可给予患者可预测的高心输出量和高灌注压。在紧急情况下,它可能拯救生命;在临界情况下,它可能降低植入术后并发症发病率。而且,对于存在瓣膜、心室、近端大血管以及心肌不可逆损伤的患者来说, 自体心室和瓣膜的原位置换提供了一种救治的手段。

患者的选择还取决于装置与受者胸廓的匹配程度。如果胸廓太小,下腔静脉(IVC)和(或)左肺静脉可能受压。充分匹配的准则包括以下内容:

- 在 T10 水平行 CT 扫描,胸骨后到脊柱前的距离为 10cm;
- 体表面积≥1.7m^2;
- 胸部正位 X 线片显示心胸比>0.5;
- 超声心动图提示左心室舒张末容积≥70mm;
- CT 扫描显示心脏体积≥1500mL。

此外,还有一些一般性准则:具有正常大小心脏的高大患者或具有较大心脏的瘦小患者很可能是良好的候选人, 而具有正常大小心脏的正常患者或瘦小患者可能不太合适。所有这些因素都需要考虑到;随着经验的增加,心脏大小问题被认为非常重要,而且外科医生也要熟练使用指南。

应用 TAH 最困难的一方面是排除那些死亡风险过大或存在致残并发症的患者。不幸的是,新研究中心选择的第一位患者往往过于乐观,最终往往以悲剧结束。这令人想起早期心脏移植的经历,那时的结果都很差。一旦应用严格的选择标准并且重视相关的禁忌证,存活率就会提高。除了不适合的匹配标准,还有一些禁忌证:恶病质、高龄、不可逆的慢性多器官功能衰竭、判定患者永远不会成为潜在心脏移植受体,以及存在高风险性大出血的情况(持续透析、既往多次手术、有肝素诱导血小板减少的病史、不能阻断旁路大出血等)。

SynCardia 全人工心脏

SynCardia 全人工心脏(TAH-t)由两个原位放置的 70mL 心室组成,它们一起能置换 400mL 血液,重 160g。它们连接到从左肋缘下方皮肤引出的管路,并通过 6 英尺(1 英尺=30.48cm)管与控制 TAH 的外部气动控制设备相连。每个心室最大存储容积约 70mL。大型控制设备包括两个完整的气动驱动器(一个起主要作用,一个备用)、两个具有足够加压空气的空气罐(每个罐能持续 2 小时)以及一组警报装置。全世界只有 36 个这样的控制设备;因此,小型的便携式驱动器成为了各大医疗机构广泛、长期的需求,到目前,这种小型的便携式驱动器才开始发挥它的功能。

气动心室装置内衬有分段聚氨酯,包括分离血液和空气的 4 层隔膜,并根据流出道的气体压力和流入道的静脉充盈压而移动。每个心室具有流入道阀门和流出道阀门。因此,在装置血液流入期间,心室在空气侧没有气压,并且通过流入道阀门充盈;而在血液流出期间,气体压力使隔膜移动,并将血液通过流出道阀门泵出。

设备运行的逻辑非常简单,即部分充盈,完全泵出(图 49.1)。这意味着该装置被设置为允许心室填充 55±5mL 血液,然后完全泵出这部分血液。控制设备上的计算机显示心室气体充盈压力、心室血液充盈速率(通过监测心室外气体的流速来测量)、心室充盈体积(充盈速率对时间的积分)、心率、大约每 1~2 秒左心室和右心室的输出量、平均输出量以及过去 8 小时的趋势。调节功能包括:每个心室的最大气体压力、心率(心室同时“搏动”)、收缩百分比(心室收缩比例)和真空压力。常规设置是:右心室压力 60mmHg,左心室压力 180mmHg,心率为 120~130 次/min,收缩百分比为 50%,真空压力约 10cmH_2O。这通常能在生理血压条件下达到 7~8L/min 的心输出量和 10~12mmHg 的中心静脉压。控制设备所选择的压力设置比预计的肺动脉压高 30mmHg,并且比预计的体循环血压高 60mmHg,因此血管阻力增加时也能完全泵出。真空绝不会在患者的心房中产生负压。它通过控制设备(距离装置 6 英尺)对气体出口施加负力,能稍微增加心室充盈速率。

外部控制设备重约 418 磅(1 磅=0.45kg),被一位患者称为“Big Blue”。携带这种控制设备的患者在移植前需留在医院,但是有两个较小类型的控制设备允许患者在医院内活动,也可出院回家。Companion Ⅱ 驱动重 55 磅。目前在美国有一种用于家庭应用的新型便携式驱动,称为 Freedom 驱动。美国 FDA 试验完成后才能广泛应用。Freedom 驱动重 13.5 磅,可以作为肩包或背包随身穿戴,患者可以回家,也可以骑自行车活动(图 49.2)。

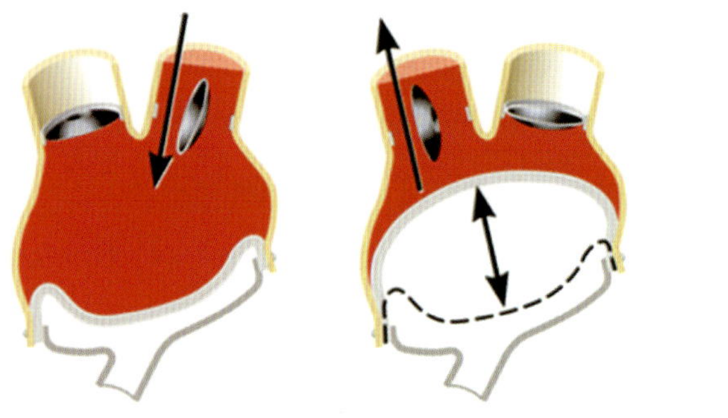

图 49.1 血液通过 SynCardia TAH-t 流动。血液通过多层聚氨酯隔膜与气体分离。血液由气压泵出,然后在静水压力下心室从心房再次充盈。

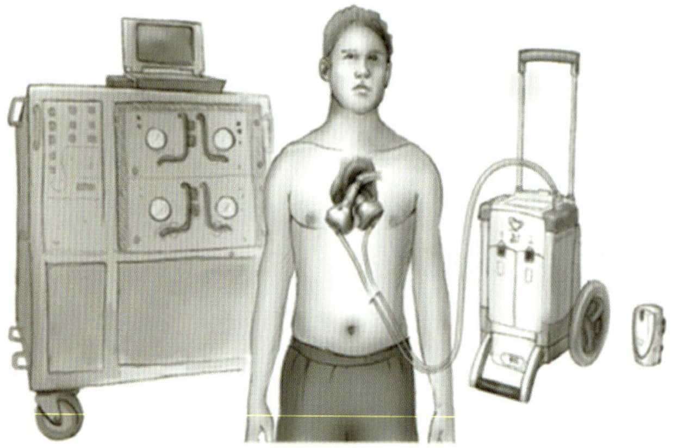

图 49.2 植入装置和三个驱动的示意图。左边的大型控制设备是“Big Blue”,重 418 磅;中间带轮子的控制设备是“Companion Ⅱ”,重 55 磅;右侧最小的是“Freedom”,重 13.5 磅。

植入和取出

装置植入与移植手术非常相似。如果外科医生在植入时不能“设计”取出方案，则装置的取出可能非常困难。

植入术的第一步是取出自身心脏。对自身心脏进行任何主要操作之前，尤其是左心室内膜可能存在附壁血栓时，应当使自身心脏停搏并且阻断主动脉。将自身心脏从房室沟的心室侧取出。保留三尖瓣和二尖瓣瓣环，以及周围 1~2mm 残余的房室瓣组织，其目的是加强心房快速连接吻合。大血管在窦管结处被离断，并充分游离以减少植入术后粘连。

阻断流出道后，连接心房，并吻合流出道。我们通常切开主动脉至快速吻合口上方 3cm，切开肺动脉至吻合口上方 6cm。将心室离断之前，构建“新心包”[10]使心室与纵隔组织分离。这样能防止严重的粘连形成，并方便移植时 TAH 的取出。我们还用聚四氟乙烯（PTFE）或其他材料松弛地悬吊上腔静脉（SVC）、IVC 和主动脉，以便在装置取出时控制这些血管（图 49.3）。

在这一点上，主要关注胸廓的排气和关闭。外科医生必须在快速连接到左心房之后，使左心室充盈，以便从左侧排出气体。其余的排气技术与常规心脏手术相似。确认匹配合适后关胸。如果装置太大，或肺水肿导致暂时的空间不足，那么关胸将立即使血泵输出下降，

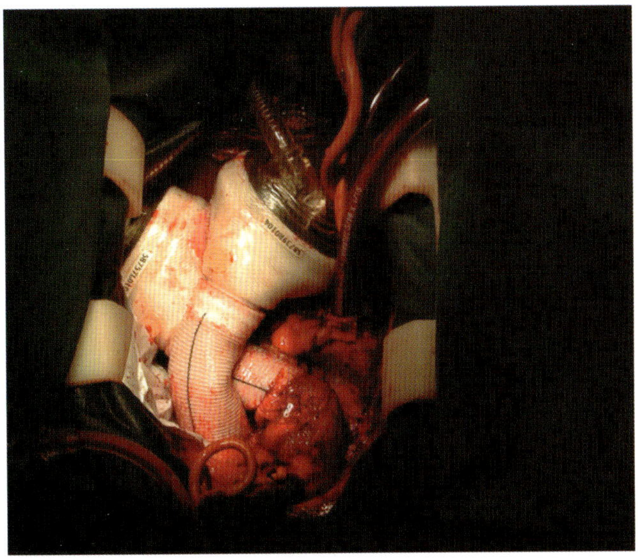

图 49.3 关胸前在原位完全植入的 SynCardia TAH-t（从患者头部观察的视图）。

必须再次开胸才能恢复。如果是这种情况，最安全的方法是将胸骨打开并用大的 Gortex 贴片关闭皮肤，同时考虑二次手术，并在纵隔炎症减少和肺顺应性增加后再次尝试关胸。

抗凝处理

TAH 患者使用抗凝和抗血小板聚集治疗后可达到凝血正常，而血小板功能中度抑制。如果 TAH 患者没有用抗凝和抗血小板聚集治疗，那么血流流经装置后，将刺激化学凝血蛋白和血小板而失去平衡，最终导致血栓形成，增加栓塞的风险。另一方面，使用当前的肝素抗凝治疗方案可能会过量而导致出血，而目前的阿司匹林方案可能不能提供足够的抗凝以抑制血小板功能，特别是预计移植后血小板增多时。因此，滴定过程中需要密切监测凝血情况和血小板功能。

我们的方法是根据血栓弹力图（TEG）和血小板功能（如血小板计数、出血时间、血小板聚集研究）来监测凝血[11]。TEG 通过测量凝血块形成期间的黏附和强度来衡量凝血块形成过程。在 TEG 中，随着凝血块的形成，存在由外来表面刺激的潜在或酶促反应。然后凝血块黏附力更强并刺激血小板黏附。数分钟后，凝血块强度变为最大，随后，如果纤维蛋白溶解系统被激活，凝血块就会被分解。

黏附性凝血块的形成速度和凝血块对外来表面的黏附具有可变性，其取决于凝血因子的活化、TEG 中初始部分因子的浓度、血小板的数量、纤维蛋白原的浓度和 TEG 中后面部分描述凝血块强度的血小板活性。在加权方程式中观察这两个特征，可以计算出凝血指数（CI）。该数值可用于定义血液“凝固性”。因此，正常范围得到确定并称为“正常凝固性”。抗凝、凝血因子耗竭和血小板减少症可导致低凝状态。在 TAH 患者中，低凝状态与出血趋势密切相关。凝血因子和血小板激活或高浓度，特别是在炎症反应增加时，将会导致高凝状态，这与装置或其他部位（静脉、病变动脉、血液淤滞或湍流区域）的凝血趋势相关。

抗凝的目的是根据 TEG 的 CI 确保患者的“正常凝固性”。该检查的优点是能安全指导医生使用抗凝剂，尤其是在植入术后的前几周。TEG 监测的肝素剂量低于它们基于部分凝血活酶时间（PTT）的剂量。使用TEG时，PTT 值甚至达不到常规使用的“治疗”水平（目标

PTT 为 45 秒)。因此,在装置植入后的最初几天几乎看不到出血。当患者从多器官功能衰竭,特别是肝衰竭恢复时,如果预计出院等待数月便能移植,那么相比肝素,可优先选择口服香豆素抗凝治疗。常规的 INR 为 2.5~3.5,联合抗血小板聚集治疗是合理的。

抗凝治疗包括阿司匹林和双嘧达莫。开始用相对高剂量(400~1000mg/d)的双嘧达莫鼻饲,在某些患者中,可静脉内给药。血小板计数至少 150 000/mm^3 后才开始使用阿司匹林,初始剂量为 81mg/d。根据血小板计数(血小板计数每增加 150 000/mm^3 需 81~162mg/d)、出血时间(目的是保持高于正常值的 1.5~2 倍)和血小板聚集(目的是保持对胶原的反应,而抑制对花生四烯酸和肾上腺素的反应),阿司匹林的剂量逐渐增加。当患者恢复并可以口服药物时,我们会给予脑康平(Aggrenox),每日 2 次口服。我们注意到,与单独使用阿司匹林或双嘧达莫相比,联合使用阿司匹林和脑康平(分别为 20mg 和 200mg)可以显著降低每种药物的使用剂量。

我们还使用潘通 400mg 每日 3 次口服用于流变效应,防止红细胞形成,降低纤维蛋白原。

术后并发症

我们最近报告了某中心 TAH 支持的连续 101 例患者 24 个患者年中的术后并发症,或者说"不良事件"[24]。主要问题是血栓栓塞、出血和感染。有 2 例患者死于三尖瓣的中心线头残留,这是可以提前预防的事件;还有 1 例死于装置故障(四个隔膜层之一穿孔)。

中风

在本报告中,出现 8 例中风(指神经功能丧失>24小时)。其中 4 例发生在术后 2 天,与植入手术有关。另 4 例发生在支持治疗(平均 87 天)后期。其中 2 例发生在状态稳定的患者中,1 例短暂的表达性失语,1 例偏瘫;2 例患者均接受了移植。另外 2 例发生在内部装置感染的患者中。1 例中风是致命的,3 例与残余缺陷相关,4 例患者存在缺陷,数天内已得到解决。因此,在稳定支持期间有 2 例中风(0.02 例事件/患者年),2 例中风仅发生在内部装置感染的 2 例患者(0.02 例事件/患者年)中。

出血

25%的患者出现出血并需要再次手术,且大多发生于植入术后 12 小时内。尽管比例似乎很高,但经验表明,对于非常严重的患者,特别是存在血小板减少和肝脏合成功能障碍的患者,装置植入后发生出血的比例相对稳定。

对这些患者出血采取的方法主要是手术。我们尝试在植入手术中做到最佳止血效果,经常耗费几个小时等待血液足够凝固,并用缝线、烧灼及局部药物控制局部出血。我们倾向于用血液和新鲜冷冻血浆替代治疗,但不愿意使用血小板,除非绝对需要。因为血小板可能携带供血者白细胞,输注血小板可能导致抗 HLA 抗体形成,从而限制随后移植的选择。我们也不愿在手术中使用浓缩的凝血因子,因为可能导致全身动脉和静脉病理性凝血的过度反应。

感染

本研究将感染定义为:任何培养阳性或疑似感染而需要使用任何抗生素治疗。64%的患者被发现患有"感染",这比例也并不意外。其中有些很严重,包括 3 例需要再次手术、引流和抗生素灌洗的纵隔感染患者,最终只有 1 例存活。

我们抗感染方法是使用规定的预防性抗生素治疗,通常只用 1~2 个剂量的万古霉素。如果已诊断为感染,就应给予特异性敏感抗生素治疗。

这三种并发症相互影响,抗凝增加了出血的风险;二次手术和出血会增加感染的风险;感染增加血液高凝及中风的风险。

死亡原因

在上述提到的连续 101 例 TAH 植入患者的报告中,有 32 例在装置支持治疗期间死亡[12]。70%患者死于术后前 2 周,这表明多数患者全身状况很差,其对存活有巨大影响。死亡原因为:13 例死于多器官功能衰竭,6 例死于肺炎和(或)肺水肿,5 例死于脓毒症,4 例死于神经损伤(1 例中风,1 例因低血压引起了低氧性损伤,2 例颅内出血),1 例为胰腺脓肿,1 例为小肠缺血,1 例为弥散性血管内凝血,1 例为弥漫性球孢子菌病。这些死亡原因与很多类型的机械装置支持治疗后的死因统计数据类似。

总结

在使用 SynCardia TAH-t 的多中心试验中，进行植入手术的患者都是经过仔细选择的，我们发现移植前过渡期的患者存活率为 80%[6,8]，移植后患者存活率为 86%。在最近的报告中[12]，因为应用的选择标准不太严格，移植的存活率降低到 70%，移植后 1 年的存活率为 77%。几个欧洲大规模中心的经验报告，通过自由选择标准，患者移植存活率为 50%~70%。无论选择偏移如何，那些被归类到“撞伤和烧伤”的患者都处于灾难性衰退的痛苦中，只有数天甚至数小时的存活时间；同时，那些不在此分类内，以及只能使用全人工心脏而没有其他解决办法的患者，通过 TAH 救助和随后的心脏移植治疗后可以存活多年。因此，任何存在严重终末期心脏病的患者均可以使用这项装置。

（杨崇威 译 向骁 朱继业 校）

参考文献

1. Akutsu T, Kolff WJ. Permanent substitutes for valves and hearts. Transactions - American Society for Artificial Internal Organs. 1958;4:240–245.
2. Cooley DA, Liotta D, Hallman GL, et al. Orthotopic cardiac prosthesis for two stage cardiac replacement. American Journal of Cardiology. 1969;24:723–730.
3. Frazier OH, Akutsu T, Cooley DA. Total Artificial Heart (TAH) utilization in man. Transactions - American Society for Artificial Internal Organs. 1982;28: 534–538.
4. Devries WC. The permanent artificial heart; four case reports. JAMA. 1988;259: 849–859.
5. Copeland JG, Levinson MM, Smith R, et al. The total artificial heart as a bridge to transplantation, a report of two cases. JAMA. 1986;256:2991–2995.
6. Copeland JG, Smith RG, Arabia FA, et al. Cardiac Replacement with a total artificial heart as a bridge to transplantation. New England Journal of Medicine. 2004;351:859–867.
7. Copeland JG, Smith RG, Arabia FA, et al. Comparison of the CardioWest total artificial heart, the Novacor left ventricular assist system and the Thoratec ventricular system in bridge to transplantation. Annals of Thoracic Surgery. 2001;71:S92–S97.
8. Kirklin JK, Naftel DC, Kormos RL, et al. Second INTERMACS annual report: more than 1,000 primary left ventricular assist device implants. Journal of Heart and Lung Transplantation. 2010;29(1):1–10.
9. Copeland JG, Smith RG, Bose RK, et al. Risk Factor analysis for bridge to transplantation with the CardioWest total artificial heart. Annals of Thoracic Surgery. 2008;85:1639–1644.
10. Copeland JG, Arabia FA, Smith RG, et al. Synthetic membrane neo-pericardium facilitates total artificial heart explantation. Journal of Heart and Lung Transplantation. 2001;20(6):654–656.
11. Copeland JG, Arabia FA, Tsau PH, et al. Total artificial hearts: bridge to transplantation. Cardiology Clinics. 2003;21:101–113.
12. Copeland JG, Copeland H, Gustafson M, et al. Experience with over 100 total artificial heart implants. Journal of Thoracic and Cardiovascular Surgery. 2012;143(3):727–734.

第 50 章
人工肺

Claire A. Watkins, Bartley P. Griffith

引言

在美国估计有 750 000 例呼吸衰竭患者，其中每年有 15 万人死亡[1]。从 1972 年最早应用心肺转流术开始，体外膜肺氧合(ECMO)技术已经发生变化，改善了生存率并减少了呼吸衰竭的发病率[2]。人工氧合器使用多孔中空纤维进行气体交换；血液通常在血泵作用下流过纤维，而气体则透过纤维(图 50.1)。早期有两项随机临床试验使用 ECMO 治疗成人呼吸窘迫综合征(RADS)患者，但存活率都较低，一项试验是在 1974 年，存活率为 10%[3]；另一项试验是在 1994 年，存活率为 33%[4]。尽管低的存活率降低了科学家对人工肺的研究兴趣，但是技术的改进，包括管路肝素涂层、聚甲基戊烯(PMP)扩散膜、离心式血泵和插管的重新设计，使结果得到改善，推动了 ECMO 更多的临床应用[5,6]。20 世纪 80 年代和 90 年代的研究[2,7,8]一致表明存活率为 40%~50%。2009 年的多中心 CESAR 试验显示，与单独通气相比，随机进行 ECMO 联合机械通气的 ARDS 患者的死亡率降低[9]。21 世纪初 H1N1 流感大流行时，使用 ECMO 的存活率>70%，在急性呼吸衰竭的治疗中有着显著效果[10]。此外，最近的研究表明，使用 ECMO 作为移植前过渡时，存活率为 50%~80%。ECMO 的成功及其适应证的扩大也促进了其他人工肺装置的发展。对于大多数生命支持的机械装置，通过选择早期行机械通气且没有其他疾病的患者，其存活率有显著改善。随着人工呼吸系统生物工程的发展，预计结果将会变得更好。

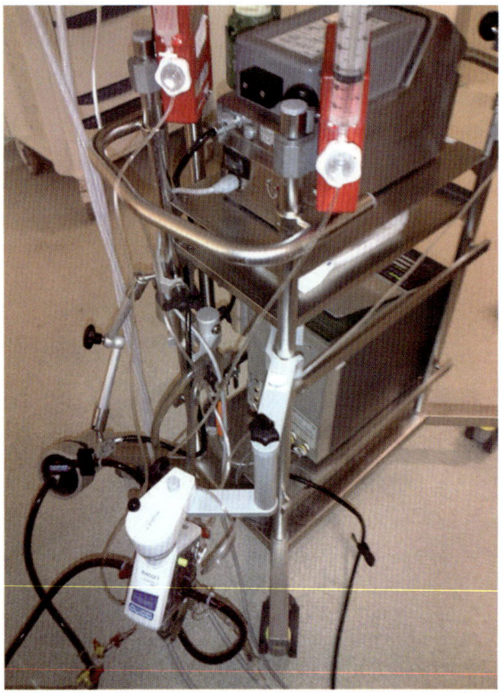

图 50.1　ECMO 回路。

广义的首字母缩略词 ECMO 通常被认为包括 $ECCO_2$-R(CO_2 清除)、ECLA(肺辅助)和 ECLS(生命支持)。然而，ECMO 最初应用在 ARDS 失代偿的缺氧患者，因为 3%~15%的呼吸衰竭是因为 ARDS[2]。根据 ARDS 临床试验协作网(ARDSNet)呼吸机管理指南，包括低潮气量(<6mL/kg)、低平台压、允许性高碳酸血症、吸入性肺血管扩张剂和合理的液体使用，ECMO 患者生存率接近 60%[11]，这可能使相当大的一部分患者从中获益。严重情况下，这种通气方法可能无法提供足够的气体交换，并且可通过诱导性气压损伤、肺泡损伤、毛细血管通透性增加、肺水肿和炎症而导致 ARDS 的进展(参见第 45 章)[2]。正如 CESAR 试验中所表明的，在 ECMO 的使用中，低频率、低潮气量的呼吸方法不仅使肺得到休息，减少呼吸机相关的肺损伤，而且还使 ARDS 患者存活率得到改善。这项多中心盲法临床试验中，严重 ARDS 患者随机接受单独常规呼吸机治疗，或联合 ECMO 治疗。本研究观察到联合 ECMO 治疗 6 个月的无病存活率有显著改善(63%对 47%)，表明严

重 ARDS 患者应优先选择 ECMO 治疗[9]。

在 ECMO 作为移植的过渡之前，它成功地用于救助移植后移植物功能障碍的患者。原发性移植物功能障碍(PGD)是肺移植后早期死亡的主要原因，约 15%~35%的患者在移植后发生，其中 7%有需要 ECMO 支持的病史[12,13]。PGD 表现为进行性缺氧、肺顺应性丧失，最终出现血流动力学不稳定。PGD 促进因子包括缺血再灌注损伤、排斥反应、缺血时间延长，以及可能的大量输血。尽管在术后无须使用 ECMO 的肺脏受体存活率更高(82%对 40%)，但研究表明移植后脱离 ECMO 的患者(67%)，其存活率与无 ECMO 对照组接近(80%对 82%)[12]。移植后 ECMO 对受体的肺功能没有长期影响。移植术后 PGD 患者脱离 ECMO 的能力在支持超过 14 天时显著降低，这种情况必须考虑再次移植[12]。ECMO 的死亡率为 25%[14]~60%[12]，在移植失败时，它能使肺功能恢复或作为再次移植的过渡救助患者。

截至 2005 年，等待肺移植的呼吸衰竭终末期患者名单中，1 年时死亡率为 20%，2 年为 40%，这明显表明需要移植前和过渡替代装置，使患者在移植前可能存活[15]。随着 ECMO 成功应用于 ARDS 患者，并实现移植前救助，它又增加了“移植前过渡”的用途。然而，由于只有短期存活率的独立报道结果，ECMO 作为移植前的过渡支持延迟使用。最初，ECMO 被认为是移植的禁忌证，因为存活率结果较差(2002 年大约为 60%)[5]。但是，有病例报道称，对于年轻急性病患者，通常患与流感相关的细菌肺炎，ECMO 能作为早期肺移植前的过渡而救助成功，这表明 ECMO 治疗对此类患者有一定帮助。ECMO 的这种适应证可应用于大量存在不可逆呼吸衰竭但不合并其他器官衰竭的患者，这些患者可能无法在等待移植名单上存活。目前报道表明 ECMO 患者存活率为 50%~80%；因此，分配肺源给 ECMO 患者是合理且常见的。

ECMO 在肺移植中的支持应用

ECMO 的适应证随着呼吸衰竭的临床紧急程度不同而变化(表 50.1)。通常情况下，对于不合并其他器官衰竭的急性或慢性呼吸功能失代偿患者，ECMO 可用作移植前的过渡支持。尽管各机构中心指南有所不同，但 PaO_2<50mmHg，$PaCO_2$>80mmHg 和(或)PaO_2/FiO_2<1 时，通常应考虑 ECMO 治疗[16]。禁忌证通常包括抗凝、不可逆的中枢神经系统(CNS)损伤、脓毒症、多器官功能衰竭和严重的外周血管疾病[6]。急性肾衰竭、高剂量血管升压素需求、年龄、肥胖和长期持续的机械通气是相对禁忌证[16]。唯一的绝对禁忌证是不可逆的 CNS 损伤。最近的数据表明，慢性严重肺功能衰竭而预计移植的患者可能因早期植入 ECMO 获益[6]。尽管出血和血栓形成在 ECMO 患者中总是能达到微妙的平衡，但是在不能抗凝或具有出血史的患者中，使用肝素结合的 ECMO 组件减弱了对 ECMO 的禁忌。虽然不是禁忌证，当出现肺炎或脓毒症时，ECMO 可能使生存率显著降低[10]。

启动 ECMO 的决定应基于呼吸受损的严重程度和患者恢复或移植前成功过渡的可能性。急性肺损伤治疗中的其他进展[例如吸入一氧化氮(iNO)、低潮气量呼吸机方案和俯卧位]可以改善一些参数，并将 ECMO 用于治疗更严重的呼吸衰竭病例[2]。此外，随着清醒和动态 ECMO 益处的发现，ECMO 在慢性疾病中的应用时机和使用正在发生变化。

作为移植前过渡的 ECMO 支持模式

临床上用于决定移植前过渡支持 ECMO 模式的因素包括：血流动力学稳定性、氧饱和度、通气失败及右心室(RV)或肺动脉(PA)衰竭。ECMO 技术可分为静脉-静脉(V-V)、静脉-动脉(V-A)和动脉静脉介入性肺辅助(iLA)ECMO(图 50.2)。因缺氧和轻度 RV 衰竭而出现的血流动力学轻微失代偿通常可以用 V-V ECMO 达到稳定的血流动力学状态，而心源性休克只能用 V-A ECMO。V-V 和 V-A 插管策略均可改善全身氧合；然而，V-A ECMO 通常能为失代偿性心力衰竭患者提供必要的即时循环支持[17]。在大多数情况下，优先选择 V-V 插管，因为其本身可降低全身血栓栓塞的风险，且不存在动脉插管相关的损伤。V-V 模式中持续性缺氧是由于再循环和(或)不能通过外周 V-V 插管将所有不饱和静脉血运送到 ECMO 通路中。如果在重置流入和流出管道后仍严重缺氧(动脉饱和度<85%)，则需考虑中心 V-V 插管或使用 V-A 模式。不伴有左心衰竭时，我们强烈建议避免使用 V-A 模式，并且通过切开胸骨上 1/3，从中央插入右心房(RA)作为流入道，插入肺动脉(PA)作为流出道。插管从右肋缘下方引出，以减少胸骨小切口的感染，而患者也能随着身体的恢复慢慢活动。在 V-V ECMO 技术中，已有其他创新的策略成功地使心力衰竭患者血流动力学达到稳定，包

表 50.1　不同移植中心的 ECMO 适应证

中心	急性标准	慢性标准
麻省总医院 宾夕法尼亚大学 彼得本特布里格姆医院 奥兰治县医疗中心 纽约西奈山医院 加州大学 北卡罗来纳大学 瑞典斯德哥尔摩卡罗林斯卡医院	在 FiO_2 为 1.0 的条件下，PaO_2<50mmHg 持续两小时以上；PEEP≥5cmH_2O	在 FiO_2 为 0.6 的条件下，PaO_2<50mmHg 持续 12 小时以上；PEEP≥5cmH_2O；最大治疗时间超过 48 小时
德国马尔堡菲利普斯大学	A-a>525mmHg；CT_{stat}30mL/cmH_2O; PIP>35cmH_2O；胸部 X 线片存在浸润；最大药物治疗时间>24 小时（急慢性标准没有区别）	
德国柏林自由大学附属夏里特医院 德国柏林洪堡大学 英国莱斯特 ECMO 中心	PaO_2/FiO_2<50mmHg 超过 2 小时；PEEP≥10cmH_2O	最大治疗时间 24~120 小时；PaO_2/FiO_2<150mmHg；PEEP≥10cmH_2O；Q_S/Q_T≥30%；EVLW≥15mL/kg；CT_{stat}≤30mL/cmH_2O 或复发性气压性创伤
法国巴黎科钦大学医院	与麻省总医院一致 评分>2.5	与麻省总医院一致 评分>2.5
密歇根大学	最佳的常规疗法；Q_S/Q_T>30%； CT_{stat}<0.5mL/(cmH_2O·kg) 胸部 X 线显示四个象限的异常弥漫影	
德国慕尼黑路德维希-马克西米利安大学	PaO_2/FiO_2<50mmHg； PEEP≥5cmH_2O 超过 2 小时 CT_{stat}≤30mL/cmH_2O	经历 48~96 小时常规治疗后：满足下面 4 个标准中的任意 3 个：PaO_2/FiO_2<150mmHg；PEEP≥5cmH_2O 持续 2 小时以上；$PaCO_2$≥60mmHg；VE≥200mL/kg；PIP≥40cmH_2O；CT_{stat}≤30mL/cmH_2O；Q_S/Q_T≥30%
加拿大多伦多综合医院 马里兰大学	危及生命的心肺功能受损；进行性呼吸衰竭；氧合不相容；使用半选择性 ECMO	
奥地利维也纳大学	PaO_2/FiO_2<70mmHg PEEP>10cmH_2O 持续 96 小时	

PaO_2，动脉血氧分压；FiO_2，吸入氧浓度；PEEP，呼气末正压；A-a，肺泡动脉血氧梯度；PIP，吸气峰压；CT_{stat}，胸肺顺应性；Q_S/Q_T，肺内分流；EVLW，血管外肺水；VE，每分通气量。

Adapted with permission from Lewandowski et al.[2] BioMed Central. Copyright © 2000.

括房间隔造口术。房间隔造口术可以将容积卸到左心室(LV)，并可通过左心房(LA)和 LV 的氧合静脉血来运输高氧饱和度的血液。另一种方法是胸骨切开术和中心二次插管，从 RA 流入并流出到 PA、LA 或主动脉。除了传统的 ECMO，无泵 iLA 已经可以使肺动脉高压患者成功过渡到移植，甚至可以拔管、下床活动[16,18]。

插管通常采用颈内静脉、股静脉和(或)动脉。虽然大多数插管可以经皮放置，但在手术期间可选择在 RA 和主动脉之间开胸插管。V-A 插管还存在由于血栓形成而导致远端肢体缺血的威胁，且需要进行频繁的肢体灌注评估[16]。在没有全身灌注时，存在血液通过回路发生回流的可能，这在插管植入过程中是非常值得考虑的重要因素。防止发生的方法是，使流入管道和流出管道末端之间保持距离。使用 V-A ECMO，可以在腹主动脉下段股动脉插管的尖端实现全身血液的充分氧合[6]。当流入管道和流出管道血氧含量高，而与患者氧合无关时，需怀疑发生了回流。V-A ECMO 股动静脉流出道插管中另一个值得注意的方面是，氧合血优先流向下

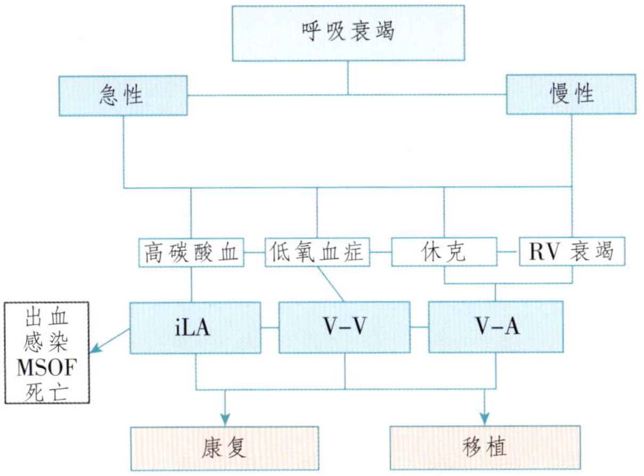

图 50.2 ECMO 的临床决策。

iLA，介入性肺辅助；V-V，静脉-静脉；V-A，静脉-动脉；MSOF，多系统器官衰竭；RV，右心室。

肢和腹部，使心脏和脑灌注依赖于心排血量。有人提出腋动脉插管，以避免上身混合血氧灌注且出现严重的外周血管疾病，同时患者也可下床活动[19]。上肢和下肢血氧饱和度存在任何差异都应得到处理，可通过通气和循环血流量进行调节[16]。只要先前的氧饱和度下降、循环回路压力增加（流入道负压、流出道正压）和溶血，都应当怀疑发生了插管相关的并发症，例如血栓形成、扭转或错位。

根据多伦多移植计划指南，ECMO 的常规治疗目标包括血氧饱和度>85%，PaO_2>100mmHg，PCO_2 为 35~45mmHg，pH 值为 7.35~7.45。为防止血栓并发症，V-V 和 V-A ECMO 支持时，活化凝固时间（ACT）应该保持在 160~200 秒。为防止出血并发症，出血时，国际标准化比率（INR）应<1.8 或<1.5，血小板应>80 000/mm^3 或>100 000/mm^3[16]（表 50.2）。可使用利尿剂控制体重，必要时行血液过滤。

表 50.2 马里兰大学 ECMO 的目标参数

血细胞比容	>35%
血小板	>20 000/μL
	>50 000/μL（输血情况下）
激活凝血时间	160~180 秒
血浆游离血红蛋白	<10mg/dL
乳酸脱氢酶	<300U/L
动脉血氧饱和度	>85%
二氧化碳分压	35~40mmHg

ECMO 过渡支持的并发症

ECMO 的缺点包括有限的持续使用时间及高并发症发生率[15]。患者使用 ECMO 作为肺移植前过渡支持可能发生的并发症包括肾衰竭（35%）、肺部感染（52%）、脓毒症（41%）、致命性脓毒症（17%）、气管切开（41%）、肠缺血（11%）、胃肠道出血（6%）和中风（6%）[20]。尽管肝素涂层管路的发展部分缓解了对高度全身性抗凝的需求，但影响死亡率的主要并发症是出血。由于血泵的剪切力作用，需要频繁监测血细胞的破坏情况，例如溶血、血小板活化，以及产生炎症反应的白细胞消耗和活化（表 50.2）。溶血不仅与细胞计数有关，而且与乳酸脱氢酶和血浆游离血红蛋白水平相关。有其他研究表明，ECMO 出血并发症发生率为 52%，血液透析发生率为 42%，神经系统事件发生率为 12%[13]。

ECMO 过渡支持的结果

尽管 ECMO 作为终末期呼吸衰竭患者肺移植前过渡支持的意义已确定，但所报道的获益情况却不尽相同。最大的一项研究调查了全美的 51 例患者的结果，研究显示，ECMO 作为移植过渡的一年存活率为 50%[21]。另外一些大型移植中心的单中心研究报道了更高的存活率：80%（汉诺威）、74%（匹兹堡）[20]和 60%（维也纳）[17]。斯堪的纳维亚两项大样本中心研究报告称，ECMO 过渡患者一年存活率为 75%，移植后一年存活率为 92%，而 10 年存活率达 50%[22]。此外，本研究中超过 60%的移植是使用国际心脏和肺移植学会（ISHLTS）标准中的边缘供体。这些结果表明，ECMO 作为移植过渡非常值得考虑。ECMO 在移植中的效果明显取决于该中心使用这项技术的经验，具有较大样本的中心结果会更好，而且随着时间的推移，所有中心的结果都能得到改善。此外，与回家等待移植的患者相比，ECMO 患者更严重且更复杂，因此 ECMO 患者报道的结果更差。应用过渡支持的 CO_2 清除装置的患者有更高的存活率，需要稳定的血流动力学状态（V-V 和 V-A ECMO 患者通常缺乏）[17]。有趣的是，在维也纳研究中，移植受者的发病率和死亡率在移植前 ECMO 的持续时间没有差异，据推测这是导致结果变化的原因。虽然 60%的存活率可能显得较低，但值得注意的是，存活 3 个月的患者中，78%能存活至 1 年，这与该机构所有其他肺移植患者 80%的存活率没有显著差异[17]。美国的经验也有类似的发现,与不用ECMO支持的移植患者相比,ECMO增加了移植早期而非晚期的死亡率风险[21]。这表明,如果濒死的ECMO患者在需要使用支持的早期失代偿中存活下来,其结果将与其他肺移植患者类似。在对匹兹堡(大型移植中心)结果的回顾中发现,移植前应用ECMO使围术期死亡率增加,但与1年内移植物功能无关(74%)[20]。本研究中,通过排除任何其他器官衰竭或全身感染的患者,以及使用标准供体,可获得更高的存活率。匹兹堡研究的其他结果包括:ECMO患者更年轻,多次移植更常见,缺血时间更长,PDG代谢率更快,并且更有可能(48%对7%)需要移植后ECMO救助[20]。美国最近通过肺移植器官分配评分(LAS)再次阐述了移植分配目标:向最紧急、最可能获得好的存活结果的患者捐献器官。同时,需要机械通气而获得高评分的ECMO患者会优先得到帮助。

ECMO移植过渡支持的新方向

肺移植前的机械通气是发生并发症的重要危险因素,例如感染、呼吸机相关的肺损伤、生理功能失调、其他系统器官功能障碍以及死亡率增加[23,24]。在ECMO作为移植前过渡支持的治疗期间,避免机械通气可能改善存活率结果,减少并发症。正如最初报道的5例肺动脉高压和右心衰竭的清醒患者,在终末期呼吸衰竭早期及机械通气前开始使用ECMO获得了满意的生存结果。在研究中,没有应用镇静剂,只在局部麻醉下进行V-A插管。2例患者死于出血并发症。3例患者恢复自主呼吸,可进食和饮水,无须补充额外营养,参与被动和主动理疗,最终完全恢复[25]。

“清醒ECMO”方法已经广泛应用到终末期呼吸衰竭患者,并取得了令人兴奋的结果。试验这种策略的最大研究中心来自汉诺威,该研究将26例清醒ECMO患者作为试验组,34例使用常规机械通气过渡的患者作为对照组[6]。清醒ECMO组患者(13例V-V和13例V-A)在过渡前具有显著更高的急性生理Ⅱ级评分和更低的氧饱和度,但移植后机械通气时间减少,6个月时死亡率降低。当清醒ECMO患者需要插管(最常继发于出血)时,存活率降至43%。而且,清醒ECMO患者入住ICU时间(P=0.07)和住院时间(P=0.06)趋于下降[6]。有趣的是,尽管通常病情很重,清醒ECMO组在等待肺捐献时没有出现更高的死亡率。清醒ECMO组作为肺移植的过渡支持有明显的生存获益,可能是因为避免了麻醉和机械通气的危险。此外,在右心衰竭的病例中,麻醉诱导和插管导致循环衰竭风险高。清醒患者可进食、饮水、自主呼吸、参与物理治疗,可能有助于改善移植后的生存结果。患有间质性肺纤维化(IPF)等严重低氧血症患者,不仅需要保证氧合的充足,而且需要保证呼吸的舒适,这导致清醒ECMO方法的应用相对困难[6]。

相比于清醒ECMO的发展,V-V ECMO技术中创建用于单一插管的双腔静脉导管推动了清醒和动态ECMO过渡支持技术的发展[26]。在超声引导下置入双腔导管(Avalon Elite Bicaval双腔导管),将流入道导管尖部的近端和远端分别置入上腔静脉(SVC)和下腔静脉(IVC),并将流出道导管置入RA。流入道导管远端应远离IVC,位于肝静脉处或经过肝静脉,以避免血液通过回路发生回流。流出道应在超声引导下指向三尖瓣。导管大小包括23F、27F和31F,并可以提供高达3.5~5L/min的血流量。使用Avalon导管,应在ECMO启动时采用全身抗凝,并在整个支持期间维持ACT在140~160秒。在最初的报告中,双腔导管能够维持氧合(使PaO_2中位值从45mmHg增加到115mmHg),稳定血流动力学状态[使平均动脉压(MAP)中位值从48mmHg增加到72mmHg],72%的患者顺利脱离支持,包括那些存在慢性阻塞性肺疾病(COPD)的患者。没有与ECMO直接相关的死亡病例(存活率55%),但是有2例的导管需要紧急重新置入,1例存在抗凝不完全导致导管血栓形成[26,27]。流入管道血液中,任何急性氧饱和度下降或氧分压增加都会引起导管并发症,需要在超声引导下重新植入。类似于清醒ECMO,步行能充分清除痰液,减少肺部感染,加快身体康复,随着恢复程度的进展,患者还可以选用跑步机和固定脚踏车来进行运动[27]。除了不能进行股动静脉插管外,这种技术可用于有IVC滤器置入等血管介入病史的患者。通过缩短导管长度及尽量减少与外来材料接触,双腔导管也可减少炎症和血栓形成[26]。尽管最开始的结果令人兴奋,但目前仍没有单一插管与传统V-V ECMO的直接比较。

人工肺清除 CO_2

Gattinoni等在1978年首次提出使用人工气体交换降低通气需求、减轻因CO_2清除产生的气压伤,从而扩展了ECMO除氧合不足之外的适应证[28]。在羊的试验中,他们应用室内空气透过硅胶膜肺,结果表明自主呼吸及机械通气的动物，通过清除 CO_2，其潮气量、呼吸速率、吸气峰压和呼气末压均下降，pH、心排血量和氧饱和度也均得到改善。此外，该研究组表明，人工 CO_2 清除可以使气道压力显著降低，足以治疗常规机械通气不能解决的严重的支气管瘘[28]。这项研究使体外气体交换应用于不同的临床病例，促进了全新改进装置的发展。

1999 年开发的 NovaLung 是一种无泵 PMP 膜肺，对于存在严重通气功能障碍，并伴有高碳酸血症和呼吸性酸中毒的患者，它能使患者 pH 值、吸气峰压和呼气末正压达到正常，也能显著改善 $PaCO_2$ 和 PaO_2[29]。这种方法类似于 ECMO 技术的肺保护性通气策略，但也应注意防止肺气压伤和呼吸机相关肺损伤的发生，这都已确定能增加远处器官衰竭的风险[30]。在患严重通气功能衰竭的成年人中，该装置能够清除多达 70%的过量 CO_2，同时能保持稳定的血流动力学状态。2005 年，NovaLung 最初用作肺移植过渡支持时，其 1 年存活率为 80%[13]。此外，有研究证明，对于肺切除术后患有 ARDS 的患者，临床状态的死亡率为 40%~60%，而 NovaLung 能提高存活率至 71.4%[31]，使患者获益。iLA 能减少进展性 COPD 患者肺通气，并增加其肺顺应性[10]。iLA 已成功用于严重的胸部损伤、ARDS、肺动脉高压、肺炎和气道阻塞的治疗[29]。

低阻抗 iLA 装置在股动脉和股静脉间植入，并通过心脏输出(而不是血泵)产生 0.5~4.5L/min 的血流量。NovaLung 缺乏人工血泵成分，这意味着只有较少的心排血量(约 20%)通过回路，因此回路可以更小，从而更加减少灌注量和异物接触面积[31]。与 ECMO 不同，CO_2 清除程度取决于扫气流量，而不是血流量。虽然在 iLA 的设置中通常由自身肺维持氧合，但是在 NovaLung 中可以使氧合轻微增加。iLA 的禁忌证包括严重缺氧、心源性休克或外周血管疾病[29]。在置入 iLA 之前，应通过超声测量股动脉直径。合适的插管尺寸应比动脉直径至少细 20%[31]。当连接两个导管并用肝素化盐水冲洗时，应使血液缓慢流入 iLA，时间至少为 2 分钟，以减少产生的 A-V 分流对血流动力学造成影响。用作流入道的动脉插管有导致肢体低灌注而缺血的额外风险，因此需要频繁评估外周肢体灌注。气体流速通常以 1L/min 开始并根据血气结果测量。治疗原则包括，在压控模式下，通过降低速率(每分钟<10 次呼吸)、潮气量(<6mL/kg)、吸气平台压(<20mmHg)及增加呼气末正压(PEEP；>10mmHg)来定期降低呼吸机参数设置，以减少呼吸机相关肺损伤。在 iLA 使用的最初 2 小时内，血流动力学尚稳定，通气设置可以降到最小，以保护肺功能。iLA 能够显著改善呼吸参数，降低炎性细胞因子的水平，并改善 Murray ARDS 评分。维持凝血酶原时间在 50~60 秒的抗凝治疗通常能防止 NovaLung 膜凝血。另外，需要使 MAP>60mmHg，以保持血流通过 NovaLung；如果必要，可使用静脉补液或血管升压素。与脱离呼吸机类似，随着呼吸功能的恢复，可以减少气流。只有当患者能够维持 3 小时以上的自主呼吸，无论有无机械通气，均没有扫气流量时，才应考虑拔除插管、移除 NovaLung。

外置人工肺

有研究表明，ECMO 能使急性肺损伤患者恢复，救助 PGD 患者，并用于移植前的过渡支持，因此将来 ECMO 的适应证可能包括外置人工肺(PAL)装置前的过渡支持，后者能像心室辅助装置模式化治疗心力衰竭患者一样，可扩大或“目的”使用[6]。目前已研发出多种 PAL，不适合移植的呼吸衰竭终末期患者及肺移植前需过渡支持的患者均为其适应证。通过使用 PAL 装置，患者能进行康复训练、下床活动，甚至离开医院，否则他们只能使用 ECMO 治疗而被限制在医院内[1]。

设计新装置和更小的装置时，必须考虑装置内血压的维持以防止凝血。尽管使用血泵是最简单的办法，但是由心脏产生血流的无泵装置也能维持装置的血流稳定[32,33]。然而，血泵或外部回路本身不应使心脏受到更大的阻力，因为这绝对会导致右心衰竭，正如在无泵装置的动物研究中所观察到的一样，尽管已增加流入道腔室或阀门以来调节心排血量达到装置需要的程度[33]。在移植前的过渡支持中，右心受到的最大阻力可能是健康肺产生的阻力[34]。选择插管方法还必须考虑到右心受到的阻力，因为串联插管可能导致右心阻力过大[33]。而并联插管存在的问题是血液未流经肺代谢和过滤，并可能存在全身性血栓栓塞的威胁。通过装置的剪切力需最优化，因为剪切力过高会导致血细胞损伤、溶血、血小板活化和消耗，但是剪切力过低会激活凝血，导致装置中纤维蛋白沉积和血栓形成[32]。炎症的激活是生物相容性问题，在用于人体之前也需要最优化。此外，尽管外置装置可以更换和维护，但其目的应是使装置在整个支持期间能持续使用。

在羊的健康和疾病模型的不同研究中发现,PAL装置能提供呼吸辅助,可持续使用长达30天[32]。早期动物研究发现,使用串联插管(PA-PA)的PAL装置,右心衰竭的发生率较高。因此,提供较低回路阻抗的并联插管(PA-LA)装置可能是PAL长期植入的首选[33]。类似于iLA,使用PA-LA导向的无泵系统进行长期气体交换是可行的,因为这项技术已应用到人体[34,35]。正如在动物试验中描述的,这项装置的风险包括栓塞事件和装置故障,后者可通过相对容易的替换修正[34]。通过使用肝素涂层组件可降低这些风险,但iLA成功的可能原因是低压导向无泵氧合器的交替使用,而不是系统性房室(A-V)导向。通过并行插管[34]和将离心泵并入PAL装置[36]的方法,初步改善了串联无泵装置[33]的不良结果和右心衰竭的发生率(图50.3)。30天的动物研究证明,整合式肺泵这样的设备可应用于人体。在RA和PA植入人工肺泵,可减轻右心前负荷,同时保持肺血流量并降低全身血栓栓塞的风险。整合式肺泵尺寸小、启动容量低,已有研究表明它能保证氧合及远处器官的正常功能,而没有显著的溶血及血小板或白细胞活化[36]。这些不错的结果及无泵PAL应用于患者的初步成功,使长期进行机械通气支持成为可能。

2008年,最初使用PAL装置作为移植前过渡支持的是一名患严重原发性肺动脉高压的患者,在肺移植前存活长达62天。胸腔PA-LA插管可使通过无泵氧合器(iLA)的并行血流速度达2~4L/min,同时避免股动静脉插管。由于该患者行胆囊切除术后出现ARDS、右心衰竭和心跳停搏,必须立即使用ECMO。9天后植入PAL装置,肝、肾衰竭也相应得到逆转,并且保护性通气使气体交换逐渐恢复正常,随后患者拔管并下床活动。因此PAL装置可成功作为双肺移植的过渡支持[1]。之后,这种用于失代偿肺动脉高压和右心衰竭的新技术也成功救助了4例肺静脉闭塞疾病(PVOD)患者。同样应用PA-LA插管和无泵膜肺氧合器,患者能在移植前支持8~21天,而且氧合、通气、心源性休克、酸中毒和肾功能和肝功能均得到改善。2例患者通过麻醉诱导简单进行V-A ECMO支持,1例患者可以脱离PAL装置,1例需要更换装置,3例完全恢复了右心功能。移植后,1例患者发生脓毒症和多器官衰竭而死亡;除此之外,没有发生其他并发症[35]。考虑到这些患者在等待移植期间的高死亡率和他们对V-A ECMO的依赖,这些移植前过渡支持的成功尝试表明,使用PAL装置能恢复右心功能并缓解难治性肺动脉高压。本研究也对ECMO技术应用于ARDS患者及V-V或RA-PA中心插管有所关注。自2009年以来,我们一共支持了57例患者,总生存率为54%。有趣的是,11例移植后存活的患者中有8例在使用ECMO平均支持53天后出院。显然,长期进行肺支持治疗越来越成为可能,过渡支持技术的应用也将越来越广泛。

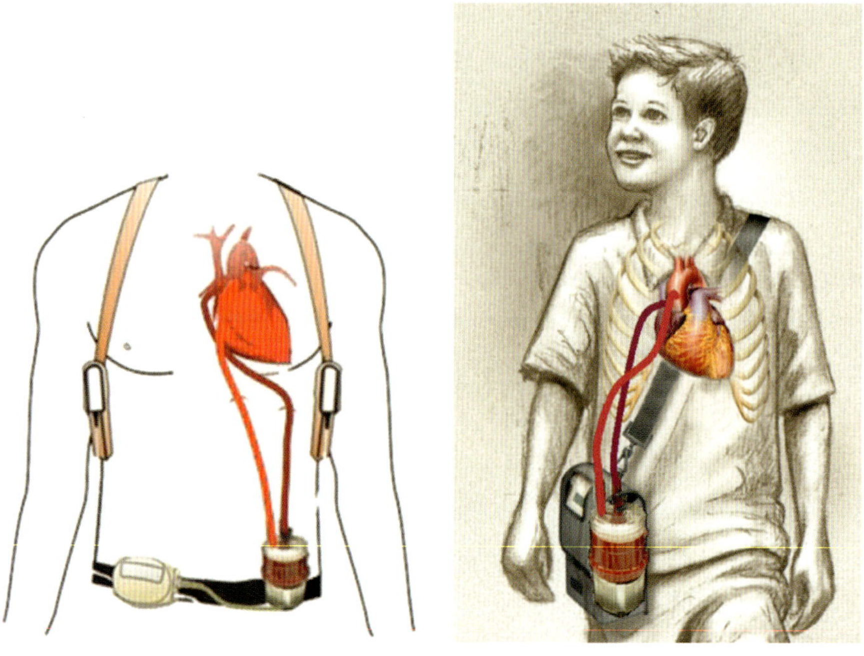

图50.3 携带式外置人工肺(PAL)。

总结

过去 20 年，包括传统 ECMO 以及协助氧气输送和清除 CO_2 的许多新型装置在内，人工肺支持技术已有显著发展。这为肺移植专家和外科医生寻求移植前、移植恢复期或再移植时的过渡支持提供了重要帮助。虽然作为目的治疗不切实际，但新型装置对患者下床活动及康复训练有显著的作用，而且永久性人工肺支持技术很可能会成为肺衰竭终末期患者的新选择。

（杨崇威 译　向骁 朱继业 校）

参考文献

1. Schmid C, Philipp A, Hilker M, et al. Bridge to lung transplantation through a pulmonary artery to left atrial oxygenator circuit. Annals of Thoracic Surgery. 2008;85(4):1202–1205.
2. Lewandowski K. Extracorporeal membrane oxygenation for severe acute respiratory failure. Critical care. 2000;4(3):156–168.
3. Zapol WM, Snider MT, Hill JD, et al. Extracorporeal membrane oxygenation in severe acute respiratory failure. A randomized prospective study. Journal of the American Medical Association. 1979;242(20):2193–2196.
4. Morris AH, Wallace CJ, Menlove RL, et al. Randomized clinical trial of pressure-controlled inverse ratio ventilation and extracorporeal CO2 removal for adult respiratory distress syndrome. American Journal of Respiratory and Critical Care Medicine. 1994;149(2 Pt 1):295–305.
5. Jackson A, Cropper J, Pye R, et al. Use of extracorporeal membrane oxygenation as a bridge to primary lung transplant: 3 consecutive, successful cases and a review of the literature. Journal of Heart and Lung Transplantation. 2008;27(3): 348–352.
6. Fuehner T, Kuehn C, Hadem J, et al. Extracorporeal membrane oxygenation in awake patients as bridge to lung transplantation. American Journal of Respiratory and Critical Care Medicine. 2012;185(7):763–768.
7. Gattinoni L, Pesenti A, Mascheroni D, et al. Low-frequency positive-pressure ventilation with extracorporeal CO2 removal in severe acute respiratory failure. Journal of the American Medical Association. 1986;256(7):881–886.
8. Bartlett D, Church DF, Bounds PL, et al. The kinetics of the oxidation of L-ascorbic acid by peroxynitrite. Free Radical Biology & Medicine. 1995;18(1):85–92.
9. Peek GJ, Mugford M, Tiruvoipati R, et al. Efficacy and economic assessment of conventional ventilatory support versus extracorporeal membrane oxygenation for severe adult respiratory failure (CESAR): a multicentre randomised controlled trial. Lancet. 2009;374(9698):1351–1363.
10. Gattinoni L, Carlesso E, Langer T. Clinical review: extracorporeal membrane oxygenation. Critical Care. 2011;15(6):243.
11. Ventilation with lower tidal volumes as compared with traditional tidal volumes for acute lung injury and the acute respiratory distress syndrome. The Acute Respiratory Distress Syndrome Network. New England Journal of Medicine. 2000;342(18):1301–1308.
12. Bermudez CA, Adusumilli PS, McCurry KR, et al. Extracorporeal membrane oxygenation for primary graft dysfunction after lung transplantation: long-term survival. Annals of Thoracic Surgery. 2009;87(3):854–860.
13. Fischer S, Bohn D, Rycus P, et al. Extracorporeal membrane oxygenation for primary graft dysfunction after lung transplantation: analysis of the Extracorporeal Life Support Organization (ELSO) registry. Journal of Heart and Lung Transplantation. 2007;26(5):472–477.
14. Aigner C, Wisser W, Taghavi S, et al. Institutional experience with extracorporeal membrane oxygenation in lung transplantation. European Journal of Cardio-Thoracic Surgery. 2007;31(3):468–473. discussion 73–74.
15. Fischer S, Gohrbandt B, Struckmeier P, et al. Lung transplantation with lungs from donors fifty years of age and older. Journal of Thoracic and Cardiovascular Surgery. 2005;129(4):919–925.
16. Cypel M, Keshavjee S. Extracorporeal life support as a bridge to lung transplantation. Clinics in Chest Medicine. 2011;32(2):245–251.
17. Lang G, Taghavi S, Aigner C, et al. Primary lung transplantation after bridge with extracorporeal membrane oxygenation: a plea for a shift in our paradigms for indications. Transplantation. 2012;93(7):729–736.
18. de Perrot M, Granton JT, McRae K, et al. Impact of extracorporeal life support on outcome in patients with idiopathic pulmonary arterial hypertension awaiting lung transplantation. Journal of Heart and Lung Transplantation. 2011;30(9): 997–1002.
19. Mangi AA, Mason DP, Yun JJ, et al. Bridge to lung transplantation using short-term ambulatory extracorporeal membrane oxygenation. Journal of Thoracic and Cardiovascular Surgery. 2010;140(3):713–715.
20. Bermudez CA, Rocha RV, Zaldonis D, et al. Extracorporeal membrane oxygenation as a bridge to lung transplant: midterm outcomes. Annals of Thoracic Surgery. 2011;92(4):1226–1231. discussion 31–32.
21. Mason DP, Thuita L, Nowicki ER, et al. Should lung transplantation be performed for patients on mechanical respiratory support? The US experience. Journal of Thoracic and Cardiovascular Surgery. 2010;139(3):765–73 e1.
22. Hammainen P, Schersten H, Lemstrom K, et al. Usefulness of extracorporeal membrane oxygenation as a bridge to lung transplantation: a descriptive study. Journal of Heart and Lung Transplantation. 2011;30(1):103–107.
23. Imai Y, Parodo J, Kajikawa O, et al. Injurious mechanical ventilation and end-organ epithelial cell apoptosis and organ dysfunction in an experimental model of acute respiratory distress syndrome. JAMA. 2003;289(16):2104–2112.
24. Smits JM, Mertens BJ, Van Houwelingen HC, et al. Predictors of lung transplant survival in Eurotransplant. American Journal of Transplantation. 2003;3(11): 1400–1406.
25. Olsson KM, Simon A, Strueber M, et al. Extracorporeal membrane oxygenation in nonintubated patients as bridge to lung transplantation. American Journal of Transplantation. 2010;10(9):2173–2178.
26. Bermudez CA, Rocha RV, Sappington PL, et al. Initial experience with single cannulation for venovenous extracorporeal oxygenation in adults. Annals of Thoracic Surgery. 2010;90(3):991–995.
27. Garcia JP, Iacono A, Kon ZN, et al. Ambulatory extracorporeal membrane oxygenation: a new approach for bridge-to-lung transplantation. Journal of Thoracic and Cardiovascular Surgery. 2010;139(6):e137–e139.
28. Gattinoni L, Kolobow T, Tomlinson T, et al. Control of intermittent positive pressure breathing (IPPB) by extracorporeal removal of carbon dioxide. British Journal of Anaesthesia. 1978;50(8):753–758.
29. Fischer S, Simon AR, Welte T, et al. Bridge to lung transplantation with the novel pumpless interventional lung assist device NovaLung. Journal of Thoracic and Cardiovascular Surgery. 2006;131(3):719–723.
30. Bartlett RH, DeLosh T, Tracey T. Extracorporeal Life Support (ECLS) for adult respiratory failure: the North American Experience. International Journal of Artificial Organs. 1995;18(10):620–623.
31. Iglesias M, Martinez E, Badia JR, et al. Extrapulmonary ventilation for unresponsive severe acute respiratory distress syndrome after pulmonary resection. Annals of Thoracic Surgery. 2008;85(1):237–244. discussion 44.
32. Nolan H, Wang D, Zwischenberger JB. Artificial lung basics: fundamental challenges, alternative designs and future innovations. Organogenesis. 2011;7(1): 23–27.
33. Alpard SK, Wang D, Deyo DJ, et al. Optional active compliance chamber performance in a pulmonary artery-pulmonary artery configured paracorporeal artificial lung. Perfusion. 2007;22(2):81–86.
34. Sato H, Hall CM, Lafayette NG, et al. Thirty-day in-parallel artificial lung testing in sheep. Annals of Thoracic Surgery. 2007;84(4):1136–1143. discussion 43.
35. Strueber M, Hoeper MM, Fischer S, et al. Bridge to thoracic organ transplantation in patients with pulmonary arterial hypertension using a pumpless lung assist device. American Journal of Transplantation. 2009;9(4):853–857.
36. Wu ZJ, Zhang T, Bianchi G, et al. Thirty-day in-vivo performance of a wearable artificial pump-lung for ambulatory respiratory support. Annals of Thoracic Surgery. 2012;93(1):274–281.

第 51 章
人工胰腺

Desmond Barry Keenan, Garry M. Steil

引言

目前还没有任何治疗方法可以预防人类 1 型糖尿病[1]。有人认为胰岛[2]或胰腺移植或者肾移植[3]是可能的治愈方法,但由于没有足够的器官供体,这两种方法都没有广泛应用。工程细胞株[4]、干细胞[5]或异种移植[6]可以克服胰岛短缺的困难,但何时才能实现仍不清楚,而且受体可能仍需终身免疫抑制治疗,相应风险也可能较大[7]。虽然血糖控制良好可使患者获益[8-10],但有研究表明,达到所需的控制水平仍较困难[11]。因此,对于想要减轻负担并改善健康的糖尿病患者,使人工胰腺(AP)形成闭环的传感器增强泵(SAP)治疗已成为该领域有力的竞争者。可以考虑在移植的教科书中将 SAP 作为该领域潜在的未来治疗方式作为介绍,因为其能减少胰腺或胰岛移植的需求,或为需要控制血糖的患者提供移植的替代方案。

设想的 AP 为全自动化系统,它通过血糖传感器将信息发送到计算程序测定胰岛素剂量,从而调节血糖[12]。近 40 年来,这项研究一直处于糖尿病研究的前沿[13]。早期 AP 闭环系统采用静脉(IV)测量血糖并输注胰岛素。Miles Laboratory(Elkhart,IN,USA)于 1979 年将第一个 AP 用于医院,使其商业化,并于 1983 年获得美国 FDA 批准。该装置称为 Biostator,它利用电化学传感器[14]通过体外在线分析进行全血测量,并使用比例微分算法的经典控制技术实现了葡萄糖调节。虽然该系统能严格控制血糖,并且对葡萄糖钳夹试验非常有效[15],但其应用仅局限于临床或实验室。目前已经出现腹膜内(IP)胰岛素输注的其他 AP 闭环系统类型,即将中心静脉血糖传感器靠近右心房的完全植入系统[16]。虽然 IP 系统能快速显示胰岛素动力学,但其控制性能却因传感器的延迟而受到影响。该系统具有全植入式 IP 胰岛素输注泵和皮下传感器的混合配置[17]。全植入式 IP 输注泵的替代品是 DiaPort (Roche Diagnostics, Mannheim,Germany)[18],即通过手术在腹壁中植入一个接口,并连接 IP 导管,利用外置泵输注胰岛素。虽然该系统发明于 1999 年,但并未被广泛使用,最近才被用于 AP 闭环研究。

目前进行的 AP 系统的研究大多是以消费者为导向的。这种装置必须方便活动且可持续佩戴,使患者能够进行日常生活。该系统可能采用间质液(ISF)葡萄糖传感[19]和连续皮下胰岛素输注(CSII)的方法。由于 ISF 和血糖之间的时间延迟[20]、测量装置本身的延迟[21]和与皮下胰岛素输注相关的延迟[22],使得 ISF 检测葡萄糖并依靠 CSII 系统的研发程序变得困难。目前已详细审查了当前市售装置中本身存在的许多问题[23]。

在本章中,讲述了基于消费者的 AP 系统在医院外的应用。AP 系统组件包括间质液和 CSII 方法的微创葡萄糖传感技术。同时讲述了每个组件特殊的系统性能和临床实用性。以下所有关于 AP 的参考文献都涉及皮下(SC)葡萄糖传感和皮下胰岛素输注(SC-SC)。用这种方法得到的结果可以与通过胰腺或胰岛移植获得的结果进行对比,这将分别在第 107 章和第 61 章中进行讨论。

葡萄糖传感

微创 SC 葡萄糖传感器通常放置于腹部,并可连续检测 ISF 葡萄糖。对于刚开始活动而没有陪护和临床监测的患者,这种技术被广泛认为是最可能被该类患者佩戴的初始动态系统。第一个由 FDA 批准可用于商业的连续葡萄糖监测(CGM)装置是 CGMS® System Gold™[24],它由 MiniMed 公司在 1999 年中期推出,也就是现在的 Medtronic Diabetes。原始 CGMS 装置能存储

3 天内连续血糖数据，测量这些数据需 5 分钟的样品采集时间。与传统心脏 Holter 监视器离线分析心电图(ECG)信号的方式类似，该装置将数据下载到电脑，然后使用软件对数据进行回顾性分析。CGM 被证明能显著捕捉到更多的血糖变化。一项研究[25]显示，使用由 Roche Diagnostics 研发的 CGM 系统，每天采集 4 份手指血糖样本的受试者遗漏了 71%的低血糖事件，而每天测量高达 7 次的受试者遗漏了 58%的低血糖事件。

随着第一个可用于商业的实时 CGM 装置(Guardian® REAL-Time)的推出，由 Medtronic Minimed 开发的这种回顾性 CGM 技术在 2005 年被批准可以实时使用[26]。它每 5 分钟就会显示血糖值，并会在低血糖或高血糖时发出警报。一项为期 12 周的多中心试验[27]，通过研究 156 例稳定的 1 型糖尿病患者[血红蛋白 A1c (HbA1c)>8.1%] 证明了该系统的作用：它能使患者 HbA1c 水平从 8.1%降至 7.0%，其中 26%的患者 HbA1c 降至 6.1%以下。尽管指尖血糖已确定，每个研究组中仍均发生过低血糖事件，并且只有 1 例患者是在穿戴装置过程中发生了低血糖。在 Guardian® REAL-Time 系统之后，由美国的 Dexcom 公司(San Diego, CA, USA)研发的 STS™ 系统获得批准。该系统的一项包括 91 名患者(一些患有 2 型糖尿病)的研究显示，使用该系统的受试者低血糖时间减少 21%，高血糖时间减少 23%，以及目标血糖范围时间增加 26%[28]。Abbott FreeStyle® Navigator®(Abbott Diabetes Care，Alameda，CA，USA)能每分钟检测葡萄糖样品 1 次，可持续 5 天，且该装置提供 FreeStyle BG 仪，于 2008 年进入市场。

所有早期研究都表明，使用改进的传感器技术能发挥 CGM 的作用。Dexcom SEVEN® Plus[29]、Abbott FreeStyle® Navigator®[30]、Guardian®和 Paradigm®[31]装置的临床精确度已在多个科学期刊上发表。然而，随着更小更舒适的传感器可以在整个血糖范围内提供更高的精确度[32]及更好的校准程序[33,34]的出现，精确度正在逐渐改善，制造过程也是如此。然而，误差低不一定保证治疗有效，相反，传感器误差不一定导致不安全的治疗，因为许多治疗程序对传感器误差可能不太敏感。

相比于闭环控制，当前的葡萄糖传感器的精确度受到质疑。一些研究小组报道称，CGM 性能的精确度足以进行闭环控制。尤其是 Hovorka 等[35]在三阶段研究中证明了在夜间能有效调节血糖，他们在一个阶段中使用 Guardian®系统，在后两个阶段中使用 Navigator®监控器。该研究报告指出 Guardian®监控器的精确度为 10%，使用 YSI 每 6 小时进行校准，而 FreeStyle®Navigator®监控器的精度为 12%，使用指尖校准。Castle 等[36]的一项类似研究表明，除了 Dexcom SEVEN Plus 系统(Dexcom，San Diego，CA，USA) 之外，Guardian®监视器也能在闭环控制期间显示出高精确度的传感器性能。使用 YSI 样品进行每 6 小时的校准时，混合数据集导致 8.7%的平均绝对相对误差(MARD)。

传感器增强泵治疗

虽然 CGM 技术没有被批准代替血糖监测，但该技术已经与胰岛素泵技术联合组成 SAP 治疗。在这种技术中，传感器仍然起辅助作用，可以发出警报由用户验证。迈向 AP 的第一个主要步骤是 Medtronic 的 Paradigm® REAL-Time 系统的推出，它使 CGM 与胰岛素泵治疗结合起来[37]。尽管该系统具有闭环控制需要的所有组件[38]，但是 CGM 和胰岛素输注子系统能自主运作。目前，CGM 和 CSII 已与全球销售的 4 种 SAP 治疗产品成功结合，最近研发的一个是 Animas® Vibe™(Animas® Corp.，West Chester，PA，USA)胰岛素泵，该产品是基于 Animas 胰岛素输注技术与葡萄糖检测可持续 7 天的 Dexcom G4™ CGM 系统的融合；另一个是 Medtronic Paradigm Veo™ 胰岛素泵，它能提供额外的功能，即在低血糖水平时增加精确度[33]，自动终止运行[39]，减少严重低血糖的发生。

几项标志性试验已成功证明 SAP 治疗的作用。STAR 1 研究[40]在 6 个月的多中心随机试验(n=146 例儿童和成人受试者)中，通过比较 SAP 和常规 CSII 治疗，发现两个 SAP 队列组 HbA1c 均有减少(成人为 0.5%)。许多研究都将 SAP 治疗与多次每日注射(MDI)治疗进行比较，包括 REAL Trend 研究，共有 115 例儿童和成人受试者[41]；Eurythmics 研究，共有 83 例成人受试者[42]；ONSET 研究，共 160 例 1~16 岁的受试者[43]；STAR 3 研究，目前为止受试者数量最大，共 485 例儿童和成人受试者[44]。REAL Trend 研究发现，治疗组HbA1c 下降近 1%，在佩戴传感器时间超过 70%的受试者中效果最好。6 个月的 Eurythmics 研究观察到，治疗组 HbA1c 下降超过 1%，对照组仅下降 0.13%——SAP 组中 34%的受试者 HbA1c 下降至推荐的 7%以下，而对照组中没有受试者达到这个目标。ONSET 研究显示，与 MDI 相比，接受 SAP 治疗的新诊断的儿童患者在 15 个月内，HbA1c 水平较低，C 肽水平下降程度较小。最后，STAR 3 研究表明，治疗组在 1 年内 HbA1c 降低 0.8%（成人为 1%），而对照组为 0.2%，同时也没有增加低血糖发生率。

Paradigm Veo™ 半闭环系统

Paradigm® Veo™ 胰岛素泵子系统之间的联系被建立。该设备于 2009 年在欧洲和除美国外的世界各地推出。Veo™ 胰岛素泵除了采用与 Paradigm® REAL-Time 胰岛素泵相同的平台，还具有其他功能，包括超过设定的低血糖阈值时，自动停止胰岛素输注，使其成为第一个利用葡萄糖传感器反馈控制胰岛素输注或停止输注的产品。

这种低血糖停止胰岛素输注（LGS）功能如图 51.1 所示，说明了传感器能降低严重低血糖的发生。此功能不是为了预防低血糖，而是为了减少用户错过任何低血糖事件时产生的影响[45]。因此，当发生低血糖事件时，系统将发出警报，必要时，可消耗碳水化合物。在受试者对低血糖事件反应不在状态或者未注意警报时，系统将暂停胰岛素输注 2 小时，之后恢复正常的基础胰岛素输注。

LGS 激活的两个示例如图 51.2 所示。在第一示例中，当两个传感器报警时，葡萄糖传感器会首先跨过在午夜和凌晨 2:00 之间的低血糖警报阈值。然而，回到正常血糖范围时，传感器会报告血糖水平。当血糖在凌晨 4:00 下降到警报阈值以下时，传感器会再次发出警报。最终，血糖降至 LGS 阈值以下，LGS 泵会在早上 5:00 之前发出警报，而当患者没有对警报做出回应时胰岛素输注会暂停。此自动暂停功能时间为 2 小时，除非有用户干预。在该段时间内，血糖水平增加。随着基础胰岛素的输注恢复，血糖水平再次下降，并且触发传感器

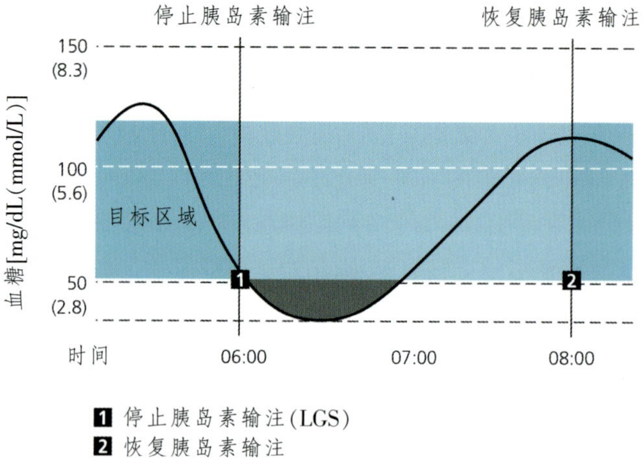

图 51.1 Paradigm®Veo™ 胰岛素泵的低血糖停止胰岛素输注（LGS）特征。（Reproduced from Keenan et al.[39], with permission from PER Medical Media.）

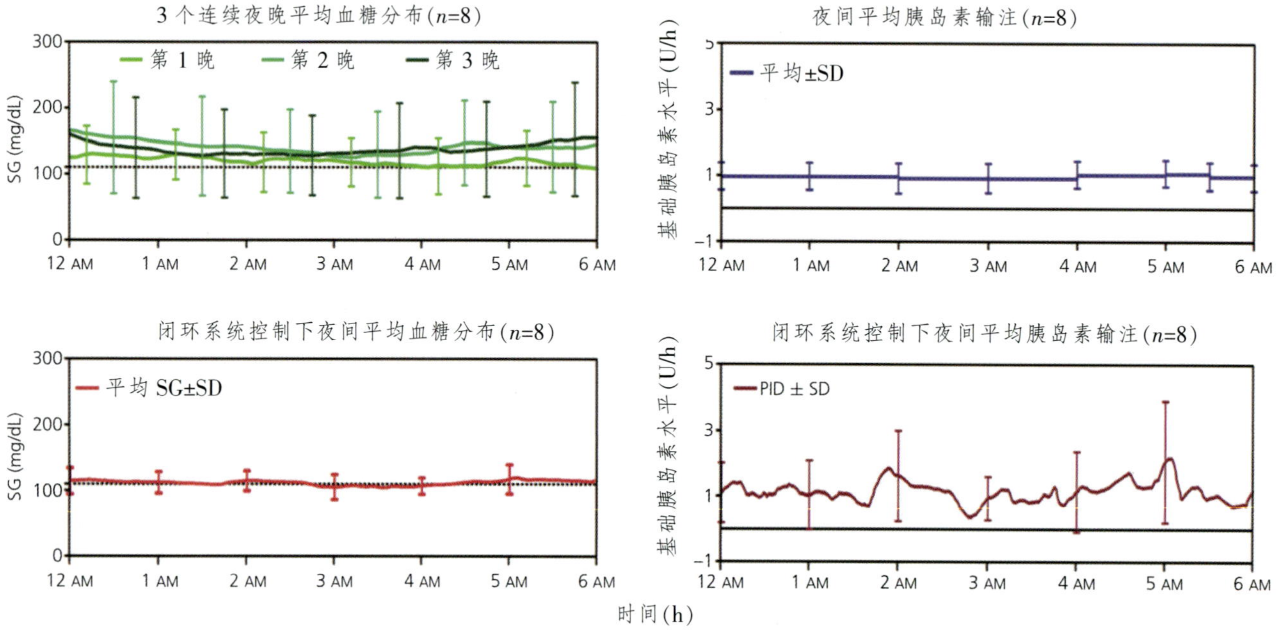

图 51.2 Paradigm® Veo™ 半闭环胰岛素泵的低血糖停止胰岛素输注（LGS）功能示例。SG，葡萄糖传感器；PID，生理胰岛素输注。

警报。最后,在上午10:30到11:00之间可激活第二个持续2小时的LGS。通过这种激活,使血糖浓度达到更安全水平。该系统的有效性已经通过一些回顾性分析[46]数据得到证明。这些数据收集了935名患者总共49 867天的情况,发现有27 216次激活LGS,60%发生在下午或晚上。一项包括21名患者的研究[47]中,Veo™胰岛素泵的功效得到证明。这项研究将LGS功能与没有LGS的对照组进行比较:表明LGS能减少低血糖偏移次数,也可减少患者在低血糖中花费的时间。

闭环研究

Medtronic Minimed通过模仿β细胞,寻求解决闭环运算程序开发问题。这种方法称为外部生理胰岛素输注(ePID),它被认为是基于β细胞应答各方面缺失而产生临床结果的最佳方法[48],例如2型糖尿病发病前经常出现第一阶段胰岛素释放的缺失。目前认为β细胞最重要的特征不仅包括第一阶段胰岛素的释放,而且包括第二阶段的释放,即预期食物消耗相关的头部阶段中胰岛素释放的缓慢上升,以及胰岛素本身能抑制胰岛素分泌的作用。其他假定的β细胞特征,例如在血糖上升前暴露以增强胰岛素反应和脉冲释放的作用,也可能在维持正常的葡萄糖耐量方面发挥重要的作用(目前还没有充分的研究)。

建立β细胞模型的早期研究主要是,通过经典的比例积分微分控制运算描述β细胞对血糖急性升高(高血糖钳夹试验)的应答观察结果。使用钳夹法计算的β细胞应答被分成三部分,并且根据存在健康β细胞的非糖尿病个体数据来估计每组的相对数量[48]。将经典控制技术与β细胞生理学相比较,发现第一阶段胰岛素释放过程非常类似于控制器衍生组件,即胰岛素输注速率与传感器葡萄糖信号的阳性变化速率成正比。控制器积分组件基本上在传感器葡萄糖测量值和血糖水平目标或期望值之间差异的平均值间移动,它能模拟第二阶段胰岛素释放或基础输注速率。将这种应答运用到SC胰岛素输注的闭合AP时,需要克服SC系统延时较长的问题。这首先需要通过调节每个阶段的相对比例来实现,即减慢积分组件的上升速率并增加衍生组件中胰岛素输注的相对量。糖尿病犬模型的初步研究显示,该方法能在夜间对合理膳食的应答做出稳定控制[49]。随后在1型糖尿病的成人受试者中的研究[50]也显示稳定的夜间控制(定义为每次80~120mg/dL),但产生胰岛素量要高于餐后2小时应答的需要量和餐后的最低需求量。

通过使用户在预计进餐前口服一小块食物丸,可将与头部相类似的阶段引入运算中[51]。Weinzimer等[52]对17位青少年进行了34小时的闭环控制,并对其进行了评估。半闭环组(n=9)的受试者在进食前15分钟接受一小剂食物丸,而剩余分配到全闭环控制组的受试者(n=8)没有进食通知。结果表明餐后平均血糖浓度显著降低(194±47mg/dL对226±51mg/dL)。半闭环组总的平均血糖浓度为135mg/dL,而全闭环组为141mg/dL。这项研究显示了严格的夜间血糖控制;然而,半闭环组出现两个低血糖事件,而全闭环组出现了一个低血糖事件,所有这些事件均发生于晚上11点至凌晨01:00之间。随后引入胰岛素反馈效应以模拟胰岛素抑制自身分泌的效果,该机制可通过使用称为“极点放置”的一项技术运用到SC胰岛素输注[53],并随后可在成人1型糖尿病的临床研究中得到评估[54]。

由于改善β细胞应答的方法很多,系统地评价每一项临床方案变得十分困难。在控制系统中,传统上解决此问题的一种常用方法是,开发受控系统的数学模型,然后使用该模型来评估所设计控制器的性能——目前称为计算机或虚拟闭环研究。这需要对受控系统的动力学有很好的理解。通过回顾这一领域代谢相关的文献发现,已有许多模型被提出,但是哪种模型最合适,仍没有达到共识[51]。而且,对于任何个体模型,其参数均需要从现有数据中获取或使用来源于不同条件和患者群体下获得的各种不同的假定数值。为了处理这样的问题,可以采用一系列公认合理的子模型技术,例如Bergman葡萄糖动力学最小模型,它是一个包含胰岛素吸收和食物吸收的简单两室模型,并将这些技术与SC-ISF葡萄糖动力学组合[54]。然后,应用加利福尼亚大学洛杉矶分校(UCLA)研究中获得的数据来鉴定这个组合模型[50]。之后在计算机(计算机模拟)中复制该研究方案。这样得到的结果与体内原始结果几乎无法区分。基于这些虚拟患者(n=10),我们模拟使用餐前食物丸来辅助控制运算的一项研究[55]。这使得餐后血糖峰值显著降低,餐后血糖最低值也得到改善。计算机模型已成功应用于调节控制运算。事实上,由弗吉尼亚大学和帕多瓦大学[56]的研究人员开发的一个模拟器已得到FDA认可,在临床研究之前它被用于测试闭环运算。剑桥大学 AP 研究所开发了一个代谢模型[57],通过许多虚拟患者测试其闭环控制运算和传感器故障,这是获得一个用于门诊研究可靠系统的必要步骤。

弗吉尼亚大学和帕多瓦大学的研究小组，通过使用 Navigator®传感器和 Omnipod(Insulet Corp.,Bedford,MA,USA)输注系统,基于模型预测控制(MPC)的运算程序,在夜间研究中测试闭环控制器。Cobelli 等[58]回顾分析了这项工作、协作及其进展。在美国一项包含 8 名受试者的研究[59]中,将闭环控制与标准开环控制进行了比较(图 51.3)。闭环控制组与开环控制组相比,平均夜间血糖和花费时间(70~180mg/dL)分别为 113.16mg/dL、111.89mg/dL 及 81.69%、96.94%。此外,平均夜间低血糖事件(1.63 对 0.13)显著减少。同样的系统正在两个欧洲中心[60]和一个美国中心进行评估,其中,美国中心正在评估 11 名青少年和 27 名成人，包含锻炼期间的 22 小时诊所内评估。被评估的控制运算使用具有不同优化水平的“控制到范围”技术。这种技术不是一种完全闭合运算,超出预定范围时它能增加胰岛素输注。在每个实施方案中,与 CSII 控制组相比,试验组控制时间增加,低血糖发生率显著降低。

迄今为止所描述的闭环控制算法和系统已经用在了胰岛素单一激素控制血糖的治疗中。用这种方法防止低血糖的唯一机制是确保最佳胰岛素输注达到安全的血糖范围，从而及时停止胰岛素输注以避免低血糖事件发生。如果输注过量，唯一的恢复方法是人为干预。因此,有人建议完全内分泌的 AP 还应该包含胰高血糖素类似物。虽然目前还不存在稳定市售的和一次性使用的 Eli-Lilly 胰高血糖素类似物，但是有两个研究小组已经成功地发明了标签外使用的胰高血糖素增强的闭环运算。

波士顿大学的研究人员开发了一种基于胰高血糖素的控制器。该系统使用两个 Cozmo 输注泵来进行胰岛素和胰高血糖素给药。GlucoScout®(International Biomedical,Austin,TX,USA)可以每 5 分钟测量一次血糖浓度。控制运算使用 MPC 计算胰岛素剂量,使用比例微分控制器确定胰高血糖素剂量[61]。在最近的一项研究中,11 名受试者在闭环控制下被研究 27 小时,期间他们接受三种高碳水化合物的食物[62]。6 名受试者的平均葡萄糖浓度达 140mg/dL，而不需要任何干预;然而,5 名受试者出现低血糖需要予以治疗。更新控制运算后,两个小组再次进行试验,均没有产生进一步的低血糖事件,平均血糖浓度为 164mg/dL。虽然该研究中没有单独应用胰岛素的对照组，但增加胰高血糖素帮助预防低血糖的同时，也应使用胰岛素进行更积极的治疗;因此,胰高血糖素的控制对于严格的血糖控制而言,它能提供的帮助依然是不明确的。

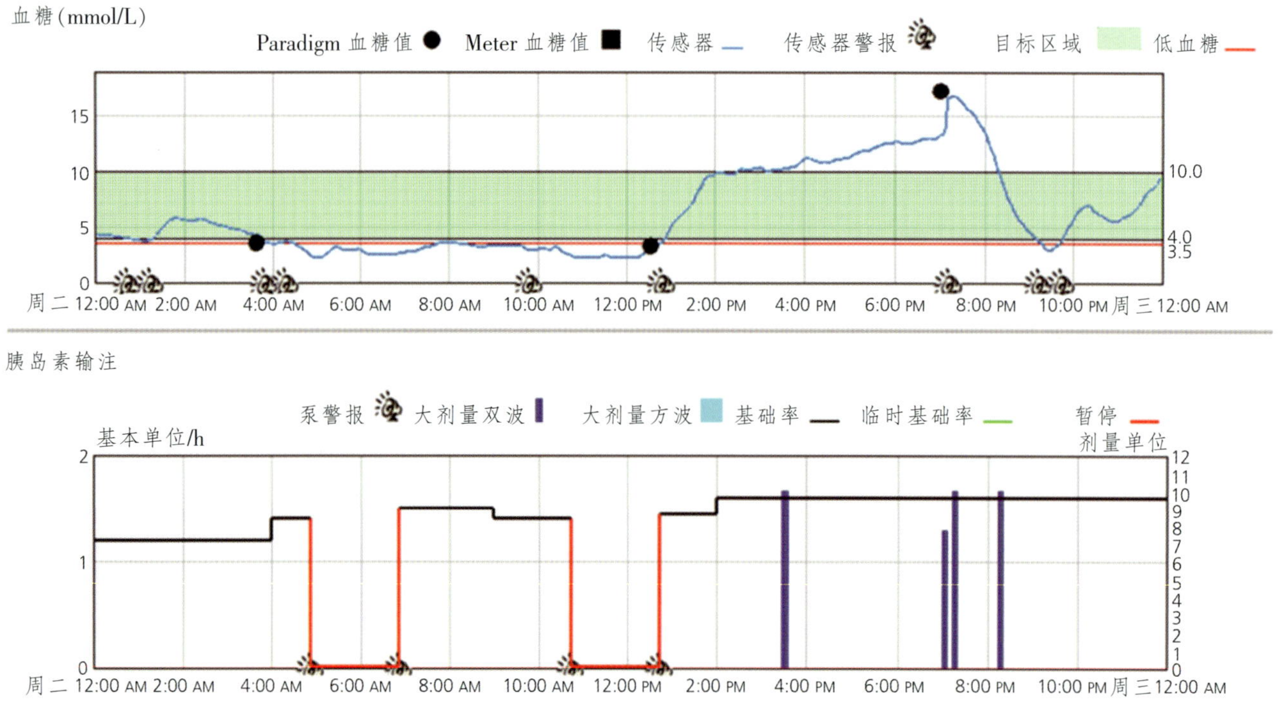

图 51.3　门诊夜间血糖和住院夜间血糖闭环控制。

俄勒冈健康与科学大学的一个研究小组，基于 Guardian® REAL-Time 或 SEVEN Plus 传感器控制，以及 Animas IR 1000 胰岛素输注泵，使用衰减记忆比例导数(FMPD)运算[63]来计算胰岛素和胰高血糖素剂量。在最近的一篇报道[64]中，对 13 名受试者进行研究，其中需要时推注胰高血糖素的 7 名受试者和长期输注胰高血糖素的 6 名受试者，与仅用胰岛素闭环加安慰剂控制组(n=8)进行比较。结果表明，与联合应用胰岛和安慰剂的对照组相比，增加胰高血糖素输注使低血糖中花费的时间减少 63%[(15±6)分钟对(40±10)分钟]，而胰高血糖素输注高增益组和安慰剂组之间的平均血糖浓度没有显著差异[(138±17)mg/dL 对(131±17)mg/dL]。但是，对于胰高血糖素输注低增益组，平均血糖浓度较高[(157±24)mg/dL 对(135±16)mg/dL]。有趣的是，研究表明，与具有更高的全胰高血糖素剂量低增益组相比，增加快速使用的 SC 大剂量胰高血糖素，更接近于生理学，能降低血糖过低的频率和时间。

剑桥大学 AP 研究所进行了随机交叉试验[35]，在一项研究中使用 Guardian® REAL-Time 系统，在后续研究中使用 FreeStyle® Navigator® CGM 系统，并每隔 15 分钟将新的输注速率手动输入 Deltec Cozmo 胰岛素泵(Smiths Medical，St.Paul，MN，USA)。总共有 17 名受试者进行标准闭环控制(n=12)或运动后闭环控制(n=9)，并将其与具有不同血糖指数的餐后控制组(n=6)进行比较。观察夜间每组努力克服基于 MPC 控制器的影响。对于控制血糖在目标范围内花费的中位时间，开环控制与标准闭环控制分别为 52%和 39%，开环控制与运动后闭环控制分别为 78%和 43%，而快速吸收食物与缓慢吸收食物分别为 53%和 55%。在运动研究期间，33 次夜间闭环控制中，仅两次血糖下降至 3mmol/L，而对照组中出现 9 次。该算法在摄入大量膳食和酒精的情况下进行了进一步的测试[65]，以进一步挑战整夜的血糖控制。与标准治疗的对照组相比，在闭环控制下，中位控制时间增加了 22%。此外，对控制良好的孕妇，还评估了控制器在妊娠糖尿病群体中维持血糖稳定的能力[66,67]。与 CSII 相比，闭环控制组的低血糖事件发生率较低。

闭环系统

前面描述的 ePID 闭环系统的开发是基于 Medtronic 技术。第一版本的 ePID 是由便携式计算机系统开发的，其间隔 1 分钟(由 5 分钟产品版本改良)就能接收葡萄糖传感器信号，基于比例积分微分控制运算计算胰岛素输注速率，并通过一系列小剂量(0.1U)药丸将胰岛素输注速率输回到泵。在 2001 年，在糖尿病犬中进行了全自动化闭环研究[49]，随后在 2003 年开始在人体进行评估[50]，这标志着第一个 SC-SC 闭环研究的出现及闭环 AP 系统应用于可活动的消费者已成功走出第一步。后来该系统在 2005 年应用到儿童群体[52]，并于 2006 年进入医院 ICU[68]。之后研究了胰岛素反馈机制来模拟胰岛素抑制自身分泌的作用[69,70]。

随后测试了许多运算方法；然而，使用这种便携式计算机系统，患者必须留在床旁。目前随着智能手机的普及，将控制从笔记本电脑系统转移到手机(如黑莓手机)是一种自然而然的进步。2011 年开展了一项由 8 位受试者组成的闭环研究试验[71]。黑莓手机拥有控制运算，并通过基于蓝牙技术的翻译器设备与胰岛素泵和传感器系统通信。启用黑莓智能手机的所有功能，每隔 1 分钟就能将实时葡萄糖和胰岛素数据传输到中央服务器。远程监控器可以登录到服务器，并在任何地方都能实时监测闭环研究。这种类型的系统主要为家庭研究提供桥梁。目前，应用智能手机技术(例如安卓手机和苹果手机)的许多类似的闭环系统正在开发。

夜间闭环系统

迄今为止，闭环血糖控制所采用的两种技术方法主导了闭环系统的研究，即经典的比例积分导数运算和基于 MPC 的更现代的方法[12]。不管采用何种控制方法，每种技术都受到同样的干扰，例如进餐和运动的问题。因此，许多研究都集中在夜间进行，这个时间段相对合理，并为完全闭环的 24 小时应用提供了中间过渡步骤。研究表明，55%的严重低血糖事件发生在睡觉期间[72]，75%的儿童癫痫发作在夜间出现[73]。因此，考虑到夜间低血糖的广泛，夜间闭环控制可以使患者显著获益。另外，Buckingham 等[74]报告 71%的夜间 CGM 警报没有引起患者反应。

任何基于消费者的闭环 AP 系统均存在大量的控制问题，其中大多问题在白天都会增多，所以第一个 AP 系统很可能仅在夜间使用。在夜间，受试者活动少，需要处理的控制问题(例如进食和大量活动)就会少得多。因此，在夜间维持严格的控制不会太困难。

总结

闭环AP得益于现代医疗装置技术，以及先进的葡萄糖传感器和胰岛素输注，已有研究报道它能实现正常的血糖控制，尤其是在夜间。虽然已经在监督的可控条件下证明了其效果，但在向消费者提供该系统之前，必须通过门诊研究证明其具有较高的安全性。目前对于系统的研究，已经从只关注控制性能转变为故障检测及处理流程。智能手机技术可以为门诊研究提供必要的桥梁，比如门诊受试者能在其家庭环境中进行监测。这是当前闭环AP系统走向商业化的必要步骤。

（杨崇威 译 向骁 朱继业 校）

参考文献

1. Devendra D, Liu E, Eisenbarth GS. Type 1 diabetes: recent developments. BMJ (Clinical Research Edition). 2004;328(7442):750–754.
2. Barshes NR, Lee T, Goodpasture S, et al. Achievement of insulin independence via pancreatic islet transplantation using a remote isolation center: a first-year review. Transplantation Proceedings. 2004;36:1127–1129.
3. Orsenigo E, Fiorina P, Cristallo M, et al. Long-term survival after kidney and kidney-pancreas transplantation in diabetic patients. Transplantation Proceedings. 2004;36:1072–1075.
4. Efrat S. Regulation of insulin secretion: insights from engineered beta-cell lines. Annals of the New York Academy of Sciences. 2004;1014:88–96.
5. Street CN, Sipione S, Helms L, et al. Stem cell-based approaches to solving the problem of tissue supply for islet transplantation in type 1 diabetes. International Journal of Biochemistry and Cell Biology. 2004;36:667–683.
6. Dufour JM, Rajotte RV, Korbutt GS, et al. Harnessing the immunomodulatory properties of Sertoli cells to enable xenotransplantation in type I diabetes. Immunological Investigations. 2003;32:275–297.
7. Rother KI, Harlan DM. Challenges facing islet transplantation for the treatment of type 1 diabetes mellitus. Journal of Clinical Investigation. 2004;114:877–883.
8. DCCT Research Group. The effect of intensive treatment of diabetes on the development and progression of long-term complications in insulin-dependent diabetes mellitus. New England Journal Medicine. 1993;329:977–986.
9. Steffes MW, Chavers BM, Molitch ME, et al. Sustained effect of intensive treatment of type 1 diabetes mellitus on development and progression of diabetic nephropathy: the Epidemiology of Diabetes Interventions and Complications (EDIC) study. JAMA. 2003;290:2159–2167.
10. Nathan DM, Lachin J, Cleary P, et al. Intensive diabetes therapy and carotid intima-media thickness in type 1 diabetes mellitus. New England Journal of Medicine. 2003;348:2294–2303.
11. Wolpert HA, Anderson BJ. Management of diabetes: are doctors framing the benefits from the wrong perspective? BMJ (Clinical Research Edition). 2001; 323(7319):994–996.
12. Bequette BW. A critical assessment of algorithms and challenges in the development of a closed loop artificial pancreas. Diabetes Technology and Therapeutics. 2005;7:28–47.
13. Albisser AM, Leibel BS, Ewart TG, et al. An artificial endocrine pancreas. Diabetes. 1974;23(5):389–396.
14. Fogt EJ, Dodd LM, Jennlng EM, et al. Development and evaluation of a glucose analyzer for a glucose-controlled insulin infusion system (Biostator®). Clinical Chemistry. 1978;24(8):1366–1372.
15. Heinemann L, Ampudia-Blasco FJ. Glucose clamps with the Biostator: a critical reappraisal. Hormone and Metabolic Research. 1994;26(12):579–583.
16. Renard E, Costalat G, Chevassus H. Artificial beta-cell: clinical experience toward an implantable closed loop insulin delivery system. Diabetes & Metabolism. 2006;32:497–502.
17. Renard E, Place J, Cantwell M, et al. Closed loop insulin delivery using a subcutaneous glucose sensor and intraperitoneal insulin delivery: feasibility study testing a new model for the artificial pancreas. Diabetes Care. 2010;33(1): 121–127.
18. Liebl A, Hoogma R, Renard E, et al. A reduction in severe hypoglycaemia in type 1 diabetes in a randomized crossover study of continuous intraperitoneal compared with subcutaneous insulin infusion. Diabetes, Obesity and Metabolism. 2009;11(11):1001–1008.
19. Steil GM, Rebrin K, Hariri F, et al. Interstitial fluid glucose dynamics during insulin-induced hypoglycemia. Diabetologia. 2005;48:1833–1840.
20. Rebrin K, Steil GM. Can interstitial glucose assessment replace blood glucose measurements? Diabetes Technology and Therapeutics. 2000;2(3):461–472.
21. Keenan DB, Voskanyan G, Mastrototaro JJ, et al. Delays in minimally invasive CGM devices: a review of the current technology. Journal of Diabetes Sciences and Technology. 2009;3(5):1207–1214.
22. Mudaliar SR, Lindberg FA, Joyce M, et al. Insulin aspart (B28 asp-insulin): a fast-acting analog of human insulin: absorption kinetics and action profile compared with regular human insulin in healthy nondiabetic subjects. Diabetes Care. 1999;22(9):1501–1506.
23. Aye T, Block J, Buckingham B. Toward closing the loop: an update on insulin pumps and continuous glucose monitoring systems. Endocrinology and Metabolism Clinics of North America. 2010;39(3):609–624.
24. Mastrototaro JJ. The MiniMed continuous glucose monitoring system. Journal of Pediatric Endocrinology and Metabolism. 1999;12:751–758.
25. Jungheim K, Wientjes KJ, Heinemann L, et al. Subcutaneous continuous glucose monitoring: feasibility of a new microdialysis-based glucose sensor system. Diabetes Care. 2001;24:1696–1697.
26. Bode B, Gross K, Rikalo N, et al. Alarms based on real-time sensor glucose values alert patients to hypo- and hyperglycemia: the guardian continuous monitoring system. Diabetes Technology and Therapeutics. 2004;6:105–113.
27. Deiss D, Bolinder J, Riveline JP, et al. Improved glycemic control in poorly controlled patients with type 1 diabetes using real-time continuous glucose monitoring. Diabetes Care. 2006;29(12):2730–2732.
28. Garg S, Zisser H, Schwartz S, et al. Improvement in glycemic excursions with a transcutaneous, real-time continuous glucose sensor: a randomized controlled trial. Diabetes Care. 2006;29(1):44–50.
29. Zisser H, Bailey TS, Schwartz S, et al. Accuracy of the SEVEN continuous glucose monitoring system: comparison with frequently sampled venous glucose measurements. Journal of Diabetes Science and Technology. 2009;3(5): 1146–1154.
30. Weinstein RL, Schwartz SL, Brazg RL, et al. Accuracy of the 5-day FreeStyle Navigator Continuous Glucose Monitoring System: comparison with frequent laboratory reference measurements. Diabetes Care. 2007;30(5):1125–1130.
31. Mastrototaro J, Shin J, Marcus A, et al. The accuracy and efficacy of real-time continuous glucose monitoring sensor in patients with type 1 diabetes. Diabetes Technology and Therapeutics. 2008;10(5):385–390.
32. Keenan DB, Mastrototaro JJ, Zisser H, et al. Accuracy of the Enlite 6-day glucose sensor with guardian and Veo calibration algorithms. Diabetes Technology and Therapeutics. 2012;14(3):225–231.
33. Keenan DB, Cartaya R, Mastrototaro JJ. Accuracy of a new real-time continuous glucose monitoring algorithm. Journal of Diabetes Science and Technology. 2010;4(1):111–118.
34. El Youssef J, Castle JR, Engle JM, et al. Continuous glucose monitoring in subjects with type 1 diabetes: improvement in accuracy by correcting for background current. Diabetes Technology and Therapeutics. 2010;12(11):921–928.
35. Hovorka R, Allen JM, Elleri D, et al. Manual closed loop insulin delivery in children and adolescents with type 1 diabetes: a phase 2 randomised crossover trial. Lancet. 2010;375:743–751.
36. Castle JR, Engle JM, El Youssef J, et al. Novel use of glucagon in a closed loop system for prevention of hypoglycemia in type 1 diabetes. Diabetes Care. 2010;33(6):1282–1287.
37. Mastrototaro J, Lee S. The integrated MiniMed Paradigm REAL-Time insulin pump and glucose monitoring system: implications for improved patient outcomes. Diabetes Technology and Therapeutics. 2009;11(1):S37–S43.
38. Hovorka R, Wilinska ME, Chassin LJ, et al. The artificial pancreas: making headway. Practical Diabetes International. 2007;24(2):56–58.
39. Keenan DB, Cartaya R, Mastrototaro JJ. The pathway to the closed loop artificial pancreas: research and commercial perspectives. Pediatric Endocrinology Reviews. 2010;7(3):445–451.
40. Hirsch IB, Abelseth J, Bode BW, et al. Sensor-augmented insulin pump therapy: results from the first randomized treat-to-target study. Diabetes Technology and Therapeutics. 2008;10:377–383.
41. Raccah D, Sulmont V, Reznik Y, et al. Incremental value of continuous glucose monitoring when starting pump therapy in patients with poorly controlled type 1 diabetes: the RealTrend study. Diabetes Care. 2009;32(12):2245–2250.
42. Hermanides J, Norgaard K, Bruttomesso D, et al. Sensor augmented pump therapy substantially lowers HbA1c; a randomized controlled trial. Diabetologia.

2009;52(1):S43.
43. Danne T. Paediatric onset study to assess the efficacy of insulin pump therapy using the MiniMed Paradigm® REAL-Time system during the first year of diabetes in children and adolescents with type 1 diabetes. 45th Annual Meeting of the European Association of the Study of Diabetes, Vienna, Austria, October 22, 2009. 2009.
44. Bergenstal RM, Tamborlane WV, Ahmann A, Buse JB, et al. Effectiveness of sensor-augmented insulin-pump therapy in type 1 diabetes. New England Journal of Medicine. 2010;363(4):311–320.
45. Choudhary P, Shin J, Wang Y, et al. Insulin pump therapy with automated insulin suspension in response to hypoglycemia: reduction in nocturnal hypoglycemia in those at greatest risk. Diabetes Care. 2011;34(9):2023–2025.
46. Agrawal P, Welsh JB, Kannard B, et al. Usage and effectiveness of the low glucose suspend feature of the Medtronic Paradigm Veo insulin pump. Journal of Diabetes Science and Technology. 2011;5(5):1137–1141.
47. Danne T, Kordonouri O, Holder M, et al. Prevention of hypoglycemia by using low glucose suspend function in sensor-augmented pump therapy. Diabetes Technology and Therapeutics. 2011;13(11):1129–1134.
48. Steil GM, Panteleon AE, Rebrin K. Closed loop insulin delivery-the path to physiological glucose control. Advanced Drug Delivery Reviews. 2004;56: 125–144.
49. Panteleon AE, Loutseiko M, Steil GM, et al. Evaluation of the effect of gain on the meal response of an automated closed loop insulin delivery system. Diabetes. 2006;55:1995–2000.
50. Steil GM, Rebrin K, Darwin C, et al. Feasibility of automating insulin delivery for the treatment of type 1 diabetes. Diabetes. 2006;55:3344–3350.
51. Steil GM, Clark B, Kanderian S, et al. Modeling insulin action for development of a closed loop artificial pancreas. Diabetes Technology and Therapeutics. 2005; 7:94–108.
52. Weinzimer SA, Steil GM, Swan KL, et al. Fully automated closed loop insulin delivery versus semiautomated hybrid control in pediatric patients with type 1 diabetes using an artificial pancreas. Diabetes Care. 2008;31:934–939.
53. Loutseiko M, Voskanyan G, Keenan DB, et al. Closed loop insulin delivery utilizing pole placement to compensate for delays in subcutaneous insulin delivery. Journal of Diabetes Science and Technology. 2011;5(6):1342–1351.
54. Steil GM, Palerm CC, Kurtz N, et al. The effect of insulin feedback on closed loop glucose control. Journal of Clinical Endocrinology and Metabolism. 2011; 96(5):1402–1408.
55. Kanderian SS, Weinzimer SA, Steil GM. The identifiable virtual patient model: comparison of simulation and clinical closed loop study results. Journal of Diabetes Science and Technology. 2012;6(2):371–379.
56. Kovatchev BP, Breton M, Man CD, et al. In silico preclinical trials: a proof of concept in closed loop control of type 1 diabetes. Journal of Diabetes Science and Technology. 2009;3(1):44–55.
57. Wilinska ME, Chassin LJ, Acerini CL, et al. Simulation environment to evaluate closed loop insulin delivery systems in type 1 diabetes. Journal of Diabetes Science and Technology. 2010;4(1):132–144.
58. Cobelli C, Renard E, Kovatchev B. Artificial pancreas: past, present, future. Diabetes. 2011;60(11):2672–2682.
59. Clarke WL, Anderson S, Breton M, et al. Closed loop artificial pancreas using subcutaneous glucose sensing and insulin delivery and a model predictive control algorithm: the Virginia experience. Journal of Diabetes Science and Technology. 2009;3(5):1031–1038.
60. Breton M, Farret A, Bruttomesso D, et al. on behalf of The International Artificial Pancreas (IAP) Study Group. Fully integrated artificial pancreas in type 1 diabetes: modular closed-loop glucose control maintains near normoglycemia. Diabetes. 2012;61(9):2230–2237.
61. El-Khatib FH, Damiano ER. A fully automated control system for type 1 diabetes. USPTO Patent Application 20080208113.
62. El-Khatib FH, Russell SJ, Nathan DM, et al. A bihormonal closed loop artificial pancreas for type 1 diabetes. Science Translational Medicine. 2010;2(27): 27ra27.
63. Gopakumaran B, Duman HM, Overholser DP, et al. A novel insulin delivery algorithm in rats with type 1 diabetes: the fading memory proportional-derivative method. Artificial Organs. 2005;29:599–607.
64. Castle JR, Engle JM, El Youssef J, et al. Novel use of glucagon in a closed loop system for prevention of hypoglycemia in type 1 diabetes. Diabetes Care. 2010;33(6):1282–1287.
65. Hovorka R, Kumareswaran K, Harris J, et al. Overnight closed loop insulin delivery (artificial pancreas) in adults with type 1 diabetes: crossover randomised controlled studies. BMJ (Clinical Research Edition). 2011;342:d1855.
66. Murphy HR, Elleri D, Allen JM, et al. Closed loop insulin delivery during pregnancy complicated by type 1 diabetes. Diabetes Care. 2011;34(2): 406–411.
67. Murphy HR, Kumareswaran K, Elleri D, et al. Safety and efficacy of 24-h closed loop insulin delivery in well-controlled pregnant women with type 1 diabetes: a randomized crossover case series. Diabetes Care. 2011;34(12): 2527–2529.
68. Wintergerst KA, Deiss D, Buckingham B, et al. Glucose control in pediatric intensive care unit patients using an insulin-glucose algorithm. Diabetes Technology and Therapeutics. 2007;9:211–222.
69. Baynes C, Anyaoku V, Johnston DG, et al. Feedback inhibition of insulin secretion in type 2 diabetes. Clinical Science. 1991;81:685–690.
70. Boden G, Chen X, DeSantis R, et al. Evidence that suppression of insulin secretion by insulin itself is neurally mediated. Metabolism. 1993;42:786–789.
71. O'Grady MJ, Retterath AJ, Keenan DB, et al. The use of an automated, ambulatory portable glucose control system for overnight glucose control in adolescents and young adults with type 1 diabetes. Diabetes Care. 2012;35(11):2182–2187.
72. Burdick J, Chase HP, Slover RH, et al. Missed insulin meal boluses and elevated hemoglobin A1c levels in children receiving insulin pump therapy. Pediatrics. 2004;113:e221–e224.
73. Davis EA, Keating B, Byrne GC, et al. Hypoglycemia: incidence and clinical predictors in a large population-based sample of children and adolescents with IDDM. Diabetes Care. 1997;20:22–25.
74. Buckingham B, Block J, Burdick J, et al. Response to nocturnal alarms using a real-time glucose sensor. Diabetes Technology and Therapeutics. 2005;7(3): 440–447.

第 52 章 组织和器官生物工程

Tracy C. Grikscheit, Erik R. Barthel

引言

一般来讲，再生医学的目的是利用身体复杂的发育、再生和愈合能力，针对受损、功能丧失或缺失的器官和器官系统性疾病进行干预治疗[1]。组织工程是再生医学的一部分，它通过构建复杂的生物结构来重现天然组织的形式和功能[2]。构建过程是利用细胞自身组织结构复杂化的能力，或者实验室中重要的结构组织构建理想的组织。

传统移植医学已成功治疗器官功能衰竭，如肝肾等实质脏器、小肠等空腔脏器、角膜等眼部组织、心脏、气道和肺，而且最近关于手和整个面部的移植也有重要的进展。鉴于此，组织工程的潜在作用可能会受到质疑。然而，正如本书中所讨论的，移植存在局限性，但也有自己的优势。实际上，所有移植治疗都非常依赖于供体器官的可用性，这也导致其使用受到限制。而且，一旦进行移植手术，移植物会被宿主排斥，患者需要终身使用昂贵而痛苦的免疫抑制药物治疗。如果患者不遵守免疫抑制方案可能会导致移植物的排斥、衰竭和丢失，然后需要再次移植和使用其他长期的过渡治疗。考虑到所有这些原因，再生医学中的组织工程是一种有吸引力的替代治疗方案，且在移植专著中也考虑必要时其可作为器官衰竭终末期患者的未来伴随或替代治疗选择。

组织工程需要跨学科的技术才能成功，需要外科医生、内科医生、材料科学家、生物工程师和其他人才的加入。20 世纪 70 年代，Green 将软骨细胞接种到骨针来产生软骨的初始试验以失败而告终，因此，很显然，用于构建组织和器官的材料和支架对于组织工程

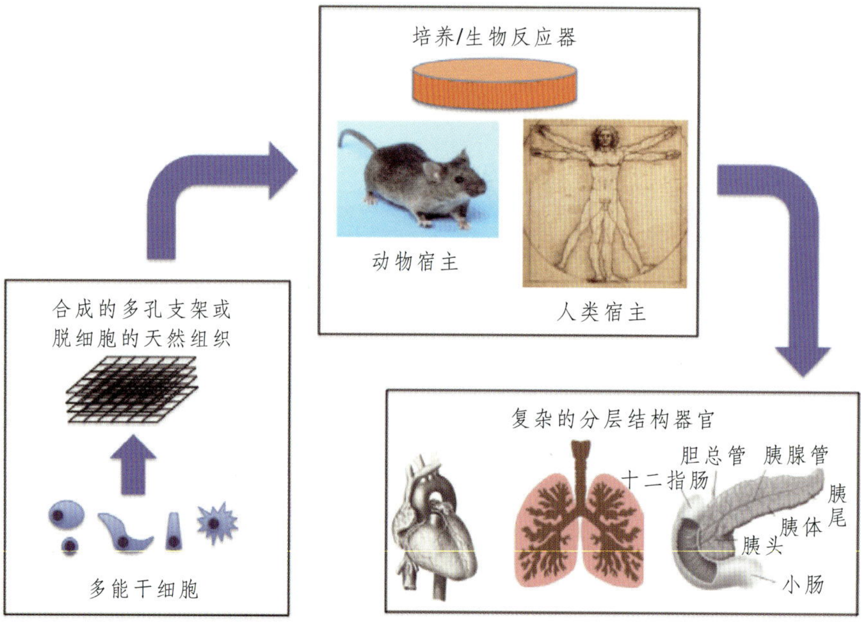

图 52.1 组织工程过程示意图。通常，可生物降解的多孔支架或脱细胞的天然组织用于支持多能干细胞群的生长。载入的支架在体外塑性或植入动物或人体宿主中，促进组织向内生长、载入细胞增殖和复杂器官的发育。

的成功是非常关键的(图52.1)。美国波士顿儿童医院和麻省理工学院(MIT)的Vacanti和Langer分别通过使用生物相容性材料制造出了适合移植的合成支架，这是生物材料方面进行移植的第一次真正尝试，他们认识到生物衍生材料本身的不可预测性和不可再生性。在20世纪80年代中期,他们开发了生物可降解聚合物支架,包括聚乙醇酸(PGA)和聚乳酸(PLA)。

组织和器官特异性技术

角膜

人的角膜是一种对视觉至关重要的透明组织,因为它会使进入眼睛的光线发生折射,从而在视网膜上聚焦并形成图像。角膜包含五层组织,总厚度约0.5mm。角膜前侧排列着复层鳞状上皮细胞作为保护，内部的内皮层细胞通过将液体连续泵出并进入前房来调节角膜的水合状态[3]。角膜内皮由高度分化的细胞群组成,不能随年龄或在损伤后自我更新[4]。因此,在角膜存在损伤、疾病或老化导致视力下降时,唯一可治愈的治疗方法就是同种异体全角膜移植[5]。1905年,Zirm[6]首次实施了角膜移植,该技术在短期内非常成功,但是据报道角膜移植物的5年和10年存活率分别仅为74%和64%[7]。此外,由于工业化国家中老年人的生存率不断增加[8],预计在21世纪角膜移植物的需求将持续增加。尽管使用微型角膜刀可以将单个角膜分成多达三部分并单独用于角膜移植[9],但几乎可以肯定的是,角膜移植的需求仍会供不应求。

虽然人类角膜内皮细胞(HCEC)在体内不会再生,但是它们在体外已成功生长。最初的分离技术需要体外培养,然后选择性迁移HCEC[10,11],随后发展为刮除法,通过该方法使HCEC首先从角膜相邻的后弹力层(DM)机械性去除[12,13]。最近,通过剥离和分解方法使这种分离技术得到改进,即分离DM和其附着的HCEC,并用胶原酶、分散酶或胰蛋白酶/乙二胺四乙酸(EDTA)酶将其分解[14-16]。然而,该方法会导致成纤维性角膜基质细胞进入培养物,这必须用合适的培养基抑制[17,18]。通过提高分离技巧和技术,如用真空吸盘进行分离,可以使角膜基质细胞的污染最小化[19,20]。一旦分离,HCEC通常就会在适当涂层覆盖的表层板面上生长以便于黏附和增殖。有效的涂层覆盖物包括胶原[14]、层粘连蛋白或硫酸软骨素[18],以及市售的含有纤连蛋白、胶原及白蛋白的FNC涂层混合物 (Biological Research Faculty&Facility,Inc,Ijamsville,MD,USA)[21]。然而,有人认为并不是一定需要涂层覆盖[16]。

心脏

为了完成将血液泵入全身循环和肺循环的功能,心脏需要复杂的结构来维持心房和心室之间的电生理和机械协调,也需要稳定的固有起搏点,其可以通过神经和循环因子以及特异的细胞群来执行这些功能[22]。心血管疾病仍然排在西方工业化国家死亡原因的第一位,其中大多数死于心肌缺血性疾病[23]。而且,先天性心脏病很常见,在新生儿中发病率接近1%[24]。传统上认为,心肌是由没有再生能力的高度分化细胞组成[25]。然而,有研究已经描述了所谓心脏祖细胞(CPC)的存在,它能表达诸如c-kit和KI-67的标志物及早期心脏谱系转录因子,例如GATA-4和Nkx2.5[26]。

不幸的是,这些细胞在体外增殖较差[27]。因此,目前已经使用其他来源的细胞来促进心肌修复和再生,包括骨髓源性成血管细胞[28]、骨骼成肌细胞[29]和新生大鼠原代心肌细胞[30]。此外,也可使用许多来源的干细胞,包括胚胎干细胞、成人骨髓干细胞和脐带干细胞[31]。还有一种方法是将心肌细胞中不同群体的单个细胞(包括心肌细胞、内皮细胞和成纤维细胞)以不同比例置于培养物中,以产生具有基本电生理特性的“心脏类器官”[32]。心肌组织工程中,这些细胞群体最初主要应用于所使用的支架材料[33,34]。包括胶原[35]、基质胶-胶原混合物[36,37]、聚乙醇酸[38]和藻酸盐[39,40]的各种支架材料都得到使用。

为寻求这种细胞和类器官技术之外的方法，并优化体外组织，有研究小组已经设计和研究了对组织工程作用下的梗死心肌进行外科手术干预的动物模型。在大鼠模型中，宿主动物的腹腔内成熟的种植藻酸盐支架，通过生物工程获得心脏补片材料。通过单独手术，将实验产生的这些补片异位移植到第二宿主的供体心脏中。超声心动图显示,修补心脏的室壁运动和功能完全正常[41]。在进一步的研究中,他们将载有新生大鼠心肌细胞、基质胶和生长因子的类似藻酸盐材料植入宿主大鼠网膜中,以诱导新生血管形成,5天后将补片移植到各自的宿主动物的梗死心肌中。结果发现,与对照组相比，心室重塑及补片与宿主动物心肌的电偶联均减少[42]。在兔子模型中，另一研究小组在猪黏膜下层植入间充质干细胞(MSC)，培养5天后移出，然后作为游离移植物植入实验产生的心肌梗死部位，之后并入心肌壁。结果表明，与对照组相比，心肌壁变薄，并且左心室扩张的程度减轻[43]。

气道和肺

气道和肺用于气体交换并与心血管系统密切相关。成人肺每天输送约10^4L或$10m^3$的空气，总表面积约$70m^2$[44]。气管和主支气管本质上是通向更深气道的传导性气道，由含有大量软骨和结缔组织的管状结构组成。气管原发性疾病很罕见，但是占位效应，损伤或甲状腺、食管、肺和纵隔肿瘤向内转移生长可使气管变窄[45]。成人气管在切除约5cm后仍可进行吻合，而儿童中5cm的长度约为气管总长度的1/3。病变范围较长时可能需要使用支架或行气管切开术。已有研究尝试行气管置换治疗气管疾病，置换材料(例如胶原支架)可通过在体外生长的硅酮支架或软骨管得到扩张[46]。然而，这些方法都没有成功，因为置换材料缺乏上皮形成导致气管狭窄，或机械强度不够导致气管塌陷或软化[47]。使用组织工程化器官进行移植的另一个问题是，器官本身没有血液供应而发生坏死，并且当组织被再吸收时软骨可能“融解”。

由于这些问题及气管和主支气管中软骨和结缔组织层次的复杂性，最初认为合成支架技术不会成功。因此，研究重点转向使用气管本身作为支架。这需要脱细胞来完成，即通过用洗涤剂溶液去除组织的细胞成分，仅留下结缔组织骨架[48]。理论上讲，原始组织的所有免疫原特征都会被去除，因此可作为生物学来源的支架支持患者自身细胞。2008年柳叶刀(*Lancet*)发表了一篇具有里程碑意义的文章，Macchiarini等为一名支气管软化终末期患者成功植入一段组织工程气管，用于替代其左主干支气管(图52.2)[49]。

鉴于组织工程气管临床试验的初步成功，其他小组也开始在人体进行肺的组织工程研究。肺的三维结构非常复杂，而且具有多个大小级别的分级关系。总之，肺具有明确的肺叶和肺段结构，这些结构与体循环和肺循环血管组织关系非常密切。中等级别的气道为隆突水平到最末端细支气管，大约有16个分叉。最小级别的气道是肺泡，其内含有气体交换结以构进行氧化和通气。因此，肺的工程面临一个重大的挑战。导致

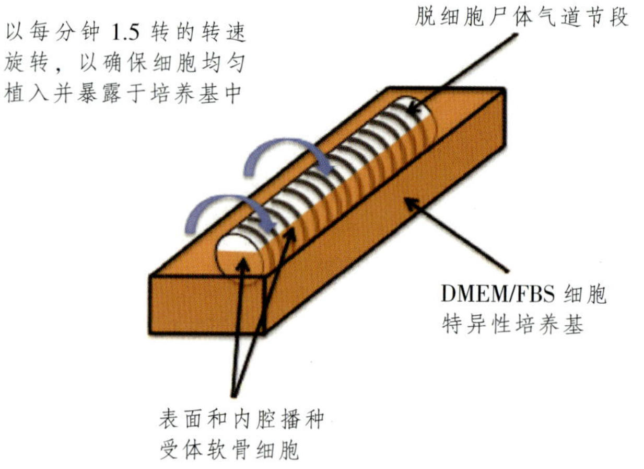

图 52.2 生物反应器系统，可用于从脱细胞尸体气道节段产生人组织工程气管。(Adapted from [49]. Copyright © 2008, with permission from Elsevier)

肺实质终末期破坏的疾病包括特发性肺纤维化(IPF)、慢性阻塞性肺疾病(COPD)、囊性纤维化和儿童的慢性肺疾病[50,51]。虽然这些患者可以通过肺叶或全肺移植获益，但是肺脏供体十分缺乏，正如实体器官和小肠一样。再生医学治疗终末期肺实质疾病的方法包括细胞治疗和组织工程。然而，前者超出了本章的范围，我们在这里只讨论组织工程。

鉴于肺脏结构的复杂性，最初该器官的组织工程方法大多集中于植入肺脏干细胞的支架研究[52]。最近

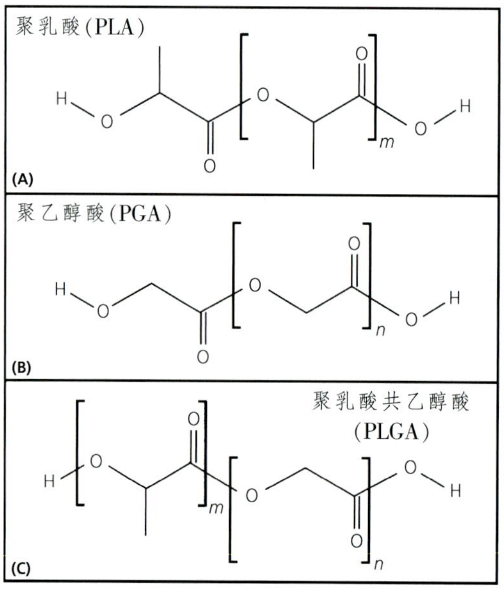

图 52.3 通常用于组织工程的可生物降解聚合物的分子结构。(A)聚乳酸(PLA)。(B)聚乙醇酸(PGA)。(C)聚乳酸共乙醇酸(PLGA)。

人体肺脏干细胞已经被鉴别，而且也表达了假定的肺脏干细胞标记物 c-kit[53]。已经用于组织工程的天然材料包括胶原[54]、基质胶[55]、吸收性明胶海绵[56]和 Englebreth-Holms 肿瘤基底膜[57]，也有合成聚合物，包括 PGA[58]、聚乳酸共乙醇酸（PLGA）和左旋聚乳酸（PLLA；图 52.3）[59]。重要的是，这些方法能将携带人体肺祖细胞（SLPC）的 PGA 复合体植入绵羊中[60]。在该项研究中，绵羊行楔形切除或全肺切除后，将携带 SLPC 的 PGA 和 Pluronic F-127（PF-127）支架植入其右上叶。6 周后，观察到支架上有部分软组织生长，并且载入的 PF-127 支架上肺泡状结构形成。另一项研究将携带胎鼠源细胞的吸收性明胶海绵植入成年大鼠的肺实质中，35~100 天后发现，在植入海绵的边缘附近有肺泡状结构形成，但在内部较少[55]。当将携带胎肺细胞（FPC）的基质胶皮下植入大鼠宿主的腹壁时，可观察到该复合体有肺上皮和血管形成[54]。

整个肺工程中还存在的一些最显著的问题包括选择用于接种的合适细胞群并确保其与潜在患者的 HLA 相容，构建具有细胞相容性的生理应力——应变特性与结构完整性结合的支架，以及合适的体外生长因子和培养条件，使所选的前体细胞群适当分化为成熟肺组织[52]。

消化道

消化道包括口咽、食管、胃、十二指肠、空肠、回肠、盲肠、升结肠、横结肠、降结肠，其功能是运输和吸收食物的营养物质，食物可以口服，也可以通过手术放置的胃造口或肠造口管给予肠内营养。消化道还有助于调节体液平衡：成人每天产生约 1L 唾液、1.5L 胃液、1L 胰液、1L 胆汁和 2L 小肠液，并且这些分泌物中的水分大部分都被结肠重吸收。当肠的大部分缺失时，无论是由于感染、创伤、缺血、肠系膜肿瘤切除术，还是其他原因，都可能发生短肠综合征（SBS）。

SBS 是切除小肠总长度的很大一部分（通常>50%~75%）后导致的疾病，其吸收能力会严重降低，患者不能从肠内营养中获得足够的营养[61-63]。儿童 SBS 的最常见原因是继发于坏死性小肠结肠炎[64]或小肠旋转不良[65]而需切除大段小肠。SBS 也可发生在成人，主要由于克罗恩病导致多次肠切除[66]，或者继发于血管疾病或创伤（例如枪伤）导致肠系膜缺血[67]，但不太常见。SBS 患者不能通过肠内吸收维持足够的营养，他们可能需要长期的全肠外营养，而儿童肝衰竭及肝硬化患者的情况会更复杂[68]。因此，SBS 患者承受着巨大的医疗费用，最近估计在 5 年内每位患者的费用约为 160 万美元[69]。当前继发性 SBS 肠衰竭的标准治疗方法是肠、肝/肠或其他多器官移植，但 5 年存活率仅为 60%，而且患者需终身进行免疫抑制治疗[70]。此外，供体器官的短缺不可避免地会导致供不应求，以及需要长时间的等待[71]。由于这些原因，患者自身小肠的自体组织工程是较为有吸引力的策略，因为它可能为 SBS 患者提供持久、长期的治疗，同时没有目前治疗方法的任何缺点[72]。

大量关于肠组织工程的研究都集中在肠上皮隐窝中的小肠干细胞群再生为正常肠上皮的过程。人体肠黏膜膜层再生周期为 3~7 天。干细胞在肠隐窝中分裂，更新自身细胞的同时，也产生短暂扩充细胞，后者能沿绒毛轴向移动并分化成各种成熟细胞，小肠中有 4 种，包括小肠细胞、潘氏细胞、杯状细胞和肠内分泌细胞；结肠中有三种，包括结肠细胞、杯状细胞和肠内分泌细胞。荷兰 Clevers 小组首先确定了小鼠等哺乳动物小肠干细胞群来自肠隐窝柱状细胞，并认为可通过亮氨酸重复序列 G 蛋白偶联受体 5（Lgr5）的表达来标记[73,74]。其他已发现的哺乳动物小肠干细胞标记物包括 DcamKL-1、Bmil、Musashi-1、CD133 和 mTert[75-79]。

肠组织工程中最成功的是类器官和多细胞单元移植，后者是自体肠组织经过接种在可生物降解的支架上，并植入宿主动物中孵育而获得。最初由 Evans 实验室进行，但目前已得到改进[80]，后续研究发现，自体肠组织经过机械性和酶消化后，肠干细胞仍然可以得到保留，因为形成的多细胞聚集体（称为器官单位）能维持隐窝中的干细胞和周围支持间质的组织学关系。这种技术已经成功应用于大鼠的食管、胃、小肠及大肠组织工程[81-85]。小鼠模型也有该技术的应用（图 52.4）[86,87]，通过获得小鼠的广泛转基因文库以更充分地理解肠组织工程类器官单元或支架技术的生化过程和详细机制。在约克猪中也有类似的结果报道，验证了该技术在大型动物中的可行性[88]。

肝脏

人体肝脏具有消化、排泄、解毒和蛋白质合成等无数功能，它还具有双重血供，门静脉系统，肝小叶与肝动脉、门静脉、胆管网状结构等复杂的结构功能关系。该器官明显供不应求：在 2008 年等待移植的患者数量

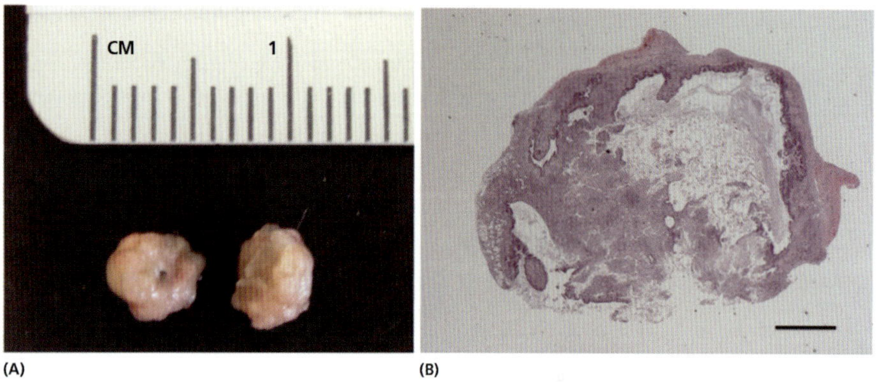

图 52.4 在小鼠宿主中产生的组织工程小肠(TESI)[86]。(A)新鲜获取的TESI,已经被分成2瓣,显示黏膜和肠腔。(B)低倍镜下小鼠TESI特征性样本组织H&E染色。放大倍数:100μm。

超过17 000例,但只有约7000例患者进行了肝移植[89]。肝移植的适应证非常多,包括慢性肝衰竭晚期、Child-Pugh-Turcotte(CPT)评分>7、适合列入终末期肝病模型(MELD)评分的进展期疾病、急性重型肝炎(病毒性或药物诱导)、胆道闭锁、家族性胆汁淤积、原发性肝脏恶性肿瘤、胆汁性肝硬化、原发性硬化性胆管炎,胆汁淤积性肝炎和Budd-Chiari综合征[90,91]。

为了充分发挥消化和排泄功能,肝脏必须与肝外胆道保持完整的连接,并与十二指肠Oddi括约肌处的肠腔保持功能连接。因此,与肺脏类似,肝脏生物工程面临的主要挑战是肝脏内部结构层次的复杂性,即从大的肝段动脉、门静脉和胆管,到中间的肝小叶,再到最小的肝窦内小胆管、门静脉和肝小动脉之间的组织关系。为了应对这一挑战,肝脏生物工程技术重点在于研究特殊的支架生物材料,以及进行体外扩增的合适的细胞群,同时,后者也显示肝细胞的功能特征[92,93]。接种肝细胞的三维微凝胶具有所需的控制导向以及组合成较大结构的特性[94,95]。另一种方法是应用微流体通道,它在细胞间相互作用、流动可溶性因子和三维机械力作用下比二维系统更精确地模拟天然肝窦[96]。去细胞化肝脏支架也被用于支持离体肝细胞,在类似于体外夹层培养基中显示出白蛋白和尿素合成,以及与正常肝组织相似的药物代谢基因表达[97]。

对于源细胞,也有肝细胞和多种干细胞的研究。成熟肝细胞可以新鲜制备,也可从冷冻保存的组织中制备,但是在直接肝细胞移植时,冷冻保存细胞比新鲜肝细胞移植结果更差[98]。此外,还有肝祖细胞的研究[99]。干细胞包括人胚胎干细胞(hESC),它可以在培养基中稳定扩增[100]。尽管最初在缺乏细胞色素P450 3A4成熟表达的胎儿肝细胞阶段,这些细胞停止分化成肝细胞,但是可以通过在培养基中适当地添加细胞因子使它们进一步分化[101]。根据诱导多能干(iPS)细胞的最新进展,可将高度分化的体细胞"重组"成多能干细胞状态的干细胞[102],因此,有人尝试将人体iPS细胞分化成肝细胞[103]。最后,对于低密度脂蛋白(LDL)受体介导的胆固醇摄取缺陷、α-1抗胰蛋白酶折叠错误和脂蛋白或糖原储存异常增加的患者,一些研究将这些患者的iPS细胞分化成肝细胞,结果发现在体外表现出与这些疾病相同的代谢紊乱特征,因而建立了患者特异性体外疾病模型[104]。

肾和尿道

肾脏是一种高度特异性器官,可进行全身体液稳态、电解质水平和血压的调节,并且将饮食或代谢的副产物——水溶性毒素排泄到尿液中。肾脏功能与输尿管、膀胱和尿道的通畅及肌肉功能有复杂的关系,以维持正常的尿排泄。终末期肾病(ESRD)的发病率持续增加,主要原因包括糖尿病、高血压和各种肾小球病[105]。虽然血液透析(HD)可作为肾脏替代治疗,但需要放置导管或制造永久性动静脉瘘[106],而且会导致显著的并发症,包括血清钙紊乱和钙过敏[107]、心血管疾病[108]、留置导管的机械并发症[109]以及瘘管失功和修复[110]。与HD相比,腹膜透析能增加患者的自主性,但是存在感染、腹膜炎[112]以及透析导管功能丧失和再次手术[113]的风险。

2007年,美国肾移植等待名单超过90 000例患者,而只有约16 000例实施了移植[114]。输尿管容易遭受放射或医源性损伤,并可以使用膀胱[115]或小肠[116]重建输尿管。在肾脏和输尿管远端,膀胱癌切除术后会引起明显的并发症,大多需要手术留置尿管[117]。

与其他器官工程方法一样，将干细胞从骨髓基质中分离[120],研究其分化过程,使这些细胞朝肾细胞系分化。这些干细胞包括胚胎干细胞(ESC)(源自胚泡早期的人胚胎干细胞[118]、诱导多能干(iPS)细胞[119]和 MSC。胚胎大鼠肾脏体外培养系统能产生分支输尿管芽和后肾间质，它们分别是集合系统和肾单位的原始成分[121]。最初的研究是将活的肾细胞载入体外合成支架中[122,123]。这种方法已经应用于动物[124]及小范围人体试验[125]。然而,这些方法本身都不是组织工程,组织工程的目的是构建整个器官或有足够功能的组织来替换衰竭器官。由于肾脏的三维结构复杂，使用完全合成材料开发肾脏支架面临巨大的挑战。因此,一些研究将研究重点集中于去细胞化支架,将其作为细胞植入的候选物,但到目前为止,只在大鼠和猴子中进行了相关实验[126,127]。在大鼠实验中，将鼠多能细胞作为异种移植物植入去细胞化肾脏,发现原始上皮分化形成原始管腔。恒河猴实验表明胎儿肾脏外植体可以移植到不同供体肾的支架上,并实现再细胞化。

相比之下，尿道和膀胱组织工程已经应用于人体治疗。早期在动物模型中已成功将聚乙醇酸网状支架用于尿道再生[128-130],后来研究重点转向膀胱和尿道来源的黏膜下层无细胞基质[131,132]。动物试验成功之后,膀胱黏膜下层复合体已经用于治疗人类的尿道狭窄[133,134]。值得注意的是，这些尿道成形术是以非种子基质覆盖方式进行的，但是如果用这种方法对整个尿道节段进行环形治疗时,术后会出现狭窄[135]。为了解决这个问题，最近主要研究正常伤口愈合对这些工程化组织反应的重要性，以及将自体或外源细胞首先接种到基质周围区段的效果[136]。

早期还使用合成材料增加人类膀胱的生产，例如聚乙烯海绵、特氟隆、胶原、聚乙醇酸和硅酮。然而,永久性材料可引起机械故障和尿石形成，而且可生物降解材料会引起成纤维细胞沉积、瘢痕形成、移植物挛缩及膀胱体积缩小[135-138]。此外,当植入各种未接种细胞的材料支架时,结果会发现尿路上皮层首先再生,其他组织层退化[139]。而支架材料首次装载或接种膀胱细胞时,肌层和其他各层发生再生[138,140]。随后在犬类模型中,切除狗的膀胱,然后植入组织工程膀胱,后者经可生物降解聚合物进行膀胱细胞接种获得。植入后膀胱容量和膀胱壁顺应性与术前相当[141]。最后,在人体初步研究(包含 7 名患者)中使用了同样的方法,但只得到初步的结果,目前还正在进行临床研究[142]。

四肢:骨、肌腱和韧带

上肢为人体提供了显著的灵活性和功能，如我们可以用完整的手臂、关节、手和手指展现高超的技术和精巧的活动。同样的,下肢为我们提供了运动,如行走、跑步、玩耍、竞赛这些经常未被充分认识的能力。反过来,轴心骨又为头部和四肢提供结构支撑和连接部位。因此,自从战争和其他重大创伤出现以来,内科医生和外科医生已经努力为失去这些功能的患者设计合适的假体。骨、结缔组织、肌肉和四肢的组织工程技术本身旨在完全恢复这些功能。在美国,每年有将近 100 万例整形手术是关于置换、创伤和发育异常的骨骼修复[143]。传统的重建方法需依赖自体或同种异体骨移植物、聚合物或金属植入物[144]。然而,因为供需不平衡和整合到周围宿主组织过程失败，尤其是同种异体移植物存在传播传染病及排斥的风险,使这些方法受到限制[145]。

众所周知,骨组织具有显著的自我更新能力,因为能够分化为成骨细胞的多能 MSC 存在于人骨髓和骨膜中[146]。骨骼发育和骨折修复都需要复杂的协调过程,包括细胞迁移、分化和激活,形成对骨组织的持续存活和再生至关重要的骨微血管系统[147,148]。之后,矿化成坚硬骨结构必须通过膜内或软骨内骨化发生[149]。

研究人员尝试植入各种材料来重现这一自然过程,目的是让相邻的骨组织长入并重塑植入物。已经采用了大量多孔支架聚合物,包括胶原[150]、PLA、PGA 和 PLGA 基质[151]。然而,这些聚合物缺乏足够的结构完整性以耐受生理压力负荷和剪切力,且骨传导性(支持天然骨细胞和组织附着的能力)受限,因此已经尝试将陶瓷材料如羟基磷灰石(HA)、磷酸钙与 PLA 或 PLGA 合并使用[152]。这些材料与人胎儿骨细胞结合组成的构建体,具有显著的骨传导性和成骨特性[153]。也有人认为,由于涉及正常骨发育以及重塑和修复的生长因子具有复杂的空间和时间分布,使用合并技术递送这些因子,包括骨形态发生蛋白(BMP)、多效生长因子(PTN)、转化生长因子-β(TGF-β)和血管内皮生长因子(VEGF),可能对于骨的原位再生非常关键[154]。

将人类运动的力和力矩从骨骼传递到肌肉和骨骼之间的结构是肌腱和韧带。在成人中,这些组织内的细胞密度低且再生能力差，如果组织的压力负荷超过临界值,会导致永久性损伤[155]。在物质含量方面,肌腱和韧带都是由55%~70%的水分组成的,其次是胶原(主要是Ⅰ型,还有一些是Ⅲ型)、弹性蛋白、蛋白聚糖、糖胺聚糖,以及糖蛋白,如纤连蛋白和血小板反应蛋白[156]。人体肌腱损伤主要是肌腱病或肌腱破裂,其愈合过程包括三个阶段:炎症期(24小时)、重塑期(3天至6周)和塑建期(6~10周)[157]。韧带损伤愈合过程类似但时间较短;最后阶段被称为重塑期并可以持续数年[158]。

已经尝试使用许多合成和生物材料来仿造肌腱和韧带的结构[159]。有研究观察到兔前交叉韧带(ACL)成纤维细胞黏附在聚ε-己内酯(PCL)、PLA和PLGA二维底物上,并进行增殖,黏附速率与附着到培养皿塑料上的速率相近[160]。为了更精确地模拟天然组织的微结构,其他小组采用具有PGA、PLGA和PLLA丝状物的三维编织支架技术进行研究,在与兔ACL成纤维细胞共培养之前用人纤维蛋白进行涂层可获得这种丝状物[161]。尽管合成材料提供了生产环境的可重复性并使制造理想的形状和尺寸更容易,但它们通常缺乏用于细胞附着的合适官能团,并且能将非生理物质洗脱进入循环[162]。因此,一些研究小组将不可降解的移植物材料功能化,研究其改善细胞融入并使失败最小化的可能性[163]。关于肌腱和韧带组织工程的其他方法主要是天然聚合生物材料,包括Ⅰ型胶原[164]、丝蛋白[165]或两者混合物[166]。切除兔的ACL后,将MSC的丝状移植物植入体内作为替代治疗,结果观察到大量的Ⅰ型和Ⅲ型胶原产生及稳定的韧带-骨附着,但其伸展强度比人体自身ACL组织小得多[167]。最后,初步研究数据表明,去细胞化天然肌腱可以从家禽供体中制备,并将其皮下植入大鼠后,可观察到宿主细胞的融入及其免疫原性的缺乏[168]。

总结

对几个器官的组织工程进行简要调查后,可以明显看到,过去20年里这个领域发展迅速。除了气管、膀胱和尿道,对于大多数器官,这些技术仍处于临床前阶段,而且目前尚未有长期结果数据的报道,但是该领域与正在尝试工程化的器官类型密切相关,其进展的速度和广度表明,组织工程最终可以通过常规植入、移植和替代方法对各种器官系统中的病变组织进行治疗。这种技术的成功意味着,供需不平衡的问题以及移植外科医生在21世纪初仍然面临的免疫障碍问题都将得到改善。

(杨崇威 译 向骁 朱继业 校)

参考文献

1. Langer R. Tissue engineering. Molecular Therapy. 2000;1:12–15.
2. Stock UA, Vacanti JP. Tissue engineering: current state and prospects. Annual Review of Medicine. 2001;52:443–451.
3. Peh GSL, Beuerman RW, Colman A, et al. Human corneal endothelial cell expansion for corneal endothelium transplantation: an overview. Transplantation. 2011;91:811–819.
4. Oh JY, Lee HJ, Khwarg SI, et al. Corneal cell viability and structure after transcorneal freezing-thawing in the human cornea. Clinical Ophthalmology. 2010;4:477–480.
5. Ritter T, Treacy M, Wilk M, et al. Novel therapeutic strategies for the induction of tolerance in cornea transplantation. Acta Ophthalmologica. 2011;89:S246.
6. Zirm EK. Eine erfolgreiche totale keratopastik. Journal of Refractive and Corneal Surgery. 1906;5:258–161.
7. Borderie VM, Boëlle P-Y, Touzeau O, et al. Predicted long-term outcome of corneal transplantation. Ophthalmology. 2009;116:2354–2360.
8. Christensen K, Doblhammer G, Rau R, et al. Ageing populations: the challenges ahead. Lancet. 2009;374:1196–1208.
9. Vajpayee RB, Sharma N, Jhanji V, et al. One donor cornea for 3 recipients: a new concept for corneal transplantation surgery. Archives of Ophthalmology. 2007;125:552–554.
10. Baum JL, Niedra R, Davis C, et al. Mass culture of human corneal endothelial cells. Archives of Ophthalmology. 1979;97:1136–1140.
11. Yue BY, Sugar J, Gilboy JE, et al. Growth of human corneal endothelial cells in culture. Investigative Ophthalmology and Visual Science. 1989;30:248–253.
12. Fabricant RN, Alpar AJ, Centifanto YM, et al. Epidermal growth factor receptors on corneal endothelium. Archives of Ophthalmology. 1981;99:305–308.
13. Tripathi RC, Tripathi BJ. Human trabecular endothelium, corneal endothelium, keratocytes, and scleral fibroblasts in primary cell culture. A comparative study of growth characteristics, morphology, and phagocytic activity by light and scanning electron microscopy. Experimental Eye Research. 1982;35:611.
14. Li W, Sabater AL, Chen Y-T, et al. A novel method of isolation, preservation, and expansion of human corneal endothelial cells. Investigative Ophthalmology and Visual Science. 2007;48:614–620.
15. Ishino Y, Sano Y, Nakamura T, et al. Amniotic membrane as a carrier for cultivated human corneal endothelial cell transplantation. Investigative Ophthalmology and Visual Science. 2004;45:800–806.
16. Chen KH, Azar D, Joyce NC. Transplantation of adult human corneal endothelium *ex vivo*: a morphologic study. Cornea. 2001;20:731–737.
17. Engelmann K, Bednarz J, Valtink M. Prospects for endothelial transplantation. Experimental Eye Research. 2004;78:573–578.
18. Engelmann K, Böhnke M, Friedl P. Isolation and long-term cultivation of human corneal endothelial cells. Investigative Ophthalmology and Visual Science. 1988;2:1656–1662.
19. Melles GR, Lander F, Rietveld FJ. Transplantation of Descemet's membrane carrying viable endothelium through a small scleral incision. Cornea. 2002;21:415–418.
20. Lie JT, Birbal R, Ham L, et al. Donor tissue preparation for Descemet membrane endothelial keratolasty. Journal of Cataract and Refractive Surgery. 2008;34:1578–1583.
21. Zhu C, Joyce NC. Proliferative response of corneal endothelial cells from young and older donors. Investigative Ophthalmology and Visual Science. 2004;45:1743–1751.
22. Zimmermann WH, Didié M, Döker S, et al. Heart muscle engineering: an update on cardiac muscle replacement therapy. Cardiovascular Research. 2006;71:419–429.
23. Nicolini F, Gherli T. Alternatives to transplantation in the surgical therapy for heart failure. European Journal of Cardio-Thoracic Surgery. 2009;35:214–228.
24. Zimmerman W-H, Cesnjevar R. Cardiac tissue engineering: implications for pediatric heart surgery. Pediatric Cardiology. 2009;30:716–723.
25. Von Harsdort R, Poole-Wilson PA, Dietz R. Regenerative capacity of the myocardium: implications for treatment of heart failure. Lancet. 2004;363:1306–1313.

26. Jawad H, Ali NN, Lyon AR, et al. Myocardial tissue engineering: a review. Journal of Tissue Engineering and Regenerative Medicine. 2007;1:327–342.
27. Messina E, De Angelis L, Frati G, et al. Isolation and expansion of adult cardiac stem cells from human and murine heart. Circulation Research. 2004;2004: 911–921.
28. Kocher AA, Scuster MD, Szabolcs MJ, et al. Neovascularization of ischemic myocardium by human bone-marrow-derived angioblasts prevents cardiomyocyte apoptosis, reduces remodeling and improves cardiac function. Nature Medicine. 2001;7:430–436.
29. Taylor DA, Atkins BZ, Hungspreugs P, et al. Regenerating functional myocardium: improved performance after skeletal myoblast transplantation. Nature Medicine. 1998;4:929–933.
30. Zimmermann WH, Fink C, Kralisch D, et al. Three-dimensional engineered heart tissue from neonatal rat cardiac myocytes. Biotechnology and Bioengineering. 2000;68:106–114.
31. Wu KH, Mo XM, Liu YL, et al. Stem cells for tissue engineering of myocardial constructs. Ageing Research Reviews. 2007;6:289–301.
32. Iyer RK, Chui J, Radisic M. Spatiotemporal tracking of cells in tissue-engineered cardiac organoids. Journal of Tissue Engineering and Regenerative Medicine. 2009;3:196–207.
33. Khait L, Birla RK. Cell-based cardiac pumps and tissue-engineered ventricles. Regenerative Medicine. 2007;4:391–406.
34. Christman KL, Lee RJ. Biomaterials for the treatment of myocardial infarction. Journal of the American College of Cardiology. 2006;48:907–913.
35. Pacak CA, Cowan DB. Fabrication of myogenic engineered tissue constructs. Journal of Visualized Experiments: JoVE. 2009;27:1137.
36. Zimmermann WH, Didie M, Wasmeier GH, et al. Cardiac grafting of engineered heart tissue in syngenic rats. Circulation. 2002;106:1151–1157.
37. Krupnick AS, Kreisel D, Engels FH, et al. A novel small animal model of left ventricular tissue engineering. Journal of Heart and Lung Transplantation. 2002;21:233–243.
38. Radisic M, Euloth M, Yang L, et al. High-density seeding of myocyte cells for cardiac tissue engineering. Biotechnology and Bioengineering. 2003;82: 403–414.
39. Dar A, Shachar M, Leor J, et al. Optimization of cardiac cell seeding and distribution in 3D porous alginate scafflolds. Biotechnology and Bioengineering. 2002;80:305–312.
40. Leor J, Aboulafia-Etzion S, Dar A, et al. Bioengineered cardiac grafts: a new approach to repair the infarcted myocardium? Circulation. 2000;102: III56–III61.
41. Amir G, Miller L, Shachar M, et al. Evaluation of a peritoneal-generated cardiac patch in a rat model of heterotopic heart transplantation. Cell Transplantation. 2009;18:275–282.
42. Dvir T, Kedem A, Ruvinov E, et al. Prevascularization of cardiac patch on the omentum improves its therapeutic outcome. Proceedings of the National Academy of Sciences of the United States of America. 2009;106:14990–14995.
43. Tan MY, Zhi W, Wei RQ, et al. Repair of infarcted myocardium using mesenchymal stem cell seeded small intestinal submucosa in rabbits. Biomaterials. 2009;30:3234–3240.
44. Moodley Y, Manuelpillai U, Weiss DJ. Cellular therapies for lung disease: a distant horizon. Respirology. 2011;16:223–227.
45. Walles T. Tracheobronchial bio-engineering: biotechnology fulfilling unmet medical needs. Advanced Drug Delivery Reviews. 2011;63:367–374.
46. Bader A, Macchiarini P. Moving towards *in situ* tracheal regeneration: the bionic tissue engineered transplantation approach. Journal of Cellular and Molecular Medicine. 2010;14:1877–1889.
47. Grillo HC. Tracheal replacement: a critical review. Annals of Thoracic Surgery. 2002;73:1995–2004.
48. Gilbert TW, Sellaro TL, Badylak SF. Decellularization of tissues and organs. Biomaterials. 2006;27:3675–3683.
49. Macchiarini P, Jungebluth P, Go T, et al. Clinical transplantation of a tissue-engineered airway. Lancet. 2008;372:2023–2030.
50. Cooper JD. The evolution of techniques and indications for lung transplantation. Annals of Surgery. 1990;212:249–256.
51. Huddleston CB, Bloch JB, Sweet SC, et al. Lung transplantation in children. Annals of Surgery. 2002;236:270–276.
52. Nichols JE, Cortiella J. Engineering of a complex organ: progress toward development of a tissue-engineered lung. Proceedings of the American Thoracic Society. 2008;5:723–730.
53. Kajstura J, Rota M, Hall SR, et al. Evidence for human lung stem cells. New England Journal of Medicine. 2011;364:1795–1806.
54. Mondrinos MJ, Koutzaki S, Lelkes PI, et al. A tissue-engineered model of fetal distal lung tissue. American Journal of Physiology. Lung Cellular and Molecular Physiology. 2007;293:736–752.
55. Mondrinos MJ, Koutzaki SH, Poblete HM, et al. In vivo pulmonary tissue engineering: contribution of donor-derived endothelial cells to construct vascularization. Tissue Engineering. 2008;14:361–368.
56. Andrade CF, Wong AP, Waddell TK, et al. Cell-based tissue engineering for lung regeneration. American Journal of Physiology. Lung Cellular and Molecular Physiology. 2007;292:L510–L518.
57. Shannon JM, Mason RJ, Jennings SD. Functional differentiation of alveolar type II epithelial cells in vitro: effects of cell shape, cell-matrix ineractions and cell-cell interactions. Biochimica et Biophysica Acta. 1987;931:143–156.
58. Shigemura N, Okumura M, Mizuno S, et al. Lung tissue engineering technique with adipose stromal cells improves surgical outcome for pulmonary emphysema. American Journal of Respiratory and Critical Care Medicine. 2006; 174:1199–1205.
59. Mondrinos MJ, Koutzaki S, Jiwanmall E, et al. Engineering three-dimensional pulmonary tissue constructs. Tissue Engineering. 2006;12:717–728.
60. Cortiella J, Nichols JE, Kojima K, et al. Tissue-engineered lung: an in vivo and in vitro comparison of polyglycolic acid and pluronic F-127 hydrogel/somatic lung progenitor cell constructs to support tissue growth. Tissue Engineering. 2006;12:1213–1225.
61. Wales PW, Christison-Lagay ER. Short bowel syndrome: epidemiology and etiology. Seminars in Pediatric Surgery. 2010;19:3–9.
62. Spencer AU, Neaga A, West B, et al. Pediatric short bowel syndrome: redefining predictors of success. Annals of Surgery. 2005;242:403–412.
63. Sukhotnik I, Coran AG, Kramer A, et al. Advances in short bowel syndrome: an updated review. Pediatric Surgery International. 2005;21:947–953.
64. Petrosyan M, Guner YS, Williams M, et al. Current concepts regarding the pathogenesis of necrotizing enterocolitis. Pediatric Surgery International. 2009;25:309–318.
65. Shew SB. Surgical concerns in malrotation and midgut volvulus. Pediatric Radiology. 2009;39:S167–S171.
66. Sampietro GM, Corsi F, Maconi G, et al. Prospective study of long-term results and prognostic factors after conservative surgery for small bowel Crohn's disease. Clinical Gastroenterology and Hepatology. 2009;7:183–191.
67. Klempnauer J, Grothues F, Bektas H, et al. Long-term results after surgery for acute mesenteric ischemia. Surgery. 1997;121:239–243.
68. Fitzgibbons SC, Jones BA, Hull MA, et al. Relationship between biopsy-proven parenteral nutrition-associated liver fibrosis and biochemical cholestasis in children with short bowel syndrome. Journal of Pediatric Surgery. 2010;45:95–99.
69. Spencer AU, Kovacevich D, McKinney-Barnett M, et al. Pediatric short bowel syndrome: the cost of comprehensive care. American Journal of Clinical Nutrition. 2008;88:1552–1559.
70. Kato T, Tzakis AG, Selvaggi G, et al. Intestinal and multivisceral transplantation in children. Annals of Surgery. 2012;243:756–766.
71. Reyes J, Bueno J, Kocoshis S, et al. Current status of intestinal transplantation in children. Journal of Pediatric Surgery. 1998;33:243–254.
72. Levin DE, Dreyfuss JM, Grikscheit TC. Tissue-engineered small intestine. Expert Review of Medical Devices. 2011;8:673–675.
73. Barker N, van Es JH, Kuipers J, et al. Identification of stem cells in small intestine and colon by marker gene Lgr5. Nature. 2007;449:1003–1008.
74. Sato T, Vries RG, Snippert HJ, et al. Single Lgr5 stem cells build crypt-villus structures in vitro without a mesenchymal niche. Nature. 2009;459:262–265.
75. May R, Sureban SM, Hoang N, et al. Doublecortin and CaM kinase-like-1 and leucine-rich-repeat-containing G-protein-coupled receptor mark quiescent and cycling intestinal stem cells, respectively. Stem Cells. 2009;27:2571–2579.
76. Sangiorgi E, Capechhi MR. Bmi1 is expressed in vivo in intestinal stem cells. Nature Genetics. 2008;40:915–920.
77. Zhu L, Gibson P, Currles DS, et al. Prominin 1 marks intestinal stem cells that are susceptible to neoplastic transformation. Nature. 2009;457:603–607.
78. Asai R, Okan H, Yasugi S. Correlation between Musashi-1 and c-hairy-1 expression and cell proliferation activity in the developing intestine and stomach of both chicken and mouse. Development, Growth and Differentiation. 2005;47: 501–510.
79. Montgomery RK, Carlone DL, Richmond CA, et al. Mouse telomerase reverse transcriptase (mTert) expression marks slowly cycling intestinal stem cells. Proceedings of the National Academy of Sciences of the United States of America. 2011;108:179–184.
80. Evans GS, Flint N, Somers AS, et al. The development of a method for the preparation of rat intestinal epithelial cell primary cultures. Journal of Cell Science. 1992;101:219–231.
81. Grikscheit TC, Ochoa ER, Srinivasan A, et al. Tissue-engineered esophagus: experimental substitution by onlay patch or interposition. Journal of Thoracic and Cardiovascular Surgery. 2003;126:537–544.
82. Grikscheit TC, Srinivasan A, Vacanti JP. Tissue-engineered stomach: a preliminary report of a versatile in vivo model with therapeutic potential. Journal of Pediatric Surgery. 2003;38:1305–1309.
83. Ramsanahie A, Duxbury MS, Grikscheit TC, et al. Effect of GLP-2 on

mucosal morphology and SGLT1 expression in tissue-engineered neointestine. American Journal of Physiology. Gastrointestinal and Liver Physiology. 2003;285:G1345–G1352.
84. Grikscheit TC, Siddique A, Ochoa ER, et al. Tissue-engineered small intestine improves recovery after massive small bowel resection. Annals of Surgery. 2004;240:748–754.
85. Grikscheit TC, Ochoa ER, Ramsanahie A, et al. Tissue-engineered large intestine resembles native colon with appropriate in vitro physiology and architecture. Annals of Surgery. 2003;238:35–41.
86. Sala FG, Matthews JA, Speer AL, et al. A multicellular approach forms a significant amount of tissue-engineered small intestine in the mouse. Tissue Engineering. Part A. 2011;17:1841–1850.
87. Speer AL, Sala FG, Matthews JA, et al. Murine tissue-engineered stomach demonstrates epithelial differentiation. Journal of Surgical Research. 2011;171(1): 6–14.
88. Sala FG, Kunisaki SM, Ochoa ER, et al. Tissue-engineered small intestine and stomach form from autologous tissue in a preclinical large animal model. Journal of Surgical Research. 2009;156:205–212.
89. O'Leary JG, Lepe R, Davis GL. Indications for liver transplantation. Gastroenterology. 2008;134:1764–1776.
90. Schuppan D, Afdhal NH. Liver cirrhosis. Lancet. 2008;371:838–851.
91. Jain A, Mazariegos G, Kashyap R, et al. Pediatric liver transplantation: a single center experience spanning 20 years. Transplantation. 2002;73: 941–947.
92. Ananthanarayanan A, Narmada BC, Mo X, et al. Purpose-driven biomaterials research in liver-tissue engineering. Trends in Biotechnology. 2011;29: 110–118.
93. Ohashi K. Liver tissue engineering: the future of liver therapeutics. Hepatology Research. 2008;38:S76–S87.
94. Du Y, Lo E, Ali S, et al. Directed assembly of cell-laden microgels for fabrication of 3D tissue constructs. Proceedings of the National Academy of Sciences of the United States of America. 2008;105:9522–9527.
95. Tsuda Y, Morimoto Y, Takeuchi S. Monodisperse cell-encapsulating peptide microgel beads for 3D cell culture. Langmuir: ACS Journal of Surfaces and Colloids. 2010;26:2645–2649.
96. Toh Y-C, Zhang C, Zhang J, et al. A novel 3D mammalian cell perfusion-culture system in microfluidic channels. Lab on a Chip. 2007;7:302–309.
97. Uygun BE, Soto-Gutierrez A, Yagi H, et al. Organ reengineering through development of a transplantable recellularized liver graft using decellularized liver matrix. Nature Medicine. 2010;16:814–820.
98. Fox IJ, Chowdhury JR. Hepatocyte transplantation. American Journal of Transplantation. 2004;4:7–13.
99. Lagasse E, Connors H, Al-Dhalimy M, et al. Purified hematopoietic stem cells can differentiate into hepatocytes in vivo. Nature Medicine. 2000;6:1229–1234.
100. Oh SK, Chen AK, Mok Y, et al. Long-term microcarrier suspension cultures of human embryonic stem cells. Stem Cell Research. 2009;2:219–230.
101. Roelandt P, Pauwelyn KA, Sancho-Bru P, et al. Human embryonic and rat adult stem cells with primitive endoderm-like phenotype can be fated to definitive endoderm, and finally hepatocyte-like cells. PLoS ONE. 2010;5:e12101.
102. Takahashi K, Yamanaka S. Induction of pluripotent stem cells from mouse embryonic and adult fibroblast cultures by defined factors. Cell. 2006; 126:663–676.
103. Si-Tayeb K, Noto FK, Nagaoka M, et al. Highly efficient generation of human hepatocyte-like cells from induced pluripotent stem cells. Hepatology. 2009; 51:297–305.
104. Rashid ST, Corbineau S, Hannan N, et al. Modeling inherited metabolic disorders of the liver using human induced pluripotent stem cells. Journal of Clinical Investigation. 2010;120:3127–3136.
105. Perin L, Da Sacco S, De Filippo RE. Regenerative medicine of the kidney. Advanced Drug Delivery Reviews. 2011;63:379–387.
106. Schwab SJ. Hemodialysis vascular access: the Achilles' heel remains. Kidney International. 2007;72:665–666.
107. Miller JE, Kovesdy CP, Norris KC, et al. Association of cumulatively low or high serum calcium levels with mortality in long-term hemodialysis patients. American Journal of Nephrology. 2010;32:403–413.
108. El-Mesallamy HO, Abdel Hamid SG, Gad MZ. Oxidative stress and asymmetric dimethylarginine are associated with cardiovascular complications in hemodialysis patients: improvements by L-arginine intake. Kidney and Blood Pressure Research. 2008;31:189–195.
109. Besarab A, Pandey R. Catheter management in hemodialysis patients: delivering adequate flow. Clinical Journal of the American Society of Nephrology: CJASN. 2011;6:227–234.
110. Schinstock CA, Albright RC, Williams AW, et al. Outcomes of arteriovenous fistula creation after the Fistula First Initiative. Clinical Journal of the American Society of Nephrology: CJASN. 2011;6:1996–2002.
111. Fan SL, Sathick I, McKitty K, et al. Quality of life of caregivers and patients on peritoneal dialysis. Nephrology, Dialysis, Transplantation. 2008;23:1713–1719.
112. Troidle L, Gorban-Brennan N, Kliger A, et al. Continuous peritoneal dialysis-associated peritonitis: a review and current concepts. Seminars in Dialysis. 2003;16:428–437.
113. Elhassan E, McNair B, Quinn M, et al. Prolonged duration of peritoneal dialysis catheter embedment does not lower the catheter success rate. Peritoneal Dialysis International. 2011;31:558–564.
114. McCullough KP, Keith DS, Meyer KH, et al. Kidney and pancreas transplantation in the United States, 1998–2007: access for patients with diabetes and end-stage renal disease. American Journal of Transplantation. 2009;9:894–906.
115. Mauck RJ, Hudak SJ, Terlecki RP, et al. Central role of Boari bladder flap and downward nephropexy in upper ureteral reconstruction. Journal of Urology. 2011;186:1345–1349.
116. Wolff B, Chartier-Kastler E, Mozer P, et al. Long-term functional outcomes after ileal ureter substitution: a single-center experience. Urology. 2011;78:692–695.
117. Daneshmand S, Bartsch G. Improving selection of appropriate urinary diversion following radical cystectomy for bladder cancer. Expert Review of Anticancer Therapy. 2011;11:941–948.
118. Batchelder CA, Lee CI, Matsell DG, et al. Renal ontogeny in the rhesus monkey (*Macaca mulatta*) and directed differentiation of human embryonic stem cells towards kidney precursors. Differentiation; Research in Biological Diversity. 2009;78:45–56.
119. Morizane R, Monkawa T, Itoh H. Differentiation of murine embryonic stem and induced pluripotent stem cells to renal lineage in vitro. Biochemical and Biophysical Research Communications. 2009;390:1334–1339.
120. Singaravelu K, Padanilam BJ. In vitro differentiation of MSC into cells with a renal tubular epithelial-like phenotype. Renal Failure. 2009;31:492–502.
121. Steer DL, Bush KT, Meyer TN, et al. A strategy for in vitro propagation of rat nephrons. Kidney International. 2002;62:1958–1965.
122. Aebischer P, Ip TK, Panol G, et al. The bioartificial kidney: progress towards an ultrafiltration device with renal epithelial cells processing. Life Support Systems. 1987;5:159–168.
123. Ip TK, Aebischer P. Renal epithelial-cell-controlled solute transport across permeable membranes as the foundation for a bioartificial kidney. Artificial Organs. 1989;13:58–65.
124. Fissell WH, Lou L, Abrishami S, et al. Bioartificial kidney ameliorates gram-negative bacteria-induced septic shock in uremic animals. Journal of the American Society of Nephrology. 2003;14:454–461.
125. Humes HD, Weitzel WF, Bartlett RH, et al. Initial clinical results of the bioartificial kidney containing human cells in ICU patients with acute renal failure. Kidney International. 2004;66:1578–1588.
126. Ross EA, Williams MJ, Hamazaki T, et al. Embryonic stem cells proliferate and differentiate when seeded into kidney scaffolds. Journal of the American Society of Nephrology. 2009;20:2338–2347.
127. Nakayama KH, Batchelder CA, Lee CI, et al. Decellularized rhesus monkey kidney as a three-dimensional scaffold for renal tissue engineering. Tissue Engineering. Part A. 2010;16:2207–2216.
128. Bazeed MA, Thuroff JW, Schmidt RA, et al. New treatment for urethral strictures. Urology. 1983;21:53–57.
129. Olsen L, Bowlad S, Busch C, et al. Urethral reconstruction with a new synthetic absorbable device: an experimental study. Scandinavian Journal of Urology and Nephrology. 1992;26:323–326.
130. Atala A, Vacanti JP, Peters CA, et al. Formation of urothelial structures *in vivo* from dissociated cells attached to biodegradable polymer scaffolds in vitro. Journal of Urology. 1992;148:658–662.
131. Chen F, Yoo JJ, Atala A. Acellular collagen matrix as a possible "off the shelf" biomaterial for urethral repair. Urology. 1999;54:407–410.
132. Sievert KD, Bakircioglu ME, Nunes L, et al. Homologous acellular matrix graft for urethral reconstruction in the rabbit: histological and functional evaluation. Journal of Urology. 2000;163:1958–1965.
133. El-Kassaby A, AbouShwareb T, Atala A. Randomized comparative study between buccal mucosal and acellular bladder matrix grafts in complex anterior urethral strictures. Journal of Urology. 2008;179:1432–1436.
134. El-Kassaby AW, Retik AB, Yoo JJ, et al. Urethral stricture repair with an off-the-shelf collagen matrix. Journal of Urology. 2003;169:170–173.
135. De Filippo RE, Yoo JJ, Atala A. Urethral replacement using cell seeded tubularized collagen matrices. Journal of Urology. 2002;168:1789–1792.
136. Atala A. Engineering Organs. Current Opinion in Biotechnology. 2009;20: 575–592.
137. Atala A. Autologous cell transplantation for urologic reconstruction. Journal of Urology. 1998;159:2–3.
138. Atala A. Commentary on the replacement of urologic associated mucosa. Journal of Urology. 1995;156:338.
139. Jayo MJ, Jain D, Wagner BJ, et al. Early cellular and stromal responses in regenera-

tion versus repair of a mammalian bladder using autologous cell and biodegradable scaffold technologies. Journal of Urology. 2008;180:392–397.
140. Yoo JJ, Meng J, Oberpenning F, et al. Bladder augmentation using allogenic bladder submucosa seeded with cells. Urology. 1998;51:221–225.
141. Oberpenning F, Meng J, Yoo JJ, et al. *De novo* reconstitution of a functional mammalian urinary bladder by tissue engineering. Nature Biotechnology. 1999;17:149–155.
142. Atala A, Bauer SB, Soker S, et al. Tissue-engineered autologous bladders for patients needing cystoplasty. Lancet. 2006;367:1241–1246.
143. Oreffo ROC, Triffitt JT. Future potentials for using osteogenic stem cells and biomaterials in orthopedics. Bone. 1999;25:5S–9S.
144. Moore WR, Graves SE, Bain GI. Synthetic bone graft substitutes. ANZ Journal of Surgery. 2001;71:354–361.
145. Kanczler JM, Oreffo ROC. Osteogenesis and angiogenesis: the potential for engineering bone. European Cells and Materials. 2008;15:100–114.
146. Fayaz HC, Giannoudis PV, Vrahas MS, et al. The role of stem cells in fracture healing and nonunion. International Orthopaedics. 2011;35:1587–1597.
147. Colnot C, Romero DM, Huang S, et al. Mechanisms of action of demineralized bone matrix in the repair of cortical bone defects. Clinical Orthopaedics and Related Research. 2005;435:69–78.
148. Schmid J, Wallkamm B, Hammerle CH, et al. The significance of angiogenesis in guided bone regeneration. A case report of a rabbit experiment. Clinical Oral Implants Research. 1997;8:244–248.
149. Tortelli F, Tasso R, Loiacono F, et al. The development of tissue-engineered bone of different origin through endochondral and intramembranous ossification following the implantation of mesenchymal stem cells and osteoblasts in a murine model. Biomaterials. 2010;31:242–249.
150. Domaschke H, Gelinsky M, Burmeister B, et al. In vitro ossification and remodeling of mineralized collagen I scaffolds. Tissue Engineering. 2006;12:949–958.
151. Agrawal CM, Ray RB. Biodegradable polymeric scaffolds for musculoskeletal tissue engineering. Journal of Biomedical Materials Research. 2001;55:141–150.
152. Popov VK, Evseev AV, Ivanov AL, et al. Laser stereolithography and supercritical fluid processing for custom-designed implant fabrication. Journal of Materials Science: Materials in Medicine. 2004;15:123–128.
153. Montjovent MO, Mathieu L, Hinz B, et al. Biocompatibility of bioresorbable poly(L-lactic acid) composite scaffolds obtained by supercritical gas foaming with human fetal bone cells. Tissue Engineering. 2005;11:1640–1649.
154. Rose FRAJ, Hou Q, Oreffo ROC. Delivery systems for bone growth factors – the new players in skeletal regeneration. Journal of Pharmacy and Pharmacology. 2004;56:415–427.
155. Kuo CK, Marturano JE, Tuan RS. Novel strategies in tendon and ligament tissue engineering: advanced biomaterials and regeneration motifs. Sports Medicine, Arthroscopy, Rehabilitation, Therapy and Technology. 2010;2:20.
156. Hoffmann A, Gross G. Tendon and ligament engineering in the adult organism: mesenchymal stem cells and gene-therapeutic approaches. International Orthopaedics. 2007;31:791–797.
157. Sharma P, Maffulli N. Biology of tendon injury: healing: modeling and remodeling. Journal of Musculoskeletal and Neuronal Interactions. 2006;6:181–190.
158. Woo SLY, Abramowitch SD, Kilger R, et al. Biomechanics of knee ligaments: injury, healing, and repair. Journal of Biomechanics. 2006;39:1–20.
159. Altman GH, Hoan L, Weitzel P, et al. The use of long-term bioresorbable scaffolds for anterior cruciate ligament repair. Journal of the American Academy of Orthopaedic Surgeons. 2008;16:177–187.
160. Ouyang HW, Goh JCH, Mo XM, et al. Characterization of anterior cruciate ligament cells and bone marrow stromal cells on various biodegradable polymeric films. Materials Science and Engineering C. 2002;20:63–69.
161. Lu HH, Cooper JA, Manuel S, et al. Anterior cruciate ligament regeneration using braided biodegradable scaffolds: in vitro optimization studies. Biomaterials. 2005;26:4805–4816.
162. Athanasiou KA, Niederauer GG, Agrawal CM. Sterilzation, toxicity, biocompatibility and clinical applications of polylactic acid/polyglycolic acid copolymers. Biomaterials. 1996;17:93–102.
163. Murphy AR, Kaplan DL. Biomedical applications of chemically-modified silk fibroin. Journal of Materials Chemistry. 2009;19:6443–6450.
164. Roeder BA, Kokini K, Sturgis JE, et al. Tensile mechanical properties of three-dimensional type I collagen extracellular matrices with varied microstructure. Journal of Biomechanical Engineering. 2002;124:214–222.
165. Altman GH, Horan RL, Lu HH, et al. Silk matrix for tissue engineered anterior cruciate ligaments. Biomaterials. 2002;23:4131–4141.
166. Chen X, Qu YY, Wang LL, et al. Ligament regeneration using a knitted silk scaffold combined with collagen matrix. Biomaterials. 2008;29:3683–3692.
167. Fan H, Liu H, Wong EJW, et al. In vivo study of anterior cruciate ligament regeneration using mesenchymal stem cells and silk scaffold. Biomaterials. 2008;29:3324–3337.
168. Whitlock PW, Smith TL, Poehling GG, et al. A naturally derived, cytocompatible, and architecturally optimized scaffold for tendon and ligament regeneration. Biomaterials. 2007;28:4321–4329.

器官接受和风险管理评估

第 53 章 标准和扩大化标准供者的器官评估及接受

Matthew Cooper, Stephen T. Bartlett

引言

器官移植的成功是从合适的供体器官开始的。如果器官是来自一个几乎没有慢性疾病的健康年轻供体,移植就有了一个良好的开端。但是,最近 20 年来,我们的器官越来越多地来自年龄更大的人群。因此,器官接受的过程就变得异常复杂,而且缺少严格系统化的、数据支持的标准,移植医生总是面临着供体和受体信息不全以及时间紧迫的压力。合适的器官与相应受体的配对受到人口老龄化和供体人群老龄化双方的影响,同样,也会受到死亡供体器官短缺的影响。

本章将会讨论捐献者的评估标准。随着器官接受的普遍化,我们将对标准捐献(SCD)供体给予简要关注。我们将更加关注对不属于理想捐献范围内供体器官的评估,即那些被指定为扩大标准捐献(ECD)供体。我们还将讨论一般情况下使用这些供体相关的预后。第 54 章将具体说明与心脏死亡(DCD)供体捐献和移植相关的程序和预后。本章将从器官特异性的角度概括性地补充操作方式和围术期管理。

标准供体:供体来源减少

在移植治疗的早期,典型的器官供体来自头部闭合性或穿透性损伤的年轻受害者。在过去 20 年里,器官供体的范围发生了巨大变化,其中最显著的变化是平均年龄。移植受体科学登记处(SRTR)的数据(表 53.1)显示,在 1991 年至 2011 年之间,来自 50 岁以上供体的尸体肾的百分比增加了 216%[1]。在此 20 年间,来自 50 岁以上供体的尸体肾从 4268 个供体的 18.2%增加到 7433 个供体的 33.1%。类似地,6~49 岁的理想年龄范围内的供体从所有供体的 76.2%减少到不足一半的 43.4%。供体老龄化的原因可能与影响美国人口的一系列公共卫生干预措施有关。

在美国,最重要的一项公共卫生成就是在各方齐心协力之下提高了道路安全水平。在 1979 年到 2010 年之间,尽管美国人口从 1979 年的 2.25 亿人显著增加到 2010 年的 3.1 亿人,但美国道路死亡人数从 51 093 人下降到 35 498 人[2]。即使在过去 10 年,车祸死亡率已经从 0.0155%下降到 0.0101%,下降了 50%。此项公共卫生成就,可以归因于汽车碰撞性能的改善、电子增强制动系统和汽车分辨性的增强。同样,人为因素还包括安全带的使用、将酒后驾车纳入违法、驾驶员教育的普及以及创伤急救水平的提高[3]。交通事故死亡率的降低

表 53.1 1991 年至 2011 年间器官供体人群的年龄变化。注意到供体人群向年龄更大的方向转变。50 岁以上的供体从占供体人群的 18.1%增加到 33.1%

1991 年和 2011 年各年龄段肾脏供体数量

年龄	1991		2011
<1	39		87
1~5	197		222
6~10	171		109
11~17	563		425
18~34	1556	3255(76.2%)	2143
35~49	965		1987
50~64	653		2039
65+	124	777(18.2%)	421
共计	4268		7433

Data from www.srtr.org

进一步减少了医院中头部损伤患者的数量，从而降低了脑死亡和器官捐献供体的数量。

在同一时期，高动能武器（高速或大规模导弹）的广泛使用导致在事故或持枪故意伤害现场死亡的受害者比例升高。值得注意的是，在过去 10 年中，美国的枪伤死亡人数并没有改变，但枪伤死亡率依然与目前的机动车事故死亡率（10/100 000）相同。其中头部中弹致死的比例接近 70%。在那些已经到达创伤中心的病例中，头部中弹致死可能是由心血管（失血）和神经方面的原因造成的。高动能武器可能导致更多的心血管疾病患者当场死亡。创伤性脑损伤的神经外科治疗方面的显著改善大大降低了死亡率[4,5]。同时进行识别和消除持续性休克以及应用减压开颅手术共同治疗脑水肿，彻底改善了闭合性和穿透性头部损伤患者的护理和预后。最后，应该注意的是，在马里兰大学休克创伤中心的因神经外科创伤入院患者的研究中，19%的患者年龄超过 75 岁，其中许多病例是因老年人跌倒造成的。这些公共卫生的发展导致捐献人群中年轻人的比例大幅度下降（Howard Eisenberg, MD, University of Maryland School of Medicine, personal. communication）。

与创伤发生率和治疗的发展一致，另一个主要导致潜在的老年器官供体数量增加的公共卫生原因是心脏停搏。以前，心脏骤停成功恢复被认为是偶然事件。如在购物中心以及机场等公共场所，公共卫生事业做出了巨大的努力，保证能对心脏骤停有组织、有计划地做出紧急处理[6]。这些紧急处理包括提供对心脏骤停的指导以及自动外部除颤器（AED）[7,8]。公众在基本生命支持方面的广泛培训促使心脏骤停患者及时就诊的概率增加。在一项具有里程碑意义的研究中，相较于在家里发生心脏骤停的患者，在公共场所发生心脏骤停的患者生存率显著提高。在研究中，出院患者的总生存率为 7%。对于在家里发生心脏骤停的患者，及时心肺复苏（CPR）患者的存活率为 10%。但在公共场所，心脏骤停患者有 20%的存活率；如果加上 AED 的应用，在公共场所心脏骤停患者的生存率为 42%[8]。心脏骤停的紧急医疗服务（EMS）的反应时间在家里是 5.6 分钟，在公共场所是 5 分钟。所以可以推断，那些没有幸存的患者或者是因为形成了不可逆脑损伤而宣布脑死亡，或者是因为没有进一步指导而抢救中断。由于公共场所对心脏骤停患者准备了紧急方案，越来越多被复苏的心脏骤停患者被积极送达医院救治。我们可以推断，最终的非存活的患者中有一些可能成为器官捐献者。因此，从 1998 年到 2011 年（图 53.1），死于脑缺氧的器官供体比例从 10%增加到 29%，而死于头部创伤的器官供体比例从 48%下降到 38%[1]。

综上所述，捐献者人口明显老龄化，随着公共卫生对于枪伤死亡的多方面控制，不难预测，器官捐献者的年龄将会继续升高[9]。

SCD 研究结果多数关注于来自 55 岁以下的供体，但这并不是近年来科研热点。最近有关肾移植的研究对象是老龄人群和近老年人群。对 SCD 结果的描述需要着重从目前关于 ECD 供体和 SCD 对照组的文献中得出推论。如结论部分所述，肾功能的保护措施被认为是对 ECD 供体移植成功的关键，应该被普遍应用，因为即使是理想的供体肾通常也不能让受体终身使用。

了解与使用 SCD 供体相关的最佳预后是至关重要的。首先，随着高风险供体肾脏使用率的升高，研究中心需要持续关注公众对于理想供体研究结果的看法，并且在某种程度上，监管机构的期望和认知可能已经落后于供者人群不断改变的现实情况。Pascual 等人[10]对于 SCD 和 ECD 移植肾的预后进行了详尽的综述。该综述概述了对于 ECD 和 SCD 肾的单中心与多中心研究的比较。来自 9 个单中心的研究表明，SCD 和 ECD 肾脏之间短期内效果相当。相比之下，39 项研究表明，正如现在广泛接受的那样，SCD 肾移植的预后优于 ECD 肾移植的预后。重要的是，对 20 项美国多中心研究和 5 项欧洲多中心研究进行回顾，每个研究结果都表明 S

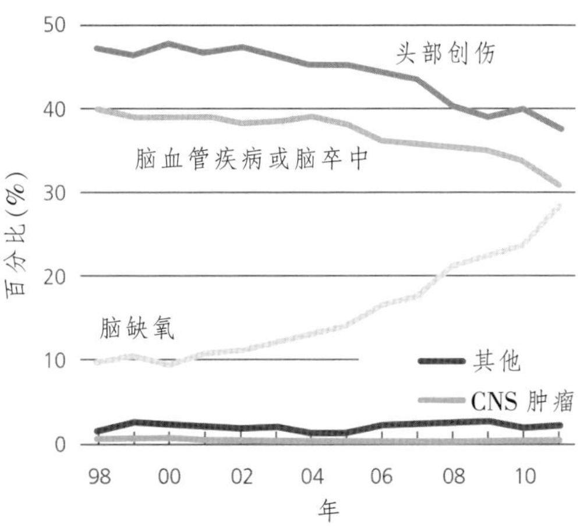

图 53.1　尸体肾捐献者的死亡原因。注意，头部创伤的供体数目急剧减少，脑缺氧的供体数目急剧增加。（Data from SRTR Annual Report 2011[1].）

CD 肾移植有显著优势。在这些研究中，最能代表当下研究的是 Andreoni 等人基于 1995 年和 2004 年之间的联合国器官共享网络(UNOS)案例的研究。SCD 肾移植的患者 1 年、3 年和 5 年的生存率分别为 96%、90%和 86%；其移植肾的存活率分别为 91%、80%和 70%。在所有对照组中，SCD 供体肾的延迟功能恢复率为 19%~50%。

BENEFIT 试验比较了基于贝拉西普和环孢霉素的免疫抑制原理，其结果阐明了在现代良好的控制条件下使用理想供体的移植预后。在这项研究中，所有患者都使用了巴利昔单抗诱导、霉酚酸酯(MMF)和皮质类固醇[11]。治疗的变量是分别使用中剂量(MI)和低剂量(LI)的贝拉西普与环孢霉素。治疗对象仅包括活体供体或 SCD 供体。这三组的 1 年内移植存活率分别为 95%、96%和 93%。计算所得每组的肾小球滤过率(GFR)分别为 65mL/(min·1.73m^2)、63mL/(min·1.73m^2)和 50mL/(min·1.73m^2)，每组的排斥反应发生率分别为 22%、17%和 7%。尽管本实验包括一些活体供体，但是对于理想的肾脏，无论是基于钙调磷酸酶的免疫抑制方案，还是无钙调磷酸酶方案，1 年后的结果都是较为理想的。这些实验随后扩展到 ECD 肾脏，其预后类似但有所下降[12]。

本章的其余部分将侧重于 ECD 供体，尤其是肾脏和肝脏。理解捐助者人群从最佳肾脏供体的改变，同时了解到理想肾脏的潜在最佳预后，有助于外科医生和移植医生做出最好的判断来进行移植的分配。如上所述，广泛应用保留肾单位的免疫抑制可以使理想和非理想的供体肾获得最佳的长期预后结果。

扩大标准肾脏捐献

关键器官供体的短缺致使移植医生去寻求更广泛的肾源进行移植。曾经被否认符合捐献标准的人群现在已经成为移植的宝贵资源，并为更多人提供了机会。否则，他们永远不会从器官移植治疗中获益。

在美国，移植的肾脏数量从 2000 年的 13 621 增加到 2010 年的 16 899，总体上绝对数量增加了 19.4%。在这 10 年期间，肾移植数量上升主要是因为死亡供体肾移植增加了 23.4%；几乎是活体供体移植的 2 倍(12.4%)。然而，在同一时期，等候肾移植治疗的患者增加了近35 000 人[13]。其他器官也出现了类似的趋势。器官捐献供与求的差距日益扩大成为当今发展的总趋势[13]。因此，增加移植手术的数量，以及降低被认为是“可移植”器官的拒绝率，这一直是研究的努力方向，并引起了大家的争议。众所周知，作为一个客观和可衡量的标准，器官的接受和移植率是对器官质量的总体主观反应。卫生资源和服务管理局(HRSA)/ OPTN 赞助的合作社试图将来自全国各地的各个专业的移植专业人员聚集在一起分享“老龄边缘人群”和来自 ECD 器官的移植经验，从而增加器官的利用度[14]。

目前和公认的 ECD 的定义来自 2001 年水晶城会议，其主题为“最大限度地利用死亡供体器官”，这是由肾移植小组提出来的[15]。在结束时，该工作组建议制定一个独立和单独的肾源分配系统，因为当时来源于死亡供体的肾脏与平均水平相比，生存率较差，但比仅透析患者的生存率稍高。该建议最终被采纳，并由 Port 等人重新修订定义了新的国家政策，即，来自相对风险较高的器官来源与参考组(10~39 岁，无高血压病史，死于非心脑血管意外)相比，其移植后肾衰竭概率高出至少 70%，不同的肾源将会按照不同的法则分配[6,7]。这项政策于 2002 年 10 月 31 日实施[8]。这个新的移植系统可以通过加速器官抵达中心的过程以减少冷缺血时间(CIT)，这些移植中心拥有移植物生存率的相关数据，并且事先让患者对接受该类型器官的移植做了知情同意。与 SCD 器官相反，ECD 肾脏的分配取决于等待时间的长短，而不需要考虑 HLA 的匹配。此外，该政策还鼓励尽可能早地进行移植前的交叉匹配。

随着 ECD 定义的建立，符合其标准的捐献肾脏数量从 1999 年的 1235 个增加到 2005 年的 1683 个，增加了 36.3%。同一时期，符合 SCD 的肾脏捐献从 6680 个增加到 7554 个，增长了 13.1%。由此反映出社会对使用 ECD 标准进行的肾脏移植有更大的兴趣。然而，到目前为止，ECD 标准下的捐献数量约占美国所有死亡捐献的 19%，仅仅比 1999 年的 15%略有增加[13]。虽然施行了非配法则以加速器官回收，但是全体 ECD 肾脏的 40%最终未被使用而浪费。我们需要认识到，ECD 定义可能明显低估了移植器官质量的极端变异性，因为>1.7 的相对危险意味着凡是满足 ECD 标准的所有器官均具有相同的相对失败风险。一些 ECD 肾脏表现出足够的长期生存，而其他的可能具有不良的预后[16-18]。

同透析比较预后

虽然一些独立的报告表明 ECD 肾移植患者的肾

存活率与 SCD 肾相当[19,20],但与 SCD 肾相比,绝大多数单中心研究、多中心研究和注册表研究报告显示,应用 ECD 肾移植的患者和移植物 1 年和 5 年生存率均有显著降低[18,21-23]。对 2007 年 SRTR 报告的回顾表明,ECD 肾受体治疗后的 1 年移植物存活率为 83.6%,而接受非 ECD 移植的患者 1 年移植物存活率为 90.4%[24]。通过对这些数据的罗列研究,Ojo 等人在 2001 年证实,经过 ECD 肾移植治疗人群的平均预期寿命较透析治疗和(或)不进行移植的患者相比,平均增加了 5 年。经研究,这种优势仅存在于某些患者群体当中,有高风险的受体并没有受益[25]。Kauffman 等人调查发现,接受 ECD 移植的 60 岁及以上患者的 1 年死亡率比接受 SCD 移植的患者高 62%(14.4%对 9.1%)[26]。此外,Merion 等人研究发现,相对于始终需要等待的 SCD 肾脏,ECD 肾脏有种种益处[27]。由于术后早期死亡率增加,我们观察到,ECD 肾受体存活并没有达到与 SCD 肾受体的相同水平,直到术后 3.5 年才达到相同的累积死亡率。因此,ECD 移植较透析而言,显然为几乎所有指定亚组提供了生存优势,尤其是那些 40 岁以上、非西班牙裔、致敏受者、糖尿病患者和等待时间较长患者(>4 年),但是 SCD 移植与 ECD 移植相比进一步提高了生存率。与 SCD 肾相比,调整后 ECD 肾移植的 1 年移植物存活率平均降低 8%,移植后 3~5 年的移植物存活率平均降低 15%~20%[7,17]。某种程度上,移植预后提示,单侧(相对于双侧)肾移植受者术后肾功能稳定在肌酐清除率(CrCl)大约为 60%的水平,且 ECD 肾受体的初始“基线”较低,其肾功能在同一测量时间点较 SCD 肾受体降低更快[14]。

受体的正确选择

由于对 ECD 移植预后的差异性存在的争议,许多研究人员建议将离散的患者群体作为死亡供体器官的适当受体。SRTR 数据显示,大部分 60 岁及以上的患者均被列为 ECD 肾移植对象。在过去 5 年中,50 岁及以上的 ECD 受体的比例从 55%增加到 81%[13]。无论在 ECD 定义建立之前还是之后,SRTR 的重复分析已经证明了 ECD 与 SCD 受体的人口统计学之间存在显著差异。这些差异不仅表现在年龄,而且表现在 HLA 匹配 (ECD 移植几乎不可能像 SCD 移植那样会出现无 HLA 匹配的情况)和终末期肾病(ESRD;相较于由肾小球肾炎引起的肾功能障碍,继发于糖尿病或高血压的 ESRD 受体更可能得到 ECD 肾移植的治疗)两个方面[17]。由群体反应性抗体(PRA)确定的血型、种族、性别和同种抗体与 ECD 分配的显著差异并无关系[18]。最令人沮丧的结果发生于再移植患者中。Miles 等人检查了 9000 多例等待再次移植患者的预后[19]。在近 3000 名最终接受新移植器官的患者中,10%接受 ECD 器官移植患者的生存率与名单上其他患者相似,但与 ESRD 治疗相关的并发症却少得多。然而,接受 SCD 移植物的患者死亡率降低了 56%。这些结果表明,如果希望再次移植的患者对供体 HLA 不存在高度敏感性,则最好选择 SCD 肾脏。

在排除再次移植可能时,接受 ECD 肾脏患者的主要选择标准是年龄> 40 岁[20]。重要的是,数据表明该标准似乎没有年龄上限,因为 70 岁或 75 岁以上的受体在使用 ECD 供体时可以获得良好的生存状况[25,28,29]。个体的生存获益一直都需要与等待移植患者名单中的死亡率进行比较。

Schold 和 Meier-Kriesche 在 2006 年根据受体存活率进一步确定了适合 ECD 移植的受体人群[30]。通过 SRTR 数据的严格审查表明,对于 40 岁以下移植受体人群,等待 4 年进行 SCD 移植的预期寿命明显大于 2 年后直接进行 ECD 移植(分别为 26.4 年和 17.6 年)。但是同样的分析结果对于 65 岁以上的受体(5.6 年对 5.3 年)并不适用。相反,研究发现糖尿病的 ECD 移植患者可以从 ECD 移植中受益。在 40 岁以下人群中,经过 2 年透析的糖尿病患者进行 ECD 移植可与等待 4 年行 SCD 移植的患者有相近的预期寿命(9.6 年对 9 年)。

也许是因为移植预后的明显差异,负责在奥地利、比利时、德国、卢森堡、荷兰和斯洛文尼亚分配器官的欧洲移植国际基金会建立了肾脏分配计划,为每个需要肾源的患者提供了合理公平的受捐机会[31,32];并且引入了欧洲移植高级计划(ESP),即 65 岁以上捐献者器官会被分配给同样年龄在 65 岁以上的受体。简单地说,ESP 试图找出每个来自供体的可用器官的最佳接受者。他们对肾移植的成功定义是移植肾的生存时间大于患者本人寿命,而生命年的损失是指移植肾功能良好而患者死亡。分配方案是基于将移植受体的代谢需求同供体器官的排泄能力匹配。为了获得一定程度的成功,研究人员努力使 CIT 最小化并降低免疫风险。以上仅对非致敏的(PRA<5%)初次移植受者。在供体 CrCl<70mL/min 的患者中包括双重移植的选择。在第 3

年时,ESP与对照移植患者的生存率分别为64%的和67%(*P*=0.04)。其来自死亡供体的移植物存活率也相似,分别为70%和71%。

许多作者描述了用于评估和选择适合ECD移植适当患者的程序[21,30,33-35]。在一篇综述里,Stratta等人描述了评估这类患者的多学科方法[36]。为了要预测并降低术后早期风险,所有患者均要接受有关医疗、社会心理和财务评估,尤其是心血管系统的综合评估。经委员会讨论,患者不论是否登记申请ECD供体,在等待名单上和已经进入随访的患者均需要进行共存疾病的风险评估。对于年龄小于30岁的患者,他们建议不要选择高度致敏(PRA>50%)、极度肥胖(BMI>35kg/m²)或再次移植的ECD肾脏。患者和主治医生都可以拒绝选择上述的供体,尤其当患者处于透析前期、对透析反应"良好",或者已经有潜在可用活体供体。如果患者本身存在乙型肝炎或丙型肝炎,且愿意接受来自乙型肝炎或丙型肝炎核抗体阳性供体器官,可以选择放弃ECD申请,因为这种移植器官的等待时间相对较短,特别是在肝炎阳性供体更常见的地方。

活检的作用

研究显示,来自不同人群供体肾的组织学检查结果存在明显差异性,例如来自老年人群和高血压人群的供体肾组织学就不一样。单一的年龄因素对肾脏组织学改变有明显影响。尸检研究显示,肾小球的数目和大小随着年龄增长进行性减少和变小。"年长"的肾脏其肾单位功能性下降,这可能不能满足受体对于肾功能的需求,不论受体年龄大小[37]。此外,来自"边缘年龄"供体的移植物可能在移植治疗的各个阶段对于缺血和容量损伤更为敏感,导致肾功能进行性下降,甚至有时会快速下降,从而导致移植物功能衰竭(图53.2)[17,38-40]。

在Sung等人的标志性论文中,他们研究了ECD肾脏未被利用的原因。他们进一步评估了其与移植功能延迟恢复(DGF)的关联。对SRTR数据的6年分析显示,在此期间内,获取的48 796个SCD肾中有8%(3887)未被利用,而12 536个ECD肾中有41%(5139)未被利用。在Logistic模型下,ECD肾未被利用的概率是SCD肾的4倍(OR=4.35;*P*<0.0001)。活检后的肾脏不被利用的可能性更大(OR=2.08)[41]。随着肾小球硬化(GS)率的增加,所有研究组的器官未利用率逐渐增加,从GS程度0~5%器官的1.5,增加到GS程度>20%器官的16.92。对ECD肾的单独分析显示,通过活检结果,未利用率从硬化程度为0~5%的0.57,增加到硬化程度超过20%的7.22(*P*<0.0001)。活检后SCD肾脏的未利用率相对于未经活检的,其OR值仅为4.21。值得注意的是,ECD肾脏的未利用率也随着ECD定义中款项的增加[年龄超过50岁,脑血管意外(CVA)死亡,高血压史(HTN),血清肌酐>1.5mg/dL]而增加[42]。

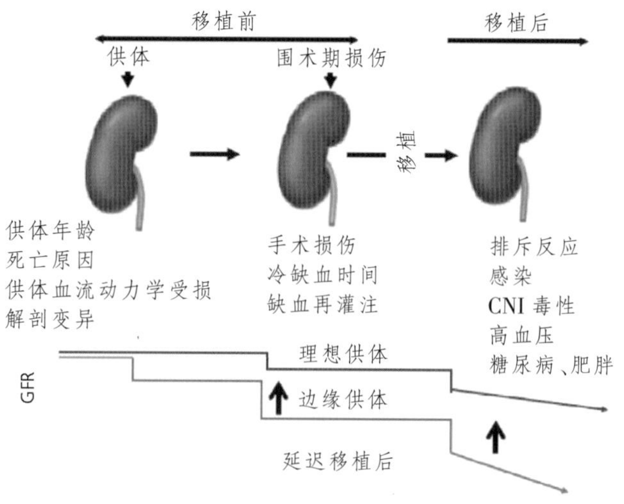

图53.2 移植前和移植后相关因素对扩大标准供体和理想供体移植结果的影响。类似的损伤对ECD器官更有影响。(Reproduced from Audard V, Matignon M, Dahan K, et al. Renal transplantation from extended criteria donors: problems and perspectives. Transplant International. 2008;21:11-17, with permission from John Wiley and Sons.)

GFR,肾小球滤过率;CNI,钙调磷酸酶抑制剂。

并发症

被谈论最多的并发症是DGF,DGF可能在ECD器官移植后导致一系列的并发症[22,23,26,43-45]。肾脏实验的异体移植模型已经证明了长期CIT、供体年龄和异体移植物功能障碍之间的强相关性。已经确定的是,器官移植有关的缺血再灌注损伤导致的DGF,与移植物的长期受损和患者生存率有关。年龄较大受者的ECD器官移植尤其如此。Remuzzi等人报道,接受ECD肾移植的60岁以上患者一旦合并DGF,则其1年死亡率显著高于移植后肾功能立即恢复的患者(7.7%对18%;*P*<0.05)(图53.3)[46]。

发展制定ECD器官分配制度的首要目的是减少CIT。据UNOS数据显示,与年轻的供体相比,年龄较大供体肾脏(51~65岁)在同等的CIT条件下DGF发生率

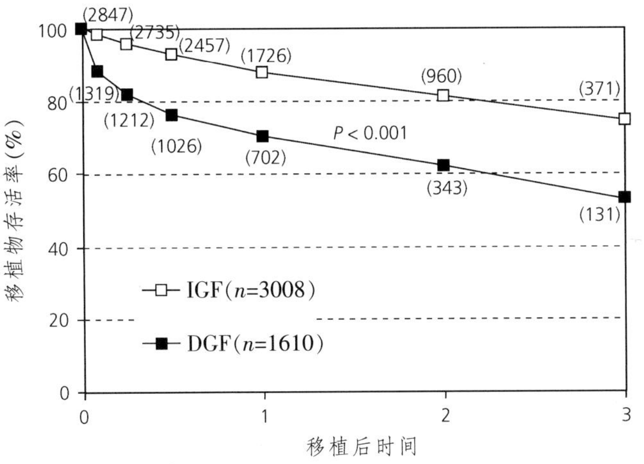

图 53.3　移植物功能延迟恢复(DGF)对 ECD 肾脏的影响,表明 DGF 显著降低长期存活率。括号中的数字表示在各个移植后随访时间点(1 个月、3 个月、6 个月和 1 年、2 年、3 年)存在风险的患者数量。(Reproduced from Matsuoka et al.[58], with permission from John Wiley and Sons.)
IGF,移植物功能立即恢复。

更高[15]。然而,在 2002 年之前或之后,美国肾脏数据系统(USRDS)的分析并没有表明小幅减短 CIT 时间能对 ECD 受体 DGF 的发展产生影响。几项研究发现,大幅缩短 CIT 可以产生有益的结果。Valcarce 等报道了一项前瞻性单中心研究的结果,其中限制 CIT<10 小时[ECD 为(9.3+2.5)小时,SCD 为(8.3+3.3)小时][47]。研究发现,两组(ECD 与 SCD)结果之间没有显著差异,例如原发性功能衰竭(4.2%对 2%)、DGF(16.7%对 10%)、手术并发症(25%对 16 %)和急性排斥反应(8.3%对 2%)。虽然两组之间的移植物 1 年存活率相似,但通过 GRF 评估,ECD 的异体移植物功能优于 SCD [ECD 为(49.4±12.5)mL/min,SCD 为(65.8±14.9)mL/min]。

经证实,50 岁以上的 ECD 肾脏受体因感染而死亡的发生率有所增加,且该组人群共存疾病种类也有所增加。据报道,接受 ECD 肾脏移植的患者手术并发症增多,尤其是尿管坏死和漏尿。然而,这些并发症没有导致移植物丢失的显著增加[34,48]。Danovitch 等人报道,ECD 肾脏受体的年死亡率为 10%,而 SCD 肾脏受体的年死亡率为 4.8%。ECD 肾脏 1 年和 5 年的调整患者生存率分别为 90.6%和 69%,而非 ECD 肾脏移植患者的则分别为 94.5%和 81.2%[49]。

特殊方案

在所有死亡供体肾中,来自边缘年龄人群的供体移植物对缺血再灌注损伤更敏感,且其修复组织和实质的能力受损[38,39,50]。防止初始肾单位数量的进一步损失是 ECD 肾脏成功的关键。所以,消除移植肾潜在的肾毒性暴露是重要的。此外,对于 ECD 移植物的老年受体,其感染、心血管并发症和恶性肿瘤的发生率有所增加。值得特别关注的是,大量报道指出,在接受 ECD 移植的患者中,巨细胞病毒(CMV)感染和多瘤病毒诱导导致肾病的发病率更高[42]。为此,医生不仅寻求降低 CIT,而且还研究特定的移植后方案,以优化移植结果并延长存活时间,同时使免疫抑制并发症降到最低。但是,很少有关于 ECD 受体的前瞻性随机多中心研究长期结果的报道;仅针对 ECD 肾脏受体的随机试验就更少了。

钙调磷酸酶抑制剂(CNI)有肾毒性,可能与短期和长期同种异体移植存活率降低有关[51–53]。ECD 肾脏尤其如此,活检证实了其薄壁组织的损伤。人们已经提出了 CNI 最小化和消除的策略来避免损伤。美国的 Stratta 等人进行的一项研究包含 101 例 ECD 受者,受者接受抗胸腺细胞球蛋白或阿仑单抗以及 MMF 和类固醇的维持免疫抑制 [20]。停用他克莫司直到血清肌酐浓度<4mg/dL,并且严格控制谷值水平,设置比较温和的剂量。4 年来的精确统计显示,患者存活率和移植物存活率分别为 93%和 74%,远远优于已公布的登记数据。一些非随机的欧洲试验在一群受者中证实了这些结果,这些受者中有 54%存在 DGF[54]。

然而,CNI 的规避没有取得类似的成功。欧洲研究人员报告显示,利用抗胸腺细胞球蛋白以及 MMF 和类固醇的双重治疗,急性排斥反应发生率为 25%,5 年的移植物存活率为 65%[55]。使用相似的方案和受者收录/排除标准,巴利昔单抗诱导产生的结果(排斥反应发生率为 45%)也令人沮丧,受者最终转为 CNI 治疗[56]。虽然基于西罗莫司的无 CNI 治疗在小型单中心试验的 SCD 移植中已经取得了一些成功,但是在更大型的随机试验中并没有得到证实。其他的单中心非随机试验在一群 ECD 受者中证实了这一发现[57]。Diekmann 等人报道,基于西罗莫司的无 CNI 治疗应用于 ECD 受者的结果与“可接受”结果相关,但是蛋白尿水平会升高。类似的免疫抑制修饰和结果以及双 ECD 肾脏的使用也已见报道[57]。

最近,Larsen 等人报道了一项前瞻性的随机多中心试验(BENEFIT-EXT)结果,比较了贝拉西普(一种用于维持免疫抑制治疗的新型生物制剂)与CNI在ECD受者中的应用[58]。该方案评估了高强度(MI)和低强度(LI)的贝拉西普方案:543名受者中有347名(64%)完成了2年的治疗。所有组的患者存活率和移植物存活率相似，但是无CNI组的肾功能得到了改善,GFR为8~10mL/min,高于接受环孢霉素的患者。在贝拉西普治疗的患者中能更频繁地观察到移植后淋巴增生性疾病(PTLD),特别是中枢神经系统PTLD,警告人们贝拉西普的使用应仅限于EB病毒(EBV)血清呈阳性的受者。

除了特异性免疫抑制方案之外，还有一些人提倡积极干预和控制ECD肾脏老年受者的共存疾病[36,59]。建议治疗高血压、高血脂、贫血、糖尿病及其他共存疾病,维持血压<140/90mmHg,空腹血清胆固醇<200mg/dL,血细胞比容>30%,空腹血糖<126mg/dL。应该对所有患者执行口服阿司匹林的抗血栓治疗以及低钠的、利于心脏健康的饮食管理，并定期评估心血管危险因素或事件,这些应该成为日常工作。定期筛查全身性或肾特异性病毒和细菌性疾病是至关重要的，因为对这些高危人群来说，早期发现可能的排斥反应可尽力避免产生淋巴消耗性抗体。

脉冲灌注

如第25章所述,脉冲灌注(PP)或“用泵灌注”已经成为用于器官评估和保存的可接受的方法，同时为ECD器官的移植决定提供了有价值的信息。PP包含供体肾的体外低温脉冲灌注，向器官供应氧和营养物同时去除废物。在灌注期间,肾脏流量和压力的常规监测提供了肾脏效用的相关信息。尝试改善肾血流量和校正酸中毒是灌注肾活动监测的重要因素。灌注液通常由标准灌注溶液组成,含有(或添加)羟乙基淀粉以防止间质性水肿;腺苷以增加ATP;磷酸盐作为质子缓冲剂;葡萄糖酸盐以减少细胞肿胀;谷胱甘肽作为抗氧化剂;以及其他各种试剂以减少新陈代谢和平衡电解质。PP被模拟用来减少血管痉挛和压力。PP期间测量到的流速下降、压力增加以及钙浓度增加与DGF有关[60,61]。

20世纪80年代的初步研究未能证明DGF的减少或显示PP相对于冷储存(CS)在移植物存活率上的优势[62-64]。此外,PP被认为增加成本过高,特别是在没有明显肾存活受益的情况下。几项研究(包括对来自相同供体的成对肾进行的研究,其中一个置于PP,另一个置于CS中)发现移植后透析率相似[61,65]。

随着可能移植的ECD肾脏数量的持续增加,利用PP来衡量肾脏“健康”的另一个客观指标的效用开始引起人们越来越多的兴趣。2003年,17.2%的移植肾来自ECD供体。其中28.4%用PP保存。在ECD-PP相对于ECD-CS肾的综述中,Matsuoka等人发现ECD-PP肾脏往往来自较年老的供体(61.1岁对59.8岁;*P*<0.001),并且末端血清肌酐增高(1.2mg/dL对1.1mg/dL;*P*=0.03)。PP供体具有统计学上升高的糖尿病发病率(12.7%对9.4%;*P*=0.003),并且更可能是DCD供体(6.5%对0.9%;*P*<0.001)。虽然CS组经历了CIT减少,但这只是两组在24小时内的结果。GS程度增加(27.3%对18.1%;*P*=0.002)和间质性纤维化(48.5%对40.5%;*P*=0.03)的肾脏更可能被置于PP中。作者指出,与ECD-PP肾相比,ECD-CS肾的原发性丧失功能的发病率没有差异,但是可以观察到DGF的发生率高出了10%(37%对26%;*P*<0.001)。虽然DGF减少,但是移植后1年内排斥反应的发生率没有差异。与DCD供体相比，大脑死亡(DBD)后的供体中DGF有所减少(34.5%对54.3%;*P*<0.001)。调整所有变量之后,PP导致DGF发展的风险与CS相比降低49%(OR=0.51;*P*<0.001)。如预期的,其他可以预测DGF的供体因素包括DCD、HTN史、升高的血清肌酐和“次优的”供体组织学。重要的是,相比于肾功能立即恢复(IGF)组,经历了DGF的ECD肾移植在1年(70.1%对87.8%)和3年(53.0%对74.4%;*P*<0.001)的存活率均具有统计学上的明显降低。保存方法对IGF肾的存活不会造成差异。总体而言,PP和CS组的移植存活率相似。

在另一篇综述中,Sung等人用相似的评估方法分析了一个后来的组群，发现ECD-PP肾的未利用率为29.7%,而使用CS保存的未利用率为43.6%[41]。此外,ECD-PP肾较高的未利用率与测出的高压力有关。末端压力<0.18mmHg/(mL·min)和压力为0.18~0.25mmHg/(mL·min)的ECD肾未利用率分别为12.6%和14.0%。相反,末端压力为0.26~0.38mmHg/(mL·min)的ECD肾具有25.7%的未利用率,而压力>0.38mmHg/(mL·min)的ECD肾具有53.1%的未利用率[分别为OR=2.50和OR=7.88,与压力<0.26mmHg/(mL·min)相比;*P*<0.0001]。有趣的是,作者还评论了器官获取组织(OPO)ECD未利用率的多变性,其范围为14%~60%。他们的数据表明,OPO的做法,包括PP和ECD肾脏的局部使用,会影响器官恢复

的速率，且是未利用率的重要决定因素。

移植程序中 ECD 肾的使用增加与 PP 的使用增加是同步的，这可以解释为需要一个额外的工具来确定相关的器官功能质量。各种测量结果，尤其是动脉内压力可用作进一步评估的数据，以确定移植的适合性。可以说，在使用 PP 作为保存技术的各种报告中，缺乏 DGF 是因为丢弃了许多器官，证明机械灌注参数十分贫乏。然而，ECD 肾脏评估中和 DGF 潜在减少中 PP 的使用，导致许多 OPO 和移植程序使用 PP。

双肾移植

由于越来越重视肾脏移植中 ECD 的使用，且器官缺乏不能满足等待移植患者的需求，移植群体开始关注使器官未利用最小化的策略，特别是考虑到捐献者人群的老龄化。从 ECD 供体获取的肾脏行双肾移植(DKT)已经被用于缓解器官短缺。最初于 1994 年在马里兰大学实施[66]，外科医生开始使用来自同一供体的两个肾脏，而这两个肾脏通常会被其他中心拒用，甚至被丢弃，因为它们被认为不适合单次移植[67,68]。DKT 的总体原则是单肾移植与经历渐进性移植物衰竭的肾单位质量重建实验模型。这些实验模型表明，初始肾单位质量是慢性同种异体移植物衰竭的决定因素。通过同时移植两个肾脏来增加可存活肾单位数量，有效地防止在单肾移植的对照受试者中出现肾功能进行性恶化[69,70]。虽然在理论上 DKT 具有增加移植的有效肾单位质量的优势，但是也存在风险，即原本适合单肾移植(SKT)的肾脏却作为 DKT 移植了，因此是减少而不是增加了移植的数量。来自单中心和登记处的 DKT 短期数据分析显示出优异的早期(1 年)存活率，但与 SKT 相比发现，其原发性丧失功能的发生率更高[67,71,72]。

Tan 等人最近的一篇论文分析了 DKT 与 SKT 的比较结果，并对其受者进行了 8 年以上的随访[72]。在这篇综述中，113 例年龄 55 岁或以上的患者进行了死亡供体的肾移植，双肾(n=39)或单肾(n=72)同种异体移植都有。有趣的是，作者注意到所有用于 DKT 的器官在移植之前都曾被其他中心拒绝。不出所料，被拒绝的最常见原因是供体年龄、供体的不稳定性、HTN 史、活检时 GS>20%，或这些因素的组合。DKT 与 SKT 的决定因素主要基于 Cockcroft-Gault 方程估计的供体 CrCl 摄取量。如果 CrCl<90mL/min，则两个肾脏都可用来移植到单个受体中。这些器官的接受下限为 45mL/min。DKT 组的平均供体年龄更大(61 岁对 48 岁；P<0.001)。在供体的末端血清肌酐、HLA 不匹配或 CIT(15 小时对 18.5 小时)上，两组之间没有统计学差异。与接受 SKT 的患者相比，接受 DKT 的患者具有明显较短的移植等待时间[(440±38)天对(664±51)天；P=0.002]，住院时间相近，在术后即刻并发症的发生方面没有差异，例如心肌梗死、感染或再次手术，发生 DGF 的比例及需要早期排斥治疗方面也无差异。DKT 与 SKT 的 5 年移植物存活率分别为 79.5%和 67%，8 年存活率分别为 69.7%和 59.4%(P=NS)。在进一步的亚分析中，供体 CrCl 估计摄入量<75mL/min 的 DKT 受者 8 年的移植物存活率为 64.3%。急性排斥反应和慢性排斥反应是致死性移植物衰竭的主要原因。DKT 与 SKT 的 5 年患者存活率分别为 82.1%和 80%，8 年存活率分别为 82.1%和 74.1%。两组中最突出的死亡原因是心血管和感染性并发症。重要的是，DKT 与 SKT 的 1 年血清肌酐中值分别为 1.45mg/dL 和 1.7mg/dL，5 年血清肌酐中值分别为 1.8mg/dL 和 1.4mg/dL(P=NS)。

在另一项类似的前瞻性病例对照研究中，Remuzzi 等人在临床或植入前组织学评估的基础上，分析了用于 ECD 分配的 SKT 或 DKT 的移植物存活率[66]。只有在宏观评估时排除主要的血管异常，才认为肾脏有资格进行 DKT。具有局部瘢痕迹象的那些器官也被排除，因为担心损伤的不均匀分布可能会影响活检的微观视图。为了使活检被认为是“完整”的，需要最少 25 个肾小球。开发基于活检的评分系统，将肾脏分配为 DKT、SKT 或直接丢弃。24 例和 48 例对照分别接受 DKT 和 SKT。DKT 供体和受者明显年长于 SKT 受者。与 SKT 受者相比，DKT 受者供体的 CrCl 明显较低[(54.5±16.0)mL/min 对(78.1±48.0)mL/min；P=0.03]，没有供体患有临床蛋白尿。其他方面，两组的受者特征类似，包括 CIT。两组的 DGF 发生率相同(20.8%)，透析需求的解决速度较快。两组在所有时间点的平均血清肌酐水平相当，DKT 与 SKT 受者 6 个月值分别为 1.48±0.54mg/dL 和 1.77±0.93mg/dL。在最后一次随访中，DKT 受者的 CrCl 平均值几乎与其相应供体相同，而接受 SKT 的受者具有比其供体明显更低的 CrCl 值。通过对减半供体 CrCl(代表单个移植肾的分裂功能)的再分析，与计算的“半”供体肌酐清除相比，SKT 受者具有明显更高的 CrCl 值(53.6±16.2mL/min 对 41.0±22.8mL/min),表明在单肾的受者中有 30%的超滤。这些结果强有力地证明了临床特征和组织学标准的组合应当同时用于 ECD 的 SKT 和 DKT 的选择。

资源利用

数据的优势证实了 ECD(和 DCD)肾脏受体具有明显较高的 DGF 发生率、血清肌酐低于 3mg/dL 的时间更长、住院时间(LOS)更长,以及因移植手术后并发症再次入院的人数增加 [23,43,45,73,74]。因此,将通常与 ECD 移植相关的财务和经济方面的内容从讨论中剔除是不完整的。在美国,医疗保险 ESRD 计划每年为移植支付超过 12 亿美元,约占所有肾移植的 70%[75]。

由马萨诸塞州总医院 Saidi 等人进行的回顾性分析中,研究者比较了 ECD 和 DCD 肾脏成人受者和 SCD 肾脏成人受者的资源利用和结果[76];分析了 271例死亡供体移植(160 例 SCD,44 例 ECD,53 例 DCD 和 11 例 ECD/DCD)。PP 通常用于所有的 ECD 和 DCD 肾脏。与 SCD 组相比,ECD、DCD 和 ECD/DCD 组 DGF 的发生率明显更高(分别为 15.1%和 35.6%、33.3%、38.2%;*P*<0.001)。所有非 SCD 组达到平台血清肌酐的时间也明显更长。非 SCD 组与 SCD 组的初始 LOS 分别为 9.8~11 天和 6.1 天(*P*<0.05)。非 SCD 组的 90 天再入院率也较高。随着 DGF 发病率的增加和住院时间的延长,非 SCD 肾脏相对也有更高的初始住院费用。ECD、ECD/DCD、DCD 和 SCD 肾脏受者的费用分别为 70 030 美元、72 438 美元、72 789 美元和 47 462 美元(*P*<0.001)。因为非 SCD 受者在护理中需要多次再入院,这些差异变得尤为明显。

Whiting 等人将 UNOS 的注册数据与近 35 000 名肾移植受者的联邦医疗保险索赔数据合并,从移植前透析期开始,预测这些相同的费用,以确定使用 ECD 肾移植受者和高风险受者 (HRR)(在本分析中定义为 60 岁以上)进行肾移植的财务"收支平衡"点[77]。利用这一定义,有 25 600 例非 HRR,其中 5718 例(22%)接受 ECD;8934 例 HRR 移植,其中 2200 例(25%)接受了 ECD。仅考虑供体来源时,与非 ECD 受者相比,ECD 受者在 5 年内具有明显更高的累积成本 (144 274 美元对 129 163 美元;*P*<0.0001)。类似地,仅评估受者风险时,与非 HRR 受者相比,HRR 受者在 5 年内具有明显更高的累积成本(145 453 美元对 124 553 美元;*P*<0.0001)。将供体和受者结合起来分析,非 ECD–非 HRR 和 ECD–HRR 组合的支付分别为 121 698 美元和 165 716 美元(*P*<0.0001)。然后绘制每一项移植成本随时间变化的曲线,并使透析的预期持续成本与移植后期成本相交,作者证实,非 ECD–非 HRR 组合的财务"收支平衡"点最早出现在 4.4 年时,而对于更昂贵的 ECD/HRR 供体–受体组合,血液透析在移植后 13 年内不会变得更昂贵(图 53.4)。

虽然许多移植中心也许完全支持 ECD 的使用,但是实际上,使用 ECD 进行移植的"成本"远远大于使用

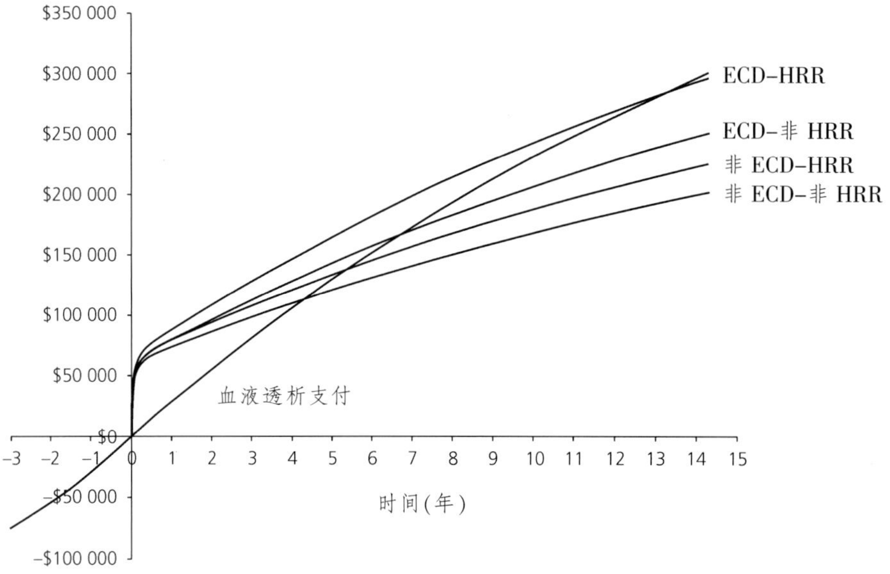

图 53.4 医疗保险支付预测和"收支平衡"点。该点表示为每个供体–受体配对穿过预期的血液透析支付线的时间点。高危受体(HRR)应用扩大化标准捐献(ECD)器官会大大增加成本。(Reproduced from Whiting et al.[78], with permission from Wolters Kluwer Health.)

SCD 的“成本”。这使得 ECD 的移植在规模较小的移植中心难以进行，因为该中心不可能建设新的基础设施容纳更多工作人员来在门诊管理 DGF 患者；所以，患者的长期住院使得 ECD 肾脏的移植不符合实际情况。许多中心已经建立了以门诊为主的方案，患 DGF 的 ECD 受体在暂无住院需求后将会出院，他们可以选择前往移植前的透析机构或到与移植机构联系的门诊部。这些策略抵消了初始成本，同时也可以在移植后的早期提供必要的提示。毫无疑问，经济水平是影响评估器官移植的另一个变量，生存结果在机构内部和外部都需要进行严格的评估。

扩大标准肝脏捐献

器官可用性方面类似的限制导致移植团队决定肝脏的优先分配不仅取决于疾病的严重程度，还取决于原发性功能障碍(PNF)或初始功能不良的高风险器官的使用[78]。包括年龄、种族、身高、死亡原因、肝细胞脂肪变性程度、劈裂移植与整体移植，以及 CIT 的一些供体的特征已被确定与肝脏同种异体移植的结果有着独立的关系[79]。

Mullhaupt 等人在文献综述中报道了供体年龄和受体移植结果之间的明确联系，尤其是 60 岁以上的供体。他们发现非裔美国人与白人相比，其相对风险为 1.19。研究表明，供体身高也与结果独立相关，但体重并没有影响。非创伤性供体死亡与 16%(CVA)和 20%(其他原因)的移植物衰竭的风险增加相关。此外，与 DBD 相比，DCD 捐献的风险相对升高 51%[79,80]。

尽管肝脏同种异体移植的总体评估对于确定是否存在严重脂肪变性是相当可靠的，但已有报告指出，其对于中度和轻度脂肪变性的检测却并不可靠[75]。此外，不同的组织处理方法和染色技术也可影响对于脂肪浸润的组织病理学评估[76]。然而，目前的共识是，由于 PNF 的增加率(13%对 SCD 的 3%)，即使是中度脂肪变性的肝脏移植也符合扩展标准[77,78]。最后，CIT>14 小时通常与长期术后病程、胆道狭窄和移植物存活降低相关的保存损伤有关[81,82]。

为了平衡这些已确定的供体危险因素，肝外科医生试图将这些风险度更高的移植物移植到患有中等严重程度疾病[终末期肝病模型(MELD)评分更低]、年龄更大(> 50 岁)并且无丙型肝炎的受体中[78,80,83,84]。

器官特异性供体风险指数

单独的 ECD 标准不能有效地确定供体质量，因为器官存活不能仅从二分变量(SCD 对 ECD)预测。器官特异性供体风险指数对器官进行了更为细致的分级评估，以预测不同特征的供体和受体组合后的移植物存活率[81-83]。Rao 等人对 1995 年到 2005 年的 SRTR 数据进行了研究，提出了肾脏供体风险指数(KDRI)，该指数提供了连续的风险评分。最终的 KDRI 包括 14 个来自供体和受体的因素，其中每一个都能独立影响移植物的结果，包括年龄、非洲裔美国人、血清肌酐、供体高血压和糖尿病、死亡原因、身高、体重、DCD、HCV、HLA 的错配、CIT、整体移植和双侧移植。将参考供体评分设为 1.00，KDRI 提供了连续的评分，可以评估同种异体移植物衰竭风险或使用未评估器官移植患者的死亡相对风险。OPTN/UNOS 已经为器官评估和潜在分配开发了一个类似的模型。肾脏供体概况指数(KDPI)是一个类似的评分，仅基于供体的特征得分，KDPI 分越低代表其预测存活时间越长。将这些器官潜在分配给那些预期移植后存活时间最长的患者，使其寿命得到最大延长，才能最大限度利用可移植器官的资源，这才是今后的发展方向[85]。

Feng 等人首次描述的肝脏供体风险指数(LDRI)确定了与肝脏同种异体移植失败显著相关的 7 个供体特征：年龄、非洲裔美国人、身高、非创伤性死亡、DCD 以及部分移植/劈裂移植。此外，CIT 和区域/国家分配作为变量也包括在最终模型中。研究表明，同种异体移植存活率与 LDRI 增加相关。作者还发现，LDRI 分数较高的移植物更适合 MELD 评分较低的受体[85]。Maluf 等人进一步通过 LDRI 检验了 ECD 肝脏移植的结果(即 LDRI≥1.7)，并且证明了随着 MELD 评分的增加，器官衰竭的相对风险也显著增加[86]。

总结

患者通过移植获得新的治疗机会，这样的机会促进了 ECD 供体死亡后移植器官的使用。虽然 ECD 器官移植患者的整体移植物存活情况不如 SCD 器官的移植人群，但数据显示，ECD 器官的使用有益于移植治疗，使患者不必继续在等待名单上排队等候器官。随着我们更多地了解到最合适移植的受体人群特征，即哪些受者可以很好地利用这些器官，以及继续制订具体的随访方案和免疫抑制治疗方案，以最好地护理这些患者和器官，这个结果将会不断改善。脉冲灌注的使用、离散病理标准和双侧器官移植使得ECD肾脏的利用率增加，同时缩短了CIT时间，并减少了器官的未利用率。ECD肝脏供体的使用已经证实了类似的结果，尤其是MELD评分较低的受体中使用更直接。由于ECD移植的机构运营成本显著增加，成本已经成为分配肾脏、计划开发和资源分配的考虑变量。在确保器官的移植利用受到伦理道德共同约束的同时，器官特异性供体风险指数的发展和不断完善为移植界提供了优化的鉴别工具，以便更好地评估来自扩大化标准供体器官的适用性和可行性。

（许庭珉 译　高鹏骥 校）

参考文献

1. Organ Procurement and Transplantation Network (OPTN) and Scientific Registry of Transplant Recipients (SRTR). OPTN/SRTR 2010 Annual Data Report. Department of Health and Human Services, Health Resources and Services Administration, American Journal of Transplantation. 2012;12(Suppl 1):1–156.
2. CDC. Injury prevention & control: Data & statistics (WISQARS). 2013 [cited February 7, 2013]; Available from: http://www.cdc.gov/injury/wisqars/fatal.html.
3. Dutton RP, et al. Trauma mortality in mature trauma systems: are we doing better? An analysis of trauma mortality patterns, 1997–2008. Journal of Trauma. 2010;69(3):620–626.
4. Hesdorffer DC, Ghajar J. Marked improvement in adherence to traumatic brain injury guidelines in United States trauma centers. Journal of Trauma. 2007; 63(4):841–847. discussion 847–848.
5. Sugerman DE, et al. Patients with severe traumatic brain injury transferred to a level I or II trauma center: United States, 2007 to 2009. Journal of Trauma and Acute Care Surgery. 2012;73, 6:1491–1499.
6. Hallstrom AP, et al. Public-access defibrillation and survival after out-of-hospital cardiac arrest. New England Journal of Medicine. 2004;351(7):637–646.
7. Girotra S, et al. Trends in survival after in-hospital cardiac arrest. New England Journal of Medicine. 2012;367(20):1912–1920.
8. Weisfeldt ML, et al. Ventricular tachyarrhythmias after cardiac arrest in public versus at home. New England Journal of Medicine. 2011;364(4):313–321.
9. Kellermann AL, Rivara FP. Silencing the science on gun research. The Journal of the American Medical Association. 2012;1–2.
10. Pascual J, Zamora J, Pirsch JD. A systematic review of kidney transplantation from expanded criteria donors. American Journal of Kidney Diseases. 2008;52(3): 553–586.
11. Vincenti F, et al. A phase III study of belatacept-based immunosuppression regimens versus cyclosporine in renal transplant recipients (BENEFIT study). American Journal of Transplantation. 2010;10(3):535–546.
12. Pestana JO, et al. Three-year outcomes from BENEFIT-EXT: a phase III study of belatacept versus cyclosporine in recipients of extended criteria donor kidneys. American Journal of Transplantation. 2012;12(3):630–639.
13. United Network of Organ Sharing. 2011; Available from: http://www.unos.org.
14. Leichtman AB, et al. Kidney and pancreas transplantation in the United States, 1997–2006: the HRSA Breakthrough Collaboratives and the 58 DSA Challenge. American Journal of Transplantation. 2008;8(4 Pt 2):946–957.
15. Rosengard BR, et al. Report of the Crystal City meeting to maximize the use of organs recovered from the cadaver donor. American Journal of Transplantation. 2002;2(8):701–711.
16. Nyberg SL, et al. Improving the prediction of donor kidney quality: deceased donor score and resistive indices. Transplantation. 2005;80(7):925–929.
17. Nyberg SL, et al. Improved scoring system to assess adult donors for cadaver renal transplantation. American Journal of Transplantation. 2003;3(6):715–721.
18. Schold JD, et al. The broad spectrum of quality in deceased donor kidneys. American Journal of Transplantation. 2005;5(4 Pt 1):757–765.
19. Morrissey PE, et al. Renal transplant survival from older donors: a single center experience. Archives of Surgery. 2004;139(4):384–389. discussion 389.
20. Stratta RJ, et al. Intermediate-term outcomes with expanded criteria deceased donors in kidney transplantation: a spectrum or specter of quality? Annals of Surgery. 2006;243(5):594–601. discussion 601–603.
21. Greenstein SM, et al. Selective use of expanded criteria donors for renal transplantation with good results. Transplantation Proceedings. 2006;38(10):3390–3392.
22. Kumar MS, et al. Long-term function and survival of elderly donor kidneys transplanted into young adults. Transplantation. 1998;65(2):282–285.
23. Matas AJ, et al. Should I accept this kidney? Clinical Transplantation. 2000;14(1):90–95.
24. Sung RS, et al. Impact of the expanded criteria donor allocation system on candidates for and recipients of expanded criteria donor kidneys. Transplantation. 2007;84(9):1138–1144.
25. Ojo AO, et al. Survival in recipients of marginal cadaveric donor kidneys compared with other recipients and wait-listed transplant candidates. Journal of the American Society of Nephrology. 2001;12(3):589–597.
26. Kauffman HM, et al. Early mortality rates in older kidney recipients with comorbid risk factors. Transplantation. 2007;83(4):404–410.
27. Merion RM, et al. Deceased-donor characteristics and the survival benefit of kidney transplantation. JAMA. 2005;294(21):2726–2733.
28. Meier-Kriesche HU, et al. Kidneys from deceased donors: maximizing the value of a scarce resource. American Journal of Transplantation. 2005;5(7): 1725–1730.
29. Rao PS, et al. Renal transplantation in elderly patients older than 70 years of age: results from the Scientific Registry of Transplant Recipients. Transplantation. 2007;83(8):1069–1074.
30. Schold JD, Meier-Kriesche HU. Which renal transplant candidates should accept marginal kidneys in exchange for a shorter waiting time on dialysis? Clinical Journal of the American Society of Nephrology. 2006;1(3):532–538.
31. Fritsche L, et al. Old-for-old kidney allocation allows successful expansion of the donor and recipient pool. American Journal of Transplantation. 2003;3(11): 1434–1439.
32. Smits JM, et al. Evaluation of the Eurotransplant Senior Program. The results of the first year. American Journal of Transplantation. 2002;2(7):664–670.
33. Alexander JW, Zola JC. Expanding the donor pool: use of marginal donors for solid organ transplantation. Clinical Transplantation. 1996;10(1 Pt 1):1–19.
34. Ratner LE, et al. Transplantation of kidneys from expanded criteria donors. Surgery. 1996;119(4):372–377.
35. Wyner LM, et al. Use of kidneys from older cadaver donors for renal transplantation. Urology. 1993;41(2):107–110.
36. Stratta RJ, et al. Increased kidney transplantation utilizing expanded criteria deceased organ donors with results comparable to standard criteria donor transplant. Annals of Surgery. 2004;239(5):688–695. discussion 695–697.
37. Karpinski J, et al. Outcome of kidney transplantation from high-risk donors is determined by both structure and function. Transplantation. 1999;67(8): 1162–1167.
38. Cicciarelli J, et al. Renal biopsy donor group: the influence of glomerulosclerosis on transplant outcomes. Transplantation Proceedings. 2005;37(2):712–713.
39. Randhawa PS, et al. Biopsy of marginal donor kidneys: correlation of histologic findings with graft dysfunction. Transplantation. 2000;69(7):1352–1357.
40. Remuzzi G, et al. Long-term outcome of renal transplantation from older donors. New England Journal of Medicine. 2006;354(4):343–352.
41. Sung RS, et al. Determinants of discard of expanded criteria donor kidneys: impact of biopsy and machine perfusion. American Journal of Transplantation. 2008; 8(4):783–792.
42. Muruve NA, Steinbecker KM, Luger AM. Are wedge biopsies of cadaveric kidneys obtained at procurement reliable? Transplantation. 2000;69(11): 2384–2388.
43. Carter JT, et al. Expanded criteria donor kidney allocation: marked decrease in cold ischemia and delayed graft function at a single center. American Journal of Transplantation. 2005;5(11):2745–2753.
44. Cho YW. Expanded criteria donors. Clinical Transplants. 1998:421–436.
45. Moreso F, et al. Donor age and delayed graft function as predictors of renal allograft survival in rejection-free patients. Nephrology, Dialysis, Transplantation. 1999;14(4):930–935.
46. Sundberg AK, et al. Safety and efficacy of valganciclovir for cmv prophylaxis in high risk kidney and pancreas transplant recipients. American Journal of Transplantation. 2003(S5);3:298.
47. Valcarcel E, et al. Cytogenetic recombinants from a female carrying a paracentric inversion of the short arm of chromosome number 5. Human Genetics. 1983;63(1):78–81.
48. Miles CD, et al. Mortality experience in recipients undergoing repeat transplantation with expanded criteria donor and non-ECD deceased-donor kidneys. Ameri-

can Journal of Transplantation. 2007;7(5):1140–1147.
49. Danovitch GM, et al. Current status of kidney and pancreas transplantation in the United States, 1994–2003. American Journal of Transplantation. 2005;5(4 Pt 2): 904–915.
50. de Fijter JW, et al. Increased immunogenicity and cause of graft loss of old donor kidneys. Journal of the American Society of Nephrology. 2001;12(7):1538–1546.
51. Bosmuller C, et al. Excellent results with calcineurin inhibitor-free initial immunosuppression in old recipients of old kidneys. Transplantation Proceedings. 2005;37(2):881–883.
52. Emparan C, et al. Long-term results of calcineurin-free protocols with basiliximab induction in "old-to-old" programs. Transplantation Proceedings. 2004;36(9): 2646–2648.
53. Meier-Kriesche HU, et al. Increased immunosuppressive vulnerability in elderly renal transplant recipients. Transplantation. 2000;69(5):885–889.
54. Donati D, et al. Calcineurin inhibitor-free immunosuppressive regimen for marginal donors/recipients of kidney transplantation. Transplantation Proceedings. 2002;34(5):1678–1680.
55. Arbogast H, et al. A calcineurin antagonist-free induction/maintenance strategy for immunosuppression in elderly recipients of renal allografts from elderly cadaver donors: long-term results from a prospective single centre trial. Clinical Transplantation. 2005;19(3):309–315.
56. Diekmann F, et al. Sequential quadruple immunosuppression including sirolimus in extended criteria and nonheartbeating donor kidney transplantation. Transplantation. 2007;84(3):429–432.
57. Matsuoka L, et al. Pulsatile perfusion reduces the incidence of delayed graft function in expanded criteria donor kidney transplantation. American Journal of Transplantation. 2006;6(6):1473–1478.
58. Larsen CP, et al. Belatacept-based regimens versus a cyclosporine A-based regimen in kidney transplant recipients: 2-year results from the BENEFIT and BENEFIT-EXT studies. Transplantation. 2010;90(12):1528–1535.
59. Bodingbauer M, et al. The advantage of allocating kidneys from old cadaveric donors to old recipients: a single-center experience. Clinical Transplantation. 2006;20(4):471–475.
60. Polyak MM, et al. The influence of pulsatile preservation on renal transplantation in the 1990s. Transplantation. 2000;69(2):249–258.
61. Polyak MM, et al. Prostaglandin E1 influences pulsatile preservation characteristics and early graft function in expanded criteria donor kidneys. Journal of Surgical Research. 1999;85(1):17–25.
62. Halloran P, Aprile M. A randomized prospective trial of cold storage versus pulsatile perfusion for cadaver kidney preservation. Transplantation. 1987;43(6): 827–832.
63. Merion RM, et al. A prospective controlled trial of cold-storage versus machine-perfusion preservation in cadaveric renal transplantation. Transplantation. 1990;50(2):230–233.
64. Polyak MM, et al. Glutathione supplementation during cold ischemia does not confer early functional advantage in renal transplantation. Transplantation. 2000;70(1):202–205.
65. Mozes MF, et al. Comparison of cold-storage and machine perfusion in the preservation of cadaver kidneys-A prospective, randomized study. Transplantation Proceedings. 1985;17:1474–1477.
66. Johnson LB, et al. Double renal allografts successfully increase utilization of kidneys from older donors within a single organ procurement organization. Transplantation. 1996;62(11):1581–1583.
67. Kuo PC, et al. Utilization of the older donor for renal transplantation. American Journal of Surgery. 1996;172(5):551–555. discussion 556–557.
68. Lu AD, et al. Excellent outcome in recipients of dual kidney transplants: a report of the first 50 dual kidney transplants at Stanford University. Archives of Surgery. 1999;134(9):971–975. discussion 975–976.
69. Mackenzie HS, et al. Renal mass as a determinant of late allograft outcome: insights from experimental studies in rats. Kidney International Supplement. 1995;52: S38–S42.
70. Taal MW, et al. An important determinant of late allograft outcome. Transplantation Reviews. 1998;12:74–84.
71. Alfrey EJ, et al. Dual-kidney transplants: long-term results. Transplantation. 2003;75(8):1232–1236.
72. Tan JC, et al. Dual-kidney transplantation with organs from expanded criteria donors: a long-term follow-up. Transplantation. 2004;78(5):692–696.
73. Jacobbi LM, et al. The risks, benefits, and costs of expanding donor criteria. A collaborative prospective three-year study. Transplantation. 1995;60(12):1491–1496.
74. Whiting JF, et al. Economic costs of expanded criteria donors in renal transplantation. Transplantation. 1998;65(2):204–207.
75. The National Institutes of Health, National Institute of Diabetes and Digestive and Kidney Diseases. USRDS 2009 Annual Report, 2009.
76. Saidi RF, et al. Outcome of kidney transplantation using expanded criteria donors and donation after cardiac death kidneys: realities and costs. American Journal of Transplantation. 2007;7(12):2769–2774.
77. Whiting JF, et al. Economic cost of expanded criteria donors in cadaveric renal transplantation: analysis of Medicare payments. Transplantation. 2000;70(5): 755–760.
78. Clavien PA. How far can we go with marginal donors? Journal of Hepatology. 2006;45(4):483–484.
79. Busuttil RW, Tanaka K. The utility of marginal donors in liver transplantation. Liver Transplantation. 2003;9(7):651–663.
80. Mullhaupt B, et al. Hot topics in liver transplantation: organ allocation–extended criteria donor–living donor liver transplantation. Journal of Hepatology. 2008;48(Suppl 1):S58–S67.
81. Briceno J, et al. Influence of marginal donors on liver preservation injury. Transplantation. 2002;74(4):522–526.
82. Ploeg RJ, et al. Risk factors for primary dysfunction after liver transplantation–a multivariate analysis. Transplantation. 1993;55(4):807–813.
83. Garcia Urena MA, et al. Hepatic steatosis in liver transplant donors: common feature of donor population? World Journal of Surgery. 1998; 22(8):837–844.
84. Imber CJ, et al. Current practice regarding the use of fatty livers: a trans-Atlantic survey. Liver Transplantation. 2002;8(6):545–549.
85. Rao PS, et al. A comprehensive risk quantification score for deceased donor kidneys: the kidney donor risk index. Transplantation. 2009;88(2): 231–236.
86. Maluf DG, et al. Impact of the donor risk index on the outcome of hepatitis C virus-positive liver transplant recipients. Liver Transplantation. 2009;15(6): 592–599.

第 54 章
心脏死亡供体的器官评估和捐献接受

Silke Niederhaus, Anthony M. D'Alessandro

引言

在美国，每天有 18 人在等待器官的过程中死亡。那些有幸进行移植手术的人接受的大多是来自脑死亡供体的器官。随着移植手术作为救命手段的成功率不断提高，器官的等候名单正在快速增长，对可移植器官的需求也正相应增加。为了缩小器官的供应缺口，对其他替代移植供体的寻求变得十分迫切。目前的替代移植供体包括活体肺移植、边缘标准供体或称之为扩大标准捐献(ECD)供体和心脏死亡(DCD)供体，其中心脏死亡供体通常是指心脏死亡后的供体或没有心跳的供体。DCD 在 20 世纪 90 年代中期被数个研究项目再次引入医学界，自那时起，其对于可用于移植的器官数量的稳定增长起到了重要作用。来自 DCD 的肾脏、肝脏、胰腺和肺的移植手术均已获得成功，有的医学中心已经开始使用 DCD 的器官进行联合移植[1,2]，其报道的结果也比较令人满意。

然而，对于 DCD 器官的使用需要在其利弊之间进行权衡：移植 DCD 器官会导致发生并发症的概率明显增高，且并发症随移植器官的不同而变化。自 1995 年以来，DCD 一直根据 Maastricht 分级进行分类[3](表 54.1)。除了少数个例以外，美国的 DCD 属于 Maastricht 3 级供体，这意味着心跳呼吸的停止和随后的器官获取都是在受控的院内环境中进行的。这些供体通常情况稳定，多数在手术室中，有时在重症监护室(ICU)中，通过有计划的生命支持的停止实现死亡。因此，供体的缺血损伤已知并被控制。欧洲的情况与美国的情况不同，其 DCD 的范围更广，各个 Maastricht 级别的供体器官都被用于移植手术。这些供体的缺血性损伤更难预料，同时学界认为，在某些病例中，这些器官的可接受性已经到达了极限。通常情况下，接受 DCD 器官的相关风险被其补偿获益抵消，获益包括器官移植的等待时间更短，以及在适当选择的环境下，终末器官衰竭的风险降低。欧洲的器官使用情况对临床医生提出了更高的要求，其既要求临床医生对于不受控制的心脏停搏和器官获取的潜在结果有深入的理解，又要求医生对接受这种器官的潜在风险有清醒的认识。在本章，我们将回顾 DCD 器官的接受标准。我们将讨论基于不同器官的 DCD 器官移植的利弊。最后，我们将说明移植后的器官功能，以及短期和长期的预后情况。针对符合标准供体和扩大标准供体的讨论见第 53 章。心脏死亡情况下供体器官的获取技术细节见第 22 章。

表 54.1 心脏死亡供体的 Maastricht 分级

1	不受控的	送至医院时已经死亡
2	不受控的	复苏不成功死亡
3	受控的	等待心脏骤停
4	受控的	脑死亡后心脏停搏
5	不受控的	住院患者意外心脏停搏

DCD 肺移植

接受标准

Hardy 和其他人于 1963 年报道了首次成功的人类肺移植手术，其使用的器官以现代标准衡量属于 DCD 肺[4]。其后不久，脑死亡的概念被提出并被确定为法定死亡标准[5]。随后，考虑到热缺血时间对供体器官的毒害效应，大部分移植改为采用脑死亡供体的器官[6]，直到 20 世纪 90 年代中期，鉴于等待名单持续增长所带来的压力，DCD 器官移植又重新进入医学界的视野[7]。自 1988 年以来，肺供体的数量显著增长，从 33 人增长到了 2010 年的 1770 人。然而和其他器官一样，器官等待名单的增长速度大于供体的增加速度。对于 DCD 肺而言，绝大多数的项目组使用国际心肺移植学会(ISHLT)的选择标准[8]。然而，考虑到热缺血时间造成的额外风险，很多中心在应用 ISHLT 标准时，相比于脑死亡供体(DBD)，对于情况相当的 DCD 的要求会更加苛刻。一些中心甚至会针对 DCD 肺采用更严格的标准。表 54.2 列举了 ISHLT 标准以及全球不同的肺移植中心针对可能的 DCD 肺的附加标准。Puri 等[9]也曾使用扩大标准供体的器官进行移植(其列于表 54.2 的括号中)。

风险与收益

实施 DCD 肺移植提高了肺移植患者获得器官的可能性，缩短了个体患者的等待时间，降低了等待死亡的风险[10]。为了使 DCD 肺移植的预后达到最优，选择合适的受体是至关重要的。患有肺动脉高压、特发性肺间质纤维化，或既往胸膜固定术后的患者在一些中心不被列入 DCD 肺移植的候选名单[9]，可能是由于接受肺切除术过程中存在可预见的困难性，也可能是由于会对肺移植物造成进一步的再灌注损伤。然而，包括我们在内的一些机构将所有的受体都列为 DCD 肺移植的潜在受体。总的来说，考虑到 DCD 肺选择标准的改变，除去某些不同点以外，DCD 肺移植的结果与 DBD 肺移植的结果相似。现针对一些重要的例外讨论如下。

DCD 肺移植术后发生原发性移植物功能障碍的概率与 DBD 肺移植的概率相似，约为 10%~18%[9,11,12]。由于原发性移植物功能障碍导致的体外膜肺氧合(ECMO)的需求相似或略小[13]。其他指标也均相似，如拔管时间、出重症监护室时间或出院时间[13]。1 级的急性排斥反应在 DCD 肺移植受体中的发生率(53.7%)比 DBD 肺移植受体(27.8%)要高[12]，但其他报告显示两种移植的排斥反应发生率相似[13]。还有的报告显示 DCD 肺移植的排斥反应发生率为 20%[11]。2 级及以上的急性排斥反应发生率相同[12]。

DCD 肺移植术后的气道并发症包括支气管狭窄、支气管裂开、支气管吻合处肉芽组织的过度生长和支气管瘘。事实上，从已报道的气道并发症发生率的数值上看，DCD 肺移植并发症发病率是 DBD 肺移植的 2 倍，分别为 27.8%和 12.8%，尽管在目前已经报告的小规模研究中，两者的差异并未达到统计学意义[12]。尽管如此，这些并发症很可能是小血管缺血和血栓生物学在循环停止期发生的结果。它们与已知的肝移植(见后述)并发症相似，可能反映了 DCD 后移植的真实结果。

移植术后感染也曾被报道，但 DCD 移植与 DBD 移植相比，术后感染发生的概率并没有增高。其他被报道的并发症包括肺炎、心房颤动(41%)、心包积液、意识错乱(23%)、急性肾损伤(12%)、血液系统异常(18%)、肠梗阻(12%)以及局部缺血(6%)[14]。与供体的情况相比，这些并发症与受体的生理功能关系更为密切。

与 DBD 肺移植一样，原发性移植物功能障碍和更长的冷缺血时间与 DCD 捐献后的早期死亡有关[9]。据报道，DCD 肺移植术后前 3 个月的死亡率为 18%[14]。

DCD 和 DBD 肺移植术后功能

只有两个研究组描述了 DCD 肺移植术后的功能情况。DeOliveira 等系统地研究了移植术后 1、6、12、24、36、48、60 个月 1 秒钟用力呼气量(FEV_1)预测百分比。肺功能在 DCD 和 DBD 肺受体之间没有差异。DCD 和 DBD 肺受体移植术后 1 个月的 FEV_1 预测百分比为 50%~60%；在术后 6~12 个月之后达到高峰，为 60%~70%；随后至移植术后 48 个月保持稳定；至术后第 60 个月，DCD 组的该值下降至预测的 40%，而 DBD 组保持在预测的 60%左右[12]。DeVleeschauwer 等评估了移植术后的最佳 FEV_1 值，并在 DCD 肺组和 DBD 肺组之间进行了比较。该研究中(两组)的 FEV_1 值也是相似的：DCD 组的最佳 FEV_1 值为 94%(78%~106%)，DBD 组为 93%(75%~112%)[13]。两组术后 30 天内均可观察到 FEV_1 的持续改善。截止术后第 30 天，DCD 肺移植组患者 FEV_1 增长 1.58L，DBD 组增长 0.84L。从更大的时间范围观察，DCD 组受体于术后 180 天可增长至 2.77L，DBD 组于术后 185 天可增长至 2.31L[14]。

肺移植中的慢性同种异体移植物损伤表现为闭塞性细支气管炎。DCD 肺移植患者术后 1 年闭塞性细支气管炎的发生率为 7%~20%，3 年可达到 20%~50%[1,12,14]。与之相比，DBD 肺移植患者术后 1 年闭塞性细支气管炎发生率为 6%，3 年为 25%。DeOliveira 等发现，如果对 DCD 肺供体和受体均进行仔细选择，DCD 肺移植组与 DBD 组之间闭塞性细支气管炎的发生率几乎相同。DeVleeschauwer 等在比利时也报道了相似的闭塞性细支气管炎发生率，在中位发病时间为 328 天的 DCD 患者中，约有 14%的患者发生闭塞性细支气

表 54.2 DCD 肺供体的选择标准

标准项目	ISHLT[8]	西班牙[66]	安大略，加拿大[11]	威斯康星大学和比利时大学[12,13]	克利夫兰医学中心，俄亥俄州[17]	Nunez 等[67]	华盛顿大学，密苏里州[9]	墨尔本，澳大利亚[10]
供体年龄(岁)	<55	<55				7~50	<55(>55 边际)	<55
ABO	相合						相合	
CXR	清晰		是		是		正常(有渗出为边界)	相对正常
PaO_2/ABG	FiO_2 为 100%且 PEEP + 5cmH$_2$O 时 > 300mmHg	PaO_2/FiO_2> 300mmHg	是		是	>300mmHg	FiO_2 为 100%且 PEEP + 5cmH$_2$O 时> 300mmHg(< 300 为边界)	FiO_2 100%时> 300mmHg
吸烟史(烟包年)	<20						(>20 为边界)	
胸部创伤	无	无				无		
吸引	无							
脓毒症	无							
心肺手术史	无							无
痰革兰染色	阴性							
支气管镜	无脓性分泌物		是		是	无损伤	正常(脓性分泌物为边界)	是
Maastricht 分级	全部	1 或 2	3	3	3	1 和 2	3	3
死亡/心脏停搏时间		已知				已知		支持停止前 2 小时小组到达
CPR 开始时间(分钟)		<15				<10		
热缺血时间(分钟)		<120	<90 >30(离体)	<60	<60			
最大冷保存时间		<240 分钟				<90 分钟		局部冷保存至心脏死亡后 6 小时
检查/可视化		无挫伤 无水肿	是		是	无损伤	尺寸符合受体	
健康史			无肿瘤等			健康，无 HIV 危险因素	无肺部疾病史，乙肝病毒和 HIV 阴性(使用吸入性药物为边界)	

ISHLT,国际心肺移植协会;CXR,胸部 X 线片;PaO_2,动脉血氧分压;ABG,动脉血气;PEEP,呼气末正压;CPR,心肺复苏。

管炎；在中位发病时间为 480 天的 DBD 患者中，约有 10%的患者发生闭塞性细支气管炎。这些数据在统计学上是相似的[13]。在近期的一篇综述中，Wigfeld 和 Love 收集并总结了不同中心的 DCD 肺移植术后的闭塞性细支气管炎病例，经汇总，191 例患者 3 年中共有 21 例(11%)患闭塞性细支气管炎[15]。

长期结果

DCD 肺移植术后的长期结果数据较少[16]，因为 DCD 肺移植是近期持续发展的领域，研究组和术后长期生存者的数量均较小。

在移植物存活方面(图 54.1)，在对 DCD 进行仔细选择的条件下，DCD 和 DBD 组表现相同。DCD 肺移植术后 1 年的移植物存活率为 69%~83%，3 年移植物存活率为 61%~77%，5 年移植物存活率为 77%(根据一项 5 年期的移植物存活率研究得出)。与之相比，DBD 肺移植术后 1 年的移植物存活率为 82%~85%，3 年移植物存活率为 68%~70%，5 年移植物存活率据报道为 60%。两者水平相当[1,9,12-14,17]。

DCD 肺移植术后 1 年患者生存率为 80%~95%，3 年为 69%~95%，5 年为 71%~82%。DBD 肺移植术后 1 年患者生存率为 78%~96%，3 年为 72%~91%，5 年为 63%~75%。同样地，在患者生存率方面两者也没有显著差异[1,9,12-14,17]。

DCD 肝移植

接受标准

与 DCD 肺移植相比，DCD 肝更为常见，对其的实践和技术改进也更加成熟。因此，其选择标准的建立也更加普遍(表 54.3)。各个中心对于 DCD 肝的选择标准不尽相同，但总体而言其比 DBD 肝的要求更加严格。大多数中心要求在血流阻断时进行肝素化冲洗，或者，更倾向于在停止生命支持之前用高剂量的静脉内肝素进行全身肝素化，其具体取决于供体所在地区或国家的法律要求。学界普遍认为，热缺血时间的上限为 30 分钟。最常用的热缺血时间的定义是指从所有生命支持措施停止至冷冲洗或血流阻断的时间，然而在某些中心，其定义被更换为从全身血压低于 50mmHg 至冷冲洗的时间，相应地，其最大允许的热缺血时间可长达 60 分钟[18]。在大多数中心，对于心脏死亡后捐献肝脏的捐献者年龄的保守上限为 40~50 岁，然而，也有项目组发表过来自

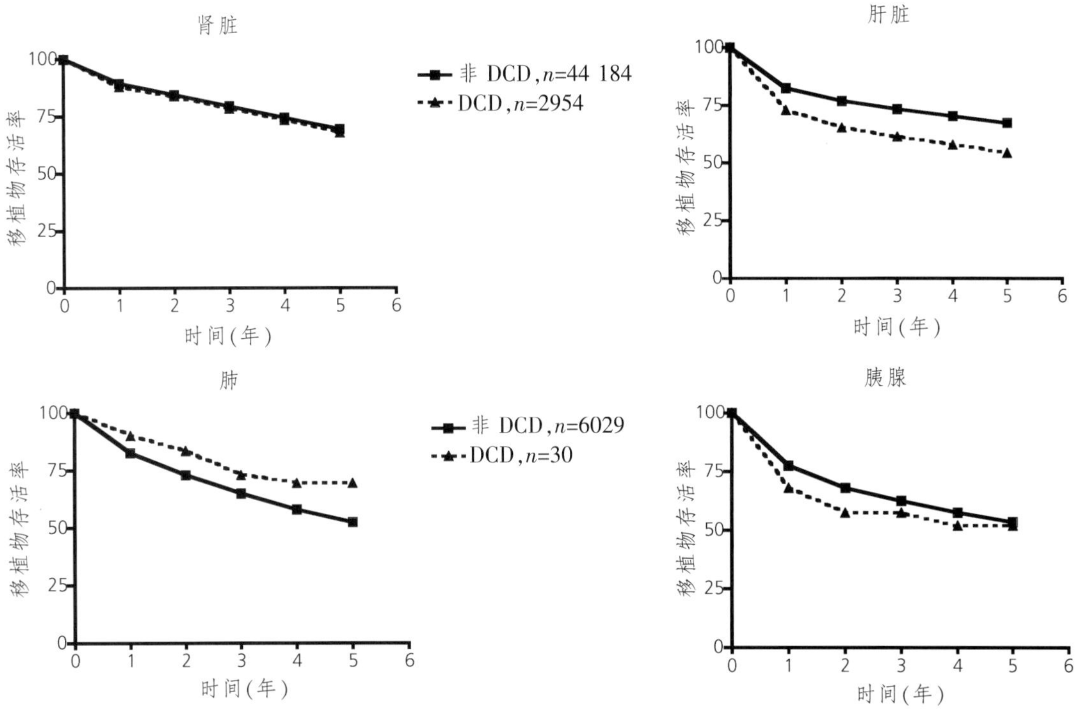

图 54.1　肾脏、肝脏、肺和胰腺移植的供体器官移植物存活率。肾脏、胰腺和肺移植后的结果没有显著差异。DCD 肝移植后的器官存活率较低，且具有统计学意义。(Based on OPTN data from 2002 to 2006.)

表 54.3　DCD 肝供体的选择标准

	荷兰[68]	英国[18]	西班牙[19]	匹兹堡[20]	洛杉矶[21]	英国[23]	威斯康星大学[63]	西班牙[69]	波士顿[70]
系统肝素化或肝素化冲洗	肝素冲洗	肝素冲洗			撤机前肝素化		撤机前肝素化	肝素 3g/kg，每 90 分钟 1.5mg/kg	
热缺血时间(从撤机到冲洗，除非另行说明)(分钟)	<30，且 MAP <50mmHg 时间<15 分钟	<60，且 SBP <50mmHg 至冲洗		<20	<30	<30，且 SBP <50mmHg 至冲洗	<30		28.6±8.8
供体年龄(岁)	1~55	<50，现为<65	<50 或<65	<60	<45	<40	<50	<60	
肝酶		好			<2 倍正常值	正常			
BMI 为 28～30kg/m² 或供体体重<100kg	<28				<30				25±5.8
住院时间(天)					<5	<5			
肉眼检查		无脂肪，灌注良好			好	好，灌注良好	无过度脂肪	无脂肪变性，灌注良好，无损伤	
组织活检(大泡性脂肪变性的百分比)		是(所有病例均需进行)					<30%~50%		
冷缺血时间(小时)				<8	<8				
无癌症病史、药物滥用史或其他生物学风险。HIV、乙肝、丙肝阴性			X					X	
腹部和股部血管正常			X					X	
心脏停搏时间 <15 分钟			X					X	
CPR 时间(分钟)			<130					<150	
NECMO(小时)			<4					<4(流速>1.7L/min 是理想的)	
Maastricht 分级	3	3	2	3	3	3	3	1、2、4	3

MAP，平均动脉压；SBP，收缩压；BMI，体重指数；CPR，心肺复苏；NECMO，常温体外膜肺氧合。

65 岁的 DCD 捐献者的肝脏成功移植的报道[18-20]。

在 DCD 肝供体中,住院治疗期间血流动力学稳定的供体或肝功能正常或接近正常的供体应当被优先选择[21]。体型较瘦的 DCD 肝较为理想,根据不同中心的标准,其体重指数(BMI)应<28~30kg/m^2 或体重<100kg。某些项目组认为住院时间较短的供体应当被优先选择[21-23]。一些机构[1,18],但不是所有机构[20,21],要求常规进行肝组织大体检查和活检以检测细胞活力,并排除肝细胞大泡性脂肪变性或纤维化。最近,一项来自英国的研究报道了一种较为激进的 DCD 肝的使用方式[24],其接受了来自扩大标准 DCD 的肝脏。扩大标准 DCD 肝的定义为满足下列标准中的一项或多项:热缺血时间>30 分钟 (但从收缩压<50mmHg 至冷冲洗或从氧饱和度<80%至冷冲洗的时间应小于 60 分钟);供体年龄超过 60 岁;供体 BMI>30kg/m^2;冷缺血时间>8 小时。通过对这些供体的仔细筛选,其效果是可接受的,即 1 年的移植物存活率与未扩大标准的 DCD 肝相似。

移植后发生移植物丢失、原发性移植物无功能、胆道并发症或受体死亡的危险因素主要包括:供体年龄超过 40~50 岁;供体体重超过 100kg;供体热缺血时间>35 分钟(相对的是<15 分钟);供体低血压时间过长[20,22,25]。冷缺血时间的延长也会对效果产生不利影响[25],冷缺血时间每延长 1 小时,异体移植物丢失发生的概率会上升 6%[20,22]。受体死亡率随供体体重和冷缺血时间的增加而增加[22]。某些中心要求预期冷缺血时间<8 小时[20,21]。器官共享会要求额外的时间将肝脏分成可用的两叶,这是引起冷缺血时间延长的潜在因素,目前已经发现器官共享与更差的 DCD 肝移植效果相关。器官受体年龄超过 60 岁、移植时肾功能障碍,以及供体丙型肝炎阳性均会导致移植效果变差[25]。

对于 DCD 肝的受体选择是优化结果的关键。年龄超过 55 岁的器官受体发生移植失败的概率比更年轻的成年受体高 26%。男性受体或非裔美国人受体的预后与女性或其他种族的受体相比更差。二次移植受体比初次 DCD 肝移植受体发生移植失败的概率高 45%。患有代谢性肝病的患者发生移植失败的概率也会升高。应用终末期肝病模型(MELD)进行评估,评分>35 分的患者比评分为 15~25 分的患者移植失败率高 47%。因此,对于年龄高于 55 岁,或等待进行二次移植,或 MELD 高评分的患者,需就等待 DBD 肝过程中的风险和接受 DCD 肝后移植失败率的升高进行仔细权衡[22]。

文献中支持 DCD 肝应用于儿童的数据非常少。然而,Gozzini 等人已经成功进行了两例全体积和两例减体积(Ⅱ~Ⅲ段)DCD 肝儿童移植术[23]。

在西班牙,DCD 肝自 2002 年起就被用于移植,其中使用的大部分器官来自未经控制的供体,且经过常温 ECMO 的保存。体外循环的流量参数已被用于判定移植物活力,理想的流量应>1.7L/min。供体排除标准包括癌症史、药物滥用史或其他生物学风险史,有犯罪史或暴力性死亡的供体也被排除。同时,要求供体人类免疫缺陷病毒(HIV)、乙型肝炎病毒(HBV)和丙型肝炎病毒(HCV)化验均为阴性,腹部和股血管正常。大体检查肉眼可见脂肪变性的器官同样被排除。其他的标准还包括无支持的心搏停止时间小于 15 分钟;呼吸机支持、心肺复苏或按压总时间<130 分钟[19];常温 ECMO 总时间<4 小时。年龄低于 55 岁的供体应被优先选择,然而在特殊情况下,年龄超过 65 岁供体的器官也曾被应用。

在荷兰,大多数 Maastricht 3 级的供体器官被用于临床。供体器官选择标准包括供体热缺血时间<30 分钟;供体年龄为 1~55 岁;BMI<28kg/m^2;平均动脉压<50mmHg 的时间<15 分钟。

风险与获益

使用 DCD 肝进行移植的唯一好处是其缓解了等待名单的持续增长,允许患者更快地获得移植。通过从 DCD 器官库中获得肝脏,患者等待期死亡的情况得到控制和改善。虽然其间接地有益于所有等待移植的患者,但是其对个体患者的益处并不明确。尤其是考虑到与其他 DCD 器官的移植相比,DCD 肝移植的风险显著高于 DBD 肝移植。原发性移植物无功能、胆道并发症(尤其是缺血性胆道狭窄)、肝动脉血栓和移植物存活时间短仍旧是 DCD 移植与 DBD 肝移植具有相似效果的障碍,该结论适用于所有 Maastricht 分级的 DCD。

以西班牙为代表的欧洲国家一直在临床中广泛地使用来自不受控制的 DCD 肝脏。一个来自西班牙的研究小组移植了 10 个 DCD 肝,这些肝脏来自通过心肺复苏或按压和常温 ECMO 维持的不受控供体。经过平均 23 个月的随访,一半的肝脏(50%)功能正常,其余移植失败的原因包括原发性移植物无功能、肝动脉血栓，或者因其他并发症或丙型肝炎复发而导致移植物功能丧失[26]。另一篇来自西班牙的报告报道了16例2级DCD肝移植的效果[19]。不受控的DCD肝的受体中发生胆道并发症的概率(42%)显著高于DBD肝受体(17%)。DCD肝移植术后发生非吻合口胆道狭窄的概率(25%)也显著高于DBD肝移植(2%)。这些并发症最终导致移植物丢失的概率升高3倍。一项欧洲国家实施的DCD器官捐献的大规模调查显示,在受控的和不受控的DCD肝移植术后1年,患者和移植物的存活率均相似[27]。

美国和欧洲的多个研究组已经开始实施受控的DCD肝移植,以降低等待期死亡率。DCD肝移植的成本比DBD肝移植高25%左右,这是因为其二次移植的数量更多(21%对7%),同时其胆道并发症发生率也更高(58%对21%)。即使排除二次移植的影响,DCD肝移植的成本仍比DBD肝移植高20%[28]。

基于更大规模数据库的研究评估了美国DCD肝移植的效果。具体来说,移植受体科学注册系统(SRTR)从1996年至2007年的数据显示,DCD器官移植组患者存活率更低,且其不随DCD器官移植术经验的增加而改善[25]。DCD肝受体需要二次移植的概率是DBD肝受体的两倍(14.7%对6.8%),且二次移植的患者生存率低于首次肝移植。DCD肝移植术后死亡率高于DBD肝移植,其证实了导致受体死亡是DCD肝移植的危险因素。

DCD肝移植术不良结果的危险因素包括：供体热缺血时间长(>20~30分钟);冷缺血时间长(>8~10小时);供体年龄大(>40~60岁)[29,30]。具体的并发症和受控的DCD肝移植的风险如下所述。

原发性移植物无功能

学界将肝移植术后原发性移植物无功能定义为严重的肝细胞损伤[谷草转氨酶(AST)≥3000U/L]、凝血因子合成功能障碍(INR>2.5)、乳酸清除功能障碍(血清乳酸盐≥4mmol/L)。DCD肝移植后原发性移植物无功能的发生率比DBD肝移植高3.6倍[31]。最近的研究显示,患者在接受受控的(Maastricht 3级)DCD肝移植后发生原发性移植物无功能的概率为0~12%[20],与之相比，患者在接受DBD肝移植后发生该症状的概率为1.4%~3%[20,32]。一项欧洲的研究显示,受控的和非受控的DCD肝移植发生原发性移植物无功能的概率相似[27]。有更大规模的研究指出,原发性移植物无功能发生的概率略低(为2.5%~3%)[29,32,33]。原发性移植物无功能的危险因素包括:将男性供体的肝脏移植给女性受体；受体年龄大 (>60岁)；受体BMI指数高(>30kg/m^2)[20]。

肝动脉血栓

肝移植后发生肝动脉血栓并不常见，但却十分棘手。DCD肝移植后,其发生的概率为0~33%,更大规模的研究报告则报道了较低的发生率(0~6%)[20,29,32,33]。与早期报告的预期状况相同[20,33,34],大型SRTR数据库统计显示DCD肝移植和DBD肝移植后出现肝动脉血栓的概率相近[31]。然而,另一项研究则称DCD肝移植后发生肝动脉血栓的概率更高。与DBD肝移植相比,DCD肝移植后发生的肝动脉血栓更易导致胆道狭窄[34]。DCD肝移植后发生的肝动脉血栓的治疗通常包括再移植[18,35]。

胆道并发症

相比于DBD肝移植，胆道并发症在DCD肝移植后更常见[30],在考虑接受DCD器官时,胆道并发症成了一个更为重要的问题。胆道并发症可能与捐献过程中热缺血时间对胆道微血管系统的不良影响有关。该影响可能与DCD肺移植过程中支气管树所出现的问题类似,如前所述。因此,尽量减少缺血时间可能有利于预防胆道并发症。此外,有人尝试了通过移植期间在肝动脉中输注组织纤溶酶原激活物(tPA)来使胆汁缺血最小化,其结果令人满意[36]。

DCD肝移植后发生胆道并发症的概率为15%~58%[18,20,21,28,29,31-33,37]。与之相比,DBD肝移植后胆道并发症的发生率明显较低(6%~21%)[18,20,21,28,29,31-35,37]。一项多国的Meta分析显示,DCD肝移植后发生胆道并发症的概率比DBD肝移植高2.4倍。供体年龄超过40岁是胆道并发症的危险因素[30]。有趣的是,供体BMI或体重较高可能会增加吻合口胆管狭窄的发生风险[30]。

胆道并发症包括多种问题，例如吻合口和非吻合口胆道狭窄、胆汁渗漏、胆汁淤积、胆泥淤积、胆汁瘤、胆道脓肿和缺血性胆管病等。一些胆道并发症可以在内镜下进行处理,其余的需要重复手术进行治疗,如二次移植[29,32]。由于胆道并发症较多发于DCD肝移植受体，这些患者更可能在术后需要后续的诊断和纠正措施，而这将降低他们的生活质量[32]。

缺血性胆管病需要特别关注。它很难治疗，通常与肝内胆汁瘤或胆源性脓毒症相关，并经常导致二次移植。与所有胆道并发症一样，其在 DCD 肝移植后的发生率显著高于 DBD 肝移植；目前报道的 DCD 肝移植后的发生率为 0~44%[28,32,33,37]，相比之下，DBD 肝移植后的发生率约为 3%[31-33]。缺血性胆管病本身表现为孤立性或弥散性的非吻合口胆管狭窄。大多数缺血性胆管病发生于移植后前 4 个月[30]。其中一些病例可以通过内镜下逆行胰胆管造影术（ERCP）或经皮肝穿刺胆管造影术（PTC）进行介入扩张治疗，但多达 50%的病例最终需要进行二次移植[30,33,37]。缺血性胆管病可导致移植物功能衰竭[21]。其危险因素包括从心搏停止至血流阻断的时间过长和受体为非裔美国人[33]。从心搏停止至血流阻断的时间每增加 1 分钟，缺血性胆管病的发生率就会提高 16%[33]。其他危险因素还包括冷缺血时间>8 小时和供体年龄超过 40 岁[30]。

其他风险

缺血-再灌注损伤在 DCD 肝移植后会加剧，其最初表现为实验室指标异常，例如移植后 1 周出现 AST 峰值升高[29]或 INR 升高[20]。一项研究探讨了 DCD 肝移植术中再灌注后综合征的发生，其发现所有患者均需要予以短暂的血管升压药支持，支持应在再灌注之前或之时开始[18]，32 例患者中有 6 例的支持持续到了手术结束。

DCD 肝移植术后恢复与 DBD 肝移植相似，其住院总时间亦相近[20,32]，尽管一项研究称 DCD 肝移植后 ICU 的停留时间会更长[20]。移植后 90 天和 1 年的排斥反应发生率相似[32,34]。

一些研究显示，DCD 肝移植短期术后移植物存活率与 DBD 肝移植相近[32,33]，但另一些研究结果则相反[30]。在对肝移植结果的 Meta 分析中发现，DCD 肝移植术后 1 年和 3 年移植失败率比 DBD 肝移植高 2 倍[31]。与 DBD 肝受体相比，DCD 肝受体发生再次移植的概率高出 2 倍以上（15%~18%对 7%），且其最常见于高龄 DCD-高龄器官受体组合[20]。供体年龄超过 40 岁、冷缺血时间>12 小时或供肝共享均会导致 DCD 肝移植结果变差。类似地，受体年龄超过 60 岁、移植时肾功能不全和供体 HCV 状态均被报道会提高 DCD 肝移植后结局不良的风险。DCD 肝移植后发生移植物丢失的危险因素包括器官受体为非白种人和二次移植，有趣的是，供体年龄过高并不会提高其风险[33]。移植物损失的原因很多，包括复发性丙型肝炎、原发性移植物无功能、肝动脉血栓和感染[21]。与 DBD 肝移植相比，DCD 肝移植后发生复发性丙型肝炎的概率相近或更高[20]。

在某些研究中，DCD 肝移植后患者生存率与 DBD 肝移植相同[32,33]。在另一些研究中，观察到 DCD 肝移植术后 1 年受体死亡率较高，但术后 3 年时两者死亡率相同[31]。根据另一项大型临床研究，DCD 肝移植受体生存率比 DBD 组差，DCD 组 1 年和 3 年患者生存率分别为 82%和 71%，DBD 组为 86%和 77%。再移植中接受 DCD 肝的患者死亡率更高（1 年和 3 年的存活率分别为 71%和 59%），其与 DBD 组相近（1 年和 3 年的存活率分别为 68%和 60%）[25]。患者死亡原因较多，包括复发性肝细胞癌、再移植并发症、术中心脏死亡和多系统器官衰竭[32,33]。值得注意的是，DCD 肝脏的分割已经被报道和实施，并取得了部分成功，其 1 年患者和移植物存活率均差强人意[18]。

长期结果

移植物存活率和再移植率

DCD 肝移植后移植物远期存活率较 DBD 肝移植差（图 54.1）。DCD 肝移植 5 年移植物存活率为 43%~53%，与之相比，DBD 肝移植为 51%~68%[19-21,30]，只有一份报告显示两者 5 年移植物存活率相近（两组均约 69%）[33]。在更远期，术后 10~20 年以上时，两组最终移植物存活率相似，10 年期均为 37.5%；20 年期 DCD 组为 29%，DBD 组为 25%[35]。由于 DCD 肝移植后移植物存活率较低，其术后再移植更为常见，概率约为 19%，而 DBD 肝移植仅为 5%~7%[30,34]。导致再移植的原因包括：缺血性胆管病（81%）；原发性移植物无功能（13%）；血管并发症（6%）[30]。

患者存活率

根据研究，DCD 肝移植后患者生存率与 DBD 肝移植相似或略低。DCD 和 DBD 肝移植后 5 年期患者生存率分别为 68%~77%和 62%~81%[19,20,30,33]。DCD 组 10 年期、15 年期和 20 年期的患者生存率分别为 43%~57%[20,30,35]、54%和 38%。DBD 组 10 年和 15 年患者生存率分别为 64%~67%和 58%[20,30]。

排斥反应和其他并发症

在免疫并发症方面,包括急性或慢性排斥反应,两组远期表现无明显差异[30]。一项研究表明,DCD肝移植后的丙型肝炎复发比DBD肝移植后更严重[38]。

DCD胰腺移植

接受标准

联合或不联合肾移植的DCD胰腺移植用于治疗严重的1型糖尿病患者在世界范围内仍然相对罕见。在美国,只有水平较高的中心会选择DCD胰腺进行移植[39]。在欧洲,目前只有英国、比利时和荷兰进行DCD胰腺移植[27]。此外,澳大利亚也有1例DCD胰腺移植的报道[40]。DCD胰腺的选择标准与DBD胰腺大致类似,但其在选择标准的定量方面更加严格。

供体的年龄范围为3~60岁[1,41],但更趋向于中间年龄,而非极端年龄,一些项目组只接受成年DCD的器官[39]。供体不应有糖尿病或胰腺炎病史。有腹内败血症史、胰腺手术史或胰腺创伤史的供体同样应被排除。供体的HIV检查必须为阴性,且应无近期恶性肿瘤史[42]。器官捐献时存在高血糖或轻度高淀粉酶血症是可接受的[41]。如果计划进行DCD胰腺移植,年轻、BMI低、血流动力学稳定的供体应被优先选择。其他影响DCD胰腺移植和术后恢复过程的因素还包括:供体器官获取是否在当地的捐献者服务区内进行;预期冷缺血时间的长短;是否能由同一个医疗组进行术后恢复期治疗;器官冲洗的操作质量和大体观察下的器官质量是否良好;若进行胰-肾联合移植,是否有可能对肾脏进行灌注[39]。热缺血时间的上限不同中心有所不同,介于20~45分钟之间,其在某种程度上取决于生命支持停止以后的处理过程[39,41]。热缺血时间的定义为从生命支持停止或低血压(系统血压<50mmHg)或缺氧(氧饱和度<70%)至冷灌注的时间[39,41]。

风险与获益

总体上讲,DCD胰腺移植和DBD胰腺移植后发生并发症的概率相似。DCD移植后1年和5年发生排斥反应的概率为14%和19%,DBD胰腺移植后为13%和15%。移植物血栓的发生较为罕见,通常发生率为2%~6%[1,41]。如果DCD胰腺移植手术最初采用的是膀胱引流,则就后期需要转换为肠引流的概率而言,DCD胰腺移植要高于DBD胰腺移植(1年期比例分别为17%和8%,5年期分别为28%和15%)。移植后1年发生胰酶渗漏的概率为4%,且此概率在接下来的5年未见增长。DBD胰腺移植后发生胰酶渗漏的概率较高,1年期为9%,5年期超过10%。移植术后发生胰腺炎的概率两组相近,DCD胰腺移植后1年期和5年期的概率分别为9%和9%,DBD组分别为9%和14%。胰腺假性囊肿和胰腺坏死在两组中均罕见(<1%)。在移植后5年内,两组约8%~10%的患者均发生胰周脓肿。

DCD胰腺移植和DBD胰腺移植的术后功能

胰腺移植包括全器官移植和胰岛移植。全器官移植的结局已经在前文进行了讨论,以下简要讨论DCD胰岛移植的结局。

DCD胰腺和DBD胰腺全器官移植后血糖的控制情况在出院时和长期时间内均相近[1,41,43]。长期来看,两组快速血糖和糖化血红蛋白(HbA1c)的数值几乎相同。移植后1年,DBD组HbAlc为(5.43±0.75)%,DCD组为(5.63±0.57)%[1,41,43]。将单纯胰腺移植和胰-肾联合移植后患者和移植物存活率进行对比,DCD与DBD相似。当不受控的供体使用体外支持原位灌注时,患者和移植物12个月的生存率均为100%[42]。受控的DCD胰腺移植后的1、3、10年患者生存率(94%、93%、87%)与DBD组(97%、94%、79%)相近。移植的胰腺1、3、10年存活率DBD组(87%、81%、61%)较DCD组(83%、78%、63%)稍低[1]。两组的大部分患者(93%)1年内都不会出现低血糖[1]。每组约9%的患者会出现移植后糖尿病[1]。两组住院时间相同[41,43]。DCD组胰腺移植物血栓的发生率为13%,DBD组为6%。DCD器官进行肾-胰联合移植后发生移植物丢失的原因包括:出血(18%);急性排斥反应(9%);慢性排斥反应(9%)。而DBD器官进行肾-胰联合移植后发生移植物丢失的原因主要是慢性排斥反应和感染。

DCD胰岛移植的临床报道主要来自日本。8个器官中有7个移植成功,胰岛质量良好,功能正常[44]。最近,另一组来自日本的研究团队报道了34例DCD胰岛移植,其从64位供体移植到18位受体。较长的停搏前低血压和较长的冷缺血时间会对胰岛质量产生不良影响，而恢复过程中应用京都方案则会有助于提高供体胰岛质量[45]。Markmann 等报道了 1 例热缺血时间更长、胰岛数量更少的移植[46]。然而，根据日本的一项研究，18 位受体中有 16 位术后立即恢复了胰岛功能，但半数在术后 1 年内失去胰岛功能。总的来说，胰岛移植后 HbA1c 的指标有改善，所有患者最终均不再会出现低血糖[45]。

长期结果

反映 DCD 胰腺移植后长期结果的数据较少。DCD 胰腺移植后 1 年期和 5 年期移植物存活率分别为 83% 和 72%，对应的 DBD 分别为 89%和 79%（图 54.1）[41,43]。使用 DCD 进行胰-肾联合移植后 1、3、5 年移植物存活率分别为 85%、80%和 74%[39]，患者存活率分别为 98%、93%和 89%[39]。DCD 胰腺移植后 1 年和 5 年患者存活率均为 92%，其与 DBD 1 年和 5 年的存活率（分别为 97%和 89%）相近[41,43]。

DCD 肾移植

肾脏是最常行 DCD 移植的器官。因此，DCD 肾的处理经验较其他器官而言更为丰富。此外，DCD 肾也最常被用于多器官移植，包括肾-胰腺联合移植和肝-肾联合移植[2]。

接受标准

除了通用的肾脏接受标准外，不同中心对于 DCD 肾的附加选择标准不尽相同，其中一些如下所述。不受控的 DCD 肾应年龄较小（60~65 岁以下），且无肾损伤、癌症、败血症或晚期糖尿病史。热缺血时间应为 40~120 分钟。大部分不受控的 DCD 肾是在急诊室复苏失败后确定的[46,47]。

在比利时，DCD 肾捐献者的最高年龄为 75 岁；热缺血时间最长为 60 分钟；冷缺血时间由于需进行 HLA 鉴定、交叉配型和分配而常超过 24 小时。所有 DCD 肾常规经机器保存[48]。

Farney 等认为冷缺血时间低于 30 小时的 DCD 肾较为理想，应将其作为标准捐献（SCD）供体，并移植给小于 60 岁的器官受体。DCD 捐献者的禁忌证包括：入院时肾小球滤过率（GFR）<70mL/min；癌症病史；HIV 阳性；冷缺血时间>45 小时；SCD 热缺血时间>90 分钟，ECD 热缺血时间>60 分钟。机器灌注标准亦被使用，流量<60mL/min 或阻力>0.4mmHg/（mL·min）是成人 DCD 肾移植的禁忌证[49]。

我们对于 DCD 肾的要求是热缺血时间<120 分钟。然而，大多数停止生命支持的患者会在 60 分钟内死亡，其符合供体要求标准。少数超过 60 分钟的供体所需的平均时间为 75 分钟。最初，我们接受的 DCD 肾的最大年龄为 65 岁；然而最近，我们尽量避免使用 DCD 或 ECD 供体，除非其血肌酐、肌酐清除率和病史均情况理想。我们会对所有的 DCD 肾进行活检并进行 Remuzzi 评分，以检查其是否有纤维蛋白血栓。Remuzzi 评分>6 的肾脏将不能被用于移植。

风险与获益

DCD 肾移植与 DBD 肾移植都是拯救患者生命的重要治疗手段。通过使用 DCD 肾进行移植，等待期死亡率得以降低[50]。移植肾功能恢复延迟（DGF）通常被定义为肾移植后 1 星期内需要透析，其在 DCD 肾移植后更为常见。DCD 肾移植后 DGF 的发生率为 28%~57%，即使其冷缺血时间相对较短（13±5 小时），也显著高于 DBD 肾移植后的发生率（19%~21%）[1,42,43,51-55]。据报道，不受控的 DCD 肾移植后发生 DGF 的概率为 93%[46,56]，可见不受控的 DCD 肾移植发生 DGF 的概率显著高于受控的 DCD 肾[27]。DGF 的平均持续时间为（13±8）天[51]，其风险因素包括供体收缩压<60mmHg 的时间> 20 分钟；供体年龄超过 50 岁[51,52]。冷缺血时间>30 小时会导致 DGF 发生率的增加[49]。DGF 常导致住院时间延长和医疗措施的增加[41,54,57]。一项 Eurotransplant 进行的的针对成对的 DCD 肾的多中心临床研究表明，脉冲灌注保存的 DCD 肾比冷储存的 DGF 的时间更短，但两者 1 年期的移植物存活率相同，分别为 94%和 95%[57]。通过脉冲灌注保存可能确实能够减少 DGF 的时间，但该结论并未受到所有研究的支持[57,58]。DGF 并不会对移植的长期结果产生不良影响，也不会影响移植物存活率[49,54]。

DCD 肾移植后发生原发性移植物无功能的概率较低（1%~5%）[43,46,47,49,51,52]，且其与 DBD 肾移植相似[55]。术中低血压（<110/80mmHg）和低中心静脉压（<6cmH$_2$O）是发生原发性移植物无功能的危险因素[59]。

DCD 肾移植后发生排斥反应的概率与 DBD 肾移植相近或略高[1,42,54,60]，急性排斥反应发生率分别为

19%~24%和10%[42,46]。其他研究报道的数据则显示DCD肾发生排斥反应的概率较脑死亡供体肾高(29%对16%)[53]。

其他并发症的发生率在两组之间没有差异，包括肾动脉狭窄或血栓形成(<2%)、输尿管并发症(<5%)和淋巴管瘤(<10%)[1,41,43,55]。

DCD肾移植和DBD肾移植的术后功能

DCD肾移植在术后短期发生DGF的概率较DBD肾移植高,但原发性移植物无功能两组均罕见。DCD肾移植后排出的肌酐浓度较DBD高(1.9mg/dL对1.7mg/dL)[43,55]。术后7天DCD肾排出的肌酐浓度也较SCD和ECD肾高[42]。DCD肾的肌酐清除率与其他相当,为112mL/min，相比之下,SCD肾为101mL/min,ECD肾为77mL/min[42]。据报道,10年期血清肌酐水平DCD肾与DBD肾相当[47,61]。荷兰的数据显示,DCD肾移植发生移植物丢失的概率较DBD高(12%对6%),但目前尚不清楚该数据是否适用于其他地区。

长期结果

DCD肾移植和DBD肾移植后长期的移植物存活率相似(图54.1)[43,53]。即使是在移植后出现DGF的DCD肾,其移植物存活率也令人满意,1年期为88%,3年期为84%,6年期为84%[45]。DCD肾移植后精确的移植物存活率1年期为89%,3年期为76%,5年期为76%。移植物衰竭的主要原因为慢性异体移植肾病和功能死亡。排除患者死亡的影响,DCD肾移植后的精确移植物存活率1年期为93%,3年期为84%,5年期为84%。对年龄超过60岁的器官受体,其1年期和3年期移植物存活率较低,分别为79%和64%[49]。一份报告显示,DCD肾在移植1年、3年和10年后的移植物存活率分别为88%、77%和44%,而DBD肾则分别为78%、69%和42%[62]；而另外一份报告的数值则较高,DCD肾移植1年、3年、10年后的移植物存活率分别为79%、70%和62%,DBD肾则分别为83%、72%和62%[47]。其他报告还显示,移植后5、10、15年后移植物存活率没有差异[55]。

DCD肾移植和DBD肾移植后患者的生存率相同,该情况甚至可延续至移植后15年[10,17,21]。移植后精确的患者生存率1年期为93%,3年期为91%,5年期为89%[49]。这些数据与报道的DCD肾移植后1年、3年和10年的患者生存率相似，分别为92%、85%和60%[1]。败血症、心血管疾病、癌症和胃肠道出血是常见的死亡原因。对于DCD肾的受体而言,年老的受体存活率较年轻者低（1年期:81%对98%;3年期:76%对97%;5年期:69%对97%)[49]。DCD-ECD受体的生存率较DCD-SCD受体的存活率低[49]。

DCD心脏和肠移植

DCD的心脏和小肠移植目前都没有被应用于临床中。然而,随着我们从临床前期的研究中获得更多的经验,这些器官可能会在未来被应用于移植。

DCD的过程

一般来说,DCD初始过程与DBD无异(图54.2)。所有格拉斯哥昏迷评分(GCS)为5分的患者均被转至器官获取组织(OPO)。所有已决定停止生命支持的患者也均被转至OPO。随后,OPO确定供体是否适用于医疗并且评估供体是否可能在2小时的时间框架内过期。接着,使用威斯康星大学(UW)DCD评估工具进行呼吸驱动评估,该工具已得到公布和验证[63]。如果供体被给予了最大供氧量或多种血管升压药，则不执行该评估工具。我们的数据显示,当我们根据评估工具的标准决定继续获取DCD时,我们在规定时间的80%内取得器官。供体的家属往往会被告知器官捐献有可能不会发生。我们的经验是,他们会对我们表示感谢,因为我们试图实现他们所爱的人捐献器官的愿望。

我们使用的DCD肾获取的指导原则是Thomas等于英国建立的[64];常规上ICU决定是否撤下生命支持。一旦撤下生命支持的决定被执行，潜在的供体会被转至OPO,并与OPO协调员进行讨论。在ICU团队的上级成员做出撤下生命支持的决定后，以及一旦患者作为候选供体的身份被确定,捐献者的家人就会被联系。从此时起,将不再允许升级治疗手段。生命支持的停止一般以ICU通常的方式进行,并由当地实践具体决定。热缺血时间被定义为从生命支持停止到器官获取完毕的时间,允许的最长时间为2小时。ICU医生在强制停止治疗5分钟后宣布患者死亡。在捐献者的遗体被带到手术室之前,家属有额外的5分钟时间。如果家属需要更多的时间，捐献就会中止。在100位潜在捐献者中,共有 29 位实现了捐献,30%拒绝了捐献。以上过程集中了很多资源,捐献过程中涉及的人尤其需要具有责任感。该原则现已被应用于肝和胰腺移植。

在英国莱斯特,3 年内共进行了 73 例 DCD 转介,其中 64 人从急诊室转介,9 人从病房转介,有 24 人成功进行了捐献(33%),共获取 44 枚肾脏。30 枚肾脏在当地进行了移植,8 枚被运出,另有 6 枚被放弃。这些 DCD 肾构成了该中心全部移植活动的 21%。与我们的经验相同,作者认为 DCD 的处理过程涉及的人员众多,需要参与的成员具有高度的责任感[65]。

相比 DBD,DCD 的处理过程需要更多资源,无论是对 OPO 还是对医院均是如此。例如,在 56 例 DCD 肺转介中,9 例在 2 小时截止时间内没有进展,13 例需要现场评估支持,只有 9 例成功进行了移植。两位医生需要在场以在 5 分钟等待期后宣布患者死亡,ICU 的工作人员需要在 ICU 或麻醉恢复室(PACU)撤下生命支持,手术室的工作人员也应就位准备开始[11]。

医院关系

目前,美国所有的可能进行 DCD 捐献的医院均需遵守由卫生保健组织认证联合委员会(JCAHO)所制定的政策和规定。此外,DCD 捐献的过程中也必须遵循器官联合共享网络(UNOS)的指南。欧洲的实施过程与美国类似。要想世界各个国家均接受 DCD 捐献,流程可能需要进行调整,以符合当地的操作要求和风俗习惯。如上文所述,DCD 捐献的过程需要更多人力,也需要更多的 OPO 资源,因为考虑到需向尚未被宣布死亡的患者负责,流程必须经过交流和跟进。我们往往会向 DCD 捐献的案件派遣两位 OPO 协调员,以确保所有的规定

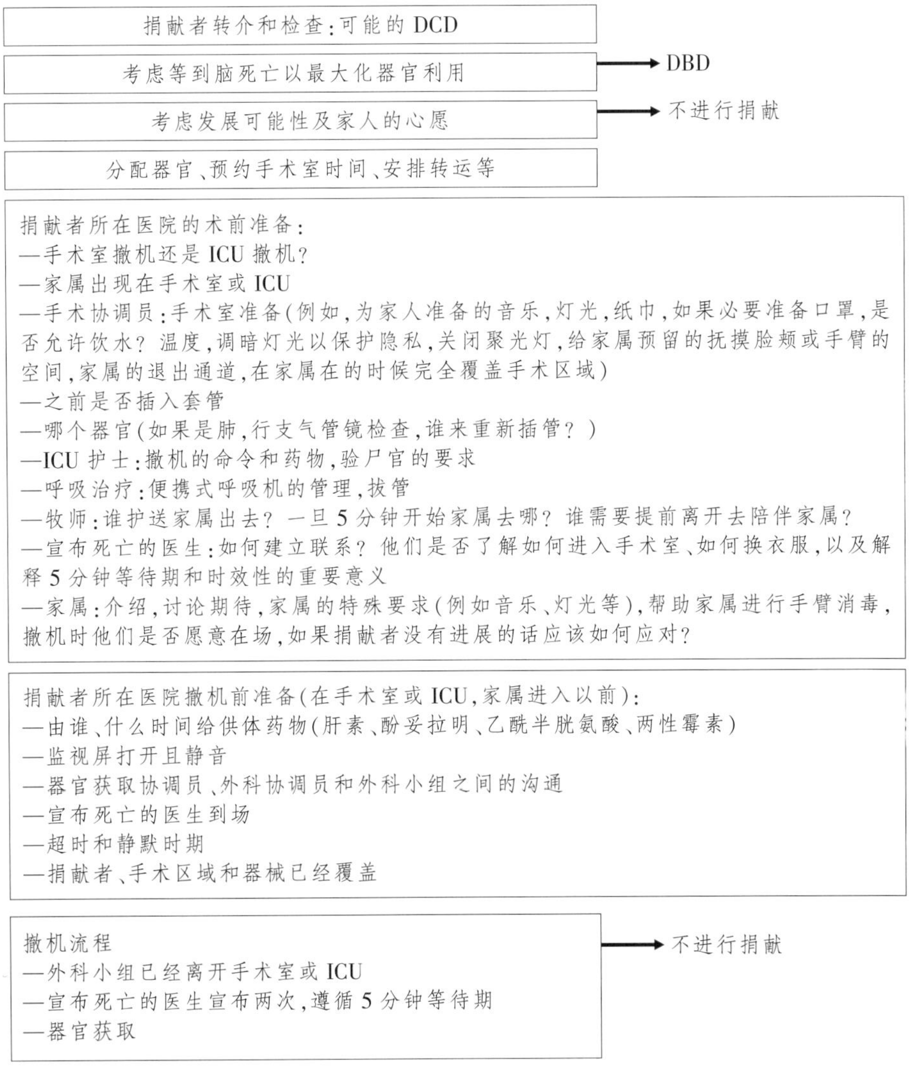

图 54.2　心脏死亡供体(DCD)的捐献流程。DBD,脑死亡供体;ICU,重症监护室。

得到遵守、家庭的需求得到满足，以及 OPO 和捐献医院的所有人员都了解他们的角色和职责。我们相信，DCD 捐献属于对患者连续的临终关爱的一部分，其为患者及其家人提供了通过捐献留下持久遗留的机会。通过照顾可能的捐献者和其家人，并提供捐献的机会，我们也为因疾病而绝望的器官候选人提供了继续生存的机会和希望。

总结

很明显，目前器官的需求量将持续超过器官供给量。因此，就尽可能满足需要移植患者的移植需求而言，额外的供体器官获得机会无疑非常重要。DCD 器官在许多情况下可作为 SCD 器官的替代物，尤其是肾移植和越来越多的肝移植中。然而，其使用需要注意风险-获益评估和适当的患者选择，以及在高度注意现有的规定与要求的前提下进行器官获取以维持整个过程专业性的敬业精神。

（彭鹏 译 高鹏骥 校）

参考文献

1. Bellingham JM, Santhanakrishnan C, Neidlinger N, et al. Donation after cardiac death: a 29-year experience. Surgery. 2011;150:692–702.
2. LaMattina JC, Mezrich JD, Fernandez LA, et al. Simultaneous liver and kidney transplantation using donation after cardiac death donors: a brief report. Liver Transplantation. 2011;17:591–595.
3. Koostra K, Daemen JHC, Oomen APA. Categories of non-heart-beating donors. Transplantation Proceedings. 1995;27(5):2893–2894.
4. Hardy JD, Webb WR, Dalton ML, et al. Lung homotransplantations in man: report of the initial case. JAMA. 1963;86:1065–1074.
5. Wijdicks EFM. The diagnosis of brain death. New England Journal of Medicine. 2001;344:1215–1221.
6. Neyrinck AP, Van De Wauwer C, Geudens N, et al. Comparative study of donor lung injury in heart-beating versus non-heart-beating donors. European Journal of Cardio-Thoracic Surgery. 2006;30(4):628–636.
7. D'Alessandro AM, Hoffmann RM, Knechtle SJ, et al. Controlled non-heart-beating donors: a potential source of extrarenal organs. Transplantation Proceedings. 1995;27(1):707–709.
8. Orens JB, Boehler A, de Perrot M, et al. A review of lung transplant donor acceptability criteria. Journal of Heart and Lung Transplantation. 2003;22(11): 1183–1200.
9. Puri V, Scavuzzo M, Guthrie T, et al. Lung transplantation and donation after cardiac death: a single center experience. Annals of Thoracic Surgery. 2009;88: 1609–1615.
10. Snell GI, Levvey BJ, Oto T, et al. Early lung transplantation success utilizing controlled donation after cardiac death donors. American Journal of Transplantation. 2008;8:1282–1289.
11. Cypel M, Sato M, Yildirim E, et al. Initial experience with lung donation after cardiocirculatory death in Canada. Journal of Heart and Lung Transplantation. 2009;28(8):753–758.
12. De Oliveira NC, Osaki S, Maloney JD, et al. Lung transplantation with donation after cardiac death donors: long-term follow up in a single center. Journal of Thoracic and Cardiovascular Surgery. 2010;139(5):1306–1315.
13. De Vleeschauwer SI, Wauters S, Dupont LJ, et al. Medium-term outcome after lung transplantation is comparable between brain-dead and cardiac-dead donors. Journal of Heart and Lung Transplantation. 2011;30(9):975–981.
14. Gomez de Antonio D, Marcos R, Laporta R, et al. Results of clinical lung transplant from uncontrolled non-heart-beating donors. Journal of Heart and Lung Transplantation. 2007;26(5):529–534.
15. Wigfield CH, Love RB. Donation after cardiac death lung transplantation outcomes. Current Opinion in Organ Transplantation 2011;16:462–468.
16. De Vleeschauwer S, Van Raemdonck D, Vandenaerde B, et al. Early outcome after lung transplantation from non-heart-beating donors is comparable to heart-beating donors. Journal of Heart and Lung Transplantation. 2009;28(4):380–387.
17. Mason DP, Thuita L, Alster JM, et al. Should lung transplantation be performed using donation after cardiac death? The United States experience. Journal of Thoracic and Cardiovascular Surgery. 2008;136(4):1061–1066.
18. Muiesan P, Girlanda R, Jassem W, et al. Single-center experience with liver transplantation from controlled non-heartbeating donors. A viable source of grafts. Annals of Surgery. 2005;242:732–738.
19. Suarez F, Otero A, Solla M, et al. Biliary complications after liver transplantation from Maastricht category-2 non-heart-beating donors. Transplantation. 2008; 85:9–14.
20. de Vera ME, Lopez-Solis R, Dvorchik I, et al. Liver transplantation using donation after cardiac death donors: long-term follow-up from a single center. American Journal of Transplantation. 2009;9:773–781.
21. Hong JC, Yersiz H, Kositamongkol P, et al. Liver transplantation using organ donation after cardiac death. Archives of Surgery. 2011;146(9):1017–1023.
22. Mathur AK, Heimbach J, Steffick DE, et al. Donation after cardiac death liver transplantation: predictors of outcome. American Journal of Transplantation. 2010;10:2512–2519.
23. Gozzini S, Perera MTPR, Mayer DA, et al. Liver transplantation in children using non-heart-beating donors. Pediatric Transplantation. 2010;14:554–557.
24. Tariciotti L, Rocha C, Perera MTPR, et al. Is it time to extend liver acceptance criteria for controlled donors after cardiac death? Transplantation. 2011; 92(10):1140–1146.
25. Jay C, Ladner D, Wang E, et al. A comprehensive risk assessment of mortality following donation after cardiac death liver transplant – An analysis of the national registry. Journal of Hepatology. 2011;55:808–813.
26. Quintela J, Gala B, Baarmonde I, et al. Long-term results for liver transplantation from non-heart-beating donors maintained with chest and abdominal compression-decompression. Transplantation Proceedings. 2005;37:3857–3858.
27. Dominguez-Gil B, Haase-Kromwijk B, Van Leiden H, et al. Current situation of donation after circulatory death in European countries. Transplant International. 2011;24:676–686.
28. Jay CL, Lyuksemburg V, Kang R, et al. The increased costs of donation after cardiac death liver transplantation. Caveat emptor. Annals of Surgery. 2010;251: 743–748.
29. Monbaliu D, Pirenne J, Talbot D. Liver transplantation using donation after cardiac death donors. Journal of Hepatology. 2012;56(2):474–485.
30. Foley DP, Fernandez LA, Leverson G, et al. Biliary complications after liver transplantation from donation after cardia death donors: an analysis of risk factors and long term outcomes from a single center. Annals of Surgery. 2011;253(4):817–825.
31. Jay CL, Lyuksemburg V, Ladner DP, et al. Ischemic cholangiopathy after controlled donation after cardiac death liver transplantation. A meta-analysis. Annals of Surgery. 2011;253:259–264.
32. Abt P, Crawford M, Desai N, et al. Liver transplantation from controlled non-heart-beating donors: an increased incidence of biliary complications. Transplantation. 2008;75:1659–1663.
33. Taner CB, Bulatao IG, Willingham DL, et al. Events in procurement as risk factors for ischemic cholangiopathy in liver transplantation using donation after cardiac death donors. Liver Transplantation. 2012;18(1):100–111.
34. Foley DP, Fernandez LA, Leverson G, et al. Donation after cardiac death. The University of Wisconsin Experience with liver transplantation. Annals of Surgery. 2005;242:734–731.
35. Yamamoto S, Wilczek HE, Duraj FF, et al. Liver transplantation with grafts from controlled donors after cardiac death: a 20-year follow-up at a single center. American Journal of Transplantation. 2010;10:602–611.
36. Hashimoto K, Eghtesad B, Gunasekaran G, et al. Use of tissue plasminogen activator in liver transplantation from donation after cardiac death donors. American Journal of Transplantation. 2010;10:2665–2672.
37. Kaczmarek B, Manas MD, Jacques BC, et al. Ischemic cholangiopathy after liver transplantation from controlled non-heart-beating donors – A single-center experience. Transplantation Proceedings. 2007;39:2793–2795.
38. Hernandez-Alejandro R, Croome KP, Quan D, et al. Increased risk of severe recurrence of hepatitis C virus in liver transplant recipients of donation after cardiac death allografts. Transplantation. 2011;92:686–689.
39. Salvalaggio PR, Davies DB, Fernandez LA, et al. Outcomes of pancreas transplantation in the United States using cardiac-death donors. American Journal of Transplantation. 2006;6:1059–1065.
40. Suh N, Ryan B, Allen R, et al. Simultaneous pancreas and kidney transplantation

from organ donation after cardiac death. ANZ Journal of Surgery. 2009;79: 245–246.
41. Fernandez LA, Di Carlo A, Odorico JS, et al. Simultaneous pancreas-kidney transplantation from donation after cardiac death. Successful long-term outcomes. Annals of Surgery. 2005;242:716–723.
42. Farney AC, Singh RP, Hines MH, et al. Experience in renal and extrarenal transplantation with donation after cardiac death donors with selective use of extracorporeal support. Journal of the American College of Surgeons. 2008;208(5):1028–1037.
43. D'Alessandro AM, Fernandez LA, Chin LT, et al. Donation after cardiac death: the University of Wisconsin Experience. Annals of Transplantation. 2004;9:68–71.
44. Nagata H, Matsumoto S, Okitsu T, et al. Procurement of the human pancreas for pancreatic islet transplantation from marginal cadaver donors. Transplantation. 2006;82:327–331.
45. Saito T, Gotoh M, Satomi S, et al. Islet transplantation using donors after cardiac death: report of the Japan Islet Transplantation Registry. Transplantation. 2010;90:740–747.
46. Markmann JF, Deng S, Desai NM, et al. The use of non-heart-beating donors for isolated pancreatic islet transplantation. Transplantation. 2008;75:1423–1429.
47. Alonso A, Fernandez-Rivera C, Villaverde P, et al. Renal transplantation from non-heart-beating donors: a single-center 10-year experience. Transplantation Proceedings. 2005;37:3658–3660.
48. Renkens JJM, Rouflat MMJ, Christiaans MHL, et al. Outcome of nonheart-beating donor kidneys with prolonged delayed graft function after transplantation. American Journal of Transplantation. 2005;5:2704–2709.
49. Farney AC, Hines MH, al-Geizawi S, et al. Lessons learned from a single center's experience with 134 donation after cardiac death donor kidney transplants. Journal of the American College of Surgeons. 2011;212(4):440–451.
50. Snoijis MG, Schaubel DE, Hene R, et al. Kidneys from donors after cardiac death provide survival benefit. Journal of the American Society of Nephrology. 2010;21:1015–1021.
51. Ho KJ, Owens CD, Johnson SR, et al. Donor postextubation hypotension and age correlate with outcome after donation after cardiac death transplantation. Transplantation. 2008;85:1588–1594.
52. Locke JE, Segev DL, Warren DS, et al. Outcomes of kidneys from donors after cardiac death: implications for allocation and preservation. American Journal of Transplantation. 2007;7:1797–1807.
53. Singh RP, Farney AC, Rogers J, et al. Kidney transplantation from donation after cardiac death donors: lack of impact on delayed graft function on post-transplant outcomes. Clinical Transplantation. 2011;25:255–264.
54. Saidi RF, Elias N, Kawai T, et al. Outcome of kidney transplantation using expanded criteria donors and donation after cardiac death kidneys: realities and costs. American Journal of Transplantation. 2007;7:2769–2774.
55. Cooper JT, Chin LT, Krieger NR, et al. Donation after cardiac death: the University of Wisconsin Experience with renal transplantation. American Journal of Transplantation. 2004;4:1490–1494.
56. Renkens JJ, Roufflart MMJ, Christiaans MHL, et al. Outcome of nonheart-beating donor kidneys with prolonged delayed graft function after transplantation. American Journal of Transplantation. 2005;5:2704–2709.
57. Jochmans I, Moers C, Smits JM, et al. Machine perfusion versus cold storage for the preservation of kidneys donated after cardiac death. Annals of Surgery. 2010;252:756–764.
58. Watson CJE, Wells AC, Roberts RJ, et al. Cold machine perfusion versus static cold storage of kidneys donated after cardiac death: a UK multicenter randomized controlled trial. American Journal of Transplantation. 2010;10:1991–1999.
59. Snoeijs MGJ, Wiermans B, Christiaans MH, et al. Recipient hemodynamics during non-heart-beating donor kidney transplantation are major predictors of primary nonfunction. American Journal of Transplantation. 2007;7:1158–1166.
60. Bains JC, Sandford RM, Brook NR, et al. Comparison of renal allograft fibrosis after transplantation from heart-beating and non-heart-beating donors. British Journal of Surgery. 2005;92:113–118.
61. Brook NR, White SA, Waller JR, et al. Non-heart beating donor kidneys with delayed graft function have superior graft survival compared with conventional heart-beating donor kidneys that develop delayed graft function. American Journal of Transplantation. 2003;3:614–618.
62. Casavilla A, Ramirez C, Shapiro R, et al. Experience with liver and kidney allografts from non-heart-beating donors. Transplantation. 1995;59(2): 197–203.
63. Lewis J, Peltier J, Nelson H, et al. Development of the University of Wisconsin donation after cardiac death evaluation tool. Progress in Transplantation. 2003;13:265–273.
64. Thomas I, Caborn S, Manara AR. Experiences in the development of non-heart beating organ donation scheme in a regional neurosciences intensive care unit. British Journal of Anaesthesia. 2008;100(6):820–826.
65. Nicholson ML, Dunlop P, Doughman TM, et al. Work-load generated by the establishment of a non-heart beating kidney transplant programme. Transplant International. 1996;9(6):603–609.
66. Chamorro C, Aparicio M, Marmisa G, et al. Organ transplantation in the Madrid Autonomous Region. Transplantation Proceedings. 2009;41:2302–2303.
67. Nunez JR, Del Rio F, Lopez E, et al. Non-heart-beating donors: an excellent choice to increase the donor pool. Transplantation Proceedings. 2005;37:3651–3654.
68. Dubbeld J, Hoekstra H, Farid W, et al. Similar liver transplantation survival with selected cardiac death donors and brain death donors. British Journal of Surgery. 2010;87:744–753.
69. Fondevila C, Hessheimer AJ, Ruiz A, et al. Liver transplant using donors after unexpected cardiac death: novel preservation protocol and acceptance criteria. American Journal of Transplantation. 2007;7:1949–1955.
70. Ho KJ, Owens CD, Johnson SR, et al. Donor postextubation hypotension and age correlate with outcome after donation after cardiac death transplantation. Transplantation. 2008;85:1588–1594.

第 5 篇

移植手术步骤和外科技术

第 55 章 肾移植手术步骤和外科技术

Paul L. Tso, Thomas C. Pearson

引言

正如诺贝尔奖得主 Joseph Murray 博士在他的获奖致辞[1]中所说,手术技术的进步,对免疫屏障理解的加深和解决方案的进展，以及开发肾脏替代治疗来支持肾衰竭患者，三者互相促进，使临床肾移植大获成功。外科手术决断是非常重要的一个环节,大批外科先驱者在实践中对移植手术的技术进行了发展和完善。影像技术、经皮内镜以及微创手术的最新进展也促进了移植后并发症的识别和管理的重大进步，这些并发症以往通常需要重新手术，同时具有更高的潜在发病率、死亡率和器官丢失的风险。目前大多数人对于肾移植是终末期肾脏疾病患者的最佳疗法已达成共识。本章将重点介绍移植手术技术以及术后并发症管理。

术前注意事项

入院进行肾移植前,需详细采集受体病史,并进行体格检查，以发现自上次评估以来影响患者健康或手术步骤的任何明显的间隔事件或体格检查结果。需要特别注意的问题包括过敏、感染和心血管储备功能的变化(参见第 37 章,其中涉及肾脏移植清单管理)。完善实验室和影像学检查、心脏功能检测、术前咨询和心理评估,以确保患者是合适的移植受体候选人,且能够耐受手术和长期的免疫抑制治疗。如第 89 章所述,需确认受体和供体器官之间的 ABO 和 HLA 相容性。检查供体肾的信息以确认器官质量（器官选择标准在第 53 章中详细讨论)。必须从患者或责任方获得知情同意。

在进行手术准备时，手术团队切皮之前应在麻醉和护理人员的指导下确认输液加热装置、静脉血栓栓塞预防设备、血液制品、术前抗生素和术中药物(包括免疫抑制剂)。对于周围静脉不畅或需侵入性血流动力学监测的患者,可留置中心静脉通路。同样,动脉导管也可以更密切地监测血压或进行频繁的血液采样。手术在全身麻醉下进行,患者取仰卧位。膀胱或输尿管内留置导管。可在输尿管重建时轻轻滴注无菌抗生素溶液(含或不含亚甲蓝)以便在手术区确定膀胱位置。需要对既往有前列腺或尿道原发病,或既往手术史,或长期无尿的萎缩性膀胱患者进行特别护理，以免在导管插入时造成医源性损伤，如形成假尿道或在灌注期间膀胱破裂。作者倾向于通过重力引流扩张膀胱,可防止萎缩性膀胱破裂，并且可了解受体膀胱的容量及其对输尿管重建的影响。

移植肾制备

肾同种异体移植物的制备在受体手术之前或与受体手术同时进行。如果担心创伤、手术损伤或异常解剖结构可能使供体器官不适合移植，在受体进入手术室之前,外科医生必须进行仔细检查。若为死亡供体的器官,主动脉 Carrel 瓣通常保留在肾动脉上,以便于更大的、技术上要求更低的血管吻合,而不涉及肾动脉口。尤其对于具有小动脉的小儿供肾[2],可减轻因吻合口导致受体和器官生长受限的影响。

多动脉较为常见,这种情况下存在多个重建选择。可牺牲小的副动脉(特别是上极)而不会产生负面影响,但要注意保存重要的辅助血管,特别是供应下极的可能对输尿管灌注至关重要的辅助血管[2,3]。多个动脉可以保留或重建在共同的主动脉 Carrel 瓣上，以便于和受体的单根动脉吻合[4,5]。相反的,根据具体情况也可以多支肾动脉分别与受体血管吻合，这样可防止临近肾静脉的张力过大、成角或压迫[3]。供体主动脉的动脉粥样硬化或肾动脉口处的动脉粥样硬化疾病可能使动脉瓣不适合使用,在这种情况下,动脉在相对无疾病且适于吻合的部位横切。在活体供体肾脏或没有合适的主动脉瓣的情况下,多个动脉可以被调配和缝合在一起形成“裤子”形状[4]以便与受体单一动脉吻合。或者也可以采用端-侧吻合方式[3]将副动脉缝合到主要动脉,或者可以将多个血管重建为由 PFTE 或自体组织形成的 Carrel 瓣(如果可用),以便于和受体血管吻合。性腺静脉、腰静脉和肾上腺静脉至肾静脉可夹闭或者用丝线结扎。因肾静脉通常有侧支连通,故小的附属肾静脉可结扎。然而,如果存在两条口径相同的主要肾脏静脉,必须保留以降低静脉血栓形成和梗死的风险[2]。死亡供体右肾移植最佳地呈现了一个完整的腔静脉腔,可以使用缝合线或吻合器形成血管导管,以有效增加肾静脉的长度[2,5]。这使得静脉吻合在技术上难度更低,并降低了撕裂脆弱的右肾静脉的可能性。同种异体移植物中的淋巴结构被认为是移植后淋巴漏和由此产生的囊状淋巴管瘤的潜在原因[3,6],因此,在后台手术分离时若发现淋巴管应仔细结扎或夹闭。注意保持足够的输尿管周围组织并保留由输尿管和肾下极(“金三角”)所界定的肾周脂肪,以减少输尿管局部缺血的可能性,这可能导致术后的尿漏或狭窄[7,8]。图 55.1 和图 55.2 分别显示了典型的左肾的和右肾重建和位置(包括腔静脉导管)。

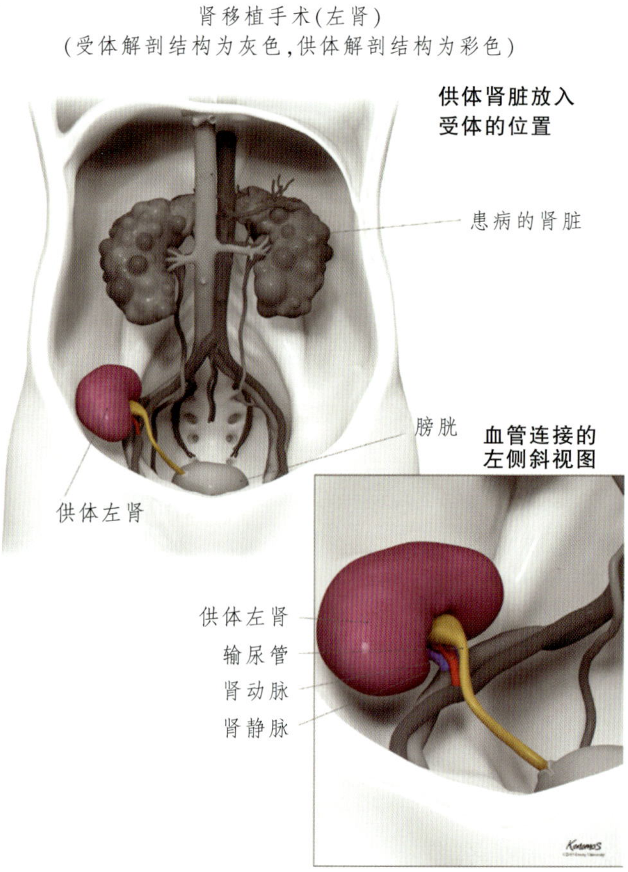

图 55.1 将左肾同种异体移植物放置在右髂窝中。这是目前为止最常见的放置方向,因为大多数活体供体肾脏是左肾(有较长的左肾静脉)。显示了肾动脉和肾静脉分别与髂外动脉和髂外静脉的典型关系。输尿管吻合术是标准的 Lich 型膀胱外输尿管膀胱吻合术。注意,当使用来自对侧的肾脏时,集合系统是内侧/前侧的,以便于在有输尿管并发症的情况下进入输尿管和集合系统。髂静脉已被横向移动以适应吻合后静脉的直接位置。

切口和显露

通常,进行斜 Gibson 切口[4]或 J 形“曲棍球球棍”形[5]右下切口,显露腹膜外结构,暴露髂外动脉和髂外静脉以备血管吻合。腹壁浅下血管和女性的圆韧带通常被结扎和分离以方便显露[5]。如果是近期同侧上腹壁血管被切断或分离(如同时进行肝移植或近期有肋缘下切口),一些外科医生建议保留腹壁下血管以避免急性腹直肌缺血。如果在后台准备时发现供体肾脏有需要保留的小的分支附属动脉或动脉分支,则可以保留或分离腹壁下动脉作为血管吻合的备选方案[2,9]。在暴露血管的过程中,要有意识地结扎、夹闭或烧灼淋巴管或淋巴结以避免淋巴漏和随后淋巴囊肿的形成[2,3,10]。

如图 55.1 和图 55.2 所示,由于右髂外血管的相对表浅和外科医生的右手优势,肾脏通常被移植到受体的右髂外血管。如果右侧被预留用于胰腺同种异体移植,或者右侧存在先前的移植物,或者右侧解剖结构不适合,则可以基于外科医生偏好来利用左外髂血管[5]。有部分外科医生主张对侧放置同种异体移植物(即右供体肾脏到受体左下象限,反之亦然),这样移植肾的肾盂和输尿管位于内侧,可以方便随后可能的尿道修复[2,4]。一般来说,髂外静脉位于髂外动脉的后方,如图 55.1 和图 55.2 所示,也可以有从外侧到内侧的变化,以适应肾静脉吻合的自然位置,对侧移植有利于髂静脉的侧向化,同侧移植有利于静脉的内侧化。如果双侧髂外血管先前已被利用,随后的移植通常通过下中线切口经腹膜进行,以便在必要时评估和接近髂血管近端或主动脉和下腔静脉用于吻合[5]。既往下肢深静脉血栓形成或血液透析的病史应进行术前成像以评估潜在的髂静脉狭窄或阻塞或者腔静脉狭窄或阻塞,以确定是否需要干预和影响同种异体移植静脉流出道的选择。如果可能,通常避

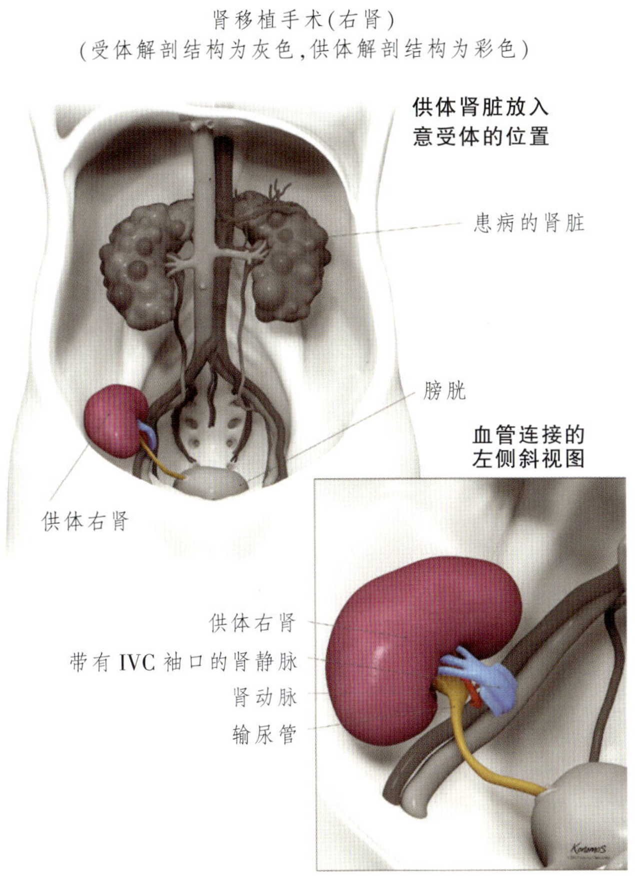

图 55.2 右肾同种异体移植物放置在右髂窝中。图中显示肾动脉和肾静脉分别与髂外动脉和髂外静脉的典型关系。输尿管吻合术是标准的 Lich 型膀胱外输尿管膀胱吻合术。注意,当使用来自同侧的肾脏时,集合系统是侧向/后向的,在发生输尿管并发症的情况下会阻碍进入输尿管和集合系统。髂静脉已经被移动到内侧以适应静脉的直接吻合位置。右肾静脉常常较短。在这种情况下,图中显示了通过吻合器穿过肾上和肾下供体腔静脉并且使用供体的左肾静脉口作为端-侧静脉吻合的最终部位而形成的腔静脉导管。

免与活动性大腿动静脉瘘同侧的移植,因为担心潜在的血管并发症,例如影响移植功能的静脉高血压。对于肾静脉过短、受体骨盆较深或垂直走行的髂静脉,髂内静脉的结扎和分离可增加髂总静脉和髂外静脉的移动性,方便吻合[2,5]。

血运重建

在吻合血管闭塞期间,部分中心使用系全身素化方法进行吻合[2,4],但该方法没有普遍实行。小心施加血管夹以获得髂血管的近端和远端血流控制。同种异体移植肾静脉通常使用细(通常为 5-0)聚丙烯缝线以端-侧吻合方式缝合到受体髂外静脉。在用细剪刀或血管穿孔机切开动脉后,通常使用细(5-0 或 6-0)聚丙烯缝合线以端-侧吻合方式将肾动脉吻合到髂外动脉。另一种选择是以端-端吻合方式将肾动脉缝合到受体髂内动脉[2]。在涉及供体多条肾动脉的情况下,可以同时利用髂外动脉和髂内动脉进行吻合[5]。如果利用髂内动脉,在其起始点应仔细检查有无动脉粥样硬化疾病,是否有危及同种异体移植灌注的风险。如果对侧髂内动脉由于阳痿、跛行或其他血管并发症的可能性增加已被分开,则不应使用髂内动脉吻合[3,4]。在处理和缝合患病的受体和供体血管时必须小心,以避免产生内膜瓣或内膜分离。小儿肾移植血管吻合应采用全部间断缝合或至少部分间断吻合术[2]以允许横截面积随时间增长。

完成血管吻合后,释放血管夹以恢复下肢流入和流出血流,以及新的血管化的肾脏血流。仔细止血。理想状态应是肾脏迅速呈现健康的粉红色、适度的充盈张力和新尿的产生。需警惕早期灌注不良。多数是由于保存时间过长或其他捐献因素,这预示移植物功能恢复缓慢或延迟。受体血流动力学或血管加压药的使用也可能在初始低灌注中起作用。在这些情况下,随着受体血流动力学和灌注被优化并且移植物血管痉挛解除,移植器官的外观往往在随后的几分钟内得到改善。若移植物出现异常搏动,而非典型的动脉搏动,表明可能有静脉流出道阻塞。如果对血管吻合手术过程存在怀疑,如血管扭曲、血栓形成、栓塞、牵开器引起血管闭塞、限流解剖(特别是在先前放置的血管夹部位)或有缺陷的缝合线,可采用手持多普勒探头检查,以便快速确认血管和肾实质中是否存在血流。如果有必要消除技术错误或血栓栓塞事件的可能性,应该有一个低阈值用于减少血管吻合。在其他复杂程序可能导致长期热缺血的情况下,最好用冷灌洗液重新冲洗肾脏,并在后台进行任何必要的技术上要求的重建,包括重建吻合口,最终确定性地建立血管通畅性。

尿路重建

在获得满意的移植物血流灌注后,下一步的关键是手术中的尿路引流。重建的类型取决于供体输尿管的长度和质量,以及受体输尿管和膀胱的状况。通常行 Lich 型膀胱外输尿管膀胱吻合术或其改进型术式(图 55.3)。与经典的 Ledbetter-Politano 经膀胱吻合术不同，膀胱外 Lich 术式不需要额外切开膀胱和长的供体输尿管。因此，后者手术时间更短，以及输尿管缺血、阻塞、血尿和尿液渗漏的发生率更低[2,8,11,12]。移植输尿管通常位于精索后方以防止精索的潜在隆起和阻塞[2]。一般来说，这也是很容易实现的，但精索分离以促进输尿管膀胱吻合在大多数情况下不会产生持久的不良后果。修剪输尿管至适当的长度并且进行调节以允许对膀胱无张力吻合。应仔细检查其远端的灌注情况，以减少缺血导致输尿管狭窄或尿漏的可能性。通过 Foley 导管灌注的亚甲蓝染料灌洗有助于在行膀胱切开术时明确膀胱位置。特别是在肥胖患者和腹膜透析患者中，腹膜可能被误认为膀胱，从而导致输尿管腹膜吻合的发生，在膀胱转移过程中应考虑到这一并发症并始终避免其发生。黏膜对黏膜输尿管膀胱吻合术通常以连续方式用细的可吸收单丝缝合线(通常为 5-0 PDS)缝合(图 55.3)。可吸收缝合线的使用对于避免持续的膀胱内异物很重要，这是结石形成和尿道感染的始动因素。根据外科医生的偏好常规使用或选择性地使用双 J 形输尿管支架。如果在吻合术完成之前存在对输尿管膀胱吻合术(或其他尿道重建)完整性的担心，可选择性使用。常规预防性输尿管支架术的应用并未普遍实施，但多项随机对照研究和病例系列的 Meta 分析发现，带有支架置入的膀胱外输尿管膀胱吻合术的肾移植患者泌尿系统的并发症发生率明显低于行非支架置入的吻合术患者[13]。通常，膀胱逼尿肌的肌肉组织在黏膜对黏膜吻合术中被重新接近(图 55.3)，以提供潜在的抗反流机制[5,9]，并且当膀胱膨胀时防止在吻合上的过度张力。注意避免产生可能导致阻塞的过紧隧道。

输尿管膀胱吻合术可以在出现需要修整的尿路引流并发症时使用自体输尿管。在受体膀胱极度萎缩、不可接近或者不适合于吻合的情况下，行输尿管输尿管吻合术可能是更好的选择的。如果供体输尿管缺血或

输尿管吻合术

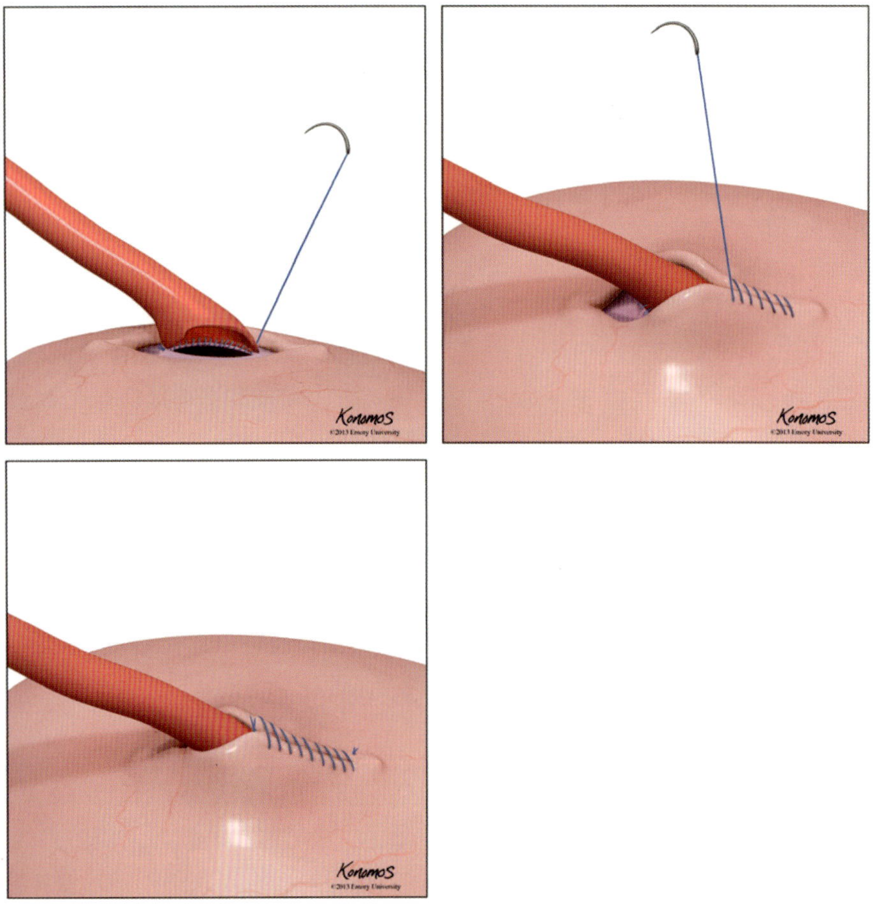

图 55.3 Lich 型输尿管膀胱吻合术。这是重建最常用的方法。在分离膀胱肌肉显露膀胱黏膜后，使用细的(5-0)可吸收缝线(如 PDS)吻合输尿管和膀胱黏膜。这种吻合在近似肌肉覆盖下形成抗反流解剖结构。一些中心留置支架(图中未显示)。

被认为不可用,可行输尿管肾盂吻合术。在准备吻合过程中,必须注意保持足够的血液供应给自体输尿管,以减少随后渗漏或狭窄的发生率。涉及自体输尿管的吻合往往在技术上要求很高,且通常留置支架进行。如果供体和受体输尿管都不适合使用,则肾盂造口术可作为一种选择。为了使膀胱和较短的输尿管或肾盂在没有张力的情况下接近,可能需要移动膀胱并行下段输尿管再建术或膀胱瓣输尿管成形术[2]。如果发现供体肾具有双输尿管,可以进行两个单独的输尿管膀胱吻合术。如果输尿管非常接近或者膀胱不适于行膀胱再次切开术,则倾向于用可吸收缝线将输尿管的内侧壁缝合一起,然后与膀胱进行单一吻合。如果受体有膀胱增大或因肠或胃产生导尿管的病史,必须充分预期导尿。还需要考虑的重要因素包括选择合适的受体组织来吻合移植输尿管、受体术后器官的血液供应情况,以及受体的哪一侧放置肾脏。一般来说,复杂的尿路重建过程是通过保护性的留置输尿管支架进行的。

关腹

腹壁闭合相对较少受到关注,但它也是手术的一个重要组成部分,可能影响长期效果。移植物的位置应避免血管或输尿管的明显扭曲、扭结或阻塞。某些情况下受体的腹膜外空间相对较小,关闭筋膜可能影响同种异体移植物灌注,此种情况可广泛地打开腹膜。手术时并不常规放置引流管,但如果对移植物周围血液、淋巴液或尿液高度担忧[2,4,9]可考虑使用引流管。

特殊情况

小儿受体

对于小儿受体,用于移植的暴露量和血管大小因患者的不同而不同。体重为 15~20kg 的受体最好选用腹部正中线切口,分离右结肠,以便靠近近端髂血管、远端主动脉和下腔静脉进行血管吻合[14,15]。手术完成后,肾脏位于腰肌上,将升结肠放回肾脏的前表面[2,5]。随着受体成长,切口应该可以选择常见的髂骨血管、主动脉或腔静脉。如果血管吻合的管腔受到儿童脉管系统小尺寸的限制,建议用间断缝合或者至少部分间断缝合,以使其与儿童一起生长并避免将来的相对狭窄[2]。

小儿整体供肾

小儿肾脏因为太小而不能作为单个肾脏移植,因此小儿整体供肾作为一个单位吻合在供体主动脉和腔静脉上。小儿血管吻合对于经验丰富的外科医生来说不是问题。但受体和肾脏生长时,原血管吻合口不太可能扩大并补偿性生长。经验表明,当整体植入而不是单独植入时,小于 15~20kg 供者的肾脏长期效果更好。通常,整体供体的主动脉和腔静脉肾上端血管闭合,主动脉和下腔静脉的肾下端血管以端-侧吻合方式缝合到受体外髂血管[2]。输尿管可以单独地植入膀胱中,或者它们可以是成型后缝合在一起。也有人报道可将整体供肾血管插入受体髂血管[16]。如果血管吻合的横截面积由于供体血管的小口径而受到限制,则应当考虑中断至少一侧吻合口,以允许移植物的生长而扩张吻合口[2]。

成人双肾移植

成人双肾移植即将边缘肾功能的死亡成年供体的两个肾放置到单个受体中,最近已经发展为一种手术方法,即将具有边缘肾单位的供体(通常来自扩大标准供体)用于需要大量透析的患者。这是对器官短缺的一种反应,并可延长移植等待时间[17]。在这个过程中,双供体肾的移植可以利用右侧和左侧受体髂骨血管通过下腹中线切口通过腹膜外或腹膜后途径或通过双侧下象限切口进行手术[18,19]。最近报道的通过 Gibson 切口将两个移植物植入同一髂窝的双肾移植技术数量和经验均有所增加。与经典的双侧双肾移植相比,这种方式可减少手术时间和创伤,并且如果需要,可使对侧髂窝完好无损,用于将来的肾移植[20]。这种方法的结果没有明确确立其优于单肾移植的好处,但是使用“两个为一个”的移植在一些中心一直具有直观的吸引力。

术后早期管理

术后立即放置 Foley 导管,常规保留 2~4 天用于膀胱减压。对于吻合困难或者存在膀胱功能障碍的非顺应性患者,新吻合的导管可能会承受过高的排尿压力,因此导尿管可能会保留较长时间。如果担心潜在的尿漏,可以在拔除导管前进行膀胱造影以明确有无外渗。输尿管支架在一些情况下与留置导尿管相连,手术后早期拔除导尿管时一并拔除。这种情况应在移植后的最初几个月内常规用膀胱镜去除。引流量降低到可接受的水平时可将引流管拔除,若有持续高渗出,应分析肌酐水平,以评估潜在的尿漏。

技术性并发症

手术技术的进步已大大降低肾移植相关的技术性并发症的发生率。肾移植后的技术相关并发症发生率远低于肝脏移植或胰腺移植。免疫抑制治疗的改善也使得急性和慢性排斥反应引起的移植物丢失减少。因此手术并发症仍然是移植后移植物丢失的相对重要的原因[21]。

早期术后问题

与其他主要腹部手术一样,存在早期术后出血的可能性,如果存在任何出血相关的典型症状和体征,如心动过速、低血压、少尿、过度疼痛、压痛、腹胀或手术部位肿块应怀疑存在出血可能。实验室检查通常会显示血红蛋白和血细胞压积降低,但急性出血早期不一定出现。因此出血主要依靠临床诊断,在血流动力学不稳定的任何情况下首先考虑出血。可能出血来源包括血管吻合口、移植物本身,如肾门或活检部位未控制的血管,或受体手术部位,如腹膜后脂肪或腹壁肌肉组织中的破裂血管。出血通常是自限性的,不会损害移植物功能,可通过保守治疗控制。但是,持续的血流动力学不稳定、持续的输血需求或由于移植物外压导致的移植物损害,则反映为明显或持续的出血,需考虑返回手术室治疗。通常,再次手术不能确定活动性出血源,但再次手术可去除血肿压迫以减轻移植物、血管和输尿管的压迫,并且去除潜在脓毒性并发症的介质。在移植物功能较差的情况下,还能检查移植物及其吻合口的完整性,并获得活检的机会。一般来说,再探查远远优于引流或大量不排血肿的长期后果。

突发的少尿或无尿在术后早期要排除血管问题,如下述的同种异体移植血栓形成,同时还应仔细评估排尿系统以诊断和治疗相对常见的机械性问题,如因扭结、移位或凝块引起的导管堵塞。导尿管堵塞患者常抱怨膀胱胀满。因此任何抱怨膀胱胀满或疼痛的患者应检查其导管通畅性。在术后早期经常发现血尿,这通常是自限性的,一般在没有干预的情况下可自行缓解。虽然经常出现肉眼血性引流,但通常不会导致大量失血或需要输血。由于凝块形成,血尿会更常见,这阻碍了尿液在导管中的流动,因此可能对新产生的输尿管吻合口造成压力。凝块通常可通过用无菌水或生理盐水灌洗 Foley 导管来进行处理。在某些情况下,可能需要更换或扩大导尿管的尺寸。在移植后的早期,尽量避免膀胱镜检查、侵入性膀胱灌洗,或不受监控的持续膀胱灌洗系统,这可能导致输尿管膀胱吻合口破裂[22]。

血管并发症

约 15%的肾移植术后患者发生血管并发症,并可能导致显著的发病率[23,24]。其包括各种复杂的问题,如同种异体移植物动脉或静脉血栓形成、移植肾动脉狭窄(TRAS)、动脉夹层、动静脉瘘和假性动脉瘤。

同种异体移植物血栓形成

约 2%的肾移植会发生早期移植物血栓形成[3,25,26],据报道,超过 1/4 的同种异体肾移植在 1 年内发生移植物丢失[27]。它通常发生在移植后 10 天内[21,26]。血栓形成的临床特征包括突发无尿、功能丧失或原发性器官无功能。受体自身肾功能检测困难,因为自体尿排出还在继续。静脉血栓更为常见,可表现为移植物肿胀变软,偶发移植物破裂[3,21,27,28]。动脉血栓形成更为隐蔽,通常无痛或无移植物肿胀[3,27]。随着病情进展,动脉和静脉都可能存在血栓形成,其起源部位可能无法辨别[27]。

唯一能够确定及时排除血栓形成以挽救肾脏的干预措施是再次探查手术。因此,任何关于动脉或静脉血栓形成的可能都应高度重视,并于评估初期与主治医生讨论是否行探查手术。若存在血栓形成的典型表现(例如在没有导管故障证据的情况下突发无尿)应立即行探查手术,而不需要额外的诊断操作。肾血栓形成后的抢救时间非常短暂,只有 1~2 小时,而确认诊断的时间通常会导致移植物丢失。

当对移植物血管通畅性存在疑问时,首选多普勒超声检查。移植肾的相对位置表浅以及正常血液流动使其有利于超声扫描。超声检查简单、快速、便携、成本低,并能避免电离辐射和肾毒性。超声技术对于诊断血管血栓形成非常准确,但是检查延迟或解读结果延迟会使其诊断能力打折扣。因此,对于怀疑血管并发症行超声检查应视为紧急程序。图 55.4 显示了正常和异常流动波的示例。

肾静脉血栓形成的超声表现通常包括肾脏水肿和

静脉血流减少。充盈缺损很少在静脉中见到。重要的是，完全静脉血栓形成患者可有动脉波形，因此动脉“流动”并不排除静脉阻塞。由于流出道阻塞，动脉波形显示具有舒张反转的高阻力指数。正确的动脉波形应伴有连续的舒张血流（图 55.4），在没有舒张血流的情况下，应考虑静脉血栓形成，并且行二次探查手术。肾动脉血栓形成时移植物充盈不佳而体积较小，且肾动脉无血流[23]。当同种异体移植物发生动脉或静脉血栓形成时，紧急手术探查取栓或导管溶栓是血栓发生后挽救移植物的唯一有效手段，但大多数情况下器官还是会丢失[21]。

导管溶栓治疗在治疗同种异体移植物血栓形成方面是成功的[29]，但因吻合口出血风险相对高，在移植术后前几周禁止应用[23,24,29]。可能仅肾动脉的分支或多个肾动脉中的一支会发生血栓形成、肾楔形缺血或输尿管缺血。这种情况临床表现不典型，如肾功能受损、高血压或尿漏[21]。同种异体移植物血栓形成的潜在技术原因包括内膜剥离、血管扭曲或扭结或缝合不佳导致

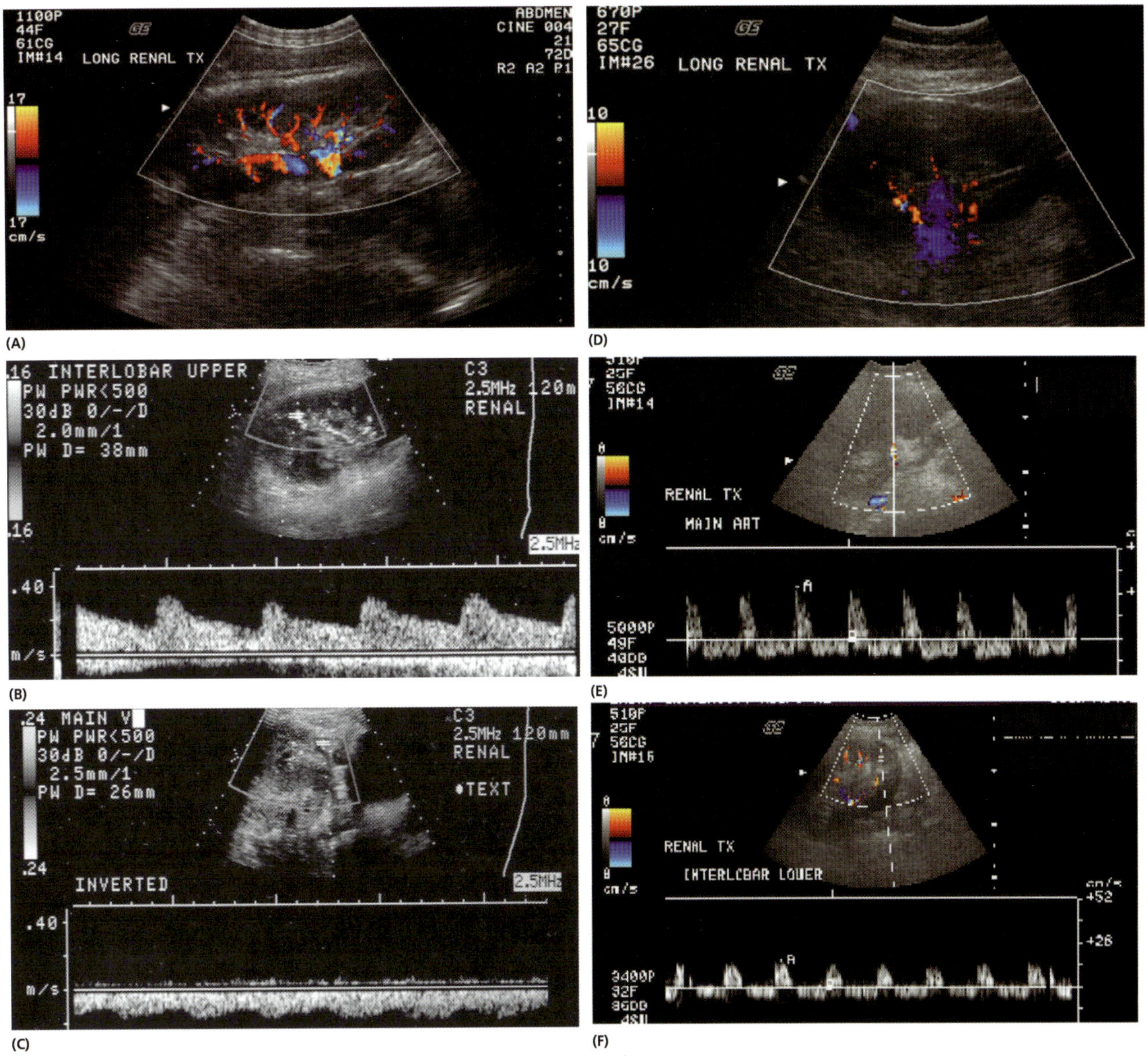

图 55.4 超声下正常血流（A，B 和 C）和静脉血栓形成（D，E 和 F）的特点。正常情况下存在（A）穿过整个肾的明亮多普勒信号，（B）具有连续流过舒张期动脉波形，以及（C）容易检测的连续静脉波形。重要的是注意到，在静脉血栓形成期间，（D）在移植物中可能仍然有一些血流可检测，但减弱，（E）可能存在动脉波形，但是动脉舒张血流反转，并且（F）没有观察到静脉的波形（在这种情况下，可看到伴有舒张血流逆转的动脉）。重要的是，没有正确波形的血流表现不能排除血管血栓形成。

的内腔损害,或者血肿或淋巴囊肿等外部压迫。供体和受体血管的大小不匹配(尤其是小儿肾移植)和复杂的多动脉重建是血栓形成的危险因素,也是低血压、急性肾小管坏死和排斥反应的危险因素[26]。通常没有技术因素或其他原因来解释这个意想不到的和看似随机的事件。

之前多篇综述报道了大量不同的移植肾血栓形成风险增加患者的标志物,包括静脉血栓形成或血管疾病、糖尿病、系统性红斑狼疮、再移植、腹膜透析或应用环孢霉素、肥胖、遗传性或获得性高凝状态。最近,明确和了解高凝状态使得大家对于血栓形成倾向导致移植物血栓形成有了良好解释[3,27]。关于所有潜在的移植受体是否应当筛选明确血栓形成因子(例如V因子 Leiden、凝血酶原基因 *20210A* 或抗磷脂抗体)仍未得到解决,并且有助于防止高危患者血栓形成的特异性治疗方案尚未得到随机对照试验验证[27,30]。至少应测试某些特定患者,如患有狼疮或有个人或家族血栓病史的患者,其临床上出现高凝状态移植物血栓形成风险增加,从而可以改善风险分层。对于高危患者,如抗磷脂抗体或具有血栓形成倾向和先前血栓形成事件的系统性红斑狼疮测试呈阳性的那些患者,包括转化为华法林和(或)阿司匹林肝素特定治疗,对于预防同种异体移植物的丢失似乎是有益的[27,31,32]。在一般移植人群中,肾脏同种异体移植血栓形成的发生率似乎可通过常规预防性使用低剂量阿司匹林降低[27,33,34]。

移植肾动脉狭窄

移植肾动脉狭窄(TRAS)可能是移植后最常见的血管并发症,报道的发生率为1%~23%[35,36]。发病率的差异较大可能是由于诊断标准以及诊断方法不同。TRAS最常见的诊断是移植后3个月至2年[3],通常发生在动脉吻合口或附近[3,24]。多种病因导致TRAS,包括移植时存在的动脉粥样硬化或移植后进展的动脉粥样硬化,以及移植时发生的血管损伤的纤维化或内膜增生,其他技术因素包括缝合技术差、钳夹损伤、限流动脉夹层或内膜瓣、肾动脉扭结或扭曲,或外在压迫[3,37]。许多非技术因素,如扩大标准供体、供体年龄和受体年龄过高、移植功能恢复延迟、免疫抑制诱导治疗、缺血性心脏病[38]和CMV感染[39],也与TRAS相关。具有典型TRAS临床表现的患者反映了肾素-血管紧张素系统激活[40]导致肾实质的低灌注。一般来说,难治性高血压、水肿、心力衰竭、在移植物杂音、移植物功能障碍均与TRAS相关。肾素-血管紧张素系统抑制剂可使肾功能恶化,从而支持该诊断[3]。值得注意的是,这些临床结果可能存在,而TRAS不是原因。相反,TRAS也可以在没有任何这些临床表现存在的情况下发生。因此,影像学检查对于诊断是必要的。

多普勒超声由于其敏感性、即时可用性和非侵入性而成为首选的诊断方式。提示TRAS包括移植肾动脉的收缩期峰值速度>2.0~2.5m/s,下游的“小慢波”波形,阻力指数、搏动指数和加速度指数减低,以及加速时间增加[23,24,41,42]。在TRAS中也可以看到动脉的狭窄和狭窄前段之间存在大于2:1的速度梯度[23,24]。MRI或CT可以更好地定位和显示病变,但需权衡使用碘化增强剂或钆的风险与明确诊断的获益。黄金标准调查研究仍然是传统的血管造影术,因为其可明确解剖结构,测量狭窄两侧的压力梯度,并可同时考虑治疗干预。对于通过非侵入性技术检测的TRAS,如果狭窄程度不超过60%,高血压可通过少剂量药物控制,并且移植物功能良好,那么无创监测TRAS并密切随访是合理可行的[3]。数据表明,选择的TRAS患者无须放射学或外科干预进行治疗就可获得良好的长期预后[43]。但目前还缺乏多中心随机前瞻性试验,因此,对于具有TRAS的任何特定患者的最佳治疗模式必须通过临床判断来调节。病情恶化,即移植物功能障碍、难以控制的高血压、明确的或进展性TRAS的超声检查结果、≥80%的狭窄、伴或不伴临床后遗症,是血管造影和干预的指征[3]。血管造影结果与血流动力学一致,管腔直径缩窄>50%或跨狭窄的压力梯度≥10~20mmHg[3,21,24]。

放置或不放置支架的经皮腔内血管成形术(PTA)是TRAS患者的主要治疗措施。TRAS-PTA的技术成功率超过80%,并发症发生率低于10%[3,23,24,44-48]。并发症包括动脉夹层、破裂、血栓形成,较少的情况下会发生移植物丢失。造影剂肾病是另一个潜在的后果,因此,仔细地规划限制造影剂负荷和建立肾脏保护措施(如足够血液容量)是非常重要的。临床成功包括肾功能改善和血压控制改善。许多研究报告了大多数患者的高血压和肾功能的短期改善,但长期随访有限[45-48]。据报道,10%~60%的患者在血管内治疗后发生再狭窄,支架置入似乎与狭窄复发减少有关[3,47,49]。复发性狭窄患者可重复PTA和支架置入。一般来说,如果在血管成形术后残留狭窄>30%或持续收缩压梯度≥

10mmHg,或者存在复发性病变或显示高弹性回缩的病变,则需要支架置入。并发症,例如肾动脉血流相关的破坏性分离或血栓形成,也可适用于经皮方法,包括支架和溶栓[3,23]。

由于动脉扭曲、复杂的动脉粥样硬化疾病或被认为不易接近或不适于 PTA 治疗的其他损伤而导致的 TRAS,外科手术可能更有利。这些患者,连同那些复发性或难治性病变血管内技术治疗失败的患者,需要外科干预作为"营救"治疗[3,24]。手术修复选择包括搭桥、切除原吻合狭窄段、放置间置移植物或贴片行血管成形。虽然有报道称手术比血管内技术有类似甚至更优的结果[37,48,49],但 TRAS 手术操作难度较大,移植物丢失率高达 20%[3,21,49]。因此,PTA 通常被认为是一线治疗方式,因其疗效较好,围术期发病率相对较低,且侵入性较手术小。PTA 通常不排除随后的外科修复。当移植肾动脉近端(即同侧髂总动脉或髂外动脉)发生血流动力学上的显著病变,限制了同种异体移植物的血流,并出现与 TRAS 相似的临床表现时,就会发生吻合前 TRAS 或假性 TRAS。据报道,近端 TRAS 的发生率高达 2.4%,而且似乎与年龄增长有关[23]。它通常适合于 PTA 或支架置入[24]。

活检后动静脉瘘和假性动脉瘤

近年来,随着经皮肾移植活检频率增加,人们已经开始认识到与这些操作相关的血管损伤。据报道,动静脉瘘(AVF)和假性动脉瘤使 15%的移植肾活检复杂化[23,24,50]。虽然通常是自限性的,大的 AVF 可以与临床相关。如果相邻的动脉和静脉撕裂,血管之间产生持续流动,则可能发生 AVF。动脉壁损伤后可能产生假性动脉瘤。这些技术并发症可能是无症状,或出现血尿。移植物上可听到杂音。由于来自动静脉分流的"窃血"现象而导致的肾脏灌注的血流动力学改变可导致移植物功能障碍。较少的情况下,患者可出现高输出性心脏衰竭。扩大的假性动脉瘤有破裂的可能。多普勒超声通常是检测这些病变的最初诊断方式。与 AVF 一致的表现包括在预期血管边界之外的高流速低阻力的湍流和扩大的引流静脉。假性动脉瘤可能表现为无回声圆形结构,流动可能是双向的[23,24]。如果超声检查不确定,磁共振血管造影可用于诊断这些病变[51]。大多数病变可以保守治疗[3]。

大多数(高达 70%)的 AVF 在数周或数月内可自行消退[52]。如果出现临床表现或逐渐扩大建议对这些医源性并发症进行干预。超选择性栓塞是治疗的一种选择[23,24]。血管造影识别 AVF 或假性动脉瘤,随后将小导管超选放置到直接供给损伤的节段或分支动脉中以限制栓塞引起的肾实质梗死的量。二氧化碳在检测小 AVF 中可能比常规造影剂更敏感[23],并可将肾毒性降到最低。虽然经导管栓塞术通常在技术上是成功的,可以改善患者的临床表现并保留移植物存活[23,53],但临床上仍存在梗死和移植物功能障碍等潜在的并发症风险[50,52]。手术通常不优先选择作为肾内 AVF 或假性动脉瘤的一线治疗方式,因为它通常需要行部分甚至全部肾切除术。

泌尿系统并发症

最常见的泌尿系统并发症是输尿管梗阻和尿漏,报道发生率约为 10%~15%[7,8,23,24,54]。这些并发症最常见的原因是缺血或技术错误,但也有其他因素的影响,包括免疫抑制治疗、炎症、感染和营养状况不佳[7,8]。移植输尿管的灌注仅由肾动脉产生,不再由腹膜后和盆腔血管供应。因此远端输尿管有灌注不良伴有泄漏或狭窄形成的风险。必须注意输尿管的血液供应,保留下极动脉和减少输尿管附近的剥离,尤其要注意输尿管和肾下极之间的"金三角"[7,8]。

输尿管梗阻

输尿管梗阻在移植受体中的发生率约为 3%[7,8,55],但是在以前的系列报道中发生率接近或超过 10%[56,57]。如前所述,远端输尿管节段或输尿管结合部的输尿管狭窄通常归因于远端移植输尿管的缺血或技术错误。输尿管梗阻还可能由其他原因引起,如淋巴囊肿、精索、管腔内结石、凝块或异物引起的外在压迫。最近,BK 多瘤病毒感染导致输尿管炎从而引起移植输尿管狭窄[7,58],所有疑似狭窄的患者均应评估 BK 病毒血症和(或)病毒尿症。输尿管梗阻导致移植物功能障碍,表现为血肌酐升高。初步评估包括同种异体移植物的超声检查,其典型表现为肾盂积水。如果还发现膀胱膨胀,应通过随访超声研究对膀胱进行减压,以消除因输尿管远端梗阻而引起的肾盂积水及相关功能障碍。膀胱减压后持续性肾盂积水提示输尿管梗阻。在疑似输尿管梗阻的情况下,顺行肾造影术可作为确诊和治疗手段。集合系统的经皮减压可缓解肾实质的阻塞并恢复肾功能。顺行肾造影可清楚描绘输尿管狭窄的位置和程度。如果阻塞导致急性上尿路感染,患者应该接受减压和抗生素治疗,并直到感染得到充分治疗后延迟注射造影剂,以降低全身性脓毒症的风险。移植物输尿管偶尔也可以逆行方式经膀胱镜检查,但膀胱前侧上的输尿管新孔口的插管通常较为困难。

由于开放式手术可能在技术上具有挑战性,内镜和经皮干预(包括球囊输尿管成形术和支架置入)通常被推荐为输尿管狭窄的一线治疗措施。病变节段较短,位于输尿管膀胱交界处或其附近,并且在移植后发生相对较早(≤3个月),通常被认为适于经皮技术,并且具有50%以上的成功率[7,24,55,59]。相比之下,较长、较近端和较晚发生的狭窄通常微创技术治疗效果不佳,成功率报告低于50%[55,59,60]。不适合或不能通过经皮介入的输尿管狭窄需要外科手术解决。如果在切除远端狭窄段后仍有足够长度的健康输尿管残留,可再次行输尿管膀胱吻合术。若膀胱具有足够的质量,如果必要的话(即行下段输尿管再建术或膀胱肌瓣输尿管成形术),它可以移动和手术修整以允许在没有紧张的情况下接近输尿管。输尿管输尿管吻合术、髓质造口术和肾盂输尿管吻合术是根据供体输尿管以及受体输尿管和膀胱的状况重建尿道的其他选择。手术通常困难,再次手术之前需充分了解移植肾肾盂(即右或左供体肾)的方向以及自体尿道结构的状态和接近度。

尿漏

肾移植后尿漏发生率3%~5%[7,8,23,24]。患者表现为排尿时盆腔疼痛、移植物区域的肿胀和压痛。手术切口可能会排出尿液,还可能发生移植物功能障碍。最常见的尿液渗漏部位包括远端输尿管和输尿管膀胱吻合口处。常见原因包括技术因素,或更常见的输尿管缺血导致的吻合失败[7,23,24]。如果是因为技术错误,在移植后的前24小时内,尿漏常常变得明显。由缺血性坏死引起的尿漏通常在最初几周内出现[7]。伤口引流可以通过其相对于血清肌酐水平升高来确定为尿。超声或CT可见移植物周围液体聚集,对液体采样可以确认是否为尿漏。在活动性尿漏的情况下,可以在逆行膀胱造影、顺行性肾盂造影或放射性核素成像中发现尿液外渗。移植后早期的尿漏常常通过手术修复,因为炎症轻且粘连少,组织结构清晰,再手术是相对容易的。如果远端输尿管灌注良好,则可通过额外缝合来简单地修复尿漏。在这些情况下,可以避免长期应用肾造口管、支架、经皮引流管和Foley导管。如果是因输尿管缺血坏死造成的尿漏,开放修复通常是必要的,以达到令人满意的长期结果。输尿管必须去除坏死组织直至显露健康的活组织,并进行适当的重建。如果认为尿漏可能无须再次手术就可愈合或者成功重新手术修复尿漏的可能性较低,应行尿路减压和(或)转向以减少尿漏的压力和尿流,促进愈合。非手术干预措施通常包括顺行肾造口术、双J形输尿管支架或肾脏输尿管支架置入术、膀胱导管引流,以及任何相关尿性囊肿的经皮引流。经皮和内镜技术通常可以成功地解决经适当选择的尿漏病例而不需再次行开放手术[7,60]。

淋巴囊肿和其他移植物周围积液

移植物周围积液在移植后很常见,发生率高达50%[61,62]。值得注意的是,大部分积液都是经常规检查(如CT或超声)偶然发现的。其中只有15%~20%具有临床意义,需要干预[23,24,62,63]。在缺乏相关临床表现的情况下,绝大多数可安全地行观察治疗,无须干预。前文已讨论过血肿和尿性囊肿的处理原则。如果患者出现感染表现,如发烧、疼痛、肿胀和该部位处的压痛,并且影像学提示积液,则考虑脓肿。如果发现壁强化或者积液内有气体,则提示感染。CT或超声引导取样,行革兰染色、培养、敏感性检测以明确诊断并指导抗感染治疗。除了抗感染治疗,对于小的积液可以穿刺引流,较大感染灶需要留置经皮引流,直到引流停止和空腔塌陷。大的、复杂的感染积液通常需要手术清创,以方便排出脓液和去除坏死组织。

淋巴囊肿是术后非上皮化的淋巴液聚集。淋巴液来源是手术区域或移植物本身中断的淋巴管[3,6]。为了减少淋巴囊肿的发生,有人建议在显露髂外血管或改变手术方式(如将淋巴管植入髂总血管或放置引流管)过程中对淋巴管进行仔细结扎[64,65]。其他因素,如同种异体免疫应答以及特异性免疫抑制剂(如西罗莫司)也报道可产生作用[6,64,66]。与血肿、尿性囊肿和感染性脓肿相比,淋巴囊肿通常在移植后较晚时出现,通常在术后数周或数月,峰值为术后6周左右[62]。它们通常位于肾移植输尿管后侧肾下极附近[3]。大的淋巴囊肿如果刺激膀胱,可引起不适,如疼痛、肿胀、尿频或尿急。髂静脉引流功能障碍可能会导致下肢水肿或深静脉血栓形成。淋巴囊肿压迫输尿管、移植血管系统或移植物本身可能导致尿液流出阻塞或损害移植物灌注，从而导致移植物功能障碍。大约 1%~26%的移植受体会出现具有明显临床意义或有症状表现的淋巴囊肿[10,67,68]。然而,如前所述,然而,如前所述,大多数淋巴囊肿常在常规影像学检查中偶然发现，一般只有在因其大小或位置引起相关症状或并发症的情况下才需要干预。若近期移植患者在输尿管支架移除后短期内发生的血清肌酐升高鉴别诊断应包括阻塞性淋巴囊肿。移植输尿管附近的积液,同时合并肾盂积水或输尿管积水,以及移植物功能障碍，提示存在具有明显临床意义的淋巴囊肿。抽吸对于诊断是有帮助的:淋巴囊肿的肌酐水平与血清肌酐水平相似,而尿性囊肿的肌酐水平通常显著升高。在抽吸液体后临床症状改善或移植物功能改善也支持淋巴囊肿的诊断。抽吸后通常容易复发,往往需要进一步治疗。最近的一项综述报告显示,单纯抽吸复发率为 59%，个别系列报告的复发率为 10%~95%[10]。经皮引流置入是治疗淋巴囊肿的唯一疗法,复发率为 50%[10]。经皮引流与硬化剂注射的成功率为 68%~100%[23,24],最近的一篇综述报道了硬化剂注射的总复发率为 31%[10]。普伐他汀碘溶液是一种常用的硬化剂[10]。已经报道了大量其他试剂的应用,如四环素，链霉素,乙醇,博莱霉素,或人纤维蛋白原、牛蛋白酶抑制剂、人凝血酶、氯化钙的混合物,以及庆大霉素作为硬化剂注入积液中。需要多种治疗方法以防止液体再积聚,并且临床治疗可能需要几周时间[10,23,24]。一些作者担心药品的潜在肾毒性,如普伐他汀碘溶液,以及与反复抽吸或导管引流延长相关的感染风险[3,10]。移植后淋巴囊肿行手术治疗通常是首选,与抽吸、引流或硬化剂相比,其成功率高,复发率低[3,10]。此外,可以避免长期经皮引流相关的不适和潜在并发症。手术包括造口术或淋巴管壁外“腹膜窗”的创建。这一方法可以作为微创腹腔镜手术进行，也可以利用先前移植切口或下中线切口作为开放手术进行。最近的一篇综述报告显示，腹腔镜手术和开放手术的总复发率分别为 8%和 16%[10]。腹腔镜手术在大多数情况下可能是首选的手术方法,因为其发病率较低且住院时间较短[10]。CT 在术前规划中是非常重要的，它可以帮助确定淋巴囊肿与相邻重要结构(如移植物、髂血管和移植输尿管)的空间关系,避免术中并发症的发生。术中使用超声检查也有助于明确淋巴囊肿的位置以及进入淋巴囊肿的安全位置。如果积液充盈且膀胱是空的,那么这一操作过程较为容易。如果可能，空腔壁中的开窗直径应该至少为 5cm。据报道,通过窗口在腔中固定网膜也有助于防止液体再积聚[3,69]。

总结

肾脏移植技术经过了时间检验已经得到认可,在过去几十年中变化相对较小。最终的成功应该是每一位患者都都有统一的预期，这在很大程度上取决于对髂血管系统和膀胱位置的共同技术问题的预期，也依赖于并发症的及时诊断和干预。对于血管并发症的识别,需要较高的怀疑指数,以便在允许的时间范围内挽救移植物,当然,外科医生在怀疑技术并发症的罕见情况下很少需要再探查。

（胡志平 译　朱继业 校）

参考文献

1. Murray JE. Nobel Prize Lecture: the first successful organ transplants in man. In: Terasaki PI, editor. History of Transplantation: Thirty-Five Recollections. Los Angeles, CA: UCLA Tissue Typing Laboratory; 1991: 123–138.
2. Barry JM, Morris PJ. Surgical techniques of renal transplantation. In: Morris PJ, Knechtle SJ, editors. Kidney Transplantation Principles and Practice, 6th edition. Philadelphia, PA: Saunders; 2008: 158–171.
3. Allen RDM. Vascular complications after kidney transplantation. In: Morris PJ, Knechtle SJ, editors. Kidney Transplantation Principles and Practice, 6th edition. Philadelphia, PA: Saunders; 2008: 439–461.
4. Barry JM. Technical aspects of renal transplantation. In: Norman DJ, Turka LA, editors. Primer on Transplantation, 2nd edition. Mt. Laurel, NJ: American Society of Transplantation; 2001: 431–439.
5. Humar A, Matas AJ. Kidney transplantation. In: Humar A, Matas AJ, Payne WD, editors. Atlas of Organ Transplantation. London: Springer; 2006: 91–131.
6. Minetti EE. Lymphocele after renal transplantation, a medical complication. Journal of Nephrology. 2011;24:707–716.
7. Shoskes D, Cranston D. Urological complications after kidney transplantation. In: Morris PJ, Knechtle SJ, editors. Kidney Transplantation Principles and Practice, 6th edition. Philadelphia, PA: Saunders; 2008: 462–468.
8. Streeter EH, Little DM, Cranston DW, et al. The urological complications of renal transplantation: a series of 1535 patients. BJU International. 2002;90: 627–634.
9. Singer J, Gritsch HA, Rosenthal JT. The transplant operation and its surgical complications. In: Danovitch G, editor. Handbook of Kidney Transplantation, 4th edition. Philadelphia, PA: Lippincott Williams and Wilkins; 2005: 193–211.
10. Lucewicz A, Wong G, Lam VW, et al. Management of primary symptomatic lymphocele after kidney transplantation: a systematic review. Transplantation. 2011;92:663–673.
11. Thrasher JB, Temple DR, Spees EK. Extravesical versus Leadbetter-Politano ureteroneocystostomy: a comparison of urological complications in 320 renal transplants. Journal of Urology. 1990;144:1105–1109.
12. Butterworth PC, Horsburgh T, Veitch PS, et al. Urological complications in renal transplantation: impact of a change of technique. British Journal of Urology. 1997;79:499–502.
13. Mangus RS, Haag BW. Stented versus nonstented extravesical ureteroneocystostomy in renal transplantation: a metaanalysis. American Journal of Transplantation. 2004;4:1889–1896.
14. Starzl TE, Marchioro TL, Morgan WW, et al. A technique for use of adult renal homografts in children. Surgery, Gynecology and Obstetrics. 1964;119:106–108.
15. Tejani A. Special considerations in pediatric kidney transplantation. In: Norman DJ, Turka LA, editors. Primer on Transplantation, 2nd edition. Mt. Laurel, NJ: American Society of Transplantation; 2001: 490–500.

16. Amante AJ, Kahan BD. En bloc transplantation of kidneys from pediatric donors. Journal of Urology. 1996;155:852–856; discussion 6–7.
17. Gill J, Cho YW, Danovitch GM, et al. Outcomes of dual adult kidney transplants in the United States: an analysis of the OPTN/UNOS database. Transplantation. 2008;85:62–68.
18. Johnson LB, Kno PC, Dafoe DC, et al. Double adult renal allografts: a technique for expansion of the cadaveric kidney donor pool. Surgery. 1996;120:580–583; discussion 3–4.
19. Haider HH, Illanes HG, Ciancio G, et al. Dual kidney transplantation using midline extraperitoneal approach: description of a technique. Transplantation Proceedings. 2007;39:1118–1119.
20. Ekser B, Furian L, Broggiato A, et al. Technical aspects of unilateral dual kidney transplantation from expanded criteria donors: experience of 100 patients. American Journal of Transplantation. 2010;10:2000–2007.
21. Humar A, Matas AJ. Surgical complications after kidney transplantation. Seminars in Dialysis. 2005;18:505–510.
22. Knechtle SJ, Pirsch JD. Early course of the patient with a kidney transplant. In: Morris PJ, Knechtle SJ, editors. Kidney Transplantation Principles and Practice, 6th edition. Philadelphia, PA: Saunders; 2008: 210–219.
23. Hedegard W, Saad WE, Davies MG. Management of vascular and nonvascular complications after renal transplantation. Techniques in Vascular and Interventional Radiology. 2009;12:240–262.
24. Kobayashi K, Censullo ML, Rossman LL, et al. Interventional radiologic management of renal transplant dysfunction: indications, limitations, and technical considerations. Radiographics. 2007;27:1109–1130.
25. Humar A, Key N, Ramcharan T, et al. Kidney retransplants after initial graft loss to vascular thrombosis. Clinical Transplantation. 2001;15:6–10.
26. Penny MJ, Nankivell BJ, Disney AP, et al. Renal graft thrombosis. A survey of 134 consecutive cases. Transplantation. 1994;58:565–569.
27. Irish A. Hypercoagulability in renal transplant recipients. Identifying patients at risk of renal allograft thrombosis and evaluating strategies for prevention. American Journal of Cardiovascular Drugs: Drugs, Devices, and Other Interventions. 2004;4:139–149.
28. Richardson AJ, Higgins RM, Jaskowski AJ, et al. Spontaneous rupture of renal allografts: the importance of renal vein thrombosis in the cyclosporin era. British Journal of Surgery. 1990;77:558–560.
29. Melamed ML, Kim HS, Jaar BG, et al. Combined percutaneous mechanical and chemical thrombectomy for renal vein thrombosis in kidney transplant recipients. American Journal of Transplantation. 2005;5:621–626.
30. Pherwani AD, Winter PC, McNamee PT, et al. Is screening for factor V Leiden and prothrombin G20210A mutations in renal transplantation worthwhile? Results of a large single-center U.K. study. Transplantation. 2003;76:603–605.
31. Friedman GS, Meier-Kriesche HU, Kaplan B, et al. Hypercoagulable states in renal transplant candidates: impact of anticoagulation upon incidence of renal allograft thrombosis. Transplantation. 2001;72:1073–1078.
32. Morrissey PE, Ramirez PJ, Gohh RY, et al. Management of thrombophilia in renal transplant patients. American Journal of Transplantation. 2002;2:872–876.
33. Murphy GJ, Taha R, Windmill DC, et al. Influence of aspirin on early allograft thrombosis and chronic allograft nephropathy following renal transplantation. British Journal of Surgery. 2001;88:261–266.
34. Robertson AJ, Nargund V, Gray DW, et al. Low dose aspirin as prophylaxis against renal-vein thrombosis in renal-transplant recipients. Nephrology, Dialysis, Transplantation. 2000;15:1865–1868.
35. Lacombe M. Arterial stenosis complicating renal allotransplantation in man: a study of 38 cases. Annals of Surgery. 1975;181:283–288.
36. Fervenza FC, Lafayette RA, Alfrey EJ, et al. Renal artery stenosis in kidney transplants. American Journal of Kidney Diseases. 1998;31:142–148.
37. Voiculescu A, Schmitz M, Hollenbeck M, et al. Management of arterial stenosis affecting kidney graft perfusion: a single-centre study in 53 patients. American Journal of Transplantation. 2005;5:1731–1738.
38. Hurst FP, Abbott KC, Neff RT, et al. Incidence, predictors and outcomes of transplant renal artery stenosis after kidney transplantation: analysis of USRDS. American Journal of Nephrology. 2009;30:459–467.
39. Audard V, Matignon M, Hemery F, et al. Risk factors and long-term outcome of transplant renal artery stenosis in adult recipients after treatment by percutaneous transluminal angioplasty. American Journal of Transplantation. 2006;6:95–99.
40. Basso N, Terragno NA. History about the discovery of the renin-angiotensin system. Hypertension. 2001;38:1246–1249.
41. Baxter GM, Ireland H, Moss JG, et al. Colour Doppler ultrasound in renal transplant artery stenosis: which Doppler index? Clinical Radiology. 1995;50: 618–622.
42. Gottlieb RH, Lieberman JL, Pabico RC, et al. Diagnosis of renal artery stenosis in transplanted kidneys: value of Doppler waveform analysis of the intrarenal arteries. AJR. American Journal of Roentgenology. 1995;165:1441–1446.
43. Geddes CC, McManus SK, Koteeswaran S, et al. Long-term outcome of transplant renal artery stenosis managed conservatively or by radiological intervention. Clinical Transplantation. 2008;22:572–578.
44. Marini M, Fernandez-Rivera C, Cao I, et al. Treatment of transplant renal artery stenosis by percutaneous transluminal angioplasty and/or stenting: study in 63 patients in a single institution. Transplantation Proceedings. 2011;43:2205–2207.
45. Beecroft JR, Rajan DK, Clark TW, et al. Transplant renal artery stenosis: outcome after percutaneous intervention. Journal of Vascular and Interventional Radiology. 2004;15:1407–1413.
46. Patel NH, Jindal RM, Wilkin T, et al. Renal arterial stenosis in renal allografts: retrospective study of predisposing factors and outcome after percutaneous transluminal angioplasty. Radiology. 2001;219:663–667.
47. Abate MT, Kaur J, Suh H, et al. The use of drug-eluting stents in the management of transplant renal artery stenosis. American Journal of Transplantation. 2011;11:2235–2241.
48. Seratnahaei A, Shah A, Bodiwala K, et al. Management of transplant renal artery stenosis. Angiology. 2011;62:219–224.
49. Bruno S, Remuzzi G, Ruggenenti P. Transplant renal artery stenosis. Journal of the American Society of Nephrology. 2004;15:134–141.
50. Dorffner R, Thurnher S, Prokesch R, et al. Embolization of iatrogenic vascular injuries of renal transplants: immediate and follow-up results. Cardiovascular and Interventional Radiology. 1998;21:129–134.
51. Bagga H, Bis KG. Contrast-enhanced MR angiography in the assessment of arteriovenous fistula after renal transplant biopsy. AJR. American Journal of Roentgenology. 1999;172:1509–1511.
52. Martinez T, Palomares M, Bravo JA, et al. Biopsy-induced arteriovenous fistula and venous aneurysm in a renal transplant. Nephrology, Dialysis, Transplantation. 1998;13:2937–2939.
53. Maleux G, Messiaen T, Stockx L, et al. Transcatheter embolization of biopsy-related vascular injuries in renal allografts. Long-term technical, clinical and biochemical results. Acta Radiologica. 2003;44:13–17.
54. Praz V, Leisinger HJ, Pascual M, et al. Urological complications in renal transplantation from cadaveric donor grafts: a retrospective analysis of 20 years. Urologia Internationalis. 2005;75:144–149.
55. Lojanapiwat B, Mital D, Fallon L, et al. Management of ureteral stenosis after renal transplantation. Journal of the American College of Surgeons. 1994;179:21–24.
56. Rigg KM, Proud G, Taylor RM. Urological complications following renal transplantation. A study of 1016 consecutive transplants from a single centre. Transplant International. 1994;7:120–126.
57. Mundy AR, Podesta ML, Bewick M, et al. The urological complications of 1000 renal transplants. British Journal of Urology. 1981;53:397–402.
58. Coleman DV, Mackenzie EF, Gardner SD, et al. Human polyomavirus (BK) infection and ureteric stenosis in renal allograft recipients. Journal of Clinical Pathology. 1978;31:338–347.
59. Bhagat VJ, Gordon RL, Osorio RW, et al. Ureteral obstructions and leaks after renal transplantation: outcome of percutaneous antegrade ureteral stent placement in 44 patients. Radiology. 1998;209:159–167.
60. Fontaine AB, Nijjar A, Rangaraj R. Update on the use of percutaneous nephrostomy/balloon dilation for the treatment of renal transplant leak/obstruction. Journal of Vascular and Interventional Radiology. 1997;8:649–653.
61. Silver TM, Campbell D, Wicks JD, et al. Peritransplant fluid collections. Ultrasound evaluation and clinical significance. Radiology. 1981;138:145–151.
62. Pollak R, Veremis SA, Maddux MS, et al. The natural history of and therapy for perirenal fluid collections following renal transplantation. Journal of Urology. 1988;140:716–720.
63. Irving HC, Kashi SH. Complications of renal transplantation and the role of interventional radiology. Journal of Clinical Ultrasound. 1992;20:545–552.
64. Tiong HY, Flechner SM, Zhou L, et al. A systematic approach to minimizing wound problems for de novo sirolimus-treated kidney transplant recipients. Transplantation. 2009;87:296–302.
65. Sansalone CV, Aseni P, Minetti E, et al. Is lymphocele in renal transplantation an avoidable complication? American Journal of Surgery. 2000;179:182–185.
66. Valente JF, Hricik D, Weigel K, et al. Comparison of sirolimus vs. mycophenolate mofetil on surgical complications and wound healing in adult kidney transplantation. American Journal of Transplantation. 2003;3:1128–1134.
67. Atray NK, Moore F, Zaman F, et al. Post transplant lymphocele: a single centre experience. Clinical Transplantation. 2004;18(Suppl. 12):46–49.
68. Chin A, Ragavendra N, Hilborne L, et al. Fibrin sealant sclerotherapy for treatment of lymphoceles following renal transplantation. Journal of Urology. 2003;170: 380–383.
69. Bry J, Hull D, Bartus SA, et al. Treatment of recurrent lymphoceles following renal transplantation. Remarsupialization with omentorplasty. Transplantation. 1990;49: 477–480.

第 56 章 肝移植手术步骤和外科技术

Joseph F. Magliocca, Steven I. Hanish, Eugenia K. Page, Stuart J. Knechtle

引言

肝脏移植是一项技术要求很高的手术，患者常合并门静脉高压、凝血功能障碍以及其他严重潜在疾病，这增加了手术的难度。因此外科手术团队必须多方面掌控，包括术中止血、避免术中失误，以及快速执行力等。团队成员之间包括麻醉师、外科医生和护士必须进行清晰有效的沟通。应用术前检查清单，在手术室预习整个手术计划，并在手术结束时回顾手术过程，都可增加手术的安全性和成功率。肝脏移植的过程漫长而复杂，包括一系列不连续的步骤，这些步骤将在下面详细描述。每个步骤的完成都必须令人满意，以确保对患者最有利的结果。

肝脏移植的手术技术在过去 30 年中有了很大的发展，包括更好的仪器、手术的标准化、术中液体管理改进、血流动力学监测的进步以及更优化的供体和受体选择方案。所有这些改进使得预后更好，1 年时预期的患者存活率大于 90%，而 20 年前为 75%。我们在这里总结了在我们中心常用的成人肝脏移植的技术方法。

同种异体肝脏的制备

供体肝脏的准备是植入手术的关键组成部分。一旦肝脏由外科医生从供体移除（参见第 19 章），它必须准备好以备移植。外科医生在获取器官的过程中一定要小心以避免损伤重要血管和实质结构。获取过程中通常保留肝脏裸露区的膈肌使主动脉保留完整，以及保留胆管和肝动脉上的胰腺组织。所有这些多余的组织必须在后台准备时去除。

同种异体移植物的准备在无菌台上进行，将供体肝脏与保存溶液置于冰盆中，用剪刀去除肝脏裸露区域的膈肌，骨骼化肝上腔静脉和肝下腔静脉，下腔静脉壁上小的穿孔用丝线结扎，解剖至肝静脉汇合处。将膈肌从肝静脉汇合处移除，并将膈静脉结扎或缝扎。肾上腺静脉进行结扎或缝扎以防开放后出血。任何剩余的心肌组织都要从腔静脉的上袖去除。

随后处理腔静脉的尾部。如果拟采用腔静脉介入技术替代肝后下腔静脉，则无须在工作台上进行额外的准备。如果采用背驮式肝移植，移植外科医生必须考虑一旦再循环开始后如何控制腔静脉的下部。可以采用多种策略，如在再循环开始后使用扎带或血管吻合器。另一种流行的方法是结扎下腔静脉，同时留置腔内导管，再循环开始后去除导管并扎紧下腔静脉。

将肝动脉从主动脉骨化到胃十二指肠动脉（GDA），在 GDA 以上部分不再进行解剖分离以避免对肝叶血管的损伤。应仔细识别任何异常的动脉解剖结构，20% 的人会存在动脉解剖结构异常[1]。最常见的两种异常是由肠系膜上动脉发出的替代肝右动脉或者由胃左动脉发出的替代肝左动脉。这些异常将在下文讨论。

门静脉骨化至门静脉分叉。去除周围的淋巴组织，并注意不要损伤肝动脉或胆管。许多外科医生在此植入硅胶管并用丝线固定，以便在器官再灌注之前进行冲洗。

胆总管此时不做处理，胆管的血供不定，但通常在三点钟和九点钟方向沿着胆管的外侧和内侧走行。因此保留胆管周围组织避免胆道缺血至关重要[2]。

如果供体肝脏预计行动脉或静脉导管血运重建，则需准备供体髂动脉或髂静脉移植物。根据需要，分支或缺损需结扎或缝扎，并用肝素盐水试漏。然后将移植物保存在冰溶液中。未使用的血管存放在标有标签的容器中，置于 4℃的溶液中。

动脉重建

肝脏的动脉解剖变化较多，彻底了解常见解剖异常能使肝脏植入更安全[1]。

替代肝右动脉

替代肝右动脉(RRHA)最常见起源于第一个空肠穿通之前的肠系膜上动脉(SMA)。因为其不与肝总动脉连续,必须重建血管,以便在手术时可以吻合单个动脉干。这种异常解剖结构有两种常见的重建方法:①RRHA 到供体胃十二指肠残端;②SMA 残端到腹腔干根部。

如前所述进行动脉重建相关的准备。为了重建 RRHA 到 GDA,修剪 GDA 的残端,保留健康组织。同样地,修剪 RRHA 到合适长度,放大镜下,使用细聚丙烯缝合线(Prolene; Ethicon Inc.,Somerville,NJ)进行端-端吻合。一旦重建完成,注意肝总动脉方向,避免扭曲(图 56.1A,选项 1)。

第二种血管重建方法只能在获取器官的外科医生在 SMA 的一个节段上提供 RRHA 时进行。在这种情况下,SMA 和 RRHA 骨化至胆总管水平。然后将腹腔干切割成适当的长度,并且用 Prolene 缝线将 SMA 残端缝到腹腔干端(图 56.1A,选项 2)。必须确保肝总动脉和 RRHA 方向正确以避免扭转。除了这两种常见的技术,RRHA 也可以缝合到脾动脉残端。脾脏和 GDA 残端植入 RRHA 的选择取决于管腔直径、血管长度和其他解剖学因素。

替代肝左动脉

替代肝左动脉(RLHA)最常源自胃左动脉。为此,获取操作时应仔细识别胃肝韧带中的动脉。获取器官的外科医生应保留胃左动脉的完整,并提供胃小网膜囊的所有组织给工作台上操作的外科医生。这种技术可以确保 RLHA 不受损害。

在工作台上,肝总动脉被骨化到 GDA。观察胃左动脉,直到 RLHA 朝向脐裂分支为止。超出 RLHA 的胃左动脉的远端用丝线结扎,并且结扎 RLHA 的剩余小分支。轻柔冲洗 RLHA 可以识别需用丝线结扎的 RLHA 小分支。仔细地修肝能防止再循环后的出血。RLHA 看起来多余,但通常不会将其缩短(图 56.1B)。

还有可能遇到其他不常见的解剖变异,每一个都应该单独处理。修肝过程中血管重建的目的是在肝脏植入时可行单个动脉吻合术。这种吻合应该足够大,以便于植入和避免血栓形成并发症。

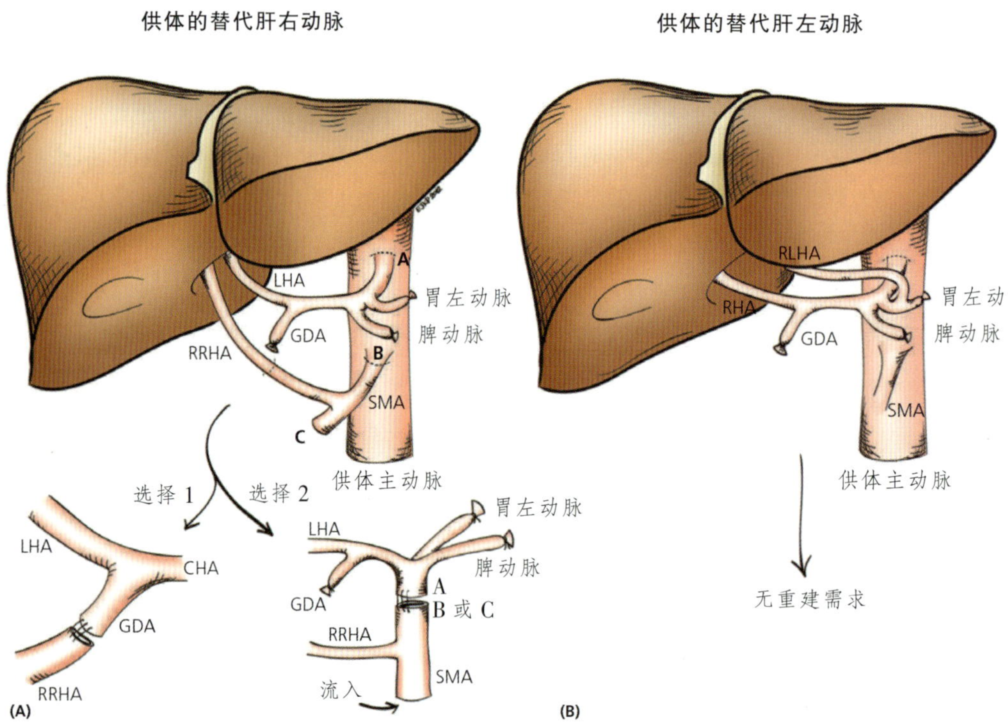

图 56.1 供体肝脏动脉解剖与重建选项。RRHA,替代肝右动脉;LHA,肝左动脉;GDA,胃十二指肠动脉;SMA,肠系膜上动脉;CHA,肝总动脉;RHA,肝右动脉;RLHA,替代肝左动脉。

受体肝切除术

出血控制

受体肝切除术通常被认为是肝脏移植中最困难的部分，该部分手术将显著影响患者的术后进程和总体结果。特别要注意减少失血和输血的需要，这些将显著影响血流动力学稳定性、肾功能、肺功能、免疫功能和医疗费用。

严重的门静脉高压患者在肝切除术过程中容易大量出血，并且因肝衰竭引起的凝血障碍以及因脾大和脾隔离引起的血小板减少会病而加重出血。减少失血量的方法包括在手术期间或至少直到肝再灌注完成维持低的中心静脉压(CVP)。当CVP<10mmHg时或者在患者的耐受度内尽可能低地维持血流动力学稳定性，出血趋于减少。术中血液回输装置可用于术中抽吸的自体血液回输。尽管血液回输可以减少对同种异体血液输注的需要，但是应当注意，回输血液必须用肝素或柠檬酸盐处理，因为清除这些抗凝血剂会导致肝脏额外的代谢需要。在任何时候精细的解剖分离以及仔细止血都可大大影响输血的需要。技术方面包括使用高频电刀和氩气刀烧灼，但要注意避免产生血管和胆管结构的热损伤。

减少出血的药理学方法包括对患有纤维蛋白溶解的患者使用氨基己酸(Amicar; Xanodyne Pharmaceuticals, Inc., Newport, KY)。抑肽酶有时可用于预防性减少失血，但在某些情况下其与弥漫性血栓形成有关[3]。研究表明，氨甲环酸可以预防性地或替代氨基己酸使用。在我们的实践中，我们一般都避免使用这些试剂，除非是在纤维蛋白溶解的情况下。患有纤维蛋白溶解的患者给予负荷剂量为5g的氨基己酸，以1g/h的速度进行静脉内输注，直到凝块溶解。在肝移植手术结束时的血红蛋白水平为8mg/dL可以提供足够的携氧能力并降低血液的黏度，使得肝动脉血栓形成可能性降到最低。只有在有过量出血的临床证据的情况下才使用血浆和血小板。除非有明显的出血，否则国际标准化比率(INR)也不会被校正，因为INR也是监测移植后肝脏合成功能的有用手段。血栓弹力图用于测量患者的术中凝血状态，可用于指导血液制品的应用[4]。

肝切除术

腹部通过双侧肋下切口(V形)打开，通常需要以垂直中线延伸至剑突以暴露肝上下腔静脉(IVC)。脐静脉被双重结扎并分开。另一种切口是右肋下“曲棍球棒”形切口，这避免了延伸至中线的左边。与T形切口相比，该切口的潜在优点是可以改善伤口愈合。将强力牵开器放置在左右肋缘之下以暴露肝脏。

用电刀分离左三角韧带，小心操作以避免对膈静脉和肝左静脉以及胃或脾造成损伤。检查胃肝韧带是否有替代肝左动脉，并用电刀分开。如果存在，变异的肝左动脉应双重结扎。既往手术或由于腹膜炎造成肝脏周围的粘连用电刀清除。这可能需要较长的时间，主要取决于粘连的严重性和密度。注意避免损伤横结肠和十二指肠。如果胆囊存在，胆囊管和胆囊动脉应分离并结扎。显露肝门，并且分离覆盖上面的腹膜和淋巴管，显露血管结构和胆总管。小心地解剖肝左动脉和肝右动脉以避免内膜损伤或分离。这些结构均应行双重结扎，并在肝脏附近分离。

在肝脏附近分离胆总管，并且注意保护受体胆总管的血液供应。分离门静脉，去除周围的结缔组织和淋巴组织，以备阻断。此时，用电刀解剖右三角形韧带，注意避免膈肌损伤或右侧肾上腺损伤。解剖应维持在右侧肾上腺前面而无须结扎进入IVC的主静脉。当在IVC附近解剖时应注意避免损伤肝右静脉。

背驮式技术

骑过结扎和分离所有的副肝静脉，尾状叶可从肝后IVC分离。这可通过旋转手术台来辅助进行。腔静脉解剖由头端向主肝静脉进行。上部IVC的暴露可以通过分离门静脉辅助完成。在与肝脏相邻的门静脉分离后，肝实质可以更容易地从IVC上剥离。在IVC的背驮式分离时要小心以避免损伤肝右静脉、肝中静脉和肝左静脉。当肝脏仅通过主肝静脉连接时，用大的Satinsky血管钳或Klintmalm钳交叉钳夹，切除肝脏，在肝实质附近切开，留下尽可能长的肝静脉。在肝脏切除和取出后，可以在植入供体肝脏之前检查后腹膜和IVC的止血情况。

腔静脉阻断技术

肝下IVC解剖到尾状叶水平以及右肾静脉和右肾

上腺静脉头侧水平，以备穿过血管环或脐带线。肝上IVC用红色橡胶Robinson导管穿过，通过夹子或手指在膈肌裂缝的IVC后面穿过。使用橡胶导管的优点是Klintmalm钳或类似钳子的钳口可以放置在导管的开口端，然后在钳子的引导下轻轻后撤并进入肝上IVC合适的位置。用大血管夹夹闭肝上和肝下IVC,与麻醉团队沟通检查患者血流动力学稳定性。如果患者能耐受,则IVC分离并尽可能靠近肝实质。这将留出足够的IVC长度用于供体吻合。

静脉旁路技术

这种方法是为了防止与门静脉和IVC阻断相关的血流动力学异常而开发的[5]。它需要一位训练有素的体外循环师进行操作，以及需要BioMedicus(Medtronic Inc,Minneapolis,MN)或具有相关管道的离心泵。所有管道用生理盐水灌注。制备"Y"形流入管,以使门静脉和肝下IVC均可插管流入。通过腋窝或颈静脉向上身放置单个流出管。导管放置可以通过经皮Seldinger技术或开放手术完成[6]。大孔径导管(例如改进的胸管)也可放置。肝下IVC通常通过股静脉或大隐静脉进入。导管头端进入IVC,留置门静脉插管并用脐带线固定。操作过程应仔细,以避免空气进入回路导致空气栓塞。回路中通过气泡检测器可除去小气泡。所有空气都从填充的管道中抽走,然后使用离心泵开始流动。旁路的最佳流速因患者而异,但通常为2~3L/min。另外,采用静脉旁路可通过回路中的热交换器加热,快速补液和补充血液制品,并可进行血液过滤,可快速调整术中容量。

静脉旁路的缺点包括手术时间长、血液制品和血小板消耗更多,以及需要减少腹股沟、腋窝或颈部静脉的通路和相关的手术并发症(如淋巴囊肿形成或淋巴水肿)。

同种异体全肝移植

目前,肝脏植入的技术和样式多种多样,每种方式都各有优缺点。肝移植外科医生需要掌握多种方法,因为某些技术在特定情况下可能应用得更好。在这里,我们讨论肝脏植入的基本步骤：腔静脉流出、门静脉流入、肝动脉流入和胆管重建。

腔静脉流出

供体腔静脉植入

在肝移植的"经典"方法中,受体肝后腔静脉与自体肝一起被切除。该方法需要在受体腔中植入供体腔静脉(图56.2A,B)。首先进行肝上腔静脉吻合术。吻合用3-0双头的Prolene缝合线。左右两侧应用角缝合,并且使血管边缘外翻以提供内膜到内膜吻合角度。将第三条牵引缝线放置在吻合中部的后壁，向前拉动后壁可提供良好视野。然后将肝脏置于肝窝中。在右叶后放置一个冷冻的剖腹垫以支撑它在适当的位置。患者左侧的缝线打结，后壁从血管内部从左到右缝合以保证良好的内膜位置。当缝合线到达时,中间牵引线被去除。缝合线在右角附近向前壁带一小段距离。然后前壁用剩余线从左到右缝合,并且缝合线被固定,留下1cm"生长因子"以防止吻合口的包绕和变窄[7]。然后固定剩余的角缝合线。

用1L含有10%人白蛋白的冷冻乳酸林格溶液经门静脉冲洗同种异体移植物，并通过移植物肝下下腔静脉排出。冲洗可以去除在冷保存期间累积的代谢废物并冲掉器官保存液。UW液含高钾,必须冲出以防再灌注时引发心脏停搏。应用肝上吻合的技术使用4-0 Prolene缝合线以端-端的方式吻合肝下腔静脉。在完成肝下腔静脉吻合之前完成冲洗。

背驮式技术

在"背驮式"肝移植中,受体肝上腔静脉、肝后腔静脉和肝下腔静脉被完全保存,只有肝静脉夹闭(图56.2C,D)。这避免了完全阻断下腔静脉。但背驮式肝移植行肝切除术时耗时更多,因为短的肝静脉必须仔细结扎[8-10]。通过从肝左静脉、肝中静脉和肝右静脉形成单一的口,产生大的肝静脉流出道，该流出道与移植肝上腔静脉吻合(图56.2D)。与腔静脉植入技术相似,角缝合线固定两端,同时使血管边缘翻转,并且中间应用牵引缝合线牵引后壁。然后将肝放置在肝窝中,固定左端角缝合线，并且从左到右缝合后壁，从而确保完好的内膜附着。如上所述,缝线围绕右角向前移动。注意缝合线缝合位置非常重要,流出阻塞是常见的错误,并且非常难以纠正。去除中间牵引缝合线。使用剩余的尾部将前壁

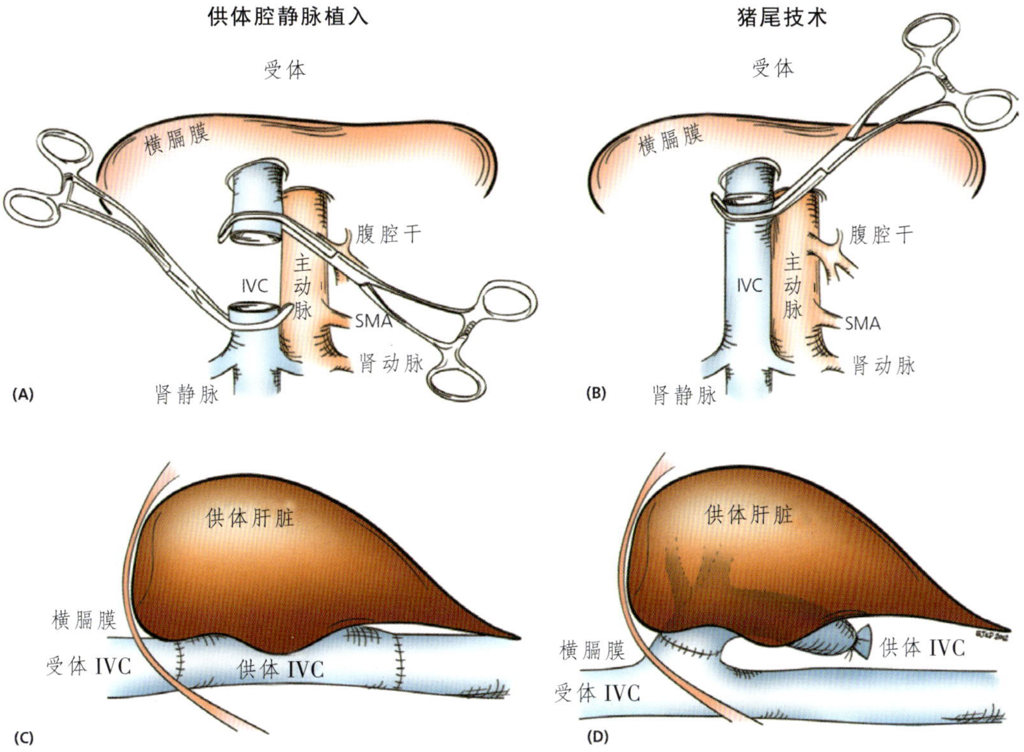

图 56.2　全肝移植中腔静脉处理。IVC，下腔静脉；SMA，肠系膜上动脉。

从左向右缝合，并固定留下 1cm 的生长因子。经门静脉注入 1L 10%人白蛋白的冷冻乳酸林格液灌洗同种异体移植物，经由移植物肝下腔静脉排出。供体肝下腔静脉用血管吻合器缝合或固定。

背驮式吻合方法的一种变化方式是侧–侧腔静脉吻合[11]。在这种技术中，用大的 Satinsky 钳或类似的钳子纵向夹住受体腔静脉。这会导致仅部分血管阻断。从受体肝中静脉和肝左静脉形成单一的孔，缝合肝右静脉有助于正确吻合，但通常肝右静脉包括在吻合中。然后将腔静脉延长轴纵向向下切开儿厘米形成一个孔以备吻合，然后将供体腔静脉的后壁切开同样的距离，在孔的上部和下部应用角缝合，再次外翻血管边缘以确定内膜对内膜吻合。肝脏放置在右肝窝内，并旋转至患者的右侧。可能需要冰纱垫来支持肝脏并保证附近无张力。吻合的右侧首先从血管内部开始。牵引缝合线位于后(右)壁头侧角和尾侧角之间，可实现较好的吻合并提供良好的视野。最下端缝合固定并且吻合时从尾侧缝合到颅侧。缝线围绕头侧角部向前移动，去除中间牵引缝合线。左侧壁从尾侧缝合到颅侧并在尾端固定。不需要留出生长因子。固定剩余的上部缝合线。然后通过门静脉注入 1L 含有 10%人白蛋白的冷冻乳酸林格液进行冲洗，再经肝下腔静脉排出，然后将肝下腔静脉用血管吻合器闭合或固定。

门静脉流入道

端–端门静脉吻合术

理想情况下，通过受体的自体门静脉提供血流流入道。绝大多数情况下可以实现，因为门静脉血栓切除术在大多数凝块的存在下均可进行。受体门静脉用血管夹夹闭，血管夹“闪烁”开闭以冲洗任何新鲜的血栓。供体门静脉应切短，以防止冗余，同时应保留受体门静脉长度，以备将来再次移植。如果供体和受体门静脉之间存在尺寸差异，则可以对较小的血管进行调节以获得良好的尺寸匹配。然后用双头 6–0 Prolene 缝合线进行吻合。外侧应用角缝全，使血管边缘外翻以确保良好的内膜贴合。后壁中间可留置牵引线以帮助对准和提供良好视野。将患者左侧的缝合线打结，由血管内部从左向右缝合后壁，确保良好的内膜贴合。缝合线围绕右角向前移动一小段距离。中间牵引缝合线被切除。前壁用剩余线从左到右缝合，留下生长因子，大约是血管直径的 75%[7]。

此时，肝脏通常要再灌注。首先取出肝上腔静脉夹，以允许用血液逆行充满肝脏，并检查吻合口的出血，然后松开肝下腔静脉夹(如果应用腔静脉植入技术)。控制任何明显的出血。然后逐步移除门静脉来。门静脉流入通过手指压迫调节，同时观察患者EKG的ST波变化以及血液温度。如果注意到显著的EKG变化或者血液温度急剧下降，则应减慢门静脉血流。门静脉血流质量有任何问题(如进行门静脉血栓切除术或搭桥移植)的情况下，首选在再灌注之前进行动脉吻合术。这将保证门静脉流入不足时的肝灌注。

门静脉血栓形成

疑似门静脉血栓形成的患者应该进行术前影像学检查，以便进行仔细的手术规划。在大多数门静脉血栓形成的患者中，可以进行门静脉腔内血栓切除术[12]。注意，应在开始植入之前进行血栓切除术，这对供体肝脏植入后具有足够的门静脉血流至关重要。在大多数情况下，门静脉血栓向下延伸至脾静脉汇合处。门静脉向下解剖至脾脏汇合处，以确保方便控制。冠状静脉和小胰腺静脉分支应小心地结扎以防止撕裂和不必要的出血。然后进行外翻性血栓切除术，其可以用Penfield分离器进行辅助。用Kocher钳抓住血栓，轻轻向内推动以将血块剥离，然后取出。在大多数情况下，可以用这种方式除去整个凝块。应特别注意防止门静脉的进一步损伤。然后，在肝移植期间如上所述执行端-端门静脉切开术。

如果不能安全地进行血栓切除术，应该使用门静脉移植物搭桥来确保足够的门静脉血流[13]。再次强调，这应在肝移植前进行。在供体肝的后台准备期间，应该准备长段的供体髂静脉，以进行预期的门静脉旁路搭桥移植。在肠系膜上动脉右侧的横结肠基底部确定肠系膜上静脉(SMV)。在血栓形成的血管区域以外进行解剖并且骨化几厘米以方便血管钳阻断。SMV纵向切开，髂静脉移植物断端呈楔形，轻柔地使移植物血管朝向头侧。用6-0 Prolene缝合线行端-侧吻合。然后将血管在横结肠系膜中间合适位置穿过。它经过胰腺前方到达肝门，然后以标准方式对门静脉进行端-端吻合(图56.3A)。如果SMV条件不足或需再次行腹部手术的情况下，可以使用粗大的门静脉侧支作为门静脉流入的最后手段。应该注意的是，这些侧支血管非常脆弱，处理时应非常小心。

在少数情况下，上述方法都不能安全地应用。在这种情况下，必须进行详细的术前成像检查，有时可以找到创造性的解决方案。例如，在门静脉血栓形成合并脾肾分流的情况下，有报道可应用左肾静脉-门静脉吻合术[14]。在完全内脏静脉血栓形成的情况下，已经描述了门腔静半转位[15]或门静脉动脉化[16]。这种技术的长期预后报告极少。

肝动脉流入道

在胃十二指肠动脉(GDA)附近小心分离受体肝动脉。将远端胃十二指肠动脉双重结扎，并用血管夹阻断肝总动脉。在受体GDA汇合处剪断形成动脉片以备吻合。在供体肝脏上，从主动脉袖切下Carrel片。如果供体主动脉存在病变，应使用供体腹腔干或远端无血管病变的部位行吻合术。我们的一般做法是留下足够长度的供体血管，以避免吻合口张力和扭转。用6-0或7-0 Prolene缝合线以连续或间断缝合进行端-端吻合术[17,18]。如果胃十二指肠动脉异常大，或者如果术前成像显示腹腔干狭窄，应保留GDA，并对受体的肝动脉进行吻合，或从受体的肝左动脉和肝右动脉汇合处形成动脉片进行吻合。或者，采用动脉导管以确保足够的动脉流入。

如果受体肝动脉由于尺寸太小或质量差而不适合植入，则应当使用供体髂动脉进行动脉吻合。这可以在上腹主动脉[19]或者肾动脉下方[20]位置进行。最好在肝移植之前放置主动脉导管以减少肝脏无动脉血流时间。

上腹主动脉在供体肝切除术后和同种异体移植物植入之前最容易接近。食管向左侧牵拉，电灼分开覆盖主动脉前方的膈肌纤维。食管旁静脉曲张必须非常小心处理。主动脉由血管环包围，在膈肌以下骨化。主动脉可以根据需要用侧壁钳或两个直角的血管钳夹紧。进行主动脉切开术并且应用5-0 Prolene缝线以连续缝合的方式对供体髂导管进行端-侧吻合。用血管钳夹住动脉导管，主动脉夹缓慢释放。在用肝素化盐水冲洗血管之前，通过短暂开放来评价其通畅性，并重新夹闭血管。随后以标准方式对供体肝血管系统进行端-端吻合(图56.3B)。

将小肠向患者右侧牵拉以检查受体肾下主动脉。无须移动降结肠，因为主动脉可通过切开后的腹膜显露。需要注意腹膜后大的侧支，并且对腹膜后仔细止血。应从头端主动脉分离到左肾静脉水平。通常需要分

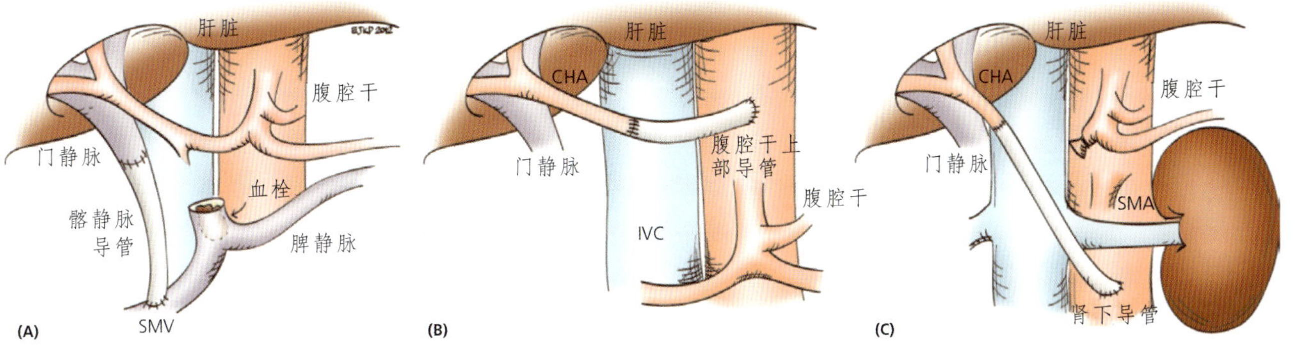

图 56.3　门静脉和肝动脉导管结构。SMV，肠系膜上静脉；CHA，肝总动脉；IVC，下腔静脉；SMA，肠系膜上动脉。

离 Treitz 韧带并将十二指肠的第四部分牵拉向患者右侧。主动脉周围环绕血管环，并根据需要用侧壁钳夹闭或用两个单独血管钳夹闭。供体髂导管吻合方式与上腹导管吻合方式相同。导管穿过横结肠系膜和小网膜囊在胃后方胰腺前方。也可以将通过 Kocher 手法移植物放置在胰头和十二指肠后方，移植物可穿通至患者右侧。随后以标准方式对供体肝血管系统进行端-端吻合(图 56.3C)。

测量肝动脉和门静脉血流

血管并发症是肝移植中最严重的并发症。到目前为止，还没有一种公认的方法可以预测哪些移植物有门静脉或肝动脉并发症的风险。外科医生手术时可采用 Medistim 超声探头(Medistim ASA，Norway)实时测量门静脉和(或)肝动脉的血流。一项研究显示，肝动脉血流速度<240mL/min 是移植物衰竭的显著预测因素[21]。有趣的是，胆道并发症的发生率不受肝动脉血流的影响。关于门静脉血流，这项相同的研究表明，门静脉血流速度<1300mL/min 在单因素分析中会影响移植物功能，但这种趋势在多变量分析中没有发现。到目前为止，外科医生之间还没有公认的处理方法，需要进行前瞻性试验以充分了解血流测量与移植物预后的关系。

胆管重建

在门静脉和肝动脉灌注建立后，可实施胆囊切除术。修剪胆管长度并用细的缝合线结扎胆管断端外侧和内侧血管以备吻合。尽可能多地保留受体胆管长度，缩短供体胆管长度，以减少冗余。这是因为供体胆管远端供血主要来自供体肝脏，避免缺血是防止胆道吻合并发症发生的关键。这通常是通过切断胆囊管插入上方胆管来实现的。但应注意，胆囊管在很高位置汇入或者非常低的位置汇入的情况下这样的操作是不能进行的。如果在胆囊管上方横切肝总管，应完全切除胆囊管，以防止黏液囊肿的形成。若胆囊管在高位置汇入，只要胆总管内引流通畅，防止黏液囊肿的形成，胆囊管即可结扎保留。

对于典型尺寸的供体胆管和受体胆管，用 6-0 聚对二氧环己酮缝线间断或连续 (PDS; Ethicon Inc., Somerville，NJ)行端-端吻合。在小管道或轻微到中等尺寸不匹配的情况下，可将其中一个或两个管道楔形切开以防止吻合口狭窄[22]。如果供体胆管较小或正常，但受体胆管很大，可以用 6-0 PDS 缝合线缝合受体部分胆管，并以标准方式对剩余的断端进行端-端吻合(图 56.4A，B)。在大多数情况下，我们不经常使用胆道支架。然而，如果认为支架有用，则可以使用合适直径的硅橡胶导管短段，并在其侧面开孔以备应用。我们不使用 T 管，而且鉴于现代内镜和介入放射学的进步[24,25]，我们认为他们的相关并发症超过了他们的作用[23]。

在供体胆管很大和受体胆管很小的情况下，或者在受体胆管不适合的情况下，可行 Roux-en-Y 肝管空肠吻合术。所有诊断为原发性硬化性胆管炎的患者均可采用 Roux-en-Y 重建，最大限度切除受体胆总管至胰头水平，以避免术后狭窄。还有一些报道是在这类患者中选择性应用胆管对胆管吻合术[26]。对于再次移植，根据受体胆管情况可采用胆管对胆管重建或 Roux-en-Y[27]。为了形成 Roux 肠袢，选择距离 Treitz 韧带远端约 30cm 处的近端空肠，用切割闭合器横切。横断点基于血管弓和切割端到肝门的距离。远断端用 3-0 丝线行 Lembert 间断缝合。然后形成 40cm 的 Roux 肠袢，进行两层手工缝合的空肠空肠端-端吻合术。内层用

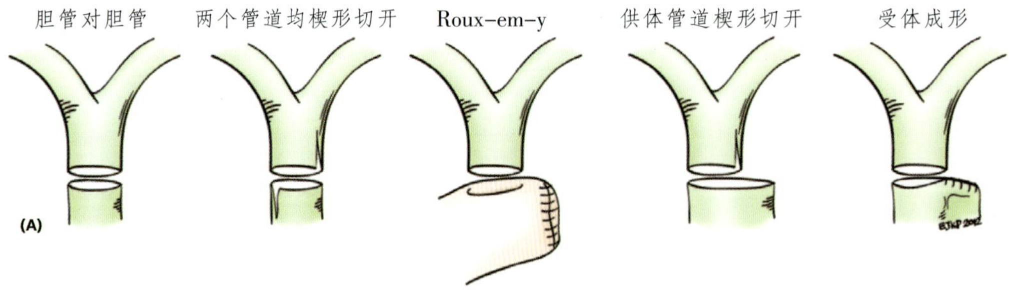

(B)

供体胆管管径	受体胆管管径	重建方式
小	小	①胆管对胆管；②双楔形切开；③Roux-en-y
小	小	①供体楔形切开；②受体成形；③Roux-en-y
大	大	Roux-en-y
大	大	胆管对胆管

图 56.4 胆管管理的选择。

4-0 PDS 缝线或 Vicryl 缝线连续缝合，外层用 3-0 丝线行 Lembert 间断缝合。亦可用吻合器吻合，但这不是我们首选的方法。然后将 Roux 肠袢通过横结肠系膜到肝门。在 Roux 肠袢末端附近进行肝管小肠吻合术，全层以 5-0 或 6-0 PDS 缝线间断缝合。然后，Roux 肠袢被固定在横结肠系膜上，用 3-0 丝线间断缝合闭合以系膜孔。

关腹

如果存在脐疝，这可以使用 1 号 PDS 缝线从腹腔内修补缝合。负压腹腔引流放置在上腹部，并可在胆管吻合口放置引流管。使用 1 号 PDS 缝线闭合筋膜，用吻合器靠近皮肤边缘。

总结

自 1967 年第一例肝移植成功以来，肝移植领域已取得了巨大的成功。肝移植已经从高发病率、高死亡率的实验过程演变成相对标准化的程序，具有优异的长期预后。这种快速进展基于外科手术器械和技术、免疫抑制方案、术前成像、术后管理和重症监护管理等方面的巨大进步。以上所描述的技术已在我们的中心常规应用，具有良好的效果，并将继续发展，从而使肝移植成为一种更安全和更普遍的技术。

（胡志平 译 朱继业 校）

参考文献

1. Hiatt JR, Gabbay J, Busuttil RW. Surgical anatomy of the hepatic arteries in 1000 cases. Annals of Surgery. 1994;220:50–52.
2. Klintmalm GB, Busuttil RW. The recipient hepatectomy and grafting. In: Busuttil RW, Klintmalm GB, editors. Transplantation of the Liver, 2nd edition. Philadelphia, PA: Elsevier Saunders; 2005: 575–587.
3. Molenaar IQ, Warnaar N, Groen H, et al. Efficacy and safety of antifibrinolytic drugs in liver transplantation: a systematic review and meta-analysis. American Journal of Transplantation. 2007;7:185–194.
4. Wang SC, Shieh JF, Chang KY, et al. Thromboelastography-guided transfusion decreases intraoperative blood transfusion during orthotopic liver transplantation: randomized clinical trial. Transplantation Proceedings. 2010;42:2590–2593.
5. Griffith BP, Shaw BW, Hardesty RL, et al. Veno-venous bypass without systemic anticoagulation for transplantation of the human liver. Surgery, Gynecology and Obstetrics. 1985;160:270–272.
6. Ozaki CF, Langnas AN, Bynon JS, et al. A percutaneous method for venovenous bypass in liver transplantation. Transplantation. 1994;57:472–473.
7. Starzl TE, Iwatsuki S, Shaw BW Jr. A growth factor in fine vascular anastomoses. Surgery, Gynecology and Obstetrics. 1984;159:164–165.
8. Lerut J, Gertsch P, Blumgart LH. "Piggy back" adult orthotopic liver transplantation. Helvetica Chirurgica Acta. 1989;56:527–530.
9. Pereira F, Herrera J, Mora NP, et al. Preservation of the recipient inferior vena cava in liver transplantation. Transplant International. 1994;7(Suppl. 1): S150–S151.
10. Tzakis A, Todo S, Starzl TE. Orthotopic liver transplantation with preservation of the inferior vena cava. Annals of Surgery. 1989;210:649–652.
11. Lerut J, Gertsch P. Side-to-side cavo-cavostomy: a useful aid in "complicated" piggy-back liver transplantation. Transplant International. 1993;6:299–301.
12. Robles R, Fernandez JA, Hernandez Q, et al. Eversion thromboendovenectomy in organized portal vein thrombosis during liver transplantation. Clinical Transplantation. 2004;18:79–84.
13. Tzakis A, Todo S, Stieber A, et al. Venous jump grafts for liver transplantation in patients with portal vein thrombosis. Transplantation. 1989;48:530–531.
14. Marubashi S, Dono K, Nagano H, et al. Living-donor liver transplantation with renoportal anastomosis for patients with large spontaneous splenorenal shunts. Transplantation. 2005;80:1671–1675.
15. Selvaggi G, Weppler D, Nishida S, et al. Ten-year experience in porto-caval hemitransposition for liver transplantation in the presence of portal vein thrombosis. American Journal of Transplantation. 2007;7:454–460.
16. Maggi U, Camagni S, Reggiani P, et al. Portal vein arterialization for hepatic artery thrombosis in liver transplantation: a case report, Doppler-ultrasound aspects, and review of the literature. Transplantation Proceedings. 2010;42:1369–1374.

17. Merion RM, Burtch GD, Ham JM, et al. The hepatic artery in liver transplantation. Transplantation. 1989;48:438–443.
18. Kalayoglu M, Belzer FO. A new technique for arterialization of the hepatic graft. Surgery, Gynecology and Obstetrics. 1987;164:564–567.
19. Shaked AA, Takiff H, Busuttil RW. The use of the supraceliac aorta for hepatic arterial revascularization in transplantation of the liver. Surgery, Gynecology and Obstetrics. 1991;173:198–202.
20. Muiesan P, Rela M, Nodari F, et al. Use of infrarenal conduits for arterial revascularization in orthotopic liver transplantation. Liver Transplantation and Surgery. 1998;4:232–235.
21. Pratschke S, Meimarakis G, Mayr S, et al. Arterial blood flow predicts graft survival in liver transplant patients. Liver Transplantation. 2011;17:436–445.
22. Belli L, De Carlis L, Del Favero E, et al. Biliary complications in orthotopic liver transplantation: experience with a modified technique of duct-to-duct reconstruction. Transplant International. 1991;4:161–165.
23. Scatton O, Meunier B, Cherqui D, et al. Randomized trial of choledochocholedochostomy with or without a T tube in orthotopic liver transplantation. Annals of Surgery. 2001;233:432–437.
24. Verdonk RC, Buis CI, Porte RJ, et al. Anastomotic biliary strictures after liver transplantation: causes and consequences. Liver Transplantation. 2006;12: 726–735.
25. Zoepf T, Maldonado-Lopez EJ, Hilgard P, et al. Balloon dilatation vs. balloon dilatation plus bile duct endoprostheses for treatment of anastomotic biliary strictures after liver transplantation. Liver Transplantation. 2006;12:88–94.
26. Esfeh JM, Eghtesad B, Hodgkinson P, et al. Duct-to-duct biliary reconstruction in patients with primary sclerosing cholangitis undergoing liver transplantation. HPB (Oxford). 2011;13:651–655.
27. Sibulesky L, Heckman MG, Perry DK, et al. A single-center experience with biliary reconstruction in retransplantation: duct-to-duct or Roux-en-Y choledochojejunostomy. Liver Transplantation. 2011;17:710–716.

第 57 章
活体肝移植手术步骤和外科技术

Sung-Gyu Lee, Deok-Bog Moon, Jung-Man Namgoong

前言

死亡供体肝移植(DDLT)成为终末期肝病(ESLD)患者的标准治疗方案后不久，死亡肝脏供体就供不应求了。为解决儿童供肝短缺问题,我们开发了减体积肝移植手术[1]。劈离式肝移植将肝脏分离开移植给一个孩子和一个成年受体[2],后来发展成为两个成年受体使用一个肝脏移植物[3]。原位劈离进一步缩短了冷缺血时间,并减少了后台手术过程中不同程度的不可避免的器官温度增高造成的损伤[4]。这些技术创新为活体肝移植(LDLT)铺平了道路。在肝脏部分切除和减体积或劈离式肝移植取得丰富经验后,1989 年第一次成功实现了将成人左肝外叶移植到儿童的 LDLT[5]。伦理理由(将在 138 章详细讨论）和这一技术的成功使其在全球广泛应用[5-7]。本章将介绍 LDLT 手术成功的关键因素。活体供肝手术在第 24 章中已有讨论。死亡供体肝移植的技术在第 56 章中有所描述。

LDLT 对成人患者影响最大的是在亚洲国家,那里的尸体器官捐献并不常见或根本不存在[8]。在日本,肝左叶用于儿童[7,9]和成人[10]的 LDLT 数量激增,但因为移植物相对较小而不能满足所有成年受体的代谢需求,故该项技术没有普遍应用。为了克服移植物体积不足和左叶移植物的成年受体预后不佳的情况,1996 年成人受体开始采用右叶肝移植术[11]。尽管这种方法迅速在全世界范围内广泛应用于成人 LDLT,但右叶肝切除术比左叶肝切除术具有更大的手术风险；其还会因供体残存的肝体积减小而增加发病率和死亡率[12]。

LDLT 中,供体的安全性至关重要,无论受体预期会有何影响,都不能损害供体安全。此外,右叶肝移植不能重建右前叶肝静脉引流，往往会导致右叶移植物淤血和功能衰竭[13]。尽管移植物尺寸对移植成功至关重要，但右叶前段实现成功的静脉引流对移植物功能最大化也是非常关键的。因此,在考虑供体和受体因素的基础上,改良右叶移植物,即重建肝中静脉或扩大右叶肝移植物（具有肝中静脉主干的右叶肝移植物),已被公认为移植物的首选。并不是所有的潜在捐献者都可以捐献他们的右半肝，因为只有当估计残余肝脏体积超过 30%时才有可能进行安全的捐献[14]。如果潜在供体右叶的体积超过全肝体积的 70%，或者如果受体需要的移植物体积比单一供体预期能提供的移植物体积要大,则双移植物 LDLT 可以作为一种替代方案,即将来自两个供体的两个移植物移植到一个受体中。

围术期注意事项

与死亡供体肝移植相比,为了获得最佳的预后,成年 LDLT 受体的术后护理更重要。门静脉高压的程度是成人活体供脏受体关键的术中危险因素。

推荐的受体皮肤切口是双侧肋缘下沿中线延伸的切口或倒 T 形切口。用于受体的手术技术是整个肝脏切除,保留下腔静脉(IVC)[15]。与 DDLT 相比,LDLT 操作更复杂,并且需要更精细地解剖肝门,同时尽可能保留更长的管道。活体肝移植物的肝动脉、肝静脉和门静脉更细,因此在技术上更具挑战性。因为肝脏解剖存在多种变化,通常可以应用多种不同的重建方式。对于技术上成功的 LDLT,我们需要满足以下 4 个条件:①足够的移植物体积以避免小肝综合征；②足够的流出道以避免淤血;③足够的门静脉血流以促进肝脏再生;④保证胆管吻合以避免胆漏(图 57.1)[16]。

手术操作步骤

受体肝切除术

外科医生必须了解受体和供体的相关解剖结构,

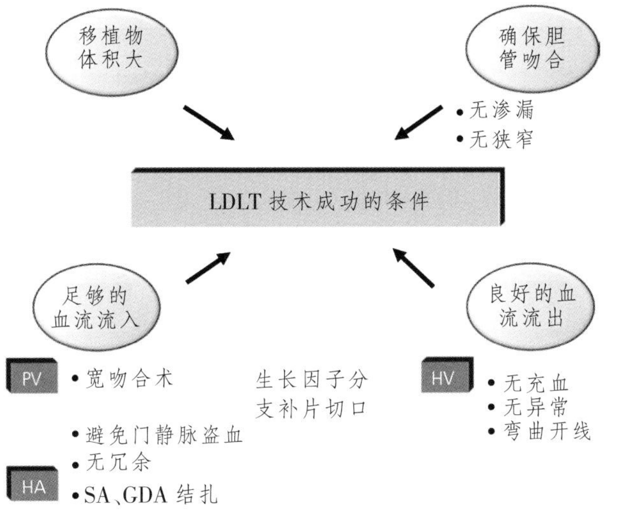

图 57.1 移植物体积、入肝血流和出肝血流与胆管吻合术之间的相互关系，以上关系决定活体肝移植（LDLT）技术上的成功。

并根据预期的移植物类型，具体制订处理受体解剖学问题的相关方案，包括肝动脉（HA）、门静脉（PV）、肝静脉（HV）和胆管（BD）。此外，在存在大的门静脉侧支、巨脾伴粗大脾动脉，以及移植物与受体重量比（GRWR）小于 1 的小尺寸移植物的情况下，必须制订具体方案以保持足够的门静脉血流，而避免发生门静脉盗血。

手术时，受体仰卧位，腹部采用中线延伸的双侧肋下切口或倒 T 形切口，需要消毒左腹股沟和大腿以便进入自体大隐静脉（GSV），GSV 壁较厚（后台准备时可用于离体操作），可用于受体的移植物植入。电灼通常用于切开皮下组织，并通过筋膜扩大切口。横向切口应当比纵向切口更早地进行，因可能需要联合应用电灼和结扎以便减少伤口的出血，肝硬化往往导致腹壁侧支静脉扩张，且走行都是纵向的。为了提供最佳的肝脏暴露，应该切断剑突，并在纵向切开时去除胸骨的远端部分。入腹腔后结扎和切断肝圆韧带和镰状韧带，但最好保留大的脐旁静脉，在完成肝切除术之前不要切断以保持血流通畅性，从而减少肠水肿和出血量，因为这些静脉是排出门脉高压血流的主要侧支路径。

切断镰状韧带，放置牵开器以最佳显露肝脏。在开始肝周游离前，检查腹腔状况，确定是否有术前操作的任务，包括脾动脉结扎、脾切除术、门静脉侧支结扎等。通常，脾动脉结扎和可能引起门静脉盗血的脾肾分流在肝移植初期进行，因为肝移植后肠和肠系膜水肿性改变可能会阻碍这些操作。其他如侧支分离和门静脉侧支结扎应在较晚阶段进行，主要在移植前或移植后。用电灼法游离冠状韧带以显露三支主要肝静脉的上表面和前表面。切断左三角韧带以便移动左肝；同样，切断右三角韧带和肝右叶上的腹膜附着。在这些操作过程中，应沿着无血管平面进行分离。我们更倾向于电凝烧灼膈肌和肝表面，以及结扎大部分膈血管以剥离肝脏包膜，从而减少肝周血管或致密粘连的术中出血，例如在进行补救肝移植时。分离肝后肾上腺附着时，应先切开覆盖 IVC 前方的腹膜，并切断数支肝短静脉。然后，应用加强缝合大面积结扎右侧肾上腺附着，包括肾上腺静脉，这一操作应在术手左手示指的指导下进行，示指应位于肾上脉后方及 IVC 上方。电凝切断肾上腺与肝脏的附着后，将 IVC 侧的肾上腺静脉缝合结扎。当分离肾上腺的止血不完全且存在困难时，我们的经验是使用 3-0 Prolene 缝线联合止血纱布，可取得较好的效果。肾上腺剥离后，肝周区域止血容易，在开始分离肝后 IVC 之前没有多少出血。因出血倾向和（或）尾叶环绕 IVC，尤其是在有尾叶增生或 Budd-Chiari 综合征的情况下，通常在分离肝后 IVC 之前分离肝门。在分离肝后 IVC 之前分离肝门和（或）肝下肾上 IVC 的环绕可有助于下一步操作，并可减少出血及控制肝短静脉撕裂的出血。

分离肝脏时预计会大量出血和（或）出现致密性粘连，特别是接受过大部分肝脏切除术的补救性 LDLT 患者，或者因反复胆道手术[如肝内胆管结石和（或）胆道狭窄]造成继发性胆汁肝硬化的患者，这些患者建议首先通过肠系膜下静脉行静脉旁路转流后再分离肝门以减少出血。

分离肝门的主要技术原则是通过保留肝门结构的长度和完整性来保证移植物植入。肝动脉的精细分离对获得足够的长度和足够的直径是非常重要的，可以保证无张力地与肝移植物的小肝动脉吻合，避免受体肝动脉的内膜剥离，这在门静脉高压受体行肝门分离时经常遇到。此外，动脉直径通常小于 3mm，与 BD 和 PV 的直径相比，其不容易有可用的替代物。首先行胆囊切除术，然后从左侧开始进行肝门分离。行胆囊切除术时，胆囊管在胆囊颈附近分离，尽可能保留足够长度以备用于胆管吻合。肝左动脉（LHA）最先在左侧肝门游离出来并切至脐部，以获得足够的长度，同时获得肝段 2 和肝段 3 肝动脉的分支补片以容纳较大的移植肝动脉。计划行右半肝移植时，该步骤是一种保险程序，并且外科医生在舒适的情况下进行分离是很重要的。分离肝中动脉和肝右动脉时应保留胆管周围结缔组织并保护胆管周围微循环，以避免发生缺血相关的移植后胆道并发症。肝右动脉(RHA)应游离至右前支和右后支，以避免移植物和受体HA之间的尺寸差异。受体肝动脉分离时不结扎比结扎要好，这样可获得更长的肝动脉并可避免内膜损伤。为了避免内膜损伤，切断受体肝动脉时采用小动脉夹夹闭切断，并且定期间断松开(通常每15分钟操作1次)以避免血栓形成。与DDLT不同，肝左动脉和肝右动脉不应向下沿肝总动脉和胃十二指肠动脉方向分离，因为肝门分离已经足够部分肝移植中小的肝门结构的重建。此外，这一操作可能不利于维持胆管的血液供应。

胆管切断位置由移植物胆管开口的尺寸和数量决定。术前和术中受体和供体的手术医生应对胆管造影进行沟通。如果移植物预计有多个胆管开口，则应在受体肝门较高水平处切开包含胆管的Glisson组织，以便产生多个胆管开口。Glisson组织断端出血明显说明受体和供体胆管血供充足。胆管成形术后移植物有两个以上胆管开口至少需要一个肝空肠吻合，而除了右前胆管、右后胆管和左胆管开口之外，多于3个胆管开口通常是不必要的。因此，获得多个胆管开口以使吻合选项最大化的技术[17-19]似乎并不实用。

肝门中最后一个结构是PV，PV周围的所有组织应被结扎并分离，包括淋巴结。然后沿PV周围向上游离，如果可以游离至右前门静脉分支、右后门静脉分支和左门静脉分支；结扎尾叶的所有后分支和侧分支并将其分离，以进行完整移动。不管近端分离的程度如何，PV从门静脉分支向胰腺上缘至少移动2cm（图57.2）。

如果选择门静脉旁路用于肝切除术和肝移植物植入，则可施行门静脉旁路移植。LDLT无肝期，门静脉旁路通常不是首选的手术方法，因为大多数受体由于要保持腔静脉血流，即使门静脉阻断也能耐受，而且不会导致血流动力学不稳定，并且肝和门静脉吻合通常少于60分钟。即使不使用门静脉旁路，肠水肿在门静脉再灌注后也会很快消退。使用右半肝移植物的LDLT(除外扩大的右叶LDLT、左叶LDLT和双叶LDLT)不需要系统旁路，因为背驮式技术可以用侧壁钳钳夹部分腔静脉，并且不会发生血流动力学不稳定。如果肝后间隙存在严重炎症或肥大的尾叶包绕IVC，预计在IVC肝后分离时会大量出血，为了促进分离可选择静脉旁路以减少出血。

下面的操作步骤是分离肝胃韧带，行左肝LDLT或双移植物LDLT时，应尽可能长地分离来自胃左动脉的LHA以利于肝移植物的动脉重建。在肝左静脉(LHV)的起始处分离静脉韧带，以便获得足够长度的喇叭状LHV和肝中静脉(MHV)残端。沿尾状叶分离IVC左侧腹膜附着点，并应用电灼和结扎所有至LHV的分支。从左侧入路使肝尾状叶与IVC完全分离，以尽可能加强肝后的剥离。然后，通过结扎和切断所有进入IVC的肝后静脉将肝右叶从IVC上剥离，这一过程是

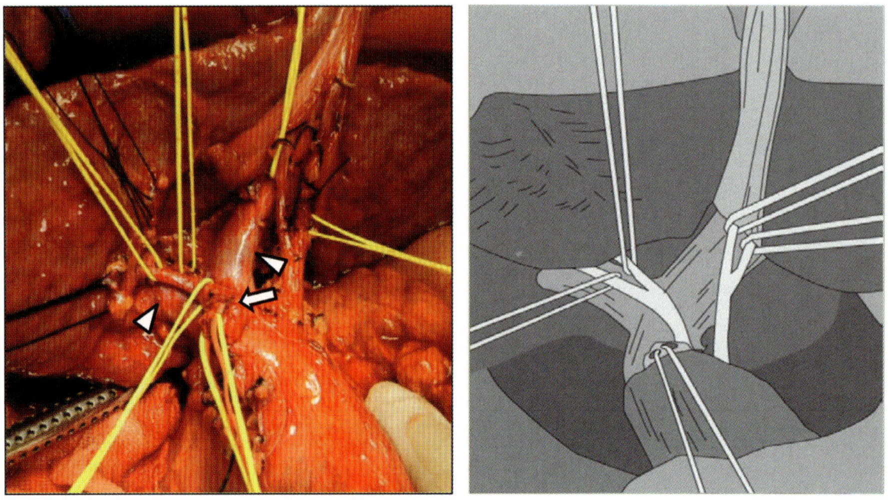

图57.2 受体肝门部分离的术中图片和操作示意图。肝动脉(HA)的二阶分支，包括HA右前分支和右后分支，以及肝中动脉和肝左动脉，分别游离出来并用黄色血管环牵拉。白色箭头指示在右侧肝管和左侧肝管的近端分离的胆管用黄色和红色的血管环牵拉。最后，门静脉(三角箭头)分离至右前门静脉分支、右后门静脉分支和左侧门静脉分支，并且门静脉主干向下游离至少2cm，向胰侧移动。

很烦琐的。如果发生出血,肝下 IVC 阻断可有助于控制出血以进行缝合结扎。此后,肝脏完全游离,仅通过 HV 根部与 PV 连接。

与供体外科医生的沟通非常重要，可以共享移植物及受体肝脏切除时有关解剖变化的信息，包括右下肝静脉(IRHV)的存在和大小及其与肝右静脉(RHV)的距离,胆管开口大小及数量,以及有关 PV 和 HA 等信息,这些信息可以帮助实现成功移植。在移除受体肝脏之前,从腹股沟取出自体 GSV 备用,通常取左侧,因为右侧腹股沟通常由麻醉师用于放置股动脉和静脉插管。GSV 通过静水压扩张并平分两段,主要用于后台重建的供体 HV。

考虑到供体移植物获取时间和后台操作持续时间，尽可能晚地移除患病肝脏以减少无肝期的时间。PV 通常分为左右两个分支，但有时会在 PV 主干分开以获得用于重建供体移植物的两个 PV 开口的 Y 形移植物。分别用血管钳夹闭切断 HV。血管吻合器吻合 HV 不是首选,因为受体的 HV 开口应该用于静脉成形术之后与移植物 HV 的吻合。

无肝期

受体准备

如果冷冻保存的髂血管或自体 GSV 尺寸不足或长度较短,PV 和 HV(少有)可从切除的肝脏游离出来,以获得自体血管移植物，可用于静脉成形术或重建 MHV 分支作为在后台操作中的血管导管。

移除受体肝脏后,应首先仔细控制出血。常见的出血位置包括肝后分离区，应特别注意膈下动脉和肾上腺静脉,因为它们在移植后难以暴露,并且这些部位是术后经常出血的位置。

理想的静脉流出道对 LDLT 的成功至关重要。在受体留置宽的 HV 开口以便与供体 HV 吻合是移植的基本准备步骤。

对于没有 MHV 主干的右叶(RL)移植物(改良的 RL 移植物)重建 MHV 分支的吻合,通常要分开受体肝中动脉和肝左动脉之间的隔膜，并且使用统一静脉成形术形成单个开口。在肝中动脉和肝左动脉残端放置多个 Allis 夹，取下之前使用的钳夹，以便在 RAV 和 IVC 前外侧壁深部放置侧咬血管钳。

移植物和受体 RHV 吻合部位的腹背侧不匹配是 RHV 狭窄的重要危险因素。降低这一危险因素的技术改进包括扩大受体的 RHV 孔[20]。在 IVC 上添加尾部腹侧切口用于 RHV 静脉成形术,同时需要侧咬钳深深地放置在 RHV 上,必要时包括 IVC 的前外侧壁。我们在 IVC 尾部的 RHV 上做形切口或单独的纵向切口,以及使用平分自体 GSV 的宽补丁成形术。这些方法可使早期 RHV 狭窄发生率降低(0~2%)[20]。

对于粗的肝短静脉(SHV)的重建,需要深且牢固的侧壁钳钳夹 IVC 以避免吻合时张力。因此,通常需要广泛游离肾上腺 IVC 的右半侧，并且右肾上腺静脉至腔静脉的一些分支需要切断[21]。

后台准备

取出供体移植物,用 4℃冷保存溶液[例如组氨酸-色氨酸-酮戊二酸(HTK)或威斯康星大学(UW)溶液]冲洗。在灌注之前测量移植物重量以确定 GRWR。移植物通过 PV 进行冲洗,直到 HV 的流出液体清澈。保存溶液也可用于冲洗清洁胆管。小心冲洗 HA 以避免内膜损伤,不能在 HA 内插管。我们通常使用 2L HTK 溶液用于这些程序。

肝移植植入的准备过程需要血管重建。移植物 MHV 的分支需要用自体 GSV、PV、扩张的脐静脉和(或)冷冻保存的髂血管进行重建。右半肝移植物的 RHV 以及左半肝移植物的肝中动脉和肝左动脉的主干可能需要使用前述血管移植物的静脉成形术，以防止肝静脉流出道阻塞（图 57.3)。当存在单个或多个主要 SHV 时,我们建议用静脉成形术指导主要 SHV 的重建(图 57.4)[21]。如果由于Ⅲ型或Ⅱ型 PV 变异,右半边肝移植物中存在两个单独的或猪鼻 PV 孔（右前分支和后分支),则可使用受体 PV 分支 Y 形移植物造一个具有足够长度的单个 PV 开口,用于在植入期间进行简单和安全的吻合[22,23]。PV 两个开口或猪鼻孔形 PV 开口的静脉成形往往会导致吻合困难和(或)术后 PV 狭窄并发症,这主要因为肝移植物的 PV 壁较弱以及肝移植物和受体之间的 PV 不匹配。当受体 PV 由于严重的 PV 狭窄引起血栓不能用于 Y 移植物时,可使用自体平分 GSV 或死亡供体 Y 移植物,新鲜髂静脉也可以作为替代。同样,如果移植物中存在两条动脉,则可以使用 Y 移植物进行动脉重建,包括适当的肝左动脉和肝右动脉[24]。然而，这种 Y 形肝动脉可能需要围绕胆管的较大范围进行分离,通常会导致胆管狭窄。另外,由于长期门静脉

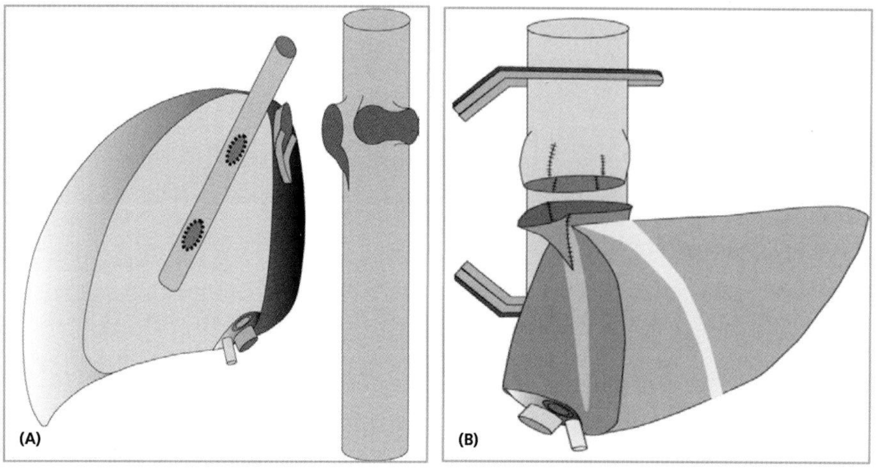

图 57.3 肝静脉成形术可形成大的流出道以防止其阻塞。(A)在右叶活体肝移植(LDLT)中,在移植物中进行尾部切口和肝右静脉(RHV)的增强补片成形术。对应于扩大的 RHV 开口,受体的 RHV 的尾部切口被延伸到 IVC。(B)在左叶 LDLT 中,受体的肝右静脉、肝中静脉和肝左静脉的隔膜分离后可形成共同的肝开口。对应于大的肝总静脉开口,切开肝中静脉的右角,并在移植物中进行增强补片成形术。

高压,供体 HA(右前分支和右后分支)和受体扩张的肝右动脉和肝左动脉之间存在严重的尺寸差异。因此,在门静脉灌注后,我们在显微镜下进行两次单独的 HA 吻合,并且主要使用受体的肝叶或 HA 段,为了获得足够长度和大小匹配的 HA,应将受体 HA 尽可能高地进行分离。

如果胆管有两个以上独立的开口且相距不太远,或者存在猪鼻孔形状的开口,可以进行统一的胆管成形术以便产生大的单个开口。

在 HV、PV 和 BD 的复杂解剖中,这些后台重建可能需要高达 2 小时的热缺血时间。因此,应该将肝移植物浸没在 4℃冷冻保存溶液中,并将其放入装满冰的容器中。在完成后台手术后,将肝移植物以在保存溶液中浸没的状态并装入冰中带到受体室。

移植物植入

肝静脉吻合

理想的静脉流出道对于 LDLT 发挥最大肝移植功能和保证移植物再生的成功是至关重要的。我们不仅要考虑吻合本身,还要考虑移植肝位置。移植物应该放置在原位,并且应该注意在腹部闭合后考虑移植物的最终位置。

由于移植肝的再生可能会引起其位置改变,从而可能产生流出道方面的问题。受体 HV 的静脉成形术延伸到 IVC 壁以形成具有足够颈部长度的椭圆形宽开口从而减少流出道并发症的发生,但即使是吻合的轻微扭曲也可导致流出道狭窄。因此,受体 HV 应该最大限度地纵向切开,然后使用具有厚壁的自体静脉补片像栅栏一样固定。最常见及应用的材料是劈开的 GSV 和受体的 PV。为了在 HV 吻合时能够正确对准,将具有双针臂的两根 5-0 不可吸收缝线置于移植物和受体 HV 的头部和尾部末端。所有缝线分别放置在供体和受体 HV 前部和后部两个角缝线的中间。缝合后壁,然后将前壁缝向中间。用肝素化盐水填充 HV 的内部,这是为了在吻合术闭合之前去除气泡。当使用 HTK 灌注溶液时,由于其钾含量较低,肝移植物在再灌注时排气通常在 LDLT 中不是必需的。

门静脉吻合

如上图 57.1 所述,足够的门静脉流量对于 LDLT 的成功是必不可少的。使用受体的 PV 主干或 PV 分支进行 PV 吻合以避免 PV 吻合的冗余。偶尔,采用受体门静脉左支或右支,因为其在尺寸上比 PV 主干更匹配,也更利于吻合对齐。PV 吻合术必须在没有张力、冗余或扭曲的情况下实施。在开始 PV 吻合术之前,应开放受体 PV 以消除夹闭期间可能形成的任何血栓。优选的缝线材料是 6-0 Prolene,通常以连续缝合的方式进行吻合,并保证留出一定的“生长因子”[25]。

PV 血栓形成的受体曾经被认为是绝对禁忌证,现

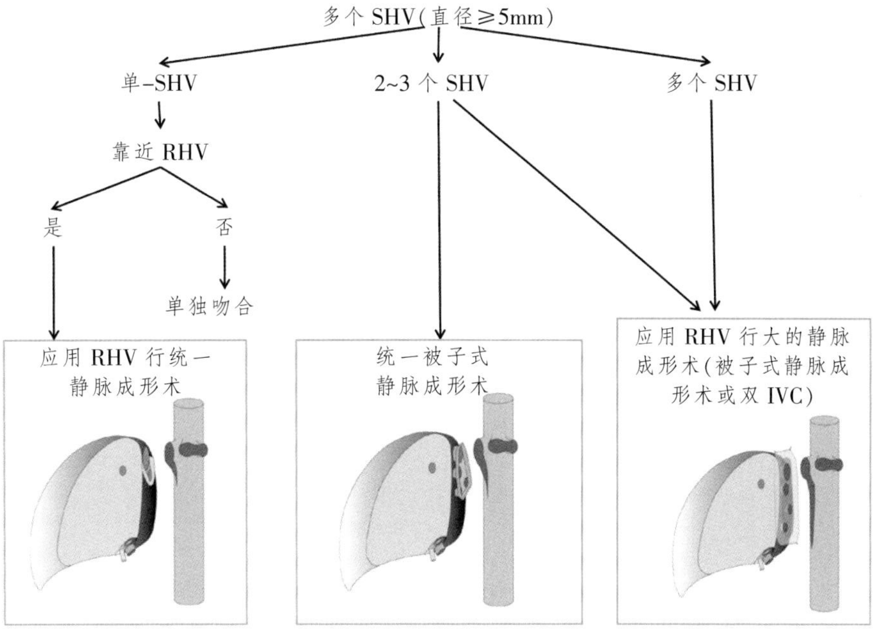

图 57.4 肝右静脉(RHV)主于及肝短静脉(SHV)重建指南。静脉成形术是一种复杂的修补手术,可用于统一多个 SHV 的尺寸,而无须应用 SHV 残端的微环境。

在也可成功实施活体肝移植[26-28]。在有严重 PV 血栓形成且不能行血栓切除术和(或)PV 成形术以扩大 PV 直径的受体中,可以使用新鲜的尸体髂静脉或聚四氟乙烯(PTFE)血管移植物连接肠系膜或肾门静脉[29]。需要 PV 的腔静脉移位或动脉化或者两者都需要的患者有更高的发病率和死亡率,并且可能不适合进行 LDLT,因为部分肝移植物再生必须有足够的门静脉血流。

对于 GRWR <0.8%,小肝综合征伴高胆红素血症、门静脉胆汁淤积、合成功能延迟、顽固性腹水较 GRWR≥0.8%更常见。门静脉高灌注可能导致重量较轻的部分肝移植物的肝窦细胞产生过大的剪切应力,这是已知的小肝综合征的主要原因[30-32]。有几种门体分流术可以减轻门静脉过度灌注并保护小尺寸移植物免受过多的 PV 流量和压力的影响[33-35]。

然而,门体分流术有一个致命性缺点,应用时应仔细考量。移植肝的门静脉盗血现象可能会导致移植物功能障碍,甚至极端情况下会导致移植物梗死,这主要是因为移植术后早期 1~2 周植入移植物内的门静脉流入不足[36]。虽然许多移植受体恢复没有发生致死性并发症,但他们会发生移植物功能延迟或失功,伴随高氨血症、肝性脑病、高胆红素血症等,引起门静脉盗血。为了解决这些可能致命的并发症,围术期精确的血流动力学监测和阻断已存在的大的门体分流侧支是必不可少的(图 57.5)[30,37]。然而,是否阻断侧支及如何阻断侧支仍然还存在争议,而且这方面的研究也还不足,因为可能还有其他重要问题需要解决,如急性排斥反应、PV 或 HV 血管并发症、小肝综合征等。用于降低门静脉高压的其他手术技术包括脾动脉结扎和脾切除术。在小移植物 LDLT 中,脾动脉结扎降低了门静脉压力,而在移植术后早期无手术相关并发症发生[38]。虽然脾切除术是减少门静脉压力的有效方法,但由于严重的脾切除术后感染的风险,很少推荐用于慢性终末期肝衰竭患者[31]。然而,在我们的临床经验中,行脾切除术是可行的程序,并且不引起脾切除术后脓毒症。至于门静脉盗血现象,对 GRWR<0.8%的小型移植物行门腔分流不是个问题,但是对于使用部分肝移植的 GRWR≥0.8%和有大量自发性门体侧支形成的受体来说,这在 LDLT 领域中是个常见问题[36,39]。

在我们的医疗中心,在具有或不具有门静脉高压的受体中,最小移植物体积应分别大于 GRWR≥0.7% 或≥0.8%,以避免小肝综合征。当移植体积小于最小标准体积时,首选的方法不是加入半门腔分流术的小体积移植物 LDLT,而是双移植物 LDLT,给予受体足够的移植物体积才能确保成功的术后结果[40-43]。与使用较大体积的全肝移植的 DDLT 不同,基本上成年受体中的大部分肝移植物都是相对小尺寸的移植物,其在术后

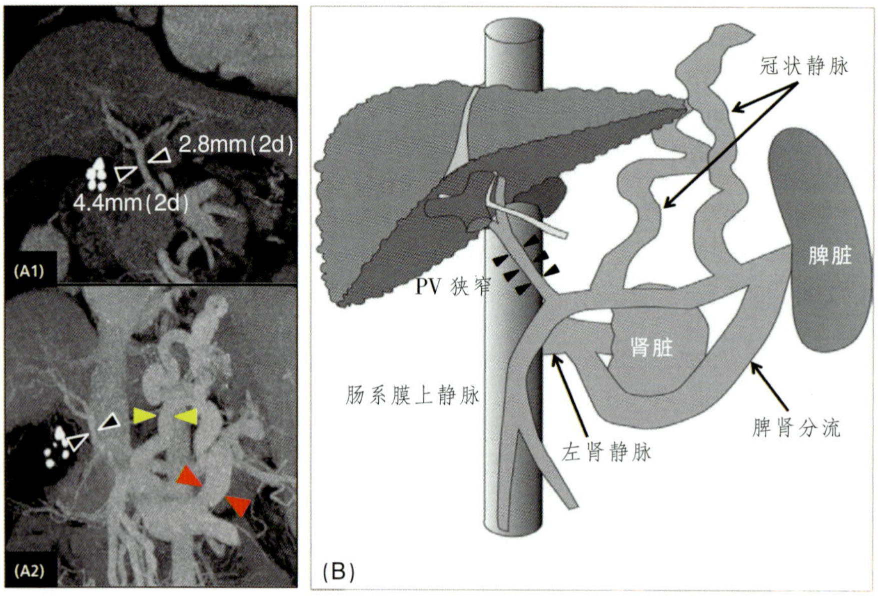

图 57.5 受体术前三维 CT(3-D CT)评估,门静脉(PV)和侧支的内脏静脉解剖结构。(A1)和(A2)为严重的 PV 狭窄(黑色三角箭头),A2 中可见冠状动脉侧支(黄色三角箭头)和脾肾侧支(红色三角箭头)。(B)图中显示严重的 PV 狭窄(多个黑色箭头),以及扩大的冠状静脉和脾肾侧支,内脏血流入左肾静脉和下腔静脉。

早期需要快速再生,即使是使用超过 GRWR≥0.8%的肝移植物进行 LDCT 也是如此。因此,预先存在的大的门体侧支导致的门静脉盗血现象可能经常引起移植物功能障碍或失功。术中切断大的门体侧支,这是术后出现门静脉盗血的可能途径，是成人 LDLT 中的一个关键步骤。手术结扎是首选,但由于它操作复杂并且很多门体侧支较深在，我们采用门静脉造影获得门体分流血流动力学的相关信息,并检查手术结扎的完整性,以及对于深部手术不能到达的大的门体侧支静脉采用“线圈栓塞”。术中动态影像不仅是重要诊断工具,而且作为门静脉狭窄和(或)血栓的治疗工具,对于伴有大型门体侧支患者，可放置血管内支架或球囊扩张（图 57.6)[39,44]。

肝动脉吻合

DDLT 的动脉吻合可以在肝移植再灌注之前或之后进行。在 LDLT 中,大多数情况下是在再灌注后进行动脉吻合,因为供体肝动脉壁薄、管腔小和血管短,吻合难度大且耗时长,需要非常小心专注才能完成。供体肝动脉的直径,特别是在亚洲人中,超过 3/4 的供体肝动脉直径小于 3mm[45,46]。这些小吻合术通常使用手术显微镜以 9-0 或 10-0 Prolene 缝线以间断缝合方式进行。应用显微外科重建技术代替手术环路放大,可使 HA 并发症发生率降低[45]。最佳的受体 HA 通常是与供体 HA 对应的 HA,但受体 HA 的选择主要通过供体和受体 HA 之间的大小匹配来决定。当存在大小差异时,使用供体或受体 HA 小分支的分补片技术对于宽的和无张力的吻合是有用的[47,48]。此外,动脉长度、动脉壁状态和吻合期间稳定定位的可行性也是影响动脉吻合的重要因素。

在许多 LDLT 中心，由整形外科医生组成的单独显微外科团队执行动脉吻合术。但他们也经常遇到技术上的挑战，因为操作领域与他们熟悉的静态情况非常不同[49,50]。最近,随着移植外科医生在大型 LDLT 移植中心进行大量 HA 吻合术，临床结果与以前相比有所改善[51]。

在许多左半肝移植和少数右半肝移植病例中，存在多条供体肝动脉。是否所有肝副动脉都需要重建仍然存在争议[52-55]。

在吻合肝移植主要肝动脉后，较小动脉发生搏动性出血，如果肝移植物没有斑块,Ikegami 等人建议结扎较小的动脉[52]。某种形式的肝门或肝内交通可以提供良好的搏动性回流，在血管造影中通常无法正常显示,除非它们是作为侧支循环发挥积极作用[56]。然而,所有肝动脉,包括替换动脉和附属动脉,基本上是必需的动脉血流，因为肝动脉是供应肝脏特定区域的末端血管。此外,在良好的搏动性回流的情况下,较小的结

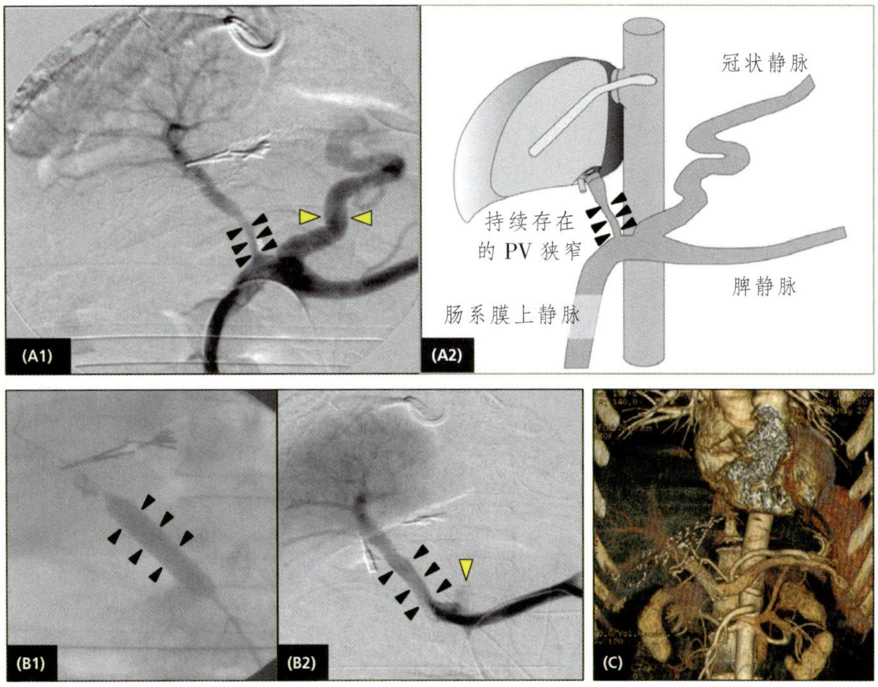

图 57.6　术中造影重要性。植入后术中造影(A1)和示意图(A2)显示胰腺内部分严重 PV 狭窄(多个黑色三角箭头),并且无论应用平分隐静脉的 PV 成形术,还是结扎左肾静脉以中断盗血血流通过脾肾分支,门静脉盗血血流都会通过冠状静脉(黄色三角箭头)。B1 提示球囊扩张(多个黑色三角箭头)和 B2 中的后续 PV 支架(多个黑色三角箭头)。最终的术中造影(B2)显示没有 PV 狭窄和门静脉盗血血流通过冠状动脉旁路(黄色三角箭头)。27 个月的随访 CT 扫描(C2)显示 PV 支架和所有侧支消失,没有门静脉高压的证据。

扎动脉对节段性胆管动脉血液供应的影响仍然不清楚[55]。因此,我们更倾向于重建所有肝动脉,以减少可能的 HA 并发症,特别是胆道并发症,它们是 LDLT 的致命弱点,因为考虑到它们之间的大小匹配,它们会使用受体 HA 的第一分支(叶;右、左)、第二分支(区;前、后、中、左外侧),甚至是第三级分支(亚段)顺序分支。当由于尺寸差异太大而几乎没有用于移植物 HA 吻合的血管时,受体的胃右动脉、胆囊动脉和肝右动脉是可用的替代物,因为这些动脉具有相对小的口径。如果 HA 口径较小(直径小于 1mm)和(或)与重建 PV 后侧短 HA 残端导致手术视野较差,HA 重建在技术上存在困难,可采用术中多普勒超声确认血流情况来决定是否需要进行额外的重建。如果血流足够则无须额外的重建。

当右半肝移植物具有两条肝动脉时,我们的标准方法是将两条供体 HA 直接与之前提到的受体 HA 分支吻合。这些吻合术在技术上要求更高,但最重要的是对受体的肝门进行细致和仔细的分离,以获得具有小口径和残端长度足够的多个分支。或者,受体有合适的 HA,将具有左 HA 和右 HA 分叉的 Y 形移植物在后台最佳条件下与移植物的两条 HA 吻合[57]。这种方法有两个潜在的缺点。首先,去除受体适当的 HA 可使近端胆管血运受影响,需要行 Roux-en-Y 胆道重建。其次,它需要三次吻合,包括后台(两个)和受体(一个)中的吻合。

与供体肝动脉相比,经多次栓塞化疗后,受体肝动脉因内膜肥大而管腔变细,但仍保持良好的搏动血流,HA 分段分支的补片技术可用来与大小匹配的 HA 吻合重建。当受体的肝门分离导致内膜剥脱或动脉被栓塞化疗破坏或在 LDLT 后发生 HA 血栓形成时,胃右动脉通常可用于替代 HA 作为动脉流入道[58-61]。原因是胃右动脉容易进行分离,其没有长度的限制,它经常作为代偿机制扩张,并且它易与移植物 HA 吻合。胃右动脉、胃十二指肠动脉、胃左动脉、脾动脉、腹壁下动脉、髂内动脉、乙状结肠动脉、肠系膜下动脉、桡动脉和隐静脉可用于 HA 重建移植物[62-68]。动脉优于隐静脉,因为隐静脉移植物容易发展成假性动脉瘤,而且长期通畅率并不理想[65]。然而,在 LDLT 中重建 HA 必须使用隐静脉移植物时,我们优选从踝部区域获取的隐静脉,以便降低并发症的可能发生率,因为它具有厚而坚固的壁，并且其口径通常可以良好地匹配移植物的HA。有时，当受体肝动脉因血栓形成或阻塞至腹腔干起始处时，使用死亡供体动脉或GSV从肾下方主动脉植入移植物是动脉重建的必要条件。

胆道重建

LDLT的胆道并发症比DDLT更常见和棘手，曾经被认为是LDLT的致命弱点[69,70]。两个最可能的原因是小尺寸和(或)多个移植物胆管开口及供体和受体肝门分离过多导致胆道吻合口血供受损。段胆管是小的，通常直径只有2~4mm，移植物在肝门部切除时有多个胆管开口，即使移植物只有一个胆管开口，其直径也仅为胆总管的一半。这些导致LDLT胆道重建比DDLT要求更高。因此，胆道并发症的发生率，包括胆漏和狭窄，在LDLT中更高。

根据我们的经验，32%的右叶和12%的左叶移植物需要重建多个胆管[71]。在32个月的随访期间，累积计算的5年胆道并发症发生率为20.2%。吻合口漏发生在第1个月内，发生率为2.9%；胆道狭窄发生在中位期6个月或平均11.7±11.8个月后，发生率为17.8%。在其他系列研究中，受体胆总管并发症的发生率为8.4%~40.6%[17,19,71-77]。自2008年以来发表的研究显示，受体胆总管并发症的总体发病率明显下降(2008年以来为8.4%~12.8%，而2008年以前为24.3%~40.6%)[78]。然而，长期研究显示，对超过200名LDLT受体进行至少2年以上的随访，胆道并发症发生率至少为20%[71,72]。在某些医疗中心，通常由独立的显微外科团队进行胆道重建，以降低胆道并发症发生率[77]。

活体供体移植物的标准胆道重建最初是具有或不具有支架的Roux-en-Y肝空肠吻合术。Roux空肠端必须具有足够的长度，从而可以在没有任何张力的情况下进行胆道吻合。

拟行肝空肠吻合时，如果只有一个供体胆管需要吻合，肠管切口应小于供体胆管的直径[79]。如果使用浆膜分裂技术，黏膜用细的可吸收缝合线黏附到浆膜[80]。为了降低狭窄的风险，应该在距离胆管边缘约5mm处行全层缝合。针距也不应太靠近，以减少缺血和随后狭窄的风险[79]。后壁可以使用6-0单丝间断缝合或连续缝合重建。根据移植物胆管的直径，我们中心采用6-0可吸收单丝缝合线间断缝合5~8根针。

完成后壁缝合后放置内、外经口支架，以降低LDLT患者胆道并发症发生率[71,81,82]。然后间断缝合前壁。如果使用外部支架，创建Witzel隧道。

目前，与Roux-en-Y肝空肠吻合术相比，胆管对胆管吻合术被认为是成人LDLT的简单和有利的方法，由于其理论优势，其也是目前的标准技术[71,72,76,83,84]。胆管对胆管吻合被认为可以保护Oddi的生理括约肌，从而防止反流性胆管炎和肠内容物的污染。它还可以减少手术时间，并为内镜处理术后胆道并发症提供良好的路径。然而，鉴于胆道狭窄的发生，胆管对胆管吻合具有比Roux-en-Y肝空肠吻合更高的胆道狭窄的风险[19,71,84]。特别是，直径<4mm的小尺寸胆管的胆管对胆管吻合术已被发现是一个重要的危险因素[71]。

在胆管对胆管吻合之前确认供体和受体胆管活性对减少胆道并发症是重要的，切割BD残端，若存在搏动性出血，说明活性良好[17]。我们喜欢比供体宽1.5倍的受体胆管以便减少吻合狭窄的可能性。胆管对胆管吻合手术技术与单层闭合肝空肠吻合术的吻合技术相同。

对于经吻合口的内、外胆道引流是否有益于降低胆道并发症的发生率还有争议。Liu等报道在右半肝LDLT无胆道支架的胆管对胆管吻合，胆道并发症的发生率与之前使用胆道支架研究中的发生率相似或略高。假设认为支架本身是异物会诱发炎症及随后的狭窄形成[85]。然而，LDLT中的经吻合口胆道支架术仍然是通常首选的方法，因为它在吻合口肿胀的情况下仍能保持胆道血流，并且在怀疑有渗漏或狭窄的情况下，它是一种很容易进行胆管造影的方法[71,75,76,81,84]。我们优选外部支架，但存在几个缺点，其中之一是需要长的等待时间，直到可以安全地移除外部支架，从而防止插入部位发生胆漏。外部支架对于减少胆道并发症(包括胆漏和狭窄)比内部支架更有效，并且危及生命的吻合口胆漏在常规使用外部胆管引流的情况下几乎已经消失。

当移植物胆管微小、壁薄、易缺血时，重建多个移植物胆管有时是LDLT面临的真正挑战。多个胆道吻合是明确的危险因素，可导致胆漏和狭窄[73,86-88]。当两个胆管相邻时，可以应用胆管成形术。虽然这种策略可以促进单一吻合操作的可行性，但这种人工操作也增加了胆管残端缺血的风险[87,88]。对于双胆管开口的移植物，根据情况选择单独的胆管对胆管吻合、单独的肝空肠吻合术，或胆管对胆管吻合和肝空肠吻合联合进行。如果肠道条件不利，如存在明显的水肿、腹膜炎引起的肠道增厚或肠系膜缩短，可以在胆管对胆管吻合和肝空肠吻合术之间取折中方案[71]。对于胆管开口 1 个以上的胆管对胆管吻合,可以使用右肝管和左肝管,或更远端的分段胆管。此外,胆囊管也可成功用于胆管对胆管吻合[89],特别是当移植物的胆管开口远离时,例如右后胆管或起源于肝总管副肝管，无法在无肝空肠吻合的情况下进行重建(图 57.7)。在重建胆囊管吻合之前,胆囊管螺旋瓣应通过金属探针探查和扩张直到其完全通过。我们常规地使用外支架经胆囊管插入胆管对胆管吻合口，以保持管腔通畅并避免纤维组织引起的阻塞[89,90]。

所有胆道吻合口应无张力,完成后应检查有无胆漏。我们使用亚甲蓝染料试漏,如果有外置支架时,应常规行胆管造影。在手术过程中最好确定和纠正胆漏[76]。

胆道并发症不仅影响受体的生活质量，有时甚至可能导致移植物的丢失和死亡[85]。避免胆道并发症是非常重要的，目前，在 LDLT 后的长期随访结果中发现,并发症发生率约为 20%,尽管有多种的预防措施,但仍无法完全避免。因此,术中和术后仔细管理减少或治疗预期的胆道并发症是必要的，以防止胆漏或狭窄造成的最坏结果。

关腹

一量所有吻合均良好完成，对肝断面和受体腹腔分离位置进行止血,包括肝周切除区域(如膈下动脉、肾上腺和肾周间隙)和肝门,因为术后出血并不是LDLT的罕见并发症。当我们插入闭式引流管,腹壁穿刺部位应选择在相对无血管区,以避免损伤腹壁血管。如果从穿刺部位的腹膜侧可以看到出血，我们用可吸收的缝合材料在穿刺部位周围进行 2/3 的圆形缝合，并注意不要缝住引流管。在腹壁肌肉完全止血后,腹部筋膜用可吸收的单丝缝合线以连续方式缝合并用间断方式缝合加强闭合腹腔。

移植物特殊类型手术操作

右肝叶无肝中静脉(MHV)主干(右叶或改良右叶移植物)

最初，一个中国香港的医生团队报道使用带有 MHV 主干(扩大的右叶移植物)的右叶移植物行成人 LDLT,因为它可以确保前部的最佳引流,从而避免静脉充血,并且它可以提供更好的移植功能,即便是受体较大[11]。但是,扩大的右叶移植物的 LDLT 增加了活体供体的风险，引发了供体安全性的一个重要的伦理问题[91]。我们只在以下两种情况使用扩大的右叶移植物。第一,供体年龄<35 岁,无脂肪变化和无血残留的左肝体积≥原肝体积的 30%。第二,如果供体年龄> 35 岁或轻度脂肪变化达 30%，无血残留左肝体积≥原始肝体积的 35%[92]。作为替代的移植类型,没有 MHV 的右叶移植物通常用于成人 LDLT。然而，引流右前叶(Couinaud 5 段和 8 段)的 MHV 分支在 1998 年之前没有被重建，当时 SG Lee 介绍了应用改良的右叶移植物,重建大尺寸(>5mm)MHV 分支到受体的肝静脉系

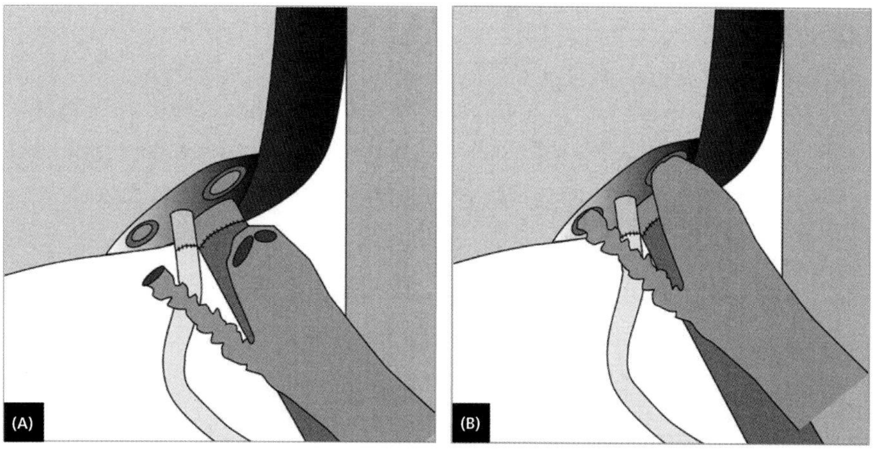

图 57.7　应用胆囊管的胆管对胆管的胆道重建。当右叶移植物分开的两条胆管间隔大于 1cm 并且在受体(A)中可获得尺寸和长度匹配的胆囊管时,我们采用胆管对胆管的胆道重建(B)。

统,以防止右前叶充血[93]。在MHV分支重建之前,5名受体中有2名术后立即发生右前叶的严重充血,早期出现长时间的大量腹水和严重的肝功能障碍。一名受体死于败血症,移植后20天移植肝功能进行性恶化[94]。Inomata等人也报道了相对较差的结果,无MHV重建的右叶移植物在LDLT后有73%的存活率[95]。在应用改良的右叶移植物后,我们中心6个月的受体生存率从71%提高到90%以上[96]。一项研究比较了三种技术下右叶移植物的再生率:①无MHV主干或MHV重建;②无MHV主干但有MHV重建(改良右叶移植物);③具有MHV主干(扩大的右叶移植物)。这项研究表明,如果不保留MHV主干,MHV重建应在所有行肝右叶LDLT的85%的病例中进行[97]。

当右叶移植物的功能性体积足够(高GRWR)而且MHV支流小(直径<5mm)时,这意味着RHV可作为前部和右叶移植物的主要流出道而无须重建MHV支流即可确保良好的移植物功能[93]。其他研究提示,右前区再生的缺乏通过右后叶的补偿性再生来解决,并且该部分中的移植物充血不会影响整个移植物再生,特别是如果GRWR是足够的[98,99]。

对于植入改良右叶(MRL)移植物,所有直径>5mm的MHV支流被保留,在供体肝切除中通过短橡皮筋或Hemolock夹闭临时阻断以备将来重建。在获得肝右叶移植物之后,打开临时闭塞的MHV支流并在后台应用保存溶液冲洗,直到灌注液清澈。最初用于MHV重建的植入材料是受体的GSV。在这种情况下,MHV支流和自体移植物之间的吻合使用连续的6-0 Prolene缝合。然而,单腔GSV移植物的小口径和来自区段5和8的较大MHV支流的尺寸差异会导致近端闭塞[93]。为克服这种尺寸差异并增加长期通畅性,同时提供直径相对较大的受体左门静脉,其他自体静脉移植物也可应用,包括脐旁静脉、肝静脉、表浅股静脉、髂外静脉或颈内静脉[93,100-103]。如果为同源静脉移植物,如髂血管、股血管和IVC或主动脉,可以从尸体器官供体获取,这在我们中心是最常应用的MHV重建的血管移植物,因为不需要耗时分离受体组织,并且有足够长的长度用于任何不同类型的MHV分支[104]。随着成人LDLT数量的增加,以及有限的尸体血管同种异体移植物数量,我们往往需要寻找新的血管替代品[43]。薄壁膨胀PTFE移植物也可用于MHV重建。MRL移植物的患者生存率和移植物存活率与扩大右叶(ERL)移植物相当,但它们的通畅率似乎很低[105]。目前我们应用环状PTFE移植物,因为其可增加通畅率,并且环状PIFE移植物6个月的通畅率(75.3%)与冷冻保存的髂静脉(76.6%)相当。因此,当另一种相当大的血管同种异体移植物不可用时,环形PTFE移植物也可以是良好的替代植入血管移植物[106]。

在受体侧,血管移植物与受体肝中静脉和肝左静脉共同开口吻合,或直接吻合在IVC,在肝移植物应用门脉血流再灌注后应用连续的6-0或5-0 Prolene缝合。受体的肝中静脉和肝左静脉主干是静脉移植物吻合的优选位点。首先,由于其解剖结构正常和技术可行性高,其吻合的走行和外形更自然。第二,植入静脉移植物流出孔的暴露更靠近负压的胸腔内压力系统,从而使肝静脉流出更平滑[107]。

有肝中静脉主干的肝右叶移植物(扩大的右叶移植物)

关于右叶移植物流出道通畅方面,如果供体对应于前述两种情况,为避免右叶移植物充血,带MHV的右叶移植物最佳[92]。尤其当GRWR不足,即<1.0%时,如果存在严重的门静脉高压,ERL移植物对于确保可靠的静脉流出而减少小肝综合征的发生起到非常重要的作用。

中国香港的医疗团队从LDLT开始一直是ERL移植物的支持者。他们的手术技术随着时间而演变。在他们的初始经验中,MHV端-端吻合到受体的肝中静脉和(或)肝左静脉开口[11]。在某些情况下,再灌注后或再生生长过程中移植物的内旋会导致MHV受压迫,这一发现改变了他们最初的重建技术。新技术包括移植物肝右静脉和肝中静脉共同开口并构成三角形。肝右静脉和肝中静脉之间的距离可通过切除中间的肝实质使其靠近,并且可以在两个相邻的壁上进行垂直切口的水平缝合[108]。在受体侧,HV吻合期间IVC的控制是必须的。将IVC从膈肌完全游离到右肾上腺静脉的水平,结扎切断数支腰静脉和膈静脉。移植物中存在>5mm的低部RHV时,要求在血管吻合时于更下方的位置游离IVC。当移植肝准备植入时,IVC在头部和尾部交叉钳夹到肝静脉。通过横向切开IVC的前壁来扩大RHV的纵向孔,其对应于移植物中的肝总静脉孔的横向尺寸。头侧和尾侧瓣被切除,从而产生大的三角形开口并与移植物相匹配[109]。该三角形开口的高度(其右侧的基部和左侧的顶部)应不超过 IVC 周长的一半,以防止其狭窄。植入开始时应用 5-0 聚丙烯缝合线以三角形方式行肝静脉吻合。在肝静脉吻合完成后,使用血管钳夹住肝移植物的门静脉,并且在 PV 吻合术之前恢复 IVC 循环以维持血流动力学稳定性[110]。

他们认为,通过静脉成形术将 RHV 和 MHV 转换为单个三角形的肝静脉成形技术缩短了腔体的交叉钳夹时间,不需要使用静脉旁路,并且可确保优良的静脉引流[11]。但是,这种方法也有几个缺点。首先,在 RHV 和 MHV 之间不使用插入性静脉补片的情况下,创建单个大的三角形静脉开口可能对肝实质产生张力,因此当 RHV 和 MHV 之间存在较宽距离时,会导致部分缺血。第二,在受体和供体侧钳夹下行 PV 吻合,以便减少 IVC 的钳夹时间是不可行的,因为移植物 PV 有时被分离得太短而无法钳夹。第三,在吻合期间,移植肝静脉的三角形开口和受体 IVC 的三角形开口之间顶点的距离很远,因为没有补片成形并且在两侧没有血管壁冗余。吻合的血管壁可能因过度紧张而撕裂,如他们最近的报告所示[111]。第四,静脉旁路的不利影响不那么令人担忧。相反,它允许内脏和腹膜后循环减压,并防止无肝期大的血流动力学变化。因此,它为我们提供了更多的时间来准备受体 IVC,例如腔成形术和进行静脉吻合,而不必着急。

在我们的医疗中心,静脉旁路用于植入 ERL 移植物。移植物的 RHV 和 MHV 通过自体隐静脉、门静脉补片,有时也通过自体冷冻保存的尸体静脉,应用被子式静脉成形术,转换为类似于穹顶的普通袖口。

同时,受体的 RHV、MHV 和 LHV 的孔径被完全打开,从而使受体的 IVC 也形成较大的口径。对切的隐静脉节段与共同开口的中部和左侧缝合以在重建时能够形成厚壁、无张力的吻合。该方法可直接应用于保留供体残肝侧 MHV 近端分支的扩大右叶移植物,因为扩大的静脉袖口可覆盖移植物 MHV 相应的缺损。

最近,由于考虑到供体的安全性,常常使用离开近端 MHV 的 ERL 移植物来保留部分 4 段到 MHV 的引流静脉[99,113,114]。在这种情况下,移植物的 MHV 和受体肝静脉之间的间隙比常规的 ERL 移植物宽,并且使用静脉移植物将 MHV 单独吻合到受体的肝中静脉和肝左静脉主干,例如无静脉旁路的改良 RL 移植物或使用被子式静脉成形术重建共同袖口后形成大的单一吻合口(图 57.8)。

带尾叶或不带尾叶的左叶移植

在成人间的 LDLT 中,左叶移植物具有有限的作用,因为移植物体积不足以避免许多患者的小肝综合征。然而,只要移植物尺寸大于受体标准肝脏体积的 40%,左叶(LL)移植物仍然是成人间 LDLT 的有用移植物[115,116]。虽然尾状叶只是整体肝脏的一小部分,但其体积在部分肝脏移植中不可忽略,其可使 LL 移植物重量增加 6%~12%[117,118]。当移植前受体的身体状况良好,没有肝硬化例如代谢性疾病(包括瓜氨酸血症或家族性淀粉样蛋白多发性神经病)时,最小成功的移植物体积可以降低至 0.6%GRWR 或受体标准肝脏体积的 30%[119]。

考虑到移植物体积相对较小,大的肝静脉流出道对于移植入受体后的功能恢复是必不可少的。在全肝切除术中,我们从腹膜后附着物上游离肝后 IVC。为了确保足够的肝静脉流出,用自体双 GSV 段对移植物肝静脉行静脉成形术。静脉成形术可以使肝静脉残端具有足够长度以制作一较宽的单个开口。仅 MHV 的右侧纵向切开,或 MHV 的右侧和 LHV 的左侧均纵向切开,并且将平分的 GSV 区段连接到肝静脉以进行静脉成形术。在受体侧,受体的 RHV、MHV 和 LHV 的孔完全打开,并且进行静脉成形术以形成足够大小的大孔,以便容纳移植物的扩大的肝静脉口(图 57.9)。在肝上 IVC 和肝下 IVC 夹闭下的静脉旁路是受体静脉成形术和植入的必要步骤(图 57.10)。

当使用具有尾状叶移植物的左叶时,尾状叶的完全血运重建可能有助于移植物再生[120]。尾状叶肝静脉切除带着 IVC 的袖口,其类似于 Carrel 补片,重建后移植物扩大的肝静脉开口,吻合到受体肝静脉大的共同开口。当尾状静脉的开口接近肝左静脉和肝中静脉时,具有 IVC 袖口的尾状静脉可以与肝中静脉和肝左静脉形成单一的共同开口,并且单个 HV 吻合口有利于流出道重建[121]。然而,在获取数百个左叶移植物的过程中,我们很少见到任何粗大的尾状静脉[117]。起源于 PV 的孤立尾状叶 PV 存在于 13%的受体中,重建大于 5mm 的 PV 是必须的[122]。然而,在我们的系列供体肝切除术中,大的、孤立的尾状 PV 是非常罕见的,我们仅决

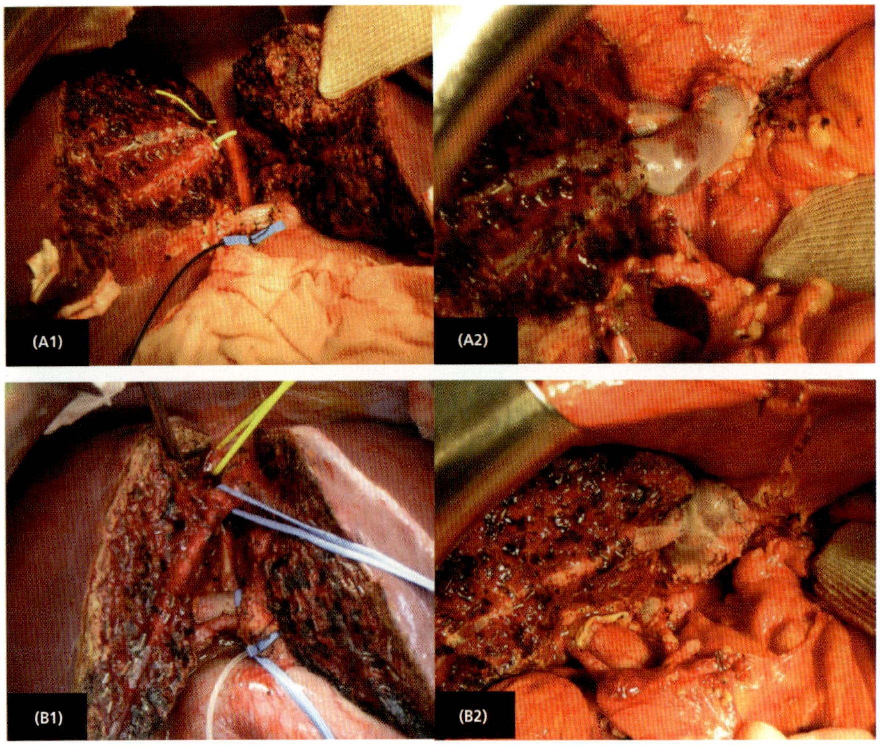

图 57.8 离开供体残留肝脏 4 段的肝中静脉分支的扩大右叶移植物。两个开口，包括肝中静脉的远端主干和肝中静脉分支的第 8 段 (V8)，预计可获取 (A1, B1)。使用静脉移植物(如改良的右叶移植物)将肝中静脉两个开口吻合于受体肝中静脉和肝左静脉主干 (A2) 或在使用静脉旁路下的被子式静脉成形术制作共同袖口后形成大的单一吻合口 (B2)。

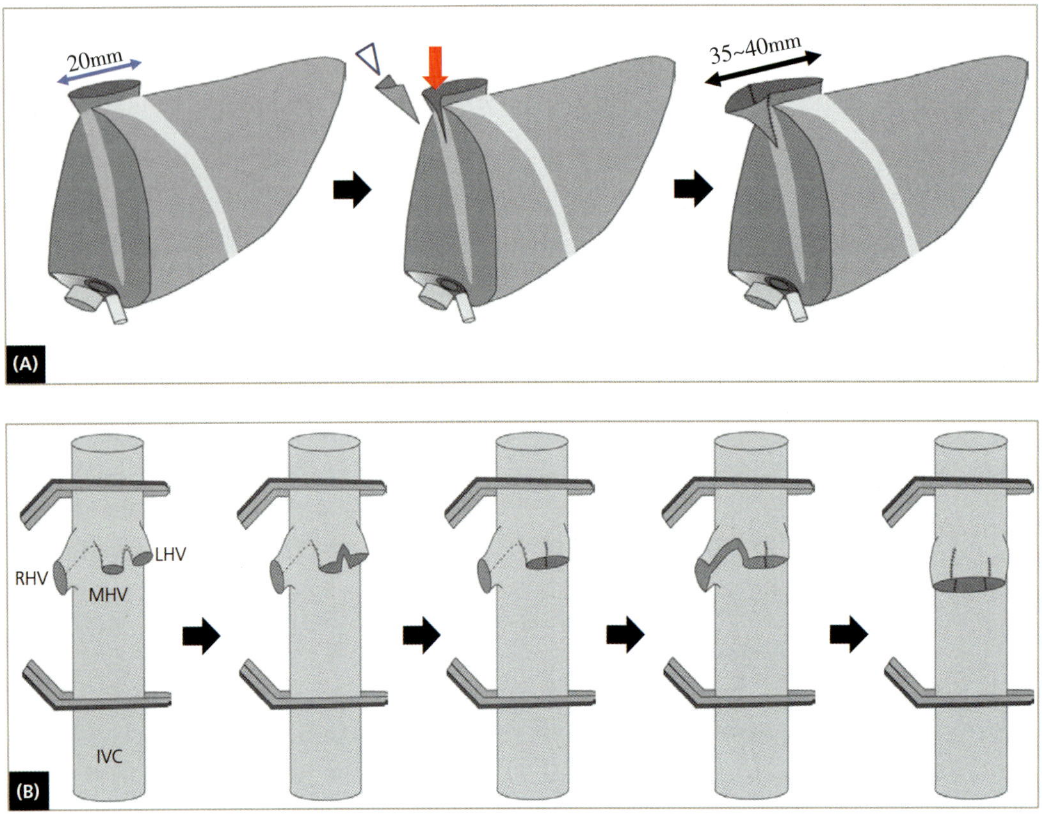

图 57.9 肝静脉成形术使左叶形成大的流出道。(A) 当移植物中的肝中静脉和肝左静脉的共同开口较小，即直径约为 20mm 时，将肝中静脉的右侧角切开(白色箭头)，并在后台中使用平分的大隐静脉(红色箭头)行补片成形术以产生大约 35~40mm 直径的扩大共同开口。(B) 在受体侧，所有 3 个肝静脉口完全打开，并且进行静脉成形术以形成适合移植物扩大的肝静脉口的大的共用开口。

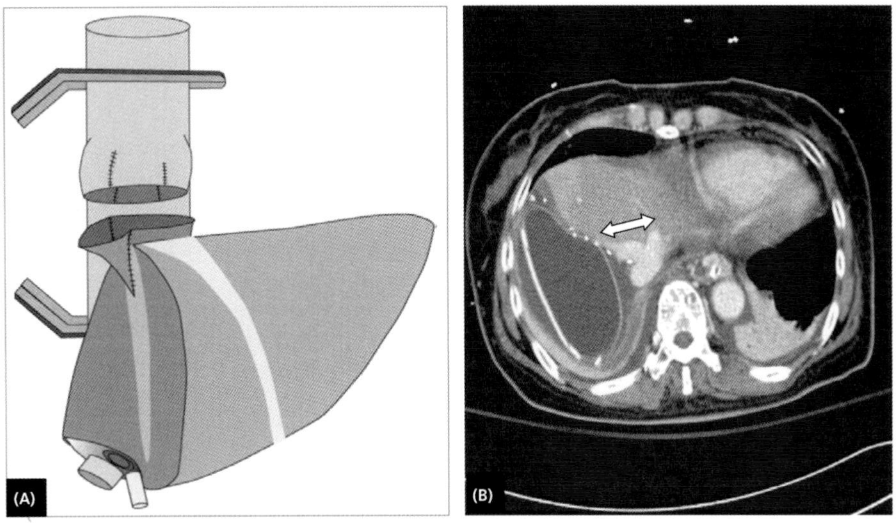

图 57.10 肝左叶静脉的重建。(A)通过夹闭肝上和肝下 IVC 以及静脉旁路进行供体和受体的扩大的肝静脉之间的吻合。(B)在术后第 7 天进行随访 CT 扫描显示,宽的肝静脉流出道和充满盐水的组织扩张器可以防止肝静脉吻合的扭转,直到植入的移植物充分再生。

定是否作为一个普通的 PV 开口仔细切除尾状叶 PV 分支或结扎它。考虑到肝动脉的重建,左叶移植物的所有肝动脉可能无法重建[52],因为肝副动脉通常与肝门的叶动脉连通[56]。然而,当存在大小和长度匹配的流入动脉时,我们重建了肝移植物的所有肝动脉,因为个体肝动脉基本上是末端动脉,并且当存在 HA 未重建时,我们有时会在移植后立即发现肝酶异常升高和左叶移植物的缺血区域。

尾状管相邻时可以重建成为单一开口,当分开时可以各自吻合[17]。但是,这是一个可选的操作,而不是必需的。选择尾状管重建,我们应特别注意确定胆管分裂位点,以避免忽略大的、分离的尾状管,包括穿过胆囊管的 9 段和 1 段的尾状管道及使用 1.5mm 的冠状动脉扩张器[117]。

双移植物活体供肝移植

来自单个供体的部分肝移植物,不管其是左叶移植物还是右叶移植物,通常不能满足体型较大受体的代谢需求或者具有门静脉高压的重症受体。作为一种替代方法,为了避免小肝综合征以及基于已建立的供体选择标准提供供体的安全性,自 2000 年以来,我们中心开始施行双移植物 LDLT,而且最近许多其他医院也开始进行双移植物 LDLT[42,123-127]。

受体手术期间,PV 和肝动脉的左右分支与周围组织分离,并且尽可能高游离,以便为将来的双侧血管吻合获得足够的长度。在全肝切除术中,受体的 IVC 应当从其腹膜后附着物游离,因为受体的肝静脉的静脉成形术和移植物植入需要阻断肝上及肝下 IVC。在大多数情况下,为了保持稳定的血流动力学及为了在无肝期避免肠系膜充血,静脉旁路是必要的。

在植入肝移植物之前,对受体肝静脉和(或)肝移植物中的肝静脉行静脉成形术以形成具有厚壁和长袖口的宽流出口。受体的 RHV 通过在下角处的纵向切开而扩大和拉长,并且用平分的 GSV 进行重建。肝中静脉和肝左静脉打开隔膜形成单个开口,然后通过在右角的横向切口和用平分 GSV 的围栏来扩大和拉长。在后台,根据受体和移植肝静脉之间的尺寸匹配来进行肝移植物肝静脉的静脉成形术。方法与前面提到的单移植物 LDLT 的方法相同。静脉成形术是重要的,以便外科医生在手术期间可以无困难地进行植入,并且还可以避免术后流出道出现问题。

使用两个左肝移植物的移植程序如下。首先,将 180°旋转的左肝置于右上象限,对受体 RHV 进行肝静脉吻合。第二,正常位置的左肝与肝中静脉和肝左静脉的共同开口吻合。第三,受体的左 PV 进行原位移植物的 PV 吻合。第四,更早地再灌注左侧(原位)移植物可以避免肠充血和减少缺血时间。在手术进行之前,血管夹应用于受体的 RHV 以防止在腔静脉夹释放后腔静脉流回右侧(异位)移植物。然后将腔静脉和主 PV 的血管夹一起移除,只夹住受体的右 PV。第五,右侧(异位)

移植物胆管对受体胆管的吻合术在PV吻合术之前以胆管对胆管的方式进行,因为胆管位于移植物逆行肝门结构的PV和肝动脉之后。第六,PV吻合在右侧移植物和受体右侧PV之间进行,并且在移除受体的RHV和右侧PV上的血管钳之后再灌注。第七,进行肝动脉吻合术,最后对左侧(原位)肝脏进行Roux-en-Y肝空肠吻合术。作为附加操作步骤,充填盐水(200~450mL)的组织扩张器插入右侧(异位)移植物下面,以减轻对肝门吻合的过度张力,因为左肝移植物总是太小而不能占据全肝切除术后的右上象限空间(图57.11)。

使用右肝移植物和左肝移植物的植入手术是分别使用右肝移植物和左肝移植物的两种单移植物LDLT的组合类型,因为两个移植物都是原位定位的。首先,将右肝移植物置于右上象限空间并进行肝静脉的重建。用静脉移植物重建供体MHV分支并与受体MHV下方的IVC前壁进行吻合。第二,左肝移植物原位放置,按肝静脉和PV顺序重建。第三,在受体右侧PV和移植物PV之间进行吻合,之后两个肝移植物同时再灌注。第四,在完成肝动脉吻合术后,仅使用Roux-en-Y肝空肠吻合术或受体胆管吻合术联合Roux-en-Y肝管空肠吻合术来对两个移植物的胆管进行重建。

如果可用的单一最大移植物不能满足受体的代谢需求,使用来自两个活体供体的左肝移植物或右肝移植物的双移植物LDLT可以通过满足受体的GRWR来扩大成人间LDLT的应用。具有双左叶LDLT(中值0.95%;范围0.59%~1.25%)的平均GRWR接近右叶移植的平均GRWR(中值0.98%;范围0.64%~1.29%)。

大多数双移植物LDLT,特别是那些使用两个左肝移植物的移植,都是为了确保供体的安全,而不是受体

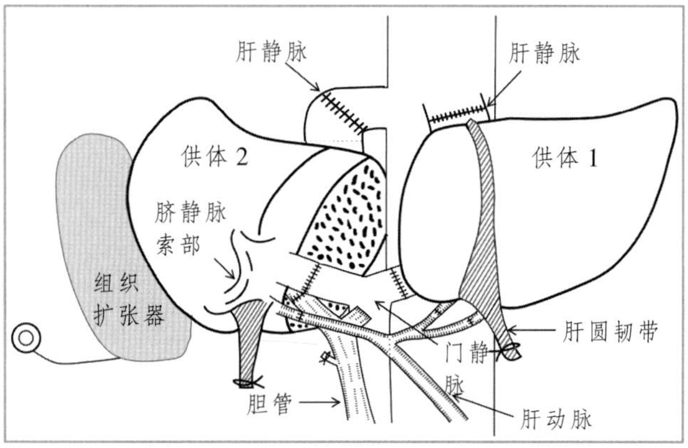

图57.11 采用双左叶移植物的LDLT。

的预后。供体并发症的发生率和严重程度低于单一右叶移植物LDLT的发生率和严重程度[92]。双移植物受体最常见的并发症是胆道狭窄(28%)和肝静脉流出道阻塞,右侧左肝移植物达到15%。肝静脉阻塞不发生在原位的左侧左肝移植物和右侧右肝移植物。这可能与通过异位定位的左肝移植物的再生过程中对肝静脉吻合的进行性压迫有关。与辅助、部分、原位肝移植(APOLT)相比,双移植物LDLT的两个肝移植物不会竞争性扩大,但在再生期间会一起扩大[128]。

在我们的医疗中心,2227名成人LDLT受体中,300名(13.5%)从2000年3月至2011年2月接受了双移植物移植(图57.12)。因暴发性肝功能衰竭行紧急双移植物移植的有18例(6.0%),因急性-慢性肝衰竭行紧急双移植物移植的有44例(14.7%)。活检证实的急性排斥反应的发生率类似于单移植物活体供体受体(17%),其中3/4在两个移植物中同时发生了急性排斥反应。院内死亡率为7.0%(21例),并且Ⅰ型和2A型患者占52%(11例)。双移植物受体和单移植物受体之间的总生存率和长期并发症的发生率及严重程度是相似的。罕见的情况下,单侧萎缩发生在两个左叶受体,但这不影响他们的肝功能或生存。

应用双左肝移植物的LDLT在技术上是复杂和精细的,但是该操作可以帮助解决与小尺寸移植物相关的问题,并且可以帮助扩大LDLT和成人受体劈离式肝移植的适应证。

右后叶移植

当满足受体的最小体积需求并且已经设定为受体的标准肝脏体积的40%时,右后叶移植物(RPS)可以是完全右叶移植物的良好替代物[129,130],并且体积大于左叶[131,132]。从技术上讲,RPS移植物的获取是最困难的,因为它需要最长时间的实质横切时间和肝门分离[130]。

Sugawara等表示,从解剖学角度看,在RPS移植物获取中没有排除标准[133]。然而,考虑到45%~50%的胆道并发症发生率,包括胆漏和狭窄,为了减少接受体的并发症,可能需要更加仔细地获取RPS移植物的供体选择标准。我们的医疗中心通常是选择性获取RPS移植物,以便在考虑包括PV、肝动脉和胆管的解剖学变化之后减少手术相关的并发症。当左叶体积不成比例地小(<30%的全肝体积)并且存在Ⅱ型或Ⅲ型PV时,成功获得RPS移植物是可能的[132]。

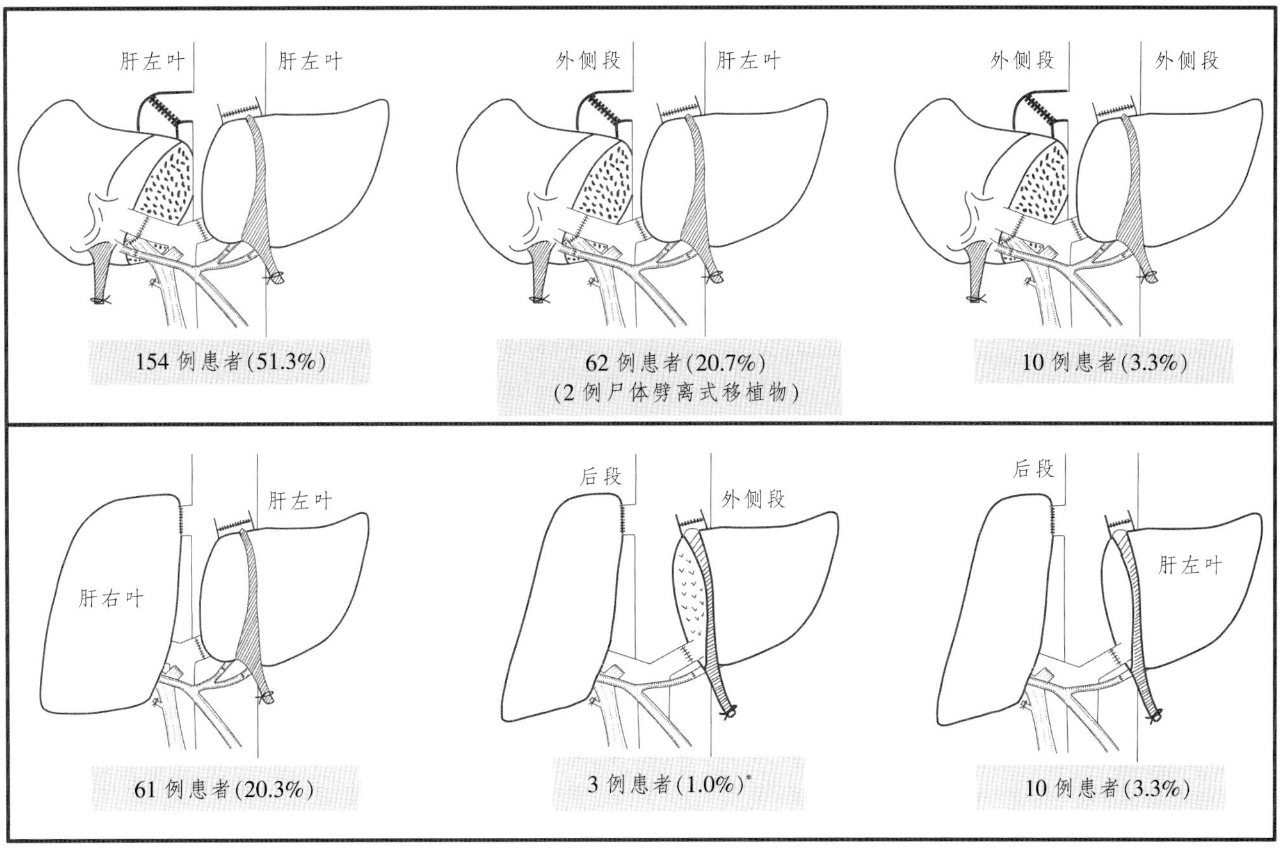

图 57.12　双移植物活体供体肝移植的各种方法。取自 2000 年 3 月至 2011 年 2 月在 Asan 医疗中心进行的 300 例双移植物移植(从 2227 位成人活体肝移植中获得的经验)的经验。

在受体手术中,应尽可能细致地进行肝门分离,以获得口径较小(直径为 1~2mm)、大小匹配的肝动脉和(或)用于胆管对胆管吻合的胆管开口。为了成功移植,准备和植入程序基本上与右叶植入相同。当 RPS 移植物的 PV 具有短的残端和(或)管壁较薄时,可以使用对分的 GSV 对移植物 PV 进行围栏,以便实现安全、广泛的吻合。当移植物的肝动脉残端过短,金属双微型血管夹不能旋转时,应当先行后壁的间断缝合修复。

总结

目前,活体供肝移植技术在全世界范围内广泛应用,但它仍然是一个技术上具有挑战性的手术,只有最有经验的团队才能执行。供体的选择对于确保供体的安全性至关重要,特别是要确保它们留有足够的(至少 30%)肝脏体积,并且术前对于受体的需要应仔细评估,确定供体肝叶的大小。如果潜在供体中右叶的体积超过全肝体积的 70%,或者如果大尺寸受体比来自单个供体的预期肝移植体积需要更多的移植体积,则双移植物 LDLT 是备选。受体的手术技术是全肝切除并保留下腔静脉。对于技术上成功的 LDLT,必须满足以下 4 个条件:①移植大体积移植物,避免小肝综合征;②良好流出道以避免充血;③足够的门静脉流入以增强移植物再生能力;④确保胆管吻合以避免胆汁渗漏。

(胡志平　译　朱继业　校)

参考文献

1. Bismuth H, Houssin D. Reduced-sized orthotopic liver graft in hepatic transplantation in children. Surgery. 1984;95:367-370.
2. Pichlmayr R, Ringe B, Gubernatis G, et al. [Transplantation of a donor liver to 2 recipients (splitting transplantation)—a new method in the further development of segmental liver transplantation]. Langenbecks Archiv fur Chirurgie. 1988;373:127-130.
3. Bismuth H, Morino M, Castaing D, et al. Emergency orthotopic liver transplantation in two patients using one donor liver. British Journal of Surgery. 1989;76:722-724.

4. Strong R, Ong TH, Pillay P, et al. A new method of segmental orthotopic liver transplantation in children. Surgery. 1988;104:104–107.
5. Strong RW, Lynch SV, Ong TH, et al. Successful liver transplantation from a living donor to her son. New England Journal of Medicine. 1990;322:1505–1507.
6. Broelsch CE, Emond JC, Whitington PF, et al. Application of reduced-size liver transplants as split grafts, auxiliary orthotopic grafts, and living related segmental transplants. Annals of Surgery. 1990;212:368–375; discussion 75–77.
7. Ozawa K, Uemoto S, Tanaka K, et al. An appraisal of pediatric liver transplantation from living relatives. Initial clinical experiences in 20 pediatric liver transplantations from living relatives as donors. Annals of Surgery. 1992;216:547–553.
8. de Villa VH, Lo CM, Chen CL. Ethics and rationale of living-donor liver transplantation in Asia. Transplantation. 2003;75(3 Suppl.):S2–S5.
9. Makuuchi M, Kawasaki S, Noguchi T, et al. Donor hepatectomy for living related partial liver transplantation. Surgery. 1993;113:395–402.
10. Hashikura Y, Makuuchi M, Kawasaki S, et al. Successful living-related partial liver transplantation to an adult patient. Lancet. 1994;343:1233–1234.
11. Lo CM, Fan ST, Liu CL, et al. Adult-to-adult living donor liver transplantation using extended right lobe grafts. Annals of Surgery. 1997;226:261–269; discussion 9–70.
12. Middleton PF, Duffield M, Lynch SV, et al. Living donor liver transplantation–adult donor outcomes: a systematic review. Liver Transplantation. 2006;12: 24–30.
13. Lee SG, Lee YJ, Park KM, et al. [Anterior segment congestion of right liver lobe graft in living donor liver transplantation and its strategy to prevent congestion] In Korean with English abstract. Journal of the Korean Society for Transplantation. 1999;13:213–219.
14. Fan ST, Lo CM, Liu CL, et al. Safety of donors in live donor liver transplantation using right lobe grafts. Archives of Surgery (Chicago, Ill.: 1960). 2000;135: 336–340.
15. Tzakis A, Todo S, Starzl TE. Orthotopic liver transplantation with preservation of the inferior vena cava. Annals of Surgery. 1989;210:649–652.
16. Moon DB, Lee SG. Liver transplantation. Gut and Liver. 2009;3:145–165.
17. Dulundu E, Sugawara Y, Sano K, et al. Duct-to-duct biliary reconstruction in adult living-donor liver transplantation. Transplantation. 2004;78:574–579.
18. Lee KW, Joh JW, Kim SJ, et al. High hilar dissection: new technique to reduce biliary complication in living donor liver transplantation. Liver Transplantation. 2004;10:1158–1162.
19. Yi NJ, Suh KS, Cho JY, et al. In adult-to-adult living donor liver transplantation hepaticojejunostomy shows a better long-term outcome than duct-to-duct anastomosis. Transplant International. 2005;18:1240–1247.
20. Hwang S, Lee SG, Ahn CS, et al. Morphometric and simulation analyses of right hepatic vein reconstruction in adult living donor liver transplantation using right lobe grafts. Liver Transplantation. 2010;16:639–648.
21. Hwang S, Ha TY, Ahn CS, et al. Reconstruction of inferior right hepatic veins in living donor liver transplantation using right liver grafts. Liver Transplantation. 2012;18:238–247.
22. Hwang S, Lee SG, Ahn CS, et al. Technique and outcome of autologous portal Y-graft interposition for anomalous right portal veins in living donor liver transplantation. Liver Transplantation. 2009;15:427–434.
23. Lee SG, Hwang S, Kim KH, et al. Approach to anatomic variations of the graft portal vein in right lobe living-donor liver transplantation. Transplantation. 2003;75(3 Suppl.):S28–S32.
24. Marcos A, Orloff M, Mieles L, et al. Reconstruction of double hepatic arterial and portal venous branches for right-lobe living donor liver transplantation. Liver Transplantation. 2001;7:673–679.
25. Starzl TE, Iwatsuki S, Shaw BW. A growth factor in fine vascular anastomoses. Surgery, Gynecology and Obstetrics. 1984;159:164–165.
26. Kim SJ, Kim DG, Park JH, et al. Clinical analysis of living donor liver transplantation in patients with portal vein thrombosis. Clinical Transplantation. 2010;25: 111–118.
27. Kadry Z, Selzner N, Handschin A, et al. Living donor liver transplantation in patients with portal vein thrombosis: a survey and review of technical issues. Transplantation. 2002;74:696–701.
28. Cho JY, Suh KS, Shin WY, et al. Thrombosis confined to the portal vein is not a contraindication for living donor liver transplantation. World Journal of Surgery. 2008;32:1731–1737.
29. Moon DB, Lee SG, Ahn CS, et al. Side-to-end renoportal anastomosis using an externally stented polytetrafluoroethylene vascular graft for a patient with a phlebosclerotic portal vein and a large spontaneous splenorenal shunt. Journal of the American College of Surgeons. 2011;212:e7–e11.
30. Sato Y, Kobayashi T, Nakatsuka H, et al. Splenic arterial ligation prevents liver injury after a major hepatectomy by a reduction of surplus portal hypertension in hepatocellular carcinoma patients with cirrhosis. Hepato-Gastroenterology. 2001;48:831–835.
31. Troisi R, Ricciardi S, Smeets P, et al. Effects of hemi-portocaval shunts for inflow modulation on the outcome of small-for-size grafts in living donor liver transplantation. American Journal of Transplantation. 2005;5:1397–1404.
32. Man K, Lo CM, Ng IO, et al. Liver transplantation in rats using small-for-size grafts: a study of hemodynamic and morphological changes. Archives of Surgery (Chicago, Ill.: 1960). 2001;136:280–285.
33. Troisi R, Cammu G, Militerno G, et al. Modulation of portal graft inflow: a necessity in adult living-donor liver transplantation? Annals of Surgery. 2003;237:429–436.
34. Boillot O, Delafosse B, Mechet I, et al. Small-for-size partial liver graft in an adult recipient; a new transplant technique. Lancet. 2002;359:406–407.
35. Takada Y, Ueda M, Ishikawa Y, et al. End-to-side portocaval shunting for a small-for-size graft in living donor liver transplantation. Liver Transplantation. 2004;10:807–810.
36. Moon DB, Lee SG, Kim KH, et al. The significance of complete interruption of large spontaneous portosystemic collaterals in adult living donor liver transplantation as a graft salvage procedure. Transplant International. 2008;21:698–700.
37. Botha JF, Campos BD, Johanning J, et al. Endovascular closure of a hemiportocaval shunt after small-for-size adult-to-adult left lobe living donor liver transplantation. Liver Transplantation. 2009;15:1671–1675.
38. Ito T, Kiuchi T, Yamamoto H, et al. Changes in portal venous pressure in the early phase after living donor liver transplantation: pathogenesis and clinical implications. Transplantation. 2003;75:1313–1317.
39. Lee SG, Moon DB, Ahn CS, et al. Ligation of left renal vein for large spontaneous splenorenal shunt to prevent portal flow steal in adult living donor liver transplantation. Transplant International. 2007;20:45–50.
40. Lee SG, Hwang S, Park KM, et al. Seventeen adult-to-adult living donor liver transplantations using dual grafts. Transplantation Proceedings. 2001;33: 3461–3463.
41. Chen Z, Yan L, Li B, et al. Prevent small-for-size syndrome using dual grafts in living donor liver transplantation. Journal of Surgical Research. 2009;155: 261–267.
42. Chen Z, Zeng Y, Wen TF, et al. Dual grafts live donor liver transplantation for acute-on-chronic hepatitis B liver failure. Transplantation Proceedings. 2010; 42:4552–4554.
43. Lee SG, Hwang S, Kim KH, et al. Toward 300 liver transplants a year. Surgery Today. 2009;39:367–373.
44. Moon DB, Lee SG, Ahn C, et al. Application of intraoperative cine-portogram to detect spontaneous portosystemic collaterals missed by intraoperative doppler exam in adult living donor liver transplantation. Liver Transplantation. 2007;13:1279–1284.
45. Inomoto T, Nishizawa F, Sasaki H, et al. Experiences of 120 microsurgical reconstructions of hepatic artery in living related liver transplantation. Surgery. 1996;119:20–26.
46. Okochi M, Ueda K, Hirose T, et al. A modified technique for hepatic artery reconstruction in living donor liver transplantation. Microsurgery. 2010;30: 541–544.
47. Aramaki O, Sugawara Y, Kokudo N, et al. Branch patch reconstruction in living donor liver transplantation: arterialization of grafts with replaced type arteries. Transplantation. 2006;82:1541–1543.
48. Di Benedetto F, Lauro A, Masetti M, et al. Use of a branch patch with the cystic artery in living-related liver transplantation. Clinical Transplantation. 2004;18:480–483.
49. Okazaki M, Asato H, Takushima A, et al. Hepatic artery reconstruction with double-needle microsuture in living-donor liver transplantation. Liver Transplantation. 2006;12:46–50.
50. Alper M, Gundogan H, Tokat C, et al. Microsurgical reconstruction of hepatic artery during living donor liver transplantation. Microsurgery. 2005;25:378–383; discussion 83–84.
51. Yan S, Zhang QY, Yu YS, et al. Microsurgical reconstruction of hepatic artery in living donor liver transplantation: experiences and lessons. Hepatobiliary and Pancreatic Diseases International. 2009;8:575–580.
52. Ikegami T, Kawasaki S, Matsunami H, et al. Should all hepatic arterial branches be reconstructed in living-related liver transplantation? Surgery. 1996;119: 431–436.
53. Sakamoto Y, Takayama T, Nakatsuka T, et al. Advantage in using living donors with aberrant hepatic artery for partial liver graft arterialization. Transplantation. 2002;74:518–521.
54. Tanaka K, Uemoto S, Tokunaga Y, et al. Surgical techniques and innovations in living related liver transplantation. Annals of Surgery. 1993;217:82–91.
55. Suehiro T, Ninomiya M, Shiotani S, et al. Hepatic artery reconstruction and biliary stricture formation after living donor adult liver transplantation using the left lobe. Liver Transplantation. 2002;8:495–499.

56. Redman HC, Reuter SR. Arterial collaterals in the liver hilus. Radiology. 1970;94:575–579.
57. Marcos A, Killackey M, Orloff MS, et al. Hepatic arterial reconstruction in 95 adult right lobe living donor liver transplants: evolution of anastomotic technique. Liver Transplantation. 2003;9:570–574.
58. Ahn CS, Lee SG, Hwang S, et al. Anatomic variation of the right hepatic artery and its reconstruction for living donor liver transplantation using right lobe graft. Transplantation Proceedings. 2005;37:1067–1069.
59. Wang CC, Lin TS, Chen CL, et al. Arterial reconstruction in hepatic artery occlusions in adult living donor liver transplantation using gastric vessels. Surgery. 2008;143:686–690.
60. Itabashi Y, Hakamada K, Narumi S, et al. A case of living-related partial liver transplantation using the right gastroepiploic artery for hepatic artery reconstruction. Hepato-Gastroenterology. 2000;47:512–513.
61. Ikegami T, Kawasaki S, Hashikura Y, et al. An alternative method of arterial reconstruction after hepatic arterial thrombosis following living-related liver transplantation. Transplantation. 2000;69:1953–1955.
62. Uchiyama H, Shirabe K, Taketomi A, et al. Extra-anatomical hepatic artery reconstruction in living donor liver transplantation: can this procedure save hepatic grafts? Liver Transplantation. 2010;16:1054–1061.
63. Katz E, Fukuzawa K, Schwartz M, et al. The splenic artery as the inflow in arterial revascularization of the liver graft in clinical liver transplantation. Transplantation. 1992;53:1373–1374.
64. Nakatsuka T, Takushima A, Harihara Y, et al. Versatility of the inferior epigastric artery as an interpositional vascular graft in living-related liver transplantation. Transplantation. 1999;67:1490–1492.
65. Mizuno S, Yokoi H, Isaji S, et al. Using a radial artery as an interpositional vascular graft in a living-donor liver transplantation for hepatocellular carcinoma. Transplant International. 2005;18:408–411.
66. Kasahara M, Sakamoto S, Ogawa K, et al. The use of a mesenteric artery of Roux-en-Y limb for hepatic arterial reconstruction after living-donor liver transplantation. Transplantation. 2005;80:538.
67. Inomoto T, Nishizawa F, Terajima H, et al. The use of the recipient sigmoid artery for a revision of hepatic arterial reconstruction after thrombosis in living related liver transplantation. Transplantation. 1995;60:881–882.
68. Asonuma K, Ohshiro H, Izaki T, et al. Rescue for rare complications of the hepatic artery in living donor liver transplantation using grafts of autologous inferior mesenteric artery. Transplant International. 2004;17:639–642.
69. Yazumi S, Chiba T. Biliary complications after a right-lobe living donor liver transplantation. Journal of Gastroenterology. 2005;40:861–865.
70. Calne RY. A new technique for biliary drainage in orthotopic liver transplantation utilizing the gall bladder as a pedicle graft conduit between the donor and recipient common bile ducts. Annals of Surgery. 1976;184:605–609.
71. Hwang S, Lee SG, Sung KB, et al. Long-term incidence, risk factors, and management of biliary complications after adult living donor liver transplantation. Liver Transplantation. 2006;12:831–838.
72. Chok KS, Chan SC, Cheung TT, et al. Bile duct anastomotic stricture after adult-to-adult right lobe living donor liver transplantation. Liver Transplantation. 2011;17:47–52.
73. Gondolesi GE, Varotti G, Florman SS, et al. Biliary complications in 96 consecutive right lobe living donor transplant recipients. Transplantation. 2004;77:1842–1848.
74. Kim SH, Lee KW, Kim YK, et al. Tailored telescopic reconstruction of the bile duct in living donor liver transplantation. Liver Transplantation. 2010;16:1069–1074.
75. Ikegami T, Shirabe K, Morita K, et al. Minimal hilar dissection prevents biliary anastomotic stricture after living donor liver transplantation. Transplantation. 2011;92:1147–1151.
76. Marubashi S, Dono K, Nagano H, et al. Biliary reconstruction in living donor liver transplantation: technical invention and risk factor analysis for anastomotic stricture. Transplantation. 2009;88:1123–1130.
77. Lin TS, Concejero AM, Chen CL, et al. Routine microsurgical biliary reconstruction decreases early anastomotic complications in living donor liver transplantation. Liver Transplantation. 2009;15:1766–1775.
78. Wang SF, Huang ZY, Chen XP. Biliary complications after living donor liver transplantation. Liver Transplantation. 2011;17:1127–1136.
79. Grussner RWG. Surgical procedures. Right lobe liver transplant. Chapter 30.3. In: Guressner RWG, Benedetti E, editors. Living Donor Organ Transplantation, 1st edition. New York, NY: McGraw-Hill Companies; 2008: 533–549.
80. Florman SS, Miller CM. Adult living donor hepatectomy and recipient operation. Chapter 45. In: Busuttil RW, Klintmalm G, editors. Transplantation of the Liver, 2nd edition. Philadelphia, PA: Elsevier Saunders; 2005: 675–702.
81. Marcos A, Ham JM, Fisher RA, et al. Surgical management of anatomical variations of the right lobe in living donor liver transplantation. Annals of Surgery. 2000;231:824–831.
82. Ishiko T, Egawa H, Kasahara M, et al. Duct-to-duct biliary reconstruction in living donor liver transplantation utilizing right lobe graft. Annals of Surgery. 2002;236:235–240.
83. Shah SA, Grant DR, McGilvray ID, et al. Biliary strictures in 130 consecutive right lobe living donor liver transplant recipients: results of a Western center. American Journal of Transplantation. 2007;7:161–167.
84. Kasahara M, Egawa H, Takada Y, et al. Biliary reconstruction in right lobe living-donor liver transplantation: comparison of different techniques in 321 recipients. Annals of Surgery. 2006;243:559–566.
85. Liu CL, Lo CM, Chan SC, et al. Safety of duct-to-duct biliary reconstruction in right-lobe live-donor liver transplantation without biliary drainage. Transplantation. 2004;77:726–732.
86. Fan ST, Lo CM, Liu CL, et al. Biliary reconstruction and complications of right lobe live donor liver transplantation. Annals of Surgery. 2002;236: 676–683.
87. Sharma S, Gurakar A, Jabbour N. Biliary strictures following liver transplantation: past, present and preventive strategies. Liver Transplantation. 2008;14: 759–769.
88. Jassem W, Heaton ND, Rela M. Reducing bile leak following segmental liver transplantation: understanding biliary anatomy of the caudate lobe. American Journal of Transplantation. 2008;8:271–274.
89. Suh KS, Choi SH, Yi NJ, et al. Biliary reconstruction using the cystic duct in right lobe living donor liver transplantation. Journal of the American College of Surgeons. 2004;199:661–664.
90. Kadry Z, Cintorino D, Foglieni CS, et al. The pitfall of the cystic duct biliary anastomosis in right lobe living donor liver transplantation. Liver Transplantation. 2004;10:1549–1550.
91. Sugawara Y, Makuuchi M. Technical advances in living-related liver transplantation. Journal of Hepato-Biliary-Pancreatic Surgery. 1999;6:245–253.
92. Hwang S, Lee SG, Lee YJ, et al. Lessons learned from 1,000 living donor liver transplantations in a single center: how to make living donations safe. Liver Transplantation. 2006;12:920–927.
93. Gyu Lee S, Min Park K, Hwang S, et al. Modified right liver graft from a living donor to prevent congestion. Transplantation. 2002;74:54–59.
94. Lee S, Park K, Hwang S, et al. Congestion of right liver graft in living donor liver transplantation. Transplantation. 2001;71:812–814.
95. Inomata Y, Uemoto S, Asonuma K, et al. Right lobe graft in living donor liver transplantation. Transplantation. 2000;69:258–264.
96. Moon DB, Lee SG. Adult-to-adult living donor liver transplantation at the Asan Medical Center. Yonsei Medical Journal. 2004;45:1162–1168.
97. Akamatsu N, Sugawara Y, Kaneko J, et al. Effects of middle hepatic vein reconstruction on right liver graft regeneration. Transplantation. 2003;76: 832–837.
98. Maetani Y, Itoh K, Egawa H, et al. Factors influencing liver regeneration following living-donor liver transplantation of the right hepatic lobe. Transplantation. 2003;75:97–102.
99. Kasahara M, Takada Y, Fujimoto Y, et al. Impact of right lobe with middle hepatic vein graft in living-donor liver transplantation. American Journal of Transplantation. 2005;5:1339–1346.
100. Cattral MS, Greig PD, Muradali D, et al. Reconstruction of middle hepatic vein of a living-donor right lobe liver graft with recipient left portal vein. Transplantation. 2001;71:1864–1866.
101. Lee KW, Lee DS, Lee HH, et al. Interpostion vein graft in living donor liver transplantation. Transplantation Proceedings. 2004;36:2261–2262.
102. Kornberg A, Heyne J, Schotte U, et al. Hepatic venous outflow reconstruction in right lobe living-donor liver graft using recipient's superficial femoral vein. American Journal of Transplantation. 2003;3:1444–1447.
103. Elola-Olaso AM, Gonzalez EM, Diaz JC, et al. Hepatic vein reconstruction in living donor liver transplantation. Transplantation Proceedings. 2005;37: 3891–3892.
104. Hwang S, Lee SG, Ahn CS, et al. Cryopreserved iliac artery is indispensable interposition graft material for middle hepatic vein reconstruction of right liver grafts. Liver Transplantation. 2005;11:644–649.
105. Yi NJ, Suh KS, Lee HW, et al. An artificial vascular graft is a useful interpositional material for drainage of the right anterior section in living donor liver transplantation. Liver Transplantation. 2007;13:1159–1167.
106. Hwang S, Jung DH, Ha TY, et al. Usability of ringed polytetrafluoroethylene grafts for middle hepatic vein reconstruction during living donor liver transplantation. Liver Transplantation. 2012;18:955–965.
107. Lee S, Park K, Hwang S, et al. Anterior segment congestion of a right liver lobe graft in living-donor liver transplantation and strategy to prevent congestion. Journal of Hepato-Biliary-Pancreatic Surgery. 2003;10:16–25.
108. Lo CM, Fan ST, Liu CL, et al. Hepatic venoplasty in living-donor liver transplantation using right lobe graft with middle hepatic vein. Transplantation. 2003;

75:358–360.
109. Liu CL, Zhao Y, Lo CM, et al. Hepatic venoplasty in right lobe live donor liver transplantation. Liver Transplantation. 2003;9:1265–1272.
110. Chan SC, Lo CM. 30.3.1b Extended right lobe transplant. In: Gruessner RWG, Benedetti E, editor. Living Donor Organ Transplantation, 1st edition. New York, NY: McGraw-Hill Companies; 2008: 549–554.
111. Chok KS, Chan SC, Lo CM, et al. Emergency re-routing of anterior sector venous outflow for right lobe living donor liver transplantation including the middle hepatic vein. Hepatobiliary and Pancreatic Diseases International. 2011;10: 325–327.
112. Hwang S, Lee SG, Ahn CS, et al. Outflow vein reconstruction of extended right lobe graft using quilt venoplasty technique. Liver Transplantation. 2006; 12:156–158.
113. Matsubara K, Cho A, Okazumi S, et al. Anatomy of the middle hepatic vein: applications to living donor liver transplantation. Hepato-Gastroenterology. 2006;53:933–937.
114. Hwang S, Lee SG, Ha TY, et al. Tailoring transection of segment V vein for optimal sharing of middle hepatic vein in right-lobe living donor liver transplantation. Hepato-Gastroenterology. 2006;53:904–908.
115. Sugawara Y, Makuuchi M, Takayama T, et al. Small-for-size grafts in living-related liver transplantation. Journal of the American College of Surgeons. 2001;192: 510–513.
116. Lo CM, Fan ST, Liu CL, et al. Minimum graft size for successful living donor liver transplantation. Transplantation. 1999;68:1112–1116.
117. Hwang S, Lee SG, Ha TY, et al. Simplified standardized technique for living donor liver transplantation using left liver graft plus caudate lobe. Liver Transplantation. 2004;10:1398–1405.
118. Akamatsu N, Sugawara Y, Tamura S, et al. Regeneration and function of hemiliver graft: right versus left. Surgery. 2006;139:765–772.
119. Ben-Haim M, Emre S, Fishbein TM, et al. Critical graft size in adult-to-adult living donor liver transplantation: impact of the recipient's disease. Liver Transplantation. 2001;7:948–953.
120. Sugawara Y, Makuuchi M, Takayama T. Left liver plus caudate lobe graft with complete revascularization. Surgery. 2002;132:904–905; author reply 5–6.
121. Sugawara Y, Makuuchi M, Kaneko J, et al. New venoplasty technique for the left liver plus caudate lobe in living donor liver transplantation. Liver Transplantation. 2002;8:76–77.
122. Kokudo N, Sugawara Y, Kaneko J, et al. Reconstruction of isolated caudate portal vein in left liver graft. Liver Transplantation. 2004;10:1163–1165.
123. Lee S, Hwang S, Park K, et al. An adult-to-adult living donor liver transplant using dual left lobe grafts. Surgery. 2001;129:647–650.
124. Lu CH, Chen TY, Huang TL, et al. Regeneration and outcome of dual grafts in living donor liver transplantation. Clinical Transplantation. 2012;26:E143–E148.
125. Dayangac M, Taner CB, Akin B, et al. Dual left lobe living donor liver transplantation using donors unacceptable for right lobe donation: a case report. Transplantation Proceedings. 2010;42:4560–4563.
126. Soejima Y, Taketomi A, Ikegami T, et al. Living donor liver transplantation using dual grafts from two donors: a feasible option to overcome small-for-size graft problems? American Journal of Transplantation. 2008;8:887–892.
127. Broering DC, Walter J, Rogiers X. The first two cases of living donor liver transplantation using dual grafts in Europe. Liver Transplantation. 2007;13:149–153.
128. Lee SG. Double liver transplant. In: Gruessner RWG, Benedetti E, editor. Living Donor Organ Transplantation, 1st edition. New York, NY: McGraw-Hill Companies; 2008: 557–560.
129. Urata K, Kawasaki S, Matsunami H, et al. Calculation of child and adult standard liver volume for liver transplantation. Hepatology (Baltimore, Md.). 1995;21: 1317–1321.
130. Kokudo N, Sugawara Y, Imamura H, et al. Tailoring the type of donor hepatectomy for adult living donor liver transplantation. American Journal of Transplantation. 2005;5:1694–1703.
131. Sugawara Y, Makuuchi M, Takayama T, et al. Right lateral sector graft in adult living-related liver transplantation. Transplantation. 2002;73:111–114.
132. Hwang S, Lee SG, Lee YJ, et al. Donor selection for procurement of right posterior segment graft in living donor liver transplantation. Liver Transplantation. 2004;10:1150–1155.
133. Sugawara Y, Makuuchi M. Right lateral sector graft as a feasible option for partial liver transplantation. Liver Transplantation. 2004;10:1156–1157.

第 58 章 心脏移植手术步骤和外科技术

John M. Craig, Soyoung Lee, Gus J. Vlahakes, Joren C. Madsen

引言

现代心脏移植外科中使用的基本外科手术都基于 Alexis Carrel 在 19 世纪 90 年代开发的血管吻合技术。在世纪之交,Carrel 首先将血管吻合技术应用于器官移植,给狗行了颈部异位心脏移植[1]。该领域经过一段沉寂后,莫斯科的 Vladimir Demikhov 开始在狗的胸腔内进行心脏移植和心–肺移植。20 世纪 40 年代末,他在狗身上成功施行了原位心脏移植,但他的大部分著作直到 20 世纪 60 年代早期才以英文发表。在那时,斯坦福大学的 Lower 和 Shumway 改进了狗的原位心脏移植的技术,并报告显著比以往的试验获得了更长的生存期[2]。利用斯坦福研究组开发的原位技术,1967 年 12月 3 日 Christiaan Barnard 在南非开普敦执行了第一次成功的人类心脏移植[3]。从那时起,最常见的移植方法是将供体心脏原位植入;然而,其他手术包括异位移植和心–肺移植,已被证明在某些情况下有用[4]。虽然自 1967 年以来在心脏移植中最显著的总体进展是效应免疫抑制的出现,但是心脏移植技术中最显著的变革是从腔静脉心房吻合到双腔。

人类心脏同种异体移植物的保存、获取和植入有许多不同的方式。下面描述的技术是马萨诸塞州总医院使用的技术。它们对我们观察到良好受体的短期和长期预后做出了贡献。然而,不同中心应用的技术不同,但也可获得良好预后。

供体手术

ICU 对供体的医疗治疗和获取期间细致的外科技术可以说是整个移植手术最重要的部分。首先,减少早期移植物功能障碍的风险,心脏必须处于高能量状态。这只能通过获取心脏的外科医生管理或优化供体血压、心排血量、体积状态、代谢参数和血细胞比容来保证。第二,因为这个时期是供体有可能被接受或排斥的时期,所有关于供体适宜性的患者数据必须谨慎获得、评估并纳入决策过程。第三,获取团队,特别是心脏和肺部团队,必须协调其各自的术中计划,以避免任何器官(最终,任何受体)处于危险中。这需要在手术开始之前进行充分沟通。最后,移植物必须被良好保存、安全移出,并且快速转运到移植设施以确保最佳结果。关于供体捐献步骤的一般性讨论参见第 21 章。

准备

供体–受体匹配的初始步骤在第 39 章中已进行了讨论。在离开供体医院之前,心脏团队必须确保所有必要的物品被包装。我们通常携带 2L 冷却的晶体停跳液(Plegisol)用作保存液。心脏保存的细节参见第 26 章。心脏停搏液放在冷冻盐水袋包围的冷却装置中运输。我们还带来了不普遍应用的物品,例如主动脉根插管、Prolene 缝线、止血带和具有必要心脏停搏适配器的管道。我们当地的器官获取组织(OPO)提供额外的心脏停搏液和胸骨牵开器。在到达供体医院时,审查患者相关医疗记录、超声心动图、胸部 X 线片和血管造影。验证患者身份和 ABO 相容性。重新评估供体的医学状况,因为生理学的快速变化并不罕见。核实正确的监测功能很重要。在最低限度,供体应该有一个大口径的外周静脉线以及动脉和中心静脉监测线。供体手术室的管理目标是保持收缩期动脉压超过 100mmHg,中心静脉压为 8~12mmHg,PaO_2>95mmHg, 血细胞比容≥30。为了最小化心室刺激和能量消耗,我们避免使用 β 激动剂,而使用去氧肾上腺素血管加压药。容量控制通常足以治疗短暂性低血压。

不同手术团队之间应该彼此熟悉,并应明确步骤,特别是那些涉及竞争关系的解剖结构。如需取左肺,心脏外科医生和肺外科医生应该一起工作以计划如何以及在何处分开肺静脉，以便为两个植入都留下适当的组织。这同样适用于分割主肺动脉,以及与肝脏外科医生讨论下腔静脉的分开。在操作之前进行几分钟的沟通可以防止错误、节省时间,并避免在操作过程中热缺血时间延长。

手术技术

在必要的“超时”之后,将供体从颈部覆盖到腹股沟,并且利用正中线切口开始多器官获取操作。严格止血很重要，即使是从暴露的胸骨表面随时间累积的缓慢渗出。胸骨用骨蜡完全密封。为了不影响腹部显露,胸骨牵开器固定杆应朝向头部。打开心包并用丝线悬吊,右下心包被游离到下腔静脉的水平以增强显露,并且当下腔静脉排出时,为血液进入右胸腔提供出口。检查心室功能是否正常,有无扩张,有无冠状动脉粥样硬化(通过视觉检查和手动触诊)、解剖变异和创伤,以及大小是否匹配。触诊主动脉震颤可能提示瓣膜疾病。做出最后供体是否适合捐献的决定，并将其与预期的钳夹时间一同与受体团队进行沟通。

虽然分离可以以各种方式进行，但我们通常以顺时针方式进行,从上腔静脉和左无名静脉开始,完全游离。向后确定奇静脉,远端结扎。如果需要,保存奇静脉可用于扩大供体的腔静脉开口。如果要获取肺,游离上腔静脉和主动脉之间的平面，相对无血管的气管前组织在无名静脉和肺动脉之间纵向分开(参见第21章和第59章)。然后打开主肺动脉窗以在随后的主动脉夹闭中防止肺动脉损伤。避免主动脉根周围的分离,以防止冠状动脉的损伤。下腔静脉沿圆周切开。

直到团队所有准备都完成才进行主动脉夹闭和插管。患者全身肝素化(300单位/kg)。然后将保存溶液从冷却器中取出并悬挂在头部的压力袋中。对于初次冲洗,我们使用冷却的Plegisol。它需要在使用前加入10mL的8.4%的碳酸氢钠溶液。将心脏停搏导管置于升主动脉中并用4-0 Prolene固定,因为其将在植入期间保留以供使用。如果要获取肺,则需增加插管,通过在远端主肺动脉上心脏和肺团队相互可接受的点进行荷包缝合,插入插管。所有颈部管线由麻醉师撤回到创伤静脉上方。一旦所有团队完成准备步骤,心脏获取就会迅速进行。心脏小组的优先级是右心室和左心室的充分减压和恰当使用保存液。以下步骤应以快速但受控的顺序执行：

1.如果要获取肺,则将500μg前列腺素E_1注射到插管附近的肺动脉或右心耳中。

2.在与无名静脉汇合处结扎上腔静脉。

3.如果要获取肺,分开左心耳或切开左心房的下壁以离开左心。如果无须获取肺,则左下肺静脉在其心包反折处切开。

4.心包内下腔静脉部分横断,血液排入右侧胸腔。

5.一旦证实有充分减压后,主动脉横向钳位应用尽可能远的位置(优选无名动脉起源处)。

6. 1L心脏停搏保存溶液用100~150mmHg的力施加于压力袋上。

7.心包充满冷保存液。

8.观察心脏是否有足够的主动脉根部压力、是否迅速停跳和变白,以及没有心室扩张。

在心脏停搏液完成后,进行供体心脏切除术。下腔静脉的后壁被分开,游离右心房下部。上腔静脉在与无名静脉汇合处分开。如果无须获取肺,则肺静脉在其心包反折处简单横切。如果需要获取肺，则心脏向左牵拉,房间沟被切开并向上延伸到左心房圆顶上,同时向下延伸到下腔静脉后方。然后心尖向头端牵拉,使两个下肺静脉进入视野。然后切口从右到左平行于房室沟,继续至左肺静脉前面。最后,心脏向头侧和前侧牵开,同时上部左心房壁被分开。在分离左心房期间肺脏和心脏团队必须频繁检查并重新评估肺静脉口。尤其在左心房的左侧，左肺静脉和供体左房室沟之间距离有限。足够的左心房袖口必须保留以备移植,而不损害或扭曲冠状动脉(参见第59章)。主动脉弓分支和近端降主动脉分开。最后,主肺动脉在其分叉处横断。然后将供体心脏带到后台进行保存并准备转运(参见下文)。

同种异体移植物的制备和转运

在捐助机构的准备

在后台上,我们将500 mL威斯康星大学(UW)溶液注入夹紧的主动脉根中，并使用剩余的溶液作为转运介质。检查移植物的解剖异常，包括卵圆孔未闭和(或)手术损伤。心麻痹插管留在原位以备后用。将心脏置于具有UW保存溶液的无菌塑料袋中，修复并用脐带胶布带绑扎。冰不直接放置与移植物接触。将该袋放入另一袋盐水冰袋中，然后将其置于塑料容器中，用最终袋包裹并放入冷却器中转运。通知受体团队交叉钳夹时间、器官的状况和到达受体医院的估计时间。有关心脏保存的更多详情请参见第 26 章。

受体医疗中心的准备

受体医疗中心，将心脏从无菌包装中取出并放置在后台上用于最终制备。获取外科医生在完成受体心脏切除术时进行这一操作。确认 ABO 匹配，分离大血管。通过连接所有四个肺静脉口并纵向切开左心房游离壁以产生单个开口而成形左心房袖口。如果存在卵圆孔未闭或左心耳开口，应牢固地闭合。如果计划行双心房吻合术，上腔静脉在窦房结上方 1~2cm 处双重结扎，右心房从外侧下腔静脉向远离窦房结的右心耳基部开放。对于双腔静脉吻合术，在奇静脉开口的水平修剪上腔静脉袖带。这可以随后用于上文提到的扩大吻合。供体主动脉和肺动脉在长度上未被修剪。供体心脏被带到手术台并用冷的、充氧的心脏搏跳液灌注。

为了扩大供体来源，有人报告了用于许多心脏缺陷供体的修复技术。然而，广泛修复的功能优势必然导致缺血时间长。二尖瓣修复术已被报道[5-7]，但是只有在高度可信的情况下，这样的修复才是必要的，并且能获得持久的功能结果时才可以进行。主动脉瓣修复也有报道，但应该由具有这些修复技术经验的外科医生进行[8]。三尖瓣血栓形成可能需要通过瓣环成形术修复，因为植入后中度三尖瓣回流的受体显示生存率降低[9]。是否所有供体心脏应进行三尖瓣瓣膜成形术是有争议的(参见下文)[10]。已经报道了室间隔缺损的闭合[11]，但是应该避免右心室切开术，因为有移植后右心室功能受损的倾向。

受体操作

时间控制

从获取团队前往供体地点之前就应开始协调工作。受体应在预计开始手术前 2 小时带到手术室，轻微镇静并插入监测管线。获取团队在主动脉横向钳夹之前与受体团队沟通以同步供体心脏移植和受体心脏切除的时间，使得受体团队在供体团队到达之前做好准备。这避免等待心脏切除手术完成时增加缺血时间。采用现有技术，缺血时间不应超过 6 小时(成人)，如果可能，应保持在 4 小时或更短时间，特别是高风险移植物(即次优供体或具有肺血管阻力增加的受体)。

受体的术前准备

受体通常服用华法林，或因药物治疗和长期心力衰竭导致的肝脏淤血而引起凝血功能障碍。在这种情况下，我们肌肉内注射或通过非常缓慢(超过 30~60 分钟)的静脉输注服用维生素 K(10mg)。鉴于其广泛的心脏病史，受体可能先前已有肝素抗体。重要的是审查既往是否使用肝素用于心肺转流。具有心室辅助装置(VAD)的患者显示，如果在移植期间避免应用肝素，并且术前抗肝素/血小板因子-4 抗体(HPF4)滴度低或不存在，在移植程序期间的再暴露与围术期并发症增加无相关[12]。但如果 HPF4 滴度升高，选择使用直接凝血酶抑制剂(如比伐卢定)或使用肝素与术中血浆置换或糖蛋白 IIBIIIA 抑制剂结合[13-15]。当患者服用阿加曲班时，我们通常在手术前 4~6 小时停止输注。我们的患者手术前口服霉酚酸酯(MMF)1000~1500mg，诱导麻醉期间给予大剂量静脉注射皮质类固醇[16]。同样，在诱导麻醉之前施用广谱预防性抗生素和抗纤维蛋白溶解剂。我们常规应用肺动脉插管、动脉监测、深静脉插管和经食管超声心动图。

受体手术

准备

永久起搏器和(或)可植入心律转复除颤器需要在现场准备。在胸骨切开术后，患者通过旁路肝素化(初始剂量为 300IU/kg)。在升主动脉上尽可能远的位置进行主动脉插管，以提供尽可能长的用于植入的长度。使用直角金属插管行双腔静脉插管，同样尽可能到血管周边。应用荷包缝合，止血带位于插管同侧，心房缝线对侧，以便保持尽可能长的长度并使随后的吻合变形最小。当获取团队到达时，启动心肺转流。一旦建立旁路，冷却至 28℃，防止供体心脏的早期恢复。所有中心静脉管路撤回上腔静脉。一旦确认心肺转流启动良好，主动脉应用横向钳夹，收紧止血带，进行受体心脏切除术。

心脏切除术

主动脉在窦管连接处横切。受体的心脏切除术以近似顺时针的方向进行。首先,通过心耳做平行于房室沟的右心房切口进入左房穹窿。右心房切口向下继续朝向下腔静脉的内侧。在腔房交界上方切断上腔静脉。受体通常有穿过上腔静脉的索,拉向心脏并且应用剪刀尽可能短地切断。分离主动脉和肺动脉直到各自的瓣膜远端,在主动脉–肺窗形成后(如果以前没有完成的话)。左房穹隆的初始切口继续沿两个方向切开。首先,房间隔间延续通过卵圆窝,向下朝向房室沟,连接先前的右心房切口,恰好位于下腔静脉内侧。然后它继续平行于房室沟,头侧朝向二尖瓣后叶。切口的另一部分越过左房穹窿,在左心耳基底和左肺静脉之间,以沿着房室沟接合先前的切口,从而完成心脏切除术。在供体心脏切除术中,非常小心地保留肺静脉口附近的左心房充盈的袖带。因为这是使后心包内容物止血的理想机会,包括烧灼左心房的自由边缘。一旦关闭旁路,在该区域的后续出血将难以纠正。一些医生通过右上肺静脉荷包缝合的方式放置通道以排出温热的肺静脉回流血。

心脏植入

植入同种异体移植物的顺序有多种,外科医生根据每个手术的需要制订策略并根据需要限制缺血时间。因为我们支持双腔技术,我们的默认吻合顺序如下:①左心房;②下腔静脉;③肺动脉;④主动脉(随后去除主动脉阻断钳;⑤上腔静脉。如果需要减少缺血时间,则将该顺序修改如下:①左心房;②主动脉(随后去除主动脉阻断钳);③肺动脉;④下腔静脉;⑤上腔静脉。后一顺序的缺点是冠状静脉回流可能部分地遮蔽肺动脉和下腔静脉吻合。在整个手术期间,应用冰纱布覆盖右心室,并且手术区域充满二氧化碳以限制心内空气聚集。注意,首选外翻的左心房缝线,是为了保持裸露的心房肌不暴露在左心房内。一般来说,肺动脉吻合口不要收紧打结直到手术结束,使得空气可以从右心脏排出。与所有开放性心脏手术一样,必须小心以确保左心已被良好除气。虽然通常定暂时的,但即使是右冠状动脉中一个小的气栓也会成为主要问题。如果在植入顺序中的早期去除阻断钳,应连续监测心脏,以确保左心室不扩张。

双腔静脉技术与双房技术

右心房吻合技术必须在植入前确定,因为这决定了心脏切除的步骤和后台准备。从心脏移植早期以来最重要的技术进步是使用全身静脉回流的双腔静脉方法。在世纪之交之前,几乎完全应用这种方法。UNOS数据表明,在2007年之前接近2/3的移植物使用了双腔静脉技术[17]。对近21 000名受试者超过10年的调查显示,在双腔静脉组放置永久性起搏器的发生率增加(OR为2.6),在30天和长期随访中存在明显的生存不利(双腔静脉死亡率OR分别为1.17和1.11),支持近10年前类似的报道[18]。双腔静脉技术也有优势,因为它保留右心房形态以及窦房结和三尖瓣功能[19,20]。三尖瓣反流在右心室功能不全的患者中不能很好地耐受,这在心脏移植后经常见到[21]。此外,双腔静脉技术与永久性起搏器植入的频率降低有关[18]。但腔静脉缝合线在早期和晚期均存在吻合口狭窄的风险,这不是技术问题。双房技术主要优点是技术上相对简单,执行吻合所必需的分离和吻合本身两方面都较为简单。但是,双房吻合有窦房结损伤的风险,并且冗余的心房组织可能对心房血流动力学不利并且导致术后心房心律失常的风险增加[22–24]。双房技术的两个窦房结的存在可能使术后确认窦房结功能和房室传导的模式方面存在困难。对41篇论文的Meta分析发现,在早期心房压力、三尖瓣反流、恢复到窦性心律,甚至围术期死亡率方面,双房技术有显著的益处。然而,长期结果在两组间差异不大[25]。

原位双腔静脉技术

左房吻合

在植入之前,偶尔需要修剪供体和(或)受体左房,以防止腔体过大存在血栓形成风险[26](图58.1A)。用长3–0聚丙烯缝合线在受体左上肺静脉和供体左心耳附近开始缝合(图58.1B)。受体左心耳和供体左心耳的部位相对应可以防止心脏旋转。缝合数针后将移植物放入心包内。缝合线首先以顺时针方向缝合,然后是逆时针,尽量用正手操作。如果心房袖口有缺陷可以使用连续缝合,但我们通常应用连续垂直褥式缝合,保证外翻和排除心房袖口的血栓性肌肉层。在冠状动脉周围区域,注意避免深部缝合。重要的是定期重新评估下腔静脉的位置，以确保其在适当的位置进行随后的双心房吻合。在房间隔右侧的中间附近打结。

另一种替代传统双腔静脉技术的是所谓的双腔静脉总技术，包括两个左心房吻合，一个到右肺静脉袖口（包括上肺静脉口和下肺静脉口），另一个到左肺静脉袖口，类似于肺移植。在这种情况下，受体的心脏切除术将包括去除除双侧肺静脉袖口之外的所有心房组织。植入时首先牵拉心脏向右侧缝合左肺静脉袖口，然后牵拉心脏回左侧行右袖口吻合[27]。

下腔静脉吻合

4–0 聚丙烯缝合线沿着后壁延伸到前壁上（图 58.1C）。为降低狭窄发生的风险，一部分受体右心房保留在下腔静脉附近以进行扩展吻合。正如我们所有的吻合，间断立式缝合放置在 3 点钟和 9 点钟位置。在供体冠状窦区域避免深度缝合。这种吻合可以通过股静脉置管和使用开放或夹闭的下腔静脉的真空辅助静脉引流来帮助实现[28]。偶尔，如果受体具有持续引流入冠状窦的左上腔静脉，则可保留左房室沟中的受体冠状窦和相关组织。当完成腔内静脉吻合术时，受体侧包括腔内静脉口和冠状窦口。在这种情况下，通常需要单独插管。

肺动脉吻合

过多的肺动脉必须修剪，因为肺动脉吻合特别容易扭结或套叠，尤其是供体心脏较大时。由于相同的原因，必须小心确保供体和受体肺动脉的几何形状良好对齐。用 4–0 聚丙烯缝合线连续缝合，在 3 点钟和 9 点钟位置间断缝合。如果需要修复缝合，将供体肺动脉修剪短，而不修剪受体血管的好处是其可以使吻合靠近并使缝合更容易。新的肺动脉长度过长可产生内陷和瓣上梯度。

主动脉吻合

与肺动脉一样，修剪主动脉以避免额外的长度，从

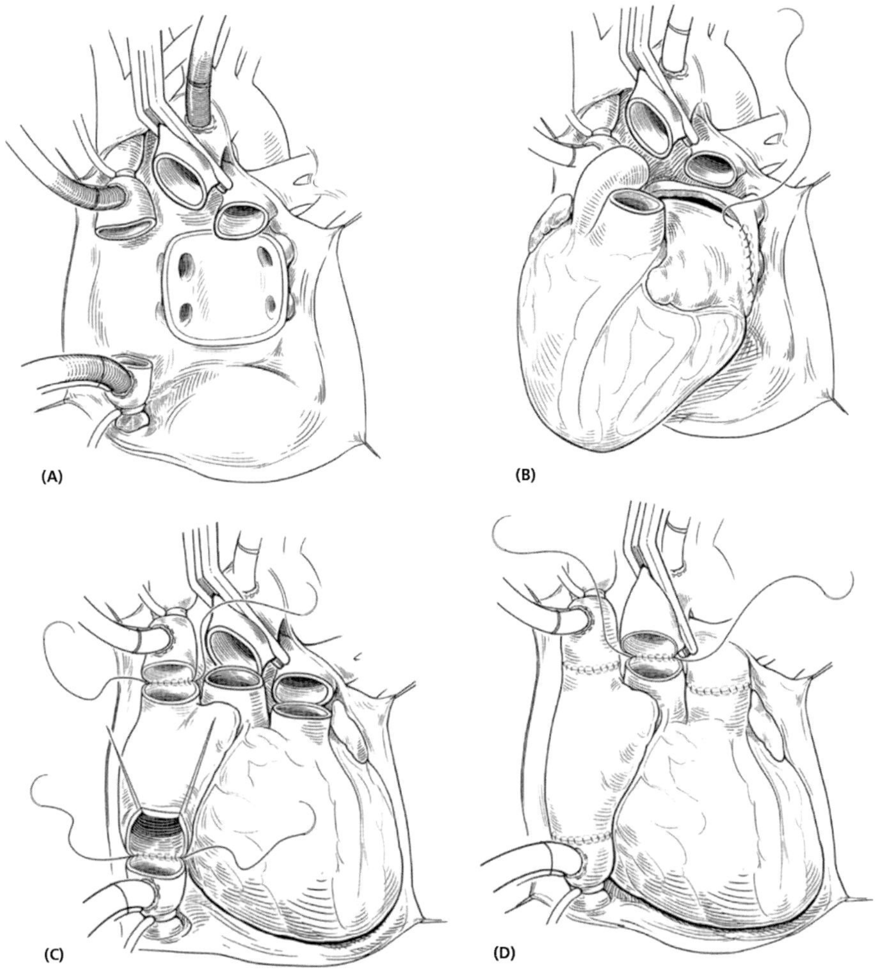

图 58.1　(A~D)心脏移植中应用双腔静脉吻合技术的详细手术步骤。

而避免随后发生扭结的可能性。这种吻合通常以与肺动脉相同的方式进行(图 58.1D)。复温重新开始。在缝合完成后,心脏被去除,并且去除主动脉阻断钳。在钳子移除后不久开始自然收缩。通过将根部通气孔抽吸进行连续主动脉根部排气。

上腔静脉吻合

实施该吻合时应注意要精细缝合以避免串线。我们在后壁上应用连续缝合，在前壁上应用 5-0 Prolene 间断缝合(图 58.1C)。在行心脏切除术时尽可能保留受体较长的上腔静脉,这样,如果供体上腔静脉较短,则可将受体上腔静脉直接缝合到腔静脉结合部。如果在移除血管阻断钳后实施该吻合,应钳夹供体上腔静脉,以防止血流模糊手术野。完成的移植描述于图 58.2,其详细描述了使用双腔静脉吻合技术的心脏前而视图和后面视图。

原位双心房技术

如同双腔静脉的方法，双房技术植入也从左心房

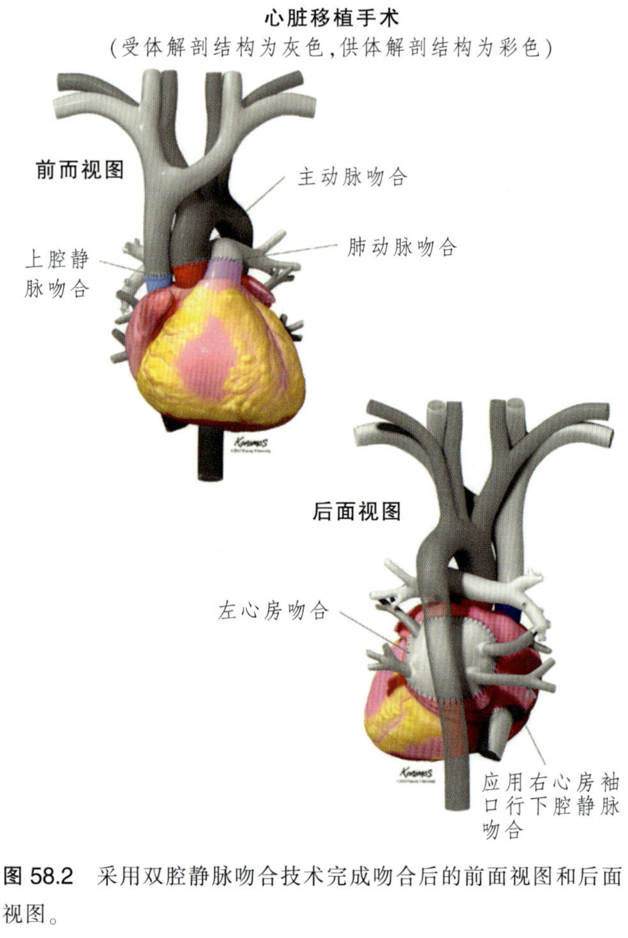

图 58.2 采用双腔静脉吻合技术完成吻合后的前面视图和后面视图。

吻合开始(图 58.3A,B)。右心房吻合通常在左心房吻合完成后进行;然而,为了减少缺血时间,主动脉吻合可以在右心房吻合之前进行。4-0 聚丙烯缝合线从房间隔的上端附近开始,并且围绕下腔静脉顺时针旋转,因为下腔静脉附近受体心房空间相对较小，这也成为吻合最困难的部分(图 58.3C)。接下来,逆时针缝合上腔静脉,并且沿右心房的游离壁打结。当缝线在供体窦房结附近时,必须小心谨慎。如上所述进行肺动脉和主动脉吻合(图 58.3D)。无论使用哪种技术,在每次吻合术完成后,给予 1L 冷的、充氧的心脏停搏液顺行灌注。

停止体外循环

一旦所有吻合完成,松开止血带,并向主动脉根部通气孔抽吸气体。随着血流流过心脏,进行更有力的除气操作。温和供氧和心脏按摩,以及左右转动心脏,可从心室和大血管排出空气。在此过程中以及以后一段时间,室颤需要迅速除颤,以避免左心室膨胀。肺动脉导管再次进入肺动脉。如果缺血时间较长,可允许移植物在从旁路分离之前存在再灌注期。给予正性肌力药物支持,通常应用米力农[0.5μg/(kg·min)]。心率应每分钟超过 100 次心跳，因为从冷缺血恢复的同种异体移植物更多地依赖于心率而不是脉搏输出量以维持心排血量[29]。再灌注期是检查所有吻合口并根据需要修补的理想时间。在从旁路分离之前,经食管超声心动图可评估心内残留的空气、瓣膜和心室功能、跨腔静脉和肺动脉吻合口梯度差以及肺静脉的通畅性。

不同程度的右心功能不全是心脏移植后的常见问题。因此,需要仔细和频繁地评估肺动脉压和右心室功能。处理右心功能不全的原则包括:①最小化右心室后负荷;②优化右心室功能,包括游离壁和室间隔;③最大化系统压力有助于灌注右心室游离壁。早期右心功能不全最好通过简单地提高全身灌注压来治疗。但是,初始肺血管扩张剂的阈值应该低。初始药物应根据其选择性作用进行选择，包括可吸入的依前列醇或一氧化氮。最可靠的是吸入一氧化氮。开始剂量从 10~20ppm 开始。在 30~35mmHg 范围内的 PCO_2 轻度过度换气，以及维持>95%的氧饱和度可辅助最小化肺血管收缩。中心静脉给予血管扩张剂(如前列腺素 E_1、前列环素或硝基甘油),或应用强心药(如米力农或多巴酚丁胺)作为替代方案[30]。如果肺动脉吻合口可触及震颤或超声提示,高度怀疑狭窄,应当直接记录压力

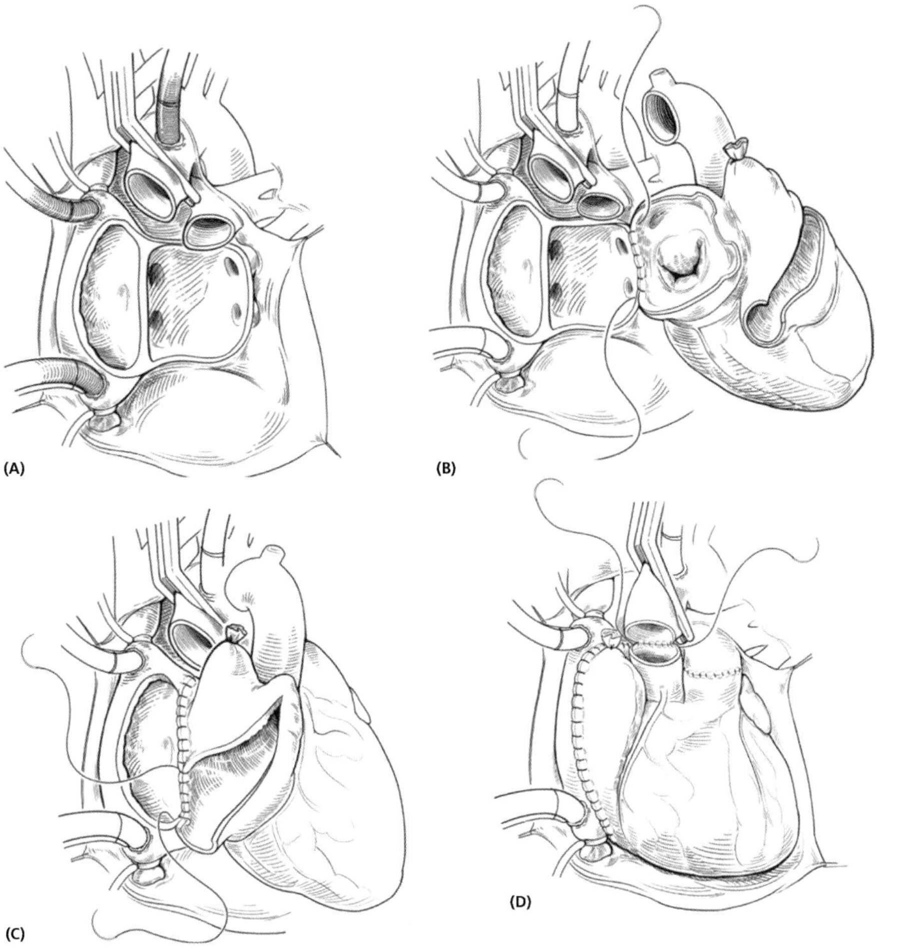

图 58.3　(A~D)心脏移植中应用双房吻合技术的详细步骤。

梯度。≥10mmHg 的梯度是重新吻合的指征[31]。最终，如果所有方法仍无法逆转而出现右心力衰竭，则需要机械辅助装置[32]。

分离转流后要特别注意三尖瓣。在双房技术中三尖瓣反流更常见，可能是由于右心房的几何变形所致[33]。手术后三尖瓣反流的严重程度与晚期存活差有关，即使只是轻度反流。三尖瓣反流与右心室功能不全相关，这些发现表明在移植时伴随的三尖瓣修复可能发挥作用[9]。一项系列研究前瞻性评估了 60 例双腔静脉移植物随机分配到接受(n=30)或不接受(n=30)植入前预性防 de Vega 三尖瓣瓣膜成形术的结果。作者报道了三尖瓣瓣膜成形术的短期和中期存活获益多，其在 1 年内显著减少了三尖瓣反流患者的严重性和数量。由于这些优点，他们在供体心脏移植的准备过程中常规施行这些处理[34]。

一旦完全复温，体外循环停止，可获得满意的血流动力学和超声影像学结果，终止主动脉根抽吸(空气)，并使用鱼精蛋白。然后去除主动脉根部通气孔。去除腔静脉插管，缝合线打结。如果使用 50%的中和剂量后没有鱼精蛋白反应，所有液体从泵返回后去除主动脉插管。

手术时打开的每个胸腔留置引流管。通常有较大的心包空间，除常用的引流管外，Blake 引流管或类似的引流管通常放置在后心包和(或)VAD 袋中以长期使用。放置临时心房和心室起搏导线。房室传导阻滞发生率约 10%，完全心脏阻塞发生率为 2%[35]。使用双腔静脉技术与术后短期起搏率较低[36]和永久性起搏器植入有关[17,18,25]。对于具自动心脏复律除颤器或永久性起搏器的患者，一旦凝血障碍纠正，就应该去除这些心脏起搏器。因为此步骤在此时不是必需的，所以如果对凝血病或稳定性有顾虑，可以在稍晚的日期进行。胸骨、软组织和皮肤在获得足够的止血和血流动力学后以常规方式闭合。

特殊情况

重新胸骨切开/重新心脏移植

双心室衰竭和右心室扩张的患者在重做胸骨切开时存在风险。在开始手术之前，谨慎地放置外部除颤器垫并通过股动静脉建立心肺旁路。胸骨切开后注意避免损伤右心室和先前的旁路移植物。操作旁路移植物时防止血栓和血流动力学损害。最先暴露主动脉插管位置，然后分开上下腔以便于双心腔插管。偶尔可能需要心肺旁路以减压心脏、限制失血，并促进暴露。

考虑到心脏同种异体移植物的中位存活率，预期许多受体最终将接受再移植[37]，特别是初次移植时年龄很小因先天性心脏病行再次移植较常见[38]。虽然技术上非常类似于前面所述的原位心脏移植，但再移植还有一些需要特别注意的事项。首先，患者通常在慢性同种异体移植物排斥反应期后进行此手术。与涉及单一炎症发作的大多数重做的心脏手术不同，用于慢性排斥反应的重新心脏移植由于长时间的炎症和在同种异体移植物分离期间的致密瘢痕和出血而复杂化。受体心脏切除术所需的分离和显露可能需要额外的时间，这可能影响与供体手术的协调。尽最大努力去除所有以前的同种异体移植物，包括所有吻合口，以及修剪自体组织。因冠状动脉疾病再移植的预后与初次移植的相似；但那些因急性移植物衰竭再次移植的预后通常较差[39]。

外植心室辅助装置

心脏供体的数量相对恒定，越来越多的患者通过心室辅助装置过渡后行移植，效果良好[40-43]。这已在第48章中详细讨论。辅助装置放置期间可采用的策略包括：

1.将流出道移植物引向右心房沟槽，以防止在胸骨切开时损伤。

2.覆盖流出道移植物额外的分层(通常应用 GorTex)，因为通常没有足够的心包用于此目的。

3.行流出道吻合尽可能靠近右侧升主动脉，从而尽可能保留尽可能多的主动脉。

4.尽可能不受干扰地分离肺动脉窗，以便于以后的分离和暴露。

5.在右心室放置保护屏障(如 GorTex、CorMatrix等)以防止在行再次切开术时的损伤。

6.避免使用脱脂棉，从而避免相关的瘢痕和纤维化。

基于这些策略，对于心室辅助装置到位的受体而言有几项需要特别注意的事项。流出道移植物的位置在切开胸骨之前必须有记录，因为它可能移位。左心室应减少操作以降低壁血栓栓塞的风险，壁血栓栓塞在该群体中更易形成。可用经食管超声心动图评估。在心肺旁路开启之前关闭该装置并且夹闭流出道，以防止功能性主动脉功能不全。由于流出道移植物缝合到升主动脉，插管和钳夹放置必须比通常更远。使用 Seldinger 技术的主动脉弓的插管在这些情况下是有用的。另外，可以使用股动脉或腋动脉插管。

先天性心脏病术后的心脏移植

心脏移植是对纠正或姑息性的先天性心脏病手术失败的公认治疗方案。虽然先天性心脏病患者接受成人心脏移植相对较少，但是这种情况在不久的将来肯定会发生变化，因为存活率和解剖范围都有一定的提高。有许多与这一群体相关的考虑。首先，肺血管疾病是常见的，并可能需要心肺移植（见下文)。第二，Fontan 手术失败的患者常表现为多器官功能不全（如肾和肝)和蛋白质丢失性肠病的营养缺乏。第三，找到合适供体可能非常困难，在某些情况下甚至是不可能的，因为患者可能高度致敏。第四，术后护理困难，因为患者易出血、合并感染和出现肺动脉高压，以及存在导致明显的左至右分流的主动脉肺动脉旁路[44]。

这类患者往往需要特别的重建，从而使移植手术可能相当复杂，特别是单心室患者[45-48]。因此，移植物带着较长的大血管移植之前不应修剪。在某些情况下需保留组织作为修复材料来完成重建。或者，可以获取原本被丢弃的自体组织(例如胸降主动脉或部分大血管)以用作补片或其他导管。移植和获取外科医生必须熟悉受体的心脏情况、血管解剖结构和既往的手术操作。

对于粘连致密、心脏扩大及大血管或导管在胸骨后位置的患者，行二次胸骨切开的风险相对大。这类患者应预先准备腹股沟区，甚至提前置管[49]。这类患者慢性发绀会增加侧支血管发生率，尤其是在纵隔后，这增加了出血的风险[50]。

最常见的情况之一是 Fontan 重建失败。该组病例移植的适应证是蛋白质丢失性肠病、顽固性心房心律失常和系统性心室功能不全[51]。获取足够长度的肺动脉和腔静脉(包括无名静脉);对于复杂的肺动脉重建,也可获取一段胸降主动脉。在受体心脏切除术期间,通过游离心外旁路移植物或者心房间隔来解构 Fontan 路径。在任一情况下,都要保留大量的上腔静脉和内腔静脉的边缘。在 Glen 通路关闭后,肺动脉循环可通过多种方法重建,包括补片或插入移植血管[48,52]。切除受体心脏和重建可能需要大量时间,以建立与供体心脏植入相容的解剖结构。最重要的是要协调供体团队与受体团队钳夹阻断的时间,以解决相关的复杂性问题,并尽可能减少缺血时间。受体解剖和重建技术的可能性是众多的,超出了本章的范围。复杂性先天性心脏病的移植应让在先天性心脏手术领域具有显著经验的外科医生进行。一般而言,该组患者心脏移植后的预后与没有先天性心脏病的患者相当,1 年存活率约为 85%,10 年存活率约为 60%~70%[50,53,54]。考虑到这些受体大多数是年轻患者,将来可能需要再次移植。

心肺移植

在过去 20 年中,随着肺移植适应证的扩大,心肺联合移植的频率有所下降[55]。但是,对于先天性心脏病[56]合并肺血管疾病和终末期心力衰竭的患者,联合移植可能是最好的治疗方案[57]。心肺获取的初始分离和暴露类似于其他章节中所描述的单独心脏和肺供体获取程序。简言之,除了供体心脏切除术的典型显露外,在主动脉和上腔静脉之间分离后心包以显露主支气管。尽量减少气管周围的分离,以保留其侧方的血液供应。心脏切除术包括分离上下腔静脉、放置主动脉阻断钳、在主动脉根部注入保存溶液和切断左心耳末端,以防止灌注液导致左心扩张。最大限度获取主动脉和腔静脉非常重要,特别是如果需要行双腔静脉吻合术时。经主动脉至少给予 1L 心脏保存溶液和至少 3L 肺保存溶液,分离肺下韧带,接着气管闭合和切断,肺部分充气以防止运输期间肺不张。肺静脉周围的心包被分离。气管从食管和后纵隔分开,注意心肺仔细止血。心肺应用与原位心脏移植类似的方式准备。根据计划实施的系统吻合方案修剪右心房或腔静脉。必须识别和控制来自心肺纵隔的潜在出血来源。受体使用主动脉和双心腔插管的完全心肺旁路。受体行心脏切除术。考虑到手术区域大小和可能的出血风险,在分离和暴露期间的止血技术是必需的。根据静脉吻合类型准备右心房和腔静脉。受体肺切除术如下。胸膜完全打开后行肺切除术,分开肺下韧带,打开膈神经后的心包窗。分离肺门,吻合器闭合气管,然后取出肺。接下来切除右肺动脉,显露隆突并分开。后纵隔仔细止血,缝合残余的左心房组织。心肺置入胸腔,肺置入膈神经血管束后面的胸膜心包窗。用连续或间断缝合技术行气管吻合术,放置侧向气管缝合线以最小化吻合的张力。接下来,应用双房技术行右心房吻合;也可采用双腔静脉技术。最后进行主动脉吻合。可根据手术需要更换吻合顺序。可在气管吻合术之后进行主动脉吻合,在心房吻合之前去除主动脉阻断钳,可以使供体缺血时间最小化。

总结

心脏移植技术的改进有助于心脏同种异体移植受体的 1 年生存率。然而,心脏受体的移植物半衰期仍然短于 11 年[58]。5 年后,心脏同种异体移植血管病变(30%)和恶性肿瘤(23%)会造成大多数心脏受体死亡[58]。这些令人警醒的统计数据说明,尽管应用了细致的外科技术,但长期应用免疫抑制对长期存活的限制是深远的。这些数据还明确指出需要采取耐受策略,在不应用长期免疫抑制的情况下实现长期的移植物存活及防止慢性排斥反应。与其他实体器官移植一样,供体器官的短缺仍然是心脏移植应用的主要限制。通过异种移植[59]、人造器官[60]和离体灌注系统[61]扩展器官来源的发展将极大地影响未来心脏移植的数量。除了供体的来源,标准化实施如上所述的手术技术是良好预后的保证。

致谢

这项工作的部分资金来自美国国立卫生研究院国家心肺研究所(PO1HL018646)、美国国立过敏与传染病研究所(U01AI094374)以及罗氏器官移植研究基金会。

(胡志平 译 朱继业 校)

参考文献

1. Cooper DK. Experimental development of cardiac transplantation. British Medical Journal. 1968;4:174–181.
2. Lower RR, Shumway NE. Studies on orthotopic homotransplantation of the canine heart. Surgical Forum. 1960;11:18–19.
3. Barnard CN. The operation. A human cardiac transplant: an interim report of a successful operation performed at Groote Schuur Hospital, Cape Town. South African Medical Journal. 1967;41:1271–1274.
4. DiBardino DJ. The history and development of cardiac transplantation. Texas Heart Institute Journal. 1999;26:198–205.
5. Antunes PE, Prieto D, Eugenio L, et al. Donor mitral valve repair in cardiac transplantation. Journal of Thoracic and Cardiovascular Surgery. 2005;129:227–228.
6. Risher WH, Ochsner JL, Van MC. Cardiac transplantation after donor mitral valve commissurotomy. Annals of Thoracic Surgery. 1994;57:221–222.
7. Massad MG, Smedira NG, Hobbs RE, et al. Bench repair of donor mitral valve before heart transplantation. Annals of Thoracic Surgery. 1996;61:1833–1835.
8. Navia JL, Atik FA, Marullo A, et al. Bench repair of donor aortic valve with minimal access orthotopic heart transplantation. Annals of Thoracic Surgery. 2005;80:313–315.
9. Anderson CA, Shernan SK, Leacche M, et al. Severity of intraoperative tricuspid regurgitation predicts poor late survival following cardiac transplantation. Annals of Thoracic Surgery. 2004;78:1635–1642.
10. Jeevanandam V, Russell H, Mather P, et al. Donor tricuspid annuloplasty during orthotopic heart transplantation: long-term results of a prospective controlled study. Annals of Thoracic Surgery. 2006;82:2089–2095.
11. Maltais S, Carrier M, Pellerin M, et al. Closure of ventricular septal defects in the donor heart before transplantation: toward expanded acceptance criteria. Journal of Thoracic and Cardiovascular Surgery. 2005;129:1187–1188.
12. Schroder JN, Daneshmand MA, Villamizar NR, et al. Heparin-induced thrombocytopenia in left ventricular assist device bridge-to-transplant patients. Annals of Thoracic Surgery. 2007;84:841–845.
13. Simsir SA, Schwarz ER, Czer LS, et al. Heart transplantation using bivalirudin as anticoagulant. Interactive CardioVascular and Thoracic Surgery. 2010;10:150–151.
14. Koster A, Meyer O, Fischer T, et al. One-year experience with the platelet glycoprotein IIb/IIIa antagonist tirofiban and heparin during cardiopulmonary bypass in patients with heparin-induced thrombocytopenia type II. Journal of Thoracic and Cardiovascular Surgery. 2001;122:1254–1255.
15. Koster A, Huebler S, Potapov E, et al. Impact of heparin-induced thrombocytopenia on outcome in patients with ventricular assist device support: single-institution experience in 358 consecutive patients. Annals of Thoracic Surgery. 2007;83:72–76.
16. Mueller XM. Drug immunosuppression therapy for adult heart transplantation. Part 2: clinical applications and results. Annals of Thoracic Surgery. 2004;77:363–371.
17. Davies RR, Russo MJ, Morgan JA, et al. Standard versus bicaval techniques for orthotopic heart transplantation: an analysis of the United Network for Organ Sharing database. Journal of Thoracic and Cardiovascular Surgery. 2010;140:700–708.
18. Meyer SR, Modry DL, Bainey K, et al. Declining need for permanent pacemaker insertion with the bicaval technique of orthotopic heart transplantation. Canadian Journal of Cardiology. 2005;21:159–163.
19. Aziz T, Burgess M, Khafagy R, et al. Bicaval and standard techniques in orthotopic heart transplantation: medium-term experience in cardiac performance and survival. Journal of Thoracic and Cardiovascular Surgery. 1999;118:115–122.
20. Traversi E, Pozzoli M, Grande A, et al. The bicaval anastomosis technique for orthotopic heart transplantation yields better atrial function than the standard technique: an echocardiographic automatic boundary detection study. Journal of Heart and Lung Transplantation. 1998;17:1065–1074.
21. Koch A, Remppis A, Dengler TJ, et al. Influence of different implantation techniques on AV valve competence after orthotopic heart transplantation. European Journal of Cardio-Thoracic Surgery. 2005;28:717–723.
22. Leyh RG, Jahnke AW, Kraatz EG, et al. Cardiovascular dynamics and dimensions after bicaval and standard cardiac transplantation. Annals of Thoracic Surgery. 1995;59:1495–1500.
23. Brandt M, Harringer W, Hirt SW, et al. Influence of bicaval anastomoses on late occurrence of atrial arrhythmia after heart transplantation. Annals of Thoracic Surgery. 1997;64:70–72.
24. Freimark D, Silverman JM, Aleksic I, et al. Atrial emptying with orthotopic heart transplantation using bicaval and pulmonary venous anastomoses: a magnetic resonance imaging study. Journal of the American College of Cardiology. 1995;25:932–936.
25. Jacob S, Sellke F. Is bicaval orthotopic heart transplantation superior to the biatrial technique? Interactive CardioVascular and Thoracic Surgery. 2009;9:333–342.
26. Riberi A, Ambrosi P, Habib G, et al. Systemic embolism: a serious complication after cardiac transplantation avoidable by bicaval technique. European Journal of Cardio-Thoracic Surgery. 2001;19:307–311.
27. Dreyfus G. Surgical technique of orthotopic heart transplantation 2: bicaval "total" approach. In: Cooper DK, Miller LW, Patterson GA, editors. The Transplantation and Replacement of Thoracic Organs: The Present Status of Biological and Mechanical Replacement of the Heart and Lungs. Lancaster, UK: Springer; 1996: 215–220.
28. Aklog L, Sepic J, Filsoufi F, et al. Open inferior vena caval anastomosis during bicaval heart transplantation. Annals of Thoracic Surgery. 2002;73:671–672.
29. Cooper DK. Surgical technique of orthotopic heart transplantation 1: standard approach. In: Cooper DK, Miller LW, Patterson GA, editor. The Transplantation and Replacement of Thoracic Organs: The Present Status of Biological and Mechanical Replacement of the Heart and Lungs. Lancaster, UK: Springer; 1996: 207–214.
30. De Wet CJ, Affleck DG, Jacobsohn E, et al. Inhaled prostacyclin is safe, effective, and affordable in patients with pulmonary hypertension, right heart dysfunction, and refractory hypoxemia after cardiothoracic surgery. Journal of Thoracic and Cardiovascular Surgery. 2004;127:1058–1067.
31. de Marchena E, Futterman L, Wozniak P, et al. Pulmonary artery torsion: a potentially lethal complication after orthotopic heart transplantation. Journal of Heart Transplantation. 1989;8:499–502.
32. Iyer A, Kumarasinghe G, Hicks M, et al. Primary graft failure after heart transplantation. Journal of Transplantation. 2011;2011:175768.
33. Park KY, Park CH, Chun YB, et al. Bicaval anastomosis reduces tricuspid regurgitation after heart transplantation. Asian Cardiovascular and Thoracic Annals. 2005;13:251–254.
34. Jeevanandam V, Russell H, Mather P, et al. A one-year comparison of prophylactic donor tricuspid annuloplasty in heart transplantation. Annals of Thoracic Surgery. 2004;78:759–766.
35. Cui G, Kobashigawa J, Margarian A, et al. Cause of atrioventricular block in patients after heart transplantation. Transplantation. 2003;76:137–142.
36. Grant SC, Khan MA, Faragher EB, et al. Atrial arrhythmias and pacing after orthotopic heart transplantation: bicaval versus standard atrial anastomosis. British Heart Journal. 1995;74:149–153.
37. Copeland H, Coelho-Anderson R, Mineburg N, et al. Elective cardiac retransplantation: a viable option that can be repeated. Journal of Thoracic and Cardiovascular Surgery. 2011;141:822–827.
38. Karamlou T, Hirsch J, Welke K, et al. A United Network for Organ Sharing analysis of heart transplantation in adults with congenital heart disease: outcomes and factors associated with mortality and retransplantation. Journal of Thoracic and Cardiovascular Surgery. 2010;140:161–168.
39. Nair RH, Pillay T, Hasan A, et al. Can cardiac re-transplantation be performed with an acceptable survival after primary graft failure? Interactive CardioVascular and Thoracic Surgery. 2005;4:41–46.
40. Russo MJ, Hong KN, Davies RR, et al. Posttransplant survival is not diminished in heart transplant recipients bridged with implantable left ventricular assist devices. Journal of Thoracic and Cardiovascular Surgery. 2009;138:1425–1432.
41. Bull DA, Reid BB, Selzman CH, et al. The impact of bridge-to-transplant ventricular assist device support on survival after cardiac transplantation. Journal of Thoracic and Cardiovascular Surgery. 2010;140:169–173.
42. Urban M, Pirk J, Dorazilova Z, et al. How does successful bridging with ventricular assist device affect cardiac transplantation outcome? Interactive CardioVascular and Thoracic Surgery. 2011;13:405–409.
43. Groetzner J, Reichart B, Roemer U, et al. Cardiac transplantation in pediatric patients: fifteen-year experience of a single center. Annals of Thoracic Surgery. 2005;79:53–60.
44. Hosseinpour AR, Cullen S, Tsang VT. Transplantation for adults with congenital heart disease. European Journal of Cardio-Thoracic Surgery. 2006;30:508–514.
45. Michielon G, Parisi F, Di CD, et al. Orthotopic heart transplantation for failing single ventricle physiology. European Journal of Cardio-Thoracic Surgery. 2003;24:502–510.
46. Simmonds J, Burch M, Dawkins H, et al. Heart transplantation after congenital heart surgery: improving results and future goals. European Journal of Cardio-Thoracic Surgery. 2008;34:313–317.
47. Jayakumar KA, Addonizio LJ, Kichuk-Chrisant MR, et al. Cardiac transplantation after the Fontan or Glenn procedure. Journal of the American College of Cardiology. 2004;44:2065–2072.
48. Kanter KR, Mahle WT, Vincent RN, et al. Heart transplantation in children with a Fontan procedure. Annals of Thoracic Surgery. 2011;91:823–829.
49. Carrel T, Neth J, Mohacsi P, et al. Perioperative risk and long-term results of heart transplantation after previous cardiac operations. Annals of Thoracic Surgery.

1997;63:1133–1137.
50. Pigula FA, Gandhi SK, Ristich J, et al. Cardiopulmonary transplantation for congenital heart disease in the adult. Journal of Heart and Lung Transplantation. 2001;20:297–303.
51. Chaudhari M, Sturman J, O'Sullivan J, et al. Rescue cardiac transplantation for early failure of the Fontan-type circulation in children. Journal of Thoracic and Cardiovascular Surgery. 2005;129:416–422.
52. Gamba A, Merlo M, Fiocchi R, et al. Heart transplantation in patients with previous Fontan operations. Journal of Thoracic and Cardiovascular Surgery. 2004; 127:555–562.
53. Jacobs JP, Asante-Korang A, O'Brien SM, et al. Lessons learned from 119 consecutive cardiac transplants for pediatric and congenital heart disease. Annals of Thoracic Surgery. 2011;91:1248–1254.
54. Patel ND, Weiss ES, Allen JG, et al. Heart transplantation for adults with congenital heart disease: analysis of the United Network for Organ Sharing database. Annals of Thoracic Surgery. 2009;88:814–821.
55. Trulock EP, Christie JD, Edwards LB, et al. Registry of the International Society for Heart and Lung Transplantation: twenty-fourth official adult lung and heart-lung transplantation report-2007. Journal of Heart and Lung Transplantation. 2007;26:782–795.
56. Januszewska K, Malec E, Juchem G, et al. Heart-lung transplantation in patients with pulmonary atresia and ventricular septal defect. Journal of Thoracic and Cardiovascular Surgery. 2009;138:738–743.
57. Deuse T, Sista R, Weill D, et al. Review of heart-lung transplantation at Stanford. Annals of Thoracic Surgery. 2010;90:329–337.
58. Stehlik J, Edwards LB, Kucheryavaya AY, et al. The registry of the International Society for Heart and Lung Transplantation: 29th official adult heart transplant report-2012. Journal of Heart and Lung Transplantation. 2012;31:1052–1064.
59. Kuwaki K, Tseng YL, Dor FJ, et al. Heart transplantation in baboons using alpha1,3-galactosyltransferase gene-knockout pigs as donors: initial experience. Nature Medicine. 2005;11:29–31.
60. Ott HC, Matthiesen TS, Goh SK, et al. Perfusion-decellularized matrix: using nature's platform to engineer a bioartificial heart. Nature Medicine. 2008; 14:213–221.
61. Ozeki T, Kwon MH, Gu J, et al. Heart preservation using continuous ex vivo perfusion improves viability and functional recovery. Circulation Journal. 2007; 71:153–159.

第 59 章 肺移植手术步骤和外科技术

R. Duane Davis，Matt Hartwig

引言

为了解决肺移植较高的排斥反应发生率和死亡率，临床实践经历了显著的变化，例如增强免疫抑制和应对非同种免疫损伤的策略，包括胃食管反流（GER）[1]。这些方案的改变，以及更精细的受体选择、器官获取和植入的技术改进和围术期护理技术的进步，使得过去 20 年患者生存率和移植物存活率得到了显著改善[2]。然而，仍然需要创新的肺移植方法来进一步改善短期和长期预后。本章将概述我们中心的技术。文献中描述的替代技术在我们的中心并不常规采用。肺获取和保存/复苏的详细信息已分别在第 21 章和第 26 章中进行讨论。

麻醉

肺移植期间的受体管理仍然是任何麻醉团队最具挑战性的任务之一[3]。呼吸窘迫和血流动力学扰动往往需要经验丰富的心胸外科麻醉工作人员进行操作以获得最佳结果。除了适当的粗大静脉通路之外，应常规地放置桡动脉和肺动脉导管以连续行血流动力学监测。由于患者需行双侧前部胸廓切开术，桡动脉监测不佳，因此我们常规放置小口径股动脉插管。其他常规使用的监测装置包括脑血氧监测和经食管超声心动图（TEE）。TEE 可以在手术期间评估心脏功能和充盈情况，而且可以在手术结束时了解血管吻合情况。我们通常在 ICU 移植后但拔管之前进行胸膜硬膜外麻醉以进行术后镇痛。

我们通常使用左侧双腔气管插管（ETT）。有时受体较小不能放置足够大小的双腔 ETT 时，手术在体外循环（CPB）进行以确保安全。我们不建议通过单管 ETT 维持单肺通气，因为它会造成气管移位或闭塞引起的气道损伤。无论选择哪种气道，应用可弯曲的支气管镜进行抽吸是必须的。这需要正确地放置 ETT，以及在整个手术过程保持其位置和通畅。手术期间的支气管操作将不可避免地导致管迁移，随后引起通气不足，这需要麻醉团队注意。

手术团队之间的有效沟通是成功肺移植的关键部分。在心脏收缩之前通知麻醉团队预先给予血管活性药物。这可以减轻团队的焦虑并避免过度反应造成干预不当。尽量减少静脉输液，同时配合大量的肌力药物支持（例如肾上腺素），有助于在手术脆弱时期保持受体血流动力学稳定。这也有助于减少植入后肺水肿的问题。应密切监测红细胞容积和凝血因子，并根据需要更换。这对于有显著出血倾向以及存在肺动脉高压或右心室功能障碍的肝脏充血患者尤其重要。

患者体位和切口选择

除了少数特殊病例，我们中心首选通过第 4 肋间的前方行横断胸骨切开术（即蛤壳切口）以进行双侧肺移植。患者仰卧位，臂轻度外展支撑在带垫的手臂板上，肘弯曲。身后垫保暖垫，从脐部向下用保暖毯覆盖受体下体。在胸部建立体外循环的血管通路，无须从腹股沟建立。女性患者的切口一般在乳房下方，并可在移植后行乳房整形。这需要在乳房两侧切开，然后向上牵拉乳房组织，再通过第 4 肋间隙进入胸膜间隙。乳房动脉通常在血管夹之间双侧分开，然后横切胸骨。值得注意的是，其他研究组报告了大量胸骨并发症的发生，包括横断胸骨后的畸形和重叠。虽然胸骨并发症的发生率在我们的中心较低，小于 5%，但对于许多患者来说，也可考虑通过胸骨双侧前胸廓切开来进行手术，而无须过多的暴露量。具有限制性肺部疾病和小胸腔的受体，肺动脉高压或需要伴随心脏手术的受体通常需要蛤壳切口。

受体移植

在横向胸骨切开术之后，在乳房静脉水平的上方分离纵隔胸膜下部到心包膜。心包不需要打开;但吻合左肺静脉显露不良时需要打开心包并且向前牵开心尖以获得更好的视野。在广泛打开胸部之前,第 4 肋间肌在第 5 肋之上分开。上面覆盖的前锯肌和背阔肌应大部分保留。对于那些存在感染性肺病或既往有胸部手术的患者,需要长时间的粘连松解。这通常是手术中最耗时的部分。高频电刀分离大部分情况下是安全的,但在沿着纵隔的膈神经附近要极度小心。膈神经附近的粘连应锐性分离。有时,膈神经附近粘连密集,需要用吻合器分离肺组织。患有限制性肺部疾病和胸腔较小的患者中，在横膈膜的纤维穹隆处放置一根 8 字形的厚丝针，并通过胁间下间隙向两侧和尾部牵拉以增强显露。

双肺从胸膜游离后,分离肺门,理想情况下,在肺切除之前游离双侧大部分肺门。这可以使一侧肺灌注到对侧肺植入之间的时间最短。哪侧肺先切除取决于几个重要因素。如果自体肺功能存在显著差异,则通常先替换较差的肺。也得考虑供体肺质量,因为明显的单侧挫伤或硬化可能导致移植肺在没有 CPB 或体外膜氧合(ECMO)支持下无法进行单肺通气。如果受体或供体肺功能没有明显的差异,应首先进行技术上更困难的一侧,以减少灌注一侧移植肺的时间。这通常是左侧。

受体肺切除术在心包外进行。用 endo-GIA 吻合器在肺动脉(PA)第一分支处或在其第一分支远端处切割闭合肺动脉。同样,上肺静脉和下肺静脉在左心房汇合之前也用吻合器分别切断。支气管在上叶起始处仍可用吻合器分开。打开心包进行心包内切开。包括右侧 Waterston 沟(房间沟),从左心房顶部和右心房后部分离肺动脉。这些操作有助于放置左心房阻断钳。左右肺动脉向近端移动。在右侧,这包括右主 PA 和上腔静脉(SVC)之间的分离。在左侧,要避免损伤喉返神经。沿左 PA 的上方分离时尽量不使用电刀。后肺门内淋巴结和支气管动脉循环较多，可能是肺移植后比较难处理的出血来源。在植入之前后方严密止血是非常有效的。同样,广泛去除剑突下淋巴结也可增加显露并避免潜在吻合口并发症。迷走神经与后门区域相邻,应避免损伤,以尽量减少移植后的胃肠动力障碍。

心包膜内分离完成后，在同种异体移植物植入之前，最后外侧预置两个 8 字形的 1 号 Maxon 缝线以备关闭胸腔。在此,我们利用在肺植入之前胸膜腔内的最佳暴露优势。同样，在肋骨沟槽中放置大孔胸腔造口管,经该管置入小口径引流管持续引流。通常,放置一个 24F Blake 引流在沟槽下部,以帮助引流液体。

单肺移植和双肺移植

许多并发症都是由自体肺引起的,包括感染、过度充气、分流和恶性肿瘤。双侧原位肺移植(BOLT)比单肺移植(SOLT)有好的长期生存获益[4,5]。因此,我们中心首选为我们大多数受体行 BOLT。但也有部分患者及某些特殊临床情况下选择 SOLT。在这些情况下,切口有多种选择。右侧 SOLT 首选的切口是前外侧胸廓切开术。这种方法可以在中心插管的情况下容易地进入肺门、主动脉和右心房。左肺移植中前外侧胸廓切开术可能会限制左心房暴露,从而影响肺静脉吻合。这在肺纤维化患者中是个较大的问题,在这种情况下,我们通常会通过标准的肌肉保留的后外侧胸廓切开术进行治疗。如果需要同时进行心脏手术,则中间胸骨切开通常为手术的两个部分提供最佳暴露。

同种异体移植

左肺和右肺移植的细节之间差别不大。但是显露左心房以备肺静脉吻合是有挑战性的，我们将在下文中讨论增强显露的方式。第一个肺叶植入之前以 80~100IU/kg 的剂量肝素化,根据外科医生的偏好,目标活化凝固时间(ACT)可以在 200~300 秒之间。

肺门结构已经如上所述被分离,参见图 59.1。将长丝线穿过 PA 和每个肺静脉分支的闭合端放置,然后将 Rummel 止血带放置在每个缝合线上之后,这些血管向前缩回,在回缩期间可以保护膈神经。Rummel 止血带可以由简单的红橡胶导管制成。为显露左肺门,将粗丝线回缩针放在心包下方、膈神经后及肺下静脉前方。丝线同样穿过粗的 Rummel 止血带，从而可以让心脏安全地向上和向右回缩，以在进一步分离肺门结构和植入供体肺时提供良好的显露。

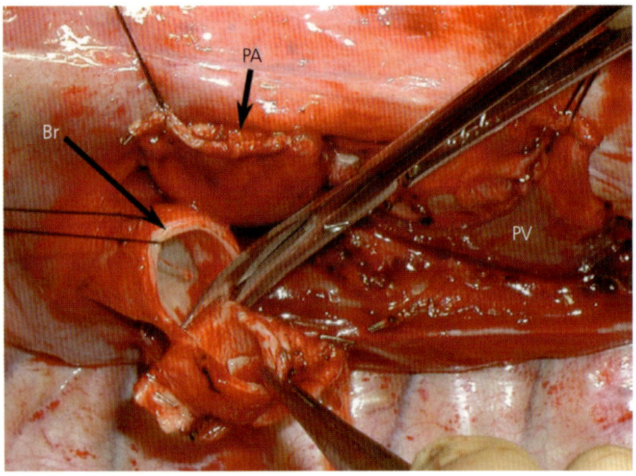

图 59.1 同种异体肺移植的肺门分离。钉住的支气管袖带被切除以备支气管吻合。Br，支气管；PA，肺动脉；LA，左心房。(Source: Hartwig et al. 2004[6].Reproduced by permission of Wolters Kluwer Health.)

首先行气道吻合。受体气管主干楔形切断，靠近上叶分叉。将丝线穿过软骨环以增加气道的可操作性。膜部横切之后应呈回缩的趋势，而且应该略长于软骨侧。吸出支气管腔分泌物，左侧 ETT 可能会略微回缩。用抗生素溶液充分冲洗胸腔，然后将 4-0 聚二恶烷酮缝合线(PDS)放置于受体膜软骨连接处的一个角上。接下来，将冰纱布垫放置在胸腔后面，供体肺原位放置在纱垫上。其他的冰浆可以保持植入期间移植物的低温状态。

支气管吻合的关键组成部分是保证膜对膜的位置对齐和软骨对软骨的位置对齐。首先用 4-0 PDS 以端-端的方式连续缝合膜部后方。在到达相对的膜软骨连接时，从较小支气管的外部到较大支气管内部行过渡缝合。通常，受体支气管略大，这会使沿支气管的前部软骨部分发生小的套叠。套叠通常为一个软骨环的深度，并且前方也以连续方式缝合。在支气管吻合术完成后，麻醉师应该从上面清除气道并准备手动为供体肺充气。完成后，将吻合口浸没在水中并试漏，同时肺轻轻地充气。

气道吻合后行肺 PA 吻合。受体主 PA 用小的 Satinsky 血管夹近端阻断，随后移除吻合钉。供体 PA 修剪至适当的长度。通常，接近第一动脉分支约 1.5~2cm，但这时需要精确测量。错误估计供体和受体 PA 长度可能会导致 PA 组织过多和吻合后扭转。我们使用 6-0 聚丙烯缝合线进行 PA 吻合。从一个角开始，后壁行连续缝合。血管对齐对于血管吻合也是至关重要的，有助于供体肺的前部和尖端节段分支可以保持正确走向。完成吻合后，将第二个血管夹放置在供体 PA 远端，同时缓慢移除近侧的 Satinsky 夹，测试 PA 吻合口，无须对供体肺过早进行再灌注。若是针孔的轻微出血则无须止血。但吻合口更大范围的出血应及时修复。

远端 PA 夹保持夹闭同时进行肺静脉左心房吻合术。应用大的 Satinsky 血管钳夹闭左心房的主体，之前闭合的肺静脉残端用 Pennington 钳夹闭。切除吻合口钉线，并横切上肺静脉口和下肺静脉口之间的左心房组织桥。可见受体左心房大的开口以备吻合。放置在该袖口前缘的 Pennington 钳向前部和内部牵拉，为随后的缝合提供最佳显露(图 59.2)。偶尔，尽管先前放置在心包边缘的回缩针向前牵拉至左肺静脉，但左肺静脉吻合暴露还是不够理想，在这种情况下，可以打开心包，用湿润海绵或用于非停跳心脏手术的可吸引牵开器将心脏保持在前正中线。在牵开期间可能影响血流动力学，在该吻合期间通常需要给予小剂量的正性肌力药物。

上肺静脉和下肺静脉的方向对于充分的吻合是极其重要的。另外，静脉袖口内膜对内膜吻合，去除大部分肌肉组织。与 PA 行类似的连续缝合，从吻合的一个角开始，先行后壁的连续缝合，再行前壁缝合。一般用 5-0 聚丙烯缝合线行肺静脉吻合，每一侧完成血管吻合术之前给予 25g 甘露醇和 500mg 甲基泼尼松龙。

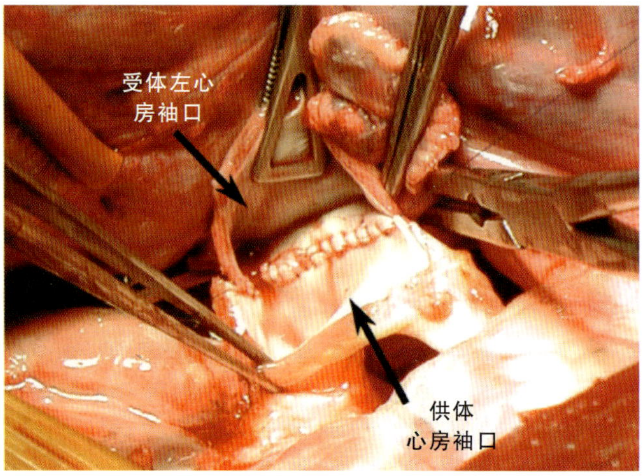

图 59.2 左心房吻合。将 Satinsky 血管夹放置在受体左心房的主体上，用 5-0 聚丙烯缝合线连续缝合吻合肺静脉，先缝合后壁，再缝合前壁。(Source: Hartwig et al. 2004 [6]. Reproduced by permission of Wolters Kluwer Health.)

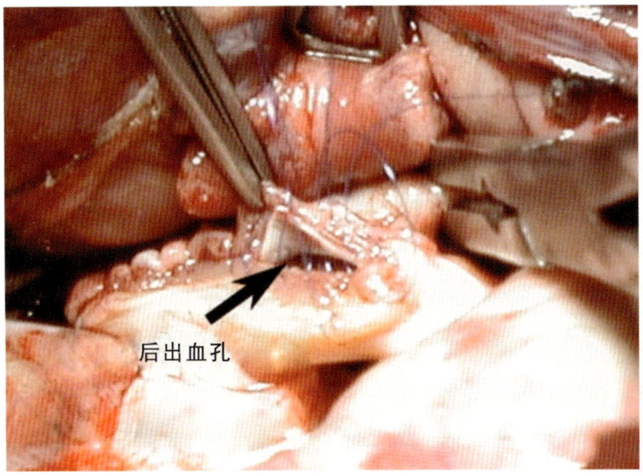

图 59.3 左心房排气。肺静脉袖口吻合的最后几针保持前部松弛，部分松开 PA 血管夹以便将肺血管内空气去除。然后放松左心房的 Satinsky 夹，排出左心房残留空气。(Source: Hartwig et al. 2004[6]. Reproduced by permission of Wolters Kluwer Health.)

再灌注

应小心控制同种异体移植物再灌注的时间，以防原发性移植物功能障碍(PGD)。左心房阻断，PA 血管夹仅部分释放时，肺静脉吻合口前壁最后几针缝线保持松弛(图 59.3)，这允许少量温血流过供体肺，以便从肺血管排出空气并开始复温。此时，左心房的 Satinsky 夹松开，以排出左心房剩余空气。在排气后，将 5-0 缝合线打结，静脉吻合完成后，完全移除左心房血管夹。

同种异体移植物的低压再灌注通过在 10~15 分钟内逐渐松弛 PA 阻断钳来实现。在这段时间内，检查 3 个吻合口、肺门分离和供体肺止血。需要注意的是，在早期再灌注期间，经常遇到低血压。在打开阻断钳之前要与麻醉师充分沟通。移植物的前列环素(PGI_2)或前列地尔(PGE_1)造成再灌注时的血流动力学扰动，血流的再分布或空气栓塞也会造成血流动力学扰动。如果低血压继发于移植物内的残留血管扩张剂或简单的再分布，它应该是自限性的。但在这段时间，麻醉团队需要提供临时的正性肌力支持和适度的容量复苏。

同种异体移植物应该在室内环境下进行轻柔的手动充气。但应在移植肺已完全复温、气道已经清除残余的血液分泌物之后进行。用手控制通气完全去除肺不张之后，可以将移植肺连通呼吸机。通常选用压力控制模式，其中正呼气末压力为 5~8cmH_2O，吸气压力小于 18~20cmH_2O，最小 FiO_2 小于 30%。随着胸膜间隙广泛开放，如在蛤壳切口的情况下，吸气压力倾向于低于胸部闭合之后所需的压力。如果肺动脉压力升高，早期肺水肿明显，或如果全身氧合不充足，则使用袢利尿剂和吸入一氧化氮。在 PA 阻断钳被完全移除时，理想状态下，PA 压力应该是正常的。异常升高的 PA 压力可能提示存在技术问题、保存不良或早期再灌注损伤，并且应对血管吻合口进行快速评估。

对侧肺大部分分离已经完成，应快速进行肺切除术。当新植入的肺行单肺通气，而对侧肺停止通气时，氧合会变差。一旦自体肺被去除，氧合会极大改善。打开心包，如上所述进行心包内分离、肺门准备和随后的肺植入。在这一部分，技术问题或早期原发性移植物功能障碍可能导致通气不足或氧合不佳。在这种情况下，可通过右心房的双插管快速施行静脉体外膜氧合(VV ECMO)[7]。详细情况如下所述。图 59.4 显示了来自双侧肺移植的前视图和后视图。

关胸

单肺移植的开胸切口以标准方式闭合。蛤壳切口的良好闭合对避免移植后的切口并发症至关重要。蛤壳式开口的前部用 3 组 5 号线重新拉近。一根线放置在胸骨的中线，另一根 8 字形线固定在中线的两边，外侧方向放置在乳房蒂的侧面。所有这三根线都穿过胸骨。有时，当胸骨被带到一起时，在第 4 和第 5 肋骨之间将存在明显的空间。这种情况可以通过在闭合之前用胸骨锯去除胸骨的小横截面来避免。蛤壳切口的其余部分可以用 1 号聚葡萄糖缝合线闭合。这些胸骨周围的缝合线在每侧肺移除之后留置。

闭合前，在前部放置双侧胸腔引流管。如果存在引流量过大（如在 CPB 之后），可在下沟中放置另外的 24F Blake 引流管。此外，对于女性患者，我们优先选择乳腺下方留置小的 Blake 引流管，接着用可吸收缝线、金属皮肤钉闭合胸膜筋膜、皮下组织和真皮层。

通常放置胸管进行抽吸；但是，如果植入的肺缺乏足够的体积以充分填充胸膜腔，在抽吸时可能发生肺的过度膨胀。如果发生这种情况，将会发展为伸展性损伤和随后的同种异体移植物功能障碍。当胸管开启和关闭吸力时，潮气量的显著差异会提醒外科医生这种情况的发生。胸部闭合后，吸气压力快速增加和潮气量

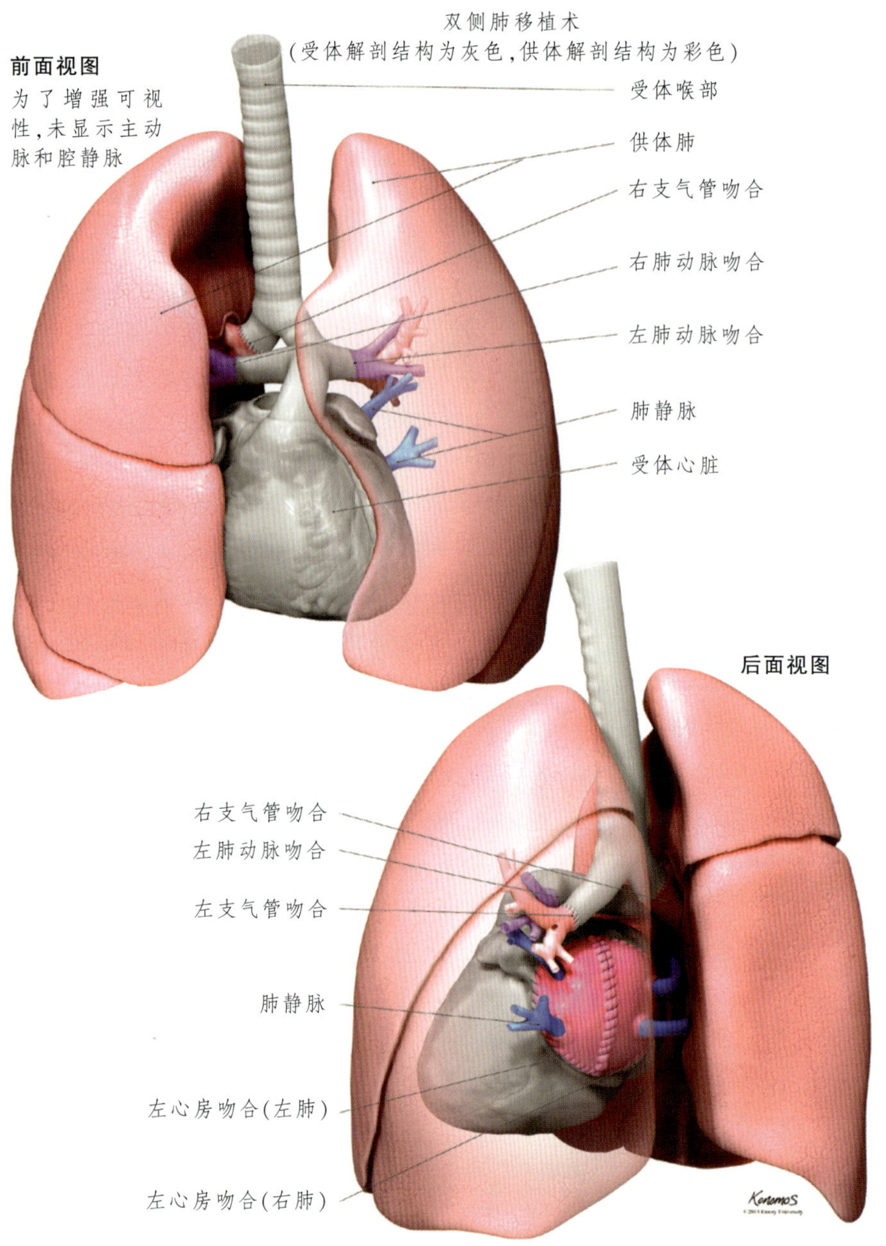

图 59.4 双侧肺移植完成的前视图和后视图。

减少可能预示同种异体移植物过大或明显的早期肺水肿。此时可行肺减容,如果可能的话,我们选择在后台修剪时去除过多的肺容积。在这些情况下,简单的右中叶切除术和对侧舌叶切除术就足够了。在极少数情况下,早期发生的肺水肿可能需要保持胸部开放。

伤口覆盖无菌敷料后,将双腔 ETT 换成单腔 ETT。在离开手术室之前进行可弯曲支气管镜检查并提供多种用途。首先,直接检查支气管吻合术的通畅性。气道的扭转或旋转不良将表现为远端气道的新月形变窄。移除残留的血液分泌物,并且任何 PGD 的发展都可能预示着泡沫性肺水肿的发展。

体外循环

在大多数情况下,双侧肺移植期间可以无须 CPB,我们约 90%的同种异体肺移植物无须心肺机。但基于受体状态和某些技术因素,非计划使用 CPB。通常需要 CPB 的情况包括:①同时进行心脏手术,例如心房或心室间隔缺损修补;②瓣膜修复;③严重肺动脉高压;④受体小气道无法行双腔 ETT 放置;⑤之前做过对侧肺切除术;⑥左心房袖口组织脆弱或不充足。在最后一种情况下，心脏停搏或纤颤停止可以无须血管阻断钳行吻合术。

行肺移植时CPB插管随显露变化。标准中线切口、蛤壳切口和右胸廓切口全部借助于右心房中心插管的双级静脉插管和升主动脉动脉回流。左侧单肺移植通常使用长的15~23号股骨静脉插管和降主动脉的标准主动脉插管。如果腹股沟不合适,则可以在胸腔中插入左肺动脉近端以便静脉回流。然而,进行左单肺移植时,通常留出同侧腹股沟区,以便在需要插管时建立血管通路。如果需要CPB的可能性较高,则可在开始手术前将小孔血管插管放置在股静脉和(或)动脉中。

如果需要,CPB可以在手术期间的任何时间启动,我们首选在CPB之前进行尽可能多的分离,包括单侧肺切除术。当CPB选择性植入时,均行肺切除,并在植入前完成双侧肺心包内切开术。随后进行后部胸廓切口的缝合和胸腔引流，并且在同种异体移植物再灌注之前如上所述植入两个肺。在植入第二个肺期间,植入的第一个肺被包裹在冰水中。在再灌注之前施用甲泼尼松龙(1g)和甘露醇(50g)。当肺部用室内空气通气时,开始逐渐再灌注,从平均PA压力的5~10mmHg开始,每5分钟增加5mmHg,直到达到正常的压力。用充氧的、低碳酸的血液再灌注肺特别有利于肺血管和肺实质恢复,而在CPB再灌注期间容易控制肺动脉压。

体外膜式氧合

体外膜式氧合(ECMO)是肺移植外科医疗设备的关键组成部分[8,9]。这种生理辅助可以在术中单肺通气不足和术后出现严重PGD时使用。在手术室中使用ECMO最常见原因是严重肺纤维化患者的自体肺不能满足单肺通气的需要。可根据基线氧需求、胸部X线片和核素肺灌注在移植前预测这种情况。在这些情况下,VV ECMO可以用双腔ECMO插管(Avalon™,Maquet Holding,Rastatt,Germany)经皮穿刺右颈内静脉建立。替代性插管方式包括通过右股静脉应用静脉导管(Bio-Medicus,Medtronic,Minneapolis,MN)和左颈内静脉应用小儿动脉导管(Medtronic,Minneapolis,MN)。在连续扩张后,应用改良的Seldinger技术在导丝上经皮放置插管。流入和流出端口的最佳放置由系统中记录的再循环水平确定,并且最初由TEE或荧光透视辅助引导。静脉插管通常靠近下腔静脉与右心房连接处,而"动脉"回流插管位于右心房。如果使用双腔ECMO插管，则应当有助于使再循环最小化，因为IVC和SVC中具有用于静脉回流的远端和近端端口，以及设置在右心房中并指向三尖瓣的"动脉"入流端口。ECMO电路由基于透明质的肝素涂覆的3/8"管与Quadrox D聚甲基戊烯(PMP)氧合器和Jostra Rotaflow泵(Maquet Cardiopulmonary,AG,Germany)组成。

在极少数情况下，同种异体移植物最初可能会立即出现功能障碍，而且在植入第二个肺期间不能充分通气或氧合。在这种情况和其他术中情况下,中心插管可以发生VV ECMO,并通常可避免全身肝素化和完全旁路。如果可以,右心房可以双重插管,静脉插管放置在IVC与右心房连接处附近,"动脉"返回插管指向三尖瓣。

潜在陷阱

从最初的肺移植经验来看,PGD会显著影响早期存活率[10]。通过使用细胞外的肺灌注溶液、加入逆行性肺灌注以保护肺脏、减少再灌注时的氧暴露、控制再灌注压力，以及通过使用氧自由基清除剂，严重的PGD发生率已从15%~25%降低至5%。PGD导致或明显促成大多数移植后的早期死亡。除非可以确定可逆的原因,否则治疗主要通过优化通气参数、提供正性肌力支持和一氧化氮来进行。最近，我们已经转向早期VV ECMO的治疗策略,当受体发展为严重的肺水肿时,需要超过0.60的FiO_2。在VV ECMO支持期间,使用保护性通气策略,包括最小氧气(FiO_2为0.30或更小)和低压通气[正呼气末正压(PEEP)小于10cmH_2O,峰值吸气压力小于25cmH_2O)柱]。最初,这可以在没有系统性肝素化的情况下完成，直到外科手术团队对止血情况满意。随后的适度抗凝可使活动凝血酶原时间保持在180~200秒,通常是足够的。撤除VV ECMO停止膜气体流动并且根据需要增加通气参数。撤除VV ECMO不需要增加抗凝。使用这种方法，患者通常在支持的3~5天内从ECMO撤除，因为ECMO和肺毛细血管渗漏解析后的肺血管阻力降低。我们中心需要VV ECMO的患者30天的存活率接近90%。

尽管PGD仍然是严重同种异体移植物功能障碍发展的最常见原因,但出现明显的缺氧、肺水肿、肺动脉压升高和顺应性差时需要立即调查可逆性原因。不对称肺水肿或月牙形气道在支气管镜评估时可能提示气道机械性问题。最重要的是需要立即识别和校正吻合或机械性病因,特别是静脉流出问题。对于静脉流出阻塞,超过4~6小时的矫正不太可能实现良好的同种异体移植物恢复。在手术室中的吻合口检查包括目视检查以评估扭转或扭结,以及应用TEE以评估湍流或有无肺静脉血流、左心房吻合质量、管腔内凝块的存在和直接测量的吻合口压力。TEE应提供所有肺静脉的最佳评估,但左下肺静脉有时很难用回声看到。

肺静脉血栓形成可在移植后的早期急性发生,并可有类似PGD的临床表现。应通过严格遵守适当的获取技术、技术上可靠的内膜-内膜吻合术和高危个体的全身抗凝治疗来预防肺静脉血栓形成。如果在手术室发现肺静脉血栓形成,应立即修复吻合。尽管在术后早期,危及生命的出血风险最高,但也可用血栓溶解剂和(或)抗凝药物治疗非闭塞性血栓。通常最安全的管理策略是在手术室中进行检查和治疗。

心脏并发症通常可由TEE识别,包括左侧瓣膜异常、左心室衰竭、心内分流和心包填塞。但是,TEE不能提供肺动脉吻合的充分评估。因此,我们常规地在移植后的最初几个小时内进行定量灌注扫描。灌注扫描上的小叶或更大的灌注缺陷通常需要进一步评估,最佳方案是手术探查。CT或常规血管造影也可以用于评估肺动脉脉管系统。在极少数的情况下,PA扭转可用腔内支架处理。

不常见的是,早期移植物功能障碍也可以由循环抗供体抗体的体液性肺损伤导致。这些抗体可通过供体和受体血清的交叉匹配来鉴定。供体特异性抗体的治疗是多模式的,包括血浆置换、免疫球蛋白(IVIG)静脉输注和抗B细胞治疗[如抗CD20(利妥昔单抗)]。

总结

在过去的20年里,肺移植取得了令人鼓舞的进展,每到一个新时期,移植物的存活率都会得到提高。最令人印象深刻的改变是早期预后,30天和1年的患者生存率和移植物存活率目前的优于肝脏移植和心脏移植[11]。患者预后的改善归功于仔细的受体选择、细致的器官获取和植入技术以及围术期护理的改进[12]。不幸的是,与所有实体器官移植一样,可用供体器官的短缺和慢性同种异体移植物损伤的发展仍然是肺移植的主要限制。毫无疑问,通过异种移植[13]、肺器官发生[14]和离体灌注系统[15,16]扩大器官来源将极大地影响未来的肺移植数量。不管在何处发现合适的供体,标准化实施如上所述的操作技术都应当获得适当的患者结果。

(胡志平 译 朱继业 校)

参考文献

1. Hartwig MG, Snyder LD, Finlen-Copeland A, et al. Lung transplantation at Duke University. Clinical Transplants. 2009:197–210.
2. Christie JD, Edwards LB, Kucheryavaya AY, et al. The registry of the international society for heart and lung transplantation: 29th adult lung and heart-lung transplant report-2012. Journal of Heart and Lung Transplantation. 2012;31:1073–1086.
3. Castillo M. Anesthetic management for lung transplantation. Current Opinion in Anaesthesiology. 2011;24:32–36.
4. Meyers BF, Lynch JP, Trulock EP, et al. Single versus bilateral lung transplantation for idiopathic pulmonary fibrosis: a ten-year institutional experience. Journal of Thoracic and Cardiovascular Surgery. 2000;120:99–107.
5. Sundaresan RS, Shiraishi Y, Trulock EP, et al. Single or bilateral lung transplantation for emphysema? Journal of Thoracic and Cardiovascular Surgery. 1996;112:1485–1494.
6. Hartwig MG, Lin SS, Simsir SA, et al. Lung transplantation. In: Kuo PC, Davis RD, editors. Comprehensive Atlas of Transplantation. Philadelphia, PA: Lippincott Williams & Wilkins; 2004.
7. Hartwig MG, Appel JZ III, Cantu E III, et al. Improved results treating lung allograft failure with venovenous extracorporeal membrane oxygenation. Annals of Thoracic Surgery. 2005;80:1872–1879.
8. Hartwig MG, Walczak R, Lin SS, et al. Improved survival but marginal allograft function in patients treated with extracorporeal membrane oxygenation after lung transplantation. Annals of Thoracic Surgery. 2012;93:366–371.
9. Hartwig MG, Appel JZ III, Cantu E III, et al. Improved results treating lung allograft failure with venovenous extracorporeal membrane oxygenation. Annals of Thoracic Surgery. 2005;80:1872–1879.
10. Meyers BF, de la Morena M, Sweet SC, et al. Primary graft dysfunction and other selected complications of lung transplantation: a single-center experience of 983 patients. Journal of Thoracic and Cardiovascular Surgery. 2005;129:1421–1429.
11. Stehlik J, Edwards LB, Kucheryavaya AY, et al. The registry of the international society for heart and lung transplantation: 29th official adult heart transplant report-2012. Journal of Heart and Lung Transplantation. 2012;31:1052–1064.
12. Hartwig MG, Davis RD. Surgical considerations in lung transplantation: transplant operation and early postoperative management. Respiratory Care Clinics of North America. 2004;10:473–504.
13. Cooper DK, Ekser B, Burlak C, et al. Clinical lung xenotransplantation—what donor genetic modifications may be necessary? Xenotransplantation. 2012;19:144–158.
14. Ott HC, Clippinger B, Conrad C, et al. Regeneration and orthotopic transplantation of a bioartificial lung. Nature Medicine. 2010;16:927–933.
15. Hartwig MG, Walczak R, Lin SS, et al. Improved survival but marginal allograft function in patients treated with extracorporeal membrane oxygenation after lung transplantation. Annals of Thoracic Surgery. 2012;93:366–371.
16. Warnecke G, Moradiellos J, Tudorache I, et al. Normothermic perfusion of donor lungs for preservation and assessment with the Organ Care System Lung before bilateral transplantation: a pilot study of 12 patients. Lancet. 2012;380:1851–1858.

第 60 章
胰腺移植手术步骤和外科技术

Dixon B. Kaufman, Jon S. Odorico, Hans W. Sollinger

引言

美国 1 型糖尿病的患者估计为 2 000 000 人，每年有超过 35 000 例新发病例[1,2]。目前，还没有一种实用的人工内分泌胰腺（与葡萄糖感受装置偶联的自动化胰岛素分泌装置）能够在一定程度上控制胰岛素，使得血糖保持在恒定状态而没有低血糖的风险。1 型糖尿病患者可通过各种形式的外源性胰岛素来手动调节血糖水平。因此，糖尿病患者会在不同小时内和不同天内产生较大的血糖值波动。严重的低血糖会危及生命，因此血糖控制必须偏高。患者必须保持慢性高血糖和高血红蛋白 A1c（HgbA1c）。

能稳定分泌胰岛素保持血糖正常、使血红蛋白 A1c 水平正常化，同时改善一些继发性并发症的进一步进展的唯一治疗手段，即用血管化的全器官胰腺移植的 β 细胞替代疗法。目前，胰岛移植是一种非常有前景的 1 型糖尿病患者的试验性治疗方法。

胰腺移植消除了对外源胰岛素治疗的需要，只要移植功能正常就可使糖化血红蛋白 A1c 水平正常化。胰腺移植还能增加胰岛素原和 C 肽释放，无须强化胰岛素治疗[3]。通过改善代谢控制，糖尿病的许多继发性并发症得到显著改善或逆转。几项开创性的研究已经证明了这些益处，包括改善糖尿病性神经病变[4]、自主神经病相关的猝死[5]、尿毒症和非尿毒症患者的糖尿病肾病[6,7]，以及稳定视力[8]。成功的胰腺移植可明显提高生活质量[9]和预期寿命[10,11]。本章主要讨论胰腺移植手术的重点内容，包括患者准备、器官获取和重建、器官植入和围术期管理。

胰腺移植类型

美国每年约进行 1100 例胰腺移植。65%~70% 是针对 1 型糖尿病和慢性肾衰竭患者的胰腺和肾同时移植（SPK）。糖尿病的尿毒症患者是 SPK 移植的极好适应证，所需的免疫抑制药物与单独的肾移植类似，而且增加胰腺移植的手术风险低。增加胰腺移植以改善糖尿病收效巨大，移植可以挽救生命[10,11]。

胰腺移植的第二类患者包括患有 1 型糖尿病已经行活体肾移植或死亡供体肾移植的患者。这组患者约占胰腺移植的 20%。重点要考虑手术风险，因为已经假定有免疫抑制风险。

胰腺移植的第三类患者是非尿毒症、非肾移植的 1 型糖尿病患者。在这种情况下，免疫抑制的风险要小于常规应用外源性胰岛素治疗的风险。其中一些糖尿病患者的病情极不稳定，常因低血糖症或糖尿病酮症酸中毒而到急诊室就诊和住院治疗。其他患者会有明显的低血糖性意识障碍，可能会在毫无征兆的情况下失去意识。对于此类患者，此类症状可能是一个毁灭性的问题，会影响他们就业和获得驾照，并可能在睡眠时产生致命性低血糖。

第 107 章详细讨论了胰腺移植的预后。

胰腺移植手术准备

时间

相对于手术获取器官时间，胰腺同种异体移植物分配到特定患者的有效协调更重要，其可减少冷缺血时间，优化移植过程。获取和移植小组与器官获取组织之间的有效沟通至关重要。确定供体 HLA 类型、感染血清学结果和 HLA 交叉匹配结果使得死亡供体胰腺（联合肾移植的 SPK 移植）在器官获取之前的分配更理想。此流程有以下优点：①允许行胰腺移植手术的中心也可选择获取胰腺；②允许患者入院、住院评估与获取器官同时进行,而不是先后进行;③减小胰腺植入前的冷缺血时间。胰腺移植与肾移植一样不耐受冷缺血。在 24 小时内对胰腺进行血运重建是最理想的方法。最后,获取前鉴定供受体 0 抗原配型,这对器官需要跨国家转运减少冷缺血时间有利。

术前移植评估

胰腺移植受体入院需再次评估,并做出是否进行手术的最终决定。再次评估过程类似于肾脏移植受体,强调对手术禁忌急性医疗问题的检查。初始评估和等待列表管理的内容在第 32 章和第 41 章中已做详细讨论。糖尿病患者有几个特别注意事项。仔细处理糖尿病患者术前不能进食或饮水的相关问题。对拟行胰脏移植肠道引流的患者行肠准备。

心脏评估是术前评估的最关键部分。事实上,所有患者都将进行广泛的心脏评估,包括胸部 X 线片、ECG、压力测试和冠状动脉造影。许多患者将通过冠状动脉介入治疗以减少移植手术的围术期风险并延长移植后的寿命。在胰腺移植之前经历长时间等待的患者应当重新评估其心脏功能。

自主神经病变很普遍,可表现为神经源性膀胱功能障碍、胃病和直立性低血压。神经源性膀胱功能障碍是接受膀胱引流胰腺移植的重要考虑因素。无法感知膀胱充盈度和排空膀胱,容易导致使尿液回流和排尿残留。这些问题可能影响移植肾功能,增加膀胱感染和肾盂肾炎的发病率,并导致移植物胰腺炎。

移植后发生胃排空障碍、胃瘫有重要意义。严重胃瘫的患者可能难以耐受口服免疫抑制药物,而口服免疫抑制药物对预防排斥反应至关重要。

血管紧张的调节异常可导致直立性低血压和卧床性高血压。这种情况对移植后的血压控制具有影响,特别是膀胱引流的胰腺移植患者,其容易产生血容量缺失。仔细评估移植后的降压药物是很重要的。

糖尿病视网膜病变在糖尿病和终末期肾病患者中常见。失明不是移植的绝对禁忌证,因为许多盲人患者生活都非常独立。虽然这不是主要问题,但应该确认视力丧失患者有足够的支持系统来确保其在出行和免疫抑制药物服用方面获得帮助。

下肢外周血管病变在糖尿病患者中很常见。尿毒症的糖尿病患者有下肢截肢的风险。这些问题通常以晚期神经性病变相关的足部溃疡开始。在长期糖尿病患者中,感觉和运动神经病的风险进一步复杂化。血管疾病可能对移植后的康复有影响,并且是对足部损伤和随后糖尿病足溃疡潜在风险的提示。

精神或情感疾病很常见,包括神经症和抑郁。诊断和治疗这类疾病非常重要,这对确保高度医疗顺从性很重要。

供体胰腺获取

确认用于胰腺移植的合适的死亡供体器官非常重要,也是经常不被重视的预后决定因素。表 60.1 列出了胰腺移植的常见禁忌证。错误判断供体器官的质量将在移植后产生严重的不良后果。移植手术从器官获取开始。

供体胰腺器官评估

确定胰腺移植的合适供体的标准比肾脏供体或肝脏供体更严格。死亡胰腺器官供体年龄通常为 10~60 岁。较低的年龄限制与儿童胰腺内分泌的代谢效率无关,主要是为了调节成人的血管控制。供体胰腺年龄限制较低说明脾动脉口径小,这可能阻碍胰腺同种异体移植物血运重建所需的 Y 型动脉移植物的成功构建。

对于年龄上限,老年供体的胰腺与因移植物血栓形成、移植后胰腺炎和胰腺移植物存活率低导致的技术失败的风险增长相关[12]。体重是死亡器官供体的一个重要考虑因素。BMI>30kg/m^2 的肥胖供体往往不是

表 60.1 胰腺移植禁忌证

1.遗漏器官捐献同意
2.血型不兼容
3.供体 HLA Ⅰ类和(或)Ⅱ类抗原免疫交叉配型阳性
4.供体 1 型或 2 型糖尿病史
5.供体有 HIV、乙型肝炎和(或)丙型肝炎病毒感染性疾病
6..供体有明显细菌和(或)真菌感染
7.供体有明显长期血流动力学不稳定
8.供体既往有胰腺手术史
9.供体胰腺腹内创伤
10.恶性肿瘤

From[19] Kaufman DB. Chapter 47. Complications of Pancreatic Transplantation, pp. 640–655. In: Complications in Surgery, 2nd edition. Ed. M. Mulholland and G. Doherty. Lippincott Williams & Wilkins, 2011. Reprinted with permission from Wolters Kluwer.

合适的胰腺供者。肥胖患者可能有 2 型糖尿病的病史，或者因胰腺的高度脂肪浸润而不适合移植。回顾性分析已经确定了许多与胰腺移植后预后差相关的供体因素，包括 BMI>30kg/m^2[13]。胰腺供体风险指数(pDRI)可用来告知器官接受决策，该指数考虑 10 个常见的供体变量和一个移植因素(缺血时间)作为与同种异体移植物衰竭风险相关的因素。

重要的是，年龄较大的供体(55~65 岁)和肥胖供体的胰腺与胰岛移植所需的胰岛分离恢复相关。因此，几乎所有死亡供体均应用 β 细胞替代疗法。

供体血流动力学稳定性和正性肌力药物支持是重要考虑因素。在 SPK 移植中，血流动力学稳定性对肾移植物功能的影响比对胰腺移植物内分泌功能影响更大。如果死亡供体心脏停搏时间很长，或者需要长期高剂量的肌力支持，供体往往会出现肾功能的缓慢恶化，这可能导致 SPK 移植受体肾功能延迟恢复。

决定胰腺是否适合移植的最重要因素是在手术获取过程中对胰腺进行直接检查。获取团队的经验非常重要。获取期间可对纤维化程度、脂肪组织浸润实质、创伤和特定血管异常做出判断。在获取期间必须准确评估重要的血管异常是否存在源自肠系膜上动脉(SMA)的异位肝右动脉或肝右副动脉。

关于采用边缘供体和心脏死亡(DCD)供体的胰腺移植已有报道[15]。如果胰腺被认为是合适的，尿毒症 SPK 移植患者需要考虑肾移植物有延迟肾功能恢复可能。根据具体情况决定是否采用边缘供体和 DCD 供体进行胰腺移植。

还描述了活体亲属和非亲属胰腺供体的应用，其中节段性胰腺移植需进行远端胰腺切除术[16]。活体供体部分胰腺切除术和肾切除术联合用于 SPK 移植的轶事病例也有报道[16]。这些操作没有广泛执行，大多是历史记录。最后，死亡供体胰腺和活体供体肾移植的同时联合使用已成功应用[17]。

胰腺十二指肠脾同种异体移植物的获取

有几种标准的手术方法用于胰腺的移植。一般原理类似，在不损害肝血管的情况下，胰腺必须有完整的血管供应。胰腺与脾脏和十二指肠一并完整获取。用保存液灌注器官并冷藏。供体髂血管用于动脉供血的血运重建，有时也用于门静脉的血运重建。

有两种一般性器官获取方法。很多中心喜欢将肝脏和胰腺整体取出后在后台处分离。还有一些中心则在保存之前通过游离相关的脉管系统进行胰腺和肝脏分离。原位分离肝脏和胰腺。下面简要介绍原位获取的相关步骤。

1.长中线切口(±十字切口)。

2.游离升结肠，控制肾下主动脉，明确肠系膜上动脉。

3.控制上腹主动脉。

4.识别肝动脉(胃十二指肠动脉结扎)、脾动脉、门静脉，以及分开胆总管。

5.识别异位肝左动脉、肝右动脉和(或)肝左副动脉、肝右副动脉。

6.胰腺前部的显露和触觉检查。

7.分开胃短血管以分离脾脏，并分离其韧带附着。

8.游离胰腺头、胰腺尾和胰腺体。

9.NG 管放置到十二指肠近端，灌注抗生素溶液。

10.移除 NG 管，分离幽门远端的近段十二指肠。

11.供体肝素化，主动脉内(±门内)灌注保存液。

12.分离胰腺钩突远端的近端空肠、结肠中血管、肠系膜上血管。

13.分离腹腔、SMA、脾动脉和门静脉。

14.肝脏、胰腺十二指肠同种异体移植物和肾的获取。

15.供体髂血管获取。

16.关闭切口。

标准供体或 DCD 供体的多器官获取中的胰腺获取已在第 21 章和第 22 章中讨论。

胰腺十二指肠同种异体移植物的后台准备

胰腺十二指肠同种异体移植物的后台准备需要细致的外科技术，以确保胰腺血运良好，并有足够的十二指肠和最小的外源性纤维和脂肪组织(图 60.1)。后台获取手术的质量对移植手术的直接结果具有最大的影响。

胰腺十二指肠同种异体移植物由外科医生从死亡供体获取后，放置在保存溶液中，并根据 UNOS 指南将其放置在冷藏容器中，以便运输到移植中心。将容器带入手术室，并且 UNOS 鉴别号与供体血型和胰移植受体相互参照。盛满冰块的凹盘上覆盖一层塑料创膜，塑料包膜中充满新鲜的冷冻保存液。然后将器官从运输容器中取出并放入冷冻保存液中。通常，两位外科医生合作行后台手术准备。

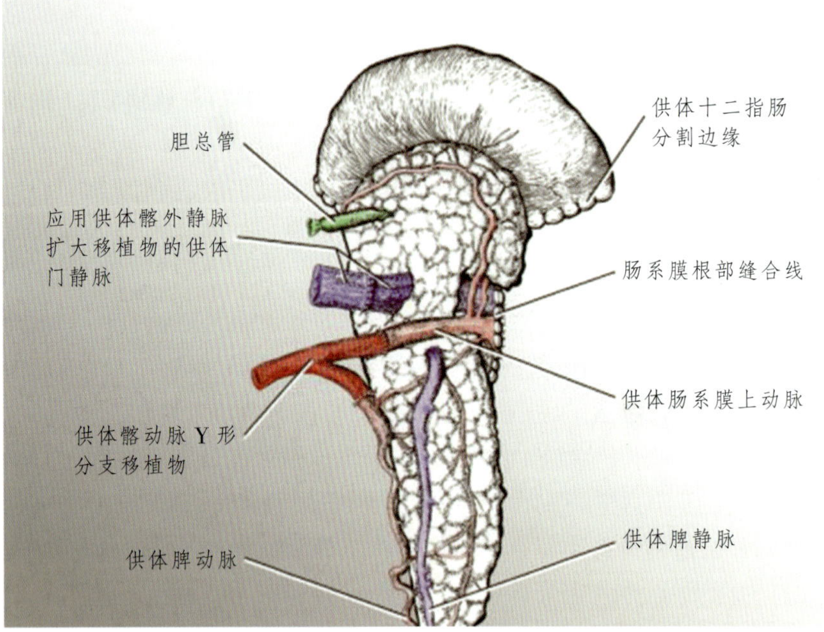

图 60.1 后台重建胰十二指肠同种异体移植物的解剖图。(Illustration by Simon Kimm MD, Department of Urologic Oncology, Memorial Sloan-Kettering Cancer Center, New York, NY.)

在最终决定进行移植之前，同种异体移植物的目视检查至关重要。应评估器官的实质脂肪浸润、纤维化或可触知的结节性病变的程度。具有脂肪重度浸润的胰腺对长期(>18 小时)的冷保存相对不耐受，并且血运重建后有高度皂化风险。这些器官可能更适合胰岛分离。

检查有无实质、血管和十二指肠损伤，以及有无血管异常。应检查断开的小肠肠系膜，确保它没有被分割得太短，保证胰腺实质和实质内的血管供应。仔细检查胰腺段门静脉，以确保其未被切割得过短，损伤连接的脾静脉。这种情况可能在肝获取期间门静脉拉伸时发生，肝侧门静脉保留过过长，特别是获取外科医生了解到肝受体是二次移植时。短(2mm)门静脉的情况可用髂外静脉供体的门静脉扩张移植来完成补救。

在获取期间必须仔细处理并在后台重新评估重要的血管异常，如源自 SMA 的异位肝右动脉或肝右副动脉。大多数情况下，存在异位肝右动脉不是胰腺移植的禁忌证。经验丰富的获取团队能够在原位或在后台成功地分离肝脏和胰腺，而不牺牲移植器官的质量。

一些重要的注意事项决定这个手术是否可行。异位肝右动脉必须能从 SMA 结合处分开。如果异位肝右动脉深入胰腺头部实质，需要行完全实质切除，这种情况无法行胰腺移植(但可适用于胰岛移植)。在这种情况下，另一种替代方案是将异位肝右动脉在胰腺实质外分开，而不进入胰腺。这样的动脉可以在不损伤胰腺的情况下安全地重建以用于肝移植，但是这需要特定重建的经验。

SMA 在异位肝右动脉起点远端分开，保留较短的 SMA 动脉片以备肝移植用。偶尔有一支较大的胰十二指肠下动脉分支供应胰腺头部，它起源于异位肝右动脉近端。胰十二指肠下动脉对于胰腺头部的血供至关重要，因为在肝移植的肝动脉分离中通常游离并结扎胃十二指肠动脉。在胰十二指肠下动脉起点的近端，将 SMA 在适应位置分离用于肝移植可能会明显损害胰腺头部的血供并使其不能用于移植。

可以通过几种方法在后台测试胰十二指肠同种异体移植物的动脉血供：①将 Renografin 注射到 SMA 或 Y 形移植物中并进行 X 线片检查；②动脉内注射荧光素，使用 Wood 灯观察；③行亚甲蓝血管造影。

十二指肠应仔细检查以排除浆膜损伤。许多移植中心在远端缝合处打开十二指肠，灌注并将内容物排出，然后关闭开口。一些中心常规培养液体和一小块十二指肠组织。

后台同种异体移植物制备的主要原理如下。首先，从胰腺尾部移除脾脏，并将大的脾脏血管缝扎。也可使用血管吻合器，而且可能更有效。接下来，切断胆总管

(CBD)并临时放置套管(5F 鼻饲管)通过触诊确定壶腹的位置。当十二指肠的近端和远端缩短到适当的长度(管被移除并且 CBD 被重新结扎)时,可用标记笔标记位置,以确保其中心位置。在幽门远端几厘米处切开十二指肠的第一段,并用吻合器切开壶腹近端。将十二指肠的第三部分从肠系膜切开,直到靠近胰腺并闭合。用 3-0 尼龙或丝线将断端缝合包埋。十二指肠的角部必须小心、充分地翻转,以避免其突出,最终发生破裂和渗漏。

通过胰腺钩突伸出的肠系膜血管可由获取器官团队吻合或单独结扎。在肠系膜根上的吻合线可用 3-0 单丝缝合线缝合加强。结肠中血管被缝合固定。

动脉系统常规重建。去除周围的神经节纤维组织,确认并准备供体脾动脉和 SMA,为重建做好准备。重建需要使用供体髂动脉复合物,常用的为髂总、髂内和髂外的 Y 形移植物。

髂动脉和静脉复合体是关键血管移植物。应仔细检查动脉复合体,以确定是否发生了内部-外部连接处的损伤(通常是在获取过程中过度收缩导致的)。修建 Y 形移植物的髂内动脉和髂外动脉长度,根据胰腺同种异体移植物的脾和肠系膜上动脉上的端-端吻合而确定长度。通常使用 7-0 单丝缝合线连续缝合,但对于小儿供体,间断缝合较为适当。若脾动脉可游离足够长度,可与肠系膜上动脉进行端-侧吻合。

有时,胰腺同种异体移植物的获取不与肝脏获取同时进行。在这种情况下,获取团队可将胰腺同种异体移植物移植到带有完全腹腔干和 SMA 及完整胃十二指肠动脉的主动脉补片上。在这些情况下,无须重建 Y 形移植物,只要保留腹腔和 SMA 动脉流入。在移植物动脉血运重建后将观察到异常的十二指肠移植物灌注。

一些中心通常会修正流出的门静脉流出血管系统。仔细游离门静脉至适当的长度,并确定是否需要使用供体髂外静脉增长短的门静脉。使用供体髂外静脉可以很容易实现门静脉延长,使用 5-0 或 6-0 单丝缝合线连续缝合。

在血管重建后,一些中心用 100~200mL 的新鲜、冷冻保存液灌注胰腺 Y 形移植物以检测实质血管是否有渗漏,如果有渗漏,可在受体血运开放之前修复。重要的是不要应用已使用的保存液冲洗,因为小颗粒物质会进入器官中,会增加血管损伤和血栓形成的风险。最后,保存溶液应更换为新鲜的溶液,并在其下方的盆中补充大量的冰。在复杂的情况下,后台工作的总操作时间可能超过 3 小时。

胰腺移植手术

准备

患者进入手术室(OR)之前所做的准备工作可优化胰腺移植手术结果:适当的抗生素预防方案;DVT 预防;根据估计失血量确认血液制品;标记手术部位。

手术室的安全和效率取决于团队成员之间的良好沟通。团队所有成员应主动介绍自己,以促进后续沟通。在开始手术之前应明确以下几个问题:确认正确的患者和移植程序;同种异体器官移植物的供体/受体 ABO 配型。外科医生应审查移植手术的关键部分、手术持续时间和估计的失血量,包括对中心静脉通路和动脉血压监测的需要。外科医生和护理人员检查外科手术设备、牵开器、电灼设备、照明等的可用性。确认给予适当的抗生素和免疫抑制治疗。

显露

胰腺移植的手术技术是多样的(图 60.2),但其原理一致,包括确保足够的动脉血流至胰腺和十二指肠,从胰腺有足够的静脉血流出,以及胰腺外分泌的安全管理。保留自体胰腺。当进行 SPK 移植手术时,还需显露腹腔内死亡供体肾脏移植的手术术野。

通过正中切口或右下象限斜切口可获得适当的显露。大多数外科医生使用正中切口,如果行 SPK 移植,两个器官移植可共用一个切口植入。胰腺优先考虑采用右侧髂血管血供。在中线切口之后,常用改良的 Cattell 手术来显露胰腺移植的受体血管。右结肠在盲肠和升结肠外侧沿 Toldt 白线向前向内分离。这可显露右侧髂血管、主动脉和下腔静脉。没有必要暴露右肾和肾血管或第四部分十二指肠。另一种方法是在不游离右结肠的情况下,通过腹膜后层分离髂血管和腔静脉远端,从而使小肠向头部回缩。为了显露用于腹内肾移植的髂血管,沿 Toldt 白线在降结肠和乙状结肠外侧向内游离降结肠和乙状结肠。

如果采用右下象限切口,与肾移植类似,需将腹膜后的髂血管分离。髂内静脉与髂动脉分离,并保持髂动脉外侧静脉的自由游离。胰腺植入头尾侧。打开腹膜,胰腺腹内旋转,胰腺的尾部固定到前腹壁,并进行十二

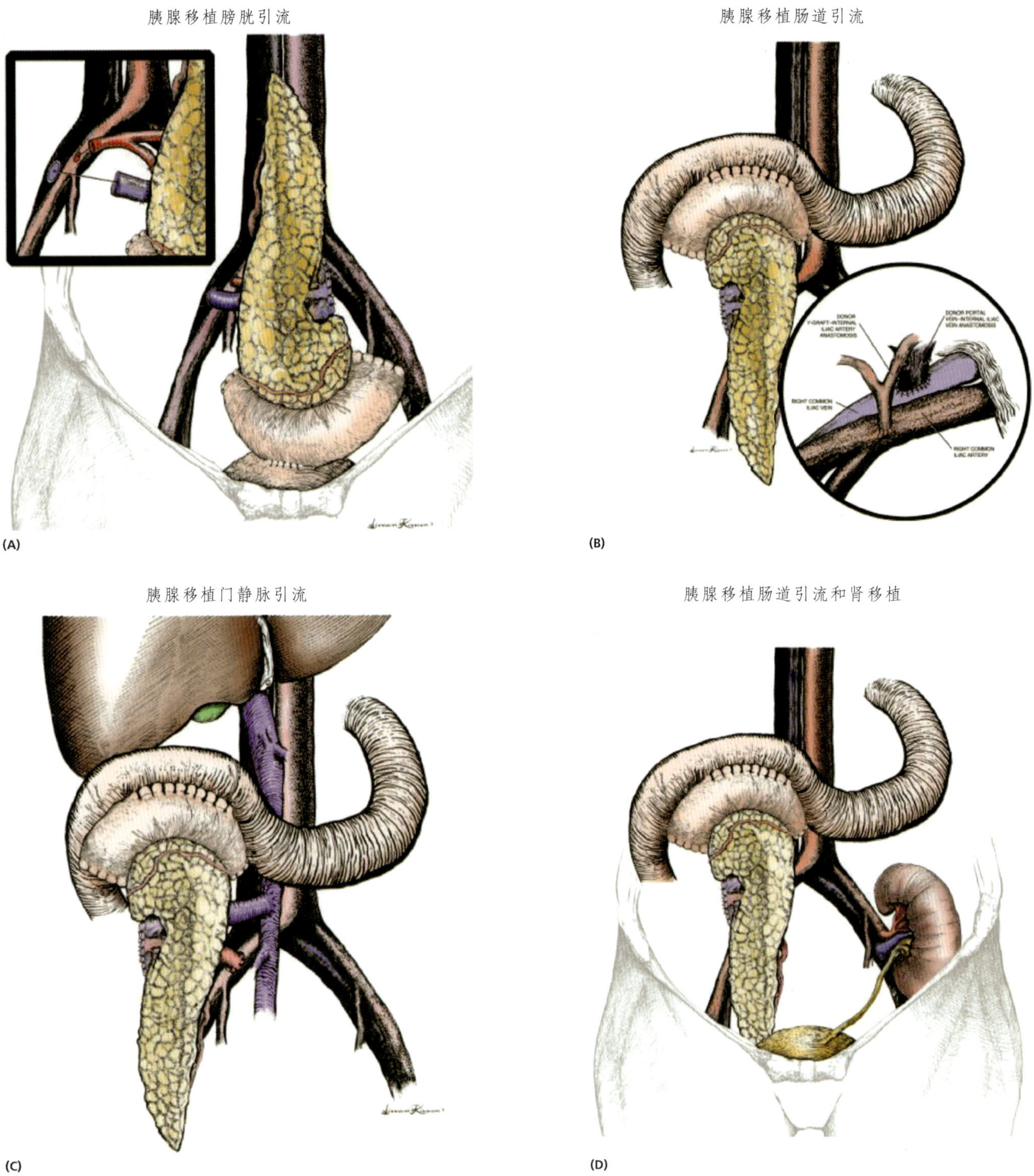

图 60.2 (A)外周静脉胰岛素输注和膀胱外分泌引流的胰十二指肠同种异体移植。(B)外周静脉胰岛素输注和肠道外分泌引流的胰十二指肠同种异体移植。(C)门静脉胰岛素输注和肠道外分泌引流的胰十二指肠同种异体移植。(D)外周静脉胰岛素输注和肠道外分泌引流的胰十二指肠同种异体移植和肾移植。(Reprinted with permission from [20] Stuart FP, Abecassis MM, Kaufman DB. Organ Transplantation, 2nd edition. Georgetown: Landes Bioscience, 2003, p. 168. Copyright © 2003, Landes Bioscience. Illustration by Simon Kimm MD, Department of Urologic Oncology, Memorial Sloan-Kettering Cancer Center, New York, NY.)

指肠造口术或十二指肠切开术。

方法

胰腺移植的手术技术根据胰岛素静脉输注和胰外分泌引流技术的方法来确定。对于腹内放置的胰腺,其可能朝向十二指肠头部或尾部。外周静脉胰岛素输注或肠分泌引流是最常用的方法,通常从胰头头侧进行。偶尔也采用门静脉胰岛素输注或肠分泌引流的方法,但只有 10%的病例会应用此种方法。在这种情况下,肠系膜上静脉用于静脉吻合。在肠系膜根部显露血管。这种技术需要更长的髂总动脉 Y 形移植物,它可以通过肠系膜下连接到受体右髂总动脉。在二次移植手术中若遇到外周静脉引流困难可采用这种方法。另一种常见的方法是外周静脉或膀胱外分泌引流(门静脉引流不可能与膀胱外分泌引流同时进行)。随着免疫抑制技术的进步,这种技术已不那么流行了。

在 SPK 移植情况下均进行肠道引流。单独进行胰腺移植的情况下偶尔使用膀胱引流,可根据尿淀粉酶监测这种类型病例的排斥反应,在此类病例中有相对较高的免疫移植物损失率。

动脉重建

通常用受体右侧髂总动脉或髂外动脉来完成胰腺移植动脉的血运重建。胰腺 Y 形移植物采用端-侧吻合。胰腺移植物头部或尾部位置与动脉血运重建无关。通常在静脉吻合后进行动脉吻合,SMV 用于门静脉引流的胰腺除外。在这种情况下,首先放置动脉移植物,常采用 Fogarty Hydragrip 血管夹夹闭动脉,对糖尿病患者的血管(通常是发生病变的)创伤较小。用 11 号刀片切开动脉,应用肝素化盐水冲洗血管。动脉打孔可用于扩张动脉切口以便匹配 Y 形移植物的髂总动脉。使用 6-0 单丝缝线连续缝合行端-侧吻合。

静脉重建

静脉血运重建有两种选择,外周静脉和门静脉。外周静脉血运重建通常包括远端腔静脉/右髂总静脉或右髂外静脉。如果使用门静脉引流,需要在肠系膜根部分离肠系膜上静脉。胰腺门静脉与肠系膜上静脉分支端-侧吻合。这种吻合方式可能影响动脉血运重建的方法,并需要使用长的 Y 形移植物以便从肠系膜到达右髂总动脉。胰腺门静脉引流相对于立即将胰岛素输注入受体肝脏而言,更具有生理学上的意义。门静脉引流方式的循环胰岛素水平相对于外周静脉引流的胰岛素水平低。静脉引流的不同路径在血糖控制方面没有临床相关差异。

常用于静脉吻合的血管夹是单个 Lambert-Kay 夹或双重无创的直 DeBakey 夹。如果需要局部阻塞静脉,若静脉切开部位是远端腔静脉并且先前行过肾同种异体移植物移植,优先选择前者。静脉切开术是用 11 号刀片或剪刀切割出椭圆开口。用肝素化盐水冲洗血管。静脉切开尺寸与门静脉或髂外静脉移植物的尺寸匹配。端-端吻合使用 6-0 单丝缝合线连续缝合。

血管再通

吻合术完成后,小心取出血管夹,先静脉后动脉。良好灌注的胰腺和十二指肠应为均匀的粉红色。十二指肠开始分泌肠液。血运重建的胰腺比肾同种异体移植物出血更多。出血血管用血管夹控制后缝合。三个最常见的出血区域是胰腺钩突肠系膜血管、胰尾的脾血管和胆总管的动脉血管。由于失血和再灌注效应,受体收缩压短暂降低是常见的。血运重建之前,与麻醉团队良好沟通至关重要,可以确保受体足够的中心静脉压、血糖稳定和电解质平衡。

根据胰头的方向仔细定位胰腺位置。如果它在头部位置,那么尾部应定位在 Douglas 窝下方或右侧的肠旁沟中的盲肠外侧,这取决于肠道之前的游离方式。旋转胰腺,脾动脉与腹膜后相邻,肠系膜血管向上定位。检查和触诊血管确认脾动脉搏动良好,以及门静脉柔软且无错位。将肠重新固定在同种异体移植物周围,其中胰腺头部朝向头侧,上部邻近空肠中部。

胰管管理

有几种处理胰腺外分泌引流的方法。胰腺外分泌引流可以通过十二指肠段与膀胱的吻合或通过小肠吻合来处理。1982 年,有人提出了膀胱引流的胰腺移植。该技术通过减少肠内引流胰腺移植物渗漏导致腹腔脓肿的发生,显著改善了手术的安全性。随着新型免疫抑制剂的成功应用,以及排斥的反应和肠漏发生率的降低,胰腺移植的肠道引流已经发生变革,并在很大程度上取代了膀胱引流。

胰腺同种异体移植物的肠内引流是关于胰酶和碳酸氢盐进入肠道进行再吸收的生理过程。胰腺肠内引流可以使用或不使用 Roux-ex-Y 肠袢构建。肠道吻合可与胰腺十二指肠段进行侧-侧吻合或端-侧吻合,可手工缝合或应用吻合器完成。前者更常见。典型的吻合术为双层吻合术,内层采用 3-0 可吸收缝合线全层缝合,外侧浆肌层应用 3-0 丝线间断缝合。

肠内引流腹腔内脓肿的危险性很低[18],避免膀胱引流潜在的并发症具有重要意义,如膀胱感染、膀胱炎、尿道炎、尿道损伤、龟头炎、血尿、代谢性酸中毒和肠内转化的需要。目前,大约 75%的胰腺移植采用肠内引流,其他采用膀胱引流。

肠内引流与膀胱引流的选择取决于静脉引流的选择和胰腺移植的临床情况。对于门静脉引流胰腺移植,无法行膀胱引流。SPK 移植的受体应选择肠道引流,因为尿液没有监测价值,并且并发症发生率很高。在 PAK 和 PTA 的情况下,膀胱引流有两个重要的优点:①排尿监测排斥反应;②移植物的放置,允许进行经皮活检以诊断排斥反应。在后一种情况下,监测的优点超过与膀胱引流相关的发病率,至少在短期内,当免疫性移植物损失的风险很高时,其具有更大优势。但许多中心也有使用肠内引流判断胰腺移植排斥反应的良好经验,如胰腺移植胰腺炎临床表现和症状,以及与活检相结合的血清淀粉酶或脂肪酶的水平。

关腹

用可吸收或不可吸收的单股 0 号、1 号或 2 号缝合线缝合筋膜。如果尿毒症患者有腹膜透析导管,可在筋膜闭合前拔除。有时可在胰腺附近 Douglas 窝放置闭式引流。皮下脂肪用 3-0 可吸收缝合线缝合,皮缘用外科缝合钉缝合并用杆菌肽软膏和敷料覆盖,或者皮下用 4-0 可吸收缝合线缝合,用二苯乙醇酮胶带黏合和敷料覆盖。

结论

手术室结束后,清点海绵、针和器械。获得适当的放射学研究。在离开 OR 前,审查患者的术后恢复和护理计划。手术结束后不久,在手术报告中应完成精确的描述性文件。与患者的家庭成员立即进行面对面沟通。

小结

自 1966 年人类第一次成功施行胰腺移植手术以来,在胰腺移植领域取得了巨大的进展。胰腺移植已经从高发病率和死亡率的实验性手术变为与肾移植良好结果类似的移植手术。该领域的兴起得益于外科技术、免疫抑制方案、供体评估、术前受体评估和术后管理的巨大进步。以上所描述的技术已在我们的中心常规使用,具有良好的效果,并继续改进,使胰腺移植成为糖尿病患者更安全、更有效的治疗选择。

(胡志平 译 朱继业 校)

参考文献

1. Centers for Disease Control and Prevention. National Diabetes Fact Sheet: National Estimates and General Information on Diabetes and Prediabetes in the United States. Atlanta, GA: U.S. Department of Health and Human Services, Centers for Disease Control and Prevention; 2011.
2. American Diabetes Association. Economic costs of diabetes in the U.S. in 2007. Diabetes Care. 2008;31:596–615.
3. Morel P, Goetz F, Moudry-Munns KC, et al. Long term metabolic control in patients with pancreatic transplants. Annals of Internal Medicine. 1991; 115:694–699.
4. Navarro X, Kennedy WR, Loewenson RB, et al. Influence of pancreas transplantation on cardiorespiratory reflexes, nerve conduction, and mortality in diabetes mellitus. Diabetes. 1990;39:802–806.
5. Kennedy WR, Navarro X, Goetz FC, et al. Effects of pancreatic transplantation on diabetic neuropathy. New England Journal of Medicine. 1990;322:1031–1037.
6. Fioretto P, Mauer SM, Bilous RW, et al. Effects of pancreas transplantation on glomerular structure in insulin-dependent diabetic patients with their own kidneys. Lancet. 1993;342:1193–1196.
7. Bilous RW, Mauer SM, Sutherland DE, et al. The effects of pancreas transplantation on the glomerular structure of renal allografts in patients with insulin-dependent diabetes. New England Journal of Medicine. 1989;321:80–85.
8. Ramsay RC, Goetz FC, Sutherland DE, et al. Progression of diabetic retinopathy after pancreas transplantation for insulin dependent diabetes mellitus. New England Journal of Medicine. 1988;318:208–214.
9. Zehr PS, Milde FK, Hart LK, et al. Pancreas transplantation: assessing secondary complications and life quality. Diabetologia. 1991;34(Suppl. 1):S138–S140.
10. Ojo AO, Meier-Kriesche HU, Hanson JA, et al. Impact of simultaneous pancreas-kidney transplantation on long-term patient survival. Transplantation. 2001;71: 82–90.
11. Mohan P, Safi K, Little DM, et al. Improved patient survival in recipients of simultaneous pancreas-kidney transplant compared with kidney transplant alone in patients with type 1 diabetes mellitus and end-stage renal disease. British Journal of Surgery. 2003;90:1137–1141.
12. Salvalaggio PR, Schnitzler MA, Abbott KC, et al. Patient and graft survival implications of simultaneous pancreas kidney transplantation from old donors. American Journal of Transplantation. 2007;7:1561–1571.
13. Humar A, Ramcharan T, Kandaswamy R, et al. Technical failures after pancreas transplants: why grafts fail and the risk factors—a multivariate analysis. Transplantation. 2004;78:1188–1192.
14. Axelrod D, Sung R, Meyer KH, et al. Systematic evaluation of pancreas allograft quality, outcomes, and geographic variation in utilization. American Journal of Transplantation. 2010;10:837–845.
15. Salvalaggio PR, Davies DB, Fernandez LA, et al. Outcomes of pancreas transplantation in the United States using cardiac-death donors. American Journal of Transplantation. 2006;6:1059–1065.
16. Humar A, Gruessner R, Sutherland D. Living related donor pancreas and pancreas-kidney transplantation. British Medical Bulletin. 1997;53:879–891.
17. Farney AC, Cho E, Schweitzer E, et al. Simultaneous cadaver pancreas living-donor kidney transplantation: a new approach for the type 1 diabetic uremic patient. Annals of Surgery. 2000;232:696–703.
18. Schnickel GT, Busuttil RW, Lipshultz GS. Improvement in short-term pancreas transplant outcome by targeted antimicrobial therapy and refined donor selection. American Surgeon. 2011;77:1407–1411.
19. Kaufman DB. Complications of pancreatic transplantation. In: Mulholland M, Doherty G, editors. Complications in Surgery, 2nd edition. Philadelphia, PA: Lippincott Williams & Wilkins; 2011: 640–655.
20. Stuart FP, Abecassis MM, Kaufman DB. Organ Transplantation, 2nd edition. Georgetown, TX: Landes Bioscience; 2003: 168.

第 61 章
胰岛细胞移植手术步骤和外科技术

A.M. James Shapiro, Camillo Ricordi

简介

在某些移植中心，临床胰岛移植(CIT)已经从一个罕见的、试验性的新奇事物迅速转变为一个合理的、常见的临床操作技术，用于治疗不稳定的1型糖尿病。全世界范围内已经进行了超过850例的胰岛移植[1]，至少在专家们眼中，胰岛移植与其他实体器官移植相比，在技术层面上安全性最高。考虑到其不断提高的短期疗效(参见第108章)，在加拿大、英国、澳大利亚、瑞士、意大利、法国及其他欧洲国家中，临床胰岛移植已经被认为是一项“非实验性”的标准临床治疗。美国食品与药品监督委员会(FDA)正在为CIT迅速申请生物认证应用(BLA)。BLA将方便通过医疗保险及医疗补助进行报销，并对未来胰岛移植产生重大影响。

本章节将讨论胰腺获取及胰岛分离和培养的外科技术，以及如何使用微创技术将胰岛通过门静脉移植至受体体内。临床药品生产质量规范(cGMP)要求在整个过程中严格关注每一个细节，保证受体在获得足够数量的高活性胰岛治疗糖尿病的同时，将相关并发症的发生风险降到最低。

胰腺的手术获取

用于临床胰岛分离、纯化及培养的cGMP要求以最大精确度获取胰腺，从而达到保证胰腺包膜完整、在主动脉夹闭前最大限度增加胰腺氧合血流量以及尽量避免发生移植物胰腺炎的目的[2]。从采用最小的血管活性药物的供体获得的胰岛最佳，理想的胰岛供体标准和全胰腺供体类似[3]。体重指数(BMI)较高的供体胰腺脂肪含量较多，易于获取，但是有潜在2型糖尿病的供体常常有胰岛素分泌缺陷，不宜用于胰岛移植[4-7]。因此，糖化血红蛋白A1c(HbA1c)水平上升超过6.5%供体的胰腺通常不能进行胰岛分离。到目前为止，从年轻的(18~30岁)理想供体中获得的胰岛数目往往较少，部分原因是年轻的腺体中胶原含量较高，纤维化较重[8-10]。目前几个临床胰岛细胞移植联合中心的成功率表明，从年轻胰腺中获得胰岛的移植成功率逐渐提高，结合出色的临床结果，这也将对未来胰腺器官的分配产生影响(是用于全胰腺移植还是用于胰岛移植)[11-15]。

最佳的胰腺获取技术原则参见表61.1。总体而言，用于胰岛移植的胰腺获取技术与用于全胰腺移植的胰腺获取技术类似，相关内容已经在第22章和第60章进行了深入探讨。UW溶液(Viaspan, Bristol-Myers-Squibb, New York, USA))最初被设计为胰腺的最佳保存溶液[16]。UW溶液一直作为标准的胰腺保存溶液，但是近年来，更多地受到节约经济成本而非直接保存

表 61.1 获取胰腺用于胰岛移植的手术原则

1.选择稳定的、需要较小剂量血管活性药物支持的供体
2.不合并糖尿病(HbA1c<6.5%)
3.获取过程中尽量少触碰胰腺组织
4.阻断前保证足够的血流供应，保持肠系膜上动脉、胃十二指肠动脉及脾动脉通畅
5.冷灌注期间避免胰腺静脉血栓(尽量避免肠系膜静脉插管，如果需要，则保证动脉和静脉导管间距离大于40cm)
6.减少热缺血时间，阻断后打开小网膜，在胰腺前后放置冰盐水冰屑，胰腺在UW或HTK保存液中温度为4℃
7.可经胰腺导管插管注射30mL UW溶液、HTK溶液或ET-Kyoto溶液
8.减少冷缺血时间(尽量少于6小时)
9.选择有经验的器官获取团队

HbA1c，糖化血红蛋白A1c；UW，威斯康星大学溶液(Viaspan, Bristol- Myers-Squibb, NY, USA)；HTK，组氨酸-色氨酸-酮戊二酸溶液(Custodiol Inc., Brantford Ontario)；ET-Kyoto溶液(Otsuka Pharmaceuticals, Tokyo, Japan)。

器官功能的影响，胰腺保存液逐渐转变为包括组氨酸-色氨酸-酮戊二酸溶液（HTK，Custodiol，Brantford，Ontario，Canada）在内的其他溶液。HTK 溶液在 20 世纪 70 年代最初作为心脏停搏液，由于其含钾量较低，其被认为是一种细胞外保存液。肝脏移植协会推动了 HTK 溶液的应用，因为其避免了使用 UW 溶液时突发高钾引发急性心脏停搏的风险。但是，在某些移植中心，HTK 溶液被认为与全胰腺移植效果较差有关[17,18]。2009 年，加拿大的一项移植项目将 UW 溶液换为 HTK 溶液作为器官保存液，令人鼓舞的是，这一改变对胰岛分离的成功率几乎没有影响。实际上，随着临床胰岛细胞移植联合中心及其分离标准操作程序（SOP）的改进，胰岛的分离至移植的成功率已经从 40%上升至接近 70%（单一供体胰岛素非依赖率水平也有上升），这明显表明 HTK 非但不会降低临床胰岛分离成功率，反而可能会有益。Caballero-Corbalan 等人比较了 HTK 溶液与 UW 溶液用于人体胰岛分离及离体功能，发现保存时间在 10 小时内时，两种溶液无明显差异[19]。

“双层技术”一直被认为可以在移植过程中更好地增加胰腺获氧。该项技术由日本的 Kuroda 及其同事首先提出，包括两层溶液，即氧化氟碳（PFC）溶液和 UW 溶液，胰腺保存在两层溶液之间[20]。随后的非对照研究表明，从使用该技术保存的胰腺中获得的胰岛质量较高[21-27]。但是，近年来，越来越多的研究对上述结论产生疑问，目前，由于该技术的复杂性及费用问题，其应用已逐年减少[28-32]。

选择合适的供体是胰岛分离及移植成功的关键[33]。多因素分析表明，供体年龄>20 岁（最好<50 岁）、供体 BMI 值较高（不伴有 2 型糖尿病）、供体血糖正常、不伴有持续的低血压或心脏停搏，以及血管活性药物支持均是胰岛分离成功的关键因素（表 61.2）[14,34-41]。明尼苏达大学的相关研究表明，年龄<50 岁及 BMI>27kg/m^2 可能是供体成功捐献的关键决定因素之一[42,43]。

获取多个器官的手术有标准的操作步骤，在动脉夹阻断腹主动脉之前尽量少触碰胰腺及分离血管。将大网膜从横结肠系膜上分离并打开小网膜囊，仔细探查胰腺前表面是否有损伤、血管损伤、胰腺炎或肿物等表现。使用 Kocher 法完全游离十二指肠。在远离幽门处及第二、三部分交界处分别使用 75mm 直线切开吻合器离断十二指肠。原位暴露脾动脉并用血管带控制。从肠系膜上动脉发出的异位肝右动脉并不是获取全胰

表 61.2 供体选择标准[33]

入选标准	排除标准
SCD 或 ECD	
多器官供体	1 型或 2 型糖尿病（HbA1c>6.5%）
男性或女性	恶性肿瘤，除外 1°脑瘤
15~75 岁	未经治疗的败血症
热缺血时间<10 分钟	病毒性肝炎
冷缺血时间<12 小时	HIV 或 AIDS
	梅毒
DCD	
可控	病毒性脑炎
热缺血时间<30 分钟	克-雅病
冷缺血时间<4 小时	狂犬病
	结核病
	持续性低血压
	血肌酐升高（大于正常值 3 倍）
	肝功能异常（大于正常值 3 倍）
	血淀粉酶或脂肪酶升高
	高危性行为（除非可以进行 NAT 监测并且监测结果为阴性）
	近期静脉药物使用

SCD，标准捐献供体；ECD，扩大标准捐献供体；DCD，循环死亡供体（无心脏搏动）；NAT，HIV 病毒核酸检测。
Data from Ponte et al.[33]

腺或胰岛分离的禁忌证，尤其是在获取胰岛分离过程中，并不需要肠系膜上动脉血管带。阻断腹主动脉之后开始显露胃十二指肠动脉，并予以分离结扎。腹主动脉夹闭并进行冰 UW 溶液或 HTK 溶液冲洗后，立即将脾、胰尾及胰体分离并翻至中线处，以便用冰盐水冲洗胰腺的前方及后方，达到迅速降温并避免热缺血损伤。理想情况下，夹闭腹主动脉并分离胆总管及门静脉后，胰腺应该是首先被获取的腹部器官（图 61.1）。这实际上便于分离肝脏血管，并提供充足的视野以避免误伤异位的肝右动脉。将胰腺与第一、二部分十二指肠整块获取并置于 4℃ UW 溶液或 HTK 溶液中，随后行三重无菌包装转运至胰岛分离中心。此时，通常留取一部分脾脏用于 HLA 配型。

Baylor 胰岛分离团队提倡在手术室里预先从 Vater 壶腹行胰管置管，并用 ET-Kyoto 溶液（Otsuka Pharm Factory Inc.，Naruto，Japan）按照每克胰腺组织 1mL 的比例进行胰管冲洗，并表示这可以保证较高的分离率[44-46]。但是这一技术并没有得到广泛推广，一部分是由于此法会增加获取后组织的准备难度，但主要

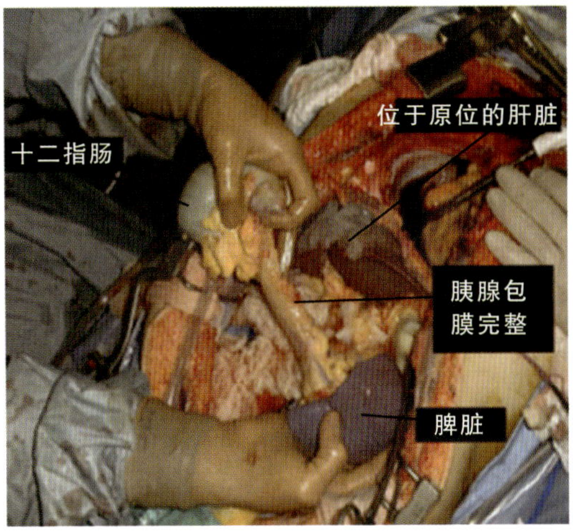

图 61.1　将胰腺与第一及第二段十二指肠、脾脏完整移除，保证胰腺包膜完整。

是由于 ET-Kyoto 溶液无法轻易获得。需要通过进一步的对照研究来证明此法的有效性。

临床胰岛分离及培养

经门静脉植入大量纯化人胰岛细胞以恢复胰岛内分泌功能这一方法的成功操作取决于6~8小时复杂的胰岛分离过程，该过程将70~100g胰腺组织中含有的1%~2%的胰岛与其他外分泌组织分离提取出来。一系列的消化、冲洗及纯化过程将60mL溶液变为5mL富含胰岛细胞的可安全注入门静脉的溶液。一般来说，受体需要5000IEQ/kg的胰岛细胞用于移植。单一供体的移植物超过6000~7000IEQ/kg则其成功率较高。20世纪70年代及80年代，由于无法提取如此高浓度的高质量人胰岛细胞，早期临床胰岛移植往往以失败告终。1986年，在圣路易斯的Paul Lacy实验室工作的Camillo Ricordi发明了一种自动分离胰岛方法，首次成功提高了胰岛分离率，成为第一例探索性临床实验成功的转折点[47,48]。尽管这一方法近年来在不断革新，Ricordi自动化方法依然十分关键，并被全球所有的临床胰岛分离实验室所采用。最近的革新主要集中于优化胶原酶混合及传递、更好的纯化原料及严格控制和记录整个cGMP过程(采用更为详细的SOP，记录过程中所有的步骤，以及用于加工临床级别胰岛产品的超净设备)。

作为CIT协作组的各中心已经将临床分离及培养过程所有步骤的详细SOP进行了更新。这些指南尚未发表，但是可以通过直接向协作组申请获得[49]。

胰管灌注及消化

消化及纯化人胰岛细胞的关键步骤参见图61.2。原理包括使用酶法、机械法及离心法纯化将胰腺逐渐分解成高浓度的完整胰岛。首先进行胰管插管(图61.3)，随后用胶原酶混合溶液浸泡胰腺。先将酶在4℃~10℃保存10分钟，随后加热4分钟至37℃，目标是释放有活性的胶原酶至胰岛-腺泡分界面[9,50]。胰腺随后被分解成几大块(常为9块)，放入含有钢珠的Ricordi舱内在500μm的筛板上进行轻柔的机械搅拌。酶的溶液在37℃条件下循环15~30分钟(图61.2A)[51]。这一过程逐渐将胰腺组织消化成更小的组分，直至含有胰岛的细胞簇通过筛板。一旦胰岛开始释放(二硫腙染色为红色)，立即将溶液冷却至4℃终止酶的消化，进行多次洗涤稀释，并加入人白蛋白溶液进一步终止酶的活性。何时停止消化需要专业的判断及技巧，因为过早或过晚的稀释会导致不当的分解片段或胰岛的不完整，从而无法产生足够的用于移植的胰岛[8,53]。

胶原酶

胶原酶混合、凝集活性、稳定性以及酶的目标位点的不稳定性在以前对大量稳定的分离胰岛带来了巨大挑战[8]。Liberase HI(Roche Diagnostic Pharmaceuticals, Indianapolis USA)的出现则对上述现象带来了极大的改观，这一更为标准的复合酶与既往类型的胶原酶相比，凝集稳定性及胰岛提取率更高[54]。Edmonton小组发现Ⅱ类胶原酶活性过高，不利于胰岛分离[55]。随后发现，Liberase HI暴露于牛生长因子提取物，其是梭状芽孢杆菌的培养层，因此临床级别的Liberase HI会给患者带来极小的感染Creutzfeld-Jacob相关朊病毒病的潜在风险[56]。尽管这一风险相当低(不到一亿分之一)，这一风险仍然被认为可以避免，研究正在寻找可作为替代的复合酶用作临床胰岛分离[56]。

Serva Inc.开发了一种不含有牛相关产物的GMP级胶原酶及中性蛋白酶NB 1 (Serva Electrophoresis GmbH, Heidelberg)，其和Liberase HI具有类似的高压液相色谱(HPLC)活性[14,57,58]。Miami小组发现使用NB 1消化胰腺的时间较Liberase HI长，并且β细胞质量及活性并非最佳[59]。Uppsala小组发现类似的使用NB 1时获得的胰岛量较低，但是胰岛纯度及血糖刺激反应

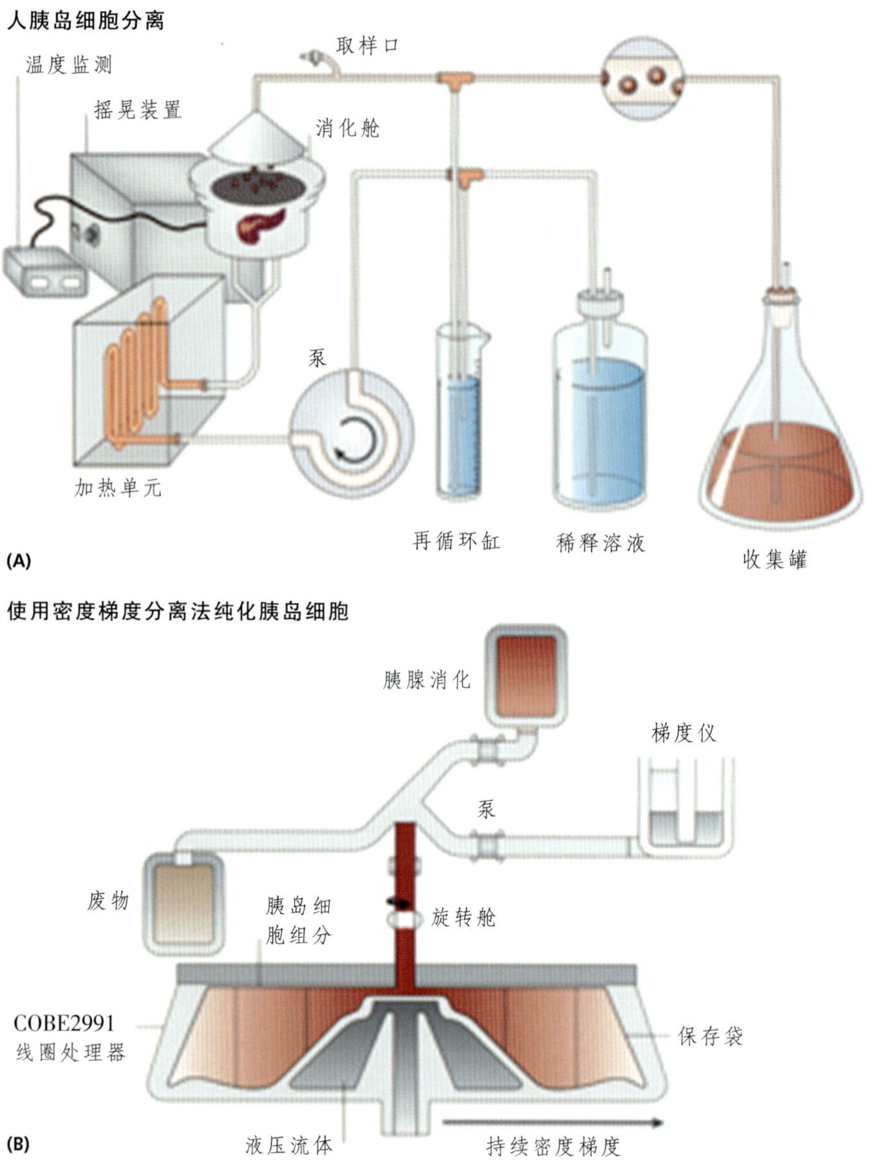

图 61.2 (A)用于胰腺消化的 Ricordi 舱、500μm 筛选、钢化大理石、再循环泵的示意图。(B)COBE2991 离心机示意图,使用持续密度梯度分离法纯化胰腺消化产物。(Reproduced from[51] Ricordi C, Strom TB. Clinical islet transplantation: advances and immunological challenges. Nature Reviews Immunology 2004;4(4):259-268. Copright © 2004, with permission from Nature Publishing Group.)

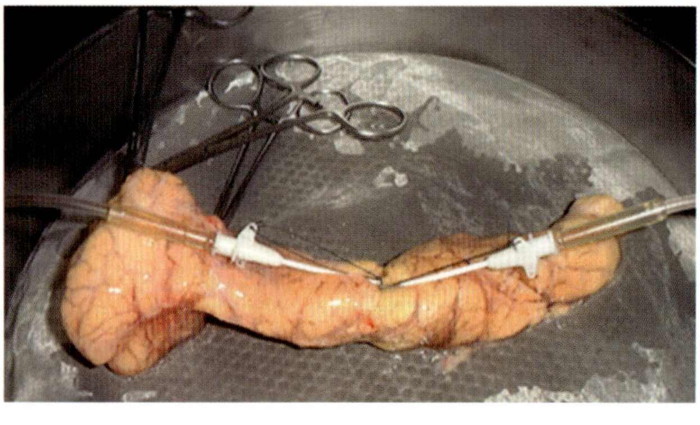

图 61.3 主胰管插管并用含有胶原酶的溶液循环灌注,扩张胰腺并将酶运送至腺泡-胰岛表面。

较高[58]。Edmonton 小组发现将 NB 1 与中性蛋白酶组分分离,分别将 NB 1 及中性蛋白酶经过胰管注入循环酶中,可以减少酶的降解,获得更多更有活力的胰岛[60]。在一部分病例报道中,并不需要在 NB 1 中加入中性蛋白酶[61]。相反地,加州大学旧金山分校(UCSF)发现,在年龄<45 岁的供体中,每克胰腺组织加入 16 单位 NB 1 及 2 单位中性蛋白酶以及 2.5mL DNAse(Pulmozyme,Genentech,San Francisco),患者的消化情况有所改善[62]。根据 UCSF 经验,12 个胰腺中有 9 个来源于年轻供体,其胰腺组织具有较高的临床功能活性[12,63]。

近年来,Roche Diagnostics Inc. 开发了新一代的Liberase无哺乳动物组织酶(MTF)。Caballero-Corbalan等发现在其中加入个体化剂量的嗜热蛋白酶时,消化时间及Ⅰ类胶原酶降解量均较前降低,表明是有益的[64]。O'Gorman等发现,MTF与NB 1具有类似的消化功能活性[14]。另一种替代胶原酶Vitacyte HA(Vitacyte LLC, Indianapolis)也可减少Ⅱ类胶原酶降解,其在临床胰岛分离中的作用正在进一步评估中[66]。

纯化

最后一个步骤即使用低温COBE2991细胞加工器进行密度梯度分离纯化胰岛消化液[66,67]。纯化过程常需要10分钟。最初使用的是不连续Ficoll梯度,但近年来,Hering等发明的碘克沙醇连续梯度(Optiprep,Axis-Shield,Oslo)具有更高的纯化效率[42]。与Ficoll梯度相比,碘克沙醇引发的炎症反应较小[68]。Barbaro等发现,在COBE2991加工器上联合使用UW溶液及碘克沙醇梯度可以增加外分泌组织与胰岛组织的密度区分度[69]。

许多小组推荐在纯化时使用挽救梯度以提高胰岛恢复率[70-72]。Vancouver小组发现,在进一步的12~36小时的培养之后,对不纯的胰岛组织进行再纯化可以提高20%的胰岛产量[70]。Miami小组发现,使用不连续梯度进行再纯化可以提高用于临床移植的胰岛细胞的数量,并且这一过程不会影响胰岛功能[72,73]。

胰岛培养

经过进一步的冲洗和再化合步骤,胰岛制备的最后一个步骤就是将其置于培养媒介中培育24~72小时,随后才可以用于临床移植。胰岛培养可以增加胰岛纯度,并可以降低胰岛移植过程中的炎症状态。除此之外,这一过程给转运、受体T细胞清除治疗等辅助治疗提供了时间,同时避免了新移植的胰岛细胞暴露于潜在有害的细胞因子风暴中,促进了患者管理[39,74-79]。胰岛培养过程中约有20%的胰岛细胞损失,根据多因素分析发现,冷缺血时间延长、胰岛纯度低和较高的胰岛功能指数均与之相关[80]。Markmann等人发现,在24℃培养胰岛细胞可以显著减少MHC抗原表达[81]。Miami小组提出可以在以CMRL为基础的培养基中加入胰岛素、转铁蛋白、锌、硒、丙酮酸及烟碱[82],近年来Little小组对其进一步改进,可以优化培养过程中胰岛细胞的存活率[83-85]。胰岛培养所需时间便于待移植的胰岛细胞在cGMP分离中心与临床移植中心之间转运,从而集中相关技术及专家,减少胰岛分离的花费[73,86,87]。

胰岛移植物评估及产物释放测试

随着胰岛移植逐步向BLA发展,FDA强调了预测胰岛效能测定与临床胰岛功能相关的必要性。该领域充满挑战,因为使用基于染料排除的膜完整性测定胰岛活性的标准测试是敏感性不高[88],而体外静态培养或胰岛细胞表面灌注评估葡萄糖刺激下胰岛素分泌试验常常无法预测体外胰岛细胞功能。为了提高这些试验的敏感性和阳性预测值,大家都在进行不断地尝试和探索。Cabrera等人研发了一种结合高通量的多个自动胰岛灌流技术和β细胞药效动力学的流成像系,有可能会填补FDA所要求的这一空白[89]。Pappas等人研发了一种耗氧率分析系统,可以预测人类胰岛移植到免疫缺陷小鼠后移植物功能以及胰岛移植后的临床结果[90]。使用流式细胞仪量化特定胰岛细胞亚群活性具有良好的发展前途。Ichii等人研发了一种利用激光扫描细胞和线粒体凋亡细胞的多参数分析系统评估β细胞含量、活性及细胞组成,目前各CIT中心正对这一系统进行详细的测试[91]。

最后,在用于临床移植之前,培养的胰岛细胞必须满足所有产物释放标准(表61.3)。这些最低标准要求保证最终的胰岛产物的无菌性和完整性,避免将感染传递给受体,同时提供一个合适的、具有足够纯度的胰岛移植物,降低门静脉血栓形成风险。

受体经皮门静脉内胰岛移植

胰岛移植与全胰腺移植最大的差别在于前者可以通过经皮经肝超声和荧光透视引导这一非手术、微创的方法,从而将胰岛细胞移植进入门静脉,至少在专业人士看来其为最安全、风险最低的移植方式之一。Weimar等人首先描述了联合使用CT和荧光透视的经皮穿刺技术[92]。Edmonton小组则使用超声联合荧光透视引导下经皮门静脉穿刺治疗其最初的7例胰岛素依赖患者[93]。不同小组间的合作促进了这一技术的进一步改进,目前该项技术允许在围移植期使用全量肝素进行治疗性抗凝,并消除操作后的出血风险。有效减少门静脉血栓发生并同时预防出血是降低该项操作并发

表61.3　胰岛细胞产物释放标准

无菌性
革兰染色:无菌
内毒素含量:根据受体体重<5EU/kg
培养:没有细菌或真菌组分(14天培养后)
潜力
静止胰岛素释放:刺激指数>1.0
体积
包裹组织体积≤5.0mL或组织体积≤7.5mL
纯度
≥30%(根据二硫腙染色)
活性
≥70%(根据膜完整性染色,使用FDA/PI或Syto绿)
最小胰岛组织(规程相关)
对于单一供体规程≥6000IEQ/kg
对于常规初始移植物≥5000IEQ/kg
对于多种输注方案的再移植物≥4000IEQ/kg
相容性
ABO血型相容
细胞毒性交叉实验为阴性(如果PRA>10%,或根据方案需要)

FDA/PI,荧光素二乙酸酯/碘化丙啶。

症发生风险的必要条件。

大多数介入科医生在进行经肝胆道造影及经肝胆管引流操作过程中均需要使用经皮经肝穿刺操作技术,该项技术被证明是安全的。

使用彩色多普勒超声可以减少肝包膜穿刺数量,避免误入胆道,并可以显著减少操作时间[94,95]。高分辨率透视C臂结合旋转数字成像便于门静脉置管。穿刺进入二级或三级门静脉分支,远离中央肝门,可及减少肝动脉损伤风险,并可提供更好的后续消融治疗路径。

在进行经皮经肝穿刺之前,患者要确定没有右肝血管瘤,并且必须经过超声检查证实,这一点非常重要。患者确定没有潜在凝血功能障碍及门静脉高压症和肝硬化。为了安全性考虑,进行该项操作前7~14天必须停用抗血小板药物(氯吡格雷、双嘧达莫等)及直接凝血酶或Xa因子的抑制剂(达比加群、利伐沙班等),意味着服用上述药物的患者将从等待名单中除名。患有已知的潜在凝血功能障碍(蛋白C、蛋白S、抗凝血酶Ⅲ、V因子Leiden缺乏症)的患者不能进行经皮门静脉内胰岛移植[96]。

经皮穿刺门静脉的显影技术已经由Owen团队、Gaba团队、Goss团队及其他团队进行了详细描述[97-102]。简单来说,穿刺部位局部浸润性麻醉后,将一根22G针头穿刺进入门静脉右支的一个外周分支内。随后一个18G导丝顺着针头进入门静脉主干。随后将导丝换成单腔4F或5F血管导管(NEFF,Cook Canada,Stouffville,Ontario)或类似导管,并将其尖端刚好置入门静脉-肠系膜静脉与脾静脉汇合的位置。随后根据门静脉血流图确认导管位置,并获得门静脉压力的基础数值。

向储存在Ricordi袋中的胰岛细胞加入肝素(每公斤受体体重70单位),并将混合液注入门静脉且随时测定门静脉压力[103]。如果基础门静脉压力高于20mmHg或者注射过程中门静脉压力高于22mmHg,则停止注射胰岛细胞直至门静脉压力恢复正常,避免产生门静脉血栓。

胰岛细胞注射完成后,缓慢将门静脉导管撤出并同时注射凝血胶。Miami小组使用D-STAT(Vascular Solutions,Minneapolis,MN)并取得了成功[104]。Edmonton小组使用Avitene胶(Medchem Products,Woburn,Massachusetts,USA),其由1g Avitene粉末加入3mL生理盐水与3mL造影剂混合而成[105]。此法制成的微纤维胶原形成一个可以在造影下显影的厚胶,可用在最小可达4cm的穿刺针道处,消除肝囊穿刺出血的风险,并已经在360余例操作中获得了验证[105,106]。其他类似措施还有使用Gelfoam塞和金属线圈,但是在我们的经验中更易发生易位,可靠性不高。

穿刺针道妥善止血后,继续进行治疗性全身肝素化治疗,剂量为每小时每公斤体重3个单位,并在病房中密切监视患者,直到其部分凝血酶原时间(PTT)为60~80秒。随后持续注射肝素48小时,可以提高单个供体胰岛细胞存活率并减少瞬时血液介导的炎症反应(IBMIR)[107,108]。患者出院后,持续使用低分子肝素(依诺肝素30mg皮下注射,每天两次,连续7天),并连用阿司匹林81mg肠溶片14天。

我们建议,在穿刺针道没有确切止血或者门静脉穿刺路径有损伤时,暂时停用术后肝素化治疗,并在操作后2小时复查多普勒超声。这将便于早期诊断潜在的腹腔出血并提供合理的肝素治疗方案。联用Avitene和治疗性肝素化,可以显著降低出血及门静脉血栓形成风险[95,105,106]。如果出血发生在肝脏表面,可直接通过腹腔镜技术进行电凝止血,因为在该种情况下出血点明确并可以通过腹腔镜技术确切止血[95]。

移植后需要密切监测血红蛋白水平及肝功能,并

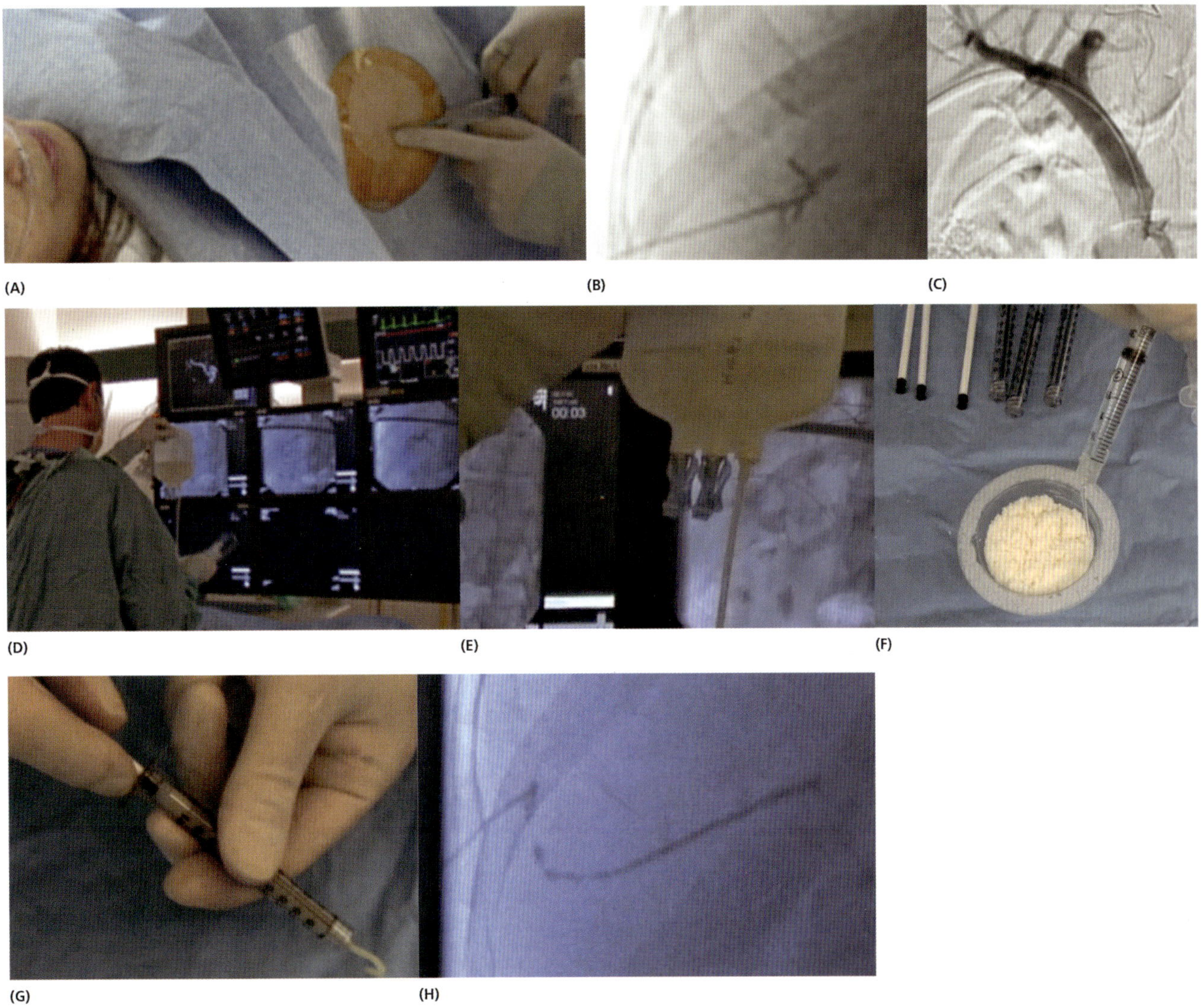

图 61.4　经皮超声引导下荧光透视胰岛移植步骤：(A)多普勒超声探查及局部麻醉。(B)直接穿刺门静脉右支的二级或三级分支，并用荧光透视明确其分支走行。(C)使用 4F 或 5F 导管在门静脉肠-系膜静脉和脾静脉汇合处进行门静脉造影。(D)将 70U/kg(根据受体体重)的肝素与胰岛细胞混合后进行注射，直接检测门静脉压力。(E)在移植组织可见的条件下关闭静脉注射管。(F)使用 1g 粉末、3mL 盐水及 3mL 对比造影剂配成微原纤维胶原胶(Avitere)。(G)将上述胶置于 1mL 注射器中。(H)在直接荧光透视条件下将导管闭塞至少 4cm。

在 24 小时及 7 天后常规进行门静脉系统和肝脏的多普勒超声检查。临床胰岛移植后发生完全门静脉系统血栓较为罕见(Edmonton 小组的 364 例患者中没有一例发生)，但是后果不堪设想[109]。外周、前支或后支门静脉血栓偶尔发生，由于该种类型血栓发生进一步蔓延的风险较低，最佳治疗方案为静脉肝素治疗加上 3 个月香豆素类药物治疗，并同时行多普勒超声评估血栓是否溶解。

经皮经肝穿刺后偶尔会发生小的动静脉瘘(发生率小于 1%)，并可以安全地通过经皮肝动脉栓塞治疗[100,110]。

通过开放技术进行门静脉穿刺

当无法进行经皮路径时(如存在较大的肝血管瘤或者当地缺少介入科医生)，则需要通过开腹路径。在大型临床中心，仅有不到 1%的病例需要通过这一方式。在这种情况下，该方式通过微创手段切开脐部，将左脐静脉再通并进入左侧门静脉系统[48,111]。或者，经腹腔镜手术方式通过大网膜或肠系膜静脉置入导管。最有效的方式是将一双腔 9F Broviac 型中心静脉导管置入，直至其尖端到达门静脉，这样可以通过较小的管腔监测门静脉压力，并通过较大的管腔注入胰岛细胞[112]。

总结

本章节详细讨论了手术获取胰腺用于胰岛分离，以及用于临床胰岛移植的cGMP人胰岛细胞的步骤。同时总结了安全进入门静脉的方式及避免门静脉血栓形成及出血的关键性步骤。需要胰岛分离准备及临床护理等各方面的专家共同合作来避免潜在并发症的发生。

致谢

AMJS和CR得到了美国全国卫生研究所(NIH)临床胰岛移植(CIT)联盟，美国全国过敏、免疫及感染疾病研究所(NIAID)及美国全国糖尿病、消化及肾脏病研究所(NIDDK)的支持。AMJS持有加拿大移植外科及再生医学研究支持，并且拥有阿尔伯塔创新医疗方案(AIHS)的临床基金支持。AMJS和CR均得到了Juvenile糖尿病研究基金(JDRF)的大力支持。阿尔伯塔大学临床胰岛移植项目得到了阿尔伯塔健康组织、阿尔伯塔政府、加拿大糖尿病研究所的支持。迈阿密大学糖尿病研究所得到了糖尿病研究所基金的支持。Edmonton及迈阿密研究中心均是糖尿病研究所的一员。AMJS和CR均是治疗联盟的一员。

(倪彦彬 译　朱继业 校)

参考文献

1. CITR. The Collaborative Islet Transplant Registry Seventh Annual Report. Bethesda, MD, 2011.
2. Kin T, Shapiro AM. Surgical aspects of human islet isolation. Islets. 2010; 2:265–273.
3. Shapiro AM, Sutherland DE. The new deceased donor pancreas allocation schema: do the recommendations go far enough? Transplantation. 2007;83: 1151–1152.
4. Kilimnik G, Zhao B, Jo J, et al. Altered islet composition and disproportionate loss of large islets in patients with type 2 diabetes. PLoS ONE. 2011;6:e27445.
5. Jurgens CA, Toukatly MN, Fligner CL, et al. Beta-cell loss and beta-cell apoptosis in human type 2 diabetes are related to islet amyloid deposition. American Journal of Pathology. 2011;178:2632–2640.
6. Loomes KM. Survival of an islet beta-cell in type-2 diabetes: curbing the effects of amyloid cytotoxicity. Islets. 2011;3:38–39.
7. Leitao CB, Bernetti K, Tharavanij T, et al. Type 2 diabetes mellitus phenotype and graft survival after islet transplantation. Transplantation. 2009;88:57–61.
8. Kin T, Johnson PR, Shapiro AM, et al. Factors influencing the collagenase digestion phase of human islet isolation. Transplantation. 2007;83:7–12.
9. Hughes SJ, Clark A, McShane P, et al. Characterisation of collagen VI within the islet-exocrine interface of the human pancreas: implications for clinical islet isolation? Transplantation. 2006;81:423–426.
10. Johnson PR, White SA, London NJ. Collagenase and human islet isolation. Cell Transplantation. 1996;5:437–452.
11. Szot GL, Lee MR, Tavakol MM, et al. Successful clinical islet isolation using a GMP-manufactured collagenase and neutral protease. Transplantation. 2009;88: 753–756.
12. Posselt AM, Szot GL, Frassetto LA, et al. Islet transplantation in type 1 diabetic patients using calcineurin inhibitor-free immunosuppressive protocols based on T-cell adhesion or costimulation blockade. Transplantation. 2010;90: 1595–1601.
13. Posselt AM, Szot GL, Frassetto LA, et al. Clinical islet transplantation at the University of California, San Francisco. Clinical Transplants. 2010:235–243.
14. O'Gorman D, Kin T, Imes S, et al. Comparison of human islet isolation outcomes using a new mammalian tissue-free enzyme versus collagenase NB-1. Transplantation. 2010;90:255–259.
15. Berney T, Johnson PR. Donor pancreata: evolving approaches to organ allocation for whole pancreas versus islet transplantation. Transplantation. 2010;90: 238–243.
16. Wahlberg JA, Love R, Landegaard L, et al. 72-hour preservation of the canine pancreas. Transplantation. 1987;43:5–8.
17. Stewart ZA, Cameron AM, Singer AL, et al. Histidine-tryptophan-ketoglutarate (HTK) is associated with reduced graft survival in pancreas transplantation. American Journal of Transplantation. 2009;9:217–221.
18. Becker T, Ringe B, Nyibata M, et al. Pancreas transplantation with histidine-tryptophan-ketoglutarate (HTK) solution and University of Wisconsin (UW) solution: is there a difference? Journal of the Pancreas. 2007;8:304–311.
19. Caballero-Corbalan J, Brandhorst H, Malm H, et al. Using HTK for prolonged pancreas preservation prior to human islet isolation. Journal of Surgical Research. 2012;175:163–168.
20. Deai T, Tanioka Y, Suzuki Y, et al. The effect of the two-layer cold storage method on islet isolation from ischemically damaged pancreas. Kobe Journal of Medical Sciences. 1999;45:191–199.
21. Kin T, Mirbolooki M, Salehi P, et al. Islet isolation and transplantation outcomes of pancreas preserved with University of Wisconsin solution versus two-layer method using preoxygenated perfluorocarbon. Transplantation. 2006;82:1286–1290.
22. Witkowski P, Liu Z, Guo Q, et al. Two-layer method in short-term pancreas preservation for successful islet isolation. Transplantation Proceedings. 2005; 37:3398–3401.
23. Kakinoki K, Fujino Y, Suzuki Y, et al. Superiority of the two-layer method before islet isolation confirmed by in vivo viability assessment. Transplantation. 2005;79:1516–1521.
24. Tsujimura T, Kuroda Y, Churchill TA, et al. Short-term storage of the ischemically damaged human pancreas by the two-layer method prior to islet isolation. Cell Transplantation. 2004;13:67–73.
25. Matsumoto S, Rigley TH, Qualley SA, et al. Efficacy of the oxygen-charged static two-layer method for short-term pancreas preservation and islet isolation from nonhuman primate and human pancreata. Cell Transplantation. 2002; 11:769–777.
26. Hering BJ, Matsumoto I, Sawada T, et al. Impact of two-layer pancreas preservation on islet isolation and transplantation. Transplantation. 2002;74: 1813–1816.
27. Lakey JR, Tsujimura T, Shapiro AM, et al. Preservation of the human pancreas before islet isolation using a two-layer (UW solution-perfluorochemical) cold storage method. Transplantation. 2002;74:1809–1811.
28. Qin H, Matsumoto S, Klintmalm GB, et al. A meta-analysis for comparison of the two-layer and university of Wisconsin pancreas preservation methods in islet transplantation. Cell Transplantation. 2011;20:1127–1137.
29. Fujino Y. Two-layer cold storage method for pancreas and islet cell transplantation. World Journal of Gastroenterology. 2010;16:3235–3238.
30. Agrawal A, Gurusamy K, Powis S, et al. A meta-analysis of the impact of the two-layer method of preservation on human pancreatic islet transplantation. Cell Transplantation. 2008;17:1315–1322.
31. Caballero-Corbalan J, Eich T, Lundgren T, et al. No beneficial effect of two-layer storage compared with UW-storage on human islet isolation and transplantation. Transplantation. 2007;84:864–869.
32. Alsaif F, Molinari M, Al-Masloom A, et al. Pancreatic islet autotransplantation with completion pancreatectomy in the management of uncontrolled pancreatic fistula after whipple resection for ampullary adenocarcinoma. Pancreas. 2006;32:430–431.
33. Ponte GM, Pileggi A, Messinger S, et al. Toward maximizing the success rates of human islet isolation: influence of donor and isolation factors. Cell Transplantation. 2007;16:595–607.
34. Lakey JR, Warnock GL, Rajotte RV, et al. Variables in organ donors that affect the recovery of human islets of Langerhans. Transplantation. 1996; 61:1047–1053.
35. Kaddis JS, Danobeitia JS, Niland JC, et al. Multicenter analysis of novel and established variables associated with successful human islet isolation outcomes.

American Journal of Transplantation. 2010;10:646–656.
36. Liu X, Matsumoto S, Okitsu T, et al. Analysis of donor- and isolation-related variables from non-heart-beating donors (NHBDs) using the Kyoto islet isolation method. Cell Transplantation. 2008;17:649–656.
37. Hanley SC, Paraskevas S, Rosenberg L. Donor and isolation variables predicting human islet isolation success. Transplantation. 2008;85:950–955.
38. Nano R, Clissi B, Melzi R, et al. Islet isolation for allotransplantation: variables associated with successful islet yield and graft function. Diabetologia. 2005; 48:906–912.
39. Fraker C, Montelongo J, Szust J, et al. The use of multiparametric monitoring during islet cell isolation and culture: a potential tool for in-process corrections of critical physiological factors. Cell Transplantation. 2004;13:497–502.
40. Kin T, O'Gorman D, Schroeder A, et al. Human islet distribution program for basic research at a single center. Transplantation Proceedings. 2011;43: 3195–3197.
41. O'Gorman D, Kin T, Murdoch T, et al. The standardization of pancreatic donors for islet isolations. Transplantation. 2005;80:801–806.
42. Hering BJ, Kandaswamy R, Ansite JD, et al. Single-donor, marginal-dose islet transplantation in patients with type 1 diabetes. Journal of the American Medical Association. 2005;293:830–835.
43. Shapiro AM, Ricordi C. Unraveling the secrets of single donor success in islet transplantation. American Journal of Transplantation. 2004;4:295–298.
44. Matsumoto S, Takita M, Chaussabel D, et al. Improving efficacy of clinical islet transplantation with iodixanol based islet purification, thymoglobulin induction and blockage of IL-1-β and TNF-α. Cell Transplantation. 2011; 20:1641–1647.
45. Noguchi H, Naziruddin B, Onaca N, et al. Comparison of modified Celsior solution and M-kyoto solution for pancreas preservation in human islet isolation. Cell Transplantation. 2010;19:751–758.
46. Matsumoto S, Noguichi H, Shimoda M, et al. Seven consecutive successful clinical islet isolations with pancreatic ductal injection. Cell Transplantation. 2010;19:291–297.
47. Ricordi C, Lacy PE, Scharp DW. Automated islet isolation from human pancreas. Diabetes. 1989;38(Suppl. 1):140–142.
48. Scharp DW, Lacy PE, Santiago JV, et al. Insulin independence after islet transplantation into type I diabetic patient. Diabetes. 1990;39:515–518.
49. Clinical Islet Transplantation (CIT) Consortium. Available from: http://www.citisletstudy.org/ (accessed Jan. 2014).
50. Lakey JR, Warnock GL, Shapiro AM, et al. Intraductal collagenase delivery into the human pancreas using syringe loading or controlled perfusion. Cell Transplantation. 1999;8:285–292.
51. Ricordi C, Strom TB. Clinical islet transplantation: advances and immunological challenges. Nature Reviews Immunology. 2004;4:259–268.
52. Latif ZA, Noel J, Alejandro R. A simple method of staining fresh and cultured islets. Transplantation. 1988;45:827–830.
53. Kin T. Islet isolation for clinical transplantation. Advances in Experimental Medicine and Biology. 2010;654:683–710.
54. Linetsky E, Bottino R, Lehmann R, et al. Improved human islet isolation using a new enzyme blend, liberase. Diabetes. 1997;46:1120–1123.
55. Kin T, Senior P, O'Gorman D, et al. Risk factors for islet loss during culture prior to transplantation. Transplant International. 2008;21:1029–1035.
56. ElSaadany S, Tyshenko MG, Oraby T, et al. The risk to human islet cell transplant recipients of acquiring variant Creutzfeldt-Jakob disease: a provisional quantitative risk assessment. Transplantation. 2011;92:e2–e4.
57. Bucher P, Mathe Z, Morel P, et al. Assessment of a novel two-component enzyme preparation for human islet isolation and transplantation. Transplantation. 2005;79:91–97.
58. Brandhorst H, Friberg A, Nilsson B, et al. Large-scale comparison of Liberase HI and collagenase NB1 utilized for human islet isolation. Cell Transplantation. 2010;19:3–8.
59. Misawa R, Ricordi C, Miki A, et al. Evaluation of viable beta-cell mass is useful for selecting collagenase for human islet isolation: comparison of collagenase NB1 and liberase HI. Cell Transplantation. 2012;21:39–47.
60. Kin T, O'Gorman D, Zhai X, et al. Nonsimultaneous administration of pancreas dissociation enzymes during islet isolation. Transplantation. 2009;87: 1700–1705.
61. Kin T, O'Gorman D, Senior P, et al. Experience of islet isolation without neutral protease supplementation. Islets. 2010;2:278–282.
62. Szot G, Lee M, Lang J, et al. Successful clinical islet isolation and purification using a bovine product-free GMP collagenase and neutral protease. University of California, San Francisco,, 2011. Available from: http://icr.coh.org/docs/Abstracts/10032008/Szot.pdf (accessed Jan. 2014).
63. Posselt AM, Bellin MD, Tavakol M, et al. Islet transplantation in type 1 diabetics using an immunosuppressive protocol based on the anti-LFA-1 antibody efalizumab. American Journal of Transplantation. 2010;10:1870–1880.
64. Caballero-Corbalan J, Brandhorst H, Asif S, et al. Mammalian tissue-free liberase: a new GMP-graded enzyme blend for human islet isolation. Transplantation. 2010;90:332–333.
65. Caballero-Corbalan J, Friberg AS, Brandhorst H, et al. Vitacyte collagenase HA: a novel enzyme blend for efficient human islet isolation. Transplantation. 2009;88:1400–1402.
66. Robertson GS, Chadwick DR, Contractor H, et al. The optimization of large-scale density gradient isolation of human islets. Acta Diabetologica. 1993;30:93–98.
67. Swift S, Kin T, Mirbolooki M, et al. Comparison of cooling systems during islet purification. Cell Transplantation. 2006;15:175–180.
68. Mita A, Ricordi C, Messinger S, et al. Antiproinflammatory effects of iodixanol (OptiPrep)-based density gradient purification on human islet preparations. Cell Transplantation. 2010;19:1537–1546.
69. Barbaro B, Salehi P, Wang Y, et al. Improved human pancreatic islet purification with the refined UIC-UB density gradient. Transplantation. 2007;84: 1200–1203.
70. Warnock GL, Meloche RM, Thompson D, et al. Improved human pancreatic islet isolation for a prospective cohort study of islet transplantation vs best medical therapy in type 1 diabetes mellitus. Archives of Surgery (Chicago, Ill.: 1960). 2005;140:735–744.
71. Miki A, Ricordi C, Messinger S, et al. Toward improving human islet isolation from younger donors: rescue purification is efficient for trapped islets. Cell Transplantation. 2009;18:13–22.
72. Ichii H, Pileggi A, Molano RD, et al. Rescue purification maximizes the use of human islet preparations for transplantation. American Journal of Transplantation. 2005;5:21–30.
73. Ichii H, Sakuma Y, Pileggi A, et al. Shipment of human islets for transplantation. American Journal of Transplantation. 2007;7:1010–1020.
74. Rabinovitch A, Suarez-Pinzon WL, Strynadka K, et al. Human pancreatic islet beta-cell destruction by cytokines is independent of nitric oxide production. Journal of Clinical Endocrinology and Metabolism. 1994;79:1058–1062.
75. Gaber AO, Fraga DW, Callicutt CS, et al. Improved in vivo pancreatic islet function after prolonged in vitro islet culture. Transplantation. 2001;72: 1730–1736.
76. Murdoch TB, McGhee-Wilson D, Shapiro AM, et al. Methods of human islet culture for transplantation. Cell Transplantation. 2004;13:605–617.
77. Berney T. Islet culture and counter-culture. Commentary on: Effect of short-term culture on functional and stress-related parameters in isolated human islets by Ihm et al. Transplant International. 2009;22:531–533.
78. Daoud J, Rosenberg L, Tabrizian M. Pancreatic islet culture and preservation strategies: advances, challenges, and future outlook. Cell Transplantation. 2010; 19:1523–1535.
79. Rabinovitch A, Sumoski W, Rajotte RV, et al. Cytotoxic effects of cytokines on human pancreatic islet cells in monolayer culture. Journal of Clinical Endocrinology and Metabolism. 1990;71:152–156.
80. Kin T, Senior P, O'Gorman D, et al. Risk factors for islet loss during culture prior to transplantation. Transplant International. 2008;21:1029–1035.
81. Markmann JF, Tomaszewski J, Posselt AM, et al. The effect of islet cell culture in vitro at 24 degrees C on graft survival and MHC antigen expression. Transplantation. 1990;49:272–277.
82. Ichii H, Wang X, Messinger S, et al. Improved human islet isolation using nicotinamide. American Journal of Transplantation. 2006;6:2060–2068.
83. Froud T, Ricordi C, Baidal DA, et al. Islet transplantation in type 1 diabetes mellitus using cultured islets and steroid-free immunosuppression: Miami experience. American Journal of Transplantation. 2005;5:2037–2046.
84. Kerr-Conte J, Vandewalle B, Moerman E, et al. Upgrading pretransplant human islet culture technology requires human serum combined with media renewal. Transplantation. 2010;89:1154–1160.
85. Clayton H, Turner J, Swift S, et al. Supplementation of islet culture medium with insulin may have a beneficial effect on islet secretory function. Pancreas. 2001;22:72–74.
86. Goss JA, Schock AP, Brunicardi FC, et al. Achievement of insulin independence in three consecutive type-1 diabetic patients via pancreatic islet transplantation using islets isolated at a remote islet isolation center. Transplantation. 2002; 74:1761–1766.
87. Goss JA, Goodpastor SE, Brunicardi FC, et al. Development of a human pancreatic islet-transplant program through a collaborative relationship with a remote islet-isolation center. Transplantation. 2004;77:462–466.
88. Barnett MJ, McGhee-Wilson D, Shapiro AM, et al. Variation in human islet viability based on different membrane integrity stains. Cell Transplantation. 2004;13:481–488.
89. Cabrera O, Jacques-Silva MC, Berman DM, et al. Automated, high-throughput assays for evaluation of human pancreatic islet function. Cell Transplantation. 2008;16:1039–1048.
90. Papas KK, Colton CK, Nelson RA, et al. Human islet oxygen consumption rate

and DNA measurements predict diabetes reversal in nude mice. American Journal of Transplantation. 2007;7:707–713.
91. Ichii H, Inverardi L, Pileggi A, et al. A novel method for the assessment of cellular composition and beta-cell viability in human islet preparations. American Journal of Transplantation. 2005;5:1635–1645.
92. Weimar B, Rauber K, Brendel MD, et al. Percutaneous transhepatic catheterization of the portal vein: a combined CT- and fluoroscopy-guided technique. Cardiovascular and Interventional Radiology. 1999;22:342–344.
93. Shapiro AM, Lakey JR, Ryan EA, et al. Islet transplantation in seven patients with type 1 diabetes mellitus using a glucocorticoid-free immunosuppressive regimen. New England Journal of Medicine. 2000;343:230–238.
94. Venturini M, Angeli E, Maffi P, et al. Technique, complications, and therapeutic efficacy of percutaneous transplantation of human pancreatic islet cells in type 1 diabetes: the role of US. Radiology. 2005;234:617–624.
95. Villiger P, Ryan EA, Owen R, et al. Prevention of bleeding after islet transplantation: lessons learned from a multivariate analysis of 132 cases at a single institution. American Journal of Transplantation. 2005;5:2992–2998.
96. Brennan DC, Shannon MB, Koch MJ, et al. Portal vein thrombosis complicating islet transplantation in a recipient with the Factor V Leiden mutation. Transplantation. 2004;78:172–173.
97. Neeman Z, Hirshberg B, Harlan D, et al. Radiologic aspects of islet cell transplantation. Current Diabetes Reports. 2006;6:310–315.
98. Gaba RC, Garcia-Roca R, Oberholzer J. Pancreatic islet cell transplantation: an update for interventional radiologists. Journal of Vascular and Interventional Radiology. 2012;23:583–594.
99. Goss JA, Soltes G, Goodpastor SE, et al. Pancreatic islet transplantation: the radiographic approach. Transplantation. 2003;76:199–203.
100. Low G, Hussein N, Owen RJ, et al. Role of imaging in clinical islet transplantation. Radiographics. 2010;30:353–366.
101. Owen RJ, Mercer JR, Al-Saif F, et al. Portal vein embolization with radiolabeled polyvinyl alcohol particles in a swine model: hepatic distribution and implications for pancreatic islet cell transplantation. Cardiovascular and Interventional Radiology. 2009;32:499–507.
102. Owen RJ, Ryan EA, O'Kelly K, et al. Percutaneous transhepatic pancreatic islet cell transplantation in type 1 diabetes mellitus: radiologic aspects. Radiology. 2003;229:165–170.
103. Baidal DA, Froud T, Ferreira JV, et al. The bag method for islet cell infusion. Cell Transplantation. 2003;12:809–813.
104. Froud T, Yrizarry JM, Alejandro R, et al. Use of D-STAT to prevent bleeding following percutaneous transhepatic intraportal islet transplantation. Cell Transplantation. 2004;13:55–59.
105. Kawahara T, Kin T, Kashkoush S, et al. Portal vein thrombosis is a potentially preventable complication in clinical islet transplantation. American Journal of Transplantation. 2011;11:2700–2707.
106. Kawahara T, Kin T, Shapiro AM. A comparison of islet autotransplantation with allotransplantation and factors elevating acute portal pressure in clinical islet transplantation. Journal of Hepatobiliary Pancreatic Sciences. 2012;19:281–288.
107. Johansson H, Lukinius A, Moberg L, et al. Tissue factor produced by the endocrine cells of the islets of Langerhans is associated with a negative outcome of clinical islet transplantation. Diabetes. 2005;54:1755–1762.
108. Koh A, Senior P, Salam A, et al. Insulin-heparin infusions peritransplant substantially improve single-donor clinical islet transplant success. Transplantation. 2010;89:465–471.
109. Hirshberg B, Rother KI, Digon BJ 3rd, et al. Benefits and risks of solitary islet transplantation for type 1 diabetes using steroid-sparing immunosuppression: the National Institutes of Health experience. Diabetes Care. 2003;26:3288–3295.
110. Suchak AA, O'Kelly K, Al Saif F, et al. Hepatic artery-portal venous fistula after percutaneous intraportal islet cell transplant. Transplantation. 2007;83:669–670.
111. Scharp DW, Lacy PE, Santiago JV, et al. Results of our first nine intraportal islet allografts in type 1, insulin-dependent diabetic patients. Transplantation. 1991; 51:76–85.
112. Turgeon NA, Avila JG, Cano JA, et al. Experience with a novel efalizumab-based immunosuppressive regimen to facilitate single donor islet cell transplantation. American Journal of Transplantation. 2010;10:2082–2091.

第 62 章

小肠移植手术步骤和外科技术

Thomas Fishbein

简介

小肠移植可以单独进行或与其他器官移植同时进行。只进行空回肠移植称为单独小肠移植[1]。该移植物的血液供应来自肠系膜上动脉，并从肠系膜上静脉回流。但是，小肠移植常根据不同患者体内其他腹腔器官的情况进行调整。有些患者曾行结肠手术（克罗恩病）或胃手术（胃旁路手术）；有些患者有慢性胰腺炎（与肠外营养相关）；还有患者患有肾衰竭（酸性结石、反复脱水）或其他与小肠功能衰竭及肠外营养相关的并发症。

结肠可以和小肠一起移植，比较少见的是，前肠也可以同时移植，如将胃、十二指肠及胰腺包括在移植物中[2,3]。多器官移植[42]包括与肝脏同时移植将在第 63 章详细讨论。选用何种移植物取决于不同供体的解剖结果及器官功能。受体的特性也决定了最常用的具体植入技术[5]。术前评估内容参见第 42 章，术后管理及预后参见第 74 章及第 109 章。

外科技术

单独小肠移植

腹腔暴露

临床最常见的单独小肠移植适应证是短肠综合征。此类患者既往常有腹部手术史，并且腹壁常有结肠造口、肠瘘、胃肠管或引流管所致瘢痕。这种情况下，单独小肠移植常选用正中切口。偶尔，使用推进皮瓣进行腹壁重建、组织缺失以及存在其他皮肤移植物时，加大了使用正中切口的难度。这种情况下，首选位于重建区域上方的脐与剑突间中点的双侧肋缘下切口。不同移植物的选择对该类手术的预后有截然不同的影响。供体的体重或体积最好为受体的 1/3 或 1/2，便于手术后能完全关闭腹腔。临时关闭腹腔有时也是必需的，但会明显增加死亡率。目前有多种方法获取小肠移植物[6-11]。极少数情况下，行小肠移植时会同时移植供体一部分腹壁。

切开腹壁后，分离腹腔内粘连以暴露腹腔及腹膜后空间。短肠综合征常造成腹腔空间减小，常需要最大限度地扩大腹腔及松解腹壁筋膜，以增强上腹壁的松弛度。可使用自动牵开器帮助暴露。受体剩余的小肠或结肠如果不切除，会显著增加受体围术期死亡率，因此必须游离这些肠道。在克罗恩病患者中，最好从盆腔中游离既往狭窄成形术区域、肠道吻合口、瘘口及狭窄，并用闭合器将其切除。自 Treitz 韧带起保留 3~5cm 空肠有利于近端肠道重建。但是，保留过多的正常肠道将对术后行肠镜检查评估移植物功能带来困难。我们建议保留的肠道不超过 20cm。同样的，保留一些自体结肠有助于关闭造口后的水分重吸收。如果远端结肠功能正常，我们尝试使用左半结肠进行肠道重建。高位结扎肠系膜血管后切除病变肠道。

短肠综合征患者的血管暴露

在大多数短肠综合征患者中，常使用肾下腹主动脉及肾下下腔静脉分别作为流入道及流出道[2]。将十二指肠从腹后附着处游离后可以很好地暴露腹主动脉。暴露左肾静脉（LRV）至足够的切除长度。结扎淋巴管预防移植术后腹腔积液及乳糜性腹水的发生。保留肠系膜下动脉尤为重要，因为在缺少侧支循环的情况下，其是供应降结肠或乙状结肠的唯一动脉。结扎一部分左肾静脉与肠系膜下动脉间的腰血管，并用 Satinsky 夹控制主动脉（图 62.1A~C）。分离右侧性腺静脉，以及一或两支腰静脉有助于暴露腔静脉。术前影像学检查必须确认是否存在变异的主动脉后左肾静脉或环主动脉型肾静脉。在暴露过程中一定要避免损伤十二指肠的第三部分或肾静脉。

小肠功能障碍患者的血管暴露

在原发性小肠功能障碍患者中，如肠道上皮细胞疾病或小肠运动障碍疾病等，受体的小肠在腹腔内几乎完整存在。此时需要行全小肠切除。这类患者腹腔内常无多余空间，尤其是在扩张型肠道运动障碍患者中，腹壁常很紧张。正中切口或双侧肋缘下切口均可。沿着与供体小肠切除术一样的血管分布行受体小肠切除术（图 62.2）。游离 Treitz 韧带，应用 Catell–Brasch 操作沿着 Toldt 白线游离右半结肠直至肠系膜血管根部。分离

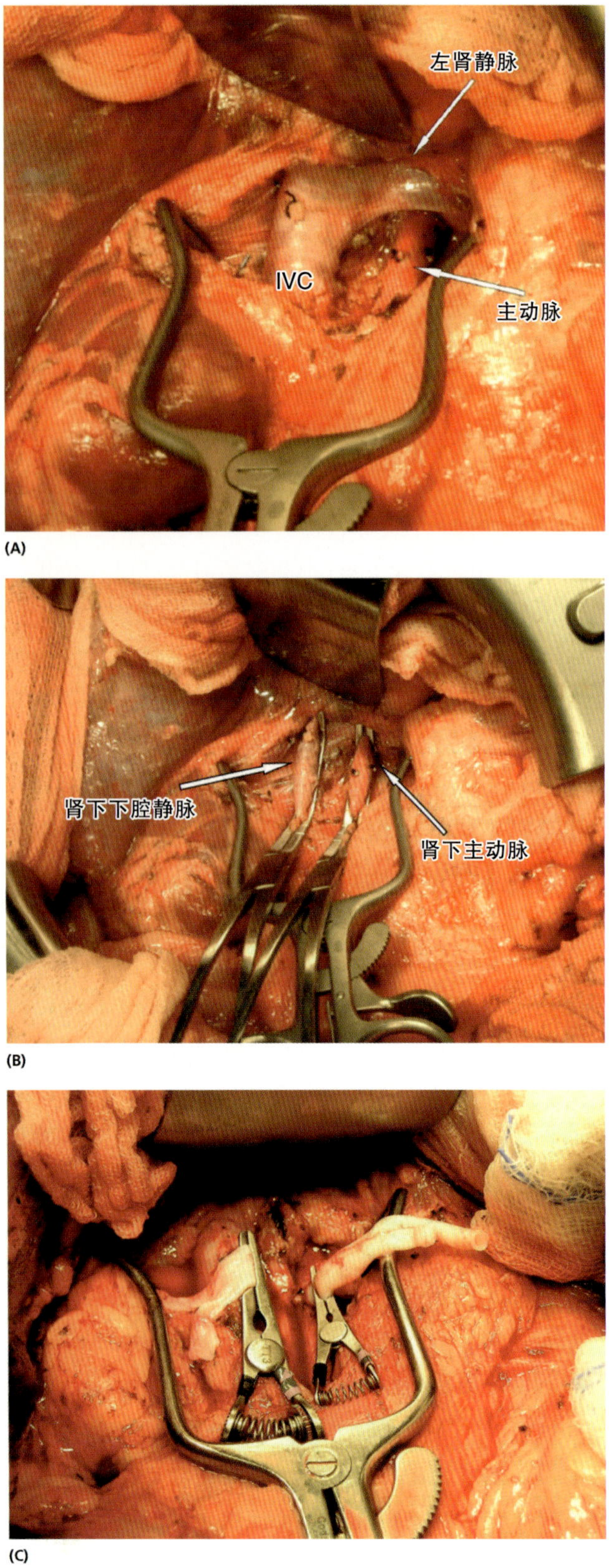

图 62.1 (A,B,C)暴露和准备肾下主动脉及腔静脉，用于放置移植物及直接吻合。

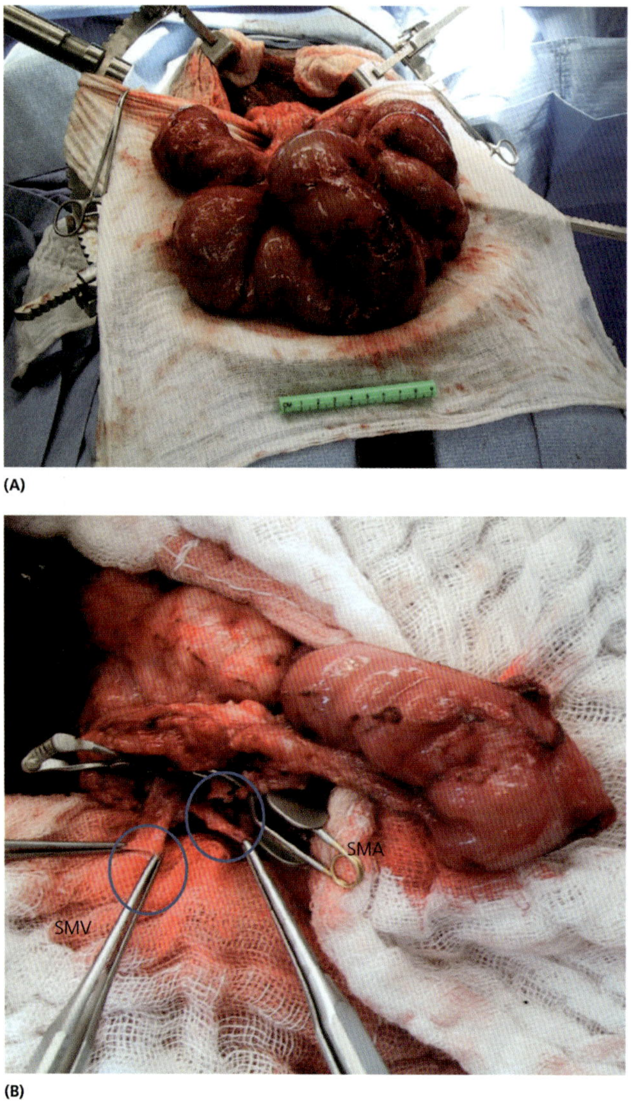

图 62.2 切除病变小肠(A)并保留肠系膜血管，横断近段空肠，为移植做准备，左侧为 SMV，右侧为 SMA(B)。

左侧横结肠，切断横结肠系膜便于游离整个小肠及右侧结肠至右下象限。这种分离空肠的方法确定了小肠系膜血管平面。我们发现，将开腹手术垫置于肠系膜血管及小肠后方可以便于分离肠系膜血管根部（图 62.2A）。结扎肠系膜脂肪及淋巴管道进行肠系膜上动脉(SMA)和肠系膜上静脉(SMV)骨骼化(图 62.2B)。熟悉近端肠系膜解剖结构尤为重要。保留近端空肠血管弓至残存的自体空肠。主要空肠静脉常位于肠系膜上动脉后方。在其与十二指肠交叉处游离 2cm 动脉及静脉便于行直接吻合。

由体循环提供移植物血供

植入移植物后，需要确保足够的血管长度。在移植物血供由体循环提供的患者中，如果移植物不包括胰腺但包括完整的 SMA 和 SMV，有些医生建议将其与主动脉直接吻合。使用特制阻断钳控制主动脉并行主动脉前切开术。但是，有些移植物的小肠袢有时会下降到腹膜后位深处，这是儿童患者的典型症状。助手轻柔地展平供体肠系膜血管根部并将其向动脉吻合处牵拉在操作中尤为重要。必须要知道，正常小肠系膜与后腹膜有一定的角度，空肠前后维度稍高，回肠稍偏后。植入移植物时，肠系膜必须展平并与后腹膜平行。即使移植物血供由体循环提供并且移植物有完整的动脉，我仍建议在将移植物从冰块中拿出前，在主动脉及下腔静脉上放置一小段间置移植物[12]。这使移植物的定位更加容易，吻合口在腹膜后的凹陷度有所降低。

动脉采用端–端吻合，并在动脉再通前使用生长因子扩张动脉。保留合适的静脉长度避免发生静脉冗长及扭转。与肝移植门静脉吻合类似的手法吻合静脉，在移除腔静脉阻断钳之前灌注器官保存液及生长因子。在行肠腔分流术时，由体循环供血的移植物有发生血管扭转和流出道吻合口关闭的风险。因此，常切除一部分静脉血管前壁。同时需要避免血管扭结。如果不存在结肠，或者供体肠道明显小于受体的肠道，移植物恢复灌注后将会沉入盆腔。如果血管长度过短将会发生血管牵拉，导致动脉狭窄。因此，必须保留适当长度的供体肠系膜上动脉便于形成与受体类似的肠系膜上动脉血管弓，同时避免过长发生扭结。

由肠系膜血管移植物血供

当使用受体自身肠系膜血管进行吻合时，使用无创血管钳控制近端血管，无须暴露主动脉或腔静脉。植入前及植入后表现参见图 62.3A 及图 62.3B。肠系膜静脉管腔需要足够大以与供体血管尺寸相匹配。由于这些血管可能从短肠综合征患者中分离，其常由于低流量状态和流量不足造成血管闭塞，引起供血不足。此时需要评估受体剩余血管的长度。供体肠道将置于十二指肠水平部下方，也就是受体自体血管旁。因此，若血管长度不足，移植物重量将会造成血管张力。在这种情况下，在其中置入髂外动脉及髂外静脉就显得尤为必要。将移植物置入腹腔右下象限，使得空肠略高于回肠，以保证合适

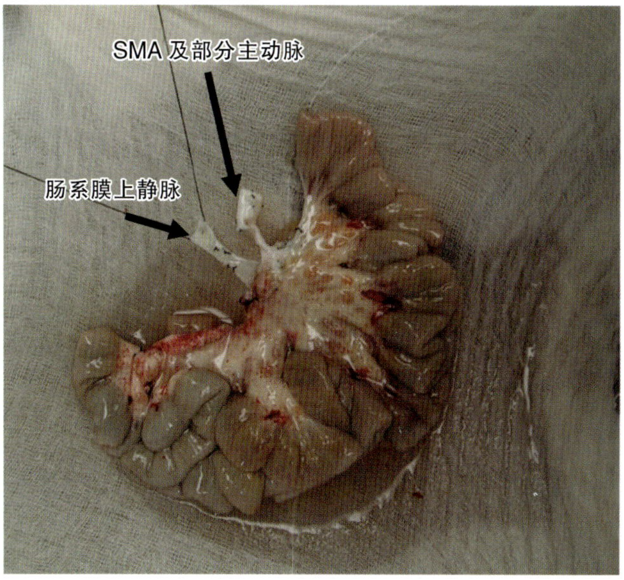

(A)

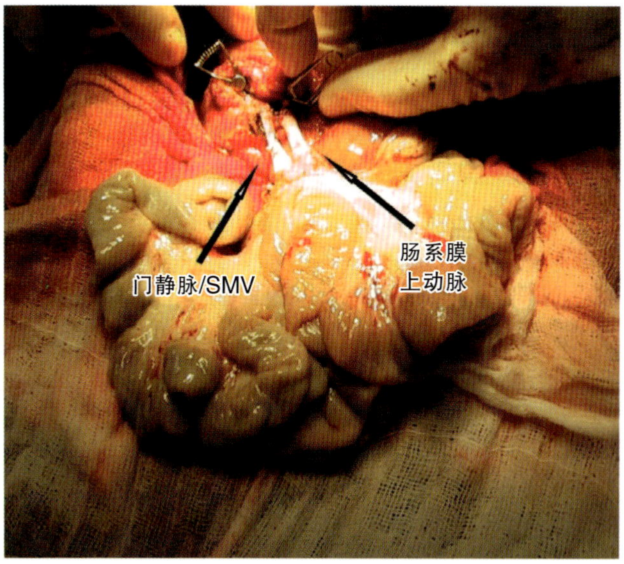

(B)

图 62.3　肠系膜引流植入前(A)、后(B)。主动脉袖口已经切除，供体和受体肠系膜血管直接行端–端吻合。

的生理角度。随后按照前述同样的步骤重建血管。

再灌注

小肠移植物再灌注时可能导致血流动力学不稳定。因此，我们常常在静脉吻合口中提前灌注生长因子。在动脉再灌注时，保持静脉吻合口开放，远端静脉夹仍保持关闭。在移除远端静脉夹前，器官保存液已经被生长因子冲出。随后收紧静脉吻合口，如果生长因子量较多，可以使用门控缝合。再灌注过程中需要进行容量复苏，避免使用任何引起内脏血管收缩的物质。肠系膜门处的小出血点必须使用单股缝线仔细结扎，避免引起主要静脉分支狭窄。

固定肠系膜

再灌注后，移植物在肠系膜门处有一处狭窄点。这有造成小肠扭转的风险，小肠会迅速发展成分泌状态并充满黏液蛋白。肠系膜根部必须与腹膜后进行间断缝合。注意不要误伤回结肠血管，并保证肠系膜两侧均需要固定。另一需要注意的是在既往多次手术患者中避免误伤输尿管。在此类患者中，我们常在术前预置输尿管支架。

重建肠道完整性

固定肠系膜后，近端空肠移植物可以按照普遍的手工缝合方式与受体原有空肠吻合。保存良好的移植物缝合效果良好，近端空肠黏膜可以为判断再灌注损伤程度提供信息。如果需要放置胃空肠营养管进行早期空肠营养，需要在吻合口后壁缝合完成后，在直视下将胃空肠营养管经胃穿入十二指肠，并越过吻合口，随后完成吻合口缝合。可根据受体剩余结肠情况进行远端肠道重建。如果保留的结肠长度不足，可以行末端回肠造口。如果保留了左半结肠，可以行端-侧吻合，并在距离吻合口约20cm处行回肠造口，或者行Santulli回肠造口。固定回肠肠系膜并关闭回肠造口附近腹壁缺损尤为重要。

小肠联合结肠移植

患者直肠功能正常，但是没有足够长度的正常结肠完成水分重吸收，此时需要在行小肠移植的同时行结肠移植。在这种情况下，移植物植入过程类似，但是没有真正的肠系膜切断边界。因此，固定肠系膜根部需要依靠后部叶状腹膜。通常需要移植右半结肠，远端横结肠必须可以抵达盆腔完成吻合以保证肠道完整性[13]。这需要游离横结肠以便升结肠横置，便于横结肠与直肠吻合，详见图62.4A。近端行回肠造口，便于监测评估移植物近端及远端结肠情况(图62.4B)。关闭肠系膜后方缺损以防止形成内疝是非常重要的。也可以在移植结肠时行末端结肠造口术，一段时间后再与直肠吻合。我个人不推荐这一方法，因为内镜医生需要通过回盲瓣进行内镜监测才能获取回肠采样。除此之外，也需要每日监测回肠黏膜情况，回肠造口排出物无法用于早期排斥反应的监测。结肠极少发生早期排斥反应。

小肠联合胰腺、胃移植

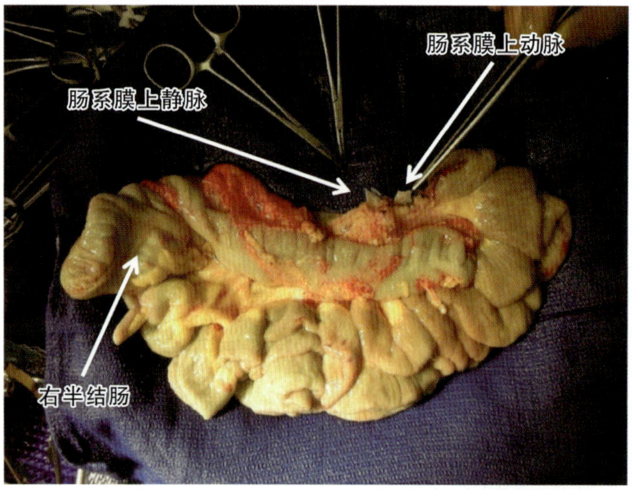

(A)

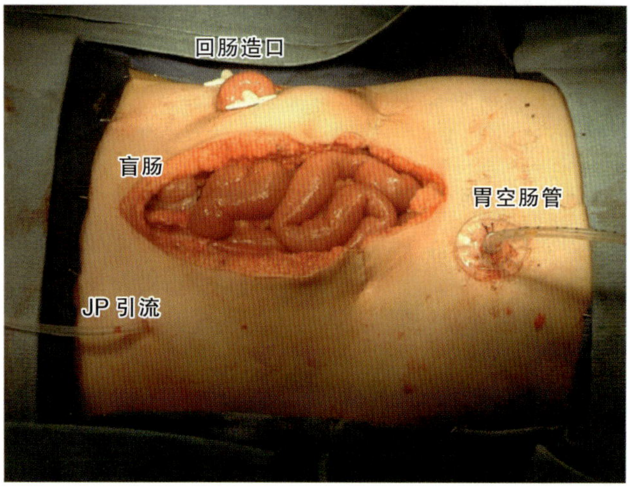

(B)

图 62.4 移植物植入前与右半结肠相连(A)。植入腹腔并且将右侧横结肠与直肠吻合后，行回肠造口术。盲肠位于左下腹(B)，引流及胃空肠管在位。右侧为患者头侧。

行小肠移植时不需要同时行肝移植的患者最好可以在小肠移植物中包括胰腺和胃。如既往行胃切除术或胰腺切除术的患者可能发生严重肠道运动功能障碍引起巨十二指肠病变，或系膜肿瘤包绕系膜血管根部并侵袭胰腺的情况。维持肝脏动脉供应的前肠清除是必需的，然后将整个胃、胰腺、空回肠移植物整体移植。这也被称为改良多器官移植[14]。简单来说，分离门静脉系统，结扎胃十二指肠动脉，并在靠近十二指肠处分离切断胆管。广泛游离十二指肠和胰头，便于从右侧确定肠系膜上动脉。骨骼化门静脉并将脾及胰尾向内侧旋转至 SMA 根部。结扎胃左动脉，确定并结扎脾动脉，仅保留腹腔干供应肝动脉。使用闭合器切断近端胃。如果保留结肠，则从侧腹壁游离左侧及右侧结肠，并向内侧旋转，保证整个小肠仅通过 SMA 与后腹壁相连。结扎 SMA，此时整个前肠(包括小肠)已经充分游离等待切除。在靠近胰管处夹闭门静脉，切断门静脉并将受体上述器官移除。随后开始进行移植物植入(图 62.5A，B)。

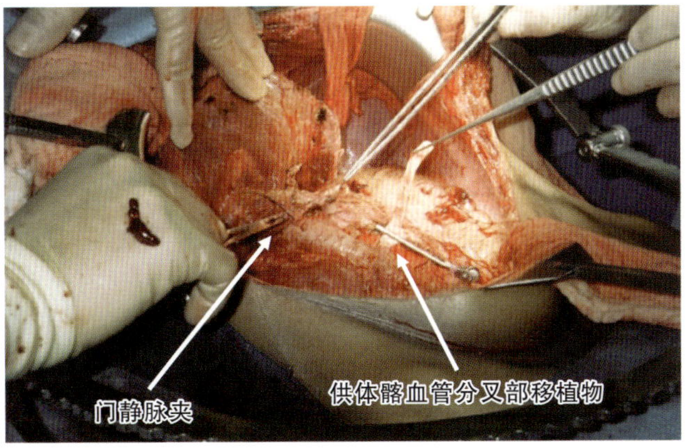

(A)

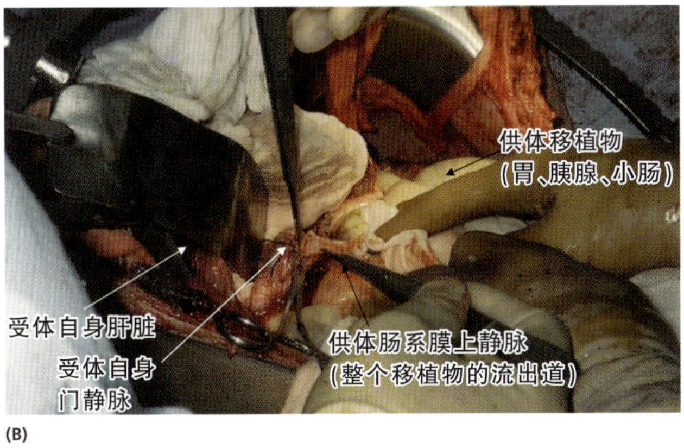

(B)

图 62.5 保留受体自身肝脏及动脉血供，夹闭门静脉(左上方)，前肠已经移除。动脉分叉移植物已经与肾下主动脉吻合(A)。移植物在助手手中，腹腔动脉及肠系膜上动脉吻合已经完成，正在重建向肝脏回流的门静脉流出道(B)。

改良的多器官联合移植

为了给移植物提供血流，在髂上主动脉或肾下主动脉上放置一个髂动脉分叉移植物。这与行单独小肠移植的手法类似。髂动脉分叉移植物的两支分别与移植物的腹腔动脉(CA)及 SMA 吻合。从十二指肠同种异体移植物发出的门静脉应用与肝移植类似的方式与受体自身门静脉行端-端吻合。本质上说，这类似于行反向肝移植。灌注时从门静脉注入生长因子冲洗器官保存液。再灌注后行胆总管端-端吻合术重建胆管。幽门是去神经的，所以行幽门成形术或幽门肌切开术便于胃排空。在鼻胃管引导下将胃缝合至食管胃交界处完成重建，并放置胃空肠营养管。将胃缝合至腹壁，将肠系膜缝合至腹膜后，如同单独的小肠移植一样，以避免移植物血管或肠道扭转。切除脾并结扎胃短血管。应用前文的方法行肠道远端重建。这种手术方式已经发展变革为可以在特定的环境下保留脾脏和(或)胰十二指肠复合体[15,16]。

罕见情形

短肠综合征，合并有因股静脉置管行肠外营养或留置下腔静脉滤器形成的肾下下腔静脉血栓

这种情况下，我们通常游离肾静脉上方下腔静脉。从肝右叶结扎肝短静脉可以暴露更长的下腔静脉。有时，可以切除右半肝帮助显露，尤其是患有肝脏疾病发生肝大时。髂总静脉可用于延长血管，结扎下腹静脉。Kocher 游离十二指肠后可以保留髂外静脉与肾下主动脉相接保证动脉供应。

因主动脉横断或其他严重血管阻塞性疾病所致短肠综合征

如果肾下主动脉无法使用，髂动脉移植物可以与如下血管吻合：①腹腔干上方主动脉；②主动脉-双股动脉弓；③与脾动脉端-端吻合；④右侧髂动脉。上述所有类型均曾实施，但是必须根据不同受体的静脉流出情况进行选择。

小肠与胰腺联合移植

在小肠功能衰竭的 1 型糖尿病患者中，可以应用

胰腺-小肠移植物复合体。髂动脉分支型移植物一侧与肾下主动脉相接，另一侧与腹腔干及肠系膜上动脉相接，保证移植物的动脉供应。使用髂静脉移植物连接受体肾下下腔静脉与移植物剩余的门静脉，保证移植物的静脉血液回流。

在胃排空障碍患者中行单独小肠移植

可以在前肠功能障碍的患者中行单独小肠移植。通常，原发性小肠运动障碍患者的胃排空障碍会在移除原有小肠后得到改善。但是，单独小肠移植需同时行空肠对空肠吻合术。在吻合口下游约20cm处行肠袢胃空肠吻合术。或者，在巨胃或严重前肠功能障碍患者中，可行近全胃切除术。此时，近端移植物可以与剩余的近端胃吻合，受体剩余空肠吻合至上述吻合口下游40cm处以避免胆汁反流。这种Roux-en-Y重建在某些患者中效果良好。

总结

小肠移植在技术上充满挑战，需要良好的空间推理、远期规划、与受体血管相吻合，以及二次手术解剖学。近20年来，血管重建的正确选择、肠道重建应保留的部分以及恢复肠道连续性的方法等已经逐步标准化。但是，手术的成功仍然面对着技术上的众多挑战，需要在合适的人群中进行多次不懈的尝试。

（倪彦彬 译 朱继业 校）

参考文献

1. Fishbein TM, Kaufman SS, Florman SS, et al. Isolated intestinal transplantation: proof of clinical efficacy. Transplantation. 2003;76:636–640.
2. Todo S, Tzakis A, Reyes J, et al. Small intestinal transplantation in humans with or without the colon. Transplantation. 1994;57:840–848.
3. Kato T, Selvaggi G, Gaynor JJ, et al. Inclusion of donor colon and ileocecal valve in intestinal transplantation. Transplantation. 2008;86:293–297.
4. Todo S, Tzakis AG, Abu-Elmagd K, et al. Intestinal transplantation in composite visceral grafts or alone. Annals of Surgery. 1992;216:223–233.
5. Sudan DL, Kaufman SS, Shaw BW Jr, et al. Isolated intestinal transplantation for intestinal failure. American Journal of Gastroenterology. 2000;95: 1506–1515.
6. Gondolesi G, Selvaggi G, Tzakis A, et al. Use of the abdominal rectus fascia as a nonvascularized allograft for abdominal wall closure after liver, intestinal, and multivisceral transplantation. Transplantation. 2009;87:1884–1888.
7. Levi DM, Tzakis AG, Kato T, et al. Transplantation of the abdominal wall. Lancet. 2003;361:2173–2176.
8. Zanfi C, Cescon M, Lauro A, et al. Incidence and management of abdominal closure-related complications in adult intestinal transplantation. Transplantation. 2008;85:1607–1609.
9. Grevious MA, Iqbal R, Raofi V, et al. Staged approach for abdominal wound closure following combined liver and intestinal transplantation from living donors in pediatric patients. Pediatric Transplantation. 2009;13:177–181.
10. Carlsen BT, Farmer DG, Busuttil RW, et al. Incidence and management of abdominal wall defects after intestinal and multivisceral transplantation. Plastic and Reconstructive Surgery. 2007;119:1247–1255.
11. Abu-Elmagd K, Fung J, Bueno J, et al. Logistics and technique for procurement of intestinal, pancreatic, and hepatic grafts from the same donor. Annals of Surgery. 2000;232:680–687.
12. Grant W, Langnas A. Pediatric small bowel transplantation: techniques and outcomes. Current Opinion Organ Transplantation. 2002;7:202–207.
13. Matsumoto CS, Kaufman SS, Fishbein TM. Inclusion of the colon in intestinal transplantation. Current Opinion Organ Transplantation. 2011;16:312–315.
14. Starzl TE, Todo S, Tzakis A, et al. The many faces of multivisceral transplantation. Surgery, Gynecology and Obstetrics. 1991;172:335–344.
15. Matsumoto CS, Fishbein TM. Modified multivisceral transplantation with splenopancreatic preservation. Transplantation. 2007;83:234–236.
16. Cruz RJ Jr, Costa G, Bond GJ, et al. Modified multivisceral transplantation with spleen-preserving pancreaticoduodenectomy for patients with familial adenomatous polyposis "Gardner's Syndrome". Transplantation. 2011;91: 1417–1423.

第 63 章

多器官移植手术步骤和外科技术

Lokesh Bathla，Alan Langnas

引言

多器官移植(MVTx)指的是行肝脏、胰十二指肠复合体及小肠整体移植[1]。本章将重点介绍 MVTx 的技术。单独小肠移植技术已经在第 62 章中进行了详细讨论。我们通常不将胃作为多器官移植的一部分，但是在其他中心，胃和(或)结肠常作为多器官移植的一部分。患有严重胃蠕动功能障碍、广泛上腹部粘连或胃外伤的患者是含胃 MVTx 的潜在受体。这种移植手术不仅仅是符合人体结构的原位移植，而且血管重建步骤简单，不需要行门腔分流。偶尔，在可能从结肠肛门成形术获益的患者中，如大肠无神经节综合征患者，结肠也可作为多器官移植物的一部分进行移植。MVTx 占所有成人小肠移植手术的 25%，占所有儿童小肠移植手术的 13%[2]。MVTx 可治疗不可逆小肠衰竭，尤其是短肠综合征合并小肠衰竭的相关肝病(IFALD)。累及整个消化道的疾病，如慢性小肠假性梗阻、严重肠粘连伴有多发肠外瘘、严重腹部外伤所致无法重建的胃肠道损伤及局部侵袭性恶性肿瘤（如硬纤维瘤）等，均是 MVTx 的适应证[3,4]。

MVTx 根据需要切除的受体器官情况不同，可分为保留前肠和不保留前肠两种方式。这主要由引起小肠衰竭的原发疾病所决定。胃受累的患者，如严重胃运动功能障碍及空腔脏器肌肉疾病等，需要行不保留前肠的器官切除术。在保留前肠的手术中，受体胃、胰腺及十二指肠(前肠)均要保留。不保留前肠的手术步骤包括切除受体大部分胃、十二指肠、胰腺及脾。两种手术方式均需切除全部小肠及直到横结肠中部的结肠。是否保留受体前肠的具体原因已经在第 33 章中进行了详细讨论。根据手术团队的习惯，胃和(或)结肠常作为移植物的一部分整体移植。常规的肝移植技术及原则(已经在第 56 章中详细讨论)通常也适用于 MVTx。这包括在移植过程中的仔细分离、细致止血及血管重建、处理凝血功能障碍。MVTx 的一个独特之处在于其难以获得足够的血管通路进行麻醉管理及复苏，这将在随后的内容中进行介绍。

麻醉注意事项

一位有经验的麻醉医师是这些复杂手术成功的关键。术前对患者详细的检查评估以及与手术医师对计划的手术方式的全面探讨是手术成功的基础。除了详细的全身病史询问及体格检查，准确评估患者血管情况、凝血状态、营养状况，以及酸碱、电解质和液体平衡尤为重要。

上文曾提到，许多需要接受 MVTx 患者的血管条件常常较差。这主要是由长期使用中心静脉输注高营养以及导管相关并发症所致静脉血栓所致。在进入手术室前需对患者进行详细评估，以便获得合适的中心静脉通路。某些特别复杂的情况下，需要介入科医生帮助从腰静脉或者奇静脉获得中心静脉通路。术前静脉图、术中血管超声往往是成功放置大口径外周静脉或者中心静脉导管的关键。如果其他方法都失败了，必须由手术医师在手术早期将大口径高容量导管直接置入下腔静脉中。除了标准麻醉输送设备之外，还需要持续监测心排出量及混合静脉氧饱和度等血流动力学参数，以及能同时显示 4 条压力通道的监测仪。对于成人患者，我们常规使用 Swan-Ganz 导管(Edward Lifesciences Corp.，Irvine，CA)监测肺动脉压、毛细血管楔压及中心静脉压。我们通常使用两条动脉通路。大多数需要接受 MVTx 的患者常为儿童，因其体型较小，难以放置动脉通路。由于这些患者需要多次监测动脉血气分析，以及需要获得准确的动脉血压监测，因此必须获得良好的动脉通路。术中经食管超声心动图使用也较为广泛,是评估前负荷及室壁运动的良好监测手段。在发生大量出血、血流动力学不稳定以及预计移植时间延长的情况下,获得合适的静脉转流循环尤为重要。密切监测电解质、动脉血气、凝血功能、血糖及红细胞比容。术中常会发生大出血,因此自体血液吸收仪器及快速输血设备作用巨大。保持患者核心体温正常有助于防止其凝血功能恶化。上半身和下半身的增强气道装置、加热毯及液体加热装置均有助于减少患者热量丧失,有时甚至需要升高手术室的温度。

从麻醉医生的角度来看,移植物再灌注是整个手术过程中最具挑战性的部分。该过程中会出现低血压、低钙血症、高钾血症、代谢性酸中毒及体温过低。需要及时进行快速液体输注及使用血管升压药物。除此之外,再灌注前应优化血钾水平,以应对移植物再灌注引起的钾离子外流。采用与纠正高钾血症一样的方法在再灌注前调节钾离子水平。如出现高钾血症,需立即输注胰岛素、葡萄糖、碳酸氢钠、袢利尿剂及钙进行纠正。极少数情况下,若出现高钾血症所致心脏停搏,需进行直流电复律。在我们中心,我们的手术野常规包括整个胸部,并且在再灌注前,术区需常规准备无菌除颤电极板。特别是对于儿童及婴儿受体,这些经验尤为重要。

手术切口

根据患者不同的体型、年龄及既往手术史,选择不同的手术切口。由于大多数患者存在手术史,手术切口的选择需要个体化。对于许多患者来说,可使用既往的正中或肋缘下切口进行移植手术,有时可以将切口顺着原切口方向延长。极少数情况下,需要沿着与原切口垂直的方向延长切口。但是,任何新切口均不能影响腹壁的血液供应。同时,切口选择也需要利于术野暴露。

切除腹腔器官

下一手术步骤为切除受体腹腔器官。近端切缘水平取决于胃是否是移植物的一部分。如果胃是移植物的一部分,近端切缘水平则为食管远端或近端胃。通常我们保留紧靠食管远端的一部分胃,便于行近端吻合术(胃胃吻合术),并降低反流或吻合口狭窄发生的风险。如果胃不是移植物的一部分,近端切缘水平取决于手术方式是保留前肠的MVTx还是不保留前肠的MVTx。首先,按照与肝移植类似的方法游离受体肝脏。这一步骤在上述两种术式中相同。切除周围韧带并确认肝门组织。根据腔静脉吻合方式(原位或背驮式)的不同,完全或部分游离腔静脉。我们中心常进行原位肝移植,所以在多器官移植中也使用同样的技术。近端小肠的切除范围将在下文中详细阐述。远切缘常在横结肠中部水平,保留左结肠动脉。

保留前肠的多器官移植

该术式保留小肠,但需要将其游离至左肾静脉及肠系膜上动脉水平。此时,需要保留胃、胰腺、脾及十二指肠的静脉回流。因此,要行门腔静脉端侧分流。门腔静脉分流后,夹闭肝下腔静脉的上部和下部并移除肝脏。

不保留前肠的多器官移植

不保留前肠的MVTx需要切除较大范围的受体器官。首先横断胃。在胃大弯侧分离大网膜上至其中部以充分游离胃。离断肝胃韧带以游离胃中部。此时便于放置吻合器横断胃中部。上述过程中应注意保留胃左动脉,因其为剩余近端胃的主要供血动脉。若需行全胃切除,需将胃及胃食管(GE)交界处游离。由于GE交界处由食管下部动脉分支供血,此时可以不保留胃左动脉。该步骤暴露了腹腔干以上的主动脉及腹腔干起始部。随后,采用Mattox手法游离脾脏及胰腺并将其向中线内侧旋转。将右半结肠从侧腹壁游离后,将剩余小肠和结肠由尾侧向头侧翻起。随后将小肠与右半结肠从后腹膜分离暴露下腔静脉与主动脉。上述分离需分离至左肾静脉,其是辨认肠系膜上动脉的重要标志。使用Kocher手法处理十二指肠,以从右侧暴露肠系膜上动脉,并游离整个肠系膜。随后使用吻合器切断左半结肠和横结肠。保留左结肠血管和肠系膜下血管,因其是剩余肠道的唯一供血来源。粘连严重会增加上述操作的难度及时间。如果操作不小心会引起大量出血,形成出血和凝血障碍的恶性循环。

完全游离上述器官后,确定SMA并用丝线双重结扎。随后确定并结扎肝总动脉及脾动脉。如上文所说,如果从中部横断胃,则保留胃左动脉。如果在GE交界处横断胃,则按照与结扎SMA类似的方法结扎腹腔干。此时，受体的前肠及中肠仅通过门静脉与肝脏相连。这时使用大的钳夹或吻合器完全横断肝门并将前肠及中肠组织完全移出腹腔。将肝脏保留在腔静脉的主要原因是其可以维持一定的血流动力学稳定性。

由于广泛的切除，腹膜后会出现一定的出血，需要仔细止血。确切止血后，分离膈肌脚以识别前腹腔干上主动脉，暴露上胸膜壁层与下腹腔轴之间的区域，用于放置主动脉管道，为移植物提供动脉血流。

在 Grant 等人之前描述的肝脏、小肠联合移植技术中，需在保持门静脉完整的同时将其骨骼化，使其成为连接肝脏及移植物小肠部分的唯一结构[2]。这主要是避免供体胰腺发生胰腺炎或胰瘘[5]。但在我中心早期实践过程中，这一技术带来了许多技术难题。首先，这增加了修整移植物的技术风险，尤其是儿童供体，可能会损伤腹腔干、肠系膜上动脉及门静脉。其次，胆肠吻合口瘘所致死亡率显著增加。最后，移植过程中门静脉扭转的发生率较高[6]。

1996 年，第一次报道了解决上述技术难题的改良方案[7]。主要的改变包括：不切除肝门，保留肝十二指肠韧带的完整性(图 63.1)。这不仅仅降低了修整移植物的难度，还避免了移植物扭转及胆肠吻合。下文对后续手术技术的描述主要基于我们的改良手术方案，参见 Sudan 等人的报道[6]。

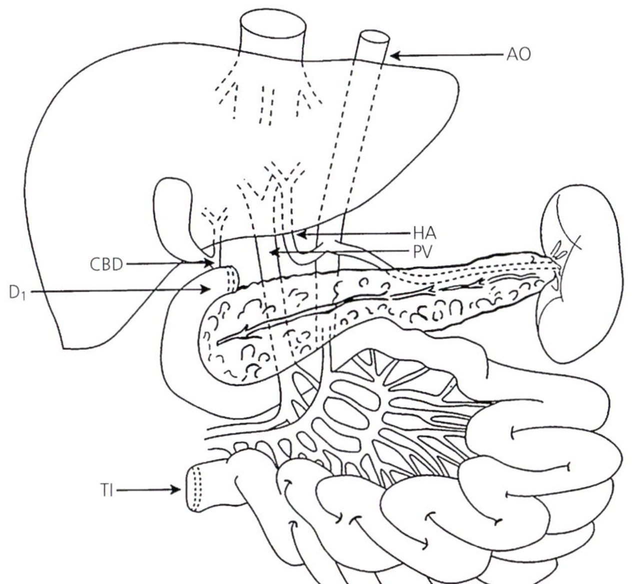

图 63.1　供体手术。注意将肝脏、小肠、胰腺及脾脏整体移除。不用切除肝门血管，并将腹腔干及 SMA 保留在主动脉上。AO，胸主动脉；HA，肝动脉；PV，门静脉；CBD，胆总管；D1，十二指肠第一段，已钉合；TI，末端回肠，已钉合。(Reproduced from[6] Sudan DL, Iyer KR, Deroover A, et al. A new technique for combined liver/small intestinal transplantation. Transplantation 2001;72(11):1846-1848, with permission from Lippincott Williams & Wilkins, Inc.)

接下来，在膈肌裂孔处进行分离，分离膈肌的脚纤维，以显露腰腔上部区域的主动脉。在显露足够空间便于留置阻断钳后，将获取的供体的一部分主动脉放置在术野(导管)中，在受体前腹腔干上主动脉留置一弯形阻断钳。供体主动脉直径可用于评估受体主动脉切开的直径大小。使用 11 号刀切开受体主动脉壁，并使用主动脉穿刺针行主动脉切开术。使用 5-0 或 6-0 聚丙烯缝合线将 4~6cm 供体主动脉回路的一部分按照端-侧吻合方式与受体主动脉吻合。吻合完成后，应用一阻断钳阻断回路，并松开前腹腔干上主动脉上的阻断钳，恢复腹腔及下肢血液灌注(图 63.2)。随后进行肝上下腔静脉试验性阻断，评估患者是否可以耐受移植过程中下腔静脉阻断操作。若血流动力学保持稳定，则阻断并分离肝上下腔静脉及肝下下腔静脉。切除肝脏及肝后方下腔静脉。此时可以行静脉转流避免患者发生肾脏及下肢血流瘀滞。在我们中心，我们在无肝期很少使用静脉转流。这些年，我们逐渐停止使用静脉转流技术，但在许多移植中心，这仍然是一项标准技术。在使用与不使用静脉转流的患者中，我们并没有发现任何显著性差异。

随后将多器官移植物置入术野。按照与肝移植类似的手法吻合肝上下腔静脉(图 63.3)。成人患者应用

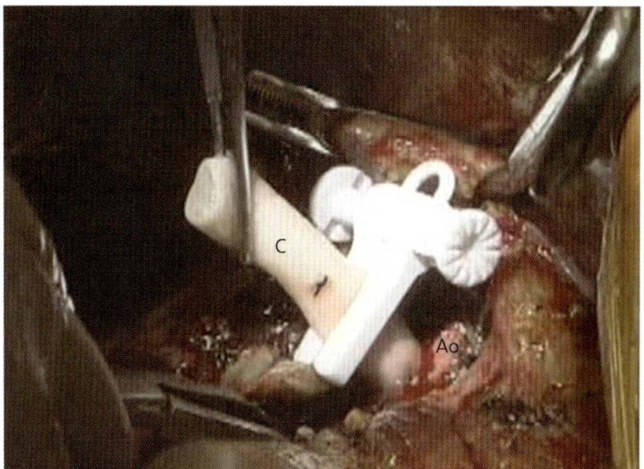

图 63.2　移除主动脉阻断钳之前迅速用哈巴狗血管夹钳夹主动脉通道。C，主动脉通道；Ao，受体主动脉。

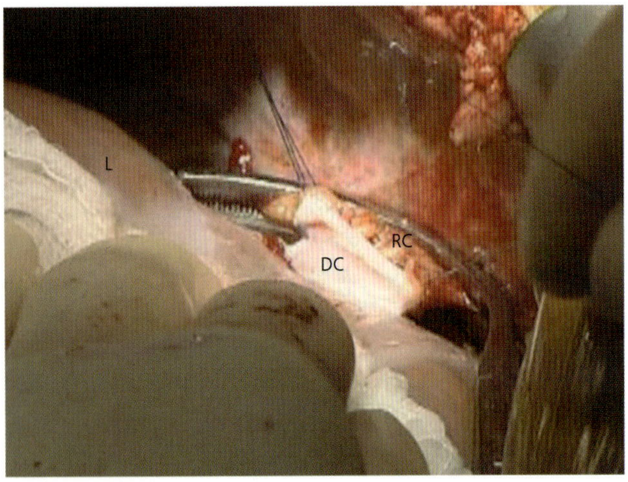

图 63.3 移植物肝上下腔静脉与钳夹的受体下腔静脉进行吻合。L,肝脏;DC,供体下腔静脉;RC,受体下腔静脉。

3-0 聚丙烯缝合线进行连续缝合，而儿童患者则使用 4-0 或 6-0 聚丙烯缝合线。随后,使用 4-0 聚丙烯缝合线将移植物肝下下腔静脉与受体肝下下腔静脉行连续缝合。已经与受体腹腔干上主动脉吻合的受体主动脉回路，与移植物主动脉使用 6-0 聚丙烯缝合线进行连续缝合(图 63.4)。

此时,首先移除肝上下腔静脉阻断钳,便于静脉回流入移植物及早期控制大出血。随后,移除肝下下腔静脉阻断钳,促进下肢血液回流,便于稳定患者血流动力学状态。最后,移除主动脉回路阻断钳,恢复移植物动脉血供。保证所有主要血管吻合口的完整性。然后,根据需要仔细缝合或烧灼供体器官上的小出血点。止血完成后,行胃肠道吻合恢复胃肠道完整性。

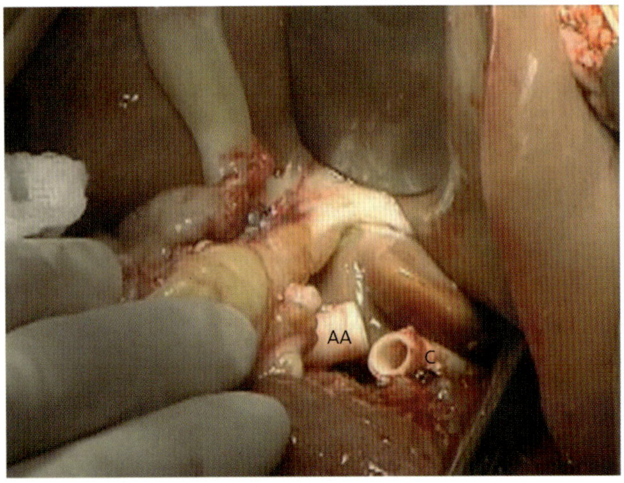

图 63.4 将移植物主动脉放置于主动脉通道旁用于吻合。AA,移植物主动脉;C,主动脉通道。

如果不移植胃，则将剩余胃与移植物的空肠行 Roux-en-Y 胃空肠吻合。通常使用双层手法吻合。Roux-en-Y 空肠空肠吻合及回肠结肠吻合也同样应用双层手法。另外,也可使用吻合器进行上述吻合,但有时会造成吻合处出血。需要注意的是,多数情况下,整个胰腺也存在于移植物中,参见图 63.5。随后切除移植物胆囊,并行回肠袢造口术。

我们通常在右下腹按照“Brooke”手法行回肠造口(图 63.6)。造口部位选择非常重要,常常因为既往手术切口、既往造口切口、造口疝、大量腹壁缺损及移植物肠系膜可拉伸长度(因供体和受体尺寸不匹配引起)等原因而增加难度，这可能会随着造口术的成熟及造口器械的应用而引起相关并发症。造口不佳不仅会造成皮肤及伤口并发症,也会影响患者心理及情感状态。术前必须邀请造口诊疗专家对患者进行详细评估，确定造口最佳部位。评估过程中需要关注患者腹部瘢痕或挛缩、既往造口部位及是否存在疝。在情况复杂的患者

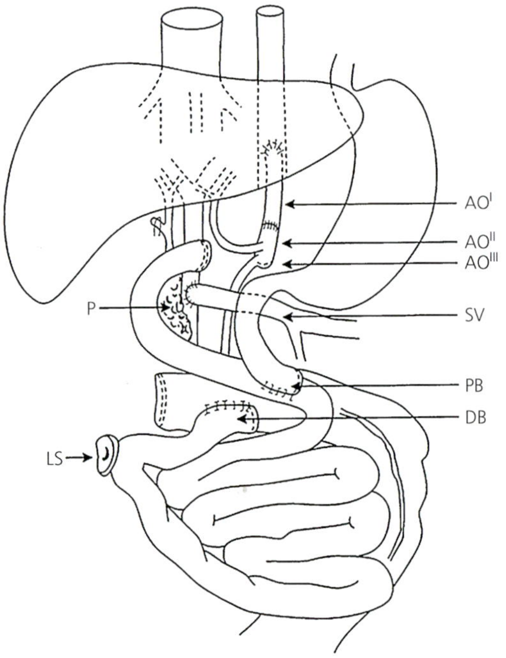

图 63.5 受体手术。AOⅠ,在位的移植物主动脉;AOⅡ,带有腹腔干及 SMA 的主动脉壁;AOⅢ,夹闭主动脉末端,切除其 SMA 下部;SV,受体自身脾静脉;P,胰管及实质边缘缝合的胰腺;PB,近端小肠;DB,远端回结肠吻合口;LS,袢回肠造口。(Reproduced from [6] Sudan DL, Iyer KR, Deroover, A et al. A New technique for combined liver/small intestinal transplantation. Transplantation 2001;72 (11):1846-1848 with permission from Lippincott Williams & Wilkins, Inc.)

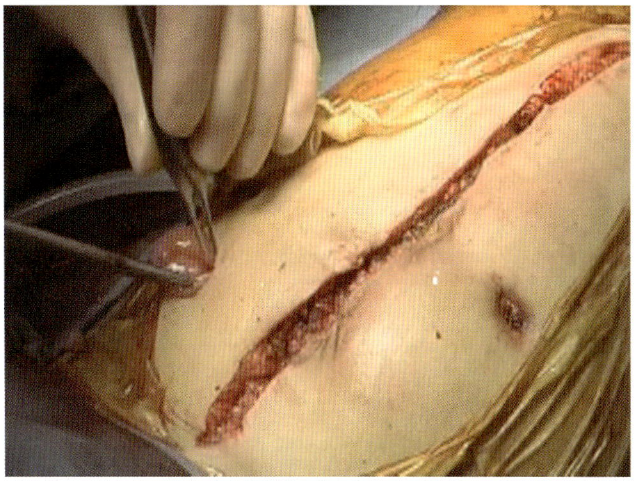

图 63.6 完成多器官移植并行 Brooke 造口术。

中需要标记多处可行的造口部位。理想情况下，常选取患者看不见的腰带下部位。除此之外，造口部位需要离切口至少 5cm。

手术中最具挑战性或最复杂的部分之一是关闭腹壁。一期筋膜缝合是最理想的目标。使用重聚丙烯缝合线连续缝合腹壁筋膜，腹壁皮肤常不关闭。但是这一方案并非适用于所有患者。必须避免吻合口存在张力，因为会：①增加切口裂开风险；②伤口张力所致腹腔压力增高会影响移植物血流灌注；③伤口张力所致气道压力增高影响患者通气功能；④移植物肿胀及第三间隙液体流失会造成腹腔间隔室综合征。有多种方案可解决上述问题，如仅仅缝合皮肤，或使用合成补片或生物补片。若使用生物补片，则在移植物水肿逐渐消退后（常为术后 48~72 小时）行二次手术评估移植物活性并尝试关闭腹壁筋膜。根据我中心的经验，最佳方案为使用生物补片，如无细胞人类真皮或可吸收补片。随后几天，患者还需行多次手术逐渐清洗并移除补片，并行腹壁筋膜缝合。在一些罕见情况下，如存在大量腹壁缺损时，需要行腹壁皮肤移植，详见下文讨论。

腹壁移植

行 MVTx 或小肠移植的患者常会遇到腹壁切口难以关闭的问题。由于既往多次腹部手术、肠瘘或造口，这些患者的腹部组织活动度有限。除此之外，这些患者既往曾行腹壁缺损修补术。并且，许多患者移除了全部中肠，剩余腹腔空间过小，无法装入移植物。腹腔空间过小需要使用较小的供体器官，除了腹壁移植，无法关闭腹腔。因此，需要考虑行腹壁移植的可能性。腹壁移植物是一个带血管复合移植物（VCA），便于在腹壁严重缺损的患者中重建及关闭腹腔。

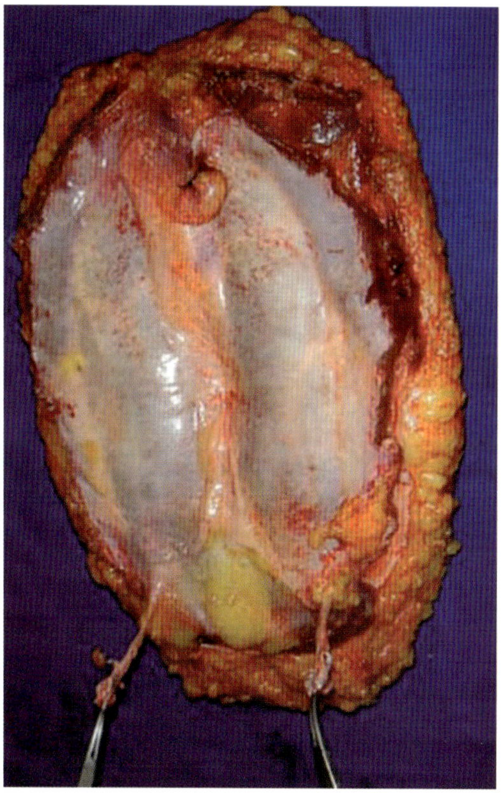

图 63.7 腹壁移植物带有两条腹壁血管蒂。（Reproduced from[8] Cipriani R, Contedini F, Santoli M, et al. Abdominal wall transplantation with microsurgical technique. American Journal of Transplantation 2007;7:1304 –1307, with permission from John Wiley and Sons Ltd.）

获取腹壁移植物是多器官移植的一部分。这一移植物包括由腹直肌、部分腹外及腹内斜肌以及一层壁腹膜所组成的一个卵圆形肌皮瓣。移植物的血管蒂来源于腹壁下血管，从髂外血管发出（图 63.7）[8]。将供体髂外动脉或静脉的左侧或右侧分别与受体髂动脉或静脉吻合获得血供。有时可以使用 10–0 不可吸收缝合线行受体–移植物腹壁血管端–端显微缝合。恢复血供后，需要注意肌肉切口处的出血。随后使用双层缝合将肌皮瓣与受体腹壁缝合。VCA 的成功移植便于减少腹壁张力并保持腹壁完整性。

减体积移植物

由于获取合适的较小供体器官非常困难，尤其是婴儿受体,通常需要在移植前减少供体器官体积。通常情况下,体积大于目标受体25%的供体需要行减体积移植术。在修整移植物时行移植物减体积术,并按照活体肝移植的相关指南进行操作(参见第57章)。通常移植左外侧段或左叶。需要移除的小肠部分不尽相同,通常为中肠的1/3。根据移植物解剖结构决定行原位或背驮式减体积移植术。

总结

多器官移植是目前最为复杂的技术。尽管我们在不断积累MVTx的经验,但是这些手术仍然具有极大风险,尤其对于病重患者。除了详细描述手术步骤之外,必须根据患者特点(如年龄、基础疾病、既往手术史及血管情况)进行个体化评估。经验丰富的团队的精细手术操作及止血、尽可能少的移植物缺血时间及有效的围术期管理对患者及移植物的良好预后十分关键。

(倪彦彬 译 朱继业 校)

参考文献

1. Tzakis AG, Kato T, Levi DM, et al. 100 multivisceral transplants at a single center. Annals of Surgery. 2005;242:480–493.
2. Grant D, Abu-Elmagd K, Reyes J, et al. 2003 report of the intestinal transplant registry: a new era has dawned. Annals of Surgery. 2005;241:607–613.
3. Loinaz C, Mittal N, Kato T, et al. Multivisceral transplantation for pediatric intestinal pseudo-obstruction: single center's experience of 16 cases. Transplantation Proceedings. 2004;36:312–313.
4. Chatzipetrou MA, Tzakis AG, Pinna AD, et al. Intestinal transplantation for the treatment of desmoid tumors associated with familial adenomatous polyposis. Surgery. 2001;129:277–281.
5. Grant D, Wall W, Mimeault R, et al. Successful small-bowel/liver transplantation. Lancet. 1990;335:181–184.
6. Sudan DL, Iyer KR, Deroover A, et al. A new technique for combined liver/small intestinal transplantation. Transplantation. 2001;72:1846–1848.
7. Langnas A, Shaw B, Antonson D, et al. Preliminary experience with intestinal transplantation in infants and children. Pediatrics. 1996;87:443–448.
8. Cipriani R, Contedini F, Santoli M, et al. Abdominal wall transplantation with microsurgical technique. American Journal of Transplantation. 2007;1304–1307.

第 64 章
带血管蒂复合移植物手术步骤和外科技术

Gerald Brandacher, Jaimie T. Shores, Chad R. Gordon, Damon S. Cooney, W.P. Andrew Lee

引言

每年，有数以万计的人们会因为受伤、肿瘤切除，或是先天性缺损而需要进行复杂的外科重建手术以修复组织缺损。然而目前，对于较大的组织缺损而开展的重建手术具有许多局限性，包括功能或美学结果差、需要多次外科手术、长期康复治疗、使用自体组织而导致的供区并发症、多次手术和住院治疗导致费用昂贵等。带血管复合移植物（VCA）提供了一种新的选择，能很好地满足治疗过程对自体组织的需求。

将身体的一部分从一个人移植到另一个人身上，这种想法可以追溯到远古时代[1]，然而，直到 20 世纪 50 年代，这一过程才通过肾脏移植得以部分实现。1962 年 5 月 23 日，Ronald Malt 在马萨诸塞州总医院执行了世界上首例手臂移植手术，VCA 的潜力第一次得到体现。在这个过程中，他彻底地改变了创伤性截肢患者和肢体丧失患者重建形式、功能和外观的方式[2]。20 世纪 80 年代和 90 年代，伴随着越来越多的显微外科手术的成功、免疫抑制药物的研发，以及实体器官的移植经验，这种开创性的手术带动了肢体及复合组织异体移植概念的兴起。终于，1998 年 9 月 23 日，在 Jean-Michel Dubernard 博士的带领下，一个外科医生团队在法国里昂成功完成了第一例基于免疫抑制的手掌移植手术[3]。

从那时起，重建手术成了一种临床现实，全世界有超过 200 种不同的 VCA 手术得以成功实施，包括手、前臂、手臂、部分面部组织和全面部、腹壁、喉部、气管、血管化的骨骼和关节、舌头，甚至是子宫和阴茎[4,5]。不断积累的经验证实，对于有组织严重损伤、不适合开展传统重建手术的患者，VCA 已经成为一种重要的治疗选择。然而，尽管外科手术已经取得了巨大成功，取得的成果也令人满意，但慢性免疫抑制相关的并发症仍然限制了这些技术更广泛的应用，且无法形成标准化的治疗方案[6]。尽管如此，如果有缜密的考量、详细的术前筛查和计划、精细的外科技术，以及细致的后续护理，依然可以实现较为理想的结果[7]。本章将重点关注 VCA 的一般步骤，每一个病例都有着技术上的独特性，它们本身就是个性化的作品。本章是第 75、87、110 章的补充，这些章节分别讲述了 VCA 排斥反应的治疗、VCA 排斥反应的组织学和 VCA 的长期预后。

受体选择、等待列表管理和供体条件

受体的选择是非常重要的，因为 VCA 手术并不是挽救生命，而是为了提高生活质量，因此必须严格按照程序进行风险-效益评估。考虑到免疫抑制药物依从性和严格的康复要求，选择合适的受体并不一定是移植重建手术取得成功最重要的影响因素。因此，受体的选择和筛查必须经历多个步骤，包括对患者过去的病史和移植前的生活进行全面的审查[8]。为此，在决定患者是否适于进行移植手术前，必须考虑和评估其解剖、生理、心理和社会因素。只有通过对潜在受体的合适性进行详尽的评估，才可能获得让患者和医生都满意的结果。值得注意的是，心理和社会因素的审查已经成为评估候选人能否适宜免疫抑制和康复治疗的关键。社会心理的审查更像是一门艺术，而非科学，它在移植学中仍在不断发展和完善[9]。众多 VCA 手术经验告诉我们，只有那些身体和精神健康、怀有期待、对技术的复杂性有足够理解能力，并能积极承受至少 6 个月至 1 年的密集康复治疗的患者，才能被视为合格的候选人。实际上，心理稳定性和对手术及术后各个方面的理解能力，需由一位独立于移植团队的精神科医生或心理学家来确定。只有满足这些心理标准，对患者下一步的筛查才可启动。根据组织缺损的不同类型，手术计划应考虑每个候选人独特的解剖状况，包括骨骼、肌肉、血管、软组织和神经状态。这通常是通过体格检查和使用各种影像设备来完成的，如CT扫描(±三维重建结构)、血管造影、CT血管造影、MRI等。肢体或解剖部位及其对侧的影像，即使是无关的，也要与重建手术技术及供体相匹配(如大小、肤色等)。为避免手术失败，备用重建方案的考虑也是至关重要的。

为了避免其他因为慢性免疫抑制(如恶性肿瘤或感染)或者手术本身而发生的并发症，潜在移植受体需要进行进一步移植相关的筛查，包括胃镜、结肠镜，以及其肾脏、心血管、肺、血液营养及牙齿状况的评估(详见表64.1)。移植相关免疫筛查包括ABO血型检查、HLA配型、自身抗体筛查及病毒筛查 [如甲型肝炎病毒、乙型肝炎病毒、丙型肝炎病毒、巨细胞病毒(CMV)、EB病毒及HIV病毒等]。如果潜在移植受体在评估过程中发现了任意一项异常，则需要进行进一步详细的检查(表64.2)。

上述检查结果也会发送至器官获取组织(OPO)以启动供体筛选。尽管目前这一过程尚无标准流程，一般来说，VCA项目的操作流程与实体器官获取流程类似[10]。VCA团队和OPO同时制订详细的入选及排除标准。从这一方面来讲，VCA的潜在供体不仅要满足常规标准，如ABO血型、年龄、血清学检查等，还要评估体型、性别、肤色及皮肤紧张度及弹性。血型必须相容。目前为止，HLA配型并不是十分必要。但是，供体与受体间的所有淋巴细胞毒性交叉配型必须均为阴性。供体与受体间的CMV病毒配型必须避免供体阳性-受体阴性这一组合，因为VCA受体中CMV感染发生率及CMV相关并发症发生率极高[11-13]。需要特别注意的是，尽管在一些国家存在“假设知情同意”这一伦理学说法，但是针对VCA捐献必须获得书面的知情同意书。这必须详细解释供体VCA获取过程及捐献后如何重建供体缺损(如藻酸盐假体、美容面具、装饰性假肢等)，以宽慰捐献者家属。最为重要的是，协调员在与潜在VCA供体家属接触时，必须保证救命的实体器官也同时捐献[10,14]。目前没有潜在VCA受体的具体排队标准及分配政策，也没有全国性的VCA等待名单。因此，每个移植中心以及当地及区域OPO仅需考虑自己的患者。直到现在，等待重建型移植的患者人数较少，因

表64.1 标准筛选检查

血液学检查
全血细胞计数、分类、网织红细胞计数、血小板计数
ABO血型、Rh分型、HLA分型
群体反应性抗体(PRA)
PT/PTT及INR
代谢检查
血清电解质及肾功能
尿液分析及肌酐清除率
肝功能
DEXA扫描(如有必要)
感染相关检查
巨细胞病毒、EB病毒、HSV、弓形虫病、VZV(IgG及IGM)、HIV抗原、HTLV Ⅰ~Ⅱ抗体，HIV 1及2抗体、丙肝病毒、梅毒、乙肝核心抗体及乙肝表面抗原
纯蛋白衍生物(PPD)/Mantous皮肤监测
心肺功能
多门控采集心电图(MUGA)或超声心动图检查心脏
DLC02测试肺功能
放射学检查
腹部超声(排除肿瘤)及手部/残余部分超声
CT扫描[CT血管造影和(或)传统血管造影]或前臂及手部骨骼肌肉MRI、功能性MRI及脑磁图(MEG)扫描
鼻窦X线片(除外感染或肿瘤)
胸片
双侧手部、腕部、前臂、手肘X线片等

表64.2 筛选咨询和评估

咨询
口腔医学
眼科学
胃肠病学[包括胃十二指肠镜(EGD)及结肠镜检查]
耳鼻喉医学(ENT)
男性患者：泌尿学(评估前列腺及睾丸肿瘤)
女性患者：妇科学(评估卵巢、子宫内膜、子宫或宫颈肿瘤)
移植心理学
移植精神病学
移植社会工作
认证的手治疗师
社会心理学筛查及功能评估工具
SF36健康调查：询问患者对其健康状况的观点
DASH手臂、肩、手功能异常评估：询问患者目前是够可以完成特定动作
采用如下问卷之一进行精神病学调查：Perlin自我掌控量表、Rosenberg自我评估量表、应对反应量表、Sherwood自我定义量表、NEO个人量表短期评估

此针对 VCA 供体的竞争较少。但是,随着 VCA 移植数量的增加(近几年来,面部及手的移植量逐年上升),制订相应的分配政策越来越重要,以促进潜在 VCA 供体信息的广泛共享。在国家层面来讲,最佳的 VCA 捐献监管机构是国家器官分配网络(UNOS),其通过器官获取移植网络(OPTN)开展工作[15-17]。目前,OPTN 进行的实体器官移植监管流程可以应用至 VCA 捐献程序中,提供相应的监督性、标准化、有效性、安全性及透明性(详细内容参见第 128 章及第 143 章)。

由于目前没有标准化的操作流程,每位 VCA 受体的手术步骤均需要制订个体化的程序。对每一位患者来说,需要制订详细的手术计划,某些情况下,需要在尸体上进行某项手术技术的训练以提高新的重建技术。

越来越多的证据表明,冷缺血及热缺血时间过长会明显影响移植物短期及长期的功能[18]。肌肉组织对缺血及损伤尤为敏感。间质水肿、微血管重建和(或)肌细胞膜损伤都会导致热缺血 2.5 小时后肌肉功能异常[19]。因此,必须避免移植物的长途转运,建议在相邻的手术室里同时进行供体移植物的获取及受体相应组织的切除。

外科技术:手、腹壁

获取供体手部的外科技术

一旦选择了一位免疫相容的合适供体,必须进一步配型,保证其肤色、年龄、性别(从全球多家移植中心的近几年的经验来看,如果皮肤纹理、毛发分布、体型等合适,也会发生性别不同的情况)、长度、周径及身体习惯相近[10]。有创监测(如动脉穿刺)可能造成的血管损伤、导致脑死亡机制所致血管损伤、血管收缩效应等都必须进行详尽的评估以保证肢体可用于移植。必须进行影像学检查评估损伤及疾病,也可帮助评估体型是否相符。

确认为合适的供体后,获取步骤与传统供体器官获取步骤类似(详见第 21 章及第 53 章)。考虑到肢体的可伸展性,也可将其单独置于手术野之外,获取肢体的过程不会影响随后其他器官的获取步骤。肢体的获取可以在获取胸腔及腹腔器官之前或者之间进行。在这两种情况下,均需在夹闭主动脉之前暴露肱动脉及肱静脉并用止血带控制肱动脉及肱静脉。这保证获取过程中与体循环不相通,减少血流动力学不稳定所致风险,并且不影响实体器官的获取。灌注导管插入肱动脉中并注入灌注液。笔者推荐注射 500~1000mL HTK 溶液及 5000 单位肝素。灌注持续至静脉引流液清亮。剩余的获取过程可以在夹闭主动脉之前,或者与获取胸腹腔器官同时进行。

取环周切口便于迅速切断伸肌或屈肌、正中神经、尺神经及桡神经。保留稍长的血管及神经便于在修整器官时辨认。从肘部切除前臂(用于远端及中前臂移植)。进行更为近端的器官获取时,则行肱骨髁上截骨术。某些情况下,需要保留足够长度的正中神经、尺神经、桡神经及肌皮神经。除此之外,需要额外切除一段贵要静脉和(或)头静脉、深静脉及肱动脉。在放置止血带之前,从近端至远端游离浅静脉。游离完成后在手臂近端上无菌止血带,便于分离近端神经及血管。在所有循环停止之前,止血带必须始终保持充气状态。与实体器官保存方法类似,灌注好保存液的肢体随后用湿毛巾包裹并置于低温无菌袋中用于转运。

受体外科技术:手移植

行上肢移植的患者准备与行肝移植类似。大口径外周静脉、中心静脉通路及动脉线被放置在远离接受 VCA 的肢体处。可以根据不同移植中心的不同经验给予免疫诱导治疗(如即复宁等)。考虑到 VCA 手术时长,必须充分估计即复宁相关细胞因子释放及相关血流动力学不稳定性。局部阻滞导管(外周神经导管)可以使用,但是不能通过其输注长效麻醉药品。术中超声评估及浅表静脉系统描图有助于静脉重建。诱导后,采用与肝移植类似的方法对患者进行全身麻醉监测。采用胶体(压积红细胞及新鲜冰冻血浆)而不是晶体进行液体复苏,以减少外周水肿。

移植物的修整及受体的准备应同时进行[20,21]。需要注意的是,所有在供体肢体进行的分离操作均需要在冰上进行,使用无菌冰块及碎冰,并且在冰块和肢体间放置毛巾以避免肢体的冷损伤。受体处的切除操作均在无菌止血带控制下进行。根据不同的移植部位水平,受体侧的皮瓣从腹侧向背侧掀起或者从桡侧向尺侧掀起,供体侧则按照相反的方向掀起。必须注意保留小静脉及其分支,其对静脉重建至关重要。避免过多地游离皮瓣及动脉蒂,以免发生无血管化和大出血等急性并发症以及进展性动脉病变,影响长期预后[22]。切除范围仅限于满足充分暴露的需要。任何影响肢体功能或软组织活性的瘢痕组织均需切除。将永久墨水写的标记条缝合在个体组织上标记其肌肉-肌腱单元,直至确认所有有名字的动脉、神经及肌肉-肌腱单元。暴露前臂骨骼,当供体肢体准备完成后再行截骨术。行单侧移植时,应与对侧前臂长度相匹配。行双侧移植时,必须保证两侧前臂具有同样长度,并且与患者身高相适应,同时保证足够的肌腱、神经、血管及软组织长度。修整供体肢体时进行同样的准备。此时释放止血带并加压包扎前臂,同时进行仔细止血。

决定好骨骼长度后,行桡骨截骨术,此时供体侧和受体侧肢体准备小组合二为一。供体肢体在血运重建之前必须始终保持在冰上。笔者常在修整台上处理桡骨和尺骨。桡骨截骨术完成后切断尺骨。使用斜行截骨术可以帮助最大化接骨面,并且限制尺骨的移动。使用3.5mm锁定加压钢板(LCP)进行刚性固定。这便于在前臂中前部区域进行负重治疗。对于前臂远部区域,笔者推荐使用桡骨远端及尺骨远端掌侧锁定延伸钢板。对于肘上移植,我们仅使用一根4.5mm LCP固定于前外侧。

进行到此,手术技术与既往所有标准复位技术有一定的差别[20,21]。如果肢体缺血时间相对较短,外科医生可以在血运重建前继续重建肌肉-肌腱单元及神经,从而缩短手术时间并减少出血。但是,什么是相对较短的缺血时间还不得而知(参见前文)。笔者通常在血运重建前完成所有伸肌肌腱重建、大部分屈肌肌腱重建及一些神经重建。

在移植中保持肌腱平衡与常规复位手术不同。复位手术中不存在相对肌腱平衡这一说法。首先重建伸肌,将手指放置于完全伸展的位置,将手腕放置于中度屈曲位置,使用手腕屈曲20°~30°位置缝合肌腱,保证手指可以完全伸展开。随后重建手腕伸肌。此时可以快速重建较大的背侧静脉。但是,如果静脉显示不清或者快速吻合重建无法进行,笔者建议直接进行屈肌肌腱重建。重建指深屈肌、表浅肌腱及拇长屈肌。手腕屈肌的重建可以在血运重建之后。此时,神经可以在没有大量出血的条件下重建,或者可以先行血运重建。分束重建神经,分别重建骨间前神经或骨间前神经群(如果可能的话)、运动束及感觉束、正中神经及尺神经。表浅的桡神经、背侧尺侧皮神经、掌侧皮神经分别进行重建。

大型静脉可以在无血状态下快速吻合。条件允许的情况下,笔者推荐使用静脉耦合装置,具有一定可靠性且可以节省时间。小静脉可以在血运重建后吻合,此时其更易识别。动脉重建时尽量保留足够多的管壁。动脉重建包括肱动脉、桡动脉、尺动脉和(或)骨间前动脉。对于前臂中远段移植,端-端吻合桡动脉、尺动脉、骨间前动脉及其伴行的静脉。对于肘上移植,无须保留受体任何远端肢体,仅需行肱动脉端-端吻合。需要注意的是,供体在ICU时曾行肱动脉置管,肱动脉很容易发生血栓。这可以导致移植物急性衰竭,但笔者曾经仅仅使用尺动脉吻合恢复动脉血供成功完成了一例此类移植[23]。动脉阻断钳开放血流恢复后,再将肢体从冰上移除。使用温盐水进行肢体复温及血管再通。可以从未缝合的静脉中放血几分钟,直至肢体发黑的部位重新恢复正常颜色。放出的血可以进行回收再利用。

移植物成功再灌注后,重建所有剩余可识别的血管及神经。这常常是手术中最耗时的部分。足够的静脉血流尤为重要,但是很难达到。笔者建议每只手至少重建4根静脉,越多越好。笔者通常使用超声多普勒探头评估哪只静脉最为可靠。移植的显微操作步骤完成后,重建表浅的屈肌肌腱-运动单元,并彻底止血。缝合重建4片皮瓣。切除任何血供不良的皮瓣组织。如果有皮肤缺损,需要从供体处获得皮肤移植物。最后,使用大量纱布及非加压夹板固定,并保证手指不被遮挡。脉搏血氧饱和度探头放置在拇指及小指上,并将血氧饱和度及波形与对侧自体手进行比较,在行双侧移植时,则与对侧移植手及另一参照测量点进行比较。

供体腹壁获取的外科技术

在获取胸腹部器官时可以同时安全获取腹壁移植物(或皮瓣),仅需改良一些手术步骤。正中切口仅延伸至剑突下,随后行双侧肋缘下切口,两侧至腹直肌鞘边缘,下至腹股沟区。随后行横行耻骨上切口[24]。完整切开腹壁,保留深部的腹壁下血管完整并将其向足侧掀开,充分显露需要获取的腹部器官。腹部器官获取完成后再继续进行后续步骤。此时,附着在髂总血管/髂外血管上的腹壁血管蒂已经游离并灌注了保存液。获取腹壁移植物的同时获取远端的腔静脉及主动脉,或者髂总血管/髂外血管的一部分,用于大血管的吻合[24]。也可以直接将腹壁移植物上的腹壁下血管从髂外血管上游离,用于显微吻合[25]。随后用湿纱布包裹腹壁移植物,三层包装,并按照标准操作步骤放在冰上进行转运。

受体外科技术：腹壁移植

腹壁移植常在腹腔多器官移植或小肠移植之后进行[26]。成功进行上述移植后，受体血管已经游离并准备完善。将获取的近端血管（远端主动脉，近端髂总血管）与受体髂总动脉/静脉或肾下主动脉、下腔静脉行端–侧吻合。有时，也可用显微外科技术将更远端、更细小的深部腹壁下血管与受体同名血管或髂血管循环行端–端吻合[24-26]。理论上可以尝试腹壁浅血管吻合及深部腹壁下血管吻合，但并没有十分必要。既往报道的病例中也无须吻合运动神经[26]。

保证腹壁足够的动脉流入及静脉流出后，缝合筋膜、皮下组织及皮肤，可以通过植入式多普勒探头、手持式多普勒探头，以及皮肤颜色、毛细血管充盈度、水肿及肿胀来监测腹壁移植物活性。

一项新技术将与肝脏相连的腹壁/筋膜移植物同时移植。腹壁后筋膜通过镰状韧带与肝脏相连并获得血供，已经在儿童肝移植受体中成功运用，尽管在报道的病例中，受体的皮肤均使用自身皮肤进行缝合，但是这一方法提供了额外的筋膜组织用于关闭手术切口。这一复合移植物称为腹直肌后鞘（PORSH）–肝脏复合带血管蒂移植物[27,28]。

外科技术：面部

移植前解剖综述

所有接受面部移植的受体都要和其他接受面部骨骼手术的患者一样进行评估[29]。手术团队记录每位受体面部各部分的骨骼缺陷尤为重要，包括：①上 1/3（颅骨）；②中 1/3；③下 1/3。以此为基础，移植团队将要为每位受体制订个体化的方案[30]。所有缺失面部结构的相对解剖及功能都将要进行详细评估，便于移植团队使用个体化自由组织移植进行预见性重建。所有已经存在的血管流入/流出通道都在移植前的头颈部筛查期进行记录[31]。详细的术前影像学评估包括三维 CT 扫描重建及血管造影（图 64.1）。需要注意的是，移植团队必须知道供体和受体两者的手术史或用药史以及明确的面部器官周围骨骼解剖结构，因为皮瓣修复及受体准备具有同等难度。

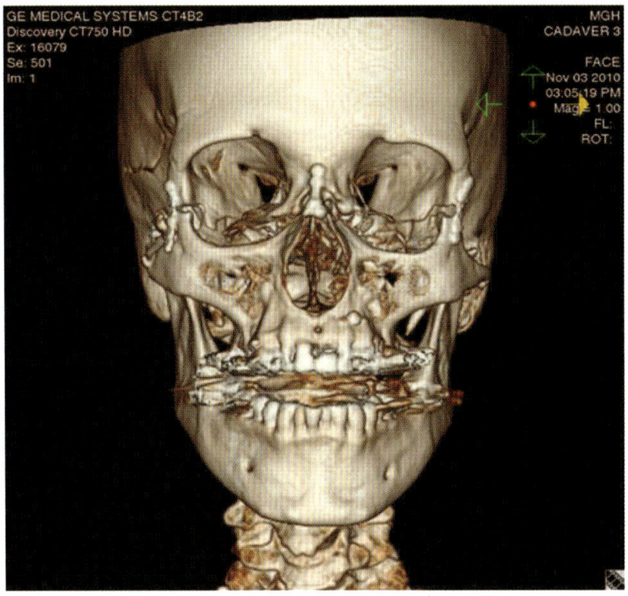

图 64.1　受体三维 CT 成像扫描（正面图）。

移植步骤：时间及逻辑

供体及受体的手术时间及协调由受体移植前解剖结构的复杂程度决定。以我们在约翰·霍普金斯大学的团队为例，整个团队包括整形及重建外科医师、颌面外科医师、显微外科医师、面部整形外科医师及头颈外科医师等。对于那些需要进行复杂截骨术的病例，我们建议将供体转运至我中心并使用相邻的两间手术室分别进行供受体手术。这便于我们协调两个团队，一个团队以颌面外科专家为基础，另一团队则以头颈外科专家和显微外科专家为基础。如果两间手术室相邻，我们则同时开始供体手术（VCA 复苏）和受体手术（移植前准备）。但是，如果受体存在大量面部瘢痕组织及复杂的微解剖结构，我们常推迟供体手术直至受体手术取得一定的进展[32]。理想情况下，皮瓣切除与目标血管及神经的标记同时结束。如果受体的分离出现延迟，仅将供体皮瓣充分游离以减少皮瓣缺血时间。但是，如果皮瓣需要在其他中心获取时，上述条件则无法达成。此时，则按照实体器官移植运输标准将皮瓣灌注，用湿纱布包裹并置于冰上保存转运。

供体面部移植物获取外科技术

移植前必须进行选择性气管切开（经皮或者开放）以保证头颈部的安全通路及维持供体稳定。某些情况下，患者可能已处于气管插管条件下。考虑到面部移植的特殊性,需要进行一些特殊的逻辑安排,在获取面部移植物的同时不影响胸腹部器官的获取。Brazio 等人对此进行了详细描述[33],参见图 64.2。按照受体缺陷及美学单位的边缘需要进行皮肤及软组织的切除。为了监测移植物活性,包括笔者团队在内,选择在皮瓣下部存留一部分皮肤便于进行皮肤活检。其他团队则获取第二个皮瓣(前哨皮瓣)以达到该目的。笔者认为保留富余的组织优于获取前哨皮瓣,因为面部皮肤排斥反应在不同的解剖部位各不相同[34]。尽可能在近端切除供体面部血管。手术用显微镜常用于显微血管神经重建。如果因为刺激颈动脉球部发生血管迷走反射,可将 1%利多卡因注射入颈动脉球部。某些情况下,暴露面部血管需要进行下颌角截骨。医生必须在移植前根据血管造影图像评估最合适的面部血管。这包括颞浅血管供应上 1/3,面横血管/颞浅血管供应中 1/3,以及同侧颈部血管供应下 1/3。

如果理想血管无法获取,则可以选择其他替代血管,如从颈外静脉和(或)颈内静脉系统发出的颈部血管分支等。发生严重面部损伤时,上述情况更为常见。这会延长手术时间,所以必须在手术前提前规划。移植前影像学检查(如超声多普勒、血管造影等)为显微手术团队提供了目标血管的重要信息,可以节省手术时间并避免移植失败。同时,皮瓣中包含的面部组织不同(软组织结合或不结合骨骼组织),其血供也不同。克利夫兰的经验表明,双侧面动脉血管可以供应大部分面部皮肤、腺体组织、肌肉及改良 Le Fort-Ⅲ颌面结构[35]。其他研究也表明,面部骨骼的骨膜血管也供应了一定的血液[36]。如果皮瓣包含一侧颈部组织、耳、头皮或者前额,则必须在复苏过程中保留颞浅血管、颌内血管和(或)面部分支。除此之外,切除颅面时需尽可能保留骨膜以保证其活性。无论选择哪支血管,需尽可能由近端切除,使得管腔足够大便于吻合,减少技术性失败风险。但是,必须避免在颈动脉分叉部切断颈动脉,以免减少颈内动脉血流引起急性脑水肿。游离切除动脉或

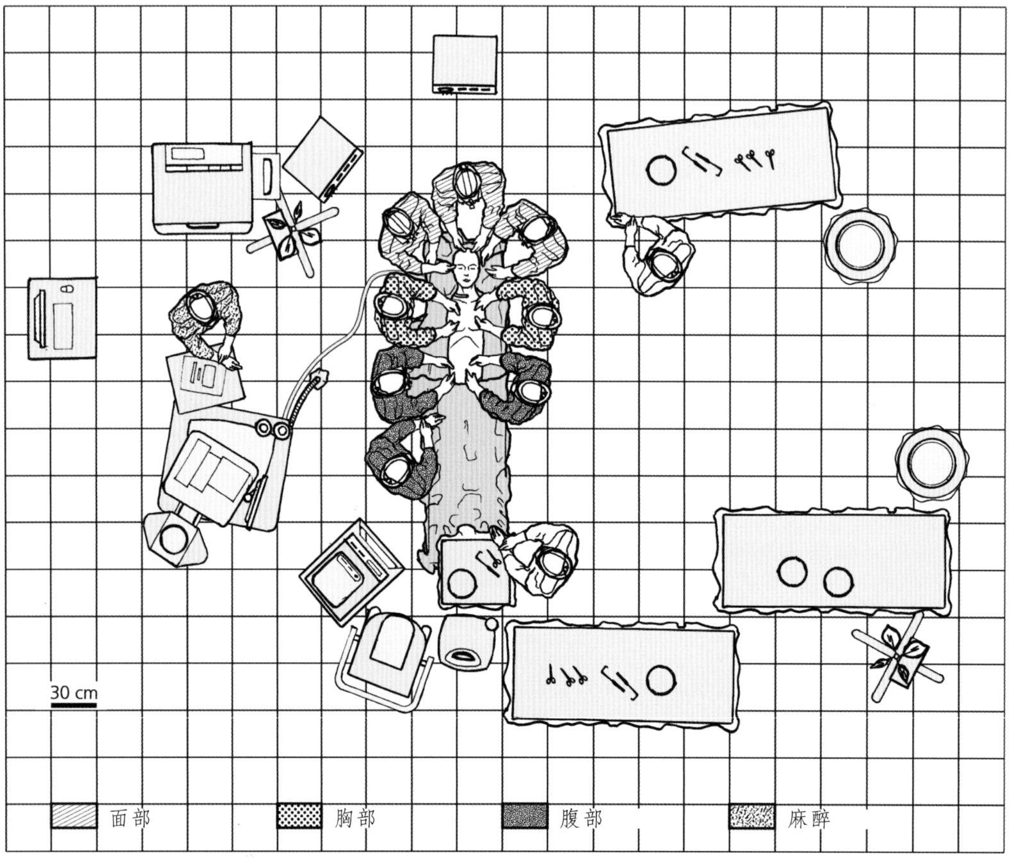

图 64.2 用于包括面部在内多器官获取的供体手术室布局。这一布局可以让面部、胸部、腹部团队同时工作。除了标准麻醉及监测的仪器外,还有两个手术灯、两个单极及一个双极点除颤仪、三个吸引器及两个头灯。手术台头侧及尾侧各有一个分别供面部及实体器官团队使用的手术台,还有一个用于器官修整的手术台。(From Brazio et al. 2013[33], with permission.)

静脉后，辨认双侧面神经分支。通常情况下，主要静脉回流进入颈外静脉系统。在茎乳孔水平游离面神经可以将皮瓣游离至供体神经主干水平。相反，波士顿小组则建议行远端神经缝合，以避免连带运动[37]。

如果条件允许，Le Fort 为基础的截骨术最好在最终皮瓣复苏前进行，以减少骨头出血。截骨范围需要按照受体需求，并最好在包裹的软组织已经切除并且标记完成后进行。颌面外科团队在 Le Fort 复苏期间要求相对低血压麻醉及反 Trendelenburg 位，以减少医源性出血。颌面部皮瓣复苏中另一重要环节是合理暴露下眶底便于行 Le Fort 截骨。可以使用小型电锯（Sonopet and Nakagawa Serrated Knife，Stryker，Inc.，Kalamazoo，ML）以保护供体眼球用于角膜捐献。如果受体颌面部缺陷主要在前部，常使用“单板法”。该法需要获取上颌骨前壁、内侧壁及外侧壁，保留上颌骨的其他部分及与其相连的软组织及韧带。

面部移植团队需要在术前与其他实体器官移植团队进行沟通协调，协调某些操作，如血管插管和血管钳夹，以免干扰获取其他救命的实体器官。每个团队都需要知道其他任何团队的手术方案及具体技术，便于统一协调。我们常在其他实体器官移植团队开始操作前复苏面部皮瓣并用专用面具覆盖。其目的是为了防止对实体器官复苏过程产生任何重大干扰，同时在将供体从手术室转运至停尸房的过程中可以保护供体身份。为保证供体遗容完整，获取完成后均需要佩戴人工面具。

受体手术技术：面部移植

供体团队在复苏面部时，受体团队同时分离并准备受体的头颈部以减少总缺血时间。仔细识别和标记可行的神经及血管末端，切除瘢痕并游离皮瓣用于缝合。所有血管神经末端都需要游离足够的长度用于吻合。移植前，将移植皮瓣中的 UW 液冲洗干净并用冰的乳酸林格液进行灌注。

与四肢重建类似，面部移植首先需要进行局部骨接合术以保持稳定，便于行血管神经重建。根据受体面部受损情况的不同，颅骨接合术包括上颌骨、眼眶、下颌骨、颧上颌复合体和（或）颅穹隆。移植皮瓣的硬质部分使用钛板或钛钉固定。某些情况下，供体面部骨骼宽度宽于或窄于受体，此时必须使用一定的手术技术（如青枝骨折等）修整供体两侧颧骨距离以与受体颧骨弓相适应[29,30]。同时，需要保证移植物的宽度和投影能在 X 轴、Y 轴和 Z 轴上准确定位，保证适当的牙齿吸合以及眼眶体积。笔者团队使用一种全新的“混合夹板”技术以及移植前头影测量预测合适的 Le Fort 插入位置。需要注意的是，如果供体和（或）受体口腔卫生条件不佳或者存在牙周疾病，往往会影响该移植步骤。进行颌面部移植前，需要进行术前口腔准备或拔牙，这会减少受体接受终身免疫治疗后发生感染并发症的风险。如果必须拔除供体上颌骨或者下颌骨的牙齿，则采用改良 Gunning 夹保证合适的上颌骨与下颌骨的位置关系。

Le Fort-Ⅲ型重建时也需要注意额鼻窦管道的位置，避免因移植引起引流阻塞而导致感染和（或）黏膜液囊肿。因此，使用高速电钻进入供体额窦黏膜时应谨慎，根据团队的需要，必要时要堵住额窦通道。单纯额鼻窦接骨术可以让微创手术团队完成单侧血管重建，并保证对侧灌注并减少缺血时间。从游离瓣分离到第一条动脉和静脉修复开通所需要的总缺血时间尤为重要。当所有面部组织灌注完成后，颌面外科医生可以根据受体稳定的骨骼继续完成剩余的接骨术，目的是使用多种适用的方法创造最佳的混合骨骼，详见上文描述（图 64.1 和图 64.3）。

接骨术及血管灌注完成后，尽可能修复面神经及感觉神经。可以游离供体的神经用于受体神经修复，如脊髓副神经、腓肠神经、迷走神经、耳大神经及舌下神经等。笔者建议使用感觉神经修复感觉神经损伤，使用运动神经修复运动神经损伤。同时也需要考虑合适的神经直径大小。根据患者损伤机制不同，有时往往难以和（或）无法修复全部的感觉神经分支。但是，需要尽可能修复三叉神经的所有分支。并且，如果面神经主干存在瘢痕，则需要行乳突切除术松解面神经。最终目的是无张力吻合双侧供受体面神经。笔者常保留供体腮腺以保证面部组织完整性，从而防止可能的同种异体皮瓣的血管损伤和（或）小的面部神经分支的医源性损伤。这会导致受体术后短期内下面部肿胀。但是，多余的组织可以用于组织活检。在后期，软组织修复阶段，所有的外部软组织均可切除以达到最佳的美学效果。

对于感觉神经长度不够的受体，可使用眶底接骨术增加眶下神经长度用于重建。仅当受体面部解剖结构完全清晰时才可行这一操作。有意思的是，由于受到近距离弹道损伤，尽管其在行移植手术时无法进行眶下神经重建，这位克利夫兰的患者仍获得了满意的两

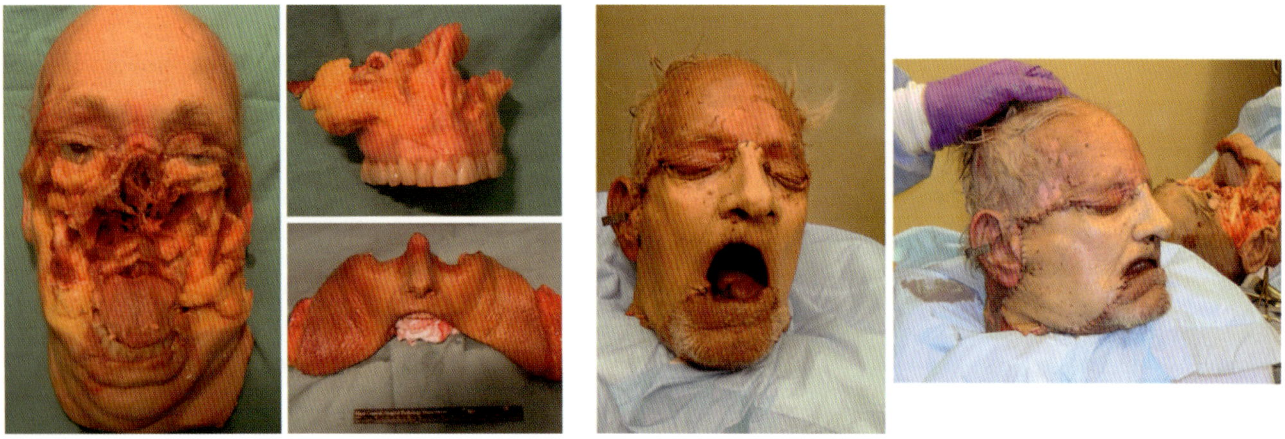

图 64.3　尸体面部移植的正面及侧面照(无牙齿技术),展示Ⅰ类骨骼关系。

点辨别能力[38]。

最后,需要使用多层缝合法缝合软组织,同时需要妥善放置和固定闭合负压引流管。在移植开始时所做的皮肤切口设计应确保供体-受体皮肤边缘的无张力闭合。更重要的是,切口应位于美学单位的交界处,并落在美学线内(如鼻唇沟)。如果皮肤覆盖不完全,则可能需要供体皮肤的移植物进行闭合。使用抗菌软膏剂及纱布覆盖伤口便于术后 1 周行物理治疗。此种类型手术后很难减少不必要的运动。因此建议使用气管切开辅助呼吸并使用胃造瘘进行营养支持。

颅颌面移植的特殊注意事项

最近的一项尸体解剖研究中,Gordon 及其同事[34]评估了保留面部骨骼系统的面部移植正颌操作的价值。关键步骤和操作(如牙弓夹板制作及头影测量)可以提高最终面部骨骼移植效果。其优点为:①优化了供体与受体间的“混合阻塞”;②为手术团队在皮瓣植入或内固定时如何达到面部-骨骼协调提供了指导;③增强了预测术中及术后供受体间硬组织不相合的能力。采用此法后,所有面部移植患者均得到了更好的混合阻塞及面部-骨骼协调。

面部游离瓣中同时包含下巴时(如颌面部移植物),必须尽全力提高受体混合阻塞(两个下巴的口腔关系)。首先,必须在移植过程中,使用“混合阻塞夹板”(供体在一侧,受体在另一侧)方法将供体上颌与受体下颌组成合适的混合阻塞。其次,在对眼眶行内固定的同时评估受体眼眶体积、颧骨突起程度及鼻额交界处。这可以帮助确定受体下颌骨的旋转程度以获得正颌效果(如Ⅰ类骨骼关系)。比如,如果受体下颌平面角陡峭,上颌骨突出(如Ⅱ类关系),则需要将面部及下巴游离瓣逆时针旋转(从右侧看),保证鼻额交界处合适的骨距。这可以使某些嵌塞从位于颧额区后外侧的受体骨中拔除,从而提升面中部及下颌部在矢状位上的投影。采用这些手段可以提高受体整体面部-骨骼形态(与移植前相比)并保证理想的眼眶体积(图 64.4)。但是,这会导致上颌后牙过度垂直几毫米以及上骨段会存在间隙。这种情况下,上颌后牙垂直过度临床表现为

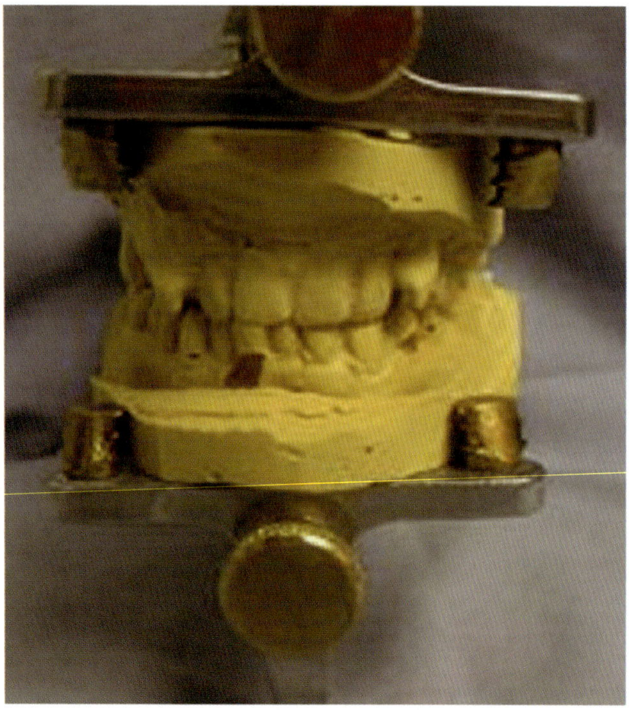

图 64.4　最佳闭合的供体上颌及受体下颌模型。

前牙区开殆。这一潜在问题可以在术前合理预测,并可以通过创造一个较小的前牙区开殆保证理想的面部-骨骼投影关系以及优化面中部凸度和眼眶体积。可以在术后采用截骨术之外的方法纠正开殆(这两项技术在伤口愈合受损、上颌截骨术后的血管生成问题及强制免疫抑制方面都具有一定挑战性)。对于移植术后开殆的矫正有两种方法。对于较小的前牙区开殆,可以通过非手术方法解决,包括后牙区调殆、磨牙压低或迷你锚固装置等。或者也可采用延迟双侧矢状劈开截骨术(BSSO),联合后期的二次美容手术[39]。第二种方法并不推荐,因其也存在前文提到的伤口难以愈合和免疫抑制等问题。但是下颌骨的血运并不会受到影响。比如,Ⅱ型骨骼形态患者可以在术后 6~12 个月进行处理,可采用 BSSO 方法及下颌前移术或后推术,并结合双侧供体腮腺切除术及皮肤剪裁术(如面部及颈部皮肤上提等)。

技术失败时的外科策略

与其他所有微创操作一样,术后早期均有发生动脉和(或)静脉并发症的风险。此时,面部移植物需要立即行血管修复,必须在 ICU 密切监测面部移植物氧合水平,至少 48 小时。如能早期诊断血运异常,往往可以挽救。但是,也有移植手术或挽救手术失败的风险,需要移除面部移植物。这种手术必须按照机构审查委员会流程进行。流程必须对挽救手术的操作技术方式进行详细描述。很多情况下,手术方式为皮肤移植和(或)自体游离组织移植。值得注意的是,我们应该考虑选用肩胛-肩胛周围游离皮瓣,因其具有较大的面积并且在面部严重畸形患者中保存较为完整。

手术技术:喉部、气管

喉部移植相关解剖注意事项

带血管喉部同种异体移植术是较为少见的一种 VCA 手术。至今为止,美国境内仅实施 2 例此类手术,其中仅有 Marshall 博士 1998 年在克利夫兰诊所实施的 1 例在文献中进行了详细的报道[40]。

尽管报道的结果(包括功能性声音、保护性咳嗽反应及没有误吸的吞咽功能)相对较好,但是喉部移植仍有一些难题。根据发布的信息,下文讨论的手术细节均出自该病例。目前仍然有其他的喉部移植方式及手术技巧,甚至有些已经成功运用于动物模型上。未来详细的喉部移植手术方式目前还没有定论[41]。

喉部自身解剖结构的复杂性决定了喉部移植手术的难度。喉部包括气道、声带及其附属肌肉组织,以及提供支撑的软骨框架。但是,这些结构与周围的组织联系紧密,包括会厌上部、气管内部、甲状腺侧叶、下咽及食管后部等。因此,实施喉部移植手术时需要考虑上述器官的切除及保留问题。此外,喉部血供来自喉上动脉及喉下动脉,这是甲状腺上动脉及下动脉的分支。其他穿入喉部的动脉来自周围的咽部及食管,并与甲状腺及咽部下方、食管的血供相关。上述因素导致很难获得带血管蒂的喉部移植物,在获取过程中必须仔细设计。

另一个需要注意的关键问题是喉部的神经。所有喉部必要功能的恢复均需要声带的感觉及运动神经完全恢复。喉上神经提供保护性咳嗽反射避免误吸,还控制环甲肌调节声带张力,从而控制声音高低。但是,单独一个环甲肌并不足以完全松弛声带用于呼吸,还依赖于喉返神经,其控制喉部其余肌肉。不幸的是,修复喉返神经,即使是独立的损伤,也往往会导致连带运动。由于无法预测移植后的声带能否恢复神经控制,因此接受该手术的患者常常需要气管切开,并且该项手术的应用也受到限制[42]。

供体手术(获取)

既往无气道外伤史、手术史或肿瘤病史的患者可以作为潜在喉部移植供体。既往行甲状腺手术、存在喉部神经损伤或神经肌肉疾病的患者是捐献的绝对禁忌证。吸烟史则为相对禁忌证。整个咽喉复合体,包括甲状腺/甲状旁腺、咽部前壁及气管上段的一部分被完整切除。这一步骤可以在血管钳夹和胸部器官获取前或获取后进行,前提是供体在行气管整体切除的平面下进行了气管造口术。可以使用标准神经监测技术识别神经,但是,重要的是要记住一旦缺少血液灌注,运动神经功能会迅速丧失。获取颈内静脉保证其静脉血供完整。动脉供应可以在甲状腺上动脉和甲状腺下动脉、颈动脉或甲状腺颈干水平获取。获取完成后,供体移植物进行灌注,并用 UW 液保存。首例移植手术缺血时间约为 10 小时。

受体手术(移植)

移植手术中需要一直保持气道通畅,如果气道不通畅出现在手术开始时应行气管切开。切开位置应位于计划行气管修复的部位。仅当移植物可以移植时才可行移植手术,受体分离操作才可进行。暴露受体剩余喉部结构,切除周围组织及瘢痕。仔细辨认所有4条神经(在第一例手术中始终无法辨认左侧喉返神经)。辨认受体血管并使用标准微创吻合技术恢复血供。尽可能修复所有可以辨认的血管。首例移植病例中,甲状腺上动脉与受体甲状腺上动脉吻合,颈内静脉与受体右侧面静脉吻合。随后行喉部切除术,完整保留甲状腺,然后将移植物旋转置入。再次连接对侧甲状腺上动脉,并按照端-侧吻合方式将左侧甲状腺中静脉与受体左侧颈内静脉吻合。甲状软骨与舌骨上部固定。后侧使用约75%的受体喉部组织。下方在气管切开水平修复气管[43]。可以根据不同受体的不同解剖结构选择不同的修复方法,但是此种修复方法已经被证明是有效的。

气管移植相关解剖注意事项

气管重建仍然是充满挑战的一个手术,目前仍然没有找到理想的重建方法。尽管已经尝试多种方式重建气管,包括自体气管、异体气管、异体材料等,但是均未取得很好的长期效果[44]。这为重建移植在推进该领域发挥重要作用提供了机会。然而,气管重建面临巨大的挑战,尤其是气管的动脉、静脉血供使得我们难以设计一个合适的血管蒂用于移植。气管的主要血供来自甲状腺下动脉的分支,其穿过甲状腺后发出极小的分支供应气管。气管下1/3由支气管动脉供应,气管后部及黏膜则由食管旁血管的穿支供应。已经设计了几种包含不同血管蒂及相关组织的气管移植物的动物模型,其中包括甲状腺及食管等。尽管在上述动物模型中可以按照带血管蒂的移植物方式进行移植,但是在人体中尚无类似技术的报道。有些团队尝试使用自体气管移植物,在受体自身血管床上进行气管移植物血运重建[45,46],包括胸锁乳突肌、大网膜及前臂桡侧皮瓣等,并可以使用原位方法进行。但是,大多数病例是在进行血运重建后使用游离组织移植法将移植物再次移植入位。最近也是最有希望的研究来自比利时的Leuven气管移植小组,其技术方案详见下文[46,47]。

供体手术(获取)

获取胸部器官后,从环状软骨以下获取8cm长的一段气管,至双肺移植的气管交汇点。需要注意在移除甲状腺及食管的同时不要损伤气管本身的其他附属结构。用UW液低温保存移植物。冷缺血时间可能高达10小时。同时从供体获取一块全层皮肤移植物并用同法保存。

受体手术(移植)

通过游离前臂桡侧皮瓣区域的皮肤,准备受体血管床用于第一阶段移植物放置。桡动脉及其筋膜用于气管移植物血运重建的血管床。按照长轴与前臂平行的方式放置移植物,并保证气管上端放在前臂近端,以便气管转入颈部后气管纤毛在位。既往手术中发现气管黏膜在血运重建前即坏死。因此在将气管放置在前臂的过程中移除气管黏膜。获取全层颊黏膜置入气管的黏膜部分。随后关闭前臂桡侧皮肤并将气管断端留在体表便于引流及观察。将供体皮肤缝合在受体耳部用于免疫监测,共监测4个月,此时免疫抑制反应逐渐变弱。当耳后的皮肤移植物完全排斥而气管移植物还存活时,可以进一步进行气管移植。这一阶段,将桡动脉及前臂筋膜共同移除并将其作为游离皮瓣。可以同时移除表面皮肤覆盖颈部或监测前哨皮瓣。否则,在提起皮瓣之前皮瓣就被分离,而前臂皮肤还留在手臂上。随后移除损毁的气道并用移植物代替。放置移植物的同时进行经口气管插管并保持在位。按照标准微创吻合手法将桡血管与受体颈部合适的血管进行吻合。建议将一部分皮瓣或筋膜暴露于皮肤表面用于监测移植物微循环状态,并可在患者离院后切除。当患者不需要接受机械通气时则可拔除气管插管,必要时可以在术后早期放置气管支架。

总结

尽管最初存在怀疑和争论,但重建性移植目前已经成为临床现实。正如本章所阐述,VCA移植手术技术已经较为成熟,已经不是该种手术应用的障碍。无可否认的是,微创手术技术仍然是各种类型重建性移植手术的重中之重。良好的结果需要高超的手术技术、有效的免疫抑制治疗、良好的患者依从性以及密切随访。随着我们经验的积累,该类手术的安全性、有效性及适用性必将逐渐提高,最终使患者受益。

(倪彦彬 译 朱继业 校)

参考文献

1. Black KS, Hewitt CW, Fraser LA, et al. Cosmas and Damian in the laboratory. New England Journal of Medicine. 1982;306:368–369.
2. Malt RA, Mckhann C. Replantation of several arms. Journal of the American Medical Association. 1964;189:716–722.
3. Dubernard JM, Owen E, Herzberg G, et al. Human hand allograft: report on first 6 months. Lancet. 1999;353:1315–1320.
4. Hewitt CW, Lee WPA, Gordon CR. Transplantation of Composite Tissue Allografts. New York, NY: Springer; 2008.
5. Swearingen B, Ravindra K, Xu H, et al. Science of composite tissue allotransplantation. Transplantation. 2008;86:627–635.
6. Schneeberger S, Landin L, Jableki J, et al. Achievements and challenges in composite tissue allotransplantation. Transplant International. 2011;24: 760–769.
7. Petruzzo P, Lanzetta M, Dubernard JM, et al. The international registry on hand and composite tissue transplantation. Transplantation. 2010;90: 1590–1594.
8. Shores JT. Recipient screening and selection: who is the right candidate for hand transplantation. Hand Clinics. 2011;27:539–543.
9. Dobbels F, Vanhaecke J, Dupont L, et al. Pretransplant predictors of posttransplant adherence and clinical outcome: an evidence base for pretransplant psychosocial screening. Transplantation. 2009;87:1497–1504.
10. McDiarmid SV, Azari KK. Donor-related issues in hand transplantation. Hand Clinics. 2011;27:545–552.
11. Schneeberger S, Lucchina S, Lanzetta M, et al. Cytomegalovirus-related complications in human hand transplantation. Transplantation. 2005;80:441–447.
12. Gordon CR, Avery R, Abouhassan W, et al. Cytomegalovirus and other infectious issues related to face transplantation: specific considerations, lessons learned, and future recommendations. Plastic and Reconstructive Surgery. 2011;127: 1515–1523.
13. Gordon CR, Abouhassan W, Avery RK. What is the true significance of donor-related cytomegalovirus transmission in the setting of facial composite tissue allotransplantation? Transplantation Proceedings. 2011;43:3516–3520.
14. Anker AE, Feeley TH. Asking the difficult questions: message strategies used by organ procurement coordinators in requesting familial consent to organ donation. Journal of Health Communication. 2011;16:643–659.
15. McDiarmid SV, Pruett TL, Graham WK. The oversight of solid organ transplantation in the United States. American Journal of Transplantation. 2008;8:739–744.
16. Cendales L, Granger D, Henry M, et al. Implementation of vascularized composite allografts in the United States: recommendations from the ASTS VCA Ad Hoc Committee and the Executive Committee. American Journal of Transplantation. 2011;11:13–17.
17. Cendales LC, Rahmel A, Pruett TL. Allocation of vascularized composite allografts: what is it? Transplantation. 2012;93:1086–1087.
18. Aravindan N, Williams MT, Riedel BJ, et al. Transcriptional responses of rat skeletal muscle following hypoxia-reoxygenation and near ischaemia-reperfusion. Acta Physiologica Scandinavica. 2005;183:367–377.
19. Nanobashvili J, Neumayer C, Fügl A, et al. Ischemia/reperfusion injury of skeletal muscle: plasma taurine as a measure of tissue damage. Surgery. 2003;133: 91–100.
20. Hartzell TL, Benhaim P, Imbriglia JE, et al. Surgical and technical aspects of hand transplantation: is it just another replant? Hand Clinics. 2011;27:521–530.
21. Azari KK, Imbriglia JE, Goitz RJ, et al. Technical aspects of the recipient operation in hand transplantation. Journal of Reconstructive Microsurgery. 2012;28:27–34.
22. Kaufman CL, Ouseph R, Blair B, et al. Graft vasculopathy in clinical hand transplantation. American Journal of Transplantation. 2012;12:1004–1016.
23. Jablecki J, Kaczmarzyk L, Domanasiewicz A, et al. First Polish forearm transplantation—final report (outcome after 4 years). Annals of Transplantation. 2010;15:61–67.
24. Levi DM, Tzakis AG, Kato T, et al. Transplantation of the abdominal wall. Lancet. 2003;361:2173–2176.
25. Cipriani R, Contedini F, Santoli M, et al. Abdominal wall transplantation with microsurgical technique. American Journal of Transplantation. 2007;7: 1304–1307.
26. Selvaggi G, Levi DM, Cipriani R, et al. Abdominal wall transplantation: surgical and immunologic aspects. Transplantation Proceedings. 2009;41:521–522.
27. Agarwal S, Dorafshar AH, Harland RC, et al. Liver and vascularized posterior rectus sheath fascia composite tissue allotransplantation. American Journal of Transplantation. 2010;10:2712–2716.
28. Lee JC, Lopez-Soler R, Renz JF, et al. Expanding the envelope: The PORSH-liver composite vascular allograft. Presented on January 16, 2012 at the American Society for Reconstructive Microsurgery 2012 Annual Meeting, Las Vegas, NV.
29. Gordon CR, Susarla S, Peacock Z, et al. Lefort-based maxillofacial transplantation: current state-of-the-art and refined technique. Journal of Craniofacial Surgery. 2012;23:81–87.
30. Gordon CR, Susarla S, Peacock Z, et al. Osteocutaneous maxillofacial allotransplantation: lessons learned from a novel cadaver study applying orthognathic principles and practice. Plastic and Reconstructive Surgery. 2011;128:465e–479e.
31. Gordon CR, Siemionow M, Coffman K, et al. The Cleveland clinic FACES score: a preliminary assessment tool for identifying the optimal face transplant candidate. Journal of Craniofacial Surgery. 2009;20:1969–1974.
32. Siemionow M, Gordon CR. Overview of guidelines for establishing a face transplant program: a work in progress. American Journal of Transplantation. 2010;10:1290–1296.
33. Brazio PS, Barth RN, Bojovis B, et al. Algorithm for Total Face and Multiorgan Procurement From a Brain-Dead Donor. American Journal of Transplantation. 2013;13:2743–2749.
34. Gordon CR, Zor F, Siemionow M. Skin area quantification in preparation for concomitant upper extremity and face transplantation: a cadaver study and literature review. Transplantation. 2011;91:1050–1056.
35. Siemionow M, Papay F, Alam D, et al. First U.S. near- total human face transplantation—a paradigm shift for massive facial injuries. Lancet. 2009; 374:203–209.
36. Lantieri L, Hivelin M, Audard V, et al. Feasibility, reproducibility, risks and benefits of face transplantation: a prospective study of outcomes. American Journal of Transplantation. 2011;11:367–378.
37. Pomahac B, Pribaz J, Eriksson E, et al. Three patients with full facial transplantation. New England Journal of Medicine. 2012;366:715–722.
38. Siemionow M, Papay F, Djohan R, et al. First U.S. near-total human face transplantation—a paradigm shift for massive complex injuries. Plastic and Reconstructive Surgery. 2010;125:111–122.
39. Meningaud JP, Hivelin M, Benjoar MD, et al. The procurement of allotransplants for ballistic trauma: a preclinical study and a report of two clinical cases. Plastic and Reconstructive Surgery. 2011;127:1892–1900.
40. Knott PD, Hicks D, Braun W, et al. A 12-year perspective on the world's first total laryngeal transplant. Transplantation. 2011;91:804–805.
41. Broumand B, Rambod M. Laryngeal transplantation: neglected Cinderella or rising phoenix? Transplantation. 2007;84:1561–1562.
42. Birchall MA, Lorenz RR, Berke GS, et al. Laryngeal transplantation in 2005: a review. American Journal of Transplantation. 2006;6:20–26.
43. Guntinas-Lichius O. Outcomes 18 months after the first human partial face transplantation. New England Journal of Medicine. 2008;358:2179–2180.
44. Smith LP, Zur KB, Jacobs IN. Single- vs double-stage laryngotracheal reconstruction. Archives of Otolaryngology—Head and Neck Surgery. 2010;136:60–65.
45. Levashov Y, Yablonsky PK, Cherny SM, et al. One-stage allotransplantation of thoracic segment of the trachea in a patient with idiopathic fibrosing mediastinitis and marked tracheal stenosis. European Journal of Cardio-Thoracic Surgery. 1993;7:383–386.
46. Klepetko W, Marta GM, Wisser W, et al. Heterotopic tracheal transplantation with omentum wrapping in the abdominal position preserves functional and structural integrity of a human tracheal allograft. Journal of Thoracic and Cardiovascular Surgery. 2004;127:862–867.
47. Bader A, Macchiarini P. Moving towards in situ tracheal regeneration: the bionic tissue engineered transplantation approach. Journal of Cellular and Molecular Medicine. 2010;14:1877–1889.

“十三五”国家重点图书出版规划项目
天津市重点出版扶持项目

Textbook of Organ Transplantation

Volume 2

器官移植学

下 卷

〔美〕艾伦·D. 柯克 等 主编
朱继业 徐 骁 李 照 主译

天津出版传媒集团
天津科技翻译出版有限公司

著作权合同登记号:图字:02-2016-05

图书在版编目(CIP)数据

器官移植学/(美)艾伦·D.柯克(Allan D. Kirk)等主编;朱继业,徐骁,李照主译.—天津:天津科技翻译出版有限公司,2020.3

书名原文:Textbook of Organ Transplantation

ISBN 978-7-5433-4014-5

Ⅰ.①器… Ⅱ.①艾… ②朱… ③徐… ④李… Ⅲ.①器官移植 Ⅳ.①R617

中国版本图书馆 CIP 数据核字(2020)第 039496 号

授权单位: John Wiley & Sons Limited
出　　版: 天津科技翻译出版有限公司
出 版 人: 刘子媛
地　　址: 天津市南开区白堤路 244 号
邮政编码: 300192
电　　话: 022-87894896
传　　真: 022-87895650
网　　址: www.tsttpc.com
印　　刷: 山东临沂新华印刷物流集团有限责任公司
发　　行: 全国新华书店
版本记录: 889mm×1194mm　16 开本　119 印张　3600 千字
2020 年 3 月第 1 版　2020 年 3 月第 1 次印刷
定价:680.00 元(上下卷)

(如有印装问题,可与出版社调换)

译者名单

主　译　朱继业　徐　骁　李　照

译校者　（按姓氏汉语拼音排序）

陈　峻　陈俊丽　陈康辰　程　倩　崔　笑　董思依　高　峰
高鹏骥　郭海军　郭颂一　郭靖珩　韩威力　胡士华　胡志平
焦守斐　柯庆宏　李　博　李　照　李仕进　李勇剑　林丽丹
林天雨　凌　琪　刘　鹏　刘　晓　刘以俊　刘原兴　刘治坤
马慧云　毛雨鸽　倪彦彬　倪一鸣　彭　鹏　秋宇典　沈　恬
汪　洋　王辉杭　王建国　王思奇　王亚洲　危荣沥　魏绪勇
文　雪　吴建永　奚　斌　肖增丽　谢文勇　向　骁　徐　骁
许庭珉　荀晓冬　杨　帆　杨崇威　杨梦凡　杨墨丹　禹　琛
张　超　张长坤　张大方　张龙辉　张云凯　赵海格　郑骏楠
周舒扬　朱凤雪　朱继业　卓建勇

主编名单

Allan D. Kirk, MD, PhD, FACS

Professor and Chairman, Department of Surgery
Duke University School of Medicine;
Surgeon-in-Chief for Duke University Health System
Duke University Medical Center
Durham, NC, USA

Stuart J. Knechtle, MD

Professor of Surgery
Emory University School of Medicine
Atlanta, GA, USA

Christian P. Larsen, MD, DPhil

Dean – Emory School of Medicine
Surgeon-in-Chief Emory Healthcare
Emory University
Atlanta, GA, USA

Joren C. Madsen, MD, DPhil

Professor of Surgery
W. Gerald and Patricia R. Austen
Distinguished Scholar in Cardiac Surgery
Massachusetts General Hospital
Boston, MA, USA

Thomas C. Pearson, MD

Emory Transplant Center
Emory University School of Medicine
Atlanta, GA, USA

Steven A. Webber, MBChB, MRCP

James C. Overall Professor and Chair, Department of Pediatrics
Monroe Carell Jr. Children's Hospital at Vanderbilt
Vanderbilt University School of Medicine
Nashville, TN, USA

编者名单

Michael Abecassis, MD, MBA
J. Roscoe Miller Distinguished Professor
Department of Surgery and
Microbiology-Immunology
Chief, Division of Organ Transplantation
Founding Director, Comprehensive Transplant Center
Northwestern University Feinberg School of Medicine
Chicago, IL, USA

Kareem M. Abu-Elmagd, MD, PhD, FACS
Professor of Surgery
Department of Surgery
Transplant Division
Intestinal Rehabilitation and Transplantation Center
University of Pittsburgh Medical Center
Pittsburgh, PA, USA

Andrew B. Adams, MD, PhD
Assistant Professor of Surgery
Emory Transplant Center
Emory University School of Medicine
Atlanta, GA, USA

Avinash Agarwal, MD, FACS
Assistant Professor of Surgery
Department of Surgery, University of Virginia
Charlottesville, VA, USA

Maria-Luisa Alegre, MD, PhD
Professor of Medicine
University of Chicago
Chicago, IL, USA

Rita R. Alloway, PharmD, FCCP
Research Professor of Medicine
Director, Transplant Clinical Research
Director, Transplant Pharmacy PGY 2 Residency and Fellowship
University of Cincinnati
Cincinnati, OH, USA

Winston A. Ally, PharmD, BCPS
Pharmacy Clinical Coordinator
Solid Organ Transplantation
Director, PGY-2 Solid Organ Transplant Pharmacy Residency
Department of Pharmacy Services
University of Virginia Health System
Charlottesville, VA;
Clinical Assistant Professor
Department of Pharmacotherapy and Outcomes Science
Virginia Commonwealth University School of Pharmacy
Richmond, VA, USA

Estella M. Alonso, MD
Professor of Pediatrics
Department of Pediatrics
Northwestern University Feinberg School of Medicine
Medical Director of Hepatology and Liver Transplantation
Ann and Robert H. Lurie Children's Hospital of Chicago
Chicago, IL, USA

Sandra Amaral, MD, MHS
Co-Director, Pediatric Kidney Transplant Program
Assistant Professor, University of Pennsylvania
The Children's Hospital of Philadelphia
Philadelphia, PA, USA

Douglas J. Anderson, MD
Senior Resident
Department of Surgery
Emory University School of Medicine
Atlanta, GA, USA

Vincent T. Armenti, MD, PhD
Principal Investigator
National Transplantation Pregnancy Registry (NTPR)
Gift of Life Institute
Philadelphia, PA;
Professor of Anatomy and Surgery
University of Central Florida College of Medicine
Orlando, FL, USA

Todd L. Astor, MD
Assistant Professor of Medicine, Harvard Medical School
Medical Director, Lung and Heart-Lung Transplant Program
Pulmonary and Critical Care Unit
Massachusetts General Hospital
Boston, MA, USA

Robin K. Avery, MD
Professor of Medicine
Johns Hopkins University School of Medicine
Infectious Disease Division
Johns Hopkins Hospital
Baltimore, MD, USA

David A. Axelrod, MD, MBA
Section Chief, Solid Organ Transplant Surgery
Dartmouth Hitchcock Medical Center
Lebanon, NH, USA

Agnes M. Azimzadeh, PhD
Assistant Professor of Surgery
University of Maryland School of Medicine
Baltimore, MD, USA

Raul Badell, MD
Chief Resident
Department of Surgery
Emory University School of Medicine
Atlanta, GA, USA

Remzi Bag, MD
McKelvey Scholar
The McKelvey Center for Lung Transplantation
Assistant Professor of Medicine, Pulmonary, Allergy and Critical Care
Emory University School of Medicine
Atlanta, GA, USA

William M. Baldwin III, MD, PhD
Staff, Department of Immunology
Cleveland Clinic
Cleveland, OH, USA

Erik R. Barthel, MD, PhD
Resident in General Surgery
Harbor-UCLA Medical Center
UCLA David Geffen School of Medicine
Los Angeles, CA, USA

Stephen T. Bartlett, MD
Peter Angelos Distinguished Professor and Chairman
Department of Surgery
University of Maryland School of Medicine
Surgeon-in-Chief, University of Maryland Medical System
Baltimore, MD, USA

Lokesh Bathla, MD
Transplant Surgeon
Methodist Specialty and Transplant Hospital
San Antonio, TX, USA

Julia B. Becker, MD
Fellow in Pulmonary and Critical Care Medicine
University of Chicago
Chicago, IL, USA

Lorraine E. Bell, MDCM, FRCPC
Associate Professor of Pediatrics, McGill University
Director, Pediatric Renal Transplant Programme
Director, Pediatric Transition to Adult Care
Montreal Children's Hospital-McGill University Health Centre
Montreal, QC, Canada

Jennifer Berumen, MD
Chief Resident, General Surgery
UC San Diego
La Jolla, CA, USA

Oriol Bestard
Renal Transplant Unit
Nephrology Department
University Hospital of Bellvitge
University of Barcelona
Barcelona, Spain

Arvind Bhimaraj, MD, MPH, FACC
Assistant Professor of Medicine
Weill Cornell Medical College, NY;
Department of Cardiology
Methodist DeBakey Heart & Vascular Center
Houston Methodist Hospital
Houston, TX, USA

Adam W. Bingaman, MD, PhD
Director, Live Donor and Incompatible Kidney Transplant Programs
Methodist Specialty and Transplant Hospital
San Antonio, TX, USA

Roy D. Bloom, MD
Professor of Medicine
Perelman School of Medicine
University of Pennsylvania
Medical Director
Penn Kidney Pancreas Transplant Program
Philadelphia, PA, USA

Emily A. Blumberg, MD
Professor of Medicine
Perelman School of Medicine
University of Pennsylvania
Philadelphia, PA, USA

J. Andrew Bradley, PhD, FRCS
Professor of Surgery
University of Cambridge
Cambridge, UK

Gerald Brandacher, MD
Associate Professor of Surgery (PAR)
Scientific Director
Reconstructive Transplantation Program
Department of Plastic and Reconstructive Surgery
Johns Hopkins University School of Medicine
Baltimore, MD, USA

Robert A. Bray, PhD
Professor of Pathology
Co-Director, Histocompatibility and Molecular Immunogenetics Laboratory
Department of Pathology
Emory University Hospital
Atlanta, GA, USA

Daniel C. Brennan, MD
Professor of Medicine
Director, Transplant Nephrology
Washington University in St. Louis
School of Medicine
St. Louis, MO, USA

Lori E. Brigham, MBA
President and CEO
Washington Regional Transplant Community
Annandale, VA, USA

Jonathan S. Bromberg, MD, PhD
Professor of Surgery and Microbiology and Immunology
University of Maryland School of Medicine
Baltimore, MD, USA

Kimberly A. Brown, MD
Chief, Gastroenterology and Hepatology
Henry Ford Hospital
Detroit, MI, USA

John C. Bucuvalas
Professor of Pediatrics
Associate Medical Director, Pediatric Liver Care Center
Cincinnati Children's Hospital Medical Center
Cincinnati, OH, USA

Deborah Budge, MD
Associate Director
UTAH Cardiac Transplant Program
Intermountain Medical Center
Salt Lake City, UT, USA

Andrew Bushell, DPhil
Senior Scientist and University Research Lecturer
Transplantation Research Immunology Group
Nuffield Department of Surgical Sciences
John Radcliffe Hospital
Oxford, UK

Chris J. Callaghan, PhD, FRCS
Consultant Transplant and Vascular Access Surgeon
Guy's Hospital
London, UK

Sir Roy Y. Calne, FRS
Emeritus Professor of Surgery
Cambridge University
Cambridge, UK;
Visiting Professor
National University of Singapore
Singapore

Esther-Marie Carmichael, MT(ASCP), CLS, PHM, BSc
Quality Assurance Manager
Keck Hospital of USC, Transplant Institute
Los Angeles, CA, USA

Kelly Carter, MS, RN, NE-BC
Virginia Commonwealth University Health System
Medical College of Virginia Hospitals
Nurse Manager
Pauley Heart Center
Richmond, VA, USA

J. Michael Cecka, PhD
Emeritus Professor
Department of Pathology and Laboratory Medicine;
Director, Clinical Research
UCLA Immunogenetics Center
David Geffen School of Medicine
University of California, Los Angeles
Los Angeles, CA, USA

Linda C. Cendales, MD
Associate Professor of Surgery
Division of Plastic and Reconstructive Surgery and Division of Transplantation (dual appointment)
Director, Vascularized Composite Allotransplantation
Duke University Medical Center
Durham, NC, USA

Ashtar Chami, MD
Assistant Professor of Medicine
Emory Transplant Center
Emory University School of Medicine
Atlanta, GA, USA

Jeremy Chapman, MD, FRCP
Director, Renal Medicine
Centre for Transplant and Renal Research
Westmead Milennium Institute
Sydney University
Westmead Hospital
Westmead, NSW, Australia

Ali H. Charafeddine, MD
General Surgery Resident
Montefiore Medical Centre
Albert Einstein College of Medicine
Bronx, New York, NY, USA

Serban Constantinescu, MD, PhD
Medical Director, Kidney Transplant Program
Associate Professor of Medicine
Temple University School of Medicine
Philadelphia, PA, USA

Damon S. Cooney, MD, PhD
Assistant Professor of Plastic Surgery
Department of Plastic and Reconstructive Surgery
Johns Hopkins University School of Medicine
Baltimore, MD, USA

Matthew Cooper, MD
Associate Professor of Surgery
Medstar Georgetown Transplant Institute
Georgetown University School of Medicine
Washington, DC, USA

Jack G. Copeland, MD
Professor of Cardiothoracic Surgery
Director of Cardiac Transplantation and Mechanical Circulatory Support
UC San Diego
La Jolla, CA, USA

Hannah Copeland, MD
Chief Resident, General Surgery
UC San Diego
La Jolla, CA, USA

A. Benedict Cosimi, MD
Claude E. Welch Distinguished Professor of Surgery
Harvard Medical School
Chief Emeritus
Division of Transplantation
Massachusetts General Hospital
Boston, MA, USA

Guilherme Costa, MD, FACS
Assistant Professor of Surgery
Department of Surgery
University of Pittsburgh
Pittsburgh, PA, USA

Peter J. Cowan, PhD
Professor, Immunology Research Centre
St Vincent's Hospital Melbourne;
Department of Medicine
University of Melbourne
Melbourne, VIC, Australia

John M. Craig, MD
Clinical Assistant Professor of Surgery
University of Tennessee Health Science Center
Baptist Memorial Hospital
Memphis, TN, USA

Josep M. Cruzado
Renal Transplant Unit
Nephrology department.
University Hospital of Bellvitge
University of Barcelona
Barcelona, Spain

Marcelo Cypel, MD, MSc
Assistant Professor of Surgery
Toronto Lung Transplant Program
University Health Network
University of Toronto
Toronto, ON, Canada

Anthony M. D'Alessandro, MD
Professor of Surgery
Director of Liver Transplantation
University of Wisconsin School of Medicine and Public Health
Madison, WI, USA

Gabriel M. Danovitch, MD
Professor of Medicine, Division of Nephrology
Medical Director, Kidney Transplant Program
Department of Medicine
David Geffen School of Medicine at UCLA
Los Angeles, CA, USA

Anthony J.F. d'Apice, MD, MBBS
Professor
Immunology Research Centre
St Vincent's Hospital Melbourne;
Department of Medicine
University of Melbourne
Melbourne, VIC, Australia

R. Duane Davis, MD, MBA
Director of Transplantation
Professor of Surgery
Duke University Medical School and Medical Center
Durham, NC, USA

John M. Davison, MD
Professor Emeritus and Consultant Obstetrician
Institute of Cellular Medicine
Newcastle University
Newcastle upon Tyne, UK

Rowena Delos Santos, MD
Assistant Professor of Medicine
Renal Division
Washington University in St. Louis
St. Louis, MO, USA

Sacha A. De Serres, MD, SM, FRCPC
Research Fellow, Brigham and Women's Hospital and Harvard Medical School
Boston, MA;
Assistant Professor of Medicine
Universite Laval
Quebec, QC, Canada

Patrick G. Dean, MD
Assistant Professor of Surgery
Division of Transplant Surgery
Mayo Clinic
Rochester, MN, USA

Francis L. Delmonico, MD
President, The Transplantation Society;
World Health Organization
Advisory for Human Transplantation;
Professor of Surgery
Harvard Medical School
Massachusetts General Hospital
Transplant Center
Boston, MA;
Medical Director
New England Organ Bank
Waltham, MA, USA

Anthony J. Demetris, MD
Starzl Professor of Liver and Transplant Pathology
Director, Division of Liver and Transplant Pathology
Department of Pathology
University of Pittsburgh Medical Center
Pittsburgh, PA, USA

Yaozhong Ding, PhD
Associate Professor (retired)
Department of Surgery
University of Maryland School of Medicine
Baltimore, MD, USA

Cinthia B. Drachenberg, MD
Professor of Pathology
Director, Electron Microscopy Laboratory
University of Maryland School of Medicine
Baltimore, MD, USA

Regina Eady
Research Data Informatics Analyst, Senior
Emory University
Atlanta, GA, USA

Bijan Eghtesad, MD
Professor of Surgery
Director, Fellowship Program
Hepato-Pancreato-Biliary/Liver Transplantation Surgery
Cleveland Clinic
Cleveland, OH, USA

Howard J. Eisen, MD
Thomas J. Vischer Professor of Medicine
Chief, Division of Cardiology
Drexel University College of Medicine
Philadelphia, PA, USA

Robert Ettenger, MD
Professor of Pediatrics
Division of Nephrology
Department of Pediatrics
David Geffen School of Medicine at UCLA;
Director of Pediatric Renal Transplant Program
Director, Pediatric Nephrology Fellowship Program
Mattel Children's Hospital, UCLA
Los Angeles, CA, USA

Richard Eliot Fagley, MD
Anesthesiologist and Intensivist
Virginia Mason Medical Center
Seattle, WA, USA

Robert L. Fairchild, PhD
Staff, Department of Immunology
Cleveland Clinic
Cleveland, OH, USA

Konrad S. Famulski, PhD, DSc
Faculty Service Officer
Manager and Lead in Transcriptomics
Alberta Transplant Applied Genomics Centre
Department of Medicine
Division of Nephrology and Transplant Immunology
Edmonton, AB, Canada

Ji Fan, MD
Instructor of Clinical Surgery
University of Miami Miller School of Medicine
Miami Transplant Institute
Miami, FL, USA

Myriam Farah, MD, FRCPC
Clinical Assistant Professor
Division of Nephrology
University of British Columbia
Vancouver, BC, Canada

Douglas G. Farmer, MD
Professor of Surgery
Director, Intestinal Transplant Program
Surgical Director, Pediatric Liver Transplant Program
Dumont-UCLA Transplant Center
David Geffen School of Medicine at UCLA
Los Angeles, CA, USA

Albert Faro, MD
Associate Professor of Pediatrics
Division of Pediatric Allergy, Immunology and Pulmonary Medicine
Washington University School of Medicine
St. Louis, MO, USA

Alton Brad Farris III, MD
Assistant Professor
Director, Laboratory of Nephropathology and Electron Microscopy
Emory University
Atlanta, GA, USA

Carol Farver, MD, MS
Section Head, Surgical Pathology
Director, Pulmonary Pathology
Pathology and Laboratory Medicine Institute
Cleveland Clinic
Cleveland, OH, USA

Sandy Feng, MD, PhD
Professor of Surgery
Division of Transplant Surgery
University of California, San Francisco
San Francisco, CA, USA

Thomas Fishbein, MD
Executive Director, Georgetown Transplant Institute
Professor of Surgery
Georgetown University School of Medicine
Washington DC, USA

Jay A. Fishman, MD
Associate Director
MGH Transplantation Center;
Director, Transplant Infectious Disease &
Compromised Host Program
Massachusetts General Hospital;
Professor of Medicine
Harvard Medical School
Boston, MA, USA

Rachel C. Forbes, MD, MBA
Assistant Professor of Surgery
Division of Kidney and Pancreas Transplantation
Department of Surgery
Vanderbilt University
Nashville, TN, USA

Mandy L. Ford, PhD
Assistant Professor
Emory Transplant Center
Department of Surgery
Emory University
Atlanta, GA, USA

Richard N. Formica Jr, MD
Associate Professor of Medicine and Surgery
Director, Transplant Nephrology
Medical Director of Adult and Pediatric Kidney
Transplantation
Medical Director of Pancreas Transplantation
Yale University School of Medicine
New Haven, CT, USA

O.H. Frazier, MD
Chief, Transplant Services
Chief, Center for Cardiac Support
Director, Cullen Cardiovascular Research Laboratory
Texas Heart Institute
Houston, TX, USA

Richard Freeman, MD
Professor of Surgery
Dartmouth Hitchcock Medical Center
Lebanon, NH, USA

Alessandrina M. Freitas, MD, MPH
Resident in General Surgery
Department of Surgery
Emory University School of Medicine
Research Fellow
Vascularized Composite Allotransplantation
Emory Transplant Center
Atlanta, GA, USA

John Fung, MD, PhD
Professor of Surgery
Cleveland Clinic Lerner College of Medicine
Case Western Reserve University;
Chairman of Digestive Disease Institute
Cleveland Clinic
Cleveland, OH, USA

Jennifer Garcia, MD
Assistant Professor of Clinical Pediatrics
Division of Gastroenterology, Hepatology, and
Nutrition
University of Miami Miller School of Medicine
Miami Transplant Institute
Miami, FL, USA

Sireesha Garikipati, MD
Fellow in Cardiology
University of Texas Medical Branch
Galveston, TX, USA

Edward R. Garrity Jr, MD, MBA
Professor of Medicine
Vice Chair for Clinical Operations
The University of Chicago Medical Center
Chicago, IL, USA

Robert S. Gaston, MD
Co-Director, Comprehensive Transplant Institute
Robert G. Luke Endowed Chair in Transplant
Nephrology
University of Alabama at Birmingham
Birmingham, AL, USA

Howard M. Gebel, PhD
Professor of Pathology
Co-Director, Histocompatibility and Molecular
Immunogenetics Laboratory
Department of Pathology
Emory University Hospital
Atlanta, GA, USA

Donna George, MS, RN, NEA-BC
Transplant Administrator & Nursing Director
The Hume-Lee Transplant Center
Virginia Commonwealth University Health System
Medical College of Virginia Hospitals
Richmond, VA, USA

John S. Gill, MD, MS, FRCP(C)
Associate Professor, Nephrology
Division of Nephrology
University of British Columbia
St. Paul's Hospital
Vancouver, BC, Canada

Alexandra K. Glazier, JD, MPH
Chair, UNOS Ethics Committee;
Vice-President and General Counsel
New England Organ Bank
Waltham, MA, USA

Denis Glotz
Department of Nephrology and Kidney
Transplantation and Research Unit INSERM U940
Hopital Saint Louis
Paris, France

Veronica Gomez-Lobo, MD
Director of Pediatric and Adolescent Obstetrics and
Gynecology
MedStar Washington Hospital Center and Children's
National Medical Center
Professor of Clinical Obstetrics and Gynecology
Department of Pediatrics, Georgetown University
Washington, DC, USA

Jeremy Goodman, MD, FACS
Assistant Professor of Surgery
Division of Transplant Surgery
University of Alabama at Birmingham
Birmingham, AL, USA

Chad R. Gordon, DO
Assistant Professor of Surgery
Department of Plastic and Reconstructive Surgery
Johns Hopkins University School of Medicine
Baltimore, MD, USA

Michael Green, MD, MPH
Professor of Pediatrics, Surgery and Clinical and
Translational Science
University of Pittsburgh School of Medicine
Division of Infectious Diseases
Children's Hospital of Pittsburgh
Pittsburgh, PA, USA

Bartley P. Griffith, MD
Thomas E. and Alice Marie Hales
Distinguished Professor in Transplantation
University of Maryland School of Medicine
Division of Cardiac Surgery
Baltimore, MD, USA

Tracy C. Grikscheit, MD, FACS
Assistant Professor of Surgery
Children's Hospital Los Angeles
Division of Pediatric Surgery
Keck University of Southern California School of
Medicine
Los Angeles, CA, USA

Josep M. Grinyó, MD
Chief of Nephrology
University Hospital of Bellvitge
University of Barcelona
Barcelona, Spain

Lakshman Gunaratnam
Assistant Professor of Medicine, Microbiology &
Immunology
University of Western Ontario
London, ON, Canada

Susan Gunderson, BSN, MHA
Chief Executive Officer
LifeSource
St. Paul, MN, USA

Divya Gupta, MD
Assistant Professor of Medicine
Division of Cardiology
Advanced Heart Failure and Transplant
Emory University School of Medicine
Atlanta, GA, USA

Philip F. Halloran, MD, PhD
Director
Alberta Transplant Applied Genomics Centre
University of Alberta
Edmonton, AB, Canada

Jenny E. Han
Assistant Professor, Division of Pulmonary and Critical Care Medicine
Department of Medicine
Emory University School of Medicine
Atlanta, GA, USA

Steven I. Hanish, MD
Assistant Professor of Surgery
Emory University School of Medicine
Atlanta, GA, USA

Douglas W. Hanto, MD, PhD
Associate Dean for Continuing Medical Education
Continuing Medical Education Office
Professor of Surgery
Washington University School of Medicine in St. Louis
St. Louis, MO, USA

Karen L. Hardinger, PharmD, BCPS
Clinical Professor of Pharmacy Practice
University of Missouri – Kansas City
School of Pharmacy
Kansas City, MO, USA

William Harmon, MD
Professor of Pediatrics
Harvard Medical School;
Pediatric Nephrology
President, Physicians' Organization
Boston Children's Hospital
Boston, MA, USA

Matt Hartwig, MD
Assistant Professor of Surgery
Duke University
Durham, NC, USA

Koji Hashimoto, MD, PhD
Assistant Professor of Surgery
Cleveland Clinic Lerner College of Medicine
Case Western Reserve University;
Digestive Disease Institute
Cleveland Clinic
Cleveland, OH, USA

Peggy B. Hasley, MD, MHSc
Associate Professor of Internal Medicine
Associate Program Director for Ambulatory Medicine
Director, Generalist Track
University of Pittsburgh Medical Center
Pittsburgh, PA, USA

Steven Head, MS
Director
Microarray and Next Generation Sequencing Core Laboratories
The Scripps Research Institute
La Jolla, CA, USA

Timm Heinbokel
Division of Transplant Surgery and Transplant Surgery Research Laboratory
Brigham and Women's Hospital
Harvard Medical School, Boston, MA;
Institute of Medical Immunology
Charité – Universitätsmedizin Berlin
Berlin, Germany

Peter Heining, PhD
Senior Toxicologist
Novartis Pharmaceuticals Corporation
East Hanover, NJ, USA

Lorna K. Henderson, MBChB, MRCP, PhD
Transplant Fellow
National Pancreas Transplant Unit
University of Sydney at Westmead Hospital
Westmead, NSW, Australia

Mitchell L. Henry, MD
Professor of Surgery
Chief, Division of Transplantation
Department of Surgery
The Ohio State University
Columbus, OH, USA

Joanna Hester, PhD
Senior Scientist
Transplantation Research Immunology Group
Nuffield Department of Surgical Sciences
John Radcliffe Hospital
Oxford, UK

J. Mark Hexham, PhD, MSc
Clinical Research Director
Novartis Pharmaceuticals Corporation
East Hanover, NJ, USA

Naim Issa, MD
Assistant Professor of Medicine
Transplant Nephrologist
Division of Renal Diseases and Hypertension
Department of Medicine
University of Minnesota
Minneapolis, MN, USA

Pamala A. Jacobson, PharmD
Associate Professor
University of Minnesota, College of Pharmacy
Minneapolis, MN, USA

Anthony M. Jevnikar, MD, MSc
Professor of Medicine, Surgery, Microbiology & Immunology
Co-Director Multi Organ Transplant Program
University of Western Ontario
London, ON, Canada

Maryl R. Johnson, MD
Professor of Medicine
Medical Director, Heart Failure and Transplantation
University of Wisconsin School of Medicine and Public Health
Madison, WI, USA

Guido Junge, MD, MBA
Vice President and Global Therapeutic Area Head
Infectious Disease and Transplantation
Novartis Pharma AG
Basel, Switzerland

Elizabeth A. Kallenborn, MSN, RN, CCTC
Clinical Manager
Liver Transplant and Hepatology
Thomas E. Starzl Transplantation Institute
University of Pittsburgh Medical Center
Pittsburgh, PA, USA

Bruce Kaplan, MD
Professor of Medicine, Microbiology, Molecular Genetics and Immunology
University of Kansas Medical Center
Kansas, MO, USA;
Adjunct Professor of Medicine
Alberta Applied Genomics and Transplant Center
University of Alberta, Canada

Dixon B. Kaufman, MD, PhD
Ray Owen Professor and Chair
Division of Transplantation
University of Wisconsin School of Medicine and Public Health
Madison, WI, USA

Daniel Kaul, MD
Associate Professor of Medicine
Director, Transplant Infectious Diseases
Division of Infectious Disease
University of Michigan School of Medicine
Ann Arbor, MI, USA

Tatsuo Kawai, MD, PhD
Associate Professor of Surgery
Harvard Medical School
A. Benedict Cosimi Endowed Chair in Transplant Surgery
Massachusetts General Hospital
Boston MA, USA

Marwan Kazimi, MD
Director
Multivisceral and Intestinal Transplantation Program
Division of Transplant Surgery
Transplant Institute
Henry Ford Hospital
Detroit, MI, USA

Desmond Barry Keenan, PhD, MBA
Research Director and Technical Fellow
Closed Loop Development
Medtronic Diabetes
Northridge, CA, USA

Shaf Keshavjee, MD, MSc, FRCSC, FACS
Surgeon-in-Chief, University Health Network
Professor, Division of Thoracic Surgery
Director, Toronto Lung Transplant Program
University of Toronto
Toronto, ON, Canada

Zain Khalpey, MD, PhD, MRCS(Eng)
Surgical Director of Heart Transplant and Mechanical Circulatory Support
Distinguished Tony Marnell Chair in Cardiothoracic Surgery
Surgical Director of Regenerative Medicine
Associate Professor of Surgery
Physiological Sciences & Biomedical Engineering
University of Arizona
Tucson, AZ, USA

Michael S. Kiernan, MD, MS
Assistant Professor of Medicine
Medical Director, Ventricular Assist Device Program
Tufts University School of Medicine
Boston, MA, USA

S. Joseph Kim
Division of Nephrology
Toronto General Hospital;
University Health Network and the Institute for Health Policy, Management and Evaluation
Faculty of Medicine
University of Toronto
Toronto, ON, Canada

Allan D. Kirk, MD, PhD, FACS
Professor and Chairman, Department of Surgery
Duke University School of Medicine;
Surgeon-in-Chief for Duke University Health System
Duke University Medical Center
Durham, NC, USA

Michelle M. Kittleson, MD, PhD
Assistant Clinical Professor of Medicine, UCLA
Director, Heart Failure Research
Director, Post-Graduate Education in Heart Failure and Transplantation
Cedars-Sinai Heart Institute
Los Angeles, CA, USA

Andrew Klein, MD, MBA, FACS
Director, Comprehensive Transplant Center
Esther and Mark Schulman Chair of Surgery and Transplant Medicine
Professor and Vice Chair
Department of Surgery
Cedars-Sinai Medical Center
Los Angeles, CA, USA

Christina L.M. Klein, MD
Assistant Professor of Medicine
Medical Director, Pancreas Transplant
Director, High Risk Kidney Transplant
Washington University in St. Louis
St. Louis, MO, USA

Stuart J. Knechtle, MD
Professor of Surgery
Emory University School of Medicine
Atlanta, GA, USA

Jon A. Kobashigawa, MD
DSL/Thomas D. Gordon Chair in Heart Transplantation Medicine
Director, Advanced Heart Disease Section
Director, Heart Transplant Program
Cedars-Sinai Heart Institute
Los Angeles, CA, USA

Chatchai Kreepala, MD
Clinical and Research Fellow
Alberta Transplant Applied Genomics Centre
Department of Medicine
Division of Nephrology and Transplant Immunology
University of Alberta
Edmonton, AB, Canada

Jill C. Krisl, PharmD
Transplant Pharmacy Fellow
Department of Surgery
Division of Transplantation
University of Cincinnati
Academic Health Center
Cincinnati, OH, USA

Aleksandra Kukla, MD
Assistant Professor of Medicine
Transplant Nephrologist;
Medical Director of Pancreas Transpant Program
Division of Renal Diseases and Hypertension
Department of Medicine
University of Minnesota
Minneapolis, MN, USA

Sunil M. Kurian, PhD
Staff Scientist
Laboratory of Functional Genomics
Department of Molecular and Experimental Medicine
The Scripps Research Institute
La Jolla, CA, USA

Keren Ladin, PhD, MSc
Director
Research on Ethics, Aging, and Community Health
Tufts University;
Assistant Professor
Department of Occupational Therapy
Tufts University
Medford, MA;
Department of Public Health and Community Medicine
Tufts University School of Medicine
Boston, MA, USA

Alan Langnas
Chief, Section of Transplant Surgery
University of Nebraska Medical Center
Omaha, NE, USA

Dianne LaPointe Rudow, ANP-BC, DNP, CCTC
Associate Professor
Department of Health Evidence and Policy
Director, Zweig Family Center for Living Donation
Medical Director of Liver and Kidney Donor Program
Recanati/Miller Transplant Institute
The Mount Sinai Medical Center
New York, NY, USA

Christian P. Larsen, MD, DPhil
Dean – Emory School of Medicine
Surgeon-in-Chief Emory Healthcare
Emory University
Atlanta, GA, USA

E. Clinton Lawrence, MD
Director, Andrew J. McKelvey Lung Transplant Center
Emory Transplant Center
Emory University Hospital;
Augustus J. McKelvey Professor of Lung Transplantation Medicine
Emory University School of Medicine
Department of Medicine
Division of Pulmonary, Allergy and Critical Care Medicine
Emory University
Atlanta, GA, USA

Daniel J. Lebovitz, MD
Associate Director, Critical Care
Akron Children's Hospital
Akron, OH;
Director, PICU
MetroHealth Medical Center
Cleveland OH;
Medical Director
Lifebanc
Cleveland, OH, USA

Sung-Gyu Lee
Professor of Surgery
Hepato-Biliary Surgery and Liver Transplantation
Department of Surgery
Asan Medical Center
University of Ulsan College of Medicine
Seoul, Korea

W.P. Andrew Lee, MD
The Milton T Edgerton, MD, Professor and Chairman
Department of Plastic and Reconstructive Surgery
Johns Hopkins University School of Medicine
Baltimore, MD, USA

Soyoung Lee, MD
Research Fellow
Massachusetts General Hospital
Boston, MA, USA

Jason R. Lees, PhD
Assistant Professor
Department of Microbiology and Immunology
Uniformed Services of Health Sciences
Bethesda, MD, USA

Carmen Lefaucheur
Department of Nephrology and Kidney Transplantation and Research Unit INSERM U940
Hopital Saint Louis
Paris, France

Henri G.D. Leuvenink, PhD
Associate Professor
Principle Investigator, Experimental Transplantation
Surgical Research Laboratory
Department of Surgery
University Medical Center Groningen
Groningen, The Netherlands

Matthew H. Levine, MD, PhD
Assistant Professor of Surgery
Division of Transplant Surgery
Perelman School of Medicine
University of Pennsylvania
Philadelphia, PA, USA

Xian C. Li, MD, PhD, ASCI
Director
Immunobiology & Transplantation Research
Houston Methodist Hospital
Texas Medical Center
Houston, Texas

Sundus A. Lodhi, MD,
Assistant Professor
Transplant Nephrology
Emory University
Atlanta, GA, USA

Marc I. Lorber, MD
Sr. Vice President and Chief Medical Officer
XenoLung Clinical Development
Lung Biotechnology, Inc
United Therapeutics Corporation
Silver Spring, MD, USA

Richard S. Luskin, MPA
President and CEO
New England Organ Bank
Waltham, MA, USA

G. Marshall Lyon, MD, MMSc
Associate Professor of Medicine
Director of Transplant Infectious Disease
Emory University School of Medicine
Atlanta, GA, USA

Joren C. Madsen, MD, DPhil
Professor of Surgery
W. Gerald and Patricia R. Austen
Distinguished Scholar in Cardiac Surgery
Massachusetts General Hospital
Boston, MA, USA

Joseph F. Magliocca, MD
Assistant Professor of Surgery
Emory University School of Medicine
Atlanta, GA, USA

Sayeed Malek, MD
Clinical Director, Division of Transplant Surgery
Brigham and Women's Hospital
Harvard Medical School
Boston, MA, USA

Roslyn B. Mannon, MD
Professor of Medicine and Surgery
University of Alabama at Birmingham
Birmingham, AL, USA

James F. Markmann, MD, PhD
Professor of Surgery
Harvard Medical School;
Chief, Division of Transplantation
Massachusetts General Hospital
Boston, MA, USA

Benjamin M. Martin, MD
Senior Resident, Department of Surgery
Emory University School of Medicine
Atlanta, GA, USA

Paulo Martins, MD, PhD
Instructor, Harvard Medical School
Clinical Fellow, Massachusetts General Hospital
Boston, MA, USA

Allan B. Massie, PhD
Department of Surgery
Johns Hopkins School of Medicine
Baltimore, MD, USA

Virginia A. McBride, RN, MPH
President
AMVAT Consulting
Grand Junction, CO, USA

Kenneth R. McCurry, MD
Staff Surgeon
CCF
Cleveland Clinic
Cleveland, OH, USA

Gwen McNatt, MS, RN, CNN, FNP-BC
Director, Operations
Kovler Organ Transplantation Center and Infectious Disease
Northwestern Memorial Hospital
Chicago, IL, USA

Mandeep R. Mehra, MD
Brigham and Women's Hospital
Harvard Medical School
Boston, MA, USA

Aneesh K. Mehta, MD
Assistant Professor of Medicine
Assistant Director of Transplant Infectious Diseases
Emory University School of Medicine
Atlanta, GA, USA

Edward A. Meister, PhD
College of Medicine
Division of Nephrology
University of Arizona
Tucson, AZ, USA

Michael H. Mengel, MD
Associate Professor
University of Alberta
Edmonton, AB, Canada

Diana Metes, MD
Associate Professor of Surgery and Immunology
Starzl Transplantation Institute
Department of Surgery and Department of Immunology
University of Pittsburgh School of Medicine
Pittsburgh, PA, USA

Charles M. Miller, MD
Professor of Surgery
Cleveland Clinic Lerner College of Medicine
Case Western Reserve University;
Director, Liver Transplant Program
Digestive Disease Institute
Cleveland Clinic
Cleveland, OH, USA

Marta I. Minervini, MD
Assistant Professor of Pathology
Department of Pathology
University of Pittsburgh Medical Center
Pittsburgh, PA, USA

Saeed Mohammad, MD, MS
Assistant Professor
Department of Pediatrics
Northwestern University Feinberg School of Medicine
Ann and Robert H. Lurie Children's Hospital of Chicago
Chicago, IL, USA

Deok-Bog Moon
Professor of Surgery
Hepato-Biliary Surgery and Liver Transplantation
Department of Surgery
Asan Medical Center
University of Ulsan College of Medicine
Seoul, Korea

Christian Morath, MD
Department of Medicine
Division of Nephrology and Hypertension
University of Heidelberg
Heidelberg, Germany

Michael J. Moritz, MD
Chief, Transplant Services
Lehigh Valley Health Network
Allentown, PA;
Professor of Surgery
University of South Florida
Morsani College of Medicine
Tampa, FL, USA

Tim Morris
Director, Research Informatics
Research and Woodruff Health Sciences IT
Emory University
Atlanta, GA, USA

Cathi L. Murphey, PhD
Director, Histocompatibility and Immunogenetics Laboratory
Southwest Immunodiagnostics, Inc.
San Antonio, TX, USA

Michael A. Nalesnik, MD
Professor of Pathology
Department of Pathology
University of Pittsburgh Medical Center
Pittsburgh, PA, USA

Jung-Man Namgoong
Clinical Instructor of Surgery
Hepato-Biliary Surgery and Liver Transplantation
Department of Surgery
Asan Medical Center
University of Ulsan College of Medicine
Seoul, Korea

Brian J. Nankivell, MD, PhD, FRACP
Transplant Physician
Department of Renal Medicine
Westmead Hospital
Sydney, NSW, Australia

Peter Neuhaus, MD, PhD
Chairman of General, Visceral, and Transplantation Surgery
Experimental Surgery and Regenerative Medicine
Charité – Campus Virchow, Universitätsmedizin Berlin
Berlin, Germany

David C. Neujahr, MD
Medical Director
Andrew McKelvey Adult Lung Transplant Program
Emory University Transplant Center
Assistant Professor of Medicine, Pulmonary, Allergy and Critical Care
Emory University School of Medicine
Atlanta, GA, USA

Kenneth A. Newell, MD, PhD
Professor of Surgery
Emory Transplant Center
Emory University School of Medicine
Atlanta, GA, USA

Silke Niederhaus, MD
Assistant Professor of Surgery
University of Maryland Medical System
Division of Transplantation
Baltimore, MD, USA

Seigo Nishida, MD
Department of Surgery, Division of Transplantation
University of Miami
Miami, FL, USA

Douglas J. Norman, MD
Professor of Medicine
Director, Transplant Medicine
Director, Laboratory of Immunogenetics and Transplantation
Oregon Health & Science University
Portland, OR, USA

Rupert Oberhuber, MD
Division of Transplant Surgery and Transplant Surgery Research Laboratory
Brigham and Women's Hospital
Harvard Medical School
Boston, MA;
Department of Visceral, Transplant and Thoracic Surgery
Medical University of Innsbruck
Innsbruck, Austria

Philip J. O'Connell, MBBS, PhD, FRACP
Professor and Director of Transplantation
University of Sydney at Westmead Hospital
Sydney, NSW, Australia

Jon S. Odorico, MD, FACS
Professor of Surgery
Director, Pancreas Transplantation
Co-director, Islet Transplantation
University of Wisconsin School of Medicine and Public Health
Madison, WI, USA

John G. O'Grady, MD, FRCPI
Professor of Hepatology
Institute of Liver Studies
King's College Hospital
London, UK

Linda Ohler, MSN, RN, CCTC, FAAN
Quality and Compliance Manager
Georgetown Transplant Institute
Georgetown University Hospital
Washington, DC, USA

Toshihiro Okamoto, MD, PhD
Department of Thoracic and Cardiovascular Surgery, Heart and Vascular Institute
Cleveland Clinic
Cleveland, OH, USA

Marc J. Overcash
Deputy Chief Information Officer
Assistant Dean, Information Technology
Emory University School of Medicine
Atlanta, GA, USA

Eugenia K. Page, MD
Surgical Resident
Emory University School of Medicine
Atlanta, GA, USA

John C. Papadimitriou, MD, PhD
Professor of Pathology
Director, Surgical Pathology
University of Maryland School of Medicine
Baltimore, MD, USA

Samir Parekh, MD
Assistant Professor of Medicine
Transplant Hepatology Fellowship Director
Emory University School of Medicine
The Emory Transplant Center
Atlanta, GA, USA

Steven M. Parnis, BS
Assistant Director, Center for Technology Development
Texas Heart Institute
Houston, TX, USA

Stephen Pastan, MD
Medical Director, Kidney and Pancreas Transplant Program
Emory Transplant Center
Associate Professor of Medicine
Emory University School of Medicine
Atlanta, GA, USA

Jignesh K. Patel, MD, PhD
Medical Director, Heart Transplant Program
Cedars-Sinai Heart Institute
Los Angeles, CA, USA

Thomas C. Pearson, MD, DPhil
Livingston Professor of Surgery
Emory University School of Medicine;
Executive Director
Director, Kidney Transplant Program
Emory Transplant Center
Atlanta, GA, USA

Alice Peng, MD
Associate Professor of Medicine
Medical Director
Pancreas Transplantation Program
Cedars-Sinai Medical Center
Los Angeles, CA, USA

Phuong-Chi T. Pham, MD
Professor of Medicine
David Geffen School of Medicine at UCLA
Olive View-UCLA-Medical Center
Chief, Division of Nephrology and Hypertension
Director, UCLA-OVMC Nephrology Training Program
Sylmar, CA, USA

Phuong-Thu T. Pham, MD
Professor of Medicine
David Geffen School of Medicine at UCLA
Department of Medicine, Nephrology Division
Director, Outpatient Services
Kidney Transplant Program
Los Angeles, CA, USA

Nicole A. Pilch, PharmD, MSCR, BCPS
Residency Program Director, PGY-2 Transplant Residency Program
Clinical Specialist, Solid Organ Transplantation
Clinical Assistant Professor, Department of Pharmacy and Clinical Sciences
South Carolina College of Pharmacy – MUSC Campus
Medical University of South Carolina
Department of Pharmacy Services
Charleston, SC, USA

Rutger J. Ploeg, MD, PhD, FRCS
Professor of Transplant Biology
University of Oxford;
Professor of Transplant Surgery
University of Groningen;
Honorary Consultant Transplant Surgeon
OUH NHS Trust
Nuffield Department of Surgical Sciences
Oxford, UK

Jennifer M. Porter, Esq
Partner, Gurne Porter, PLLC
Washington, DC, USA

Luke Preczewski
Administrative Director
Comprehensive Transplant Center
Northwestern University Feinberg School of Medicine
Chicago, IL, USA

Timothy L. Pruett, MD
John S. Najarian Clinical Chair
Professor of Surgery and Internal Medicine
University of Minnesota
Minneapolis, MN, USA

Cristiano Quintini, MD
Assistant Professor of Surgery
Cleveland Clinic Lerner College of Medicine
Case Western Reserve University
Liver Transplant Program
Digestive Disease Institute
Cleveland Clinic
Cleveland, OH, USA

Giorgio Raimondi, PhD
Department of Plastic and Reconstructive Surgery
Johns Hopkins School of Medicine
Baltimore, MD, USA

Raja Rajalingam, PhD
Professor of Clinical Surgery
Director of Immunogenetics and Transplantation Laboratory
University of California, San Francisco
San Francisco, CA, USA

Parmjeet Randhawa, MD
Professor of Pathology
Department of Pathology
University of Pittsburgh Medical Center
Pittsburgh, PA, USA

Nathanael Raschzok, MD
General, Visceral, and Transplantation Surgery
Experimental Surgery and Regenerative Medicine
Universitätsmedizin Berlin
Berlin, Germany

Elaine F. Reed, PhD
Professor
Department of Pathology and Laboratory Medicine;
Director, UCLA Immunogenetics Center
David Geffen School of Medicine
University of California, Los Angeles
Los Angeles, CA, USA

John Adam Reich, MD
Instructor of Anesthesiology
Tufts University
Staff Anesthesiologist
Director, Post Anesthesia Care Unit
Tufts Medical Center
Boston, MA, USA

Scott A. Reule, MD
Nephrology Fellow
Division of Renal Diseases and Hypertension
Department of Medicine
University of Minnesota
Minneapolis, MN, USA

Camillo Ricordi, MD
Stacy Joy Goodman Professor of Surgery
Director, Cell Transplant Center and Diabetes Research Institute
University of Miami
Miami, FL, USA

E. Rene Rodriguez, MD
Professor of Pathology
Director, Cardiovascular Pathology
Director, Autopsy Pathology
Department of Anatomic Pathology/L25
The Cleveland Clinic
Cleveland, OH, USA

Christin C. Rogers, PharmD, FCCP, BCPS
Clinical Pharmacy Coordinator – Solid Organ Transplant
Beth Israel Deaconess Medical Center
Boston, MA, USA

Erin Rubin, MD
Associate Professor of Pathology
Department of Pathology
University of Pittsburgh Medical Center
Pittsburgh, PA, USA

Phillip Ruiz Jr, MD, PhD
Professor of Pathology and Surgery
Medical Director, Transplant Laboratories
University of Miami Miller School of Medicine
Miami, FL, USA

David H. Sachs, MD
Scientific Director, Transplantation Biology Research Center
Massachusetts General Hospital;
Paul S Russel/Warner-Lambert Professor of Surgery
Harvard Medical School
Boston, MA, USA

Daniel R. Salomon, MD
Professor, Department of Molecular and Experimental Medicine
Program Medical Director, Scripps Center for Organ Transplantation
The Scripps Research Institute
La Jolla, CA, USA

Alberto Sánchez-Fueyo, MD, PhD
Institute of Liver Studies
School of Medicine
King's College London
Denmark Hill
London, UK

Chandrasekar Santhanakrishnan, MD
Assistant Professor of Clinical Surgery
Division of Transplant Surgery
Department of Surgery
University of California Davis Medical Center
Sacramento, CA, USA

Eizaburo Sasatomi, MD, PhD
Assistant Professor of Pathology
Department of Pathology
University of Pittsburgh Medical Center
Pittsburgh, PA, USA

Igor M. Sauer, MD
Chairman of Research
General, Visceral, and Transplantation Surgery
Experimental Surgery and Regenerative Medicine
Charité – Campus Virchow, Universitätsmedizin Berlin
Berlin, Germany

Deirdre Sawinski, MD
Assistant Professor of Medicine
Department of Medicine
University of Pennsylvania Perelman School of Medicine
Philadelphia, PA, USA

Birgit Sawitzki
Institute of Medical Immunology
Charite University Medicine
Berlin, Germany

Franz Schaefer, MD
Professor of Pediatrics
Center for Pediatrics and Adolescent Medicine
University of Heidelberg
Heidelberg, Germany

Margaret Schaeffer, MS, MSHA, RN
Virginia Commonwealth University Health System
Medical College of Virginia Hospitals
Nurse Manager
Hume-Lee Transplant Center
Richmond, VA, USA

Peter Schemmer, MD, MBA
Department of Surgery
Division of Visceral and Transplantation Surgery
University of Heidelberg
Heidelberg, Germany

Stefan Schneeberger, MD
Department of Visceral, Transplant and Thoracic Surgery
Innsbruck Medical University
Innsbruck, Austria;
Department of Plastic and Reconstructive Surgery
Johns Hopkins University School of Medicine
Baltimore, MD, USA

Jesse D. Schold, PhD
Associate Staff
Department of Quantitative Health Sciences
Cleveland Clinic
Cleveland, OH, USA

Kristine S. Schonder, PharmD
Assistant Professor
Pharmacy and Therapeutics
Clinical Pharmacist, Transplant
University of Pittsburgh School of Pharmacy
Thomas E. Starzl Transplantation Institute
Pittsburgh, PA, USA

Kathy Schwab, RN, BSN, CCTC
Compliance Coordinator
Mayo Clinic
Rochester, MN, USA

Dorry L. Segev, MD, PhD
Associate Vice Chair of Research
Associate Professor of Surgery
Associate Professor of Epidemiology
Johns Hopkins University
Baltimore, MD, USA

Gennaro Selvaggi, MD
Associate Professor of Clinical Surgery
University of Miami Miller School of Medicine
Miami Transplant Institute
Miami, FL, USA

Keyur B. Shah, MD
Virginia Commonwealth University;
Medical College of Virginia Hospital
Richmond, VA, USA

A.M. James Shapiro, MD, PhD, FRCS(Eng), FRCSC, MSM, DSc, FRS(Canada)
Canada Research Chair in Transplantation Surgery and Regenerative Medicine
Director, Clinical Islet Transplant Program
University of Alberta
Edmonton, AB, Canada

Ron Shapiro, MD
Professor of Surgery
Robert J. Corry Chair in Transplantation Surgery
University of Pittsburgh Medical Center
Thomas E. Starzl Transplantation Institute
Pittsburgh, PA, USA

Chris Shay-Downer, RN, BSN, CCTC
Transplant & Cardiac Program Director
BioScrip, Inc.
Elmsford, NY, USA

Jaimie T. Shores
Assistant Professor of Plastic Surgery
Department of Plastic and Reconstructive Surgery
Johns Hopkins University School of Medicine
Baltimore, MD, USA

William D. Simmons, RPh
US Medical
Novartis Pharmaceuticals Corporation
Madison, WI, USA

Daniel B. Sims, MD
Assistant Professor
Montefiore Medical Center
Albert Einstein College of Medicine
Bronx, NY, USA

Alan Slade, PharmD
Translational Medicine Director, Transplantation
Novartis Pharmaceuticals Corporation
East Hanover, NJ, USA

Richard G. Smith, MSEE
Director, Marshall Foundation Artificial Heart Laboratory
University Medical Center
Tucson, AZ, USA

Andrew L. Smith, MD
Professor of Medicine
Medical Director, Heart Failure and Transplantation
Division of Cardiology
Emory University School of Medicine
Atlanta, GA, USA

Lonnie D. Smith, PharmD
Manager, Department of Solid Organ Transplant
Director, PGY-2 Pharmacy Residency – Transplant
University of Utah Hospitals and Clinics
Salt Lake City, UT, USA

Mark Schnitzler, PhD
Professor
St. Louis University School of Medicine
St. Louis, MO, USA

Hans W. Sollinger, MD, PhD
Folkert Belzer Professor
Division of Transplantation
University of Wisconsin School of Medicine and Public Health
Madison, WI, USA

Lisa G. Sorensen, PhD
Assistant Professor of Clinical Psychiatry and Behavioral Sciences
Northwestern University Feinberg School of Medicine;
Ann and Robert H. Lurie Children's Hospital of Chicago
Chicago, IL, USA

James R. Spivey, MD
Associate Professor of Medicine and Surgery
Director of Hepatology
Medical Director, Liver Transplantation
Emory University School of Medicine
The Emory Transplant Center
Atlanta, GA, USA

Mark D. Stegall
Professor of Surgery and Immunology
Mayo Clinic
Rochester, MN, USA

Josef Stehlik, MD, MPH
Associate Professor of Medicine
University of Utah School of Medicine
Salt Lake City, UT, USA

Garry M. Steil, PhD
Research Scientist, Division of Medicine Critical Care
Boston Children's Hospital;
Assistant Professor of Pediatrics
Harvard Medical School
Boston, MA, USA

Neema Stephens, MD
Assistant Professor
Transplant Nephrology
University of Texas – San Antonio
San Antonio, TX, USA

Peter G. Stock, MD, PhD
Division of Transplant Surgery
University of California, San Francisco
San Francisco, CA, USA

Margaret L. Stuber, MD
Assistant Dean of Student Affairs for Career Development and Well-Being
Vice Chair for Education in Psychiatry
Daniel X. Freedman Professor, Psychiatry and Biobehavioral Sciences
David Geffen School of Medicine at UCLA
Los Angeles, CA, USA

Charles A. Su, BS
Graduate Student
Department of Immunology
Cleveland Clinic
Cleveland, OH, USA

Ram M. Subramanian
Assistant Professor of Medicine and Surgery
Emory University School of Medicine
Atlanta, GA, USA

Stuart C. Sweet, MD, PhD
W. McKim Marriott Professor of Pediatrics
Division of Pediatric Allergy, Immunology and Pulmonary Medicine
Washington University School of Medicine
St. Louis, MO, USA

David J. Taber, PharmD, BCPS
Assistant Professor
Division of Transplant Surgery
Department of Surgery
Medical University of South Carolina
Charleston, SC, USA

Carmela D. Tan, MD
Assistant Professor
Department of Anatomic Pathology
The Cleveland Clinic
Cleveland, OH, USA

Akin Tekin, MD
Assistant Professor of Clinical Surgery
University of Miami Miller School of Medicine
Miami Transplant Institute
Miami, FL, USA

Paul I. Terasaki, PhD
Professor Emeritus
University of California, Los Angeles;
Terasaki Foundation
Los Angeles, CA, USA

Angus W. Thomson, PhD, DSc
Distinguished Professor of Surgery and Immunology
Starzl Transplantation Institute;
Department of Surgery and Department of Immunology
University of Pittsburgh School of Medicine
Pittsburgh, PA, USA

Eric M. Tichy, PharmD, FCCP, BCPS
Clinical Pharmacy Specialist
Solid Organ Transplant
Director, PGY-2 Residency – Transplant
Yale-New Haven Hospital
Department of Pharmacy
New Haven, CT, USA

Paul L. Tso, MD
Associate Professor of Surgery
Emory University School of Medicine
Atlanta, GA, USA

Stefan G. Tullius, MD, PhD, FACS
Professor of Surgery, Harvard Medical School
Chief, Division of Transplant Surgery & Director,
Transplant Surgery Research Laboratory,
Brigham and Women's Hospital
Boston, MA, USA

Nicole A. Turgeon, MD, FACS
Assistant Professor of Surgery
Emory University Hospital
Atlanta, GA, USA

Alexandra P. Turner, MD
Abdominal Transplant Fellow
Emory Transplant Center
Department of Surgery
Emory University School of Medicine
Atlanta, GA, USA

Heth R. Turnquist, PhD
Assistant Professor of Surgery and Immunology
Starzl Transplantation Institute
Department of Surgery and Department of Immunology
University of Pittsburgh School of Medicine
Pittsburgh, PA, USA

Andreas Tzakis, MD, PhD, Dhc
Director of Liver and Kidney Transplant
Cleveland Clinic Florida
Weston, FL, USA

Simon Urschel, MD
Assistant Professor of Pediatrics and Immunology
Department of Pediatrics
Alberta Transplant Institute
University of Alberta
Edmonton, AB, Canada

Parsia A. Vagefi, MD
Division of Transplant Surgery
Massachusetts General Hospital;
Harvard Medical School
Boston, MA, USA

Anna Valujskikh, PhD
Associate Staff, Department of Immunology
Cleveland Clinic
Cleveland, OH, USA

Ronald G. Van Valen
Sr. Global Program
Regulatory Director/Transplantation
Novartis Pharmaceuticals
East Hanover, NJ, USA

Robert S. Venick, MD
Assistant Professor of Pediatrics
David Geffen School of Medicine at UCLA
Los Angeles, CA, USA

Flavio Vincenti, MD
Professor of Clinical Medicine
University of California
San Francisco, CA, USA

Gus J. Vlahakes, MD
Professor of Surgery
Massachusetts General Hospital
Boston, MA, USA

Philip Y. Wai, MD
Assistant Professor of Surgery
Division of Intra-abdominal Transplantation
Department of Surgery
Loyola University Medical Center
Maywood, IL, USA

W. Dean Wallace, MD
Associate Professor
Chief, Pulmonary Pathology
Department of Pathology and Laboratory Medicine
David Geffen School of Medicine at UCLA
Los Angeles, CA, USA

Candace Wang, MD
Novartis Pharmaceuticals Corporation
East Hanover, NJ, USA

Rui Wang
The Transplant Institute and Center for Transplant Outcomes and Quality Improvement
Beth Israel Deaconess Medical Center;
Harvard Medical School
Boston, MA, USA

Claire A. Watkins, MD, MS
Resident Physician in Cardiothoracic Surgery
University of Maryland School of Medicine
Division of Cardiac Surgery
Baltimore, MD, USA

Melissa Watson, MD
Clinical Fellow
Abdominal Multiorgan Transplantation Surgery
Cleveland Clinic
Cleveland, OH, USA

Jeff Weaver, MBA
Director, Data Solutions
Research and Woodruff Health Sciences IT
Emory University
Atlanta, GA, USA

Steven A. Webber, MBChB, MRCP
James C. Overall Professor and Chair
Department of Pediatrics
Vanderbilt University School of Medicine
Nashville, TN, USA

Allison B. Webber, MD
Assistant Clinical Professor of Medicine
University of California
San Francisco, CA, USA

Lori J. West, MD, DPhil, FRCPC
Professor of Pediatrics, Surgery and Immunology
Department of Pediatrics
Alberta Transplant Institute
University of Alberta
Edmonton, AB, Canada

David Wheeler, RRT
Anesthesia Institute
Cleveland Clinic
Cleveland, OH, USA

Marissa B. Wilck, MBChB
Assistant Professor
Department of Medicine
University of Pennsylvania
Philadelphia, PA, USA

Kathryn J. Wood, DPhil
Professor of Immunology
Transplantation Research Immunology Group
Nuffield Department of Surgical Sciences
John Radcliffe Hospital
Oxford, UK

E. Steve Woodle, MD, FACS
William A. Altemeier Chair in Surgery
Professor of Surgery
Director, Division of Transplantation
Director, Isreal Penn International Tranasplant Tumor Registry
University of Cincinnati
Cincinnati, OH, USA

Jiangnan Xu, MD
Associate Professor
Capital Medical University
Beijing, China

Heidi Yeh, MD
Surgical Director
Pediatric Transplantation;
Instructor, Harvard Medical School
Assistant in Surgery, Massachusetts General Hospital
Boston, MA, USA

Jonathan C. Yeung, MD, PhD
Fellow in Thoracic Surgery
Toronto Lung Transplant Program
University Health Network
University of Toronto
Toronto, ON, Canada

Melissa Y. Yeung, MD, FRCPC
Instructor in Medicine
Transplantation Research Center
Brigham and Women's Hospital and Harvard Medical School
Boston, MA, USA

Martin G. Zeier, MD, FASN
Head, Division of Nephrology
Heidelberg University Hospital
Heidelberg, Germany

Qiuheng Zhang, PhD
Assistant Professor
Department of Pathology and Laboratory Medicine;
Associate Director
UCLA Immunogenetics Center
David Geffen School of Medicin,
University of California, Los Angeles
Los Angeles, CA, USA

Shelley Zomak, RN MS CCTC
Unit Director, Cardiothoracic Transplant
University of Pittsburgh Medical Center
Pittsburgh, PA, USA

中文版序言

经历半个多世纪的探索与发展，在全球范围内，以心脏、肝脏、肾脏等大器官移植为代表的器官移植技术已经挽救了近百万罹患各类终末期疾病患者的生命，器官移植技术已经成为治疗终末期器官衰竭的最佳手段。在我国器官移植工作者数十载孜孜以求的不懈努力下，中国器官移植无论在实施数量还是临床疗效方面，都取得了令国人鼓舞、国际瞩目的巨大成就，成千上万的终末期疾病患者获得了新生。为了更好地推进健康中国建设，一个重大且亟待解决的现实问题摆在我们面前：我们应当为器官移植事业的人才培养做些什么？要培养未来一流的临床医生、医学科学家，必须以一流的医学教育作为基础。

因此，编撰一本适应当前器官移植教育教学需求的《器官移植学》教材是人才培养的要求、国家的需求、时代的需求。

由美国 Wiley Blackwell 出版社出版的 *Textbook of Organ Transplantation* 一书内容新颖、丰富，紧跟科学技术前沿，不仅涵盖医学专业领域知识，还包括相关移植国家政策的介绍与解读，是国际移植学术界经典的参考用书，广受好评。此书的中文版由北京大学人民医院朱继业教授和浙江大学医学院附属第一医院徐骁教授领衔翻译，50 余位移植临床、教学和科研一线且经验丰富的专家学者共同努力，同心同德，群策群力，在尊重原文的前提下，灵活解读，用词精准，文笔简练，使读者更易于理解与阅读。因此，我相信本书不仅可作为器官移植专科医师的培训教材，也是研究生科研与创新的参考书，更是广大奋战于器官移植一线工作者的工具书，同时也可为国家器官移植相关政策制定与修改提供重要借鉴。

器官移植学是生物医学学科领域中一门年轻活跃、发展迅速的新兴学科。随着分子生物学与基因工程技术逐步介入移植及其相关研究领域，器官移植面临着前所未有的挑战与机遇。我能为此书作序，感到十分的荣幸，愿借此书以启发广大从事器官移植专业的医务工作者们，更好地服务于健康中国建设。

中国工程院院士
中华医学会副会长
中国医师协会副会长
鄭樹森

中文版前言

器官移植作为20世纪最伟大的医学成果之一，经过半个多世纪的发展，已经成为终末期器官功能衰竭患者的有效治疗手段。我国器官移植始于20世纪70年代，几经波折，但经过老一辈移植工作者的不懈努力，目前已经发展成为世界器官移植第二大国，其数量和质量都居于国际领先水平。由黄洁夫部长推动的器官移植改革已经使得国际社会彻底接受和承认中国在器官移植领域所取得的成就，我国提出的器官捐献的“中国模式”、肝癌肝移植的“杭州标准”已经被世界所认同，中国正以崭新的姿态站在世界器官移植的舞台上。

器官移植学是一门新兴学科，涉及多个学科的交叉和融合，新概念和新技术不断涌现，为了更好地与国际移植学界接轨，培养我国优秀的器官移植人才，特组织工作在移植一线的专家学者翻译了此部由美国艾伦·D.柯克等教授所著的《器官移植学》上下卷。

本书内容全面丰富，除了囊括了器官移植历史、基础理论、手术技术、术后管理、器官分配等各个方面，同时还涵盖了移植伦理、移植研究设计、移植政策制定等非临床相关内容，是一本不可多得的器官移植教学参考书。

由于时间仓促和水平有限，本书翻译过程中难免有疏漏之处，恳请广大读者给予批评指正。

目 录

上卷

第 6 篇

移植后管理

第 65 章 诱导性免疫抑制治疗

Ali H. Charafeddine, Allan D. Kirk

引言

免疫调节药物的使用和进步为器官移植治疗大多数原因导致的器官衰竭铺平了道路。几十年来,用于器官移植的免疫调节疗法逐渐演变出三个一般分类:诱导、维持或抢救治疗。免疫诱导治疗是一种当移植受体的免疫系统首次接触供体器官时使用的高强度预防性治疗。它包括用于免疫诱导的特殊药物(这些药物在长期使用中采用低剂量,而在免疫诱导时使用高剂量)以及其他免疫调节手段(如供体特异性输血)来促进受体初步接受异体移植物。该法来源于经验主义观察,认为早期对免疫调节的要求超过移植后的后期要求。随着时间的推移,这个观察显示出日益明显的生物学基础并与许多免疫活化机制相关联。

一般来说,免疫诱导治疗持续时间越久,毒性越大,往往会导致感染性疾病的发生和伤口愈合延迟。然而,适当地使用免疫诱导治疗可以降低早期急性排斥反应的发生率,并避免移植术后缺血性损伤恢复期(最脆弱的时期)的新器官受到免疫损伤。这种避免早期排斥反应发生的方法简化了移植受体的早期免疫管理;而是否能改善移植长期预后仍需进一步研究。无论如何,2010 年移植受体科学注册表显示免疫诱导治疗的使用越来越普遍。在 2010 年,超过 80%的肾移植受体除了接受作为大多数免疫诱导方案基础的单剂甲泼尼龙注射外,还接受了某种形式的免疫诱导治疗。更具体地说,58%的肾移植受体接受了 T 细胞消耗抗体治疗,21%接受了 IL-2RA(白介素 2 受体抗体)治疗,4%同时接受了以上两种治疗(表 65.1 和图 65.1)。

由于免疫调节的需求降低,免疫诱导治疗逐渐过渡到维持治疗——长期使用使用效力较低而耐受性更好的药物。对于维持治疗期间出现的急性排斥反应应采用抢救疗法。抢救疗法与诱导疗法类似,是一种高强度短期疗法。本章将介绍诱导治疗的新生物学基础,并回顾目前临床使用的专业免疫诱导治疗药物。免疫维持治疗及挽救治疗的一般临床原理及组成将在第 66 章和第 67 章以及“临床同种异体移植物排斥反应综合征:诊断和处理”(其包含器官特异性急性排斥反应的临床诊断和治疗部分内容)部分介绍。

免疫诱导治疗的生物学基础

受体移植器官首先遇到由两种非生理环境的不利因素支持的病理性免疫应答。第一种是受体的胸腺和造血系统选择了适合他们的淋巴细胞族群,这些族群有相对低的自体反应细胞[细胞响应自体 MHC 和(或)自体多肽]前体频率。那些具有自体反应潜能的细胞一般依赖于辅助信号(下文将讨论)激活。第二种非生理因素导致的器官特异性免疫反应与移植过程中不可避免的缺血、再灌注及相关的组织损伤有关(图 65.2)。这些因素改变抗原递呈的机制,改变 T 细胞和 B 细胞的活化阈值,并改变细胞转运,从而促进同种免疫反应(表 65.2)。因此,导致同种免疫过程源于器官在非生理条件下(高同种特异性前体频率内损伤)的生理免疫。这形成了同种免疫的基础,并为同种免疫排斥反应的初始免疫调节方法提供了适当的概念框架。在第 11 章可以找到这些概念的额外细节。在本节中,我们将涉及免疫诱导疗法成为器官移植的必要治疗手段的免疫学基础。目前临床上常见的免疫诱导方案主要针对 T 细胞介导的排斥反应(主要基于目前可用的药物,而非忽

表 65.1 1994—2009 年免疫诱导治疗：接受某种形式的专门(不包括甲泼尼龙单次注射)免疫诱导治疗的不同器官受体百分比

	专用的诱导治疗药物使用比例 (%)		
	年份		
移植器官	1994	2003	2009
肾脏	25	70	82.8
胰腺	30	79	81.4
肝脏	13	20	24.6
小肠	13	74	56.7
心脏	36	48	49.5
肺	25	44	59.7

Data from the Scientific Registry of Transplant Recipients (SRTR) and Organ Procurement and Transplantation Network (OPTN). SRTR/OPTN 2010 Annual Data Report. Department of Health and Human Services, Health Resources and Services Administration, Healthcare System Bureau, Division of Transplantation. Am J Transplant 2012; 12(Suppl. 1).

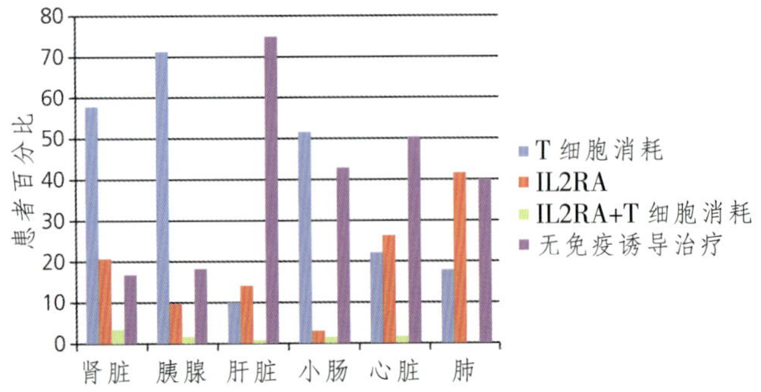

图 65.1 不同器官移植受体接受不同种类免疫诱导治疗药物百分比。Data from the Scientific Registry of Transplant Recipients (SRTR)and Organ Procurement and Transplantation Network (OPTN). SRTR/OPTN 2010 Annual Data Report. Department of Health and Human Services, Health Resources and Services Administration, Healthcare System Bureau, Division of Transplantation. Am J Transplant 2012; 12(Suppl. 1).

视移植后同种抗体的产生的重要性)。

免疫诱导治疗需求相关免疫学概念

几个基本概念共同决定了受体对同种免疫的反应初始能力。由于诱导免疫抑制是建立在阻断初始应答的基础上的，且其风险-收益评估的前提是受体需要使用这种强效免疫抑制方法，一般来说，我们需要了解影响这种应答真实性和效果的因素。我们可以通过了解那些常规因素来对上述因素进行灵活定义，常规因素包括：决定受体T细胞活化阈值、其同种特异性前体频率、全体T细胞中有记忆的T细胞处于非幼稚状态的程度、损伤伴随抗原暴露的数量以及被移植器官的整体易感性。下面将对这些因素进行简要总结。

活化阈值：免疫应答的三种信号模型

理论上，免疫活化的三种信号模型对于理解T细胞活化是有用的(图 65.3)。事实上，那些最常用的免疫抑制药物的目标特异性通路都在这个框架内。

同种抗原刺激活化在很大程度上是一个发生在次级淋巴组织内的过程。供体树突状细胞在移植时被激活，而且迁移至次级淋巴器官T细胞区域(图 65.1)。来自新近再灌注器官的趋化信号也吸引受体树突状细胞和其他具有移动抗原递呈功能的细胞（如单核细胞和巨噬细胞)前往可摄取供体抗原的移植物。这些细胞也迁移到二级淋巴组织。由此导致的情况是，次级淋巴组织内大量的供体抗原被递呈，而且被递呈给同种特异性T细胞。在这个位置，产生抗体的树突状细胞非生理性地吸引了大量幼稚T细胞和中央记忆T细胞。

当抗原递呈细胞(APC)表面的抗原通过CD3复合物触发T细胞相应的受体时，“信号1”被传送。其中T细胞响应供体衍生抗原递呈细胞的过程被称为直接抗原递呈；而T细胞响应受体衍生抗原递呈细胞的过程则被称为间接抗原递呈(图 65.4)。此外，当T细胞表达的CD28接触树突状细胞表面的CD80和CD86时，抗原递呈细胞可提供共同刺激，也被称为“信号2”。有许多共同刺激通路，其中许多(例如CD152，也称为CTLA-4)提供下调信号。因此，信号1和信号2的组合可以导致抗原特异性活化或抗原特异性无应答。详细内容已在第5章中描述。在移植时，CD28衍生共刺激活化信号往往占主导地位。因此，信号1和2激活三个T细胞内的信号转导通路：钙-钙调蛋白和钙调磷酸酶通路、RAS-MAP激酶通路和核因子kappa-B(NFκB)通路。这些通路导致许多新分子的表达，包括IL-2、CD154和CD25。最终，JAK-STAT依赖的信号通路通过IL-15和IL-2(以及其他)细胞因子受体共同γ链形成的“信号3”激活了西罗莫司(TOR)通路，引发了更多细胞的募集，增强了细胞增殖，从而导致大量的效应T细胞出现[1]。

值得注意的是，当抗原在淋巴滤泡或滤泡外区域(例如脾脏红髓)与抗原受体结合时，B细胞也将被激

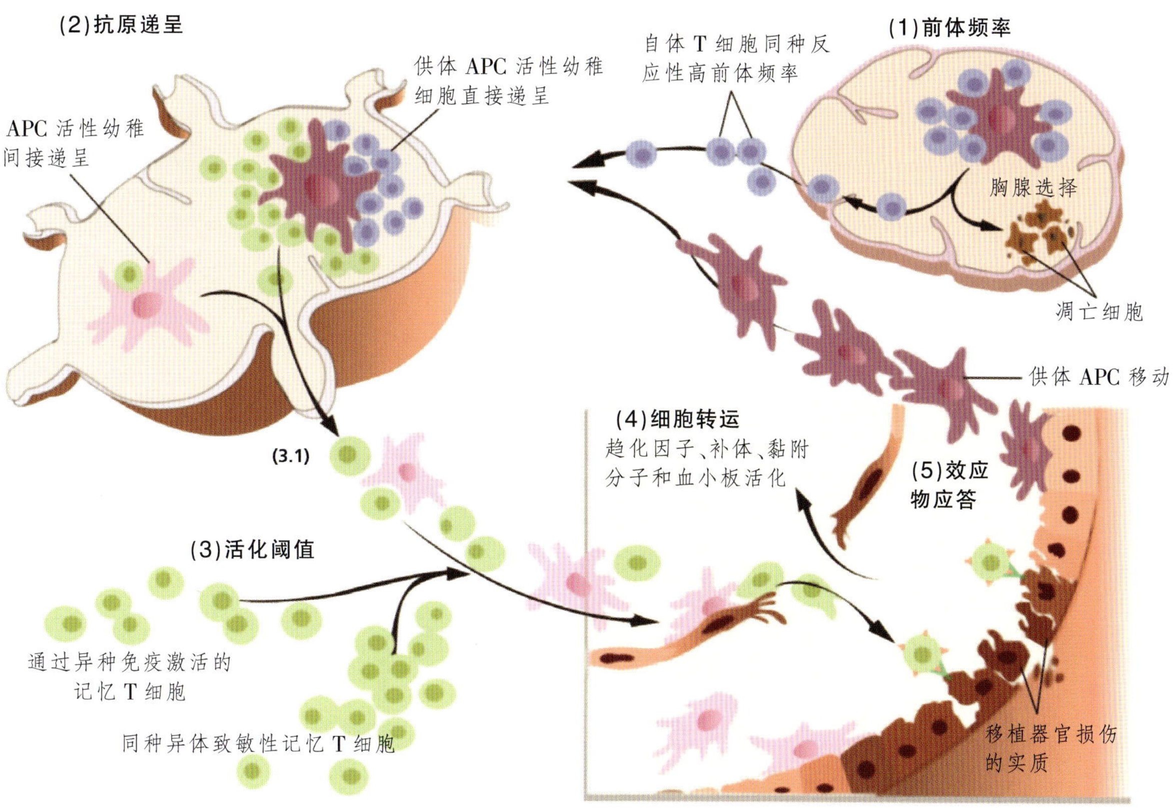

图 65.2 免疫诱导治疗的必要性因素。(1)前体频率。在胸腺选择时,自体胸腺中同种抗原缺失导致 T 细胞的释放,而不考虑同种异体 MHC,进而导致非生理性的幼稚 T 细胞池中高前体频率的产生。这受到 MHC 错配的影响,而且从理论上,讲可以通过将供体抗原引入受体胸腺来操作。(2)抗原递呈。同种特异性抗原递呈(直接通过供体抗原递呈细胞迁移到淋巴结或脾脏以及间接通过自体抗原递呈细胞进行抗原摄取和递呈)发生在次级淋巴组织(如周围淋巴结和脾脏)。它可以被共刺激阻断剂(如贝拉西普)、T 细胞消耗,类固醇、抗白介素 2 抗体等操纵。改变 T 细胞活化阈值(钙调神经磷酸酶抑制剂,西罗莫司靶蛋白)或细胞分裂(抗代谢物)的策略也影响 T 细胞对抗原递呈的接受能力。(3)活化阈值。T 细胞可以在淋巴结(3.1)或在移植物周围激活。记忆 T 细胞可绕过淋巴结的递呈需求。(4)细胞转运。受体抗原递呈细胞和活化的 T 细胞被趋化因子和黏附分子吸引到达新近受损的移植物。再灌注损伤促进供体抗原递呈细胞迁移到淋巴结进行直接递呈。(5)效应物应答。环境中强化了的 T 细胞衍生细胞因子(白介素 2)加强供体特异性细胞毒性,通过细胞的直接效应和促炎细胞因子的间接效应损害移植物。

表 65.2 诱导治疗的生物学基础

	前体频率	抗原递呈	活化阈值	细胞转运
生物学因素	MHC 错配	IRI,APC 活化	致敏,稳态	IRI,内皮损伤
治疗措施	OKT3,ATG,阿仑单抗,DST,mTOR	激素,贝拉西普	mTOR,CNI,MMF,激素,抗 IL2R,ATG	激素

IRI,缺血再灌注损伤;DST,供体特异性输血;mTOR,西罗莫司靶蛋白;CNI,钙调神经磷酸酶抑制剂;MMF,霉酚酸酯;ATG,抗胸腺细胞球蛋白。

活。这个治疗途径的具体操作虽然重要,但一般来说,不可在临床运用。因此,在很短的时间内自然的免疫反应可以调动效应 T 细胞和同种抗体。

前体频率

同种特异性 T 细胞前体频率是在宿主的免疫系统中通过直接或间接方式能够响应供体同种抗原的 T 细胞数量。不幸的是,对于临床医生来说,大多数受体这种供体特异性前体频率可以比任何自体 MHC 上的抗原递呈前体频率高几个数量级。换句话说,受体中响应供体抗原的 T 细胞数量远远高于生理情况下响应一种典型病毒感染的 T 细胞数量。要记住,免疫反应在本质上是指数级别的,初始供体特异性前体频率的一个细微变化可以造成免疫反应整体的巨大改变,而且现在迅速升级的免疫力已超过了为更受限制的反应而进化的监管控制。图 65.5 详细描绘了前体频率的概念,阐明了前体频率对临床免疫反应的影响[2]。

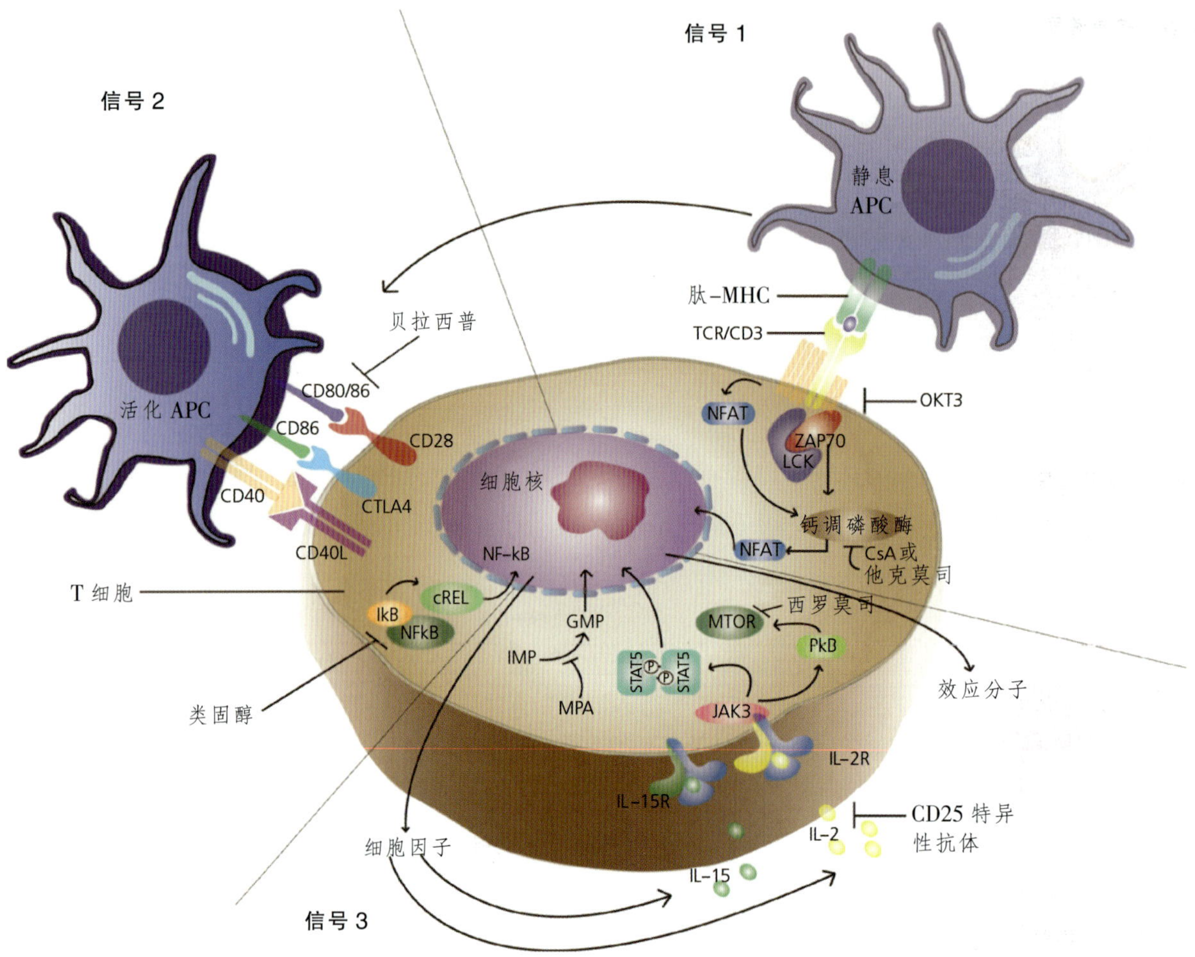

图 65.3 T细胞活化的3种信号模型。信号1是由TCR赋予的抗原特异性信号。信号2是由共刺激分子接收,信号3来自激活后细胞因子。OKT3、CsA 和他克莫司作用于信号1;贝拉西普和类固醇作用于信号2(并且在某种程度上通过限制MHC表达作用于信号1);CD25特异性单克隆抗体和西罗莫司阻断信号3。APC,抗原递呈细胞;CTLA-4,细胞毒性T细胞抗原4;GMP,单磷酸鸟苷;IκB,抑制性κB;IMP,肌苷一磷酸;JAK3,Janus 激酶3;L,配体;mTOR,西罗莫司靶蛋白;NFAT,活化T细胞的核因子;NF-κB,核因子κB;PKB,蛋白激酶B;R,受体;STAT5,信号转导和转录激活因子5;TCR,T细胞受体;TLR4,Toll样受体4;ZAP70,ζ链相关蛋白70。

有效的前体频率在不同受体之间有很大的不同,主要是受到MHC在供体和受体之间错配程度的影响。MHC匹配,实际上是将受体的胸腺选择更紧密地匹配供体的MHC,而且在这一过程中,要保证引入的移植物有一个更合适的T细胞前体频率。其他影响受体前体频率的因素包括既往免疫历史和MHC敏化(图65.6)。受体大约10%的免疫系统组成对移植物具有同种反应性。由此,在次级淋巴组织内发生的活化过程被大大(而且是非生理性的)促进,使生产性APC-T细胞相互作用变得不可避免,并大大降低通过自我平衡监管进行恢复的可能性。

记忆性 T 细胞

免疫记忆是哺乳动物适应性免疫应答的一个重要特征,一般来说,它使二次应答比初次应答更高效。记忆性T细胞对诱导免疫耐受构成重大障碍(图65.7)。它们是之前抗原暴露的产物,在有足够的共刺激背景下诱导细胞分裂,并作为长寿的抗原特异性细胞池持续生存[3]。记忆性T细胞根据表面表型不同,分为中央记忆型(Tcm)和效应记忆型(Tem)。中央记忆细胞(Tcm)迁移到二级淋巴器官(淋巴结、脾脏),而且从这些位置通过记忆暴发产生新的效应T细胞。效应记忆细胞(Tem)迁移到外周非淋巴区域,并针对外来抗原(例如,器官移植后同种抗原)提供即刻效应功能[3]。二者的共同特点是再激活时对共刺激及重复MHC-TCR绑定的需求大幅减少。因此,适合幼稚细胞的治疗在针对记忆细胞时可能有所欠缺。值得注意的是,记忆细胞一旦再次激活可能会降低增殖能力和减少存活能力。

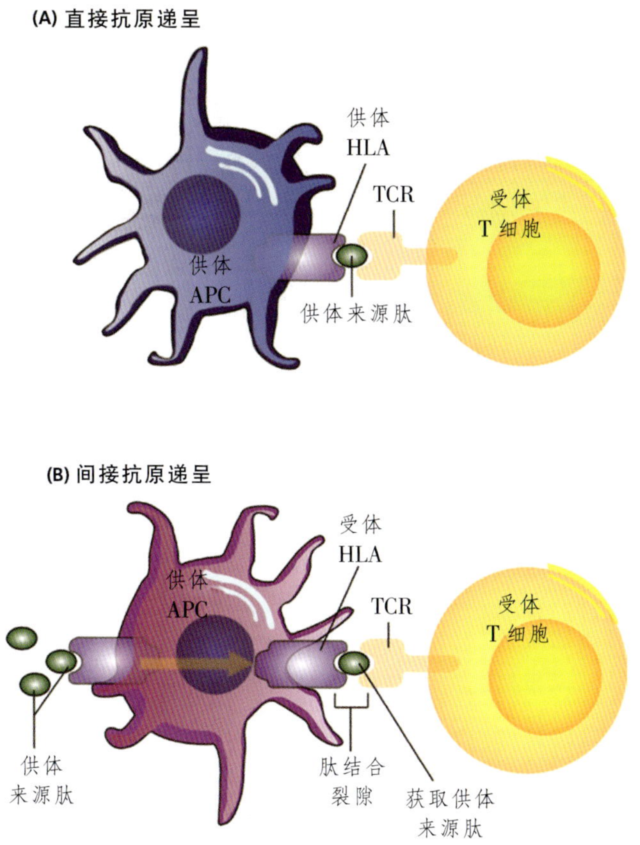

图 65.4 (A) 直接同种识别。响应供体来源的抗原递呈细胞(APC) 直接递呈抗原后,T 细胞可识别同种异体 HLA 分子的决定因素以及结合肽的结构。(B)间接同种识别。间接识别需要抗原加工和来自受体 APC 的递呈。HLA,人白细胞抗原;TCR,T 细胞受体。

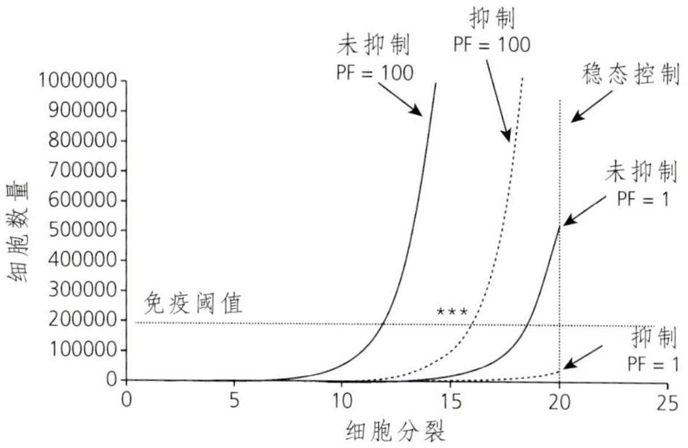

图 65.5 前体频率对临床相关免疫反应的影响。以低前体频率(PF)开始的有效(或未抑制)免疫应答可以被从高前体频率开始的低效(抑制)免疫应答所超越。为了产生有效的适应性免疫应答,T 细胞必须达到"免疫阈值"(理论上一定数量或活性水平),而不超过稳态控制。在正常生理条件下(前体频率为 1 且无免疫抑制)的最佳免疫应答期间,T 细胞分裂和增殖(约 20 个细胞分裂;y = 0.5e0.69x 时的细胞倍增)以达到免疫阈值并产生免疫应答。稳态控制标记 T 细胞增殖的结束。当 T 细胞失去其共刺激(抑制;PF = 1;y = 0.03e69x 时的细胞倍增)时,将在活化阈值之前达到稳态控制点,并且该免疫活性不能作为免疫表型登记。另一方面,将前体频率提高到 100(在 y = 50e0.69x 时未抑制的细胞倍增)将极大地帮助免疫活性达到免疫阈值以在稳态控制点之前建立免疫应答。即使在抑制时,前体频率为 100 的那些细胞仍然比在 PF 为 1 时未抑制的细胞更有效地达到活化阈值。

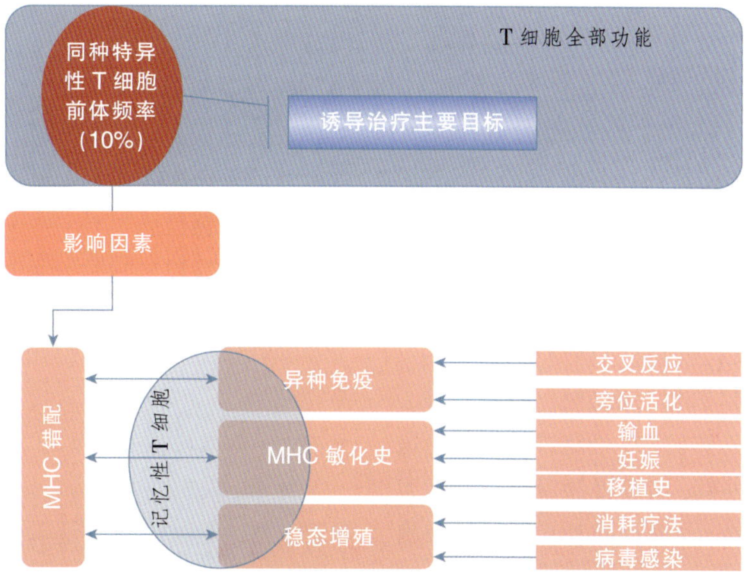

图 65.6 同种特异性前体频率是诱导免疫抑制的主要目标。

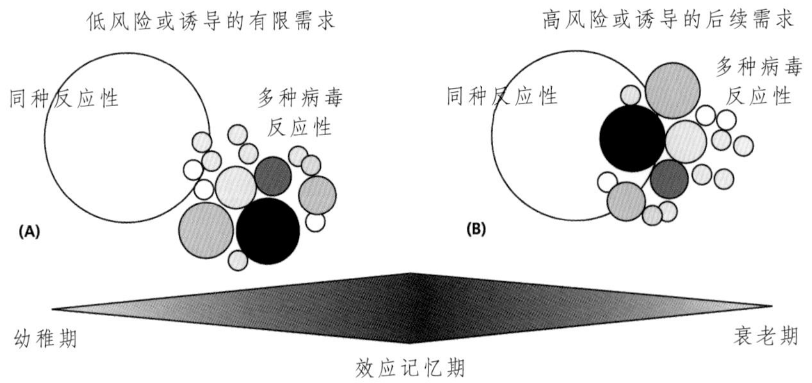

图 65.7 免疫诱导的概念图。幼稚 T 细胞谱通过扩增的活化效应记忆状态，过渡到衰老期，其显示在图的底部。观察在成熟的不同阶段同种反应性和多种病毒反应性组成成分，我们假设具有非常低程度的异源交叉反应性(A)的个体将处于低排斥风险中，并且具有高度交叉反应性的个体(B)(具有大量扩增的活化群体，其实际上并入同种免疫谱系中，由黑色圆圈表示)将具有非常高的排斥风险。因此，如果我们能够区分 A 个体和 B 个体，就可以定制免疫管理策略，从而避免并发症和不必要的风险。

因此，该障碍虽然巨大，但可以用简短的疗法瞬间消除，这也是免疫诱导治疗的原理之一。

阻断共刺激的效果可以在实验上证实对记忆的影响。在啮齿类动物模型中，在抗原递呈时剥夺共刺激中的 T 细胞可成功诱导移植耐受[4]。然而，这种方法在远系繁殖模型(如人类)中不太成功，而且记忆性 T 细胞被认为是罪魁祸首。具体来说，在特定的无菌条件下生长的年轻实验室小鼠的记忆性 T 细胞仅占总 T 细胞群的 5%~10%。另一方面，超过 50%的人类和其他非人类灵长类动物的 T 细胞群由记忆性 T 细胞组成。这种差异可以解释为不同环境暴露和免疫历史的结果。因此，人类和群居的非人类灵长类动物拥有强有力的记忆性 T 细胞，从某种意义上说，其为诱导移植耐受设置了障碍[3]。

除了在成年人中广泛存在以外，记忆性 T 细胞对消耗性治疗也表现出更强的抗性，对调节性 T 细胞的活性所致的抑制作用也强于幼稚 T 细胞。成年人类的庞大记忆性 T 细胞群随机包含高比例的供体反应性记忆性 T 细胞，而这是诱导移植免疫耐受方案能否成功的一个主要决定因素[5]。

开发人类受体免疫耐受诱导策略时，必须同时考虑同种免疫的幼稚细胞成分和记忆细胞成分，无论这些记忆细胞生成的途径如何，这都是很重要的。事实上，已经有几种机制解释了供体反应性记忆性 T 细胞的生成，包括异种免疫、稳态增殖、前期 MHC 敏化，以及 T 细胞双受体。下文将简要描述记忆性和同种免疫性的关系，而第 9 章中已作详细阐述。

异种免疫

未来对完全无关刺激的反应过程会受到前期免疫暴露的影响。至少有两种机制可以解释这一现象:T 细胞交叉反应性和旁位活化[6]。当抗原递呈细胞在二级淋巴器官处理病毒蛋白并递呈抗原肽与自体-MHC 分子复合物时会发生一个正常的针对病原体(比如病毒)的免疫反应。分子模拟导致 T 细胞交叉反应，它是指病毒抗原-自体-MHC 复合物模拟包含自体肽的外来 MHC 分子。另外，通过旁位活化可能发生异种反应，当病毒特异性 T 细胞释放生长因子、细胞因子和炎症介质后，通过非特异性的方式激活旁位同种反应性 T 细胞[6](图 65.8)。

稳态增殖

在淋巴细胞减少的条件下，T 细胞可以广泛增殖，这是一个被称为自我平衡增殖的过程。这个过程显示了对共刺激阻断的强大抵抗，而且产生了同种反应性记忆性 T 细胞对诱导耐受的抵抗力。临床上，淋巴细胞减少可以通过病毒或治疗性的 T 细胞损耗诱导来治疗自身免疫性疾病或器官移植。剩余的 T 细胞进行快速分裂并获得记忆表型，因此构成针对移植耐受的强大障碍[7]。

前期 MHC 敏化及其他机制

怀孕、输血和移植均可发生前期抗原暴露。最近，研究发现，显然存在其他可能生成供体反应性记忆性 T 细胞的机制。在某些情况下，针对病原体衍生表位的记忆性 T 细胞显示表达第二种 T 细胞受体，这种受体可以发生同种异体反应[8]。

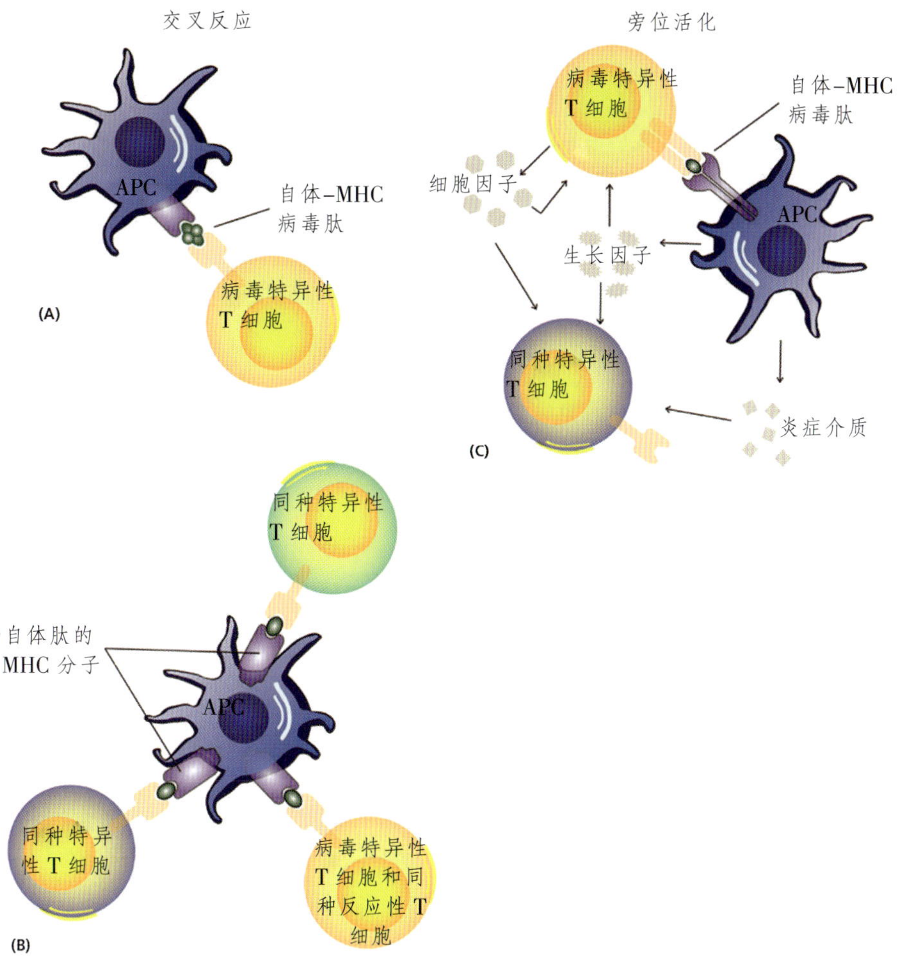

图 65.8　异种免疫应答。(A)正常免疫应答。APC 处理病毒蛋白并递呈给自体-MHC 复合的抗原肽。(B)通过“分子模拟”的交叉反应性。(C)旁位活化。

需要免疫诱导治疗的组织损伤机制

损伤和免疫密切相关，损伤导致组织暴露于病原体，病原体本身最终导致组织破坏，这是一个恶性循环。损伤的类型包括内皮损伤、补体激活、缺血和再灌注、受体手术损伤、供体损伤、脑死亡，这些都会影响免疫反应的强度。这些因素通过增加抗原递呈的有效性，以及通过转运细胞到移植器官及其引流淋巴结，从而推进免疫[9]。对损伤的识别和反应，通常被视为免疫系统(已在第 7 章中深度介绍)的一种先天性作用。

损伤的其他几个方面协同促进了同种免疫反应。例如，再灌注的移植器官内的补体可以促进幼稚 T 细胞活化。缺血和再灌注被认为可以增加共刺激分子的表达，从而导致残留和迁移过来的抗原递呈细胞效率提高，也改善了 T 细胞的反应。此外，再灌注后出现的细胞因子环境强烈支持激活，而且与移植数月后明显不同[9]。受损的内皮细胞和实质分泌趋化因子吸引效应细胞到达器官；与此同时，再灌注损伤启动 APC 移动到淋巴结和脾脏。这两个事件都增加了特异性 T 细胞遇到合适的 APC 或目标抗原的可能性，从而创造了一个局部增强的 T 细胞前体频率[9]。

器官敏感性是免疫诱导治疗需求的变量

重要的是要记住，不同移植器官对损伤的敏感性显著不同。例如，心脏及时和持续的工作依赖于传导系统(小体积组织)的电活动；它也容易受到局部负性肌力作用细胞因子的影响。与之相比，肾脏即使在明显损伤后失功好几周，仍然可以再生肾小管和肾功能，而肝脏可以再生超过一半的体积以应对损伤。此外，年老器官由于自身已存在损伤，更加需要避免免疫损伤。因此，器官可接受的免疫损伤的量级变化很大，不仅仅基于损伤反应的大小，还取决于器官承受免疫损伤后仍然能在足够的时间内恢复功能的能力。总之，不同受体、不同供体以及不同器官之间的可承受同种免疫反应的程度均不同。因此,围术期为获得良好预后而对免疫抑制的需求也不同[9]。

将上述因素与临床情况联系起来是复杂的，还需要找到一种前瞻性的量化途径。但是,广义上,我们仍然可以发现有多种因素在共同起作用。需要考虑的因素有年龄、怀孕史、EB病毒感染情况、器官移植史、MHC匹配、供体的临床状况以及缺血时间。理想情况下，诱导治疗将根据供受体的具体特点个体化实行[9]。然而在实践中，一种经过精确协调的以定量比例方式来评估各种情况的方法尚未开发。因此,常规方法被用于早期免疫激活的一般情况，诱导的药物使用基于经验性的或以人口统计为基础的指导方针。

初始免疫应答的特定目标组成

免疫抑制这个词意义广泛且无法提供患者发生排斥反应风险的具体信息。由于每个受体接受的器官都有其独特的免疫经历,且每个移植物有其独有的缺陷，免疫诱导疗法应该根据所需的强度、持续时间和目标不同而有所变化。最合理的方法是观察这些影响诱导治疗的变量因素，然后选择专门针对这些因素的药物(表65.3)。

针对前体频率

消耗性的诱导药物可以无差别地降低前体频率。消耗性药物包括多克隆抗T淋巴细胞/胸腺细胞制剂(胸腺球蛋白、抗胸腺球蛋白、免疫球蛋白)以及针对常见的淋巴细胞决定因子的特定单克隆制剂，比如CD3(OKT3)和CD52(阿仑单抗)。这些药物介导不同程度持久性和耐受性的快速T细胞消耗。在这一过程中,它们能够减少会损害移植物的细胞数目,更理想的是,其以一种更加近似生理性免疫反应的方式减少了同种特异性T细胞的频率。一项重要的观察项目指出,并不是所有的T细胞都以同样的程度消耗。针对抗体介导的消耗,有记忆表型的T细胞(仍然易感但比例更低)比幼稚T细胞(它们可以耐受,但T细胞计数明显减少)。同样重要的是,在T细胞消耗后,剩余的T细胞将进行维持稳态的增殖，从而生成一个有记忆表型的T细胞群。这大大降低了活化每个细胞的阈值,剩下的细胞相对更加活跃和有效。所以消耗治疗后,受体只需很少的T细胞就会发生排斥反应。因此,由于受体接受了消耗治疗,总是需要额外的免疫抑制治疗。临床试验中,如果采用OKT3、阿仑单抗、胸腺细胞球蛋白进行高强度消耗治疗而没有额外的维持性免疫抑制，当T细胞重新开始增殖后,即使T细胞计数不到10个/μl,也会产生排斥反应。

为了避免消耗治疗后T细胞自我平衡活化这种批量激活的影响，一种理论上的方法是特异性地针对活化的T细胞。IL-2受体(CD25)特异性单克隆抗体(达利珠单抗和巴利昔单抗)设计时就考虑到了这一点。虽然设计时希望可以选择性消耗，但它们的临床效果有限,很少或几乎没有消耗治疗的能力。

当与促进活化-诱导细胞死亡(AICD)的药物联合使用时,供体特异性输血(血液或骨髓)已被证明能够促进同种特异性T细胞消耗。从理论上讲,提供供体抗原来激活细胞,同时剥夺它的信号3(促进其分裂所需的细胞因子),将导致细胞凋亡。这一方法使用的药物是mTOR抑制剂(西罗莫司和依维莫司)。供体特异性输血起作用的可能机制包括克隆缺失、调节性T细胞活化、失能和嵌合现象。无论如何,虽然在实验模型中效果很明显,但还未被证明在临床上是实际有效的。

表65.3 可降低T细胞活化阈值的免疫抑制药物

免疫抑制剂	作用机制
钙调磷酸酶抑制剂	减少信号转导
抗T细胞受体抗体	限制T细胞受体的绑定效率
mTOR抑制剂	限制活化细胞因子的作用
IL-2R拮抗剂	限制活化细胞因子的作用
糖皮质激素	改变T细胞受体对应的核蛋白
共刺激拮抗剂	阻止CD28的参与

针对抗原递呈

正如本章前文所提到的，器官移植后两代不同的抗原递呈细胞可以启动排斥反应:一些来自供体(参与直接递呈),一些来自受体(参与间接递呈)(图65.4)。两者都可以导致排斥反应;然而,由于供体衍生抗原递呈细胞进入了大部分同种反应性T细胞群，它们最有可能影响初始排斥反应的风险。

有无数措施可以用来限制APC的移动,首先是良好的保存技术和快速的移植。已经显示氧化应激这种限制因素可影响APC活化和功能。从药物治疗的角度来看，甲泼尼龙几乎无一例外地在器官再灌注时使用，并能减少 APC 转运。虽然通常因为没有“真正”进行诱导而撤除单剂激素的使用，但实际上，它是更有效的诱导策略之一，并已被接受为移植过程的一部分，而不是一种特殊的诱导方法。

多克隆抗体制剂有抗黏附效果。因此他们可能阻止 APC 活化和转运，而且这可以用来区分多克隆制剂和单克隆制剂，因为前者在机制上超越了消耗的范畴。脱氧精胍菌素（DSG）在实验中也被发现能阻止 APC 活化，在此基础上非正式地使用，但是还没有实质性的效果[10]。共刺激分子在 APC 功能方面至关重要。最突出的是 B7 分子、CD80 和 CD86。已有专门设计的生物制剂来阻断这个通路，其中最先进的是贝拉西普[11]。贝拉西普已被作为一种维持治疗药品来研究，但可能对最初的 APC 功能有一些影响。即使在移植时使用，还没有数据显示它具有超越一般维持治疗药物的实质性效果。

针对活化阈值

许多因素参与 T 细胞活化。由于标记抗原的亲和力、过度的抗原递呈或弱抗原表达辅以最佳共刺激，甚至在 T 细胞的直接环境中有大量的刺激性细胞因子，使 T 细胞达到活化阈值。鉴于 T 细胞对器官排斥反应至关重要，大多数商用免疫抑制药物改变了 T 细胞活化的事件序列（表 65.3）。这些影响已在第 17 章中进行了深度介绍。关于标准免疫抑制药物在免疫诱导中的使用，大多数临床医生认为实现移植后早期的治疗药物水平是一个重要的目标。因此，大剂量的钙调磷酸酶抑制剂、抗代谢物和 mTOR 抑制剂都被研究过了。总的来说，这些药物的可耐受剂量都被毒性反应限制，因此，使用高“诱导剂量”的药物来改变 T 细胞活化是受到限制的。此外，糖皮质激素可以诱导核结合蛋白的变化，而这种蛋白可以通过 T 细胞受体传输信号，因此，可能通过影响这个机制增加其作为诱导药物的功效。

针对细胞转运

缺血和再灌注促进细胞通过多因子途径（包括黏附受体上调、内皮收缩或损坏、趋化细胞因子释放）转运到移植器官[12]。这个阶段的同种免疫应答被广泛认为是具有价值的特定目标。一般来说，糖皮质激素限制黏附分子表达，而多克隆抗淋巴细胞药物也有抗黏附分子的效果。因此，这种机制被认为是甲泼尼龙和（或）多克隆抗体用于免疫诱导阶段的部分原因。然而，基于再灌注阶段转运的重要性，大量试验药物被纳入考虑范围。

整合素在白细胞活化和转运至炎症区域中发挥了至关重要的作用。整合素存在于多种免疫细胞上，包括 T 细胞、B 细胞、中性粒细胞和巨噬细胞，它是异质二聚体的细胞表面受体，调节这些细胞和在它们周围环境中其他细胞之间的黏附，特别是白细胞功能关联抗原-1（LFA-1）和极迟抗原-4（VLA-4），其是研究最多的整合素。LFA-1 在 T 细胞和抗原递呈细胞之间免疫突触的形成中起着至关重要的作用，而且 LFA-1 和 VLA-4 已被证明在阻止炎症区域的淋巴细胞滚动和 T 细胞迁移到炎症区域中发挥作用。整合素拮抗剂将在后面讨论。

有一类药物专门针对在细胞归巢和转运中至关重要的趋化因子通路。特别是，鞘氨醇-1-磷酸盐（S1P）是调节趋化因子敏感性的一个关键因素，而且在理论上其代表一个有趣的阻断靶点。芬戈莫德（FTY720）旨在结合 S1P 并导致这种分子的内化，从而抑制淋巴细胞从二级淋巴器官迁移。它已经被证明可以降低复发-缓解型多发性硬化症的复发率。不幸的是，芬戈莫德被发现具有首剂心动过缓的作用，限制了其在移植领域的发展。

特异性免疫诱导药物的临床效果

临床上有许多可用的针对移植后不久被放大的同种免疫成分的药物。几种药物已经在临床试验中与标准维持治疗方案联合使用并被证明是有效的，但很少有前瞻性研究对较为突出的几种药物进行比较，而且没有药物能在所有情况下都显示出明显的优越性。大多数研究都采用早期急性排斥反应，而不是更明确的受体或移植物的存活作为研究终点。几乎所有的试验都在以单剂甲泼尼龙为基础的诱导治疗上分列了几种“特异的”诱导药物。

在肾移植中，与单剂甲泼尼龙的标准诱导治疗相比，特异的诱导药物作为一个整体，被证实能够减少受体中可经活检证实的早期急性排斥反应（BPAR）的发生率，特别是那些对标准的环孢素（CsA）、硫唑嘌呤（AZA）和泼尼松具有同种敏化作用的患者[13,14]。胰肾联合移植的诱导治疗显示出排斥反应适度减少的趋势[15,16],但其在心脏移植中的疗效仍有争议[17]。诱导治疗没有显示能使肝移植获益。远期研究在肾移植后5年未能显示出可观的效果[13],可能是因为维持治疗的影响,以及受体的共存疾病随着时间的推移开始占主导地位。

与所有形式的强力免疫抑制一样,诱导治疗与感染和恶性并发症的发生率增加有关。诱导治疗的获益与其所致的更高的技术性并发症并不匹配[18]。然而,当联合常规维持性免疫抑制治疗时,一些诱导策略大大增加了移植后淋巴增殖性疾病(PTLD)和恶性肿瘤死亡的风险[19,20]。具体来说,未接受专门的免疫诱导治疗或接受CD25特异性治疗的受体,其预期的PTLD发病率是0.5%。OKT3诱导治疗将风险增加到了0.85%,多克隆损耗治疗将风险增加到0.81%,尤其是新近暴露于EB病毒的移植受体。权衡这种情况,目前尚不清楚诱导治疗是否提高了远期疗效。无论如何,减少早期排斥反应的发生确实使移植受体的早期管理更容易,这已总体提高了诱导治疗的使用率。表65.4总结了诱导治疗中使用的单克隆抗体和多克隆抗体。

莫罗单抗-OKT3

OKT3(莫罗单抗-CD3;Orthoclone OKT3,Janssen-Cilag)是一种鼠源性IgG2a抗人类CD3抗体,是第一个获批准的用于诱导治疗的单克隆抗体。OKT3与CD3蛋白质ε链结合,导致循环T细胞的瞬时激活并释放细胞因子(IL-2、IL-3、IL-6,IFN-γ);最终,使T细胞大规模裂解并从循环中消失[21]。

莫罗单抗最初是在20世纪80年代初引入的,很快就证明其能有效治疗急性排斥反应。尽管临床应用成功,但其引起的副作用也是具有挑战性的,主要由于T细胞释放大量细胞因子导致临床上的细胞因子释放症候群,包括低血压、发烧、恶心、呕吐、肺水肿。极少的情况下,OKT3可导致无菌性脑膜炎或移植物内血栓形成。此外,作为一种鼠源性抗体,受体在首剂使用后可能产生抗鼠类抗体,限制了OKT3的有效性。OKT3其他主要的副作用有移植后淋巴细胞增生性疾病、真菌感染和巨细胞病毒感染。因此,OKT3远离了市场,这里提到是为了解历史[21]。为了在不释放细胞因子的情况下达到抗排斥反应的效果,已经开发了很多人源化的OKT3 Fc变异体;然而,没有一种已被证明能用于移植诱导。

表65.4 单克隆抗体和多克隆抗体

名称	形式	来源	作用
抗胸腺细胞球蛋白(ATGAM)	多克隆	马	抗CD2,CD3,CD4,CD8,CD11a,CD18,CD25,CD44,CD45,HLA-DR1
抗胸腺细胞球蛋白(即复宁)	多克隆	兔	
莫罗单抗(OKT3)*	单克隆	鼠	抗CD3
巴利昔单抗(舒莱)	单克隆	重组物(嵌合体)	抗CD25
达利珠单抗(赛尼哌)#	单克隆	重组物(人源化)	抗CD25
阿仑单抗(Campath)	单克隆	重组物(人源化)	抗CD52

*2009年退出全球市场;#2009年退出美国市场。

抗CD-25抗体

莫罗单抗全消耗的副作用刺激了耐受性更好的诱导免疫抑制剂的发展。由于IL-2是公认有效的T细胞生长因子,巴利昔单抗与达利珠单抗这两种针对IL-2受体(CD25)的α亚基的单克隆抗体得到了开发。这两种抗体竞争性抑制IL-2绑定并阻止T细胞扩张[21]。最重要的是,与马、老鼠、兔蛋白衍生的单克隆抗体相关的血清病及加快药物清除的问题在巴利昔单抗(嵌合体化的)和达利珠单抗(人源化的)中并不存在。理论上的优势在于,这些单克隆抗体仅针对在活化的T细胞表达的受体。

达利珠单抗与肾移植。达利珠单抗是人源化的IgG1单克隆抗体,1998年经前瞻性安慰剂对照试验证明在肾移植中安全有效后被引入临床[22]。在三联疗法(AZA、CsA、类固醇)或二联疗法(CsA、类固醇)的背景下,达利珠单抗已被证明在6个月时可适度减少BPAR[23]。在其他研究中,与安慰剂相比,应用达利珠单抗治疗的受体,其移植肾有类似的移植后淋巴增殖性疾病发生率,但是有更好的功能,且巨细胞病毒感染率降低[24-26]。重要的是,达利珠单抗并未引起全身炎症反应综合征(SIRS)或其相关的症状。

采用达利珠单抗诱导联合三联疗法,使用较低剂量的CsA显示出与采用标准剂量的CsA效果大致相当;不幸的是,完全撤除 CsA 可导致 BPAR 发生率显著上升[27-29]。达利珠单抗诱导方案联合霉酚酸酯(MMF)、皮质类固醇、低剂量他克莫司(TAC)三联疗法,相比达利珠单抗诱导联合低剂量的 CsA 或低剂量的西罗莫司,或单用标准剂量 CsA,其在肾功能、移植物存活和急性排斥反应发生率方面有优势[30]。

对高危患者——既往失去过移植物或具有同种抗体(不是供者特异性的),采用消耗性药物兔源抗胸腺细胞免疫球蛋白(RATG)诱导联合三联疗法(TAC、MMF、类固醇)相比采用达利珠单抗诱导在激素抵抗性排斥反应及 BPAR 发生率方面明显更有效[31]。

达利珠单抗与其他实体器官。达利珠单抗在肝脏、心脏和肺移植领域的应用也有一些研究。在肝移植中,达利珠单抗应用二剂疗法方案也有与其在肾移植中应用类似的效果[32]。几项研究显示达利珠单抗联合传统 MMF 和 TAC 方案具有较低的急性排斥反应发生率,最近的几项研究表明,皮质类固醇可以安全地从这个方案中撤除[33-35]。

在心脏移植受体中,达利珠单抗的标准五剂方案与传统免疫抑制方案相比,其可减少急性排斥反应发生率。最终,在心脏移植受体中,达利珠单抗的二剂方案被证明与五剂方案效果相当[36-39]。至于肺移植受体,两项对照研究都显示达利珠单抗效果略优于 RATG[40,41]。

尽管达利珠单抗上市已有大约 10 年,但其于 2009 年 9 月已停止使用。这在很大程度上是由于同一代的巴利昔单抗竞争市场份额所致,而非生物学差异的原因。达利珠单抗与巴利昔单抗最显著的区别就是诱导治疗推荐剂量不同(分别为 5 和 2),而且这种差异产生了有利于巴利昔单抗的影响。

巴利昔单抗在肾移植中的应用。1997 年的一项随机前瞻性试验将巴利昔单抗诱导联合 CsA 和类固醇治疗与安慰剂治疗进行了比较,巴利昔单抗治疗的受体 6 个月的 BPAR 较低,耐激素性排斥反应发生率较低,没有细胞因子释放综合征的证据,同时类似的感染和 PTLD 发生率也很低[42]。这些结果在其他三个不同机构的不同试验中获得再次证实;巴利昔单抗诱导联合三联疗法(CsA、AZA 和泼尼松)也显示移植后 6 个月急性排斥反应发生率较低[43-46]。着眼于单剂与双剂巴利昔单抗的试验显示单剂治疗(术后第 1 天 40mg)有略好的 BPAR 和急性排斥反应发生率[47-49]。最重要的是,几项试验表明,在包含巴利昔单抗诱导的免疫抑制方案中,撤除钙调磷酸酶抑制剂可提高耐受性[50-52]。

此外,另一项研究对比了 RATG+延迟 CsA 与巴利昔单抗 + CsA 诱导联合 MMF 和类固醇。结果两组移植物存活率、受体生存率和 BPAR 结果类似[53]。

巴利昔单抗与其他实体器官移植。两剂巴利昔单抗诱导治疗在肝移植受体的临床试验中能被良好耐受并有效减少 BPAR(但在 HCV 阳性受体中降低幅度较小)[54-56]。有趣的是,巴利昔单抗允许 TAC 延迟使用并能使肝移植患者获得更好的肾功能[57]。最重要的是,在 HCV 阳性受体中,巴利昔单抗诱导联合无激素免疫抑制方案具有更高的 BPAR(巴利昔单抗联用类固醇者为 24.3%,巴利昔单抗不联用类固醇者为 39.4%),但其受体生存率更高(使用类固醇者为 61.0%,不使用类固醇者为 84.3%)。此外,巴利昔单抗诱导联合无激素免疫抑制方案中 HCV 复发率较低[58-60]。

巴利昔单抗在心脏移植受体中的效果目前仍无定论。在一项试验中,巴利昔单抗诱导用于促进延迟 CsA 使用,从而减少其对于心脏移植受体的肾毒性[61]。而它与 RATG 的比较研究仍有争议[62,63]。最近的一项关于几项较小研究的 Meta 分析发现,几乎没有证据证明 IL-2R 特异性治疗可以改善结果[64]。

在肺移植领域,最近关于国际心脏和肺移植注册中心的数据分析显示,IL-2R 特异性治疗对单肺和双肺移植受者是有益的[65]。

阿仑单抗

CD52 是一种功能未知的膜糖蛋白,主要出现在 T 细胞、B 细胞、巨噬细胞、单核细胞、嗜酸性粒细胞和男性生殖系统细胞中。阿仑单抗是一种特异作用于人类 CD52 的人源化 IgG2b,已用于诱导和抢救治疗[66-69]。其可以导致快速和有效的 T 细胞和 B 细胞消耗,以及某种程度的单核细胞消耗。它可用于治疗淋巴系统恶性肿瘤,而且正被研究治疗多发性硬化症。虽然不是专门用于诱导移植免疫耐受,但它一直被标签外应用于该治疗,目前美国大约有 10%的肾移植患者使用该药物。深入讨论该药品的标签外说明使用详见第 101 章。

由于可促进肾移植中低剂量 CsA 单药疗法,阿仑单抗获得了移植界的关注[67]。随后的研究探索了其作为耐受原的应用[68],明确显示尽管其可以带来深度的损耗,但阿仑单抗并没有诱导耐受,而是促进了低剂量的维持治疗。后来的研究将它与更传统的免疫抑制疗法联合,使得该药物能够合理地常规使用[69-71],显示它可以有效地降低BPAR,并提供几个月的窗口期以减少免疫抑制的需求,但缺少足够的维持免疫抑制可能出现晚期急性排斥反应。

比较研究。几乎没有进行过关于阿仑单抗良好对照的比较研究,这反映了其缺乏在移植中的具体适应证及实验实施的财务可行性。一项早期使用历史对照的试验在使用MMF和TAC的背景下比较了阿仑单抗与巴利昔单抗。在这项大型的单中心研究中,阿仑单抗治疗的受体在3个月时有较低的排斥反应发生率,不过1年时排斥反应发生率相似[70]。其他后续的小型研究中,短期随访表明阿仑单抗诱导可有获益[71,72]。

最重要的关于阿仑单抗作为诱导剂的研究是一项多中心随机对照试验,它将受体根据发生排斥反应的风险(定义为重复移植、群体反应性抗体的峰值超过20%,或黑种人群)分层并与低危受体比较,其中低危组随机选用巴利昔单抗或阿仑单抗进行比较,高危组随机选用RATG或阿仑单抗[73]。阿仑单抗组的BPAR在6个月(3%对15%,$P<0.001$)及12个月(5%对17%,$P<0.001$)都明显较低。3年BPAR,低危组使用阿仑单抗的患者低于使用巴利昔单抗的患者(10%对22%,$P=0.003$),但在高危组中,使用阿仑单抗的患者与使用RATG的患者之间无显著差异(18%对15%,$P=0.63$)。不良事件发生率在所有组中都是相似的。本研究做了大量工作证明阿仑单抗是诱导治疗一个可行的选择,但未能说服它的制造者——Sanofi,去探求其在移植中的适应证。

阿仑单抗并没有系统地或广泛地在肾外器官进行研究。一项研究比较了阿仑单抗联合低剂量的TAC与传统的TAC联合类固醇在肝移植受体中的应用。使用阿伦单抗治疗的受体进行维持治疗需要的类固醇更少,肾毒性更小,最重要的是,1年的急性排斥反应发生率更低且距发生排斥反应的中位时间间隔更长[74]。患有难治性急性排斥反应或闭塞性细支气管炎综合征的肺移植受体接受了阿仑单抗治疗。排斥的组织学评分有所改善,且在2年的随访期内未发生细支气管炎[75]。这些关于肝脏和肺的研究表明,阿仑单抗可能对肾外器官也有益处。

多克隆抗体

从移植时代早期开始,已经研发出了一些多克隆抗体制剂。多克隆抗体是由不同动物的全细胞免疫产生的一种抗体制剂,而临床使用的制剂源自兔子(RATG)或马(ATGAM)。总的来说,兔源制剂被认为在多药肾移植免疫抑制方案中是最有效的[76,77]。多克隆抗体包含与多种细胞抗原特异性结合的抗体,包括参与抗原识别、T细胞黏附和共刺激的TCR细胞表面标记物(如CD2、CD3、CD4、CD8、CD11a、CD18、CD25、CD44、CD45),以及MHC分子和非T细胞分子。

多克隆抗体制剂的亲和谱多样而可变,即便是临床批准的只含有IgG的RATG和ATGAM药物仍然是多样化的,这样的高免疫原性导致大量不良反应,包括全血细胞减少症[78,79]。目前,有3种制剂应用于临床:抗胸腺细胞免疫球蛋白-R(ATG-R或RATG)、抗胸腺细胞球蛋白-费森尤斯(ATG-F)和ATGAM(马源性)。尽管每一种都是在某种程度上才被使用,但目前最为常用的是RATG,对比试验的结果显示其在肾移植中疗效更高[80]。多克隆制剂的主要作用机制目前未知,但已经推断与前体频率减少、抑制白细胞黏附、阻断淋巴细胞激活所需的辅助分子信号的共同作用有关。

多克隆抗体诱导的副作用是有据可查的。细胞因子释放综合征往往是治疗中观察到的最常见的不良反应,大约影响到20%的接受治疗的受体。这种生理现象被认为是由与前文所讨论的莫罗单抗类似的方法所导致,但总的来说并不严重。另外,这些药物通常需要通过中央静脉给药以使血栓性静脉炎的发生风险最小化。其他不良反应主要与其强有力的免疫抑制效果有关,包括PTLD、机会性感染、潜伏的疱疹病毒再激活。剂量依赖的副作用主要包括白细胞减少和血小板减少、血清病和过敏反应。

多克隆抗体在肾移植中的应用。在美国,大约50%的肾移植受体接受多克隆抗体制剂免疫诱导。欧洲和世界其他地区使用率低一些。迄今为止,大多数试验旨在评估将多克隆抗体添加到一个原本严格的维持治疗方案中,而且,正如预期的,这种强力的方法减少了急性排斥反应发生率,但同时也增加了感染的发生率[81,82]。考虑到多克隆抗体以许多机制为靶点,在CD4消耗和细胞表面分子调节方面具有良好的诱导作用和持久效果,最近试验旨在减少维持治疗的需求。两项初步研究表明,RATG促进了单药维持性免疫抑制治疗在选定的受体中获得与当前标准相似的移植物和受体存活率[83,84]。更长时间的随访表明,由于淋巴细胞的再增殖,可以观察到晚期排斥反应,因此,这种方法是否可取仍然有争议。

追溯到前 CsA 时代的试验表明,RATG 诱导可延迟早期急性排斥反应的发生[76]。更多当代的试验显示,RATG 在大多数情况下比 ATGAM 更有效且耐受性更好[85,86]。随着现代所关心的问题转向成本分析,证据表明,多克隆诱导所带来的长期利益可能不敌其购买和使用的相关额外成本[87]。

一项随机前瞻性的试验提供了正确使用多克隆诱导药物的最坚实证据,它比较了 RATG 与巴利昔单抗对急性排斥反应或移植物功能延迟恢复的高危受体的作用[88]。在这项研究中,278 名患者随机接受 RATG 或巴利昔单抗治疗。RATG 组较少发生 BPAR (15.6%对 25.5%,P=0.02),且较少发生耐激素性排斥反应(1.4%对 8.0%,P=0.005),但两组的移植物失功发生率(分别为 9.2%和 10.2%)、移植物功能延迟恢复发生率(分别为 40.4%和 44.5%)和死亡率(分别为 4.3%和 4.4%)无明显差异。不良事件、严重不良事件和癌症发生率无明显差别,但是 RATG 组感染发生率较高(85.8%对 75.2%,P=0.03),矛盾的是,其巨细胞病毒感染率较低(7.8%对 17.5%,P=0.02)。因此,多克隆诱导药物可用于高危受体的管理,因为它减少了 BPAR,但是这并没有减少移植物功能延迟恢复发生率或改善长期结果。

多克隆抗体的肾外使用。ATG-R 和 ATG-F 已被前瞻性地证明了在心脏移植中能降低急性排斥反应的发生率且预后优于 OKT3[89,90]。比较研究发现,在心脏移植中它们的效果相当[91]。诱导治疗似乎最有利于排斥风险最高的受体(非裔美国人、同种致敏的患者、依赖于心室辅助装置的患者);否则,接受多克隆抗体诱导治疗的心脏移植受体会有更高的概率发生感染性并发症及恶性肿瘤[21]。多克隆诱导药物还没有被证明可用于肝移植[92],但对于已有肾衰竭的受体接受 RATG 诱导可延迟钙调磷酸酶抑制剂的使用[93]。

在肺移植领域,RATG 联合三联疗法被认为可减少排斥反应发生而不影响闭塞性细支气管炎综合征的发生率[94]。国际心肺移植注册协会的分析表明,RATG 诱导治疗对双肺移植受者有明显益处[65]。

值得关注的试验性药物

抗黏附药物

由于黏附分子在淋巴细胞转运至移植物及二级引流淋巴器官的过程中具有明确的作用,抗黏附在概念上一直是有吸引力的诱导策略。目前已经开发了几种方法,并保持了潜在的重要性。

LFA-1(白细胞功能相关抗原 1),一种 B2 整合素,主要存在于 T 细胞的表面,有两种独特的功能:①对表面表达一个 LFA-1 配体 (细胞内黏附分子-1,ICAM-1)的细胞阻滞和迁移;②接触 APC 并稳定免疫突触。LFA-1 帮助 T 细胞抵抗血液流动的剪切力,并帮助 T 细胞牢固黏附和移行进入损伤处[95]。

依法利珠单抗(Raptiva;Genentech)是一个人源化的 LFA-1 IgG1 抗体,最初在 2003 年被批准用于牛皮癣的治疗。Vincenti 等人研究了 38 例接受依法利珠单抗诱导联合标准三联维持性免疫抑制治疗的肾移植受体[96]。研究证明了该方案在抗排斥方面的有效性,但其添加到一个已经有效的免疫抑制方案会带来过度免疫抑制,导致 PTLD 的发生。随后的两项初步研究证实了依法利珠单抗在胰岛移植中应用具有显著的耐受性和疗效[97,98]。这些研究激发了人们的研究兴趣,但不幸的是,由于 2009 年依法利珠单抗退出银屑病治疗市场,这一研究方向由此中止。由于该药物唯一的适应证是银屑病,因此在移植领域的标签外应用已经停止。

阿法赛特(Amevive;Astellas)是一个 LFA-3/IgG1 融合蛋白,就像依法利珠单抗一样,其适应证为银屑病。灵长类动物的临床前数据表明,由于其可以消耗记忆性 T 细胞并由此促进以共刺激阻断为基础的免疫抑制,所以阿法赛特是一种有前景的药物[99]。而其应在上述背景下合理应用,如将阿法赛特引入临床并添加到以 TAC 为基础的治疗方案中,但并无效果。无论如何,就像依法利珠单抗,阿法赛特已经退出了银屑病治疗市场,使其难以在移植领域进行标签外应用研究。

TNF 抑制剂

使用 TNF 特异性单抗英夫利西单抗或者最近使用的 TNF 受体拮抗剂依那西普进行 TNF 阻断,常用于炎症性肠病,并已明确证实其有效性。在移植领域,TNF 特异性治疗已经作为诱导剂用于胰岛细胞移植。虽然它已被证明在啮齿动物模型中是有效的[100],但其在胰岛中的应用是基于无对照的经验用法。

依那西普与抗胸腺细胞球蛋白和达利珠单抗一起用于单供体边缘剂量胰岛移植的 8 例人类受体。所有受体都脱离了胰岛素依赖且并未发生低血糖[101]。依那西普还被研究用于接受补充胰岛移植的受体(这些受体接受同种异体胰岛细胞移植并发生进行性移植物失功)。尽管样本量小并缺乏随机性,研究结果还是提示能改善移植成功率、移植物长期存活率和功能[102]。最近,依那西普被用于17例接受补充性胰岛输注的移植物失功受体。13例受体采用抗胸腺细胞球蛋白联合依那西普诱导治疗,而4例受者接受达利珠单抗诱导。维持性治疗采用西罗莫司联合TAC或TAC联合MMF。两组之间的胰岛素脱离率及持续时间都没有差别[103]。

总结

诱导治疗目前在美国是大多数移植手术程序中的一种常见做法(如果包括单剂甲泼尼龙那就是在所有移植中)。正如本章详细阐述的,前体频率、天然免疫、移植中组织损伤和缺血再灌注损伤是导致使用诱导疗法的主要因素。它的好处主要是可以降低早期急性排斥反应的发生率和总体简化早期受体围术期免疫管理、代偿早期免疫药物的浓度,并在当非排斥反应相关原因导致的功能障碍更常见时(如再灌注损伤、技术问题)降低排斥反应的可能性。此后,诱导所带来的好处仍没有非常明确,但可能包括逐渐减少排斥反应,同时增加感染(病毒和真菌)和恶性肿瘤(病毒诱发的癌症、PTLD)的风险。因此,使用诱导治疗应考虑受体的个体风险和他们特定的器官,并选择匹配最有可能影响这些风险的生物因素。

(陈峻 译 徐骁 校)

参考文献

1. Halloran PF. Immunosuppressive drugs for kidney transplantation. New England Journal of Medicine. 2004;351:2715–2729.
2. Ford ML, Koehn BH, Wagener ME, et al. Antigen-specific precursor frequency impacts T cell proliferation, differentiation, and requirement for costimulation. Journal of Experimental Medicine. 2007;204:299–309.
3. Page AJ, Ford ML, Kirk AD. Memory T-cell-specific therapeutics in organ transplantation. Current Opinion in Organ Transplantation. 2009;14: 643–649.
4. Larsen CP, Elwood ET, Alexander DZ, et al. Long-term acceptance of skin and cardiac allografts after blocking CD40 and CD28 pathways. Nature. 1996;381:434–438.
5. Ford ML, Kirk AD, Larsen CP. Donor-reactive T-cell stimulation history and precursor frequency: barriers to tolerance induction. Transplantation. 2009; 87(9 Suppl.):S69–S74.
6. Adams AB, Pearson TC, Larsen CP. Heterologous immunity: an overlooked barrier to tolerance. Immunological Reviews. 2003;196:147–160.
7. Wu Z, Bensinger SJ, Zhang J, et al. Homeostatic proliferation is a barrier to transplantation tolerance. Nature Medicine. 2004;10:87–92.
8. Padovan E, Casorati G, Dellabona P, et al. Expression of two T cell receptor alpha chains: dual receptor T cells. Science. 1993;262:422–424.
9. Kirk AD. Induction immunosuppression. Transplantation. 2006;82:593–602.
10. Kirk AD, Mannon RB, Kleiner DE, et al. Results from a human renal allograft tolerance trial evaluating T-cell depletion with alemtuzumab combined with deoxyspergualin. Transplantation. 2005;80:1051–1059.
11. Vincenti F, Larsen CP, Alberu J, et al. Three-year outcomes from BENEFIT, a randomized, active-controlled, parallel-group study in adult kidney transplant recipients. American Journal of Transplantation. 2012;12:210–217.
12. Wood KJ, Goto R. Mechanisms of rejection: current perspectives. Transplantation. 2012;93:1–10.
13. Szczech LA, Berlin JA, Aradhye S, et al. Effect of anti-lymphocyte induction therapy on renal allograft survival: a meta-analysis. Journal of the American Society of Nephrology. 1997;8:1771–1777.
14. Szczech LA, Berlin JA, Feldman HI, et al. The effect of antilymphocyte induction therapy on renal allograft survival. A meta-analysis of individual patient-level data. Anti-Lymphocyte Antibody Induction Therapy Study Group. Annals of Internal Medicine. 1998;128:817–826.
15. Kaufman DB, Burke GW III, Bruce DS, et al. Prospective, randomized, multi-center trial of antibody induction therapy in simultaneous pancreas-kidney transplantation. American Journal of Transplantation. 2003;3:855–864.
16. Burke GW III, Kaufman DB, Millis JM, et al. Prospective, randomized trial of the effect of antibody induction in simultaneous pancreas and kidney transplantation: three-year results. Transplantation. 2004;77:1269–1275.
17. Higgins R, Kirklin JK, Brown RN, et al. To induce or not to induce: do patients at greatest risk for fatal rejection benefit from cytolytic induction therapy? Journal of Heart and Lung Transplantation. 2005;24:392–400.
18. Humar A, Ramcharan T, Denny R, et al. Are wound complications after a kidney transplant more common with modern immunosuppression? Transplantation. 2001;72:1920–1923.
19. Meier-Kriesche HU, Arndorfer JA, Kaplan B. Association of antibody induction with short- and long-term cause-specific mortality in renal transplant recipients. Journal of the American Society of Nephrology. 2002;13:769–772.
20. Cherikh WS, Kauffman HM, McBride MA, et al. Association of the type of induction immunosuppression with posttransplant lymphoproliferative disorder, graft survival, and patient survival after primary kidney transplantation. Transplantation. 2003;76:1289–1293.
21. Mahmud N, Klipa D, Ahsan N. Antibody immunosuppressive therapy in solid-organ transplant: part I. mAbs. 2010;2:148–156.
22. Vincenti F, Kirkman R, Light S, et al. Interleukin-2-receptor blockade with daclizumab to prevent acute rejection in renal transplantation. Daclizumab Triple Therapy Study Group. New England Journal of Medicine. 1998;338: 161–165.
23. Vincenti F, Nashan B, Light S. Daclizumab: outcome of phase III trials and mechanism of action. Double Therapy and the Triple Therapy Study Groups. Transplantation Proceedings. 1998;30:2155–2158.
24. Ferran C, Dy M, Merite S, et al. Reduction of morbidity and cytokine release in anti-CD3 MoAb-treated mice by corticosteroids. Transplantation. 1990;50: 642–648.
25. Nashan B, Light S, Hardie IR, et al. Reduction of acute renal allograft rejection by daclizumab. Daclizumab Double Therapy Study Group. Transplantation. 1999;67:110–115.
26. Hengster P, Pescovitz MD, Hyatt D, et al. Cytomegalovirus infections after treatment with daclizumab, an anti IL-2 receptor antibody, for prevention of renal allograft rejection. Roche Study Group. Transplantation. 1999;68:310–313.
27. Pescovitz MD, Knechtle S, Alexander SR, et al. Safety and pharmacokinetics of daclizumab in pediatric renal transplant recipients. Pediatric Transplantation. 2008;12:447–455.
28. Carswell CI, Plosker GL, Wagstaff AJ. Daclizumab: a review of its use in the management of organ transplantation. Biodrugs: Clinical Immunotherapeutics, Biopharmaceuticals and Gene Therapy. 2001;15:745–773.
29. Ekberg H, Grinyó J, Nashan B, et al. Cyclosporine sparing with mycophenolate mofetil, daclizumab and corticosteroids in renal allograft recipients: the CAESAR study. American Journal of Transplantation. 2007;7:560–570.
30. Ekberg H, Tedesco-Silva H, Demirbas A, et al. Reduced exposure to calcineurin inhibitors in renal transplantation. New England Journal of Medicine. 2007; 357:2562–2575.
31. Noel C, Abramowicz D, Durand D, et al. Daclizumab versus antithymocyte globulin in high-immunological-risk renal transplant recipients. Journal of the American Society of Nephrology. 2009;20:1385–1392.
32. Schuller S, Wiederkehr JC, Coelho-Lemos IM, et al. Daclizumab induction therapy associated with TAC-MMF has better outcome compared with TAC-MMF alone in pediatric living donor liver transplantation. Transplantation Proceedings. 2005;37:1151–1152.
33. Figueras J, Prieto M, Bernardos A, et al. Daclizumab induction and maintenance steroid-free immunosuppression with mycophenolate mofetil and TAC to prevent acute rejection of hepatic allografts. Transplant International. 2006; 19:641–648.

34. Becker T, Foltys D, Bilbao I, et al. Patient outcomes in two steroid-free regimens using TAC monotherapy after daclizumab induction and TAC with mycophenolate mofetil in liver transplantation. Transplantation. 2008;86:1689–1694.
35. Boillot O, Mayer DA, Boudjema K, et al. Corticosteroid-free immunosuppression with TAC following induction with daclizumab: a large randomized clinical study. Liver Transplantation. 2005;11:61–67.
36. Beniaminovitz A, Itescu S, Lietz K, et al. Prevention of rejection in cardiac transplantation by blockade of the interleukin-2 receptor with a monoclonal antibody. New England Journal of Medicine. 2000;342:613–619.
37. Hershberger RE, Starling RC, Eisen HJ, et al. Daclizumab to prevent rejection after cardiac transplantation. New England Journal of Medicine. 2005;352: 2705–2713.
38. Ortiz V, Almenar L, Martínez-Dolz L, et al. Induction therapy with daclizumab in heart transplantation–how many doses? Transplantation Proceedings. 2006;38:2541–2543.
39. Potter BJ, Giannetti N, Routy JP, et al. CD25 saturation rate in heart transplant patients receiving two-dose daclizumab induction. Transplantation. 2005;79: 857–858.
40. Mullen JC, Oreopoulos A, Lien DC, et al. A randomized, controlled trial of daclizumab vs anti-thymocyte globulin induction for lung transplantation. Journal of Heart and Lung Transplantation. 2007;26:504–510.
41. Lischke R, Simonek J, Davidová R, et al. Induction therapy in lung transplantation: initial single-center experience comparing daclizumab and antithymocyte globulin. Transplantation Proceedings. 2007;39:205–212.
42. Nashan B, Moore R, Amlot P, et al. Randomised trial of basiliximab versus placebo for control of acute cellular rejection in renal allograft recipients. CHIB 201 International Study Group. Lancet. 1997;350:1193–1198.
43. Kahan BD, Rajagopalan PR, Hall M. Reduction of the occurrence of acute cellular rejection among renal allograft recipients treated with basiliximab, a chimeric anti-interleukin-2-receptor monoclonal antibody. United States Simulect Renal Study Group. Transplantation. 1999;67:276–284.
44. Mulloy LL, Wright F, Hall ML, et al. Simulect (basiliximab) reduces acute cellular rejection in renal allografts from cadaveric and living donors. Transplantation Proceedings. 1999;31:1210–1213.
45. Sheashaa HA, Bakr MA, Ismail AM, et al. Basiliximab reduces the incidence of acute cellular rejection in live-related-donor kidney transplantation: a three-year prospective randomized trial. Journal of Nephrology. 2003;16: 393–398.
46. Ponticelli C, Yussim A, Cambi V, et al. A randomized, double-blind trial of basiliximab immunoprophylaxis plus triple therapy in kidney transplant recipients. Transplantation. 2001;72:1261–1267.
47. Matl I, Bachleda P, Lao M, et al. Safety and efficacy of an alternative basiliximab (Simulect) regimen after renal transplantation: administration of a single 40-mg dose on the first postoperative day in patients receiving triple therapy with azathioprine. Transplant International. 2003;16:45–52.
48. Matl I, Bachleda P, Michalsky R, et al. Basiliximab can be administered safely and effectively in a single dose on day 1 postrenal transplantation in patients receiving triple therapy with azathioprine. Transplantation Proceedings. 2001; 33:3205–3206.
49. Baquero A, Pérez J, Rizik N, et al. Basiliximab: a comparative study between the use of the recommended two doses versus a single dose in living donor kidney transplantation. Transplantation Proceedings. 2006;38:909–910.
50. Flechner SM, Kurian SM, Solez K, et al. De novo kidney transplantation without use of calcineurin inhibitors preserves renal structure and function at two years. American Journal of Transplantation. 2004;4:1776–1785.
51. Emparan C, Laukötter M, Wolters H, et al. Calcineurin-free protocols with basiliximab induction allow patients included in "old to old" programs achieve standard kidney transplant function. Transplantation Proceedings. 2003;35: 1326–1327.
52. Tojimbara T, Sato S, Koyama I, et al. Cyclosporine-sparing effect of basiliximab in renal transplant recipients with mycophenolate mofetil. Transplantation Proceedings. 2005;37:895–898.
53. Lebranchu Y, Bridoux F, Büchler M, et al. Immunoprophylaxis with basiliximab compared with antithymocyte globulin in renal transplant patients receiving MMF-containing triple therapy. American Journal of Transplantation. 2002; 2:48–56.
54. Neuhaus P, Clavien PA, Kittur D, et al. Improved treatment response with basiliximab immunoprophylaxis after liver transplantation: results from a double-blind randomized placebo-controlled trial. Liver Transplantation. 2002;8:132–142.
55. Calmus Y, Scheele JR, Gonzalez-Pinto I, et al. Immunoprophylaxis with basiliximab, a chimeric anti-interleukin-2 receptor monoclonal antibody, in combination with azathioprine-containing triple therapy in liver transplant recipients. Liver Transplantation. 2002;8:123–131.
56. Marino IR, Doria C, Scott VL, et al. Efficacy and safety of basiliximab with a TAC-based regimen in liver transplant recipients. Transplantation. 2004;78: 886–891.
57. Lin CC, Chuang FR, Lee CH, et al. The renal-sparing efficacy of basiliximab in adult living donor liver transplantation. Liver Transplantation. 2005;11: 1258–1264.
58. Filipponi F, Callea F, Salizzoni M, et al. Double-blind comparison of hepatitis C histological recurrence rate in HCV+ liver transplant recipients given basiliximab + steroids or basiliximab + placebo, in addition to cyclosporine and azathioprine. Transplantation. 2004;78:1488–1495.
59. Llado L, Fabregat J, Castellote J, et al. Impact of immunosuppression without steroids on rejection and hepatitis C virus evolution after liver transplantation: results of a prospective randomized study. Liver Transplantation. 2008;14: 1752–1760.
60. Marubashi S, Dono K, Amano K, et al. Steroid-free living-donor liver transplantation in adults. Transplantation. 2005;80:704–706.
61. Rosenberg PB, Vriesendorp AE, Drazner MH, et al. Induction therapy with basiliximab allows delayed initiation of cyclosporine and preserves renal function after cardiac transplantation. Journal of Heart and Lung Transplantation. 2005;24:1327–1331.
62. Flaman F, Zieroth S, Rao V, et al. Basiliximab versus rabbit anti-thymocyte globulin for induction therapy in patients after heart transplantation. Journal of Heart and Lung Transplantation. 2006;25:1358–1362.
63. Carrier M, Leblanc MH, Perrault LP, et al. Basiliximab and rabbit anti-thymocyte globulin for prophylaxis of acute rejection after heart transplantation: a non-inferiority trial. Journal of Heart and Lung Transplantation. 2007;26:258–263.
64. Møller CH, Gustafsson F, Gluud C, et al. Interleukin-2 receptor antagonists as induction therapy after heart transplantation: systematic review with meta-analysis of randomized trials. Journal of Heart and Lung Transplantation. 2008;27:835–842.
65. Hachem RR, Edwards LB, Yusen RD, et al. The impact of induction on survival after lung transplantation: an analysis of the International Society for Heart and Lung Transplantation Registry. Clinical Transplantation. 2008;22:603–608.
66. Calne R, Moffatt SD, Friend PJ, et al. Campath IH allows low-dose cyclosporine monotherapy in 31 cadaveric renal allograft recipients. Transplantation. 1999;68:1613–1616.
67. Basu A, Ramkumar M, Tan HP, et al. Reversal of acute cellular rejection after renal transplantation with Campath-1H. Transplantation Proceedings. 2005;37: 923–926.
68. Kirk AD, Mannon RB, Kleiner DE, et al. Results from a human renal allograft tolerance trial evaluating the humanized CD52-specific monoclonal antibody Campath-1H. Transplantation. 2003;76:120–129.
69. Barth RN, Janus CA, Lillesand CA, et al. Outcomes at 3 years of a prospective pilot study of Campath-1H and sirolimus immunosuppression for renal transplantation. Transplant International. 2006;19:885–892.
70. Kaufman DB, Leventhal JR, Axelrod D, et al. Alemtuzumab induction and prednisone-free maintenance immunotherapy in kidney transplantation: comparison with basiliximab induction–long-term results. American Journal of Transplantation. 2005;5:2539–2548.
71. Tan HP, Kaczorowski D, Basu A, et al. Steroid-free TAC monotherapy after pretransplantation thymoglobulin or Campath and laparoscopy in living donor renal transplantation. Transplantation Proceedings. 2005;37:4235–4240.
72. Thomas PG, Woodside KJ, Lappin JA, et al. Alemtuzumab (Campath 1H) induction with TAC monotherapy is safe for high immunological risk renal transplantation. Transplantation. 2007;83:1509–1512.
73. Hanaway MJ, Woodle ES, Mulgaonkar S, et al. Alemtuzumab induction in renal transplantation. New England Journal of Medicine. 2011;364:1909–1919.
74. Tzakis AG, Tryphonopoulos P, Kato T, et al. Preliminary experience with alemtuzumab (Campath-1H) and low-dose TAC immunosuppression in adult liver transplantation. Transplantation. 2004;77:1209–1214.
75. Reams BD, Musselwhite LW, Zaas DW, et al. Alemtuzumab in the treatment of refractory acute rejection and bronchiolitis obliterans syndrome after human lung transplantation. American Journal of Transplantation. 2007;7: 2802–2808.
76. Wechter WJ, Brodie JA, Morrell RM, et al. Antithymocyte globulin (ATGAM) in renal allograft recipients. Multicenter trials using a 14-dose regimen. Transplantation. 1979;28:294–302.
77. Webster A, Pankhurst T, Rinaldi F, et al. Polyclonal and monoclonal antibodies for treating acute rejection episodes in kidney transplant recipients. Cochrane Database of Systematic Reviews. 2006;(9):CD004756.
78. Bonnefoy-Berard N, Vincent C, Revillard JP. Antibodies against functional leukocyte surface molecules in polyclonal lymphocyte and antithymocyte globulins. Transplantation. 1992;59:669.
79. Rebellato LM, Gross U, Verbanac KM, et al. A comprehensive definition of the major antibody specificities in polyclonal rabbit antithymocyte globulin. Transplantation. 1994;57:685.

80. Hardinger KI, Schnitzler MA, Miller B, et al. Five year follow up of thymoglobulin versus ATGAM induction in adult renal transplantation. Transplantation. 2004;78:136–141.
81. Mourad G, Garrigue V, Squifflet JP, et al. Induction versus noninduction in renal transplant recipients with tacrolimus-based immunosuppression. Transplantation. 2001;72:1050–1055.
82. Charpentier B, Rostaing L, Berthoux F, et al. A three-arm study comparing immediate tacrolimus therapy with antithymocyte globulin induction therapy followed by tacrolimus or cyclosporine A in adult renal transplant recipients. Transplantation. 2003;75:844–851.
83. Swanson SJ, Hale DA, Mannon RB, et al. Kidney transplantation with rabbit antithymocyte globulin induction and sirolimus monotherapy. Lancet. 2002;360:1662–1664.
84. Starzl TE, Murase N, Abu-Elmagd K, et al. Tolerogenic immunosuppression for organ transplantation. Lancet. 2003;361:1502–1510.
85. Hardinger KL, Rhee S, Buchanan P, et al. A prospective, randomized, double-blinded comparison of thymoglobulin versus Atgam for induction immunosuppressive therapy: 10-year results. Transplantation. 2008;86:947–952.
86. Brennan DC, Flavin K, Lowell JA, et al. A randomized, double-blinded comparison of Thymoglobulin versus Atgam for induction immunosuppressive therapy in adult renal transplant recipients. Transplantation. 1999;67:1011–1018.
87. Morton RL, Howard K, Webster AC, et al. The cost-effectiveness of induction immunosuppression in kidney transplantation. Nephrology, Dialysis, Transplantation. 2009;24:2258–2269.
88. Brennan DC, Daller JA, Lake KD, et al. Rabbit antithymocyte globulin versus basiliximab in renal transplantation. New England Journal of Medicine. 2006;355:1967–1977.
89. Griffith BP, Kormos RL, Armitage JM, et al. Comparative trial of immunoprophylaxis with RATG versus OKT3. Journal of Heart Transplantation. 1990;9:301–305.
90. Bock HA, Gallati H, Zurcher RM, et al. A randomized prospective trial of prophylactic immunosuppression with ATG-fresenius versus OKT3 after renal transplantation. Transplantation. 1995;59:830–840.
91. Schnetzler B, Leger P, Volp A, et al. A prospective randomized controlled study on the efficacy and tolerance of two antilymphocytic globulins in the prevention of rejection in first-heart transplant recipients. Transplant International. 2002;15:317–325.
92. Neuhaus P, Klupp J, Langrehr JM, et al. Quadruple tacrolimus-based induction therapy including azathioprine and ALG does not significantly improve outcome after liver transplantation when compared with standard induction with tacrolimus and steroids: results of a prospective, randomized trial. Transplantation. 2000;69:2343–2353.
93. Tector AJ, Fridell JA, Mangus RS, et al. Promising early results with immunosuppression using rabbit anti-thymocyte globulin and steroids with delayed introduction of TAC in adult liver transplant recipients. Liver Transplantation. 2004;10:404–407.
94. Palmer SM, Miralles AP, Lawrence CM, et al. Rabbit antithymocyte globulin decreases acute rejection after lung transplantation: results of a randomized, prospective study. Chest. 1999;116:127–133.
95. Hogg N, Patzak I, Willenbrock F. The insider's guide to leukocyte integrin signalling and function. Nature Reviews Immunology. 2011;11:416–426.
96. Vincenti F, Mendez R, Pescovitz M, et al. A phase I/II randomized open-label multicenter trial of efalizumab, a humanized anti-CD11a, anti-LFA-1 in renal transplantation. American Journal of Transplantation. 2007;7:1770–1777.
97. Posselt AM, Szot GL, Frassetto LA, et al. Islet transplantation in type 1 diabetics using an immunosuppressive protocol based on the anti-LFA-1 antibody efalizumab. American Journal of Transplantation. 2010;10:1870–1880.
98. Turgeon NA, Avila JG, Cano JA, et al. Experience with a novel efalizumab-based immunosuppressive regimen to facilitate single donor islet cell transplantation. American Journal of Transplantation. 2010;10:2082–2091.
99. Weaver TA, Charafeddine AH, Agarwal A, et al. Alefacept promotes co-stimulation blockade based allograft survival in nonhuman primates. Nature Medicine. 2009;15:746–749.
100. McCall M, Pawlick R, Kin T, et al. Anakinra potentiates the protective effects of etanercept in transplantation of marginal mass human islets in immunodeficient mice. American Journal of Transplantation. 2012;12:322–329.
101. Hering BJ, Kandaswamy R, Ansite JD, et al. Single-donor, marginal-dose islet transplantation in patients with type 1 diabetes. JAMA. 2005;293:830–835.
102. Faradji RN, Tharavanij T, Messinger S, et al. Long-term insulin independence and improvement in insulin secretion after supplemental islet infusion under exenatide and etanercept. Transplantation. 2008;86:1658–1665.
103. Koh A, Imes S, Kin T, et al. Supplemental islet infusions restore insulin independence after graft dysfunction in islet transplant recipients. Transplantation. 2010;89:361–365.

第 66 章
维持性免疫抑制治疗

Karen L. Hardinger, Daniel C. Brennan, Christina L.M. Klein

引言

免疫抑制策略在过去的几十年中已推动实体器官移植领域的重大进步。环孢素在 20 世纪 80 年代通过降低急性排斥反应发生率和改善短期移植物存活率彻底改革了移植实践(参见第 1 章)。在 20 世纪 90 年代,他克莫司和霉酚酸改善了移植效果。尽管有这些进展,但尚缺乏有利于长期移植物存活率的明确证据,尤其是在肾移植领域。此外,早期移植物存活率的显著改善是以相关不良反应为代价的,包括增加心血管和脑血管疾病风险的代谢副作用。新免疫抑制剂的使用,包括哺乳动物西罗莫司靶蛋白(mTOR)抑制剂和贝拉西普,已被纳入减少钙调磷酸酶抑制剂和皮质类固醇的终身暴露及提高长期生存率的发展战略。

为了改善结果,临床医生使用了多种适用于各种器官移植的常规维持性免疫抑制策略。有一种关于评估受体发生排斥反应危险因素的方法。高危受体可能接受强力的免疫抑制(更大剂量或更长时间的治疗),而低危受体可能接受较弱的免疫抑制。免疫抑制也可能根据移植后的时间调整。术后即刻的治疗需求不同于长期维持的治疗需求。其他管理策略包括病毒感染监测,这似乎是过度免疫抑制的迹象,并可指导免疫抑制的调整和降低。同样,调整维持性免疫抑制可能对恶性肿瘤或疾病复发的受体有益。

一份理想的免疫抑制方案能限制毒性和延长移植物的功能存活时间。本章将回顾维持性免疫抑制策略并对肾脏、胰腺、肺、肝脏、心脏和小肠移植的关键试进行概述。

维持性治疗的动态和类型

移植受体的免疫抑制方案在不同时代和不同中心有所不同。目前,包含维持性治疗的 5 类药物有钙调磷酸酶抑制剂(环孢素和他克莫司)、mTOR 抑制剂(西罗莫司和依维莫司)、抗增殖剂(硫唑嘌呤和霉酚酸)、共刺激阻断剂(贝拉西普)和皮质类固醇(表 66.1 和表 66.2)。这些药物的机制在第 17 章中已作详细介绍,它们获审批的适应证在第 98 章中已作详细介绍。在过去的 20 年里,他克莫司已经取代环孢素,霉酚酸已取代硫唑嘌呤,并已在大多数美国移植中心作为首选治疗,使他克莫司+霉酚酸酯/霉酚酸钠联合皮质类固醇成为最常见维持性免疫抑制方案(图 66.1A~F)。当考虑来自美国移植受体科学注册中心(SRTR)的数据时,常规的实体器官移植中用药方案很少有差异(图 66.2)。目前,大多数肺移植受体接受他克莫司+霉酚酸酯治疗,但 20%的受体接受他克莫司和硫唑嘌呤治疗[1]。其次,大多数小肠移植受体接收他克莫司单药治疗,而不联合霉酚酸酯主要是因为霉酚酸酯的胃肠道副作用[1]。最后,大约有 20%的心脏移植受体接受环孢素治疗,而绝大多数都接受他克莫司治疗[1]。

维持性免疫抑制治疗可分为四联、三联、二联,或单药疗法。四联疗法治疗过程包括一种移植时使用的诱导药物,以及之后的三联维持性治疗。三联疗法包含三种药物的治疗方案,是最常用的维持性治疗方案,因为它针对免疫反应的不同位点,且药物协同作用可以使毒性最小化。历史上,免疫抑制治疗的主要目的是为了防止急性排斥反应和移植物失功。这些目标的相对实现已将重点转移到在不损害疗效的情况下尽量减少免疫抑制治疗及其相关感染及药物毒性。因此,一些中心使用皮质类固醇或钙调磷酸酶抑制剂减量方案,以期实现这些目标。有两种主要的激素减量方案:①激素撤除或停用;②无激素。这些方案分别包括移植后短时间内应用皮质类固醇或不使用皮质类固醇。根据当前的数据,在肾、肝和胰腺移植中,有停用皮质类固醇的

表 66.1 FDA 批准用于移植的免疫抑制药物

药物	剂量	副作用
泼尼松	维持治疗:2.5~10mg/d 排斥反应治疗:250~1000mg/d,持续3日,静脉输注	情绪不稳,精神异常,白内障,高血压,液体潴留,消化性溃疡,骨质疏松症,肌肉无力,切口愈合不良,葡萄糖不耐受,体重增加
环孢素	4~5mg/kg,口服,每日2次	神经毒性,牙龈增生,多毛症,高血压,高脂血症,葡萄糖不耐受,肾毒性,电解质紊乱
他克莫司	0.05~0.075mg/kg,口服,每日2次	神经毒性,脱发,高血压,高脂血症,葡萄糖不耐受,肾毒性,电解质紊乱
西罗莫司	2~10mg,每日口服	高甘油三酯血症,贫血,血小板减少,口腔溃疡,高胆固醇血症,胃肠功能紊乱,骨髓抑制,切口愈合不良,水肿,胸腔积液,心包积液
依维莫司	0.75~1.5mg,口服,每日2次	高甘油三酯血症,贫血,血小板减少,口腔溃疡,高胆固醇血症,胃肠功能紊乱,骨髓抑制,切口愈合不良,水肿,胸腔积液,心包积液
硫唑嘌呤	每日1~2.5mg/kg,口服	白细胞减少,血小板减少,胃肠功能紊乱,胰腺炎,肝毒性
霉酚酸酯	500~1500mg,口服,每日2次	白细胞减少,血小板减少,胃肠功能紊乱
霉酚酸钠	360~1080mg,口服,每日2次	白细胞减少,血小板减少,胃肠功能紊乱
贝拉西普	在供体器官植入前,移植后第5天,第2、4、8、12周末给药10mg/kg,然后每4周(±3天)给药5mg/kg	急性排斥反应增加,移植后淋巴组织增生性疾病,进行性多灶性脑白质病,结核病

表 66.2 免疫抑制剂分类

分类	药物(通用名)	药物(商品名)	剂型
皮质类固醇	甲泼尼龙	Solumedrol®(Pfizer, New York, NY)	针剂,口服
	泼尼松	Deltasone®(Pfizer, New York, NY)	口服
	泼尼松龙		口服
钙调磷酸酶抑制剂	环孢素,CsA	Sandimmune®(Novartis, East Hanover, NJ)	针剂,口服
	环孢素微乳剂	Neoral®(Novartis, East Hanover, NJ) GenGraf®(AbbVie, Chicago, IL)	针剂,口服
	他克莫司,FK506	Prograf®(Astellas, Northbrook, IL)	口服
	Astragraf(安斯泰来)	Hecoria®(Novartis, East Hanover, NJ)	
mTOR抑制剂	西罗莫司,雷帕霉素	Rapamune®(Pfizer, New York, NY)	口服
	依维莫司	Zortress®(Novartis, East Hanover, NJ) Certican®(Novartis, East Hanover, NJ)	口服
抗增殖剂	硫唑嘌呤,AZA	Imuran®(GlaxoSmithKline, Mississauga, Ontario, Canada)	针剂,口服
	霉酚酸酯,MMF	Cellcept®(Genentech, San Francisco, CA)	针剂,口服
	霉酚酸钠,EC-MPS	Myfortic®(Novartis, East Hanover, NJ)	口服
共刺激信号阻断剂	贝拉西普	Nulojix®(Bristol-Myers Squibb, New York, NY)	针剂

趋势,而大多数心脏、小肠和肺移植受体仍然接受皮质类固醇治疗(图 66.3)[1]。这些方案中的大多数都包括两种维持性治疗药物或二联维持性治疗。目前正在研究减量或避免应用钙调磷酸酶抑制剂的治疗方案,但并未常规使用。最后一种维持性治疗是单药疗法,除了临床试验很少使用[2,3]。单药疗法或二联疗法的候选人包括可能具有较低潜在免疫原性及较低免疫风险的器官移植受体。两组受体的确定主要根据流行病学数据,而不是免疫学数据,如人类白细胞抗原(HLA)匹配情况(参见第 36 章),尽管其在肾移植中使用,但在其他实体器官移植中不常用或无法确定[4-7]。

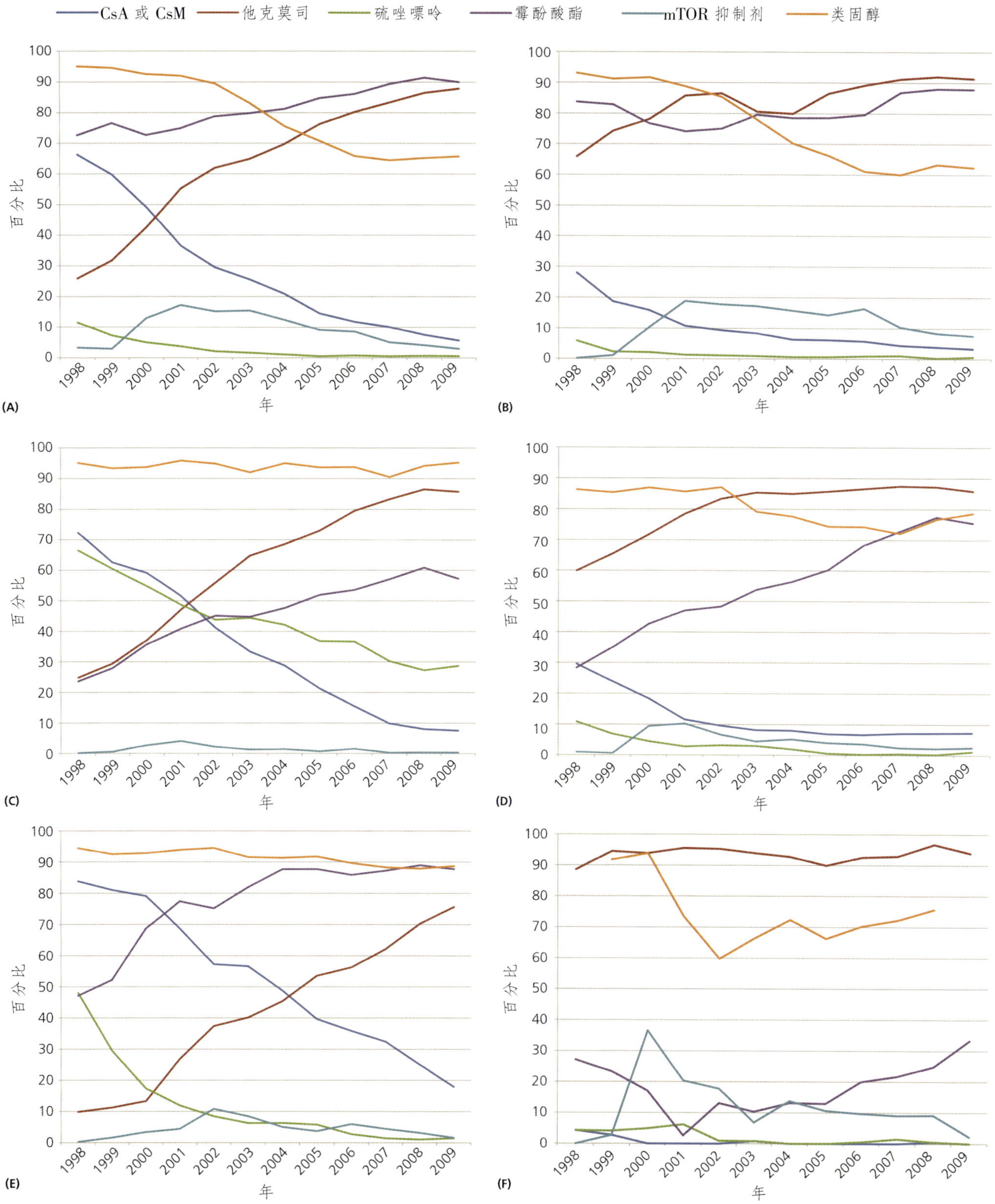

图 66.1　移植免疫抑制随着时间变化的趋势：(A)肾移植；(B)胰腺移植；(C)肺移植；(D)肝移植；(E)心脏移植；(F)小肠移植。

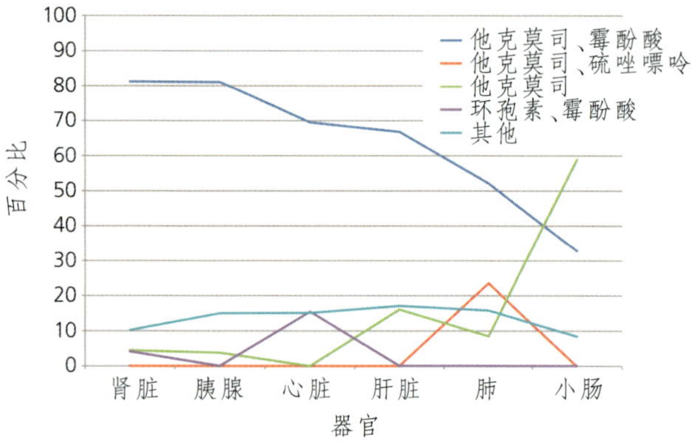

图 66.2 移植时的维持性免疫抑制方案。

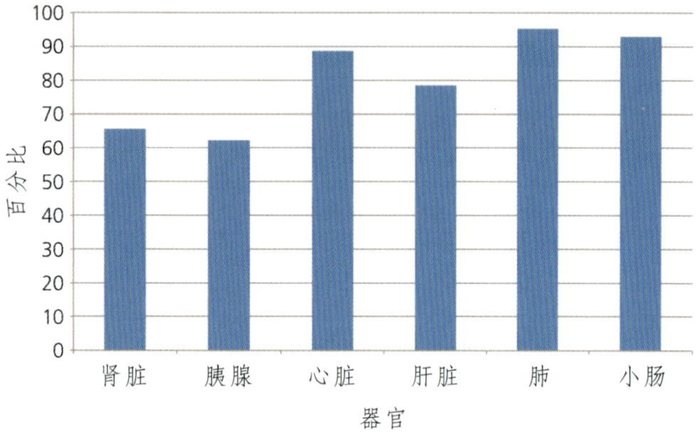

图 66.3 根据器官类型在移植术后患者出院时应用皮质类固醇的情况。

维持性免疫抑制与危险因素

具有较高急性排斥反应风险的受体可能会接受更强力的维持性免疫抑制方案。这些危险因素有不同程度的效用，但总的来说，没有明确的指标能够验证免疫抑制治疗的必要性。免疫、供体和受体的危险因素将在下文讨论。

免疫的危险因素

移植前可能会进行多个测试来评估受体急性排斥反应的风险，包括群体反应性抗体、免疫学的交叉配型、HLA 匹配和血液/组织分型。这些测试的方法和原理已在第 36 章中作深度介绍。高度致敏的受体，即那些具有直接针对供体 HLA 抗原的同种抗体的受体，具有较高的急性排斥反应发生风险。血液循环中具有针对供体抗原的抗体可能是由于之前的移植、怀孕或多次输血所致。随着群体反应性抗体水平上升，B 细胞或 T 细胞交叉配型阳性及免疫不相容移植的机会增加。在一项关于致敏作用对单倍体相合亲体移植移植物存活率影响的研究中，具有高于 50%的群体反应性抗体滴度的受体发生移植物衰竭的时间明显较短[8]。T 细胞毒性交叉配型阳性而没有有效"脱敏"，由此导致的相关超急性排斥反应和移植物失功的风险是肾移植禁忌证。B 细胞交叉配型阳性的受体具有加速急性排斥反应发生的风险，因此会使用更强力的免疫抑制方案，但这种做法还没有得到充分的研究。虽然不是移植手术的禁忌证，交叉配型阳性也与更差的移植物预后相关，并可能需要增强的免疫抑制或更严格的移植后监测[9]。总的来说，供体特异性是高风险抗体的基本特征，而非供体特异性的同种抗体的风险性较差。

人类白细胞抗原匹配

在肾移植中，HLA 抗原是重要的确定排斥反应发生风险因素，特别是当未使用强有力的免疫抑制剂时。供体和受体间错配抗原的数目越多，受体发生排斥反应的风险越大。许多研究表明，更好的 HLA 匹配会带来更高的移植物存活率[10,11]。尽管如此，一项关于美国肾脏数据系统（USRDS）数据库的研究分析了 23 443 例 1995 年至 2002 年间移植的病例，发现与 DR 错配组相比，术后 6 个月免疫抑制剂霉酚酸酯和他克莫司的使用率在"非 HLA ABDR 错配组"仅低 4%~8%。因此，基于 HLA 配型的免疫抑制调节为免疫抑制的"定制"提供了一个可能的机会，而免疫抑制是基于免疫，而非未充分利用的排斥反应的流行病学风险。

研究表明，HLA 错配在非肾移植中也与排斥反应和移植物预后相关。HLA 错配影响肝移植急性排斥反应发生率，但不影响 1 年的肝移植物存活率[12]。在肺移植中，HLA 错配与急性排斥反应和闭塞性细支气管炎综合征(BOS)的发展相关，并且会降低患者生存率[13,14]。关于 HLA 配型对心脏移植影响的研究结果是矛盾的，最近较大的单中心研究证明，HLA 配型对生存率无影响[15]。对于非肾实体器官的移植，关于移植器官大小与受体大小相匹配和冷缺血时间限制等的考虑，已经超过了对常规的 HLA 配型的使用，但由于使用移植前单珠抗 HLA 抗体评估重新计算的群体反应性抗体(cPRA)，HLA 配型可能对所有器官维持性免疫抑制治疗的指导都是有用的。

其他免疫学评估

已经研究了其他的检测方法和标记物来识别预先形成的 T 细胞记忆，从而能够进一步评估移植前的风险或用于移植后监测。这些内容将在第 89 章、第 90 章和第 91 章详细介绍。理想情况下，这可以为个性化治疗提供信息，即那些具有高排斥反应发生风险的患者接受增强的免疫抑制治疗，而那些具有低排斥反应发生风险的患者施行药物剂量最小化的治疗[16]。干扰素(IFN)-γ 酶联免疫斑点试验是一项检测同种抗原特异性记忆性 T 细胞的技术。有证据表明，高频的供体反应记忆性 T 细胞与移植物不良预后相关[17]，群体反应记忆性 T 细胞的反应性独立于 PRA[18]。反映总体免疫激活水平的标记物也被检查，如可溶性 CD30，其由活化 T 细胞的膜结合 CD30 蛋白水解生成[19]。尽管可溶性 CD30 水平被用来预测移植后供体特异性抗体的产生[20]，但是高水平的 CD30 并不与排斥反应必然相关[21]。ImmuKnow 检测(Cylex，Inc.，Columbia，MD)，从分离的多克隆刺激 $CD4^+$ T 细胞检测体外释放的 ATP(iATP)，也被作为区分免疫抑制程度过度或不足的一个方法。Meta 分析表明，这种检测对排斥反应或感染的预测能力很差，并且用它直接管理患者的结果通常是令人失望的[22]。总的来说，在推荐这些检测用于常规临床应用来指导免疫抑制治疗前，其在不同患者群体和免疫抑制方案中的临床效用的进一步前瞻性信息是有保证的。

供体和受体特征

急性排斥反应的供体危险因素包括冷缺血时间、移植物功能延迟恢复[23-26]。冷缺血时间和移植物功能延迟恢复也影响预后。据报道，在多中心研究中，冷缺血与移植物功能延迟恢复密切相关，每 6 小时的冷缺血使移植物功能延迟恢复的风险增加 23%。急性排斥反应更常发生于功能延迟恢复(其是 5 年移植物失功的独立预测因素)的移植物中[27]。移植肾功能延迟恢复与环孢素时代前后移植肾存活率显著降低相关[28]。对移植物功能延迟恢复的受体使用强有力的免疫抑制在临床实践中是常见的，但这种做法尚未得到充分研究。通过其对细胞增殖的抑制作用，西罗莫司可能会延长移植物功能延迟恢复的时间[29]。

受体排斥反应的风险特征包括年龄、移植前透析和再次移植。老龄化由于会使 T 细胞产物与反应性普遍下降而与免疫抑制需求下降相关[30,31]。然而，“贝拉西普的肾功能保护评估和作为一线免疫保护药物的有效性试验”(BENEFIT-EXT)显示，排斥反应在接受扩大选择标准供肾的年长受体中更常见[32]。由于扩大选择标准的供肾具有更多的组织学损伤，这可能代表排斥反应的“启动”或反映年老的供体器官具有与急性排斥反应相似的组织学变化。关于老年患者的免疫抑制管理的随机临床试验是必要的。有报道认为，依赖透析进行更长时间的移植前等待和再次移植的状态也对术后受体和移植物的生存具有重要的负面影响[33]。从历史上看，再次移植是不成功的。然而，最近，强有力的免疫抑制方案提高了成功率[1]。虽然对具有这些危险因素的患者使用更强有力的免疫抑制剂是常见的，但这种做法并没有得到充分的研究。

种族

从历史上看，非洲裔美国人和白种人之间的肾移植结果存在差异[34-37]。非洲裔美国人有更高的排斥反应发生风险，即使是接受具有两个单倍型匹配的活体移植的受体[38]，并可能受益于更积极的免疫抑制策略[39]。尽管在环孢素时代，1 年期移植物存活率有了整体改善，非洲裔美国人患者的生存率仍低于白种人[40-43]，而且尽管基于环孢素的四联免疫抑制方案据报道能够提高非裔美国人及白种人受体的短期移植物存活率，但非裔美国人患者的长期结果没有得到改善[44,45]。应用他克莫司和霉酚酸的结果显示了更好的前言。与环孢素相比，特别是在非裔美国人的受体中，基于他克莫司的免疫抑制联合抗体诱导可以降低移植后 1 年急性排斥反应的发生率及其严重程度[46]。尽管非裔美国人肾移植受体可能需要比白种人更高的剂量，但报道也显示了应用霉酚酸酯的有利结果。一项关于硫唑嘌呤和霉酚酸酯的比较研究结果显示，非裔美国人肾移植受体接受霉酚酸酯治疗的急性排斥反应发生率低于接受硫唑嘌呤治疗的受体，接受每天 3g 霉酚酸酯治疗的非裔美国人和接受每天 2g 霉酚酸酯治疗的白种人急性排斥反应发生率是相似的[39]。这项研究还显示，在非裔美国人以外的人群中没有剂量效应，而且在非裔美国人以外的人群中移植后 6 个月活检证实的急性排斥反应和治疗失败的联合研究终点在硫唑嘌呤和霉酚酸酯之间没有显著差异。

依从性

依从性差与排斥反应、移植物失功、移植后不良预后相关，特别是在青少年当中[47-50]。这部分内容将在第120章中深入介绍。新的免疫抑制治疗可以为已知依从性差的患者提供替代治疗。西罗莫司半衰期很长，可以方便地每天给药一次。相比其他每天口服给药一次或两次的治疗方案，贝拉西普由于具有更低的给药频率（每月给药一次）而具有更高的患者依从性，因此可能对依从性差的患者有效。然而，对那些没有社会支持的患者、那些具有困难静脉通路的患者，或者那些难以到达输液中心的患者而言，它可能反而被视作一种障碍。

妊娠

妊娠可能增加急性排斥反应和移植物失功的发生风险。妊娠移植的影响将在第97章中阐述。为了降低这种风险，谨慎的免疫抑制选择和药物监测是必要的。霉酚酸、西罗莫司和依维莫司可能对胎儿有害，应该避免使用。尽管被列为妊娠期D类药物，硫唑嘌呤自20世纪50年代起已安全应用于妊娠期移植患者。药物动力学在妊娠期也有所改变，如免疫抑制剂的分布容积与代谢，因此需要监控和调整。

总结

由于免疫抑制药物的毒性，不同维持治疗方案正在被探索以减少短期和长期的副作用。然而，引导这些策略的仍只是被认识到的免疫风险而非严格验证的客观指标。具有排斥反应发生风险的患者可能需要更强有力的免疫抑制治疗、更多的药物和更高的剂量。具有较低排斥反应发生风险的患者可能需要较温和的治疗、更低的药物浓度和剂量，或者单药治疗或二联治疗。目前，强有力的证据只存在于基于HLA错配和预先形成的同种抗体的风险分层，而不存在于流行病学风险。

感染与维持性免疫抑制

新型免疫抑制方案已经彻底改变了移植，降低排斥反应发生率并提高移植物的存活率，但代价是更高的感染风险。病毒利用目标宿主细胞的结构进行复制，而有效的抗病毒免疫反应取决于先天（如自然杀伤细胞）和获得性（例如T细胞）反应。为了保护移植物而抑制宿主的免疫系统，病毒感染的风险有所增加。移植固有的感染性疾病风险将在第92章、第93章和第94章中详细介绍。本部分将关联病毒感染与免疫抑制管理。一般来说，病毒复制提示强有力的，或许是过度的免疫抑制，提示应该考虑降低维持性免疫抑制。

对普通人群相对温和的高度血清阳性率的病毒可以威胁到免疫抑制的移植受体，导致移植物损伤和恶性肿瘤。造成临床威胁最大的病毒包括人类疱疹病毒（HHV）1和2，水痘带状疱疹病毒（VZV），EB病毒（EBV），巨细胞病毒（CMV），HHV6、7、8，丙型肝炎病毒（HCV），乙肝病毒（HBV），BK病毒（BKV），人类免疫缺陷病毒（HIV），人类乳头状瘤病毒（HPV）和细小病毒。虽然许多免疫抑制剂已经被证明具有体外抗病毒效果，但临床观察结果可能不同（表66.3）。已对移植后病毒感染高危或确诊患者的维持性免疫抑制管理策略进行讨论，主要集中在BK病毒、CMV、乙肝病毒、丙肝病毒、EB病毒。

BK病毒

BK病毒是人类实体器官移植后激活的最常见的多瘤病毒。健康献血者的BK病毒血清阳性率是82%；病毒潜伏在肾皮质、髓质和尿路上皮细胞。尽管免疫抑制引起BK病毒特异性T细胞减少[51]，但因为BK病毒肾病（BKVN）主要是由于移植器官内潜伏的BK被激活，所以BKVN很少发生在非肾实体器官移植受体的自体肾脏[52]。因此，BKVN主要见于肾移植受体（1%~10%）。临床表现包括无症状病毒传染、膀胱炎、肾小管间质肾炎、肾病综合征、输尿管狭窄和移植物失功。

BKV感染和免疫抑制的整体程度之间存在相关

表66.3 维持性免疫抑制对病毒感染的影响

	BKV	CMV	HCV	HBV	EBV
环孢素	—	↑↑↑	↓↓↓	↓↓	↑↑↑
他克莫司	↑↑↑	—	↑	—	—
硫唑嘌呤	↓	↓↓	—	↑↑	↑
霉酚酸	↑	↓↓	↓↓	↓↓	↓
mTOR抑制剂	↓	↓↓	↓	↓	↓↓

↓已证实的抗病毒治疗活性；↑已证实的有害影响（例如增加病毒复制）；—已证实没有影响。

BKV，BK病毒；CMV，巨细胞病毒；HCV，丙肝病毒；HBV，乙肝病毒；EBV，EB病毒。

性。抗排斥治疗和累积类固醇暴露是 BKVN 的危险因素。几项研究表明,基于他克莫司的免疫抑制方案与更高的 BKVN 风险有关[53-55]。然而,没有特定的诱导或维持性免疫抑制剂或其组合与 BKVN 的发展唯一相关。

80%的 BK 病毒血症在移植后 3 月内发生[56]。幸运的是,BKV 在发展成肾病之前就可以在血浆中检测到[57]。因此,共识建议受体移植后每 1~3 个月筛查病毒血症[58]。由于 BK 病毒血症代表 BKV 再激活和 BKV 特异性细胞免疫之间的失衡以及缺乏有效的抗病毒药物,降低免疫抑制以发展 BKV 特异性免疫仍然是治疗的基础。在那些存在病毒血症(> 10 000copies/mL)的患者中减少免疫抑制可以避免损害肾脏的组织和功能。尽管尚未进行比较试验,但应用筛查和预防策略的结果很可能优于治疗现有肾病的结果。

本章描述了两种检测病毒血症后降低免疫抑制水平的方法。在第一种方法中,钙调磷酸酶抑制剂减少 25%~50%,然后减少抗增殖剂[59,60]。另一种方法是首先减少或消除抗代谢物,然后在必要时减少钙调磷酸酶抑制剂,从而实现对病毒血症的清除[54]。这两种方法的直接比较尚未完成。一项单中心研究报道了采用停止抗代谢物联合后续减少钙调磷酸酶抑制剂来治疗 BK 病毒血症的长期结果。在 200 名患者中,术后 1 年的病毒尿和病毒血症发生率分别为 35%和 12%。降低免疫抑制后,95%的患者病毒血症得到了解决。5 年患者总体生存率为 91%,移植物存活率为 84%。BK 病毒血症的发展没有影响患者生存率或移植物存活率[61]。

对移植物功能障碍的患者,应进行移植物活检以指导治疗。由于 BKVN 活检时看起来与炎症有关,BK 病毒肾病可能被误诊为排斥反应,也可能与排斥反应同时发生。动脉内膜炎、纤维素样血管壁坏死、肾小球炎或肾小管周围毛细血管 C4d 阳性的存在支持并发排斥反应的诊断[62]。SV40 染色可以证实 BKVN 的存在。针对同时发生 BKVN 和排斥反应的治疗是有争议的,一种方法是抗排斥反应治疗联合后续的减少维持性免疫抑制治疗。由于静脉注射免疫球蛋白(IVIG)也被用于治疗排斥反应,IVIG 的使用对 BK 肾病和排斥反应难以鉴别的患者可能特别有益。对于通过降低免疫抑制而清除 BK 病毒血症后发生急性排斥反应而采用传统抗排斥反应治疗的患者,应在治疗后每 2 周仔细监测 BK 病毒血症复发。对于已确诊的 BKVN,其他的维持性免疫抑制策略也已被描述,例如环孢素代替具有额外降低霉酚酸浓度作用的他克莫司[57]。可以考虑把钙调磷酸酶抑制剂转换为 mTOR 抑制剂[63],只是这种策略仅适用于那些肾功能尚好而无蛋白尿的患者。虽然体外研究和最初的小型研究表明,来氟米特(一种氨基丙二腈)可以抑制 BKV 复制[64,65],但系统性回顾未能确认添加来氟米特对发生 BKVN 后移植物存活有任何益处[66]。此外,一项关于采用 FK778(一种来氟米特衍生物)治疗合并 BKVN 的肾移植受体的研究没能证明患者能从中获益[67]。

对因 BKVN 导致移植物失功的受体进行再次移植能够获得成功[68]。虽然有对具有活跃的病毒血症的受体进行再次移植的个案报告,但一般共识认为再次移植应延迟到病毒血症被清除后。在对器官获取与移植网络(OPTN)数据库进行的分析中,确定了 126 例由于 BKVN 导致移植物失功而进行再次肾移植的患者。其中 80%的再次移植使用了免疫诱导药物,而且他克莫司+霉酚酸酯是最常见的维持性免疫抑制方案(57%)。在这些患者中,17.5%接受了 BKV 治疗且只有 1 例 BKVN 导致的移植物失功,而术后 1 年移植物存活率为 98.5%[68]。

巨细胞病毒

与 BK 病毒相反,CMV 在所有实体器官移植受体中都具有很高的感染率和死亡率[69]。CMV 的临床表现变化可以从无症状的病毒血症到感染(发热、关节痛、白细胞减少症、血小板减少症)再到器官侵袭性疾病(肺炎、胃肠炎、结肠炎、肝炎、脑炎)。血清阳性率在那些 20 岁以上的人群中大约为 60%,且在感染后病毒将终身潜伏。因此,CMV 感染或移植后的疾病代表宿主体内潜伏病毒的再激活或来自供体器官的原发感染。除了供体和受体 CMV 血清状态,宿主先天免疫力和净免疫抑制的状态是感染的主要危险因素,因此采用免疫抑制来预防和治疗急性排斥反应后感染的风险是最大的。没有采取预防措施的情况下,超过 50%的实体器官移植受体将发生 CMV 感染,提前采取措施可以使 CMV 疾病的发病率显著降低。预防,或者在最大感知风险时给予受体抗病毒药物,以及在检测到巨细胞病毒抗原血症后采取预防治疗或直接开始治疗,这两种方法都已成功得到应用[69,70]。

虽然没有一种免疫抑制剂确定与 CMV 感染相关,但淋巴细胞消耗性药物[71,72]和钙调磷酸酶抑制剂(特别是环孢素)[73,74] 的使用似乎与风险增加有关,而mTOR抑制剂西罗莫司和依维莫司的使用可能具有保护作用[75-78]。关于应用霉酚酸和硫唑嘌呤导致CMV发病率的临床研究是有争议的[79],部分但不是全部研究显示,霉酚酸酯的使用可能会导致更高的发病率和疾病严重程度。这些研究之间的差异可能反映了霉酚酸酯和硫唑嘌呤使用剂量的不同。此外,许多早期的研究是在预防性更昔洛韦常规使用之前进行的。总的来说,鉴于CMV抗病毒药物的预防和治疗疗效,目前没有足够的证据支持任何单个或联合使用的维持性免疫抑制剂能预防CMV。对于复发性或难治性CMV疾病的患者可以考虑转换为应用mTOR抑制剂[80]。

使用抗病毒药物治疗CMV感染和疾病,特别是证实已累及器官时,降低免疫抑制的整体水平应考虑作为辅助疗法。通常,这可以通过减少或停用抗代谢物(霉酚酸酯或硫唑嘌呤)实现,但在重症病例中可能还需要额外减少钙调磷酸酶抑制剂的使用[81]。在比较缬更昔洛韦和静脉注射更昔洛韦治疗CMV的试验中,二联维持性免疫抑制方案组和低剂量钙调磷酸酶抑制剂组比三联维持性免疫抑制方案组和高剂量钙调磷酸酶抑制剂组观察到更高的21天CMV病毒血症根除率。然而,组间的长期根除率和疾病复发风险相当[82]。目前,尚不清楚成功的CMV治疗后是否应该重新启用抗代谢物,最好应该在免疫风险预测结果的指导下进行决定。

丙肝病毒

丙型肝炎患病率在实体器官移植组之间存在着很大的差别,在肝脏和肾脏移植人群中患病率更高。HCV引起的肝硬化仍然是肝移植的主要适应证之一[83]。此外,HCV在肾移植受体的患病率由于地域差异在5%~46%之间。移植后病毒复发几乎是普遍的,将导致肝纤维化加速,而移植物存活率和患者生存率的降低主要是由于肝硬化和肝癌[84]。

移植肝纤维化加速发展、肝硬化的发生率上升和纤维化淤胆型肝炎表明免疫抑制可导致疾病进展[85]。广泛的体外证据已经表明,环孢素具有抗HCV活性的作用[86,87],因此无免疫抑制作用的环孢素类似物作为HCV的治疗药物正在进行研究[88]。然而,与他克莫司相比,临床研究并未显示出环孢素在复发率或对抗病毒治疗的反应方面具有明显优势。一项Meta分析比较了基于环孢素与基于他克莫司的免疫抑制方案,显示两种方案在肝移植术后死亡率、移植物存活率和纤维化淤胆型肝炎发病率等方面无显著差异[89]。同样,一项随机对照试验表明随机使用环孢素或他克莫司方案的肝移植受体在生存率和HCV严重复发率方面没有差异[90]。然而,环孢素组具有更长的组织学复发平均时间间隔。回顾性研究表明,环孢素可提高抗病毒治疗疗效并改善持续病毒学应答率[85];尚缺乏确定性的前瞻性数据。

使用皮质类固醇对HCV复发及对抗病毒治疗反应的影响也是有争议的。激素使用通常被视为有害的。到目前为止,激素撤除及无激素方案尚未显示能够改善生存率或延缓纤维化进展[91,92]。两种抗代谢物硫唑嘌呤和霉酚酸酯在体外都显示了抗HCV效果[93]。总的来说,临床研究没能证明使用基于抗代谢药物的免疫抑制方案在HCV复发方面始终具有有效性,虽然有系统性回顾表明在肝移植受体中,相比霉酚酸酯,使用硫唑嘌呤的患者HCV复发的严重程度较低[94]。关于mTOR抑制剂对HCV阳性肝移植受体效用的数据是有限的和矛盾的。在一项研究中,接受或不接受西罗莫司的患者,其HCV复发时间和严重程度相似[95],而在另一项研究中,西罗莫司的使用对1年和2年最低限度纤维化是一个独立的预测因素[96]。

乙肝病毒

由于免疫抑制治疗,HBV复制可能发生在实体器官移植之后。复制再激活更可能发生在移植前HBeAg阳性或HBV DNA检测阳性的受体中,再激活极少在HBcAb阳性而HBsAg阴性的患者中观察到[97]。类似于CMV预防,防止移植后HBV再活化的两种方法是预防(最大激活风险期间抗病毒药物管理)和包含移植后病毒血症监测的预防策略。在抗病毒治疗取得进展(包括拉米夫定、乙肝免疫球蛋白)之前,肝移植术后HBV再活化几乎是普遍的[98]。

虽然免疫抑制可能导致HBV复制,但尚缺乏信息指导针对当前抗病毒药物可用性和有效性的维持性免疫抑制管理。目前的建议支持基于个体免疫风险评估的最小化免疫抑制方案。例如,对于HBsAg阳性肝移植受体,可考虑激素撤除方案,因为使用皮质类固醇被证明在体外能增加HBV DNA合成[99]。虽然体外研究表明霉酚酸酯对HBV复制具有抑制作用,但一项小型研究中使用霉酚酸酯在拉米夫定耐药的 HBV 再激活后并不能改善肝移植受体的预后[100]。慢性肝炎可能会增加硫唑嘌呤或环孢素的肝毒性风险。

EB 病毒

临床上,实体器官移植后 EBV 感染的最重要表现是 EBV 感染的 B 细胞不受控制地增生,这是导致移植后淋巴增殖性疾病(PTLD)的部分原因。PTLD 的发病率呈现双峰形态。移植后第 1 年发病的病例往往发生在 EBV 血清学阴性的受体接受了 EBV 血清学阳性器官的病例中,绝大多数表现为表达 CD20 的 B 细胞淋巴瘤。PTLD 的风险取决于所移植的器官,心肺移植受体是风险最高的(图 66.4)[101],且器官类型之间的差异可能反映了所使用的免疫抑制强度、器官的免疫原性程度和移植器官内的淋巴组织数量[102]。免疫诱导和(或)治疗排斥反应所用的消耗性抗体确定与 PTLD 发生的风险增加相关,特别是移植后早期[101,103]。然而,维持性免疫抑制剂的使用和整体的免疫抑制程度也通过抑制 EBV 特异性 T 细胞的反应而增加 PTLD 的风险。移植失败后停用免疫抑制淋剂可使巴瘤的风险降至移植前的水平[104]。与使用二联或三联免疫抑制剂的患者相比,使用四联免疫抑制剂的患者风险最高[103]。

注册表分析显示,采用基于钙调磷酸酶疗法的患者 PTLD 的风险增加,尤其是那些使用他克莫司的患者[101,103]。然而,这种风险的增加主要在未接受诱导治疗的患者中可以观察到[103,105],提示最初诱导治疗的强有力的免疫抑制效果超过任何钙调磷酸酶抑制剂的效果差异。而且,钙调磷酸酶抑制剂的使用可能会影响后期 PTLD 的发病率[104]。关于他克莫司的任何风险差异可能是由于他克莫司相对于环孢素提供了更高水平的免疫

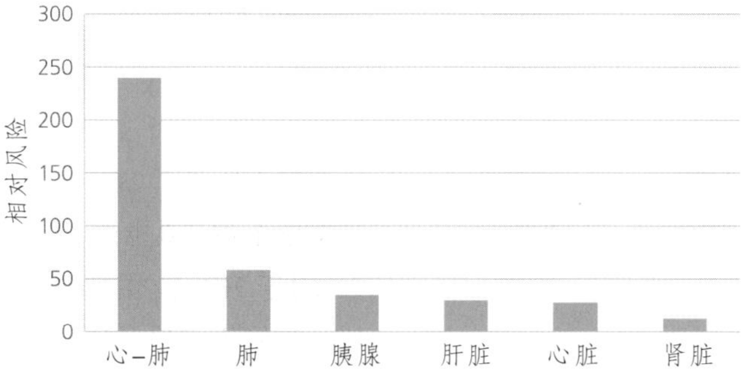

图 66.4 器官移植后 5 年不同器官类型发生移植后淋巴增生性疾病(PTLD)的相对风险。

抑制。相比钙调磷酸酶抑制剂,抗代谢物的使用并不与 PTLD 相关,一些研究认为其还能稍微降低发病风险。霉酚酸在体外能抑制人类 B 细胞淋巴瘤的增殖[106]。在注册表分析[104]、病例对照[107]和前瞻性队列研究[108]中,霉酚酸酯与 PTLD 风险增加无关,并具有降低恶性肿瘤发生风险的趋势,而且可以延缓恶性肿瘤的发生。在一项大型注册表分析中,霉酚酸酯与硫唑嘌呤相比,它们对于 PTLD 的影响没有差别;然而,使用硫唑嘌呤的患者比例较低[105]。

mTOR 抑制剂西罗莫司和依维莫司对 PTLD 的影响尚不清楚。使用 mTOR 抑制剂与移植后总体新发恶性肿瘤的发病率降低有关[109]。已发现这些药物能抑制 EBV 阳性 B 细胞淋巴瘤细胞的增殖[110]。关于 25 000 例联邦医疗保险的移植受体的分析显示,PTLD 的发生与西罗莫司的应用无关[103];然而,这个组中只有 665 名患者接受了西罗莫司治疗。在肾移植受体的 ELITE-Symphony 试验中(该试验是一个比较低剂量他克莫司、低剂量环孢素、标准剂量环孢素和基于西罗莫司的维持性免疫抑制的随机对照试验),所有的 PTLD 及非霍奇金淋巴瘤病例均发生在西罗莫司组。而急性排斥反应发生率,也是西罗莫司组最高;因此使用 T 细胞消耗性药物可能导致更高的淋巴瘤发生率[74]。

新的药物——贝拉西普是一种选择性阻断 T 细胞共刺激信号的融合蛋白,在Ⅲ期试验中,与标准环孢素方案相比,其具有更高的 PTLD 发生风险,尤其是那些具有 EBV 血清学阳性供体的 EBV 血清学阴性受体[111,112]。有趣的是,贝拉西普组排斥反应的发生率也更高,当使用维持性药物时,这一发现使较高程度的免疫抑制是增加 PTLD 发生风险的唯一原因的概念更具挑战性。目前推荐 EBV 血清学阳性的患者限制使用贝拉西普。

PTLD 的治疗包括减少免疫抑制、抗病毒治疗(EBV 相关的)、化疗、放疗和局部切除。单独减少免疫抑制约 25%~50%的基线水平,可以有效地治疗限制性多态 PTLD。更多的病例可能需要更积极地减少免疫抑制;然而,排斥反应和移植物失功的发生风险必须仔细考虑[113]。一项包括 19 例来自欧洲中心的肾移植患者的研究中,当发生 PTLD 后,将患者的钙调磷酸酶抑制剂停用或降到最低剂量,并转而使用西罗莫司或依维莫司[114]。15 例患者的 PTLD 得到缓解;其中 6 例患者同时接受利妥昔单抗治疗,而另外 6 例患者接受 CHOP(环

磷酰胺、阿霉素、长春新碱和泼尼松)方案治疗,使得mTOR抑制剂的效果难以辨别。最近,通过注入自体细胞毒性T细胞重组EBV特异性免疫的策略越来越受到关注[115]。

癌症与维持性免疫抑制

移植后免疫抑制剂的使用增加了实体器官移植后恶性肿瘤的远期风险。这种风险将在第95章中深入介绍。在一项大型队列研究中,使用了来自美国科学移植受体注册中心和13个州及地方注册中心的关联数据,统计了1987年至2008年间超过175 000例移植(肾、肝、心脏和肺)患者的恶性肿瘤发病率。在研究期间,共报告了10 656例恶性肿瘤,与普通人群相比,相关标准化发病率比为2.1。与一般人群相比,卡波西肉瘤、非霍奇金淋巴瘤、皮肤癌、唇部肿瘤、会阴部肿瘤、肛门部肿瘤和肝癌的发生风险增加了5倍或更高,说明特定病毒感染的致癌潜力。一般人群常规筛查的癌症,包括宫颈癌、乳腺癌、前列腺癌,在移植受体中的发生风险没有明显增加[116]。

消耗性抗体治疗显然与PTLD的风险增加有关,通常与EBV感染有关(如上文所述)。除此之外,没有确凿证据表明特定的免疫抑制剂与特定的恶性肿瘤的发生有关。而且免疫抑制总体程度与风险相关,并有一些观察支持这一结论。不同实体器官移植受体恶性肿瘤的发生风险也不同,那些接受更强免疫抑制治疗(如心、肺移植)的受体癌症发生的风险最大[101]。此外,某些癌症(如PTLD)的发生风险在移植后第1年的高免疫抑制环境下最大[101]。排斥反应的发生会增加恶性肿瘤的风险,或许是由于消耗性抗体和(或)维持性免疫抑制的增强[117]。所使用的免疫抑制药物的数量与癌症发生风险有关[103]。某些恶性肿瘤(如卡波西肉瘤、多态PTLD)可能随着免疫抑制的降低完全消退[113]。最后,移植物失功后停用免疫抑制剂可使恶性肿瘤的发生风险显著下降[104]。免疫抑制可能导致恶性肿瘤发生的机制包括损伤针对致癌病毒的免疫活性、降低针对肿瘤细胞的免疫监视、直接损伤DNA和破坏DNA修复机制、上调促进肿瘤形成的细胞因子[118]。

单个免疫抑制剂的致癌潜力是否独立于它们的免疫抑制效果是有争议的。迄今为止的研究受限于效力不足,特别是一些恶性肿瘤的发病率较低。此外,免疫抑制剂的使用数据可能只代表移植时使用的药物,而没有记录长期管理中的情况变化。此外,尽管使用类似的方案,免疫抑制的程度可能因药物浓度的不同而有所不同[119]。然而,有些实验和临床研究结果值得进一步讨论。环孢素和他克莫司可以通过产生转化生长因子-β(TGF-β)、血管内皮生长因子(VEGF)和白细胞介素-6(IL-6)促进癌症进展[120,121]。较低浓度的钙调磷酸酶抑制剂与癌症风险降低相关[122]。在肾移植受体中,观察到与使用环孢素者相比,使用他克莫司者新发肿瘤(包括PTLD)发生率增加;然而,这种观察报告仅限于那些没有接受诱导治疗的受体[105]。硫唑嘌呤被认为与皮肤[123]和唇部[124]鳞状细胞癌的发生风险增加有关,可能是通过紫外线A辐射的光敏作用引起[125]。相反,霉酚酸酯似乎并没有增加恶性肿瘤风险[108,123]。西罗莫司在动物模型中的抗肿瘤效应的证据正在增加,其抑制肿瘤生长的机制包括抑制p70 S6激酶(抑制细胞增殖)、IL-10(Jak/STATs活动)、细胞周期蛋白(阻断细胞周期活动)以及VEGF信号(阻碍淋巴管生成)[120,126]。在雷帕鸣维持性治疗方案研究中,肾移植患者随机分配到泼尼松+环孢素+西罗莫司组或西罗莫司单药组中,环孢素撤除组恶性肿瘤的风险几乎低两倍[127]。在CONVERT试验中,转换为西罗莫司治疗的患者相比继续使用钙调磷酸酶抑制剂者,其非黑色素瘤皮肤癌发病率更低[128]。

虽然减少免疫抑制在已确诊的恶性肿瘤治疗中可能是有用的,但这种方法主要对肾移植受体有用,因为排斥反应导致的移植物失功并不是致命的。减少免疫抑制可能对治疗淋巴瘤、皮肤癌和卡波西肉瘤特别有效[129]。将肾移植受体的环孢素替换为西罗莫司可使卡波西肉瘤完全消退[130,131]。对于恶性肿瘤患者,无论是处于缓解期还是正在治疗中,都可以考虑改用以西罗莫司为基础的治疗方案。然而,无论是否有恶性肿瘤史,应用西罗莫司的患者全因死亡率的风险会增加2倍以上[132]。在接受化疗的患者中,应当最小化或中止使用维持性药物,直到治疗完成;特别是硫唑嘌呤可以增加骨髓抑制的严重程度。环孢素是一种ATP结合盒式B亚科成员1基因(*ABCB1*)编码的流出p-糖蛋白的有效抑制剂,可能会受到与p-糖蛋白相互作用的各种化疗药物的影响[133]。

移植后不同时期的维持性免疫抑制

移植后早期管理

移植后早期优化免疫抑制管理对实现长期的移植物功能和存活具有重要意义。早期移植经验表明,在移植后早期使用诱导药物和(或)更高剂量的维持性免疫抑制剂使得移植后数月内急性排斥反应发生率升高,这一做法已经逐渐改变[134]。特定的免疫诱导治疗已在第 65 章深入介绍。环孢素的引入彻底改变了移植,急性排斥反应发生率和术后 1 年的移植物存活率得到显著改善。环孢素最初设想是作为一种预防排斥反应并替代激素的药物。然而,单独使用环孢素被证明是有问题的,因为预防排斥反应所需的大剂量环孢素会引起显著的毒性,尤其是肾毒性[135]。因此三联疗法,或联合使用钙调磷酸酶抑制剂、泼尼松、硫唑嘌呤,已成为一个最大化免疫抑制效应同时最小化毒性的策略。尽管他克莫司和霉酚酸在很大程度上取代了环孢素和硫唑嘌呤作为初始维持性免疫抑制剂,但三联疗法仍然是在实体器官移植后应用的主要方法[1]。由于急性排斥反应的发生风险在移植后前 3 个月最高,在此期间使用高剂量,然后情况稳定的患者减少剂量以降低毒性。

即使在移植后早期,人们仍然对最小化免疫抑制感兴趣。钙调磷酸酶抑制剂问世以来,目标剂量水平得到降低,从而在降低肾毒性效果的同时可以保持可接受的急性排斥反应发生率。无钙调磷酸酶抑制剂方案并未广泛使用,因为急性排斥反应发生率高,尤其是在免疫原性更强的实体器官移植中。人们关注的还是尽量减少和避免使用类固醇。然而,尽管同时使用钙调磷酸酶抑制剂,但在这些方案中还是观察到了较高的排斥反应发生率[136],这在一定程度上阻止了这些方案的广泛应用。

关于术后立即使用维持性药物的特殊问题需要进一步回顾。在肾移植中,mTOR 抑制剂西罗莫司和依维莫司的使用与移植肾功能延迟恢复相关,因此,“肾脏疾病:改善全球的结果(KDIGO)”临床实践指南建议,如果使用 mTOR 抑制剂,应该直到移植肾功能建立和手术伤口愈合后再开始使用[58]。虽然西罗莫司具有相对较低的传统输入小动脉收缩肾毒性的风险,但同时应用血管紧张素转换酶抑制剂(ACEI)可能会导致急性肾衰竭[137]或过敏反应[138]。西罗莫司在肺移植后早期未能广泛使用,主要是因为支气管吻合口有裂开的风险[139,140]。它也与肝移植后肝动脉血栓形成有关[141]。

移植后中期到长期管理

移植后中期到长期管理着重于预防慢性排斥反应和减少药物毒性。药物毒性和管理选择的总结见表 66.4。钙调磷酸酶抑制剂往往伴随着剂量依赖的毒性反应。多毛症、牙龈肥大、高血压、高脂血症在环孢素治疗中比他克莫司更常见,而神经毒性、脱发和潜在的移植后糖尿病在他克莫司治疗中比环孢素更常见。

应用他克莫司存在的一个问题是可能会相对增加糖尿病的发病率,这已在单独接受肾移植的受体中发现[142]。几项研究报道他克莫司在胰腺移植受体中并没有增加糖尿病发病率[143–146]。相比更高剂量的他克莫司,低剂量他克莫司降低了移植后新发糖尿病(NODAT)的风险[147]。钙调磷酸酶抑制剂也可能导致肾毒性。低剂量

表 66.4　针对免疫抑制不良事件的治疗方案调整

不良事件	免疫抑制相关诱因	免疫抑制方案调整
移植后新发糖尿病	皮质类固醇、他克莫司、环孢素、mTOR 抑制剂	避免使用,降低剂量
血脂异常	皮质类固醇、环孢素、西罗莫司、依维莫司	避免使用,降低剂量,改用他克莫司
高血压	皮质类固醇、环孢素、他克莫司、mTOR 抑制剂	避免使用,降低剂量
骨质疏松	皮质类固醇	避免使用,降低剂量,应用维生素 D
骨髓抑制	霉酚酸、硫唑嘌呤、西罗莫司、依维莫司、他克莫司	降低剂量
切口愈合延迟	西罗莫司、依维莫司	避免使用
胃肠道不良反应	霉酚酸酯、他克莫司、西罗莫司	改用霉酚酸钠肠溶片,降低剂量,改用硫唑嘌呤
蛋白尿	西罗莫司、依维莫司	避免使用
肾毒性	环孢素、他克莫司、西罗莫司	避免使用,降低剂量,改用贝拉西普

或无钙调磷酸酶方案将在后面的器官部分讨论。然而，即使患者从未接受钙调磷酸酶抑制剂治疗也可能会在肾脏活检中出现与钙调磷酸酶抑制剂毒性反应一致的组织学变化[148]。

皮质类固醇具有包括高血压、血脂异常、葡萄糖耐受不良、骨质疏松症等副作用。许多新的方案试图撤除皮质类固醇以规避这些不良反应。这些方案将在后面不同类型器官的皮质类固醇撤除部分讨论。

抗代谢药物与骨髓抑制和胃肠道副作用有关。密切监测血常规在移植后是必要的。胃肠道副作用将在后面的肾移植抗代谢物部分中讨论。

西罗莫司和依维莫司可能具有许多不良反应，包括白细胞减少、血小板减少、贫血、黏膜炎、高胆固醇血症、高甘油三酯血症、胸腔积液、心包积液、卵巢囊肿和水肿。首次使用西罗莫司可出现伤口愈合延迟和淋巴囊肿形成，延长移植肾功能延迟恢复时间。

移植物失功

针对移植物失功的合适的免疫抑制方案尚不明确。因为尚无可用的支持性疗法，而再次移植是唯一的选择，这对于实体器官移植受体来说很复杂。然而，左心室辅助装置的逐渐普及及其功效使得针对心脏移植受体的再次移植成为潜在的可行选择。在肾移植中，许多医生会降低钙调磷酸酶抑制剂的剂量，或将其替换为mTOR抑制剂。然而COVERT研究表明，当估计的肾小球滤过率<40mL/min时，用西罗莫司替代钙调磷酸酶抑制剂是不安全的；当估计肾小球滤过率>40mL/min时，这将是无效和危险的，尿蛋白超过100mg/d限制了其在这种情况下的有效性[149]。当患者回到透析状态后，合适的免疫抑制方案也是未知的。当患者回到透析状态后，血清肌酐水平不再是识别排斥反应的有效标志，而且钙调磷酸酶抑制剂减少了急性排斥反应的常见症状和体征。一些中心撤除抗代谢物以减少感染的发生风险，当患者每日尿量超过500mL时减少钙调磷酸酶抑制剂用量和泼尼松至每天5mg[150]。当患者出现无尿后，持续免疫抑制的风险是毫无根据的，钙调磷酸酶抑制剂应撤除，泼尼松也应逐渐减量。如果患者症状和体征的发展符合急性排斥反应，治疗可能包括激素和可能的移植肾切除术。移植物失功后撤除免疫抑制剂的一个例外情况是当后续的移植（例如活体肾移植）迫在眉睫。在这种情况下，维持性免疫抑制可能是有益的，以避免提高同种抗体水平。考虑到越来越多的患者回到透析状态并寻求再次移植，移植物失功后亟须相对无毒的免疫抑制策略来避免同种致敏作用。

原发病复发

原发病复发是一个已知的影响移植物存活的因素。然而，各种免疫抑制方案对原发病复发的发生、严重程度和进展的影响往往知之甚少。总的来说，具有免疫介导的原发疾病（如自身免疫性肝炎和狼疮性肾炎）的患者需使用更高剂量的免疫抑制治疗，包括皮质类固醇，而具有感染问题（如HCV）的患者可能受益于较温和的免疫抑制方案。这将根据不同器官类型在本书其他部分详细讨论（参见第77~80章）。

通用的免疫抑制剂

成本可能是选择维持性免疫抑制剂时一个重要的因素。环孢素、他克莫司、泼尼松、霉酚酸酯、霉酚酸钠和硫唑嘌呤是可供选择的通用产品。为了让FDA批准，通用产品必须包含相同的活性成分，相同的强度、剂型和给药途径，具有相同的使用指征，具有生物等效性，满足与品牌药品相同批次的标识、强度纯度和质量要求。通用药物不需要被证明对治疗人群（例如移植受体）是有效和安全的。总的来说，通用药物在各移植领域的使用日益频繁，他们很可能成为未来10年维持性免疫抑制的主要形式。药品性能存在一定的差异，但不太可能进行系统的确定。

肾移植受体的维持性治疗

目前的肾移植通过钙调磷酸酶抑制剂、抗代谢物和皮质类固醇的使用，移植物1年存活率超过90%[1]。药物机制和用法分别在第17章和第98章中额外讨论。

钙调磷酸酶抑制剂

在过去20年中，钙调磷酸酶抑制剂已广泛用于移植后免疫抑制方案中，并且今天的实体器官移植已经确保其预防急性排斥反应和改善移植物存活的重要地位。几项标志性的试验比较了可用的钙调磷酸酶抑制剂、环孢素和他克莫司。前两项多中心研究，使用钙调磷酸酶抑制剂（环孢素微乳剂对他克莫司）联合硫唑嘌呤和皮质类固醇的方案，结果显示使用他克莫司的急性排斥反应发生率显著降低，但移植后患者生存率或移植物存活率没有差异[151,152]。随后的研究将尸体供肾受体随机分配到3种免疫抑制方案之一（均包括皮质类固醇）：①他克莫司与硫唑嘌呤；②他克莫司与霉酚酸酯；③环孢素微乳剂和霉酚酸酯[153]。每组的急性排斥反应发生率相似(<20%)，但他克莫司组的耐激素性排斥反应发生率较低。3年随访发现肾功能、患者或整体移植物存活没有统计学差异，但在他克莫司组的移植肾功能延迟恢复受体的移植物存活率更高[153]。一项Meta分析报道与这些数据一致，对于每100名接受他克莫司而不是环孢素治疗患者来说，第1年中，预防了12例急性排斥反应，以及2例移植物失功，但增加了5例移植后新发糖尿病[154]。最近，ELITE Symphony试验证明，低剂量环孢素方案不如低剂量他克莫司方案有效[74]。由于这些试验的结果，KDIGO临床实践指南建议，他克莫司应作为肾移植受体的一线钙调磷酸酶抑制剂[58]。

皮质类固醇

皮质类固醇是大多数免疫抑制方案的关键组成部分。然而，它也具有相关副作用，包括高脂血症、葡萄糖耐受不良和骨质疏松等。为了减少不良事件并改善移植物存活，关于无皮质类固醇或皮质类固醇撤除的试验显示出不同的结果。一项双盲随机安慰剂对照多中心的5年试验比较了早期皮质类固醇撤除(移植后7天)与皮质类固醇维持治疗，研究人员报道皮质类固醇撤除组的急性排斥反应发生率更高。试验包括了移植物功能立即恢复的患者，并且免疫抑制由每个当地移植中心的诱导治疗、他克莫司和霉酚酸酯组成。大多数患者接受了抗兔淋巴细胞球蛋白的抗淋巴细胞诱导治疗。在试验结束时，皮质类固醇快速停药的患者血清甘油三酯较低，体重增加较少，并且需要使用胰岛素的移植后新发糖尿病的发病率较低。在高密度脂蛋白、低密度脂蛋白、血压或糖尿病方面没有观察到差异[136]。活检证实的急性排斥反应和慢性同种异体移植肾病的发生率是皮质类固醇快速停药组的两倍。相比之下，一项Meta分析显示，在无皮质类固醇或皮质类固醇撤除患者中，这些心血管危险因素显著降低[155]。皮质类固醇撤除的三项联合研究表明，尽管在撤除组中急性排斥反应的发生率增加，但短期结果显示患者生存率和移植物存活率相似[156-158]。

具有皮质类固醇并发症的低免疫风险患者如果接受抗淋巴细胞诱导治疗，可能是皮质类固醇撤除的最佳候选人。高风险受体，如非洲裔美国人，可能不是皮质类固醇撤除的最佳候选人，然而这仍有争议[159,160]。另一个要考虑的因素是皮质类固醇撤除的时间。长期使用皮质类固醇可导致依赖性，因此晚期撤除可能与排斥反应的风险增加相关。如果在移植后泼尼松使用超过1周，则应该继续使用而不是撤除。考虑到缺乏定义皮质类固醇撤除最佳时机的长期数据、可继续使用适当的维持性药物以及可接受实践的患者群体，皮质类固醇长期使用的理想方法仍有待确定。

抗代谢药物

抗代谢药物通常被认为是三联免疫抑制方案中的“第三药物”，提供加成效应，但必要性低于钙调磷酸酶抑制剂或皮质类固醇。硫唑嘌呤和霉酚酸是该类别中常用的药剂。目前，市场上有两种形式的霉酚酸，霉酚酸酯和肠溶霉酚酸钠。一些设计良好的试验已经报道过霉酚酸酯在肾移植中的功效[161-163]。霉酚酸酯治疗组与使用低剂量硫唑嘌呤的他克莫司+皮质类固醇/环孢素+皮质类固醇的治疗方案相比，早期排斥反应的发生率和严重性均有降低[161]。这些研究的3年随访发现，霉酚酸酯组早期排斥反应的发生率降低并未转化为移植物功能或存活率的显著改善[162,163]。一项使用环孢素微乳剂和皮质类固醇的尸体供体肾移植受体的意大利试验也表明，霉酚酸酯与硫唑嘌呤相比没有益处[164,165]。虽然可能有争议，但由于这些试验的总结性证据，KDIGO临床实践指南建议霉酚酸盐可作为一线抗代谢药物[58]。

霉酚酸酯经常与剂量相关的上消化道和下消化道副作用有关。肠溶霉酚酸钠已被开发以通过促进在小肠中释放来帮助规避上消化道副作用[166]。两项大型临床试验表明，肠溶霉酚酸钠在治疗上与霉酚酸酯相当，两种药物的副作用发生率和严重程度相似[167,168]。当给予等量的霉酚酸酯或肠溶霉酚酸钠时，这些试验没有表现出总体胃肠道症状的统计学差异。上市后的研究试图探索两种霉酚酸制剂的胃肠道特征[169-181]。许多试验已证明肠溶霉酚酸钠的有利效果[169-177]，而其他人没有报道胃肠相关不良反应的差异[178-181]。在myTIME、Progris和myGAIN[171,180,181]研究中，通过自填胃肠道症状的量表问卷、胃肠道症状总体治疗效果(OTE)量表以及与健康相关的生活质量OTE量表问卷,患者报告转换为肠溶霉酚酸钠后自觉胃肠道症状改善。

胃肠道事件可能是多因素的(感染性病因,与胃瘫或其他伴随药物有关),肠溶霉酚酸钠可能对特定人群有益。如果患者由于胃肠道副作用而不耐受霉酚酸酯,则患者可能因换用肠溶霉酚酸钠而受益。此外,如果患者易患胃肠道疾病,则肠溶霉酚酸钠可能是患者更好的初始选择。然而,肠溶衣不太可能影响药物的全身效应,包括对肠上皮细胞增殖和病毒感染的影响,这可能是胃肠道副作用的原因。

药物相互作用也可以在同时使用质子泵抑制剂和霉酚酸酯时发生。研究表明,霉酚酸酯与泮托拉唑或奥美拉唑的组合可导致霉酚酸酯在胃中的溶解减少,导致生物利用度减少和系统性霉酚酸暴露降低。相比之下,霉酚酸的肠溶衣制剂可以通过胃的酸性环境,并在达到小肠的中性pH值环境后溶解[182]。

mTOR抑制剂

由钙调神经磷酸酶抑制剂、皮质类固醇和抗代谢物组成的治疗方案已经达到了良好的排斥反应发生率。尽管钙调磷酸酶抑制剂可显著降低急性排斥反应发生率,但其具有直接肾毒性,并可引起其他一些副作用。历史上,防止急性排斥反应是移植的主要任务。目前,慢性移植肾肾病是移植物丢失的最常见原因,且这已成为临床医生主要关心的问题。无钙调神经磷酸酶抑制剂方案是一种有吸引力的免疫抑制方案,可将长期移植物丢失的风险降至最低,同时维持低的急性排斥反应发生率。基于钙调磷酸酶抑制剂方案的替代方案是使用mTOR抑制剂。西罗莫司和依维莫司这两种药物已经被开发并获得FDA批准,以期实现这一目标。

西罗莫司可能在无钙调磷酸酶抑制剂的维持性治疗中具有良好的作用[183,184],但是在钙调磷酸酶抑制剂减量方案中仍需谨慎,因为肾毒性和排斥反应仍然需要关注。在Spare-the-Nephron试验中,将西罗莫司和霉酚酸酯的无钙调磷酸酶方案与环孢素和霉酚酸酯方案相比较。在2年的随访中,两组的肾功能没有不同[185]。ORION(优化肾移植免疫抑制以克服肾毒性),另一项钙调磷酸酶减量试验,由于在他克莫司撤除组的高急性排斥反应发生率而于最近被终止了。这项试验[186]包含3组共450例新移植患者的研究,比较了西罗莫司/霉酚酸酯/皮质类固醇方案、西罗莫司/他克莫司在第12周停用/皮质类固醇方案以及标准方案(包括他克莫司/霉酚酸酯/皮质类固醇)。本研究中所有患者均接受达利珠单抗诱导治疗。在2年后,患者生存率、移植物存活率以及肾小球滤过率在3组之间没有差异,并且与他克莫司组相比,含有西罗莫司的2组中尿蛋白肌酐比值显著升高。依维莫司也已在钙调磷酸酶减量方案中得到了研究。

在钙调磷酸酶减量方案中,有人对联合诱导治疗(巴利昔单抗,n=256)或不联合诱导治疗(n=237)下依维莫司1.5mg/d+皮质类固醇+低剂量环孢素以及依维莫司3mg/d+皮质类固醇+低剂量环孢素两种方式进行了比较[187]。在本研究中,使用诱导药物消除了对高剂量依维莫司的需求。在6个月时,无诱导组中应用依维莫司1.5mg/d和3mg/d的患者发生活检证实的急性排斥反应的比例分别为25%和15.2%,而在诱导组分别为13.7%和15.1%。计算的肾小球滤过率(62~67mL/min)和不良事件发生率在所有组中结果相似。

钙调磷酸酶抑制剂到西罗莫司的转换已获得有限的成功。CONVERT试验研究了830名接受环孢素或他克莫司治疗6~120个月的肾移植患者。参与者被随机分配至持续钙调磷酸酶抑制剂组(n=275)或从钙调磷酸酶抑制剂转换为西罗莫司组(n=555)[149]。仅在具有基线肾小球滤过率>40mL/min和尿蛋白肌酐比值≤0.11的亚组患者中观察到西罗莫司的成功。在经过筛选的患者中将钙调磷酸酶抑制剂早期撤除转换为基于依维莫司的免疫抑制方案可以改善肾功能,同时保持安全有效的结果。在随后的一项研究中,对平均肾小球滤过率高于60mL/min的患者,在移植后4~5月用依维莫司替代钙调磷酸酶抑制剂[188]。在这项欧洲多中心开放性研究(ZEUS)中,300例低、中危肾移植患者最初接受了巴利昔单抗诱导治疗以及环孢素、肠溶霉酚酸钠和皮质类固醇治疗。在12个月时,与环孢素方案相比,依维莫司方案显著改善了肾小球滤过率(平均差异+9.8mL/min)。在随机化后,依维莫司组的活检证实急性排斥反应发生率比环孢素组高(10%对3%),但在研究期结束时相似(15%对15%)。与环孢素方案相比,依维莫司方案具有更高的平均血脂浓度,尿蛋白排泄略有增加,血红蛋白浓度较低;血小板减少、阿弗他口腔炎和腹泻也在依维莫司组中更常见。

在最近一项试验中,依维莫司与环孢素和皮质类固醇联合应用，被用作霉酚酸酯的替代物(n=583)[189]。依维莫司(1.5mg/d 或 3mg/d)与霉酚酸酯一样有效，但不良事件有所增加。由于不良事件(溶血尿毒综合征、淋巴增殖性疾病、蛋白尿和血清肌酐水平升高)导致的治疗的停止在依维莫司组比在霉酚酸酯组更频繁。

总之，重新应用西罗莫司已被证明与钙调磷酸酶抑制剂效果相似，但它也与移植后早期不良事件有关，包括淋巴囊肿、延长的移植功能延迟恢复时间和伤口愈合不良[183,184]。同样地，重新应用依维莫司联合诱导治疗具有可接受的急性排斥反应发生率，但常会发生不良事件[187,189]。似乎，西罗莫司转换仅在基线肾小球滤过率>40mL/min 且尿蛋白肌酐比值≤0.11 的患者亚组中可成功应用[149]。同样，ZEUS 研究证明，在具有正常肾功能的低、中危患者中，依维莫司的转换是可能的，但这可能以较高的急性排斥反应发生率为代价。使用 mTOR 抑制剂的钙调磷酸酶撤除的最佳证据存在于已经选择的患者中。密切监测药物浓度水平和不良事件是有必要的。使用 mTOR 抑制剂的无钙调磷酸酶抑制剂方案或钙调磷酸酶减量方案的维持治疗是否长期有效仍然是未知的。因此，目前，KDIGO 临床实践指南建议钙调磷酸酶抑制剂应继续使用而不是撤除[58]。

贝拉西普

贝拉西普是第一个被证明肾获益优于基于钙调磷酸酶抑制剂方案的免疫抑制剂。它是第 2 代共刺激阻滞剂，在 2011 年 6 月获得 FDA 批准用于肾移植。在第 1 个偏盲、平行组的Ⅱ期研究中，对更高强度的贝拉西普、较低强度的贝拉西普和环孢素的给药方案进行了比较[190]。所有患者接受了巴利昔单抗、霉酚酸酯和皮质类固醇治疗(n=218)。在 6 个月时，每个组的急性排斥反应发生率和移植物失功率类似，而两个贝拉西普组中的肾小球滤过率在统计学上更高。贝拉西普组中较少出现慢性移植肾病、糖尿病、高血压和高脂血症。

随后，两项 3 年期Ⅲ期随机多中心研究，即贝拉西普肾脏保护和作为一线免疫保护试验功效评价(BENEFIT)和 BENEFIT 扩大标准供体(BENEFIT-EXT)，测试了贝拉西普在成年新肾移植患者中的功效和安全性[32,190,191]。在两项试验中，患者被随机分为 3 组：高强度的贝拉西普组，较低强度的贝拉西普组和环孢素联合巴利昔单抗、霉酚酸酯和皮质类固醇组。BENEFIT-EXT 的设计类似于 BENEFIT 试验，包括扩大标准的供体。在 BENEFIT 试验中，尽管贝拉西普组的急性排斥反应发生率较高，但在第 1 年结束时，贝拉西普组的肾功能更好(高强度组 65mL/min，低强度组 63mL/min，环孢素组 50mL/min)。相反，在 BENEFIT-EXT 试验中，急性排斥反应发生率相似，但高强度贝拉西普组患者的比低强度组更好(高强度组 18%，低强度组 18%，环孢素组 14%)[191]。这些试验的 3 年随访表明，肾功能在持续改善(在 BENEFIT 中的平均变化为+21mL/min，而在 BENEFIT-EXT 中为+10mL/min)[112]。由这些试验引发的一个主要问题是，在贝拉西普治疗的同时，EB 病毒血清学阴性受体组中的移植后淋巴增殖性疾病的高发病率。因此，该药物在 EB 病毒血清阴性的患者中是禁用的。

BENEFIT 和 BENEFIT-EXT 试验的一个局限是环孢素(一种不太现代的免疫抑制剂)在高剂量和浓度下的应用。最近，报道了一项包含一种更现代的免疫抑制方案的试验。在一项Ⅱ期 1 年随机研究中，比较了贝拉西普/霉酚酸酯、贝拉西普/西罗莫司和他克莫司/霉酚酸酯联合兔抗胸腺细胞球蛋白而不含皮质类固醇的 3 种组合(n=89)[192]。在贝拉西普/霉酚酸酯组中急性排斥反应发生率最高，在他克莫司/霉酚酸酯组中移植物失功率最低，同时贝拉西普组中的肾功能更好。

最近进行了一项转换试验，以验证基于贝拉西普的方案可能为基于钙调磷酸酶的维持性免疫抑制提供不同选择的假设。将移植后具有稳定肾功能(计算的肾小球滤过率≥35mL/min 和≤75mL/min)的超过 6 个月但不到 36 个月的患者随机分入转换贝拉西普组(n=84)或继续钙调磷酸酶抑制剂治疗组(n=89)[193]。在第 12 个月，贝拉西普组与钙调神经磷酸酶抑制剂组相比，从基线开始计算的肾小球滤过率的平均变化更大。贝拉西普组的 6 名患者发生了急性排斥反应，所有排斥反应均发生在转换后的 6 个月内;所有病例都得到解决而没有移植物失功。在第 24 个月，贝拉西普组的平均计算肾小球滤过率为 62.0mL/min，而钙调磷酸酶抑制剂组的平均计算肾小球滤过率为 55.4mL/min [194]。在贝拉西普组中计算的肾小球滤过率从基线开始的平均变化为+8.8mL/min，在钙调磷酸酶抑制剂组中为±0.3mL/min。从环孢素(+7.8mL/min)或他克莫司(+ 8.9mL/min)转换的患者中，不管其基线肾功能如何，都观察到了贝拉西普对肾脏的益处。患者生存率、移植物存活率和总体安全性在不同组之间相似。

贝拉西普是第一个显示出对肾小球滤过率的改善超过基于钙调磷酸酶抑制剂方案的免疫抑制剂。长期静脉给药和药物成本可能影响处方模式和患者依从性。贝拉西普的另一个特殊问题是它具有相对较长的半衰期,并且在严重感染的情况下不能中断。需要进一步的试验来探索其长期结果、EB病毒对移植后淋巴增殖性疾病的影响,以及贝拉西普对慢性移植肾病发展的影响。这些试验应包括更现代的免疫抑制方案。

总结

KDIGO临床实践指南建议联合应用免疫抑制药物作为维持性治疗,包括钙调磷酸酶抑制剂和抗增殖剂,联用或不用皮质类固醇[58]。他们建议他克莫司作为一线钙调磷酸抑制剂,霉酚酸酯作为一线抗增殖剂。在低免疫风险和接受诱导治疗的患者中,皮质类固醇可在移植后第1周停用。

胰腺移植受体的维持性治疗

在临床实践中,包含钙调磷酸酶抑制剂、霉酚酸和皮质类固醇的维持性免疫抑制方案是胰腺移植受体的优选方案。循证医学已经支持在过去15~20年从环孢素到他克莫司和从硫唑嘌呤到霉酚酸的过渡。一项多中心随机试验(n=205)已经证明他克莫司可减少急性排斥反应的发生率(中度至重度;他克莫司3%对环孢素28%),并具有更好的胰腺移植物存活率(89.2%对72.4%)[145,195]。同样,霉酚酸酯也显示可改善胰腺移植后的早期结果。在一项开放性随机多中心研究中,患者在移植后1年接受每日1.5g霉酚酸酯(n=74)或每日1~3mg/kg的硫唑嘌呤(n=76)[196]。在6个月时,生存率或排斥反应发生率之间没有差异,但是与硫唑嘌呤相比,接受霉酚酸酯治疗的患者出现排斥反应或治疗失败的时间明显更长。接受霉酚酸酯与硫唑嘌呤治疗的患者1年急性排斥反应发生率相似(分别为35%和47%)。

支持在胰腺移植中使用皮质类固醇撤除和mTOR抑制剂的证据较少。根据SRTR数据,38%的胰腺移植受体接受皮质类固醇撤除[1]。几项非随机研究[197-205]和一项随机单中心研究[206]调查了胰腺移植的受体的皮质类固醇撤除。在随机研究中,50例胰腺-肾脏同时移植的受体接受无皮质类固醇或在3个月时撤除皮质类固醇联合兔抗胸腺细胞球蛋白、环孢素和霉酚酸酯治疗。急性排斥反应发生率(两组都是4%)、患者生存率和移植物存活率相似,但是无皮质类固醇组1年随访后血清肌酐水平明显更高(1.50mg/dL对1.30mg/dL)。总之,早期激素撤除联合强效诱导剂、钙调磷酸酶抑制剂和霉酚酸可能在胰移植受体中是安全的,但需要长期随访。皮质类固醇撤除的代谢益处可能仅限于胰腺-肾脏同时移植的受体,因为在一项研究中肾移植受体术后胰腺并未改善血脂水平[207]。关于mTOR抑制剂在胰腺移植受体中的使用了解甚少。西罗莫司似乎能预防胰腺移植受体的排斥反应,但只有少数小型非随机研究已见报道[156,157,208-212]。

肺移植受体的维持性治疗

在过去的二三十年里,肺移植受体最常用的免疫抑制方案包括钙调磷酸酶抑制剂联合抗代谢物和皮质类固醇[1],特别是环孢素、硫唑嘌呤和泼尼松。支持在肺移植中使用他克莫司的证据较少,因此与其他移植器官相比,环孢素向他克莫司的转换被延迟了(图66.3)。目前,基于SRTR的统计,86%的初次肺移植受体在出院时应用他克莫司处方[1]。关于肺移植中他克莫司的许多试验受到单中心非随机设计的限制。大多数比较他克莫司与环孢素的研究表明,使用他克莫司治疗的患者100天内的急性排斥反应发生率较低[213-216],而有一项试验则未显示急性排斥反应发生率的差异[217]。类似地,许多肺移植中心没有从硫唑嘌呤转换成霉酚酸。基于目前的SRTR数据,55%的肺移植受体在移植时接受了霉酚酸,30%的肺移植受体接受了硫唑嘌呤[1],也许是因为已发表的文献表明霉酚酸酯可增加感染和胃肠道毒性的发生率[217-220]。两项非随机研究比较了硫唑嘌呤与霉酚酸酯分别联合环孢素和泼尼松的临床试验,结果表明霉酚酸酯治疗的患者排斥反应发生率降低[218,221],而随访1年时FEV_1的降低更少[218],而使用类似免疫抑制方案的试验显示急性排斥反应发生率没有差异[219,220]。此外,在一项研究中,术后3年时无闭塞性细支气管炎的患者数量没有差异(75%对73%)[220]。最后,几乎所有的肺移植受体都接受了皮质类固醇的维持性治疗[1]。一项使用强效诱导剂的小型非随机试验显示在肺移植受体中有可能避免应用皮质类固醇[222]。

西罗莫司不常用或未得到FDA批准用于肺移植,因为其在移植后早期的使用与几例致死性支气管吻合口裂开[139,140]及间质性肺炎[223,224]相关。相比之下，依维莫司在肺移植中的应用更加成功。在一项随机双盲试验中，213 名肺移植受体被分配接受依维莫司联合环孢素和皮质类固醇或硫唑嘌呤联合环孢素和皮质类固醇[225]。虽然依维莫司治疗显示第 1 年的急性排斥反应发作和 FEV_1 恶化均更少，但是 2 年后仅急性排斥反应的发生率仍然更低。不幸的是，依维莫司治疗可能会导致更严重的不良事件和血清肌酐水平升高。将肺移植受体(移植后大于 1 年)转换为依维莫司联合低剂量钙调磷酸酶抑制剂显示出肾脏获益 (+3.2mL/min 对-2.4mL/min)并维持到转换后 2 年[226]。

肝移植受体的维持性治疗

根据联合器官分配网络(UNOS)的注册数据，患者原位肝移植术后的 1 年和 5 年生存率分别为 88%和 74%，移植物存活率分别为 83%和 67%[1]。这些结果部分是由于免疫抑制剂的最新进展。对于肝移植受体，在移植时最常使用的方案是他克莫司+霉酚酸+皮质类固醇，但皮质类固醇撤除越来越常见[1]。虽然许多患者在移植时接受三联免疫抑制治疗，但是在移植初期过后，一些药物最终停用，常常只剩二联或单药治疗。

在初次接受肝移植患者的两项具有里程碑意义的随机多中心试验中(美国试验 n=529，欧洲试验 n=545)中，他克莫司治疗比环孢素的排斥反应发生率更低[227]。他克莫司与急性或难治性排斥反应显著减少相关，但实际上有更多的不良事件需要停药。这些研究使用 Sandimmune®，其吸收需要胆汁，而许多方案历史上在肝移植时需要使用胆汁引流管。然而，也已经报道了环孢素微乳剂(环孢素 USP 修饰，其吸收不依赖胆汁)取得类似结果。在一项英国和爱尔兰的包括 606 名肝移植受体的随机试验中，他克莫司治疗患者的主要结果(包括死亡、再移植或免疫原因导致的治疗失败的总体发生率)在统计学上较低(他克莫司 21%对环孢素微乳剂 32%)[228]。3 年随访的复合主要终点相似；然而，存活率或非再次移植不再具有统计学意义[229]。一项最近的 Meta 分析证实了这些发现[230]。结论是，用他克莫司代替环孢素治疗 100 名受体，可分别减少 9 例和 7 例排斥反应和耐皮质类固醇抵抗性排斥反应病例，可分别减少 5 例和 2 例移植物失功和死亡病例，但增加了 4 例肝移植后糖尿病病例[230]。

尽管霉酚酸与硫唑嘌呤作用类似，但它是更有效的免疫抑制剂，具有较少的副作用，包括较小的肝毒性，导致硫唑嘌呤在肝移植中的使用减少。霉酚酸酯也已经显示可降低肝移植受体急性排斥反应的发生率[231]。在一项随机双盲比较研究中，肝移植受体接受霉酚酸酯或硫唑嘌呤治疗，均联合环孢素和皮质类固醇[232]。术后 1 年急性排斥反应发生率(霉酚酸酯 68%对硫唑嘌呤 76%)和耐激素性排斥反应发生率(霉酚酸酯 19%对硫唑嘌呤 36%)在 6 个月时明显较低，而患者生存率和移植物存活率相似。

在不同肝移植方案之间，皮质类固醇的使用也有所不同。已经尝试在肝移植受体中使用无皮质类固醇或皮质类固醇撤除方案，以减少不良事件，并最小化后续的 HCV 复发[233,234]。3 项 Meta 分析结果表明，当皮质类固醇被其他药物取代时，急性排斥反应发生率降低[92,235,236]，而无皮质类固醇方案有利于降低胆固醇[92,235]、巨细胞病毒感染[92,235]、高血压病[92]和新发糖尿病[209,235]。

西罗莫司的术后副作用包括肝动脉血栓形成、伤口愈合延迟和切口疝，而长期使用与高脂血症、骨髓抑制、口腔溃疡、皮疹、白蛋白尿和肺炎有关。2002 年，FDA 警告移植界关于对肝移植受体使用西罗莫司的两项研究[237]。在一项关于初次肝移植受体的研究中，西罗莫司与额外的死亡和移植物失功相关(联合应用为 22%，单用他克莫司为 9%)。在这项研究和另一项研究中，重新应用西罗莫司与肝动脉血栓形成增加相关(联合应用为 7%，对照组为 2%)；大多数肝动脉血栓形成的病例发生在移植后 30 天内，导致移植物失功或死亡。2009 年 6 月，美国 FDA 发布了另一项基于一项未发表的研究的警告，发现在将基于钙调磷酸酶抑制剂的免疫抑制方案转换为西罗莫司后，稳定的肝移植患者的死亡率增加[237]。在本研究中，稳定的肝移植患者在移植后至少 6 个月，与继续使用基于钙调磷酸酶抑制剂方案的组相比，在转换为基于西罗莫司方案的组中观察到死亡数目的增加，但并无统计学意义 (3.8%对 1.4%)。这些警告导致西罗莫司在肝移植受体中的使用减少，但几个研究已经探索了其应用。在一项包括 11 项研究的系统性综述中发现，西罗莫司使用 1 年后，由于肾功能不全接受西罗莫司作为初始免疫抑制剂或由于肾毒性转换为西罗莫司的肝移植患者，肾小球滤过率有较小的非显著性增加(3.4mL/min)[238]。然而，西罗莫司使用与更高的感染率、皮疹、溃疡和停药相关。

依维莫司也在肝移植受体中进行了研究。在一些小型非随机研究中，肝移植患者由于肾功能不全转换为依维莫司，其肌酐水平和肾小球滤过率得到显著改善[239]。一项为期15个月的回顾性研究发现，在240例肝移植术后转换为依维莫司维持治疗的患者中，发现使用依维莫司患者的排斥反应发生率较低[239]。由于不良事件，47名患者(20%)中停用依维莫司，59名(25%)患者降低剂量。

心脏移植受体的维持性治疗

自1967年实施第1例心脏移植以来，免疫抑制已经发生显著改变。2000年以来，他克莫司的使用稳定增加[1]。目前，他克莫司是最广泛使用的钙调磷酸酶抑制剂(75%)，霉酚酸酯是主要的抗代谢药物(88%的患者)，而且西罗莫司和依维莫司的使用率仍然很低。大多数患者(89%)在移植后1年仍保持应用低剂量的糖皮质激素。

已经有多个关于在心脏移植后重新应用他克莫司和环孢素的单中心和多中心随机比较的报道[240,241]。这些试验显示了与他克莫司类似的患者生存率和更有利的副作用。在最大的试验中(n=314)，初次心脏移植受体被随机分配到他克莫司组或环孢素微乳剂组并分别与硫唑嘌呤、糖皮质激素和诱导治疗联用[240]。在6个月时，他克莫司组中度至重度急性细胞排斥反应的发生率较低(他克莫司组28%对环孢素组42%，P=0.013)，更少的高血压(66%对78%)和血脂异常(29%对40%)，以及更多的新发糖尿病(20%对11%)。

用霉酚酸酯取代硫唑嘌呤可以减少心脏移植后第1年的死亡率和排斥反应发生率。在一项双盲阳性对照试验中，除了环孢素和皮质类固醇外，28个中心将650例首次心脏移植受体随机分为接受霉酚酸酯(3000mg/d)组或硫唑嘌呤[1.5~3mg/(kg·d)]组，并分别联用环孢素和皮质类固醇。尽管入组患者的生存率和排斥反应发生率相似，但是治疗组患者在1年时死亡率显著降低(6.2%对11.4%)，并且排斥反应的治疗需求显著降低(65.7%对73.7%)。机会性感染，主要是单纯疱疹，在霉酚酸酯组中更常见(53.3%对43.6%)。肠溶霉酚酸钠和霉酚酸酯似乎是相似的，但在治疗期间需要减少剂量的肠溶霉酚酸钠患者明显更少[175,242]。

mTOR抑制剂通常用于患有心脏移植物血管病变(CAV)或肾功能不全的患者，因为它们对平滑肌增殖有抑制作用并且不存在固有的肾毒性[226,243]。不良反应的高发生率，包括下肢水肿和伤口愈合不良，可能会限制这些药物的普遍使用。

在两种可用的mTOR抑制剂中，依维莫司具有最多的证据支持在心脏移植中使用。在一项包括634名初次心脏移植受体的随机双盲试验中，将两种剂量的依维莫司(1.5mg/d和3.0mg/d)与硫唑嘌呤进行比较。所有患者均接受环孢素和皮质类固醇。在移植后6个月，相比硫唑嘌呤组，1.5mg依维莫司组(36%对47%)和3.0mg依维莫司组(27%对47%，P<0.001)中的患者达到主要功效复合终点（包括死亡、移植物失功或再移植、随访丧失、活检证实的中度至重度急性细胞排斥反应、具有血流动力学损伤的排斥反应)者明显更少。组间的功效差异几乎完全是由于依维莫司组中急性细胞排斥反应的发生率降低所致。在这项研究中，依维莫司治疗与硫唑嘌呤相比血清肌酐浓度显著增加，这可能是由于依维莫司对环孢素肾毒性的增强作用[244]。依维莫司对排斥反应发生率、移植物血管病变和肾功能的影响在24个月时持续[245]。

在Nordic Certican试验的心脏和肺移植亚组研究中，111例维持性治疗的心脏移植受体被随机分配到依维莫司+低剂量钙调磷酸酶抑制剂组或标准钙调磷酸酶抑制剂组[246]。在治疗组之间，CAV进展无显著差异。然而，其他免疫抑制治疗也是重要的，因为硫唑嘌呤+依维莫司治疗的患者表现出CAV进展减弱和炎症标记物下降，而相反的情况见于依维莫司+霉酚酸酯组。

术后早期，皮质类固醇在大多数心脏移植受体中以相对较高的剂量使用，然后逐渐减至低剂量或在移植第1年完全停止使用[247,248]。低风险患者可以较早(移植后1~2个月内）耐受皮质类固醇撤除而无长期不良后果[249,250]。一项澳大利亚的研究将112名患者随机分为兔抗胸腺细胞球蛋白诱导+环孢素+硫唑嘌呤+皮质类固醇组和兔抗胸腺细胞球蛋白诱导+环孢素+硫唑嘌呤组[251]。在皮质类固醇撤除组中，3个月的排斥反应发生率和经历耐皮质类固醇性排斥反应患者的数量更多。在皮质类固醇维持组中，3年时使用抗高血压药物和胆固醇水平较高的患者明显更多。值得注意的是，在皮质类固醇撤除组中，47%的患者在随访期间需要添加维持性皮质类固醇，这主要是由于排斥反应的发生率增加所致。

小肠移植受体的维持性治疗

由于肠的高免疫原性，小肠移植受体具有最高的排斥反应发生率和最低的移植物存活率。更新的免疫抑制药物在 20 世纪 90 年代中期以来的移植成功中发挥了重要作用。目前，大多数肠移植受体接受他克莫司和皮质类固醇作为维持性免疫抑制方案。每年进行的小肠移植不到 200 例，因此免疫抑制的临床试验数量很少[252]。

总结

在过去的 10~20 年，他克莫司和霉酚酸已成为免疫抑制治疗的基础。在等待免疫抑制药物进一步发展的同时，我们应该通过定制可用的诱导和维持性治疗方案来改善大多数移植物的功能寿命。为了保持免疫抑制治疗的有效性，我们需要将治疗方法从“一刀切”转变为定制或个体化策略。定制的免疫抑制治疗应防止免疫抑制不足（排斥反应）和免疫抑制过度（相关的感染和癌症）。因此，对移植患者持续的警惕性监测应该与对维持性免疫抑制治疗的改变以应对排斥反应或感染相结合。通过进一步研究这些复杂的方案所获得的信息应提供创新的策略和新的免疫抑制剂，以用于延长移植物的功能寿命而无毒性或感染。

（陈峻 译　徐骁 校）

参考文献

1. Organ Procurement and Transplantation Network (OPTN) and Scientific Registry of Transplant Recipients (SRTR). SRTR/OPTN 2010 Annual Data Report. Department of Health and Human Services, Health Resources and Services Administration, Healthcare Systems Bureau, Division of Transplantation. American Journal of Transplantation. 2012;12(Suppl. 1):1–156.
2. Sansone F, Rinaldi M. Cyclosporine monotherapy in cardiac transplantation: review of the literature. Transplantation Reviews (Orlando, Fla.). 2011;25:131–135.
3. Kamphues C, Bova R, Rocken C, et al. Safety of mycophenolate mofetil monotherapy in patients after liver transplantation. Annals of Transplantation. 2009;14:40–46.
4. Aydingoz SE, Takemoto SK, Pinsky BW, et al. The impact of human leukocyte antigen matching on transplant complications and immunosuppression dosage. Human Immunology. 2007;68:491–499.
5. Krishnan N, Buchanan PM, Dzebisashvili N, et al. Monozygotic transplantation: concerns and opportunities. American Journal of Transplantation. 2008;8:2343–2351.
6. Squifflet JP, Moudry K, Sutherland DE. Is HLA matching relevant in pancreas transplantation? A registry analysis. Transplant International. 1988;1:26–29.
7. Opelz G, Wujciak T, Dohler B, et al. HLA compatibility and organ transplant survival. Collaborative Transplant Study. Reviews in Immunogenetics. 1999;1:334–342.
8. Barama A, Oza U, Panek R, et al. Effect of recipient sensitization (peak PRA) on graft outcome in haploidentical living related kidney transplants. Clinical Transplantation. 2000;14:212–217.
9. Ilham MA, Winkler S, Coates E, et al. Clinical significance of a positive flow crossmatch on the outcomes of cadaveric renal transplants. Transplantation Proceedings. 2008;40:1839–1843.
10. Doxiadis II, Smits JM, Schreuder GM, et al. Association between specific HLA combinations and probability of kidney allograft loss: the taboo concept. Lancet. 1996;348:850–853.
11. Takemoto SK, Terasaki PI, Gjertson DW, et al. Twelve years' experience with national sharing of HLA-matched cadaveric kidneys for transplantation. New England Journal of Medicine. 2000;343:1078–1084.
12. Lan X, Zhang MM, Pu CL, et al. Impact of human leukocyte antigen mismatching on outcomes of liver transplantation: a meta-analysis. World Journal of Gastroenterology. 2010;16:3457–3464.
13. Brugiere O, Thabut G, Suberbielle C, et al. Relative impact of human leukocyte antigen mismatching and graft ischemic time after lung transplantation. Journal of Heart and Lung Transplantation. 2008;27:628–634.
14. van den Berg JW, Hepkema BG, Geertsma A, et al. Long-term outcome of lung transplantation is predicted by the number of HLA-DR mismatches. Transplantation. 2001;71:368–373.
15. Tenderich G, Zittermann A, Prohaska W, et al. No evidence for an improvement of long-term survival by HLA matching in heart transplant recipients. Transplantation Proceedings. 2007;39:1575–1579.
16. Sawitzki B, Schlickeiser S, Reinke P, et al. Pretransplant immune risk assessment. Current Opinion in Organ Transplantation. 2009;14:650–655.
17. Augustine JJ, Poggio ED, Heeger PS, et al. Preferential benefit of antibody induction therapy in kidney recipients with high pretransplant frequencies of donor-reactive interferon-gamma enzyme-linked immunosorbent spots. Transplantation. 2008;86:529–534.
18. Andree H, Nickel P, Nasiadko C, et al. Identification of dialysis patients with panel-reactive memory T cells before kidney transplantation using an allogeneic cell bank. Journal of the American Society of Nephrology. 2006;17:573–580.
19. Saini D, Ramachandran S, Nataraju A, et al. Activated effector and memory T cells contribute to circulating sCD30: potential marker for islet allograft rejection. American Journal of Transplantation. 2008;8:1798–1808.
20. Vaidya S, Partlow D, Barnes T, et al. Pretransplant soluble CD30 is a better predictor of posttransplant development of donor-specific antibodies and acute vascular rejection than panel reactive antibodies. Transplantation. 2006;82:1606–1609.
21. Platt RE, Wu KS, Poole K, et al. Soluble CD30 as a prognostic factor for outcome following renal transplantation. Journal of Clinical Pathology. 2009;62:662–663.
22. Ling X, Xiong J, Liang W, et al. Can immune cell function assay identify patients at risk of infection or rejection? A meta-analysis. Transplantation. 2012;93:737–743.
23. Pallardo Mateu LM, Sancho Calabuig A, Capdevila Plaza L, et al. Acute rejection and late renal transplant failure: risk factors and prognosis. Nephrology, Dialysis, Transplantation. 2004;19(Suppl. 3):iii38–iii42.
24. Mota A, Figueiredo A, Cunha MF, et al. Risk factors for acute rejection in 806 cyclosporine-treated renal transplants: a multivariate analysis. Transplantation Proceedings. 2003;35:1061–1063.
25. Boom H, Mallat MJ, de Fijter JW, et al. Delayed graft function influences renal function, but not survival. Kidney International. 2000;58:859–866.
26. Oien CM, Reisaeter AV, Leivestad T, et al. Living donor kidney transplantation: the effects of donor age and gender on short- and long-term outcomes. Transplantation. 2007;83:600–606.
27. Ojo AO, Wolfe RA, Held PJ, et al. Delayed graft function: risk factors and implications for renal allograft survival. Transplantation. 1997;63:968–974.
28. Cacciarelli T, Sumrani N, Delaney V, et al. The influence of delayed renal allograft function on long-term outcome in the cyclosporine era. Clinical Nephrology. 1993;39:335–339.
29. Stallone G, Di Paolo S, Schena A, et al. Addition of sirolimus to cyclosporine delays the recovery from delayed graft function but does not affect 1-year graft function. Journal of the American Society of Nephrology. 2004;15:228–233.
30. Castle SC. Clinical relevance of age-related immune dysfunction. Clinical Infectious Diseases. 2000;31:578–585.
31. Yung RL. Changes in immune function with age. Rheumatic Diseases Clinics of North America. 2000;26:455–473.

32. Larsen CP, Grinyo J, Medina-Pestana J, et al. Belatacept-based regimens versus a cyclosporine A-based regimen in kidney transplant recipients: 2-year results from the BENEFIT and BENEFIT-EXT studies. Transplantation. 2010;90:1528–1535.
33. Meier-Kriesche HU, Port FK, Ojo AO, et al. Effect of waiting time on renal transplant outcome. Kidney International. 2000;58:1311–1317.
34. Opelz G, Mickey MR, Terasaki PI. Influence of race on kidney transplant survival. Transplantation Proceedings. 1977;9:137–142.
35. Butkus DE, Meydrech EF, Raju SS. Racial differences in the survival of cadaveric renal allografts. Overriding effects of HLA matching and socioeconomic factors. New England Journal of Medicine. 1992;327:840–845.
36. Young CJ, Gaston RS. Renal transplantation in black Americans. New England Journal of Medicine. 2000;343:1545–1552.
37. Kasiske BL, Neylan JF 3rd, Riggio RR, et al. The effect of race on access and outcome in transplantation. New England Journal of Medicine. 1991;324:302–307.
38. Ojo AO, Port FK, Held PJ, et al. Inferior outcome of two-haplotype matched renal transplants in blacks: role of early rejection. Kidney International. 1995;48:1592–1599.
39. Neylan JF. Immunosuppressive therapy in high-risk transplant patients: dose-dependent efficacy of mycophenolate mofetil in African-American renal allograft recipients. U.S. Renal Transplant Mycophenolate Mofetil Study Group. Transplantation. 1997;64:1277–1282.
40. Valente JF, Hariharan S, Peddi VR, et al. Causes of renal allograft loss in black vs. white transplant recipients in the cyclosporine era. Clinical Transplantation. 1997;11:231–236.
41. Isaacs RB, Nock SL, Spencer CE, et al. Racial disparities in renal transplant outcomes. American Journal of Kidney Diseases. 1999;34:706–712.
42. Dawidson IJ, Coorpender L, Fisher D, et al. Impact of race on renal transplant outcome. Transplantation. 1990;49:63–67.
43. Koyama H, Cecka JM, Terasaki PI. Kidney transplants in black recipients. HLA matching and other factors affecting long-term graft survival. Transplantation. 1994;57:1064–1068.
44. Light JA, Kelly JL, Aquino A, et al. Improving renal transplant outcomes in African Americans with OKT3 induction therapy. Transplantation Proceedings. 1993;25:2436–2438.
45. Gaston RS, Hudson SL, Deierhoi MH, et al. Improved survival of primary cadaveric renal allografts in blacks with quadruple immunosuppression. Transplantation. 1992;53:103–109.
46. Neylan JF. Racial differences in renal transplantation after immunosuppression with tacrolimus versus cyclosporine. FK506 Kidney Transplant Study Group. Transplantation. 1998;65:515–523.
47. Vlaminck H, Maes B, Evers G, et al. Prospective study on late consequences of subclinical non-compliance with immunosuppressive therapy in renal transplant patients. American Journal of Transplantation. 2004;4:1509–1513.
48. Jarzembowski T, John E, Panaro F, et al. Impact of non-compliance on outcome after pediatric kidney transplantation: an analysis in racial subgroups. Pediatric Transplantation. 2004;8:367–371.
49. Yen EF, Hardinger K, Brennan DC, et al. Cost-effectiveness of extending Medicare coverage of immunosuppressive medications to the life of a kidney transplant. American Journal of Transplantation. 2004;4:1703–1708.
50. Butler JA, Roderick P, Mullee M, et al. Frequency and impact of nonadherence to immunosuppressants after renal transplantation: a systematic review. Transplantation. 2004;77:769–776.
51. Egli A, Kohli S, Dickenmann M, et al. Inhibition of polyomavirus BK-specific T-Cell responses by immunosuppressive drugs. Transplantation. 2009;88:1161–1168.
52. Bohl DL, Storch GA, Ryschkewitsch C, et al. Donor origin of BK virus in renal transplantation and role of HLA C7 in susceptibility to sustained BK viremia. American Journal of Transplantation. 2005;5:2213–2221.
53. Prince O, Savic S, Dickenmann M, et al. Risk factors for polyoma virus nephropathy. Nephrology, Dialysis, Transplantation. 2009;24:1024–1033.
54. Brennan DC, Agha I, Bohl DL, et al. Incidence of BK with tacrolimus versus cyclosporine and impact of preemptive immunosuppression reduction. American Journal of Transplantation. 2005;5:582–594.
55. Hirsch HH, Randhawa P. BK virus in solid organ transplant recipients. American Journal of Transplantation. 2009;9(Suppl. 4):S136–S146.
56. Bressollette-Bodin C, Coste-Burel M, Hourmant M, et al. A prospective longitudinal study of BK virus infection in 104 renal transplant recipients. American Journal of Transplantation. 2005;5:1926–1933.
57. Hirsch HH, Knowles W, Dickenmann M, et al. Prospective study of polyomavirus type BK replication and nephropathy in renal-transplant recipients. New England Journal of Medicine. 2002;347:488–496.
58. Kidney Disease: Improving Global Outcomes (KDIGO) Transplant Work Group. KDIGO clinical practice guideline for the care of kidney transplant recipients. American Journal of Transplantation. 2009;9(Suppl. 3):S1–S155.
59. Vasudev B, Hariharan S, Hussain SA, et al. BK virus nephritis: risk factors, timing, and outcome in renal transplant recipients. Kidney International. 2005;68:1834–1839.
60. Saad ER, Bresnahan BA, Cohen EP, et al. Successful treatment of BK viremia using reduction in immunosuppression without antiviral therapy. Transplantation. 2008;85:850–854.
61. Hardinger KL, Koch MJ, Bohl DJ, et al. BK-virus and the impact of pre-emptive immunosuppression reduction: 5-year results. American Journal of Transplantation. 2010;10:407–415.
62. Hirsch HH, Brennan DC, Drachenberg CB, et al. Polyomavirus-associated nephropathy in renal transplantation: interdisciplinary analyses and recommendations. Transplantation. 2005;79:1277–1286.
63. Wali RK, Drachenberg C, Hirsch HH, et al. BK virus-associated nephropathy in renal allograft recipients: rescue therapy by sirolimus-based immunosuppression. Transplantation. 2004;78:1069–1073.
64. Farasati NA, Shapiro R, Vats A, et al. Effect of leflunomide and cidofovir on replication of BK virus in an in vitro culture system. Transplantation. 2005;79:116–118.
65. Williams JW, Javaid B, Kadambi PV, et al. Leflunomide for polyomavirus type BK nephropathy. New England Journal of Medicine. 2005;352:1157–1158.
66. Johnston O, Jaswal D, Gill JS, et al. Treatment of polyomavirus infection in kidney transplant recipients: a systematic review. Transplantation. 2010;89:1057–1070.
67. Guasch A, Roy-Chaudhury P, Woodle ES, et al. Assessment of efficacy and safety of FK778 in comparison with standard care in renal transplant recipients with untreated BK nephropathy. Transplantation. 2010;90:891–897.
68. Dharnidharka VR, Cherikh WS, Neff R, et al. Retransplantation after BK virus nephropathy in prior kidney transplant: an OPTN database analysis. American Journal of Transplantation. 2010;10:1312–1315.
69. Fisher RA. Cytomegalovirus infection and disease in the new era of immunosuppression following solid organ transplantation. Transplant Infectious Disease. 2009;11:195–202.
70. De Keyzer K, Van Laecke S, Peeters P, et al. Human cytomegalovirus and kidney transplantation: a clinician's update. American Journal of Kidney Diseases. 2011;58:118–126.
71. Jamil B, Nicholls KM, Becker GJ, et al. Influence of anti-rejection therapy on the timing of cytomegalovirus disease and other infections in renal transplant recipients. Clinical Transplantation. 2000;14:14–18.
72. Humar A, Snydman D. Cytomegalovirus in solid organ transplant recipients. American Journal of Transplantation. 2009;9(Suppl. 4):S78–S86.
73. Kanter J, Pallardo L, Gavela E, et al. Cytomegalovirus infection renal transplant recipients: risk factors and outcome. Transplantation Proceedings. 2009;41:2156–2158.
74. Ekberg H, Tedesco-Silva H, Demirbas A, et al. Reduced exposure to calcineurin inhibitors in renal transplantation. New England Journal of Medicine. 2007;357:2562–2575.
75. Brennan DC, Legendre C, Patel D, et al. Cytomegalovirus incidence between everolimus versus mycophenolate in de novo renal transplants: pooled analysis of three clinical trials. American Journal of Transplantation. 2011;11:2453–2462.
76. Buchler M, Caillard S, Barbier S, et al. Sirolimus versus cyclosporine in kidney recipients receiving thymoglobulin, mycophenolate mofetil and a 6-month course of steroids. American Journal of Transplantation. 2007;7:2522–2531.
77. Vigano M, Dengler T, Mattei MF, et al. Lower incidence of cytomegalovirus infection with everolimus versus mycophenolate mofetil in de novo cardiac transplant recipients: a randomized, multicenter study. Transplant Infectious Disease. 2010;12:23–30.
78. San Juan R, Aguado JM, Lumbreras C, et al. Impact of current transplantation management on the development of cytomegalovirus disease after renal transplantation. Clinical Infectious Diseases. 2008;47:875–882.
79. Vanrenterghem Y, van Hooff JP, Squifflet JP, et al. Minimization of immunosuppressive therapy after renal transplantation: results of a randomized controlled trial. American Journal of Transplantation. 2005;5:87–95.
80. Ozaki KS, Camara NO, Nogueira E, et al. The use of sirolimus in ganciclovir-resistant cytomegalovirus infections in renal transplant recipients. Clinical Transplantation. 2007;21:675–680.
81. Kotton CN, Kumar D, Caliendo AM, et al. International consensus guidelines on the management of cytomegalovirus in solid organ transplantation. Transplantation. 2010;89:779–795.
82. Asberg A, Jardine AG, Bignamini AA, et al. Effects of the intensity of immunosuppressive therapy on outcome of treatment for CMV disease in organ transplant recipients. American Journal of Transplantation. 2010;10:1881–1888.
83. Thuluvath PJ, Guidinger MK, Fung JJ, et al. Liver transplantation in the United States, 1999-2008. American Journal of Transplantation. 2010;10:1003–1019.

84. Fabrizi F, Martin P, Dixit V, et al. Hepatitis C virus antibody status and survival after renal transplantation: meta-analysis of observational studies. American Journal of Transplantation. 2005;5:1452–1461.
85. Berenguer M. Hot topic in hepatitis C virus research: the type of immunosuppression does not matter. Liver Transplantation. 2011;17(Suppl. 3):S24–S28.
86. Watashi K, Hijikata M, Hosaka M, et al. Cyclosporin A suppresses replication of hepatitis C virus genome in cultured hepatocytes. Hepatology (Baltimore, Md.). 2003;38:1282–1288.
87. Fernandes F, Ansari IU, Striker R. Cyclosporine inhibits a direct interaction between cyclophilins and hepatitis C NS5A. PLoS ONE. 2010;5:e9815.
88. Gallay PA. Cyclophilin inhibitors. Clinics in Liver Disease. 2009;13:403–417.
89. Berenguer M, Royuela A, Zamora J. Immunosuppression with calcineurin inhibitors with respect to the outcome of HCV recurrence after liver transplantation: results of a meta-analysis. Liver Transplantation. 2007;13:21–29.
90. Berenguer M, Aguilera V, San Juan F, et al. Effect of calcineurin inhibitors in the outcome of liver transplantation in hepatitis C virus-positive recipients. Transplantation. 2010;90:1204–1209.
91. Vivarelli M, Burra P, La Barba G, et al. Influence of steroids on HCV recurrence after liver transplantation: a prospective study. Journal of Hepatology. 2007;47:793–798.
92. Segev DL, Sozio SM, Shin EJ, et al. Steroid avoidance in liver transplantation: meta-analysis and meta-regression of randomized trials. Liver Transplantation. 2008;14:512–525.
93. Stangl JR, Carroll KL, Illichmann M, et al. Effect of antimetabolite immunosuppressants on Flaviviridae, including hepatitis C virus. Transplantation. 2004;77:562–567.
94. Germani G, Pleguezuelo M, Villamil F, et al. Azathioprine in liver transplantation: a reevaluation of its use and a comparison with mycophenolate mofetil. American Journal of Transplantation. 2009;9:1725–1731.
95. Asthana S, Toso C, Meeberg G, et al. The impact of sirolimus on hepatitis C recurrence after liver transplantation. Canadian Journal of Gastroenterology. 2011;25:28–34.
96. McKenna GJ, Trotter JF, Klintmalm E, et al. Limiting hepatitis C virus progression in liver transplant recipients using sirolimus-based immunosuppression. American Journal of Transplantation. 2011;11:2379–2387.
97. Duhart BT Jr, Honaker MR, Shokouh-Amiri MH, et al. Retrospective evaluation of the risk of hepatitis B virus reactivation after transplantation. Transplant Infectious Disease. 2003;5:126–131.
98. Murray KF, Carithers RL Jr. AASLD practice guidelines: Evaluation of the patient for liver transplantation. Hepatology (Baltimore, Md.). 2005;41:1407–1432.
99. Tur-Kaspa R, Shaul Y, Moore DD, et al. The glucocorticoid receptor recognizes a specific nucleotide sequence in hepatitis B virus DNA causing increased activity of the HBV enhancer. Virology. 1988;167:630–633.
100. Ben-Ari Z, Zemel R, Tur-Kaspa R. The addition of mycophenolate mofetil for suppressing hepatitis B virus replication in liver recipients who developed lamivudine resistance–no beneficial effect. Transplantation. 2001;71:154–156.
101. Opelz G, Dohler B. Lymphomas after solid organ transplantation: a collaborative transplant study report. American Journal of Transplantation. 2004;4:222–230.
102. Stojanova J, Caillard S, Rousseau A, et al. Post-transplant lymphoproliferative disease (PTLD): pharmacological, virological and other determinants. Pharmacological Research. 2011;63:1–7.
103. Caillard S, Dharnidharka V, Agodoa L, et al. Posttransplant lymphoproliferative disorders after renal transplantation in the United States in era of modern immunosuppression. Transplantation. 2005;80:1233–1243.
104. van Leeuwen MT, Grulich AE, Webster AC, et al. Immunosuppression and other risk factors for early and late non-Hodgkin lymphoma after kidney transplantation. Blood. 2009;114:630–637.
105. Bustami RT, Ojo AO, Wolfe RA, et al. Immunosuppression and the risk of posttransplant malignancy among cadaveric first kidney transplant recipients. American Journal of Transplantation. 2004;4:87–93.
106. Vegso G, Sebestyen A, Paku S, et al. Antiproliferative and apoptotic effects of mycophenolic acid in human B-cell non-Hodgkin lymphomas. Leukemia Research. 2007;31:1003–1008.
107. Funch DP, Ko HH, Travasso J, et al. Posttransplant lymphoproliferative disorder among renal transplant patients in relation to the use of mycophenolate mofetil. Transplantation. 2005;80:1174–1180.
108. Robson R, Cecka JM, Opelz G, et al. Prospective registry-based observational cohort study of the long-term risk of malignancies in renal transplant patients treated with mycophenolate mofetil. American Journal of Transplantation. 2005;5:2954–2960.
109. Kauffman HM, Cherikh WS, Cheng Y, et al. Maintenance immunosuppression with target-of-rapamycin inhibitors is associated with a reduced incidence of de novo malignancies. Transplantation. 2005;80:883–889.
110. Majewski M, Korecka M, Kossev P, et al. The immunosuppressive macrolide RAD inhibits growth of human Epstein-Barr virus-transformed B lymphocytes in vitro and in vivo: a potential approach to prevention and treatment of posttransplant lymphoproliferative disorders. Proceedings of the National Academy of Sciences of the United States of America. 2000;97:4285–4290.
111. Vincenti F, Larsen CP, Alberu J, et al. Three-year outcomes from BENEFIT, a randomized, active-controlled, parallel-group study in adult kidney transplant recipients. American Journal of Transplantation. 2012;12:210–217.
112. Pestana JO, Grinyo JM, Vanrenterghem Y, et al. Three-year outcomes from BENEFIT-EXT: a phase III study of belatacept versus cyclosporine in recipients of extended criteria donor kidneys. American Journal of Transplantation. 2012;12:630–639.
113. Parker A, Bowles K, Bradley JA, et al. Management of post-transplant lymphoproliferative disorder in adult solid organ transplant recipients—BCSH and BTS guidelines. British Journal of Haematology. 2010;149:693–705.
114. Pascual J. Post-transplant lymphoproliferative disorder–the potential of proliferation signal inhibitors. Nephrology, Dialysis, Transplantation. 2007;22(Suppl. 1):i27–i35.
115. Nourse JP, Jones K, Gandhi MK. Epstein-Barr Virus-related post-transplant lymphoproliferative disorders: pathogenetic insights for targeted therapy. American Journal of Transplantation. 2011;11:888–895.
116. Engels EA, Pfeiffer RM, Fraumeni JF Jr, et al. Spectrum of cancer risk among US solid organ transplant recipients. JAMA. 2011;306:1891–1901.
117. Caforio AL, Fortina AB, Piaserico S, et al. Skin cancer in heart transplant recipients: risk factor analysis and relevance of immunosuppressive therapy. Circulation. 2000;102(Suppl. 3):III222–III227.
118. Rama I, Grinyo JM. Malignancy after renal transplantation: the role of immunosuppression. Nature Reviews. Nephrology. 2010;6:511–519.
119. Vajdic CM, van Leeuwen MT. Cancer incidence and risk factors after solid organ transplantation. International Journal of Cancer. 2009;125:1747–1754.
120. Guba M, Graeb C, Jauch KW, et al. Pro- and anti-cancer effects of immunosuppressive agents used in organ transplantation. Transplantation. 2004;77:1777–1782.
121. Maluccio M, Sharma V, Lagman M, et al. Tacrolimus enhances transforming growth factor-beta1 expression and promotes tumor progression. Transplantation. 2003;76:597–602.
122. Dantal J, Hourmant M, Cantarovich D, et al. Effect of long-term immunosuppression in kidney-graft recipients on cancer incidence: randomised comparison of two cyclosporin regimens. Lancet. 1998;351:623–628.
123. Buell JF, Gross TG, Woodle ES. Malignancy after transplantation. Transplantation. 2005;80(2 Suppl.):S254–S264.
124. van Leeuwen MT, Grulich AE, McDonald SP, et al. Immunosuppression and other risk factors for lip cancer after kidney transplantation. Cancer Epidemiology, Biomarkers and Prevention. 2009;18:561–569.
125. Perrett CM, Walker SL, O'Donovan P, et al. Azathioprine treatment photosensitizes human skin to ultraviolet A radiation. British Journal of Dermatology. 2008;159:198–204.
126. Andrassy J, Graeb C, Rentsch M, et al. mTOR inhibition and its effect on cancer in transplantation. Transplantation. 2005;80(1 Suppl.):S171–S174.
127. Campistol JM, Eris J, Oberbauer R, et al. Sirolimus therapy after early cyclosporine withdrawal reduces the risk for cancer in adult renal transplantation. Journal of the American Society of Nephrology. 2006;17:581–589.
128. Alberu J, Pascoe MD, Campistol JM, et al. Lower malignancy rates in renal allograft recipients converted to sirolimus-based, calcineurin inhibitor-free immunotherapy: 24-month results from the CONVERT trial. Transplantation. 2011;92:303–310.
129. Euvrard S, Kanitakis J, Claudy A. Skin cancers after organ transplantation. New England Journal of Medicine. 2003;348:1681–1691.
130. Campistol JM, Gutierrez-Dalmau A, Torregrosa JV. Conversion to sirolimus: a successful treatment for posttransplantation Kaposi's sarcoma. Transplantation. 2004;77:760–762.
131. Stallone G, Schena A, Infante B, et al. Sirolimus for Kaposi's sarcoma in renal-transplant recipients. New England Journal of Medicine. 2005;352:1317–1323.
132. Cortazar F, Molnar MZ, Isakova T, et al. Clinical outcomes in kidney transplant recipients receiving long-term therapy with inhibitors of the mammalian target of rapamycin. American Journal of Transplantation. 2012;12:379–387.
133. Foxwell BM, Mackie A, Ling V, et al. Identification of the multidrug resistance-related P-glycoprotein as a cyclosporine binding protein. Molecular Pharmacology. 1989;36:543–546.
134. Kahan BD. Fifty years in the vineyard of transplantation: looking back. Transplantation Proceedings. 2011;43:2853–2859.
135. Johnson CP, Simmons RL, Sutherland DE, et al. A randomized trial comparing cyclosporine with antilymphoblast-globulin-azathioprine for renal allograft recipients. Results at 2 1/2-6 years. Transplantation. 1988;45:380–385.
136. Woodle ES, First MR, Pirsch J, et al. A prospective, randomized, double-blind, placebo-controlled multicenter trial comparing early (7 day) corticosteroid cessation versus long-term, low-dose corticosteroid therapy. Annals of Surgery.

2008;248:564–577.
137. Sabbatini M, Sansone G, Uccello F, et al. Acute effects of rapamycin on glomerular dynamics: a micropuncture study in the rat. Transplantation. 2000;69: 1946–1990.
138. Burdese M, Rossetti M, Guarena C, et al. Sirolimus and ACE-inhibitors: a note of caution. Transplantation. 2005;79:251–252.
139. Groetzner J, Kur F, Spelsberg F, et al. Airway anastomosis complications in de novo lung transplantation with sirolimus-based immunosuppression. Journal of Heart and Lung Transplantation. 2004;23:632–638.
140. King-Biggs MB, Dunitz JM, Park SJ, et al. Airway anastomotic dehiscence associated with use of sirolimus immediately after lung transplantation. Transplantation. 2003;75:1437–1443.
141. Massoud O, Wiesner RH. The use of sirolimus should be restricted in liver transplantation. Journal of Hepatology. 2012;56:288–290.
142. Vincenti F, Friman S, Scheuermann E, et al. Results of an international, randomized trial comparing glucose metabolism disorders and outcome with cyclosporine versus tacrolimus. American Journal of Transplantation. 2007;7: 1506–1514.
143. Gruessner RW, Burke GW, Stratta R, et al. A multicenter analysis of the first experience with FK506 for induction and rescue therapy after pancreas transplantation. Transplantation. 1996;61:261–273.
144. Jordan ML, Shapiro R, Gritsch HA, et al. Long-term results of pancreas transplantation under tacrolius immunosuppression. Transplantation. 1999;67: 266–272.
145. Saudek F, Malaise J, Boucek P, et al. Efficacy and safety of tacrolimus compared with cyclosporin microemulsion in primary SPK transplantation: 3-year results of the Euro-SPK 001 trial. Nephrology, Dialysis, Transplantation. 2005; 20(Suppl. 2):ii3–ii10, ii62.
146. Dieterle CD, Schmauss S, Veitenhansl M, et al. Glucose metabolism after pancreas transplantation: cyclosporine versus tacrolimus. Transplantation. 2004; 77:1561–1565.
147. Maes BD, Kuypers D, Messiaen T, et al. Posttransplantation diabetes mellitus in FK-506-treated renal transplant recipients: analysis of incidence and risk factors. Transplantation. 2001;72:1655–1661.
148. Snanoudj R, Royal V, Elie C, et al. Specificity of histological markers of long-term CNI nephrotoxicity in kidney-transplant recipients under low-dose cyclosporine therapy. American Journal of Transplantation. 2011;11:2635–2646.
149. Schena FP, Pascoe MD, Alberu J, et al. Conversion from calcineurin inhibitors to sirolimus maintenance therapy in renal allograft recipients: 24-month efficacy and safety results from the CONVERT trial. Transplantation. 2009;87:233–242.
150. Miller B, Brennan DC Withdrawal of Immunosuppression after Renal Transplant, 2012 (accessed Jan. 2014). Available from: http://www.uptodate.com.
151. Johnson C, Ahsan N, Gonwa T, et al. Randomized trial of tacrolimus (Prograf) in combination with azathioprine or mycophenolate mofetil versus cyclosporine (Neoral) with mycophenolate mofetil after cadaveric kidney transplantation. Transplantation. 2000;69:834–841.
152. Margreiter R. Efficacy and safety of tacrolimus compared with ciclosporin microemulsion in renal transplantation: a randomised multicentre study. Lancet. 2002;359:741–746.
153. Gonwa T, Johnson C, Ahsan N, et al. Randomized trial of tacrolimus + mycophenolate mofetil or azathioprine versus cyclosporine + mycophenolate mofetil after cadaveric kidney transplantation: results at three years. Transplantation. 2003;75:2048–2053.
154. Webster AC, Woodroffe RC, Taylor RS, et al. Tacrolimus versus ciclosporin as primary immunosuppression for kidney transplant recipients: meta-analysis and meta-regression of randomised trial data. BMJ (Clinical Research Ed.). 2005;331:810.
155. Knight SR, Morris PJ. Steroid avoidance or withdrawal after renal transplantation increases the risk of acute rejection but decreases cardiovascular risk. A meta-analysis. Transplantation. 2010;89:1–14.
156. Knight RJ, Kerman RH, McKissick E, et al. Selective corticosteroid and calcineurin-inhibitor withdrawal after pancreas-kidney transplantation utilizing thymoglobulin induction and sirolimus maintenance therapy. Clinical Transplantation. 2008;22:645–650.
157. Knight RJ, Podder H, Kerman RH, et al. Comparing an early corticosteroid/late calcineurin-free immunosuppression protocol to a sirolimus-, cyclosporine A-, and prednisone-based regimen for pancreas-kidney transplantation. Transplantation. 2010;89:727–732.
158. Schold JD, Santos A, Rehman S, et al. The success of continued steroid avoidance after kidney transplantation in the US. American Journal of Transplantation. 2009;9:2768–2776.
159. Boardman RE, Alloway RR, Alexander JW, et al. African-American renal transplant recipients benefit from early corticosteroid withdrawal under modern immunosuppression. American Journal of Transplantation. 2005;5:356–365.
160. Hricik DE, Augustine JJ, Knauss TC, et al. Long-term graft outcomes after steroid withdrawal in African American kidney transplant recipients receiving sirolimus and tacrolimus. Transplantation. 2007;83:277–281.
161. Halloran P, Mathew T, Tomlanovich S, et al. Mycophenolate mofetil in renal allograft recipients: a pooled efficacy analysis of three randomized, double-blind, clinical studies in prevention of rejection. The International Mycophenolate Mofetil Renal Transplant Study Groups. Transplantation. 1997;63:39–47.
162. Mathew TH. A blinded, long-term, randomized multicenter study of mycophenolate mofetil in cadaveric renal transplantation: results at three years. Tricontinental Mycophenolate Mofetil Renal Transplantation Study Group. Transplantation. 1998;65:1450–1454.
163. Miller J, Mendez R, Pirsch JD, et al. Safety and efficacy of tacrolimus in combination with mycophenolate mofetil (MMF) in cadaveric renal transplant recipients. FK506/MMF Dose-Ranging Kidney Transplant Study Group. Transplantation. 2000;69:875–880.
164. Remuzzi G, Lesti M, Gotti E, et al. Mycophenolate mofetil versus azathioprine for prevention of acute rejection in renal transplantation (MYSS): a randomised trial. Lancet. 2004;364:503–512.
165. Remuzzi G, Cravedi P, Costantini M, et al. Mycophenolate mofetil versus azathioprine for prevention of chronic allograft dysfunction in renal transplantation: the MYSS follow-up randomized, controlled clinical trial. Journal of the American Society of Nephrology. 2007;18:1973–1985.
166. Bjarnason I. Enteric coating of mycophenolate sodium: a rational approach to limit topical gastrointestinal lesions and extend the therapeutic index of mycophenolate. Transplantation Proceedings. 2001;33:3238–3240.
167. Budde K, Curtis J, Knoll G, et al. Enteric-coated mycophenolate sodium can be safely administered in maintenance renal transplant patients: results of a 1-year study. American Journal of Transplantation. 2004;4:237–243.
168. Salvadori M, Holzer H, de Mattos A, et al. Enteric-coated mycophenolate sodium is therapeutically equivalent to mycophenolate mofetil in de novo renal transplant patients. American Journal of Transplantation. 2004;4: 231–236.
169. Chan L, Mulgaonkar S, Walker R, et al. Patient-reported gastrointestinal symptom burden and health-related quality of life following conversion from mycophenolate mofetil to enteric-coated mycophenolate sodium. Transplantation. 2006; 81:1290–1297.
170. Darji P, Vijayaraghavan R, Thiagarajan CM, et al. Conversion from mycophenolate mofetil to enteric-coated mycophenolate sodium in renal transplant recipients with gastrointestinal tract disorders. Transplantation Proceedings. 2008;40:2262–2267.
171. Bolin P, Tanriover B, Zibari GB, et al. Improvement in 3-month patient-reported gastrointestinal symptoms after conversion from mycophenolate mofetil to enteric-coated mycophenolate sodium in renal transplant patients. Transplantation. 2007;84:1443–1451.
172. Pelletier RP, Soule J, Henry ML, et al. Clinical outcomes of renal transplant recipients treated with enteric-coated mycophenolic acid vs. mycophenolate mofetil as a switch agent using a primary steroid-free rapamune and microemulsion cyclosporine protocol. Clinical Transplantation. 2007;21:532–535.
173. Hardinger KL, Hebbar S, Bloomer T, et al. Adverse drug reaction driven immunosuppressive drug manipulations: a single-center comparison of enteric-coated mycophenolate sodium vs. mycophenolate mofetil. Clinical Transplantation. 2008;22:555–561.
174. Gozdowska J, Urbanowicz A, Baczkowska T, et al. Safety and tolerance of sodium mycophenolate in patients after renal transplantation–an observational study. Transplantation Proceedings. 2009;41:3016–3018.
175. Kobashigawa JA, Renlund DG, Gerosa G, et al. Similar efficacy and safety of enteric-coated mycophenolate sodium (EC-MPS, myfortic) compared with mycophenolate mofetil (MMF) in de novo heart transplant recipients: results of a 12-month, single-blind, randomized, parallel-group, multicenter study. Journal of Heart and Lung Transplantation. 2006;25:935–941.
176. Burg M, Saemann MD, Wieser C, et al. Enteric-coated mycophenolate sodium reduces gastrointestinal symptoms in renal transplant patients. Transplantation Proceedings. 2009;41:4159–4164.
177. Sollinger HW, Sundberg AK, Leverson G, et al. Mycophenolate mofetil versus enteric-coated mycophenolate sodium: a large, single-center comparison of dose adjustments and outcomes in kidney transplant recipients. Transplantation. 2010;89:446–451.
178. Kamar N, Oufroukhi L, Faure P, et al. Questionnaire-based evaluation of gastrointestinal disorders in de novo renal-transplant patients receiving either mycophenolate mofetil or enteric-coated mycophenolate sodium. Nephrology, Dialysis, Transplantation. 2005;20:2231–2236.
179. Minz M, Sharma A, Heer M. Comparison of enteric-coated mycophenolate sodium with mycophenolate mofetil in living renal allograft transplantation. Transplantation Proceedings. 2006;38:2041–2043.
180. Chang HR, Lin CC, Lian JD. Early experience with enteric-coated mycophenolate sodium in de novo kidney transplant recipients. Transplantation Proceedings.

2005;37:2066–2068.
181. Langone AJ, Chan L, Bolin P, et al. Enteric-coated mycophenolate sodium versus mycophenolate mofetil in renal transplant recipients experiencing gastrointestinal intolerance: a multicenter, double-blind, randomized study. Transplantation. 2011;91:470–478.
182. Kofler S, Wolf C, Shvets N, et al. The proton pump inhibitor pantoprazole and its interaction with enteric-coated mycophenolate sodium in transplant recipients. Journal of Heart and Lung Transplantation. 2011;30:565–571.
183. MacDonald AS. A worldwide, phase III, randomized, controlled, safety and efficacy study of a sirolimus/cyclosporine regimen for prevention of acute rejection in recipients of primary mismatched renal allografts. Transplantation. 2001; 71:271–280.
184. Kahan BD. Efficacy of sirolimus compared with azathioprine for reduction of acute renal allograft rejection: a randomised multicentre study. The Rapamune US Study Group. Lancet. 2000;356:194–202.
185. Weir MR, Mulgaonkar S, Chan L, et al. Mycophenolate mofetil-based immunosuppression with sirolimus in renal transplantation: a randomized, controlled Spare-the-Nephron trial. Kidney International. 2011;79:897–907.
186. Flechner SM, Glyda M, Cockfield S, et al. The ORION study: comparison of two sirolimus-based regimens versus tacrolimus and mycophenolate mofetil in renal allograft recipients. American Journal of Transplantation. 2011;11:1633–1644.
187. Vitko S, Tedesco H, Eris J, et al. Everolimus with optimized cyclosporine dosing in renal transplant recipients: 6-month safety and efficacy results of two randomized studies. American Journal of Transplantation. 2004;4:626–635.
188. Budde K, Becker T, Arns W, et al. Everolimus-based, calcineurin-inhibitor-free regimen in recipients of de-novo kidney transplants: an open-label, randomised, controlled trial. Lancet. 2011;377:837–847.
189. Lorber MI, Mulgaonkar S, Butt KM, et al. Everolimus versus mycophenolate mofetil in the prevention of rejection in de novo renal transplant recipients: a 3-year randomized, multicenter, phase III study. Transplantation. 2005;80: 244–252.
190. Vincenti F, Charpentier B, Vanrenterghem Y, et al. A phase III study of belatacept-based immunosuppression regimens versus cyclosporine in renal transplant recipients (BENEFIT study). American Journal of Transplantation. 2010;10: 535–546.
191. Durrbach A, Pestana JM, Pearson T, et al. A phase III study of belatacept versus cyclosporine in kidney transplants from extended criteria donors (BENEFIT-EXT study). American Journal of Transplantation. 2010;10: 547–557.
192. Ferguson R, Grinyo J, Vincenti F, et al. Immunosuppression with belatacept-based, corticosteroid-avoiding regimens in de novo kidney transplant recipients. American Journal of Transplantation. 2011;11:66–76.
193. Rostaing L, Massari P, Garcia VD, et al. Switching from calcineurin inhibitor-based regimens to a belatacept-based regimen in renal transplant recipients: a randomized phase II study. Clinical Journal of the American Society of Nephrology. 2011;6:430–439.
194. Vincenti F, Blancho G, Durrbach A, et al. Five-year safety and efficacy of belatacept in renal transplantation. Journal of the American Society of Nephrology. 2010;21:1587–1596.
195. Bechstein WO, Malaise J, Saudek F, et al. Efficacy and safety of tacrolimus compared with cyclosporine microemulsion in primary simultaneous pancreas-kidney transplantation: 1-year results of a large multicenter trial. Transplantation. 2004;77:1221–1228.
196. Merion RM, Henry ML, Melzer JS, et al. Randomized, prospective trial of mycophenolate mofetil versus azathioprine for prevention of acute renal allograft rejection after simultaneous kidney-pancreas transplantation. Transplantation. 2000;70:105–111.
197. Thai NL, Khan A, Tom K, et al. Alemtuzumab induction and tacrolimus monotherapy in pancreas transplantation: one- and two-year outcomes. Transplantation. 2006;82:1621–1624.
198. Kaufman DB, Leventhal JR, Koffron AJ, et al. A prospective study of rapid corticosteroid elimination in simultaneous pancreas-kidney transplantation: comparison of two maintenance immunosuppression protocols: tacrolimus/mycophenolate mofetil versus tacrolimus/sirolimus. Transplantation. 2002;73: 169–177.
199. Muthusamy AS, Vaidya AC, Sinha S, et al. Alemtuzumab induction and steroid-free maintenance immunosuppression in pancreas transplantation. American Journal of Transplantation. 2008;8:2126–2131.
200. Axelrod D, Leventhal JR, Gallon LG, et al. Reduction of CMV disease with steroid-free immunosuppresssion in simultaneous pancreas-kidney transplant recipients. American Journal of Transplantation. 2005;5:1423–1429.
201. Gruessner RW, Sutherland DE, Parr E, et al. A prospective, randomized, open-label study of steroid withdrawal in pancreas transplantation-a preliminary report with 6-month follow-up. Transplantation Proceedings. 2001;33: 1663–1664.
202. Tanchanco R, Krishnamurthi V, Winans C, et al. Beneficial outcomes of a steroid-free regimen with thymoglobulin induction in pancreas-kidney transplantation. Transplantation Proceedings. 2008;40:1551–1554.
203. Kaufman DB, Leventhal JR, Gallon LG, et al. Alemtuzumab induction and prednisone-free maintenance immunotherapy in simultaneous pancreas-kidney transplantation comparison with rabbit antithymocyte globulin induction - long-term results. American Journal of Transplantation. 2006;6:331–339.
204. Aoun M, Eschewege P, Hamoudi Y, et al. Very early steroid withdrawal in simultaneous pancreas-kidney transplants. Nephrology, Dialysis, Transplantation. 2007;22:899–905.
205. Malheiro J, Martins L, Fonseca I, et al. Steroid withdrawal in simultaneous pancreas-kidney transplantation: a 7-year report. Transplantation Proceedings. 2009;41:909–912.
206. Cantarovich D, Karam G, Hourmant M, et al. Steroid avoidance versus steroid withdrawal after simultaneous pancreas-kidney transplantation. American Journal of Transplantation. 2005;5:1332–1338.
207. Gruessner RW, Kandaswamy R, Humar A, et al. Calcineurin inhibitor- and steroid-free immunosuppression in pancreas-kidney and solitary pancreas transplantation. Transplantation. 2005;79:1184–1189.
208. Gallon LG, Winoto J, Chhabra D, et al. Long-term renal transplant function in recipient of simultaneous kidney and pancreas transplant maintained with two prednisone-free maintenance immunosuppressive combinations: tacrolimus/mycophenolate mofetil versus tacrolimus/sirolimus. Transplantation. 2007;83: 1324–1329.
209. Knight RJ, Kerman RH, Zela S, et al. Pancreas transplantation utilizing thymoglobulin, sirolimus, and cyclosporine. Transplantation. 2006;81:1101–1105.
210. Girman P, Lipar K, Koznarova R, et al. Similar early complication rate in simultaneous pancreas and kidney recipients on tacrolimus/mycophenolate mofetil versus tacrolimus/sirolimus immunosuppressive regimens. Transplantation Proceedings. 2010;42:1999–2002.
211. Laham G, Sleiman S, Soler Pujol G, et al. Conversion to sirolimus allows preservation of renal function in kidney and kidney-pancreas allograft recipients. Transplantation Proceedings. 2010;42:309–313.
212. Matias P, Araujo MR, Romao JE Jr, et al. Conversion to sirolimus in kidney-pancreas and pancreas transplantation. Transplantation Proceedings. 2008;40:3601–3605.
213. Treede H, Klepetko W, Reichenspurner H, et al. Tacrolimus versus cyclosporine after lung transplantation: a prospective, open, randomized two-center trial comparing two different immunosuppressive protocols. Journal of Heart and Lung Transplantation. 2001;20:511–517.
214. Griffith BP, Bando K, Hardesty RL, et al. A prospective randomized trial of FK506 versus cyclosporine after human pulmonary transplantation. Transplantation. 1994;57:848–851.
215. Keenan RJ, Konishi H, Kawai A, et al. Clinical trial of tacrolimus versus cyclosporine in lung transplantation. Annals of Thoracic Surgery. 1995;60:580–584; discussion 4–5.
216. Hachem RR, Yusen RD, Chakinala MM, et al. A randomized controlled trial of tacrolimus versus cyclosporine after lung transplantation. Journal of Heart and Lung Transplantation. 2007;26:1012–1018.
217. Zuckermann A, Reichenspurner H, Birsan T, et al. Cyclosporine A versus tacrolimus in combination with mycophenolate mofetil and steroids as primary immunosuppression after lung transplantation: one-year results of a 2-center prospective randomized trial. Journal of Thoracic and Cardiovascular Surgery. 2003;125:891–900.
218. Ross DJ, Waters PF, Levine M, et al. Mycophenolate mofetil versus azathioprine immunosuppressive regimens after lung transplantation: preliminary experience. Journal of Heart and Lung Transplantation. 1998;17:768–774.
219. Palmer SM, Baz MA, Sanders L, et al. Results of a randomized, prospective, multicenter trial of mycophenolate mofetil versus azathioprine in the prevention of acute lung allograft rejection. Transplantation. 2001;71:1772–1776.
220. McNeil K, Glanville AR, Wahlers T, et al. Comparison of mycophenolate mofetil and azathioprine for prevention of bronchiolitis obliterans syndrome in de novo lung transplant recipients. Transplantation. 2006;81:998–1003.
221. Zuckermann A, Klepetko W, Birsan T, et al. Comparison between mycophenolate mofetil- and azathioprine-based immunosuppressions in clinical lung transplantation. Journal of Heart and Lung Transplantation. 1999;18:432–440.
222. McCurry KR, Iacono A, Zeevi A, et al. Early outcomes in human lung transplantation with Thymoglobulin or Campath-1H for recipient pretreatment followed by posttransplant tacrolimus near-monotherapy. Journal of Thoracic and Cardiovascular Surgery. 2005;130:528–537.
223. Morelon E, Stern M, Israel-Biet D, et al. Characteristics of sirolimus-associated interstitial pneumonitis in renal transplant patients. Transplantation. 2001;72: 787–790.
224. Lennon A, Finan K, FitzGerald MX, et al. Interstitial pneumonitis associated with

sirolimus (rapamycin) therapy after liver transplantation. Transplantation. 2001;72:1166–1167.
225. Snell GI, Valentine VG, Vitulo P, et al. Everolimus versus azathioprine in maintenance lung transplant recipients: an international, randomized, double-blind clinical trial. American Journal of Transplantation. 2006;6:169–177.
226. Gullestad L, Mortensen SA, Eiskjaer H, et al. Two-year outcomes in thoracic transplant recipients after conversion to everolimus with reduced calcineurin inhibitor within a multicenter, open-label, randomized trial. Transplantation. 2010;90:1581–1589.
227. Collins RH. Tacrolimus (FK506) versus cyclosporin in prevention of liver allograft rejection. Lancet. 1994;344:949.
228. O'Grady JG, Burroughs A, Hardy P, et al. Tacrolimus versus microemulsified ciclosporin in liver transplantation: the TMC randomised controlled trial. Lancet. 2002;360:1119–1125.
229. O'Grady JG, Hardy P, Burroughs AK, et al. Randomized controlled trial of tacrolimus versus microemulsified cyclosporin (TMC) in liver transplantation: poststudy surveillance to 3 years. American Journal of Transplantation. 2007; 7:137–141.
230. McAlister VC, Haddad E, Renouf E, et al. Cyclosporin versus tacrolimus as primary immunosuppressant after liver transplantation: a meta-analysis. American Journal of Transplantation. 2006;6:1578–1585.
231. Wiesner RH. A long-term comparison of tacrolimus (FK506) versus cyclosporine in liver transplantation: a report of the United States FK506 Study Group. Transplantation. 1998;66:493–499.
232. Wiesner R, Rabkin J, Klintmalm G, et al. A randomized double-blind comparative study of mycophenolate mofetil and azathioprine in combination with cyclosporine and corticosteroids in primary liver transplant recipients. Liver Transplantation. 2001;7:442–450.
233. Tisone G, Angelico M, Palmieri G, et al. A pilot study on the safety and effectiveness of immunosuppression without prednisone after liver transplantation. Transplantation. 1999;67:1308–1313.
234. Washburn K, Speeg KV, Esterl R, et al. Steroid elimination 24 hours after liver transplantation using daclizumab, tacrolimus, and mycophenolate mofetil. Transplantation. 2001;72:1675–1679.
235. Sgourakis G, Radtke A, Fouzas I, et al. Corticosteroid-free immunosuppression in liver transplantation: a meta-analysis and meta-regression of outcomes. Transplant International. 2009;22:892–905.
236. Knight SR, Morris PJ. Steroid sparing protocols following nonrenal transplants; the evidence is not there. A systematic review and meta-analysis. Transplant International. 2011;24:1198–1207.
237. US Food and Drug Administration. Information for Healthcare Professionals: Sirolimus (marketed as Rapamune). 2009 Accessed Jan., 2014. Available from: http://www.fda.gov/Drugs/DrugSafety/PostmarketDrugSafetyInformationforPatientsandProviders/DrugSafetyInformationforHeathcareProfessionals/ucm165015.htm.
238. Asrani SK, Leise MD, West CP, et al. Use of sirolimus in liver transplant recipients with renal insufficiency: a systematic review and meta-analysis. Hepatology (Baltimore, Md.). 2010;52:1360–1370.
239. Saliba F, Dharancy S, Lorho R, et al. Conversion to everolimus in maintenance liver transplant patients: a multicenter, retrospective analysis. Liver Transplantation. 2011;17:905–913.
240. Grimm M, Rinaldi M, Yonan NA, et al. Superior prevention of acute rejection by tacrolimus vs. cyclosporine in heart transplant recipients–a large European trial. American Journal of Transplantation. 2006;6:1387–1397.
241. Kobashigawa JA, Miller LW, Russell SD, et al. Tacrolimus with mycophenolate mofetil (MMF) or sirolimus vs. cyclosporine with MMF in cardiac transplant patients: 1-year report. American Journal of Transplantation. 2006;6: 1377–1386.
242. Lehmkuhl H, Hummel M, Kobashigawa J, et al. Enteric-coated mycophenolate-sodium in heart transplantation: efficacy, safety, and pharmacokinetic compared with mycophenolate mofetil. Transplantation Proceedings. 2008;40: 953–955.
243. Topilsky Y, Hasin T, Raichlin E, et al. Sirolimus as primary immunosuppression attenuates allograft vasculopathy with improved late survival and decreased cardiac events after cardiac transplantation. Circulation. 2012; 125:708–720.
244. Eisen HJ, Tuzcu EM, Dorent R, et al. Everolimus for the prevention of allograft rejection and vasculopathy in cardiac-transplant recipients. New England Journal of Medicine. 2003;349:847–858.
245. Vigano M, Tuzcu M, Benza R, et al. Prevention of acute rejection and allograft vasculopathy by everolimus in cardiac transplants recipients: a 24-month analysis. Journal of Heart and Lung Transplantation. 2007;26:584–592.
246. Arora S, Ueland T, Wennerblom B, et al. Effect of everolimus introduction on cardiac allograft vasculopathy–results of a randomized, multicenter trial. Transplantation. 2011;92:235–243.
247. Miller LW, Wolford T, McBride LR, et al. Successful withdrawal of corticosteroids in heart transplantation. Journal of Heart and Lung Transplantation. 1992; 11:431–434.
248. Teuteberg JJ, Shullo M, Zomak R, et al. Aggressive steroid weaning after cardiac transplantation is possible without the additional risk of significant rejection. Clinical Transplantation. 2008;22:730–737.
249. Taylor DO, Bristow MR, O'Connell JB, et al. Improved long-term survival after heart transplantation predicted by successful early withdrawal from maintenance corticosteroid therapy. Journal of Heart and Lung Transplantation. 1996; 15:1039–1046.
250. Renlund DG, O'Connell JB, Gilbert EM, et al. Feasibility of discontinuation of corticosteroid maintenance therapy in heart transplantation. Journal of Heart Transplantation. 1987;6:71–78.
251. Keogh A, Macdonald P, Mundy J, et al. Five-year follow-up of a randomized double-drug versus triple-drug therapy immunosuppressive trial after heart transplantation. Journal of Heart and Lung Transplantation. 1992;11:550–555.
252. Pirenne J, Kawai M. Intestinal transplantation: evolution in immunosuppression protocols. Current Opinion in Organ Transplantation. 2009;14: 250–255.

第 67 章
免疫抑制的挽救治疗

Mark D. Stegall, Patrick G. Dean

引言

“挽救治疗”在本文中定义为任何用于解决导致急性或慢性同种异体移植物损伤的特异性同种异体介导的移植后过程的治疗性干预。它具有足够的效力来逆转出现的急性过程，但是被禁止用于长时间免疫抑制耐受。经典的挽救治疗是临床上显著的急性细胞排斥反应(ACR)治疗。历史上，早期 ACR 的管理是移植治疗的中心问题之一。更有效的免疫抑制方案的发展已经大大地解决了这个曾经不可克服的问题；然而，其管理仍然重要，我们将在下面讨论这个问题。

在过去的 10 年中，急性抗体介导的排斥反应(AMR)在急性同种异体移植物损伤中的作用已经越来越受到重视。通过供体特异性同种异体抗体(DSA)介导，AMR 可以与 ACR 同时发生或以更纯粹的形式发生，特别是在致敏受体中。下面详细讨论这些临床情况的管理方法。

随着早期移植后管理的改进，长期同种异体移植物丢失已经成为移植受体面临的主要问题。事实上，肾移植术后 1 年以上的移植物丢失率几十年来都保持相对恒定[1]。我们已提出，改善长期同种异体移植物存活的路径是详细的患者随访以确定晚期肾同种异体移植物丢失的具体原因，以及设计发展用于在同种异体移植物损伤变得不可逆之前解决这些问题的新疗法[2]。我们将讨论临床情况，包括遇到的慢性同种异体移植损伤，并解决亚临床炎症和慢性损伤，特别是在挽救治疗的背景下。

关于排斥反应的临床诊断和治疗的器官特异性指南在第 69~76 章中讨论，同时定义器官各种形式排斥反应的组织病理学标准将在第 81~87 章中详细描述。本章将概述器官特异性治疗的共同原则，并在大体上为读者适当介绍排斥反应的治疗。

在开始讨论这些主题之前，重要的是要注意，大多数数据没有达到Ⅰ级有效性证据，最广泛使用的做法仅基于Ⅲ级证据[3]。这对于慢性损伤尤其如此，其中对于主要机制(其中可能有许多机制)仍然存在争议，并且对其可能指示什么治疗没有共识。

急性肾同种异体移植物功能障碍

虽然急性同种异体移植物功能障碍的定义不是标准化的，但是良好的工作定义可能与用于其他形式的急性肾损伤的定义类似：肾功能的突然(在 48 小时内)降低 [目前定义为血清肌酐的绝对值增加≥0.3mg/dL(≥26.4mmol/L)]，血清肌酐从基线增加≥50%，或尿量减少[记录的少尿少于 0.5mL/(kg·h)超过 6 小时][4]。移植后早期急性肾同种异体移植物功能障碍的鉴别诊断是广泛的，并且与原发性肾脏的急性肾损伤类似，包括肾前、肾内和肾后病因(表 67.1)。本章的大部分将集中于移植物功能障碍的免疫原因；然而，移植实施者也应该熟悉并能够识别非免疫原因。

具有急性同种异体移植物功能障碍移植受体的评估应包括以下内容：详细的病史和体格检查以评估血压和容受状态；尿分析(特别注意蛋白尿或肾炎性沉积物的存在)和尿培养，如果检测到脓尿，测量血浆神经钙调蛋白抑制剂(CNI)浓度(接受 CNI 的患者)；测量血浆多瘤病毒拷贝数；用于检测肾动脉狭窄、尿渗漏、淋巴细胞或尿道梗阻的同种异体移植物超声；通过单抗原珠测定来测量血清同种抗体水平；并且如果怀疑膀胱功能障碍或出口阻塞，放置导尿管。如果从上述干预中没有鉴定到同种异体移植物功能障碍的确定性原因，则应进行肾同种异体移植活检。该活检应进行常规光学显微镜检查以及 IgG、IgA、IgM、C3、白蛋白和纤维

表 67.1 急性和慢性同种异体移植肾功能障碍或损伤的鉴别诊断

急性同种异体移植肾功能障碍或损伤
肾前因素
移植肾血栓形成
移植肾动脉粥样硬化栓子形成
血容量不足
低血压
肾性因素
急性细胞排斥反应
急性抗体介导(体液)排斥反应
原发肾脏疾病复发
多瘤病毒肾病
急性钙调磷酸酶抑制剂毒性反应
移植肾肾盂肾炎
移植后淋巴组织增生性疾病
肾后因素
输尿管梗阻
膀胱功能障碍
膀胱出口梗阻
慢性同种异体移植肾功能障碍或损伤
慢性抗体介导排斥反应
慢性细胞炎症
原发肾脏疾病复发
慢性药物毒性反应(如钙调磷酸酶抑制剂)
多瘤病毒肾病

蛋白的免疫荧光检查。如果怀疑多瘤病毒肾病或移植后淋巴增殖性疾病,应行免疫过氧化物酶研究。如果怀疑是新生的或复发性肾小球疾病,应用电子显微镜检测。肾同种异体移植物活检目前根据肾脏同种异体移植物病变的 Banff'07 分类进行分级和评分,这是一种基于共识的诊断系统,将在第 81 章中详细讨论[5]。

急性细胞排斥反应

急性细胞排斥反应发作可以分为临床或亚临床,这取决于发作时是否伴随同种异体移植物功能障碍。本部分将重点介绍支持临床急性细胞排斥反应治疗的明显证据,亚临床炎症将在本章的后面进行讨论。

在临床肾移植的前 30 年,多达 80%的受体发现有 ACR,并且是早期同种异体移植物功能障碍的常见原因[6]。此外,ACR 的单发作预示同种异体移植物的长期存活[7-10]。最近,移植后 6 个月内 ACR 的发生率从 1995 年的大约 40%显著降低到小于 15%,但是这种降低没有使移植物的长期存活率显著增加,表明早期 ACR 和长期结局之间的联系可能没有以前提议的那么紧密[1,11]。与以前的报道[12,13]相似,这些登记数据的分析表明,如果在 ACR 治疗后达到完全功能恢复,似乎对长期结果没有不良影响。然而,那些受体的移植物功能(由 Cockroft-Gault 估计)在 ACR 治疗后没有恢复到基线 75%以内的,与功能恢复到基线的相比,6 年移植物损失的风险增加了 5 倍[10]。虽然 ACR 发生的频率比以前少,影响也更小,这并不意味着 ACR 是良性的,而是它的识别和及时治疗已经成为移植中心的常规实践。事实上,在减轻 ACR 的影响中所实现的进展强调了在诊断时及时和适当地治疗 ACR 的重要性。以下各部分将讨论治疗 ACR 最常用的两种药物(类固醇和针对淋巴细胞的抗体)的应用理由和证据。讨论将以肾脏为中心的角度进行,因为在历史上,ACR 的管理最初是在肾移植中建立的,而目前由于其他器官的移植越来越普遍,ACR 的管理也在很大程度上适应了其他器官。本章末尾将介绍器官移植的特定注意事项。

类固醇治疗

从早期的临床移植开始,皮质类固醇已被用作 ACR 的维持治疗和辅助治疗[14,15]。部分是由于这些年肾移植领域的快速发展以及未治疗已发 ACR 的严重影响,尚未进行比较使用类固醇治疗 ACR 和不治疗 ACR 的随机试验。因此,关于这些药物治疗 ACR 的有效性的共识仅仅来自Ⅲ级数据。然而,这种"基于经验"的方法确实使人们广泛使用类固醇来治疗 ACR,这种做法持续到今天。对于临床上明显的、活检证实的 ACR 治疗,多数当前的治疗方案要求对有临界改变、活检分数为 Banff 1A 或 Banff 1B 的受体使用大剂量甲泼尼龙治疗(图 67.1)。应当注意,使用糖皮质激素而不是盐皮质激素治疗排斥反应,因为它们可以发挥实质性和广泛的免疫抑制作用。甲泼尼龙的理想剂量尚未建立,并且因移植中心不同而存在较大差异,从每剂 100mg 至 1000mg(或至多 15mg/kg)不等,持续时间也有从 3 天至几周的变化,有或没有剂量逐渐减少。持续时间和强度通常随组织病理学等级而变化,但还没有支持特异性变异的数据。

耐激素性排斥反应定义为临床上对类固醇治疗无反应,但其精确的定义有很大不同。大多数试验需要使

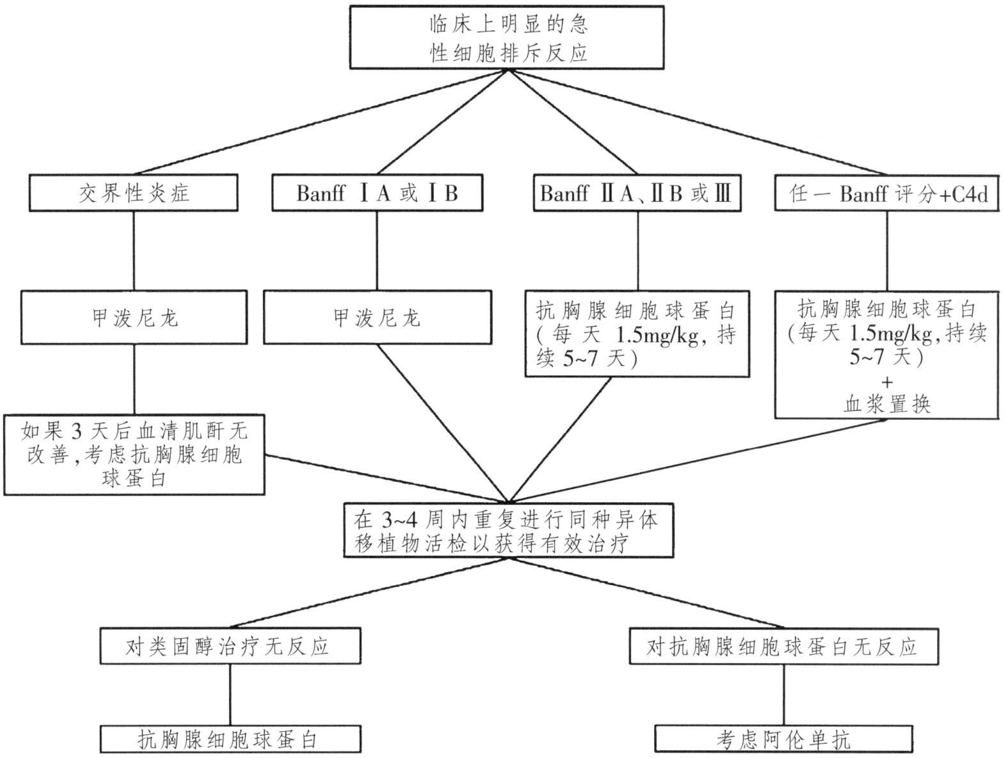

图 67.1 临床可见的急性细胞介导肾同种异体移植排斥的诊疗方案。

用整整 3 天的大剂量甲泼尼龙，且没有符合这一定义的临床改善。

抗淋巴细胞治疗

与使用皮质类固醇治疗 ACR 相反，使用针对淋巴细胞的单克隆抗体和多克隆抗体制剂的治疗已经进行了随机临床试验(Ⅰ级证据)。这些试验检查了几种不同抗体制剂的作用[16-36]，并报道了在小鼠、兔子或马中产生的多种抗淋巴细胞制剂对 ACR 的第一次发作或在耐激素性 ACR 治疗中的作用。这 21 项试验（包括 1394 名参与者）的性质、结果和局限性已在 Cochrane 综述中详细描述[37]。数据的总和表明抗体治疗在逆转第一次排斥反应时优于类固醇治疗，并且没有一种抗体制剂在逆转耐激素性排斥反应方面在统计学上更有效。

虽然令人鼓舞的是看到这些试验已经进行，但是其中许多试验仍有一些局限性，在解释结果时无法让读者信服。这些缺陷在上述 Cochrane 综述中得到了很好的描述[37]，但主要涉及用于诊断排斥反应的标准，以及定义排斥反应发作的“逆转”。在大多数研究中，主要基于临床、实验室和影像标准来诊断排斥反应，而不需要同种异体移植物活检。没有一项研究是重复活检以验证炎症过程得到缓解，并确定显示排斥反应逆转。最后，没有一项研究检查了这些药物在接受更多现代免疫抑制治疗的患者队列中的作用（例如他克莫司和霉酚酸酯±类固醇±诱导治疗）。因此，这些药物在当前免疫抑制时代中治疗 ACR 的真正疗效可以从先前结果推断，但是目前尚不清楚。这些限制说明，如果免疫抑制剂对排斥发作和长期结果的真正影响是有效的，则需要精心设计的临床试验，包括严格的入选标准、仔细定义的终点和全面随访（包括重复同种异体移植物活检）来确定。然而，鉴于这些注意事项，我们的方法是使用抗淋巴细胞球蛋白[特别是抗胸腺细胞球蛋白(Thymoglobulin®，Genzyme，Cambridge，MA)] 来治疗临床上明显的 Banff ⅡA、Banff ⅡB 或 Banff Ⅲ级急性排斥反应，或与具有“混合”急性细胞和急性抗体介导排斥反应受体的血浆交换相结合(图 67.1)。与使用类固醇一样，抗体制剂作为一线治疗的使用、在耐激素性排斥反应中的使用以及治疗的持续时间，在很大程度上仍然是中心特异性的。这些政策由效力和成本考虑驱动，要知道抗体制剂通常是昂贵的。

急性抗体介导的排斥反应

在过去的10年中,同种异体抗体在急性肾同种异体移植物损伤中的作用越来越受到重视。根据Banff分类的急性AMR的诊断标准是:①在血清中检测到DSA;②管周毛细血管C4d染色;③急性组织损伤的形态学证据,包括肾小球微血栓、肾小球膜炎、肾小球炎和(或)涉及嗜中性粒细胞、巨噬细胞和淋巴细胞的毛细血管炎[38]。再次,急性移植物功能障碍有临床与亚临床形式的区别。双层肾小球基底膜(移植肾病)的存在表明更多的慢性病变(见下文)。早期AMR可以与急性细胞排斥反应(联合ACR和AMR)的特征相关联或者可以单独发生("纯"AMR)。虽然同种异体抗体的重新发展可能是T细胞依赖性的,并因此意味着在某一水平的T细胞活化,但是由于未知原因,这不总是在同种异体移植物中显示。T细胞在致敏患者抗体应答中的作用也不清楚。

纯抗体介导的排斥反应

在移植前具有高水平DSA的肾移植受体中,足以引起阳性交叉匹配(+XMKTx;关于DSA检测的完整讨论参见第36章),前3个月临床AMR报告的发病率很高,为10%~43%[39]。在许多这样的情况下,AMR是"纯"的形式,并且不涉及急性细胞排斥反应的组织学特征。假定存在DSA、典型的活检结果和常见的严重移植物功能障碍,AMR的诊断相对容易。根据梅奥诊所的经验,我们使用血浆置换(PE)和PE后低剂量(100mg/kg)静脉注射免疫球蛋白(IVIG)脱敏;在+XMKTx后急性AMR的平均时间为10天,并且所有发作均在移植后3个月内发生[40]。这项研究表明,早期AMR的发生率与AMR时存在的DSA水平相关,而不是基线DSA水平。因此,高水平DSA(持续性DSA或"记忆"反应)的患者会发展为AMR,而移植后DSA保持低水平的患者通常不会发生AMR。在这种情况下,AMR的发生是相当快的,并且如果不积极治疗,可能导致移植物丢失。关于脱敏步骤的完整讨论参见第68章。

令人惊讶的是,急性AMR通常是可接受治疗的,并且在实际的AMR发作期间使用当前治疗几乎没有移植物丢失。因为大多数临床可用的免疫抑制药物靶向T细胞,所以它们在治疗AMR中无效。目前,急性AMR的治疗包括被认为影响抗体水平的方法(PE、IVIG、硼替佐米和利妥昔单抗)和(或)通过阻断末端补体激活(依库珠单抗或皮质类固醇)来改善同种异体移植物损伤的药剂。我们会在下面讨论这些治疗,并应认识到挽救治疗这一领域可能会继续迅速发展。此外,作为研究终点的AMR逆转有时难以评估。以下讨论的研究超出了FDA批准的药物适应证的范围,并且被称为"标签外"使用。其使用得到了新出现数据的支持,这些数据受到受试者人数少、非随机设计和多种治疗方式联合应用的限制,使我们难以单独评估任何一种药剂的影响。关于移植中标签外药物使用的深入讨论参见第101章。

AMR治疗的主要方法是多重PE治疗联合低剂量IVIG或高剂量(1~2g/kg)IVIG单独应用(表67.2)。在更严重的情况下,例如具有DSA增加和频繁血浆交换仍无法解决的严重移植物功能障碍,可使用脾切除术进行解决[41]。一些报告中建议应用利妥昔单抗[42]。Cedars-Sinai集团报道了使用高剂量IVIG作为主要治疗和保留PE用于抗性发作的两级方案[43]。在超过90%的病例中,基于PE和高剂量IVIG的方案似乎都能解决AMR[40]。最近的一项回顾性分析表明,用PE、低剂量IVIG和利妥昔单抗联合治疗急性AMR优于高剂量IVIG,因为DSA水平在3个月时较低,36个月时的移植物存活率较高(91.7%对50%,P=0.02)[44]。

使用依库珠单抗的末端补体抑制已经显示能够减轻抗体介导的损伤,甚至在移植后DSA水平非常高时

表67.2 急性抗体介导排斥反应的治疗选择

影响抗体水平的药物
血浆置换
大剂量IVIG
硼替佐米
利妥昔单抗
改善移植物损害的药物
依库丽单抗(末端补体封闭)
皮质类固醇
针对顽固性或严重抗体介导排斥反应行脾切除术

* 目前梅奥诊所用于急性抗体介导排斥反应(AMR)的方案包括应用依库丽单抗和皮质类固醇来改善持续的损伤,以及应用血浆交换和低剂量IVIG来降低供体特异性同种抗体水平。当DSA水平非常高时(例如B流式细胞术交叉匹配通道转换>400或单抗原粒上的平均荧光指数>10 000),加入硼替佐米(1.5mg/kg×4剂)。

也有效[45]。依库珠单抗也已被用于治疗 AMR[46]。在早期严重 AMR 发作期间使用依库珠单抗的优点是其可以显著阻断进行中的补体激活,并可减轻进一步的损伤。缺点是,由于它是人源化单克隆抗体,它将在 PE 期间与同种异体抗体一起被去除,并且在每次 PE 治疗后需要被替换。尽管用依库珠单抗治疗仍然可以发生急性 AMR,这表明存在 C5 独立的 AMR 机制,但这些对 PE 的反应良好[45]。我们目前治疗急性 AMR 的方案包括依库珠单抗(每剂 600mg)和大剂量皮质类固醇联合每日 PE 和低剂量 IVIG。虽然没有关于这种治疗的控制研究,但该方案确实提供了移植保护的结合,同时初始治疗是为了降低 DSA 水平。

蛋白酶体抑制剂硼替佐米也已经用于治疗急性 AMR,主要与 PE 结合[47-50]。使用硼替佐米的理由是其可能在体外[47]和体内[50]从骨髓中消耗抗体分泌细胞。它可能对新激活的淋巴细胞有额外的影响。硼替佐米的一个可能的缺点是其生物利用度较低,可能需要多个剂量才能产生疗效。硼替佐米单药治疗在急性 AMR 中的研究是罕见的，其对治疗 AMR 的贡献仍不清楚。Walsh 等报道了 87%的早期 AMR 患者对硼替佐米、利妥昔单抗和 PE 的联合治疗有反应[51]。

联合的急性细胞排斥反应和抗体介导的排斥反应

在移植时具有负交叉匹配的常规肾移植中，最常见的 AMR 形式是与 ACR 联合发生[48]。与在+ XMKTx 中观察到的急性纯 AMR 相反,这种 AMR 和 ACR 的组合倾向于在移植后数月至数年发生，并且与非依从性药物治疗相关。

鉴于其在晚期出现，这种形式的 ACR 和 AMR 通常在已经患有慢性损伤的移植物中见到。治疗应该解决免疫过程中的细胞和体液组分。因此,应当给予大剂量皮质类固醇和（或）抗 T 细胞抗体以治疗 T 细胞组分。PE 和(或)硼替佐米以治疗体液组分。PE 和(或)硼替佐米的持续时间没有明确定义，但是已发表的报告使用了一个 4 剂量硼替佐米“周期”[48]。无论采用何种治疗，移植后晚期联合 ACR 和 AMR 的长期预后似乎相当差，超过一半的移植物在治疗后 4 年内发展成慢性损伤或移植物丢失。

亚临床炎症和慢性损伤

上述讨论集中在与显示细胞和(或)体液同种异体反应性特征的活检相关的早期移植物功能障碍的临床情况。有关这些实体管理的数据正在出现,并且其结果至少在一定程度上通过移植物功能的急性改善而得到改进。在活检中发现的亚临床炎症,虽然不明显表现为移植功能障碍,但仍令人不安。

然而,在过去 10 年中已经清楚的是,移植中主要未解决的问题是慢性同种异体移植物丢失，并且提出了是否可以应用挽救疗法来预防慢性损伤的想法。针对这个问题的建议需要引入两个重要问题：①如何定义或诊断慢性损伤;②慢性炎症(通常在功能良好的器官中早期存在,例如亚临床炎症)在病因学上与慢性损伤和移植物退化的相关程度。虽然对慢性损伤的发病机制进行详细讨论超出了本章的范围，但是为了理解未来在该临床情况下可能采取挽救疗法的理论基础,需要对其进行简要总结。

通常从功能或组织学角度定义慢性损伤。功能定义通常涉及代表同种异体移植物慢性损伤的某些肌酸酐或肾小球滤过率(GFR)。由于同种异体移植物功能广泛,因此在以前功能良好的同种异体移植物中,肾功能的下降也可能是一个有用的指标。有趣的是,很少有研究通过功能下降来研究慢性损伤。目前最常见的是通过组织学定义慢性损伤。一般来说,功能不良伴随间质性纤维化是慢性损伤的可接受定义[52]。慢性抗体介导的损伤通常由移植肾小球病变的存在来定义[53]。

在移植的早期应注意到 ACR 和间质纤维化之间的关联。然而,Rush 等人明确提出亚临床排斥反应与随后间质性纤维化之间的联系[52]。在一项随机试验中，他们发现，用皮质类固醇治疗亚临床排斥反应增加了移植物存活率,并可能引起更少的纤维化。这项早期研究来自环孢素-硫唑嘌呤时代的移植，亚临床 ACR 发生率为 30%,基于他克莫司方案的亚临床 ACR 比率似乎低得多，而在当前的免疫抑制时代中没有进行随机化的治疗试验。几项移植项目,包括我们的项目,常规地对功能良好的肾同种异体移植物进行监测活检。我们还发现移植后 1 年的亚临床炎症与随后低移植功能和生存率之间存在联系（图 67.2)[53]。因为其不满足 ACR 的标准,在活检中发现的大多数炎症处于“边界”

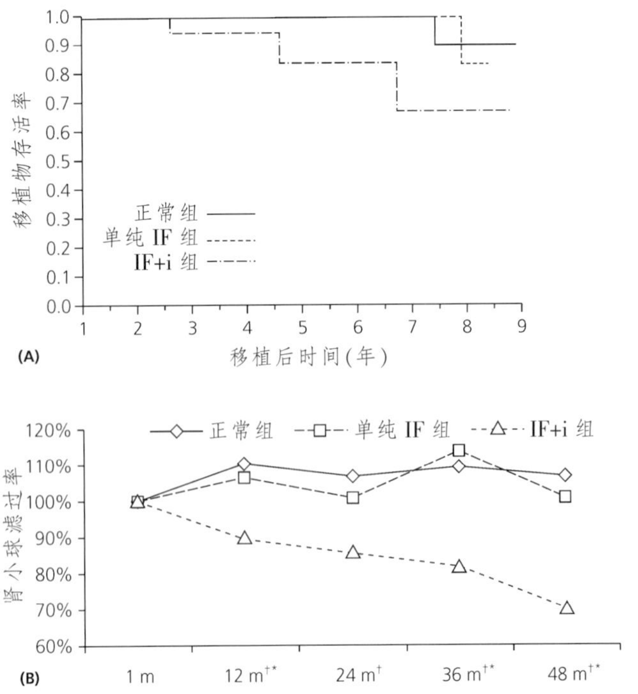

图 67.2 (A)与活检正常和活检提示单纯纤维化(单纯 IF)的患者相比,1 年活检显示间质性纤维化加亚临床炎症(IF +i)的患者移植物存活率降低。(B)IF+i 患者的肾小球滤过率(GFR)随时间降低 (+正常组对 IF+i 组,$P\leq0.05$;* 单纯 IF 组对 IF+i 组,$P\leq0.05$)。(Reprinted with permission from the American Society of Nephrology, from [53] Park WD, Griffin MD, Cornell LD, Cosio FG, Stegall MD. Fibrosis with inflammation at one year predicts transplant functional decline. J Am Soc Nephrol 2010; 21: 1987-1997.)

状态。边界变化的意义仍不清楚,近来有更多人研究这一问题 [54]。我们和其他执行监测活检的中心倾向于治疗亚临床炎症,其满足 ACR 快速推注皮质类固醇的 Banff 标准。然而,治疗对功能良好的移植物预后的影响尚不清楚,并且需要考虑除了移植功能变化外额外免疫抑制的潜在感染风险。

功能不断下降移植物的治疗方法

常见的临床情况是同种异体移植功能逐渐下降,例如肾小球滤过率从移植后 1 年的 60mL/min 降至移植后 5 年的 40mL/min。GFR 的下降速率如此缓慢,可能使得临床医生认为这并非急性变化。对这些患者进行治疗干预的作用尚不清楚,但可以概述一般的临床方法。

首先,为了排除非免疫原因(例如,部分输尿管梗阻、多发性骨髓瘤病毒肾病等),与对急性功能障碍的同种异体移植物进行详细评估一样,应当对这些衰竭的同种异体移植物进行类似的评估(表 67.1)。此外,还应该使用固相单抗原珠对 DSA 水平进行评估。因此,同种异体移植物活检应是下一个步骤。活检的可能结果可能包括原发性肾脏疾病的复发和慢性组织学损伤,伴或不伴活动性炎症的证据。

然而,如上所述,在这种情况下的组织活检也可能显示满足 Banff 标准的急性细胞排斥反应的间质淋巴细胞浸润。虽然关于此有一个新兴的共识,即亚临床排斥与慢性损伤相关联,但并没有关于其治疗的共识。我们的治疗方案包括推注甲基泼尼松龙,类似于临床急性细胞排斥反应的治疗;然而,没有证据表明这种治疗或任何其他治疗可以预防慢性损伤的进展。在一些情况下,近期随着免疫抑制治疗(无论是处方的还是其他方式)亚临床排斥的发现率减少,可谨慎尝试恢复以前的药物治疗方案和水平。与 ACR 的情况类似,关于建立亚临床排斥反应治疗成功的适当终点的共识甚至更少。我们的方法是在治疗后 1 个月重复肾活检,以证明浸润严重程度的改善。

第二种常见的组织学发现提示慢性抗体介导的损伤。与慢性抗体介导的损伤最密切相关的组织病变是移植肾小球病(TG)。然而,TG 也可能代表复发性的原发性肾脏疾病[55]。肾小球炎和(或)管周毛细血管炎也可提示慢性活性抗体介导的损伤[56,57]。细胞浸润不仅在位置上不同于细胞排斥反应,而且其更易出现巨噬细胞和嗜中性粒细胞。与急性抗体介导的排斥反应相反,在慢性 AMR 中,管周毛细血管通常 C4d 染色阴性。新 DSA 的存在提示肾小球损伤可能是由于慢性 AMR 引起的。

TG 的预后似乎很差,诊断明确后 5 年内超过 50% 的同种异体移植物会出现衰竭[58,59]。遗憾的是,几乎没有报道过经过证实的慢性 AMR 治疗方法。我们使用多重 PE 来降低 DSA 水平,但是 DSA 在治疗结束后又会很快回复。高剂量 IVIG、利妥昔单抗和(或)硼替佐米也可以考虑,但没有一种被证明能减缓 TG 的进展。鉴于慢性 AMR 可能占晚期移植物损失的一半以上[60],需要更多的对照试验来为该临床类别发展有效的挽救疗法。

避免或戒断钙调磷酸酶抑制剂作为挽救疗法

过去几年中,越来越多的人使用新药来避免 CNI[61-66]。

这些方案的主要目标是避免长期肾毒性。然而，过去 10 年中呈现的大部分数据没有证明慢性 CNI 毒性是晚期肾同种异体移植物损失的主要原因[55]。无 CNI 方案的主要终点是移植后 1 年或 2 年肾功能的改善。然而，尚缺乏证明改善整个肾移植人群中的肾功能将防止注定失败的患者移植物丢失的数据。甚至使用无 CNI 方案的早期，改善的肾功能的替代终点也难以证明，特别是与基于他克莫司的免疫抑制相比[61]。最近 10 年的肾活检研究同样显示使用组织学将晚期损伤归因于 CNI 十分困难[67,68]。

当移植物发展成慢性损伤时，从 CNI 到无 CNI 方案的转变可能会改善 GFR，但是不清楚这是否会确实增加移植物存活率[69-71]。单纯提高血清肌酸酐水平可能轻微延长移植物的存活时间，但考虑到潜在的病理很可能不是由于 CNI 引起的，同种异体移植物的命运可能不会改变。

终末期肾同种异体移植物

挽救治疗在功能极差的同种异体移植物(例如GFR <25mL/min)和严重的不可逆组织学变化中的作用可能是轻微的。大多数临床医生试图通过控制血压和优化血管内容积状态来使医疗管理最大化。还有人提出改变免疫抑制方案，包括降低 CNI 的靶水平或在停止应用 CNI，转换为西罗莫司。如果存在满足 ACR 标准的活动性炎症，可以考虑使用皮质类固醇治疗；然而，严重(Banff ci3)纤维化的存在表明没有哪种治疗能影响这种移植的结果。晚期移植物损伤的患者应进行再移植评估。

评估同种异体移植物的新方法

尽管肾脏功能和组织学已经成为几十年来同种异体移植物评估的基础，但是目前也在尝试应用新的方法来提供侵入性较小和(或)更详细的移植物内事件概况。尿液细胞因子和其他炎症标志物的测定作为 ACR 的早期检测正在接受测试[72-74]。这些测定侵袭性更小，并且可以更频繁地进行。此外，外周血或同种异体移植物活检的基因组谱开始帮助区分不同类型的炎症[53,75-79]。在未来，基因表达谱可用于决定哪些移植物需要治疗，并且也可以用作治疗功效的替代标志物。因此，在将来，“挽救疗法”可能会基于尿液测定和(或)基因表达谱的结果。

其他实体器官移植的挽救疗法

一般来说，在非肾实体器官移植中 ACR 和 AMR 的治疗已经沿着与肾移植相同的方向发展，并且与肾移植类似，大多数没有Ⅰ级证据支持的治疗方案已经被采用。然而，心脏移植和肝移植中急性和慢性同种异体移植物损伤的影响和治疗是独一无二的。考虑到这些器官的生命支持性质，在这些类型的移植中同种免疫介导的同种异体移植物损伤的管理值得关注。

肝移植

肝移植中 ACR 的发生率约为 24%~80%[80,81]。用推注皮质类固醇治疗和增强基线免疫抑制强度(特别是他克莫司)治疗 ACR 通常会导致同种异体移植物的损伤(至少在生化上)。对于那些耐激素性的患者，往往应用单克隆抗淋巴细胞制剂或这个时代更常见的多克隆抗淋巴细胞制剂[82,83]。肝脏的恢复力大大超过肾脏，因为肝脏具有显著的再生能力，使得 ACR 的快速逆转不那么紧迫。然而，在感染丙型肝炎病毒(HCV)的受体中，ACR 的管理中出现了特别困难的情况。虽然 ACR 的轻度发作似乎与非 HCV 感染的受体中移植物丢失或死亡的风险增加无关，但是 HCV 感染的受体中 ACR 治疗的确导致了 HCV 复发、移植物丢失和死亡的风险增加[84-89]。目前，在 HCV 存在时对于 ACR 的最适当治疗方案尚未达成共识，表明需要在该领域进行前瞻性试验[90]。因此，对于 HCV 感染的肝移植受体最适当的“挽救疗法”可能很少或根本没用。

心脏移植

与肝移植一样，心脏移植中同种异体移植物损伤引起的移植物衰竭的意义是深刻的。ACR 或 AMR 的治疗强度通常由受体的血流动力学状态决定，并且可以从维持免疫抑制的剂量增加或推注皮质类固醇治疗无症状(亚临床)ACR，变化到血浆交换±硼替佐米联合血流动力学支持来治疗严重发作的导致心源性休克的 AMR[91,92]。

与肾移植相似，关于同种抗体在急性和慢性心脏同种异体移植物损伤中作用的数据有所增加。更具体地，有新证据支持早期同种异体移植物损伤和CAV发展之间的联系，CAV是心外膜冠状动脉病变，其特征是内皮细胞浸润、血管平滑肌细胞增殖和随后管腔狭窄[93]。CAV的特异性治疗将在第79章中详细讨论。经历心脏同种异体移植ACR或AMR的患者更可能发生CAV[94-96]。直到最近，虽然经皮支架和优化药物治疗可以延缓病情，但严重CAV唯一明确的治疗疗法是再移植[93]。

CAV的不良预后和生存影响已开始引起了人们对预防和挽救策略的研究。在这一领域最有希望的免疫抑制剂似乎是增殖抑制剂(依维莫司和西罗莫司)。尽管确切的作用机制尚未被完全理解，但转换或重新应用增殖抑制剂已显示能降低同种异体移植物血管病变的发生率和严重程度[97-100]。应用这样的方案可能对改善慢性心脏同种异体移植物损伤的长期生存有重要影响。

“挽救疗法”对改善移植物长期存活的未来作用

我们处理急性免疫并发症的能力(例如ACR，甚至AMR)使肾移植几乎成为一项常规操作。然而，很明显，尽管早期移植物丢失几乎已经消失，但是在过去20年中，晚期肾同种异体移植物存活几乎没有改善。

我们认为，改善长期同种异体移植物存活的方法应包括详细的患者随访，以确定晚期肾同种异体移植物丢失的具体原因，并在同种异体移植损伤变得不可逆之前找到解决这些问题的新方法。不幸的是，关于晚期肾同种异体移植物丢失原因的数据很少，这阻碍了我们设计合理方法以改善结果。我们最近的程序性活检研究表明，从1998年到2004年的肾同种异体移植显示在移植后前5年进展性组织学变化比早期时代报道更少[101,102]。例如，中度至重度纤维化的患病率在移植后5年时仅为17%(60/343)，并且在移植后1年活检存在轻度纤维化时，其在5年时发展为更严重形式的仅占23%。事实上，5年所有同种异体移植物中的2/3对于慢性组织学变化(cg、ci、ct、cv和ah)显示0(无)或1(轻度)的Banff评分。

基于这些数据，我们提出了一种新方法以改善移植物长期存活[2]。我们建议优化随访方案，并且验证晚期移植物丢失原因的近期研究。血清测试(DSA水平和多瘤病毒测试)和程序性组织活检的联合可能是最好的方法。密集随访的目的是在移植物仍然功能良好的情况下识别具有特定问题的患者。活检的原因可能是时间太晚，无法成功干预。

因此，我们相信，如果挽救疗法能够从对临床变化的反应转变为预防性治疗，它将在改善移植物长期存活中起重要作用。例如，对于新生DSA出现的监测可能在慢性抗体介导的损伤发展之前建立“挽救疗法”。类似地，使用常规光学显微镜或基因表达分析来监测肾同种异体移植物活检可用于鉴定具有慢性损伤风险的同种异体移植物。

总结

挽救疗法的概念在移植中根深蒂固。用于ACR的治疗已经确立。单独或与ACR联合的急性AMR治疗方案可能在尝试新疗法时继续发展。亚临床过程中挽救疗法的作用仍不清楚，但我们认为，这些将成为干预最重要的新领域，因为我们开始了解慢性同种异体移植物损伤的发病机制。

(陈峻 译　徐骁 校)

参考文献

1. Lodhi SA, Lamb KE, Meier-Kriesche HU. Solid organ allograft survival improvement in the United States: the long-term does not mirror the dramatic short-term success. American Journal of Transplantation. 2011;11:1226–1235.
2. Stegall MD, Park WD, Dean PG, et al. Improving long-term renal allograft survival via a road less traveled by. American Journal of Transplantation. 2011;11:1382–1387.
3. Guyatt G, Schunëmann H, Cook D, et al. American College of Chest Physicians. Grades of recommendation for antithrombotic agents. Chest. 2001;119:3S–7S.
4. Mehta RL, Kellum JA, Shah SV, et al. Acute Kidney Injury Network: report of an initiative to improve outcomes in acute kidney injury. Critical Care (London, England). 2007;11:R31.
5. Solez K, Colvin RB, Racusen LC, et al. Banff 07 classification of renal allograft pathology: updates and future directions. American Journal of Transplantation. 2008;8:753–760.
6. Matas AJ, Tellis VA, Quinn T, et al. ALG treatment of steroid-resistant rejection in patients receiving cyclosporine. Transplantation. 1986;41:579–583.
7. Tesi RJ, Elkhammas EA, Henry ML, et al. Acute rejection episodes. Best predictor of long-term primary cadaveric renal transplant survival. Transplantation Proceedings. 1993;25:901–902.
8. Pirsch JD, Ploeg RJ, Gange S, et al. Determinants of graft survival after renal transplantation. Transplantation. 1996;61:1581–1586.
9. Almond PS, Matas A, Gillingham K, et al. Risk factors for chronic rejection in renal allograft recipients. Transplantation. 1993;55:752–756.
10. Ferguson RM. Acute rejection episodes—best predictor of long-term primary cadaveric renal transplant survival. Clinical Transplantation. 1994;8:328–331.
11. Meier-Kriesche H-U, Schold JD, Srinivas TR, et al. Lack of improvement in renal allograft survival despite a marked decrease in acute rejection rates over the most recent era. American Journal of Transplantation. 2004;4:378–383.
12. Vereerstraeten P, Abramowicz D, De Pauw L, et al. Absence of deleterious effect on long-term kidney graft survival of rejection episodes with complete functional recovery. Transplantation. 1997;63:1739–1743.
13. Madden RL, Mulhern JG, Benedetto BJ, et al. Completely reversed acute rejection

is not a significant risk factor for the development of chronic rejection in renal allograft recipients. Transplant International. 2000;13:344–350.
14. Bell PR, Briggs JD, Calman KC, et al. Reversal of acute clinical and experimental organ rejection using large doses of intravenous prednisolone. Lancet. 1971;1: 876–880.
15. Woods JE, Anderson CF, DeWeerd JH, et al. High-dosage intravenously administered methylprednisolone in renal transplantation. A preliminary report. JAMA. 1973;223:896–899.
16. Birkeland SA. A controlled clinical trial of treatment with ALG in established rejection of renal allografts. Acta Medica Scandinavica. 1975;198:489–496.
17. Howard RJ, Condie RM, Sutherland DE, et al. The use of antilymphoblast globulin in the treatment of renal allograft rejection: a double-blind, randomized study. Transplantation. 1977;24:419–423.
18. Baldi A, Malaise J, Mourad M, et al. A prospective randomized study comparing poly-ATG to mono-OKT3 clonal antibodies for the first rejection therapy after kidney transplantation: long-term results. Transplantation Proceedings. 2000;32:429–431.
19. Spieker C, Barenbrock M, Buchholz B, et al. Cardiovascular effects of ATG and OKT3 in renal allograft recipients. Transplantation Proceedings. 1992;24: 2594–2595.
20. Casadei D, Rial M, Argento J, et al. Preliminary results from a randomized and prospective study of high-dose immunoglobulin versus monoclonal antibody in the rescue of steroid-resistant rejections. Transplantation Proceedings. 1998; 30:2164.
21. Filo RS, Smith EJ, Leapman SB. Therapy of acute cadaveric renal allograft rejection with adjunctive antithymocyte globulin. Transplantation. 1980;30: 445–449.
22. Gaber AO, First MR, Tesi RJ, et al. Results of the double-blind, randomized, multicenter, phase III clinical trial of Thymoglobulin versus Atgam in the treatment of acute graft rejection episodes after renal transplantation. Transplantation. 1998;66:29–37.
23. Glass NR, Miller DT, Sollinger HW, et al. A comparative study of steroids and heterologous antiserum in the treatment of renal allograft rejection. Transplantation Proceedings. 1983;15:617–621.
24. Hesse UJ, Wienand P, Baldamus C, et al. Preliminary results of a prospectively randomized trial of ALG vs OKT3 for steroid-resistant rejection after renal transplantation in the early postoperative period. Transplantation Proceedings. 1990;22:2273–2274.
25. Goldstein G, Schindler J, Tsai H, et al. A randomized clinical trial of OKT3 monoclonal antibody for acute rejection of cadaveric renal transplants. Ortho Multicenter Transplant Study Group. New England Journal of Medicine. 1985;313:337–342.
26. Hilbrands LB, Hoitsma AJ, Koene RA. Methylprednisolone versus ATG as initial treament for acute rejections after renal transplantation. Nephrology, Dialysis, Transplantation. 1996;11:1675.
27. Hoitsma AJ, Reekers P, Kreeftenberg JG, et al. Treatment of acute rejection of cadaveric renal allografts with rabbit antithymocyte globulin. Transplantation. 1982;33:12–16.
28. Hourmant M, Soulillou JP, Remi JP, et al. Use of cyclosporin A after antilymphocyte serum in renal transplantation [French]. La Presse Medicale. 1985;14:2093–2096.
29. Johnson K, Niblack G, Richie R, et al. Multicenter comparison of rejection reversal: rabbit anti-human lymphocyte serum (ATS) versus horse anti-human lymphocyte globulin (ATGAM). Transplantation Proceedings. 1989;21: 1734–1735.
30. Mariat C, Alamartine E, Diab N, et al. A randomized prospective study comparing low-dose OKT3 to low-dose ATG for the treatment of acute steroid-resistant rejection episodes in kidney transplant recipients. Transplant International. 1998;11:231–236.
31. Midtvedt K, Tafjord AB, Hartmann A, et al. Half dose of OKT3 is efficient in treatment of steroid-resistant renal allograft rejection. Transplantation. 1996; 62:38–42.
32. Midtvedt K, Fauchald P, Lien B, et al. Individualized T cell monitored administration of ATG versus OKT3 in steroid-resistant kidney graft rejection. Clinical Transplantation. 2003;17:69–74.
33. Shield CF 3rd, Cosimi AB, Tolkoff-Rubin N, et al. Use of antithymocyte globulin for reversal of acute allograft rejection. Transplantation. 1979;28:461–464.
34. Streem SB, Novick AC, Braun WE, et al. Low-dose maintenance prednisone and antilymphoblast globulin for the treatment of acute rejection. A steroid-sparing approach to immunosuppressive therapy. Transplantation. 1983;35:420–424.
35. Waid TH, Lucas BA, Thompson JS, et al. Treatment of renal allograft rejection with T10B9.1A31 or OKT3: final analysis of a phase II clinical trial. Transplantation. 1997;64:274–281.
36. Theodorakis J, Schneeberger H, Illner WD, et al. Aggressive treatment of the first acute rejection episode using first-line anti-lymphocytic preparation reduces further acute rejection episodes after human kidney transplantation. Transplant International. 1998;11(Suppl. 1):S86–S89.
37. Webster A, Pankhurst T, Rinaldi F, et al. Polyclonal and monoclonal antibodies for treating acute rejection episodes in kidney transplant recipients. Cochrane Database of Systematic Reviews. 2006;(2):CD004756.
38. Sis B, Mengel M, Haas M, et al. Banff '09 meeting report: antibody mediated graft deterioration and implementation of the Banff working groups. American Journal of Transplantation. 2010;10:464.
39. Raghavaiah S, Stegall MD. New therapeutic approaches to antibody-mediated rejection in renal transplantation. Clinical Pharmacology and Therapeutics. 2011;90:310–315.
40. Burns JM, Cornell LD, Perry DK, et al. Alloantibody levels and antibody mediated rejection early after positive crossmatch kidney transplantation. American Journal of Transplantation. 2008;8:2684–2694.
41. Locke JE, Zachary AA, Mohammed BS, et al. Rescue splenectomy for severe acute antibody-mediated rejection. Clinical Transplants. 2006:518–520.
42. Kaposztas Z, Podder H, Mauiyyedi S, et al. Impact of rituximab therapy for the treatment of acute humoral rejection. Clinical Transplantation. 2009;23:63–73.
43. Vo AA, Lukovsky M, Toyoda M, et al. Rituximab and intravenous immune globulin for desensitization during renal transplantation. New England Journal of Medicine. 2008;359:242–251.
44. Lefaucheur C, Nochy D, Andrade J, et al. Comparison of combination plasmapheresis IVIg/anti-CD20 versus high-dose IVIg in the treatment of antibody mediated rejection. American Journal of Transplantation. 2009;9:1099–1107.
45. Stegall MD, Diwan T, Cornell LD, et al. Terminal complement blockade decreases early acute rejection in sensitized renal transplant recipients. American Journal of Transplantation. 2011;11:2405–2413.
46. Locke JE, Magro CM, Singer AL, et al. The use of antibody to complement protein C5 for salvage treatment of severe antibody-mediated rejection. American Journal of Transplantation. 2009;9:231–235.
47. Perry DK, Burns JM, Pollinger HS, et al. Proteasome inhibition causes apoptosis of normal human plasma cells preventing alloantibody production. American Journal of Transplantation. 2009;9:201–209.
48. Everly MJ, Everly JJ, Susskind B, et al. Bortezomib provides effective therapy for antibody and cell-mediated rejection. Transplantation. 2008;86:1754–1761.
49. Everly MJ. An updated on antibody reduction and rejection reversal following bortezomib use: a report of 52 cases across 10 centers. Clinical Transplants. 2010:353–362.
50. Diwan T, Raghavaiah S, Burns JM, et al. The impact of proteasome inhibition on alloantibody-producing plasma cells in vivo. Transplantation. 2011;91:536–541.
51. Walsh RC, Brailey P, Girnita A, et al. Early and late antibody mediated rejection differ immunologically and in response to proteasome inhibition. Transplantation. 2011;91:1218.
52. Rush D, Nickerson P, Gough J, et al. Beneficial effects of treatment of early subclinical rejection: a randomized study. Journal of the American Society of Nephrology. 1998;9:2129.
53. Park WD, Griffin MD, Cornell LD, et al. Fibrosis with inflammation at one year predicts transplant functional decline. Journal of the American Society of Nephrology. 2010;21:1987–1997.
54. de Freitas DG, Sellares J, Mengel M, et al. The nature of biopsies with "borderline rejection" and prospects for eliminating this category. American Journal of Transplantation. 2012;12:191–201.
55. El-Zoghby ZM, Stegall MD, Lager DJ, et al. Identifying specific causes of kidney allograft loss. American Journal of Transplantation. 2009;9:527–535.
56. Loupy A, Suberbielle-Boissel C, Hill GS, et al. Outcome of subclinical antibody-mediated rejection in kidney transplant recipients with preformed donor-specific antibodies. American Journal of Transplantation. 2009;9:2561–2570.
57. Haas M, Montgomery RA, Segev DL, et al. Subclinical acute antibody-mediated rejection in positive crossmatch renal allografts. American Journal of Transplantation. 2007;7:576–585.
58. Cosio FG, Grande JP, Wadei H, et al. Predicting subsequent decline in kidney allograft function from early surveillance biopsies. American Journal of Transplantation. 2005;5:2464–2472.
59. Issa N, Cosio FG, Gloor JM, et al. Transplant glomerulopathy: risk and prognosis related to anti-human leukocyte antigen Class II antibody levels. Transplantation. 2008;15:681–685.
60. Gaston RS, Cecka JM, Kasiske BL, et al. Evidence for antibody-mediated injury as a major determinant of late kidney allograft failure. Transplantation. 2010;90:68.
61. Larson TS, Dean PG, Stegall MD, et al. Complete avoidance of calcineurin inhibitors in renal transplantation: a randomized trial comparing sirolimus and tacrolimus. American Journal of Transplantation. 2006;6:514–522.
62. Dean PG, Grande JP, Sethi S, et al. Kidney transplant histology after one year of continuous therapy with sirolimus compared with tacrolimus. Transplantation. 2008;85:1212–1215.

63. Weir MR, Mulgaonkar S, Chan L, et al. Mycophenolate mofetil-based immunosuppression with sirolimus in renal transplantation: a randomized, controlled Spare-the-Nephron trial. Kidney International. 2011;79:897–907.
64. Vincenti F, Blacho G, Durrbach A, et al. Five-year safety and efficacy of belatacept in renal transplantation. Journal of the American Society of Nephrology. 2010;21:1587–1596.
65. Vicenti F, Chapentier B, Vanrenterghem Y, et al. A phase III study of belatacept-based immunosuppression regiments versus cyclosporine in renal transplant recipients (BENEFIT study). American Journal of Transplantation. 2010;10: 535–546.
66. Williams D, Haragism L. Calcineurin nephrotoxicity. Advances in Chronic Kidney Disease. 2006;13:47–55.
67. Snandoudj R, Royal V, Elle C, et al. Specificity of histologic markers of long-term CNI nephrotoxicity in kidney transplant recipients under low-dose cyclosporine therapy. American Journal of Transplantation. 2011;11:2635–2646.
68. Mengel M, Mihatsch M, Halloran PF. Histologic characteristics of calcineurin inhibitor toxicity—there is no such thing as specificity! American Journal of Transplantation. 2011;12:2549–2550.
69. Holdaas H, Rostaing L, Serón D, et al. Conversion of long-term kidney transplant recipients from calcineurin inhibitor therapy to everolimus: a randomized, multicenter, 24-month study. Transplantation. 2011;92:410–418.
70. Egbuna OI, Davis RB, Chudinski R, et al. Outcomes with conversion from calcineurin inhibitors to sirolimus after renal transplantation in the context of steroid withdrawal or steroid continuation. Transplantation. 2009;88: 684–692.
71. Schena FP, Pascoe MD, Alberu J, et al. Conversion from calcineurin inhibitors to sirolimus maintenance therapy in renal allograft recipients: 24-month efficacy and safety results from the CONVERT trial. Transplantation. 2009; 87:233–242.
72. Afaneh C, Muthukumar T, Lubetzky M. Urinary levels of mRNA for OX40, OX40L, PD-1, PD-L1, or PD-L2 and acute rejection of human renal allografts. Transplantation. 2010;90:1381–1387.
73. Ho J, Rush DN, Karpinski M, et al. Validation of urinary CXCL10 as a marker of borderline, subclinical, and clinical tubulitis. Transplantation. 2010;92:878–882.
74. Jackson JA, Kim EJ, Begley B, et al. Urinary chemokines CXCL9 and CXCL10 are noninvasive markers of renal allograft rejection and BK viral infection. American Journal of Transplantation. 2011;10:2228–2234.
75. Eineke G, Sis B, Reeve J, et al. Antibody mediated microcirculation is the major cause of late kidney transplant failure. American Journal of Transplantation. 2009;9:2520–2531.
76. Robison EH, Mondala TS, Williams AR, et al. Whole genome transcript profiling from fingerstick blood samples: a comparison and feasibility study. BMC Genomics. 2009;10:617.
77. Mas VR, Mueller TF, Archer KJ, et al. Identifying biomarkers as diagnostic tools in kindey transplantation. Expert Review of Molecular Diagnostics. 2011;2:183–196.
78. Ozluk Y, Blanco PL, Mengel M, et al. Superiority of virtual microscopy versus light microscopy in transplantation pathology. Clinical Transplantation. 2012;26:336–344.
79. Naesens M, Khatri P, Li L. Progressive histologic damage in renal allografts is associated with expression of innate and adaptive immunity genes. Kidney International. 2011;80:1363–1376.
80. Fisher LR, Henley KS, Lucey MR. Acute cellular rejection after liver transplantation: variability, morbidity, and mortality. Liver Transplantation and Surgery. 1995;1:10–15.
81. Wiesner RH, Demetris AJ, Belle SH, et al. Acute hepatic allograft rejection: incidence, risk factors and impact on outcome. Hepatology (Baltimore, Md.). 1998;28:638–645.
82. Bijleveld CG, Klompmaker IJ, van den Berg AP, et al. Incidence, risk factors, and outcome of antithymocyte globulin treatment of steroid-resistant rejection after liver transplantation. Transplant International. 1996;9:570–575.
83. Schmitt TM, Phillips M, Sawyer RG, et al. Anti-thymocyte globulin for the treatment of acute cellular rejection following liver transplantation. Digestive Diseases and Sciences. 2010;55:3224–3234.
84. Sheiner PA, Schwartz ME, Mor E, et al. Severe or multiple rejection episodes are associated with early recurrence of hepatitis C after orthotopic liver transplantation. Hepatology (Baltimore, Md.). 1995;21:30–34.
85. Charlton M, Seaberg E. Impact of immunosuppression and acute rejection on recurrence of hepatitis C: results of the National Institute of Diabetes and Digestive and Kidney Diseases Liver Transplant Database. Liver Transplantation and Surgery. 1999;5:S107–S114.
86. Prieto M, Berenguer M, Rayon JM, et al. High incidence of allograft cirrhosis in hepatitis C virus genotype 1b infection following transplantation: relationship with rejection episodes. Hepatology (Baltimore, Md.). 1999;29:250–256.
87. Neumann UP, Berg T, Bahra M, et al. Long-term outcome of liver transplants for chronic hepatitis C: a 10-year follow-up study. Transplantation. 2004;77: 226–231.
88. Rosen HR, Shackleton CR, Higa L, et al. Use of OKT3 is associated with early and severe recurrence of hepatitis C after liver transplantation. American Journal of Gastroenterology. 1997;92:1453–1457.
89. Berenguer M, Prieto M, Cordoba J, et al. Early development of chronic active hepatitis in recurrent hepatitis C virus infection after liver transplantation: association with treatment of rejection. Journal of Hepatology. 1998;28: 756–763.
90. Burton JR, Rosen HR. Acute rejection in HCV-infected liver transplant recipients: the great conundrum. Liver Transplantation. 2006;12:S38–S47.
91. Patel JK, Kittleson M, Kobashigawa JA. Cardiac allograft rejection. Surgeon. 2011;9:160–167.
92. Uber WE, Self SE, Van Bakel AB, et al. Acute antibody-mediated rejection following heart transplantation. American Journal of Transplantation. 2007; 7:2064–2074.
93. Lee MS, Finch W, Kirtane AS. Cardiac allograft vasculopathy. Reviews in Cardiovascular Medicine. 2011;12:143–152.
94. Raichlin E, Edwards BS, Kremers WK, et al. Acute cellular rejection and the subsequent development of allograft vasculopathy after cardiac transplantation. Journal of Heart and Lung Transplantation. 2009;28:320–327.
95. Kirklin JK. Is biopsy-proven cellular rejection an important clinical consideration in heart transplantation? Current Opinion in Cardiology. 2005;20:127–131.
96. Wu GW, Kobashigawa JA, Fishbein MC, et al. Asymptomatic antibody-mediated rejection after heart transplantation predicts poor outcomes. Journal of Heart and Lung Transplantation. 2009;28:417–422.
97. Raichlin E, Khalpey Z, Kremers WK, et al. Conversion to sirolimus as primary immunosuppression attenuates the progression of allograft vasculopathy after cardiac transplantation. Circulation. 2007;116:2726–2733.
98. Keogh A, Richardson M, Ruygrok P, et al. Sirolimus in de novo heart transplant recipients reduces acute rejection and prevents coronary artery disease at 2 years: a randomized clinical trial. Circulation. 2004;110:2694–2700.
99. Eisen HJ, Tuzcu EM, Dorent R, et al. Everolimus for the prevention of allograft rejection and vasculopathy in cardiac-transplant recipients. New England Journal of Medicine. 2003;349:847–858.
100. Topilsky Y, Hasin T, Raichlini E, et al. Sirolimus as primary immunosuppression attenuates allograft vasculopathy with improved late survival and decreased cardiac events following cardiac transplantation. Circulation. 2012;125: 708–720.
101. Stegall MD, Park WD, Larson TS, et al. The histology of solitary renal allografts at 1 and 5 years after transplantation. American Journal of Transplantation. 2011;11:698–707.
102. Nankivell BJ, Borrows RJ, Fung CL-S, et al. The natural history of chronic allograft nephropathy. New England Journal of Medicine. 2003;349:2326–2333.

第 68 章

器官移植的脱敏治疗方案

Carmen Lefaucheur, Denis Glotz

引言

脱敏可以定义为旨在减少移植前同种致敏患者中同种抗体的预处理治疗。同种致敏作用是指针对另一个遗传学上不同个体存在的同种异体抗体。虽然患者可能是B细胞或T细胞致敏的，一般来说，该术语通常被看作B细胞同种致敏并推断存在针对特定供体的同种抗体。脱敏方法的目的是消除供体导向的同种抗体以达到阴性或足够低的交叉匹配，并且使得先前不相容的供体–受体对可以进行移植。关于阳性交叉匹配的解释详见第36章。目前，关于脱敏的绝大多数数据来自肾移植文献。因此，本章将仅专注于肾移植前的脱敏治疗。

在当前环境中肾移植的脱敏治疗

脱敏方案的成功与肾移植治疗终末期肾病(ESRD)的全球性成功密切相关。移植提供了扩大准入及降低成本以成功治疗ESRD的机制，并超越了透析治疗的生存质量和数量以及成本效益[1-3]。目前肾移植率的主要限制是捐赠器官的短缺。器官可用性的危机与需要肾移植的患者数量超过可用器官数量的现实有关，在大多数高收入国家，供体和潜在受体比例低于1:3[4,5]。世界范围内，肾脏替代治疗的潜在候选人的数量正在迅速增长，并且几乎在所有国家中，移植只能满足全球需求的10%[6]。

当前的进展主要集中于基于ABO血型不相容移植的优异结果使供体库增加以及致敏患者移植取得的进展。高滴度的供者特异性HLA抗体也具有有限的移植个体前景，尽管现在更佳的脱敏方案和配对的肾交换程序为那些原先被认为不适合移植的患者提供了真实可行的机会。

用于跨HLA抗体屏障的肾移植脱敏方案

故意跨越HLA屏障是与用于检测和表征抗HLA抗体的方法的发展以及潜在有效治疗的可用性相关的相对较新的现象。脱敏治疗领域在过去10年中取得了巨大的进步。虽然脱敏实践的扩展促进了对可行性、临床疗效、移植物功能的耐久性和与其使用相关的患者安全性的关注[7-12]，然而，最近的研究表明，与等待相容器官相比，患者脱敏后移植具有更显著的生存获益[12]。因此，这些治疗越来越多地被认为是有价值的策略，可以使进行移植的患者大大增加。

针对HLA致敏的脱敏策略：严重的公共健康问题

HLA致敏的患者由于等待时间延长或限制了移植的机会而处于不利境地，难以匹配和(或)被认为是高度HLA致敏的患者尤其如此[4,5,13]。因此，这些患者因潜在匹配供者数量不足而注定要在等待名单上滞留更长时间，只能接受透析治疗，这是死亡和移植物失功的另一个危险因素[8,12]。

HLA特异性抗体通过先前的输血、怀孕和移植而产生；曾接受移植目前被认为是肾移植候选者致敏的主要原因。使用单一HLA表型和单一HLA抗原检测抗HLA抗体的固相测试的增加使得可能建立计算的群体反应性抗体(CPRA)称为评估对HLA抗原敏的新方法。这一过程的细节见第36章。CPRA定义为预期具有一种或多种在等待名单上的候选受者不可接受的HLA抗原的潜在捐赠者比例。CPRA代表了分配政策的根本性转变，替代了PRA，在2009年7月应用于法国移植候选人，在2009年10月应用于美国移植候选人[14-16]。它提供了一个更一致和负责任的肾移植候选人的致敏衡量措施。在实施CPRA之前,移植中心和实验室可以基于敏感性和特异性范围较广的多种测试中的任何一种报告PRA值。目前,CPRA政策要求实验室在国家计算机系统上输入其移植候选人特定的可接受的HLA。

CPRA的引入增加了致敏患者中器官分配的效率[15]。然而,CPRA不能解决高度致敏患者在移植中出现的所有问题。此外,它导致了新的问题,如等待名单上的高度致敏患者越来越多，以及他们越来越难以获得移植机会。目前，我们的动态候选名单上有35%~50%的注册人有致敏的证据[15,16]。大约1/4的移植候选者广泛致敏:器官获取和移植网络(OPTN)中15.8%的注册者和法国国家名单上23%的患者的PRA/CPRA>80%，并且这一比例可能因为广泛使用的单抗原测定而继续升高。几乎所有的增加都发生于PRA/CPRA>95%的注册者中。2009年(5.3%)至2010年(10.2%),PRA/CPRA> 95%的注册者的比例翻了一番。因此,我们可能看到具有超高CPRA值的患者累积下降，并且未接受任何治疗。超过95%的PRA/CPRA候选者的移植率从97/1000人年降至69/1000人年[15]。对于对HLA广泛致敏的患者,目前存在的移植选择很少。

致敏患者的移植准入可以通过特异性策略来降低HLA特异性抗体水平并提高移植率。脱敏方案将接受移植患者的比例增加到80%[20例患者中有16例接受静脉免疫球蛋白（IVIG）及利妥昔单抗脱敏后在平均12个月内接受肾移植][11]或更高(一组患者中98%脱敏后接受活体肾移植)[12]。因此,脱敏方案有可能极大地增加移植候选人中这些不成比例的弱势群体获得移植的机会(框68.1)。

框68.1 要点:敏化作用与肾移植

- 基于固相测定的HLA抗体表征的引入改善了供体特异性抗体(DSA)的检测和定量。
- 移植候选者的新的敏感性测定是计算基于等待名单上候选者的不相容的HLA抗原的群体反应性抗体(CPRA)。
- 在过去10年中，非常广泛致敏患者的比例增加(>80% CPRA),移植率下降。
- 供体特异性抗HLA抗体的消耗和移植前调节改善了移植率。
- 脱敏后移植与等待相容器官相比,为HLA敏化的患者提供了显著的生存获益。

脱敏疗法的治疗选择

高剂量静脉免疫球蛋白是脱敏治疗的主体

静脉注射免疫球蛋白(IVIG)产品具有强大的免疫调节效应[17]。联用或不联用血浆置换是脱敏方案的主要组成部分。IVIG是指正常多克隆多特异性Ig的商业制剂，主要由从数千个健康供者来源的血浆库制备的IgG同种型抗体组成。IVIG由超过97%的IgG分子组成，其中IgG1、IgG2、IgG3和IgG4同种型的比例与人血清相当。制剂含有针对外来(非自身)抗原、自身抗原(天然自身抗体)和其他抗体(独特型抗体)的抗体。

已经提出了几种非互斥机制来解释IVIG在患者中的有益效果。没有一种被证明在所有环境中都有效,并且很可能在IVIG的有益效果中都发挥一定作用。

1.抗独特型抗体的设计[17,18]。抗独特型抗体是对另一抗体的抗原结合部分具有特异性的抗体。当结合时,这些抗体抑制其靶抗体的有效性。

2. IVIG对细胞功能的影响。施用的IgG的一些有益效果延长到超过其半衰期，表明这些作用不仅仅是由于被动清除或与致病抗体的竞争。这些观察提出IVIG治疗导致免疫系统的细胞区室的显著改变的可能性[17,19,20]。最近几项观察研究强调了IVIG治疗对树突状细胞、单核细胞/巨噬细胞系统、粒细胞、自然杀伤细胞和各种T细胞亚群，特别是调节性T细胞(Treg)亚群和B细胞的影响。

3.补体片段的清除。IgG分子与潜在有害的补体片段(C3b、C4b、C2a和C5a)的结合阻断这些片段沉积到其靶抗体,并防止随后的免疫损伤[21-24]。

4.唾液酸化IgG的免疫调节。Ravetch等人提出[25],IVIG的有益效果主要由在IgG的恒定Fc链的297位置(Asn 297)处与天冬酰胺连接的聚糖处具有末端唾液酸的抗体的部分介导。通过增强抑制性IgG Fc受体,ⅡB的表达,富含这些含唾液酸抗体的IVIG的部分显示出抗炎作用，酶促去除唾液酸残基消除了该抗炎作用。最近的数据表明,IVIG的抗炎特性可以用适当唾液酸化的IgG Fc片段的完全重组制备[26]。这些和其他类似的机制可能涉及维持一般免疫球蛋白稳态的方法。

这些研究结果表明已经在了解 IVIG 的作用机制方面取得了相当大的进展，并且可能影响器官移植中 Ig 治疗领域的未来前景。

血浆置换和免疫吸附

血浆置换(PP)和免疫吸附(IA)是分别用于去除血浆蛋白和特异性蛋白质类似于同种抗体的技术。这些疗法的终点是在移植前后消除 HLA 供者特异性抗体。PP 并非特异性地去除 Ig,其可导致所有血浆蛋白(包括凝血因子)的降低,并且需要用新鲜冷冻的血浆和白蛋白替换。IA 包括琼脂糖结合的葡萄球菌蛋白 A 柱，对结合所有 IgG 具有高亲和力,而不仅仅是针对同种抗体。抗 HLA 抗体滴度反弹并在 PP 或 IA 完成后回到基线水平[27]。这涉及用于调节生理性 Ig 水平的一般体内平衡机制，使得生理学上的低 Ig 水平实际上可以促进抗体产生。因此，这些技术不会导致 HLA 抗体的持久减少,除非患者在最后一次治疗后的几天内进行移植。

一些研究表明,紧急移植前 IA 可能会导致致敏的尸体供体异体肾移植受体中补体依赖细胞毒性交叉匹配由阳性转为阴性,从而允许移植。然而,这种经验仍然非常有限。1996 年,Higgins 等人首次进行了移植前紧急使用 IA 的研究,针对 12 例细胞毒性或流式细胞术交叉匹配阳性患者，排斥率 (9 例患者发生了 13 次排斥)以及移植物失功率(26.8 个月时为 53.8%)较高[28]。此后,Lorenz 等人报道了更好的结果。针对 40 例尸体供体异体肾移植受体的结果，包括 9 例通过单次移植前 IA 使交叉匹配阳性转阴性的患者。在交叉匹配阳性和交叉匹配阴性的患者中,3 年移植物存活率 (78%比 71%)、急性排斥反应(11%比 20%)和 C4d 阳性移植物功能障碍(33%比 32%)都是相当的[29]。

利妥昔单抗的争论

对器官移植中 B 细胞和抗体的新的关注刺激了新药的研究。利妥昔单抗是一种嵌合鼠/人单克隆抗体，与 CD20 抗原反应并选择性消耗 B 细胞[30]。表面蛋白 CD20 在幼稚和记忆 B 细胞上表达，在活化的 B 细胞中快速下调，并且在前 B 细胞和浆细胞上不存在[31,32]。因此,利妥昔单抗对抗体分泌细胞没有直接影响。

该药物最初由 FDA 批准用于治疗难治性或复发性 B 细胞淋巴瘤，并且已经广泛用于实体器官移植领域中的 ABO 血型不相容移植[33,34]、排斥治疗[35,36]及其预防[37]和脱敏方案[10,38-40]。不幸的是,描述利妥昔单抗用于移植的研究的规模较小,通常无对照。这是关键点,并且在脱敏方案中添加利妥昔单抗的价值仍然受到质疑。

利妥昔单抗可能通过两种潜在的方法在脱敏方案中起作用[41]:

1.利妥昔单抗可能耗尽特定的抗供体抗体,尽管这种情况发生的机制是未知的。这种效果的数据是稀少的。在一项小型 1 期研究中,应用单剂量利妥昔单抗治疗 9 例致敏的透析患者，只有 1 例患者的活体捐赠者的特异性交叉匹配转化为阴性，并成功接受了肾移植[39]。在大多数患者中,群体反应性抗体水平或抗体特异性没有显著降低。在使用单抗原珠的更详细分析中，Pescovitz 发现在利妥昔单抗治疗后特异性滴度较低的下降可能性更大[38]。其他研究已经证明,用于抗体介导的排斥(ABMR)的利妥昔单抗治疗与多种其他治疗的联合导致供体特异性抗体减少或消失[36,42]。利妥昔单抗的使用据说可干扰 B 细胞的流式细胞交叉匹配和补体依赖细胞毒性交叉匹配[11]。

2.利妥昔单抗可以通过消除 B 细胞起作用,并且这样做可阻断 B 细胞的非抗体分泌功能,如抗原呈递。支持 B 细胞在排斥中的直接作用是 Sarwal 等人的结论,其显示 CD20 基因表达和 $CD20^+$ 浸润与不良预后相关[43]。具有 CD20 阳性排斥的受试者的移植物长期存活率更低[44]。应用利妥昔单抗治疗这些患者是成功的[45]。

这两个理念都是有问题的。首先,抗 CD20 活性对长寿 $CD138^+$浆细胞没有影响,而这是急性抗体产生的主要来源[46,47]。其次,利妥昔单抗对循环抗体水平没有即时或强大的影响。这些问题可以解释当利妥昔单抗单药治疗时评估其功效的困难。然而,与包括 IVIG 和(或)多克隆兔抗胸腺细胞球蛋白的其他治疗联合使用可以构成管理同种致敏的改良方法。这些组合方案可以减少长寿浆细胞的抗体分泌和数量。利妥昔单抗可能减少或消除沉默静息幼稚和记忆性同种反应性 B 细胞以及早期记忆反应的短寿命 $CD20^+$活化浆母细胞。

新型药物

两种新药正在考虑用于高致敏性患者的移植前管理。两者都属于药品核准标示外使用(参见第 101 章),因此在常规效能的随机试验中均未显示有效。

硼替佐米是一种蛋白酶体抑制剂，其针对所有具有高水平蛋白质翻转的细胞，包括浆细胞。该药物被FDA批准用于多发性骨髓瘤患者，并且传闻证据表明通过许多机制对移植患者有效[48]。硼替佐米的免疫调节作用包括对正常浆细胞的活性，如动物模型[49-51]所示，以及诱导正常人浆细胞凋亡以阻止同种抗体的产生[52]。此外，蛋白酶体抑制剂已显示出抑制T细胞功能[53]和抑制抗原呈递细胞的功能[54,55]。

在移植的环境中，硼替佐米已被用于急性ABMR的一线治疗[56]或挽救策略[48]。硼替佐米还被用于在急性排斥之外消除HLA特异性抗体，以试图改善移植物的长期存活率[57]。所有这些临床经验突出了硼替佐米快速降低抗体水平(通过Luminex测定法)的能力。在这些基于蛋白酶体抑制剂的治疗中，硼替佐米与PP联用。由于PP提供了能消除先前筛选的抗体的优点，由此循环抗体水平更准确地反映了残留浆细胞群的当前产生速率，而不是硼替佐米治疗之前的抗体产生速率[56]。这些考虑导致了关于评估硼替佐米在脱敏过程中的功效的前瞻性临床试验的建议，如Woodle及其同事(俄亥俄州辛辛那提大学)所提出的。硼替佐米的严重副作用的发生率，最值得注意的是神经性副作用，也必须在数量有意义的移植前患者中探讨。

依库丽单抗是针对补体蛋白C5的人源化单克隆抗体，是另一种正在研究的药物。通过作用于补体级联的终端组分，依库丽单抗作用于储存抗体的继发效应，因此本身不依赖于抗体清除。在急性ABMR的预致敏小鼠模型中，C5阻断与常规免疫抑制联合显示可以防止抗体介导的移植物损伤，延长移植物存活期[58]。正如Mayo Clinic小组提出的，末端补体激活对ABMR的发展至关重要。依库丽单抗降低了致敏移植受者中早期急性ABMR的风险。急性ABMR的发生率从对照组(51例接受基于血浆置换的方案而非依库丽单抗治疗的致敏患者)的41.2%下降到治疗组(26例依库丽单抗治疗的致敏患者)的7.7%[59]。

成功脱敏方案的入选标准

脱敏方案准入标准以及脱敏方案完成后接受供体的标准是各不相同的。这反映了在移植前评估免疫风险的概念的发展。当前，用于定义这种风险的技术不同于经典的补体依赖性细胞毒交叉匹配和T细胞抗体球蛋白增强的补体依赖性细胞毒测定，而是发展为更敏感的固相测定技术，其中基于Luminex的测定是最常用的(详见第36章)。虽然这些测定中更先进的是定量的潜力，但是目前它们仅被批准为定性测定，并且这实质上限制了临床医生客观确定患者ABMR风险的能力。

在尸体供体脱敏方案的第一次实施中，准入和成功标准完全基于细胞毒性测试：细胞毒性PRA>50%或80%作为准入标准，并且交叉匹配阴性的患者才有资格接受肾移植[7,8]。对于活体供体，脱敏治疗的目标是在移植前将交叉匹配转换为阴性[9]。

近年来，移植准入的政策已经取得进展，且供体HLA特异性抗体的交叉匹配强度在较低的反应性水平上稳定：对补体细胞毒性测定的效价<1:8[12]或T细胞供体特异性流式细胞术交叉匹配<250平均流道位移[11]。约翰·霍普金斯关于活体肾移植的经验清楚地揭示了这一概念。在本研究中，HLA不相容性的定义包括三种非重叠类型的抗体强度：阳性补体依赖性细胞毒性或流式细胞术交叉匹配或仅在Luminex测定中可检测的供体特异性抗HLA抗体。所有三类HLA不相容的生存获益与脱敏相关。这项研究还表明，供体特异性水平的增加是移植物存活率降低的预测因素：在串珠测定中阳性结果的患者具有最短的随访期，在48个月时的存活率为90.8%；在流式细胞术交叉匹配阳性的脱敏患者中，1年存活率为92.2%，3年为85.5%，8年为79.8%，在补体依赖性细胞毒测定中交叉匹配阳性的脱敏患者中分别为87.7%、82%和78%[12]。其他研究显示，急性ABMR的风险与脱敏后供体特异性抗体水平之间存在强相关性，由通过流式细胞仪交叉匹配的平均流道位移和Luminex测定的平均荧光强度来定义[60,61]。

特异性脱敏方案

目前存在三种临床功效已经被证明的脱敏方案：①大剂量IVIG；②利妥昔单抗联合大剂量IVIG(R/IVIG)；③血浆置换术(或免疫吸附)联合低剂量IVIG(PP/IVIG)。目前还没有比较其临床疗效的随机前瞻性研究。此外，迄今为止来自各种研究的数据难以进行解释或比较，这是由包括脱敏方案、组织相容性测试技术、供体特异性抗HLA抗体水平以及供体和受体人群的人口统计学和临床特征的准入标准和成功标准的异质性所致(表68.1)。

主要出于逻辑原因，脱敏方案的选择依赖于供体的来源，即活体或尸体供体。在活体供体情况下，一旦抗体水平的降低达到预期就可以进行移植，联用 PP/IVIG 是首选的治疗方案，无论是否加入利妥昔单抗。当在必须等待死亡供体的未知时间段里时，首选单独使用大剂量 IVIG 或与利妥昔单抗联用，因为抗体水平降低的时间段更长，因此与等待器官的时间段匹配。

大剂量 IVIG 方案

大剂量 IVIG 方案适用于活体和尸体移植，该方法的主要优点是适用于尸体供体肾移植候选人。它包括每个月 2g/kg 体重的 IVIG，直到交叉匹配被认为是安全的或完全阴性的[7,8,18]。

大剂量 IVIG 方案的效果由 1997—2000 年由 NIH（NIH IG02 研究）进行的随机多中心安慰剂对照试验得以证明[8]。该研究是脱敏治疗唯一的对照临床试验，旨在确定 IVIG 是否可在难以移植组中降低 PRA 水平并改善移植率，增加移植物失功的风险。IVIG 在降低 HLA 特异性抗体水平和改善移植速率方面优于安慰剂（图 68.1）。3 年随访显示，IVIG 组的预计平均移植等待时间为 4.8 年，而安慰剂组为 10.3 年（P=0.02）。移植后 2 年的中位随访时间里，存活的移植物的平均血清肌

表 68.1　已报道的脱敏方案及其临床结果的总结

作者/年份	患者人数	供体类型	CXM 技术	诱导药物	平均随访时间（月）	AR/ABMR（%）	患者存活率	移植物存活率
移植前 IA								
Higgins 1996[28]	13	尸体	CDC; FCXM	Thymo	26	69/–	92	54
Lorenz 2005[29]	40	尸体	CDC	Thymo	CXM 阳性	44/33	–	78
					(n=9)32	52/32	–	71
					CXM 阴性			
					(n=31)34			
PP/低剂量 IVIG								
Schweitzer 2000[63]	11	活体	CDC	OKT3	13	36/27	100	100
Montgomery 2000[68]	4	活体	CDC	达利珠单抗	14	100/100	100	100
Gloor 2003[64]	14	活体	CDC	Thymo/利妥昔单抗/SPL	15	43/43	86	78
Magee 2008[65]	28	活体	CDC	Thymo/巴利昔单抗/利妥昔单抗	22	71/39	93	89
Thielke 2009[66]	51	活体	FCXM	Thymo/利妥昔单抗	23	33/24	95	93
Haririan 2009[67]	41	活体	FCXM	OKT3 或 Thymo	47	24/12	78	66
Montgomery 2011[12]	211	活体	CDC;FCXM	达利珠单抗或 Thymo	96	–	81	–
高剂量 IVIG								
Glotz 2002[7]	13	尸体	CDC	Thymo	12	8/8	85	85
Jordan 2003[18]	42	尸体，活体	CDC	达利珠单抗 24	31/31	98	89	
Jordan 2004[8]	17	尸体，活体	CDC		24	53/–	76	80
Vo 2006[62]	97	尸体，活体	CDC	达利珠单抗（n=58）	24	36/22	96	84
				Thymo（n=39）	24	31/21	100	90
高剂量 IVIG/利妥昔单抗								
Vo 2008[11]	16	尸体，活体	CDC;FCXM	阿仑单抗	12	50/31	100	94
Vo 2010[95]	76	尸体，活体	CDC;FCXM	阿仑单抗	24	37/29	95	84
高剂量 IVIG 比 PP/低剂量 IVIG/利妥昔单抗								
Stegall 2006[10]	59	活体	CDC	Thymo	12			82

CXM，细胞毒交叉匹配；FCXM，流式细胞术交叉匹配；CDC，补体依赖性细胞毒性；AR，急性排斥反应；ABMR，抗体介导的排斥；IA，免疫吸附；IVIG，静脉注射免疫球蛋白；PP，血浆置换；SPL，脾切除术；Thymo，抗胸腺细胞球蛋白。

酐为 1.68±0.28(IVIG),而安慰剂组为 1.28±0.13mg/dL(P=0.29)。IVIG 组 3 年的移植物存活率也较高。从这项多中心双盲安慰剂对照试验中,我们得出结论,IVIG 在减少 HLA 特异性抗体水平和改善高致敏性终末期肾病患者的移植率方面优于安慰剂。

脱敏患者的急性排斥反应率仍然很高(35%~50%)。虽然观察到更多急性的 ABMR 发作(20%~38%),3 年同种异体移植存活率令人满意:在法国经验中为 78%,在 NIH IG02 研究中为 80%[7,8]。作者没有报道供体特异性 HLA 特异性抗体的特异性和强度。

高剂量 IVIG 方案中诱导治疗使用抗胸腺细胞球蛋白[7]或达利珠单抗[18],两者具有类似的结果。诱导治疗的效果并不明显,如西达-赛奈中心的经验所示,其诱导治疗从达利珠单抗转换为抗胸腺细胞球蛋白[62]。达利珠单抗组(58 例)和抗胸腺细胞组(39 例)的 2 年移植存活率分别为 84%和 90%,而急性排斥率分别为 36%(22%为 ABMR)和 31%(21%为 ABMR)。

利妥昔单抗联合大剂量 IVIG 方案

西达-赛奈中心组在每月 IVIG 方案(第 0 天和 30 天 2g/kg 体重)中给予两次(第 7 天和第 22 天分别给予 1g)的利妥昔单抗,在 20 例患者中达到 80%的移植率,1 年时患者和移植物存活率为 94%[11]。然而,急性排斥率非常高(50%),其中 31%为 ABMR。

PRA 的减少类似于 NIH IG02 研究,并且仍不清楚利妥昔单抗是否在 IVIG 方案中起作用(图 68.2)。

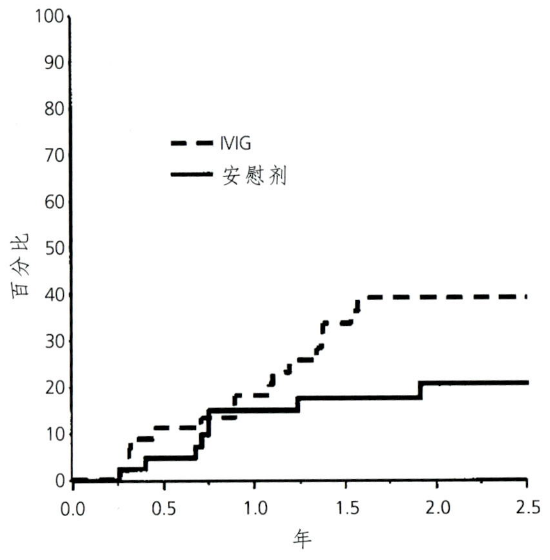

图 68.1 移植前的累积时间。与安慰剂相比,经静脉注射免疫球蛋白(IVIG)显著(P<0.05)缩短移植前时间。IVIG 组的移植率是安慰剂组的两倍,在再次移植的受体中两者差距更大。(Source:Jordan et al. 2004[8]。Reproduced with permission of Massachusetts Medical Society.)

血浆置换联合低剂量 IVIG 方案

该方案使抗 HLA 滴度的快速降低,其允许在 3~5 次 PP 治疗后移植,这取决于移植前 HLA 特异性抗体的强度。添加低剂量 IVIG 增加了免疫调节效应机制,其可能有利于保持抗体低滴度。

1998 年,PP /低剂量 IVIG 方案首先在约翰霍普金斯医院应用,其用于交叉匹配不相容的活体供体肾移植候选人[9]。患者在移植后 2~3 周开始,在每个 PP 之后给予 100mg/kg PP 和 IVIG 以及他克莫司和霉酚酸酯。根据对患者 ABMR 风险的评估,治疗计划是个体化的[9]。Montgomery 等人报道了他们一项长达 11 年的大型的囊括 211 个活体捐赠者的研究经验。他们清楚地证明相比等待相容器官,脱敏后的活体供体移植为 HLA 致敏的患者提供了显著的生存获益。到 8 年时,生存率优势增加了一倍(80.6%比仅透析组的患者的 30.5%)[12](图 68.3)。

类似的 PP /低剂量基于 IVIG 的脱敏方案被其他几个团队使用[63-67]。在这些研究中,诱导治疗是极富异质性的,包括达利珠单抗[68]、OKT3[63]或抗胸腺细胞球蛋白/巴利昔单抗和利妥昔单抗[65,66],或与利妥昔单抗和脾切除相关的抗胸腺细胞[64]。尽管做了这些改变,排斥率仍然较高(33%~100%),但短期移植物存活良好,移

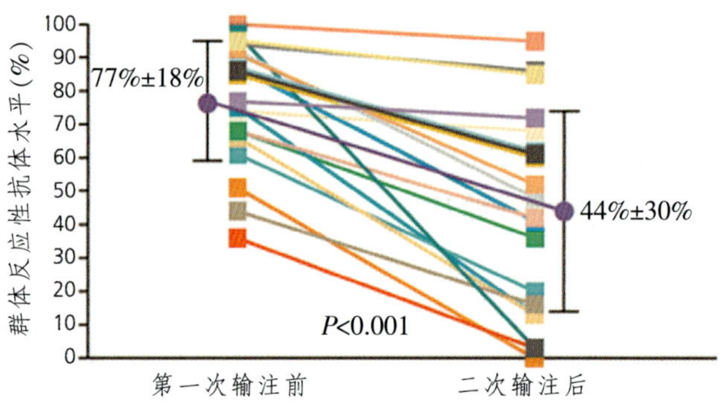

图 68.2 群体反应性抗体水平。显示了第一次经静脉输注免疫球蛋白之前和第二次输注后患者的个体数据。还显示了预处理和后处理方法,如用 T 细胞补体依赖性细胞毒性群体反应性抗体测定所确定。平均值显著性差异(P<0.001)。条表示标准偏差。(Source:Vo et al. 2008 [11]. Reproduced with permission of Massachusetts Medical Society.)

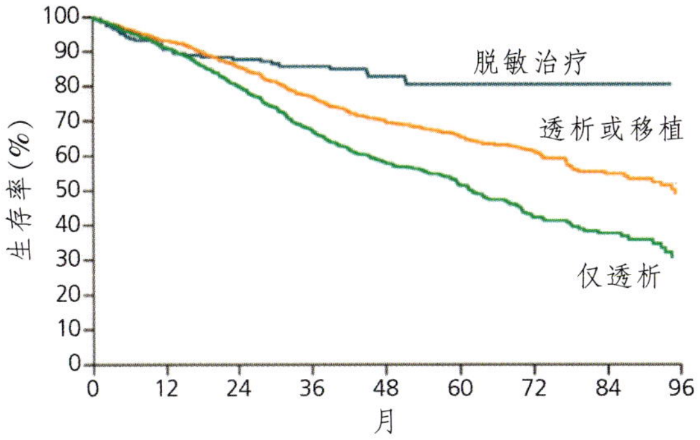

风险患者数量

脱敏治疗	210	170	143	110	75	58	42	28	14
双重疗法	1027	854	688	497	321	230	157	96	41
仅透析	1012	822	626	419	250	159	93	54	17

图 68.3　HLA 不相容肾脏受体的存活率。Kaplan-Meier 患者存活率评估显示了在肾移植之前接受脱敏治疗的患者（治疗组），与肾脏等候名单上的持续接受透析（仅透析组）及继续进行透析或进行 HLA 相容性移植（透析或移植或双重疗法组）的两个匹配对照组患者的存活率。(Source：Montgomery et al. 2011[12]。Reproduced with permission of Massachusetts Medical Society.)

植后 2 年存活率为 78%~100%。马里兰大学报道了其在使用 PP /低剂量 IVIG 与 OKT3 或抗胸腺细胞球蛋白诱导治疗治疗 41 例流式细胞术交叉匹配阳性患者的长期经验。与上述研究相比，患者的急性 ABMR 较低(12%)，但患者 4 年生存率和移植物存活率分别为 78%和 66%[67]。要点见框 68.2。

脱敏方案的安全性

静脉免疫球蛋白的特异性副作用

有许多 IVIG 产品具有产品特异性副作用，这取决于个体制剂的渗透压、pH 值和钠或糖含量。西达-赛奈小组表示，他们检查了 279 例脱敏患者的 IVIG 副作用[69]，大多数患者对 IVIG 的不良反应轻微，包括头痛、恶心、肌痛、背痛和血压升高，这些都可以通过降低输注速率或用抗组胺药物预处理来解决。已报道的 IVIG 罕见严重副作用包括：抗体介导的(Coombs 阳性)溶血[70]、急性无菌性脑膜炎[71]和急性肾衰竭(ARF)。IVIG 输注后 ARF 已知的主要机制是与含蔗糖制剂相关的近端肾小管上皮的渗透损伤。血栓性事件如急性心肌梗死、深静脉血栓形成和卒中与高渗透压有关，并且可以通过预防性抗凝来解决。IgA 缺乏的患者可能发生严重过敏反应，这是非常罕见的。

框 68.2　要点：脱敏方案

- 通过免疫吸附或血浆置换去除 DSA，使用大剂量经静脉免疫球蛋白的 DSA 失活是脱敏治疗的主体，其具有良好的短期至中期效果。
- 添加利妥昔单抗的价值仍有争议。
- 使用补体阻断以预防抗体介导的同种异体移植物损伤的新干预措施，或使用蛋白酶体抑制剂介导的浆细胞耗竭的 DSA 合成抑制似乎很有前景。应用蛋白酶体抑制剂硼替佐米正成为一种潜在的新策略。

血浆置换相关的不良事件

约翰·霍普金斯小组评估了经 PP/IVIG 方案(215 例)脱敏的最大队列活体移植患者的 PP 相关不良事件[12]：轻微反应(10.9%)；主要事件包括伴有低血压和气道水肿的过敏反应 (1.4%)；手术部位出血或活检后出血，因为 PP 消耗凝血因子，其中一些可能与 PP 相关。

感染和恶性肿瘤的风险

脱敏患者比非致敏患者接受更多的免疫抑制，这混淆了脱敏方案的任何组成部分与感染风险的直接关联。无论如何，脱敏方法的总体影响之一是大量的免疫抑制，而且其必须与透析和未能进行移植的风险相平衡。

进行性多发性脑白质病(PML)的发展是由潜伏性 JC 多瘤病毒的再活化引起的。FDA 和 WHO 发布安全警告，描述了应用利妥昔单抗治疗的系统性红斑狼疮患者的 PML 病例。在肾移植患者中没有归因于利妥昔单抗的病例报道[72]。

类风湿关节炎和淋巴瘤治疗的对照临床试验已经证明利妥昔单抗的安全性，而感染率没有显著增加[73,74]。此外，关于脱敏患者的三项研究中报道的感染发病率并未超过移植患者平均值[11,66,75]。Kamar 等[76]报道了使用利妥昔单抗和移植后感染相关性死亡风险显著增加(利妥昔单抗治疗组为 9.1%，回顾性对照组为 1.6%)，其关联令人不安。然而，在该报道中给出的利妥昔单抗的剂量比脱敏方案中使用的剂量高 4 倍。

总之，严重的感染并发症可能发生在脱敏方案治疗后。应该考虑病毒聚合酶链反应(PCR)监测，特别是那些接受除利妥昔单抗外改变 T 细胞功能的药物治疗的患者[77]。与其他免疫抑制剂一样，必须寻找最有效和安全的剂量。

针对 ABO 血型抗体屏障的肾移植脱敏方案

在肾移植中使用 ABO-血型不相容的供体已经不是一种新情况[78],其由 Guy Alexander 开创并随后在日本得到发展，后者由缺乏脑死亡的定义及其所产生的 ABO 相容性供体短缺所驱动。一般来说,由 ABO 特异性抗体呈现的屏障似乎在质量上不如由 HLA 特异性抗体呈现的屏障强大。1989—2005 年间,日本进行了超过 850 例来自活体捐献者的 ABO 血型不相容肾移植[79],并获得了优异的短期和长期结果,目前 1 年移植物存活率超过 95%。

常用的脱敏方案与用于 HLA 不相容移植的方案几乎没有不同,并且基于使用 PP 或 IA 的抗体去除[34],以及最初通过脾切除术实现而现在由利妥昔单抗替代的抗体再合成预防联合常规免疫抑制。多年来,免疫抑制方案已经改变，对移植前 PP 的实施数量加以限制,使用利妥昔单抗替代脾切除术[80],并停止移植后 PP,从而限制了免疫抑制的总量而没有增加排斥率。

ABO 不相容移植后的急性 ABMR 发生率为 15%~33%[81,82],并对移植物存活有负面影响。所有方案都基于通过 PP 或最近的 IA 的移植前抗体去除[34]。然而,极高的血浆凝集素滴度可能需要多次的 PP,与体液排斥的高发病率相关[83],并且可能出现禁忌证[84]。

在北美中心的调查中,80%使用血浆置换和 IVIG 的组合[85]。从这些移植中获得了两个开创性的观察结果:①血浆凝集素(即抗供体抗体)的移植前滴度不需要降至零,表明尽管存在低水平的抗供体抗体,仍可进行成功的移植;此外,排斥的风险以及移植物存活与移植前血浆凝集素水平密切相关[81,86],这一发现也存在于 HLA 不相容的移植物中;②尽管抗供体抗体持续存在,但长期移植物仍然可以实现功能良好并且没有组织学损伤,这是一种适应性现象[87],但在 HLA 不相容移植中有待验证。

总结:脱敏方案中的突出问题

关于脱敏方案的恰当部署仍然存在许多问题。这些已经在最近由 FDA 赞助的 ABMR 研讨会上得到了总结[88]。

谁能够获益于脱敏方案?

所有公开的方案都基于细胞测定选择其患者,即用于活体移植的阳性交叉匹配测定（细胞毒性或通过流式细胞术）或用于尸体移植的高细胞毒性群体反应性抗体。然而,在尸体供体等待名单上的患者的移植准入在许多国家(如美国或法国)依赖于 CPRA(计算的群体反应性抗体),基于通过 Luminex 测定禁止的 HLA 抗原的定义[15,16]。不幸的是,越来越多的患者仅通过新型高度敏感的技术如 Luminex 测定来免疫，几乎没有细胞毒性群体反应性抗体。这些患者可能具有高 CPRA,从而阻止他们接受移植却不能参加基于细胞毒性试验的规范脱敏方案。因此,我们需要重新评估脱敏方案的准入标准，并基于目前的敏化测量技术和用于检测 HLA 特异性抗体的敏感技术。

移植前免疫学风险评估：阈值是重要的且在不可接受的抗原方面又意味着什么?

固相抗体测试方法如 Luminex 技术对禁止抗原的定义还没有达成共识。至于临床相关性,我们已经了解到，仅仅存在仅由 Luminex 单一抗原检测的针对供体(供体特异性抗体或 DSA）的给定 HLA 特异性抗体不再是移植的禁忌,因为尽管存在这些抗体,但移植物存活率仍然优良[88-90]。因此,定量方法是强制的,但是目前每个实验室已经定义了自己的平均荧光强度（MFI)阈值来定义禁止抗原,范围为 500~3000。在我们的机构,我们回顾性研究了 402 例在 T 细胞细胞毒交叉匹配阴性后进行的尸体供体移植[91]。在其中 83 例患者中,使用 Luminex 单一抗原测定法检测出了 DSA。尽管急性体液排斥反应的发生率随着 DSA 的 MFI 增加而显著增加,但 3000 的 MFI 阈值与移植物失功增加相关。我们今后几年的主要挑战是对排斥和移植物损失的免疫风险精确分级，考虑可接受和禁止抗原的临床相关定义,进而精确评估移植的可行性,最终获得真正需要脱敏方案的患者群体的最佳定义。

等待名单管理的积极政策需求

从我们的观点来看，患者在等待过长时间（5~10年)后转向脱敏方案是一种不可接受的方法。我们需要预测高度致敏的患者移植的可能性，以便早期识别能从脱敏方案中获益的患者[16]。模拟程序应该允许我们检查国家分配系统是否为这些高度致敏患者提供了现实的移植可能性。我们需要在其进入等待名单时尽早确定哪些患者没有足够的捐助者，并且不会从国家优先程序中受益，以便为其分配特定的脱敏方案。

将配对捐赠整合到脱敏方案中

难以匹配并难以脱敏的非常广泛致敏并具有高HLA反应性的患者，可以通过联用肾脏配对供体(KPD)及脱敏治疗进行移植，以在KPD池中发现低免疫风险供体，从而增加脱敏的实用性和成功率。然后可以将KPD和脱敏治疗作为互补形式来合理地做出关于特定供体/受体表型的最佳移植选择的决定。

脱敏患者移植物长期存活的挑战

施用目前用于脱敏的预处理方案，其近期目标是防止急性抗体介导的损伤。然而，目前可清楚地认识到，预先形成DSA的患者不仅存在急性或加速ABMR的风险，而且还存在移植功能恢复延迟和在没有临床ABMR的情况下发生移植物长期存活受损事件的风险[91]。这些研究已经导致冰山的“水下”部分的发现，代表导致慢性体液排斥和晚期移植物失功的病变的进展[92-94]。主要问题是，我们如何防止或阻止这种抗体介导的损伤的进展？因此，脱敏方案后的移植受体需要具有单独的具有互补目的的移植前和移植后干预。

(陈峻 译 徐骁 校)

参考文献

1. Evans RW, Manninen DL, Garrison LP Jr, et al. The quality of life of patients with end-stage renal disease. New England Journal of Medicine. 1985;312:553–559.
2. Port FK, Wolfe RA, Mauger EA, et al. Comparison of survival probabilities for dialysis patients vs cadaveric renal transplant recipients. JAMA. 1993;270:1339–1343.
3. Russell JD, Beecroft ML, Ludwin D, et al. The quality of life in renal transplantation–a prospective study. Transplantation. 1992;54:656–660.
4. Organ Procurement and Transplantation Network. Scientific Registry of Transplant Recipients. Accessed Jan., 2014. Available at: http://optn.transplant.hrsa.gov/.
5. Agence de la Biomédecine. Rapport annuel de l'Agence de la biomédecine 2012. 2013 Accessed Jan., 2014. Available at: http://www.agence-biomedecine.fr/rapport-annuel2012.
6. Garcia GG, Harden P, Chapman J. The global role of kidney transplantation. Lancet. 2012;379:e36–38.
7. Glotz D, Antoine C, Julia P, et al. Desensitization and subsequent kidney transplantation of patients using intravenous immunoglobulins (IVIg). American Journal of Transplantation. 2002;2:758–760.
8. Jordan SC, Tyan D, Stablein D, et al. Evaluation of intravenous immunoglobulin as an agent to lower allosensitization and improve transplantation in highly sensitized adult patients with end-stage renal disease: report of the NIH IG02 trial. Journal of the American Society of Nephrology. 2004;15:3256–3262.
9. Montgomery RA, Zachary AA. Transplanting patients with a positive donor-specific crossmatch: a single center's perspective. Pediatric Transplantation. 2004;8:535–542.
10. Stegall MD, Gloor J, Winters JL, et al. A comparison of plasmapheresis versus high-dose IVIG desensitization in renal allograft recipients with high levels of donor specific alloantibody. American Journal of Transplantation. 2006;6:346–351.
11. Vo AA, Lukovsky M, Toyoda M, et al. Rituximab and intravenous immune globulin for desensitization during renal transplantation. New England Journal of Medicine. 2008;359:242–251.
12. Montgomery RA, Lonze BE, King KE, et al. Desensitization in HLA-incompatible kidney recipients and survival. New England Journal of Medicine. 2011;365:318–326.
13. Gebel HM, Bray RA, Nickerson P. Pre-transplant assessment of donor-reactive, HLA-specific antibodies in renal transplantation: contraindication vs. risk. American Journal of Transplantation. 2003;3:1488–1500.
14. Cecka JM. Calculated PRA (CPRA): the new measure of sensitization for transplant candidates. American Journal of Transplantation. 2010;10:26–29.
15. Cecka JM, Kucheryavaya AY, Reinsmoen NL, et al. Calculated PRA: initial results show benefits for sensitized patients and a reduction in positive crossmatches. American Journal of Transplantation. 2011;11:719–724.
16. Lefaucheur C, Antoine C, Suberbielle C, et al. Mastering the risk of HLA antibodies in kidney transplantation: an algorithm based on pretransplant single-antigen flow bead techniques. American Journal of Transplantation. 2011;11:1592–1598.
17. Kazatchkine MD, Kaveri SV. Immunomodulation of autoimmune and inflammatory diseases with intravenous immune globulin. New England Journal of Medicine. 2001;345:747–755.
18. Jordan SC, Vo A, Bunnapradist S, et al. Intravenous immune globulin treatment inhibits crossmatch positivity and allows for successful transplantation of incompatible organs in living-donor and cadaver recipients. Transplantation. 2003;76:631–636.
19. Nimmerjahn F, Ravetch JV. Anti-inflammatory actions of intravenous immunoglobulin. Annual Review of Immunology. 2008;26:513–533.
20. Conley ME, Dobbs AK, Farmer DM, et al. Primary B cell immunodeficiencies: comparisons and contrasts. Annual Review of Immunology. 2009;27:199–227.
21. Basta M, Langlois PF, Marques M, et al. High-dose intravenous immunoglobulin modifies complement-mediated in vivo clearance. Blood. 1989;74:326–333.
22. Basta M, Kirshbom P, Frank MM, et al. Mechanism of therapeutic effect of high-dose intravenous immunoglobulin. Attenuation of acute, complement-dependent immune damage in a guinea pig model. Journal of Clinical Investigation. 1989;84:1974–1981.
23. Basta M. Modulation of complement-mediated immune damage by intravenous immune globulin. Clinical and Experimental Immunology. 1996;104(Suppl. 1):21–25.
24. Basta M, Van Goor F, Luccioli S, et al. F(ab)′2-mediated neutralization of C3a and C5a anaphylatoxins: a novel effector function of immunoglobulins. Nature Medicine. 2003;9:431–438.
25. Samuelsson A, Towers TL, Ravetch JV. Anti-inflammatory activity of IVIG mediated through the inhibitory Fc receptor. Science. 2001;291:484–486.
26. Anthony RM, Nimmerjahn F, Ashline DJ, et al. Recapitulation of IVIG anti-inflammatory activity with a recombinant IgG Fc. Science. 2008;320:373–376.
27. Hakim RM, Milford E, Himmelfarb J, et al. Extracorporeal removal of anti-HLA antibodies in transplant candidates. American Journal of Kidney Diseases. 1990;16:423–431.
28. Higgins RM, Bevan DJ, Carey BS, et al. Prevention of hyperacute rejection by removal of antibodies to HLA immediately before renal transplantation. Lancet. 1996;348:1208–1211.
29. Lorenz M, Regele H, Schillinger M, et al. Peritransplant immunoadsorption: a strategy enabling transplantation in highly sensitized crossmatch-positive cadaveric kidney allograft recipients. Transplantation. 2005;79:696–701.
30. Reff ME, Carner K, Chambers KS, et al. Depletion of B cells in vivo by a chimeric mouse human monoclonal antibody to CD20. Blood. 1994;83:435–445.
31. Loken MR, Shah VO, Dattilio KL, et al. Flow cytometric analysis of human bone marrow. II. Normal B lymphocyte development. Blood. 1987;70:1316–1324.
32. Zand MS, Vo T, Huggins J, et al. Polyclonal rabbit antithymocyte globulin triggers B-cell and plasma cell apoptosis by multiple pathways. Transplantation. 2005;79:1507–1515.
33. Sonnenday CJ, Warren DS, Cooper M, et al. Plasmapheresis, CMV hyperimmune globulin, and anti-CD20 allow ABO-incompatible renal transplantation without splenectomy. American Journal of Transplantation. 2004;4:1315–1322.
34. Tyden G, Kumlien G, Genberg H, et al. ABO incompatible kidney transplantations without splenectomy, using antigen-specific immunoadsorption and rituximab. American Journal of Transplantation. 2005;5:145–148.
35. Becker YT, Becker BN, Pirsch JD, et al. Rituximab as treatment for refractory kidney transplant rejection. American Journal of Transplantation. 2004;4:996–1001.

36. Lefaucheur C, Nochy D, Andrade J, et al. Comparison of combination Plasmapheresis/IVIg/anti-CD20 versus high-dose IVIg in the treatment of antibody-mediated rejection. American Journal of Transplantation. 2009;9: 1099–1107.
37. Loupy A, Suberbielle-Boissel C, Zuber J, et al. Combined posttransplant prophylactic IVIg/anti-CD 20/plasmapheresis in kidney recipients with preformed donor-specific antibodies: a pilot study. Transplantation. 2010;89:1403–1410.
38. Pescovitz M, Book B, Rahman A, et al. Measurement of HLA antibody specificity by single antigen beads and MESF quatitation demonstrates efficacy of rituximab desensitization. American Journal of Transplantation. 2005;5(Suppl. 11):324.
39. Vieira CA, Agarwal A, Book BK, et al. Rituximab for reduction of anti-HLA antibodies in patients awaiting renal transplantation: 1. Safety, pharmacodynamics, and pharmacokinetics. Transplantation. 2004;77:542–548.
40. Balfour IC, Fiore A, Graff RJ, et al. Use of rituximab to decrease panel-reactive antibodies. Journal of Heart and Lung Transplantation. 2005;24: 628–630.
41. Pescovitz MD. Rituximab, an anti-cd20 monoclonal antibody: history and mechanism of action. American Journal of Transplantation. 2006;6:859–866.
42. Faguer S, Kamar N, Guilbeaud-Frugier C, et al. Rituximab therapy for acute humoral rejection after kidney transplantation. Transplantation. 2007;83:1277–1280.
43. Sarwal M, Chua MS, Kambham N, et al. Molecular heterogeneity in acute renal allograft rejection identified by DNA microarray profiling. New England Journal of Medicine. 2003;349:125–138.
44. Hippen BE, DeMattos A, Cook WJ, et al. Association of CD20+ infiltrates with poorer clinical outcomes in acute cellular rejection of renal allografts. American Journal of Transplantation. 2005;5:2248–2252.
45. Alausa M, Almagro U, Siddiqi N, et al. Refractory acute kidney transplant rejection with CD20 graft infiltrates and successful therapy with rituximab. Clinical Transplantation. 2005;19:137–140.
46. Angelin-Duclos C, Cattoretti G, Lin KI, et al. Commitment of B lymphocytes to a plasma cell fate is associated with Blimp-1 expression in vivo. Journal of Immunology. 2000;165:5462–5471.
47. Ramos EJ, Pollinger HS, Stegall MD, et al. The effect of desensitization protocols on human splenic B-cell populations in vivo. American Journal of Transplantation. 2007;7:402–407.
48. Everly MJ, Everly JJ, Susskind B, et al. Bortezomib provides effective therapy for antibody- and cell-mediated acute rejection. Transplantation. 2008;86: 1754–1761.
49. Palombella VJ, Conner EM, Fuseler JW, et al. Role of the proteasome and NF-kappaB in streptococcal cell wall-induced polyarthritis. Proceedings of the National Academy of Sciences of the United States of America. 1998;95: 15671–15676.
50. Luo H, Wu Y, Qi S, et al. A proteasome inhibitor effectively prevents mouse heart allograft rejection. Transplantation. 2001;72:196–202.
51. Zollner TM, Podda M, Pien C, et al. Proteasome inhibition reduces superantigen-mediated T cell activation and the severity of psoriasis in a SCID-hu model. Journal of Clinical Investigation. 2002;109:671–679.
52. Perry DK, Burns JM, Pollinger HS, et al. Proteasome inhibition causes apoptosis of normal human plasma cells preventing alloantibody production. American Journal of Transplantation. 2009;9:201–209.
53. Wang X, Luo H, Chen H, et al. Role of proteasomes in T cell activation and proliferation. Journal of Immunology. 1998;160:788–801.
54. Sun K, Welniak LA, Panoskaltsis-Mortari A, et al. Inhibition of acute graft-versus-host disease with retention of graft-versus-tumor effects by the proteasome inhibitor bortezomib. Proceedings of the National Academy of Sciences of the United States of America. 2004;101:8120–8125.
55. Nencioni A, Garuti A, Schwarzenberg K, et al. Proteasome inhibitor-induced apoptosis in human monocyte-derived dendritic cells. European Journal of Immunology. 2006;36:681–689.
56. Walsh RC, Everly JJ, Brailey P, et al. Proteasome inhibitor-based primary therapy for antibody-mediated renal allograft rejection. Transplantation. 2010;89: 277–284.
57. Trivedi HL, Terasaki PI, Feroz A, et al. Abrogation of anti-HLA antibodies via proteasome inhibition. Transplantation. 2009;87:1555–1561.
58. Rother RP, Arp J, Jiang J, et al. C5 blockade with conventional immunosuppression induces long-term graft survival in presensitized recipients. American Journal of Transplantation. 2008;8:1129–1142.
59. Stegall MD, Diwan T, Raghavaiah S, et al. Terminal complement inhibition decreases antibody-mediated rejection in sensitized renal transplant recipients. American Journal of Transplantation. 2011;11:2405–2413.
60. Reinsmoen NL, Lai CH, Vo A, et al. Acceptable donor-specific antibody levels allowing for successful deceased and living donor kidney transplantation after desensitization therapy. Transplantation. 2008;86:820–825.
61. Gloor JM, Winters JL, Cornell LD, et al. Baseline donor-specific antibody levels and outcomes in positive crossmatch kidney transplantation. American Journal of Transplantation. 2010;10:582–589.
62. Vo AA, Toyoda M, Peng A, et al. Effect of induction therapy protocols on transplant outcomes in crossmatch positive renal allograft recipients desensitized with IVIG. American Journal of Transplantation. 2006;6:2384–2390.
63. Schweitzer EJ, Wilson JS, Fernandez-Vina M, et al. A high panel-reactive antibody rescue protocol for cross-match-positive live donor kidney transplants. Transplantation. 2000;70:1531–1536.
64. Gloor JM, DeGoey SR, Pineda AA, et al. Overcoming a positive crossmatch in living-donor kidney transplantation. American Journal of Transplantation. 2003;3:1017–1023.
65. Magee CC, Felgueiras J, Tinckam K, et al. Renal transplantation in patients with positive lymphocytotoxicity crossmatches: one center's experience. Transplantation. 2008;86:96–103.
66. Thielke JJ, West-Thielke PM, Herren HL, et al. Living donor kidney transplantation across positive crossmatch: the University of Illinois at Chicago experience. Transplantation. 2009;87:268–273.
67. Haririan A, Nogueira J, Kukuruga D, et al. Positive cross-match living donor kidney transplantation: longer-term outcomes. American Journal of Transplantation. 2009;9:536–542.
68. Montgomery RA, Zachary AA, Racusen LC, et al. Plasmapheresis and intravenous immune globulin provides effective rescue therapy for refractory humoral rejection and allows kidneys to be successfully transplanted into cross-match-positive recipients. Transplantation. 2000;70:887–895.
69. Vo AA, Cam V, Toyoda M, et al. Safety and adverse events profiles of intravenous gammaglobulin products used for immunomodulation: a single-center experience. Clinical Journal of the American Society of Nephrology. 2006;1:844–852.
70. Kahwaji J, Barker E, Pepkowitz S, et al.Acute hemolysis after high-dose intravenous immunoglobulin therapy in highly HLA sensitized patients. Clinical Journal of the American Society of Nephrology. 2009;4:1993–1997.
71. Sekul EA, Cupler EJ, Dalakas MC. Aseptic meningitis associated with high-dose intravenous immunoglobulin therapy: frequency and risk factors. Annals of Internal Medicine. 1994;121:259–262.
72. Carson KR, Evens AM, Richey EA, et al. Progressive multifocal leukoencephalopathy after rituximab therapy in HIV-negative patients: a report of 57 cases from the Research on Adverse Drug Events and Reports project. Blood. 2009; 113:4834–4840.
73. McLaughlin P, Grillo-Lopez AJ, Link BK, et al. Rituximab chimeric anti-CD20 monoclonal antibody therapy for relapsed indolent lymphoma: half of patients respond to a four-dose treatment program. Journal of Clinical Oncology. 1998;16:2825–2833.
74. Nam JL, Winthrop KL, van Vollenhoven RF, et al. Current evidence for the management of rheumatoid arthritis with biological disease-modifying antirheumatic drugs: a systematic literature review informing the EULAR recommendations for the management of RA. Annals of the Rheumatic Diseases. 2010;69:976–986.
75. Akalin E, Dinavahi R, Friedlander R, et al. Addition of plasmapheresis decreases the incidence of acute antibody-mediated rejection in sensitized patients with strong donor-specific antibodies. Clinical Journal of the American Society of Nephrology. 2008;3:1160–1167.
76. Kamar N, Milioto O, Puissant-Lubrano B, et al. Incidence and predictive factors for infectious disease after rituximab therapy in kidney-transplant patients. American Journal of Transplantation. 2010;10:89–98.
77. Jordan SC, Glotz D. Is rituximab safe to use in kidney transplant patients? American Journal of Transplantation. 2010;10:8–9.
78. First International Symposium and Workshop on ABO Incompatibility and Transplantation. Combined proceedings of conferences held in Philadelphia, Pennsylvania, USA and Gothenburg, Sweden (the Third Tore Nilson Symposium). March 29–31, 1987, and June 8–10, 1987. Transplantation Proceedings. 1987;19: 4397–4642.
79. Tanabe K. Japanese experience of ABO-incompatible living kidney transplantation. Transplantation. 2007;84:S4–S7.
80. Gloor J, Stegall M. ABO-incompatible kidney transplantation with and without splenectomy. Transplantation. 2006;82:720.
81. Toki D, Ishida H, Setoguchi K, et al. Acute antibody-mediated rejection in living ABO-incompatible kidney transplantation: long-term impact and risk factors. American Journal of Transplantation. 2009;9:567–577.
82. Fidler ME, Gloor JM, Lager DJ, et al. Histologic findings of antibody-mediated rejection in ABO blood-group-incompatible living-donor kidney transplantation. American Journal of Transplantation. 2004;4:101–107.
83. Gloor JM, Lager DJ, Fidler ME, et al. A comparison of splenectomy versus intensive posttransplant antidonor blood group antibody monitoring without splenectomy in ABO-incompatible kidney transplantation. Transplantation. 2005; 80:1572–1577.
84. Lawrence C, Galliford JW, Willicombe MK, et al. Antibody removal before ABO-incompatible renal transplantation: how much plasma exchange is therapeutic? Transplantation. 2011;92:1129–1133.
85. Garonzik Wang JM, Montgomery RA, Kucirka LM, et al. Incompatible live-donor

kidney transplantation in the United States: results of a national survey. Clinical Journal of the American Society of Nephrology. 2011;6:2041–2046.
86. Shimmura H, Tanabe K, Ishikawa N, et al. Role of anti-A/B antibody titers in results of ABO-incompatible kidney transplantation. Transplantation. 2000; 70:1331–1335.
87. Park WD, Grande JP, Ninova D, et al. Accommodation in ABO-incompatible kidney allografts, a novel mechanism of self-protection against antibody-mediated injury. American Journal of Transplantation. 2003;3:952–960.
88. Archdeacon P, Chan M, Neuland C, et al. Summary of FDA antibody-mediated rejection workshop. American Journal of Transplantation. 2011;11:896–906.
89. Amico P, Honger G, Mayr M, et al. Clinical relevance of pretransplant donor-specific HLA antibodies detected by single-antigen flow-beads. Transplantation. 2009;87:1681–1688.
90. Lefaucheur C, Suberbielle-Boissel C, Hill GS, et al. Clinical relevance of preformed HLA donor-specific antibodies in kidney transplantation. American Journal of Transplantation. 2008;8:324–331.
91. Lefaucheur C, Loupy A, Hill GS, et al. Preexisting donor-specific HLA antibodies predict outcome in kidney transplantation. Journal of the American Society of Nephrology. 2010;21:1398–1406.
92. Mauiyyedi S, Pelle PD, Saidman S, et al. Chronic humoral rejection: identification of antibody-mediated chronic renal allograft rejection by C4d deposits in peritubular capillaries. Journal of the American Society of Nephrology. 2001;12: 574–582.
93. Regele H, Bohmig GA, Habicht A, et al. Capillary deposition of complement split product C4d in renal allografts is associated with basement membrane injury in peritubular and glomerular capillaries: a contribution of humoral immunity to chronic allograft rejection. Journal of the American Society of Nephrology. 2002;13:2371–2380.
94. Loupy A, Suberbielle-Boissel C, Hill GS, et al. Outcome of subclinical antibody-mediated rejection in kidney transplant recipients with preformed donor-specific antibodies. American Journal of Transplantation. 2009;9:2561–2570.
95. Vo AA, Jordan S, Peng A, et al. Use of intravenous immune globulin and rituximab for desensitization of highly HLA-sensitized patients awaiting kidney transplantation. Transplantation. 2010;89:1095–1102.

第 69 章 肾移植临床排斥反应综合征

Brian J. Nankivell

引言

免疫反应所导致的移植物损伤

两个基因型不同的供受体之间，受体针对供体抗原启动的免疫反应表现为移植物排斥。预存的免疫记忆主要指残留的异源免疫，包括既往感染导致的交叉反应或以前的免疫刺激，与排斥和移植物的丢失密切相关[1]。组织或三级移植淋巴结构里的记忆 T 细胞也能外围地被激活[2-4]。排斥反应会唤醒由特异性 T 淋巴细胞、B 细胞和分泌抗体的浆细胞组成的适应性免疫，同时也涉及由补体、NK 细胞和巨噬细胞组成的固有免疫。对于移植肾来说，同种异体免疫反应才是最首要的威胁，未经控制的排斥反应会导致移植物彻底失功[5]。

随着强有力的神经钙调磷酸酶抑制剂(CNI)药物的面世和更好的免疫学配对，急性排斥反应的临床综合征也发生了变化。早期在硫唑嘌呤/激素抗排斥时代，急性排斥非常常见，比例达 70%~80%，表现为发热、移植物胀痛、少尿和血清肌酐升高。目前移植后 1 年内排斥的发生率已经降至 15%以下，但是这些排斥都是临床上较为严重的类型。遗憾的是，正如第 103 章所述，长期丢失率并没有得到明显改善。

由于排斥的严重程度、发生时间、持续时间和组织病理类型的不同，功能受损程度及对治疗的反应也不尽相同，因此免疫反应导致的移植物损伤程度相差较大。急性间质性 T 细胞介导的排斥反应通过迅速的糖皮质激素冲击治疗可以得到很好的治愈而不留下后遗症。相反，血管性的、激素抵抗或者抗体介导的急性排斥反应的治疗会更加困难，除此之外，伴随复发性的排斥反应、未经治疗的亚临床排斥、慢性排斥，或者后续新发的急性排斥，都会对移植物造成不可逆的损害，需要强有力的对症治疗。不同的免疫介导机制和类型的排斥也可能同时发生在一个个体身上，尤其是那些表现为进展性的或迟发型的急性移植物功能不全的受体。排斥导致的损伤会通过调整自身的免疫抑制来刺激移植肾产生愈合反应[6-9]。

根据排斥反应发生的时间可以将排斥反应分为超急性(立即至几分钟)、急性(术后早期至几天)、亚急性或慢性(术后几个月到几年)排斥；根据组织病理学分类(间质/细胞、血管性和抗体介导/内皮细胞介导的排斥)；根据组织学程度分类(取决于炎症和损伤的范围、Banff 方案的评分和等级[10])；根据治疗反应分类(是否激素敏感或抵抗)；以及根据肾功能受损情况(急性排斥和亚临床排斥)和免疫生物学分类(T 细胞及抗体介导的适应性免疫系统和补体、巨噬细胞及固有免疫系统途径)。通过穿刺活检对排斥进行不同的病理类型分类诊断，可以指导治疗并且影响其预后[11,12]。

本章将移植后功能不全分为 4 类进行阐述，包括排斥的类型、非免疫性的鉴别诊断和即刻、早期、晚期排斥。主要集中在临床实际管理，包括免疫学机制、组织病理学发现、治疗以及第 5 至 9 章、第 67 章和第 81 章中提到的特殊鉴别诊断方法。

原发性移植肾无功能

临床定义：移植的肾脏植入之初即无功能。

通常移植物在开放血管灌注后能立即获得功能(IGF)，在肾移植里表现为尿液的产生和血清肌酐的进行性下降。原发性移植肾无功能的特点为移植后少尿，并且对输液及利尿剂无反应，同时伴有血清肌酐水平的上升。最常见的原因是缺血–再灌注损伤；而输尿管梗阻、血管损伤和超急性排斥反应，都是重要的鉴别诊断。

超急性排斥反应

超急性排斥反应是由受体体内预存的抗供体的特异性细胞毒抗体（DSA）介导的，通常是直接针对供肾内皮细胞上的Ⅰ型 HLA 抗原而做出的强烈排斥反应[13–15]。大多数的移植受体体内并不存在预先生成的针对 HLA 分子的抗体，除非先前通过妊娠、输血或既往移植接触过表达 HLA 的异体细胞，这些都是增加致敏的危险因素。可以分别回顾第 36 章和第 89 章中对 HLA 抗体的描述和临床检测方法。

超急性排斥反应通常在血管夹松开的一瞬间发生，移植肾表现为松弛和花斑状表面，而不是正常灌注所呈现的粉红色表面。随着微血管 DSA 的沉积，经典的补体级联反应、固有免疫和凝集旁路均被迅速激活。急性炎症白细胞紧接着附着在肾小球（肾小球炎症）和管周毛细血管（PTC）的内皮细胞上。一旦这样的机制开始启动就很难被逆转。内皮细胞的坏死、血小板和纤维素的沉积和局部凝集造成了局部皮质坏死和严重的急性肾小管坏死[13]。在这个过程中移植肾都是无尿的，随着大血管的血栓增多，使得移植肾表面逐渐变黑，同时伴随着血小板的持续性消耗性减少和移植肾缺血。这样的过程通常会导致移植肾最后被切除。

超急性排斥反应最早描述于补体依赖的淋巴毒交叉试验（CDC）阳性的移植[16]，随后 CDC 交叉试验阳性成为绝对禁忌证。特异性和敏感性更高的交叉检测技术（包括抗人球蛋白 CDC 交叉试验、流式细胞术或固相血清电泳；见第 89 章）用来明确移植前就存在的 DSA，从而消除超急性排斥反应的发生[15]。目前，由于未能检测到的非 HLA DSA（如抗内皮细胞抗体）而导致早期超急性排斥反应的发生较为少见[17]。

ABO 血型不相容的肾移植

超急性排斥反应在 ABO 血型不相容时也会发生。抗 A 和抗 B 抗体（同族血细胞凝集素）是会直接针对内皮细胞和红细胞表面血型抗原的同种抗体，目前仍然是移植的壁垒。1 个世纪之前发现 ABO 血型的不相容性（表现为大量溶血、无胆色素尿性黄疸、血红蛋白尿和肾衰竭），在 20 世纪 50 年代又得到重新认知，ABO 不相容的肾移植通常会发生超急性排斥反应，由于凝固性坏死导致移植肾迅速失功。因此，目前的肾移植都是通过 ABO 血型是否兼容而进行分配。

尽管如此，通过在围术期给予去除抗体的试验性的方法，越来越多 ABO 血型不相容的肾脏被移植给受体而不发生超急性排斥反应[18]。术前和术后的血浆置换或免疫吸附[固定 A 和（或）B 抗原并去除血浆抗体]能够降低抗体滴度，通常还要结合静脉输注免疫球蛋白、脾切除术或者使用利妥昔单抗，以及应用抗细胞增殖的药物来防止抗体的回升[19]。循环抗体滴度在移植后会回升，并且吸附在内皮细胞上，激活补体（合并 C4d 的阳性），由于微循环的"适应"现象[20]，又或许是因为内皮细胞保护基因的上调，通常不会导致发生毛细血管炎或明显的损害。如果发生了，由于同族血细胞凝集素不同导致的急性抗体介导的排斥反应同样也具备以下特征：如早期肾小球囊的节段性栓塞、肾小球膜溶解和多形核细胞的募集。长期随访显示，与血型匹配的受体的结果相似[21]，通过和抗 HLA 抗体进行对照可以发现持续性的抗体介导的排斥会明显影响移植物的生存率。第 68 章对脱敏的方案有进一步的介绍。

原发性无功能的鉴别诊断

缺血再灌注损伤

移植肾延迟复功（DGF）指的是植入的肾脏可以排出尿液，但是最初并没有功能，原因包括供体因素相关的缺血再灌注损伤、器官获取技术和缺血时间较长。DGF 通常的定义是指移植术后 7 天内需要行透析治疗过渡，但是也有其他功能性的定义（每天血清肌酐下降值小于 10%超过 3 天），与移植是否成功相关（HR 为 1.47；95%CI 为 1.06~2.03）[22]。由于器官的短缺，近 20 年来采用有血管并发症的老年供体（扩大标准的供体，ECD），以及因循环系统导致死亡的供体（DCD 或心脏停搏的供体），使得 DGF 的发生率从 14.7%上升到 21%~23%[23]。虽然采用边缘供肾的受体基础肾功能、存活率和移植物的存活率比不上使用标准供体的受体，但与继续透析相比，其生存率明显改善[24]。系统性的荟萃分析显示 DGF 使移植物丢失的比例增加至 41%（RR 为 1.41；95%CI 为 1.27~1.56）[25]。其他增加 DGF 的因素包括供体年龄、器官大小和质量（年老的供体、低血压、糖尿病、供肾本身损害和高血压)和“运送”时间过长导致的缺血性损害[26,27]。尸体供体器官的这些应激损害和不利因素都可以通过理想的供体ICU管理、供肾体外机械灌注[28,29]、快速的供肾运输和植入得到改善[30]。供体器官的质量与其应激反应能力相关,并最终且影响到它的寿命。

新陈代谢旺盛的肾小管上皮细胞对于缺血较为敏感,因其会导致氧的耗尽、减弱细胞的新陈代谢和Na/K ATP泵的交换功能。再灌注之后由于含氧血液生成了包括超氧化物、一氧化氮和过氧硝酸物等大量活性氧物质,导致DNA断裂、脂质过氧化、细胞凋亡和坏死。血管内皮细胞的缺血性损伤会导致脂质磷酸分解、凝血酶介导的纤维沉积、P选择素受体、β-整合素和趋化因子的表面信号上调以及白细胞的黏附[23]。

供体脑死亡或围术期的缺血再灌注损伤也会刺激趋化因子,前炎症因子(IL-6、TNF-α、IFN-γ)和黏附分子[CD54(ICAM-1)、VCAM-1、CD18/11a(LFA-1)]引起级联反应,使移植肾内MHC抗原的表达上调。损伤的组织会表达天然危险受体或Toll受体系统配体(对于感染病原体的正常保护反应)[31],以促进免疫细胞的成熟、活化和排斥的发生[32]。组织免疫原性的增强增加了发生细胞浸润和排斥的概率[32,33]。

对于无尿的移植肾,手术台上灌注后立即穿刺或术后早期穿刺可以明确急性肾小管坏死以及排除未知的排斥(在一些罕见的病例中,有DSA存在的体液性排斥只表现为急性肾小管坏死和C4d阳性)。通常,相比细胞内的增生增厚异常,由于缺血所导致的非特异性的小管改变在光镜下很容易被发现。DGF使得临床排斥的发生率增高(合并发生49%比35%,RR为1.38;95%CI为1.29~1.47),因此需要密切的观察和调整免疫抑制方案(CNI类药物有时候会减量来提高移植物功能)[25]。对于没有恢复功能同时未确诊排斥的患者需要行透析治疗过渡(数天至数周),此时行程序性活检(每隔5~7天)比利用血清肌酐评估更可靠。尿量排出的增加(1~1.5L/d才可暂停透析)、透析前血清肌酐的下降至稳定阶段都预示着移植肾功能的恢复,可以逐渐脱离透析。高达3%的移植肾植入后永远没有功能[6]。

动静脉血管受累

外科血管受累(副肾动脉缝合灌注不理想或肾血管扭转)或者明显的血栓形成(临床上立即显现或不久以后完全无尿)都是少见的鉴别诊断,并且需要急诊行多普勒超声评估。对于液体负荷、血压和心脏排出量的评估在临床上也很重要。在临床某些特殊阶段,需要注意通过尿量来评估受体是否有血管并发症并不可靠,因为原有肾脏可能还能产生尿液,此时应当提高警觉,尽早行急诊彩超或手术探查来明确是否有血管受累。

移植肾输尿管梗阻

超声显示移植肾肾盂积水可确诊输尿管梗阻。利用输尿管支架可以减少其作为早期并发症的发生率。

早期移植肾功能不全

临床定义:在移植早期最初有功能的移植肾表现为功能不全和肌酐的升高。

早期移植肾功能监测

移植肾功能的评估是反映移植物病理状态首要的监测工具。定期的血清肌酐监测在移植后应当立即开始(缺血性DGF和早期排斥需要每日监测),稳定的患者在此后1年的时间里逐渐降低到每月检测[34]。恒定的每日肌酐生成率意味着血清肌酐水平对个体移植物功能的相对变化是敏感的。血清肌酐检测是一种快速的实验室检测方法,具有费用低、便捷、操作简单等优点,同时有良好的测量精度(实验室内部差异小于3%)和准确度(10~20μmol/L或0.10~0.20mg/dL)。血清肌酐在个体内有一定范围的波动,其检测对于急性排斥的发现较为敏感(亚临床排斥会遗漏),生物变异性适中(患者间CV为7%)但是特异性相对会低,因为一些物理性因素如脱水和血压变化也会影响到肾小球滤过率(GFR)。

通常血清肌酐在手术后2周内会下降至基线值,取决于早期的缺血损伤、供体质量、供受体表面积匹配程度、神经钙调磷酸酶抑制剂的浓度和受体本身的肌肉肌酐生成情况。早期肌酐的急性增高(如高于基线值25%以上),甚至不能降低,应当立即给予重复的充足补液水化,同时排除一些可逆性因素(利用多普勒彩超检查血供和是否有肾盂积水)。诊断性的移植肾活检可以显示排斥、急性肾小管坏死或者接近正常(急性CNI

毒性可以推断，特别是均匀等长的管腔空泡变性和血清 CNI 浓度过高)(表 69.1)

早期急性抗体介导的排斥

抗体介导的排斥(AMR)是由于致病抗体介导的直接针对特异性供体分子发生的反应。虽然大多数 DSA 都是 HLA-特异性,也有非 HLA 介导的如抗 ABO 血型抗原和抗其他生物多态性抗原的抗体。针对生物多态性 MICA (表达在内皮细胞的 MHC Ⅰ A 类)[35,36]、AT_1 受体或抗内皮细胞的抗体很少在超急性、急性和慢性移植物排斥中出现。作用于血管 AT_1 受体的 IgG 抗体在一些难治性血管性排斥的病例中被提及 [组织结构上表现为动脉内膜炎和(或)纤维样坏死],通常合并恶性高血压,并且对血管紧张素受体拮抗剂(ARB)治疗有反应(如氯沙坦)[37]。

DSA 是由先前存在的浆细胞或记忆 B 细胞转换成新的浆细胞产生,介导 AMR 的发生。这些曾暴露于既往抗原的有免疫反应的"有记忆的"或"存在回忆"的抗体可以迅速生成高滴度的补体固定 HLA 抗体[15],直接针对供体内皮细胞表达的 MHC 抗原(图 69.1)。受损的内皮细胞分泌血管性血友病(von Willebrand)因子和 P 选择素(促进血小板凝集)、炎症分子(如 IL-1α、IL-8 和 CCL-2),以及趋化因子(C3a 和 C5a),引起肾小球白细胞黏附(肾小球炎症)[38]或管周毛细血管的扩张(俗称管周炎)[13]。C5b-9 膜攻击复合物的聚集会导致局限性的内皮细胞坏死和凋亡、基底膜细胞的脱离和毛细血管纤维微血栓的沉积。在一些严重的病例中,会发生动脉血管壁的出血和坏死或远端局部末梢血管内栓塞的生成[13]。

表 69.1　移植肾功能异常的临床思路

1.临床检查包括血压、水负荷程度、移植肾的软硬度触诊和杂音听诊
2.检查药物的依从性和肾毒性,以及是否在服用会改变 CNI 药物浓度的药物
3.予以充分水化以及消除可逆转因素后再次复查肌酐
4.检查 CNI 药物的血药浓度是否已达中毒浓度(过高的浓度会导致肾毒性的风险增加,不稳定的浓度意味着排斥风险的增加需要调整剂量)
5.应用多普勒超声评估移植肾的动脉流速,同时排除输尿管梗阻,B 超不能确定的时候可以用锝(^{99m}Tc)巯替肽造影
6.血液核酸试验评估是否有 BK 病毒感染,结果为阳性时需要行定量检查
7.尿液分析蛋白尿和血尿(提示肾小球肾炎或者移植肾肾小球疾病)
8.移植肾行穿刺来明确特殊诊断
9.DSA 检测(如果怀疑抗体介导的排斥反应)

急性 AMR 表现为早期的炎性移植肾功能不全(发生在移植后的几天内，会因为抗淋巴细胞诱导治疗而推迟)和急性少尿性移植肾失功,有时候也表现为低热和移植物变软。多普勒成像证实舒张期血流量减少、移植物肿胀和高阻力指数。急诊的病理组织学检查显示,炎性的微血管损伤伴随着多形核细胞或单核细胞黏附在管周和肾小球毛细血管的内皮细胞上[38],可见 C4d的沉积和管腔损害[14]。

组织病理学上对于移植肾功能不全的急性 AMR[9,13]的三个诊断依据如下：

1.急性组织损伤的形态学证据(肾小球或管周毛细血管白细胞浸润内皮炎，动脉炎症或急性小管损

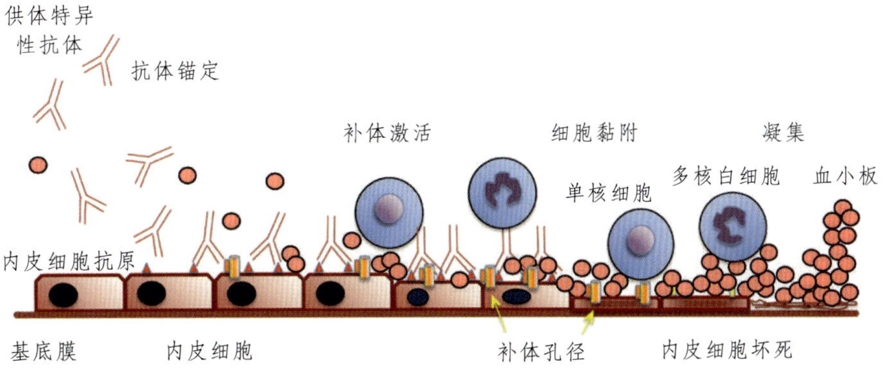

图 69.1　急性抗体介导排斥反应的病理生理学示意图。供体特异性抗体锚定于上皮细胞表达的抗原,紧接着补体活化、细胞黏附、血小板沉积和凝集导致内皮的损伤。

伤)。皮质、小管周围和肾小球毛细血管白细胞聚集(PAS 染色)是重要的诊断特征,意味着需要开始激素冲击治疗来抗排斥反应发生。

2.抗体活动的组织病理学的证据(C4d 染色阳性,经典的定义是“强染色的、弥漫的包括至少 50%以上的PTC”,但是临床上符合的只有不到 10%)。

3.循环 DSA 直接针对 HLA Ⅰ类和(或)Ⅱ分子或其他(较少)已经明确的多态性特异抗原。

C4d 是经典补体激活途径的诊断性标志物,经常出现在管周毛细血管,但缺乏敏感性[40],C4d 偶然见于仅表现为内皮炎症的早期体液性排斥的活检(随后变成明确的阳性)[13]。C4d 能在内皮上形成稳定并长期存在的共价键,在成功地进行 AHR 治疗后几天至几周持续阳性(可以观察到残余的 PTC 空泡变性)。“仅 C4d 沉积而并没有活动性排斥的形态学依据”已作为一个新的亚分类纳入 Banff 系统。C4d(23%~95%)与急性 AHR 的标志物(如 DSA)的敏感性有所差异,主要体现在技术不同(利用蜡块切片法会使免疫组织化学敏感性变差,但是可以使肾小球 C4d 结构清晰且不影响检测,但是利用间接免疫荧光法观察临时冰冻样本会有更高的敏感性)、使用不同的抗体(单克隆或多克隆抗体)、阈值设定不同(管周毛细血管炎的 10%比 50%)和穿刺时间不同[41]。局灶范围内的 C4d(管周毛细血管炎的 10%~50%伴强线性染色)和毛细血管炎、肾小球炎相关,其中期预后也是差的[39,42]。C4d 阳性是极好的体液免疫特异性指标(93%~96%),尤其是在已经证实有 DSA、内皮细胞炎症和特定的临床环境下(如再次移植、高敏受体、明确的移植前 DSA)[40,43-46]。

早期诊断和积极治疗是挽救这些肾脏的关键。治疗措施包括糖皮质激素冲击治疗、血浆置换去除循环抗体(同时也会去除凝血因子,因此穿刺后的第一次血浆置换应该补充新鲜冰冻血浆来避免出血,并且在随后补充白蛋白)、低剂量静注免疫球蛋白(血浆置换后 100mg/kg 至累积剂量达到 1~2g/kg),以及应用抗细胞增殖的药物(如吗替麦考酚酯)来抑制 B 细胞和 T 细胞的增殖并限制抗体合成的恢复。通过监测肾功能、连续的 DSA 水平和最近一次复查的肾活检来评估治疗效果。

补充疗法包括利妥昔单抗,是一种针对 CD20+的 B 淋巴细胞嵌合单克隆抗体,可以快速清除 B 细胞并维持长达 1 年的时间(单次 375mg/m^2 的静脉剂量)。利妥昔单抗通过抗体依赖的细胞介导的细胞毒性、补体介导的细胞毒性和 B 细胞的凋亡(不包括浆细胞)途径发挥作用。通常耐受性良好,偶然出现急性输液反应,轻度增加细菌感染风险和潜在的病毒激活(引起低丙球蛋白血症程度很轻微)[47]。在 B 细胞浸润的小儿急性排斥的随机试验中,利妥昔单抗可以改善移植肾功能,降低程序性活检的排斥分数,阻止 C4d 的再现,不依赖于 DSA 水平[48]。在已知的观察研究中,由于治疗方法比较混杂,利妥昔单抗作为急性 AHR 的辅助治疗的作用并不明确。抗淋巴细胞抗体(有抗 CD20 特性)有时候也会被用于 T 细胞共存的排斥(混合排斥)[11]。

其他一些试验性药物包括依库丽单抗(人源化补体 C5 终未复合物活化抑制剂),可以快速阻止补体小孔形成,使得 AMR 的治疗富有前景[49,50]。硼替佐米(直接针对浆细胞的蛋白酶抑制剂)可以直接影响 DSA 的合成来缓慢降低 DSA 水平(IgG 的半衰期是 7~21 天,取决于不同的亚型)。在给予血浆置换的同时输注 3~5 次 1.3mg/m^2 剂量(每一个骨髓瘤治疗周期的剂量)的硼替佐米作为挽救治疗,可以成功地降低 DSA 水平并逆转 AMR。副作用包括周围神经病变(约 30%)、骨髓抑制和疱疹病毒的激活[50]。目前并没有关于使用硼替佐米或者依库丽单抗的随机试验数据。

在等待二次移植的名单里,首次移植 HLA 错配强烈提示着会有更高滴度的 HLA Ⅱ抗体[51]。1/3 的受体因为抗体滴度过高暂缓移植而延长了透析等待时间[52]。DSA 阳性的高致敏受体会经常发生急性和(或)慢性的抗体介导的排斥反应,会减少移植物的功能和生存率。许多中心会避免这样的配对情况,转而寻找更合适的供体。不管如何,去除预存的抗体和增强免疫抑制能使移植成功,同时会有增加感染和慢性抗体介导的排斥反应(CAMR)的潜在发生机会[53]。活体交换计划很好地解决了诸如受体 ABO 血型不相容或存在供体特异性抗 HLA 抗体的问题。对于敏感个体的综合处理详见第 68 章。

早期急性 T 细胞介导的排斥

急性细胞性排斥是由于 T 淋巴细胞最早介导侵入肾间质和肾小管上皮细胞;临床主要表现为血清肌酐上升,需要通过移植肾活检来确诊[5]。树突状细胞直接向淋巴器官里的幼稚 T 细胞提呈供体抗原,从而使其激活、分化和复制出辅助 T 细胞和有破坏效应的 T 淋巴细胞[55]。急性细胞性排斥发生时,循环中淋巴细胞会锚定内皮细胞,越过管周毛细血管网[31],进而聚集在间质部分,产生炎症细胞因子和趋化因子(例如 TNF-α、TNF-β、CCL5/RANTES、CCL3/MIP-1α 和 IFN-γ),诱导移植物里的 IFN-γ 基因表达 (图 69.2)[56,57]。CD4 和 CD8 T 细胞可能同时伴有 B 细胞 (通过基因表达标志物检测和 CD20 的组织化学反应)[58]或嗜酸性粒细胞;B 细胞和嗜酸性细胞的存在与严重的激素抵抗的细胞性排斥相关。活化的巨噬细胞分泌促炎症细胞因子(例如 IL-1、IL-12 和 IL-18、TNF-α 和 IFN-γ),与功能性损害和残留的 T 细胞排斥有关[59]。

分泌的趋化因子(CCL2、CCL5 和 CX3CL1)[60]会吸引同种特异 CD8 T 淋巴细胞攻击肾小管 (小管炎),通过直接接触(细胞介导的细胞毒性)、局部区域的细胞因子释放或间接的炎症细胞活化导致局部的小管损伤。CD8 T 细胞释放穿孔素(允许颗粒酶 A 和 B 通过细胞膜孔进入) 和 Fas 自由基的 Fas 凋亡受体相互作用,导致细胞蛋白凋亡酶介导凋亡(图 69.2)[61]。效应 CD4 T 细胞可以通过 TNF 的释放介导细胞毒性至次级抗原[62]。受损的小管细胞会转化为较为原始的间充质肌成纤维细胞,或者进展为上皮细胞坏死伴基底膜破裂造成尿液外渗、移植物功能不全和小管萎缩引起严重损伤[63]。

临床上发生急性排斥的高危免疫风险包括 HLA 错配、无亲缘关系的供肾、预存的抗体,尤其是供体存在特殊情况、再次移植、供肾缺血(特别是缺血时间长或者供体标准扩大),会通过增强损伤分子的表达及固有免疫系统对其的识别和应答来增加移植的免疫原性[64]。在随机对照实验中,他克莫司(与环孢霉素相比)、吗替麦考酚酯(与硫唑嘌呤相比)以及诱导治疗都可以降低急性排斥的风险。移植后 1 年内的排斥发生率已经降低至 10%~15%,但和以前相比都是严重的和难治性的排斥。更好的 HLA 匹配、DSA 的检测技术(减少排斥风险)和有效的 CMV 预防、抗感染治疗(允许安全范围内的免疫抑制剂量增加)都起到了作用。目前仍有近 4%的肾脏由于早期的排斥而丢失[64]。

急性 T 细胞介导排斥的病理学诊断关键是间质和肾小管可见单核细胞的炎性浸润,其相对比例和范围程度决定了严重等级。Banff 急性 T 细胞介导的排斥(TCMR)[9]分级如下(也可见于第 81 章):

临界“可疑”排斥。局灶小管炎(t1、t2 或 t3)伴轻度间质浸润(i0 或 i1 间质浸润 10%~25%的皮质)或中度间质浸润(i2、i3)伴随轻度(t1)小管炎(无动脉内膜炎)。

ⅠA 级排斥。明显的间质浸润(大于 25%的实质影响,i2 或 i3 评分)和中度小管炎(t2)。

ⅠB 级排斥。明显的间质浸润(大于 25%的实质)和严重的小管炎(t3)。

Banff 标准的排斥严重程度主要取决于小管炎分值。小管炎症分值决定了最终的排斥级别及最严重的损伤。局部严重的小管炎(不恰当的说法)即使局限在单一的小管会使得排斥级别上升。如果某些区域因为炎症导致小管破坏而没有 PAS 着色,就很难评价小管炎。间质炎症范围(Banff 分值)在临床上对于随后小管间质性破坏的诊断和预测非常有用[65]。之前的 CCTT 系统根据至少 5%皮质淋巴细胞性炎症和两个损伤标志物(水肿、小管变性/损伤或有反应的淋巴母细胞)以及小管炎(最少三个小管受到最大程度的浸润)来定义排斥。临床上一些患者血清肌酐上升,同时超过 10%的皮质区域发生了伴有小管炎的间质淋巴细胞炎症,则需要当作临床排斥来处理,直至证实是由其他原因引起。

活检可以诊断排斥,同时可以根据组织学类型和严重程度进行分类,从而决定治疗。单纯的细胞性排斥的基础治疗是激素冲击 (如 500mg 的甲泼尼静脉滴注 3 天)或者短期口服大剂量治疗(如每天 100mg 然后逐渐减量),之后观察血清肌酐是否下降至基础值。从已登记的研究来看,成功治疗急性细胞性排斥后不会遗留组织学影响或额外的移植物丢失。然而,复发或严重的急性排斥可能引起部分遗留移植肾功能不全[64]。严重的、复发的、反复发作的或激素抵抗的细胞性排斥应该再次行活检同时行 C4d 染色、DSA 测定、药物依从性确定和加强免疫抑制方案,同时考虑抗胸腺细胞的治疗。

血管性排斥

血管性排斥(术语称为动脉炎或者动脉内膜炎)是一种严重的、激素无反应的排斥类型,特征是血管的单核细胞浸润、内膜肌成纤维细胞分泌基质蛋白和胶原以及内皮细胞凋亡。CD4 和 CD8 T 细胞和巨噬细胞在活化的内皮细胞表达的黏附分子(ICAM-1 或 VCAM)和趋化因子(CCL4、CCL5 和 CXCL8)的帮助下侵入内皮下层和小动脉的内膜[66]。在实验研究中,抗 MHC 抗体、细胞介导对次级抗原的免疫、NK 细胞通路和 IFN-γ 导致病理生理学改变。

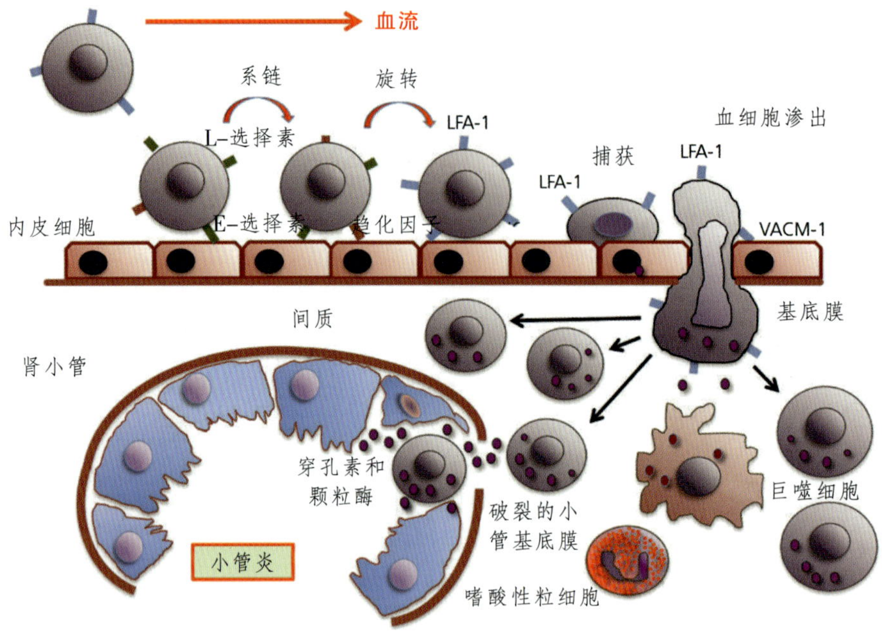

图 69.2 肾移植 T 细胞介导排斥反应的机制和细胞运输交换示意图。随着最初的效应淋巴细胞的系链、旋转、捕获、锚定内皮细胞表达整合素和选择素，淋巴细胞和其他免疫细胞进入间质并且进攻小管，使得局部组织发生破坏。

血管性排斥最初归类于 Banff T 细胞介导排斥下，排斥分级如下(详见第 81 章)：

ⅡA 级排斥。轻到中度的动脉内膜炎(v1 动脉炎评分)。

ⅡB 级排斥。严重的动脉内膜炎(大于 25%的细胞腔内狭窄，v2)。

Ⅲ级排斥。透壁动脉炎、潜在的纤维变性和中间层平滑肌细胞坏死，同时伴随动脉的淋巴性炎症(v3)。

血管性排斥临床上表现主要是进行性的移植肾功能不全，活检有典型的动脉炎表现，对糖皮质激素冲击治疗部分有效或无效。血管性排斥会引起慢性间质纤维化，进而导致不可逆的小管丢失，治疗后也通常不会恢复所有的功能，有很大的移植物丢失风险(HR 为 2.07；95%CI 为 1.60~2.68)[14]。血管性排斥有时也会表现为孤立性的动脉炎，通常会伴随间质细胞浸润，一般推荐抗胸腺细胞球蛋白和糖皮质激素冲击等强有力的免疫抑制方案。动脉炎通常是由体液机制介导，较差的移植物结局往往与严重的动脉炎、高 DSA 水平和间质性炎症有关[67]。对致病的 DSA 进行强有力的治疗包括血浆置换、IVIG 和利妥昔单抗都是有据可循的。

亚临床排斥

亚临床细胞性排斥

亚临床排斥(SCR)是指程序性活检提示组织学急性 T 细胞介导的排斥(急性或临界)但临床上没有肾功能恶化表现[68]。亚临床排斥会损害移植物的组织学结构，进而降低移植物的生存率，其中一部分还会进展为慢性排斥。亚临床排斥会引起小管间质的损害，主要是因为先前的间质性炎症合并损伤前的亚临床排斥，亚临床排斥的强度与慢性损害的严重程度有关（“剂量-反应”），其生物学依据在许多移植人群中被证实。

在一项使用环孢霉素作为基础免疫抑制剂的随机试验中(背景发病率为 30%)，通过糖皮质激素冲击来治疗亚临床排斥可以降低急性排斥的发生率、6 个月时的小管间质慢性评分和 2 年时的血清肌酐，并且有更好的生存率趋势[69]。另一项激素治疗亚临床排斥的试验(使用环孢霉素或他克莫司，亚临床排斥发病率为 28%)显示在移植后的 6 个月和 12 个月，更佳 eGFR[70]，但是在第三项利用他克莫司治疗低免疫风险患者的试验中(SCR 的发病率仅为 4.7%)并没有明显获益[71]。

亚临床抗体介导的排斥

亚临床抗体介导的排斥(SAMR)在程序性活检中显示为与 DSA 相关的 C4d 阳性的毛细血管炎。小管周围白细胞聚集是一个敏感又实用的提示 DSA 存在的标志，但是并非特异地存在于 T 细胞介导的排斥反应中。早期 SAMR 在“交叉配型阳性”或致敏的受体或者晚期发生的抗体介导的排斥治疗后相当常见，据报道,其发生在 10%的标准风险的个体中[7,72,73]。循环DSA 导致的持续性的亚致死的微循环损伤会刺激肾小球内皮细胞以及内皮下的肾小球基底膜(GBM)增生,进而发展成慢性移植性肾病，或者伴随 PTC 基底膜增生、小管间质炎损伤、肾功能损害、蛋白尿和移植物生存率下降[72,74-77]。

移植肾的诊断性活检

移植肾功能不全在排除了可逆性的因素后才考虑行诊断性移植肾活检(图 69.3)。组织学仍然是急性排斥的关键性诊断证据,虽然在将来,疾病的基因转录组测序数据可能会对组织学的分类和预测起到很好的补充[58,78]。大多数的活检都是有指征的(有原因),但是程序性的活检能够定期执行以监测一些肾功能稳定但是有高危因素的受体发生排斥,高危因素包括移植肾延迟复功、DSA 风险较高、ABO 不相容或者其他需要监测亚临床排斥发生的情况,尤其是一些临床试验的参与者[68]。

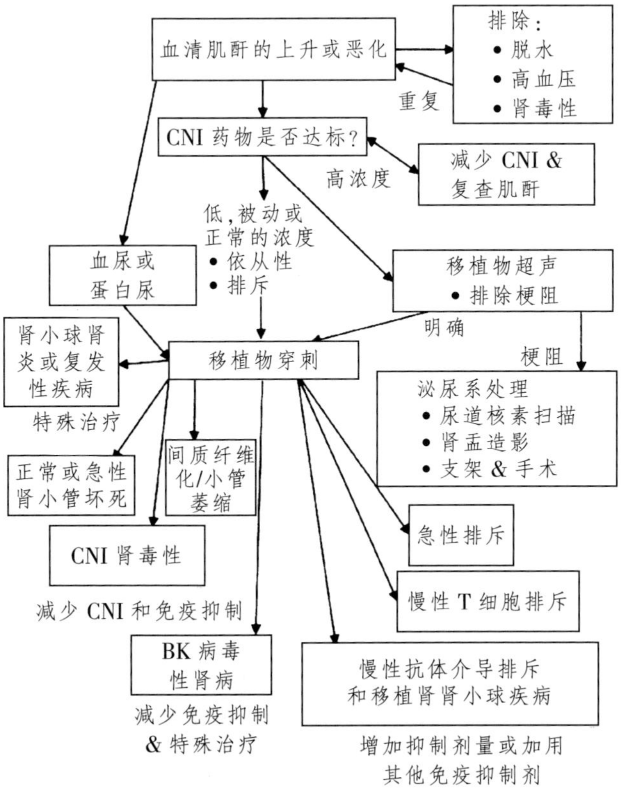

图 69.3　移植肾功能不全的诊断性评价。CNI,神经钙调蛋白抑制剂。

进行活检需要局麻，然后使用一个自动弹簧针装置来完成。主要的活检并发症(如肉眼可见的血尿和输尿管的梗阻)的发生率为 1%,移植物丢失的发生率为 0.03%[68]。次要的并发症(不需要介入解决)包括 3.5%的明显血尿、2.5%的肾周血肿、7.3%无症状的动静脉瘘和 0.5%的血管迷走神经性反应[10]。若有以下因素:有指征的活检(与程序性活检相比)婴儿腹膜外或经腹膜移植成人肾,或者使用更粗的针(16g 或以上),会使风险增大[11]。一个熟练的操作者在彩超引导下操作能确保最大限度的安全。一些高血压控制不佳的、正在进行抗凝治疗的和一些由于尿毒症导致血小板功能不良的患者在穿刺后需要给予特殊观察和护理。

病理学可以证实排斥的存在(通常临床表现更加明显),另外一个重要的用途是组织学分类和严重等级的划分,从而决定二线治疗和预测移植物的预后。排斥也许是不均匀的，因此至少需要行两次活检并且穿刺两条肌性动脉。管周和肾小球的毛细血管炎的评估、小动脉和 C4d 染色对于排除抗体或血管性排斥亚型非常重要。

早期移植肾功能不全的鉴别诊断

缺血再灌注损伤所致的移植肾延迟复功

缺血再灌注损伤会导致早期移植物功能不全,包括一些供体因素(冷、热缺血时间过长,脑死亡供体炎症指标高)和受体因素(再灌注损伤,心血管受累)。我们可以通过诊断性活检来明确急性肾小管坏死和排除急性排斥。

急性移植物血栓形成

早期技术性并发症是由移植肾动脉损伤（通常在血管吻合处)或静脉扭转或外部受压导致梗阻引起,可导致 2%~7%的早期成人移植肾丢失和 12%~35%的儿童和婴儿移植肾丢失,通常发生在移植后的 1 周以内,在第 2 天发生的可能性最大[79]。主要的原因是“Virchow 三因素”:①血管壁因素(细小、女性、尸体供体、血管壁粥样硬化、儿童受体或糖尿病受体、多支或重建的血管、小的肾副动脉、血管钳损伤或灌流套管损伤);②移植血管血流因素(低血压、心力衰竭、灌注不足);③凝血功能障碍(预先存在的高凝状态、V因子突变、狼疮抗凝物、抗心磷脂综合征、红细胞比容高)。临床上若出现导尿管突然无尿(通常自体肾脏无功能,大多数DGF的肾脏是少尿的)和急性的移植肾变软伴消耗性的血小板减少等情况,需要警惕,可通过立即进行多普勒超声和(或)紧急探查或放射介入行血栓去除或血栓溶解术来确诊。通常被挽救的肾脏由于经历过长的热缺血会导致严重急性肾小管坏死,遗留较差的肾功能并且发展成小管萎缩、间质纤维化。

输尿管梗阻

移植肾B超显示典型的肾盂积水。但部分梗阻如中度的淋巴囊肿压迫导致的积水并不明显。

尿漏

移植肾的肾盂肾盏或者输尿管都可能漏尿表现为:①外渗(可以通过引流液肌酐较血清升高诊断);②被腹膜吸收的内渗(当出现不能解释的血清肌酐升高,同时移植物组织学正常时应怀疑),通过移植肾放射性核素扫描进行腹部延迟影像可以确诊。

急性间质性肾炎

预防性使用复方新诺明很少会导致急性间质性肾炎,通常会表现为亚急性移植物功能不全、嗜酸细胞增多症以及活检病理表现为嗜酸性肾小管间质性肾炎。治疗主要为停复方新诺明和激素冲击治疗。病毒导致的急性间质性肾炎(如BK病毒、CMV或者腺病毒肾盂肾炎)在病理学上表现不尽相同。

早期复发性肾病

溶血性尿毒综合征(HUS)或原发性高草酸尿症复发极少会导致早期的急性移植肾失功。复发的局灶节段性肾小球硬化(FSGS)一般最先表现为孤立性的蛋白尿,随后才出现进行性的肾功能不全(见下文)。

溶血性尿毒综合征

经典的HUS包含3个临床诊断表现:微血管溶血性贫血、血小板减少和肾损害,肾衰竭与腹泻有关(通常由0157:H7大肠杆菌内毒素引起),这一过程中会生成志贺毒素促进内皮损伤。不典型的HUS是由于补体旁路基因调节障碍(偶尔来自自身抗体)引起补体过度活动和慢性移植肾失功。不典型的HUS在移植前通常被漏诊,表现为突发的移植后HUS和移植肾功能不全,尤其是同时存在CFH和CFI(与低MCP风险相比)突变[80]。治疗方法是利用新鲜冰冻血浆进行血浆置换、应用,依库丽单抗(针对PNH开发的一种抗C5抑制剂,同时也对非典型和志贺毒素HUS有效)和避免使用CNI。联合肝移植可以纠正遗传性的补体通路缺陷,但是会增加受体风险[80]。

原发性高草酸尿症

原发性高草酸尿症(Ⅰ型更为常见)是隐性的常染色体肝细胞丙氨酸乙醛酸转氨酶缺陷,引起全身草酸盐生成过多,导致尿液中大量排泄草酸(代谢终产物),不能溶解的草酸钙在肾脏沉积,导致肾结石和进行性肾脏失功(原因未知)。由于循环中草酸钙在肾小管沉积,引起移植肾亚急性失功,在偏振光显微镜下呈现出明显的草酸钙晶体双折光现象。治疗包括水化、柠檬酸钠和(或)磷酸盐,对敏感个体使用血液透析和维生素B6可以减少系统性的草酸盐和限制进一步的沉积,但是效果并不理想[81]。由于高剂量的维生素C会导致透析患者的二次草酸盐沉积,应当避免使用。

复发性局灶节段性肾小球硬化

局灶节段性肾小球硬化是一种足细胞疾病(肾小球脏层上皮细胞),由下列任一原因引起:①足细胞某些关键蛋白的基因突变(如通过DNA分析证实的膜蛋白),表现为家族性或散发性肾病综合征;②由于一种公认的30~50kDa的循环蛋白(FSGS因子或毒性渗透性因子)损伤足细胞,升高肾小球的通透性。特发性的局灶节段性肾小球硬化在20%~50%的移植肾中会复发,近一半会在5年内失功[82]。复发的高危因素包括儿童时期发病(年龄<15岁)、弥漫性的肾小球系膜增生或肾小球塌陷型,以及原发性肾病快速进入透析阶段,或者上一次移植迅速复发[83]。

临床上,每周尿的蛋白肌酐比值升高需要怀疑复发(原肾的蛋白尿会在肾移植后逐渐减少),在电镜下看到足细胞足突融合则可以明确诊断,这比在光镜下看到节段性的肾小球硬化更早。

通过血浆置换可以去除循环中的致病蛋白(由最初的每周3次减少到每月1次,持续6个月),高剂量的环孢霉素(初始环孢霉素2小时目标浓度为1200~

1400ng/mL,可以稳定足突细胞的肌动蛋白细胞骨架),糖皮质激素[初期 1mg/(kg·d)逐渐减量至 10mg/d],以及 ACEI(或者 ARB)减少蛋白尿的措施,可以使 80%~90%的患者达到完全或部分缓解,偶尔晚期复发[84]。mTOR 抑制剂(西罗莫司和依维莫司)会影响足细胞而引起蛋白尿,应该避免使用。

Alport 综合征受体抗基底膜病的重新发作

比较少见的是,Alport 综合征(X 染色体男性 GBM 胶原的 *COL4A5* 基因突变)的受体在肾移植术后会产生针对“新的”α5 链(再隐性遗传个体中是 α3)的抗 GBM 抗体,这对于受体的免疫系统来说是外来物[85]。早期就会有所表现(数周或数月),表现为急性肾功能不全、坏死性和新月体性肾小球肾炎,以及活检可见 IgG 免疫荧光线性沉积的 Goodpastures 病。治疗方法包括血浆置换和环磷酰胺冲击。

慢性移植物功能缓慢衰退

临床定义(场景):肾功能逐渐衰退表现为血清肌酐逐年累月缓慢而不可逆的上升。

移植物功能长期监测和进行性移植物功能不全

因为 GFR 与肾小管间质损伤有关,规律的血清肌酐测定是保证移植肾健康的主要方法[86]。血清肌酐水平的相对变化都是有意义的,除生物学正常范围内的波动外,进行性移植肾功能不全是移植肾失功的征兆。

通过公式计算出来的 GFR 估计值(eGFR)(如简略的 MDRD、Nsnkivell 或者 CKD-EPI 公式)比未修正的血清肌酐评估更加精确;要注意血肌酐受到许多因素影响,如肌肉总量、肌酐产生量、小管肌酐分泌和实验室校正系数不同[87,88]。甲氧苄啶通常与磺胺甲恶唑联用来预防尿路感染和肺囊虫感染,同时也会抑制小管肌酐分泌,最终导致血清肌酐的无害性升高。血清胱抑素 C 反映出 GFR 不受肌肉量的影响,但比较昂贵,需要优化公式,并没有明显优于基于肌酐计算得出的 eGFR。碘海醇(“冷的”)或者 ^{99m}Tc 同位素的 DTPA、Cr^{51}EDTA 或 ^{125}I 碘海醇盐来计算血浆清除率是比较精确的方法(代替菊粉清除率),但因给患者带来不便且花费较贵而不常使用。

因为与 GFR 呈对数线性关系,血清肌酐在移植物损伤较多的情况下才会明显上升,并且会由于剩余肾单位的高滤过而减缓上升趋势。移植肾 GFR 随时间变化曲线取决于基线水平(决定于供体质量和早期是否有排斥等事件发生)和肾功能损耗的速率(“斜率”是由于持续性的损伤)(图 69.4)。肌酐倒数的下降(下降 30%,RR 为 2.56)或肌酐的上升(OR 为 2.2/1mg/dL=88.4μmol/L)都与移植肾失功有关[13];通过一些前瞻性的试验,它们对随后移植肾的失功有着一定的提示意义[89,90]。很多个体的 GFR 随时间变化的曲线并不是线性的,当发生新的病理状态时(肾小球肾炎、急性排斥或者 BK 病毒性肾病)会出现转折点而后突然下降。此外,即使早期有严重的移植肾缺血性损伤,移植肾在功能上也可以保持数年稳定。因此,虽然队列研究中移植肾的功能在统计学意义上与移植肾丢失有关,但是对于个体的预测能力仍比较弱。

尿液检测和移植肾影像学

尿液试纸分析可以反映移植肾肾小球疾病。尿蛋白肌酐比或者 24 小时尿蛋白可以用来评估尿蛋白量。蛋白尿是移植物失功和患者生存率的强有力的独立相关因素,即使 0.5g/d 的蛋白尿也有意义[91]。血尿和蛋白尿都提示着肾病复发或者新发的肾小球肾炎。

最初的超声诊断需要排除诸如输尿管梗阻或者动

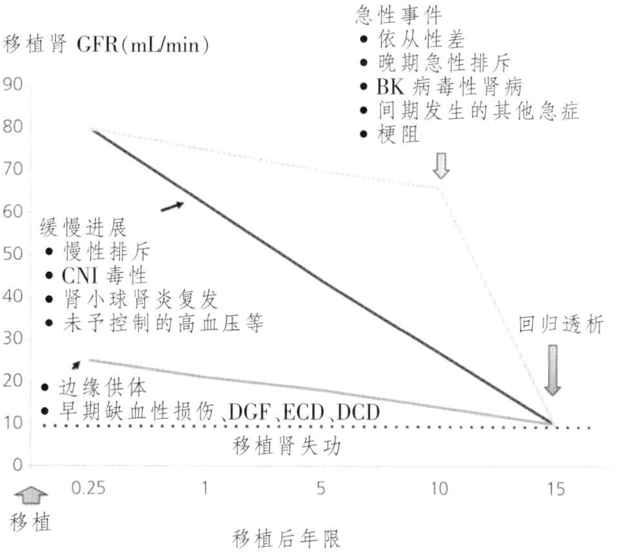

图 69.4 依据不同的病理生理学事件,移植肾肾小球滤过率和进展到移植物失功的时间变化图。CNI,钙调神经蛋白抑制剂。GFR,肾小球滤过率。DGF,移植肾延迟复功。ECD,扩大标准的供体。DCD,心脏死亡的供体。

脉血管狭窄等引起移植物功能不全的潜在原因。完全性和急性输尿管梗阻一般较为少见，可表现为移植物功能不全、无尿和肾盂积水。梗阻一般需要通过顺行或者逆行肾盂造影来证实和定位，通过输尿管导管可以暂时缓解，最终需要外科手术治疗来纠正。慢性和部分输尿管梗阻诊断上存在一定的难度，因为轻度的移植肾肾盂积水较为常见。泌尿系同位素造影利用锝(^{99m}Tc)巯替肽，不依赖于肾功能的好坏都能从小管分泌，有良好的敏感性和特异性[92]。未经治愈的移植肾膀胱输尿管反流是否会导致不可逆的实质瘢痕形成目前尚未被证实[93-95]。

多普勒的“阻力指数”与肾内血管顺应性、间质纤维化、随后的移植肾失功(≥0.8则风险升高9倍)以及受体的死亡率相关(反映受体的脉管系统顺应性)[96,97]。移植肾的血管阻力、MR或钆增强动态序列都是相对不敏感的影像学方法，只有存在明显的实质损伤才会有异常的表现[98]。

慢性移植肾失功的诊断步骤

当血清肌酐逐渐恶化或者持续性升高时，需要对其进行评估分析。可逆性因素包括脱水(液体负荷状态检查、腹泻、使用利尿剂)、急性CNI毒性(检测药物浓度)、肾毒性药物(ACEI、ARB、NSAID或者COXⅡ抑制剂)都会导致GFR下降，早期肾小球疾病复发(尿常规)和输尿管梗阻或者血管损伤(影像学)应该逐一排除(表69.1)。

排除了这些可逆性因素(表69.3)后，需要立即考虑移植肾活检，否则会使严重的移植肾损伤失去诊断的特异性且治疗反应较差。一份合格的组织样本需要进行免疫荧光(肾小球肾炎)、光镜和电镜观察以及C4d染色。详细的组织学和临床评估应该能够确定移植肾功能不全的原因。临床医生(评估免疫风险，抗体状态，既往是否排斥，目前治疗方案和并发症，供体质量和移植肾功能)和病理学家的联合诊断可合理解释这些发现(见第81章)。针对移植肾功能不全的病理生理学原因进行合理治疗需要特性的病因学诊断(表69.2和表69.3)[86,99]。

慢性细胞性间质性排斥

慢性活动性T细胞介导的排斥包含了由于维持性免疫抑制剂控制残余同种异体免疫反应失效而造成的持久的免疫性移植物损伤。进行性的移植物功能下降与间质T淋巴细胞浸润有关，通常还伴随着B细胞和巨噬细胞的浸润以及肾小管炎。偶尔能看到小肌性动脉的血管内膜纤维增生(平滑肌细胞的增殖和增生造成局灶性的内弹力层破坏并形成新的内膜)，发展为血管闭塞[10]。

治疗方法包括加强免疫抑制剂，如将环孢霉素替换成他克莫司(初始目标浓度为10ng/mL)[100]，硫唑嘌呤替换成吗替麦考酚[101]以及增加激素用量。同时进行药物依从性检查，回顾是否达到合适的血药浓度，以及排除干扰浓度的药物(如金丝桃或苯妥英会诱导产生代谢酶，从而降低CNI药物浓度)。

表69.2 慢性移植肾功能不全的鉴别诊断

结构性/感染性因素
输尿管梗阻或下尿路梗阻
复发性移植肾肾盂肾炎和(或)输尿管反流
BK病毒性肾病
移植肾动脉狭窄
免疫损伤
晚期急性排斥(医源性或患者依从性差)
慢性T细胞介导的排斥
慢性抗体介导的排斥
混合型急性或慢性排斥
其他原因
非特异性硬化性肾小管间质的损害(正式名称为慢性移植肾肾病)
慢性CNI毒性
复发性血栓性微血管病
急性间质性肾炎
复发或新发的肾小球肾炎
疾病的复发(如糖尿病肾病)
高血压未予控制和高血压肾病
代谢紊乱(未控制的高钙血症或高糖血症)
同时服用的药物：肾毒性(如NSAID或COX-Ⅱ抑制剂、造影剂)，影响肾小球血流和GFR类药(如ACE-Ⅰ、ARB、钙通道阻滞剂)或影响CNI的代谢(苯妥英、地尔硫䓬、维拉帕米和氟康唑、酮康唑等唑类抗真菌药物)
其他重大疾病导致的急性肾损伤

慢性抗体介导的排斥

慢性抗体介导的排斥(CAMR)的发生是由于一些未识别的预先存在的低滴度DSA(移植前CDC交叉试

表 69.3 慢性移植物损伤的管理

预防和筛查
缺血再灌注损伤最小化(最短的缺血时间,最佳获取、保存和运输方法)
供-受体组织不相容性最小化
急性排斥的快速病理学诊断和有效的治疗
早期最佳的免疫抑制方案(对于中至高敏的受体应用包括IL2R阻滞剂或抗胸腺细胞诱导的方案,视临床具体情形而定)
适当的免疫抑制来控制早期的亚临床排斥 (只有通过程序性活检诊断发现)
使用更昔洛韦或伐昔洛韦来早期预防CMV感染
早期BK病毒筛查(特别是使用高剂量的免疫抑制剂)
血清肌酐的定期检测
定期检查尿液和泌尿系影像(排除泌尿系梗阻)
必要时进行定期的依从性回顾和宣教
进展因素的控制
控制高血压(观念上倾向于钙通道阻滞剂,理论上使用ACEI或ARB能够获益),也可以使用利尿剂
低盐饮食,戒烟,控制脂肪,限制体重,改变生活方式(防止代谢综合征)
控制好糖尿病和尿路感染(如果发生的话)
对于低-中等免疫风险的受体,考虑减少CNI的长期剂量,或者对于已经发生慢性移植物损伤或CNI毒性的受体,考虑停用CNI或更换为其他药物
避免免疫抑制剂不足(会发生亚临床排斥或后期的急性排斥)
对免疫抑制方案进行个体化(根据HLA错配、既往排斥病史、是否二次移植和DSA)
处理受体的应急情况 (如败血症导致的急性肾小管坏死),等急性期过后再调整回合理的免疫抑制方案

验遗漏的)或者移植后新出现的抗体导致的[50,102]。后期的抗HLA抗体与慢性体液性排斥、移植肾肾病与移植物失功有关[45,102,103]。移植后数年出现的晚期新发DSA与早期细胞性或者混合排斥发生(通常与PTC黏附有关)以及HLA错配、服药的依从性差有关,使得移植物功能不全缓慢进展[77]。

CAMR主要临床表现为进行性的功能下降、高血压和日益加重的蛋白尿。慢性持续性DSA主要影响移植物的微循环,特别是肾小球和肾小管周围毛细血管,通过改变基膜下物质,产生特征性的变化。亚致死性的DSA与毛细血管内皮相互作用,使得肾小球内皮细胞增生和活化,内皮下因纤维化增宽和(或)GBM成双轨。管周毛细血管细胞产生多层的基底膜 (诊断学上一般定义为至少5层,正常状态只有1层)[9]。肾小球毛细血管增厚、系膜细胞的插入,通过亚甲胺银染色,显示为"双轨症",这是移植肾肾小球病的特征性标志。鉴别诊断包括血栓性微血管病(通过血涂片、结合珠蛋白和乳酸脱氢酶水平排除诊断)和丙肝膜增殖性肾小球肾炎(通过血清学、血病毒核酸试验和GBM沉积)[104]。作为CAMR肾小球表现的移植肾小球病,据报道,在正在逐渐失功和已经失功的移植物中的比例为5%~15%[6,45,50,105],在程序性活检中高达20%,而且大多表现为亚临床性[50,106]。

目前CAMR的诊断包括以下三个特征:①循环DSA(通常是Ⅱ型抗HLA抗体);②毛细血管C4d沉积,管周毛细血管抗体激活的经典补体通路的痕迹(但相对不敏感且通常呈阴性);③在器官功能不全时,通过光镜观察到的移植肾肾小球疾病。

电镜下表现为肾小球内皮肿胀、内皮下增宽和GBM双轨和(或)PTC基底膜成多层,可以证实CAMR诊断。管周白细胞炎和肾小球炎支持DSA介导的微循环损伤。CAMR导致的进行性的动脉内膜增生纤维化相当少见。通常,CAMR与进行性的移植物功能不全、顽固性的间质细胞排斥与肾小管间质损伤(间质纤维化和肾小管萎缩,IF/TA)有关,证明了这是一种不可控的广泛的自身免疫反应[77]。

目前的治疗方法的证据仅限于一些非随机队列研究,源于急性AMR治疗,包括加强基础免疫抑制剂、加大他克莫司和吗替麦考酚酯的剂量(抑制B细胞和T细胞的增殖)以及激素的剂量(如果不含类固醇重新加药)以及ACEI或者ARB来控制蛋白尿[13,50]。积极治疗如血浆置换联合静脉注射球蛋白去除循环中DSA和利妥昔单抗应用可以产生不一样的结局。硼替佐米(浆细胞蛋白酶体抑制剂)和依库丽单抗(抗C5抗体抑制剂)对CAMR的治疗效果并不明确,需要进一步临床评估[13,50]。

慢性移植物功能恶化的鉴别诊断

间质纤维化和肾小管萎缩

移植物缓慢、进行性失功最常见的病理类型是慢性IF/TA,伴有血管改变和肾小球硬化[12]。晚期移植肾失功患者中有27%~45%存在IF/TA[6,7],在大多数晚期诊断性活检或者程序性活检中均有表现。它被正式定义为硬化性“慢性移植物肾病”(CAN)[111],代表了肾单位损伤后通过纤维修复形成瘢痕组织的共同结局,而并不是某一类特殊的诊断[112]。多种潜在的病因和致病途径都可能导致IF/TA,同种免疫反应是最常见和最重要的病因[12,65]。

早期的肾小管损害始于缺血再灌注损伤,随后的急性或亚临床排斥加重了原先存在的供体疾病。IF/TA合并炎症预示着更差的预后[65,108,113]。在晚期活检中一种原因不明的非特异性类型被分类为“IF/TA未另行规定类”[112]。随后在CNI的毒性、高血压、糖尿病和高血脂等作用下,移植肾逐渐发生微血管异常和肾小球硬化等病变,同时可能混有一些特殊的诊断,如复发性肾小球肾炎或者晚期同种免疫损伤[12]。

IF/TA-CAN类型的一种治疗策略是将CNI药物减量到最低(假设最先的病理学原因是由CNI肾毒性引起的)。在一项随机对照试验中,减少CNI剂量同时增加吗替麦考酚酯的用量,可以提高移植肾GFR(4.4mL/min;95%CI为2.9~5.9),同时可以提高移植物生存率(OR为0.72;95%CI为0.52~1.01)。只有在完全去除CNI的试验中,急性排斥发生率才有所上升。但即使去除CNI仍不能避免移植物功能不全发生[114]。在移植肾功能不全(CAN证实为91.3%)的大型CONVERT随机试验中,从CNI替换为西罗莫司(“替换”),与继续使用CNI相比,主要终点eGFR并没有不同。在严重的移植肾功能不全(eGFR<40mL/min)或蛋白尿大于0.5g/d的患者中,替换西罗莫司无效[110]。在其他对照试验中,去除CNI(西罗莫司替换或者初始未使用)可以减少血管和肾小管间质损伤[109,115]。

对于肾功能逐渐下降的IF/TA患者,应该从可能存在免疫或者非免疫介导的病因开始考虑,并结合临床、生物学和组织学的信息[86]。IF/TA从病理生理学上分类应该主要归因于:①早期的非免疫因素如供体疾病或者缺血再灌注的肾小管损伤;②免疫损伤,包括急性的、严重的、持续的或者后期发生的排斥和(或)③其他特异性的诊断存在,包括复发的疾病、BK病毒、高血压或者CNI中毒。一些损伤的因素可能会同时存在,或者在移植物存活期中分别出现(表69.2)。

移植物失功伴IF/TA的治疗的方法需要考虑受体先前是否有排斥和非依从性病史、是否为高敏患者、HLA错配情况,和循环中DSA状态,这些都能帮助在考虑CNI减量时量化评估免疫风险。最近的移植物病理类型对于排除活动性的同种免疫活动非常重要(组织学的线索包括小动脉的血管内膜纤维增生、间质淋巴细胞浸润、管周毛细血管淋巴细胞、移植肾肾小球病,或者C4d沉积阳性)。通过连续性活检配对[65]可以评估亚临床间质性排斥导致的渐进性的IF/TA,此时免疫抑制剂需要加强。

BK病毒肾病

BK病毒是一种流行性多瘤病毒,在儿童中会引起轻症的原发性感染,其血清学阳性率为60%~80%。残留的病毒可以在强有力的免疫抑制状态下被激活,通常在移植后的1年内保持无症状性的病毒血症。严重的BK病毒肾病会发展成肾小管间质性肾炎,进而导致进行性移植肾功能不全和移植物丢失(发生率为5%,其中46%会失功)[116]。移植物活检显示出有诊断价值的核内包涵体,同时肾小管细胞内病毒复制形成增大的核染色体,通过SV40T病毒免疫染色阳性可以证实。移植物的BK病毒感染可以导致肾小管细胞的退化、凋亡和脱落(形成有诊断意义的尿液“诱饵”细胞)和间质单核细胞性炎症[117]。

目前的抗病毒药物对BK病毒无效。通过避免过度的免疫抑制进行预防是最好的策略,同时加上定期的常规病毒性监测(通过血液核酸检测或者PCR检测)。在移植物功能不全前,早期病毒血症(病毒载量定量)检测和谨慎地降低CNI治疗剂量(通常减少50%的CNI剂量和降低或去除抗代谢类药物),可以有效减少或消除循环中病毒量,防止具有破坏性的实质感染。

移植物BK病毒肾病一旦确诊,则是一种严重的威胁,并且很难被根除[116,117]。给予环丙沙星(使用1个月),低剂量的西多福韦(0.5mg/kg,静脉输注,每两周予以生理盐水水化),去除MMF或者替换为来氟米特(具有比较弱的抗病毒功能)或者AZA,他克莫司转化为低剂量的环孢素A(C2目标浓度是500ng/mL)或者CNI剂量减少,或者静脉内使用丙种球蛋白治疗(一种非清除性的免疫调节药,在BK病毒合并排斥时使用),在小样本的队列研究中都仅是有限的获益[34,118]。

钙调神经磷酸酶抑制剂的肾毒性

对于移植领域来说,环孢霉素及随后他克莫司的发现大幅减少了早期急性排斥反应的发生,带来了良好的移植肾1年存活率并且奠定了现代免疫抑制基础。但是 CNI 类药物具有肾毒性,这是这一类药物最主要的缺点[119]。CNI 的肾毒性对随后的移植物损伤可以从以下几点推断:①急性排斥得到控制后,移植物长期丢失率仍没有改变;②纵向的组织病理学研究中发现存在特征性的毒性损伤[120];③临床试验如 CNI 不使用、早期撤除(避免毒性)、剂量减少或者随后撤除(针对已经确立的 CNI 损伤),显示功能或结构得到改善[109,115,121,122,];④非肾脏的实体器官移植患者或者自身免疫疾病患者使用 CNI 治疗后自体肾可能表示出经典的 CNI 组织学表现和肾功能不全[123]。

进行性小动脉透明样变性是慢性 CNI 毒性的最可靠的诊断标志,与下游肾小球硬化有关,也是 30%的"预后不佳的移植"患者中的第二常见诊断[7]。小动脉透明样变性随着持续的慢性 CNI 暴露和移植年限的增长会变得越来越普遍,大多数的受体在移植后 10 年均会存在,但是严重程度各不相同(提示不同个体的差异和易感性)[12,120]。小动脉透明变性不仅仅源于 CNI 毒性,同样也可以来源于供肾本身[124](供体年龄较大、患者血管疾病或者吸烟,此时基线植入活检可以对随后的组织学解释有所帮助),或者随后其他并发症的进展如糖尿病(表现为活检标本符合糖尿病肾小球疾病伴基底膜增厚和蛋白尿)。

单纯的 CNI 肾中毒(环孢霉素介导的急性肾小球血管收缩或者非排斥的慢性改变),如果能够早期识别可有较好的预后,而且通过 CNI 减量很容易得到缓解[7]。在一些队列研究和非随机试验中,移植肾功能不全患者撤除 CNI 药物后可以逆转功能下降并且提高 eGFR[115]。在随机试验中,通过减少或撤除 CNI,可以提高 90%受体的肾功能,同时发生移植物排斥和丢失的风险较小[121]。虽然从环孢霉素替换为低剂量的他克莫司,受体显示出了更好的肾功能、血脂水平、血压和心血管标志物,但是 5 年移植物生存率并没有改变[125]。

当低免疫风险的患者由于 CNI 毒性导致功能恶化(同时通过活检排除亚临床排斥),则需要撤除 CNI 并保持 MMF 浓度和激素应用[126]。对于高免疫风险、再次移植或者既往发生排斥的患者,如果发现 CNI 中毒,可以对 CNI 药物减量或者更换(西罗莫司或依维莫司),仔细监测血清肌酐变化(完全撤药后排斥风险接近 10%)[34]。mTOR 抑制剂是一种相对弱的免疫抑制药物,并且给予高剂量时患者很难耐受,有 30%~40%的患者因为口腔溃疡、外周水肿、蛋白尿、贫血或者血小板减少等副作用而停药[127,128]。当活动性的排斥和慢性 CNI 毒性一起发生时,应当优先治疗同种免疫反应,因为这是对移植肾更大的威胁(表 69.3)。

新型的非肾毒性免疫抑制药物带来了一些希望,但是临床数据并不完整。根据 CNI 减量的荟萃分析实验,Belatacept(作用于 CD28-CD80/86 通路和 T 细胞的共同刺激)和托法替尼(JAK 激酶 1/3 抑制剂)联合吗替麦考酚酯可以减少移植物失功的风险(OR 为 0.61;95%CI 为 0.39~0.96)[129]。Voclosporine(一种环孢霉素的类似物,免疫效应不亚于他克莫司)声称可以减少肾毒性。此外,CD2 特别融合蛋白 alefacept(作用于 LFA3-CD2 通路并且选择性地去除记忆 T 细胞,对银屑病有效)和 sotrastaurin(AEB071,蛋白激酶 C 抑制剂,减少 T-淋巴细胞的活化和细胞因子的释放)正在进行临床前的试验。

后期发生的肾小球疾病

10 年内,高达 8.4%移植物失功是因为复发或新发肾小球肾炎[130-132]。临床线索是血尿或蛋白尿,通过移植肾病理来确诊。在现代免疫抑制剂应用下,很少有因早期排斥而失功,但产生了更多"处于风险状态"的患者,然而他们由于肾小球肾炎复发所导致的后期移植物失功并没有增加[133]。移植后的免疫抑制剂能够控制大多数免疫介导的肾脏疾病,包括 ANCA 相关性血管炎、狼疮性肾炎、膜性肾病和 Goodpasture 病。IgA 肾病通常会复发但是临床表现较轻[130]。根据已经登记的资料分析,糖皮质激素的使用与 IgA 复发减少相关(亚风险比为 0.50;95%CI 为 0.30~0.84)[133]。吗替麦考酚酯(在原发的 IgA 肾病中显示有获益)也有助于避免后期的复发。

大多数的轻链沉积病都会复发,50%~90%的重链沉积病会复发并且导致移植物失功(有一些病例报道使用依库丽单抗可以获益)。Fabry 病复发时间较晚,需要特殊的半乳糖苷酶治疗。移植肾糖尿病肾病同样也会复发,表现为蛋白尿移植肾功能不全和典型的病理表现。血压控制和肾素-血管紧张素系统的阻滞在队列研究中显示获益,建议使用。

移植后高血压和血脂异常

70%~90%的受体都会出现高血压,与移植物的丢失和存活相关。如此高的发病率和移植前高血压以及受体血管疾病,糖皮质激素、环孢霉素的治疗和移植肾功能不全相关，仅少数由于移植肾动脉狭窄所引起[134]。在荟萃分析中显示，钙离子通道阻滞剂（对抗环孢霉素引起的血管收缩）耐受性好，并且有效减少了移植物失功（RR 为 0.75；95%CI 为 0.57~0.99）并提高了 GFR（与安慰剂组相比提高了 4.5mL/min）[135]。虽然肾素-血管紧张素系统阻滞剂在理论上可以减少移植物纤维化、蛋白尿产生以及移植肾失功的比例[136]，但是实际上对移植物的预后的好处并没有被证实。ACEI 会减轻 GFR 下降（约 8.1mL/min）、蛋白尿（每天 0.28g）和血红蛋白（每天 0.28g），但是会加重高钾血症[135]。袢利尿剂对于系统性的水肿或者由于移植肾无法清除盐分、水分引起的高血压是比较有效的。建议目标血压为 130/80mmHg[34]。

HMG 辅酶 A 还原酶抑制剂（他汀类药物）耐受性好，除了明显改善高脂血症外，随机对照试验还证明它可以有效减少患者心血管事件的发生[137]。血脂紊乱的受体心血管事件接近 3.5%~5.0%/年，因此应该提倡治疗血脂紊乱，健康的饮食、生活方式和恰当的控制糖尿病[34]。

晚期输尿管狭窄和梗阻

见尿液检测和移植肾成像章节。

晚期急性移植肾失功

临床表现：与之前基线相比，移植患者出现（有时会长时间的无任何表现）更加严重的移植肾功能丧失和血清肌酐显著升高。

晚期急性排斥

晚期急性排斥是指移植后超过 3 个月发生的急性排斥，由于依从性差或者医源性导致的免疫抑制过低而引起，表现为亚急性的或急性移植肾功能不全。它也可以发生在对移植肾有高免疫活动的致敏受体，但更多的是由于患者的药物依从性差（见下文）或者医源性导致的低免疫抑制状态（由于诊断为癌症或者严重的感染而减药）引起[77]。有研究表明，在临床医师指导下减少吗替麦考酚酯剂量来缓解腹泻与急性排斥相关[128]。

晚期发生的急性排斥通常都较为严重，大多数患者表现为激素抵抗，很难逆转，同时伴随广泛的肾小管间质损害[46]。维持性免疫抑制治疗的完全或部分停药（不可控的）会导致移植物排斥，其涉及获得性和固有免疫系统，抗体的产生，T 细胞和 B 细胞、嗜酸性粒细胞、浆细胞和巨噬细胞的混合性浸润。慢性移植物排斥的开始可能也会伴随着持续的细胞间质浸润和（或）新发 DSA 的产生（通常为Ⅱ级抗体）[77]。诊断性活检通常会有明确的急性排斥表现：间质大量淋巴细胞浸润和水肿，慢性间质纤维化，管腔破坏和肾小球硬化。其中，抗体介导的排斥（循环 DSA/内皮细胞炎症和 C4d 沉积）和血管性排斥都很常见[6,7,77]。

利用激素冲击和加强基础免疫抑制方案进行早期治疗效果有限，移植肾功能会继续下降，最终发展为移植物失功。移植物通常会由于晚期的排斥发作造成不可逆的损伤，表现为严重的 IF/TA（2 级包括 25%~50% 或更多皮质），从而限制功能的恢复。还有一个很重要的治疗相关问题，进行强有力的二线治疗方案需要医生对每一个个体通过治疗获得的利弊进行仔细的评估。而是否使用抗胸腺细胞球蛋白和（或）联合静脉应用免疫球蛋白血浆置换或利妥昔单抗取决于以下几点：①潜在肾单位不可逆丢失的严重程度（最佳评估方法为 IF/TA 的穿刺评估分数，移植肾功能下降的持续时间和趋势）；②预期的治疗反应（抗体、血管性和混合性排斥均为难治性；③受体对于强有力的免疫抑制药物的耐受程度（年龄较大，合并一些并发症的脆弱患者，顽固性的慢性感染如支气管扩张是相对禁忌证）；④潜在的一些情况（短期内可逆性的或存在更多慢性疾病因素的急性排斥和无法更改的药物因素）。

通过肾小管间质炎损害的范围来判断整体肾单位丢失是最好的方法，对预后有指导意义（肾小球硬化并不可靠并且容易误导，某些肾小球表现为管状）。应当仔细分析移植肾的病理（不仅仅是通过阅读报告来估计），以评估免疫细胞浸润的潜在可逆转性。需要精确的临床判断来平衡受体免疫抑制的风险（首要死因是控制不好的细菌性败血症、浸润性真菌感染、迟发的 CMV 或淋巴细胞增生性疾病等）和拯救受损的移植肾（尽可能稳定或提高移植肾的功能）。首选的保守治疗是激素冲击治疗，增强基础免疫治疗和（或）IVIG，同时也要让受体接受治疗失败并重新回到透析的治疗可能性。

药物依从性差

23%~50%的受体在某段时间存在药物依从性差[139]，包括：间断性地遗漏某些药片（单纯或故意的遗忘、酗酒或滥用药物、混乱的生活方式，痴呆或健忘），暗中减少药物剂量或避免服用某类药物(由于副作用或其他顾虑)或完全的停药,最终引发急性排斥[77,140]。较差的药物依从性会使得急性排斥和移植物丢失的风险升高 7 倍,在某些研究中造成了 36%的肾脏丢失[139]。药物依从性差对高免疫风险的受体如既往排斥,HLA 错配、已知 DSA 存在或再次移植造成的影响有所不同,但结局相似。

危险因素包括透析时依从性差、精神方面的疾病或人格障碍、滥用药物、危险行为,贫穷或社会经济支持不完善。将儿童移植给成人或青少年的肾脏都比较脆弱,一些衔接工作能够有所帮助。随着移植年限的增长和患者的疏忽会使药物依从性变差[141]。

临床提示线索包括错过约定的就诊,CNI 血药浓度的波动或未检测,药物的发放和实际使用不符合,或尽管表面上的治疗很到位,却发生了无法预期的急性排斥。但在实际操作中,却很难实现把握线索,不规律地服用药物可以被明确的否认所掩盖(避免临床医生的不悦),被临床药生的药物审查所质疑,或监护人自我承认(某些时候是护士)。临床工作中应当间接询问患者,避免提出恐吓性的问题,并且仔细聆听患者的反应(“医学沟通的艺术”)。同时应该理解患者因为个人原因和所处环境压力导致的药物依从性差,能够帮助整体治疗策略的构想,最终避免这种情况再次发生。

除了肾毒性,免疫抑制治疗还有其他非肾脏毒性的副作用,影响着它们的使用和误用。影响容貌的副作用,如年轻女性使用环孢霉素导致的多毛症(可以使用他克莫司替代),使用激素导致的满月脸和痤疮(可以局部治疗或使用多西环素)使人不安并且导致依从性变差。激素撤销或最少化可以减少糖尿病、白内障、骨质疏松症、骨折、儿童发育迟缓和血脂紊乱的发生,同时能改善高血压和高脂血症的控制、减少糖尿病的发作,但会增加排斥的概率(试验中与继续使用激素相比升高 10%~15%)并导致移植肾功能变差,与获益旗鼓相当[142,143]。环孢霉素会引起牙龈增生和血脂紊乱,与环孢霉素相比,他克莫司会引起更多的移植后糖尿病、震颤、头痛、神经症状和腹泻。mTOR 抑制剂(西罗莫司或依维莫司)通常存在剂量依赖的副作用,如水肿和口腔溃疡。

预防性的策略包括专业的移植药物药剂师通过个体化和重复的告知,最大限度减小药物副作用、复杂程度和花费,以及给予患者更多临床上的支持来消除顾虑[34,144]。

晚期急性移植肾功能不全的鉴别诊断

其他相关疾病引起的急性肾损伤

移植肾急性功能损伤可能由于药物或手术因素引起,如心肌梗死、败血症、晚期 CMV、急腹症等。特殊的治疗取决于潜在的急症、对心血管药物的最优化、严重威胁生命感染时暂时减少免疫抑制药物(痊愈后恢复剂量)和必要时进行支持性的静脉水化。移植肾功能不全通常能够治愈恢复功能;但是,不完全的恢复也会出现严重的急症(表 69.3)。

晚期移植肾输尿管狭窄

如前所述,晚期移植肾输尿管狭窄会在排斥复发之后发作,导致远端输尿管的缺血性损伤。BK 病毒也是引起输尿管狭窄的潜在原因。

晚期新发或晚期复发的肾小球肾炎

在晚期发生的肾小球疾病章节中有所描述。

晚期移植物血栓

极其少见,与潜在的高凝状态或者严重的系统性灌注不足有关。

移植肾失功受体的管理

慢性的移植肾失功通常是隐蔽的,并且在很多时候是难以预计。许多肾脏功能能够在到达 5 期 [$<15mL/(min\cdot 1.73m^2)$] 透析治疗开始之前保持中等或严重的慢性肾脏疾病水平并维持多年。许多受体移植肾失功时年龄较大(15%等待名单里的患者超过 65 岁)并且合并有心血管疾病、糖尿病、移植前肿瘤或慢性肺部疾病,这些都会增加死亡率[145,146]。移植物功能不良的受体通常患有尿毒症、贫血、营养不良,临床上容易感染,有着较高的死亡率(失功后第一个星期的 HR 为 13.6,但是有患者甚至可以存活 10 年)[146]。由于免疫抑制所导致的晚期机会性感染通常表现为 CMV 和细菌性或真菌性疾病,需要特殊的抗菌治疗。外科急症或心血管急症会引起急性肾脏损伤和突然的移植物失功,特别是较差的移植肾基础功能。

慢性肾脏失功的并发症需要早期干预。通过促红细胞生成素来纠正贫血，通过磷酸盐结合剂和维生素D类似物来治疗高磷酸盐血症和继发性甲状旁腺功能亢进，合理营养纠正低蛋白血症，给予合适的抗高血压药物来控制血压[147,148]。提前的透析进入计划，合适的心理支持、谨慎地应用逐渐减量的免疫抑制剂，以及利用多学科专业的治疗，可以减少过渡期间的发病率和死亡率。

总结

移植肾功能不全有许多的鉴别诊断，早期更侧重于技术和缺血等相关问题，术后短期内需要考虑免疫排斥，晚期主要是复发疾病和免疫抑制的平衡。熟练的临床评估、诊断方法的准确应用（包括活检）和移植病理学家的合作，可以缓和许多会潜在导致移植肾失功的病因。急性排斥是移植肾特殊的诊断，在增强免疫抑制方案之前需要考虑并排除其他的病因。

（吴建永 译　吴建永 校）

参考文献

1. Bestard O, Nickel P, Cruzado JM, et al. Circulating alloreactive T cells correlate with graft function in longstanding renal transplant recipients. Journal of the American Society of Nephrology. 2008;19:1419–1429.
2. Nasr IW, Reel M, Oberbarnscheidt MH, et al. Tertiary lymphoid tissues generate effector and memory T cells that lead to allograft rejection. American Journal of Transplantation. 2007;7:1071–1079.
3. Valujskikh A, Lakkis FG. In remembrance of things past: memory T cells and transplant rejection. Immunological Reviews. 2003;196:65–74.
4. Dai Z, Konieczny BT, Lakkis FG. The dual role of IL-2 in the generation and maintenance of CD8+ memory T cells. Journal of Immunology. 2000;165: 3031–3036.
5. Nankivell BJ, Alexander SI. Rejection of the kidney allograft. New England Journal of Medicine. 2010;363:1451–1462.
6. El-Zoghby ZM, Stegall MD, Lager DJ, et al. Identifying specific causes of kidney allograft loss. American Journal of Transplantation. 2009;9:527–535.
7. Gourishankar S, Leduc R, Connett J, et al. Pathological and clinical characterization of the 'troubled transplant': data from the DeKAF study. American Journal of Transplantation. 2010;10:324–330.
8. Nankivell BJ, Chapman JR. Chronic allograft nephropathy: current concepts and future directions. Transplantation. 2006;81:643–654.
9. Sis B, Mengel M, Haas M, et al. Banff '09 meeting report: antibody mediated graft deterioration and implementation of Banff working groups. American Journal of Transplantation. 2010;10:464–471.
10. Solez K, Colvin RB, Racusen LC, et al. Banff 07 classification of renal allograft pathology: updates and future directions. American Journal of Transplantation. 2008;8:753–760.
11. Halloran PF. Immunosuppressive drugs for kidney transplantation. New England Journal of Medicine. 2004;351:2715–2729.
12. Nankivell BJ, Borrows RJ, Fung CL, et al. The natural history of chronic allograft nephropathy. New England Journal of Medicine. 2003;349:2326–2333.
13. Colvin RB. Antibody-mediated renal allograft rejection: diagnosis and pathogenesis. Journal of the American Society of Nephrology. 2007;18:1046–1056.
14. Halloran PF, Wadgymar A, Ritchie S, et al. The significance of the anti-class I antibody response. I. Clinical and pathologic features of anti-class I-mediated rejection. Transplantation. 1990;49:85–91.
15. Terasaki PI. Humoral theory of transplantation. American Journal of Transplantation. 2003;3:665–673.
16. Patel R, Terasaki PI. Significance of the positive crossmatch test in kidney transplantation. New England Journal of Medicine. 1969;280:735–739.
17. Jackson AM, Kuperman MB, Montgomery RA. Multiple hyperacute rejections in the absence of detectable complement activation in a patient with endothelial cell reactive antibody. American Journal of Transplantation. 2012;12: 1643–1649.
18. Warren DS, Montgomery RA. Incompatible kidney transplantation: lessons from a decade of desensitization and paired kidney exchange. Immunologic Research. 2010;47:257–264.
19. Fidler ME, Gloor JM, Lager DJ, et al. Histologic findings of antibody-mediated rejection in ABO blood-group-incompatible living-donor kidney transplantation. American Journal of Transplantation. 2004;4:101–107.
20. Lynch RJ, Platt JL. Accommodation in organ transplantation. Current Opinion in Organ Transplantation. 2008;13:165–170.
21. King KE, Warren DS, Samaniego-Picota M, et al. Antibody, complement and accommodation in ABO-incompatible transplants. Current Opinion in Immunology. 2004;16:545–549.
22. Moore J, Shabir S, Chand S, et al. Assessing and comparing rival definitions of delayed renal allograft function for predicting subsequent graft failure. Transplantation. 2010;90:1113–1116.
23. Siedlecki A, Irish W, Brennan DC. Delayed graft function in the kidney transplant. American Journal of Transplantation. 2011;11:2279–2296.
24. Rao PS, Schaubel DE, Guidinger MK, et al. A comprehensive risk quantification score for deceased donor kidneys: the kidney donor risk index. Transplantation. 2009;88:231–236.
25. Yarlagadda SG, Coca SG, Formica RN Jr, et al. Association between delayed graft function and allograft and patient survival: a systematic review and meta-analysis. Nephrology, Dialysis, Transplantation. 2009;24:1039–1047.
26. Danovitch GM, Cecka JM. Allocation of deceased donor kidneys: past, present, and future. American Journal of Kidney Diseases. 2003;42:882–890.
27. Stratta RJ, Sundberg AK, Rohr MS, et al. Optimal use of older donors and recipients in kidney transplantation. Surgery. 2006;139:324–333.
28. Matsuoka L, Almeda JL, Mateo R. Pulsatile perfusion of kidney allografts. Current Opinion in Organ Transplantation. 2009;14:365–369.
29. Moers C, Smits JM, Maathuis MH, et al. Machine perfusion or cold storage in deceased-donor kidney transplantation. New England Journal of Medicine. 2009;360:7–19.
30. Gasser M, Waaga AM, Laskowski IA, et al. The influence of donor brain death on short and long-term outcome of solid organ allografts. Annals of Transplantation: Quarterly of the Polish Transplantation Society. 2000;5:61–67.
31. Alegre ML, Leemans J, Le Moine A, et al. The multiple facets of toll-like receptors in transplantation biology. Transplantation. 2008;86:1–9.
32. Kim IK, Bedi DS, Denecke C, et al. Impact of innate and adaptive immunity on rejection and tolerance. Transplantation. 2008;86:889–894.
33. Briscoe DM, Alexander SI, Lichtman AH. Interactions between T lymphocytes and endothelial cells in allograft rejection. Current Opinion in Immunology. 1998;10:525–531.
34. Kasiske BL, Zeier MG, Chapman JR, et al. KDIGO clinical practice guideline for the care of kidney transplant recipients: a summary. Kidney International. 2010;77:299–311.
35. Sumitran-Holgersson S. Relevance of MICA and other non-HLA antibodies in clinical transplantation. Current Opinion in Immunology. 2008;20: 607–613.
36. Zou Y, Stastny P, Susal C, et al. Antibodies against MICA antigens and kidney-transplant rejection. New England Journal of Medicine. 2007;357: 1293–1300.
37. Dragun D, Muller DN, Brasen JH, et al. Angiotensin II type 1-receptor activating antibodies in renal-allograft rejection. New England Journal of Medicine. 2005;352:558–569.
38. Gibson IW, Gwinner W, Brocker V, et al. Peritubular capillaritis in renal allografts: prevalence, scoring system, reproducibility and clinicopathological correlates. American Journal of Transplantation. 2008;8:819–825.
39. Crary GS, Raissian Y, Gaston RC, et al. Optimal cutoff point for immunoperoxidase detection of C4d in the renal allograft: results from a multicenter study. Transplantation. 2010;90:1099–1105.
40. Loupy A, Hill GS, Suberbielle C, et al. Significance of C4d Banff scores in early protocol biopsies of kidney transplant recipients with preformed donor-specific antibodies (DSA). American Journal of Transplantation. 2011;11:56–65.
41. Batal I, Girnita A, Zeevi A, et al. Clinical significance of the distribution of C4d deposits in different anatomic compartments of the allograft kidney. Modern Pathology. 2008;21:1490–1498.
42. Mengel M, Bogers J, Bosmans JL, et al. Incidence of C4d stain in protocol biopsies from renal allografts: results from a multicenter trial. American Journal of Transplantation. 2005;5:1050–1056.
43. Cohen D, Colvin RB, Daha MR, et al. Pros and cons for C4d as a biomarker.

Kidney International. 2012;81:628–639.
44. Worthington JE, McEwen A, McWilliam LJ, et al. Association between C4d staining in renal transplant biopsies, production of donor-specific HLA antibodies, and graft outcome. Transplantation. 2007;83:398–403.
45. Sis B, Campbell PM, Mueller T, et al. Transplant glomerulopathy, late antibody-mediated rejection and the ABCD tetrad in kidney allograft biopsies for cause. American Journal of Transplantation. 2007;7:1743–1752.
46. Sun Q, Liu ZH, Ji S, et al. Late and early C4d-positive acute rejection: different clinico-histopathological subentities in renal transplantation. Kidney International. 2006;70:377–383.
47. Pescovitz MD. Rituximab, an anti-cd20 monoclonal antibody: history and mechanism of action. American Journal of Transplantation. 2006;6:859–866.
48. Zarkhin V, Li L, Kambham N, et al. A randomized, prospective trial of rituximab for acute rejection in pediatric renal transplantation. American Journal of Transplantation. 2008;8:2607–2617.
49. Locke JE, Magro CM, Singer AL, et al. The use of antibody to complement protein C5 for salvage treatment of severe antibody-mediated rejection. American Journal of Transplantation. 2009;9:231–235.
50. Stegall MD, Gloor JM. Deciphering antibody-mediated rejection: new insights into mechanisms and treatment. Current Opinion in Organ Transplantation. 2010;15:8–10.
51. Scornik JC, Kriesche HU. Human leukocyte antigen sensitization after transplant loss: timing of antibody detection and implications for prevention. Human Immunology. 2011;72:398–401.
52. Meier-Kriesche HU, Scornik JC, Susskind B, et al. A lifetime versus a graft life approach redefines the importance of HLA matching in kidney transplant patients. Transplantation. 2009;88:23–29.
53. Vo AA, Lukovsky M, Toyoda M, et al. Rituximab and intravenous immune globulin for desensitization during renal transplantation. New England Journal of Medicine. 2008;359:242–251.
54. Roodnat JI, Kal-van Gestel JA, Zuidema W, et al. Successful expansion of the living donor pool by alternative living donation programs. American Journal of Transplantation. 2009;9:2150–2156.
55. Larsen CP, Morris PJ, Austyn JM. Migration of dendritic leukocytes from cardiac allografts into host spleens. A novel pathway for initiation of rejection. Journal of Experimental Medicine. 1990;171:307–314.
56. Hoffmann SC, Hale DA, Kleiner DE, et al. Functionally significant renal allograft rejection is defined by transcriptional criteria. American Journal of Transplantation. 2005;5:573–581.
57. Akalin E, Hendrix RC, Polavarapu RG, et al. Gene expression analysis in human renal allograft biopsy samples using high-density oligoarray technology. Transplantation. 2001;72:948–953.
58. Sarwal M, Chua MS, Kambham N, et al. Molecular heterogeneity in acute renal allograft rejection identified by DNA microarray profiling. New England Journal of Medicine. 2003;349:125–138.
59. Wyburn KR, Jose MD, Wu H, et al. The role of macrophages in allograft rejection. Transplantation. 2005;80:1641–1647.
60. Robertson H, Kirby JA. Post-transplant renal tubulitis: the recruitment, differentiation and persistence of intra-epithelial T cells. American Journal of Transplantation. 2003;3:3–10.
61. Barry M, Bleackley RC. Cytotoxic T lymphocytes: all roads lead to death. Nature Reviews. Immunology. 2002;2:401–409.
62. Zorn E, Miklos DB, Floyd BH, et al. Minor histocompatibility antigen DBY elicits a coordinated B and T cell response after allogeneic stem cell transplantation. Journal of Experimental Medicine. 2004;199:1133–1142.
63. Bonsib SM, Abul-Ezz SR, Ahmad I, et al. Acute rejection-associated tubular basement membrane defects and chronic allograft nephropathy. Kidney International. 2000;58:2206–2214.
64. McDonald S, Russ G, Campbell S, et al. Kidney transplant rejection in Australia and New Zealand: relationships between rejection and graft outcome. American Journal of Transplantation. 2007;7:1201–1208.
65. Nankivell BJ, Borrows RJ, Fung CL, et al. Delta analysis of posttransplantation tubulointerstitial damage. Transplantation. 2004;78:434–441.
66. Middleton J, Patterson AM, Gardner L, et al. Leukocyte extravasation: chemokine transport and presentation by the endothelium. Blood. 2002;100:3853–3860.
67. Lefaucheur C, Loupy A, Vernerey D, et al. Antibody-mediated vascular rejection of kidney allografts: a population-based study. Lancet. 2012;381:313–319.
68. Nankivell BJ, Chapman JR. The significance of subclinical rejection and the value of protocol biopsies. American Journal of Transplantation. 2006;6:2006–2012.
69. Rush D, Nickerson P, Gough J, et al. Beneficial effects of treatment of early subclinical rejection: a randomized study. Journal of the American Society of Nephrology. 1998;9:2129–2134.
70. Kurtkoti J, Sakhuja V, Sud K, et al. The utility of 1- and 3-month protocol biopsies on renal allograft function: a randomized controlled study. American Journal of Transplantation. 2008;8:317–323.
71. Rush D, Arlen D, Boucher A, et al. Lack of benefit of early protocol biopsies in renal transplant patients receiving TAC and MMF: a randomized study. American Journal of Transplantation. 2007;7:2538–2545.
72. Lerut E, Naesens M, Kuypers DR, et al. Subclinical peritubular capillaritis at 3 months is associated with chronic rejection at 1 year. Transplantation. 2007;83:1416–1422.
73. Sis B, Jhangri GS, Bunnag S, et al. Endothelial gene expression in kidney transplants with alloantibody indicates antibody-mediated damage despite lack of C4d staining. American Journal of Transplantation. 2009;9:2312–2323.
74. Haas M, Montgomery RA, Segev DL, et al. Subclinical acute antibody-mediated rejection in positive crossmatch renal allografts. American Journal of Transplantation. 2007;7:576–585.
75. Loupy A, Suberbielle-Boissel C, Hill GS, et al. Outcome of subclinical antibody-mediated rejection in kidney transplant recipients with preformed donor-specific antibodies. American Journal of Transplantation. 2009;9:2561–2570.
76. Wavamunno MD, O'Connell PJ, Vitalone M, et al. Transplant glomerulopathy: ultrastructural abnormalities occur early in longitudinal analysis of protocol biopsies. American Journal of Transplantation. 2007;7:2757–2768.
77. Wiebe C, Gibson IW, Blydt-Hansen TD, et al. Evolution and clinical pathologic correlations of de novo donor-specific HLA antibody post kidney transplant. American Journal of Transplantation. 2012;12:1157–1167.
78. Reeve J, Einecke G, Mengel M, et al. Diagnosing rejection in renal transplants: a comparison of molecular- and histopathology-based approaches. American Journal of Transplantation. 2009;9:1802–1810.
79. Ponticelli C, Moia M, Montagnino G. Renal allograft thrombosis. Nephrology, Dialysis, Transplantation. 2009;24:1388–1393.
80. Kavanagh D, Richards A, Goodship T, et al. Transplantation in atypical hemolytic uremic syndrome. Seminars in Thrombosis and Hemostasis. 2010;36:653–659.
81. Cochat P, Fargue S, Harambat J. Primary hyperoxaluria type 1: strategy for organ transplantation. Current Opinion in Organ Transplantation. 2010;15:590–593.
82. Hickson LJ, Gera M, Amer H, et al. Kidney transplantation for primary focal segmental glomerulosclerosis: outcomes and response to therapy for recurrence. Transplantation. 2009;87:1232–1239.
83. Shimizu A, Higo S, Fujita E, et al. Focal segmental glomerulosclerosis after renal transplantation. Clinical Transplantation. 2011;25(Suppl. 23):6–14.
84. Canaud G, Zuber J, Sberro R, et al. Intensive and prolonged treatment of focal and segmental glomerulosclerosis recurrence in adult kidney transplant recipients: a pilot study. American Journal of Transplantation. 2009;9:1081–1086.
85. Wang XP, Fogo AB, Colon S, et al. Distinct epitopes for anti-glomerular basement membrane alport alloantibodies and goodpasture autoantibodies within the non-collagenous domain of alpha3(IV) collagen: a janus-faced antigen. Journal of the American Society of Nephrology. 2005;16:3563–3571.
86. Nankivell BJ, Kuypers DR. Diagnosis and prevention of chronic kidney allograft loss. Lancet. 2011;378:1428–1437.
87. White CA, Akbari A, Doucette S, et al. Estimating glomerular filtration rate in kidney transplantation: is the new chronic kidney disease epidemiology collaboration equation any better? Clinical Chemistry. 2010;56:474–477.
88. White CA, Huang D, Akbari A, et al. Performance of creatinine-based estimates of GFR in kidney transplant recipients: a systematic review. American Journal of Kidney Diseases. 2008;51:1005–1015.
89. Mariat C, Degauque N, Balasubramanian S, et al. Tim-1 signaling substitutes for conventional signal 1 and requires costimulation to induce T cell proliferation. Journal of Immunology. 2009;182:1379–1385.
90. Kaplan B, Schold J, Meier-Kriesche HU. Poor predictive value of serum creatinine for renal allograft loss. American Journal of Transplantation. 2003;3:1560–1565.
91. Cherukuri A, Welberry-Smith MP, Tattersall JE, et al. The clinical significance of early proteinuria after renal transplantation. Transplantation. 2010;89:200–207.
92. Nankivell BJ, Cohn DA, Spicer ST, et al. Diagnosis of kidney transplant obstruction using Mag3 diuretic renography. Clinical Transplantation. 2001;15:11–18.
93. Akioka Y, Chikamoto H, Horita S, et al. Screening of vesicoureteral reflux in pediatric patients with kidney transplantation showing non-specific interstitial fibrosis and tubular atrophy with interstitial Tamm-Horsfall protein deposits in protocol allograft biopsy. Clinical Transplantation. 2009;23(Suppl. 20):2–5.
94. Dupont PJ, Psimenou E, Lord R, et al. Late recurrent urinary tract infections may produce renal allograft scarring even in the absence of symptoms or vesicoureteric reflux. Transplantation. 2007;84:351–355.
95. Mathew TH, Kincaid-Smith P, Vikraman P. Risks of vesicoureteric reflux in the transplanted kidney. New England Journal of Medicine. 1977;297:414–418.
96. Bergmann IP, Boger RH, Marti E, et al. Renal resistance index in renal allograft recipients: a role for ADMA. American Journal of Kidney Diseases. 2009;54:327–333.
97. Radermacher J, Mengel M, Ellis S, et al. The renal arterial resistance index and renal allograft survival. New England Journal of Medicine. 2003;349:115–124.
98. de Vries AP, van Son WJ, van der Heide JJ, et al. The predictive value of renal

vascular resistance for late renal allograft loss. American Journal of Transplantation. 2006;6:364–370.
99. Mengel M. The kidney transplant: new horizons. Current Opinion in Nephrology and Hypertension. 2010;19:260–265.
100. Webster AC, Woodroffe RC, Taylor RS, et al. Tacrolimus versus ciclosporin as primary immunosuppression for kidney transplant recipients: meta-analysis and meta-regression of randomised trial data. BMJ (Clinical Research Ed.). 2005;331:810.
101. Knight SR, Russell NK, Barcena L, et al. Mycophenolate mofetil decreases acute rejection and may improve graft survival in renal transplant recipients when compared with azathioprine: a systematic review. Transplantation. 2009;87: 785–794.
102. Terasaki PI, Cai J. Human leukocyte antigen antibodies and chronic rejection: from association to causation. Transplantation. 2008;86:377–383.
103. Lee PC, Zhu L, Terasaki PI, et al. HLA-specific antibodies developed in the first year posttransplant are predictive of chronic rejection and renal graft loss. Transplantation. 2009;88:568–574.
104. Haas M. Transplant glomerulopathy: it's not always about chronic rejection. Kidney International. 2011;80:801–803.
105. Matas AJ, Leduc R, Rush D, et al. Histopathologic clusters differentiate subgroups within the nonspecific diagnoses of CAN or CR: preliminary data from the DeKAF study. American Journal of Transplantation. 2010;10:315–323.
106. Sacks S, Lee Q, Wong W, et al. The role of complement in regulating the alloresponse. Current Opinion in Organ Transplantation. 2009;14:10–15.
107. Mengel M, Sis B, Haas M, et al. Banff 2011 Meeting Report: new concepts in antibody-mediated rejection. American Journal of Transplantation. 2012; 12:563–570.
108. Cosio FG, Grande JP, Wadei H, et al. Predicting subsequent decline in kidney allograft function from early surveillance biopsies. American Journal of Transplantation. 2005;5:2464–2472.
109. Mota A, Arias M, Taskinen EI, et al. Sirolimus-based therapy following early cyclosporine withdrawal provides significantly improved renal histology and function at 3 years. American Journal of Transplantation. 2004;4:953–961.
110. Schena FP, Pascoe MD, Alberu J, et al. Conversion from calcineurin inhibitors to sirolimus maintenance therapy in renal allograft recipients: 24-month efficacy and safety results from the CONVERT trial. Transplantation. 2009;87: 233–242.
111. Solez K, Axelsen RA, Benediktsson H, et al. International standardization of criteria for the histologic diagnosis of renal allograft rejection: the Banff working classification of kidney transplant pathology. Kidney International. 1993;44: 411–422.
112. Solez K, Colvin RB, Racusen LC, et al. Banff '05 Meeting Report: differential diagnosis of chronic allograft injury and elimination of chronic allograft nephropathy ('CAN'). American Journal of Transplantation. 2007;7:518–526.
113. Mengel M, Reeve J, Bunnag S, et al. Scoring total inflammation is superior to the current Banff inflammation score in predicting outcome and the degree of molecular disturbance in renal allografts. American Journal of Transplantation. 2009;9:1859–1867.
114. Moore J, Middleton L, Cockwell P, et al. Calcineurin inhibitor sparing with mycophenolate in kidney transplantation: a systematic review and meta-analysis. Transplantation. 2009;87:591–605.
115. Flechner SM, Kobashigawa J, Klintmalm G. Calcineurin inhibitor-sparing regimens in solid organ transplantation: focus on improving renal function and nephrotoxicity. Clinical Transplantation. 2008;22:1–15.
116. Johnston O, Jaswal D, Gill JS, et al. Treatment of polyomavirus infection in kidney transplant recipients: a systematic review. Transplantation. 2010;89:1057–1070.
117. Nickeleit V, Singh HK, Mihatsch MJ. Polyomavirus nephropathy: morphology, pathophysiology, and clinical management. Current Opinion in Nephrology and Hypertension. 2003;12:599–605.
118. Hilton R, Tong CY. Antiviral therapy for polyomavirus-associated nephropathy after renal transplantation. Journal of Antimicrobial Chemotherapy. 2008;62: 855–859.
119. Naesens M, Kuypers DR, Sarwal M. Calcineurin inhibitor nephrotoxicity. Clinical Journal of the American Society of Nephrology. 2009;4:481–508.
120. Nankivell BJ, Borrows RJ, Fung CL, et al. Calcineurin inhibitor nephrotoxicity: longitudinal assessment by protocol histology. Transplantation. 2004;78: 557–565.
121. Abramowicz D, Del Carmen Rial M, Vitko S, et al. Cyclosporine withdrawal from a mycophenolate mofetil-containing immunosuppressive regimen: results of a five-year, prospective, randomized study. Journal of the American Society of Nephrology. 2005;16:2234–2240.
122. Weir MR, Blahut S, Drachenburg C, et al. Late calcineurin inhibitor withdrawal as a strategy to prevent graft loss in patients with suboptimal kidney transplant function. American Journal of Nephrology. 2004;24:379–386.
123. Ojo AO, Held PJ, Port FK, et al. Chronic renal failure after transplantation of a nonrenal organ. New England Journal of Medicine. 2003;349:931–940.
124. Brocker V, Schubert V, Scheffner I, et al. Arteriolar lesions in renal transplant biopsies: prevalence, progression, and clinical significance. American Journal of Pathology. 2012;180:1852–1862.
125. Shihab FS, Waid TH, Conti DJ, et al. Conversion from cyclosporine to tacrolimus in patients at risk for chronic renal allograft failure: 60-month results of the CRAF Study. Transplantation. 2008;85:1261–1269.
126. Hazzan M, Labalette M, Copin MC, et al. Predictive factors of acute rejection after early cyclosporine withdrawal in renal transplant recipients who receive mycophenolate mofetil: results from a prospective, randomized trial. Journal of the American Society of Nephrology. 2005;16:2509–2516.
127. Diekmann F, Budde K, Oppenheimer F, et al. Predictors of success in conversion from calcineurin inhibitor to sirolimus in chronic allograft dysfunction. American Journal of Transplantation. 2004;4:1869–1875.
128. Smith KD, Wrenshall LE, Nicosia RF, et al. Delayed graft function and cast nephropathy associated with tacrolimus plus rapamycin use. Journal of the American Society of Nephrology. 2003;14:1037–1045.
129. Sharif A, Shabir S, Chand S, et al. Meta-analysis of calcineurin-inhibitor-sparing regimens in kidney transplantation. Journal of the American Society of Nephrology. 2011;22:2107–2118.
130. Briganti EM, Russ GR, McNeil JJ, et al. Risk of renal allograft loss from recurrent glomerulonephritis. New England Journal of Medicine. 2002;347:103–109.
131. Golgert WA, Appel GB, Hariharan S. Recurrent glomerulonephritis after renal transplantation: an unsolved problem. Clinical Journal of the American Society of Nephrology. 2008;3:800–807.
132. Ivanyi B. A primer on recurrent and de novo glomerulonephritis in renal allografts. Nature Clinical Practice. Nephrology. 2008;4:446–457.
133. Clayton P, McDonald S, Chadban S. Steroids and recurrent IgA nephropathy after kidney transplantation. American Journal of Transplantation. 2011;11: 1645–1649.
134. Tedla F, Hayashi R, McFarlane SI, et al. Hypertension after renal transplant. Journal of Clinical Hypertension (Greenwich, Conn.). 2007;9:538–545.
135. Cross NB, Webster AC, Masson P, et al. Antihypertensive treatment for kidney transplant recipients. Cochrane Database of Systematic Reviews. 2009;(3): CD003598.
136. Heinze G, Mitterbauer C, Regele H, et al. Angiotensin-converting enzyme inhibitor or angiotensin II type 1 receptor antagonist therapy is associated with prolonged patient and graft survival after renal transplantation. Journal of the American Society of Nephrology. 2006;17:889–899.
137. Navaneethan SD, Perkovic V, Johnson DW, et al. HMG CoA reductase inhibitors (statins) for kidney transplant recipients. Cochrane Database of Systematic Reviews. 2009;(2):CD005019.
138. Bunnapradist S, Ambuhl PM. Impact of gastrointestinal-related side effects on mycophenolate mofetil dosing and potential therapeutic strategies. Clinical Transplantation. 2008;22:815–821.
139. Butler JA, Roderick P, Mullee M, et al. Frequency and impact of nonadherence to immunosuppressants after renal transplantation: a systematic review. Transplantation. 2004;77:769–776.
140. Prendergast MB, Gaston RS. Optimizing medication adherence: an ongoing opportunity to improve outcomes after kidney transplantation. Clinical Journal of the American Society of Nephrology. 2010;5:1305–1311.
141. Morrissey PE, Flynn ML, Lin S. Medication noncompliance and its implications in transplant recipients. Drugs. 2007;67:1463–1481.
142. Knight SR, Morris PJ. Steroid avoidance or withdrawal after renal transplantation increases the risk of acute rejection but decreases cardiovascular risk. A meta-analysis. Transplantation. 2010;89:1–14.
143. Pascual J, Zamora J, Galeano C, et al. Steroid avoidance or withdrawal for kidney transplant recipients. Cochrane Database of Systematic Reviews. 2009;(1): CD005632.
144. Fine RN, Becker Y, De Geest S, et al. Nonadherence consensus conference summary report. American Journal of Transplantation. 2009;9:35–41.
145. Kauffman HM, McBride MA, Cors CS, et al. Early mortality rates in older kidney recipients with comorbid risk factors. Transplantation. 2007;83:404–410.
146. Rao PS, Schaubel DE, Jia X, et al. Survival on dialysis post-kidney transplant failure: results from the Scientific Registry of Transplant Recipients. American Journal of Kidney Diseases. 2007;49:294–300.
147. Ansell D, Udayaraj UP, Steenkamp R, et al. Chronic renal failure in kidney transplant recipients. Do they receive optimum care?: data from the UK renal registry. American Journal of Transplantation. 2007;7:1167–1176.
148. Marcen R, del Castillo D, Capdevila L, et al. Achieving chronic kidney disease treatment targets in renal transplant recipients: results from a cross-sectional study in Spain. Transplantation. 2009;87:1340–1346.

第 70 章 肝移植临床排斥反应综合征

Matthew H. Levine, Sandy Feng

引言

肝硬化患者出现急性不可逆性肝损伤、慢性终末期肝病、某些代谢性疾病和肝细胞肝癌时,肝移植被公认为理想的治疗标准。在过去的 40 年里,肝移植已经从高风险的试验性手术发展成为遍及世界的具有极好预后的治疗方法,患者的 1 年、5 年生存率分别超过 90%和 75%[1]。肾移植预后的改善很大程度上归因于早期急性排斥率的显著降低,但肝移植中没有出现类似情况,系列报道和数据集显示其急性排斥率仍超过 30%[2-5]。多数急性排斥反应发生在肝移植术后 3 个月内,但急性和慢性排斥反应均可于移植手术 3 个月后出现[6]。肝移植慢性排斥反应的发生率比其他实体器官移植低,可能是因为肝脏本身具有再生性质,不随时间积累损伤,而是利用保留的结构和功能有效修复损伤[7]。肝脏再生修复损伤的能力或许解释了同种异体移植肝生存期短与急性排斥反应无关,这在实体器官移植中是特有的[3,8-10]。移植肝排斥反应与其他移植物排斥反应的另一个不同点在于 HLA 抗体介导过程相对不重要[11,12]。除肝脏移植外,所有实体器官移植通常需要进行交叉配型[4,12]。绝大多数急性排斥反应可成功被逆转,无须考虑或使用抗体介导治疗。肝脏吸收抗体使其能够抵抗抗体介导损害,这种内在特性也许能保护同源脏器,如易受抗体介导损害的肾脏[4]。最近有报道移植肝功能丧失和慢性排斥反应中存在抗体介导排斥反应[13-16]。

前述章节已描述器官排斥反应的细胞分子基础原理,本章将在此基础上按照排斥反应出现时间和类型概述同种异体移植肝排斥反应的临床表现。本章也将介绍同种异体移植肝功能不全的鉴别诊断及肝脏排斥反应的治疗策略。最后,我们将概述肝脏排斥反应诊断与管理中的争议、个案及未来方向。

排斥反应的细胞基础

第 5~7 章已详细探讨了排斥反应的细胞和分子基础原理以及组织病理学方面的内容,第 81~87 章将涉及组织病理学的内容。肝脏排斥反应最常见的类型是急性排斥反应,组织学显示汇管区(胆管、门静脉及肝动脉)淋巴细胞浸润,伴或不伴中央静脉浸润[17-20]。浸润的淋巴细胞大多是 $CD4^+$和 $CD8^+$ T 细胞,伴随巨噬细胞,称为急性细胞性排斥反应(ACR)。$CD4^+$ T 细胞是主要的浸润细胞,但临床排斥反应中可见更多活化 $CD8^+$ T 细胞[2,21]。嗜酸性粒细胞浸润常伴自然杀伤细胞(NK)[17,18]。根据 Banff 标准将 ACR 严重程度分为轻度、中度、重度三级(表 70.1)[17,18]。

尽管人类白细胞抗原(HLA)的匹配程度不能够预测肝移植排斥反应发生的风险,但 ACR 抗原靶点可能

表 70.1 同种异体移植肝急性排斥反应分级

整体评估*	标准
不确定	汇管区炎性浸润,不符合急性排斥反应诊断标准(见文中)
轻度	排斥性浸润见于少数汇管区,浸润轻微且仅限于汇管区内
中度	排斥性浸润累及大部分或全部汇管区
重度	除中度外,炎细胞侵入汇管区周围区,并有中度到重度静脉周围炎症。炎症侵入肝实质并有静脉周围肝细胞坏死

注意:活检回顾及排斥反应诊断后建立排斥反应整体评估分级模式。

*轻度、中度、重度急性排斥反应可分别口头描述为Ⅰ级、Ⅱ级、Ⅲ级。

Source: Banff Schema Group 1997[17]. Reproduced with permission from John Wil and Sons.

与供体细胞表面结合的主要组织相容性(MHC)抗原不相匹配,在其他移植器官中也可见[2,4,22,23]。肝细胞和胆管上皮细胞通常只表达低水平 MHC Ⅰ类分子。然而,胆管上皮细胞受炎症影响增强 MHC Ⅰ类和Ⅱ类抗原表达[4]。肝窦内皮细胞(LSEC)是主要的肝脏非实质细胞,表达 MHC Ⅱ类分子和共刺激信号分子,实验中可向 $CD4^+$和 $CD8^+$ T 细胞提呈抗原[4,24-27]。但是供体 LSEC 可能通过形成有效连续的肝窦内层阻止淋巴细胞浸润。实验通过 MHC Ⅰ类复合体上的内源性抗原交叉提呈导致克隆缺失和 T 细胞失能,显示供体 LSEC 和受体 T 细胞之间存在耐受作用。因此,LSEC 可能在肝移植耐受中起作用[25,28]。另外一种肝脏非实质细胞 Kupffer 细胞由大量巨噬细胞组成,Kupffer 细胞也可向受体 T 细胞提呈抗原。Kupffer 细胞诱导 T 细胞凋亡与实验系统移植肝耐受相关[29,30]。

排斥反应的抗体基础

肝脏能够相对耐受抗体介导超急性排斥反应[31-34]。移植肝超急性排斥反应可在致敏动物模型发生,但临床上很少见到。因此,绝大多数肝移植中心在移植前不进行交叉配型,许多中心甚至不确认供受者 HLA 类型[35,36]。在 ABO 血型不合肝移植,特别是在成人受体中,抗供体血型抗原的预存抗体可诱导早期严重的排斥反应,伴更高的胆道和血管并发症发生率。这表明抗体可致移植肝损伤[37-40]。ABO 血型不合的障碍能够在低抗体效价背景下(多见于婴幼儿)通过加强抗细胞及抗体液免疫性疗法被克服,如交换输血、血浆置换、亲和柱抗体吸附、静脉输注免疫球蛋白、脾切除和(或)抗 CD20 抗体疗法[38,41-44]。

移植肝对同种抗体介导损伤相对抵抗的生物学机制无法明确定义。假设机制包括肝脏具有再生能力,LSEC 和其他内皮细胞构成肝实质屏障,分泌可溶性 MHC Ⅰ类分子结合并清除抗体,肝脏对免疫细胞有潜在的直接影响[45,46]。这些假设在临床上全部未被证实,有待进一步研究。辅助性肝移植能够保护交叉配型阳性的同一供体肾脏移植,该事实证明肝脏可影响抗体发病机制[47]。但是保护性作用并不广泛,肝脏或肾脏发生抗体介导排斥反应(AMR)可伴随高效价的抗体[4,48-50]。

最近有病例报道可用抗体液免疫性药剂和疗法成功治疗 ABO 血型不合肝移植急性 AMR[11,13,36,48,51,52]。过去的几十年里,对于应用抗体检测,肝脏受体检测及 AMR 是否随时发生存在诸多争议[51,53-58]。一项前瞻性研究发现,抗肝窦内皮细胞抗体与迟发急性排斥反应高度相关,认为该抗体可能改变肝脏 TGF-β 表达量并且增强肝脏 T 细胞应答[59]。争论持续至今,焦点在于移植肝 C4d 染色以及 C4d 染色与移植肝生存期较短之间的关联[14,15,54,60-67]。而且,另有资料显示初次和再次肝移植出现供体特异性抗体后移植肝生存期较短[34,68-70]。

最近被关注的假设认为同种抗体促进肝脏慢性排斥反应的发生。慢性排斥反应病例稀少大大增加了阐述相关机制的难度[4]。许多研究表明 C4d 染色及供体特异性抗体的出现预示慢性排斥反应的发生。有趣的是,研究者未能解释慢性排斥反应在分子细胞水平的发生过程[11,14,60,66,67,71]。最后在免疫抑制最小化或撤除过程中也要考虑供体特异性抗体[4,72,73]。免疫抑制剂剂量减少时出现供体特异性抗体可能引发抗供体应答,从而阻碍免疫抑制剂减少。但是在肝移植同种抗体功能重要性未被研究透彻前,尤其是在移植肝功能正常的情况下,这些关注点仍只是假设。

肝移植中同种抗体与体液性排斥反应通路的临床重要性仍然存在争议。同种抗体至少在某些急性和慢性排斥反应病例中可能起作用。但是需要更多的临床及病理学研究证实存在同种抗体,并评估其在移植肝功能正常或异常的受体中的重要性。

排斥反应诊断中的组织病理学和分子病理学

同种异体移植肝功能不全的鉴别诊断随肝移植后时间而变化,但肝脏组织病理学直接分析确定移植肝排斥反应[17,19,74]。肝移植后有多种方法进行移植肝活检。最直接的方法通常是超声引导下经皮肝穿刺活检,并发症包括出血、胆漏、肝内血管漏和相邻结构损伤[75-78]。过去 10 年里,经颈静脉肝穿刺活检作为一种放射介入的方法使用逐渐增多,特别是患者存在凝血障碍或腹水时。排除肝被膜或主胆管结构被刺破,这种方法主要的优势在于减少血管内出血。缺点是组织样本采集量较少,操作过程烦琐[79]。当患者因其他原因或无其他安全活检方法时,可通过楔形或细针进行开放式肝活检。细针穿刺(FNA)活检无法得到细胞结构,目前不适合用来评估排斥反应[80]。但是如果能用分子而不是组织学分析诊断急性排斥反应，那么细针穿刺可能作为一种可行的替代方法[81]。最后，有人尝试运用胆汁细胞学诊断排斥反应，但技术上还不可实现[82,83]。

1997 年，Banff 共识会议确定肝脏 ACR 组织病理学特征分类[17]。ACR 根据三部分的炎症——汇管区炎症、胆管炎症和损伤、静脉内皮炎症，分别进行评分，为 0~3 分（无、轻度、中度、重度）。三项分数相加得到总数 0~9 分，即排斥活动指数（RAI）。RAI≤4 诊断为轻度急性排斥反应，不强烈推荐治疗。中度或重度急性排斥反应 RAI≥6（图 70.1；可见 82 章细胞浸润的特性），常伴肝功能异常，建议免疫抑制剂治疗（表 70.1 和表 70.2，均来自 1997 年 Banff 标准；可见于 82 章 Banff 分级系统的附加特征）。共识会议认为保存、缺血及病毒性疾病复发导致移植肝早期损伤，特别是当多个影响因素同时存在时，可能混淆排斥反应的诊断。

病毒血症患者进行肝移植时感染丙肝病毒（HCV）的现象很常见[84]。HCV 复发和急性排斥反应的组织学表现非常相似，难以辨别两者表型的差异。同一受体可同时出现 HCV 复发和急性排斥反应。但两者治疗方案不同，这是临床上一个重要的区别。HCV 感染复发的特征包括肝脏脂肪变性、肝小叶炎症、点状坏死和嗜酸性小体形成[17,85,86]。

2000 年新版 Banff 标准包含移植肝慢性排斥反应的组织病理学特征[18]。分级标准强调慢性排斥反应不是一个迟发过程，慢性排斥反应可在移植后数月内被观察到，偶尔可能快速发展导致移植肝衰竭。急性排斥反应未被治愈常发展成为慢性排斥反应，可导致严重的胆管损伤，最终造成胆管、肝动脉分支和终末肝微静脉消失。急性排斥反应的重要诊断依据是典型的汇管区坏死性炎症浸润，慢性排斥反应中汇管区坏死性炎症浸润常常减少或消失。出现活动性炎症时可通过免疫抑制调控逆转，但不存在炎症的情况下胆管等结构消失，此时不能逆转（表 70.3[84]；也可见第 82 章）[18,87]。最近有人指出急慢性排斥反应，特别是慢性排斥反应的组织病理学分析中是否需要考虑到 C4d 染色和供体特异性抗体效价[11,14,15,60,61,65,67,88]。

利用外周血转录标志物和血清 miRNA 进行无创分子式诊断肝脏排斥反应效果显著。这些方法可能简化了排斥反应的诊断，尚待统计学验证。而且，经过验证的标记物有利于持续监测排斥反应和抗排斥治疗反

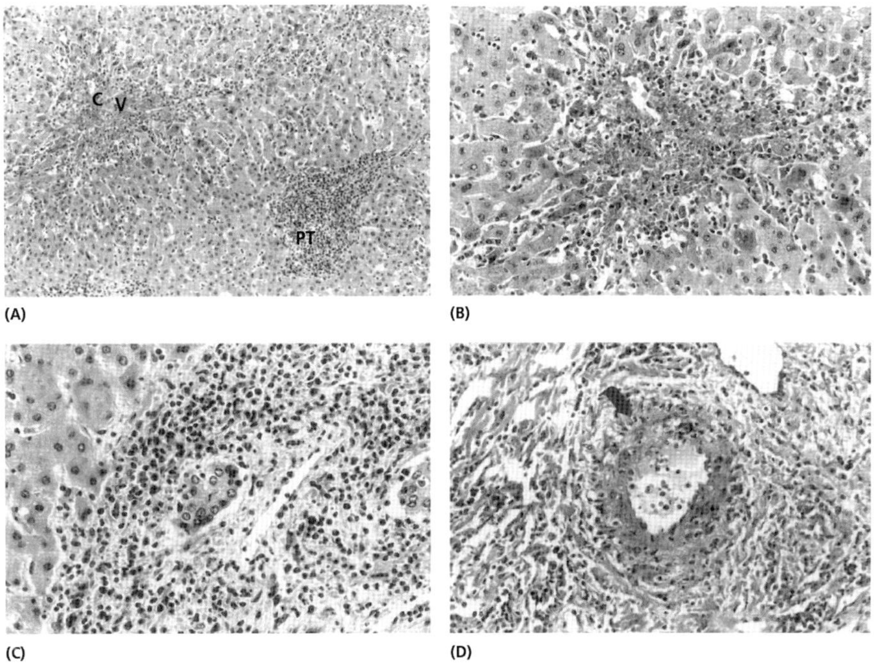

图 70.1　(A)低倍镜显示移植肝失功伴重度急性排斥反应，标注明显的汇管区（PT）和中央静脉（CV）炎症，(B)高倍镜显示伴有中央静脉周围融合性坏死，这些结果可诊断重度急性排斥反应。(C)同一移植肝中胆管的炎症和损伤广泛分布，局部管腔破坏，胆管损伤 RAI 评分 3 分，汇管区小静脉和静脉内皮炎症程度评为重度，或评为 3 分，RAI 总评分为 9/9。(D)失功移植肝的核心显示界限清楚的坏死性动脉炎（箭头），穿刺活检时很少被发现。（Source: Banff Schema Group 1997[17]. Reproduced with permission from John Wiley and Sons.）

表 70.2 排斥活动指数评分

分类	标准	评分
汇管区炎症	淋巴细胞性炎症为主，累及少数汇管区，无明显扩散	1
	累及大部或全部汇管区，炎症细胞为混合性，包括淋巴母细胞、中性和嗜酸性粒细胞	2
	明显累及大部或全部汇管区，混合性炎症细胞包括淋巴母细胞和嗜酸性粒细胞，炎症累及汇管区周围肝实质	3
胆管炎症和损伤	少数胆管炎症细胞浸润，胆管上皮轻微反应性改变，如核质比增加	1
	大部或全部胆管炎症细胞浸润，一个以上胆管上皮变性，如核多形性，细胞极性紊乱，胞质空泡形成	2
	同上，大部或全部胆管变性或灶性管腔破坏	3
静脉内皮炎症	少数汇管区小静脉或肝静脉内皮下淋巴细胞浸润	1
	大部或全部汇管区小静脉或肝静脉内皮下炎症浸润	2
	除上述病变外，还有中度或重度静脉周围炎症，累及静脉周围肝实质且伴肝细胞坏死	3

注意：总评分=各项评分之和，标准可评估移植肝活检急性排斥反应程度，世界胃肠病学共识定义。

Source: Banff Schema Group 1997[17]. Reproduced with permission from John Wiley and Sons.

应，可用于制订个体化免疫抑制方案，包括药物剂量最小化和（或）完全撤除[89-94]。

肝脏排斥反应的临床表现

移植后6个月作为早期和迟发急性排斥反应的分界，我们将分别讨论两者的临床表现。患者出现转氨酶、碱性磷酸酶和（或）胆红素升高，常怀疑存在排斥反应，尚未有单一的指标异常被证实可做出诊断[95,96]。排斥反应发生时，血清总胆红素、直接胆红素和转氨酶升高，排斥反应组织学越严重，但是与血清碱性磷酸酶或γ-谷氨酰基转移酶水平无关[6]。临床体征包括发热、精神萎靡、腹痛和肝大，但是这些较少见，不能个体化诊断[6]。

表 70.3 移植肝早期和迟发慢性排斥反应(chronic rejection, CR)特征

结构	早期慢性排斥反应	迟发性慢性排斥反应
小胆管(<60μm)	大多数胆管上皮细胞变性：胞质嗜酸性改变；核质比增加；核深染；胆管仅由部分上皮细胞构成 <50%的汇管区胆管丧失	残余胆管变性 ≥50%的汇管区胆管丧失
终末支肝静脉和第3区肝细胞	内膜/管腔炎症 第3区坏死溶解和炎症，轻度静脉周围纤维化	灶性闭锁 不同程度的炎症 严重(桥接)纤维化
汇管区肝小动脉	偶有丧失，累及<25%的汇管区	丧失累及>25%的汇管区
其他	所谓"过渡性"肝炎，伴肝细胞点状坏死	肝窦泡沫细胞聚集；显著胆汁淤积
肝门周围大的肝动脉分支	内膜炎症，泡沫细胞灶性沉积，未累及管腔	内膜下的泡沫细胞致管腔狭窄 纤维内膜增生
肝门周围大的胆管	炎症损害和泡沫细胞灶性沉积	管壁纤维化

Source: Demetris et al. 2000[18]. Reproduced with permission from John Wiley and Sons.

早期急性排斥反应

鉴别诊断

早期急性排斥反应标准不一，我们将其定义为发生在肝移植后6个月内[97]。最近报道早期急性排斥反应的发生率大约为25%，尸体肝移植和活体肝移植早期急性排斥反应发生率没有统计学差异(图 70.2)[5]。肝功能检查异常可发现移植肝失功，但存在许多不同的诊断标准。基于移植后的时间和临床表现，图 70.3 显示了流程示意图指导诊断。在移植术后，初期需要评估血管和胆管并发症。患者移植后初期由于侧支循环尚未形成，肝动脉血栓形成(HAT)会出现转氨酶显著升高，接近急性肝衰竭的重度移植肝功能障碍、胆管坏死和（或）肝脓肿形成，因此可能需要再次移植。目前的器官分配政策适用于移植等待状态或终末期肝病模型(MELD)，如果患者在移植后2周内确诊 HAT 可适用

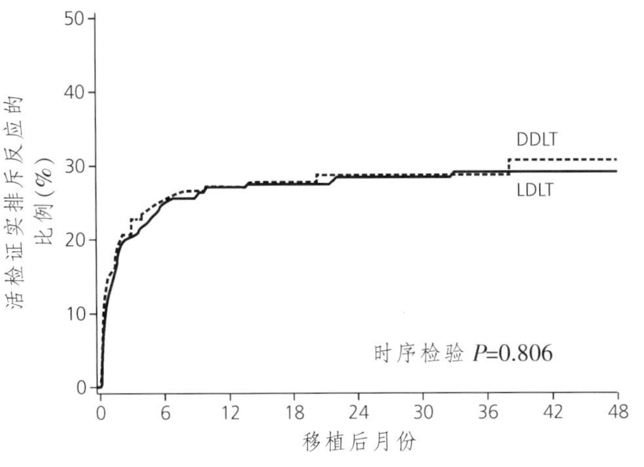

图 70.2 早期急性排斥反应发生率。DDLT,尸体肝移植;LDLT,活体肝移植。(Source: Shaked et al. 2009[5]. Reproduced with permission from John Wiley and Sons.)

分配政策的特例。如果在 2 周以后,根据临床情况诊断 HAT 则要求进行额外的评分。少见的血管并发症也有不同情况,如门静脉血栓形成或肝静脉梗阻,每种情况需要通过血管造影多普勒超声明确诊断。

肝功能异常需要鉴别是否继发于胆道并发症,这将决定下一步进行胆道检查或是移植肝活检。如果超声检查显示胆道系统扩张,尽管在移植后早期不常见,需要胆道影像学用于经内镜逆行胰胆管造影胆管间重建和经皮经肝胆管造影(PTC)进行 Roux-en-Y 重建。这些有创方法也为介入治疗提供了可能性。或者,利用磁共振胰胆管造影术(MRCP)或计算机断层扫描胆管造影术,这类诊断方法是无创的,依靠胆汁分泌成像。胆管炎或胆汁瘤也可能伴发胆漏和(或)胆道狭窄,需要特殊治疗。利用胆道吻合术干预治疗的时机和种类——手术或介入——可能因个人判断而不同。

如果不疑似胆道并发症或者胆道成像不能确定是否存在并发症,下一步诊断需要进行移植肝活检。肝活检前需要检查有无胆道并发症,因为活动性胆管炎是

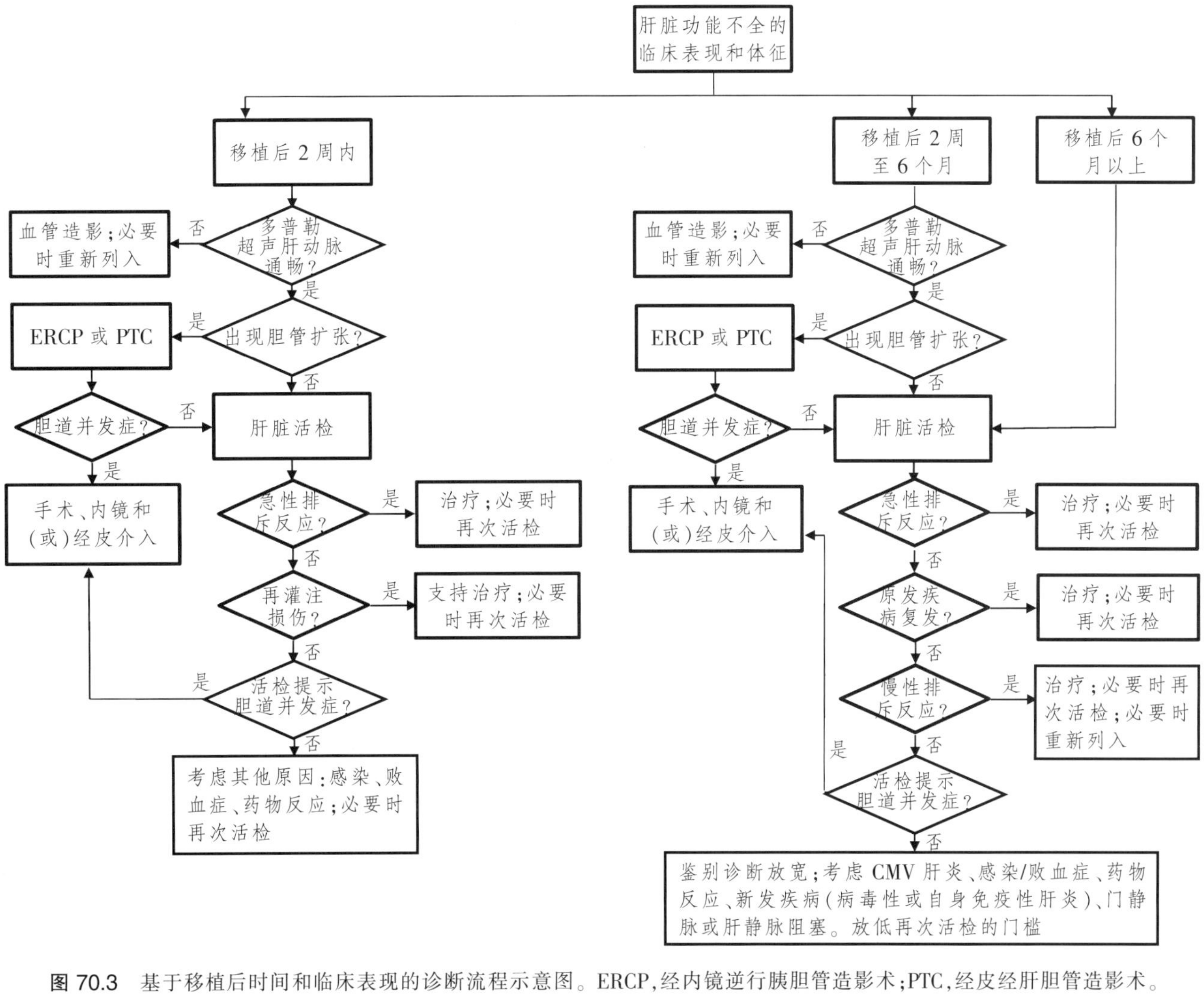

图 70.3 基于移植后时间和临床表现的诊断流程示意图。ERCP,经内镜逆行胰胆管造影术;PTC,经皮经肝胆管造影术。

肝活检的相对禁忌证。活检组织可说明存在急性排斥反应、保存损伤、原发疾病复发或感染[病毒性肝炎或巨细胞病毒(CMV)]和(或)慢性排斥反应。组织学分析也可提示存在血管或胆道并发症。两种病理过程也可能同时存在,如丙型肝炎复发伴急性排斥反应。如果初次活检未能做出诊断或是为了评估治疗疗效，需要进行随访活检。若患者出现感染或发热,移植肝早期功能不全的辅助性诊断包括获取HCV患者的丙型肝炎RNA病毒载量,CMV病毒DNA效价、血培养和横断面成像。第78章可见鉴别诊断和疾病复发的讨论。

免疫抑制方案与排斥反应

多项研究根据不同免疫抑制治疗方案推断出ACR和激素抵抗型排斥反应的发生率。一项包含16组随机试验的概述比较了以环孢素为主和以他克莫司为主的免疫抑制治疗方案，发现使用后者的移植术后第1年,患者ACR的风险降低了20%,激素抵抗型排斥反应的风险降低了50%[98,99]。霉酚酸酯和他克莫司均可作为救援剂,用来治疗难治性排斥反应,初期治疗效果良好[100-102],霉酚酸酯比硫唑嘌呤更加有效,特别是与环孢素联用时[103,104]。目前可用药物中,标准方案是由糖皮质激素和他克莫司、含或不含霉酚酸酯衍生物构成二联或三联方案，伴相应的早期ACR发生率[105,106]。进一步完全撤除糖皮质激素或者糖皮质激素和(或)他克莫司剂量最小化应用最多的方案是用抗IL-2受体抗体或兔抗胸腺细胞球蛋白诱发免疫抑制。这种方案相比标准非诱发方案，早期ACR的发生率相似或偏低[107-109]。钙调磷酸酶抑制剂(CNI)的毒性作用包括肾脏功能不全和肿瘤恶化的风险增加，维持免疫抑制治疗方案中使用m-TOR抑制剂可结合CNI的毒性作用。移植受者出现肾功能减退时,把以CNI为主的治疗方案转换成以m-TOR为主的方案可以稳定甚至改善肾功能[110,111]。m-TOR抑制剂也可用于有肝癌病史或丙型肝炎感染的受体,源于m-TOR抑制剂具有抗增殖作用,可阻止恶性肿瘤复发或移植肝纤维化[112]。在美国,西罗莫司和依维莫司是两类经批准用于预防移植肾排斥反应的m-TOR抑制剂。现在依维莫司被批准用于肝移植,但需要注意的是,西罗莫司会增加肝动脉血栓形成的风险[113]。

早期急性排斥反应的治疗

ACR一经确诊，需要马上根据多种因素制订治疗方案。首先需要考虑急性排斥反应的临床和组织学的严重程度。其次,原发性肝病很重要。肝病的自身免疫病因包括自身免疫性肝炎、原发性胆汁性肝硬化和原发性硬化性胆管炎,会增加排斥反应的风险,需要更加强效的治疗。与此相反,丙型肝炎需要的免疫抑制治疗效能较低,因为过度免疫抑制会刺激丙型肝炎复发。其他临床疾病和(或)实验室检查异常会影响治疗方案的选择,包括肾功能不全、蛋白尿、糖尿病、高血压、高脂血症和血细胞减少症。再次,急性排斥反应发生时需要考虑免疫抑制的强度。因为急性排斥反应发作,特别是对于非丙型肝炎受体,不会对长期预后产生消极影响。选择一种适当不过度的治疗策略是非常值得的。但是急性排斥反应治疗不彻底会演变成慢性排斥反应,慢性排斥反应非常难以逆转,而且会威胁移植肝的存活。急性排斥反应较稳妥的治疗策略是实验室异常指标逐步正常化,要求密切监测和频繁评估直至完全缓解。更多免疫抑制援救的讨论见第67章。

急性排斥反应的治疗选择如同阶梯从少到多逐层递进(图70.4)。最低一级的是强化基础免疫抑制治疗,增加一种或多种已有药物的剂量。第二级是转换,把低效的药物换成相同类别的强效药物，包括环孢素替换

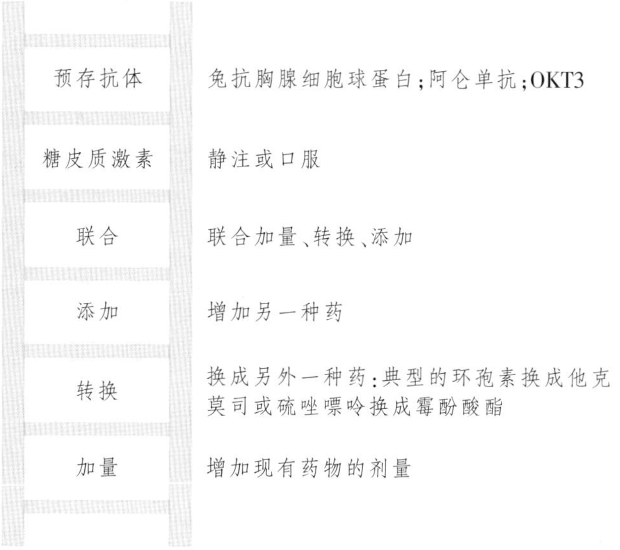

图70.4　肝移植急性排斥反应的治疗阶梯。

成他克莫司，硫唑嘌呤替换成霉酚酸酯或 mTOR 抑制剂[989,101,102]。急性排斥反应治疗的第三级是添加，在现有的治疗方案中加入一类新药，从一种或两种药物变成两药或三药联用。这些方法适用于组织学轻度改变和肝功能轻微升高的患者。第四步，过去治疗 ACR 的起点是糖皮质激素，起始给药量为二或三倍剂量的糖皮质激素静脉推注，之后口服激素，逐渐减量。或者单独口服糖皮质激素循环疗程。糖皮质激素会增加丙型肝炎复发的侵略性，在丙肝肝炎患者群体中需要慎重考虑风险/获益比。

排斥反应对糖皮质激素无应答称为激素抵抗型排斥反应。T 细胞介导的抗体疗法已经全部被使用，如单克隆抗 IL-2 受体抗体（巴利昔单抗）、单克隆抗 CD52 抗体（阿仑单抗）和多克隆兔抗胸腺细胞球蛋白（rATG），rATG 是最常见的选择[114-119]。总的来说，60%~75%的激素难治性排斥反应可以成功被逆转，且肝移植早期进行治疗易于移植晚期。

上述策略是治疗 ACR 的标准方法。如果诊断为体液性排斥反应，要考虑到会存在和产生不同的治疗靶点抗体。AMR 介导的疗法包括先后使用血浆置换和 IVIG、单克隆抗 CD20 抗体（利妥昔单抗），B 细胞是利妥昔单抗主要的靶点。因为这种药不会明显改变记忆 B 细胞（血浆细胞）的储存，药物在肾移植受体体内对血浆细胞有积极作用，但是在肝移植中还未被检测。

早期急性排斥反应治疗选择中的影响因素

受体丙型肝炎状态是决定肝移植早期 ACR 治疗策略的主要考虑因素。丙型肝炎感染复发的侵略性和速度取决于供体、受体和病毒多重因素[120-122]。受体的免疫状态在丙肝控制中起重要作用。例如，糖皮质激素冲击，特别是抗体制备治疗 ACR，会使丙肝复发更迅速且更加严重[1072,13-125]。ACR 和 HCV 复发组织学区分模糊，可能会导致诊断错误[86,1262,127]。患者存在丙型肝炎病毒支持均衡的 ACR 治疗方法，鼓励选择治疗阶梯中尽可能低一级的方案。鼓励进行重复活检来监测排斥反应发生的进程、对治疗的反应和病毒介导损害的程度[86,127-129]。患者出现 ACR 时可能伴发丙型肝炎，强化肝移植早期输送及维持充足的免疫抑制剂可使 ACR 的风险最小。

此外，肾功能不全也是选择抗排斥反应治疗方案的主要考虑因素。进行 MELD 分配增加了肾功能不全，特别是在移植早期的患病率和严重程度，常常限制了 CNI 的剂量。伴肾功能不全的受体经常在维持糖皮质激素和霉酚酸酯治疗的基础上可加入一种 CNI 类药物完善免疫抑制治疗方案。因此，甚至是 HCV 受体，若出现早期 ACR，也需要降低激素静注剂量。因为替代方案（加量、转换、添加）不可能或不太可能控制 ACR。

移植早期发生骨髓抑制是选择抗排斥治疗方案的另一个考虑因素，通常会出现相对中性粒细胞减少症及血小板减少症。影响因素包括残余的脾功能亢进、抗 CMV 药物（缬更昔洛韦）和（或）免疫抑制药物（霉酚酸酯、m-TOR 抑制剂或硫唑嘌呤）的影响。血细胞降低需要减少免疫抑制剂剂量，受体更易发生 ACR。目前暂无有效治疗血小板减少的方法，但是非格司亭可用于治疗白细胞减少/中性粒细胞减少。与肾功能不全类似，血细胞降低减少了抗排斥反应治疗的替代方案，但可能加用静注糖皮质激素[130,131]。

早期急性排斥反应的特殊病例

成人 ABO 血型不合（ABOi）肝移植比 ABO 血型相同或相容肝移植预后较低且排斥反应的发生率较高[42,44]。肝内弥散性血管内凝固是 ABOi 移植肝排斥反应标志性的组织学特征，会导致血栓形成和坏死[41,132]。这种情况与肾移植体液性排斥反应的组织学特征相似。并非抗 HLA 抗体，而是抗血型抗体造成了病理学改变。由于日本尸体肝移植稀缺，活体肝移植成为许多 ABOi 肝移植研究及实践的来源。辅助性治疗已经代表性地用于多途径联合缓解 ABOi 移植肝抗体介导的排斥反应，包括血浆置换/交换血液、静脉注射免疫球蛋白、抗 CD20 单克隆抗体、脾切除和门静脉和（或）肝动脉多药输注，如大剂量的糖皮质激素、前列腺素 E1（血管扩张剂）和甲磺酸加贝酯（一种蛋白酶抑制剂预防血小板聚集）[37-40]。此外，标准免疫抑制方案加四药维持方案是治疗 ABOi 移植经常使用的独特方法。

肝脏再次移植发生 ACR 的风险相对于首次肝移植的风险未被完整记录[133,134]。据报道，再次肾移植发生排斥反应的风险更高[135-137]。一项单中心研究显示，32 例再次肝移植患者的 1 年总生存率很低，但并未发生 ACR[138]。旨在预测再次肝移植术后生存的模型并没有把首次肝移植的排斥反应作为预示移植肝预后的因素纳入[134,139,140]。总之，尚未有足够的数据表明首次和非首次肝移植排斥反应的发生率有差异。

早期急性排斥反应的预后

肝移植不像其他器官移植，早期ACR排斥反应不太可能对移植肝和患者的长期生存产生影响[8]。事实上，单因素分析已经显示，早期ACR排斥反应与移植后病死率较低显著相关[6]。相比无排斥反应的受体，相关性归因于排斥反应的受体有较好的总体健康状态。需要指出的是，这项研究是在数十年以前进行的，还未接受MELD分配时代的检验。但减少早期急性排斥反应的发生率并不意味着提高长期预后，需要更多的证据说明早期ACR相比其他因素（如丙型肝炎状态）对长期预后重要性较低[141]。

迟发性急性排斥反应

定义

迟发性急性排斥反应（LAR）按急性排斥反应出现时间的不同有多种定义，可出现在移植后1、3、6或12个月，通常6个月是临界值。据报道，迟发性急性排斥反应的发生率为7%~23%，取决于诊断时间、诊断严格性（是否活检证明）以及随访时间[142-145]。尽管已被报道可利用全国注册中心数据进行广泛评估[104]，迟发性急性排斥反应的文献仍以单中心研究居多，试图阐明诱发和（或）决定因素，临床和组织学的严重程度，治疗方法与应答以及患者与移植肝的预后[142-144]。

迟发性急性排斥反应的危险因素

受体诱发迟发性急性排斥反应的特征包括肝病的人口统计学和病因学特征。受体年龄越小，与其相关性越一致[97,142,144,145]。肝病的自身免疫性病因是一个极大的危险因素，如自身免疫性肝炎、原发性胆汁性肝硬化或原发性硬化性胆管炎[97,143]。有趣的是，早期急性排斥反应的发生与此没有较强的相关性。

至于免疫抑制的应用，发生迟发性急性排斥反应无疑意味着此时患者免疫抑制治疗不够充分。据文献报道，LAR极有可能与无法依从治疗相关[146,147]。但是与现有的数据相矛盾，可能某种特定药物或维持免疫抑制总体强度增加了LAR的风险。一些研究显示，发生LAR的患者与没有发生LAR的患者相比，更加频繁地维持三倍治疗以及使用相应的CNI剂量[97,142]。相反，其他研究显示，发生LAR的患者相比LAR的患者，可能把他克莫司转换成环孢素维持免疫抑制治疗[142]，或更可能减弱了免疫抑制治疗（如移植后淋巴组织异常增生时停用糖皮质激素或大剂量减少）[97,144]。按患者肝病病因分组的注册中心分析根据移植治疗出院时的免疫抑制治疗方案评估LAR的风险。按患者的出院用药分组比较，一组使用糖皮质激素和他克莫司组成的二联药物维持治疗，一组使用二联方案加霉酚酸酯组成三联药物维持治疗。多因素分析发现，每个诊断组（丙型肝炎组、乙型肝炎组和非病毒性肝病组）中三联方案组比二联方案组LAR发生率较低[145]。

迟发性急性排斥反应的诊断、严重程度和治疗

迟发性急性排斥反应通常发生在移植受体不再进行高频率或高强度的随访时，可能会延误诊断。移植后肝功能指标升高超过6个月，尤其是近期免疫抑制剂量减少或免疫抑制不充分时，肝脏活检是首先需要进行的检查（图70.3）。发生迟发性急性排斥反应时，组织学的严重程度不同，一项研究显示以轻度ACR居多（79%），另一项研究显示中度至重度ACR居多（51%）[143]。迟发性急性排斥反应的治疗原则上与早期急性排斥反应相似，都进行分阶梯治疗。但是很少使用低阶治疗，如加量及转换。更加强效的治疗反映了迟发性急性排斥反应已经被延误诊断，更难以治疗。因此，大多数患者需要静脉输注和（或）口服糖皮质激素[142-144]。预存抗体治疗严重的和（或）激素抵抗型的迟发性排斥反应也并不罕见。

迟发性急性排斥反应的预后

相比早期急性排斥反应，迟发性急性排斥反应会降低移植肝及患者的存活率被广泛认可。主要的机制是诱发慢性排斥反应（胆管或血管消失），迫使二次移植和（或）导致患者死亡。据报道，LAR出现慢性排斥反应的发生率各不相同（4.1%~16.3%）[974,13,144]，但活体肝移植受体发生LAR后并未出现慢性排斥反应[142]。注册中心检测了移植术后1年生存的患者的移植肝的4年生存率[145]。定义ACR发生在移植后6个月内为早期，发生在移植后6~12个月为迟发性，所有患者被分成四组（早期ACR组、LAR组、两者均无组、两者均有组）（图70.5）。Cox回归分析显示，两者均无组患者迟发性

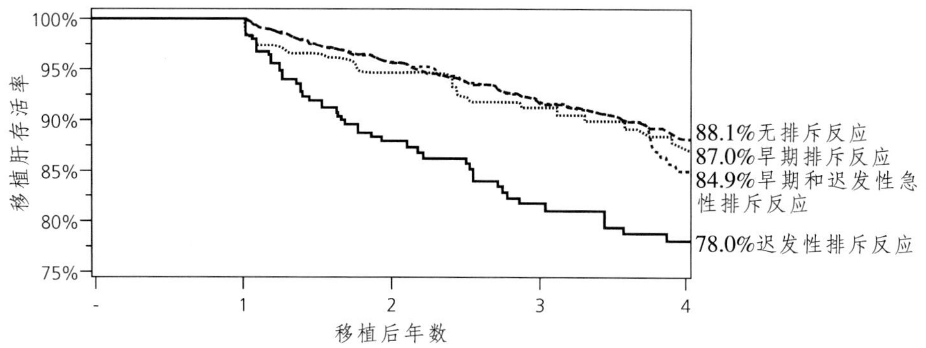

早期排斥反应(0~6 个月)	451	451	426	248	246
迟发性排斥反应(6~12 个月)	255	255	217	143	107
早期和迟发性急性排斥反应	261	261	243	165	121
无排斥反应(0~12 个月)	3742	3742	3614	2613	1893

图 70.5　迟发性急性排斥反应的不利影响。(Source: Wiesner et al. 2006[145]. Reproduced with permission from John Wiley and Sons.)

移植肝功能丧失的风险比为 0.99(95%CI 为 0.75~1.31),两者均有组的风险比为 1.5 (95%CI 为 1.09~2.07),LAR 组的风险比为 1.99(95%CI 为 1.5~2.66)。两者均无组与早期 ACR 组患者的 4 年生存率相似 (88.1%和 87.0%);两者均有组与 LAR 组患者的 4 年生存率分别为 84.9%和 78.0%。

慢性排斥反应

慢性排斥反应背景

广泛认为所有实体移植器官中,肝脏最能耐受慢性排斥反应。在 20 世纪 80 年代的环孢素时代,慢性排斥反应的发生率高达 20%~40%[7,148-152]。20 世纪 90 年代起使用他克莫司,慢性排斥反应发生率降至 2%~5%[87,150,152-155]。病程进展也随之变化。以前同种移植肝慢性排斥反应常常在移植后 1 年内发生,迅速发展,3~6 个月可致移植肝功能丧失。在免疫抑制的时代,慢性排斥反应更晚发生,且进展缓慢[61,156]。肾脏、心脏和肺移植发生慢性排斥反应会逐渐不可逆转地发展至移植物功能丧失,但肝移植不同,如果早期诊断,慢性排斥反应可经强化免疫抑制治疗被逆转[18,61,154,157-160]。然而慢性排斥反应仍是迟发性移植肝功能不全的重要原因,可导致肝移植受体的发病率和死亡率较高。

慢性排斥反应的危险因素

慢性排斥反应最大的危险因素普遍认为是 ACR 发生次数和严重程度[6,9,87,97,148-150,152,153,161]。在不发生 ACR 的情况下,患者可频繁出现耐受激素治疗和治疗不充分的慢性排斥反应[18,61,148,150,152]。相比以他克莫司为主的免疫抑制方案,以环孢素为主的免疫抑制治疗方案是慢性排斥反应的第二个危险因素[87,150,152,153,162]。三条直接或间接的证据证实了这一关联。他克莫司预防急性细胞性排斥反应效果优于环孢素[98,162]。将环孢素更换为他克莫司,可有效治疗受体慢性排斥反应[157,163]。此外,匹兹堡大学组报道指出,他克莫司可预防成人和小儿受体首次肝移植术后的慢性排斥反应[153,164]。另一个增加慢性排斥反应风险的因素是自身免疫性疾病(自身免疫性肝炎、原发性胆汁性肝硬化和原发性硬化性胆管炎),需要再次肝移植[87,150,152,153,165]。由于常规治疗方案,或出现免疫抑制治疗的禁忌证,或者是患者依从性差,减弱免疫抑制治疗随后可能发生慢性排斥反应[150,152,153,166]。

最近,慢性排斥反应与干扰素和利巴韦林治疗复发 HCV 之间的潜在关联被提出并引起争论。普遍认为干扰素会刺激肾移植受体的急性和慢性排斥反应[167,168]。但干扰素与移植肝急慢性排斥反应的关联仍有诸多争议[169]。多种因素混淆两者间的关联,包括 ACR 发生率随移植术后时间的变化而变化,干扰素疗法的初始时机和免疫抑制强度多变,以及异常肝功能可能减少肝活检次数。而且包括聚乙二醇在内的多种配伍在理论和实践上均会造成不同比例的风险。最后,影响排斥反应与治疗间关联的另一个因素可能是辅助性使用免疫调节药物利巴韦林。

除了上述情况,几项详细的单中心分析显示以干扰素为主的治疗方案可能会诱发慢性排斥反应[170-173]。许多患者是在肝移植多年后开始接受干扰素治疗，所以慢性排斥反应的发生率非常高(8.7%~17%)。通常在干扰素治疗开始后的数周到数月，慢性排斥反应迅速发展，做出了进一步佐证。有意思的是，病毒清除被认为是慢性排斥反应发展的一个危险因素[170-172]。现有假设认为，成功治疗是指通过提高免疫清除病毒的机制产生有效的抗病毒反应。

慢性排斥反应的诊断与治疗

在可治疗阶段，尤其是在病程早期，诊断慢性排斥反应非常困难[18,96,149,152,154,158]。临床医生需要放宽鉴别范围，任何ACR发作伴有不良表现(如组织学分级为重度或者激素抵抗型)出现时都应考虑到即将出现或已经出现慢性排斥反应。潜在的终末表现是大于50%的汇管区有胆管丧失或者出现闭塞性泡沫细胞动脉病，意味着需要再次移植[18,61,149,152,154,158-160,174]。而且众所周知，细针活检标本提供有限，这些特征很难被发现[18,62,154,160]。胆管消失不能被准确量化，除非活检包含足够数量的汇管区。泡沫细胞动脉病主要发生在比活检样本更大的动脉里。

然而，多篇文献共同报道了慢性排斥反应的早期组织学特征[18,61,87,154,157,158,161,175]。胆道的早期改变主要表现为退化伴发育异常或萎缩，存在不同程度的炎症，而非胆管消失。这些改变被认为由直接免疫攻击胆管上皮细胞以及小动脉分支消失诱导间接缺血引起。动脉组织学检查暗示早期的慢性排斥反应包括炎症损伤，出现淋巴细胞和富脂巨噬细胞。肝小叶中央区域也发现早期排斥反应的特征，出现中央静脉周围炎症、细胞气球样变、肝小叶中央细胞脱落，导致静脉周围轻度纤维化。通常慢性排斥反应过程中会出现炎症减轻、胆管消失、动脉闭塞、严重的纤维化及胆汁淤积。

最近，慢性排斥反应进展被认为与体液性机制存在潜在的关联 [14,15,58]。虽然两个抗体介导反应的标志物——供体特异性抗体[14,58]和C4d染色[14,15]——在慢性排斥反应中可能会增加，但相关的生物学意义仍不清楚。迄今为止，在正常同种异体移植肝或含有其他病程的移植肝中，包括急性排斥反应和复发疾病，尚未前瞻性地收集大量受体横向或纵向的数据来计算这两个标志物的阳性率。

慢性排斥反应治疗的重点在增强免疫抑制治疗。首先考虑若存在急性炎性物质，需要口服糖皮质激素或预存抗体——治疗选项通常用于急性排斥反应。如前所述，炎性变化通常出现在慢性排斥反应早期，进展过程中会减弱。除此之外，治疗选择大多取决于发生慢性排斥反应时所采用的免疫抑制方案。对于环孢素治疗的患者，根据现有的资料强烈建议替换成他克莫司治疗[157]。据报道，霉酚酸酯也是一种潜在的解救药物，作为新增药物或者硫唑嘌呤的强效替代剂使用[101,176-178]。近来，西罗莫司被报道可能因其抗纤维化特性对慢性排斥反应也有效果[113]。

慢性排斥反应的预后

慢性排斥反应的预后往往取决于早期可逆阶段的及时诊断和治疗。预后较好的临床因素包括谷草转氨酶和血清胆红素水平较低[153,154,157]。预后较好的组织学因素包括胆管和动脉的丧失减少，泡沫细胞聚集减少，严重的静脉周围纤维化减轻[153,154,157,158]。总之，20%~70%的慢性排斥反应可自愈或长期的移植肝功能维持治疗有效[87,113,152,153,157,158,177]。慢性排斥反应不被逆转通常会导致移植肝功能丧失，需要再次移植，或者患者因感染或移植肝功能不全死亡。

总结

同种异体肝移植排斥反应的临床表现不同于其他器官的同种免疫表现，其结果相对良好且同种抗体依赖机制参与有限。但是，预后较好的临床表现通常依赖于及时准确的诊断和适当的治疗。病毒性肝炎容易混淆排斥反应的诊断，影响治疗策略，要防止过度免疫抑制治疗。为极大提高现代肝移植预后，必须适当地革新治疗方案。

(徐骁 译　徐骁 校)

参考文献

1. Desai M, Neuberger J. Chronic liver allograft dysfunction. Transplantation Proceedings. 2009;41:773-776.
2. Sanchez-Fueyo A, Strom TB. Immunologic basis of graft rejection and tolerance following transplantation of liver or other solid organs. Gastroenterology. 2011;140:51-64.
3. Jain A, Reyes J, Kashyap R, et al. What have we learned about primary liver transplantation under tacrolimus immunosuppression? Long-term follow-up of the first 1000 patients. Annals of Surgery. 1999;230:441-448; discussion 448-449.
4. Knechtle SJ, Kwun J. Unique aspects of rejection and tolerance in liver transplan-

tation. Seminars in Liver Disease. 2009;29:91-101.
5. Shaked A, Ghobrial RM, Merion RM, et al. Incidence and severity of acute cellular rejection in recipients undergoing adult living donor or deceased donor liver transplantation. American Journal of Transplantation. 2009;9: 301-308.
6. Wiesner RH, Demetris AJ, Belle SH, et al. Acute hepatic allograft rejection: incidence, risk factors, and impact on outcome. Hepatology (Baltimore, Md.). 1998;28:638-645.
7. Demetris AJ, Murase N, Lee RG, et al. Chronic rejection. A general overview of histopathology and pathophysiology with emphasis on liver, heart and intestinal allografts. Annals of Transplantation. 1997;2:27-44.
8. Seiler CA, Renner EL, Czerniak A, et al. Early acute cellular rejection: no effect on late hepatic allograft function in man. Transplant International. 1999;12: 195-201.
9. Dousset B, Conti F, Cherruau B, et al. Is acute rejection deleterious to long-term liver allograft function? Journal of Hepatology. 1998;29:660-668.
10. Neuberger J, Adams DH. What is the significance of acute liver allograft rejection? Journal of Hepatology. 1998;29:143-150.
11. Watson R, Kozlowski T, Nickeleit V, et al. Isolated donor specific alloantibody-mediated rejection after ABO compatible liver transplantation. American Journal of Transplantation. 2006;6:3022-3029.
12. Michaels PJ, Fishbein MC, Colvin RB. Humoral rejection of human organ transplants. Springer Seminars in Immunopathology. 2003;25:119-140.
13. Schadde E, d'Alessandro AM, Musat AI, et al. Donor-specific HLA-antibody-mediated humoral rejection in a liver transplant recipient fully reversed with plasmapheresis and immunoglobulin. Clinical Transplants. 2006;479-482.
14. Musat AI, Agni RM, Wai PY, et al. The significance of donor-specific HLA antibodies in rejection and ductopenia development in ABO compatible liver transplantation. American Journal of Transplantation. 2011;11:500-510.
15. Martelius T, Halme L, Arola J, et al. Vascular deposition of complement C4d is increased in liver allografts with chronic rejection. Transplant Immunology. 2009;21:244-246.
16. Lunz J, Ruppert KM, Cajaiba MM, et al. Re-examination of the lymphocytotoxic crossmatch in liver transplantation: can C4d stains help in monitoring? American Journal of Transplantation. 2011.
17. Banff schema for grading liver allograft rejection: an international consensus document. Hepatology (Baltimore, Md.). 1997;25:658-663.
18. Demetris A, Adams D, Bellamy C, et al. Update of the International Banff Schema for Liver Allograft Rejection: working recommendations for the histopathologic staging and reporting of chronic rejection. An International Panel. Hepatology (Baltimore, Md.). 2000;31:792-799.
19. Demetris AJ, Ruppert K, Dvorchik I, et al. Real-time monitoring of acute liver-allograft rejection using the Banff schema. Transplantation. 2002;74:1290-1296.
20. Racusen LC, Colvin RB, Solez K, et al. Antibody-mediated rejection criteria— an addition to the Banff 97 classification of renal allograft rejection. American Journal of Transplantation. 2003;3:708-714.
21. Strom TB, Tilney NL, Carpenter CB, et al. Identity and cytotoxic capacity of cells infiltrating renal allografts. New England Journal of Medicine. 1975;292: 1257-1263.
22. Toyokawa H, Nakao A, Bailey RJ, et al. Relative contribution of direct and indirect allorecognition in developing tolerance after liver transplantation. Liver Transplantation. 2008;14:346-357.
23. Afzali B, Lechler RI, Hernandez-Fuentes MP. Allorecognition and the alloresponse: clinical implications. Tissue Antigens. 2007;69:545-556.
24. Knolle PA, Schmitt E, Jin S, et al. Induction of cytokine production in naive CD4(+) T cells by antigen-presenting murine liver sinusoidal endothelial cells but failure to induce differentiation toward Th1 cells. Gastroenterology. 1999;116:1428-1440.
25. Knolle PA, Limmer A. Neighborhood politics: the immunoregulatory function of organ-resident liver endothelial cells. Trends in Immunology. 2001;22: 432-437.
26. Limmer A, Knolle PA. Liver sinusoidal endothelial cells: a new type of organ-resident antigen-presenting cell. Archivum Immunologiae et Therapiae Experimentalis. 2001;49(Suppl. 1):S7-S11.
27. Ge X, Nowak G, Ericzon BG, et al. Liver sinusoidal endothelial cell function in rejected and spontaneously accepted rat liver allografts. Transplant International. 2008;21:49-56.
28. Limmer A, Ohl J, Kurts C, et al. Efficient presentation of exogenous antigen by liver endothelial cells to CD8+ T cells results in antigen-specific T-cell tolerance. Nature Medicine. 2000;6:1348-1354.
29. Chen Y, Liu Z, Liang S, et al. Role of Kupffer cells in the induction of tolerance of orthotopic liver transplantation in rats. Liver Transplantation. 2008;14: 823-836.
30. Crispe IN. The liver as a lymphoid organ. Annual Review of Immunology. 2009;27:147-163.
31. Knechtle SJ, Kolbeck PC, Tsuchimoto S, et al. Hepatic transplantation into sensitized recipients. Demonstration of hyperacute rejection. Transplantation. 1987;43:8-12.
32. Bird G, Friend P, Donaldson P, et al. Hyperacute rejection in liver transplantation: a case report. Transplantation Proceedings. 1989;21:3742-3744.
33. Starzl TE, Demetris AJ, Todo S, et al. Evidence for hyperacute rejection of human liver grafts: the case of the canary kidneys. Clinical Transplantation. 1989;3:37-45.
34. Demetris AJ, Nakamura K, Yagihashi A, et al. A clinicopathological study of human liver allograft recipients harboring preformed IgG lymphocytotoxic antibodies. Hepatology (Baltimore, Md.). 1992;16:671-681.
35. Knechtle SJ, Kolbeck P, Tsuchimoto S, et al. Hyperacute rejection of liver transplants in rats. Current Surgery. 1986;43:303-305.
36. Ratner LE, Phelan D, Brunt EM, et al. Probable antibody-mediated failure of two sequential ABO-compatible hepatic allografts in a single recipient. Transplantation. 1993;55:814-819.
37. Usuda M, Fujimori K, Koyamada N, et al. Successful use of anti-CD20 monoclonal antibody (rituximab) for ABO-incompatible living-related liver transplantation. Transplantation. 2005;79:12-16.
38. Tanabe M, Kawachi S, Obara H, et al. Current progress in ABO-incompatible liver transplantation. European Journal of Clinical Investigation. 2010;40: 943-949.
39. Egawa H, Ohmori K, Haga H, et al. B-cell surface marker analysis for improvement of rituximab prophylaxis in ABO-incompatible adult living donor liver transplantation. Liver Transplantation. 2007;13:579-588.
40. Egawa H, Teramukai S, Haga H, et al. Present status of ABO-incompatible living donor liver transplantation in Japan. Hepatology (Baltimore, Md.). 2008;47:143-152.
41. Demetris AJ, Jaffe R, Tzakis A, et al. Antibody-mediated rejection of human orthotopic liver allografts. A study of liver transplantation across ABO blood group barriers. American Journal of Pathology. 1988;132:489-502.
42. Farges O, Kalil AN, Samuel D, et al. The use of ABO-incompatible grafts in liver transplantation: a life-saving procedure in highly selected patients. Transplantation. 1995;59:1124-1133.
43. Gugenheim J, Samuel D, Reynes M, et al. Liver transplantation across ABO blood group barriers. Lancet. 1990;336:519-523.
44. Stewart ZA, Locke JE, Montgomery RA, et al. ABO-incompatible deceased donor liver transplantation in the United States: a national registry analysis. Liver Transplantation. 2009;15:883-893.
45. Kamada N, Goto S, Kobayashi E, et al. Release of soluble MHC class I antigens before and after orthotopic liver retransplantation in the rat. Transplantation Proceedings. 1993;25:2857.
46. Kamada N, Sumimoto R, Baguerizo A, et al. Mechanisms of transplantation tolerance induced by liver grafting in rats: involvement of serum factors in clonal deletion. Immunology. 1988;64:315-317.
47. Olausson M, Mjornstedt L, Norden G, et al. Successful combined partial auxiliary liver and kidney transplantation in highly sensitized cross-match positive recipients. American Journal of Transplantation. 2007;7:130-136.
48. Hadaya K, Ferrari-Lacraz S, Giostra E, et al. Humoral and cellular rejection after combined liver-kidney transplantation in low immunologic risk recipients. Transplant International. 2009;22:242-246.
49. Reichman TW, Marino SR, Milner J, et al. Acute humoral rejection in an ABO compatible combined liver-kidney transplant-the kidney is not always protected. American Journal of Transplantation. 2009;9:1957-1960.
50. Dar W, Agarwal A, Watkins C, et al. Donor-directed MHC class I antibody is preferentially cleared from sensitized recipients of combined liver/kidney transplants. American Journal of Transplantation. 2011;11:841-847.
51. Manez R, Kobayashi M, Takaya S, et al. Humoral rejection associated with antidonor lymphocytotoxic antibodies following liver transplantation. Transplantation Proceedings. 1993;25:888-890.
52. Wilson CH, Agarwal K, Carter V, et al. Late humoral rejection in a compliant ABO-compatible liver transplant recipient. Transplantation. 2006;82: 988-989.
53. Kasahara M, Kiuchi T, Takakura K, et al. Postoperative flow cytometry crossmatch in living donor liver transplantation: clinical significance of humoral immunity in acute rejection. Transplantation. 1999;67:568-575.
54. Charco R, Vargas V, Balsells J, et al. Influence of anti-HLA antibodies and positive T-lymphocytotoxic crossmatch on survival and graft rejection in human liver transplantation. Journal of Hepatology. 1996;24:452-459.
55. Neumann UP, Lang M, Moldenhauer A, et al. Significance of a T-lymphocytotoxic crossmatch in liver and combined liver-kidney transplantation. Transplantation. 2001;71:1163-1168.
56. Furuya T, Murase N, Nakamura K, et al. Preformed lymphocytotoxic antibodies: the effects of class, titer and specificity on liver vs. heart allografts. Hepatology (Baltimore, Md.). 1992;16:1415-1422.

57. Terasaki PI. Humoral theory of transplantation. American Journal of Transplantation. 2003;3:665–673.
58. O'Leary JG, Kaneku H, Susskind BM, et al. High mean fluorescence intensity donor-specific anti-HLA antibodies associated with chronic rejection postliver transplant. American Journal of Transplantation. 2011;11:1868–1876.
59. Sumitran-Holgersson S, Ge X, Karrar A, et al. A novel mechanism of liver allograft rejection facilitated by antibodies to liver sinusoidal endothelial cells. Hepatology (Baltimore, Md.). 2004;40:1211–1221.
60. Ali S, Ormsby A, Shah V, et al. Significance of complement split product C4d in ABO-compatible liver allograft: diagnosing utility in acute antibody mediated rejection. Transplant Immunology. 2011;26:62–69.
61. Neil DA, Hubscher SG. Current views on rejection pathology in liver transplantation. Transplant International. 2010;23:971–983.
62. Adeyi O, Fischer SE, Guindi M. Liver allograft pathology: approach to interpretation of needle biopsies with clinicopathological correlation. Journal of Clinical Pathology. 2010;63:47–74.
63. Urbani L, Mazzoni A, De Simone P, et al. Treatment of antibody-mediated rejection with high-dose immunoglobulins in ABO-incompatible liver transplant recipient. Transplant International. 2007;20:467–470.
64. Fung J, Kelly D, Kadry Z, et al. Immunosuppression in liver transplantation: beyond calcineurin inhibitors. Liver Transplantation. 2005;11:267–280.
65. Colvin RB. C4d in liver allografts: a sign of antibody-mediated rejection? American Journal of Transplantation. 2006;6:447–448.
66. Feucht HE. Complement C4d in graft capillaries—the missing link in the recognition of humoral alloreactivity. American Journal of Transplantation. 2003;3:646–652.
67. Sakashita H, Haga H, Ashihara E, et al. Significance of C4d staining in ABO-identical/compatible liver transplantation. Modern Pathology. 2007;20:676–684.
68. Castillo-Rama M, Castro MJ, Bernardo I, et al. Preformed antibodies detected by cytotoxic assay or multibead array decrease liver allograft survival: role of human leukocyte antigen compatibility. Liver Transplantation. 2008;14:554–562.
69. Goh A, Scalamogna M, De Feo T, et al. Human leukocyte antigen crossmatch testing is important for liver retransplantation. Liver Transplantation. 2010;16:308–313.
70. Takaya S, Duquesnoy R, Iwaki Y, et al. Positive crossmatch in primary human liver allografts under cyclosporine or FK 506 therapy. Transplantation Proceedings. 1991;23:396–399.
71. Li F, Atz ME, Reed EF. Human leukocyte antigen antibodies in chronic transplant vasculopathy-mechanisms and pathways. Current Opinion in Immunology. 2009;21:557–562.
72. Thomson AW, Mazariegos GV, Reyes J, et al. Monitoring the patient off immunosuppression. Conceptual framework for a proposed tolerance assay study in liver transplant recipients. Transplantation. 2001;72(8 Suppl.):S13–S22.
73. Feng S, Ekong UD, Lobritto SJ, et al. Complete immunosuppression withdrawal and subsequent allograft function among pediatric recipients of parental living donor liver transplants. JAMA. 2012;307:283–293.
74. Hubscher SG. Transplantation pathology. Seminars in Liver Disease. 2009;29:74–90.
75. Vijayaraghavan GR, David S, Bermudez-Allende M, et al. Imaging-guided parenchymal liver biopsy: how we do it. Journal of Clinical Imaging Science. 2011;1:30.
76. Rockey DC, Caldwell SH, Goodman ZD, et al. Liver biopsy. Hepatology (Baltimore, Md.). 2009;49:1017–1044.
77. Papini E, Pacella CM, Rossi Z, et al. A randomized trial of ultrasound-guided anterior subcostal liver biopsy versus the conventional Menghini technique. Journal of Hepatology. 1991;13:291–297.
78. Bravo AA, Sheth SG, Chopra S. Liver biopsy. New England Journal of Medicine. 2001;344:495–500.
79. Kalambokis G, Manousou P, Vibhakorn S, et al. Transjugular liver biopsy—indications, adequacy, quality of specimens, and complications—a systematic review. Journal of Hepatology. 2007;47:284–294.
80. Kwekkeboom J, Zondervan PE, Kuijpers MA, et al. Fine-needle aspiration cytology in the diagnosis of acute rejection after liver transplantation. British Journal of Surgery. 2003;90:246–247.
81. Warle MC, Metselaar HJ, Hop WC, et al. Early differentiation between rejection and infection in liver transplant patients by serum and biliary cytokine patterns. Transplantation. 2003;75:146–151.
82. Kubota K, Ericzon BG, Reinholt FP. Diagnosis of liver transplant rejection by bile cytology. Transplantation Proceedings. 1990;22:1521–1523.
83. Roberti I, Lieberman KV, Manzarbeitia C, et al. Evidence that the systematic analysis of bile cytology permits monitoring of hepatic allograft rejection. Transplantation. 1992;54:471–474.
84. Firpi RJ, Abdelmalek MF, Soldevila-Pico C, et al. Combination of interferon alfa-2b and ribavirin in liver transplant recipients with histological recurrent hepatitis C. Liver Transplantation. 2002;8:1000–1006.
85. Khettry U, Anand N, Gordon FD, et al. Recurrent hepatitis B, hepatitis C, and combined hepatitis B and C in liver allografts: a comparative pathological study. Human Pathology. 2000;31:101–108.
86. Petrovic LM, Villamil FG, Vierling JM, et al. Comparison of histopathology in acute allograft rejection and recurrent hepatitis C infection after liver transplantation. Liver Transplantation and Surgery. 1997;3:398–406.
87. Blakolmer K, Jain A, Ruppert K, et al. Chronic liver allograft rejection in a population treated primarily with tacrolimus as baseline immunosuppression: long-term follow-up and evaluation of features for histopathological staging. Transplantation. 2000;69:2330–2336.
88. Schmeding M, Dankof A, Krenn V, et al. C4d in acute rejection after liver transplantation—a valuable tool in differential diagnosis to hepatitis C recurrence. American Journal of Transplantation. 2006;6:523–530.
89. Berstad AE, Brabrand K, Foss A. Clinical utility of microbubble contrast-enhanced ultrasound in the diagnosis of hepatic artery occlusion after liver transplantation. Transplant International. 2009;22:954–960.
90. Brouard S, Mansfield E, Braud C, et al. Identification of a peripheral blood transcriptional biomarker panel associated with operational renal allograft tolerance. Proceedings of the National Academy of Sciences of the United States of America. 2007;104:15448–15453.
91. Farid WR, Pan Q, van der Meer AJ, et al. Hepatocyte-derived micrornas as serum biomarker of hepatic injury and rejection after liver transplantation. Liver Transplantation. 2011;18:290–297.
92. Feng S. Long-term management of immunosuppression after pediatric liver transplantation: is minimization or withdrawal desirable or possible or both? Current Opinion in Organ Transplantation. 2008;13:506–512.
93. Martinez-Llordella M, Lozano JJ, Puig-Pey I, et al. Using transcriptional profiling to develop a diagnostic test of operational tolerance in liver transplant recipients. Journal of Clinical Investigation. 2008;118:2845–2857.
94. Martinez-Llordella M, Puig-Pey I, Orlando G, et al. Multiparameter immune profiling of operational tolerance in liver transplantation. American Journal of Transplantation. 2007;7:309–319.
95. Abraham SC, Furth EE. Receiver operating characteristic analysis of serum chemical parameters as tests of liver transplant rejection and correlation with histology. Transplantation. 1995;59:740–746.
96. Batts KP. Acute and chronic hepatic allograft rejection: pathology and classification. Liver Transplantation and Surgery. 1999;5(4 Suppl. 1):S21–S29.
97. Uemura T, Ikegami T, Sanchez EQ, et al. Late acute rejection after liver transplantation impacts patient survival. Clinical Transplantation. 2008;22:316–323.
98. Haddad EM, McAlister VC, Renouf E, et al. Cyclosporin versus tacrolimus for liver transplanted patients. Cochrane Database of Systematic Reviews. 2006;(4):CD005161.
99. Perry I, Neuberger J. Immunosuppression: towards a logical approach in liver transplantation. Clinical and Experimental Immunology. 2005;139:2–10.
100. Aw MM, Verma A, Rela M, et al. Long-term outcome of mycophenolate mofetil rescue therapy for resistant acute allograft rejection in pediatric liver transplant recipients. Liver Transplantation. 2008;14:1303–1308.
101. Hebert MF, Ascher NL, Lake JR, et al. Four-year follow-up of mycophenolate mofetil for graft rescue in liver allograft recipients. Transplantation. 1999;67:707–712.
102. Klein A. Tacrolimus rescue in liver transplant patients with refractory rejection or intolerance or malabsorption of cyclosporine. The US Multicenter FK506 Liver Study Group. Liver Transplantation and Surgery. 1999;5:502–508.
103. Fisher RA, Ham JM, Marcos A, et al. A prospective randomized trial of mycophenolate mofetil with neoral or tacrolimus after orthotopic liver transplantation. Transplantation. 1998;66:1616–1621.
104. Wiesner R, Rabkin J, Klintmalm G, et al. A randomized double-blind comparative study of mycophenolate mofetil and azathioprine in combination with cyclosporine and corticosteroids in primary liver transplant recipients. Liver Transplantation. 2001;7:442–450.
105. Neuhaus P, Langrehr JM, Williams R, et al. Tacrolimus-based immunosuppression after liver transplantation: a randomised study comparing dual versus triple low-dose oral regimens. Transplant International. 1997;10:253–261.
106. Serrano J, Garcia Gonzalez M, Gomez M, et al. Tacrolimus is effective in both dual and triple regimens after liver transplantation. Transplantation Proceedings. 2002;34:1529–1530.
107. Klintmalm GB, Davis GL, Teperman L, et al. A randomized multicenter study comparing steroid-free and standard immunosuppression for liver transplant recipients with chronic hepatitis C. Liver Transplantation. 2011;17:1394–1403.
108. Lupo L, Panzera P, Tandoi F, et al. Basiliximab versus steroids in double therapy immunosuppression in liver transplantation: a prospective randomized clinical trial. Transplantation. 2008;86:925–931.
109. Uemura T, Schaefer E, Hollenbeak CS, et al. Outcome of induction immunosuppression for liver transplantation comparing anti-thymocyte globulin, daclizumab, and corticosteroid. Transplant International. 2011;24:640–650.

110. Asrani SK, Leise MD, West CP, et al. Use of sirolimus in liver transplant recipients with renal insufficiency: a systematic review and meta-analysis. Hepatology (Baltimore, Md.). 2010;52:1360–1370.
111. Heffron TG, Smallwood GA, Davis L, et al. Sirolimus-based immunosuppressive [correction of immunosuppresive] protocol for calcineurin sparing in liver transplantation. Transplantation Proceedings. 2002;34:1522–1523.
112. Massoud O, Wiesner RH. The use of sirolimus should be restricted in liver transplantation. Journal of Hepatology. 2010;56:288–290.
113. Neff GW, Montalbano M, Slapak-Green G, et al. A retrospective review of sirolimus (Rapamune) therapy in orthotopic liver transplant recipients diagnosed with chronic rejection. Liver Transplantation. 2003;9:477–483.
114. Aw MM, Taylor RM, Verma A, et al. Basiliximab (Simulect) for the treatment of steroid-resistant rejection in pediatric liver transplant recipients: a preliminary experience. Transplantation. 2003;75:796–799.
115. Bijleveld CG, Klompmaker IJ, van den Berg AP, et al. Incidence, risk factors, and outcome of antithymocyte globulin treatment of steroid-resistant rejection after liver transplantation. Transplant International. 1996;9:570–575.
116. Dhesi S, Boland B, Colquhoun S. Alemtuzumab and liver transplantation: a review. Current Opinion in Organ Transplantation. 2009;14:245–249.
117. Orr DW, Portmann BC, Knisely AS, et al. Anti-interleukin 2 receptor antibodies and mycophenolate mofetil for treatment of steroid-resistant rejection in adult liver transplantation. Transplantation Proceedings. 2005;37:4373–4379.
118. Schmitt TM, Phillips M, Sawyer RG, et al. Anti-thymocyte globulin for the treatment of acute cellular rejection following liver transplantation. Digestive Diseases and Sciences. 2010;55:3224–3234.
119. Kirk AD, Cherikh WS, Ring M, et al. Dissociation of depletional induction and posttransplant lymphoproliferative disease in kidney recipients treated with alemtuzumab. American Journal of Transplantation. 2007;7:2619–2625.
120. Wali M, Harrison RF, Gow PJ, et al. Advancing donor liver age and rapid fibrosis progression following transplantation for hepatitis C. Gut. 2002;51:248–252.
121. Perez-Daga JA, Ramirez-Plaza C, Suarez MA, et al. Impact of donor age on the results of liver transplantation in hepatitis C virus-positive recipients. Transplantation Proceedings. 2008;40:2959–2961.
122. Alonso O, Loinaz C, Moreno E, et al. Advanced donor age increases the risk of severe recurrent hepatitis C after liver transplantation. Transplant International. 2005;18:902–907.
123. Klintmalm GB, Washburn WK, Rudich SM, et al. Corticosteroid-free immunosuppression with daclizumab in HCV(+) liver transplant recipients: 1-year interim results of the HCV-3 study. Liver Transplantation. 2007;13:1521–1531.
124. Bahra M, Neumann UP, Jacob D, et al. Repeated steroid pulse therapies in HCV-positive liver recipients: significant risk factor for HCV-related graft loss. Transplantation Proceedings. 2005;37:1700–1702.
125. Sheiner PA, Schwartz ME, Mor E, et al. Severe or multiple rejection episodes are associated with early recurrence of hepatitis C after orthotopic liver transplantation. Hepatology (Baltimore, Md.). 1995;21:30–34.
126. Moreira RK. Recurrent hepatitis C and acute allograft rejection: clinicopathologic features with emphasis on the differential diagnosis between these entities. Advances in Anatomic Pathology. 2011;18:393–405.
127. Regev A, Molina E, Moura R, et al. Reliability of histopathologic assessment for the differentiation of recurrent hepatitis C from acute rejection after liver transplantation. Liver Transplantation. 2004;10:1233–1239.
128. Watt K, Veldt B, Charlton M. A practical guide to the management of HCV infection following liver transplantation. American Journal of Transplantation. 2009;9:1707–1713.
129. Burton JR Jr, Rosen HR. Acute rejection in HCV-infected liver transplant recipients: the great conundrum. Liver Transplantation. 2006;12(11 Suppl. 2):S38–S47.
130. Atici AE, Bostanci EB, Ozer I, et al. Use of granulocyte colony-stimulating factor for neutropenia after orthotopic liver transplantation: report of two cases. Transplantation Proceedings. 2011;43:909–911.
131. Page AV, Liles WC. Granulocyte colony-stimulating factor, granulocyte-macrophage colony-stimulating factor, and other immunomodulatory therapies for the treatment of infectious diseases in solid organ transplant recipients. Current Opinion in Organ Transplantation. 2008;13:575–580.
132. Haga H, Egawa H, Shirase T, et al. Periportal edema and necrosis as diagnostic histological features of early humoral rejection in ABO-incompatible liver transplantation. Liver Transplantation. 2004;10:16–27.
133. Marudanayagam R, Shanmugam V, Sandhu B, et al. Liver retransplantation in adults: a single-centre, 25-year experience. HPB (Oxford). 2010;12:217–224.
134. Rosen HR, Prieto M, Casanovas-Taltavull T, et al. Validation and refinement of survival models for liver retransplantation. Hepatology (Baltimore, Md.). 2003;38:460–469.
135. Horovitz D, Caumartin Y, Warren J, et al. Outcome of third renal allograft retransplants versus primary transplants from paired donors. Transplantation. 2009;87:1214–1220.
136. Kienzl-Wagner K, Mark W, Maglione M, et al. Single-center experience with third and fourth kidney transplants. Transplant International. 2011;24:780–786.
137. Delmonico FL, Tolkoff-Rubin N, Auchincloss H Jr, et al. Second renal transplantations. Ethical issues clarified by outcome; outcome enhanced by a reliable crossmatch. Archives of Surgery (Chicago, Ill.: 1960). 1994;129:354–360.
138. Chen GH, Fu BS, Cai CJ, et al. A single-center experience of retransplantation for liver transplant recipients with a failing graft. Transplantation Proceedings. 2008;40:1485–1487.
139. Rosen HR, Madden JP, Martin P. A model to predict survival following liver retransplantation. Hepatology (Baltimore, Md.). 1999;29:365–370.
140. Yao FY, Saab S, Bass NM, et al. Prediction of survival after liver retransplantation for late graft failure based on preoperative prognostic scores. Hepatology (Baltimore, Md.). 2004;39:230–238.
141. Lodhi SA, Lamb KE, Meier-Kriesche HU. Solid organ allograft survival improvement in the United States: the long-term does not mirror the dramatic short-term success. American Journal of Transplantation. 2011;11:1226–1235.
142. Akamatsu N, Sugawara Y, Tamura S, et al. Late-onset acute rejection after living donor liver transplantation. World Journal of Gastroenterology. 2006;12: 6674–6677.
143. Florman S, Schiano T, Kim L, et al. The incidence and significance of late acute cellular rejection (>1000 days) after liver transplantation. Clinical Transplantation. 2004;18:152–155.
144. Ramji A, Yoshida EM, Bain VG, et al. Late acute rejection after liver transplantation: the Western Canada experience. Liver Transplantation. 2002;8: 945–951.
145. Wiesner RH, Steffen BJ, David KM, et al. Mycophenolate mofetil use is associated with decreased risk of late acute rejection in adult liver transplant recipients. American Journal of Transplantation. 2006;6:1609–1616.
146. Berquist RK, Berquist WE, Esquivel CO, et al. Adolescent non-adherence: prevalence and consequences in liver transplant recipients. Pediatric Transplantation. 2006;10:304–310.
147. Berquist RK, Berquist WE, Esquivel CO, et al. Non-adherence to post-transplant care: prevalence, risk factors and outcomes in adolescent liver transplant recipients. Pediatric Transplantation. 2008;12:194–200.
148. Freese DK, Snover DC, Sharp HL, et al. Chronic rejection after liver transplantation: a study of clinical, histopathological and immunological features. Hepatology (Baltimore, Md.). 1991;13:882–891.
149. Lowes JR, Hubscher SG, Neuberger JM. Chronic rejection of the liver allograft. Gastroenterology Clinics of North America. 1993;22:401–420.
150. Neuberger J. Incidence, timing, and risk factors for acute and chronic rejection. Liver Transplantation and Surgery. 1999;5(4 Suppl. 1):S30–S36.
151. Neuhaus P, Blumhardt G, Bechstein WO, et al. Comparison of FK506- and cyclosporine-based immunosuppression in primary orthotopic liver transplantation. A single center experience. Transplantation. 1995;59:31–40.
152. Wiesner RH, Batts KP, Krom RA. Evolving concepts in the diagnosis, pathogenesis, and treatment of chronic hepatic allograft rejection. Liver Transplantation and Surgery. 1999;5:388–400.
153. Jain A, Demetris AJ, Kashyap R, et al. Does tacrolimus offer virtual freedom from chronic rejection after primary liver transplantation? Risk and prognostic factors in 1,048 liver transplantations with a mean follow-up of 6 years. Liver Transplantation. 2001;7:623–630.
154. Neil DA, Hubscher SG. Histologic and biochemical changes during the evolution of chronic rejection of liver allografts. Hepatology (Baltimore, Md.). 2002;35: 639–651.
155. Starzl TE, Todo S, Fung J, et al. FK 506 for liver, kidney, and pancreas transplantation. Lancet. 1989;2(8670):1000–1004.
156. Sebagh M, Rifai K, Feray C, et al. All liver recipients benefit from the protocol 10-year liver biopsies. Hepatology (Baltimore, Md.). 2003;37: 1293–1301.
157. Sher LS, Cosenza CA, Michel J, et al. Efficacy of tacrolimus as rescue therapy for chronic rejection in orthotopic liver transplantation: a report of the U.S. Multicenter Liver Study Group. Transplantation. 1997;64:258–263.
158. Blakolmer K, Seaberg EC, Batts K, et al. Analysis of the reversibility of chronic liver allograft rejection implications for a staging schema. American Journal of Surgical Pathology. 1999;23:1328–1339.
159. Sebagh M, Blakolmer K, Falissard B, et al. Accuracy of bile duct changes for the diagnosis of chronic liver allograft rejection: reliability of the 1999 Banff schema. Hepatology (Baltimore, Md.). 2002;35:117–125.
160. Demetris AJ, Adeyi O, Bellamy CO, et al. Liver biopsy interpretation for causes of late liver allograft dysfunction. Hepatology (Baltimore, Md.). 2006;44: 489–501.
161. Gouw AS, van den Heuvel MC, van den Berg AP, et al. The significance of parenchymal changes of acute cellular rejection in predicting chronic liver graft rejection. Transplantation. 2002;73:243–247.
162. A comparison of tacrolimus (FK 506) and cyclosporine for immunosuppression in liver transplantation. The U.S. Multicenter FK506 Liver Study Group. New

England Journal of Medicine. 1994;331:1110–1115.
163. Demetris AJ, Fung JJ, Todo S, et al. Conversion of liver allograft recipients from cyclosporine to FK506 immunosuppressive therapy—a clinicopathologic study of 96 patients. Transplantation. 1992;53:1056–1062.
164. Jain A, Mazariegos G, Pokharna R, et al. The absence of chronic rejection in pediatric primary liver transplant patients who are maintained on tacrolimus-based immunosuppression: a long-term analysis. Transplantation. 2003;75: 1020–1025.
165. Hayashi M, Keeffe EB, Krams SM, et al. Allograft rejection after liver transplantation for autoimmune liver diseases. Liver Transplantation and Surgery. 1998;4:208–214.
166. Soin AS, Rasmussen A, Jamieson NV, et al. CsA levels in the early posttransplant period-predictive of chronic rejection in liver transplantation? Transplantation. 1995;59:1119–1123.
167. Magnone M, Holley JL, Shapiro R, et al. Interferon-alpha-induced acute renal allograft rejection. Transplantation. 1995;59:1068–1070.
168. Rostaing L, Modesto A, Baron E, et al. Acute renal failure in kidney transplant patients treated with interferon alpha 2b for chronic hepatitis C. Nephron. 1996;74:512–516.
169. Samuel D. Hepatitis C, interferon, and risk of rejection after liver transplantation. Liver Transplantation. 2004;10:868–871.
170. Fernandez I, Ulloa E, Colina F, et al. Incidence, risk factors, and outcome of chronic rejection during antiviral therapy for posttransplant recurrent hepatitis C. Liver Transplantation. 2009;15:948–955.
171. Stanca CM, Fiel MI, Kontorinis N, et al. Chronic ductopenic rejection in patients with recurrent hepatitis C virus treated with pegylated interferon alfa-2a and ribavirin. Transplantation. 2007;84:180–186.
172. Stravitz RT, Shiffman ML, Sanyal AJ, et al. Effects of interferon treatment on liver histology and allograft rejection in patients with recurrent hepatitis C following liver transplantation. Liver Transplantation. 2004;10:850–858.
173. Saab S, Kalmaz D, Gajjar NA, et al. Outcomes of acute rejection after interferon therapy in liver transplant recipients. Liver Transplantation. 2004;10:859–867.
174. Demetris AJ, Seaberg EC, Batts KP, et al. Chronic liver allograft rejection: a National Institute of Diabetes and Digestive and Kidney Diseases interinstitutional study analyzing the reliability of current criteria and proposal of an expanded definition. National Institute of Diabetes and Digestive and Kidney Diseases Liver Transplantation Database. American Journal of Surgical Pathology. 1998;22:28–39.
175. Lunz JG 3rd, Contrucci S, Ruppert K, et al. Replicative senescence of biliary epithelial cells precedes bile duct loss in chronic liver allograft rejection: increased expression of p21(WAF1/Cip1) as a disease marker and the influence of immunosuppressive drugs. American Journal of Pathology. 2001;158:1379–1390.
176. Detry O, de Roover A, Delwaide J, et al. The use of mycophenolate mofetil in liver transplant recipients. Expert Opinion on Pharmacotherapy. 2003;4: 1949–1957.
177. Pfitzmann R, Klupp J, Langrehr JM, et al. Mycophenolatemofetil for immunosuppression after liver transplantation: a follow-up study of 191 patients. Transplantation. 2003;76:130–136.
178. Klupp J, Pfitzmann R, Langrehr JM, et al. Indications of mycophenolate mofetil in liver transplantation. Transplantation. 2005;80(1 Suppl.):S142–S146.

第71章 心脏移植临床排斥反应综合征

Matthew H. Levine，Sandy Feng

引言

Christiaan Barnard医生在完成他个人的第二例心脏移植手术后，在一篇术后早期报道中将同种异体排斥反应归纳为如下一系列临床表现。

器官受体对于移植器官的免疫排斥反应的临床表现包括：①发热、心动过速、厌食等系统性反应；②导致移植器官增大的局部表现；③移植器官功能减退相关的临床表现或实验室结果；④脏器实质破坏相关证据；⑤同种异体器官移植导致的人体免疫学改变[1]。

随着心脏移植在临床上的开展，我们必须认识到，移植物排斥反应无法通过单一实验室检查结果或临床表现来诊断，而是需要综合分析患者的症状、体格检查结果、心电图结果以及反映免疫反应和肌肉损伤相关的实验室结果才得以明确诊断[1-4]。随着免疫抑制剂的研发和应用，心脏移植排斥反应的表现也在发生变化。目前，我们可以得出的明确结论是，不同患者同种异体器官移植排斥反应的临床表现和组织病理学表现可能存在较大的差异，其表现可以是急性、隐匿性或慢性的，可能是细胞排斥介导的或抗体排斥介导的，可能是症状明确或是表现隐匿的。

近年来，许多新研发上市的免疫抑制剂都针对细胞介导的排斥反应，但临床上我们较少见到单一由细胞介导的排斥反应。更多的是其同抗体介导的免疫过程（AMR）相结合起到免疫排斥作用。目前，移植物排斥反应仍是一个我们需要关注的重点问题，因此，免疫监视、移植物临床状态评估及心脏移植物组织学检测等多渠道联合的免疫排斥反应监测仍是目前临床心脏移植的重要工作内容。

在本章中，我们综述了诊断细胞和抗体介导的排斥反应的方法和预防高危人群排斥反应的新疗法，并简要讨论了不同类型排斥反应的治疗。

细胞排斥

急性细胞排斥反应（ACR）是指T细胞介导的机体对移植物组织的攻击，该反应在移植后初期比较普遍（见第5章）。细胞排斥反应在组织病理学上（见第83章）表现为淋巴细胞浸润，发生轻度排斥反应时，这种淋巴细胞较多局限于血管周围区域。排斥反应较严重时，淋巴细胞浸润将更为严重，并可能进展至心肌间质。此外，除了心肌细胞损伤、心肌内出血和（或）血管炎相关证据之外，还可以观察到其他的炎性细胞，包括中性粒细胞和嗜酸粒细胞。

心肌细胞损伤同最严重程度的排斥反应，即在心内膜心肌活检标本中表现为肌质扇形展开、嗜酸细胞过多以及核固缩的排斥反应，有密切联系。

1990年，国际心肺移植协会（ISHLT）对细胞排斥反应的病例诊断和分级进行了标准的制定（表71.1）[5]。最初的标准包括7个大类。但该标准因不同观察者间差异较大，没有受到广泛认可[6]。并且，该标准中的部分亚分类的临床相关性受到了质疑。其中，对于“局灶性中度排斥”（2级）的概念被频繁应用到Quilty病变的诊断中，而其本身却没有任何的临床相关性[7]。轻度弥漫性排斥反应（1级）诊断较罕见，且该诊断同中度弥漫性排斥（3B级）的定义上划分不清。该病理诊断标准最终于2004年被重新修订，原有的1A、1B和2级统一合并为修订后的1R级，原3A级改为修订后的2R级，原严重排斥反应的3B级和4级统一合并为修订后的3R级（图71.1和图71.2）[8]。

危险因素

心脏移植研究数据库（CTRD）所报道的一篇分析

表 71.1 细胞排斥的病理学诊断标准

ISHLT 1990 年分级	病理学表现	ISHLT 2004 年分级	病理学表现
0 级	没有细胞排斥的证据	0R 级	没有细胞排斥的证据
1A 级(局灶轻度急性排斥)	局灶炎性细胞浸润,不伴坏死	1R 级(轻度、低级别的急性排斥反应)	间质或血管周围单核细胞浸润,至多 1 个病灶的心肌细胞损伤,或正常心肌细胞结构
1B 级(弥漫轻度急性排斥)	弥漫的,但较稀疏的炎性细胞浸润,不伴坏死		
2 级(局灶中度急性排斥)	单病灶的炎性细胞侵袭性浸润,常有局部心肌细胞损伤		
3A 级(多发中度排斥)	多病灶炎性细胞侵袭性浸润,常有局部心肌细胞损伤	2R 级(中度、中等级别的急性排斥反应)	两个及以上病灶浸润及相关心肌细胞损伤,病灶间正常心肌
3B 级 (弥漫边界重度急性排斥)	弥漫性炎性细胞浸润,伴心肌损伤的证据	3R 级(重度、高级别的急性排斥反应)	弥漫性浸润,伴多病灶心肌细胞损伤, 可伴有水肿、出血和(或)血管炎
4 级(重度急性排斥)	弥漫性炎性细胞浸润,含浸润物、心肌损伤及水肿、出血和(或)血管炎中的多种成分		

ISHLT,国际心肺移植协会。

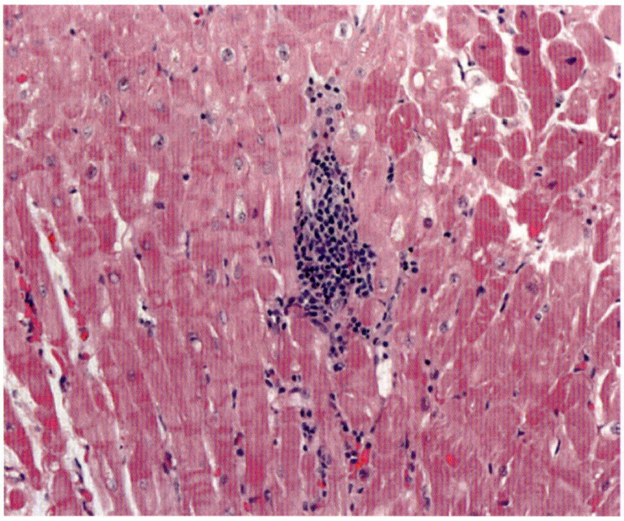

图 71.1 HE 染色显示,1R 级(原 2 级)排斥反应,单区域侵袭性浸润。(Image provided by Dr. Margaret M. Grimes, Richmond, VA.)

表明, 急性细胞排斥反应的危险度在移植术后 1 个月达到顶峰,之后开始下降,到 1 年后处于稳定水平。排斥反应的危险因素包括女性受体、低龄、黑色人种、巨细胞病毒感染、女性供体、机械灌注支持以及较高程度的供体-受体人白细胞抗原(HLA)不匹配[9-11]。

类似于肾移植,心脏移植供体-受体人白细胞抗原匹配程度很可能影响移植后排斥发生概率, 以及移植物的存活, 但目前就这方面的研究数据仍存在一定争议。部分小样本研究表明,人白细胞抗原匹配度同移植术后安全性无明显联系。但 Opelz 和 Wujcik 发表的《器官移植联合分析》,纳入了 8000 多例患者,表明供体和受体在 HLA-A、HLA-B 或 DR 位点上若仅有 2 个或以下的错配, 其移植后移植器官功能和存活率将明显提

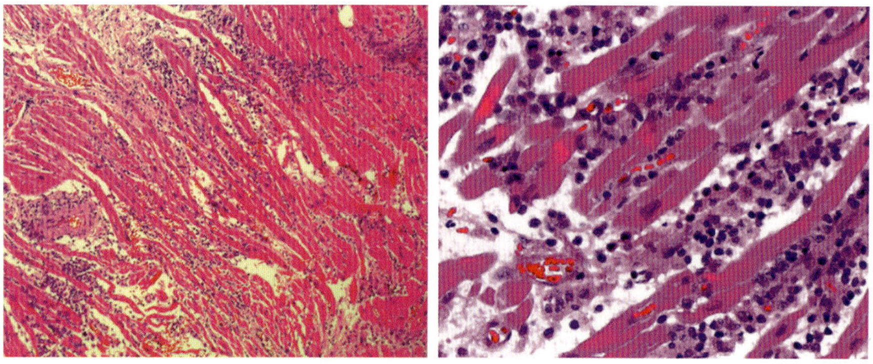

(A) (B)

图 71.2 (A)低倍镜和(B)高倍镜下 HE 染色显示 3R 级(原 3B 级)排斥反应,弥漫性浸润、心肌细胞坏死、心肌结构损坏。(Image provided by Dr. Margaret M. Grimes, Richmond, VA.)

高[12-14]。在该研究中,存活率的改善主要是在移植后的前 3~6 个月,提示 HLA 匹配对急性移植物排斥反应的保护作用[12]。心脏移植研究数据库的一项对 1200 例患者的分析显示,仅有 2 个及以下 HLA 错配的患者,术后第 1 年均无排斥相关死亡,或需要再次移植[10]。并且,在移植术后的第 1 个月,人体组织相容性复合物Ⅱ的 DR 位点上有 2 个位点错配的患者,其移植物排斥反应(2 级或以上)的发生概率显著升高(65%比 40%)[15]。OKT3 或 IL-2 抑制剂诱导治疗对于 HLA-DR 相关的排斥反应的发生并没有作用。但是,抗胸腺细胞球蛋白在诱导治疗中的应用,以及他克莫司在维持治疗过程中替代环孢霉素,均可使这种排斥的发生概率降低[16-18]。尽管有上述发现,心脏移植患者的 HLA 匹配在实施上受到诸多限制。考虑到手术时间窗狭窄、供体器官紧缺、受体一般情况不稳定等问题,HLA 匹配算法目前在临床上并未广泛开展。

心脏移植术后巨细胞病毒(CMV)感染将会增加急、慢性移植排斥反应。活动性巨细胞病毒具有促炎症反应、激活免疫反应的作用。特定患者进行巨细胞病毒感染的预防能够有效降低急、慢性排斥反应的发生[19]。一般情况下,在巨细胞病毒感染期间,可能会因控制病毒感染的需要而降低免疫抑制剂的使用量,常常会导致巨细胞病毒感染后恢复期时细胞排斥反应风险大大上升。

不同人种患者对于免疫抑制治疗可能有不同的反应。有研究报道显示,黑色人种受体相比高加索人种受体,移植器官衰竭、移植物排斥反应概率升高,因此生存率相应降低[20]。需要进行进一步的研究来验证这种现象产生的人口统计学或生物学机制。针对黑色人种心脏移植受体患者采用更加精准靶向的免疫抑制治疗,可能可以降低不良事件发生的风险[21]。

也有研究表明,女性受体患者相比男性,移植排斥反应发生的概率更高。妊娠史是排斥反应发生的一个明确的危险因素,除此之外,可能也有其他性别特异性的机制对抑制排斥的发生产生影响。有学者研究指出,性别匹配可能可以降低排斥反应的发生,且其作用与受体-供体体重是否匹配无关[22]。

诊断

症状

心脏移植排斥反应没有特异性的症状和体征。因此,对于排斥反应的诊断,通常是由根据心内膜心肌活检的组织学结果得出的。大多数急性排斥反应的症状通常在移植术后 3~6 个月内发生,大多数症状较轻或无临床症状。

重度排斥反应患者的心力衰竭症状,表现为运动耐量降低、气急、液体潴留、端坐呼吸、夜间阵发性呼吸困难和疲乏等。临床医生应该时刻警惕胃肠道反应,包括腹部右上象限疼痛、恶心及呕吐,这些现象可能是右室功能减退、中心静脉压升高的表现。若有如上任一反应,尤其是在移植后的早期,或是在患者依从性不强的情况下,因经验性给予静脉糖皮质激素治疗,并尽早行心内膜心肌活检。

自从经静脉活检术首次由日本开创并由斯坦福大学的 Caves 团队改良以来,心肌活检一直是受体对于移植物的免疫反应监测的金标准[23,24]。评估性心内膜心肌活检对于心脏移植的成功来说,可谓功不可没。但是,尽管心内膜心肌活检的并发症发生率较低,该技术因为高成本、患者不适、临床实用性不确切等问题,其临床应用在目前这个现代免疫抑制治疗时代,受到诸多质疑和限制。在免疫抑制治疗下,评估性心内膜炎活检所检测到的无症状排斥反应的发生率低于 2%。不仅如此,评估性心内膜心肌活检所发现的低、中级别的排斥反应并不一定完全准确,因为接近 85%的心内膜心肌活检显示为低、中级别排斥反应的患者,在没有任何医学干预的情况下,这些细胞排斥反应的组织病理表现能自发消失[25]。其他问题,如心肌中发现的炎症细胞很有可能是其他途径来源的,因此可能造成假阳性结果[26]。即便有足够多的样本量,不同组织标本观察者的对于中度排斥反应的诊断和解读也可能造成较大的差异[7]。

但即使是有如上诸多限制,由于其他工具缺乏足够的特异性和敏感性,心内膜心肌活检依然是目前诊断、评估移植排斥反应的主要工具。但是,如上诸多顾虑和关注点已促进进一步的无创的、基于实验室的排斥反应评估手段的研发。

心电图

心电图有助于识别重度急性心脏排斥反应相关的传导、节律异常,但心电图缺乏特异性。此外,心电图对于早期、中度排斥反应,尤其是正在接受免疫抑制治疗的患者,敏感性不高。急性排斥反应发生时,由炎症和细胞浸润造成的心肌水肿将会改变心肌传导的特点。QRS 波右偏、心电图电压降低是急性排斥反应的典型心电图表现。

超声心动图

移植心脏的 2D 或多普勒超声可以发现心肌结构或同急性排斥反应相关的功能上的改变。

为了了解排斥反应的超声心动图表现，我们首先有必要了解患者心脏移植术后的正常超声必动图表现。相比年龄匹配的正常对照组，移植心脏有如下几个特征。左室重量上升，心室壁在术后达到最厚，并接下来逐步变薄。移植术后左室大小以及收缩功能通常正常，而右室可能出现扩大，收缩功能降低。部分受体在移植术后早期右室功能的降低可能与右室心肌对缺血性损伤更为敏感、脑死亡介导的儿茶酚胺通路受损、肺动脉阻力上升等有关。通常情况下，早期右室功能减退是一过性的，会在移植术后数周至一个月内得到改善。

若移植手术时行双房吻合，心房将会呈瘦长、漏斗形，超声可以看到缝线。移植心脏同本体心脏不同，不附着于后胸壁。室间隔也会因此因为移植心脏的前向摆动而出现矛盾运动[29-32]。

心脏移植术后三尖瓣彩超血流信号将于短时间内频繁显示三尖瓣反流[33]。随着移植心脏的右室功能得到改善，受体患者的肺血管阻力将会降低，三尖瓣反流也将得到改善。由肺动脉高压、心内膜心肌活检所致腱索损伤、术后瓣环结构重构或右室功能减退所导致的术后持续三尖瓣反流则预示预后不良[24]。

2D 超声心动图可以发现心脏结构和功能上的改变，但是这些参数对于早期排斥反应的检测缺乏特异性(<50%)，这使得将超声心动图作为移植术后常规检查变得性价比不高[35]。排斥反应将造成心室质量的急性升高以及心室壁的增厚[4,36]。左室收缩功能的降低通常在重度排斥时才出现。右室功能减退可能在发生轻度排斥反应时显得尤为突出，随着排斥所带来的炎症反应常常会出现心包积液的情况[31,37,38]。

在排斥反应出现期间，心脏舒张功能减退将比收缩功能减退更迅速。心超中反应心室舒张充盈特性的指标有助于发现早期急性排斥。多普勒信号所体现的血流特性可以反映出患者类似限制型心肌病样的改变。急性排斥反应还可以表现为等容舒张时间(IVRT)缩短、早期二尖瓣压力减半时间(PHT)降低、早晚期二尖瓣血流速度(Em)峰值比值升高、肺静脉心房部分血流的持续倒流[37-42]。但是，参数受到心脏负荷状态的影响，其可靠性有限[42]。而组织多普勒成像则较少受到血流动力学的影响，并在急性排斥反应期间测量二尖瓣瓣环及左室后壁收缩及舒张期血流速度的降低[43]。但这些指标的特异性因移植心脏的收缩特性受到其他因素的影响而受到限制，这些因素包括免疫抑制相关的高血压、左室肥厚、既往排斥发作所致纤维化等。相应的，不同研究所表明的超声心对移植排斥反应的诊断准确性参差不齐，动图在移植排斥评估中的作用相关的研究目前仍没有明确结果[40,44-48]。

磁共振成像

心脏磁共振成像(CMR)已逐渐成为心脏疾病有力的诊断工具。CMR 具有图像质量高、空间分辨率高的特点，已经成为评估心室质量和收缩功能的参考标准[49]。CMR 也已经成为冠状动脉疾病患者评估局部心室壁活动、心肌活性和缺血情况的有力工具[50-52]。

CMR 对于心脏移植患者的实用价值目前尚无定论。CMR 相比超声心动图，其在移植心脏质量、收缩射血分数和心室体积方面具有较高的可重复性[53]。然而，这些参数的改变通常只反映迟发、重度的排斥反应[54]。在急性移植排斥中，心肌中升高的水含量连同炎症反应，会延长 T2 弛豫时间(由自旋回波技术测定)。早期动物试验表明，在没有接受免疫治疗的严重排斥反应的心脏移植狗受体中，T2 弛豫时间明显延长，心室壁明显增厚[55]。但是，利用现代免疫抑制技术治疗移植患者后，却得出了同动物试验相矛盾的结果，这一结果从一定程度上阻碍了这一技术在临床上的应用[56-59]。

磁共振成像技术能够发现移植心脏内标记免疫细胞的累积，对于这种技术的研究目前正在进行中[60,61]。

生物指标

在发生多种移植心脏排斥反应时，心肌损伤指标，包括肌酸激酶同工酶异构体和肌钙蛋白，将有不同程度的升高[62]。所有移植患者在心脏移植术后早期都一致地出现了这些指标水平的上升，其原因可能同术前缺血时间有关[63,64]。那些持续存在肌钙蛋白阳性或指标升高的患者，很可能存在微血管病变或心肌坏死，这些患者更容易出现早期的移植心脏冠状动脉病变或是移植心脏衰竭[63]。

总的来说，心肌坏死的指标多见于程度较严重的移植排斥反应，而对常规移植排斥评估来说，敏感性不够高[65,66]。而超敏肌钙蛋白测定可能具有更高的临床实用价值，但其具体效果还有待进一步研究评估。

B 型脑钠肽(BNP)是由心肌伸展后刺激心肌细胞分泌的一种氨基酸多肽。BNP 以及氨基末端 BNP(NT-BNP) 对于心力衰竭患者的诊断和预后判断来说是有用的指标。有研究表明，移植术后早期 BNP 含量升高，在术后 4~6 个月达到平台期[67,68]。

BNP 水平的升高与急性排斥反应时心脏超声的结果通常一致，这些结果包括心室壁增厚、心室质量增加、右室舒张增加、右室功能减退等[69]。对于心室收缩功能正常患者，BNP 水平与心脏充盈压力升高、心排血量降低、限制充盈像等血流动力学紊乱有关[69,70]。然而，BNP 升高也可独立于超声心动图血流动力学测量结果，说明多肽分泌中存在同心肌伸展无关的信号通路[71]。实际上，心脏移植患者 BNP 的分泌与其他心肌伸展敏感的指标，包括心房利钠因子等无关[72]。

一项对于心功能、心充盈压力等临床情况稳定的心脏移植受体患者的外周基因表达相关研究表明，那些具有上调免疫功能，以及与 HLA 系统、肥大细胞、热休克蛋白及 B 细胞系相关的基因，同 BNP 水平有密切联系[73]。细胞因子介导的 BNP 分泌可能从一条共同通路，即连结心脏多肽分泌和炎症的 p38 通路[74]。综上，这些数据表明，除血流动力学紊乱及心肌排斥反应外，炎症过程也会调节并上调 BNP 的分泌。

BNP 水平的升高预示着术后 1 年或更久的移植心脏功能不全[75,76]。心脏移植术后 BNP 水平升高与急性移植排斥反应的发生有关，但该研究循证证据不足(曲线下面积：0.71~0.76)，其证据力度比主诉呼吸困难的患者诊断为急性心力衰竭的证据要低很多[77,78]。因此，BNP 并没有替代心内膜心肌活检成为新的移植评估工具。

有创血流动力学

移植术后早期，利用有创血流动力学检测，患者常呈现充盈压力升高的限制性充盈现象。不顺应的右心室可能表现出 Kussmaul 征(吸气时右房压力升高)，且右房压力可能升高并伴随持续的“a”“v”型偏离或快速的“y”型下降。这些早期的血流动力学异常可能与心肌顿抑、排斥、先前就存在的受体肺动脉高压、供体儿茶酚胺波动和(或)术中扩容等情况有关[79-82]。尽管心脏内压力通常在术后几个月内都接近正常范围，但即便心肌活检没有排斥反应或纤维化的证据，心脏内压力很可能也无法完全恢复到正常水平[81]。这种限制性充盈现象通常在移植术后数月内消失，但是一旦容量负荷增加则又会出现[82]。

在急性排斥反应发生期间，室壁较薄的右心室因为功能储备较少，更易受损伤，并出现水肿及不可膨胀现象。血流动力学检测易发现与限制型充盈相关的证据。有创血流动力学常常可以发现充盈压力升高。重度排斥反应时，心排血量降低。排斥反应经治疗后，急性炎症反应缓解，充盈压力往往可以得到改善。但是，血流动力学的异常可能依然存在，其机制可能与心肌损伤和纤维化的不可逆过程有关[83,84]。

基因表达谱

基因表达谱指的是通过较多基因的 mRNA 的产生以识别与特定疾病的进展或某个临床事件相关的特定基因的激活模式。一些研究通过分析移植器官组织以及外周血标本发现，急性排斥相关的诸多信号通路中的基因表达量得到了上调[85-89]。利用基因芯片分析技术进行特定基因的探索，目前已开发出一套实用的评分系统及商业检测手段，可以用于对心脏移植排斥反应的发生进行预测。目前已研发出 1 组包含 11 个基因的基因芯片，利用该芯片可以对巨噬细胞的激活、皮质激素应答反应、血小板生产功能、造血作用、T 细胞激活以及细胞形态进行识别，并进而研发出一套评分系统，利用该评分系统可以对基因的表达进行验证，从而预测移植排斥反应的发生[90]。

目前，与心内膜心肌活检相比，基因表达谱是一种非创伤性移植排斥监测策略。“利用基因表达减少创伤性监测”(IMAGE) 临床试验项目对该监测策略进行了评估[91]。IMAGE 试验评估了一部分低风险心脏移植患者，这些患者在原位心脏移植术后 1 年情况显著改善，且没有排斥反应、血管病变或移植器官功能不全病史。对于患者人群的分析发现，两组患者在多种主要试验终点上发生概率相似(14.5%比 15.3%)，这些试验终点包括左室射血分数下降 25%以上、任何伴随血流动力学改变的排斥反应或全因死亡。

该研究是第一个将替代排斥评估方案与已被长期接受的心内膜心肌活检进行比较的临床试验。然而，仍需要针对高风险患者、更接近移植时间点进行进一步的研究。该试验的评分系统对于心脏移植术后情况稳定的患者的监测评估效果较明确，但对于短时间内输血或近期针对排斥进行治疗的患者，其应用仍缺乏证据。并且，该方法因具有激素敏感的特点，其对于接受过每天20mg以上糖皮质激素治疗的患者，效果不确切。进一步针对基因表达谱与心内膜心肌活检的对比研究或许可以验证该方法对于医生（减少创伤）和患者（减少费用）的双重优点。

抗体介导的移植排斥

非细胞的、由抗体驱动的心脏移植排斥反应的概念的提出已有许多年，该话题自从产生至今，一直存在争论。1983年，Hess和Mohanakumar观察到，抗体能够作用于B细胞，并在加速移植心脏的粥样硬化的过程中起到重要的作用[92]。Herskowitz等进一步观察到，有一种排斥反应与移植器官衰竭患者的心内膜心肌活检发现的小动脉血管炎有关[93]。接下来，Hammond等介绍了一种新的移植排斥模式，这种排斥与免疫病理学发现的免疫球蛋白沉积、补体的免疫荧光结合以及组织病理学发现的心内膜水肿、常规光镜下发现的心肌间质水肿现象相一致。与病理学检查发现，与"体液"排斥现象相比细胞排斥，患者生存率下降的结果有直接联系。这些以及其他早期的工作引起了学界多年的争论，但最终还是得到了越来越多的对于抗体介导的排斥反应（AMR）概念的认同。

在抗体介导排斥反应期间，针对供体同种异体移植物的特异性抗体通过与同种异体移植物结合并增强其免疫反应，从而造成急性排斥反应（见第6章）。在部分严重案例中，这种反应将会导致急性移植器官功能不全，并增加移植心脏冠状动脉血管病变的风险。

由于目前尚缺乏针对排斥反应评估和诊断的实践指南，抗体介导的排斥反应对于心脏移植来说，仍是一个诊断和治疗上的难题。抗体介导的排斥反应的流行病学特点，包括疾病发生率、流行特点、进展率，由于目前评估模式、组织病理学诊断标准、活检标本组织病理学和免疫病理学技术等方面的不同，目前仍没有统一的定论。由于临床、组织病理学诊断标准的不同，文献报道的"非细胞"排斥反应或抗体介导排斥反应的发生率有很大差异。但是，该发生率为8%~20%，而且在心脏移植术后的前6个月，其发生率相对较高[95,96]。不同于学者所观察到的细胞排斥反应发生率逐年降低的现象，抗体介导排斥反应的发生率和患病率随着时间延长依然没有明显改变[97]。

对于具有预敏化事件史的患者，其抗体介导排斥反应的发生率较高。例如，抗体介导排斥反应在女性患者、错配阳性受体患者和（或）群体反应性抗体水平升高患者中发生率较高[95,96]。其他抗体介导排斥反应发生的危险因素包括血液制品输注、机械灌注循环支持、怀孕和感染等。

诊断

移植物抗体介导排斥反应的临床和诊断标准正在逐步演变。早期研究报告的入组标准差异较大。大多数研究报道纳入的是具有心内膜心肌活检表明抗体介导损伤、移植器官功能不全的临床诊断和（或）循环中自身抗体的血清指标等相关证据的患者。与细胞免疫相似，ISHLT提出的现行指南中，考虑到临床上无症状的体液排斥反应，因此将抗体介导排斥列为单纯的病理学诊断（表71.2）。

临床表现

通常受体血流动力学改变或无法解释的移植器官功能不全的患者需要考虑抗体介导排斥反应的诊断。早期抗体介导排斥反应的症状和体征可能是隐匿的、非特异性的、容易被忽视的。患者可以表现为疲劳、虚弱、恶心或呕吐，可有因肝淤血引起肝包膜疼痛导致的右上腹疼痛。然而，由于更有效的组织病理学生物标志物的应用，对于早期或无症状抗体介导排斥反应的认识正在逐步改善。虽然这一现象的本质同临床的相关性尚未确定，目前已有越来越多的数据表明，早期无症状、由心内膜心肌活检发现的抗体介导排斥反应患者，其发生移植心脏血管病变及移植心脏相关死亡的发生风险升高[98,99]。

循环中人白细胞抗原（HLA）及非抗HLA抗体

受体循环血液中供体特异性自身抗体（见第36章）的检测结果对于抗体介导排斥反应的诊断具有参考价值，但并不是必需的。然而，抗供体HLA抗体的阳性检测结果与心脏移植术后抗体介导排斥的发生以及移植心脏血管病变的发生有一定关联[100-102]。

表 71.2　抗体介导排斥反应的组织病理学诊断标准

ISHLT 2004 年标准	病理学表现	2011 年标准	病理学表现
0 级抗体介导排斥反应	无抗体介导排斥相关证据	0 级病理学抗体介导排斥反应	无抗体介导排斥相关证据
1 级抗体介导排斥反应	组织学标准：心内膜组织水肿、血管内巨噬细胞聚集相关证据；严重病例可能出现中性粒细胞侵犯以及间质出血。 免疫病理学标准：毛细血管的免疫球蛋白或补体染色阳性(IC)，或毛细血管巨噬细胞及补体沉积的 CD68 染色阳性(IF)，或血管纤维染色阳性	1 级(1+级)病理学抗体介导排斥：单纯组织病理学抗体介导的排斥反应	抗体介导排斥反应仅符合组织学标准。尽管无特异性定义，可能包括：内皮水肿、血管内巨噬细胞聚集、间质水肿、出血、血管内栓塞、心肌细胞坏死等
		1 级(1+级)病理学抗体介导排斥：单纯免疫病理学抗体介导的排斥反应	抗体介导排斥反应仅符合免疫病理学标准。虽然尚无定论，但可能包括免疫球蛋白、补体、巨噬细胞的 IC、IF 染色阳性
		2 级病理学抗体介导排斥反应：病理学抗体介导排斥反应	既符合组织学标准又符合免疫病理学标准
		3 级病理学抗体介导排斥反应：重度抗体介导排斥反应	组织病理学上表现为显著水肿、间质出血、毛细血管碎片、混合炎性细胞浸润、上皮细胞固缩或核破裂

随着固相分析的广泛应用，循环中供体特异性 HLA 抗体的检测和定量技术目前已比较成熟。然而定量技术目前仍没有统一的标准，其应用目前还有待验证。基于细胞的分析检测方法可以作为辅助检测手段，用于评估抗体是否具有供体抗原反应活性，从而具有实际临床应用价值。

循环抗体中有一部分是针对非 HLA 抗原的，这部分抗体的存在会对诊断提出难题，尤其是一些难以解释的移植器官功能不全的情况。在组织相容性复合物 I 类链相关基因 A 抗体(MICA)、抗磷脂抗体、内膜细胞抗体、波形抗体、核抗体及肌球蛋白重链、轻链抗体等方面已有报道[102-106]。目前阶段仍不推荐非 HLA 抗体常规检测在临床中的应用，但在不可解释的移植器官功能不全的情况下可以进行应用。

心内膜心肌活检

早期的抗体介导排斥反应与毛细血管损伤、伴核扩大的内皮细胞肿大以及脉管系统内巨噬细胞沉积等现象有关。血管内巨噬细胞依附以及血管上皮水肿等表现(图 71.3A，B)，若单独作为评估性检测，其敏感性过低[107]。血管内栓塞、纤维沉积、心肌细胞坏死、间质出血以及内皮细胞退行性变等表现通常只有在最严重程度的抗体介导的排斥反应中才能观察到。其他的免疫病理学检测方法在对组织的抗体介导的排斥反应进行常规评估时可以应用。目前被最广泛接受的免疫表型的标准是心肌毛细血管中补体碎片(C3d、C4d)的染色

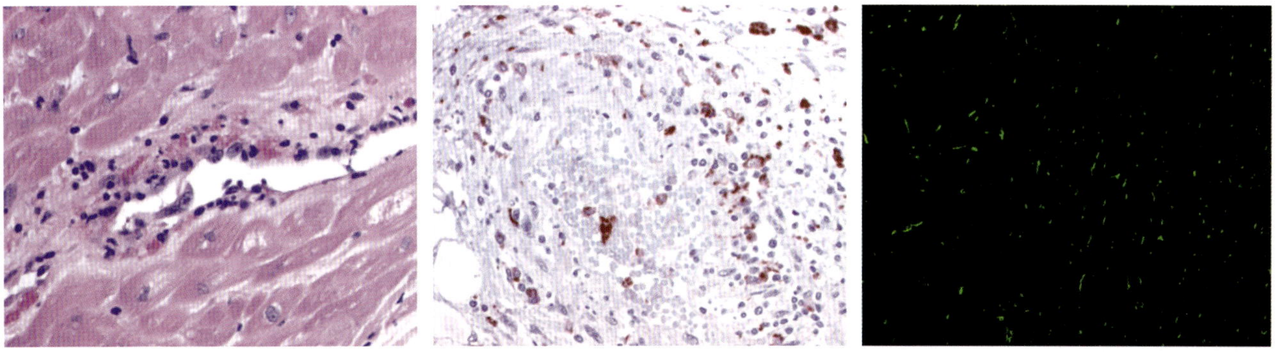

(A)　(B)　(C)

图 71.3　(A)HE 染色示抗体介导排斥相关组织学证据：心内膜水肿、中性粒细胞等炎性表现。(B)抗体介导排斥标本中，免疫过氧化物酶染色示 CD68 阳性细胞，提示这些血管内细胞为巨噬细胞。(C)抗体介导排斥标本中，免疫荧光法示 C4d 阳性，提示毛细血管壁上补体沉积。(Images provided by Dr. Margaret M. Grimes, Richmond, VA.)

阳性，但部分中心也有采用对 CD68 阳性巨噬细胞和免疫球蛋白进行染色的方法(图 71.3C)。

尽管经历了多年的争论,ISHLT 仅在 2005 年将抗体介导的排斥反应归为一个组织学上的概念[8]。到了 2011 年,ISHLT 针对抗体介导的排斥反应修订了病理学诊断标准,并提出了一个初步的评分系统。该工作组将移植器官功能不全或循环中供体特异性抗体检测指标排除在抗体介导排斥反应的诊断标准之外，从而将其纯粹定义为病理学诊断[108]。该初步模型目前在临床使用上尚缺乏验证。该模型下,0 级定义为该活检样本目前无任何抗体介导排斥反应的组织学或免疫病理学证据。1 级定义为该活检标本仅有抗体介导排斥反应的组织病理学或免疫病理学两者其中之一的证据。2 级定义为该标本既具有抗体介导排斥反应的组织学证据,也有免疫病理学证据。3 级是程度最严重的病理学分级,该分级下,可有心肌间质出血、炎性浸润、内皮细胞增厚、显著水肿等表现。

对于无症状患者的基于活检标本的评估检测,目前在频率、时间点、实用性等方面尚无统一的定论。早期对于补体和免疫球蛋白的免疫病理学染色在已接受过免疫球蛋白介导的诱导治疗的患者中可能会出现假阳性结果，因此在临床解释其结果的时候应注意到这些问题。

治疗策略(见第 67 章)

临床“静止”的急性细胞排斥

对于无症状的 1R 级细胞排斥患者,在进行常规评估性活检时一般仅予以严密观察，而并不增强免疫调节治疗力度。1R 级排斥通常能够自行缓解,一般不会进展,或对移植器官存活产生重大影响。Winters 等观察到,85%单病灶的轻度移植排斥在没有任何干预的情况下能够自行缓解。而 Loveras 等发现,对于轻到中度移植排斥患者，应用泼尼松激素治疗后并无明显治疗效果[25,109]。然而,如果某个病灶有心肌细胞损伤、坏死的情况出现(原 2 级),那么患者可能较易进展成为具有临床意义的移植排斥,对于这部分患者,需要加强移植监测评估力度[10]。

若心内膜心肌活检结果提示多病灶炎性细胞浸润且伴心肌损害证据(2R 级),一般给予小脉冲剂量的口服或静脉注射类固醇，并可以考虑在维持剂量免疫抑制方案上适当加强。不同中心对于泼尼松的应用剂量存在差异,通常在前几天给予总剂量 3~5mg/kg 的泼尼松,并在之后将剂量降低至基线水平。Park 等进行了一个纳入 100 例中度排斥反应患者的回顾性分析研究，研究发现，给予 3 天 100mg 冲击剂量泼尼松后，大约 75%的患者的改善在组织学上得到证实[111]。并在接下来 1~2 周进行重复心内膜心肌活检。若排斥未缓解,那么建议给予静脉冲击剂量的甲泼尼治疗。

急性细胞排斥的血流动力学改变

有病理学或临床排斥反应证据且伴心肌功能下降的患者,应最优先给予治疗。因为有报道表明,这部分患者在 3 个月后的死亡率可以接近 40%。而那些主要表现为细胞排斥的患者的相对预后较好,2 年生存率接近 84%[112]。早期需要应用血流动力学支持比如静脉强心剂、变时性药物、主动脉内球囊泵或心室辅助装置的设置作为保障。除静脉皮质激素注射外,也可以应用去淋巴细胞的抗体对患者进行治疗。目前,鼠单克隆抗体 OKT3 的应用已很大程度上被抗胸腺细胞球蛋白(ATG)所替代。OKT3 能够同 T 细胞表面的 CD3 抗原相结合，且与血清病高发以及阻止药物的重复剂量起效的致敏作用有关。抗胸腺细胞球蛋白是针对 T 细胞表面不同抗原的一种多克隆制剂。尽管相比 OKT3, ATG 的耐受性更好,但 ATG 同药物输注过程中过敏反应介导的免疫反应有关。患者一般在输注前,先进行皮质激素、按组胺药物以及利尿药物治疗。CD3 细胞数量监测可用于指导 ATG 的用量，目标将 CD3 含量降至 25 个细胞/μL[113]。在治疗过程中,患者应接受抗真菌药、抗生素以及预防抗病毒治疗,并给予严密的血流动力学监测。排斥反应后的几周应进行重复心内膜心肌活检,以确保排斥反应的缓解。复发或持续存在的症状可应用重复静脉内皮质激素以及抗胸腺细胞抗体进行治疗,并且,临床医生必须警惕与去淋巴细胞相关的恶性肿瘤发生率升高的风险。

伴血流动力学改变的抗体介导排斥反应或混合排斥(急性细胞排斥加上抗体介导排斥)

表现出抗体介导排斥临床证据的患者，若同时存在细胞排斥或移植心脏功能不全时，应在治疗上依照消除或抑制循环中的抗体，并抑制抗体进一步生成。利用静脉皮质激素进行初始治疗可能从多种途径起到有利的疗效。利用血浆单采或血浆置换等够将抗体迅速地从循环中去除。针对这两种方法，目前有多种途径及操作方法。然而，即便如此，仍应尽早开始对抗体水平进行监测评估，并进一步重启并加强免疫调节治疗，以防临床上较多见的抗体再生成发生。

静脉注射免疫球蛋白(IVIG)或巨细胞病毒高免疫球蛋白常常同血浆单采联用进行抗体介导排斥反应的治疗。IVIG 法有多种抗炎及免疫调节作用，对于抗体介导的排斥反应来说，常有不错的疗效。从血浆中浓缩提取 IgG 作为抗体准备。IVIG 是通过从血液循环中去除可能进入循环的自体抗体，并下调炎症因子而发挥作用。因为该方法的不良反应较少，目前临床上已广泛开展利用该方法进行抗体介导排斥反应的治疗。但是，目前还没有针对心脏移植后急性抗体介导排斥反应下 IVIG 治疗有效性展开的系统性研究。

除上述耗尽抗体的方法之外，临床上也常常利用增加维持免疫药物或 ATG 剂量的方法，通过 T 淋巴细胞介导的抑制起到治疗效果。

对于标准治疗方案效果不明显的患者，可以考虑采用去除 B 淋巴细胞或抑制浆细胞的治疗方法。利妥昔单抗是一种抗 B 细胞表面 CD20 蛋白的单克隆抗体。利妥昔单抗能够针对实质脏器移植前已经进行致敏化的患者，降低其机体中群体反应性抗体的水平。对于利妥昔单抗的应用，目前有越来越多的有关其在心脏移植患者抗体介导排斥反应中治疗效果的文献[114–116]。然而，针对利妥昔单抗的边缘效应，目前的研究仍不是很清楚，因为上述多项研究中多种背景治疗方法可能会造成干扰。对于这些药物，目前仍缺乏随机对照研究。并且，由于这些药物的作用主要局限于去除记忆 B 细胞，而对浆细胞无明显作用，因此目前对这方面的研究开展得并不广泛。

硼替佐米是一种蛋白酶体抑制剂，它能够同 26S 蛋白酶的催化位点相结合，从而调节蛋白质表达，并防止促凋亡因子的降解，进而促进浆细胞凋亡的活化。该药物对治疗包括 AL 型淀粉样变及多发性骨髓瘤在内的浆细胞病，有不俗的疗效。并且，目前也已有越来越多的证据证实该药物在实质器官移植后血管排斥及脱敏化中的治疗效果[117–119]。硼替佐米常见的不良反应有血小板减少症、胃肠道反应及感觉异常。

进一步的针对抗体介导排斥反应的治疗方案正在逐步进入我们的视野。例如，利用依库丽单抗进行补体抑制以及利用贝利木单抗和依帕珠单抗进行 B 细胞抑制等。

临床“静止”的抗体介导排斥反应

目前，已有越来越多的学者认同临床上无表现的或是亚临床的抗体介导排斥反应实际上具有一定的临床意义。Kfoury 等对近 900 例患者进行研究，研究发现，对于无症状抗体介导排斥反应的患者，不论是否合并细胞排斥反应，均具有较高的心血管相关死亡的风险[98]。Wu 等研究表明，临床“静止”的抗体介导排斥反应患者具有较高的发生移植心脏血管病变的风险[99]。虽然无症状抗体介导排斥反应患者的活检标本的组织病理学和免疫病理学均证实，这部分患者具有较高的发病风险，但针对这部分患者，目前仍无替代方案以供进一步的治疗或移植检测评估。

复发性或顽固排斥性反应（抗体介导排斥反应或急性细胞排斥反应）

复发性排斥反应(尽管加强免疫抑制力度仍反复发作)或顽固性排斥反应(持续的病理学提示的排斥)临床上较少见，但却是临床上的难题。全身淋巴组织放疗(TLI)作为难治性排斥反应的治疗手段已有几十年的历史。临床应用表明，该方法对治疗心脏移植后持续性细胞排斥反应具有良好的疗效[120,121]。全身淋巴组织放疗将所有的淋巴结、胸腺、脾脏暴露于高剂量辐射之下，目的是为了改变 T 淋巴细胞介导的免疫作用。由于近年来 TLI 治疗后复发性排斥反应比例上升，脊髓发育不良及白血病的发病率升高，目前对于该方法的研究有降温趋势[122]。

体外光分离置换疗法是一种免疫调节治疗，该方法利用具有光活性的药物以及随后的紫外光照射对白细胞进行处理，使得快速增殖的 T 淋巴细胞受到损伤。光分离置换对于反复发作难治性细胞排斥反应的患者具有良好的治疗效果，且其不良反应较小[123–125]。

由于大多数浆细胞在迁移到骨髓之前存在于脾脏之中，脾切除术对于抗体介导排斥反应的患者具有一定的治疗效果。脾切除术目前已被应用于 ABO 血型不匹配的器官移植患者以及肾移植术后急性重度抗体介导排斥反应患者[126]。

类似移植排斥反应

临床医生必须对可能会被误诊为移植排斥反应的病理学过程有清楚的认识，特别是由于免疫抑制治疗的加强，可能会加剧造成类似移植排斥反应的疾病过程。由肠道病毒引起的心肌炎可能会导致移植器官功能不全的发生。巨细胞病毒性心肌炎是心脏移植术后的并发症之一，利用显微镜能够观察到由大的嗜碱性细胞核及周围淡色的人造光环所组成的核内含体，并可以借此将其与排斥反应相区别[127,128]。随着对高危患者群体的预防性抗病毒治疗的实施，巨细胞病毒性心肌炎的发生率正逐年降低。弓形虫感染的激活或传递可以导致暴发性散播，也可仅局限于1~2个器官系统[129]。当心脏移植术后，寄生虫导致心肌炎发生时，进行心内膜心肌活检往往可以观察到非特异性的炎症细胞浸润，伴或不伴心肌细胞内弓形虫孢囊。免疫化学染色以及电镜发现的囊内卵形的、双层薄膜的、前端圆锥形的微生物能够明确诊断[130]。移植后的累及心脏的淋巴增生性障碍(PTLD)的典型表现为淋巴细胞的不典型浸润。利用原位杂交技术有助于识别EB病毒感染并明确诊断[131]。

结论

免疫抑制治疗的进展一定程度上降低了传统细胞排斥的发生率，且将目前的关注点逐渐转移到重要性正被逐步发掘的抗体介导排斥反应上来。尽管基于非创伤性的基因和生物标记物的监测评估策略正被逐步开发和应用，相应的新近定义的抗体介导排斥反应的流行病学在诊断领域的应用还不够成熟。病理学上的共识正逐步成为诊断临床抗体介导排斥反应的标准，且其对于长、短期预后的预测效果也正被逐步开发。针对抗体抑制和清除方面的治疗难题依然困扰着临床医生，但利用新的分子和通路的治疗策略也正逐步进入我们的视野[132]。

致谢

感谢NHLB和NIAID的PO/HL18646和U01AI 094374的资金支持。

（赵海格 倪一鸣 郑骏楠 译 倪一鸣 校）

参考文献

1. Barnard CN. Human heart transplantation. The diagnosis of rejection. American Journal of Cardiology. 1968;22:811–819.
2. Cooley DA, Hallman GL, Bloodwell RD, et al. Human heart transplantation. Experience with twelve cases. American Journal of Cardiology. 1968;22:804–810.
3. Lower RR, Kontos HA, Kosek JC, et al. Experiences in heart transplantation. Technic, physiology and rejection. American Journal of Cardiology. 1968;22:766–771.
4. Schroeder JS, Popp RL, Stinson EB, et al. Acute rejection following cardiac transplantation. Phonocardiographic and ultrasound observations. Circulation. 1969;40:155–164.
5. Billingham ME, Cary NR, Hammond ME, et al. A working formulation for the standardization of nomenclature in the diagnosis of heart and lung rejection: Heart Rejection Study Group. The International Society for Heart Transplantation. Journal of Heart Transplantation. 1990;9:587–593.
6. Winters GL, McManus BM. Consistencies and controversies in the application of the International Society for Heart and Lung Transplantation working formulation for heart transplant biopsy specimens. Rapamycin Cardiac Rejection Treatment Trial Pathologists. Journal of Heart and Lung Transplantation. 1996;15:728–735.
7. Marboe CC, Billingham M, Eisen H, et al. Nodular endocardial infiltrates (Quilty lesions) cause significant variability in diagnosis of ISHLT Grade 2 and 3A rejection in cardiac allograft recipients. Journal of Heart and Lung Transplantation. 2005;24:S219–S226.
8. Stewart S, Winters GL, Fishbein MC, et al. Revision of the 1990 working formulation for the standardization of nomenclature in the diagnosis of heart rejection. Journal of Heart and Lung Transplantation. 2005;24:1710–1720.
9. Kubo SH, Naftel DC, Mills RM, et al. Risk factors for late recurrent rejection after heart transplantation: a multiinstitutional, multivariable analysis. Cardiac Transplant Research Database Group. Journal of Heart and Lung Transplantation. 1995;14:409–418.
10. Jarcho J, Naftel DC, Shroyer TW, et al. Influence of HLA mismatch on rejection after heart transplantation: a multiinstitutional study. The Cardiac Transplant Research Database Group. Journal of Heart and Lung Transplantation. 1994;13:583–595.
11. Kobashigawa JA, Kirklin JK, Naftel DC, et al. Pretransplantation risk factors for acute rejection after heart transplantation: a multiinstitutional study. The Transplant Cardiologists Research Database Group. Journal of Heart and Lung Transplantation. 1993;12:355–366.
12. Opelz G, Wujciak T. The influence of HLA compatibility on graft survival after heart transplantation. The Collaborative Transplant Study. New England Journal of Medicine. 1994;330:816–819.
13. Almenar L, Maeso M, Martinezdolz L, et al. Influence of HLA matching on survival in heart transplantation. Transplantation Proceedings. 2005;37:4001–4005.
14. Mascaretti L, Poli F, Scalamogna M, et al. HLA-DR matching defined by DNA typing in heart transplantation. Transplantation Proceedings. 1997;29:1464–1466.
15. Kerman RH, Kimball P, Scheinen S, et al. The relationship among donor-recipient HLA mismatches, rejection, and death from coronary artery disease in cardiac transplant recipients. Transplantation. 1994;57:884–888.
16. Costanzo-Nordin MR, Fisher SG, O'Sullivan EJ, et al. HLA-DR incompatibility predicts heart transplant rejection independent of immunosuppressive prophylaxis. Journal of Heart and Lung Transplantation. 1993;12:779–789.
17. Lietz K, John R, Beniaminovitz A, et al. Interleukin-2 receptor blockade in cardiac transplantation: influence of HLA-DR locus incompatibility on treatment efficacy. Transplantation. 2003;75:781–787.
18. Herzberg GZ, Rossi AF, Courtney M, et al. The effects of HLA mismatching and immunosuppressive therapy on early rejection outcome in pediatric heart transplant recipients. Journal of Heart and Lung Transplantation. 1998;17:1195–1200.
19. Potena L, Holweg CTJ, Chin C, et al. Acute rejection and cardiac allograft vascular disease is reduced by suppression of subclinical cytomegalovirus infection. Transplantation. 2006;82:398–405.
20. Liu V, Bhattacharya J, Weill D, et al. Persistent racial disparities in survival after heart transplantation. Circulation. 2011;123:1642–1649.
21. Mehra MR, Uber PA, Scott RL, et al. Ethnic disparity in clinical outcome after heart transplantation is abrogated using tacrolimus and mycophenolate mofetil-based immunosuppression. Transplantation. 2002;74:1568–1573.
22. Patel ND, Weiss ES, Nwakanma LU, et al. Impact of donor-to-recipient weight ratio on survival after heart transplantation: analysis of the United Network for

Organ Sharing Database. Circulation. 2008;118:S83-S88.
23. Sakakibara S, Konno S. Endomyocardial biopsy. Japanese Heart Journal. 1962;3:537-543.
24. Caves PK, Stinson EB, Billingham M, et al. Percutaneous transvenous endomyocardial biopsy in human heart recipients. Experience with a new technique. Annals of Thoracic Surgery. 1973;16:325-336.
25. Winters GL, Loh E, Schoen FJ. Natural history of focal moderate cardiac allograft rejection. Is treatment warranted? Circulation. 1995;91:1975-1980.
26. Wu YL, Ye Q, Sato K, et al. Noninvasive evaluation of cardiac allograft rejection by cellular and functional cardiac magnetic resonance. JACC. Cardiovascular Imaging. 2009;2:731-741.
27. Cooper DK, Charles RG, Rose AG, et al. Does the electrocardiogram detect early acute heart rejection. Journal of Heart Transplantation. 1985;4:546-549.
28. Locke TJ, Karnik R, McGregor CG, et al. The value of the electrocardiogram in the diagnosis of acute rejection after orthotopic heart transplantation. Transplant International. 1989;2:143-146.
29. Gorcsan J, Snow FR, Paulsen W, et al. Echocardiographic profile of the transplanted human heart in clinically well recipients. Journal of Heart and Lung Transplantation. 1992;11:80-89.
30. Hosenpud JD, Norman DJ, Cobanoglu MA, et al. Serial echocardiographic findings early after heart transplantation: evidence for reversible right ventricular dysfunction and myocardial edema. Journal of Heart Transplantation. 1987;6: 343-347.
31. Almenar L, Osa A, Martínez-Dolz L, et al. Echocardiographic evaluation of the evolutionary changes after heart transplantation. Transplantation Proceedings. 2006;38:2575-2576.
32. Thorn EM, de Filippi CR. Echocardiography in the cardiac transplant recipient. Heart Failure Clinics. 2007;3:51-67.
33. Cladellas M, Oriol A, Caralps JM. Quantitative assessment of valvular function after cardiac transplantation by pulsed Doppler echocardiography. American Journal of Cardiology. 1994;73:1197-1201.
34. Aziz TM, Saad RA, Burgess MI, et al. Clinical significance of tricuspid valve dysfunction after orthotopic heart transplantation. Journal of Heart and Lung Transplantation. 2002;21:1101-1108.
35. Angermann CE, Nassau K, Stempfle H, et al. Recognition of acute cardiac allograft rejection from serial integrated backscatter analyses in human orthotopic heart transplant recipients: comparison with conventional echocardiography. Circulation. 1997;95:140-150.
36. Sagar KB, Hastillo A, Wolfgang TC, et al. Left ventricular mass by M-mode echocardiography in cardiac transplant patients with acute rejection. Circulation. 1981;64:II217-II220.
37. Sun JP, Abdalla IA, Asher CR, et al. Non-invasive evaluation of orthotopic heart transplant rejection by echocardiography. Journal of Heart and Lung Transplantation. 2005;24:160-165.
38. Ciliberto GR, Mascarello M, Gronda E, et al. Acute rejection after heart transplantation: noninvasive echocardiographic evaluation. Journal of the American College of Cardiology. 1994;23:1156-1161.
39. Desruennes M, Corcos T, Cabrol A, et al. Doppler echocardiography for the diagnosis of acute cardiac allograft rejection. Journal of the American College of Cardiology. 1988;12:63-70.
40. Valantine HA, Fowler MB, Hunt SA, et al. Changes in Doppler echocardiographic indexes of left ventricular function as potential markers of acute cardiac rejection. Circulation. 1987;76:V86-V92.
41. Amende I, Simon R, Seegers A, et al. Diastolic dysfunction during acute cardiac allograft rejection. Circulation. 1990;81:III66-III70.
42. Grodecki PV, Klein AL. Pitfalls in the echo-Doppler assessment of diastolic dysfunction. Echocardiography (Mount Kisco, NY). 1993;10:213-234.
43. Aranda JM, Weston MW, Puleo JA, et al. Effect of loading conditions on myocardial relaxation velocities determined by Doppler tissue imaging in heart transplant recipients. Journal of Heart and Lung Transplantation. 1998;17: 693-697.
44. Dandel M, Hummel M, Müller J, et al. Reliability of tissue Doppler wall motion monitoring after heart transplantation for replacement of invasive routine screenings by optimally timed cardiac biopsies and catheterizations. Circulation. 2001;104:I184-I191.
45. Mankad S, Murali S, Kormos RL, et al. Evaluation of the potential role of color-coded tissue Doppler echocardiography in the detection of allograft rejection in heart transplant recipients. American Heart Journal. 1999;138:721-730.
46. Puleo JA, Aranda JM, Weston MW, et al. Noninvasive detection of allograft rejection in heart transplant recipients by use of Doppler tissue imaging. Journal of Heart and Lung Transplantation. 1998;17:176-184.
47. Stengel SM, Allemann Y, Zimmerli M, et al. Doppler tissue imaging for assessing left ventricular diastolic dysfunction in heart transplant rejection. Heart (British Cardiac Society). 2001;86:432-437.
48. Boyd SY, Mego DM, Khan NA, et al. Doppler echocardiography in cardiac transplant patients: allograft rejection and its relationship to diastolic function. Journal of the American Society of Echocardiography. 1997;10:526-531.
49. Bellenger N, Burgess M, Ray S, et al. Comparison of left ventricular ejection fraction and volumes in heart failure by echocardiography, radionuclide ventriculography and cardiovascular magnetic resonance. Are they interchangeable? European Heart Journal. 2000;21:1387-1396.
50. Fieno DS, Kim RJ, Chen EL, et al. Contrast-enhanced magnetic resonance imaging of myocardium at risk: distinction between reversible and irreversible injury throughout infarct healing. Journal of the American College of Cardiology. 2000;36:1985-1991.
51. Kwong RY, Schussheim AE, Rekhraj S, et al. Detecting acute coronary syndrome in the emergency department with cardiac magnetic resonance imaging. Circulation. 2003;107:531-537.
52. Nagel E, Lehmkuhl HB, Bocksch W, et al. Noninvasive diagnosis of ischemia-induced wall motion abnormalities with the use of high-dose dobutamine stress MRI: comparison with dobutamine stress echocardiography. Circulation. 1999;99:763-770.
53. Bellenger NG, Marcus NJ, Davies C, et al. Left ventricular function and mass after orthotopic heart transplantation: a comparison of cardiovascular magnetic resonance with echocardiography. Journal of Heart and Lung Transplantation. 2000;19:444-452.
54. Walpoth BH, Muller MF, Celik B, et al. Assessment of cardiac rejection by MR-imaging and MR-spectroscopy. European Journal of Cardio-Thoracic Surgery. 1998;14:426-430.
55. Aherne T, Tscholakoff D, Finkbeiner W, et al. Magnetic resonance imaging of cardiac transplants: the evaluation of rejection of cardiac allografts with and without immunosuppression. Circulation. 1986;74:145-156.
56. Almenar L, Igual B, Martínez-Dolz L, et al. Utility of cardiac magnetic resonance imaging for the diagnosis of heart transplant rejection. Transplantation Proceedings. 2003;35:1962-1964.
57. Marie PY, Angioï M, Carteaux JP, et al. Detection and prediction of acute heart transplant rejection with the myocardial T2 determination provided by a black-blood magnetic resonance imaging sequence. Journal of the American College of Cardiology. 2001;37:825-831.
58. Smart FW, Young JB, Weilbaecher D, et al. Magnetic resonance imaging for assessment of tissue rejection after heterotopic heart transplantation. Journal of Heart and Lung Transplantation. 1993;12:403-410.
59. Wisenberg G, Pflugfelder PW, Kostuk WJ, et al. Diagnostic applicability of magnetic resonance imaging in assessing human cardiac allograft rejection. American Journal of Cardiology. 1987;60:130-136.
60. Kanno S, Wu YJ, Lee PC, et al. Macrophage accumulation associated with rat cardiac allograft rejection detected by magnetic resonance imaging with ultrasmall superparamagnetic iron oxide particles. Circulation. 2001;104: 934-938.
61. Wu YL, Ye Q, Sato K, et al. Noninvasive evaluation of cardiac allograft rejection by cellular and functional cardiac magnetic resonance. JACC. Cardiovascular Imaging. 2009;2:731-741.
62. Dengler TJ, Zimmermann R, Braun K, et al. Elevated serum concentrations of cardiac troponin T in acute allograft rejection after human heart transplantation. Journal of the American College of Cardiology. 1998;32:405-412.
63. Labarrere CA, Nelson DR, Cox CJ, et al. Cardiac-specific troponin I levels and risk of coronary artery disease and graft failure following heart transplantation. JAMA. 2000;284:457-464.
64. Mullen JC, Bentley MJ, Scherr KD, et al. Troponin T and I are not reliable markers of cardiac transplant rejection. European Journal of Cardio-Thoracic Surgery. 2002;22:233-237.
65. Wang CW, Steinhubl SR, Castellani WJ, et al. Inability of serum myocyte death markers to predict acute cardiac allograft rejection. Transplantation. 1996;62: 1938-1941.
66. Alexis JD, Lao CD, Selter JG, et al. Cardiac troponin T: a noninvasive marker for heart transplant rejection? Journal of Heart and Lung Transplantation. 1998; 17:395-398.
67. Arnau-Vives MA, Almenar L, Hervas I, et al. Predictive value of brain natriuretic peptide in the diagnosis of heart transplant rejection. Journal of Heart and Lung Transplantation. 2004;23:850-856.
68. Bader FM, Rogers RK, Kfoury AG, et al. Time-dependent changes in B-type natriuretic peptide after heart transplantation: correlation with allograft rejection and function. Congestive Heart Failure (Greenwich, Conn.). 2009;15: 63-67.
69. Almenar L, Arnau MA, Martínez-Dolz L, et al. Is there a correlation between brain naturietic peptide levels and echocardiographic and hemodynamic parameters in heart transplant patients? Transplantation Proceedings. 2006;38: 2534-2536.
70. Park MH, Scott RL, Uber PA, et al. Usefulness of B-type natriuretic peptide levels in predicting hemodynamic perturbations after heart transplantation despite

preserved left ventricular systolic function. American Journal of Cardiology. 2002;90:1326–1329.
71. Talha S, Di Marco P, Doutreleau S, et al. Does circulating BNP normalize after heart transplantation in patients with normal hemodynamic and right and left heart functions? Clinical Transplantation. 2008;22:542–548.
72. Masters RG, Davies RA, Veinot JP, et al. Discoordinate modulation of natriuretic peptides during acute cardiac allograft rejection in humans. Circulation. 1999;100:287–291.
73. Mehra MR, Uber PA, Walther D, et al. Gene expression profiles and B-type natriuretic peptide elevation in heart transplantation: more than a hemodynamic marker. Circulation. 2006;114:I21–I26.
74. Meirovich YF, Veinot JP, de Bold MLK, et al. Relationship between natriuretic peptides and inflammation: proteomic evidence obtained during acute cellular cardiac allograft rejection in humans. Journal of Heart and Lung Transplantation. 2008;27:31–37.
75. Martinez-Dolz L, Almenar L, Moro J, et al. Prognostic value of brain natriuretic peptide in heart transplant patients. Journal of Heart and Lung Transplantation. 2007;26:986–991.
76. Mehra MR, Uber PA, Potluri S, et al. Usefulness of an elevated B-type natriuretic peptide to predict allograft failure, cardiac allograft vasculopathy, and survival after heart transplantation. American Journal of Cardiology. 2004;94:454–458.
77. Garrido IP, Pascual-Figal DA, Nicolás F, et al. Usefulness of serial monitoring of B-type natriuretic peptide for the detection of acute rejection after heart transplantation. American Journal of Cardiology. 2009;103:1149–1153.
78. Hammerer-Lercher A, Mair J, Antretter H, et al. B-type natriuretic peptide as a marker of allograft rejection after heart transplantation. Journal of Heart and Lung Transplantation. 2005;24:1444.
79. Corcos T, Tamburino C, Léger P, et al. Early and late hemodynamic evaluation after cardiac transplantation: a study of 28 cases. Journal of the American College of Cardiology. 1988;11:264–269.
80. Davies RA, Koshal A, Walley V, et al. Temporary diastolic noncompliance with preserved systolic function after heart transplantation. Transplantation Proceedings. 1987;19:3444–3447.
81. Greenberg ML, Uretsky BF, Reddy PS, et al. Long-term hemodynamic follow-up of cardiac transplant patients treated with cyclosporine and prednisone. Circulation. 1985;71:487–494.
82. Young JB, Leon CA, Short HD, et al. Evolution of hemodynamics after orthotopic heart and heart-lung transplantation: early restrictive patterns persisting in occult fashion. Journal of Heart Transplantation. 1987;6:34–43.
83. Skowronski EW, Epstein M, Ota D, et al. Right and left ventricular function after cardiac transplantation. Changes during and after rejection. Circulation. 1991;84:2409–2417.
84. Wilensky RL, Bourdillon PD, O'Donnell JA, et al. Restrictive hemodynamic patterns after cardiac transplantation: relationship to histologic signs of rejection. American Heart Journal. 1991;122:1079–1087.
85. Fahmy NM, Yamani MH, Starling RC, et al. Chemokine and receptor-gene expression during early and late acute rejection episodes in human cardiac allografts. Transplantation. 2003;75:2044–2047.
86. Horwitz PA, Tsai EJ, Putt ME, et al. Detection of cardiac allograft rejection and response to immunosuppressive therapy with peripheral blood gene expression. Circulation. 2004;110:3815–3821.
87. Schoels M, Dengler TJ, Richter R, et al. Detection of cardiac allograft rejection by real-time PCR analysis of circulating mononuclear cells. Clinical Transplantation. 2004;18:513–517.
88. de Groot-Kruseman HA, Mol WM, Niesters HGM, et al. Differential intragraft cytokine messenger RNA profiles during rejection and repair of clinical heart transplants. A longitudinal study. Transplant International. 2003;16: 9–14.
89. Lin D, Hollander Z, Ng RT, et al. Whole blood genomic biomarkers of acute cardiac allograft rejection. Journal of Heart and Lung Transplantation. 2009;28:927–935.
90. Deng MC, Eisen HJ, Mehra MR, et al. Noninvasive discrimination of rejection in cardiac allograft recipients using gene expression profiling. American Journal of Transplantation. 2006;6:150–160.
91. Pham MX, Teuteberg JJ, Kfoury AG, et al. Gene-expression profiling for rejection surveillance after cardiac transplantation. New England Journal of Medicine. 2010;362:1890–1900.
92. Hess ML, Hastillo A, Mohanakumar T, et al. Accelerated atherosclerosis in cardiac transplantation: role of cytotoxic B-cell antibodies and hyperlipidemia. Circulation. 1983;68:II94–II101.
93. Herskowitz A, Soule LM, Ueda K, et al. Arteriolar vasculitis on endomyocardial biopsy: a histologic predictor of poor outcome in cyclosporine-treated heart transplant recipients. Journal of Heart Transplantation. 1987;6:127–136.
94. Hammond EH, Yowell RL, Nunoda S, et al. Vascular (humoral) rejection in heart transplantation: pathologic observations and clinical implications. Journal of Heart Transplantation. 1989;8:430–443.
95. Lones MA, Czer LS, Trento A, et al. Clinical-pathologic features of humoral rejection in cardiac allografts: a study in 81 consecutive patients. Journal of Heart and Lung Transplantation. 1995;14:151–162.
96. Michaels PJ, Espejo ML, Kobashigawa J, et al. Humoral rejection in cardiac transplantation: risk factors, hemodynamic consequences and relationship to transplant coronary artery disease. Journal of Heart and Lung Transplantation. 2003;22:58–69.
97. Subherwal S, Kobashigawa JA, Cogert G, et al. Incidence of acute cellular rejection and non-cellular rejection in cardiac transplantation. Transplantation Proceedings. 2004;36:3171–3172.
98. Kfoury AG, Hammond MEH, Snow GL, et al. Cardiovascular mortality among heart transplant recipients with asymptomatic antibody-mediated or stable mixed cellular and antibody-mediated rejection. Journal of Heart and Lung Transplantation. 2009;28:781–784.
99. Wu GW, Kobashigawa JA, Fishbein MC, et al. Asymptomatic antibody-mediated rejection after heart transplantation predicts poor outcomes. Journal of Heart and Lung Transplantation. 2009;28:417–422.
100. Petrossian GA, Nichols AB, Marboe CC, et al. Relation between survival and development of coronary artery disease and anti-HLA antibodies after cardiac transplantation. Circulation. 1989;80:III122–III125.
101. Reed EF, Hong B, Ho E, et al. Monitoring of soluble HLA alloantigens and anti-HLA antibodies identifies heart allograft recipients at risk of transplant-associated coronary artery disease. Transplantation. 1996;61:566–572.
102. McKenna RM, Takemoto SK, Terasaki PI. Anti-HLA antibodies after solid organ transplantation. Transplantation. 2000;69:319–326.
103. Dunn MJ, Rose ML, Latif N, et al. Demonstration by western blotting of antiheart antibodies before and after cardiac transplantation. Transplantation. 1991;51: 806–812.
104. Jurcevic S, Ainsworth ME, Pomerance A, et al. Antivimentin antibodies are an independent predictor of transplant-associated coronary artery disease after cardiac transplantation. Transplantation. 2001;71:886–892.
105. Laguens RP, Argel MI, Chambó JG, et al. Anti-skeletal muscle glycolipid antibodies in human heart transplantation as markers of acute rejection. Correlation with endomyocardial biopsy. Transplantation. 1996;62:211–216.
106. Fredrich R, Toyoda M, Czer LS, et al. The clinical significance of antibodies to human vascular endothelial cells after cardiac transplantation. Transplantation. 1999;67:385–391.
107. Hammond MEH, Stehlik J, Snow G, et al. Utility of histologic parameters in screening for antibody-mediated rejection of the cardiac allograft: a study of 3,170 biopsies. Journal of Heart and Lung Transplantation. 2005;24:2015–2021.
108. Berry GJ, Angelini A, Burke MM, et al. The ISHLT working formulation for pathologic diagnosis of antibody-mediated rejection in heart transplantation: evolution and current status (2005-2011). Journal of Heart and Lung Transplantation. 2011;30:601–611.
109. Lloveras JJ, Escourrou G, Delisle MB, et al. Evolution of untreated mild rejection in heart transplant recipients. Journal of Heart and Lung Transplantation. 1992;11:751–756.
110. Brunner-La Rocca HP, Sütsch G, Schneider J, et al. Natural course of moderate cardiac allograft rejection (International Society for Heart Transplantation grade 2) early and late after transplantation. Circulation. 1996;94:1334–1338.
111. Park MH, Starling RC, Ratliff NB, et al. Oral steroid pulse without taper for the treatment of asymptomatic moderate cardiac allograft rejection. Journal of Heart and Lung Transplantation. 1999;18:1224–1227.
112. Mills RM, Naftel DC, Kirklin JK, et al. Heart transplant rejection with hemodynamic compromise: a multiinstitutional study of the role of endomyocardial cellular infiltrate. Cardiac Transplant Research Database. Journal of Heart and Lung Transplantation. 1997;16:813–821.
113. Uber WE, Uber LA, VanBakel AB, et al. CD3 monitoring and thymoglobulin therapy in cardiac transplantation: clinical outcomes and pharmacoeconomic implications. Transplantation Proceedings. 2004;36:3245–3249.
114. Kaczmarek I, Deutsch M, Sadoni S, et al. Successful management of antibody-mediated cardiac allograft rejection with combined immunoadsorption and anti-CD20 monoclonal antibody treatment: case report and literature review. Journal of Heart and Lung Transplantation. 2007;26:511–515.
115. Garrett HE, Duvall-Seaman D, Helsley B, et al. Treatment of vascular rejection with rituximab in cardiac transplantation. Journal of Heart and Lung Transplantation. 2005;24:1337–1342.
116. Keren A, Hayes HM, O'Driscoll G. Late humoral rejection in a cardiac transplant recipient treated with the anti-CD20 monoclonal antibody rituximab. Transplantation Proceedings. 2006;38:1520–1522.
117. Everly MJ, Everly JJ, Susskind B, et al. Proteasome inhibition reduces donor-specific antibody levels. Transplantation Proceedings. 2009;41:105–107.
118. Trivedi HL, Terasaki PI, Feroz A, et al. Abrogation of anti-HLA antibodies via proteasome inhibition. Transplantation. 2009;87:1555–1561.

119. Patel J, Everly M, Chang D, et al. Reduction of alloantibodies via proteosome inhibition in cardiac transplantation. Journal of Heart and Lung Transplantation. 2011;30:1320–1326.
120. Pelletier MP, Coady M, Macha M, et al. Coronary atherosclerosis in cardiac transplant patients treated with total lymphoid irradiation. Journal of Heart and Lung Transplantation. 2003;22:124–129.
121. Ross HJ, Gullestad L, Pak J, et al. Methotrexate or total lymphoid radiation for treatment of persistent or recurrent allograft cellular rejection: a comparative study. Journal of Heart and Lung Transplantation. 1997;16:179–189.
122. Tallaj JA, Pamboukian SV, George JF, et al. Total lymphoid irradiation in heart transplantation: long-term efficacy and survival-an 18-year experience. Transplantation. 2011;92:1159–1164.
123. Costanzo-Nordin MR, Hubbell EA, O'Sullivan EJ, et al. Photopheresis versus corticosteroids in the therapy of heart transplant rejection. Preliminary clinical report. Circulation. 1992;86:II242–II250.
124. Dall'Amico R, Montini G, Murer L, et al. Benefits of photopheresis in the treatment of heart transplant patients with multiple/refractory rejection. Transplantation Proceedings. 1997;29:609–611.
125. Giunti G, Schürfeld K, Maccherini M, et al. Photopheresis for recurrent acute rejection in cardiac transplantation. Transplantation Proceedings. 1999;31:128–129.
126. Locke JE, Zachary AA, Haas M, et al. The utility of splenectomy as rescue treatment for severe acute antibody mediated rejection. American Journal of Transplantation. 2007;7:842–846.
127. Gonwa TA, Capehart JE, Pilcher JW, et al. Cytomegalovirus myocarditis as a cause of cardiac dysfunction in a heart transplant recipient. Transplantation. 1989;47:197–199.
128. Millett R, Tomita T, Marshall HE, et al. Cytomegalovirus endomyocarditis in a transplanted heart. A case report with in situ hybridization. Archives of Pathology and Laboratory Medicine. 1991;115:511–515.
129. Hermanns B, Brunn A, Schwarz ER, et al. Fulminant toxoplasmosis in a heart transplant recipient. Pathology, Research and Practice. 2001;197:211–215.
130. Wagner FM, Reichenspurner H, Uberfuhr P, et al. Toxoplasmosis after heart transplantation: diagnosis by endomyocardial biopsy. Journal of Heart and Lung Transplantation. 1994;13:916–918.
131. Eisen HJ, Hicks D, Kant JA, et al. Diagnosis of posttransplantation lymphoproliferative disorder by endomyocardial biopsy in a cardiac allograft recipient. Journal of Heart and Lung Transplantation. 1994;13:241–245.
132. Nair N, Ball T, Uber PA, et al. Current and future challenges in therapy for antibody-mediated rejection. Journal of Heart and Lung Transplantation. 2011;30:612–617.

第72章 肺移植临床排斥反应综合征

David C. Neujahr

引言

类似于其他实体器官移植，肺移植受体面临着移植物遭受重复免疫攻击的困境。在约30年的临床经验中已发生各种类型的肺移植排斥反应。相比其他器官移植,肺移植物更容易遭受免疫损伤。肺移植受体发生排斥反应的风险极高,原因可能有如下几点:首先,肺组织通过呼吸道直接与外界环境相接触，因此肺组织容易直接遭受如病毒、真菌、细菌等病原微生物感染。此外,作为呼吸器官,肺部易受到空气污染等刺激,从而触发免疫反应。第二,肺脏在胚胎发育过程中为前肠来源,出生后气道与消化道直接连通,因此容易受到吸入口腔或胃内容物的损伤，此外误吸也可触发并激活免疫反应。第三,移植肺易遭受缺血再灌注损伤,导致炎症细胞与介质浸润到移植物内。最后,外科吻合会破坏呼吸道黏膜上纤毛运动功能，致使其清除致病菌的能力下降。本章回顾了肺移植后出现的各种排斥反应的临床表现及其潜在的免疫病理学机制。急性与慢性排斥反应将被分开探讨，但不可忽视这两个过程之间存在的相关性。急性与慢性排斥反应发生的相关危险因素同样有所涉及。在本章最后,将提出针对不同类型排斥的治疗对策。

急性排斥反应

急性排斥诊断

急性与慢性移植排斥反应的组织病理学改变将在第84章详述。肺活检急性细胞性排斥病理学评分主要由血管周成分(A级)和细支气管成分(B级)组成,其由肺移植排斥研究组(LRSG)制订。目前肺移植未解决的主要问题为如何将该广泛使用的组织病理学评分系统应用于临床。其中具体问题包括何时进行肺组织活检以及当排斥发生时如何针对性治疗。

应用可屈光导纤维支气管镜可定期获取小块蜂窝状肺泡组织用于组织病理学评价，镜下钳夹单块或多块肺泡组织,发生并发症风险较低。已报道的经支气管肺活检的副反应包括肺炎(8%)、气胸(<3%)、轻微可逆性血氧不足(10%),以及临床显性出血,且出血量大于100mL(10%)[1-4]。支气管镜在肺移植应用中目前无死亡病例报道，在普通人群中总体死亡风险亦较低(<0.02%)[5]。肺移植中心采用的检测排斥发生的策略有两种:定期计划性肺穿刺检查(又称为监视性活检)或仅在临床进展时进行活检(又称为查因活检)。监视性活检的优势在于可早期发现亚临床急性排斥，且被认为可能提高远期结果,如生存改善与肺功能维持等,但未被证实。查因活检的理论优势在于只有当患者出现阳性表现[ACR和(或)感染],才会进行该侵入性检查。因此,可以减少患者费用以及可能的副反应发生。值得注意的是,在最近一项研究中,共分析了224例监视性支气管镜活检患者,发现A2和更高级别排斥反应发生的概率为18.7%。此外,活检结果改变了32%的临床管理方案[1]。这些发现表明即使在病情较平稳患者中,移植后排斥发生可能性仍较高。然而,一项小规模前期研究结果显示,即使存在较高的验前排斥与感染概率,患者采用查因活检方案与监视性活检方案具有较接近的中期结果。因此,到目前为止,是否监视性活检或者查因活检可提高患者移植后结果仍未可知。

肺移植患者临床功能出现下降时，须考虑进行查因肺组织活检。下降的功能指标包括肺活量(后文讨论)、呼吸急促、放射性浸润如毛玻璃影、胸腔积液、全身炎性表现如发烧等。实际上,采用经支气管镜肺活检的诊断结果包括急性细胞性排斥和肺部感染。

采用监视性或者查因经支气管肺活检均可获取多块蜂窝状肺泡组织。这需要使用支气管镜下钳夹技术以及单水平实时透视技术引导。尽管急性细胞性排斥可发生于肺脏的任何区域，但不少临床医生均发现在肺依赖部位发生率最高[6]，因此肺活检组织至少需要包括其中一个部位。但一次支气管镜下活检具体须采集多少个部位组织目前仍不确定。肺移植研究排斥研究组建议采集5处以上蜂窝状肺组织，至少包含100个肺泡囊结构，取下后需要立刻用福尔马林处理保存。而Snell等通过文献查询建议至少采集10处以上活检样本，才足够用于病因诊断[7,8]。据一项较早的肺移植研究报道，用于诊断急性细胞性排斥平均需要17处活检样本，其敏感性可达94%，特异性可达90%[7]，且未考虑采样问题。不同病理学专家们对组织病理解读的一致性较高，使得经支气管镜下活检成为移植排斥诊断的金标准。至今为止，最大的一项关于不同机构对组织病理学评价一致性的研究表明，A级排斥的诊断kappa值达到0.426（kappa=0表示一致性最低，kappa=1表示一致性最高）[9]。但前提是需要有只有足够活检组织用于排斥诊断，才可达到该一致程度。此外，另有小样本研究也证实了该一致性程度[10-12]。因此，当急性细胞排斥的验前概率很高，但肺活检报告显示急性细胞排斥呈阴性时，仍不能完全排除排斥发生可能，尤其是取样质量不高时。

抗体介导排斥诊断

肺移植中体液排斥的诊断定义不明，相比心脏与肾脏等其他器官移植存在更多争议。在实体器官移植中，普遍共识是抗体介导排斥一般表现为毛细血管内皮损伤。因此，有大量研究工作致力于理解内皮抗原是如何促进与抗体结合、激活补体以及导致后续组织损伤[13,14]。越来越多的研究者认为，免疫系统中有体液成分参与并导致肺移植物失功。目前存在的主要争议包括如何通过活检样本准确地发现抗体介导排斥以及是否存在完全区别于细胞性排斥的急性抗体介导排斥。抗体反应对于移植物功能是否极其重要仍不确切，在汇总所有证据后，结果较令人信服。首先，在少数病例中，移植前预先存在且未被察觉的针对供体的特异性抗体，导致超急性排斥反应发生，其临床特征表现为呼吸衰竭和肺水肿[15-18]。其次，心脏和肺移植中抗体介导排斥在本书已有详细描述。抗体介导排斥反应已确认可导致心脏与肾脏移植物失功，因此在肺移植过程中也可能介导相似的作用。第三，已有不少研究发现移植前存在的群体反应性抗HLA抗体（PRA）水平与肺移植效果相关。在一项纳入656个研究对象的大规模回顾性研究中，不存在或仅有较低群体反应性抗体水平的移植患者，其移植物平均生存时间为5.2年，而25%存在较高群体反应性抗体水平的移植患者，其移植物平均生存时间仅有1.5年[19]。基于UNOS肺移植登记系统的另一项研究共分析了10 000例以上肺移植病理，同样发现了类似结果。该研究结果显示高水平的群体反应性抗体可使30天死亡风险升至2.6倍[20]。第四，不少研究发现移植后群体反应性抗体水平增加，与急性细胞性排斥、淋巴性细支气管炎，支气管闭塞综合征发生相关。最后，还有研究报道了移植后供体特异性抗HLA抗体（DSA）产生与之后的支气管闭塞综合征存在极强的相关性[21]。此外，患者在移植前成功降低DSA水平可改善移植后生存。

考虑到抗HLA抗体水平与肺移植后效果之间存在较强的相关性，大量研究致力于发现肺活检样本中抗体介导的直接损伤，并制订了病理分级系统，用于评价抗体介导排斥（AMR）。到目前为止，肺移植排斥研究组还未明确抗体介导排斥的具体类型，其中最大的困难在于C4d在肺移植组织中的沉积缺乏特异性。肺移植抗体介导排斥的诊断早期依赖于冰冻肺组织的免疫荧光技术。少数具有较大活检样本的研究发现，急性细胞性排斥患者的毛细血管内同样都有一定的C4d沉积[22]。但这些结果难以被其他研究所证实。在一项纳入68例肺移植受者的研究中，对先前包埋的肺移植石蜡标本应用免疫组化技术后证实抗体介导排斥，同时伴有少量的毛细血管内C4d沉积和散在的静脉或动脉内皮，与急性细胞性排斥反应发生无关。此外，在非移植的肺组织内同样发现了一定程度的C4d弥散性沉积，表明该现象并非抗体介导排斥反应的特征性表现[23]。

尽管缺乏明确的肺移植后抗体介导排斥诊断标准，不少病例均报道了排斥反应发生时的临床特征表现。Girnita等对两例产生供体特异性抗HLA抗体的患者行支气管镜肺活检后发现，毛细血管内皮内有C4d沉积[24]。两例患者的移植物生存情况均逐渐恶化，在加强免疫抑制剂使用后最终仍完全丧失移植物功能。Morrell也报道了例类似病例，该患者在移植后产生供体特异性抗体，移植物功能早期即出现恶化。肺组织病理结果显示内皮下C4d沉积，抗体清除治疗包括IVIG、血浆置换和抗CD20单克隆抗体治疗，对该患者有一定治疗效果[25]。最后，Astor报道了1例儿童肺移植患者，该患者肺活检显示C4d沉积，同时伴有明显B细胞浸润，以及血液循环中较高的DSA水平。该患者同样对抗体清除治疗有效果[26]。总的来说，尽管通过组织学明确抗体介导排斥十分困难，但是当患者出现较高DSA水平、逐渐加重的临床表现、对传统排斥治疗方法无反应，以及肺活检病理未表现为典型的急性细胞排斥时，须考虑抗体介导排斥的发生。

急性排斥的危险因素

大量文献已发现了不少与急性细胞性排斥发生相关的危险因素，包括免疫抑制、基因变异、供受体间的抗原差异以及移植后临床相关因素。关于免疫抑制，绝大多数肺移植受体接受包括钙调磷酸酶抑制的维持性免疫抑制治疗。两项研究均证实了对于预防急性细胞性排斥发生风险，他克莫司(TAC)比环孢霉素(CSA)治疗更具有优势，但优势不十分显著，移植后1年急性细胞性排斥发生率下降7%~22%[27,28]。肺移植中心目前仍未解决的问题是移植后如何进行最佳的淋巴细胞清除治疗。不同移植中心使用不同方式的诱导治疗，包括多克隆抗胸腺球蛋白、选择性抗IL-2受体单克隆抗体如巴利西单抗和达克西单抗，以及强效的多淋巴细胞清除药物阿伦单抗。部分中心不使用任何诱导治疗。关于急性细胞性排斥风险，不少研究支持诱导治疗可降低急性细胞性排斥发生风险[29-32]，ISHLT登记数据显示，相比不接受诱导治疗的患者，接受抗IL-2受体抗体诱导治疗的患者具有相对较低的急性细胞排斥发生风险[33]。与其他实体器官移植类似，绝大多数肺移植供受体之间的HLA抗原差异性亦较大。供受体间HLA A、HLA B和DR等位基因错配程度与急性细胞性排斥发生相关[34-36]。普通人群中也有不少高频基因多态性也与急性细胞性排斥发生相关。其中有TLR4、CD14脂多糖受体、CCL4L趋化因子、细胞因子IL-10多态性均与急性细胞性排斥反应风险相关[37-40]。最后，已有证据表明，胃食管反流疾病(GERD)不仅与慢性排斥相关，还可能增加急性细胞性排斥反应发生风险[41]。

急性排斥治疗

绝大多数发生急性细胞性排斥的患者可通过加强免疫抑制治疗进行成功管理。对于A2或更高程度的急性细胞性排斥，几乎每个中心均会进行治疗，而对于A1程度的排斥患者是否需要治疗存在一定争议。考虑到即使最轻微的排斥也与慢性肺失功相关，部分中心对于轻微的排斥反应亦采用较为积极的治疗策略。一线治疗方案包括甲泼尼龙，10~15mg/(kg·d)，持续3天。虽然该方案被全世界范围内多个中心广泛使用，但仍未有足够证据表明这是最合适的剂量。一项前瞻性研究结果显示，移植后糖皮质激素使用时间与其效果呈负相关：85%患者在移植后1年内应用高剂量糖皮质激素具有明显效果，而在移植2年后发生的急性细胞性排斥患者中，只有55%对糖皮质激素治疗有反应[42]。该糖皮质激素冲击治疗最主要的副作用为短暂性高血糖，可能需要胰岛素治疗，以及暂时性的潜伏巨细胞病毒激活。大多数方案会针对糖皮质激素冲击治疗后的高风险患者，同时加入巨细胞病毒预防性疗法。

顽固性急性细胞性排斥，其定义为常规大剂量糖皮质激素使用后仍存在的任何程度的排斥，可采用多种治疗策略，包括二次高剂量糖皮质激素治疗。其他治疗方案包括使用多克隆抗胸腺细胞球蛋白(ATG)、CD3单克隆抗体(OKT3)，以及人源化CD52单克隆抗体(阿仑单抗)，都有望成为正规治疗策略。由于所有关于治疗难治性急性细胞性排斥的报道都只纳入少量患者，因此目前仍未有标准的抗急性细胞性排斥的二线治疗药物。除了靶向淋巴细胞治疗方案以外，部分临床医生推荐对于难治性急性细胞性排斥患者，改变基线免疫抑制方案：例如，将环孢霉素替换为他克莫司，或者把硫唑嘌呤替换为霉酚酸酯[43,44]。而对于极严重的难治性排斥，补救治疗方案则包括全身淋巴结照射以及体外光分离自治疗方法[45,46]。

慢性移植排斥

绝大多数患者行肺移植后生活质量明显提高，其与呼吸困难程度减轻和外源性氧治疗需求解除有关。肺活量测定是肺移植受体最主要的肺功能检测手段，主要包括两个特异性测量指标：一秒用力呼气容积(FEV_1)和用力肺活量(FVC)。25%~75%用力呼气容积($FEV_{25\sim75}$)为第三个常用的测量指标。大多数肺移植受体的肺功能在移植后6~12个月达到峰值。慢性排斥发生于肺功能由顶峰开始下降之后。慢性排斥的典型病理学改变为呼吸道末端管腔闭塞，被命名为闭塞性细支气管炎(BO)。闭塞性细支气管炎的病理表现不同于A级或B级急性细胞性排斥。闭塞性细支气管炎在解剖学上仅累及末端气道,而不累及较大的软骨气道、肺泡及肺间质。此外,急性细胞性排斥的特征表现为血管周或者细支气管周淋巴细胞浸润，而闭塞性细支气管炎则仅有较少的淋巴细胞浸润。闭塞性细支气管炎的阻塞部位可以是同轴的,也可以是散在的。此外,闭塞性细支气管炎还可伴有泡沫性巨噬细胞浸润。由于广泛纤维化是闭塞性细支气管炎的特殊表现，因此大量研究致力于查明肺内纤维原细胞来源，有时会因其延长的细胞结构以及增加的肌动蛋白成分被认为是肌成纤维细胞。理论上说，肌成纤维细胞可有多个不同来源。首先,肌成纤维细胞可来自供体器官内定居的纤维原细胞。其次,可来源于受体血液循环内骨髓来源的前体纤维原细胞。第三,由于它们存在的部位先前可能已存在气道损伤，因此它们可能来自细支气管上皮间质转分化。肌成纤维细胞多个潜在来源之间并不矛盾,证据表明可能涉及上述所有可能的过程。

闭塞性细支气管炎病变部位有时可在支气管镜肺活检时被发现，因此肺移植排斥研究组制订了相应评级模式。但需要注意,闭塞性细支气管炎的病理表现差异较大。因此,支气管镜下肺活检用于诊断闭塞性细支气管炎的阴性预测价值较低。需要有更好的临床替代指标,用于细支气管闭塞综合征的诊断。由 ISHLT 制订的细支气管闭塞综合征分级系统已修改过两次，最近于 2003 年制订。

如表 72.1 所示,当移植后一秒用力呼气容积下降到低于最高值的 80%时，即可诊断为闭塞性细支气管炎综合征。由于闭塞性细支气管炎综合征早期会导致

表 72.1　闭塞性细支气管炎综合征分级标准

级别	标准
BOS 0	FEV_1>90%基线水平,$FEV_{25\sim75}$>75%基线水平
BOS 0p	FEV_1 处于 81%~90%基线水平和(或)$FEV_{25\sim75}$<75%基线水平
BOS 1	FEV_1 处于 66%~80%基线水平
BOS 2	FEV_1 处于 51%~65%基线水平
BOS 3	FEV_1<50%基线水平

BOS,闭塞性细支气管炎综合征;FEV_1,用力一秒呼气容积;$FEV_{25\sim75}$,25%~75%用力呼气容积。

部分管腔狭窄，一秒用力呼气容积下降通常与用力肺活量改变不成比例，用力肺活量改变对气道阻力改变相对不敏感。因此,一秒用力呼气容积逐渐下降可提示闭塞性细支气管炎综合征的进展，表现为向内弯曲的呼气量环(图 72.1)。很多不同于纤维性气道闭塞的过程也可引起一秒用力呼气容积下降。因此,为更好地诊断细支气管闭塞综合征,还须排除其他病因。常见的可导致气道阻塞的原因包括急性细胞性排斥以及感染性因素。因此,气道通气障碍患者的标准检查手段包括放射性检查与支气管镜检查。后者可用于查明感染性病因以及移植排斥。谨记很多其他病因也可导致气道通气功能的丧失，需要在诊断为闭塞性细支气管炎综合征前首先被考虑。气道硬化性病变,主要发生于支气管吻合处,可导致一秒用力呼气容积下降。肺移植受体在支气管吻合处有较高风险发展为局限性狭窄，因为在移植时该区域的血管未很好地进行吻合。这种吻合处狭窄可在 CT 以及支气管镜下发现(图 72.2)。体重也可改变患者的呼吸状况，肥胖患者一秒用力呼气容积明显降低。恶性肥胖导致的呼吸功能损伤包括用力肺活量和一秒用力呼气容积同时下降，且程度相同，但 25%~

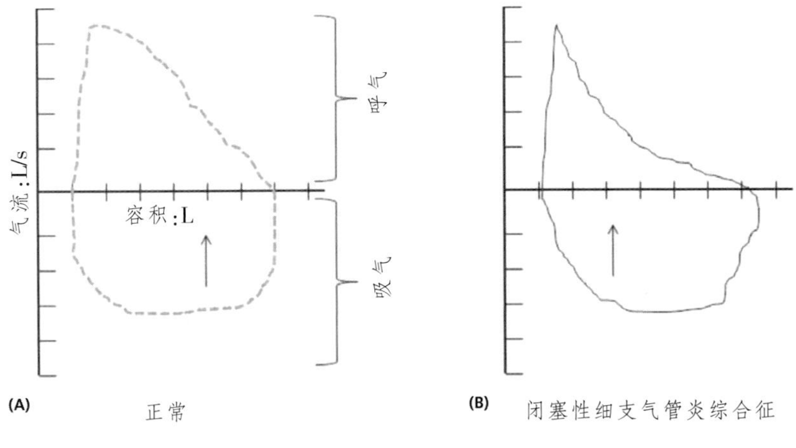

图 72.1　移植后呼吸功能改变趋势。气流/容积环比较了肺容量(X 轴)与气流功能(Y 轴)。X 轴以上代表呼气,X 轴以下代表吸气。正常患者(A),FEV_1(箭头)发生于肺容积相对较高时。在小气道闭塞的情况下，见于闭塞性细支气管炎综合征(B),气道功能紊乱性丧失,FEV_1(箭头)发生于肺容积较小时。气道功能进行性下降,呼气形态由凸面状转变为凹面状。

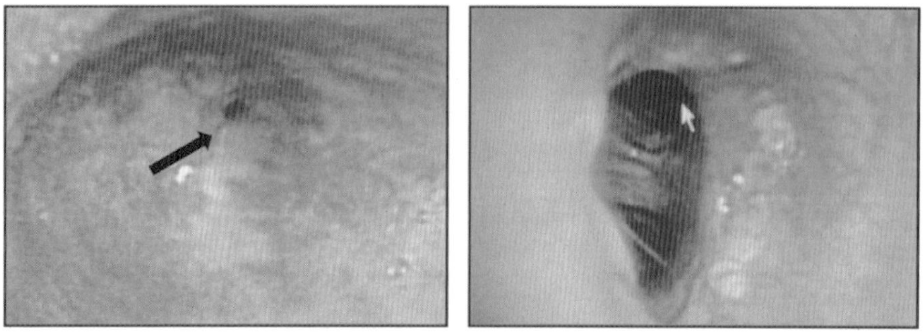

(A) (B)

图 72.2 局限性气道狭窄。一例肺移植受体表现为 FEV_1 无规则下降。支气管镜活检发现右主支气管吻合处针尖样狭窄，如(A)箭头所示。支气管镜下球囊扩张后，气道扩大(B)，FEV_1 恢复到基础水平。

75%用力呼气容积无改变。25%~75%用力呼气容积是察觉气道阻力最为敏感的指标。如表 72.1 所示，一种额外的分类被命名为 BOS0p（适用于潜在 BOS）。BOS0p 标准于 2002 年制订，具体为 FEV_1 下降 10%或者 $FEV_{25\sim75}$ 下降 25%。将 BOS0p 纳入分级标准的目的在于提醒临床医生还存在一群肺功能处于下降的特殊患者。一项回顾性研究评价了 BOS0p 的两个变量，FEV_1 和 $FEV_{25\sim75}$，结果表明只有 FEV_1 下降对于单肺移植受体具有正确的预后价值[48]。另一项回顾性研究也发现了类似的结果，结合使用 FEV_1 和 $FEV_{25\sim75}$ 比单独 FEV_1 具有更好的预后价值[49]。考虑到绝大多数肺移植受体最终将达到闭塞性细支气管炎综合征的诊断标准，但治疗手段仍十分有限，除了作为调查研究的终点指标以外，BOS0p 的临床使用价值还未可知。

闭塞性细支气管炎综合征的临床表现

每个肺移植受体都有发展为闭塞性细支气管炎综合征的风险。基于最近更新的 ISHLT 登记系统，追踪全世界范围内最大的肺移植队列研究，结果显示 1 年后未发生闭塞性细支气管炎综合征的概率为 90%，5 年后为 51%，而 10 年后则为 25%[33]。总的来说，数据表明肺移植后闭塞性细支气管炎综合征总体发生率很高，大都发生于移植后数年内。闭塞性细支气管炎综合征的临床表现差异较大。大多数患者开始为无明显症状，仅有呼吸功能的改变，但有部分患者表现为急性呼吸困难，类似于典型的呼吸道感染。有研究者将闭塞性细支气管炎综合征根据疾病进展速度分类。在一项纳入 204 例肺移植受体的研究中，FEV_1 快速下降患者的中位生存时间为 29 个月，相比下降速度较为缓慢的患者，其中位生存时间为 58 个月[50]。截至目前，最大的一项研究显示，大多数病例中，闭塞性细支气管炎综合征随时间进展过程中，FEV_1 下降速度在开始 6 个月内最快。而在之后的 18 个月内，下降速度较为缓慢[51]。而评价闭塞性细支气管炎综合征的治疗效果时，还须考虑 FEV_1 下降与时间之间的非线性关系。对于更早符合诊断标准的患者，2 年后 FEV_1 下降速度也更快[51]。

针对闭塞性细支气管炎综合征患者的放射学相关研究普遍比较微妙。典型的肺部平片表现为正常到高度肿胀的肺脏而无明显模糊影。高分辨率 CT 研究可提供更多细节。例如，比较吸气相和呼气相时 CT 图像可显示。此外，由于涉及末端细支气管，闭塞性细支气管炎综合征患者在肺部外周可出现树芽征。但需要注意的是，很多导致细支气管炎的感染性疾病也可表现出树芽征模糊影。

慢性移植排斥的其他临床表现

慢性移植排斥的典型表现包括末端气道腔内纤维黏液样物质聚集，导致气流阻塞；其他表现之前已有描述，包括限制性移植综合征(RAS)、中性粒细胞可逆性移植功能减退(NRAD)和滤泡性细支气管炎。RAS 的特征表现为出现 FEV_1(>20%)和肺活量(TLC，>10%)的同时下降。部分 RAS 患者表现为肺上叶纤维化，包括射线下蜂窝状改变和胸膜增厚(图 72.4)，但这个改变并未在所有患者中出现。NRAD 的表型特征包括：①FEV_1 下降；②支气管肺泡灌洗液内中性粒细胞增多；③阿奇霉素治疗后 FEV_1 明显改善[52]。滤泡性细支气管炎是一种少见的小气道疾病，可见于非移植患者。其特征表现为气道周围淋巴细胞增生，并逐渐进展为支气管扩张。目前已有两篇滤泡性细支气管炎发生于肺移植受体的病例报道，其与先前的霉菌属真菌感染、气

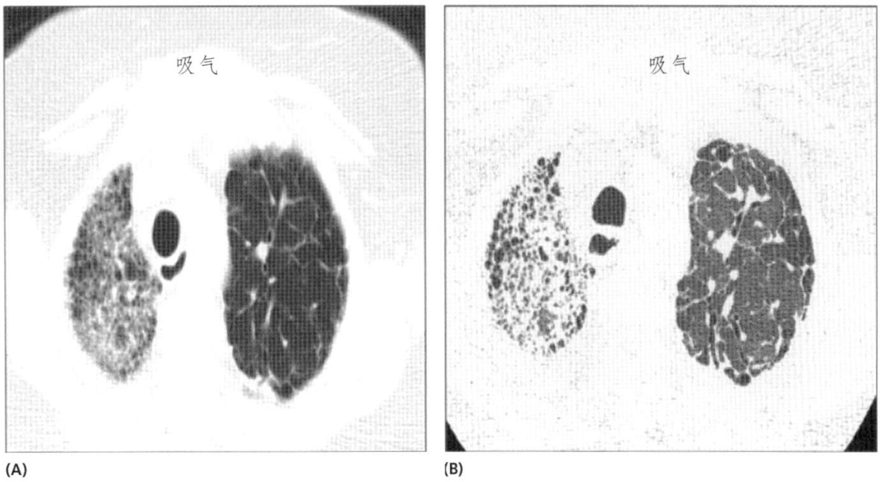

图 72.3　闭塞性细支气管的放射线下表现。单肺移植 7 年受体伴有 FEV_1 下降；(A)吸气相左肺出现一定程度的模糊影衰减；(B)同一部位呼气相，二级肺小叶空气滞留衰减变异。

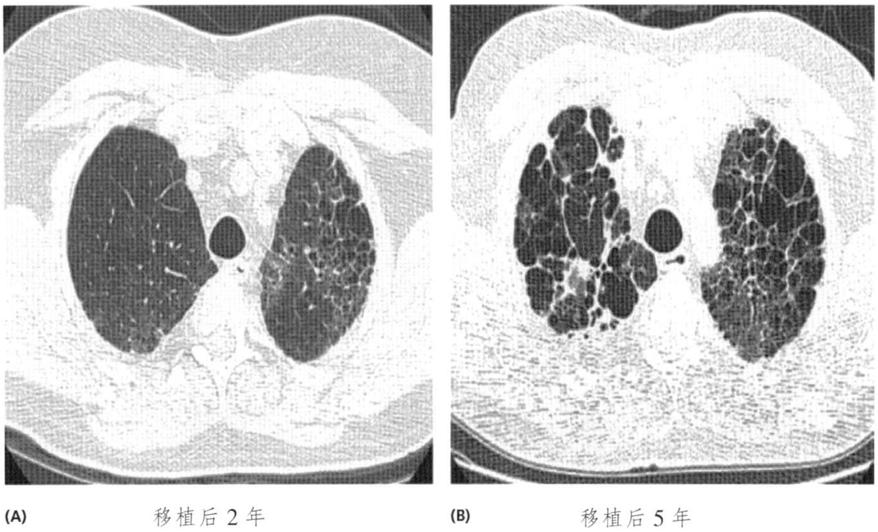

图 72.4　限制性移植综合征的射线下表现。患者出现进行性肺活量下降，移植 2 年后肺总量下降 10%，5 年后下降 40%。肺总量下降与随时间进展的顶部蜂窝状改变相关。

道中性粒细胞增加和阿奇霉素治疗后病情改善强烈相关[53,54]。总的来说，慢性肺移植失功包括其中一种表现，也有作者将闭塞性细支气管炎(OB)命名为慢性肺移植失功(CLAD)。对慢性肺移植失功不同分型间比较后发现，同时伴有闭塞性细支气管炎综合征的患者要比同时伴有限制性移植综合征的患者有更好的生存结果。

闭塞性细支气管炎综合征的危险因素

闭塞性细支气管炎综合征的病理生理学机制涉及多方面因素。多种危险因素与闭塞性细支气管综合征的发展有关，相关机制研究已进展到研究这些危险因素是如何影响闭塞性细支气管炎综合征的。不少研究报道认为，急性细胞性排斥为闭塞性细支气管炎综合征的强烈危险因素[55-59]。研究证实，即使是轻微的排斥反应，也与闭塞性细支气管炎综合征发生风险相关。今后的研究工作着重于淋巴性细支气管炎与 B 级程度的急性细胞性排斥性之间的相关性。原因在于淋巴性细支气管炎病变与闭塞性细支气管炎病变涉及相似的解剖部位，尽管它们在组织病理学上表现不一。在动物气管移植模型中也得到进一步支持，淋巴性细支气管炎与之后的气道堵塞存在短暂紧密的联系[61-63]。最近，Glanbille 对 341 例肺移植受体就淋巴性细支气管炎与闭塞性细支气管炎综合征间的相关性做了一项随访调查[64]。结果发现,在多变量回归模型中,最高B级评分排斥与之后的闭塞性细支气管炎综合征和死亡发生相关。单变量模型中A级评分(血管性)与闭塞性细支气管炎综合征风险相关,而在多变量模型中则不再有相关性[64]。

并非每个发生急性细胞性排斥的患者最终都会发展为闭塞性细支气管炎综合征,也并非所有闭塞性细支气管炎综合征患者都有前驱急性细胞性排斥反应发生。因此,即使急性细胞性排斥诊断不够明确,也可能有其他因素参与闭塞性细支气管炎综合征的发生过程。这些因素为非免疫相关,包括缺血再灌注损伤[又称为原发性移植物功能障碍 (PED)]、胃食管反流病(GERD)、呼吸道感染。

原发性移植物功能障碍

对移植物的损伤早于移植完成前就已发生。脑死亡可导致神经免疫轴激活,继而引发亚临床上皮与内皮损伤。此外,机械通气导致移植肺供体误吸和损伤的风险增加。还有之后发生的冷,热缺血过程。因此,很多正常的肺脏在移植后1天内就出现明显的非心源性水肿。目前已有相关指南用于原发性移植物功能障碍分级[65]。如表72.2所示,原发性移植物功能障碍根据四个时间点(0~6、24、48、72小时)进行病理分级。当然,符合原发性移植物功能障碍的患者还须排除心源性水肿可能。

不少研究者将该病理分级系统用于评价原发性移植物功能障碍对闭塞性细支气管炎综合征的发生影响风险。在一项单中心的回归性研究中,共纳入337例肺移植受体,研究发现原发性移植物功能障碍的严重性与之后闭塞性细支气管炎综合征发生相关,不管是在移植后早期还是后期。一项大规模国际登记研究发现,

表72.2 原发性移植物失功分级方案共识

级别	PaO_2/FiO_2	放射性浸润改变伴有肺水肿
0	>300	无
1	>300	有
2	200~300	有
3	<200	有

除了0~3级,原发性移植物失功患者还可根据移植后不同时间点分级。分别为肺移植后0~6h,24h,48h,72h。

原发性移植物功能障碍存活者的死亡率增加,即使是生存时间超过1年的患者,尽管原发性移植物功能障碍患者存在增加闭塞性细支气管炎综合征的趋势。原发性移植物功能障碍是如何导致闭塞性细支气管炎综合征发生目前仍不清楚,两者发生于移植后不同时间点,近期Bharat等发现患有原发性移植物功能障碍的患者出现直接靶向MHC二类表位的抗供体HLA抗体的风险明显增高。可能是由于在原发性移植物功能障碍发生过程中肺上皮损伤而导致肺抗原性增加。此外,也有可能是因为在此过程中隐藏的自身抗原暴露到免疫系统中。V型胶原是其中一种抗原。V型胶原是胶原组成成分中较少的一种,通常呈胶原束,因此可免于T细胞监视。在缺乏抗原错配的啮齿类动物移植中,V型胶原释放进入气道,导致移植物内特异性T细胞浸润[68]。据一项单中心研究报道,特发性肺纤维化患者在移植前可出现大量V型胶原特异性T淋巴细胞 (55%比22%)[69]。因此,原发性移植物功能障碍促进闭塞性细支气管炎综合征发展的另一可能机制为早期肺组织损伤导致隐藏的自身抗原暴露,触发后续的免疫反应,即使是发生在移植物功能障碍恢复后。

胃食管反流病

许多因素会导致肺移植受体发生胃食管反流病和误吸风险增高。外科和手术后进程均会损伤正常吞咽过程。Atkins等对移植后患者进行吞咽评价后发现,1/3患者出现喉部渗漏或吸入稀液[70]。临床上很多患者存在隐性误吸。此外,患者还有较高的胃瘫发生率。影响胃食管运动,可引起退化性胃反流的因素包括术中迷走神经损伤以及使用钙调磷酸酶抑制剂,可导致胃排空延迟。黏膜纤毛清除功能降低,迟钝的反射性咳嗽和吻合口处瘢痕组织形成均会导致肺上皮细胞暴露于胃内容物的风险增加。目前发现至少有50%患者存在胃食管反流病[73]。此外,在移植患者肺泡灌洗液中发现胃蛋白酶、胆盐等胃液成分存在[74,75]。胃食管反流病患者存在更高的急性细胞性排斥发生风险[41]。由于这些相关性的存在,部分研究中心开始在移植后早期常规进行外科修复手术。由于未设对照组,相比以往研究,该方法可提高移植后结果。有趣的是,一项小规模肺移植队列研究发现,经外科手术改进后,移植肺内激活的CD8 T淋巴细胞数量明显减少[76]。因此,胃食管反流病伴有误吸可诱导损伤反应,增加对移植物的免疫排斥。

一项肺移植前后生存对比研究发现胃食管反流病患者体内对 V 型胶原的 T 淋巴细胞反应性增加。移植后，胃食管反流同时伴有 V 型胶原特异性 T 淋巴细胞增加的患者发生闭塞性细支气管炎综合征发的风险增加[77]。这些发现提示误吸可能与自身免疫反应发展相关。

感染

由于大量免疫抑制剂应用以及肺易受外界环境的影响，肺移植受体发生多呼吸道感染的风险很高。移植后发生感染风险详见第 92~94 章。多种病原微生物感染与之后的闭塞性细支气管炎综合征发生相关，包括假单胞菌感染[78]、非典型细菌如衣原体[79]、真菌感染[80,81]、社区获得性呼吸道病毒(CARV)[82,83]、巨细胞病毒感染激活等[84,85]。社区获得性呼吸道病毒感染后遗症已有大量研究。其一般包括流感病毒、副流感病毒、呼吸道合胞病毒、偏肺病毒、腺病毒和鼻病毒。目前为止，几乎所有报道社区获得性呼吸道病毒与移植后结果相关性的研究都是单中心回顾性研究。根据这些研究可知，社区获得性呼吸道病毒与呼吸道症状如咳嗽、呼吸困难强烈相关。而关于社区获得性呼吸道病毒感染与急性细胞性排斥或者闭塞性细支气管炎综合征发生之间的相关性却未有统一结果。在一项大规模前瞻性单中心研究中，呼吸道病毒感染经敏感的分子学手段检测后，结果显示社区获得性呼吸道病毒感染与 A2 级排斥有极强相关性，但是未发现与其他级别的排斥存在相关性。关于社区获得性呼吸道病毒感染与闭塞性细支气管炎综合征的发生风险，大多数研究报道病例数较少，尽管 3/4 研究均发现两者有关。一篇荟萃分析研究了社区获得性呼吸道病毒与肺移植的相关性，发现各研究间异质性很大，没有合适的统计学方法进行合并计算。总的来说，社区获得性呼吸道病毒感染对于肺移植受体来说是有害的，但相关风险仍需要更多对照研究来分析。关于病毒感染，须明确的一个问题是目前可以用来治疗绝大多数感染的药物很少。流感病毒可以使用奥司他韦等药物治疗，可减少病毒释放；呼吸道合胞病毒可以使用利巴韦林治疗(吸入或者而口服)，对病毒感染的一般管理还包括减少基础免疫抑制以及增加支持治疗。2009 年，新型 H1N1 流感病毒大流行，澳大利亚等地学者认为该次爆发与闭塞性细支气管炎综合征的总发生率增加有关[87]。

除了社区获得性呼吸道病毒，其最终可被感染者所清除，对于肺移植受体，另一潜在的威胁是宿主体内潜伏的病毒激活。其中获得最广泛研究的是巨细胞病毒，其为乙型疱疹病毒家族成员之一。大约 80%的普通人群的血清内巨细胞病毒检查呈阳性，因此当应用免疫抑制后存在再激活和病毒复制的风险。在所有潜伏病毒中，巨细胞病毒最容易在肺内复制。在肺移植后前几年，巨细胞病毒感染可使闭塞性支气管炎综合征的风险明显增加。一项国际性注册数据结果显示，相比巨细胞病毒感染阳性的移植受体，巨细胞病毒感染阴性患者，在接受阳性移植肺后，闭塞性支气管炎综合征的发生风险更高。肺内巨细胞病毒感染可引发巨细胞病毒性肺炎，引起肺内炎症细胞浸润，同时呼吸道上皮细胞免疫原性增加。因此，巨细胞病毒感染导致闭塞性细支气管炎综合征的机制可能与呼吸道慢性损伤有关。一项基于人移植肺的机制性研究显示，巨细胞病毒性肺炎患者的支气管灌洗液内 CCL2、MCP-1 水平升高—(两种已知与闭塞性支气管综合征发生风险相关的细胞因子)[88]。

在过去的几十年，巨细胞病毒治疗已标准化。最常使用的是口服更昔洛韦，其可有效抑制病毒复制。对于巨细胞病毒感染高风险患者，在移植后 3~12 个月内使用更昔洛韦可明显减少闭塞性细支气管炎综合征发生风险。最近，一项基于 ISHLT 注册登记数据的研究比较了供受体之间不同的巨细胞病毒感染状态，以及移植后死亡发生风险的差异。在巨细胞病毒预防的新时代，供受体间巨细胞病毒感染错配(D+/R-)与不错配的生存情况已无统计学差异。但这不代表巨细胞病毒复制为良性表现，另一项近期数据显示，巨细胞病毒性肺炎与之后的闭塞性细支气管炎综合征发生风险相关。Snyder 在一项大规模回顾性队列研究中纳入 231 例肺移植受体，结果显示巨细胞病毒感染后之后，闭塞性细支气管炎综合征发生风险增至 2 倍[89]。同样的，Paraskeva 应用敏感 PCR 技术，对肺泡灌洗液内巨细胞病毒复制呈阳性的 192 例移植患者进行检测后发现，巨细胞病毒阳性者闭塞性支气管炎综合征发生风险增至 2 倍[90]。基于这些发现，大量研究工作致力于为肺移植受体找到最佳的巨细胞病毒预防策略。在一项由美国 11 个中心参与的安慰剂对照研究中，比较了口服更昔洛韦 3 个月与 6 个月的预防效果。该研究发现，患者接受更长时间的预防治疗可明显降低移植后 13 个月的巨细胞病毒感染风险(4%比 32%)[91]。移植后更长时间的预防治疗是否可以进一步降低闭塞性细支气管炎综合征发生风险,仍需要前瞻性试验来回答该问题。

慢性排斥的治疗策略

鉴于肺移植受体的闭塞性细支气管炎综合征发生率很高,导致死亡风险明显增加,目前针对慢性排斥的治疗方案仍难以令人满意。急性细胞性排斥与闭塞性细支气管炎综合征发生有关,不少研究者通过调整标准免疫抑制方案来降低闭塞性细支气管炎综合征发生风险,如将硫唑嘌呤替换为霉酚酸酯,环孢霉素替换为他克莫司[92-96],或者采用细胞溶解治疗方案[97-99]。目前为止,并没有确切结果显示,在闭塞性细支气管炎综合征诊断后肺功能可得到明显改善,但在部分患者中,肺功能可维持较稳定水平。由于都是非对照或者回顾性研究,这些发现是否仅与闭塞性细支气管炎综合征的病程特点有关而未可知。

肺移植受体患闭塞性细支气管炎的组织学特征与一种少见的肺部疾病——弥漫性细支气管炎(DPB)类似。弥漫性细支气管炎最终可导致终末期肺病。大环内脂类抗生素为其最有效的治疗药物之一[100]。关于囊性纤维化的研究结果显示,应用阿奇霉素可有效改善病情[101]。基于这些发现,为验证阿奇霉素是否可用于移植后发生闭塞性细支气管炎综合征患者的肺功能维持,已进行前期研究。第一个病例研究结果显示5/6已有闭塞性细支气管炎综合征的移植患者接受阿奇霉素治疗后 FEV_1 趋向于稳定水平[102]。在其后一项更大的单中心研究中,81例闭塞性细支气管炎综合征患者经阿奇霉素治疗后,24例患者出现 FEV_1 提高10%[103]。此外,被发现有效果者较无效果者治疗前肺泡灌洗液内有更高水平的中性粒细胞。有学者建议,将阿奇霉素治疗有效的患者从其他闭塞性细支气管炎综合征患者中区分出来,归为另一亚型,并将其命名为中性粒细胞可逆性移植功能障碍。在一项随机前瞻性试验中,共纳入40例阿奇霉素治疗组患者,43例安慰剂对照组患者,研究者对阿奇霉素可能发挥的作用进行评估。结果发现,移植时即开始使用阿奇霉素较移植2年后使用阿奇霉素的患者,闭塞性细支气管炎综合征的发生率下降3倍,但两者生存无明显差异[104]。考虑到患者对阿奇霉素耐受性较好,目前也无其他治疗闭塞性细支气管炎综合征的有效方法,应用阿奇霉素治疗气道阻塞患者也较为合理。

目前已有多种治疗闭塞性细支气管炎综合征的方法被提出,这些方法可能具有一定治疗效果,但仍没有足够强有力的实验证据支持,包括使用抗体清除治疗降低DSA水平、环孢霉素雾化、光分离置换法,以及供体造血干细胞输注。如前所述,在一项单中心研究中发现移植后新产生DSA的患者,在利妥昔单抗和静脉免疫球蛋白联合治疗成功清除DSA后,患者发生闭塞性细支气管炎综合征的概率降低[21]。由此可以推测对于新产生DSA患者使用抗体清除治疗,可以使闭塞性细支气管炎综合征发生风险减降。吸入性环孢霉素被认为可用于治疗减少特异气道反应。在一项单中心前瞻性研究中,把急性细胞性排斥减轻作为主要研究终点,结果显示吸入性环孢霉素对急性细胞性排斥并没有治疗效果。有趣的是,另一回顾性分析研究的结果显示,患者接受吸入性环孢霉素治疗后,生存率提高,闭塞性细支气管炎综合征发生率降低[105]。因此,将来仍需要更多关于吸入性环孢霉素应用效果的研究。体外光分离置换法(ECP)是指在使用光敏感药物后,从外周血中分离白细胞,体外经紫外线处理后,最终将白细胞回输至患者体内。该方法对于同种异体骨髓移植并伴有闭塞性支气管炎的患者有一定治疗潜力。而在肺移植中,一项研究结果显示,应用体外光分离置换法可稳定移植后发生闭塞性细支气管炎综合征患者的肺功能,但该研究并未设置对照组[106]。混合造血嵌合可能是诱导特异性耐受的策略之一。在一项临床研究中,26例患者同时接受肺移植与供体骨髓细胞输注,13例患者仅接受肺移植。在同时输注骨髓细胞组中,5%的患者发生闭塞性细支气管炎,而在未输注组中,33%的患者发生闭塞性细支气管炎[107]。嵌合程度会在移植后1年时衰退到检测阈值,因此是否能达到稳定的嵌合水平仍不可知。在输注供体骨髓细胞成为预防闭塞性细支气管炎综合征的有效手段前,该结果仍需要有大量研究验证。

总结

急性与慢性排斥均常发生于肺移植受体,需要主动监督管理,包括计划性活检和高度怀疑后活检。将免疫排斥导致的移植炎症从其他疾病中区分诊断,需要有专业病理科医师的紧密合作,同时还需要恰当的治疗以及积极的随访。

(韩威力 译 韩威力 校)

参考文献

1. McWilliams TJ, Williams TJ, Whitford HM, et al. Surveillance bronchoscopy in lung transplant recipients: risk versus benefit. Journal of Heart and Lung Transplantation. 2008;27:1203–1209.
2. Valentine VG, Gupta MR, Weill D, et al. Single-institution study evaluating the utility of surveillance bronchoscopy after lung transplantation. Journal of Heart and Lung Transplantation. 2009;28:14–20.
3. Hopkins PM, Aboyoun CL, Chhajed PN, et al. Prospective analysis of 1,235 transbronchial lung biopsies in lung transplant recipients. Journal of Heart and Lung Transplantation. 2002;21:1062–1067.
4. Chan CC, Abi-Saleh WJ, Arroliga AC, et al. Diagnostic yield and therapeutic impact of flexible bronchoscopy in lung transplant recipients. Journal of Heart and Lung Transplantation. 1996;15:196–205.
5. Jin F, Mu D, Chu D, et al. Severe complications of bronchoscopy. Respiration; International Review of Thoracic Diseases. 2008;76:429–433.
6. Hasegawa T, Iacono AT, Yousem SA. The anatomic distribution of acute cellular rejection in the allograft lung. Annals of Thoracic Surgery. 2000;69:1529–1531.
7. Scott JP, Fradet G, Smyth RL, et al. Prospective study of transbronchial biopsies in the management of heart-lung and single lung transplant patients. Journal of Heart and Lung Transplantation. 1991;10:626–636; discussion 36–37.
8. Trulock EP, Ettinger NA, Brunt EM, et al. The role of transbronchial lung biopsy in the treatment of lung transplant recipients. An analysis of 200 consecutive procedures. Chest. 1992;102:1049–1054.
9. Arcasoy SM, Berry G, Marboe CC, et al. Pathologic interpretation of transbronchial biopsy for acute rejection of lung allograft is highly variable. American Journal of Transplantation. 2011;11:320–328.
10. Stephenson A, Flint J, English J, et al. Interpretation of transbronchial lung biopsies from lung transplant recipients: inter- and intraobserver agreement. Canadian Respiratory Journal: Journal of the Canadian Thoracic Society. 2005;12:75–77.
11. Chakinala MM, Ritter J, Gage BF, et al. Reliability for grading acute rejection and airway inflammation after lung transplantation. Journal of Heart and Lung Transplantation. 2005;24:652–657.
12. Colombat M, Groussard O, Lautrette A, et al. Analysis of the different histologic lesions observed in transbronchial biopsy for the diagnosis of acute rejection. Clinicopathologic correlations during the first 6 months after lung transplantation. Human Pathology. 2005;36:387–394.
13. Colvin RB, Smith RN. Antibody-mediated organ-allograft rejection. Nature Reviews. Immunology. 2005;5:807–817.
14. Takemoto SK, Zeevi A, Feng S, et al. National conference to assess antibody-mediated rejection in solid organ transplantation. American Journal of Transplantation. 2004;4:1033–1041.
15. Frost AE, Jammal CT, Cagle PT. Hyperacute rejection following lung transplantation. Chest. 1996;110:559–562.
16. Bittner HB, Dunitz J, Hertz M, et al. Hyperacute rejection in single lung transplantation—case report of successful management by means of plasmapheresis and antithymocyte globulin treatment. Transplantation. 2001;71:649–651.
17. Masson E, Stern M, Chabod J, et al. Hyperacute rejection after lung transplantation caused by undetected low-titer anti-HLA antibodies. Journal of Heart and Lung Transplantation. 2007;26:642–645.
18. de Jesus Peixoto Camargo J, Marcantonio Camargo S, Marcelo Schio S, et al. Hyperacute rejection after single lung transplantation: a case report. Transplantation Proceedings. 2008;40:867–869.
19. Hadjiliadis D, Chaparro C, Reinsmoen NL, et al. Pre-transplant panel reactive antibody in lung transplant recipients is associated with significantly worse post-transplant survival in a multicenter study. Journal of Heart and Lung Transplantation. 2005;24(7 Suppl.):S249–S254.
20. Shah AS, Nwakanma L, Simpkins C, et al. Pretransplant panel reactive antibodies in human lung transplantation: an analysis of over 10,000 patients. Annals of Thoracic Surgery. 2008;85:1919–1924.
21. Hachem RR, Yusen RD, Meyers BF, et al. Anti-human leukocyte antigen antibodies and preemptive antibody-directed therapy after lung transplantation. Journal of Heart and Lung Transplantation. 2010;29:973–980.
22. Magro CM, Pope Harman A, Klinger D, et al. Use of C4d as a diagnostic adjunct in lung allograft biopsies. American Journal of Transplantation. 2003;3:1143–1154.
23. Wallace WD, Reed EF, Ross D, et al. C4d staining of pulmonary allograft biopsies: an immunoperoxidase study. Journal of Heart and Lung Transplantation. 2005;24:1565–1570.
24. Girnita AL, McCurry KR, Yousem SA, et al. Antibody-mediated rejection in lung transplantation: case reports. Clinical Transplants. 2006:508–510.
25. Morrell MR, Patterson GA, Trulock EP, et al. Acute antibody-mediated rejection after lung transplantation. Journal of Heart and Lung Transplantation. 2009;28:96–100.
26. Astor TL, Weill D, Cool C, et al. Pulmonary capillaritis in lung transplant recipients: treatment and effect on allograft function. Journal of Heart and Lung Transplantation. 2005;24:2091–2097.
27. Hachem RR, Yusen RD, Chakinala MM, et al. A randomized controlled trial of tacrolimus versus cyclosporine after lung transplantation. Journal of Heart and Lung Transplantation. 2007;26:1012–1018.
28. Zuckermann A, Reichenspurner H, Birsan T, et al. Cyclosporine A versus tacrolimus in combination with mycophenolate mofetil and steroids as primary immunosuppression after lung transplantation: one-year results of a 2-center prospective randomized trial. Journal of Thoracic and Cardiovascular Surgery. 2003;125:891–900.
29. Ailawadi G, Smith PW, Oka T, et al. Effects of induction immunosuppression regimen on acute rejection, bronchiolitis obliterans, and survival after lung transplantation. Journal of Thoracic and Cardiovascular Surgery. 2008;135:594–602.
30. Swarup R, Allenspach LL, Nemeh HW, et al. Timing of basiliximab induction and development of acute rejection in lung transplant patients. Journal of Heart and Lung Transplantation. 2011;30:1228–1235.
31. Shyu S, Dew MA, Pilewski JM, et al. Five-year outcomes with alemtuzumab induction after lung transplantation. Journal of Heart and Lung Transplantation. 2011;30:743–754.
32. Burton CM, Andersen CB, Jensen AS, et al. The incidence of acute cellular rejection after lung transplantation: a comparative study of anti-thymocyte globulin and daclizumab. Journal of Heart and Lung Transplantation. 2006;25:638–647.
33. Christie JD, Edwards LB, Kucheryavaya AY, et al. The registry of the international society for heart and lung transplantation: twenty-eighth adult lung and heart-lung transplant report–2011. Journal of Heart and Lung Transplantation. 2011;30:1104–1122.
34. Wisser W, Wekerle T, Zlabinger G, et al. Influence of human leukocyte antigen matching on long-term outcome after lung transplantation. Journal of Heart and Lung Transplantation. 1996;15:1209–1216.
35. Schulman LL, Weinberg AD, McGregor C, et al. Mismatches at the HLA-DR and HLA-B loci are risk factors for acute rejection after lung transplantation. American Journal of Respiratory and Critical Care Medicine. 1998;157:1833–1837.
36. Quantz MA, Bennett LE, Meyer DM, et al. Does human leukocyte antigen matching influence the outcome of lung transplantation? An analysis of 3,549 lung transplantations. Journal of Heart and Lung Transplantation. 2000;19:473–479.
37. Palmer SM, Burch LH, Trindade AJ, et al. Innate immunity influences long-term outcomes after human lung transplant. American Journal of Respiratory and Critical Care Medicine. 2005;171:780–785.
38. Palmer SM, Klimecki W, Yu L, et al. Genetic regulation of rejection and survival following human lung transplantation by the innate immune receptor CD14. American Journal of Transplantation. 2007;7:693–699.
39. Zheng HX, Burckart GJ, McCurry K, et al. Interleukin-10 production genotype protects against acute persistent rejection after lung transplantation. Journal of Heart and Lung Transplantation. 2004;23:541–546.
40. Colobran R, Casamitjana N, Roman A, et al. Copy number variation in the CCL4L gene is associated with susceptibility to acute rejection in lung transplantation. Genes and Immunity. 2009;10:254–259.
41. Shah N, Force SD, Mitchell PO, et al. Gastroesophageal reflux disease is associated with an increased rate of acute rejection in lung transplant allografts. Transplantation Proceedings. 2010;42:2702–2706.
42. Fuehner T, Simon A, Dierich M, et al. Indicators for steroid response in biopsy proven acute graft rejection after lung transplantation. Respiratory Medicine. 2009;103:1114–1121.
43. Vitulo P, Oggionni T, Cascina A, et al. Efficacy of tacrolimus rescue therapy in refractory acute rejection after lung transplantation. Journal of Heart and Lung Transplantation. 2002;21:435–439.
44. Sarahrudi K, Estenne M, Corris P, et al. International experience with conversion from cyclosporine to tacrolimus for acute and chronic lung allograft rejection. Journal of Thoracic and Cardiovascular Surgery. 2004;127:1126–1132.
45. Villanueva J, Bhorade SM, Robinson JA, et al. Extracorporeal photopheresis for the treatment of lung allograft rejection. Annals of Transplantation. 2000;5:44–47.
46. Valentine VG, Robbins RC, Wehner JH, et al. Total lymphoid irradiation for refractory acute rejection in heart-lung and lung allografts. Chest. 1996;109:1184–1189.
47. Estenne M, Maurer JR, Boehler A, et al. Bronchiolitis obliterans syndrome 2001: an update of the diagnostic criteria. Journal of Heart and Lung Transplantation. 2002;21:297–310.
48. Hachem RR, Chakinala MM, Yusen RD, et al. The predictive value of bronchiolitis obliterans syndrome stage 0-p. American Journal of Respiratory and Criti-

cal Care Medicine. 2004;169:468–472.
49. Lama VN, Murray S, Mumford JA, et al. Prognostic value of bronchiolitis obliterans syndrome stage 0-p in single-lung transplant recipients. American Journal of Respiratory and Critical Care Medicine. 2005;172:379–383.
50. Jackson CH, Sharples LD, McNeil K, et al. Acute and chronic onset of bronchiolitis obliterans syndrome (BOS): are they different entities? Journal of Heart and Lung Transplantation. 2002;21:658–666.
51. Lama VN, Murray S, Lonigro RJ, et al. Course of FEV(1) after onset of bronchiolitis obliterans syndrome in lung transplant recipients. American Journal of Respiratory and Critical Care Medicine. 2007;175:1192–1198.
52. Verleden GM, Vos R, De Vleeschauwer SI, et al. Obliterative bronchiolitis following lung transplantation: from old to new concepts? Transplant International. 2009;22:771–779.
53. Vos R, Vanaudenaerde BM, De Vleeschauwer SI, et al. Follicular bronchiolitis: a rare cause of bronchiolitis obliterans syndrome after lung transplantation: a case report. American Journal of Transplantation. 2009;9:644–650.
54. McManus TE, Milne DG, Whyte KF, et al. Exudative bronchiolitis after lung transplantation. Journal of Heart and Lung Transplantation. 2008;27: 276–281.
55. Burton CM, Iversen M, Scheike T, et al. Minimal acute cellular rejection remains prevalent up to 2 years after lung transplantation: a retrospective analysis of 2697 transbronchial biopsies. Transplantation. 2008;85:547–553.
56. Kroshus TJ, Kshettry VR, Savik K, et al. Risk factors for the development of bronchiolitis obliterans syndrome after lung transplantation. Journal of Thoracic and Cardiovascular Surgery. 1997;114:195–202.
57. Hopkins PM, Aboyoun CL, Chhajed PN, et al. Association of minimal rejection in lung transplant recipients with obliterative bronchiolitis. American Journal of Respiratory and Critical Care Medicine. 2004;170:1022–1026.
58. Khalifah AP, Hachem RR, Chakinala MM, et al. Minimal acute rejection after lung transplantation: a risk for bronchiolitis obliterans syndrome. American Journal of Transplantation. 2005;5:2022–2030.
59. Hachem RR, Khalifah AP, Chakinala MM, et al. The significance of a single episode of minimal acute rejection after lung transplantation. Transplantation. 2005;80:1406–1413.
60. Boehler A, Chamberlain D, Kesten S, et al. Lymphocytic airway infiltration as a precursor to fibrous obliteration in a rat model of bronchiolitis obliterans. Transplantation. 1997;64:311–317.
61. Yousem SA. Lymphocytic bronchitis/bronchiolitis in lung allograft recipients. American Journal of Surgical Pathology. 1993;17:491–496.
62. El-Gamel A, Sim E, Hasleton P, et al. Transforming growth factor beta (TGF-beta) and obliterative bronchiolitis following pulmonary transplantation. Journal of Heart and Lung Transplantation. 1999;18:828–837.
63. Ross DJ, Marchevsky A, Kramer M, et al. "Refractoriness" of airflow obstruction associated with isolated lymphocytic bronchiolitis/bronchitis in pulmonary allografts. Journal of Heart and Lung Transplantation. 1997;16:832–838.
64. Glanville AR, Aboyoun CL, Havryk A, et al. Severity of lymphocytic bronchiolitis predicts long-term outcome after lung transplantation. American Journal of Respiratory and Critical Care Medicine. 2008;177:1033–1040.
65. Christie JD, Carby M, Bag R, et al. Report of the ISHLT Working Group on Primary Lung Graft Dysfunction part II: definition. A consensus statement of the International Society for Heart and Lung Transplantation. Journal of Heart and Lung Transplantation. 2005;24:1454–1459.
66. Daud SA, Yusen RD, Meyers BF, et al. Impact of immediate primary lung allograft dysfunction on bronchiolitis obliterans syndrome. American Journal of Respiratory and Critical Care Medicine. 2007;175:507–513.
67. Huang HJ, Yusen RD, Meyers BF, et al. Late primary graft dysfunction after lung transplantation and bronchiolitis obliterans syndrome. American Journal of Transplantation. 2008;8:2454–2462.
68. Haque MA, Mizobuchi T, Yasufuku K, et al. Evidence for immune responses to a self-antigen in lung transplantation: role of type V collagen-specific T cells in the pathogenesis of lung allograft rejection. Journal of Immunology. 2002;169:1542–1549.
69. Bobadilla JL, Love RB, Jankowska-Gan E, et al. Th-17, monokines, collagen type V, and primary graft dysfunction in lung transplantation. American Journal of Respiratory and Critical Care Medicine. 2008;177:660–668.
70. Atkins BZ, Trachtenberg MS, Prince-Petersen R, et al. Assessing oropharyngeal dysphagia after lung transplantation: altered swallowing mechanisms and increased morbidity. Journal of Heart and Lung Transplantation. 2007;26: 1144–1148.
71. Berkowitz N, Schulman LL, McGregor C, et al. Gastroparesis after lung transplantation. Potential role in postoperative respiratory complications. Chest. 1995;108:1602–1607.
72. Young LR, Hadjiliadis D, Davis RD, et al. Lung transplantation exacerbates gastroesophageal reflux disease. Chest. 2003;124:1689–1693.
73. Davis CS, Shankaran V, Kovacs EJ, et al. Gastroesophageal reflux disease after lung transplantation: pathophysiology and implications for treatment. Surgery. 2010;148:737–744; discussion 44–45.
74. Blondeau K, Dupont LJ, Mertens V, et al. Gastro-oesophageal reflux and aspiration of gastric contents in adult patients with cystic fibrosis. Gut. 2008;57:1049–1055.
75. D'Ovidio F, Mura M, Tsang M, et al. Bile acid aspiration and the development of bronchiolitis obliterans after lung transplantation. Journal of Thoracic and Cardiovascular Surgery. 2005;129:1144–1152.
76. Neujahr DC, Mohammed A, Ulukpo O, et al. Surgical correction of gastroesophageal reflux in lung transplant patients is associated with decreased effector CD8 cells in lung lavages: a case series. Chest. 2010;138:937–943.
77. Bobadilla JL, Jankowska-Gan E, Xu Q, et al. Reflux-induced collagen type v sensitization: potential mediator of bronchiolitis obliterans syndrome. Chest. 2010;138:363–370.
78. Botha P, Archer L, Anderson RL, et al. Pseudomonas aeruginosa colonization of the allograft after lung transplantation and the risk of bronchiolitis obliterans syndrome. Transplantation. 2008;85:771–774.
79. Glanville AR, Gencay M, Tamm M, et al. Chlamydia pneumoniae infection after lung transplantation. Journal of Heart and Lung Transplantation. 2005;24: 131–136.
80. Weigt SS, Elashoff RM, Huang C, et al. Aspergillus colonization of the lung allograft is a risk factor for bronchiolitis obliterans syndrome. American Journal of Transplantation. 2009;9:1903–1911.
81. Valentine VG, Gupta MR, Walker JE Jr, et al. Effect of etiology and timing of respiratory tract infections on development of bronchiolitis obliterans syndrome. Journal of Heart and Lung Transplantation. 2009;28:163–169.
82. Kumar D, Husain S, Chen MH, et al. A prospective molecular surveillance study evaluating the clinical impact of community-acquired respiratory viruses in lung transplant recipients. Transplantation. 2010;89:1028–1033.
83. Gottlieb J, Schulz TF, Welte T, et al. Community-acquired respiratory viral infections in lung transplant recipients: a single season cohort study. Transplantation. 2009;87:1530–1537.
84. Heng D, Sharples LD, McNeil K, et al. Bronchiolitis obliterans syndrome: incidence, natural history, prognosis, and risk factors. Journal of Heart and Lung Transplantation. 1998;17:1255–1263.
85. Smith MA, Sundaresan S, Mohanakumar T, et al. Effect of development of antibodies to HLA and cytomegalovirus mismatch on lung transplantation survival and development of bronchiolitis obliterans syndrome. Journal of Thoracic and Cardiovascular Surgery. 1998;116:812–820.
86. Neurohr C, Huppmann P, Leuchte H, et al. Human herpesvirus 6 in bronchalveolar lavage fluid after lung transplantation: a risk factor for bronchiolitis obliterans syndrome? American Journal of Transplantation. 2005;5:2982–2991.
87. Ng BJ, Glanville AR, Snell G, et al. The impact of pandemic influenza A H1N1 2009 on Australian lung transplant recipients. American Journal of Transplantation. 2011;11:568–574.
88. Weigt SS, Elashoff RM, Keane MP, et al. Altered levels of CC chemokines during pulmonary CMV predict BOS and mortality post-lung transplantation. American Journal of Transplantation. 2008;8:1512–1522.
89. Snyder LD, Finlen-Copeland CA, Turbyfill WJ, et al. Cytomegalovirus pneumonitis is a risk for bronchiolitis obliterans syndrome in lung transplantation. American Journal of Respiratory and Critical Care Medicine. 2010; 181:1391–1396.
90. Paraskeva M, Bailey M, Levvey BJ, et al. Cytomegalovirus replication within the lung allograft is associated with bronchiolitis obliterans syndrome. American Journal of Transplantation. 2011;11:2190–2196.
91. Palmer SM, Limaye AP, Banks M, et al. Extended valganciclovir prophylaxis to prevent cytomegalovirus after lung transplantation: a randomized, controlled trial. Annals of Internal Medicine. 2010;152:761–769.
92. Speich R, Boehler A, Thurnheer R, et al. Salvage therapy with mycophenolate mofetil for lung transplant bronchiolitis obliterans: importance of dosage. Transplantation. 1997;64:533–535.
93. Whyte RI, Rossi SJ, Mulligan MS, et al. Mycophenolate mofetil for obliterative bronchiolitis syndrome after lung transplantation. Annals of Thoracic Surgery. 1997;64:945–948.
94. Sarahrudi K, Carretta A, Wisser W, et al. The value of switching from cyclosporine to tacrolimus in the treatment of refractory acute rejection and obliterative bronchiolitis after lung transplantation. Transplant International. 2002;15:24–28.
95. Cairn J, Yek T, Banner NR, et al. Time-related changes in pulmonary function after conversion to tacrolimus in bronchiolitis obliterans syndrome. Journal of Heart and Lung Transplantation. 2003;22:50–57.
96. Borro JM, Bravo C, Sole A, et al. Conversion from cyclosporine to tacrolimus stabilizes the course of lung function in lung transplant recipients with bronchiolitis obliterans syndrome. Transplantation Proceedings. 2007;39:2416–2419.
97. Snell GI, Esmore DS, Williams TJ. Cytolytic therapy for the bronchiolitis oblit-

erans syndrome complicating lung transplantation. Chest. 1996;109:874–878.
98. Kesten S, Rajagopalan N, Maurer J. Cytolytic therapy for the treatment of bronchiolitis obliterans syndrome following lung transplantation. Transplantation. 1996;61:427–430.
99. Reams BD, Musselwhite LW, Zaas DW, et al. Alemtuzumab in the treatment of refractory acute rejection and bronchiolitis obliterans syndrome after human lung transplantation. American Journal of Transplantation. 2007;7:2802–2808.
100. Kudoh S, Azuma A, Yamamoto M, et al. Improvement of survival in patients with diffuse panbronchiolitis treated with low-dose erythromycin. American Journal of Respiratory and Critical Care Medicine. 1998;157:1829–1832.
101. Wolter J, Seeney S, Bell S, et al. Effect of long term treatment with azithromycin on disease parameters in cystic fibrosis: a randomised trial. Thorax. 2002;57: 212–216.
102. Gerhardt SG, McDyer JF, Girgis RE, et al. Maintenance azithromycin therapy for bronchiolitis obliterans syndrome: results of a pilot study. American Journal of Respiratory and Critical Care Medicine. 2003;168:121–125.
103. Gottlieb J, Szangolies J, Koehnlein T, et al. Long-term azithromycin for bronchiolitis obliterans syndrome after lung transplantation. Transplantation. 2008;85: 36–41.
104. Vos R, Vanaudenaerde BM, Verleden SE, et al. A randomised controlled trial of azithromycin to prevent chronic rejection after lung transplantation. European Respiratory Journal. 2011;37:164–172.
105. Iacono AT, Johnson BA, Grgurich WF, et al. A randomized trial of inhaled cyclosporine in lung-transplant recipients. New England Journal of Medicine. 2006;354:141–150.
106. Morrell MR, Despotis GJ, Lublin DM, et al. The efficacy of photopheresis for bronchiolitis obliterans syndrome after lung transplantation. Journal of Heart and Lung Transplantation. 2010;29:424–431.
107. Pham SM, Rao AS, Zeevi A, et al. Effects of donor bone marrow infusion in clinical lung transplantation. Annals of Thoracic Surgery. 2000;69:345–350.

第 73 章

胰腺和胰岛移植临床排斥反应综合征

Parsia A. Vagefi，Peter G. Stock

胰腺移植物的免疫原性——历史回顾

现代胰腺移植始于1966年12月17日，美国明尼苏达大学的William Kelly和Richard Lillehei医生将一个胰管结扎过的部分胰腺和一个肾脏同时移植给一例28岁女性患者[1]。在过去的40年来，胰腺移植已成为糖尿病或糖尿病伴有终末期肾病患者的一种有效治疗选择。截至2010年12月，国际胰腺移植注册中心登记35 000例以上胰腺移植，其中美国例数最多（24 000例）[2]。在这些胰腺移植中，胰肾联合移植（SPK）占75%、肾移植后胰腺移植（PAK）占18%、单纯胰腺移植（pancreas transplant alone，PTA）占7%（图73.1）。

手术技术和患者护理管理的改进，以及新型免疫抑制药物的研发应用使得患者存活率和移植物存活率都有了明显改善。由于手术技术原因所导致的术后早期胰腺移植物失功比率已下降到8%。然而，移植效果的改善更多的是得益于对同种异体免疫和自体免疫反应的控制。由于免疫原因所导致的1年移植物失功比率为：SPK 1.8%；PAK 3.7%；PTA 6.0%。这些结果反映了对于高免疫原性的胰腺移植术后的免疫调节已经有了显著的控制[2,3]。所有这些改善胰腺移植效果的努力已经使得移植术后患者1年存活率达到95%，5年存活率达83%。其中，SPK受体存活率最好，1年移植物存活率分别为胰腺86%和肾脏93%。PAK移植术后1年胰腺存活率达到80%，PTA为78%。胰腺移植的远期效果将在第107章中详述。

无论受体敏感性如何，绝大多数胰腺移植都使用T细胞耗竭剂阿仑单抗（alemtuzumab）或抗胸腺细胞球蛋白（thymoglobulin）来抗体诱导治疗（图73.2）。这也反映出了早期胰腺移植后非常高的排斥反应发生率。与T细胞耗竭类药物同时使用的维持治疗药物一般包括类固醇激素、霉酚酸酯（MMF）和他克莫司（图73.3）。目前许多中心对非致敏SPK受体采用移植术后一周内

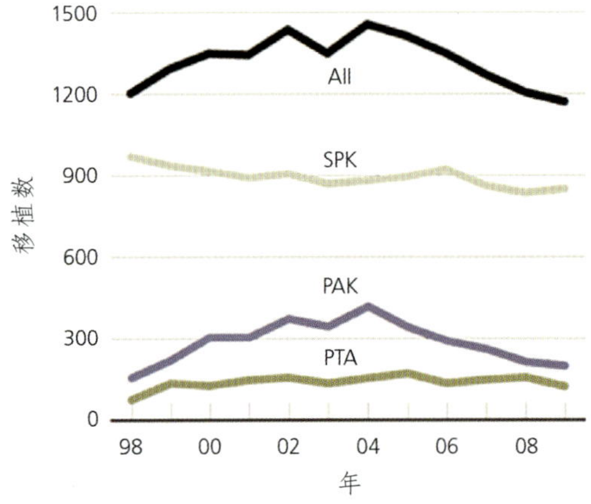

图 73.1　成人胰腺移植总数。（From: Organ Procurement and Transplantation Network (OPTN) and Scientific Registry of Transplant Recipients (SRTR). OPTN/SRTR 2010 Annual Data Report. Rockville, MD: Department of Health and Human Services, Health Resources and Services Administration, Healthcare Systems Bureau, Division of Transplantation, 2011.）

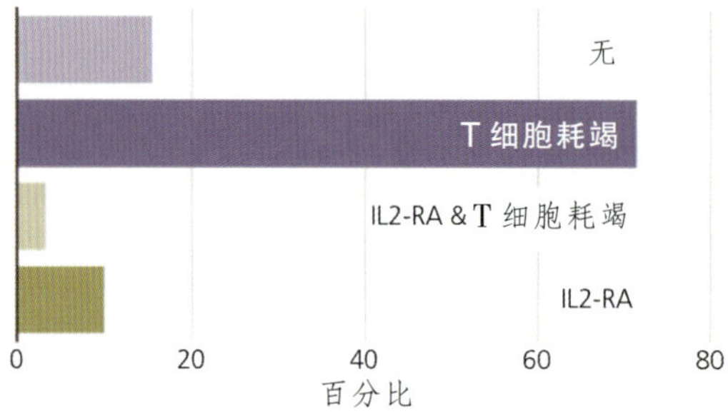

图 73.2　在胰腺移植时使用的诱导剂，成年患者，2009年。（From: Organ Procurement and Transplantation Network (OPTN) and Scientific Registry of Transplant Recipients (SRTR). OPTN/SRTR 2010 Annual Data Report. Rockville, MD: Department of Health and Human Services, Health Resources and Services Administration, Healthcare Systems Bureau, Division of Transplantation, 2011.）

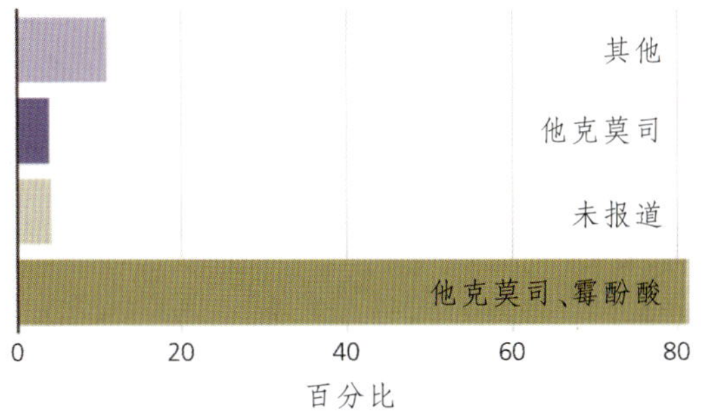

图 73.3　成年胰腺移植受体的初始免疫抑制方案,2009 年(不考虑类固醇)。(From: Organ Procurement and Transplantation Network (OPTN) and Scientific Registry of Transplant Recipients (SRTR). OPTN/SRTR 2010 Annual Data Report. Rockville, MD: Department of Health and Human Services, Health Resources and Services Administration, Healthcare Systems Bureau, Division of Transplantation, 2011.)

激素迅速减量联合他克莫司和 MMF 二联维持用药。针对有较高免疫风险的受体, 包括致敏的 SPK,PAK 或 PTA,维持治疗通常采用包括激素在内的三联用药。而针对早期就出现排斥反应或具有高排斥风险的受体,有时则需要采用包括西罗莫司在内的四联治疗。

临床表现:胰腺移植物功能障碍

胰腺移植物功能障碍常无临床症状, 常因血清淀粉酶、脂肪酶变化,或因血糖升高而偶然发现。导致移植物失功的病因学因素有很多(表 73.1),首要的是对所有胰腺移植的受体进行临床评估, 其中应包括移植物多普勒超声或者 CT、磁共振的检查,完善包括淀粉酶和脂肪酶检测在内的实验室检查。对于 SPK 受体,应检查肾脏超声。此外,糖化血红蛋白、C-肽、肌酐水平(SPK 受体) 以及免疫抑制血药浓度的检查也很有必要。同时如果高度怀疑有病原菌感染,则应进行全身体检、血培养和 CMV 检测。考虑到患者免疫抑制状态常常会掩盖其典型的症状和体征, 因此阳性的检测结果常常有用,而阴性的结果往往不能够排除诊断。对于严重的高血糖的患者,有必要予以补液及胰岛素治疗。

胰腺移植术后各种特异性或非特异性炎症反应、受体的易感状态、吻合口漏或药物诱导的毒性均可以导致血清淀粉酶和(或)脂肪酶升高。在胰腺排斥反应中, 血清淀粉酶和脂肪酶的值分别平均升高了 3.6 倍和 8.3 倍,其中 80%与活检证实的排斥反应相关[4]。其他实验室检查结果,如血清 HbA1c 的水平升高也对胰腺移植物排斥有一定的预警作用。在 SPK 移植受体中,肾脏移植物的免疫状态也能够从一定程度上反映胰腺排斥的情况, 特别是当在血清肌酸酐和胰腺腺泡细胞损伤的血清标志物同时升高时。在 SPK 排斥反应中,双器官同时出现排斥的比例占 73%。而单独的胰腺或者肾脏移植排斥反应发生率则分别为 3%和 23%[5]。

胰腺移植的超声评估一般包括胰腺实质的检查、胰周积液和渗出,以及胰腺动静脉血流的探查,同时可以通过超声引导行经皮胰腺穿刺活检[6](图 73.4A)。用超声评估胰腺移植物血管可避免使用静脉注射造影的 CT(图 73.4B)和 MRI 成像,但超声也有其局限性,如检查结果受操作者的主观影响,同时胰腺位于后腹膜,其前方的肠道气体也常给胰腺的评估带来困难。

也许对胰腺移植受体来说, 超声最大的作用是引导经皮穿刺活检[7]。由于缺乏血清学诊断胰腺移植功能障碍的特异性指标, 移植物活检已经成为胰腺移植受体的一项基本辅助检查。胰腺移植物活检通常在超声引导下, 经腹膜直接将 18 号或 20 号活检针插入胰腺体部或尾部。多普勒成像可显示胰腺周围的血管结构。同时在活检后, 超声检查可以立即早期评估有无任何活检相关的并发症。胰移植物活检具有较高的成功率,88%的样本足够进行组织病理学评价。超声引导穿刺有较低的并发症发生率(2.8%),其中包括活检后出血、生化指标检测发现的活检后胰腺炎, 以及误检到相邻的组织器官[8,9]。肠道气体感染所致胰腺显示不清、患者的体型以及小的胰腺移植物常常增加超声引导穿刺的难度。如果因为肠道气体干扰无法获得一个良好的超声穿刺窗口, 可以短时间后重复探查直到找到合适的活检窗口。此外,CT 引导下穿刺活检仍可作为备选。作为最后的手段, 也可以通过开腹或腹腔镜手术进行胰腺移植物活检[10]。

需要指出,胰腺移物膀胱引流和小肠引流术式对排斥反应的监测和诊断存在差异。目前虽然大多数移植物通过肠道引流(80%),但另外 20%经膀胱引流的病例则可以通过尿淀粉酶水平来评估移植物功能。事实上,有人认为稳定的尿淀粉酶水平能够可靠地排除排斥反应,但这一观点目前仍有争议。虽然,尿淀粉酶的下降可以作为急性排斥的指标, 但却不具有特异性,而且需要胰腺移植物活检来辅助诊断。相比在超声引导下经皮穿刺活检胰腺移植物,膀胱引流术式更

表 73.1 胰腺穿刺活检中除排斥反应以外的病理改变

诊断	主要组织病理学研究	临床表现
移植后缺血性胰腺炎	炎症:中性粒细胞,泡沫状的巨噬细胞	血清淀粉酶和脂肪酶的增加
	位置:轻度呈间隔状,严重的呈弥漫性	尿淀粉酶下降*
	其他特征:脂肪坏死、水肿和间质性出血	如果有广泛的坏死,表现为高血糖
	胰腺腺泡细胞可能存在团块状凝固性坏死	
	无纤维化,脓腔可能因水肿、脂肪坏死而扩大	
胰腺周围炎/胰周积液	炎症:混合(淋巴细胞、浆细胞、嗜酸性粒细胞、中性粒细胞)	局部或全身性感染症状,腹痛,腹膜炎
	位置:小叶间隔和外周	
	其他特征:活跃的成纤维细胞增殖束填塞间隔结构	胰周积液
	小叶中心相对保留("硬化的表现")	血清淀粉酶和脂肪酶的增加
巨细胞病毒性胰腺炎	炎症:主要是单核细胞	血清淀粉酶和脂肪酶的增加
	位置:间隔和腺泡、呈片状	尿淀粉酶减少*
	其他特征:巨细胞病毒导致腺泡、内皮细胞和基质细胞发生变化	如果为广义的疾病,则存在全身性症状 其他:十二指肠穿孔
移植后淋巴组织增生失调	炎症:从多形态,如低级别病变中的淋巴母细胞、浆细胞、嗜酸性粒细胞,到单一形态,主要为高级别病变(淋巴瘤)中的淋巴细胞	无症状,或血清淀粉酶和脂肪酶增加 淋巴结病变
	其他特征:淋巴增殖呈结节状、膨胀	肿瘤
	可能发生坏死	可能合并急性排斥反应
细菌或真菌感染	炎症:多变的;急性、慢性、化脓性、坏死性(脓肿)、肉芽肿	全身性和(或)局部感染性症状
	位置:随机	腹膜炎、十二指肠穿孔
	其他特征:与其他器官的细菌和真菌感染相同	血清淀粉酶和脂肪酶的增加
反复的自身免疫性疾病/糖尿病	炎症:胰岛中心的淋巴细胞性炎	
	β细胞消失后的晚期,无炎症	随着对胰岛素需求的增加,糖代谢急性或慢性恶化
	其他特征:胰岛素和胰高血糖素的免疫组织化学染色	即使没有体征,胰岛细胞自身抗体也通常存在
	在某些或所有胰岛中产生胰岛素的β细胞缺失,要视疾病的早期或晚期	(即 GAD 65、IA-2 等)
钙调磷酸酶抑制剂的急性中毒	无炎症	急性高血糖
	胰岛细胞损伤程度[胞质肿胀,空泡形成,胰岛细胞脱落形成空洞(腔隙),凋亡片段]	随着血糖回到正常值,高浓度的环孢霉素或他克莫司调整药物剂量或停药
	免疫过氧化物酶染色:与胰高血糖素染色相比,胰岛素染色显著减少	
	电子显微镜:缺失致密核心颗粒的胰岛素与存在致密核心颗粒的胰高血糖素	

* 膀胱移植物。

Reproduced from [16] Drachenberg et al. American Journal of Transplantation 2008;8:1237, with permission from Wiley.

适合进行膀胱镜下经十二指肠的胰腺移植物活检[11]。

急性胰腺排斥反应

胰腺移植受体中出现急性胰腺排斥反应可高达35%[12,13]。胰腺移植排斥反应的组织病理学诊断将在第85章详细说明。虽然胰腺移植排斥反应的临床表现有其特点,但病理生理则与其他移植器官排斥相似,治疗方法也和肾移植排斥治疗相似,同时在胰腺移植排斥反应中往往治疗升级速度更快。在第67章中可以找到关于移植排斥反应的治疗的总论。移植1年后,胰肾联合移植患者表现出较低的急性排斥反应发生率(25%),

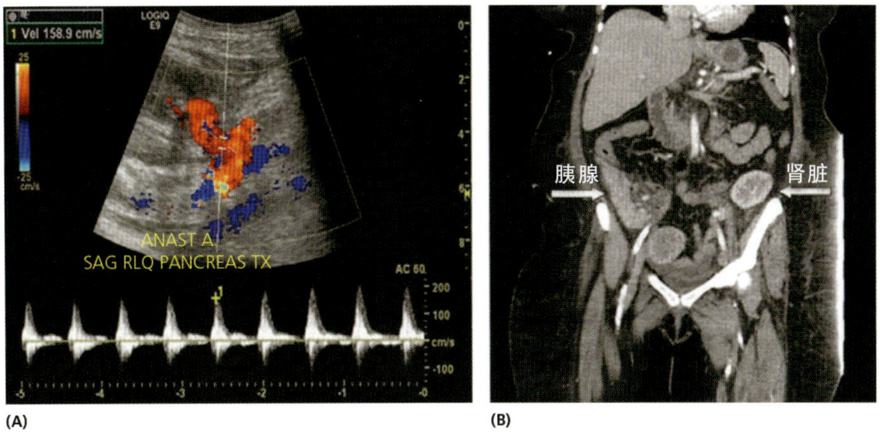

图 73.4　(A)胰腺移植血管系统的超声评估。(B)同时肾移植受体的计算机断层扫描。

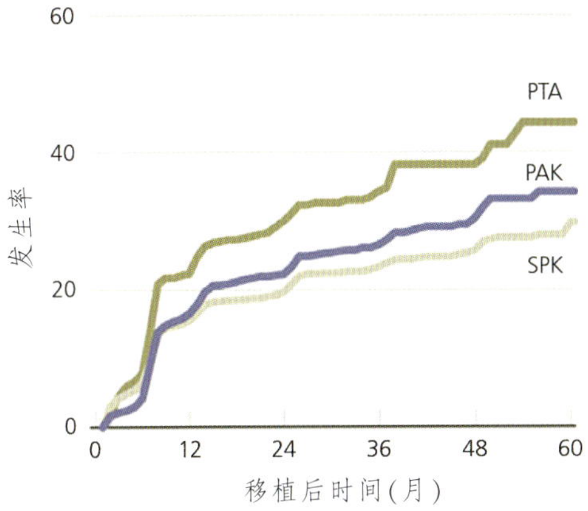

图 73.5　2005–2009 年接受胰腺移植的成年患者首例急性排斥反应发生率。(From: Organ Procurement and Transplantation Network (OPTN) and Scientific Registry of Transplant Recipients (SRTR). OPTN/SRTR 2010 Annual Data Report. Rockville, MD: Department of Health and Human Services, Health Resources and Services Administration, Healthcare Systems Bureau, Division of Transplantation, 2011.)

而 PAK 受体为 36%,PTA 受体为 40%(图 73.5)。虽然这些排斥反应分析表明，大多数发生在移植后的前 6 个月内，而后期(>6 个月)的排斥反应发生主要发生在 PAK 和 PTA 的人群。事实上，胰肾联合移植受体急性排斥反应导致的移植失败率为 0.3%，而 PAK 和 PTA 组分别为 1.8%和 2.9%。那些有多个急性排斥反应的受体，发生慢性排斥的风险显著增加。所以适当和及时地通过医疗机构给予胰腺移植受体抗排斥治疗很有必要。因为 PTA 和 PAK 受体增加了急性排斥反应概率，因此和胰肾联合移植患者相比有较高的风险发生慢性排斥反应。后者可能由于缺少像 PTA 和 PAK 受体中排斥反应的标记物，相比在 SPK 受体肾移植中，可以更敏感地提示急性排斥，从而防止延误诊断或治疗。尽管提高免疫抑制方案，减少了单独胰腺移植受体排斥反应发生率，急性排斥反应的累积效应在慢性排斥反应中的发展已被证明[14]。这类患者被认为可以受益于前瞻性监测活组织切片检查，可早期检测移植排斥反应，从而使移植物和受体长期共存[15]。虽然活组织切片检查时间在不同机构间不尽相同，一般认为可以在 3 个月、6 个月和 12 个月时进行活检。

细胞介导排斥反应

依据组织病理学评估，2008 年专家共识将胰腺移植中细胞介导的急性排斥反应程度分为轻度（Ⅰ级)、中度(Ⅱ级)或重度(Ⅲ级)[16]。在获得组织病理学结果之前，最初治疗需要达到钙调蛋白抑制剂和 MMF 的最大药物浓度，以免延误治疗。明确发生了急性细胞排斥反应后，针对Ⅱ级和Ⅲ级排斥可以用 T 细胞耗竭疗法，而对于Ⅰ级排斥，可以首先采用激素冲击治疗。在后一种情况下，冲击治疗失败应及时转而利用 T 细胞耗竭疗法来治疗Ⅰ级排斥。排斥反应相关或医源性高剂量类固醇给药相关的高血糖患者，应予以饮食调整和胰岛素治疗。达到正常的血糖浓度，血清淀粉酶/脂肪酶标准水平，以及排斥反应额外的相关症状(移植的疼痛、肿胀、发热)，可作为有效的治疗干预的指标。Ⅰ级急性细胞排斥反应患者的治疗有效率接近 90%，Ⅱ级排斥反应下降到 71%~85%，Ⅲ级排斥反应小于 50%。症状无缓解或仅有局部效果的患者，应及时做进一步处理：①考虑抗体介导的排斥反应(见下文)；②进一步升级免疫抑制和(或)③再次行胰腺移植物活检。

抗体介导排斥反应

不仅对于胰腺移植,同时在其他实体器官移植中,抗体介导的排斥反应越来越受到广泛重视。胰腺排斥Banff分级模式在2011年进行了更新，引入了抗体介导排斥反应 [17](见85章)。常规术前交叉配型和ABO血型匹配，基本上消除了抗体介导的超急性和迟发性超急性排斥反应。更令人关注的是抗体介导的急性排斥反应,通常在移植最初的几周以内[18]。存在:①同种异体移植物功能障碍；②在受体血清中供体特异性抗体;③毛细血管C4d沉积(与补体沉积一致)可用于诊断抗体介导的急性排斥反应。当不存在移植物功能障碍时，分离供体特异性抗体或分离C4d沉积的重要性仍待明确。目前,满足两个及以上标准的患者应该予以治疗。

一旦诊断明确，应制订减少抗体介导的移植损伤的治疗。目前的治疗通常包括:用抗胸腺细胞球蛋白加强T细胞耗竭、抗体介导治疗联合血浆置换、静脉注射免疫球蛋白和利妥昔单抗。其他抗体介导的治疗(硼替佐米、依库丽单抗、贝拉西普)仍需获得更广泛的认可[19]。在急性抗体介导排斥反应救治之后,应在6个月或1年期间内,连续监测供体特异性抗体的复发,同时应作移植肾活检和C4d沉积的评估。

慢性胰腺排斥反应

细胞介导排斥反应

外科技术的改善减少了因并发症导致的移植物失功,改善了胰腺移植后的存活率,同时逐步细化的免疫抑制方案和术后管理也减少了急性排斥反应发作。因此,越来越多的胰腺移植患者能长期存活,这使得慢性排斥导致的胰腺移植物丢失逐渐受到重视[12]。慢性排斥反应的临床表现常为移植后晚期出现血糖控制失调。与急性胰腺排斥反应不同,血清淀粉酶/脂肪酶升高较为少见[13]。糖化血红蛋白水平的增高和C肽水平下降常预示移植慢性丢失。同种异体移植物活检能够发现慢性排斥反应中移植物硬化和实质细胞功能性损伤。移植后再次出现高血糖状态,即使移植物未发生纤维化,但如果存在胰岛炎症和β细胞丢失的证据,仍可预示复发性自身免疫性疾病和移植物丧失。一项单中心研究报道了通过强化免疫抑制来临时缓解胰腺移植物反复受到的自身免疫性疾病的影响[20],但目前仍无能够逆转慢性排斥反应的有效方法。后者更需要通过激进的方案来控制急性排斥反应，因为急性排斥的发作次数及严重程度与发生慢性排斥反应的风险及移植失败相关[13]。

抗体介导的排斥反应

抗体介导的胰腺移植物慢性排斥反应的机制可以通过移植物组织病理学检查发现的纤维化、间质毛细血管C4d染色阳性及出现供体特异性抗体等来明确[17]。临床表现类似于通过细胞介导的慢性排斥反应，常常是患者逐渐再次出现高血糖状态。不幸的是,像细胞介导的慢性排斥反应一样，抗体介导的排斥反应目前还没有有效的治疗方法，目前的预防手段仍以积极检测和控制急性排斥反应为主。

同种异体胰岛移植的免疫原性——历史的视角

糖尿病患者胰岛替代的起源始于19世纪末，有报道将羊胰腺提取物进行移植,但未取得临床成功[21]。虽然当前的胰岛移植的临床发展与胰腺移植相接近,但它的临床应用仍相对缓慢和有限。1972年,Ballinger等人通过胰岛异种移植逆转了链脲佐菌素诱导的大鼠糖尿病,奠定了现代胰岛替代治疗的基础[22]。明尼苏达大学随后在临床上对一例几乎全胰腺切除的患者进行了成功的自体胰岛移植[23,24]。接着依靠无类固醇免疫抑制方案(埃德蒙顿方案)带来的优势,同种异体移植也有了成功的报道[25]。但仍须获得多个胰腺供体才能使受体摆脱胰岛素依赖[26]。不幸的是,长期随访中,在最初不依赖胰岛素的胰岛移植受体中,2年内有超过80%的受体转变为胰岛素依赖。此外,许多受体变得高敏,可能是由于接受多个供体的同种异体移植而排斥的结果。进一步优化合适的供体选择和胰岛分离的技术改进将有助于依靠单个胰腺供体来实现非胰岛素依赖的成功。此外,不采用钙调神经磷酸酶抑制剂和类固醇激素的共刺激分子联合阻断方案 (贝拉西普或依法利珠单抗)被证实不但可促进胰岛细胞长期存活,同时与钙调神经磷酸酶抑制剂对β细胞和肾脏毒性无关[27]。后一个方案包括在胰岛移植时采用 T 细胞耗竭疗法，后续用霉酚酸酯或西罗莫司免疫抑制，联合共刺激分子阻断抗体。胰岛移植更全面的讨论见第 61 章。

胰岛移植物失功能——排斥与胰岛“耗尽”

虽然胰岛移植的临床成功，可以由糖尿病状态的逆转来评估，但门静脉注射后的胰岛移植物的组织病理学评估仍然比较困难。胰岛移植后经皮肝穿刺活检是可行的，但其实际应用价值有限，因为只有在 31%的活检标本中可以识别出胰岛细胞[28]。与胰岛功能或排斥反应相关的移植后胰岛移植物的非侵入性成像目前尚未正式确立[29]。因为无法通过组织病理学评估确认胰岛移植是否成功，所以移植后胰岛素需求的程度，以及血清 C 肽、糖化血红蛋白、葡萄糖水平等均作为间接指标。

由于无法准确将输入到门脉系统的胰岛细胞成像，难以确定胰岛移植物失功的原因是排斥反应还是非免疫介导的损失(即“耗尽”)。有人推测，胰岛失功可能与胰岛在缺乏前体细胞或干细胞的情况下难以更替 β 细胞有关。然而，最近通过胰岛移植后诱导淋巴细胞耗竭取得了移植物长期存活，表明早期埃德蒙顿研究中移植物失功可能是由于免疫抑制治疗不充分，而不是早期胰岛“耗尽”。事实上，利用更为严格的免疫抑制方案的单中心研究结果发现，高达 66%的胰岛移植受体脱离胰岛素依赖的平均时间达到 3 年以上[30]。目前大多数的临床胰岛试验使用了诱导淋巴细胞耗竭和更积极免疫抑制方案，反映了对控制 Ⅰ 型糖尿病患者 β 细胞替代治疗后免疫反应的顾虑。这预示着胰腺实体器官移植后免疫抑制方案向着更积极转变，并有必要同时控制同种免疫和自身免疫反应。采用淋巴细胞耗竭策略的胰岛移植的长期胰岛素依赖率和胰腺移植相近。

胰岛排斥反应

虽然有大量文献报道了啮齿动物和大型动物模型有关胰岛移植和排斥反应的，但是有关人类急性或慢性排斥反应的组织病理学评价的信息却非常有限。基于鼠胰岛移植的研究，似乎胰岛排斥是通过抗原呈递的间接通路驱动的(参见第 5 章关于间接通路的详细论述)。虽然明显缺乏关于人类胰岛移植排斥反应途径的研究数据，但在胰岛移植临床病例中仍可看到同种免疫反应发挥着作用[31]。

临床胰岛排斥反应的诊断，无论是急性还是慢性排斥反应，完全是基于一个复发的高血糖状态，根据其程度确定是急性或慢性的过程。增强免疫抑制是必要的，考虑到治疗针对的是抗体介导的排斥反应，应在术后检测供体特异性抗体[32]。

总结

全胰腺移植是治疗糖尿病安全且持久的治疗方法。持续且积极地监测、治疗急性排斥反应是应对慢性排斥反应导致移植失败的唯一策略，特别是具有高排斥风险的单一胰腺移植。虽然胰岛移植还处于实验阶段，而且缺乏组织病理学检查手段以评估移植后胰岛细胞，但仍可通过限定单一供体来源、积极的免疫抑制治疗达到长期疗效。在未来，胰岛细胞分离的改进、对各种胰岛细胞来源的研究(干细胞来源 β 细胞)、新的安全有效的免疫抑制剂都将会为胰岛细胞移植带来更多的治疗选择。

(刘原兴 译　刘原兴 校)

参考文献

1. Kelly WD, Lillehei RC, Merkel FK, et al. Allotransplantation of the pancreas and duodenum along with the kidney in diabetic nephropathy. Surgery. 1967;61:827–837.
2. Gruessner AC. 2011 update on pancreas transplantation: comprehensive trend analysis of 25,000 cases followed up over the course of twenty-four years at the International Pancreas Transplant Registry (IPTR). Review of Diabetic Studies. 2011;8:6–16.
3. Gruessner AC, Sutherland DE. Pancreas transplant outcomes for United States (US) cases as reported to the United Network for Organ Sharing (UNOS) and the International Pancreas Transplant Registry (IPTR). Clinical Transplants. 2008:45–56.
4. Klassen DK, Hoen-Saric EW, Weir MR, et al. Isolated pancreas rejection in combined kidney pancreas transplantation. Transplantation. 1996;61:974–977.
5. Hawthorne WJ, Allen RD, Greenberg ML, et al. Simultaneous pancreas and kidney transplant rejection: separate or synchronous events? Transplantation. 1997;63:352–358.
6. Dachman AH, Newmark GM, Thistlethwaite JR Jr, et al. Imaging of pancreatic transplantation using portal venous and enteric exocrine drainage. AJR. American Journal of Roentgenology. 1998;171:157–163.
7. Gaber DO, Gaber LW, Shokouh-Amiri MR, et al. Percutaneous biopsy of pancreas transplants. Transplantation. 1992;54:548–550.
8. Klassen DK, Weir MR, Cangro CB, et al. Pancreas allograft biopsy: safety of percutaneous biopsy-results of a large experience. Transplantation. 2002;73:553–555.
9. Malek SK, Potdar S, Martin JA, et al. Percutaneous ultrasound-guided pancreas allograft biopsy: a single-center experience. Transplantation Proceedings. 2005;37:4436–4437.
10. Kayler LK, Merion RM, Rudich SM, et al. Evaluation of pancreatic allograft dysfunction by laparoscopic biopsy. Transplantation. 2002;74:1287–1289.
11. Benedetti E, Najarian JS, Gruessner AC, et al. Correlation between cystoscopic biopsy results and hypoamylasuria in bladder-drained pancreas transplants. Surgery. 1995;118:864–872.

12. Humar A, Khwaja K, Ramcharan T, et al. Chronic rejection: the next major challenge for pancreas transplant recipients. Transplantation. 2003;76:918–923.
13. Papadimitriou JC, Drachenberg CB, Klassen DK, et al. Histological grading of chronic pancreas allograft rejection/graft sclerosis. American Journal of Transplantation. 2003;3:599–605.
14. Odorico JS, Becker YT, Groshek M. Improved solitary pancreas transplant graft survival in the modern immunosuppressive era. Cell Transplantation. 2000;9: 919–927.
15. Stratta RJ, Taylor RJ, Grune MT, et al. Experience with protocol biopsies after solitary pancreastransplantation. Transplantation. 1995;60:1431–1437.
16. Drachenberg CB, Odorico J, Demetris AJ, et al. Banff schema for grading pancreas allograft rejection: working proposal by a multi-disciplinary international consensus panel. American Journal of Transplantation. 2008;8:1237–1249.
17. Drachenberg CB, Odorico J, Demetris AJ, et al. Guidelines for the diagnosis of antibody-mediated rejection in pancreas allografts-updated Banff grading schema. American Journal of Transplantation. 2011;11:1792–1802.
18. Melcher ML, Olson JL, Baxter-Lowe LA, et al. Antibody-mediated rejection of a pancreas allograft. American Journal of Transplantation. 2006;6:423–428.
19. Stegall MD, Gloor JM. Deciphering antibody-mediated rejection: new insights into mechanisms and treatment. Current Opinion in Organ Transplantation. 2010;15:8–10.
20. Burke GW 3rd, Vendrame F, Pileggi A, et al. Recurrence of autoimmunity following pancreas transplantation. Current Diabetes Reports. 2011;11:413–419.
21. Williams PW. Notes on diabetes treated with extract and by grafts of sheep's pancreas. British Medical Journal. 1894;2:1303–1304.
22. Ballinger WF, Lacy PE. Transplantation of intact pancreatic islets in rats. Surgery. 1972;72:175–186.
23. Sutherland DE, Matas AJ, Goetz FC, et al. Transplantation of dispersed pancreatic islet tissue in humans: autografts and allografts. Diabetes. 1980;29(Suppl. 1):31–44.
24. Najarian JS, Sutherland DE, Baumgartner D, et al. Total or near total pancreatectomy and islet autotransplantation for treatment of chronic pancreatitis. Annals of Surgery. 1980;192:526–542.
25. Largiader F, Kolb E, Binswanger U. A long-term functioning human pancreatic islet allotransplant. Transplantation. 1980;29:76–77.
26. Shapiro AMJ, Lakey JRT, Ryan EA, et al. Islet transplantation in seven patients with type 1 diabetes mellitus using a glucocorticoid-free immunosuppressive regimen. New England Journal of Medicine. 2000;343:230–238.
27. Posselt AM, Szot GL, Frassetto LA, et al. Islet transplantation in type 1 diabetic patients using calcineurin inhibitor-free immunosuppressive protocols based on T-cell adhesion or costimulation blockade. Transplantation. 2010;90: 1595–1601.
28. Toso C, Isse K, Demetris AJ, et al. Histologic graft assessment after clinical islet transplantation. Transplantation. 2009;88:1286–1293.
29. Gaglia JL. Noninvasive imaging of islet transplantation and rejection. Current Diabetes Reports. 2007;7:309–313.
30. Bellin MD, Kandaswamy R, Parkey J, et al. Prolonged insulin independence after islet allotransplants in recipients with type 1 diabetes. American Journal of Transplantation. 2008;8:2463–2470.
31. Naziruddin B, Wease S, Stablein D, et al. HLA class I sensitization in islet transplant recipients—report from the collaborative islet transplant registry. Cell Transplantation. 2012;21:901–908.
32. Kessler L, Parissiadis A, Bayle F, et al. Evidence for humoral rejection of a pancreatic islet graft and rescue with rituximab and IV immunoglobulin therapy. American Journal of Transplantation. 2009;9:1961–1966.

第 74 章
小肠移植临床排斥反应综合征

Andreas Tzakis, Gennaro Selvaggi, Akin Tekin, Jennifer Garcia, Ji Fan, Phil Ruiz Jr

引言

排斥反应是小肠移植后的重要并发症之一，是导致术后死亡率、发病率、移植物功能丧失的主要原因，仅次于败血症(常继发于移植反应的治疗)[1-5]。严重的急性排斥反应可以呈剥脱样进展：由于广泛上皮损伤导致大段小肠黏膜剥脱[6,7]。这种形式的严重排斥反应与患者不良预后密切相关。

小肠移植物易产生排斥反应的原因多种多样，包括小肠壁组织与细胞具有多样性、肠系膜和肠道黏膜下层聚集大量具有免疫功能的造血细胞与淋巴细胞，以及肠腔内细菌对免疫应答的激活[8,9]。此外，排斥反应继发肠道黏膜上皮完整性的破坏可使肠道细菌异位，并进一步发展为败血症，后者曾是急性排斥期的唯一先兆[10]。排斥反应还阻碍对药物浓度的控制，因此治疗效果欠佳。

小肠移植物的急性排斥反应可发生于术后任何时间，表现为细胞排斥或体液排斥。慢性排斥反应可发展为意想不到的长期并发症，更常见于急性排斥反应反复发作后。本文将讨论不同形式小肠移植排斥反应的临床表现及治疗。有关小肠移植排斥反应的组织病理学内容详见第 86 章。

急性细胞排斥

小肠移植受体最常见的排斥反应是急性细胞排斥反应(ACR)，早期文献指出，高达 60%~70%的患者至少经历一个阶段的急性细胞排斥反应[1,2,5]。近期文献指出，诱导治疗后排斥率可降至 30%[3,4]。ACR 可发生于术后任何时间段，移植后多年仍可出现，但最常见于术后早期。早期急性排斥反应通常见于术后 2~4 周，70%以上的各期排斥反应发生于移植后 1 年内[11]。据报道，肝-小肠联合移植较单独的小肠移植发生 ACR 的概率降低[2,4,12,13]。有证据表明，即使在没有肝脏保护的情况下，多器官移植也可以提供一些保护[3,11]。

ACR 的严重程度可根据病理分为轻度、中度和重度[14,15]。病理诊断为“可疑排斥反应”(可疑但不符合轻度 ACR 的诊断标准) 则需要结合内镜检查及临床表现，必要时可再次行内镜下活检以明确诊断，患者无内镜表现和临床症状而仅有病理改变，可诊断为“亚临床排斥反应”，该情况须引起重视，若不进行治疗则与不良预后相关[16]。

排斥反应的病程与其严重程度相关。轻度排斥反应通常持续约 1 周，程度加重则病程加倍，即中度 ACR 持续约 2 周，重度 ACR 持续约 1 个月[11]。病程延长超过 45 天与移植物功能丧失密切相关[11]。

症状

早期小肠移植排斥反应常缺乏症状，症状通常于进展期出现，包括造口输出增加、腹胀、腹痛、发热及败血症。造口输出不仅可出现体积增加，并且可出现性状改变，即呈水样。造口输出减少和血性造口输出是晚期的严重征象。严重的剥脱样排斥反应中，凝胶状纤维蛋白和肠道黏膜可经吻合口排出。腹痛剧烈，呈持续性，并对止痛药反应欠佳。腹胀通常出现于回肠、肠系膜、小肠壁水肿的患者。发热几乎与 ACR 伴随出现，与全身性的炎症反应或细菌异位导致的重叠感染有关。发热患者不可忽视，需要立即行内镜检查，延误治疗 24 小时即可显著影响预后。感染期，尤其是病毒性肠炎亦可出现发热，因此及早行内镜检查及活检明确诊断十分重要。

诊断

ACR 的诊断金标准为内镜下肠黏膜评估及多点病

理活检[1-5,8,11]。根据移植后时间长短的不同，患者应通过回肠造口或消化道自然开口行内镜检查。其目标是尽可能到达并评估回肠末端黏膜，因为回肠是ACR最容易累及的部位。胃肠道不同部位发生排斥反应的概率各不相同。一篇有关多器官移植标本排斥反应的相对频率的报道显示，ACR在小肠的检出率为25.5%，胃为12.2%，大肠为16%。ACR患者在小肠检出的相对频率为80.0%，胃为38.5%，大肠为33.3%[17]。若内镜不能到达回肠末端，可取邻近空肠标本代替。

即使排斥反应已累及回肠末端，仍可有某些区域不受累（"跳过区域"），因此回肠镜检须覆盖一定长度（至少15~20cm），并在不同水平行多点活检。所见异常区域均应取样，并取所见正常区域样本用于对照。溃疡区域应在边缘处取活检，效果优于在溃疡中心取样。单纯内镜诊断有助于排除肠黏膜的大体改变。可适应大范围镜检的患者，使用肠黏膜放大内镜可更深层次评估患者的小肠绒毛长度、形状变化，以及黏膜红斑及脆性[18]。

干血斑检测血清瓜氨酸值有助于ACR诊断。移植后约3个月，瓜氨酸值从一个稳定的基线水平[19,20]突然降至基线值以下或绝对值低于13~15μmol/L与中度和重度的排斥反应密切相关[19,21]。血清瓜氨酸值与肾移植后的血清尿素氮、肌酐值和肝移植后的肝功能指标相似，这些指标并不是ACR的特异性指标，因为它们可能与感染、缺血等其他原因有关，所以需要通过内镜检查及活检进一步确诊。此外，钙卫蛋白也可作为替代非侵入性标记帮助诊断[22]。

近期相关分析表明，供者特异性抗体（DSA）和群体反应性抗体（PRA）的变化趋势与急性细胞排斥反应、混合细胞排斥反应和体液排斥反应的存在以及对治疗的反应有关[23,24]。

近期研究在外周血与小肠移植受体的黏膜活检中寻找排斥反应的替代标志物[25,26]。在外周血的相关研究中，取排斥反应不同时期的外周血标本与同时期的黏膜标本进行比较，作者发现多种翻译相关的蛋白质基因有明显的表达下调，其中核糖体蛋白L13a（RPL13a）在排斥反应中变化最为明显[25]。假说认为该反应可能发生于排斥反应早期，该试验可作为排斥反应的潜在非侵入性标志。

另一项研究中，将病理确认患有或未患有ACR患者的组织标本，通过福尔马林固定后进行石蜡切片。通过基因芯片（SAM）证实，排斥组和非排斥组的患者在基因模式上存在差异。在排斥组，患者体内特异性白细胞表面标记物及某些化学因子和共刺激因子相对过表达[26]。

至今尚缺乏高度特异性的标志物可代替病理诊断作为诊断的金标准。

ACR须与由病毒或细菌引起的感染性肠炎相鉴别，在这类疾病中，病理只能作为鉴别的辅助手段。须进行病毒，感染检测包括全身性病毒（EB病毒、巨细胞病毒）、呼吸道病毒和肠道病毒，并收集粪便标本检测常规病原体如艰难梭状芽孢杆菌、隐孢子虫、鞭毛虫和其他寄生虫。

ACR的最终诊断应结合临床指标、症状及病理。一旦确诊，应及时治疗。

治疗

ACR的经验治疗可选用糖皮质激素制剂，适用于暂时无条件转送移植中心或行内镜检查的患者。

ACR的规范治疗基于三大原则：逐渐加量的免疫抑制治疗、类固醇和抗淋巴细胞药物治疗及抗生素治疗预防机会性感染。

一线免疫抑制药物（常为他克莫司）从初始低剂量逐渐加量至移植后即刻水平（15~20ng/mL）。必须指出的是，移植排斥反应出现后，肠黏膜对药物的吸收能力增强，肠上皮细胞对药物代谢能力降低，可导致患者体内他克莫司水平急剧升高。

其次，戒断性使用类固醇激素用于控制轻度排斥反应，抗淋巴细胞药物如球蛋白、阿伦单抗则用于中、重度排斥反应，疗程作用几天至2~3周不等，直至ACR获得临床及病理缓解。耐激素治疗的排斥反应可选用抗肿瘤坏死因子单克隆抗体（英夫利昔单抗）[27]。有血管形成的排斥反应及有抗体调节的排斥反应（常伴DSA/PRA比值升高）可通过抑制体液免疫进行干预：如B细胞CD20单克隆抗体利妥昔单抗，血浆置换清除循环抗体并静脉注射免疫球蛋白（IVIG）、蛋白酶体抑制剂硼替佐米等[28,29]。此外，二线免疫抑制药物如西罗莫司可抑制成纤维细胞增殖并延缓损伤移植物的纤维化进程，可用于需要长时间高水平免疫抑制治疗和可能出现慢性排斥反应的患者[30]。

ACR的第三个治疗原则是使用足量抗生素，小肠黏膜完整性破坏细菌移位发生率升高，强免疫抑制剂的作用使得患者暴露于机会性感染，接受抗淋巴细胞药物治疗的患者须经验性使用抗真菌和抗病毒药物预防巨细胞病毒或 EB 病毒感染或复发，以及针对肠道厌氧菌和耐药菌，如耐万古霉素肠球菌(VRE)的抗生素。值得注意的是，败血症是许多患者发生 ACR 的最初征兆，因此经验性抗生素治疗常先于 ACR 的诊断。

排斥反应无法控制且情况不断恶化的患者可选择移植物切除术，切除导致细菌移位及继发感染的无功能移植物，迅速脱离免疫抑制状态，改善患者状况，为再次移植提供机会[4,7]。但在肝-小肠联合移植及其他多器官联合移植的病例中，完整切除移植物并不可行，单独切除小肠保留其余异体移植物(肝-小肠联合移植保留肝脏，肝-胃-胰腺联合移植保留其余脏器)排斥反应发生率较低。移植小肠切除后仍可成功进行小肠再移植。移植小肠切除术前，通过介入放射学对移植物动脉进行有效的术前栓塞，可减少术中出血，并有助于明确移植物与固有小肠的分界线[31]。

预后

轻度排斥反应可短期内治愈，移植小肠一般不残留功能障碍。重度 ACR、长时间中度 ACR 及反复发作的 ACR 移植物与患者生存预后明显不佳[11]。重度排斥反应中最恶性的剥脱性排斥反应的移植物功能丧失发生率超过 50%，患者发病率与死亡率显著升高[4,6,7]。

并发感染是导致接受治疗的 ACR 患者最常见的直接死亡原因。常见的有肺部的病毒性或细菌性感染(儿童尤为多见)、中心静脉导管感染和(或)细菌移位导致的感染。

虽然 ACR 可以被成功治愈，其中期与长期预后仍令人担忧：治疗后数周乃至数月，病毒感染发生率极高，若患者出现 EB 病毒复发则可能发生移植后淋巴增生性疾病(PTLD)。

ACR 可导致慢性移植排斥反应，相关内容将在其他章节详述。

其他类型的急性排斥反应

抗体介导的急性排斥反应

抗体介导的急性排斥反应由特异性抗体介导，主要攻击移植小肠内皮，导致微血栓和血栓形成，导致移植物缺血损伤[32]。18%~30%等待小肠移植的患者的特异性抗体呈高水平[33]，以及移植后新增供体特异性抗体(DSA)的患者有发生体液或混合细胞/体液排斥反应的倾向。因移植物功能丧失而再次接受移植的患者为曾致敏的患者，其预成型抗体或 DSA 滴度较高[34,35]。

术中超急性排斥反应表现为移植小肠的突然淤血、变色、水肿及动脉搏动消失，移植后数分钟内发生典型超急性排斥反应综合征十分罕见，少数病例报道变色、淤血及移植物快速功能丧失。作者曾目睹一例相关的体液排斥反应，阿仑单抗、利妥昔单抗和血浆置换治疗疗效较好，患者后续恢复平稳，移植 5 年后移植物功能仍旧完善[36]。

移植后数天至数周出现的快速进展的细胞排斥反应更常见，也越来越被人们所熟知，并伴有 PRA、DSA 的升高及特征性病理变化。加速急性排斥反应可在移植后数天内出现，伴有腹胀、无力、血性造口输出或无造口输出，内镜下可见黏膜淤血、红斑及脆性增加。

体液排斥反应(急性抗体介导的排斥反应)的病理表现不如 ACR 明确，但有越来越多的病理学证据显示体液介导的排斥反应通过破坏小、中血管而破坏移植物，可加速同期 ACR 进展或单独引起移植物亚临床损伤并导致慢性排斥反应。体液排斥反应尚无明确的临床症状或体征，病理出现淤血、血管固有层内 C4d、C3d 复合物沉积，可提示病情进展，尤其是患者 DSA、PRA 滴度持续升高[34]。

第三种综合征表现为抗体水平逐渐升高但无排斥反应证据，对于此种情况目前尚无标准化治疗方案，应密切观察抗体水平，对曾致敏患者或有反复排斥反应病史的患者进行治疗。

抗体液排斥反应的治疗常与抗 ACR 治疗同时进行，增加针对体液免疫机制的治疗方法如联合血浆置换、静脉注射免疫球蛋白、利妥昔单抗或硼替佐米。持续性细胞排斥反应或高抗体滴度为不良预兆。

在罕见的超急性或加速急性排斥反应病例中，移植物切除往往难以避免，药物治疗应积极使用抗胸腺蛋白，联合血浆置换、利妥昔单抗及其他针对抗体介导的免疫应答的治疗。

慢性排斥反应

约 15%接受小肠移植的患者会出现慢性排斥反应[4]。

危险因素包括既往 ACR 发生的次数及病程，尤其为中、重度 ACR，病毒感染及既往 PTLD 病史[4,37]。

慢性排斥反应的症状和体征不容易被发现，患者常出现慢性吸收不良伴排便增加，偶有脂肪泻，需要频繁补液的脱水及反复腹胀、腹痛。患者小肠绒毛平坦，内镜下黏膜正常或基本正常。小肠吸收功能异常需肠外营养。慢性排斥反应可导致移植肠道狭窄及反复小肠梗阻。

影像学显示肠道肥厚、黏膜皱襞减少，肠蠕动减弱、呈铅管样外观，少数病例可出现术中包裹性腹膜硬化。由于小肠黏膜活检标本过于浅表，难以评估黏膜基层小、中型血管情况[38]。大多数关于慢性排斥反应的研究以死亡后的外植体和切除后的移植物为对象进行组织病理分析[17,27]。这是由于肠黏膜活检过于浅表难以评估位于肠壁的黏膜肌层内的较小和中等尺寸的血管。故慢性排斥反应仅能通过黏膜纤维化、隐窝缺失间接诊断，或移植物切除后对肠壁全层进行分析[39]。

部分患者有局部肠梗阻，以回肠末端多见。少数病例可尝试切除局部受累肠段以保留剩余肠段及其余移植脏器，但更多情况下需要完整切除移植物。完整切除移植物术前建议先行栓塞术，有助于明确移植物与固有肠段分界、减少出血[31]。

总结

排斥反应是所有小肠移植患者术后管理的重要问题，排斥反应造成显著发病率、死亡率，且会导致患者长期生存率降低。近年来，取得的医疗进步已大大降低了排斥反应发生率。移植后 1 年内使用抗胸腺蛋白或白细胞介素-2 受体抑制剂予以诱导治疗已成为广泛共识，临床高度怀疑的病例则须行维持治疗。各种排斥反应均须通过内镜检查和病理活检明确诊断，非侵入性标志物仅具有参考价值。排斥反应的早期积极治疗可预防病情进展和移植物功能丧失，注意还应同时处理并发的感染。目前预防慢性排斥反应及治疗抗体介导的排斥反应的方法尚未明确，监测及调节受体体液免疫应答日益重要，DSA/PRA 水平分析、移植交叉配型、致敏患者的脱敏治疗及利妥昔单抗和硼替佐米等药物治疗应成为目前小肠移植后患者的标准治疗。

（周舒扬 杨梦凡 译 周舒扬 校）

参考文献

1. Todo S, Reyes J, Furukawa H, et al. Outcome analysis of 71 intestinal transplantations. Annals of Surgery. 1995;222:270–282.
2. Abu-Elmagd K, Reyes J, Bond G, et al. Clinical intestinal transplantation: a decade of a single center experience. Annals of Surgery. 2001;234:404–417.
3. Tzakis AG, Kato T, Levi DM, et al. 100 multivisceral transplants at a single center. Annals of Surgery. 2005;242:480–493.
4. Abu-Elmagd K, Costa G, Bond GJ, et al. Five hundred intestinal and multivisceral transplantations at a single center. Annals of Surgery. 2009;250:567–581.
5. Grant D, Abu-Elmagd K, Reyes J, et al. Report of the intestine transplant registry: a new era has dawned. Annals of Surgery. 2005;241:607–613.
6. Kato T, Ruiz P, Tzakis A. Exfoliative bowel rejection–a dangerous loss of integrity. Pediatric Transplantation. 2004;8:426–427.
7. Ishii T, Mazariegos GV, Bueno J, et al. Exfoliative rejection after intestinal transplantation in children. Pediatric Transplantation. 2003;7:185–191.
8. Fishbein TM. Intestinal transplantation. New England Journal of Medicine. 2009;361:998–1008.
9. Iwaki Y, Starzl TE, Yagihashi A, et al. Replacement of donor lymphoid tissue in small-bowel transplants. Lancet. 1991;337:818–819.
10. Cicalese L, Sileri P, Green M, et al. Bacterial translocation in clinical intestinal transplantation. Transplantation. 2001;71:1414–1417.
11. Selvaggi G, Gaynor JJ, Moon J, et al. Analysis of acute cellular rejection episodes in recipients of primary intestinal transplantation: a single center, 11 year experience. American Journal of Transplantation. 2007;7:1249–1257.
12. Calne RY, Sells RA, Pena JR, et al. Induction of immunological tolerance by porcine liver allografts. Nature. 1969;223:472.
13. Calne R, Davis H. Organ graft tolerance: the liver effect. Lancet. 1994;343:67–68.
14. Ruiz P, Bagni A, Brown R, et al. Histological criteria for the identification of acute cellular rejection in human small bowel allografts: results of the pathology workshop at the VIII International Small Bowel Transplant Symposium. Transplantation Proceedings. 2004;36:335–337.
15. Ruiz P, Takahashi H, Delacruz V, et al. International grading scheme for acute cellular rejection in small-bowel transplantation: single center experience. Transplantation Proceedings. 2010;42:47–53.
16. Takahashi H, Kato T, Selvaggi G, et al. Subclinical rejection in the initial postoperative period in small intestinal transplantation: a negative influence on graft survival. Transplantation. 2007;84:689–696.
17. Takahashi H, Kato T, Delacruz V, et al. Analysis of acute and chronic rejection in multiple organ allografts from retransplantation and autopsy cases of multivisceral transplantation. Transplantation. 2008;85:610–616.
18. Kato T, Gaynor JJ, Nishida S, et al. Zoom endoscopic monitoring of small bowel allograft rejection. Surgical Endoscopy. 2006;20:773–782.
19. David AI, Selvaggi G, Ruiz P, et al. Blood citrulline level is an exclusionary marker for significant acute rejection after intestinal transplantation. Transplantation. 2007;84:1077–1081.
20. Pappas PA, Tzakis AG, Gaynor JJ, et al. An analysis of the association between serum citrulline and acute rejection among 26 recipients of intestinal transplant. American Journal of Transplantation. 2004;4:1124–1132.
21. Ruiz P, Tryphonopoulos P, Island E, et al. Citrulline evaluation in bowel transplantation. Transplantation Proceedings. 2010;42:54–56.
22. Mercer DF, Vargas L, Sun Y, et al. Stool calprotectin monitoring after small intestine transplantation. Transplantation. 2011;91:1166–1171.
23. Tsai HL, Island ER, Chang JW, et al. Association between donor-specific antibodies and acute rejection and resolution in small bowel and multivisceral transplantation. Transplantation. 2011;92:709–715.
24. Gonzalez-Pinto IM, Tzakis AG, Tsai HL, et al. Association between panel reactive antibodies and acute small bowel rejection: analysis of a series of 324 intestinal transplants. Transplantation Proceedings. 2010;42:4269–4271.
25. Andreev VP, Tryphonopoulos P, Blomberg BB, et al. Peripheral blood gene expression analysis in intestinal transplantation: a feasibility study for detecting novel candidate biomarkers of graft rejection. Transplantation. 2011;92:1385–1391.
26. Asaoka T, Island ER, Tryphonopoulos P, et al. Characteristic immune, apoptosis and inflammatory gene profiles associated with intestinal acute cellular rejection in formalin-fixed paraffin-embedded mucosal biopsies. Transplant International. 2011;24:697–707.
27. Gerlach UA, Koch M, Muller HP, et al. Tumor necrosis factor alpha inhibitors as immunomodulatory antirejection agents after intestinal transplantation. American Journal of Transplantation. 2011;11:1041–1050.
28. Island ER, Gonzalez-Pinto IM, Tsai HL, et al. Successful treatment with bortezomib of a refractory humoral rejection of the intestine after multivisceral trans-

plantation. Clinical Transplants. 2009;465–469.
29. Gerlach UA, Schoenemann C, Lachmann N, et al. Salvage therapy for refractory rejection and persistence of donor-specific antibodies after intestinal transplantation using the proteasome inhibitor bortezomib. Transplant International. 2011;24:e43–e45.
30. Fishbein TM, Florman S, Gondolesi G, et al. Intestinal transplantation before and after the introduction of sirolimus. Transplatation. 2002;73:1538–1542.
31. Fan J, Tekin A, Nishida S, et al. Preoperative embolization of the graft superior mesenteric artery assists graft enterectomy in intestinal transplant recipients. Transplantation. 2012; 94:89–91.
32. Terasaki PI, Cai J. Humoral theory of transplantation: further evidence. Current Opinion in Immunology. 2005;17:541–545.
33. Wu T, Abu Elmagd K, Bond G, et al. A clinicopathologic study of isolated intestinal allografts with preformed IgG lymphocytotoxic antibodies. Human Pathology. 2004;35:1332–1339.
34. Ruiz P, Carreno M, Weppler D, et al. Immediate antibody-mediated (hyperacute) rejection in small-bowel transplantation and relationship to cross-match status and donor-specific C4d-binding antibodies: case report. Transplantation Proceedings. 2010;42:95–99.
35. Kato T, Mizutani K, Terasaki P, et al. Association of emergence of HLA antibody and acute rejection in intestinal transplant recipients: a possible evidence of acute humoral sensitization. Transplantation Proceedings. 2006;38:1735–1737.
36. Ruiz P, Carreno M, Weppler D, et al. Immediate antibody-mediated (hyperacute) rejection in small bowel transplantation and relationship to cross-match status and donor-specific C4d-binding antibodies: case report. Transplantation Proceedings. 2010;42:95–99.
37. Parizhskaya M, Redondo C, Demetris A, et al. Chronic rejection of small bowel grafts: pediatric and adult study of risk factors and morphologic progression. Pediatric and Developmental Pathology. 2003;6:240–250.
38. Ramos E, Molina M, Sarria J, et al. Chronic rejection with sclerosing peritonitis following pediatric intestinal transplantation. Pediatric Transplantation. 2007; 11:937–941.
39. Tryphonopoulos P, Weppler D, Nishida S, et al. Mucosal fibrosis in intestinal transplant biopsies correlates positively with the development of chronic rejection. Transplantation Proceedings. 2006;38:1685–1686.

第 75 章

同种异体复合组织移植临床排斥反应综合征

Matthew H. Levine，Sandy Feng

引言

约 100 例手和面部移植病例证实，即使移植物中含有具有高度免疫原性的组织如皮肤，移植后手部和面部亦不会出现不可逆排斥[1-8]。1 年后移植物存活率与其他脏器移植基本一致。单克隆或多克隆抗体联合三联免疫抑制方案的诱导治疗可预防早期的移植物功能丧失。但患者急性皮肤排斥反应发生率高于其他器官移植，而此类排斥反应可导致移植物功能丧失，曾有报道停用免疫抑制治疗后晚期急性排斥反应（AR）导致的一只手移植物功能丧失，另一只手因未进一步说明的“皮肤炎症”继发功能丧失[1,8,9]。此外，激素抵抗的排斥反应须应用抗胸腺蛋白（ATG）、巴利昔单抗或阿伦单抗治疗[1,8-10]。据报道，移植后 1 年，多数患者至少经历一次 AR，而皮肤是免疫应答的主要靶点[1-10]。某些患者移植 1 年后还可出现反复 AR[1,5-10]。

手移植 AR 的频率较高和程度严重，可归因于皮肤的高免疫原性，而皮肤是移植物的一个主要组成部分。皮肤的高抗原性在一定程度上与其高比例的有效抗原呈递细胞（朗格汉斯细胞）和角化细胞相关，二者表达 MHC Ⅰ、MHC Ⅱ、ICAM-Ⅰ，刺激后表达细胞因子[11-20]。此外，病毒感染尤其是巨细胞病毒感染也是排斥反应的诱因[21]。有假说认为，手移植的 AR 发生率高是由于观察检测相对容易而导致阳性率增高。因为移植手取样方便，活检可作为常规检查，临床疑似出现排斥反应可立即行病理组织活检以确诊。而此类情况在器官移植中可能被忽视。

临床同种异体移植物排斥反应综合征是对一个或多个组织形成的同种异体复合组织移植（VCA）免疫应答的结果。尽管皮肤排斥反应是手部和面部移植较常见的形式，也有针对组织而非皮肤免疫应答的相关报道[22-24]。

移植后 1 年内，约 85%的患者经历过至少一次急性皮肤排斥[1]。皮肤排斥反应对移植物生存率及功能的临床相关及长期影响依然未知。对来自 5 例接受手或前臂移植的患者的超过 170 例标本进行皮肤活检，发现大部分皮肤排斥反应的组织学为轻度（Ⅰ级）[25]。

本章描述了 VCA 移植后皮肤排斥反应的临床表现、诊断及治疗。由于迄今为止病例数量较少，尚不能与其他器官移植数据进行比较。组织学表现详见第 87 章。

诊断、定义及机制

皮肤排斥反应

最初 10 年，普遍认为皮肤是手部和面部移植排斥反应的主要靶点[1-10]。近期研究认为，移植物的血管亦是排斥的靶点，并可能出现肌内膜增生[23]。实际上，血管效应可能与移植物长期生存率更为相关。皮肤排斥反应常表现为局部或弥漫移植物的斑丘疹，其颜色、位置各异，伴或不伴有水肿、无甲[5,10,26]。不同于实体器官移植，有皮肤的 VCA 排斥反应可通过肉眼检查初步诊断，并可结合皮肤病理活检快速诊断。某些非排斥反应如真菌感染、自身免疫性疾病亦可出现皮疹，应注意鉴别。皮肤排斥反应的主要病理表现为免疫细胞浸润，其位置、分布、范围与排斥反应的严重程度相关。进展期还可能出现凋亡和坏死细胞/组织[9,22,26]。

手移植皮肤排斥反应的“典型”病变累及前臂和手腕的背侧和掌侧，某些病例亦可累及手背。皮肤排斥反应的表现因个体而异，同一个体的表现随病变时期不同亦有不同（图 75.1）。AR 一般表现为斑丘疹红斑皮疹，可呈弥漫性、斑片状或局灶性，伴或不伴有灼痛。病变的位置、颜色、大小随病情进展发生变化。

尽管排斥反应一般不累及手掌和指甲，但在 4 例“非典型”病例中，患者手掌皮肤与指甲有受累[10]。这些病例患者均为年轻患者，且手掌有反复、持续受压史。病变特征包括掌心皮肤干燥、红色丘疹、脱屑与苔藓样变，伴有指甲营养不良、变性、变形或脱落。该类型的排斥反应与手掌皮肤及其附属物指甲的排斥反应模式不同，通过削弱甲板使其从甲床松动脱落。此类排斥反应激素耐受的发生率高于其他排斥反应。皮肤和甲床的病理提示有大量淋巴细胞与 T 细胞（CD3+、CD4+、CD8+）与少量 B 细胞（CD20+、CD79a+）和少量 FOXP3+细胞浸润。病变可持续数周或数月，激素治疗基本无效，须使用抗胸腺细胞球蛋白、阿仑单抗和（或）强化维持免疫抑制治疗。

重复和显著的压力作用可导致手掌皮肤出现皮肤炎症和免疫应答，可能与中性粒细胞介导的免疫应答及 AR 相关[27]。

任何 VCA 上的特定大小、位置与进展方式的皮肤红斑在未确诊时都应排除排斥反应。鉴别诊断包括皮肤感染、类天疱疮、其他皮肤炎症和充血（通常不伴有皮疹），应进行皮肤活检。

皮肤排斥反应的机制

根据实验、临床和病理学评估，VCA 的 AR 主要针对皮肤，尤其是表皮的细胞介导的免疫应答，主导细胞为 CD4+、CD8+或 CD3+ T 细胞目前仍有争议，VCA 皮肤排斥反应中细胞浸润的原型主要为 CD3 T 细胞[28-30]。轻度至中度皮肤排斥反应的细胞浸润中巨噬细胞可占 10%~50%，Ⅳ级排斥反应的主要浸润细胞为 CD68+巨噬细胞。

对手部及面部移植物的深入病理学分析显示，皮肤排斥是一个动态的、多步骤的过程，T 细胞（主要为 CD3+ T 细胞）穿过血管壁后形成皮肤免疫细胞浸润，位于血管周围区域[29]。炎症细胞扩散至真皮层。在多种细胞因子的作用下，细胞开始向表皮浸润。激活的角化细胞可分泌大量促炎症因子，进一步募集炎症细胞。单个角化细胞坏死及凋亡[29]，可导致真皮-表皮的脱离及表皮脱落，是皮肤排斥反应的最终级联步骤[9,26,29]。在动物模型中，因为移植物和皮肤缺损的大小有限，移植物边缘皮肤可再生，使得缺损皮肤得以重建[30]。

人类移植手的黏附分子的研究表明，E 选择素、P

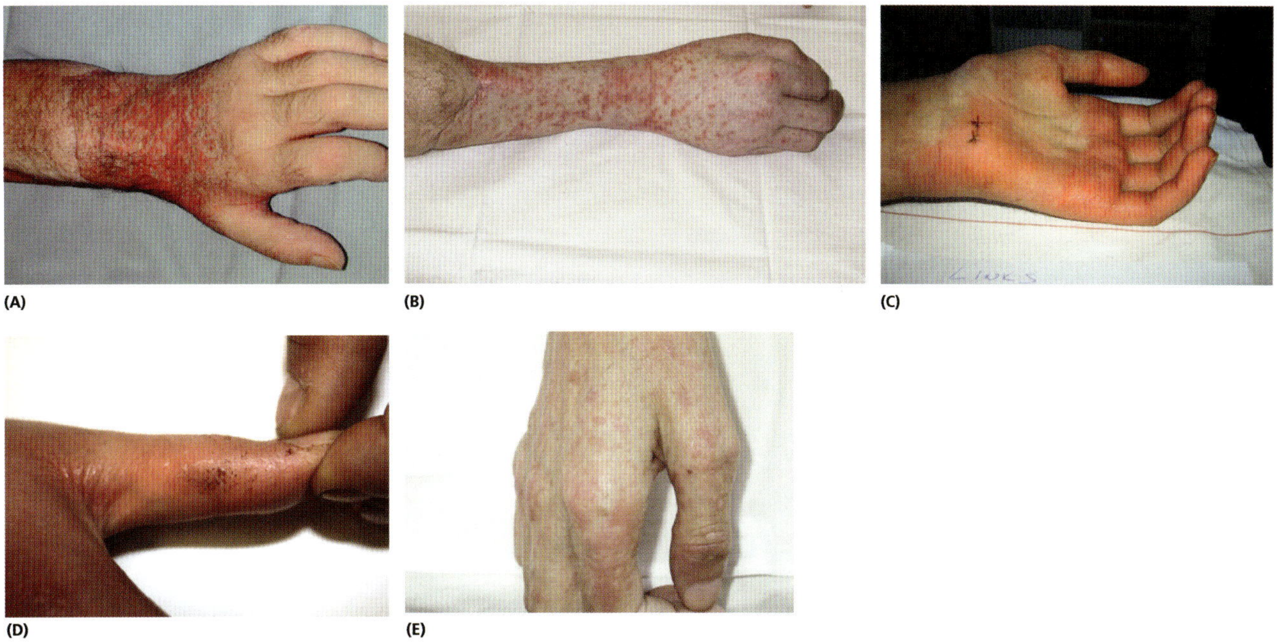

图 75.1　手移植皮肤排斥反应的不同表现。通常，不同的排斥反应可表现为前臂背侧与移植物交界处的斑丘疹（A）。病变可广泛分布于移植物（B）。或局限于手掌（C）。排斥反应也可发生在压力和刺激作用的部位（D）。随着时间延长，病变较移植后早期黯淡平坦（E）。

选择素表达上调,该上调与白细胞附壁滚动、血管内皮细胞ICAM-1及其对应的淋巴细胞LFA-1受体有关,使得细胞黏附于血管壁[29]。在重度排斥反应中,几乎所有黏附分子的表达均会上调,表明黏附分子调节真皮层白细胞和淋巴细胞滚动与血管壁黏附是皮肤排斥反应的初始步骤之一[29]。

抗体介导的排斥反应(AMR)在VCA中的临床意义尚不明确[31]。两项不同的研究和一项大样本的人类手部及面部移植物病理活检均提示,CD20⁺ B细胞稀少或缺如[29,31,32]。仅有1例重度排斥反应病例发现B细胞在真皮层及皮下组织聚集[28]。

在2例手移植患者的毛细血管中发现有C4d沉积,患者出现细胞排斥反应[33],但无临床表现。对存在排斥反应的6例双手或双前臂移植的患者进行皮肤病理活检发现,50%的标本呈C4d染色阳性[29]。而这些病例中,供体特异性抗体(DSA、HLA Ⅰ/Ⅱ类)为阴性[28,33,34]。

Ⅰ级皮肤排斥反应

轻度皮肤排斥反应是VCA的一个特殊问题。虽然常被发现,但是其临床相关性并不明确。轻度排斥反应的病理与免疫组化分析显示其存在大量CD8⁺细胞浸润,以及少量CD20⁺B淋巴细胞和CD68⁺巨噬细胞浸润。黏附分子LFA-1、ICAM-1,选择素E、选择素P和VE-钙黏蛋白表达上调,移植后1年,样本C4d染色大多呈阳性,此后吲哚胺2,3-双加氧酶(IDO)表达及Foxp3⁺阳性细胞增加[25]。Ⅰ级排斥反应中,浸润的细胞中(有IDO或Foxp3⁺表达)可发现耐受性表型,且其比例随时间增加。这一观察表明,调节机制存在于同种异体移植物的皮肤内并可能有助于限制免疫性应答[25]。

皮肤排斥反应评价

基于肢体移植的实验观察,移植第一只手时皮肤可能是AR的主要靶点,因此无论有无临床指征,我们会定期或在临床需要时对皮肤进行活检。第一只手移植后,可发现皮肤斑丘疹,红斑病变是排斥反应的宏观表现,并与组织形态学明确相关[2-10]。

排斥反应会导致不同的皮肤表现,靠近病变区域但未完全来自病变区域的活检样本的病理学表现可能显示正常。因此,选择正确的活检位置非常重要,活检应按照指南或临床指示收集。在手和手臂的同种异体移植中,前臂与上臂活检的解剖学问题较少,但是任何情况下,活检均须从病变区取样。对于面部移植的患者,活检可从"定点皮瓣"处取材,但定点皮瓣与面部移植物排斥反应的相关性须进一步明确,才可使远离病变部位取材的活检令人信服。皮肤样本的病理学及免疫组化检查应根据2007版Banff皮肤VCA分类进行(参见87章)。

综上所述,皮肤是手移植后早期排斥反应免疫应答的主要对象,其他部位如神经束膜和结缔组织也有一些较小的单核细胞浸润。同种抗体的作用仍不清楚,但随着更多临床证据的出现,可能会进一步明确。无论是细胞介导还是抗体介导的血管损伤,与预后意义和活检直接评估活性有关。

急性皮肤排斥反应分级

目前,皮肤状况监测是VCA排斥反应的重要组成部分。移植手出现不规则红斑性斑丘疹病变是AR的临床标志。目前,红斑与病理上单核细胞浸润有关。但在我们的经验中,没有宏观病变并不一定意味着皮肤病理表现正常,这种情况称为"亚临床排斥反应",此概念已在肾移植章节中有所描述。

细胞排斥反应的主要病理特征是单核细胞浸润,其首先出现于真皮层血管周围,若排斥反应继续进展,浸润将扩散至真皮与表皮间和(或)附件结构。表皮内细胞浸润常出现于中度排斥反应免疫应答累及最外层,若此阶段排斥反应未能成功治疗,炎症介质将进一步造成破坏。单个角化细胞坏死可导致局灶性的真皮-表皮分离,随着进一步进展,皮肤排斥反应的最终阶段将出现不可逆的坏死与表皮脱落。

浸润细胞的组成无法鉴别排斥反应与皮炎,但临床上若病变局限于移植物,则可认为是排斥反应。此外,在免疫抑制的情况下,非特异性皮炎发生概率极低。

除皮肤外其他组织的排斥反应

AR中其他组织参与的排斥反应的相关资料比较有限,临床上不常规进行骨、血管、神经或肌肉活检,据临床研究报道,除皮肤外的其他组织受累程度较轻,但可能存在抽样选择偏倚[1,3-6,8,9,22]。

最好的个例是里昂的一例手移植2.5年后截肢患者的系统化病理评估。尽管患者皮肤已糜烂坏死,但肌肉、肌腱仅有轻度的炎症反应,而骨与关节无明显变化[22]。另一深部组织活检证实,免疫应答主要发生在皮肤,但肌肉和结缔组织亦可能出现细胞浸润,浸润发生在较大血管和血管周围肌肉、肌腱和神经,并有骨髓淋巴细胞浸润,表明其他组织亦有某种程度的累及[22-24]。轻度淋巴细胞活动的长期潜在影响尚不明确,须采用活检外的检测手段监测这些组织的情况。有些患者的血管病变会导致移植手功能丧失,证实内膜增生导致的血管病变与排斥反应有关[23]。

总之,有强烈证据表明,相比单组织移植,VCA 移植后引起的免疫排斥更小,皮肤引起的免疫排斥最为强烈。少量证据表明组织对异体移植排斥反应也有影响。

慢性排斥反应

手移植后,移植物 1 年存活率可达 100%,远高于其他实体器官移植,然而结合实际情况来看,其他器官移植的存活是以其功能来定义的。对于 VCA 来说,功能评估与神经重新支配滞后、移植物远端缺乏肌肉功能有关。这样的高存活率与规范的免疫抑制治疗和早期通过肉眼检查发现 AR 有关。实验证据显示,长期移植物存活率受到 VCA 血管病变和退化的影响,但目前仍不清楚。

Unadkat 等人发表了大鼠原位后肢异体移植模型系统分析,其中多个 AR 发作时期导致肌内膜增生,并出现慢性排斥反应(CR)的形态学改变[35]。在这个模型中,反复发作 AR 应用环孢素 A 和地塞米松治疗。在术后第一天(POD),90 只动物发生 19 次 AR 后出现肌内膜增生、血管闭塞及血管周围纤维组织改变类似于心脏移植后血管病变。

在血管蒂骨瓣移植中,有 6 例患者的同种异体移植膝盖都在头 56 个月内丧失功能,最新的组织形态学评估检测到弥散的血管纤维内膜增生和移植物血管闭塞[36],其结果与心脏移植物血管病变(CAV)相似。骨移植中,骨反复发生 AR 缺乏适当的监测排斥反应的手段,最终导致肌内膜增生及移植物血管闭塞。

手移植中,最近一例病例描述了因无法控制缺血而导致截肢,肢体的病理发现移植物动脉有显著肌内膜增生,增生局限于供体动脉。

对于实体器官(如心、肾)的移植,肌内膜增生和移植物血管闭塞可作为 CR 的标志,最早可在移植后 1 年出现,某中心应用高分辨超声检测发现手移植术后患者也有相似发现。由此产生假设,VCA 中移植物血管可能是 CR 的主要靶点。但在其他中心,超声、血管造影和 CT-造影扫描联合皮肤病理活检未发现官腔变窄或闭塞的早期迹象。总之,少数手移植患者可出现肌内膜增生和灌注损伤,所以手部、面部移植后对血管的监测仍十分重要。关于 CR 的药物预防,据报道,雷帕有积极作用[37],因此有可能将其纳入长期免疫抑制治疗方案中。

管理

排斥反应预防

临床治疗

由于 VCA 来自基因完全不同的死亡供体,受者需要终身接受免疫抑制治疗防止排斥反应。VCA 作为移植物,不同于实体器官移植,是由多种组织成分如肌肉、肌腱、神经、血管、骨骼和皮肤组成的,而皮肤具有高免疫原性,所以历史上,VCA 移植被认为是免疫学领域的挑战[38]。皮肤的高免疫原性主要归因于表皮特异性皮肤抗原和大量抗原呈递细胞(APC),可直接提呈同种抗原参与免疫应答[39]。因此,皮肤的强免疫排斥使手异体移植难以广泛开展,需要进行长期大剂量多药物免疫抑制维持治疗,这些免疫抑制药物副作用须引起关注。风险包括但不限于感染、糖尿病、高脂血症、肾毒性或恶性肿瘤,上述仍然是临床常规应用移植重建的最大障碍。

目前用于手移植的免疫抑制治疗方案来源于实体器官移植方案,其维持免疫抑制治疗的深入介绍可参见第 66 章。但目前移植重建暂无标准化免疫抑制治疗方案。免疫抑制剂的总剂量须确保移植物存活或稍高于肾移植所需剂量。如前所述,手移植使用免疫抑制维持治疗后可达到第一年高移植物存活率(患者使用免疫抑制药物治疗的情况下)[1]。常规免疫抑制治疗方案多数情况下可停止对移植物的非特异性免疫排斥。根据国际手和复合组织移植组织报道,广大手移植患者均接受多克隆(抗胸腺细胞球蛋白,ATG)或单克隆(阿伦单抗、巴利昔单抗)抗体制剂作为诱导剂,继而使用高剂量的三联药物维持治疗,如他克莫司、霉酚酸酯(MMF)和类固醇[1,40]。他克莫司剂量头 1~3 个月为 10~15ng/mL,此后为 5~10ng/mL,而类固醇,如泼尼松,大多数患者移植后早期使用高剂量,然后低剂量维持(5~15mg/d)6~12个月。根据最近的33例国际登记处病例,所有受体均使用他克莫司作为基础免疫抑制剂,26例患者使用霉酚酸酯,27例患者使用类固醇。随访期间,8例患者停用他克莫司改用mTOR抑制剂西罗莫司以减少肾毒性,改善血糖,避免潜在的慢性血管改变(肌内膜增生)和神经毒性[41]。其中5例患者停用类固醇,2例患者使用类固醇和低剂量他克莫司、依维莫司治疗,2例患者使用西罗莫司和MMF[4,40]。没有接受诱导治疗(n=2)或三联免疫抑制治疗方案(n=2)的患者除使用全身免疫抑制药物外,还应用外用类固醇和他克莫司软膏。截至目前,诱导治疗之后的维护免疫抑制与最佳剂量的双药物组合被认为是移植重建最广泛使用的治疗方案。

总体而言,常规方案已被证明可防止早期免疫移植物功能丧失,但不能防止AR,85%~90%手移植受体在移植后1年内至少发生一次AR。发生率显著高于实体器官移植,在肾移植病例中,移植后1年内AR发生率低于10%[41]。可能是由于移植重建时移植物是可见的,所以即使是微小的外观变化也可立即诊断排斥反应,AR的特征是可见的不规则分布的红斑、斑丘疹病变,与病理学单核细胞浸润相关[43]。

皮肤排斥反应中异体移植手的其他组织如肌肉、神经、肌腱和骨骼并未受到显著破坏。然而,这些组织参与免疫排斥的资料仍十分有限,仍须更多数据说明皮肤是移植重建排斥反应的唯一的和重要的靶点(参见除皮肤外组织的排斥反应)。

慢性多药免疫抑制是昂贵的,造成巨大的长期花销。此外,每天口服药物较多,患者负担较大,导致其依从性较差。考虑到多药物免疫抑制治疗的缺点明显,有时还有明显的副作用,VCA排斥反应的预防迫切需要新的全身免疫抑制理念。在此方面,手移植有其独特的优点,相比实体器官移植而言,手移植的连续监测可通过对皮肤的简单视检来实现,而皮肤是排斥反应的主要靶点。直接活检和病理确诊可证实AR早期,并及时干预、治疗并根据个人情况精确调节免疫抑制剂剂量。如果治疗充分有效,AR并不影响移植物功能或其长期存活率。因此,尽量减少免疫抑制的新的治疗策略,甚至实现以诱导免疫耐受的终极临床目标,在手移植和VCA中很有前景。我们的小组研究表明,相比单组织移植,全肢体同种异体移植后引起的免疫排斥反应更小,取决于其组织抗原性的相对比例[44]。此外,某些VCA含有免疫活性成分如骨髓或淋巴结可能会加速排斥反应进程或导致移植物抗宿主病(GVHD)。这些因素不仅影响同种异体组织的免疫反应,同时也影响潜在的不同于目前用于实体器官移植的免疫调节策略。

实验治疗

历史上,常规治疗(如前所述)为非特异性的多药物抑制疗法,用于抑制受体的免疫系统。其副作用包括机会性感染风险增加、代谢障碍和恶性肿瘤。因此,目前研究主要集中于研发针对特异性通路与T细胞活化受体的新药物和生物制剂,为了避免对其他免疫谱系的副作用,可在保证移植物存活的情况下显著减少不良并发症[45]。

此外,手部和面部移植免疫抑制方案多年来经过多次修改,如类固醇限制/避免疗法、阿仑单抗诱导、基于细胞的免疫调节疗法,从他克莫司转为mTOR抑制剂西罗莫司长期治疗,或外用类固醇和他克莫司软膏,以减少全身性免疫抑制剂剂量[46]。

有趣的是,有少数器官移植受体出现对移植物的免疫耐受,可停止免疫抑制治疗而不发生排斥反应[47]。自发供体抗原特异性免疫耐受现象使人们认识到存在克服组织相容性障碍的可行性方法,可以不通过免疫抑制,而是免疫调节。此外,在实验器官移植模型中实现的自发免疫耐受,通常是耗尽宿主抗移植物的免疫应答的结果。介导排斥反应的特异性细胞克隆被删除,对移植物的免疫应答耗尽,达到操作耐受状态。此外,少量供体白细胞长期存在于受体(微嵌合)中被认为有利于移植物的存活[48]。该疗法在VCA领域特别有吸引力,因为此类移植虽然能显著提高生活质量,但并非用于挽救生命,并有与生俱来的独特生物学特征。尽管如此,VCA的"风险收益平衡"比其他任何类型的实体器官移植更需要小心把握。迄今,一些小型和大型动物研究显示,移植血管复合同种异体移植物无须长期免疫抑制维持,其结果十分令人鼓舞[49,50]。这些实验中使用的方案包括全淋巴组织放疗,共刺激阻断剂(CD28/B7和CD154/CD40途径),选择性消耗同种反应性受体T细胞和B细胞(如αβ T细胞和CD20-特异性单克隆抗体),抑制移植淋巴细胞迁移,输注$CD4^+$ $CD25^+$ $Foxp3^+$调节性T细胞和免疫耐受的APC,以及输注供者骨髓以及嵌合体诱导[29,51-57]。采用免疫调节概念,完全MHC错配的猪异位后肢移植模型采用供体骨髓细胞实现了无须长期全身免疫移植治疗的不确定移植物存活[58,59]。此概念被约翰霍普金斯大学医学院和匹兹堡大学联合研究小组转化为移植重建的以细胞治疗为基础的新治疗方案[60]。在最初的试验中,5 例接受阿仑单抗诱导治疗和他克莫司单药免疫抑制维持治疗的患者同时输注了未经修改的供体骨髓细胞。这项研究目前正在进行,至今该方案可行,并可使用低剂量的他克莫司单药治疗上肢截肢者重建移植。

沿着这些实验思路,Mathes 等人开发出一种结合非脊髓清除诱导方法和 VCA 的犬的模型,可在无须长期免疫抑制维持的情况下对 VCA 的所有组织产生免疫耐受[61]。因此,由于 VCA 的独特性,考虑开发新治疗策略以减少或避免免疫抑制维持,细胞治疗方案如供体骨髓细胞或干细胞都是非常有前景的。实体器官移植取得的新进步进一步证明了这一治疗趋势的可行性,在研究中,细胞疗法和非细胞疗法均可减少或避免长期免疫抑制治疗[62–64]。VCA 中可包含血管化骨和骨髓,其本身可充当骨髓移植[65],可持续提供供体来源的干细胞,而在动物模型中已证实,供体来源的干细胞可以有效调节受体免疫应答[66]。在此实验中,供体特异性的免疫耐受归因于骨髓移植。近期引起了对优化以骨髓移植为基础的疗法的探寻,以延长 VCA 生存期并诱导供体抗原特异性免疫耐受。沿着这些实验思路,Barth 等人应用选择性错配食蟹猴面部异种移植模型来说明伴血管骨髓的 VCA 独特的病理生理学、免疫原性特征和免疫抑制需求[67]。对于伴有血管化骨的面部异位移植 VCA,给予他克莫司和 MMF 治疗,未给予化疗或 T 细胞耗竭治疗诱导,其无排斥生存期为 205~430 天,而没有血管骨髓的 VCA 在术后 7~15 天即出现早期排斥反应和移植物功能丧失[67]。尽管 VCA 的血管化骨髓表现为少量低层次的吻合,免疫抑制维持治疗停药后仍有 AR、CR 和移植物功能丧失发生。然而放射学、免疫表型、组织学和基因型证据均支持供体骨髓移植可在移植的血管化骨内持续存在,此模型中血管化骨髓在停用免疫抑制治疗后仍可抑制同种致敏及 IgM、IgG 抗体的增加[67]。此研究数据进一步证实血管化骨髓在 VCA 中免疫调节的重要作用及其减少免疫抑制药物的作用。

尽管取得了这些进展,CR 在实体器官中仍难以解决,并持续影响预后。但迄今为止,在 VCA 的前瞻性队列研究中,只有少数患者随访超过 10 年,但 VCA 的 CR 发病率较低。国际上只有 1 例在免疫抑制治疗后出现血管病变如血管内膜增生导致 VCA 移植物功能丧失的报道,其病变与实体器官移植的 CR 相似。随着越来越多实验性的免疫抑制剂减量和诱导耐受方案的出现,VCA 的长期密切随访和标准化后续治疗非常重要。

排斥反应的治疗

临床治疗

几乎所有手部和面部移植受体,无论使用何种诱导或维持免疫抑制治疗方案,均经历过 AR 发作。其皮肤排斥反应的发生率高于肾脏、肝脏和心脏移植后,所有临床诊断的皮肤排斥反应均由皮肤穿刺活检确诊。为维持免疫抑制治疗方案,AR 的治疗方案来源于实体器官移植方案。其他补救治疗方案可参见第 67 章。据国际手和复合组织移植组织,60%的病例的急性排斥反应的治疗包括高剂量静脉注射类固醇,30%的受体增加口服类固醇即生效,只有 7.5%的患者呈类固醇耐受,须考虑给予抗胸腺细胞球蛋白、巴利昔单抗、阿仑单抗治疗[1]。除全身治疗以外,由于皮肤排斥反应的特殊性,可局部使用软膏(他克莫司、皮质类固醇或氟轻松)。目前认为免疫抑制剂量不足是持续排斥反应的重要原因,因此多数病例也会同时增加免疫抑制剂量。

当出现第二次排斥反应,局部使用或不使用软膏的患者都需要静脉注射类固醇,只有少数患者使用 ATG、巴利昔单抗或外用药物。1 例类固醇和 ATG 耐受的病例中,使用阿仑单抗(Campath-1H,Genzyme,美国马萨诸塞州剑桥市)后皮肤病理完全恢复正常。迄今为止,移植重建中尚无因不可逆急性排斥反应导致的移植物功能丧失。而 VCA 相关的移植物功能的定义与心脏不同,心脏的轻微损伤即可产生严重的临床症状。

应用上述方法,手移植的多数排斥反应可成功治疗。1998 年,法国的第一例手移植病例中,不规范的免疫抑制治疗下进展的 AR 导致皮肤的苔藓样病变和功能丧失,尽管据推测排斥反应是可逆的,类固醇和抗 CD25 抗体不能阻止排斥反应进展。移植后 2 年 4 个月时患者要求手截肢[22]。另一个病例中,患者出现耐受"任何"治疗的严重的"皮肤炎症",移植后 3 年行手截肢[1]。

实验疗法

手移植 AR 治疗中,局部使用免疫抑制剂已常规用于免疫抑制维持治疗[1–10]。有趣的是,1951 年,局部免疫抑制治疗概念最先被提出，Billingham 等人在兔模型中发现，在全身给药的情况下，局部使用一定量醋酸可的松对移植物生存无效[68]。当时除局部放疗外，其余局部免疫抑制治疗的研究停滞了近 20 年。随着给药系统的进步及对异体移植物排斥反应中细胞作用机制和靶点治疗药物动力学的深入理解，这些治疗策略在移植重建领域重新兴起。

多种给药技术，包括药物调控释放微米和纳米颗粒或其他生物工程粒子、脂质体、转基因和细胞联合移植已在实验移植模型中直接介导免疫抑制药物和分子作用于移植物靶点[69]。Hautz 等人发现人类手部和前臂移植的急性皮肤排斥皮肤活检标本中存在细胞浸润和细胞迁移[29]。样本组中，ICAM-1 和选择素 E 的表达与排斥反应的严重程度密切相关。轻度排斥反应和晚期排斥反应中，选择素 E 都主要见于血管壁内皮细胞。内皮选择素 E 和选择素 P 可介导免疫细胞沿血管壁牵引和滚动，作为复杂的多步骤级联反应的一部分，募集 T 细胞和其他免疫细胞至皮肤。治疗靶向黏附分子的概念也被用于皮肤炎性疾病，如依法珠单抗，已成功用于治疗银屑病[70]。一项小型动物研究证明，局部使用特定选择阻滞剂(efomycine M)联合肌萎缩侧索硬化症(ALS)的诱导和低剂量他克莫司维持治疗可显著延长肢体移植存活期。淋巴细胞耗竭联合针对 VCA 皮肤淋巴细胞迁移的靶向治疗是治疗 AR 和减少/避免免疫移植维持的有吸引力的方法。然而外用制剂存在如下缺点：无法控制 VCA 其他组织的排斥反应，深部组织如肌肉、骨的免疫排斥可能进一步进展。尽管局限于移植物的免疫抑制制剂有可取之处，但是排斥反应是全身性的，单独的局部治疗并不足以防治。因此，尽管前景较好，采用局部用药治疗移植重建的急性皮肤排斥的治疗策略在安全应用于人类前，仍须在动物实验中进一步评估。

理想的免疫抑制治疗

移植医学的理想情况和最终临床目标是诱导供体抗原特异性免疫耐受的能力，避免使用免疫抑制剂并可显著改善长期预后[46]。免疫耐受的机制和临床实现的完整介绍可参见第 11 章和第 76 章。然而，免疫耐受诱导至今尚未实现，未来临床上也难以广泛实现，但最近推出的新的方案显示有机会实现患者避免免疫维持药物治疗或将长期的免疫抑制剂量降至最低水平。然而，这样的致免疫耐受方案对 VCA 是否有效仍有待证明。

目前，多个免疫抑制方案的优劣对比只能从前瞻性随机临床试验中获得，然而对于尚处于起步阶段的手部和面部移植，这样的数据可能要几十年才能获得。因此，免疫抑制方案的制订需要结合从前患者的治疗经验，参考实体器官移植获取的进展以及 VCA 实验研究中获得的数据。由于这些原因，实行规范法随访和预后评价十分重要，可以对不同的研究机构的不同方案数据进行对比，在患者数量有限的情况下进行多中心前瞻性试验。

设计 VCA 优化免疫抑制方案时，须考虑其与实体器官移植的区别：①除了截肢或颅面组织损伤外，VCA 患者也是健康的受体，通常没有可能增加感染和恶性肿瘤风险的疾病；②手部或面部移植不属于挽救生命的移植，也不影响患者的长期存活；③VCA 的皮肤是可见的，多数情况下排斥反应可通过简单的肉眼观察判断，活检也可在直视下从病变部位取材；④反复急性皮肤排斥反应若得到充分治疗，对移植物长期功能几乎没有影响；⑤目前与 DSA 和 AMR 的关联没有实体器官移植紧密；⑥VCA 中几乎所有的 AR 均在术后第一年内发作。

制订 VCA 的新治疗策略或理想方案时应考虑这些相关因素，因此基于移植重建的经验和可用的数据，我们对 VCA 的免疫抑制方案的制订提出如下建议：

1.使用消耗性生物制剂，如 ATG 或阿仑单抗诱导治疗，可能有助于预防早期排斥反应并降低免疫抑制维持治疗所需的剂量。

2.免疫抑制治疗方案应包含他克莫司，且术后至少使用 2 年，他克莫司可通过刺激生长相关蛋白(GAP-43)合成促进神经再生。

3.术后 2 年内的三联疗法应包括类固醇和霉酚酸，对预防 AR 有效。类固醇应逐渐减量至停药。

4.移植后 2~3 年，可以用 TOR 抑制剂代替钙调神经磷酸酶抑制剂，因为其对 CR 有抗增殖和潜在的保护作用，以及抗肿瘤作用。

总结

总之，设计新的免疫抑制方案时须考虑上述 VCA 的具体要求，尽管在从多种可用药物中选择最有利的药物组合以预防实体器官异体移植排斥方面取得了巨大进展，但由于本章概述中提出的独特的生物学/免疫学特征，重建移植中使用或尝试相同方案时，该方案并不总是最佳的。此外，设计用于实体器官移植的免疫抑制最小化方案用于 VCA 时须谨慎。

因为目前的常规免疫抑制治疗没有重大突破，我们仍须继续优化目前的药物组合方案，并参考其他研究中心数据，开发具有抑制肌内膜增生和 CR 的低毒性治疗方案。只要坚持这些指南，终将改变移植的风险-收益平衡，并推进移植的新时代。

（周舒扬　杨梦凡　译　周舒扬　校）

参考文献

1. Petruzzo P, Lanzetta M, Dubernard JM, et al. The international registry on hand and composite tissue transplantation. Transplantation. 2010;90:1590–1594.
2. Jones JW, Gruber SA, Barker JH, et al. Successful hand transplantation. One-year follow-up. Louisville Hand Transplant Team. New England Journal of Medicine. 2000;343:468–473.
3. Margreiter R, Brandacher G, Ninkovic M, et al. A double-hand transplant can be worth the effort! Transplantation. 2002;74:85–90.
4. Schneeberger S, Zelger B, Ninkovic M, et al. Transplantation of the hand. Transplantation Reviews. 2005;19:100–107.
5. Schneeberger S, Ninkovic M, Piza-Katzer H, et al. Status 5 years after bilateral hand transplantation. American Journal of Transplantation. 2006;6:834–841.
6. Schneeberger S, Ninkovic M, Gabl M, et al. First forearm transplantation: outcome after 3 years. American Journal of Transplantation. 2007;7:1753–1762.
7. Dubernard JM, Lengele B, Morelon E, et al. Outcomes 18 months after the first human partial face transplantation. New England Journal of Medicine. 2007;357:2451–2460.
8. Schuind F, Abramowicz D, Schneeberger S. Hand transplantation: the state-of-the-art. Journal of Hand Surgery (Edinburgh, Lothian). 2007;32:2–17.
9. Schneeberger S, Kreczy A, Brandacher G, et al. Steroid- and ATG-resistant rejection after double forearm transplantation responds to Campath-1H. American Journal of Transplantation. 2004;4:1372–1374.
10. Schneeberger S, Gorantla VS, van Riet RP, et al. Atypical acute rejection after hand transplantation. American Journal of Transplantation. 2008;8:688–696.
11. Steinmuller D, Wakely E, Landas SK. Evidence that epidermal alloantigen Epa-1 is an immunogen for murine heart as well as skin allograft rejection. Transplantation. 1991;51:459–463.
12. Fuchimoto Y, Gleit ZL, Huang CA, et al. Skin-specific alloantigens in miniature swine. Transplantation. 2001;72:122–126.
13. Volc-Platzer B, Majdic O, Knapp W, et al. Evidence of HLA-DR antigen biosynthesis by human keratinocytes in disease. Journal of Experimental Medicine. 1984;159:1784–1789.
14. Dustin ML, Singer KH, Tuck DT, et al. Adhesion of T lymphoblasts to epidermal keratinocytes is regulated by interferon gamma and is mediated by intercellular adhesion molecule 1 (ICAM-1). Journal of Experimental Medicine. 1988;167:1323–1340.
15. Simon M Jr, Hunyadi J. Expression of OKM5 antigen on human keratinocytes in positive intracutaneous tests for delayed-type hypersensitivity. Dermatologica. 1987;175:121–125.
16. Luger TA, Stadler BM, Katz SI, et al. Epidermal cell (keratinocyte)-derived thymocyte-activating factor (ETAF). Journal of Immunology. 1981;127:1493–1498.
17. Aragane Y, Riemann H, Bhardwaj RS, et al. IL-12 is expressed and released by human keratinocytes and epidermoid carcinoma cell lines. Journal of Immunology. 1994;153:5366–5372.
18. Partridge M, Chantry D, Turner M, et al. Production of interleukin-1 and interleukin-6 by human keratinocytes and squamous cell carcinoma cell lines. Journal of Investigative Dermatology. 1991;96:771–776.
19. Barker JN, Jones ML, Mitra RS, et al. Modulation of keratinocyte-derived interleukin-8 which is chemotactic for neutrophils and T lymphocytes. American Journal of Pathology. 1991;139:869–876.
20. Richters CD, van Pelt AM, van Geldrop E, et al. Migration of rat skin dendritic cells. Journal of Leukocyte Biology. 1996;60:317–322.
21. Schneeberger S, Lucchina S, Lanzetta M, et al. Cytomegalovirus-related complications in human hand transplantation. Transplantation. 2005;80:441–447.
22. Kanitakis J, Jullien D, Petruzzo P, et al. Clinicopathologic features of graft rejection of the first human hand allograft. Transplantation. 2003;76:688–693.
23. Kaufman CL, Breidenbach W. World experience after more than a decade of clinical hand transplantation: update from the Louisville hand transplant program. Hand Clinics. 2011;27:417–421.
24. Wang HJ, Ding YQ, Pei GX, et al. A preliminary pathological study on human allotransplantation. Chinese Journal of Traumatology. 2003;6:284–287.
25. Hautz T, Zelger B, Brandacher G, et al. Histopathologic characterization of mild rejection (grade I) in skin biopsies of human hand allografts. Transplant International. 2012;25:56–63.
26. Cendales LC, Kanitakis J, Schneeberger S, et al. The BANFF 2007 working classification of skin-containing composite tissue allograft pathology. American Journal of Transplantation. 2008;8:1396–1400.
27. Morita K, Miura M, Paolone DR, et al. Early chemokine cascades in murine cardiac grafts regulate T cell recruitment and progression of acute allograft rejection. Journal of Immunology. 2001;167:2979–2984.
28. Cendales LC, Kirk AD, Moresi JM, et al. Composite tissue allotransplantation: classification of clinical acute skin rejection. Transplantation. 2006;81:418–422.
29. Hautz T, Zelger B, Grahammer J, et al. Molecular markers and targeted therapy of skin rejection in composite tissue allotransplantation. American Journal of Transplantation. 2010;10:1200–1209.
30. Petruzzo P, Kanitakis J, Badet L, et al. Long-term follow-up in composite tissue allotransplantation: in-depth study of five (hand and face) recipients. American Journal of Transplantation. 2011;11:808–816.
31. Russell PS, Chase CM, Colvin RB. Alloantibody- and T cell-mediated immunity in the pathogenesis of transplant arteriosclerosis: lack of progression to sclerotic lesions in B cell-deficient mice. Transplantation. 1997;64:1531–1536.
32. Kanitakis J, Badet L, Petruzzo P, et al. Clinicopathologic monitoring of the skin and oral mucosa of the first human face allograft: report on the first eight months. Transplantation. 2006;82:1610–1615.
33. Landin L, Cavadas PC, Nthumba P, et al. Preliminary results of bilateral arm transplantation. Transplantation. 2009;88:749–751.
34. Kanitakis J, McGregor B, Badet L, et al. Absence of c4d deposition in human composite tissue (hands and face) allograft biopsies: an immunoperoxidase study. Transplantation. 2007;84:265–267.
35. Unadkat JV, Schneeberger S, Horibe EH, et al. Composite tissue vasculopathy and degeneration following multiple episodes of acute rejection in reconstructive transplantation. American Journal of Transplantation. 2009;10:251–261.
36. Diefenbeck M, Nerlich A, Schneeberger S, et al. Allograft vasculopathy after allogeneic vascularized knee transplantation. Transplant International. 2010;24:e1–e5.
37. Viganò M, Tuzcu M, Benza R, et al. Prevention of acute rejection and allograft vasculopathy by everolimus in cardiac transplants recipients: a 24-month analysis. Journal of Heart and Lung Transplantation. 2007;26:584–592.
38. Murray JE. Organ transplantation (skin, kidney, heart) and the plastic surgeon. Plastic and Reconstructive Surgery. 1971;47:425–431.
39. Siemionow M, Nasir S. Immunologic responses in vascularized and nonvascularized skin allografts. Journal of Reconstructive Microsurgery. 2008;24:497–505.
40. Petruzzo P, Lanzetta M, Dubernard JM, et al. The international registry on hand and composite tissue transplantation. Transplantation. 2008;86:487–492.
41. Ravindra KV, Ildstad ST. Immunosuppressive protocols and immunological challenges related to hand transplantation. Hand Clinics. 2011;27:467–749.
42. Kaufman DB, Leventhal JR, Axelrod D, et al. Alemtuzumab induction and prednisone-free maintenance immunotherapy in kidney transplantation: comparison with basiliximab induction–long-term results. American Journal of Transplantation. 2005;5:2539–2548.
43. Schneeberger S, Gorantla VS, Hautz T, et al. Immunosuppression and rejection in human hand transplantation. Transplantation Proceedings. 2009;41:472–475.
44. Lee WP, Yaremchuk MJ, Pan YC, et al. Relative antigenicity of components of a vascularized limb allograft. Plastic and Reconstructive Surgery. 1991;87:401–411.
45. Lechler RI, Sykes M, Thomson AW, et al. Organ transplantation—how much of the promise has been realized? Nature Medicine. 2005;11:605–613.
46. Hautz T, Brandacher G, Engelhardt TO, et al. How reconstructive transplantation is different from organ transplantation—and how it is not. Transplantation Proceedings. 2011;43:3504–3511.
47. Ashton-Chess J, Giral M, Brouard S, et al. Spontaneous operational tolerance after immunosuppressive drug withdrawal in clinical renal allotransplantation. Transplantation. 2007;84:1215–1219.
48. Starzl TE, Lakkis FG. The unfinished legacy of liver transplantation: emphasis on immunology. Hepatology (Baltimore, MD). 2006;43:S151–S163.
49. Siemionow M, Klimczak A. Tolerance and future directions for composite tissue allograft transplants: part II. Plastic and Reconstructive Surgery. 2009;123:7e–17e.
50. Bozulic LD, Breidenbach WC, Ildstad ST. Past, present, and future prospects for inducing donor-specific transplantation tolerance for composite tissue allotransplantation. Seminars in Plastic Surgery. 2007;21:213–225.

51. Siemionow MZ, Izycki DM, Zielinski M. Donor-specific tolerance in fully major histocompatibility major histocompatibility complex-mismatched limb allograft transplants under an anti-alphabeta T-cell receptor monoclonal antibody and cyclosporine A protocol. Transplantation. 2003;76:1662–1668.
52. Foster RD, Ascher NL, McCalmont TH, et al. Mixed allogeneic chimerism as a reliable model for composite tissue allograft tolerance induction across major and minor histocompatibility barriers. Transplantation. 2001;72:791–797.
53. Larsen CP, Pearson TC, Adams AB, et al. Rational development of LEA29Y (belatacept), a high-affinity variant of CTLA4-Ig with potent immunosuppressive properties. American Journal of Transplantation. 2005;5:443–453.
54. Issa F, Hester J, Goto R, et al. Ex vivo-expanded human regulatory T cells prevent the rejection of skin allografts in a humanized mouse model. Transplantation. 2010;90:1321–1327.
55. Ezzelarab M, Thomson AW. Tolerogenic dendritic cells and their role in transplantation. Seminars in Immunology. 2011;23:252–263.
56. Pilat N, Sayegh MH, Wekerle T. Costimulatory pathways in transplantation. Seminars in Immunology. 2011;23:293–303.
57. Siemionow M, Klimczak A, Unal S, et al. Hematopoietic stem cell engraftment and seeding permits multi-lymphoid chimerism in vascularized bone marrow transplants. American Journal of Transplantation. 2008;8:1163–1176.
58. Hettiaratchy S, Melendy E, Randolph MA, et al. Tolerance to composite tissue allografts across a major histocompatibility barrier in miniature swine. Transplantation. 2004;77:514–521.
59. Schneeberger S, Wachtman G, Gorantla VS, et al. Utilization of bone marrow cells for immunomodulation in transplantation. American Journal of Transplantation. 2010;10 (Suppl. s4):116.
60. Brandacher G, Gorantla VS, Schneeberger S, et al. Hand/forearm transplantation using a novel cell-based immunomodulatory protocol—experience with five patients. American Journal of Transplantation. 2011;11(Suppl. s2):190.
61. Mathes DW, Hwang B, Graves SS, et al. Tolerance to vascularized composite allografts in canine mixed hematopoietic chimeras. Transplantation. 2011;92: 1301–1308.
62. Starzl TE, Murase N, Abu-Elmagd K, et al. Tolerogenic immunosuppression for organ transplantation. Lancet. 2003;361:1502–1510.
63. Kawai T, Cosimi AB, Spitzer TR, et al. HLA-mismatched renal transplantation without maintenance immunosuppression. New England Journal of Medicine. 2008;24:353–361.
64. Scandling JD, Busque S, Dejbakhsh-Jones S, et al. Tolerance and chimerism after renal and hematopoietic-cell transplantation. New England Journal of Medicine. 2008;24:362–368.
65. Taieb A, Clavijo-Alvarez JA, Hamad GG, et al. Immunologic approaches to composite tissue allograft. Journal of Hand Surgery. 2007;32:1072–1085.
66. Siemionow M, Nasir S. Impact of donor bone marrow on survival of composite tissue allografts. Annals of Plastic Surgery. 2008;60:455–462.
67. Barth RN, Rodriguez ED, Mundinger GS, et al. Vascularized bone marrow-based immunosuppression inhibits rejection of vascularized composite allografts in non-human primates. American Journal of Transplantation. 2011;11:1407–1416.
68. Billingham RE, Krohn PL, Medawar PB. Effect of locally applied cortisone acetate on survival of skin homografts in rabbits. British Medical Journal. 1951; 2(4739):1049–1053.
69. Gruber SA. Locoregional immunosupression in composite tissue allografting. In: Transplantation of Composite Tissue Allografts. Gordon CR, Hewitt CW, Lee WPA, eds. New York, NY: Springer; 2008;164–171.
70. Lebwohl M, Tyring SK, Hamilton TK, et al. A novel targeted T-cell modulator, efalizumab, for plaque psoriasis. New England Journal of Medicine. 2003; 349:2004–2013.

第 76 章

临床移植耐受

Tatsuo Kawai, David H. Sachs, A. Benedict Cosimi

引言

临床耐受广泛定义为在没有进行免疫抑制的情况下异体移植物有功能，自从 Medawar 的初步研究提出其在异体移植的可能性后，成为移植的根本目标（见 11 章），广泛认为诱导免疫耐受可促进器官移植的长期预后。然而直到最近这个目标才能预期实现。显然，免疫耐受需要患者接受超出预防移植排斥反应的所需的治疗，所以这些治疗的短期和长期风险不能超过当前护理标准下免疫耐受所赋予的优势。本章节总结了临床器官移植中诱导免疫耐受的相关伦理学因素、适应证与治疗策略。

长期免疫抑制的风险

自从 1956 年 Murray 等人成功进行了第一例肾移植，多种免疫抑制方案已进入临床应用[1]。有效的免疫抑制药物联合治疗已成功预防或治疗急性排斥反应，器官移植的短期生存有了显著的改善，实体器官移植已成为很多终末期器官疾病的首选治疗[2,3]。

长期使用免疫抑制剂可导致心血管疾病[4-6]、感染[7-9]和恶性肿瘤[10-13]风险显著增加，还可导致多种副作用，如肾毒性、新发糖尿病[14-16]、血脂异常[17-20]和神经毒性[21,22]，其中心血管疾病是主要致死原因，导致肾移植后 30%~48%的死亡[10]。感染在移植后致死原因中排名第二[11,23]。长期使用免疫抑制剂的移植患者中常见肿瘤的发生率增高，其中非黑色素瘤皮肤癌和黑色素瘤/白血病多见，分别比一般人群高 30 倍和 3 倍。一些研究报告显示，肾移植患者持续 20 年免疫抑制治疗后，其肿瘤的总发病率高达 40%，而对照的年龄匹配的非移植对照群体肿瘤发病率仅为 6%[13,24]。由于各种并发症存在，肾移植后 10 年内移植物功能完善时患者死亡占移植物功能丧失的 16%[25]。调神经磷酸酶抑制剂（CNI）的慢性肾毒性也是严重的副作用，不仅损伤移植肾，还会损伤肾外移植患者的自身的肾脏。非肾移植患者 CNI 慢性肾毒性发生率高达 18%，其中一半患者进展至明显的肾衰竭，需要在 10 年内进行替代治疗[26]。尽管当前的治疗方案有强大的免疫调节作用，但并不能预防慢性排斥反应。15%~30%（取决于测量方法）接受免疫抑制维持治疗的肾移植患者最终会形成 HLA 抗体[27]。慢性排斥反应，通常与新产生的抗体检测相关，导致肾移植后 10 年内 20%的移植物功能丧失[25]。总而言之，目前采用的长期免疫抑制疗法的种种限制不可避免的导致每年 5%~7%的移植物功能丧失[28]，在过去 10 年中无明显改善[3,29]（图 76.1）。

诱导耐受的原因

诱导免疫耐受被认为是改善移植器官长期结果的一种策略。术后 4~10 年 20%完全停用免疫抑制的肝移植受者可出现操纵耐受（在不进行免疫抑制的情况对移植组织无破坏性免疫应答）[30,31]。然而，这种自发性免疫耐受在肾移植患者中十分罕见，在心脏或肺移植患者中更为罕见，说明对于主要组织相容性复合物（MHC）屏障需要额外的调节或治疗以持续诱导耐受，为了证明临床应用的合理性，这种另外的调节/治疗方案的短期和长期风险不能超过当前护理标准下的优势。如果能持续诱导耐受可消除慢性排斥反应，并最小化心血管疾病、感染、恶性肿瘤和其他药物相关并发症的风险。这些优势必须与移植后早期潜在增加的感染和治疗相关疾病的风险相比较，诱导耐受方案导致的风险可能更高，还必须考虑原发性自身免疫性疾病患者复发的可能性，对于这些患者，移植后免疫抑制可能带来

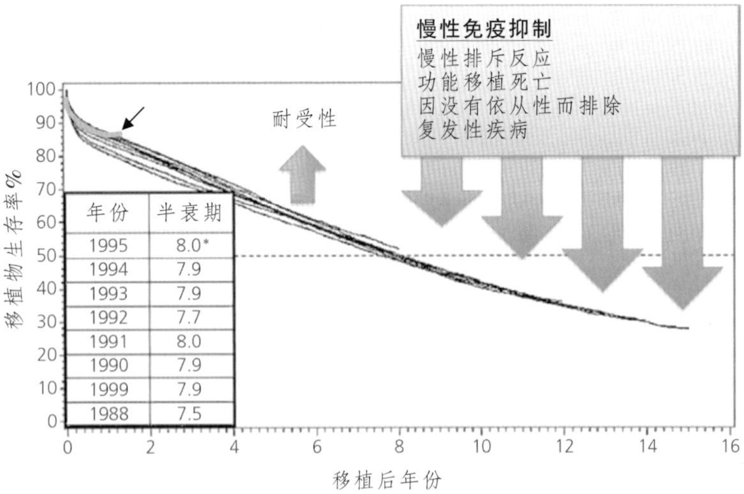

图 76.1 目前采用的长期免疫抑制疗法的种种限制不可避免地导致每年 5%~7%的移植物功能丧失，其半衰期在过去 10 年中无明显改善（黑色的较低的生存曲线）。在移植物功能丧失的主要原因中，如能实现持续诱导耐受，则急性细胞排斥反应、慢性排斥反应和依从性差导致的排斥反应均可被排除（预测的灰色曲线，细箭头所示），慢性排斥反应可排除，并可最小化心血管疾病、感染和恶性肿瘤的风险。* 生存率为 51.8%（Medified from [36] Meier-Kriesche HU et al., Am J Transplant 2004; 4:1289, with permission from Wiley）。

超出其同种免疫要求的益处。

从联合肾和骨髓移植的经验看，这些需求是可行的，表明在某些情况下免疫耐受是可行的。根据我们的诱导方案，抗第三方应答在 6 个月内完全恢复，且无持续供体特异性应答[32]。此外，在随访 13 年的非人灵长类动物受体和随访 9 年的人类受体（尚未发布）中均未出现严重的感染并发症。此外还须考虑耐受调节后潜在的恶性肿瘤风险，并关注免疫调节期间电离辐射的副作用。例如，诱导方案中包括全身照射（TBI）或总淋巴细胞照射（TLI），辐射诱发的恶性肿瘤发生率应与长期免疫抑制治疗导致的恶性肿瘤风险比较。流行病学研究认为，低剂量 TBI（2~2.5Gy）与未暴露于辐射的对照人群相比，其恶性肿瘤发生风险增加 1.2 倍[33]。相比之下，长期免疫抑制治疗的恶性肿瘤风险增加 3~30 倍，该数据可支持低剂量辐射用于耐受诱导。此外需要关注的是供体骨髓移植（DBMT）方案，除非患者正在接受恶性肿瘤治疗，否则发生在器官移植受体的任何水平的移植物抗宿主病（GVHD）都不可接受[34,35]。

诱导耐受指征

何种患者是最合适的诱导耐受候选人？诱导耐受有什么具体的禁忌证？近 10 年来，死亡供体移植肾的半衰期无明显改善，为 9~10 年[3,36]。年轻的肾移植受体终身可能需要多次重新移植。然而供体有限，先前移植 HLA 的致敏作用使再次移植变得十分困难。对于移植后药物治疗依从性较差的儿童患者，在不影响诱导耐受方案所需随访的情况下，可作为诱导耐受的高度合适候选者，5%~80%的儿童受体存在依从性差的情况，其中青少年比例最高[37-40]。因此，青少年组的长期预后差于其他年龄组[41,42]。成功的耐受诱导对青少年受体十分有利。此外，由于长期免疫抑制治疗，受体患恶性肿瘤的风险显著增加，有恶性肿瘤史或家族史的患者也将从诱导耐受中额外获益。对 HLA 预先致敏的患者行诱导耐受十分困难[43]。初始临床试验中，ELISA 检测到高反应性抗体（PRA）但无供体特异性抗体（DSA）的患者在移植术后 2 周内发生强烈的体液排斥[32]。因此，目前排除具有可检测出 PRA 的患者参与诱导耐受临床试验。

原发疾病复发率高的患者是否适合诱导耐受尚待确定[25]。在斯坦福临床试验 HLA 匹配的肾移植受体中，1 例患者出现疾病复发，导致研究者停止计划继续免疫抑制治疗[44]。在我们的临床试验中，1 例患者停止免疫抑制治疗 7 年后出现膜性增生性肾小球性肾炎的复发，需要重新使用低剂量免疫抑制治疗。尽管针对异体抗原的诱导耐受也可能抑制自身免疫，但在这些传闻病例中，诱导耐受并不增强或降低原发疾病复发的概率。目前尚未有评估自身免疫的非人灵长类动物（NHP）模型，但有正在进行的关于机制的研究，如 Tregs（调节性 T 细胞），有助于评估诱导耐受的潜在障碍。

诱导耐受的方案

Billingham、Brent 和 Medawar 成功实现新生儿耐受的标志性研究[45]，为啮齿动物模型提供了许多诱导耐受方案[46-53]，但仅少数能成功用于 NHP[54-62]，能用于人类的方案数量更少[32,44,63-66]。啮齿动物和灵长类动物模型之间诱导耐受的差异可归因于 MHC 抗原,特别是Ⅱ型的表达差异[67,68],以及受体异源性免疫性 T 细胞不在环境控制的情况下存在[69-71]。最新研究表明,异体记忆性 T 细胞可通过阻断共刺激[72]或混合嵌合[69]抑制诱导耐受。不过近期非鼠模型中取得了与 NHP 甚至人类受体诱导耐受一致的观察结果。迄今,已用于临床移植的耐受诱导方案包括:①T 细胞清除;②共刺激阻断;③DBM 注射/移植。这些方案来源于三种主要的诱导耐受途径:①T 细胞清除;②无反应;③调节(图 76.2)。这些途径组合的一个实例是混合嵌合体诱导耐受,通过抗 T 细胞抗体清除 T 细胞[73],该方法已被报道用于扩增调节性 T 细胞,已成为非清髓性调节方案的必要部分[74]。临床试验中机制研究也提示,调节性 T 细胞通过瞬时混合嵌合在诱导耐受中发挥关键作用。

T 细胞清除

实现供体反应性 T 细胞清除可通过:①电离辐射;②有效的抗 T 细胞抗体或重组蛋白。

1.总淋巴照射(TLI)。大型动物模型和人类 TLI 诱导耐受研究最早始于 20 世纪 80 年代。斯坦福研究小组在犬类实验中应用 TLI,其累积剂量为 2800~4500cGy[70]。Myburgh 等人随后提出在狒狒实验中,TLI 累积剂量减至 1600cGy 即可延长肾和肝移植的生存期[77],在该研究中,一些受体接受 DBM 注射,但其存活期与未接受 DBM 注射的受体无差异。斯坦福研究小组随后在临床肾移植试验中使用累积剂量为 2000gGy 的 TLI 评估,最初报道 3 例成功停用免疫抑制治疗的病

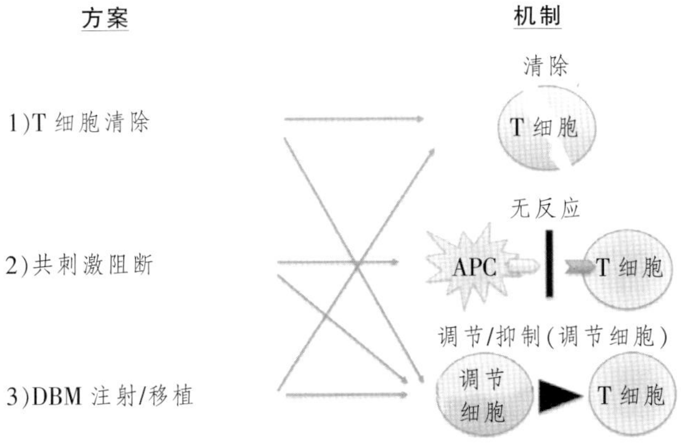

图 76.2 已用于临床移植的耐受诱导方案包括:①T 细胞清除;②共刺激阻断;③DBM(供体骨髓)注射/移植。有效的治疗方案主要来源于三种主要的诱导耐受机制:清除、无反应和调节。APC,抗原提呈细胞。

例[65],但其中 2 例因输尿管狭窄和慢性排斥,导致移植物功能丧失[66]。接受该方案的患者 1 年肾异体移植存活率为 76%[78],低于常规免疫抑制的移植物存活率。因为方案的复杂性,且未能改善移植物生存率,直到近期该研究才能进一步进行(见下文)。

2-抗 T 细胞疗法。抗 CD3(分化簇 3)免疫毒素(IT),是与突变白喉毒素蛋白(CRM9)[79]偶联的抗恒河猴 CD3 单克隆抗体(mAb),能清除恒河猴外周血和淋巴结 T 细胞,延长移植肾生存期[59,60,80]。但 IT 不防止 DSA 产生,肾脏还是会出现抗体介导的排斥反应[60]。Calne 等人基于诱导耐受的临床试验指出,人肾移植受者用阿仑单抗[Campath-1H(Genzyme,马萨诸塞州剑桥市),抗-CD52mAb]清除 T 细胞后,可处于“前(几乎)耐受”状态[81,82]。这些患者使用低剂量环孢素单一疗法,仅观察到少量排斥反应的证据,但并没有尝试完全停用免疫抑制。Starzl 等人尝试在 90 例肾移植受体中应用阿仑单抗或兔血清球蛋白进行诱导耐受[83]。在这些研究中,尽管完全停用免疫抑制治疗不成功,但在特定患者中实行间断停用免疫抑制,与历史对照相比,患者或移植物生存期无改善,两组患者慢性移植肾肾病进展相同[84]。使用阿仑单抗尝试诱导耐受的结果与其他试验也不一致。Kirk 等人在 T 细胞显著清除的情况下,用阿仑单抗治疗患者时出现急性排斥反应,移植物中单核细胞和巨噬细胞浸润,淋巴细胞排斥反应明显[85]。基于 NHP[86]的喜人结果,Kirk 等人随后在阿仑单抗方案[88]的基础上加用脱氧精胍菌素(DSG,单核细胞活化抑制剂)[87],但尽管 T 细胞清除及治疗性 DSG 给药,所有使用阿仑单抗/DSG 并尝试中断免疫抑制治疗的患者的可逆性排斥反应发生率与单独使用阿仑单抗组相似[88]。移植物活检中可观察到多种趋化因子基因转录产物增加,可能与导致淋巴细胞残留、肾移植排斥反应有关。目前多数研究认为,单独的 T 细胞清除不能诱导人类的免疫耐受。

共刺激阻断

在已确定的共刺激信号中,CD28/CD80-CD86[89,90],CD40/CD154[61,62,91]和淋巴细胞功能相关抗原(LFA)-1/ICAM-1[92]阻断已在 NHP 中测试,尽管阻断 CD80 和 CD86 未能显著延长猴的移植物生存期[90],但用人源化抗 CD154 mA6(人源化 5c8)阻断 CD40/CD154 通路后,超过一半的停止免疫抑制治疗的患者移植物生存期延

长[58,61,62]。这些实验结果均表明该方法有望用于人肾移植试验。但在该方案的唯一临床试验中,并没有观察到类似的免疫抑制效应，并且7例患者中有5例出现了排斥反应[93]。该疗法还被发现与高血栓栓塞并发症发病率相关,该抗体的进一步临床试验被暂停[94]。因此，抗CD154单克隆抗体的临床应用仍待商榷。

CTLA4Ig[由与人IgG1的Fc段融合的CTLA4细胞(细胞毒性T淋巴细胞相关蛋白-4)的外结构域组成的蛋白]用于阻断CD28/CD80-CD86通路,该试剂仅能中度延长NHP中异体移植物生存期[95,96],修饰后的CT-LA4Ig,即LEA29Y(贝拉西普),取代了其中两个氨基酸,与CD80和CD86配体解离率更低,在NHP和人类的免疫抑制作用更强[97-101],近期被批准用于临床。尽管LEA29Y的效果令人鼓舞，但其完全中止免疫抑制治疗的尝试并不成功[102]。贝拉希普是第一种被认可用于临床新型肾移植制剂,并即将用于临床诱导耐受试验。我们近期的混合嵌合方案用贝拉希图替代CD40L单克隆抗体,希望能开发出临床应用的共刺激阻断方案,且初步结果令人鼓舞(Kawai等人,仍在制备)。

在一项离体使用共刺激阻断治疗的复杂试验中，Bashuda等人报道了接受抗CD80/CD86抗体存在情况下，与供体异体抗原共同诱导培养的过度转移的致敏T细胞后,6只猴子受体中有3只的移植肾诱导耐受成功[103]。然而,移植物诱导耐受不是持续的,是第一次在NHP肾异体移植中由过度转移的致敏T细胞诱导的耐受。然而在随后的临床试验中,该方案治疗的患者未能成功停止免疫抑制治疗[104]。

供体骨髓注射/移植

DBM方案可分为仅能通过分子水平测定的微小嵌合和宏观水平易检测的混合嵌合。这两种方法通过不同的免疫机制实现。微小嵌合途径中,无论有无T细胞清除,DBM与常规免疫抑制剂一起注射，诱导的嵌合体水平最小(<0.1%),且仅通过聚合酶链反应(PCR)检测(因此称为“微小嵌合体”)[105-108]。相比之下,混合嵌合途径中,更强效的细胞毒性药物和(或)电离辐射被用于T细胞完全清除,植入DBM并诱导更高水平的嵌合体,应用流式细胞术检测。

微小嵌合方案

20世纪70年代,Monaco等人首次报道了通过注射DBM和抗淋巴细胞血清(ALS)来尝试诱导耐受[46,109]。该方案随后应用于NHP[110]和人类[111]试验,尽管在NHP研究中获得了有利结果，但初期临床试验中,57例受试者均未成功终止免疫抑制治疗，且未评价这些患者的嵌合情况。1992年,Starzl等人首先提出微小嵌合概念，用于解释使用常规免疫抑制治疗而不注射骨髓的患者出现的移植物耐受。该研究中,研究人员使用敏感细胞染色和PCR技术监测到30例移植后停用免疫抑制治疗，移植物功能仍长期稳定的肝脏或肾脏受体的少量供体白细胞(微小嵌合体)[105]。于是假设供体和受体细胞共存使其相互的克隆清除，导致外周供体反应性克隆缺失[107]。基于动物研究和Starzl的观察,已经在多种临床器官移植方案中试验了常规免疫抑制治疗联合DBM注射疗法[111-114]。到目前为止,尽管该疗法降低了急性排斥反应发生率，减少了免疫抑制药物维持剂量，但暂无证据表明其有益于患者或移植物生存期[111-113,115]。

混合嵌合

与DBMT治疗恶性肿瘤时的清髓性方案不同,用于诱导混合嵌合的治疗方案通常是非清髓性的，所以受体即使未接受DBM移植,其诱导治疗导致的全血细胞减少亦可恢复。这种非清髓性方案诱导的嵌合体为“混合嵌合体”，指供体和受体造血细胞稳定共存的状态[47,50,74,116-121]。宿主和供体来源的淋巴造血细胞成分的存在将混合造血嵌合体与清髓后的完全(即100%)嵌合体区分开来。混合嵌合的优点在于保留受体的免疫功能,且发生GVHD的概率小[117]。

HLA错配肾移植的混合嵌合

斯坦福研究小组报道了使用TLI和DBMT诱导的HLA同种异体肾移植受体成功诱导稳定的混合嵌合及移植物耐受[44,64]。该方案包括TLI(80~120cGy×10)、抗兔胸腺细胞球蛋白(1.5mg/kg×5,第0~4天)和第11天注射HLA匹配的外周血$CD34^+$干细胞。患者接受霉酚酸酯(MMF)治疗1个月,环孢菌素从第0天开始使用并持续至少6个月。接受该方案的12例患者均出现持续混合嵌合,8例患者已完全停用抑制药物,移植物最长存活期超过3年。4例患者继续接受免疫抑制药物治疗，其中1例患者出现局灶性节段性肾小球硬化复发,其余3例患者在环孢菌素减量时出现排斥反应。到目前为止,该方案尚未成功用于HLA不匹配的肾移植(见下文)。该方案中的所有治疗均始于器官移植后,可用于死亡供体移植。

马萨诸塞总医院的 10 例多发性骨髓瘤继发性肾衰竭患者接受非清髓方案和 HLA 同种异体肾移植和骨髓移植(CKBMT)治疗,后续注射供体淋巴细胞以提供额外的抗骨髓瘤效应,随访 3~14 年。方案包括环磷酰胺(60mg/kg×2)、局部胸腺照射 700cGy、马抗胸腺细胞球蛋白(ATG)和移植后 60 天环孢菌素治疗[34,35,122,123]。10 例患者全部出现混合嵌合体,其中 4 例患者接受 CKBMT 治疗 100 天后无法检测。其中 6 例患者骨髓瘤稳定缓解,4~7 年后,有 3 例患者因骨髓瘤复发死亡,2 例存活患者须针对复发性骨髓瘤行持续性治疗。在骨髓瘤稳定缓解的 6 例患者中,4 例已成功停止所有免疫抑制治疗,其余 2 例具有稳定嵌合体的患者须行低剂量免疫抑制以控制慢性轻度 GVHD 症状。尽管骨髓瘤的早期复发导致 1 例患者无法完成治疗,所有移植肾均被接受且无排斥反应的证据。

HLA 错配肾移植的混合嵌合

斯坦福研究小组尝试对 HLA 不匹配的肾移植受体使用基于 TLI 的 DBMT 方案,在该临床试验中,4 例受体中的 3 例出现了暂时多线性嵌合现象,但在尝试终止免疫抑制治疗时出现排斥反应。该研究表明,尽管该方案可成功应用于 HLA 相合的肾移植受体,但不能诱导 HLA 不匹配受体的移植物耐受。

马萨诸塞总医院基于 NHP[54,56,125,126]的研究和 HLA 匹配的 CKBMT 骨髓瘤的经验[34,122,123],对 HLA 不匹配的肾移植受体应用非清髓性疗法[32]。与骨髓瘤患者情况不同,我们认为 GVHD 对于没有潜在恶性疾病的肾移植受体是不可接受的并发症。因此,用于 HLA 匹配患者(如上所述)和用于骨髓瘤和淋巴瘤患者[127]DBMT 的 ATG 被抗 CD2 单克隆抗体 (Medi507) 取代。已知 CD2 单抗具有强效 T 细胞清除及共刺激阻断作用[128,129],且在接受不匹配 DBM 治疗恶性肿瘤的患者中不导致 GVHD[130]。当一例患者发生抗体介导的排斥反应后(见上文),HLA 不匹配移植受体的治疗方案中还增加了 CD20 单抗(利妥昔单抗)防止体液排斥反应。共有 10 例受试者被纳入这项研究,移植后 8~14 个月,有 8 例患者的免疫抑制维持剂量成功减量。8 例患者中有 1 例患者在终止免疫抑制治疗后 7 周出现急性细胞排斥反应。随着免疫抑制的重建,该患者的移植肾的功能虽然有一定程度的改善但仍有受损,该患者 3 年后接受了再移植。2 例受体不能按照计划终止免疫抑制治疗,其原因十分复杂[32]。如前所述,尽管第 1 例患者高度致敏(PRA>40%),移植前未能通过 ELISA 检测到 DSA,移植后 2 周出现不可逆的体液排斥。随后 Luminex 试验表明,该患者对供体 HLA 特异性预致敏。第 2 例患者出现了进行性血栓性微血管病变,可能是他克莫司毒性所导致,然而不能排除其他细胞排斥的原因。尽管停用钙调神经磷酸酶抑制剂,该患者在移植 6 个月后最终移植失败,恢复透析。其余已终止免疫抑制治疗的 7 例患者的肾功能保持稳定,已随访 2.5~9 年。7 例患者中有 1 例患者在移植后 7 年出现原发疾病 (Ⅰ型膜性增生性肾小球肾炎)复发,尽管该患者的肾功能保持稳定,但仍加用低剂量 MMF 以延迟复发疾病的进展。另一例患者终止免疫抑制治疗后出现短暂的抗供者 HLA Ⅱ类抗体,但连续活检未显示慢性排斥反应的证据,直到终止免疫抑制 5 年后,活检提示基底膜增厚,提示早期慢性排斥反应。尽管患者的肾功能稳定,无蛋白尿,6 年后仍重新开始免疫抑制治疗。这些患者成功终止免疫治疗,体外免疫测定法显示供体特异性无反应。然而,这种诱导耐受方法的机制尚未完全阐明,因此这些患者中诱导的混合嵌合体是短暂的,仅持续 2~3 周,假设嵌合体消失后,外周耐受机制参与维持其耐受性[32,75]。仍需进一步阐明耐受机制并修改治疗方案,以降低治疗过程中的发病率,从而加强此方法的临床实用性。

HLA 不匹配肾移植中的完全异体嵌合

直接证据表明持续性供体嵌合体可使初始条件为接受清髓性 HLA 匹配骨髓移植的血液疾病患者或肾衰竭持续多年、需要肾移植的患者成功完成器官移植。在肾脏供体与骨髓供体是同一人的情况下,成功的肾移植不需要免疫抑制治疗,证实供体嵌合体可为同供体移植组织或器官提供耐受[131]。然而,供体细胞完全取代受体骨髓和淋巴谱系可能损伤受体的免疫功能并有引起 GVHD 的风险,完全嵌合体直到最近才被认为不具有诱导异体移植物耐受的临床实用性。然而,Leventhal 等人近期报道了联用全身照射(200Gy)、阿达加滨和环磷酰胺的调节方案,联合供体造血干细胞治疗 8 例 HLA 错配肾移植受体[132]。该方案与清髓性方案相似,所有受体出现完全异体嵌合体,但可能由于运用了新的"致耐受性 $CD8^+$/TCR 促进细胞",故无 GVHD 的报道。虽然该研究的随访期较短,但其结果是惊人的;1 个月时,所有受试者均出现多谱系完全供体嵌合体;并且在8例患者中有5例患者长期维持，并完全终止免疫抑制维持1年，肾功能维持4~18个月，且尚无明显的排斥反应或GVHD证据。未能成功导致耐受的3例病例中，第1例因膜性肾病发展导致暂停终止免疫抑制，第2例出现可疑的排斥反应，第3例出现移植肾血栓形成，认为是败血症发作。最后一例患者表现出高水平嵌合，并且其败血症伴随一过性皮疹，也可能是GVHD导致的结果。

Leventhal等人报道的显著结果可归因于骨髓来源的“促进细胞“群，包括前体浆细胞样突状细胞[133]。在动物模型中发现，这些细胞可以通过诱导调节性T细胞来改善移植并避免GVHD[134,135]。

肝移植中的手术耐受性

自1969年Calne等人首次报道异体肝移植的自发性耐受以来[136]，已有许多关于异体肝移植耐受性的实验和临床研究，研究中使用的猪是远系繁殖的，未输入MHC抗原，随后的MHC特异的微型猪肝移植数据表明，这种自发性耐受只在动物MHC匹配时发生[137]，Calne的农场繁殖的猪可能有相同的MHC抗原。肝脏通常被认为是移植中最容易产生耐受性的器官，据推测，其致耐受性是多因素的，但尚不明确。由异体移植肝诱导耐受性的假说包括：①肝脏产生的可溶性MHC Ⅰ类抗原，可潜在中和移植物特异性抗体或抑制移植物反应性细胞毒性T细胞[138,139]；②移植肝中来自供体淋巴细胞的微嵌合体的存在，引起有限的移植物抗宿主反应，抵消了排斥反应[105]；③T细胞快速活化在肝脏中引起异体反应细胞的克隆缺失/凋亡；④大量的抗原提呈细胞，如肝窦状内皮细胞、Kupffer细胞和肝脏树突状细胞(DC)，以耐受的方式向初始T细胞提呈抗原[143,145]；⑤肝脏生成的调节性T细胞增殖[146]。

1997年，匹兹堡首次报道了有关肝移植耐受的大型临床研究[30]。该研究中，95例受体(64例成人和31例儿童)在移植后5年临床表现稳定，被选择终止免疫抑制治疗。其中18/95(19%)的患者成功终止免疫抑制治疗长达10个月至4.8年，18/95(19%)的患者在停用免疫抑制治疗期间出现排斥反应。伦敦国王学院研究小组尝试对18例成年受体终止免疫抑制治疗，最初报道显示，18例受体中有5例患者成功停用免疫抑制治疗，最长可达3年[147]，但后来的研究显示，10年后仅有2/18的患者可持续停用免疫抑制治疗，在丙型肝炎阳性患者的研究中，7/34(20%)的受体获得了长期(最长可达6.5年)稳定的肝功能[149,150]。

京都大学最初报道显示，在儿科患者中，较高比例的患者(38%)达到免疫抑制状态[151]，但在近期的更大样本的研究中，约15%(87/581)的患者停用免疫抑制治疗[31]。此外，最新研究显示，尽管停用免疫抑制患者无排斥反应的临床指标，但其活检标志纤维化发生率较高[152]。京都大学的研究对象中包括年龄较大的儿童患者(最大为18岁，中位年龄为12岁)，UCSF的Feng等人试图对更年轻的肝移植受体进行研究（移植后5.5~5.9个月，加入研究6~11年)，这些患者接受了父母活体供肝[153]。与京都大学研究的其他差异包括该研究移植时间更长(4年比2年)，且纳入研究前需要进行正常活检。免疫抑制治疗在最少36个月内逐渐减量，60%(12/20)的受体成功终止免疫抑制治疗，并维持正常的移植肝功能，中位值约为3年。尽管在一些耐受性受体中可检测到新的供体特异性抗体，但超过2年的随访活检显示，终止免疫抑制治疗后的病理结果与基线活检病理结果无明显变化。该研究中，虽然HLA不匹配、致敏状态和供体特异性抗体的存在与手术耐受性不相关，但是与非耐受性患者相比，耐受性患者在移植后开始终止免疫抑制治疗的时间较晚（中位值为100.6个月比73个月)。

如上所述，Starzl等人报道了使用大剂量(5mg/kg)兔抗胸腺球蛋白清除T细胞后，肾、肝和胰腺移植受体成功终止免疫抑制治疗[83]。该研究中，约70%(14/17)的受体实现最小剂量他克莫司单一疗法。但胸腺球蛋白诱导治疗未能实现完全终止免疫抑制。Eason等人尝试对18例移植后6个月的患者终止免疫抑制治疗，但只有1例患者成功终止免疫抑制治疗，大多数患者(14/18)出现排斥反应。基于微嵌合体通过克隆缺失/耗尽诱导耐受的假说[105]，迈阿密研究小组尝试通过围术期注射供体骨髓细胞(DBMC)诱导肝异体耐受[113]。尽管DBMC受体排斥反应发生率显著降低，但移植物总体生存期无明显差异。该研究中，约20%的患者成功终止免疫抑制治疗1~3年，与是否接受DBMC无关。

总之，与肾异体移植受体相比，有20%的肝异体移植受体可实现终止免疫抑制治疗后的自发性诱导耐受。尝试终止免疫抑制治疗后未出现耐受性患者的长期预后仍有待研究。到目前为止，尚无临床研究试图证明或诱导心脏或肺移植受体的手术耐受性。

耐受性生物学标志物

能准确鉴定仍处于免疫抑制状态的患者是否出现免疫耐受性的生物标志物有很高的价值，既可帮助识别哪些患者须减量或停用免疫抑制药物，还有助于探究耐受性诱导的机制。

肝移植

大多数关于耐受性生物学标志物的研究均在肝移植受体中进行，因为如上所述，肝移植终止免疫抑制治疗后出现耐受的概率高于其他器官移植。Mazariegos 等人的早期研究表明，与健康志愿者和正在进行免疫抑制维持治疗或正在经历排斥反应的受体相比，手术耐受性受体的某些淋巴细胞亚群数量增加，在终止免疫抑制治疗且移植物存活的受体中，相对于单核细胞 DC（DC1 或 $CD11c^+$ $CD123^{-/lo}$）的频率，其浆细胞样 DC 前体（DC2 或 $CD11c^-$ $CD123^{hi}$）的数量增加。其他研究表明，与非耐受性受体或健康志愿者相比，儿童和成人手术耐受性肝移植受体的外周血 $CD4^+$ $CD25^{high}$ T 细胞和 γδT 细胞（Vδ1/Vδ2 比）比例更高[155,156]。后续研究还表明，相比产生排斥反应的患者，终止免疫抑制治疗的肝移植患者 $FOXP3^+$ $CD4^+$ $CD25^{high}$ T 细胞水平显著升高[157]。近期，手机耐受性肝移植受体的基因谱证明，自然杀伤细胞、自然杀伤 T 细胞和 γδT 细胞中优先表达独特的基因组标志[156,158]。

肾移植

与肝移植的情况相反，肾移植发生自发性手术耐受性病例稀缺，难以确定其耐受性生物标志物。Brouard 等人分析了 5 例手术耐受性肾移植受体血液中的全体 T 细胞，发现与正常对照和接受常规免疫抑制治疗的稳定受体相比，其 Vβ 家族有较高 CDR3 长度分布（LD）。低剂量类固醇单一疗法的受体 TCR Vβ 也显示出类似的高 CDR3-LD[159]，但其他研究小组未得出相似结论。同一研究小组随后分析了肾移植耐受性受体的外周淋巴细胞，显示 B 细胞、$CD25^{high}$ $CD4^+$细胞绝对数显著减少，而慢性排斥反应受体 Foxp3 转录物的水平低于耐受性受体[160]。该研究小组进一步对这 5 例耐受性受者的外周血进行微阵列分析，以鉴定耐受性受体是否存在特异性基因表达模式。通过对 33 种区分耐受性和慢性排斥反应的基因进行微阵列分析后发现一个耐受性受体 49 个特异性基因[161]。然而，一例完全符合手术耐受性全面临床描述的患者随后出现了抗供体抗体，出现了排斥反应。作者认为，手术耐受性基因表达可能表现为亚稳态而并非永久状态。

近期，两项研究报道了肾移植耐受性个体的基因生物标志物，在由免疫耐受网络（ITN）赞助并在美国进行的第一项研究中，对 25 例停止免疫抑制治疗但未发生排斥反应的肾移植受体的遗传和细胞特征进行研究[162]。研究发现一组三个 B 细胞分化基因在耐受性与非耐受性受体中存在差异，尽管不是来自正常个体，但这些基因在非耐受性受体中的低表达是否与正在进行的免疫抑制有关，仍须进一步研究。这种 B 细胞特性与耐受性受体的外周血幼稚和过渡性 B 细胞数量升高有关，该结果由 ITN 资助在欧洲进行独立验证。欧洲的研究也证实了 B 细胞相关基因的差异表达的偏向，其与外周血 B 细胞和自然杀伤细胞百分比的显著升高相关。该研究还显示耐受性受体循环活化的 $CD4^+$ CD25 低表达细胞百分比显著降低，循环 $CD4^+$ $CD25^{high}$ 细胞则无显著差异，α-1、2-甘露糖苷酶基因的转录因子 Foxp3 在外周血中表达明显升高[163]。关于肾异体移植耐受性的生物学标志的研究基于有限的肾移植手术耐受性的病例，初始结果仍须更大样本的研究的进一步验证，以显示正常个体与耐受性个体生物标志物的差异。

总结

目前已有肝移植甚至停止服用免疫抑制药物的肾移植异体移植患者出现自发性耐受的报道[159,164,165]，然而，在过去的 10 年中，有意识诱导同种异体移植物耐受性的目标已经从动物模型转向 HLA 匹配和不匹配的临床肾移植。目前联合肾和 DBMT 诱导耐受是临床上诱导耐受性的唯一有效方法，还须进一步通过基础实验和临床前研究不断修改方案并研究新的方法，以降低发病率并制订常规诱导移植物耐受性的护理标准。

（周舒扬　杨梦凡　译　周舒扬　校）

参考文献

1. Murray JE, Merrill JP, Harrison JH. Kidney transplantation between seven pairs of identical twins. Annals of Surgery. 1958;148:343–359.
2. Lodhi SA, Lamb KE, Meier-Kriesche HU. Solid organ allograft survival improvement in the United States: the long-term does not mirror the dramatic short-term success. American Journal of Transplantation. 2011;11:1226–1235.
3. Meier-Kriesche HU, Schold JD, Srinivas TR, et al. Lack of improvement in renal allograft survival despite a marked decrease in acute rejection rates over the most recent era. American Journal of Transplantation. 2004;4:378–383.
4. Lentine KL, Brennan DC, Schnitzler MA. Incidence and predictors of myocardial infarction after kidney transplantation. Journal of the American Society of Nephrology. 2005;16:496–506.
5. Miller LW. Cardiovascular toxicities of immunosuppressive agents. American Journal of Transplantation. 2002;2:807–818.
6. Morales JM, Dominguez-Gil B. Cardiovascular risk profile with the new immunosuppressive combinations after renal transplantation. Journal of Hypertension. 2005;23:1609–1616.
7. Dharnidharka VR, Caillard S, Agodoa LY, et al. Infection frequency and profile in different age groups of kidney transplant recipients. Transplantation. 2006;81:1662–1667.
8. Alangaden GJ, Thyagarajan R, Gruber SA, et al. Infectious complications after kidney transplantation: current epidemiology and associated risk factors. Clinical Transplantation. 2006;20:401–409.
9. Snyder JJ, Israni AK, Peng Y, et al. Rates of first infection following kidney transplant in the United States. Kidney International. 2009;75:317–326.
10. Marcen R. Immunosuppressive drugs in kidney transplantation: impact on patient survival, and incidence of cardiovascular disease, malignancy and infection. Drugs. 2009;69:2227–2243.
11. Rama I, Grinyo JM. Malignancy after renal transplantation: the role of immunosuppression. Nature Reviews. Nephrology. 2010;6:511–519.
12. Adami J, Gabel H, Lindelof B, et al. Cancer risk following organ transplantation: a nationwide cohort study in Sweden. British Journal of Cancer. 2003;89: 1221–1227.
13. London NJ, Farmery SM, Will EJ, et al. Risk of neoplasia in renal transplant patients. Lancet. 1995;346:403–406.
14. Scantlebury V, Shapiro R, Fung J, et al. New onset of diabetes in FK 506 vs cyclosporine-treated kidney transplant recipients. Transplantation Proceedings. 1991;23:3169–3170.
15. Jindal RM, Sidner RA, Milgrom ML. Post-transplant diabetes mellitus. The role of immunosuppression. Drug Safety. 1997;16:242–257.
16. Marchetti P, Navalesi R. The metabolic effects of cyclosporin and tacrolimus. Journal of Endocrinological Investigation. 2000;23:482–490.
17. Jevnikar AM, Petric R, Holub BJ, et al. Effect of cyclosporine on plasma lipids and modification with dietary fish oil. Transplantation. 1988;46:722–725.
18. Nemunaitis J, Deeg HJ, Yee GC. High cyclosporin levels after bone marrow transplantation associated with hypertriglyceridaemia. Lancet. 1986;2(8509): 744–745.
19. Abouljoud MS, Levy MF, Klintmalm GB. Hyperlipidemia after liver transplantation: long-term results of the FK506/cyclosporine A US Multicenter Trial. US Multicenter Study Group. Transplantation Proceedings. 1995;27: 1121–1123.
20. McCune TR, Thacker LR II, Peters TG, et al. Effects of tacrolimus on hyperlipidemia after successful renal transplantation: a Southeastern Organ Procurement Foundation multicenter clinical study. Transplantation. 1998;65:87–92.
21. Ponticelli C, Campise MR. Neurological complications in kidney transplant recipients. Journal of Nephrology. 2005;18:521–528.
22. Wijdicks EF. Neurotoxicity of immunosuppressive drugs. Liver Transplantation. 2001;7:937–942.
23. Kasiske BL, Snyder JJ, Gilbertson DT, et al. Cancer after kidney transplantation in the United States. American Journal of Transplantation. 2004;4: 905–913.
24. Wimmer CD, Rentsch M, Crispin A, et al. The janus face of immunosuppression - de novo malignancy after renal transplantation: the experience of the Transplantation Center Munich. Kidney International. 2007;71:1271–1278.
25. Briganti EM, Russ GR, McNeil JJ, et al. Risk of renal allograft loss from recurrent glomerulonephritis. New England Journal of Medicine. 2002;347:103–109.
26. Lonze BE, Warren DS, Stewart ZA, et al. Kidney transplantation in previous heart or lung recipients. American Journal of Transplantation. 2009;9:578–585.
27. Terasaki PI, Ozawa M. Predicting kidney graft failure by HLA antibodies: a prospective trial. American Journal of Transplantation. 2004;4:438–443.
28. Lodhi SA, Meier-Kriesche HU. Kidney allograft survival: the long and short of it. Nephrology, Dialysis, Transplantation. 2011;26:15–17.
29. Pascual M, Theruvath T, Kawai T, et al. Strategies to improve long-term outcomes after renal transplantation. New England Journal of Medicine. 2002;346: 580–590.
30. Mazariegos GV, Reyes J, Marino IR, et al. Weaning of immunosuppression in liver transplant recipients. Transplantation. 1997;63:243–249.
31. Koshiba T, Li Y, Takemura M, et al. Clinical, immunological, and pathological aspects of operational tolerance after pediatric living-donor liver transplantation. Transplant Immunology. 2007;17:94–97.
32. Kawai T, Cosimi AB, Spitzer TR, et al. HLA-mismatched renal transplantation without maintenance immunosuppression. New England Journal of Medicine. 2008;358:353–361.
33. Kellerer AM. Risk estimates for radiation-induced cancer–the epidemiological evidence. Radiation and Environmental Biophysics. 2000;39:17–24.
34. Spitzer TR, Delmonico F, Tolkoff-Rubin N, et al. Combined histocompatibility leukocyte antigen-matched donor bone marrow and renal transplantation for multiple myeloma with end stage renal disease: the induction of allograft tolerance through mixed lymphohematopoietic chimerism. Transplantation. 1999;68:480–484.
35. Spitzer TR, Sykes M, Tolkoff-Rubin N, et al. Long-term follow-up of recipients of combined human leukocyte antigen-matched bone marrow and kidney transplantation for multiple myeloma with end-stage renal disease. Transplantation. 2011;91:672–676.
36. Meier-Kriesche HU, Schold JD, Kaplan B. Long-term renal allograft survival: have we made significant progress or is it time to rethink our analytic and therapeutic strategies? American Journal of Transplantation. 2004;4:1289–1295.
37. Fredericks EM, Dore-Stites D. Adherence to immunosuppressants: how can it be improved in adolescent organ transplant recipients? Current Opinion in Organ Transplantation. 2010;15:614–620.
38. Aujoulat I, Deccache A, Charles AS, et al. Non-adherence in adolescent transplant recipients: the role of uncertainty in health care providers. Pediatric Transplantation. 2011;15:148–156.
39. Dobbels F, Ruppar T, De Geest S, et al. Adherence to the immunosuppressive regimen in pediatric kidney transplant recipients: a systematic review. Pediatric Transplantation. 2011;14:603–613.
40. Dobbels F, Van Damme-Lombaert R, Vanhaecke J, et al. Growing pains: non-adherence with the immunosuppressive regimen in adolescent transplant recipients. Pediatric Transplantation. 2005;9:381–390.
41. Smith JM, Ho PL, McDonald RA. Renal transplant outcomes in adolescents: a report of the North American Pediatric Renal Transplant Cooperative Study. Pediatric Transplantation. 2002;6:493–499.
42. Ishitani M, Isaacs R, Norwood V, et al. Predictors of graft survival in pediatric living-related kidney transplant recipients. Transplantation. 2000;70: 288–292.
43. Levesque V, Bardwell PD, Shimizu I, et al. B-cell-dependent memory T cells impede nonmyeloablative mixed chimerism induction in presensitized mice. American Journal of Transplantation. 2011;11:2322–2331.
44. Scandling JD, Busque S, Shizuru JA, et al. Induced immune tolerance for kidney transplantation. New England Journal of Medicine. 2011;365:1359–1360.
45. Billingham RE, Brent L, Medawar PB. Activity acquired tolerance of foreign cells. Nature. 1953;172:603–606.
46. Monaco AP, Wood ML. Studies on heterologous antilymphocyte serum in mice. VII. Optimal cellular antigen for induction of immunologic tolerance with antilymphocyte serum. Transplantation Proceedings. 1970;2:489–496.
47. Ildstad ST, Sachs DH. Reconstitution with syngeneic plus allogeneic or xenogeneic bone marrow leads to specific acceptance of allografts or xenografts. Nature. 1984;307:168–170.
48. Cobbold S, Waldmann H. Infectious tolerance. Current Opinion in Immunology. 1998;10:518–524.
49. Waldmann H, Cobbold S. Exploiting tolerance processes in transplantation. Science. 2004;305:209–212.
50. Sykes M. Chimerism and central tolerance. Current Opinion in Immunology. 1996;8:694–703.
51. Azuma H, Chandraker A, Nadeau K, et al. Blockade of T-cell costimulation prevents development of experimental chronic renal allograft rejection. Proceedings of the National Academy of Sciences of the United States of America. 1996;93:12439–12444.
52. Hancock WW, Sayegh MH, Zheng XG, et al. Costimulatory function and expression of CD40 ligand, CD80, and CD86 in vascularized murine cardiac allograft rejection. Proceedings of the National Academy of Sciences of the United States of America. 1996;93:13967–13972.
53. Sayegh MH, Akalin E, Hancock WW, et al. CD28-B7 blockade after alloantigenic challenge in vivo inhibits Th1 cytokines but spares Th2. Journal of Experimental Medicine. 1995;181:1869–1874.
54. Kawai T, Cosimi AB, Colvin RB, et al. Mixed allogeneic chimerism and

renal allograft tolerance in cynomolgus monkeys. Transplantation. 1995;59: 256–262.
55. Kawai T, Poncelet A, Sachs DH, et al. Long-term outcome and alloantibody production in a non-myeloablative regimen for induction of renal allograft tolerance. Transplantation. 1999;68:1767–1775.
56. Kawai T, Sogawa H, Boskovic S, et al. CD154 blockade for induction of mixed chimerism and prolonged renal allograft survival in nonhuman primates. American Journal of Transplantation. 2004;4:1391–1398.
57. Yamada Y, Boskovic S, Aoyama A, et al. Overcoming memory T-cell responses for induction of delayed tolerance in nonhuman primates. American Journal of Transplantation. 2012;12:330–340.
58. Preston EH, Xu H, Dhanireddy KK, et al. IDEC-131 (anti-CD154), sirolimus and donor-specific transfusion facilitate operational tolerance in non-human primates. American Journal of Transplantation. 2005;5:1032–1041.
59. Knechtle SJ, Vargo D, Fechner J, et al. FN18-CRM9 immunotoxin promotes tolerance in primate renal allografts. Transplantation. 1997;63:1–6.
60. Knechtle SJ, Kirk AD, Fechner JH Jr, et al. Inducing unresponsiveness by the use of anti-CD3 immunotoxin, CTLA4-Ig, and anti-CD40 ligand. Transplantation Proceedings. 1999;31(3B Suppl.):27S–28S.
61. Kirk AD, Harlan DM, Armstrong NN, et al. CTLA4-Ig and anti-CD40 ligand prevent renal allograft rejection in primates. Proceedings of the National Academy of Sciences of the United States of America. 1997;94:8789–8794.
62. Kirk AD, Burkly LC, Batty DS, et al. Treatment with humanized monoclonal antibody against CD154 prevents acute renal allograft rejection in nonhuman primates. Nature Medicine. 1999;5:686–693.
63. Millan MT, Shizuru JA, Hoffmann P, et al. Mixed chimerism and immunosuppressive drug withdrawal after HLA-mismatched kidney and hematopoietic progenitor transplantation. Transplantation. 2002;73:1386–1391.
64. Scandling JD, Busque S, Dejbakhsh-Jones S, et al. Tolerance and chimerism after renal and hematopoietic-cell transplantation. New England Journal of Medicine. 2008;358:362–368.
65. Strober S, Dhillon M, Schubert M, et al. Acquired immune tolerance to cadaveric renal allografts. A study of three patients treated with total lymphoid irradiation. New England Journal of Medicine. 1989;321:28–33.
66. Strober S, Benike C, Krishnaswamy S, et al. Clinical transplantation tolerance twelve years after prospective withdrawal of immunosuppressive drugs: studies of chimerism and anti-donor reactivity. Transplantation. 2000;69:1549–1554.
67. Pescovitz MD, Sachs DH, Lunney JK, et al. Localization of class II MHC antigens on porcine renal vascular endothelium. Transplantation. 1984;37:627–630.
68. Pescovitz MD, Thistlethwaite JR Jr, Auchincloss H Jr, et al. Effect of class II antigen matching on renal allograft survival in miniature swine. Journal of Experimental Medicine. 1984;160:1495–1508.
69. Adams AB, Pearson TC, Larsen CP. Heterologous immunity: an overlooked barrier to tolerance. Immunological Reviews. 2003;196:147–160.
70. Wu Z, Bensinger SJ, Zhang J, et al. Homeostatic proliferation is a barrier to transplantation tolerance. Nature Medicine. 2004;10:87–92.
71. Nadazdin O, Boskovic S, Murakami T, et al. Phenotype, distribution and alloreactive properties of memory T cells from cynomolgus monkeys. American Journal of Transplantation. 2010;10:1375–1384.
72. Valujskikh A, Fedoseyeva EV, Benichou G, et al. Development of autoimmunity following skin graft rejection via an indirect alloresponse. Transplantation. 2002;73:1130–1137.
73. Feng X, Kajigaya S, Solomou EE, et al. Rabbit ATG but not horse ATG promotes expansion of functional CD4+CD25highFOXP3+ regulatory T cells in vitro. Blood. 2008;111:3675–3683.
74. Sharabi Y, Sachs DH. Mixed chimerism and permanent specific transplantation tolerance induced by a nonlethal preparative regimen. Journal of Experimental Medicine. 1989;169:493–502.
75. Andreola G, Chittenden M, Shaffer J, et al. Mechanisms of donor-specific tolerance in recipients of haploidentical combined bone marrow/kidney transplantation. American Journal of Transplantation. 2011;11:1236–1247.
76. Slavin S, Gottlieb M, Strober S, et al. Transplantation of bone marrow in outbred dogs without graft-versus-host disease using total lymphoid irradiation. Transplantation. 1979;27:139–142.
77. Myburgh JA, Smit JA, Stark JH, et al. Total lymphoid irradiation in kidney and liver transplantation in the baboon: prolonged graft survival and alterations in T cell subsets with low cumulative dose regimens. Journal of Immunology. 1984;132:1019–1025.
78. Saper V, Chow D, Engleman ED, et al. Clinical and immunological studies of cadaveric renal transplant recipients given total-lymphoid irradiation and maintained on low-dose prednisone. Transplantation. 1988;45:540–546.
79. Neville DM Jr, Scharff J, Srinivasachar K. In vivo T-cell ablation by a holo-immunotoxin directed at human CD3. Proceedings of the National Academy of Sciences of the United States of America. 1992;89:2585–2589.
80. Knechtle SJ, Fechner JH Jr, Dong Y, et al. Primate renal transplants using immunotoxin. Surgery. 1998;124:438–446; discussion 46–47.
81. Calne R, Friend P, Moffatt S, et al. Prope tolerance, perioperative campath 1H, and low-dose cyclosporin monotherapy in renal allograft recipients. Lancet. 1998;351:1701–1702.
82. Knechtle SJ, Fernandez LA, Pirsch JD, et al. Campath-1H in renal transplantation: The University of Wisconsin experience. Surgery. 2004;136:754–760.
83. Starzl TE, Murase N, Abu-Elmagd K, et al. Tolerogenic immunosuppression for organ transplantation. Lancet. 2003;361:1502–1510.
84. Shapiro R, Basu A, Tan H, et al. Kidney transplantation under minimal immunosuppression after pretransplant lymphoid depletion with thymoglobulin or Campath. Journal of the American College of Surgeons. 2005;200:505–515; quiz A59–61.
85. Kirk AD, Hale DA, Mannon RB, et al. Results from a human renal allograft tolerance trial evaluating the humanized CD52-specific monoclonal antibody alemtuzumab (CAMPATH-1H). Transplantation. 2003;76:120–129.
86. Thomas JM, Contreras JL, Jiang XL, et al. Peritransplant tolerance induction in macaques: early events reflecting the unique synergy between immunotoxin and deoxyspergualin. Transplantation. 1999;68:1660–1673.
87. Nicoletti F, Borghi MO, Barcellini W, et al. Immunosuppressive activity of 15-deoxyspergualin on normal and autoimmune peripheral blood mononuclear cells. European Journal of Pharmacology. 1996;311:213–220.
88. Kirk AD, Mannon RB, Kleiner DE, et al. Results from a human renal allograft tolerance trial evaluating T-cell depletion with alemtuzumab combined with deoxyspergualin. Transplantation. 2005;80:1051–1059.
89. Poirier N, Azimzadeh AM, Zhang T, et al. Inducing CTLA-4-dependent immune regulation by selective CD28 blockade promotes regulatory T cells in organ transplantation. Science Translational Medicine. 2010;2:17ra10.
90. Kirk AD, Tadaki DK, Celniker A, et al. Induction therapy with monoclonal antibodies specific for CD80 and CD86 delays the onset of acute renal allograft rejection in non-human primates. Transplantation. 2001;72:377–384.
91. Kenyon NS, Chatzipetrou M, Masetti M, et al. Long-term survival and function of intrahepatic islet allografts in rhesus monkeys treated with humanized anti-CD154. Proceedings of the National Academy of Sciences of the United States of America. 1999;96:8132–8137.
92. Badell IR, Russell MC, Thompson PW, et al. LFA-1-specific therapy prolongs allograft survival in rhesus macaques. Journal of Clinical Investigation. 2010;120:4520–4531.
93. Kirk ADKS, Sollinger HW, Vincenti F, et al. Preliminary results of the use of humanized anti-CD154 in human renal allotransplantation. American Journal of Transplantation. 2001;1:S191.
94. Kawai T, Andrews D, Colvin RB, et al. Thromboembolic complications after treatment with monoclonal antibody against CD40 ligand. Nature Medicine. 2000;6:114.
95. Levisetti MG, Padrid PA, Szot GL, et al. Immunosuppressive effects of human CTLA4Ig in a non-human primate model of allogeneic pancreatic islet transplantation. Journal of Immunology. 1997;159:5187–5191.
96. Krieger NR, Yuh D, McIntyre WB, et al. Prolongation of cardiac graft survival with anti-CD4Ig plus hCTLA4Ig in primates. Journal of Surgical Research. 1998;76:174–178.
97. Larsen CP, Pearson TC, Adams AB, et al. Rational development of LEA29Y (belatacept), a high-affinity variant of CTLA4-Ig with potent immunosuppressive properties. American Journal of Transplantation. 2005;5:443–453.
98. Vincenti F, Larsen C, Durrbach A, et al. Costimulation blockade with belatacept in renal transplantation. New England Journal of Medicine. 2005;353:770–781.
99. Vincenti F, Charpentier B, Vanrenterghem Y, et al. A phase III study of belatacept-based immunosuppression regimens versus cyclosporine in renal transplant recipients (BENEFIT study). American Journal of Transplantation. 2010;10: 535–546.
100. Durrbach A, Pestana JM, Pearson T, et al. A phase III study of belatacept versus cyclosporine in kidney transplants from extended criteria donors (BENEFIT-EXT study). American Journal of Transplantation. 2010;10:547–557.
101. Larsen CP, Grinyo J, Medina-Pestana J, et al. Belatacept-based regimens versus a cyclosporine A-based regimen in kidney transplant recipients: 2-year results from the BENEFIT and BENEFIT-EXT studies. Transplantation. 2010;90:1528–1535.
102. Kirk ADMS, Xu H, Mehta A, et al. Kidney transplantation using alemtuzumab induction and belatacept/sirolimus maintenance therapy. American Journal of Transplantation. 2011;11(Suppl. 2):45.
103. Bashuda H, Kimikawa M, Seino K, et al. Renal allograft rejection is prevented by adoptive transfer of anergic T cells in nonhuman primates. Journal of Clinical Investigation. 2005;115:1896–1902.
104. Koyama KBH, Seino KI, Yagi J, et al. Induction of donor specific hyporesponsiveness by adoptive transfer of ex vivo expanded anergic cells. American Journal of Transplantation. 2011;11(Suppl. 2):77.
105. Starzl TE, Demetris AJ, Trucco M, et al. Systemic chimerism in human female recipients of male livers. Lancet. 1992;340:876–877.

106. Starzl TE, Demetris AJ, Trucco M, et al. Cell migration and chimerism after whole-organ transplantation: the basis of graft acceptance. Hepatology (Baltimore, Md.). 1993;17:1127–1152.
107. Starzl TE, Demetris AJ. Transplantation tolerance, microchimerism, and the two-way paradigm. Theoretical Medicine and Bioethics. 1998;19:441–455.
108. Starzl TE. Chimerism and tolerance in transplantation. Proceedings of the National Academy of Sciences of the United States of America. 2004;101(Suppl. 2):14607–14614.
109. Gozzo JJ, Wood ML, Monaco AP. Use of allogenic, homozygous bone marrow cells for the induction of specific immunologic tolerance in mice treated with antilymphocyte serum. Surgical Forum. 1970;21:281–284.
110. Thomas JM, Carver FM, Cunningham PR, et al. Kidney allograft tolerance in primates without chronic immunosuppression–the role of veto cells. Transplantation. 1991;51:198–207.
111. Barber WH, Mankin JA, Laskow DA, et al. Long-term results of a controlled prospective study with transfusion of donor-specific bone marrow in 57 cadaveric renal allograft recipients. Transplantation. 1991;51:70–75.
112. Ciancio G, Burke GW, Garcia-Morales R, et al. Effect of living-related donor bone marrow infusion on chimerism and in vitro immunoregulatory activity in kidney transplant recipients. Transplantation. 2002;74:488–496.
113. Tryphonopoulos P, Tzakis AG, Weppler D, et al. The role of donor bone marrow infusions in withdrawal of immunosuppression in adult liver allotransplantation. American Journal of Transplantation. 2005;5:608–613.
114. Light J, Salomon DR, Diethelm AG, et al. Bone marrow transfusions in cadaver renal allografts: pilot trials with concurrent controls. Clinical Transplantation. 2002;16:317–324.
115. Delis S, Burke GW 3rd, Ciancio G. Bone marrow-induced tolerance in the era of pancreas and islets transplantation. Pancreas. 2006;32:1–8.
116. Sharabi Y, Aksentijevich I, Sundt TM 3rd, et al. Specific tolerance induction across a xenogeneic barrier: production of mixed rat/mouse lymphohematopoietic chimeras using a nonlethal preparative regimen. Journal of Experimental Medicine. 1990;172:195–202.
117. Sykes M, Sachs DH. Mixed allogeneic chimerism as an approach to transplantation tolerance. Immunology Today. 1988;9:23–27.
118. Wekerle T, Sachs DH, Sykes M. Mixed chimerism for the induction of tolerance: potential applicability in clinical composite tissue grafting. Transplantation Proceedings. 1998;30:2708–2710.
119. Wekerle T, Kurtz J, Bigenzahn S, et al. Mechanisms of transplant tolerance induction using costimulatory blockade. Current Opinion in Immunology. 2002;14: 592–600.
120. Wekerle T, Sayegh MH, Ito H, et al. Anti-CD154 or CTLA4Ig obviates the need for thymic irradiation in a non-myeloablative conditioning regimen for the induction of mixed hematopoietic chimerism and tolerance. Transplantation. 1999;68:1348–1355.
121. Tomita Y, Khan A, Sykes M. Role of intrathymic clonal deletion and peripheral anergy in transplantation tolerance induced by bone marrow transplantation in mice conditioned with a nonmyeloablative regimen. Journal of Immunology. 1994;153:1087–1098.
122. Buhler LH, Spitzer TR, Sykes M, et al. Induction of kidney allograft tolerance after transient lymphohematopoietic chimerism in patients with multiple myeloma and end-stage renal disease. Transplantation. 2002;74:1405–1409.
123. Fudaba Y, Spitzer TR, Shaffer J, et al. Myeloma responses and tolerance following combined kidney and nonmyeloablative marrow transplantation: in vivo and in vitro analyses. American Journal of Transplantation. 2006;6: 2121–2133.
124. Millan MTSJ, Shizuru J, Lowsky R, et al. Studies of tolerance and chimerism after combined blood stem cell and kidney transplantation in humans. American Journal of Transplantation. 2005;5(Suppl. 11):544.
125. Kimikawa M, Sachs DH, Colvin RB, et al. Modifications of the conditioning regimen for achieving mixed chimerism and donor-specific tolerance in cynomolgus monkeys. Transplantation. 1997;64:709–716.
126. Kawai T, Wee SL, Bazin H, et al. Association of natural killer cell depletion with induction of mixed chimerism and allograft tolerance in non-human primates. Transplantation. 2000;70:368–374.
127. Sykes M, Preffer F, McAfee S, et al. Mixed lymphohaemopoietic chimerism and graft-versus-lymphoma effects after non-myeloablative therapy and HLA-mismatched bone-marrow transplantation. Lancet. 1999;353:1755–1759.
128. Latinne D, De La Parra B, Nizet Y, et al. An anti-CD2 mAb induces immunosuppression and hyporesponsiveness of CD2+ human T cells in vitro. International Immunology. 1996;8:1113–1119.
129. Xu Y, Kolber-Simonds D, Hope JA, et al. The anti-CD2 monoclonal antibody BTI-322 generates unresponsiveness by activation-associated T cell depletion. Clinical and Experimental Immunology. 2004;138:476–483.
130. Spitzer TR, McAfee SL, Dey BR, et al. Nonmyeloablative haploidentical stem-cell transplantation using anti-CD2 monoclonal antibody (MEDI-507)-based conditioning for refractory hematologic malignancies. Transplantation. 2003;75: 1748–1751.
131. Sayegh MH, Fine NA, Smith JL, et al. Immunologic tolerance to renal allografts after bone marrow transplants from the same donors. Annals of Internal Medicine. 1991;114:954–955.
132. Leventhal J, Abecassis M, Miller J, et al. Chimerism and tolerance without GVHD or engraftment syndrome in HLA-mismatched combined kidney and hematopoietic stem cell transplantation. Science Translational Medicine. 2012;4:124ra28.
133. Kaufman CL, Colson YL, Wren SM, et al. Phenotypic characterization of a novel bone marrow-derived cell that facilitates engraftment of allogeneic bone marrow stem cells. Blood. 1994;84:2436–2446.
134. Fugier-Vivier IJ, Rezzoug F, Huang Y, et al. Plasmacytoid precursor dendritic cells facilitate allogeneic hematopoietic stem cell engraftment. Journal of Experimental Medicine. 2005;201:373–383.
135. Huang Y, Bozulic LD, Miller T, et al. CD8α+ plasmacytoid precursor DCs induce antigen-specific regulatory T cells that enhance HSC engraftment in vivo. Blood. 2011;117:2494–2505.
136. Calne RY, Sells RA, Pena JR, et al. Toleragenic effects of porcine liver allografts. British Journal of Surgery. 1969;56:692–693.
137. Flye MW, Pennington L, Kirkman R, et al. Spontaneous acceptance or rejection of orthotopic liver transplants in outbred and partially inbred miniature swine. Transplantation. 1999;68:599–607.
138. Davies HS, Pollard SG, Calne RY. Soluble HLA antigens in the circulation of liver graft recipients. Transplantation. 1989;47:524–527.
139. Zavazava N, Fandrich F, Ott KA, et al. Rat MHC class I peptides are immunogenic. Transplant International. 1996;9(Suppl. 1):S337–S339.
140. Ansari AA, Sundstrom JB, Kanter K, et al. Cellular and molecular mechanisms of human cardiac myocyte injury after transplantation. Journal of Heart and Lung Transplantation. 1995;14:102–112.
141. Bishop GA, Wang C, Sharland AF, et al. Spontaneous acceptance of liver transplants in rodents: evidence that liver leucocytes induce recipient T-cell death by neglect. Immunology and Cell Biology. 2002;80:93–100.
142. Crispe IN, Giannandrea M, Klein I, et al. Cellular and molecular mechanisms of liver tolerance. Immunological Reviews. 2006;213:101–118.
143. Thomson AW, Knolle PA. Antigen-presenting cell function in the tolerogenic liver environment. Nature Reviews. Immunology. 2010;10:753–766.
144. Thomson AW, Lu L, Wan Y, et al. Identification of donor-derived dendritic cell progenitors in bone marrow of spontaneously tolerant liver allograft recipients. Transplantation. 1995;60:1555–1559.
145. Thomson AW, Mazariegos GV, Reyes J, et al. Monitoring the patient off immunosuppression. Conceptual framework for a proposed tolerance assay study in liver transplant recipients. Transplantation. 2001;72(8 Suppl.):S13–S22.
146. Nafady-Hego H, Li Y, Ohe H, et al. The generation of donor-specific CD4+CD25++CD45RA+ naive regulatory T cells in operationally tolerant patients after pediatric living-donor liver transplantation. Transplantation. 2010;90:1547–1555.
147. Devlin J, Doherty D, Thomson L, et al. Defining the outcome of immunosuppression withdrawal after liver transplantation. Hepatology (Baltimore, Md.). 1998;27:926–933.
148. Girlanda R, Rela M, Williams R, et al. Long-term outcome of immunosuppression withdrawal after liver transplantation. Transplantation Proceedings. 2005; 37:1708–1709.
149. Tisone G, Orlando G, Cardillo A, et al. Complete weaning off immunosuppression in HCV liver transplant recipients is feasible and favourably impacts on the progression of disease recurrence. Journal of Hepatology. 2006;44:702–709.
150. Orlando G, Manzia T, Baiocchi L, et al. The Tor Vergata weaning off immunosuppression protocol in stable HCV liver transplant patients: the updated follow up at 78 months. Transplant Immunology. 2008;20:43–47.
151. Takatsuki M, Uemoto S, Inomata Y, et al. Weaning of immunosuppression in living donor liver transplant recipients. Transplantation. 2001;72:449–454.
152. Yoshitomi M, Koshiba T, Haga H, et al. Requirement of protocol biopsy before and after complete cessation of immunosuppression after liver transplantation. Transplantation. 2009;87:606–614.
153. Feng S, Ekong UD, Lobritto SJ, et al. Complete immunosuppression withdrawal and subsequent allograft function among pediatric recipients of parental living donor liver transplants. JAMA. 2012;307:283–293.
154. Mazariegos GV, Zahorchak AF, Reyes J, et al. Dendritic cell subset ratio in peripheral blood correlates with successful withdrawal of immunosuppression in liver transplant patients. American Journal of Transplantation. 2003;3: 689–696.
155. Li Y, Koshiba T, Yoshizawa A, et al. Analyses of peripheral blood mononuclear cells in operational tolerance after pediatric living donor liver transplantation. American Journal of Transplantation. 2004;4:2118–2125.
156. Martinez-Llordella M, Puig-Pey I, Orlando G, et al. Multiparameter immune profiling of operational tolerance in liver transplantation. American Journal of

Transplantation. 2007;7:309–319.

157. Pons JA, Revilla-Nuin B, Baroja-Mazo A, et al. FoxP3 in peripheral blood is associated with operational tolerance in liver transplant patients during immunosuppression withdrawal. Transplantation. 2008;86:1370–1378.
158. Martinez-Llordella M, Lozano JJ, Puig-Pey I, et al. Using transcriptional profiling to develop a diagnostic test of operational tolerance in liver transplant recipients. Journal of Clinical Investigation. 2008;118:2845–2857.
159. Brouard S, Dupont A, Giral M, et al. Operationally tolerant and minimally immunosuppressed kidney recipients display strongly altered blood T-cell clonal regulation. American Journal of Transplantation. 2005;5:330–340.
160. Louis S, Braudeau C, Giral M, et al. Contrasting CD25hiCD4+T cells/FOXP3 patterns in chronic rejection and operational drug-free tolerance. Transplantation. 2006;81:398–407.
161. Brouard S, Mansfield E, Braud C, et al. Identification of a peripheral blood transcriptional biomarker panel associated with operational renal allograft tolerance. Proceedings of the National Academy of Sciences of the United States of America. 2007;104:15448–15453.
162. Newell KA, Asare A, Kirk AD, et al. Identification of a B cell signature associated with renal transplant tolerance in humans. Journal of Clinical Investigation. 2010;120:1836–1847.
163. Sagoo P, Perucha E, Sawitzki B, et al. Development of a cross-platform biomarker signature to detect renal transplant tolerance in humans. Journal of Clinical Investigation. 2010;120:1848–1861.
164. Braud C, Baeten D, Giral M, et al. Immunosuppressive drug-free operational immune tolerance in human kidney transplant recipients: part I. Blood gene expression statistical analysis. Journal of Cellular Biochemistry. 2008;103:1681–1692.
165. Sivozhelezov V, Braud C, Giacomelli L, et al. Immunosuppressive drug-free operational immune tolerance in human kidney transplants recipients. Part II. Non-statistical gene microarray analysis. Journal of Cellular Biochemistry. 2008;103:1693–1706.

第 77 章
肾和胰腺移植术后复发性疾病

Lorna K. Henderson，Philip J. O'Connell

引言

器官移植的目标是为了实现患者和移植物的长期生存，且最大限度地减少与免疫抑制剂相关的副反应。免疫抑制剂和抗感染预防的进步对短期生存产生了有利的影响，早期急性排斥率低于 15%，移植物 1 年存活率超过 90%[1]。然而，对长期移植物功能的影响一直令人失望，晚期移植物功能衰竭目前是终末期肾病(ESKD)的主要原因。导致移植物功能不全的原因很多，复发性疾病是一个重要的却在很大程度上被忽略的原因。

随着对疾病的发病机制的深入了解和诊断水平的提高，肾脏复发性疾病比先前了解的更具挑战性。据报道，复发性疾病是移植物功能不全的一个重要原因，是导致移植物失功的第三个最常见原因（前两个是移植物带功能死亡和间质纤维化、肾小管萎缩）[2]。此外，定期活检监测研究的数据表明，真正的复发性疾病的发病率可能更大，因许多移植物功能逐渐恶化的患者可能从未接受活检却被错误地诊断为“慢性排斥反应”。复发性疾病的挑战不仅在于准确的诊断。对于许多原发性肾小球疾病，移植物复发是不可预测的，一旦诊断明确，其治疗选择也非常有限。此外，在许多情况下，复发性疾病对移植物生存的真正影响并不明确。有些可能会导致移植物功能迅速恶化，导致早期移植物衰竭，而另一些则似乎对移植物长期存活很少或根本没有影响。

胰肾联合移植(SPK)对某些 1 型糖尿病所致 ESKD 患者是一种治疗选择。在过去的 30 年中，胰腺和肾脏移植物的存活率稳步提高，注册和结果研究数据表明，1 型糖尿病患者接受胰肾联合移植的生存率高于仅接受尸体肾移植患者[3-5]。在保护移植肾避免复发糖尿病肾病的同时，胰腺仍然易患复发性自身免疫性疾病，是公认的移植物衰竭的原因。虽然有关报道认为，胰腺衰竭罕见原因，由于明确诊断依赖于胰腺活检，而大多数移植中心并不常规开展胰腺活检，所以其真正的患病率并不清楚。

本章将回顾移植后病因学、临床表现、肾脏和胰腺移植物复发性疾病的调查研究。特殊类型的肾小球肾炎的复发和胰腺自身免疫性疾病单独罗列，同时回顾当下对疾病发病机制的理解和对当前治疗方案的评价。

肾移植后复发性疾病

背景

移植是大多数终末期肾病患者选择的治疗方式，包括原发性或者特发性肾小球肾炎(GN)。然而，这种方法通常不能消除发生肾衰竭的根本原因，因此应当被视为治疗而不是治愈。

近年来，移植物短期生存率大幅改善，在于早期急性排斥率的显著改善[1]。尽管对长期生存的影响并不令人印象深刻[6]，但是整体移植物存活率提高，疾病的复发可能性也随之提高。对肾脏和胰腺长期生存的具体讨论分别参见第 103 章和 107 章。

自移植成功开始，原发性 GN 的复发就一直被纳入讨论[7,8]。先前被认为只在移植物衰竭中起很小的作用，随着移植物生存率的提高和诊断水平的提高，揭示了 GN 的复发是影响移植物的结局和生存期的一个重要因素。

复发的风险和随之而来对移植物生存的影响因不

同种类的 GN 而不同。据报道,复发率为 10%~20%,在长期随访中,高达 50%移植物失功[2,9]。这些概率可能被低估,因为许多疾病是亚临床的,免疫荧光和电子显微镜方法并不常规用于移植物活检。此外,近年来,快速类固醇的戒断或者完全禁用也导致 GN 的复发率提高,据报道,复发风险增至 3 倍[10]。

流行病学

为了更好地理解移植后 GN 的复发，了解原发性 GN 导致肾脏疾病的流行病学是非常重要的。ESKD 的原因中有 10%~25%是 GN,白种人的发病率更高[11]。儿童 GN 发病率高可能是由于 ESKD 中糖尿病肾病患病率低，而登记中心之间的种族分布差异可能部分解释肾脏疾病类型的差异。例如,与澳大利亚和新西兰透析和移植登记系统(ANZDATA)相比,美国肾脏病数据系统(USRDS)包括一大群黑种人患者。在黑种人患者中,报道的 GN 低患病率在某种程度上可能与缺乏活检信息相关，同时也与高血压肾病和糖尿病肾病的高发病率相关。

根据美国和澳大利亚登记系统分析,原发性 GN 移植后复发率为 2.9%~12.1%,与受体的年龄呈反比,与随访时间呈正比[11]。美国应用肾移植疾病登记(RADR)来更好地了解免疫性及代谢疾病的复发率，以及对移植肾功能的影响。报道证实随着时间的推移,疾病复发的风险也随之增加,从 2 年的 2.8%上升至 5 年的 9.8%和 8 年的 18.5%[12]。自从肾移植疾病登记系统建立后,在复发或者新发 GN 中,移植物存活率下降行更快。在美国的一项研究中，复发性疾病移植物的中位生存时间为 1360 天，而没有复发的移植物的中位生存时间为 3382 天($P<0.0001$)[13]。

复发性 GN 的真实发病率很难确定。分析后的数据报道受到以下因素影响:随访时间、患者疾病是否复发,有功能的移植物包括失功的移植物。复发率也可能被低估,因为许多疾病是亚临床疾病。定期活检监测研究证实,某种 GN 的患病率高于先前的报道[14,15]。此外,许多患者可能缺乏准确的诊断，因复发性疾病并未被病理证实或被误诊。

复发性疾病的定义和分类

复发和新发肾小球疾病按照临床和组织学标准进行分类(表 77.1)。为了建立准确的移植后 GN 复发的诊断,确定个准确的原发性疾病诊断和排除供体的疾病是至关重要的。这需要原位肾的活检(或植入物活检,如果 GN 不是主诊断)和移植肾的活检。文献中引用的许多瘢不符合这些标准。因此,一些患者被假定患 GN(活检来证实),移植后患上了活检证实的 GN,因而被贴上 GN 复发的标签,然而其有可能是复发或者新发 GN。此外,一些患者肾功能恶化和移植后出现蛋白尿可能永远不被活检,而被误诊为“慢性排斥反应”。当描述随后的移植物活检时,植入时活检的信息同样非常有用，未被怀疑的供体原发性 GN 也该被纳

表 77.1 复发性肾小球疾病的分类

临床分类	
真正的复发性肾小球肾炎	组织学证实的原位肾和移植肾同时为相同肾小球肾炎
新发肾小球肾炎	活检证实的肾小球疾病只出现在移植肾,而原位肾无此表现
未知原发病的移植物肾小球病	活检证实的移植肾的复发或者新发肾小球疾病,而无法取得原位肾的病理来证实诊断
供体肾小球病	活检证实的移植肾的肾小球疾病,在移植时就已经存在(经植入物活检证实)
组织学分类	
复发性原发性肾小球肾炎	局灶性节段性肾小球硬化
	IgA 肾病
	膜性肾病
	膜增生性肾小球肾炎
	抗 GBM 病
复发性继发性肾小球肾炎	狼疮性肾炎
	紫癜性肾炎
	溶血尿毒综合征(HUS)
	ANCA 相关性血管炎
	硬皮病
新发疾病	溶血尿毒综合征
	移植物肾小球病
	抗 GBM 病合并 Alport 综合征
	膜性肾小球肾炎
复发性代谢性或贮积性障碍/肾小球沉积病	糖尿病肾病
	草酸盐沉着症
	胱氨酸贮积症
	淀粉样变性
	Fabry 病
	纤维性或免疫腺泡性肾小球肾炎

ANCA,抗中性粒胞浆抗体;GBM,肾小球基底膜。

入考虑。

因此,复发的诊断可以通过以下四种方法分类:

1.真性复发性 GN: 组织学证实的原位肾和移植肾为相同的肾小球肾炎。

2.新发 GN:活检证实的肾小球疾病只出现在移植肾,而原位肾无此表现。

3.移植物肾小球病(未知原发病):因为无法取得原位肾的病理诊断,活检证实的移植肾肾小球病可能是复发或者新发的。

4.供体肾小球病:活检证实的移植肾肾小球病,在移植时就已经存在(经植入物活检证实)。

临床特征

临床诊断通常是基于新发血尿和(或)蛋白尿。血肌酐升高通常伴随着异常的尿液分析,然而疾病复发时肾功能可能是正常的或者稳定的。肾脏疾病的进展速度取决于潜在的疾病、隐匿的共存的病理改变,如间质纤维化和小管萎缩或者同样影响移植物功能的钙调蛋白抑制剂(CNI)的毒性。

除狼疮性肾炎和血管炎外,因其同时也被肾移植免疫抑制剂所控制,复发性疾病的临床过程和严重程度通常与原始疾病相似。复发时间和对移植物结局的影响也因原发病的不同而不同。移植后,局灶性节段性肾小球硬化症(FSGS)可能在几天到几周内复发,而其他肾小球肾炎如 IgA 肾病,可能在移植许多年后才复发,对移植物的结果影响很小或者没有影响。

肾外的特征和原发性疾病有关,可能伴随着疾病复发而发生。例如,复发性韦格纳肉芽肿累及肺,复发性 HUS 出现溶血、血小板减少。

检查

尿液分析

新发和持续蛋白尿,或者血尿和蛋白尿(排除感染和机械性因素),提示新发或复发性 GN,应该做进一步检查。高达 45%的移植受体存在蛋白尿(点蛋白尿或者 24 小时蛋白尿),不管是什么原因导致的,蛋白尿是移植物失功和影响患者生存的强有力的独立危险因素[16]。它代表了许多可能疾病的复合终点,包括移植物肾小球病,非特异性间质纤维化/小管萎缩(IF/TA)、小管性蛋白尿,以及新发或复发性 GN 肾小球性蛋白尿。随着高滤过、肥胖、高血压、医源性 mTOR 的使用,蛋白尿排出随之增多。相反,通过肾素-血管紧张素抑制,CNI 的治疗和因缺血、肾功能差导致的低肾小球滤过率,可以使蛋白尿减少。

移植肾病理性蛋白尿的范围不如原位肾的明确。许多中心认为 0.5g/24h 或者更高 (可能延误诊断和干预的时机), 而其他中心认为 0.15g/24h 预示着更差的结局[17]。程序性和诊断性活检研究中越来越多的证据表明,绝大多数患者的蛋白尿和特定疾病相关[18]。因此,推荐预防性处理蛋白尿,允许早期诊断和及时管理。

血清学

血清学可以支持复发性疾病的诊断,如治疗古氏病的抗肾小球基角膜(GBM)抗体和抗中性粒细胞胞浆抗体(ANCA)与韦格纳肉芽肿有关的,以及显微镜下多血管炎。其他如抗 dsDNA 则意义较小。HBV 或者 HCV 抗原有助于诊断膜增生性肾小球肾炎或者膜性肾病复发。乳酸脱氢酶升高、触珠蛋白偏低和血涂片微血管病性溶血有助于诊断 HUS 复发,但是缺乏这些证据并不能完全排除。

肾活检

对病理学家而言,鉴别诊断移植后 GN 充满着挑战,因为移植物往往存在许多潜在的组织学结果和许多共存的病理学表现,包括许多重叠的组织学特征。

肾活检对复发性 GN 的诊断至关重要。全面的组织学评估,包括光镜、免疫荧光和电子显微镜检查。可靠的移植物病理标本应包含至少 10 个肾小球和两条动脉。有些病理特征往往呈斑片状,因此建议包含至少两个皮质核。组织学的处理应等同于原位活检,光镜有助于区分新发还和复发性 GN、急性排斥反应、BK 病毒相关性肾病(BKVAN)、肾小球肾炎、CNI 肾毒性和高血压肾病,同时还能明确移植物慢性损害的程度。PAS 染色法可用于区分基底膜,银染检测可明确移植物肾小球病和膜性肾病的双重轮廓,而三色染色检测可确定胶原沉积和确定纤维化程度。光学显微镜下的特点,如肾小球基底膜的复制,可能出现在移植肾小球疾病中,使得与膜增生性肾小球肾炎(MCGN)的鉴别较为困难。免疫组化(检测免疫复合物沉积)和(或)电子显微镜(评估基底膜和沉积)的使用对明确诊断是必不可少的。

复发性肾小球肾炎的临床特征和鉴别诊断

局灶性阶段性肾小球硬化

背景和发病机制

在成年患者中，原发性 FSGS 导致 ESKD 比例很高，且其是儿童获得性肾病中导致 ESKD 的首要原因[19-22]。据报道，移植后复发风险高，为 20%~50%[23-25]，如果因为 FSGS 复发导致第一次移植失功，第二次移植时复发风险将上升到 80%~100%[26]。如果不干预，有 13%~20% 的移植物会在 10 年内失功，预后不容乐观[2]（表 77.2）。临床表现主要有两种形式，第一种（也是最常见的）发生在移植后数小时到数天，特征为早期肾病范围蛋白尿。第二种较为隐匿，发生在移植后数月甚至数年。复发风险因素包括原发病迅速恶化，发展为终末期肾病、患者年龄小、白种人、移植后复发病史。

主要临床表现为蛋白尿，且可能先于生化证据反映移植物功能不全。组织学表现为肾小球节段性硬化，电子显微镜下表现为足突消失和足突融合。在疾病复发的早期阶段，光镜结果可能是正常的，在这种情况下，电子显微镜对明确诊断是至关重要的（图 77.1）。

原发性 FSGS 的病理生理机制仍不清楚，但越来越多的证据表明，某一循环因素损害了肾小球的通透性。检测这种通透性因子的体外试验显示，具有高水平通透性因子活性的患者可能更易复发[27]。证据支持循环因子的作用包括：将复发 FSGS 的患者血清注射到大

表 77.2　疾病复发和移植失功的风险

原发性肾小球肾炎	复发率(%)	因复发导致移植失功率(%)
FSGS	20~50	13~20‡
IgA	9~61	9.7‡
膜性肾病	10~30	10~15‡
Ⅰ型膜增生性肾小球肾炎	20~50	15‡~40
Ⅱ型膜增生性肾小球肾炎	50~100	15~30§
ANCA 相关性肾小球肾炎	7*	罕见
抗 GBM		
组织学复发	15~50	罕见
临床复发	罕见*	罕见
狼疮性肾炎	2~9	2~4
溶血尿毒综合征		
所有	4~60	31
H 因子突变	80~100	74~100
I 因子突变	80~100	100
MCP 突变	罕见	罕见
硬皮病	1.9~20	20~21
纤维样肾小球肾炎	50†	罕见
Fabry 病	罕见*	罕见

FSGS，局灶性节段性肾小球硬化；IgA，免疫球蛋白 A；MCGN，系膜毛细血管性肾小球肾炎；ANCA，抗中性粒细胞胞浆抗体；GN，肾小球肾炎；GBM，肾小球基底膜；HUS，溶血尿毒综合征；MCP，膜共因子蛋白。

* 移植时疾病处于缓解期。

† 组织学诊断。

‡ 随访 10 年。

§ 随访 5 年。

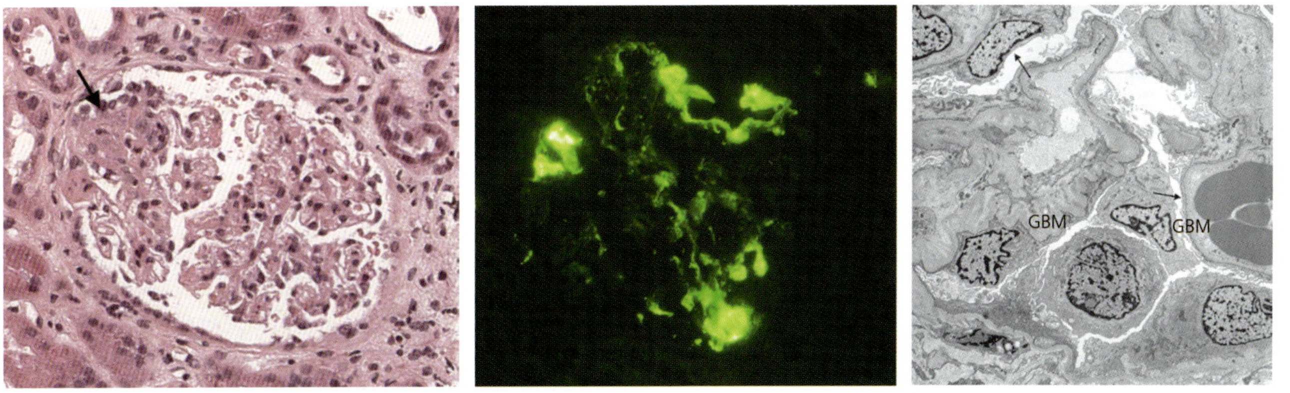

(a)　(b)　(c)

图 77.1　复发性 FSGS 患者的移植肾活检。(a)光学显微镜下显示节段性硬化症（黑色箭头）和肾小球系膜扩张（H&E）。(b)免疫荧光检查显示硬化区域内 IgM 沉积（用荧光素标记的抗 IgM 抗体的免疫荧光）。C3 和 IgG 偶尔也可能沉积在肾小球硬化节段内，可能代表非特异性血清蛋白沉积。(c)电子显微镜显示足突细胞融合（黑色箭头），肾小球基底膜（GBM）稀薄。所有病理照片由澳大利亚悉尼 Westmead 医院临床病理和医学研究所制备。

鼠,诱发大鼠产生蛋白尿[28];观察到FSGS女性患者的胎儿出现一过性肾病综合征[29];使用已知的除去循环中大分子蛋白质的方法,如血浆置换或免疫吸附,可以使疾病缓解[30,31]。多年来,通透性因子的鉴定和特性仍难以实现。其分子量为30~50kDa,这取决于糖基化和蛋白水解裂解[32,33]。假定一种蛋白质可以改变肾小球通透性,FS渗透性因子(FSPS)蛋白,已显示与半乳糖有高亲和力,并且可以被半乳糖亲和柱清除[34]。血清可溶性尿激酶受体(suPAR)已被证实为一种循环因子,可能导致FSGS[35]。2/3原发性FSGS证实suPAR的浓度升高。高血清浓度的suPAR和移植后复发相关,在实验模型中,发现suPAR可以激活足突β3整合素,导致足突消失,引起蛋白尿和FSGS样肾小球病,为疾病提供了理论基础[35]。虽然这种研究提供了明确的证据表明suPAR与疾病相关,然而以往也曾提出了一些可溶性因子作为FSGS的介质。这些来自前瞻性多中心研究的证据,将用来诊断和监测原发性FSGS[36]。

尽管大部分针对T细胞(抗CD3、CNI、抗CD53)来预防或治疗FSGS复发的处理并不成功,但关于特发性肾病综合征(INS)的人类研究和实验动物模型表明,淋巴细胞功能不全在疾病发病机制中起作用[31]。虽然缺乏直接证据,但在应用抗CD20人源化单克隆抗体、利妥昔单抗治疗复发FSGS时获得了缓解,提示B淋巴细胞参与的可能性[37]。虽然明确的发病机制仍不清楚,但足细胞损伤在疾病发病机制中的作用似乎已明确。足细胞损伤似乎是这个复杂的病理生理过程的终点,有人认为循环因子(有或没有免疫细胞的参与)与足细胞相互作用,导致nephrin和(或)podocin的丢失与足细胞的消失[31]。

治疗策略和结局

特发性FSGS通常早期出现,其中80%出现在移植后4周内[38]。原发病为FSGS的患者应在移植后早期频繁地监测蛋白尿(表77.3)。对移植前蛋白尿的了解可以解释移植后早期蛋白尿。虽然可以接受原位肾仍有尿液排出(与蛋白尿相关),但肾移植后尿液减少至消失的时间是不一定的[38]。

近几年出现了支持成功治疗复发FSGS的证据。非对照研究和病例报道显示血浆置换可以减少蛋白尿[39-41]。血浆置换可能对疾病早期复发有一定治疗作用,尽管停止治疗后蛋白尿可能会再次出现。长期使用血浆置换,无论加入或不加入环孢素或环磷酰胺,都有可能阻止疾病复发。环孢素直接作用于足细胞,阻断了钙调神经磷酸酶介导的触突去磷酸化,稳定了细胞支骨架[42]。一项小规模回顾性非随机对照研究显示,静脉用大剂量激素后口服环孢素并进行强化的、长时间的血浆置换,使90%患者获得完全缓解,而对照组用常规联合治疗使仅27%患者获得完全缓解[43]。

据小样本非随机对照研究显示,围术期预进行血浆置换可以减少儿童[44]和成人FSGS的复发[41]。但是,这种方法对尸体移植是巨大的挑战,因其增加低凝和术中、术后出血风险。

一系列案例报道利妥昔单抗已被用于治疗血浆置换难治的复发性FSGS。案例报道描述了不同的方案,结果好坏参半,从完全和持久的缓解到无反应和早期移植失功[45-48]。这些治疗在调节疾病中的作用被清楚地阐明之前,需要具有足够样本量的随机对照研究。

其他治疗这种疾病的新疗法包括抗TNF-α疗法和抗CTLA4疗法。临床试验正在进行评估维A酸(NCT00098020)和半乳糖(NCT00814255)治疗原位肾的原发性FSGS的作用。

IgA肾病

背景和发病机制

IgA肾病(IgAN)是世界上最常见的GN[49],随访25年,有30%~50%导致ESKD,也是移植后最常见的复发性GN[50]。发病机制复杂,目前对其了解仍不完全。目前认为原发病患者的链接改变产生了异常糖基化IgA1,如果沉积在肾小球系膜区(图77.2)可引起肾小球炎症和损伤。

最近的文献回顾显示复发率约为30%,各研究报道的发病率为9%~61%[51](表77.2)。随访时间不同,活检阈值不同,包括是否进行程序性活检,以及种族和地域差异,可以解释报道复发率的明显差异。程序性活检报道指出,在没有临床症状的患者中,复发率为50%~60%[52,53]。

临床表现类似于原发性IgA肾病,最常见的症状为镜下血尿、轻度蛋白尿和肾功能缓慢下降。发病可能出现在移植后早期(在这样的情况下,植入物活检是必要的,用于排除供肾IgA)。更常见的是在移植后3年复发[9]。一旦诊断建立,疾病进展通常是良性的,至少在最初是这样的。事实上,原发病为IgA肾病的患者进行肾移植,与其他疾病相比,移植物5年生存率似乎更

表 77.3　筛查复发性疾病和潜在治疗方法(adapted from Kidney Disease: Improving Global Outcomes Guidelines)

疾病	额外筛查[*]	最低筛查频率	诊断试验[†]	潜在治疗方法
FSGS	蛋白尿	每天(1 周)每周(4 周)每 3 个月(1 年)然后每年		血浆置换,糖皮质激素,环孢素,环磷酰胺,利妥昔单抗[‡] 如果有蛋白尿,AECI/ARB
IgA	蛋白尿,镜下血尿	第一个月 1 次,第一年每 3 个月 1 次,然后每年		没有有效的治疗方法 如果有蛋白尿,AECI/ARB
MN				没有有效的治疗方法 如果有蛋白尿 ,AECI/ARB
MCGN			C3,C4 水平	没有有效的治疗方法,排除治疗继发性原因(乙肝或丙肝)
ANCA 相关性 GN			ANCA	推迟移植直到临床缓解 环磷酰胺,糖皮质激素 考虑额外的治疗方法(血浆置换,利妥昔单抗)[‡]
抗 GBM		未知	抗 GBM 抗体	推迟移植直到临床缓解 环磷酰胺,糖皮质激素,血浆置换[§]
狼疮性肾炎		未知	抗 dsDNA,C3,C4	推迟移植直到临床缓解 没有有效的治疗方法 MMF[‡]
HUS	蛋白尿,血小板计数	移植物功能不全期间	血小板计数,LDH,结合珠蛋白,血涂片	使用 FFP 血浆置换 IVIG 或者利妥昔单抗[‡] 依库珠单抗[‡]

FSGS, 局灶性节段性肾小球硬化症; IgA, 免疫球蛋白 A; MCGN, 肾小球膜毛细血管性肾小球肾炎; ANCA, 抗中性粒细胞质抗体; GBM,肾小球基底膜; HUS,溶血性尿毒症综合征; LDH,乳化剂; ACEI,血管紧张素转化酶抑制剂; ARB,血管紧张素受体阻断剂; MMF,吗替麦考酚酯; FFP,新鲜冰冻血浆

[*] 除血清肌酐外。

[†] 排除肾活检。

[‡] 仅限于单一病例报道的证据。

[§] 复发伴高抗 GBM 强度和活检时细胞增多。

好[54-56]。原因尚不清楚,但可能的机制包括保护性的同种异体反应性的抗 HLA 的 IgA 抗体阻断了致病的 IgG 和 IgM 抗体对移植物的影响，或保护了 IgA 患者免疫功能的畸变[57,58]。移植物 10 年以上存活率相当或劣于其他原发性疾病。疾病的复发导致移植失功可能是部分原因,由于疾病复发导致的 10 年移植失功率估计为 9.7%[2]。

如果第一次移植后几年内，因 IgA 肾病复发而失功,第二次移植的复发风险很高(20%~100%)[51,59,60]。在这种情况下,活体移植应予以考虑。因 IgA 复发,移植物超过 10 年失功的患者应视为低风险，在这种情况下,活体移植不应该被排除。虽然复发往往频繁发生在年轻供体或那些最初呈现更严重的肾病患者，然而没有其他独立因子来预测复发性疾病的发生。虽然有假设认为复发的风险更多发生在接收活体肾的患者;然而,这是毫无事实依据的,也是相互矛盾的。

治疗策略和结局

并没有特别有效的方法来防止 IgA 肾病的复发。治疗应注重使用抑制肾素-血管紧张素来控制血压。较新的免疫抑制剂似乎对疾病的复发没有作用,据报道,霉酚酸酯(MMF)治疗后有较低的复发率,这是未经证实的。虽然据报道不用类固醇激素或迅速撤离类固醇,不会影响复发的危险[61],然而 ANZDATA 最近的生存分析报道使用类固醇与降低 IgA 肾病复发[62]的风险相关。ACEI 和 ARB 可减少蛋白尿,可能保护复发 IgA 肾病的肾功能[63]。

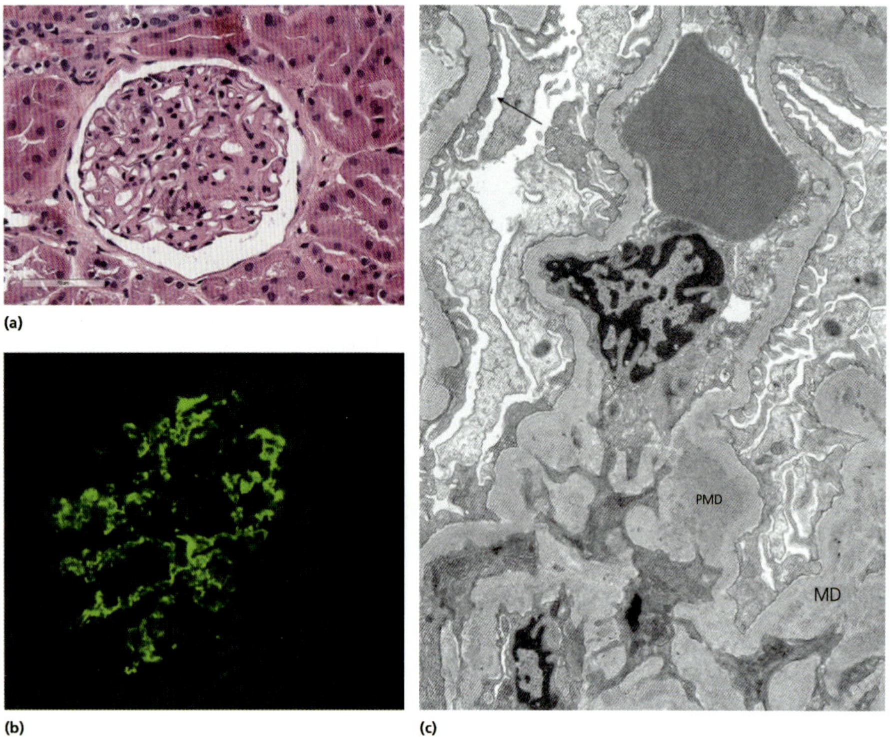

图 77.2　复发性 IgA 肾病。(a)光镜下显示系膜扩张和细胞轻度增多(HE 染色)。(b)免疫荧光显示系膜区弥漫性 IgA 染色(用荧光素标记的抗 IgA 抗体的免疫荧光)。(c)电子显微镜显示肾小球系膜区(MD)和系膜旁区(PMD)电子致密物沉积,局灶性足突融合(黑色箭头)。所有病理照片由澳大利亚悉尼 Westmead 医院临床病理和医学研究所制备。

膜性肾小球肾炎

背景和发病机制

膜性肾小球肾炎(MN)是成人肾病综合征的常见原因,导致多达 50%的患者发生 ESKD。据报道,10%~30%的患者移植后复发[64],复发率的准确评估受到 MN 的新发频率和不同中心之间活检阈值的差异的影响。定期监测活检表明 MN 复发率可能比先前估计的更高[14]。

原发性 MN 患者的移植物存活率似乎类似于具有不同肾病的(包括其他 GN)移植患者。MN 移植后复发的预后,目前还不太清楚,据报道,60%~65%的复发患者经过 4 年的时间发展到 ESKD[65,66],而在其他报道中,MN 复发和无复发患者的移植物功能衰竭、死亡或肾功能无显著差异[67]。据澳大利亚和新西兰透析和移植登记报道,10 年时移植物功能衰竭[2](见表 77.2)。

迄今为止，没有临床或组织学因子能可靠地预测复发风险。虽然一些团队已经报道活体移植[68,69]更易复发,而另一些报道却相反[70]。

临床表现通常出现在移植后第 1~2 年，并且通常以蛋白尿作为表现(经常在肾病范围),有或无肾功能不全。表现可能更早就出现了,定期监测活检表明蛋白尿或肌酐升高可能在疾病复发的初期轻度地表现或者不出现[14]。肾活检的特征是肾小球基底膜(GBM)的均匀增厚,是由于免疫复合物沉积在 GBM 外表面或上皮表面。鉴别新发 MN 和复发 MN 需要对原发肾病的准确诊断和回顾受体的原位肾活检,以协助诊断。支持新发 MN 的临床线索包括移植肾小球病、毛细血管炎、小管周围毛细血管的 C4d 沉积的组织学特征，以及供体特异性抗体的存在，所有这些都是从急性或慢性的抗体介导的排斥反应中产生的，而不是原发性 MN 复发的结果。

虽然原发性 MN 的病理生理学仍然不确定，有证据表明,针对足细胞酶 M 型磷脂酶-2 受体、锰超氧化物歧化酶和醛糖还原酶产生的自身循环抗体可能在疾病的发病机制中起作用。上皮下免疫复合物,其中含有终端补体，沉积在足细胞膜上，导致亚溶解型细胞活化,以及氧化剂和蛋白酶的生产,从而破坏潜在的肾小球基底膜。特发性 MN 患者复发的数据很少,但最近的临床观察表明自身循环抗体抗磷脂酶 A2 受体,以及供体肾暴露表位相互作用[71]。

治疗策略和结局

没有任何证据支持任意一种免疫抑制剂的治疗优势。明确地说,环孢霉素和 MMF(这已被证明治疗原发性 MN 是有益的)不能阻止或改变复发性疾病的病程。利妥昔单抗治疗复发性 MN 的报道较少，仅限于病例报道或系列研究。结果是多变的,样本量太小以至于无法达成任何确切的结论来证实其部分或完全缓解的功效。非免疫抑制疗法包括 ACEI 和 ARB，以减少蛋白尿,降脂药、利尿药用于治疗症状性水肿,以及重症肾病性蛋白尿的抗凝治疗。

系膜毛细血管性或者膜性增生性肾小球肾炎

背景和发病机制

膜性增生性肾小球肾炎(MCGN)描述了一种组织学损伤的模式,而不是一个特定的疾病。特点包括系膜细胞增多,毛细血管内增生,沿肾小球毛细血管壁双层轮廓的形成,复发性 MCGN 应该有别于新发移植物肾小球病,但这二者组织学特征相似。在这样的情况下,复发性 MCGN 在光学显微镜下有新月体,C3 染色强阳性和电子显微镜下有致密的内皮下层沉积[72],而移植物肾小球病表现为 C4d 染色和循环的供体特异性抗体存在。原发性 MCGN 可能是特发的,但通常继发于一系列潜在原因包括感染(2 型肝炎和丙型肝炎的最常见的感染原因)、自身免疫疾病(全身性红斑狼疮、干燥综合征和类风湿关节炎)和蛋白异常血症。

Ⅰ型 MCGN

疾病的发病机制是系膜和肾小球内皮下 IgG 和 C3 的沉积，可能是暴露于内源性自身抗原（SLE 的 DNA）或外源性非自身抗原（乙型肝炎或丙型肝炎抗原)产生的免疫复合物。这些抗原在移植后不被清除,可以预见复发率很高(20%~50%)[58,73,74],据报道,在这些复发患者中,移植物失功达 40%[73,74](表 77.2)。临床表现包括移植肾功能异常、镜下血尿、蛋白尿等。复发相关的危险因素包括原位肾组织学病变的严重程度、活体移植(HLA 匹配的受体似乎特别危险)、HLA-B8DR3 和既往因复发导致移植失功（其中风险上升到约 80%)[73,75]。虽然Ⅰ型 MCGN 的根本原因可能影响治疗,但是没有恰当的治疗被证明是有用的。与乙型肝炎抗原血症相关的复发性疾病可能对抗病毒治疗有反应,然而对于丙型肝炎相关的 MCGN,肝移植治疗只带来短期的成功。Ⅰ型 MCGN 的其他类型接受的免疫抑制剂伴或不伴血浆置换治疗，所有这些治疗仅带来有限的成功。

Ⅱ型 MCGN

Ⅱ型 MCGN(或致密沉积物病)表现为肾小球基底膜内电子密度形成和 C3(和其他补体蛋白)的沉积,但没有 IgG 的沉积。据说其移植物复发率更高,为 50%~100%,通常在移植后第一年内表现为非肾病范围的蛋白尿、血尿,并逐渐出现移植物肾功能不全。因复发导致移植物失功时间在 5 年以上的概率为 15%~30%[76](表 77.2)。男性、大量蛋白尿和活检显示细胞性新月体似乎与较差的结果和移植物失功高风险相关。有报道提出了细胞性新月体、间质纤维化和系膜增生(即疾病的严重程度)的叠加比疾病亚型本身更好地解释了复发的高风险[75]。无论如何,Ⅱ型 MCGN 似乎比Ⅰ型呈现出更具侵略性的组织学特征，可能解释了这组患者复发风险更大和预后更差的原因。病例报道已使用免疫抑制剂和血浆置换,但没有成功治疗的案例。

Ⅲ型 MCGN

通常被认为是Ⅰ型 MCGN 的一个变型,组织学诊断表现为内皮下和上皮下的沉积物。本病亚型复发风险或者预后的数据过于稀少而不可靠，一例成功移植后 13 个月出现复发,经历 7 年后出现移植物失功[77]。

血栓性微血管病

背景和发病机制

血栓性微血管病(TMA)的特征在于组织学表现为内皮损伤和内膜细胞增生,血管壁增厚和坏死,管腔变窄和肾小球、小动脉或小叶间动脉血栓形成。溶血性尿毒综合征(HUS)或血栓性血小板减少性紫癜(TTP)患者的肾活检中可以看到典型表现。疾病复发须与移植后继发于感染(如多瘤病毒)、医源性(和钙调磷酸酶抑制剂、mTORi 或 OKT3 相关)或免疫原因(急性体液排斥)的新发 TMA 相鉴别。

复发型 TMA 通常发生在非腹泻型 HUS 发展至肾衰竭的患者。它尤其频繁地出现在常染色体隐性或显性遗传的或非典型 HUS(aHUS)患者中,aHUS 产生于编码补体调节蛋白因子 H(CFH)、膜辅助因子蛋白(MCP)和因子 I(FI)的基因突变或多态性。据目前的研究显示，患者补体活化组分因子 B 及 C3 突变也存在复发的风险。循环补体因子蛋白、H 因子(最常见的突变)、因子 I、因子 B 及 C3,全部由肝脏产生的,解释了肾移植患者复发率高的原因。与此相反,MCP是一种膜相关的调节因子,在细胞表面限制补体活性。它普遍表达于肾同种异体移植物内的内皮细胞。出于这个原因,MCP突变的患者很少复发TMA。

aHUS患者补体缺乏或抗CFH自身抗体的肾脏内皮细胞被认为早期更容易受到缺血性损伤,引发补体激活和血栓性微血管病。移植后的病毒或细菌的感染激活补体,损伤可能加重炎症反应,如急性排斥反应,也可以进一步增加触发复发TMA的风险。

历史报道HUS患者进行肾移植后复发率为4%~60%。有些报道复发率低可能是排除了腹泻引发的HUS肾移植,而且是产生志贺毒素大肠埃希菌(STEC)相关HUS(Stx-HUS)的肾移植。STEC释放的毒素是Stx-HUS的原因,而且再次接触毒素时将诱发复发。由于大多数患者产生了中和Stx的抗体,所以复发较罕见。

一项回顾了118例腹泻引发的HUS(其中大部分应该是Stx-HUS)儿童患者接受了137次肾移植的研究中,只有1例复发。另一项纳入62例Stx-HUS儿童的研究中,没有HUS的复发,且和其他原因相比,HUS移植物的10年存活率更长[78,79]。

相反,非典型HUS(STEC感染除外)移植后结果欠佳。Bresin等人回顾,发现约60%患者经历了病情复发,91.6%进展为移植物功能衰竭。接受DCD移植的移植物的1年存活率为32%,活体移植的为50%。CFH或FI突变的存在与移植物功能衰竭的高发生率(分别为74%和100%)相关[80]。USRDS数据证实预后差,3年的存活率只有50%[81]。复发时间从几天到几年不等,但多数(60%)出现在第一个月内[79]。

临床表现从移植物轻度功能不全到缺乏肾外表现的快速进展的肾功能不全,有或无微血管病性贫血和血小板减少。应在非典型HUS患者肾功能不全期间密切监测血小板计数,应以较低阈值来评估外周血涂片(破碎细胞)、结合球蛋白和乳酸脱氢酶来寻找溶血的证据(表77.3)。在严重的血小板减少的情况下须谨慎,肾活检总是用来明确诊断。

治疗策略和结局

没有证据表明,避免使用TMA相关的药物,如CNI和mTOR抑制剂,可减少复发的风险。一些研究已经表明,早期使用环孢素增加TMA复发的风险[82],而其他研究发现没有此作用[83]。虽然有些主张避免移植后早期使用CNI[84],但是有报道指出HUS复发出现在不使用CNI免疫抑制剂的CFH或CFI突变的患者。积极治疗策略包括应用新鲜冰冻血浆(FFP)的血浆置换(增加因子H和因子I水平)、IVIG和利妥昔单抗[85,86]。成功的报道仅限于个案报道,结果不一。进行肝肾联合移植,围术期采用肝素和FFP血浆置换,已经在H因子突变的棘手案例中取得成功[87-89]。数据显示,使用人源化抗C5单克隆抗体依库珠单抗治疗原位肾的非典型HUS和挽救治疗复发性HUS已取得成功。使用依库珠单抗治疗移植后复发性疾病的5项报道中,4项完全恢复,1项部分恢复[90](表77.3)。

ANCA相关性肾炎

背景和发病机制

早期识别和治疗ANCA相关性肾炎的研究进展改善了患者的生存期和肾脏疾病的发展。尽管这样,仍然有部分患者进展至ESKD。假设已经达到和维持临床缓解,移植是安全的且疾病的复发风险很低。真正的复发率尚不清楚,数据依然稀少。一项1999年出版的汇总分析报道复发率为17%,随访时间为4~89个月。其中,57%表现为肾脏受累,但只有两例因复发而移植失功[91]。在基于他克莫司和MMF免疫抑制的时代,最近的分析报道指出复发率较低,为7%,5年移植物存活率为94%[92]。Briganti等人报道ANCA相关性血管炎10年的移植失功发生率为7.7%,但并不是所有这些移植失功都归结于疾病复发[2](表77.2)。

临床表现通常表现为移植肾功能异常伴有血尿和蛋白尿。组织学特征包括寡免疫复合物型坏死性血管炎的变化,急性动脉炎也可能存在,肉芽肿性血管炎导致输尿管狭窄阻塞也有报道。

除了移植前临床活动性疾病的证据,没有明确的因子来预测移植后疾病的复发。移植前疾病病程、疾病亚型(韦格纳肉芽肿,显微镜下多血管炎、Churg-Strauss)、cANCA或pANCA亚型和移植前抗体滴度(无临床疾病)、供体类型或随访的持续时间全都不能可靠地预测复发。

治疗策略和结局

目前用于治疗原位肾血管炎的方法对移植物似乎也有效。汇总分析和一系列病例表明复发性疾病对环磷酰胺治疗的反应良好[93]。病例报道和少量的病例系列也报道了使用其他治疗,包括血浆置换、利妥昔单抗和静脉注射免疫球蛋白,也取得成功缓解[94-98]。

抗肾小球基底膜病

早期系列病例报道移植后的复发率很高（高达50%)[99]。尽管 Goodpasture 病的复发是罕见的,但目前的治疗方法和延迟移植直到几个月检测不到抗肾小球基底膜抗体的策略,或许可以解释在过去的 15 年只有 1 例抗 GBM 病复发[100]。据报道,使用类固醇激素的冲击治疗、环磷酰胺和血浆置换可以获得良好的治疗反应。

狼疮性肾炎

背景和发病机制

5%~10%的患者从诊断狼疮性肾炎发展至 ESKD 须经历 10 年时间[101],在所有需移植的 ESKD 患者中占 1%~2%[102]。关于移植后复发率没有明确的共识。传统上认为复发率是低的，最近的数据报道复发率为 2%~9%[2,103](表 77.2)。组织学数据(包括来自定期活检监测的报道)报道的复发率为 30%~54%,但移植物失功是罕见的[15,102]。平均复发时间大约是 3 年,但也可能发生在移植后的几天内。没有标志能可靠地预测复发。尤其是血清学和移植前透析时间不能预测复发。狼疮性肾炎患者的移植物存活率报道是有争论的。汇总的数据表明三项研究的结局相当,有 6 项报道狼疮性肾炎患者结果糟糕,尽管他们的年龄较小[103]。然而,由于狼疮性肾炎复发导致移植失功并不常见(2%~4%),越来越多的数据显示,与其他不同疾病的受体相比,患者和移植物存活率相似[102,104](表 77.2)。应注意,在有已知的抗磷脂抗体的狼疮患者中,发生血栓性事件(包括移植物血栓形成)的风险更大。

治疗策略和结局

复发性狼疮性肾炎的处理还未正式定论。移植后的免疫抑制治疗和常规标准治疗没有不同。有一些报道 MMF 治疗复发性狼疮性肾炎的传闻;然而,这些目前都仅限于个案报道[105,106]。

系统性硬化症/硬皮病

背景及发病机制

约 10%硬皮病患者发生硬皮病肾危象，不论当前疗法如何,导致许多患者肾疾病进展。尽管如此,近年来存活率有所提高，肾移植可以为进展为 ESKD 的患者提供一个治疗选择。

以前认为复发的风险较高,为 20%~50%,复发患者最终移植物失功占 20% [107]。相比之下,来自美国器官共享网络(UNOS)的最新数据报道,1987—2004 年间移植的 260 例硬皮病或进行性系统性硬化症患者的复发率为 1.9%。1 年移植物存活率为 79%,5 年为 57%,10 年为 27%[108]。复发率差异的原因可能包括早期病例更为复杂的发表偏倚，同时 UNOS 复发性疾病的发病率可能未报道(不是所有的移植物失功都被报道和在 UNOS 研究中有 32%的病例移植物失功的原因是未知的)。

原位肾的硬皮病肾危象的危险因素包括使用类固醇、病程小于 4 年、进行性皮肤增厚、新发贫血、心包积液或充血性心力衰竭。没有对移植肾进行这样的风险因素研究，因此不知道使用类固醇是否会加速疾病复发。

治疗策略和结局

硬皮病复发的时间是未知的。然而,有限的数据显示复发通常出现在移植后的几个月至第二年，晚期复发是罕见的。没有很好的方法来处理复发性硬皮病。使用 ACE 抑制剂治疗高血压似乎合理,但没有证据清楚地表明这组患者是否受益。

纤维性肾小球肾炎或免疫腺泡样肾小球病

纤维性 GN 是一种公认的组织学诊断的疾病,来自西方国家研究显示,其约占原位肾脏活检的 1%。它的特点是无序排列的纤维丝积累于肾小球，其和淀粉样蛋白的大小不同,且刚果红反应呈阴性。和免疫腺泡样 GN(组织学类似)相反,纤维性 GN 很少与潜在全身性疾病相关。约 50%的患者在诊断后几年内进展为 ESKD,并且没有有效的干预治疗措施被试验。许多患者已成功地进行移植。尽管复发性疾病似乎遵循着相对良性的过程，但 50%以上的移植肾有纤维素沉积[109](表 77.2)。

法布里病

背景和发病机制

法布里病是因溶酶体酶 α 半乳糖苷酶 A 缺陷而引起的罕见的 X-连锁糖脂贮积症。它导致各种细胞和组织,包括肾上皮细胞的溶酶体内糖脂的逐渐累积,产生蛋白尿,发生肾功能不全,最终大多数受影响的患者进展成 ESKD。尽管缺乏关于疾病复发率、移植物存活率和移植后酶替代疗法疗效的数据，但肾移植是这些患者可以选择的治疗方式。美国器官获取和移植网络登记研究调查了 197 例法布里病的肾移植受体，结果发现 5 年移植物存活率为 74%，而因其他原因而移植的患者 5 年存活率为 64%[110]。同样，分析来自欧洲透析和移植协会/欧洲肾脏协会注册的数据发现，33 例法布里病的 3 年移植生存率与其他不同肾病患者相似(72%比 69%)[111]。

移植后疾病复发的证据稀少，仅限于病例报道，这些报道显示疾病移植后 6~8 个月内可能复发[112]，而在肾小管上皮细胞和内皮细胞的糖脂沉积在移植后长达 14 年被证实[113]。这些病变的存在似乎不足以损害肾功能。

治疗策略和结局

酶替代疗法(ERT)已被证明有效，半乳糖苷酶-α 或半乳糖苷酶-β 可以减慢原位肾的肾功能下降速度。然而，目前还不清楚治疗是否能改善移植存活率或降低移植相关法布里病并发症的发生率。最近的一项欧洲研究表明，ERT 是安全的，耐受性良好，在 2 年研究期间移植肾功能保持稳定。是否影响移植远期存活仍不清楚[114]。

胰腺移植后复发性疾病

背景和发病机制

胰腺移植后糖尿病复发最早在 20 世纪 80 年代由 David Sutherland 团队报道。他们报道了 10 例活体胰腺尾部移植病例。其中 5 例供体器官来自 HLA 匹配的双胞胎，另 5 例来自非孪生兄弟姐妹。当术后免疫抑制药物减量或停药时，糖尿病会快速复发。移植物病理提示胰岛炎症和选择性 β 细胞的破坏，证实了糖尿病的复发[115-117]。

然而，对于 SPK 或肾移植后胰腺移植(PAK)的受体，他们的供体并不是 HLA 匹配的，但这些受体却能获得长期的免疫抑制。这种协同作用被认为可以使大多数胰腺移植后患者避免糖尿病的复发。缺乏 MHC 匹配性意味着记忆性 CD4 和 CD8 T 细胞对新移植 β 细胞的亲和力有限。这种自体反应激活减弱看起来足以被用于防止排斥反应的联合免疫抑制作用。对于大多数胰腺移植后患者，他们的临床数据似乎可以支持这个假设。一旦移植胰腺能免于早期的技术相关并发症，远期移植物的存活情况往往比较理想。在我们中心，同一供体的移植胰腺的 20 年存活率超过移植肾，说明自身免疫疾病的复发并不会对移植物存活产生很大的影响。并且移植物可以很好地长期存活，糖耐量试验正常，糖化血红蛋白维持稳在 10 年以上且无功能减退[118]。探索胰腺移植后自身免疫复发的许多研究给出了不同的结果。一项包含了 100 例胰腺移植受体的回顾性分析研究，结合了病理组织样本、胰腺切除术、尸检等结果，并没有得出明确的自身免疫复发的证据[119]。在 HLA 不匹配的胰腺移植物中，胰岛炎症在 19%移植物中确认存在，但这种情况只存在于相关移植排斥反应发生时。尽管疾病复发无法证实，但这些受体都没有复发糖尿病[119,120]。这个团队额外随访了 200 例胰腺移植患者，他们也无法找出一例与移植物 MHC 不匹配及受体存在免疫抑制有关的自身免疫糖尿病复发病例[117]。因此，他们认为疾病复发主要发生于接受了 HLA 匹配的节段胰腺移植物及那些较低剂量或没有免疫抑制的患者。

最近，有证据显示自身免疫疾病复发是一部分胰腺移植受体移植物丧失的一个原因。首先，已有 2 例已经被组织病理学证实的自身免疫性复发性糖尿病的报道[121]。这 2 例受体接受了 HLA 匹配胰腺移植物，并且术后应用环孢素、硫唑嘌呤及糖皮质激素维持。经过最初的移植物正常期间，移植后 29 个月，胰腺失功而移植肾功能仍完好[121]。组织病理学显示，非排斥相关的胰岛炎及 β 细胞选择性丢失与免疫抑制损伤一致。另一项研究主要探究了胰岛自身抗原和胰腺移植物结局的关系[122]。他们研究了 110 例受体的胰岛自身免疫抗体并且随访了其中 75 例，最长达 11.2 年(中位随访时间为 6.3 年)。他们发现，移植物存活和移植前 GAD 或 IA-2A 抗体的出现无关。大部分(59%)患者的自身免疫抗体处于阴性状态；移植后 34%的患者自身抗体稳定或处于较低水平，而这并不能成为移植物功能丧失的一个预测因子。但是，有 5 例(7%)患者出现了 IgG1 抗体的升高并且 4 例移植物功能最终丧失，这说明小部分患者出现胰岛抗体的持续升高是移植物失功和糖尿病的非常强的预测因子[122]。

糖尿病复发最强有力的证据是由迈阿密大学的研究人员提出的。他们通过对少数患者进行很复杂的研究，发现了自身免疫性复发导致了移植物失功。他们发现 3 例移植物失功患者存在下列现象：非排斥性高血糖症、胰岛炎症伴随选择性 β 细胞减少、胰岛抗体的持续出现和再次出现，以及血液循环内存在自身反应性 CD4 和 CD8 T 细胞[123-125]。证实特异性胰岛细胞自身抗体的试验室检查非常困难，全世界只有少数研究中心才具备这项技术。因此，这不适合作为常规筛查试验。然而，这些研究证实了无论免疫抑制与否，自身免疫复发确实存在于 HLA 不匹配性胰腺移植。这种情况可能并不常见，但这会发生于高达 5%受体中[126]。目前还需要更多的研究探索这些问题，以寻找一种在移植物失功前便能诊断的标志性方法。

临床特点

临床上，当排斥反应发生伴随 C 肽减少应高度怀疑自身免疫疾病复发(表 77.4)。在 SPK 患者中这个结论非常容易证实，因为排斥诊断依赖于肾功能检测，肾活检是标准的排斥反应诊断方法。对于仅行胰腺移植或者肾移植后行胰腺移植患者，这个操作就非常困难，因为胰腺排斥可以发生在肾脏排斥时，而胰腺穿刺活检对于确定自身免疫复发和胰腺排斥是非常必要的。

检查

自身免疫糖尿病的早期特征是单核细胞浸润的胰岛炎和选择性 β 细胞减少[127]。随着时间推移，如 α 细胞在内的其他细胞也会发生不同程度的减少，但 β 细胞的减少是持续的。此外，胰腺腺泡组织和血管是正常的，无炎症细胞浸润。相反，当排斥发生时，单核细胞浸润可存在于胰腺各个部位(腺泡、胰岛和血管)，伴或不伴血管内膜炎。尽管胰腺排斥也可发生胰岛单核细胞浸润，但却不存在 β 细胞的选择性丢失，其他胰腺成分，如腺泡组织受累程度相似[119]。

表 77.4　胰腺移植后复发性 1 型糖尿病的特征

	复发性 1 型糖尿病的特征
发病率	不常见 高达小于 5%
临床特征	在无排斥情况，C 肽逐渐下降和糖尿病复发
病理	胰岛炎、β 细胞选择性损失，而腺泡和血管组织病理学正常
诊断	抗 GAD 和抗 IA2 抗体滴度再现或升高 胰腺活检
治疗	未证实有获益 如果存在免疫抑制能最大化免疫抑制

尽管证实自身免疫复发取决于组织病理学诊断，但其他实验室检查也可一定程度上提示复发的可能性。疾病复发导致持续性移植物功能丧失以及 C 肽的逐渐减少[125]。此外，抗 GAD 抗体和抗 IA2 抗体的再次出现或者升高被认为与复发相关。但是自身免疫性糖尿病是否会在自身抗体出现时复发是不确定的，许多患者能在自身抗体持续存在时长期存活。因此，诊断要依靠长期自身抗体滴度的纵向衡量，而这一指标往往不是常规检测的。

治疗策略和结局

自身免疫相关的 1 型糖尿病还没有有效的治疗方法。不同的免疫抑制或短期 T 细胞耗竭疗法在进行不断尝试，但往往效果不确切[128,129]。一项小规模临床研究旨在 1 型糖尿病发生时行自体造血干细胞移植[130]。虽然有证据显示这个方法有其益处，但是长期情况以及合适的风险评估还不确定。目前还未将其引入移植中，因为会增加已经接收长期免疫移植患者的风险，其在移植中的应用也将比较困难。

由于胰腺移植后糖尿病复发的诊断仅局限于若干病例报道，因此很难明确其疗效。对于已经长期接受免疫抑制治疗的患者，应该进行回顾分析并且确认其使用足够的免疫抑制治疗。这是一个可行的方法，因为先前的报道都是 HLA 匹配的非孪生兄弟姐妹之间移植的病例，这些病例很少应用免疫抑制治疗甚至不应用。一些中心在诊断时采用 T 细胞或 B 细胞清除性抗体，虽然这种方法可以暂时减少自身反应性 T 细胞及维持 C 肽稳定，但最终自身反应 T 细胞仍会复发并且最终导致移植物功能丧失。由于存在潜在的风险，这一方法无法被推荐用作常规治疗手段。

胰腺移植后复发性糖尿病的总结

胰腺移植后，1 型糖尿病可能复发，其是成功的胰腺移植后移植物失功和糖尿病复发的原因。对于移植后 C 肽成年累月地进行性减少，在肾脏移植物功能稳定时应高度怀疑 1 型糖尿病复发。抗 GAD 和抗 IA2 抗体滴度再次出现或升高时，也高度提示该诊断，但最终确诊需要胰腺病理活检。尽管该病不常见，但实际发病率目前尚不清楚。很明显，这个领域需要更多的实验和研究去探索。

总结

尽管肾脏和胰腺移植的研究已经有了很大的突破，但我们对于两种器官复发疾病的诊断以及真实发病情况仍然不清楚，并且治疗干预措施受限。

其中一部分问题主要在于我们对于相关器官的原发性疾病尚缺乏足够的认知。但是与其把它作是一种障碍，不如把它视为一种机会，可以为我们制订不同维持免疫移植方案提供一个新的视角。此外，新的分子方法的出现，最初目的是允许对移异体植物进行侵入性病理可以将诸如基因序列、蛋白组学和代谢组学的技术，用于研究可发生于非移植物的原发疾病的病因和发病机制。

由于病例数量相对缺乏，为了更好地预防和治疗干预方法，更大的多中心合作试验是非常有必要的。这样可以更清楚地了解复发性疾病的发病情况、复发风险及对移植物存活的影响。

（刘原兴 译 刘原兴 校）

参考文献

1. Meier-Kriesche HU, Schold JD, Kaplan B. Long-term renal allograft survival: have we made significant progress or is it time to rethink our analytic and therapeutic strategies? American Journal of Transplantation. 2004;4:1289–1295.
2. Briganti EM, Russ GR, McNeil JJ, et al. Risk of renal allograft loss from recurrent glomerulonephritis. New England Journal of Medicine. 2002;347:103–109.
3. Becker BN, Brazy PC, Becker YT, et al. Simultaneous pancreas-kidney transplantation reduces excess mortality in type 1 diabetic patients with end-stage renal disease. Kidney International. 2000;57:2129–2135.
4. Ojo AO, Meier-Kriesche HU, Hanson JA, et al. The impact of simultaneous pancreas-kidney transplantation on long-term patient survival. Transplantation. 2001;71:82–90.
5. Smets YF, Westendorp RG, van der Pijl JW, et al. Effect of simultaneous pancreas-kidney transplantation on mortality of patients with type-1 diabetes mellitus and end-stage renal failure. Lancet. 1999;353:1915–1919.
6. McDonald S, Russ G, Campbell S, et al. Kidney transplant rejection in Australia and New Zealand: relationships between rejection and graft outcome. American Journal of Transplantation. 2007;7:1201–1208.
7. Hume DM, Merrill JP, Miller BF, et al. Experiences with renal homotransplantation in the human: report of nine cases. Journal of Clinical Investigation. 1955;34:327–382.
8. Glassock RJ, Feldman D, Reynolds ES, et al. Human renal isografts: a clinical and pathologic analysis. Medicine. 1968;47:411–454.
9. Hariharan S, Savin VJ. Recurrent and de novo disease after renal transplantation: a report from the Renal Allograft Disease Registry. Pediatric Transplantation. 2004;8:349–350.
10. Kukla A, Chen E, Spong R, et al. Recurrent glomerulonephritis under rapid discontinuation of steroids. Transplantation. 2011;91:1386–1391.
11. Golgert WA, Appel GB, Hariharan S. Recurrent glomerulonephritis after renal transplantation: an unsolved problem. Clinical Journal of the American Society of Nephrology. 2008;3:800–807.
12. Hariharan S, Peddi VR, Savin VJ, et al. Recurrent and de novo renal diseases after renal transplantation: a report from the renal allograft disease registry. American Journal of Kidney Diseases. 1998;31:928–931.
13. Hariharan S, Adams MB, Brennan DC, et al. Recurrent and de novo glomerular disease after renal transplantation: a report from Renal Allograft Disease Registry (RADR). Transplantation. 1999;68:635–641.
14. Dabade TS, Grande JP, Norby SM, et al. Recurrent idiopathic membranous nephropathy after kidney transplantation: a surveillance biopsy study. American Journal of Transplantation. 2008;8:1318–1322.
15. Norby GE, Strom EH, Midtvedt K, et al. Recurrent lupus nephritis after kidney transplantation: a surveillance biopsy study. Annals of the Rheumatic Diseases. 2010;69:1484–1487.
16. Cherukuri A, Welberry-Smith MP, Tattersall JE, et al. The clinical significance of early proteinuria after renal transplantation. Transplantation. 2010;89:200–207.
17. Keane WF, Eknoyan G. Proteinuria, albuminuria, risk, assessment, detection, elimination (PARADE): a position paper of the National Kidney Foundation. American Journal of Kidney Diseases. 1999;33:1004–1010.
18. Nankivell BJ, Borrows RJ, Fung CL, et al. The natural history of chronic allograft nephropathy. New England Journal of Medicine. 2003;349:2326–2333.
19. Filler G, Young E, Geier P, et al. Is there really an increase in non-minimal change nephrotic syndrome in children? American Journal of Kidney Diseases. 2003;42:1107–1113.
20. Kitiyakara C, Eggers P, Kopp JB. Twenty-one-year trend in ESRD due to focal segmental glomerulosclerosis in the United States. American Journal of Kidney Diseases. 2004;44:815–825.
21. Artero M, Biava C, Amend W, et al. Recurrent focal glomerulosclerosis: natural history and response to therapy. American Journal of Medicine. 1992;92:375–383.
22. Tejani A, Nicastri AD, Sen D, et al. Long-term evaluation of children with nephrotic syndrome and focal segmental glomerular sclerosis. Nephron. 1983;35:225–231.
23. Couser W. Recurrent glomerulonephritis in the renal allograft: an update of selected areas. Experimental and Clinical Transplantation. 2005;3:283–288.
24. Tejani A, Stablein DH. Recurrence of focal segmental glomerulosclerosis posttransplantation: a special report of the North American Pediatric Renal Transplant Cooperative Study. Journal of the American Society of Nephrology. 1992;2(12 Suppl.):S258–S263.
25. Vincenti F, Ghiggeri GM. New insights into the pathogenesis and the therapy of recurrent focal glomerulosclerosis. American Journal of Transplantation. 2005;5:1179–1185.
26. Newstead CG. Recurrent disease in renal transplants. Nephrology, Dialysis, Transplantation. 2003;18(Suppl. 6):vi68–vi74.
27. Savin VJ, Sharma R, Sharma M, et al. Circulating factor associated with increased glomerular permeability to albumin in recurrent focal segmental glomerulosclerosis. New England Journal of Medicine. 1996;334:878–883.
28. Zimmerman SW. Increased urinary protein excretion in the rat produced by serum from a patient with recurrent focal glomerular sclerosis after renal transplantation. Clinical Nephrology. 1984;22:32–38.
29. Lagrue G, Branellec A, Niaudet P, et al. [Transmission of nephrotic syndrome to two neonates. Spontaneous regression]. La Presse Medicale. 1991;20:255–257.
30. Dantal J, Godfrin Y, Koll R, et al. Antihuman immunoglobulin affinity immunoadsorption strongly decreases proteinuria in patients with relapsing nephrotic syndrome. Journal of the American Society of Nephrology. 1998;9:1709–1715.
31. Canaud G, Martinez F, Noel LH, et al. Therapeutic approach to focal and segmental glomerulosclerosis recurrence in kidney transplant recipients. Transplantation Reviews (Orlando, Fla.). 2010;24:121–128.
32. Blasi F, Carmeliet P. uPAR: a versatile signalling orchestrator. Nature Reviews. Molecular Cell Biology. 2002;3:932–943.
33. Smith HW, Marshall CJ. Regulation of cell signalling by uPAR. Nature Reviews. Molecular Cell Biology. 2010;11:23–36.
34. Savin VJ, McCarthy ET, Sharma R, et al. Galactose binds to focal segmental glomerulosclerosis permeability factor and inhibits its activity. Translational Research. 2008;151:288–292.
35. Wei C, El Hindi S, Li J, et al. Circulating urokinase receptor as a cause of focal segmental glomerulosclerosis. Nature Medicine. 2011;17:952–960.
36. Parikh SM. Circulating mediators of focal segmental glomerulosclerosis: soluble urokinase plasminogen activator receptor in context. American Journal of Kidney Diseases. 2012;59:336–339.
37. Pescovitz MD, Book BK, Sidner RA. Resolution of recurrent focal segmental glomerulosclerosis proteinuria after rituximab treatment. New England Journal of Medicine. 2006;354:1961–1963.
38. Myslak M, Amer H, Morales P, et al. Interpreting post-transplant proteinuria in patients with proteinuria pre-transplant. American Journal of Transplantation. 2006;6:1660–1665.
39. Davenport RD. Apheresis treatment of recurrent focal segmental glomerulosclerosis after kidney transplantation: re-analysis of published case-reports and case-

series. Journal of Clinical Apheresis. 2001;16:175–178.
40. Matalon A, Markowitz GS, Joseph RE, et al. Plasmapheresis treatment of recurrent FSGS in adult renal transplant recipients. Clinical Nephrology. 2001;56: 271–278.
41. Gohh RY, Yango AF, Morrissey PE, et al. Preemptive plasmapheresis and recurrence of FSGS in high-risk renal transplant recipients. American Journal of Transplantation. 2005;5:2907–2912.
42. Faul C, Donnelly M, Merscher-Gomez S, et al. The actin cytoskeleton of kidney podocytes is a direct target of the antiproteinuric effect of cyclosporine A. Nature Medicine. 2008;14:931–938.
43. Canaud G, Zuber J, Sberro R, et al. Intensive and prolonged treatment of focal and segmental glomerulosclerosis recurrence in adult kidney transplant recipients: a pilot study. American Journal of Transplantation. 2009;9: 1081–1086.
44. Ohta T, Kawaguchi H, Hattori M, et al. Effect of pre-and postoperative plasmapheresis on posttransplant recurrence of focal segmental glomerulosclerosis in children. Transplantation. 2001;71:628–633.
45. Yabu JM, Ho B, Scandling JD, et al. Rituximab failed to improve nephrotic syndrome in renal transplant patients with recurrent focal segmental glomerulosclerosis. American Journal of Transplantation. 2008;8:222–227.
46. Hristea D, Hadaya K, Marangon N, et al. Successful treatment of recurrent focal segmental glomerulosclerosis after kidney transplantation by plasmapheresis and rituximab. Transplant International. 2007;20:102–105.
47. Gossmann J, Scheuermann EH, Porubsky S, et al. Abrogation of nephrotic proteinuria by rituximab treatment in a renal transplant patient with relapsed focal segmental glomerulosclerosis. Transplant International. 2007;20:558–562.
48. Kamar N, Faguer S, Esposito L, et al. Treatment of focal segmental glomerular sclerosis with rituximab: 2 case reports. Clinical Nephrology. 2007;67:250–254.
49. Barratt J, Feehally J. IgA nephropathy. Journal of the American Society of Nephrology. 2005;16:2088–2097.
50. Furness PN, Roberts IS, Briggs JD. Recurrent glomerular disease in transplants. Transplantation Proceedings. 2002;34:2422.
51. Ponticelli C, Traversi L, Banfi G. Renal transplantation in patients with IgA mesangial glomerulonephritis. Pediatric Transplantation. 2004;8:334–338.
52. Berger J, Noel LH, Nabarra B. Recurrence of mesangial IgA nephropathy after renal transplantation. Contributions to Nephrology. 1984;40:195–197.
53. Odum J, Peh CA, Clarkson AR, et al. Recurrent mesangial IgA nephritis following renal transplantation. Nephrology, Dialysis, Transplantation. 1994;9:309–312.
54. Kessler M, Hiesse C, Hestin D, et al. Recurrence of immunoglobulin A nephropathy after renal transplantation in the cyclosporine era. American Journal of Kidney Diseases. 1996;28:99–104.
55. Andresdottir MB, Hoitsma AJ, Assmann KJ, et al. Favorable outcome of renal transplantation in patients with IgA nephropathy. Clinical Nephrology. 2001; 56:279–288.
56. Choy BY, Chan TM, Lo SK, et al. Renal transplantation in patients with primary immunoglobulin A nephropathy. Nephrology, Dialysis, Transplantation. 2003;18: 2399–2404.
57. Lim EC, Chia D, Gjertson DW, et al. In vitro studies to explain high renal allograft survival in IgA nephropathy patients. Transplantation. 1993;55:996–999.
58. Choy BY, Chan TM, Lai KN. Recurrent glomerulonephritis after kidney transplantation. American Journal of Transplantation. 2006;6:2535–2542.
59. Ohmacht C, Kliem V, Burg M, et al. Recurrent immunoglobulin A nephropathy after renal transplantation: a significant contributor to graft loss. Transplantation. 1997;64:1493–1496.
60. Bumgardner GL, Amend WC, Ascher NL, et al. Single-center long-term results of renal transplantation for IgA nephropathy. Transplantation. 1998;65: 1053–1060.
61. Ibrahim H, Rogers T, Casingal V, et al. Graft loss from recurrent glomerulonephritis is not increased with a rapid steroid discontinuation protocol. Transplantation. 2006;81:214–219.
62. Clayton P, McDonald S, Chadban S. Steroids and recurrent IgA nephropathy after kidney transplantation. American Journal of Transplantation. 2011;11: 1645–1649.
63. Oka K, Imai E, Moriyama T, et al. A clinicopathological study of IgA nephropathy in renal transplant recipients: beneficial effect of angiotensin-converting enzyme inhibitor. Nephrology, Dialysis, Transplantation. 2000;15:689–695.
64. Couchoud C, Pouteil-Noble C, Colon S, et al. Recurrence of membranous nephropathy after renal transplantation. Incidence and risk factors in 1614 patients. Transplantation. 1995;59:1275–1279.
65. Cosyns JP, Couchoud C, Pouteil-Noble C, et al. Recurrence of membranous nephropathy after renal transplantation: probability, outcome and risk factors. Clinical Nephrology. 1998;50:144–153.
66. Josephson MA, Spargo B, Hollandsworth D, et al. The recurrence of recurrent membranous glomerulopathy in a renal transplant recipient: case report and literature review. American Journal of Kidney Diseases. 1994;24:873–878.
67. Sprangers B, Lefkowitz GI, Cohen SD, et al. Beneficial effect of rituximab in the treatment of recurrent idiopathic membranous nephropathy after kidney transplantation. Clinical Journal of the American Society of Nephrology. 2010;5:790–797.
68. Wang AY, Lai FM, Yu AW, et al. Recurrent IgA nephropathy in renal transplant allografts. American Journal of Kidney Diseases. 2001;38:588–596.
69. Andresdottir MB, Haasnoot GW, Doxiadis II, et al. Exclusive characteristics of graft survival and risk factors in recipients with immunoglobulin A nephropathy: a retrospective analysis of registry data. Transplantation. 2005;80:1012–1018.
70. Ponticelli C, Traversi L, Feliciani A, et al. Kidney transplantation in patients with IgA mesangial glomerulonephritis. Kidney International. 2001;60:1948–1954.
71. Stahl R, Hoxha E, Fechner K. PLA2R autoantibodies and recurrent membranous nephropathy after transplantation. New England Journal of Medicine. 2010;363: 496–498.
72. Andresdottir MB, Assmann KJ, Koene RA, et al. Immunohistological and ultrastructural differences between recurrent type I membranoproliferative glomerulonephritis and chronic transplant glomerulopathy. American Journal of Kidney Diseases. 1998;32:582–588.
73. Andresdottir MB, Assmann KJ, Hoitsma AJ, et al. Recurrence of type I membranoproliferative glomerulonephritis after renal transplantation: analysis of the incidence, risk factors, and impact on graft survival. Transplantation. 1997;63:1628–1633.
74. Chadban S. Glomerulonephritis recurrence in the renal graft. Journal of the American Society of Nephrology. 2001;12:394–402.
75. Little MA, Dupont P, Campbell E, et al. Severity of primary MPGN, rather than MPGN type, determines renal survival and post-transplantation recurrence risk. Kidney International. 2006;69:504–511.
76. Braun MC, Stablein DM, Hamiwka LA, et al. Recurrence of membranoproliferative glomerulonephritis type II in renal allografts: The North American Pediatric Renal Transplant Cooperative Study experience. Journal of the American Society of Nephrology. 2005;16:2225–2233.
77. Morales JM, Martinez MA, Munoz de Bustillo E, et al. Recurrent type III membranoproliferative glomerulonephritis after kidney transplantation. Transplantation. 1997;63:1186–1188.
78. Ferraris JR, Ramirez JA, Ruiz S, et al. Shiga toxin-associated hemolytic uremic syndrome: absence of recurrence after renal transplantation. Pediatric Nephrology (Berlin, Germany). 2002;17:809–814.
79. Noris M, Remuzzi G. Thrombotic microangiopathy after kidney transplantation. American Journal of Transplantation. 2010;10:1517–1523.
80. Bresin E, Daina E, Noris M, et al. Outcome of renal transplantation in patients with non-Shiga toxin-associated hemolytic uremic syndrome: prognostic significance of genetic background. Clinical Journal of the American Society of Nephrology. 2006;1:88–99.
81. Reynolds JC, Agodoa LY, Yuan CM, et al. Thrombotic microangiopathy after renal transplantation in the United States. American Journal of Kidney Diseases. 2003;42:1058–1068.
82. Artz MA, Steenbergen EJ, Hoitsma AJ, et al. Renal transplantation in patients with hemolytic uremic syndrome: high rate of recurrence and increased incidence of acute rejections. Transplantation. 2003;76:821–826.
83. Quan A, Sullivan EK, Alexander SR. Recurrence of hemolytic uremic syndrome after renal transplantation in children: a report of the North American Pediatric Renal Transplant Cooperative Study. Transplantation. 2001;72:742–745.
84. Ponticelli C, Banfi G. Thrombotic microangiopathy after kidney transplantation. Transplant International. 2006;19:789–794.
85. Banerjee D, Kupin W, Roth D. Hemolytic uremic syndrome after multivisceral transplantation treated with intravenous immunoglobulin. Journal of Nephrology. 2003;16:733–735.
86. Yassa SK, Blessios G, Marinides G, et al. Anti-CD20 monoclonal antibody (Rituximab) for life-threatening hemolytic-uremic syndrome. Clinical Transplantation. 2005;19:423–426.
87. Remuzzi G, Ruggenenti P, Codazzi D, et al. Combined kidney and liver transplantation for familial haemolytic uraemic syndrome. Lancet. 2002;359:1671–1672.
88. Jalanko H, Peltonen S, Koskinen A, et al. Successful liver-kidney transplantation in two children with aHUS caused by a mutation in complement factor H. American Journal of Transplantation. 2008;8:216–221.
89. Saland JM, Shneider BL, Bromberg JS, et al. Successful split liver-kidney transplant for factor H associated hemolytic uremic syndrome. Clinical Journal of the American Society of Nephrology. 2009;4:201–206.
90. Kavanagh D, Goodship TH. Atypical hemolytic uremic syndrome, genetic basis, and clinical manifestations. Hematology the Education Program of the American Society of Hematology.. 2011;2011:15–20.
91. Nachman PH, Segelmark M, Westman K, et al. Recurrent ANCA-associated small vessel vasculitis after transplantation: a pooled analysis. Kidney International. 1999;56:1544–1550.
92. Gera M, Griffin MD, Specks U, et al. Recurrence of ANCA-associated vasculitis

following renal transplantation in the modern era of immunosupression. Kidney International. 2007;71:1296–1301.
93. Geetha D, Seo P. Renal transplantation in the ANCA-associated vasculitides. American Journal of Transplantation. 2007;7:2657–2662.
94. Rosenstein ED, Ribot S, Ventresca E, et al. Recurrence of Wegener's granulomatosis following renal transplantation. British Journal of Rheumatology. 1994; 33:869–871.
95. Nyberg G, Akesson P, Norden G, et al. Systemic vasculitis in a kidney transplant population. Transplantation. 1997;63:1273–1277.
96. Lobbedez T, Comoz F, Renaudineau E, et al. Recurrence of ANCA-positive glomerulonephritis immediately after renal transplantation. American Journal of Kidney Diseases. 2003;42:E2–E6.
97. Geetha D, Seo P, Specks U, et al. Successful induction of remission with rituximab for relapse of ANCA-associated vasculitis post-kidney transplant: report of two cases. American Journal of Transplantation. 2007;7:2821–2825.
98. Hermle T, Goestemeyer AK, Sweny P, et al. Successful therapeutic use of rituximab in refractory Wegener's granulomatosis after renal transplantation. Clinical Nephrology. 2007;68:322–326.
99. Wilson CB, Dixon FJ. Anti-glomerular basement membrane antibody-induced glomerulonephritis. Kidney International. 1973;3:74–89.
100. Khandelwal M, McCormick BB, Lajoie G, et al. Recurrence of anti-GBM disease 8 years after renal transplantation. Nephrology, Dialysis, Transplantation. 2004;19:491–494.
101. Houssiau FA, Vasconcelos C, D'Cruz D, et al. The 10-year follow-up data of the Euro-Lupus Nephritis Trial comparing low-dose and high-dose intravenous cyclophosphamide. Annals of the Rheumatic Diseases. 2010;69:61–64.
102. Goral S, Ynares C, Shappell SB, et al. Recurrent lupus nephritis in renal transplant recipients revisited: it is not rare. Transplantation. 2003;75:651–656.
103. Stone JH, Millward CL, Olson JL, et al. Frequency of recurrent lupus nephritis among ninety-seven renal transplant patients during the cyclosporine era. Arthritis and Rheumatism. 1998;41:678–686.
104. Moroni G, Tantardini F, Gallelli B, et al. The long-term prognosis of renal transplantation in patients with lupus nephritis. American Journal of Kidney Diseases. 2005;45:903–911.
105. Denton MD, Galvanek EG, Singh A, et al. Membranous lupus nephritis in a renal allograft: response to mycophenolate mofetil therapy. American Journal of Transplantation. 2001;1:288–292.
106. Ahuja TS, Boughton J, Weiss V, et al. Late recurrence of lupus nephritis in a renal transplant recipient: response to mycophenolate mofetil. American Journal of the Medical Sciences. 2001;322:166–169.
107. Kotanko P, Pusey CD, Levy JB. Recurrent glomerulonephritis following renal transplantation. Transplantation. 1997;63:1045–1052.
108. Pham PT, Pham PC, Danovitch GM, et al. Predictors and risk factors for recurrent scleroderma renal crisis in the kidney allograft: case report and review of the literature. American Journal of Transplantation. 2005;5:2565–2569.
109. Samaniego M, Nadasdy GM, Laszik Z, et al. Outcome of renal transplantation in fibrillary glomerulonephritis. Clinical Nephrology. 2001;55:159–166.
110. Shah T, Gill J, Malhotra N, et al. Kidney transplant outcomes in patients with Fabry disease. Transplantation. 2009;87:280–285.
111. Tsakiris D, Simpson HK, Jones EH, et al. Report on management of renale failure in Europe, XXVI, 1995. Rare diseases in renal replacement therapy in the ERA-EDTA Registry. Nephrology, Dialysis, Transplantation. 1996; 11(Suppl. 7):4–20.
112. Alroy J, Sabnis S, Kopp JB. Renal pathology in Fabry disease. Journal of the American Society of Nephrology. 2002;13(Suppl. 2):S134–S138.
113. Gantenbein H, Bruder E, Burger HR, et al. Recurrence of Fabry's disease in a renal allograft 14 years after transplantation. Nephrology, Dialysis, Transplantation. 1995;10:287–289.
114. Cybulla M, Walter KN, Schwarting A, et al. Kidney transplantation in patients with Fabry disease. Transplant International. 2009;22:475–481.
115. Sutherland DE, Sibley R, Xu XZ, et al. Twin-to-twin pancreas transplantation: reversal and reenactment of the pathogenesis of type I diabetes. Transactions of the Association of American Physicians. 1984;97:80–87.
116. Sibley RK, Sutherland DE, Goetz F, et al. Recurrent diabetes mellitus in the pancreas iso- and allograft. A light and electron microscopic and immunohistochemical analysis of four cases. Laboratory Investigation. 1985;53:132–144.
117. Sutherland DE, Goetz FC, Sibley RK. Recurrence of disease in pancreas transplants. Diabetes. 1989;38(Suppl. 1):85–87.
118. Nankivell BJ, Chapman JR, Bovington KJ, et al. Glucose homeostasis standards for pancreas transplantation. Clinical Transplantation. 1998;12:434–438.
119. Sibley RK, Sutherland DE. Pancreas transplantation. An immunohistologic and histopathologic examination of 100 grafts. American Journal of Pathology. 1987;128:151–170.
120. Drachenberg CB, Papadimitriou JC, Weir MR, et al. Histologic findings in islets of whole pancreas allografts: lack of evidence for recurrent cell-mediated diabetes mellitus. Transplantation. 1996;62:1770–1772.
121. Tyden G, Reinholt FP, Sundkvist G, et al. Recurrence of autoimmune diabetes mellitus in recipients of cadaveric pancreatic grafts. New England Journal of Medicine. 1996;335:860–863.
122. Braghi S, Bonifacio E, Secchi A, et al. Modulation of humoral islet autoimmunity by pancreas allotransplantation influences allograft outcome in patients with type 1 diabetes. Diabetes. 2000;49:218–224.
123. Vendrame F, Pileggi A, Laughlin E, et al. Recurrence of type 1 diabetes after simultaneous pancreas-kidney transplantation, despite immunosuppression, is associated with autoantibodies and pathogenic autoreactive CD4 T-cells. Diabetes. 2010;59:947–957.
124. Laughlin E, Burke G, Pugliese A, et al. Recurrence of autoreactive antigen-specific CD4+ T cells in autoimmune diabetes after pancreas transplantation. Clinical Immunology (Orlando, Fla.). 2008;128:23–30.
125. Pugliese A, Reijonen HK, Nepom J, et al. Recurrence of autoimmunity in pancreas transplant patients: research update. Diabetes Management(London, England). 2011;1:229–238.
126. Gruessner RW, Pugliese A, Reijonen HK, et al. Development of diabetes mellitus in living pancreas donors and recipients. Expert Review of Clinical Immunology. 2011;7:543–551.
127. Foulis AK. The pathology of islets in diabetes. Eye (Lond). 1993;7:197–201.
128. Bonifacio E. Immunotherapy in type 1 diabetes: a shorter but more winding road? Diabetes. 2012;61:2214–2215.
129. Chatenoud L, Warncke K, Ziegler AG. Clinical immunologic interventions for the treatment of type 1 diabetes. Cold Spring Harbor Perspectives in Medicine. 2012;2:a007716.
130. Voltarelli JC, Couri CE, Stracieri AB, et al. Autologous nonmyeloablative hematopoietic stem cell transplantation in newly diagnosed type 1 diabetes mellitus. JAMA. 2007;297:1568–1576.

第 78 章
肝移植后复发性疾病

Samir Parekh, James R. Spivey

引言

对于许多慢性肝病患者，原位肝移植(OLT)提供了最佳的术后生存率和较高的长期生活质量。对于一些患者来说，肝移植可以治愈困扰已久的肝病，帮助受体摆脱复发的风险；而对另一些患者来说，原有疾病仍可能复发，或者显示患者之前未被确诊的疾病，这些都是术后可能出现阻碍康复的困难与挑战。本章我们将着重讨论肝移植后的复发性疾病：医生对复发性疾病的诊断不一定正确，如原发性硬化性胆管炎的复发与特殊的缺血性胆管疾病尤其难以鉴别、原发性自身免疫性疾病本身不断演变导致难以做出正确的诊断。或许受到这些疾病的低存活率所影响，科学家目前正致力于丙型肝炎复发问题的研究。另一方面，曾经一度令人恐惧的乙型肝炎复发问题可能很快就将成为一段历史。本章涵盖了肝移植受体常见的复发风险，同时叙述了这些复发疾病的鉴别诊断和治疗，也对第 70 章的临床鉴别和肝移植同种异体排斥的管理进行了补充，并为第 82 章对肝移植组织病理学的深入探讨提供了临床背景。

病毒性疾病

丙型肝炎病毒

丙型肝炎病毒(HCV)的再感染是原位肝移植术后造成 HCV 患者免疫排斥和死亡的主要原因[1]。Forman 回顾了器官共享联合网络(UNOS)数据库中超过 11 000 例原位肝移植病例，比较了 HCV 阳性和 HCV 阴性患者的预后，发现 HCV 阳性患者的移植死亡率和器官排斥率比 HCV 阴性患者更高；但这项结果与其他移植中心的小型研究结果相反[2-5]。移植后 HCV 再感染的患者再行移植的成功率比初次移植要低[6,7]，也就导致了一些移植中心拒绝为患者实施再次肝移植术，尤其是肾脏功能不全的患者。当 HCV 阴性患者的肝功能不全程度、体能状态与 HCV 阳性患者相似时，HCV 阳性患者再移植的预后与 HCV 阴性患者相比可能并不会出现显著差异[8]。

病毒动力学

原位肝移植后，丙肝感染的复发通常发生得十分迅速，尤其是在患者术中感染 HCV 病毒血症的病例中。丙肝病毒 RNA 水平在无肝期和再灌注后短期内显著下降[9]，高达 90%的患者在 OLT 后一周内会患上病毒血症，7~8 周内病毒载量达到峰值，却又不易被医务工作者所发现。移植受体的平均病毒载量高于移植之前应用免疫抑制剂阶段。Gane 等[10]指出，为防止急性细胞排斥反应而应用的大剂量激素冲击疗法与高病毒载量和严重的组织病理损伤密切相关。

病程

一旦移植物发生感染，临床过程就变得变化多端。5%~7%的患者会发展成严重的纤维化淤胆性肝炎，这些患者通常携带高载量的病毒，表现为肝坏死和黄疸。病理检查发现包括小叶中心的肝细胞球囊性肝细胞变性、胆汁淤积和小叶炎(图 78.1)。该疾病进展迅速而且预后较差，或许可以由此证明病毒对肝移植物的损伤作用[11]。大多数患者在肝移植 3~6 个月内出现小叶性肝炎，约 25%的患者在 3~5 年内经历了严重的复发疾病，导致了移植肝硬化或晚期纤维化。Ciccorossi 等[12]认为行 OLT 1 周后携带高病毒载量会导致疾病的预后较差。Sreekumar 等[13]注意到，在行 OLT 4 个月后，丙肝病毒 RNA 水平更高(大于 10^9/mL 或大于 log 1meq/mL)，

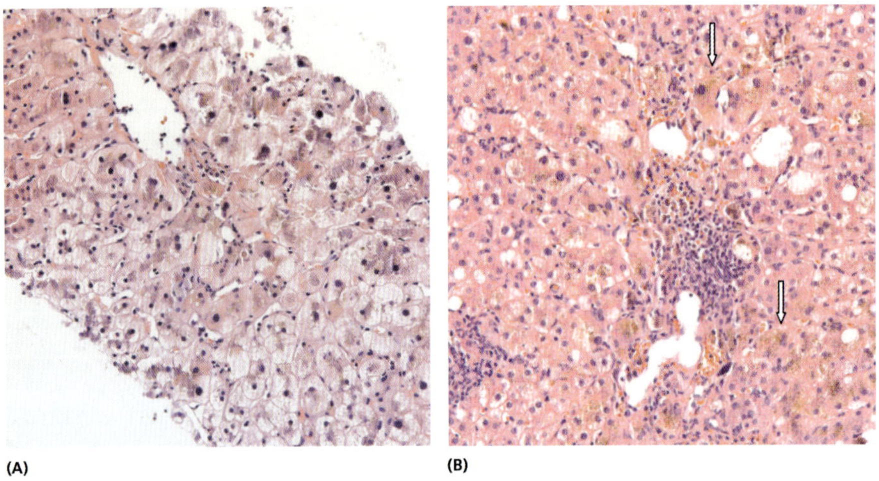

图 78.1 (A)纤维化淤胆型丙型肝炎(HCV)复发导致球囊样肝细胞变性;(B)胆代淤积(箭头)与纤维化淤胆性 HCV 复发相关胆。

OLT 后炎症水平和纤维化的程度也更严重。大约有 2/3 的患者会有不同程度的病毒载量增高,但很少会发生纤维化或者仅发生轻度的肝纤维化。典型的疾病过程包括:移植物感染的数月内发生轻度肝小时炎(图 78.2),随后是镜下表现更明显的淋巴细胞汇管区浸润和慢性活动性肝炎(图 78.3)。OLT 后丙肝病毒复发感染常常使得肝移植患者的生活质量下降和身体功能受损[14]。丙肝病毒复发感染的病理诊断容易被急性细胞排斥反应的病理表现所干扰[15]。患者发生急性细胞排斥反应时,通常大剂量地应用激素,这也导致了 HCV 复发感染的组织学表现更加明显。表 78.1 概括了 HCV 严重复发感染的预测因素。

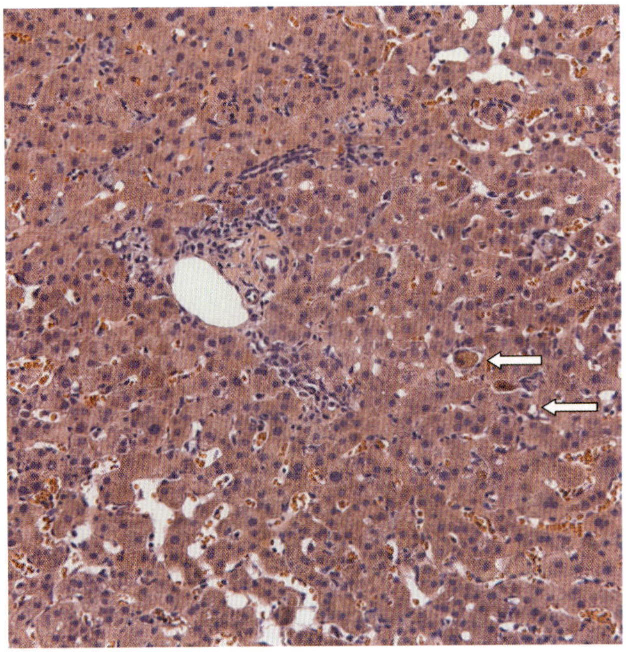

图 78.2 HCV 早期复发伴小叶炎和康氏小体(箭头)。

受体因素和病毒特征

容易导致 HCV 感染患者在 OLT 术后预后较差的因素包括移植前病毒载量、受体年龄、性别、种族和丙肝病毒基因型[1,10,12,16]。在上述因素中,移植前高病毒载量最容易导致移植物失功和死亡[1]。病毒基因型和病毒异质性等特点可能与疾病的严重程度相关,但这些发现实际应用很少,因为 OLT 前的病毒基因型不一定与

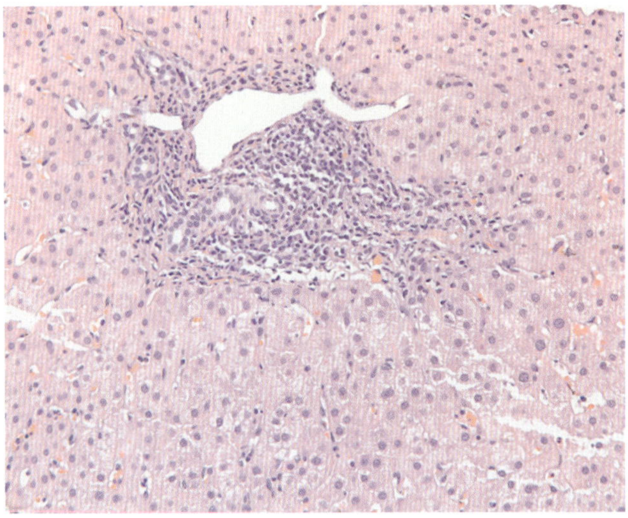

图 78.3 淋巴细胞汇管区浸润和 HCV 复发引起的交界性肝炎。

表 78.1　复发性 HCV 更严重感染的危险因素

因素	证据强度
移植前	
供体年龄(大于 35 岁呈线性相关)	+++
活体捐献	+
供体/受体 HLA 匹配	+
1B 基因型	
HIV 共感染	+++
女性	+
时代(最近)	+
供体脂肪变性	+
手术因素	
更长的冷缺血时间(>12 小时)	++
供体遗传因素	+
移植后受体因素	
年龄大于 50 岁	+++(患者/移植物生存率)
非白色人种/种族	+++(患者生存率)
胆道并发症	++
病毒性指标	
移植前更高的病毒载量	+++
移植后更高的病毒载量	+++
免疫抑制	
OKT3,糖皮质激素冲击疗法	+++
早期复发	+++
已治疗的巨细胞病毒感染	+++

(Adapted from [49] Watt et al.(2009),with permission from John Wiley and Sons Ltd.)

OLT 后感染的病毒基因型一致[17]。有研究表明,HCV 基因型 1b 可能会导致 OLT 后严重的 HCV 感染[10],但在其他研究中并未验证这种差异[3,18,19]。在一项小样本研究中,HCV 基因型 4 感染的患者纤维化进展更快,预后更差,其他预后结果与其他基因型相比没有明显差异[20]。另一项来自澳大利亚的研究提示,HCV 基因型 4 病毒感染的患者相比其他类型的患者,预后相对较差[21]。在上述诸多的因素中,患者群体的异质性和免疫抑制方案的差异使得数据分析尤为困难。

供体因素

供体年龄是供体因素中与 HCV 复发程度相关性最强的。在欧洲和北美,无论是活体捐献还是遗体捐献器官,但凡供体年龄大于 50 岁,特别是大于 65 岁,已被明确证实更容易导致预后不良[22-24]。供体器官脂肪变性可能导致 OLT 后更早和更频繁的 HCV 复发感染[25],但由于脂肪变性导致的不良预后,必须首先排除长时间缺血和再灌注损伤的干扰[26]。

其他因素

为了让肝移植后 HCV 感染的受体有更好的预后,我们需要防治众多并发症。过度的免疫抑制必须避免,虽然 HCV 阴性的受体发生急性排斥反应并不会产生巨大影响,但急性排斥反应会使得 HCV 阳性受体产生更差的预后[27]。如何在 HCV 感染的患者中最合理地使用免疫抑制剂是移植领域的难点,引起专家们的密切关注。巨细胞病毒(CMV)感染是与免疫抑制水平直接相关的又一因素,可以导致复发疾病的迅速进展,但它与移植物存活率的关联仍有待考察[28,29]。尽管很难排除缺血再灌注损伤的干扰,但可以知道的是胆道并发症的发生预示着 HCV 感染患者的预后将更加糟糕。一项来自两个中心的纳入 700 例患者的回顾性研究显示,虽然胆道并发症可能降低移植物 1 年存活率,但是患胆道并发症合并 HCV 感染并不会影响移植物纤维化的发生率[30]。

治疗挑战

实施后续免疫抑制治疗的初始目的是通过治疗持续清除 HCV 感染,但是现有大量的数据证明,通过 OLT 前期和后期的免疫抑制治疗,针对病毒的持续免疫应答(SVR)可能持续存在[31-33]。研究者担心,先前患有肝炎的患者在接受肝移植后会重新感染[34]。然而,上述观点需要针对病毒载量和病毒检测的现代实验室检查以及合理的随访来支撑[35]。个别学者报道,在忽略患者肝硬化评分的前提下,针对 HCV 复发感染的早期治疗手段有导致肝硬化进展和门脉高压的风险[36]。由于某些丙型肝炎患者在原位肝移植术后病情并没有快速进展,以及考虑到可能由治疗干预引起的慢性排斥反应和自体免疫现象,有研究项目仅在患者病情恶化必须接受治疗时,启动治疗方案[37,38]。那些使用抗病毒治疗而产生不良后果的案例报道一般只涉及个别患者,需要谨慎对待的同时,一般不需要采取过激的治疗方案。与直接的抗病毒疗法相比,目前用于移植后 HCV 复发感染的公认的治疗方案是聚乙二醇干扰素(长效干扰素)和利巴韦林。移植后的患者更不易耐受上述治疗方案,且常常由于并发贫血,治疗剂量通常需要减量。病毒的持续免疫应答的比率在不同个体间差异巨大，但在许多研究中大约30%的患者可以获得持续免疫应答,并且当治疗不足48周时很少发现[39]。在2005年时,仍没有OLT后HCV治疗的前瞻性随机试验。在一项多中心研究中,Chalasani等人设计了两组随机对照试验,一组行预防试验和另一组行治疗试验,用于评估聚乙二醇干扰素α-2a治疗OLT后丙肝病毒复发的安全性和有效性。应用干扰素α-2a治疗的患者HCV的RNA水平明显降低,肝组织学特点也发生改善。然而,在预防试验中只有2例患者(8%),在治疗试验中只有3例患者(12%)获得了持续的病毒免疫应答。在预防性试验中,使用长效干扰素α-2a的患者中有8例(31%),未治疗组中有9例(32%)退出实验;而在治疗性试验中，使用长效干扰素α-2a的患者中有10例(30%),未治疗组中有6例(19%)也退出实验。在预防性试验(12%比21%;P=0.5)和治疗性试验(12%比0%，P=0.1)中,治疗组和非治疗组的急性排斥反应发生率相似[40]。IL28B基因型在其中扮演角色的重要性以及患者在OLT后对治疗的敏感性尚不确定。而近期一项来自巴塞罗那的研究表明，决定OLT后HCV感染的患者治疗成功与否的主要因素是受体和供体的IL28B基因表型[41]。

对于治疗药物导致的移植物排斥的担忧仍然存在,而且各种数据彼此矛盾[42]。在一项研究中,干扰素导致的排斥反应出现时可以被轻松治愈[43],而在法国的某项研究中,70例患者在使用干扰素治疗时，其中21%发生排斥反应,5例反应程度较轻微,9例反应程度适中以及1例十分严重。另一项研究中,几乎所有患者在治疗中发生排斥反应，但是却没有发生移植物功能丢失[44]。具有排斥反应病史的患者在使用长效干扰素时十分容易产生排斥反应。最终,Berardi等人发现,尽管体内病毒被清除，但干扰素和利巴韦林联合的抗病毒疗法导致了44例中的9例患者患上原发性自身免疫性肝炎[45]。自身免疫性肝炎和(或)浆细胞性肝炎的发生将在后文介绍。

新型病毒特异性药物(波普瑞韦和特拉匹韦)的出现提供了更安全有效的治疗选择，在减少并发症的同时提高疗效。尽管目前用于移植后的新型病毒特异性药物和其他药品的检测数据仍然有限，但可以预见的是，特异性抗病毒药物将会在未来占据治疗丙肝患者移植后复发疾病的大部分的药品市场。

浆细胞性肝炎

Ward和其他学者引起了人们对在原位肝移植后复发HCV感染的患者身上出现的浆细胞性肝炎的关注[46]。对于其属于自身免疫性疾病还是排斥反应的特殊类型,人们尚未知晓。所有的问题都集中在一个更大的挑战上:HCV患者肝脏移植物活检特征的具体含义是什么？当两种疾病都具有肝小叶汇管区炎症和淋巴细胞浸润的胆管炎等共同特征时，丙肝复发与急性排斥反应的鉴别就显得十分困难。Demetris和Sebagh发现,对急性排斥反应的治疗可能导致HCV的表现更加显著[47]。他们在2008年的评论着重强调小叶中央的细胞坏死、与急性和慢性排斥反应的联系、浆细胞浸润和自身免疫现象的重要性。在普通人群中,HCV患者出现自身免疫现象被研究得十分透彻，包括冷球蛋白血症和血管炎、自身抗体和血清中类风湿因子的生成、干燥综合征、肾炎和B细胞淋巴瘤[48]。尽管既往的经验清楚地表明,具有自身免疫特征的HCV阳性肝移植患者使用糖皮质激素经常有效，但在一些研究中对肝移植患者使用糖皮质激素的治疗方案已被弃用。然而,个别具有自身免疫特征的HCV阳性移植患者可能会经历更加严重的疾病过程和更糟糕的预后结果。每个个体的移植后疾病进程、组织活检特征和HCV阳性的移植物受体对糖皮质激素和抗病毒治疗的敏感性都不会完全一致，也就要求我们注意这些患者病程中的不同特性,认识到不能以同样的方治疗每个患者。然而,一般的治疗方案都会有效[42,49]。

免疫抑制的注意事项

他克莫司和丙型肝炎病毒抗体检测在20世纪90年代早期进入临床。从那时起,研究者就对免疫抑制对于原位肝移植后丙肝病毒复发感染的严重程度的影响产生了强烈兴趣。Berenguer等人[50]在2000年报道,最近几年肝移植后HCV复发感染导致的肝硬化进展的比率正在逐年增加,表明了或许可以通过改变免疫抑制状态来改善患者的转归。基于体外实验的两组数据显示,环孢霉素对丙肝病毒[51,52]可能有抑制作用,而这种理念并没有得到临床数据的支持。1998年,Wiesner[53]证明,接受他克莫司治疗的丙肝病毒感染受体的5年生存率明显高于接受环孢霉素治疗的受体。最近,Irish WD等人检索了UNOS/OPTN(器官供应和移植网络)数据库,在 2000—2007 年间随访了 8809 例服用了环孢霉素或者他克莫司的患者，发现服用环孢霉素的患者在移植后 2 年内患有移植器官衰竭或者死亡的概率更大[54]。研究者认为,考察不同类型的免疫抑制剂的作用,需要随访 1 年以上的患者的生存率。而某些移植项目会在丙肝病毒感染的受体开始抗病毒治疗时，停用环孢霉素而改用他克莫司。这样的换药可能是合理的,但只有非常成功的抗病毒治疗方案才可以停用他克莫司而选择环孢霉素。Manousou 等人前瞻性地比较了他克莫司的单药疗法和他克莫司、咪唑硫嘌呤和短期的泼尼松三药联合疗法，并发现在三药联合的治疗方案中,患者肝纤维化的比例更低。Jain 等人[56]前瞻性地比较了他克莫司和泼尼松联合方案与他克莫司、泼尼松和麦考酚酯三联用药(MMF),发现两种方案的移植物生存率或患者生存率，排斥反应或者 HCV 复发率没有显著差异。最近,McKenna 等人[57]在一项回顾性研究中发现,服用西罗莫司的患者比没有服用西罗莫司的对照组患者的移植后纤维化比例更低。但是相反的是,Watt 等人[58]对移植受体科学注册系统(SRTR)中的超过 26 000 例患者进行回顾性的分析,其中有超过 12 000 例 HCV 感染患者，发现 HCV 感染患者在肝移植后服用西罗莫司会导致移植物丢失和死亡的风险增加,非 HCV 感染的肝移植患者则没有上述风险。作者认为,他克莫司可以改善预后，但丙肝病毒感染的移植受体应当谨慎使用。在多中心 HCV3 的前瞻性试验中,患者随机服用三种药物组合:他克莫司/糖皮质激素;他克莫司/糖皮质激素/ MMF;他克莫司/MMF 和达利珠单抗诱导[59]。经过 2 年的实验,他克莫司/MMF 和达利珠单抗诱导被证明是安全可行的，也更少发生糖尿病并发症,但对于丙肝病毒重度复发感染的患者而言,三组治疗方案没有显著区别。因此,避免对这些患者使用类固醇激素是可取的。另一方面,考虑到应当规避急性排斥反应(ACR)和原发性自身免疫性疾病,类固醇不应刻意禁用。

总之，与丙肝病毒感染的严重程度相关的免疫抑制问题仍然吸引着人们的关注,但是,很难得出一致性的结论。

乙型肝炎病毒

肝移植早期发生乙型肝炎病毒(HBV)感染并不像普通病毒复发那么乐观,其经常伴随着不良的预后。目前，纤维化淤胆型肝炎更多地与原位肝移植后丙肝病毒复发感染相关，但曾经也被用来描述一些移植后乙肝病毒感染的病例。一旦可靠且敏感的化验可以检测 HBV，在行 OLT 之前体内有无 HBV DNA 的不同患者的预后的差异也变得显而易见。对乙型肝炎病毒活动期的移植患者行肝脏移植尤其应谨慎,直到 Samuel 等人[60]证明了对这类患者使用乙型肝炎免疫球蛋白(HBIg)这种被动免疫方式十分有效。欧洲多中心试验测试了 334 例患者，经抗病毒治疗的患者的病毒复发率为 36%,未经治疗的患者的复发率为 75%。在那之后不久，弗吉尼亚大学和加州旧金山大学组成的团队证明了在维持乙型肝炎表面抗体阈值浓度的条件下,乙型肝炎免疫球蛋白疗效的可信度进一步提高[61,62]。使用这些剂量方案同时监测抗体浓度，项目开始证明使用乙型肝炎免疫球蛋白只有罕见的病毒学突破，包括行 OLT 前乙型肝炎 E 抗原阳性的患者。一直以来,肌注乙型肝炎免疫球蛋白虽然有效,但费用昂贵,且使用不方便。最终证据表明,肌注和静脉输注乙型肝炎免疫球蛋白一样有效能够解决移植领域的担忧[63,64]。随着拉米夫定和阿德福韦等口服药物上市,这些药物可以和乙型肝炎免疫球蛋白联合使用来减少病毒学突破的风险[65]。使用拉米夫定单独在预防 OLT 后乙肝复发效果不佳[66]。然而，同时使用拉米夫定和乙型肝炎免疫球蛋白在突然停药的情况下也不会造成病毒毒血症的复发。联用恩曲他滨/富马酸替诺福韦酯(FTC/TDF)对于合并艾滋病病毒感染和乙肝病毒的患者也非常有效，为研究者提供了充足的信心来考虑乙型肝炎免疫球蛋白的撤销协议。Teperman 等人[67]用乙型肝炎免疫球蛋白和富马酸替诺福韦酯(FTC/TDF)治疗 40 例感染乙型肝炎病毒的移植患者长达 24 周,一旦病毒水平下降,患者会被 1:1 随机分配,一组进行药物治疗,另一组撤回乙型肝炎免疫球蛋白。实验经过 48 周后,没有患者发生病毒突破。Stravitz 等人[68]对乙型肝炎患者行免疫球蛋白治疗 6 个月,6 个月后 21 例患者停用了乙型肝炎免疫球蛋白改用富马酸替诺福韦酯(FTC/TDF),患者的预后依旧良好，可以为每例患者每年节省下 12 469 美元。

最近，肝脏移植项目在原位肝移植术后早期已经开始更有把握地使用替诺福韦或者恩替卡韦取代乙型肝炎免疫球蛋白。

自身免疫性疾病

自身免疫性肝炎

自身免疫性肝炎(AIH)是病因未明的慢性坏死炎性肝病,其特征性表现为存在循环自身抗体、高γ-球蛋白血症和淋巴浆细胞性界面性肝炎的组织学证据。免疫抑制治疗通常为泌尼松和硫唑嘌呤,可有效预防疾病进展。但10%的患者药物治疗无效,需肝移植。相对而言,AIH不是肝移植的常见适应证,在欧洲和美国占儿童肝移植的2%~3%和成人肝移植的4%~5%[69]。肝移植后的总体预后令人满意,患者5年和10年生存率约为75%[69]。

尽管移植术后使用免疫抑制药物,AIH的发生率为12%~46%[1]。复发率的范围宽泛可能是由不同诊断标准、免疫抑制方案、随访长度和肝脏活检的操作方法导致的。Gautman等人[70]回顾25篇文献研究发现,经过26个月的中位时间后,23%的患者出现AIH复发。尽管AIH可发生在移植术后早期,但最多的是在移植后12个月,发生频率随移植后时间的推移而增加。

因为没有特异性诊断标志物,AIH的诊断基于一个特征群,其也适用于AIH复发(表78.2)。美国肝脏疾病研究协会(AASLD)提出下列AIH复发的诊断标准:

1.血清AST或ALT水平升高。

2.存在自身性抗体。

3.高γ-球蛋白血症。

4.相应的组织病理学发现

5.排除其他病因。

6.激素治疗有反应[69]。

因为移植后残留高丙种球蛋白血症和自身抗体并不意味着复发,所以对于AIH复发的正确诊断尤为困难。因此,有研究指出,组织病理学是诊断AIH复发最适当的标志。复发性AIH相应的组织学证据包括淋巴浆细胞浸润的汇管区和(或)小叶性肝炎,且没有其他组织病理学改变提示其他鉴别诊断。AIH复发的组织学特征改变出现时间早于临床或实验室证据,可在肝脏生化正常的患者中被发现,提示移植后肝活检可能有助于早期发现AIH复发[71,72]。

虽然AIH发病机制尚不明确,多项研究已经发现AIH复发的危险因素;但是多数未被验证,仍存有争议。有研究发现HLA DRB1*03或HLA DRB1*04可作为危险因素[71,73-77]。供受体之间HLA-DR基因不匹配也被认为是复发风险[70,76]。回顾89例患者发现,相比2型

表78.2 肝移植后复发性自身免疫性疾病的诊断标准

	诊断标准	排除标准
自身免疫性肝炎	• 转氨酶升高 • 高丙种球蛋白血症 • 可能存在以下病理学证据: -淋巴浆细胞性浸润 -界面性肝炎 -类固醇治疗缓解	• 病毒性肝炎 • 药源性肝损伤 • 急性细胞性排斥反应
原发性胆汁性肝硬化	• 碱性磷酸酶升高(波动) • 血清AMA阳性 • 病理学证据: -典型病变:旺炽性胆管病变(肉芽肿性胆管炎) -可能存在淋巴浆细胞性浸润或淋巴细胞性胆管炎	• 急性或慢性排斥反应 • 药源性肝损伤 • 胆管梗阻
原发性硬化性胆管炎	• 胆管造影显示肝内和(或)肝外的胆管狭窄 • 或胆管不规则充盈 • 肝移植后90天或更长 • 病理学证据: -纤维性胆管炎 -纤维素性血栓,伴有或不伴有胆管缺失、胆管纤维化或肝硬化	• 急性或慢性排斥反应 • 肝动脉血栓形成或者狭窄 • 吻合口狭窄 • 非吻合口狭窄,肝移植后90天内 • ABO血型不合

AMA,抗线粒体抗体;LT,肝移植。

AIH,1 型 AIH 复发率增加 7 倍[74,77-79]。AIH 移植的患者不仅发生急性和慢性排斥反应的风险更高,而且急性细胞性排斥反应也可能与 AIH 复发风险的增加有关[72,80]。移植物炎症严重程度的增加与移植前血清 IgG 高水平是强烈的复发预测因素[72,81]。13 项研究的系统回顾报道,尽管免疫抑制方案不同,使用初始免疫抑制药物环孢素或他克莫司对疾病复发的影响没有显著差异[70]。对 AIH 患者移植术后停用糖皮质激素仍有争议。数项研究表明疾病复发与停用激素相关,因此认为移植后需要维持低剂量激素治疗[74,78]。相反,另有研究报道成功撤除激素而不引起复发,但是这些研究缺乏肝脏活检标准方案,无症状的疾病也可能被漏诊[82,83]。

AIH 复发的主要治疗方法仍是加强免疫抑制;但是缺乏随机对照试验。多数患者对重新使用激素或增加激素剂量有反应[73,75,78]。优化钙调磷酸酶抑制剂剂量并加用硫唑嘌呤或霉酚酸酯可能获得额外的疗效。免疫抑制治疗无应答的病例中,将环孢素换成他克莫司或者将钙调磷酸酶抑制剂换成西罗莫司可能会有效[84,85]。鉴于存在移植肝功能丧失的风险,不推荐成功治疗 AIH 复发后停用激素。在多数情况下,AIH 复发可被免疫抑制有效治疗,且对移植肝或患者的预后影响有限。尽管复发造成移植肝功能丧失的准确发生率仍未明确,但是部分患者将发展为肝硬化、移植肝功能丧失,需要再次移植[86]。

原发性胆汁性肝硬化

原发性胆汁性肝硬化(PBC)是一种胆汁淤积性自身免疫性肝病,其特点是存在高度特异的抗线粒体抗体(AMA)和中小胆管的淋巴细胞性胆管炎,最终可发展为胆汁性肝硬化。熊去氧胆酸(UDCA)被证明可延长患者生存期,并使其免于肝移植;但是大约 1/3 的患者对熊去氧胆酸治疗没有反应,其中部分患者需要肝移植。在 20 世纪 80 年代,PBC 是肝移植的主要适应证,但是 PBC 患者需要移植的数量在过去 10 年下降了 20%,部分原因可能是增加了 UDCA 的使用[87]。PBC 患者移植术后的预后佳,5 年生存率达 85%[81]。

PBC 复发(rPBC)在 1982 年首次被报道,随后的研究表明,复发率在 9%~35%[88-96]。复发平均时间为 3~5.5 年[88-90,95,96]。复发率随着时间推移增加,10 年的累积发生率为 21%~37%,15 年为 43%[88,89,95]。

与原生肝 PBC 不同,rPBC 的实验室检查不是可靠的诊断标志物(表 78.2)。多数患者就诊时,肝酶水平正常或者没有临床意义上的增高[89,90,95,96]。其次,移植术后 AMA 水平不可预测,可能下降或升高,或者消失后再次出现[97,98]。血清 AMA 与 rPBC 的发生没有明显关联。诊断 rPBC 取决于肝脏活检和组织病理学分析。rPBC 的诊断标志是大约 60%的首次诊断性活检中呈,肉芽肿性胆管炎现炽旺性胆管病变[89]。其他特异性较弱的特征包括汇管区淋巴浆细胞浸润或者淋巴细胞性胆管炎,这些特征或许可以预测最后疾病的复发[91,93,94,97,99]。尽管具有挑战性,rPBC 的组织学改变与胆管损伤的其他原因之间的鉴别很重要,如急性和慢性排斥反应、缺血性胆管病或者药物肝毒性。

rPBC 的危险因素仍不明确,几项研究试图找出危险因素,但结果却互相矛盾。常见的危险因素有供体与受体年龄增加、男性受体、热缺血和冷缺血时间延长和 HLA 不匹配[76,88,89,95,96]。多项研究表明,与环孢素为主的方案相比,他克莫司可使疾病复发的风险增加。他克莫司也与出现复发的时间显著缩短有关,一项研究报道减少 50%[88-90,99]。另一方面,对 16 项研究中共 1241 例因 PBC 接受肝移植的患者进行系统回顾,发现受体中位生存时间为 46.5 个月,PBC 的总体复发率为 16% 。尽管与环孢霉素相比,他克莫司治疗复发趋势增加,但其没有统计学意义。而且到目前为止,相比他克莫司,环孢霉素为主的免疫抑制对 PBC 肝移植患者的长期生存没有影响[89,96]。没有研究发现使用硫唑嘌呤、霉酚酸酯或糖皮质激素与 rPBC 有明确的关系。

尽管还没有治疗指南,UDCA 由于移植前疗效、副作用最少,以及在疾病早期有机会进行初始治疗,被广泛用于治疗 rPBC。UDCA 疗效的评估仍有挑战,因为许多 rPBC 患者的肝酶正常或接近正常;但是,Guy 等[100]发现 75%的 rPBC 患者接受 UDCA 治疗后可出现碱性磷酸酶水平升高。相似的,Charatcharoenwitthaya 等[89]发现有 52%的 rPBC 患者接受 UDCA 治疗后肝酶恢复正常,而未接受 UDCA 治疗的概率只有 22%。但这些研究样本量较小,还没有决定性的数据表明 UDCA 会影响患者或移植肝的生存期。

幸运的是,rPBC 几乎不影响患者或移植肝的生存;但是,rPBC 在少数情况下可导致移植肝衰竭,进而需要再次肝移植。一项研究表明,在英国伯明翰进行肝移植的 PBC 患者中,所有移植肝失功的患者中有 5.4%是由复发性疾病造成的。从确诊复发到移植肝失功的中位时间为7.8年(22~181个月)[86]。

原发性硬化性胆管炎

原发性硬化性胆管炎(PSC)是一种慢性胆汁淤积性肝病，其特征是肝内和肝外胆管的炎症和纤维化导致胆管阻塞和胆汁性肝硬化。没有任何的药物、内镜或手术治疗能够影响PSC的进展。对于PSC导致终末期肝病的患者，OLT仍是唯一有效的方法。目前，在欧洲和美国，PSC肝移植占成人肝移植的4%~5%[101]。与PBC相似，PSC移植术后的预后非常好，患者5年生存率大约是80%[102-104]。

1988年，Lerut首次报道了在OLT后出现PSC复发[105]，现在移植术后5~10年PSC的整体复发率为20%~25%[102,106,107]。rPSC的诊断还没有金标准，仍然具有挑战性，1999年梅奥诊所提出的rPSC的定义被广泛接受：

1.移植前确实存在PSC。

2.胆道造影显示肝内和(或)肝外胆管狭窄、串珠状以及移植后异常至少超过90天；和(或)

3.组织学结果显示纤维化胆管炎和(或)纤维化闭塞性病变伴或不伴胆管消失、胆汁性纤维化或肝硬化。

4.排除其他诊断(肝动脉血栓形成或狭窄、胆管消失性排斥反应、供受体ABO血型不匹配、孤立性吻合口狭窄、缺血性狭窄、细菌或真菌性胆管炎伴狭窄和CMV或隐孢子虫感染)(表78.2)[102]。

多个rPSC的危险因素被报道，包括受体年龄、男性、供受体性别不同、HLA DRB1*08、移植前存在活动性溃疡性结肠炎、特别需要激素、发生急性细胞性排斥反应、激素抵抗型急性细胞性排斥反应、激素抵抗型急性细胞性排斥反应需要OKT3、存在胆管癌、糖皮质激素维持和使用扩大供体标准的移植肝[107-115]。

rPSC对移植肝生存的影响仍存在争议。Campsen等[106]发现，rPSC受体接受再移植前的中位生存时间为39.1个月。在一项来自UNOS数据库包括3309例PSC肝移植患者的分析中，Maheshwari等[116]发现，与PBC肝移植的患者相比，再次移植比例较高并且生存率较低，在行OLT后7年更加明显。也就是说，大多数已发表的研究未能表明rPSC对患者生存有影响[106,107,111-115]。对于原始肝脏，还没有明确的药物疗法用于治疗rPSC。尽管许多中心使用UDCA，但并没有已发表的资料显示UDCA对治疗rPSC有效益。治疗rPSC仍聚焦于缓解胆管狭窄的症状，疾病复发导致移植肝衰竭的患者需要考虑再次移植。

酒精性肝病

酒精性肝脏疾病(ALD)是西方国家第二常见的肝移植适应证，约占肝移植总例数的20%[117]。医学界对于ALD肝移植仍有争议，认为ALD是自身造成的疾病，存在移植后复饮或无法依从的风险，这些情况会增加对供体器官的需求。事实上，约95%伴有酒精性终末期肝病的患者从未正式评估肝移植[118]。尽管最初报道表明，移植后患者生存率低(3年20%)，与那些因其他指征进行肝移植的患者相比，最近的数据显示即便没有更好的生存率，其1年和5年生存率分别是86%和74%[119,120]。

不幸的是，酗酒是一种会故态复萌且缓解与复饮相交替的疾病，频繁复饮会导致移植后原病复发。所报道，原位肝移植后复饮率有显著的差异，为10%~90%[121]。对酒精复饮的定义不同和难以获取患者酒精摄入量的准确数据，导致了复饮率的高度变异性。关于复饮率的许多数据把酒精复饮定义为任意酒精摄入，而非更加适当地区分为偶然饮酒或有害饮酒或成瘾[122]。估计有20%的ALD肝移植患者重新开始有害饮酒，然而，多数患者保持戒酒状态或只偶尔少量饮酒[123,124]。这是一个重要的区分因素，因为重度饮酒与患者长期生存率的降低有关[125]。早期研究没有显示复饮对患者或者移植肝生存的影响，这些研究普遍是随访时间短暂的小样本研究[126,127]。延长随访时间显示，在重新饮酒的患者中，研究者发现越来越多更差预后的证据[125,128,129]。Pfitzmann等[130]表明，与那些保持戒酒或偶尔饮酒的患者相比，重新酗酒的患者的生存期显著降低。在重新酗酒患者中，ALD的复发导致多数受体死亡(87.5%)。然而，那些维持戒酒的ALD肝移植患者通常死于心血管疾病或恶性肿瘤，在移植后重新酗酒的受体中，多数是由ALD复发导致死亡[128,129]。

多个因素与肝移植后酒精复饮相关(表78.3)。其中一个仍有严重争议的因素是移植前戒酒时间。较长的戒酒时间与较低的移植术后复饮率相关，但是最佳的时间间隔还未被确定[131,132]。在美国，85%的移植中心要求患者在进入移植列表之前的至少戒酒6个月，称为“6个月规则”[131]。然而，研究指出，仅靠戒酒6个月来预测移植术后再饮酒并不充分，需要5年时间完成真

表 78.3　肝移植术后酒精复饮的危险因素

低危	高危
• 诊断为酒精滥用	• 诊断为酒精依赖
• 社会支持良好	• 社会支持匮乏
• 坚持治疗、服药和复诊	• 无法坚持模式
• 低危的社会心理危险因素	• 高危的社会心理危险因素
–治疗下心境障碍	–精神病性障碍
–康复药物滥用	–人格障碍

(Reproduced by permission of Robert Weinrieb, MD.)

实的预测[131,132,134]。移植前的饮酒模式显示在复饮风险中起作用,有酒精滥用史的受体与有酒精依赖史的受体相比,复饮风险更低[131]。社会支持的不满足始终与酒精复饮有关联，最常见的是没有配偶或婚姻关系差[130,131,135]。其他移植术后复饮的危险因素包括年龄较轻、无法坚持酗酒治疗、不依从药物治疗、酗酒家族史、多种药物滥用、伴发精神病(人格障碍、精神病性障碍、抑郁障碍)[136-138]。可惜的是,研究得出多种关于复饮风险的结论，而且迄今没有一个预测指标能可靠识别酒精复饮。

由于长期预后不良与肝移植术后再酗酒相关,移植中心须采取必要的措施预防患者再次饮酒。措施从移植评估阶段开始，通过社会工作人员对复饮风险进行谨慎的社会心理评估,以及培训精神健康专家。有复饮风险的患者可于肝移植术前进行适当的药物滥用或者精神科咨询和治疗。肝移植术后发现酒精复饮非常有挑战性。已经提出诸干策略用来监测和识别肝移植术后酒精饮用,包括生物化学标志物、精神科谈话、问卷调查和筛查工具[122,139,140]。许多移植中心有精神健康专家会随访移植术后患者，持续预防患者复饮以及提供支持。没有一种识别复饮的方法是真正具有特异性的。因此,建议联合使用多种方法来增加酒精复饮患者的探查。当发现患者再次饮酒时,应该迅速实施治疗计划;但是文献中缺乏治疗肝移植术后复饮的相关信息。Weinrieb 等[141]认为,让患者参与复饮治疗很困难,也不能招募到肝移植后酗酒患者参与纳屈酮治疗的试验。患者不仅认为他们不需要治疗，而且不愿意服用有潜在肝毒性的药物。Bjornsson 等[142]能够成功实施移植酒精治疗计划，其中设置技术娴熟的精神科医生对患者进行评估，鼓励患者参与励志活动，以及签订戒酒合约。结果显示,在超过 4 年的时间里,患者对任何酒类的复饮率均降低(22%比历史控制的 48%)。尽管治疗肝移植术后酒类复饮有重大障碍，但是为了限制 ALD 的复发，移植中心必须采取行动预防、发现和治疗复饮。

非酒精性脂肪性肝病

非酒精性脂肪性肝病(NAFLD)在发展中国家是慢性肝病最常见的病因,影约 1/3 的普通人群[143]。NAFLD 包含的范围包括从单纯性肝脂肪变性到伴有不同程度的坏死性炎症和纤维化或非酒精性脂肪性肝炎(NASH)的脂肪变性。发达国家中,大约有 3%的人群患 NASH,其中 20%的人可能发展成肝硬化[144,145]。而且,1/3 的 NASH 患者将死于肝病并发症或者需要 OLT。NAFLD 与肥胖、血脂异常和糖尿病有关,被认为是肝脏代谢综合征的临床表现[146]。每年 NAFLD 移植占 OLT 的 5%~10%,预计在未来将超过 HCV 感染,成为 OLT 的主要并发症[147,148]。通常,NAFLD 移植预后较好,与其他移植适应证的预后相似，患者的 1 年和 5 年生存率分别为 86%和 71%[149]。

1992 年,第一例 OLT 后脂肪性肝病复发被报道,随后多项研究证实 NAFLD 复发是常见的[150]。移植术后 NAFLD 的复发率为 25%~60%,但多数研究随访有限[151-155]。在一项前瞻性研究中,Maor-Kendler 等[155]报道了 60%的 NASH 移植受体有 2 级及以上的脂肪变性,其中半数患者满足 NASH 的组织学诊断标准。另一项类似研究显示，在 18 个月的平均随访时间里,70%的患者出现复发的脂肪变性,25%的患者发展为 NASH,接近 20%的患者发展为肝纤维化 2 期及以上[156]。最近一项研究报道了较低的脂肪变性复发率，移植术后 1 年、5 年和 10 年的复发率分别为 8%、25%和 33%[149]。已有报道称约 10%的 NASH 移植患者复发并导致肝硬化,其中约有半数发展为移植肝衰竭,尽管最近更多的研究显示,移植肝功能丧失与 NASH 复发无关[157,158]。

已发现数个危险因素与 OLT 后 NAFLD 的复发有关。意料之中的是,许多危险因素与代谢综合征密切相关,包括肥胖、糖尿病、血脂异常和移植前后高血压[156,159,160]。OLT 术后免疫抑制也可能影响疾病复发,因为激素、钙调素磷酸酶抑制剂和西罗莫司与肥胖、高血压和胰岛素抵抗的增加有关;但是,还没有一种特定的免疫抑制方案可以预防 NAFLD 的复发。越来越多的证据显示，避免激素或钙调素磷酸酶抑制剂剂量最小化是安全的，且可减少移植术后代谢并发症的发生率[161,162]。至今尚未确定这些策略能否降低 NAFLD 的复发率。

诊断复发性 NAFLD 与诊断原发性肝脏 NAFLD 相似。肝脏生化检查没有特异性，1/3 的 NASH 复发患者的肝酶可正常[156]。尽管放射影像学可发现存在脂肪变性，但它不能区分脂肪肝的其他病因或者判断其严重程度。因此，肝脏活检可用来明确诊断、判定疾病程度、排除其他病因。遗憾的是，与原发性肝脏 NAFLD 相似，还没有安全有效治疗复发性 NAFLD 的药物。主要治疗聚集在改善代谢综合征相关的症状。其中包括改变生活方式、减轻体重以及严格的针对糖尿病和血脂异常的药物治疗。可以预见的是，目前用于原发性肝脏 NAFLD 治疗有效的方案会被用于治疗复发性 NAFLD，但是到目前为止，仍缺乏预防和治疗复发疾病的数据。

肝细胞癌

肝细胞癌(HCC)是世界上第六大常见的实体恶性肿瘤，占肿瘤原因死亡率的第三位[163]。大部分 HCC 是在肝硬化的基础上发展形成的，在美国，通常与 HCV 感染有关，全球范围内则与 HBV 感染有关。据报道，在接下来的几十年里，由于 HCV 和 NASH 的患病率居高不下，美国 HCC 的发生率仍会继续上升[164]。最近几年，在治疗 HCC 方面有重大进展，包括局部消融治疗及使用化疗药物，如索拉菲尼；然而，HCC 的有效治疗方法主要还是手术治疗。由于肿瘤累及范围和肝硬化时肝功能储备差，80%的 HCC 患者不可切除肿瘤[165]。因此，对大多数患者而言，肝移植是最佳的手术治疗方法，能够完全切除肿瘤及移除病肝。

最初的 HCC 肝移植是在不可切除的进展期大肝癌患者上施行的，由于 HCC 复发率高，导致患者生存率低，预后非常差[166,167]。1996 年，Mazzafero 等[168]的里程碑式的研究显示，对早期肝癌患者和符合特定选择标准的患者进行肝移植，可提高受体生存期。这个标准现在被称为米兰标准，包括单个肿瘤直径≤5cm 或多发肿瘤少于 3 个且最大直径≤3cm，没有大血管侵犯和肝外转移。这一标准导致其预后与其他原位肝移植良性适应证相似，5 年生存率达 70%，HCC 复发率为 8%。米兰标准的积极影响被 UNOS 数据库的一个分析证实，该数据库纳入 1987—2001 年的 985 例接受肝癌肝移植的患者。在这项研究中，Yoo 等[167]采用了米兰标准(5 年生存率：使用米兰标准前 25%比使用米兰标准后 61%，P=0.001)，移植后患者生存率有极大的提高。最近，一些移植中心因米兰标准太严格而提出质疑，主张扩大标准使更多患者能够进行原位肝移植，且不增加 HCC 复发风险或死亡率。在这些扩大标准中，最确定的是来自加州大学旧金山分校的 UCFS 标准，其允许单个肿瘤直径≤6.5cm，或多发肿瘤少于 3 个且最大直径≤4.5cm，总的肿瘤直径不超过 8cm[169]。报道称使用该标准 5 年生存率为 75%，HCC 复发率为 11%。然而，扩大标准还未被广泛接受，仍有争论，需要更多的前瞻性研究验证。

各项报道的原位肝移植后 HCC 复发率略有不同，为 6%~56%，主要是由于患者移植的选择标准不同[170-173]。尽管有 10%~43%的案例报道原位肝移植后 HCC 的复发最初表现为肝外复发，但是大多数均为肝内复发[174-181]。HCC 复发的肝外部分通常是肺和骨转移，但在腹部淋巴结、肾上腺和腹膜也有发现。HCC 复发的机制可能是由于移植时淋巴结或远处脏器存在微小的恶性病灶，以及血源性或腹膜肿瘤种植。复发的风险在原位肝移植后两年内最高，但移植后超过 5 年的晚期复发也有报道[174-181]。

尽管 HCC 的复发率在各个移植中心有所不同，但数个预示肿瘤复发的因素已经被发现。最强有力预示 HCC 复发的因素是受体存在大血管或微血管侵犯，提示预后极差[182,183]。肿瘤直径大于 5cm、肿瘤灶总数量和双叶疾病与复发风险增加相关，可替代微血管侵犯的预示作用[184-186]。相似的，不良的肿瘤分化分型可预示微血管侵犯，其也是肿瘤复发的独立危险因素。然而，肿瘤分级评估需要经皮肝活检确认，不排除活检通道肿瘤种植的风险，其发生在 3%的病例中[187-190]。肿瘤组织学测定的价值需要更多的研究予以确认，因为有学者提出低分化可更好地预示复发，不论是否符合或者超出米兰标准[191]。许多研究尝试发现可替代的分子标志物，以预测微血管侵犯和复发，而无肿瘤种植风险。运用最广泛的标志物是血清甲胎蛋白(AFP)，与 HCC 复发相关。但是，AFP 的作用有限，因为 30%~40%的 HCC 患者的 AFP 水平是正常的[192]。其他许多的分子标志物——细胞增殖、细胞黏附、细胞外基质，血管生成、细胞表面标志物和转录因子，仍处于研究阶段。

患者在等待原位肝移植过程中避免被排除（如肝

癌进展超出移植标准,从移植等待列表中移除患者),推荐局部消融治疗以减慢 HCC 的进展。为此,治疗分析显示这一过渡治疗对移植等待时间超过 6 个月的患者有效,但局部疗法能否在移植后减少复发和提高生存率仍不得而知[193-197]。局部治疗也可用于米兰标准之外的肿瘤患者进行降期治疗,进而符合 OLT 标准。有证据表明,减小肿瘤负荷以满足米兰标准,能成功进行肝移植而不会增加 HCC 复发风险。并且,肿瘤对降期的应答可用于预测移植预后,帮助选择移植患者[193,194,198]。新辅助化疗还未被证明对 HCC 肝移植前或移植后的治疗有所裨益。但是,近来显示多重激酶抑制剂、索拉菲尼,可显著提高进展期 HCC 患者的总体生存率[199]。像索拉菲尼这类药物能否降低肝移植后 HCC 复发的风险及在怎样的情况下使用,仍需要进一步研究。

免疫抑制通常与移植后恶性肿瘤的风险增加相关,且可成为 HCC 复发和肿瘤进展的影响因素。Vivarelli 等[200]观察到移植后 1 年内较高的环孢霉素累积剂量和较低的 5 年 HCC 无复发生存率之间有直接关系。该观察在对 70 例 HCC 肝移植患者的回顾性分析中被验证,发现肝移植后 HCC 复发与较高的环孢霉素水平有统计学意义上的关联[201]。随后同一团队报道发现较高剂量的环孢霉素和他克莫司可作为肝移植后 HCC 复发的独立危险因素[202]。相似的,激素也可在 HCC 复发中产生负向调节作用,肝移植后早期撤除激素可减少肝癌复发的风险[209]。m-TOR(哺乳动物西罗莫司靶点)抑制剂在 HCC 背景中可起到相当大的作用。加上强效免疫抑制的活动,m-TOR 抑制剂显示出潜在的抗肿瘤作用,可损伤血管内皮细胞生长因子(VEGF)产物。西罗莫司可诱导细胞循环停止,阻滞 HCC 细胞系的增殖[203]。在一个匹配的病例对照研究中,肝移植后患者维持西罗莫司治疗与维持他克莫司标准治疗相比,3 年无复发生存率高 30%[204]。Toso 等[205]分析了美国移植受体科学注册系统中的数据,提出更加有前景的临床数据,以判断所使用的免疫抑制剂类型是否会影响 HCC 患者肝移植后的生存。研究者得出的结论是以西罗莫司为主的维持治疗方案可提高生存率。尽管如此,一种特定免疫抑制方案与肝移植后 HCC 复发之间仍没有明确的关联。但现有数据提示最小化钙调磷酸酶抑制剂剂量或转换成 mTOR 抑制剂对 HCC 复发的高危患者有益。

很少有公开出版的数据用于指导最有效且合算的策略去监测肝移植后 HCC 的复发,且各大移植中心的监视方法也不尽相同[206]。曾经有报道发现,OLT 后转移性 HCC 复发的 5 年生存率为 13%~35%[175-181]。不幸的是,许多患者出现播散性病变时,在当前仅可获得有限的 HCC 复发治疗选择。尽管数据有限,特定的局部复发患者可考虑积极的手术干预治疗。Regallia 等[175]首次报道在小样本的移植后患者研究中,对患者肝、肺、骨和皮肤的孤立性复发病灶进行手术切除。这些患者的 4 年生存率为 57%,相比之下,那些因病灶无法切除而未接受手术干预的患者的 4 年生存率为 14%。最近一篇来自西奈山医疗中心的研究报道了相似的优势,接受根治性手术切除局部 HCC 复发灶的患者生存期增加[181]。多因素分析显示,除了无骨转移及术后复发时间大于 1 年以外,手术治疗与延长生存期无关。基于移植前 HCC 患者人群经验,肝移植术后复发的其他潜化治疗包括局部消融治疗或局部化疗,如索拉菲尼。然而,在移植后的背景下仍缺乏充足的数据得出确切的结论。最后,作为一种治疗选择,放射治疗可用来减以轻肝外病变和骨转移为主的患者的症状[207,208]。减少肝移植后的 HCC 复发率及其相关死亡率需要谨慎考虑移植前因素和移植后免疫抑制,以及运用患者护理的多学科交叉方法,包括肝脏病学、移植手术、放射学和肿瘤学。

总结

肝移植仍是多数终末期肝病的主要治疗手段。不像在其他器官移植中那样,排斥反应成为影响生存的根本问题,肝脏移植更多的是受病毒复发和自身免疫性疾病的影响。因此,临床医生必须要经常意识到疾病复发的风险,熟悉诊断流程和可用于准确诊断的处理选择,以及控制与治疗这些复发疾病。免疫控制应该联合使用病毒特异性治疗,以获得最理想的结果且尽量减少再次移植的需求。

(徐骁 译 徐骁 校)

参考文献

1. Charlton M, Seaberg E, Wiesner R, et al. Predictors of patient and graft survival following liver transplantation for hepatitis C. Hepatology (Baltimore, Md.). 1998;28:823-830.
2. Forman LM, Lewis JD, Berlin JA, et al. The association between hepatitis C infection and survival after orthotopic liver transplantation. Gastroenterology. 2002;122:889-896.
3. Boker KHW, Dalley G, Bahr MJ, et al. Long-term outcome of hepatitis C virus infection after liver transplantation. Hepatology (Baltimore, Md.). 1997;25: 203-210.
4. Feray C, Gigou M, Samuel D, et al. The course of hepatitis C virus infection after liver transplantation. Hepatology (Baltimore, Md.). 1994;20:1137-1143.
5. Ghobrial RM, Farmer DG, Baquerizo A, et al. Orthotopic liver transplantation for hepatitis C: outcome, effect of immunosuppression, and causes of retransplantation during an 8-year single-center experience. Annals of Surgery. 1999;229:824-833.
6. Pelletier SJ, Schaubel DE, Punch JE, et al. Hepatitis C is a risk factor for death after liver retransplantation. Liver Transplantation. 2005;11:434-440.
7. Thuluvath PJ, Krok KL, Segev DL, et al. Trends in post-liver transplant survival in patients with hepatitis C between 1991 and 2001 in the United States. Liver Transplantation. 2007;13:719-724.
8. McCashland T, Watt K, Lyden E, et al. Retransplantation for hepatitis C: results of a U.S. multicenter retransplant study. Liver Transplantation. 2007;13: 1246-1253.
9. Garcia-Retortillo M, Forns X, Feliu A, et al. Hepatitis C virus kinetics during and immediately after liver transplantation. Hepatology (Baltimore, Md.). 2002;35:680-687.
10. Gane EJ, Nikolai VN, Ke-Ping Q, et al. A longitudinal analysis of hepatitis C virus replication following liver transplantation. Gastroenterology. 1996;110:167-177.
11. Taga SA, Washington MK, Terrault N, et al. Cholestatic hepatitis C in liver allografts. Liver Transplantation and Surgery. 1998;4:304-310.
12. Ciccorossi P, Maina AM, Oliveri F, et al. Viral load 1 week after liver transplantation, donor age and rejections correlate with the outcome of recurrent hepatitis C. Liver International. 2007;27:612-619.
13. Skreekumar R, Gonzalez-Koch A, Maor-Kendler Y, et al. Early identification of recipients with progressive histologic recurrence of hepatitis C after liver transplantation. Hepatology (Baltimore, Md.). 2000;32:1125-1130.
14. Paterson DL, Gayowski T, Wannstedt CF, et al. Quality of life in long-term survivors after liver transplantation: impact of recurrent viral hepatitis C virus hepatitis. Clinical Transplantation. 2000;14:48-54.
15. Regev A, Molina E, Moura R, et al. Reliability of histopathologic assessment for the differentiation of recurrent hepatitis C from acute rejection after liver transplantation. Liver Transplantation. 2004;10:1233-1239.
16. Charlton M. Liver biopsy viral kinetics, and the impact of viremia on severity of hepatitis C virus recurrence. Liver Transplantation. 2003;9:S58-S62.
17. Pelletier SJ, Raymond DP, Crabtree TD, et al. Pretransplantation hepatitis C virus quasispecies may be predictive of outcome after liver transplantation. Hepatology (Baltimore, Md.). 2000;32:375-381.
18. Zhou S, Terrault NA, Ferrell L, et al. Severity of liver disease in liver transplantation recipients with hepatitis C virus infection: relationship to genotype and level of viremia. Hepatology (Baltimore, Md.). 1996;24:1041-1046.
19. Vargas HE, Laskus T, Wang L-F, et al. The influence of hepatitis C virus genotypes on the outcome of liver transplantation. Liver Transplantation and Surgery. 1998;4:22-27.
20. Wali MH, Heydtmann M, Harrison RF. Outcome of liver transplantatioin for patients infected by hepatitis C, including those infected by genotype 4. Liver Transplantation. 2003;9:796-804.
21. Zekry A, Whiting P, Crawford DH, et al. Liver transplantation for HCV associated liver cirrhosis: predictors of outcomes in a population with significant genotype 3 and 4 distribution. Liver Transplantation. 2003;9:339-347.
22. Machicao V, Bonatti H, Krishna M, et al. Donor age affects fibrosis progression and graft survival after liver transplantation for hepatitis C. Transplantation. 2004;77:84-92.
23. Wiesner RH, Sorrell M, Villamil F. Report of the first International Liver Transplantation Society expert panel consensus conference on liver transplantation and hepatitis C. Liver Transplantation. 2003;9:S1-S9.
24. Selzner N, Girgrah N, Lilly L, et al. The difference in the fibrosis progression of recurrent hepatitis C after live donor liver transplantation versus deceased donor liver transplantation is attributable to the difference in donor age. Liver Transplantation. 2008;14:1778-1786.
25. Brinceno J, Ciria R, Pleguezuelo M, et al. Impact of donor graft steatosis on overall outcome and viral recurrence after liver transplantation for hepatitis C virus cirrhosis. Liver Transplantation. 2008;15:37-48.
26. Yilmaz N, Schiffman ML. Impact of the donor liver with steatosis in patients with hepatitis C virus: not so FAsT. Liver Transplantation. 2009;15:4-6.
27. Charlton M, Seaberg E. Impact of immunosuppression and acute rejection on recurrence of hepatitis C: results of the National Institute of Diabetes and Digestive and Kidney Diseases Liver Transplantation Database. Liver Transplantation and Surgery. 1999;5:S107-S114.
28. Razonable RR, Burak KW, van Cruijsen H, et al. The pathogenesis of hepatitis C virus is influenced by cytomegalovirus. Clinical Infectious Diseases. 2002;35: 974-981.
29. Singh N, Wannstedt C, Keyes L, et al. Indirect outcomes associated with cytomegalovirus (opportunistic infections, hepatitis C *virus* sequelae, and mortality) in liver-transplant recipients with the use of preemptive therapy for 13 years. Transplantation. 2005;79:1428-3144.
30. Verna EC, De Martin E, Burra P, et al. The impact of hepatitis C and biliary complications on patient and graft survival following liver transplantation. American Journal of Transplantation. 2009;9:1398-1405.
31. Everson G. Treatment of patients with hepatitis C virus on the waiting list. Journal of Hepatology. 2005;42:456-462.
32. Forns X, Navasa M, Rodes J. Treatment of HCV infection in patients with advanced cirrhosis. Hepatology (Baltimore, Md.). 2004;40:498.
33. Terrault NA. Hepatitis C therapy before and after liver transplantation. Liver Transplantation. 2008;14:S58-S66.
34. Hoare M, Gelson WTH, Rushbrook S, et al. Histologic changes in HCV antibody positive, HCV RNA negative subjects suggest persistent viral infection. Hepatology (Baltimore, Md.). 2008;48:1737-1745.
35. Wiesner RH. Is there disease progression in patients who are hepatitis C virus antibody-positive and hepatitis C virus RNA-seronegative? Hepatology (Baltimore, Md.). 2008;48:1734-1736.
36. Carrión JA, Navasa M, Garcia-Retortillo M, et al. Efficacy of antiviral therapy on hepatitis c recurrence after liver transplantation: a ramdomized controlled study. Gastroenterology. 2007;132:1746-1756.
37. Mukherjee S. Fatal liver disease despite sustained eradication of recurrent hepatitis C virus requiring liver transplantation. Transplantation. 2006;82: 286-288.
38. Hitomi S, Arase Y, Tsubota A, et al. Type C-chronic hepatitis patients who had autoimmune phenomenon and developed jaundice during interferon therapy. Journal of Gastroenterology. 2003;38:493-500.
39. Terrault NA, Berenguer M. Treating hepatitis C infection in liver transplant recipients. Liver Transplantation. 2006;12:1192-1204.
40. Chalasani N, Manzarbeitia C, Ferenci P, et al. Peginterferon alfa-2a for hepatitis C after liver transplantation: two randomized, controlled trials. Hepatology (Baltimore, Md.). 2005;41:289-298.
41. Coto-Llerena M, Perez-del-Pulgar S, Crespo G, et al. Donor and recipient IL28B polymorphisms in HCV-infected patients undergoing antiviral therapy before and after liver transplantation. American Journal of Transplantation. 2011;11: 1051-1057.
42. Brown RS. Hepatitis C and liver transplantation. Nature. 2005;436:973-978.
43. Jain A, Demetris AJ, Manez R, et al. Incidence and severity of acute allograft rejection in liver transplant recipients treated with alfa interferon. Liver Transplantation and Surgery. 1998;4:197-203.
44. Ferray C, Samuel D, Gigou M, et al. An open trial of interferon alfa recombinant for hepatitis C after transplantation: antiviral effects and risk of rejection. Hepatology (Baltimore, Md.). 1995;22:1084-1089.
45. Berardi S, Lodato F, Gramenzi A, et al. High incidence of allograft dysfunction in liver transplanted patients treated with pegylated-interferon alpha-2b and ribavirin for hepatitis C recurrence; possible de novo autoimmune hepatitis? Gut. 2007;56:237-242.
46. Ward SC, Schiano TD, Thung SN, et al. Plasma cell hepatitis in hepatitis c virus patients post-liver transplantation: case-con troll study showing poor outcome and predicative features in the liver explants. Liver Transplantation. 2009;15: 1826-1833.
47. Demetris AJ, Sebagh M. Plasma cell hepatitis in liver allografts: variant of rejection or autoimmune hepatitis? Liver Transplantation. 2008;14:750-755.
48. Czaja AJ, Carpenter HA. Histological findings in chronic hepatitis C with autoimmune features. Hepatology (Baltimore, Md.). 1997;26:459-466.
49. Watt K, Veldt B, Charlton M. A practical guide to the management of HCV infection following liver transplantation. American Journal of Transplantation. 2009;9:1707-1713.
50. Berenguer M, Ferrell L, Watson J, et al. HCV-related fibrosis progression following liver transplantation: increase in recent years. Journal of Hepatology. 2000;32:673-684.
51. Firpi RJ, Shu H, Morelli G, et al. Cyclosporine suppresses hepatitis C virus in vitro and increases the chance of a sustained virological response after liver

transplantation. Liver Transplantation. 2006;12:51–57.
52. Nagagawa M, Sakamoto N, Enomoto N, et al. Specific inhibition of hepatitis C virus replication by cyclosporine A. Biochemical and Biophysical Research Communications. 2004;313:42–47.
53. Wiesner RH. A long-term comparison of tacrolimus (FK506) versus cyclosporine in liver transplantation: a report of the United States FK506 Study Group. Transplantation. 1998;66:493–499.
54. Irish WD, Arcona S, Bowers D, et al. Cyclosporine versus tacrolimus treated liver transplant recipients with chronic hepatitis C: outcomes analysis of the UNOS/OPTN database. American Journal of Transplantation. 2011;11: 1676–1685.
55. Manousou P, Samonakis D, Cholongitas E, et al. Outcome of recurrent hepatitis C virus after liver transplantation in a randomized trial of tacrolimus monotherapy versus triple therapy. Liver Transplantation. 2009;15:1783–1791.
56. Jain A, Kashyap R, Demetris AJ, et al. A prospective randomized trial of mycophenolate mofetil in liver transplant recipients with hepatitis C. Liver Transplantation. 2002;8:40–46.
57. McKenna GJ, Trotter JF, Klintmalm E, et al. Limiting hepatitis C virus progression in liver transplant recipients using sirolimus-based immunosuppression. American Journal of Transplantation. 2011;11:2379–2387.
58. Watt KD, Dierkhising R, Heimbach JK, et al. Impact of sirolimus and tacrolimus on mortality and graft loss in liver transplant recipients with or withour hepatitis C virus: an analysis of the Scientific Registry of Transplant Recipients Database. Liver Transplantation. 2012;18:1029–1036.
59. Klintmalm GB, Davis GL, Tepperman L, et al. A randomized, multicenter study comparing steroid-free immunosuppression and standard immunosuppression for liver transplant recipients with chronic hepatitis C. Liver Transplantation. 2011;17:1394–1403.
60. Samuel D, Bismuth A, Mathieu D, et al. Passive immunoprophylaxis after liver transplantation in HBsAg-positive patients. Lancet. 1991;337:813–815.
61. McGory RW, Ishitani MB, Oliveira WM, et al. Improved outcome of orthotopic liver transplantation for chronic hepatitis B cirrhosis with aggressive passive immunization. Transplantation. 1996;61:1358–1364.
62. Terrault NA, Zhou S, Combs C, et al. Prophylaxis in liver transplantrecipients using a fixed dosing schedule of hepatitis B immunoglobulin. Hepatology (Baltimore, Md.). 1996;24:1327–1333.
63. Yao FY, Osorio RW, Roberts JP, et al. Intramuscular hepatitis B immune globulin combined with lamivudine for prophylaxis against hepatitis B recurrence after liver transplantation. Liver Transplantation. 1999;5:491–496.
64. Faust D, Rabenau HF, Allwinn R, et al. Cost-effective and safe ambulatory long-term immunoprophylaxis with intramuscular instead of intravenous hepatitis B immunoglobulin to prevent reinfection after orthotopic liver transplantation. Clinical Transplantation. 2003;17:254–258.
65. Steinmuller T, Seehofer D, Rayes N, et al. Increasing applicability of liver transplantation for patients with hepatitis B-related liver disease. Hepatology (Baltimore, Md.). 2002;35:1528–1535.
66. European Association for the Study of the Liver. EASL Clinical Practice Guidelines: management of chronic hepatitis B. Journal of Hepatology. 2009;50: 227–242.
67. Teperman LW, Poordad F, Bzowej N, et al. A randomized trial of emtricitabine/tenofovir disoproxil fumarate after hepatitis B immunoglobulin withdrawal post-liver transplant. Liver Transplantation. 2013;19:594–601.
68. Stravitz RT, Shiffman ML, Kimmel M, et al. Substitution of tenofovir/emtricitabine for hepatitis B immune globulin prevents recurrence of hepatitis B after liver transplantation. Liver International. 2012;32:1138–1145.
69. Manns MP, Czaja AJ, Gorham JD, et al. Diagnosis and management of autoimmune hepatitis. Hepatology (Baltimore, Md.). 2010;51:2193–2213.
70. Gautman M, Cheruvattath R, Balan V. Recurrence of autoimmune liver disease after liver transplantation: a systematic review. Liver Transplantation. 2006;12: 1813–1824.
71. Duclos-Vallee JC, Sebagh M, Rifai K, et al. A 10 year follow up study of patients transplanted for autoimmune hepatitis: histological recurrence precedes clinical and biochemical recurrence. Gut. 2003;52:893–897.
72. Ayata G, Gordon FD, Lewis WD, et al. Liver transplantation for autoimmune hepatitis: a long-term pathologic study. Hepatology (Baltimore, Md.). 2000;32:185–192.
73. Gonzalez-Koch A, Czaja AJ, Carpenter HA, et al. Recurrent autoimmune hepatitis after orthotopic liver transplantation. Liver Transplantation. 2001;7: 302–310.
74. Milkiewicz P, Hubscher SG, Skiba G, et al. Recurrence of autoimmune hepatitis after liver transplantation. Transplantation. 1999;68:253–256.
75. Wright HL, Bou-Abboud CF, Hassanein T, et al. Disease recurrence and rejection following liver transplantation for autoimmune chronic active liver disease. Tranplantation. 1992;53:136–139.
76. Balan V, Ruppert K, Demetris AJ, et al. Long-term outcome of human leukocyte antigen mismatching in liver transplantatioin: results of the National Institute of Diabetes and Digestive and Kidney Diseases Liver Transplantation Database. Hepatology (Baltimore, Md.). 2008;48:878–888.
77. Hubscher SG. Recurrent autoimmune hepatitis after liver transplantation: diagnostic criteria, risk factors, and outcome. Liver Transplantation. 2001;7: 285–291.
78. Prados E, Cuervas-Mons V, de la Mata A, et al. Outcomes of autoimmune hepatitis after liver transplantation. Transplantation. 1998;66:1645–1650.
79. Ratzui V, Samuel D, Sebagh M, et al. Long-term follow-up after liver transplantation for autoimmune hepatitis: evidence of recurrence of primary disease. Journal of Hepatology. 1999;30:131–141.
80. Molmenti EP, Netto GJ, Murray NG, et al. Incidence and recurrence of autoimmune/alloimmune hepatitis in liver transplant recipients. Liver Transplantation. 2002;8:519–526.
81. Kashyap R, Safadjou S, Chen R, et al. Living donor and deceased donor liver transplantation for autoimmune and cholestatic liver diseases- an analysis of the UNOS Database. Journal of Gastrointestinal Surgery. 2010;14:1362–1369.
82. Campsen J, Zimmerman MA, Trotter JF, et al. Liver transplantation for autoimmune hepatitis and the success of aggressive corticosteroid withdrawal. Liver Transplantation. 2008;14:1281–1286.
83. Heffron TG, Smallwood GA, Oakley B, et al. Autoimmune hepatitis following liver transplantation: relationship to recurrent disease and steroid weaning. Transplantation Proceedings. 2002;34:3311–3312.
84. Hurtova M, Duclos-Vallee JC, Johanet C, et al. Successful tacrolimus therapy for a severe recurrence of type 1 autoimmune hepatitis in a liver graft recipient. Liver Transplantation. 2001;7:556–558.
85. Kerkar N, Dugan C, Rumbo C, et al. Rapamycin successfully treats post-transplant autoimmune hepatitis. American Journal of Transplantation. 2005;5: 1085–1089.
86. Rowe IA, Webb K, Gunson BK, et al. The impact of disease recurrence on graft survival following liver transplantation: a single center experience. Transplant International. 2008;5:459–465.
87. Lee J, Belanger A, Douchette JT, et al. Transplantation trends in primary biliary cirrhosis. Clinical Gastroenterology and Hepatology. 2007;5:1313–1315.
88. Liermann Garcia RF, Evangelista Garcia C, McMaster P, et al. Transplantation for primary biliary cirrhosis: retrospective analysis of 400 patients in a single center. Hepatology (Baltimore, Md.). 2001;33:22–27.
89. Charatcharoenwitthaya P, Pimentel S, Talwalker JA, et al. Long-term survival and impact of ursodeoxycholic acid treatment for recurrent primary biliary cirrhosis after liver transplantation. Liver Transplantation. 2007;13:1236–1245.
90. Sanchez EQ, Levy MF, Goldstein RM, et al. The changing clinical presentation of recurrent primary biliary cirrhosis after liver transplantation. Transplantation. 2003;76:1583–1588.
91. Khettry U, Anand N, Faul PN, et al. Liver transplantation for primary biliary cirrhosis: a long-term pathologic study. Liver Transplantation. 2003;9: 87–96.
92. Levitsky J, Hart J, Cohen SM, et al. The effect of immunosuppressive regimen on the recurrence of primary biliary cirrhosis after liver transplantation. Liver Transplantation. 2003;9:733–736.
93. Sebagh M, Farges O, Dubel L, et al. Histological features predictive of recurrence of primary biliary cirrhosis after liver transplantation. Transplantation. 1998;65:1328–1333.
94. Jacob DA, Bahra M, Schmidt SC, et al. Mayo risk score for primary biliary cirrhosis: a useful tool for the prediction of course after liver transplantation? Annals of Transplantation. 2008;13:35–42.
95. Abu-Elmagd K, Demetris J, Rakela J, et al. Tranplantation for primary biliary cirrhosis: disease recurrence and outcome in 421 patients. Hepatology (Baltimore, Md.). 1997;26:176A.
96. Neuberger J, Portmann B, Macdougall BR, et al. Recurrence of primary biliary cirrhosis after liver transplantation. New England Journal of Medicine. 1982;106:1–4.
97. Sylvestre PB, Batts KP, Burgart LJ, et al. Recurrence of primary biliary cirrhosis after liver transplantation: histologic estimate of incidence and natural history. Liver Transplantation. 2003;9:1086–1093.
98. Dubel L, Farges O, Bismuth H, et al. Kinetics of anti-M2 antibodies after liver transplantation for primary biliary cirrhosis. Journal of Hepatology. 1995;15: 674–680.
99. Mells G, Mann C, Hubscher S, et al. Late protocol liver biopsies in the liver allograft: a neglected investigation? Liver Transplantation. 2009;15: 931–938.
100. Guy JE, Qian P, Lowell PA, et al. Recurrent primary biliary cirrhosis: pretransplant factors and ursodeoxycholic acid treatment post-liver transplant. Liver Transplantation. 2005;11:1252–1257.
101. LaRusso NF, Shneider BL, Black D, et al. Primary sclerosing cholangitis: summary

of a workshop. Hepatology (Baltimore, Md.). 2006;44:746–764.
102. Graziadei IW, Wiesner RH, Marotta PJ, et al. Long-term results of patients undergoing liver transplantation for primary sclerosing cholangitis. Hepatology (Baltimore, Md.). 1999;30:1121–1127.
103. Roberts MS, Angus DC, Bryce CL, et al. Survival after liver transplantation in the United States: a disease-specific analysis of the UNOS database. Liver Transplantation. 2004;10:886–897.
104. Wiesner RH. Liver transplantation for primary sclerosing cholangitis: timing, outcome, impact of inflammatory bowel disease and recurrence of disease. Best Practice and Research. Clinical Gastroenterology. 2001;15:667–680.
105. Lerut J, Demetris AJ, Stieber AC, et al. Intrahepatic bile duct strictures after human orthotopic liver transplantation. Recurrence of primary sclerosing cholangitis or unusual presentation of allograft rejection. Transplant International. 1988;1:127–130.
106. Campsen J, Zimmerman MA, Trotter JF, et al. Clinically recurrent primary sclerosing cholangitis following liver transplantation: a time course. Liver Transplantation. 2008;14:138–143.
107. Alabraba E, Nightingale P, Gunson B, et al. A re-evaluation of the risk factors for the recurrence of primary sclerosing cholangitis in liver allografts. Liver Transplantation. 2009;15:330–340.
108. Jeyarajah DR, Netto GJ, Lee SP, et al. Recurrent primary sclerosing cholangitis after orthotopic liver transplantation: is chronic rejection part of the disease process? Transplantation. 1998;66:1300–1306.
109. Vera A, Moledina S, Gunson B, et al. Risk factors for recurrence of primary sclerosing cholangitis of liver allograft. Lancet. 2002;360:1943–1944.
110. Khettry U, Keaveny A, Goldar-Najafi A, et al. Liver transplantation for primary sclerosing cholangitis: a long-term clinicopathologic study. Human Pathology. 2003;34:1127–1136.
111. Alexander J, Lord JD, Yeh MM, et al. Risk factors for recurrence of primary sclerosing cholangitis after liver transplantation. Liver Transplantation. 2008;14:245–251.
112. Cholongitas E, Shusang V, Papatheodordis GV, et al. Risk factors for primary sclerosing cholangitis recurrence of after liver transplantation. Liver Transplantation. 2008;14:138–143.
113. Moncrief KJ, Savu A, Ma MM, et al. The natural history of inflammatory bowel disease and primary sclerosing cholangitis after living donor liver transplantation: a single-centre experience. Canadian Journal of Gastroenterology. 2010;24:40–46.
114. Brandsaeter B, Schrumpf E, Bentdal O, et al. Recurrent primary sclerosing cholangitis after liver transplantation: a magnetic resonance cholangiography study with analyses of predictive factors. Liver Transplantation. 2005;11:1361–1369.
115. Kuglemas M, Spiegelman P, Osgood MJ, et al. Different immunosuppressive regimens and recurrence of primary sclerosing cholangitis after liver transplantation. Liver Transplantation. 2003;9:727–732.
116. Maheshwari A, Yoo HY, Thuluvath PJ. Long-term outcome of liver transplantation in patients with PSC: a comparative analysis with PBC. American Journal of Gastroenterology. 2004;99:538–542.
117. United Network for Organ Sharing. OPTN & SRTR Annual Data Report 2011. Available from: http://www.unos.org.
118. O'Grady JG. Liver transplantation alcohol related liver disease: (deliberately) stirring the hornet's nest! Gut. 2006;55:1529–1531.
119. European Liver Transplant Registry. 2012; Available from: http://www.eltr.org.
120. Scharschmmidt BF. Human liver transplantation: analysis of data on 540 patients from four centers. Hepatology (Baltimore, Md.). 1984;4:95S–101S.
121. Tome S, Lucey MR. Timing of liver transplantation in alcoholic cirrhosis. Journal of Hepatology. 2003;39:302–307.
122. Fuller RK. Definition and diagnosis of relapse to drinking. Liver Transplantation and Surgery. 1997;3:258–262.
123. DiMartini A, Dew MA, Day N, et al. Trajectories of alcohol consumption following liver transplantation. American Journal of Transplantation. 2010;10:2305–2312.
124. Tang H, Boulton R, Gunson B, et al. Patterns of alcohol consumption after liver transplantation. Gut. 1998;43:140–145.
125. Cuardrado A, Fabrega E, Casafont F, et al. Alcohol recidivism impairs long-term patient survival after orthotopic liver transplantation for alcoholic liver disease. Liver Transplantation. 2005;11:420–426.
126. Fabrega E, Crespo J, Casafont F, et al. Alcoholic recidivism after liver transplantation for alcoholic cirrhosis. Journal of Clinical Gastroenterology. 1998;26:204–206.
127. Pageaux GP, Michel J, Coste V, et al. Alcoholic cirrhosis is a good indication for livertransplatation, even for cases of recidivism. Gut. 1999;45:421–426.
128. Pageaux GP, Bisumuth M, Perney P, et al. Alcohol relapse after liver transplantation for alcoholic liver disease: does it matter? Journal of Hepatology. 2003;38:629–634.
129. Conjeevaram HS, Hart J, Lissoos TW, et al. Rapidly progressively liver injury and fatal alcoholic hepatitis occurring after liver transplantation in alcoholic patients. Transplantation. 1999;67:1562–1568.
130. Pfitzmann R, Schwenzer J, Rayes N, et al. Long-term survival and predictors of relapse after orthotopic liver transplantation for alcoholic liver disease. Liver Transplantation. 2007;13:197–205.
131. DiMartini A, Day N, Dew MA, et al. Alcohol consumption patterns and predictors of use following liver transplantation for alcoholic liver disease. Liver Transplantation. 2006;12:813–820.
132. Foster PF, Fabrega F, Karademir S, et al. Prediction of abstinence from ethanol in alcoholic recipients following liver transplantation. Hepatology (Baltimore, Md.). 1997;25:1469–1477.
133. Everhart JE, Beresford TP. Liver transplantation for alcoholic liver disease: a survey of transplantation programs in the United States. Liver Transplantation and Surgery. 1997;3:220–226.
134. Vaillant GE. The natural history of alcoholism and its relationship to liver transplantation. Liver Transplantation and Surgery. 1997;3:304–310.
135. Coffman KL, Hoffman A, Sher L, et al. Treatment of the postoperative alcoholic liver transplant recipient with other addictions. Liver Transplantation and Surgery. 1997;3:322–327.
136. McCallum S, Masterton G. Liver transplantation for alcoholic liver disease: a systematic review of psychosocial selection criteria. Alcohol and Alcoholism. 2006;41:358–363.
137. Kotlyar DS, Burke A, Campbell MS, et al. A critical review of candidacy for orthotopic liver transplantation in alcoholic liver disease. American Journal of Gastroenterology. 2008;103:734–743.
138. Jauhar S, Talwalkar JA, Schneekloth T, et al. Analysis of factors that predict alcohol relapse following liver transplantation. Liver Transplantation. 2004;10:408–411.
139. Everson G, Bharadhwaj G, House R, et al. Long-term follow-up of patients with alcoholic liver disease whi underwent hepatic transplantation. Liver Transplantation and Surgery. 1997;3:263–274.
140. Pereira SP, Williams R. Alcohol relapse and functional outcome after liver transplantation for alcoholic liver disease. Liver Transplantation. 2001;7:204–205.
141. Weinrieb RM, Van Horn DH, McLellan AT, et al. Drinking behavior and motivation for treatment among alcohol-dependent liver transplant candidates. Journal of Addictive Diseases. 2001;20:105–119.
142. Bjornsson E, Olsson J, Rydell A, et al. Long-term follow-up of patients with alcoholic liver disease after liver transplantation in Sweden: impact of structured management on recidivism. Scandinavian Journal of Gastroenterology. 2005;40:206–216.
143. Browning JS, Szczepaniak LS, Dobbin LS, et al. Prevalence of hepatic steatosis in an urban population in the United States: impact of ethnicity. Hepatology (Baltimore, Md.). 2004;40:1387–1395.
144. Neuschwander-Tetri BA, Caldwell SH. Nonalcoholic steatohepatitis: summary of an AASLD single topic conference. Hepatology (Baltimore, Md.). 2003;37:1202–1219.
145. Ong JP, Younossi ZM. Epidemiology and natural history of NAFLD and NASH. Clinics in Liver Disease. 2007;11:1–16.
146. Marchesini G, Brizi M, Bianchi G, et al. Nonalcoholic fatty liver disease: a feature of the metabolic syndrome. Diabetes. 2001;50:1844–1850.
147. Koehler E, Watt K, Charlton M. Fatty liver and liver transplantation. Clinics in Liver Disease. 2009;13:621–630.
148. Charlton M. Nonalcoholic fatty liver disease: a review of current understanding and future impact. Clinical Gastroenterology and Hepatology. 2004;2:1048–1058.
149. Yalamanchili K, Saadeh S, Klintmalm GB, et al. Nonalcoholic fatty liver disease after liver transplantation for cryptogenic cirrhosis or nonalcoholic fatty liver disease. Liver Transplantation. 2010;16:431–439.
150. Burke GW, Cirocco R, Hensley G, et al. Liver transplantation for cirrhosis following jejuno-ileal bypass-regional cytokine differences associated with pathological changes in the transplant liver. Transplantation. 1992;54:374–377.
151. Bhagat V, Mindikoglu AL, Nudo CG, et al. Outcomes of liver transplantation in patients with cirrhosis due to nonalcoholic steatohepatitis versus patients with cirrhosis due to alcoholic liver disease. Transplantation. 2009;15:1814–1820.
152. Contos MJ, Cales W, Sterling RK, et al. Development of nonalcoholic fatty liver disease after orthotopic liver transplantation for cryptogenic cirrhosis. Liver Transplantation. 2001;7:363–373.
153. Molloy RM, Komorowski R, Varma RR. Recurrent nonalcoholic steatohepatitis and cirrhosis after liver transplantation. Liver Transplantation and Surgery. 1997;3:177–178.
154. Kim WR, Poterucha JJ, Porayko MK, et al. Recurrence of nonalcoholic steatohepatitis following liver transplantation. Transplantation. 1996;62:1802–1805.
155. Maor-Kendler Y, Batts KP, Burgart LJ, et al. Comparative allograft histology after

liver transplantation for cryptogenic cirrhosis, alcohol, hepatitis C, and cholestatic liver disease. Transplantation. 2000;70:292–297.
156. Malik SM, deVera ME, Fontes P, et al. Recurrent disease following liver transplantation for nonalcoholic steatohepatitis cirrhosis. Liver Transplantation. 2009;15:1843–1851.
157. Malik SM, deVera ME, Fontes P, et al. Outcome after liver transplantation for NASH cirrhosis. American Journal of Transplantation. 2009;9:782–793.
158. Charlton M, Kasparova P, Weston S, et al. Frequency of nonalcoholic steatohepatitis as a cause of advanced liver disease. Liver Transplantation. 2001;7:608–614.
159. Cauble MS, Gilroy R, Sorrell MF, et al. Lipoattrophic diabetes and end-stage liver disease secondary to nonalcoholic steatohepatitis with recurrence after transplantation. Tranplantation. 2001;71:829–895.
160. Ong J, Younossi ZM, Reddy V, et al. Cryptogenic cirrhosis and posttransplantation nonalcoholic fatty liver disease. Liver Transplantation. 2001;7:797–801.
161. Lerut J, Bonaccorsi-Riani E, Finet P, et al. Minimization of steroids in liver transplantation. Transplant International. 2009;22:2–19.
162. Farkas SA, Schnitzbauer AA, Kirchner G, et al. Calcineurin inhibitor minimization protocols in liver transplantation. Transplant International. 2009;22:49–60.
163. Ferlay J, Shin HR, Bray F, et al. Estimates of worldwide burden of cancer in 2008: GLOBOCAN 2008. International Journal of Cancer. 2010;127:2893–2917.
164. Altekruse SF, McGlynn KA, Reichman ME. Hepatocellular carcinoma incidence, mortality, and survival trends in the United States from 1975 to 2005. Journal of Clinical Oncology. 2009;27:1485–1491.
165. Thomas MB, Jaffe D, Choti MM, et al. Hepatocellular carcinoma: consensus recommendations of the National Cancer Institute Clinical Trials Planning Meeting. Journal of Clinical Oncology. 2010;28:3994–4005.
166. Penn I. Hepatic transplantation for primary and metastatic cancers of the liver. Surgery. 1991;110:726–735.
167. Yoo HY, Patt CH, Geschwind JF, et al. The outcome of liver transplantation in patients with hepatocellular carcinoma in the United States between 1988 and 2001: 5-year survival has improved significantly with time. Journal of Clinical Oncology. 2003;21:4329–4335.
168. Mazzaferro V, Regalia E, Doci R, et al. Liver transplantation for the treatment of small hepatocellular carcinomas in patients with cirrhosis. New England Journal of Medicine. 1996;334:693–699.
169. Yao FY, Ferrell L, Bass NM, et al. Liver transplantation for hepatocellular carcinoma: expansion of the tumor size limits does not adversely impact survival. Hepatology (Baltimore, Md.). 2001;33:1394–1403.
170. Zavaglia C, De Carlis L, Alberti AB, et al. Predictors of long-term survival after liver transplantation for hepatocellular carcinoma. American Journal of Gastroenterology. 2005;100:2708–2716.
171. Marsh JW, Dvorchik I, Subotin M, et al. The prediction of risk of recurrence and time to recurrence of hepatocellular carcinoma after orthotopic liver transplantation: a pilot study. Hepatology (Baltimore, Md.). 1997;26:444–450.
172. Hemming AW, Cattral MS, Reed AI, et al. Liver transplantation for hepatocellular carcinoma. Annals of Surgery. 2001;233:652–659.
173. Shimoda M, Ghobrial RM, Carmody IC, et al. Predictors of survival after liver transplantation for hepatocellular carcinoma associated with Hepatitis C. Liver Transplantation. 2004;10:1478–1486.
174. Schlitt HJ, Neipp M, Weimann A, et al. Recurrence patterns of hepatocellular and fibrolamellar carcinoma after liver transplantation. Journal of Clinical Oncology. 1999;17:324–331.
175. Regalia E, Fassati LR, Valente U, et al. Pattern and management of recurrent hepatocellular carcinoma after liver transplantation. Journal of Hepato-Biliary-Pancreatic Surgery. 1998;5:29–34.
176. Chok KS, Chan SC, Cheung TT, et al. Late recurrence of hepatocellular carcinoma after liver transplantation. World Journal of Surgery. 2011;35:2058–2062.
177. Kornberg A, Kupper B, Tannapfel A, et al. Long-term survival after recurrent hepatocellular carcinoma in liver transplant patients: clinical patterns and outcome variables. European Journal of Surgical Oncology. 2010;36:275–280.
178. Shin WY, Suh KS, Lee HW, et al. Prognostic factors affecting survival after recurrence in adult living donor liver transplantation for hepatocellular carcinoma. Liver Transplantation. 2010;16:678–684.
179. Valdivieso A, Bustamante J, Gastaca M, et al. Management of hepatocellular carcinoma recurrence after liver transplantation. Transplantation Proceedings. 2010;42:660–662.
180. Taketomi A, Fukuhara T, Morita K, et al. Improved results of a surgical resection for the recurrence of hepatocellular carcinoma after living donor liver transplantation. Annals of Surgical Oncology. 2010;17:2283–2289.
181. Roayaie S, Schwartz JD, Sung MW, et al. Recurrence of hepatocellular carcinoma after liver transplant: patterns and prognosis. Liver Transplantation. 2004;10:534–540.
182. Jonas S, Bechstein WO, Steinmüller T, et al. Vascular invasion and histopathologic grading determine outcome after liver transplantation for hepatocellular carcinoma in cirrhosis. Hepatology (Baltimore, Md.). 2001;33:1080–1086.
183. Plessier A, Codes L, Consigny Y, et al. Underestimation of the influence of satellite nodules as a risk factor for post-transplantation recurrence in patients with small hepatocellular carcinoma. Liver Transplantation. 2004;10:S86–S90.
184. Löhe F, Angele MK, Gerbes AL, et al. Tumour size is an important predictor for the outcome after liver transplantation for hepatocellular carcinoma. European Journal of Surgical Oncology. 2005;31(9):994–999.
185. Todo S, Furukawa H. Living donor liver transplantation for adult patients with hepatocellular carcinoma: experience in Japan. Annals of Surgery. 2004;240(3):451–459.
186. Bismuth H, Chiche L, Adam R, et al. Liver resection versus transplantation for hepatocellular carcinoma in cirrhotic patients. Annals of Surgery. 1993;218(2):145–151.
187. Cillo U, Vitale A, Bassanello M, et al. Liver transplantation for the treatment of moderately or well-differentiated hepatocellular carcinoma. Annals of Surgery. 2004;239:150–159.
188. Silva M, Moya A, Berenguer M, et al. Expanded criteria for liver transplantation in patients with cirrhosis and hepatocellular carcinoma. Liver Transplantation. 2008;14:1449–1460.
189. Esnaola NF, Lauwers GY, Mirza NQ, et al. Predictors of microvascular invasion in patients with hepatocellular carcinoma who are candidates for orthotopic liver transplantation. Journal of Gastrointestinal Surgery. 2002;6:224–232.
190. Silva MA, Hegab B, Hyde C, et al. Needle track seeding following biopsy of liver lesions in the diagnosis of hepatocellular cancer: a systematic review and meta-analysis. Gut. 2008;57:1592–1596.
191. DuBay D, Sandroussi C, Sandhu L, et al. Liver transplantation for advanced hepatocellular carcinoma using poor tumor differentiation on biopsy as an exclusion criterion. Annals of Surgery. 2011;253:166–172.
192. Tateishi R, Yoshida H, Matsuyama Y, et al. Diagnostic accuracy of tumor markers for hepatocellular carcinoma: a systematic review. Hepatology International. 2008;2:17–30.
193. Otto G, Herber S, Heise M, et al. Response to transarterial chemoembolization as a biological selection criterion for liver transplantation in hepatocellular carcinoma. Liver Transplantation. 2006;12:1260–1267.
194. Yao FY, Kerlan RK Jr, Hirose R, et al. Excellent outcome following down-staging of hepatocellular carcinoma prior to liver transplantation: an intention-to-treat analysis. Hepatology (Baltimore, Md.). 2008;48:819–827.
195. Zimmerman MA, Trotter JF, Wachs M, et al. Predictors of long-term outcome following liver transplantation for hepatocellular carcinoma: a single-center experience. Transplant International. 2007;20:747–753.
196. Graziadei IW, Sandmueller H, Waldenberger P, et al. Chemoembolization followed by liver transplantation for hepatocellular carcinoma impedes tumor progression while on the waiting list and leads to excellent outcome. Liver Transplantation. 2003;9:557–563.
197. Llovet JM, Mas X, Aponte JJ, et al. Cost effectiveness of adjuvant therapy for hepatocellular carcinoma during the waiting list for liver transplantation. Gut. 2002;50:123–128.
198. Millonig G, Graziadei IW, Freund MC, et al. Response to preoperative chemoembolization correlates with outcome after liver transplantation in patients with hepatocellular carcinoma. Liver Transplantation. 2007;13:272–279.
199. Llovet JM, Ricci S, Mazzaferro V, et al. Sorafenib in advanced hepatocellular carcinoma. New England Journal of Medicine. 2008;359:378–390.
200. Vivarelli M, Bellusci R, Cucchetti A, et al. Low recurrence rate of hepatocellular carcinoma after liver transplantation: better patient selection or lower immunosuppression? Transplantation. 2002;74:1746–1751.
201. Vivarelli M, Cucchetti A, Piscaglia F, et al. Analysis of risk factors for tumor recurrence after liver transplantation for hepatocellular carcinoma: key role of immunosuppression. Liver Transplantation. 2005;11:497–503.
202. Vivarelli M, Cucchetti A, La Barba G, et al. Liver transplantation for hepatocellular carcinoma under calcineurin inhibitors: reassessment of risk factors for tumor recurrence. Annals of Surgery. 2008;248:857–862.
203. Wang Z, Zhou J, Fan J, et al. Sirolimus inhibits the growth and metastatic progression of hepatocellular carcinoma. Journal of Cancer Research and Clinical Oncology. 2009;135:715–722.
204. Vivarelli M, Dazzi A, Zanello M, et al. Effect of different immunosuppressive schedules on recurrence-free survival after liver transplantation for hepatocellular carcinoma. Transplantation. 2010;89:227–231.
205. Toso C, Merani S, Bigam DL, et al. Sirolimus-based immunosuppression is associated with increased survival after liver transplantation for hepatocellular carcinoma. Hepatology (Baltimore, Md.). 2010;51:1237–1243.
206. Roberts JP. Tumor surveillance: what can and should be done? Screening for recurrence of hepatocellular carcinoma after liver transplantation. Liver Transplantation. 2005;11:S45–S46.

207. Seong J, Koom WS, Park HC. Radiotherapy for painful bone metastases from hepatocellular carcinoma. Liver International. 2005;25:261–265.
208. Kaizu T, Karasawa K, Tanaka Y, et al. Radiotherapy for osseous metastases from hepatocellular carcinoma: a retrospective study of 57 patients. American Journal of Gastroenterology. 1998;93:2167–2171.
209. Chen ZS, He F, Zeng FJ, et al. Early steroid withdrawal after liver transplantation for hepatocellular carcinoma. World Journal of Gastroenterology. 2007;13: 5273–5276.

第 79 章

心脏移植后复发性疾病

Jignesh K. Patel, Jon A. Kobashigawa

引言

心脏移植术后疾病复发的风险同移植前的实际病因有关。幸运的是,对绝大多数心脏移植患者而言,疾病复发的可能性较小。扩张型心肌病及冠状动脉疾病是最常见的两种需要进行心脏移植手术治疗的疾病。大多数扩张性心肌病的病因不外乎特发性、病毒感染相关以及家族性三种,且这三种情况不会影响移植后的病程。有一小部分心肌病患者,其病因可能同部分浸润性疾病有关,如特殊类型的心肌炎、肉瘤或查加斯病,这部分患者在移植术后有一定复发的可能。最常见的导致远期移植心脏功能不全及移植心脏衰竭的病因可能是移植心脏血管病变(CAV)——一种复发性疾病,其机制可能与移植受体本身存在的动脉粥样硬化有关。大约一半的心脏移植患者最终因冠状动脉疾病导致终末期移植心脏疾病。然而,在 CAV 的发生过程中,免疫系统起到了重要的作用,因此,可以将其看作是一种慢性的移植心脏排斥反应。

心脏移植患者术后第一年内死亡通常与排斥风险增加、高强度免疫抑制相关的感染有密切联系(参见第 105 章)。然而,在第一年之后,决定长期移植心脏生存率的一个重要因素就是 CAV 是否发生。CAV 最初在心脏移植动物实验中被发现,随着时间的进展,CAV 的程度逐渐加重,并表现出类似动脉粥样硬化的血管内膜增厚的组织学表现。对于 CAV 的患者,在移植术后早期,对移植心脏进行组织学检测可以发现冠状动脉广泛性病变,而这种病变在移植术前行血管造影时一般无明显表现。尽管在 20 世纪 80 年代,引入了环孢素作为新型免疫抑制剂,该药物能够显著降低移植心脏排斥反应发生率,并改善预后,但对 CAV 的发生并没有明显的改善作用[1]。

注册临床试验数据表明,心脏移植 1 年后,每年新增死亡率约为 4%(图 79.1)[2]。在移植术后的前 3 年,急性排斥反应导致的死亡率约为 9%。3 年后,由急性排斥反应所致的死亡率明显下降。移植术后第 1 年内的死亡患者中,大约有 20%死于非特异性移植心脏衰竭,对于这部分患者,其具体死亡原因尚不明确。这些患者的死亡原因很可能与未被诊断的移植心脏排斥反应或复发后遗症或低级别的排斥反应,如小血管 CAV、限制性生理学等有关;很多患者对于其导致移植心脏衰竭的疾病原因和过程,目前仍知之甚少。心脏移植术后 1 年后,抗体介导性排斥反应和 CAV 可导致移植心脏的衰竭。术后 1~3 年的死亡患者中,大约 10%与 CAV 有关,术后第 3 年时该概率达到 20%,第 5 年达到 30%,第 8 年达到 45%。新型免疫抑制剂对于 CAV 发生的改善作用相当有限,对于 2001—2009 年行心脏移植术的患者,相比 1994—2000 年行心脏移植术的患者,其 CAV 的发生仅下降 2%~4%(图 79.1)。

病理学

非移植动脉粥样硬化表现为以包括巨噬细胞、T 细胞和平滑肌细胞在内的多种细胞累及血管壁的慢性炎症过程。Ross 等[3]提出,该过程是血管内皮损伤的一种应答反应。CAV 的发生可能与这种过程有一定的联系。但一般认为,血管内皮的初始损伤是由心脏移植相关的多种因素共同作用导致的,这些因素包括缺血再灌注损伤、免疫应答反应、供体因素以及常见的动脉粥样硬化的危险因素。

CAV 的病理学表现与非移植患者的动脉粥样硬化有许多不同(参见第 83 章)(表 79.1)。在 CAV 中,疾病的病理学表现为更具弥散性,可能表现为血管的向心性狭窄,不仅累及大血管和中血管,也常累及微血管[4]。

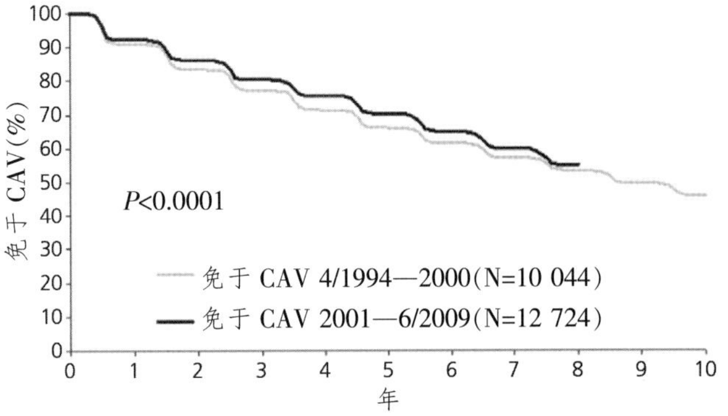

图 79.1 成年心脏移植患者免于心脏移植血管病变的曲线图(1994—2009 年行移植手术)。(Reproduced from [2] Stehlik et al., Journal of Heart and Lung Transplantation 2011;30:1078-1094 with permission from Elsevier. Copyright 2011, Elsevier.)

表 79.1 非移植动脉粥样硬化与心脏移植血管病变的典型特征

非移植动脉粥样硬化	移植心脏血管病变
大多影响心外膜血管	泛血管疾病,包括微血管病变
进展缓慢	快速进展
偏心性病灶	向心性病灶
一般富含脂质	脂质含量较低
钙化常见	钙化少见
代偿性扩张(Glagov 现象)	动脉收缩

CAV 的向心性、弥散性病变的特征使其在血管造影中不常被发现[4],反而利用血管内超声(TVUS),检测效果更佳。然而,也有许多患者可能表现出与非移植动脉粥样硬化患者相类似的典型的局灶性病变,尽管这些病变中脂质成分可能变化较大,且若发生钙化也多较晚[5]。对于冠状动脉钙化同 CAV 之间的关系,目前还存在争论。早期研究表明,利用电子束 CT 成像评估血管钙化程度同血管造影或血管内超声发现的病变程度有明显关联[6,7]。而近期的研究则表明,冠状动脉钙化同 CAV 的严重程度并没有明显联系。最近的一项研究表明[8],在 11 例冠状动脉造影证实为重度 CAV 的患者中仅有 4 例患者钙化评分为 0 分。该诊断的精确度低于 60%。其作者假设,CAV 患者出现冠状动脉钙化可能同既往疾病或传统冠状动脉粥样硬化的发生有关。

血管内膜向心性增厚主要由平滑肌细胞和细胞外基质构成,其内、外弹力膜一般完整。CAV 常常不仅侵犯内膜,还可能造成中膜与外膜纤维浸润。因此,动脉代偿性重构减少(非移植动脉粥样硬化患者中可见的 Glagov 现象),且动脉甚至可能出现收缩[9]。一般情况下,术后第 1 年内多见由内膜增生导致的管腔狭窄,并在此之后出现收缩性的血管重构[10,11]。

移植心脏血管病变的免疫学机制

获得性免疫

移植心脏,作为一个富血管的器官,大量内膜同受体血液相接触,造成抗原刺激,而受体免疫应答主要通过识别外来主要组织相容性抗原来激活。循环中的宿主 T 淋巴细胞和树突状细胞的抗原识别(详见第 5 章)将导致免疫应答的增强,并进一步产生多种细胞因子,包括白介素、γ-干扰素、肿瘤坏死因子 α。这些细胞因子进一步促进免疫效应机制的发生, 包括细胞毒 T 细胞、巨噬细胞浸润和抗体的产生(详见第 5-7 章)。尽管这种免疫应答一般在急性排斥反应时发生, 其对于 CAV 的发生可能也起到了同样重要的作用。CAV 作为慢性排斥反应的诸多表现之一,不仅见于移植心脏,在移植肾脏、肺和肝脏中也有表现。事实上,其他移植器官中一定程度的纤维变性可能在一定程度上同下游血管缺血性萎缩伴进行性血管病变有关。在移植肺脏中,慢性排斥反应可以表现为闭塞性细支气管炎, 在移植肝脏中,相应的病理过程称为胆管消失综合征。

直接同种异体识别反应, 通过利用受体树突状细胞来识别供体细胞上的外来人白细胞抗原 (HLA),这种反应是急性排斥反应发生的主要原因。相对地,间接同种异体识别反应,即当供体抗原被内化、处理并以多肽的形式呈递给宿主的树突状细胞, 可能为慢性排斥反应以及 CAV 的发生原因[12,16]。重度 CAV 的发生同 HLA 错配的程度以及供体特异性抗体的生成呈正相关(参见第 6 章和第 30 章)[14]。无论是有症状还是无症状的抗体介导性排斥反应,都倾向于促进 CAV 的发生和发展。

传统的免疫抑制治疗主要通过作用于 T 细胞以防止急性细胞排斥反应的发生,而近年来,利用钙调磷酸酶抑制剂(特别是他克莫司)和霉酚酸酯(MMF)能够显著降低排斥反应的发生率[15]。然而,这些药物对于 CAV 发生的预防作用十分有限[2]。这些药物虽然在抑制 Th-1 细胞因子的产生以及限制 T 细胞活化方面有显著效果,但对抗体产生的限制作用却比较有限[16]。实质器官移植之后, 有相当一部分患者会继续对移植心脏产生抗体。移植受体体内抗 HLA 抗体的产生会在一定程度上提高死亡率[17]和 CAV 发生率[18,19]。因此,同种异体免疫反应是区别 CAV 和一般的进行性动脉粥样硬化性血管病的重要因素,且一定程度上会加速 CAV 的进展。

另一方面,非 HLA 抗体的产生也会引起 CAV(参见第 36 章)。这些抗体对人体自身心肌病的进展并没有显著作用。循环中抗内皮抗体的存在与 CAV 的发生有关[20]。波形蛋白产生于内皮细胞,但不局限于内皮细胞,是一种具有媒介作用的纤维蛋白,其抗体的产生可能是 CAV 发生的独立危险因素[21]。波形蛋白在正常和病变冠状动脉的内、中膜中都有弥散性表达。因此,移植术后早期损伤,如缺血和再灌注,可使波形蛋白释放进入循环中。由于波形蛋白一般不与免疫系统接触,而是进一步被抗原提呈细胞(APC)所摄取,并作为自抗原进行提呈。有趣的是,体外实验表明,这些细胞似乎并不介导内皮细胞的补体介导性细胞毒反应,而补体介导性细胞毒反应与超急性排斥反应相关。抗波形蛋白抗体可能从更细微的层面发挥低级别的损伤作用,而这种损伤与 CAV 发展的慢性进展型病程是一致的。并且,采用他克莫司进行移植术后免疫抑制的患者与于采用环孢素的患者,以及霉酚酸酯与硫唑嘌呤的患者相比,他们产生抗波形蛋白抗体的水平相对较低[22,23]。

除了波形蛋白之外,内皮细胞多种抗原的抗体,如血管紧张素Ⅱ1 型受体及抗主要组织匹配性复合物Ⅰ链相关蛋白 A(MICA)或 B 抗体,在实质脏器移植受体中都有表达,且其预后均较差[24,25]。MICA 抗原是 HLA 相关的多态性糖蛋白,它表达于人内皮细胞、上皮细胞和成纤维细胞表面。应激环境会诱导 MICA 的表达。这些蛋白作为自然杀伤细胞(NK 细胞)以及 CD8 阳性 T 细胞的活化受体 NKG2D 的配体起作用。MICA 在内皮细胞表面表达,却不在淋巴细胞上表达,这可能可以用于解释为何部分受体与供体淋巴细胞间交叉配型结果阴性,但却造成移植器官功能丧失。

抗 MICA 抗体的存在以及移植心脏心内膜心肌活检发现的 MICA 表达与急性移植心脏排斥反应的发生相关[26]。抗 MICA 抗原的抗体的产生可以诱导补体依赖的细胞毒反应的产生[27]。心脏移植受体中的 MICA 抗体与急性排斥反应和 CAV 进展相关[28]。

固有免疫

尽管传统免疫抑制剂能够有效作用于获得性免疫系统,这些药物很大程度上并不作用于固有免疫系统。完整功能的固有免疫应答可能既刺激获得性免疫,又促进 CAV 的远期进展(参见第 7 章)。在固有免疫系统中,目前被研究的最多的可能是 toll 样受体(TLR),多种细胞上表达的跨膜蛋白家族,包括上皮细胞、树突状细胞、巨噬细胞、T 和 B 细胞。TLR 及免疫系统进化中最保守的蛋白家族之一,与微生物抗原表皮保守的配体,如革兰阴性菌表面的脂多糖相结合。然而,一般认为 TLR 既可以被外源性配体,也可以被内源性配体所激活[29]。供体心脏移植后的缺血再灌注损伤常导致一系列内源性配体的释放,包括直接组织损伤的产物,如细胞外基质中的透明质酸多糖。研究表明透明质酸能通过与 TLR 相结合以激活树突状细胞[30]。其他缺血再灌注产物,如热休克蛋白 70[31]及同种异体移植炎症因子 1(AIF-1),可能导致固有免疫系统的激活。TLR 的激活会导致一系列炎症级联反应的激活,这些炎症反应很有可能影响急性移植器官排斥的发生及 CAV 的进展。在心脏移植患者中,AIF-1、TLR-2 及白介素 18 表达谱与移植器官排斥相关,这一结果已被外周血和活检组织结果所证实[32]。以冠状动脉血流储备受损为表征的动脉内皮功能不全的移植患者,其体内 TLR-4 的 mRNA 转录水平、TLR-4 表达水平及 TLR 下游信号成分如 B7-1、白介素 12 及 TNF-α 表达均有所增加[33]。

内皮活化

内皮细胞在介导急性和慢性排斥反应中发挥关键作用[34]。由于内皮细胞构成供体与宿主循环中淋巴细胞之间的第一级交界线,对防止炎症细胞进入血管间质的屏障具有稳定作用,因此内皮损伤及功能不全被认为是 CAV 发展[35]中的前哨性事件。内皮细胞对细胞因子[36]具有高反应性,并表达Ⅱ型抗原,尤其在微脉管系统[37,38]和冠状动脉中。内皮细胞也能够发挥 APC[39,40]的作用。人类冠状动脉内皮细胞能在体外刺激异基因 T 细胞[41]。

内皮细胞高渗性可能是移植心脏血管壁内脂质浸润增加的机制,从而导致 CAV 的发生[42]。血管内皮生长因子(VEGF)是一种潜在的血管通透性诱导剂,且在出现急性排斥反应的人类移植心脏中表达上调。因此,VEGF 的出现与 CAV 的发生相关[44,45]。

移植心脏血管内皮细胞表达Ⅱ型 HLA 抗原及黏附分子如细胞间黏附分子 1(ICAM-1)及血管细胞黏附

分子(VCAM)[46,47]。上述分子在内皮的表达反映了内皮的活化。在正常心脏的内皮中,上述分子一般不表达。

尽管内皮黏附分子的表达也是非移植动脉粥样硬化的特征之一,HLA 抗原的诱导表达则是移植心脏内皮所特有的。将内皮细胞与 $CD4^+$ T 淋巴细胞共培养能引起内皮细胞增殖,并合成白介素-2[46],这是内皮活化的结果。供体内皮慢性活化能对受体淋巴细胞形成持续性刺激,从而维持慢性免疫反应。研究表明,移植心脏血管内皮表达 ICAM-1 和 HLA-DR 能够引起移植器官血管病变,但也有证据表明,供体心脏中的特定 ICAM-1 对 CAV 的发生具有保护作用[49],这也许与降低和 B 细胞结合的 ICAM-1 的等位基因改变相关。

内皮细胞活化可由许多因素引起,且能用于区别加速型 CAV 的表型和自体动脉粥样硬化(图 79.2)。急性排斥反应引起炎症细胞释放细胞因子,可激活内皮细胞,而 CAV 的发生与急性移植器官排斥反应的发作频率有关[50]。除此之外,内皮特异性 T 淋巴细胞损伤或受体抗供体内皮抗体的产生,如抗波形蛋白抗体,也可引发内皮激活。移植术中的缺血再灌注损伤也可引起内皮激活。实验研究表面,人内皮细胞在缺氧状态下可有 ICAM-1 上调[51]。在动物模型中,移植前黏附分子对移植心脏内皮的诱导也与后续 CAV 的发生有关[52]。在移植后评估人体循环中可溶性 ICAM-1 可作为 CAV 后续发展的标志[53]。IFN-γ 在其中发挥关键作用,能够激活巨噬细胞,促进炎症细胞募集,并增强免疫应答[54]。即便是在急性排斥反应过程中,若缺少 IFN-γ,则可阻止 CAV 的发展[55]。

整合素与趋化因子

有证据表明,整合素和趋化因子也在移植器官血管病变中发挥作用。研究显示,玻璃黏附蛋白受体(整合素 α-V、β-3)的持续表达与 IVUS 检出的 CAV 进展相关[56]。移植术中的心肌缺血性损伤与 α-V、β-3、组织因子的上调,以及基质金属蛋白酶系统的激活有关[57]。有趣的是,供体的死亡原因也可影响整合素的调节。供体颅内出血死亡与移植术后 CAV 的发生相关[58],且这与 α-V、β-3 的全身激活有关[59]。巨细胞病毒(CMV)感染与移植心脏血管病变密切相关,可能与内皮细胞增殖与迁移引起的血管源性反应有关。CMV 诱导的血管源性反应可能是由于病毒与整合素 β1、β3 及表皮生长因子受体相结合,并参与其信号转导,由此激活磷脂酰肌醇 3-激酶和丝裂素活化蛋白激酶信号通路[60]。

除了易化内皮细胞相互作用,淋巴细胞整合素还可在抗原提呈过程中发挥共刺激的作用。在实验模型中,阻断 ICAM-1 和白细胞功能相关性抗原-1(LFA-1)之间的相互作用能够诱导移植器官的免疫耐受[61],并

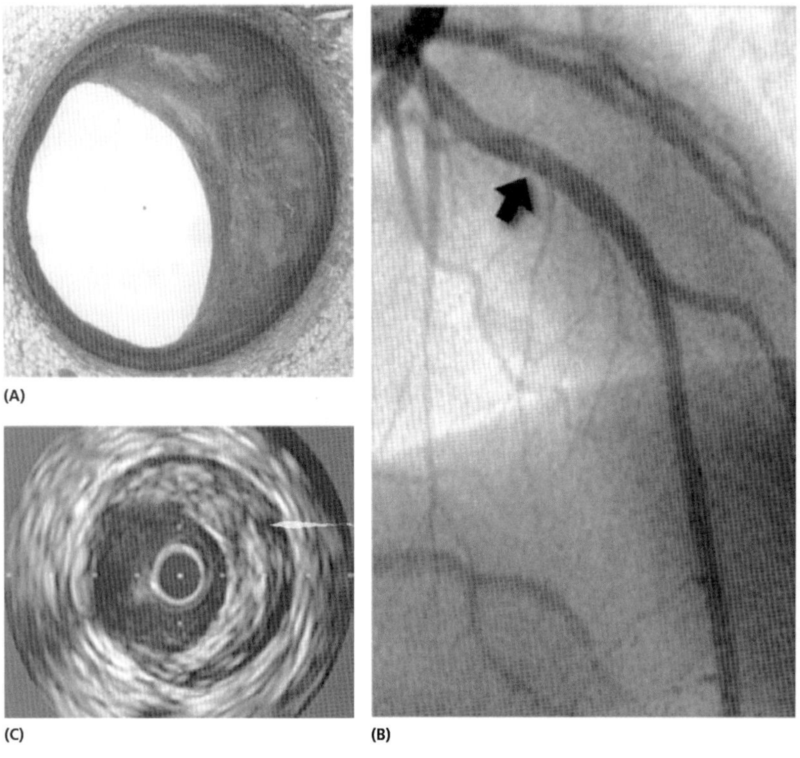

图 79.2 组织学检测可见 CAV 向心性或偏心性内膜下增殖(A),而其病变严重程度在血管造影中被低估(B),但 IVUS 对其显示较佳(C)。[Reproduced with permission from [219]: Patel JK, Kobashigawa JA. Cardiac allograft vasculopathy. In: Ahsan N, ed. Chronic Allograft Failure: Natural History, Pathogenesis, Diagnosis and Management. Austin: Landes Bioscience, 2008:65 (Figure 3).]

显著减少 CAV 的发生[62]。

RANTES 是一种对 T 淋巴细胞、NK 细胞、单核细胞及嗜酸性粒细胞存在选择性趋化作用的趋化因子，在人类 CAV 中存在表达[63]。在动物模型中，单核细胞的募集与内膜增厚需要 $CD4^{+}$细胞及 RANTES 的持续合成[64]。在人体中，外周血 CCR3 趋化因子 ITAC/CXCL11 水平的升高与重度 CAV 相关[65]。在该项研究中，CCR3 趋化因子的配体 ITAC/CXCL11 位于 CAV 病变区域的内皮表面，而其下浸润的单个核炎症细胞表达 CCR3。在小鼠模型中，阻断趋化因子受体 CCR1 和 CCR5 可抑制 CAV 的发展[66]。在大鼠模型中，有证据表明他汀可通过调控趋化因子及其受体而发挥保护作用[66]。低剂量与高剂量的辛伐他汀都能显著降低 CAV 评分，抑制 T 淋巴细胞和巨噬细胞的募集，降低移植器官内单核细胞趋化蛋白 1 (MCP-1)RANTES 和干扰素诱导蛋白 10(IP-10)的水平，并下调趋化因子受体 CCR2 和 CCR5 的表达。

内膜下平滑肌细胞增殖是 CAV 病变的典型特征。最初，这一病理改变被认为是源于供体本身。但性别错配心脏移植和 Y 染色体原位杂交显示了受体来源的平滑肌细胞，提示宿主来源的干细胞可能在 CAV 的发展中发挥重要作用[68,69]。

凝血功能紊乱

弥散性是 CAV 的标志性表现之一，不仅影响动脉系统，还累及毛细血管网和静脉系统[70]，表明这确实是一种泛血管性疾病。在正常情况下，心脏微血管系统处于高度抗血栓状态。然而，在心脏移植后的 1 个月内，心内膜心肌活检显示微血管存在纤维蛋白沉积，这与后续 CAV 的发生密切相关[71]。微血管血栓形成也可引起心肌缺血，造成急性心肌细胞损伤。肌钙蛋白作为心肌损伤的敏感指标，在存在微血管纤维蛋白沉积的心脏移植患者的心内膜心肌活检中明显升高[72]。此外，移植术后 1 年内，若患者存在肌钙蛋白持续性升高，则其移植发生心脏衰竭或重度 CAV 的可能性大大增加。心脏移植术后 1 个月内，肌钙蛋白升高，可能是由于移植术中的缺血再灌注损伤。然而，一些患者在移植术后数月仍有肌钙蛋白的持续性升高，这可能与移植器官排斥反应等更持久的促血栓形成的损伤所引起的进行性微血管血栓形成有关。时间依赖性因素可能参与微血管损伤，缺血再灌注损伤在移植术后早期发挥重要作用，而抗体或细胞因子依赖性内皮细胞活化在之后的过程中更为关键。一些早期变化，如在缺血再灌注损伤过程中，体液免疫应答达到顶峰，波形蛋白等内皮细胞抗原释放，可能会进一步扩大慢性损伤。

血管血栓形成的风险取决于促凝血因子和内源性纤溶活性之间的平衡。纤溶活性降低会抑制促凝血微血管系统中纤维蛋白的清除，并易化凝血酶和纤维蛋白的生成。血浆纤维蛋白原浓度升高和血浆纤溶活性降低都与心脏移植患者动脉内膜增厚有关[47,73]。心脏移植患者心内膜心肌活检显示的组织型纤溶酶原激活物(t-PA)水平越低，血管造影显示的冠状动脉病变发生率越高[47]。这些患者与小动脉血管 t-PA 水平正常的患者相比，发病更早且更重。循环中 t-PA 和纤溶酶原激活物抑制剂-1(PAI-1)的水平同样与 CAV 的发生相关[74]。

CAV 的发生还与移植后凝血系统异常有关。移植后早期微血管抗凝血酶消耗可引起 CAV。抗凝血酶表达恢复的移植心脏不易发生 CAV[75]。引起抗凝血酶表达改变的机制尚未明确，可能包括排斥反应后的细胞因子释放，或是与抗凝血酶相结合的分子的表达或有效性改变，如硫酸乙酰肝素蛋白多糖分子[76]。缺血和再灌注可导致受募集的中性粒细胞释放特定酶类，包括中性粒细胞弹性蛋白酶和乙酰肝素酶。缺乏硫酸乙酰肝素所导致的抗凝血酶结合减少可促进凝血酶的产生，进一步引起硫酸乙酰肝素蛋白多糖的丢失，从而形成微血管系统内持续性促凝环境。

非免疫因素在 CAV 的发展中的影响

尽管同种异体免疫反应是决定移植器官短期和长期转归的主导因素，一些非免疫因素同样参与 CAV 的发生。从时间上而言，免疫反应在 CAV 早期发挥重要作用，而非免疫因素则决定了移植后晚期 CAV 的严重程度[77]。

供体相关性因素

尸体来源的器官往往存在严重的生理紊乱。极其严重的中枢神经系统损伤常伴有血压不稳定，且常需正性肌力药物的持续支持(参见第 20 章)。循环中的神经内分泌激素水平可能升高，而一些其他激素的水平则会降低[78]。细胞因子和黏附分子等炎症标志物可有上调，引起凋亡和心功能不全[79]。器官在其获取和转运过程中可发生缺血性损伤，而在其植入和再灌注过程中可进一步受到干扰。自发性或非创伤性颅内出血占脑死亡供体的40%，其短期转归较差，多在移植后5年内发生CAV[80]。

缺血再灌注时内皮损伤所引起的改变对随后数年内CAV的发生非常关键[81]。早期的表现包括内皮脱落和回缩，引起内皮通透性增加。缺氧能诱导一系列内皮细胞基因的表达，包括VEGF、碱性成纤维细胞生长因子(b-FGF)和血小板源性生长因子(PDGF)[82-84]。PDGF和b-FGF能诱导内膜平滑肌细胞增殖迁移，而VEGF能刺激内皮细胞增殖，提高血管通透性[85]。血管紧张素Ⅱ作为潜在的有丝分裂原，经实验证实能够促进平滑肌细胞增殖，且抑制其功能可有效阻止CAV的发展[86,87]。实验表明，血管受损时，血管紧张素转化酶(ACE)表达升高，而对其进行抑制能够减轻CAV。因此，ACE抑制剂可能存在潜在的保护作用[86]。

一项长期随访的多机构研究分析表明[88]，致命性CAV的危险因素包括供体年龄较大、男性供体、受体年龄较小、移植较早、缺血性病因、受体有吸烟史、痛风性关节炎史、黑色人种受体，以及供体CMV血清学阳性。此前的另一项研究表明[89]，早发性CAV与自体动脉粥样硬化具有许多共同的危险因素，包括供体年龄较大、男性供体、高血压病供体、男性受体，以及黑色人种受体。移植术后重度冠心病的5年发病率为9%，且死亡率非常高。一项关于心脏移植受体心血管疾病危险因素的多中心回顾性分析研究发现，高脂血症和糖尿病与非致命性主要不良心脏结局有关，而高肌酐和BMI则与移植物失功有关[90]。有趣的是，在该研究中没有发现对CAV有意义的协变量。研究表明，供体传播性冠心病可增加CAV进展的风险[91,92]，且患有自体冠心病的患者发生心肌梗死、心力衰竭、猝死等心脏事件的风险可升高3~5倍[93,94]。然而，其他研究表明，CAV是一种多因素疾病，供体心脏中的粥样斑块并不一定会进展为CAV[95]。Li等人[96]利用IVUS检测技术发现，事先存在的供体粥样硬化病变并不会加速原动脉粥样硬化灶或同一血管其他部位CAV的发生。

高脂血症

缺血性心肌病是终末期心脏疾病的常见病因，约占心脏移植病因的一半。这些患者中大多数有高脂血症病史，且在移植术后普遍存在高脂血症[97]。移植术后高脂血症与一些因素有关。类固醇能够增加载脂蛋白B的合成，也可导致移植术后肥胖症的发生。环孢素可提高肝酯酶活性，降低脂蛋白酯酶活性[98]，导致极低密度脂蛋白(VLDL)和低密度脂蛋白(LDL)的清除功能受损。他克莫司的使用可引起极轻的血脂异常[99,100]。

高脂血症是非移植心脏动脉粥样硬化的明确危险因素。临床和实验研究的结果都表明高脂血症是引起CAV的重要因素[101-103]。在一项研究中，移植术后6个月脂质水平升高对术后3年CAV的发生具有重要的预测意义[102]。另一项研究则表明移植术后1年LDL水平升高是IVUS检测到CAV发生或进展的唯一预测因素[104]。早期的实验研究发现，兔心脏移植术后高脂饮食可加速CAV发展。高脂血症可增强移植术后的内皮活化效应[105]。在动物模型中，与自体血管相比，当暴露于相同的高血脂水平，移植器官血管系统会出现更显著的内膜增厚、内膜血管形成及T细胞聚集[106,107]。然而，尽管免疫抑制对血脂存在影响，但其对CAV的净效应可能依赖于其对同种异体免疫应答和对平滑肌增殖的抑制作用。因此，尽管可引起血脂升高，但免疫抑制剂作为增殖信号抑制剂，能够减少CAV的发生[108]。

有趣的是，有一类药物对移植心脏特别有益，不但能有效降低血脂，还能减少同种异体免疫反应。在移植术后两周内开始使用羟甲基戊二酰辅酶A (HMG Co-A)还原酶抑制剂(他汀类)不但能够减少冠状动脉内膜增厚的发生，还能减少有血流动力学改变的排斥反应发作，从而改善生存率[109]。这类药物具有免疫抑制的作用，这在心脏移植术后的重要性不亚于降脂作用。他汀类具有多重功效。研究显示，他汀类能减少患者细胞因子的合成，改善冠状动脉内皮功能[110]，抑制IFN-γ诱导的Ⅱ型MHC在血管内皮细胞中的表达[111]，减少NK细胞的细胞毒性[109,112]，通过抑制单核细胞组织因子降低移植术后高凝状态[113]，并调节趋化因子和趋化因子受体的功能(见前文)。

高血压

高血压是非移植冠状动脉粥样硬化的明确危险因素。心脏移植术后常出现高血压，其原因包括糖皮质激素的使用、体重增加以及钙调磷酸酶抑制剂的影响。移植术后1年高血压的发病率为74%，而至术后10年则升高至98%[114]。少数研究发现，移植术后高血压与CAV存在联系[115]，但目前大多数研究尚未证实两者的相关性[89,90,116]。

然而，有资料显示，抗高血压药物具有减少 CAV 发生的作用。在一项研究中[117]，随机选取患者应用地尔硫䓬治疗，分别通过定量冠状动脉造影（QCA）测量 1 年和 5 年时冠状动脉管径，结果发现治疗组与基线相比管径显著减小。移植术后 5 年，地尔硫䓬治疗组与对照组相比，在死亡和 CAV 方面也有显著性差异。在大鼠异位移植模型中，氨氯地平能够显著降低移植器官血管病变的发生率[118]。体外实验显示，钙离子通道阻滞剂能够稳定内皮细胞功能，抑制血小板聚集，并减少血小板源性生长因子的释放[119]。

一项研究表明，使用钙离子通道阻滞剂或 ACE 抑制剂 1 年后，通过 IVUS 检测发现冠状动脉内膜增厚明显减少[120]；单用钙离子通道阻滞剂或与 ACE 抑制剂合用时都具有这一效应。钙离子通道阻滞剂或 ACE 抑制剂治疗存在此类效应。另一项研究表明，根据移植术后 1 年 IVUS 检测结果显示，钙离子通道阻滞剂和 ACE 抑制剂对减少移植器官血管病变的发生率具有协同作用[121]。

心脏移植实验模型发现，血管紧张素受体阻滞剂氯沙坦在预防移植器官血管病变方面的效果优于依那普利[122]。血管紧张素受体组织减轻平滑肌细胞新生内膜增殖的作用可能是通过减少外周单个核细胞向平滑肌细胞表型的分化[123]，或与抑制过氧化物酶体增生物激活受体 γ（PPAR-γ）相关[124]。

糖尿病

超过 30%的成年心脏移植受体在移植术后 1 年出现糖尿病[114]。引起移植术后新发糖尿病的主导因素包括移植前 BMI 增加[125]和免疫抑制治疗，尤其是糖皮质激素和钙调磷酸酶抑制剂的应用[126]。在一项回顾性研究中，移植前葡萄糖不耐受、糖尿病家族史、移植术后胰岛素使用超过 24 小时等因素都与移植术后糖尿病相关[127]。糖皮质激素是移植术后新发糖尿病的最高危因素。大剂量应用泼尼松是心脏移植术后新发糖尿病的危险因素之一[127]。他克莫司比环孢素更易引起糖尿病[126,128]。然而，一项研究通过检测糖化血红蛋白 A1c 监测血糖控制情况发现，血糖控制对 CAV 严重程度的影响比致糖尿病性免疫抑制剂的累积剂量更为重要[129]。一项研究对 20 000 例来自器官共享联合网（UNOS）数据库的心脏移植受体展开分析，结果同样显示糖尿病可增加 CAV 的风险[130]。

大多数心脏移植受体存在严重的胰岛素抵抗，具有代偿性高胰岛素血症的多种表现，包括动脉粥样硬化和促炎效应[131,132]。即便采用他汀类治疗，胰岛素抵抗和促炎状态仍可引起 CAV[133]。免疫抑制剂的使用以及移植术后肥胖等因素是引起胰岛素抵抗综合征的主要原因，与 CAV 的发生相关[134]。

巨细胞病毒

人巨细胞病毒在全球广泛分布（参见第 94 章）。随着年龄增长，CMV 暴露相应增加，至 60 岁时，大多数人群都存在既往暴露的证据。所幸的是，对绝大多数免疫系统健全的人而言，CMV 感染一般只引起轻微的亚临床疾病，几乎不构成威胁。然而，对于免疫缺陷的患者，如 AIDS 患者、肿瘤化疗患者和器官移植受体等，CMV 感染可以是致命的，可引起全身病毒血症、肝炎、肺炎、肾炎、结肠炎及其他临床表现。CMV 感染与心脏移植受体 CAV 的发生有关。一些临床研究表明，CMV 感染与 CAV 的发生存在相关性[135-139]。25%~50%的心脏移植受体存在 CMV 感染。抗淋巴细胞诱导治疗和急性排斥反应发作可增加 CMV 感染[1]。此前有研究显示，未感染 CMV 的心脏移植受体的 5 年生存率为 70%，而这一数据在 CMV 感染者中仅为 30%[136]。

CMV 感染引起 CAV 的机制尚不明确。心内膜心肌活检表明，与未感染 CMV 的患者相比，感染 CMV 的心脏移植受体行血管造影显示的冠心病更严重，且内膜增厚、血管平滑肌细胞增殖、血管周围炎性反应等均更明显。移植术后 CMV 感染通过特定通路引起内皮一氧化氮合成功能受损，从而导致慢性内皮功能不全[143]。

在大鼠主动脉移植模型的动物研究中，移植术中 CMV 感染可引起新生内膜增殖[144]。内皮细胞感染可通过合成白介素-1β 的旁分泌作用介导感染和非感染细胞的黏附分子上调[145]。共培养实验显示，T 细胞的 CMV 感染可通过旁分泌作用诱导 IFN-γ 和 TNF-α 的合成，继而诱导Ⅰ型和Ⅱ型抗原、VCAM-1 和 ICAM-1 的表达。CMV 感染还可通过抑制平滑肌细胞凋亡引起新生内膜增殖[146]。

临床评估

由于心脏去神经支配，CAV 可能直至极晚期才出现症状，且已错过治疗干预的时机。因此，多数项目通过一定的监测手段对CAV进行监测。尽管按照传统常采用冠状动脉造影或IVUS等有创手段,然而近年来一些无创检查方式逐渐被接受。典型的无创检查手段包括心脏负荷试验,但由于依赖于血流动力学的严重受损,其应用受到一定限制。多巴酚丁胺负荷超声心动图(DSE)在检测CAV方面的敏感性和特异性不稳定,对心脏不良事件有较好的预测性。该方法可能会受到一些与CAV无关的异常改变的限制,如移植心脏静息室壁运动异常和多普勒组织成像等特定参数异常[149,150]。然而,定量技术和心肌声学造影[151,152]的应用使DSE对CAV的检测能力得到了很大改进,甚至是检测血管造影无法检出的病变[153]。

心肌灌注显像(MPI)具有同时检测心外膜大血管和微脉管系统灌注情况的优点。MPI能够可靠地分辨出CAV病例中可能发生心脏事件的高危患者,且其阴性预测值很高[154-156]。心肌血流及血液储备的定量检测和正电子发射断层扫描(PET)在确定微血管性移植器官血管病变作为疾病早期标志以及检测疾病进展方面具有重要作用[157]。

超快速计算机断层扫描(CT)被用于冠状动脉钙化的检测,也可用于CAV的检测[158],但无法提供关于管腔或管壁的详细信息。CT血管成像(CTA)逐渐成为冠心病无创评估的有效手段。64排、双源、ECG门控技术使CTA能够在辐射量较低的条件下对冠状动脉管腔和管腔外细节进行检测。CTA对CAV的检测准确度与IVUS相当[159],且能详细评估斑块的成分[160]。或许能将系列CTA作为许多患者替代的传统有创性冠状动脉造影随访方式[161]。

磁共振成像(MRI)在心脏结构和功能的评估方面很有前景。MRI可评估心脏移植的急性移植器官排斥反应,并能对已经过活检证实的排斥反应进行进一步的无创心功能、早期对比剂增强及心肌水肿的评估[162]。检测磷酸肌酐/三磷酸腺苷比值的 ^{31}P 磁共振化学位移成像能够预测血管成像显示的CAV[163]。MRI的心肌应变与灌注储备定量分析也与CAV[164]相关,或许可用于微血管疾病的评估。

有创检查是评估CAV的传统标志。冠状动脉造影需要辨别血管的正常节段与病变节段。然而,由于缺乏正常管径作为参照,CAV的全血管情况常被低估。血管造影显示的管腔轻微异常往往提示既往病史,这一点已在前文中有所介绍。与既往检查结果进行对照有助于判断疾病的进展,但需要在每次检查时使用具有可比性的造影图像并放大倍率以供精确评估对比。此外,还能通过计算机辅助QCA增加CAV检测的敏感性。然而,QCA无法评估血管壁,对于血管代偿性扩张以维持管腔的早期病变可能漏诊。有趣的是,冠状动脉造影能够对微血管病变进行一定的评估。造影频繁显示血管远端参差不齐提示弥漫性小血管受累。冠状动脉侧支伴心肌灌注与微血管疾病相关[165]。根据心肌梗死溶栓(TIMI)的心肌灌注分级,移植患者通常存在微循环异常,而其严重程度与心外膜病变及生存率相对应[166]。近期的心肌灌注造影定量评估显示对移植受体的生存率具有预测意义,且有助于识别灌注储备受损但不伴动脉粥样硬化的造影证据的早期CAV患者[167]。

冠状动脉造影是评估冠心病的金标准,但由于内膜下细胞增殖往往使病灶呈向心性,故传统的冠状动脉造影常会低估病变的范围。而IVUS能够对血管壁直接显影,从而确定内膜和中膜病变的范围(图79.2)。通过面积测量法定量评估内膜和中膜的面积,甚至能够发现血管造影无法检测的早期斑块负荷。通过自动导管撤回能够获得血管壁病变范围的序列图像[168-170]。多项研究肯定了IVUS在检测CAV方面具有比血管造影更高的敏感性。系列IVUS评估具有强大的统计功能,可检测到细微的病变,并确定粥瘤体积变化的百分比。因此,该项技术被常规应用于评估新兴CAV治疗方法的疗效。IVUS提示在移植术后1年内,内膜增厚的速度最快,此后进展逐渐减缓但难以阻止[171]。IVUS检测到的内膜进行性增厚对血管造影明显的CAV具有预测意义。若存在快速进展的CAV,即移植术后1年内最大内膜厚度增加≥0.5mm,则患者有发生各种原因的死亡、心肌梗死和血管造影显示的重度CAV的风险明显增加[171,172]。因此,IVUS越来越多地被应用于移植术后的评估,在术后1个月和12个月时行IVUS检查能够识别心血管事件的高危人群,且有助于免疫抑制治疗方案的调整。最近,IVUS技术得到了进一步发展,能够利用波普频率分析对斑块成分进行评估[173,174]。该技术又称为虚拟组织学,在该领域内极具前景,不但能够定量分析斑块负荷,还能确定斑块成分的变化或对疾病预后具有指导意义[173,175]。

尽管得到了上述具有前景的发展,IVUS技术也存在一些局限性:高度有创性、需要抗凝、需使用昂贵的一次性导管，以及对病变的评估主要局限于心外膜大血管。此外，由于心脏移植受体存在持续性内皮功能不全，导管引起的冠状动脉痉挛也受到了特别的关注。

利用冠状动脉内多普勒血流测量检测冠状动脉血流储备对 CAV 的评估具有一定作用，尽管这一指标的临床意义尚不明确，且 PET 心肌灌注成像或心脏超声等无创性检查也可提供类似的信息。利用安装在导丝上的多普勒传感器能够测定冠状动脉内的血流速度。利用腺苷或双嘧达莫等药物干预能够测量最大冠状动脉血流，并计算血流储备。在 CAV 患者中，冠状动脉血流储备降低，且随移植术后的时间推移而进一步恶化[178]。冠状动脉血流储备测量可反映微脉管系统和心外膜血管的变化，且与 IVUS 检出的斑块负担具有相关性。

不幸的是，CAV 的定义具有多样性，目前尚无统一的国际标准能将这一范畴命名。然而，国际心肺移植协会对血管造影、IVUS、微血管功能、移植心脏组织学、循环免疫标志物、无创性影像学检查以及基于基因和蛋白质的生物标志物等相关资料进行严格分析，得到高级别证据与临床共识，并在此基础上发表了一份共识文件[179]。该文件为 CAV 国际化命名的工作指南，与移植心脏排斥反应的组织学判定系统的制订相似(表 79.2)。

表 79.2 移植心脏血管病变的推荐命名法

ISHLT CAV0(不明显)：血管造影未显示病变

ISHLT CAV1(轻度)：血管造影显示左主干(LM)<50%，或主干血管最大病变<70%，或任一分支狭窄<70%(包括弥漫性狭窄)，不伴移植心脏功能障碍

ISHLT CAV2(中度)：血管造影显示左主干(LM)<50%；单一的主干血管狭窄≥70%，或两条系统的独立分支狭窄≥70%，不伴移植心脏功能障碍

ISHLT CAV3(重度)：血管造影显示左主干(LM)≥50%，或两条及以上主干血管狭窄≥70%，或三条系统的独立分支狭窄≥70%；或 ISHLT CAV1 或 CAV2 伴移植心脏功能障碍(定义为 LVEF≤45%，通常伴有局部心壁运动异常)或具有显著限制性生理学的证据(常见但非特异性；详见定义)

定义

(a)主干血管是指左前降支的近端及中 33%部、左旋支、下颌支，以及右优势型或均衡型中的右冠状动脉后降支和后外侧支

(b) 二级分支血管包括主干血管远端 33%或间隔穿通血管的任何节段、对角支和钝缘支，或左优势型中右冠状动脉的任何部分

(c)移植心脏生理受限定义为有症状的心力衰竭，伴心脏超声 E 到 A 速度比>2(儿童为>1.5)，等容舒张时间缩短(<60ms)，减速时间缩短(<150ms)，或限制性血流动力学表现[右房压力>12mmHg，肺毛细血管楔压>25mmHg，心脏指数<2L/(min/m^2)]

ISHLT，国际心肺移植协会。

药物治疗

免疫抑制剂对 CAV 的疗效很复杂（详见第 98 章至第 102 章）。长期类固醇治疗脂质代谢的间接影响已被阐明。环孢素会进一步增强这一影响，而环孢素的替代物他克莫司似乎能够减轻血脂的升高[100]。CAV 的发生与急性排斥反应的发作次数和严重程度有关[50,77]，即便是无症状的抗体介导性排斥反应也是移植器官血管病变的危险因素[180]。因此，更有效的免疫抑制剂可能对防治移植器官血管病变有益。

他克莫司在预防肝移植后慢性排斥反应方面优于环孢素[181]，但心脏移植患者的资料十分有限。尽管与环孢素相比，他克莫司改善血压血脂的疗效更佳[100]，但接受他克莫司治疗的患者的糖尿病患病率增加。一项为期 5 年的随机试验对他克莫司和微乳化环孢素进行了对比，结果显示，两者对 CAV 的疗效相当[182]。

MMF 是一种嘌呤生物合成新通路的抑制剂，能够更加有效地减少移植心脏排斥反应和移植术后死亡率[183]。MMF 还能更有效地减少移植器官血管病变的发生[184]。其作用可能与降低 B 细胞应答有关，因为接受 MMF 治疗的患者抗波形蛋白抗体滴度较低，而与之相应的是 IVUS 测得的 CAV 发生率较低。IVUS 显示，与硫唑嘌呤相比，MMF 能够减少内膜增厚[185]，尽管应用 MMF 可增加 CMV 的感染率，而后者则是 CAV 的危险因素之一[186]。

增殖信号抑制剂(PSI)西罗莫司和依维莫司的应用是 CAV 治疗的一大进展。其是一种抗增殖药物，能够在体外和血管损伤实验动物模型中抑制平滑肌细胞增殖，后者是 CAV 发生的重要因素之一。上述药物在临床上具有减少自体冠心病支架内再狭窄的作用[187,188]。一项随机临床试验纳入了 136 例患者[189]，在近期心脏移植患者中使用西罗莫司，其移植术后 2 年的 CAV 发生率低于使用硫唑嘌呤的患者。在随后的定点多中心研究中[190]，超过 600 例患者被随机分组，分别在心脏移植术后 72 小时内接受依维莫司或硫唑嘌呤治疗。IVUS 显示，12 个月时依维莫司治疗组患者的平均最大内膜增厚程度显著低于硫唑嘌呤治疗组。由于移植术后 1 年最大内膜增厚程度与移植术后 5 年死亡率相关，故上述结果

具有重要意义[172]。

治疗

临床表现明显的病变往往预后较差,因此对移植器官血管病变的预防非常重要。除了应用抗增殖性免疫抑制剂,还可通过防治自体冠心病治疗CAV。阿司匹林因其在非移植性冠心病中的广泛应用而同样广泛应用于CAV的防治,它可能在预防CAV持续性内皮功能不全和促凝环境引起的血栓形成中发挥重要作用。血压和血脂的控制也已被讨论。使用他汀类药物尤其重要,因为有助于预防免疫排斥反应。与自体动脉粥样硬化相比,补充维生素C和E可能减少CAV的发生[191]。

一旦病变出现明显的临床表现,可通过一系列方法缓解缺血。尽管冠状动脉再狭窄在心脏移植患者中较常见,尤其是使用切割球囊技术的病例[193],但经皮冠状动脉干预(PCI)及气囊血管成形术仍能够有效治疗局灶性病变[192]。支架植入有助于解决上述问题,尤其是药物涂层支架的应用能够显著降低再狭窄发生率[194,195]。目前尚无研究表明PCI能够改变CAV的预后,且由于许多具有明显病变的患者并无临床症状,因此是否进行干预常成为一个难以抉择的问题。此外,PCI术后出现支架内再狭窄的患者可在未干预的血管内出现进展性病变,且具有更高的心肌梗死或死亡风险[196],提示免疫应答的增强作为一种全血管性现象可加速CAV的进展[197]。

存在多血管局灶性病变且具备合适的远端目标血管的患者可考虑接受冠状动脉旁路手术(CABG)。由于目前报道的相关病例很少,很难确定该手术的有效性,这也反映了许多患者并不具备合适的目标血管或更倾向于接受PCI。对于具备合适的目标血管的CAV患者,血运重建术是一个安全有效的选择[198,199]。

对于许多PCI或CABG无法挽救的进展性CAV患者,再移植或许是唯一的选择。据多项研究报道,再移植后的生存率普遍低于初次移植。其中一项研究表明,再移植与初次移植的1年生存率相近[200]。该研究还发现,接受二次移植并不会增加发生CAV的风险。最近的数据显示,由于CAV或慢性移植心脏衰竭而接受再移植的患者的长期结局较为可观,其中位生存期超过10年[201]。

浸润性心肌病的心脏移植及复发风险

许多浸润性病变可导致终末期心脏病,需要实施心脏移植。上述疾病包括心脏结节病、心肌炎(巨细胞性、淋巴细胞性、嗜酸性粒细胞性或病毒性)、自身免疫性疾病如狼疮和淀粉样变。其诊断常常仅基于移植心脏的组织学检查。多数情况下,除部分心内膜心肌活检显示的复发病例报道外,移植术后患者的转归与因其他病因而接受心脏移植的患者相当[202]。

心脏结节病

一些病例报道心脏移植术后多年移植心脏复发性心脏结节病的病例[203-207]。有一篇报道了4例因心脏结节病而接受心脏移植的病例,移植术后均未出现复发[208]。仅有的少量资料表明,肺移植术后肺结节病的复发率高达50%,而心脏移植术后复发心脏结节病的风险则显著低于这一数据。心脏移植术后的疾病复发可通过免疫抑制疗法加以治疗,尤其是应用糖皮质激素。

巨细胞病毒性心肌炎

巨细胞病毒性心肌炎能引起不可逆的暴发性左室功能不全伴传导功能异常及充血性心力衰竭。其对免疫抑制治疗的反应性较差[209],心脏移植是唯一的治疗选择。巨细胞病毒性心肌炎的组织学特征包括多形性免疫反应,表现为呈地图样的大量多核巨细胞聚集和心肌细胞坏死。根据巨细胞病毒性心肌炎注册项目登记,在38例因巨细胞病毒性心肌炎接受心脏移植的患者中,有9例的移植心脏出现复发。考虑到其高复发率,有专家学者认为,移植心脏巨细胞病毒性心肌炎的复发或许是心脏移植的禁忌证。在克利夫兰诊所的5例病例中[210],有1例患者在移植术后早期即出现疾病复发,且合并细胞性排斥反应发作,经相应治疗后好转。尽管巨细胞病毒性心肌炎的复发率很高,但不接受心脏移植的患者死亡率更高,因此心脏移植仍然被认为是合理的治疗方案。有趣的是,虽然该疾病本身对免疫抑制治疗的反应性不佳,移植术后的复发更易用免疫抑制疗法控制。这可能是因为移植心脏的疾病往往比在自体心脏中发现得早,也可能与移植心脏中的免疫抑制环境有关。疾病对治疗的良好反应性提示巨细胞病毒性心肌炎的复发不应成为心脏移植的障碍。

查加斯病

查加斯病是拉美疫区心脏病的重要原因之一，由克氏锥虫感染引起。如今，由于移民因素，这一疾病也开始出现于非疫区，且逐渐成为美国终末期心脏病的重要病因之一。虽然克氏锥虫很少发生本地传播，在美国，浣熊依然是克氏锥虫的主要宿主[211]。捐赠器官中的传染性病原体也成为值得关注的问题，要求对潜在感染的供体进行充分筛查。血清学检查的可靠性有限，而准确的诊断取决于组织样本、组织学或聚合酶链反应(PCR)，因此供体病原体的筛查相当复杂。查加斯病的典型心脏表现包括扩张性心肌病、充血性心力衰竭、心律失常、心源性栓塞及脑卒中。

在巴西，查加斯病作为心脏移植的第三大指征，占所有移植病例的 15%~20%[212]。其复发率约为 40%[212,213]，但近来也有证据表明，通过最小剂量的免疫移植治疗、密切监测及恰当的治疗，复发率明显降低[212]。一项研究对 1985—2010 年间巴西圣保罗[212]的 107 例因查加斯病行心脏移植的病例进行了分析，结果显示，住院死亡率为 17.7%(n=19)，死因包括感染(n=6;31.5%)、移植心脏功能不全(n=6;31.5%)、排斥反应(n=4;21.1%)、心搏骤停(n=2;10.5%)及 ABO 血型不相容(n=1;5.3%)。有 27 例(25.2%)患者出现晚期死亡。其主要死因包括排斥反应 (n=6;22.2%)、感染 (n=6;22.2%)、淋巴瘤 (n=4;14.8%)、肉瘤(n=2;7.4%)、心包炎(n=2;7.4%)及中枢神经系统查加斯病再活化(n=1;7.1%)。由于大剂量免疫抑制治疗，在疾病早期更易发生恶性肿瘤[214]。而随着免疫移植治疗剂量的降低，尤其是类固醇停药[212]，以及 MMF 的停药或减量[215,216]，患者生存率有所改善，且疾病再活化率降低。有排斥反应或恶性肿瘤病史的患者更易出现再活化。目前监测疾病再活化的方法主要为血样 PCR 检测[217]，该技术也可用于疗效监测。寄生虫血症、心肌炎及查加斯病再活化须以 5mg/(kg·d)剂量持续应用苄硝唑治疗 60 天。硝呋替莫也可用于治疗疾病再活化，有报道称还可使用大剂量别嘌呤醇[214,218]。

总结

CAV 是心脏移植的重要并发症，大大限制了移植心脏的长期存活率。该病与自体非移植冠状动脉粥样硬化有许多相似之处，同时也存在其独特的病理学改变和病变分布特征。CAV 的发生与许多因素有关，包括传统动脉粥样硬化的危险因素、移植术中缺血再灌注损伤、宿主同种异体免疫反应、凝血因子以及移植术后药物治疗的影响。由于手术去神经化，CAV 的临床表现往往不典型。以往主要通过有创技术对疾病进行诊断和监测，而近期出现的无创技术也许能在将来减少常规有创检查的使用。CAV 的预后较差，因而对其进行预防十分重要。对 CAV 病理学的深入研究带动了许多有应用前景的免疫抑制药物的研发，如 PSI。抗体介导性排斥反应在 CAV 的发展中发挥作用，关于这一现象的深入认识有利于研发以抑制体液免疫为靶点的治疗手段。同时，对于已有症状的患者，可以通过传统的血管再通技术进行姑息治疗，而对于一些特定的患者也可考虑再移植。

对于少数因浸润性病变行心脏移植的患者，其复发查加斯病和巨细胞病毒性心肌炎的风险最高。对疾病复发的密切监测和适当的治疗有助于改善其结局。

(赵海格 倪一鸣 郑骏楠 译 倪一鸣 校)

参考文献

1. Gao SZ, Schroeder JS, Alderman EL, et al. Prevalence of accelerated coronary artery disease in heart transplant survivors: comparison of cyclosporine and azathioprine regimens. Circulation. 1989;80:III100–III105.
2. Stehlik J, Edwards LB, Kucheryavaya AY, et al. The registry of the international society for heart and lung transplantation: twenty-eighth adult heart transplant report, 2011. Journal of Heart and Lung Transplantation. 2011;30:1078–1094.
3. Ross R, Glomset J, Harker L. Response to injury and atherogenesis. American Journal of Pathology. 1977;86:675–684.
4. Arbustini E, Roberts WC. Morphological observations in the epicardial coronary arteries and their surroundings late after cardiac transplantation (allograft vascular disease). American Journal of Cardiology. 1996;78:814–820.
5. Rickenbacher PR, Pinto FJ, Chenzbraun A, et al. Incidence and severity of transplant coronary artery disease early and up to 15 years after transplantation as detected by intravascular ultrasound. Journal of the American College of Cardiology. 1995;25:171–177.
6. Ludman PF, Lazem F, Barbir M, et al. Incidence and clinical relevance of coronary calcification detected by electron beam computed tomography in heart transplant recipients. European Heart Journal. 1999;20:303–308.
7. Knollmann FD, Bocksch W, Spiegelsberger S, et al. Electron-beam computed tomography in the assessment of coronary artery disease after heart transplantation. Circulation. 2000;101:2078–2082.
8. Nickel T, Bigdeli A, von Ziegler F, et al. Coronary dilatation after heart transplantation. Transplantation. 2011;92:697–702.
9. Kobashigawa J, Wener L, Johnson J, et al. Longitudinal study of vascular remodeling in coronary arteries after heart transplantation. Journal of Heart and Lung Transplantation. 2000;19:546–550.
10. Li H, Tanaka K, Chhabra A, et al. Vascular remodeling 1 year after cardiac transplantation. Journal of Heart and Lung Transplantation. 2007;26:56–62.
11. Li H, Tanaka K, Oeser B, et al. Vascular remodelling after cardiac transplantation: a 3-year serial intravascular ultrasound study. European Heart Journal. 2006;27:1671–1677.
12. Rogers NJ, Lechler RI. Allorecognition. American Journal of Transplantation. 2001;1:97–102.
13. Weis M, von Scheidt W. Coronary artery disease in the transplanted heart. Annual Review of Medicine. 2000;51:81–100.

14. Kaczmarek I, Deutsch MA, Kauke T, et al. Donor-specific HLA alloantibodies: long-term impact on cardiac allograft vasculopathy and mortality after heart transplant. Experimental and Clinical Transplantation. 2008;6:229–235.
15. Subherwal S, Kobashigawa JA, Cogert G, et al. Incidence of acute cellular rejection and non-cellular rejection in cardiac transplantation. Transplantation Proceedings. 2004;36:3171–3172.
16. Han CW, Imamura M, Hashino S, et al. Differential effects of the immunosuppressants cyclosporin A, FK506 and KM2210 on cytokine gene expression. Bone Marrow Transplantation. 1995;15:733–739.
17. Suciu-Foca N, Reed E, Marboe C, et al. The role of anti-HLA antibodies in heart transplantation. Transplantation. 1991;51:716–724.
18. Rose EA, Pepino P, Barr ML, et al. Relation of HLA antibodies and graft atherosclerosis in human cardiac allograft recipients. Journal of Heart and Lung Transplantation. 1992;11:S120–S123.
19. Valantine H. Cardiac allograft vasculopathy after heart transplantation: risk factors and management. Journal of Heart and Lung Transplantation. 2004;23(Suppl):S187–S193.
20. Dunn MJ, Crisp SJ, Rose ML, et al. Anti-endothelial antibodies and coronary artery disease after cardiac transplantation. Lancet. 1992;339:1566–1570.
21. Jurcevic S, Ainsworth ME, Pomerance A, et al. Antivimentin antibodies are an independent predictor of transplant- associated coronary artery disease after cardiac transplantation. Transplantation. 2001;71:886–892.
22. Jurcevic S, Dunn MJ, Crisp S, et al. A new enzyme-linked immunosorbent assay to measure anti-endothelial antibodies after cardiac transplantation demonstrates greater inhibition of antibody formation by tacrolimus compared with cyclosporine. Transplantation. 1998;65:1197–1202.
23. Rose ML, Smith J, Dureau G, et al. Mycophenolate mofetil decreases antibody production after cardiac transplantation. Journal of Heart and Lung Transplantation. 2002;21:282–285.
24. Zwirner NW, Marcos CY, Mirbaha F, et al. Identification of MICA as a new polymorphic alloantigen recognized by antibodies in sera of organ transplant recipients. Human Immunology. 2000;61:917–924.
25. Dragun D, Muller DN, Brasen JH, et al. Angiotensin II type 1-receptor activating antibodies in renal-allograft rejection. New England Journal of Medicine. 2005;352:558–569.
26. Suarez-Alvarez B, Lopez-Vazquez A, Gonzalez MZ, et al. The relationship of anti-MICA antibodies and MICA expression with heart allograft rejection. American Journal of Transplantation. 2007;7:1842–1848.
27. Zhang Y, Stastny P. MICA antigens stimulate T cell proliferation and cell-mediated cytotoxicity. Human Immunology. 2006;67:215–222.
28. Kauke T, Kaczmarek I, Dick A, et al. Anti-MICA antibodies are related to adverse outcome in heart transplant recipients. Journal of Heart and Lung Transplantation. 2009;28:305–311.
29. Chao W. Toll-like receptor signaling: a critical modulator of cell survival and ischemic injury in the heart. American Journal of Physiology, Heart and Circulatory Physiology. 2009;296:H1–H12.
30. Shirali AC, Goldstein DR. Activation of the innate immune system by the endogenous ligand hyaluronan. Current Opinion Organ Transplantation. 2008;13:20–25.
31. Zou N, Ao L, Cleveland JC Jr, et al. Critical role of extracellular heat shock cognate protein 70 in the myocardial inflammatory response and cardiac dysfunction after global ischemia-reperfusion. American Journal of Physiology, Heart and Circulatory Physiology. 2008;294:H2805–H2813.
32. Barker AK, McDaniel DO, Zhou X, et al. Combined analysis of allograft inflammatory factor-1, interleukin-18, and Toll-like receptor expression and association with allograft rejection and coronary vasculopathy. American Surgeon. 2010;76:872–878.
33. Methe H, Zimmer E, Grimm C, et al. Evidence for a role of toll-like receptor 4 in development of chronic allograft rejection after cardiac transplantation. Transplantation. 2004;78:1324–1331.
34. Rose ML. Role of endothelial cells in allograft rejection. Vascular Medicine (London, England). 1997;2:105–114.
35. Valantine HA. Cardiac allograft vasculopathy: central role of endothelial injury leading to transplant "atheroma". Transplantation. 2003;76:891–899.
36. Shirwan H. Chronic allograft rejection: do the Th2 cells preferentially induced by indirect alloantigen recognition play a dominant role? Transplantation. 1999;68:715–726.
37. Daar AS, Fuggle SV, Fabre JW, et al. The detailed distribution of MHC Class II antigens in normal human organs. Transplantation. 1984;38:293–298.
38. Page C, Rose M, Yacoub M, et al. Antigenic heterogeneity of vascular endothelium. American Journal of Pathology. 1992;141:673–683.
39. Rose ML, Page C, Hengstenberg C, et al. Identification of antigen presenting cells in normal and transplanted human heart: importance of endothelial cells. Human Immunology. 1990;28:179–185.
40. Rose ML. Endothelial cells as antigen-presenting cells: role in human transplant rejection. Cellular and Molecular Life Sciences. 1998;54:965–978.
41. McDouall RM, Page CS, Hafizi S, et al. Alloproliferation of purified CD4+ T cells to adult human heart endothelial cells, and study of second-signal requirements. Immunology. 1996;89:220–226.
42. Wong BW, Rahmani M, Luo Z, et al. Vascular endothelial growth factor increases human cardiac microvascular endothelial cell permeability to low-density lipoproteins. Journal of Heart and Lung Transplantation. 2009;28:950–957.
43. Bayliss J, Maguire JA, Bailey M, et al. Increased vascular endothelial growth factor mRNA in endomyocardial biopsies from allografts demonstrating severe acute rejection: a longitudinal study. Transplant Immunology. 2008;18:264–274.
44. Bayliss J, Bailey M, Leet A, et al. Late onset antibody-mediated rejection and endothelial localization of vascular endothelial growth factor are associated with development of cardiac allograft vasculopathy. Transplantation. 2008;86: 991–997.
45. Wong BW, Wong D, Luo H, et al. Vascular endothelial growth factor-D is overexpressed in human cardiac allograft vasculopathy and diabetic atherosclerosis and induces endothelial permeability to low-density lipoproteins in vitro. Journal of Heart and Lung Transplantation. 2011;30:955–962.
46. Salomon RN, Hughes CC, Schoen FJ, et al. Human coronary transplantation-associated arteriosclerosis. Evidence for a chronic immune reaction to activated graft endothelial cells. American Journal of Pathology. 1991;138:791–798.
47. Labarrere CA, Pitts D, Nelson DR, et al. Vascular tissue plasminogen activator and the development of coronary artery disease in heart-transplant recipients. New England Journal of Medicine. 1995;333:1111–1116.
48. Labarrere CA, Nelson DR, Faulk WP. Endothelial activation and development of coronary artery disease in transplanted human hearts. JAMA: Journal of the American Medical Association. 1997;278:1169–1175.
49. Borozdenkova S, Smith J, Marshall S, et al. Identification of ICAM-1 polymorphism that is associated with protection from transplant associated vasculopathy after cardiac transplantation. Human Immunology. 2001;62:247–255.
50. Kobashigawa JA, Miller L, Yeung A, et al. Does acute rejection correlate with the development of transplant coronary artery disease? A multicenter study using intravascular ultrasound. Sandoz/CVIS Investigators. Journal of Heart and Lung Transplantation. 1995;14:S221–S226.
51. Zund G, Uezono S, Stahl GL, et al. Hypoxia enhances induction of endothelial ICAM-1: role for metabolic acidosis and proteasomes. American Journal of Physiology. 1997;273:C1571–C1580.
52. Poston RS Jr, Billingham ME, Pollard J, et al. Effects of increased ICAM-1 on reperfusion injury and chronic graft vascular disease. Annals of Thoracic Surgery. 1997;64:1004–1012.
53. Labarrere CA, Nelson DR, Miller SJ, et al. Value of serum-soluble intercellular adhesion molecule-1 for the noninvasive risk assessment of transplant coronary artery disease, posttransplant ischemic events, and cardiac graft failure. Circulation. 2000;102:1549–1555.
54. Tellides G, Pober JS. Interferon-gamma axis in graft arteriosclerosis. Circulation Research. 2007;100:622–632.
55. Nagano H, Mitchell RN, Taylor MK, et al. Interferon-gamma deficiency prevents coronary arteriosclerosis but not myocardial rejection in transplanted mouse hearts. Journal of Clinical Investigation. 1997;100:550–557.
56. Yamani MH, Masri S, Ratliff NB, et al. The role of vitronectin receptor and tissue factor in the pathogenesis of transplant coronary vasculopathy. Journal of Heart and Lung Transplantation. 2001;20:185.
57. Yamani MH, Tuzcu EM, Starling RC, et al. Myocardial ischemic injury after heart transplantation is associated with upregulation of vitronectin receptor (alpha(v) beta3), activation of the matrix metalloproteinase induction system, and subsequent development of coronary vasculopathy. Circulation. 2002;105:1955–1961.
58. Mehra MR, Uber PA, Ventura HO, et al. The impact of mode of donor brain death on cardiac allograft vasculopathy: an intravascular ultrasound study. Journal of the American College of Cardiology. 2004;43:806–810.
59. Yamani MH, Cook DJ, Tuzcu EM, et al. Systemic activation of integrin alphaV-beta3 in donors with spontaneous intracerebral hemorrhage is associated with subsequent development of vasculopathy in the heart transplant recipient. Journal of Heart and Lung Transplantation. 2005;24:1014–1018.
60. Bentz GL, Yurochko AD. Human CMV infection of endothelial cells induces an angiogenic response through viral binding to EGF receptor and beta1 and beta3 integrins. Proceedings of the National Academy of Sciences of the United States of America. 2008;105:5531–5536.
61. Isobe M, Yagita H, Okumura K, et al. Specific acceptance of cardiac allograft after treatment with antibodies to ICAM-1 and LFA-1. Science. 1992;255:1125–1127.
62. Suzuki J, Isobe M, Yamazaki S, et al. Inhibition of accelerated coronary atherosclerosis with short-term blockade of intercellular adhesion molecule-1 and lymphocyte function-associated antigen-1 in a heterotopic murine model of heart transplantation. Journal of Heart and Lung Transplantation. 1997; 16:1141–1148.
63. Pattison JM, Nelson PJ, Huie P, et al. RANTES chemokine expression in

transplant-associated accelerated atherosclerosis. Journal of Heart and Lung Transplantation. 1996;15:1194–1199.
64. Yun JJ, Fischbein MP, Laks H, et al. Rantes production during development of cardiac allograft vasculopathy. Transplantation. 2001;71:1649–1656.
65. Kao J, Kobashigawa J, Fishbein MC, et al. Elevated serum levels of the CXCR3 chemokine ITAC are associated with the development of transplant coronary artery disease. Circulation. 2003;107:1958–1961.
66. Yun JJ, Whiting D, Fischbein MP, et al. Combined blockade of the chemokine receptors CCR1 and CCR5 attenuates chronic rejection. Circulation. 2004;109: 932–937.
67. Yin R, Zhu J, Shao H, et al. Inhibition of chemokine receptor CCR2 and CCR5 expression contributes to simvastatin-induced attenuation of cardiac allograft vasculopathy. Journal of Heart and Lung Transplantation. 2007;26:485–493.
68. Shimizu K, Mitchell RN. Stem cell origins of intimal cells in graft arterial disease. Current Atherosclerosis Reports. 2003;5:230–237.
69. Hillebrands J, van den Hurk BM, Klatter FA, et al. Recipient origin of neointimal vascular smooth muscle cells in cardiac allografts with transplant arteriosclerosis. Journal of Heart and Lung Transplantation. 2000;19:1183–1192.
70. Oni AA, Ray J, Hosenpud JD. Coronary venous intimal thickening in explanted cardiac allografts. Evidence demonstrating that transplant coronary artery disease is a manifestation of a diffuse allograft vasculopathy. Transplantation. 1992;53:1247–1251.
71. Labarrere CA, Nelson DR, Faulk WP. Myocardial fibrin deposits in the first month after transplantation predict subsequent coronary artery disease and graft failure in cardiac allograft recipients. American Journal of Medicine. 1998;105: 207–213.
72. Labarrere CA, Nelson DR, Cox CJ, et al. Cardiac-specific troponin I levels and risk of coronary artery disease and graft failure following heart transplantation. JAMA: Journal of the American Medical Association. 2000;284: 457–464.
73. Meckel CR, Anderson TJ, Mudge GH, et al. Hemostatic/fibrinolytic predictors of allograft coronary artery disease after cardiac transplantation. Vascular Medicine (London, England). 1997;2:306–312.
74. Warshofsky MK, Wasserman HS, Wang W, et al. Plasma levels of tissue plasminogen activator and plasminogen activator inhibitor-1 are correlated with the presence of transplant coronary artery disease in cardiac transplant recipients. American Journal of Cardiology. 1997;80:145–149.
75. Labarrere CA. Early risk factors for transplant coronary artery disease and cardiac allograft failure. Italian Heart Journal. 2001;2(Suppl 3):26S–8S.
76. Labarrere CA, Abellada GC. Vascular anticoagulation and transplant coronary artery disease. Zeitschrift fur Kardiologie. 2000;89(Suppl 9):IX/32–IX/35.
77. Hornick P, Smith J, Pomerance A, et al. Influence of acute rejection episodes, HLA matching, and donor/recipient phenotype on the development of 'early' transplant- associated coronary artery disease. Circulation. 1997;96(Suppl): II-148–II-153.
78. Arita K, Uozumi T, Oki S, et al. The function of the hypothalamo-pituitary axis in brain dead patients. Acta Neurochirurgica. 1993;123:64–75.
79. Birks EJ, Yacoub MH, Burton PS, et al. Activation of apoptotic and inflammatory pathways in dysfunctional donor hearts. Transplantation. 2000;70:1498–1506.
80. Tsai FC, Marelli D, Bresson J, et al. Use of hearts transplanted from donors with atraumatic intracranial bleeds. Journal of Heart and Lung Transplantation. 2002;21:623–628.
81. Day JD, Rayburn BK, Gaudin PB, et al. Cardiac allograft vasculopathy: the central pathogenetic role of ischemia-induced endothelial cell injury. Journal of Heart and Lung Transplantation. 1995;14:S142–S149.
82. Kourembanas S, Hannan RL, Faller DV. Oxygen tension regulates the expression of the platelet-derived growth factor-B chain gene in human endothelial cells. Journal of Clinical Investigation. 1990;86:670–674.
83. Levy AP, Levy NS, Wegner S, et al. Transcriptional regulation of the rat vascular endothelial growth factor gene by hypoxia. Journal of Biological Chemistry. 1995;270:13333–13340.
84. Lindner V, Reidy MA. Proliferation of smooth muscle cells after vascular injury is inhibited by an antibody against basic fibroblast growth factor. Proceedings of the National Academy of Sciences of the United States of America. 1991; 88:3739–3743.
85. Dvorak HF, Brown LF, Detmar M, et al. Vascular permeability factor/vascular endothelial growth factor, microvascular hyperpermeability, and angiogenesis. American Journal of Pathology. 1995;146:1029–1039.
86. Furukawa Y, Matsumori A, Hirozane T, et al. Angiotensin II receptor antagonist TCV-116 reduces graft coronary artery disease and preserves graft status in a murine model: a comparative study with captopril. Circulation. 1996;93: 333–339.
87. Richter M, Skupin M, Grabs R, et al. New approach in the therapy of chronic rejection? ACE- and AT1-blocker reduce the development of chronic rejection after cardiac transplantation in a rat model. Journal of Heart and Lung Transplantation. 2000;19:1047–1055.
88. Costanzo MR, Eisen HJ, Brown RN, et al. Are there specific risk factors for fatal allograft vasculopathy? An analysis of over 7000 cardiac transplant patients. Journal of Heart and Lung Transplantation. 2001;20:152.
89. Costanzo MR, Naftel DC, Pritzker MR, et al. Heart transplant coronary artery disease detected by coronary angiography: a multiinstitutional study of preoperative donor and recipient risk factors. Cardiac Transplant Research Database. Journal of Heart and Lung Transplantation. 1998;17:744–753.
90. Kobashigawa JA, Starling RC, Mehra MR, et al. Multicenter retrospective analysis of cardiovascular risk factors affecting long-term outcome of de novo cardiac transplant recipients. Journal of Heart and Lung Transplantation. 2006;25: 1063–1069.
91. Gao HZ, Hunt SA, Alderman EL, et al. Relation of donor age and preexisting coronary artery disease on angiography and intracoronary ultrasound to later development of accelerated allograft coronary artery disease. Journal of the American College of Cardiology. 1997;29:623–629.
92. Wong CK, Yeung AC. The topography of intimal thickening and associated remodeling pattern of early transplant coronary disease: influence of pre-existent donor atherosclerosis. Journal of Heart and Lung Transplantation. 2001; 20:858–864.
93. Uretsky BF, Kormos RL, Zerbe TR, et al. Cardiac events after heart transplantation: incidence and predictive value of coronary arteriography. Journal of Heart and Lung Transplantation. 1992;11:S45–S51.
94. Uretsky BF, Murali S, Reddy PS, et al. Development of coronary artery disease in cardiac transplant patients receiving immunosuppressive therapy with cyclosporine and prednisone. Circulation. 1987;76:827–834.
95. Botas J, Pinto FJ, Chenzbraun A, et al. Influence of preexistent donor coronary artery disease on the progression of transplant vasculopathy: an intravascular ultrasound study. Circulation. 1995;92:1126–1132.
96. Li H, Tanaka K, Anzai H, et al. Influence of pre-existing donor atherosclerosis on the development of cardiac allograft vasculopathy and outcomes in heart transplant recipients. Journal of the American College of Cardiology. 2006; 47:2470–2476.
97. Stamler JS, Vaughan DE, Rudd MA, et al. Frequency of hypercholesterolemia after cardiac transplantation. American Journal of Cardiology. 1988;62: 1268–1272.
98. Superko HR, Haskell WL, Di Ricco CD. Lipoprotein and hepatic lipase activity and high-density lipoprotein subclasses after cardiac transplantation. American Journal of Cardiology. 1990;66:1131–1134.
99. Penson MG, Winter WE, Fricker FJ, et al. Tacrolimus-based triple-drug immunosuppression minimizes serum lipid elevations in pediatric cardiac transplant recipients. Journal of Heart and Lung Transplantation. 1999;18:707–713.
100. Taylor DO, Barr ML, Radovancevic B, et al. A randomized, multicenter comparison of tacrolimus and cyclosporine immunosuppressive regimens in cardiac transplantation: decreased hyperlipidemia and hypertension with tacrolimus. Journal of Heart and Lung Transplantation. 1999;18:336–345.
101. Kobashigawa JA, Kasiske BL. Hyperlipidemia in solid organ transplantation. Transplantation. 1997;63:331–338.
102. Eich D, Thompson JA, Ko DJ, et al. Hypercholesterolemia in long-term survivors of heart transplantation: an early marker of accelerated coronary artery disease. Journal of Heart and Lung Transplantation. 1991;10:45–49.
103. Esper E, Glagov S, Karp RB, et al. Role of hypercholesterolemia in accelerated transplant coronary vasculopathy: results of surgical therapy with partial ileal bypass in rabbits undergoing heterotopic heart transplantation. Journal of Heart and Lung Transplantation. 1997;16:420–435.
104. Kapadia SR, Nissen SE, Ziada KM, et al. Impact of lipid abnormalities in development and progression of transplant coronary disease: a serial intravascular ultrasound study. Journal of the American College of Cardiology. 2001;38: 206–213.
105. Alonso DR, Starek PK, Minick CR. Studies on the pathogenesis of atheroarteriosclerosis induced in rabbit cardiac allografts by the synergy of graft rejection and hypercholesterolemia. American Journal of Pathology. 1977;87:415–442.
106. Tanaka H, Sukhova GK, Libby P. Interaction of the allogeneic state and hypercholesterolemia in arterial lesion formation in experimental cardiac allografts. Arteriosclerosis and Thrombosis: A Journal of Vascular Biology. 1994;14:734–745.
107. Raisanen-Sokolowski A, Tilly-Kiesi M, Ustinov J, et al. Hyperlipidemia accelerates allograft arteriosclerosis (chronic rejection) in the rat. Arteriosclerosis and Thrombosis: A Journal of Vascular Biology. 1994;14:2032–2042.
108. Eisen H, Kobashigawa J, Starling RC, et al. Improving outcomes in heart transplantation: the potential of proliferation signal inhibitors. Transplantation Proceedings. 2005;37(Suppl):4S–17S.
109. Kobashigawa JA, Katznelson S, Laks H, et al. Effect of pravastatin on outcomes after cardiac transplantation. New England Journal of Medicine. 1995;333: 621–627.

110. Weis M, Pehlivanli S, Meiser BM, et al. Simvastatin treatment is associated with improvement in coronary endothelial function and decreased cytokine activation in patients after heart transplantation. Journal of the American College of Cardiology. 2001;38:814–818.
111. Kwak B, Mulhaupt F, Veillard N, et al. The HMG-CoA reductase inhibitor simvastatin inhibits IFN-gamma induced MHC class II expression in human vascular endothelial cells. Swiss Medical Weekly. 2001;131:41–46.
112. Katznelson S, Kobashigawa JA. Dual roles of HMG-CoA reductase inhibitors in solid organ transplantation: lipid lowering and immunosuppression. Kidney International. Supplement. 1995;52:S112–S115.
113. Holschermann H, Hilgendorff A, Kemkes-Matthes B, et al. Simvastatin attenuates vascular hypercoagulability in cardiac transplant recipients. Transplantation. 2000;69:1830–1836.
114. Taylor DO, Stehlik J, Edwards LB, et al. Registry of the international society for heart and lung transplantation: twenty-sixth official adult heart transplant report, 2009. Journal of Heart and Lung Transplantation. 2009;28:1007–1022.
115. Radovancevic B, Poindexter S, Birovljev S, et al. Risk factors for development of accelerated coronary artery disease in cardiac transplant recipients. European Journal of Cardio-Thoracic Surgery. 1990;4:309–312.
116. Caforio AL, Tona F, Fortina AB, et al. Immune and nonimmune predictors of cardiac allograft vasculopathy onset and severity: multivariate risk factor analysis and role of immunosuppression. American Journal of Transplantation. 2004;4:962–970.
117. Schroeder JS, Gao SZ, Alderman EL, et al. A preliminary study of diltiazem in the prevention of coronary artery disease in heart-transplant recipients. New England Journal of Medicine. 1993;328:164–170.
118. Atkinson JB, Wudel JH, Hoff SJ, et al. Amlodipine reduces graft coronary artery disease in rat heterotopic cardiac allografts. Journal of Heart and Lung Transplantation. 1993;12:1036–1043.
119. Betz E, Weiss HD, Heinle H, et al. Calcium antagonists and atherosclerosis. Journal of Cardiovascular Pharmacology. 1991;18(Suppl 10):S71–S75.
120. Mehra MR, Ventura HO, Smart FW, et al. An intravascular ultrasound study of the influence of angiotensin-converting enzyme inhibitors and calcium entry blockers on the development of cardiac allograft vasculopathy. American Journal of Cardiology. 1995;75:853–854.
121. Erinc K, Yamani MH, Starling RC, et al. The effect of combined angiotensin-converting enzyme inhibition and calcium antagonism on allograft coronary vasculopathy validated by intravascular ultrasound. Journal of Heart and Lung Transplantation. 2005;24:1033–1038.
122. Richter MH, Richter HR, Olbrich HG, et al. Two good reasons for an angiotensin-II type 1 receptor blockade with losartan after cardiac transplantation: reduction of incidence and severity of transplant vasculopathy. Transplant International. 2003;16:26–32.
123. Yamamoto T, Sata M, Fukuda D, et al. The angiotensin II type 1 receptor blocker valsartan attenuates graft vasculopathy. Basic Research in Cardiology. 2005; 100:84–91.
124. Kosuge H, Ishihara T, Haraguchi G, et al. Treatment with telmisartan attenuates graft arteriosclerosis in murine cardiac allografts. Journal of Heart and Lung Transplantation. 2010;29:562–567.
125. Kahn J, Rehak P, Schweiger M, et al. The impact of overweight on the development of diabetes after heart transplantation. Clinical Transplantation. 2006;20: 62–66.
126. Lindenfeld J, Miller GG, Shakar SF, et al. Drug therapy in the heart transplant recipient: part II: immunosuppressive drugs. Circulation. 2004;110:3858–3865.
127. Depczynski B, Daly B, Campbell LV, et al. Predicting the occurrence of diabetes mellitus in recipients of heart transplants. Diabetic Medicine. 2000;17:15–19.
128. Heisel O, Heisel R, Balshaw R, et al. New onset diabetes mellitus in patients receiving calcineurin inhibitors: a systematic review and meta-analysis. American Journal of Transplantation. 2004;4:583–595.
129. Kato T, Chan MC, Gao SZ, et al. Glucose intolerance, as reflected by hemoglobin A1c level, is associated with the incidence and severity of transplant coronary artery disease. Journal of the American College of Cardiology. 2004;43: 1034–1041.
130. Russo MJ, Chen JM, Hong KN, et al. Survival after heart transplantation is not diminished among recipients with uncomplicated diabetes mellitus: an analysis of the United Network of Organ Sharing database. Circulation. 2006;114: 2280–2287.
131. Valantine H, Rickenbacker P, Kemna M, et al. Metabolic abnormalities characteristic of dysmetabolic syndrome predict the development of transplant coronary artery disease : a prospective study. Circulation. 2001;103:2144–2152.
132. Biadi O, Potena L, Fearon WF, et al. Interplay between systemic inflammation and markers of insulin resistance in cardiovascular prognosis after heart transplantation. Journal of Heart and Lung Transplantation. 2007;26:324–330.
133. Raichlin ER, McConnell JP, Lerman A, et al. Systemic inflammation and metabolic syndrome in cardiac allograft vasculopathy. Journal of Heart and Lung Transplantation. 2007;26:826–833.
134. Potena L, Valantine HA. Cardiac allograft vasculopathy and insulin resistance: hope for new therapeutic targets. Endocrinology and Metabolism Clinics of North America. 2007;36:965–981, ix.
135. McDonald K, Rector TS, Braulin EA, et al. Association of coronary artery disease in cardiac transplant recipients with cytomegalovirus infection. American Journal of Cardiology. 1989;64:359–362.
136. Grattan MT, Moreno-Cabral CE, Starnes VA, et al. Cytomegalovirus infection is associated with cardiac allograft rejection and atherosclerosis. JAMA: Journal of the American Medical Association. 1989;261:3561–3566.
137. Loebe M, Schuler S, Zais O, et al. Role of cytomegalovirus infection in the development of coronary artery disease in the transplanted heart. Journal of Heart Transplantation. 1990;9:707–711.
138. Gao SZ, Hunt SA, Schroeder JS, et al. Early development of accelerated graft coronary artery disease: risk factors and course. Journal of the American College of Cardiology. 1996;28:673–679.
139. Hussain T, Burch M, Fenton MJ, et al. Positive pretransplantation cytomegalovirus serology is a risk factor for cardiac allograft vasculopathy in children. Circulation. 2007;115:1798–1805.
140. Koskinen PK, Krogerus LA, Nieminen MS, et al. Quantitation of cytomegalovirus infection-associated histologic findings in endomyocardial biopsies of heart allografts. Journal of Heart and Lung Transplantation. 1993;12:343–354.
141. Petrakopoulou P, Kubrich M, Pehlivanli S, et al. Cytomegalovirus infection in heart transplant recipients is associated with impaired endothelial function. Circulation. 2004;110(Suppl 1):II207–II212.
142. Simmonds J, Fenton M, Dewar C, et al. Endothelial dysfunction and cytomegalovirus replication in pediatric heart transplantation. Circulation. 2008;117: 2657–2661.
143. Weis M, Cooke JP. Cardiac allograft vasculopathy and dysregulation of the NO synthase pathway. Arteriosclerosis, Thrombosis, and Vascular Biology. 2003;23: 567–575.
144. Lemstrom KB, Bruning JH, Bruggeman CA, et al. Cytomegalovirus infection enhances smooth muscle cell proliferation and intimal thickening of rat aortic allografts. Journal of Clinical Investigation. 1993;92:549–558.
145. Dengler TJ, Raftery MJ, Werle M, et al. Cytomegalovirus infection of vascular cells induces expression of pro-inflammatory adhesion molecules by paracrine action of secreted interleukin-1beta. Transplantation. 2000;69:1160–1168.
146. Zhu H, Shen Y, Shenk T. Human cytomegalovirus IE1 and IE2 proteins block apoptosis. Journal of Virology. 1995;69:7960–7970.
147. Akosah KO, Olsovsky M, Kirchberg D, et al. Dobutamine stress echocardiography predicts cardiac events in heart transplant patients. Circulation. 1996;94(Suppl 9):II283–II288.
148. Spes CH, Angermann CE. Stress echocardiography for assessment of cardiac allograft vasculopathy. Zeitschrift fur Kardiologie. 2000;89(Suppl 9):IX/50–IX/53.
149. Sade LE, Sezgin A, Eroglu S, et al. Dobutamine stress echocardiography in the assessment of cardiac allograft vasculopathy in asymptomatic recipients. Transplantation Proceedings. 2008;40:267–270.
150. Nguyen T, Ahmadie R, Fang T, et al. Stress echocardiography: abnormal tissue doppler imaging in the absence of cardiac allograft vasculopathy in heart transplant recipients. Echocardiography (Mount Kisco, N.Y.). 2008;26:182–188.
151. Hacker M, Hoyer HX, Uebleis C, et al. Quantitative assessment of cardiac allograft vasculopathy by real-time myocardial contrast echocardiography: a comparison with conventional echocardiographic analyses and [Tc99m]-sestamibi SPECT. European Journal of Echocardiography. 2008;9:494–500.
152. Rodrigues AC, Bacal F, Medeiros CC, et al. Noninvasive detection of coronary allograft vasculopathy by myocardial contrast echocardiography. Journal of the American Society of Echocardiography. 2005;18:116–121.
153. Eroglu E, D'Hooge J, Sutherland GR, et al. Quantitative dobutamine stress echocardiography for the early detection of cardiac allograft vasculopathy in heart transplant recipients. Heart (British Cardiac Society). 2008;94:e3.
154. Verhoeven PP, Lee FA, Ramahi TM, et al. Prognostic value of noninvasive testing one year after orthotopic cardiac transplantation. Journal of the American College of Cardiology. 1996;28:183–189.
155. Elhendy A, van Domburg RT, Vantrimpont P, et al. Prediction of mortality in heart transplant recipients by stress technetium-99m tetrofosmin myocardial perfusion imaging. American Journal of Cardiology. 2002;89:964–968.
156. Hacker M, Tausig A, Romuller B, et al. Dobutamine myocardial scintigraphy for the prediction of cardiac events after heart transplantation. Nuclear Medicine Communications. 2005;26:607–612.
157. Wu YW, Chen YH, Wang SS, et al. PET assessment of myocardial perfusion reserve inversely correlates with intravascular ultrasound findings in angiographically normal cardiac transplant recipients. Journal of Nuclear Medicine.

2010;51:906–912.
158. Farzaneh-Far A. Electron-beam computed tomography in the assessment of coronary artery disease after heart transplantation. Circulation. 2001; 103:E60.
159. Schepis T, Achenbach S, Weyand M, et al. Comparison of dual source computed tomography versus intravascular ultrasound for evaluation of coronary arteries at least one year after cardiac transplantation. American Journal of Cardiology. 2009;104:1351–1356.
160. Ballesteros Pradas SM, Romero Rodriguez N, Lage Galle E, et al. Cardiac allograft vasculopathy: coronary computed tomography and virtual histology assessment. Transplantation Proceedings. 2010;42:3175–3177.
161. Rohnean A, Houyel L, Sigal-Cinqualbre A, et al. Heart transplant patient outcomes: 5-year mean follow-up by coronary computed tomography angiography. Transplantation. 2011;91:583–588.
162. Taylor AJ, Vaddadi G, Pfluger H, et al. Diagnostic performance of multisequential cardiac magnetic resonance imaging in acute cardiac allograft rejection. European Journal of Heart Failure. 2010;12:45–51.
163. Caus T, Kober F, Marin P, et al. Non-invasive diagnostic of cardiac allograft vasculopathy by 31P magnetic resonance chemical shift imaging. European Journal of Cardio-Thoracic Surgery. 2006;29:45–49.
164. Korosoglou G, Osman NF, Dengler TJ, et al. Strain-encoded cardiac magnetic resonance for the evaluation of chronic allograft vasculopathy in transplant recipients. American Journal of Transplantation. 2009;9:2587–2596.
165. Bajaj S, Shah A, Crandall C, et al. Coronary collateral circulation in the transplanted heart. Circulation. 1993;88:II263–II269.
166. Potluri SP, Mehra MR, Uber PA, et al. Relationship among epicardial coronary disease, tissue myocardial perfusion, and survival in heart transplantation. Journal of Heart and Lung Transplantation. 2005;24:1019–1025.
167. Korosoglou G, Riedle N, Erbacher M, et al. Quantitative myocardial blush grade for the detection of cardiac allograft vasculopathy. American Heart Journal. 2010;159:643–51 e2.
168. Kapadia SR, Nissen SE, Ziada KM, et al. Development of transplantation vasculopathy and progression of donor- transmitted atherosclerosis: comparison by serial intravascular ultrasound imaging. Circulation. 1998;98:2672–2678.
169. Rickenbacher PR, Kemna MS, Pinto FJ, et al. Coronary artery intimal thickening in the transplanted heart: an in vivo intracoronary untrasound study of immunologic and metabolic risk factors. Transplantation. 1996;61:46–53.
170. Konig A, Theisen K, Klauss V. Intravascular ultrasound for assessment of coronary allograft vasculopathy. Zeitschrift fur Kardiologie. 2000;89(Suppl 9): 45–49.
171. Tuzcu EM, Kapadia SR, Sachar R, et al. Intravascular ultrasound evidence of angiographically silent progression in coronary atherosclerosis predicts long-term morbidity and mortality after cardiac transplantation. Journal of the American College of Cardiology. 2005;45:1538–1542.
172. Kobashigawa JA, Tobis JM, Starling RC, et al. Multicenter intravascular ultrasound validation study among heart transplant recipients: outcomes after five years. Journal of the American College of Cardiology. 2005;45:1532–1537.
173. Hernandez JM, de Prada JA, Burgos V, et al. Virtual histology intravascular ultrasound assessment of cardiac allograft vasculopathy from 1 to 20 years after heart transplantation. Journal of Heart and Lung Transplantation. 2009;28:156–162.
174. Konig A, Kilian E, Rieber J, et al. Assessment of early atherosclerosis in de novo heart transplant recipients: analysis with intravascular ultrasound-derived radiofrequency analysis. Journal of Heart and Lung Transplantation. 2008; 27:26–30.
175. Sarno G, Lerman A, Bae JH, et al. Multicenter assessment of coronary allograft vasculopathy by intravascular ultrasound-derived analysis of plaque composition. Nature Clinical Practice. Cardiovascular Medicine. 2009;6:61–69.
176. Mullins PA, Chauhan A, Sharples L, et al. Impairment of coronary flow reserve in orthotopic cardiac transplant recipients with minor coronary occlusive disease. British Heart Journal. 1992;68:266–271.
177. Mazur W, Bitar JN, Young JB, et al. Progressive deterioration of coronary flow reserve after heart transplantation. American Heart Journal. 1998;136:504–509.
178. Lee CM, Wu YW, Jui HY, et al. Intravascular ultrasound correlates with coronary flow reserve and predicts the survival in angiographically normal cardiac transplant recipients. Cardiology. 2008;109:93–98.
179. Mehra MR, Crespo-Leiro MG, Dipchand A, et al. International Society for Heart and Lung Transplantation working formulation of a standardized nomenclature for cardiac allograft vasculopathy, 2010. Journal of Heart and Lung Transplantation. 2010;29:717–727.
180. Wu GW, Kobashigawa JA, Fishbein MC, et al. Asymptomatic antibody-mediated rejection after heart transplantation predicts poor outcomes. Journal of Heart and Lung Transplantation. 2009;28:417–422.
181. Williams R, Neuhaus P, Bismuth H, et al. Two-year data from the European multicentre tacrolimus (FK506) liver study. Transplant International. 1996;9(Suppl 1):S144–S150.
182. Kobashigawa JA, Patel J, Furukawa H, et al. Five-year results of a randomized, single-center study of tacrolimus vs microemulsion cyclosporine in heart transplant patients. Journal of Heart and Lung Transplantation. 2006;25:434–439.
183. Kobashigawa J, Miller L, Renlund D, et al. A randomized active-controlled trial of mycophenolate mofetil in heart transplant recipients. Mycophenolate Mofetil Investigators. Transplantation. 1998;66:507–515.
184. Rose ML, Danskine A, Smith JD, et al.. Mycophenolate mofetil (MMF) depresses antibody production after cardiac transplantation [abstract]. Circulation. 2000; 102:II-490.
185. Kobashigawa JA, Tobis JM, Mentzer RM, et al. Mycophenolate mofetil reduces intimal thickness by intravascular ultrasound after heart transplant: reanalysis of the multicenter trial. American Journal of Transplantation. 2006;6:993–997.
186. Giesler G, Espejo M, Kubak B, et al. Increased risk of CMV infection in heart transplant patients on mycophenolate mofetil. Journal of Heart and Lung Transplantation. 2001;20:178.
187. Morice MC, Serruys PW, Sousa JE, et al. A randomized comparison of a sirolimus-eluting stent with a standard stent for coronary revascularization. New England Journal of Medicine. 2002;346:1773–1780.
188. Stone GW, Rizvi A, Newman W, et al. Everolimus-eluting versus paclitaxel-eluting stents in coronary artery disease. New England Journal of Medicine. 2010;362:1663–1674.
189. Keogh A, Richardson M, Ruygrok P, et al. Sirolimus in de novo heart transplant recipients reduces acute rejection and prevents coronary artery disease at 2 years: a randomized clinical trial. Circulation. 2004;110:2694–2700.
190. Eisen HJ, Tuzcu EM, Dorent R, et al. Everolimus for the prevention of allograft rejection and vasculopathy in cardiac-transplant recipients. New England Journal of Medicine. 2003;349:847–858.
191. Fang JC, Kinlay S, Beltrame J, et al. Effect of vitamins C and E on progression of transplant-associated arteriosclerosis: a randomised trial. Lancet. 2002;359: 1108–1113.
192. Dempsey SJ, D'Amico C, Weintraub WS, et al. Angiographic and clinical follow-up of percutaneous revascularization for transplant coronary artery disease. Journal of Invasive Cardiology. 2000;12:311–315.
193. Takano Y, Currier JW, Yeatman LA, et al. Cutting balloon angioplasty for cardiac transplant vasculopathy. Journal of Heart and Lung Transplantation. 2002;21: 910–913.
194. Zakliczynski M, Lekston A, Osuch M, et al. Comparison of long-term results of drug-eluting stent and bare metal stent implantation in heart transplant recipients with coronary artery disease. Transplantation Proceedings. 2007;39: 2859–2861.
195. Lee MS, Kobashigawa J, Tobis J. Comparison of percutaneous coronary intervention with bare-metal and drug-eluting stents for cardiac allograft vasculopathy. JACC: Cardiovascular Interventions. 2008;1:710–715.
196. Jonas M, Fang JC, Wang JC, et al. In-stent restenosis and remote coronary lesion progression are coupled in cardiac transplant vasculopathy but not in native coronary artery disease. Journal of the American College of Cardiology. 2006;48:453–461.
197. Kobashigawa JA. Cardiac allograft vasculopathy in heart transplant patients: pathologic and clinical aspects for angioplasty/stenting. Journal of the American College of Cardiology. 2006;48:462–463.
198. Goerler H, Simon A, Warnecke G, et al. Cardiac surgery late after heart transplantation: a safe and effective treatment option. Journal of Thoracic and Cardiovascular Surgery. 2010;140:433–439.
199. Bhama JK, Nguyen DQ, Scolieri S, et al. Surgical revascularization for cardiac allograft vasculopathy: is it still an option? Journal of Thoracic and Cardiovascular Surgery. 2009;137:1488–1492.
200. Smith JA, Ribakove GH, Hunt SA, et al. Heart retransplantation: the 25-year experience at a single institution. Journal of Heart and Lung Transplantation. 1995;14:832–839.
201. Copeland H, Coelho-Anderson R, Mineburg N, et al. Elective cardiac retransplantation: a viable option that can be repeated. Journal of Thoracic and Cardiovascular Surgery. 2011;141:822–827.
202. Moloney ED, Egan JJ, Kelly P, et al. Transplantation for myocarditis: a controversy revisited. Journal of Heart and Lung Transplantation. 2005;24: 1103–1110.
203. Yager JE, Hernandez AF, Steenbergen C, et al. Recurrence of cardiac sarcoidosis in a heart transplant recipient. Journal of Heart and Lung Transplantation. 2005;24:1988–1990.
204. Oni AA, Hershberger RE, Norman DJ, et al. Recurrence of sarcoidosis in a cardiac allograft: control with augmented corticosteroids. Journal of Heart and Lung Transplantation. 1992;11:367–369.
205. Muller C, Briegel J, Haller M, et al. Sarcoidosis recurrence following lung transplantation. Transplantation. 1996;61:1117–1119.

206. Luk A, Lee A, Ahn E, et al. Cardiac sarcoidosis: recurrent disease in a heart transplant patient following pulmonary tuberculosis infection. Canadian Journal of Cardiology. 2010;26:e273–e275.
207. Khan R, Tweedie EJ, Pflugfelder PW, et al. Cardiac sarcoid in a heart transplant recipient: detection with cardiac magnetic resonance imaging. Transplantation Proceedings. 2010;42:1976–1978.
208. Milman N, Andersen CB, Mortensen SA, et al. Cardiac sarcoidosis and heart transplantation: a report of four consecutive patients. Sarcoidosis, Vasculitis, and Diffuse Lung Diseases. 2008;25:51–59.
209. Cooper LT Jr, Berry GJ, Shabetai R; Multicenter Giant Cell Myocarditis Study Group Investigators. Idiopathic giant-cell myocarditis: natural history and treatment. New England Journal of Medicine. 1997;336:1860–1866.
210. Scott RL, Ratliff NB, Starling RC, et al. Recurrence of giant cell myocarditis in cardiac allograft. Journal of Heart and Lung Transplantation. 2001;20:375–380.
211. Milei J, Guerri-Guttenberg RA, Grana DR, et al. Prognostic impact of Chagas disease in the United States. American Heart Journal. 2009;157:22–29.
212. Fiorelli AI, Santos RH, Oliveira JL Jr, et al. Heart transplantation in 107 cases of Chagas' disease. Transplantation Proceedings. 2011;43:220–224.
213. Godoy HL, Guerra CM, Viegas RF, et al. Infections in heart transplant recipients in Brazil: the challenge of Chagas' disease. Journal of Heart and Lung Transplantation. 2009;29:286–290.
214. Bacal F, Silva CP, Pires PV, et al. Transplantation for Chagas' disease: an overview of immunosuppression and reactivation in the last two decades. Clinical Transplantation. 2010;24:E29–E34.
215. Bacal F, Silva CP, Bocchi EA, et al. Mychophenolate mofetil increased chagas disease reactivation in heart transplanted patients: comparison between two different protocols. American Journal of Transplantation. 2005;5:2017–2021.
216. Campos SV, Strabelli TM, Amato Neto V, et al. Risk factors for Chagas' disease reactivation after heart transplantation. Journal of Heart and Lung Transplantation. 2008;27:597–602.
217. Diez M, Favaloro L, Bertolotti A, et al. Usefulness of PCR strategies for early diagnosis of Chagas' disease reactivation and treatment follow-up in heart transplantation. American Journal of Transplantation. 2007;7:1633–1640.
218. Almeida DR, Carvalho AC, Branco JN, et al. Chagas' disease reactivation after heart transplantation: efficacy of allopurinol treatment. Journal of Heart and Lung Transplantation. 1996;15:988–992.
219. Patel JK, Kobashigawa JA. Cardiac allograft vasculopathy. In: Ahsan N, editor. Chronic Allograft Failure: Natural History, Pathogenesis, Diagnosis and Management. Austin, TX: Landes Bioscience; 2008: 65.

第 80 章
肺移植后复发性疾病

Todd L. Astor

引言

肺移植已经成为多种不同的晚期肺疾病的决定性治疗手段。尽管外科技术(参见第59章)和供体器官保存的进展使得早期移植后生存率大为改善,但感染(参见第93和94章)和闭塞性细支气管炎综合征(BOS,参见第72章)依然是患者长期生存的主要障碍。因此,有大量的研究正围绕这些移植相关并发症开展。

然而,原发性肺疾病作为肺移植后移植物失功的潜在病因,目前仍未得到足够的重视。已经有一系列肺移植后疾病复发的报道,从偶然的活检发现、移植物失功到死亡(框80.1)。在本章中,我们关注肺移植后原发性疾病复发,并研究原发性疾病复发对移植物功能的影响,讨论疾病复发的原因,并探讨实施肺移植的决策时对潜在原发性疾病复发的考量。

结节病

结节病是一种不明原因的多器官肉芽肿性疾病。结节病最有可能的病因是,巨噬细胞或树突状细胞递呈不明抗原给初始T淋巴细胞(主要是CD4$^+$),导致异常的Th1免疫反应,进而引起一系列临床表现。上述反应最终导致肉芽肿的形成,表现为上皮样组织细胞和多核巨细胞与CD4$^+$淋巴细胞混合。诊断结节病需要排除其他一系列疾病,一般需要结合临床以及多个器官的影像学和(或)组织学表现[1]。

框 80.1 肺移植后原发性肺部疾病复发的报道

- 结节病[15-22]
- 淋巴管平滑肌瘤病[47-53]
- 朗格汉斯细胞组织细胞增生症[79-81]
- 细支气管肺泡癌[100-105]
- 继发于α1-抗胰蛋白缺乏症的肺气肿[140,141]
- 肺泡蛋白沉积症[122,123]
- 脱屑性间质性肺炎[148-150]
- 巨细胞间质性肺炎[153]
- 弥漫性泛细支气管炎[155]

肺脏是结节病最常见的受累器官[2,3]。肉芽肿可发生于肺实质和气道,并导致限制性和阻塞性肺疾病[4,5]。肺疾病的严重程度可以从孤立的影像学发现而无临床症状到需要肺移植的终末期肺病。肺结节病的治疗目前包括糖皮质激素的剂量递增应用[6,7]、非类固醇药物(氨甲蝶呤、硫唑嘌呤、来氟米特、麦考酚酯)[8-11],以及可阻断肿瘤坏死因子的生物制剂(英夫利昔单抗)[12,13]。

肺移植目前已成为继发于结节病重症难治性肺疾病患者的决定性疗法。1995—2010年,共有783例肺移植(236例单肺移植和547例双肺移植)在结节病患者中进行,占具有肺移植适应证病例的2.6%。肺移植治疗结节病患者的中位生存期是5.3年,囊性纤维化为7.4年,α-1抗胰蛋白酶缺乏症为6.3年,慢性阻塞性肺疾病(COPD)为5.3年,特发性肺纤维化为4.5年,特发性肺动脉高压为4.9年[14]。

结节病是最常见的肺移植后复发性肺疾病,报道的移植后发病率为30%~80%[15-22]。尽管一些早期的报道了肺结节病患者肺移植后局部非干酪性肉芽肿活检结果[18-20],无一例表现出符合结节病的症状或影像学表现。有趣的是,其中1例报道描述了肺移植后移植肺复发结节病性肉芽肿,以及再次移植后对侧移植肺闭塞性细支气管炎[20]。

Martinez 等[21]报道了第一例肺移植受体出现相应的症状、CT影像学改变,以及活检病理,均符合结节病的诊断。该例患者在肺移植后13个月出现呼吸困难和疲劳,高分辨率CT(HRCT)扫描显示上叶结节性浸润。随后支气管镜肺活检显示非干酪性肉芽肿。该患者的症状和影像学异常经口服糖皮质激素治疗得到缓解，但在随后的3、6和9个月行活检时均发现干酪性肉芽肿持续存在。

此后，一系列报道共描述了31例患者肺移植后结节病复发。Milman等[17]报道了7例肺结节病患者行肺移植后的长期预后。这些患者的术后随访中位时间为31个月(12~136个月)。仅1例患者的影像学检查结果与肺结节病一致。3例患者分别在移植后第2、5和6个月时经活检证实结节病。Ionescu等[15]描述了8例结节病肺移植后复发病例。2例患者在前6个月经组织学证实结节病性肉芽肿，2例在6~12个月时确诊，其他4例在1~2年确诊。

这些报道所累积的研究结果表明，复发性结节病通常是支气管活检偶然发现非干酪性肉芽肿而确诊性的。临床症状和体征通常不存在，一旦存在，通常较原发性疾病的程度轻。影像学异常通常罕见，但可能出现淋巴结肿大、孤立或多发结节，以及弥漫性网状结节浸润[23,24]。移植物功能障碍相关的肉芽肿较为罕见。与原发疾病相比，这种轻微的复发性疾病可能是由于移植后的免疫抑制治疗所导致的。有趣的是，移植后结节病复发的患者出现急性排斥反应的机会要大得多[15,16,18,21,24]。基于这一观察，有理由认为排异和结节病可能存在共同免疫途径[17,21,25]。

移植肺内复发性结节病性肉芽肿来自受体或供体细胞，或两者兼而有之，目前尚不明确。供体来源结节病的观点已经被提出，即肺移植后结节病来源于未确诊结节病的供体[16]。然而，很少有数据可以支持已知结节病供体导致“正常”器官移植受体发生显著的结节病。Heatly等[26]报道了肺结节病的供体(移植时未知)移植肺给一例原发性肺动脉高压受体，后者无已知的结节病病史。在移植后16个月的随访期内，没有组织学、影像学、临床证据表明移植后发生肺结节病。Ionescu等[15]通过聚合酶链反应(PCR)DNA分析了3例肺移植后复发结节病患者的受体的肺样本、移植肺样本和复发性结节病肉芽肿移植肺样本，表明肉芽肿内上皮样细胞团中受体DNA的百分比增高。Milman等[22]应用荧光原位杂交(FISH)技术分析一例女性肺移植后结节病复发患者的复发性肉芽肿内的免疫细胞，该女性患者接受了男性供者的肺，研究发现此类免疫细胞X染色体阳性且Y染色体阴性。这些结果表明复发性肉芽肿来源于受体，且有可能浸润到移植肺受体的巨噬细胞，而非供体组织细胞对受体抗原的反应。

淋巴管平滑肌瘤病

淋巴管平滑肌瘤病(LAM)是一种罕见的特发性疾病，主要发生于育龄期妇女，仅有少数男性患病的报道，且与结节性硬化症相关[27-29]。LAM的特点是肺、肾、肝、脾、子宫、卵巢和腹膜后淋巴管平滑肌增生和薄壁囊肿的形成。肺是最常见的受累器官，且由于肺实质、气道、血管和淋巴管内平滑肌细胞增殖和囊肿形成导致肺功能不全[30]。症状包括进行性呼吸困难、破裂的囊肿所致的气胸、闭塞的淋巴管所致的乳糜胸，以及肺出血。HRCT扫描显示均匀分布的大小不等的薄壁囊肿[31]。组织学特点是囊肿被增殖的平滑肌样梭形细胞所包绕，可以通过免疫染色确定黑色素瘤相关的标记物(HMB-45)[32]。

LAM自然病程具有非常缓慢和渐进的特点，10年生存率约为70%[30]。治疗策略主要围绕防止平滑肌样细胞进一步扩散，既往主要依赖外科手术或药物减少雌激素的产生。最近的研究发现，LAM中存在结节性硬化症的基因TSC1和TSC2，因而利用哺乳动物西罗莫司靶蛋白(mTOR)抑制剂西罗莫司，成功治疗LAM[36-42]。

尽管对LAM的理解有所加深，且治疗有所进展，但肺移植仍然是唯一明确的决定性治疗手段。1995—2010年间，共进行了308例肺移植（101例单侧，207例双侧），占所有具有肺移植适应证的LAM患者的1%[14]。基于已经发表的美国和欧洲LAM肺移植数据，1年生存率为79%~86%，3年为73%~76%，5年为65%[43,44]。术后LAM相关并发症包括显著的胸膜粘连和出血、乳糜胸，以及自身肺的气胸[43,45,46]。

已证实的关于移植后复发的LAM至少有7篇已发表的报道[47-53]。早期的LAM复发的报道主要是基于尸检结果。然而，LAM一般具有阻塞性肺功能检查结果的特点，肺移植后复发可能会被误诊为BOS。

O'Brein等[48]报道了第一例复发性LAM，一例38岁的女性肺LAM患者接受右侧单肺移植后，LAM复发。肺移植术后1个月，患者的肺功能开始下降，开肺活检显示中度急性细胞性排异反应和淋巴细胞性细支气管炎。肺活检及之后的支气管活检没有发现LAM的证据。尽管行强化免疫抑制治疗，患者的肺功能未见改善，最终在18个月后死于浸润性曲霉病。尸检没有发现排异或闭塞性支气管炎，但表现出平滑肌细胞与梭形细胞的结节性增生增殖，这与 LAM 的组织学特性一致。这些结果提示 LAM 在早期移植物失功方面可能有重要作用。

目前临床上鉴别 LAM 和 BOS 存在巨大的挑战，Bittman 等[50,51]的报道强调了这一情况。作者描述了一例 31 岁的女性肺 LAM 患者接受右单肺移植治疗，移植后 1 年肺功能显著下降。开肺活检显示闭塞性细支气管炎，但当时没有 LAM 复发的组织学证据。在随后数月，她的肺功能可能由于渐进性闭塞性细支气管炎而持续下降。该患者在移植 3 年后出现右肺气胸，并死于相关并发症。正如预期的那样，尸检发现闭塞性细支气管炎的组织学证据，同时也表现出增殖平滑肌细胞染色 HMB45 强阳性。此外，原先肺活检标本重新进行免疫组织化学染色，显示平滑肌细胞增殖及 HMB-45 染色阳性。这些组织学结果和气胸的临床并发症，突出强调了该患者存在潜在的复发性 LAM。

复发性 LAM 也在活体供体肺叶移植中有所报道。Chen 等[52,53]描述了一例 20 岁女性肺和腹部 LAM 患者接受活体肺叶移植，患者在移植后第一年出现复发性乳糜胸和气胸。HRCT 显示肺气肿改变和肺浸润，左肺支气管活检显示 LAM 的组织学证据。在治疗上，以西罗莫司取代了硫唑嘌呤，随后更换为他克莫司。该患者的症状、HRCT 表现和肺功能检查逐渐改善，并在移植后 2 年内保持稳定。

我们最近对一例复发性 LAM 患者进行了双肺移植[54]。患者为 34 岁的女性肺、腹盆腔 LAM 患者，最初接受了活体供体肺叶移植，6 年后 HRCT 发现多发双侧肺囊肿，符合复发性 LAM 的诊断。该患者的肺功能可能由于复发性 LAM 和闭塞性细支气管炎综合征的混合情况而逐渐恶化，9 年时再次接受了双侧肺移植。取出移植肺叶的组织学分析发现肌样梭形细胞和狭缝状淋巴管，以及 HMB-45 免疫染色阳性，符合 LAM 的诊断(图 80.1)。我们同样发现斑片状的闭塞性细支气管炎和慢性排异反应。移植后 5 个月开始给予西罗莫司，以防止新移植肺的 LAM 复发。虽然在随后 2 年的随访期内未检测到复发性 LAM，但肝、肾病变在此期间显著恶化。

肺移植后 LAM 复发的起源存在争议。早期报道利用人类 X 和 Y 染色体探针的非同位素原位杂交技术(NISH)研究提示细胞来源于供体[46,50]。然而，同时也发现，受体 LAM 细胞往往与供体来源细胞密切相关，导致错误的 NISH 信号。使用 NISH 分析和免疫组织化学染色同步分析，提示 LAM 细胞其实源于受体，而非供体[51]。Karbowniczek 等[47]利用微卫星标记指纹技术和 TSC2 突变分析表明，接受单肺移植出现复发性 LAM 的患者移植物内的 LAM 细胞源于自身肺和淋巴结。这些研究结果支持了以下假设，LAM 细胞可能从自身的肺、淋巴管或腹盆腔病灶迁移或转移而来。

我们认识到 LAM 可以在移植肺中复发，以及常规移植肺支气管活检监测的开展，为早期治疗性干预创造了机会。LAM 存在 TSC2 突变的发现，提示 mTOR 信号通路在 LAM 发生中的重要作用。这一发现引发了 mTOR 信号通路抑制剂西罗莫司的在 LAM 中的应用[36-42]。Chen 等[52,53]报道了一例西罗莫司成功治疗肺移植后复发性 LAM 患者的乳糜胸。其他 3 个报道表明，西罗莫司治疗可以改善肺移植后肺和后腹膜 LAM 复发患者的病情[55-57]。我们已经成功利用西罗莫司抑制再

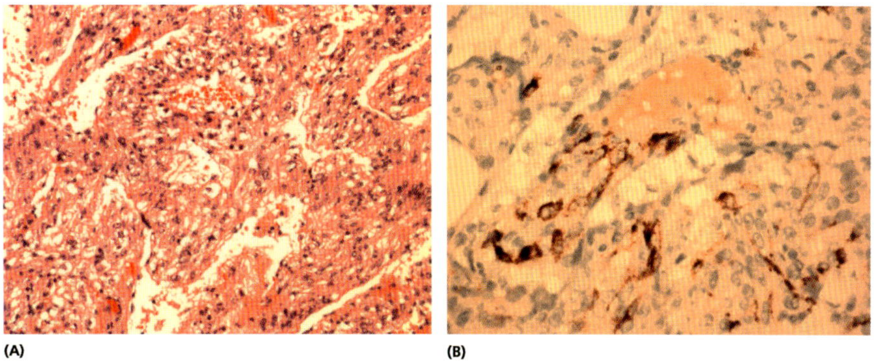

图 80.1 肺表现为肌样梭形细胞和狭缝状淋巴管替代正常肺泡间质(A)。HMB-45 免疫染色显示浸润的梭形细胞。结果显示为淋巴管平滑肌瘤病(B)，H&E，原始放大率为 250 倍。(Courtesy of Dr. Richard Kradin.)

次肺移植后LAM复发[54]。然而,西罗莫司治疗可导致肝肾功能的恶化。

肺朗格汉斯细胞组织细胞增生症

肺朗格汉斯细胞组织细胞增生症(PLCH)是一种罕见的疾病,表现为朗格汉斯细胞[58],一种骨髓来源的树突状细胞,在肺泡和间质的浸润。虽然朗格汉斯细胞组织细胞增生症(LCH)可以影响肺外器官,如骨骼、皮肤和垂体(特别是儿童),大多数受累的成年患者存在孤立性肺疾病[59-61]。PLCH与吸烟存在很强的相关性,90%的患者在确诊时是吸烟者[59,60,62,63]。PLCH患者可能出现轻微的呼吸困难或咳嗽,或在某些情况下出现自发性气胸。许多患者是无症状的,仅通过胸片偶然发现。胸部HRCT扫描显示特征性上肺和中肺囊肿合并结节[64-66]。支气管镜活检对PCLH的诊断敏感性较低,一般依赖手术活检做出诊断[67]。组织学分析发现,LCH细胞病变特征较容易识别,表现为肾形和豆形的细胞核,CD1a免疫组织化学染色,以及电镜下发现Birbeck小粒(细胞质包涵体)[68-70]。

PLCH的临床病程多变。一些患者在没有任何治疗的情况下可以自行改善,而其他一些患者尽管给予免疫抑制治疗仍出现渐进性疾病。由于与吸烟关系密切,戒烟被认为是一个重要的干预措施。事实上,戒烟已被一些研究证明能有效减少疾病临床表现,同时也有一些研究表明即使戒烟,病情依旧会恶化[71-73]。糖皮质激素治疗依然应用于有症状的患者,尽管缺乏文献的证据支持[60,74,75]。全身化疗,如给予细胞毒性药物,如环磷酰胺、氨甲蝶呤、长春碱,已用于治疗多系统LCH,但这些药物在治疗中的作用目前还不清楚[76-78]。

肺移植已成为少部分因为严重的囊性肺破坏和(或)重度肺动脉高压引发难治性呼吸衰竭的PLCH患者的最终治疗手段[58,79-81]。虽然许多移植中心具备有限的PLCH患者肺移植经验,但目前很少有公开发表的肺移植后的短期和长期数据。Dauriat等[58]在法国进行了一项多中心的回顾性研究,入组了39例接受肺移植的终末期PLCH患者(单肺移植15例,双肺移植15例,心肺联合移植9例)。除2例患者以外,其他均为既往或目前吸烟者。大多数患者在术前有中重度肺动脉高压,约1/3有LCH肺外受累。结果显示,肺移植后1年存活率为76.9%,2年为63.6%,5年为57.2%年,10年为53.7%。尽管该中心没有其他更常见肺移植适应证的生存数据公布,但这些生存率与同时期国际心脏和心脏协会肺移植登记的数据具有可比性[82]。此外,相关生存率在肺移植类型之间(即单、双、心肺联合)无显著差异。急性细胞性排异反应和闭塞性支气管炎综合征的发生率与其他接受肺移植患者的人群也相似。

PLCH的临床和影像学证据,伴随或不伴随组织学确认,已经在一系列肺移植中被报道[79-81]。Gabbay等[79]报道了第一例肺移植后PLCH复发病例,一例32岁的男性患者,存在尿崩症病史(可能源于垂体LCH)和渐进性肺衰竭。在双肺移植后第24个月和30个月,在肺活检监测中发现朗格汉斯细胞浸润、间质纤维化,以及终末期支气管朗格汉斯细胞聚集。同时,患者出现呼吸困难和限制性肺功能障碍,与间质纤维化相符。患者在移植前后均不抽烟。有趣的是,在这一时期,患者的尿崩症恶化,需要增加吸入用去氨加压素剂量,在环孢素和糖皮质激素免疫抑制治疗基础上增加环磷酰胺,患者症状、肺功能和尿崩症得到改善。同样在这份报道中,作者还提到了其他4例PLCH患者在其中心接受移植,只有1例患者通过活检发现朗格汉斯细胞。

Habib等[81]报道了1例27岁接受双侧肺移植后PLCH复发的亚裔男性患者。该患者术前吸烟,但移植后未吸烟。约2年后,该患者呼吸功能恶化,伴随HRCT上中下肺广泛的囊性改变。这种分布于下肺的疾病(与LCH特征性分布于上肺相反)的罕见性还在于,患者自身的下肺也有相关病灶。右下叶支气管镜活检标本组织学分析显示在间质和血管周围聚集了朗格汉斯细胞,该患者无法耐受阿霉素、长春新碱和依托泊苷的联合化疗,免疫抑制治疗基础上加用环磷酰胺无效。

Etienne等[80]报道了他们关于肺移植后PLCH复发的单中心经验,7例接受肺移植的患者(6例单肺,1例心肺联合)行随访发现,5例患者没有复发的证据,而且生存时间为15~90个月。2例的移植肺出现LCH复发,均出现影像学、组织学和肺功能异常。这两例患者分别在移植后3个月和6个月恢复吸烟。

目前最大的肺移植后PLCH复发的研究是前文提到的法国的多中心研究[58]。在这项研究中,39例接受肺移植的PLCH患者中,8例(20.5%)出现复发,其中2例患者在之前被Etienne等所描述[80]。除了这2例患者,研究中仅有1例患者在术后恢复吸烟。复发在肺外受累的患者中比在单纯肺受累的患者中更常见(41.7%比

11.1%)。

虽然这些报道中仅有 10 例复发发生于移植肺,但这些发现强调了一些肺移植后 LCH 复发的病因。首先,只有 3 例患者在移植后恢复吸烟。因此,吸烟似乎不是导致疾病复发的单一因素。如前文所述,吸烟与移植前 PLCH 发病密切相关。已经发现烟草损害支气管上皮,导致特定的细胞表面抗原改变,进而募集朗格汉斯细胞,且此类细胞递呈更多的抗原给 $CD4^+$ T 淋巴细胞[59,83]。可以说,肺移植后 PLCH 复发率相对较低很大程度上是由于吸烟复吸率较低。其次,LCH 肺外受累似乎是复发的重要危险因素。这一观察表明疾病的复发可能是源于供体肺内受体朗格汉斯细胞的再聚集。可以想象的是,这个过程可能通过烟草对支气管上皮损伤和(或)其他环境刺激(即呼吸道病毒)被强化。

尽管肺移植后存在 PLCH 复发的可能性,临床上显著疾病的发病率是相对较低的。因此,肺移植仍然是难治性进行性肺功能恶化的患者可行的治疗选择,特别是对那些合并重症继发性肺动脉高压的患者。应反复建议患者避免肺移植后再次吸烟。肺移植术后监测包括肺功能测试、HRCT 和肺活检。如果经支气管肺活检无法明确的话,对于可疑的病例应进行手术肺活检。肺外 LCH 患者应密切监测。

细支气管肺泡癌

细支气管肺泡癌(BAC)是一种罕见的肺部肿瘤,以高分化肿瘤细胞沿着肺泡壁生长而不破坏或侵犯肺部组织、不出现淋巴或全身性转移为特征[84,85]。BAC 是一种原位癌,然而一些被分类为混合型腺癌的肿瘤伴随有 BAC 特征和局部侵袭性的特点更为常见[84,86,87]。BAC 仅占所有非小细胞肺癌的 5%,腺癌合并 BAC 特征占非小细胞肺癌的 20%[86,87]。BAC 通常表现为孤立性结节,常偶然通过胸片或 HRCT 发现。BAC 也可以表现为多发结节或弥漫性实质性疾病,虽然这种形式通常见于腺癌合并 BAC。BAC 结节在 HRCT 上多为毛玻璃样改变,然而也经常观察到实变[88-92]。治疗孤立性 BAC 肿瘤通常采取亚肺叶或肺叶手术切除,多发性 BAC 通常需要所有病灶的亚肺叶切除,可伴或不伴全身化疗[85,93-96]。表皮生长因子受体(EGFR)突变在 BAC 在比其他肺部肿瘤中更常见,因此 EGFR 受体酪氨酸激酶抑制剂(TKI)可应用于晚期或复发性 BAC 患者的治疗[97-99]。

肺移植已成为少数复发或不可切除的 BAC 患者的一种治疗方式,特别是那些弥漫性肺疾病患者[100]。由于复发的风险大,BAC 被认为是肺移植有争议的适应证[101-105]。阿拉巴马大学在 BAC 患者肺移植方面具有最丰富的经验。Garver 等在该中心最早报道了一小部分进展期 BAC 患者接受肺移植治疗。7 例接受单、双肺移植的 BAC 患者中有 4 例出现术后移植肺复发,尽管这些患者中有 2 例无复发时间长达 39 个月和 48 个月。该中心随后又报道了一项研究结果,以确定是否可将肺移植作为 BAC 患者的治疗[100]。8 例确诊为 BAC 的患者接受肺移植,虽然目前还不清楚这些患者是否包括原来的报道中的患者。其中 6 例患者术后复发,时间是移植后 12~75 个月。2 例患者局部复发,其中 1 例接受左下叶切除及右中下叶楔形切除术,另一例患者接受左肺全肺切除术。其他 4 例为弥漫性复发。4 例患者中有 2 例死于肺衰竭,第三例接受再次移植后不久死亡,第四例复发后 39 个月依然生存。尽管该小队中复发率很高,但 5 年生存率为 52%,与作者所在中心总体移植后 5 年生存率相似。然而,基于达到 75%的高复发率,作者决定终止这项研究。

在移植肺内复发的 BAC 的来源目前存在争议。大多数报道支持多灶性 BAC 来源于单克隆肿瘤沿着肺泡内、淋巴管或气道扩散[101,106,107]。在阿拉巴马大学的研究队列中,3 例移植肺内的复发性肿瘤表现出与原发性肿瘤相似的影像学和组织学特征。3 例患者中,对复发病灶 DNA 进一步 PCR 扩增表现出与原发性肿瘤类似的结果[103,104]。这些研究结果支持这一假设,复发的 BAC 来源于移植后受体的肿瘤细胞。这一假设进一步通过已发表的病例报道得到证实,该病例通过分析原发性和复发性肿瘤 DNA 分子指纹图谱得出研究结论[101]。15 例病例的肿瘤细胞基因多态性分析显示,原发性肿瘤与复发性肿瘤相似。

淋巴扩散是肺移植后 BAC 复发的最常见的机制。然而,因为大多数肺移植后复发 BAC 病例没有发现淋巴结转移的证据,无论是在移植时或在复发肿瘤切除时,这种解释似乎并不合理。因此,可能由于肿瘤细胞沿着气道播散到移植肺这一观点被提出、进而通过细致外科手术和气道灌洗在预防 BAC 复发方面发挥作用[101,102]。尽管在 BAC 和 BAC 患者肺移植围术期和手术后的外科介入措施有所进展,肺移植应用于 BAC 仍然存在争议。

肺泡蛋白沉积症

肺泡蛋白沉积症(PAP)是一种罕见的以表面活性蛋白在肺泡间隙累积为特征的肺部疾病。虽然过去10年间在治疗方面有显著进步,但我们对PAP的发病机制仍知之甚少。PAP可能涉及Ⅱ型肺泡细胞表面活性物质产生异常,以及肺泡巨噬细胞清除表面活性物质的功能受损[108-112]。PAP一般有三种不同类型:

1.一组先天性疾病,由表达表面活性蛋白和(或)粒细胞巨噬细胞集落刺激因子(GM-CSF)的基因发生突变。

2.某些化学或矿物粉尘暴露,或某些血液系统恶性肿瘤和免疫缺陷疾病。

3.特发性或原发性PAP,无明显病因。

第三种类型最常见,占所有PAP病例的90%[111,113]。全肺灌洗是唯一有效的治疗方法,主要用于治疗特发性病例[114-116]。GM-CSF被认为在PAP发病机制中发挥重要作用,在大多数特发性病例中可发现抗GM-CSF自身抗体。这些结果导致外源性GM-CSF治疗可应用于PAP,但其有效性尚不确定[116-120]。

肺移植很少应用于PAP继发性肺衰竭[121-125]。已经有肺移植后PAP复发的报道[122,123]。Parker等[123]报道了一例44岁女性PAP患者,双侧肺移植术后3年出现PAP复发。患者出现疲劳和呼吸困难,胸片显示新的浸润。经支气管镜活检组织学分析显示,肺泡间隙充满嗜酸性致密絮状物质,以及散在分布的泡沫细胞和胆固醇结晶。电镜证实存在表面活性物质的堆积。

Santamaria等[122]随后报道了一例曾接受心肺联合移植的继发于赖氨酸尿性蛋白不耐症(LPI)的PAP患儿发生致命性PAP复发。患者为3岁男孩,曾被诊断患有LPI,一种由质膜阳离子氨基酸转运蛋白缺陷引起的罕见的遗传性疾病。肺部症状主要表现为移植前一年严重的PAP。全肺灌洗治疗和GM-CSF的应用并不成功,该患儿最终接受心肺联合移植。移植后18个月,患儿出现严重的呼吸困难和低氧血症,推测可能继发于严重的病毒性肺炎。然而,随后的支气管镜检查显示在移植肺出现PAP,没有感染或排异的证据。无论是全肺灌洗,还是GM-CSF治疗未见任何改善,患儿最终在移植后26个月死亡。

我们对肺移植术后PAP复发的发病机制知之甚少。针对GM-CSF的循环抗体的存在被认为是移植后PAP发生的潜在的机制。第二种假设是PAP源于骨髓来源的单个核细胞的缺陷,如GM-CSF受体的异常。在这种情况下,肺移植可能是无法获益的,因为移植后不成熟的肺泡巨噬细胞依然无法有效清除表面活性物质[122,126-128]。

既往发表的报道阐述了肺移植受体发生初始PAP,这对PAP的发病机制是一种佐证[129,130]。Yousem等[129]描述了3例肺移植或心肺联合移植后发生PAP的病例,移植前无PAP的证据。作者作出假设,原发性移植肺损伤、排异反应和感染,再加上长期糖皮质激素治疗,导致肺泡间隙过多表面活性物质的产生。Gal等[130]报道了一例患者在单肺移植后66天出现初始肺纤维化。基于支气管肺泡灌洗(BAL)持续发现无定形、脱细胞、细颗粒做出PAP的诊断。患者35个月后死于渐进的BOS和巨细胞病毒性肺炎。两肺尸检证实PAP存在于自身肺中,而不是移植肺中。作者提出,免疫抑制药物可能会抑制肺泡巨噬细胞清除表面活性物质的能力。他们还认为,仔细检查BAL液可能是诊断肺移植后PAP最敏感的方法。

继发于α1-抗胰蛋白酶缺乏症的肺气肿

α1-抗胰蛋白酶缺乏症(ATD)是一种遗传性疾病,全球近340万人受累,在美国最高占到所有慢性阻塞性肺病的2%。最常见的受累器官是肝和肺[131,132]。肝脏疾病往往进展为肝硬化,可能由α1-抗胰蛋白酶结构改变后累积在肝脏导致[133]。对于肺部疾病,在最初的第4或第5年主要是全小叶肺气肿,是由循环中α1-抗胰蛋白酶减少导致的。肺气肿源于蛋白酶-抗蛋白酶的失衡,导致蛋白水解酶的活性增强。炎症反应增加似乎也是一个重要的共同因素,吸烟在疾病发展中也有重要作用[134,135]。治疗ATD主要集中在α1-抗胰蛋白酶替代治疗,通过静脉滴注人血浆、吸入疗法、重组治疗或抑制合成弹性蛋白酶进行[136-139]。

肺移植对于α1-ATD继发晚期肺气肿是一种成功的治疗方法。自1995年以来,已对α1-ATD患者进行了近2000例肺移植(728例单肺,1225例双肺),约占所有肺移植的6.5%[14]。α1-ATD患者接受肺移植术后中位生存期为6.3年,仅次于囊性纤维化患者(7.4年)[14]。

事实上,肺移植主要针对自体肺的肺气肿损害。然而,在 α1-抗胰蛋白酶系统性缺乏的情况下,肺移植并不针对疾病的病因。肺移植后复发肺气肿也是很常见的。然而,在 2002 年之前,没有继发于 α1-ATD 的肺气肿的报道。Glanville 等[140]在 2002 年报道了 2 例肺移植后尸检病理确诊 α1-ATD 的患者。这两例患者在尸检前都没有被怀疑有疾病复发。

Mal 等[14]随后发表了一份报道,描述了一例 α1-ATD 患者单肺移植后 10 年肺气肿复发。当时胸部 CT 提示移植肺肺气肿,在接下来的 2 年里,患者的肺功能逐渐恶化。有趣的是,患者在移植后的前 18 个月经历了一些急性排异反应,并在肺气肿之前约 3 年恢复吸烟。作者假设重复急性排异反应导致的初始炎症,再加上吸烟,可能触发了肺气肿复发。此外,该患者 BAL 液和血清中发现高水平的弹性蛋白酶活性。既往研究表明,肺移植后受体在显著的移植物排异反应或感染所致的炎症期间,BAL 液会出现高水平弹性蛋白酶活性[142,143]。

在 α1-ATD 肺移植后弹性蛋白酶活性增加的情况下,研究表明移植后补充 α1-抗胰蛋白可能是有益的[142-145]。Mal 等[141]建议,α1-抗胰蛋白酶替代治疗对患者有益,尤其是 BOS。BOS 与气道和肺实质中的中性粒细胞数量增加有关,可能会导致弹力蛋白酶相关损伤的显著增加。许多肺移植方案都针对具有 BOS 迹象的患者采用静脉置换 α1-抗胰蛋白酶。一些中心甚至在移植后对所有 α1-ATD 肺移植患者迅速开始 α1-抗胰蛋白酶替代治疗,尽管目前还缺乏支持这种做法的证据。

其他移植后肺部疾病复发

已经有多个案例报道描述了肺移植术后移植肺疾病复发,大多数情况下涉及非常罕见的肺移植适应证。

脱屑性间质性肺炎

脱屑性间质性肺炎(DIP)是一种罕见的间质性肺炎,其特点是大量的巨噬细胞在肺泡间隙累积,可能是肺泡上皮受损的一种反应。DIP 与吸烟有很强的相关性,其他药物和吸入剂也与疾病的发展有关。虽然大多数 DIP 患者通过免疫抑制治疗可改善病情,一小部分发展为不可逆的肺纤维化,需要行肺移植[146,147]。

肺移植术后 DIP 复发已有报道[148,149]。King 等[148]报道了一例 50 岁接受左单肺移植的 DIP 女性患者。移植后 1 个月,患者在影像学检查没有异常的情况下,出现咳嗽和呼吸困难,胸腔镜肺活检证实 DIP。尽管给予高剂量糖皮质激素重复治疗,其病情仍持续恶化,最终死于呼吸衰竭。尸检结果证实了移植肺存在弥漫性 DIP。Verleden 等[149,150]随后发表了第二例肺移植术后 DIP 复发的病例。在该病例中,DIP 在肺移植 1 年后通过支气管镜检查发现特征性的组织学改变而被证实。相比 King 等[148]报道的难治性病程,最终导致死亡,本报道中患者通过增加糖皮质激素治疗完全恢复。

巨细胞间质性肺炎

巨细胞间质性肺炎(GIP)是一种罕见的间质性肺炎,与暴露于某些重金属有关,其特征是通过巨大多核巨噬细胞和矿物颗粒在肺泡累积[151,152]。Frost 等[153]报道了一例 GIP 患者在肺移植后出现 GIP 复发,该患者因钴暴露导致 GIP 而接受了单肺移植。之后患者没有进一步接触到钴。此外,最终尸检发现移植肺有特征性的 GIP 改变,但没有证据表明无机颗粒的存在。作者提出假设,认为自身免疫性因素导致疾病复发。可以想象的是,在自身肺存在的或者肺外来源的无机颗粒可能诱发自身免疫反应。

弥漫性泛细支气管炎

弥漫性泛细支气管炎是一种常见的复杂的遗传肺疾病,几乎只影响东亚人群,与 Ⅰ 类 HLA-b54 和 HLA-A11 关系密切。它的特点是呼吸性细支气管内慢性炎症,以及呼吸道和鼻窦慢性细菌性感染。肺功能检测提示气道阻塞和过度通胀。肺组织病理学分析显示淋巴细胞和泡沫样巨噬细胞浸润在呼吸性细支气管周围。使用大环内酯类药物治疗能显著改善弥漫性泛细支气管炎患者的预后,虽然对其作用机制知之甚少。有些患者治疗无效并进展为肺衰竭,很少需要考虑肺移植[154]。

仅有一例肺移植后弥漫性泛细支气管炎复发的报道。Baz 等[155]描述了一例弥漫性泛细支气管炎患者在双肺移植后 10 周,出现非常迅速的移植肺功能恶化。通过红霉素治疗,移植肺功能在之后数周显著改善。虽然这是一个孤立的报道,仅描述了一个罕见的肺移植适应证,但研究结果提示弥漫性泛细支气管炎患者在肺移植术后使用大环内酯类抗生素可能获益。

肺毛细血管瘤病

肺毛细血管瘤病(PCH)是肺动脉高压的一种罕见的病因,以不受控制的毛细血管在肺间质和血管,以及肺泡壁增殖为特征。HRCT 表现包括小叶中心结节、间隔线、胸腔积液、淋巴结肿大,这些表现与肺静脉闭塞性疾病类似。PCH 病情进展迅速,肺移植目前仍然是唯一的治疗手段[156-159]。

关于 PCH 肺移植,没有已发表的数据,但 PCH 移植后复发的病例有所报道。作者首次报道了一例肺气肿患者双肺移植术后 3 个月发生 PCH[160]。作者提出假设,认为初发的 PCH 是由于从感染或炎症触发血管生成失控导致的。

Lee 等[161]随后报道了唯一一例 PCH 肺移植术后复发的病例。该 PCH 患者在双肺移植术后 6 个月发生肺气肿,临床和组织学符合 PCH 的诊断。有趣的是,其术后早期合并了反复急性细胞排异反应、闭塞性细支气管炎和机化性肺炎。患者在移植后 8 个月死亡,尸检分析显示,两移植肺广泛发生 PCH 相关的静脉闭塞性疾病。作者提出假设,认为早期移植肺损伤,导致循环上皮细胞的被招募沉积并增殖,进而导致 PCH 复发。

Williams-Campbell 综合征

Williams-Campbell 综合征是影响儿童的一种罕见疾病,其特征是亚段气管软骨缺乏,导致气道塌陷和支气管扩张。临床病程多变,部分患儿迅速进展为呼吸衰竭,而其他患儿则可生存到成年,发生反复的感染和气道阻塞[162,163]。尽管缺乏治疗手段,但依然有一个报道涉及此类疾病的肺移植。Palmer 等[164]描述了一例 28 岁男性 Williams-Campbell 综合征患者由于呼吸衰竭而接受双侧肺移植。该患者经历了移植后并发症,严重的近端主支气管软化,导致反复感染,最终在移植后 1 年死亡。作者提出假设,认为尽管软骨缺陷主要累及远端气道,有可能存在潜在的近端气道软骨缺陷,导致更容易出现移植后气道缺血。移植后气道灌注受损与支气管扩张并导致阻塞性支气管炎相关[165]。基于该病例气道早期并发症的发生,作者认为双侧肺移植不应该作为本病的适应证,但双肺移植可能是一个可行的选择。

结论

各种原发性肺疾病肺移植后复发均有所报道(框 80.1)。结节病复发是最常见的,复发率高达 80%。然而,大多数情况下,复发是活检偶然发现的,对移植肺功能影响不大。这种复发性疾病的温和特性,在很大程度上可能是由于移植后使用免疫抑制剂导致的。BAC 在肺移植后多有复发,报道的复发率高达 75%。尽管有显著的发病率和移植术后复发导致的再次外科介入,移植后生存率与其他适应证类似。LAM 和 PLCH 也常在移植后复发,由于阻塞性特点而容易被误诊为 BOS。肺泡蛋白沉积症和 DIP 是非常罕见的适应证,但可能有较高的复发率。α1-抗胰蛋白酶缺乏症移植后再发肺气肿的情况,可能被低估,但可能随着受体移植后生存时间延长而更为普遍。

原发性疾病的复发更突出了移植后监测的重要性和实用性。常规胸部 X 线及 HRCT 可以识别特定的与复发性疾病相一致的结果,特别是对于 BAC、PLCH 和 LAM。复发性疾病的影像学表现经常与原有疾病相似。肺功能检查可以检测出阻塞性缺陷特征如结节病、LAM、PLCH 和肺气肿,虽然这一手段难以单独区分移植排斥反应或感染。经纤维支气管镜或手术活检仍然是确认疾病复发的金标准,并强调了移植后监测性肺活检的重要性。

对于大多数类型的原发性肺疾病移植后复发的发病机制仍然知之甚少。在结节病和 LAM 中,原位杂交和免疫组织化学研究表明,复发性疾病可能源于受体免疫细胞浸润到移植肺。肺外受累 LCH 和 PLCH 移植后复发的相关性研究也支持一个可能,就是受体免疫细胞(朗格汉斯细胞)的转移和浸润机制。复发性 BAC 可能源于原生肺中的肿瘤细胞经气道播散,也许就是在移植的时候。在复发 PAP、DIP 和 GIP 中,没有公布的数据研究复发机制,尽管有假设认为这些疾病的异常受体免疫细胞(单个核细胞/巨噬细胞)可能发挥显著的作用。类似的机制可能会发生在复发 PCH 的受体招募循环中异常的内皮细胞。α1-抗胰蛋白酶缺乏导致的肺气肿复发可能是由于面对移植相关炎症(如继发于 BOS)时缺乏保护。

原发性疾病可能复发的认识促进了移植后使用预防和(或)早期治疗干预的实施。mTOR 抑制剂药物能有效预防或治疗 LAM 移植后复发。对于增强免疫抑制或系统性化疗多复发性 PLCH 和结节病有效。α1-抗胰蛋白酶替代疗法可以预防复发性肺气肿的发生或进展。肺移植术后戒烟的作用不像肝移植后戒酒那样明确。然而,戒烟可能在预防 PLCH、DIP 和 α1-抗胰蛋白酶缺乏导致肺气肿的复发方面发挥重要作用。精细的移植技术和仔细的自身肺气道灌注可有助于防止肿瘤细胞经气道播散和污染移植肺。

考虑到某些潜在的肺疾病在肺移植后复发的可能性，也许会对是否应该将这些疾病作为肺移植的适应证提出质疑。虽然部分疾病的复发率可能相当高,肺移植后肺失功的概率和死亡率是比较低的。BAC 就是重要代表,其复发是很常见的,常导致须反复行放疗或手术干预。在这种可能下,BAC 接受肺移植仍存在争议。重要的是,须再次指出,尽管 BAC 容易复发,移植后的存活率仍有改善。

总之,原发性肺疾病可能会在移植后复发,导致移植肺功能受到不同程度的影响。复发性肺疾病也是较为罕见的肺移植适应证。在大多数情况下,复发的可能性不应作为不行移植的理由。然而,移植受体和移植医生或外科医生应该了解潜在的疾病复发的临床症状和表现。特异性预防措施、药物治疗和早期治疗干预措施应该整合纳入临床规范。

(韩威力 译　韩威力 校)

参考文献

1. Baughman RP, Culver DA, Judson MA. A concise review of pulmonary sarcoidosis. American Journal of Respiratory and Critical Care Medicine. 2011;183:573–581.
2. Baughman RP, Teirstein AS, Judson MA, et al. Clinical characteristics of patients in a case control study of sarcoidosis. American Journal of Respiratory and Critical Care Medicine. 2001;164:1885–1889.
3. Hunninghake GW, Costabel U, Ando M, et al. ATS/ERS/WASOG statement on sarcoidosis. American Thoracic Society/European Respiratory Society/World Association of Sarcoidosis and other Granulomatous Disorders. Sarcoidosis, Vasculitis, and Diffuse Lung Diseases. 1999;16:149–173.
4. Harrison BD, Shaylor JM, Stokes TC, et al. Airflow limitation in sarcoidosis: a study of pulmonary function in 107 patients with newly diagnosed disease. Respiratory Medicine. 1991;85:59–64.
5. Handa T, Nagai S, Fushimi Y, et al. Clinical and radiographic indices associated with airflow limitation in patients with sarcoidosis. Chest. 2006;130:1851–1856.
6. Gibson GJ, Prescott RJ, Muers MF, et al. British Thoracic Society Sarcoidosis study: effects of long term corticosteroid treatment. Thorax. 1996;51:238–247.
7. McKinzie BP, Bullington WM, Mazur JE, et al. Efficacy of short-course, low-dose corticosteroid therapy for acute pulmonary sarcoidosis exacerbations. American Journal of the Medical Sciences. 2010;339:1–4.
8. Baughman RP, Winget DB, Lower EE. Methotrexate is steroid sparing in acute sarcoidosis: results of a double blind, randomized trial. Sarcoidosis, Vasculitis, and Diffuse Lung Diseases. 2000;17:60–66.
9. Muller-Quernheim J, Kienast K, Held M, et al. Treatment of chronic sarcoidosis with an azathioprine/prednisolone regimen. European Respiratory Journal. 1999;14:1117–1122.
10. Baughman RP, Lower EE. Leflunomide for chronic sarcoidosis. Sarcoidosis, Vasculitis, and Diffuse Lung Diseases. 2004;21:43–48.
11. Kouba DJ, Mimouni D, Rencic A, et al. Mycophenolate mofetil may serve as a steroid-sparing agent for sarcoidosis. British Journal of Dermatology. 2003;148:147–148.
12. Baughman RP, Drent M, Kavuru M, et al. Infliximab therapy in patients with chronic sarcoidosis and pulmonary involvement. American Journal of Respiratory and Critical Care Medicine. 2006;174:795–802.
13. Rossman MD, Newman LS, Baughman RP, et al. A double-blinded, randomized, placebo-controlled trial of infliximab in subjects with active pulmonary sarcoidosis. Sarcoidosis, Vasculitis, and Diffuse Lung Diseases. 2006;23:201–208.
14. Christie JD, Edwards LB, Kucheryavaya AY, et al. The registry of the International Society for Heart and Lung Transplantation: twenty-eighth adult lung and heart-lung transplant report, 2011. Journal of Heart and Lung Transplantation. 2011;30:1104–1122.
15. Ionescu DN, Hunt JL, Lomago D, et al. Recurrent sarcoidosis in lung transplant allografts: granulomas are of recipient origin. Diagnostic Molecular Pathology. 2005;14:140–145.
16. Padilla ML, Schilero GJ, Teirstein AS. Sarcoidosis and transplantation. Sarcoidosis, Vasculitis, and Diffuse Lung Diseases. 1997;14:16–22.
17. Milman N, Burton C, Andersen CB, et al. Lung transplantation for end-stage pulmonary sarcoidosis: outcome in a series of seven consecutive patients. Sarcoidosis, Vasculitis, and Diffuse Lung Diseases. 2005;22:222–228.
18. Johnson BA, Duncan SR, Ohori NP, et al. Recurrence of sarcoidosis in pulmonary allograft recipients. American Review of Respiratory Disease. 1993;148:1373–1377.
19. Scott J, Higenbottam T. Transplantation of the lungs and heart and lung for patients with severe pulmonary complications from sarcoidosis. Sarcoidosis. 1990;7:9–11.
20. Bjortuft O, Foerster A, Boe J, et al. Single lung transplantation as treatment for end-stage pulmonary sarcoidosis: recurrence of sarcoidosis in two different lung allografts in one patient. Journal of Heart and Lung Transplantation. 1994;13:24–29.
21. Martinez FJ, Orens JB, Deeb M, et al. Recurrence of sarcoidosis following bilateral allogeneic lung transplantation. Chest. 1994;106:1597–1599.
22. Milman N, Andersen CB, Burton CM, et al. Recurrent sarcoid granulomas in a transplanted lung derive from recipient immune cells. European Respiratory Journal. 2005;26:549–552.
23. Kazerooni EA, Cascade PN. Recurrent miliary sarcoidosis after lung transplantation. Radiology. 1995;194:913.
24. Kazerooni EA, Jackson C, Cascade PN. Sarcoidosis: recurrence of primary disease in transplanted lungs. Radiology. 1994;192:461–464.
25. Nunley DR, Hattler B, Keenan RJ, et al. Lung transplantation for end-stage pulmonary sarcoidosis. Sarcoidosis, Vasculitis, and Diffuse Lung Diseases. 1999;16:93–100.
26. Heatly T, Sekela M, Berger R. Single lung transplantation involving a donor with documented pulmonary sarcoidosis. Journal of Heart and Lung Transplantation. 1994;13:720–723.
27. Urban T, Lazor R, Lacronique J, et al. Pulmonary lymphangioleiomyomatosis: a study of 69 patients. Groupe d'Etudes et de Recherche sur les Maladies "Orphelines" Pulmonaires (GERM"O"P). Medicine (Baltimore). 1999;78:321–337.
28. Kitaichi M, Nishimura K, Itoh H, et al. Pulmonary lymphangioleiomyomatosis: a report of 46 patients including a clinicopathologic study of prognostic factors. American Journal of Respiratory and Critical Care Medicine. 1995;151:527–533.
29. Muzykewicz DA, Sharma A, Muse V, et al. TSC1 and TSC2 mutations in patients with lymphangioleiomyomatosis and tuberous sclerosis complex. Journal of Medical Genetics. 2009;46:465–468.
30. Johnson SR. Lymphangioleiomyomatosis. European Respiratory Journal. 2006;27:1056–1065.
31. McCormack FX. Lymphangioleiomyomatosis: a clinical update. Chest. 2008;133:507–516.
32. Zhe X, Schuger L. Combined smooth muscle and melanocytic differentiation in lymphangioleiomyomatosis. Journal of Histochemistry and Cytochemistry. 2004;52:1537–1542.
33. Johnson SR, Tattersfield AE. Decline in lung function in lymphangioleiomyomatosis: relation to menopause and progesterone treatment. American Journal of

Respiratory and Critical Care Medicine. 1999;160:628-633.
34. Taylor JR, Ryu J, Colby TV, et al. Lymphangioleiomyomatosis: clinical course in 32 patients. New England Journal of Medicine. 1990;323:1254–1260.
35. Oh YM, Mo EK, Jang SH, et al. Pulmonary lymphangioleiomyomatosis in Korea. Thorax. 1999;54:618–621.
36. Taille C, Borie R, Crestani B. Current management of lymphangioleiomyomatosis. Current Opinion in Pulmonary Medicine. 2011;17:374–378.
37. Goncharova EA, Goncharov DA, Spaits M, et al. Abnormal growth of smooth muscle-like cells in lymphangioleiomyomatosis: role for tumor suppressor TSC2. American Journal of Respiratory Cell and Molecular Biology. 2006;34:561–572.
38. Taille C, Debray MP, Crestani B. Sirolimus treatment for pulmonary lymphangioleiomyomatosis. Annals of Internal Medicine. 2007;146:687–688.
39. Bissler JJ, McCormack FX, Young LR, et al. Sirolimus for angiomyolipoma in tuberous sclerosis complex or lymphangioleiomyomatosis. New England Journal of Medicine. 2008;358:140–151.
40. Davies DM, Johnson SR, Tattersfield AE, et al. Sirolimus therapy in tuberous sclerosis or sporadic lymphangioleiomyomatosis. New England Journal of Medicine. 2008;358:200–203.
41. Davies DM, de Vries PJ, Johnson SR, et al. Sirolimus therapy for angiomyolipoma in tuberous sclerosis and sporadic lymphangioleiomyomatosis: a phase 2 trial. Clinical Cancer Research. 2011;17:4071–4081.
42. McCormack FX, Inoue Y, Moss J, et al. Efficacy and safety of sirolimus in lymphangioleiomyomatosis. New England Journal of Medicine. 2011;364: 1595–1606.
43. Benden C, Rea F, Behr J, et al. Lung transplantation for lymphangioleiomyomatosis: the European experience. Journal of Heart and Lung Transplantation. 2009;28:1-7.
44. Kpodonu J, Massad MG, Chaer RA, et al. The US experience with lung transplantation for pulmonary lymphangioleiomyomatosis. Journal of Heart and Lung Transplantation. 2005;24:1247–1253.
45. Boehler A. Lung transplantation for cystic lung diseases: lymphangioleiomyomatosis, histiocytosis x, and sarcoidosis. Seminars in Respiratory and Critical Care Medicine. 2001;22:509–516.
46. Boehler A, Speich R, Russi EW, et al. Lung transplantation for lymphangioleiomyomatosis. New England Journal of Medicine. 1996;335:1275–1280.
47. Karbowniczek M, Astrinidis A, Balsara BR, et al. Recurrent lymphangiomyomatosis after transplantation: genetic analyses reveal a metastatic mechanism. American Journal of Respiratory and Critical Care Medicine. 2003;167: 976–982.
48. O'Brien JD, Lium JH, Parosa JF, et al. Lymphangiomyomatosis recurrence in the allograft after single-lung transplantation. American Journal of Respiratory and Critical Care Medicine. 1995;151:2033–2036.
49. Nine JS, Yousem SA, Paradis IL, et al. Lymphangioleiomyomatosis: recurrence after lung transplantation. Journal of Heart and Lung Transplantation. 1994;13: 714–719.
50. Bittmann I, Dose TB, Muller C, et al. Lymphangioleiomyomatosis: recurrence after single lung transplantation. Human Pathology. 1997;28:1420–1423.
51. Bittmann I, Rolf B, Amann G, et al. Recurrence of lymphangioleiomyomatosis after single lung transplantation: new insights into pathogenesis. Human Pathology. 2003;34:95–98.
52. Chen F, Bando T, Fukuse T, et al. Recurrent lymphangioleiomyomatosis after living-donor lobar lung transplantation. Transplantation Proceedings. 2006;38:3151–3153.
53. Chen F, Omasa M, Kondo N, et al. Sirolimus treatment for recurrent lymphangioleiomyomatosis after lung transplantation. Annals of Thoracic Surgery. 2009;87: e6–7.
54. Astor TL, Wain J. Unpublished data, 2011.
55. Ohara T, Oto T, Miyoshi K, et al. Sirolimus ameliorated post lung transplant chylothorax in lymphangioleiomyomatosis. Annals of Thoracic Surgery. 2008;86:e7–8.
56. Morton JM, McLean C, Booth SS, et al. Regression of pulmonary lymphangioleiomyomatosis (PLAM)-associated retroperitoneal angiomyolipoma post-lung transplantation with rapamycin treatment. Journal of Heart and Lung Transplantation. 2008;27:462–465.
57. Sugimoto R, Nakao A, Yamane M, et al. Sirolimus amelioration of clinical symptoms of recurrent lymphangioleiomyomatosis after living-donor lobar lung transplantation. Journal of Heart and Lung Transplantation. 2008;27:921–924.
58. Dauriat G, Mal H, Thabut G, et al. Lung transplantation for pulmonary Langerhans' cell histiocytosis: a multicenter analysis. Transplantation. 2006;81: 746–750.
59. Juvet SC, Hwang D, Downey GP. Rare lung diseases III: pulmonary Langerhans' cell histiocytosis. Canadian Respiratory Journal. 2010;17:e55–62.
60. Vassallo R, Ryu JH, Schroeder DR, et al. Clinical outcomes of pulmonary Langerhans'-cell histiocytosis in adults. New England Journal of Medicine. 2002;346:484–490.
61. Watanabe R, Tatsumi K, Hashimoto S, et al. Clinico-epidemiological features of pulmonary histiocytosis X. Internal Medicine. 2001;40:998–1003.
62. Basset F, Corrin B, Spencer H, et al. Pulmonary histiocytosis X. American Review of Respiratory Disease. 1978;118:811–820.
63. Travis WD, Borok Z, Roum JH, et al. Pulmonary Langerhans cell granulomatosis (histiocytosis X). A clinicopathologic study of 48 cases. American Journal of Surgical Pathology. 1993;17:971–986.
64. Moore AD, Godwin JD, Muller NL, et al. Pulmonary histiocytosis X: comparison of radiographic and CT findings. Radiology. 1989;172:249–254.
65. Koyama M, Johkoh T, Honda O, et al. Chronic cystic lung disease: diagnostic accuracy of high-resolution CT in 92 patients. AJR. American Journal of Roentgenology. 2003;180:827–835.
66. Brauner MW, Grenier P, Tijani K, et al. Pulmonary Langerhans cell histiocytosis: evolution of lesions on CT scans. Radiology. 1997;204:497–502.
67. Housini I, Tomashefski JF Jr, Cohen A, et al. Transbronchial biopsy in patients with pulmonary eosinophilic granuloma: comparison with findings on open lung biopsy. Archives of Pathology and Laboratory Medicine. 1994;118:523–530.
68. Myers JL. Other diffuse lung diseases. In: Chung AM, Myers JL, Tazelaar HD, et al. editors. Thurlbeck's Pathology of the Lung, 3rd edition. New York: Thieme; 2005: 601–673.
69. Lieberman PH, Jones CR, Steinman RM, et al. Langerhans cell (eosinophilic) granulomatosis: a clinicopathologic study encompassing 50 years. American Journal of Surgical Pathology. 1996;20:519–552.
70. Emile JF, Wechsler J, Brousse N, et al. Langerhans' cell histiocytosis: definitive diagnosis with the use of monoclonal antibody O10 on routinely paraffin-embedded samples. American Journal of Surgical Pathology. 1995;19:636–641.
71. Mogulkoc N, Veral A, Bishop PW, et al. Pulmonary Langerhans' cell histiocytosis: radiologic resolution following smoking cessation. Chest. 1999;115:1452–1455.
72. Von Essen S, West W, Sitorius M, et al. Complete resolution of roentgenographic changes in a patient with pulmonary histiocytosis X. Chest. 1990;98:765–767.
73. Tazi A, Montcelly L, Bergeron A, et al. Relapsing nodular lesions in the course of adult pulmonary Langerhans cell histiocytosis. American Journal of Respiratory and Critical Care Medicine. 1998;157:2007–2010.
74. Schonfeld N, Frank W, Wenig S, et al. Clinical and radiologic features, lung function and therapeutic results in pulmonary histiocytosis X. Respiration; International Review of Thoracic Diseases. 1993;60:38–44.
75. Delobbe A, Durieu J, Duhamel A, et al. Determinants of survival in pulmonary Langerhans' cell granulomatosis (histiocytosis X). Groupe d'Etude en Pathologie Interstitielle de la Societe de Pathologie Thoracique du Nord. European Respiratory Journal. 1996;9:2002–2006.
76. Arico M, Girschikofsky M, Genereau T, et al. Langerhans cell histiocytosis in adults. Report from the International Registry of the Histiocyte Society. European Journal of Cancer. 2003;39:2341–2348.
77. Giona F, Caruso R, Testi AM, et al. Langerhans' cell histiocytosis in adults: a clinical and therapeutic analysis of 11 patients from a single institution. Cancer. 1997;80:1786–1791.
78. Tsele E, Thomas DM, Chu AC. Treatment of adult Langerhans cell histiocytosis with etoposide. Journal of the American Academy of Dermatology. 1992; 27:61–64.
79. Gabbay E, Dark JH, Ashcroft T, et al. Recurrence of Langerhans' cell granulomatosis following lung transplantation. Thorax. 1998;53:326–327.
80. Etienne B, Bertocchi M, Gamondes JP, et al. Relapsing pulmonary Langerhans cell histiocytosis after lung transplantation. American Journal of Respiratory and Critical Care Medicine. 1998;157:288–291.
81. Habib SB, Congleton J, Carr D, et al. Recurrence of recipient Langerhans' cell histiocytosis following bilateral lung transplantation. Thorax. 1998;53: 323–325.
82. Trulock EP, Edwards LB, Taylor DO, et al. The registry of the International Society for Heart and Lung Transplantation: twentieth official adult lung and heart-lung transplant report, 2003. Journal of Heart and Lung Transplantation. 2003;22:625–635.
83. Tazi A. Adult pulmonary Langerhans' cell histiocytosis. European Respiratory Journal. 2006 ;27:1272–1285.
84. Travis WD, Colby TV, Corrin B, et al. Histological typing of lung and pleural tumors. In: Colby TV, Corrin B, Shimosato Y, et al., editors. International Histological Classification of Tumors. 3rd ed. Berlin: Springer; 1999: 36–38.
85. Raz DJ, Kim JY, Jablons DM. Diagnosis and treatment of bronchioloalveolar carcinoma. Current Opinion in Pulmonary Medicine. 2007;13:290–296.
86. Raz DJ, He B, Rosell R, et al. Bronchioloalveolar carcinoma: a review. Clinical Lung Cancer. 2006;7:313–322.
87. Read WL, Page NC, Tierney RM, et al. The epidemiology of bronchioloalveolar carcinoma over the past two decades: analysis of the SEER database. Lung Cancer. 2004;45:137–142.
88. Raz DJ, Glidden DV, Odisho AY, et al. Clinical characteristics and survival of patients with surgically resected, incidentally detected lung cancer. Journal of

Thoracic Oncology. 2007;2:125–130.
89. Carretta A, Canneto B, Calori G, et al. Evaluation of radiological and pathological prognostic factors in surgically-treated patients with bronchoalveolar carcinoma. European Journal of Cardio-Thoracic Surgery. 2001;20:367–371.
90. Okada M, Nishio W, Sakamoto T, et al. Correlation between computed tomographic findings, bronchioloalveolar carcinoma component, and biologic behavior of small-sized lung adenocarcinomas. Journal of Thoracic and Cardiovascular Surgery. 2004;127:857–861.
91. Jung JI, Kim H, Park SH, et al. CT differentiation of pneumonic-type bronchioloalveolar cell carcinoma and infectious pneumonia. British Journal of Radiology. 2001;74:490–494.
92. Takashima S, Li F, Maruyama Y, et al. Discrimination of subtypes of small adenocarcinoma in the lung with thin-section CT. Lung Cancer. 2002;36:175–182.
93. Watanabe S, Watanabe T, Arai K, et al. Results of wedge resection for focal bronchioloalveolar carcinoma showing pure ground-glass attenuation on computed tomography. Annals of Thoracic Surgery. 2002;73:1071–1075.
94. Yamato Y, Tsuchida M, Watanabe T, et al. Early results of a prospective study of limited resection for bronchioloalveolar adenocarcinoma of the lung. Annals of Thoracic Surgery. 2001;71:971–974.
95. West HL, Crowley JJ, Vance RB, et al. Advanced bronchioloalveolar carcinoma: a phase II trial of paclitaxel by 96-hour infusion (SWOG 9714): a Southwest Oncology Group study. Annals of Oncology. 2005;16:1076–1080.
96. Scagliotti GV, Smit E, Bosquee L, et al. A phase II study of paclitaxel in advanced bronchioloalveolar carcinoma (EORTC trial 08956). Lung Cancer. 2005;50: 91–96.
97. Marchetti A, Martella C, Felicioni L, et al. EGFR mutations in non-small-cell lung cancer: analysis of a large series of cases and development of a rapid and sensitive method for diagnostic screening with potential implications on pharmacologic treatment. Journal of Clinical Oncology. 2005;23:857–865.
98. Miller VA, Hirsch FR, Johnson DH. Systemic therapy of advanced bronchioloalveolar cell carcinoma: challenges and opportunities. Journal of Clinical Oncology. 2005;23:3288–3293.
99. Miller VA, Kris MG, Shah N, et al. Bronchioloalveolar pathologic subtype and smoking history predict sensitivity to gefitinib in advanced non-small-cell lung cancer. Journal of Clinical Oncology. 2004;22:1103–1109.
100. Zorn GL Jr, McGiffin DC, Young KR Jr, et al. Pulmonary transplantation for advanced bronchioloalveolar carcinoma. Journal of Thoracic and Cardiovascular Surgery. 2003;125:45–48.
101. Gomez-Roman JJ, Del Valle CE, Zarrabeitia MT, et al. Recurrence of bronchioloalveolar carcinoma in donor lung after lung transplantation: microsatellite analysis demonstrates a recipient origin. Pathology International. 2005;55: 580–584.
102. Paloyan EB, Swinnen LJ, Montoya A, et al. Lung transplantation for advanced bronchioloalveolar carcinoma confined to the lungs. Transplantation. 2000;69: 2446–2448.
103. Shin MS, Ho KJ. Recurrent bronchioloalveolar carcinoma after lung transplantation: radiographic and histologic features of the primary and recurrent tumors. Journal of Thoracic Imaging. 2004;19:79–81.
104. Garver RI Jr, Zorn GL, Wu X, et al. Recurrence of bronchioloalveolar carcinoma in transplanted lungs. New England Journal of Medicine. 1999;340:1071–1074.
105. Etienne B, Bertocchi M, Gamondes JP, et al. Successful double-lung transplantation for bronchioalveolar carcinoma. Chest. 1997;112:1423–1424.
106. Barsky SH, Grossman DA, Ho J, et al. The multifocality of bronchioloalveolar lung carcinoma: evidence and implications of a multiclonal origin. Modern Pathology. 1994;7:633–640.
107. Shin SW, Breathnach OS, Linnoila RI, et al. Genetic changes in contralateral bronchioloalveolar carcinomas of the lung. Oncology. 2001;60:81–87.
108. Seymour JF, Presneill JJ. Pulmonary alveolar proteinosis: progress in the first 44 years. American Journal of Respiratory and Critical Care Medicine. 2002;166: 215–235.
109. Shah PL, Hansell D, Lawson PR, et al. Pulmonary alveolar proteinosis: clinical aspects and current concepts on pathogenesis. Thorax. 2000;55:67–77.
110. Rosen SH, Castleman B, Liebow AA. Pulmonary alveolar proteinosis. New England Journal of Medicine. 1958;258:1123–1142.
111. Trapnell BC, Whitsett JA, Nakata K. Pulmonary alveolar proteinosis. New England Journal of Medicine. 2003;349:2527–2539.
112. Gonzalez-Rothi RJ, Harris JO. Pulmonary alveolar proteinosis: further evaluation of abnormal alveolar macrophages. Chest. 1986;90:656–661.
113. Huizar I, Kavuru MS. Alveolar proteinosis syndrome: pathogenesis, diagnosis, and management. Current Opinion in Pulmonary Medicine. 2009;15:491–498.
114. Wasserman K, Blank N, Fletcher G. Lung lavage (alveolar washing) in alveolar proteinosis. American Journal of Medicine. 1968;44:611–617.
115. Ben-Abraham R, Greenfeld A, Rozenman J, et al. Pulmonary alveolar proteinosis: step-by-step perioperative care of whole lung lavage procedure. Heart and Lung: Journal of Critical Care. 2002;31:43–49.
116. Yamamoto H, Yamaguchi E, Agata H, et al. A combination therapy of whole lung lavage and GM-CSF inhalation in pulmonary alveolar proteinosis. Pediatric Pulmonology. 2008;43:828–830.
117. Bonfield TL, Kavuru MS, Thomassen MJ. Anti-GM-CSF titer predicts response to GM-CSF therapy in pulmonary alveolar proteinosis. Clinical Immunology. 2002;105:342–350.
118. Seymour JF, Begley CG, Dirksen U, et al. Attenuated hematopoietic response to granulocyte-macrophage colony-stimulating factor in patients with acquired pulmonary alveolar proteinosis. Blood. 1998;92:2657–2667.
119. Bonfield TL, Raychaudhuri B, Malur A, et al. PU.1 regulation of human alveolar macrophage differentiation requires granulocyte-macrophage colony-stimulating factor. American Journal of Physiology. Lung Cellular and Molecular Physiology. 2003;285:L1132–1136.
120. Seymour JF, Presneill JJ, Schoch OD, et al. Therapeutic efficacy of granulocyte-macrophage colony-stimulating factor in patients with idiopathic acquired alveolar proteinosis. American Journal of Respiratory and Critical Care Medicine. 2001;163:524–531.
121. Tagawa T, Yamasaki N, Tsuchiya T, et al. Living-donor lobar lung transplantation for pulmonary alveolar proteinosis in an adult: report of a case. Surgery Today. 2011;41:1142–1144.
122. Santamaria F, Brancaccio G, Parenti G, et al. Recurrent fatal pulmonary alveolar proteinosis after heart-lung transplantation in a child with lysinuric protein intolerance. Journal of Pediatrics. 2004;145:268–272.
123. Parker LA, Novotny DB. Recurrent alveolar proteinosis following double lung transplantation. Chest. 1997;111:1457–1458.
124. Murata H, Hara T, Matsumoto S, et al. Anesthetic management of a patient with a double inferior vena cava and pulmonary alveolar proteinosis who underwent bilateral living-donor lobar lung transplantation. Journal of Anesthesia. 2009; 23:583–586.
125. Huddleston CB, Bloch JB, Sweet SC, et al. Lung transplantation in children. Annals of Surgery. 2002;236:270–276.
126. Nishinakamura R, Wiler R, Dirksen U, et al. The pulmonary alveolar proteinosis in granulocyte macrophage colony-stimulating factor/interleukins 3/5 beta c receptor-deficient mice is reversed by bone marrow transplantation. Journal of Experimental Medicine. 1996;183:2657–2662.
127. Martinez-Moczygemba M, Doan ML, Elidemir O, et al. Pulmonary alveolar proteinosis caused by deletion of the GM-CSFRalpha gene in the X chromosome pseudoautosomal region 1. Journal of Experimental Medicine. 2008;205: 2711–2716.
128. Notarangelo LD, Pessach I. Out of breath: GM-CSFRalpha mutations disrupt surfactant homeostasis. Journal of Experimental Medicine. 2008;205: 2693–2697.
129. Yousem SA. Alveolar lipoproteinosis in lung allograft recipients. Human Pathology. 1997;28:1383–1386.
130. Gal AA, Bryan JA, Kanter KR, et al. Cytopathology of pulmonary alveolar proteinosis complicating lung transplantation. Journal of Heart and Lung Transplantation. 2004;23:135–138.
131. de Serres FJ. Worldwide racial and ethnic distribution of alpha1-antitrypsin deficiency: summary of an analysis of published genetic epidemiologic surveys. Chest. 2002;122:1818–1829.
132. Lieberman J, Winter B, Sastre A. Alpha 1-antitrypsin Pi-types in 965 COPD patients. Chest. 1986;89:370–373.
133. Carlson JA, Rogers BB, Sifers RN, et al. Accumulation of PiZ alpha 1-antitrypsin causes liver damage in transgenic mice. Journal of Clinical Investigation. 1989;83:1183–1190.
134. Kelly E, Greene CM, Carroll TP, et al. Alpha-1 antitrypsin deficiency. Respiratory Medicine. 2010;104:763–772.
135. Piitulainen E, Eriksson S. Decline in FEV1 related to smoking status in individuals with severe alpha1-antitrypsin deficiency (PiZZ). European Respiratory Journal. 1999;13:247–251.
136. Seersholm N, Wencker M, Banik N, et al. Does alpha1-antitrypsin augmentation therapy slow the annual decline in FEV1 in patients with severe hereditary alpha1-antitrypsin deficiency? Wissenschaftliche Arbeitsgemeinschaft zur Therapie von Lungenerkrankungen (WATL) alpha1-AT study group. European Respiratory Journal. 1997;10:2260–2263.
137. Wencker M, Banik N, Buhl R, et al. Long-term treatment of alpha1-antitrypsin deficiency-related pulmonary emphysema with human alpha1-antitrypsin. Wissenschaftliche Arbeitsgemeinschaft zur Therapie von Lungenerkrankungen (WATL)-alpha1-AT-study group. European Respiratory Journal. 1998;11: 428–433.
138. Hubbard RC, McElvaney NG, Sellers SE, et al. Recombinant DNA-produced alpha 1-antitrypsin administered by aerosol augments lower respiratory tract antineutrophil elastase defenses in individuals with alpha 1-antitrypsin deficiency. Journal of Clinical Investigation. 1989;84:1349–1354.
139. Birrer P, McElvaney NG, Gillissen A, et al. Intravenous recombinant secretory

leukoprotease inhibitor augments antineutrophil elastase defense. Journal of Applied Physiology. 1992;73:317-323.
140. Glanville AR, Hopkins PM, Aboyoun CL, et al. Recurrent emphysema after lung transplantation for alpha-1 antitrypsin deficiency (abstract). American Journal of Respiratory and Critical Care Medicine. 2002;165.
141. Mal H, Guignabert C, Thabut G, et al. Recurrence of pulmonary emphysema in an alpha-1 proteinase inhibitor-deficient lung transplant recipient. American Journal of Respiratory and Critical Care Medicine. 2004;170:811-814.
142. King MB, Campbell EJ, Gray BH, et al. The proteinase-antiproteinase balance in alpha-1-proteinase inhibitor-deficient lung transplant recipients. American Journal of Respiratory and Critical Care Medicine. 1994;149:966-971.
143. Meyer KC, Nunley DR, Dauber JH, et al. Neutrophils, unopposed neutrophil elastase, and alpha1-antiprotease defenses following human lung transplantation. American Journal of Respiratory and Critical Care Medicine. 2001;164:97-102.
144. Trulock EP. Lung transplantation for alpha 1-antitrypsin deficiency emphysema. Chest. 1996;110(Suppl):284S-94S.
145. American Thoracic Society/European Respiratory Society. American Thoracic Society/European Respiratory Society statement: standards for the diagnosis and management of individuals with alpha-1 antitrypsin deficiency. American Journal of Respiratory and Critical Care Medicine. 2003;168:818-900.
146. Tazelaar HD, Wright JL, Churg A. Desquamative interstitial pneumonia. Histopathology. 2011;58:509-516.
147. Carrington CB, Gaensler EA, Coutu RE, et al. Natural history and treated course of usual and desquamative interstitial pneumonia. New England Journal of Medicine. 1978;298:801-809.
148. King MB, Jessurun J, Hertz MI. Recurrence of desquamative interstitial pneumonia after lung transplantation. American Journal of Respiratory and Critical Care Medicine. 1997;156:2003-2005.
149. Verleden GM, Sels F, Van Raemdonck D, et al. Possible recurrence of desquamative interstitial pneumonitis in a single lung transplant recipient. European Respiratory Journal. 1998;11:971-974.
150. Verleden GM. Recurrence of desquamative interstitial pneumonia after lung transplantation. American Journal of Respiratory and Critical Care Medicine. 1998;157:1349-1350.
151. Paris C, Pairon JC, Billon-Galland MA, et al. Giant cell interstitial pneumonia: report of two cases with high titanium concentration in the lung. American Journal of Respiratory and Critical Care Medicine. 2011;184:1315-1317.
152. Nemery B, Abraham JL. Hard metal lung disease: still hard to understand. American Journal of Respiratory and Critical Care Medicine. 2007;176:2-3.
153. Frost AE, Keller CA, Brown RW, et al. Giant cell interstitial pneumonitis: disease recurrence in the transplanted lung. American Review of Respiratory Disease. 1993;148:1401-1404.
154. Keicho N, Hijikata M. Genetic predisposition to diffuse panbronchiolitis. Respirology. 2011;16:581-588.
155. Baz MA, Kussin PS, Van Trigt P, et al. Recurrence of diffuse panbronchiolitis after lung transplantation. American Journal of Respiratory and Critical Care Medicine. 1995;151:895-898.
156. Eltorky MA, Headley AS, Winer-Muram H, et al. Pulmonary capillary hemangiomatosis: a clinicopathologic review. Annals of Thoracic Surgery. 1994;57:772-776.
157. Lippert JL, White CS, Cameron EW, et al. Pulmonary capillary hemangiomatosis: radiographic appearance. Journal of Thoracic Imaging. 1998;13:49-51.
158. Dufour B, Maitre S, Humbert M, et al. High-resolution CT of the chest in four patients with pulmonary capillary hemangiomatosis or pulmonary venoocclusive disease. American Journal of Roentgenology. 1998;171:1321-1324.
159. Tron V, Magee F, Wright JL, et al. Pulmonary capillary hemangiomatosis. Human Pathology. 1986;17:1144-1150.
160. de Perrot M, Waddell TK, Chamberlain D, et al. De novo pulmonary capillary hemangiomatosis occurring rapidly after bilateral lung transplantation. Journal of Heart and Lung Transplantation. 2003;22:698-700.
161. Lee C, Suh RD, Krishnam MS, et al. Recurrent pulmonary capillary hemangiomatosis after bilateral lung transplantation. Journal of Thoracic Imaging. 2010;25:W89-92.
162. Williams H, Campbell P. Generalized bronchiectasis associated with deficiency of cartilage in the bronchial tree. Archives of Disease in Childhood. 1960;35:182-191.
163. Newman KB, Beam WR. Congenital bronchiectasis in an adult. American Journal of Medicine. 1991;91:198-201.
164. Palmer SM Jr, Layish DT, Kussin PS, et al. Lung transplantation for Williams-Campbell syndrome. Chest. 1998;113:534-537.
165. Novick RJ, Ahmad D, Menkis AH, et al. The importance of acquired diffuse bronchomalacia in heart-lung transplant recipients with obliterative bronchiolitis. Journal of Thoracic and Cardiovascular Surgery. 1991;101:643-648.

第 81 章 肾移植排斥反应和复发疾病的组织病理学综合征

Alton Brad Farris, III, Michael H. Mengel

引言

在过去近 50 年中,肾移植的成功率已有了显著提高[1]。自从 1954 年第一例肾移植成功以来,免疫抑制剂已经能够有效控制和治疗急性排斥反应, 特别是发生于移植后 1 年内的早期排斥反应[2]。然而,挑战仍然存在,如后期的细胞性和体液性排斥反应(AMR)的治疗,以及慢性排斥反应及复发性肾病的预防[1]。

肾活检是临床医生一项行之有效的辅助诊断手段。肾活检为近 40%的患者的治疗方案的改变提供证据,导致近 20%的患者的免疫抑制剂的使用剂量减少[3-5]。大部分移植肾活检主要是常规光镜下组织病理学表现的评估,而免疫荧光和电子显微镜(EM)等技术对移植肾活检病理诊断也是至关重要的。如今,分子学评估等新技术也正在迅速兴起。肾活检作为重要的诊断手段贯穿于肾移植的整个过程。在移植前,供肾活检用于评估和筛选供肾; 在移植后早期, 用于确诊移植肾的排斥反应;在移植后晚期,当考虑慢性排斥反应、复发和(或)新发疾病及感染时,则须行移植肾活检[3]。本章主要阐述移植排斥反应的主要类型、移植肾其他相关疾病、以及可能出现的新发和复发性肾病。

移植肾排斥反应

1991 年,在 Kim Solez 博士建立 Banff 分类标准之前,并没有统一的排斥反应的诊断标准。排斥反应的诊断主要是依据各地的临床经验和病理学家的个人判断[6-12]建立。自 20 世纪 90 年代初以来,共识标准由专家小组开发并不断细化[9]。它最初用于肾移植病理,然后推广至其他实体器官移植病理[9]。移植肾排斥反应通常可以归因于细胞介导或抗体(体液因素)介导的机制,或者两者同时存在[5,13]。

急性排斥反应是指由于移植肾的免疫损伤而引起相对快速的肾功能恶化,通常发生在几天内。虽然使用了“急性”这个词,但移植肾急性排斥反应在移植后的几个小时内或者几年内都有可能发生。而急性排斥反应的进展通常是在短时间内发生的[14]。相反,慢性排斥反应是指潜在的移植肾损伤引起的肾功能缓慢恶化,发生和进展的时间通常达几个月甚至几年 [14]。此外,“慢性”这个词也适用于各种移植物组织结构重塑后观察到的形态学改变 (如动脉内膜的纤维化或肾小球基底膜双轨化)。在这些过程中有着不同的临床表现,而诊断依赖于移植肾穿刺活检。

依据 Banff 1997 定义的标准,一份“合格”活检标本至少应包括 10 个肾小球和 2 条动脉,而一份“最小”标本应该包括 7 个肾小球和 1 条动脉。推荐至少两份穿刺标本。此外,建议同一份穿刺标本至少有两个不同区域的皮质。移植肾活检的病理评估最好是有 7 份组织切片,包含多个连续厚 3~4μm 的组织,并按如下染色:3 份切片使用苏木精和伊红(HE)染色,3 份使用过碘酸雪夫(PAS)染色或银染色,以及一份进行三色染色[7,15]。此外,由于 C4d 是目前 Banff 分类标准中重要的一部分,C4d 染色通常使用荧光免疫或免疫组化法[8]。根据组织学活检的评分标准, 将肾脏组织各部分形态进行病理半定量评分。参照 Banff 统一的诊断标准(表

81.1 和表 81.2)，得出最终的病理诊断。值得注意的是，不同观察者间的组织学评分是存在差异的，而这种局限性的存在也为未来的改进和技术进步提供了可能[16]。排斥反应的效应机制同样作用在其他免疫介导的肾脏疾病中，因此一些相关的组织学表现也值得关注。

细胞介导排斥反应

细胞介导排斥反应(CMR)，在大多数情况下，是由来自淋巴器官的效应 T 细胞浸润移植物所导致的炎症反应(参见第 5 章)。因此，“细胞介导排斥反应”一词通常是指 T 细胞介导的排斥反应(TCMR)。T 细胞主要是针对供体抗原而引起反应的[14,17]。间质由 T 细胞浸润，最终导致小管炎改变（即肾小管上皮细胞间的 T 细胞浸润）。其中，小管炎是许多排斥反应的早期标志(图 81.1)[5,18]。而间质浸润的大部分细胞是由 $CD4^+$、$CD8^+$ T 细胞和 $CD68^+$ 单核巨噬细胞组成。嗜酸性粒细胞有时也会存在，它可能提示更差的预后[13,19]。肾小管也会上调 HLA-DR 的表达[20]。然而，尽管小管炎常被认为是 TCMR 的特异性表现，但最近的研究表明小管炎可能是上皮损伤导致的结果，而非引起上皮损伤的原因[21]。此外，小管炎也可能出现在移植肾的其他疾病或原位肾的肾脏疾病中。

急性肾小管间质排斥反应包括间质水肿与单核细胞浸润，并伴有小管炎病变。对满足 Banff 诊断标准的急性 CMR(表 81.1)，分别使用“i”和“t”评分评估间质

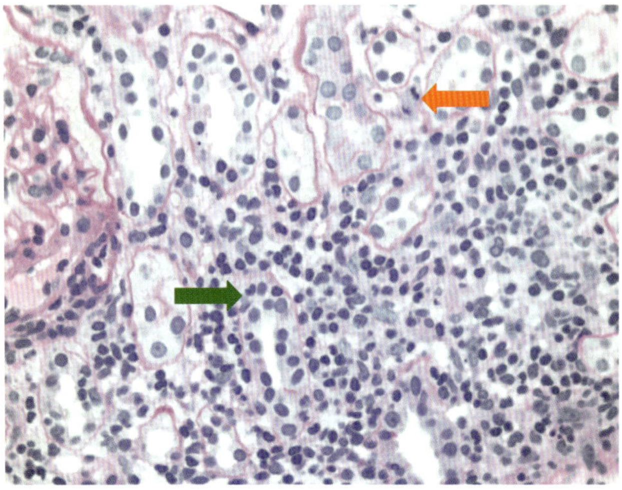

图 81.1 间质炎症和小管炎。在急性细胞性排斥反应Ⅰ型中，间质炎症伴随“活跃”浸润，表现为明显的有丝分裂活动(橙色箭头)和小管炎(绿色箭头)。

淋巴细胞浸润和小管炎的程度(表 81.2)。急性 CMR 的 IA 型表现为“中度”(t2，或 5~10 个炎细胞/肾小管切面)的移植肾小管炎，并伴有“显著”炎性浸润(i2 或 i3，>25%的非瘢痕的肾皮质区域受累)。如果急性小管间质排斥反应的程度更剧烈，病理学表现为更严重的小管炎(t3)，则诊断为急性 CMR 的 IB 型，其预后将会更差。严重的肾小管间质急性 CMR 表现为肾小管基底膜的多灶破坏，提示发生了肾单位不可逆的损伤[8,22]。

在急性小管间质性排斥反应分类中，存在一个“灰色地带”，表现为小管炎(t1、t2 或 t3)却没有实质性的炎细胞间质浸润(只有 i0 或 i1)或者有间质浸润但仅伴有轻微的小管炎(t1)。这种情况被称为“临界”或“可疑”的急性 CMR[8]。对于这种病变的解释仍存在争议，往往取决于不同中心或研究原则。一些临床中心认为这种临界改变是排斥反应，而其他中心却认为不是[5]。最近的一项研究用基因表达来分析临界改变，显示 1/3 的病例表现为分子表型与“真实”的 TCMR 一致，而 2/3 的病例没有证据表明排斥反应[23]。过去的研究也表明，对某些病例进行保守治疗可能是恰当的[24]。因此，希望未来的研究和指南可以明确临界改变的定义范畴，最终有助于消除这种模糊的灰色地带[23]。

浆细胞为主的急性排斥反应类型表现为间质大量的浆细胞浸润。此外，某些情况下可能表现为显著的水肿。以上这种形式的急性排斥反应往往伴有一个急进性的过程，可能提示预后较差。然而，前文提到的这些情况是基于抗体检测和多瘤病毒筛查阴性而言的。实际上有可能存在潜在的 AMR 或多瘤病毒相关性肾病(PVAN)。有时可以发现 C4d 在管周毛细血管(PTC)沉积。然而，在许多情况下，尤其是排斥后期，AMR 成分可能并不明显，并同时存在细胞成分。PVAN 也经常表现为浆细胞的间质浸润、水肿和小管炎，因此诊断常常难以鉴别。同时，浆细胞的浸润需鉴别是否存在移植后淋巴细胞增殖性疾病(PTLD)，还可以通过对 κ 轻链和 λ 轻链染色，检测是否存在单克隆浆细胞[25-27]。

此外，血管可能由炎细胞浸润而导致内皮细胞的破坏。这个过程被称为内皮炎、血管性排斥，或者更准确地说是动脉内膜炎(图 81.2)[5]。如果存在轻到中度动脉内膜炎(特指 V1)，根据 Banff 标准可诊断为急性 CMR 的ⅡA 型。如果严重动脉炎(v2)，可以诊断急性 CMR 的ⅡB 型[8]。若出现ⅡB，则其预后较 Banff 分类的ⅡA 型差[28]。如出现透壁性动脉炎和(或)动脉纤维素样改

表 81.1 移植肾病理 Banff 分类标准:最新的诊断分类摘要

分类	特征
一类	正常
二类	抗体介导的改变(可与三、四、五和六类同时存在)
	(一)急性/活动性抗体介导排斥反应(诊断需同时具备以下 3 个条件)[a,b]
	1.急性组织损伤的组织学证据(包括以下 1 个或多个表现)
	(1)微血管炎症[g>0[c] 和(或)ptc>0]
	(2)内膜或者透壁性动脉炎(v>0)[d]
	(3)急性微血栓性血管病,无其他病因存在
	(4)急性肾小管损伤,无其他明显病因
	2.当前/近期存在抗体与血管内皮细胞相互作用的证据(包括以下至少一种)
	(1)管周毛细血管 C4d 呈线性沉积(冰冻切片免疫荧光染色 C4d 评分为 2 分或 3 分,或石蜡切片免疫组化染色 C4d 评分>0)
	(2)中度以上微血管炎症[(g+ptc)>2][e]
	(3)明确证实活检组织中内皮细胞损伤相关的转录因子表达增加[f]
	3.供体特异性抗体的血清学证据(HLA 或其他抗原)
	(二)慢性活动性抗体介导排斥反应(诊断须同时具备以下 3 个条件)[a,g]
	1.性组织损伤的形态学证据(包括以下 1 个或多个)
	(1)移植肾小球病(cg>0)[h],无慢性血栓性微血管病(TMA)证据
	(2)严重的管周毛细血管基膜多层化(需电镜诊断)[i]
	(3)排除其他原因引起的新发生的动脉内膜纤维化
	2.当前/近期抗体与血管内皮相互作用的证据(包括以下至少 1 点)
	(1)管周毛细血管 C4d 线性沉积(冰冻切片免疫荧光染色 C4d 评分为 2 分或 3 分,或石蜡切片免疫组化染色 C4d 评分>0)[*]
	(2)中度以上微血管炎症[(g+ptc)>2][e]
	(3)明确证实活检组织中内皮细胞损伤相关的转录因子表达增加
	3.供体特异性抗体的血清学证据(HLA 或其他抗原)
	(三)无排斥反应证据的 C4d 沉积(诊断需同时包括以下 3 个特点)[j]
	1.肾小管周围毛细血管 C4d 线性沉积(冰冻切片免疫荧光染色 C4d 评分为 2 分或 3 分,或石蜡切片免疫组化染色 C4d 评分>0)[*]
	2. g=0,ptc=0,cg=0(光镜和电镜),v = 0;无血栓性微血管病,无肾小管周围毛细血管基膜多层化,无肾小管急性损伤(无其他明显原因)
	3.无 T 细胞介导的急性排斥反应(Banff 97 分级ⅠA 及以上)或者交界性改变
三类	临界病变,指"可疑"T 细胞介导的急性排斥反应(可与二、五和六类同时存在)
	无动脉内膜炎(v 0),但有灶性肾小管炎(t1、t2 或 t3)伴轻度间质炎(i0 或 i1),或者间质炎(i2 或 i3)伴轻度肾小管炎(t1)
四类	T 细胞介导的排斥反应(可与二、五和六类同时存在)
	(一)T 细胞介导的急性/活动性排斥反应(类型/级别)
	ⅠA:间质显著炎性浸润(>25%肾皮质区域,i2 或 i3),灶性中度肾小管炎(t2)
	ⅠB:间质显著炎性浸润(>25%肾皮质区域,i2 或 i3),灶性重度肾小管炎(t3)
	ⅡA:轻至中度动脉内膜炎(v1)
	ⅡB:重度动脉内膜炎,>25%管腔(v2)
	Ⅲ:"透壁性"动脉炎和(或)动脉纤维素样变性及中膜平滑肌坏死伴淋巴细胞浸润(v3)
	(二)T 细胞介导的慢性活动性排斥反应
	慢性移植物动脉病变(动脉内膜纤维化伴单核细胞浸润,新生内膜形成)
五类	肾小管萎缩-间质纤维化(无任何特异性病因证据),可包括非特异性血管硬化和肾小球硬化,但仅根据肾小管-间质病变程度进行分级
	Ⅰ级:轻度肾小管萎缩-间质纤维化(<25%肾皮质)
	Ⅱ级:中度肾小管萎缩-间质纤维化(26%~50%肾皮质)
	Ⅲ级:重度肾小管萎缩-间质纤维化(>50%肾皮质)

(待续)

表 81.1 移植肾病理 Banff 分类标准:最新的诊断分类摘要(续)

分类	特征
六类	其他 与急性和(或)慢性排斥反应无关的病变,单独出现 g、cg 或 cv 病变,或与二、三、四和五类同时存在

Source: Sis et al. 2010[8] and Haas et al. 2014[36]. Adapted with permission from John Wiley and Sons.

Ab,抗体;ABMR,抗体介导排斥反应;C4d+,按表 81.2 描述,C4d 在管周毛细血管内皮下沉积;Cat.,类别;EM,电镜;cg,Banff 慢性移植肾小球病评分;g,Banff 小球炎评分;i,Banff 间质炎症评分;IFTA,间质纤维化/小管萎缩;ptc,Banff 管周毛细血管炎评分;TCMR,T 细胞介导的排斥反应,±表示可能共存;v,Banff 动脉炎评分。

[*] 只要存在中度以上微血管炎症([g + ptc]>2)或内皮细胞损伤相关的转录因子表达增加,都可用来替代 C4d 沉积的指标用于诊断 ABMR。

[a] 所有的 ABMR 诊断都应该标明是 C4d 阳性(冰冻切片免疫荧光染色 C4d 评分为 2 分或 3 分,或石蜡切片免疫组化染色 C4d 评分>0),还是 C4d 阴性(冰冻切片免疫荧光染色 C4d 评分 0 或 1 分,或石蜡切片免疫组化染色 C4d 评分=0)。

[b] 这些病变可能是临床上急性或是亚临床的。活检显示已具备三个条件中的两个,则需要"怀疑"是急性/活动性 ABMR。也存在有特殊情况(见下文脚注 k):循环抗体存在和 C4d 阳性,却没有 ABMR 或 TCMR 相关的组织学证据(C4d 阳性却无排斥证据)。

[c] 复发的及新发的肾小球肾炎须排除。

[d] 动脉病变可能预示着 ABMR、TCMR 或是两者同时存在。"V"的评分须在动脉的两个或两个以上连续平滑肌层评估。

[e] 在存在急性 T 细胞介导排斥反应、临界改变或感染的情况下,单纯 ptc 评分≥2 不足以诊断中度以上微血管炎症,而必须同时具备 g 评分≥1。

[f] 目前符合标准被证实的分子标志物只有 ENDAT 的表达,而这也只在一个中心(Alberta 大学)被证实。若其他中心开展使用 ENDAT 表达或其他基因表达指标作为 ABMR 诊断证据,需要首先由 Sis 等进行独立的 ENDAT 表达验证。

[g] 慢性活动性 ABMR 病变可以只有电镜下早期移植肾小球病(cg 1a)的轻微活动病变,也可以表现为严重的移植肾小球病(TG)和其他慢性改变加上活动性微血管炎症。若缺乏现存的抗体与内皮相互作用的证据,则不应该诊断为"活动性"。这些抗体可能在活检时存在也可能在移植后早期即存在。

[h] 包括电镜下肾小球基底膜(GBM)分层(cg 1a)或光镜下 GBM 双轨表现。

[i] 一条皮质管周毛细血管≥7 层,合并另外两条毛细血管≥5 层,须避免部分横切。

[j] 在纤维内膜层中存在白细胞更倾向慢性排斥反应,可能是慢性 TCMR 或是慢性 ABMR。只有在既往没有发生过 TCMR 的情况下更有意义。虽然没有明确,弹力层染色或有助于鉴别,弹力层没有折光晶片更像是典型的慢性排斥反应,而有多层折光晶片存在则更倾向于动脉粥样硬化诊断。

[k] 在 ABO 血型不合肾移植中,移植肾与血型抗体间相关作用没有组织学损伤表现,而是表现为免疫适应状态。而 HLA 抗体的相关表现还需要更多临床数据。

变(考虑 v3),则可诊断为急性 CMR 的Ⅲ型;然而,这种情况通常伴有抗体介导参与其中[5,8]。值得注意的是,"血管排斥"这个词常用于异种移植中单纯的 AMR。研究表明存在动脉内膜炎往往提示更差的预后[29]。

Banff 2011 会议资料表明,"孤立性血管病变"(即有动脉内膜炎而没有显著的小管间质炎或毛细血管炎)实际上可能代表的是一个疾病过程。一项多中心回顾性队列研究显示,除了 AMR 外,另外两种类型的孤立性血管病变还包括 TCMR 相关和移植肾功能延迟恢复(DGF)相关。因此,针对动脉内膜炎,需要更加细化的诊断和个体化的治疗方法[30]。

间质纤维化和肾小管萎缩(IFTA)是慢性 CMR 和 AMR 最终共同的非特异性表现,也存在于移植肾退化的其他类型中[31]。然而,在 Banff 分类中,慢性 CMR 唯一公认的诊断标准是慢性移植物动脉病变,包括动脉内膜的纤维化伴有单核细胞浸润和新生动脉内膜的形成[8]。在 IFTA 中,肾小管萎缩、小管基底膜变厚皱缩,并伴有炎细胞浸润。根据目前的评分标准,IFTA 区域的炎症并不适用于 Banff 分类的 i 评分;然而,最近的研究表明,纤维化区域的炎症反应在慢性排斥反应和最终移植肾退化中有着关键作用,也是一个重要预后指标[32-34]。因此,一项新的评分体系被提出,用于总的间质炎症评分(ti 评分),目前正在进行观察者间重复性和临床实用性的评估[11,35]。为了明确硬化区域的炎症反应和 ti 评分的重要性,Banff 委员会成立了工作组来评估 T 细胞介导排斥反应的相关问题,包括"临界"浸润的

表 81.2 基于量化指标的 Banff 评分标准(data from [7] and [36])

病变	简写符号	Banff 评分			
		0	1	2	3
间质炎[a]	i	非瘢痕皮质区域中间质单核炎细胞浸润<10%	非瘢痕皮质区域中间质单核炎细胞浸润<10%~25%	非瘢痕皮质区域中间质单核炎细胞浸润<25%~50%	非瘢痕皮质区域中间质单核炎细胞浸润>50%
肾小管炎[b]	t	无	1~4 个单核炎细胞/小管横切面	5~10 个单核炎细胞/小管横切面	>10 个单核炎细胞/小管横切面,或者出现至少 2 个肾小管基膜损伤并伴有 i2/i3 和 t2
内膜动脉炎[c]	v	无	内皮下单核炎细胞累及管腔面积<25%	内皮下单核炎细胞累及管腔面积>25%,无坏死	透壁性炎症和(或)动脉纤维素样坏死伴单核细胞浸润
小球炎[d]	g	无	<25%肾小球有单核细胞浸润	26%~75%肾小球有单核细胞浸润	>75%肾小球有单核细胞浸润
管周毛细血管炎[e]	ptc	无或<10%皮质管周毛细血管有毛细血管炎	≥10%皮质管周毛细血管腔内 3~4 个炎性细胞	≥10%皮质管周毛细血管腔内 5~10 个炎性细胞	≥10%皮质管周毛细血管腔内炎性细胞>10 个
移植肾小球病[f]	cg	受累最重肾小球的血管袢双轨化区域<10%	受累最重肾小球的血管袢双轨化区域 10%~25%	受累最重肾小球的血管袢双轨化区域 26%~50%	受累最重肾小球的血管袢双轨化区域>50%
肾小球系膜基质增生[g]	mm	肾小球内无系膜基质增生	25%非硬化肾小球出现系膜基质增生	26%~50%非硬化肾小球出现系膜基质增生	50%以上非硬化肾小球出现系膜基质增生
间质纤维化	ci	肾皮质纤维化区域 0~5%	肾皮质纤维化区域 6%~25%	肾皮质纤维化区域 26%~50%	肾皮质纤维化区域> 50%
肾小管萎缩	ct	无肾小管萎缩	皮质肾小管萎缩区域≤25%	皮质肾小管萎缩区域 26%~50%	质肾小管萎缩区域>50%
动脉内膜纤维样增厚[h]	cv	无动脉内膜纤维样增厚	动脉内膜纤维样增厚导致管腔狭窄 1%~25%	动脉内膜纤维样增厚导致管腔狭窄 26%~50%	动脉内膜纤维样增厚导致管腔狭窄 > 50%
小动脉透明变性	ah	无小动脉透明变性	至少一条小动脉轻-中度透明变性	至少一条小动脉中-重度透明变性	许多小动脉重度透明变性
管周毛细血管基底膜多层化*	ptcml	电镜下 PTC 基底膜 1~2 层	电镜下 PTC 基底膜 3~4 层	电镜下 PTC 基底膜 5~6 层	电镜下 PTC 基底膜>6 层
总体间质炎症	ti	无或轻微(<10%实质)	10%~25%皮层实质	25%~50%皮层实质	>50%皮层实质
小动脉透明样增厚[k]	aah	无典型的 CNI 小动脉病变	仅 1 支小动脉病变,不伴有周围组织损伤	> 1 支,不伴有周围组织损伤	小动脉病变,伴有周围组织损伤,不计动脉的数量
PTC 的 C4d 免疫荧光染色[k]	C4d(IF)	0%活检区域内 PTC 环周线性染色,阴性	1 <10%活检区域内 PTC 环周线性样染色,轻微/阴性	10%~50%活检区域内 PTC 环周线性样染色,局灶未知	>50%活检区域内 PTC 环周线性样染色,弥漫阳性

(待续)

表 81.2 基于量化指标的 Banff 评分标准(data from [7] and [36])(续)

病变	简写符号	Banff 评分			
		0	1	2	3
PTC 的 C4d 免疫组化染色[k]	C4d(IHC)	0%活检区域内PTC 环周线性样染色,阴性	1 <10% 活检区域内PTC 环周线性样染色,轻微/未知	10%~50%活检区域内PTC 环周线性样染色,局灶阳性	>50%活检区域内 PTC 环周线性样染色,弥漫阳性

[a] 如果有"大量"的嗜酸性粒细胞、中性粒细胞或浆细胞须记录,用星号表示。

[b] 适用于不超过轻度萎缩的肾小管。

[c] 记录动脉的数量和受影响动脉的数量;用星号标注梗死和(或)间质出血。

[d] 因白细胞浸润和内皮细胞增大导致≥1条肾小球毛细血管完全或部分阻塞。

[e] 注明细胞成分(单核细胞和中性粒细胞)和程度(局灶≤50%;弥漫>50%)。

[f] 指受累最严重的肾小球;记录数量和硬化百分比。cg1a 指光镜下没有 GBM 双轨表现但电镜下可见 GBM 双轨表现,内皮肿胀和(或)内皮下电子透亮度增宽;cg1b 指≥1个非硬化的肾小球中存在≥1个双轨化表现,最好是电镜证实。

[g] 指至少中度增生,即至少相邻两个毛细血管间的系膜基质中>2个系膜细胞。

[h] 是慢性排斥反应的特征表现(纤维内膜增厚/新生内膜生成±内弹力层破口或存在单核细胞或泡沫细胞,±内弹力层破裂)。

[i] 提示动脉炎用星号标记。

[j] 可选的间质炎症评分,不常用于诊断。

[k] 可选的评分用于钙调磷酸酶抑制剂(CNI)引起的小动脉透明增厚(不常用于诊断)。

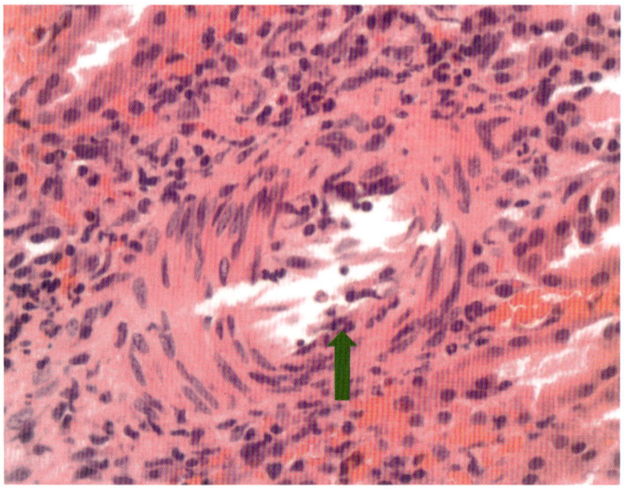

图 81.2 动脉炎。急性细胞性排斥反应 2 型的动脉内膜炎中,内皮下可以观察单核细胞浸润(绿色箭头)。

意义[36]。

急性 CMR,特别是在早期 CMR 仅伴有少量 IFTA 时,炎症反应在治疗后明显减轻。然而,有将近 50%的急性 CMR 在 1~2 个月后,活检组织中仍显示存在持续的炎症。在这些活检组织中,炎症主要仍存在于纤维化的区域内。某些情况下,当炎症细胞存在于血管内膜中或嵌入疏松的基质内,则可能是移植动脉病变的前驱表现[13]。这些表现增加了损伤相关的炎症反应与浸润介导的急性排斥反应相鉴别的难度。

抗体介导的排斥反应

自从第一例肾移植后的 50 年里,除了预存供体特异性抗体(DSA)介导的超急性排斥反应[37,38]外,T 细胞被认为是移植排斥的主要决定因素。然而,20 多年的时间里,我们逐渐认识到,移植物损伤很多是由抗体介导(体液)的排斥反应引起的,且主要是针对供体 HLA 的抗体[14]。因此,在 2001 年,AMR 作为诊断类别被纳入 Banff 分类标准中[6]。AMR 在移植肾失功的早期和晚期都有影响,特别是对晚期移植物失功影响更明显[39,40]。抗体损伤是通过补体激活,引起组织损伤,同时通过中性粒细胞和巨噬细胞募集,最终导致内皮损伤。水肿是由肥大细胞释放组胺引起的。内皮细胞黏附分子(如 E 选择蛋白、细胞黏附分子 1 和血管黏附分子 1)通过补体的作用而上调。最终,膜攻击复合 C5b-9 导致内皮细胞溶解。这个过程是复杂的,可能并不总是依赖于补体途径,已有研究表明,AMR 可以直接由 NK 细胞介导而独立于补体作用[3,14,41,42]。

临床上,AMR 大体可以分为两类:一类是发生在预存 DSA 而未完全脱敏患者的移植后早期;另一类是发生在移植后期,伴有新生 DSA 的产生。急性 AMR 在形态学上可表现为以下三种类型:

1 型/Ⅰ级，急性肾小管坏死（ATN）样的微炎症类型。

2 型/Ⅱ级，包含 PTC 和（或）肾小球炎（=微循环炎症）（图 81.3），有时伴有血栓。

3 型/Ⅲ级，血管纤维素样坏死（v3）。

根据当前的 Banff 共识标准，诊断 AMR 除了具备以上三类组织损伤其中一项证据外，还需要满足其他两个标准：循环中存在 DSA 和补体裂解产物 C4d 在 ptc 内皮的沉积（图 81.4）[8]。显微结构中，管周和肾小球毛细血管的内皮细胞出现损伤，表现为细胞增大、窗孔结构缺失、基底膜分离、溶解和细胞凋亡[43]。

慢性抗体介导排斥反应（CAMR）表现为肾脏微循环结构的重塑，也可表现为较大动脉内膜的增生，并继发 IFTA，最终导致移植肾功能下降。临床上，CAMR 可能伴有蛋白尿[13,44]。在显微结构中，肾小球基底膜增厚重叠导致“双轨化”的过程称为移植肾小球病[44]。在 Banff 标准中，CAMR 的诊断必须具备形态学上慢性结构重塑的证据、PTC 内皮上 C4d 沉积以及循环中 DSA 存在的证据[8]。慢性抗体介导的损伤在形态学上的证据包括：肾小球基底膜双轨化（图 81.5）、PTC 基底膜多层样表现、IFTA、动脉纤维层增厚[8]。至少需具备以上 4 项形态学损伤中的 2 项方可诊断 CAMR[5]。肾小球和 PTC 基底膜多层化被认为是诊断慢性移植肾排斥反应

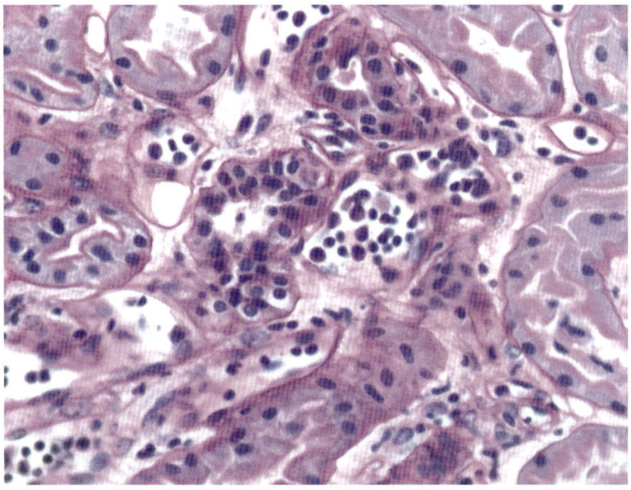
(A)

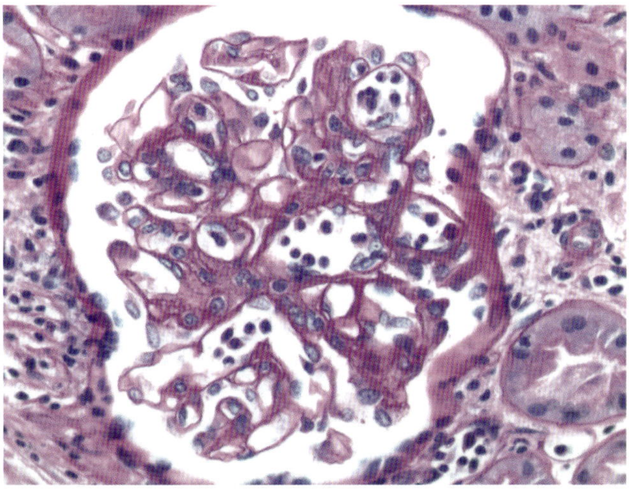
(B)

图 81.3 急性抗体介导排斥反应。在急性抗体介导排斥反应中可以看到（A）管周毛细管炎和（B）肾小球炎。

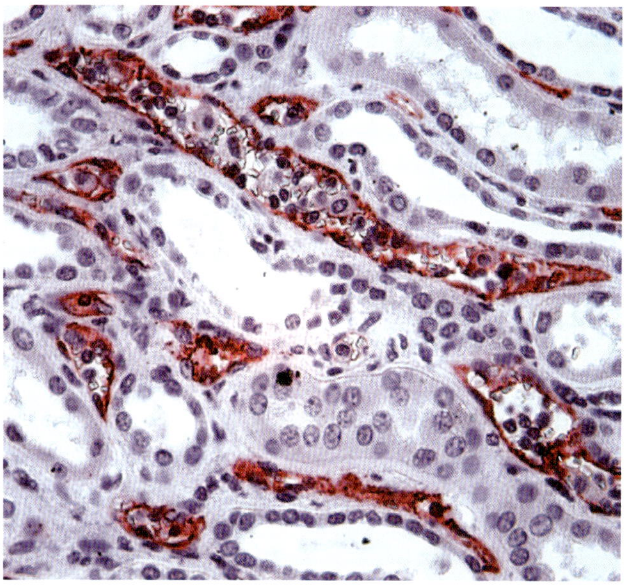
(A)

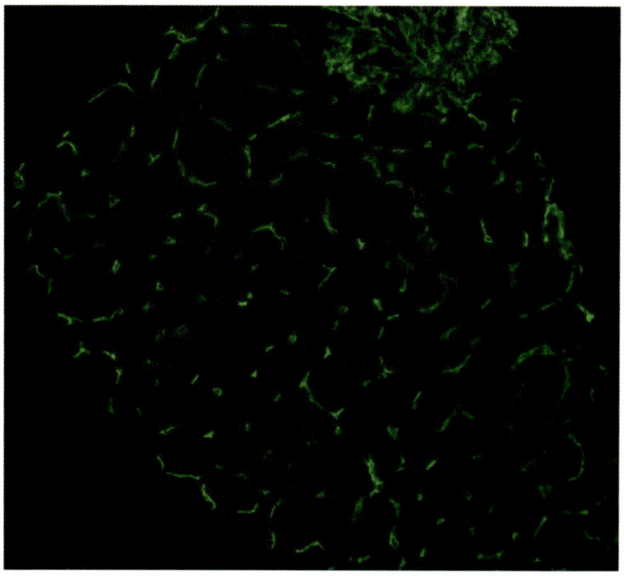
(B)

图 81.4 C4d 染色。在急性抗体介导排斥反应中，（A）C4d 在管周毛细血管内皮上呈线性、环形染色，（A）免疫组织化学（红发色体）和（B）免疫荧光（绿色荧光团）。

最有价值的证据[45]。此外，和急性 AMR 一样，典型的肾小球炎和管周毛细管炎也会在大多数 CAMR 的活检标本中出现。这些发现可以解释为，这是持续的疾病活动并进展的征象。肾小球炎细胞主要是由 $CD68^+$ 单核细胞、少量 $CD3^+$ T 细胞和偶尔出现的中性粒细胞组成。在 CAMR 中 ptc 有 C4d 沉积，而 C4d 染色也可以是肾小球双轨化的一种非特异性表现。CAMR 很可能发生在多个阶段，这个理论已经在非人灵长类动物模型中证实[46]。CAMR 最初被认为是由 DSA 产生引起，伴随 C4d 在 ptc 上的沉积，以及随后的急性和慢性形态学上微循环损伤，最终导致移植物功能异常。C4d 和 DSA 可以间歇性地出现在整个过程中。这些阶段可以发生

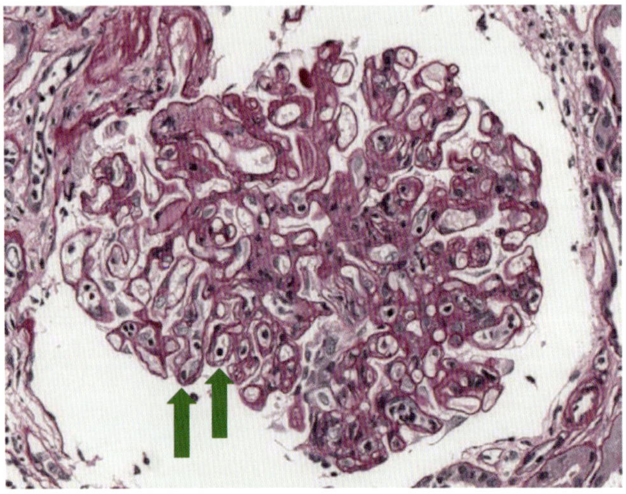

(A)

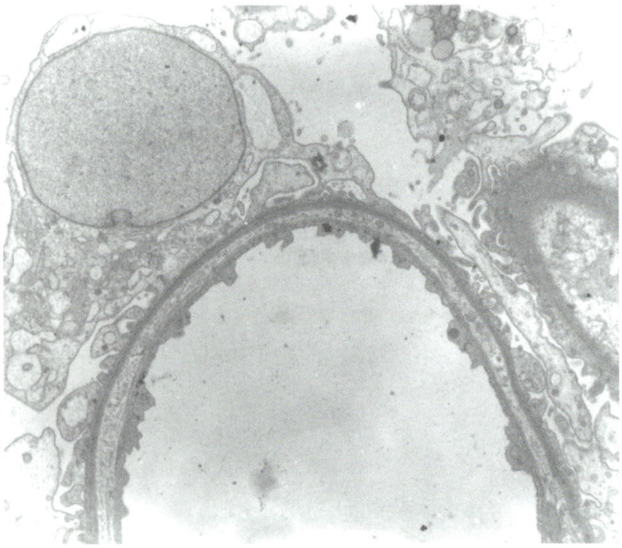

(B)

图 81.5 移植肾小球病。在慢性抗体介导排斥反应中，移植肾小球病在光镜上表现为肾小球基底膜分层(绿色箭头)。(B)电镜上，肾小球基底膜重分层更明显。

在几个月内或者持续存在数年，这主要取决于患者的依从性和免疫抑制状态[13,47]。

至于 AMR，最近 C4d 阴性的 AMR 引起了关注。是指有血清 DSA 证据和形态学上抗体介导损伤的证据，但在 PTC 内皮上 C4d 染色阴性。C4d 阴性的 AMR 可有以下多种解释：独立补体的抗体介导损伤；染色方法的敏感性和重复性差；"阳性" 定义标准的随意性；C4d 沉积在微循环中消退具有时间依赖性。分子学研究表明，存在 DSA 和有抗体介导损伤的形态学特征的情况下，存在内皮细胞相关转录因子表达增加，是内皮细胞应激的表现[48]。这些研究数据表明，根据当前 Banff 标准有 50%~60%的 AMR 因 C4d 染色阴性而无法诊断。目前，在 Banff 专门工作小组的努力下，C4d 阴性的 AMR 已经被纳入 Banff 诊断分类[30,36,49]。

AMR 与 CMR 可能同时存在，特别是发生在依从性差的患者中。存在大量间质炎性浸润和小管炎表现则倾向于诊断急性 CMR。单核细胞小管炎存在于 30%~80% 的急性 AMR 中，也被认为是并发 TCMR 的证据[5,50–52]。HLA-DR 的表达也提示并发 T 细胞和抗体介导排斥反应[5,53]。

免疫适应

有一种 AMR 相关的特殊状态被称为免疫适应。免疫适应是指存在 C4d 在 PTC 沉积的证据，但缺乏抗体介导损伤表现的一种状态。它被认为是内皮细胞与抗体及补体相适应的过程。在这些情况下，DSA 可以被检测到，然而没有形态学上组织损伤的证据。缺乏急性或慢性的 TCMR 或 AMR 的征象；更确切地说，是没有 ATN 样的微炎症，没有肾小球炎(g0)，没有慢性移植肾小球病(cg0)，没有管周毛细管炎(ptc0)和 PTC 基底膜多层化(电子显微镜下< 5 层)。根据目前 Banff 标准，这些情况被认为是 "C4d 沉积而没有急性排斥反应"，即使同时有临界改变，诊断也是不确定的[8]。免疫适应在 ABO 不相容移植中常被提及。这种情况相对少见，其长期意义仍在研究之中[13,54,55]。

不典型排斥反应综合征

新型免疫抑制方案会导致新的排斥反应类型。例如，阿仑单抗(CAMPATH-1H)可引起明显淋巴细胞耗竭[56–58]。以单核细胞占优势的急性 CMR(即急性单核细

胞的排斥反应）被认为与阿仑单抗引起的淋巴细胞耗竭有关。在以上排斥反应中，大部分的间质浸润以CD68 染色细胞为主,表现为相关肾脏功能异常和肾小管损伤,伴有 HLA-DR 染色。而 T 细胞在这种情况下与肾脏功能异常或 HLA-DR 染色无关[56]。

最近有研究提出骨髓和肾脏联合移植方案以诱导移植器官的免疫耐受。肾骨髓联合移植患者在 HLA 错配的肾移植后，保证肾功能正常的情况下撤除了维持免疫抑制剂[59]。而这些患者在非清髓的肾骨髓联合移植后 10 天左右出现了毛细血管渗漏或植入综合征。“植入综合征”表现为 ptc 充满了单核细胞和红细胞,并伴有急性肾小管损伤(ATI)。免疫组织化显示,这些细胞大多是 CD68$^+$ MPO$^+$的单核细胞和 CD3$^+$ CD8$^+$的 T 细胞，后者具有高增殖指数（Ki67$^+$）。荧光原位杂交(FISH)表明,ptc 的这些细胞来自受体。同时,嵌合性研究表明,这个时间段内供体循环细胞下降,受体循环细胞恢复。电子显微镜(EM)发现了 PTC 内皮细胞的损伤[59,60]。然而其他肾骨髓联合移植的患者并没有出现这种现象,该综合征的病因仍未明确[61]。

致敏患者尽管进行了脱敏治疗,但仍存在较高的AMR 风险。抑制补体级联反应被作为一种新的治疗选择。使用依库丽单抗的患者早期活检表明,存在广泛的 C4d 阳性但没有形态学上 AMR 的征象,也缺乏电镜下内皮细胞激活证据。事实证明,依库丽单抗靶目标——补体成分 C5 是处于 C4d 的下游。这就解释了弥漫的 C4d 阳性,却缺乏相应的病理学表现。这说明依库丽单抗同时保护了内皮。然而,少数患者尽管使用了依库丽单抗还是发生了 AMR，特别是慢性AMR 移植肾小球病(TG)[62]。这就说明,单单抑制补体并不能阻止慢性抗体介导微循环损伤的进展。此外,这些观察结果也说明使用 C4d 和 DSA 作为诊断依据的可靠性存在一定限制,需要更为细化的诊断标准。

移植肾常见其他疾病

排斥反应的鉴别诊断应考虑以下多种疾病（表81.1),包括各种感染、药物相关、外科问题[7]。后文讨论的急性肾小管损伤或坏死(ATI / ATN)也是一个常见的问题[7]。

在诊断急性排斥反应之前应首先排除感染[7]。移植肾也可能出现肾盂肾炎。通常,肾盂肾炎表现为更明显的中性粒细胞浸润,有时可出现中性粒细胞管型(图 81.8)。临床上尿常规检查和尿培养有助于诊断[5]。此外,很多病毒感染也会出现在肾移植中,其中一些将在后文讨论[7]。

有部分药物可能会影响到移植肾功能，如稍后讨论的钙调磷酸酶抑制剂(CNI)类免疫抑制剂在这方面的影响就很明显(图 81.6)。还有,移植肾中出现的急性间质性肾炎可能往往是由药物引起的。

肾移植中也常常会碰到尿路外科问题，其中包括尿路梗阻、反流和尿漏。尽管在过去的几十年中,外科技术的提高已经使外科并发症的发生率明显降低,但是外科并发症仍然是无法避免的。其主要原因还是与手术技术有关，包括输尿管缝合错位、输尿管长度不足、输尿管或肾盂撕裂。大部分输尿管并发症发生在术后第一周,与输尿管缺血性损伤有关。在这些情况下,吻合不当可能导致反流和(或)尿漏[5,63-66],其在移植肾病理活检相关的形态学特征与原位肾相似。有局部的肾小管扩张形成,偶尔可以看到肾小管基底膜破裂,并伴有局部炎症反应。

框 81.1　非排斥反应的鉴别诊断考虑

- 外科解剖性
  - 血管性(血管吻合问题、血栓形成、移植前急性内皮损伤)
  - 尿路性(梗阻/反流、尿漏)
- 感染性
  - 多瘤病毒肾病
  - 巨细胞病毒
  - 腺病毒
- 药物性
  - 钙调磷酸酶抑制剂作用
  - 药物相关或其他原因引起的急性间质性肾炎
- 移植后淋巴细胞增殖性疾病
- 急性肾小管损伤/坏死(各种病因,包括上述几种)
- 肾乳头坏死
- 非特异性
  - 局灶间质性炎症,无小管炎
  - 血管反应性改变
  - 小静脉炎
- 包膜下损伤或“愈合中”
- 复发/新发肾小球病

Adapted from [7] Racusen LC, Solez K, Colvin RB, et al. The Banff 97 working classification of renal allograft pathology. Kidney International. 1999;55:713-723 by permission from Macmillan Publishers ⓒ copyright 1999.

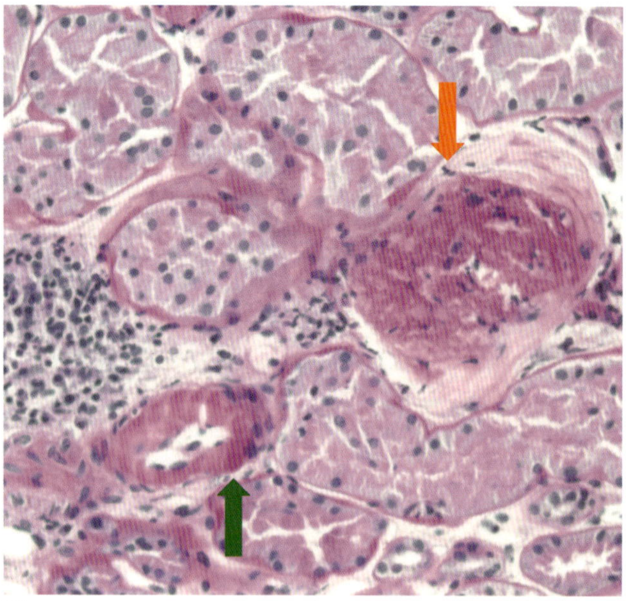

(A)

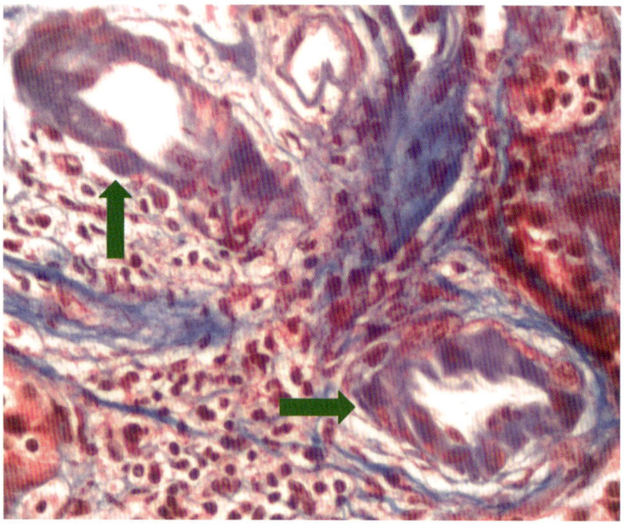

(B)

图81.6 小动脉透明变性。与慢性CNI毒性相关的小动脉透明变性类型在(A)PAS染色和(B)三色染色(绿色箭头)中都可以观察到。透明变性局部有结节,硬化的肾小球也可以看到(橙色箭头)。

血管相关外科问题也可能会发生，包括吻合不当导致的肾动脉狭窄[7,67–70]。血管问题可由器官获取时血管内膜的损伤、吻合口狭窄、严重创伤和肾静脉缩窄、受压或扭曲引起。这些问题在高凝状态的患者中,如V因子相关的Leiden病、抗磷脂抗体病、肾病综合征中显得更为复杂[13]。移植肾动脉狭窄可能是由于动脉粥样硬化、内膜肿胀、扭曲和移植后期慢性排斥反应引起的。肾动脉狭窄可引起肾素分泌增加,导致难治性高血压[71–73]。血管血栓形成可能会导致肾脏功能异常和肾实质的损伤[7,71–73]。因淋巴管处理不当所致的淋巴囊肿会引起轻度炎症反应,这可能达到"临界/可疑"急性CMR的诊断标准,而被错误地归类为CMR[74–76]。

血管问题可能存在非特异性的组织学变化，必须与排斥反应相鉴别。小静脉炎并不认为是特殊的移植肾排斥反应。此外,包膜下组织往往存在IFTA、炎症和肾小球硬化症;可是,包膜下组织的病理学表现的解释必须谨慎,因为包膜下的损伤或"修复"在移植肾中是一个相当常见的非特异性表现，不考虑特殊的排斥反应[5,7]。

急性肾小管损伤

肾单位的上皮细胞是影响肾脏功能和预后的关键因素[77–79]。然而,严重损伤的无功能肾脏的活检病理仍显示"正常"组织学表现或非特异性损伤,如刷状缘脱落、上皮细胞坏死和细胞变性。这突显了光学显微镜评估能力的局限性，尤其是在上皮损伤的潜在可逆的早期阶段。此外,肾单位去分化是从急性可逆损伤到慢性不可逆萎缩的一个连续过程。从形态学上,仍无法确定一个确切的转折时间点来判定损伤的肾小管何时萎缩。因此,大量的研究通过原位损伤标记物(如Kim-1、波形蛋白和整合素β6)来加强光学显微镜对上皮损伤的评估[80,81]。大量分子学、机械和成像数据证明,上皮细胞对任何类型的损伤表现为高度一致的反应[82,83]。这包括胚胎及发育途径的再表达；上皮细胞呈现出更多的间充质去分化表型,通常代表着一个暂时状态[84,85]。间充质表型的表达经常与邻近间质的炎症反应和基质产生增加共存。但是,至少在移植肾中,并没有令人信服的证据表明,纤维化是来源于迁移的去分化上皮细胞,还是来源于邻近的间质细胞（即没有证据证明上皮间充质转化(EMT))。相反,这个过程可能仅仅代表一个上皮向间充质转化表型(EMP)[86]。因此,上皮细胞损伤原位标记在临床上将非常有应用前景。它可以反映肾脏的早期潜在可逆性损伤，也可以反映后期肾脏上皮细胞的去分化和萎缩。

多瘤病毒肾病

目前药物所致的强力免疫抑制状态下，病毒感染可能是一个棘手的问题。临床上,患者可以出现与排斥相似的肾功能不全表现。多瘤病毒中,BK病毒占PVAN病例的80%左右。多瘤病毒中,JC病毒占近

20%,也会引起 PVAN;然而,JC 病毒引起的表现通常是轻微的。PVAN 导致肾小管间质性肾炎,肾小管上皮细胞感染,核包涵体形成(图 81.7)。炎性浸润通常有大量浆细胞,有时还可以看到浆细胞小管炎[13],也可以看到免疫复合物沿着肾小管基底膜沉积,最终 IFTA 到晚期移植肾功能丧失,预后相对较差[13,87-89]。有人认为,急性 CMR 和多瘤病毒感染可以同时存在,这两者间的鉴别是困难的[90]。

免疫组织化学可针对多瘤病毒的 SV40 大 T 抗原,用于检测病毒感染的细胞,从而明确诊断。尽管在多瘤病毒肾炎的肾小管间质炎症中有一些典型的形态学改变[91],考虑多瘤病毒肾炎或肾病时,特别是轻度炎性浸润或“临界改变”状态下[87,92],推荐低阈值的 SV40 检测。病毒感染的细胞也可用原位杂交或电镜检测,可以显示为病毒颗粒类晶状的排列[13,87-89]。

腺病毒

腺病毒可以感染移植肾。但腺病毒感染是非常罕见的 (< 1%的移植患者), 通常在移植后 1~3 个月出现。患者可能会出现发热、出血性膀胱炎引起的血尿。组织学检查表现为肾小管坏死(图 81.7)和肉芽肿性炎症。肾小管上皮可出现污秽细胞和含有嗜碱性的核内包涵体。免疫组织化学有助于诊断病毒感染细胞[13,93-95]。

巨细胞病毒

巨细胞病毒(CMV)感染虽然在实体器官受体中常见, 但很少引起移植肾肾炎。患者往往重度免疫力低下,表现为流感样症状和肾功能异常。在使用更昔洛韦等药物预防后,移植肾巨细胞病毒感染已不常见。巨细胞病毒包涵体偶尔在肾小管上皮细胞、肾小球毛细血管和(或)PTC 内皮细胞上可以看到(图 81.7),可伴有间质炎症。特殊染色,如巨细胞病毒的免疫组织化,可以帮助识别受感染的细胞[13,96-98]。

钙调磷酸酶抑制剂的毒性

钙调磷酸酶抑制剂(如环孢霉素和他克莫司)有助于预防肾移植排斥反应[17];然而,钙调磷酸酶抑制剂可引起急性和慢性肾毒性。急性毒性可能与近端小管的空泡化引起的肾小管损伤坏死相关。入球小动脉可出现平滑肌细胞坏死,最终透明样变。少见的血栓性微血管病(TMA)也可能发生。长期钙调磷酸酶抑制剂对平滑肌细胞的毒性会导致广泛的透明样变, 常表现为串珠样和突向动脉外膜(图 81.6)。间质也可能表现为条纹样纤维化和肾小管萎缩[99]。

然而, 这些组织学表现并非钙调磷酸酶抑制剂的肾毒性所特有, 也可在从未接受钙调磷酸酶抑制剂的肾病患者中观察到[100]。因此,钙调磷酸酶抑制剂对移植肾失功的实际影响, 以及关于钙调磷酸酶抑制剂的风险–收益分析,仍是一个争论的话题。

移植后淋巴细胞增殖性疾病

PTLD 是由于移植后强有力的免疫抑制状态和相关 EB 病毒(EBV)再激活,进而出现的淋巴细胞增殖性疾病。PTLD 在实体器官移植或骨髓移植患者中可以看到。据报道,淋巴瘤最终可能导致 40%~60%的死亡率。大多数(85%~90%)的 PTLD 是 B 细胞来源,伴 CD20 表达。很多情况下是由 EBV 引起,移植前 EBV 血清学阴性是发生 PTLD 的一个危险因素。形态学上,大多数情况下由“激活”单核细胞组成,表现为核增大,核仁明显和频繁的有丝分裂活动。免疫组织化可有助于发现 B 细胞或 T 细胞抗原和 EBV 相关抗原 (如 EBV 潜在膜蛋白), 原位杂交则有助于寻找 EBV 编码 的 RNA (EBER)。在世界卫生组织(WHO)的推动下,PTLD 分类已建立,其分类主要有四个主要类别:早期病变、多形性 PTLD (浆细胞增生和传染性单核细胞增多样 PTLD)、单形性 PTLD(B 细胞、T 细胞和 NK 细胞)和经典霍奇金淋巴瘤[13,101]。PTLD 的治疗包括减少免疫抑制剂、抗病毒药物、CD20 单抗(利妥昔单抗,如果 B 细胞表型)、化疗和放疗。

复发和新发疾病

随着急性移植肾排斥反应的有效治疗, 移植肾存活更为长久, 而复发性疾病也已成为影响移植肾预后的重要因素(表 81.3)。大量研究表明,移植肾功能下降的明确病因包括非免疫机制和免疫机制。肾小球病理包括了一部分复发性疾病的患者[102]。大约 40%的肾移植受体出现临床相关的蛋白尿最常见原因是 CAMR, 其后是移植后肾小球肾炎[103,104]。

研究表明, 肾病复发可能是肾小球肾炎患者移植失败的第三大主要原因。可能影响移植肾存活的肾脏疾病主要包括:复发性局灶性节段性肾小球硬化症(FS-

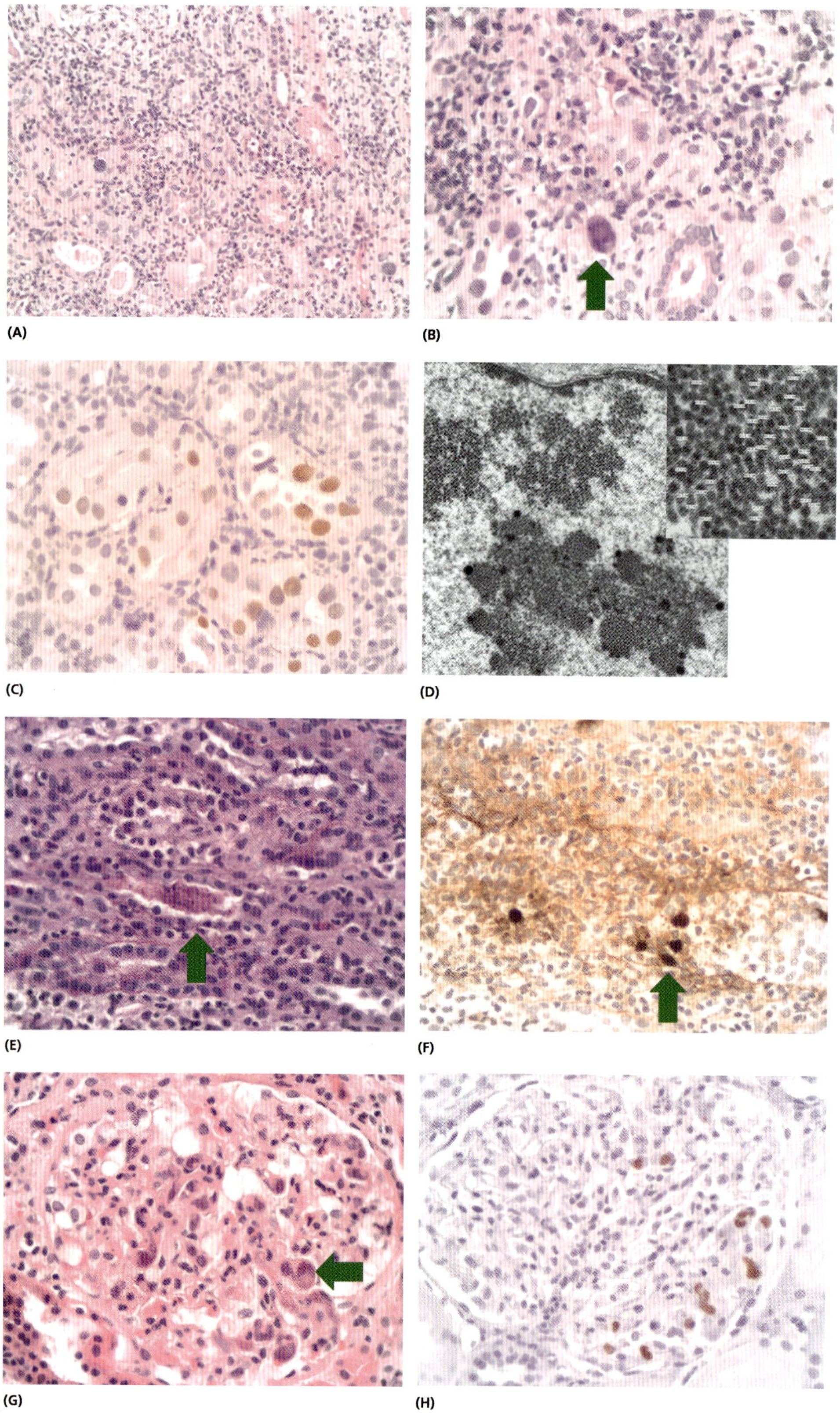

图 81.7 病毒相关性肾炎。在多瘤病毒肾炎中，通常是(A)大量淋巴浆细胞浸润和(B)明显可以看到增大的管状上皮细胞(箭头所示)。(C)SV40免疫组织化可以用来确认细胞为多瘤病毒感染，(D)可以看到电镜下测量多瘤病毒的颗粒为40~50nm(插图)。在腺病毒肾炎中，(E)常常可以看到肾小管坏死物质(箭头所示)和(F)腺病毒免疫组织化可以确认存在的腺病毒感染(箭头所示)。(G)巨细胞病毒的龙包涵体有时可能会出现在肾小球内(箭头所示)，使用巨细胞病毒免疫组织化学染色可以证实(H)。

GS)[105-107]、非典型的溶血性尿毒症综合征(HUS)[103]、狼疮性肾炎[108]、膜增生性肾小球肾炎(MPGN)[103,109,110]。其他值得注意的移植后复发性疾病还包括膜性肾病(MGN)、抗肾小球基底膜(GBM)肾炎、抗中性粒细胞胞浆抗体(ANCA)相关性肾炎[13,111]和感染后肾炎[112]。

一般来说，复发和新发肾病的表现与原位肾一样有相同的形态学特点和临床症状。移植肾活检标本的C4d常规染色可以作为筛选试验。通过免疫荧光和免疫组织化，发现颗粒状C4d沉积(特别是在肾小球基底膜上)则很有可能是新发或复发性的肾小球肾炎。免疫荧光发现系膜区的C4d是正常的表现[13]。一些疾病复发较快，而有些疾病，如糖尿病肾病等可能需要多年时间才表现为复发性肾病[13,111]。

免疫荧光和电镜检查对复发性肾病的诊断是至关重要的(图 81.8)。复发性疾病的表现可能和急性或慢性排斥反应或药物毒性相重叠，这明显增加了鉴别诊断的难度。复发性疾病应与新发性肾病相鉴别，因此，在识别和解释相关移植肾病理时，原发病的相关病史信息显得尤为重要。因为新发和复发性肾病在形态学特性上是相同的。然而，这种明确鉴别常常是不可能的，因为只有少数的肾移植受体进行过原位肾的活检。一般来说，对于早期发生的肾病(< 6 个月)通常倾向于考虑复发性肾病。

原发性FSGS可以在移植后(几分钟内)迅速复发，导致大量蛋白尿，出现类似微小病变病理的足细胞足突广泛融合，并最终产生节段硬化性病变[105,106]。儿童的复发率比成人高5倍[13]。一些队列研究显示，根据FSGS的Columbia分类的一些FSGS复发患者具有相同的形态学表现[113,105]，但是其他的研究未能证明这一点。有研究表明，使用血浆置换加强治疗是有效的[13,103,107,114]。

FSGS也可能是一种新发的肾病。它有时是塌陷型，可表现为肾小球毛细血管袢塌陷和上覆足突细胞的肥大。新发的FSGS也可表现为蛋白尿。塌陷型可能是由严重的血管疾病和钙调磷酸酶抑制剂的毒性引起的。新发FSGS和塌陷型FSGS的5年移植肾存活率分别为约60%和50%[13,115-117]。FSGS也经常是各种肾小球疾病和肾移植高血压受体的继发病变。

肾小球基底膜双轨征在移植(即移植肾小球病)中

表 81.3　复发性疾病(data from [102,103])

疾病	复发率(受者比率/%)	5~10 年移植肾失功(受者比率/%)	备注
原发性侵犯肾小球的疾病			
FSGS	20~40	20	典型的伴有蛋白尿和塌陷型表现
MPGN，Ⅰ型	20~33	高	
MPGN，Ⅱ型(DDD)	67~100	34~66	
膜性肾病	10~30	50	复发性MGN以IgG4亚型为主，而新发膜性肾病以IgG1为主
IgA肾病/HSP	7~10	3~16	可表现为新月体型肾小球肾炎
狼疮性肾炎	30	<5	可表现为足细胞病或FSGS
抗GBM肾病	<5	少见	
ANCA相关新月体肾炎	0~20	10	
纤丝性肾小球肾炎	50	20	
触须样免疫性肾小球病	少见	不确定	
系统性/代谢性疾病			
糖尿病肾病	>50	5	
HUS(先天性D-)	33~82	90	
淀粉样变AL型	10~30	35	
淀粉样变AA型	<10	5	
单克隆免疫球蛋白沉积病	70~85	>50	
Fabry病	低	少见	酶替代疗法可降低发生率
原发性高草酸尿症	90~100	80~100	
胱氨酸病	少见	0	
镰状细胞肾病	少见	未知	

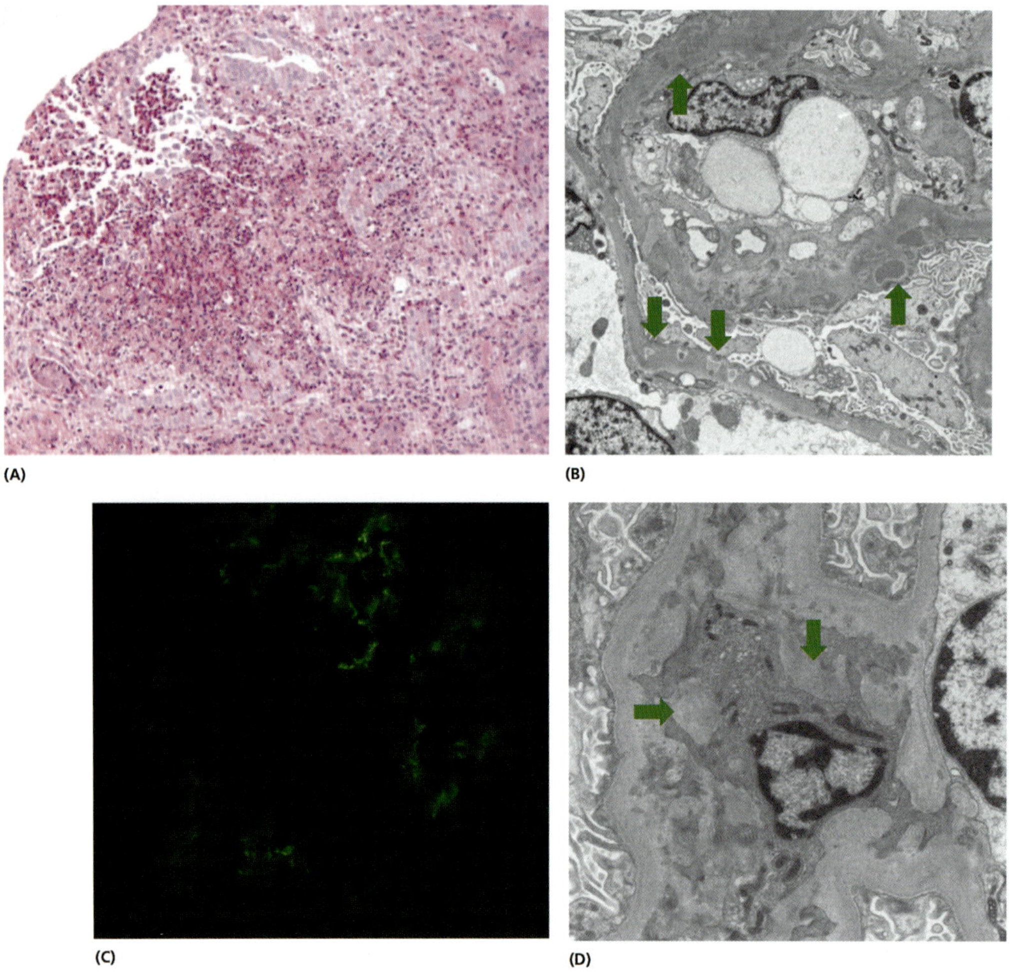

图 81.8 非排斥反应的疾病举例,包括复发性/新发的肾小球肾炎。(A)移植肾盂肾炎中,通常是以中性粒细胞为主的大量炎细胞浸润。(B)新发膜性肾病电镜显示上皮下许多免疫复合物沉积(箭头所示)。(C)IgA 肾病复发,IgA 免疫荧光显示系膜区颗粒样物质染色,(D)电镜显示相应系膜细胞电子密度物沉积(箭头所示)。

通常表现为 CAMR。30%~40%的肾小球基底膜双轨征在活检时并没有检测到 C4d 和 DSA [118]。在这些情况下,复发或新发的肾小球疾病必须纳入考虑。最有可能的病变是 TMA 和 MPGN,特别是在有病毒性肝炎的患者中[119,120]。MPGN 通常可以看到免疫荧光下免疫球蛋白和 C3 的沉积,电镜下大量的电子致密物沉积在内皮下,其 ptc 上 C4d 阴性[13]。

膜性肾病(MGN)复发在大量蛋白尿的病例中约占 30%,多发生在移植后 1 周[13,121]。在膜性肾病中,可以看到肾小球基底膜增厚、空泡化,以及钉突的形成,同时有膜性肾病典型的电镜和免疫荧光征象 (图 81.8)[13]。有时,膜性肾病可能是一种特殊的体液排斥反应,可并发 C4d 沉积[13,122-125]。

在复发性狼疮性肾炎中,可以看到系膜细胞增生或硬化表现,也可以观察到新月体形成和纤维素样坏死。节段性硬化或明显的足细胞损伤有时也会出现[13,108]。

复发性 IgA 肾病/ 过敏性紫癜(HSP)可出现在移植肾中。同原位肾 IgA 肾病一样,可能会有不同程度的系膜内细胞增生和新月体的形成,在荧光显微镜和电镜下会有特征性表现(图 81.8)[13,126-128]。

血清学检查在 ANCA 相关相肾炎或抗 GBM 肾炎复发的监测中是至关重要的。而血清和(或)尿蛋白电泳检查在诊断复发性或新发的免疫球蛋白沉积病或淀粉样变也是重要的[13]。

在原发病 Alport 综合征的肾移植受体中,抗 GBM 相关疾病可能在肾移植后出现。在这种疾病中,会出现针对移植肾Ⅳ型胶原 α-3、α-4 或 α-5 链的抗体,因为受体之前从未接触到这些胶原蛋白。Alport 综合征患者的 COL4A5 基因相对地缺失被认为更容易发生抗 GBM 肾炎。X 染色体连锁的 Alport 综合征患者是针对

COL4A5 的 NC1 域，而其他常染色体隐性的 Alport 综合征患者是针对 COL4A3 或 COL4A4 的 NC1 域。3%~5%的 Alport 综合征患者在肾移植后会出现新发的抗 GBM 肾炎。约 75%的抗 GBM 肾炎发生在移植后第一年，而约 90%的移植肾在发生抗 GBM 肾炎的几个月内失功。抗 GBM 肾炎表现为血尿。显微镜下，有细胞新月体形成和(或)> 80%肾小球的纤维素样坏死。免疫荧光下，可以看到沿着 GBM 分布 IgG 染色强阳性。血浆置换是常规的治疗方案；免疫抑制剂如环磷酰胺、大剂量糖皮质激素、抗胸腺细胞免疫球蛋白、霉酚酸酯也被使用[13,129-135]。

一些代谢性和其他家族性疾病也可能在肾移植后复发。对于原发性高草酸尿症，肝移植是可以治愈的，而肾移植后复发却无法避免。草酸的排泄可能刺激疾病复发[13]。Fabry 疾病的复发率随着酶替代疗法的发展而下降。在胱氨酸病中，巨噬细胞吞噬胱氨酸晶体后可能积聚在肾间质或肾小球系膜；半胱氨酸也可能沉积在其他器官[13]。因为补体因子 H 和 I 的突变，家族性、非典型或非志贺杆菌毒素相关 HUS 也有很高的复发率；有 20%的复发是由于 CD46 变异[13,136,137]。在肾移植后，镰状细胞肾病也可能复发[13,138]。

未来活检评估的发展方向

随着分子和图像分析技术的发展，活检评估工作将有更大的进步空间。将“组学”技术应用于移植肾活检已经取得了显著的成效[77,78]。移植肾活检的分子表型已被广泛的定义和认知。下一步工作将进一步验证其临床效用性(即明确在哪些方面和疾病中，分子评估优于组织病理学评估)。此外，进一步优化的流程时间，形成高维“组学”数据的报告格式和降低成本是分子活检评估未来应用于临床所必须解决的问题。因此，为了推动分子标记物的应用，新的 Banff 工作小组已成立，以制订共识指南[36]。

此外，数码显微镜的出现(即整个病理切片扫描)为活检评估的改进提供了巨大的潜力。组织学活检标本的数码扫描文件提供了前所未有的细节和丰富的图像信息，而一些重要的信息可以被计算机图像分析技术提取。例如，在接下来的几年中，间质性纤维化的评估将很有可能实现自动化。过去 10 年的研究已证明了这种方法的实用性。在一些情况下[139-161]，如间质性纤维化的抑制治疗研究和移植肾程序性活检比较的研究中，间质性纤维化均需要精确测量技术[162-165]。此外，彩色免疫荧光技术与数码显微镜相结合，以及相应的图像分析技术，将使活检免疫病理学中相关蛋白的定量和重复性评估成为可能。

结论

移植肾排斥反应和复发性疾病在肾移植中值得重点关注。特别是，AMR 和肾小球疾病是相关的，因为它们是晚期移植肾失功的两个主要的原因[39,40,102]。通过活检，80%的移植肾功能异常和 IFTA 患者可以明确导致慢性组织损伤的潜在疾病过程[102]。我们希望根据活检以明确诊断，而非特异性诊断名称，如“慢性移植物肾病”(CAN)概括地解释多种病理学机制[12]。常见的组织学表现如 IFTA 和间质炎症大多是潜在特定疾病的非特异性表象。仔细观察形态学表现，整体分析血清学、实验室和临床特征，对制订合理的治疗决策至关重要。移植肾活检分子表型评估的最新进展，为移植肾相关发病机制研究提供了重要手段。可以预期，分子学分析在病情评估和组织病理学研究方面[36,77-79]会有更大的发展空间，最终可能减少一些活检的必要性。

(吴建永 译 吴建永 校)

参考文献

1. Nankivell BJ, Alexander SI. Rejection of the kidney allograft. New England Journal of Medicine. 2010;363:1451–1462.
2. Morris PJ. Transplantation: a medical miracle of the 20th century. New England Journal of Medicine. 2004;351:2678–2680.
3. Williams WW, Taheri D, Tolkoff-Rubin N, et al. Clinical role of the renal transplant biopsy. Nature Reviews Nephrology. 2012;8:110–121.
4. Pascual M, Vallhonrat H, Cosimi AB, et al. The clinical usefulness of the renal allograft biopsy in the cyclosporine era: a prospective study. Transplantation. 1999;67:737–741.
5. Colvin RB, Nickeleit V. Renal transplant pathology. In: Jennette JC, Olson JL, Schwartz MM, et al., editors. Heptinstall's Pathology of the Kidney, 6th edn. Philadelphia, PA: Lippincott Williams and Wilkins; 2006: 1347–1490.
6. Racusen LC, Colvin RB, Solez K, et al. Antibody-mediated rejection criteria: an addition to the Banff 97 classification of renal allograft rejection. American Journal of Transplantation. 2003;3:708–714.
7. Racusen LC, Solez K, Colvin RB, et al. The Banff 97 working classification of renal allograft pathology. Kidney International. 1999;55:713–723.
8. Sis B, Mengel M, Haas M, et al. Banff '09 meeting report: antibody mediated graft deterioration and implementation of Banff working groups. American Journal of Transplantation. 2010;10:464–471.
9. Solez K. History of the Banff classification of allograft pathology as it approaches its 20th year. Current Opinion in Organ Transplantation. 2010;15:49–51.
10. Solez K, Axelsen RA, Benediktsson H, et al. International standardization of criteria for the histologic diagnosis of renal allograft rejection: the Banff working classification of kidney transplant pathology. Kidney International. 1993;44:

411–422.
11. Solez K, Colvin RB, Racusen LC, et al. Banff 07 classification of renal allograft pathology: updates and future directions. American Journal of Transplantation. 2008;8:753–760.
12. Solez K, Colvin RB, Racusen LC, et al. Banff '05 meeting report: differential diagnosis of chronic allograft injury and elimination of chronic allograft nephropathy ('CAN'). American Journal of Transplantation. 2007;7:518–526.
13. Colvin RB, Chang A, Farris AB, et al. Diagnostic Pathology: Kidney Diseases. Salt Lake City, UT: Amirsys; 2011.
14. Colvin RB, Smith RN. Antibody-mediated organ-allograft rejection. Nature Reviews. Immunology. 2005;5:807–817.
15. McCarthy GP, Roberts IS. Diagnosis of acute renal allograft rejection: evaluation of the Banff 97 guidelines for slide preparation. Transplantation. 2002;73: 1518–1521.
16. Furness PN, Taub N, Assmann KJ, et al. International variation in histologic grading is large, and persistent feedback does not improve reproducibility. American Journal of Surgical Pathology. 2003;27:805–810.
17. Halloran PF. Immunosuppressive drugs for kidney transplantation. New England Journal of Medicine. 2004;351:2715–2729.
18. Halloran PF. T cell-mediated rejection of kidney transplants: a personal viewpoint. American Journal of Transplantation. 2010;10:1126–1134.
19. Emovon OE, King JA, Smith SR, et al. Clinical significance of eosinophils in suspicious or borderline renal allograft biopsies. Clinical Nephrology. 2003;59: 367–372.
20. Nickeleit V, Zeiler M, Gudat F, et al. Histological characteristics of interstitial renal allograft rejection. Kidney and Blood Pressure Research. 1998;21: 230–232.
21. Einecke G, Broderick G, Sis B, et al. Early loss of renal transcripts in kidney allografts: relationship to the development of histologic lesions and alloimmune effector mechanisms. American Journal of Transplantation. 2007;7:1121–1130.
22. Minervini MI, Torbenson M, Scantlebury V, et al. Acute renal allograft rejection with severe tubulitis (Banff 1997 grade IB). American Journal of Surgical Pathology. 2000;24:553–558.
23. de Freitas DG, Sellares J, Mengel M, et al. The nature of biopsies with "borderline rejection" and prospects for eliminating this category. American Journal of Transplantation. 2012;12:191–201.
24. Meehan SM, Siegel CT, Aronson AJ, et al. The relationship of untreated borderline infiltrates by the Banff criteria to acute rejection in renal allograft biopsies. Journal of the American Society of Nephrology. 1999;10:1806–1814.
25. Desvaux D, Le Gouvello S, Pastural M, et al. Acute renal allograft rejections with major interstitial oedema and plasma cell-rich infiltrates: high gamma-interferon expression and poor clinical outcome. Nephrology, Dialysis, Transplantation. 2004;19:933–939.
26. Charney DA, Nadasdy T, Lo AW, et al. Plasma cell-rich acute renal allograft rejection. Transplantation. 1999;68:791–797.
27. Meehan SM, Domer P, Josephson M, et al. The clinical and pathologic implications of plasmacytic infiltrates in percutaneous renal allograft biopsies. Human Pathology. 2001;32:205–215.
28. Haas M, Kraus ES, Samaniego-Picota M, et al. Acute renal allograft rejection with intimal arteritis: histologic predictors of response to therapy and graft survival. Kidney International. 2002;61:1516–1526.
29. Nickeleit V, Vamvakas EC, Pascual M, et al. The prognostic significance of specific arterial lesions in acute renal allograft rejection. Journal of the American Society of Nephrology. 1998;9:1301–1308.
30. Mengel M, Sis B, Haas M, et al. Banff 2011 meeting Report: new concepts in antibody-mediated rejection. American Journal of Transplantation. 2012;12: 563–570.
31. Sellares J, de Freitas DG, Mengel M, et al. Inflammation lesions in kidney transplant biopsies: association with survival is due to the underlying diseases. American Journal of Transplantation. 2011;11:489–499.
32. Mannon RB, Matas AJ, Grande J, et al. Inflammation in areas of tubular atrophy in kidney allograft biopsies: a potent predictor of allograft failure. American Journal of Transplantation. 2010;10:2066–2073.
33. Moreso F, Ibernon M, Goma M, et al. Subclinical rejection associated with chronic allograft nephropathy in protocol biopsies as a risk factor for late graft loss. American Journal of Transplantation. 2006;6:747–752.
34. Shishido S, Asanuma H, Nakai H, et al. The impact of repeated subclinical acute rejection on the progression of chronic allograft nephropathy. Journal of the American Society of Nephrology. 2003;14:1046–1052.
35. Mengel M, Reeve J, Bunnag S, et al. Scoring total inflammation is superior to the current Banff inflammation score in predicting outcome and the degree of molecular disturbance in renal allografts. American Journal of Transplantation. 2009;9:1859–1867.
36. Haas M, Sis B, Racusen LC, et al.; Banff Meeting Report Writing Committee. Banff 2013 meeting report: inclusion of C4d-negative antibody-mediated rejection and antibody-associated arterial lesions. American Journal of Transplantation. 2014;14:272–283.
37. Kissmeyer-Nielsen F, Olsen S, Petersen VP, et al. Hyperacute rejection of kidney allografts, associated with pre-existing humoral antibodies against donor cells. Lancet. 1966;2:662–665.
38. Ahern AT, Artruc SB, DellaPelle P, et al. Hyperacute rejection of HLA-AB-identical renal allografts associated with B lymphocyte and endothelial reactive antibodies. Transplantation. 1982;33:103–106.
39. Einecke G, Sis B, Reeve J, et al. Antibody-mediated microcirculation injury is the major cause of late kidney transplant failure. American Journal of Transplantation. 2009;9:2520–2531.
40. Gaston RS, Cecka JM, Kasiske BL, et al. Evidence for antibody-mediated injury as a major determinant of late kidney allograft failure. Transplantation. 2010;90:68–74.
41. Cornell LD, Smith RN, Colvin RB. Kidney transplantation: mechanisms of rejection and acceptance. Annual Review of Pathology. 2008;3:189–220.
42. Hirohashi T, Chase CM, Della Pelle P, et al. A novel pathway of chronic allograft rejection mediated by NK cells and alloantibody. American Journal of Transplantation. 2012;12:313–321.
43. Liptak P, Kemeny E, Morvay Z, et al. Peritubular capillary damage in acute humoral rejection: an ultrastructural study on human renal allografts. American Journal of Transplantation. 2005;5:2870–2876.
44. Colvin RB. C4d in liver allografts: a sign of antibody-mediated rejection? American Journal of Transplantation. 2006;6:447–448.
45. Ivanyi B. Transplant capillaropathy and transplant glomerulopathy: ultrastructural markers of chronic renal allograft rejection. Nephrology, Dialysis, Transplantation. 2003;18:655–660.
46. Smith RN, Kawai T, Boskovic S, et al. Chronic antibody mediated rejection of renal allografts: pathological, serological and immunologic features in nonhuman primates. American Journal of Transplantation. 2006;6:1790–1798.
47. Sellares J, de Freitas DG, Mengel M, et al. Understanding the causes of kidney transplant failure: the dominant role of antibody-mediated rejection and nonadherence. American Journal of Transplantation. 2012;12:388–399.
48. Sis B, Jhangri GS, Bunnag S, et al. Endothelial gene expression in kidney transplants with alloantibody indicates antibody-mediated damage despite lack of C4d staining. American Journal of Transplantation. 2009;9:2312–2323.
49. Haas M. C4d-negative antibody-mediated rejection in renal allografts: evidence for its existence and effect on graft survival. Clinical Nephrology. 2011;75: 271–278.
50. Trpkov K, Campbell P, Pazderka F, et al. Pathologic features of acute renal allograft rejection associated with donor-specific antibody, analysis using the Banff grading schema. Transplantation. 1996;61:1586–1592.
51. Mauiyyedi S, Crespo M, Collins AB, et al. Acute humoral rejection in kidney transplantation: II. Morphology, immunopathology, and pathologic classification. Journal of the American Society of Nephrology. 2002;13:779–787.
52. Regele H, Exner M, Watschinger B, et al. Endothelial C4d deposition is associated with inferior kidney allograft outcome independently of cellular rejection. Nephrology, Dialysis, Transplantation. 2001;16:2058–2066.
53. Nickeleit V, Mihatsch MJ. Kidney transplants, antibodies and rejection: is C4d a magic marker? Nephrology, Dialysis, Transplantation. 2003;18: 2232–2239.
54. Takahashi K. Recent findings in ABO-incompatible kidney transplantation: classification and therapeutic strategy for acute antibody-mediated rejection due to ABO-blood-group-related antigens during the critical period preceding the establishment of accommodation. Clinical and Experimental Nephrology. 2007;11:128–141.
55. Haas M, Rahman MH, Racusen LC, et al. C4d and C3d staining in biopsies of ABO- and HLA-incompatible renal allografts: correlation with histologic findings. American Journal of Transplantation. 2006;6:1829–1840.
56. Girlanda R, Kleiner DE, Duan Z, et al. Monocyte infiltration and kidney allograft dysfunction during acute rejection. American Journal of Transplantation. 2008;8:600–607.
57. Kirk AD, Hale DA, Mannon RB, et al. Results from a human renal allograft tolerance trial evaluating the humanized CD52-specific monoclonal antibody alemtuzumab (CAMPATH-1H). Transplantation. 2003;76:120–129.
58. Kirk AD, Mannon RB, Kleiner DE, et al. Results from a human renal allograft tolerance trial evaluating T-cell depletion with alemtuzumab combined with deoxyspergualin. Transplantation. 2005;80:1051–1059.
59. Kawai T, Cosimi AB, Spitzer TR, et al. HLA-mismatched renal transplantation without maintenance immunosuppression. New England Journal of Medicine. 2008;358:353–361.
60. Farris AB, Taheri D, Kawai T, et al. Acute renal endothelial injury during marrow recovery in a cohort of combined kidney and bone marrow allografts. American Journal of Transplantation. 2011;11:1464–1477.

61. Leventhal J, Abecassis M, Miller J, et al. Chimerism and tolerance without GVHD or engraftment syndrome in HLA-mismatched combined kidney and hematopoietic stem cell transplantation. Science Translational Medicine. 2012;4:124-128.
62. Stegall MD, Diwan T, Raghavaiah S, et al. Terminal complement inhibition decreases antibody-mediated rejection in sensitized renal transplant recipients. American Journal of Transplantation. 2011;11:2405-2413.
63. Wieczorek G, Bigaud M, Menninger K, et al. Acute and chronic vascular rejection in nonhuman primate kidney transplantation. American Journal of Transplantation. 2006;6:1285-1296.
64. Karam G, Maillet F, Parant S, et al. Ureteral necrosis after kidney transplantation: risk factors and impact on graft and patient survival. Transplantation. 2004;78:725-729.
65. Jefferson RH, Burns JR. Urological evaluation of adult renal transplant recipients. Journal of Urology. 1995;153:615-618.
66. Hakim NS, Benedetti E, Pirenne J, et al. Complications of ureterovesical anastomosis in kidney transplant patients: the Minnesota experience. Clinical Transplantation. 1994;8:504-507.
67. Audard V, Matignon M, Hemery F, et al. Risk factors and long-term outcome of transplant renal artery stenosis in adult recipients after treatment by percutaneous transluminal angioplasty. American Journal of Transplantation. 2006;6:95-99.
68. Beecroft JR, Rajan DK, Clark TW, et al. Transplant renal artery stenosis: outcome after percutaneous intervention. Journal of Vascular and Interventional Radiology. 2004;15:1407-1413.
69. Bruno S, Remuzzi G, Ruggenenti P. Transplant renal artery stenosis. Journal of the American Society of Nephrology. 2004;15:134-141.
70. Buturovic-Ponikvar J. Renal transplant artery stenosis. Nephrology, Dialysis, Transplantation. 2003;18(Suppl 5):v74-v77.
71. Aschwanden M, Thalhammer C, Schaub S, et al. Renal vein thrombosis after renal transplantation: early diagnosis by duplex sonography prevented fatal outcome. Nephrology, Dialysis, Transplantation. 2006;21:825-826.
72. Osman Y, Shokeir A, Ali-el-Dein B, et al. Vascular complications after live donor renal transplantation: study of risk factors and effects on graft and patient survival. Journal of Urology. 2003;169:859-862.
73. Bakir N, Sluiter WJ, Ploeg RJ, et al. Primary renal graft thrombosis. Nephrology, Dialysis, Transplantation. 1996;11:140-147.
74. Krol R, Kolonko A, Chudek J, et al. Did volume of lymphocele after kidney transplantation determine the choice of treatment modality? Transplantation Proceedings. 2007;39:2740-2743.
75. Friedewald SM, Molmenti EP, Friedewald JJ, et al. Vascular and nonvascular complications of renal transplants: sonographic evaluation and correlation with other imaging modalities, surgery, and pathology. Journal of Clinical Ultrasound. 2005;33:127-139.
76. Goel M, Flechner SM, Zhou L, et al. The influence of various maintenance immunosuppressive drugs on lymphocele formation and treatment after kidney transplantation. Journal of Urology. 2004;171:1788-1792.
77. Halloran PF, de Freitas DG, Einecke G, et al. An integrated view of molecular changes, histopathology and outcomes in kidney transplants. American Journal of Transplantation. 2010;10:2223-2230.
78. Halloran PF, de Freitas DG, Einecke G, et al. The molecular phenotype of kidney transplants. American Journal of Transplantation. 2010;10:2215-2222.
79. Einecke G, Reeve J, Sis B, et al. A molecular classifier for predicting future graft loss in late kidney transplant biopsies. Journal of Clinical Investigation. 2010;120:1862-1872.
80. Hertig A. Epithelial-mesenchymal transition of the renal graft. Nephrologie and Therapeutique. 2008;4(Suppl 1):S25-S28.
81. Bonventre JV. Kidney Injury Molecule-1 (KIM-1): a specific and sensitive biomarker of kidney injury. Scandinavian Journal of Clinical and Laboratory Investigation Supplement. 2008;241:78-83.
82. Koesters R, Kaissling B, Lehir M, et al. Tubular overexpression of transforming growth factor-beta1 induces autophagy and fibrosis but not mesenchymal transition of renal epithelial cells. American Journal of Pathology. 2010;177:632-643.
83. Famulski KS, Broderick G, Einecke G, et al. Transcriptome analysis reveals heterogeneity in the injury response of kidney transplants. American Journal of Transplantation. 2007;7:2483-2495.
84. von Toerne C, Schmidt C, Adams J, et al. Wnt pathway regulation in chronic renal allograft damage. American Journal of Transplantation. 2009;9:2223-2239.
85. Einecke G, Kayser D, Vanslambrouck JM, et al. Loss of solute carriers in T cell-mediated rejection in mouse and human kidneys: an active epithelial injury-repair response. American Journal of Transplantation. 2010;10:2241-2251.
86. Kriz W, Kaissling B, Le Hir M. Epithelial-Mesenchymal Transition (EMT) in kidney fibrosis: fact or fantasy? Journal of Clinical Investigation. 2011;121:468-474.
87. Drachenberg CB, Hirsch HH, Ramos E, et al. Polyomavirus disease in renal transplantation: review of pathological findings and diagnostic methods. Human Pathology. 2005;36:1245-1255.
88. Hirsch HH, Brennan DC, Drachenberg CB, et al. Polyomavirus-associated nephropathy in renal transplantation: interdisciplinary analyses and recommendations. Transplantation. 2005;79:1277-1286.
89. Fishman JA. Infection in solid-organ transplant recipients. New England Journal of Medicine. 2007;357:2601-2614.
90. Nickeleit V, Mihatsch MJ. Polyomavirus allograft nephropathy and concurrent acute rejection: a diagnostic and therapeutic challenge. American Journal of Transplantation. 2004;4:838-839.
91. Mengel M, Marwedel M, Radermacher J, et al. Incidence of polyomavirus-nephropathy in renal allografts: influence of modern immunosuppressive drugs. Nephrology, Dialysis, Transplantation. 2003;18:1190-1196.
92. Nickeleit V, Mihatsch MJ. Polyomavirus nephropathy in native kidneys and renal allografts: an update on an escalating threat. Transplant International. 2006;19:960-973.
93. Varma MC, Kushner YB, Ko DS, et al. Early onset adenovirus infection after simultaneous kidney-pancreas transplant. American Journal of Transplantation. 2011;11:623-627.
94. Lim AK, Parsons S, Ierino F. Adenovirus tubulointerstitial nephritis presenting as a renal allograft space occupying lesion. American Journal of Transplantation. 2005;5:2062-2066.
95. Ito M, Hirabayashi N, Uno Y, et al. Necrotizing tubulointerstitial nephritis associated with adenovirus infection. Human Pathology. 1991;22:1225-1231.
96. Cathro HP, Schmitt TM. Cytomegalovirus glomerulitis in a renal allograft. American Journal of Kidney Diseases. 2008;52:188-192.
97. Humar A, Asberg A, Kumar D, et al. An assessment of herpesvirus co-infections in patients with CMV disease: correlation with clinical and virologic outcomes. American Journal of Transplantation. 2009;9:374-381.
98. Kliem V, Fricke L, Wollbrink T, et al. Improvement in long-term renal graft survival due to CMV prophylaxis with oral ganciclovir: results of a randomized clinical trial. American Journal of Transplantation. 2008;8:975-983.
99. Liptak P, Ivanyi B. Primer: histopathology of calcineurin-inhibitor toxicity in renal allografts. Nature Clinical Practice Nephrology. 2006;2:398-404. quiz following 404.
100. Mengel M, Mihatsch M, Halloran PF. Histological characteristics of calcineurin inhibitor toxicity: there is no such thing as specificity! American Journal of Transplantation. 2011;11:2549-2550.
101. Swerdlow SH, Webber SA, Chadburn A, et al. Posttransplant lymphoproliferative disorders. In: Swerdlow SH, Campo E, Harris NL, et al., editors. WHO Classification of Tumours of Haematopoietic and Lymphoid Tissues. Lyon: IARC; 2008: 343-348.
102. El-Zoghby ZM, Stegall MD, Lager DJ, et al. Identifying specific causes of kidney allograft loss. American Journal of Transplantation. 2009;9:527-535.
103. Ivanyi B. A primer on recurrent and de novo glomerulonephritis in renal allografts. Nature Clinical Practice Nephrology. 2008;4:446-457.
104. Choy BY, Chan TM, Lai KN. Recurrent glomerulonephritis after kidney transplantation. American Journal of Transplantation. 2006;6:2535-2542.
105. IJpelaar DH, Farris AB, Goemaere N, et al. Fidelity and evolution of recurrent FSGS in renal allografts. Journal of the American Society of Nephrology. 2008;19:2219-2224.
106. Canaud G, Dion D, Zuber J, et al. Recurrence of nephrotic syndrome after transplantation in a mixed population of children and adults: course of glomerular lesions and value of the Columbia classification of histological variants of focal and segmental glomerulosclerosis (FSGS). Nephrology, Dialysis, Transplantation. 2010;25:1321-1328.
107. Canaud G, Zuber J, Sberro R, et al. Intensive and prolonged treatment of focal and segmental glomerulosclerosis recurrence in adult kidney transplant recipients: a pilot study. American Journal of Transplantation. 2009;9:1081-1086.
108. Meehan SM, Chang A, Khurana A, et al. Pauci-immune and immune glomerular lesions in kidney transplants for systemic lupus erythematosus. Clinical Journal of the American Society of Nephrology. 2008;3:1469-1478.
109. Little MA, Dupont P, Campbell E, et al. Severity of primary MPGN, rather than MPGN type, determines renal survival and post-transplantation recurrence risk. Kidney International. 2006;69:504-511.
110. Braun MC, Stablein DM, Hamiwka LA, et al. Recurrence of membranoproliferative glomerulonephritis type II in renal allografts: the North American Pediatric Renal Transplant Cooperative Study experience. Journal of the American Society of Nephrology. 2005;16:2225-2233.
111. Joshi K, Nada R, Minz M, et al. Recurrent glomerulopathy in the renal allograft. Transplantation Proceedings. 2007;39:734-736.
112. Casquero A, Ramos A, Barat A, et al. Recurrent acute postinfectious glomerulonephritis. Clinical Nephrology. 2006;66:51-53.

113. D'Agati VD, Fogo AB, Bruijn JA, et al. Pathologic classification of focal segmental glomerulosclerosis: a working proposal. American Journal of Kidney Diseases. 2004;43:368–382.
114. Ponticelli C, Glassock RJ. Posttransplant recurrence of primary glomerulonephritis. Clinical Journal of the American Society of Nephrology. 2010;5:2363–2372.
115. Swaminathan S, Lager DJ, Qian X, et al. Collapsing and non-collapsing focal segmental glomerulosclerosis in kidney transplants. Nephrology, Dialysis, Transplantation. 2006;21:2607–2614.
116. Nadasdy T, Allen C, Zand MS. Zonal distribution of glomerular collapse in renal allografts: possible role of vascular changes. Human Pathology. 2002;33:437–441.
117. Meehan SM, Pascual M, Williams WW, et al. De novo collapsing glomerulopathy in renal allografts. Transplantation. 1998;65:1192–1197.
118. Sis B, Campbell PM, Mueller T, et al. Transplant glomerulopathy, late antibody-mediated rejection and the ABCD tetrad in kidney allograft biopsies for cause. American Journal of Transplantation. 2007;7:1743–1752.
119. Baid-Agrawal S, Farris AB 3rd, Pascual M, et al. Overlapping pathways to transplant glomerulopathy: chronic humoral rejection, hepatitis C infection, and thrombotic microangiopathy. Kidney International. 2011;80:879–885.
120. Haas M. Transplant glomerulopathy: it's not always about chronic rejection. Kidney International. 2011;80:801–803.
121. Truong L, Gelfand J, D'Agati V, et al. De novo membranous glomerulonephropathy in renal allografts: a report of ten cases and review of the literature. American Journal of Kidney Diseases. 1989;14:131–144.
122. Poduval RD, Josephson MA, Javaid B. Treatment of de novo and recurrent membranous nephropathy in renal transplant patients. Seminars in Nephrology. 2003;23:392–399.
123. Lal SM. De novo membranous nephropathy in renal allografts with unusual histology. Archives of Pathology and Laboratory Medicine. 2007;131:17.
124. Monga G, Mazzucco G, Basolo B, et al. Membranous glomerulonephritis (MGN) in transplanted kidneys: morphologic investigation on 256 renal allografts. Modern Pathology. 1993;6:249–258.
125. Schwarz A, Krause PH, Offermann G, et al. Impact of de novo membranous glomerulonephritis on the clinical course after kidney transplantation. Transplantation. 1994;58:650–654.
126. Jeong HJ, Park SK, Cho YM, et al. Progression of renal allograft histology after renal transplantation in recurrent and nonrecurrent immunoglobulin A nephropathy. Human Pathology. 2008;39:1511–1518.
127. Kowalewska J, Yuan S, Sustento-Reodica N, et al. IgA nephropathy with crescents in kidney transplant recipients. American Journal of Kidney Diseases. 2005;45:167–175.
128. Soler MJ, Mir M, Rodriguez E, et al. Recurrence of IgA nephropathy and Henoch-Schonlein purpura after kidney transplantation: risk factors and graft survival. Transplantation Proceedings. 2005;37:3705–3709.
129. Kashtan CE. Renal transplantation in patients with Alport syndrome. Pediatric Transplantation. 2006;10:651–657.
130. Byrne MC, Budisavljevic MN, Fan Z, et al. Renal transplant in patients with Alport's syndrome. American Journal of Kidney Diseases. 2002;39:769–775.
131. Rutgers A, Meyers KE, Canziani G, et al. High affinity of anti-GBM antibodies from Goodpasture and transplanted Alport patients to alpha3(IV)NC1 collagen. Kidney International. 2000;58:115–122.
132. Ding J, Zhou J, Tryggvason K, et al. COL4A5 deletions in three patients with Alport syndrome and posttransplant antiglomerular basement membrane nephritis. Journal of the American Society of Nephrology. 1994;5:161–168.
133. Gobel J, Olbricht CJ, Offner G, et al. Kidney transplantation in Alport's syndrome: long-term outcome and allograft anti-GBM nephritis. Clinical Nephrology. 1992;38:299–304.
134. Peten E, Pirson Y, Cosyns JP, et al. Outcome of thirty patients with Alport's syndrome after renal transplantation. Transplantation. 1991;52:823–826.
135. Kashtan CE, Butkowski RJ, Kleppel MM, et al. Posttransplant anti-glomerular basement membrane nephritis in related males with Alport syndrome. Journal of Laboratory and Clinical Medicine. 1990;116:508–515.
136. Saunders RE, Abarrategui-Garrido C, Fremeaux-Bacchi V, et al. The interactive factor H-atypical hemolytic uremic syndrome mutation database and website: update and integration of membrane cofactor protein and factor I mutations with structural models. Human Mutation. 2007;28:222–234.
137. Kavanagh D, Goodship TH. Membrane cofactor protein and factor I: mutations and transplantation. Seminars in Thrombosis and Hemostasis. 2006;32:155–159.
138. Kim L, Garfinkel MR, Chang A, et al. Intragraft vascular occlusive sickle crisis with early renal allograft loss in occult sickle cell trait. Human Pathology. 2011;42:1027–1033.
139. Cosio FG, Grande JP, Wadei H, et al. Predicting subsequent decline in kidney allograft function from early surveillance biopsies. American Journal of Transplantation. 2005;5:2464–2472.
140. Diaz Encarnacion MM, Griffin MD, Slezak JM, et al. Correlation of quantitative digital image analysis with the glomerular filtration rate in chronic allograft nephropathy. American Journal of Transplantation. 2004;4:248–256.
141. Kostadinova-Kunovska S, Petrusevska G, Jovanovic R, et al. Histomorphometric analysis of fibrosis in the renal interstitial compartment. Prilozi. 2005;26:51–59.
142. Servais A, Meas-Yedid V, Buchler M, et al. Quantification of interstitial fibrosis by image analysis on routine renal biopsy in patients receiving cyclosporine. Transplantation. 2007;84:1595–1601.
143. Servais A, Meas-Yedid V, Toupance O, et al. Interstitial fibrosis quantification in renal transplant recipients randomized to continue cyclosporine or convert to sirolimus. American Journal of Transplantation. 2009;9:2552–2560.
144. Servais A, Meas-Yedid V, Noel LH, et al. Interstitial fibrosis evolution on early sequential screening renal allograft biopsies using quantitative image analysis. American Journal of Transplantation. 2011;11:1456–1463.
145. De Heer E, Sijpkens YW, Verkade M, et al. Morphometry of interstitial fibrosis. Nephrology, Dialysis, Transplantation. 2000;15(Suppl 6):72–73.
146. Vleming LJ, Baelde JJ, Westendorp RG, et al. Progression of chronic renal disease in humans is associated with the deposition of basement membrane components and decorin in the interstitial extracellular matrix. Clinical Nephrology. 1995;44:211–219.
147. Abrass CK, Berfield AK, Stehman-Breen C, et al. Unique changes in interstitial extracellular matrix composition are associated with rejection and cyclosporine toxicity in human renal allograft biopsies. American Journal of Kidney Diseases. 1999;33:11–20.
148. Verkade MA, Bajema IM, De Heer E, et al. Decorin and TGF-beta-1 protein expression in renal disease: a morphometric analysis (abstract). Journal of the American Society of Nephrology. 1999;10:584.
149. Grimm PC, Nickerson P, Gough J, et al. Computerized image analysis of Sirius Red-stained renal allograft biopsies as a surrogate marker to predict long-term allograft function. Journal of the American Society of Nephrology. 2003;14:1662–1668.
150. Pape L, Henne T, Offner G, et al. Computer-assisted quantification of fibrosis in chronic allograft nephropaty by picosirius red-staining: a new tool for predicting long-term graft function. Transplantation. 2003;76:955–958.
151. Sund S, Grimm P, Reisaeter AV, et al. Computerized image analysis vs semiquantitative scoring in evaluation of kidney allograft fibrosis and prognosis. Nephrology, Dialysis, Transplantation. 2004;19:2838–2845.
152. Bains JC, Sandford RM, Brook NR, et al. Comparison of renal allograft fibrosis after transplantation from heart-beating and non-heart-beating donors. British Journal of Surgery. 2005;92:113–118.
153. Hunter MG, Hurwitz S, Bellamy CO, et al. Quantitative morphometry of lupus nephritis: the significance of collagen, tubular space, and inflammatory infiltrate. Kidney International. 2005;67:94–102.
154. Masseroli M, O'Valle F, Andujar M, et al. Design and validation of a new image analysis method for automatic quantification of interstitial fibrosis and glomerular morphometry. Laboratory Investigation. 1998;78:511–522.
155. Moreso F, Seron D, Vitria J, et al. Quantification of interstitial chronic renal damage by means of texture analysis. Kidney International. 1994;46:1721–1727.
156. Pape L, Mengel M, Offner G, et al. Renal arterial resistance index and computerized quantification of fibrosis as a combined predictive tool in chronic allograft nephropathy. Pediatric Transplantation. 2004;8:565–570.
157. Nicholson ML, Bailey E, Williams S, et al. Computerized histomorphometric assessment of protocol renal transplant biopsy specimens for surrogate markers of chronic rejection. Transplantation. 1999;68:236–241.
158. Nicholson ML, McCulloch TA, Harper SJ, et al. Early measurement of interstitial fibrosis predicts long-term renal function and graft survival in renal transplantation. British Journal of Surgery. 1996;83:1082–1085.
159. Ruiz P, Kolbeck PC, Scroggs MW, et al. Associations between cyclosporine therapy and interstitial fibrosis in renal allograft biopsies. Transplantation. 1988;45:91–95.
160. Ruiz P, Kolbeck PC, Scroggs MW, et al. Cyclosporine therapy and the development of interstitial fibrosis in renal allografts. Transplantation Proceedings. 1988;20(Suppl 3):807–811.
161. Farris AB, Adams CD, Brousaides N, et al. Morphometric and visual evaluation of fibrosis in renal biopsies. Journal of the American Society of Nephrology. 2011;22:176–186.
162. Liu Y. Renal fibrosis: new insights into the pathogenesis and therapeutics. Kidney International. 2006;69:213–217.
163. Liu Y, Yang J. Hepatocyte growth factor: new arsenal in the fights against renal fibrosis? Kidney International. 2006;70:238–240.
164. Vilayur E, Harris DC. Emerging therapies for chronic kidney disease: what is their role? Nature Reviews Nephrology. 2009;5:375–383.
165. Boor P, Sebekova K, Ostendorf T, et al. Treatment targets in renal fibrosis. Nephrology, Dialysis, Transplantation. 2007;22:3391–3407.

第 82 章 肝移植排斥反应和复发疾病的组织病理学综合征

Anthony J. Demetris, Marta I. Minervini, Michael A. Nalesnik, Erin Rubin, Parmjeet Randhawa, Eizaburo Sasatomi

引言

肝移植广泛用于终末期肝病的治疗。在北美、欧洲、南美,肝移植的主要病因为丙型肝炎病毒(HCV)、酒精性和非酒精性脂肪肝病导致的肝硬化,而亚洲则以乙型肝炎病毒(HBV)相关肝硬化为主。

这一章着重讲解肝移植常见适应证,以及特异性并发症,如排斥反应、小肝综合征、缺血再灌注损伤的独特组织病理学特征。我们制作了众多图表便于更为直观的解读,其中包括由 Banff 工作组制订的急性和慢性排斥反应和晚期移植物功能障碍的简易图表。本章与讲述肝移植复发性疾病临床管理的 78 章和讲述移植物排斥的 70 章互为补充。

死亡供肝活检评估

冰冻组织切片最好是在阅片的病理学医生在场的情况下获取,选取典型部位并且及时送检。如果移植物大体外形一致,我们通常会取三个组织样本:用 16G 针芯在左右半肝各取一个长 2.0cm 的肝组织,肝右叶被膜下取一块 $2cm^2$ 的楔形肝组织。针芯获取的样本用于评估肝硬化的程度;楔形样本还可以用于评估动脉或小动脉疾病以及脂肪变性的程度。

在组织样本过程中要避免晾晒以及用生理盐水存储,这会导致肝细胞出现萎缩或坏死。此外,吸附剂会将组织中的脂肪析出,可能导致病理检验时低估组织的脂肪变性程度。因此,组织活检应置于组织固定液浸润的纸巾上或塑料标本容器中,并迅速运送至冰冻室。

病理医生应警惕肝细胞中潜在的脂肪变。我们可以通过增加伊红染色时间,使得坏死的肝细胞发生嗜酸性变,从而识别肝细胞脂肪变的程度。此外,该方法也可以辨认出早期的核破裂。

当组织活检结果和患者现病史或既往史不符时,病理医生应要求获取额外的临床信息。但是,捐献者活检评估终究只是一项简便的实验室检查,病理学医生并不能在缺少重要组织病理学变化证据的时候仅仅基于切片报告来预测移植后器官功能。

如果活检发现弥漫的肝细胞坏死、严重的大泡性脂肪变(定义见后文)、高级别的肝内动脉粥样硬化和明确的桥接坏死[1-4]等病变,医生通常会取消该供器官的移植手术。偏光显微镜可以快速而准确地评估肝纤维化程度,有效地辅助诊断。

大泡性脂肪变通常是细胞内出现典型的大型脂肪空泡(通常大于核直径的 1/2),并伴随细胞核被挤压到细胞边缘,反之,小泡性脂肪变则是出现多个小的脂肪空泡(小于 1/2 核直径),同时细胞核仍在中心。大泡性脂肪变(大于 30%)的肝脏对保存再灌注损伤的易感性增加,细胞再生受损,可能导致移植物存活率降低[5-7]。短期的热缺血经常导致小泡性脂肪变,但通常不产生不利影响。然而,有一项研究认为"高级别的"小泡性脂肪变可以导致移植物功能恢复延迟[8]。我们建议,可以通过苏木精和伊红染色粗略评估大泡性脂肪变的严重程度。

我们中心指定的评估方案如下:供肝轻度的大泡性脂肪变(小于 10%)不会造成影响。发生中度大泡性脂肪变(10%~30%)的肝脏仍可使用,但在考虑器官是否符合标准的决策过程中也需要参考其他因素(如扩大标准的器官捐献(ECD)指标)。肝脏脂肪变性大于 30%或更加严重者,只在特殊情况下允许使用,比如冷缺血时间保持在最低限度(通常是小于 8~9 小时)并且没有或几乎没有其他ESD风险因素。只有在这种情况下的手术结果才可以和无脂肪变性的供体肝脏相提并论[9,10]。

在某些情况下，供体肝脏组织活检可能发现肝组织坏死，对移植手术结果会产生不良影响[11,12]。但并不是所有的研究都是如此[8,13]。以我们的经验，如果肝细胞坏死大于10%，而且坏死范围包括活检组织，那么该肝脏通常是不合格的；评估结果不应该仅依赖于孤立的被膜下肝叶坏死程度的判定，而应与捐赠者肝损伤测试结果相联系。

我们对机构内的HCV阳性的活体捐献肝脏进行了冰冻切片检查。充分告知患者后，没有桥接纤维化[Ishak评分系统小于3分(满分6分)]的肝脏被提供给受体。其他情况的供肝组织报道应选择Ishak评分小于2分的肝脏[14]。

各种肿瘤、感染性和代谢性疾病可能偶然地从供体转移到受体[15]。病理医生可能发现的病变包括各种癌症、淀粉样变、血色沉着病、真菌、病毒和寄生虫疾病[15]。代谢疾病，如家族性淀粉样多发性神经病[16]、草酸盐沉着症[17]，甚至α_1-抗胰蛋白酶缺乏症[18]都可能不经意间通过器官移植进行转移传播。

活体供体活检评估

目前，活体肝脏捐献手术仅占北美和欧洲移植数量的5%以下，但在亚洲占据了绝大多数[19]。由于肝切除术具有一定的风险(死亡率约为2:700[20])，一部分移植中心例行对活体捐献者的肝脏进行活检从而规避风险[21-24]；20%~50%的捐献肝脏活体切片检查显示肝脏轻度异常。

病理检查中最常见的病变是不同程度的大泡性脂肪变(14%~53%)，这也是器官捐献被取消资格最常见的原因[21-27]。大多数移植手术要求捐献肝脏的脂肪变程度应小于30%，因为这种水平的脂肪变性一般不会对供肝或肝脏受体产生不良影响[23]，也有其他移植项目要求脂肪变性的程度要求小于10%或20%[26,27]。

其他活检结果包括低评分的不明原因的慢性肝炎、肉芽肿和各种意外的病变发现[如意外发现的早期原发性胆汁性肝硬化(PBC)][24]。约17%的男性器官捐献者中会出现汇管区的肝细胞含铁血黄素沉积，但这种亚临床的发现并不会妨碍移植进行。活检中在汇管区也曾偶尔发现不明原因的嗜酸性粒细胞，但不影响供体以及受体术后恢复[24]。

移植后器官功能障碍的病因诊断(表82.1)

移植后移植物穿刺活检

同种异体移植物移植后活体组织检查的适应证包括：①检测肝脏功能障碍的原因；②评估治疗的效果和(或)疾病的进展；③记录免疫状态来帮助指导免疫抑制的治疗(IS)。由于小样本活检(长度小于20mm)容易产生抽样误差，美国肝脏疾病研究协会推荐16G针穿刺两块组织样本用于评估肝纤维化程度；此外，那些取样少于11个门管区的样本可能不具有代表性[28]。移植肝脏活组织检查也应遵循其他类似的指南，特别是包含移植后评估肝纤维化程度的指南。

大多数组织病理学检查常规通过甲醛固定石蜡包埋切片来完成。在对包含抗体介导的急性排斥反应(AMR)等在内的并发症进行临床鉴别诊断时，推荐使用冰冻组织来对免疫球蛋白和补体进行免疫荧光染色，而非染色敏感性较差的甲醛固定石蜡包埋样本。甲醛固定石蜡包埋切片也可以用于C4d染色[29,30]。常用的特殊染色法，只有在HE染色切片检查后才可以使用，主要包括三色染色法、铁染色法、铜染色法来检测慢性胆汁淤积。怀疑患者发生胆管缺失或者慢性炎症时，还可以使用细胞角蛋白7或19来定位胆管细胞和向胆管细胞化生的肝细胞[31]。

最好一次性完成切片检查，然后将切片检查结果与患者的既往史和实验室检查结果相结合，也可常规将当前切片与既往同种切片进行对比，再做出鉴别诊断。这有助于病因解释，评估治疗干预效果和疾病进展。每周临床病理会议上复核所有的肝脏移植物活检结果，并向临床医生和病理医生进行反馈，这是保障评估质量的重要方法。

失功移植物的评估

同种异体移植物衰竭的大体病理检查应当遵循标准化方法[32]，尤其关注各级胆管、肝动脉、门静脉和肝静脉。有时需要主刀外科医生的援助，帮助解释外科解剖的问题。常规组织取样应包括：①血管吻合口(如果存在的话)；②肝左叶和肝右叶浅表和深部的组织；③至

表 82.1　常见的移植脏器综合征发生的时间估算

综合征	临床相关性/观察	高峰时段
“缺血”再灌注损伤	冷缺血时间>12 小时或热缺血时间>120 分钟；年龄>60 岁，血流动力学不稳定，DCD，吻合术再行；胆汁分泌匮乏；胆汁淤积期延长导致的胆汁淤积综合征	主要在再灌注后或移植术(OLTx)后几周内的活检中确诊。根据初次损伤的严重程度不同，再灌注损伤可能持续数月
AMR	ABO 血型不符的捐献者；高滴度(>1:32)的淋巴毒实验 DSA；移植后初期出现持续低水平的血小板和补体	移植后早期的数周至数月；后期新发比较少见或者未得到诊断
急性细胞排斥反应	更年轻的“更健康的”女性，免疫抑制程度不足的受体；长时间的冷缺血，以及免疫失调(如 PSC，AIH，PBC)	高峰阶段取决于免疫抑制方案，通常是 3~40 天；后期的发作主要与免疫抑制治疗不合理相关
慢性排斥反应	通常出现在免疫抑制程度不同的患者(如感染、肿瘤、PTLD)和有急性排斥反应既往史和依从性差的患者	双峰分布：第一个高峰通常在 0~4 周，第二个高峰通常在 18~36 个月(详见正文)
肝动脉血栓形成	非最优吻合；儿童的或者小口径的血管；器官供体和(或)受体动脉粥样硬化；动脉吻合不理想或困难，吻合口血管管径差异明显；高凝状态；动脉供血不足(小肝综合征的血管痉挛)	
胆道梗阻或者狭窄	动脉供血不足或血栓形成；长时间的冷缺血，DCD，困难的胆道吻合；AMR；PSC 等原发病	没有固定规律，但是发病的时间可以用于病因学检测：<6 个月的通常是机械性的缺血-再灌注损伤引起的(缺血性胆管病)或者 AMR；>6 个月的通常是复发疾病或者机械性损伤
静脉流出道梗阻	困难的“背驮式”肝静脉重建；心力衰竭	通常是早期数月内
机会性感染病毒(CMV，EBV，腺病毒等)和真菌感染(见正文)	血清反应阳性的供体向阴性受体捐献（通常是儿童）；过度免疫抑制	0~8 周内，在这之后除了 EBV 相关的 PTLD 及其他 EBV 相关的肿瘤(详见正文)，其余不常见
病毒性肝炎（如 AIH，HCV，HEV）复发或新发	HBV、HCV 原发性感染或者患者通过与动物接触或饮食不洁导致的获得性 HEV 肝炎	通常在移植后 4~6 周首次诊断并持续存在；进展迅速的案例可 2 周内初次确诊
HIV，PBC，PSC 再发	原发性 AIH、PBC、PSC(危险因素详见正文)	通常是移植后 6 个月后发现；移植后复发率随时间增加而增加
酗酒	精神病共患率/社会动乱；治疗依从性差；γ-GTP：ALP 比值>1.4(危险因素详见正文)	常常大于 6 个月
NASH	原发性 NASH 或病因未明的肝硬化；一般人群中 NASH 危险因素持续存在或加剧	通常是 3~4 周后发现并且随着危险因素的持续存在而增加

AIH，自身免疫性肝炎；ALP，碱性磷酸酶；AMR，抗体介导的排斥反应；CMV，巨细胞病毒；DCD，遗体捐献；DSA，供体特异性抗体；EBV，EB 病毒；γ-GTP，γ-谷酰胺转肽酶；HBV，乙型肝炎病毒；HCV，丙型肝炎病毒；HEV，戊型肝炎病毒；HLA，人类白细胞抗原；HSV，单纯性疱疹病毒；IS，免疫抑制；NASH，非酒精性脂肪性肝炎；PBC，原发性胆汁性肝硬化；PSC，原发性硬化性胆管炎；PTLD，移植后淋巴组织增生性疾病；VZ，水痘带状疱疹病毒。

少一处小叶中央深部取样同时包含中型胆管和动脉；④任何明显的大体异常。

移植后早期移植物衰竭的主要原因为缺血再灌注损伤或原发性的移植物无功能、血管血栓形成和患者死亡[33,34]，有少部分则是因为急性排斥反应(ACR)或抗体介导的排斥反应所导致[35,36]。复发性疾病，技术失误所导致的并发症(如血管血栓形成或胆泥)以及患者死亡，是远期移植物衰竭(大于 1 年)最常见的原因[37,38]。慢性排斥反应并不是导致移植物衰竭的常见原因[37,39]，复发性 HCV 导致的肝硬化是移植物衰竭的主要原因，并为器官合理分配制造了障碍[40]。

小体积活体供肝的特别注意事项

正常的肝性结构和功能依靠门静脉和肝动脉血液流入以及肝静脉流出与胆道引流胆汁。肝脏部分移植必须包括至少一个上述的管道系统，尤其是在残余肝脏的切缘。因此对于病理医生来说，必须知晓手术操作的技术细节和术后活检组织来源，因为非典型的组织取样可能误导移植肝段的选取。例如，在手术切缘的组织样本中可以观察到肝实质梗死或高位胆道或静脉流出阻塞，而实际上受试者肝损伤测试结果可以正常或接近正常，因此病理医生必须知晓手术操作的技术细节和术后活检组织来源。

移植后早期，活体供肝的肝细胞通常持续再生，也就意味着更容易被穿刺活检[41]和抗体介导的排斥反应损伤[42]。移植后晚期，门静脉病变、低级别胆管细胞化生和结节状增生在小体积活体肝移植中则相当常见[43]。

缺血再灌注损伤

缺血再灌注损伤是由器官捐献时的热缺血、冷缺血、血液再灌注和各种围术期事件效应累积而导致的供肝损伤[44,45]。心脏死亡器官捐献(DCD)尤其值得一提，因为这些器官都会经历长时间的缺血性损伤。即使最好的医生主刀，移植手术也会因为缺血再灌注损伤而造成胆管周围血管丛大量的血液成分梗阻和术后损伤，进而更容易诱发缺血性胆管病[46-48]。

临床表现

缺血再灌注损伤的早期症状包括胆汁生成减少和血清中乳酸持续提升，通常同时伴随移植后开始几天内血清丙谷转氨酶(ALT)和谷草转氨酶(AST)显著升高(大于2500IU/mL)[3]，其次是在首周内ALT /AST比值迅速恢复正常以及长期的“淤胆阶段”——总胆红素和γ-GTP持续攀升。随着肝脏损伤测试的异常指标不断恢复正常，器官功能也逐渐复苏，但是缺血性胆管病和胆汁综合征的发生风险仍会增加[49,50]。

组织病理学结果

血管再生后数个小时内获得再灌注后穿刺活检样本可以有效地评估缺血再灌注损伤的程度[3,51]。轻微损伤十分常见，如小泡性脂肪变、肝细胞聚集(即肝细胞相互分离和细胞质的“聚集”)和肝细胞肿胀[3,32]。重度损伤的特点是汇管区坏死、桥接坏死和伴有严重嗜中性炎症的带状或融合性的凝固坏死[3,51]。

轻微损伤后常伴随肝细胞有丝分裂、细胞核扩大和骨小梁增厚。持续的损伤表现为持续几个星期的典型的小叶中心轻度肝细胞肿胀和肝内毛细胆管胆汁淤积并存，而严重的损伤通常伴随着显著的小叶中心肝细胞肿胀和肝内毛细胆管胆汁淤积，这种损伤可能会持续1~2个月[3,32]。胆小管增生通常由汇管区和伴随网状结构破坏的大片桥接坏死所触发[3,32]。随着肝脏功能的复苏，正常的结构可以修复，但缺血性胆管病的风险仍然存在。

大泡性脂肪变比例大于20%的移植肝中发生缺血再灌注损伤，可能导致含有脂质的肝细胞死亡，并将脂质释放到血窦中去。这些脂肪滴聚集成更大的脂肪球，引发局部的纤维蛋白沉积，中性白细胞增多，淤血以及局部的肝窦阻塞[1]。如果肝脏开始复苏，这种脂肪球会被巨噬细胞包绕，经过数周的吞噬最终被分解。

肝细胞会在4~6小时执行一次完整的凋亡循环，如果在移植完成数天后在组织活检中发现肝细胞凋亡或者凝固性坏死，则应怀疑移植物受到了新的损伤(通常是器官缺血)[52]。

鉴别诊断

胆道梗阻及其引起的胰腺炎、败血症、抗体介导排斥反应和淤胆型肝炎可以引起类似缺血再灌注损伤的组织病理学改变。详尽的供体临床资料可以帮助寻找可能的病因[35]。而移植手术后早期肝损伤最常见的原因就是缺血再灌注损伤和手术中的技术瓶颈带来的并发症。

对胆道和毛细胆管的检查可以为区分缺血再灌注损伤和胆道阻塞或狭窄提供有用的线索。胆道阻塞通常会造成一定程度的胆管周围水肿或者中隔胆管管腔内或管壁内中性粒细胞浸润。相反，缺血再灌注损伤通常不会导致胆道发生变化，实际上只会导致中性粒细胞围绕毛细胆管分布。而二者都会导致小叶中心的肝内毛细胆管胆汁淤积和小叶内中性粒细胞聚集。

缺血损伤导致的急性排斥反应的特征是汇管区和血管周围出现“典型的排斥反应型细胞浸润”：即再结晶的和小淋巴细胞，尤其是嗜酸性粒细胞浸润，这是早期出现排斥反应的重要标志，可以用于确诊淋巴细胞性胆管炎和淋巴细胞浸润的中央静脉周围炎(CP)。

淤胆型肝炎在缺乏临床资料支持的情况下，难以与缺血损伤相区别。淤胆型肝炎只在感染乙型肝炎病毒或丙肝病毒的患者有过报道，移植后的 3~4 周会有特殊表现。除非患者进行逐渐减量的免疫抑制或者抗病毒治疗，淤胆型肝炎患者的病情通常会随着时间的推移不断恶化。

门静脉过度灌注/小肝综合征

病理生理学

过量的静脉血流可以损伤小叶中央静脉和中央静脉周围的肝窦内皮细胞[43,53]，进而导致移植物的功能障碍，这就是小叶中央静脉过度灌注(PHP)或小肝综合征(SFSS)。中央静脉血流增加可以导致腺苷流失和动脉收缩，又反过来导致动脉血栓和缺血性胆管炎。

肝细胞再生[43]依赖于门脉血液供应，门脉血供太少会阻碍细胞再生，导致移植物脂肪变性[54,55]。除非肝静脉流出受阻，肝细胞再生障碍一般来说不是肝移植的主要问题[56]。

临床表现

Dahm 等人[57]将 PHP/SFSS 定义为移植早期连续 3 天出现至少两个下列并发症：排除技术、免疫、感染并发症之后的胆红素升高(大于 100μmol/L)，INR>2 和 3~4 级肝性脑病。PHP/SFSS 可能也会导致所谓的技术并发症，在小体移植物中较为常见[43]。

组织病理学结果

小叶中央静脉和中央静脉周围的肝窦内皮细胞剥脱最早在移植后 5 分钟时就发生[43,53,58-60]。严重时，在中央静脉肝窦连接处微血管破裂可能会导致小叶中央间质出血，渗入肝实质[61,62]。移植后肝脏可能出现内皮细胞肥大、皮下水肿、肌成纤维细胞增生和血管内皮细胞纤维增生/内膜增厚和血管闭塞或栓塞血管再通，如果移植物从最初的这些风险中存活下来，那么肝脏就会开始自我修复。活检中静脉病变并不常见。相反，活检中可以经常观察到非特异性的小叶中心胆汁淤积，小叶中心的肝细胞脂肪变性与伴随肝窦扩张的肝细胞萎缩和(或)小叶中心的肝细胞坏死以及低位的胆管反应。

衰竭移植物的肝门切片经常表现出中央静脉内皮创伤，分支静脉局灶性纤维增生，动脉血管痉挛以及某些情况下会发生缺血性胆管炎，尤其在肝动脉形成血栓的情况下[43]。随着移植物功能逐渐复苏，门脉高压和腹水几周后就会缓解，这一过程通常会伴随着正常结构的恢复，然而也有个别移植物会因门静脉病变最终发展成结节性再生[43]。

鉴别诊断

动脉血栓、动脉狭窄、败血症、低血压、胆道阻塞或狭窄和缺血性胆管炎都会导致类似于 PHP/SFSS 的病理变化，可能需要与缺血再灌注损伤相鉴别，但活体捐献的器官通常不会产生这种影响。胆道阻塞或者狭窄本身通常不会导致汇管区周围结缔组织出血或者小叶中心的肝细胞缺血性改变或明显的结节状增生。

血管并发症

肝动脉血栓

病理生理学

肝动脉血栓形成(HAT)是最常见的主要血管并发症，2%~20%的受体通常在移植后 30 天内发生[63,64]。由于肝动脉为肝外和肝内胆管、肝门、汇管区结缔组织以及肝门淋巴结提供营养，所以肝动脉血栓形成后这些结构更易受到破坏。这种损伤形式通常被称为是“缺血性胆管炎”[32,49]或“缺血性胆管病变”[50]，表现为显著的坏死，伤口/吻合愈合不良、胆漏和胆管脓肿，进而导致胆汁综合征[65]。

临床表现

肝动脉血栓形成早期临床表现主要包括发热、白细胞升高、肝损伤测试评分显著升高和脓毒性休克[63,64]。晚期则可能无症状或者仅表现为隐匿性胆管炎、反复发热，以及与肝梗死、肝脓肿、缺血性胆道病变相关的败血症和随后出现的胆汁分泌减少[63,64]。超声检查可用于监测肝动脉血流情况，但是血管造影术才是明确诊断最可靠的途径。

组织病理学发现

肝细针穿刺活检可用于诊断肝动脉血栓形成，但由于活检组织取自被膜下肝实质，而该区域肝组织很容易受到各种因素影响产生取样误差，因此这一方法并非完全可靠[32,66]。此外，肝门旁组织和大胆管这类最常发生缺血损伤的结构，常常无法进行例行检查。

肝细针穿刺活检可以显示小叶中央凝固性坏死或显著的小叶中央肝细胞水肿以及胆道并发症，如胆管增生、急性毛细胆管炎、阻塞或狭窄。有时由于患者血管侧支循环的建立或继发于胆汁淤积的肝门部胆管坏死还未侵及周围组织，活检结果也可能不明显。肝动脉血栓形成偶尔与急性病毒性肝炎相似，也可表现为肝细胞点状嗜酸性坏死或“缺血性坏死”。慢性动脉血流不足则会导致小叶中央肝细胞肥大以及肝血窦扩张。

失败的同种异体移植案例中，若移植肝发生过肝动脉血栓形成，则多有以下表现：肝门部或门周胆管坏死合并胆漏且漏入周围结缔组织，胆汁淤积，合并真菌和细菌播散的胆道脓肿，肝门淋巴结梗死以及斑片状肝实质梗死。

鉴别诊断

由于肝动脉血栓形成或狭窄几乎与每一种肝脏同种异体移植物综合征都有相似之处，应时刻保持高度警惕。小叶中央的缺血性坏死是肝动脉血栓形成最可靠的证据，但应注意血流不足也会造成小叶中央肝细胞水肿、胆道梗阻和胆管炎。慢性动脉血流不足会使胆管内皮细胞发生老化，其改变与慢性排斥反应相似。“缺血性肝炎”(点状肝细胞凋亡)几乎无法与急性病毒性肝炎的小叶阶段相鉴别。动脉血栓形成和胆道并发症之间的联系紧密，因此出现胆道并发症时应常规检测肝动脉通畅率。

门静脉血栓形成

病理生理学

1%~2%的受体会发生门静脉并发症，相比动脉并发症较为少见[67]。长期存活的同种异体肝移植患者若疾病复发或再次出现硬化，则与肝硬化患者一样容易形成门静脉血栓[67]。

临床表现

门静脉血栓形成会造成非硬化性同种异体移植肝广泛性坏死，患者则出现静脉曲张出血，爆发性肝衰竭以及肝硬化伴大量腹水和水肿[67]。如果梗阻不完全，将会发生小梗死或由于肠道菌群播散至肝脏引起反复发热。

组织病理学发现

移植术后早期的完全性门静脉梗阻常造成大片凝固性坏死。血管狭窄、扭曲或持续性侧支循环引起的门静脉血流不足可导致门静脉周围或中心性肝细胞萎缩、凝固性坏死、无法解释的条带状或全小叶型脂肪变性、结节性再生性增生[68]，或者肝脏脂肪变性。局部门静脉血栓的细菌或真菌感染会引起粟粒状播散的肝脏小脓肿。

鉴别诊断

门静脉血流不足与肝静脉引流不充分很难鉴别。前者易发生线性缺血坏死和肝细胞萎缩，而后者多出现中央静脉和小叶中心肝血窦内红细胞淤积以及闭塞性中央静脉病变。为明确血管异常的原因，必须进行超声波检查和血管造影。因门静脉血流不足而发生肝内脂肪变性者应该与复发或新发的脂肪变性或脂肪型肝炎相鉴别。

肝静脉和腔静脉并发症

肝静脉流出道相关的并发症相当少见。大部分流出道的显著狭窄或血栓形成都没有显著的临床或组织病理学表现。

临床表现

静脉严重狭窄或血栓形成表现为布加综合征（肝大、压痛、腹水和水肿）；轻度狭窄最先可能仅有组织病理学表现或门静脉-腔静脉压力梯度升高。

组织病理学发现

累及肝小静脉和静脉周围肝血窦的淤血及出血是静脉引流不畅最为可靠的组织病理学证据，常表现为轻微的小叶中心肝细胞坏死和脱落。慢性改变包括结节性再生性增生、静脉周围纤维化、中央静脉闭塞(尤其是当流出道梗阻严重或长时间梗阻）以及中央静脉硬化。慢性病变会伴随着界板区和静脉周围显著胆管反应而发生，使得结构标志不易辨认而难以排除胆道梗阻。

鉴别诊断

如果上述的改变均无显著炎性反应，则应该怀疑存在机械性或流出道梗阻的因素。相反的，如果小叶中央改变伴随显著的淋巴细胞、组织细胞或淋巴浆细胞性炎症，则应该考虑发生了免疫介导的损伤，如急性或慢性排斥反应、自身免疫性肝炎（AIH）或药物性肝损伤（可能性较小）。然而，一些“免疫介导的”小叶中心损伤会出现短暂的静脉周围炎症，而且其后期表现无法与机械性静脉流出道梗阻相鉴别[69]。回顾临床病史和先前的组织活检有助于确定潜在病因。

胆道并发症

胆管系统一直是肝移植术最为脆弱的部分，约20%的受体会出现相关并发症——在小体肝移植中发生率更高。供体肝外胆管的末梢部分最容易发生缺血，而周围胆管丛容易同时发生缺血–再灌注损伤和手术损伤[70]。

胆管狭窄是最常见的并发症，可以根据移植术后的时间（早期或晚期）和位置（吻合口–非吻合口或肝内）进行细分[71–75]。肝内狭窄可进一步分为肝门部或周围性狭窄。早期（<1 年）非吻合口狭窄常与缺血–再灌注损伤有关[74,76]，且多发生在门周胆管。晚期（>1 年）非吻合口狭窄多为周围性且与免疫风险因素相关，如患者的基础疾病为原发性硬化性胆管炎（PSC）。

组织病理学改变

同种异体肝移植胆道并发症与受体原肝脏的胆道病变在组织病理上表现一致。狭窄性或梗阻性胆管病变典型表现常包括肝门部和胆管周围水肿、门部显著中性粒细胞性炎症、胆管上皮内或管腔内的中性粒细胞浸润、不同严重程度的界板区胆管反应、小叶中心毛细胆管胆汁淤积以及全小叶的中性粒细胞簇集。慢性胆道狭窄或间歇性梗阻常常与混合型或显著的慢性门静脉炎相关，小胆管则常发生胆道内皮细胞的衰老以及低级别胆管缺失。移植术后一年以上，除了上述典型特征之外，胆道狭窄也是门静脉嗜酸性变性较为常见的原因。

胆道管腔内出现红细胞或血管中出现胆结石提示发生了胆道–脉管瘘，有时也会表现为血清胆红素过高（超出病理生理范围）。相比较而言，无症状患者接受肝胆管造影术后一天左右进行组织活检，理论上不应该出现小叶内胆管周围出血[77]。

鉴别诊断

最初几周内胆道梗阻或胆管炎很难与缺血–再灌注损伤以及急性细胞排斥反应相鉴别，尤其是组织活检之前进行过加大剂量的免疫抑制（IS）治疗的患者。

移植术后早期胆道梗阻或狭窄与急性细胞排斥反应相比更容易出现显著门静脉中性粒细胞浸润，胆管周围水肿，细胞核结构无异常——正常核浆比、正常胆管上皮细胞、中央静脉周围无单核细胞炎症。而混合型门静脉周围浸润如幼稚细胞、小淋巴细胞、浆细胞和嗜酸性粒细胞、淋巴细胞胆管炎和增大的细胞核（胆道上皮细胞核浆比增加）以及静脉周围炎症则容易继发急性排斥反应。早期急性排斥反应引起的门静脉周围嗜酸性粒细胞增多非常显著，尤其是在进行节制性免疫抑制治疗的患者[78]。

迟发性和慢性胆道并发症偶尔表现为显著的门静脉单核细胞炎症、胆管内皮细胞衰老和低级胆管缺失[79]；这些并发症也可造成单独的门静脉嗜酸性粒细胞增多——这与急性和慢性排斥反应、病毒性肝炎以及复发性功能紊乱如原发性硬化性胆管炎类似。

胆道狭窄或原发性硬化性胆管炎复发与慢性排斥反应相比更易有以下表现：有胆道并发症或原发性硬化性胆管炎病史、胆管周围片状水肿、门静脉放射状扩张、门静脉中性粒细胞增多症、胆管反应以及门静脉周围肝细胞铜或铜相关蛋白沉积。而容易发生急性或慢性排斥反应者则多有以下特点：有排斥反应或免疫抑制治疗不充分病史、淋巴浆细胞性门静脉炎、小门脉系统、胆管反应缺失、活跃的中央静脉炎和静脉周围纤维化。

同种异体移植失败案例的其他发现也可用于鉴别胆道狭窄或原发性硬化性胆管炎复发与慢性排斥反应[80]。发生慢性排斥反应的肝脏质量通常正常或轻度增加，而伴有梗阻性胆管病变的肝脏则显著增大。梗阻性胆管病变常造成门部淋巴结的肝静脉窦胆汁染色组织细胞增多症，而慢性排斥反应时淋巴结通常萎缩或纤维化。门周动脉可正常或者有轻度局灶性偏心性血管内膜纤维增生，而慢性排斥反应典型表现为动脉泡沫细胞病变和显著的中心性血管纤维增生。发生梗阻性胆管病变时，肝外及大的肝内胆管常出现局灶性溃疡、胆管周围淋巴浆细胞性炎症和纤维化，而在慢性排斥反应中溃疡很少见。如果浸润部位周围穿刺活检和肝门部周围大胆管组织培养切片检查都发现显著的浆细胞浸润，则应该考虑原发疾病复发或IgG4硬化性疾病[81]。

胆道并发症多为胆管炎，而毛细胆管炎与小叶结构紊乱多发生于慢性肝炎。除非是胆汁淤积性病毒性肝炎患者，梗阻性胆管病变多表现为胆汁淤积性肝损伤测试结果异常。慢性排斥反应时不会单独出现汇管区周围肝细胞铜和铜相关蛋白沉积。

排斥反应

抗体介导的排斥反应

受体进行ABO血型交叉配型时，高滴度的同族凝集素将造成严重同种异体移植肝损伤[82]，导致强烈抗体的介导排斥反应并使移植失败的发生率升高（约60%）[83]，而大部分的北美移植中心可以避免这种情况。由于供体器官库受到更多限制，亚洲移植中心仍会进行ABO血型不符的同种异体肝移植。在上述情况下应该采取血浆净化、强力的抗排斥治疗和微循环保护疗法以获得预期效果[84,85]。尽管如此，ABO-Ⅰ型受体仍然有发生晚期并发症如缺血性胆管炎的风险[83,86]。

临床表现

避免进行未经预治疗的ABO-Ⅰ型移植，能在很大程度上减轻强烈的抗体介导的排斥反应[84,85]。而不幸发生时，超急性排斥反应往往在再灌注之后迅速出现，并且这一时期持续数小时到数天(而不是数分钟到数小时)，这在其他同种异体移植类型中同样存在[83]。手术过程中血液循环完全重建后的几分钟内发生不均匀的再灌注、水肿、边界表面模糊以及最先开始分泌胆汁的肝叶突然停止分泌胆汁——这些都是功能障碍的最初标志。上述症状常伴有凝血功能障碍[82]。突然发生的同种异体移植失败非常少见。

临床上更为常见的是：移植术后几天至几周内血清胆红素和ALT/AST突然增加或持续上升，往往伴随持续的交叉配型和(或)供体特异性抗体阳性(DSA)、无法解释的难治性血小板减少症以及血清补充不足[30,87,88]。严重病例会出现动脉痉挛，肝血管造影显示节段性狭窄[83]。

组织病理学发现

抗体介导的排斥反应有多种组织病理学表现，与抗人类白细胞抗原或淋巴浆细胞毒性抗体引起的AMR相比，伴有同族凝集素反应的AMR会造成更多的损伤(图82.1和图82.2)。

高滴度的同族凝集素(>1:64)[82,89,90]常造成显著的肝血窦红细胞增多，局灶性中性粒细胞沉积、门周血窦、门静脉以及中央静脉血小板纤维蛋白栓塞。未经过治疗的受体再灌注后2~6小时可出现肝细胞嗜酸性坏死，在这之后通常很快会发生门静脉或门静脉周围水肿、坏死、局灶性出血、门周间质C4d沉积[89]以及门静脉、毛细血管和肝血窦内皮弥散性C4d沉积[35,89]。移植术后1~5天进行周围肝组织细针穿刺活检可以发现融合性凝固性坏死、显著肝血窦和静脉淤积、水肿以及汇管区结缔组织淤血(图82.1)[35,82,89]。门静脉常出现纤维蛋白沉积。穿刺活检时通常无法取到中动脉组织，若能取到则常显示内皮细胞肥大和动脉痉挛，如血管壁肌细胞空泡形成、血管弹力膜皱缩和血管壁脆性增加伴管腔狭窄。偶尔能观察到中性粒细胞性坏死性动脉炎。门静脉中性粒细胞浸润、毛细胆管增生和小面积融合性肝坏死常在第2~3天发生。如果不进行治疗，ABO血型不合的器官将在极短的时间内(1~2周)出现进行性出血梗死。

抗体介导的排斥反应造成ABO-Ⅰ型同种异体移植失败的案例中，移植肝大体上表现为体积增大、发绀以及花斑状地图样坏死。在极严重的病例中可以观察到被膜破裂、肝动脉或门静脉血栓形成。门部和门周区域的改变对诊断抗体介导的排斥反应有极大的帮助，这些改变包括周围胆管血管丛发生白细胞凝集和边集、动脉分支部分栓塞、局灶性小叶间隔内胆管管壁坏死以及动脉炎症和(或)坏死。抗体介导的排斥反应的远期后遗症包括胆汁淤积、胆道狭窄伴梗阻性毛细胆管病变、闭塞性动脉病变以及小胆管缺失或慢性排斥反应[82,84,86,91,92]。

对高淋巴浆细胞毒性抗体滴度(>1:32)的患者进

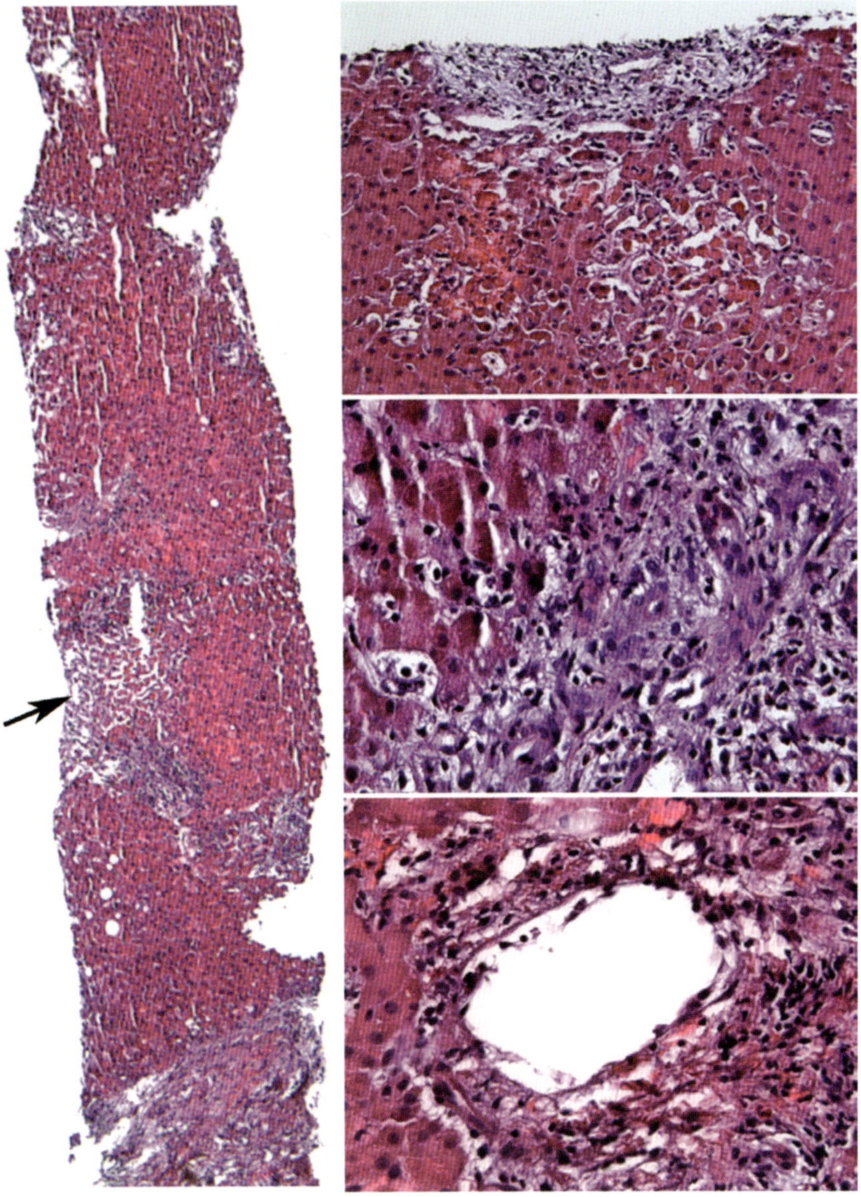

图 82.1　急性抗体介导的排斥反应。该组织活检样本取自一例移植术后 8 天的 ABO 血型不合的同种异体移植肝。组织活检显示斑片状融合坏死(箭头所示),右上方图片是其高倍镜视野下的组织图像。该标本也展示了轻度混合性中性粒细胞性门静脉炎(右侧中间图片)和显著的末梢小静脉内皮/肥大反应(右下方图片)。实际上与淋巴浆细胞抗体相比,ABO 血型不合的同种异体移植肝更容易引起抗体介导的排斥反应。

行再灌注组织活检，结果显示门静脉或中央静脉中出现血小板凝聚体的频率远大于交叉配型阴性的对照组[2,87]。在高滴度患者中,伴有胆小管增生和肝小管胆汁淤积的肝细胞点状嗜酸性坏死以及水肿往往在移植术后首周内发生。标本中很少出现动脉炎症或坏死,一旦出现则具有诊断意义。这些组织病理学改变与缺血-再灌注损伤的组织病理学改变非常相似。为了确定和验证诊断，需要通过与临床病理相联系并对 C4d 以及其他免疫沉积物进行染色，从而排除其他原因引起的功能障碍(图 82.2)[29,30,35,93]。

诊断同种异体肝移植发生免疫介导的排斥反应要符合以下所有标准：

1.仔细对组织活检进行审查,结果与 AMR 损伤的任意一种形式相符。

2.临床病理学联系可排除其他损伤因素。

3.供体特异性抗体的血清学证据。

4.有证据证明在受损的同种异体移植肝脏内存在高滴度而广泛分布的抗体和(或)补体(C4d)沉积[35,82,87]。

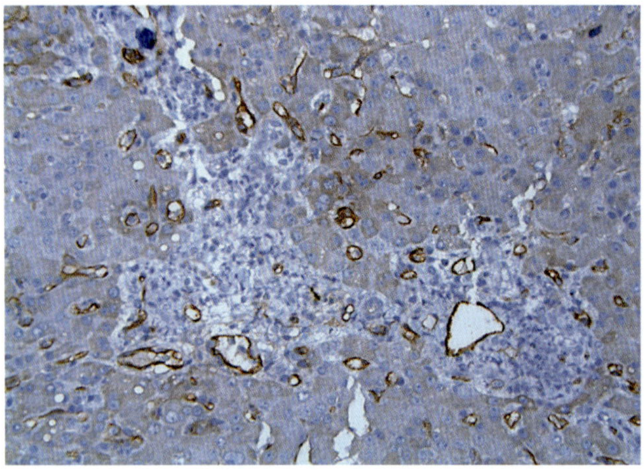

图 82.2 对图 82.1 中同一组织活检进行 C4d 染色。结果显示门脉系统中毛细血管和末梢静脉以及肝血窦内皮细胞中出现显著的 C4d 染色。C4d 染色也可用于检测甲醛固定石蜡包埋组织的补体沉积。

最后一项是指累及大多数门脉系统的门静脉、毛细血管以及汇管区肝血窦内皮深染。

然而与其他同种异体移植物相比，由抗人类白细胞抗原(anti-HLA)抗体引起的单纯同种异体肝移植 AMR 很难证实。诊断时遇到的困难如下：

1.同种异体移植肝体积较大,会吸收高载量抗体尤其是Ⅰ类抗人类白细胞抗原(anti-class Ⅰ HLA)[94],此抗原可以抵抗抗体介导的排斥反应相关性损伤[3,83,87,95,96]。

2.免疫沉积标志着潜在的损伤,其原因包括:(a)存在时间短暂[82,87];(b)与其他损伤有关(见下文);(c)更容易在冷冻切片中发现[97]。

3.抗体介导的排斥反应与缺血-再灌注损伤、败血症和胆道或血管并发症的临床病理学表现相似[82,87]。

抗体介导的排斥反应发生时，肝内免疫沉积物存在时间很短，即使是对冷冻组织采用更为敏感的免疫荧光染色检验技术也无法提高检出率[30,82,87]。在严重的病例中,IgG 和(或)IgM 以及 C4 选择性沉积分散在肝血窦、门周动脉、门静脉以及周围胆管丛,这些沉积物很容易被检测出来[30,82,87]。此后,免疫沉积物会呈现斑片状分布而且除非抗体滴度非常高，否则很难与背景染色相区分。无论如何,如果怀疑发生了抗体介导的排斥反应，留取冷冻组织用于免疫荧光染色检测有助于诊断。

对同种异体移植肝进行 C4d 染色和结果分析比同种异体移植肾更具有挑战性[89,98-105]。Bellamy 最近对这篇文献进行了回顾[29]。正常肝脏和同种异体移植肝组织活检常表现为 C4d 阴性。与交叉配型 (XM) 阴性(XM-)的对照组[97,105]和单纯发生抗体介导的排斥反应的受体相比,交叉配型阳性(XM+)的受体更容易在门静脉、动脉、门静脉毛细血管和肝血窦内皮检测到 C4d。内皮细胞 C4d 染色对抗体介导的排斥反应最具有特异性,但是 ABO 血型不符的抗体介导的排斥反应[89]、急性细胞排斥反应[103]和慢性排斥反应[93,106]也可出现“门静脉基质 C4d”染色。

在其他的同种异体移植中,C4d 沉积常伴随急性细胞排斥反应[35,89,93,98-105],而且在一些研究中这种沉积与 Banff 评分[89,98-105]相对应。坏死和脂肪变性的肝细胞表现为非特异性 C4d 染色。

在其他情况下也可以检测到门静脉和毛细血管 C4d 沉积,包括胆道梗阻[98]、HBV 感染复发[99]、HCV 感染复发[101]以及 AIH 复发[107]。此外,门静脉、毛细血管、肝血窦、中央静脉、动脉内皮细胞、淋巴结以及患有 HBV、HCV、AIH 和 AIH/PSC 重叠综合征的小儿自体肝脏的胆管周围和门静脉基质细胞中也可出现 C4d 染色[108]。与非排斥反应相关的同种异体移植疾病相比,严重 ACR 和 AMR 的内皮细胞 C4d 沉积更为广泛。与同种异体移植肾脏和心脏相似，同种异体移植肝脏出现 C4d 沉积也可伴有巨噬细胞和浆细胞浸润[100]。

鉴别诊断

供体特异性抗体或淋巴细胞毒性抗体高滴度的女性同种异体移植肝受体中,供体肝冷缺血的时间较短,但如果在移植后抗体持续存在、最初几周内发生了移植物功能障碍、出现难治的或者无法解释的血小板减少症以及循环中低补体水平,则应该怀疑发生了 AMR[30,35,87,88]。

若随后的组织病理学检测有以下表现时，发生 AMR 的可能性高于缺血-再灌注损伤：①管腔面以及门静脉和中央静脉分支发生中性粒细胞、单核细胞以及小范围的淋巴细胞边集,同时伴有显著且分散的内皮细胞肥大/增殖活跃;②水肿、嗜酸性变以及微血管炎;③微血管系统分散性C4d 染色[35]。门静脉周围水肿、坏死和出血则高度提示 ABO 血型不符的可能性。

除了 ABO-Ⅰ型移植肝以外，目前抗体介导的排斥反应很少造成突发性同种异体移植失败。然而一旦发生,将很难将其与门脉高压和灌注不足、败血症或血管血栓引起的出血性肝坏死相鉴别。若果没有检测到明确的 AMR 证据如动脉炎或动脉坏死和(或)弥漫性免疫球蛋白、补体和 C4d 沉积并结合抗供者抗体的血清学证据,同种异体移植失败的原因将极难确定。许多对 AMR 具有诊断意义的常规改变没有列出,若要进行诊断,则要求有完整的临床病理学联系。

急性(细胞性或 T 细胞介导的)排斥反应

急性(细胞性)排斥反应(ACR)是指“由于供体和受体之间的遗传差异引起的同种异体移植物炎症,主要累及小叶间胆管和血管内皮,包括门静脉和肝静脉,有时也发生于肝动脉及其分支”[109]。早期 ACR 极少导致同种异体移植物衰竭或永久性破坏[39,110],而晚期 ACR 更容易引起永久性同种异体移植物破坏,——很可能是治疗不及时引起的[111,114]。

临床表现

临床上 ACR 通常在移植术后 5~30 天发生。目前约有 30%的肝移植受体受到 ACR 的影响[111]。预先致敏或未接受最佳基础性免疫抑制治疗的受体早期出现 ACR,而使用淋巴细胞消耗抗体治疗或未进行重复免疫抑制治疗的患者出现 ACR 的时间较迟。早期组织破坏轻微时,往往没有临床表现。晚期或严重的急性排斥反应可能出现发热、同种异体移植物肿大、发绀以及压痛。移植术后早期 T 管在位时常出现胆汁减少、稀薄以及白胆汁。有时会因肝内静水压升高而出现腹水[115]。

组织学病理学发现和分级

ACR 有以下特征:

1.显著的单核细胞门静脉炎,但多混合幼稚细胞或活化的淋巴细胞、中性粒细胞以及嗜酸性细胞。

2.门静脉和(或)末梢肝小静脉内皮下炎症。

3.胆道炎症和损伤[115,116]。

建立急性排斥反应诊断的最低标准应至少包括上述两条组织病理学发现。如果有超过 50%的胆管/末梢肝静脉被破坏或者门静脉/终末肝静脉分支有明确的内皮炎症,则诊断更为明确。组织严重损伤的病理学证据如静脉周围炎症、小叶中央坏死、动脉炎和炎症(多为中心到中心和桥接炎症以及坏死)用于进行组织病理学分级[110,115]。

上述急性“排斥型”浸润几乎都出现在汇管区(图 82.3 和图 82.4),有时也累及中央静脉。内皮炎是指门静脉和中央静脉内皮下的炎症(图 82.3)。急性排斥反应的这一特征性表现也可出现在其他原因导致功能障碍的同种异体移植物中[117]。正如我们所预期的,急性排斥反应的浸润细胞免疫表型分析通常显示为 T 淋巴细胞,其中 $CD8^+$ T 细胞常包围并侵入被破坏的胆道[118,119]。B 细胞在浸润中通常占次要地位。在严重的急性排斥反应中也可见到巨噬细胞和其他白细胞,甚至由这些细胞占主导地位[118-120]。除用于区分急性排斥反应(T 细胞介导的)和移植后淋巴细胞增殖失调疾病(B 细胞介导的;在鉴别诊断中也提及)外,对浸润移植物的淋巴细胞进行常规的免疫表型分析对建立急性排斥反应的诊断没有意义。

累及小胆管(直径<30μm)的淋巴细胞性胆管炎具有重要诊断价值。胆管基底膜内可发现与胆管内皮细胞损伤相关及应答相关损伤的淋巴细胞。组织病理学表现还包括核周空泡、凋亡小体以及细胞核(核浆比,有丝分裂,核仁)体积增大。细胞质嗜酸性变和多核化通常是衰老相关改变和慢性损伤的标志[79]。基底膜破裂标志着严重的胆管损伤。门静脉和胆道周围肉芽肿既不是急性也不是慢性排斥反应的特征。

炎症性动脉炎或坏死性动脉炎是严重急性排斥反应的特征性表现,但是细针穿刺活检很难检出,而且很难再生[121],因此分级标准中通常不包括这一条。典型早期轻度和中度 ACR 的界板区通常无明显改变。发生重度急性排斥反应时,门静脉炎症浸润常侵入门脉周围肝血窦[113]。

排斥反应型炎症也可发生于结缔组织和终末肝静脉周围的肝血窦——也称为“中央周围静脉炎”[113],高达 30%的 ACR 发作时会出现排斥性炎症。这在移植术后晚期(>100 天)更为常见。仅有在门静脉发生典型 ACR 性改变合并静脉周围炎症并伴有小叶中央条带状淤血、出血以及肝细胞坏死脱落时才能诊断为严重的 ACR(图 82.5)。

Banff 急慢性排斥反应分级的数据来源可靠,这些数据由肝脏移植病理学、肝脏学领域公认的专家以及北美、欧洲和亚洲多家肝脏移植中心的外科医生提供(表 82.2 和表 82.3)。由于简单、易于使用、可重复[123]、经科学矫正且在前瞻性和回顾性研究中有重要预测意义[110,124],该分级被广泛使用[122]。

Banff 分级包括未确定、轻度、中度和重度四个等

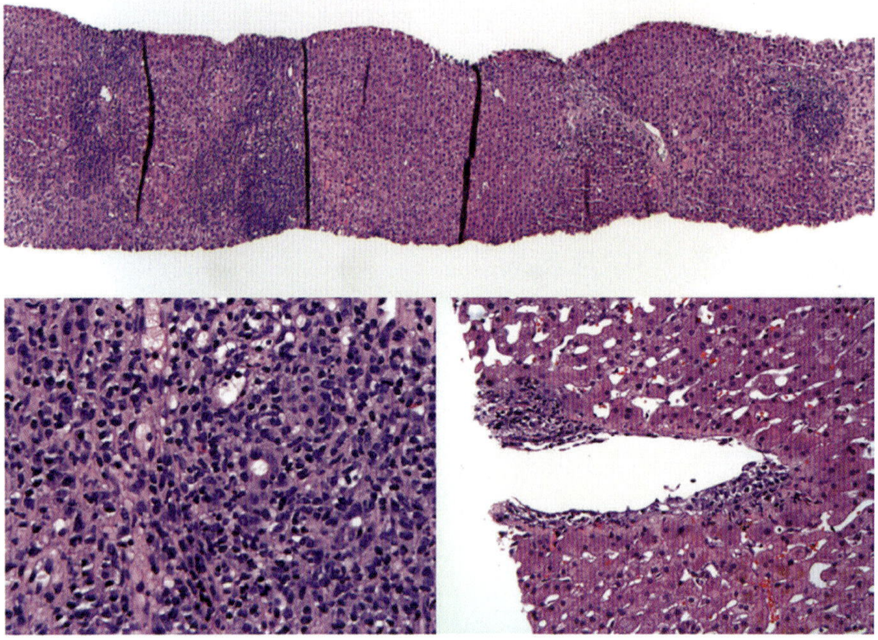

图 82.3 中度急性T细胞介导的(细胞性)排斥反应。这张显微镜图片显示,大部分汇管区都出现强烈的"排斥型"门静脉浸润合并胆道炎症和损伤(左图)。右图则解释了典型的"内皮炎",或炎症细胞浸润至内皮下间隙。

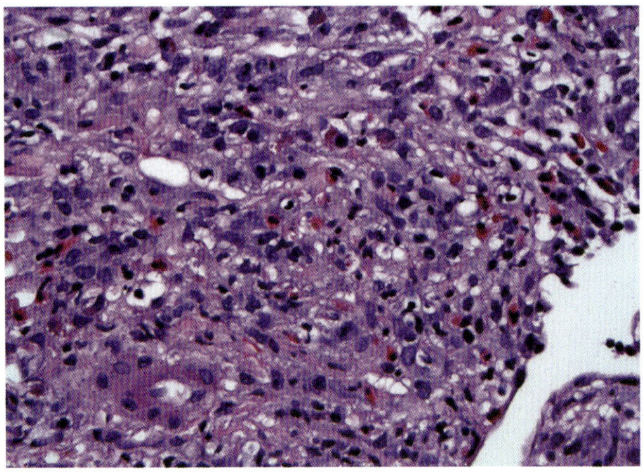

图 82.4 典型的多样性"排斥型"浸润,包括幼稚细胞、小淋巴细胞、嗜酸性粒细胞和中性粒细胞。这一活检组织与图 82.3 为同一样本。

级描述(表 82.2)以及一项半定量的排斥反应指数(RAI)(表 82.3)[116]:它是欧洲分级标准[125]的一部分且与肝炎活动指数[126]在概念上等价。RAI 半定量地对三个独立的组织病理学特征(门静脉炎,胆管破坏以及内皮下炎症)的分布范围和严重程度进行评分,每项分值均为 0~3 分,每项得分相加即为总 RAI 评分。

总 RAI 评分与描述性排斥反应等级、急性排斥反应持续性和复发性慢性排斥反应以及移植失败的风险有直接关联[110]。常规的 RAI 等级划分包括未确定(1~2)、轻度(3~4)、中度(5~6)和重度(>6)。总 RAI 的最大分值为 9,但是组织活检结果极少会达到这一分数[110]。相反的,由于增量的免疫抑制治疗后有应答,大部分活检结果,总 RAI<6,而且在晚期或随后的组织活检中不会引起明显的纤维化、胆管缺失或血管病变[110]。

在组织活检取样之前进行免疫抑制治疗会使组织病理学结果解读更加困难,因为一些特征性症状将会缓解,如静脉的内皮下浸润在 24 小时内就会出现。组织活检之前的治疗还会导致小叶中心肝细胞肿胀和肝毛细胆管胆汁淤积,进一步增加了不确定性。一般来说,治疗后 7~10 天,排斥相关性改变才会完全缓解。

迟发型急性排斥反应(>100 天)与早期急性排斥反应有很多相似之处,但也可出现轻度非典型表现(回顾见[113]):幼稚淋巴细胞较少、界板区中性粒细胞炎性反应明显、静脉内皮下炎症轻微、静脉周围炎症发生率高以及轻度增多的小叶活动性炎症,这会导致组织活检结果与慢性肝炎更为相似(回顾见[113])。

迟发型急性排斥反应也可以表现为单一的或显著的周围静脉炎症以及肝细胞脱落,且极少或不伴有门脉管道改变(单纯的中央静脉周围炎)[127-129]。这些病例

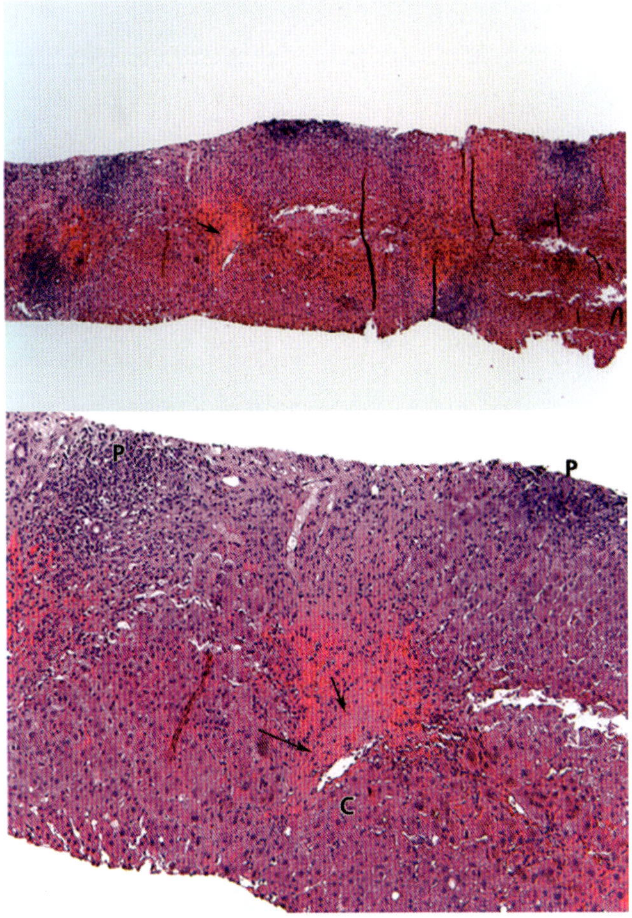

图 82.5　这一严重急性 T 细胞介导的(细胞性)排斥反应样本显示由显著“排斥型”浸润引起的全部汇管区扩张。也有显著的中央静脉周围炎伴随静脉周围肝细胞坏死和脱落(箭头所示),底部是高倍镜视野下的组织(P,汇管区;C,中央静脉)

表 82.2　同种异体肝移植急性排斥反应 Banff 分级(data from [261])

整体评估*	标准
未确定	汇管区炎症细胞浸润,未达到急性排斥反应诊断标准(见文中)
轻度	排斥性浸润见于少数汇管区,浸润轻微且仅限于汇管区内
中度	排斥性浸润累及大部分或全部汇管区
重度	除中度标准外,炎细胞侵入汇管区周围区,并有中度到重度静脉周围炎症。炎症侵入肝实质并有静脉周围肝细胞坏死

注:排斥反应分级整体评价的前提是对所有已经确诊排斥反应的研究对象的组织活检结果进行回顾,当排斥反应的诊断还未确立时,该排斥反应分级不适用。

表 82.3　急性排斥反应指数(RAI)(data from [261])

分类	标准	评分
汇管区炎症	少量汇管区炎症细胞浸润,以淋巴细胞为主,无明显扩散	1
	炎症累及几乎所有汇管区,炎症细胞为混合性,包括淋巴母细胞、中性和嗜酸性粒细胞	2
	在上述基础上出现大量转化淋巴细胞为主的混合性炎症细胞浸润,累及汇管区周围肝实质	3
胆管炎症和损伤	少数胆管炎症细胞浸润,胆管上皮细胞核浆比例轻度增加	1
	几乎所有胆管炎症细胞浸润,至少一个胆管上皮有变性,如核多形性,极向改变和胞浆空泡化	2
	在上述基础上所有胆管变性或局灶性管腔破坏	3
静脉内膜炎	部分汇管区中央静脉或肝静脉内皮下淋巴细胞浸润	1
	几乎所有汇管区中央静脉或肝静脉内皮下炎症浸润	2
	除上述病变外,还有中度或重度静脉周围炎症,累及静脉周围肝实质且伴肝细胞坏死	3

注:总 RAI 评分=门静脉炎症、胆道炎症/损伤和静脉内皮炎症的评分之和。

之后会发展为典型的慢性排斥反应,表现为胆管缺失和周围静脉纤维化,然而并非所有病例都会发生门静脉或中央静脉内皮下炎症。严重的周围静脉损伤会导致周围静脉纤维化和布加综合征或静脉闭塞性临床综合征[69,130]。Banff 工作团队提出用框 82.1 中的描述来对这一反应进行分级[113]:框 82.1 中描述的“最低”和“轻度”病例有自发恢复的可能,而严重的静脉周围改变则预示着可能需要更积极的治疗,但是目前还没有对已实施的治疗的效果进行前瞻性分析的研究。

鉴别诊断

如前文所述,移植术后的最初几个月中,ACR 应该与保存损伤、梗阻性胆管病变以及胆管炎相区分。

急性细胞排斥反应与 HBV、HCV 和 AIH 复发极难鉴别,只有对胆道破坏的累及范围和严重程度、界板区活动性炎症、小叶改变、周围静脉炎症以及肝细胞脱落进行极为细致的检查才能完成[131]。继发于 ACR 的病变

框 82.1 首先发生在静脉周围区域的排斥反应的 Banff 描述性分级

描述	表现
最轻微/不明确	累及大部分终末肝静脉的静脉周围炎症,伴静脉周围斑片状肝细胞缺失,不伴静脉周围融合性坏死
轻度	上述表现累及大部分终末肝静脉
中度	符合轻度表现且至少伴有局灶性静脉周围肝细胞融合性脱落以及轻中度炎症,但不伴桥接坏死
重度	符合中度表现且伴有融合性静脉周围肝细胞脱落和炎症,累及大部分肝毛细血管的中心性桥接坏死

包括胆道炎症性损伤、累及大部分胆道和中央静脉的静脉周围炎症;低级别或小叶结构缺失及界板区中性粒细胞炎症。相对的,当胆道破坏和周围静脉改变以界板区或小叶中性粒细胞炎症反应为主时,则更容易发生复发/新发病毒感染或 AIH。

同种异体移植 AIH(回顾见[132])在很多方面与病毒性肝炎相似,只是在 AIH 中,浸润的主要成分为大量浆细胞且大多显示出剧烈的界板区炎性反应。累及大部分中央静脉的富含浆细胞的中央静脉周围炎也会出现在发生 AIH 的同种异体移植受体中,这与发生 AIH 的自体肝表现一致。在这类病例中,AIH 与急性排斥反应相比更容易发生重度界板区炎性反应、浆细胞为主的浸润以及相对轻微的胆道破坏。

慢性排斥反应

慢性排斥反应(CR)的定义是:常继发于有严重或持续急性排斥反应且可能导致胆道和动静脉不可逆破坏的免疫损伤(回顾见[133])。"慢性"是一个没有严格界限的时间范围[115],因为慢性排斥反应可在移植术后几个月内发生且可在移植术后第一年内出现同种异体移植物衰竭(回顾见[133])。目前,3%~5%的同种异体肝移植患者在移植术后 5 年内发生传统意义上的慢性排斥反应,与 20 世纪 80 年代的发生率(15%~20%)相比显著降低[133]。除患有特发性移植前肝炎(IPTH)的受体外,慢性排斥反应的发生率不会随着移植术后时间推移而升高。

然而,慢性排斥反应持续出现并且可能成为同种异体移植晚期肝功能障碍和衰竭的重要原因,尤其是患有 IPTH 的受体。绝大多数慢性排斥反应见于依从性差、接受药物治疗如 α 干扰素[134,135]的 HCV 阳性以及因副作用而进行减量免疫抑制治疗的受体[136]。

临床表现

慢性排斥反应通常出现在有显著急性排斥反应病史的患者,这类患者有进行性胆汁淤积而且其体内对于抗排斥治疗无效的微管蛋白酶增加[115]。标准肝脏损伤测试通常显示 γ-谷氨酰转肽酶和碱性磷酸酶首先升高[115,137,138]。谷氨酸转移酶(ALT)和总胆红素的持续升高通常标志着急性排斥反应向慢性排斥反应转化,同时也可能提示同种异体移植物衰竭[127,136,139]。如果 CR 出现临床症状,在移植物功能障碍严重到能引起黄疸之前,都与急性排斥反应相似。胆汁淤积、胆道狭窄、肝梗死以及合成功能丧失在临床上表现为凝血功能障碍和营养不良,这些晚期症状也可能提示移植物衰竭[115]。肝脏血管造影常显示肝内动脉不显影伴周围静脉充盈不良以及节段性狭窄[115,140]。

组织病理学发现和分期

慢性排斥反应首先累及汇管区以及静脉周围区域,Banff 分级(表 82.4)[133]将其分为"早期"和"晚期"(图 82.6)。早期 CR 的标志包括:轻度门静脉炎症伴有淋巴细胞性胆管炎、累及大多数小胆管的胆管内皮细胞衰老改变以及累及 50%以下汇管区的各种小胆管缺失(图 82.6)。与急性排斥反应相比,慢性排斥反应炎症和嗜酸性粒细胞较少,其炎性浸润以淋巴细胞、浆细胞和肥大细胞为主[141]。

辨识胆道内皮细胞衰老改变对于诊断早期慢性排斥反应极为重要[79]:细胞核体积增大、染色过深、与细胞发育不良相似的空间分布不均;多核巨细胞形成;细胞质嗜酸性变;胆道大部分内皮细胞缺失(图 82.6)。细胞衰老的免疫组化标志物如 p16[142]、不同时表达 Ki-67 的 p21WAF1/Cip1 均有上调[79]。由于间叶细胞蛋白上调,内皮连接蛋白发生下调,这可能属于人体损伤后的应激反应[143]。晚期慢性排斥反应的特征性表现为累及>50%汇管区的胆道缺失;此外,还可出现动脉缺失。

Crawford 等人[144]将汇管区定义为"含有结缔组织的实质(Masson 三色染色法)与至少两条嵌入结缔组织(Masson 三色染色法)的管道(其中每条管道都被连续的结缔组织包绕)的交点"。在正常的肝脏,汇管区可检

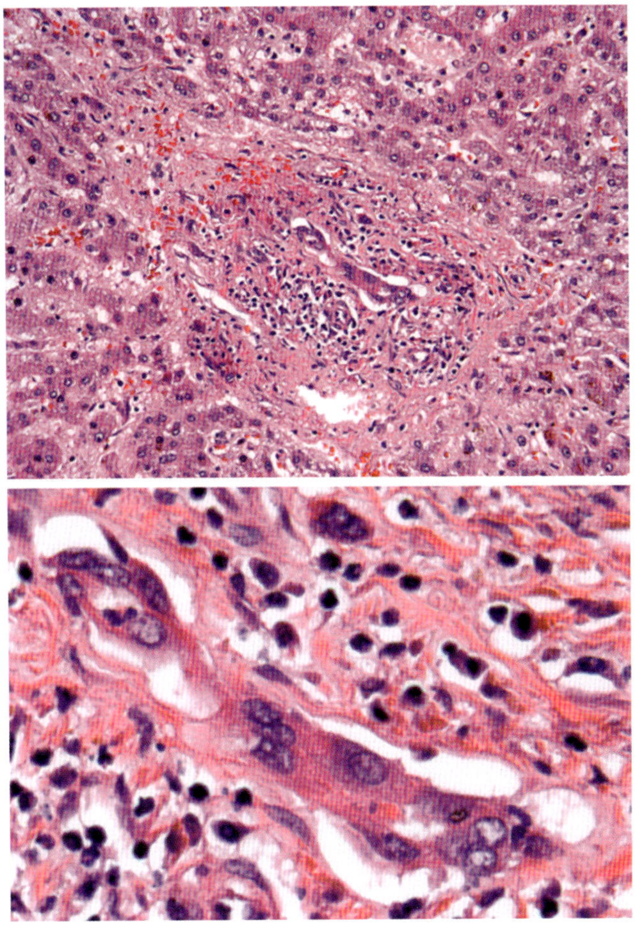

图 82.6　早期慢性排斥反应以累及大多数胆管的胆管内皮细胞衰老所引起的胆管破坏为特征。如果出现门静脉单核细胞炎症，组织活检显示其通常聚集于小胆管。如果发生胆管缺失，则累及50%以下的汇管区。高倍镜视野下（底部）的胆管内皮细胞衰老表现包括：细胞质的嗜酸性变，细胞核体积增大——包括核质比改变和细胞核分布不均。

测到的胆管和肝动脉分支分别占其总数的 93%±6%和 91%±7%[144]。下方的图片由其他人用更大的组织样本制作而成[145]。以正常均值加减两个标准差为界，当含有胆管的汇管区<80%时认为出现了胆管缺失，而当含有肝动脉分支的汇管区<77%时说明发生了动脉缺失。最近提倡应用一种类似的方法进行评估，即采用胆管-动脉相对应的概念：胆管缺失被定义为>10%的汇管区至少有一条动脉无胆管伴行或两个不同的汇管区都出现无胆管伴行的动脉[146]。无伴行动脉是指自动脉边缘起以 10 个肝动脉直径之和为半径的范围内没有伴行的胆管。

然而，晚期慢性排斥反应会导致胆管和动脉同时缺失[145,147]，这就使得上述评估办法很难应用。判断汇管区情况应首先基于公认的解剖结构——慢性排斥反应的胆汁淤积发生在小叶中央。

如果肝脏正处于慢性排斥反应的恢复期，那么界板区胆管反应很少见[139,148,149]。细胞角蛋白 19 和角蛋白 7 可以用于证明胆管缺失，随后进行染色可以观察到汇管区周围肝细胞向胆管上皮化生[31]。然而，若常规光镜检查很容易发现胆管反应，则标志着胆管再生[139,148,149]或潜在的胆管狭窄。后者可以通过汇管区周围肝细胞铜沉积进行证实——慢性排斥反应没有这一表现。

末梢肝静脉和静脉周围肝实质的早期慢性排斥反应的特征性表现为内皮炎和（或）静脉周围单核细胞炎症（图 82.6）。静脉周围浸润往往由淋巴细胞、深染的巨噬细胞和浆细胞组成[133,150]，常伴有静脉周围肝细胞脱落及轻度纤维化[133]。慢性排斥反应由早期向晚期转化的进程中，可以发现点状肝细胞嗜酸性变或“过渡期肝炎”[151]。

晚期 CR 的静脉周围改变的特点是严重（桥接）静脉周围纤维化，且至少伴有局灶性中心-中心或中心-汇管区的桥接以及终末肝静脉闭塞[133]。在进入终末期之前，由 CR 引起的进展良好的肝硬化很少见，此时静脉闭塞会导致实质区域消失和静脉中心硬化[152]。真性“再生性”结节也不常见，这可能是由于静脉病变与闭塞性动脉病变之间的联合作用削弱了所有的再生反应[153]。此外，静脉周围肝细胞空泡化和脱落、小叶中央毛细胆管胆汁淤积、非结节型纤维增生性再生改变以及肝血窦内泡沫细胞簇集也是 CR 的常见表现。

典型慢性排斥反应的最终诊断应该建立在临床、影像学、实验室以及组织病理学发现之上。在组织活检样本中，慢性排斥反应的最低标准应该包括：

1.累及大部分胆管的衰老病变，伴或不伴胆管缺失。

2.明确的泡沫细胞性闭塞性动脉病变。

3.胆管缺失累及超过 50%的汇管区[94]。

衰竭的同种异体移植肝的慢性排斥反应很容易诊断，因为特征性的诊断依据在第一、二、三级肝动脉树分支以及肝门部可以直接地观察到。除了部分以单纯胆管缺失或静脉周围纤维化为特征的病例以外，闭塞性动脉病变至少会累及一些门周动脉。泡沫巨噬细胞簇集通常最先累及内膜，这会激发内膜增生和供者源性的肌成纤维细胞向内侧迁移。为了增加并代偿减少的动脉血流，最终将导致内膜变脆/管腔狭窄以及动脉管壁肌层变薄。然而当代偿失败且整个血管壁完全被泡沫细胞取代之后，会形成动脉血栓，导致大胆管的坏

表 82.4 同种异体移植肝早期和晚期慢性排斥反应的特点(Reproduced from [133] with permission from John Wiley and Sons. Copyright © 2000 American Association for the Study of Liver Diseases)

结构	早期慢性排斥反应	迟发性慢性排斥反应
小胆管 (<60μm)	<50%的汇管区胆管丧失 大多数汇管区小叶间胆管上皮细胞变性：胞质嗜酸性改变；核深染；核内空泡；局部胆管上皮细胞崩解胆管仅由部分上皮细胞构成	残余胆管变性 ≥50%的汇管区胆管丧失
终末支肝静脉和第3区肝细胞	血管内膜炎 第3区肝组织溶解性坏死及炎性浸润，轻度静脉周围纤维化	终末肝静脉血管管腔局部闭塞 血管内膜不同程度的炎性浸润 严重的或桥接纤维化
汇管区肝小动脉	<25%的汇管区肝小动脉消失	>25%的汇管区肝小动脉消失
其他	所谓“过渡期”肝炎*伴肝细胞点状坏死	肝窦泡沫细胞聚集；显著淤胆
肝门周围大的肝动脉分支	内膜炎症，泡沫细胞灶性沉积，未累及管腔	内膜下的泡沫细胞致管腔狭窄 管腔纤维内膜增生
肝门周围大胆管	炎症损害和泡沫细胞灶性沉积	管壁纤维化

*“过渡期”肝炎。慢性排斥反应病情进展或从早期过渡到晚期过程中出现的轻度小叶结构紊乱和点状肝细胞嗜酸性坏死。

死以及缺血性毛细胆管病变。

周围结缔组织中的胆管和静脉内也可发现泡沫巨噬细胞。大的肝门部胆管可能出现局灶性内皮脱落、乳头状增生、管壁纤维化以及急性或慢性炎症。

正确的诊断是慢性排斥反应(CR)分期的前提[133]。早期CR提示若免疫反应的源头或病因能够被控制或逆转，则有较大的恢复潜能。晚期CR则提示恢复潜能有限，而且如果有临床适应证的话需要考虑再次移植。并非所有患者都会按照循序渐进的方式由早期进展到晚期，此时很难明确诊断。一些患者的急性或早期阶段持续数月或数年，而其他患者则在移植后的第一年内或初次发病后的几周或几个月内迅速发生纤维化并进展为晚期。也有部分患者以胆管缺失或动脉病变为主或仅表现为其中一种，但是通常情况下两者一起出现[133]。

组织病理学无法明确在什么样的情况下移植物失去恢复能力，而CR分期的重要实际意义就在于此。事实上它们提供与疾病逆转可能性相关的信息，这些信息与其他临床和实验室指标联系密切，如血清胆红素持续升高(>20mg/dL)，进行性合成功能下降、肝动脉栓塞以及胆管坏死或胆汁淤积。

鉴别诊断

在组织穿刺活检样本中，CR的诊断首先基于小胆管破坏、缺失以及静脉周围纤维化。穿刺活检的组织样本中很少出现具有特征性病理改变的动脉[133]。胆管损伤和缺失也可由非排斥反应相关性并发症引起，如梗阻性毛细胆管病变、肝动脉狭窄或栓塞、药物引起的“胆管炎性”肝脏损伤以及CMV感染。肝静脉引流不充分和其他原因造成的周围静脉损伤也可引起静脉周围纤维化。因此，基于单纯的胆管内皮细胞衰老、缺失或周围静脉纤维化进行CR诊断之前，应该首先排除其他非排斥反应性病因引起的相同病变。

CR很难与胆道梗阻或狭窄相鉴别，包括PSC复发[80]。梗阻性毛细胆管病变好发于下列情况：

1.部分汇管区发生胆管缺失并伴有其他汇管区胆管反应。

2.小叶内中性粒细胞簇集。

3.胆汁性梗死。

4.汇管区周围肝细胞内铜或铜相关蛋白沉积。

5.与胆管缺失(<50%)不成比例(超出)的肝毛细胆管胆汁淤积。

CR则容易出现以下特征：①与中央静脉炎和(或)纤维化相关的胆管改变；②没有典型的PSC复发改变(在前文中描述过)。在部分病例中需要进行胆管造影术和(或)血管造影术来鉴别CR和胆道梗阻。CR病例通常会显示“不显影”或周围充盈不足。

肝损伤测试得分无显著升高的患者可发生单纯的胆管缺失，其累及小于50%的汇管区，目前还无法确定这些罕见的病例是否由早期CR引起。很多原因都可引起单纯的静脉周围纤维化，包括机械性流出道梗阻、药物引起的肝脏损伤、所有引起静脉阻塞的疾病以及自体肝的布加综合征。

在任何情况下，诊断 CR 最可靠的方法是回顾之前的组织活检结果并将组织病理学发现与临床进展紧密联系，通常情况下，这些患者在组织病理学发现符合 CR 表现之前都有严重或未治愈的急性排斥反应病史。

细菌和真菌感染

对于移植术后两个月内为预防急性排斥反应而采取大剂量免疫抑制治疗的受体，由于合并手术引起的应激和组织损伤，发生严重“机会性”真菌和病毒感染的风险极高。移植完成 6 个月之后，会发生更多具有代表性的细菌感染。临床出现包括发热、吻合口或伤口裂开、再次移植、持续腹部疼痛以及血管栓塞的症状体征时都应高度怀疑严重感染。

细菌和真菌感染常出现在无活性的组织，因此大部分坏死组织应该常规进行细菌和真菌的特殊染色。急慢性炎症以及肉芽肿同时存在通常是感染的另一指征，但是这在高强度的免疫抑制治疗之后可能不会出现。大部分病理学家很熟悉深部真菌和细菌感染，这不在本章的讨论范围内。

“机会性”肝炎病毒

巨细胞病毒性肝炎

临床表现

任何器官系统都可能被巨细胞病毒累及，其程度具体取决于病毒传播的范围，但是活跃的 CMV 感染或 CMV 病通常首先出现胃肠道症状和体征，包括发热、腹泻、胃肠道溃疡、白细胞减少症和轻度肝炎伴肝损伤测试结果轻度升高[154,155]。呼吸功能不全、肺炎和视网膜炎标志着严重感染性疾病。CMV 有时也可产生与 EB 病毒感染相似的移植后淋巴细胞增殖疾病（PTLD），表现为淋巴结病变、发热和非典型性淋巴细胞增生症（回顾见[156]）。

组织病理学发现

由于血清学检测、预防性和积极的抗病毒治疗，CMV 肝炎目前很少见[154,155]。CMV 肝炎的特征性表现通常包括小叶点状坏死、Kupffer 细胞肥大、小叶结构紊乱以及小叶斑片状炎症（后文进行描述）。过度免疫抑制治疗、监测不力或治疗不充分的患者，其内涵体的形成受到抑制。任何类型的细胞都可能被 CMV 感染。诊断性特征包括细胞核内大嗜酸性包涵体（周围被一个清晰的环包围），伴小嗜碱性或双嗜性胞质内涵体。单纯的 CMV 不会造成亚大块或大块坏死[156]。

被 CMV 感染的细胞通常被中性粒细胞性微脓肿或巨噬细胞以及淋巴细胞集簇——微肉芽肿包围。CMV 肝炎也和轻度淋巴浆细胞性门静脉炎症有关，表现为胆管浸润和破坏，表面上与急性或早期 CR 相似，实际上认为胆管缺失和 CR 与持续的同种异体移植物 CMV 感染有关（回顾见[154，155]）。

经过治疗后，只能看见“碎片状的”细胞核 CMV 包涵体，这些包涵体在不用免疫染色或原位杂化技术检测病毒抗原或核酸的情况下很难辨认。迅速分化的组织如新生肉芽组织、增生的毛细胆管、梗死边缘组织、脓肿或其他受到感染的软组织是 CMV 生长的沃土。

鉴别诊断

CMV 肝炎较少引起小叶结构紊乱和肝细胞水肿——这类细微变化使其能够与早期急性 HBV 或 HCV 相区别。除此之外，早期或小叶期 HBV 或 HCV 一般很少出现微脓肿或微肉芽肿。明确诊断 CMV 肝炎要求至少有特征性包涵体（极少出现）或检测到特异性病毒抗原或病毒核酸。

CMV 肝炎表面上与 EBV 肝炎很相似，因为二者均有轻度淋巴浆细胞性门静脉和小叶炎症，且都可能出现幼稚或不典型淋巴细胞。在这些病例中，EBV 肝炎通常有更显著的淋巴浆细胞性细胞异型变化，而 CMV 肝炎则常造成更显著的小叶内炎症（例如微肉芽肿和微脓肿）。对二者进行鉴别时，常需要对深部组织切片进行染色以寻找 EBV 和 CMV 病毒抗原以及应用 EBV 核酸的原位杂交技术进行检测。

单纯疱疹病毒和水痘-带状疱疹病毒

组织病理学发现

通过细针穿刺活检发现 HSV 和 VZ 肝炎并进行报告非常重要，因为诊断后采取治疗往往有效，如果不进行治疗,则病情会迅速向致命性感染发展。HSV肝炎有两种分型:局限型和弥漫型[157]。两种都会造成特征性的局部区域凝固性坏死,这类坏死不受小叶结构的限制(回顾见[156,157])。坏死中心区域被肝细胞"影"占据,其内混合有中性粒细胞和细胞核碎片,而环绕在周围区域的多种肝细胞内通常可见HSV或VZ包涵体。被感染的细胞通常有轻度体积增大且包含有"污浊的"磨玻璃样细胞核或特征性Cowdry A型嗜酸性包涵体。HE染色切片上常可见多核细胞,但是很多情况下无法找到有诊断意义的HSV或VZ包涵体。

根据我们的经验,用于检测HSV Ⅰ和HSV Ⅱ以及VZ的抗体制剂之间会发生交叉反应,这使得病毒鉴别变得很困难。在这种情况下,检测VZ前体和成熟糖蛋白的抗体更具有鉴别意义。

鉴别诊断

如果HE切片的组织病理学诊断为HSV或VZ肝炎,无论该诊断是否确立,应该立即通知临床医生[158],这样做能够提供有效的抗病毒治疗,而且即使经免疫学染色后诊断不成立也可中断治疗。通过检测坏死斑边缘的活细胞以寻找特征性病毒包涵体,可以对HSV和VZ肝炎造成的坏死斑和梗死进行鉴别。然而多数情况下,该区域内只能看见含有磨玻璃状细胞核染色质的细胞。针对HE切片"过度诊断"HSV肝炎的问题,我们的解决策略是随后进行HSV Ⅰ、HSV Ⅱ和VZ的免疫学染色以明确诊断。

CMV和HSV肝炎的组织病理学鉴别诊断前文已经讨论过。

人类疱疹病毒-6

人类疱疹病毒-6(HHV-6)是β-疱疹病毒科人类疱疹病毒亚科的一员,是一种几乎无处不在的病毒。15%~80%的同种异体肝移植受体发生此类病毒感染,感染通常在移植术后2~8周出现,多由大剂量免疫抑制治疗引起。

引起HHV-6的间接因素包括CMV病加重、复发性HCV病情严重、其他机会性感染风险增加、移植物功能障碍以及ACR[159]。

HHV-6感染的同种异体移植肝组织活检结果呈多样化:中度淋巴细胞性门静脉和斑片状小叶炎症、微脓肿[160,161]、合胞体巨细胞肝炎[162]。该疾病常合并有ACR[160,161]。在HHV-6的个案报告中,单核炎症细胞[160]和肝细胞合胞体巨细胞内HHV-6病毒抗原的免疫过氧化物酶染色显著[162],这与病毒已知的生物学特性一致。

人类疱疹病毒-8

人类疱疹病-8(HHV-8)是嗜淋巴细胞的γ-疱疹病毒家族的一员,该病毒在卡波西肉瘤、多中心的卡斯尔曼病以及巨大淋巴结增生症和原发性渗出性淋巴瘤中均发挥致病作用[163-165]。

HHV-8原发感染可能更为严重且其造成的病变呈多样化,包括肝功能障碍、多器官衰竭、多中心的卡斯尔曼病和卡波西肉瘤[163-165]。急性病毒性肝炎的典型肝脏活检发现包括:小叶结构紊乱、气球样变、肝细胞水肿、细胞凋亡以及多种胆管反应。当多中心的卡斯尔曼病、卡波西肉瘤或无法解释的急性肝炎发生时,应该考虑对HHV-6和HHV-8进行鉴别诊断。

EB病毒

EBV感染使B淋巴细胞"永生化"并潜伏于B细胞或一些上皮细胞内[166-168]。高强度的免疫抑制剂增加了多种EBV疾病的风险,它们表现不一,从自限性传染性单核细胞增多症样综合征到强烈的移植后克隆性淋巴细胞增殖以及明显的淋巴瘤[166-168]。目前把EBV疾病归入PTLD的范围之内。

组织病理学发现

"典型的"EBV肝炎表现为轻度门静脉淋巴浆细胞性炎症,合并小淋巴细胞或轻度不典型淋巴细胞组成的肝血窦淋巴细胞增多症。肝血窦内淋巴细胞"堆积"提示EBV相关性疾病,在自体肝内也是如此。小叶改变包括局灶性肝细胞水肿、肝细胞轻度嗜酸性坏死、轻度小叶结构紊乱以及再生反应。

PLTD在肝脏常表现为细胞学上非典型性淋巴浆细胞门静脉浸润。在早期或多形性病变中,不典型细胞常与小淋巴细胞、幼稚淋巴细胞、类浆细胞以及浆细胞相混杂。由于不典型免疫母细胞覆盖在正常的门部结构上,导致其标志性结构难以辨别,因此EBV多形性病变以不典型细胞为主,并伴有汇管区的地图样扩张。部分病例伴有显著的肝坏死。霍奇金淋巴瘤相似性PTLD有经典的R-S细胞,并且与胆管缺失有关,在自体肝中也是如此。门静脉或中央静脉内皮的淋巴细胞定位则与急性排斥反应相似。

EBV RNA 原位杂交检测技术(原位杂交序列)可以证实 EBV 相关性疾病的诊断,可用于检查任何可疑的浸润。我们的常规病情检查也包括对 κ 和 γ 轻链以及 CD20 进行免疫组化染色或原位杂交技术检测,可以确定对于抗-CD20 抗体的反应程度[168]。有时我们也会检测 EBV 的抗原表达,如果有足够的新鲜组织,也会取一部分进行流式细胞术和核型分析,这有助于深入研究表型特征和免疫球蛋白基因重组。

鉴别诊断

支持急性排斥反应诊断的病理表现包括:多种“排斥反应型”汇管区和(或)静脉周围炎症,其中嗜酸性粒细胞浸润明显;以及严重且广泛的胆道破坏——与炎症相符。EB 病毒性肝炎引起的汇管区炎症相对单一,以具有免疫母细胞特性的活化单核细胞浸润为主,其中多数细胞有浆细胞分化特征,部分表现出非典型细胞学特征;胆道破坏局灶或轻微,与严重的汇管区炎症并不相称。

丙型肝炎和 EB 病毒性肝炎都可表现为窦间隙淋巴细胞增生,但后者通常可见少数非典型细胞。此外,丙型肝炎的淋巴细胞通常小而圆,且不活跃,往往在汇管区聚成结节[169-172]。外周血 EB 病毒水平升高,也有助于二者的鉴别。

确诊往往依赖于 EB 病毒 RNA 的原位杂交(E-BER),但对检测结果要谨慎解读[173];因为即使在普通人群淋巴组织中,EBER 阳性细胞也不少见。通常认为,EBER 阳性细胞聚集成群,或是 EBER 阳性细胞和 EB 病毒性肝炎病理表现同时存在,往往预示 EB 病毒复制增强,而患该病的风险也相应升高。

腺病毒性肝炎

病理生理学

发生于肝移植后的腺病毒性肝炎在成人中偶有报道[176,177],但主要见于有原发感染的小儿移植受体[174,175]。

组织病理学发现

腺病毒性肝炎并不多见,加上典型的核内包涵体难以识别,所以病理诊断需要有丰富的经验。典型者可见巨噬细胞构成的“痘样”肉芽肿,伴或不伴中性粒细胞随机浸润;不典型者则表现为肉芽肿包绕小片“地图样”坏死区[174-176]。腺病毒感染后,细胞十分“杂乱”——大量染色质挤向核膜,胞核像“烘烤过的松饼”;而典型核内包涵体多见于坏死区或肉芽肿边缘的残存肝细胞。确诊常需借助免疫组化染色,且多采用抗六邻体蛋白抗体——该抗体存在于腺病毒所有血清型中(共 52 种)(例如,MAB805,克隆体 20/11 和 1/6 的混合物,加利福尼亚州特曼库拉,CHEMICON)。

鉴别诊断

特征性包涵体可将腺病毒性肝炎与其他病变相鉴别,如单纯疱疹病毒(HSV)、带状疱疹病毒(VZ)、梗死,以及深部真菌或结核分枝杆菌感染。单纯疱疹或带状疱疹病毒性肝炎和巨细胞病毒性肝炎分别可引起肉芽肿性炎和局灶性坏死。然而,腺病毒引起的坏死相比单纯疱疹或带状疱疹病毒程度要轻。巨细胞病毒多形成“微小肉芽肿”,而腺病毒形成的肉芽肿更大,且罕有多核巨细胞。此外,巨细胞病毒性肝炎病理可见巨大细胞,并有嗜碱性或嗜两色性小胞质包涵体,以及周围伴清晰光晕的嗜酸性核内包涵体生成。而腺病毒性肝炎无巨大细胞形成,也无胞质包涵体,且胞核“松散”。

但往往需要借助免疫染色或腺病毒抗原检测来确诊,并联合其他检测方法以排外单纯或带状疱疹病毒、巨细胞病毒等。

评估晚期移植肝失功能和程序性活检的注意事项

导致移植肝失功能的因素多种多样,且很多在临床、血清学和组织病理学上表现出相同特征。对此,从事肝移植病理学研究工作的 Banff 工作组制订过一份共识文件,以指导解读活检结果(表 82.5 和表 82.6)[113]。

活检发现,导致晚期移植肝失功能的首要原因包括原发病复发和梗阻性胆管疾病[137,178],而急性和(或)慢性移植排斥反应只占 4%~38%。肝功能检查异常或有临床症状,且存活超过一年的移植受体,大部分(约 75%)活检结果都存在明显异常[113,137,178]。这些异常通常归因于疾病复发或胆管狭窄,但有些在临床上是隐匿的。无症状且肝功能正常的长期存活受体中,约 25%发现有明显异常,尤其原发病属于常见复发类型者(如丙型肝炎、原发性胆汁性肝硬化、自身免疫性肝炎[113,137,178])。

60%~70%有症状受体中、即使无复发性疾病且肝功能正常或接近正常，也可发现组织病理学有轻微异常。常见的轻微病变包括门静脉病变、结节性再生性增生、肝动脉小分支管壁增厚和磨玻璃样变,以及汇管区和肝小叶的“非特异性”炎症;但目前这些无法解释的病变都在仔细审查中。

移植后晚期肝活检发现，很多受体都存在主要累及汇管区的单核细胞性炎症，伴有类型不一的坏死性炎型界板区炎症，甚至无慢性坏死性炎性疾病复发者也存在[113];但是这些炎症产生的原因仍然不清楚。所以确诊可能很难,尤其是病变尚处于早期时。这时,可利用早期特征性表现做出初步诊断[113]。

移植前用于辅助诊断的实验室检查，移植后可能不那么有意义[113]。移植后 PBC 或 AIH 复发——甚至病理上无复发证据的受体，其体内抗线粒体抗体(AMA)和抗核抗体(ANA)通常暂时消失,而后又低滴度形式再次出现。移植前无自身免疫性肝炎的患者,移植后也可发现自身抗体——这可能是不典型排斥反应的并发症表现[179-181],也可能与新发自身免疫性肝炎有关[113,132]。

复发性疾病和移植诱发性疾病

原发病复发是造成晚期移植肝损伤和失功能最常见且最重要的原因,第 78 章已有详细介绍。复发性疾病包括感染性疾病(如甲、乙、丙、丁、戊型肝炎)、免疫失调性疾病(如 AIH、PBC、PSC、重叠综合征)、恶性肿瘤(肝细胞癌、胆管细胞癌)、中毒性损伤(如药物和酒精滥用引起的肝损伤),以及肝脏本身因素引起的代谢性疾病(如 α_1-抗胰蛋白酶缺乏症、Wilson 病)和肝外因素引起的代谢性疾病(如代谢综合征、血色素沉着症、戈谢病)。

很多病因不明的少见疾病在肝移植后同样可能复发,包括结节病[182,183]、特发性肉芽肿性肝炎[137]、婴儿巨细胞性肝炎[184]和 Budd-Chiari 综合征[185-187]。供肝基因型异常时,肝移植可能传播相应疾病,如家族性淀粉样变性、多发性神经病[16],以及草酸盐沉着症[17];但供肝表型多为正常,可用于“多米诺”移植。

肝炎病毒感染

甲型肝炎

有报道显示,肝移植后甲型肝炎病毒(HAV)的残存或复发——从瞬态移植物功能障碍受者肝组织、血清或粪便中通过逆转录-聚合酶链反应(RT-PCR)检测到甲肝病毒 RNA 即可说明。HAV 引起的常见病理学改变包括:类型不一的肝细胞凋亡,肝细胞变性伴胆汁淤积,轻度汇管区炎症合并胆道破坏,以及胆管胆汁淤积[188,189]。然而,对于发生不典型急性或慢性排斥反应的受体,其组织中也可检测到甲肝病毒 RNA[188-191]。因此,诊断移植后 HAV 残存或复发,都应综合分析血清学与临床病理学资料。

乙型肝炎和丁型肝炎

临床表现

资料显示,移植后若不进一步治疗,受体短时间内即会再次感染 HBV。随着 ALT 和 AST 水平不明原因的升高,6~8 周后临床表现也开始明显[192,193],较重者表现为恶心、呕吐、黄疸,少数病例甚至发生暴发性肝衰竭。肝移植后,若 IS(免疫抑制)治疗过度,受体会发生纤维化淤胆性肝炎并进一步恶化。但 HBV 复制活跃者要避免 IS 减量过快,特别是突然停药,否则会促使免疫系统“重建”,导致严重的免疫介导性肝损伤和暴发性肝衰竭。

组织病理学发现

除罕见型——纤维化淤胆性肝炎[193,194],HBV 感染后,移植肝和自体肝的病理表现通常类似,而此罕见型也因为有效的治疗而被大量消除。

HBV 感染后通常表现为急性肝炎,移植后 4~6 周内多可识别。若不处理,少部分受体——尤其是 IS 治疗减量过快者,会发生融合性或桥接坏死,甚至亚大块坏死[192]。而且还可检测到 Delta 抗原,提示合并 HDV 感染[195]。其余受体在移植后 12~18 个月内可快速发

表 82.5 各种引起晚期移植肝失功能因素的常见组织病理学发现 *(Reproduced from [113] with permission from John Wiley and Sons. Copyright ⓒ 2006 American Association for the Study of Liver Diseases)

组织病理学发现	AIH†	急性排斥反应	慢性排斥反应	慢性乙型肝炎和丙型肝炎	PBC	PSC/胆管狭窄
汇管区炎症的范围，程度及组成	通常弥漫；程度不一；单个核细胞浸润为主，其中浆细胞多明显	通常弥漫；程度不一；"排斥反应型"——混合性浸润(见正文)	局灶；通常轻微或极轻微；淋巴浆细胞浸润	局灶；程度不一；单核细胞浸润为主；有结节形成	十分局灶；程度不一；单核细胞浸润为主；有结节和肉芽肿形成	局灶或弥漫（取决于病程）；炎症轻微；中性或嗜酸性粒细胞，偶为单核细胞浸润为主
有无界板区炎症及其类型	典型特征：坏死性炎型；通常富含浆细胞	局灶且轻微，坏死性炎型	无或极轻微	通常不明显：坏死性炎型，伴或不伴胆管型	疾病后期重要的病理特征：胆管型和坏死性炎型，并伴铜沉积	典型特征：胆管型，并伴汇管区和汇管区周围水肿
胆管炎症和胆道损伤	无或仅累及小部分胆管	存在，常累及大部分胆管	局灶进行性淋巴细胞性胆道损伤；炎症随胆管缺失而减轻	无或仅累及小部分胆管	肉芽肿性或局灶重度淋巴细胞性胆管炎（一定条件下，极具诊断价值）	胆管周围片状水肿，"纤维性胆管炎"，急性胆管炎，汇管区胆管病变多样
胆管上皮衰老和小胆管缺失	不存在；或仅累及少数胆管或汇管区，局灶但可能严重	不存在，或仅累及少数胆管	衰老、萎缩或不典型病变累及大部分残存胆管(见正文)	不存在，或仅累及少数胆管	小胆管缺失(与胆管反应有关)	小胆管缺失（与胆管反应有关）
静脉周围单个核细胞性炎和(或)肝细胞脱落	类型不一，可累及大部分静脉周围区，类似排斥反应（见正文）；可能富含浆细胞	类型不一，重者累及大部分静脉周围区；有时可见静脉内皮下炎(见正文)	通常存在，但类型不一	类型不一，但大多轻微，仅累及少数静脉周围区	类型不一，但大多轻微，仅累及少数静脉周围区	不存在
肝小叶病变和坏死性炎	程度不一；且可见"玫瑰花环"，但程度不一	类型不一；若存在，集中于静脉周围区	类型不一；若存在，集中于静脉周围区	类型不一	轻度肝小叶紊乱；有肉芽肿形成；汇管区周围铜沉积和胆汁淤积为晚期表现	小叶紊乱不常见；中性粒细胞簇状聚集，伴或不伴胆汁淤积
肝纤维化类型	常见大结节，肝炎后型	罕见	少见，若存在常为中央静脉型；后期可能进展为胆汁型	常见大结节，肝炎型；也可见小结节型（见正文）	胆汁型	胆汁型

注：AIH，自身免疫性肝炎；BD，胆管；PBC，原发性胆汁性肝硬化；PSC，原发性硬化性胆管炎。

*最后确诊应该综合此表组织病理学发现和临床、血清学、放射影像学表现以及表 82.2 的重要鉴别标准。

† 适用于复发性和新发 AIH。

表 82.6 肝移植后复发性和新发慢性坏死性炎性疾病的诊断和鉴别诊断标准，以及肝功能检查异常的起始时间和类型 *(data from [113] and [260])

诊断	原发病	血清学/分子学检测 †	肝功能检查异常的起始时间和类型 ‡	重要鉴别标准
复发性 AIH	AIH	自身抗体(ANA,ASMA,ALKM)常为高滴度(>1:80);血清 IgG 水平升高	>6 个月 肝细胞型	急性和慢性排斥反应,HBV、HCV、HEV 感染；第三代 ELISA 阵列检测和(或)血清/组织 PCR 检测可鉴别
浆细胞性肝炎(新发 AIH)	除外 AIH	同上	>6 个月 肝细胞型	同上
复发性乙型肝炎或丙型肝炎	HBV 或 HCV 引起的肝硬化	HBV 或 HCV：标准第三代血清学检测和（或）核酸分子学检测阳性	通常 6~8 周，早的仅需 10 天;通常为肝细胞型,偶见淤胆型	急性和慢性排斥反应,AIH
复发性 PBC	PBC	AMA 阳性，但额外作用不大,因为大部分受者移植后 AMA 依旧高水平	>1 年 淤胆型	胆管梗阻或狭窄
复发性 PSC	PSC	正常	通常>1 年 淤胆型	肝动脉血栓或狭窄,慢性(胆管缺失性)排斥反应,外科解剖异常,单纯吻合性狭窄，原位肝移植(OLTx)术后 90 天内非吻合性狭窄,以及 ABO 血型不符
急性排斥反应	无（正文见危险因素）	正常	见于任何时候 通常为肝细胞型；若合并慢性排斥反应,可见混合型	常有 IS 治疗不充分，但不总存在（见正文） 重点鉴别:胆管梗阻或狭窄、HBV、HCV、AIH
慢性排斥反应	无（正文见危险因素）	正常	见于任何时候，但通常<1 年;淤胆型;肝细胞型罕见于静脉闭塞者(见正文)	常有 IS 治疗不充分，但不总存在（见正文） 重点鉴别:胆管梗阻或狭窄、HBV、HCV、AIH
特发性移植后肝炎	除外病毒感染和 AIH	HBV、HCV、HEV 感染和自身抗体检测皆阴性	>1 年 通常为肝细胞型	急性和慢性排斥反应,合理排除所有其他慢性肝炎，胆管梗阻或狭窄；做出该诊断须排除所有其他可能

注:AIH,自身免疫性肝炎;ALKM,抗肝肾微粒体抗体;AMA,抗线粒体抗体;ANA,抗核抗体;ASMA,抗平滑肌抗体;HBV,乙型肝炎病毒;HCV,丙型肝炎病毒;HEV,戊型肝炎病毒;IS,免疫抑制;PBC,原发性胆汁性肝硬化;PCR,聚合酶链式反应;PSC,原发性硬化性胆管炎。

* 组织病理学发现见表 82.5。

† 起始时间,即开始出现的时间。

‡ 结果持续升高超过一个月:肝细胞型即 ALT 和(或)AST>ALP 和(或)GGTP;淤胆型即 ALP 和(或)GGTP>AST 和(或)ALT。

展为肝硬化[192,193]。肝小叶慢性期病理表现通常远不如急性期明显，包括磨玻璃样肝细胞或含泥沙样核肝细胞(染色检测分别为乙肝表面抗原阳性,乙肝核心抗原阳性),轻度肝小叶紊乱,以及轻度坏死性炎症。

因过度免疫抑制,以及供受体间 MHC(主要组织相容性复合物)不相容,HBV 将大量复制,进而导致纤维化淤胆型肝炎；有些病毒突变后也可诱发此病变[193,196]。纤维化淤胆型肝炎的病理表现包括肝细胞明显肿胀、肝小叶紊乱、胆汁淤积,以及严重的胆管型和纤维化型界板区炎症，且常合并轻微或极轻微汇管区和肝小叶炎症。肿胀和变性肝细胞常高表 HBV C 抗原和(或)S 抗原,表明 HBV 可直接导致细胞病变[193,197]。

HDV 和 HBV 双重感染——尤其是接受了 HBV 相关治疗的受体,原发病的复发风险低于单纯 HBV 感染者[198]。而双重感染后的病理表现,移植受体估计和普通人群类似[199]。

鉴别诊断

急性乙型肝炎须和其他因素诱发的急性肝炎相鉴别,包括病毒类型如巨细胞病毒、丙肝病毒、EB 病毒性肝炎,其他类型如"缺血性"肝炎以及急性排斥反应到慢性排斥反应这一过渡期形成的"过渡期"肝炎。而最可靠的鉴别方法,就是对临床、组织病理学、免疫组化和血清学等资料综合分析。

慢性乙型肝炎须和其他慢性肝炎疾病相鉴别,如慢性丙型肝炎、自身免疫性肝炎以及药物性肝损伤。发现磨玻璃样肝细胞或在血液/肝组织中检测到 HBV 抗原或核酸,如没有其他原因提示慢性乙型肝炎。若不仅 HBV 抗原或核酸阳性,同时病理学发现有活动性小叶性肝炎,则提示复发性乙型肝炎,但尚不能排除其他疾病[193]。

急性排斥反应与急性或慢性肝炎的鉴别在前面章节已具体描述(见急性排斥反应,鉴别诊断部分)。

丙型肝炎病毒

复发性丙型肝炎引起的肝损伤是病毒复制和免疫介导共同作用的结果,二者任一都可单独诱发肝损伤[200]。IS 治疗减药过快,一方面可诱发严重的免疫介导性肝炎[201-203],类似数十年前 HBV 引起的慢性肝病。另一方面,减药过快可引起 HCV 高度复制,继而促使免疫系统"重建",并最终导致复发性丙型肝炎急剧进展[201-203]。因此,对于肝移植受体,尤其是对长期存活受体,免疫抑制剂治疗应缓慢减量[201-203]。

根据肝纤维化模型[200],不只是 HCV,其他任何损伤性因素(包括脂肪变性、病毒高容量复制、氧化应激、铁沉积、缺血-再灌注损伤、胆道重建、急性排斥反应等)都会加速疾病的进展。因此,超标准供体的使用会抵消部分疗效;尽管近年来 HCV 的临床治疗已有较明显进展,但受体的长期预后却无明显改善[200,204,205]。

临床表现

移植人群丙型肝炎的临床表现和普通人群类似,绝大部分患者发生急性肝炎,但一般没有症状,多因 ALT 和 AST 水平升高到基线的 4~8 倍而被发现[200]。此临床表现通常在肝移植后 3~6 周发生,若早至 10~14 天内发生,则很可能预示更严重的疾病。

HCV 引起的纤维化淤胆性肝炎和"过度免疫抑制治疗"有关,其临床表现以乏力、黄疸、胆红素和碱性磷酸酶(AKP)以及 γ-GTP 水平显著升高为特征。

组织病理学

常见型。移植肝的常见病理表现及演变与自体肝通常类似。然而,急性期移植肝的汇管区和肝小叶炎症通常更轻,慢性期主要浸润汇管区的淋巴细胞很少聚成结节;但移植肝的胆管型界板区炎症更明显[200,206]。

病理学可见炎性胆道破坏,但只累及少部分胆管,损伤轻且局灶,也无胆管缺失。少数肝小叶可见中央静脉及周围炎性病变。然而,对于丙型肝炎复发的受体,中央静脉周围炎既不严重,也不广泛。

富含浆细胞的"自身免疫"型。类似自身免疫性肝炎,复发性慢性丙型肝炎表现为富含浆细胞的侵袭性界板区和静脉周围坏死性炎(图 82.7)[132,200,207]。但这一类型尚不能明确,可能是"HCV 的自身免疫型",也可能是急性排斥反应,或者自身免疫性肝炎,甚至可能是这几种的综合[132,200,207]。

IS 治疗可减轻 HCV 引起的肝脏损害[207,208,209],但也会促使其复制增强进而妨碍病毒的彻底清除[208]。

急性排斥反应和自身免疫性肝炎都可见广泛的中央静脉周围坏死性炎,伴或不伴大量浆细胞浸润,但复发性丙型肝炎则无此病理表现。无论是否感染 HCV,也无论是否是肝移植受体,中央静脉周围炎大多对强化 IS 治疗敏感[132,200,207]。

纤维化淤胆性肝炎型。过度 IS 治疗后,HCV 诱发的纤维化淤胆性肝炎通常发生于移植后一年内,典型者以外周血高滴度 HCV RNA (通常>$3\sim5\times10^7$ IU/mL)为特征。FCH 最多见的病理表现包括胆汁淤积、肝细胞气球样变、纤维化(汇管区周围、汇管区,以及桥接性)和胆管反应[210]。肝细胞点状凋亡或坏死,以及轻度混合性——甚至以中性粒细胞浸润为主的汇管区炎症也很常见。HCV 引起的 FCH 轻重程度不一,轻型仅表现为细胞轻度肿胀,轻微或极轻微胆管反应,以及稍重的汇管区单核细胞性炎。

共存病变的诊断

丙型肝炎复发情况下,病理上往往很难诊断急性

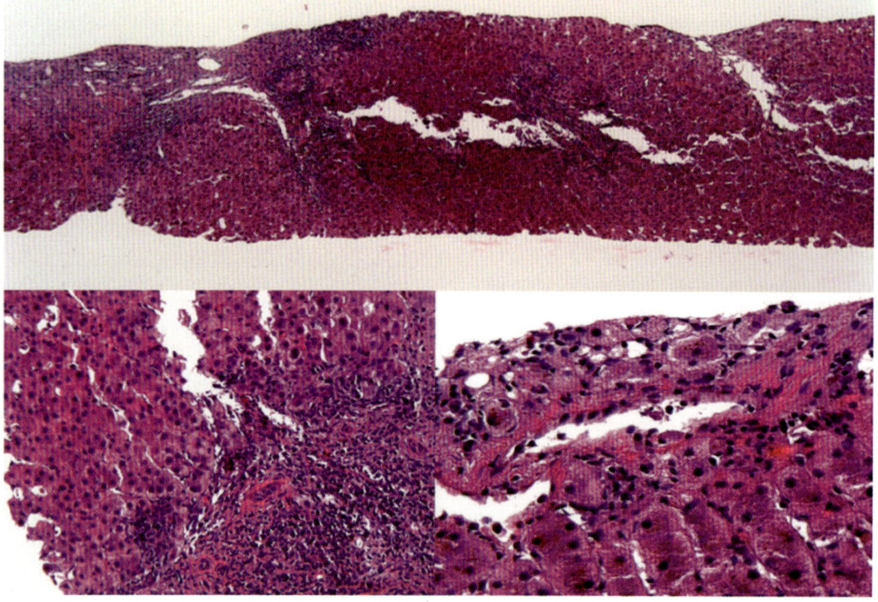

图 82.7 移植肝复发性丙型肝炎病理表现通常和自体肝类似。然而,部分可见“自身免疫”特征,如富含浆细胞的汇管区炎症,侵袭性界板区炎症(左下图),以及富含浆细胞的静脉周围炎(右下图)。此活检取自一位肝移植后约26个月的女性受体,HCV RNA 阳性,且血清学证据表明同时存在自身免疫反应。这种病例很难鉴别是急性排斥反应还是自身免疫反应,二者都对强化 IS 治疗敏感,但 HCV RNA 水平往往也升高。

或慢性排斥反应。最常见的错误是过多诊断 ACR,导致 IS 治疗过度强化[131,200]。急性和慢性排斥反应的特征性表现包括:

1.分别为单核细胞炎性胆道破坏和(或)胆管上皮细胞衰老。

2.分别为中央静脉周围炎和纤维化,累及大部分胆管或肝静脉终末分支。

复发性或新发丙型肝炎特征性表现包括肝小叶坏死性炎,以及胆管型和坏死性炎型界板区炎症,而确诊的关键在于明确哪种病变占主导。

丙型肝炎复发下的大多数临床“重度”移植排斥反应,按 Banff 标准评分都仅属于“中度”[116]。大部分胆管上皮细胞衰老往往提示慢性排斥反应,其发生通常与免疫抑制剂减量或免疫刺激物(如 α-干扰素)治疗有关[200,211]。无论是急性排斥还是慢性排斥是主要过程,此改变都应该是明显的。此外,丙型肝炎复发基础上发生的重度排斥反应多和外周血 HCV RNA 相对低水平($<1\sim5\times10^6$ IU/mL)相关,这表明移植免疫也有助于病毒清除[131,205]。

鉴别诊断

需要与急性、慢性丙型肝炎进行鉴别的疾病包括急性和慢性排斥反应,非 HCV 诱发的复发性肝炎(如 HBV、巨细胞病毒、EB 病毒),复发或新发 AIH、PBC 和 PSC,以及胆管梗阻或狭窄[200,206]。C4d 的沉积,HCV 蛋白和核酸检测都可辅助鉴别,但作用有限[200,206]。移植后最初几周内,HCV 通常不会引起移植肝失功能,大多是在移植后 3~8 周,但有极少数例外——可早至移植后 10~14 天。而相比之下,多数急性排斥反应发生于移植后最初 30 天内,中位数为 8 天[212]。

慢性丙型肝炎和其他慢性肝炎的鉴别,须综合临床、生化和血清学资料。病毒抗原和(或)核酸检测、磨玻璃样肝细胞,以及泥沙样核都有助于乙型肝炎和丙型肝炎的鉴别。融合性坏死极少单独见于丙肝病毒;而复发或新发 AIH,尤其合并有自身抗体和高丙种球蛋白血症时,可见浆细胞大片浸润于汇管区和静脉周围,并伴静脉周围融合性坏死。而汇管区周围和中央区轻度脂肪变性,以及汇管区淋巴细胞聚集则支持复发性丙型肝炎的诊断。

HCV 诱发的 FCH 与胆管梗阻、肝动脉血栓可能很难鉴别。胆管梗阻和急性胆管炎常可见汇管区水肿,以及汇管区或周围中性粒细胞浸润;而对于非梗阻性淤胆型肝炎,其特征性表现为显著的胆管反应和不伴汇管区水肿的急性胆管炎。病毒性肝炎常见肝小叶紊乱和肝细胞明显肿胀,而单纯性胆管梗阻并不多见。

戊型肝炎病毒

戊型肝炎病毒(HEV)是单链 RNA 嗜肝病毒,无包膜,主要流行于南亚和非洲。肝移植受体感染 HEV 后可发展为急性或慢性肝炎[213-220]。部分患者肝炎可自行消退,但超过 60%的慢性感染者(定义为粪便或血清中 HEV RNA 阳性长达 6 个月)将转为慢性肝炎,而其中 15%将发展成肝硬化[217]。重要的是,免疫抑制剂减量有利于慢性戊型肝炎和其他感染[217],对药量最小化试验也具有潜在意义。

组织病理学发现和鉴别诊断

与乙肝、丙肝类似,丙肝的急、慢性期描述详见下文[213,215,218,220]。急性戊型肝炎主要以肝小叶炎症、肝细胞点状坏死和凋亡为特征;汇管区可见以淋巴细胞浸润为主的轻、中度炎症,以及轻度坏死性炎型界板区炎症[213]。

慢性戊型肝炎则表现为典型的慢性病毒性肝炎,可见类型不一的汇管区淋巴细胞和淋巴浆细胞炎性浸润,且合并多种坏死性炎型界板区炎症和进行性纤维化[213,215,218,220]。慢性乙型或丙型肝炎与急、慢性排斥反应的鉴别标准,同样适用于戊型肝炎。

免疫失调性疾病

肝移植后免疫失调复发很常见,5 年发生率约为 25%。然而,复发后疾病进展的速度可能慢于移植前[221,222]。疾病复发率有随时间增长而快速升高的迹象;因此,尽管尚未发现,但复发性疾病很可能对远期发病率和死亡率有不良影响[222]。

原发性胆汁性肝硬化

临床表现

程序性活检项目中,疾病复发最常见于无症状且肝功能检查大多正常(或接近正常)的患者[223]。Mayo 中心大量临床数据显示,仅 12%的 PBC 复发患者出现过症状,以乏力和皮肤瘙痒最常见[223]。然而对于指征性活检项目,一旦血清学常规监测指标 AKP 和 γ-GTP 水平升高,往往首先怀疑 PBC 复发。

尽管移植后复发性 PBC 可持续发展,但受体和移植肝的远期预后仍然良好[223],而因 PBC 复发导致再次肝移植的情况十分罕见。抗线粒体抗体(AMA)对诊断 PBC 复发帮助不大,因为绝大多数受体的 AMA 水平在肝移植后不久会暂时下降,而后又回升,甚至无 PBC 复发者也是如此。

组织病理学发现

移植后复发性 PBC 的病理诊断标准基于移植前,其特征性病变包括非感染、非干酪样肉芽肿性胆道破坏,或是导致胆小管基底膜断裂的重型淋巴细胞性胆管炎——也被称为旺炽性胆道破坏[223]。肝移植后 1 年,若发现浆细胞灶状密集浸润汇管区,往往预示后期将进展为严重疾病[224]。

病理上常可见汇管区局灶性单核细胞性炎,以及局灶性淋巴细胞性胆管炎(伴汇管区淋巴细胞结节状聚集和显著的胆管型界板区炎症)。胆管型界板区炎症形成“胆管完整形态格式塔”,其病理表现包括界板区的胆管反应,汇管区周围“透明”或水肿,胆汁淤积,汇管区周围肝细胞铜或铜相关色素沉积,以及灶状小胆管缺失。相应处出现这些情况则“强烈暗示”PBC 的复发,其中包含 PBC 原发病的胆道病理和 GTP 与 AKP 的升高没有其他合理解释。

肝组织活检若未发现明显的淋巴细胞性胆管炎或“胆管完整形态格式塔”,则不能轻易诊断为复发性 PBC。活检未取到含胆道破坏的组织,或是患者患有重叠综合征(有 1 例为 AIH)[225]或只是单纯的 AIH[226],都会让“潜在”复发性 PBC 类似不明原因的慢性肝炎[137,225]。

与自体肝类似,移植肝复发性 PBC 通常呈轻微肝小叶病变。

鉴别诊断

需要与复发性 PBC 相鉴别的疾病包括急性和慢性排斥反应,慢性梗阻性胆管疾病,慢性病毒性、自身免疫性或特发性肝炎,以及药物性肝损伤;但这些病变也可与复发性 PBC 同时存在。其他可引起肉芽肿性胆管炎的因素,如真菌或抗酸杆菌、丙型肝炎病毒等,也都应该合理排除。

关于胆管病变和其他导致肝脏失功能病变的鉴别,“胆管完整形态格式塔”(前文已有描述)最具作用。

急性和慢性排斥反应都没有明显的胆管反应、胆汁性纤维化或肝硬化表现。移植排斥反应导致的汇管区炎症和淋巴细胞性胆管炎通常累及大部分汇管区，尤其是小胆管(最小直径<20μm)。相比之下,PBC引起的汇管区炎症和淋巴细胞性胆管炎更具局灶性，且主要累及中等大小的胆管(最小直径>40~50μm)。

肝移植后,PBC患者也可能合并新发自身免疫性肝炎或重叠综合征[226]。移植前用于诊断自身免疫性肝炎和重叠综合征的临床、血清学及组织病理学标准也可用于移植后的诊断,但更难应用。

复发性PBC和梗阻性胆管疾病很难鉴别,因为二者都可形成“胆管格式塔”。支持梗阻性胆管疾病诊断的组织病理学发现包括：

1.汇管区结缔组织内胆管和胆管周围水肿和(或)中性粒细胞性炎症。

2.肝小叶中央区胆汁淤积。

3.胆管梗死。

4.肝小叶内中性粒细胞簇状聚集。

某些情况下，可能仍须利用胆管造影来排除胆管机械性梗阻。

PBC和慢性病毒性肝炎、自身免疫性肝炎难以鉴别,特别是复发性HCV(因为也可有显著的胆管反应)。这时须仔细检查胆管、小胆管缺失,以及淋巴细胞性或肉芽肿性胆道破坏都明显有助于鉴别诊断。有报道显示复发性HCV也可存在汇管区肉芽肿[227],但并不多见,而且这种肉芽肿很少引起明显、严重的胆道破坏。最后可通过铜和铜相关蛋白染色，将慢性胆汁淤积引起的胆管反应与其他因素引起的疾病相区别。

复发性和新发“自身免疫性”肝炎

移植后诊断复发或新发自身免疫性肝炎甚至比移植前更难,因为:①血清学异常要么持续存在,要么短暂消失而后又重新出现——与疾病复发毫无关联;②其他因素引起的肝损伤病理表现和AIH很相似[228,229]。Banff团队主张以更严格的标准[113]诊断移植后AIH,但解决这一问题仍需更多研究。

组织病理学和鉴别诊断

对于自体肝,新发和复发性AIH难以区分,典型者表现为富含浆细胞的侵袭性坏死性炎型界板区炎症和类型不一的静脉周围坏死性炎症。部分AIH复发患者可见富含浆细胞的的中央静脉周围炎(见急性排斥反应部分)。这时,要对急性排斥反应(主要累及小叶中央)和AIH做出鉴别是有难度的。高百分比浆细胞(>30%)支持AIH的诊断,而累及大部分胆管的炎性胆道破坏或胆管上皮衰老则支持急性排斥反应。

胆盐输出泵(BSEP)抗体阳性的受体病理表现为胆汁淤积,多核或巨核肝细胞形成,界板区胆管反应明显,以及肝纤维化,这些可导致移植肝功能丧失。而富含浆细胞的侵袭性界板区炎症、静脉周围坏死性炎症,或炎性胆道破坏,都尚无报道[230-232]。

一旦确定为“肝炎性”损伤,须进行临床病理学和血清学相关检查:①作为支撑自身免疫性肝炎诊断的证据[如抗核抗体(ANA)、抗平滑肌抗体(ASMA),肝肾微粒体(LKM)、血清γ微球蛋白];②排除其他慢性肝炎,如HBV、HCV、HEV、PBC,以及梗阻性胆管疾病[178,228,229]。

病毒性肝炎与急性和慢性排斥反应的鉴别诊断标准(见丙型肝炎病毒部分)同样适用于AIH与急性和慢性排斥反应的鉴别。而AIH与梗阻性胆管疾病及PBC的鉴别已分别在胆道并发症和原发性胆汁性肝硬化部分描述。

复发性原发性硬化性胆管炎

早期复发性原发性硬化性胆管炎(复发性PSC)通常发生在肝移植后6~9个多月，因AKP和γ-GTP水平升高才开始引起医生的注意。非吻合性肝内胆管狭窄若发生在肝移植后90天内,通常认为不是由复发性PSC引起的,而应该考虑其他因素。

组织病理学发现

复发性PSC的组织病理学发现与发生于自体肝的并无明显不同，且难以与引起胆管梗阻或狭窄的其他病变鉴别。典型的早期表现包括轻度非特异性急性和慢性胆管周围炎，以及类型不一的轻微界板区胆管反应。疾病充分进展后,可形成胆管格式塔,包括大部分汇管区星形纤维紊乱增生(伴类型不一的汇管区水肿),胆管周围片状水肿,胆管星形管腔,胆管上皮或胆管腔内中性粒细胞浸润,纤维性胆管炎,局灶小胆管缺失,汇管区结缔组织内巨噬细胞色素沉着,伴外周水肿带的胆管型界板区炎症,以及汇管区周围金黄色素、铜和铜相关蛋白沉积。扩张的汇管区和中央静脉的空间位置关系将长期保持，直至进展为肝硬化。

复发性 PSC 早期肝小叶病变包括类型不一的胆汁淤积，小叶内中性粒细胞簇状聚集，以及轻度结节性再生性增生。而晚期特征性表现包括胆汁淤积、肝小叶内泡沫细胞簇集、铜和铜相关蛋白显著沉积、结节边缘 Mallory 小体，以及胆汁性肝硬化。

鉴别诊断

“胆管格式塔”，γ-GTP 和 AKP 升高，都提示“胆管”病变。然而，还须充分结合临床病理学和放射影像学资料，以明确胆管病变是由复发性 PSC 还是其他因素引起。鉴别诊断不能只依赖组织活检，必须综合分析临床、组织病理学以及放射影像学表现，并辅以重要的排除标准。

代谢性疾病和中毒性损伤

为清楚肝移植对代谢性疾病进展和复发的影响，Jaffe 等[233]将代谢性疾病分为三类（表 82.7）。随着更多治疗方法的出现，肝脏移植的需求正逐渐减少——但依旧十分有效[234]。内科治疗或其他外科治疗失败后，第一组患者将是肝移植治疗的首选受体，因为病肝将替换成基因型和表型都正常的肝脏，疾病通常可达到治愈。然而，随供肝引入的变异蛋白会刺激新生抗体形成，而该抗体又将导致部分受体家族性肝内胆汁淤积综合征复发（见自身免疫性肝炎部分）[230-232]。

第二组患者肝脏表型正常或接近正常。由于移植后代谢紊乱持续存在，第三组患者原发病很容易复发。尽管如此，生存期延长和（或）生活质量的提高，都说明肝移植治疗仍然合理且有必要[233]。

复发性酒精性肝病

临床表现

疾病复发被发现的常见原因包括：肝功能检查（常规监测项目）异常[235]，未定期复查[236]，社交活动不恰当[137]，以及免疫抑制治疗不依从[235,237]。γ-GTP/AKP 比值升高或许可作为提示复发的生化依据[137,235]，但相比而言，血液酒精浓度更具诊断价值。由于脂肪性肝炎复发，少数受体的病情会出现一段急剧加重期[238-240]。然而，绝大部分受体并不因此进展为严重的酒精性肝病。

组织病理学发现和鉴别诊断

酒精性肝病在移植肝的组织病理学发现和自体肝并无不同，此处不详述。最常见病理表现为大泡性和小泡性肝细胞脂肪变性，且主要见于小叶中央肝细胞；

表 82.7　基于肝脏移植治疗的代谢性疾病的 Jaffe 分类[233]（见正文）

先天性代谢缺陷来自肝脏，且肝脏表型多有异常（见正文）	先天性代谢缺陷来自肝脏，但肝脏表型通常正常或接近正常	先天性代谢缺陷很可能来自肝外，且肝移植可降低肝脏疾病的发病率和死亡率
α_1-抗胰蛋白酶缺乏症[234,262]	支链氨基酸缺乏[234]	胱氨酸沉积症[233]。一般不引起肝脏疾病；但目前有 1 例报道肝内胱氨酸结晶沉积并伴静脉周纤维化，且肝移植后疾病复发[233]
胆汁酸合成缺陷[234]	Crigler-Najjar 综合征[263,264]	囊性纤维化；肝移植可治愈原发性肝病，且若移植及时，可改善肺功能[234]
碳水化合物代谢缺陷[234]	FAP[265]。肝脏轻微异常：淀粉样蛋白沉积于汇管区和神经干；作为供肝的使用尚有争议	卟啉病[266,267]
		血色素沉着症（或意外接受血色素沉着症患者的肝脏）[268]
家族性肝内胆汁淤积综合征[234]	家族性高胆固醇血症[233]	Niemann-Pick 病[233,234]
糖原累积病，Ⅰ、Ⅰb、Ⅲ、Ⅳ型[234,269,270]	血友病 A，B[233]	海蓝组织细胞综合征[271]
新生儿血色素沉着症[234]	草酸尿症Ⅰ型[233,234]	
线粒体缺陷（累及肝脏部分）[234]	尿素循环酶缺乏[233,234]	
酪氨酸血症[234,272]		
Wilson 病[234,273]		

注：FAP，家族性淀粉样变多发性神经病。

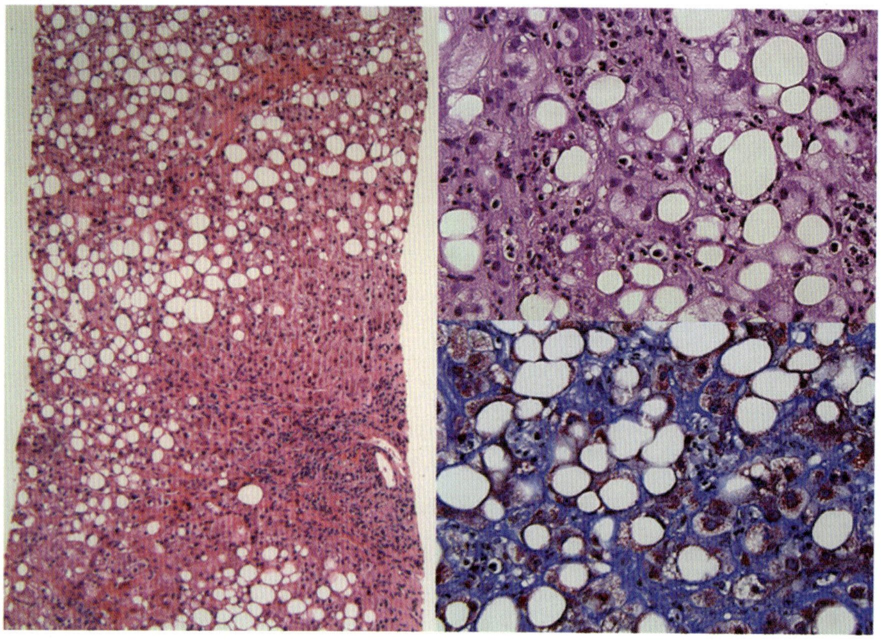

图 82.8 复发性酒精性肝损伤导致移植肝严重受损相对少见。酒精性肝病和非酒精性脂肪性肝病难以鉴别，但病理表现——中性粒细胞性炎，肝细胞"泡沫样变"（图右上方），脂肪变性严格分布于静脉周围（图左），窦周纤维化（图右下方），更多见于复发性酒精性肝病。

脂肪变性呈带状分布更是其特征性表现（图82.8）。更严重时可导致所谓的小叶中央肝细胞"泡沫样变"，随后可见充分进展的"酒精性肝炎"（伴 Mallory 小体出现），以及肝细胞气球样变且合并相应肝小叶中性粒细胞性炎。

鉴别诊断，见非酒精性脂肪性肝炎部分。

复发性非酒精性脂肪性肝炎

临床表现

在美国，非酒精性脂肪性肝病（NAFLD）目前是肝移植第三大适应证，并正逐渐成为最常见适应证[241]。因 NAFLD 行肝移植治疗的患者多为老年、女性和高体重指数者。

因隐源性肝硬化行肝移植的患者中，很大一部分移植后存在非酒精性脂肪性肝病[242-245]。据推测，很可能这些患者在移植前也患有 NAFLD，但病肝的相关病理表现并不明显。

复发性 NAFLD 通常首先发现于无症状受者活检时，且大多患者都存在多种 NAFLD 的危险因素。然而，少部分相对健康的受体在移植后也出现原因不明的 NAFLD，这类患者须进行胰岛素抵抗试验并进一步研究以明确病因。

组织病理学和鉴别诊断

病理学家基本都熟知肝脂肪变性和脂肪性肝炎的具体病理表现，与发生于自体肝的并无不同[246]。

存在小部分很难明确脂肪性肝炎的潜在病因的受体。与自体肝类似，移植肝的脂肪性肝炎最常见于合并病态性肥胖、糖尿病、胰岛素抵抗，以及酒精滥用者。然而，脂肪性肝炎还可能和很多其他因素有关。例如，肝血流异常——尤其是在移植后几个月内就开始出现，是诱发肝脂肪变性和脂肪性肝炎的重要因素。

酒精性肝病和非酒精性脂肪性肝病的鉴别，需要密切结合临床和病理。对原发病的认识，详细的病史——包括近期饮酒情况，血液酒精浓度以及 γ-GTP/AKP 比值，都有助于鉴别诊断。

特发性移植后肝炎

病理生理学和临床表现

特发性移植后肝炎这一诊断术语由 Hubscher 命

名[247],用于描述移植肝活检发现的慢性肝炎样病变(如汇管区单核细胞性炎症并伴类型不一的界板区炎症),该病变无临床或血清学证据表明是由病毒感染、自身免疫,或药物引起[113,248]。根据定义,用于诊断急性排斥反应的特征都不剧烈也不普遍,如胆道破坏和静脉内皮炎症[113,248]。

与其他特发性疾病类似,预计随着潜在病因被发现,IPTH 的诊断会逐渐减少:如前文所述,部分病例重新明确为慢性 HEV 感染。少部分病例很可能就是复发性 AIH[247],尽管不一定严格符合 AIH 诊断标准。大部分慢性肝炎的潜在病因仍然不明确,对此仍须进一步研究;然而,目前主流观点是大部分 IPTH 可能是不典型的迟发性急性排斥反应[113,178,248,249]。

组织病理学和鉴别诊断

IPTH 病理表现以慢性汇管区炎症、类型不一的界板区和小叶坏死性炎症为特征,但是不存在明显、广泛的胆道破坏或中央静脉周围炎。广泛的淋巴细胞性胆管炎和中央静脉周围炎往往提示急性排斥反应;而浆细胞丰富浸润(占比>30%)的炎症——多提示复发性或新发 AIH,但不多见。而引起慢性肝炎的其他病因,如 HBV、HCV、HEV,以及复发或新发 AIH,需要结合临床、血清学和分子诊断学资料鉴别。

IPTH 的鉴别诊断与 HBV、HCV 及 AIH 相同(见前文)。

免疫抑制方案最优化的注意事项

临床表现

关于免疫抑制治疗最小量或最优化,包括严格选择小部分受体完全停药,活检结果评估扮演了重要角色[113,178,248,250]。相比其他器官,这是肝移植独有的,因为①相比其他实体器官移植,肝移植更易"免疫耐受"[111];②如果减药期间或是减药后发生排斥反应,继续当前 IS 治疗,通常可快速逆转而不发生明显的肝纤维化或肝衰竭[111,113,178,248,250]。

组织病理学和鉴别诊断

对于 IS 最小量试验,通常认为减药前活检必不可少[248]。减药成功的活检结果包括:①汇管区炎症减轻[251,252];②小叶内 $CD3^+$ 和 $CD8^+$ 淋巴细胞减少,而 $CD45RO^+$ 淋巴细胞增多[6,252],HCV^+ 受体汇管区纤维化增强[253],以及微血管 C4d 沉积减轻[251]。

后续活检通常在减药期间或是减药后进行,并由肝功能检查异常触发[248,250]。然而,肝功能检查异常是非特异性的,而且减药可使潜在的原发病复发并进展[248,250]。γ-GTP 升高,可能是提示减药后 ACR 最具特异性和敏感性的指标[254,255]。

IS 减量期间的 ACR,常规病理表现往往类似"典型"ACR;但是不典型或不完全者也很常见[113,248,250],包括:①局灶、轻微的炎性胆道破坏;②更广泛、严重的界板区和小叶坏死性炎症;③较轻微的汇管区静脉内皮下炎症(见不典型者)。病理学表现类似轻度慢性肝炎[248,250],难以鉴别诊断,尤其是合并潜在 AIH 或 PBC 的受体减药后出现界板区炎症时(很可能是疾病复发的表现)。

对于 HCV^+ [203]和部分接受淋巴细胞耗竭型抗体治疗的 HCV^- 患者[256],减药过早过快会引起免疫"重建"综合征[203],该综合征表现为急进性纤维化的侵袭性肝炎[203]。

排斥反应相关的进行性纤维化备受关注[113,248],为监测此并发症,对于没有症状和肝损伤生化依据的患者,Banff 团队提倡在大幅减药或完全停药后第 1、3、5、10 年,要完成合乎要求的(两个大于:>20mm 的 16 号针和 >11 个汇管区[28])程序性活检。

后续活检应重视并密切随访的病变包括:明显加重的炎症、胆管上皮细胞损伤、肝纤维化、静脉周围坏死性炎症,以及闭塞性动脉病变。

复发性疾病难以解释的长期病变

生存期长的移植肝发生的某些病变无法归因于某一疾病复发,可能是药物不良反应,也可能是长期植入引起的机体反应[113,137,178]。这类病变包括门静脉病变,结节性再生性增生,肝动脉小分支管壁增厚和磨玻璃样变[137,257],窦周纤维化,以及"非特异性"汇管区和肝小叶炎症[113,137,178]。年长者的供肝将保持原速甚至加速衰老(此观察尚未发表),而不会因为植入年轻受体而"返老还童"[258]。移植后 4 年内出现结节性再生性增生样变,预示疾病朝门静脉高压进展[259]。肝移植受体预后日益改善，而诸多相关问题亦须进一步研究、攻克。

结论

对于肝移植，肝脏的病理表现尤其“复杂多变”，故病理学家是临床肝移植团队不可或缺的成员。为指导受体的临床治疗，须行实时肝活检并贯穿移植肝整个存活期，包括必要时的再移植。移植后常见损伤包括缺血-再灌注损伤、小肝综合征，以及排斥反应，并逐渐替代为复发性疾病和病毒性肝炎。而免疫治疗方案改变，也会引起肝脏病理改变。通常，移植肝出现任何异常都应行组织活检，并由对肝移植相关疾病有丰富经验的病理学家解读和评估。

致谢

在此，对编辑 Linda Askren 给予的帮助表示衷心感谢。同时，因排版限制，本书未引用原始文献而是参考综述性文献，对此，向原著作者与广大读者表示诚挚歉意。

（徐骁 危荣沥 杨墨丹 译 徐骁 校）

参考文献

1. Todo S, Demetris AJ, Makowka L, et al. Primary nonfunction of hepatic allografts with preexisting fatty infiltration. Transplantation. 1989;47:903–905.
2. Kakizoe S, Yanaga K, Starzl TE, et al. Frozen section of liver biopsy for the evaluation of liver allografts. Transplantation Proceedings. 1990;22:416–417.
3. Kakizoe S, Yanaga K, Starzl TE, et al. Evaluation of protocol before transplantation and after reperfusion biopsies from human orthotopic liver allografts: considerations of preservation and early immunological injury. Hepatology. 1990;11:932–941.
4. Zamboni F, Franchello A, David E, et al. Effect of macrovescicular steatosis and other donor and recipient characteristics on the outcome of liver transplantation. Clinical Transplantation. 2001;15:53–57.
5. Alkofer B, Samstein B, Guarrera JV, et al. Extended-donor criteria liver allografts. Seminars in Liver Disease. 2006;26:221–233.
6. Busuttil RW, Tanaka K. The utility of marginal donors in liver transplantation. Liver Transplantation. 2003;9:651–663.
7. Spitzer AL, Lao OB, Dick AA, et al. The biopsied donor liver: incorporating macrosteatosis into high-risk donor assessment. Liver Transplantation. 2010;16:874–884.
8. Sharkey FE, Lytvak I, Prihoda TJ, et al. High-grade microsteatosis and delay in hepatic function after orthotopic liver transplantation. Human Pathology. 2011;42:1337–1342.
9. McCormack L, Petrowsky H, Jochum W, et al. Use of severely steatotic grafts in liver transplantation: a matched case-control study. Annals of Surgery. 2007;246:940–946, discussion 6–8.
10. Angele MK, Rentsch M, Hartl WH, et al. Effect of graft steatosis on liver function and organ survival after liver transplantation. American Journal of Surgery. 2008;195:214–220.
11. D'Alessandro AM, Kalayoglu M, Sollinger HW, et al. The predictive value of donor liver biopsies for the development of primary nonfunction after orthotopic liver transplantation. Transplantation. 1991;51:157–163.
12. Markin RS, Wisecarver JL, Radio SJ, et al. Frozen section evaluation of donor livers before transplantation. Transplantation. 1993;56:1403–1409.
13. Fiorentino M, Vasuri F, Ravaioli M, et al. Predictive value of frozen-section analysis in the histological assessment of steatosis before liver transplantation. Liver Transplantation. 2009;15:1821–1825.
14. Ballarin R, Cucchetti A, Spaggiari M, et al. Long-term follow-up and outcome of liver transplantation from anti-hepatitis C virus-positive donors: a European multicentric case-control study. Transplantation. 2011;91:1265–1272.
15. Ison MG, Nalesnik MA. An update on donor-derived disease transmission in organ transplantation. American Journal of Transplantation. 2011;11:1123–1130. [Review.]
16. Adams D, Lacroix C, Antonini T, et al. Symptomatic and proven de novo amyloid polyneuropathy in familial amyloid polyneuropathy domino liver recipients. Amyloid. 2011;18(Suppl 1):169–172.
17. Aziz S, Callen PW, Vincenti F, et al. Rapidly developing nephrocalcinosis in a patient with end-stage liver disease who received a domino liver transplant from a patient with known congenital oxalosis. Journal of Ultrasound in Medicine. 2005;24:1449–1452. [Case reports.]
18. Lee SM, Speeg KV, Pollack MS, et al. Progression of morphological changes after transplantation of a liver with heterozygous alpha-1 antitrypsin deficiency. Human Pathology. 2012;43:753–756.
19. Tanaka K, Kiuchi T. Living-donor liver transplantation in the new decade: perspective from the twentieth to the twenty-first century. Journal of Hepato-Biliary-Pancreatic Surgery. 2002;9:218–222.
20. Trotter JF, Wachs M, Everson GT, et al. Adult-to-adult transplantation of the right hepatic lobe from a living donor. New England Journal of Medicine. 2002;346:1074–1082.
21. Nadalin S, Malago M, Valentin-Gamazo C, et al. Preoperative donor liver biopsy for adult living donor liver transplantation: risks and benefits. Liver Transplantation. 2005;11:980–986.
22. Tran TT, Changsri C, Shackleton CR, et al. Living donor liver transplantation: histological abnormalities found on liver biopsies of apparently healthy potential donors. Journal of Gastroenterology and Hepatology. 2006;21:381–383.
23. Ryan CK, Johnson LA, Germin BI, et al. One hundred consecutive hepatic biopsies in the workup of living donors for right lobe liver transplantation. Liver Transplantation. 2002;8:1114–1122.
24. Minervini MI, Ruppert K, Fontes P, et al. Liver biopsy findings from healthy potential living liver donors: reasons for disqualification, silent diseases and correlation with liver injury tests. Journal of Hepatology. 2009;50:501–510.
25. Lee JY, Kim KM, Lee SG, et al. Prevalence and risk factors of non-alcoholic fatty liver disease in potential living liver donors in Korea: a review of 589 consecutive liver biopsies in a single center. Journal of Hepatology. 2007;47:239–244.
26. Rinella ME, Alonso E, Rao S, et al. Body mass index as a predictor of hepatic steatosis in living liver donors. Liver Transplantation. 2001;7:409–414. [Comparative study.]
27. Fan ST, Lo CM, Liu CL, et al. Safety of donors in live donor liver transplantation using right lobe grafts. Archives of Surgery. 2000;135:336–340.
28. Rockey DC, Caldwell SH, Goodman ZD, et al. Liver biopsy. Hepatology. 2009;49:1017–1044. [Practice guideline.]
29. Bellamy CO. Complement C4d immunohistochemistry in the assessment of liver allograft biopsy samples: applications and pitfalls. Liver Transplantation. 2011;17:747–750. [Editorial.]
30. Kozlowski T, Rubinas T, Nickeleit V, et al. Liver allograft antibody-mediated rejection with demonstration of sinusoidal C4d staining and circulating donor-specific antibodies. Liver Transplantation. 2011;17:357–368.
31. Bellizzi AM, LeGallo RD, Boyd JC, et al. Hepatocyte cytokeratin 7 expression in chronic allograft rejection. American Journal of Clinical Pathology. 2011;135:238–244.
32. Demetris AJ, Jaffe R, Starzl TE. A review of adult and pediatric post-transplant liver pathology. Pathology Annual. 1987;22:347–386.
33. Sieders E, Peeters PM, TenVergert EM, et al. Graft loss after pediatric liver transplantation. Annals of Surgery. 2002;235:125–132.
34. Kashyap R, Jain A, Reyes J, et al. Causes of retransplantation after primary liver transplantation in 4000 consecutive patients: 2 to 19 years follow-up. Transplantation Proceedings. 2001;33:1486–1487.
35. Lunz J, Ruppert KM, Cajaiba MM, et al. Re-examination of the lymphocytotoxic crossmatch in liver transplantation: can C4d stains help in monitoring? American Journal of Transplantation. 2012;12:171–182.
36. Ruiz R, Tomiyama K, Campsen J, et al. Implications of a positive crossmatch in liver transplantation: a 20-year review. Liver Transplantation. 2012;18:455–460.
37. Jain A, Reyes J, Kashyap R, et al. Long-term survival after liver transplantation in 4,000 consecutive patients at a single center. Annals of Surgery. 2000;232:

490–500.
38. Rabkin JM, de La Melena V, Orloff SL, et al. Late mortality after orthotopic liver transplantation. American Journal of Surgery. 2001;181:475–479.
39. Jain A, Demetris AJ, Kashyap R, et al. Does tacrolimus offer virtual freedom from chronic rejection after primary liver transplantation? Risk and prognostic factors in 1,048 liver transplantations with a mean follow-up of 6 years. Liver Transplantation. 2001;7:623–630.
40. McCashland T, Watt K, Lyden E, et al. Retransplantation for hepatitis C: results of a U.S. multicenter retransplant study. Liver Transplantation. 2007;13:1246–1253.
41. Kim KR, Ko GY, Sung KB, et al. Transjugular liver biopsy in patients with living donor liver transplantation: comparison with percutaneous biopsy. Liver Transplantation. 2008;14:971–979. [Comparative study.]
42. Astarcioglu I, Cursio R, Reynes M, et al. Increased risk of antibody-mediated rejection of reduced-size liver allografts. Journal of Surgical Research. 1999;87:258–262.
43. Demetris AJ, Kelly DM, Eghtesad B, et al. Pathophysiologic observations and histopathologic recognition of the portal hyperperfusion or small-for-size syndrome. American Journal of Surgical Pathology. 2006;30:986–993.
44. Abu-Amara M, Yang SY, Tapuria N, et al. Liver ischemia/reperfusion injury: processes in inflammatory networks: a review. Liver Transplantation. 2010;16:1016–1032.
45. de Rougemont O, Dutkowski P, Clavien PA. Biological modulation of liver ischemia-reperfusion injury. Current Opinion in Organ Transplantation. 2010;15:183–189. [Review.]
46. Foley DP, Fernandez LA, Leverson G, et al. Biliary complications after liver transplantation from donation after cardiac death donors: an analysis of risk factors and long-term outcomes from a single center. Annals of Surgery. 2011;253:817–825.
47. Hong JC, Yersiz H, Kositamongkol P, et al. Liver transplantation using organ donation after cardiac death: a clinical predictive index for graft failure-free survival. Archives of Surgery. 2011;146:1017–1023.
48. de Vera ME, Lopez-Solis R, Dvorchik I, et al. Liver transplantation using donation after cardiac death donors: long-term follow-up from a single center. American Journal of Transplantation. 2009;9:773–781.
49. Ludwig J, Batts KP, MacCarty RL. Ischemic cholangitis in hepatic allografts [see comments]. Mayo Clinic Proceedings. 1992;67:519–526.
50. Cameron AM, Busuttil RW. Ischemic cholangiopathy after liver transplantation. Hepatobiliary and Pancreatic Diseases International. 2005;4:495–501.
51. Kocbiyik A, Demirhan B, Sevmis S, et al. Role of postreperfusion subcapsular wedge biopsies in predicting initially poor graft function after liver transplantation. Transplantation Proceedings. 2009;41:2747–2748.
52. Kukan M, Haddad PS. Role of hepatocytes and bile duct cells in preservation-reperfusion injury of liver grafts. Liver Transplantation. 2001;7:381–400.
53. Man K, Fan ST, Lo CM, et al. Graft injury in relation to graft size in right lobe live donor liver transplantation: a study of hepatic sinusoidal injury in correlation with portal hemodynamics and intragraft gene expression. Annals of Surgery. 2003;237:256–264.
54. Starzl TE, Fung JJ. Themes of liver transplantation. Hepatology. 2010;51:1869–1884.
55. Hessheimer AJ, Fondevila C, Taura P, et al. Decompression of the portal bed and twice-baseline portal inflow are necessary for the functional recovery of a "small-for-size" graft. Annals of Surgery. 2011;253:1201–1210.
56. Fukuhara T, Umeda K, Toshima T, et al. Congestion of the donor remnant right liver after extended left lobe donation. Transplant International. 2009;22:837–844.
57. Dahm F, Georgiev P, Clavien PA. Small-for-size syndrome after partial liver transplantation: definition, mechanisms of disease and clinical implications. American Journal of Transplantation. 2005;5:2605–2610. [Review.]
58. Kelly DM, Demetris AJ, Fung JJ, et al. Porcine partial liver transplantation: a novel model of the "small-for-size" liver graft. Liver Transplantation. 2004;10:253–263.
59. Man K, Lo CM, Ng IO, et al. Liver transplantation in rats using small-for-size grafts: a study of hemodynamic and morphological changes. Archives of Surgery. 2001;136:280–285.
60. Asakura T, Ohkohchi N, Orii T, et al. Portal vein pressure is the key for successful liver transplantation of an extremely small graft in the pig model. Transplant International. 2003;16:376–382.
61. Ayata G, Pomfret E, Pomposelli JJ, et al. Adult-to-adult live donor liver transplantation: a short-term clinicopathologic study. Human Pathology. 2001;32:814–822.
62. Pantanowitz L, Pomfret EA, Pomposelli JJ, et al. Pathologic analysis of right-lobe graft failure in adult-to-adult live donor liver transplantation. International Journal of Surgical Pathology. 2003;11:283–294.
63. Bekker J, Ploem S, de Jong KP. Early hepatic artery thrombosis after liver transplantation: a systematic review of the incidence, outcome and risk factors. American Journal of Transplantation. 2009;9:746–757.
64. Gunsar F, Rolando N, Pastacaldi S, et al. Late hepatic artery thrombosis after orthotopic liver transplantation. Liver Transplantation. 2003;9:605–611.
65. Demetris AJ, Fontes P, Lunz JG 3rd, et al. Wound healing in the biliary tree of liver allografts. Cell Transplantation. 2006;15(Suppl 1):S57–S65.
66. Demetris AJ. The pathology of liver transplantation. Progress in Liver Diseases. 1990;9:687–709.
67. Ponziani FR, Zocco MA, Campanale C, et al. Portal vein thrombosis: insight into physiopathology, diagnosis, and treatment. World Journal of Gastroenterology. 2010;16:143–155. [Review.]
68. Zahmatkeshan M, Geramizadeh B, Eshraghian A, et al. De novo fatty liver due to vascular complications after liver transplantation. Transplantation Proceedings. 2011;43:615–617.
69. Sebagh M, Debette M, Samuel D, et al. "Silent" presentation of veno-occlusive disease after liver transplantation as part of the process of cellular rejection with endothelial predilection. Hepatology. 1999;30:1144–1150.
70. Demetris A, Crawford J, Nalesnik M, et al. Transplantation pathology of the liver. In: Odze R, Goldblum J, Crawford JM, editors. Surgical Pathology of the GI Tract, Liver, Biliary Tract, and Pancreas. Philadelphia, PA: WB Saunders; 2004:909–966.
71. Verdonk RC, Buis CI, Porte RJ, et al. Anastomotic biliary strictures after liver transplantation: causes and consequences. Liver Transplantation. 2006;12:726–735.
72. Verdonk RC, Buis CI, Porte RJ, et al. Biliary complications after liver transplantation: a review. Scandinavian Journal of Gastroenterology Supplementum. 2006;243:89–101.
73. Verdonk RC, Buis CI, van der Jagt EJ, et al. Nonanastomotic biliary strictures after liver transplantation, part 2: management, outcome, and risk factors for disease progression. Liver Transplantation. 2007;13:725–732.
74. Buis CI, Verdonk RC, Van der Jagt EJ, et al. Nonanastomotic biliary strictures after liver transplantation, part 1: radiological features and risk factors for early vs. late presentation. Liver Transplantation. 2007;13:708–718.
75. Pascher A, Neuhaus P. Bile duct complications after liver transplantation. Transplant International. 2005;18:627–642.
76. Foley DP, Fernandez LA, Leverson G, et al. Donation after cardiac death: the University of Wisconsin experience with liver transplantation. Annals of Surgery. 2005;242:724–731.
77. Hartshorne N, Hartman G, Markin RS, et al. Bile duct hemorrhage: a biopsy finding after cholangiography or biliary tree manipulation. Liver. 1992;12:137–139.
78. Nagral A, Ben-Ari Z, Dhillon AP, et al. Eosinophils in acute cellular rejection in liver allografts. Liver Transplantation and Surgery. 1998;4:355–362.
79. Lunz JG 3rd, Contrucci S, Ruppert K, et al. Replicative senescence of biliary epithelial cells precedes bile duct loss in chronic liver allograft rejection: increased expression of p21(WAF1/Cip1) as a disease marker and the influence of immunosuppressive drugs. American Journal of Pathology. 2001;158:1379–1390.
80. Demetris AJ. Distinguishing between recurrent primary sclerosing cholangitis and chronic rejection. Liver Transplantation. 2006;12(Suppl 2):S68–S72.
81. Clendenon JN, Aranda-Michel J, Krishna M, et al. Recurrent liver failure caused by IgG4 associated cholangitis. Annals of Hepatology. 2011;10:562–564. [Case reports.]
82. Demetris AJ, Jaffe R, Tzakis A, et al. Antibody-mediated rejection of human orthotopic liver allografts. A study of liver transplantation across ABO blood group barriers. American Journal of Pathology. 1988;132:489–502.
83. Demetris AJ, Murase N, Nakamura K, et al. Immunopathology of antibodies as effectors of orthotopic liver allograft rejection. Seminars in Liver Disease. 1992;12:51–59. [Review.]
84. Wu J, Ye S, Xu X, et al. Recipient outcomes after ABO-incompatible liver transplantation: a systematic review and meta-analysis. PLoS ONE. 2011;6:e16521.
85. Raut V, Uemoto S. Management of ABO-incompatible living-donor liver transplantation: past and present trends. Surgery Today. 2011;41:317–322.
86. Kawagishi N, Takeda I, Miyagi S, et al. Long-term outcome of ABO-incompatible living-donor liver transplantation: a single-center experience. Journal of Hepato-Biliary-Pancreatic Surgery. 2009;16:468–472.
87. Demetris AJ, Nakamura K, Yagihashi A, et al. A clinicopathological study of human liver allograft recipients harboring preformed IgG lymphocytotoxic antibodies. Hepatology. 1992;16:671–681.
88. Manez R, Kelly RH, Kobayashi M, et al. Immunoglobulin G lymphocytotoxic antibodies in clinical liver transplantation: studies toward further defining their significance. Hepatology. 1995;21:1345–1352.
89. Haga H, Egawa H, Fujimoto Y, et al. Acute humoral rejection and C4d immunostaining in ABO blood type-incompatible liver transplantation. Liver Transplantation. 2006;12:457–464.
90. Egawa H, Teramukai S, Haga H, et al. Present status of ABO-incompatible living

donor liver transplantation in Japan. Hepatology. 2008;47:143–152.
91. Takeda K, Tanaka K, Morioka D, et al. Pathogenesis in ABO incompatible liver transplantation: a clinicohistological evaluation of four patients. Clinical Transplantation. 2010;24:747–751.
92. Sanchez-Urdazpal L, Sterioff S, Janes C, et al. Increased bile duct complications in ABO incompatible liver transplant recipients. Transplantation Proceedings. 1991;23:1440–1441.
93. Musat AI, Agni RM, Wai PY, et al. The significance of donor-specific HLA antibodies in rejection and ductopenia development in ABO compatible liver transplantation. American Journal of Transplantation. 2011;11:500–510.
94. Dar W, Agarwal A, Watkins C, et al. Donor-directed MHC class I antibody is preferentially cleared from sensitized recipients of combined liver/kidney transplants. American Journal of Transplantation. 2011;11:841–847.
95. Furuya T, Murase N, Nakamura K, et al. Preformed lymphocytotoxic antibodies: the effects of class, titer and specificity on liver vs. heart allografts. Hepatology. 1992;16:1415–1422.
96. Nakamura K, Murase N, Becich MJ, et al. Liver allograft rejection in sensitized recipients. Observations in a clinically relevant small animal model. American Journal of Pathology. 1993;142:1383–1391.
97. Kozlowski T, Rubinas T, Nickeleit V, et al. Liver allograft antibody-mediated rejection with demonstration of sinusoidal C4d staining and circulating donor-specific antibodies. Liver Transplantation. 2011;17:357–368.
98. Bellamy CO, Herriot MM, Harrison DJ, et al. C4d immunopositivity is uncommon in ABO-compatible liver allografts, but correlates partially with lymphocytotoxic antibody status. Histopathology. 2007;50:739–749.
99. Bu X, Zheng Z, Yu Y, et al. Significance of C4d deposition in the diagnosis of rejection after liver transplantation. Transplantation Proceedings. 2006;38:1418–1421.
100. Dankof A, Schmeding M, Morawietz L, et al. Portal capillary C4d deposits and increased infiltration by macrophages indicate humorally mediated mechanisms in acute cellular liver allograft rejection. Virchows Archive. 2005;447:87–93.
101. Jain A, Mohanka R, Orloff M, et al. Characterization of CD4, CD8, CD56 positive lymphocytes and C4d deposits to distinguish acute cellular rejection from recurrent hepatitis C in post-liver transplant biopsies. Clinical Transplantation. 2006;20:624–633.
102. Krukemeyer MG, Moeller J, Morawietz L, et al. Description of B lymphocytes and plasma cells, complement, and chemokines/receptors in acute liver allograft rejection. Transplantation. 2004;78:65–70.
103. Sakashita H, Haga H, Ashihara E, et al. Significance of C4d staining in ABO-identical/compatible liver transplantation. Modern Pathology. 2007;20:676–684.
104. Sawada T, Shimizu A, Kubota K, et al. Lobular damage caused by cellular and humoral immunity in liver allograft rejection. Clinical Transplantation. 2005;19:110–114.
105. Troxell ML, Higgins JP, Kambham N. Evaluation of C4d staining in liver and small intestine allografts. Archives of Pathology and Laboratory Medicine. 2006;130:1489–1496.
106. Martelius T, Halme L, Arola J, et al. Vascular deposition of complement C4d is increased in liver allografts with chronic rejection. Transplant Immunology. 2009;21:244–246.
107. Aguilera I, Sousa JM, Gavilan F, et al. Complement component 4d immunostaining in liver allografts of patients with de novo immune hepatitis. Liver Transplantation. 2011;17:779–788.
108. Bouron-Dal Soglio D, Rougemont AL, Herzog D, et al. An immunohistochemical evaluation of C4d deposition in pediatric inflammatory liver diseases. Human Pathology. 2008;39:1103–1110.
109. Terminology of chronic hepatitis, hepatic allograft rejection, and nodular lesions of the liver: summary of recommendations developed by an international working party, supported by the World Congresses of Gastroenterology, Los Angeles, 1994. American Journal of Gastroenterology. 1994;89(Suppl):S177–S181.
110. Demetris AJ, Ruppert K, Dvorchik I, et al. Real-time monitoring of acute liver-allograft rejection using the Banff schema. Transplantation. 2002;74:1290–1296.
111. Knechtle SJ, Kwun J. Unique aspects of rejection and tolerance in liver transplantation. Seminars in Liver Disease. 2009;29:91–101.
112. Uemura T, Ikegami T, Sanchez EQ, et al. Late acute rejection after liver transplantation impacts patient survival. Clinical Transplantation. 2008;22:316–323.
113. Banff Working Group, Demetris AJ, Adeyi O, et al. Liver biopsy interpretation for causes of late liver allograft dysfunction. Hepatology. 2006;44:489–501.
114. Neil DA, Hubscher SG. Delay in diagnosis: a factor in the poor outcome of late acute rejection of liver allografts. Transplantation Proceedings. 2001;33:1525–1526.
115. Anonymous. Terminology for hepatic allograft rejection. International working party. Hepatology. 1995;22:648–654. [Review.]
116. Anonymous. Banff schema for grading liver allograft rejection: an international consensus document. Hepatology. 1997;25:658–663.
117. Yeh MM, Larson AM, Tung BY, et al. Endotheliitis in chronic viral hepatitis: a comparison with acute cellular rejection and non-alcoholic steatohepatitis. American Journal of Surgical Pathology. 2006;30:727–733.
118. Demetris AJ, Lasky S, Thiel DHV, et al. Induction of DR/IA antigens in human liver allografts: an immunocytochemical and clinicopathologic analysis of twenty failed grafts. Transplantation. 1985;40:504–509.
119. McCaughan GW, Davies JS, Waugh JA, et al. A quantitative analysis of T lymphocyte populations in human liver allografts undergoing rejection: the use of monoclonal antibodies and double immunolabeling. Hepatology. 1990;12:1305–1313.
120. Steinhoff G, Behrend M, Wonigeit K. Expression of adhesion molecules on lymphocytes/monocytes and hepatocytes in human liver grafts. Human Immunology. 1990;28:123–127.
121. Demetris AJ, Belle SH, Hart J, et al. Intraobserver and interobserver variation in the histopathological assessment of liver allograft rejection. The Liver Transplantation Database (LTD) investigators. Hepatology. 1991;14:751–755.
122. Cong WM, Zhang SY, Wang ZL, et al. Pathologic diagnosis of 1123 post-transplant liver biopsies from 665 liver transplant patients. Zhonghua Bing Li Xue Za Zhi. 2005;34:716–719.
123. Netto GJ, Watkins DL, Williams JW, et al. Interobserver agreement in hepatitis C grading and staging and in the Banff grading schema for acute cellular rejection: the "hepatitis C 3" multi-institutional trial experience. Archives of Pathology and Laboratory Medicine. 2006;130:1157–1162.
124. Demirhan B, Bilezikci B, Haberal AN, et al. Hepatic parenchymal changes and histologic eosinophilia as predictors of subsequent acute liver allograft rejection. Liver Transplantation. 2008;14:214–219.
125. Hubscher S. Diagnosis and grading of liver allograft rejection: a European perspective. Transplantation Proceedings. 1996;28:504–507.
126. Ishak K, Baptista A, Bianchi L, et al. Histological grading and staging of chronic hepatitis. Journal of Hepatology. 1995;22:696–699.
127. Demetris AJ, Fung JJ, Todo S, et al. Conversion of liver allograft recipients from cyclosporine to FK506 immunosuppressive therapy: a clinicopathologic study of 96 patients. Transplantation. 1992;53:1056–1062.
128. Tsamandas AC, Jain AB, Felekouras ES, et al. Central venulitis in the allograft liver: a clinicopathologic study. Transplantation. 1997;64:252–257.
129. Krasinskas AM, Ruchelli ED, Rand EB, et al. Central venulitis in pediatric liver allografts. Hepatology. 2001;33:1141–1147.
130. Sanei MH, Schiano TD, Sempoux C, et al. Acute cellular rejection resulting in sinusoidal obstruction syndrome and ascites postliver transplantation. Transplantation. 2011;92:1152–1158.
131. Demetris AJ, Eghtesad B, Marcos A, et al. Recurrent hepatitis C in liver allografts: prospective assessment of diagnostic accuracy, identification of pitfalls, and observations about pathogenesis. American Journal of Surgical Pathology. 2004;28:658–669.
132. Guido M, Burra P. De novo autoimmune hepatitis after liver transplantation. Seminars in Liver Disease. 2011;31:71–81.
133. Demetris A, Adams D, Bellamy C, et al. Update of the international Banff schema for liver allograft rejection: working recommendations for the histopathologic staging and reporting of chronic rejection. An international panel. Hepatology. 2000;31:792–799.
134. Walter T, Dumortier J, Guillaud O, et al. Rejection under alpha interferon therapy in liver transplant recipients. American Journal of Transplantation. 2007;7:177–184.
135. Stanca CM, Fiel MI, Kontorinis N, et al. Chronic ductopenic rejection in patients with recurrent hepatitis C virus treated with pegylated interferon alfa-2a and ribavirin. Transplantation. 2007;84:180–186.
136. Blakolmer K, Jain A, Ruppert K, et al. Chronic liver allograft rejection in a population treated primarily with tacrolimus as baseline immunosuppression: long-term follow-up and evaluation of features for histopathological staging. Transplantation. 2000;69:2330–2336.
137. Pappo O, Ramos H, Starzl TE, et al. Structural integrity and identification of causes of liver allograft dysfunction occurring more than 5 years after transplantation. American Journal of Surgical Pathology. 1995;19:192–206.
138. Demetris AJ, Seaberg EC, Batts KP, et al. Chronic liver allograft rejection: a National Institute of Diabetes and Digestive and Kidney Diseases interinstitutional study analyzing the reliability of current criteria and proposal of an expanded definition. National Institute of Diabetes and Digestive and Kidney Diseases Liver Transplantation Database. American Journal of Surgical Pathology. 1998;22:28–39.
139. Blakolmer K, Seaberg EC, Batts K, et al. Analysis of the reversibility of chronic liver allograft rejection implications for a staging schema. American Journal of Surgical Pathology. 1999;23:1328–1339.
140. White RM, Zajko AB, Demetris AJ, et al. Liver transplant rejection: angiographic

findings in 35 patients. AJR. American Journal of Roentgenology. 1987;148: 1095–1098.
141. O'Keeffe C, Baird AW, Nolan N, et al. Mast cell hyperplasia in chronic rejection after liver transplantation. Liver Transplantation. 2002;8:50–57.
142. Sasaki M, Ikeda H, Haga H, et al. Frequent cellular senescence in small bile ducts in primary biliary cirrhosis: a possible role in bile duct loss. Journal of Pathology. 2005;205:451–459.
143. Rygiel KA, Robertson H, Willet JD, et al. T cell-mediated biliary epithelial-to-mesenchymal transition in liver allograft rejection. Liver Transplantation. 2010;16:567–576.
144. Crawford AR, Lin XZ, Crawford JM. The normal adult human liver biopsy: a quantitative reference standard. Hepatology. 1998;28(2):323–331.
145. Oguma S, Belle S, Starzl TE, et al. A histometric analysis of chronically rejected human liver allografts: insights into the mechanisms of bile duct loss: direct immunologic and ischemic factors. Hepatology. 1989;9:204–209.
146. Moreira RK, Chopp W, Washington MK. The concept of hepatic artery-bile duct parallelism in the diagnosis of ductopenia in liver biopsy samples. American Journal of Surgical Pathology. 2011;35:392–403.
147. Matsumoto Y, McCaughan GW, Painter DM, et al. Evidence that portal tract microvascular destruction precedes bile duct loss in human liver allograft rejection. Transplantation. 1993;56:69–75.
148. Freese DK, Snover DC, Sharp HL, et al. Chronic rejection after liver transplantation: a study of clinical, histopathological and immunological features. Hepatology. 1991;13:882–891.
149. Hubscher SG, Buckels JA, Elias E, et al. Vanishing bile-duct syndrome following liver transplantation: is it reversible? Transplantation. 1991;51:1004–1010.
150. Neil DA, Hubscher SG. Histologic and biochemical changes during the evolution of chronic rejection of liver allografts. Hepatology. 2002;35:639–651.
151. Quaglia AF, Del Vecchio Blanco G, Greaves R, et al. Development of ductopaenic liver allograft rejection includes a "hepatitic" phase prior to duct loss. Journal of Hepatology. 2000;33:773–780.
152. Nakazawa Y, Jonsson JR, Walker NI, et al. Fibrous obliterative lesions of veins contribute to progressive fibrosis in chronic liver allograft rejection. Hepatology. 2000;32:1240–1247.
153. Wanless I. Physioanatomic considerations. In: Schiff ER, Sorrell MF, Maddrey WC, editors. Diseases of the Liver. 8th ed. Philadelphia, PA: Lippincott Williams & Wilkins; 1999: 3–37.
154. Lautenschlager I. CMV infection, diagnosis and antiviral strategies after liver transplantation. Transplant International. 2009;22:1031–1040. [Review.]
155. Razonable RR. Cytomegalovirus infection after liver transplantation: current concepts and challenges. World Journal of Gastroenterology. 2008;14:4849–4860. [Editorial review.]
156. Demetris AJ, Nalesnik M, Randhawa P, et al. Histologic patterns of rejection and other causes of liver dysfunction. In: Busuttil RW, Klintmalm GB, editors. Transplantation of the Liver. Philadelphia, PA: Elsevier Saunders; 2005: 1057–1128.
157. Kusne S, Schwartz M, Breinig MK, et al. Herpes simplex virus hepatitis after solid organ transplantation in adults. Journal of Infectious Diseases. 1991;163: 1001–1007.
158. Riediger C, Sauer P, Matevossian E, et al. Herpes simplex virus sepsis and acute liver failure. Clinical Transplantation. 2009;23(Suppl 21):37–41. [Review.]
159. Abdel Massih RC, Razonable RR. Human herpesvirus 6 infections after liver transplantation. World Journal of Gastroenterology. 2009;15:2561–2569.
160. Lautenschlager I, Hockerstedt K, Linnavuori K, et al. Human herpesvirus-6 infection after liver transplantation. Clinical Infectious Diseases. 1998;26:702–707.
161. Lautenschlager I, Harma M, Hockerstedt K, et al. Human herpesvirus-6 infection is associated with adhesion molecule induction and lymphocyte infiltration in liver allografts. Journal of Hepatology. 2002;37:648–654.
162. Potenza L, Luppi M, Barozzi P, et al. HHV-6A in syncytial giant-cell hepatitis. New England Journal of Medicine. 2008;359:593–602.
163. Andreoni M, Goletti D, Pezzotti P, et al. Prevalence, incidence and correlates of HHV-8/KSHV infection and Kaposi's sarcoma in renal and liver transplant recipients. Journal of Infection. 2001;43:195–199.
164. Pietrosi G, Vizzini G, Pipitone L, et al. Primary and reactivated HHV8 infection and disease after liver transplantation: a prospective study. American Journal of Transplantation. 2011;11:2715–2723.
165. Aseni P, Vertemati M, Minola E, et al. Kaposi's sarcoma in liver transplant recipients: morphological and clinical description. Liver Transplantation. 2001;7:816–823. [Case reports.]
166. Nourse JP, Jones K, Gandhi MK. Epstein–Barr virus-related post-transplant lymphoproliferative disorders: pathogenetic insights for targeted therapy. American Journal of Transplantation. 2011;11:888–895.
167. Cesarman E. Gammaherpesvirus and lymphoproliferative disorders in immunocompromised patients. Cancer Letters. 2011;305:163–174.
168. Nalesnik MA. Clinicopathologic characteristics of post-transplant lymphoproliferative disorders. Recent Results in Cancer Research. 2002;159:9–18.
169. Randhawa PS, Markin RS, Starzl TE, et al. Epstein–Barr virus-associated syndromes in immunosuppressed liver transplant recipients: clinical profile and recognition on routine allograft biopsy. American Journal of Surgical Pathology. 1990;14:538–547.
170. Randhawa PS, Jaffe R, Demetris AJ, et al. The systemic distribution of Epstein–Barr virus genomes in fatal post-transplantation lymphoproliferative disorders: an in situ hybridization study. American Journal of Pathology. 1991;138:1027–1033.
171. Randhawa PS, Jaffe R, Demetris AJ, et al. Expression of Epstein–Barr virus-encoded small RNA (by the EBER-1 gene) in liver specimens from transplant recipients with post-transplantation lymphoproliferative disease. New England Journal of Medicine. 1992;327:1710–1714.
172. Randhawa P, Blakolmer K, Kashyap R, et al. Allograft liver biopsy in patients with Epstein–Barr virus-associated posttransplant lymphoproliferative disease. American Journal of Surgical Pathology. 2001;25:324–330.
173. Hubscher SG, Williams A, Davison SM, et al. Epstein–Barr virus in inflammatory diseases of the liver and liver allografts: an in situ hybridization study. Hepatology. 1994;20:899–907.
174. Koneru B, Jaffe R, Esquivel CO, et al. Adenoviral infections in pediatric liver transplant recipients. Journal of the American Medical Association. 1987;258:489–492.
175. Michaels MG, Green M, Wald ER, et al. Adenovirus infection in pediatric liver transplant recipients. Journal of Infectious Diseases. 1992;165:170–174.
176. Saad RS, Demetris AJ, Lee RG, et al. Adenovirus hepatitis in the adult allograft liver. Transplantation. 1997;64:1483–1485.
177. Perez D, McCormack L, Petrowsky H, et al. Successful outcome of severe adenovirus hepatitis of the allograft following liver transplantation. Transplant Infectious Disease. 2007;9:318–322.
178. Hubscher SG. What is the long-term outcome of the liver allograft? Journal of Hepatology. 2011;55:702–717.
179. Dubel L, Farges O, Johanet C, et al. High incidence of antitissue antibodies in patients experiencing chronic liver allograft rejection. Transplantation. 1998;65:1072–1075.
180. Duclos-Vallee JC, Johanet C, Bach JF, et al. Autoantibodies associated with acute rejection after liver transplantation for type-2 autoimmune hepatitis. Journal of Hepatology. 2000;33:163–166.
181. Shinkura N, Ikai I, Egawa H, et al. Presence of anti-FKBP12 autoantibodies in patients with liver allografts: its association with allograft rejection. Transplantation. 1997;64:1336–1342.
182. Hunt J, Gordon FD, Jenkins RL, et al. Sarcoidosis with selective involvement of a second liver allograft: report of a case and review of the literature. Modern Pathology. 1999;12:325–328.
183. Vanatta JM, Modanlou KA, Dean AG, et al. Outcomes of orthotopic liver transplantation for hepatic sarcoidosis: an analysis of the United Network for Organ Sharing/Organ Procurement and Transplantation Network data files for a comparative study with cholestatic liver diseases. Liver Transplantation. 2011;17: 1027–1034.
184. Pappo O, Yunis E, Jordan JA, et al. Recurrent and de novo giant cell hepatitis after orthotopic liver transplantation. American Journal of Surgical Pathology. 1994;18:804–813.
185. Starzl TE, Demetris AJ. Liver transplantation: a 31-year perspective. Part I. Current Problems in Surgery. 1990;27:55–116.
186. Starzl TE, Demetris AJ. Liver transplantation: a 31-year perspective. Part II. Current Problems in Surgery. 1990;27:117–178. [Review.]
187. Starzl TE, Demetris AJ. Liver transplantation: a 31-year perspective. Part III. Current Problems in Surgery. 1990;27:187–240.
188. Eisenbach C, Longerich T, Fickenscher H, et al. Recurrence of clinically significant hepatitis A following liver transplantation for fulminant hepatitis A. Journal of Clinical Virology. 2006;35:109–112. [Case reports.]
189. Park GC, Hwang S, Yu YD, et al. Intractable recurrent hepatitis A virus infection requiring repeated liver transplantation: a case report. Transplantation Proceedings. 2010;42:4658–4660.
190. Gane E, Sallie R, Saleh M, et al. Clinical recurrence of hepatitis A following liver transplantation for acute liver failure. Journal of Medical Virology. 1995; 45:35–39.
191. Fagan E, Yousef G, Brahm J, et al. Persistence of hepatitis A virus in fulminant hepatitis and after liver transplantation. Journal of Medical Virology. 1990;30: 131–136.
192. Demetris AJ, Jaffe R, Sheahan DG, et al. Recurrent hepatitis B in liver allograft recipients. Differentiation between viral hepatitis B and rejection. American Journal of Pathology. 1986;125:161–172.
193. Demetris AJ, Todo S, Van Thiel DH, et al. Evolution of hepatitis B virus liver disease after hepatic replacement. Practical and theoretical considerations. American Journal of Pathology. 1990;137:667–676.

194. Harrison RF, Davies MH, Goldin RD, et al. Recurrent hepatitis B in liver allografts: a distinctive form of rapidly developing cirrhosis. Histopathology. 1993;23:21–28.
195. Thung SN. Histologic findings in recurrent HBV. Liver Transplantation. 2006;12(11 Suppl 2):S50–S53.
196. Davies SE, Portmann BC, O'Grady JG, et al. Hepatic histological findings after transplantation for chronic hepatitis B virus infection, including a unique pattern of fibrosing cholestatic hepatitis. Hepatology. 1991;13:150–157.
197. O'Grady JG, Smith HM, Davies SE, et al. Hepatitis B virus reinfection after orthotopic liver transplantation. Serological and clinical implications. Journal of Hepatology. 1992;14:104–111.
198. Pascarella S, Negro F. Hepatitis D virus: an update. Liver International. 2011;31:7–21. [Review].
199. Yurdaydin C, Idilman R, Bozkaya H, et al. Natural history and treatment of chronic delta hepatitis. Journal of Viral Hepatitis. 2010;17:749–756. [Review.]
200. Demetris AJ. Evolution of hepatitis C virus in liver allografts. Liver Transplantation. 2009;15(Suppl 2):S35–S41.
201. Berenguer M, Aguilera V, Prieto M, et al. Significant improvement in the outcome of HCV-infected transplant recipients by avoiding rapid steroid tapering and potent induction immunosuppression. Journal of Hepatology. 2006;44: 717–722.
202. Marcos A, Eghtesad B, Fung JJ, et al. Use of alemtuzumab and tacrolimus monotherapy for cadaveric liver transplantation: with particular reference to hepatitis C virus. Transplantation. 2004;78:966–971.
203. Eghtesad B, Fung JJ, Demetris AJ, et al. Immunosuppression for liver transplantation in HCV-infected patients: mechanism-based principles. Liver Transplantation. 2005;11:1343–1352.
204. Gane EJ. The natural history of recurrent hepatitis C and what influences this. Liver Transplantation. 2008;14(Suppl 2):S36–S44.
205. McCaughan GW, Shackel NA, Bertolino P, et al. Molecular and cellular aspects of hepatitis C virus reinfection after liver transplantation: how the early phase impacts on outcomes. Transplantation. 2009;87:1105–1111.
206. Moreira RK. Recurrent hepatitis C and acute allograft rejection: clinicopathologic features with emphasis on the differential diagnosis between these entities. Advances in Anatomic Pathology. 2011;18:393–405. [Review.]
207. Demetris AJ, Sebagh M. Plasma cell hepatitis in liver allografts: variant of rejection or autoimmune hepatitis? Liver Transplantation. 2008;14:750–755.
208. Schiano TD, Te HS, Thomas RM, et al. Results of steroid-based therapy for the hepatitis C-autoimmune hepatitis overlap syndrome. American Journal of Gastroenterology. 2001;96:2984–2991.
209. Fiel MI, Agarwal K, Stanca C, et al. Posttransplant plasma cell hepatitis (de novo autoimmune hepatitis) is a variant of rejection and may lead to a negative outcome in patients with hepatitis C virus. Liver Transplantation. 2008;14: 861–871.
210. Narang TK, Ahrens W, Russo MW. Post-liver transplant cholestatic hepatitis C: a systematic review of clinical and pathological findings and application of consensus criteria. Liver Transplantation. 2010;16:1228–1235.
211. Selzner N, Guindi M, Renner EL, et al. Immune-mediated complications of the graft in interferon-treated hepatitis C positive liver transplant recipients. Journal of Hepatology. 2011;55:207–217. [Review].
212. Wiesner RH, Demetris AJ, Belle SH, et al. Acute hepatic allograft rejection: incidence, risk factors, and impact on outcome. Hepatology. 1998;28:638–645.
213. Kamar N, Selves J, Mansuy JM, et al. Hepatitis E virus and chronic hepatitis in organ-transplant recipients. New England Journal of Medicine. 2008;358: 811–817.
214. Haagsma EB, Niesters HG, van den Berg AP, et al. Prevalence of hepatitis E virus infection in liver transplant recipients. Liver Transplantation. 2009;15: 1225–1228.
215. Pischke S, Suneetha PV, Baechlein C, et al. Hepatitis E virus infection as a cause of graft hepatitis in liver transplant recipients. Liver Transplantation. 2010; 16:74–82.
216. Pischke S, Wedemeyer H. Chronic hepatitis E in liver transplant recipients: a significant clinical problem? Minerva Gastroenterologica E Dietologica. 2010;56:121–128.
217. Kamar N, Garrouste C, Haagsma EB, et al. Factors associated with chronic hepatitis in patients with hepatitis E virus infection who have received solid organ transplants. Gastroenterology. 2011;140:1481–1489.
218. Haagsma EB, Riezebos-Brilman A, van den Berg AP, et al. Treatment of chronic hepatitis E in liver transplant recipients with pegylated interferon alpha-2b. Liver Transplantation. 2010;16:474–477.
219. Kamar N, Abravanel F, Selves J, et al. Influence of immunosuppressive therapy on the natural history of genotype 3 hepatitis-E virus infection after organ transplantation. Transplantation. 2010;89:353–360.
220. Halac U, Beland K, Lapierre P, et al. Chronic hepatitis E infection in children with liver transplantation. Gut. 2012;61:597–603.
221. Faust TW. Recurrent primary biliary cirrhosis, primary sclerosing cholangitis, and autoimmune hepatitis after transplantation. Liver Transplantation. 2001;7(Suppl 1):S99–S108.
222. Gautam M, Cheruvattath R, Balan V. Recurrence of autoimmune liver disease after liver transplantation: a systematic review. Liver Transplantation. 2006;12:1813–1824.
223. Silveira MG, Talwalkar JA, Lindor KD, et al. Recurrent primary biliary cirrhosis after liver transplantation. American Journal of Transplantation. 2010;10: 720–726.
224. Sebagh M, Farges O, Dubel L, et al. Histological features predictive of recurrence of primary biliary cirrhosis after liver transplantation. Transplantation. 1998;65:1328–1333.
225. Hubscher SG, Elias E, Buckels JA, et al. Primary biliary cirrhosis. Histological evidence of disease recurrence after liver transplantation. Journal of Hepatology. 1993;18:173–184.
226. Jones DE, James OF, Portmann B, et al. Development of autoimmune hepatitis following liver transplantation for primary biliary cirrhosis. Hepatology. 1999;30:53–57.
227. Vakiani E, Hunt KK, Mazziotta RM, et al. Hepatitis C-associated granulomas after liver transplantation: morphologic spectrum and clinical implications. American Journal of Clinical Pathology. 2007;127:128–134.
228. Mendes F, Couto CA, Levy C. Recurrent and de novo autoimmune liver diseases. Clinics in Liver Disease. 2011;15:859–878.
229. Czaja AJ, Manns MP. Advances in the diagnosis, pathogenesis, and management of autoimmune hepatitis. Gastroenterology. 2010;139:58–72 e4. [Review.]
230. Maggiore G, Gonzales E, Sciveres M, et al. Relapsing features of bile salt export pump deficiency after liver transplantation in two patients with progressive familial intrahepatic cholestasis type 2. Journal of Hepatology. 2010;53:981–986.
231. Jara P, Hierro L, Martinez-Fernandez P, et al. Recurrence of bile salt export pump deficiency after liver transplantation. New England Journal of Medicine. 2009;361:1359–1367.
232. Siebold L, Dick AA, Thompson R, et al. Recurrent low gamma-glutamyl transpeptidase cholestasis following liver transplantation for bile salt export pump (BSEP) disease (posttransplant recurrent BSEP disease). Liver Transplantation. 2010,16.856–863. [Multicenter study.]
233. Jaffe R. Liver transplant pathology in pediatric metabolic disorders. Pediatric and Developmental Pathology. 1998;1:102–117.
234. Hansen K, Horslen S. Metabolic liver disease in children. Liver Transplantation. 2008;14:713–733.
235. Bellamy CO, DiMartini AM, Ruppert K, et al. Liver transplantation for alcoholic cirrhosis: long term follow-up and impact of disease recurrence. Transplantation. 2001;72:619–626.
236. Abosh D, Rosser B, Kaita K, et al. Outcomes following liver transplantation for patients with alcohol- versus nonalcohol-induced liver disease. Canadian Journal of Gastroenterology. 2000;14:851–855.
237. Lucey MR. Liver transplantation in patients with alcoholic liver disease. Liver Transplantation. 2011;17:751–759. [Review.]
238. Conjeevaram HS, Hart J, Lissoos TW, et al. Rapidly progressive liver injury and fatal alcoholic hepatitis occurring after liver transplantation in alcoholic patients. Transplantation. 1999;67:1562–1568.
239. Molloy RM, Komorowski R, Varma RR. Recurrent nonalcoholic steatohepatitis and cirrhosis after liver transplantation. Liver Transplantation and Surgery. 1997;3:177–178.
240. Tang H, Boulton R, Gunson B, et al. Patterns of alcohol consumption after liver transplantation. Gut. 1998;43:140–145.
241. Charlton MR, Burns JM, Pedersen RA, et al. Frequency and outcomes of liver transplantation for nonalcoholic steatohepatitis in the United States. Gastroenterology. 2011;141:1249–1253.
242. Contos MJ, Cales W, Sterling RK, et al. Development of nonalcoholic fatty liver disease after orthotopic liver transplantation for cryptogenic cirrhosis. Liver Transplantation. 2001;7:363–373.
243. Ayata G, Gordon FD, Lewis WD, et al. Cryptogenic cirrhosis: clinicopathologic findings at and after liver transplantation. Human Pathology. 2002;33: 1098–1104.
244. Kim WR, Poterucha JJ, Porayko MK, et al. Recurrence of nonalcoholic steatohepatitis following liver transplantation. Transplantation. 1996;62:1802–1805.
245. Ong J, Younossi ZM, Reddy V, et al. Cryptogenic cirrhosis and posttransplantation nonalcoholic fatty liver disease. Liver Transplantation. 2001;7:797–801.
246. Brunt EM, Tiniakos DG. Histopathology of nonalcoholic fatty liver disease. World Journal of Gastroenterology. 2010;16:5286–5296.
247. Hubscher SG. Recurrent autoimmune hepatitis after liver transplantation: diagnostic criteria, risk factors, and outcome. Liver Transplantation. 2001;7: 285–291.

248. Group BW. Importance of liver biopsy findings in immunosuppression management: biopsy monitoring and working criteria for patients with Operational Tolerance (OT). Liver Transplantation. 2012;18:1154–1170.
249. Shaikh OS, Demetris AJ. Idiopathic posttransplantation hepatitis? Liver Transplantation. 2007;13:943–946.
250. Demetris AJ, Lunz JG 3rd, Randhawa P, et al. Monitoring of human liver and kidney allograft tolerance: a tissue/histopathology perspective. Transplant International. 2009;22:120–141.
251. Feng S, Ekong UD, Lobritto SJ, et al. Complete immunosuppression withdrawal and subsequent allograft function among pediatric recipients of parental living donor liver transplants. Journal of the American Medical Association (in press). 2012;307:283–293.
252. Wong T, Nouri-Aria KT, Devlin J, et al. Tolerance and latent cellular rejection in long-term liver transplant recipients. Hepatology. 1998;28:443–449.
253. Tisone G, Orlando G, Cardillo A, et al. Complete weaning off immunosuppression in HCV liver transplant recipients is feasible and favourably impacts on the progression of disease recurrence. Journal of Hepatology. 2006;44:702–709.
254. Takatsuki M, Uemoto S, Inomata Y, et al. Weaning of immunosuppression in living donor liver transplant recipients. Transplantation. 2001;72:449–454.
255. Ramos HC, Reyes J, Abu-Elmagd K, et al. Weaning of immunosuppression in long-term liver transplant recipients. Transplantation. 1995;59:212–217.
256. Eason JD, Cohen AJ, Nair S, et al. Tolerance: is it worth the risk? Transplantation. 2005;79:1157–1159.
257. Gane E, Portmann B, Saxena R, et al. Nodular regenerative hyperplasia of the liver graft after liver transplantation. Hepatology. 1994;20:88–94.
258. Eguchi S, Takatsuki M, Hidaka M, et al. Lack of grafted liver rejuvenation in adult-to-pediatric liver transplantation. Digestive Diseases and Sciences. 2011;56:1542–1547.
259. Devarbhavi H, Abraham S, Kamath PS. Significance of nodular regenerative hyperplasia occurring de novo following liver transplantation. Liver Transplantation. 2007;13:1552–1556.
260. Demetris AJ, Crawford JM, Minvervini MI, et al. Transplantation pathology of the liver. In: Odze R, Goldblum J, Crawford JM, editors. Surgical Pathology of the GI Tract, Liver, Biliary Tract, and Pancreas. Philadelphia, PA: Saunders Elsever; 2008.
261. Harada K, Ozaki S, Gershwin ME, et al. Enhanced apoptosis relates to bile duct loss in primary biliary cirrhosis. Hepatology. 1997;26:1399–1405.
262. Kemmer N, Kaiser T, Zacharias V, et al. Alpha-1-antitrypsin deficiency: outcomes after liver transplantation. Transplantation Proceedings. 2008;40:1492–1494.
263. Wolff H, Otto G, Giest H. Liver transplantation in Crigler-Najjar syndrome. A case report. Transplantation. 1986;42:84.
264. Kaufman SS, Wood RP, Shaw BW Jr, et al. Orthotopic liver transplantation for type I Crigler-Najjar syndrome. Hepatology. 1986;6:1259–1262.
265. Yamashita T, Ando Y, Okamoto S, et al. Effect of liver transplantation on the survival of patients with ordinary onset familial amyloid polyneuropathy in Japan. Amyloid. 2011;18(Suppl 1):180–181.
266. Seth AK, Badminton MN, Mirza D, et al. Liver transplantation for porphyria: who, when, and how? Liver Transplantation. 2007;13:1219–1227. [Review.]
267. Wahlin S, Stal P, Adam R, et al. Liver transplantation for erythropoietic protoporphyria in Europe. Liver Transplantation. 2011;17:1021–1026.
268. Brandhagen DJ. Liver transplantation for hereditary hemochromatosis. Liver Transplantation. 2001;7:663–672.
269. Maheshwari A, Rankin R, Segev DL, et al. Outcomes of liver transplantation for glycogen storage disease: a matched-control study and a review of literature. Clinical Transplantation. 2012;26:432–436.
270. Matern D, Starzl TE, Arnaout W, et al. Liver transplantation for glycogen storage disease types I, III, and IV. European Journal of Pediatrics. 1999;158(Suppl 2):S43–S48.
271. Gartner JC Jr, Bergman I, Malatack JJ, et al. Progression of neurovisceral storage disease with supranuclear ophthalmoplegia following orthotopic liver transplantation. Pediatrics. 1986;77:104–106.
272. Arnon R, Annunziato R, Miloh T, et al. Liver transplantation for hereditary tyrosinemia type I: analysis of the UNOS database. Pediatric Transplantation. 2011;15:400–405. [Evaluation studies.]
273. Arnon R, Annunziato R, Schilsky M, et al. Liver transplantation for children with Wilson disease: comparison of outcomes between children and adults. Clinical Transplantation. 2011;25:E52–E60. [Comparative study.]

第 83 章 心脏移植排斥反应和复发疾病的组织病理学综合征

E. Rene Rodriguez, Carmela D. Tan

引言

原位心脏移植是治疗冠状动脉及非冠状动脉病变引起的终末期心脏疾病的有效手段。患者的存活率随时间推移得到了不断的提高。近三十年来，心脏移植最常见指征没有很大的变化，主要包括非缺血性心肌病(53.3%)与缺血性心脏病(37.7%)[1]。儿童人群中，先天性心脏病为 1 岁以下患儿最主要的手术指征，而超过半数的 1 岁及以上患者被诊断为心肌病[2]。目前，心脏移植后 10 年生存率约为 50%，这一数据在大规模医疗中心则更高[1,2]。

本章节着重介绍心脏移植技术、移植器官的形态及解剖病理学等内容。在此围绕移植器官活检病理学评估，对国际心肺移植协会分别于 1990 年、2005 年及 2011 年所制定的指南(ISHLT-WF-1990、ISHLT-WF-2005 及 ISHLT-WF-2011)的进展及现状展开讨论。针对上述指南，也有学者提出了一些可能存在的缺陷与警示，以及心脏移植排斥反应诊断过程中的争议性问题。本章节是对第 71 章和第 79 章的补充，这两章分别详细介绍了心脏移植排斥反应及复发疾病的临床诊断与处理。

心内膜心肌活检

心内膜心肌活检(EMB)一直是诊断心脏移植患者免疫排斥反应的金标准。该诊断手段对急性细胞性排斥反应具有很高的敏感性及特异性[3,4]。当前尚无其他敏感性及特异性更高且检测周转时间更短的心脏成像技术、血清标志物或分子诊断技术，因而监测性心内膜心肌活检在心脏移植术后患者的护理与治疗中的地位尚无可取代[5]。尽管分子检测技术的发展有助于心脏移植排斥反应的诊断，心内膜心肌活检在目前的实时临床决策中仍具有更高的可行性。

活检时机。理想状况下应在移植时对供体进行基线活检，以评估供体器官状况，并排除心肌炎、缺血性损伤及其他病理性改变。大多数心脏移植中心都在移植术后进行计划性监测活检，其频率为：术后第一个月每周一次，第二个月每两周一次，第 3~12 个月每 4~8 周一次。

组织的获取。通常用活检刀经颈静脉或股静脉于右心室间隔壁采样。活检刀有各种尺寸(图 83.1)，故所获组织的大小也略有不同。成人用活检刀的常用尺寸为 7F(French)及 9F，儿童用活检刀的常用尺寸则为 3F、5F 及 7F[6]。通常用剪切钳钳夹适量室间隔部的心内膜下心肌作为样本。

组织样本最少数量。心脏移植急性细胞性排斥反应并非均匀分布，故在活检过程中多点采样尤为重要。Pomerance 和 Stovin[7]研究发现，若三个活检样本均未显示排斥反应改变，则漏检轻度排斥反应及中重度排斥反应的概率分别为 5%及 0%。然而，若将样本数增加至四个，则能将轻度排斥反应的假阳性率降至 2%[8]。此外，其他研究还强调了浸润范围的重要性。这些研究发现，若四个活检样本中至少有三个被各自归为轻度排斥反应，实际这种情况的发生概率为 13.57%，那么在这种情况下，漏检中重度排斥反应的概率则高达 25%[9]。

根据国际心肺移植协会 1990 年指南(ISHLT-WF-1990)，每次活检必须检测至少四个样本，必要时可额外分别取一个样本进行冰冻及电镜检测[10]。与之不同的是，国际心肺移植协会 2005 年指南(ISHLT-WF-

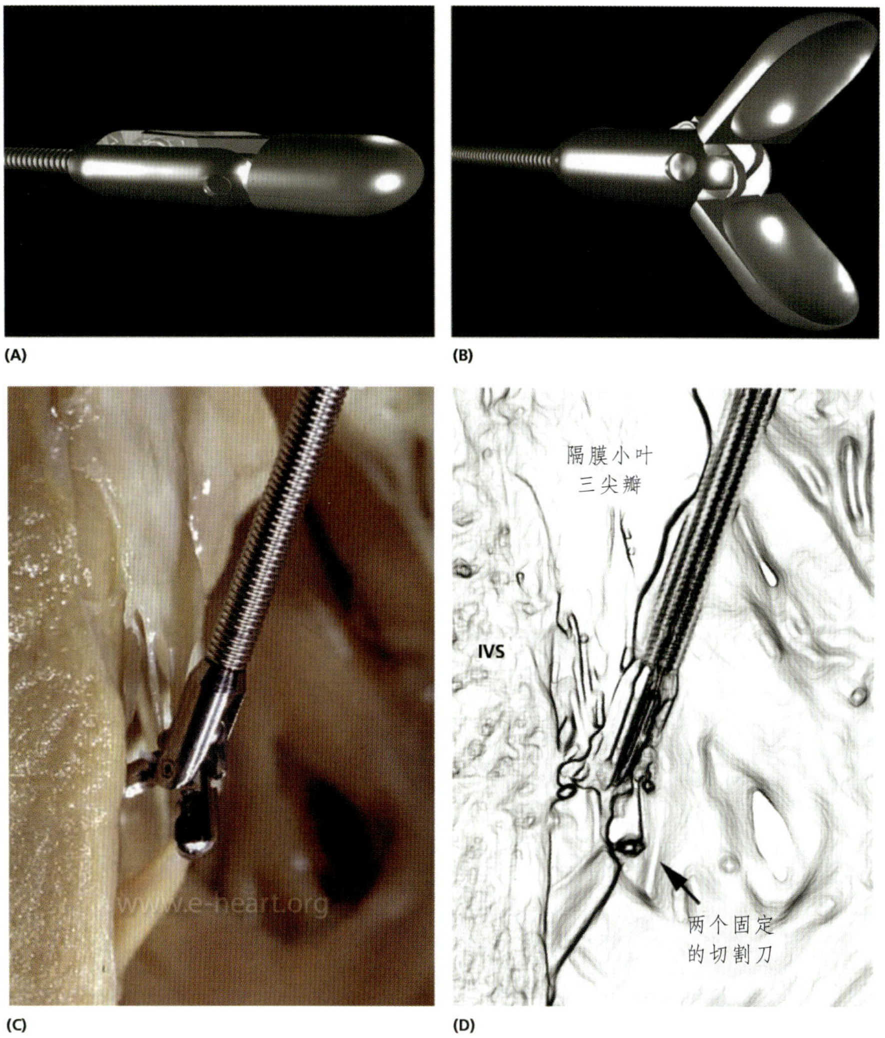

图 83.1　活检刀(A,B)是用于获取心内膜心肌活检组织的器械。在北美,大多数心内膜心肌活检采用经颈静脉右心途径,活检部位为室间隔部心肌(C,D)。用两个匙状切割刀获取充足的心肌样本并尽可能避免人为改变。

2005)要求至少检测三个心肌样本,并建议检测四个及以上样本,且 50%的样本必须为具可评估性的心肌组织,而不是活检位点或瘢痕[11]。未达上述标准的样本应诊断为“不充分活检”[10]。修订版指南未对冰冻组织或电镜检测作出要求[11]。

活检病理学评估。在心脏活检室内能够达到组织诊断分析的最佳保存条件。对于能够存放于室温(25℃)的固定剂,应立即将组织固定在相应的固定剂中。冷的固定剂会增加收缩带的人为改变。勿将组织长时间放置于滤纸、纱布或其他经生理盐水浸润的表面,因为生理盐水不仅不利于心肌组织形态的维持,且易引起人为改变。必要时也可使用其他有助于维持组织抗原稳定性的固定剂或防腐剂以进行免疫组化或免疫荧光检测。当科研需要时,可取一块或以上组织样本进行快速冰冻以用于分子检测。

大体检查。样本的大体描述应包括患者的基本资料、组织样本数、样本平均大小及颜色等。更为详细的大体检查还应提供有关心肌、增厚的心内膜、脂肪组织、腱索[12]及血凝块或心内膜小栓子等的重要信息。笔者所在的机构要求依照固定格式说明组织样本的数量,在大体标本上进行确认,并始终确保其与镜检标本上标注的组织数量一致。

组织处理。在大体检查过程中,处理组织样本需要小心操作,避免使用镊子等。可将标本从标本容器安全转移至网袋中,再小心折叠置入处理盒中。不应对组织进行分类挑选。活检组织镜检能够提供一些有价值的信息,因此应该提交活检获得的所有组织。白色的组织提示由较厚的心内膜组成,有时可能卷曲,从而可在组织切片上暴露出部分心肌组织(详见“缺陷与警示”部分)。同样的,部分外形类似血凝块的组织可能内含心肌组织。

本中心为美国第三大心脏移植中心，在这里所有活检组织(即所有四个或更多组织样本)都被处理为冰冻切片标本。这一过程有助于评估所有组织样本中急性细胞性排斥反应及抗体介导的排斥反应(AMR),而这两者的检测周转时间仅有数小时。小心处理标本能够避免冰冻产物,如心肌细胞肌质内冰晶的产生。

心脏移植排斥反应:形态学特征

在2001年举行的Banff移植病理学学组会议心脏分会上,对广泛沿用了十余年的ISHLT-WT-1990指南进行了修订。此次会议达成了一项共识,即尽管该指南历经了时间的考验，细胞性排斥反应的分级方法仍有待改进,且尚无抗体介导的排斥反应的诊断标准。正式修订版于2005年出版,是目前急性细胞性排斥反应的指南。同时,ISHLT-WT-2005首次为抗体介导的排斥反应的诊断提供了指南（表83.1)[11,14]。2011年出版的ISHLT-WT-2011又在急性细胞性排斥反应的诊断方面对ISHLT-WT-2005进行了修订[15]。与其他实体器官一样，心脏移植排斥反应可分为体液排斥反应与细胞排斥反应。其又可根据机制与病程进一步分为超急性、急性及慢性排斥反应。

超急性排斥反应是对移植器官产生的补体介导的强烈免疫攻击，由预先形成的抗体所触发，故非常迅速,通常在移植后数分钟至数小时内发生。超急性排斥反应的具体机制详见第6章。可能的诱发因素包括预先形成的ABO及人白细胞抗原(HLA)系统抗原表位的相应抗体、多次妊娠、多次手术并输注血制品,以及以往心脏移植手术史等。补体的级联激活可引起严重的内皮细胞损伤及血小板活化，进而引起凝血级联反应及血栓形成。形态学改变包括内皮细胞肿胀(光镜下不易观察)、微血栓、红细胞漏出,甚至镜下出血、间质水肿,从而引起多形核细胞炎性浸润,进而导致组织坏死。大体检查可无显著改变,也可有出血或同时存在苍白与出血。免疫组化试验可显示血管壁及间质纤维蛋白中的IgM、IgG和补体沉积。不幸的是,针对此类排斥反应的病理学检查通常在尸检时进行[16]。

表83.1 急性细胞性排斥反应[10,11]

ISHLT-WF-1990	ISHLT-WF-2005
0级(无急性排斥反应)	0R级
1A级(局部轻度急性排斥反应) 1B级(弥漫性轻度急性排斥反应) 2级(局部中度急性排斥反应)	1R级 轻度[间质和(或)血管周围浸润伴不多于1处的心肌损伤]
3A级(多灶性中度排斥反应)	2R级 中度(2处或以上的浸润灶伴心肌损伤)
3B级(弥漫性、交界性重度急性排斥反应) 4级(重度急性排斥反应)	3R级 重度(弥漫性浸润伴多灶性心肌损伤,伴或不伴水肿、出血或血管炎)

急性细胞性排斥反应:效应细胞。从形态学角度而言,急性细胞性排斥反应是一种以淋巴细胞为主,针对心脏移植的单个核细胞炎症反应。其具体机制详见第5章。在严重的排斥反应病例中还可有粒细胞的参与。排斥反应的分级与反应的严重程度相关。指南推荐的排斥反应分级系统主要基于炎性浸润程度和肌细胞损伤情况,而炎性浸润的形式则并非主要因素。有研究将心脏活检组织中淋巴细胞的表型进行分类，并对移植器官中T淋巴细胞的浸润程度及细胞组成(CD4/CD8比值)和排斥反应的组织学分级进行了相关性分析,结果显示两者并无良好相关性[17,18]。然而,也有研究表明,$CD8^+$ T细胞的平均数量与排斥反应严重程度之间存在良好的相关性[19]。上述研究结果之间的差异可能是因为移植器官免疫反应是一个不断变化的连续过程,而相关的病理学研究往往将其分隔为小的“时间片段”进行研究分析。支持这一观点的研究声称,根据是否存在幼稚细胞(CD45RA)、记忆细胞或活化细胞(CD45RO)将T淋巴细胞进一步分类，可在轻度排斥反应的活检组织中观察到大量幼稚的CD4细胞;而在中度排斥反应中,主要细胞类型则向活化的CD8细胞转变[20]。在重度排斥反应中亦可观察到抗原提呈细胞（即巨噬细胞和树突状细胞)数量的增加[21-24]。调节T细胞在人类心脏移植排斥反应中的作用尚未被阐明。但近年来随着活检组织定量研究技术的发展，心脏移植器官中调节T细胞的特征也将得到更深入的研究[25]。

在轻度排斥反应中,B细胞浸润极为罕见。但在中度排斥反应中可见大量活化的B淋巴细胞和NK细胞，提示其在细胞性排斥反应过程中发挥重要的促进和效应作用[24]。

心内膜心肌活检的急性细胞性排斥反应分级

ISHLT-WF-2005 的排斥反应分级将各等级添加后缀“R”(表 83.1),以示修订(revised)[11]:

0R 级(**无急性细胞性排斥反应**)。在 0R 级中,不存在单个核细胞(淋巴细胞/巨噬细胞)炎症或肌细胞损伤(图 83.2)。

1R 级(**轻度急性细胞性排斥反应**)。轻度排斥反应可有以下两点表现:①血管周围和(或)间质出现单个核细胞(淋巴细胞/组织细胞)。上述细胞一般沿肌细胞的边界分布,既不侵犯相邻肌细胞,又不引起正常结构变形(图 83.3)。②可出现一个单个核细胞浸润灶,并伴有相应的肌细胞损伤。

2R 级(**中度急性细胞性排斥反应**)。当出现两个或以上的单个核细胞(淋巴细胞/巨噬细胞)浸润灶,并伴有相应的肌细胞损伤时,则为 2R 级。有时可见嗜酸性

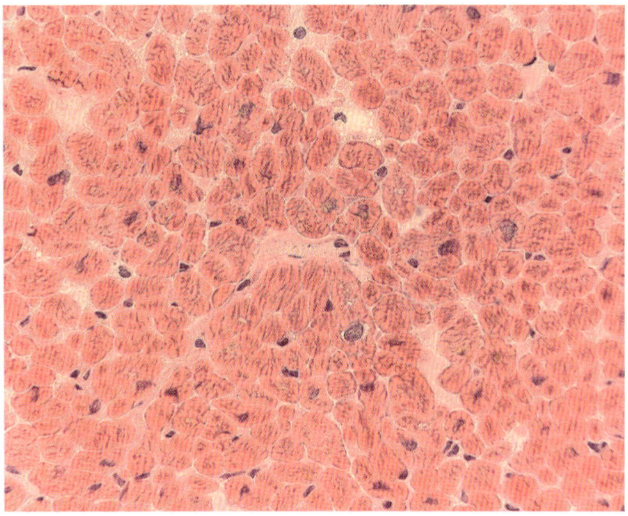

图 83.2 心脏移植器官心内膜心肌活检排斥反应 0R 级。肌细胞轻微肥大,核深染增大,但间质或小动脉(图片正中)周围无炎性浸润(HE 染色,×400)。

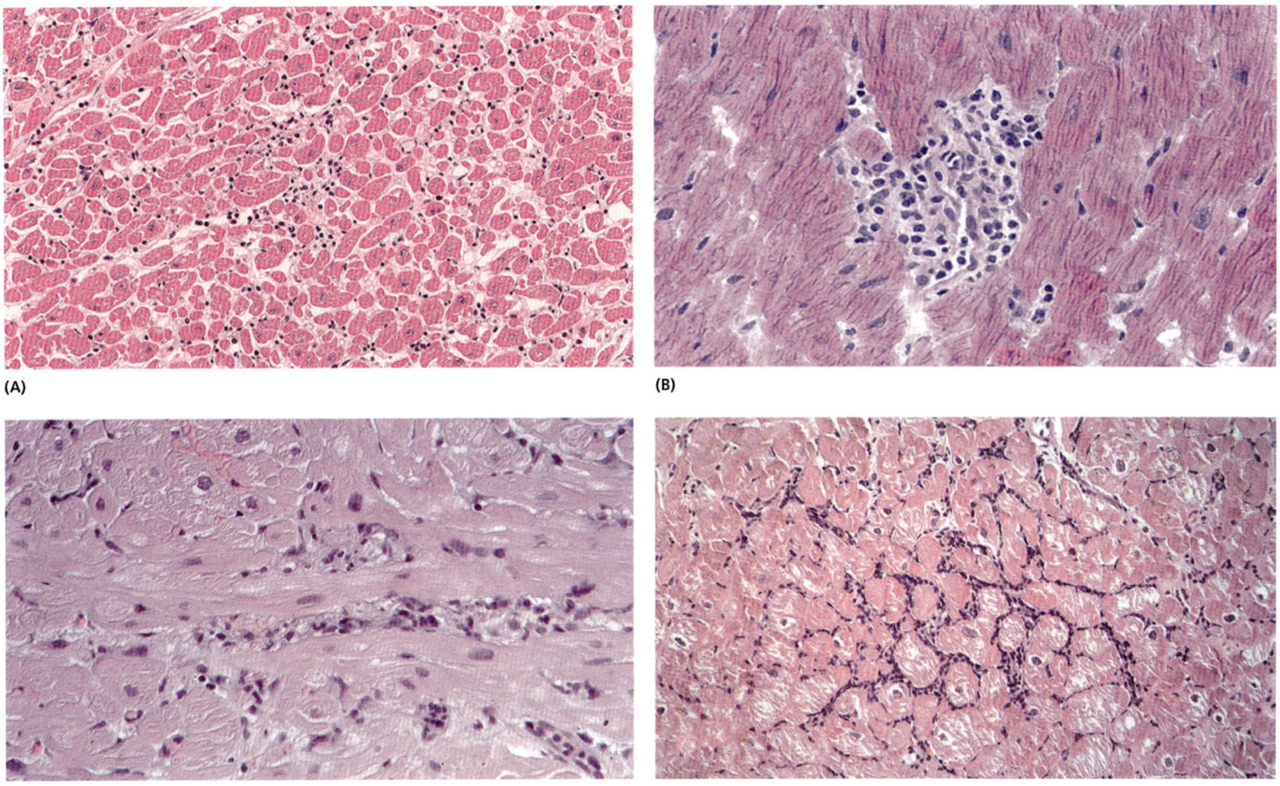

(A) (B) (C) (D)

图 83.3 1R 级排斥反应。(A)该光镜照片中可见心肌间质内少量明显的淋巴细胞浸润,无肌细胞坏死、损伤或丢失(HE 染色,×100)。(B)淋巴细胞围绕小动脉簇状浸润,并向间质间隙延伸。细胞浸润呈非连续性,且以血管为中心(HE 染色,×200)。(C)以血管周围及间质淋巴细胞浸润为特征,与前者稍有区别(HE 染色,×200)。(D)该光镜照片所示为更大量的细胞浸润,各个肌细胞周围的肌束膜间隙内存在明显的淋巴细胞浸润。这种铁丝网样改变属于 ISHLT-WF-1990 分级系统中的 1B 级改变(HE 染色,×150)。

粒细胞。浸润灶可出现在一个或多个活检组织中。排斥反应病灶之间被未受累的心肌组织分隔(图 83.4)。在其他活检标本中也可同时存在轻度排斥反应病灶。

3R 级(**重度急性细胞性排斥反应**)。出现以淋巴/巨噬细胞为主或多形细胞浸润为特征的弥漫性炎症过程(图 83.5)。活检样本多均受累,但样本间的浸润程度可不等。可见多处肌细胞损伤。最严重的细胞(及体液)排斥反应中还可见水肿、间质出血及血管炎。

活检报告中的附加信息 (非排斥反应性表现)(表 83.2)

活检充分性说明。若活检标本少于三个,则为不充分活检[10,11]。此外,有时活检标本数达到了四个,但有一个或以上标本中的心肌比例少于 50%,则仍属于不充分活检。不充分活检的标本通常主要包含或仅包含心内膜、血栓、既往活检部位肉芽组织或脂肪组织。不过不可否认的是,有时其他充分活检的标本仍能提供排斥反应等有用信息。尽管无法用于排斥反应的诊断,这些相关信息可作为组织学描述的一部分或备注记录在活检报告中。

围术期缺血性损伤。这是缺血性损伤的早期过程,与缺血时间过长有关,以收缩带坏死或凝固性坏死为特征(图 83.6A,B)。早期围术期坏死可能与影响供体的因素相关,如儿茶酚胺释放、急症监护中的加压疗法、严重供体创伤、再植损伤或早期围术期损伤[26]。在移植时行室间隔活检,尽管其病理改变可能极其轻微,但仍能提供许多信息。指南中介绍了在移植器官监测过程中可能出现的两种不同的缺血性损伤:一种常见于移植后 3 周内,标志着围术期损伤;另一种为迟发型缺血,一般见于 3 个月之后。典型的形态学改变为肌细

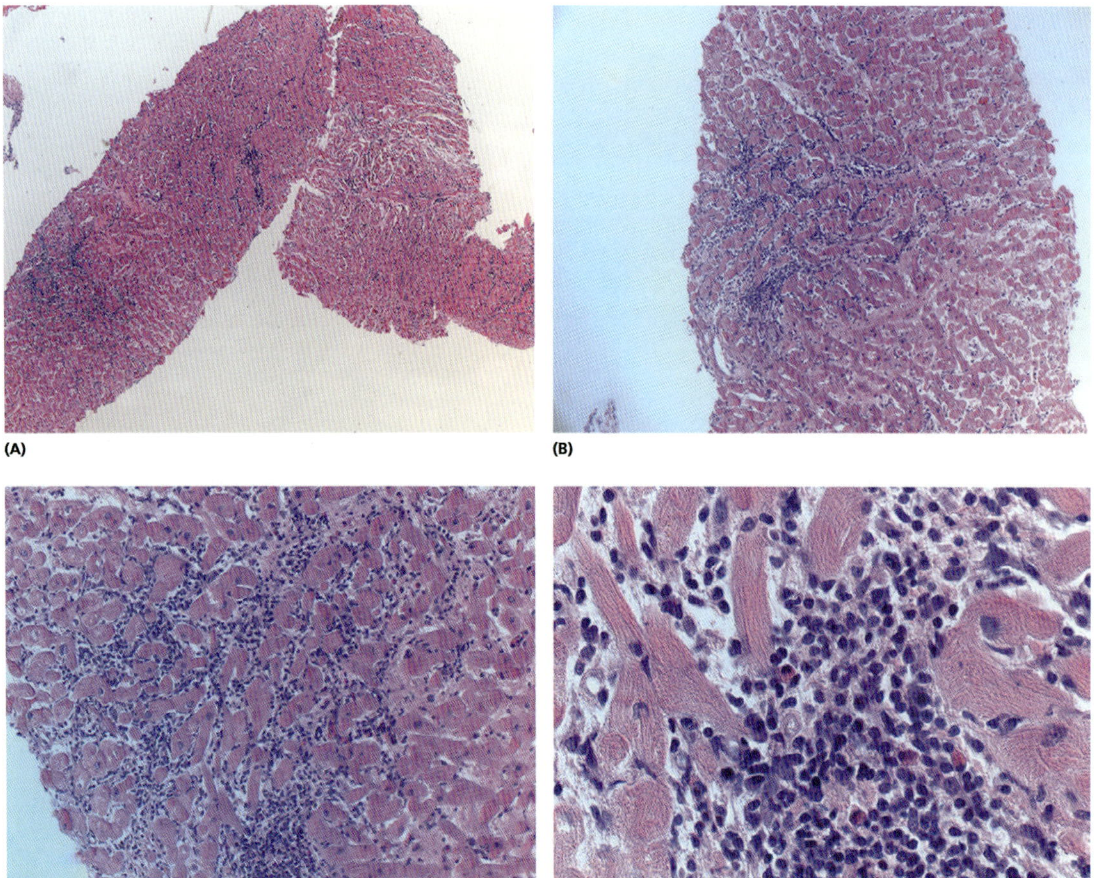

图 83.4 2R 级排斥反应。(A)该活检标本中可见多个淋巴细胞浸润灶,并向间质间隙延伸。图中可见两处明显的炎性浸润灶,两者之间为正常心肌组织分隔(HE 染色,×20)。(B,C)可见明显的肌细胞丢失及淋巴细胞侵犯(B,HE 染色,×40;C,HE 染色,×200)。(D)为图 C 的局部放大,可明显观察到炎性浸润扩张并替代肌细胞(丢失),且出现嗜酸性粒细胞(HE 染色,×400)。

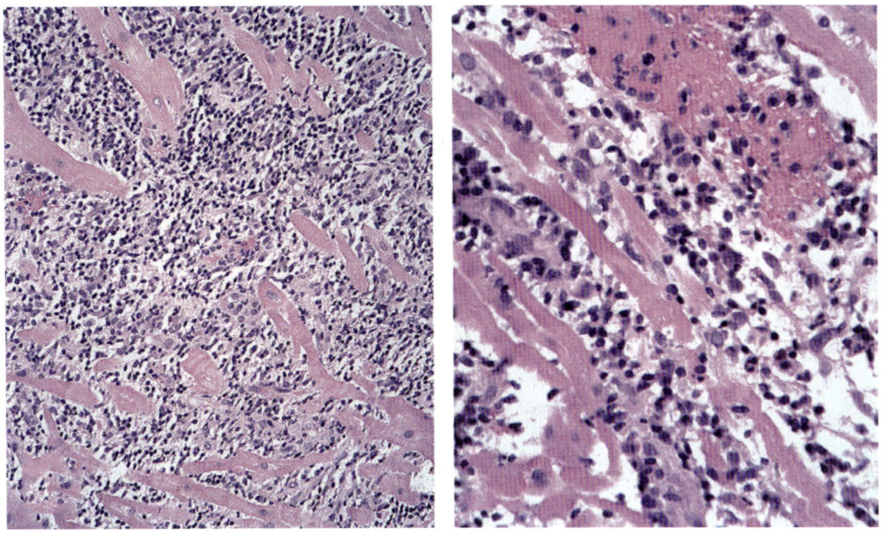

图 83.5　3R 级排斥反应。(A)心肌组织被密集的单个核细胞广泛性弥漫性浸润。这一改变对应 ISHLT-WF-1990 分级系统中的 3B 级改变(HE 染色,×100)。(B)广泛性炎症可进一步进展,出现中性粒细胞,甚至引起血管坏死。此外,炎性浸润还伴有显著的间质水肿(HE 染色,×400)。

表 83.2　非排斥反应性表现

ISHLT-WF-1990	ISHLT-WF-2005
缺血性损伤	缺血性损伤
A=移植后 3 周内	早期:移植后 6 周内
B=迟发型缺血	晚期:与移植器官冠状动脉疾病相关
Quilty 效应	Quilty 效应
A=无肌细胞受累	
B=肌细胞受累	
感染	感染
淋巴细胞增殖性疾病	淋巴细胞增殖性疾病

胞坏死,通常为凝固性坏死,伴有肌细胞嗜酸性增强、核固缩,甚至核碎裂。肌细胞坏死的程度通常与炎性浸润程度不成比例;有时可见肌细胞空泡形成。免疫抑制可能延迟组织的修复[26]。尽管这类坏死可无任何临床表现,严重的病理改变仍可对移植器官的功能造成损害。病变区域往往较为明显,尤其是经 Masson 三色染色后。有时可出现肌细胞钙化(图 83.7)。有时也可见肌细胞空泡形成或脂肪坏死[26]。随着损伤的修复,活检标本可表现为混合性炎性细胞浸润,包括中性粒细胞、淋巴细胞、巨噬细胞及嗜酸性粒细胞。这一现象可见于移植后 6 周之内的活检标本。肌细胞的损伤程度高于病灶内炎性浸润的程度[11]。

移植器官间质纤维化是围移植期早期损伤的可能原因之一[27]。能够确定围移植期缺血性损伤是否为纤维化的原因的唯一方法是在心脏移植时进行基线活检。关于纤维化还需注意的一点是心肌标本的大小可能会影响纤维化病灶的检出数量[28]。

迟发型缺血性损伤。活检标本中的血管往往较小,不足以评估移植器官血管病变的动脉改变。然而,继发性心肌病变,比如液化性肌细胞溶解及凝固性坏死,则较容易检出。在移植心脏血管病变中,缺血灶与显著单个核细胞浸润无明显相关性。但迟发型缺血性损伤的诊断可在移植受体心力衰竭的鉴别诊断中排除其他潜在可治疗的病因,如急性细胞性排斥反应或抗体介导的排斥反应[11]。

心内膜淋巴细胞浸润(Quilty 效应)。心内膜淋巴细胞浸润[29],又称“Quilty 效应”[30],是移植心脏心内膜 T 细胞、B 细胞及组织细胞的聚集(图 83.8)[31]。约半数上述病变中存在浆细胞[32]。有时也会出现嗜酸性粒细胞和中性粒细胞。浸润灶中可见毛细血管,内有红细胞,有时也可见突起的内皮细胞。毛细血管管径为 0.007~1.89mm^2[29]。一些假说解释了上述浸润的病理机制,包括环孢素的使用[33]、伴随感染 EB 病毒[34]、Quilty 效应发生区域心内膜局部环孢素低浓度[35]、对环孢素的特殊体质[33]等,但上述假说尚未得到证实。然而,令人惊讶的是,Quilty 效应并不出现在因其他器官移植(如肝、肾)而使用环孢素的患者心脏中[36],而仅仅出现在移植

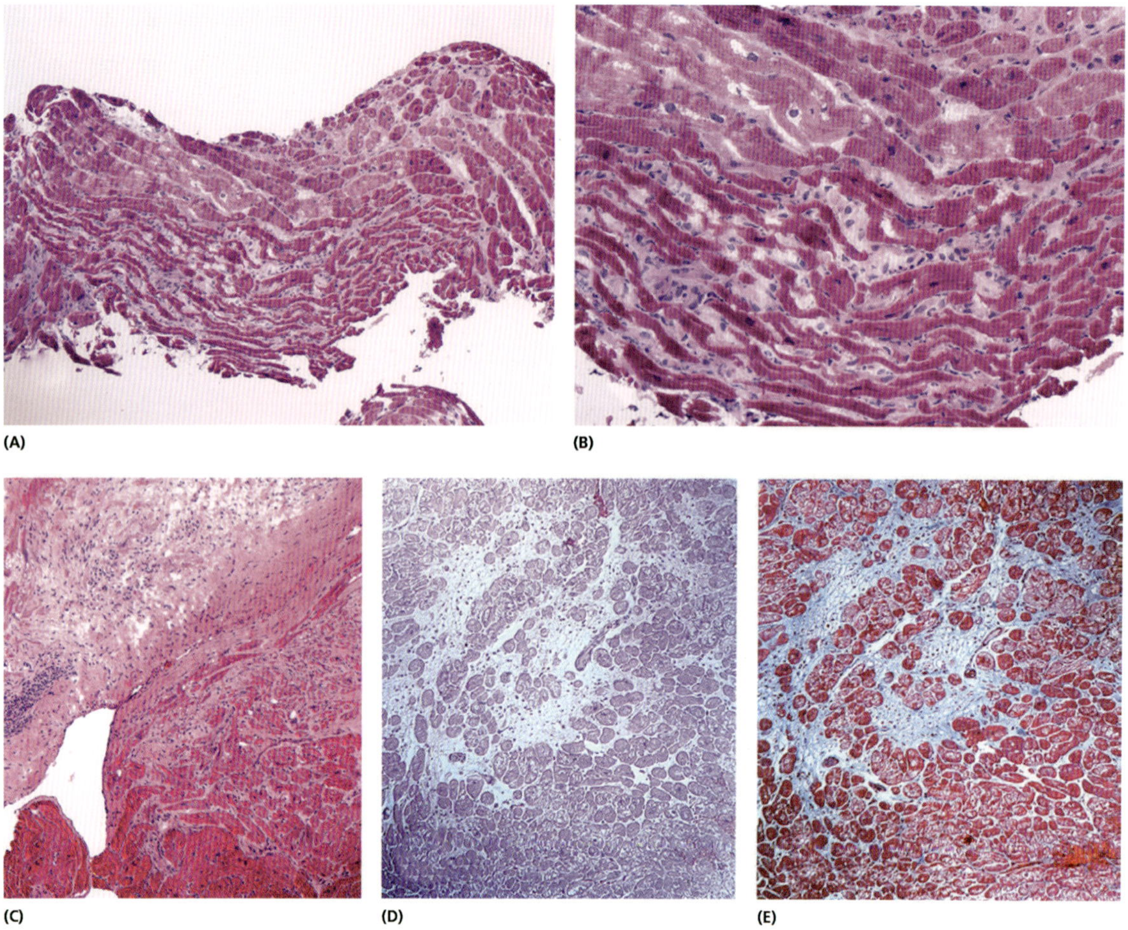

图 83.6 缺血性损伤。(A,B)肌细胞嗜酸性增高,呈波浪形变薄,出现核固缩和(或)核丢失,并伴有急性缺血性损伤(HE 染色,A,×40;B,×200)。(C)缺血修复灶伴疏松肉芽组织,轻度淋巴细胞浸润(HE 染色,×40)。(D,E)图示为已修复的缺血灶,存在替代细胞及间质纤维化。当移植后出现上述病理改变时,应怀疑移植器官血管病变的可能(D,Masson 三色染色,×40)。

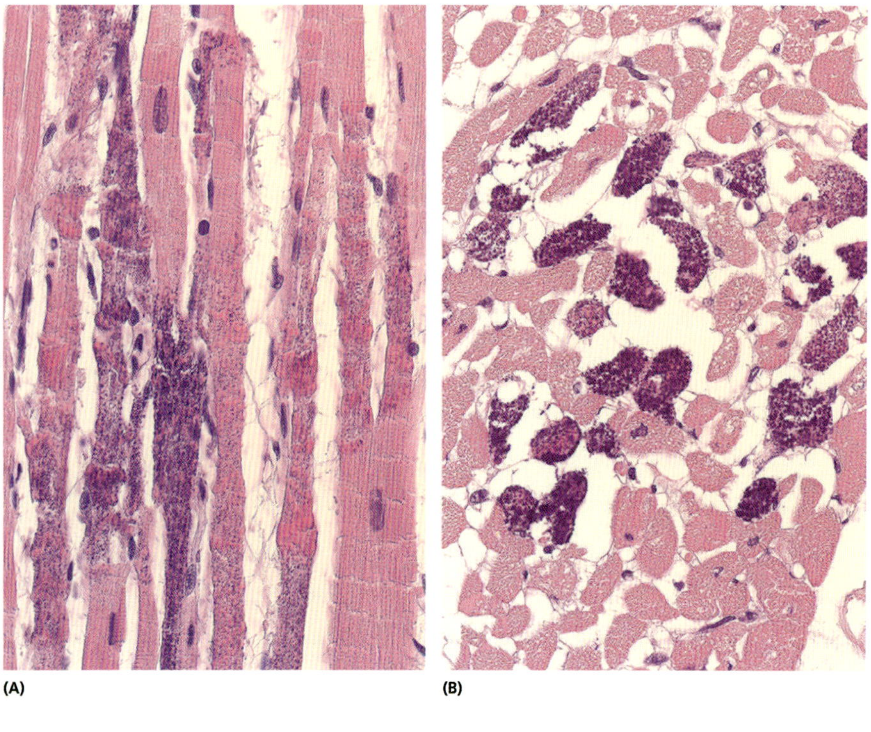

图 83.7 缺血性损伤肌细胞线粒体钙化。坏死肌细胞肌质内嗜碱性颗粒为线粒体钙化的典型表现。(A)肌细胞纵切面示嗜碱性线粒体沿肌质纹理排列(HE 染色,×400)。(B)横切面示肌质内钙化线粒体的排列方式较为杂乱无章(HE 染色,×400)。随着时间推移,肌细胞渐渐完全钙化(图 83.12)。

心脏的心内膜中。

Quilty 效应浸润与排斥反应可能相关，也可能无关。浸润灶的大小差异很大，小至一小簇单个核细胞，大至 2mm 肉眼可见的病损。ISHLT–WF–1990 中提到两种形态学改变：A 型及 B 型。A 型局限于心内膜，而 B 型则累及相邻的心肌(图 83.8C，D)[10]。ISHLT–WF–2005 不再要求将 Quilty 效应病损分类为 A 型与 B 型，因为两者的分类与临床并无明确相关性[11]。然而，还发现了第三种罕见的类型，即除了典型的心内膜淋巴细胞浸润之外，还在心肌深层出现与 Quilty 效应病损相同的病理改变。

Quilty 效应与中度排斥反应。Quilty 浸润与排斥反应[37]的区别影响临床治疗指征，因而两者的鉴别是病理学家面前的一个难题。可以想象，倘若仅对活检标本中深层心肌的少数层面进行检测，则所示的炎性浸润可能与排斥反应表现相似。然而，若对更深层面进行检测，或更佳的是对整个标本组织进行检测，则较易将心肌的炎性浸润与心内膜 Quilty 病损相联系。

Quilty 效应与淋巴性肿瘤。根据细胞成分与位置可将明显的 Quilty 病损与淋巴性肿瘤相区别。据报道，6%的移植患者可发生淋巴性肿瘤[38]。研究发现，EB 病毒在移植后淋巴增生紊乱(PTLD)中发挥一定作用[39–42]，但并不是其必要因素[43,44]。其中，多数为单克隆 B 细胞性肿瘤[45]，其临床表现包括淋巴结、中枢神经系统、全身器官或移植器官受累[39]。然而，也存在 T 细胞淋巴瘤[46]，但其原发性心脏表现并不多见[39]。多发性骨髓瘤较少见[47]。PTLD 及移植后恶性肿瘤将分别在第 93 章及第 95 章详述。

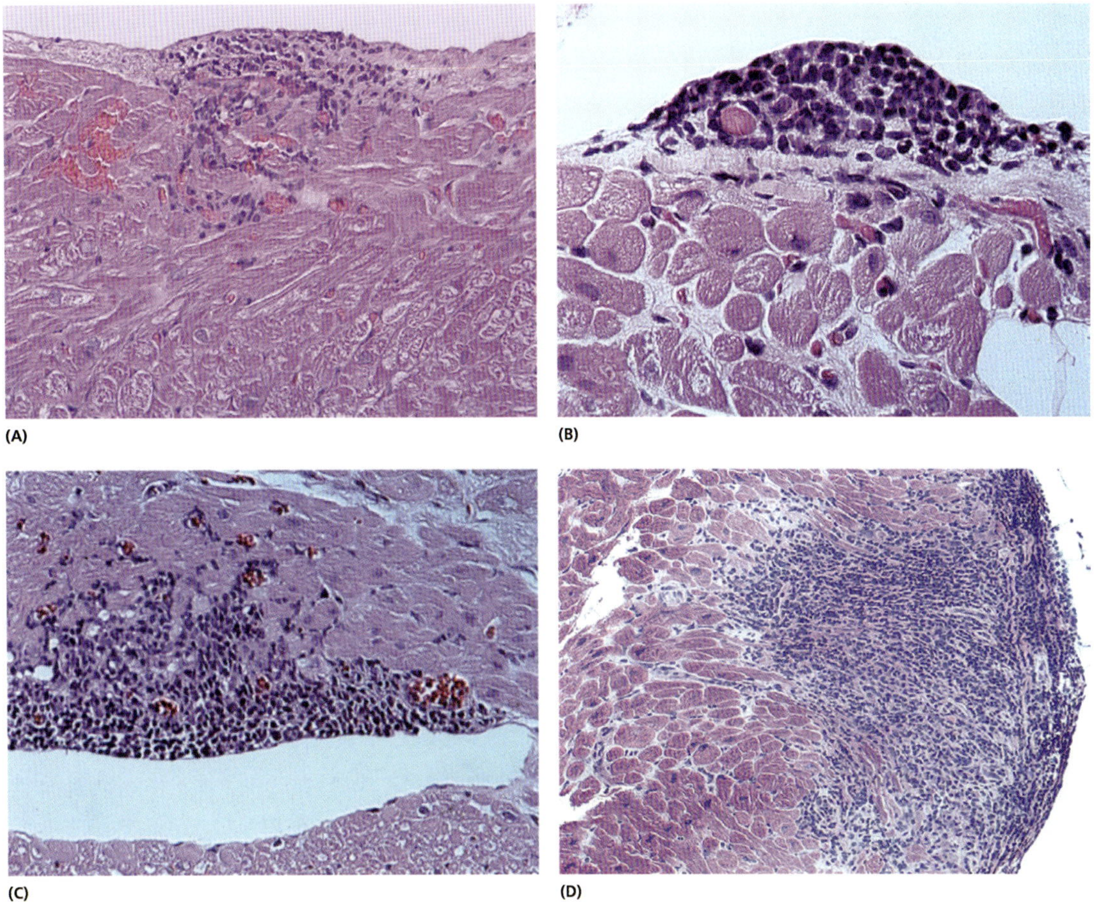

图 83.8　心内膜淋巴细胞浸润(Quilty 病损)。(A)图示活检标本心内膜及延伸至心肌的淋巴细胞浸润(HE 染色，×150)。(B)图示明显的心内膜 Quilty 病损，并不穿透相邻的心肌。以往在 ISHLT–WF–1990 中将该病损称为 Quilty A 型(HE 染色，×400)。(C)心内膜内可见明显的浸润，心肌内存在早期浸润改变。此外，还可见明显的充满红细胞的血管。上述为 Quilty 病损常见的特征性改变。然而，在冰冻切片中，血管可能不明显(HE 染色，×200)。(D)在该活检标本中，显著的淋巴细胞浸润延伸至相邻的心肌组织，呈指状突起。以往在 ISHLT-WF-1990 中将该病损称为 Quilty B 型(HE 染色，×100)。

总体而言,心内膜淋巴细胞浸润(Quilty 效应)是心脏移植活检标本中常见的病损,但目前缺乏临床相关资料。最近的一项为期 10 年的研究纳入了 217 名成人与 22 名儿童,结果显示,其中有 49%的成人与 68%的儿童存在心内膜淋巴浸润[30]。该研究的重点在于心内膜浸润与以下几点似乎并无关联:①排斥分级;②继发性血管病变(血管慢性排斥反应);③淋巴瘤的发生;④病毒感染(巨细胞病毒或 EB 病毒)。最后,由于 A 型与 B 型浸润并无区别,ISHLT-WF-2005 中对其分类不再要求[11]。

缺陷与警示

尽管专家学者们一直致力于制订关于排斥反应分级的标准指南[10,11],病理学家和心脏病学家们在使用工作指南时仍提出了一些争议。

肌细胞损伤。人类移植器官心内膜活检的解读是一个难点,导致许多经验丰富的心脏病学病理学家在肌细胞损伤的定义问题上难以达成共识[13]。在 2001 年 Banff 会议上针对精确术语的制订(如肌细胞损伤)提出了建议[13]。光镜检查下,此类损伤可能由一系列轻微、先兆性的病理改变组成。对于非专业观察者,上述轻微改变极易被漏检。严格来说,肌细胞内的单纯改变,如空泡变性、水样变性、核周晕环[48]等,是上述改变中最为轻微的;而凝固性坏死、肌细胞溶解及核固缩则是上述改变中最为严重的。因此,损伤这个词较为模棱两可。除非肌细胞内存在明确的凝固性坏死、肌质裂解或核固缩等典型核改变,通过 HE 染色石蜡切片对“受损”细胞特征的观察是一个主观过程。对超微结构的研究可以清晰地显示轻微的肌细胞损伤[49]。肌细胞变性与坏死很容易区分。内皮细胞、基底层或其他血管结构的损伤也很容易辨认[50]。根据超微结构标准定义的肌细胞坏死在体液排斥反应中较常见,而在细胞性排斥反应中更为常见的则是肌细胞变性,后者具有恢复的潜能[51]。超微结构研究提示,部分排斥反应中的肌细胞损伤实际上可能是可逆的[49,52]。然而,在光镜下,部分代表肌细胞亚损伤的改变与早期坏死难以区分。

既往活检灶。这在移植监测活检中较常见(图 83.9),在活检中的发生率为 53%~69%[53,54]。其发生率之所以如此之高,是因为对于一名特定的患者,其心脏流入道至右心室的解剖结构是连续的。在经颈静脉活检过程中,心房吻合处的嵴、右心室小梁和节制索均为在室间隔原杂交位置进行活检提供了指导。对生前在心脏移植后存活数月至数年的患者尸体进行尸检,大体检查可能显示右心室间隔部中 1/3 心内膜上存在局部片状增厚,直径为 1~2cm。

机会性感染。众所周知,长期使用免疫抑制剂的移植受体易受病毒、细菌、真菌及原虫的机会性感染。相关内容详见第 92~94 章。其中最常见的是细菌感染[55],病毒感染次之,其余分别为真菌和原虫[56,57]。心内膜心肌活检标本中最常见的引起机会性感染的病原体是弓形虫和巨细胞病毒[58-60]。其他见于心脏移植患者的病原体包括:

病毒:乙肝病毒[61]、丙肝病毒[62]、肠病毒、细小病毒 B19[63]、EB 病毒[63]及其他疱疹病毒和腺病毒。

细菌及分枝杆菌[64-66]。

真菌:曲霉菌[67-68]、念珠菌[68]、诺卡菌[55]、毛霉菌[69](图 83.10A,B)。

原虫:肺孢子虫[70]、弓形虫(图 83.10C)[71]、利什曼原虫[72]、锥虫病的重新激活[73]。

在接受心脏移植的儿童中,引起机会性感染的病原体包括病毒(巨细胞病毒、单纯疱疹病毒、水痘-带状疱疹病毒、呼吸道病毒及 EB 病毒)、细菌(分枝杆菌、革兰阳性细菌及革兰阴性细菌)、弓形虫和肺孢子虫[68,74,75]。

值得注意的是,在心内膜心肌活检标本中很难辨认微生物,因此不应将这一点作为排除感染的依据。活检时必须留意提示感染的线索,如异常的炎性浸润。此处的异常是指在无肌细胞坏死或替代的部位出现炎症,伴有粒细胞、浆细胞和(或)巨噬细胞的存在。此类病灶可能含有大量胞内寄生虫(如弓形虫)或真菌,而这两者在 HE 染色下不易检出,因此需进行特殊染色。病理学家还应在内皮细胞、平滑肌细胞或各类血管周细胞的细胞核内寻找病毒包涵体。心肌细胞内的病毒包涵体很难用光镜观察到。

脂肪组织:穿孔与浸润。脂肪细胞是组成心脏的正常细胞之一,主要位于心外膜。脂肪组织的显微灶通常位于心内膜下及心肌内。上述显微灶可见于各个心房心室,但主要见于肥胖患者或服用类固醇患者的右心室壁。因此,病理学家应注意,心脏脂肪组织本身并非病理性的。由于脂肪组织也可源于心外膜,在心内膜心肌活检时应尽量判断检出的脂肪组织是否为心室壁的一部分(图 83.11)。尽管右心室活检的目的在于获得室间隔右侧的标本,也可用活检刀在右心室游离壁取样。

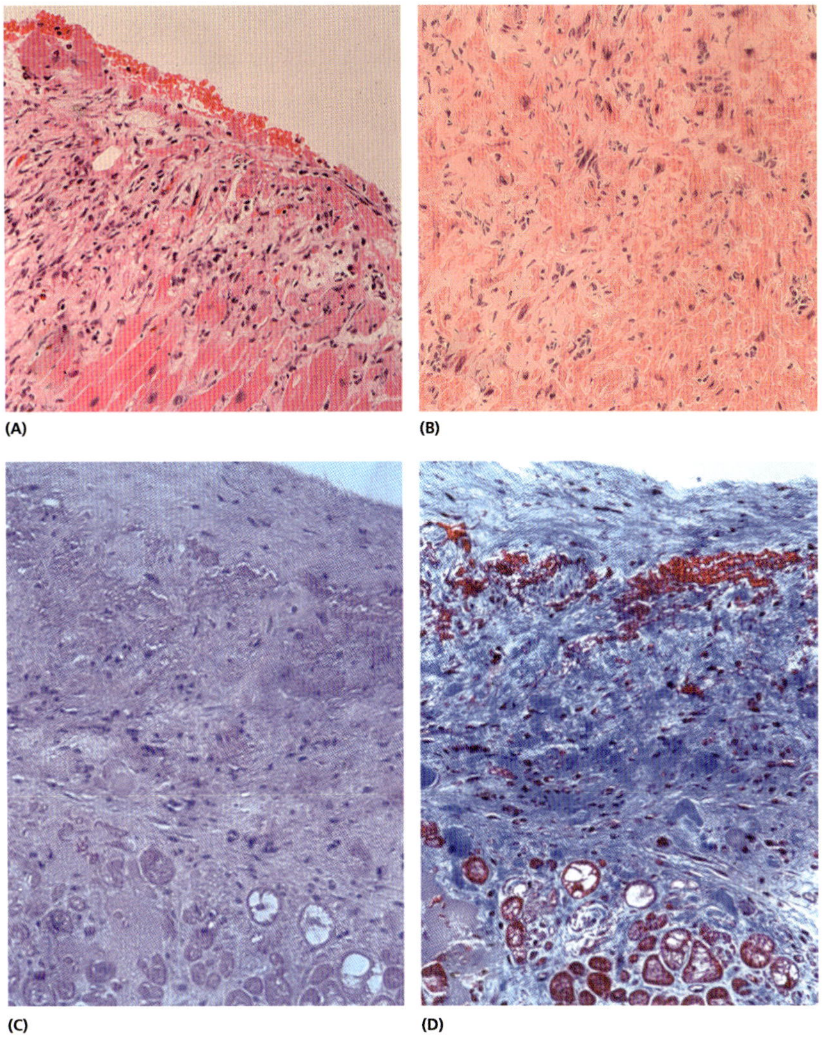

图 83.9　既往活检灶。(A)该图所示为心内膜肉芽组织，富含成纤维细胞，表面存在红细胞，纤维组织尚较疏松。上述改变代表修复中的近期活检灶(约 1 周)(HE 染色，×100)。(B)此处的肉芽组织内成纤维细胞较少，纤维组织与图 A 相比明显更为成熟致密，表明处于进一步修复状态。注意视野中瘢痕组织内杂乱排列的肌细胞。该病理改变可能代表活检后 2~3 周的修复灶(HE 染色，×200)。(C，D)这两张图所示的是完全修复的活检灶，伴有心内膜的增厚及周边的瘢痕。图 D 使用三色染色，显示明显增加的致密纤维组织形成瘢痕（C，HE 染色，×200；D，Masson 三色染色，×200)。

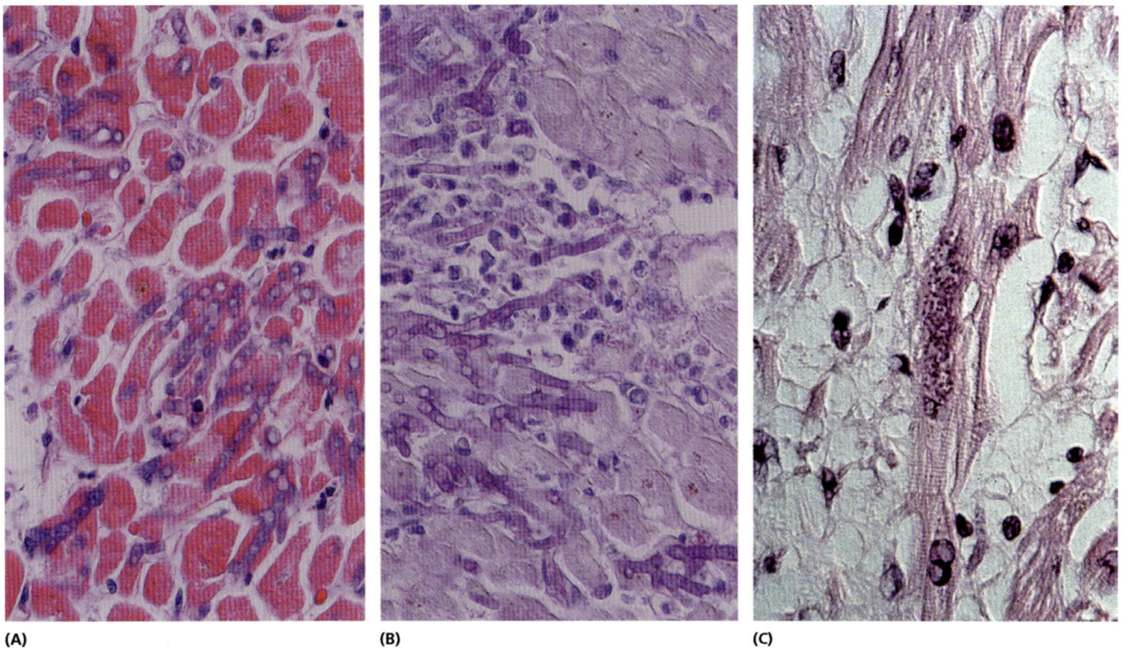

图 83.10　心内膜心肌活检中的检出物。(A，B)心肌内生长的曲霉菌菌丝(A，HE 染色，×400；B，PAS 染色，×400)。(C)该活检标本所示为一个肌细胞，表现为一个充满弓形虫缓殖子的肌质囊(HE 染色，×800)。

因此，当在心内膜心肌活检标本中发现脂肪组织时，病理学家应尽量判断这是心内膜下还是心外膜下的脂肪组织。有时这一判断较为简单，只需寻找间皮细胞层，后者是心外膜的标志(图 83.11B)。节细胞或神经的出现并不代表心脏穿孔。然而，移植后通常会出现纤维蛋白性心包炎，并最终演变成纤维性心包炎，可能会对寻找间皮细胞层造成困难。在后一种情况下，神经和节细胞的存在可能提示心外膜的位置，因为该类周围神经组织多见于心外膜。然而，在移植后几周，机化的心包炎通常会在心肌周围形成致密的保护层，能够防止心脏穿孔时心包压塞的发生。已有研究对非移植患者心内膜心肌活检标本中存在的脂肪组织进行了报道[76]与分类[77]。其中一项研究表明，有 4.62%的移植患者活检标本中存在脂肪组织[77]。在移植活检标本中发现，既往活检灶或可能的缺血性损伤修复病灶中也可存在脂肪沉积。目前尚未证实服用类固醇防治排斥反应会增加心内膜中的脂肪组织。

其他人为改变：收缩带。这是移植和非移植心脏活检中非常常见的人为改变。某些因素可导致活检标本中收缩带的产生(图 83.12A)。这可能是活检刀切割组织时损伤心肌所造成的，也可能由标本固定前或固定时的介质渗透压过低或固定剂介质温度过低(如 4℃或 22℃)引起。由于收缩带的检出率很高，收缩带本身不应作为诊断肌细胞坏死或缺血性损伤的唯一标准。

钳夹引起的人为改变：这提示操作不当引起的组织机械性扭曲(图 83.12B)。活检刀本身能够造成此类人为改变，尤其是当刀刃不够锋利时(活检刀反复利用的情况下)。在病理学实验室处理组织的过程中也可引起这类改变。在处理组织时应尽量小心，因为人为造成的组织变形可能增加解读活检标本的难度。

异物。有时在活检标本中可见移植时带入的异物，如凝胶海绵等。有时活检刀钳取的可能是留置导管片段或起搏器电极的塑料软外壳。

假性出血。在活检过程中，活检刀的匙状切割刀可阻挡红细胞，并通过活检刀对组织的压力将红细胞植入心肌内(图 83.12C)。这会人为形成血池，与出血相似。通常不伴有心肌炎症细胞浸润或病理改变，因此易与排斥反应相鉴别。

小动脉"望远镜样"改变或套叠。当活检刀采样的组织内有肌性小动脉时可出现这种现象。活检刀切割组织前，小动脉处于伸展状态；而切割时小动脉则卷缩入管腔内。因此，标本中的小动脉多表现为血管阻塞或小动脉血管病变。然而，当小动脉出现套叠时，可见标志性的弹性膜，因此这一点可用于其与血管病变的鉴别。细小动脉的这类改变较为罕见(图 83.12D)。

萎缩性钙化。据报道，移植后的心脏可出现多种形

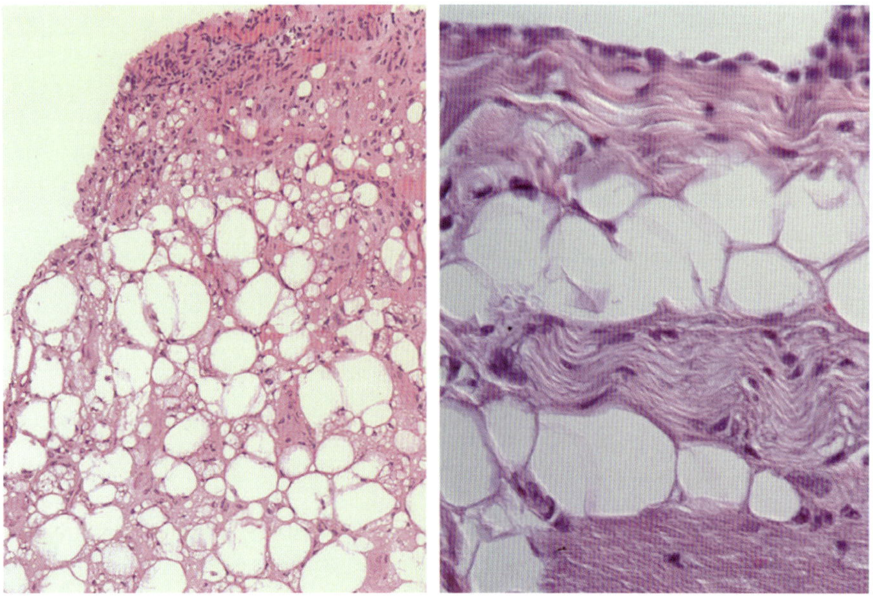

(A) (B)

图 83.11 心肌心内膜活检标本内的脂肪组织。(A)心肌心内膜活检显示大量脂肪组织与巨噬细胞(HE 染色，×100)。(B)活检标本中可见立方形间皮细胞(上方)及脂肪组织与神经纤维。上述改变明确提示心肌壁穿孔，且标本中还包括了间皮细胞及心外膜神经纤维等心外膜结构(HE 染色，×400)。

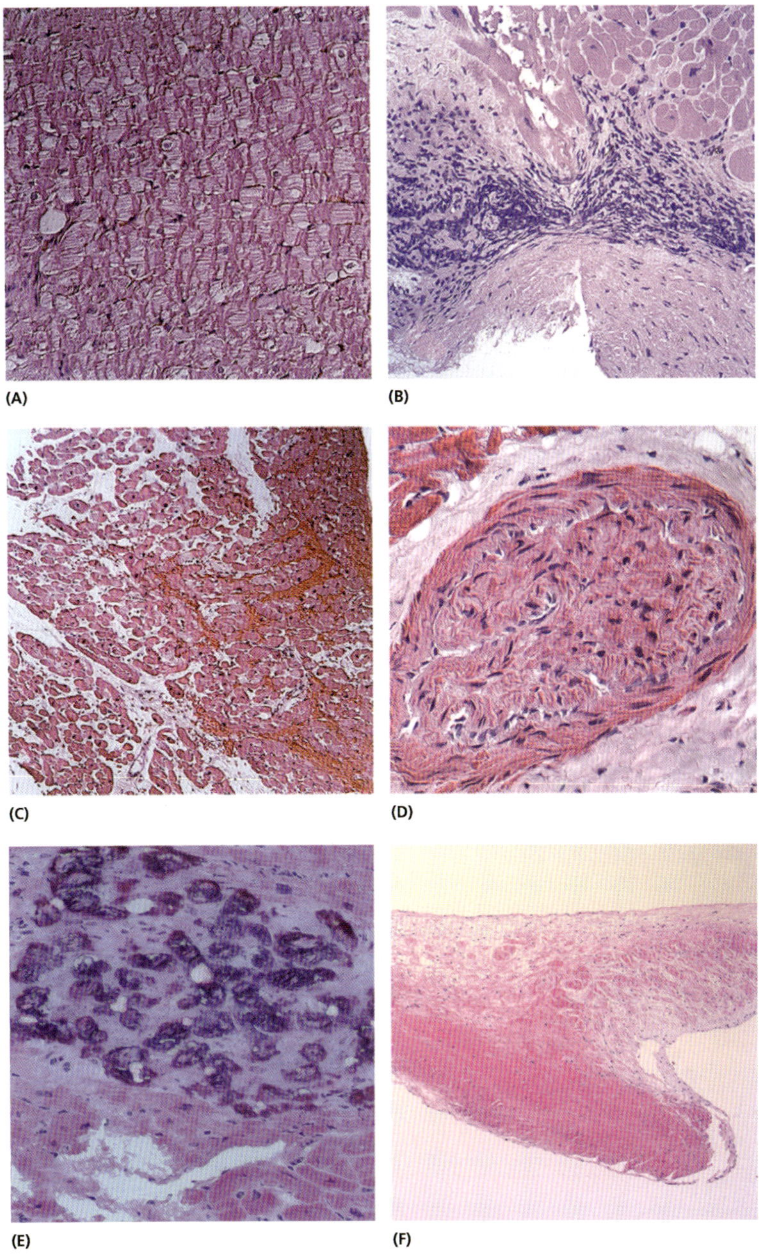

图 83.12　心内膜心肌活检的各种人为改变。(A)收缩带改变在心内膜心肌活检中较为常见(HE 染色，×100)。(B)活检时若用活检刀压迫组织而并非剪切组织，则可出现钳夹不当引起的组织扭曲。该图所示为心内膜 Quilty 病损的严重扭曲，可见 Quilty 病损灶中受挤压的淋巴细胞(HE 染色，×200)。(C)假性出血。活检刀可阻碍血液流动，并将血细胞压入心肌内，造成出血的假象(HE 染色，×100)。(D)有时活检刀可采到细小动脉和小动脉。在某些情况下，上述动脉可在活检标本切割过程中被过度牵拉，从而缩入自身管腔内，形成套叠或“望远镜样”改变。该现象不应被误认为移植器官血管病变(HE 染色，×400)。(E)有时可见整个肌细胞的萎缩性钙化(HE 染色，×300)。(F)由于许多三尖瓣隔瓣腱索直接嵌入室间隔，活检时可能切割到腱索组织(HE 染色，×20)。

式的钙化(图 83.12E)。部分患者的 X 线片显示原生心房[78,79]和活检组织[78]中都存在钙化的征象。根据笔者的经验，活检标本中心室部心肌的萎缩性钙化较为少见(图 83.7)。在文献报道中，钙化最常见于肌细胞，尤其是线粒体内。光镜下可见肌细胞内深蓝色颗粒状物质，即线粒体萎缩性钙化。上述颗粒直径为 1~2.5μm，可见于核周或沿肌节分布。大量颗粒可沿整个肌细胞轮廓分布。一些病例表明线粒体钙化可能与环孢素治疗存在关联[80]。与萎缩性钙化相关的因素包括脓毒症、一过性尿毒症、低镁血症、使用类固醇、酗酒[78]以及缺血性损伤。

腱索和瓣膜组织。活检标本中有时可见腱索片段(图 83.12F)[32]。应将这些组织与活检标本一同处理，并对其加以描述。腱索断裂引起的三尖瓣功能不全可有不同的临床表现[12,81]。

活检阴性移植器官功能不全。近年来，一些关于心脏移植的文献提出了活检阴性排斥反应或活检阴性移植器官功能不全的概念。这是指临床出现移植器官功能不全，但活检结果显示并无相应的细胞性排斥反应。因此，这些移植器官功能不全可能是由抗体介导的排斥反应引起的[82]。而在那些常规进行活检对细胞性和抗体介导的排斥反应进行评估的医学中心[83]，严格意义上的活检阴性移植器官功能不全通常是指由移植心脏血管病变引起的功能不全，而并非细胞性或抗体介导的排斥反应引起的。

抗体介导的排斥反应（体液性排斥免疫应答）

抗体介导的排斥反应(AMR)是供体特异性抗体与移植器官内的抗原相结合，引起补体系统激活从而造成移植器官损伤的免疫病理过程(详见第6章)。这类排斥反应作为一个明确的临床病理学概念，最早发现于肾脏移植患者中，表现为急性移植器官排斥反应，伴有抗供体的反应性抗体，预后差[84]。由于传统免疫抑制治疗是针对细胞免疫应答的，故AMR对传统免疫抑制治疗反应不良。有学者提出假说，即同种异体识别和抗体的合成可发生于任何器官移植，且其表现可由亚临床至临床显著的AMR[85]。以往心脏移植的文献中常提到血管性排斥反应、微血管性排斥反应及体液性排斥反应等术语应加以避免，以免引起歧义。AMR是目前公认的术语。多年来的观点认为，AMR出现在移植后早期(前3个月内)，而ISHLT-WF-1990也推荐仅需在移植术后6个月内通过活检标本免疫荧光试验监测AMR。这一观点显然是错误的，因为现在发现AMR主要发生于移植后数月甚至数年[83,86,87]。

AMR发生的危险因素包括妊娠、既往移植手术史、输血史、OKT3诱导治疗敏感、使用心室辅助装置、婴儿期同种移植史、流式细胞检测B细胞交叉配对阳性，以及群体反应性抗体升高[11,88,89]。目前心脏移植AMR的远期转归尚未被完全阐明，但研究表明移植心脏血管病变(CAV)可降低患者生存率[90,91]。

ISHLT-WF-1990并未对活检标本中所谓的“体液性排斥反应”加以详细的病理学分类(表83.3)。因此，AMR的发生原因尚未被阐明，对于AMR是一个独立概念的观点也未被广泛接受。在Banff移植器官病理学组敦促制定AMR的定义标准之前，在AMR方面并无可用于指导不同移植项目的统一诊断标准[13]，这样的状况持续了十余年。ISHLT-WF-2005中制定了AMR心内膜心肌活检评估标准，为全球范围内的心脏移植中心提供了指南(表83.3)。这套标准包括组织学和免疫病理学特征。指南建议，在活检中应对AMR的组织学特征(见下文“AMR的诊断标准”)加以辨认，并应促进免疫病理学检查的运用[11,14]。然而，ISHLT-WF-2005发布后不久就有研究表明AMR组织学标准的敏感性和特异性都偏低[92]。

在AMR的诊断方面，有许多抗体可用于免疫荧光试验，包括检测IgG、IgM、C3、C1q、纤维蛋白原、纤维蛋白及HLA-DR的抗体。但这些抗体的存在并不一定与血流动力学受损或CAV的发生有关，因此这项试验的有效性并不高[93]。此外，在AMR的诊断方面，最近一项来自北美的多中心调查研究显示，大量使用敏感性或特异性未经大样本队列研究评估的免疫病理学标志物可造成混乱状况的出现[94]。北美多家大规模心脏移植中心的研究表明，尽管在活检标本中能够检测到许多标志物，诸如免疫球蛋白和一些补体成分(C3、C3c、C1q)，由于其敏感性及特异性较低，这些标志物不适合作为AMR的诊断[86]和预后标志物[95,96]。

AMR的诊断标准。ISHLT-WF-2005中定义了AMR心内膜心肌活检的组织学特征，而其关于AMR的配套文章[11,14,32]也包括了内皮细胞肿胀、血管内巨噬细胞聚集等毛细血管损伤。间质水肿和出血可同时出现，并伴有毛细血管内及管周中性粒细胞浸润。有时也可见到血管内血栓和肌细胞坏死，但无细胞浸润[11,14]。

表83.3 抗体介导的排斥反应(AMR)[10,11,15]

ISHLT-WF-1990	ISHLT-WF-2005	ISHLT-WF-2011
体液性排斥反应	抗体介导的排斥反应	抗体介导的排斥反应
免疫荧光阳性，血管炎或严重水肿，无细胞浸润	AMR 0=无急性AMR	pAMR 0=无病理性AMR：组织学与免疫病理学试验均阴性
	AMR 1=AMR阳性	pAMR 1(H+)=仅有组织病理性AMR：组织学表现阳性，免疫病理学表现阴性
	AMR的组织学特征	pAMR 1(I+)=仅有免疫病理性AMR：免疫病理学表现阳性，组织学表现阴性
	AMR免疫荧光或免疫过氧化物酶染色阳性(CD68，C4d阳性)	pAMR 2=病理性AMR：组织学及免疫病理学表现均为阳性
		pAMR 3=严重的病理性AMR：罕见，伴间质出血、毛细血管破裂、混合性炎症、内皮细胞固缩、核碎裂及显著水肿等严重AMR的组织病理学表现

然而，组织学标准（光镜镜检表现，如内皮细胞肿胀、血管内巨噬细胞等）的敏感性很低，因此不适合用于 AMR 的筛查[92]。因此，笔者推荐在原标准的基础上增加免疫染色，以用于筛查 AMR。

ISHLT-AMR-WF-2011 中推荐对心内膜心肌活检标本进行免疫组化染色[15]：最新的指南推荐在对石蜡包埋的组织进行免疫组化检测（IHC）时，单独或合并使用 C4d 和 CD68（或其他适当的巨噬细胞标志物）。需注意的是，关于 AMR 标本中 CD68 表达情况的说明对于缺乏经验的病理学家可能存在难度，这是因为仅有血管内巨噬细胞才提示 AMR，而间质内巨噬细胞不应作为 AMR 的标志。

一些大型移植中心的研究表明，C4d 和 C3d 的免疫荧光检测结果与 AMR[83]存在很好的相关性（图83.13）。而许多大规模中心尚未进一步评估上述两个标志物在免疫组化检测中的运用情况[15]。

ISHLT-AMR-WF-2011 中提出，移植后 2 周内不应进行免疫染色，因为从理论上而言，围术期可能出现坏死的肌细胞和缺血性损伤，这可能会造成补体系统的激活，因此在移植术后早期，坏死肌细胞与补体可相结合[97]。然而，AMR 中毛细血管的染色表现与肌细胞坏死的肌质染色明显不同。因此在移植后早期，尤其是高度敏感的患者，不应进行免疫荧光检测。

最新指南中的分级系统 pAMR 0。无病理性 AMR：组织学与免疫病理学试验均为阴性。

pAMR 1（H+）。仅有组织病理性 AMR：组织学表现阳性，免疫病理学表现阴性。

pAMR 1（I+）。仅有免疫病理性 AMR：免疫病理学表现阳性，组织学表现阴性。

pAMR 2。病理性 AMR：组织学及免疫病理学表现均为阳性。

pAMR 3。严重的病理性 AMR：罕见，伴间质出血、毛细血管破裂、混合性炎症、内皮细胞固缩、核碎裂及显著水肿等严重 AMR 的组织病理学表现。

ISHLT-WF-2005 建议患者对抗 HLA Ⅰ或Ⅱ及非 HLA 供体抗原的循环抗体进行检测，而 ISHLT-WF-2011 并未对组织学或免疫病理学表现与供体特异性抗体或移植器官功能不全之间的相关性作出要求。若心内膜心肌活检未发现 AMR 的组织学或免疫病理学表现，则为 0 级（pAMR 0）。若活检免疫荧光或免疫组化染色结果符合 AMR 的组织学特征，则为阳性（pAMR 2）。若仅存在组织学或免疫病理学改变中的任一项，则为 pAMR 1 H+或 I+。需注意的是，严重的病理性 AMR 或 pAMR 3 在目前的临床工作中极其罕见。上述病理分级所对应的准确临床表现有待进一步研究确定。

混合性急性细胞性排斥反应与 AMR。尽管大部分 AMR 不与急性细胞性排斥反应同时出现，或至多伴有轻度急性细胞性排斥，然而据报道混合性排斥反应的死亡率很高[98,99]。混合性排斥反应可出现在移植的早期或晚期[100]，且可引起移植器官功能不全。

AMR 诊断的实际问题。一些有关 AMR 诊断的观点认为有必要对补体裂解产物进行检测。近十年来，免疫荧光在 AMR 检测方面得到了很大的发展。一些补体成分，特别是 C3d 和 C4d，比抗体更易检出，且具有诸多优点，因而成了心内膜心肌活检检测排斥反应非常敏感的标志物[101]。各种抗体与抗原结合的亲和力各不相同，并通过以不同速率解离或以脱落或内化的形式被消除。与之相对应，补体系统的激活能够产生 C4 和 C3 的裂解产物，后者能与补体激活处的组织相结合。这能够通过延长补体半衰期来提高补体检测的敏感性。血清中浓度最高的补体成分是 C3，其次是 C4，因此其裂解产物在组织中的含量也是最高的（图 83.14）[32]。此外，补体系统的级联放大机制也产生更多的 C3 裂解产物[102]。

尽管补体系统可通过经典途径由抗体激活，仍必须牢记体外循环等术中操作[104,104]、缺血再灌注损伤及移植前抗胸腺细胞球蛋白诱导疗法[97]等也能够激活补体系统。因此，仅仅在毛细血管内检测到 C4d 或 C3d 并不等同于 AMR。

根据笔者的经验，仅采用 C4d 免疫染色并不可靠。要评估 AMR 的心内膜心肌活检，应同时进行 C4d 和 C3d 的免疫染色[83,86]，因为两者同时存在与移植器官功能不全及供体特异性抗体升高有很高的相关性。

病理结果与临床表现的矛盾。通过 C4d 和（或）C3d 免疫染色检测到补体系统级联激活并不一定伴有移植器官功能不全。一些学者在动物模型[105]和 ABO 血型不合的肾脏移植病例[106]中将这种存在补体激活而缺乏移植器官损伤的现象称为“适应”。一个可能的原因是宿主中的补体激活过程被一些保护机制所干扰阻断。这提示除非补体级联激活形成了攻膜复合物（MAC），否则就不会出现移植器官损伤。攻膜复合物能

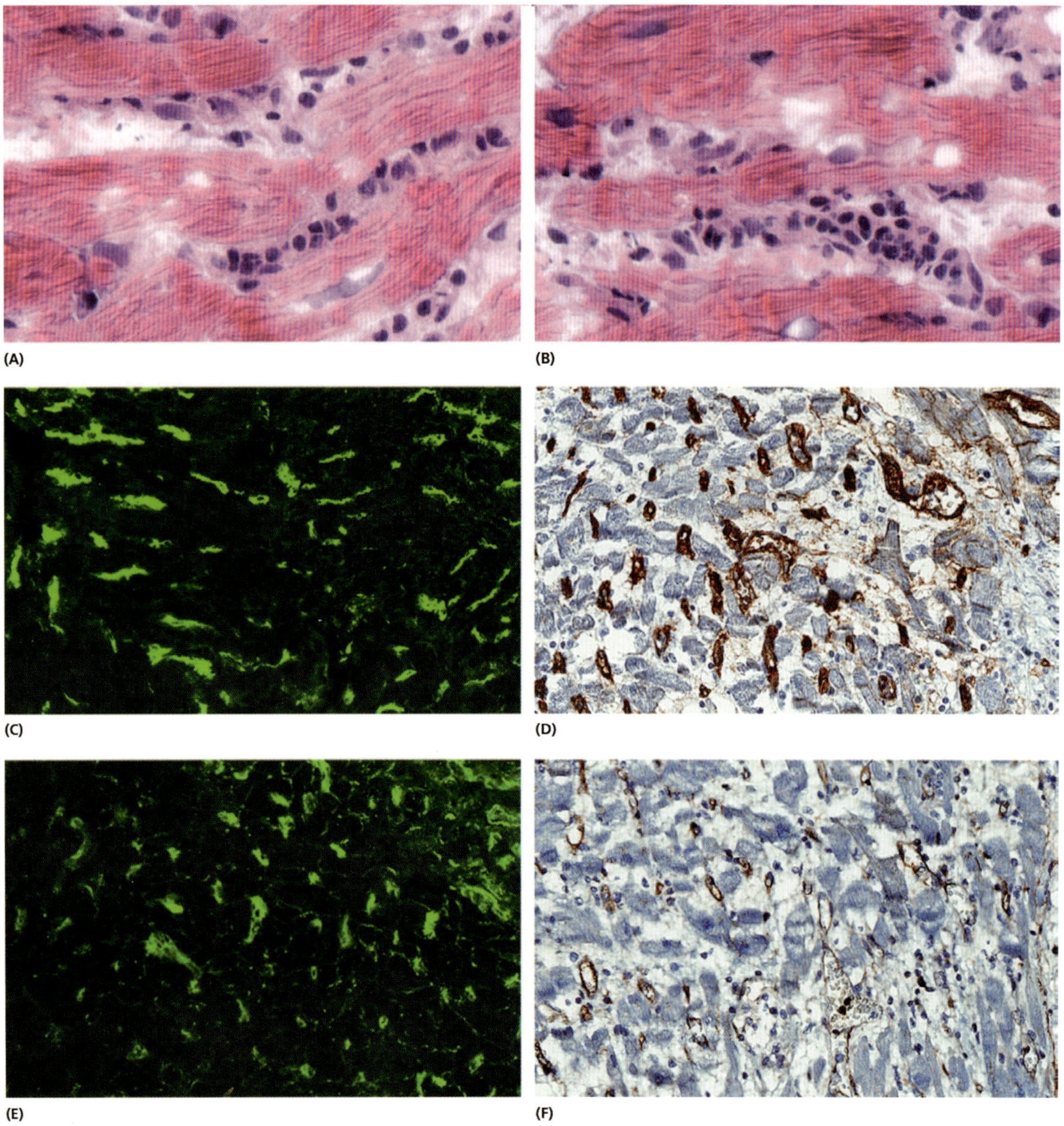

图 83.13 抗体介导的排斥反应。(A)该活检所示为内皮细胞肿胀与少量血管内巨噬细胞(HE 染色,×600)。(B)该视野内可见一细小动脉存在明显的血管内巨噬细胞聚集(HE 染色,×600)。(C)用免疫荧光染色检测心内膜心肌活检冰冻标本内的 C4d,显示 C4d 沿毛细血管致密沉积(C4d 免疫荧光,×300)。(D)检测福尔马林固定的活检标本内的 C4d。该图所示的 C4d 沉积形式(沿毛细血管排列)与免疫荧光的表现相同(C4d 免疫组化,×300)。(E,F)这两个活检标本中 C3d 表现为相同的毛细血管染色线性排列形式。(E)C3d 免疫荧光(×300)。(F)C3d 免疫组化(×300)。

够在细胞膜上形成小孔,从而使细胞膜的完整性受损。众所周知,人体中存在补体激活调节物(RCA),能够在补体激活的各个阶段阻止补体级联反应的进行。

补体激活的调控。不论补体系统通过经典途径、替代途径或甘露糖结合凝集素途径激活,RCA 都能在补体级联激活的各个阶段发挥作用。上述途径在形成酶复合物,即 C3 转化酶时汇合,并依次激活形成 MAC 所需的其余补体成分。调控补体激活的蛋白主要分为两类:膜结合性和可溶性。人类中的膜结合性调节物为 CD35 或补体受体 1 (CR1)、CD46 或膜共因子蛋白(MCP)、CD55 或促衰变因子 (DAF)、CD59 或保护素(protectin),以及 C8 结合蛋白或同源性限制因子(C8bp/HRF)[107,108]。可溶性因子包括 C1 抑制剂、C4 结合蛋白(C4bp)、I 因子、H 因子、丛生因子,以及 S 蛋白(玻连蛋白)。上述蛋白的作用点详见图 83.14[32]。

关于 RCA 在人类心脏移植中表达情况的研究很

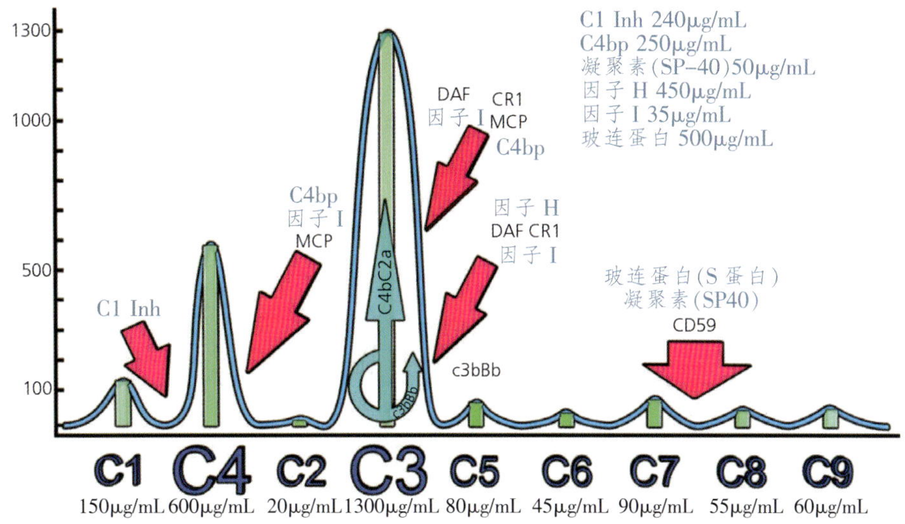

图 83.14 各类补体以及补体的拮抗剂的血清浓度。如图所示，不同补体成分在血清中的浓度单位是 μg/mL。C3 的激活尤为重要，因为它可以促进细胞和体液性免疫反应。经典途径的 C4b2a 和旁路途径的 C3bBb 正反馈途径可以介导 C3 补体的分裂和活化。C3 的活化需要通过显著的扩大效应，因为 C3 分子在体内的存量相当巨大，一旦激活，可以通过级联反应迅速增加活化程度。补体激活过程的拮抗剂主要有血清蛋白(蓝色字体)和膜蛋白(黑色字体)，可以抑制 C3 激活的经典途径和旁路途径，从而阻止补体结合膜攻击复合物。C1 Inh，C1 抑制剂；C4bp，C4 结合蛋白；CR1，补体受体 1；DAE，衰变加速因子；MCP，膜辅助因子。

少。近期的一项研究表明，DAF 或 CD55 在心脏移植患者的心肌内存在局部表达[109]，其中对心内膜心肌活检中存在补体沉积的患者进行了研究。活检标本通过免疫荧光染色检测 C4d、C3d 和 DAF 的表达。根据是否存在移植器官功能不全将患者分为两个亚组。所有患者的活检标本都被证实存在 C4d 和 C3d 沉积。治疗反应性良好且出现 AMR 消退的患者，移植心脏内皮组织中存在 CD55 高表达。而转归不良的患者则在组织中低表达 CD55。因此，即便毛细血管内存在 C4d 和 C3d 沉积，DAF 局部低表达的患者不易出现移植器官功能不全(图 83.15)。

补体染色的人为改变。移植器官活检免疫荧光染色显微镜检的常见人为改变包括脂褐质自发荧光及与间质胶原和动脉内弹力层的非特异性结合。相似地，坏死的肌细胞也可与补体结合。

排斥反应中的血小板和凝血因子。抗体和补体与炎症细胞结合，可对移植器官的血管内皮细胞和平滑肌细胞造成损伤[110]。众所周知，IgG 受体或补体裂解产物可刺激并活化巨噬细胞，而这两者的共同刺激存在协同作用。因此，抗体和补体能有效激活内皮细胞、血小板和巨噬细胞[110]。

同种异体抗体能够诱导内皮细胞外分泌血管假性血友病因子和 P-选择素，在数分钟内诱导血小板黏附。因此，血小板也能黏附并刺激白细胞，而补体激活能够增强这一效应。黏附后的血小板发生脱颗粒，并释放预先合成并储存于颗粒中的介质，如血小板因子 4 和 CXCL4[111]。这一效应也可参与 CAV 的发生(详见下文中 CAV 部分)。

溶栓因子与凝血因子也与移植器官排斥反应及 CAV 密切相关。研究发现，人类心脏移植早期组织因子和纤维蛋白水平升高，而组织型纤溶酶原激活物(tPA)和抗凝血酶水平下降，这与 CAV 的发病、严重程度及移植器官衰竭存在相关性，这一发现有力支持了高凝状态在 CAV 中的作用。按照预期，纤溶系统受损也与 CAV 相关[112]。

移植心脏血管病变

移植器官血管病变是影响心脏移植长期转归的最主要因素[32]。CAV 的临床表现详见第 79 章。CAV 并非心脏移植所特有，在任何实体器官移植后都可出现[113]。实际上，随着时间的推移，所有的移植器官都会发生移植器官血管疾病(又称慢性排斥反应、移植器官动脉硬化加速，或移植冠状动脉疾病)。一些患者可能在数月内就出现 CAV，而也有患者可能在数年后才出现。引起该血管病变的原因很复杂，包括：供体自身动

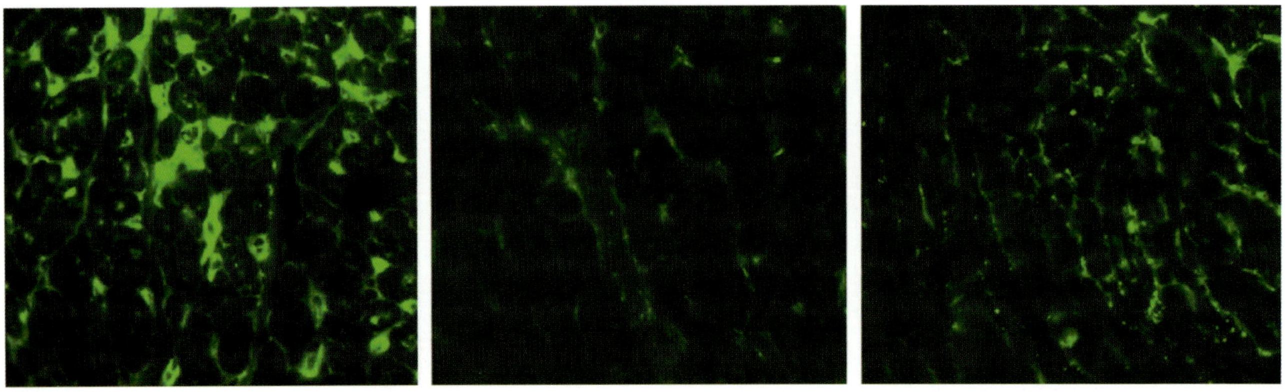

(A) (B) (C)

图 83.15 仅有 C4d 阳性并不能说明存在抗体介导的排斥反应。(A)该活检标本显示毛细血管内存在明显的致密线性 C4d 免疫荧光(C4d 免疫荧光,×400)。(B)C3d 染色阴性,毛细血管无染色(C3d 免疫荧光,×400)。(C)该显微照片显示毛细血管及肌细胞内存在促衰变因子(CD55)(CD55 免疫荧光,×400)。CD55 的出现可阻断活化型 C4 向活化型 C3 的进程,阻止补体级联系统的激活,从而避免了攻膜复合物的激活。

脉粥样硬化[114]、移植器官缺血时间[115]、各种原因引起的内皮损伤[116,117]、组织相容性[118]、动脉炎[119]、慢性体液性与细胞性免疫攻击[120-123]、纤溶[124,125]、病毒感染[126]、血清脂质[127],以及激素[128]。儿童人群中也存在该血管病变,且与成人的病程类似[129,130]。

CAV 可累及心外膜及心壁冠状动脉[32]。为了更好地理解其发病机制,需了解冠状动脉的结构分为外膜、中膜和内膜三层。每一层都包含许多不同的细胞和细胞外成分。研究表明,在血管病变的发展过程中,会发生一系列变化,对血管的各结构(内膜、中膜、外膜及营养血管)造成损伤。

大体检查可见排斥反应区的心肌呈浅棕色或红色,因而易于辨认。检查心外膜冠状动脉可发现,一些部位存在局部偏心性病损,另一些部位则出现管壁向心性增厚(图 83.16)。然而,有时即便肉眼观察不到心外膜冠状动脉血管病变,心肌内血管也可能存在大量病理改变。仔细检查心室切面往往能发现增厚的动脉壁(直径为 0.2~0.5mm),并伴有大量管周纤维化。这些血管在大体检查中十分明显(图 83.16A~C)。在部分移植器官中可见到明显的心外膜冠状动脉硬化,且供体在移植前就已出现上述病变(图 83.16D~G)[32,114,131]。在这种情况下,移植器官在动脉粥样硬化的基础上又叠加了移植器官血管病变。若事先存在动脉粥样硬化斑块,则病变形态可呈偏心性,且具有粥样斑块的特征,如内弹性膜破坏、无定形脂质斑块及胆固醇结晶。心外膜冠状动脉的长期损伤可最终与传统的动脉粥样硬化具有相似的外观,两者难以区分。

光镜观察下,心外膜血管病变引起的损伤形态与中膜或小动脉存在细微差别[32,132]。若不存在动脉粥样硬化斑块,典型的血管病变损伤表现为内膜内平滑肌细胞及低分化细胞(肌纤维母细胞或称"肌内膜"细胞)向心性增殖(图 83.17)。病灶内存在胶原及蛋白聚糖等结缔组织成分的沉积。心壁冠状动脉通常表现为由增殖的内膜平滑肌细胞组成的均质向心性病损,伴或不伴增殖细胞内脂蛋白沉积。内弹性膜多保持完整性,或仅有局部结构紊乱;中膜无或仅有少量脂蛋白沉积;外膜常可出现袖套样纤维组织,伴或不伴单个核细胞炎症浸润。儿童 CAV 也具有基本相同的病理表现[133]。

部分患者存在明显的血管炎(图 83.18)[120]。这主要影响远端冠状动脉。活动性血管炎可出现淋巴细胞、浆细胞,有时也可出现多形核白细胞。病变早期可有纤维素性坏死。血管栓塞后再通表明伴血栓形成的血管炎痊愈(图 83.19)。虽然在心内膜心肌活检标本中可见小动脉或细小动脉的血管病变,但与心外膜冠状动脉的解剖结构或功能状态无明确相关性[134]。尽管如此,若在活检标本中发现血管病变,仍需在病理报告中加以记录。

移植后复发疾病

一部分移植后的心脏会反复出现一些病变,包括感染[73]和淀粉样变[135]。第 79 章对这一部分做了详细的

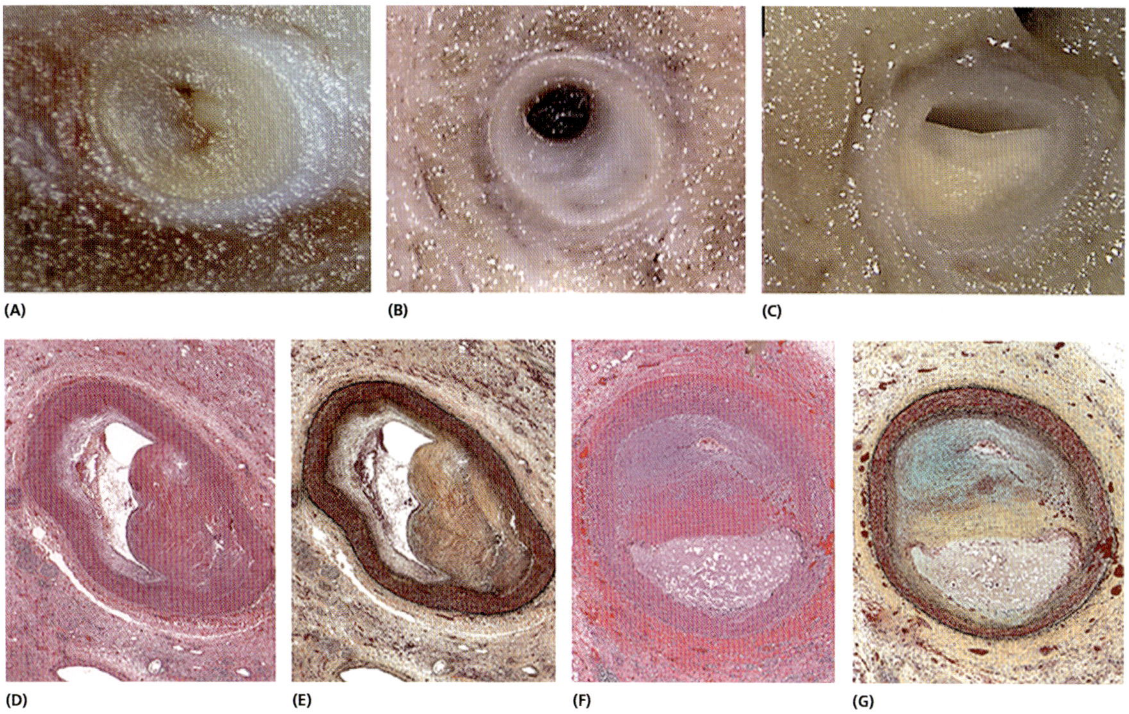

图 83.16　移植心脏血管病变(CAV)Ⅰ。(A)心外膜冠状动脉显示由内膜增殖引起的典型的管腔向心性狭窄。(B)偏心性病损也很常见。注意内膜中珍珠白色的黏液样基质。(C)若供体存在冠状动脉粥样硬化，则 CAV 病损(珍珠白色)往往叠加于粥样斑块(黄色)之上。(D)偏心斑块镜检示血管右半部内膜增殖(HE 染色，×10)。(E)该病例的内膜增殖由成熟的纤维组织构成(黄色)。内弹性膜(黑色)和中膜(深红色)均完整(Movat 五色染色，×10)。(F)光镜图显示同时存在粥样斑块(下半部)与叠加的 CAV，造成管腔近乎完全阻塞(HE 染色，×10)。(G)与上图为同一条动脉，经 Movat 五色染色可见粥样斑、纤维帽(黄色)及 CAV 引起的新生内膜增殖，细胞外基质中富含蛋白聚糖(绿色)(Movat 五色染色，×10)。

介绍。许多心脏移植病例是由于铁过载，而持续存在引起铁过载的因素可能引起移植器官铁过载复发[137]。尽管处于免疫抑制状态[140]，仍偶有巨细胞性心肌炎[138,139]和结节病[141,142]的复发病例。移植前应用胺碘酮可引起移植心脏 QT 间期延长[143]。曾有学者报道凝血酶原 G20210A 单核苷酸多态性纯合子患者复发血栓性并发症[144]，以及马方综合征患者于心脏移植后复发主动脉夹层的病例[145]，介绍了遗传性全身疾病的复发。以往有病例报道过伴有主动脉吻合口处巨大假性动脉瘤的白塞病患者在移植术后并发血管病变[146]。对于难以切除的原发性心脏肉瘤患者是否应进行心脏移植仍存在争议，因为存在局部复发和转移的风险。例如，据报道，原发性心脏肉瘤可在原生右心房[147]和左肺动脉[148]出现局部复发。此外，也有关于年轻患者复发性 EB 病毒相关性平滑肌肉瘤的报道[149]。

移植器官衰竭的检查

大体检查。可在再次移植时或尸检时进行。这两者提供的标本有所不同。再次移植过程中的标本包括心室、心房、主动脉、肺动脉的一小部分，有时也含有既往吻合口。应在报告中对这些内容进行相应的描述。下面以尸检为例介绍笔者目前采用的心脏检查方法。应根据死亡时间判断组织适用于细胞培养或核酸提取。大部分尸检标本可用于 DNA 提取，但 RNA 则在死亡后迅速降解。

心包与心脏、胸骨及纵隔胸膜之间常有致密的纤维粘连，因此解剖员在取样时应尽量避免切断上述组织。这只需多花几分钟仔细分离。应先检查心脏和纵隔的原始结构，再分离和切断下列血管：

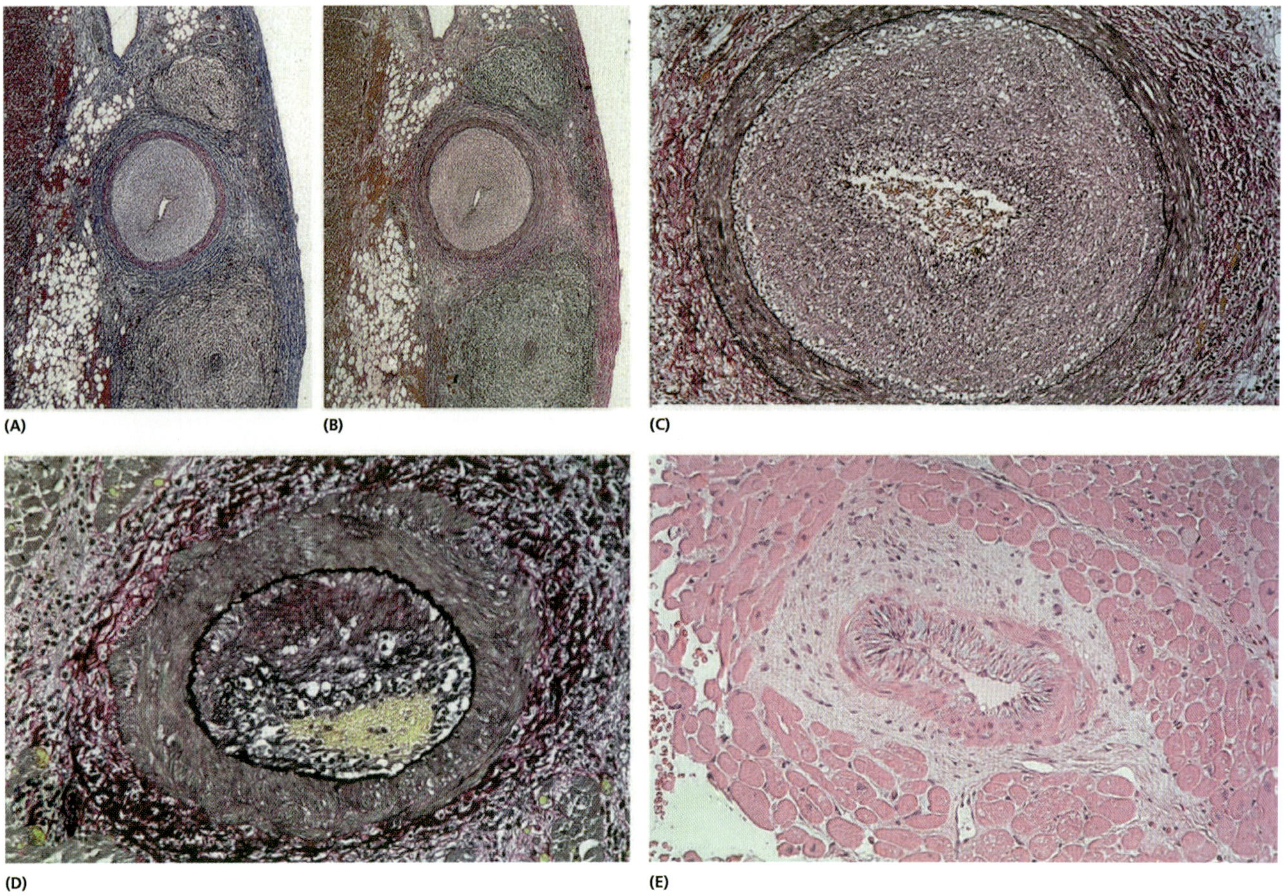

图 83.17 移植心脏血管病变Ⅱ。(A)光镜图显示心外膜冠状动脉内膜细胞增殖及结缔组织沉积(红色-蓝色),造成管腔明显狭窄。外膜因纤维化而呈蓝色。中膜平滑肌及心肌(左侧)呈红色。该冠状动脉两侧分别有一个巨大的淋巴细胞浸润灶(Masson 三色染色,×1.25)。(B)与上图相邻切面所示的中膜和内膜之间的境界更为清楚(中膜呈深红色,内膜呈浅粉色)(Verhoeff-Van Gieson 弹性纤维染色,×1.25)。(C)高倍镜下的内膜、中膜与外膜。内膜细胞增殖明显,管腔近乎完全性狭窄。注意弹性膜完整(Verhoeff-Van Gieson 弹性纤维染色,×4)。(D)图示一条心脏内小冠状动脉存在内膜离心性病损,造成管腔部分性阻塞(>60%)。动脉管腔下部存在小栓子,并捕获了红细胞(黄色细胞)(Verhoeff-Van Gieson 弹性纤维染色,×10)。(E)心脏内小冠状动脉显示内膜早期增殖性病变及大量蛋白聚糖聚集(内皮细胞旁色泽改变,呈浅蓝色)。注意外膜大量纤维化(HE 染色,× 20)。

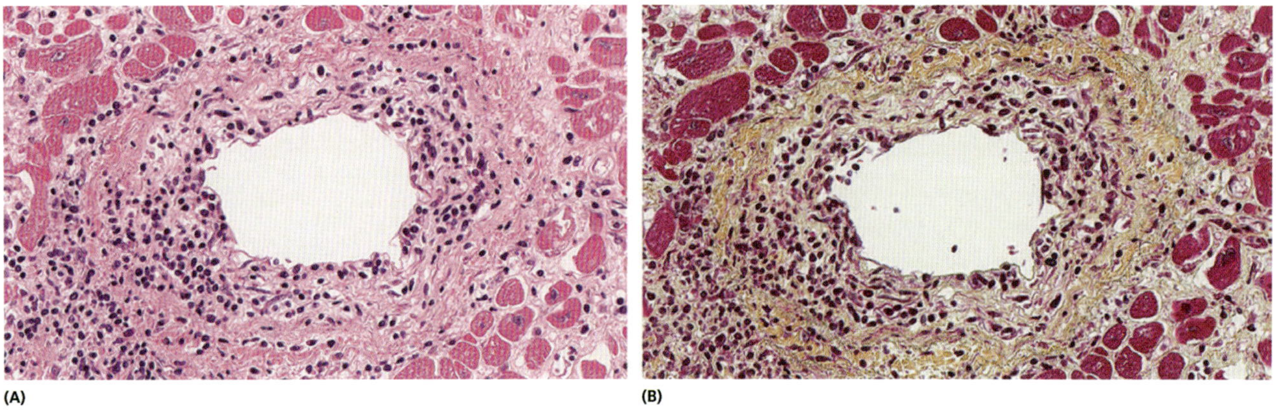

图 83.18 伴有明显血管炎的移植器官血管病变。有时,细胞性排斥反应可显著影响动脉各层。(A)可见单个核细胞透壁性浸润(偶有嗜酸性粒细胞),累及心壁冠状动脉外膜、中膜及内膜(HE 染色,×40)。(B)与上图为同一动脉,可见中膜因炎性浸润而结构紊乱。由于结缔组织呈黄色,故外膜纤维化尤其醒目(Movat 五色染色,×40)。

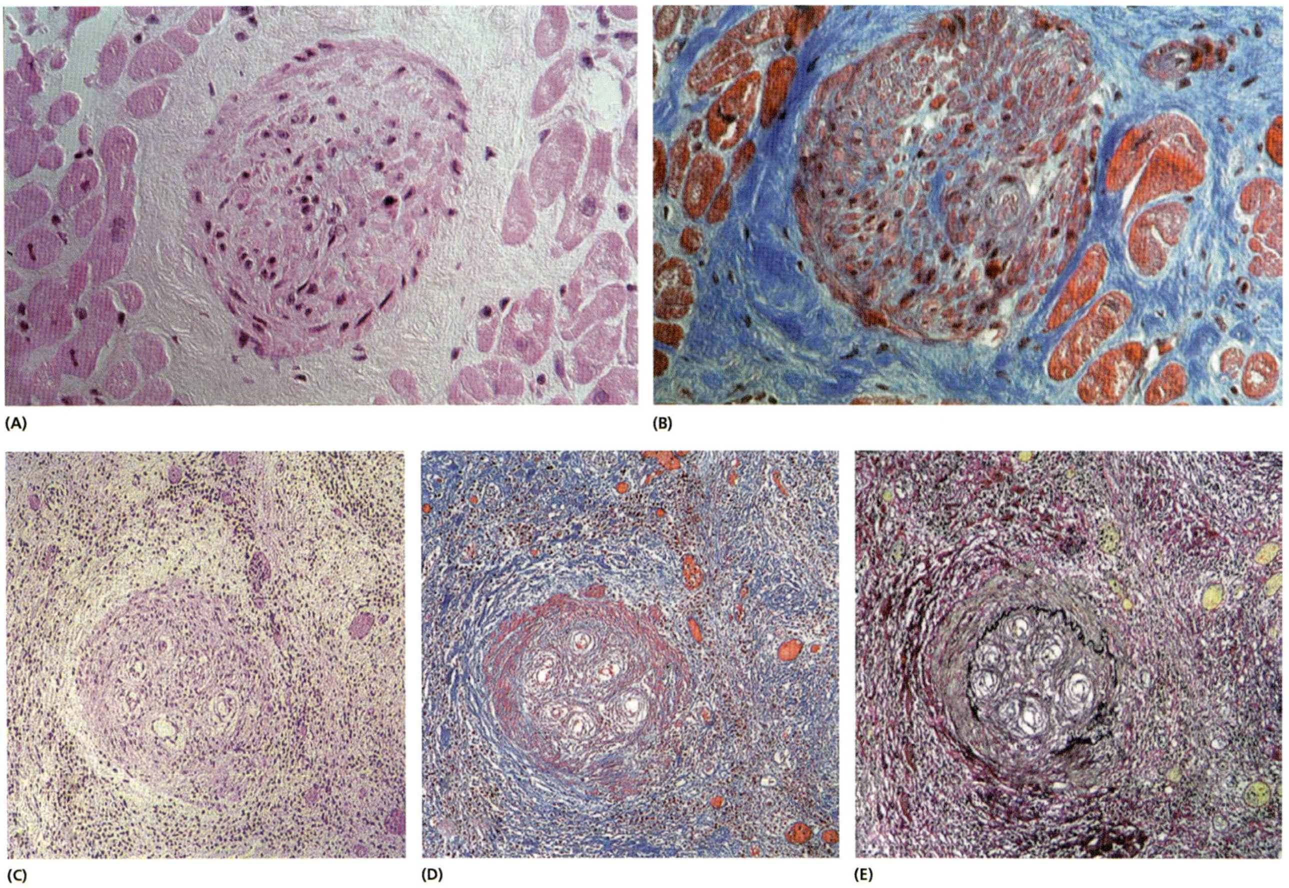

图 83.19　心壁冠状动脉的移植器官血管病变。(A)心壁小冠状动脉的平滑肌细胞增殖引起血管阻塞。注意外膜纤维化(HE 染色，×40)。(B)该染色证实管腔狭窄主要是由于平滑肌增殖(红色细胞)和少量胶原聚集。也可明确观察到外膜纤维化(Masson 三色染色，×40)。(C)心壁冠状动脉的再通可能是由于伴血栓形成的血管炎痊愈(HE 染色，×20)。(D)与上图为同一条动脉，可见显著的外膜和管腔内纤维组织聚集(Masson 三色染色，×20)。(E)弹性纤维染色可见弹性膜碎片，提示既往血管炎(Verhoeff-Van Gieson 弹性纤维染色，×20)。

1.至少在颈外静脉水平以上切断上腔静脉；

2.至少在颈总动脉及双侧锁骨水平以上切断主动脉弓分支；

3.在靠近膈肌处横断主动脉胸段；

4.在左右肺动脉入肺处切断其叶支；

5.在肺静脉出肺叶处将其切断；

6.在膈肌处切断下腔静脉并尽可能靠近肝脏。

若心脏内存在导管或起搏器电极，每个电极都可以固定于其相应进入心脏时的血管（缝合固定更佳），并在必要时切下。这样解剖员就不会改变上述装置在心脏内的位置。或者解剖员可以在分离和切断所有血管时将其结扎。这样可以保持工作区域的清洁，尤其当尸检同意书仅限于手术切口或心脏时，能保证成功获取心脏。

切断上述大血管后，即可取回心脏。去除血管结扎线，然后将标本置于 10%缓冲福尔马林中过夜，注意容器应比标本体积大 10 倍以上(12L 的水桶最佳)。次日早晨继续进行解剖。壁层心包与脏层心包(心外膜)之间可见不同程度的粘连(图 83.20)。从前壁开始向心尖进行钝性分离，然后向两侧心室分离，最后分离心脏膈面。这样能将心室和部分心房周围的心包囊游离。然后分离大血管和原生心房。一旦确定吻合口的位置，解剖上述结构通常与解剖正常心脏并无差别。不同病例中切开心脏的方法可有不同。

为了观察到预期中的病理变化，可能需要通过传统的“血流”途径切开心脏。或者也可采用四腔切面甚至横切面(图 83.20)。笔者所在的实验室常采用四腔切面观，因为这样便于快速而彻底地检查各个心腔、瓣膜、房间隔、室间隔以及吻合口缝合线。此外，这样还易于获得高质量的照片，便于记录及教学。需注意心内膜

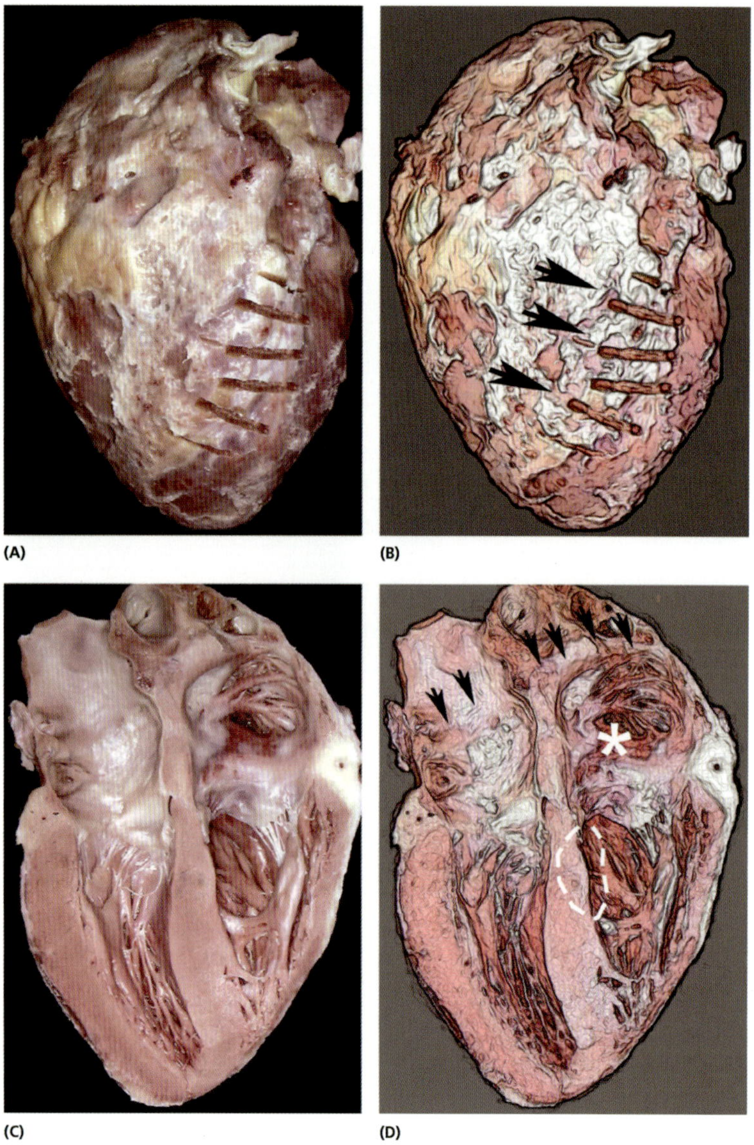

图 83.20 移植器官衰竭。(A,B)一名 16 岁的患者于心脏移植术后 15 个月猝死，尸检显示纤维机化性心包炎。对冠状动脉进一步采样(箭头)。(C,D)四腔切面观示心房吻合口已完全内皮化。由于供体与受体的心房相吻合，故可见心房明显增大。心内膜局部增厚(白色斑片)，代表既往右心室(虚线)小梁活检灶。供体右心房(星号)处可见瘀斑。左心室轻度肥厚。

色泽改变、血栓形成、赘生物或纤维蛋白沉积等情况。记录任何导管或起搏器电极的位置。检查吻合口（近期、愈合的、内皮化的)是否存在扭结或狭窄。描述心肌切面的色泽改变(局部、弥漫性、大小、位置)、出血或瘢痕(血管周围、心内膜下、透壁)。记录既往室间隔活检或附壁血栓形成引起的心内膜瘢痕。检查瓣膜完整性，以及是否存在感染、纤维化或腱索断裂。然后可详细检查心室，必要时可做横切面。当临床病史、冠状动脉检查或心室切面提示缺血性疾病时，我们倾向于行心室横切。这样可展示坏死区域、出血或再灌注损伤的情况。冠状动脉和任何旁路血管都应密集切片，检查有无狭窄、血栓栓塞及钙化。

病理学家有时会面临一些特殊的手术操作，需要在尸检时调整解剖方式。比如，若要检查双心室辅助装置植入患者的胸腔，则需扩大原位解剖范围，且需调整心脏大体检查的方法，以便于病理变化的展示、相关研究的开展以及标本的保存。在这种情况下，很有必要延长心脏原位观察的时间。为取出心脏和相连装置，应制订相应的解剖方式。一旦取得心脏，通常即可对其进行彻底的检查。我们发现，在获取心脏后至少有效固定 18~24 小时，并由此开始将检查过程分为不同阶段，这一点非常实用。用照片记录解剖的各个阶段。有时在解剖过程中会有特殊的发现，应在拍摄高质量的照片后再继续解剖。大多数学术中心都具备高质量的数字图库，因此不必耗费过多时间用于拍照。

总结

组织病理学诊断对心脏移植受体的合理治疗至关重要。事实上,移植器官损伤早期临床表现的缺乏及其后果的严重性说明没有哪个器官移植的术后治疗如此依赖于病理学。因此,活检规范的说明是所有医学中心移植后治疗的重要组成部分。活检是连接病理机制与临床表现的桥梁与纽带，其相关研究有助于深入了解影响移植转归的生物学因素，也有助于指导临床医生根据患者的具体情况进行免疫抑制治疗方案的决策。

(赵海格 倪一鸣 郑骏楠 译 倪一鸣 校)

参考文献

1. Stehlik J, Edwards LB, Kucheryavaya AY, et al. The Registry of the International Society for Heart and Lung Transplantation: twenty-eighth adult heart transplant report, 2011. Journal of Heart and Lung Transplantation. 2011;30:1078–1094.
2. Kirk R, Edwards LB, Kucheryavaya AY, et al. The Registry of the International Society for Heart and Lung Transplantation: fourteenth pediatric heart transplantation report, 2011. Journal of Heart and Lung Transplantation. 2011;30:1095–1103.
3. Zerbe TR, Arena V. Diagnostic reliability of endomyocardial biopsy for assessment of cardiac allograft rejection. Human Pathology. 1988;19:1307–1314.
4. Wagner K, Oliver MC, Boyle GJ, et al. Endomyocardial biopsy in pediatric heart transplant recipients: a useful exercise? (Analysis of 1169 biopsies). Pediatric Transplantation. 2000;4:186–192.
5. Mehra MR, Uber PA, Uber WE, et al. Anything but a biopsy: noninvasive monitoring for cardiac allograft rejection. Current Opinion in Cardiology. 2002;17:131–136.
6. Balzer D, Moorhead S, Saffitz JE, et al. Pediatric endomyocardial biopsy performed solely with echocardiographic guidance. Journal of the American Society of Echocardiography. 1993;6:510–515.
7. Pomerance A, Stovin PG. Heart transplant pathology: the British experience. Journal of Clinical Pathology. 1985;38:146–159.
8. Spiegelhalter DJ, Stovin PG. An analysis of repeated biopsies following cardiac transplantation. Statistics in Medicine. 1983;2:33–40.
9. Sharples LD, Cary NR, Large SR, et al. Error rates with which endomyocardial biopsy specimens are graded for rejection after cardiac transplantation. American Journal of Cardiology. 1992;70:527–530.
10. Billingham ME, Cary NR, Hammond ME, et al. A working formulation for the standardization of nomenclature in the diagnosis of heart and lung rejection: Heart Rejection Study Group. The International Society for Heart Transplantation. Journal of Heart Transplantation. 1990;9:587–593.
11. Stewart S, Winters GL, Fishbein MC, et al. Revision of the 1990 working formulation for the standardization of nomenclature in the diagnosis of heart rejection. Journal of Heart and Lung Transplantation. 2005;24:1710–1720.
12. Wiklund L, Suurkula MB, Kjellstrom C, et al. Chordal tissue in endomyocardial biopsies. Scandinavian Journal of Thoracic and Cardiovascular Surgery. 1994;28:13–18.
13. Rodriguez ER, International Society for Heart and Lung Transplantation. The pathology of heart transplant biopsy specimens: revisiting the 1990 ISHLT working formulation. Journal of Heart and Lung Transplantation. 2003;22:3–15.
14. Reed EF, Demetris AJ, Hammond E, et al. Acute antibody-mediated rejection of cardiac transplants. Journal of Heart and Lung Transplantation. 2006;25:153–159.
15. Berry GJ, Angelini A, Burke MM, et al. The ISHLT working formulation for pathologic diagnosis of antibody-mediated rejection in heart transplantation: evolution and current status (2005–2011). Journal of Heart and Lung Transplantation. 2011;30:601–611.
16. Rose AG, Cooper DK, Human PA, et al. Histopathology of hyperacute rejection of the heart: experimental and clinical observations in allografts and xenografts. Journal of Heart and Lung Transplantation. 1991;10:223–234.
17. Schuurman HJ, Gmelig Meyling FH, Wijngaard PL, et al. Lymphocyte status in endomyocardial biopsies and blood after heart transplantation. Journal of Pathology. 1989;159:197–203.
18. van Besouw NM, Balk AH, Mochtar B, et al. Phenotypic analysis of lymphocytes infiltrating human cardiac allografts during acute rejection and the development of graft vascular disease. Transplant International. 1996;9(Suppl 1):S234–S236.
19. Higuchi ML, de Assis RV, Sambiase NV, et al. Usefulness of T-cell phenotype characterization in endomyocardial biopsy fragments from human cardiac allografts. Journal of Heart and Lung Transplantation. 1991;10:235–242.
20. Ibrahim S, Dawson DV, Van Trigt P, et al. Differential infiltration by CD45RO and CD45RA subsets of T cells associated with human heart allograft rejection. American Journal of Pathology. 1993;142:1794–1803.
21. Mues B, Brisse B, Steinhoff G, et al. Diagnostic assessment of macrophage phenotypes in cardiac transplant biopsies. European Heart Journal. 1991;12(Suppl D):32–35.
22. Hoshinaga K, Mohanakumar T, Goldman MH, et al. Clinical significance of in situ detection of T lymphocyte subsets and monocyte/macrophage lineages in heart allografts. Transplantation. 1984;38(6):634–637.
23. Gassel AM, Hansmann ML, Radzun HJ, et al. Human cardiac allograft rejection: correlation of grading with expression of different monocyte/macrophage markers. American Journal of Clinical Pathology. 1990;94:274–279.
24. Sorrentino C, Scarinci A, D'Antuono T, et al. Endomyocardial infiltration by B and NK cells foreshadows the recurrence of cardiac allograft rejection. Journal of Pathology. 2006;209:400–410.
25. Takahashi H, Ruiz P, Ricordi C, et al. Quantitative in situ analysis of FoxP3+ T regulatory cells on transplant tissue using laser scanning cytometry. Cell Transplantation. 2012;21:113–125.
26. Fyfe B, Loh E, Winters GL, et al. Heart transplantation-associated perioperative ischemic myocardial injury: morphological features and clinical significance. Circulation. 1996;93:1133–1140.
27. Pickering JG, Boughner DR. Fibrosis in the transplanted heart and its relation to donor ischemic time: assessment with polarized light microscopy and digital image analysis. Circulation. 1990;81:949–958.
28. Meckel CR, Wilson JE, Sears TD, et al. Myocardial fibrosis in endomyocardial biopsy specimens: do different bioptomes affect estimation? American Journal of Cardiovascular Pathology. 1989;2:309–313.
29. Kottke-Marchant K, Ratliff NB. Endomyocardial lymphocytic infiltrates in cardiac transplant recipients. Incidence and characterization. Archives of Pathology and Laboratory Medicine. 1989;113:690–698.
30. Joshi A, Masek MA, Brown BW Jr, et al. "Quilty" revisited: a 10-year perspective. Human Pathology. 1995;26:547–557.
31. Luthringer DJ, Yamashita JT, Czer LS, et al. Nature and significance of epicardial lymphoid infiltrates in cardiac allografts. Journal of Heart and Lung Transplantation. 1995;14:537–543.
32. Tan CD, Baldwin WM 3rd, Rodriguez ER. Update on cardiac transplantation pathology. Archives of Pathology and Laboratory Medicine. 2007;131:1169–1191.
33. Suit PF, Kottke-Marchant K, Ratliff NB, et al. Comparison of whole-blood cyclosporine levels and the frequency of endomyocardial lymphocytic infiltrates (the Quilty lesion) in cardiac transplantation. Transplantation. 1989;48:618–621.
34. Nakhleh RE, Copenhaver CM, Werdin K, et al. Lack of evidence for involvement of Epstein–Barr virus in the development of the "Quilty" lesion of transplanted hearts: an in situ hybridization study. Journal of Heart and Lung Transplantation. 1991;10:504–507.
35. Freimark D, Czer LS, Aleksic I, et al. Pathogenesis of Quilty lesion in cardiac allografts: relationship to reduced endocardial cyclosporine A. Journal of Heart and Lung Transplantation. 1995;14:1197–1203.
36. Barone JH, Fishbein MC, Czer LS, et al. Absence of endocardial lymphoid infiltrates (Quilty lesions) in nonheart transplant recipients treated with cyclosporine. Journal of Heart and Lung Transplantation. 1997;16:600–603.
37. Marboe CC, Billingham M, Eisen H, et al. Nodular endocardial infiltrates (Quilty lesions) cause significant variability in diagnosis of ISHLT Grade 2 and 3A rejection in cardiac allograft recipients. Journal of Heart and Lung Transplantation. 2005;24(7 Suppl):S219–S226.
38. Gao SZ, Chaparro SV, Perlroth M, et al. Post-transplantation lymphoproliferative disease in heart and heart-lung transplant recipients: 30-year experience at Stanford University. Journal of Heart and Lung Transplantation. 2003;22:505–514.
39. Eisen HJ, Hicks D, Kant JA, et al. Diagnosis of posttransplantation lymphoproliferative disorder by endomyocardial biopsy in a cardiac allograft recipient. Journal of Heart and Lung Transplantation. 1994;13:241–245.
40. Hanasono MM, Kamel OW, Chang PP, et al. Detection of Epstein–Barr virus in

cardiac biopsies of heart transplant patients with lymphoproliferative disorders. Transplantation. 1995;60:471–473.
41. Schwend M, Tiemann M, Kreipe HH, et al. Rapidly growing Epstein-Barr virus-associated pulmonary lymphoma after heart transplantation. European Respiratory Journal. 1994;7:612–616.
42. Montone KT, Friedman H, Hodinka RL, et al. In situ hybridization for Epstein–Barr virus NotI repeats in posttransplant lymphoproliferative disorder. Modern Pathology. 1992;5:292–302.
43. Lager DJ, Burgart LJ, Slagel DD. Epstein–Barr virus detection in sequential biopsies from patients with a posttransplant lymphoproliferative disorder. Modern Pathology. 1993;6:42–47.
44. Ohta H, Fukushima N, Ozono K. Pediatric post-transplant lymphoproliferative disorder after cardiac transplantation. International Journal of Hematology. 2009;90:127–136.
45. Hanto DW, Birkenbach M, Frizzera G, et al. Confirmation of the heterogeneity of posttransplant Epstein–Barr virus-associated B cell proliferations by immunoglobulin gene rearrangement analyses. Transplantation. 1989;47:458–464.
46. Kemnitz J, Cremer J, Gebel M, et al. T-cell lymphoma after heart transplantation. American Journal of Clinical Pathology. 1990;94:95–101.
47. Chucrallah AE, Crow MK, Rice LE, et al. Multiple myeloma after cardiac transplantation: an unusual form of posttransplant lymphoproliferative disorder. Human Pathology. 1994;25:541–545.
48. Kemnitz J, Cohnert T, Schafers HJ, et al. A classification of cardiac allograft rejection: a modification of the classification by Billingham. American Journal of Surgical Pathology. 1987;11:503–515.
49. Myles JL, Ratliff NB, McMahon JT, et al. Reversibility of myocyte injury in moderate and severe acute rejection in cyclosporine-treated cardiac transplant patients. Archives of Pathology and Laboratory Medicine. 1987;111:947–952.
50. Hammond EH, Yowell RL. Ultrastructural findings in cardiac transplant recipients. Ultrastructural Pathology. 1994;18:213–220.
51. Hook S, Caple JF, McMahon JT, et al. Comparison of myocardial cell injury in acute cellular rejection versus acute vascular rejection in cyclosporine-treated heart transplants. Journal of Heart and Lung Transplantation. 1995;14: 351–358.
52. McMahon JT, Ratliff NB. Regeneration of adult human myocardium after acute heart transplant rejection. Journal of Heart Transplantation. 1990;9: 554–567.
53. Foerster A, Simonsen S, Froysaker T. Heart transplantation in Norway. Morphological monitoring of cardiac allograft rejection: a 3-year follow-up. APMIS: Acta Pathologica, Microbiologica, et Immunologica Scandinavica. 1988;96:14–24.
54. Sibley RK, Olivari MT, Ring WS, et al. Endomyocardial biopsy in the cardiac allograft recipient: a review of 570 biopsies. Annals of Surgery. 1986;203: 177–187.
55. Haddad F, Deuse T, Pham M, et al. Changing trends in infectious disease in heart transplantation. Journal of Heart and Lung Transplantation. 2010;29:306–315.
56. Miller LW, Naftel DC, Bourge RC, et al. Infection after heart transplantation: a multiinstitutional study. Cardiac Transplant Research Database Group. Journal of Heart and Lung Transplantation. 1994;13:381–392, discussion 393.
57. Smart FW, Naftel DC, Costanzo MR, et al. Risk factors for early, cumulative, and fatal infections after heart transplantation: a multiinstitutional study. Journal of Heart and Lung Transplantation. 1996;15:329–341.
58. Arbustini E, Grasso M, Diegoli M, et al. Histopathologic and molecular profile of human cytomegalovirus infections in patients with heart transplants. American Journal of Clinical Pathology. 1992;98:205–213.
59. Holliman R, Johnson J, Savva D, et al. Diagnosis of toxoplasma infection in cardiac transplant recipients using the polymerase chain reaction. Journal of Clinical Pathology. 1992;45:931–932.
60. Wagner FM, Reichenspurner H, Uberfuhr P, et al. Toxoplasmosis after heart transplantation: diagnosis by endomyocardial biopsy. Journal of Heart and Lung Transplantation. 1994;13:916–918.
61. Drescher J, Wagner D, Haverich A, et al. Nosocomial hepatitis B virus infections in cardiac transplant recipients transmitted during transvenous endomyocardial biopsy. Journal of Hospital Infection. 1994;26:81–92.
62. Fishman JA, Rubin RH, Koziel MJ, et al. Hepatitis C virus and organ transplantation. Transplantation. 1996;62:147–154.
63. Breinholt JP, Moulik M, Dreyer WJ, et al. Viral epidemiologic shift in inflammatory heart disease: the increasing involvement of parvovirus B19 in the myocardium of pediatric cardiac transplant patients. Journal of Heart and Lung Transplantation2010;29:739–746.
64. Peters M, Schurmann D, Mayr AC, et al. Immunosuppression and mycobacteria other than Mycobacterium tuberculosis: results from patients with and without HIV infection. Epidemiology and Infection. 1989;103:293–300.
65. Patel R, Roberts GD, Keating MR, et al. Infections due to nontuberculous mycobacteria in kidney, heart, and liver transplant recipients. Clinical Infectious Diseases. 1994;19:263–273.
66. LeMense GP, VanBakel AB, Crumbley AJ 3rd, et al. Mycobacterium scrofulaceum infection presenting as lung nodules in a heart transplant recipient. Chest. 1994;106:1918–1920.
67. Morio F, Treilhaud M, Lepelletier D, et al. Aspergillus fumigatus endocarditis of the mitral valve in a heart transplant recipient: a case report. Diagnostic Microbiology and Infectious Disease. 2008;62:453–456.
68. Zaoutis TE, Webber S, Naftel DC, et al. Invasive fungal infections in pediatric heart transplant recipients: incidence, risk factors, and outcomes. Pediatric Transplantation. 2011;15:465–469.
69. Almyroudis NG, Sutton DA, Linden P, et al. Zygomycosis in solid organ transplant recipients in a tertiary transplant center and review of the literature. American Journal of Transplantation. 2006;6:2365–2374.
70. Montoya JG, Giraldo LF, Efron B, et al. Infectious complications among 620 consecutive heart transplant patients at Stanford University Medical Center. Clinical Infectious Diseases. 2001;33:629–640.
71. Hermanns B, Brunn A, Schwarz ER, et al. Fulminant toxoplasmosis in a heart transplant recipient. Pathology, Research and Practice. 2001;197:211–215.
72. Golino A, Duncan JM, Zeluff B, et al. Leishmaniasis in a heart transplant patient. Journal of Heart and Lung Transplantation. 1992;11:820–823.
73. Fiorelli AI, Santos RH, Oliveira JL Jr, et al. Heart transplantation in 107 cases of Chagas' disease. Transplantation Proceedings. 2011;43:220–224.
74. Deen JL, Blumberg DA. Infectious disease considerations in pediatric organ transplantation. Seminars in Pediatric Surgery. 1993;2:218–234.
75. Braunlin EA, Canter CE, Olivari MT, et al. Rejection and infection after pediatric cardiac transplantation. Annals of Thoracic Surgery. 1990;49:385–390.
76. Cladellas M, Abadal ML, Ballester M, et al. Endomyocardial diagnosis of cardiac lipomatosis. Catheterization and Cardiovascular Diagnosis. 1987;13:269–270.
77. Bonacina E, Recalcati F, Mangiavacchi M, et al. Interstitial myocardial lipomatosis: a morphological study on endomyocardial biopsies and diseased hearts surgically removed for heart transplantation. European Heart Journal. 1989;10(Suppl D):100–102.
78. Cohnert TR, Kemnitz J, Haverich A, et al. Myocardial calcification after orthotopic heart transplantation. Journal of Heart Transplantation. 1988;7:304–308.
79. Florence SH, Hutton LC, McKenzie FN, et al. Cardiac transplantation: postoperative chest radiographs. Canadian Association of Radiologists Journal. 1988;39: 115–117.
80. Millane T, Wilson AJ, Patel MK, et al. Mitochondrial calcium deposition in association with cyclosporine therapy and myocardial magnesium depletion: a serial histologic study in heart transplant recipients. Journal of Heart and Lung Transplantation. 1994;13:473–480.
81. Yankah AC, Musci M, Weng Y, et al. Tricuspid valve dysfunction and surgery after orthotopic cardiac transplantation. European Journal of Cardio-Thoracic Surgery. 2000;17:343–348.
82. Fishbein MC, Kobashigawa J. Biopsy-negative cardiac transplant rejection: etiology, diagnosis, and therapy. Current Opinion in Cardiology. 2004;19:166–169.
83. Tan CD, Sokos GG, Pidwell DJ, et al. Correlation of donor-specific antibodies, complement and its regulators with graft dysfunction in cardiac antibody-mediated rejection. American Journal of Transplantation. 2009;9:2075–2084.
84. Racusen LC, Colvin RB, Solez K, et al. Antibody-mediated rejection criteria: an addition to the Banff 97 classification of renal allograft rejection. American Journal of Transplantation. 2003;3:708–714.
85. Takemoto SK, Zeevi A, Feng S, et al. National conference to assess antibody-mediated rejection in solid organ transplantation. American Journal of Transplantation. 2004;4:1033–1041.
86. Rodriguez ER, Skojec DV, Tan CD, et al. Antibody-mediated rejection in human cardiac allografts: evaluation of immunoglobulins and complement activation products C4d and C3d as markers. American Journal of Transplantation. 2005;5:2778–2785.
87. Tan CD, Rodriguez ER. Diagnosis of antibody-mediated rejection in cardiac transplantation: a call for standardization. Current Opinion in Organ Transplantation. 2010;15:769–773.
88. Hammond EH, Wittwer CT, Greenwood J, et al. Relationship of OKT3 sensitization and vascular rejection in cardiac transplant patients receiving OKT3 rejection prophylaxis. Transplantation. 1990;50:776–782.
89. Bishay ES, Cook DJ, Starling RC, et al. The clinical significance of flow cytometry crossmatching in heart transplantation. European Journal of Cardio-Thoracic Surgery. 2000;17:362–369.
90. Michaels PJ, Espejo ML, Kobashigawa J, et al. Humoral rejection in cardiac transplantation: risk factors, hemodynamic consequences and relationship to transplant coronary artery disease. Journal of Heart and Lung Transplantation. 2003;22:58–69.
91. Taylor DO, Yowell RL, Kfoury AG, et al. Allograft coronary artery disease: clinical correlations with circulating anti-HLA antibodies and the immunohistopathologic pattern of vascular rejection. Journal of Heart and Lung Transplantation. 2000;19:518–521.

92. Hammond ME, Stehlik J, Snow G, et al. Utility of histologic parameters in screening for antibody-mediated rejection of the cardiac allograft: a study of 3,170 biopsies. Journal of Heart and Lung Transplantation. 2005;24: 2015–2021.
93. Bonnaud EN, Lewis NP, Masek MA, et al. Reliability and usefulness of immunofluorescence in heart transplantation. Journal of Heart and Lung Transplantation. 1995;14:163–171.
94. Kucirka LM, Maleszewski JJ, Segev DL, et al. Survey of North American pathologist practices regarding antibody-mediated rejection in cardiac transplant biopsies. Cardiovascular Pathology. 2011;20:132–138.
95. Revelo MP, Stehlik J, Miller D, et al. Antibody testing for cardiac antibody-mediated rejection: which panel correlates best with cardiovascular death? Journal of Heart and Lung Transplantation. 2011;30:144–150.
96. Rodriguez ER, Tan CD. Pathologic evaluation for antibody-mediated rejection: prognostic vs diagnostic markers? Journal of Heart and Lung Transplantation. 2011;30:136–138.
97. Baldwin WM 3rd, Samaniego-Picota M, Kasper EK, et al. Complement deposition in early cardiac transplant biopsies is associated with ischemic injury and subsequent rejection episodes. Transplantation. 1999;68:894–900.
98. Hammond EH, Yowell RL, Nunoda S, et al. Vascular (humoral) rejection in heart transplantation: pathologic observations and clinical implications. Journal of Heart Transplantation. 1989;8:430–443.
99. Lones MA, Czer LS, Trento A, et al. Clinical-pathologic features of humoral rejection in cardiac allografts: a study in 81 consecutive patients. Journal of Heart and Lung Transplantation. 1995;14:151–162.
100. Loupy A, Cazes A, Guillemain R, et al. Very late heart transplant rejection is associated with microvascular injury, complement deposition and progression to cardiac allograft vasculopathy. American Journal of Transplantation. 2011;11:1478–1487.
101. Baldwin WM, Ota H, Rodriguez ER. Complement in transplant rejection: diagnostic and mechanistic considerations. Springer Seminars in Immunopathology. 2003;25:181–197.
102. Baldwin WM 3rd, Kasper EK, Zachary AA, et al. Beyond C4d: other complement-related diagnostic approaches to antibody-mediated rejection. American Journal of Transplantation. 2004;4:311–318.
103. Mollnes TE. Complement and biocompatibility. Vox Sanguinis. 1998;74(Suppl 2):303–307.
104. Mollnes TE. Biocompatibility: complement as mediator of tissue damage and as indicator of incompatibility. Experimental and Clinical Immunogenetics. 1997;14:24–29.
105. Williams JM, Holzknecht ZE, Plummer TB, et al. Acute vascular rejection and accommodation: divergent outcomes of the humoral response to organ transplantation. Transplantation. 2004;78:1471–1478.
106. Haas M, Rahman MH, Racusen LC, et al. C4d and C3d staining in biopsies of ABO- and HLA-incompatible renal allografts: correlation with histologic findings. American Journal of Transplantation. 2006;6:1829–1840.
107. Kirschfink M. Targeting complement in therapy. Immunological Reviews. 2001;180:177–189.
108. Kim DD, Song WC. Membrane complement regulatory proteins. Clinical Immunology (Orlando, Fla.). 2006;118:127–136.
109. Gonzalez-Stawinski GV, Tan CD, Smedira NG, et al. Decay-accelerating factor expression may provide immunoprotection against antibody-mediated cardiac allograft rejection. Journal of Heart and Lung Transplantation. 2008;27: 357–361.
110. Wehner J, Morrell CN, Reynolds T, et al. Antibody and complement in transplant vasculopathy. Circulation Research. 2007;100:191–203.
111. Kuo HH, Morrell CN, Baldwin WM 3rd. Alloantibody induced platelet responses in transplants: Potent mediators in small packages. Human Immunology. 2012;73:1233–1238.
112. Labarrere CA, Woods JR, Hardin JW, et al. Early prediction of cardiac allograft vasculopathy and heart transplant failure. American Journal of Transplantation. 2011;11:528–535.
113. Libby P, Pober JS. Chronic rejection. Immunity. 2001;14:387–397.
114. Tuzcu EM, Hobbs RE, Rincon G, et al. Occult and frequent transmission of atherosclerotic coronary disease with cardiac transplantation: insights from intravascular ultrasound. Circulation. 1995;91:1706–1713.
115. Gaudin PB, Rayburn BK, Hutchins GM, et al. Peritransplant injury to the myocardium associated with the development of accelerated arteriosclerosis in heart transplant recipients. American Journal of Surgical Pathology. 1994;18: 338–346.
116. Koskinen P, Lemstrom K, Bruggeman C, et al. Acute cytomegalovirus infection induces a subendothelial inflammation (endothelialitis) in the allograft vascular wall: a possible linkage with enhanced allograft arteriosclerosis. American Journal of Pathology. 1994;144:41–50.
117. Hosenpud JD, Morris TE, Shipley GD, et al. Cardiac allograft vasculopathy: preferential regulation of endothelial cell-derived mesenchymal growth factors in response to a donor-specific cell-mediated allogeneic response. Transplantation. 1996;61:939–948.
118. Petrossian GA, Nichols AB, Marboe CC, et al. Relation between survival and development of coronary artery disease and anti-HLA antibodies after cardiac transplantation. Circulation. 1989;80:III122–III125.
119. Smith SH, Kirklin JK, Geer JC, et al. Arteritis in cardiac rejection after transplantation. American Journal of Cardiology. 1987;59:1171–1173.
120. Foerster A. Vascular rejection in cardiac transplantation: a morphological study of 25 human cardiac allografts. APMIS: Acta Pathologica, Microbiologica, et Immunologica Scandinavica. 1992;100:367–376.
121. Hengstenberg C, Hufnagel G, Haverich A, et al. De novo expression of MHC class I and class II antigens on endomyocardial biopsies from patients with inflammatory heart disease and rejection following heart transplantation. European Heart Journal. 1993;14:758–763.
122. Hosenpud JD, Everett JP, Morris TE, et al. Cardiac allograft vasculopathy: association with cell-mediated but not humoral alloimmunity to donor-specific vascular endothelium. Circulation. 1995;92:205–211.
123. Duquesnoy RJ, Kaufman C, Zerbe TR, et al. Presence of CD4, CD8 double-negative and T-cell receptor-gamma-delta-positive T cells in lymphocyte cultures propagated from coronary arteries from heart transplant patients with graft coronary disease. Journal of Heart and Lung Transplantation. 1992;11:S83–S86.
124. Faulk WP, Labarrere CA, Nelson DR, et al. Coronary artery disease in cardiac allografts: association with arterial antithrombin. Transplantation Proceedings. 1995;27:1944–1946.
125. Labarrere CA, Pitts D, Nelson DR, et al. Coronary artery disease in cardiac allografts: association with depleted arteriolar tissue plasminogen activator. Transplantation Proceedings. 1995;27:1941–1943.
126. Koskinen PK. The association of the induction of vascular cell adhesion molecule-1 with cytomegalovirus antigenemia in human heart allografts. Transplantation. 1993;56:1103–1108.
127. Dong C, Redenbach D, Wood S, et al. The pathogenesis of cardiac allograft vasculopathy. Current Opinion in Cardiology. 1996;11:183–190.
128. Herrington DM, Nanjee N, Achuff SC, et al. Dehydroepiandrosterone and cardiac allograft vasculopathy. Journal of Heart and Lung Transplantation. 1996;15: 88–93.
129. Denfield SW. Cardiac transplant coronary allograft vasculopathy in children: Achilles' heel. Congenital Heart Disease. 2012;7:301.
130. Jeewa A, Dreyer WJ, Kearney DL, et al. The presentation and diagnosis of coronary allograft vasculopathy in pediatric heart transplant recipients. Congenital Heart Disease. 2012;7:302–311.
131. Billingham ME. Histopathology of graft coronary disease. Journal of Heart and Lung Transplantation. 1992;11:S38–S44.
132. Pucci AM, Forbes RD, Billingham ME. Pathologic features in long-term cardiac allografts. Journal of Heart Transplantation. 1990;9:339–345.
133. Berry GJ, Rizeq MN, Weiss LM, et al. Graft coronary disease in pediatric heart and combined heart-lung transplant recipients: a study of fifteen cases. Journal of Heart and Lung Transplantation. 1993;12:S309–S319.
134. Clausell N, Butany J, Molossi S, et al. Abnormalities in intramyocardial arteries detected in cardiac transplant biopsy specimens and lack of correlation with abnormal intracoronary ultrasound or endothelial dysfunction in large epicardial coronary arteries. Journal of the American College of Cardiology. 1995;26: 110–119.
135. Luk A, Ahn E, Lee A, et al. Recurrent cardiac amyloidosis following previous heart transplantation. Cardiovascular Pathology. 2010;19:e129–e133.
136. Caines AE, Kpodonu J, Massad MG, et al. Cardiac transplantation in patients with iron overload cardiomyopathy. Journal of Heart and Lung Transplantation. 2005;24:486–488.
137. Kuppahally SS, Hunt SA, Valantine HA, et al. Recurrence of iron deposition in the cardiac allograft in a patient with non-HFE hemochromatosis. Journal of Heart and Lung Transplantation. 2006;25:144–147.
138. Scott RL, Ratliff NB, Starling RC, et al. Recurrence of giant cell myocarditis in cardiac allograft. Journal of Heart and Lung Transplantation. 2001;20: 375–380.
139. Chung L, Berry GJ, Chakravarty EF. Giant cell myocarditis: a rare cardiovascular manifestation in a patient with systemic lupus erythematosus. Lupus. 2005;14: 166–169.
140. Kong G, Madden B, Spyrou N, et al. Response of recurrent giant cell myocarditis in a transplanted heart to intensive immunosuppression. European Heart Journal. 1991;12:554–557.
141. Strecker T, Zimmermann I, Wiest GH. Pulmonales und kardiales Rezidiv einer Sarkoidose nach Herztransplantation [Pulmonary and cardiac recurrence of sarcoidosis in a heart transplant recipient]. Deutsche Medizinische Wochenschrift. 2007;132:1159–1162.
142. Luk A, Lee A, Ahn E, et al. Cardiac sarcoidosis: recurrent disease in a heart

transplant patient following pulmonary tuberculosis infection. Canadian Journal of Cardiology. 2010;26:e273–e275.

143. Schwarz ER, Czer LS, Simsir SA, et al. Amiodarone-induced QT prolongation in a newly transplanted heart associated with recurrent ventricular fibrillation. Cardiovascular Journal of Africa. 2010;21:109–112.

144. Miriuka SG, Langman LJ, Evrovski J, et al. Thromboembolism in heart transplantation: role of prothrombin G20210A and factor V Leiden. Transplantation. 2005;80:590–594.

145. Mullen JC, Lemermeyer G, Bentley MJ. Recurrent aortic dissection after orthotopic heart transplantation. Annals of Thoracic Surgery. 1996;62:1830–1831.

146. Hollander SA, Yasnovsky JR, Reinhartz O, et al. Behcet's disease and heart transplantation: a word of caution. Journal of Heart and Lung Transplantation. 2010;29:1306–1308.

147. Akhter SA, McGinty J, Konys JJ, et al. Recurrent primary cardiac malignant fibrous histiocytoma following orthotopic heart transplantation. Journal of Heart and Lung Transplantation. 2004;23:1447–1450.

148. Myruski KS, Manecke GR Jr, Kotzur A, et al. Late recurrence of cardiac sarcoma presenting as giant pulmonary artery aneurysm. Journal of Heart and Lung Transplantation. 2004;23:1445–1446.

149. Bonatti H, Hoefer D, Rogatsch H, et al. Successful management of recurrent Epstein–Barr virus-associated multilocular leiomyosarcoma after cardiac transplantation. Transplantation Proceedings. 2005;37:1839–1844.

第 84 章 肺移植排斥反应和复发疾病的组织病理学综合征

Carol Farver, W. Dean Wallace

引言

肺移植排斥反应是临床上一常见的、严重的问题。与其他器官相比，肺移植急性细胞性排斥反应的发生率相当高。移植后第一年发病率为 36%[1,2]~55%[3]，而心脏和肾脏移植的发病率则为 40%[4]和 11%[5]。这些发作很少是致命的，但其对肺部的累积影响将会导致血管甚至气道的慢性排斥反应，最终导致移植失败。关于肺移植排斥反应的临床表现和鉴别诊断的详细资料详见第 72 章和第 80 章。

因排斥相关的移植物损伤有持续进展的可能，故常规监测肺移植受体急性排斥反应的临床和病理标志。支气管镜活检是用来评估移植急性排斥反应的主要诊断工具，其灵敏度大于 80%[6]。通过该过程可以获得组织学和细胞学标本，进而用于急性排斥反应的形态学证据的评估。为了最佳的患者管理，全面的肺移植团队与其他移植团队一样，需与病理团队保持紧密联系。本章回顾了肺移植排斥反应特异的组织病理学特征，这对肺移植的内外科医生在临床和病理服务中的相互理解及进一步的交流是重要的。

肺移植排斥反应的组织学分级

这个用于活检组织排斥反应分级的分类系统是由国际心肺移植学会（ISHLT）于 1990 年首次提出，现在是它的第三次更新[7]。肺移植中心中该机构的病理学家间频繁比对结果数据，使得初步的工作分类逐渐发展成一个简单的、可重复的、易教的系统。这种使用 A 和 C 于血管排斥反应以及 B 和 D 于气道排斥反应的原始分级模式，在后续的 5 年被大多数的中心采用并取得较大成功。由于这一领域的发展，1995 年召集了更多的病理学家来进一步完善这个分级模式。1996 年发表的以多中心公布的数据及实际经验为基础的第二版工作分类，强调为了提供最佳的患者护理，这些病理学资料需在一个广泛的临床背景下去解读。更具体地说，为了更准确和可重复的分级[7]，活检组织中的感染及其他来源的炎症需要被临床排除。

该评分系统最新的修订版本于 2007 年发表，并一直沿用至今（表 84.1）。该文件的主要变化在于急性气道排斥反应分级系统从四级体系（B1~B4）修订成含低等和高等的二级体系以及慢性气道排斥反应（C），未提及炎症反应的存在。最终，尽管提出了用于抗体介导排斥反应（AMR）病理评估的推荐规范，但关于它在肺移

表 84.1 肺移植排斥反应分类及分级工作分类 2007 年修订版

A.急性排斥反应	0 级——无
	1 级——最低限度
	2 级——轻度
	3 级——中度
	4 级——重度
B.气道炎症反应——淋巴细胞细支气管炎	0 级——无
	1R 级——低级
	2R 级——高级
	X 级——未分级
C.慢性气道排斥反应——闭塞性细支气管炎	0 级——无
	1 级——有
D.慢性血管排斥反应——加速的移植物血管硬化	

Based on [7] Stewart S, Fishbein MC, Snell GI, et al. Revision of the 1996 Working Formulation for the standardization of nomenclature in the diagnosis of lung rejection. *J Heart Lung Transplant* 2007;26: 1229–1242. Copyright 2007, with permission from Elsevier.

植排斥反应中的作用或诊断标准还未达成共识[7]。

通用推荐规范

为了从组织中获得最佳信息，对移植活检组织进行适当的技术处理是重要的，ISHLT 分类标准对于其技术处理规范进行了标准化[7]。需对活检组织进行甲醛固定及石蜡包埋。石蜡切片放置于显微镜载玻片上(2~3 块切片/每块玻片；总共 3 块玻片)并进行常规苏木精和伊红染色。另有两块玻片一块用于镀银染色来评估真菌生物，包括耶氏肺孢子虫；另一块用于弹性纤维染色以显示纤维化(慢性排斥反应的一个标志，尤其在气道)的证据。若临床需要，还可以对其他感染生物进行研究，包括对巨细胞病毒(CMV)和 EB 病毒(EBV)的免疫组化研究。

充分评估有无排斥反应需要多少活检组织切片在肺移植排斥研究小组(LRSG)最新(2007)修订的工作分类中还未最终确定。最初的 1990 年工作分类及之后 1997 年的分类推荐需 5 片蜂窝状肺组织或至少 100 个肺泡用于评估有无排斥反应，并且被多中心沿用至今[8]。对于那些无法充分评估的活检组织，还未给出有无排斥反应的明确诊断(见后文)。

急性排斥反应的组织学特征

肺急性细胞排斥反应用两种评分来分级：A 用于血管排斥反应，B 用于气道炎症反应，后者未明确标示为排斥反应可能因其可以是气道急性排斥反应的结果，但也可有其他病因。血管排斥反应常伴随着气道排斥反应，尤其在中、重度血管排斥反应[9]，但即使无气道排斥反应，血管排斥反应也是及时治疗的临床触发点。

急性血管排斥反应由 A0~A4 评分系统分级，评分愈高表明炎症反应愈重，由最初的血管旁逐渐浸润至肺泡壁。渗透物包括淋巴细胞、一些微嗜酸性粒细胞或者“转化的”细胞核、巨噬细胞、嗜酸性粒细胞以及中性粒细胞，后两种急性炎症细胞一般仅见于 A2 级及以上血管排斥反应。急性排斥反应的诊断未对涉及血管的最低数量作出要求，只要单一血管有排斥反应的组织学证据即可做出诊断。相对动脉和小动脉而言，静脉和小静脉发生排斥反应更常见。最后，尽管血管排斥反应可能包含了整个分级谱，但是活检组织的分级代表的是组织中出现的最高分级。

A0 级(无急性排斥反应)是指有充足的组织用于分级，且未见急性血管排斥反应的活检组织。

A1 级(最低限度的急性排斥反应)表明血管外膜有 2~3 层淋巴细胞环绕(图 84.1)。尽管先前的工作分类承认不完整的血管套与排斥反应一致，但是最新的工作分类表明渗透物必须完整地环绕于血管周围[7]。不同于分级高的急性排斥反应，该分级可无嗜酸性粒细胞或中性粒细胞。尽管很细微，但在组织无误差前提下这一病理改变在低倍镜下仍可见。

A2 级(轻度急性排斥反应)中血管周围也存在单核细胞浸润，包括淋巴细胞、许多活化的类浆细胞变异体及嗜酸性粒细胞。渗透物比 A1 级更显著，在低倍镜下易见 3~5 层细胞环绕(图 84.2)。内皮下也可能见到这些单核细胞(内皮炎)。另外，尽管在 A1 级不常见气道炎症反应，但是在 A2 级常见两者共存[10]。在这一分级中单核细胞浸润未扩散至肺泡，这一点可用于同 A3、A4 级区分。

A3 级(中度急性排斥反应)包含致密的单核细胞浸润血管套及常见的嗜酸性粒细胞、中性粒细胞和显著的内皮炎。当然，渗透物会扩散至邻近肺泡壁的空泡及隔膜；在某些情况下还可出现早期急性肺损伤的特征，即 2 型肺泡细胞反应性增生和肺泡内纤维蛋白。肺部空泡浸润导致肺巨噬细胞团及淋巴细胞，偶尔可见局灶纤维素沉积，加剧肺实质肿胀及肺膨胀不全(图 84.3)。

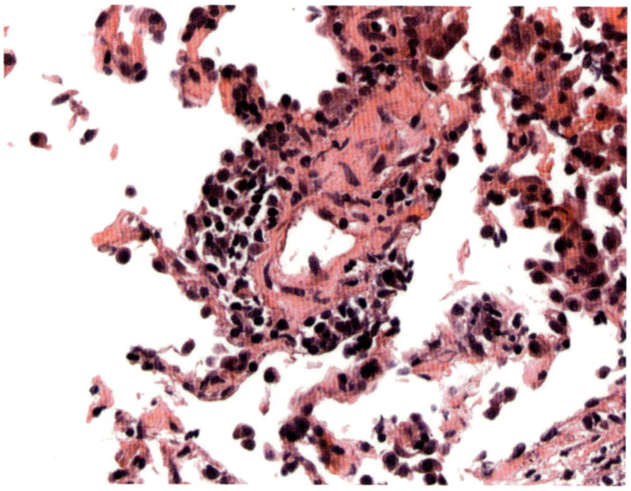

图 84.1 A1 级急性细胞排斥反应(最低限度)。小血管周围被类浆细胞及 2~3 层变异淋巴细胞环绕(HE 染色)。

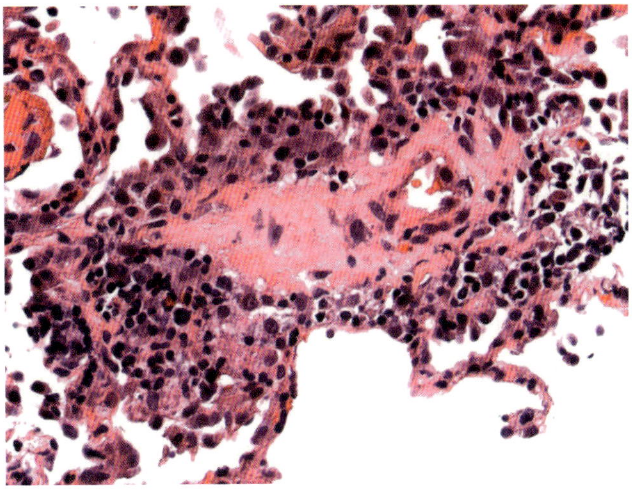

图 84.2　A2 级急性细胞排斥反应(轻度)。小血管被超过 3 层炎症细胞环绕。渗出物含淋巴细胞、分散的嗜酸性粒细胞及中性粒细胞(HE 染色)。

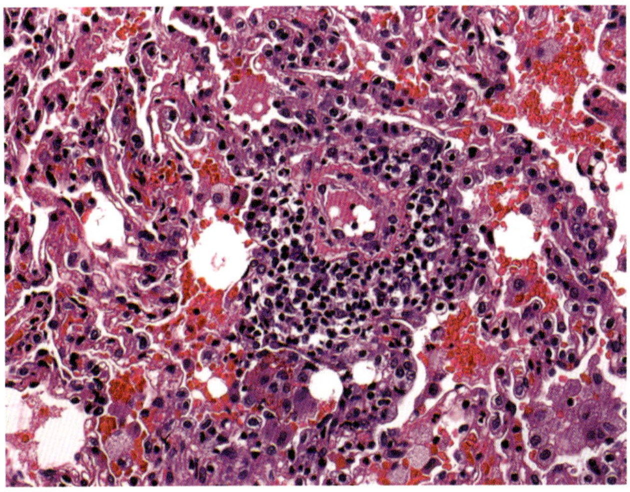

图 84.3　A3 级急性细胞排斥反应(中度)。淋巴细胞、嗜酸性粒细胞、中性粒细胞等炎症细胞浸润至肺泡隔(HE 染色)。

A4 级(重度急性排斥反应),经支气管镜活检较少见这一分级,定义为弥漫性肺血管受累、肺泡单核细胞浸润及严重急性肺损伤。组织学特征有弥漫性间质性肺炎及肺泡内巨噬细胞、纤维蛋白、血管周围炎、实质坏死及血管纤维素样坏死(图 84.4)。A4 级排斥反应主要特征为肺泡内充满巨噬细胞、纤维蛋白、出血、透明膜及大量的中性粒细胞。血管炎及显著的血管周围炎有助于鉴别 A4 级急性排斥反应和弥漫性肺泡损伤,后者由感染或移植后期即时的再灌注损伤等多病因造成[11]。2 型肺泡细胞反应性增生及内皮炎均较 A3 级更显著。A4 级急性排斥反应,炎症反应常扩散至邻近大小气

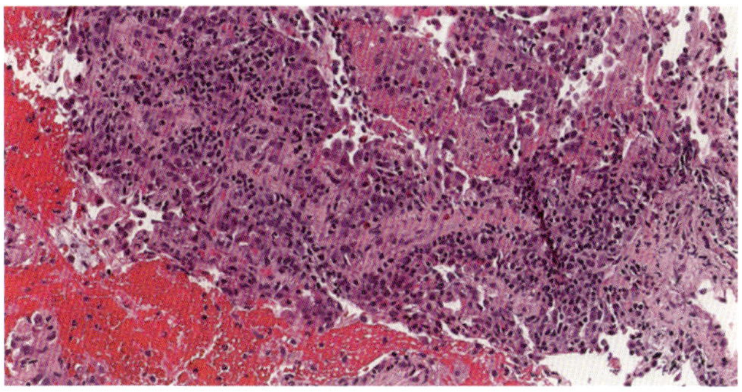

图 84.4　A4 级急性细胞排斥反应(重度)。血管周扩散、肺间质及空泡渗出物表明急性肺损伤和出血(HE 染色)。

道,导致上述炎症细胞浸润至上皮及溃疡[12]。由于大量的急性炎症包括中性粒细胞,A4 级排斥反应主要的鉴别诊断特征常在于一个感染的过程。生物染色和临床资料对于得出正确的诊断是必要的。

对于少于 5 片的组织或不足以用于评估排斥反应的活检组织,定义为 AX 级。

小气道急性排斥反应的分级基于气道淋巴细胞浸润及上皮损伤的程度,且仅适用于小气道[7]。在最初的 1990 年的工作分类中,急性气道排斥反应由各机构自行判定有或无[12]。在 1996 年的修订版中,对于气道炎症反应的分级扩展到 B0(无炎症反应)至 B4(严重气道炎症反应)[12]。但是,不是所有的 LRSG 成员相信仅用炎症反应来进行排斥反应的分级, 因为它可以在其他情况中出现(尤其是感染)[13],因此,最终达成的共识是这一模式尚需进一步研究。在 2007 年的修订版本中,因在识别炎症反应(显著排斥反应或感染)原因存在难点,该分级模式正式引入了"气道炎症反应"这一专业术语。另外,该共识还未达标准的水平,因此将气道炎症反应分成 4 级, 将评分模式分成 2 级, 即 B1R 和 B2R(R 用于修订的分级),保留 B0 定义无炎症反应和 BX 用于定义因众多因素不足以评估炎症反应的活检组织。包括无气道用于评估、其他有炎症反应的炎症过程(例如感染),避开正切面的组织或人工挤压变形掩盖了小气道[7]。

在 B1R 级气道中单核细胞块状分布,或在更显著的病例,可于小气道黏膜下层带状分布。渗透物可扩散至细支气管肌层但未达细支气管覆盖上皮, 且无显著的上皮损伤(图 84.5)。B2R 级更多活化的巨噬细胞、类浆细胞变异体及嗜酸性粒细胞及中性粒细胞, 形成更显著的致密带状渗出。炎症反应浸润至细支气管覆盖

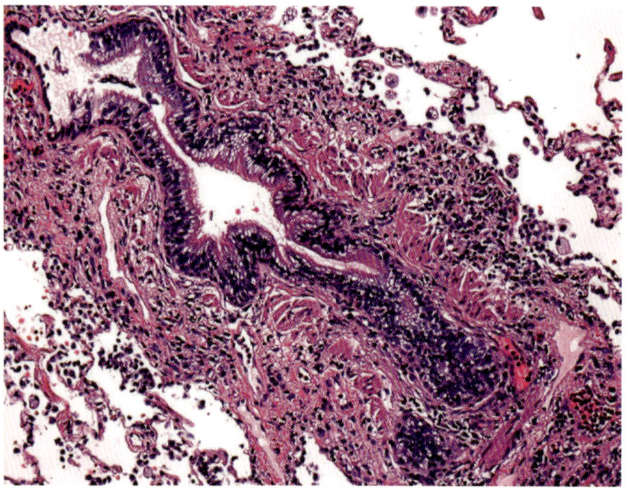

图 84.5 B1R 级低级淋巴细胞性细支气管炎。淋巴细胞带状浸润黏膜下层且单细胞渗透至细支气管覆盖上皮(HE 染色)。

上皮引起明显的上皮损伤，呈现细胞凋亡及溃疡处的大量细胞碎屑(图 84.6)。这些急性炎症细胞使得难以区别高级的排斥反应与感染；但是，上皮及气道管腔中大量中性粒细胞更多提示炎症反应而非排斥反应。病毒性细支气管炎可引起相似程度的气道周围炎症及上皮损伤。在这种情况下，仔细观察损伤的上皮细胞可见病毒包涵体；免疫组化研究，尤其是对巨细胞病毒及单纯疱疹病毒，可能见到相应的病毒包涵体。

经支气管镜活检对于评估排斥反应及指导治疗较重要，所以评估那些通过分析观察者差异进而分析目前分类系统有效性及重现性的研究也很重要。研究显示专业肺部病理学家对于急性排斥反应的一致性从低(κ 0.183)[13]到中(κ 0.47~0.79)[8,14,15]，大部分差异性出现在 A1 级(最低限度急性排斥反应)，而大部分一致性在 A2 级(轻度急性排斥反应)。对于气道炎症反应，有显著的低观察者差异性(κ 0.035~0.25)[14,16]，而在 B0 级(无气道炎症反应)有明显的一致性。为提高诊断的可重复性[13]，需继续研究这些数据进而优化和提高急性排斥反应病理分级的一致性以及持续细化该标准。

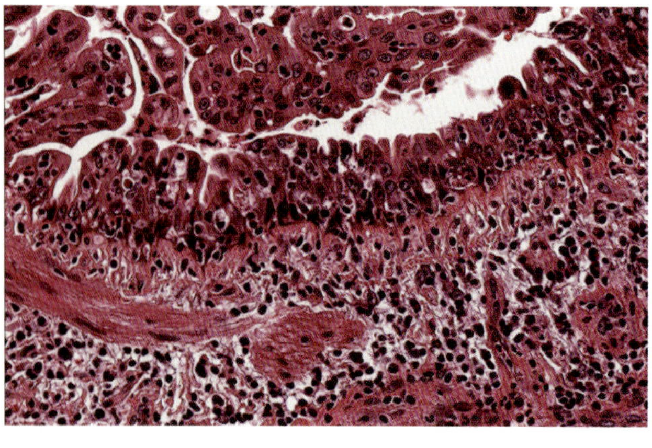

图 84.6 B2R 级高级淋巴细胞性细支气管炎。黏膜下层可见淋巴细胞及广泛浸润至覆盖上皮细胞，导致广泛上皮损伤(HE 染色)。

慢性排斥反应

相比急性排斥反应，肺移植慢性排斥反应组织学特征明确定义在血管及气道，后者被认为是目前最具临床意义的。慢性气道排斥反应，或者闭塞性细支气管炎(OB)，是小气道胶原型纤维化的一个过程，作为淋巴细胞性细支气管炎的一个后遗症，或者作为急性排斥反应中气道炎症的一个结果[17-19]。这一异常修复反应可能是由急性损伤及炎症反应导致转化生长因子-β(TGF-β)过度表达介导的[19]。气道纤维化可于移植后数月或数年出现在任何部位。出现的中位时间为 16~20 个月[20]。因移植物中其不均匀性，在大部分中心经支气管镜活检（TBB）监测慢性气道排斥反应的敏感性为 15%~40%[3,21]。其敏感性可因组织碎片的数量、支气管镜检者及病理学者的经验而提高，但相比于肺功能检查，敏感性仍不高且更昂贵、有创[20]。因此，大部分临床移植中心不再使用经支气管镜活检监测闭塞性细支气管炎。ISHLT 提出了一个基于肺功能检查结果的闭塞性细支气管炎或闭塞性细支气管炎综合征诊断标准化规范，用于指导治疗[22]。

慢性气道排斥反应最重要的组织学标志是细支气管黏膜上皮下区由 3 型胶原蛋白形成的致密的透明变性纤维化[19]。它可是同心或偏心的且逐渐变窄(图84.7)，最终造成小气道闭塞(图 84.8)。随着纤维化的进展，细支气管上皮逐渐消失，闭塞的气道变得难以辨认。靠近肺动脉或管壁残余的平滑肌有助于辨认它。当然，结缔组织染色如弹性纤维染色或 Movat 五色染色有助于闭塞气道弹性膜显现及识别早期纤维化证据。尽管先前的工作分类中考虑了该模式中慢性炎症反应的数量，但是最新的分级系统未包含该问题且仅由两级组成：C0 级(无)和 C1 级(有)。

对于有急慢性小气道排斥反应的肺移植，有时可见大气道慢性炎症反应、纤维化及最终支气管扩张。这

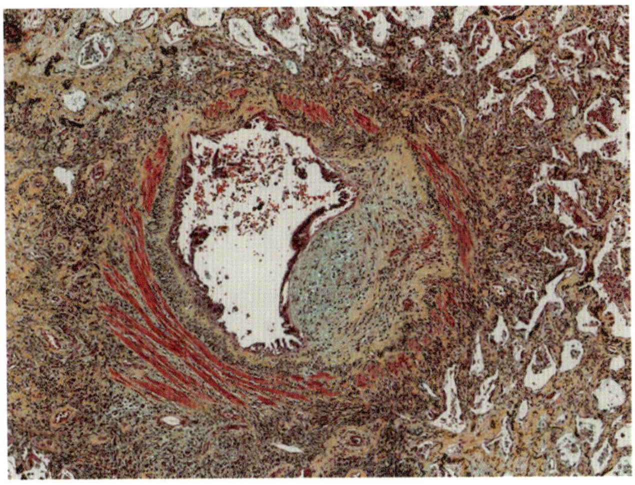

图 84.7　C1 级慢性气道排斥反应-闭塞性细支气管炎。小气道早期纤维化及管腔不对称性狭窄(Movat 染色)。

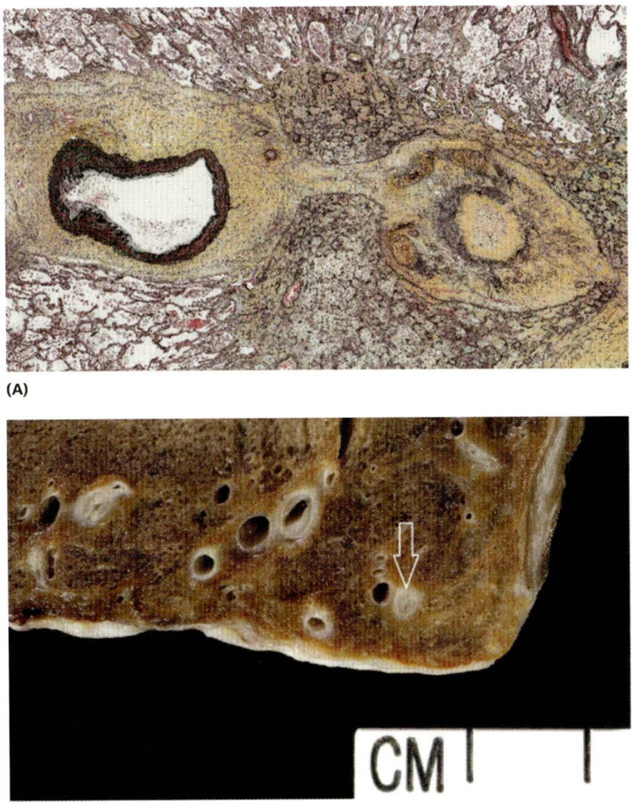

(A)

(B)

图 84.8　(A)C1D 级慢性气道排斥反应-闭塞性细支气管炎及早期慢性血管排斥反应。气道软骨残余(右),在弹性纤维染色下显现轮廓(黑色),完全被胶原纤维阻塞。肺动脉(左)可见内膜纤维化,提示早期慢性血管排斥反应(Movat 染色)。(B)慢性气道排斥反应。在因慢性气道排斥反应切除的移植肺上可见部分狭窄的小气道及因纤维化完全闭塞的气道(箭头)(Gross)。

些组织学特征表明移植物可能受到一些慢性损害,包含感染、误吸及排斥反应。因这些病理学发现非排斥反应所特有,故未将其纳入 2006 年的工作分类且不认为是慢性气道排斥反应。

慢性血管排斥反应的病理学特征无太多关注,因经支气管镜活检未采集到这些病变可靠样本且其病理的临床意义尚未明了。慢性血管排斥反应病理学特征未被很好的记录。描述的特征有内膜纤维化及变异的跨壁慢性炎症浸润(图 84.8 和图 84.9)。报道显示内膜增生可以是非层偏心及同心,血管中层示轻度细胞外基质沉积及平滑肌萎缩[23]。慢性血管排斥反应分级与慢性气道排斥反应类似,仅有 D0(无)和 D1(有)分级。

由慢性气道和慢性血管排斥反应的一致性,推测两者之间存在着因果关系[24]。近期研究表明,慢性血管排斥反应病理所见的供应气道小血管的内膜纤维化可能与 OB 的存在有关[25,26]。因供给肺组织氧气的高压支气管循环,在移植过程中未重新连接,故肺组织包括小气道更易受缺氧损害[27]。这些研究表明慢性血管排斥反应的病理改变可能会进一步危及移植肺小气道的氧合,导致上皮损伤、纤维化及最终导致 OB。早期的研究表明,在支气管循环已重新连接的肺部,OB 的发生率会降低[28]。目前还需进一步研究慢性血管变化及其对移植肺的影响来阐明这些发现。

抗体介导的排斥反应

抗体介导的排斥反应(AMR)是由移植后供体特异性抗 HLA 抗体介导的移植物损伤[29]。这一形式的移植物排斥反应临床上在其他实心器官移植(如肾脏、心脏)

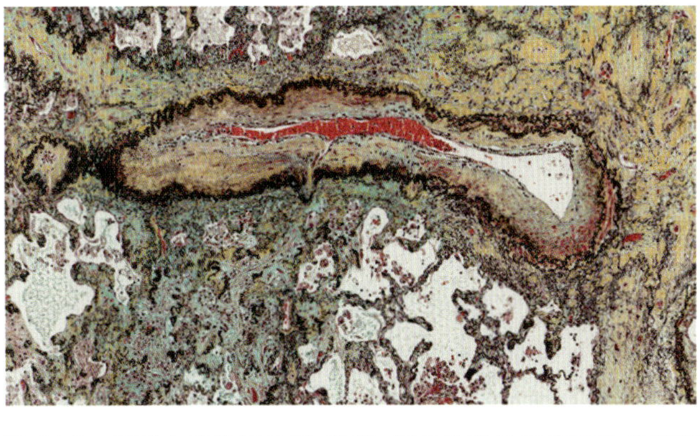

图 84.9　慢性血管排斥反应:静脉。因慢性排斥反应切除的移植肺叶间隔中一较大静脉显示内膜纤维化(Movat 染色)。

较重要[30]。但是,其在肺移植上的临床意义包括其对移植物存活率的影响尚未明了。肺移植受体中检测到HLA抗体者移植肺存活率更低[31,32],且受体已存在的抗供体HLA抗原的抗体介导的体液排斥,即所谓的肺超急性排斥反应,已充分证明其存在[33]。后者以弥漫性肺泡损伤(DAD)为最常见的损伤形式,也揭示了血管损伤证据,如血管血栓形成、肺泡隔毛细血管中性粒细胞及坏死[30,34]。在前两个工作分类中,AMR未用于肺排斥反应的分类或分级[12],尽管最新工作分类讨论了AMR,但它推断肺部AMR的病理学特征尚不明确,还需进一步研究。再者,它引入了"毛细血管损伤"这一专业术语(代替"毛细血管炎")且表明这可能是AMR损伤的一种形式,但可能有一个更广的病因谱,包含感染及高级细胞排斥反应[7]。

目前,关于肺部AMR的研究定义了其临床和病理学的特征。国际评估实体器官移植抗体介导反应会议工作小组提出了用于体液排斥反应的通用分类系统,提出体液排斥反应必备四个特征:检测到循环HLA或供体特有抗体;移植组织C4d沉积;组织存在病理改变;以及移植物功能障碍[30]。关于已发现的组织病理学变化定义的研究发现,若无明确的坏死或肺出血的证据,它一般包括肺泡隔毛细血管中性粒细胞(图84.10),特征至少提示了肺部毛细血管炎[35];但未进行C4d染色。在进行了C4d染色的研究中,其结果与前者稍有差异。一些研究发现这种形式的损伤中移植肺有C4d沉积的证据[36-39],然而其他研究并未发现毛细血管炎有C4d沉积[40]。这些差异可能是由于方法的不同、弹性结缔组织和纤维蛋白非特异性染色以及移植肺活检组织极低的毛细血管特异性C4d阳性发生率。目前正在进行的大范围多机构的标准化协议,包括那些用于C4d组织染色、利于收集更多决定性证据作为肺部AMR的病理特征[41]。

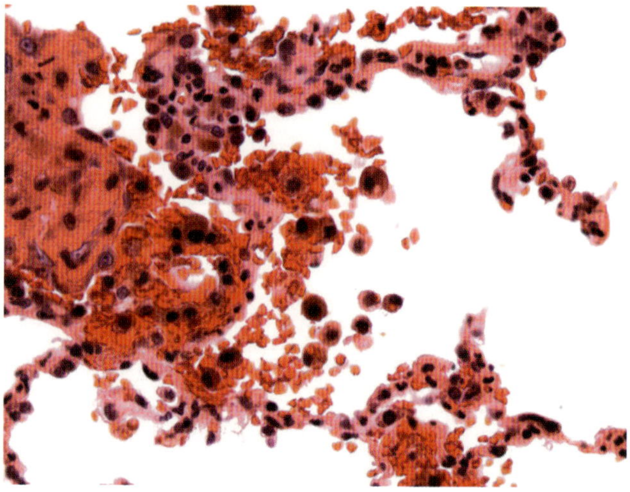

(A)

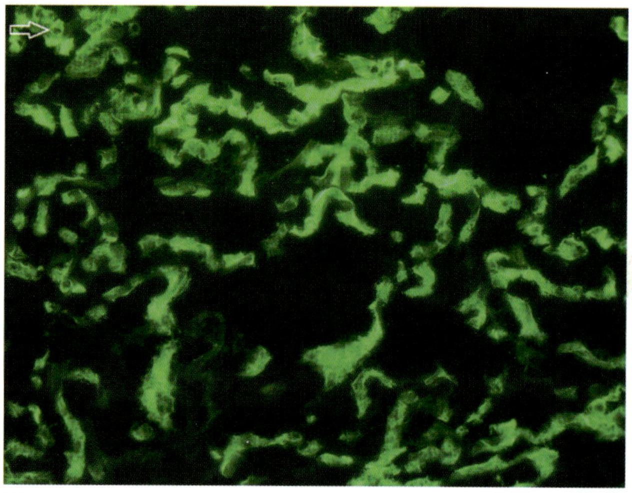

(B)

图84.10　(A)抗体介导排斥反应。肺实质显示急性肺损伤特征,含活化的肺泡壁细胞及肺泡内纤维蛋白。肺泡隔毛细血管可见中性粒细胞(HE染色)。(B)抗体介导排斥反应。免疫荧光染色示毛细血管C4d线状沉积,横断面血管染色示特征性圆环状(箭头)(偏光)。

支气管肺泡灌洗液在肺移植排斥反应诊断中的作用

支气管肺泡灌洗液(BALF)分析用于监测肺移植排斥反应尚存在争议。通过支气管镜及支气管肺泡灌洗(BAL)技术进而对支气管肺泡灌洗液(BALF)中炎症细胞进行计数及免疫分型,使得监测肺实质包括肺泡、肺间质及大小气道的活化细胞动力学变为可能。通过灌洗移植肺,估计可采集超过100万的肺泡[42],同经支气管镜活检(TBB)相比是一个相当大范围的肺组织。因排斥反应的不均匀性,BAL似乎比TBB具有更大的优势。但是,尽管BAL为评估肺部感染的主要方法[43],当怀疑肺移植患者感染时常用该方法[44],由于一些原因,关于BAL作为诊断排斥反应更敏感方法的前景还未得到证实。

首先,移植后BALF中的细胞成分会改变。在手术后即刻,总细胞数升高,尤其是中性粒细胞,可能是炎症损害及再灌注损伤造成的[44,45]。细胞计数可能几年都持续升高,因此难以建立稳固的基线用于后期样本的比较。其次，尽管肺移植急性排斥反应主要特征是间质及空泡单核炎症细胞增多及更高级的急性血管和气道排斥反应[7]，但粒细胞（嗜酸性粒细胞和中性粒细胞）增多[46]使得区分感染与排斥反应存在困难。研究表明，对比 TBB 样本中与 BALF 中的炎症细胞，TBB 样本中炎症细胞对排斥反应具有高度特异性。然而，在有排斥反应的肺部 BALF 中，排斥反应早期淋巴细胞增加，而后期的中性粒细胞增加，但是对于排斥反应不是特异的[47,48]。

为了评估 BALF 中 AMR 的特征，一项研究评估了可溶解 C4d 和 C4d 片段酶免疫分析及与其相关的组织 C4d 沉积、抗 HLA 供体特异性抗体。研究发现可溶解 C4d 与组织 C4d 沉积、供体特异性抗体正相关，但是该发现非特异且在 CMV 感染时发现高假阳性结果[49]。

最后，考虑到 T 细胞在排斥反应中的重要性[50]，关于 BALF 中 T 细胞亚型的研究表明，$CD4^+$和 $CD8^+$比值与移植肺急性细胞排斥反应的存在[51]和慢性气道排斥反应的进展[43,52]具有一定的关联。但是，在 BALF 用于临床诊断排斥反应之前，需进一步的研究来证实这些发现。

总结

肺移植患者的一生都在遭受同种免疫介导排斥反应的风险。表现为显著的急性排斥反应或进展缓慢的以 OB 及其相关 BOS 形式的慢性损害。使用组织病理学诊断或者 BALF 分析连续监测患者仍是肺移植的重要组成部分。

（韩威力 译 韩威力 校）

参考文献

1. Hopkins PM, Aboyoun CL, Chhajed PN, et al. Prospective analysis of 1,235 transbronchial lung biopsies in lung transplant recipients. Journal of Heart and Lung Transplantation. 2002;21:1062–1067.
2. Christie JD, Edwards LB, Kucheryavaya AY, et al. The Registry of the International Society for Heart and Lung Transplantation: twenty-eighth adult lung and heart-lung transplant report, 2011. Journal of Heart and Lung Transplantation. 2011;30:1104–1122.
3. Trulock EP, Christie JD, Edwards LB, et al. Registry of the International Society for Heart and Lung Transplantation: twenty-fourth official adult lung and heart-lung transplantation report, 2007. Journal of Heart and Lung Transplantation. 2007;26:782–795.
4. Patel JK, Kittleson M, Kobashigawa JA. Cardiac allograft rejection. The Surgeon. 2011;9:160–167.
5. Perkins D, Verma M, Park KJ. Advances of genomic science and systems biology in renal transplantation: a review. Seminars in Immunopathology. 2011;33:211–218.
6. Hopkins PM, Aboyoun CL, Chhajed PN, et al. Association of minimal rejection in lung transplant recipients with obliterative bronchiolitis. American Journal of Respiratory and Critical Care Medicine. 2004;170:1022–1026.
7. Stewart S, Fishbein MC, Snell GI, et al. Revision of the 1996 working formulation for the standardization of nomenclature in the diagnosis of lung rejection. Journal of Heart and Lung Transplantation. 2007;26:1229–1242.
8. Chakinala MM, Ritter J, Gage BF, et al. Yield of surveillance bronchoscopy for acute rejection and lymphocytic bronchitis/bronchiolitis after lung transplantation. Journal of Heart and Lung Transplantation. 2004;23:1396–1404.
9. Husain AN, Siddiqui MT, Montoya A, et al. Post-lung transplant biopsies: an 8-year Loyola experience. Modern Pathology. 1996;9:126–132.
10. Marboe CC. Pathology of lung transplantation. Seminars in Diagnostic Pathology. 2007;24:188–198.
11. Sato M, Hwang DM, Ohmori-Matsuda K, et al. Revisiting the pathologic finding of diffuse alveolar damage after lung transplantation. Journal of Heart and Lung Transplantation. 2012;31:354–363.
12. Yousem SA, Berry GJ, Cagle PT, et al. Revision of the 1990 working formulation for the classification of pulmonary allograft rejection: Lung Rejection Study Group. Journal of Heart and Lung Transplantation. 1996;15:1–15.
13. Arcasoy SM, Berry G, Marboe CC, et al. Pathologic interpretation of transbronchial biopsy for acute rejection of lung allograft is highly variable. American Journal of Transplantation. 2011;11:320–328.
14. Stephenson A, Flint J, English J, et al. Interpretation of transbronchial lung biopsies from lung transplant recipients: inter- and intraobserver agreement. Canadian Respiratory Journal. 2005;12:75–77.
15. Colombat M, Groussard O, Lautrette A, et al. Analysis of the different histologic lesions observed in transbronchial biopsy for the diagnosis of acute rejection. Clinicopathologic correlations during the first 6 months after lung transplantation. Human Pathology. 2005;36:387–394.
16. Chakinala MM, Ritter J, Gage BF, et al. Reliability for grading acute rejection and airway inflammation after lung transplantation. Journal of Heart and Lung Transplantation. 2005;24:652–657.
17. Sharples LD, McNeil K, Stewart S, et al. Risk factors for bronchiolitis obliterans: a systematic review of recent publications. Journal of Heart and Lung Transplantation. 2002;21:271–281.
18. Husain AN, Siddiqui MT, Holmes EW, et al. Analysis of risk factors for the development of bronchiolitis obliterans syndrome. American Journal of Respiratory and Critical Care Medicine. 1999;159:829–833.
19. Corris PA. Lung transplantation. Bronchiolitis obliterans syndrome. Chest Surgery Clinics of North America. 2003;13:543–557.
20. Boehler A, Estenne M. Obliterative bronchiolitis after lung transplantation. Current Opinion in Pulmonary Medicine. 2000;6:133–139.
21. Woo MS. Overview of lung transplantation. Clinical Reviews in Allergy and Immunology. 2008;35:154–163.
22. Cooper JD, Billingham M, Egan T, et al. A working formulation for the standardization of nomenclature and for clinical staging of chronic dysfunction in lung allografts. International Society for Heart and Lung Transplantation. Journal of Heart and Lung Transplantation. 1993;12:713–716.
23. Saggar R, Ross DJ, Saggar R, et al. Pulmonary hypertension associated with lung transplantation obliterative bronchiolitis and vascular remodeling of the allograft. American Journal of Transplantation. 2008;8:1921–1930.
24. Jiang X, Khan MA, Tian W, et al. Adenovirus-mediated HIF-1α gene transfer promotes repair of mouse airway allograft microvasculature and attenuates chronic rejection. Journal of Clinical Investigation. 2011;121:2336–2349.
25. Langenbach SY, Zheng L, McWilliams T, et al. Airway vascular changes after lung transplant: potential contribution to the pathophysiology of bronchiolitis obliterans syndrome. Journal of Heart and Lung Transplantation. 2005;24:1550–1556.
26. Dhillon GS, Zamora MR, Roos JE, et al. Lung transplant airway hypoxia: a diathesis to fibrosis? American Journal of Respiratory and Critical Care Medicine. 2010;182:230–236.
27. Nicolls MR, Zamora MR. Bronchial blood supply after lung transplantation without bronchial artery revascularization. Current Opinion in Organ Transplantation. 2010;15:563–567.
28. Pettersson GB, Yun JJ, Nørgaard MA. Bronchial artery revascularization in lung transplantation: techniques, experience, and outcomes. Current Opinion in Organ Transplantation. 2010;15:572–577.
29. Montgomery RA, Cozzi E, West LJ, et al. Humoral immunity and antibody-mediated rejection in solid organ transplantation. Seminars in Immunology. 2011;23:224–234.
30. Takemoto SK, Zeevi A, Feng S, et al. National conference to assess antibody-mediated rejection in solid organ transplantation. American Journal of Transplantation. 2004;4:1033–1041.
31. Girnita AL, Duquesnoy R, Yousem SA, et al. HLA-specific antibodies are risk

factors for lymphocytic bronchiolitis and chronic lung allograft dysfunction. American Journal of Transplantation. 2005;5:131–138.
32. Girnita AL, McCurry KR, Zeevi A. Increased lung allograft failure in patients with HLA-specific antibody. Clinical Transplants. 2007;231–239.
33. Masson E, Stern M, Chabod J, et al. Hyperacute rejection after lung transplantation caused by undetected low-titer anti-HLA antibodies. Journal of Heart and Lung Transplantation. 2007;26:642–645.
34. Dilling DF, Glanville AR. Advances in lung transplantation: the year in review. Journal of Heart and Lung Transplantation. 2011;30:247–251.
35. Astor TL, Weill D, Cool C, et al. Pulmonary capillaritis in lung transplant recipients: treatment and effect on allograft function. Journal of Heart and Lung Transplantation. 2005;24:2091–2097.
36. Magro CM, Pope Harman A, Klinger D, et al. Use of C4d as a diagnostic adjunct in lung allograft biopsies. American Journal of Transplantation. 2003;3: 1143–1154.
37. Morrell MR, Patterson GA, Trulock EP, et al. Acute antibody-mediated rejection after lung transplantation. Journal of Heart and Lung Transplantation. 2009;28: 96–100.
38. Girnita AL, McCurry KR, Yousem SA, et al. Antibody-mediated rejection in lung transplantation: case reports. Clinical Transplants. 2006;508–510.
39. Magro CM, Deng A, Pope-Harman A, et al. Humorally mediated posttransplantation septal capillary injury syndrome as a common form of pulmonary allograft rejection: a hypothesis. Transplantation. 2002;74:1273–1280.
40. Wallace WD, Reed EF, Ross D, et al. C4d staining of pulmonary allograft biopsies: an immunoperoxidase study. Journal of Heart and Lung Transplantation. 2005;24:1565–1570.
41. Mengel M, Sis B, Haas M, et al. Banff 2011 meeting report: new concepts in antibody-mediated rejection. American Journal of Transplantation. 2012;12: 563–570.
42. Hunninghake GW, Gadek JE, Kawanami O, et al. Inflammatory and immune processes in the human lung in health and disease: evaluation by bronchoalveolar lavage. American Journal of Pathology. 1979;97:149–206.
43. Meyer KC. Bronchoalveolar lavage as a diagnostic tool. Seminars in Respiratory and Critical Care Medicine. 2007;28:546–560.
44. Tiroke AH, Bewig B, Haverich A. Bronchoalveolar lavage in lung transplantation: state of the art. Clinical Transplantation. 1999;13:131–157.
45. Zheng L, Orsida B, Whitford H, et al. Longitudinal comparisons of lymphocytes and subtypes between airway wall and bronchoalveolar lavage after human lung transplantation. Transplantation. 2005;80:185–192.
46. Vos R, Vanaudenaerde BM, Verleden SE, et al. Bronchoalveolar lavage neutrophilia in acute lung allograft rejection and lymphocytic bronchiolitis. Journal of Heart and Lung Transplantation. 2010;29:1259–1269.
47. Clelland C, Higenbottam T, Stewart S, et al. Bronchoalveolar lavage and transbronchial lung biopsy during acute rejection and infection in heart-lung transplant patients: studies of cell counts, lymphocyte phenotypes, and expression of HLA-DR and interleukin-2 receptor. American Review of Respiratory Disease. 1993;147:1386–1392.
48. Tikkanen J, Lemström K, Halme M, et al. Cytological monitoring of peripheral blood, bronchoalveolar lavage fluid, and transbronchial biopsy specimens during acute rejection and cytomegalovirus infection in lung and heart–lung allograft recipients. Clinical Transplantation. 2001;15:77–88.
49. Girnita AL, Lee TM, McCurry KR, et al. Anti-human leukocyte antigen antibodies, vascular C4d deposition and increased soluble C4d in broncho-alveolar lavage of lung allografts. Transplantation. 2008;86:342–347.
50. Wood KJ. Regulatory T Cells in Transplantation. Transplantation Proceedings. 2011;43:2135–2136.
51. Gregson AL, Hoji A, Saggar R, et al. Bronchoalveolar immunologic profile of acute human lung transplant allograft rejection. Transplantation. 2008;85:1056–1059.
52. Slebos D-J, Postma DS, Koëter GH, et al. Bronchoalveolar lavage fluid characteristics in acute and chronic lung transplant rejection. Journal of Heart and Lung Transplantation. 2004;23:532–540.

第 85 章
胰腺和胰岛移植排斥反应和复发疾病的组织病理学综合征

Cinthia Beskow Drachenberg, John C. Papadimitriou

引言

目前认为Ⅰ型糖尿病患者可以通过全胰腺移植(WPnTx)或胰岛移植(IT)来实现胰岛素自主性分泌。移植后β细胞的成功替代明显改善了糖尿病患者的生活质量[1],如果能长期维持正常血糖浓度,那么以前认为不可逆的继发性糖尿病病变也将得到改善[2,3]。

1966年,人类实施了首例胰腺移植手术。然而,由于一系列技术限制和免疫学发展滞后的问题,胰腺移植手术发展一直比较缓慢[4,8]。自20世纪90年代以来,全胰腺移植患者的预后明显改善;目前认为对于一些符合条件的患者,大多采用全胰腺移植的方案[9]。胰腺移植活检常规组织学评价和标准化的病理判读在全胰腺移植中发挥重要作用[5,10-15]。有关胰腺移植进展、长期益处及预后详见第107章。

自从2000年报道首批成功的胰岛移植(IT),胰岛移植已经获得良好的短期效果。然而,很多患者在胰腺移植术后5年内仍需要胰岛素治疗。尽管胰岛移植有很多不足,但是,它可以使患者低血糖症状消失,并能长期有效控制血糖浓度[16,17]。有关胰岛移植效果详见第108章。

与其他类型的移植术相比,全胰腺移植和胰岛移植系统性的组织病理分析很大程度上受到经皮活检获取合适移植胰腺组织的技术限制。胰腺活检结果判读仍处于发展阶段,但不断的研究有助于我们理解移植胰腺功能丢失机制。虽然这两种移植方式移植物功能丢失的基本途径可能不同,但是最终都会出现持续的和不可逆转的移植胰腺功能退化,这种移植胰腺功能退化与全胰腺移植中的进行性移植胰腺纤维化和硬化以及胰岛移植中缺少足够的胰岛有关[14,16-18]。这两种移植方式中,胰岛的主要组成部分Langerhans细胞,易受到一些常见疾病发展过程的影响(如移植排斥反应、Ⅰ型糖尿病复发、淀粉样物沉积,巨细胞病毒感染)[18-21]。

全胰腺移植中移植排斥反应的组织病理诊断原则和实践应用

免疫排斥反应

胰腺急性移植排斥反应的组织病理学特征与其他实体器官移植病理学特征相比没有什么不同[6,8,22-24]。急性T细胞介导的排斥反应(ACMR)及抗体介导的排斥反应(AMR)的病理特征:前者表现为胰腺组织内炎性细胞浸润;后者表现为血管壁抗体和补体沉积。这些基本发病机制将分别在第5章和第6章中讨论。在这两种排斥反应中,移植胰腺损伤通常由于抗原特异性免疫损伤及其他非特异性因素引起[22-24]。

移植胰腺排斥反应高度依赖于受体和供体之间主要组织相容性复合体(MHC)抗原不相容的程度[24]。在正常和炎症条件下,MHCⅠ类和Ⅱ类在胰腺外分泌和内分泌组织中表达存在差异(表85.1)[13,25-27]。MHC差异,尤其是MHCⅡ类,一直与发生AMR和移植胰腺功能丢失的高风险相关[28]。

在胰腺移植后初期,组织病理学表现主要与缺血、手术创伤相关[24,29-31]。ACMR的发生和发展在各种动物模型中已有描述。ACMR表现为胰腺间质、小静脉及不同种类的导管炎症细胞浸润[32-39]。腺泡炎症和腺泡细胞损伤,包括凋亡,都是急性排斥反应的特征[5,12 32,35-39]。重度或较晚期的ACMR主要表现为动脉内膜炎、坏死性

表 85.1 正常和异常胰腺组织内 I 类和 II 类 HLA 的表达

	正常胰腺的组织学切片		组织背景–炎症环境(β–IFN,γ–IFN,IL–2)		糖尿病(DM)	
细胞类型	分类 I	分类 II	分类 I	分类 II	分类 I	分类 II
腺泡细胞	–	–	+,异常表达	+,异常表达	n/a	n/a
导管细胞	++	–	++	+,异常表达	n/a	n/a
胰岛细胞	+/–(弱)	–	++,过表达	++,异常表达	++,全胰岛细胞过表达(伴胰岛素炎–早期 DM)	+,β 细胞异常表达(+/–胰岛素炎)
毛细血管						
内皮细胞	++	++	n/a	n/a	n/a	n/a
大的血管						
内皮细胞	++	不确定	n/a	n/a	n/a	n/a

n/a,数据不可用。

Adapted from[13] Drachenberg et al. *American Journal of Transplantation.* 2011;11:1792–1802, with permission from Wiley.

血管炎、血栓形成和最终导致胰腺实质坏死[14,36,39]。

虽然胰岛不是 ACMR 主要靶点,但是重度排斥反应导致的广泛胰腺实质坏死与继发性胰岛损伤或坏死以及高血糖症发生有关[40]。此外,复发或未经治疗的 ACMR 发作可导致慢性胰腺损伤,表现为腺泡破坏或丢失、慢性血管损伤。这些病变引起胰腺的纤维化反应,从而破坏胰腺正常结构并且导致继发性大部分胰岛功能丢失。移植胰腺硬化体现了慢性排斥反应主要特征[41–42]。

在 AMR 中,抗体血管壁沉积造成血管壁直接损伤的原因是激活补体级联反应以及抗体依赖的细胞介导毒性(ADCC)[28,43,44]。因此,血管损伤及坏死、血栓形成、继发缺血性胰腺实质坏死都是急性 AMR 典型特征;超急性排斥反应是急性 AMR 中最极端的例子[24,43,45,46]。虽然最初认为即发的移植胰腺丢失仅与超急性排斥反应相关,但现在认为其与急性和慢性活动性 AMR 也相关。AMR 内可见大量巨噬细胞和中性粒细胞聚集;然而,这类细胞也可出现在重度 T 细胞介导的排斥反应以及其他类型的重度胰腺实质损伤[11,45,47–49]。一些 AMR 患者出现高血糖症,提示胰岛功能损伤可能与血管壁抗体沉积造成的微血管损伤有关[11,47,50,51]。

移植排斥反应组织学诊断

随着非侵袭性生物标志物的发展,可有效避免移植胰腺活检[52–54]。然而,组织样本评估仍然是诊断急性胰腺排斥反应的金标准。仅依靠临床资料很难区别 ACMR 和 AMR。有关胰腺移植和胰岛移植排斥反应的临床认知讨论详见第 73 章。在这两种移植中,患者通常表现为胰腺外分泌功能异常或外分泌和内分泌功能联合异常;移植物内仅出现内分泌功能障碍(高血糖)并不常见,所占比例<10%[10,11,47,55,56]。

理想的移植胰腺活检组织至少包括三个胰腺小叶结构及相应的导管、静脉和小动脉分支,这些结构在 T 细胞介导的排斥反应中常常受累(图 85.1)。动脉分支越大,样本采集越困难。病理报告中应提出活检内有无动脉分支,因为动脉病变对于病理诊断尤为重要[14]。

首先低倍镜下观察活检标本内整个胰腺小叶结构,如果间隔和腺泡间存在胶原蛋白(纤维化),则需半定量的评估。低倍镜下很容易识别胰腺小叶间隔内炎症。然而,腺泡炎症需要更具体、系统性评估混杂

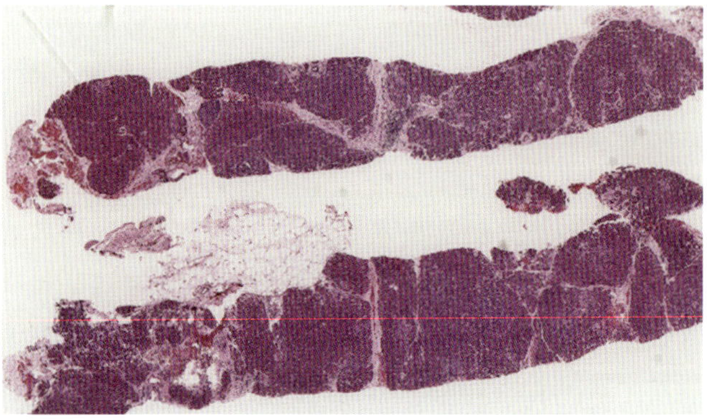

图 85.1 移植胰腺活检低倍镜下 HE 染色,显示活检组织样本主要由薄的结缔组织分割的外分泌胰腺(腺泡小叶)组成。本例活检中可见极少量甚至可忽略的胰腺小叶间隔纤维化(即移植胰腺硬化)(分级 0)。

在腺泡细胞内的炎症细胞类型，尤其在早期排斥反应中[51,57]。

活检类型

经皮粗针(直径 18G 或 20G)穿刺活检通常在超声或 CT 引导下完成[12,15,58-63]。88%~90%的病例能获得足够的胰腺组织[15,58-61,64-66],2%~3%的病例出现明显并发症(例如,出血、轻度胰腺炎),但无一例导致移植胰腺丢失[59,60]。

当经皮穿刺活检难以取得满意的胰腺组织时,尤其是通过肠道引流的移植胰腺，可进行胰腺腹腔镜活检[67,68]。然而,采用腹膜后门静脉引流的移植胰腺,通过经皮穿刺活检效果可能更好[69,70]。

过去,胰液膀胱内引流的移植胰腺患者中,通常采用膀胱镜经十二指肠进行胰腺活检。然而,仅在 57%~80%的病例活检中可获得胰腺组织,因此,活检组织病理特征也依靠通过活检移植十二指肠吻合口处的十二指肠黏膜来判读[71-74]。同样地,对于通过肠道引流的胰腺移植患者，也可以使用上消化道胃肠内镜对十二指肠吻合口黏膜活检,进行病理评估[75]。有关内容将在十二指肠移植病理学中叙述。

手术活检增加胰液漏出和发生相应并发症的风险，所以仅在其他方法难以提供足够的活检样本时使用[76]。

组织学评价:技术指导

通常，显微镜下 HE 染色切片需要评估至少 2 个不同穿刺位点的组织,有时采用 C4d 染色(参见后面的抗体介导排斥反应诊断)和 Masson 三色染色作为辅助诊断(图 85.2)。Masson 染色是胶原纤维染色,用于纤维化的定量研究，同时也有助于辨认特殊的组织结构或病理改变(如动脉壁、纤维素样坏死物等)[13,14]。通过石蜡包埋/免疫组织化学和冰冻切片/免疫荧光方法,可获得相对应的 C4d 染色结果(图 85.3)[13]。

对于高血糖症患者的移植胰腺活检，需要进行胰岛素和胰高血糖素染色以排除选择性 β 细胞丢失[77-79]。其他染色应根据评估需要进行选择(例如 EB 病毒、巨细胞病毒染色等)[80,81]。

淀粉样物(胰岛淀粉样蛋白)需用刚果红染色鉴别[82](参阅“Banff 胰腺移植排斥反应”部分)。

如果有冷冻组织，采用免疫荧光染色方法容易显

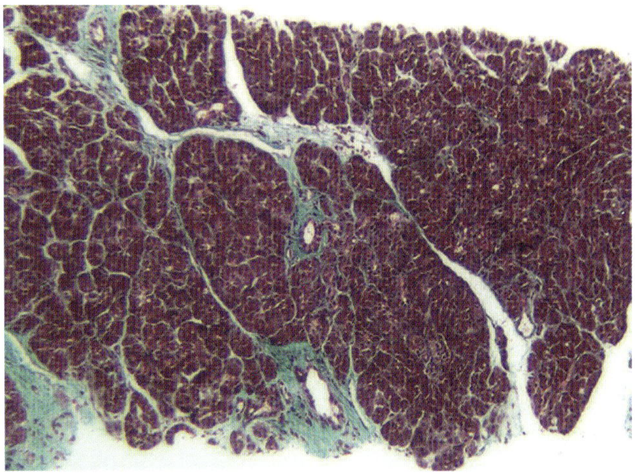

图 85.2　Masson 三色染色显示每个纤细的纤维间隔内均含有胰腺导管分支。

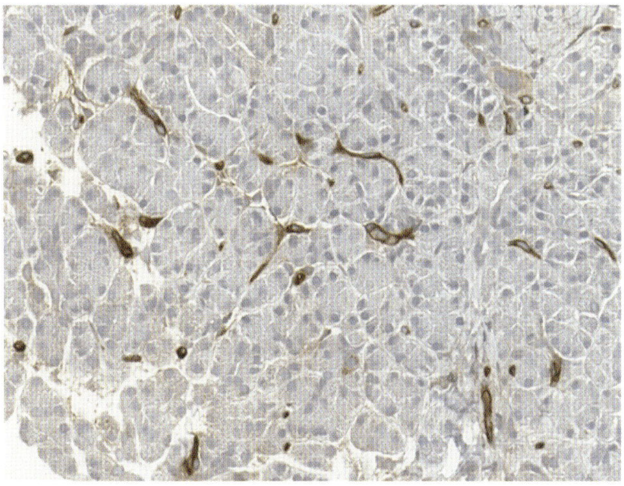

(A)

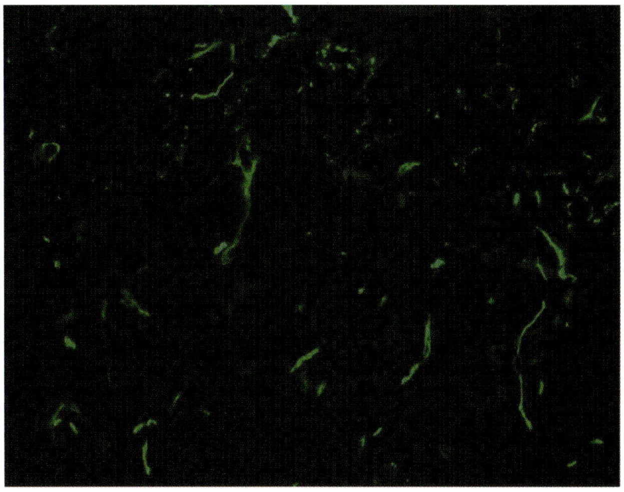

(B)

图 85.3　C4d 免疫组织化学染色(A)及免疫荧光染色(B)显示抗体介导的排斥反应(AMR)中胰腺腺泡间相同区域的毛细血管染色。

示沉积在血管壁内的免疫球蛋白和补体；尤其当怀疑胰腺移植患者出现超急性或暴发性急性 AMR 时，免疫荧光染色更有利于鉴别[42]。电子显微镜可用于观察Ⅰ型糖尿病复发时选择性 β 细胞丢失或钙调磷酸酶抑制剂毒性中 β 细胞变性[83]。

急性 T 细胞介导的移植排斥反应

急性 T 细胞介导的移植排斥反应(ACMR)主要特征包括胰腺小叶间隔内炎症和水肿、小静脉炎、导管炎及局灶炎症细胞弥漫浸润到相邻或不相邻的腺泡内(腺泡炎)[10,12,14,61]。形态学上，胰腺 ACMR 中发生的动脉性病变也会出现在其他实体移植器官中，并且与即发性或迟发性移植胰腺血栓形成相关。因此，动脉性病变被划归为重度排斥反应[14,84]。

在典型的 ACMR 中，胰腺腺泡间毛细血管(≥5%)不表达 C4d 染色[11]。

ACMR 中炎症细胞类型

ACMR 主要表现为 T 细胞浸润。ACMR 较轻时，胰腺小叶间隔区出现比较密集的 T 细胞聚集(图 85.4A)；而较严重时，胰腺实质可见弥漫性 T 细胞浸润(图 85.4B)；急性 ACMR 中嗜酸性粒细胞较常见，在某些病例中甚至占主导地位[85]。类似于肾移植的 ACMR，胰腺移植 ACMR 中也可见巨噬细胞，但通常不占主导地位，除非伴发其他病变，如缺血性胰腺炎和胰周脓肿[86]。急性 ACMR 早期，浆细胞常常难以觅见；但在长期或部分治疗后或迟发的急性-慢性排斥反应中，浆细胞常与其他单核细胞混杂聚集。胰腺移植后早期阶段，B 细胞浸润不是 ACMR 的特征，但在慢性移植胰腺炎内常常出现并聚集。B 细胞随时间推移而增加，特别是患者原先有排斥反应发作或进行性 ACMR。B 细胞在肾脏移植中的意义和机制是复杂和难以解释的；在胰腺移植中也没有系统性研究[87-89]。

治疗的影响

大多数 ACMR 患者使用标准化抗排斥反应(如脉冲式类固醇、抗淋巴细胞抗体)可获得良好的治疗效果。早期一系列研究发现，大部分出现胰腺实质和血管坏死的重度 ACMR 排斥反应患者表现出抗排斥反应治疗无应答，这些相互矛盾的结果可能表明患者实

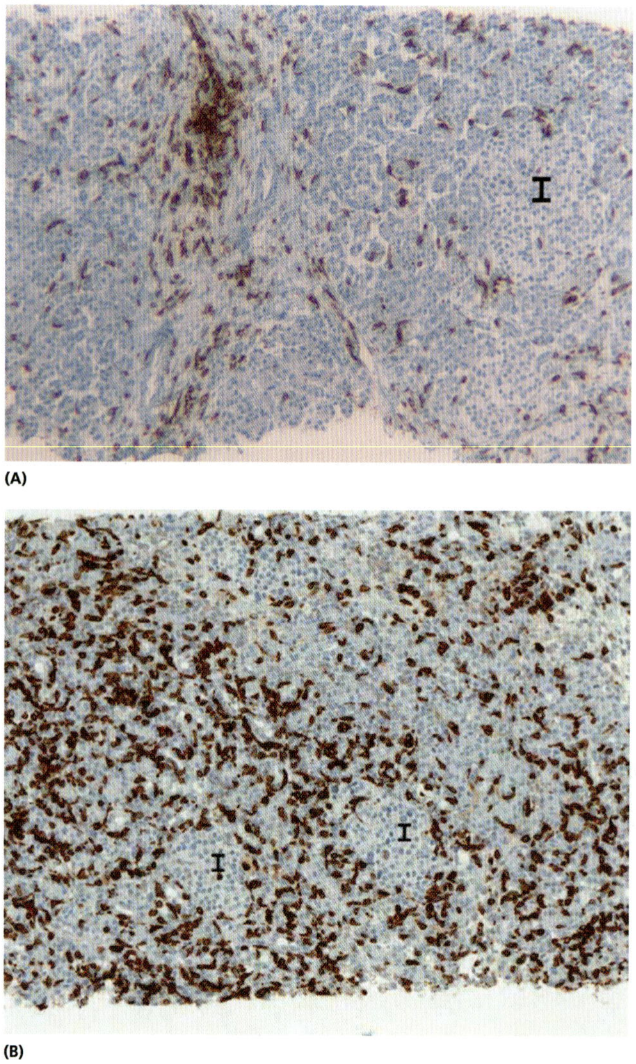

图 85.4 (A)轻度急性细胞介导的排斥反应(ACMR)(Banff 分级：Ⅰ级)。CD3 染色显示胰腺小叶间隔内大量 T 细胞浸润，而腺泡间仅见少量 T 细胞浸润。(B)重度 ACMR(Banff 分级：Ⅲ级)表现为各种类型的病理改变(Banff 体系)。本例中 CD3 染色显示弥漫的 T 细胞腺泡炎症。这两张图中胰岛内(Ⅰ)CD3 染色分布较广，但量较少，因为在 ACMR 中胰岛不是炎症细胞的靶点。

际上出现了急性 AMR[65,90]。关于一般的挽救治疗及胰腺急性排除反应治疗的讨论在第 67 章和第 73 章中分别介绍。

ACMR 的鉴别诊断

阴性或微小病灶

移植胰腺功能障碍的活检标本缺少具有诊断意义的明显炎症成分，这可能是因为错误的取样造成的。一些特殊的轻度 ACMR 活检标本可表现出胰腺小叶间

隔内没有炎症，或低倍镜下容易被忽略的局灶腺泡炎症[8,14]。类似的，早期轻度 AMR 可表现为极轻微的腺泡炎症，有时也难以分辨[13,91]。

不同于 ACMR 的胰腺小叶间隔和(或)腺泡炎症特征

主要的鉴别诊断包括胰腺周围炎、巨细胞病毒感染和移植后淋巴组织增生性疾病(PTLD)。

感染性胰腺周围炎、胰腺周围积液或胰腺周围脓肿是胰腺移植相对常见的早期并发症，常常继发于缺血性移植胰腺炎[92,93]。移植后剖腹探查术中细针穿活检发现移植胰腺内可见不同程度混合性炎症反应，主要位于胰腺小叶间隔。最重要的组织学特征是胰腺组织内出现大量增生活跃的成纤维细胞呈束状生长。这些纤维带在胰腺外分泌小叶之间穿行，使得活检组织出现“硬化”的表现(图 85.5)。随着时间的推移，如果胰腺周围感染积液持续存在，胰腺小叶间隔纤维化变得更加明显。移植物伴有腹腔内及胰腺周围脓肿主要鉴别诊断是移植物伴有急、慢性排斥反应。综合分析组织学及临床信息，包括影像学和微生物学对于区别上述病变是有帮助的。从形态学角度考虑，急性 ACMR 通常不出现胰腺小叶明显的纤维化(或明确的纤维间隔)，除非有潜在慢性炎的成分。胰腺周围炎中一般胰腺外分泌小叶保存完整，而在慢性排斥反应或移植胰腺硬化中胰腺外分泌小叶的中央区易出现广泛萎缩[14,41,86]。虽然胰腺小叶间隔纤维化的程度需要患者一次或多次剖腹探查活检证实，但是这些病理改变通常只能确定移植胰腺周围(表面)组织情况，因此表浅的移植胰腺纤维活检不能代表整个器官的纤维化状态。与 ACMR 相比，胰腺周围炎通常表现为腺泡实质内少量炎症和腺泡破坏[86]。

伴脓肿形成的坏死性感染性十二指肠胰腺炎可出现在移植后任何时间，但通常发生于移植后第一个月。各种生物可以在移植物内繁殖，最常见的是肠杆菌和耐甲氧西林金黄色葡萄球菌(MRSA)。Candida sp 源性真菌感染，以及细菌和真菌混合感染并不少见[94,95]。

广泛使用抗病毒药物预防移植胰腺感染，巨细胞病毒移植胰腺炎已非常罕见。Klassen 等[80]报道 4 例患者在胰腺移植术后 18 周至 44 个月活检诊断为 CMV 胰腺炎。随着更昔洛韦治疗时间延长，巨细胞病毒感染患者的临床症状和病理学组织特征均消退[80]。经皮穿刺活检中，ACMR 和轻度 CMV 胰腺炎可能表现出温和

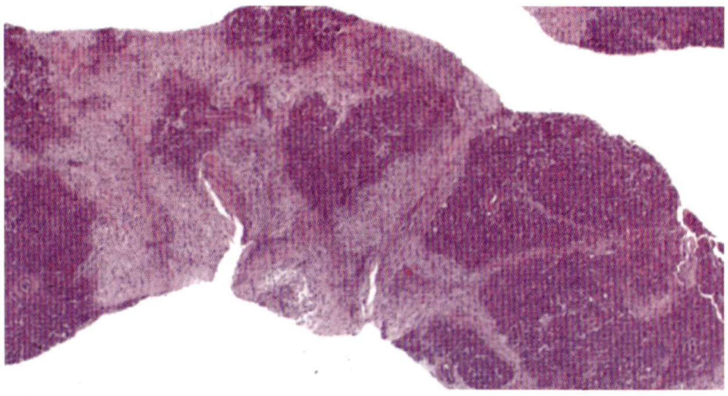

(A)

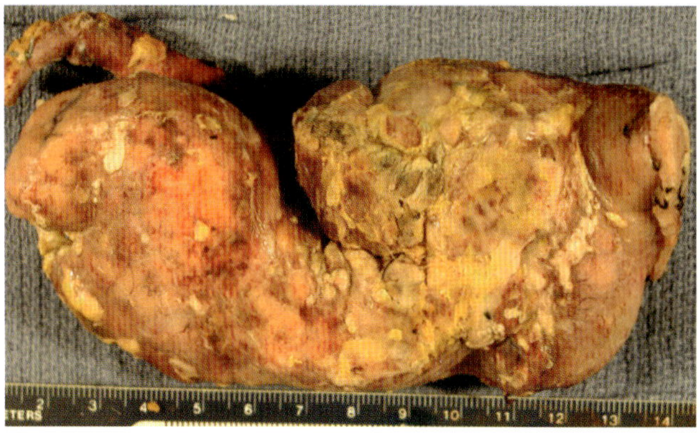

(B)

图 85.5 (A)胰腺移植后周围胰腺炎显微镜下病理特征表现为混合性炎症，以胰腺小叶间隔炎症为主，并见增生的间隔纤维化。纤维带在胰腺外分泌腺小叶间穿行，活检组织呈现“硬化”的表现。移植胰腺周围可见炎症和纤维化改变。(B)由于移植术后周围胰腺炎，移植胰腺切除标本的大体形态。胰腺表面部分区域可见脓性分泌物覆盖。

的、淋巴细胞为主的腺泡炎症(图 85.6)。嗜酸性粒细胞在排斥反应中比较常见，但也可在小部分巨细胞病毒感染患者中出现。在排斥反应及巨细胞病毒胰腺炎内均可见中性粒细胞，这可能与区域坏死或腺泡细胞损伤有关。如果需要排除病毒感染，则可多次组织切片和进行巨细胞病毒染色[80,86]。

巨细胞病毒感染的移植胰腺炎的临床表现与急性排斥反应的临床表现无法区分(例如，血清淀粉酶和脂肪酶的增加)。严重的巨细胞病毒感染患者可出现顽固性消化道出血或十二指肠吻合口穿孔[96-100]。伴脓肿形成的坏死性巨细胞病毒感染及与巨细胞病毒感染相关的动静脉瘘已有文献报道[101-103]。

移植后淋巴组织增生性疾病

移植后淋巴组织增生性疾病(PTLD)在胰腺移植患者中的发病率为 1%~3%[81,104-106]。绝大多数 PTLD 与 EBV 相关且主要来源于 B 细胞谱系。EBV 相关 PTLD

包括一个广泛的从良性增生到恶性淋巴增生的范围。在大部分良性谱系末端(浆细胞增生)中,移植胰腺活检通常不具有诊断价值。移植胰腺受累在其他类型的PTLD是比较常见的(多形性B细胞增生/淋巴瘤、免疫母细胞淋巴瘤)[81,107,108]。早期阶段诊断PTDL问题较多,特别是如果同时伴发急性排斥反应。T细胞和B细胞标志物评估(如CD3、CD20)可以帮助鉴别浸润细胞类型。急性排斥反应的特点是T细胞占主导(通常是75%以上)和少量直径不超过几百微米的B细胞群。相比之下,出现大片的相互融合结节状的B淋巴细胞聚集则提示PTLD累及移植胰腺。若出现以免疫母细胞和浆细胞样细胞浸润为主的显著异型细胞,也支持PTLD诊断(图85.7)。数量不等的嗜酸性粒细胞可出现在急性排斥反应和PTLD中,而免疫球蛋白轻链限制通常在淋巴瘤中出现[81,107,108]。应用原位杂交EBV编码的RNA(EBER)技术有助于确诊EBV相关PTLD和标记出非典型细胞所占的比例。另外,LMP-1(EBV潜在膜蛋白)染色在不同比例的细胞内阳性表达。相对于Ⅲ级(重度)细胞介导急性排斥反应中胰腺实质出现的弥漫

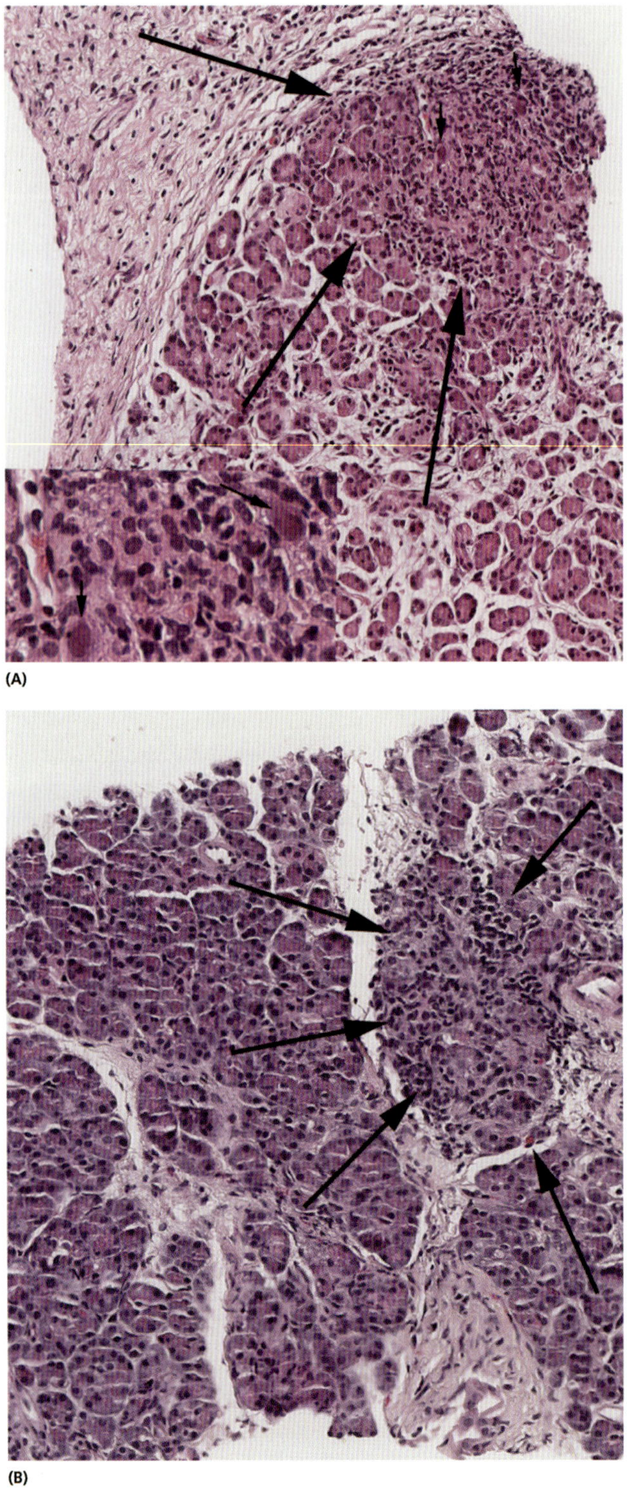

图85.6 (A)巨细胞病毒感染的炎性病灶(大箭头)。(A)小箭头及(B)内显示伴有巨细胞病毒(CMV)感染的大细胞的细胞病理改变。(B)注意与AMCR引起的局灶腺泡炎症整体相似(大箭头)。

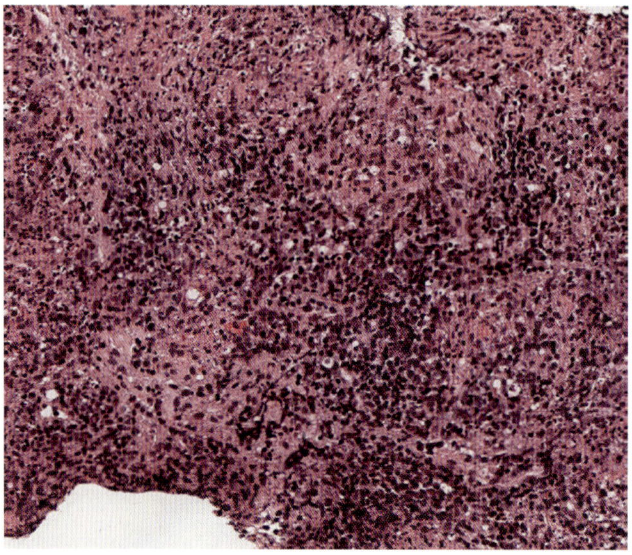

图85.7 胰腺移植后淋巴组织增生性疾病的病理特征:胰腺实质内可见细胞学上非典型的免疫母细胞或浆细胞样细胞以破坏性、膨胀性浸润生长。本例HE视野中坏死区域染色较浅,常见于侵袭性PTLD。

性炎症反应，随机研究病例发现 PTLD 患者移植胰腺实质中可完全没有炎症反应[5,81,107]。

急性抗体介导的排斥反应

急性抗体介导的排斥反应(AMR)包括广泛的组织学改变，从极轻微的炎症反应到弥漫性凝固性坏死出现[43]。动脉内膜炎，被认为是 ACMR 的典型病变，也是目前公认的与急性 AMR 有关的病变[48,109,110]。

急性 AMR 患者中>5%的胰腺腺泡间毛细血管阳性表达 C4d(图 85.3)。根据胰腺腺泡间毛细血管 C4d 染色范围占胰腺小叶的面积百分比，C4d 染色可分为局灶性(> 5%~50%)或弥漫性(> 50%)[11,13]。

急性 AMR 炎症细胞类型

在急性 AMR 中，单核–巨噬细胞类的单核细胞作为最主要的炎症细胞类型。中性粒细胞也普遍存在，并与组织损伤或坏死的程度成正比。T 淋巴细胞分散在整个实质组织，但仅有少量浸润。嗜酸性粒细胞罕见(框 85.1)[13,14,39,86,91]。

治疗的影响

根据胰腺腺泡间炎症浸润的范围或毛细血管炎和组织损伤情况，急性 AMR 组织学分为三级（轻度、中度、重度)(表 85.2)[13]。重度急性 AMR 伴发弥漫性血管血栓形成和胰腺实质坏死基本上是无法治愈的[5]。早期轻度或较惰性的急性 AMR 可能更适合治疗，但与其他实质性器官相比，疗效差异较大。移植胰腺中 AMR 仍然是一个难以攻克的治疗性难题[18]。

急性 AMR 的鉴别诊断

阴性或微小病灶

早期微小的 AMR 很轻微，活检可能会错误地认为“没有诊断意义”；除非样本高度怀疑受体胰腺小叶炎细胞浸润，这时可做 C4d 染色及供体特异性抗体相关性(DSA)检查[13]。

当活检组织内没有或仅有轻微的炎症反应，或出现孤立的胰岛炎，应该考虑自身免疫性糖尿病复发[111]或其他胰岛相关疾病[83]，特别是高血糖症患者[112]。

移植后胰腺炎

AMR 中胰腺小叶出现混合性炎反应，伴或不伴隐性渗血或明显出血，或者血管栓塞形成，都需要与缺血性胰腺炎相鉴别。区别这些病理特征需对样本进行严格评估[42]。

轻度缺血再灌注损伤的特点是点状腺泡细胞丢失或凋亡、腺泡细胞变扁平及其他轻微炎症反应（图 85.8)[30,113,114]。没有 AMR 发生时，缺血性胰腺炎活检组

框 85.1　急性抗体介导的排斥反应(AMR)组织学严重程度分级(详见框 85.2 Banff 分级体系的其他诊断)

轻度急性 AMR(Ⅰ级)

胰腺整体结构完整，轻度单核–巨噬细胞或混合性炎症(单核–巨噬细胞/中性粒细胞)细胞浸润，腺泡细胞损伤罕见

中度急性 AMR(Ⅱ级)

胰腺整体结构完整，胰腺小叶腺泡间单核–巨噬细胞或混合性炎症(单核–巨噬细胞/中性粒细胞)细胞浸润，毛细血管扩张充血，毛细血管炎，多灶腺泡细胞丢失，红细胞外渗

重度急性 AMR(Ⅲ级)

胰腺结构紊乱，胰腺小叶间隔内出血伴散在分布的炎症细胞浸润，多灶和融合的胰腺实质坏死，动脉和静脉壁坏死、血栓形成

表 85.2　急性 T 细胞介导的排斥反应(ACMR)和抗体介导的排斥反应(AMR)的形态学特征

	ACMR	AMR
小叶间隔炎症	+++	–到+
嗜酸性粒细胞	+到+++	–到+
中性粒细胞	–到++	+/–到+++
T 淋巴细胞	++到+++	+/–到+
巨噬细胞	++	++++
静脉炎	++	–
导管炎	++	–
腺泡细胞损伤	+/–到++	+++
腺泡细胞炎症	–到+++	+到+++
腺泡炎(个别腺泡基底膜单核细胞浸润)	+到+++	–到+/–
腺泡间毛细血管炎	–到+/–	+到+++
动脉内膜炎	+	+
坏死性血管炎/血栓形成	–到+	+++
融合出血性坏死	–到++	+++

Adapted from[13] Drachenberg et al. *American Journal of Transplantation*. 2011;11:1792–1802, with permission from Wiley.

织内胰腺腺泡间毛细血管不表达 C4d 蛋白。C4d 染色常常非特异地突出坏死细胞和坏死组织，但这不是诊断 AMR 的依据[13]。缺血性胰腺炎另一个表现是胰腺腺泡和胰岛细胞明显的胞浆肿胀和空泡变性，这些应与药物毒性胰岛病变相区别。

移植胰腺炎的发生率及严重程度与冷缺血时间的长短以及缺血再灌注期微循环重新分布直接相关[29,92,94,115]。

移植胰腺血栓形成

移植胰腺血栓形成发生在不同的阶段，包括以下几方面：

• 早期移植胰腺血栓形成(真正的技术失败)通常发生在胰腺移植术后的 1 周内[42]。移植胰腺出现的唯一的病理改变包括新近形成的血管血栓及轻度缺血性胰腺实质坏死。没有潜在的血管病变或任何其他特殊的组织学改变(图 85.9A)。围术期炎症反应及水肿、微血管及内皮损伤与供者、器官获取及保存等因素均相关,这些因素均能增加早期移植胰腺血栓形成的发病率[42,116]。

• 与急性排斥反应相关的血栓形成可出现在移植后任何时期,这通常是急性或慢性血管损伤的结果(如动脉内膜炎、透壁性动脉炎、移植动脉病变等)。AMR 和 ACMR 均可出现坏死性动脉炎(图 85.9B)。透壁性

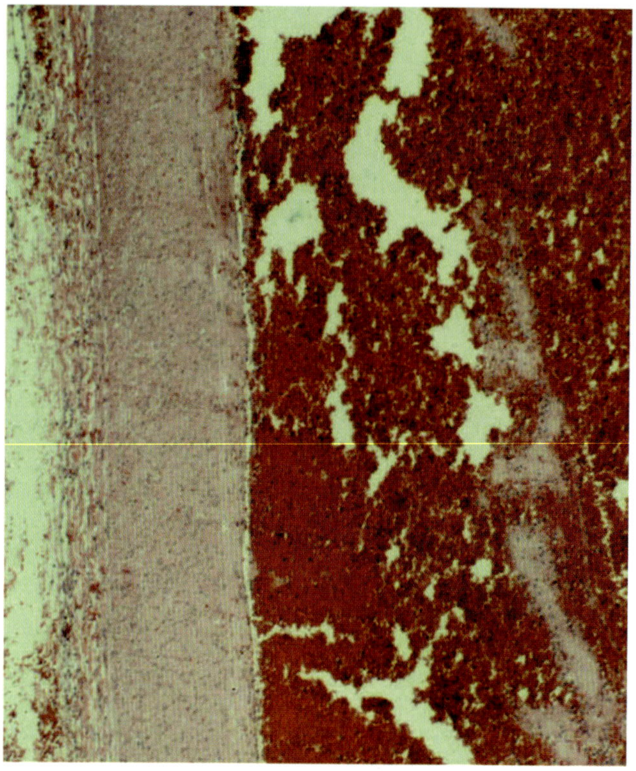

(A)

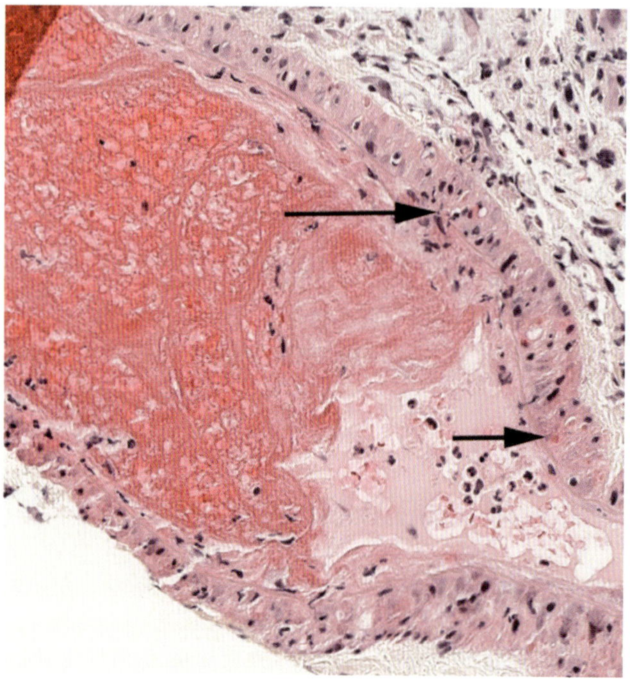

(B)

图 85.9 (A)由于"技术性原因",HE 染色显示大血管内血栓,动脉壁结构完全正常。(B)与重度排斥反应相关的动脉血栓。动脉壁 HE 染色显示区域细胞核消失(坏死,下箭头)和血管腔内炎症细胞浸润(上箭头)。

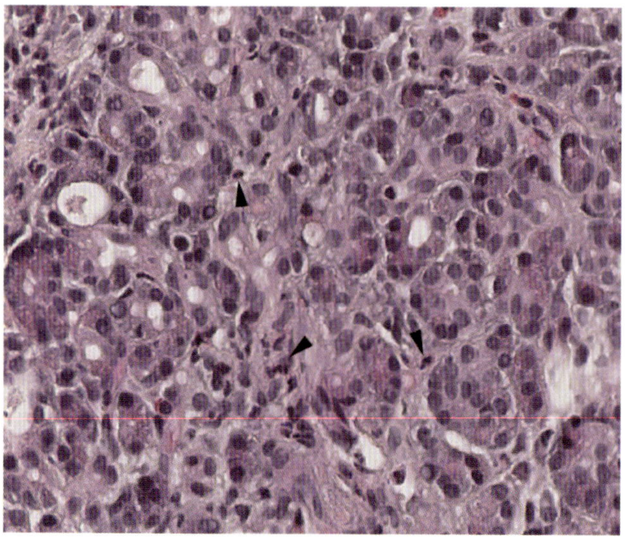

图 85.8 轻度缺血性胰腺炎的特点是腺泡细胞损伤（如细胞肿胀、单个或多个细胞丢失)、少量中性粒细胞(箭头)和巨噬细胞浸润。整体特征需与急性 AMR 相鉴别。

炎症和不同程度的动脉内膜炎在 ACMR 中更常见。移植物丢失需进行系统性组织学评估，分析移植物丢失的确切原因，评估内容包括大血管、胰腺实质应该足够多的中、小血管和 C4d 染色[8,13,14,42,86]。回顾性分析发现血清中 PRA 及 DSA 升高多见于早期伴有暴发性移植胰腺血栓形成的重度 AMR 患者[5,42]。

• 后期移植胰腺血栓形成是移植胰腺丢失的一个公认的原因。这个过程也与基本血管病变相关，这种病变可能是免疫介导的（急性或慢性活动性移植排斥反应）或者可能是非免疫性的（如动脉粥样硬化）[42,84]。

全胰腺移植中慢性排斥反应和移植胰腺硬化

尽管有良好的、及时的抗排斥反应治疗，急性 ACMR 发生后胰腺实质仍然可见不同程度的不可逆纤维化改变。纤维瘢痕生成与炎症细胞浸润范围、腺泡细胞损伤严重程度成正比。胰腺小叶间隔单纯的炎性细胞浸润（轻度或 Banff 分级Ⅰ级 ACMR）可能完全消失并且腺泡功能不受影响；而融合的胰腺腺泡炎症反应和坏死促使胰腺腺泡间质胶原化，最终导致受影响的胰腺外分泌区消失[41]。

难治性急性 AMR 导致短期内（几周或几个月）移植胰腺功能丧失，主要原因是广泛的微血管和大血管闭塞及血栓形成。重度急性 AMR 中血栓形成和缺血性坏死主要由于弥漫性动脉和静脉坏死[43]。在较长期的 AMR 中，由于急性或慢性免疫球蛋白和补体诱导的微血管损伤及重塑，导致移植胰腺纤维化[13,117]，最终引起胰腺移植失败。

一般来说，慢性排斥反应的组织学表现为进行性的胰腺实质硬化，定义为胰腺小叶间的结缔组织间隔进行性纤维增宽和不同程度的腺泡小叶萎缩。所有外分泌组织最终消失，一些区域变得面目全非的，除了极少量残留在致密瘢痕组织内的胰岛。胰腺腺泡消失预示着胰岛逐渐消失，最终导致血糖控制失调[41,118]。在慢性排斥反应中，由于增生性动脉内膜炎或移植动脉病变可导致动脉分支狭窄[32,34,41,42]。

胰腺移植患者长期使用抑制钙调磷酸酶的免疫抑制剂（环孢素、他克莫司），可能会出现广泛的小动脉玻璃样变性，但不清楚这是否影响移植胰腺硬化过程[8]。此外，全身动脉粥样硬化的患者，移植胰腺粥样硬化栓塞滞留可引起迟发性胰腺炎并且进一步引起缺血性损害[119]。慢性排斥反应和移植胰腺纤维化分期标准如下（Banff 分级体系的诊断分类 6）（框 85.2）。

十二指肠移植病理学

在全胰腺移植中胰腺外分泌物引流术通过移植十二指肠段引流完成[4]。各种病理过程可能会影响十二指肠移植段，包括技术问题（如缺血、吻合口瘘）、巨细胞病毒感染及排斥反应。

活检类型

20 世纪 90 年代常使用膀胱镜下十二指肠活检，当时移植胰腺外分泌物常通过膀胱引流排出。这段时期，人们从这些病例的研究中积累了许多重要的经验[34,66,71,73,74,120,121]。十二指肠组织偶然也可以通过经皮活检获得。

最近，对于移植胰腺与邻近空肠吻合的患者，人们又重新通过上消化道胃肠内镜获得十二指肠活检样本进行评估。Margreiter 等[75]研究中详细介绍了肠镜下移植胰腺活检技术。这些学者研究发现，75%的患者（76/102 病例）可经上消化道胃肠内镜获得移植胰腺与十二指肠吻合口处合格的样本，而 25%的患者无法通过上消化道胃肠内镜获得。约 1/3 活检样本病理学特征表现为从不明确意义的炎症反应到严重排斥反应。每一例均需评估 CMV 感染肠炎和（或）Giardia 鞭毛虫感染。这样可以在 65%的十二指肠样本中确认患者是否有排斥反应[75]。

移植十二指肠吻合口病理发现

技术问题（十二指肠漏）：感染

缺血和不完善的手术方式可能会导致十二指肠和膀胱或小肠之间的吻合口破裂[94]。基于这些因素进行的移植胰腺活检病理学特征可能表现为一些特定的病变，如 CMV 感染相关穿孔或可能仅表现出一些非特异性病变，如吻合口周围组织坏死和急性炎症反应等。邻近腹膜表面常常可见急性纤维素性渗出或化脓性浆膜炎[122]。

框 85.2 Banff 胰腺移植排斥反应分级模式，2011 更新诊断类别*

1.正常

小叶间隔内无炎症或非活跃性间隔、单核细胞炎症不累及导管、静脉、动脉或腺泡。没有移植物纤维化表现。纤维组织局限于正常小叶间隔且纤维组织的量与小叶结构的大小成比例(导管和静脉)。胰腺实质显示无萎缩或损伤的迹象

2.不确定的排除反应

小叶间隔内活动性炎症，但整体特征未达到轻度细胞介导的急性排斥反应的诊断标准

3.急性T细胞介导的排斥反应‡

Ⅰ级，轻度急性T细胞介导的排斥反应

小叶间隔内活化的炎症细胞浸润(浸润细胞包括活化母细胞样淋巴细胞±嗜酸性粒细胞)：小叶间隔小静脉炎(静脉内皮下炎性细胞聚集和静脉内皮损伤)，胰腺小叶间导管炎(胰腺小叶间导管上皮炎症细胞浸润和导管损伤)和(或)局灶性腺泡炎症。每个小叶不超过2个炎症病灶伴或不伴轻微的小叶腺泡细胞损伤

Ⅱ级，中度急性T细胞介导的排斥反应(需要与AMR鉴别)

多灶性腺泡炎症(但不融合性或弥漫性)(每个小叶≥3)伴灶性(个别)腺泡细胞损伤和丢失

和(或)轻度动脉内膜炎(极少量，<25%黏膜固有层)

Ⅲ级，重度急性T细胞介导的排斥反应(需要与AMR鉴别)

弥漫性(广泛而密集的)腺泡炎症伴有局灶性或弥漫性多细胞/融合的腺泡细胞坏死

和(或)中度或重度动脉内膜炎(>25%黏膜固有层)

和(或)透壁性炎症-坏死性动脉炎

4.抗体介导的排斥反应(见下文诊断要素*)

*确定血清内供体特异性抗体

*组织损伤的形态学证据(胰腺腺泡间炎症/毛细血管炎、腺泡细胞损伤肿胀/坏死/凋亡/脱落、血管炎、血栓形成)

*腺泡间毛细血管C4d染色阳性(≥5%腺泡小叶表面积)

- 急性AMR：具备三条诊断依据*
- 符合急性AMR：具备三条诊断依据中的两条*
- 需要排除AMR：仅具备三条诊断依据中的一条*

详见急性AMR组织学分级表†

慢性活性抗体介导的排斥反应

具备类别4*和6的特征而没有类别3的特征

5.慢性移植动脉病

动脉内膜纤维化伴单核细胞纤维内浸润

6.慢性移植排斥反应/移植物纤维化

Ⅰ期(轻度移植物纤维化)

纤维间隔增宽；纤维化范围累及活检组织条的范围<30%，腺泡小叶结构出现紊乱，但多数小叶中心区结构正常

Ⅱ期(中度移植物纤维化)

纤维化范围累及活检组织条的范围30%~60%。多数小叶周围外分泌腺出现萎缩(不规则轮廓)并且小叶中心区出现纤细的纤维组织穿插分割

Ⅲ期(重度移植物纤维化)

纤维化占主导，纤维化范围累及活检组织条的范围超过60%，仅剩残留腺泡组织和(或)胰岛细胞

7.胰岛病理

自身免疫性糖尿病复发

- 胰岛炎
- 选择性的β细胞缺失
- 胰岛淀粉样蛋白沉积(淀粉样物)
- 胰岛细胞药物毒性

8.其他组织学诊断

排除了急性和(或)慢性排斥反应的病变(如CMV胰腺炎、PTLD)

AMR，抗体介导排斥反应；CMV，巨细胞病毒；PTLD，移植后淋巴增生性疾病。

*考虑到临床病理意义的重要性，类别2~8可同时诊断，并应列在诊断报告中。

†急性AMR组织学分级(见框85.1)。

‡典型ACMR和AMR的组织学特征(见表85.2)。

参见框85.3的特定病变的形态定义和表85.3的其他组织学诊断。

急性移植排斥反应

胰腺移植引流的早期经验表明(胰腺移植经皮十二指肠造瘘术)：移植十二指肠的裸露部分炎症反应与胰腺的急性排斥反应相关[123]。十二指肠和胰腺的样本早期研究证实十二指肠急性排斥反应通常伴发胰腺排斥反应(72%~100%的一致性)[71,73]；但每个器官排斥反应，甚至CMV感染各不相同[71,124]。

在一些狗[125]、猪[126]和啮齿类动物[127]的研究表明，十二指肠和胰腺中的排斥反应高度一致，但是，有趣的是，在啮齿类动物研究中也发现针对十二指肠排斥反应的治疗效果要较胰腺排斥反应治疗效果好[127]。

十二指肠吻合口黏膜移植排斥反应的分级标准还没有确立。一般来说，轻度急性排斥反应表现为十二指肠固有层中包括中性粒细胞在内的炎症细胞增加，黏膜绒毛变平和黏膜上皮细胞凋亡(图85.10)。重度排斥反应中出现融合上皮坏死及整个黏膜上皮层缺失。坏死可扩展到全层，包括黏膜固有肌层。动脉受累(如动

脉内膜炎、坏死性动脉炎),作为移植胰腺排斥反应的一个病理特征,也会出现在十二指肠[71]。急性排斥反应引起的十二指肠穿孔已有 1 例报道[128]。

慢性排斥反应和移植胰腺纤维化

伴发进展性慢性排斥反应和纤维化的胰腺移植失败患者,胰腺-十二指肠吻合口活检表现出类似的硬化性改变(图 85.11)。后者典型特征为十二指肠黏膜明显变得平坦、萎缩甚至减少,使得反应性增生的上皮细胞厚度减少。深层肌肉和结缔组织被纤维组织不规则取代并且常伴有散在的炎症细胞浸润,类似于出现在胰腺实质本身的病变。

十二指肠吻合口急、慢性移植排斥反应的特定的病理特征仍然不清。对移植十二指肠的 ACMR 及 AMR 的病理特征进行系统性研究是必要的,以便确定这类组织是否可以替代胰腺活检组织。目前,这方面的研究作为 Banff 2013 胰腺工作组的一部分正在进行中[129]。

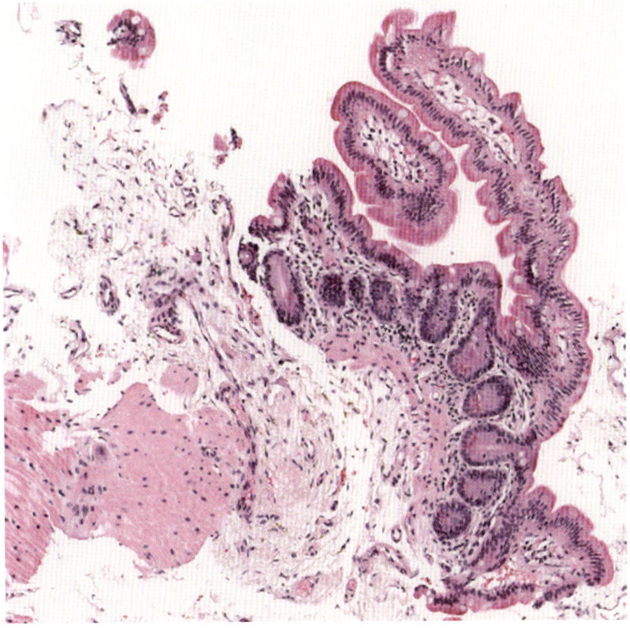

(A)

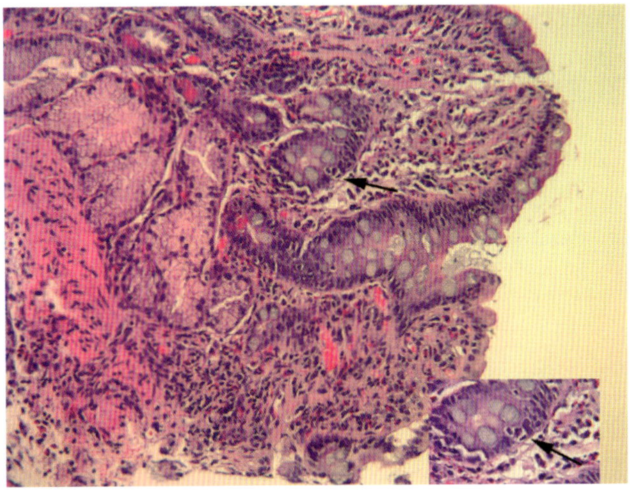

(B)

图 85.10 (A)一名移植物功能正常的患者十二指肠吻合口处十二指肠黏膜活检。十二指肠黏膜显示保存完整的小肠绒毛和固有层内常见的炎症细胞,没有出现急性排斥反应的特征。(B)十二指肠黏膜吻合口轻度急性排斥反应表现为变钝的小肠绒毛,固有层内炎症细胞增加,包括大量的嗜酸性粒细胞,以及偶然出现肠上皮凋亡细胞(箭头)。

Banff 胰腺移植排斥反应:Banff 分级体系(2011 年更新版,表 85.2)

诊断类别:特别考虑的内容

Banff 分级体系包含 8 个诊断类别,涵盖了胰腺移植中出现的一系列组织病理变化。类似于其他移植器官,已获认可的两种主要的移植排斥反应包括 T 淋巴细胞介导的排斥反应和抗体介导的排斥反应[13,14,22,23,45]。对于每一种排斥反应,已经认识急、慢性病变的组织学特征,并且提出了界定严重程度分级的标准。在 Banff 胰腺移植体系中使用的特定的组织学特征见框 85.3。

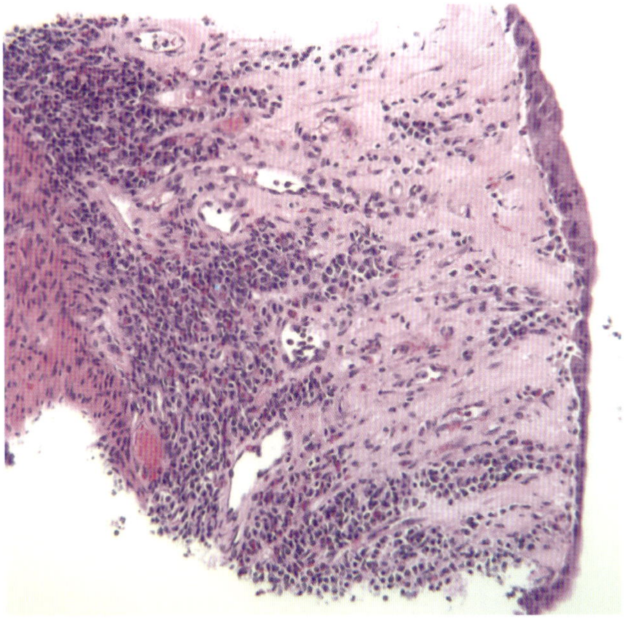

图 85.11 十二指肠吻合口重度慢性排斥反应。小肠黏膜绒毛变平坦、明显纤维化和固有层硬化以及伴随大量浆细胞的慢性炎症细胞浸润。

框 85.3 推荐的移植胰腺活检排斥反应组织病理学诊断

1.**腺泡细胞损伤/坏死** 腺泡细胞肿胀、空泡化和(或)核固缩以及出现凋亡小体,甚至可见因腺泡细胞溶解性坏死而出现所谓的细胞丢失现象
2.**腺泡炎症** 外分泌腺泡内与小叶间隔相似的炎性细胞浸润
3.**腺泡炎性损伤/局灶性** 1个腺泡区域内≥10个淋巴细胞/嗜酸性粒细胞浸润
4.**"活动性"的移植物动脉血管病变** 在移植胰腺内动脉分支内膜内由于成纤维细胞、肌成纤维细胞和平滑肌细胞增生使动脉管腔狭窄的同时仍可见内膜下T淋巴细胞和巨噬细胞在内的单核炎症细胞浸润
5.**毛细血管炎** 胰腺腺泡间和胰岛细胞周围毛细血管扩张伴有中性粒细胞和单核细胞浸润
6. **C4d 半定量分级** 弥漫性阳性:≥50%的腺泡间毛细血管内皮细胞呈阳性;局灶性阳性:5%~50%的腺泡间毛细血管内皮细胞呈阳性;弱阳性/阴性:<5%的腺泡间毛细血管内皮细胞呈阳性
7.**胰腺小叶间导管炎** 胰腺小叶间胰腺导管出现单核细胞和(或)嗜酸性粒细胞浸润伴有导管上皮细胞损伤甚至引起导管上皮细胞脱落
8.**局灶性腺泡炎症** 每个小叶内≤2个局灶性炎性浸润灶但没有胰腺腺泡细胞损伤表现
9.**轻微的动脉内膜炎** 罕见的、偶然出现的、动脉分支内皮下(内膜下)单核细胞浸润
10.**中-重度动脉内膜炎** 动脉内肌壁间易见(多达6~8个)淋巴细胞浸润伴有以下任何内膜损伤特点:内皮细胞肥大、纤维蛋白渗出、中性粒细胞和(或)巨噬细胞黏附和渗出以及内膜肌成纤维细胞增生
11.**多细胞/融合性胰腺腺泡细胞损伤/坏死** 呈簇的胰腺腺泡细胞损伤/坏死
12.**多灶性腺泡炎症** 每个胰腺小叶内≥3个局灶性炎性细胞浸润伴随单个孤立的腺泡细胞损伤或坏死,炎性浸润灶之间可有正常腺泡
13.**坏死性动脉炎** 动脉分支管壁局灶性或全周纤维素样坏死,伴或不伴有透壁性炎性细胞浸润
14.**神经纤维和神经纤维周围炎症** 胰腺小叶间隔内神经纤维分支周围或内部炎性细胞浸润(注:由于活检组织的局限性,这一病变在穿刺活检中罕见)
15.**胰腺小叶间隔内炎性细胞浸润** 以单核细胞为主的炎性细胞浸润,包括活化的淋巴细胞和数量不定的嗜酸性粒细胞,有时也以嗜酸性粒细胞为主要的炎性细胞
16.**严重/广泛的腺泡炎症** 均匀弥漫而广泛的小叶内腺泡炎性细胞浸润伴有灶性或弥漫性多细胞/融合性腺泡细胞损伤/坏死,可有或无正常的腺泡组织
17.**单个细胞/零星的腺泡细胞损伤/坏死** 仅累及孤立的腺泡细胞,而周边绝大多数细胞正常。
18.**移植动脉血管病** 移植胰腺内动脉分支纤维内膜增生导致管腔变窄。其狭窄程度依据动脉管腔截面积丧失的程度分级:轻度,<25%的管腔截面积丧失;中度,26%~50%的管腔截面积丧失;重度,> 50%的管腔截面积丧失
19.**小静脉炎** 胰腺小叶间隔内细小静脉血管周围袖套状炎性细胞浸润,伴有血管内皮下炎性细胞黏附和内皮细胞损伤

Adapted from[14] Drachenberg et al. *American Journal of Transplant*. 2008;8:1237 with permission from Wiley.

正常特征

在正常的胰腺组织中,炎症细胞浸润是罕见的,或是非常稀疏的、失活的单核细胞(如小淋巴细胞、浆细胞罕见)浸润。如果有轻微的炎症,那也是局灶的或者局限于小叶间隔而不会累及任何间隔组织(如血管、导管、神经)(图 85.2)。

足量样本且均含有以上组织学特征实际上排除了ACMR的诊断。因此,这些组织学特征往往会在功能良好的移植胰腺活检中遇到[65,90,130]。活检中出现"正常"的组织学特征也可能在其他临床情况下遇到,特别是患有高血糖症的患者中。鉴别诊断包括:

1.复发性自身免疫性疾病的晚期阶段(如胰岛炎溶解以后)[111];

2.药物毒性,以胰岛细胞的损伤或空泡化为特征[83];

3.早期或轻度 AMR[51]。

不确定的排斥反应

病理学特征:胰腺小叶间隔可见局灶活动性炎性细胞浸润(活动性改变±嗜酸性粒细胞),但总体特征未达到轻度排斥反应标准(如部分小叶间隔内静脉或导管受累,但缺乏任何内皮细胞或上皮细胞受累证据)(图 85.12)。

这些组织学特征在移植胰腺功能良好和功能障碍的活检中均可以看到。类似于肾脏移植的"交界性"分类,这些组织学特征可能表示早期或治疗过的急性排斥反应,或者是完全非特异性的排斥反应[90,130]。

活检组织成分内出现"不确定"排斥反应改变与患者治疗相关,而治疗方案的制订最终取决于临床判断。相对于治疗效果好的急性细胞介导的排斥反应,由于"不确定"排斥反应的组织学异质性特点,患者相应的治疗效果明显不同[90]。

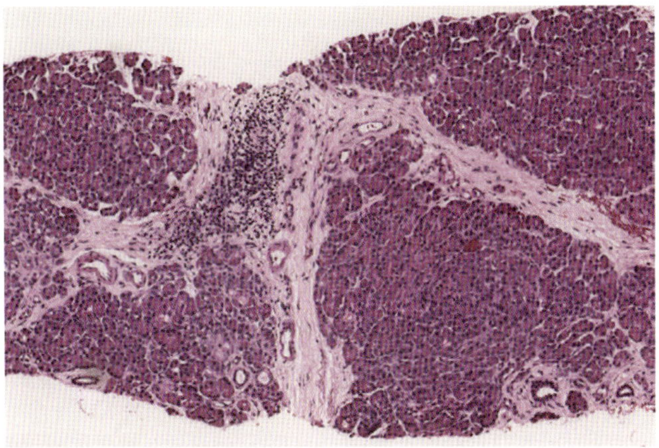

图 85.12　Banff 分级中不确定的排斥反应。图像显示胰腺小叶间隔内灶性单核细胞浸润，但没有累犯腺泡、脉管或导管。

急性 T 淋巴细胞介导的排斥反应

基于病变严重程度，ACMR 分为轻度、中度和重度（分别为Ⅰ级、Ⅱ级和Ⅲ级）[5,24,32,33,36-40,131]。急性期 ACMR 诊断前提是同时行 C4d 染色以排除 AMR 成分[13,14]。

Ⅰ级/轻度 ACMR

病理学特征：胰腺小叶间隔内不仅出现炎性细胞（如母细胞样淋巴细胞，不同程度嗜酸性粒细胞）浸润，而且出现小静脉血管炎、导管炎和（或）局灶腺泡炎症。这些组织学特征在不同的小叶间隔区域可能会有所不同，然而，出现任何程度的小静脉血管炎（静脉血管内皮细胞下炎症细胞聚集伴有静脉内皮损伤）或小叶间隔导管炎（胰腺导管上皮炎性细胞浸润和损伤）都足以诊断Ⅰ级/轻度 T 细胞介导的排斥反应（图 85.13）。胰腺实质中周围神经束支炎性细胞浸润也是Ⅰ级 ACMR 的特征。

在移植胰腺活检中，出现Ⅰ级排斥反应的局灶性腺泡炎症并不少见，而且，通常在小叶间隔结缔组织和腺泡小叶之间的交界处出现（例如，外分泌区周围）。

Ⅰ级排斥反应，也包括由于取样原因，在活检标本中未见受累小叶间隔成分，仅见局灶性腺泡炎症的病例。

在任何情况下，在Ⅰ级排斥反应中，腺泡炎症反应应该是局灶性的（即每个小叶内不超过 2 个微小炎症性病灶但未见腺泡细胞损伤现象——凋亡或坏死）。腺泡炎症成分通常类似于小叶间隔炎症细胞浸润的成分。

具有Ⅰ级排斥反应的活检标本偶尔会出现在移植胰腺功能良好的患者中[130]，然而，在移植胰腺功能不全的活检标本往往比较容易发现（通常情况下，血清中淀粉酶/脂肪酶的比例增加，或者膀胱引流的胰腺移植患者尿淀粉酶减少）[12,36,65]。

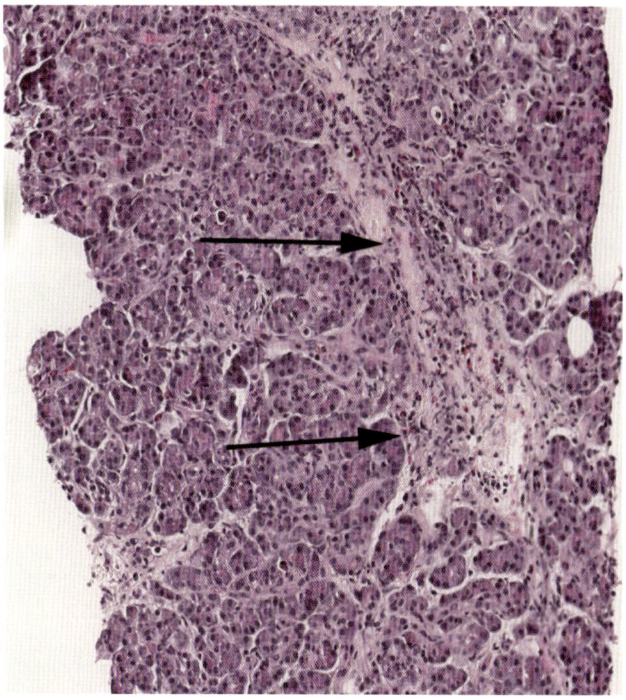

(A)

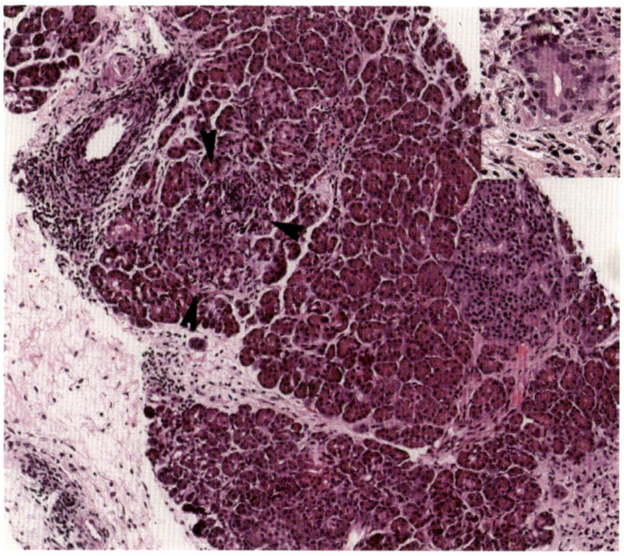

(B)

图 85.13　(A,B)轻度 ACMR（Banff 分级：Ⅰ级）。ACMR 的病理特征表现为胰腺小叶间隔炎症和水肿（长箭头）、小静脉炎及腺泡炎症（箭头）。右上图显示的导管炎也是 ACMR 的一个常见特征。

Ⅱ级/中度 ACMR

典型的胰腺小叶间隔炎性细胞浸润上文已有描述。ACMRⅡ级除Ⅰ级的特征外，还有 2 个额外的组织学特征，即多灶性胰腺腺泡炎症和轻微的动脉内膜炎，这些特征可以单独存在或同时存在。

多灶性胰腺腺泡炎症。Ⅱ级最常见的组织学特征是多灶腺泡炎症(每个小叶内≥3个病灶)且伴随单个孤立的腺泡细胞损伤或丢失。尽管ACMRⅡ级中腺泡炎症容易发现；但是，腺泡炎症不融合或弥漫成片。从实用的角度来看，在炎症病灶之间完全非炎症性腺泡或外分泌区很容易辨别。缺乏融合炎症病灶有助于区别中度与重度排斥反应(见下文)。明显的腺泡炎症常常与腺泡细胞损伤有关，但在中度(II级)的腺泡细胞损伤应该是点状的(单个的)(图85.14)。具体来说，腺泡细胞损伤可能出现以下特征：细胞丢失(等同于单个细胞大小的空的空间)、细胞胞浆肿胀和空泡化、核固缩、凋亡小体出现或单个细胞溶解性坏死。

轻微的动脉内膜炎。由于活检取样不同，当出现单一轻度局灶性动脉内膜炎（内膜下出现极少量但清晰可辨的单核细胞）时，便可归为中度排斥性反应(Ⅱ级)(图85.15)。后者的变化可能伴或不伴前面描述的小叶间隔内完整的炎症细胞群浸润。

从临床角度来看，中度排斥反应通常发生在移植胰腺功能障碍患者的活检中(血清中的淀粉酶或脂肪酶的升高或者膀胱引流的患者中尿淀粉酶降低)[12,36,65]。

III级/重度ACMR

重度ACMR有三个组织学特征，这些特征可以单独出现也可以同时出现。这些形态学特征也需要与中度或重度AMR相鉴别；后者通常表现为更加明显的间质性出血和局灶性或广泛性血管血栓形成。

严重的胰腺腺泡炎症和腺泡细胞损伤。病理特征：融合的或弥漫性(普遍的、广泛的)腺泡炎症伴局灶性或者弥漫性的多细胞或者融合性腺泡细胞坏死(图85.14B)。炎症反应细胞可能以淋巴样细胞为主导或者可能含有丰富的嗜酸性粒细胞或数量不等的中性粒细胞。根据定义，几乎整个胰腺腺泡或外分泌实质均有炎症反应，而且C4d染色阴性。

中度或重度动脉内膜炎。病理特征：肌动脉内膜内出现容易辨认(如超过6~8个)的淋巴细胞，这个特征本身足以诊断为Ⅲ级/重度ACMR。中度或重度动脉内膜炎通常与一些内膜损伤特征有关[即内皮细胞肥大、纤维蛋白渗漏、中性粒细胞和(或)巨噬细胞包被、血管内膜肌成纤维细胞激活]。

坏死性动脉炎。导致完全或部分动脉环周坏死的透壁性动脉炎症反应也归为重度ACMR(图85.9B)。然而，透壁性纤维素样动脉坏死也常常与AMR有关。因此，如果出现坏死性动脉炎，为了排除AMR，有必要进行C4d染色和DSA检测。

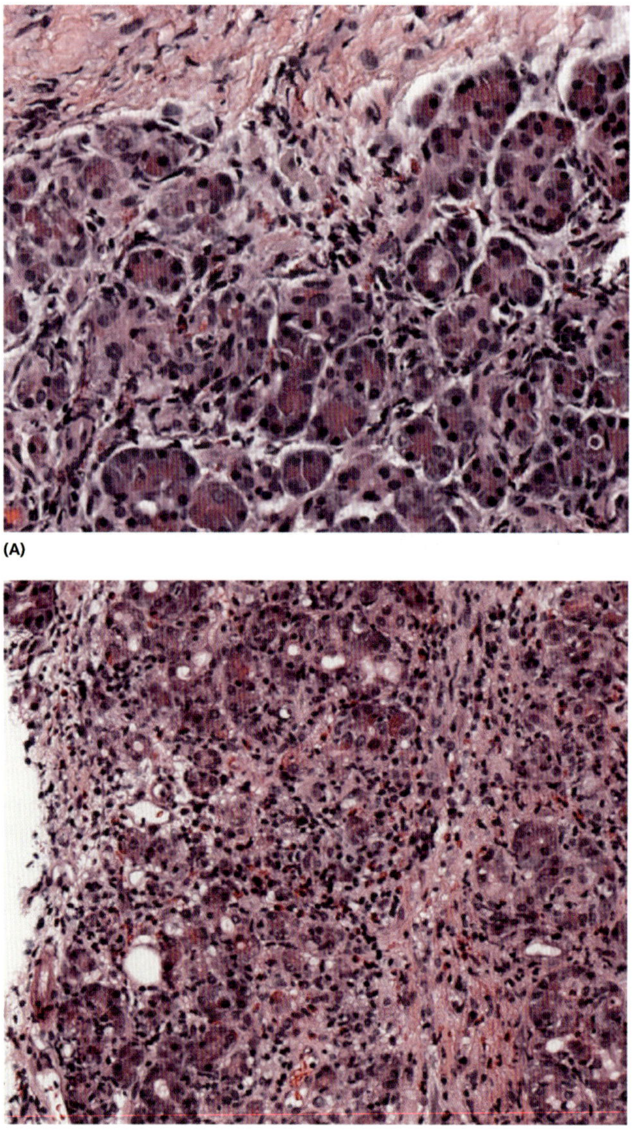

(A)

(B)

图85.14 (A)胰腺外分泌腺泡边缘区腺泡细胞炎症反应。虽然炎症细胞浸润导致腺泡排列结构紊乱，但仅有少量腺泡损伤。(B)广泛弥漫的腺泡炎症反应伴多处区域腺泡细胞损伤和丢失(如腺泡细胞质肿胀且透明、点状细胞丢失留下空洞样区域)。

以上三个病变出现其中一个便可诊断为重度ACMR，并预示移植胰腺效果不佳，因为它们与不可逆的胰腺实质损害有关，或者直接导致后者发生。对移植胰腺短期和长期的影响取决于腺泡损伤程度和出现动脉内膜炎或坏死的动脉大小和数量。类似于其他实体器官移植，动脉内膜炎增加了患急性或迟发性血栓形

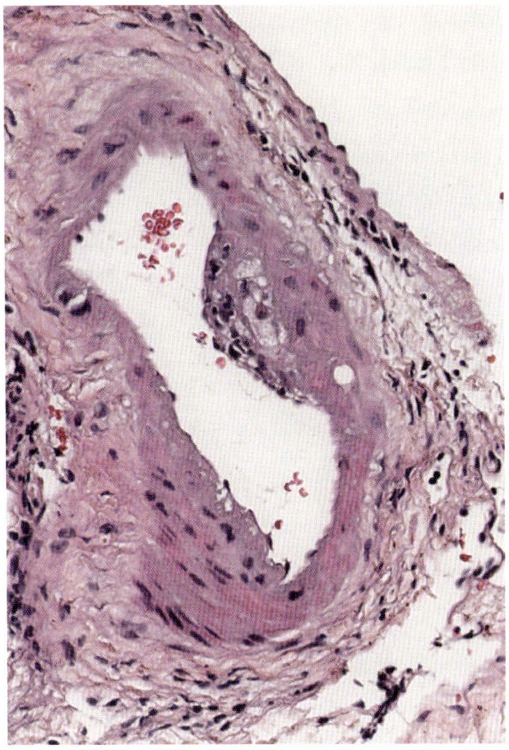

图 85.15 HE 显示小灶动脉内膜炎，其可划归为中度 ACMR (Banff 分级：Ⅱ级，详见 Banff 分级体系)。灶性泡沫样巨噬细胞动脉内膜下聚集提示移植动脉病变发展的可能，特别是若伴有持续的血管炎症。

成的风险(图 85.9B)。这种病变的出现也预示着移植胰腺血管病变[42,132]。

此类活检组织学特征与典型的移植胰腺功能障碍和失败相关，通常包括高血糖症[37,65,90]。

急性抗体介导的排斥反应

近年来，随着对人们胰腺 AMR 的了解，已经熟悉了其病理过程[56,133-135]。基于我们掌握的 AMR 相关知识，AMR 的 Banff 体系诊断标准包括三个要素(框 85.2)：外周血中的供体特异性抗体(DSA)、移植胰腺组织损伤的形态学特征和移植胰腺腺泡间毛细血管(IAC)阳性表达 C4d。值得注意的是，相当比例的 AMR 患者不可能同时出现以上三个特征；这可能与我们不能证实 DSA(即非 HLA 抗体)或者移植胰腺内没有足够的血管补体沉积有关(即 C4d 阴性的 AMR)。

因此，当三个诊断要素中出现两个时，可诊断为疑似急性 AMR；并且应该立即开始急性 AMR 治疗，特别是移植胰腺功能障碍的患者。

急性 AMR 的形态学特征包括不同程度的炎症反应和组织损伤(下文详述)。

在轻度的急性 AMR 中，胰腺腺泡或腺泡间表现为轻度的炎症反应，且常伴有轻微的点状腺泡细胞丢失或凋亡(图 85.16)。

在轻度胰腺炎的活检中出现腺泡细胞损伤，病理学家应警惕腺泡间炎症或毛细血管炎出现的可能，则需做 C4d 染色和 DSA 相关的检查以帮助鉴别。更明显的炎症反应导致腺泡间毛细血管炎，如在扩张和充血的 IAC 内出现的炎症细胞边集和血管腔内炎性细胞浸润(图 85.17)。腺泡间毛细血管炎形态和可能的发病机制类似于肾移植的肾小管周围毛细血管炎；但相对于肾小管周围毛细血管炎，胰腺 IAC 分布难以预测和相对稀疏。重度急性 AMR 可见广泛的微血管损伤并导致局灶性或融合性间质出血、水肿以及间质和腺泡细胞的多细胞性细胞坏死，使得腺泡间的毛细血管炎更难辨别。研究发现，与腺泡间炎症细胞浸润相关的

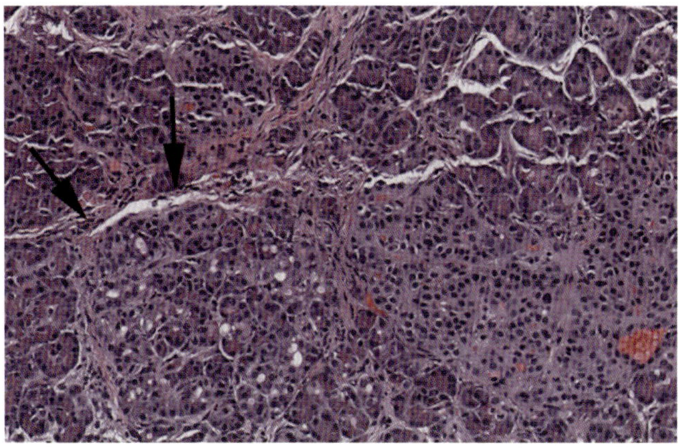

(A)

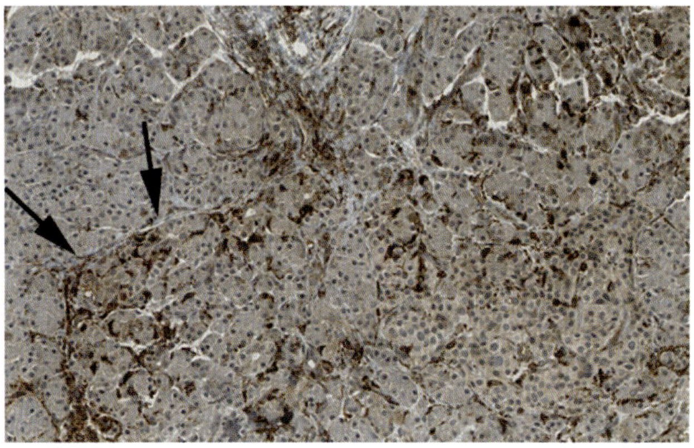

(B)

图 85.16 轻度急性 AMR。(A)在常规的 HE 染色中只有轻度的腺泡炎症；然而，腺泡细胞损伤比较局限(箭头)。(B)活检标本内多灶腺泡细胞损伤明显的区域，CD68 染色显示巨噬细胞增多(箭头)。

腺泡间毛细血管炎过度表达 C4d 蛋白，并且外周血中出现 DSA[11,56]。

非常严重或进展的急性 AMR 形态学特征接近于超急性排斥反应。这些特征包括在小或大血管内广泛的血管坏死和血栓形成，以及出现较小的或融合性胰腺实质坏死灶(图 85.18)。

急性 AMR 组织学分级(轻度、中度、重度)基于腺泡间炎症细胞浸润范围或毛细血管炎和胰腺组织损伤程度(框 85.1)。

慢性活动性 AMR

慢性活动性 AMR 组织学诊断包括以下三个特点：

1.出现急性 AMR 的特点(也见框 85.2 AMR 诊断)；

2.缺少急性 T 细胞介导的排斥反应(ACMR)特征；

3.移植胰腺纤维化[Banff 诊断分类 5 和(或)6]。

应用此诊断标准提示：持续的 AMR 是移植胰腺纤维化的主要原因，因此需要排除其他原因造成的移植胰腺纤维化或硬化，如急性 T 细胞介导的排斥反应前驱期。在临床实践中，当获得足够多的评估样本时，这一结论将是最准确的。

慢性移植胰腺动脉病变

病理诊断特征是出现活动性移植胰腺动脉病变，即移植胰腺动脉分支内膜下由于成纤维细胞、肌成纤维细胞和平滑肌细胞增生使动脉管腔狭窄；同时，内膜下可见 T 淋巴细胞和巨噬细胞在内炎性细胞浸润(图 85.19)。最初认为慢性移植胰腺动脉病变是 T 细胞介导的排斥反应[14,22,23,45]，但最近研究表明急性和慢性动脉病变也可能与 DSA 和 AMR 相关[48,109,110]。因此，这种病变被列为一个单独的形态学分类，以区别急性细胞介导的排斥反应和抗体介导的排斥反应。

由于取样原因，这种病变尽管很少在细针穿刺活检中发现，但常常出现在因慢性排斥反应导致胰腺移植失败的标本中[14,41,42]。

在临床上，识别活检样本中的慢性移植胰腺动脉病变是重要的。因为它表明有持续性或慢性同种免疫性损伤，而且慢性移植胰腺动脉病变与移植胰腺后期的血栓形成有关[42]。

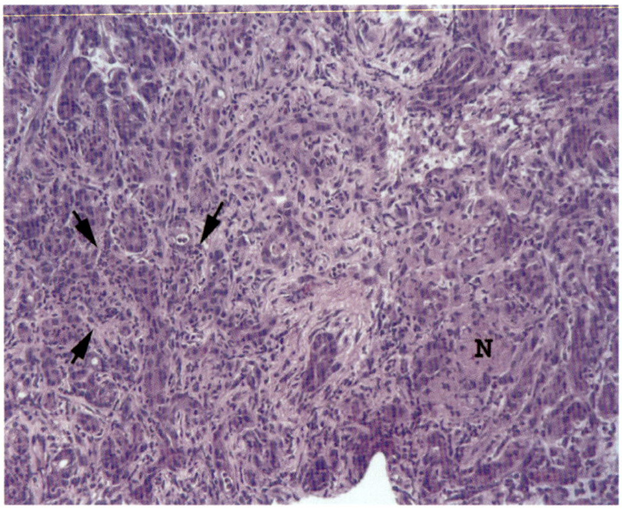

图 85.17 1 例中度急性 AMR 显示腺泡间大量炎症细胞浸润，包括中性粒细胞(箭头)；以及灶性坏死区出现(N)。

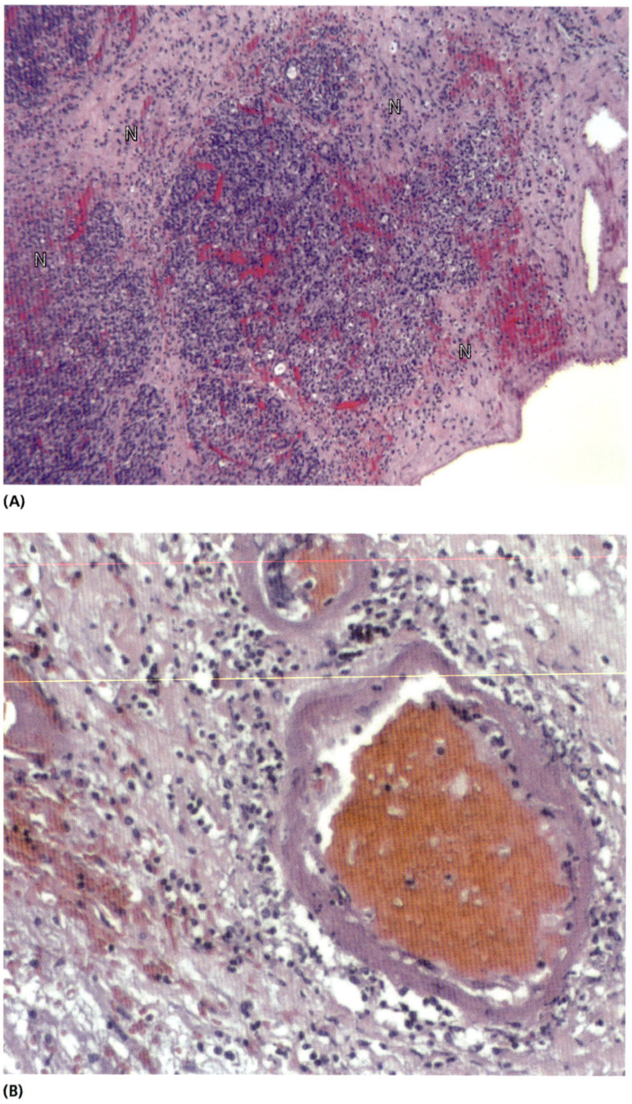

图 85.18 (A)中至重度急性 AMR：因微血管损伤而继发明显的组织损伤。此外，在严重充血和红细胞外渗的片状区域，胰腺实质出现地图样坏死区域(N)。(B)重度暴发性急性 AMR 与超急性排斥反应有重叠性特征。HE 显示整个血管壁纤维素样坏死。

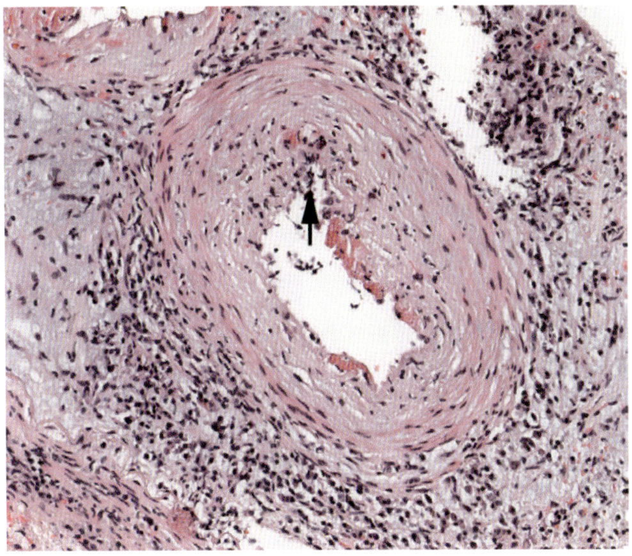

图 85.19　活化性移植动脉病变特征是：内膜下梭形细胞增生形成的纤维化和硬化导致动脉管腔狭窄。此外，纤维化区域有单核炎症细胞（偶尔出现嗜酸性粒细胞）浸润。箭头显示一个局灶动脉内膜炎以及黏附于右侧和左下方的动脉内膜小栓子。

移植胰腺慢性排斥反应和移植胰腺纤维化

在胰腺活检中，移植胰腺纤维化分期按照胰腺纤维化替代小叶成分的比例进行，可分为Ⅰ期/轻度（≤30%）、Ⅱ期/中度（≥30%但<60%）和Ⅲ期/重度（> 60%）（框 85.2 和图 85.20）[14,41]。

胰岛病理

由于逐渐认识到胰岛完整性对于移植胰腺功能的影响，在 2011 年版 Banff 分级体系中，对特别涉及这些特征的病变提出一个单独的分类[13]。这个分类的主要目的是认识以胰岛炎和（或）选择性 β 细胞丢失为特征的复发性自身免疫性糖尿病、胰岛淀粉样蛋白沉积以及胰岛细胞毒性药物（稍后讨论）。

目前，仍然不清楚抗体介导的排斥反应是如何影响胰腺胰岛功能的。在早期抗体介导的排斥反应研究报道中发现患者有高血糖症[51]，然而，在随后更多的活检研究中发现，早期介导的排斥反应的患者较少出现高糖血症[11,47,55,56]。大约 20%的患者样本中胰岛毛细血管内皮细胞表达 C4d 且外周血出现 DSA，但这些与高血糖症并不相关[11]。在重度坏死性抗体介导的排斥反应以及重度急性细胞介导的排斥反应中出现的高血糖症与胰腺实质坏死程度有关。

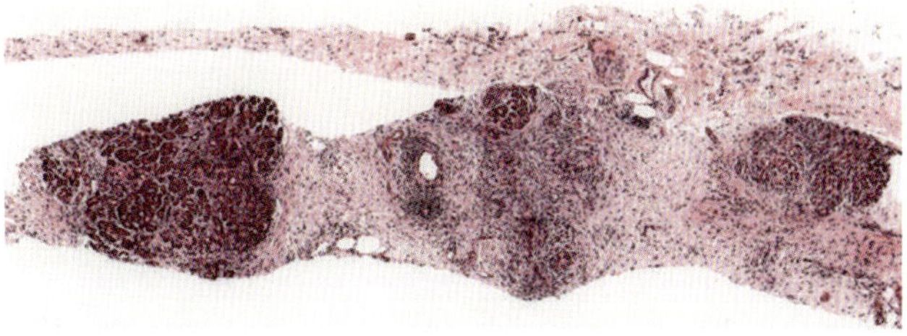

(A)

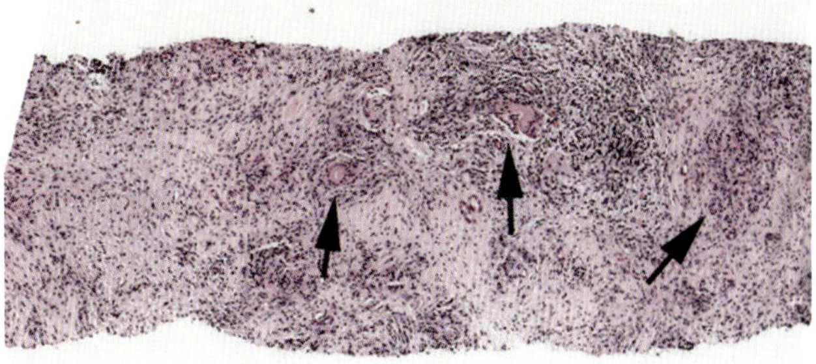

(B)

图 85.20　慢性移植排斥和移植物纤维化。由于结缔组织的显著增加和相应的外分泌（腺泡）实质丢失，胰腺结构明显紊乱。（A）可辨别三个萎缩性小叶，此被显著扩大的纤维间隔分离。（B）胰腺实质完全被结缔组织所取代。可见少量导管和腺泡结构（箭头）。注意：在两张图中，结缔组织中大量炎症细胞浸润表明持续性排斥反应（慢性 T 细胞介导的排斥反应的急性期）。

其他组织学诊断

目前免疫抑制治疗后，急性排斥反应发作已不多见。在移植胰腺功能障碍的患者活检中可以出现其他病理过程。这些特征可以单独或同时出现在其他诊断内（表 85.3）。

胰岛功能障碍的组织病理学特征

全胰腺移植中胰岛非特异的病理特征

即使 Langerhans 胰岛在正常胰腺实质中分布不均，绝大多数（95%）胰腺移植活检中仍能发现有一个或多个 Langerhans 胰岛[136]。

没有实验或临床证据表明，WPnTx 患者内分泌胰岛是同种免疫排斥反应的特定靶器官。在急性和慢性同种移植排斥反应中，胰岛病理变化似乎本质上是非特异性的，常继发于急性胰腺实质损伤并且随之引起胰腺纤维化或硬化。在这些病变中，病理特征包括胰岛炎性细胞浸润和偶尔出现坏死，这种坏死与胰岛急性

表 85.3 移植胰腺活检组织排斥反应以外其他的组织学诊断:Banff 诊断分类 8

病理诊断	主要病理组织学特征	临床表现
移植后缺血性胰腺炎	炎性细胞浸润:中性粒细胞和泡沫性巨噬细胞 浸润部位:轻微的炎性浸润常局限于小叶间隔内;严重的炎性浸润常常为弥漫性的 其他特征:脂肪坏死、水肿和间质出血。也可出现成簇的腺泡细胞凝固性坏死;小叶间隔由于水肿或(和)脂肪坏死而变宽,但不出现纤维化	血清淀粉酶和脂肪酶升高 尿淀粉酶下降* 如果有广泛的坏死,则可出现高血糖
胰腺周围炎/胰周积液	炎性细胞浸润:混合性(淋巴细胞、浆细胞、嗜酸性粒细胞和中性粒细胞) 浸润部位:小叶间隔和小叶周边 其他病变:不连续的纤维组织增生至小叶腺泡范围缩小,但小叶中央尚保持正常("硬化性外观")	局部或全身性感染性症状,腹痛、腹膜炎、胰周积液,血清淀粉酶和脂肪酶升高
巨细胞病毒性胰腺炎	炎性细胞浸润:主要是单核细胞 浸润部位:小叶间隔和腺泡内局灶性浸润 其他病变:腺泡细胞、血管内皮细胞或基质细胞胞浆巨细胞样改变	血清淀粉酶和脂肪酶升高 尿淀粉酶下降* CMV 病时的全身性感染症状,甚至十二指肠穿孔
移植后淋巴细胞异常增生性紊乱	炎性细胞浸润:低级别病变时包括淋巴母细胞、浆细胞、嗜酸性粒细胞等在内的多形性细胞;高级别病变时以淋巴细胞为主的单形性细胞(如淋巴瘤) 其他病变:淋巴细胞增生可为结节样和弥漫性,可出现坏死	早期可无症状,或仅表现为血清淀粉酶和脂肪酶升高 淋巴结肿大 出现肿瘤结节 可与急性排斥反应并存
细菌或真菌感染	炎性细胞浸润:可出现急性、慢性、化脓性、坏死性(脓肿性)以及肉芽肿形成 浸润部位:机体任意部位 其他病变:与其他器官的细菌和真菌感染相同	系统和(或)局部感染性症状 腹膜炎、十二指肠穿孔,血清淀粉酶和脂肪酶升高

*胰腺移植患者膀胱引流术时。

排斥反应的严重程度成一定比例。因而,炎症反应是随机的且浸润胰岛的炎性细胞与浸润周围的炎性细胞类似,或多或少地体现了一种"溢出"现象[5,33,37,39,136,137]。

胰腺移植时间较长的患者,胰岛分布和形态在很大程度上反映了持续的损伤和修复。慢性排斥反应中的广泛纤维化导致外分泌小叶结节状改变,以及引起胰岛的形状改变或胰岛可能仅由少数几个不规则分布的细胞簇构成,但仍含有能分泌胰岛素和胰高血糖素的细胞。相反,在一些移植胰腺中,大而似乎正常的胰岛细胞聚集也反映了胰岛代偿性增生[136,137]。在不到5%病因不明的病例中,若不考虑活检因素和一些未知的病因或意义,可以看到胰岛细胞的异型性、细胞核深染[136]。

胰岛细胞增生症,即在成人胰腺导管上皮细胞中出现分泌胰岛素细胞,似乎代表胰岛细胞异常分化而本身最有可能是胰岛细胞再生。动物胰腺移植模型已经证实了胰岛细胞增生症[138],而且在约4%的胰腺穿刺活检样品中也会出现,不论是否有移植胰腺排斥反应。胰岛细胞增生并没有显著的临床意义[136,137]。仅1例胰腺移植患者出现明显的胰岛细胞增生与低血糖发生有关[139]。

胰岛移植的病理组织学研究

在胰岛移植病例中,获得具有诊断价值的移植胰腺样品是困难的,因为注入的供体胰岛(通常总重为5~10g)分布于受体的整个肝脏(平均1.5kg)。Toso等人[140]分别研究了16例经皮肝穿刺活检标本和2例尸检标本中胰岛及邻近肝组织的形态学变化。31%的肝穿活检组织内可见到胰岛细胞,其能否识别与活检组织大小直接相关。一般情况下,尸检时肝脏组织中可以发现多处移植胰岛灶,相邻的肝实质往往表现出局部脂肪变性[140]。总的来说,移植的胰岛细胞有类似于正常胰岛的细胞成分，在组织活检时，少数病例表现为微小的炎症反应（胰岛炎），而与临床表现无关[140]。在 1 例胰岛移植失败后再次胰岛移植的患者尸体解剖中，肝脏组织内发现了类似的缺乏免疫损伤（异体或自体免疫）表现，并能看见能正常产生胰岛素的胰岛细胞[141]。C4d 染色在移植胰岛组织活检中一直是阴性的[21]，尽管有许多胰岛移植患者出现了 DSA[140,141]。

形态学研究匮乏明显限制了我们对胰岛移植失败原因的理解。胰岛丢失的原因可能与代谢或微环境应急有关的胰岛局部缺血、毒性损伤、胰岛再生破坏等相关。同时可能与轻度免疫排斥反应有关，但其真正的原因目前还不清楚[140-142]。监测胰岛移植非侵入性技术目前正在研发中[143,144]。

移植后糖尿病

技术上成功且移植胰腺功能良好也会出现移植后糖尿病（PTDM），可能是由于过量的胰岛素需求超过了全胰腺移植（WPnTx）中功能良好的胰腺生成量[145]。尽管 PTDM 在胰腺移植患者中更常见，但也与高比例的排斥反应相关，然而，系统性临床病理研究很难实现，从而导致目前对 PTDM 发病的机制仍然不清楚[145,146]。

在一项大数据的胰腺移植患者的队列研究中，PTDM 发病率在移植后 3、5 和 10 年后分别为 14%、17%和 25%[146]。发生 PTDM 的危险相关因素包括老年的捐赠者、单独胰腺移植（P=0.01）、较高的受体体重指数（BMI）、供体阳性而受体阴性 CMV 感染、移植后体重增加、较高的 6 个月空腹血糖、糖化血红蛋白和甘油三酯相对于高密度脂蛋白比值以及较高的术前 BMI 和胰岛素需求[145,146]。

自身免疫性Ⅰ型糖尿病复发

定义：全胰腺或胰岛成功移植的患者在经过一段时间胰岛素非依赖期后，由于自身免疫，患者出现 β 细胞破坏、胰岛素分泌减少并且重新依赖胰岛素。尽管有免疫抑制和忽视 HLA 匹配，Ⅰ型糖尿病仍然出现复发[77,111]。

复发性Ⅰ型糖尿病的基本临床和病理特征包括：在没有排斥反应的临床或病理特征的情况下胰岛素分泌选择性丢失，组织表现为胰岛炎和（或）β 细胞选择性丢失的组织学证据，以及复发之前自身抗体谷氨酸脱羧酶（GAD）持续升高[77]。Vendrame 等[147]研究 3 例糖尿病患者，发现明显的复发性自身免疫性疾病的证据：①自身反应性 T 细胞；②胰腺炎；③β 细胞群破坏[147]。

据估计，至少有 5%的全胰腺移植患者会出现复发性Ⅰ型糖尿病；然而，Ⅰ型糖尿病复发的准确诊断需要详尽的随访，随访困难一定程度上导致我们对这个过程认识不足[77,137]。

复发性Ⅰ型糖尿病的主要组织学特征是胰岛炎和选择性 β 细胞丢失（图 85.21）。这两个过程在胰岛中序贯性发生，但在整个胰腺实质中发生的时间并不统一。胰岛炎特点是选择性胰岛周围和胰岛内淋巴细胞浸润，明显不涉及其他胰腺实质区域（图 85.22）。炎症细胞分布与胰腺特征性的 ACMR 内炎症细胞分布相反。Ⅰ型糖尿病复发的进展导致选择性 β 细胞破坏，当 β 细胞完全消失时，受影响的胰岛中炎症反应也被清除。复发的Ⅰ型糖尿病导致胰腺移植失败的患者，HE 染色显示胰腺结构正常，且具有相对应的外分泌和内分泌成分。然而，胰岛素和胰高血糖素免疫组织化学染色结果证实选择性 β 细胞丢失[77,111,147,148]。由于胰岛炎病变是短暂的，炎症阶段很难看到。Ishida-Oku 等[149]报道，1 例患者胰腺移植 48 个月后发生血清抗 GAD 抗体阳性，同时出现突发的高血糖。组织样本发现 β 细胞丢失与胰岛炎和胰腺周围炎有关。炎症细胞主要包括 T 淋巴细胞和巨噬细胞[149]。

胰岛淀粉样变

胰腺移植胰岛内可出现刚果红染色阳性的胰淀粉素，也被称为胰岛淀粉样多肽（IAPP）。几十年来，人们已经发现许多Ⅱ型糖尿病患者胰岛中可出现淀粉样蛋白沉积，但其在疾病发展中的意义仍然不清楚[82]。

在正常情况下，胰岛淀粉样多肽（IAPP）是胰岛 β 细胞分泌胰岛素时分泌的蛋白质，与 C 肽和其他物质主要位于胰岛 β 细胞分泌颗粒周围[82]。在病理情况下，特别是高血糖时（如Ⅱ型糖尿病），IAPP 过度或异常表达形成含有淀粉样蛋白结构特征的不溶性聚合体。IAPP 淀粉样蛋白积聚导致胰岛细胞损伤和分泌胰岛素的细胞数量减少。导致 IAPP 积聚的机制仍然未明，但是已经明确 IAPP 和其他有助于淀粉样蛋白生成的物质的比例异常会影响淀粉样蛋白形成。在移植胰腺的胰岛，出现胰淀粉素沉积通常与血糖控制功能丧失有关（如高血糖）[19,82,150,151]。

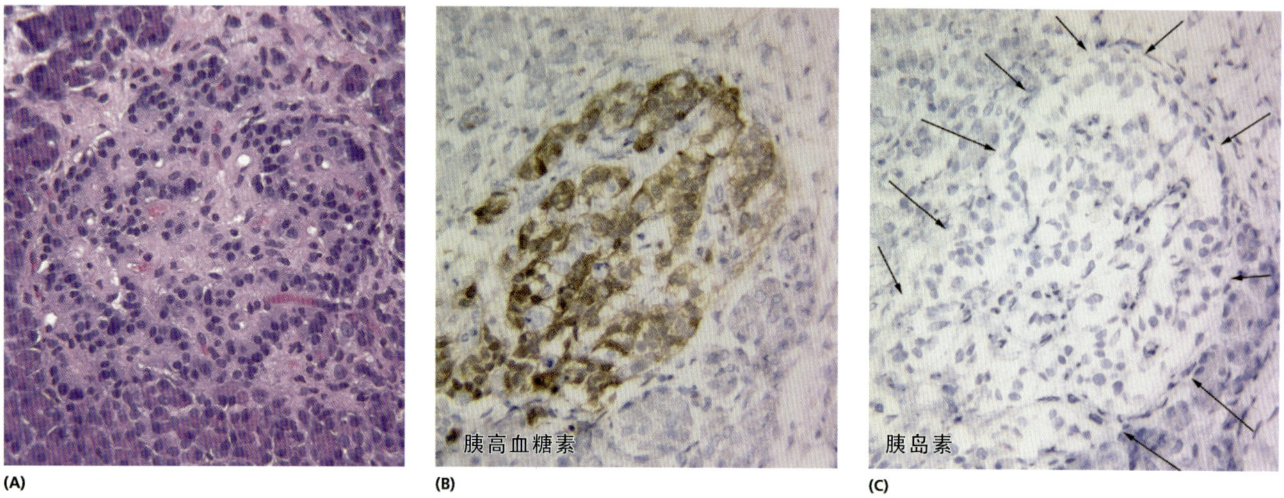

图 85.21 Ⅰ型糖尿病复发。(A)HE 图像显示一个全胰腺移植失败的 Langerhans 胰岛。在这个视野,胰岛缺乏任何具体的病理特征,虽然可见微小病灶,但相邻外分泌实质在正常范围内[即缺乏可以解释移植失败的慢性排斥反应和(或)移植纤维化特征]。(B)胰高血糖素染色显示许多胰高血糖素产生细胞(α 细胞)。(C)胰岛素染色显示 β 细胞完全缺失。

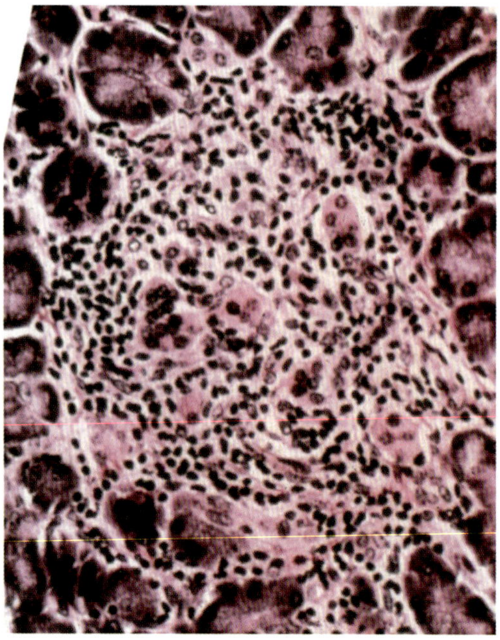

图 85.22 复发型Ⅰ型糖尿病早期表现为选择性胰岛及胰岛周围淋巴细胞浸润(胰岛炎)。

3 例接受门静脉胰岛注射的患者,其中 1 例 5 年后死于心肌梗死,在其胰岛中发现 IAPP 广泛沉积[150]。4 例胰岛移植的患者尸检中发现 3 例肝脏胰岛移植区有胰岛淀粉样蛋白沉积, 进一步研究表明淀粉样蛋白沉积可能是移植胰岛 β 细胞功能衰退的主要原因[19]。淀粉样蛋白沉积出现在 WPnTx 患者的胰岛中比较罕见(图 85.23)。

胰岛细胞药物毒性

动物研究表明,口服环孢霉素与胰岛素分泌减少、β 细胞密度降低、胰岛素合成减少和胰岛素分泌缺陷有关。类似的形态学结果也可以在口服他克莫司动物中发现[152]。

在临床表现为钙调磷酸酶抑制剂药物毒性的患者中,胰腺活检显示嗜酸性腺泡周围胰岛结构清晰;其形态学结果包括:胰岛细胞质肿胀和空泡化。在比较严重的病例中,如果有融合胰岛细胞丢失,那么可以看到胰岛细胞丢失形成空的区域(空洞)。偶尔也可看到胰岛内细胞凋亡产生的细胞碎片[83]。

胰岛素和胰高血糖素的免疫过氧化物酶染色显示:与对照组比较,胰岛细胞中胰岛素染色减少。电子显微镜可以观察到胰岛细胞中胰岛素致密核颗粒明显丢失。在药物减量或停药后胰岛组织学变化和临床表现是可逆的。在同时使用脉冲类固醇治疗急性排斥反应中,高血糖和药物毒性的组织学特征变得更严重[83]。

病毒感染与胰岛

感染巨细胞病毒(CMV)在 PTDM 发生和Ⅰ型糖尿病复发中的意义目前还不清楚,但研究发现 CMV 供体阳性而受体阴性与 PTDM 发生密切相关[146]。我们将在第 94 章中继续讨论巨细胞病毒和其他病毒感染。啮齿类动物模型研究发现,β 细胞易受 CMV 感染并且

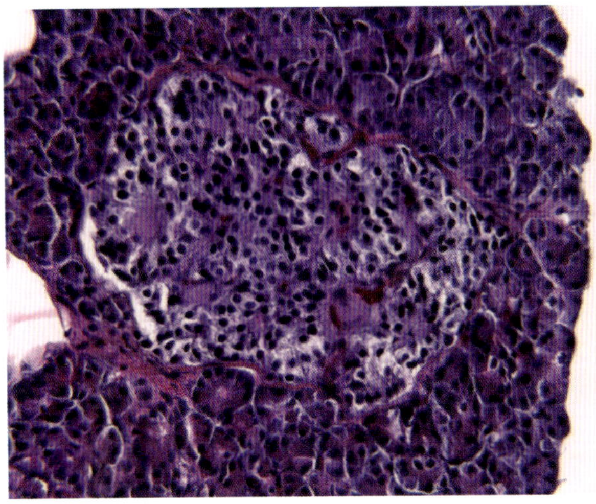

(A)

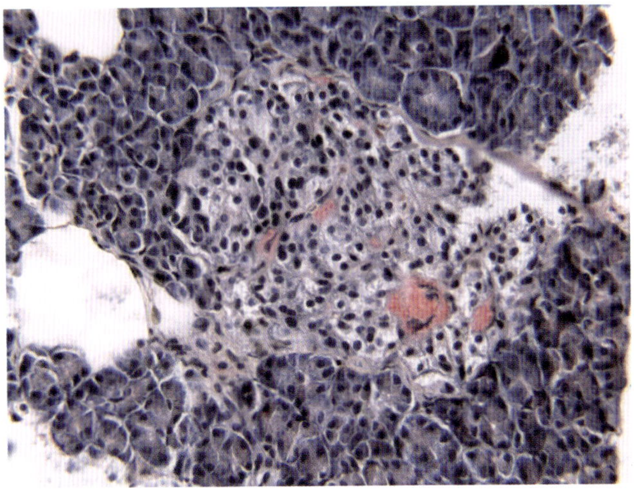

(B)

图 85.23 HE 染色显示在全胰腺移植中胰岛淀粉样蛋白沉积(A)和刚果红染色显示淀粉样蛋白细胞外沉积(B)。

能维持持续的低水平病毒基因表达[153]。感染 CMV 后，β 细胞免疫原性明显增强，并且促使更多的细胞表达免疫细胞激活配体[20,153,154]。

因此，在全胰腺移植或胰岛移植患者中，巨细胞病毒感染可影响 β 细胞活性和排斥反应的发展或糖尿病的复发。1 例胰腺移植患者临床研究发现，复发的 CMV 感染与针对胰岛自身抗原的体液和细胞自身免疫复发有关[155]。

最近研究表明，通过分子模拟病毒抗原表位和胰岛自身抗原，轮状病毒可能通过激活自身反应性 T 细胞从而引起胰岛细胞破坏。因此，这种病毒被认为是 I 型糖尿病的一个潜在病因[156]。在全胰腺移植或胰岛移植患者中，应进一步研究病毒感染与移植胰岛患者有限生存期的潜在关系。

总结

全胰腺和胰岛移植易受同种/自身免疫、炎症反应、代谢性疾病和技术不完善等因素影响，而且确切的系统性组织病理学诊断有助于临床医生制订合适的手术方案。人们已经研究了很多关于如何获取组织的方法，然而，相比其他形式的同种异体移植术，胰腺(特别是胰岛)移植获得组织是比较困难的。尽管如此，临床医生应该寻求明确的诊断并与病理学家合作共同关注这些 β 细胞替代治疗的患者。

(文雪 译 徐骁 校)

参考文献

1. Robertson P, Davis C, Larsen J, et al. Pancreas transplantation in type 1 diabetes. Diabetes Care. 2004;27(Suppl 1):S105.
2. Fioretto P, Caramori ML, Mauer M. The kidney in diabetes: dynamic pathways of injury and repair. The Camillo Golgi Lecture 2007. Diabetologia. 2008;51: 1347–1355.
3. Gremizzi C, Vergani A, Paloschi V, et al. Impact of pancreas transplantation on type 1 diabetes-related complications. Current Opinion in Organ Transplantation. 2010;15:119–123.
4. Sollinger HW, Odorico JS, Becker YT, et al. One thousand simultaneous pancreas-kidney transplants at a single center with 22-year follow-up. Annals of Surgery. 2009;250:618–630.
5. Sibley RK. Pancreas Transplantation. In: Sale GE, editor. Boston, MA: Butterworth Publishers; 1990.
6. Gruessner R, Sutherland D. Transplantation of the Pancreas; History of Pancreas Transplantation, 1st ed. New York, NY: Springer; 2004.
7. Gruessner AC, Sutherland DE, Gruessner RW. Pancreas transplantation in the United States: a review. Current Opinion in Organ Transplantation. 2010;15: 93–101.
8. Drachenberg C, Papadimitriou J. Pancreas Transplantation Pathology. In: Ruiz P, editor. New York, NY: Cambridge University Press; 2009.
9. Paraskevas S. Pancreas transplantation: in for the long run. Current Opinion in Organ Transplantation. 2012;17:71–72.
10. Troxell ML, Koslin DB, Norman D, et al. Pancreas allograft rejection: analysis of concurrent renal allograft biopsies and posttherapy follow-up biopsies. Transplantation. 2010;90:75–84.
11. Torrealba JR, Samaniego M, Pascual J, et al. C4d-positive interacinar capillaries correlates with donor-specific antibody-mediated rejection in pancreas allografts. Transplantation. 2008;86:1849–1856.
12. Gaber LW. Pancreas allograft biopsies in the management of pancreas transplant recipients: histopathologic review and clinical correlations. Archives of Pathology and Laboratory Medicine. 2007;131:1192–1199.
13. Drachenberg CB, Torrealba JR, Nankivell BJ, et al. Guidelines for the diagnosis of antibody-mediated rejection in pancreas allografts-updated Banff grading schema. American Journal of Transplantation. 2011;11:1792–1802.
14. Drachenberg CB, Odorico J, Demetris AJ, et al. Banff schema for grading pancreas allograft rejection: working proposal by a multi-disciplinary international consensus panel. American Journal of Transplantation. 2008;8:1237–1249.
15. Allen RD, Wilson TG, Grierson JM, et al. Percutaneous biopsy of bladder-drained pancreas transplants. Transplantation. 1991;51:1213–1216.
16. Shapiro AM. Strategies toward single-donor islets of Langerhans transplantation. Current Opinion in Organ Transplantation. 2011;16:627–631.
17. Ryan EA, Paty BW, Senior PA, et al. Five-year follow-up after clinical islet transplantation. Diabetes. 2005;54:2060–2069.
18. Waki K, Terasaki PI, Kadowaki T. Long term pancreas allograft survival in simultaneous pancreas kidney transplantation by Era: UNOS Registry Analysis. Diabetes Care. 2010;33:1789–1791.

19. Westermark GT, Davalli AM, Secchi A, et al. Further evidence for amyloid deposition in clinical pancreatic islet grafts. Transplantation. 2012;93:219–223.
20. Smelt MJ, Faas MM, de Haan BJ, et al. Susceptibility of human pancreatic beta cells for cytomegalovirus infection and the effects on cellular immunogenicity. Pancreas. 2012;41:39–49.
21. Campbell PM, Senior PA, Salam A, et al. High risk of sensitization after failed islet transplantation. American Journal of Transplantation. 2007;7:2311–2317.
22. Solez K, Colvin RB, Racusen LC, et al. Banff '05 Meeting Report: differential diagnosis of chronic allograft injury and elimination of chronic allograft nephropathy ('CAN'). American Journal of Transplantation. 2007;7:518–526.
23. Solez K, Colvin RB, Racusen LC, et al. Banff 07 classification of renal allograft pathology: updates and future directions. American Journal of Transplantation. 2008;8:753–760.
24. Dallman M. Immunobiology of Graft Rejection. In: Ginns LC, Cosimi AB, Morris PJ, editors. Malden, MA: Blackwell Science; 1988.
25. Steiniger B, Klempnauer J, Wonigeit K. Altered distribution of class I and class II MHC antigens during acute pancreas allograft rejection in the rat. Transplantation. 1985;40:234–239.
26. Daar AS, Fuggle SV, Fabre JW, et al. The detailed distribution of HLA-A, B, C antigens in normal human organs. Transplantation. 1984;38:287–292.
27. Daar AS, Fuggle SV, Fabre JW, et al. The detailed distribution of MHC Class II antigens in normal human organs. Transplantation. 1984;38:293–298.
28. Pelletier RP, Hennessy PK, Adams PW, et al. Clinical significance of MHC-reactive alloantibodies that develop after kidney or kidney-pancreas transplantation. American Journal of Transplantation. 2002;2:134–141.
29. Troppmann C, Gruessner AC, Papalois BE, et al. Delayed endocrine pancreas graft function after simultaneous pancreas-kidney transplantation: incidence, risk factors, and impact on long-term outcome. Transplantation. 1996;61:1323–1330.
30. Benz S, Schnabel R, Morgenroth K, et al. Ischemia/reperfusion injury of the pancreas: a new animal model. Journal of Surgical Research. 1998;75:109–115.
31. Benz S, Pfeffer F, Adam U, et al. Impairment of pancreatic microcirculation in the early reperfusion period during simultaneous pancreas-kidney transplantation. Transplant International. 1998;11(Suppl 1):S433–S435.
32. Steiniger B, Klempnauer J. Distinct histologic patterns of acute, prolonged, and chronic rejection in vascularized rat pancreas allografts. American Journal of Pathology. 1986;124:253–262.
33. Dietze O, Konigsrainer A, Habringer C, et al. Histological features of acute pancreatic allograft rejection after pancreaticoduodenal transplantation in the rat. Transplant International. 1991;4:221–226.
34. Carpenter HA, Engen DE, Munn SR, et al. Histologic features of rejection in cystoscopically directed needle biopsies of pancreatoduodenal allografts in dogs and humans. Transplantation Proceedings. 1990;22:707–708.
35. Severyn W, Olson L, Miller J, et al. Studies on the survival of simultaneous canine renal and segmental pancreatic allografts. Transplantation. 1982;33:606–612.
36. Nakhleh RE, Sutherland DE. Pancreas rejection: significance of histopathologic findings with implications for classification of rejection. American Journal of Surgical Pathology. 1992;16:1098–1107.
37. Nakhleh RE, Gruessner RW, Swanson PE, et al. Pancreas transplant pathology: a morphologic, immunohistochemical, and electron microscopic comparison of allogeneic grafts with rejection, syngeneic grafts, and chronic pancreatitis. American Journal of Surgical Pathology. 1991;15:246–256.
38. Dubernard JM, Traeger J, Touraine JL, et al. Rejection of human pancreatic allografts. Transplantation Proceedings. 1980;12(4 Suppl 2):103–106.
39. Drachenberg CB, Papadimitriou JC, Klassen DK, et al. Evaluation of pancreas transplant needle biopsy: reproducibility and revision of histologic grading system. Transplantation. 1997;63:1579–1586.
40. Sibley RK, Sutherland DE. Pancreas transplantation: an immunohistologic and histopathologic examination of 100 grafts. American Journal of Pathology. 1987;128:151–170.
41. Papadimitriou JC, Drachenberg CB, Klassen DK, et al. Histological grading of chronic pancreas allograft rejection/graft sclerosis. American Journal of Transplantation. 2003;3:599–605.
42. Drachenberg CB, Papadimitriou JC, Farney A, et al. Pancreas transplantation: the histologic morphology of graft loss and clinical correlations. Transplantation. 2001;71:1784–1791.
43. Hawthorne WJ, Griffin AD, Lau H, et al. Experimental hyperacute rejection in pancreas allotransplants. Transplantation. 1996;62:324–329.
44. Feucht HE, Opelz G. The humoral immune response towards HLA class II determinants in renal transplantation. Kidney International. 1996;50:1464–1475.
45. Sis B, Mengel M, Haas M, et al. Banff '09 meeting report: antibody mediated graft deterioration and implementation of Banff working groups. American Journal of Transplantation. 2010;10:464–471.
46. Loupy A, Hill GS, Suberbielle C, et al. Significance of C4d Banff scores in early protocol biopsies of kidney transplant recipients with preformed donor-specific antibodies (DSA). American Journal of Transplantation. 2011;11:56–65.
47. Torrealba JR, Odorico J. Antibody-mediated rejection of the pancreas allograft. Transplantation. 2009;88:292–293.
48. Sis B, Einecke G, Chang J, et al. Cluster analysis of lesions in nonselected kidney transplant biopsies: microcirculation changes, tubulointerstitial inflammation and scarring. American Journal of Transplantation. 2010;10:421–430.
49. Papadimitriou JC, Drachenberg CB, Munivenkatappa R, et al. Glomerular inflammation in renal allografts biopsies after the first year: cell types and relationship with antibody-mediated rejection and graft outcome. Transplantation. 2010;90:1478–1485.
50. Pascual J, Samaniego MD, Torrealba JR, et al. Antibody-mediated rejection of the kidney after simultaneous pancreas-kidney transplantation. Journal of the American Society of Nephrology. 2008;19:812–824.
51. Melcher ML, Olson JL, Baxter-Lowe LA, et al. Antibody-mediated rejection of a pancreas allograft. American Journal of Transplantation. 2006;6:423–428.
52. Heidt S, San Segundo D, Shankar S, et al. Peripheral blood sampling for the detection of allograft rejection: biomarker identification and validation. Transplantation. 2011;92:1–9.
53. Fattahi R, Modanlou KA, Bieneman BK, et al. Magnetic resonance imaging in pancreas transplantation. Topics in Magnetic Resonance Imaging. 2009;20:49–55.
54. Cashion AK, Sabek O, Driscoll C, et al. Serial analysis of biomarkers of acute pancreas allograft rejection. Clinical Transplantation. 2010;24:E214–E222.
55. Rangel EB, Malheiros DM, de Castro MC, et al. Antibody-mediated rejection (AMR) after pancreas and pancreas-kidney transplantation. Transplant International. 2010;23:602–610.
56. de Kort H, Munivenkatappa RB, Berger SP, et al. Pancreas allograft biopsies with positive C4d staining and anti-donor antibodies related to worse outcome for patients. American Journal of Transplantation. 2010;10:1660–1667.
57. Munivenkatappa RB, Philosophe B, Papadimitriou JC, et al. Interacinar C4d staining in pancreas allografts. Transplantation. 2009;88:145–146.
58. Kuo PC, Johnson LB, Schweitzer EJ, et al. Solitary pancreas allografts: the role of percutaneous biopsy and standardized histologic grading of rejection. Archives of Surgery (Chicago, Ill.: 1960). 1997;132:52–57.
59. Klassen DK, Weir MR, Cangro CB, et al. Pancreas allograft biopsy: safety of percutaneous biopsy-results of a large experience. Transplantation. 2002;73:553–555.
60. Klassen DK, Hoen-Saric EW, Weir MR, et al. Isolated pancreas rejection in combined kidney pancreas tranplantation. Transplantation. 1996;61:974–977.
61. Gaber AO, Gaber LW, Shokouh-Amiri MH, et al. Percutaneous biopsy of pancreas transplants. Transplantation. 1992;54:548–550.
62. Atwell TD, Gorman B, Larson TS, et al. Pancreas transplants: experience with 232 percutaneous US-guided biopsy procedures in 88 patients. Radiology. 2004;231:845–849.
63. Aideyan OA, Schmidt AJ, Trenkner SW, et al. CT-guided percutaneous biopsy of pancreas transplants. Radiology. 1996;201:825–828.
64. Stratta RJ, Taylor RJ, Grune MT, et al. Experience with protocol biopsies after solitary pancreas transplantation. Transplantation. 1995;60:1431–1437.
65. Papadimitriou JC, Drachenberg CB, Wiland A, et al. Histologic grading of acute allograft rejection in pancreas needle biopsy: correlation to serum enzymes, glycemia, and response to immunosuppressive treatment. Transplantation. 1998;66:1741–1745.
66. Kuhr CS, Davis CL, Barr D, et al. Use of ultrasound and cystoscopically guided pancreatic allograft biopsies and transabdominal renal allograft biopsies: safety and efficacy in kidney-pancreas transplant recipients. Journal of Urology. 1995;153:316–321.
67. Kayler LK, Merion RM, Rudich SM, et al. Evaluation of pancreatic allograft dysfunction by laparoscopic biopsy. Transplantation. 2002;74:1287–1289.
68. Silver JM, Vitello JM, Benedetti E. Laparoscopic-guided biopsy of pancreatic transplant allograft. Journal of Laparoendoscopic and Advanced Surgical Techniques. Part A. 1997;7:319–322.
69. Boggi U, Vistoli F, Signori S, et al. Outcome of 118 pancreas transplants with retroperitoneal portal-enteric drainage. Transplantation Proceedings. 2005;37:2648–2650.
70. Boggi U, Vistoli F, Del Chiaro M, et al. Retroperitoneal pancreas transplantation with portal-enteric drainage. Transplantation Proceedings. 2004;36:571–574.
71. Nakhleh RE, Benedetti E, Gruessner A, et al. Cystoscopic biopsies in pancreaticoduodenal transplantation: are duodenal biopsies indicative of pancreas dysfunction? Transplantation. 1995;60:541–546.
72. Lowell JA, Bynon JS, Nelson N, et al. Improved technique for transduodenal pancreas transplant biopsy. Transplantation. 1994;57:752–753.
73. Carpenter HA, Engen DE, Munn SR, et al. Histologic diagnosis of rejection by using cystoscopically directed needle biopsy specimens from dysfunctional pancreatoduodenal allografts with exocrine drainage into the bladder. American

Journal of Surgical Pathology. 1990;14:837-846.
74. Laftavi MR, Gruessner AC, Bland BJ, et al. Diagnosis of pancreas rejection: cystoscopic transduodenal versus percutaneous computed tomography scan-guided biopsy. Transplantation. 1998;65:528-532.
75. Margreiter C, Aigner F, Resch T, et al. Enteroscopic biopsies in the management of pancreas transplants: a proof of concept study for a novel monitoring tool. Transplantation. 2012;93:207-213.
76. Kitada H, Sugitani A, Okabe Y, et al. Availability of pancreatic allograft biopsies via a laparotomy. Transplantation Proceedings. 2009;41:4274-4276.
77. Pugliese A, Reijonen HK, Nepom J, et al. Recurrence of autoimmunity in pancreas transplant patients: research update. Diabetes Management (London, England). 2011;1:229-238.
78. Petruzzo P, Andreelli F, McGregor B, et al. Evidence of recurrent type I diabetes following HLA-mismatched pancreas transplantation. Diabetes and Metabolism. 2000;26(3):215-218.
79. Burke GW 3rd, Vendrame F, Pileggi A, et al. Recurrence of autoimmunity following pancreas transplantation. Current Diabetes Reports. 2011;11: 413-419.
80. Klassen DK, Drachenberg CB, Papadimitriou JC, et al. CMV allograft pancreatitis: diagnosis, treatment, and histological features. Transplantation. 2000;69:1968-1971.
81. Drachenberg CB, Abruzzo LV, Klassen DK, et al. Epstein-Barr virus-related posttransplantation lymphoproliferative disorder involving pancreas allografts: histological differential diagnosis from acute allograft rejection. Human Pathology. 1998;29(6):569-577.
82. Westermark P, Andersson A, Westermark GT. Islet amyloid polypeptide, islet amyloid, and diabetes mellitus. Physiological Reviews. 2011;91:795-826.
83. Drachenberg CB, Klassen DK, Weir MR, et al. Islet cell damage associated with tacrolimus and cyclosporine: morphological features in pancreas allograft biopsies and clinical correlation. Transplantation. 1999;68:396-402.
84. Racusen LC, Solez K, Colvin RB, et al. The Banff 97 working classification of renal allograft pathology. Kidney International. 1999;55:713-723.
85. Weir MR, Bartlett ST, Drachenberg CB. Eosinophilia as an early indicator of pancreatic allograft rejection. Clinical Transplantation. 2011;26:238-241.
86. Drachenberg CB, Papadimitriou JC. The inflamed pancreas transplant: histological differential diagnosis. Seminars in Diagnostic Pathology. 2004;21:255-259.
87. Bagnasco SM, Tsai W, Rahman MH, et al. CD20-positive infiltrates in renal allograft biopsies with acute cellular rejection are not associated with worse graft survival. American Journal of Transplantation. 2007;7:1968-1973.
88. Cheng J, Torkamani A, Grover RK, et al. Ectopic B-cell clusters that infiltrate transplanted human kidneys are clonal. Proceedings of the National Academy of Sciences of the United States of America. 2011;108:5560-5565.
89. Thaunat O. Pathophysiologic significance of B-cell clusters in chronically rejected grafts. Transplantation. 2011;92:121-126.
90. Papadimitriou JC, Wiland A, Drachenberg CB, et al. Effectiveness of immunosuppressive treatment for recurrent or refractory pancreas allograft rejection: correlation with histologic grade. Transplantation Proceedings. 1998;30:3945.
91. Papadimitriou JC, Drachenberg CB. Distinctive morphological features of antibody-mediated and T-cell-mediated acute rejection in pancreas allograft biopsies. Current Opinion in Organ Transplantation. 2012;17:93-99.
92. Busing M, Hopt UT, Quacken M, et al. Morphological studies of graft pancreatitis following pancreas transplantation. British Journal of Surgery. 1993;80:1170-1173.
93. Knight RJ, Bodian C, Rodriguez-Laiz G, et al. Risk factors for intra-abdominal infection after pancreas transplantation. American Journal of Surgery. 2000; 179:99-102.
94. Troppmann C, Gruessner AC, Dunn DL, et al. Surgical complications requiring early relaparotomy after pancreas transplantation: a multivariate risk factor and economic impact analysis of the cyclosporine era. Annals of Surgery. 1998; 227:255-268.
95. Letourneau JG, Hunter DW, Crass JR, et al. Percutaneous aspiration and drainage of abdominal fluid collections after pancreatic transplantation. AJR. American Journal of Roentgenology. 1988;150:805-809.
96. Keay S. CMV infection and disease in kidney and pancreas transplant recipients. Transplant Infectious Disease. 1999;1(Suppl 1):19-24.
97. Lo A, Stratta RJ, Egidi MF, et al. Patterns of cytomegalovirus infection in simultaneous kidney-pancreas transplant recipients receiving tacrolimus, mycophenolate mofetil, and prednisone with ganciclovir prophylaxis. Transplant Infectious Disease. 2001;3:8-15.
98. Ishibashi M, Bosshard S, Fukuuchi F, et al. Incidence of CMV infection in simultaneous pancreas and kidney transplantation: comparative study of two surgical procedures of segmental pancreas versus whole bladder-drained pancreas. Transplantation Proceedings. 1996;28:2859-2860.
99. Humar A, Uknis M, Carlone-Jambor C, et al. Cytomegalovirus disease recurrence after ganciclovir treatment in kidney and kidney-pancreas transplant recipients. Transplantation. 1999;67:94-97.
100. Backman L, Brattstrom C, Reinholt FP, et al. Development of intrapancreatic abscess: a consequence of CMV pancreatitis? Transplant International. 1991;4:116-121.
101. Backman L, Brattstrom C, Reinholt FP, et al. Development of intrapancreatic abscess: a consequence of CMV pancreatitis? Transplant International. 1991;4: 116-121.
102. Fernandez-Cruz L, Sabater L, Gilabert R, et al. Native and graft pancreatitis following combined pancreas-renal transplantation. British Journal of Surgery. 1993;80:1429-1432.
103. Fernandez JA, Robles R, Ramirez P, et al. Arterioenteric fistula due to cytomegalovirus infection after pancreas transplantation. Transplantation. 2001;72: 966-968.
104. Paraskevas S, Coad JE, Gruessner A, et al. Posttransplant lymphoproliferative disorder in pancreas transplantation: a single-center experience. Transplantation. 2005;80:613-622.
105. Issa N, Amer H, Dean PG, et al. Posttransplant lymphoproliferative disorder following pancreas transplantation. American Journal of Transplantation. 2009;9: 1894-1902.
106. Caillard S, Lamy FX, Quelen C, et al. Epidemiology of posttransplant lymphoproliferative disorders in adult kidney and kidney pancreas recipients: report of the French Registry and analysis of Subgroups of Lymphomas. American Journal of Transplantation. 2012;12:682-693.
107. Randhawa PS, Magnone M, Jordan M, et al. Renal allograft involvement by Epstein-Barr virus associated post-transplant lymphoproliferative disease. American Journal of Surgical Pathology. 1996;20:563-571.
108. Paya CV, Fung JJ, Nalesnik MA, et al. Epstein-Barr virus-induced posttransplant lymphoproliferative disorders. ASTS/ASTP EBV-PTLD Task Force and The Mayo Clinic Organized International Consensus Development Meeting. Transplantation. 1999;68:1517-1525.
109. Shimizu T, Ishida H, Shirakawa H, et al. Clinicopathological analysis of acute vascular rejection cases after renal transplantation. Clinical Transplantation. 2010;24(Suppl 22):22-26.
110. Hirohashi T, Uehara S, Chase CM, et al. Complement independent antibody-mediated endarteritis and transplant arteriopathy in mice. American Journal of Transplantation. 2010;10:510-517.
111. Assalino M, Genevay M, Morel P, et al. Recurrence of type 1 diabetes after simultaneous pancreas-kidney transplantation in the absence of GAD and IA-2 autoantibodies. American Journal of Transplantation. 2012;12:492-495.
112. Drachenberg CB, Papadimitriou JC. Graft dysfunction in pancreas and islet transplantation: morphological aspects. Current Opinion in Organ Transplantation. 2011;16:106-109.
113. Benz S, Schnabel R, Morgenroth K, et al. Ischemia/reperfusion injury of the pancreas: a new animal model. Journal of Surgical Research. 1998;75:109-115.
114. Schulak JA, Franklin WA, Stuart FP, et al. Effect of warm ischemia on segmental pancreas transplantation in the rat. Transplantation. 1983;35:7-11.
115. Gruessner RW, Dunn DL, Tzardis PJ, et al. Complications occurring after whole organ duodenopancreatic transplantation: relation to the allograft duodenal segment. Transplantation Proceedings. 1990;22:578-579.
116. Muthusamy AS, Giangrande PL, Friend PJ. Pancreas allograft thrombosis. Transplantation. 2010;90:705-707.
117. Einecke G, Sis B, Reeve J, et al. Antibody-mediated microcirculation injury is the major cause of late kidney transplant failure. American Journal of Transplantation. 2009;9:2520-2531.
118. Humar A, Khwaja K, Ramcharan T, et al. Chronic rejection: the next major challenge for pancreas transplant recipients. Transplantation. 2003;76:918-923.
119. Matsukuma S, Suda K, Abe H. Histopathological study of pancreatic ischemic lesions induced by cholesterol emboli: fresh and subsequent features of pancreatic ischemia. Human Pathology. 1998;29:41-46.
120. Benedetti E, Najarian JS, Gruessner AC, et al. Correlation between cystoscopic biopsy results and hypoamylasuria in bladder-drained pancreas transplants. Surgery. 1995;118:864-872.
121. Jones JW, Nakhleh RE, Casanova D, et al. Cystoscopic transduodenal pancreas transplant biopsy: a new needle. Transplantation Proceedings. 1994;26:527-528.
122. Nath DS, Gruessner A, Kandaswamy R, et al. Late anastomotic leaks in pancreas transplant recipients: clinical characteristics and predisposing factors. Clinical Transplantation. 2005;19:220-224.
123. Lillehei RC, Simmons RL, Najarian JS, et al. Pancreatico-duodenal allotransplantation: experimental and clinical experience. Annals of Surgery. 1970;172: 405-436.
124. Nakhleh RE, Sutherland DE, Benedetti E, et al. Diagnostic utility and correlation of duodenal and pancreas biopsy tissue in pancreaticoduodenal transplants with emphasis on therapeutic use. Transplantation Proceedings. 1995;27:1327-1328.
125. Carpenter HA, Barr D, Marsh CL, et al. Sequential histopathologic changes in

pancreaticoduodenal allograft rejection in dogs. Transplantation. 1989;48: 764–768.
126. Nakhleh RE, Sutherland DE, Tzardis P, et al. Correlation of rejection of the duodenum with rejection of the pancreas in a pig model of pancreaticoduodenal transplantation. Transplantation. 1993;56:1353–1356.
127. Mark W, Hechenleitner P, Dietze O, et al. Duodenal histology for monitoring treatment of acute rejection in pancreaticoduodenal allografts in rats. Transplantation. 2002;73:198–203.
128. Esterl RM, Stratta RJ, Taylor RJ, et al. Rejection with duodenal rupture after solitary pancreas transplantation: an unusual cause of severe hematuria. Clinical Transplantation. 1995;9:155–159.
129. Mengel M, Sis B, Haas M, et al. Banff 2011 meeting report: new concepts in antibody-mediated rejection. American Journal of Transplantation. 2012;12: 563–570.
130. Drachenberg CB, Papadimitriou JC, Schweitzer E, et al. Histological findings in "incidental" intraoperative pancreas allograft biopsies. Transplantation Proceedings. 2004;36:780–781.
131. Nakhleh RE, Gruessner RW, Tzardis PJ, et al. Pancreas transplant pathology: an immunohistochemical comparison of allografts with rejection, syngeneic grafts, and chronic pancreatitis. Transplantation Proceedings. 1991;23: 1598–1599.
132. Wieczorek G, Bigaud M, Menninger K, et al. Acute and chronic vascular rejection in nonhuman primate kidney transplantation. American Journal of Transplantation. 2006;6:1285–1296.
133. Cantarovich D, De Amicis S, Akl A, et al. Posttransplant donor-specific anti-HLA antibodies negatively impact pancreas transplantation outcome. American Journal of Transplantation. 2011;11:2737–2746.
134. Colvin RB. Dimensions of antibody-mediated rejection. American Journal of Transplantation. 2010;10:1509–1510.
135. Prikis M, Norman D, Rayhill S, et al. Preserved endocrine function in a pancreas transplant recipient with pancreatic panniculitis and antibody-mediated rejection. American Journal of Transplantation. 2010;10:2717–2722.
136. Drachenberg CB, Papadimitriou JC, Klassen DK, et al. Distribution of alpha and beta cells in pancreas allograft biopsies: correlation with rejection and other pathologic processes. Transplantation Proceedings. 1998;30:665–666.
137. Drachenberg CB, Papadimitriou JC, Weir MR, et al. Histologic findings in islets of whole pancreas allografts: lack of evidence for recurrent cell-mediated diabetes mellitus. Transplantation. 1996;62:1770–1772.
138. Dudek RW, Lawrence IE Jr, Hill RS, et al. Induction of islet cytodifferentiation by fetal mesenchyme in adult pancreatic ductal epithelium. Diabetes. 1991;40: 1041–1048.
139. Semakula C, Pambuccian S, Gruessner R, et al. Clinical case seminar: hypoglycemia after pancreas transplantation – association with allograft nesidiodysplasia and expression of islet neogenesis-associated peptide. Journal of Clinical Endocrinology and Metabolism. 2002;87:3548–3554.
140. Toso C, Isse K, Demetris AJ, et al. Histologic graft assessment after clinical islet transplantation. Transplantation. 2009;88:1286–1293.
141. Smith RN, Kent SC, Nagle J, et al. Pathology of an islet transplant 2 years after transplantation: evidence for a nonimmunological loss. Transplantation. 2008;86:54–62.
142. Davalli AM, Maffi P, Socci C, et al. Insights from a successful case of intrahepatic islet transplantation into a type 1 diabetic patient. Journal of Clinical Endocrinology and Metabolism. 2000;85:3847–3852.
143. Jirak D, Kriz J, Strzelecki M, et al. Monitoring the survival of islet transplants by MRI using a novel technique for their automated detection and quantification. Magma (New York, NY). 2009;22:257–265.
144. Kriz J, Jirak D, Berkova Z, et al. Detection of pancreatic islet allograft impairment in advance of functional failure using magnetic resonance imaging. Transplant International. 2012;25:250–260.
145. Dean PG, Kudva YC, Larson TS, et al. Posttransplant diabetes mellitus after pancreas transplantation. American Journal of Transplantation. 2008;8: 175–182.
146. Neidlinger N, Singh N, Klein C, et al. Incidence of and risk factors for posttransplant diabetes mellitus after pancreas transplantation. American Journal of Transplantation. 2010;10:398–406.
147. Vendrame F, Pileggi A, Laughlin E, et al. Recurrence of type 1 diabetes after simultaneous pancreas-kidney transplantation, despite immunosuppression, is associated with autoantibodies and pathogenic autoreactive CD4 T-cells. Diabetes. 2010;59:947–957.
148. Tyden G, Reinholt FP, Sundkvist G, et al. Recurrence of autoimmune diabetes mellitus in recipients of cadaveric pancreatic grafts. New England Journal of Medicine. 1996;335:860–863.
149. Ishida-Oku M, Iwase M, Sugitani A, et al. A case of recurrent type 1 diabetes mellitus with insulitis of transplanted pancreas in simultaneous pancreas-kidney transplantation from cardiac death donor. Diabetologia. 2010;53:341–345.
150. Westermark GT, Westermark P, Berne C, et al. Widespread amyloid deposition in transplanted human pancreatic islets. New England Journal of Medicine. 2008;359:977–979.
151. Westermark P. Amyloid in the islets of Langerhans: thoughts and some historical aspects. Upsala Journal of Medical Sciences. 2011;116:81–89.
152. Hirano Y, Fujihira S, Ohara K, et al. Morphological and functional changes of islets of Langerhans in FK506-treated rats. Transplantation. 1992;53:889–894.
153. Smelt MJ, Faas MM, de Haan BJ, et al. Rat pancreatic beta cells and cytomegalovirus infection. Pancreas. 2010;39:47–56.
154. Smelt MJ, de Haan BJ, Faas MM, et al. Effects of acute cytomegalovirus infection on rat islet allograft survival. Cell Transplantation. 2011;20:1271–1283.
155. Zanone MM, Favaro E, Quadri R, et al. Association of cytomegalovirus infections with recurrence of humoral and cellular autoimmunity to islet autoantigens and of type 1 diabetes in a pancreas transplanted patient. Transplant International. 2010;23:333–337.
156. Honeyman MC, Stone NL, Falk BA, et al. Evidence for molecular mimicry between human T cell epitopes in rotavirus and pancreatic islet autoantigens. Journal of Immunology. 2010;184:2204–2210.

第 86 章 小肠移植排斥反应和复发疾病的组织病理学综合征

Phillip Ruiz, Jennifer Garcia, Akin Tekin, Seigo Nishida, Andreas Tzakis

引言

小肠(ITx)和器官移植(MVTx)领域的成熟在治疗短肠综合征(SGS)和继发于灾难性腹腔损伤、内科疾病和某些肿瘤的难治性胃肠道损伤方面取得了可喜的进展[1-4]。小肠移植和多器官移植失败的主要原因为小肠吸收功能缺失,最终导致患者营养不良。这些情况部分列于表 86.1,其详细信息详见第 33 章和第 117 章。尽管有上述问题,儿童和成人患者仍可接受消化道移植[5],并且消化道功能因为年龄不同而显著不同(表 86.1)。大多数患者相较于移植更依赖肠外营养。短肠综合征的药物管理与同种异体移植相比已经得到加强[6],但慢性肠外营养致命的并发症、高额的费用和生命质量变差等问题对患者造成严重影响。相反,小肠移植和多器官移植有助于患者恢复消化道功能,避免或最小化饮食限制,促进生长和发育,改善和独立的生活方式[7]。

小肠移植的手术步骤根据肠道功能和移植候选患者的基本情况确定。肠道同种异体移植可为单独移植或者多器官移植的一部分;后者是腹腔器官整体移植,包括胃、小肠、大肠、肝脏、胰腺和脾脏[8,9]。(注:无肝移植被称为改良多器官移植。)步骤的技术细节详见第 62 章和第 117 章。单独小肠移植或多器官移植取决于受体的潜在病理学情况。最近几年,与单独小肠移植相比,多器官移植的应用逐渐增多,而其移植物和患者的存活率则与之相当[9]。

原位和异位小肠移植的大型和小型动物模型的实验经验有助于人类移植治疗和操作的进步[10,11]。例如,单纯小肠移植或多器官移植已经显著促进了移植前评估、合适供体和受体的选择、手术技术、肠道生理和黏膜免疫的知识的迅猛增长以及整体移植后维护,因此促进了移植小肠和受体生存的改善。移植病理学家是监测团队的关键成员,一名经认证的专家应结合解剖病理学、临床检验和实质性器官移植或骨髓移植相关的基本科学知识。因此,胃肠道移植病理学家是临床队伍的关键成员,其通过结合活检评估、常规和专门的临床检验分析、与移植小肠和其他移植腹腔脏器相关的病理生理学机制来监测移植后并发症[12]。

尽管取得了这些进展,小肠移植给受体带来了含同种抗原的淋巴造血细胞和实质细胞团,其介导了强力的宿主效应免疫反应,并需要强力持久的免疫抑制试剂来不断地调节和中断。随着介导和维持免疫移植的方案发展,新的靶点药物复合物和抗体介导的免疫抑制试剂也在不断发展[13],宿主来源的免疫反应[14]以及对宿主的移植免疫反应[15](如移植物抗宿主病),仍为小肠移植和多器官移植的重要并发症。免疫抑制的水平和类型不是对宿主同种免疫反应有害的唯一因素,因为静止的免疫系统(在适当免疫抑制范围)也可能为许多因素的结果,如可能影响宿主反应水平的宿主先天基因多态性的类型[16]、效应细胞和调节细胞的比值[17],以及受体和供体的基因不一致的程度和类型。无论如何,小肠和多器官移植受体多半表现出严重的临床或“亚临床”基于免疫的急性排斥期[18,19]。数据显示,与其他实质性器官移植不同,急性排斥仍为小肠移植和多器官移植的主要移植后并发症。

和其他接受强力免疫抑制的患者一样,严格的调节免疫反应使小肠移植和多器官移植的患者感染和恶性肿瘤风险增加[20]。而且,药物的毒性通常直接作用于多种器官系统(如肾脏、神经系统)(见第 94 章和第 95 章)[21,22]。除了免疫系统相关并发症,小肠移植和多器官

表 86.1 接受小肠或多器官移植的患者移植小肠功能丧失的结构和功能原因

儿童	成年人
腹裂	缺血(静脉或动脉梗塞)
中肠扭转	克罗恩病
坏死性肠炎	外伤
假性肠梗阻	肠扭转
肠闭锁	动力障碍
再次移植	再次移植
微绒毛包涵体病	放射性肠炎
吸收不良	其他肿瘤
	Gardner 综合征

框 86.1 小肠和多器官移植患者的并发症及病理过程

1.供体器官病理及保存损伤
2.急性排斥反应
  a.抗体介导的排斥反应(AMR)
    i.超急性和加速急性排斥反应
    ii.急性抗体介导的排斥反应(AAMR)
  b.急性T细胞介导(细胞)的排斥反应(ACR)*
    i.无急性排斥反应,0级
    ii.急性排斥反应不确定,IND级
    iii.急性T细胞介导的急性排斥反应(ACR),轻度,1级
    iv.急性T细胞介导的急性排斥反应(ACR),中度,2级
    v.急性T细胞介导的急性排斥反应(ACR),严重,3级
  c.结肠和胃的ACR
  d."混合"急性排斥反应-伴发ACR和AAMR
3.慢性排斥反应
4.感染
  a.病毒(如轮状病毒、腺病毒、杯状病毒、巨细胞病毒、单纯疱疹病毒和EB病毒)
  b.杂项(如细菌、真菌、隐孢子虫、分枝杆菌)
5.复发性疾病
  a.胃肠道疾病,肿瘤
6.其他项目
  a.病因不明的持续性溃疡
  b.病因不明的活动性肠炎
  c.病因不明的嗜酸性粒细胞综合征
7.再生变化
8.自体组织移植物抗宿主病(GVHD)
9.移植后淋巴组织增生性疾病(PTLD)

* Grading of ACR performed based on [60] Ruiz et al. *Transplantation Proceedings*. 2004;36:335-337.

移植受体也易感其他并发症，如与移植前和移植后营养计划、既往腹部手术史或受体并发的潜在疾病相关的并发症。移植后并发症见框 86.1。

在过去的25年中,移植后不断检查小肠移植和多器官移植手术后早期和后期的小肠功能及患者状态均得到了加强。多器官移植评估需要移植病理学家了解自体器官的组织病理学和同种异体移植不典型的变化(如胃、结肠)且知道不同取材部位(十二指肠和回肠)的病理学变化可能性。例如,监测多器官移植患者需要同时进行原组织活检(如食管、直肠、皮肤)和移植组织(胃、小肠、结肠和肝)活检。自体和移植组织的比较在许多情况下是有价值的,例如,试图辨别某种变化是否是同种免疫(如排斥反应)、一般病理(如感染、移植后淋巴增生性疾病(PTLD)或移植物衍生变化(GVHD、保存性损伤)所特有的。

组织病理学评估

同种异体移植的病理学评估包括小肠移植和多器官移植的全部阶段和存活移植器官的长期评估。根据活检的组织学评估仍然是移植物病理学评估的金标准;然而,组织辅助检查和系统性生物标志物评估在这些复杂的评估过程中常见。小肠移植和多器官移植活检必须与同期的受体医学检测值相联系。移植病理学家需要了解受体的病史(如移植时间、原发疾病或需要移植的原因及临床表现)、以前的活检结果及内镜检查结果。活检获取部位(病灶、病灶周围或非相关部位)的描述是至关重要的。多数的小肠移植和多器官移植组织样本是在内镜直视下通过表面黏膜活检获取的。通常不提倡通过造瘘术(如回肠造瘘或结肠造瘘)获取活检组织，因为可能存在与手术切口愈合相关的炎症反应,如组织炎症过程、纤维化和变形结构[23]。

由于提供给病理学家的改变水平通常局限于胃肠道部位及黏膜和黏膜下层，内镜操作者根据移植胃肠道的经验来决定哪个部位活检是至关重要的。内镜操作者和病理学家应不断交流内镜观察到的黏膜正常和异常的变化。如果为异常的变化,则应描述移植物位置和分布、原始组织的受累情况以及特征（如红斑性黏膜、溃疡)。移植的胃肠道全层评估非常规检查,当手术检查问题区域或移植器官被移除时才需要。

大多数胃肠道移植的并发症为临床紧急情况,且

能快速导致移植器官功能异常和功能丧失。因此,提供移植病理学支持的组织学实验室和病理学服务必须每周 7 天提供特别快速的周转时间，并具有纳入专门的免疫组化(IHC)、免疫荧光(IF)和原位杂交(ISH)技术的能力。另外,现代实验室也适当开展移植器官来源的分子检测,如感染介质的定量评估和特殊基因排列。

将 1~2 个胃肠道移植组织碎片迅速置入适合的固定液(如福尔马林缓冲液)且至少持续 1 小时。多个切片通常每 0.5cm 切割,苏木精和伊红(HE)染色用于初步评估。小肠移植和多器官移植需要多种特殊的染色方法,例如免疫组织化学(例如检测感染源如巨细胞、腺病毒);原位杂交检测病毒如 EB 病毒、病毒载量检测(如 EB 病毒)和其他分子检测如 T 细胞和 B 细胞抗原受体重新分布检测（当评估移植后淋巴组织增生性疾病的可能性时)。最终,移植病理学家应该能获取,最好参与小肠移植或多器官移植患者的其他关键实验室检验的解读,如瓜氨酸水平免疫功能检测(如 Cylex、酶联免疫分析、细胞因子)、供体和受体的人类白细胞抗原类型以及同种抗体检测。因为小肠移植和多器官移植管理的不断进步,特定基因检测(如 MBL-2 或 NOD 多态性）和其他潜在生物标志物检测目前被用于评估且为患者组织病理和临床表现的有用补充。

病理学步骤

多种与移植过程相关的并发症可能发生于小肠移植和多器官移植受体。如表 86.1,许多这些并发症能同时发生,这就需要特定的鉴别方法,因为治疗方法不同或主要问题有负面影响（治疗移植后淋巴组织增生性疾病或者感染和排斥的治疗方法差异巨大)。

供体器官病理学和保存性损伤

供移植的小肠或多腹腔器官的成功获取依赖复杂的、协调的系统,其通过纳入各种因素包括大小(受体腹腔的大小、患儿年龄)、供体临床相配和消除大部分危险因素的算法来识别潜在的供体[24]。实验室检测必须迅速评估供体内感染病原，临床队伍必须评估供体器官的状态如缺血性损伤、可能的肿瘤和危害肠道功能的状况。通常,供体器官的大体检查足以评估可能的损伤。小肠移植和多器官移植极少需要冰冻切片评估。因此,不同于其他异体移植如肾脏和肝脏,当移植器官有可疑的病史时需要行移植前活检，在移植前供体胃或肠道则不需要病理学家评估。残余供体组织的病理学评估除了有少量的缺血性损伤外，没有任何显著的病理学变化。

绝大多数移植器官在不同时间内保存于低温液体(取决于移植的器官)中,血管吻合后受体血液重新温灌注移植器官。胃肠道移植没有足够的冷缺血时间。无论如何，移植器官的保存相关损伤或缺血再灌注损伤起通常由血管再生引起[25]。缺血再灌注损伤可发生于肠道[26],并能导致一系列可能影响功能的病理学改变。在大多数病例中,缺血再灌注改变为轻度,且对器官的短期功能没有太大的影响，尽管可能对移植器官免疫介导的损伤和生理功能有显著的影响。越来越多的证据表明，非炎症尸体器官的许多基因在转录水平有巨大的变化,包括炎症相关基因[27,28]。这些供体肠道的转录变化的意义仍然未知，这些器官变化是否会影响移植物的长期功能仍然是推测。存在早期缺血再灌注损伤的长期存活的移植器官未发现有特定的变化。“边缘”供体的使用不是现在小肠移植和多器官移植的主要问题[29],其被认为会使受体更易出现缺血再灌注损伤、移植器官无功能或功能延迟、并发症(如排斥)。

形态学。绝大多数小肠移植和多器官移植有“规定”的活检,尤其在移植后最初的几周内。例如,在移植后早期获取黏膜活检来验证保存性损伤变化并不罕见[30]。轻度保存性损伤的移植小肠和大肠表现出弥漫性缺血和绒毛水肿，无浸润的炎性细胞显著增多、血管堵塞以及上皮细胞和其下固有层分离(图 86.1)。随着缺血再灌注损伤加重,会发生额外的变化如上皮细胞坏死从黏膜表面扩展到黏膜下层。这些变化已经在对照环境下的缺血再灌注损伤实验模型中进行了描述。例如，一些鼠类模型表明，可分级和进展的变化从黏膜最终进展到小肠透壁性坏死[31,32]。临床上,后者的这种变化在显微镜下不明显，除非有严重的缺血再灌注损伤合并长时间的血管堵塞。在这些情况下,异体移植组织表现出与自体肠道缺血相似的缺血性改变。目前有缺血再灌注损伤的移植胃的形态学未得到很好的描述。

急性排斥

受体同种免疫效应细胞群体（细胞介导的排斥或 T 细胞排斥),受体 B 细胞来源的同种抗体(体液或抗体介导的排斥)的起始和增值,合并非特异性的固有免

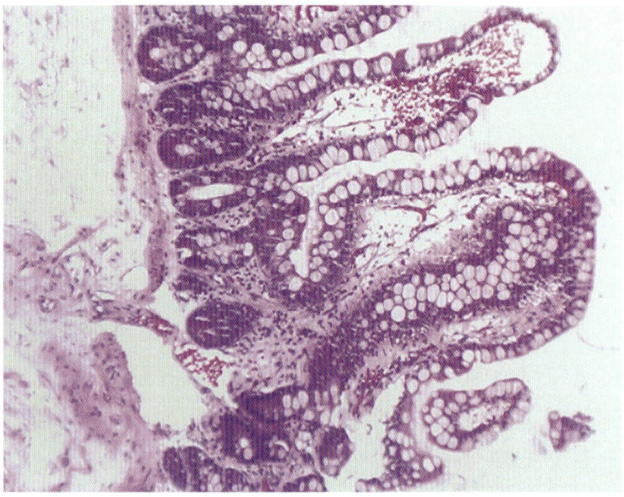

图 86.1 保存性损伤。移植后几天小肠活检显示绒毛水肿，但无炎症细胞的显著性增加，一些血管堵塞，变面上皮细胞和下面的固有层分离（HE 染色，×200）。

疫机制构成抗移植物炎性急性反应，定义为急性排斥[17]。这些情况基本的作用方式详见第5~7章。免疫细胞群和可溶分子的这种有效组合可以协同作用，也可以单独作用，以表现不同形式的损伤。这些损伤在形态学上被经典地描述，有时表现为急性排斥反应的不同形式。急性排斥很有可能会降低移植器官功能并导致器官功能丧失，与其他实体器官移植一样，在小肠移植和多器官移植受体中检测和有效干预急性排斥富有挑战性，并且是移植医生的目标。然而，尽管有强力免疫抑制的应用，异体移植急性排斥仍为胃肠道移植的常见并发症。其机制包括T细胞介导的和基于抗体的急性排斥，与其他器官系统类似，其超过了本章节的讨论范围。受体来源的B细胞和T细胞（其代表适应性免疫反应），与固有免疫细胞群体，包括自然杀伤细胞、树突状细胞、巨噬细胞和免疫分子混合物[33]有复杂的相互影响关系，其主要参与识别异体基因胃肠道组织的免疫通路的起源和高潮。有多种潜在刺激目标在胃肠道驻足免疫效应细胞和分子，包括薄壁组织或上皮细胞（如肠上皮细胞、潘氏细胞）、血管上皮细胞、肌肉、内分泌和神经细胞。肠道中这类目标细胞群的急性排斥介导的损伤或死亡可导致的临床结果包括发热、吸收不良、动力障碍和缺血[7,24,34]。肠道的急性排斥能快速进展，因为显著的抗原性和肠道巨大的细胞量在某些情况下能导致黏膜和黏膜下层脱落[35,36]、透壁性缺血和肠道菌群移位[37,38]，移位会进展为脓毒血症。因此，在小肠移植和多器官移植中迅速准确地诊断出急性排斥以防止排斥的临床后果至关重要。

当考虑诊断可能为急性排斥时，临床和内镜相结合是十分重要的。肠道急性排斥与包括排便增加（从造口早期排便）、发热和水肿在内的症状有关[9]。这些症状非特异性且其他情况如感染也能导致相似的效果。就这一点而言，内镜下获取的胃肠道活检术通常是鉴别这些情况的关键。缺乏临床症状情况下形态学定义急性排斥为亚临床排斥，其已在肠道移植[18]、肝脏移植和肾脏移植中描述过[19,39,40]。通常亚临床排斥在临床稳定的患者进行活检时被发现。亚临床排斥有潜在的重要性，因为患者最终发展为移植器官功能丧失的危险性很高。一些医疗方案通过额外的免疫抑制来治疗亚临床排斥。其他非侵入性实验室检查和生物标志物检测，虽然现在缺少最佳的特异度和敏感度，但越来越多地用于进一步支持根据活检的形态学来诊断急性排斥[41]。这些检查包括外周免疫细胞群落[42]、细胞因子谱和特定基因的定量分析[33]。外周血瓜氨酸水平的系列检查，虽然为非特异性排斥，可显示肠道肿块，这项分析为我们协会检测小肠移植和多器官移植后患者的常规检查。

形态学。小肠移植或多器官移植后与急性排斥相关的活检组织病理学变化范围较大，并且根据移植受体、移植器官和移植后的时间存在不同变化。小肠移植和多器官移植中，急性排斥的分类和其他的实体器官移植分类一样，采用了来源于基础免疫学的术语（如超急性排斥、加速排斥、急性血管排斥）；后来这些术语慢慢得到规范。与这些急性排斥亚型有关的形态学改变能同时共存（如混合性排斥）。我们使用了基于排斥的潜在病因学的常规分类：抗体介导的或T细胞介导的排斥（框86.1）。

抗体介导的排斥

超急性和加速急性排斥

超急性和加速急性排斥定义为移植器官暴露于极高水平的与器官的抗原起交叉反应的抗体（如供体特异性抗体），并且移植后数分钟至数小时内（超急性排斥）或数天内（加速急性排斥）发生严重排斥[46,47]。这些潜在的严重急性排斥发生于预先致敏的患者（如已存在抗体），并且继发严重的以血管内皮为主要目标的抗体介导的反应，组织学上表现为血管损伤、栓塞和缺血性损伤。存在肠道移植物排斥形式的实验证据，但是小肠移植或多器官移植的超急性排斥有记录的临床案例描述极少。以往不常规开展移植交叉前配对，但这种方法正在改变，因为已经有报道肠道超急性反应期与移植前供体特异性抗体的存在相关[49-51]。大体上，供体器官吻合性颜色迅速变暗并且充血，类似的变化也可见于其他存在超急性排斥的实质性器官。

形态学上，有大量的黏膜淤血及坏死、中性粒细胞且着边于血管周围(图 86.2)。后续的血管堵塞从黏膜扩展到移植器官的全层(透壁性)。原生组织不明显。令人好奇的是，通过血浆置换的强力干预，抗 CD20 抗体(其他免疫抑制剂)的治疗和密切监测，这些患者有克服这些严重的抗体介导的急性排斥能力[48,50]。我们描述了 1 例发生超急性排斥的患者，其表现出正常的肠道功能(正常的外观且无症状)，抗供体抗体滴度减少合并正常内镜表现的发展[48]。我们中心对于小肠移植和多器官移植的患者常规开展交叉配对。

有时，我们也发现加速抗体介导的排斥反应发生于多器官移植后最初的几天，受体因预先存在同种抗体而致敏，其大体上表现为如下描述的抗体介导的排斥反应特点，但未达到超急性排斥程度。

急性抗体介导的(体液)排斥

直到现在，人类小肠和多器官移植中急性抗体介导的排斥的发生率和严重程度没有被很好地阐述。其病理生理学为抗体直接作用于同种抗原，然后导致各种后果[49,52]。相应地，没有额外的技术和移植前/移植后抗体的证据，急性抗体介导的排斥不能被识别。血管炎症为这一过程的组织学部分。然而，这是抗体的非特异性，因为细胞介导的免疫反应(T 细胞介导血管炎)也可能为移植肠道内血管炎的潜在原因。一些小肠移植中急性抗体介导的排斥已经被报道，与受体同种抗体对供体抗原的移植后敏感化作用有关，移植前抗体非常低的滴度随后上升。移植器官常表现出广泛的炎症改变，大动脉一直到小动脉分枝出现血管炎(图 86.3)。血管炎表现为在动脉内膜有急性和慢性炎症细胞浸润，伴随内膜水肿和上皮细胞反应。补充的 C4d 和 C3d 成分常出现于固有层和大血管；检测这些分子免疫组织化学表达的变化并将之分级是对病理学家一项重要的要求。血管炎包括透壁炎症纤维蛋白沉积和动脉坏死，造成移植器官严重的缺血性损伤。有时，移植器官中选择动脉比其他器官更易受血管炎的影响。比如，肠系膜动脉可发生急性抗体介导的排斥，其可导致硬化性肠系膜炎[53]。这种不常见的现象与升高的抗体有关。胃和结肠异体移植也可出现严重的血管炎，见于小肠移植。当考虑这种严重血管炎的诊断时，其他原因如感染(如真菌或病毒感染)也应考虑到。其他导致血管炎的原因如肿瘤形成、药物和同种免疫不是常见的原因，且在原生器官和移植器官中均有分布。

大血管的血管炎常见于外植体或排斥的器官或尸检。这样，在小肠移植中，黏膜活检时急性抗体介导的排斥和严重血管炎的诊断具有挑战性，其常常伴有大

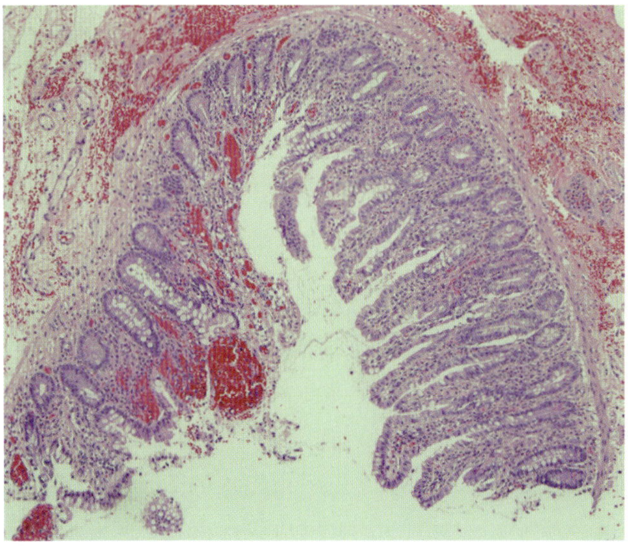

图 86.2　超急性排斥。移植后 1 天小肠活检发现严重血管堵塞、中性粒细胞、早期血管炎和坏死(HE 染色，×200)。

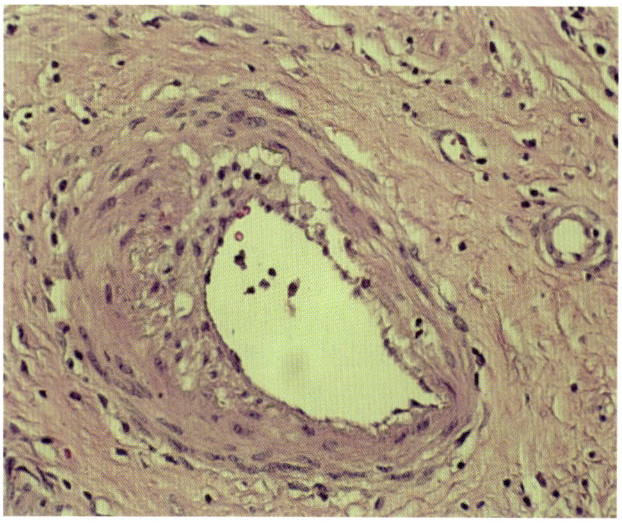

图 86.3　急性抗体介导的排斥。小肠活检显示大动脉炎(HE 染色，×400)。

体坏死的证据。

然而,轻度急性抗体介导的排斥也可发生于小肠、胃和结肠移植,其发生频率比以前认为的高。我们已经描述了识别早期、轻度或进展中的急性抗体介导的排斥变化,这些变化可能单独发生或与 T 细胞介导的急性排斥反应相关[52]。这些早期和(或)轻度急性抗体介导的排斥表现为黏膜大体改变,且在许多病例中与已存在的或移植后的同种抗体形成有关。这些改变尤其在移植后早期易发生。移植器官黏膜的微血管表现为弥漫性显著的血管堵塞合并红细胞外渗(图 86.4)。绒毛区域和固有层微血管主要受影响,且没有血管炎的证据。慢性炎症细胞不一定增多,通常有上皮细胞的保留。辅助实验有助于评估急性排斥的液体形式,例如,在疑似急性抗体介导排斥的患者中,免疫荧光用于检测免疫球蛋白的存在(IgG,IgA,IgM)和补充成分(C3,C4,C1q);纤维蛋白原、C3d 和 C4d 在我们实验室中通过免疫组织化学检测。在急性抗体介导排斥中,免疫球蛋白能沉积于血管,与补充成分于间质。和其他发生严重急性抗体介导排斥(如前所述)的移植器官和胃肠道移植一样,我们在发生轻度和进展急性抗体介导排斥患者的小动脉和小毛细血管中发现 C4d 和 C3d。有更多不易察觉的急性抗体介导排斥形式没有特异性组织病理学表现,其中一些改变可在缺血、非特异性肠炎、病毒感染和急性心血管问题中见到。因此,需要将临床病史与实验室检查结果(如同种抗体抗供体的滴定度)、损伤分布(移植器官和原生组织)、其他形态学发现(如急性炎症细胞浸润或表面上皮细胞随肠炎改变)以及培养结果相关联。

急性 T 细胞介导的(细胞)排斥

急性 T 细胞介导的排斥(ACR)是胃肠道移植中急性排斥最常见的类型,且可与急性抗体介导的排斥、移植后淋巴组织增生性疾病、感染或其他并发症同时存在。最主要的病理生理过程为受体 T 细胞介导的对供体同种抗原的反应。组织学上,多种类的富含淋巴细胞的慢性炎症细胞浸润分散于移植器官的小肠区域,并伴有特定实质部分浸润和损伤[54]。这些胃肠道成分是陷窝、腺体结构、表面上皮的重要细胞;然而,肌肉、内皮和神经细胞也可能被影响。实质损伤存在一些功能和结构的后遗症,如化生、凋亡和细胞通路调节的变化。

同种免疫效应细胞对血管损伤的血管损伤尤其具有破坏性(如 AAMR),因为血管损伤随后导致广泛坏死。胃肠道移植中的急性 T 细胞介导的排斥是一个复杂的、多因素($CD4^+$和 $CD8^+$ T 细胞)参与的过程(图 86.5),这与其他类型的移植排斥相似。隐窝上皮细胞凋亡是与移植小肠中急性 T 细胞介导的排斥有关的主要特征之一[55],由于 $CD8^+$通过粒酶 B-穿孔素的颗粒胞吐途径和 Fas、Fas 配体介导的细胞毒性来诱导目的细胞的凋亡[33]。有趣的是,在实验动物模型中非 $CD8^+$ T 细胞也参

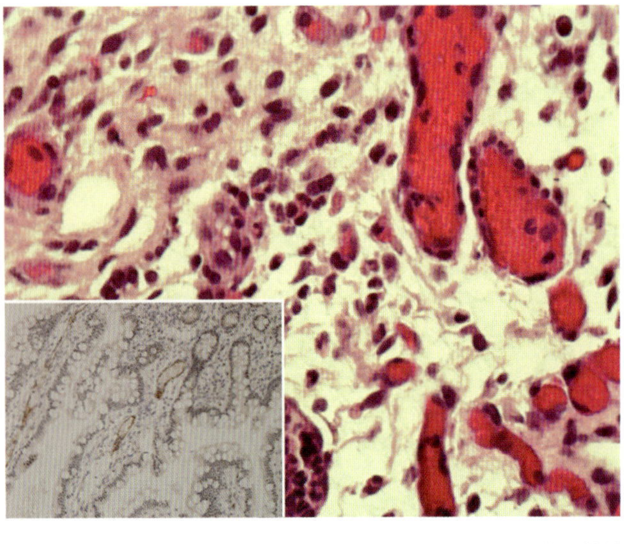

图 86.4 AAMR。抗体介导的排斥的小肠活检显示黏膜血管被附壁中性粒细胞、间隙和混合性慢性炎症细胞浸润急性堵塞(HE 染色,×400)。(插图)固有层脉管系统被 C4d 染色(C4d 免疫组织化学染色,×200)。

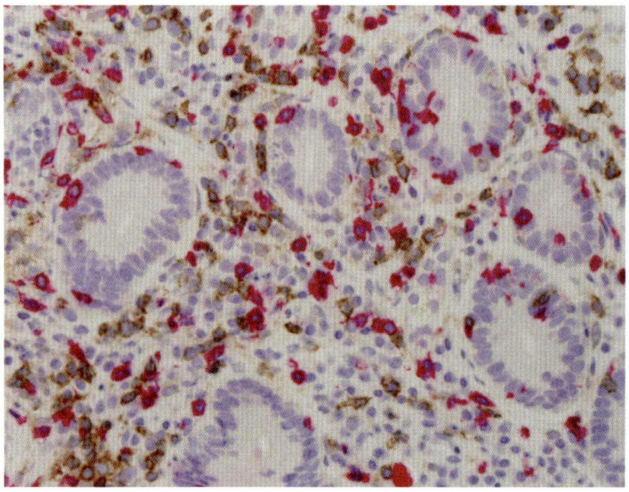

图 86.5 发生急性 T 细胞介导的排斥的移植结肠,轻度(1 级)伴随间隙和陷窝内显著出现混合性 $CD4^+$和 $CD8^+$细胞(两种颜色的免疫组织化学染色,×400,$CD4^+$=褐色,$CD8^+$=红色)。

与了隐窝上皮细胞的凋亡和急性移植器官排斥。

一些小肠和结肠移植的急性排斥分类系统，同胃移植道一起已经被报道过。在 2003 年第 18 届国际小肠移植研讨会上，来自不同国家的病理学家和临床医生提出了一项统一小肠移植中急性 T 细胞介导的排斥分级方案(框 86.1)，该方案已得到了广泛应用，并已在我们机构进行了 4000 多次活检。迄今，形态学分级系统和受体的临床症状的关系显著，并且不同机构(数据未发表)的观察者间研究同样如此。

没有急性排斥的证据，0 级

这一级别的急性排斥的变化是极小的或不存在(如组织形态学不能与正常肠道区分开)；然而，其他并存的情况(非排斥)可能会存在变化。

不确定急性排斥，不确定级

这一级别活检中形态学的变化可见于任何阶段，包括急性 T 细胞介导的排斥的早期和恢复期，其有极小的上皮细胞损伤，但实质内浸润的细胞增多。炎症细胞包括淋巴细胞、嗜酸性粒细胞、免疫母细胞、一些浆细胞和偶尔可见的中性粒细胞，各细胞所占的比例不同，但弥漫或局限的密度均高于正常值。也常见绒毛变平、水肿和血管堵塞，但这些特征对于诊断不是必需的。隐窝炎、淋巴细胞或嗜酸性粒细胞及上皮凋亡小体均可见。然而，凋亡小体的数量未达到 1 级(轻度)急性 T 细胞介导的排斥。

T 细胞介导的急性排斥，轻度，1 级

轻度 T 细胞介导的急性排斥是国际分级方案规定的以 6 个凋亡小体或超过 10 个陷窝细胞作为最小的分界值。其他典型特征包括水肿、堵塞及变化的结构如绒毛变平。陷窝细胞损伤、炎症和其他不确定级的改变也可见于 1 级 T 细胞介导的急性排斥，但水平更高，包括凋亡水平。轻度到中度混合性慢性炎症细胞浸润趋向于弥漫性分布(图 86.6)，浸润往往深至黏膜下层并可累及肌肉。这些形态学特征，尤其是浸润的特点和程度，会因移植后时间的变动而波动。也可见再生的特点如黏蛋白的丢失、上皮细胞细核增大和染色过深，取决于排斥持续的时间长短。血管堵塞和内皮炎也伴随出现于这一级或更高级的 T 细胞介导的急性排斥。

急性 T 细胞介导的急性排斥，中度，2 级

2 级 T 细胞介导的急性排斥中，存在轻度 T 细胞介导的急性排斥特征，但也存在更大程度的陷窝细胞损伤，有时在单一的隐窝内有融合的凋亡小体。可能存

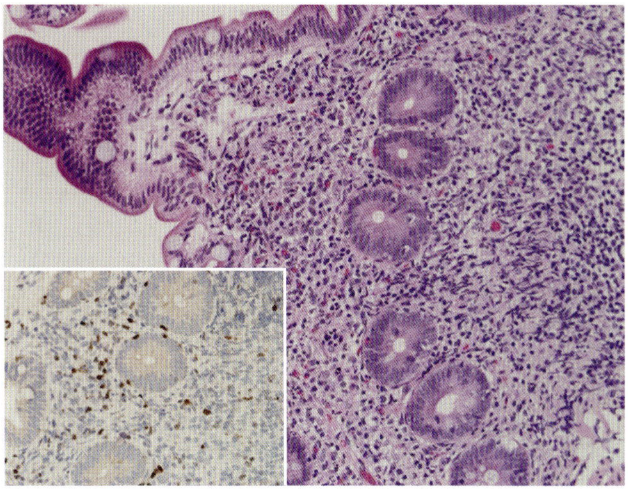

图 86.6　急性 T 细胞介导的排斥，轻度。隐窝内见混合性炎性浸润合并许多凋亡小体(10 个隐窝内可见超过 6 个凋亡小体)(HE 染色，×200)。(插图)Tbet+T 细胞(Th1 细胞)增多(Tbet 免疫组织化学染色，HE 染色，×400)(HE 染色，×400)。

在全部腺体坏死和陷窝脓肿。炎症浸润至固有层和黏膜下层且比表现为混合性但主要为单核细胞浸润(包括淋巴母细胞或激活的淋巴细胞、黏膜结构改变)的轻度 T 细胞介导的急性排斥程度更大。中至重度浸润受移植后时间的影响更小，绒毛变平，水肿和血管堵塞比 1 级排斥分布更广。

急性 T 细胞介导的急性排斥，严重，3 级

急性 T 细胞介导的急性排斥(3 级)是临床和形态学上有显著变化的类型。这常常也是混合性急性排斥(T 细胞介导的急性排斥加上急性抗体介导的排斥)，可发现同种抗体。陷窝细胞损伤和凋亡、腺体破坏和相关的黏膜溃疡无所不在。陷窝上皮凋亡的水平是可变动的。事实上，在存活的陷窝中也可能存在正常水平的凋亡。可发现显著的炎症浸润，包括淋巴母细胞或激活的淋巴细胞，嗜酸性粒细胞和中性粒细胞。内镜医生常能发现易碎的组织，这样就能获取有显著结构改变的组织的碎片。持久的严重排斥常导致肠道组织结构的完全丧失，可有肉芽组织和(或)纤维脓性(假膜)渗出及黏膜脱落(图 86.7)。黏膜溃疡在没有活动性隐窝细胞损伤的情况下，不应被归为 3 级 ACR，而应归为“与 ACR 一致，严重”级别，因为缺血和感染过程也可导致黏膜坏死。严重的长期急性排斥的结果——仅对坏死组织有效——也被称为剥脱性排斥。

因此，获取来自累及较少的区域的组织是非常有用的。严重的 T 细胞介导的急性排斥能导致小肠失去功

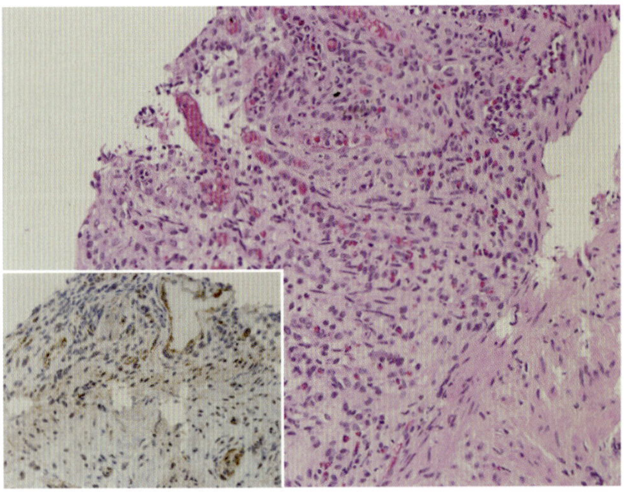

图 86.7 急性T细胞介导的排斥/急性抗体介导的排斥(混合性排斥),严重。移植小肠的黏膜结构变化巨大且被肉芽组织替代。因为陷窝的完全丧失导致陷窝上皮细胞凋亡很难评估。可见致密炎症浸润,其由混合性但主要为单核细胞和激活的淋巴母细胞;嗜酸性粒细胞和中性粒细胞构成(HE染色,×200)。(插图)脉管系统被C4d染色。患者同样有供体特异的同种抗体(C4d免疫组织化学染色,×400)。

能。通常,小肠内部分区域较易发生T细胞介导的急性排斥;例如,回肠比十二指肠和空肠更易发生更严重的T细胞介导的急性排斥[63]。强力免疫抑制治疗T细胞介导的急性排斥,同种免疫介导的损伤和黏膜屏障功能(小肠上皮细胞、胞间紧密连接和基膜)的损伤有可能导致严重的感染并发症,从而使细菌移位进入腹腔内[38,64]。

结肠和胃的T细胞介导的急性排斥

在多器官移植的患者中,除小肠外移植的消化道也能发生急性和慢性排斥。移植结肠的T细胞介导的急性排斥中可见与移植小肠相似的变化。我们关于移植结肠的活检经验正逐渐增加,因为结肠移植越来越多见于多器官移植[65]。结肠T细胞介导的急性排斥浸润其炎症细胞的构成和方法与小肠类似,同时也有隐窝中上皮细胞损伤、结构扭曲、杯状细胞丢失和上皮细胞变薄。我们在结肠中使用和小肠一样的标准和分级系统[60,61,66]。在多器官移植的患者中,常常同时存在原生结肠;这样,同时获取原生和移植器官的组织对于病理学家鉴别同种反应和其他炎症反应是很有用的。

移植胃内全部区域都能发生T细胞介导的急性排斥,单独或合并其他炎症反应(如各种慢性胃炎或感染性疾病)。上皮损伤以凋亡或反应性变化的方式发生,这与小肠和结肠移植类似。胃部急性排斥的炎症程度比小肠轻,胃部急性排斥程度不代表对应程度的小肠、结肠炎症和上皮细胞损伤程度。然而,我们已经发现许多仅有移植胃排斥或胃排斥的程度超过小肠或结肠的情况。生成数值评分,以提供不同T细胞介导的急性排斥水平的分级方案,成为评估同种异体胃移植病理学的有用方法[59]。

慢性排斥

随着小肠移植和多器官移植的存活率显著增加,慢性同种移植排斥肠病或小肠移植的慢性排斥发生率正在增加[2,34]。事实上,其正成为胃肠道移植中移植器官失去功能的主要原因。肠道慢性排斥的病理生理学和其他器官系统一样,受非免疫[67]和免疫因素[68-71]相互作用的影响。慢性同种移植排斥肠病的临床症状趋向于非特异性(如蛋白丢失性肠病),内镜信息包括绒毛结构丢失、变平;这些发现对于整合黏膜活检的病理发现非常有用。因严重的慢性排斥而移除的肠道大体,存在丰富的浆膜附着并显示出导致暗淡的缠结的器官团,伴随透壁性增厚、不规则的扁平黏膜表面和间断性溃疡。

肠道慢性排斥有特殊病征的损伤为动脉同心圆型内膜增厚及纤维改变、平滑肌细胞内侧肥大、夹杂着泡沫细胞及外膜纤维化。小肠黏膜活检常局限于仅能发现大血管的慢性排斥变化[72,73],因为这些动脉不常规见于内镜下活检。在各期中动脉分支的血栓有时能同内膜间慢性炎症细胞一起被发现,后者与活动性慢性肾脏移植动脉病相同。黏膜层、黏膜下层和肌层纤维化,伴随陷窝丢失、陷窝分离、绒毛变平、黏膜萎缩和出现移植动脉病的小动脉分支。神经节细胞破坏和增生,以及可能存在纤维蛋白性浆膜炎。慢性炎症细胞浸润也常见,并可能有溃疡和叠加的急性排斥。

发生慢性同种移植排斥肠病的胃肠移植黏膜活检对于鉴别慢性损伤非常有用(如纤维化、陷窝丢失和变形、结构改变),结合临床病史及内镜检查也对鉴别慢性排斥有用(图86.8)。对比邻近的原生组织是非常有用的,因为原生组织是普通的。结合淋巴细胞和巨噬细胞的免疫组织化学特点可用于黏膜活检评估慢性排斥。半定量评分系统对于鉴别和预测慢性同种移植排斥肠病也同样有用[73]。

感染

与小肠移植和多器官移植有关的严重副反应包括

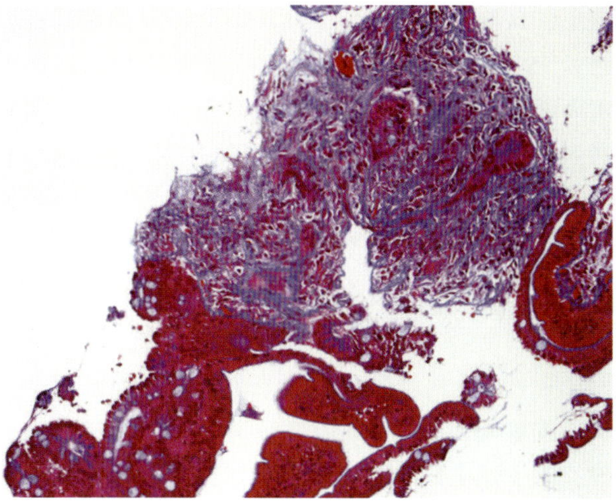

图 86.8 慢性排斥。三色排斥显示黏膜下层和固有层存在显著的纤维化(三色染色,×200)。

机会性感染和并发症[74-76]。这些感染系统性或局限性出现于移植器官和邻近原生组织(如感染性胃炎、肠炎或结肠炎)。感染病原体可危害移植器官的功能并使受体在没有鉴别和治疗的情况下发生死亡的危险。因为胃肠道感染的症状有时和急性排斥的症状相似(如腹泻、发热),这些诊断必须通过培养和(或)活检来区分,因为治疗常包括降低免疫抑制水平。

许多病毒可参与肠道移植并且能被形态学改变所辨别,被免疫组织化学或分子技术或培养所证实。这些病毒包括轮状病毒、腺病毒、杯状病毒 (人类杯状病毒)、巨细胞病毒、单纯疱疹病毒和 EB 病毒。这些病毒出现于胃肠道组织,伴随着由急性和慢性炎症细胞和混合性构成并有局限或弥漫性上皮损伤、细胞增生改变和细胞学改变的肠道炎症(如胃炎、肠炎)[77]。更严重的病例可出现局部坏死。也可见急性排斥相伴随。因此,当分析组织学时移植病理学家获取患者的临床病史和培养及分子检测结果仍然十分重要。

腺病毒感染对于胃肠道移植患者是复杂且危险的,在小肠移植和多器官移植病例报道不一[78,79]。可发现有陷窝细胞凋亡和混合性的慢性炎症细胞浸润,并合并增大深染的表面上皮细胞。也存在嗜酸性核合并破碎细胞、增大的嗜碱性细胞核和肠表面细胞的增生[80]。检测组织中病毒的免疫染色、电子显微镜和聚合酶链反应分析对于检测病原体十分有用。一些与腺病毒感染有关的组织病理学变化在急性排斥中也明显存在。因此通过各种工具来鉴别是十分重要的。腺病毒性肠炎的快速诊断是必要的,因为没有适当的治疗,患者的临床状况往往迅速恶化。

儿童普遍有轮状病毒感染史,其也可发生于小肠移植和多器官移植的患者。与病毒有关的组织病理学变化不明显,活检不常规用于鉴别轮状病毒。上皮内有表面增生变化,混合性黏膜表面中心粒细胞和细胞碎片炎症浸润。深部的隐窝不受上皮损伤的影响。急性排斥和轮状病毒感染也可能同时存在[81,82]。

杯状病毒感染由两条病原链构成:类诺瓦克病毒和札幌病毒。杯状病毒是人群中轻度胃肠道炎和(或)长期的大量腹泻的常见原因,通过排泄物样本中反式聚合酶链反应检测发现。组织病理学改变包括绒毛变钝变细、混合性淋巴浆细胞性浸润、固有层少量中性粒细胞浸润、表面上皮活动性变化,包括细胞极性的丢失、表面上皮细胞和隐窝中凋亡、固有层巨噬细胞增多[83]。

胃肠道移植受体中常见巨细胞病毒感染[84-87],呈系统性或局限性分布。巨细胞病毒性肠炎也表现为腹泻、上腹痛和腹部不适。胃和小肠的内镜检查中常发现黏膜侵蚀和溃疡。典型的巨细胞病毒感染表现为被明显的光环包绕的细胞核内含嗜酸性物质和细胞膜增厚。这些细胞表现为慢性炎症浸润,包括淋巴细胞和组织细胞,有时固有层内可观察到中性粒细胞。孤立的细胞核内容物隐藏于慢性炎症浸润中很难发现。巨细胞的免疫组织化学染色及组织的聚合酶链反应分析检测对于确诊巨细胞病毒性肠炎也是有帮助的,其有时在严重炎症细胞浸润中不明显。

在移植患者中,单纯疱疹病毒感染(HSV)最常见于口腔、食管、肛周区域和直肠,但单纯疱疹病毒性肠炎相对少见。内镜检查时,单纯疱疹病毒性肠炎表现为口疮和坏死性溃疡、黏膜红斑易碎以及炎症性损伤。显微镜下,可发现淋巴浆细胞性炎性改变合并分散的嗜酸性粒细胞。病毒感染细胞可表现为嗜酸性核内包涵体和多核化。活检样本的培养和免疫组织化学对于确诊单纯疱疹病毒十分有用。

小肠移植和多器官移植中少见 EB 病毒急性感染,但与移植后淋巴组织增生性疾病相关的(见下文)慢性感染常见。

可以发现肠道移植的细菌过度增生 (与正常群体相比),病理学家应当就这些信息进行交流。在这些肠道移植的潜在重要的细菌感染中,不典型的分枝杆菌可导致移植器官功能显著异常[89]。同样,一些真菌和寄生病原体,包括假丝酵母和隐孢子虫[90],存在于胃肠道且可累及胃肠道移植物。

复发性疾病及其他肠炎

有少部分的小肠移植和多器官移植患者,其原发的系统性或小肠疾病有可能复发于移植的器官。一般而言,胃肠道移植的疾病复发不如其他实质性器官移植(如肝脏、肾脏)频繁。炎症性肠病(如克罗恩病)[91,92]患者可能重新累及移植的肠道且可能明显存在于黏膜活检中。炎症性肠病合并特定的系统性疾病如硬化性胆管炎[93]也可能发生于胃肠道移植中。原发性疾病为特定腹腔肿瘤(如韧带样瘤)的多器官移植患者[94,95],移植后即可能出现肿瘤复发。这些肿瘤复发可出现在腹腔内,也可发生在胃肠道外或腹腔外。

胃肠道移植可发生炎性损伤且来源模糊或无法解释。在治疗的过程中,一些小肠移植和多器官移植的患者可进展,发生持续的同时累及移植器官和原生胃肠道组织的溃疡[96,97]。这些溃疡的发生有多种原因,包括EB病毒阳性的移植物抗宿主病(最常见的原因)、急性排斥、感染和一些原因不明的病例。

除了同种免疫反应,也存在其他影响移植小肠和原生小肠的炎症[98,99]。病因未明的活动性肠炎以固有层和(或)表面上皮的急性炎症(如多晶型中心粒细胞浸润)为特征,伴有局灶性溃疡和隐窝脓肿。一些可能的致病机制已经被提出,包括血行停滞、改变的菌群、缺血、下垂、黏液溶解。富嗜酸性粒细胞肠炎和结肠炎有时是一种与变应性致敏相关的炎症状态。一些NOD2基因多态性与改变的细菌清除和增多的炎症浸润有关[16,91,100,101]。

再生性变化的出现是由于急性排斥后的愈合、感染性肠炎。

移植物抗宿主病可发生在小肠移植和包含皮肤、原生消化道和其他系统的多器官移植患者中[15,102-104]。移植物抗宿主病在原生胃肠道组织中的组织病理学特点与急性T细胞介导的(细胞)排斥相似,其陷窝上皮细胞凋亡且炎症浸润增多。了解临床病史和组织样本的来源(来自移植器官或原生器官)对于诊断移植物抗宿主病十分重要。移植后淋巴组织增生性疾病在小肠移植和多器官移植患者中发生率高。因为长期的免疫抑制,这些常见的并发症发生率随着移植后时间的增加而上升[20,87,105,106]。虽然EB病毒阴性移植后淋巴组织增生性疾病也会发生,但EB病毒感染常与移植后淋巴组织增生性疾病相关。肠道移植后淋巴组织增生性疾病的组织病理学包括增生性浆细胞(损伤早期)、多态的移植后淋巴组织增生性疾病,单态的移植后淋巴组织增生性疾病和淋巴瘤。随着移植后时间延长,移植后淋巴组织增生性疾病的可疑前驱损伤、淋巴浆细胞性浸润(如增生性浆细胞的)常见于肠道移植活检,上皮结构可能被浸润所影响(图86.9)。依靠EB早期基因产物的EB病毒染色和免疫组织化学检测浸润的B和T细胞的出现和构成,对于评估可疑的移植后淋巴组织增生性疾病十分有用[109]。基于石蜡块的T和B细胞抗原受体的基因重排研究,对于评估潜在的单克隆性十分有用[107,108]。单形态的移植后淋巴组织增生性疾病可能为T或B细胞来源[110,111],被认为是肿瘤。根据结构和细胞学特点与发生于原生组织的淋巴瘤相同,移植后淋巴组织增生性淋巴瘤被分为一类[109]。

总结

过去20年间小肠移植和多器官移植的成功有多种原因,病理学对移植内脏的评估也取得了显著进展。对影响这些特殊移植器官同种异体移植的多个病理实体进行了精确的描述,开发了几种情况下的分级方案。而且,额外生物标志物正在更多地用于系统组织的评估,这对于完善活检的形态学描述有帮助。未来临床和

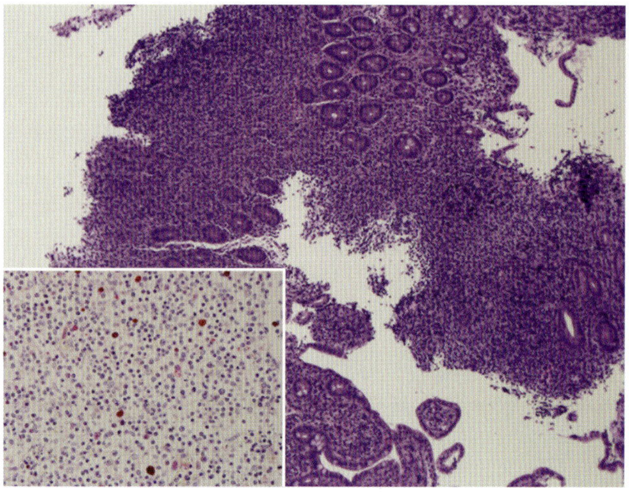

图86.9 移植后淋巴组织增生性疾病。病灶非典型性扩张的轻度淋巴浆细胞性浸润(HE染色,×40)。(插图)EB病毒原位杂交染色。EB病毒阳细胞浸润(HE染色,×400)。

科学发现能进一步加强移植器官的诊断能力。

（周舒扬 杨梦凡 译 周舒扬 校）

参考文献

1. LaRosa C, Baluarte HJ, Meyers KEC. Outcomes in pediatric solid-organ transplantation. Pediatric Transplantation. 2011;15:128–141.
2. Mazariegos GV. Intestinal transplantation: current outcomes and opportunities. Current Opinion in Organ Transplantation. 2009;14:515–521.
3. Avitzur Y, Grant D. Intestine transplantation in children: update 2010. Pediatric Clinics of North America. 2010;57:415–431.
4. Fishbein TM. Intestinal transplantation. New England Journal of Medicine. 2009;361:998–1008.
5. Sauvat F, Fusaro F, Lacaille F, et al. Is intestinal transplantation the future of children with definitive intestinal insufficiency? European Journal of Pediatric Surgery. 2008;18:368–371.
6. Gupte GL, Beath SV. Update on intestinal rehabilitation after intestinal transplantation. Current Opinion in Organ Transplantation. 2009;14:267–273.
7. Sudan D. Long-term outcomes and quality of life after intestine transplantation. Current Opinion in Organ Transplantation. 2010;15:357–360.
8. Ruiz P, Kato T, Tzakis A. Current status of transplantation of the small intestine. Transplantation. 2007;83:1–6.
9. Tzakis AG, Kato T, Levi DM, et al. 100 multivisceral transplants at a single center. Annals of Surgery. 2005;242:480–490; discussion 491–493. [see comment].
10. D'Alessandro AM, Rankin MA. Heterotopic rat intestinal transplantation: effect of cyclosporine and RS-61443 on graft-vs-host disease and rejection. Transplantation Proceedings. 1994;26:1611–1612.
11. Zhong R, Grant D, Sutherland F, et al. Refined technique for intestinal transplantation in the rat. Microsurgery. 1991;12:268–274.
12. Ruiz P. Transplantation Pathology, 1st ed. In: Ruiz P, editor. Vol. 1, New York, NY: Cambridge University Press; 2009.
13. Nayyar NS, McGhee W, Martin D, et al. Intestinal transplantation in children: a review of immunotherapy regimens. Paediatric Drugs. 2011;13:149–159.
14. Sirinek LP, O'Dorisio MS, Dunaway DJ. Accumulation of donor-specific cytotoxic T cells in intestinal lymphoid tissues following intestinal transplantation. Journal of Clinical Immunology. 1995;15:258–265.
15. Wu G, Selvaggi G, Nishida S, et al. Graft-versus-host disease after intestinal and multivisceral transplantation. Transplantation. 2011;91:219–224.
16. Fishbein T, Novitskiy G, Mishra L, et al. NOD2-expressing bone marrow-derived cells appear to regulate epithelial innate immunity of the transplanted human small intestine. Gut. 2008;57:323–330.
17. Wood KJ, Goto R. Mechanisms of rejection: current perspectives. Transplantation. 2012;93:1–10.
18. Takahashi H, Kato T, Selvaggi G, et al. Subclinical rejection in the initial postoperative period in small intestinal transplantation: a negative influence on graft survival. Transplantation. 2007;84:689–696.
19. Mengel M. What is the significance of subclinical inflammation in human renal allografts? It depends! Transplantation. 2012;93:22–23.
20. Abu-Elmagd KM, Mazariegos G, Costa G, et al. Lymphoproliferative disorders and de novo malignancies in intestinal and multivisceral recipients: improved outcomes with new outlooks. Transplantation. 2009;88:926–934.
21. Wallemacq PE, Reding R. FK506 (tacrolimus), a novel immunosuppressant in organ transplantation: clinical, biomedical, and analytical aspects. Clinical Chemistry. 1993;39:2219–2228.
22. Cardenas ME, Zhu D, Heitman J. Molecular mechanisms of immunosuppression by cyclosporine, FK506, and rapamycin. Current Opinion in Nephrology and Hypertension. 1995;4:472–477.
23. Konigsrainer A, Ladurner R, Iannetti C, et al. The 'Blind Innsbruck Ostomy', a cutaneous enterostomy for long-term histologic surveillance after small bowel transplantation. Transplant International. 2007;20:867–874.
24. Ueno T, Fukuzawa M. Current status of intestinal transplantation. Surgery Today. 2010;40:1112–1122.
25. Eltzschig HK, Eckle T. Ischemia and reperfusion: from mechanism to translation. Nature Medicine. 2011;17:1391–1401.
26. Mallick IH, Yang W, Winslet MC, Seifalian AM. Protective effects of ischemic preconditioning on the intestinal mucosal microcirculation following ischemia-reperfusion of the intestine. Microcirculation. 2005;12:615–625.
27. Akalin E, O'Connell PJ. Genomics of chronic allograft injury. Kidney International. 2010;78(Suppl 119):S33–S37.
28. Naito Y, Mizushima K, Yoshikawa T. Global analysis of gene expression in gastric ischemia-reperfusion: a future therapeutic direction for mucosal protective drugs. Digestive Diseases and Sciences. 2005;50(Suppl 1):S45–S55.
29. Stallone G, Infante B, Gesualdo L. Older donors and older recipients in kidney transplantation. Journal of Nephrology. 2010;23(Suppl 15):S98–S103.
30. Quaedackers JS, Beuk RJ, Bennet L, et al. An evaluation of methods for grading histologic injury following ischemia/reperfusion of the small bowel. Transplantation Proceedings. 2000;32:1307–1310.
31. Wasserberg N, Tzakis AG, Santiago SF, Ruiz P, Salgar SK. Anastomotic healing in a small bowel transplantation model in the rat. World Journal of Surgery. 2004;28:69–73.
32. Beuk RJ, Tangelder GJ, Maassen RL, et al. Leucocyte and platelet adhesion in different layers of the small bowel during experimental total warm ischaemia and reperfusion. British Journal of Surgery. 2008;95:1294–1304.
33. Asaoka T, Island ER, Tryphonopoulos P, et al. Characteristic immune, apoptosis and inflammatory gene profiles associated with intestinal acute cellular rejection in formalin-fixed paraffin-embedded mucosal biopsies. Transplant International. 2011;24:697–707.
34. Nayyar N, Mazariegos G, Ranganathan S, et al. Pediatric small bowel transplantation. Seminars in Pediatric Surgery. 2010;19:68–77.
35. Kato T, Ruiz P, Tzakis A. Exfoliative bowel rejection: a dangerous loss of integrity. Pediatric Transplantation. 2004;8:426–427.
36. Park KT, Berquist WL, Pai R, Triadafilopoulos G. Exfoliative rejection in intestinal transplantation. Digestive Diseases and Sciences. 2010;55:3336–3338.
37. Berney T, Kato T, Nishida S, et al. Portal versus systemic drainage of small bowel allografts: comparative assessment of survival, function, rejection, and bacterial translocation. Journal of the American College of Surgeons. 2002;195:804–813.
38. Cicalese L, Sileri P, Green M, et al. Bacterial translocation in clinical intestinal transplantation. Transplantation. 2001;71:1414–1417.
39. Seron D, Moreso F. Protocol biopsies in renal transplantation: prognostic value of structural monitoring. Kidney International. 2007;72:690–697.
40. Choi BS, Shin MJ, Shin SJ, et al. Clinical significance of an early protocol biopsy in living-donor renal transplantation: ten-year experience at a single center. American Journal of Transplantation. 2005;5:1354–1360.
41. Mercer DF. Hot topics in postsmall bowel transplantation: noninvasive graft monitoring including stool calprotectin and plasma citrulline. Current Opinion in Organ Transplantation. 2011;16:316–322.
42. Sageshima J, Ciancio G, Gaynor JJ, et al. Addition of anti-CD25 to thymoglobulin for induction therapy: delayed return of peripheral blood CD25-positive population. Clinical Transplantation. 2011;25:E132–E135.
43. Ruiz P, Tryphonopoulos P, Island E, et al. Citrulline evaluation in bowel transplantation. Transplantation Proceedings. 2010;42:54–56.
44. David AI, Selvaggi G, Ruiz P, et al. Blood citrulline level is an exclusionary marker for significant acute rejection after intestinal transplantation. Transplantation. 2007;84:1077–1081.
45. Pappas PA, Tzakis A, Gaynor JJ, et al. An analysis of the association between serum citrulline and acute rejection among 26 recipients of intestinal transplant. American Journal of Transplantation. 2004;4:1124–1132.
46. Rose AG. Understanding the pathogenesis and the pathology of hyperacute cardiac rejection. Cardiovascular Pathology. 2002;11:171–176.
47. Terasaki PI, Cai J. Humoral theory of transplantation: further evidence. Current Opinion in Immunology. 2005;17:541–545.
48. Ruiz P, Carreno M, Weppler D, et al. Immediate antibody-mediated (hyperacute) rejection in small-bowel transplantation and relationship to cross-match status and donor-specific C4d-binding antibodies: case report. Transplantation Proceedings. 2010;42:95–99.
49. Tsai HL, Island ER, Chang JW, et al. Association between donor-specific antibodies and acute rejection and resolution in small bowel and multivisceral transplantation. Transplantation. 2011;92:709–715.
50. Gerlach UA, Schoenemann C, Lachmann N, Koch M, Pascher A. Salvage therapy for refractory rejection and persistence of donor-specific antibodies after intestinal transplantation using the proteasome inhibitor bortezomib. Transplant International. 2011;24:e43–e45.
51. Kato T, Mizutani K, Terasaki P, et al. Association of emergence of HLA antibody and acute rejection in intestinal transplant recipients: a possible evidence of acute humoral sensitization. Transplantation Proceedings. 2006;38:1735–1737.
52. Ruiz P, Garcia M, Pappas P, et al. Mucosal vascular alterations in isolated small-bowel allografts: relationship to humoral sensitization. American Journal of Transplantation. 2003;3:43–49.
53. Ruiz P, Suarez M, Nishida S, et al. Sclerosing mesenteritis in small bowel transplantation: possible manifestation of acute vascular rejection. Transplantation Proceedings. 2003;35:3057–3060.
54. Lee RG, Nakamura K, Tsamandas AC, et al. Pathology of human intestinal transplantation. Gastroenterology. 1996;110:1820–1834.
55. Delacruz V, Garcia M, Mittal N, et al. Immunoenzymatic and morphological detection of epithelial cell apoptotic stages in gastrointestinal allografts from

multivisceral transplant patients. Transplantation Proceedings. 2004;36:338-339.
56. Krams SM, Hayashi M, Fox CK, et al. CD8+ cells are not necessary for allograft rejection or the induction of apoptosis in an experimental model of small intestinal transplantation. Journal of Immunology. 1998;160:3673-3680.
57. Ogura Y, Martinez OM, Villanueva JC, et al. Apoptosis and allograft rejection in the absence of CD8+ T cells. Transplantation. 2001;71:1827-1834.
58. Wu T, Abu-Elmagd K, Bond G, et al. A schema for histologic grading of small intestine allograft acute rejection. Transplantation. 2003;75:1241-1248.
59. Garcia M, Delacruz V, Ortiz R, et al. Acute cellular rejection grading scheme for human gastric allografts. Human Pathology. 2004;35:343-349.
60. Ruiz P, Bagni A, Brown R, et al. Histological criteria for the identification of acute cellular rejection in human small bowel allografts: results of the pathology workshop at the VIII International Small Bowel Transplant Symposium. Transplantation Proceedings. 2004;36:335-337.
61. Ruiz P, Takahashi H, Delacruz V, et al. International grading scheme for acute cellular rejection in small-bowel transplantation: single-center experience. Transplantation Proceedings. 2010;42:47-53.
62. Ishii T, Mazariegos GV, Bueno J, et al. Exfoliative rejection after intestinal transplantation in children. Pediatric Transplantation. 2003;7:185-191.
63. Takahashi H, Selvaggi G, Nishida S, et al. Organ-specific differences in acute rejection intensity in a multivisceral transplant. Transplantation. 2006;81:297-299.
64. Zou Y, Hernandez F, Burgos E, et al. Bacterial translocation in acute rejection after small bowel transplantation in rats. Pediatric Surgery International. 2005;21:208-211.
65. Kato T, Selvaggi G, Gaynor JJ, et al. Inclusion of donor colon and Ileocecal valve in intestinal transplantation. Transplantation. 2008;86:293-297.
66. Ruiz P, Weppler D, Nishida S, et al. International grading scheme for acute rejection in small bowel transplantation: implementation and experience at the University of Miami. Transplantation Proceedings. 2006;38:1683-1684.
67. Murphy SP, Porrett PM, Turka LA. Innate immunity in transplant tolerance and rejection. Immunological Reviews. 2011;241:39-48.
68. Baluja P, Haragsim L, Laszik Z. Chronic allograft nephropathy. Advances in Chronic Kidney Disease. 2006;13:56-61.
69. Colvin RB, Hirohashi T, Farris AB, et al. Emerging role of B cells in chronic allograft dysfunction. Kidney International. 2010;78(Suppl 119):S13-S17.
70. Thaunat O, Patey N, Caligiuri G, et al. Chronic rejection triggers the development of an aggressive intragraft immune response through recapitulation of lymphoid organogenesis. Journal of Immunology. 2010;185:717-728.
71. Takeda A, Horike K, Ohtsuka Y, et al. Current problems of chronic active antibody-mediated rejection. Clinical Transplantation. 2011;25(Suppl 23):2-5.
72. Tryphonopoulos P, Weppler D, Nishida S, et al. Mucosal fibrosis in intestinal transplant biopsies correlates positively with the development of chronic rejection. Transplantation Proceedings. 2006;38:1685-1686.
73. Perez MT, Garcia M, Weppler D, et al. Temporal relationships between acute cellular rejection features and increased mucosal fibrosis in the early posttransplant period of human small intestinal allografts. Transplantation. 2002;73:555-559.
74. Fryer JP. The current status of intestinal transplantation. Current Opinion in Organ Transplantation. 2008;13:266-272.
75. Dijkstra G, Rings EH, van Dullemen HM, et al. Small bowel transplantation as a treatment option for intestinal failure in children and adults [in Dutch]. Nederlands Tijdschrift Voor Geneeskunde. 2005;149:391-398.
76. Abu-Elmagd K, Reyes J, Bond G, et al. Clinical intestinal transplantation: a decade of experience at a single center. Annals of Surgery. 2001;234:404-416; discussion 416-417.
77. Ziring D, Tran R, Edelstein S, et al. Infectious enteritis after intestinal transplantation: incidence, timing, and outcome. Transplantation. 2005;79:702-709.
78. McLaughlin GE, Delis S, Kashimawo L, et al. Adenovirus infection in pediatric liver and intestinal transplant recipients: utility of DNA detection by PCR. American Journal of Transplantation. 2003;3:224-228.
79. Pinchoff RJ, Kaufman SS, Magid MS, et al. Adenovirus infection in pediatric small bowel transplantation recipients. Transplantation. 2003;76:183-189.
80. Berho M, Torroella M, Viciana A, et al. Adenovirus enterocolitis in human small bowel transplants. Pediatric Transplantation. 1998;2:277-282.
81. Giovanelli M, Gupte GL, Sharif K, et al. Chronic rejection after combined liver and small bowel transplantation in a child with chronic intestinal pseudo-obstruction: a case report. Transplantation Proceedings. 2008;40:1763-1767.
82. Ziring D, Tran R, Edelstein S, et al. Infectious enteritis after intestinal transplantation: incidence, timing, and outcome. Transplantation Proceedings. 2004;36:379-380.
83. Kaufman SS, Chatterjee NK, Fuschino ME, et al. Calicivirus enteritis in an intestinal transplant recipient. American Journal of Transplantation. 2003;3:764-768.
84. Pascher A, Klupp J, Schulz RJ, et al. CMV, EBV, HHV6, and HHV7 infections after intestinal transplantation without specific antiviral prophylaxis. Transplantation Proceedings. 2004;36:381-382.
85. Bueno J, Green M, Kocoshis S, et al. Cytomegalovirus infection after intestinal transplantation in children. Clinical Infectious Diseases. 1997;25:1078-1083.
86. Furukawa H, Kusne S, Abu-Elmagd K, et al. Effect of CMV serology on outcome after clinical intestinal transplantation. Transplantation Proceedings. 1996;28:2780-2781.
87. Kocoshis SA. Small bowel transplantation in infants and children. Gastroenterology Clinics of North America. 1994;23:727-742.
88. Gourishankar S, McDermid JC, Jhangri GS, Preiksaitis JK. Herpes zoster infection following solid organ transplantation: incidence, risk factors and outcomes in the current immunosuppressive era. American Journal of Transplantation. 2004;4:108-115.
89. Kato T, Dowdy L, Weppler D, et al. Non-tuberculous mycobacterial associated enterocolitis in intestinal transplantation. Transplantation Proceedings. 1998;30:2537-2538.
90. Delis SG, Tector J, Kato T, et al. Diagnosis and treatment of cryptosporidium infection in intestinal transplant recipients. Transplantation Proceedings. 2002;34:951-952.
91. Ningappa M, Higgs BW, Weeks DE, et al. NOD2 gene polymorphism rs2066844 associates with need for combined liver-intestine transplantation in children with short-gut syndrome. American Journal of Gastroenterology. 2011;106:157-165.
92. Sustento-Reodica N, Ruiz P, Rogers A, et al. Recurrent Crohn's disease in transplanted bowel. Lancet. 1997;349:688-691.
93. Knight C, Murray KF. Hepatobiliary associations with inflammatory bowel disease. Expert Review of Gastroenterology and Hepatology. 2009;3:681-691.
94. Chatzipetrou MA, Tzakis AG, Pinna AD, et al. Intestinal transplantation for the treatment of desmoid tumors associated with familial adenomatous polyposis. Surgery. 2001;129:277-281.
95. Moon JI, Selvaggi G, Nishida S, et al. Intestinal transplantation for the treatment of neoplastic disease. Journal of Surgical Oncology. 2005;92:284-291.
96. Sarkar S, Selvaggi G, Mittal N, et al. Gastrointestinal tract ulcers in pediatric intestinal transplantation patients: etiology and management. Pediatric Transplantation. 2006;10:162-167.
97. Turner D, Martin S, Ngan BY, et al. Anastomotic ulceration following small bowel transplantation. American Journal of Transplantation. 2006;6:236-240.
98. Martland GT, Shepherd NA. Indeterminate colitis: definition, diagnosis, implications and a plea for nosological sanity. Histopathology. 2007;50:83-96.
99. Goldstein N, Dulai M. Contemporary morphologic definition of backwash ileitis in ulcerative colitis and features that distinguish it from Crohn disease. American Journal of Clinical Pathology. 2006;126:365-376.
100. Fritz T, Niederreiter L, Adolph T, et al. Crohn's disease: NOD2, autophagy and ER stress converge. Gut. 2011;60:1580-1588.
101. Janse M, Weersma RK, Sudan DL, et al. Association of Crohn's disease-associated NOD2 variants with intestinal failure requiring small bowel transplantation and clinical outcomes. Gut. 2011;60(6):877-878; author reply 878-879.
102. Zhang Y, Ruiz P. Solid organ transplant-associated acute graft-versus-host disease. Archives of Pathology and Laboratory Medicine. 2010;134:1220-1224.
103. Andres AM, Santamaría ML, Ramos E, et al. Graft-vs-host disease after small bowel transplantation in children. Journal of Pediatric Surgery. 2010;45:330-336.
104. Triulzi DJ, Nalesnik MA. Microchimerism, GVHD, and tolerance in solid organ transplantation. Transfusion. 2001;41:419-426.
105. Pirenne J, Koshiba T, Geboes K, et al. Complete freedom from rejection after intestinal transplantation using a new tolerogenic protocol combined with low immunosuppression. Transplantation. 2002;73:966-968.
106. Ruiz P, Soares MF, Garcia M, et al. Lymphoplasmacytic hyperplasia (possibly pre-PTLD) has varied expression and appearance in intestinal transplant recipients receiving Campath immunosuppression. Transplantation Proceedings. 2004;36:386-387.
107. Blaes AH, Morrison VA. Post-transplant lymphoproliferative disorders following solid-organ transplantation. Expert Review of Hematology. 2010;3:35-44.
108. Nourse JP, Jones K, Gandhi MK. Epstein-Barr Virus-related post-transplant lymphoproliferative disorders: pathogenetic insights for targeted therapy. American Journal of Transplantation. 2011;11:888-895.
109. Parker A, Bowles K, Bradley JA, et al. Diagnosis of post-transplant lymphoproliferative disorder in solid organ transplant recipients: BCSH and BTS Guidelines. British Journal of Haematology. 2010;149:675-692.
110. Berho M, Viciana A, Weppler D, et al. T cell lymphoma involving the graft of a multivisceral organ recipient. Transplantation. 1999;68:1135-1139.
111. Sivaraman P, Lye WC. Epstein-Barr virus-associated T-cell lymphoma in solid organ transplant recipients. Biomedicine and Pharmacotherapy. 2001;55:366-368.

第 87 章 同种异体复合组织移植排斥反应和复发疾病的组织病理学综合征

Alexandra P. Turner, Alton Brad Farris, III, Alessandrina M. Freitas, Linda C. Cendales

引言

同种异体复合组织移植(VCA)是指不同胚胎来源的组织作为一个功能单位的非自体转移，常见于手移植。VCA 常用于一些不可再生组织的重建。不同于其他多种富含血管的组织嫁接,VCA 移植还包括皮肤的嫁接。迄今为止,根据国际登记处的手和复合组织移植记录,已有 90 名患者接受 VCA,其中包括 51 例四肢,7 例面部,9 例腹壁,6 例膝关节,3 例股骨干,2 例手指,1 例下肢和 1 例喉[1]。

实际上,所有接受过 VCA 的患者都有免疫排斥反应。在撰写本章时,85%接受了 VCA 的患者在第一年发生了急性排斥反应[2]。正如第 110 章中指出,高发病率可能由多种因素引起；其中一个因素是抗皮肤基因的存在可能上调同种免疫应答。作为一个暴露在外部环境中的器官，皮肤在肉眼上的病理改变并不一定是由同种免疫排斥引起的，但目前认为同种免疫本质上对皮肤是排斥的。这就涉及一个独特细微的病理学诊断,而这在其他器官移植中往往是不明显的。

虽然已经认为 VCA 的排斥反应与其他器官的排斥反应机制类似,但尚未确定在 VCA 发生免疫排斥反应时组织中是否存在不同程度的同种特异性浸润,或者组织中是否有部分结构没有发生排斥反应。临床前模型的研究表明,相比于单组织移植,多个组织移植时不同组织间的浸润程度和存活时间均有所不同[3]。由于 VCA 本身不常应用,因此尚无研究小组有足够的经验来确定其免疫排斥的病理学类型。因此,本章着重于讨论移植排斥中 VCA 发展的早期组织病理学。我们也回顾了主要由 Banff 工作组[4]提供的 VCA 病理学特征,并探讨非同种免疫的病理学特点。

背景

关于 VCA 的描述最早可追溯到公元 348 年,来自阿拉伯的双胞胎兄弟,Saint Cosmas 和 Damian 进行了下肢移植(图 87.1)。近年来,外科手术、免疫学和移植技术的发展使得 VCA 成为可能。1964 年,Joseph Murray 在同卵双胞胎中首次成功进行肾移植后，又在厄瓜多尔进行了第一例手移植术。然而由于免疫抑制治疗不足,2 周后移植物出现免疫排斥反应[5]。随后大型动物 VCA 研究出现,在这些研究中应用了人类抑制中没有使用的免疫系统干预[6]。随着 20 世纪 80 年代初环孢素的问世,VCA 再次引起人们的兴趣。灵长类动物和小型猪的大型动物模型研究显示，使用钙调磷酸酶抑制剂可改善同种移植的存活率，这些研究同时显示皮肤是发生免疫排斥反应最主要的部位[7]。1998 年，法国里昂实施了单纯手移植手术，开启了环孢素问世后 VCA 的新时代。

大型动物模型已经表明免疫排斥的速度和性质对人类 VCA 排斥反应的分类有着重要意义。在早期小型猪模型免疫排斥研究中，对排斥反应的评估主要根据以下组织中血管外细胞的外渗:真皮结缔组织、皮肤附件和上皮细胞。在猪前肢骨肌游离皮瓣移植后,对肉眼和组织学上的特点进行了研究。根据肤色、活检点出血情况及水泡形成情况将肉眼评分分为 0~4 分。组织学评分主要基于血管炎、毛囊炎、皮肤炎症及表皮变性的程度[9]。有趣的是,研究结果表明肉眼评估 1 分的排斥反应往往在病理学上并无免疫排斥反应，与肉眼评分相比,病理学评分有±1 分的偏差。在主要组织相容性

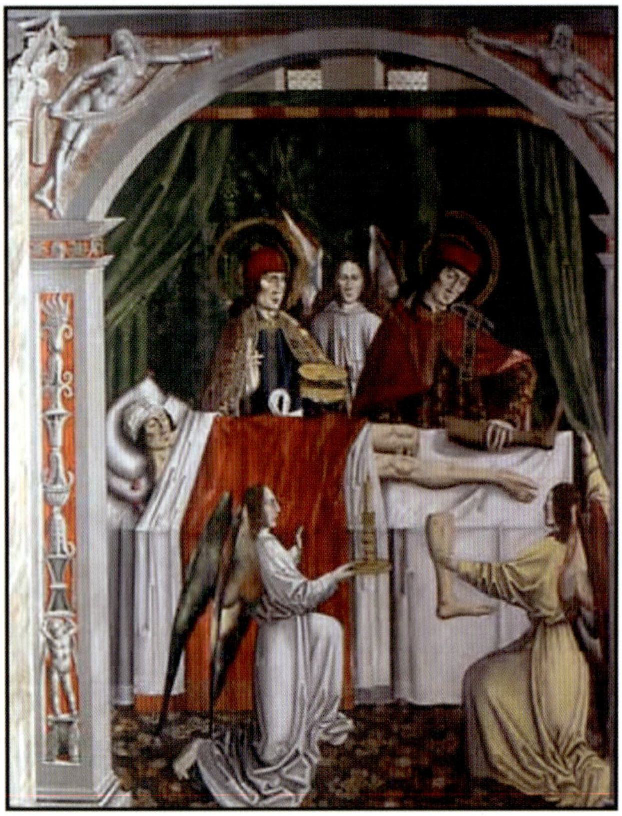

图 87.1 Saint Cosmas 和 Damian 进行肢体移植。[Source：A Verger's dream: Saint Cosmas and Damian performing miraculous cure by transplantation of a leg. Oil painting attributed to the Master of Los Balbases, ca. 1495. http://www.wdl.org/en/item/3251/(last accessed 23 January 2014).]

复合体(MHC)的相匹配小型猪研究者中,后腿在异位移植后发生了急性排斥反应。术后即刻接受 12 天的环孢素治疗，所发生的急性排斥反应表现为与组织学表皮细胞浸润有关的皮肤红斑硬结外观，随后表皮层完全脱落。尽管排斥引起了表皮坏死,但真皮、肌肉和骨并没有组织学排斥的迹象。随后真皮层能再次生发出上皮层[3]。

非人灵长类动物包括一个含有骨骼、肌肉和皮肤[10]等组织的面部 VCA 模型和一个使用可感觉骨骼肌前臂皮瓣模型[11]。在面部 VCA 模型中,真皮的排斥反应主要通过焦痂形成来表现，从而揭示了骨骼和肌肉移植的潜在可行性(图 87.2)。免疫抑制的动物在可感觉骨骼肌前臂皮瓣移植的急性免疫排斥反应中，皮肤变化主要是非烫伤样斑块状红斑疹皮疹，有时有水泡形成。活检显示皮肤周围血管、淋巴滤泡以及真皮-表皮交界处有淋巴细胞浸润。骨骼肌可出现多灶性坏死区

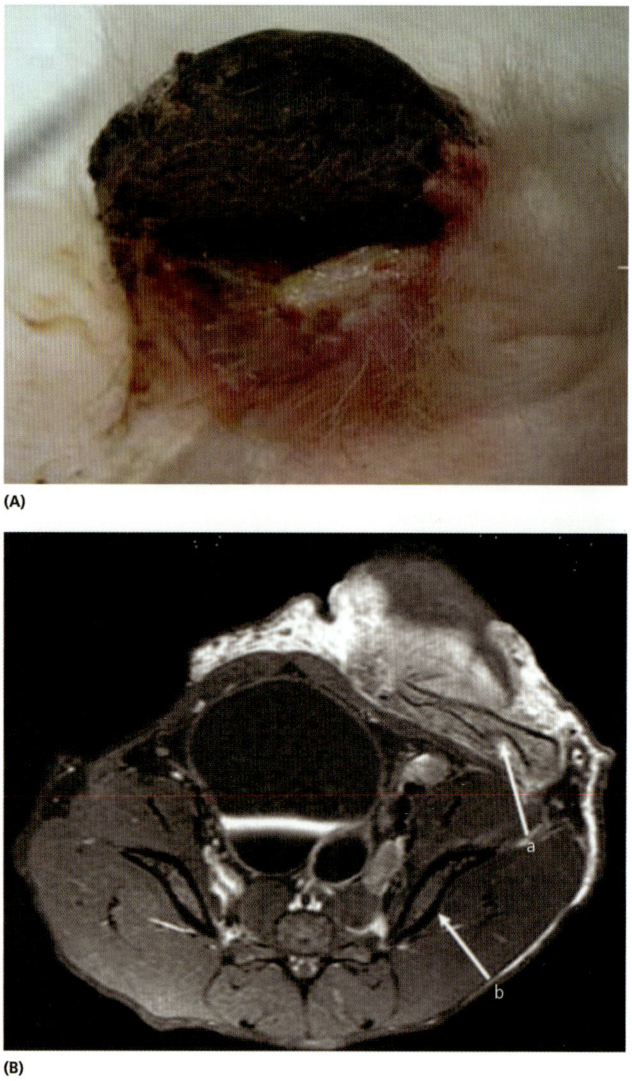

图 87.2 非人类灵长类动物带血管蒂的同种异体面部移植的差异性排斥反应:(A)焦痂形成;(B)有活力的肌肉和骨骼的影像学表现。(Reproduced from [10] Barth R, Nam AJ, Stanwix MG, et al. Prolonged survival of composite facial allografs in non-human primates associated with posttransplant lymphoproliferative disorder. Transplantation. 2009;88:1242-1250, from Wolters Kluwer Health.)

域以及血管周围淋巴浸润。神经、动脉和静脉的切片显示中度淋巴细胞浸润。排斥反应的组织学机制与 VCA 受体排斥反应发作时的机制相似(图 87.3)。

与所有移植器官的情况一样，组织病理学对于 VCA 在诊断排斥、理解排斥的病理生理学和促进管理方面具有关键作用。标准化对于报告临床结果和建立临床试验的客观终点是必要的。2005 年,全世界具有 VCA 临床经验的研究者之间建立了协作关系，以启动普遍认可的组织学分类基础。2007 年,在第九届同种异体移植病理学 Banff 会议上发表了第一个关于 VCA

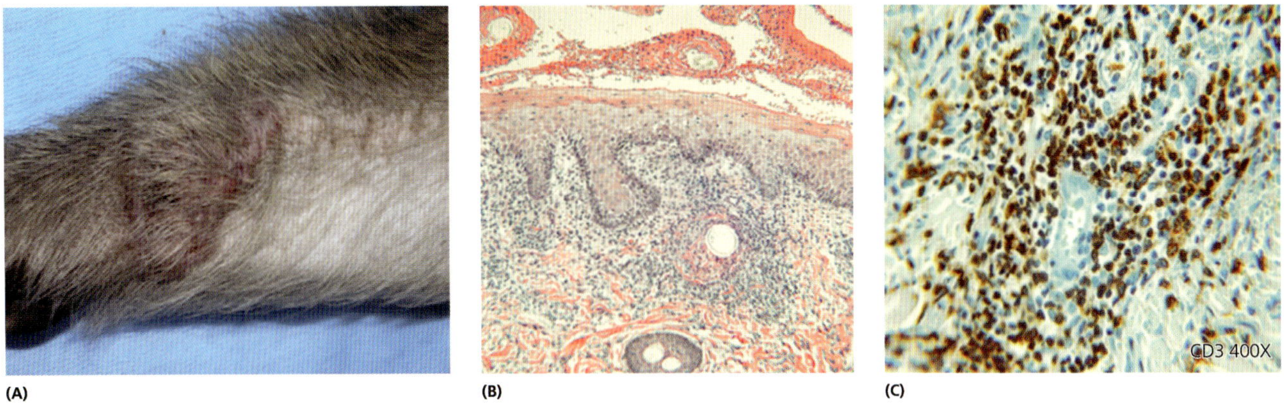

图 87.3 非人类灵长类动物带血管蒂的同种异体复合移植(VCA)的皮肤排斥反应。(A)局限于同种异体移植物的皮疹。(B)角化不全性角化过度伴浆细胞外壳明显。中度真皮、滤泡周围和血管周围单核细胞浸润(血红素和伊红,×100 倍)。(C)淋巴细胞浸润 CD3 免疫染色阳性 (×400)。(Reproduced from [11] Cendales L, Xu H, Bacher J, et al. Composite tissue allotransplantation: development of a preclinical model in non-human primates. Transplantation. 2005;80:1447–1457, from Wolters Kluwer Health.)

排斥的工作分类国际会议共识[4]。VCA 小组参加同种异体移植物病理学 Banff 会议是该领域第一次作为移植的一个分支被公众认识。VCA 会议总结了四个已公布的关于人类 VCA 排斥的分级系统,并且强调了它们的相似之处: 血管周围淋巴细胞进行性浸润的严重程度(与排斥的严重程度相似);若炎症累及真皮基底、表皮及附件为中度排斥; 严重排斥则包括表皮凋亡和坏死。其中一个系统基于血管浸润的程度对排斥进行评分:<10%为轻度排斥,>50%为严重排斥[12]。

Banff 会议试图回答关于 VCA 受体急性排斥诊断的几个问题:①标本充足性和活检准备;②急性排斥诊断所需的特征;③急性排斥的分级严重性;④慢性排斥诊断所需的特征;⑤体液排斥的诊断。目前,VCA 排斥的治疗与其他实体器官排斥的治疗相同。

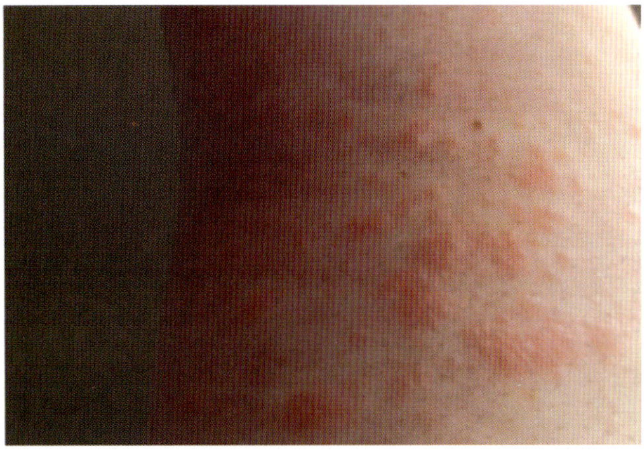

图 87.4 手移植。同种异体移植的局部红斑。(Courtesy of the Emory Transplant Center, Atlanta, Georgia, USA.)

标本充足性

含有皮肤的同种异体移植物是独特的, 因为排斥可以通过视觉检查和临床医生对病变的触觉来观察。目前在移植物中出现排斥的视觉特征的时效尚未被确定。已经将 VCA 的这一独特特征并入评分系统,并评价其在区分 VCA 与实体器官同种异体移植中的作用。临床记录排斥区域为<10%、10%~50%、>50%或没有可见的变化(图 87.4)。排斥的大体特征包括溃疡、皮疹、水肿、红斑、囊泡、脱屑和坏死。在移植物最严重的皮肤变化区域进行活检。与其他器官(例如肾)相反,并且考虑到排斥可能是可见的,因此建议通过 4mm 穿刺活检进行诊断。虽然活检的部位是可见的,但是仍然要排除取样偏差。一些中心已经移植了血管化的前哨皮肤移植物(由供体前臂组成),其可作为面部移植物和手部移植物的活检位点,以避免破坏同种异体移植[13]。此非通用方法,故尚未有验证研究的报道。

活检应包含表皮及其附属结构、真皮、皮下组织和脉管系统。载玻片应该用苏木精和伊红(HE)、高碘酸(PAS)染料制备。根据 HE 结果或者研究目的,可以进行免疫组织化学染色:CD3、CD4、CD8、CD19、CD20、CD68、HLA-DR 和 C4d。三色染色也可根据需要进行,但是目前尚不用于诊断。

急性细胞介导的排斥反应：VCA Banff评分系统

急性排斥反应的组织病理学诊断依据为淋巴细胞炎性浸润逐渐累及真皮小血管、皮肤附件和表皮。浸润细胞包括淋巴细胞和中性粒细胞，其细胞密度及位置也需记录。与肾同种异体移植急性排斥反应的Banff分类相似，排斥反应的严重程度与血管周围浸润程度呈正相关。

Banff 2007年VCA病理学分级按排斥反应严重程度分为0~Ⅳ级。0级表示没有浸润或罕见的炎性浸润。Ⅰ级或轻度排斥为轻度的血管周围浸润，不累及上覆表皮。Ⅱ级或中度排斥为中度至重度的血管周围受累，伴或不伴轻度表皮或附件受累。Ⅲ级或严重排斥为表皮受累的致密炎性浸润，并出现上皮细胞凋亡、角化不良或角质溶解。Ⅳ级或坏死性急性排斥为表皮或附件坏死(图87.5)[4]。

血管炎可出现于除排斥反应外的其他病理过程，特别是存在溃疡及坏死的情况下。排斥反应介导的血管炎，其特征在于活检中可见真皮层不同深度和不同大小的多个血管受累、单个血管多灶性受累、受累血管远离溃疡病灶、脉管炎且无创伤史。与实体器官急性排斥反应的诊断相似，排斥反应与其他病理过程的组织病理学表现可有重叠，在鉴别诊断时应加以考虑[4]。

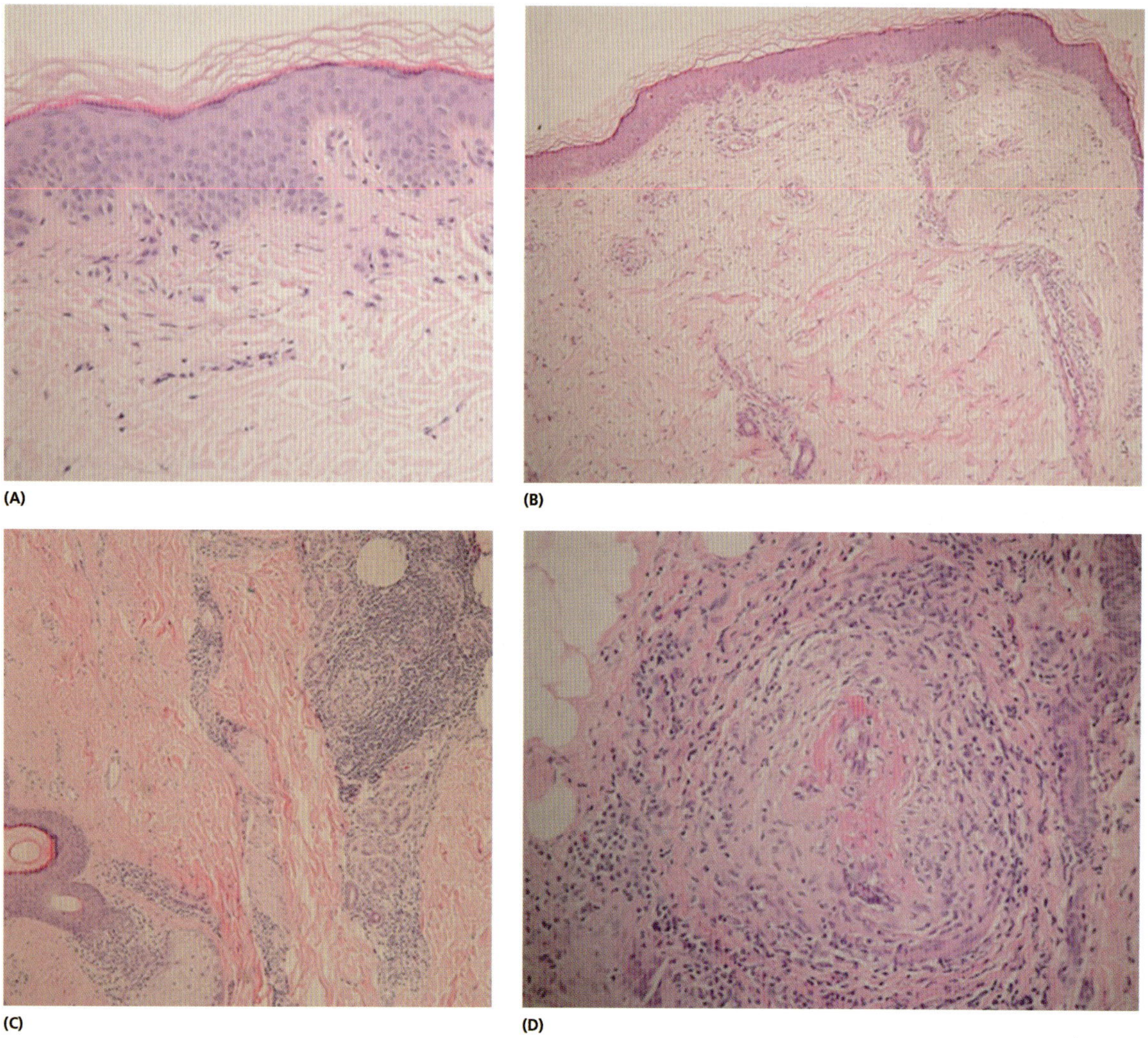

图87.5 包含皮肤的同种异体复合组织移植物的Banff分类系统。(A)Banff 0级：没有浸润或罕见炎性浸润。(B)Banff Ⅰ级：轻度血管周围浸润，无上覆表皮受累。(C)Banff Ⅱ级：中度至重度的血管周围受累，伴或不伴有轻度表皮和(或)附件受累。无表皮角化不良或细胞凋亡。(D)Banff Ⅲ级：严重排斥反应伴纤维蛋白样变性。[Reproduced with permission from [30] Liapis H, Wang HL (eds.) Pathology of Solid Organ Transplantation. Springer, 2011, pp.393-399.]

非异体免疫病理学

包含皮肤的 VCA 持续接触外界环境，皮肤可发生与异体免疫过程无关的变化。活检时，皮肤变化可表现为淋巴细胞浸润，不一定为排斥反应的特异性表现；因此须考虑广泛的鉴别诊断：感染、药物毒性、淋巴增生性疾病、昆虫叮咬、移植物抗宿主病（GVHD）和过敏性或刺激性接触性皮炎[4]。

排斥反应的临床特征表现为红斑，若不治疗可进展为大片融合的紫癜性苔藓样丘疹[14]。Ⅰ级排斥反应的临床表现为散布在移植物上的红斑或一般的皮疹，此阶段的临床表现可能类似于病毒感染。Ⅰ级排斥反应的组织学表现与病毒感染类似，表现为集中于上层真皮的淋巴细胞性血管周围浸润。Ⅱ级排斥反应临床上可表现为鳞状红斑。组织学上，血管周围浸润更致密，可延伸至真皮中间层，并出现表皮胞吐和海绵样血管。此阶段的鉴别诊断较广泛，包括病毒和药物相关性反应、接触性皮炎、皮肤真菌感染和昆虫叮咬。排斥反应与其他原因导致的炎症相鉴别时，需考虑详细的病史、体格检查与病理检查。病毒感染和药物反应病变通常不局限于移植物。病理也与异体免疫反应不同，样本真皮层中可出现外渗的红细胞。接触性皮炎可与排斥反应的临床和病理表现类似，二者需通过病史和正常皮肤的临床检查加以鉴别。皮肤真菌感染的临床特征是 Eczematiform 皮肤改变，病理学特征是血管周围真皮浸润，其他培养和染色（如 PAS）也有助于鉴别诊断。昆虫叮咬表现为真皮层中致密的嗜酸性粒细胞，一般在 VCA 排斥反应早期不可见[15]。

更严重的排斥反应可表现为类苔藓样斑块和丘疹。病理学上，真皮浸润更加致密，可延伸至表皮、周围血管和附件。鉴别诊断包括皮肤淋巴瘤、假性淋巴瘤、苔藓样皮肤病（如 GVHD 和多形性红斑）。皮肤 B 细胞淋巴瘤的特征为真皮层中主要为 B 细胞浸润、表皮保护和存在 Epstein-Barr 病毒（EBV）。皮肤假性淋巴瘤则表现为 T 细胞、B 细胞以及嗜酸性粒细胞的混合性淋巴细胞浸润。具有嗜酸性粒细胞增多和全身症状综合征的药疹也应纳入鉴别诊断。许多皮肤病如多形性红斑、扁平苔藓、苔藓样红斑狼疮和 GVHD 病理上出现黑色素失禁，可与排斥反应相鉴别。

最严重的排斥反应表现为致密的真皮-表皮淋巴细胞浸润，与Ⅲ级排斥反应类似，并伴有表皮及表皮附件坏死。临床表现可与中毒性表皮坏死松解症类似[14,15]。鉴别诊断的重要线索为排斥反应病变局限于移植物。目前 VCA 的动物模型正在研究通过不同的细胞因子鉴别排斥和非排斥相关的炎症[16]。

我们小组在 VCA 的非人类灵长动物模型中观察到移植物和原生磨损区域均存在花边状的粉色扁平疹（图 87.6）。未经排斥反应治疗的皮疹可从移植物和原生皮肤消失。其他病变包括移植物上发展为增厚瘢痕的红斑。全身皮肤检查发现在原生皮肤上有几处类似的痂，最初被认为是药物错误地注射到移植物皮肤上造成的排斥反应的先兆，后被确定为药物注射的局部反应（图 87.7）。

慢性排斥反应

正如预期的那样，在肢体移植后报道的慢性排斥反应随着随访的延长数量增加。实体器官移植中的慢性排斥反应表现为移植功能逐渐丧失，且伴随移植血管病变或内膜增生，通常存在 C4d 沉积和循环供体特异性抗体[17,18]。同种异体移植物的慢性损伤可能由非免疫机制引起，并且其常见表型病因多样。VCA 慢性排斥的病理表现为血管狭窄、皮肤肌肉萎缩、附件结构损伤、深部组织纤维化、肌内膜增生及指甲变化[4]。纤维化和萎缩可影响运动和强度的范围，并且长期的神经炎可导致感觉变化。然而，复合移植物的预后数据较少，与已进行半个多世纪的内脏器官移植相比，其已进行的移植病例数有限，随访时间较短。

许多人和动物复合移植模型中可观察到移植物血管病变主要由血管内膜增生引起[19-22]。其结果与其他器官移植（如心脏移植血管病变）中的肌内膜增生类似[21]。来源于 6 名手移植受体的数据显示，动脉与静脉均为排斥反应的靶点[19]。移植物血管病变应与供者动脉硬化相鉴别。若早期活检中发现动脉硬化，则可以认为预先存在的供体动脉硬化是引起血管变化的原因。

除血管变化之外，其他组织亦有改变。肌肉和肌腱可出现轻度的慢性炎症[23]，肌肉肥大主要影响深层肌肉[24]。可继发缓慢的神经再生，并伴有脂肪变性[24]。一些研究者报道骨髓、关节未受慢性排斥影响[25]，但滑膜组织显示存在排斥反应。动物模型中对短串联重复基因型分析显示供体骨髓被受体骨髓替代[20]。供体和受体

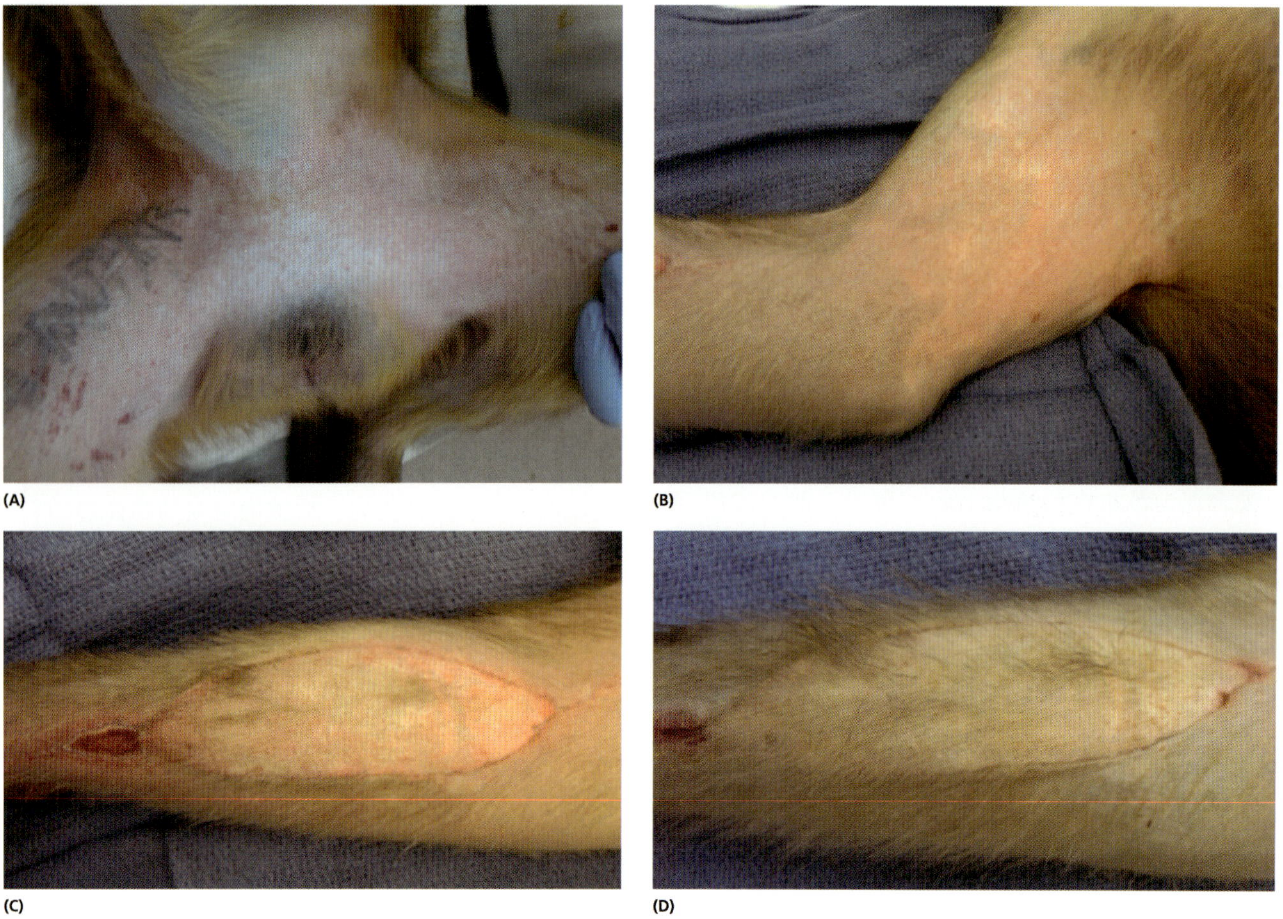

图 87.6 非人灵长类动物同种异体复合组织移植后的非特异性皮炎：(A)腹股沟原生皮肤；(B)腋窝原生皮肤；(C)移植物皮肤的皮疹；(D)未治疗的移植物皮疹。(Source：Emory Transplant Center.)

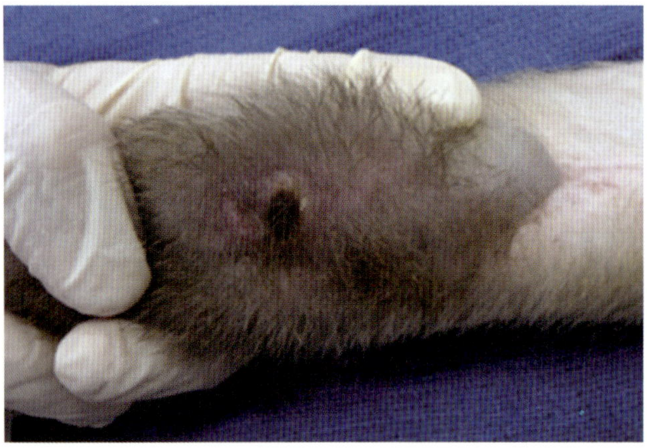

图 87.7 在非人灵长类动物中的同种异体移植皮肤上的注射部位反应。(Source：Emory Transplant Center.)

组织之间均可观察到骨连接[20]，但移植物骨小梁密度降低[24]，尤其可出现在受体胫骨与移植物桡骨。移植物桡骨变化还可影响皮质[24]。

中国对15例手移植患者进行了1~9年的随访并描述了慢性排斥的临床表现，如皮肤红斑、指甲不均匀、移植物僵硬、肌肉萎缩和功能丧失、不耐冷和疼痛。这些症状大多随时间推移出现。这些患者的慢性排斥反应病理学表现为表皮、表面真皮及血管内皮的基质水肿，伴有血管周围淋巴细胞浸润及血管狭窄[26]。一些患者在移植前接受了移植物照射，以减少骨髓中供体来源的淋巴细胞。放射损伤的病理特征与慢性排斥反应相似，如基质纤维化、表皮萎缩及血管炎，因此该队列患者的慢性排斥反应与放射损伤诊断上难以鉴别[26]。

影像和其他辅助技术表现

放射学方法可用于评估VCA的慢性改变。超声生物显微镜可评估移植物血管壁增厚的血管病变[19]。磁共振成像[24]、生物力学分析、血管造影[20]和高分辨率超声检查[24,31]有助于评估，但通过影像检测到的变化可能不可逆。

抗体介导的排斥反应

抗体介导的排斥反应(AMR)在多种器官中以急性和慢性的形式存在。移植时存在或移植后产生的供者特异性人白细胞抗原(HLA)抗体是排斥反应的危险因素。因此,针对抗原的糖体检测对移植物存活至关重要[27,28]。使用免疫荧光和免疫组织化学的 C4d 染色是抗体介导排斥反应的标志，但在当前数据有限的情况下,VCA 中 C4d 染色尚未出现特征性染色[11,29]。据报道,VCA 受体手移植物功能丧失后同时存在供体特异性抗体与血管病变[19]。目前为止,尚没有足够的信息得出有关 VCA 受体 AMR 的结论，应假设收集临床与组织学资料以帮助诊断 VCA 中的 AMR,包括 VCA 活检标本中的 C4d 沉积,伴或不伴有血清供体特异性(抗 HLA)抗体。此外,应注意是否存在慢性损伤如血管炎、血栓形成、中性粒细胞迁移和坏死的病理标志物,以及移植前患者的致敏史,包括 PRA(群体反应性抗体)、妊娠、输血与同种异体移植史。移植前还应进行 T 细胞和 B 细胞交叉匹配。

总结

VCA 的基础生物学与其他实体器官类似，随着临床经验的增长其他表型将被发现。含有皮肤的 VCA 移植候选物应进行详细的皮肤病学检查，包括先前存在的皮肤病史和详细的家族史，因为一些皮肤病和恶性肿瘤在移植后将变得明显或进展。作为一个还在发展的领域,VCA 中仍有许多问题未得到解答。VCA 的 Banff 分类是一个国际性的分类方法，为促进对 VCA 病理学的理解和研究奠定了基础。类似于其他 Banff 分类,VCA 评分系统是一个时刻变化的数据库,随着更多的数据变得可用。需要通过分析系统数据和临床试验来进一步改进诊断标准。

(周舒扬　杨梦凡　译　周舒扬　校)

参考文献

1. www.handregistry.com [Accessed December 2012]; Available from: http://www.handregistry.com.
2. Petruzzo P, Lanzetta M, Dubernard JM, et al. The international registry on hand and composite tissue transplantation. Transplantation. 2010;90:1590–1594.
3. Mathes DW, Randolph MA, Solari MG, et al. Split tolerance to a composite tissue allograft in a swine model. Transplantation. 2003;75:25–31.
4. Cendales LC, Kanitakis J, Schneeberger S, et al. The Banff 2007 working classification of skin-containing composite tissue allograft pathology. American Journal of Transplantation. 2008;8:1396–1400.
5. Thaunat O, Badet L, El-Jaafari A, et al. Composite tissue allograft extends a helping hand to transplant immunologists. American Journal of Transplantation. 2006;6:2238–2242.
6. Kann BR, Furnas DW, Hewitt CW. Past, present, and future research in the field of composite tissue allotransplantation. Microsurgery. 2000;20:393–399.
7. Lapchinsky AG, Eingorn AG, Uratkov EF. Homotransplantation of extremities in tolerant dogs observed up to seven years. Transplantation Proceedings. 1973;5:773–779.
8. Dubernard JM, Owen E, Lefrancois N, et al. First human hand transplantation: case report.. Transplant International. 2000;13(Suppl 1):S521–S524.
9. Zdichavsky M, Jones J, Ustuner T, et al. Scoring rejection in a swine composite tissue allograft model. Journal of Surgical Research. 1999;85:1–8.
10. Barth R, Nam AJ, Stanwix MG, et al. Prolonged survival of composite facial allografts in non-human primates associated with posttransplant lymphoproliferative disorder. Transplantation. 2009;88:1242–1250.
11. Cendales LC, Xu H, Bacher J, et al. Composite tissue allotransplantation: development of a preclinical model in nonhuman primates. Transplantation. 2005;80:1447–1454.
12. Bejarano PA, Levi D, Nassiri M, et al. The pathology of full-thickness cadaver skin transplant for large abdominal defects: a proposed grading system for skin allograft acute rejection. American Journal of Surgical Pathology. 2004;28:670–675.
13. Kanitakis J, Badet L, Petruzzo P, et al. Clinicopathologic monitoring of the skin and oral mucosa of the first human face allograft: report on the first eight months. Transplantation. 2006;82:1610–1615.
14. Kanitakis J, Jullien D, Nicolas JF, et al. Sequential histological and immunohistochemical study of the skin of the first human hand allograft. Transplantation. 2000;69:1380–1385.
15. Kanitakis J. The challenge of dermatopathological diagnosis of composite tissue allograft rejection: a review. Journal of Cutaneous Pathology. 2008;35:738–744.
16. Starzl R, Brandacher G, Lee WP, et al. Review of the early diagnoses and assessment of rejection in vascularized composite allotransplantation. Clinical and Developmental Immunology. 2013;2013:402980.
17. Kouwenhoven EA, IJzermans JN, de Bruin RW. Etiology and pathophysiology of chronic transplant dysfunction. Transplant International. 2000;13:385–401.
18. Solez K, Colvin RB, Racusen LC, et al. Banff '05 Meeting Report: differential diagnosis of chronic allograft injury and elimination of chronic allograft nephropathy ('CAN'). American Journal of Transplantation. 2007;7:518–526.
19. Kaufman CL, Ouseph R, Blair B, et al. Graft vasculopathy in clinical hand transplantation. American Journal of Transplantation. 2012;12:1004–1016.
20. Mundinger GS, Nam AJ, Hui-Chou HG, et al. Nonhuman primate model of fibula vascularized composite tissue allotransplantation demonstrates donor–recipient bony union. Plastic and Reconstructive Surgery. 2011;128:1193–1204.
21. Diefenbeck M, Nerlich A, Schneeberger S, et al. Allograft vasculopathy after allogeneic vascularized knee transplantation. Transplant International. 2011;24:e1–e5.
22. Wang HJ, Ding YQ, Pei GX, et al. A preliminary pathological study on human allotransplantation. Chinese Journal of Traumatology. 2003;6:284–287.
23. Siemionow MZ, Kulahci Y, Bozkurt M. Composite tissue allotransplantation. Plastic and Reconstructive Surgery. 2009;124(6 Suppl):e327–e339.
24. Petruzzo P, Kanitakis J, Badet L, et al. Long-term follow-up in composite tissue allotransplantation: in-depth study of five (hand and face) recipients. American Journal of Transplantation. 2011;11:808–816.
25. Kanitakis J, Jullien D, Petruzzo P, et al. Clinicopathologic features of graft rejection of the first human hand allograft. Transplantation. 2003;76:688–693.
26. Pei G, Xiang D, Gu L, et al. A report of 15 hand allotransplantations in 12 patients and their outcomes in China. Transplantation. 2012;94:1052–1059.
27. Gebel HM, Bray RA. Sensitization and sensitivity: defining the unsensitized patient. Transplantation. 2000;69:1370–1374.
28. Gebel HM, Bray RA, Nickerson P. Pre-transplant assessment of donor-reactive, HLA-specific antibodies in renal transplantation: contraindication vs. risk. American Journal of Transplantation. 2003;3:1488–1500.
29. Kanitakis J, McGregor B, Badet L, et al. Absence of c4d deposition in human composite tissue (hands and face) allograft biopsies: an immunoperoxidase study. Transplantation. 2007;84:265–267.
30. Liapis H, Wang HL, editors. Pathology of Solid Organ Transplantation. Berlin: Springer; 2011: 393–399.
31. Ostermann S, Loizides A, Spiss V, et al. Notable features in composite tissue allografts: value of high-resolution ultrasonography as a first-line imaging modality. Ultraschall in Der Medizin (Stuttgart, Germany: 1980). 2011;32(Suppl 2):E1–E7.

第 88 章 器官移植后的心血管疾病及预防保健

Stephen Pastan, Divya Gupta

引言

心血管疾病(CVD),包括心肌梗死(MI)、心力衰竭、心脏骤停及外周血管疾病,是总人群发病率及死亡率重要组成部分[1-3]。随着免疫抑制剂、外科技术的进步以及对感染控制认识的改善,移植术后患者生存时间越来越长,心血管疾病逐渐成为实体器官移植(SOT)患者中发病率及死亡率排名前列的并发症[4-6]。如图 88.1 所示,以肾移植患者为例,心血管疾病在实体器官移植患者中的发病率明显高于同龄的对照组[7,8]。即使引起心血管疾病发病率升高的因素尚未完全明确,移植界普遍认为免疫抑制剂治疗带来的副作用确实可增加心血管风险,部分通过经典风险因素的放大来实现[5,6,9]。本章将回顾实体器官移植患者的心血管疾病,并讨论普通人群心血管疾病风险因素的识别及处理,以及移植受体的特殊风险因素。本章将完善第 37~42 章关于器官特定的移植受体等待名单管理的相关讨论。

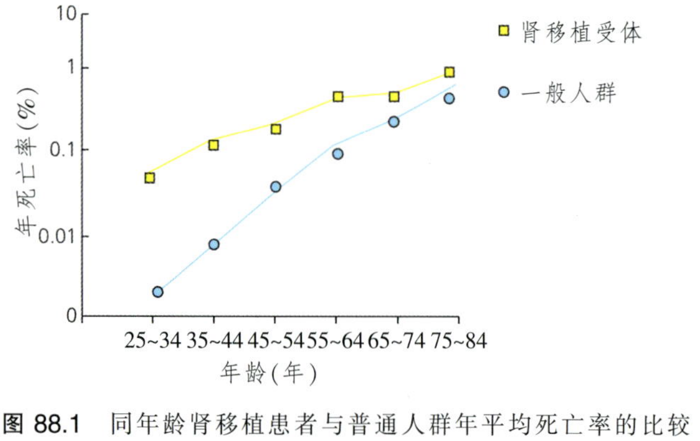

图 88.1 同年龄肾移植患者与普通人群年平均死亡率的比较(Reproduced Foley et al.[7],with permission from Elsevier. Copyright ⓒ,1998,Elsevier.)

实体器官移植受体及其独立风险因素

心血管疾病是肾脏及心脏移植受体的首要死因,也是肝脏及胰腺移植患者在术后第一年死亡的主要原因之一[4,5,10-13]。肺移植受体的移植物衰竭和死亡率明显高于其他实体器官移植患者[13,14],其相对较短的生存期与低心血管病症死亡率相关[5,14,15]。

许多心血管疾病的独立危险因素在移植前已经存在,或者由免疫抑制剂诱发甚至是恶化,包括高血压、脂代谢紊乱、糖尿病、肥胖以及代谢综合征[3,13]。相比普通人群,器官移植等待者和受体的心血管疾病发生率和死亡率都更高[12,16]。为减少移植术后心血管疾病的发生,术前应采用影像学(超声心动图)、应激测试(运动或药物应激)以及心血管介入技术对受体进行全面的评估[12,16]。

高血压

移植受体的高血压通常定义为血压>140/90mmHg,或者需要降压药物控制的血压升高[3,17]。在普通人群中,高血压与心血管事件的发生相关[18],认为是心血管疾病最常见、最易辨认并且可逆的危险因素[18]。在移植患者中,高血压不仅与心血管疾病发病率和死亡率升高相关,同时也与移植物功能障碍和受体生存率有关[3,19]。

心血管疾病危险因素常在移植前已经存在,免疫抑制剂尤其是钙调蛋白磷酸酶抑制剂(CNI)和类固醇皮质激素的使用会增加高血压的发生率[3,4,20];但也有例外,例如西罗莫司和霉酚酸酯(MMF)[3]。降血压药物应将血压控制在<140/90mmHg;钙通道阻滞剂是常用

的降压药[20],其不仅能控制血压,还能拮抗 CNI 相关肾血管收缩[3]。血管紧张素转化酶(ACE)抑制剂和β受体阻滞剂在普通人群的血压控制中发挥了重要作用,能降低心肌梗死后患者心血管事件的发生率和死亡率,但在实体器官移植人群中的作用仍存在争议。在实验模型中,ACE 抑制剂和血管紧张素受体阻滞剂(ARB)能减缓移植术后动脉粥样硬化和慢性排斥反应的发生[3,21];同时还可降低蛋白尿。然而,ACE 阻滞剂和 ARB 会降低肾小球滤过率(GFR),造成接受免疫抑制治疗的患者肾功能损伤[3,22]。对已存在冠状动脉粥样硬化的患者,部分医务工作者建议使用β受体阻滞剂作为控制移植术后高血压的一线药物[23]。但是,β受体阻滞剂相关的高甘油三酯血症及高密度脂蛋白(HDL)降低,意味着其可能并不适用于移植受体[3,21,24]。特定器官移植人群的高血压控制将在后续小节中详述。

脂代谢异常/高脂血症

已经明确在普通人群中,脂代谢异常与心血管疾病的发生存在强相关,实体器官移植患者同样存在这一联系[3]。25%~50%的患者移植术后存在脂代谢异常[25]。免疫抑制剂治疗已被认为是脂代谢异常/高脂血症发生及恶化的病因学因素[3,25]。现已证明,移植术后患者及非移植手术患者使用环孢素 A(CyA)会增加脂质及脂蛋白的水平(见下文)[3,26-28]。联合使用类固醇皮质激素则进一步促进 CyA 升血脂作用[3,29]。使用他克莫司的患者,脂代谢谱优于 CyA 患者,而且 MMF 对血脂无不良影响[3,30,31]。西罗莫司对胆固醇和甘油三酯升高的效果最明显[3,32,33]。

移植术后人群的脂代谢异常需要药物干预[3];具体建议将在后续章节介绍。免疫抑制剂对脂质水平的影响各不相同,如药物治疗高脂血症效果不明显,更换免疫抑制剂治疗方案也可能获益[3]。对于心脏移植患者,早期应用降血脂药物不仅对控制脂质水平有利,还可以减少移植物血管病变、减少排斥发生、降低最大血管内膜厚度,同时增加总体移植物存活率[34-36]。

糖尿病

心血管相关并发症发病率及死亡率显著增加被认为与移植术后糖尿病(DM)有关[37,38]。目前报道的移植术后糖尿病发病率为 3%~19%,肾移植患者的发病率为 25%[39-41]。免疫抑制剂对移植术后糖尿病的发病率有极其重要的影响,CNI、CyA 及他克莫司通过减少胰岛素合成和分泌诱导 DM 的发生[39,42]。皮质激素也可通过诱导胰岛素抵抗使移植或非移植患者糖尿病恶化[39,42]。不过这一效应呈现剂量反应关系,随着皮质激素使用剂量的减少而减轻[3,43,44]。当皮质激素与 CNI 联合使用时,促尿糖的效应互相叠加。此外,西罗莫司也与糖尿病的发生存在相关性[45]。未发现 MMF 与血糖升高相关。

移植术后糖尿病的治疗将在后续章节中讨论,其总体方案与普通人群的糖尿病治疗方案相似。根据美国糖尿病协会(ADA)的推荐,建议减少碳水化合物的摄入,同时使用口服降糖药和(或)胰岛素。对于部分实体器官移植患者,可以考虑减少诱导糖尿病产生的药物剂量,但这一方案需仔细平衡排斥反应的风险。

肥胖

移植术后营养情况改善,激素和 CNI 等免疫抑制剂的使用与体重增加存在相关性[46-48]。相较于心脏移植、肝移植及肺移植患者,肾移植患者的体重增加更为显著[49]。据报道,高达 50%的肾移植患者出现肥胖,或者在术后第一年内体重平均增加超过 10kg[50]。对肝移植患者的研究同样发现体重指数(BMI)在术后第一年显著增加;移植数年后,20%~40%的患者最终进展为肥胖 ($BMI>30kg/m^2$)[46,51-53]。有趣的是,BMI 似乎并不是肝移植患者术后心血管事件发生的一项独立危险因素[46,51-53]。

普遍认为普通人群中肥胖与心血管疾病的几个危险因素存在相关性。高血压、糖尿病及高脂血症会随着体重增加而恶化,随着体重减轻而改善。肥胖与炎症的发生同样存在相关性,而炎症最近被认为是心血管疾病的危险因素(见下文"慢性炎症"部分)[54]。由此可以推断,在移植患者中,肥胖与心血管风险事件同样存在相关性。因此,需要采取措施来优化营养结构,减少能量摄入,增加运动量,以减少肥胖对心血管疾病的影响[50,55]。

慢性炎症

动脉粥样硬化是一种慢性炎症过程。在普通人群中,C 反应蛋白(CRP)水平能预测心血管事件发生、心血管疾病死亡率及脑血管事件的发生[54,56]。这些表现对器官移植患者同样适用,尤其是肾脏移植和心脏移植患者[5,57]。有证据表明,移植术后早期炎症水平会升高,但大部分患者会随时间进展而逐渐缓解[9];另外,肝移植患者炎症标志物的水平在众多器官移植中处于最低水平[9]。在移植和非移植患者中,吸烟和肥胖均能加剧炎症程度,但移植患者还存在其他促炎因素[58]。虽然在普通人群中,巨细胞病毒(CMV)感染与心血管疾病是否存在相关性仍有争论,但在心脏移植患者中,巨细胞病毒滴度升高与心血管疾病的发生高度相关[57]。排斥反应也被认为在促进全身炎症状态中发挥重要作用,并可增加心脏移植患者的心血管疾病风险[5,57]。因此,减少排斥反应的发生并对巨细胞病毒进行预防性治疗可降低全身慢性炎症状态和心血管疾病风险(见下文"心脏移植"部分)。

免疫抑制剂引起心血管副作用的机制

现代免疫抑制剂的出现使得器官功能衰竭患者的移植治疗得以进行。然而,免疫抑制剂的使用需要以感染、恶性肿瘤及心血管疾病等风险增加作为代价。本章节将回顾免疫抑制剂增加心血管疾病风险的机制,而心血管疾病的临床表现将在后续章节中讨论。免疫抑制药物的机制详见第17章。

钙调蛋白磷酸酶抑制剂

虽然CNI、CyA及他克莫司的化学结构各不相同,但都通过抑制钙调蛋白磷酸酶活性发挥免疫抑制效应。阻止活化T细胞核因子(NF-AT)进入细胞核,从而阻断IL-2的转录。这一过程抑制了T细胞的激活,阻止细胞毒性T细胞的生成,并抑制Th细胞依赖的B细胞扩增,有效地阻断了免疫应答[59]。然而,这些药物的作用并不局限于免疫系统,目前已知这些药物能通过升高血压、增加血脂含量以及损害糖代谢等途径增加心血管风险。因为钙调蛋白磷酸酶在全身各组织中均有表达[61],可推测钙调蛋白磷酸酶抑制剂的副作用效果远超其作用于T细胞的效果[60,61]。

尽管机制尚未完全明确,CNI可通过多种途径来影响血压[62,63],CyA的心血管副作用较他克莫司更强。CNI诱发高血压主要是基于广泛的动脉收缩,导致总外周阻力增加[64]。血管收缩效果作用于肾脏则促进钠重吸收,引起血容量增加。CyA可直接作用于球旁细胞激活RAS系统,并且可通过收缩肾血管床间接激活[65]。另外,CyA也扩大了血管紧张素Ⅱ的收缩血管效应[64]。CyA影响了血管紧张素及花生四烯酸产生的血管舒张产物之间的平衡,其净作用为肾血管收缩[60];CyA能增加局部血管内皮细胞血栓素介导的收缩血管效应,并减少前列腺素介导的扩张血管效应[66]。Wadei等研究了肝移植患者[64],发现术后2年CyA及他克莫司都持续抑制了前列环素的舒张血管效应。他们还发现尿中的内皮素在这段时间内显著增加,并与肾血流及GFR的减少有关[64]。这些证据支持两种CNI在引起肾血管收缩中的重要作用。进一步研究表明,在动物模型中,内皮素受体拮抗剂能改善肾血管血流及血压[64]。研究报道CyA及他克莫司均能抑制一氧化氮的产生[60]。

有研究假设交感神经活性增加是引起CNI相关高血压的重要机制,但尚未被证明。另一项研究[67]证明,肾移植患者的交感神经系统被激活,且可能不通过CyA的作用来介导。近期交感神经活性的相关研究表明,在正常志愿者中,CyA会引起血压升高和交感神经张力增加,而他克莫司则不能[62]。CNI介导高血压的机制见表88.1。

尽管不同患者之间的高脂血症脂代谢谱存在较大差异,但总体上CNI可升高总胆固醇及LDL胆固醇、降低HDL胆固醇及增加甘油三酯血症水平,是影响肾移植患者脂质代谢异常的重要因素。大鼠的同位素示踪研究表明,CNI能降低LDL胆固醇清除率,并增加胆固醇生成率[68]。后者可能与肝脏超低密度脂蛋白(VLDL)清除率下降相关,从而引起LDL转化率升高[69,70]。Rayyes等[71]的研究表明,CyA减少肝细胞25%的LDL摄取和降解,这一效应可能由LDL受体合成数量减少引起;CyA减少了约40%的LDL mRNA水平。CyA被发现具有损害人皮肤成纤维细胞对LDL颗粒的内化作用[72]。这些发现可以推断,细胞LDL摄取减少可能引起其血浆水平升高。另外,Vaziri等对大鼠的研究发现,CyA能降低胆固醇7α羟化酶活性,因其为胆固醇转化

表88.1 文献报道的有关钙调神经素抑制剂诱发高血压的机制

- 肾素-血管紧张素系统的激活
- 血管紧张素Ⅱ增加诱发的血管收缩
- 肾血管收缩-钠重吸收-容量增加
- 血栓素产生增加
- 前列环素产生下降
- 内皮素产生增加
- 交感神经活性增加

为胆酸的限速酶；胆酸生成减少可促进总胆固醇水平的升高[73]。CyA 同样能抑制胆酸合成中其他酶(如 27-羟化酶),可引起细胞内胆固醇含量升高,形成负反馈导致 LDL 受体合成减少[69,74]。CyA 治疗的其他研究表明,胆固醇酯转移蛋白(CETP)水平会升高,CETP 与 HDL 循环结合，促使胆固醇酯从 HDL 向含脂蛋白 B 的颗粒(VLDL 及 LDL)转移,并伴有甘油三酯的相互转移[74]。富含胆固醇酯的 VLDL 及 LDL 会促进动脉粥样硬化斑块形成。Tory 等通过对血清的体外研究验证了 CyA 能引起 CETP 升高，但他克莫司并不会引起这种改变[75]。然而,CyA 和他克莫司均能显著抑制脂蛋白脂肪酶(LPL)活性,这解释了部分 CNI 治疗的移植患者甘油三酯水平升高的原因。随访研究验证他克莫司治疗的肾移植患者与 LPL 水平降低及甘油三酯水平升高之间的联系。总的来说,HDL、LDL 胆固醇及血浆 CETP 水平没有明显改变。在他克莫司治疗的患者中,实际胆固醇水平变化并未像 CyA 治疗的患者那么明显(见“肾移植”章节)。动物实验同样表明 CNI 引起的 LPL 活性降低[73](见上文)。

Le Go 等[76]报道,在大鼠中 CyA 会抑制 ATP 结合盒式转运子 ABCA1,ABCA1 能辅助胆固醇和磷脂转运至低脂质含量的 HDL,在清除动脉壁巨噬细胞的胆固醇中发挥重要作用[77]。这一效应可能是某些肾移植患者低 HDL 胆固醇的机制,导致动脉粥样硬化风险增加。Kockx 等报道,CyA 通过钙调蛋白磷酸酶抑制巨噬细胞分泌 apoE，但这一效应不依赖 ABCA1 途径[77]。ApoE 能直接将脂质从外周转移至肝脏，肝脏通过 ApoE 与 LDL 受体的结合来摄取脂蛋白颗粒，达到动脉粥样硬化的保护效应。尽管有了这些研究,但 CNI 影响脂质代谢和心血管风险的机制仍只有部分得到明确。

长期以来 CNI 都被认为是引起糖代谢损伤的因素之一,会促进移植术后新发糖尿病(NODAT)的发展[78,79]。CNI 削弱胰岛素分泌[80],而他克莫司对胰岛素分泌的削弱程度较 CyA 更强,并与 NODAT 的高发病率相关[81]。Heit 等的研究表明,钙调蛋白磷酸酶/NF-AT 信号转导对胰腺 β 细胞增殖和功能发挥起到重要作用[82],而 CNI 可阻断 β 细胞的信号转导通路[83]。他克莫司也能可逆性抑制胰岛素基因转录，造成胰岛素基因 mRNA 水平降低,使胰岛素合成和释放减少[84]。一项关于肾移植患者使用他克莫司和 CyA 的随机试验研究表明,发生 NODAT 的患者较血糖正常的肾移植患者胰岛素分泌明显减少，且服用他克莫司组减少程度更严重[81]。对胰腺移植物做进一步活检,发现服用他克莫司的患者较服用 CyA 的患者胰岛细胞损伤的程度和频率都更严重[85]。

糖皮质激素

激素是移植免疫治疗的中流砥柱，而这一类药物的副作用也是显而易见的，尤其是可影响血压和血糖升高,引起脂质代谢异常,造成心血管风险增加等。

激素引起高血压的最重要机制是其对盐皮质激素受体的交叉激活[86],引起水钠潴留,进而扩张容量。这种情况多在长期使用泼尼松和甲泼尼龙等激素过程中发生,这些激素混杂有盐皮质激素及糖皮质激素活性。但早期出现的激素诱导高血压不能归因于肾脏钠重吸收的增加[86,87],而且螺内酯并不能阻断应用糖皮质激素造成的高血压[87]。外周血管收缩,造成外周阻力增加,一直都被认为是糖皮质激素诱导的外周血压升高的机制之一[86-88]。研究表明血管内皮细胞和平滑肌细胞均表达糖皮质激素受体,糖皮质受体能介导细胞水平的钠钙摄取[89]。糖皮质激素还能上调血管紧张素Ⅱ受体[90]。Mangos 等阐述了胆碱能药物扩张前臂血流的效应被糖皮质激素阻断，推断可能存在内皮 NO 通路损伤[91]。Goodwi 等敲除了小鼠血管平滑肌细胞的糖皮质激素受体，发现糖皮质激素引起的急性期血压升高得到了极大的缓解[86]。上述这些研究揭示,糖皮质激素存在多种介导高血压的机制。

无论患者是否移植器官，糖皮质激素与血脂异常之间的联系是明确存在的,可能出现总胆固醇、LDL 胆固醇及甘油三酯水平升高[92],以及 HDL 胆固醇水平下降[93]。皮质激素相关的体重增加、高胰岛素血症及胰岛素抵抗是脂代谢改变的重要机制[94]。动物试验显示 LDL 胆固醇和甘油三酯升高是由肝脏 VLDL 合成升高引起[95]。胰岛素抵抗同样增加肝脏摄取游离脂肪酸的量,进而导致 VLDL 生成增加[92]。LPL 活性抑制引起血浆甘油三酯的增加。其他一些研究发现 LDL 受体减少和 3-羟基-3 甲基戊二酸单酰辅酶 A 还原酶(HMG-CoA)活性升高[93]也会导致血浆 LDL 含量增加。

皮质激素在糖尿病患者和进展为 NODAT 患者的血糖恶化中发挥关键作用，这一效应有两个机制。首先,皮质激素会产生胰岛素抵抗,造成外周血糖利用减少以及肝脏糖生成增加[96]。因此,葡萄糖摄取和肌肉组织的糖原合成均减少。胰岛素抵抗也导致了胰岛素分泌增加和空腹高胰岛素血症。其次,皮质激素能引起胰岛β细胞功能障碍[96]。

西罗莫司

西罗莫司导致40%~60%的肝移植和肾移植患者的高脂血症[97,98]。常发生高甘油三酯血症和(或)高胆固醇血症，并伴有LDL水平升高。Hoogeveen等研究表明,西罗莫司可显著减少含有apoB 100的脂蛋白分解代谢[99]。LDL apoB 100降解分数减少会恶化高胆固醇血症并提高LDL水平。高甘油三酯血症与基线LPL活性无关,但与VLDL apoB 100的清除分数减少显著相关,导致VLDL清除下降。同时,在体外试验中,西罗莫司使LDL受体基因转录下降，引起LDL细胞摄取减少[97,100]。这一发现可能部分解释了观察到的脂蛋白降解下降的现象[98]。Morrisett等进一步研究表明,西罗莫司治疗的肾移植患者出现了游离脂肪酸含量增加[101]。$^{13}C_4$棕榈酸与甘油三酯的结合减少提示西罗莫司可能干扰了胰岛素对脂肪细胞储存甘油三酯的刺激,造成肝脏摄取脂肪酸和合成甘油三酯的增加,进而导致高甘油三酯血症。近期有关大鼠的研究表明,多个关于脂质清除、脂肪酸转运及脂肪组织甘油三酯合成和沉积的基因一致下调[102],可能是临床上观察到血脂升高的原因。西罗莫司引起高脂血症的病理基础仅有部分被研究清楚。

早期,西罗莫司被认为不会引起糖代谢受损[103];然而，近期更多的研究表明西罗莫司与肾移植患者发生的NODAT相关[45]。Johnston等研究了美国肾脏数据系统(USRDS)超过20 000例患者,发现当西罗莫司联合一种CNI(CyA或者他克莫司)使用时,NODAT风险升高约60%;而联合使用一种抗代谢药物(霉酚酸酯或咪唑硫嘌呤)时,风险升高约40%[45]。其他研究也证实西罗莫司的促糖尿病效应[104,105]。西罗莫司影响糖代谢的机制仍未完全明确[45]。目前提出的可能机制包括胰岛素受体下游信号转导通路损伤[106]、胰岛素抵抗引起异位甘油三酯沉积[45,107],以及西罗莫司对胰腺β细胞的毒性作用[45,108]。近期的一项研究发现,西罗莫司能直接诱导大鼠生糖基因的转录和激活,引起糖耐量的损害[102]。

心脏移植患者的心血管疾病

心脏移植患者的平均生存期大约为10年[5]。心血管疾病,尤其是缺血性心脏病,在心脏移植患者中的患病率较同龄普通人群明显更高，相关的发病率及死亡率也较高[109]。心血管死亡是心脏移植患者三大死因之一，部分研究报道认为心血管死亡是心脏移植术后第一年的首要死因[5,110]。受限于患者群体较小,风险因素调控所获收益的研究存在局限性，关于预防和治疗经典心血管疾病的风险因素的数据大多是从普通人群的数据中推断而来。

血脂异常

血脂异常是少数几个长期被认为是心脏移植物血管病变(CAV)的危险因素之一[109-111]。其发生率在心脏移植术后第一年高达57.6%，术后第10年时达93.3%[5]。Sanchez Lazaro等发现68.3%的心脏移植患者有移植物血管异常[110]。移植前的血脂异常并不会影响术后CAV的发生;但是,术后总胆固醇、LDL和甘油三酯的升高,以及HDL水平降低均与CAV显著相关[111]。移植术后血脂异常发病率和死亡率增加主要是使用皮质激素、CNI和(或)西罗莫司等部分免疫抑制剂造成的(见上文)。

血脂异常的治疗需要采取多因素措施。美国心脏协会(AHA)推荐普通人群的低饱和脂肪酸和胆固醇摄入的饮食结构调整[25]。已证明鱼油等含Ω-3不饱和脂肪酸的食物对实体器官移植患者有益，这一建议可推广至心脏移植患者[25]。HMG-CoA还原酶抑制剂是治疗血脂异常最有潜力的药物[25]。对于严重血脂异常的患者,推荐加用非诺贝特(fenofibrate)的双重疗法[25]。当服用CNI和(或)非诺贝特的患者同时使用HMG-CoA还原酶抑制剂时，应仔细评估潜在的横纹肌溶解或肌病可能[25]。移植术后早期即开始采用他汀类治疗,尤其是普伐他汀和辛伐他汀能提高生存率并预防CAV的发生[35,36,109]。

高血压

高血压是心脏移植患者最常见的心血管疾病经典危险因素之一。根据国际心肺移植注册中心的最新数据，大约 73.3%的患者在术后第一年出现高血压，而在第 10 年这一数据上升到 97.4%[5]。在普通人群中，高血压和心血管疾病之间存在明显的相关性，但这一数据可能混合了高血压和 CAV 的发生。部分研究发现高血压和 CAV 之间存在明显的联系，而一些其他研究则并未显示这种显著的关系[109-113]。心脏移植患者术后高血压发病率的升高水平与其他实体器官移植患者类似，部分原因是免疫抑制剂治疗存在副作用。然而，心脏容量受体的去神经支配也可导致心脏移植患者高血压的高发[109]。

心脏移植患者的高血压可能需要多种降压药治疗[109]。已证明 ACEI 和钙通道阻滞剂均能使心脏移植患者受益[109]。这些药物不仅能分别通过拮抗肾素-血管紧张素-醛固酮系统减轻肾脏入球小动脉血管收缩作用来降压，而且小型研究发现这些药物能减轻心脏移植患者的冠状动脉内膜增厚情况，达到减轻 CAV 严重程度的作用[3,109,112,113]。总体上两种药物均能改善心脏移植患者的移植物和患者生存情况。

糖尿病

15%~27%的心脏移植患者在术后第一年出现糖尿病[5,109]。在术后第 10 年，这一数值升高到接近 40%[5]。糖皮质激素和 CNI 的使用与心血管疾病危险因素强烈相关，其他相关因素还包括移植前的血糖升高、移植前的代谢综合征、家族性糖尿病病史以及术后第二天胰岛素使用[109,114]。糖尿病对这类患者心血管疾病的风险仍有争论。部分研究认为，糖尿病是 CAV 的显著危险因素，而其他研究则显示糖尿病是引起感染增加和排斥反应的独立危险因素，并伴随血流动力学恶化及生存率下降[111,115-117]。其他研究发现，糖尿病对患者结局几乎没有影响[118]。Czerny 等的报道表明，心脏移植患者合并糖尿病的 10 年存活率较没有合并糖尿病的患者下降了 18%[116]。有意思的是，该研究还表明，两组之间 CAV 的发生率没有显著差异[116]。相比之下，Valantine 等发现血糖升高较血糖正常的患者动脉内膜显著增厚，并且会降低 CAV 免疫率(56%对 81%；$P<0.01$)和实际存活率(60%对 92%；$P<0.005$)[117]。

心脏移植患者糖尿病的治疗与普通人群的治疗方案类似。采用低碳水化合物饮食，以及使用胰岛素和(或)口服降糖药可以保持血糖正常[109]。糖皮质激素和 CNI 的减量有助于减少高血糖，但血糖水平控制需要与早期免疫抑制剂浓度降低导致的排斥风险增加之间进行平衡[3]。尽管糖尿病与生存率下降、感染增加及 CAV 风险增加之间可能存在联系，糖尿病的治疗是否最终能改善并发症发病率和(或)死亡率仍未可知[109]。

代谢综合征

AHA 定义代谢综合征(MS)为向心性肥胖、甘油三酯升高、低高密度脂蛋白、血压升高及空腹血糖升高(表 88.2)[119]。通常认为 MS 通过促炎、促高凝状态引起心血管功能障碍，并且在普通人群中与心血管疾病发病率和死亡率升高相关[120,121]。研究表明，MS 及 CAV 的发生存在联系[117,121,122]。普通人群中，MS 发生率为 18%~39%；而在心脏移植患者中发病率大约为 43%，其中很大一部分归功于免疫抑制剂治疗[121,123]。Sanchez-Gomez 等发现随着 MS 的因素数量增加，CAV 的发生率也随之增加(图 88.2)[121]。通过血管内超声(IVUS)评估冠状动脉时，约 67%的心脏移植合并 MS 患者在术后第一年即发现有 CAV 的出现[121,123]。

心脏移植物血管病变

心脏移植患者心血管疾病的发生主要由于 CAV 或排斥反应，是这一类人群的主要死亡原因。CAV 是心脏移植术后第一年的首要死亡原因，并且造成术后 5 年内 7%的死亡或再次移植[5,57,109]。心绞痛的典型症状在这一类去神经支配的心脏中很少出现（再神经化非常罕见）。CAV 和排斥反应都可以表现为心力衰竭引起的疲劳和气短，可能表现为室性心律失常和(或)心源性猝死。如果两者均难以通过症状识别，需定期通过右心导管评估血流动力学、左心导管评估冠状动脉解剖结构以及心内膜活检来评估排斥反应。

CAV 是冠状动脉疾病(CAD)的一种加速形式。心脏移植患者终身大约有 50%会发生 CAV，其广泛作用于冠状动脉树的动脉、毛细血管及静脉[111,124,125]。心脏移植术后一年内，5.5%~7.8%的患者被诊断为 CAV[121,126]。其独立危险因素范围包含 CAD 典型的危险因素（高脂血症、DM 以及高血压等）及一些不典型因素，例如 CMV 血清学排斥反应发作等（表 88.3 及下文）[121]。目前有数个心脏移植患者的回顾性研究正在进行，以寻求发现 CAV 发展过程中众多 CAD 及非 CAD 相关的风险因素[110,111]。一些研究证明，供体年龄>50 岁是 CAV 发生的独立危险因素[121,127]。CMV 血清学阳性是血

表 88.2 美国全胆固醇教育计划的代谢综合征诊断标准

腹型肥胖	男性腰围>102cm 或女性腰围>88cm
糖耐量受损	空腹血糖≥100mg/dL(5.6mmol/L)或需降糖药治疗
高甘油三酯血症	甘油三酯水平≥150mg/dL(1.7mmol/L)或需要药物控制
低 HDL 水平	男性 HDL 水平<40mg/dL(1mmol/L),女性<50mg/dL(1.3mmol/L)或需要药物治疗
高血压	血压≥130/85mmHg 或需要药物治疗

说明:患者需要符合至少 3 条及以上标准。国际糖尿病联盟采用相同的标准但根据人种的不同细分腰围水平(南亚、中国和南/中美,男性腰围 90cm,女性 80cm;在日本,男性 85cm,女性 90cm;其他地区,男性 94cm,女性 80cm)。根据国际糖尿病联盟标准,BMI>30kg/m^2,可认为是中心性肥胖,此时不需要测量腰围。

Data from watt et al.[365]

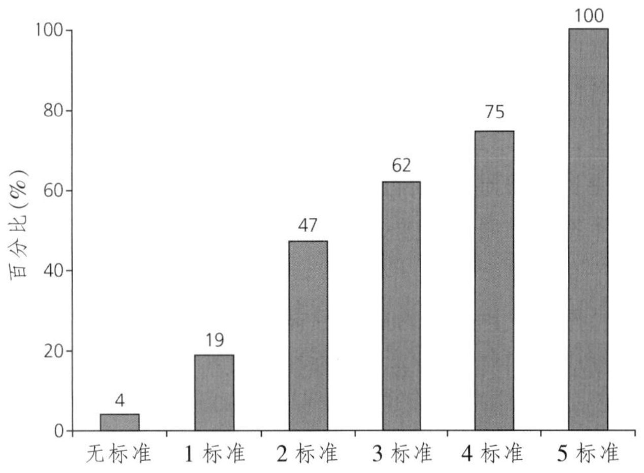

图 88.2 基于代谢综合征诊断标准数量的心脏同种异体移植物血管病变发生率。(Reproduced from Sanchez-Gomez et al.[121], with permission of Wolters Kluwer Health.)

管病变的一个非典型危险因素,也与 CAV 发生率升高存在联系[128,129]。在 CMV 阳性的心脏移植受体或接受 CMV 阳性心脏的患者中使用预防 CMV 药物后可以观察到 CAV 的发生率下降[128]。血脂异常、糖尿病及吸烟是 CAD 的典型危险因素,在心脏移植患者中与 CAV 的发生关系最为密切[110,111,121]。他汀类药物不仅有助于治疗血脂异常,同时在降低 IgG 自身抗体水平、减少 CAV 的发生方面也起作用[111]。心脏移植术后关于 CAV 的详细描述参见第 79 章。

同种异体移植物排斥反应

排斥反应在移植术后第一年发生率最高,是移植

表 88.3 慢性同种移植物血管病变发展的患者特点

- 移植前:
  - 体重指数
- 移植后:
  - 总胆固醇
  - 低密度脂蛋白
  - 高密度脂蛋白
  - 甘油三酯
  - 糖尿病

Reproduced from Chamorro et al.[111], with permission from Elsevier. Copyright 2006, Elsevier.

术后死亡的首要原因之一。频繁的心内膜活检及供体特异性抗体(DSA)血样检测是筛选细胞介导的排斥反应和抗体介导的排斥反应的重要方式。同种异体移植物排斥反应可表现为心力衰竭,伴收缩功能下降和心电图改变,传导时间延长或室上性心动过速(房颤、房扑、房室结折返性心动过速等)室性心律失常或心源性猝死[130,131]。这一诊断的关键在于意识到采用合适的免疫抑制治疗,包括高剂量的糖皮质激素冲击、血浆置换及静脉免疫球蛋白(IVIG)或胸腺球蛋白的使用。采取的具体方法可基于血流动力学恶化情况和各中心采用的治疗方案。有血流动力学改变的细胞介导的排斥反应和(或)抗体介导的排斥反应发作会使总体生存率降低 8%~15%,无 CAV 患者的发生率减少 9%~15%,术后 5 年无致命性心血管并发症患者的发生率减少 2%~18%[132]。

传导系统异常和房颤

传导系统异常在心脏移植术后较为常见;然而,造成心脏移植术后节律异常的原因尚无法完全明确。大约 70%的心脏移植术后心内膜 ECG 存在异常,最常见的是右束支传导阻滞[133,134]。Leonelli 等发现供体心脏缺血时间和移植术后早期在院期间的排斥反应与最初的 ECG 变化有关[133]。ECG 随时间呈进展性传导系统损伤或初始即呈现并保持异常的患者,其左室功能恶化的可能性增加,死亡率也更高[135]。进展性传导系统异常的患者,其心源性猝死的可能性更高,可能的原因是完全性传导阻滞或室性心律失常[135]。ECG 表现并维持正常状态的移植患者结局一般也最好[135]。

Cui 等对超过 1000 例心脏移植患者的研究表明,大约 11%的患者初始心电图有房室阻滞的一些表现[131]。

其中,部分房室传导阻滞与房性心动过速有关[131]。大约 88%是由排斥反应导致的。当房室传导阻滞不合并房性心动过速时,排斥的发生率只有 36%,且程度较轻[131]。Ⅱ度传导阻滞(包括莫氏Ⅰ型及Ⅱ型)和完全性心脏传导阻滞更为罕见(2%);这些情况多在冠状动脉介入或心内膜活检期间发生[131]。窦房结功能异常亦有报道。DiBiase 报道了一系列病例,发现窦房结功能异常的发生率在 7%左右,排斥及窦房结血管病变是引起这类心律失常的常见原因[136]。出现窦房结功能异常、有症状的心脏传导阻滞或怀疑存在无症状的心脏传导阻滞(莫氏Ⅱ型或完全性心脏传导阻滞)时,需安装永久性起搏器。若潜在的病因为排斥反应时,需采用更积极的免疫抑制方案。

脑血管事件

根据 Mayo Clinic 的综述,有 18%的心脏移植患者出现了神经系统事件[137]。80%的缺血性脑血管事件出现在移植术后 60 天内,并导致了 11%的神经系统事件;然而,仅考虑围术期脑血管事件,术后 1 年死亡率危害比高达 4.17(P=0.04)[137,138]。在脑血管风险最高的围术期过后,心脏移植患者 5 年的脑血管风险为 4.1%[138]。大约 40%发生缺血性脑血管意外的患者因诊断为特发性扩张性心肌病而行心脏移植术,而因其他诊断行心脏移植术的患者仅有 12%发生这一情况[137]。这些比例相较 1993 年之前的心脏移植患者增加了大约 10 倍[137,139]。在 20 世纪 80 年代,缺血性事件与心脏低灌注或房颤高度相关[139]。近年来,缺血性事件发生率增加则与选择高风险的患者进行心脏移植有关,比如严重的心肌病患者。栓子可能形成于受体心脏,或者可能因术中操作和(或)对动脉粥样硬化的主动脉钳夹引起[137]。既往卒中病史、血流动力学不稳定、体外循环时间超过 2 小时、心脏骤停及颈动脉狭窄>50%被认为是围术期神经系统事件的高危因素[138]。而围术期以外发生卒中的患者,危险因素包括卒中病史、缺血及出血引起卒中的风险最高[138]。Mayo Clinic 的综述表明,所有发生神经系统事件的心脏移植患者均能完全或近乎完全恢复,并且有“良好的生活质量及结局”[137]。

肺移植患者的心血管疾病

肺移植患者在术后第一年的死亡率最高,生存率术后第一年为 84%,第 5 年下降到 49%。肺移植患者的移植物衰竭、感染及死亡率远高于其他实体器官移植患者[13,14,140],而且随着时间在不断改善。有多种因素可导致肺移植患者死亡率相对较高(表 88.4)。心血管疾病相关的死亡率在术后 30 天内最高,随后显著下降(表 88.4)[141]。然而,心血管疾病并不是肺移植患者的首要死亡原因。有趣的是,现代免疫抑制剂的使用导致心血管疾病危险因素(高血压、糖尿病及高脂血症)的发生更早,且在肺移植中比其他实体器官移植中发生更为频繁[13,142]。

心血管死亡率与其他因素死亡率的比较

与其他实体器官移植的患者不同,肺移植患者的心血管事件发生率(大约 30%)和死亡率(大约 10%)都低得多[5,14,15,142,143]。Christie 等发现造成肺移植患者 5 年死亡率升高的因素包括糖尿病病史、HLA 配对等级、造成供体死亡的原因及一些移植术后结局(表 88.4)[140,141]。Plantier 等研究了肺移植术后患者终身死因的分布情况:首因是感染(34.6%),其次是闭塞性细支气管综合征 (18.5%)、原发性移植物功能障碍(11.7%)及出血性并发症(8.6%)[143]。Vadnerkar 等发现年龄大于 60 岁的患者有类似的结果[144]。有意思的是,Aratari 等对 73 例需要双侧序贯肺移植并且其中 3 例需要再次移植的患者的研究发现,闭塞性细支气管炎而非败血症才是长期死亡的主要原因[145]。为降低闭塞性细支气管炎发生率,采用改善的免疫抑制剂方案能取得良好的预后[141,144,145]。肺移植术后心血管事件最常发生于血管事件(8.9%)、心力衰竭(7.4%)以及房颤(4.7%)[141,143]。血管事件发生的中位时间通常更长,急性冠状动脉综合征的中位时间为 1227 天,而伴有症状的严重外周动脉疾病(2 级以上)为 1490 天,两者的终身发病率均为 2%[143]。卒中是另一个血管事件,移植术后早期的发病率中位时间为 191 天,在血管事件中发生率最高(5%)[143]。移植术前与移植术后发生血管事件联系最紧密的因素是糖尿病、颈动脉粥样硬化,以及动脉粥样硬化血栓形成,其危险比(HR)分别为 4.06、3.05 及 7.7[143]。Plantier 等对肺移植术后患者终身的研究表明心力衰竭的发生率为每年 2.08/100 人[143]。这一发生率远高于 50~59 岁的非移植患者的发生率[143]。

表 88.4 成人肺移植患者死亡原因

死因	0~30 天 (n=1622)	31 天~1 年 (n=2781)	>1~3 年 (n=2481)	>3~5 年 (n=1445)	5~10 年 (n=1592)	>10 年 (n=310)
细支气管炎	8(0.5%)	129(4.6%)	648(26.1%)	412(28.5%)	394(24.7%)	62(20.0%)
急性排斥反应	70(4.3%)	50(1.8%)	40(1.6%)	10(0.7%)	11(0.7%)	0
肿瘤						
淋巴瘤	1(0.1%)	74(2.7%)	56(2.3%)	26(1.8%)	41(2.6%)	15(4.8%)
其他	2(0.1%)	71(2.6%)	145(5.8%)	114(7.9%)	151(9.5%)	22(7.1%)
感染						
巨细胞病毒	0 86(3.1%)	25(1.0%)	5(0.3%)	3(0.2%)	0	
非巨细胞病毒	330(20.3%)	1011(36.4%)	578(23.3%)	278(19.2%)	292(18.3%)	59(19.0%)
移植物失功	458(28.2%)	504(18.1%)	462(18.6%)	274(19.0%)	286(18.0%)	61(19.7%)
心血管相关	180(11.1%)	109(3.9%)	77(3.1%)	63(4.4%)	76(4.8%)	17(5.5%)
医源性并发症	134(8.3%)	63(2.3%)	16(0.6%)	4(0.3%)	11(0.7%)	4(1.3%)
其他	439(27.1%)	684(24.6%)	434(17.5%)	259(17.9%)	327(20.5%)	70(22.6%)

肺移植术后的危险因素

免疫抑制剂的进展使肺移植术后第一年新发高血压、糖尿病及高脂血症的发病率增加[13,141,142,146]。在全球范围内，无论是否移植的患者，每个因素都是心血管疾病的独立危险因素。大约 90%的肺移植患者术后有一种心血管疾病危险因素，并且大约 40%的患者会在术后 3 年内出现两种及以上的危险因素[146]。然而，直到现在，高脂血症或高血压与心血管事件增加或肺移植患者的死亡率关系仍没有明确的记录[13,141-143]。术前糖尿病可导致移植术后心血管疾病相关死亡率明显恶化[143]。低心脏指数、房颤及术前收缩期肺动脉压升高同样与心血管疾病死亡率升高有关[143]。

糖尿病

6%~32%的肺移植患者在移植术后第一年会出现新发糖尿病[13,141,146]。发病率会随着时间延长而增加。Christie 等发现，肺移植术后第一年发病率为 26%，而第 5 年发病率则为 36%[141,146]。在经典的心血管疾病危险因素中，糖尿病与心血管事件和肺移植患者的死亡率相关性最强。存活超过 1 年的患者中，移植术后糖尿病与术后 5 年内死亡率的危险比为 1.24 ($P<0.05$)[141]。Silverborn 等报道了与肺移植术后糖尿病发生最相关的危险因素，包括血药浓度不相关的高剂量 CyA[7.2±3.9mg/(kg·d)对 5.2±2.0mg/(kg·d)；$P=0.006$]、囊性纤维化的诊断($P=0.01$)以及移植前血糖水平升高($P=0.02$)[146]。

移植术前的糖尿病史也会增加术后早期(HR 2.3；CI 1.2~4.4)及术后 5 年死亡(RR 1.15；$P<0.05$)风险[141,143]。生存率较非糖尿病的肺移植患者显著降低，其 5 年的生存率从大约 50%降低到 10%[143]。移植前糖尿病同样与动脉粥样硬化性斑块事件风险增加及心血管疾病死亡率相关[143]。有意思的是，糖尿病对肺移植患者总生存率的负性作用不仅仅是其为心血管疾病的危险因素，其同样参与了诱发及恶化感染的过程。

目前尚没有数据表明肺移植患者发病率和(或)死亡率的改善与良好的血糖控制有关。然而，与其他实体器官移植患者相似，通过饮食及运动控制糖尿病，同时使用口服降糖药及必要时使用胰岛素同样被推荐，从而降低糖尿病相关的死亡率、糖尿病的心血管并发症及所有原因引起的死亡率。

高血压

在三大经典心血管疾病危险因素中，高血压是肺移植患者中发生率最高的(图 88.3)[146]。50%~60%的肺移植患者在术后第一年出现新发高血压。Silverborn 等的研究表明 69%的患者在移植术后出现了高血压，平均初发时间为 16±13 个月[13,141,146]。在移植术后 7 年里，75%~85%的存活患者出现了高血压[13,141,147,148]。这类患者高血压的发生机制与其他实体器官移植的患者相似：血管

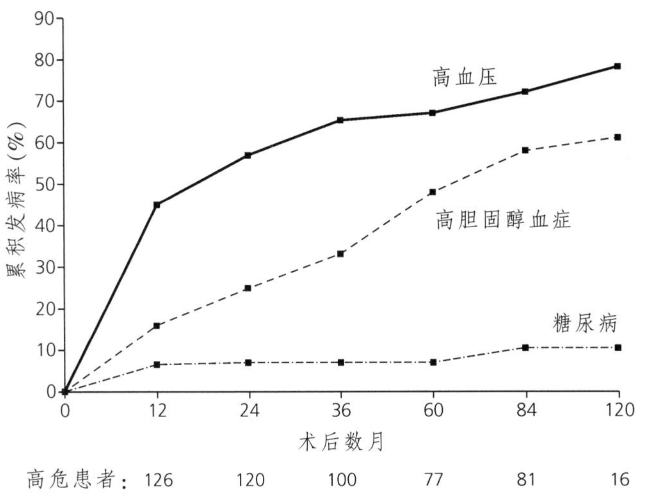

图 88.3　肺移植术后患者心血管疾病风险因素(高血压、高胆固醇血症及糖尿病)的累积发病率(Reproduced from Silverborn et al. [146], with permission from Elsevier. Copyright ⓒ 2005, Elsevier.)

收缩、慢性血管结构改变及继发于 CNI 和激素的水钠潴留[13,148]。有趣的是,尽管高血压的发病率与其他实体器官移植类似,其首发时间通常较其他实体器官移植患者更晚,但并发症情况仍类似[148]。实体器官移植患者的生理血压特征存在异常,这类患者并不会出现夜间血压生理性下降,或存在夜间高血压[13,149]。Vandergheynst 等研究了肺移植患者的这种现象,发现这种现象在很长的一段时间里都会存在[149]。相比对照组,肺移植患者的确不存在夜间收缩期和舒张期血压下降($P<0.01$ 和 $P<0.001$)这一现象[149]。

Silverborn 等报道了引起移植术后高血压的危险因素,单因素分析提示移植前收缩期血压和移植前血糖水平显著性升高($P<0.05$),多因素分析仅提示移植前收缩期血压显著性升高($P=0.005$)[146]。有意思的是,CyA 或泼尼松使用的剂量或血清浓度与高血压的发生之间并没有发现存在相关性[146]。相比血压正常的患者,高血压患者的平均 [41±15mL/(min·1.73^2)对 47±13mL/(min·1.73^2);$P<0.05$]及最低 GFR[33±14mL/(min·1.73^2)对 38±15mL/(min·1.73^2);$P<0.05$]均下降[146]。奇怪的是,Silverborn 等还发现急性排斥发作在没有高血压的患者中发生率更低(每年随访为 0.6±0.6 对 1.0±0.8;$P=0.002$)[146]。

目前没有研究证明肺移植患者的高血压与心血管疾病发生的关系[143]。然而,基于我们对其他实体器官移植和普通人群的心血管疾病进展的理解,肺移植患者同样应遵循高血压治疗的标准指南。当然,这一患者群更需要多种降压药联治疗[13,148]。

高脂血症

高脂血症是普通人群中为人熟知的心血管疾病危险因素。基于共存的心血管疾病危险因素的目标导向治疗已被证明能减少心血管疾病相关的并发症发生率和死亡率[150]。因免疫抑制剂,尤其是西罗莫司和泼尼松造成的升血脂效应,大约 20%的患者在肺移植术后第一年会出现新发高脂血症,5 年内大约为 50%,而 10 年内为 62%,其平均出现时间为移植术后 27±21 个月(图 88.3)[3,13,146]。尽管高脂血症与 CyA 之间存在相关性,有研究并未能发现血清 CyA 或泼尼松浓度与高脂血症发生率之间的联系[146,151]。Silverborn 等报道,在单因素分析中,年龄增加、收缩期血压升高、BMI 及术前血清甘油三酯、血清胆固醇水平与术后高脂血症存在显著联系;然而,在多因素分析中仅有血清胆固醇水平具有预测效力[146]。他们同样发现,血脂越高,患者的排斥发生次数就越少[146]。有趣的是,因囊性纤维化行肺移植的患者与其术后高脂血症的出现存在联系[146,151]。

尽管肺移植术后高脂血症的患病率和发病率逐渐升高,至今尚没有研究表明肺移植患者中高脂血症的发生与心血管疾病事件或死亡率增加有关[141,146,151,152]。术前高脂血症情况与术后心血管疾病的发生同样不存在联系[143]。类似地,移植术后高脂血症同样未发现能降低这类患者的心血管疾病事件发生率及死亡率。但有报道表明高脂血症与肺移植术后慢性肾脏病的加速进展存在联系[153]。这类人群使用他汀类药物较不适合使用他汀药物的患者能降低慢性肾脏病的风险[153]。尽管不能减少心血管疾病相关的生存率,但肺移植患者使用他汀类药物能降低总体死亡率[153]。

高脂血症和高甘油三酯血症的处理方式与普通人群的处理方式类似。可使用他汀类、烟酸类、Ω-3 不饱和脂肪酸及非诺贝特等药物来改善血糖。这些药物的选择及联合应用需注意药物相互作用,因其部分降脂药和免疫抑制剂通过肝脏进行代谢。

心血管疾病的术前评估

肺移植中心应该常规对年龄超过 60 岁的患者进行心血管疾病风险评估[141]。然而,对于术前冠状动脉疾病与移植术后结局是否有关联尚有争议。Vadnerkar

等发现年龄大于60岁的患者，术前冠状动脉疾病是移植术后死亡率的危险因素，5年HR为2.43[144]。然而，Sherman等却发现移植术前有冠状动脉疾病的患者较对照组在肺移植术后同期的心血管疾病（包括脑血管疾病和心肌梗死）或生存率没有差异[154]，但大于60岁的患者肺移植术后发生血栓性事件的风险增加[144]。

肺移植术后房颤

房颤能使普通人群的死亡率增加，忽略年龄时，HR为1.5~1.9[155]。在术前有房颤的肺移植患者中，HR升高到3.1，并且大部分事件发生于移植术后早期[143]。Isiadinso等对137例肺移植患者的研究发现，术后200天内发生房颤的患者，其死亡率高达43.5%[156]。大约20%的肺移植患者可出现新发房颤，既往存在房颤病史时，HR高达12.2[157]。Plantier等的研究表明，可能由于心律失常而予抗凝处理的患者出现大咯血是有房颤病史的肺移植患者的主要死因之一[143]。

尽管房颤属于室上性心动过速且主要发生于移植术后早期，肺移植12个月以后的房性心动过速的发生率仍会升高[158]。高龄、原发性肺动脉高压及肥胖或过瘦都会增加发生房颤的可能性[157]。Mason等的一项研究表明，房颤在移植术后2天时发生率最高，平均时间为11±9天，而房性心动过速发生的平均时间为1486±2462天[157]。由于房颤起源于肺静脉周围组织的异常电活动，且会受肺动脉压升高的诱发，双肺移植带来的肺动脉压降低对肺移植术后房颤的发生可起保护作用[159]。

可采用不同的方案来治疗肺移植术后房颤，包括药物及电复律。电复律能快速恢复患者的窦性节律[157]。胺碘酮是最常用的控制心律的药物，可达到化学性电复律。需要注意的是，有研究表明胺碘酮的使用与死亡率的升高相关[156]。Isiadinso等观察到房颤患者单独使用胺碘酮治疗时死亡率升高[156]；而不适用胺碘酮的患者死亡率则与没有发生房颤的患者类似[156]。这一死亡率的升高常被归因于使用胺碘酮造成的肺毒性[156]。应考虑采用预防性消融以减少房性心律失常带来的心脏负担，从而提高肺移植患者的存活率[159]。

其他并发症

心包缩窄

心包缩窄在普通人群中极其罕见，发生率仅有0.1%[160]，而在肺移植患者中的发生率甚至更低。心包缩窄患者的心包膜增厚，造成心腔血液不足、舒张末期容积降低、心搏降低及心排血量减少。舒张期左室和右室压力相等，心室间相互依赖，以及腔静脉波形x轴及y轴极度下降是心包缩窄的特点。Sever等对肾移植患者进行了回顾性研究，发现心包缩窄在这一人群中的发生率为2.4%，远高于有记录的肺移植患者的发生率[161]。为了减少排斥反应的发生，肺移植术后会使用更大剂量的免疫抑制剂维持。很可能大剂量的免疫抑制剂减轻了促心包缩窄的炎症反应，使得肺移植术后心包缩窄的发生率极低[160]。

支气管–肺静脉瘘导致空气栓塞

术后粘连是所有手术的常见术后并发症。肺移植术后，感染和解剖性并发症是支气管及邻近血管形成瘘管的主要原因[162]。这一内瘘可出现在移植术后的早期或者晚期，并能导致气体栓塞。尽管被认为极其罕见，但支气管–肺静脉瘘的实际发生率很可能并没有那么低[162]。肺移植患者出现心肌梗死或周围性缺血表现时，必须考虑这一可能。及时评估并诊断支气管–肺静脉瘘引起的空气栓塞对患者的结局很重要[162]。支气管镜、经食管超声心动图和(或)心脏CT可用于诊断支气管–肺静脉瘘[162]。

右冠状动脉损伤

单肺移植的患者会出现纵隔移位，术后立即或较晚发生。据报道，1例急性纵隔移位患者术后出现了右冠状动脉的“手风琴”征。尽管冠状动脉内血流尚好，其近端的扭曲导致了心电图下导联的形状改变[163]。对此，已成功运用经皮介入技术来恢复右冠状动脉血流量[163]。

肾移植患者的心血管疾病

患者常在经过一段较长时间的CKD期或需肾脏替代治疗的ESRD期后进行肾移植。高血压和糖尿病史是引起ESRD的主要原因，且在其他病因引起的肾衰竭患者中也常见。此外，高脂血症和肥胖在此类人群中也高发。这些及其他相关的因素造成动脉粥样硬化性CVD进展的同时也造成了心肌功能障碍。这些原因导致CKD患者的死亡率增加了30%~120%[164,165]，透析患者心血管死亡风险增加了10倍[166]。尽管肾移植的总体生存率几乎已经翻倍,但 CVD 仍然是肾移植患者的首要死因(图 88.4)[166]。幸运的是,肾移植术后心血管死亡的比例似乎在降低[167];然而,在肾移植中,其风险仍然是普通人群的 3~5 倍[7],并且仍然是长期生存的主要限制因素[168]。本章将回顾已知的肾移植术后心血管风险因素,以及相应风险管理的指南。

充血性心力衰竭

移植曾被称为“心力衰竭加速状态”[168,169]。充血性心力衰竭(CHF)和心肌梗死是肾移植患者最常见的心血管并发症,在医疗保险覆盖的患者中,移植术后第一年大约每 100 例患者中有 15 例因心血管原因入院[166]。CHF 是最常见的原因,占前两年心血管因素入院患者的 25%,其次是冠状动脉粥样硬化或急性心肌梗死,占 17%。近期 Lentine 等研究了 1995—2004 年肾移植等待名单中的 67 000 多例患者,表明在移植术后早期(<90 天)患者发生 CHF 的风险是移植等待者的 2 倍以上。然而,这一风险在迅速降低[170]。Rigatto 等[169]研究了 1969—1999 年移植术后 1 年内没有发生 CVD 的患者,在随访的 7 年内,新发 CHF 的频率与新发 IHD 的频率接近,且死亡率也相近。Framingham 人群 IHD 发病率与上述相似,而 CHF 的发病率明显更低。在后续的研究中,Rigatto 等发现移植术后 5 年左心室肥大(LVH)与 CHF、死亡率存在较强联系[171];高血压是预测左心室肥大的主要指标。尽管 CHF 的发病风险在移植

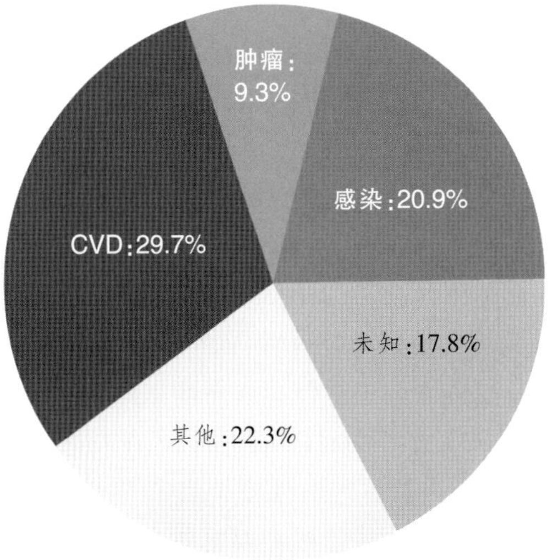

图 88.4 2005—2009 年年龄大于 18 岁,首次单独肾脏移植,且肾功能正常发挥的肾移植患者死亡原因。[Reproduced from United States Renal Data System (USRDS) [256].]

术后一直都存在,Lentine 等研究发现肾移植术后长期 CHF 风险较等待名单上的患者更低;而活体肾移植受体和非肥胖患者的发病风险最低[170]。移植被认为能改善“尿毒症状态”,如透析增加的体重、容量负荷过重、高血压、与心血管疾病死亡率相关的高磷酸血症和贫血[172]、LVH 以及“尿毒症性心肌病”[173,174]。更重要的是,大多数研究都揭示了患者在肾移植后左室收缩期功能改善[175],以及 LVH 病情减轻[176-178]。一项随机试验以肾移植术后 1 年内血压控制良好的患者为研究对象,发现赖诺普利和硝苯地平对减轻 LVH 有相似的效果[178]。值得注意的是,Patel 等对 25 例肾移植术后 2.5 年的患者进行心脏磁共振检测 (敏感性优于超声心动图),并与透析患者对比, 发现两组之间 LVH 并没有明显差异;然而这一发现仍有待证实[179]。通常建议密切监控肾移植患者的血压和血容量情况, 这些控制正常后将有助于改善左室功能,以及降低 CHF 的发生[176]。

冠状动脉性心脏病

缺血性心脏病(IHD)是肾移植患者发病率和死亡率的常见原因。尽管相较 CHF 更少见,急性心肌梗死(AMI)是移植术后早期或晚期的常见并发症[168]。Kasiske 等[180]研究了 1995—2002 年移植列表上有医疗保险的超过 53 000 例患者,移植术后 3 年内 AMI 的累积发病率在尸体供体移植组为 6.1%,而在活体供体移植组为 4.2%。总的来说,移植患者较仍在等待名单上的患者,AMI 的发生率减少了 17%。有趣的是,即使冠状动脉血管再通且术前进行了筛查,但 AMI 的发病率在移植后早期仍然是最高的。下一小节将讨论对肾移植患者较重要的冠状动脉性心脏病的风险因素。

非典型风险因素

高血压、高脂血症及糖尿病(可能术前即已存在),在肾移植患者中很常见, 并且是 CVD 的重要风险因素。这些典型的风险因素将在后续详细叙述。然而,一直以来这些风险因素都被认为并不足以预测肾移植患者的心血管风险[38,181]。这一结论是 1996 年 Kasiske 等在研究了 Hennepin 郡医学中心的 1000 例肾移植患者后得出的[38,181]。他们发现预先存在的脑血管、外周血管及 CHD 与心血管事件增加(最高可达 9 倍)有关,而吸烟、高血压及高脂血症并不能预测这一复合终点(CHD、MI 及心源性猝死或冠状动脉介入)。他们随后

报道 Framingham 评分低估了肾移植术后 IHD 风险，尤其是对糖尿病患者[181]。

后续研究发现非典型危险因素与肾移植受体的心脏事件高度相关(表 88.5)[169,182-184]。在近期，肾移植患者结局(PORT)研究详细评估了非典型风险因素。PORT 分析了来自全球 14 个移植中心超过 24 000 例患者[185]。传统的 Framingham 心脏研究变量，包括胆固醇、高血压及降压药的使用都单独与超过 1 年的肾移植患者相关，但是都没能提高其模型对 CHD 事件的预测能力(表 88.5)。这一研究确认了移植前并发的心脏状况与移植后 CHD 事件存在相关性。对非典型风险因素的研究则确认了肥胖[183]、透析持续时间[184]、糖尿病及高血压是 ESRD 的相关因素[182]，以及与移植物功能不佳相关的危险因素，比如尸体供体对比于活体供体[169]、急性排斥发作[169]以及移植物功能延迟恢复[182]。CKD 分期是公认的 CKD 人群 CVD 的风险因素(见下文)[186]。根据既往的报道，合并有 NODAT 的患者，心血管事件增加可达 70%[187]。这一点在 PORT 研究中得到了确认，尽管移植前合并有糖尿病的患者可能糖尿病暴露更久进而风险更高。

心脏疾病的非典型因素很可能反映了与 CKD 进展、透析相关的心血管系统受损。众所周知，透析时间长短与移植结局强烈相关。有趣的是，心血管死亡率在 21 世纪前就一直下降，而感染相关的死亡率却几乎保持不变[188]。这可能说明，对更年轻、暴露于尿毒症相关的心脏风险时间更短的人群来说，存在一个持续的移植后感染环境。这一发现直接与 PORT 以及其他一些报道肾移植长期存活群体的高 CVD 发生率、高死亡率的研究相对立[189]。

表 88.5 移植术后冠状动脉性心脏病的非经典风险因素

• 受体年龄
• 男性
• 白人
• 体重指数>35kg/m^2
• 群反应抗体(PRA)>10%
• 移植术前透析时间
• 死亡供体移植
• 移植物功能延迟恢复
• 急性排斥反应
• 移植前肿瘤病史
• 移植后淋巴增生性疾病
• 移植术后新发糖尿病
• 肾功能不全
• 移植前并存的心血管风险数目*

*包括急性心肌梗死、充血性心力衰竭、冠状动脉再血管化、脑血管意外及外周动脉再通操作。

Data from Israni et al.[185].

PORT 的研究人员提出很多非典型风险因素都可以改善，包括 BMI、透析期时长、急性排斥反应、移植术后淋巴组织增生性疾病(PTLD)、移植术后新发糖尿病以及移植术后肾衰竭。同样重要的是，能够认识到在回顾性研究中，典型风险因素绝不是不能识别和治疗的[185]。

已发现的肾移植术后与 CVD 相关的其他非典型风险因素，包括贫血[184]、CRP 升高[190]以及同型半胱氨酸升高[191]。叶酸改善移植术后血管结局这一临床试验(FAVORIT)[192]纳入了超过 4000 例肾移植患者，随机分为叶酸组和安慰剂组，最后发现虽然叶酸能降低同型半胱氨酸水平，但并不能减少心血管事件的发生。关于血红蛋白浓度升高对心血管事件影响的研究有不同结论。Heinze 等[193]回顾性分析了约 1800 例肾移植患者，发现使用促红细胞生成素治疗的患者和血红蛋白值更高的患者其生存率反而降低。另一方面[194]，近期一项关于 128 例肾移植患者的小型随机对照研究采用 β-促红细胞生成素治疗肾移植患者，一组用药至血红蛋白水平恢复正常 13~15g/dL，与部分纠正血红蛋白至 10.5~11.5g/dL 对比，发现用药至正常血红蛋白水平组 CKD 进展的速度显著减慢，生活质量提高，并且两组的心血管事件发生率都较低。尽管规模较小，这一研究并未发现高心血管事件发生率与促红细胞生成素使用相关[193]或者与 CKD 患者相关，这一结论与既往的一些研究一致，包括纠正血红蛋白水平对肾功能不全患者结局影响研究 (CHOIR)、β-促红细胞生成素治疗早期贫血减少心血管事件研究(CREATE)，以及 Aranesp 治疗减少心血管事件研究(TREAT)试验[195-198]。可能慢性移植物功能异常的患者及自身肾脏合并 CKD 患者，其对促红细胞生成素的反应存在本质的不同。

在普通人群中，GFR 降低的 CKD 与高心血管危险因素发生率、心血管事件发生风险及总体死亡率增加相关[186,199,200]。在肾移植患者中的研究同样得到了类似的结果；肌酐升高及 GFR 估计值降低的肾移植患者，心源性猝死和总体死亡率风险均升高[201,202]。因此，通过保持肾功能，例如避免排斥反应发生、减少肾毒性药物的使用以及控制高血压等或许可以降低心血管风险。

高脂血症

高脂血症在肾移植患者中很常见。高胆固醇血症发生率约为 40%，高甘油三酯血症则为 60%[203];HDL 水平多为正常,但也可能观察到低 HDL 水平。这些血清脂质水平异常不仅与心血管风险升高有关，还与肾移植物存活率下降相关[204,205]。对于高血脂的控制,需对患者可使用药物控制的病因进行评估，包括肾病综合征、甲状腺功能减退、酗酒及肝脏疾病[206]。肥胖和糖尿病常见，但免疫抑制剂使用是导致脂代谢异常的主要因素。CNI、mTOR 抑制剂及糖皮质激素对血脂的影响已在上文中叙述。值得注意的是,CyA 对脂代谢谱的副作用较他克莫司更大，而西罗莫司则是最可能引起总胆固醇和甘油三酯极度升高的药物[207]。理论上来说,西罗莫司的抗增殖作用可能缓解部分其对血管内皮细胞的损伤[203,208];但实际上,对短期内患者的随访表明,对比 CyA 治疗的患者,使用包含西罗莫司药物方案的患者并未使心血管事件发生率显著升高[207]。其他已知的导致高脂血症的药物包括利尿剂、β-受体阻滞剂、口服避孕药及高效抗逆转录药物[206]。

药物方案及生活方式调整

LEscol 肾移植评估(ALERT)临床试验[209]发表于 2003 年,是唯一的他汀类药物治疗肾移植患者的大型随机对照临床试验，并对此类患者的降脂治疗产生了持续的影响。在这一试验中,2102 例总胆固醇为 4.0~9.0mmol/L(150~350mg/dL)的肾移植患者被随机分为氟伐他汀(来适可)组和安慰剂组,并进行 6 年的随访。总胆固醇及 LDL 胆固醇都出现了显著的降低(降低了 32%)。尽管在重大心脏事件副作用(定义为心源性猝死、非致命性 MI 或冠状动脉血管再通)这一主要终点上有 17%的降低,但尚未达到统计学意义(相对危险度 0.83;95% CI 0.64~1.06;P=0.139)。部分原因可能是预期事件的发生率更低；回顾性研究发现，若研究纳入 6800 例患者，可充分显示出主要终点的显著性差异。然而,氟伐他汀仍能显著降低次要终点的发生情况,包括 38%的心源性猝死和 32%的非致命性 MI。后续又延长了 2 年的 ALERT 研究，也表明主要终点-重大心脏事件发生率降低了 21%(P=0.036)(图 88.5)[210]。已经有一系列的研究表明没有 CKD 的患者其心血管和脑血管的发病率和死亡率更低[211],心脏保护研究(SHARP)临床试验[212]也说明了辛伐他丁和依折麦布联合用药在减少晚期 CKD 患者的主要动脉粥样硬化事件的效果，ALERT 试验为积极处理肾移植患者的高脂血症提供了强有力的证据[203]。

尽管大部分他汀类药物总体在降胆固醇上安全有效[213],仍需要认识到很多他汀类药物(包括辛伐他汀、阿托伐他汀及洛伐他汀)通过同样代谢 CyA 的细胞色素 P450 同工酶(CP3A4)代谢,造成血浆他汀类水平升高,并且横纹肌溶解的风险大大升高[214]。辛伐他汀的包装说明书中表明其不适用于服用 CyA 的患者，同样地,尽管罗苏伐他汀清除不依赖于 3A4 通路,制造商仍然建议 CyA 服用剂量限制在 5mg/d，以避免药物浓度过高。普伐他汀和氟伐他汀通过不同的途径代谢,可能在正常剂量范围内是安全的。他克莫司和他汀类药物也可能存在显著的药物相互作用,以及贝特类及烟酸类衍生物,都可能增加肌肉溶解的风险[214,215]。除了普伐他汀和洛伐他汀主要通过肾脏分泌，大多数他汀类药物在肝脏代谢。尽管大多数他汀类药物不通过肾脏排泄,通常仍建议这类药物在 CKD 患者中从小剂量开始服用[216]。所有的肾移植患者服用他汀类药物都应高度警惕出现横纹肌溶解,应检测基线 CPK 水平,并且出现任何肌肉相关症状时及时复查。

2003 版肾脏病与透析患者生存质量指导(KDOQI)的脂代谢异常指南,在 2009 年更新为改善全球肾脏病患者生存质量(KDIGO)指南,是目前最常用的关于评

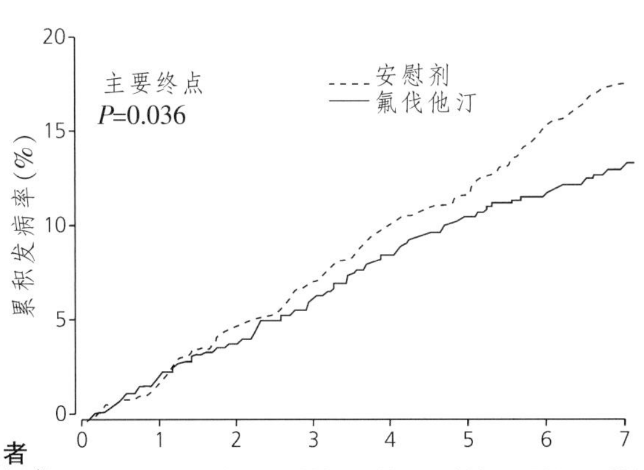

高危患者								
氟伐他汀组	1050	1009	974	930	885	836	755	691
安慰剂组	1052	1018	972	929	878	846	743	679

时间(年)

图 88.5 基于意向治疗(ITT)组的主要心脏负性事件累积发病率（Kaplan-Meier 估计)。(Reproduced with from Holdaas et al. [210], with permission from John Wiley & Sons.)

价及治疗肾移植患者脂代谢异常的指南[206,213]。这些指南与美国胆固醇教育项目对普通人群胆固醇控制的建议存在不同[217]。尽管脂代谢异常与CVD的联系从普通人群中拓展而来，检测及处理肾移植患者脂代谢异常的手段与普通CKD患者一样，都视其为心血管疾病最高风险因素。KDIGO指南推荐应在移植术前、术后2~3个月及服用免疫抑制剂数年内监测脂质水平。对于LDL胆固醇水平在100~129mg/dL，且治疗性生活方式调整3个月仍无效的患者，建议开始服用他汀类药物，并在服药过程中每2~3个月复查脂质水平。

尽管肾移植患者CVD的患病率高，他汀类药物仍未被充分利用。Pilmore等报道仅62%既往发作过MI的PORT患者使用了他汀类治疗[218]，Gaston等发现，在肾移植术后远期肾功能恶化的研究中，既往有CVD病史的患者仅有59%开始服用他汀类药物[219]。同样，阿司匹林在上述两组患者中的使用率分别仅为75%和59%。这些发现说明仍有机会通过使用降脂药物和其他心血管药物来改善移植患者的治疗。

免疫抑制剂的调整

激素撤药或避免使用激素可能改善血脂水平。Vincenti等[220]近期发表的研究发现，术后避免使用激素或早期撤除激素使用的患者，其体重增量减少、降脂药物使用剂量及甘油三酯水平降低。一项循证医学综述回顾了30例关于激素减少策略的随机对照研究，发现避免使用激素与术后服用CyA和他克莫司的患者胆固醇水平更低有关，尽管降脂药物需求减少仅出现于服用他克莫司的患者[221]。

高血压

高血压几乎发生于所有肾移植患者，50%~90%的患者血压高于140/90mmHg或需要服用降压药[10,64]。对未治疗的患者进行动态血压监测，确认95%的患者血压超过130/80mmHg[222]。与前述相同，高血压是肾移植患者重要的CVD危险因素[223]。协同移植研究等报道了超过24 000例实体肾移植患者，发现血压升高是造成移植物衰竭的主要决定因素(图88.6)[19]。

后续对这一人群的研究表明，移植术后1年收缩压超过140mmHg，并最终将血压控制在140mmHg以下的患者，移植物存活率较仍处于高血压状态的患者高；对于50岁以下的患者，心血管因素死亡率也可下降[224]。

众所周知，对于刚完成移植手术的患者，CNI和激素是引起血压情况恶化的主要原因。然而，许多其他因素导致了肾移植患者高血压高发(表88.6)[225]。造成高血压的重要的供体因素包括供体死亡背景；在CyA出现前的时期，Guidi等的研究发现，受体接受了有高血压家族史的供肾后更易发展为高血压[226]。受体接受年龄较大的供体后也更易发展为高血压[227,228]；受体接受相对于受体体积较小的肾脏后，需要使用更大剂量的降压药[229]。受体因素同样重要：多达90%的肾移植等待者术前即存在高血压[164]。而血管钙化、动脉僵硬等证据在术后更易长期出现血压升高[230,231]。肥胖在这类患者中同样高发。CKD移植肾功能异常同样可因急性排斥发作、慢性移植物功能异常或肾脏疾病复发引起。偶然情况下，特殊解剖结构异常，例如移植肾动脉狭窄或输尿管狭窄造成的阻塞以及外部受压，可能需要通过适当的试验进行诊断(见下文)。加重肾移植患者高血压的重要的特殊因素将在后续章节中讨论。

钙调蛋白磷酸酶抑制剂

在肾移植患者中，钙调蛋白磷酸酶抑制剂相关高血压较CNI广泛使用前已经明显减少[168,232]，且免疫抑制剂引起的血压升高起主要作用。CNI在一系列骨髓、肝脏及心脏移植以及自身免疫疾病患者中的使用也与高血压发生率增加相关[225]。已注意到他克莫司治疗的患者较CyA治疗的患者高血压发生率明显更低[233]。正常志愿者使用常规剂量CyA治疗，表现为血压升高及GFR和肾脏血流减少，而他克莫司治疗的患者并未出现这一情况[234]。这些交叉研究表明，将CyA改用他克

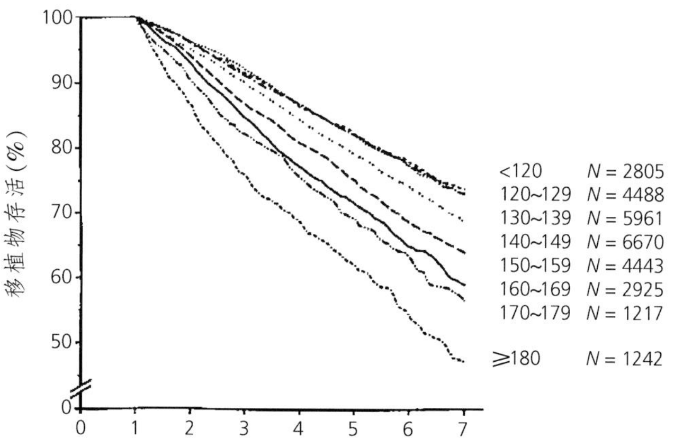

图88.6 死亡供体移植术后1年血压与后续肾移植物存活情况($P<0.001$)。(Reproduced from Opelz et al.[19]: with permission of Macmillan Publishers Ltd. Copyright 1998.)

表 88.6 肾移植术后高血压因素

- 供体因素:
  - 年龄
  - 高血压
  - 家族史
  - 肾脏体积
- 受体因素:
  - 移植前已存在的高血压
  - 肥胖
  - 基础肾脏疾病
  - 睡眠呼吸障碍
- 免疫抑制剂治疗:
  - 钙调蛋白磷酸酶抑制剂
  - 糖皮质激素
- 移植输尿管阻塞
- 移植肾动脉狭窄
- 移植肾功能障碍:
  - 急性排斥反应
  - 抗体介导的排斥反应
  - 血栓性微血管病变
  - 慢性移植物功能障碍伴慢性肾病
  - 肾脏疾病复发

莫司治疗会显著改善高血压情况，但在重新使用 CyA 时情况会逆转[235]。

尽管仍未完全明确,CNI 能通过多重途径引起血压升高[62,63]。CNI 引起血压升高的机制已在上文中详述。

糖皮质激素

长期以来,糖皮质激素都被认为能引起高血压。激素引起血压升高的机制已在上文中叙述,主要是通过血管收缩,引起外周血管阻力增加。尽管有一项随机临床试验并未说明 CyA 治疗的患者给予泼尼松治疗或采取激素撤药或不适用激素治疗等情况下并未出现血压的显著差异[220],对 30 项随机对照试验的系统性回顾表明，激素减量或激素撤药策略能减少降压药的使用[221]。激素类药物使用在过去的 20 年里显著减少；1995 年超过 90%的肾移植患者仍需要使用,而到 2007 年,使用激素的患者减少了约 60%[236]。

移植后肾脏血管疾病

因肾灌注不足造成的高血压可能由肾主动脉阻塞或肾脏微血管疾病引起。移植肾动脉狭窄(TRAS)估计发生于多达 12%的高血压肾移植患者[225],常表现为高血压和不同程度的肾衰竭。移植手术中对器官的操作引起的血管外伤和移植物位置放置不当可能是引起移植术后 TRAS 的原因。移植术后可能造成 TRAS 的原因包括 CMV 感染、排斥及冷缺血时间[237]。多普勒超声是筛选 TRAS 的合适方案，但可能会过度估计动脉阻塞导致的血流动力学改变。在某项研究中[238],仅有 25%出现动脉收缩峰值速度升高的患者经血管成像确认了狭窄的存在。磁共振血管成像(MRA)使用现代技术,同样可用于辨认移植肾动脉的解剖异常[239,240]。血管成像技术仍是诊断的金标准,并且血管成形术多能在技术上取得成功;尽管如此,并非所有的患者血压都能够得到改善[241,242]。TRAS 对移植结果似乎有负面影响[237]。

血栓性微血管病可能与 CNI 治疗、恶性高血压或移植肾肾小球病变等并存，或由凝血系统疾病如抗磷脂抗体综合征导致[243],也可由复发性疾病如溶血性尿毒症综合征或硬皮病导致[244]。临床情况包括肾缺血及其所导致的高血压或肾功能衰竭，可能包括血小板减少和溶血造成的血液系统异常。这一情况的治疗需基于潜在的病理生理,建议避免使用 CNI。肾移植预后往往不良[245]。

Dragun 等描述了一种肾移植患者难治性血管性排斥导致的恶性高血压综合征，不存在抗 HLA 抗体,却存在血管紧张素Ⅱ1 型受体相关的抗体[246]。血浆置换和 ARB 药物氯沙坦对这些患者有效,并能延长移植物的存活时间。在大鼠中,这些抗体的输注会导致高血压伴内膜炎病变。后续的研究证明高亲和性的血管紧张素Ⅱ1 型受体抗体与临床诊断为抗体介导的排斥反应有很强的相关性,且在抗 HLA 抗体不存在时也是如此[247],尽管恶性高血压在这一研究中发病率并不高。这些抗体仅能在 3%~4%的移植等待患者中被识别;这类激活性自身抗体是否有临床显著意义目前仍未知[248]。

移植后治疗

目前暂无大型随机研究能指导肾移植受体的高血压治疗。基于其他高 CVD 风险人群的指南,KDIGO 指南建议将目标血压制定在 130/80mmHg 或以下，如高血压、糖尿病或 CKD 患者[213]。这可能是一个合理的治疗目标;它与第七次美国高血压委员会(JNC 7)对高血压预防、检测、评估及治疗的建议一致[249]。控制血压可降低预期心血管事件,并预防移植物功能损害[225]。

生活方式调整诸如饮食、锻炼及减少钠和酒精摄入是高血压治疗的第一步，可能改善血压的控制[250]；但通常仍需要使用降压药。尽管一些小型研究对降血压药物类型进行过比较[251]，未有大型研究清楚地表明无论何种降压药均比不用药收益更大。降压药的选择通常由患者共存疾病和移植中心的经验决定。单纯肾移植患者，除内皮素受体阻滞剂，CyA 能造成其肝脏代谢减少，导致血浓度过高以外[64]，其他降压药不存在禁忌情况[213]。二氢吡啶类钙通道阻滞剂因其明确的有效性和安全性而较为常用，且它们在理论上有抵消 CNI 的收缩血管作用的优势（见上文）[64]。应谨慎使用非二氢吡啶类钙阻滞剂维拉帕米和地尔硫䓬，因为它们有效地抑制细胞色素 P450 3A4 同工酶，使他克莫司和 CyA 血药浓度升高。钙通道阻滞剂也可加重 CNI 引起的牙龈增生[64]。肾移植受体常会给予 β-受体阻滞剂，这尤其对于存在 CVD 的患者更为有利。利尿剂在移植后血容量过高时可发挥重要作用；然而，利尿剂引起的容量减少及肾前性氮质血症可能导致血清肌酸酐水平升高。ACE 抑制剂和 ARB 阻滞剂也是有效的抗高血压药物，证明能减少移植后蛋白尿[252]；这些药物一直被认可为心脏保护剂使用[219]。目前没有明确的数据表明肾素-血管紧张素系统抑制剂较其他降压药物更佳；ACEI 和 ARB 在移植人群中的不良反应包括贫血和高钾血症。近期关于肾移植患者高血压管理方面的综述可见这些文章[63,64,225]。

糖尿病

在美国，糖尿病是导致 ESRD 的首要原因；它是造成 46%的 ESRD 患者进行透析的原因[253]，并发生在其他原因引起 ESRD 的患者中。近 24%的移植患者的首要肾脏诊断为糖尿病[254]。糖尿病一直被认为是 CVD 的危险因素，许多移植项目通过前瞻性地对糖尿病肾移植受体进行额外的检查，以期在进入名单前便发现存在 CVD 的证据。例如，Cosio 等报道 1998—2006 年在梅奥诊所的 933 例首次移植患者[187]。在 46 个月的随访中，移植时有糖尿病的患者心血管事件（25%）、心管死亡率（12%）和全因死亡率（19.3%）均较没有糖尿病的患者（分别为 7.4%、1.1%和 6.1%；$P<0.0001$）更高；意料之中，糖尿病患者的 CVD 发病率也高得多。近期，Kuo 等从器官获取和移植网络/美国器官共享网络（OPTN/UNOS）数据库获取了 2004—2007 年 37 448 例移植术后存活 1 年以上的患者[255]。他们发现，移植前有糖尿病的患者，心血管疾病死亡率增加了 89%（$P<0.001$）。

NODAT 已越来越多地被认为是一个严重的问题。最近 USRDS 数据报告显示，成人移植后糖尿病的累积发病率在 1 年时约为 30%，在 3 年时>40%，而对小于 18 岁的年轻患者，移植后 3 年的糖尿病累积发病率则>10%[256]。然而，NODAT 的发病率可能被过度报道，因其用于 NODAT 诊断的标准未知。Valderhaug 等[257]对连续的 1410 例首次且无糖尿病的肾移植患者进行了研究，并在术后第 10 周对尚未发展为 NODAT 的患者进行口服葡萄糖耐量检测。使用当前 ADA 标准，他们发现 17%的患者发展为 NODAT，22%的患者糖耐量受损。NODAT 的高发基于 90%的患者使用他克莫司作为其初始 CNI 治疗方案[236]；他克莫司的使用与 NODAT 的发生强烈相关（见上文）[78]。目前 ADA 和 WHO 对糖尿病的诊断的现行标准列于表 88.7。

肾移植后新发糖尿病长期以来一直被认为是死亡的危险因素。Kasiske 等[78] 研究了 1996—2000 年报道至 USRDS 的 11 659 例没有糖尿病的首次肾移植患者。在这些患者中，24%的患者在 36 个月发展为 NODAT，与 CVD 的死亡率增长 47%存在相关性（$P=0.0140$），同时与各种原因导致的总体死亡率增加 87%相关联（$P<0.0001$）。Cole 等[258]报道了 1995—2002 年 USRDS 数据库的 27 707 首次非联合肾移植，他们发现 NODAT 的患者在移植物功能发挥状态下死亡的相对危险度为 1.41（1.25~1.59），这一情况被认为可能由 CVD 引起。在 Valderhaug 等的研究中[257]，移植后糖尿病患者出现心血管死亡的风险相对增加 80%（$P<0.05$），全因死亡率相对增加 54%（$P<0.05$）。空腹血糖每增加 1mmol/L（18mg/dL），心血管死亡风险增加 19%（$P<0.05$）。有趣

表 88.7 当前 ADA 和 WHO 定义的糖尿病诊断标准

1. 空腹血糖≥126mg/dL(7.0mmol/L)。空腹血糖定义为至少 8 小时未进食
2. 高血糖症状及随机血糖≥200mg/dL(11.1mmol/L)。随机血糖定义为不受进食时间限制的任意时间内的血糖测量，典型的高血糖症状包括糖尿、多尿及无法解释的体重下降。

或者

3. 口服糖耐量测试中，餐后 2 小时血糖≥200mg/dL(11.1mmol/L)。检测需根据 WHO 的描述进行，使用含糖当量为 75g 的无水葡萄糖溶解于水中*

*若无含糖当量测定条件，这一标准可通过不同日期的反复测定来确定。

的是，Kuo 等关于超过 35 000 例患者的研究中，患有 NODAT 的患者心血管疾病死亡的风险增加 15%，但其统计学差异尚不显著[255]。这一结果可能与其仅有 1.5年的随访期有关，也可能因为 NODAT 的报道不完整（仅 6.6%的患者移植 1 年后发病）。与 NODAT 相关风险的发病率和死亡率仍需要进一步研究。

NODAT 的危险因素

肾移植患者 NODAT 许多重要的危险因素是无法改变的，包括族裔是非洲裔和西班牙裔、受体或供体为男性、数目越来越多的 HLA 不匹配，以及一级亲属糖尿病家族史；感染丙型肝炎病毒（HCV）或巨细胞病毒也会增加风险[78,103,142,259]。年龄的增加是一个重要的危险因素，患者超过 45 岁较年轻患者 NODAT 的风险增加 2 倍以上[78]。常染色体显性多囊肾病已被报道与 NODAT 风险增加有关[260]；然而，最近的研究还没有证实这一发现[261,262]。潜在可改变的危险因素包括肥胖，其在人群中越来越普遍；高达 60%的肾移植受体已被报道为超重或肥胖[263]。根据 Shah 等的报道，超重患者（体重指数 25~30kg/m^2）风险增加 1.5 倍，而那些肥胖（BMI>30kg/m^2）NODAT 的患者风险则上升 1.8 倍[261]。其他潜在改变的危险因素包括急性排斥发作（可能与类固醇治疗有关）、CNI 使用、mTOR 抑制剂以及皮质类固醇[103]。特别是，使用他克莫司比 CyA 更容易发生 NODAT[78,79]。糖耐量受损有关的免疫抑制药物的机理如上所述。

肾移植后管理

免疫抑制剂方案调整

糖皮质激素、CNI 及西罗莫司损害糖耐量的机制已在上文回顾。这些药物剂量减少或某些情况下停药必须将血糖改善与排斥风险进行平衡。关于类固醇停药或避免使用研究，Pascual 等在 Cochrane 回顾中进行了总结[221]，表明其能降低 NODAT 发生率，尤其是服用环孢素 A 的患者；服用他克莫司的患者似乎不能从类固醇停药中受益。为了确认这些观测，近期进行了两项类固醇避免使用或早期撤药的随机研究，但未发现服用他克莫司和小剂量泼尼松的患者 NODAT 的发病率下降[220,264]；然而，无类固醇使用组的确需要更少的降糖药物。在 NODAT 高危的患者，即使无类固醇方案并不是标准方案，仍需要考虑快速类固醇减量或撤药。尽管存在高血压和高脂血症恶化的可能性，并且心血管疾病风险总体的变化尚未可知；但类似的，他克莫司改用 CyA 后，特定患者仍可能受益[263]。移植术后早期他克莫司浓度高于 15ng/mL 可能会造成永久性血糖控制能力受损的风险增加，故应避免[265]。

生活方式改变及药物治疗

生活方式改变着眼于改善饮食结构和增加运动量，这是控制移植和非移植患者糖尿病的重要内容。坚持调整为积极的生活方式已被证实可以改善 NODAT 高危患者的血糖控制[266]。然而，许多患者会持续需要使用降糖药物。目前尚无关于肾移植后糖尿病患者的随机研究来提供药物选择的依据；KDIGO 等实践指南只是针对一般人群提供建议[213]。在全体人群中，阶梯式口服单药开始的，并最终通过联合胰岛素治疗的糖尿病管理方案一直都为大家认同[263,267]。Yates 等最近的一篇综述建议，无论生活方式是否改善，如果血红蛋白 $A1_c$（$HbA1_c$）保持 7.0%以上都应开始控制血糖[263]。KDIGO 指南建议 $HbA1_c$ 应在 7.0%~7.5%，以避免严重低血糖反应，严重低血糖反应被认为是肾移植患者中积极血糖控制方案更常见的情况[268]。所有类别的降糖药都曾被用于这一类患者。考虑到许多格列吡嗪属磺酰脲类药物会升高移植患者 CyA 水平，使用这类药物时应仔细监测，不过这种效果不会在格列吡嗪中出现，故可以优先考虑[263,269]。使用二甲双胍可造成胃肠道不适，特别是在服用霉酚酸酯的患者中问题可能更严重；噻唑烷二酮被报道可能增加水肿和心血管事件[263]。如果需要胰岛素治疗，很多内分泌专家建议上午使用 NPH 胰岛素，其作用时间与口服糖皮质激素的药代动力学特性相匹配。近期发表了更多关于肾移植患者的糖尿病管理，其国际指南共识在 2003 年发表[103,142,263]。

新型免疫抑制剂

贝拉西普（belatacept）是一类新型免疫抑制剂，通过阻断 T 细胞和抗原呈递细胞之间的共刺激信号（第二信号），从而阻止 T 细胞活化[270]。贝拉西普是一种替代 CNI 的融合蛋白。每月静脉注射一次。在 BENEFIT 临床试验中，1209 例接受了贝拉西普与 CyA 的患者随机分组，并同时服用 MMF 和泼尼松，并未使用 CNI 情况下得到了更低的收缩压和舒张压，非 HDL 胆固醇和甘油三酯水平的下降[271]。此外，使用基于贝拉西普方案治疗的患者，3 年后的 GFR 预测值为 21mL/(min·1.73m^2)，较 CyA 组高[272]。尽管尚未证明服用贝拉西普的患者移植物和生存率更高，但这类药物显著降低了心血管风险，改善了肾功能，这为 CVD 发生率减少、提高患者及移植物的生存提供了保证。目前，现有的肾移植患者或CVD高危患者，能否从转换到基于贝拉西普的方案中获益尚未明确。

托法替尼(Tofacitinib)是Janus激酶(JAK)抑制剂，JAK是一种酪氨酸激酶，参与多个细胞表面受体的信号转导通路，以及T细胞、B细胞和自然杀伤细胞的正常功能发挥[273,274]。在肾移植患者中，一项研究初步比较了托法替尼与CyA，发现托法替尼治疗的患者肾功能改善，NODAT的发生率较低；但托法替尼组存在更高的严重感染、血液学异常和PTLD的发病率[274]。在未来，这类药物不仅能作为备选方案，并且具有更低的心脏风险。

胰腺移植患者的心血管疾病

胰腺移植是一种能够成功治疗糖尿病的方法；肾脏和胰腺联合移植(SPK)占胰腺移植的70%以上[275]。尽管1型糖尿病历来被认为是胰腺移植的唯一对象，越来越多的2型糖尿病患者从这种方法中受益[276]。

相比仅行供体肾移植，成功的SPK移植患者生存率有显著的改善。值得注意的是，1型糖尿病SPK与活体供体肾移植患者的存活率和移植物存活率同样显著[277]。由于活体供体和SPK受体特点不同，两组之间是很难精确比较的：活体供体的患者年龄通常较大，伴发心脏疾病的可能性更高，接受较老供体肾脏的患者中非洲裔美国人的可能性更低，可能已经接受过移植，并且较SPK患者相比HLA配型更好[277]。最近的多因素分析研究试图把这些差异考虑在内，并得出了不同的结论。Young等分析了UNOS数据库，发现活体移植受体具有更好的结局[278]。然而，Weiss等检索了SRTR上的数据，报道活体供体肾移植患者结局的优势集中在移植后第一年；胰腺移植物功能正常超过一年的患者长期存活率和移植物存活率是最高的[277]。活肾移植后接受胰腺移植的患者同样有很好的长期结局[279]。胰腺移植受体结局的改善可能是由于长期血糖正常引起的良好效果。

胰腺移植后血糖恢复正常已被证明能减慢并最终停止糖尿病性视网膜病[280]和糖尿病性神经病的进展[281,282]，且能防止糖尿病性肾病在共存的移植肾中复发[282]。糖尿病性肾病的病理学改变已被发现在单纯接受胰腺移植的患者中逆转[282]。

已有报道胰腺移植患者的心脏风险因素得到了改善，包括总胆固醇和血清甘油三酯减少，以及收缩压和舒张压降低[283,284]；但并非所有的研究都发现了这些进展。胰腺移植也被认为能改善大血管疾病。Larsen等研究了胰腺移植前和移植后2年的患者，他们发现超声显示颈动脉内膜中层厚度(IMT)改善，与心血管事件的风险相关[285]。在一项横断面研究中，Fiorina等同样发现IMT改善，并进一步报道了血管内皮细胞功能改善；肱动脉内皮依赖性舒张被发现在SPK患者中正常，而在单纯肾移植的患者中则未发现[286]。Jukema等对26例SPK且胰腺移植物功能正常的患者和6例胰腺移植物功能丧失的患者进行了定量冠状动脉造影[287]。平均3.9年后，移植物功能正常的患者冠状动脉粥样硬化进展显著减慢；38%的患者病变消退，而胰腺移植物功能丧失的患者则无病变消退。左心室收缩和舒张功能改善程度在SPK患者中同样更大[288,289]。同样有报道表明，胰肾联合移植的患者急性心肌梗死[288,290]和充血性心力衰竭[288]的发生率也较单纯接受肾脏移植的患者更低。

总之，这些数据强有力地表明胰腺移植改善了微血管和大血管疾病，并改善了心血管疾病的发病率和死亡率。尽管如此，CVD仍是这一人群发病和死亡的首要原因之一[288,291]。

肝移植患者的心血管疾病

原位肝移植(OLT)的改进使患者较以往生存期更长。目前1年和5年生存率分别为85%和67%，10年生存率超过50%[292]。患者存活率稳步提高与外科手术技术的改进，以及对这些患者术前及术后的医疗管理有关。虽然CVD明显的患者不被考虑肝移植，近来CVD患者存活时间延长已成为这类患者发病率和死亡率的重要原因[293]。此外，CVD的危险因素(例如高血压、高血脂、糖尿病和代谢综合征)在OLT术后患病率越来越高。心脏并发症也是术后早期死亡的常见病因[294]。据报道，肝移植患者相比一般人群心血管死亡率更高[295]。值得注意的是，肝移植受体正在逐年变老，最近的数据显示平均年龄已经从2000年的46岁上升到2009年的将近50岁[292]；65岁以上的患者是发展最为快速的，OLT从2000年的7%提高到2009年的11%以上。随着年龄的增加，心脏危险因素也不断增加。虽然相比肾移植或心脏移植，肝移植患者CVD的发病率相对较低，但这可能是无法识别的。本节将回顾肝移植术后导致心血管疾病的危险因素,并讨论管理指南。

术后心血管并发症

接受肝移植的患者在移植术后的数天和数周内处于心血管并发症的高发期；心脏并发症是围术期死亡的主要原因[294]。

虽然有潜在 CHD 的患者数量相对较少（见下文),肝硬化性心肌病仍是一种常见的情况[296]。肝硬化患者心脏功能异常的识别应归功于 Kowalski 和 Abelmann [297]；后来 Regan 等[298]和 Gould 等[299]的经典研究发现左心室舒张末压异常增高，以及肝硬化患者在使用血管紧张素或运动时心脏收缩力显著下降。目前普遍认为肝硬化性心肌病在酒精性和非酒精性肝硬化患者中均会发生[296]。在临床上,患者会表现为应激状态下收缩和舒张功能异常;然而,肝病患者在外周血管扩张及后负荷降低状态下则会阻止 CHF 的临床表现。

这些潜在的心脏异常导致患者在肝移植术中及术后心脏不良事件的风险升高。在手术过程中,出血、第三间隙液体量变化以及持续产生的腹水可导致前负荷明显下降，而过度使用液体或血液制品扩容则可能导致术后容积超负荷[296]。潜在的心肌舒张和收缩功能损伤会增加心排血量减少和低血压的风险,以及肺水肿。肺水肿是一种常见的情况，有报道 22%~56%的 OLT 受体在术后第 1 个月会发生肺水肿[294]。移植术后血压和体循环血管阻力的迅速增加会对心脏产生负担,在液体管理时,可能导致肺水肿高发;大多数有临床症状的肺水肿发作可通过适当治疗缓解[296,300]。即使在缺乏潜在心脏疾病或相关危险因素的情况下,Eimer 等仍报道在 86 例心脏导管和超声心动图正常的患者中,7%在肝移植术后出现了严重的心力衰竭[301]。至关重要的是,围术期需仔细监测血流动力学状态,保持细致的体液和电解质平衡,以减少急性心血管并发症。

Sampathkumar 等报道了肝移植术后早期罕见的扩张型心肌病(754 例患者中的 7 例),不过心功能得到了改善[302]。Torregrosa 等的研究表明肝硬化性心肌病患者的心脏结构和功能异常通常会在 OLT 术后 9~12 个月缓解[300,303]。

再灌注后综合征(PRS)是另一个可在术后极早期发生的并发症。它最初是由 Aggarwal 等在 1987 年报道[304],定义为平均动脉压降低至少 30%,且在再灌注 5 分钟内出现 1 分钟的心律下降。相关的血流动力学表现包括肺动脉压升高、中心静脉和肺毛细血管楔压以及全身血管阻力下降[305]。对于这一综合征尚不完全了解,其归因于术后代谢异常,例如代谢性酸中毒和高钾血症,以及从同种异体移植物释放血管活性物质。大约 30%的肝移植患者可发生 PRS[306]。Hilmi 等回顾了匹兹堡大学 2002—2003 年的 338 例移植患者，发现 PRS 更严重的患者情况更差，需要更长的重症监护和住院时间,并可能需要再次移植。然而,这些患者 5 年生存率并未降低[307]。

术后出现的其他心脏并发症包括房性和室性心律失常、心肌梗死、空气栓塞[308]、心内和肺栓塞[309],以及心脏骤停[294,310]。Fouad 等报道了 2002—2007 年的 324 例40 岁以上 OLT 患者,23 例患者存在术中心血管事件,包括 2 例患者死于 PRS。21 例患者在术后的前 6 个月内死亡,5 例（23%）由于直接心脏原因死亡，使得 CVD 成为这项研究中死亡的首要原因[294]。其他研究估计心血管并发症占移植后死亡人数的 7%~15%[296,311]。

长期心血管死亡情况及冠状动脉性心脏疾病

目前肝移植患者术后死于 CVD 是一种常见的情况[294]。虽然早期的报道认为 CVD 是造成死亡的非常见原因[312-314],近年来的数据表明 CVD 死亡是一个越来越重要的问题。Abbasoglu 等前瞻性地收集了 1985—1995 年的 1174 例 OLT 患者的数据,发现 17% 存活>1 年的患者死于 CVD 或平均在术后 5 年发生卒中[315]。Kashyap 等报道 CVD 导致匹兹堡大学 4000 例连续的肝移植患者中 8.3%的死亡，其平均随访时间为 9.4 年[316]。Pruthi 等报道 CVD 造成 1977—1984 年肝移植术后 299 例存活至少 3 年的成人患者中 21%的死亡；大多数患者存在此前公认的冠心病或已知的心脏危险因素[317]。Rabkin 等报道了 1991—2000 年的 459 移植患者,13%的晚期死亡率与复发性肝病无关,是由心血管原因造成[318]。Johnston 等研究了 110 例连续的 OLT 患者,发现与年龄相匹配的人群相比,心血管死亡的相对风险为 2.56;16%的患者在 3.9 年的平均随访期内因心血管疾病死亡[295]。Albeldawi 等报道克利夫兰诊所 1996—2008 年的 775 例肝移植患者的心血管事件;83 例患者(10.7%)在 40 个月的平均随访期内因心血管相关原因死亡，是继肝功能衰竭和感染之后的第三大常见死亡原因[319]。Watt 等最近报道了来自 NIDDK数据库的数据，1990—1994 年间在多个中心进行移植且中位随访时间为 10 年的 798 例患者[320]，近 20%与肝脏疾病无关的死亡由心血管原因导致[320]。糖尿病、高血压、肾功能不全及患者年龄是移植术后 1 年和 5 年死亡的重要因素[320]。对这些研究的回顾表明，与肝脏疾病、感染和恶性肿瘤一样，CVD 可引起显著比例的肝移植术后死亡，是一个越来越重要的问题。

已报道冠状动脉疾病(CAD)在肝移植患者中发病率较高，但常无法识别。Carey 等研究了克利夫兰诊所连续的 37 例 50 岁以上的 OLT 且行冠状动脉造影的患者[321]。虽然 30 例患者均无心脏疾病病史，10 例(27%)有中重度的 CAD，其中 6 例(16.2%)为严重 CAD；糖尿病被认为是最显著的危险因素。最近，Tiukinhoy-Laing 等报道 2000—2003 年间 45 岁以上、连续的 174 例因终末期肝病(ESLD)而行 OLT 患者的心导管检查结果[322]。风险因素在这些患者中很普遍；一半的患者有高血压或糖尿病，1/3 的患者吸烟或有吸烟史。60%的患者有血管造影证实的病灶；26%的患者既往无中、重度冠状动脉疾病史。已有 CHD 的患者 OLT 术后发病率和死亡率显著增加[323,324]。死亡率的增加可通过 Yo 和 Thuluvath 对 UNOS 数据库的分析加以说明：预先记录患者既往是否有 CAD 和糖尿病(图 88.7)后，对 1988—2001 年间的 18 044 例 OLT 患者进行分析发现，CAD 或糖尿病史都是 5 年生存率降低约 40%的独立危险因素；两个危险因素共存的患者表现为存活率下降 60%[324]。

移植后心脏事件

尽管移植患者会对心血管疾病进行常规筛查，肝移植术后心血管事件仍很常见[319]。

在 Johnston 等的研究中[295]，在 OLT 术后中位时间 3.9 年时对 110 例患者进行检查，发现 25 例缺血性和 32 例非缺血性心血管事件(术后早期事件被排除在外)[295]。缺血性心脏事件的相对危险度与匹配人群的预期风险相比为 3.07。Mazuelos 等发现在 5 年的随访中，170 例 OLT 患者中有 9.4%发生心血管并发症[53]。Al-beldawi 等的研究中，83 例患者在 40 个月的随访中发生一次或多次心血管事件，其 5 年的累积事件发生率为 13.5%。多因素分析发现，包括移植后的代谢综合征(PTMS)、年龄、男性，以及移植后的糖尿病和高血压是独立的危险因素。MMF 也被发现是一个危险因素，但被认为是因在肾功能衰竭 CNI 会造成副作用增加而必须降低浓度时采用的替代药物导致的[319]。Laryea 等报道 118 例 1998—2004 年间加拿大大西洋移植登记处的肝脏移植患者[325]。在超过 58 个月的随访中，发生了 25 例主要血管事件，包括急性冠状动脉综合征、心肌梗死、短暂性脑缺血发作(TIA)和卒中。PTMS 患者的事件显著更多(21 对 4；P=0.003)。Laish 等回顾了 1991—2007 年接受肝移植的 248 例患者，并报道了类似的结果。23 例患者在超过 6.2 年的随访中经历了主要血管事件；PTMS 患者的发生率显著更高(17 对 6，P=0.027)[326]。梅奥诊所最近的一项报道说明了心血管事件的发生情况，1998—2001 年的 230 名移植患者，中位时间为 8.2 年，其中发生了 59 次心脏事件，包括临床记录的 CAD(心绞痛或造影显著狭窄)、充血性心力衰竭、脑卒中、周围血管疾病或心血管死亡[293]。尽管这一人群中普遍存在多个危险因素，多因素分析证实移植前糖尿病、吸烟史及既往心脏疾病是独立的危险因素。此外，肌钙蛋白 I 水平升高能预测心血管事件，可能反映潜在心脏微血管病变或无法识别的左心功能不全。

心血管危险因素

心脏危险因素在 OLT 患者中很常见。单中心的观

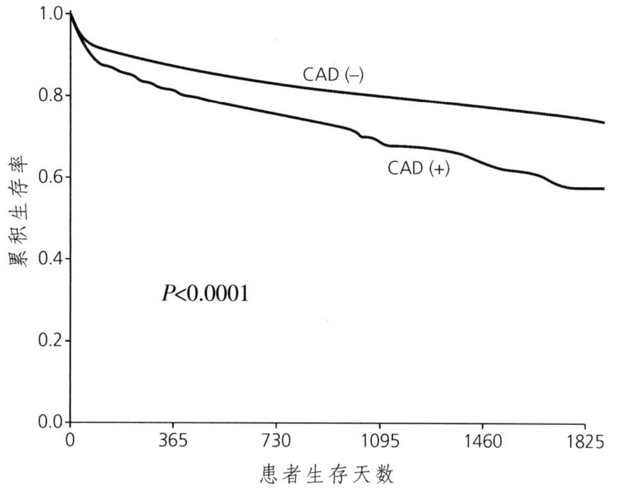

高危人数

CAD	441	272	196	125	76	28
没有	17603	11972	7752	5109	3012	1053

图 88.7 Kaplan-Meier 法分析肾移植术后有无 CHD 患者的生存率。(Reproduced from Yoo et al. [324], with permission of Wolters Kluwer Health.)

察性研究患者数量相对较少，如上所述，可能证据并不足以确认普通人群中心脏风险因素与肝移植患者的相关性。Framingham 风险因素，包括高血压和高脂血症，以及糖尿病和肥胖，可以在移植前就已存在，但在 OLT 后则越来越普遍。可以推测，它们对于肝移植患者的心血管发病率和死亡率有重要作用。

心脏危险因素在这一人群中的患病率较高，很大程度上是由于对免疫抑制剂的暴露。CNI 和皮质激素在升高血压和血糖，以及导致血脂异常（见上文“免疫抑制药物的心血管副作用机制”）中起重要作用；西罗莫司也可能加重心脏病风险。队列期间吸烟可以增加心脏病死亡率[327]。其他引起 CVD 风险的因素包括患者年龄、移植前既往心脏疾病史、CKD 及非酒精性脂肪肝（NAFLD）（表 88.8）[328]。部分有多种危险因素的患者表现为代谢综合征，也在肝移植后越来越普遍[329]。下一节将介绍选择重要的危险因素在肝移植患者中的作用。

高血压

高血压在肝移植患者中很常见；估计发病率在 30%~80%[330]。CNI 的使用在新发高血压中发挥重要的作用；这一发病率在使用 CyA 治疗的患者中要比使用他克莫司的患者高（图 88.8）[331,332]。糖皮质激素的使用也加重了高血压。OLT 患者不使用或后续停止使用固醇类激素经研究证实能改善血压[333,334]。

其他促进高血压高发病的因素包括肝移植术后常见的肥胖（见下文）和 CKD 的进展，5 年内累积发生率约为 20%[335]。

尚无特定的用于肝移植受体高血压管理的循证医学指南。近期一些综述建议以 130/80mmHg 为目标血压[330,336,337]。与普通人群中的高血压一样，推荐改变的生活方式包括减肥、锻炼以及减少钠摄入，但如果没有成功则需要使用降压药物。肝移植受体可以使用各类药物进行治疗，目前尚无对这一人群基于何种降压药物的大型研究，尽管可使用一般人群和肾移植高血压治疗指南[213,249]。钙通道阻滞剂因其出色的安全性和药理优势，即可抵消 CNI 药物引起的血管收缩效应而被推荐[338,339]。建议谨慎使用非二氢吡啶类钙通道阻滞剂、地尔硫䓬和维拉帕米，因其通过与竞争细胞色素 P450 3A4 而升高 CNI 水平。β-受体阻滞剂是 CHD 患者的首选，且大多数患者都能耐受这一药物。ACEI 和 ARB 建议在 CKD 伴有蛋白尿的患者中使用。一项小型随机研究比较了硝苯地平与卡维地洛在 OLT 术后新发高血压患者中的作用，发现卡维地洛耐受性更好，但两种药物都只能在一少部分患者中凭自身效应降低至目标血压[340]。事实上，许多患者需要降压药的联合使用。可考虑对特定的患者更换免疫抑制剂。皮质激素可减少或停用。使用 CyA 的患者可以改为他克莫司，或其他基于 MMF 或西罗莫司的方案。

高脂血症

虽然 ESLD 患者血清胆固醇较低，但由于肝胆固醇的合成和酯化受损，高脂血症也常发生于肝移植后[341]。

表 88.8　肝移植术后患者心血管疾病危险因素

- 患者年龄
- 男性
- 移植前或移植后糖尿病
- 移植前或移植后高血压
- 血脂异常
- 肥胖
- 移植术后代谢综合征
- 非酒精性脂肪肝
- 吸烟
- 移植术前心血管疾病
- 慢性肾脏疾病
- 肌钙蛋白 I

Modified from Watt et al.[320], with permission from John Wiley and Sons.

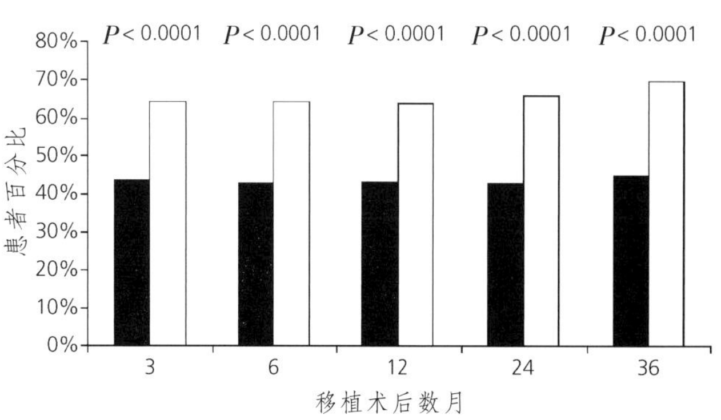

图 88.8　肝移植术后随访 3~36 个月，他克莫司和环孢素治疗的患者需要降压药比例的比较。(Reproduced from Lucey et al. [332], reproduced with permission from John Wiley & Sons.)

大约一半的OLT患者有高脂血症,虽然这部分患者随着时间的推移会逐渐减少[342]。例如,Laryea等研究了118例随访至少18个月的肝移植患者,发现46%的患者出现血脂异常,45%的患者甘油三酯异常[325]。Johnston等研究了1999年110例患者,中位随访时间为3.9年,发现44%的患者血清胆固醇升高,52%的患者HDL水平低,以及8%的患者甘油三酯水平升高[295]。Neal等回顾了1994—1999年181例接受OLT的患者,中位随访时间为54个月[343]。术前仅16%的患者存在高胆固醇血症,移植后则为60%,高甘油三酯患者的比例从10%提高到40%。混合性高脂血症在移植后最常见,但单独胆固醇或甘油三酯升高也可以出现。

与高血压类似,免疫抑制药物在脂质代谢异常中发挥重要作用。CNI、西罗莫司和皮质激素都会导致血脂异常;其发生的机制已在上文中详细讨论。饮食、肥胖和糖尿病也会加重血脂异常(见下文)。CyA已被认为较他克莫司更易造成血脂异常,CyA更换为他克莫司可降低胆固醇[344]。然而,最近的研究报道了不同的发现;一项比较这两种药物的研究发现,无基线血脂异常的患者,肝移植术后1年总胆固醇和甘油三酯水平是相似的[345];这个观察同样被其他研究证实[346]。

饮食调整通常不足以使血脂正常化,通常需要增加降脂药物。他汀类药物是OLT后安全有效的药物,常能良好地耐受,且副反应发生率较低[347]。各种他汀类药物已在移植患者中安全使用。从较低初始剂量开始可能更佳,例如从20mg/d阿托伐他汀或20mg/d普伐他汀开始,两者均已在肝脏移植患者中验证[348,349]。他汀类药物和CNI之间的药物相互作用已在上文中讨论。目前尚无循证医学证据指导来选择一个胆固醇阈值进行治疗。我们建议CVD高危的肝移植患者使用他汀类药物,并控制LDL胆固醇低于100mg/dL(2.6mmol/L)。如果他汀类药物无法降低LDL至目标值或药物不耐受,可安全地加入依折麦布[350]。鱼油和纤维酸衍生物可用于治疗甘油三酯升高,且通常是安全的。

有趣的是,肝移植已被用于治疗纯合子家族性高胆固醇血症,包括在发展为重症CVD之前[204]。

糖尿病

糖尿病在肝脏移植后越来越普遍。移植前患病率约为15%,移植后则为30%~40%[351]。早期的研究报道患病率为13%~27%[352],但最近的研究发现其发病率更高。例如,Larea等报道糖尿病的患病率从13%增加至61%,而Laish等则报道增幅从之前的14.4%至肝移植之后的39.6%[325,326]。患病率增加部分原因可能是由于采用了较低的临界值来诊断糖尿病,即ADA推荐的空腹126mg/dL(表88.7)[325,352,353]。肝移植患者导致NODAT发展的危险因素包括年龄>50岁、男性[354]、BMI>30kg/m^2[355]、使用他克莫司(相比于CyA)[355]以及巨细胞病毒感染[356]。HCV感染是肝移植和肾移植受体NODAT发展的一个重要危险因素[259,355],而且与非移植患者2型糖尿病的发展有关[355,357]。HCV感染会导致胰岛素抵抗[358,359];该病毒还可以感染胰岛β细胞,可能导致胰岛素生成减少[360]。在肝移植和肾脏移植患者中,HCV似乎比CyA更常在服用他克莫司患者中导致NODAT[259,355]。移植肝去神经支配本身可能导致胰岛素抵抗,并有助于NODAT的发展[361]。如上所述,肝移植患者糖尿病的发生与CHD、心血管事件及心源性猝死有关[293,319-321]。

与其他移植患者一样,肝脏移植后糖尿病患者的治疗与一般人群的治疗类似[351]。应注意,肝代谢大部分磺酰脲类和噻唑烷二酮类药物;这些药物应谨慎且仅于移植物功能正常稳定的情况下用[362]。激素的用量应尽量降到最低[330];在特定的患者中,从他克莫司更换为CyA或其他无CNI的方案被认为能改善糖耐量[363,364]。

肥胖和代谢综合征

PTMS日益成为肝移植受体的重要问题。我们已经讨论了许多MS的成分,包括高甘油三酯血症、低LDL水平、高血压及糖耐量受损(表88.2)[351]。腹型肥胖也在普通人群中尤其是肝移植患者中高发。腹水的存在可以使中心性肥胖更难以评估[351],因此有些项目采用BMI大于30kg/m^{2}作为用于MS的附加判断标准[325]。肥胖发生于超过1/3的ESLD患者和非酒精性脂肪性肝炎(NASH)需要移植治疗患者。MS的总发病率在肝移植前为5%~29%,在肝移植后为43%~58%[365]。PTMS已被证明是肝脏移植后大血管和心脏事件的重要危险因素,虽然尚未证明会增加心脏病死亡率[319,325,326]。PTMS可通过寻找导致心脏风险的各个成分进行管理。除了饮食和锻炼,使用奥利司他已被发现是肝移植患者减轻体重的安全辅助手段[366]。

总结

移植患者与普通人群一样经历同样的心血管疾病，但因存在原发性疾病和需要免疫抑制药物治疗等情况而更加严重。随着整体移植效果逐渐改善，患者享有更长的移植后寿命，心血管相关情况成为目前对长期结果的最显著的威胁。因此，所有的移植医生应认真应对可改变的危险因素，并努力寻求减少获得性风险，以避免过早的 CVD 发病率和死亡率。这应与更广泛认可的免疫抑制剂药物管理方案齐头并进。

（凌琪 译 凌琪 校）

参考文献

1. Yusuf S, Reddy S, Ounpuu S, et al. Global burden of cardiovascular diseases: part I: general considerations, the epidemiologic transition, risk factors, and impact of urbanization. Circulation. 2001;104(22):2746–2753.
2. Deaton C, Froelicher ES, Wu LH, et al. The global burden of cardiovascular disease. Journal of Cardiovascular Nursing. 2011;26(4 Suppl):S5–S14.
3. Fellstrom B. Risk factors for and management of post-transplantation cardiovascular disease. Biodrugs: Clinical Immunotherapeutics, Biopharmaceuticals and Gene Therapy. 2001;15(4):261–278.
4. Rabkin JM, Corless CL, Rosen HR, et al. Immunosuppression impact on long-term cardiovascular complications after liver transplantation. American Journal of Surgery. 2002;183(5):595–599.
5. Ghods AJ. Risk factors profile and cardiovascular events in solid organ transplant recipients. Iranian Journal of Kidney Diseases. 2012;6(1):9–13.
6. Mehra MR. Contemporary concepts in prevention and treatment of cardiac allograft vasculopathy. American Journal of Transplantation. 2006;6(6):1248–1256.
7. Foley RN, Parfrey PS, Sarnak MJ. Clinical epidemiology of cardiovascular disease in chronic renal disease. American Journal of Kidney Diseases. 1998;32(5 Suppl 3):S112–S119.
8. Mells G, Neuberger J. Long-term care of the liver allograft recipient. Seminars in Liver Disease. 2009;29(1):102–120.
9. Levitsky J, Freifeld A, Lyden E, et al. Evaluation of the coagulation and inflammatory responses in solid organ transplant recipients and donors. Clinical Transplantation. 2009;23(6):943–950.
10. Ojo AO. Cardiovascular complications after renal transplantation and their prevention. Transplantation. 2006;82(5):603–611.
11. Guckelberger O, Mutzke F, Glanemann M, et al. Validation of cardiovascular risk scores in a liver transplant population. Liver Transplantation. 2006;12(3):394–401.
12. Diaz G, O'Connor M. Cardiovascular and renal complications in patients receiving a solid-organ transplant. Current Opinion in Critical Care. 2011;17(4):382–389.
13. De Vito Dabbs A, Song MK. Risk profile for cardiovascular morbidity and mortality after lung transplantation. Nursing Clinics of North America. 2008;43(1):37–53, vi.
14. Trulock EP, Edwards LB, Taylor DO, et al. Registry of the International Society for Heart and Lung Transplantation: twenty-third official adult lung and heart-lung transplantation report–2006. Journal of Heart and Lung Transplantation. 2006;25(8):880–892.
15. Sekine Y, Waddell TK, Matte-Martyn A, et al. Risk quantification of early outcome after lung transplantation: donor, recipient, operative, and post-transplant parameters. Journal of Heart and Lung Transplantation. 2004;23(1):96–104.
16. Findlay JY, Wen D, Mandell MS. Cardiac risk evaluation for abdominal transplantation. Current Opinion in Organ Transplantation. 2010;15(3):363–367.
17. Zeier M, Mandelbaum A, Ritz E. Hypertension in the transplanted patient. Nephron. 1998;80(3):257–268.
18. Braunwald E, Bonow RO. Braunwald's Heart Disease: A Textbook of Cardiovascular Medicine, 9th ed. Philadelphia, PA: Saunders; 2012. xxiv, 1961.
19. Opelz G, Wujciak T, Ritz E. Association of chronic kidney graft failure with recipient blood pressure. Collaborative Transplant Study. Kidney International. 1998;53(1):217–222.
20. Curtis JJ. Posttransplant hypertension. Transplantation Proceedings. 1998;30(5):2009–2011.
21. Elliott WJ. Traditional drug therapy of hypertension in transplant recipients. Journal of Human Hypertension. 1998;12(12):845–849.
22. Olyaei AJ, deMattos AM, Bennett WM. A practical guide to the management of hypertension in renal transplant recipients. Drugs. 1999;58(6):1011–1027.
23. Rao VK. Posttransplant medical complications. Surgical Clinics of North America. 1998;78(1):113–132.
24. Donahoo WT, Kosmiski LA, Eckel RH. Drugs causing dyslipoproteinemia. Endocrinology and Metabolism Clinics of North America. 1998;27(3):677–697.
25. Jindal RM. Post-transplant hyperlipidaemia. Postgraduate Medical Journal. 1997;73(866):785–793.
26. Hilbrands LB, Demacker PN, Hoitsma AJ, et al. The effects of cyclosporine and prednisone on serum lipid and (apo)lipoprotein levels in renal transplant recipients. Journal of the American Society of Nephrology. 1995;5(12):2073–2081.
27. Raine AE, Carter R, Mann JI, et al. Adverse effect of cyclosporin on plasma cholesterol in renal transplant recipients. Nephrology, Dialysis, Transplantation. 1988;3(4):458–463.
28. Ballantyne CM, Podet EJ, Patsch WP, et al. Effects of cyclosporine therapy on plasma lipoprotein levels. JAMA. 1989;262(1):53–56.
29. Vathsala A, Weinberg RB, Schoenberg L, et al. Lipid abnormalities in cyclosporine-prednisone-treated renal transplant recipients. Transplantation. 1989;48(1):37–43.
30. Jensik SC. Tacrolimus (FK 506) in kidney transplantation: three-year survival results of the US multicenter, randomized, comparative trial. FK 506 Kidney Transplant Study Group. Transplantation Proceedings. 1998;30(4):1216–1218.
31. Satterthwaite R, Aswad S, Sunga V, et al. Incidence of new-onset hypercholesterolemia in renal transplant patients treated with FK506 or cyclosporine. Transplantation. 1998;65(3):446–449.
32. Groth CG, Backman L, Morales JM, et al. Sirolimus (rapamycin)-based therapy in human renal transplantation: similar efficacy and different toxicity compared with cyclosporine. Sirolimus European Renal Transplant Study Group. Transplantation. 1999;67(7):1036–1042.
33. Kahan BD, Podbielski J, Napoli KL, et al. Immunosuppressive effects and safety of a sirolimus/cyclosporine combination regimen for renal transplantation. Transplantation. 1998;66(8):1040–1046.
34. Kato T, Tokoro T, Namii Y, et al. Early introduction of HMG-CoA reductase inhibitors could prevent the incidence of transplant coronary artery disease. Transplantation Proceedings. 2000;32(2):331–333.
35. Kobashigawa JA, Katznelson S, Laks H, et al. Effect of pravastatin on outcomes after cardiac transplantation. New England Journal of Medicine. 1995;333(10):621–627.
36. Wenke K, Meiser B, Thiery J, et al. Simvastatin reduces graft vessel disease and mortality after heart transplantation: a four-year randomized trial. Circulation. 1997;96(5):1398–1402.
37. Lindholm A, Albrechtsen D, Frodin L, et al. Ischemic heart disease–major cause of death and graft loss after renal transplantation in Scandinavia. Transplantation. 1995;60(5):451–457.
38. Kasiske BL, Guijarro C, Massy ZA, et al. Cardiovascular disease after renal transplantation. Journal of the American Society of Nephrology. 1996;7(1):158–165.
39. Jindal RM, Sidner RA, Milgrom ML. Post-transplant diabetes mellitus. The role of immunosuppression. Drug Safety. 1997;16(4):242–257.
40. Jindal RM. Posttransplant diabetes mellitus–a review. Transplantation. 1994;58(12):1289–1298.
41. Arner P, Gunnarsson R, Blomdahl S, et al. Some characteristics of steroid diabetes: a study in renal-transplant recipients receiving high-dose corticosteroid therapy. Diabetes Care. 1983;6(1):23–25.
42. Boudreaux JP, McHugh L, Canafax DM, et al. The impact of cyclosporine and combination immunosuppression on the incidence of posttransplant diabetes in renal allograft recipients. Transplantation. 1987;44(3):376–381.
43. Hricik DE, Bartucci MR, Mayes JT, et al. The effects of steroid withdrawal on the lipoprotein profiles of cyclosporine-treated kidney and kidney-pancreas transplant recipients. Transplantation. 1992;54(5):868–871.

44. Schulak JA, Hricik DE. Steroid withdrawal after renal transplantation. Clinical Transplantation. 1994;8(2 Pt 2):211–216.
45. Johnston O, Rose CL, Webster AC, et al. Sirolimus is associated with new-onset diabetes in kidney transplant recipients. Journal of the American Society of Nephrology. 2008;19(7):1411–1418.
46. Everhart JE, Lombardero M, Lake JR, et al. Weight change and obesity after liver transplantation: incidence and risk factors. Liver Transplantation and Surgery. 1998;4(4):285–296.
47. Ward HJ. Nutritional and metabolic issues in solid organ transplantation: targets for future research. Journal of Renal Nutrition. 2009;19(1):111–122.
48. Reuben A. Long-term management of the liver transplant patient: diabetes, hyperlipidemia, and obesity. Liver Transplantation. 2001;7(11 Suppl 1): S13–S21.
49. Guida B, Trio R, Nastasi A, et al. Body composition and cardiovascular risk factors in pretransplant hemodialysis patients. Clinical Nutrition. 2004;23(3): 363–372.
50. Armstrong KA, Campbell SB, Hawley CM, et al. Obesity is associated with worsening cardiovascular risk factor profiles and proteinuria progression in renal transplant recipients. American Journal of Transplantation. 2005;5(11): 2710–2718.
51. Stegall MD, Everson G, Schroter G, et al. Metabolic complications after liver transplantation. Diabetes, hypercholesterolemia, hypertension, and obesity. Transplantation. 1995;60(9):1057–1060.
52. Munoz SJ, Deems RO, Moritz MJ, et al. Hyperlipidemia and obesity after orthotopic liver transplantation. Transplantation Proceedings. 1991;23(1 Pt 2): 1480–1483.
53. Mazuelos F, Abril J, Zaragoza C, et al. Cardiovascular morbidity and obesity in adult liver transplant recipients. Transplantation Proceedings. 2003;35(5): 1909–1910.
54. Ross R. Atherosclerosis–an inflammatory disease. New England Journal of Medicine. 1999;340(2):115–126.
55. Johnson DW, Isbel NM, Brown AM, et al. The effect of obesity on renal transplant outcomes. Transplantation. 2002;74(5):675–681.
56. Ridker PM. High-sensitivity C-reactive protein: potential adjunct for global risk assessment in the primary prevention of cardiovascular disease. Circulation. 2001;103(13):1813–1818.
57. Bostom AD, Brown RS Jr, Chavers BM, et al. Prevention of post-transplant cardiovascular disease–report and recommendations of an ad hoc group. American Journal of Transplantation. 2002;2(6):491–500.
58. van Ree RM, de Vries AP, Oterdoom LH, et al. Abdominal obesity and smoking are important determinants of C-reactive protein in renal transplant recipients. Nephrology, Dialysis, Transplantation. 2005;20(11):2524–2531.
59. Rowe IAN, Neuberger JM. Pharmacology of transplantation. In: Hricik D, editor. Primer on Transplantation, 3rd ed. Oxford: Wiley-Blackwell; 2011: 18–34.
60. Naesens M, Kuypers DR, Sarwal M. Calcineurin inhibitor nephrotoxicity. Clinical Journal of the American Society of Nephrology. 2009;4(2):481–508.
61. Liu EH, Siegel RM, Harlan DM, et al. T cell-directed therapies: lessons learned and future prospects. Nature Immunology. 2007;8(1):25–30.
62. Klein IH, Abrahams AC, van Ede T, et al. Differential effects of acute and sustained cyclosporine and tacrolimus on sympathetic nerve activity. Journal of Hypertension. 2010;28(9):1928–1934.
63. Chatzikyrkou C, Menne J, Gwinner W, et al. Pathogenesis and management of hypertension after kidney transplantation. Journal of Hypertension. 2011; 29(12):2283–2294.
64. Wadei HM, Textor SC. Hypertension in the kidney transplant recipient. Transplantation Reviews. 2010;24(3):105–120.
65. Lassila M. Interaction of cyclosporine A and the renin-angiotensin system; new perspectives. Current Drug Metabolism. 2002;3(1):61–71.
66. Van Buren DH, Burke JF, Lewis RM. Renal function in patients receiving long-term cyclosporine therapy. Journal of the American Society of Nephrology. 1994;4(8 Suppl):S17–S22.
67. Hausberg M, Lang D, Levers A, et al. Sympathetic nerve activity in renal transplant patients before and after withdrawal of cyclosporine. Journal of Hypertension. 2006;24(5):957–964.
68. Lopez-Miranda J, Vilella E, Perez-Jimenez F, et al. Low-density lipoprotein metabolism in rats treated with cyclosporine. Metabolism: Clinical and Experimental. 1993;42(6):678–683.
69. Ginsberg HN. Cyclosporine, plasma lipids, and organ transplantation. Hepatology. 1996;24(3):735–736.
70. Kaptein A, de Wit EC, Princen HM. Cotranslational inhibition of apoB-100 synthesis by cyclosporin A in the human hepatoma cell line HepG2. Arteriosclerosis and Thrombosis. 1994;14(5):780–789.
71. Rayyes OA, Wallmark A, Floren CH. Cyclosporine inhibits catabolism of low-density lipoproteins in HepG2 cells by about 25%. Hepatology. 1996;24(3): 613–619.
72. Wasan KM, Donnachie EM, Seccombe DW, et al. Effect of cyclosporine A on the binding affinity and internalization of low-density lipoproteins in human skin fibroblasts. Journal of Pharmaceutical Sciences. 2002;91(12): 2520–2524.
73. Vaziri ND, Liang K, Azad H. Effect of cyclosporine on HMG-CoA reductase, cholesterol 7alpha-hydroxylase, LDL receptor, HDL receptor, VLDL receptor, and lipoprotein lipase expressions. Journal of Pharmacology and Experimental Therapeutics. 2000;294(2):778–783.
74. Gueguen Y, Ferrari L, Batt AM. [Dyslipidaemia and its management after immunosuppressive treatment]. Therapie. 2004;59(4):463–469.
75. Tory R, Sachs-Barrable K, Hill JS, et al. Cyclosporine A and Rapamycin induce in vitro cholesteryl ester transfer protein activity, and suppress lipoprotein lipase activity in human plasma. International Journal of Pharmaceutics. 2008;358(1–2):219–223.
76. Le Goff W, Peng DQ, Settle M, et al. Cyclosporin A traps ABCA1 at the plasma membrane and inhibits ABCA1-mediated lipid efflux to apolipoprotein A-I. Arteriosclerosis, Thrombosis, and Vascular Biology. 2004;24(11):2155–2161.
77. Kockx M, Guo DL, Traini M, et al. Cyclosporin A decreases apolipoprotein E secretion from human macrophages via a protein phosphatase 2B-dependent and ATP-binding cassette transporter A1 (ABCA1)-independent pathway. Journal of Biological Chemistry. 2009;284(36):24144–24154.
78. Kasiske BL, Snyder JJ, Gilbertson D, et al. Diabetes mellitus after kidney transplantation in the United States. American Journal of Transplantation. 2003; 3(2):178–185.
79. Woodward RS, Schnitzler MA, Baty J, et al. Incidence and cost of new onset diabetes mellitus among U.S. wait-listed and transplanted renal allograft recipients. American Journal of Transplantation. 2003;3(5):590–598.
80. Duijnhoven EM, Boots JM, Christiaans MH, et al. Influence of tacrolimus on glucose metabolism before and after renal transplantation: a prospective study. Journal of the American Society of Nephrology. 2001;12(3):583–588.
81. Vincenti F, Friman S, Scheuermann E, et al. Results of an international, randomized trial comparing glucose metabolism disorders and outcome with cyclosporine versus tacrolimus. American Journal of Transplantation. 2007; 7(6):1506–1514.
82. Heit JJ, Apelqvist AA, Gu X, et al. Calcineurin/NFAT signalling regulates pancreatic beta-cell growth and function. Nature. 2006;443(7109):345–349.
83. Heit JJ. Calcineurin/NFAT signaling in the beta-cell: from diabetes to new therapeutics. Bioessays: News and Reviews in Molecular, Cellular and Developmental Biology. 2007;29(10):1011–1021.
84. Redmon JB, Olson LK, Armstrong MB, et al. Effects of tacrolimus (FK506) on human insulin gene expression, insulin mRNA levels, and insulin secretion in HIT-T15 cells. Journal of Clinical Investigation. 1996;98(12):2786–2793.
85. Drachenberg CB, Klassen DK, Weir MR, et al. Islet cell damage associated with tacrolimus and cyclosporine: morphological features in pancreas allograft biopsies and clinical correlation. Transplantation. 1999;68(3):396–402.
86. Goodwin JE, Zhang J, Geller DS. A critical role for vascular smooth muscle in acute glucocorticoid-induced hypertension. Journal of the American Society of Nephrology. 2008;19(7):1291–1299.
87. Mangos GJ, Whitworth JA, Williamson PM, et al. Glucocorticoids and the kidney. Nephrology. 2003;8(6):267–273.
88. Kelly JJ, Tam SH, Williamson PM, et al. The nitric oxide system and cortisol-induced hypertension in humans. Clinical and Experimental Pharmacology & Physiology. 1998;25(11):945–946.
89. Kornel L. The role of vascular steroid receptors in the control of vascular contractility and peripheral vascular resistance. Journal of Steroid Biochemistry and Molecular Biology. 1993;45(1–3):195–203.
90. Provencher PH, Saltis J, Funder JW. Glucocorticoids but not mineralocorticoids modulate endothelin-1 and angiotensin II binding in SHR vascular smooth muscle cells. Journal of Steroid Biochemistry and Molecular Biology. 1995;52(3): 219–225.
91. Mangos GJ, Walker BR, Kelly JJ, et al. Cortisol inhibits cholinergic vasodilation in the human forearm. American Journal of Hypertension. 2000;13(11): 1155–1160.
92. Olyaei AJ, Demattos AM, Bennett WM. Cardiovascular complications of immunosuppressive agents in renal transplant recipients. Expert Opinion on Drug Safety. 2005;4(1):29–44.
93. Kobashigawa JA, Kasiske BL. Hyperlipidemia in solid organ transplantation. Transplantation. 1997;63(3):331–338.
94. Chan MK, Varghese Z, Moorhead JF. Lipid abnormalities in uremia, dialysis, and transplantation. Kidney International. 1981;19(5):625–637.
95. Becker DM, Chamberlain B, Swank R, et al. Relationship between corticosteroid

exposure and plasma lipid levels in heart transplant recipients. American Journal of Medicine. 1988;85(5):632–638.
96. van Raalte DH, Nofrate V, Bunck MC, et al. Acute and 2-week exposure to prednisolone impair different aspects of beta-cell function in healthy men. European Journal of Endocrinology. 2010;162(4):729–735.
97. Ma KL, Ruan XZ, Powis SH, et al. Sirolimus modifies cholesterol homeostasis in hepatic cells: a potential molecular mechanism for sirolimus-associated dyslipidemia. Transplantation. 2007;84(8):1029–1036.
98. Kasiske BL, de Mattos A, Flechner SM, et al. Mammalian target of rapamycin inhibitor dyslipidemia in kidney transplant recipients. American Journal of Transplantation. 2008;8(7):1384–1392.
99. Hoogeveen RC, Ballantyne CM, Pownall HJ, et al. Effect of sirolimus on the metabolism of apoB100- containing lipoproteins in renal transplant patients. Transplantation. 2001;72(7):1244–1250.
100. Sharpe LJ, Brown AJ. Rapamycin down-regulates LDL-receptor expression independently of SREBP-2. Biochemical and Biophysical Research Communications. 2008;373(4):670–674.
101. Morrisett JD, Abdel-Fattah G, Hoogeveen R, et al. Effects of sirolimus on plasma lipids, lipoprotein levels, and fatty acid metabolism in renal transplant patients. Journal of Lipid Research. 2002;43(8):1170–1180.
102. Houde VP, Brule S, Festuccia WT, et al. Chronic rapamycin treatment causes glucose intolerance and hyperlipidemia by upregulating hepatic gluconeogenesis and impairing lipid deposition in adipose tissue. Diabetes. 2010;59(6): 1338–1348.
103. Pham PT, Pham PM, Pham SV, et al. New onset diabetes after transplantation (NODAT): an overview. Diabetes, Metabolic Syndrome and Obesity: Targets and Therapy. 2011;4:175–186.
104. Sulanc E, Lane JT, Puumala SE, et al. New-onset diabetes after kidney transplantation: an application of 2003 International Guidelines. Transplantation. 2005;80(7):945–952.
105. Teutonico A, Schena PF, Di Paolo S. Glucose metabolism in renal transplant recipients: effect of calcineurin inhibitor withdrawal and conversion to sirolimus. Journal of the American Society of Nephrology. 2005;16(10): 3128–3135.
106. Di Paolo S, Teutonico A, Leogrande D, et al. Chronic inhibition of mammalian target of rapamycin signaling downregulates insulin receptor substrates 1 and 2 and AKT activation: a crossroad between cancer and diabetes? Journal of the American Society of Nephrology. 2006;17(8):2236–2244.
107. Lewis GF, Carpentier A, Adeli K, et al. Disordered fat storage and mobilization in the pathogenesis of insulin resistance and type 2 diabetes. Endocrine Reviews. 2002;23(2):201–229.
108. Bussiere CT, Lakey JR, Shapiro AM, et al. The impact of the mTOR inhibitor sirolimus on the proliferation and function of pancreatic islets and ductal cells. Diabetologia. 2006;49(10):2341–2349.
109. Valantine H. Cardiac allograft vasculopathy after heart transplantation: risk factors and management. Journal of Heart and Lung Transplantation. 2004;23(5 Suppl):S187–S193.
110. Sanchez Lazaro IJ, Almenar Bonet L, Moro Lopez J, et al. Influence of traditional cardiovascular risk factors in the recipient on the development of cardiac allograft vasculopathy after heart transplantation. Transplantation Proceedings. 2008; 40(9):3056–3057.
111. Chamorro CI, Almenar L, Martinez-Dolz L, et al. Do cardiovascular risk factors influence cardiac allograft vasculopathy? Transplantation Proceedings. 2006;38(8):2572–2574.
112. Mehra MR, Ventura HO, Smart FW, et al. An intravascular ultrasound study of the influence of angiotensin-converting enzyme inhibitors and calcium entry blockers on the development of cardiac allograft vasculopathy. American Journal of Cardiology. 1995;75(12):853–854.
113. Schroeder JS, Gao SZ, Alderman EL, et al. A preliminary study of diltiazem in the prevention of coronary artery disease in heart-transplant recipients. New England Journal of Medicine. 1993;328(3):164–170.
114. Depczynski B, Daly B, Campbell LV, et al. Predicting the occurrence of diabetes mellitus in recipients of heart transplants. Diabetic Medicine. 2000; 17(1):15–19.
115. Mills RM, Naftel DC, Kirklin JK, et al. Heart transplant rejection with hemodynamic compromise: a multiinstitutional study of the role of endomyocardial cellular infiltrate. Cardiac Transplant Research Database. Journal of Heart and Lung Transplantation. 1997;16(8):813–821.
116. Czerny M, Sahin V, Fasching P, et al. The impact of diabetes mellitus at the time of heart transplantation on long-term survival. Diabetologia. 2002;45(11): 1498–1508.
117. Valantine H, Rickenbacker P, Kemna M, et al. Metabolic abnormalities characteristic of dysmetabolic syndrome predict the development of transplant coronary artery disease: a prospective study. Circulation. 2001;103(17):2144–2152.
118. Lang CC, Beniaminovitz A, Edwards N, et al. Morbidity and mortality in diabetic patients following cardiac transplantation. Journal of Heart and Lung Transplantation. 2003;22(3):244–249.
119. Grundy SM, Cleeman JI, Daniels SR, et al. Diagnosis and management of the metabolic syndrome: an American Heart Association/National Heart, Lung, and Blood Institute Scientific Statement. Circulation. 2005;112(17):2735–2752.
120. Mottillo S, Filion KB, Genest J, et al. The metabolic syndrome and cardiovascular risk a systematic review and meta-analysis. Journal of the American College of Cardiology. 2010;56(14):1113–1132.
121. Sanchez-Gomez JM, Martinez-Dolz L, Sanchez-Lazaro I, et al. Influence of metabolic syndrome on development of cardiac allograft vasculopathy in the transplanted heart. Transplantation. 2012;93(1):106–111.
122. Raichlin ER, McConnell JP, Lerman A, et al. Systemic inflammation and metabolic syndrome in cardiac allograft vasculopathy. Journal of Heart and Lung Transplantation. 2007;26(8):826–833.
123. Cordero DR, Goldberg Y, Basel D, et al. Prenatal sonographic diagnosis of Grebe syndrome. Journal of Ultrasound in Medicine. 2006;25(1):115–118; quiz 9–21.
124. Kobashigawa J. What is the optimal prophylaxis for treatment of cardiac allograft vasculopathy? Current Controlled Trials in Cardiovascular Medicine. 2000;1(3):166–171.
125. Labarrere CA. Relationship of fibrin deposition in microvasculature to outcomes in cardiac transplantation. Current Opinion in Cardiology. 1999;14(2):133–139.
126. Stehlik J, Edwards LB, Kucheryavaya AY, et al. The Registry of the International Society for Heart and Lung Transplantation: twenty-seventh official adult heart transplant report–2010. Journal of Heart and Lung Transplantation. 2010; 29(10):1089–1103.
127. Nagji AS, Hranjec T, Swenson BR, et al. Donor age is associated with chronic allograft vasculopathy after adult heart transplantation: implications for donor allocation. Annals of Thoracic Surgery. 2010;90(1):168–175.
128. Potena L, Holweg CT, Chin C, et al. Acute rejection and cardiac allograft vascular disease is reduced by suppression of subclinical cytomegalovirus infection. Transplantation. 2006;82(3):398–405.
129. Grattan MT, Moreno-Cabral CE, Starnes VA, et al. Cytomegalovirus infection is associated with cardiac allograft rejection and atherosclerosis. JAMA. 1989; 261(24):3561–3566.
130. Chang AC, Hruban RH, Levin HR, et al. Comparison of rejection in the atrioventricular node and bundles with the working myocardium in transplanted hearts. Journal of Heart and Lung Transplantation. 1991;10(6):915–920.
131. Cui G, Kobashigawa J, Margarian A, et al. Cause of atrioventricular block in patients after heart transplantation. Transplantation. 2003;76(1):137–142.
132. Czer L, Patel J, Kittleson M, et al. Consequences of first-year rejection after heart transplantation: is the worse yet to come? Journal of Heart and Lung Transplantation. 2012;31(4):S25.
133. Leonelli FM, Pacifico A, Young JB. Frequency and significance of conduction defects early after orthotopic heart transplantation. American Journal of Cardiology. 1994;73(2):175–179.
134. Sandhu JS, Curtiss EI, Follansbee WP, et al. The scalar electrocardiogram of the orthotopic heart transplant recipient. American Heart Journal. 1990; 119(4):917–923.
135. Leonelli FM, Dunn JK, Young JB, et al. Natural history, determinants, and clinical relevance of conduction abnormalities following orthotopic heart transplantation. American Journal of Cardiology. 1996;77(1):47–51.
136. DiBiase A, Tse TM, Schnittger I, et al. Frequency and mechanism of bradycardia in cardiac transplant recipients and need for pacemakers. American Journal of Cardiology. 1991;67(16):1385–1389.
137. Jarquin-Valdivia AA, Wijdicks EF, McGregor C. Neurologic complications following heart transplantation in the modern era: decreased incidence, but postoperative stroke remains prevalent. Transplantation Proceedings. 1999; 31(5):2161–2162.
138. van de Beek D, Kremers W, Daly RC, et al. Effect of neurologic complications on outcome after heart transplant. Archives of Neurology. 2008;65(2):226–231.
139. Andrews BT, Hershon JJ, Calanchini P, et al. Neurologic complications of cardiac transplantation. Western Journal of Medicine. 1990;153(2):146–148.
140. Weiss ES, Allen JG, Merlo CA, et al. Factors indicative of long-term survival after lung transplantation: a review of 836 10-year survivors. Journal of Heart and Lung Transplantation. 2010;29(3):240–246.
141. Christie JD, Edwards LB, Aurora P, et al. Registry of the International Society for Heart and Lung Transplantation: twenty-fifth official adult lung and heart/lung transplantation report–2008. Journal of Heart and Lung Transplantation. 2008;27(9):957–969.
142. Davidson J, Wilkinson A, Dantal J, et al. New-onset diabetes after transplantation: 2003 International consensus guidelines. Proceedings of an international expert panel meeting. Barcelona, Spain, 19 February 2003. Transplantation. 2003;75(10 Suppl):SS3–SS24.
143. Plantier L, Skhiri N, Biondi G, et al. Impact of previous cardiovascular disease on the outcome of lung transplantation. Journal of Heart and Lung Transplanta-

tion. 2010;29(11):1270–1276.
144. Vadnerkar A, Toyoda Y, Crespo M, et al. Age-specific complications among lung transplant recipients 60 years and older. Journal of Heart and Lung Transplantation. 2011;30(3):273–281.
145. Aratari MT, Venuta F, De Giacomo T, et al. Lung transplantation for cystic fibrosis: ten years of experience. Transplantation Proceedings. 2008;40(6): 2001–2002.
146. Silverborn M, Jeppsson A, Martensson G, et al. New-onset cardiovascular risk factors in lung transplant recipients. Journal of Heart and Lung Transplantation. 2005;24(10):1536–1543.
147. Rutherford RM, Fisher AJ, Hilton C, et al. Functional status and quality of life in patients surviving 10 years after lung transplantation. American Journal of Transplantation. 2005;5(5):1099–1104.
148. Morrison RJ, Short HD, Noon GP, et al. Hypertension after lung transplantation. Journal of Heart and Lung Transplantation. 1993;12(6 Pt 1):928–931.
149. Vandergheynst A, Van de Borne P, Melot C, et al. High prevalence of nocturnal arterial hypertension and non-dipping in lung transplant recipients. Acta Cardiologica. 2010;65(4):395–400.
150. Raza JA, Babb JD, Movahed A. Optimal management of hyperlipidemia in primary prevention of cardiovascular disease. International Journal of Cardiology. 2004;97(3):355–366.
151. Nash EF, Stephenson A, Helm EJ, et al. Impact of lung transplantation on serum lipids in adults with cystic fibrosis. Journal of Heart and Lung Transplantation. 2011;30(2):188–193.
152. Kesten S, Mayne L, Scavuzzo M, et al. Lack of left ventricular dysfunction associated with sustained exposure to hyperlipidemia following lung transplantation. Chest. 1997;112(4):931–936.
153. Stephany BR, Alao B, Budev M, et al. Hyperlipidemia is associated with accelerated chronic kidney disease progression after lung transplantation. American Journal of Transplantation. 2007;7(11):2553–2560.
154. Sherman W, Rabkin DG, Ross D, et al. Lung transplantation and coronary artery disease. Annals of Thoracic Surgery. 2011;92(1):303–308.
155. Benjamin EJ, Wolf PA, D'Agostino RB, et al. Impact of atrial fibrillation on the risk of death: the Framingham Heart Study. Circulation. 1998;98(10):946–952.
156. Isiadinso I, Meshkov AB, Gaughan J, et al. Atrial arrhythmias after lung and heart-lung transplant: effects on short-term mortality and the influence of amiodarone. Journal of Heart and Lung Transplantation. 2011;30(1):37–44.
157. Mason DP, Marsh DH, Alster JM, et al. Atrial fibrillation after lung transplantation: timing, risk factors, and treatment. Annals of Thoracic Surgery. 2007; 84(6):1878–1884.
158. See VY, Roberts-Thomson KC, Stevenson WG, et al. Atrial arrhythmias after lung transplantation: epidemiology, mechanisms at electrophysiology study, and outcomes. Circulation. Arrhythmia and Electrophysiology. 2009;2(5):504–510.
159. Lee G, Wu H, Kalman JM, et al. Atrial fibrillation following lung transplantation: double but not single lung transplant is associated with long-term freedom from paroxysmal atrial fibrillation. European Heart Journal. 2010;31(22):2774–2782.
160. Afshar K, Cunningham MJ, Barbers RG, et al. Pericardial constriction after lung transplantation. Annals of Thoracic Surgery. 2010;90(4):1361–1363.
161. Sever MS, Steinmuller DR, Hayes JM, et al. Pericarditis following renal transplantation. Transplantation. 1991;51(6):1229–1232.
162. Johnston SL, Halabi S, Cohoon K, et al. Stroke and myocardial infarction as late complications of lung transplantation. Journal of Heart and Lung Transplantation. 2007;26(10):1065–1068.
163. Melby SJ, Larue SJ, Lasala JM, et al. Anatomic distortion of the right coronary artery as a complication of lung transplantation. Annals of Thoracic Surgery. 2010;89(6):2000–2001.
164. Young JB, Neumayer HH, Gordon RD. Pretransplant cardiovascular evaluation and posttransplant cardiovascular risk. Kidney International. 2010;118 (Suppl): S1–S7.
165. Culleton BF, Wilson PW. Cardiovascular disease: risk factors, secular trends, and therapeutic guidelines. Journal of the American Society of Nephrology. 1998;9(12 Suppl):S5–S15.
166. Sarnak MJ. Cardiovascular complications in chronic kidney disease. American Journal of Kidney Diseases. 2003;41(5 Suppl):11–17.
167. Pilmore H, Dent H, Chang S, et al. Reduction in cardiovascular death after kidney transplantation. Transplantation. 2010;89(7):851–857.
168. Gill JS. Cardiovascular disease in transplant recipients: current and future treatment strategies. Clinical Journal of the American Society of Nephrology. 2008;3(Suppl 2):S29–S37.
169. Rigatto C, Parfrey P, Foley R, et al. Congestive heart failure in renal transplant recipients: risk factors, outcomes, and relationship with ischemic heart disease. Journal of the American Society of Nephrology. 2002;13(4):1084–1090.
170. Lentine KL, Xiao H, Brennan DC, et al. The impact of kidney transplantation on heart failure risk varies with candidate body mass index. American Heart Journal. 2009;158(6):972–982.
171. Rigatto C, Foley R, Jeffery J, et al. Electrocardiographic left ventricular hypertrophy in renal transplant recipients: prognostic value and impact of blood pressure and anemia. Journal of the American Society of Nephrology. 2003;14(2):462–468.
172. Kalantar-Zadeh K, Regidor DL, Kovesdy CP, et al. Fluid retention is associated with cardiovascular mortality in patients undergoing long-term hemodialysis. Circulation. 2009;119(5):671–679.
173. Patel RK, Oliver S, Mark PB, et al. Determinants of left ventricular mass and hypertrophy in hemodialysis patients assessed by cardiac magnetic resonance imaging. Clinical Journal of the American Society of Nephrology. 2009;4(9):1477–1483.
174. Borrows R, Loucaidou M, Chusney G, et al. Anaemia and congestive heart failure early post-renal transplantation. Nephrology, Dialysis, Transplantation. 2008; 23(5):1728–1734.
175. Wali RK, Wang GS, Gottlieb SS, et al. Effect of kidney transplantation on left ventricular systolic dysfunction and congestive heart failure in patients with end-stage renal disease. Journal of the American College of Cardiology. 2005;45(7):1051–1060.
176. Ferreira SR, Moises VA, Tavares A, et al. Cardiovascular effects of successful renal transplantation: a 1-year sequential study of left ventricular morphology and function, and 24-hour blood pressure profile. Transplantation. 2002;74(11): 1580–1587.
177. Montanaro D, Gropuzzo M, Tulissi P, et al. Effects of successful renal transplantation on left ventricular mass. Transplantation Proceedings. 2005;37(6): 2485–2487.
178. Midtvedt K, Ihlen H, Hartmann A, et al. Reduction of left ventricular mass by lisinopril and nifedipine in hypertensive renal transplant recipients: a prospective randomized double-blind study. Transplantation. 2001;72(1):107–111.
179. Patel RK, Mark PB, Johnston N, et al. Renal transplantation is not associated with regression of left ventricular hypertrophy: a magnetic resonance study. Clinical Journal of the American Society of Nephrology. 2008;3(6):1807–1811.
180. Kasiske BL, Maclean JR, Snyder JJ. Acute myocardial infarction and kidney transplantation. Journal of the American Society of Nephrology. 2006;17(3): 900–907.
181. Kasiske BL, Chakkera HA, Roel J. Explained and unexplained ischemic heart disease risk after renal transplantation. Journal of the American Society of Nephrology. 2000;11(9):1735–1743.
182. Lentine KL, Brennan DC, Schnitzler MA. Incidence and predictors of myocardial infarction after kidney transplantation. Journal of the American Society of Nephrology. 2005;16(2):496–506.
183. Aker S, Ivens K, Grabensee B, et al. Cardiovascular risk factors and diseases after renal transplantation. International Urology and Nephrology. 1998; 30(6):777–788.
184. Vanrenterghem YF, Claes K, Montagnino G, et al. Risk factors for cardiovascular events after successful renal transplantation. Transplantation. 2008;85(2): 209–216.
185. Israni AK, Snyder JJ, Skeans MA, et al. Predicting coronary heart disease after kidney transplantation: Patient Outcomes in Renal Transplantation (PORT) Study. American Journal of Transplantation. 2010;10(2):338–353.
186. Weiner DE, Tabatabai S, Tighiouart H, et al. Cardiovascular outcomes and all-cause mortality: exploring the interaction between CKD and cardiovascular disease. American Journal of Kidney Diseases. 2006;48(3):392–401.
187. Cosia FG, Hickson LJ, Griffin MD, et al. Patient survival and cardiovascular risk after kidney transplantation: the challenge of diabetes. American Journal of Transplantation. 2008;8(3):593–599.
188. Foster BJ, Dahhou M, Zhang X, et al. Change in mortality risk over time in young kidney transplant recipients. American Journal of Transplantation. 2011; 11(11):2432–2442.
189. Matas AJ, Gillingham KJ, Humar A, et al. 2202 kidney transplant recipients with 10 years of graft function: what happens next? American Journal of Transplantation. 2008;8(11):2410–2419.
190. Winkelmayer WC, Lorenz M, Kramar R, et al. C-reactive protein and body mass index independently predict mortality in kidney transplant recipients. American Journal of Transplantation. 2004;4(7):1148–1154.
191. Winkelmayer WC, Kramar R, Sunder-Plassmann G, et al. Effects of single-nucleotide polymorphisms in MTHFR and MTRR on mortality and allograft loss in kidney transplant recipients. Kidney International. 2005;68(6): 2857–2862.
192. Bostom AG, Carpenter MA, Kusek JW, et al. Homocysteine-lowering and cardiovascular disease outcomes in kidney transplant recipients: primary results from the Folic Acid for Vascular Outcome Reduction in Transplantation trial. Circulation. 2011;123(16):1763–1770.
193. Heinze G, Kainz A, Horl WH, et al. Mortality in renal transplant recipients given erythropoietins to increase haemoglobin concentration: cohort study. BMJ (Clinical Research Edition). 2009;339:b4018.

194. Choukroun G, Kamar N, Dussol B, et al. Correction of postkidney transplant anemia reduces progression of allograft nephropathy. Journal of the American Society of Nephrology. 2012;23(2):360–368.
195. Singh AK, Szczech L, Tang KL, et al. Correction of anemia with epoetin alfa in chronic kidney disease. New England Journal of Medicine. 2006; 355(20):2085–2098.
196. Drueke TB, Locatelli F, Clyne N, et al. Normalization of hemoglobin level in patients with chronic kidney disease and anemia. New England Journal of Medicine. 2006;355(20):2071–2084.
197. Pfeffer MA, Burdmann EA, Chen CY, et al. A trial of darbepoetin alfa in type 2 diabetes and chronic kidney disease. New England Journal of Medicine. 2009;361(21):2019–2032.
198. McMurray JJ, Uno H, Jarolim P, et al. Predictors of fatal and nonfatal cardiovascular events in patients with type 2 diabetes mellitus, chronic kidney disease, and anemia: an analysis of the Trial to Reduce cardiovascular Events with Aranesp (darbepoetin-alfa) Therapy (TREAT). American Heart Journal. 2011;162(4): 748–755, e3.
199. Sarnak MJ, Levey AS, Schoolwerth AC, et al. Kidney disease as a risk factor for development of cardiovascular disease: a statement from the American Heart Association Councils on Kidney in Cardiovascular Disease, High Blood Pressure Research, Clinical Cardiology, and Epidemiology and Prevention. Hypertension. 2003;42(5):1050–1065.
200. Shastri S, Sarnak MJ. Cardiovascular disease and CKD: core curriculum 2010. American Journal of Kidney Diseases. 2010;56(2):399–417.
201. Soveri I, Holdaas H, Jardine A, et al. Renal transplant dysfunction–importance quantified in comparison with traditional risk factors for cardiovascular disease and mortality. Nephrology, Dialysis, Transplantation. 2006;21(8):2282–2289.
202. Kasiske BL, Israni AK, Snyder JJ, et al. The relationship between kidney function and long-term graft survival after kidney transplant. American Journal of Kidney Diseases. 2011;57(3):466–475.
203. Shirali AC, Bia MJ. Management of cardiovascular disease in renal transplant recipients. Clinical Journal of the American Society of Nephrology. 2008;3(2): 491–504.
204. Maiorana A, Nobili V, Calandra S, et al. Preemptive liver transplantation in a child with familial hypercholesterolemia. Pediatric Transplantation. 2011; 15(2):E25–E29.
205. Carvalho MF, Soares V. Hyperlipidemia as a risk factor of renal allograft function impairment. Clinical Transplantation. 2001;15(1):48–52.
206. Kidney Disease Outcomes Quality Initiative (K/DOQI) Group. K/DOQI clinical practice guidelines for management of dyslipidemias in patients with kidney disease. American Journal of Kidney Diseases. 2003;41(4 Suppl 3):I–IV, S1–91.
207. Chueh SC, Kahan BD. Dyslipidemia in renal transplant recipients treated with a sirolimus and cyclosporine-based immunosuppressive regimen: incidence, risk factors, progression, and prognosis. Transplantation. 2003;76(2):375–382.
208. Blum CB. Effects of sirolimus on lipids in renal allograft recipients: an analysis using the Framingham risk model. American Journal of Transplantation. 2002;2(6):551–559.
209. Holdaas H, Fellstrom B, Jardine AG, et al. Effect of fluvastatin on cardiac outcomes in renal transplant recipients: a multicentre, randomised, placebo-controlled trial. Lancet. 2003;361(9374):2024–2031.
210. Holdaas H, Fellstrom B, Cole E, et al. Long-term cardiac outcomes in renal transplant recipients receiving fluvastatin: the ALERT extension study. American Journal of Transplantation. 2005;5(12):2929–2936.
211. Baigent C, Keech A, Kearney PM, et al. Efficacy and safety of cholesterol-lowering treatment: prospective meta-analysis of data from 90,056 participants in 14 randomised trials of statins. Lancet. 2005;366(9493):1267–1278.
212. SHARP Collaborative Group. Study of Heart and Renal Protection (SHARP): randomized trial to assess the effects of lowering low-density lipoprotein cholesterol among 9,438 patients with chronic kidney disease. American Heart Journal. 2010;160(5):785–794, e10.
213. Kidney Disease: Improving Global Outcomes (KDIGO) Transplant Work Group. KDIGO clinical practice guideline for the care of kidney transplant recipients. American Journal of Transplantation. 2009;9(Suppl 3):S1–S155.
214. Nogueira J, Weir M. The unique character of cardiovascular disease in chronic kidney disease and its implications for treatment with lipid-lowering drugs. Clinical Journal of the American Society of Nephrology. 2007;2(4):766–785.
215. Zhao YY, Weir MA, Manno M, et al. New fibrate use and acute renal outcomes in elderly adults: a population-based study. Annals of Internal Medicine. 2012;156(8):560–569.
216. Sica DA, Gehr TW. 3-Hydroxy-3-methylglutaryl coenzyme A reductase inhibitors and rhabdomyolysis: considerations in the renal failure patient. Current Opinion in Nephrology and Hypertension. 2002;11(2):123–133.
217. National Cholesterol Education Program (NCEP) Expert Panel on Detection, Evaluation, and Treatment of High Blood Cholesterol in Adults (Adult Treatment Panel III). Third Report of the National Cholesterol Education Program (NCEP) Expert Panel on Detection, Evaluation, and Treatment of High Blood Cholesterol in Adults (Adult Treatment Panel III) final report. Circulation. 2002;106(25): 3143–3421.
218. Pilmore HL, Skeans MA, Snyder JJ, et al. Cardiovascular disease medications after renal transplantation: results from the Patient Outcomes in Renal Transplantation study. Transplantation. 2011;91(5):542–551.
219. Gaston RS, Kasiske BL, Fieberg AM, et al. Use of cardioprotective medications in kidney transplant recipients. American Journal of Transplantation. 2009; 9(8):1811–1815.
220. Vincenti F, Schena FP, Paraskevas S, et al. A randomized, multicenter study of steroid avoidance, early steroid withdrawal or standard steroid therapy in kidney transplant recipients. American Journal of Transplantation. 2008;8(2):307–316.
221. Pascual J, Zamora J, Galeano C, et al. Steroid avoidance or withdrawal for kidney transplant recipients. Cochrane Database of Systematic Reviews. 2009;(1): CD005632.
222. Paoletti E, Gherzi M, Amidone M, et al. Association of arterial hypertension with renal target organ damage in kidney transplant recipients: the predictive role of ambulatory blood pressure monitoring. Transplantation. 2009;87(12): 1864–1869.
223. Kasiske BL, Anjum S, Shah R, et al. Hypertension after kidney transplantation. American Journal of Kidney Diseases. 2004;43(6):1071–1081.
224. Opelz G, Dohler B. Improved long-term outcomes after renal transplantation associated with blood pressure control. American Journal of Transplantation. 2005;5(11):2725–2731.
225. Mangray M, Vella JP. Hypertension after kidney transplant. American Journal of Kidney Diseases. 2011;57(2):331–341.
226. Guidi E, Menghetti D, Milani S, et al. Hypertension may be transplanted with the kidney in humans: a long-term historical prospective follow-up of recipients grafted with kidneys coming from donors with or without hypertension in their families. Journal of the American Society of Nephrology. 1996;7(8):1131–1138.
227. Cosio FG, Henry M, Pesavento TE, et al. The relationship between donor age and cadaveric renal allograft survival is modified by the recipient's blood pressure. American Journal of Transplantation. 2003;3(3):340–347.
228. Hariharan S, McBride MA, Cherikh WS, et al. Post-transplant renal function in the first year predicts long-term kidney transplant survival. Kidney International. 2002;62(1):311–318.
229. Giral M, Foucher Y, Karam G, et al. Kidney and recipient weight incompatibility reduces long-term graft survival. Journal of the American Society of Nephrology. 2010;21(6):1022–1029.
230. Bahous SA, Stephan A, Blacher J, et al. Aortic stiffness, living donors, and renal transplantation. Hypertension. 2006;47(2):216–221.
231. Delahousse M, Chaignon M, Mesnard L, et al. Aortic stiffness of kidney transplant recipients correlates with donor age. Journal of the American Society of Nephrology. 2008;19(4):798–805.
232. First MR, Neylan JF, Rocher LL, et al. Hypertension after renal transplantation. Journal of the American Society of Nephrology. 1994;4(8 Suppl):S30–S36.
233. Margreiter R. Efficacy and safety of tacrolimus compared with ciclosporin microemulsion in renal transplantation: a randomised multicentre study. Lancet. 2002;359(9308):741–746.
234. Klein IH, Abrahams A, van Ede T, et al. Different effects of tacrolimus and cyclosporine on renal hemodynamics and blood pressure in healthy subjects. Transplantation. 2002;73(5):732–736.
235. Ligtenberg G, Hene RJ, Blankestijn PJ, et al. Cardiovascular risk factors in renal transplant patients: cyclosporin A versus tacrolimus. Journal of the American Society of Nephrology. 2001;12(2):368–373.
236. National Institutes of Health. USRDS 2011 Annual Data Report: Atlas of Chronic Kidney Disease and End-Stage Renal Disease in the United States. Bethesda, MD: National Institutes of Health, National Institute of Diabetes and Digestive and Kidney Diseases, 2011;2:255, Figure 27ii.
237. Audard V, Matignon M, Hemery F, et al. Risk factors and long-term outcome of transplant renal artery stenosis in adult recipients after treatment by percutaneous transluminal angioplasty. American Journal of Transplantation. 2006;6(1):95–99.
238. Halimi JM, Al-Najjar A, Buchler M, et al. Transplant renal artery stenosis: potential role of ischemia/reperfusion injury and long-term outcome following angioplasty. Journal of Urology. 1999;161(1):28–32.
239. Lanzman RS, Voiculescu A, Walther C, et al. ECG-gated nonenhanced 3D steady-state free precession MR angiography in assessment of transplant renal arteries: comparison with DSA. Radiology. 2009;252(3):914–921.
240. Ismaeel MM, Abdel-Hamid A. Role of high resolution contrast-enhanced magnetic resonance angiography (HR CeMRA) in management of arterial complications of the renal transplant. European Journal of Radiology. 2011;79(2):e122–e127.
241. Hagen G, Wadstrom J, Magnusson M, et al. Outcome after percutaneous trans-

luminal angioplasty of arterial stenosis in renal transplant patients. Acta Radiologica. 2009;50(3):270–275.
242. Henning BF, Kuchlbauer S, Boger CA, et al. Percutaneous transluminal angioplasty as first-line treatment of transplant renal artery stenosis. Clinical Nephrology. 2009;71(5):543–549.
243. Hadaya K, Ferrari-Lacraz S, Fumeaux D, et al. Eculizumab in acute recurrence of thrombotic microangiopathy after renal transplantation. American Journal of Transplantation. 2011;11(11):2523–2527.
244. Pham PT, Pham PC, Danovitch GM, et al. Predictors and risk factors for recurrent scleroderma renal crisis in the kidney allograft: case report and review of the literature. American Journal of Transplantation. 2005;5(10):2565–2569.
245. Forman JP, Lin J, Pascual M, et al. Significance of anticardiolipin antibodies on short and long term allograft survival and function following kidney transplantation. American Journal of Transplantation. 2004;4(11):1786–1791.
246. Dragun D, Muller DN, Brasen JH, et al. Angiotensin II type 1-receptor activating antibodies in renal-allograft rejection. New England Journal of Medicine. 2005;352(6):558–569.
247. Reinsmoen NL, Lai CH, Heidecke H, et al. Anti-angiotensin type 1 receptor antibodies associated with antibody mediated rejection in donor HLA antibody negative patients. Transplantation. 2010;90(12):1473–1477.
248. Xia Y, Kellems RE. Receptor-activating autoantibodies and disease: preeclampsia and beyond. Expert Review of Clinical Immunology. 2011;7(5):659–674.
249. Chobanian AV, Bakris GL, Black HR, et al. The Seventh Report of the Joint National Committee on Prevention, Detection, Evaluation, and Treatment of High Blood Pressure: the JNC 7 report. JAMA. 2003;289(19):2560–2572.
250. Guida B, Trio R, Laccetti R, et al. Role of dietary intervention on metabolic abnormalities and nutritional status after renal transplantation. Nephrology, Dialysis, Transplantation. 2007;22(11):3304–3310.
251. Midtvedt K, Hartmann A, Foss A, et al. Sustained improvement of renal graft function for two years in hypertensive renal transplant recipients treated with nifedipine as compared to lisinopril. Transplantation. 2001;72(11): 1787–1792.
252. Hiremath S, Fergusson D, Doucette S, et al. Renin angiotensin system blockade in kidney transplantation: a systematic review of the evidence. American Journal of Transplantation. 2007;7(10):2350–2360.
253. National Institutes of Health. USRDS 2011 Annual Data Report: Atlas of Chronic Kidney Disease and End-Stage Renal Disease in the United States. Bethesda, MD: National Institutes of Health, National Institute of Diabetes and Digestive and Kidney Diseases, 2011;2:190, Table dii.
254. National Institutes of Health. USRDS 2011 Annual Data Report: Atlas of Chronic Kidney Disease and End-Stage Renal Disease in the United States. Bethesda, MD: National Institutes of Health, National Institute of Diabetes and Digestive and Kidney Diseases, 2011;2:191, Table eii.
255. Kuo HT, Sampaio MS, Vincenti F, et al. Associations of pretransplant diabetes mellitus, new-onset diabetes after transplant, and acute rejection with transplant outcomes: an analysis of the Organ Procurement and Transplant Network/United Network for Organ Sharing (OPTN/UNOS) database. American Journal of Kidney Diseases. 2010;56(6):1127–1139.
256. National Institutes of Health. USRDS 2011 Annual Data Report: Atlas of Chronic Kidney Disease and End-Stage Renal Disease in the United States. Bethesda, MD: National Institutes of Health, National Institute of Diabetes and Digestive and Kidney Diseases, 2011;2:254.
257. Valderhaug TG, Hjelmesaeth J, Hartmann A, et al. The association of early post-transplant glucose levels with long-term mortality. Diabetologia. 2011;54(6): 1341–1349.
258. Cole EH, Johnston O, Rose CL, et al. Impact of acute rejection and new-onset diabetes on long-term transplant graft and patient survival. Clinical Journal of the American Society of Nephrology. 2008;3(3):814–821.
259. Bloom RD, Rao V, Weng F, et al. Association of hepatitis C with posttransplant diabetes in renal transplant patients on tacrolimus. Journal of the American Society of Nephrology. 2002;13(5):1374–1380.
260. de Mattos AM, Olyaei AJ, Prather JC, et al. Autosomal-dominant polycystic kidney disease as a risk factor for diabetes mellitus following renal transplantation. Kidney International. 2005;67(2):714–720.
261. Shah T, Kasravi A, Huang E, et al. Risk factors for development of new-onset diabetes mellitus after kidney transplantation. Transplantation. 2006;82(12): 1673–1676.
262. Ruderman I, Masterson R, Yates C, et al. New onset diabetes after kidney transplantation in autosomal dominant polycystic kidney disease: a retrospective cohort study. Nephrology. 2012;17(1):89–96.
263. Yates CJ, Fourlanos S, Hjelmesaeth J, et al. New-onset diabetes after kidney transplantation-changes and challenges. American Journal of Transplantation. 2012;12(4):820–828.
264. Woodle ES, First MR, Pirsch J, et al. A prospective, randomized, double-blind, placebo-controlled multicenter trial comparing early (7 day) corticosteroid cessation versus long-term, low-dose corticosteroid therapy. Annals of Surgery. 2008;248(4):564–577.
265. Maes BD, Kuypers D, Messiaen T, et al. Posttransplantation diabetes mellitus in FK-506-treated renal transplant recipients: analysis of incidence and risk factors. Transplantation. 2001;72(10):1655–1661.
266. Sharif A, Moore R, Baboolal K. Influence of lifestyle modification in renal transplant recipients with postprandial hyperglycemia. Transplantation. 2008;85(3): 353–358.
267. Nathan DM, Buse JB, Davidson MB, et al. Medical management of hyperglycaemia in type 2 diabetes mellitus: a consensus algorithm for the initiation and adjustment of therapy: a consensus statement from the American Diabetes Association and the European Association for the Study of Diabetes. Diabetologia. 2009;52(1):17–30.
268. Barbosa J, Steffes MW, Sutherland DE, et al. Effect of glycemic control on early diabetic renal lesions. A 5-year randomized controlled clinical trial of insulin-dependent diabetic kidney transplant recipients. JAMA. 1994;272(8): 600–606.
269. Sagedal S, Asberg A, Hartmann A, et al. Glipizide treatment of post-transplant diabetes does not interfere with cyclosporine pharmacokinetics in renal allograft recipients. Clinical Transplantation. 1998;12(6):553–556.
270. Larsen CP, Knechtle SJ, Adams A, et al. A new look at blockade of T-cell costimulation: a therapeutic strategy for long-term maintenance immunosuppression. American Journal of Transplantation. 2006;6(5 Pt 1):876–883.
271. Vanrenterghem Y, Bresnahan B, Campistol J, et al. Belatacept-based regimens are associated with improved cardiovascular and metabolic risk factors compared with cyclosporine in kidney transplant recipients (BENEFIT and BENEFIT-EXT studies). Transplantation. 2011;91(9):976–983.
272. Vincenti F, Larsen CP, Alberu J, et al. Three-year outcomes from BENEFIT, a randomized, active-controlled, parallel-group study in adult kidney transplant recipients. American Journal of Transplantation. 2012;12(1):210–217.
273. Vincenti F. Are calcineurin inhibitors-free regimens ready for prime time? Kidney International. 2012;82(10):1054–1060.
274. Vincenti F, Tedesco Silva H, Busque S, et al. Randomized phase 2b trial of tofacitinib (CP-690,550) in de novo kidney transplant patients: efficacy, renal function and safety at 1 year. American Journal of Transplantation. 2012;12(9):2446–2456.
275. Hoshino J. An analysis of long-term survival and renal function in simultaneous pancreas and kidney transplantation from the OPTN/UNOS registry. Clinical Transplants. 2011:17–28.
276. Wiseman AC, Gralla J. Simultaneous pancreas kidney transplant versus other kidney transplant options in patients with type 2 diabetes. Clinical Journal of the American Society of Nephrology. 2012;7(4):656–664
277. Weiss AS, Smits G, Wiseman AC. Twelve-month pancreas graft function s ignificantly influences survival following simultaneous pancreas-kidney transplantation. Clinical Journal of the American Society of Nephrology. 2009; 4(5):988–995.
278. Young BY, Gill J, Huang E, et al. Living donor kidney versus simultaneous pancreas-kidney transplant in type I diabetics: an analysis of the OPTN/UNOS database. Clinical Journal of the American Society of Nephrology. 2009; 4(4):845–852.
279. Poommipanit N, Sampaio MS, Cho Y, et al. Pancreas after living donor kidney versus simultaneous pancreas-kidney transplant: an analysis of the organ procurement transplant network/united network of organ sharing database. Transplantation. 2010;89(12):1496–1503.
280. Shipman KE, Patel CK. The effect of combined renal and pancreatic transplantation on diabetic retinopathy. Clinical Ophthalmology. 2009;3:531–535.
281. Navarro X, Sutherland DE, Kennedy WR. Long-term effects of pancreatic transplantation on diabetic neuropathy. Annals of Neurology. 1997;42(5):727–736.
282. Fioretto P, Mauer M. Effects of pancreas transplantation on the prevention and reversal of diabetic nephropathy. Contributions to Nephrology. 2011;170: 237–246.
283. Davenport C, Hamid N, O'Sullivan EP, et al. The impact of pancreas and kidney transplant on cardiovascular risk factors (analyzed by mode of immunosuppression and exocrine drainage). Clinical Transplantation. 2009;23(5):616–620.
284. Luan FL, Miles CD, Cibrik DM, et al. Impact of simultaneous pancreas and kidney transplantation on cardiovascular risk factors in patients with type 1 diabetes mellitus. Transplantation. 2007;84(4):541–544.
285. Larsen JL, Colling CW, Ratanasuwan T, et al. Pancreas transplantation improves vascular disease in patients with type 1 diabetes. Diabetes Care. 2004;27(7): 1706–1711.
286. Fiorina P, La Rocca E, Venturini M, et al. Effects of kidney-pancreas transplantation on atherosclerotic risk factors and endothelial function in patients with uremia and type 1 diabetes. Diabetes. 2001;50(3):496–501.
287. Jukema JW, Smets YF, van der Pijl JW, et al. Impact of simultaneous pancreas and kidney transplantation on progression of coronary atherosclerosis in patients

with end-stage renal failure due to type 1 diabetes. Diabetes Care. 2002;25(5): 906–911.

288. La Rocca E, Fiorina P, di Carlo V, et al. Cardiovascular outcomes after kidney-pancreas and kidney-alone transplantation. Kidney International. 2001;60(5): 1964–1971.
289. Fiorina P, La Rocca E, Astorri E, et al. Reversal of left ventricular diastolic dysfunction after kidney-pancreas transplantation in type 1 diabetic uremic patients. Diabetes Care. 2000;23(12):1804–1810.
290. Biesenbach G, Konigsrainer A, Gross C, et al. Progression of macrovascular diseases is reduced in type 1 diabetic patients after more than 5 years successful combined pancreas-kidney transplantation in comparison to kidney transplantation alone. Transplant International. 2005;18(9):1054–1060.
291. Gruessner RW, Sutherland DE, Gruessner AC. Mortality assessment for pancreas transplants. American Journal of Transplantation. 2004;4(12): 2018–2026.
292. Organ Procurement and Transplantation Network (OPTN) and Scientific Registry of Transplant Recipients (SRTR). OPTN/SRTR 2010 Annual Data Report. Rockville, MD: Department of Health and Human Services, Health Resources and Services Administration, Healthcare Systems Bureau, Division of Transplantation; 2011.
293. Coss E, Watt KD, Pedersen R, et al. Predictors of cardiovascular events after liver transplantation: a role for pretransplant serum troponin levels. Liver Transplantation. 2011;17(1):23–31.
294. Fouad TR, Abdel-Razek WM, Burak KW, et al. Prediction of cardiac complications after liver transplantation. Transplantation. 2009;87(5):763–770.
295. Johnston SD, Morris JK, Cramb R, et al. Cardiovascular morbidity and mortality after orthotopic liver transplantation. Transplantation. 2002;73(6):901–906.
296. Alqahtani SA, Fouad TR, Lee SS. Cirrhotic cardiomyopathy. Seminars in Liver Disease. 2008;28(1):59–69.
297. Kowalski HJ, Abelmann WH. The cardiac output at rest in Laennec's cirrhosis. Journal of Clinical Investigation. 1953;32(10):1025–1033.
298. Regan TJ, Levinson GE, Oldewurtel HA, et al. Ventricular function in noncardiacs with alcoholic fatty liver: role of ethanol in the production of cardiomyopathy. Journal of Clinical Investigation. 1969;48(2):397–407.
299. Gould L, Shariff M, Zahir M, et al. Cardiac hemodynamics in alcoholic patients with chronic liver disease and a presystolic gallop. Journal of Clinical Investigation. 1969;48(5):860–868.
300. Liu H, Lee SS. What happens to cirrhotic cardiomyopathy after liver transplantation? Hepatology. 2005;42(5):1203–1205.
301. Eimer MJ, Wright JM, Wang EC, et al. Frequency and significance of acute heart failure following liver transplantation. American Journal of Cardiology. 2008;101(2):242–244.
302. Sampathkumar P, Lerman A, Kim BY, et al. Post-liver transplantation myocardial dysfunction. Liver Transplantation and Surgery. 1998;4(5):399–403.
303. Torregrosa M, Aguade S, Dos L, et al. Cardiac alterations in cirrhosis: reversibility after liver transplantation. Journal of Hepatology. 2005;42(1):68–74.
304. Aggarwal S, Kang Y, Freeman JA, et al. Postreperfusion syndrome: cardiovascular collapse following hepatic reperfusion during liver transplantation. Transplantation Proceedings. 1987;19(4 Suppl 3):54–55.
305. Ramsay M. The reperfusion syndrome: have we made any progress? Liver Transplantation. 2008;14(4):412–414.
306. Nanashima A, Pillay P, Crawford M, et al. Analysis of postrevascularization syndrome after orthotopic liver transplantation: the experience of an Australian liver transplantation center. Journal of Hepato-Biliary-Pancreatic Surgery. 2001; 8(6):557–563.
307. Hilmi I, Horton CN, Planinsic RM, et al. The impact of postreperfusion syndrome on short-term patient and liver allograft outcome in patients undergoing orthotopic liver transplantation. Liver Transplantation. 2008;14(4):504–508.
308. Prager MC, Gregory GA, Ascher NL, et al. Massive venous air embolism during orthotopic liver transplantation. Anesthesiology. 1990;72(1):198–200.
309. Gologorsky E, De Wolf AM, Scott V, et al. Intracardiac thrombus formation and pulmonary thromboembolism immediately after graft reperfusion in 7 patients undergoing liver transplantation. Liver Transplantation. 2001;7(9):783–789.
310. Dec GW, Kondo N, Farrell ML, et al. Cardiovascular complications following liver transplantation. Clinical Transplantation. 1995;9(6):463–471.
311. Therapondos G, Flapan AD, Plevris JN, et al. Cardiac morbidity and mortality related to orthotopic liver transplantation. Liver Transplantation. 2004;10(12): 1441–1453.
312. Asfar S, Metrakos P, Fryer J, et al. An analysis of late deaths after liver transplantation. Transplantation. 1996;61(9):1377–1381.
313. Iwatsuki S, Starzl TE, Gordon RD, et al. Late mortality and morbidity after liver transplantation. Transplantation Proceedings. 1987;19(1 Pt 3):2373–2377.
314. Backman L, Gibbs J, Levy M, et al. Causes of late graft loss after liver transplantation. Transplantation. 1993;55(5):1078–1082.
315. Abbasoglu O, Levy MF, Brkic BB, et al. Ten years of liver transplantation: an evolving understanding of late graft loss. Transplantation. 1997;64(12): 1801–1807.
316. Kashyap R, Jain A, Reyes J, et al. Causes of death after liver transplantation in 4000 consecutive patients: 2 to 19 year follow-up. Transplantation Proceedings. 2001;33(1–2):1482–1483.
317. Pruthi J, Medkiff KA, Esrason KT, et al. Analysis of causes of death in liver transplant recipients who survived more than 3 years. Liver Transplantation. 2001;7(9):811–815.
318. Rabkin JM, de La Melena V, Orloff SL, et al. Late mortality after orthotopic liver transplantation. American Journal of Surgery. 2001;181(5):475–479.
319. Albeldawi M, Aggarwal A, Madhwal S, et al. Cumulative risk of cardiovascular events after orthotopic liver transplantation. Liver Transplantation. 2012;18(3): 370–375.
320. Watt KD, Pedersen RA, Kremers WK, et al. Evolution of causes and risk factors for mortality post-liver transplant: results of the NIDDK long-term follow-up study. American Journal of Transplantation. 2010;10(6):1420–1427.
321. Carey WD, Dumot JA, Pimentel RR, et al. The prevalence of coronary artery disease in liver transplant candidates over age 50. Transplantation. 1995;59(6): 859–864.
322. Tiukinhoy-Laing SD, Rossi JS, Bayram M, et al. Cardiac hemodynamic and coronary angiographic characteristics of patients being evaluated for liver transplantation. American Journal of Cardiology. 2006;98(2):178–181.
323. Diedrich DA, Findlay JY, Harrison BA, et al. Influence of coronary artery disease on outcomes after liver transplantation. Transplantation Proceedings. 2008;40(10):3554–3557.
324. Yoo HY, Thuluvath PJ. The effect of insulin-dependent diabetes mellitus on outcome of liver transplantation. Transplantation. 2002;74(7):1007–1012.
325. Laryea M, Watt KD, Molinari M, et al. Metabolic syndrome in liver transplant recipients: prevalence and association with major vascular events. Liver Transplantation. 2007;13(8):1109–1114.
326. Laish I, Braun M, Mor E, et al. Metabolic syndrome in liver transplant recipients: prevalence, risk factors, and association with cardiovascular events. Liver Transplantation. 2011;17(1):15–22.
327. Leithead JA, Ferguson JW, Hayes PC. Smoking-related morbidity and mortality following liver transplantation. Liver Transplantation. 2008;14(8):1159–1164.
328. Targher G, Day CP, Bonora E. Risk of cardiovascular disease in patients with nonalcoholic fatty liver disease. New England Journal of Medicine. 2010; 363(14):1341–1350.
329. Satapathy SK, Charlton MR. Posttransplant metabolic syndrome: new evidence of an epidemic and recommendations for management. Liver Transplantation. 2011;17(1):1–6.
330. Desai S, Hong JC, Saab S. Cardiovascular risk factors following orthotopic liver transplantation: predisposing factors, incidence and management. Liver International. 2010;30(7):948–957.
331. Rabkin JM, Rosen HR, Corless CL, et al. Tacrolimus is associated with a lower incidence of cardiovascular complications in liver transplant recipients. Transplantation Proceedings. 2002;34(5):1557–1558.
332. Lucey MR, Abdelmalek MF, Gagliardi R, et al. A comparison of tacrolimus and cyclosporine in liver transplantation: effects on renal function and cardiovascular risk status. American Journal of Transplantation. 2005;5(5):1111–1119.
333. Llado L, Xiol X, Figueras J, et al. Immunosuppression without steroids in liver transplantation is safe and reduces infection and metabolic complications: results from a prospective multicenter randomized study. Journal of Hepatology. 2006;44(4):710–716.
334. Stegall MD, Everson GT, Schroter G, et al. Prednisone withdrawal late after adult liver transplantation reduces diabetes, hypertension, and hypercholesterolemia without causing graft loss. Hepatology. 1997;25(1):173–177.
335. Ojo AO, Held PJ, Port FK, et al. Chronic renal failure after transplantation of a nonrenal organ. New England Journal of Medicine. 2003;349(10):931–940.
336. Guckelberger O. Long-term medical comorbidities and their management: hypertension/cardiovascular disease. Liver Transplantation. 2009;15(Suppl 2): S75–S78.
337. Stravitz RT, Carl DE. Biskobing DM. Medical management of the liver transplant recipient. Clinics in Liver Disease. 2011;15(4):821–843.
338. Textor SC, Burnett JC Jr, Romero JC, et al. Urinary endothelin and renal vasoconstriction with cyclosporine or FK506 after liver transplantation. Kidney International. 1995;47(5):1426–1433.
339. Ruggenenti P, Perico N, Mosconi L, et al. Calcium channel blockers protect transplant patients from cyclosporine-induced daily renal hypoperfusion. Kidney International. 1993;43(3):706–711.
340. Galioto A, Semplicini A, Zanus G, et al. Nifedipine versus carvedilol in the treatment of de novo arterial hypertension after liver transplantation: results of a controlled clinical trial. Liver Transplantation. 2008;14(7):1020–1028.
341. Lim KB, Schiano TD. Long-term outcome after liver transplantation. Mount Sinai Journal of Medicine, New York. 2012;79(2):169–189.

342. Guckelberger O, Byram A, Klupp J, et al. Coronary event rates in liver transplant recipients reflect the increased prevalence of cardiovascular risk-factors. Transplant International. 2005;18(8):967–974.
343. Neal DA, Tom BD, Luan J, et al. Is there disparity between risk and incidence of cardiovascular disease after liver transplant? Transplantation. 2004;77(1):93–99.
344. Roy A, Kneteman N, Lilly L, et al. Tacrolimus as intervention in the treatment of hyperlipidemia after liver transplant. Transplantation. 2006;82(4):494–500.
345. Levy G, Grazi GL, Sanjuan F, et al. 12-month follow-up analysis of a multicenter, randomized, prospective trial in de novo liver transplant recipients (LIS2T) comparing cyclosporine microemulsion (C2 monitoring) and tacrolimus. Liver Transplantation. 2006;12(10):1464–1472.
346. Sanchez Perez B, Aranda Narvaez JM, Suarez Munoz MA, et al. Adverse effects on the lipid profile of immunosuppressive regimens: tacrolimus versus cyclosporin measured using C2 levels. Transplantation Proceedings. 2009;41(3):1028–1029.
347. Martin JE, Cavanaugh TM, Trumbull L, et al. Incidence of adverse events with HMG-CoA reductase inhibitors in liver transplant patients. Clinical Transplantation. 2008;22(1):113–119.
348. Imagawa DK, Dawson S 3rd, Holt CD, et al. Hyperlipidemia after liver transplantation: natural history and treatment with the hydroxy-methylglutaryl-coenzyme A reductase inhibitor pravastatin. Transplantation. 1996;62(7):934–942.
349. Taylor PJ, Kubler PA, Lynch SV, et al. Effect of atorvastatin on cyclosporine pharmacokinetics in liver transplant recipients. Annals of Pharmacotherapy. 2004;38(2):205–208.
350. Almutairi F, Peterson TC, Molinari M, et al. Safety and effectiveness of ezetimibe in liver transplant recipients with hypercholesterolemia. Liver Transplantation. 2009;15(5):504–508.
351. Watt KD, Charlton MR. Metabolic syndrome and liver transplantation: a review and guide to management. Journal of Hepatology. 2010;53(1):199–206.
352. Pagadala M, Dasarathy S, Eghtesad B, et al. Posttransplant metabolic syndrome: an epidemic waiting to happen. Liver Transplantation. 2009;15(12):1662–1670.
353. Report of the expert committee on the diagnosis and classification of diabetes mellitus. Diabetes Care. 2003;26(Suppl 1):S5–S20.
354. Saab S, Shpaner A, Zhao Y, et al. Prevalence and risk factors for diabetes mellitus in moderate term survivors of liver transplantation. American Journal of Transplantation. 2006;6(8):1890–1895.
355. Saliba F, Lakehal M, Pageaux GP, et al. Risk factors for new-onset diabetes mellitus following liver transplantation and impact of hepatitis C infection: an observational multicenter study. Liver Transplantation. 2007;13(1):136–144.
356. Driscoll CJ, Cashion AK, Hathaway DK, et al. Posttransplant diabetes mellitus in liver transplant recipients. Progress in Transplantation. 2006;16(2):110–116.
357. Zein CO, Levy C, Basu A, et al. Chronic hepatitis C and type II diabetes mellitus: a prospective cross-sectional study. American Journal of Gastroenterology. 2005;100(1):48–55.
358. Delgado-Borrego A, Casson D, Schoenfeld D, et al. Hepatitis C virus is independently associated with increased insulin resistance after liver transplantation. Transplantation. 2004;77(5):703–710.
359. Shintani Y, Fujie H, Miyoshi H, et al. Hepatitis C virus infection and diabetes: direct involvement of the virus in the development of insulin resistance. Gastroenterology. 2004;126(3):840–848.
360. Masini M, Campani D, Boggi U, et al. Hepatitis C virus infection and human pancreatic beta-cell dysfunction. Diabetes Care. 2005;28(4):940–941.
361. Colle I, Van Vlierberghe H, Troisi R, et al. Transplanted liver: consequences of denervation for liver functions. Anatomical Record. Part A, Discoveries in Molecular, Cellular, and Evolutionary Biology. 2004;280(1):924–931.
362. Marchetti P. New-onset diabetes after liver transplantation: from pathogenesis to management. Liver Transplantation. 2005;11(6):612–620.
363. Dumortier J, Bernard S, Bouffard Y, et al. Conversion from tacrolimus to cyclosporine in liver transplanted patients with diabetes mellitus. Liver Transplantation. 2006;12(4):659–664.
364. Herrero JI, Quiroga J, Sangro B, et al. Conversion from calcineurin inhibitors to mycophenolate mofetil in liver transplant recipients with diabetes mellitus. Transplantation Proceedings. 2003;35(5):1877–1879.
365. Watt KD. Metabolic syndrome: is immunosuppression to blame? Liver Transplantation. 2011;17(Suppl 3):S38–S42.
366. Cassiman D, Roelants M, Vandenplas G, et al. Orlistat treatment is safe in overweight and obese liver transplant recipients: a prospective, open label trial. Transplant International. 2006;19(12):1000–1005.

第89章 器官移植后HLA抗体监测

Robert A. Bray, Howard M. Gebel

引言

能提供同种异体移植物状态信息，特别是与免疫抑制程度相关的外周生物标志物，对任何器官移植都是非常需要的，尤其是对无可替代的器官如心脏等，但目前这样的生物标志物尚不存在。尽管许多生物标志物在一定程度上已经过测试，但是供体特异性抗体(DSA)仍是目前最广泛且最有效的生物标志物。事实上，对所有移植受体进行术后DSA监控逐渐被认为是术后管理的一个重要组成部分。随着DSA监测与临床结局的关系被认可，临床医生应该意识到其存在的细微差别，并以严谨的态度去对待移植受体。本章将介绍移植术后DSA监测的现有方案。用于检测DSA和组织相容性实验室操作的专业信息已在第36章中叙述。

合理性

确定临床上排斥信息的生物标志物的原因有许多；包括亚临床排斥反应的检测、区分因过度免疫抑制导致的排斥反应，以及判断患者的免疫抑制是否可以减弱或停止。毫无疑问，移植术后出现DSA的患者，其预后肯定较缺乏DSA的患者更差。这一点适用于肾、心脏、肺移植，且可能也适用于肝移植，这将在下文中讨论[1-4]。如果要监测HLA，有必须解决的几个问题：

- 什么时候需要监控，需要怎样的频率？
- 用什么方法监测DSA能最有效提供信息？
- 当DSA存在且预测预后不良时应如何判断？反之，什么时候DSA消失提示免疫耐受状态？
- 对获得的信息应该做什么？

DSA和移植结局

肾移植

在一项纳入了1329例死亡供体肾移植受体的多中心回顾性研究中，Terasaki等报道移植后新发现HLA抗体的患者其4年移植物存活率仅为58%，而未出现HLA抗体的患者存活率为81%[5]。受体HLA阳性的移植物失功相对危险度为3.3。这项研究存在一些局限性，包括排斥分级和移植物失功原因不完整，其包含了患者在移植物功能正常时死亡，因而这些结果有待商榷。然而，这些数据支持早期的设想，即HLA DSA和移植排斥之间存在显著关联[6]，并明确了新发HLA抗体与临床的联系，尽管其平均发生率小于20%。Lee等[9]随后的研究显示术后1年新发DSA预示着更严重的预后。Li等[8]的研究也发现了类似的结果，活体供体移植HLA抗体阴性患者的5年移植物生存率为96%，而新发HLA DSA患者的5年移植物生存率为69%。Lee等[9]随后更长期的研究表明，从未检测到新发DSA的肾移植患者的5年、10年和15年肾移植物存活率分别为85%、75%和56%；而检测到新发HLA DSA的患者生存率分别为65%、53%和28%。这些差异非常显著。Lachmann等[1]同样证明，即使新发DSA较晚出现，即移植后超过5年，也会减少长期移植物存活率(DSA阳性49%对DSA阴性83%；$P<0.0001$)。一些独立研究对DSA进行了补充，Lachmann等的数据也表明联合DSA和移植物功能，如GFR测定，可以更好地辨认长期移植物存活率降低的患者。虽然DSA自身与长期生存率降低相关，但显著性仍不如DSA与GFR降低的联合。有趣的是，Lachmann等同样发现，非DSA HLA抗体阳性的患者也出现了移植物存活率小幅下降。这

是一个有趣的现象,可能有多种解释。但鉴于这些患者仅在移植后单一时间点进行评估,可能出现的情况是DSA被吸附在移植物内,不能在血清中检测到,或被检测出的HLA抗体可能只是更广泛的免疫反应的一部分,即交叉反应簇。有越来越多的文献表明,在未检测出HLA DSA时,其他非DSA HLA在移植物失功中发挥重要作用[10,11]。在未来,移植后的监测方案很有可能需要纳入这一检测。

早期,Terasaki和Ozawa等[12]的研究建立了血清肌酐、HLA DSA和移植结局之间的关联。对于新发DSA阳性且血清肌酐<2.0mg/dL的患者,2年移植物存活率与无DSA的患者没有显著差异。然而,对于DSA阳性的患者,肌酐值>2.0mg/dL或>3.0mg/dL时,移植物失功率显著升高到17.9%和16.3%。

因此,Terasaki和Lachmann的数据表明单独DSA是重要的,但其重要性不及DSA和一个功能性参数的组合,如血清肌酐或GFR。这些数据还表明,并非所有的DSA都会立即造成有害的后果。众所周知,部分DSA阳性的患者仍能长期保持良好的移植肾功能。因此,我们面临的挑战应是明确为何一组DSA阳性的患者会出现早期移植物失功,而另一组患者却似乎无肾功能损伤。

为了解决其中的一些问题,调查人员还使用了其他一些参数,如C4d的沉积[13]、可溶性CD30[14]和移植肾病(TG)的程度,以补全HLA DSA的效能[15]。例如,Sis等[15]表明,73%存在TG的患者表现出移植肾抗体介导的损伤。同样,Eng等[16]报道,在61例移植后活检证实为TG的患者中,>50%的患者有Ⅰ类和(或)Ⅱ类HLA DSA的证据。在这项研究中,TG联合DSA与移植物存活率降低显著相关;但单独TG而无DSA则与移植物存活率降低没有显著联系。显然,TG和DSA之间的关系存在多种机制,并需要进一步研究。

其他研究集中在将DSA的精细特异性作为附加的生物标志物与临床进行联系。Kobayashi等[17]对586例肾移植患者进行了一系列中位时间为5.9年的随访,注意到针对HLA-DRB1抗体,至少在中高滴度时与慢性抗体介导的排斥反应(CAMR)有紧密联系。与此相反,HLA-DQB1抗体与CAMR的紧密程度则不及DRB抗体。这些有趣的数据表明,DSA反应作为免疫目标可能存在一定的重要性。例如,某些目标抗体可能不会在血管内皮细胞表达,或较其他目标的表达显著降低。因此,可能不会出现抗体的结合,或亲和力可能不足以引起显著的病理变化。Wiebe等[18]的对比研究发现,患者出现抗体介导的移植肾急性功能障碍(DSA阳性,血清肌酐迅速上升)或抗体介导的无痛性移植物功能障碍(DSA阳性,血清肌酐缓慢上升)呈现截然不同的HLA抗体分布情况,包括Ⅰ类和Ⅱ类。尽管Ⅱ类抗体(DRB和DQB)较Ⅰ类抗体更多,但后者与功能障碍的相关性似乎更明显。与Kobayashi等[17]的研究形成对比的是,Wiebe发现受影响的患者大多存在HLA-DQB1*抗体,虽然也观察到针对DRB1、DRB3、DRB4、DRB5和DPB1基因的抗体。新发DSA的存在也与HLA-DRB匹配程度下降及早期的急性排斥反应发作有关。新发DSA阳性患者与DSA阴性患者的10年生存率分别为57%和96%(P<0.0001)。有趣的是,有稳定移植肾功能的DSA阳性患者,其HLA分布较为相似,单独检测新发DSA可能是以偏概全的。

如前所述,单独DSA可能不足以预测移植物功能恶化。然而令人吃惊的是,上述几乎所有的研究都发现,移植后新发HLA DSA与移植物存活率差具有独立且显著的联系。这些数据表明,排斥的临床表现由多种病理损伤过程介导。HLA DSA显然是一个重要的组成部分,但并不一定是独立的生物标志物。未来的研究将需要把重点放在阐述临床、免疫学和(或)DSA存在时移植物功能异常的生理学因素[18,19]。

心脏移植

Smith等研究了224例心脏移植患者,并对新发DSA的患者随访了13年[20]。相比没有出现DSA阳性的移植患者,无论是一过性DSA阳性或持续性DSA阳性患者,生存率都显著降低(危险比4.351,P<0.001)。在这项研究中,研究者还考察了补体结合抗体的影响。令他们惊讶的是,DSA固定补体的能力不如单独DSA对移植的影响大。然而,尽管统计学差异不显著,但出现补体结合抗体的患者发生冠状动脉疾病的风险更大。Nath等在心脏移植患者中进行了类似的研究,新发DSA阳性与AMR和冠状动脉疾病相关[21]。除了HLA DSA,Smith等的研究还涉及MHCⅠ类相关链A(MICA)抗体。在大多数情况下,HLA DSA在MICA之前出现。单独MICA出现是否是心脏或肾移植预后不良的独立生物标志物仍存在争议[22-25]。

肺移植

肺移植患者接受 DSA 监测的重要性也已明确,尽管其不如肾或心脏移植重要性高[26]。部分原因可能在于对抗体介导的肺损伤的机制了解较少，且没有明显可依赖的组织学图像用于诊断抗体介导的同种异体移植物排斥[27,28]。相反,AMR 倾向于表现为闭塞性细支气管炎综合征(BOS),这是一种渐进的气道阻塞过程,也是肺移植术后死亡的主要原因之一。活检发现 C4d 或 C3d 的染色是肺移植中 AMR 的诊断标志物[29];然而,染色过程具有挑战性[27],且无法在所有移植中心常规开展。尽管如此,仍有研究确定移植后的 HLA DSA(伴或不伴补体沉积)是 BOS 的危险因素[26]。Girnita 等[30]早期的研究发现联合 DSA、血管 C4d 的沉积及支气管肺泡灌洗液中可溶性的 C4d 构成了肺移植受体 AMR 的诊断方案。Hachem 等[31]报道,HLA DSA 在移植后是相当普遍的。在 116 例平均随访时间为 1.67 年的肺移植患者中,65 例患者(56%)出现了新发 HLA DSA。在这项研究中，有些患者接受降低 DSA 滴度的尝试性治疗，其 BOS 的发病率与无 DSA 患者的发病率类似,并显著低于未治疗的 DSA 阳性患者。总之,这些数据表明频繁监测 DSA 并联合积极治疗可以降低 BOS 的发病率，至少在理论上能提高移植物和患者的存活率。Saini 等[32]对 42 例肺移植患者的同种异体免疫和自身免疫之间的关系进行了回顾性研究。发现 HLA DSA、自身抗体以及 BOS 之间有明显的相关性。与之前的研究类似,HLA DSA 的发生率为 42.7%。在 HLA DSA 阳性患者中，大约 30%产生了 K-α1 微管蛋白和胶原蛋白 V 的抗体。基于这些发现,作者提出 HLA DSA 的产物会造成血管损伤，导致自身抗体的产生并最终引起 BOS 的病理表现。由于 HLA DSA 先于自身抗体和 BOS 出现，采取监测并减少 HLA DSA 的策略可有效减少 BOS 的发病率。

肝脏移植

术后 DSA 在肝移植中的作用已成为一个新的且不断增长的关注点[33,34]。曾经 HLA DSA 被认为在肝移植中没有临床意义[35,36],现在却已成为极度关心的话题。移植术后 DSA 监测与 C4d 沉积的联系已被用来鉴别排斥和丙型肝炎复发。最近,两项研究表明,移植术后 DSA 的出现与 ABO 血型相同/兼容的肝脏移植预后不良有关[4,37]。Musat 等[4]研究了 43 例肝移植患者,发现 17 例(40%)移植后产生 DSA 的患者与弥散性门静脉 C4d 沉积相关。这组患者急性细胞性排斥和激素抵抗的发病率显著更高。其中 3 例患者接受了治疗性 DSA 清除疗法并挽救了移植肝功能。与肾移植中的情况相同，肝移植的 AMR 可能在接受适当的治疗后完全可逆[4,38]。因此,对于肝移植,移植后 DSA 的产生可能与不良预后显著相关。

DSA 的生物学特性

将要详细研究的 DSA 的一个方面是其内在的生物学性质是否会使移植结局更差。移植后 DSA 出现可以对肾、心脏、肺以及肝造成有害影响。一些研究已评估了移植前的同型免疫球蛋白和 DSA 结合补体的能力,以及其对移植物结局的影响。然而,迄今取得的结果是不一致的,部分研究显示其会导致排斥/移植物失功,而其他一些研究则发现其没有显著临床效果[39-42]。最近一项关于 1016 例患者的研究发现，移植后出现 C1q 阳性的 DSA 与增加抗体介导的排斥反应和移植肾失功的发病率有关。尽管 C1q 的阳性率与移植后结局相关，作为移植前的结局预测项目,C1q 提供的信息仍不够翔实。因此,对于这项特殊检查的信心可能被减弱[43,44]。然而,耐人寻味的是,要猜测 DSA 的功能特性对临床结局预测的重要性。显然,这一领域仍需要开展更多的工作。

移植术后 DSA 监测策略

在纳入移植后的监测策略之前，理解哪些患者需要移植并将这些患者进行分类是很重要的[45]。根据患者移植时的病史,术后予监测的方案存在很大的变化。图 89.1 列出了一些潜在可能遇到的不同患者人群。虽然大多数患者在移植时是低风险的(即没有 DSA),但许多中心的临床实践可能使患者在移植时转变为高风险,高风险定义为移植时存在 DSA。交叉配型阳性的患者,或者交叉配型阴性但存在 DSA 的患者术前需要进行脱敏治疗以清除 DSA。因此,移植后的 DSA 阳性患者可分为三组：

- 第 1 组:患者移植前存在 DSA,无论交叉配型阴性或阳性,均需要接受脱敏治疗。此类患者可列为“永久性”抗体。

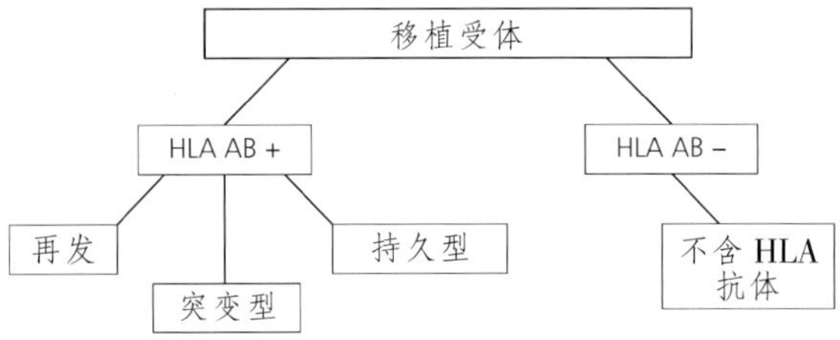

图 89.1　移植术后患者潜在的分类方案。移植术后患者可根据供体特异性(HLA Ab 阳性)或阴性抗体分类。对 HLA Ab 阳性患者,至少存在 3 种可能的亚型:再发,即患者移植时 DSA 阴性但有明显致敏病史,如移植术前怀孕;永久性,即移植时患者已经存在 DSA;新发,即 DSA 阴性且没有致敏病史的患者出现新发的 DSA。对最初归类为 DSA 阴性且移植术后未产生 DSA 抗体的患者,仍存在产生非 HLA 的 DSA 的可能性。

• 第 2 组:患者移植前已知既往有 DSA 病史,接受交叉配型阴性移植。这一组患者,移植后 DSA 的出现可能是身体的记忆反应,而非真正的新发 DSA。

• 第 3 组:患者移植前完全没有 DSA,无论是病史还是在移植时,但移植后出现了 DSA。被认为是真正的新发 DSA。

重要的是,不同组的监测策略存在显著区别。致敏和(或)DSA 阳性患者早期 AMR 的风险增加,且可能可以从移植后更早期且更频繁的监测中受益。另外,第 3 组患者术后发展为 DSA 的可能性较低,可能简单到只需单份 HLA 抗体筛查。如果筛查结果为阳性,则继续随后的监测以确认 DSA 的存在。

一旦 DSA 被确认,需要注意以下几个重要问题:

• 更频繁的 DSA 监测是否有益?

• 如果存在功能不全的迹象,治疗是否有用?

• 如果没有移植物功能障碍,是否有必要治疗?

这些问题都需要一个明确的答案。

移植时伴有 DSA 的患者

相比第 3 组,第 1 组和第 2 组的患者提出了更大的挑战,并且可能需要独特和个体化的方案[2,46,47]。对于移植时存在 DSA 的患者(1 组和 2 组),应该进行敏感性检测明确 DSA,并试图量化抗体存在的滴度,以评估移植术后 DSA 反应的程度[48]。这两个方面可能对规划移植后初期治疗方案和监测患者术后进展情况有利。DSA 的鉴别具有很大的挑战性,因大多数受体存在非供体特异性 HLA 抗原。首先,必须确保目标抗原(DSA)存在于珠板上。这种评估必须在抗原水平进行,而且越来越多的 HLA 等位基因抗体被发现[49]。如未能鉴别,则可能导致 DSA 假阳性或假阴性评估。随后,需要考虑是否存在抑制 DSA 检测的任何因素。IgM 和补体成分已被证明会干扰抗原珠上 IgG HLA 抗体对单体抗原的结合[50–52]。在测试之前除去这些干扰因素可能有利于检测。特殊的处理方案如二硫苏糖醇(DTT)、热灭活或低渗处理等,已被证明能去除干扰因素,完成 HLA 抗体检测[50–52]。最后,还必须要考虑监测的频率。对于高风险患者,移植后频繁的监测可能提示记忆效应的发生。对于低危患者,移植后最初几年监测频率应稍高,并在随后的几年里逐渐减少。重要的是,若采用抗排斥治疗,监测的频率则至关重要。一些抗排斥治疗可以干扰 HLA 抗体的监测,即使采用固相测定法。例如,高剂量静脉注射免疫球蛋白(IVIG 2g/kg)可显著干扰 HLA 抗体的检测。因此,建议注射高剂量 IVIG 与固相检测的时间间隔为 30 天左右。兔抗胸腺细胞球蛋白和其他多克隆抗体制剂,以及其他治疗药物也能干扰 HLA 抗体的检测。这些试剂包含大量不同特异性的抗体,如抗 HLA 和抗 β2 微球蛋白抗体[53]。当滴度较高时,固相测定会受到干扰。因此,实验室明确每位患者移植时注射的药物是至关重要的。

为明确地识别 DSA,迫切需要 HLA DSA 的定量监测。不幸的是,根据最近 FDA 关于抗体介导的排斥反应的专题报道[54],目前的测定方法都不是定量检测,而且通过中值荧光强度(MFI)水平定量抗体是不可靠的。许多因素可影响抗体测定的表观量。首先,患者的 HLA 抗体表现为多克隆应答。这意味着所观察到的 HLA 特异性是许多不同的免疫球蛋白分子的总和。对于大多数患者,有多少不同的 HLA 表观位点能被单一的多克隆血清辨别,或者有多少特异性抗体存在于这份血清中,目前还不清楚。这些差异明显可以改变这一测试"检测出"的 DSA 的量。例如,某一制造商当前的Ⅰ类单体抗原,HLA 抗体检测产品的配置中,有 31 个珠子表达 Bw4 表位,但只有一个珠子表达了 HLA-B7 或 HLA-B8。如果一位患者拥有特定滴度的 Bw6 抗体,而第二位患者有同样滴度的 B7 抗体,在固相测试中观察到的谱图将是明显不同的。对于第二位患者,所有的 B7 抗体都被结合到单个珠子上。与此相反,对于 Bw6 的个体,抗体在 31 个不同珠粒之间分布。因此,每个珠测得的荧光强度将是 B7 珠测定的荧光强度的 3%。

其次,如果患者有针对多个不同的供体特异性

HLA 抗原的抗体，所有的 DSA 累积的荧光值比单个珠 DSA 的荧光值能提供更多的信息。上述仅仅是两个针对 DSA 解读及其存在的挑战的例子。这也突出了检测技术方面的重要性，以及它们如何影响抗体的数量和强度的感知。

检测 HLA DSA 的方法

第 36 章更为详细地讨论了用于检测 HLA 同种抗体的方法。当前最先进的方法是使用固相法来确定 HLA 抗体的存在，以及辨别抗体的精细特异性。与 HLA 分型的分子手段相结合，明确地证实或否定某个 DSA 存在的能力比过去任何时代都强。直接孤立特定供体的 HLA 作为检测目标[55-58]来个体化地评估 DSA 的方法已经在研发中，其实用性也有待进一步研究。

总结

术后 HLA DSA 是一个与移植物损伤、移植物功能障碍以及加速移植物失功的重要生物标志物。虽然监测 DSA 并不能一致地预测即将到来的移植物失功，DSA 的存在显然预示着比无 DSA 的患者更差的预后。当与其他生物标志物[侵入性和(或)非侵入性]联合时，其与移植物失功的临床相关性显著增加。许多受体存在 DSA 且移植物功能并不恶化，表明一些 DSA 可能并非有害，或者并非所有的片段都被识别。其他研究描述了 DSA 的生物学活性联合其他组学评估获得的信息，可能可以提供完整的画面。最后，目前尚不能明确术后早期可发现 DSA 或其他排斥生物标志物是否能转化为有效的治疗措施。一些研究表明，移植术后减少 DSA 可能改善移植物存活[59-62]，但样本量较少且没有长期随访。但是，无论在什么情况下，移植术后 HLA DSA 的监测都是移植临床医生的一个重要工具。

（凌琪 译　凌琪 校）

参考文献

1. Lachmann N, Terasaki P, Budde K, et al. Anti-human leukocyte antigen and donor-specific antibodies detected by luminex posttransplant serve as biomarkers for chronic rejection of renal allografts. Transplantation. 2009;87:1505–1513.
2. Zeevi A, Lunz JG, Shapiro R, et al. Emerging role of donor-specific anti-human leukocyte antigen antibody determination for clinical management after solid organ transplantation. Human Immunology. 2009;70:645–650.
3. Mangi AA, Mason DP, Nowicki ER, et al. Predictors of acute rejection after lung transplantation. Annals of Thoracic Surgery. 2011;91:1754–1762.
4. Musat AI, Agni RM, Wai PY, et al. The significance of donor-specific HLA antibodies in rejection and ductoopenia development in ABO compatible liver transplantation. American Journal of Transplantation. 2011;11:500–510.
5. Terasaki PT, Ozawa M, Castro R. Four-year follow-up of a prospective trial of HLA and MICA antibodies on kidney graft survival. American Journal of Transplantation. 2007;7:408–415.
6. Terasaki PI, Cai J. Human leukocyte antigen antibodies and chronic rejection: from association to causation. Transplantation. 2008;86:377–383.
7. Lee PC, Zhu L, Teraski PI, et al. HLA-specific antibodies developed in the first year posttransplant are predictive of chronic rejection and renal graft loss. Transplantation. 2009;88:568–574.
8. Li X, Ishida H, Yamaguchi Y, et al. Poor graft outcome in recipients with de novo donor-specific anti-HLA antibodies after living related kidney transplantation. Transplant International. 2008;21:1145–1152.
9. Lee PC, Ozawa M, Hung CJ, et al. Eighteen-year follow-up of a retrospective study of HLA antibody on kidney graft survival. Transplantation Proceedings. 2009;41:121–123.
10. Dragun D. Humoral responses directed against non-human leukocyte antigens in solid-organ transplantation. Transplantation. 2008;86:1019–1025.
11. Zhang Q, Reed EF. Non-MHC antigenic targets of the humoral immune response in transplantation. Current Opinion in Immunology. 2010;22:682–688.
12. Terasaki PI, Ozawa M. Predictive value of HLA antibodies and serum creatinine in chronic rejection: results of a 2-year prospective trial. Transplantation. 2005; 80:1194–1197.
13. Scornick JC, Guerra G, Schold JD, et al. Value of post-transplant antibody tests in the evaluation of patients with renal graft dysfunction. American Journal of Transplantation. 2007;7:1808–1814.
14. Solgi G, Furst D, Mytillineos J, et al. Clinical relevance of pre and post-transplant immune markers in kidney allograft recipients: anti-HLA and MICA antibodies and serum levels of sCD30 and sMICA. Transplant Immunology. 2012;26(2–3): 81–87.
15. Sis B, Campbell PM, Mueller T, et al. Transplant glomerulopathy, late antibody-mediated rejection and the ABCD tetrad in kidney allograft biopsies for cause. American Journal of Transplantation. 2007;7:1743–152.
16. Eng HS, Bennett G, Chang SH, et al. Donor human leukocyte antigen specific antibody predicts the development and defines prognosis in transplant glomerulopathy. Human Immunology. 2011;72:386–391.
17. Kobayashi T, Maruya E, Niwa M, et al. Significant association between chronic antibody-mediated rejection and donor-specific antibodies against HLA-DRB rather than DQB in renal transplantation. Human Immunology. 2011;72:11–17.
18. Wiebe C, Gibson IW, Blydt-Hansen TD, et al. Evolution and clinical pathologic correlations of de novo donor specific HLA antibody post kidney transplant. American Journal of Transplantation. 2012;12(5):1157–1167.
19. Turgeon NA, Kirk AD, Iwakoshi NN. Differential effects of donor-specific alloantibody. Transplantation Reviews. 2009;23:25–33.
20. Smith JD, Banner NR, Mamour IM, et al. De novo donor HLA-specific antibodies after heart transplantation are an independent predictor of poor patient survival. American Journal of Transplantation. 2011;11:312–319.
21. Nath DS, Angaswamy N, Basha HI, et al. Donor-specific antibodies to human leukocyte antigens are associated with and precede antibodies to major histocompatibility complex class I-related chain A in antibody-mediated rejection and cardiac allograft vasculopathy after human cardiac transplantation. Human Immunology. 2010;71:1191–1196.
22. Kauke T, Kaczmarek I, Dick A, et al. Anti-MICA antibodies are related to adverse outcome in heart transplant recipients. Journal of Heart and Lung Transplantation. 2009;28:305–311.
23. Smith JD, Brunner VM, Jigjidsuren S, et al. Lack of effect of MICA antibodies on graft survival following heart transplantation. American Journal of Transplantation. 2009;9:1912–1919.
24. Zou Y, Stastny P, Susal C, et al. Antibodies against MICA antigens and kidney transplant rejection. New England Journal of Medicine. 2007;357:1293–1300.
25. Lemy A, Andrien M, Wissing KM, et al. Major histocompatibility complex Class I chain related antigen A antibodies: sensitizing events and impact on renal graft outcomes. Transplantation. 2010;90:168–174.
26. Reinsmoen NL, Nelson K, Zeevi A. Anti-HLA antibody analysis and crossmatching in heart and lung transplantation. Transplant Immunology. 2004;13:63–71.
27. Glanville AR. Antibody-mediated rejection in lung transplantation: myth or reality? Journal of Heart and Lung Transplantation. 2010;29:395–400.
28. Martinu T, Howell DN, Palmer SM. Acute cellular and humoral sensitization in lung transplant recipients. Seminars in Respiratory and Critical Care Medicine. 2010;31:179–188.
29. Westall GP, Snell GI, McLean C, et al. C3d and C4d deposition early after lung transplantation. Journal of Heart and Lung Transplantation. 2008;27:722–728.

30. Girnita AL, Lee TM, McCurry KR, et al. Anti-human leukocyte antigen antibodies, vascular C4d deposition and increased soluble C4d in broncho-alveolar lavage of lung allografts. Transplantation. 2008;86:342–347.
31. Hachem RR, Yusen RD, Myers BF, et al. Anti-human leukocyte antigen antibodies and preemptive antibody-directed therapy after lung transplantation. Journal of Heart and Lung Transplantation. 2010;29:973–980.
32. Saini D, Weber J, Ramachandran S, et al. Alloimmunity-induced autoimmunity as a potential mechanism in the pathogenesis of chronic rejection of human lung allografts. Journal of Heart and Lung Transplantation. 2011;30:624–631.
33. Castillo-Rama M, Castro MJ, Bernardo I, et al. Preformed antibodies detected by cytotoxic assay or multi-bead array decrease liver allograft survival: role of human leukocyte antigen compatibility. Liver Transplantation. 2008;14:554–562.
34. Goh A, Scalamogna M, De Feo T, et al. Human leukocyte antigen crossmatch testing is important for liver transplantation. Liver Transplantation. 2010;16: 308–313.
35. Colvin RB. C4d in liver allografts: a sign of antibody-mediated rejection? American Journal of Transplantation. 2006;6:447–448.
36. Michaels PJ, Fishbein MC, Colvin RB. Humoral rejection of human organ transplants. Springer Seminars in Immunopathology. 2003;25:119–140.
37. Sakashita H, Haga H, Ashihara E, et al. Significance of C4d staining in ABO-identical/compatible liver transplantation. Modern Pathology. 2007;20: 676–684.
38. Schadde E, d'Alessandro AM, Musat AI, et al. Donor-specific HLA antibody mediated humoral rejection in a liver recipient fully reversed with plasmapheresis and immunoglobulin. Clinical Transplants. 2006:479–482.
39. Honger G, Wahrman M, Amico P, et al. C4d-fixing capability of low-level donor-specific HLA antibodies is not predictive for early antibody-mediated rejection. Transplantation. 2010;89:1471–1475.
40. Chen G, Sequeria F, Tyan DB. Novel C1q assay reveals a clinically relevant subset of human leukocyte antigen antibodies independent of immunoglobulin G strength on single-antigen beads. Human Immunology. 2011;72:849–858.
41. Otten HG, Vehaar MC, Borst HPE, et al. Pretransplant donor-specific HLA class I and –II antibodies are associated with an increased risk for kidney graft failure. American Journal of Transplantation. 2012;12:1618–1623.
42. Lachmann N, Todorova K, Schulze H, Schonemann C. Systemic comparison of four cell- and Luminex-based methods for assessment of complement-activating HLA antibodies. Transplantation. 2013;95:694–700.
43. Tincam KJ, Heeger PS. Complement donor-specific antibody testing. Nature Reviews Nephrology. 2013;9:713–714.
44. Rascusen LC, Leffell MS. C1q-binding antibodies in kidney transplantation. New England Journal of Medicine. 2013;369(13):1266–1267.
45. Bray RA, Gebel HM. Strategies for human leukocyte antigen antibody detection. Current Opinion in Organ Transplantation. 2009;14:392–397.
46. Leffell MS, Zachary AA. The role of the histocompatibility laboratory in desensitization for transplantation. Current Opinion in Organ Transplantation. 2009; 14:398–402.
47. Lai CH, Cao K, Ong G, et al. Antibody testing strategies for deceased donor kidney transplantation after immunomodulatory therapy. Transplantation. 2011;92: 48–53.
48. Gloor JM, Winters JL, Comell LD, et al. Baseline donor-specific antibody levels and outcomes in positive crossmatch kidney transplantation. American Journal of Transplantation. 2010;10:582–589.
49. Gebel HM, Moussa O, Eckels DD, et al. Donor-reactive HLA antibodies in renal allograft recipients: considerations, complications and conundrums. Human Immunology. 2009;70:610–617.
50. Kosmoliaptsis V, Bradley JA, Peacok S, et al. Detection of immunoglobulin G human leukocyte antigen-specific alloantibodies in renal transplant patients using single antigen beads is compromised by the presence of immunoglobulin M human leukocyte antigen specific alloantibodies. Transplantation. 2009;87: 813–820.
51. Zachary AA, Lucas DP, Detrick B, et al. Naturally occurring interference in Luminex assays for HLA-specific antibodies: characteristics and resolution. Human Immunology. 2009;70:496–501.
52. Schnaidt M, Weinstock C, Jurisic M, et al. HLA antibody specification using single-antigen-beads: a technical solution for the prozone effect. Transplantation. 2011;92:510–515.
53. Popow I, Leitner J, Majdic O, et al. Assessment of batch-to-batch variation in polyclonal anti-thymocyte globulin preparations. Transplantation. 2012;93: 32–40.
54. Archdeacon P, Chan M, Neuland C, et al. Summary of FDA antibody-mediate rejection workshop. American Journal of Transplantation. 2011;11:896–806.
55. Billen EVA, Christiaans HML, ven den Berg-Loonen EM. Clinical relevance of Luminex donor-specific crossmatches: data from 165 renal transplants. Tissue Antigens. 2009;74:205–212.
56. Fujiwara K, Shimano K, Tanaka H, et al. Application of bead array technology to simultaneous detection of human leukocyte antigen and human platelet antigen antibodies. Vox Sanguinis. 2009;96:244–251.
57. Everly M, Reballato LM, Ozawa M, et al. Beyond histology: lowering human leukocyte antigen antibody to improve renal allograft survival in acute rejection. Transplantation. 2010;89:962–967.
58. Morrow WR, Frazier EA, Mahle WT, et al. Rapid reduction in donor-specific anti-human leukocyte antigen antibodies and reversal of antibody-mediated rejection with bortezomib in pediatric heart transplant patients. Transplantation. 2012;93(3):319–324.
59. Sebastiaan H, San Segundo D, Shankar S, et al. Peripheral blood sampling for the detection of allograft rejection: biomarker identification and validation. Transplantation. 2011;98:1–9.
60. Roedder S, Vitalone M, Kharti P, et al. Biomarker in solid organ Transplantation: establishing personalized transplantation medicine. Genome Medicine. 2011;3: 37–49.
61. Bestard O, Cruzado JM, Franquesa M, et al. Biomarkers in renal transplantation. Current Opinion in Organ Transplantation. 2010;15:467–473.
62. Nickerson P. Post-transplant monitoring of renal allografts: are we there yet? Current Opinion in Immunology. 2009;21:563–568.

第 90 章 器官移植后的生物标志物和同种免疫监测

Oriol Bestard, Birgit Sawitzki, Alberto Sánchez-Fueyo

引言

感染、恶性肿瘤和心血管及代谢并发症是器官移植后死亡的主要原因。这些并发症可由慢性暴露于免疫抑制剂引起。由于免疫抑制药物的治疗窗口较窄以及移植患者个体差异显著，量化免疫抑制剂对个体的影响一直是移植领域的重点。除了对这一领域的兴趣和临床相关性，临床免疫抑制的监测仍几乎完全通过药代动力学指标完成。这种方案目前仍被沿用，即使目前使用的药动学指南从未被长期临床试验所验证。另外，免疫抑制剂的药物动力学特征并不能准确地反映其生物学作用(或药效学)[1,2]，并且不能被用来评估特定受体的实际免疫抑制的需要。

受体的免疫状况和供体特异性免疫活性对移植结局有很大的影响。因此，使用免疫监测方案来评估移植受体的最佳免疫抑制水平有着直观的吸引力。细胞和分子分析技术的最新进展使得许多生物标志物得以鉴定，以及评判其潜在的对免疫学和移植的价值。这些标志物的发展有望通过促进移植的个性化医疗来改善患者的治疗。此外，通过临床试验测量生物标志物可以探索临床反应的细胞和分子机制。不幸的是，在移植临床实践中，实现这些生物标志物的检测并不简单，需要面临各种科学、技术、金融和监管方面的挑战(图 90.1)。因此，尽管大量的生物标志物研究已实施并且发表了很多器官移植领域的文章，其有效性和标准化仍处于起步阶段。因此，迄今为止只有两个生物标志物的诊断测试通过了监管部门的批准，并已进入市场[3-6]。即使是这两个商业化的试验仍未能对常规临床实践产生足够的影响。显然，器官移植中基于生物标志物的诊断及个性化用药距离实现仍很远。要注意的是，供体特异性同种抗体的检测是不受控制的同种免疫的明确指标，可被认为是重要的生物标志物。这些单独在第 89 章介绍。

鉴别和评价移植相关的生物标志物

生物标志物是生物标志物工作组定义为“正常生物学过程、病理过程或对治疗干预的药理应答等情况下可客观测量并评估的指示性物质”[7]。对于移植来说，生物标志物被研发用来监控干预性治疗，以及作为诊断和预后判断的工具。可用于临床终点替代的生物标志被称为替代终点。生物标志物作为替代终点要求临床试验和(或)流行病学研究证明该生物标志物的确能准确且重复地预测临床收益[7]。在生物标志物发现的整体考虑将在这里叙述。有关本次讨论更深入的统计学和临床试验设计问题将在第 134 章介绍。

生物标志物研发过程中的第一步是确定临床问题和研究对象(图 90.1)[8-10]。需要选择的方面包括采用的技术、样品类型(血液、同种异体移植组织、尿等)以及用于对比的最适当的金标准。生物标志物的发现阶段会伴随一个或多个验证阶段。在发现阶段常会采用高通量的“组学”技术，以同时评估大量的潜在生物标志物的候选对象。在发现阶段，需要评估候选生物标志物的诊断/预后性能。检测的最低性能阈值取决于可用的金标准的性质以及检测预期的使用方案。后续对患者独立队列中验证性试验样本量的估计可以根据这些评估来确定。通常，最初的验证基于样本的回顾性研究。随后需要前瞻性验证研究，更理想的是在多中心进行验证。为确保生物标志物验证使用的患者队列能忠实代表其测试的目标人群，需要仔细辨别临床和技术的混杂因素对结果的影响。如果发现阶段采用了高通量平台，技术平台的转移还需要实现应用于更广泛临床情况的目标。

(A)研究目标的明确
- 临床应用的明确
- 靶向患者的明确
- 生物标本类型的明确
- 生物标志物鉴定技术平台
- 评估研究的可行性
- 鉴别潜在的临床混淆因素

(B)生物标本收集

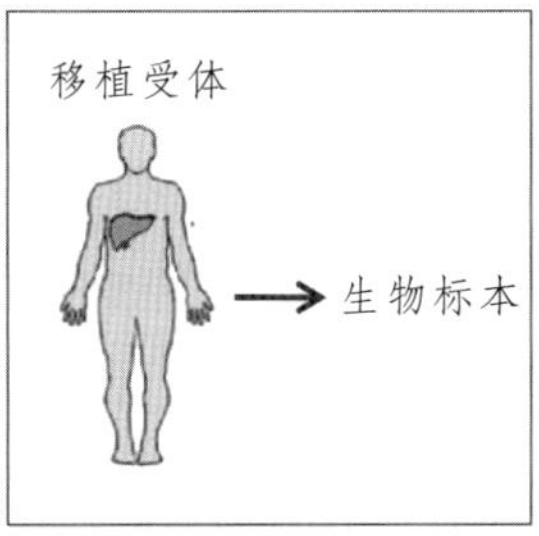

(C)生物标志物的发现
- 高通量生物标志物综合分析
- 鉴别候选生物标志物
- 诊断算法的形成
- 生物标志物诊断表现的评估
- 生物标记技术重复
- 混杂因素分析
- 估计用于临床验证的样本量

(D)生物标志物验证
- 回顾性(研究)
- 前瞻性单中心(研究)
- 前瞻性多中心(研究)
- 生物标志物的最终诊断性能评估
- 确认技术再现性/可变性

图 90.1 建立移植生物标志物的方法。第一步包括仔细确定针对的临床问题、目标人群、标本类型及检测平台和总体研究设计。关键步骤在于发现潜在的标志物并对其进行验证。

在涉及移植受体的介入临床试验中，使用如受体存活和(或)不可逆的移植物衰竭等终点事件是不切实际的。鉴于临床器官移植能取得良好的短期结果,若使用这些终点,势必会导致样本量不切实际地增加,或进行非常长的随访。因此,寻找充分替代终点在加速新疗法评价中至关重要。目前在常规临床实践中所用的主要替代终点是同种异体移植物功能障碍(如血清肌酐、肾小球滤过率、肝功能试验)或移植活检得到的病理改变。这些标志物不能预测同种异体移植组织开始破坏，故其几乎无法提供预测信息[11](图 90.2)。此外,它们并非一定与长期效果相关，且不能提供受体的整体免疫状态的信息。由于移植患者的临床复杂性,从各种不同的平台获得的不同的生物标志物的组合，可能需要体现医疗干预的整体效果。

在移植中,免疫相关的生物标志物已开始研发,以试图解决移植患者四个主要方面的情况：

- 辨别患者移植前是否对有供体特异性致敏,导致容易出现排异反应；
- 出现明显的临床损伤前检测与排斥相关的炎症改变；
- 预测免疫抑制药物剂量最小化或成功停药；
- 评估免疫抑制的净状态，以便确定可能发展成

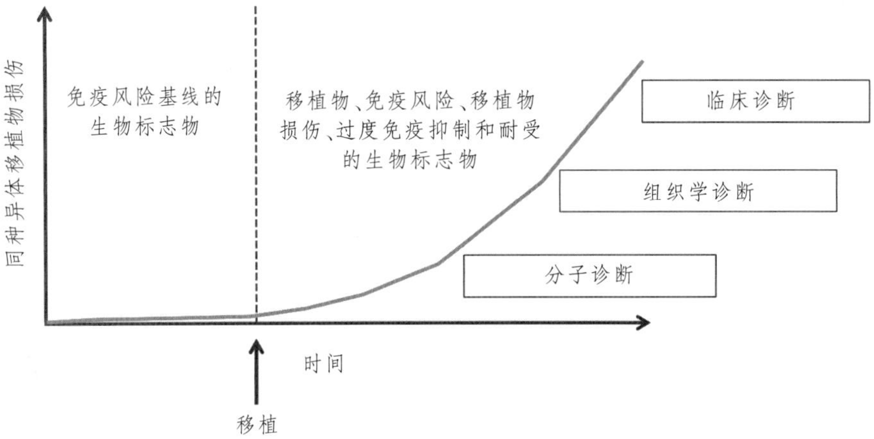

图 90.2 移植免疫监测标志物的应用。标志物在移植中的使用与时间相关。移植前强调评估基础移植免疫风险。移植术后目标在于确定移植物排斥反应和(或)移植物损伤的风险,以及尽早监测移植物损伤。此处假设移植物损伤的分子标志物先于组织学表现和临床表现出现。(Adapted from Anglicheau et al. [210] and Roedder et al. [9].)

机会性感染或恶性肿瘤的过度免疫抑制受体。

细胞同种免疫监测原则

受体对供体致敏从开始使用移植相关药物时就被认为是移植成功的一个障碍。尽管 T 细胞在同种异体移植物排斥中建立了中心作用，通过同种抗体测定装置评估体液致敏已常规在临床实践中开展。这部分内容已在第 89 章中详细介绍。同种抗体检测目前已是临床移植基本决策工具，与其相对的，目前尚没有试验能评估同种异体移植物细胞免疫效应机制。这可归因于 T 细胞亚群的异质性及其参与免疫应答的复杂性(T 细胞介导免疫的详细讨论见第 5 章)。T 细胞受体复合物通过两个不同的途径辨别供体抗原：①直接途径，供体肽与供体抗原提呈细胞(APC)表面的主要组织相容性复合体(MHC)结合，并被受体 T 细胞识别；②间接途径，即供体肽结合到受体 APC 上的 MHC，并由受体 T 细胞识别。大量的研究[12-15]已表明移植术后前几个月中，直接途径占主导地位，因其成熟的供体 APC 仍存在；而间接途径则与慢性免疫介导的移植物损伤相关[16-18]。最近一种新的途径被称为第三或半直接抗原呈递途径，在实验动物模型中被确定，表现为受体的 APC 获取供体的 MHC-肽复合物，从而直接和间接激发受体 T 细胞同种异体识别途径[19]。

通过 MHC-肽链-T 细胞受体复合物的结合以及适当的共刺激因子的共同作用，幼稚 T 细胞被激活。引起细胞内产生三磷酸腺苷(ATP)、钙内流以及蛋白质磷酸化，这些因素都被用于量化 T 细胞激活。激发的幼稚 T 细胞随后增殖，合成细胞因子，并分化为效应 T 细胞，这个过程需要数天的时间。一些效应 T 细胞最终分化为记忆性 T 细胞。与幼稚 T 细胞相反，再度激活的记忆性 T 细胞的激活阈值较低，需要更少的共刺激，并只需数小时而非数天便能产生效应细胞因子。目前已明确供体再度活化的 $CD4^+$ T 细胞通过识别供体特异性抗原在炎症中发挥重要作用。基于淋巴细胞激活微环境的细胞因子情况，幼稚 $CD4^+$ T 辅助细胞可以引起各种细胞病变和(或)出现多种免疫调节表型[20]。因此，当在富含白介素(IL)-12(通常由活化的成熟树突状细胞产生的)的微环境中激活时，$CD4^+$ T 细胞会启动一种产生组织破坏性干扰素(IFN)-γ 的 Th1 程序。与此相反，在富含 IL-4 环境中激活的 $CD4^+$ T 细胞分化为产生 IL-4 和 IL-5 的 Th2 细胞。在促炎细胞因子缺乏的环境中，肿瘤生长因子（TGF）引导 $CD4^+$ T 细胞转变为 $Foxp3^+$ 诱导的调节性 T 细胞表型。直接进行比较时，TGF-β 伴 IL-6 和（或)IL-21 表达会阻止向移植保护性调节性 T 细胞分化，而这些抗原反应性 $CD4^+$ T 细胞会向导致高度细胞病变的 IL-17 T 细胞表型分化(Th17 细胞)[20-23]。

直到最近，人们都认为抗原激活的 T 辅助细胞最终只会向 Th1 或 Th2 细胞分化，并且这些 T 细胞亚群引起 Th1 依赖性细胞病变或 Th2 依赖性细胞保护作用。Th1/Th2 这种分类模式并不正确，因为两者都可以导致移植排斥[24,25]，调节性 T 细胞而不是 Th2 细胞才是抑制细胞病变同种异体性免疫应答的关键[26-28]。最近同样发现，无论是 Th17 还是调节性 T 细胞都不是终末分化的表型，这两种细胞亚型实际上密切相关，且表现出显著的可塑性[29]。目前认为同种异体移植物在停用免疫抑制剂后的反应模式、排斥或耐受，是通过细胞病变 Th1 和 Th17 $CD4^+$ T 细胞之间的平衡决定的，这一平衡极度依赖于 T 细胞活化过程所处微环境中炎症状态的细微变化。

用于评估同种异体免疫应答的细胞学检验依赖淋巴细胞亚群和(或)总体情况，涉及 T 细胞活化事件(例如，关于活化、增殖、细胞因子的产生、细胞毒性等细胞内标志物)的测量，或移植物损伤的检测。另外，随着高通量的“多组学”技术(转录组学、蛋白质组学、代谢组学等)的出现，系统生物学方法已经开始尝试在一次检测中捕捉免疫细胞效应和同种异体移植物产生的影响。

同种异体特异性抗原检测

对比慢性免疫介导疾病，其产生免疫性抗原原因未知，在移植中获得供体组织使检测导致细胞免疫应答的同种异体特异性抗原成为可能。这些检测方法原则上应能提供对实际移植物排斥风险更准确且个性化的评估。此外，这些方法还可能需要辨别产生了移植耐受的患者。但另一方面，这些技术昂贵、劳动密集且难以标准化。经典同种异体特异性抗原的细胞学检测评估细胞增殖、细胞毒性和(或)细胞因子的产生，包括混合性白细胞反应(MLR)测定法、细胞毒性 T 淋巴细胞前体(CTLp)测定以及有限稀释分析(LDA)。虽然 MLR 测定法已被证明在移植中几乎没有预测能力[30]，CTLp

检测和 LDA 对效应 T 细胞功能的检测可以为临床提供更多可重复的信息，如同种反应性相关的增殖和细胞因子生成的检测[31-33]。然而，这些检测的应用主要局限于骨髓移植中，CTLP 发生率是良好的移植物抗宿主疾病的预测指标[34,35]。与此相反，在实体器官移植中报道的数据存在矛盾，这些检测的临床效果仍不清楚[36-38]。最近一种同种异体特异性抗原测定方法更适合于常规临床使用，即酶链免疫斑点(ELISPOT)测定法[32,36,39,40]。在该试验中，分泌细胞因子的幼稚或效应/记忆受体 T 细胞在体外受供者抗原刺激后定量，供体抗原通常是血液、脾脏或淋巴结单核细胞。如果短刺激期(<24 小时)后分析，只有记忆/效应 T 细胞能被检测到，故而能估计已致敏的抗供体 T 细胞数量。该测定法已被用于 IL-2、IFN-γ、IL-10，或产颗粒酶 B 性 T 细胞的定量。其限制是无法同时分析不同淋巴细胞亚群和(或)细胞因子，但更新的双色分析正在开发中。近期的研究致力于该技术的标准化，以提高其可靠性[41-44]。

多参数流式细胞仪具有同时分析多种细胞表型标志物的优点。此外，最近的技术改进使其也可以提供细胞内信号传导途径、细胞因子释放以及抗原特异性等信息。通过联合细胞内和细胞表面标记染色，流式细胞仪分析 T 细胞细胞因子生成已被研发作为一种替代技术用于评估供体特异性 T 细胞反应[45,46]。然而，该检测方法对产细胞因子的淋巴细胞计数比 ELISPOT 灵敏度低[39]。基于使用羧基琥珀酰亚胺酯(CFSE)标记法，流式细胞仪还可以在供体抗原刺激后用于评估 T 细胞的有丝分裂活性，但是这一方法在肾移植中预测效力较小[36]。

非同种异体特异性抗原检测

获取供体材料可能较为困难，特别是在死者捐赠时，这些方法不需提供供体材料。而且，这些技术往往容易标准化和(或)比特异性功能抗原检测更容易应用于临床。此外，通过提供免疫抑制净状态(即一般的免疫能力)的信息，它们不仅可用于预测移植物结局，也能预测过度免疫抑制造成的并发症。

流式细胞技术对循环淋巴细胞进行免疫分型已被广泛用于辨别移植相关的生物标志物。大量的流式检测结果显示，经历急性排斥的患者其激活和(或)效应记忆性 T 细胞亚群数量升高(如评估细胞表面标志物 CD45RA、CCR7、CD62L、CD69 或 CD38 等)[47-52]。这些检测的问题在于缺乏特异性，近似的细胞表面标志物活化水平可在其他炎性情况中观察到。例如，巨细胞病毒(CMV)感染的肾移植患者表明 $CD8^+$ T 细胞表面的活化标记水平升高，其与 CMV 病毒血症而不是急性排斥反应相关[40,53,54]。使用定量聚合酶链反应(qPCR)对移植器官或白细胞源性基因转录组进行量化一直是最能提供信息的非特异性抗原方法之一[55,56]。反应白细胞和(或)非免疫细胞活化的转录水平改变这一技术可用来分析免疫应答的质量和程度，所有可能的成分如外周血、移植组织和引流液等均可用于检测。

近期小型调节性 RNA 分子的发现(microRNA、miRNA)开创了一组新的、潜在的移植诊断和预后生物标志物。免疫细胞活化也可通过分析免疫细胞衍生的可溶性产物如 CD30、CXC 配体以及受体趋化因子进行评估[57-62]。这是一种分析 T 细胞群体与耐受性和(或)移植排斥相关的特殊模式的方法[63-65]。另一种非抗原特异性测量 T 细胞总体功能的方法是对植物血凝素(PHA)刺激后的全血 $CD4^+$ T 细胞内三磷酸腺苷(iATP)含量定量。此法已获得美国食品和药物管理局(FDA)认可，用于检测 ATP 含量，并可商业化提供(ImmuKnow® assay；Cylex Inc.，Columbia，MD，USA)。然而，它尚未在临床实践中被验证为有效。

基于调节性 $CD4^+$ $CD25^+$ $Foxp3^+$ T 细胞(Treg)在自身免疫疾病中的预防和(或)发展，以及在移植动物模型中的关键作用[66,67]，对这一 T 细胞亚群在血液和(或)同种移植物浸润中的量化方案获得了极大关注。不过，对比啮齿类动物，活化的人 T 细胞也可以短暂表达细胞内转录因子 Foxp3[68-70]。基于这个原因，通过流式细胞仪分析细胞表面 CD25 和细胞内 Foxp3 标记并不能精确量化人 Treg 细胞。加用 CD127 标记能部分解决这一限制，因 Treg 细胞多为激活的淋巴细胞[71,72]。然而，最可靠的识别人 Treg 细胞的方法是评估 Foxp3 基因第一内含子保守区的甲基化水平，这一区域被称为 Treg 细胞特异性去甲基化区域(TSDR)的。这种方法可以对分群的 T 细胞、全血甚至石蜡包埋的活检组织进行定量检测[73-75]。表现为慢性移植物损伤或移植耐受患者循环 Treg 细胞之间的差异，或受体接受的不同免疫抑制方案的差异越来越受到关注[76-81]。此外，有报道发现，急性同种异体移植物排斥反应的肾移植患者，尿和移植物内发现了高水平的 Foxp3 转录[56,82-85]。然而，这些观察结果及其与临床结局的关联目前仍未知。

移植前生物标志物：移植受体的基础免疫风险评估

受体血清中供体特异性 HLA 抗体的检测广泛用于辨别处于致敏状态、体液排斥反应的高危患者，并在第 89 章详细介绍。本章将集中一些新技术，实现 T 细胞致敏化和(或)活化状态的检测，并且已显示出潜在的临床意义。

IFN-γ ELISPOT 检测

Heeger 等[32,36,39,40]首次描述了在 24 小时 ELISPOT 检测中受体 T 细胞对供体细胞进行免疫应答产生的 IFN-γ，并将这一方案作为主要供体特异性免疫的一部分，且与肾移植术后急性细胞排斥的风险相关。众多团队后续的研究证实，移植前供体来源反应性 T 细胞产 IFN-γ 增加与早期肾同种异体移植物急性排斥反应之间存在相关性[43,44,86,87]。重要的是，这些研究发现相当一部分患者可在术前表现为细胞致敏，但群体反应性抗体(PRA)评分较低。即使在使用包含 CNI 类药物的强效免疫抑制移植方案的情况下，其中一些患者可出现移植后早期严重的排斥反应和移植物失功[86,87]。另一项研究表明，移植前 IFN-γ 的 ELISPOT 活性与透析治疗的累积持续时间相关[88]，提示细胞致敏程度增加会降低长期透析患者的移植物存活率。

在无法获取供体细胞时，群体反应性 T 细胞(PRT)检测被开发用来评估移植前细胞致敏水平[89,90]。PRT 检测使用最常见的 HLA 抗原刺激群体细胞，测定 IFN-γ ELISPOT 反应水平。值得注意的是，PRT 反应被证明与 PRA 评分相独立[91]。更进一步地，PRT 反应性与既往移植、HLA 错配及女性性别相关，并能够预测移植后急性排斥反应和 6 个月的肾功能情况，且相关性比 PRA 更好[91]。为了使供体刺激细胞能重复用于 ELISPOT 和 PRT 实验，Zand 等[92]描述了使用 CD40L 刺激供体的 $CD19^+$ B 细胞的方案。综上，IFN-γ ELISPOT 检测成为评估肾移植前免疫风险最有前途的测试之一。在其他器官移植中的适用性还有待探索。

可溶性 CD30

CD30 分子属于肿瘤坏死因子受体(TNF-R)的超家族。在激活的 T 细胞中，与膜结合 CD30 分子被蛋白水解而产生可溶性 CD30，进而可以在血清中被检测[93,94]。健康人往往血清 CD30 水平较低，而在一些炎症情况下 sCD30 血清浓度增加[95]。在移植中，假设sCD30 可反映移植前 T 细胞的激活状态，由此可鉴别出高免疫风险的受体[93,96]。事实上，一些研究表明，无论移植前还是移植后的 sCD30 水平都能预测急性同种异体移植物排斥的发生，且与 PRA 检测独立[57-59]。然而，Altermann 等发现潜在的肾移植受体血清sCD30 水平存在较大的个体差异。因此，对等待移植的肾病患者，sCD30 的水平随着时间的推移存在大幅度波动[95]，妨碍了其作为移植前风险分层的标记。此外，进一步的研究表明，尽管移植前低水平的 sCD30 发生急性细胞或体液排斥风险较低，这一检测方法仍无法对高危患者进行准确判断[97,98]。sCD30 作为预测性移植生物标志物的精确度被证明在诱导治疗[58,99]或经历急性病毒或细菌感染[100]患者中的效力进一步减小。

趋化因子和趋化因子受体血清水平

IFN-γ 诱导的 CXC 趋化因子配体 9(CXCL9；MIG)和 10(CXCL10；干扰素 γ 诱导蛋白-10)聚集 CXC 趋化因子受体 3(CXCR3)阳性 T 细胞至移植物。一些研究发现移植前血清 CXCL10 和 CXCL9 水平高能预测移植肾失功，以及心脏和肾同种异体移植物的早期急性排斥[60,61]。然而，这些结果与后续研究结果并不一致[62]，后续研究发现移植前 CXCL9 和 CXCL10 血清水平在接受阿仑单抗或巴利昔单抗诱导治疗的患者中预测效力并不强，可能是由于 $CXCR3^+$ T 细胞被耗竭或被灭活导致。

ImmuKnow® 检测

这一检测的目标是测定植物血凝素刺激后全血的 $CD4^+$ T 细胞 iATP 含量，以提供有关受体的一般免疫状态信息，而非具体的同种异体特异性 T 细胞的反应活性。该测定法已被用于定量肺、小肠、肝和肾移植移前及移植后的免疫状态[101]。无对照的数据用于探索感染性疾病风险与 iATP 水平之间的联系，通常异常低的 iATP 水平与不良后果之间的联系不紧密[102,103]。然而，目前尚没有前瞻性对照数据支持使用这一工具进行免疫管理。

移植后的生物标志物：急性同种异体排斥反应和慢性同种异体肾移植损伤

IFN-γ ELISPOT 检测

在肾移植中，多项研究采用 IFN-γ ELISPOT 检测血中同种异体反应性 T 细胞的数量对临床结局的影响[42-44,86,88,104-106]。Hricik 等[86]首次描述了移植后直接诱导的抗供体抗体水平和在 6 个月和 12 个月时与血清肌酐水平呈正相关的第三方反应。因其高灵敏度，IFN-γ ELISPOT 测定也被用于测量间接同种异体反应性识别途径引发的同种异体记忆/效应 T 细胞的应答。出现间接同种异体反应的肾移植患者，其肾功能比未出现的患者更差[104-106]。因此，直接诱导的记忆/效应 T 细胞在长期预后中有较高价值，至少在使用 IFN-γ ELISPOT 评估时[106]。ELISPOT 和（或）流式细胞术/胞内染色技术也被用于量化移植后抗病毒 T 细胞应答的频率。病毒特异性 T 细胞高频率针对包括 LT 和 VP1 BK 病毒（BKV）的重复肽抗原库，与 BKV 病毒复制的控制相关[107-109]。与此类似，在心肺联合移植和肾移植患者中，针对包含 CMV IE-1 蛋白的重复肽抗原库的产 IFN-γ T 细胞数量与针对巨细胞病毒病的保护、移植物功能的改善呈正相关[110,111]。

趋化因子和趋化因子受体血清水平

在肝移植中，CXCL10 血清水平与丙型肝炎病毒复发导致的肝移植早期纤维化相关[112]。此外，不同的报道都显示在肾移植术后尿 CXCL10 水平高与急性排斥、亚临床排斥反应甚至 BKV 感染增加相关[113-115]。

移植组织样品中 mRNA 和 miRNA 的表达

首次利用基因表达标记来辨别肾移植急性排斥反应的研究出现在 20 世纪 90 年代早期。T.B. Strom 的团队首次证实在急性肾移植物排斥反应发生时，组织内细胞毒性 T 淋巴细胞（CTL）转录组明显升高，如颗粒酶 B 和穿孔素[116-120]。在后续的研究中，CTL 转录物组在治疗抗抵抗、敏感的急性期排斥发作[121]以及临床和亚临床排异斥反应中均存在差异[122]。更全面的转录谱方法使用了芯片技术，揭示了排斥反应不同的免疫学和组织学亚型，以及各不相同的临床结局[123-127]。肝脏、心脏和胰腺移植中也进行了类似的研究，发现特定的 mRNA 表达印记与急性排斥反应、组织学和临床结局存在联系[128-130]。移植组织样品中 miRNA 定量也被证明可以鉴别稳定的患者和不同程度的移植物内炎症的患者[131-133]。Anglicheau 等[134]首次报道了 miRNA 表达谱可以作为预测人类移植肾状况的工具。一组 miRNA 的表达，包括 miR-142-5p、miR-155 和 miR-223，在急性排斥反应患者的活检组织中存在显著的改变[134]。其他团队的研究确定了与肾或肠道急性细胞排斥反应相关[135,136]或与肝移植治疗肝癌预后相关[137,138]的 miRNA 印记。

外周血中 mRNA 和 miRNA 的表达

为了避免移植术后有创性的免疫反监测，研究人员研究了其他成分如外周血中 mRNA 表达的诊断潜力[139]。首次采用从急性排斥和非急性排斥肾移植患者中提取外周血单核细胞的研究报道，CTL 转录组的增加如穿孔素和颗粒酶 B 也与排斥反应相关[140-142]。这些转录组情况可在临床出现明显的急性排斥反应时甚至之前检测到[140-142]。随着全血稳定剂的发展，这些检测可以更标准化的方式进行，从而识别更多的与排斥相关的转录标志物，如共刺激基因 CD154 和 ICOS[143]。在动物肾脏、心脏和肝脏移植模型中，Toag-1 的表达最初被认为是一个排斥相关生物标志物[139]；对肾移植前及移植后人全血的检测同样发现，其与移植物功能和急性/慢性排斥相关[144,145]。在心脏移植中，采用外周血单核细胞对 11 个转录组的检测已经商业化，可非侵入性地辨别可能出现中度至重度排斥反应的心脏移植患者[3,4,146]。FDA 批准的这项测试（Allomap，XDX）被设计用于减少监视性心内膜活检。但是，这项检测表现出很高的阴性预测值和非常低的阳性预测值。如下文所述，外周血 mRNA 表达的分析也用于识别“可操作”的移植耐受患者，这些患者即使停止所有的免疫抑制药物也能具有稳定的移植物功能。使用血液来检测 mRNA 因其方便性被寄予高度期望，但也可能会有技术问题。外周血单核细胞被采集后，使用 Ficoll 分离法在不同实验室间可能存在明显差异。尽管减少球蛋白 mRNA 能稳定全血 mRNA，并且严格的样品处理方案能解决这一问题，然而在转录水平发现的差异比移植物本身所发现的差异更弱[139,147]。这可能会破坏表达模型预测能力的重现。目前尚没有关于血细胞亚群的异质性[148]对移植影响的研究，这个变量也可以是变异性的来源。显然，采用“去卷积”生物信息学算法需要进一步推敲[149]。其他代替的方案包括外周血单核细胞亚群的转录分析，这个方案已经证明在自身免疫疾病诊疗中有效[150]，应该进一步开发以便于对表达谱印记进行更强效的预测。有趣的是，miRNA 在血清中很稳定，这使得血清分析 miRNA 水平很适合作为诊断性工具用于监测移植患者的免疫反应。事实上，Farid 等最近发现，肝源性 miRNA 能作为肝移植患者肝细胞损伤和排斥反应的血清标志物[151]。不过血清 miRNA 水平是否同样是其他器官移植排斥和(或)耐受性的标志物仍有待验证。

移植物引流液中 mRNA 和 miRNA 的表达

肾、肺和肝移植术后对引流液，如尿、支气管肺泡灌洗液(BAL)和胆汁的分析使得对局部免疫反应的研究成为可能。肾同种异体移植物上皮有经由尿直接与外界之间通信的优点，一些研究者通过非侵入性方法研究了尿中趋化因子和细胞因子检测急性排斥反应。鉴于活化的淋巴细胞对肾小管上皮细胞的浸润和急性排斥反应的诊断之间的基本关系，尿中的生物标志物已在概念上具有了吸引力。Suthanthiran 等首次描述了通过检测尿中穿孔素和颗粒酶 B 的信使 RNA 水平来非侵入性诊断肾同种异体移植物排斥的可能性[55]。

如上所述，为保持血清样品中的干扰素 γ 轴，CXCL9、CXCL10(IP-10)及其受体的转录和蛋白尿水平升高与短期及长期移植物功能受损相关，并且与 T 细胞介导的肾脏炎症事件(包括急性排斥反应和 BKV 肾病)相关[114,115,155,156]。许多其他团队已证实，这些标记不仅能诊断排斥反应，还能预测长期的移植物功能[56,152-154]。在肺移植中，类似的转录分析已应用在 BAL 灌洗液中。在这一背景下，Madsen 等发现在急性排斥反应中 BAL 而非血的 CTLA-4、Foxp3 及颗粒酶 B 的转录水平升高[157]。

尿 miRNA 印记也被提出可作为肾移植排斥生物标志物[158]。这种方案中，出现急性排斥反应患者的尿液中 miR-10b 和 miR-210 表达下调、miR-10a 表达上调，同时 miR-210 的表达水平能预测移植后 1 年肾小球滤过率下降的长期移植物功能[158]。

过度免疫抑制的生物标志物

移植受体需要频繁的监测免疫应答，以避免免疫抑制不足造成排斥反应，也需要避免全局性非特异性过度免疫抑制可能导致的危及生命的并发症[145]。不幸的是，目前尚无法确定免疫抑制针对个体移植受体的“适当”水平。同样，对于“过度免疫抑制”也没有达成共识，也不是通过其常见表现即机会性感染和恶性肿瘤的发生来定义[159]。反映总体适应性和(或)固有免疫能力及其移植医学相关的生物标志物的例子将在这里讨论。

评估 T 细胞的功能容量

ImmuKnow®试验作为一种标准化检测，用于衡量免疫抑制患者的淋巴细胞反应，以区分免疫不足与过度免疫[101,160,161]。在一些研究中，高 iATP 水平与急性排斥反应相关性较差[101]，而 iATP 水平非常低的患者则有出现移植后感染并发症和较高短期死亡的风险[162,163]。但是，单个时间点的 iATP 水平分析在后续的研究中显示其对机会性感染或急性排斥的预测不准确，表明试验应在纵向水平上进行顺序采样[164-168]。最近的结果表明，iATP 水平受到患者年龄和免疫抑制方案的影响，低于 12 岁的受体表现出较低的免疫应答水平[167,169-171]。最近的一项研究还表明，ImmuKnow®水平降低在肾移植后的前 6 个月是很常见的，但这种降低并不表明其与过度免疫抑制有关[172]，而在第 12 个月，其低水平则与 BKV 感染有关。总体而言，纵向分析时，ImmuKnow®检测被设想将患者分层为低危及高危人群，以指导免疫抑制的用量。然而，一些临床应用的关键问题仍然悬而未决(例如，不同的时间点、不同器官的受体理想的免疫应答是什么?HLA 不匹配、器官的种类或免疫抑制治疗的影响是什么?)。因此，对公布的数据应持谨慎态度，直至大型前瞻性研究表明基于 ImmuKnow®读数调整免疫抑制剂治疗能改善临床结果。

血清水平的补体途径因子

补体是移植相关的主要炎症介质之一[173-176]。除了经典和替代补体激活途径，甘露糖结合凝集素(MBL)的途径在移植中也起着重要作用;MBL 与受伤组织的结合会放大炎症反应。一些研究表明,移植前的MBL血浆水平能预测移植结局。Berger等发现,移植前低MBL血清水平与患者和移植物存活率增加相关[177],胰肾联合移植亦然[178]。此外,血浆MBL水平在肺移植后增加,这种情况下,持续升高MBL水平与较差的长期预后存在明显联系[179]。血浆MBL浓度同样与感染发生相关联。在肾移植中,移植后的血浆MBL缺乏(<500ng/mL)会增加CMV病的风险[180181]。与此相反,肾移植前血浆MBL水平不与CMV病相关[182,183],而高水平的MBL还能防止尿道感染及尿脓毒症,胰肾移植亦然[183]。关于BKV感染,肾移植后血浆MBL水平似乎不影响BKV病毒血症的发展[184]。总的来说,数据表明测量血浆MBL浓度可识别过度免疫抑制或者免疫抑制不足,尽管MBL水平预测临床结果根据病毒感染的类型和该标志物移植前后是否进行分析不是一成不变的。

单核细胞的HLA-DR表达

另一种评估过度免疫抑制或者免疫抑制不足的方法是评估移植患者循环单核细胞的MHCⅡ类分子HLA-DR的表达水平[185,186]。单核细胞等APC上的MHCⅡ类分子的表达是受到严格调控的。炎症介质如IFN-γ和粒细胞巨噬细胞集落刺激因子(GM-CSF)会增加MHCⅡ类分子在单核细胞的表达[187-189],而抗炎介质如IL-10、TGF-β、应激激素、免疫抑制药物如类固醇和调节性T细胞则会减少MHCⅡ类分子的水平[190-195]。因此,研究每个循环单核细胞的HLA-DR表达可以揭示个体全身炎症和抗炎介质之间的平衡。在大手术、外伤或全身性感染时,循环单核细胞发展为功能性无应答或脱敏的状态,特征为低MHCⅡ类分子表达,以及抗原提呈能力的受损[196,197]。此外,单核细胞的低HLA-DR表达与手术或外伤后感染的风险增加有关[198]。实体器官移植后,循环单核细胞持续性低HLA-DR表达预示着细菌或真菌败血症[185,198-200]。因此,单核细胞HLA-DR水平的测量是可用的,以确定严重过度免疫抑制并评估感染的风险。这在移植中可能会特别重要,目前越来越多的T细胞清除药物和记忆性T细胞的生物靶向药物正在进入临床。同样地,这个参数也可能是一个重要的安全性生物标志物,以确定临床试验中采用细胞疗法的患者的整体免疫抑制状态,例如选择性转移多克隆调节性T细胞。为确定这些安全性生物标志物的临床应用,它们需要被纳入未来的临床试验中。为了让患者分层到低危和高危人群,需要建立不同实验室或不同的流式细胞仪间标准化的流式细胞分析和在可接受范围内的差异(<30%)。这已经在商业化开发的BD Quantibrite HLA-DR/单核细胞分析中实现,它能根据所提供的标准定量检测每个单核细胞的HLA-DR分子。在多中心的临床试验中获得了非常低的变异系数(4%~25%)[201]。

移植物适应和移植耐受的生物标志物

偶尔有肝、肾移植受者可以停止所有的免疫抑制药物而不发生排斥反应。这些特定的患者能保持稳定的移植功能,没有临床显著的有害性免疫应答,这种免疫缺损通常称为"可操作的"耐受。尽管只有非常少的一部分移植受体,可操作的耐受受到越来越多的研究团队的关注。这些患者可能表现出耐受印记,用于选择免疫抑制剂剂量最小化或停药的患者。此外,与耐受分子表型相关的分子通路的明确,可能为治疗提供卓越的靶点。这些研究主要使用流式细胞免疫分型和转录组技术,集中于外周血样品的分析。另外,肝移植受体中,移植物组织的分子分析也已在进行。

在肝移植中,首次鉴定耐受生物标志物的研究采用了流式细胞免疫分型和(或)血样基因表达分析[79,80,202-204]。这些回顾性横断面研究中,耐受可操作的受体(较长时间内未使用免疫抑制剂且肝功能稳定患者)与被认为未耐受的、仍需要免疫抑制剂维持治疗的患者进行对比(尽管并非所有的患者都已尝试通过停止免疫抑制明确不存在免疫耐受)。Mazariegos等[202]量化了6个耐受受体(移植后0.8~7.9年完全停止免疫抑制)的单核状细胞(mDC)和浆细胞样(PDC)外周血树突状细胞前体的频率,并对23例受体进行了前瞻性药物降级(但在血液收集时仍有最低剂量的免疫移植),以及维持11例受体的常规免疫抑制(药物停用失败或从未尝试)。两组耐受的患者和接受最低剂量免疫抑制的患者pDC/mDC的比例较免疫抑制维持的受体或健康人的比例要显著升高。Li等[79]评估了12例耐受(移植后2~6年完整停止免疫抑制)和19例非耐受的(需免疫抑制剂维持)儿童活供体肝移植的外周血B细胞、自然杀伤(NK)细胞和一些T细胞亚群的频率。耐受受体表现为:①B细胞和$CD4^+$ $CD25^+$ T细胞数量增加;②NK细胞数量降低；以及③耐受患者的 γδ T 细胞两个主要的外周血细胞亚群(即 δ1 和 δ2)分布改变，即 δ1 T 细胞比例增加，以及 δ1/δ2 T 细胞比例升高。Martínez-Llordella 等[80]首次采用了全基因组 Affymetrix 芯片彻底分析耐受表型相关的血细胞分子模式。耐受患者的血液样本 γδ T 细胞和 NK 细胞转录组较为富集。可操作耐受及非耐受患者在循环 γδ T 细胞亚群和 $CD4^+$ $CD25^+$ $Foxp3^+$的 T 细胞亚群的分布也不同。在耐受患者中这些细胞亚群增加，即使耐受和非耐受受体之间的 $Foxp3^+$转录水平没有差异。

Martínez-Llordella 等随后扩展了他们最初的观测人群(28 例操作性耐受和 33 例非耐受受体)[203]。耐受相关的表达数据位于 NK 及 γδ T 细胞相关的转录组，与循环 NK 细胞 γδ(但不是 $CD4^+$ $CD25^+$ $Foxp3^+$)T 细胞的频率显著相关[203]。耐受及非耐受受体间显著的转录差异同样在磁性分离的外周血单核细胞(PBMC)亚群中被观察到。此外，血样本具有预测效应的三种基因表达特征(含有 2~7 个基因)被鉴定出来。

Böhne 等近期报道在肝移植受体中首个暂停免疫抑制的试验，转录生物标志物分析采用了血液和肝脏组织[147]。这项研究中，98 例肝移植患者中 75 例完成了试验，57 发生了排斥反应，41 例成功停药。随后使用全基因组微阵列和 qPCR 分析了 75 例患者的系列血液和(或)肝组织样品。Martínez-Llordella 等[203]发现 PBMC NK 相关的转录富集在入组之初就已被观测到(免疫抑制药物停止试验之前)，从而证实先前的回顾性研究的结果。与此相反，Foxp3 的转录水平或 $CD4^+$ $Foxp3^+$ T 细胞水平在耐受和非耐受患者之间无显著差异。转录的差异同样也在移植物自身被验证。然而，移植物内的基因表达谱主要为参与铁稳态基因的富集，并且未显示出与 PBMC 衍生的表达标志物之间的重叠。这些标记被认为是独立于所有其他临床参数以外的与停药成功相关联的免疫类型。与血液的结果一致，入组时耐受和不耐受患者在移植物内的表达无差异，并对 $CD4^+$ $Foxp3^+$的 T 细胞或 Foxp3 mRNA 水平进行了检测。重要的是，侧面之间的比较发现肝组织来源的转录印记比 PBMC 来源的印记在预测药物戒断方面更准确，且重复性更好[147]。

总体上，这些研究表明可耐受的肝移植患者的血液和肝组织具有独特的基因表达模式，在区分耐受和非耐受患者中有重要作用。NK 细胞和相关的转录组似乎是可耐受患者最强的血液标志，因其在免疫抑制药停止使用之前已经出现在可耐受患者的血中。由于不同免疫抑制药物的影响，$CD4^+$ $CD25^+$ $Foxp3^+$ T 细胞的作用还不太清楚。重要的是，血细胞和转录标志物似乎不反映移植物内免疫反应的性质。此外，肝组织来源的生物标志物比预测停药方案是否成功的血液相关的标志物更准确。

Brouard 等[205]首次进行了可耐受的肾移植患者的分子分析。这项研究纳入 17 例可耐受患者(2 年以上未使用免疫抑制剂且移植物功能稳定)、22 例慢性排斥患者、10 例皮质类固醇单药治疗患者、12 例稳定的标准免疫抑制治疗患者及 14 例急性排斥反应患者。定制免疫方向的 cDNA 芯片(Lymphochip)被用于分析 5 例可耐受患者、11 慢性排斥患者和 8 例年龄匹配的健康受试者的血样。一组 49 个基因的系列能够区分可耐受患者与健康受试者，并分辨慢性排斥患者。首次分析[205]发现，耐受相关的表达模式在 T 细胞相关基因和参与细胞周期调控的基因中富集，但对相同的数据集的后续再分析显示 B 细胞相关转录组明显富集[206,207]。可耐受的肾移植患者表现为循环 B 细胞频率和绝对数量增加，以及存在潜在的抑制模式[207]。

在可耐受的肾移植患者中，B 细胞循环对血基因表达存在显著的作用同样被另外两个大型多中心研究明确[208,209]。Newell 等报道了美国免疫耐受网络(ITN)多中心研究的结果，对 25 例可耐受肾移植患者(至少 1 年无免疫抑制使用且肾功能稳定)和 33 例三重免疫抑制治疗的肾功能稳定的患者进行了分析。全血 Affymetrix 芯片实验检测了其中 19 例可耐受肾移植患者、27 例免疫抑制状态下稳定的肾移植患者和 12 例健康对照患者的血样。30 个基因中有 22 个基因在耐受患者和免疫抑制患者之间的差异超过 2 倍，并且这些基因是 B 细胞特异性。这些在可耐受患者与健康对照患者之间没有观察到差异。B 细胞和可操作耐受之间的关联，可进一步由免疫抑制患者和健康个体的尿液样本 CD20 转录水平之间的比较证明。欧洲多中心研究(RISET)[209]评估了 11 例可耐受患者、11 例皮质类固醇单药治疗稳定的患者、10 例无 CNI 免疫抑制治疗的患者、30 例基于 CNI 治疗的患者、59 例慢性排斥反应患者及 19 例健康对照患者的全血样本。可耐受患者较健康对照组和其他研究组表现出更高的循环 B 细胞和 NK 细胞数量。B 细胞数量的扩大主要是由于幼稚和过渡B细胞亚群的数量增加。可耐受患者表达独特的一组基因，这组基因不由其他对照组共有且与B细胞相关通路富集有关。在这项研究中，Foxp3转录并未在耐受患者中显著上升，但综合分析计算Foxp3与MAN1A1转录的比例则能区分可耐受患者、稳定的肾移植患者和发生慢性排斥的患者。这些结果同样由ITN研究得出。

这些研究存在一些方法学的局限性。在肾移植中，上述回顾性横断面研究发现基因印记耐受特性是难以建立的。其主要的问题来源于缺乏适当的比较。事实上，没有足够的对照组能表现出正常的肾功能，尽管没有完全停止免疫抑制剂使用。缺少耐受患者的活检组织是另一个潜在的问题。首先，"微小型"的亚临床排斥反应是无法被排除的。其次，外周血标本的分析是否能用于替代移植物内发生的免疫反应目前还不清楚。肾脏耐受相关印记的稳定性和预后价值也是未知的，并且需要在长期的纵向研究中验证。在肝移植的前瞻性免疫抑制暂停试验中[147]，联合肝活检的方案部分解决了一些肾脏研究中方法学的局限性。然而，预测性基因特征来源的肝移植受体的人群仍较小。因此，这些特征的强度和稳定性在很大程度上无法得到保证，不能理所当然地利用这些特征。此外，肝移植免疫抑制剂停药的远期疗效和总体临床获益仍是未知数。

总结

人们普遍认为进行移植的患者个体存在广泛的免疫能力差异，以及他们免疫抑制的需求，无论是数量和类型方面同样存在差异。目前，尚没有前瞻性试验基于排斥风险或免疫抑制剂相关并发症情况对患者进行分层，只有一般性标志物检测与患者结局之间的关联。因此，免疫抑制剂的管理仍然针对并发症的反应而非采取强制性措施。然而，对于排斥反应总体机制的理解在过去的二十年中得到了极其显著的提升，也使当下监测工具能基于排斥反应的机制进行设计。这些因素的发展和验证将在移植的改善中发挥极其重要的作用，这些进展也无疑将是未来移植临床医生对患者诊疗护理的坚实基础。

（凌琪 译 凌琪 校）

参考文献

1. Nickerson P. Post-transplant monitoring of renal allografts: are we there yet? Current Opinion in Immunology. 2009;21(5):563–568.
2. Millan O, Urtasun N, Brunet M. Biomarkers of the immunomodulatory effect of immunosuppressive drugs in transplant recipients. Transplantation Reviews. 2009;23(2):120–128.
3. Pham MX, Teuteberg JJ, Kfoury AG, et al. Gene-expression profiling for rejection surveillance after cardiac transplantation. New England Journal of Medicine. 2010;362(20):1890–1900.
4. Deng MC, Eisen HJ, Mehra MR, et al. Noninvasive discrimination of rejection in cardiac allograft recipients using gene expression profiling. American Journal of Transplantation. 2006;6(1):150–160.
5. Ashton-Chess J, Giral M, Mengel M, et al. Tribbles-1 as a novel biomarker of chronic antibody-mediated rejection. Journal of the American Society of Nephrology. 2008;19(6):1116–1127.
6. Ashton-Chess J, Giral M, Brouard S, et al. Spontaneous operational tolerance after immunosuppressive drug withdrawal in clinical renal allotransplantation. Transplantation. 2007;84(10):1215–1219.
7. Biomarkers Definition Working Group Biomarkers and surrogate endpoints: preferred definitions and conceptual framework. Clinical Pharmacology and Therapeutics. 2001;69(3):89–95.
8. Simon R. Roadmap for developing and validating therapeutically relevant genomic classifiers. Journal of Clinical Oncology. 2005;23(29):7332–7341.
9. Roedder S, Vitalone M, Khatri P, et al. Biomarkers in solid organ transplantation: establishing personalized transplantation medicine. Genome Medicine. 2011; 3(6):37.
10. Ransohoff DF. How to improve reliability and efficiency of research about molecular markers: roles of phases, guidelines, and study design. Journal of Clinical Epidemiology. 2007;60(12):1205–1219.
11. Hartono C, Muthukumar T, Suthanthiran M. Noninvasive diagnosis of acute rejection of renal allografts. Current Opinion in Organ Transplantation. 2010; 15(1):35–41.
12. Lechler RI, Batchelor JR. Immunogenicity of retransplanted rat kidney allografts. Effect of inducing chimerism in the first recipient and quantitative studies on immunosuppression of the second recipient. Journal of Experimental Medicine. 1982;156(6):1835–1841.
13. Batchelor JR, Lechler RI. Why MHC incompatible grafts induce strong primary alloimmunity. Transplantation Proceedings. 1982;14(3):535–537.
14. Lechler RI, Batchelor JR. Restoration of immunogenicity to passenger cell-depleted kidney allografts by the addition of donor strain dendritic cells. Journal of Experimental Medicine. 1982;155(1):31–41.
15. van Besouw NM, Zuijderwijk JM, Vaessen LM, et al. The direct and indirect allogeneic presentation pathway during acute rejection after human cardiac transplantation. Clinical and Experimental Immunology. 2005;141(3):534–540.
16. Baker RJ, Hernandez-Fuentes MP, Brookes PA, et al. Loss of direct and maintenance of indirect alloresponses in renal allograft recipients: implications for the pathogenesis of chronic allograft nephropathy. Journal of Immunology. 2001;167(12):7199–7206.
17. Vella JP, Spadafora-Ferreira M, Murphy B, et al. Indirect allorecognition of major histocompatibility complex allopeptides in human renal transplant recipients with chronic graft dysfunction. Transplantation. 1997;64(6):795–800.
18. Sayegh MH, Carpenter CB. Role of indirect allorecognition in allograft rejection. International Reviews of Immunology. 1996;13(3):221–229.
19. Domenig C, Sanchez-Fueyo A, Tian Y, et al. The role of immunoregulatory networks in tolerant mixed chimeras induced by a non-myeloablative irradiation free protocol. American Journal of Transplantation. 2003;3(Suppl 5):156.
20. Strom TB, Koulmanda M. Recently discovered T cell subsets cannot keep their commitments. Journal of the American Society of Nephrology. 2009;20(8): 1677–1680.
21. Korn T, Bettelli E, Gao W, et al. IL-21 initiates an alternative pathway to induce proinflammatory T(H)17 cells. Nature. 2007;448(7152):484–487.
22. Bettelli E, Carrier Y, Gao W, et al. Reciprocal developmental pathways for the generation of pathogenic effector TH17 and regulatory T cells. Nature. 2006;441(7090):235–238.
23. Weaver CT, Hatton RD. Interplay between the TH17 and TReg cell lineages: a (co-)evolutionary perspective. Nature Reviews. Immunology. 2009;9(12):883–889.
24. Strom TB, Roy-Chaudhury P, Manfro R, et al. The Th1/Th2 paradigm and the

allograft response. Current Opinion in Immunology. 1996;8(5):688–693.
25. Li XC, Zand MS, Li Y, et al. On histocompatibility barriers, Th1 to Th2 immune deviation, and the nature of the allograft responses. Journal of Immunology. 1998;161(5):2241–2247.
26. Hall BM, Pearce NW, Gurley KE, et al. Specific unresponsiveness in rats with prolonged cardiac allograft survival after treatment with cyclosporine. III. Further characterization of the CD4+ suppressor cell and its mechanisms of action. Journal of Experimental Medicine. 1990;171(1):141–157.
27. Sakaguchi S, Sakaguchi N, Asano M, et al. Immunologic self-tolerance maintained by activated T cells expressing IL-2 receptor alpha-chains (CD25). Breakdown of a single mechanism of self-tolerance causes various autoimmune diseases. Journal of Immunology. 1995;155(3):1151–1164.
28. Waldmann H, Chen TC, Graca L, et al. Regulatory T cells in transplantation. Seminars in Immunology. 2006;18(2):111–119.
29. Mitchell P, Afzali B, Lombardi G, et al. The T helper 17-regulatory T cell axis in transplant rejection and tolerance. Current Opinion in Organ Transplantation. 2009;14(4):326–331.
30. Segall M, Noreen H, Edwins L, et al. Lack of correlation of MLC reactivity with acute graft-versus-host disease and mortality in unrelated donor bone marrow transplantation. Human Immunology. 1996;49(1):49–55.
31. Hernandez-Fuentes MP, Warrens AN, Lechler RI. Immunologic monitoring. Immunological Reviews. 2003;196:247–264.
32. van Besouw NM, Zuijderwijk JM, de Kuiper P, et al. The granzyme B and interferon-gamma enzyme-linked immunospot assay as alternatives for cytotoxic T-lymphocyte precursor frequency after renal transplantation. Transplantation. 2005;79(9):1062–1066.
33. Hernandez-Fuentes MP, Salama A. In vitro assays for immune monitoring in transplantation. Methods in Molecular Biology. 2006;333:269–290.
34. Kaminski E, Hows J, Man S, et al. Prediction of graft versus host disease by frequency analysis of cytotoxic T cells after unrelated donor bone marrow transplantation. Transplantation. 1989;48(4):608–613.
35. Spencer A, Brookes PA, Kaminski E, et al. Cytotoxic T lymphocyte precursor frequency analyses in bone marrow transplantation with volunteer unrelated donors. Value in donor selection. Transplantation. 1995;59(9):1302–1308.
36. Kreijveld E, Koenen HJ, van Cranenbroek B, et al. Immunological monitoring of renal transplant recipients to predict acute allograft rejection following the discontinuation of tacrolimus. PLoS ONE. 2008;3(7):e2711.
37. van der Mast BJ, Rischen-Vos J, de Kuiper P, et al. Calcineurin inhibitor withdrawal in stable kidney transplant patients decreases the donor-specific cytotoxic T lymphocyte precursor frequency. Transplantation. 2005;80(9): 1220–1225.
38. Steinmann J, Kaden J, May G, et al. Failure of in vitro T-cell assays to predict clinical outcome after human kidney transplantation. Journal of Clinical Laboratory Analysis. 1994;8(3):157–162.
39. Heeger PS, Greenspan NS, Kuhlenschmidt S, et al. Pretransplant frequency of donor-specific, IFN-gamma-producing lymphocytes is a manifestation of immunologic memory and correlates with the risk of posttransplant rejection episodes. Journal of Immunology. 1999;163(4):2267–2275.
40. Karpinski M, Rush D, Jeffery J, et al. Heightened peripheral blood lymphocyte CD69 expression is neither sensitive nor specific as a noninvasive diagnostic test for renal allograft rejection. Journal of the American Society of Nephrology. 2003;14(1):226–233.
41. van Besouw NM, van de Wetering J, van der Mast BJ, et al. After discontinuation of calcineurin inhibitors, tapering of mycophenolate mofetil further impairs donor-directed cytotoxicity. Clinical Transplantation. 2008;22(2):129–135.
42. Gebauer BS, Hricik DE, Atallah A, et al. Evolution of the enzyme-linked immunosorbent spot assay for post-transplant alloreactivity as a potentially useful immune monitoring tool. American Journal of Transplantation. 2002;2(9): 857–866.
43. Nather BJ, Nickel P, Bold G, et al. Modified ELISPOT technique–highly significant inverse correlation of post-Tx donor-reactive IFNgamma-producing cell frequencies with 6 and 12 months graft function in kidney transplant recipients. Transplant Immunology. 2006;16(3–4):232–237.
44. Bestard O, Stein M, Roelen R, et al. Interlab crossvalidation of IFN-γ Elispot assay for measuring alloreactive memory/effector T-cell responses in renal transplant recipients. Abstract. Transplant International. 2011;24(s3):1–67.
45. Volk HD, Kern F. Insights into the specificity and function of (allo)antigen-reactive T cells. American Journal of Transplantation. 2001;1(2):109–114.
46. Couzi L, Thiebaut R, Carron JC, et al. Immunological monitoring of calcineurin inhibitors for predicting cytomegalovirus infection in kidney transplant recipients. Transplantation. 2008;86(8):1060–1067.
47. Creemers P, Brink J, Wainwright H, et al. Evaluation of peripheral blood CD4 and CD8 lymphocyte subsets, CD69 expression and histologic rejection grade as diagnostic markers for the presence of cardiac allograft rejection. Transplant Immunology. 2002;10(4):285–292.
48. Lanio N, Sarmiento E, Gallego A, et al. The potential role of T-cell memory distribution as predisposing factor for rejection in heart transplant recipients. Transplantation Proceedings. 2009;41(6):2480–2484.
49. Posselt AM, Vincenti F, Bedolli M, et al. CD69 expression on peripheral CD8 T cells correlates with acute rejection in renal transplant recipients. Transplantation. 2003;76(1):190–195.
50. Trzonkowski P, Zilvetti M, Chapman S, et al. Homeostatic repopulation by CD28-CD8+ T cells in alemtuzumab-depleted kidney transplant recipients treated with reduced immunosuppression. American Journal of Transplantation. 2008;8(2):338–347.
51. Trzonkowski P, Zilvetti M, Friend P, et al. Recipient memory-like lymphocytes remain unresponsive to graft antigens after CAMPATH-1H induction with reduced maintenance immunosuppression. Transplantation. 2006;82(10): 1342–1351.
52. Pearl JP, Parris J, Hale DA, et al. Immunocompetent T-cells with a memory-like phenotype are the dominant cell type following antibody-mediated T-cell depletion. American Journal of Transplantation. 2005;5(3):465–474.
53. Belles-Isles M, Houde I, Lachance JG, et al. Monitoring of cytomegalovirus infections by the CD8+CD38+ T-cell subset in kidney transplant recipients. Transplantation. 1998;65(2):279–282.
54. Ticha O, Stouracova M, Kuman M, et al. Monitoring of CD38high expression in peripheral blood CD8+ lymphocytes in patients after kidney transplantation as a marker of cytomegalovirus infection. Transplant Immunology. 2010;24(1): 50–56.
55. Li B, Hartono C, Ding R, et al. Noninvasive diagnosis of renal-allograft rejection by measurement of messenger RNA for perforin and granzyme B in urine. New England Journal of Medicine. 2001;344(13):947–954.
56. Muthukumar T, Dadhania D, Ding R, et al. Messenger RNA for FOXP3 in the urine of renal-allograft recipients. New England Journal of Medicine. 2005; 353(22):2342–2351.
57. Cinti P, Pretagostini R, Arpino A, et al. Evaluation of pretransplant immunologic status in kidney-transplant recipients by panel reactive antibody and soluble CD30 determinations. Transplantation. 2005;79(9):1154–1156.
58. Pelzl S, Opelz G, Wiesel M, et al. Soluble CD30 as a predictor of kidney graft outcome. Transplantation. 2002;73(1):3–6.
59. Vaidya S, Partlow D, Barnes T, et al. Soluble CD30 concentrations in ESRD patients with and without panel reactive HLA antibodies. Clinical Transplantation. 2006;20(4):461–464.
60. Lazzeri E, Rotondi M, Mazzinghi B, et al. High CXCL10 expression in rejected kidneys and predictive role of pretransplant serum CXCL10 for acute rejection and chronic allograft nephropathy. Transplantation. 2005;79(9):1215–1220.
61. Crescioli C, Buonamano A, Scolletta S, et al. Predictive role of pretransplant serum CXCL10 for cardiac acute rejection. Transplantation. 2009;87(2): 249–255.
62. Heidt S, Shankar S, Muthusamy AS, et al. Pretransplant serum CXCL9 and CXCL10 levels fail to predict acute rejection in kidney transplant recipients receiving induction therapy. Transplantation. 2011;91(8):e59–e61.
63. Alvarez CM, Opelz G, Giraldo MC, et al. Evaluation of T-cell receptor repertoires in patients with long-term renal allograft survival. American Journal of Transplantation. 2005;5(4 Pt 1):746–756.
64. Brouard S, Dupont A, Giral M, et al. Operationally tolerant and minimally immunosuppressed kidney recipients display strongly altered blood T-cell clonal regulation. American Journal of Transplantation. 2005;5(2):330–340.
65. Miqueu P, Degauque N, Guillet M, et al. Analysis of the peripheral T-cell repertoire in kidney transplant patients. European Journal of Immunology. 2010;40(11):3280–3290.
66. Wood KJ, Sakaguchi S. Regulatory T cells in transplantation tolerance. Nature Reviews. Immunology. 2003;3(3):199–210.
67. Bennett CL, Christie J, Ramsdell F, et al. The immune dysregulation, polyendocrinopathy, enteropathy, X-linked syndrome (IPEX) is caused by mutations of FOXP3. Nature Genetics. 2001;27(1):20–21.
68. Walker MR, Kasprowicz DJ, Gersuk VH, et al. Induction of FoxP3 and acquisition of T regulatory activity by stimulated human CD4+CD25- T cells. Journal of Clinical Investigation. 2003;112(9):1437–1443.
69. Roncador G, Brown PJ, Maestre L, et al. Analysis of FOXP3 protein expression in human CD4+CD25+ regulatory T cells at the single-cell level. European Journal of Immunology. 2005;35(6):1681–1691.
70. Ziegler SF. FOXP3: not just for regulatory T cells anymore. European Journal of Immunology. 2007;37(1):21–23.
71. Seddiki N, Santner-Nanan B, Martinson J, et al. Expression of interleukin (IL)-2 and IL-7 receptors discriminates between human regulatory and activated T cells. Journal of Experimental Medicine. 2006;203(7):1693–1700.
72. Liu W, Putnam AL, Xu-Yu Z, et al. CD127 expression inversely correlates with FoxP3 and suppressive function of human CD4+ T reg cells. Journal of Experimental Medicine. 2006;203(7):1701–1711.

73. Baron U, Floess S, Wieczorek G, et al. DNA demethylation in the human FOXP3 locus discriminates regulatory T cells from activated FOXP3(+) conventional T cells. European Journal of Immunology. 2007;37(9):2378–2389.
74. Sehouli J, Loddenkemper C, Cornu T, et al. Epigenetic quantification of tumor-infiltrating T-lymphocytes. Epigenetics. 2011;6(2):236–246.
75. Bestard O, Cunetti L, Cruzado JM, et al. Intragraft regulatory T cells in protocol biopsies retain foxp3 demethylation and are protective biomarkers for kidney graft outcome. American Journal of Transplantation. 2011;11(10):2162–2172.
76. Akl A, Jones ND, Rogers N, et al. An investigation to assess the potential of CD25highCD4+ T cells to regulate responses to donor alloantigens in clinically stable renal transplant recipients. Transplant International. 2008;21(1):65–73.
77. Louis S, Braudeau C, Giral M, et al. Contrasting CD25hiCD4+T cells/FOXP3 patterns in chronic rejection and operational drug-free tolerance. Transplantation. 2006;81(3):398–407.
78. Braudeau C, Racape M, Giral M, et al. Variation in numbers of CD4+CD25highFOXP3+ T cells with normal immuno-regulatory properties in long-term graft outcome. Transplant International. 2007;20(10):845–855.
79. Li Y, Koshiba T, Yoshizawa A, et al. Analyses of peripheral blood mononuclear cells in operational tolerance after pediatric living donor liver transplantation. American Journal of Transplantation. 2004;4(12):2118–2125.
80. Martinez-Llordella M, Puig-Pey I, Orlando G, et al. Multiparameter immune profiling of operational tolerance in liver transplantation. American Journal of Transplantation. 2007;7(2):309–319.
81. van de Wetering J, Koumoutsakos P, Peeters A, et al. Discontinuation of calcineurin inhibitors treatment allows the development of FOXP3+ regulatory T-cells in patients after kidney transplantation. Clinical Transplantation. 2011;25(1):40–46.
82. Yang H, Ding R, Sharma VK, et al. Hyperexpression of Foxp3 and IDO during acute rejection of islet allografts. Transplantation. 2007;83(12):1643–1647.
83. Mansour H, Homs S, Desvaux D, et al. Intragraft levels of Foxp3 mRNA predict progression in renal transplants with borderline change. Journal of the American Society of Nephrology. 2008;19(12):2277–2281.
84. Veronese F, Rotman S, Smith RN, et al. Pathological and clinical correlates of FOXP3+ cells in renal allografts during acute rejection. American Journal of Transplantation. 2007;7(4):914–922.
85. Bunnag S, Allanach K, Jhangri GS, et al. FOXP3 expression in human kidney transplant biopsies is associated with rejection and time post transplant but not with favorable outcomes. American Journal of Transplantation. 2008;8(7):1423–1433.
86. Hricik DE, Rodriguez V, Riley J, et al. Enzyme linked immunosorbent spot (ELISPOT) assay for interferon-gamma independently predicts renal function in kidney transplant recipients. American Journal of Transplantation. 2003;3(7): 878–884.
87. Nickel P, Presber F, Bold G, et al. Enzyme-linked immunosorbent spot assay for donor-reactive interferon-gamma-producing cells identifies T-cell presensitization and correlates with graft function at 6 and 12 months in renal-transplant recipients. Transplantation. 2004;78(11):1640–1646.
88. Augustine JJ, Poggio ED, Clemente M, et al. Hemodialysis vintage, black ethnicity, and pretransplantation antidonor cellular immunity in kidney transplant recipients. Journal of the American Society of Nephrology. 2007;18(5): 1602–1606.
89. Andree H, Nickel P, Nasiadko C, et al. Identification of dialysis patients with panel-reactive memory T cells before kidney transplantation using an allogeneic cell bank. Journal of the American Society of Nephrology. 2006;17(2):573–580.
90. Poggio ED, Clemente M, Hricik DE, et al. Panel of reactive T cells as a measurement of primed cellular alloimmunity in kidney transplant candidates. Journal of the American Society of Nephrology. 2006;17(2):564–572.
91. Poggio ED, Augustine JJ, Clemente M, et al. Pretransplant cellular alloimmunity as assessed by a panel of reactive T cells assay correlates with acute renal graft rejection. Transplantation. 2007;83(7):847–852.
92. Zand MS, Bose A, Vo T, et al. A renewable source of donor cells for repetitive monitoring of T- and B-cell alloreactivity. American Journal of Transplantation. 2005;5(1):76–86.
93. Spiridon C, Hunt J, Mack M, et al. Evaluation of soluble CD30 as an immunologic marker in heart transplant recipients. Transplantation Proceedings. 2006; 38(10):3689–3691.
94. Saini D, Ramachandran S, Nataraju A, et al. Activated effector and memory T cells contribute to circulating sCD30: potential marker for islet allograft rejection. American Journal of Transplantation. 2008;8(9):1798–1808.
95. Schlaf G, Altermann WW, Rothhoff A, et al. Soluble CD30 serum level–an adequate marker for allograft rejection of solid organs? Histology and Histopathology. 2007;22(11):1269–1279.
96. Rodriguez LM, Paris SC, Arbelaez M, et al. Kidney graft recipients with pretransplantation HLA CLASS I antibodies and high soluble CD30 are at high risk for graft loss. Human Immunology. 2007;68(8):652–660.
97. Platt RE, Wu KS, Poole K, et al. Soluble CD30 as a prognostic factor for outcome following renal transplantation. Journal of Clinical Pathology. 2009;62(7): 662–663.
98. Slavcev A, Honsova E, Lodererova A, et al. Soluble CD30 in patients with antibody-mediated rejection of the kidney allograft. Transplant Immunology. 2007;18(1):22–27.
99. Kovac J, Arnol M, Vidan Jeras B, et al. Pretransplant soluble CD30 serum concentration does not affect kidney graft outcomes 3 years after transplantation. Transplantation Proceedings. 2010;42(10):4043–4046.
100. Spiridon C, Nikaein A, Lerman M, et al. CD30, a marker to detect the high-risk kidney transplant recipients. Clinical Transplantation. 2008;22(6): 765–769.
101. Kowalski RJ, Post DR, Mannon RB, et al. Assessing relative risks of infection and rejection: a meta-analysis using an immune function assay. Transplantation. 2006;82(5):663–668.
102. Bhorade SM, Janata K, Vigneswaran WT, et al. Cylex ImmuKnow assay levels are lower in lung transplant recipients with infection. Journal of Heart and Lung Transplantation. 2008;27(9):990–994.
103. Reinsmoen NL, Cornett KM, Kloehn R, et al. Pretransplant donor-specific and non-specific immune parameters associated with early acute rejection. Transplantation. 2008;85(3):462–470.
104. van Besouw NM, Vaessen LM, Zuijderwijk JM, et al. The frequency of interferon-γ producing cells reflects alloreactivity against minor histocompatibility antigens. Transplantation. 2003;75(8):1400–1404.
105. Poggio ED, Clemente M, Riley J, et al. Alloreactivity in renal transplant recipients with and without chronic allograft nephropathy. Journal of the American Society of Nephrology. 2004;15(7):1952–1960.
106. Bestard O, Nickel P, Cruzado JM, et al. Circulating alloreactive T cells correlate with graft function in longstanding renal transplant recipients. Journal of the American Society of Nephrology. 2008;19(7):1419–1429.
107. Hammer MH, Brestrich G, Andree H, et al. HLA type-independent method to monitor polyoma BK virus-specific CD4 and CD8 T-cell immunity. American Journal of Transplantation. 2006;6(3):625–631.
108. Binggeli S, Egli A, Schaub S, et al. Polyomavirus BK-specific cellular immune response to VP1 and large T-antigen in kidney transplant recipients. American Journal of Transplantation. 2007;7(5):1131–1139.
109. Zhou W, Sharma M, Martinez J, et al. Functional characterization of BK virus-specific CD4+ T cells with cytotoxic potential in seropositive adults. Viral Immunology. 2007;20(3):379–388.
110. Bunde T, Kirchner A, Hoffmeister B, et al. Protection from cytomegalovirus after transplantation is correlated with immediate early 1-specific CD8 T cells. Journal of Experimental Medicine. 2005;201(7):1031–1036.
111. Nickel P, Bold G, Presber F, et al. High levels of CMV-IE-1-specific memory T cells are associated with less alloimmunity and improved renal allograft function. Transplant Immunology. 2009;20(4):238–242.
112. Berres ML, Trautwein C, Schmeding M, et al. Serum chemokine CXC ligand 10 (CXCL10) predicts fibrosis progression after liver transplantation for hepatitis C infection. Hepatology. 2011;53(2):596–603.
113. Jackson JA, Kim EJ, Begley B, et al. Urinary chemokines CXCL9 and CXCL10 are noninvasive markers of renal allograft rejection and BK viral infection. American Journal of Transplantation. 2011;11(10):2228–2234.
114. Schaub S, Nickerson P, Rush D, et al. Urinary CXCL9 and CXCL10 levels correlate with the extent of subclinical tubulitis. American Journal of Transplantation. 2009;9(6):1347–1353.
115. Matz M, Beyer J, Wunsch D, et al. Early post-transplant urinary IP-10 expression after kidney transplantation is predictive of short- and long-term graft function. Kidney International. 2006;69(9):1683–1690.
116. Strehlau J, Pavlakis M, Lipman M, et al. Quantitative detection of immune activation transcripts as a diagnostic tool in kidney transplantation. Proceedings of the National Academy of Sciences of the United States of America. 1997;94(2): 695–700.
117. Strehlau J, Pavlakis M, Lipman M, et al. The intragraft gene activation of markers reflecting T-cell-activation and -cytotoxicity analyzed by quantitative RT-PCR in renal transplantation. Clinical Nephrology. 1996;46(1):30–33.
118. Pavlakis M, Strehlau J, Lipman M, et al. Intragraft IL-15 transcripts are increased in human renal allograft rejection. Transplantation. 1996;62(4):543–545.
119. Lipman ML, Stevens AC, Strom TB. Heightened intragraft CTL gene expression in acutely rejecting renal allografts. Journal of Immunology. 1994;152(10): 5120–5127.
120. Lipman ML, Stevens AC, Bleackley RC, et al. The strong correlation of cytotoxic T lymphocyte-specific serine protease gene transcripts with renal allograft rejection. Transplantation. 1992;53(1):73–79.
121. Nickel P, Lacha J, Ode-Hakim S, et al. Cytotoxic effector molecule gene expression in acute renal allograft rejection: correlation with clinical outcome; histopathol-

ogy and function of the allograft. Transplantation. 2001;72(6):1158–1160.
122. Hoffmann SC, Hale DA, Kleiner DE, et al. Functionally significant renal allograft rejection is defined by transcriptional criteria. American Journal of Transplantation. 2005;5(3):573–581.
123. Mengel M, Reeve J, Bunnag S, et al. Scoring total inflammation is superior to the current Banff inflammation score in predicting outcome and the degree of molecular disturbance in renal allografts. American Journal of Transplantation. 2009;9(8):1859–1867.
124. Reeve J, Einecke G, Mengel M, et al. Diagnosing rejection in renal transplants: a comparison of molecular- and histopathology-based approaches. American Journal of Transplantation. 2009;9(8):1802–1810.
125. Perco P, Kainz A, Wilflingseder J, et al. Histogenomics: association of gene expression patterns with histological parameters in kidney biopsies. Transplantation. 2009;87(2):290–295.
126. Sarwal M, Chua MS, Kambham N, et al. Molecular heterogeneity in acute renal allograft rejection identified by DNA microarray profiling. New England Journal of Medicine. 2003;349(2):125–138.
127. Viklicky O, Hribova P, Volk HD, et al. Molecular phenotypes of acute rejection predict kidney graft prognosis. Journal of the American Society of Nephrology. 2010;21(1):173–180.
128. Barker AK, McDaniel DO, Zhou X, et al. Combined analysis of allograft inflammatory factor-1, interleukin-18, and Toll-like receptor expression and association with allograft rejection and coronary vasculopathy. American Surgeon. 2010;76(8):872–878.
129. Luan FL, Trillsch F, Henger A, et al. A pilot study of gene expression-based categorization of pancreas transplant biopsies. Transplantation. 2009;87(2): 222–226.
130. Minisini R, Giarda P, Grossi G, et al. Early activation of interferon-stimulated genes in human liver allografts: relationship with acute rejection and histological outcome. Journal of Gastroenterology. 2011;46(11):1307–1315.
131. Anglicheau D, Muthukumar T, Suthanthiran M. MicroRNAs: small RNAs with big effects. Transplantation. 2010;90(2):105–112.
132. Harris A, Krams SM, Martinez OM. MicroRNAs as immune regulators: implications for transplantation. American Journal of Transplantation. 2010;10(4): 713–719.
133. Shan J, Feng L, Luo L, et al. MicroRNAs: potential biomarker in organ transplantation. Transplant Immunology. 2011;24(4):210–215.
134. Anglicheau D, Sharma VK, Ding R, et al. MicroRNA expression profiles predictive of human renal allograft status. Proceedings of the National Academy of Sciences of the United States of America. 2009;106(13):5330–5335.
135. Asaoka T, Sotolongo B, Island ER, et al. MicroRNA signature of intestinal acute cellular rejection in formalin-fixed paraffin-embedded mucosal biopsies. American Journal of Transplantation. 2011.
136. Sui W, Dai Y, Huang Y, et al. Microarray analysis of MicroRNA expression in acute rejection after renal transplantation. Transplant Immunology. 2008;19(1): 81–85.
137. Barry CT, D'Souza M, McCall M, et al. Micro RNA expression profiles as adjunctive data to assess the risk of hepatocellular carcinoma recurrence after liver transplantation. American Journal of Transplantation. 2012;12(2):428–437.
138. Chen HY, Han ZB, Fan JW, et al. miR-203 expression predicts outcome after liver transplantation for hepatocellular carcinoma in cirrhotic liver. Medical Oncology. 2012;29(3):1859–1865.
139. Sawitzki B, Bushell A, Steger U, et al. Identification of gene markers for the prediction of allograft rejection or permanent acceptance. American Journal of Transplantation. 2007;7(5):1091–1102.
140. Sabek O, Dorak MT, Kotb M, et al. Quantitative detection of T-cell activation markers by real-time PCR in renal transplant rejection and correlation with histopathologic evaluation. Transplantation. 2002;74(5):701–707.
141. Simon T, Opelz G, Wiesel M, et al. Serial peripheral blood perforin and granzyme B gene expression measurements for prediction of acute rejection in kidney graft recipients. American Journal of Transplantation. 2003;3(9):1121–1127.
142. Vasconcellos LM, Schachter AD, Zheng XX, et al. Cytotoxic lymphocyte gene expression in peripheral blood leukocytes correlates with rejecting renal allografts. Transplantation. 1998;66(5):562–566.
143. Alakulppi NS, Kyllonen LE, Partanen J, et al. Diagnosis of acute renal allograft rejection by analyzing whole blood mRNA expression of lymphocyte marker molecules. Transplantation. 2007;83(6):791–798.
144. Hutchinson JA, Riquelme P, Sawitzki B, et al. Cutting Edge: immunological consequences and trafficking of human regulatory macrophages administered to renal transplant recipients. Journal of Immunology. 2011;187(5):2072–2078.
145. Sawitzki B, Reinke P, Pascher A, et al. State of the art on the research for biomarkers allowing individual, tailor-made minimization of immunosuppression. Current Opinion in Organ Transplantation. 2010. Oct 7 [Epub ahead of print]
146. Mehra MR, Kobashigawa JA, Deng MC, et al. Transcriptional signals of T-cell and corticosteroid-sensitive genes are associated with future acute cellular rejection in cardiac allografts. Journal of Heart and Lung Transplantation. 2007; 26(12):1255–1263.
147. Bohne F, Martinez-Llordella M, Lozano JJ, et al. Intra-graft expression of genes involved in iron homeostasis predicts the development of operational tolerance in human liver transplantation. Journal of Clinical Investigation. 2012;122(1): 368–382.
148. Watkins NA, Gusnanto A, de Bono B, et al. A HaemAtlas: characterizing gene expression in differentiated human blood cells. Blood. 2009;113(19):e1–e9.
149. Shen-Orr SS, Tibshirani R, Khatri P, et al. Cell type-specific gene expression differences in complex tissues. Nature Methods. 2010;7(4):287–289.
150. McKinney EF, Lyons PA, Carr EJ, et al. A CD8+ T cell transcription signature predicts prognosis in autoimmune disease. Nature Medicine. 2010;16(5):586–591.
151. Farid WR, Pan Q, van der Meer AJ, et al. Hepatocyte-derived microRNAs as serum biomarker of hepatic injury and rejection after liver transplantation. Liver Transplantation. 2012;18(3):290–297.
152. Seiler M, Brabcova I, Viklicky O, et al. Heightened expression of the cytotoxicity receptor NKG2D correlates with acute and chronic nephropathy after kidney transplantation. American Journal of Transplantation. 2007;7(2):423–433.
153. Ho J, Rush DN, Gibson IW, et al. Early urinary CCL2 is associated with the later development of interstitial fibrosis and tubular atrophy in renal allografts. Transplantation. 2010;90(4):394–400.
154. Kotsch K, Mashreghi MF, Bold G, et al. Enhanced granulysin mRNA expression in urinary sediment in early and delayed acute renal allograft rejection. Transplantation. 2004;77(12):1866–1875.
155. Hu H, Kwun J, Aizenstein BD, et al. Noninvasive detection of acute and chronic injuries in human renal transplant by elevation of multiple cytokines/chemokines in urine. Transplantation. 2009;87(12):1814–1820.
156. Tatapudi RR, Muthukumar T, Dadhania D, et al. Noninvasive detection of renal allograft inflammation by measurements of mRNA for IP-10 and CXCR3 in urine. Kidney International. 2004;65(6):2390–2397.
157. Madsen CB, Norgaard A, Iversen M, et al. Elevated mRNA levels of CTLA-4, FoxP3, and granzyme B in BAL, but not in blood, during acute rejection of lung allografts. Transplant Immunology. 2010;24(1):26–32.
158. Lorenzen JM, Volkmann I, Fiedler J, et al. Urinary miR-210 as a mediator of acute T-cell mediated rejection in renal allograft recipients. American Journal of Transplantation. 2011;11(10):2221–2227.
159. Budde K, Matz M, Durr M, et al. Biomarkers of over-immunosuppression. Clinical Pharmacology and Therapeutics. 2011;90(2):316–322.
160. Sottong PR, Rosebrock JA, Britz JA, et al. Measurement of T-lymphocyte responses in whole-blood cultures using newly synthesized DNA and ATP. Clinical and Diagnostic Laboratory Immunology. 2000;7(2):307–311.
161. Kowalski RJ, Zeevi A, Mannon RB, et al. Immunodiagnostics: evaluation of functional T-cell immunocompetence in whole blood independent of circulating cell numbers. Journal of Immunotoxicology. 2007;4(3):225–232.
162. Sanchez-Velasco P, Rodrigo E, Valero R, et al. Intracellular ATP concentrations of CD4 cells in kidney transplant patients with and without infection. Clinical Transplantation. 2008;22(1):55–60.
163. Berglund D, Bengtsson M, Biglarnia A, et al. Screening of mortality in transplant patients using an assay for immune function. Transplant Immunology. 2011; 24(4):246–250.
164. Sommerer C, Giese T, Meuer S, et al. Pharmacodynamic monitoring of calcineurin inhibitor therapy: is there a clinical benefit? Nephrology, Dialysis, Transplantation. 2009;24(1):21–27.
165. Millan O, Sanchez-Fueyo A, Rimola A, et al. Is the intracellular ATP concentration of CD4+ T-Cells a predictive biomarker of immune status in stable transplant recipients? Transplantation. 2009;88(3 Suppl):S78–S84.
166. Kobashigawa JA, Kiyosaki KK, Patel JK, et al. Benefit of immune monitoring in heart transplant patients using ATP production in activated lymphocytes. Journal of Heart and Lung Transplantation. 2010;29(5):504–508.
167. Serban G, Whittaker V, Fan J, et al. Significance of immune cell function monitoring in renal transplantation after Thymoglobulin induction therapy. Human Immunology. 2009;70(11):882–890.
168. Huskey J, Gralla J, Wiseman AC. Single time point immune function assay (ImmuKnow) testing does not aid in the prediction of future opportunistic infections or acute rejection. Clinical Journal of the American Society of Nephrology. 2011;6(2):423–429.
169. Hooper E, Hawkins DM, Kowalski RJ, et al. Establishing pediatric immune response zones using the Cylex ImmuKnow assay. Clinical Transplantation. 2005;19(6):834–839.
170. Israeli M, Klein T, Sredni B, et al. ImmuKnow: a new parameter in immune monitoring of pediatric liver transplantation recipients. Liver Transplantation. 2008;14(6):893–898.

171. Rossano JW, Denfield SW, Kim JJ, et al. Assessment of the Cylex ImmuKnow cell function assay in pediatric heart transplant patients. Journal of Heart and Lung Transplantation. 2009;28(1):26–31.
172. Gralla J, Huskey J, Wiseman AC. Trends in immune function assay (ImmuKnow; Cylex™) results in the first year post-transplant and relationship to BK virus infection. Nephrology, Dialysis, Transplantation. 2011;27(6):2565–2570.
173. Li K, Patel H, Farrar CA, et al. Complement activation regulates the capacity of proximal tubular epithelial cell to stimulate alloreactive T cell response. Journal of the American Society of Nephrology. 2004;15(9):2414–2422.
174. Peng Q, Li K, Patel H, et al. Dendritic cell synthesis of C3 is required for full T cell activation and development of a Th1 phenotype. Journal of Immunology. 2006;176(6):3330–3341.
175. Raedler H, Yang M, Lalli PN, et al. Primed CD8(+) T-cell responses to allogeneic endothelial cells are controlled by local complement activation. American Journal of Transplantation. 2009;9(8):1784–1795.
176. Zhou W, Medof ME, Heeger PS, et al. Graft-derived complement as a mediator of transplant injury. Current Opinion in Immunology. 2007;19(5):569–576.
177. Berger SP, Roos A, Mallat MJ, et al. Association between mannose-binding lectin levels and graft survival in kidney transplantation. American Journal of Transplantation. 2005;5(6):1361–1366.
178. Berger SP, Roos A, Mallat MJ, et al. Low pretransplantation mannose-binding lectin levels predict superior patient and graft survival after simultaneous pancreas-kidney transplantation. Journal of the American Society of Nephrology. 2007;18(8):2416–2422.
179. Carroll KE, Dean MM, Heatley SL, et al. High levels of mannose-binding lectin are associated with poor outcomes after lung transplantation. Transplantation. 2011;91(9):1044–1049.
180. Manuel O, Pascual M, Trendelenburg M, et al. Association between mannose-binding lectin deficiency and cytomegalovirus infection after kidney transplantation. Transplantation. 2007;83(3):359–362.
181. Manuel O, Tarr PE, Venetz JP, et al. Meningococcal disease in a kidney transplant recipient with mannose-binding lectin deficiency. Transplant Infectious Disease. 2007;9(3):214–218.
182. Sagedal S, Thiel S, Hansen TK, et al. Impact of the complement lectin pathway on cytomegalovirus disease early after kidney transplantation. Nephrology, Dialysis, Transplantation. 2008;23(12):4054–4060.
183. Verschuren JJ, Roos A, Schaapherder AF, et al. Infectious complications after simultaneous pancreas-kidney transplantation: a role for the lectin pathway of complement activation. Transplantation. 2008;85(1):75–80.
184. Liman P, Babel N, Schachtner T, et al. Mannose-binding lectin deficiency is not associated with increased risk for polyomavirus nephropathy. Transplant Immunology. 2012;26:123–127.
185. Reinke P, Volk HD. Diagnostic and predictive value of an immune monitoring program for complications after kidney transplantation. Urologia Internationalis. 1992;49(2):69–75.
186. Hummel M, Docke WD, Friedel N, et al. Monitoring of the cellular immune system in patients with biventricular assist devices awaiting cardiac transplantation. Clinical Transplantation. 1994;8(1):59–66.
187. Docke WD, Randow F, Syrbe U, et al. Monocyte deactivation in septic patients: restoration by IFN-gamma treatment. Nature Medicine. 1997;3(6):678–681.
188. Smith PD, Lamerson CL, Wong HL, et al. Granulocyte-macrophage colony-stimulating factor stimulates human monocyte accessory cell function. Journal of Immunology. 1990;144(10):3829–3834.
189. Hornell TM, Beresford GW, Bushey A, et al. Regulation of the class II MHC pathway in primary human monocytes by granulocyte-macrophage colony-stimulating factor. Journal of Immunology. 2003;171(5):2374–2383.
190. Crockard AD, Treacy MT, Droogan AG, et al. Methylprednisolone attenuates interferon-beta induced expression of HLA-DR on monocytes. Journal of Neuroimmunology. 1996;70(1):29–35.
191. Koppelman B, Neefjes JJ, de Vries JE, et al. Interleukin-10 down-regulates MHC class II alphabeta peptide complexes at the plasma membrane of monocytes by affecting arrival and recycling. Immunity. 1997;7(6):861–871.
192. Randow F, Syrbe U, Meisel C, et al. Mechanism of endotoxin desensitization: involvement of interleukin 10 and transforming growth factor beta. Journal of Experimental Medicine. 1995;181(5):1887–1892.
193. Rigby WF, Waugh M, Graziano RF. Regulation of human monocyte HLA-DR and CD4 antigen expression, and antigen presentation by 1,25-dihydroxyvitamin D3. Blood. 1990;76(1):189–197.
194. Tiemessen MM, Jagger AL, Evans HG, et al. CD4+CD25+Foxp3+ regulatory T cells induce alternative activation of human monocytes/macrophages. Proceedings of the National Academy of Sciences of the United States of America. 2007;104(49):19446–19451.
195. Yonish-Rouach E, Fischer DG, Rubinstein M. Cyclosporin A regulates the expression of HLA-DR on human monocytes by two different mechanisms. Cellular Immunology. 1991;134(2):402–413.
196. Wolk K, Docke WD, von Baehr V, et al. Impaired antigen presentation by human monocytes during endotoxin tolerance. Blood. 2000;96(1):218–223.
197. Wolk K, Kunz S, Crompton NE, et al. Multiple mechanisms of reduced major histocompatibility complex class II expression in endotoxin tolerance. Journal of Biological Chemistry. 2003;278(20):18030–18036.
198. van den Berk JM, Oldenburger RH, van den Berg AP, et al. Low HLA-DR expression on monocytes as a prognostic marker for bacterial sepsis after liver transplantation. Transplantation. 1997;63(12):1846–1848.
199. Haveman JW, van den Berg AP, van den Berk JM, et al. Low HLA-DR expression on peripheral blood monocytes predicts bacterial sepsis after liver transplantation: relation with prednisolone intake. Transplant Infectious Disease. 1999;1(3):146–152.
200. Hoffman JA, Weinberg KI, Azen CG, et al. Human leukocyte antigen-DR expression on peripheral blood monocytes and the risk of pneumonia in pediatric lung transplant recipients. Transplant Infectious Disease. 2004;6(4):147–155.
201. Docke WD, Hoflich C, Davis KA, et al. Monitoring temporary immunodepression by flow cytometric measurement of monocytic HLA-DR expression: a multicenter standardized study. Clinical Chemistry. 2005;51(12):2341–2347.
202. Mazariegos GV, Zahorchak AF, Reyes J, et al. Dendritic cell subset ratio in peripheral blood correlates with successful withdrawal of immunosuppression in liver transplant patients. American Journal of Transplantation. 2003;3(6):689–696.
203. Martinez-Llordella M, Lozano JJ, Puig-Pey I, et al. Using transcriptional profiling to develop a diagnostic test of operational tolerance in liver transplant recipients. Journal of Clinical Investigation. 2008;118(8):2845–2857.
204. Li Y, Zhao X, Cheng D, et al. The presence of Foxp3 expressing T cells within grafts of tolerant human liver transplant recipients. Transplantation. 2008;86(12):1837–1843.
205. Brouard S, Mansfield E, Braud C, et al. Identification of a peripheral blood transcriptional biomarker panel associated with operational renal allograft tolerance. Proceedings of the National Academy of Sciences of the United States of America. 2007;104(39):15448–15453.
206. Braud C, Baeten D, Giral M, et al. Immunosuppressive drug-free operational immune tolerance in human kidney transplant recipients: part I. Blood gene expression statistical analysis. Journal of Cellular Biochemistry. 2008;103(6):1681–1692.
207. Pallier A, Hillion S, Danger R, et al. Patients with drug-free long-term graft function display increased numbers of peripheral activated and memory B cells with an inhibitory phenotype. Kidney International. 2010;78(5):503–513.
208. Newell KA, Asare A, Kirk AD, et al. Identification of a B cell signature associated with renal transplant tolerance in humans. Journal of Clinical Investigation. 2010;120(6):1836–1847.
209. Sagoo P, Perucha E, Sawitzki B, et al. Development of a cross-platform biomarker signature to detect renal transplant tolerance in humans. Journal of Clinical Investigation. 2010;120(6):1848–1861.
210. Anglicheau D, Suthanthiran M. Noninvasive prediction of organ graft rejection and outcome using gene expression patterns. Transplantation. 2008;86(2):192–199.

第 91 章
器官移植后的免疫保护能力

Aneesh K. Mehta

引言

免疫抑制药物和多学科临床护理的进展显著改善了移植受体的短期结局。然而,长期预后的改善受到阻碍主要原因在于免疫抑制药物的副作用, 包括代谢异常、感染和恶性肿瘤等[1,2]。移植后感染的种类及其流行病学在持续变化,原因是更新的免疫抑制方案、扩大的供体和受体标准、受体寿命改善,以及提供预防、接种疫苗并监测移植受体的免疫状态等[3]。因此,移植传染病领域会继续随着传统和新型病原体相关的发病率模式变迁。移植传染病的动态改变将在第 92~94 章中介绍。

实现免疫调节的最佳平衡受到无法表征个体患者免疫抑制净状态的限制。造成评估保护性免疫能力更复杂化的原因在于, 个体的免疫系统针对不同的病原体识别和应对模式存在不同。因此,在移植患者同种异体免疫和保护性免疫之间的平衡比双极的简单平衡更为复杂,它更类似于互相作用、互相影响的网络。

理想情况下, 简单的非侵入性获得性生物标志物或一系列的生物标志物与某个特定的临床结局存在联系,会被允许有针对性地、个性化地应用于移植受体的治疗方案。Dinavahi 和 Heeger 回顾了众多方法和能满足这一要求的早期研究结论[4]。这项工作大部分都集中在对淋巴细胞进行分型并分辨与同种异体免疫相关的功能。所采用的方法包括 ELISPOT、流式细胞术、抗体检测、基因表达及“组学”检测。这些方法及其应用因与同种异体免疫相关, 故而在第 13 章和第 90 章中详细叙述。最近,该领域已经开始推断这些技术及其数据用以评估保护性免疫状态。然而,从这些更广泛的实验中解读数据需要面临每次检测的差异和缺乏标准化等情况。本章将介绍可能可用于评估患者保护性免疫能力的方法,并探讨其转化为更广泛的临床使用的可能性。

保护性免疫

前面章节中已详细讨论了免疫系统的生物学(见第 2 章和第 5~7 章),因其面临对同种异体移植物的暴露以及用于调节这些反应的治疗方法 (见第 17 章、第 98 章和第 101 章)。然而,这些非特异性免疫调节同样很大程度上阻碍了受体免疫系统适当识别和处理病原体的能力。因此,理解这种关系是关键,在此简要地强调保护性免疫和同种异体免疫成分之间的相互作用[5,6]。

初次免疫应答

固有免疫系统是原发感染的第一线防御, 实际上加强了适应性免疫系统以产生有效的免疫应答。自然杀伤(NK)细胞和树突细胞(DC)是组成固有免疫系统的主要细胞组分。NK 细胞对感染的细胞有直接细胞毒作用,也能分泌细胞因子,例如干扰素-γ(IFN-γ),其能激活并协调适应性免疫成分。树突细胞通过模式识别受体(PRR)识别外来病原体,包括 Toll 样受体(TLR)、甘露糖凝集素受体、整合素、NOD 样受体,并且随后将抗原呈递给适应性免疫系统[7]。PRR 不针对任何特定的病原体,而是专门的非自身抗原。依据病原体类型和固有免疫接触的情况(例如 TLR 被激活),这些细胞将表达细胞因子和共刺激分子, 以诱导促炎或免疫应答耐受[5,8]。经过固有免疫系统的细胞增强,适应性免疫系统的抗原特异性 T 细胞和 B 细胞分化为效应细胞, 散播于整个机体并最终通过分化为记忆细胞使细胞总量减少。这一话题更深入的讨论参见第 7 章。

免疫记忆

免疫记忆包含记忆 B 细胞、抗体分泌的浆细胞

(ASC)、抗体和记忆CD4和CD8 T细胞。抗体直接与病原体或外源蛋白结合,可能中和或促进病原体的调理作用以辅助控制感染。记忆B细胞在应对这些抗原时能迅速再活化并分化成ASC,以增加抗体滴度。记忆T细胞通过迅速增殖、分泌细胞因子及表达细胞毒性酶等方法提供快速细胞免疫应答,以辅助快速清除感染。

记忆细胞响应的机制仍在探索中。维持B细胞记忆最有效的方法是反复暴露于该抗原。然而,即使在不存在抗原暴露的情况下,记忆B细胞仍可以持续几十年;疫苗特异性抗体和记忆B细胞在使用天花疫苗接种50年后仍能被检测到[10]。对于抗原特异性T细胞而言,在效应反应之后,大约90%会在收缩阶段被消除。剩余的大部分细胞会被转换成长寿命的记忆T细胞[5]。最近的数据表明,记忆T细胞实际上是异质的细胞群体,在后续的病原体感染中发挥特定的作用。感染的类型、潜在的遗传学和并发的疾病可显著影响这些病原体特异性细胞群的相对频率[10]。重要的是,新兴的免疫抑制剂的细胞学效应研究似乎表明,每种药物都可能不同地抑制或提高这些记忆细胞群的发展[11,12]。关于细胞记忆的详细讨论参见第9章,因其涉及同种异体免疫谱。

移植前免疫能力

移植前免疫偏移

慢性肾脏病(CKD)会形成慢性炎症状态,从而增加ESRD患者的并发症发病率[13]。有研究表明,CKD患者的炎症生物标志物如C反应蛋白增加,并且循环炎性细胞因子的水平也增加[13-15]。Kimmel等证明了促炎细胞因子水平增加,如肿瘤坏死因子(TNF)和白介素(IL)-1与透析患者的死亡率增加存在相关性,并且与这些患者感染增加也可能有关[15]。这些数据表明,在某些CKD患者中,细胞免疫功能障碍参与了其疾病的进展。

慢性肝病患者出现免疫损害与肝功能异常和黏膜免疫功能丧失均存在相关性[16]。肝硬化患者的肠道屏障减弱,可能是由于细胞内通道和细胞完整性改变,引起病原体通过肠壁移位至肠系膜和淋巴循环系统[17,18]。进而导致细菌内毒素和抗菌反应,引起系统性炎性细胞因子升高[19]。细菌易位一个最显著的后果是肿瘤坏死因子浓度增加,这是造成肝细胞损伤反应的重要组成部分,并且通常促进肝细胞增殖[20]。然而,在肝硬化患者中,过高的肿瘤坏死因子诱导会增加IL-1、IL-6和IL-8的分泌并激活下游激酶和蛋白酶,导致固有免疫系统功能失调[19]。

肝硬化患者的免疫功能异常有很大一部分发生于细胞免疫系统内。特别是慢性肝功能异常导致中性粒细胞、单核细胞和巨噬细胞功能异常,并且对病原体的调理作用降低[21-25]。功能障碍最严重的是在网状内皮系统(RES),网状内皮系统是血液中病原体的主要防御系统,大约90%的免疫细胞位于肝脏内[26]。RES活性降低的患者发生细菌感染的风险较正常RES的患者更高[27]。随着肝功能障碍的恶化,RES功能持续丧失,这是进展性肝硬化患者感染高发的主要原因[28]。

因此,患者需要进行器官移植的潜在的病理学常导致患者保护性免疫功能的显著缺陷,引起移植后感染性疾病发病率增加。

移植前保护性免疫评估

在评估过程中,潜在的移植受体需要进行额外的感染风险和感染暴露的评估,这些内容在第28~33章中详细叙述。一般情况下,大多数移植中心通过血清学评估病原体暴露史,包括巨细胞病毒(CMV)、EB病毒(EBV)、人免疫缺陷病毒(HIV)和肝炎病毒[29]。虽然病原体血清学阳性提示某种程度的保护性免疫,这种保护性免疫与移植术后足够强度的保护性免疫并不存在相关性[30]。这些筛选试验同时促进疫苗接种策略的发展,以提高保护性免疫。虽然大多数疫苗在维持术后保护性免疫方面并没有充分的研究,有限的数据和专家意见表明移植前使用疫苗可增加功效,而且可以充分增强免疫力以扩大供体范围,例如乙肝供体[31,32]。完成这些评估和疫苗接种会为患者提供保护性免疫能力,并且能明确挑战净免疫抑制状态的因素。

保护性免疫"净"状态的评估

移植患者的"免疫抑制净状态",包括所有可能引起感染的危险因素,对理解监测这些患者的免疫情况并进行治疗是非常重要的[3,33,34]。这种状态通常受到免疫抑制药物使用、疾病特异性免疫缺陷(如上所述)、骨髓功能(例如保持正常白细胞数量的能力)、围术期并发症、同种异体移植/器官功能障碍、代谢紊乱、抗菌药物的使用以及感染并发的影响[3,34]。这一概念被用于归因有相似并发症患者的流行病学风险是非常有用的。然而，这些因素量化的困难造成无法量化特定的免疫抑制净状态，医生已努力在为患者提供个体化的风险评估。近期新的个体化移植后风险评估监测工具已经被引入临床。

移植免疫细胞功能测定

在过去的十年中，移植界见证了生物标志物和免疫检测发展的巨大成果，以帮助指导临床决策和辅助移植受体的个体化护理，即使可能不是伟大的进步。ImmuKnow®检测（Cylex Inc.，Columbia，MD，USA）是目前第一个且唯一的商用检测方案，可直接检测整体免疫系统的反应。这一免疫检测方案也被称为移植免疫细胞功能测定（ICFA），用于体外测定 $CD4^+$ T 细胞响应促细胞分裂剂刺激后产生 ATP 的情况[35]。由于 ATP 是包括淋巴细胞在内的所有细胞的主要能量来源，并且目前越来越多的免疫抑制剂作用于调节 T 细胞的功能，该试验被设计用于量化 T 辅助细胞的应答，以评估细胞介导免疫功能的总能力[35]。FDA 声明 ICFA 用于评估免疫抑制治疗的实体器官移植人群的细胞内 ATP 含量。报告表明，基于所检测的 ATP 含量的免疫反应有："低"（≤225ng/mL），"中等"（226~524ng/mL），或"强"（≥525ng/mL）。这一检测尚未被批准专门用于评估患者的免疫抑制需求，并且没有相关应用指南。

已有几项研究验证该检测可预测细胞性排斥反应和（或）感染。总的来说，尚没有这一研究的前瞻性随机对照数据，因此其效用仍然有待验证。当然，也尚未证实其在某种环境下能预测排斥反应。然而，这一检测的数据用于感染风险评估还存在一些特殊情况。Kowalski 等报道了一项多中心的研究，回顾分析了 504 例实体器官移植受体（心脏、肾脏、胰肾、肝脏和小肠）的排斥风险，这些患者在不同的时间点进行了 ICFA 前瞻性观察评估[35]。免疫反应值 ATP 为 25ng/mL 的患者进展为感染的可能性较反应更强的患者高 12 倍（95% CI，4~36）。有趣的是，这组数据表明排斥反应和感染的相对危险度曲线相交于 280ng/mL，提示对实体器官受体来说这可能是合理的目标免疫范围[35]。后续的一些研究表明低 ICFA 值与高感染风险存在相关性[36,37]，包括一些特殊病原体感染：BK 病毒（BKV）[38,39]、巨细胞病毒、EBV[40,41]、移植后丙型肝炎病毒（HCV）[42-44]和侵袭性真菌感染[45]。然而，转化应用这些数据至一般的患者受到限制，因素包括患者样本量较少、免疫移植方案的异质性、单中心的实验设计，以及更重要的是目标免疫区范围过大造成感染的风险。有两项研究表明，校正其他临床和人口统计学因素后，患者种族也会影响 ICFA 值[46,47]。此外，许多研究显示，ICFA 值与传染病风险的相关性并不表明更高的 ICFA 值与细胞性排斥之间存在强联系[38,48-50]。因此，对于单个患者的单一 ICFA 值（无论是对感染还是排斥事件），在短期内的预测值都不高。同样，数项针对 ICFA 的研究以及近期的一项荟萃分析都表明，ICFA 在一般人群的检测中并未显示明显的有效性[52-54]。

使用 ICFA 方案一个有意思的方面是监测减少免疫抑制剂后感染[55,56]和恶性肿瘤[57]的控制情况。Gautam 等利用 ICFA 来减少免疫抑制剂的使用，在联合抗病毒药的情况下，在 12 例移植后各类病毒感染的患者中未观察到任何相关排斥反应[55]。然而，虽然发生感染时平均 ICFA 为 56.8ng/mL，降低免疫抑制后平均为 194.5ng/mL，ICFA 范围仍存在显著重叠，两者分别为 3~178ng/mL 和 53~409ng/mL[55]。Lee 等比较了 18例儿科肝脏移植患者的 EBV 病毒载量与 ICFA 值，以及 3 例持续高 EBV 病毒载量的患者，以确定 ICFA 值在减少免疫抑制中的作用[56]。这些患者均未出现移植后淋巴组织增生性疾病（PTLD）；然而，尽管 ICFA 值均增加，只有 2 例患者 EBV 病毒载量下降[56]。这些研究受限于较小的样本量，但是鉴于 T 辅助细胞功能的至关重要性，这种方法显示了难治性感染个体化降低免疫抑制的前景。

总之，在移植后患者 ICFA 监测的有效性仍有待明确。可以确定的是患者年龄和种族、移植器官、免疫抑制方案的不同，尤其是采用清除性诱导或挽救方案时淋巴细胞计数异常都会影响风险阈值和相应的监测方案。此外，仍需要进行临床试验比较 ICFA 和其他常规监测，以充分理解这一方案对患者风险评估的效用。

监测免疫球蛋白

过去十几年里，抗体介导的排斥反应的重要性越来越显现，同时，记忆 B 细胞、抗体分泌细胞和抗体在移植中的研究也越来越多。随着病原体特异性血清学效价检测的研究表明其没有预测移植后保护性免疫的能力，一些研究推断免疫球蛋白水平可能有助于保护性免疫的预测。探讨保护性免疫净状态的第一个大型研究是 Goldfarb 等对 67 例肺移植患者的研究[58]。这组患者表现为移植后低丙球蛋白血症(70%)和严重的低丙球蛋白血症(37%)(定义为 IgG 水平<400mg/dL)发生率显著升高[58]。感染,包括细菌、病毒和真菌,在低丙球蛋白血症患者中显著增加(总体感染 P=0.006)[58]。严重低丙球蛋白血症与侵袭性曲菌(发病率 44%)和患者死亡率相关[58]。Yamani 等报道了连续 111 例心脏移植患者,术后 3 个月和术后 6 个月的免疫球蛋白(IgG)水平,发现队列中 10%的患者移植后发生严重的低丙球蛋白血症(定义为 IgG<350mg/dL)[59]。严重低丙球蛋白血症的患者较 IgG>350mg/dL 的患者机会性感染的风险显著增加,相对风险为 22.8[59]。这些患者被诊断为多种细菌、病毒和真菌感染,未发生主要的综合征[59]。他们还发现,移植后的低丙球蛋白血症与排斥治疗高度相关,增加了一种排斥可以诱导感染风险的途径[59]。Sarmiento 等对 41 例心脏移植患者的研究同样得出了类似的结论,并且还发现移植前 IgG 表现,尤其是 IgG1 与机会性感染风险增加相关[60]。这项研究也表明低丙球蛋白血症患者,CMV 病为优势感染。调整临床预测变量后,IgG 预测值尽管有所减少,但仍然显著[60]。这一团队试图通过他们中心 46 例连续的肝移植拓展这一结论[61]。然而,与心脏移植的研究相对,在这项研究中,移植前高 IgG 血症和 IgA 球蛋白血症与移植后感染存在相关性,相对危险度分别为 2.78 和 2.77[61]。移植后的免疫球蛋白水平在有无感染的患者之间没有显著差异[61]。这些发现归因于慢性肝脏疾病的免疫刺激,如上所述,肝脏疾病严重程度增加与抗体水平升高相关[61,62]。近期,Fernández-Ruiz 等分析了 226 例肾移植患者低丙球蛋白血症对传染病风险的影响,血清免疫球蛋白水平在基线,移植术后 1 个月和 6 个月定量。低丙球蛋白血症在这个队列中的患病率在 1 个月和 6 个月时分别为 52%和 31%,与感染的发病率升高相关,尤其是细菌感染[63]。这些数据并不表明移植术后前 6 个月 CMV 病毒或其他机会性感染病毒与低丙球蛋白血症相关[63]。

这些研究初步表明,监测移植前和移植后的免疫球蛋白水平可能在预测移植受体的感染风险中发挥作用。移植前免疫球蛋白水平的改变似乎与保护性免疫无关,而移植后出现低丙球蛋白血症则增加感染风险。直观来看,体液免疫在机体感染时有中和、调理并激活补体的作用,其改变可能与细菌感染相关[63]。基于 T 细胞免疫在控制大部分病毒感染中的首要地位,许多研究没有发现低丙球蛋白血症与 CMV 感染之间存在联系也就不足为奇了。再次,现有的数据可能不能在移植中大范围推广。这些研究大多数为单中心或回顾性分析。低丙球蛋白血症的定义以及用于评估的测定方案因研究不同而不同。此外,这些研究采用不同的免疫抑制方案、传染病诊断方案和随访持续时间,以及不同的感染谱监测。基于这些差异,获得性低丙球蛋白血症或严重低丙球蛋白血症与感染风险之间可能不存在因果关系,因为很多感染可诱导免疫失调,导致 B 细胞功能改变。然而,鉴于在大多数移植中心检测方便且检测成本低,血清免疫球蛋白水平应尽量保证在精心设计的多中心并行,特别是在新的免疫抑制剂方案基础上进行。

病原体分子监测作为免疫抑制净状态监测的替代方案

病原体分子监测,特别是定量聚合酶链反应(PCR)测定病毒病原体,已在移植中心司空见惯。许多专家认为,这些病原体的监测工具可以用作保护性免疫能力净状态的标志[64]。这个想法主要从预防 BK 肾病时监测 BKV 多瘤病毒的经验中产生。BKV 会造成肾同种异体移植物的肾小管性肾炎和肾病,且 BK 病毒滴度与多瘤病毒相关性肾病(PVAN)发生率存在相关性,PCR 监测 BKV 复制应用于肾移植受体变得越来越普遍[65-67]。这一经验很大程度表明响应 BKV 病毒血症时减少免疫抑制剂可能的方案[68-70]。Ginevri 等发表了第一项根据 BKV 血症情况减少免疫抑制剂来预防 PVAN 的报道,研究纳入 62 例儿童肾移植受体[71]。这个前瞻性队列采用定量 PCR 对血液和尿液样本的 BK 病毒进行监测。该队列的 4 级免疫抑制降级过程表明,在所有病毒血症患者中都达到了 BK 病毒的清除,而没有发生任何相关的排斥反应[71]。BKV 特异性 ELISPOT 分析用于监测病毒特异性 T 细胞应答,并证明与 BKV 病毒血症风险无相关性(第 13 章介绍了 ELISPOT 测定法)。重要的是,表明预期免疫抑制降级能改善病毒特异性应答,且这些应答的改善与病毒清除相关[71]。一些研究进一步证明了伴有 BK 病毒血症的肾移植患者的预期免疫抑制降级与病毒清除、预防 PVAN、低后期排斥发生率以及良好的长期肾功能存在相关性[67,72-76]。因此,在伴有 BKV 病毒血症的肾移植患者中,BKV PCR 检测能对免疫抑制净状态进行良好评估,可用于指导保护性免疫和同种异体免疫之间的平衡。

最近,许多人推测 EBV 监测可能提示免疫抑制净状态监测适用于所有实体器官移植。为明确 EBV PCR 在这些方面的应用，Ahya 等使用 EBV PCR 对 31 例长达 2 年时间进行血浆和全血化验的肺移植患者进行了回顾性分析[77]。可检测到 EBV 病毒载量的患者比没有检出 EBV 的患者发生 2 级或以上排斥的发病率显著降低(83%对45%，OR 为 0.17)[77]。重要的是，检测出的 EBV 并不与其他感染的风险相关(OR 为 1.6)[77]。Doesch 等报道了一项类似的研究数据，评估 EBV PCR 作为发展为 PTLD 的预后工具用于检测 172 例成年稳定心脏移植受体[78]。36 例(21%)患者可持续检测出 EBV，但并不与 PTLD 的风险相关，而与免疫抑制水平相关[78]。一项对 41 例儿童心脏移植受体的研究也发现免疫抑制类型和数量与 EBV 病毒载量增加之间有较强的联系[79]。Bakker 等前瞻性地评估了 75 例肺移植患者，证明利用 EBV 监测指导免疫抑制治疗的能力[80]。该中心的患者每年接受至少两次 EBV 病毒载量监测，并且测试结果为阳性的至少 1 个月内或当呈现上升斜率时，其免疫抑制降低[80]。其中 26 例(35%)患者被检测出 EBV，19 例患者减少了免疫抑制并出现 EBV 病毒载量迅速且持续的下降，且没有发生排斥反应或闭塞性细支气管炎[80]。

这些数据使得已用于监测患者病毒活性的病毒 PCR 检测作为免疫抑制净状态的评估成为可能。目前这一转变受到的广泛限制在于这些数据在不同的检测方案中存在很大的差异，且其灵敏度和动态范围都太宽泛[81-83]。一些 PCR 检测的变体正在被世界卫生组织(WHO)作为 CMV 和 EBV 的标准所采用。然而，病原体暴露程度的高度差异率以及各类型器官移植的独特生物学特性使单一病毒 PCR 检测的应用存在困难。一些专家认为同时定量多种病毒将使病毒检测作为评估免疫抑制水平的替代方案的特异性得到改善[64]。鉴于 PCR 检测的易用性、技术费用逐渐降低以及通过国际通用标准可提高重复性，无论是在单一或多重病毒，PCR 检测对免疫抑制的评估都应进一步在大型临床研究中评估。

病原体特异性保护性免疫的评估

上述免疫抑制和整体保护性免疫的评估为个体水平上的传染病风险提供了深入了解，并可能极大地影响临床治疗。然而，仍然可观察到一些患者在成功地控制其他病原体同时，对消除特定的感染存在困难。因此，对免疫抑制净状态的理解仍无法使临床医生明确患者对哪种特定的病原体易感。越来越多的研究评估了特定的病原体，这些数据可用于对特定病原体的具体评估。另外，监测有效免疫应答参数的能力可用于确定监测和治疗传染病的类型和持续时间。

免疫测试

普遍认为在免疫抑制患者中监测特异性病原体抗体滴度不能充分定量该病原体的风险，特别是需要 T 细胞帮助和(或)细胞毒活性辅助的病原体，如病毒[84,85]。T 细胞活化是免疫抑制药物的主要目标，其最佳的活化要求精细的信号网络，并最终使免疫记忆形成[86]。记忆性 T 细胞的划分包含 CD4 和 CD8 T 细胞，可以快速增殖，分泌炎性细胞因子并杀死被感染的细胞以消除病原体。近期检测病原体特异性免疫的技术发展，包括病原体肽/主要组织相容性复合体(MHC)的多聚体、肽增殖测定法以及 ELISPOT 细胞因子测定法和流式细胞术，使得病原体特异性 T 细胞的量化、表征和监控成为可能[87-90]。MHC 多聚体通常是四聚体，对病毒蛋白来源的单个 HLA 限制性表位的 $CD8^+$或 $CD4^+$ T 细胞进行应答。器官移植的几项研究已经利用包括巨细胞病毒、EBV 和 BKV 的病毒多聚体来探测跟踪移植后病原体特异性 T 细胞群。这些测定法一致表明免疫抑制的移植患者仍能够产生并扩大病毒特异性 T 细胞，以及病毒血症过程相关动力学情况[91-93]。但是这些数据表明单独病原体特异性 T 细胞计数并不能用于预测对患者的保护水平，可能是由于缺乏功能质量和细胞增殖能力等数据造成的。

有效的记忆性 T 细胞应答的标志为快速细胞因子分泌。由 T 细胞分泌的细胞因子混合物影响这一病原体特异性应答的特性。例如，Th1 细胞因子(TNF、IFN-γ、IL-2)对细胞内病原体的免疫应答极其重要，如 EBV 和巨细胞病毒；而 Th2 细胞因子(IL-4 和 IL-10)则对细胞外感染产生的免疫应答非常关键。Egli 等回顾发现，这些特性反应的检测被证明在预测移植受体的保护效应中极其重要，特别是对巨细胞病毒[90]。这些测定通常涉及使用单个肽链或肽链组合、重叠肽池或者特定的病毒的全部裂解物在体外对全血或 PBMC 淋巴细胞刺激。HLA 特异性表位刺激 $CD8^+$和(或)$CD4^+$ T 细胞产生细胞因子，然后由流式细胞仪、ELISPOT 或酶联免疫吸附试验(ELISA)检测(图 91.1)。正如预期的那样，基线免疫功能与血清状态相关[93]。几项研究的数据表明，体外病毒抗原刺激产生细胞因子(通常为 IFN-γ)，与抗病毒复制和病毒疾病的保护能力相关[94-98]。然而，这些反应的预测能力可能并不适合于所有人群。高风险巨细胞病毒感染的移植受体，定义为供体 CMV 血清阳性受体与受体血清学阴性配对，似乎能刺激出现一群 CMV 特异性 T 细胞，但这些应答并不能预测不发生 CMV 病[99,100]。抗病毒治疗下 CMV 病毒血症不清除可能与功能特异性 T 细胞缺陷以及无法产生抵抗病毒血症相关[93]。这些应答测定的另一个应用可能是决定是否进行抗病毒治疗[90]。例如，正在进行抗病毒药物治疗且病毒特异性 T 细胞功能改善的患者，可早于没有功能性反应的同类患者停止治疗。这些数据预测感染风险和控制感染的能力也是非常有趣的，但需要在更大的研究中来评估。

这些枚举特定病原体的免疫功能的研究具有巨大的科研潜力，但它们应用到临床上的可行性是有限的[90]。这些检测多需要专门的设备、昂贵或不稳定的试剂，或需要专家或者时间。最重要的是，这些试验缺乏跨实验室标准，从而阻碍创建参考值或分层值。然而，在近期开发的试验中，QuantiFERON-CMV® (Cellestis Ltd., Valencia, CA, USA)解决了许多 CMV 免疫监测的限制。该测定法采用全血与不同 CMV 病毒来源的特异性针对 20 个 HLA Ⅰ类位点的 21 个肽链组合培养过夜，与无抗原(阴性对照)或植物血凝素(PHA；阳性分裂原对照)一同孵育 24 小时[101]。通过 ELISA 定量测定每个管的 IFN-γ 产量。CMV 肽段响应组减去阴性对照组后 IFN-γ≥0.2IU/mL 为阳性[101]。该测试在检测健康对照组的 CMV 免疫力时高敏感且高特异[101]。这一检测对 CMV 病的预测值不尽相同。在一项 39 例肺移植受体 297 个支气管镜检查样本的研究中，QuantiFERON®不能预测肺移植的 CMV 发作，不过该研究没有评估病毒血症[102]。在一项设计更完善的预测病毒血症的研究中，Kumar 等评估了单中心 108 例肺、肾、肝及胰肾联合移植术后 1、2 及 3 个月的结果[103]。35.2%的患者检测到了 CMV 免疫力，但这一研究采用了 0.1IU/mL 的 IFN-γ 截止值[103]。5.3%的患者发生了 CMV 病且有可检测的 CMV 应答，而 22.9%的 CMV 病没有免疫响应(*P*=

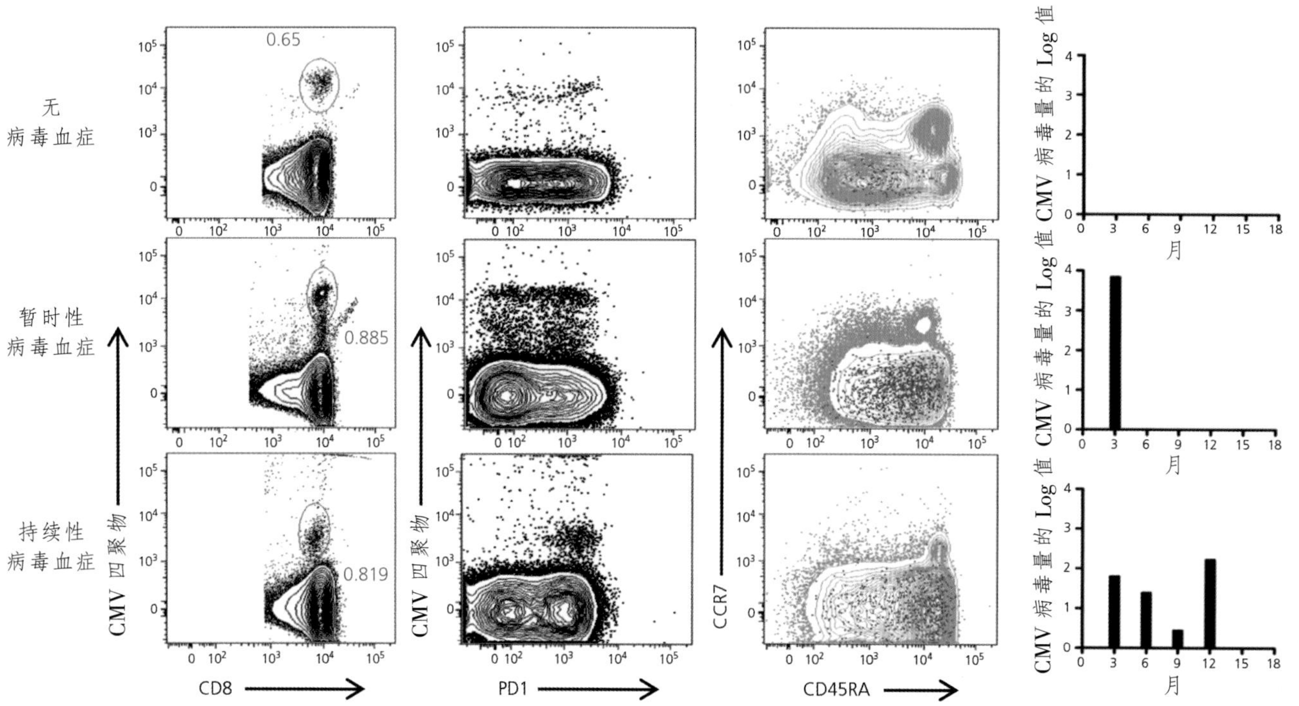

图 91.1 整合的流式细胞仪细胞分型距离。根据 MHC 四聚体和 PCR 病毒监测列举了病毒特异性 T 细胞。3 例患者的数据展示于此，1 例无病毒血症的健康对照及 2 例移植患者在第 18 个月的情况。第二栏表明 CMV 病毒血症的持续时间与 CMV 特异性 $CD8^+$ T 细胞的 PD-1 表达增加相关。第三栏说明 CMV 四聚体染色阳性细胞位于 $CD8^+$ T 细胞群体中，同时说明了持续 CMV 病毒血症在总体 $CD8^+$ T 细胞和 CMV 特异性 $CD8^+$ T 细胞中的滞后性。

0.038)[103]。因此,阳性结果有无疾病的高度预测值,但阴性测试不能预测 CMV。Lisboa 等根据这一研究对 37 例低病毒血症移植患者的 QuantiFERON-CMV®进行了前瞻性研究[104]。发病时测试结果阳性的患者,自发清除病毒的频率为 92.3%,而结果为阴性的患者清除率为 45.5%(P=0.004)[104]。这些有限的研究数据说明这种方法在确定 CMV 病毒血症风险及不使用抗病毒药物控制低水平的病毒血症中的预测作用。然而,这一测试受到较多无法判定的结果的限制,即高达 30%的移植患者有丝分裂原和 CMV 结果都<0.2IU/mL[102,103]。此外,0.2IU/mL 的阳性阈值没有在实体器官移植受体中进行验证[90]。然而,由于该检测的易用性和结果解读的简便性,一些中心已经开始在临床监测中使用该项测试。预计更多类似性质的测定将来可用于移植患者的研究中,这些研究和正在进行的研究也会在未来几年里对移植中心明确其效用。

总结

引入新的免疫抑制方案和更好的临床监测工具,在过去三十年中稳步提高了移植患者的存活率。但是,患者的长期存活率仍然受制于感染的发病率,甚至在一些患者中的影响超过了急性排斥反应[105]。即使免疫抑制净状态和病原体特异性保护性免疫的模型已被接受,明确量化这些概念并将其应用于患者具体的风险仍难以执行。基于解剖学、外部和无菌内部环境的暴露,每一种类型的同种异体移植都有其独特的传染病风险。最近,从临床试验中获得的数据表明,特定的免疫抑制剂有独特的传染疾病风险。药物特异性的例子可见 mTOR 抑制剂的使用和 CMV 感染风险降低的相关性[106-109],以及 EBV 相关 PTLD 在共刺激阻断的患者中发病率增加[110]。这些试验和机制方面的数据表明每种药物和方案都对保护性免疫的生成、维护和质量产生特定的影响[11,12]。因此,保护性免疫能力的评估和感染的概率根据年龄、种族、器官类型和免疫抑制方案进行分层是非常合理的。尽管移植患者保护性免疫的状态极其复杂,但若本章提供的近期数据能作为新兴的一个指示,便可为临床医生提供跨世纪的工具,用于个体化的保护性免疫能力的具体预测评估。

(凌琪 译 凌琪 校)

参考文献

1. Lodhi SA, Lamb KE, Meier-Kriesche HU. Solid organ allograft survival improvement in the United States: the long-term does not mirror the dramatic short-term success. American Journal of Transplantation. 2011;11(6):1226-1235.
2. Zand MS. Immunosuppression and immune monitoring after renal transplantation. Seminars in Dialysis. 2005;18(6):511-519.
3. Fishman JA, the ASTIDCoP. Introduction: infection in solid organ transplant recipients. American Journal of Transplantation. 2009;9:S3-S6.
4. Dinavahi R, Heeger PS. T-cell immune monitoring in organ transplantation. Current Opinion in Organ Transplantation. 2008;13(4):419-424.
5. Gangappa S, Kokko KE, Carlson LM, et al. Immune responsiveness and protective immunity after transplantation. Transplant International. 2008;21(4):293-303.
6. Dallman MJ. Immunology of graft rejection. In: Morris PJ, Knechtle SJ, editors. Kidney Transplantation: Principles and Practice, 6th ed. Philadelphia, PA: Saunders Elsevier; 2008: 9-31.
7. Akira S, Takeda K, Kaisho T. Toll-like receptors: critical proteins linking innate and acquired immunity. Nature Immunology. 2001;2(8):675-680.
8. Pulendran B. Modulating Th1/Th2 responses with microbes, dendritic cells, and pathogen recognition receptors. Immunologic Research. 2004;29(1-3):187-196.
9. Crotty S, Felgner P, Davies H, et al. Cutting edge: long-term B cell memory in humans after smallpox vaccination. Journal of Immunology. 2003;171(10):4969-4973.
10. Seder RA, Darrah PA, Roederer M. T-cell quality in memory and protection: implications for vaccine design. Nature Reviews. Immunology. 2008;8(4):247-258.
11. Araki K, Turner AP, Shaffer VO, et al. mTOR regulates memory CD8 T-cell differentiation. Nature. 2009;460(7251):108-112.
12. Turner AP, Shaffer VO, Araki K, et al. Sirolimus enhances the magnitude and quality of viral-specific CD8+ T-Cell responses to vaccinia virus vaccination in rhesus macaques. American Journal of Transplantation. 2011;11(3):613-618.
13. Meuwese CL, Stenvinkel P, Dekker FW, et al. Monitoring of inflammation in patients on dialysis: forewarned is forearmed. Nature Reviews Nephrology. 2011;7(3):166-176.
14. Yilmaz MI, Carrero JJ, Axelsson J, et al. Low-grade inflammation in chronic kidney disease patients before the start of renal replacement therapy: sources and consequences. Clinical Nephrology. 2007;68(1):1-9.
15. Kimmel PL, Phillips TM, Simmens SJ, et al. Immunologic function and survival in hemodialysis patients. Kidney International. 1998;54(1):236-244.
16. Chavez-Tapia NC, Torre-Delgadillo A, Tellez-Avila FI, et al. The molecular basis of susceptibility to infection in liver cirrhosis. Current Medicinal Chemistry. 2007;14(28):2954-2958.
17. Campillo B, Pernet P, Bories PN, et al. Intestinal permeability in liver cirrhosis: relationship with severe septic complications. European Journal of Gastroenterology and Hepatology. 1999;11(7):755-759.
18. Liu H, Zhang S, Yu A, et al. Studies on intestinal permeability of cirrhotic patients by analysis lactulose and mannitol in urine with HPLC/RID/MS. Bioorganic & Medicinal Chemistry Letters. 2004;14(9):2339-2344.
19. Tilg H, Diehl AM. Cytokines in alcoholic and nonalcoholic steatohepatitis. New England Journal of Medicine. 2000;343(20):1467-1476.
20. Diehl AM, Yin M, Fleckenstein J, et al. Tumor necrosis factor-alpha induces c-jun during the regenerative response to liver injury. American Journal of Physiology. Gastrointestinal and Liver Physiology. 1994;267(4):G552-G561.
21. Rajkovic IA, Williams R. Abnormalities of neutrophil phagocytosis, intracellular killing and metabolic activity in alcoholic cirrhosis and hepatitis. Hepatology. 1986;6(2):252-262.
22. Clapperton M, Rolando N, Sandoval L, et al. Neutrophil superoxide and hydrogen peroxide production in patients with acute liver failure. European Journal of Clinical Investigation. 1997;27(2):164-168.
23. Gomez F, Ruiz P, Schreiber AD. Impaired function of macrophage Fc gamma receptors and bacterial infection in alcoholic cirrhosis. New England Journal of Medicine. 1994;331(17):1122-1128.
24. Guarner C, Runyon BA. Macrophage function in cirrhosis and the risk of bacterial infection. Hepatology. 1995;22(1):367-369.
25. Runyon BA. Patients with deficient ascitic fluid opsonic activity are predisposed to spontaneous bacterial peritonitis. [Erratum appears in Hepatology 1988 Sep-Oct;8(5):1184]. Hepatology. 1988;8(3):632-635.
26. Navasa M. Bacterial infections in patients with cirrhosis: reasons, comments and suggestions. Digestive and Liver Disease. 2001;33(1):9-12.
27. Rimola A, Soto R, Bory F, et al. Reticuloendothelial system phagocytic activity in cirrhosis and its relation to bacterial infections and prognosis. Hepatology.

1984;4(1):53–58.
28. Borzio M, Salerno F, Piantoni L, et al. Bacterial infection in patients with advanced cirrhosis: a multicentre prospective study. Digestive and Liver Disease. 2001;33(1):41–48.
29. Fischer SA, Avery RK, the ASTIDCoP. Screening of donor and recipient prior to solid organ transplantation. American Journal of Transplantation. 2009;9: S7–S18.
30. Falagas ME, Snydman DR, Griffith J, et al. Effect of cytomegalovirus infection status on first-year mortality rates among orthotopic liver transplant recipients. The Boston Center for Liver Transplantation CMVIG Study Group. Annals of Internal Medicine. 1997;126(4):275–279.
31. Foster WQ, Murphy A, Vega DJ, et al. Hepatitis B vaccination in heart transplant candidates. Journal of Heart and Lung Transplantation. 2006;25(1):106–109.
32. Danzinger-Isakov L, Kumar D, the ASTIDCoP. Guidelines for vaccination of solid organ transplant candidates and recipients. American Journal of Transplantation. 2009;9:S258–S262.
33. Fishman JA, Rubin RH. Infection in organ-transplant recipients. New England Journal of Medicine. 1998;338(24):1741–1751.
34. Fishman JA, Issa NC. Infection in organ transplantation: risk factors and evolving patterns of infection. Infectious Disease Clinics of North America. 2010; 24(2):273–283.
35. Kowalski RJ, Post DR, Mannon RB, et al. Assessing relative risks of infection and rejection: a meta-analysis using an immune function assay. Transplantation. 2006;82(5):663–668.
36. Xue F, Zhang J, Han L, et al. Immune cell functional assay in monitoring of adult liver transplantation recipients with infection. Transplantation. 2010;89(5): 620–626.
37. Israeli M, Ben-Gal T, Yaari V, et al. Individualized immune monitoring of cardiac transplant recipients by noninvasive longitudinal cellular immunity tests. Transplantation. 2010;89(8):968–976.
38. Batal I, Zeevi A, Heider A, et al. Measurements of global cell-mediated immunity in renal transplant recipients with BK virus reactivation. American Journal of Clinical Pathology. 2008;129(4):587–591.
39. Moon HH, Kim TS, Roh YN, et al. Can immune function assay predict infection or recovery? Transplantation Proceedings. 2012;44(4):1048–1051.
40. Macedo C, Zeevi A, Bentlejewski C, et al. The impact of EBV load on T-cell immunity in pediatric thoracic transplant recipients. Transplantation. 2009;88(1): 123–128.
41. Elidemir O, Kancherla BS, Schecter MG, et al. Post-transplant lymphoproliferative disease in pediatric lung transplant recipients: recent advances in monitoring. Pediatric Transplantation. 2009;13(5):606–610.
42. Mendler M, Kwok H, Franco E, et al. Monitoring peripheral blood CD4+ adenosine triphosphate activity in a liver transplant cohort: insight into the interplay between hepatitis C virus infection and cellular immunity. Liver Transplantation. 2008;14(9):1313–1322.
43. Cabrera R, Ararat M, Soldevila-Pico C, et al. Using an immune functional assay to differentiate acute cellular rejection from recurrent hepatitis C in liver transplant patients. Liver Transplantation. 2009;15(2):216–222.
44. Alkhouri N, Hanouneh IA, Lopez R, et al. Monitoring peripheral blood CD4+ adenosine triphosphate activity in recurrent hepatitis C and its correlation to fibrosis progression. Liver Transplantation. 2010;16(2):155–162.
45. Zhou T, Xue F, Han LZ, et al. Invasive fungal infection after liver transplantation: risk factors and significance of immune cell function monitoring. Journal of Digestive Diseases. 2011;12(6):467–475.
46. Bhorade SM, Janata K, Vigneswaran WT, et al. Cylex ImmuKnow assay levels are lower in lung transplant recipients with infection. Journal of Heart and Lung Transplantation. 2008;27(9):990–994.
47. Gupta S, Mitchell JD, Markham DW, et al. Utility of the Cylex assay in cardiac transplant recipients. Journal of Heart and Lung Transplantation. 2008;27(8): 817–822.
48. Helantera I, Koskinen P. Association of immune cell function assay with protocol biopsy findings and viral infections in well matched kidney transplant recipients. Clinical Nephrology. 2010;74(2):123–131.
49. De Paolis P, Favaro A, Piola A, et al. "Immuknow" to measurement of cell-mediated immunity in renal transplant recipients undergoing short-term evaluation. Transplantation Proceedings. 2011;43(4):1013–1016.
50. Torio A, Fernández EJ, Montes-Ares O, et al. Lack of association of immune cell function test with rejection in kidney transplantation. Transplantation Proceedings. 2011;43(6):2168–2170.
51. Huskey J, Gralla J, Wiseman AC. Single time point immune function assay (ImmuKnow) testing does not aid in the prediction of future opportunistic infections or acute rejection. Clinical Journal of the American Society of Nephrology. 2011;6(2):423–429.
52. Ling X, Xiong J, Liang W, et al. Can immune cell function assay identify patients at risk of infection or rejection? A meta-analysis. Transplantation. 2012;93(7): 737–743.
53. Rossano JW, Denfield SW, Kim JJ, et al. Assessment of the Cylex ImmuKnow cell function assay in pediatric heart transplant patients. Journal of Heart and Lung Transplantation. 2009;28(1):26–31.
54. Serban G, Whittaker V, Fan J, et al. Significance of immune cell function monitoring in renal transplantation after Thymoglobulin induction therapy. [Erratum appears in Human Immunology. 2010;71(9):929]. Human Immunology. 2009; 70(11):882–890.
55. Gautam A, Fischer SA, Yango AF, et al. Cell mediated immunity (CMI) and post transplant viral infections–role of a functional immune assay to titrate immunosuppression. International Immunopharmacology. 2006;6(13–14): 2023–2026.
56. Lee TC, Goss JA, Rooney CM, et al. Quantification of a low cellular immune response to aid in identification of pediatric liver transplant recipients at high-risk for EBV infection. Clinical Transplantation. 2006;20(6):689–694.
57. Uemura T, Riley TR, Khan A, et al. Immune functional assay for immunosuppressive management in post-transplant malignancy. Clinical Transplantation. 2011;25(1):E32–E37.
58. Goldfarb NS, Avery RK, Goormastic M, et al. Hypogammaglobulinemia in lung transplant recipients. Transplantation. 2001;71(2):242–246.
59. Yamani MH, Avery RK, Mawhorter SD, et al. Hypogammaglobulinemia following cardiac transplantation: a link between rejection and infection. Journal of Heart and Lung Transplantation. 2001;20(4):425–430.
60. Sarmiento E, Rodríguez-Molina J, Muñoz P, et al. Decreased levels of serum immunoglobulins as a risk factor for infection after heart transplantation. Transplantation Proceedings. 2005;37(9):4046–4049.
61. Carbone J, Micheloud D, Salcedo M, et al. Humoral and cellular immune monitoring might be useful to identify liver transplant recipients at risk for development of infection. Transplant Infectious Disease. 2008;10(6):396–402.
62. Maruyama S, Hirayama C, Horie Y, et al. Serum immunoglobulins in patients with chronic hepatitis C: a surrogate marker of disease severity and treatment outcome. Hepatogastroenterology. 2007;54(74):493–498.
63. Fernández-Ruiz M, López-Medrano F, Varela-Peña P, et al. Monitoring of immunoglobulin levels identifies kidney transplant recipients at high risk of infection. American Journal of Transplantation. 2012;12(10):2763–2773.
64. Fishman JA. Infection in solid-organ transplant recipients. New England Journal of Medicine. 2007;357(25):2601–2614.
65. Randhawa PS, Finkelstein S, Scantlebury V, et al. Human polyoma virus-associated interstitial nephritis in the allograft kidney. Transplantation. 1999; 67(1):103–109.
66. Nickeleit V, Klimkait T, Binet IF, et al. Testing for polyomavirus type BK DNA in plasma to identify renal-allograft recipients with viral nephropathy. New England Journal of Medicine. 2000;342(18):1309–1315.
67. Hirsch HH, Randhawa P, the ASTIDCoP. BK virus in solid organ transplant recipients. American Journal of Transplantation. 2009;9:S136–S146.
68. Vats A, Shapiro R, Singh Randhawa P, et al. Quantitative viral load monitoring and cidofovir therapy for the management of BK virus-associated nephropathy in children and adults. Transplantation. 2003;75(1):105–112.
69. Ramos E, Drachenberg CB, Papadimitriou JC, et al. Clinical course of polyoma virus nephropathy in 67 renal transplant patients. Journal of the American Society of Nephrology: JASN. 2002;13(8):2145–2151.
70. Vasudev B, Hariharan S, Hussain SA, et al. BK virus nephritis: risk factors, timing, and outcome in renal transplant recipients. Kidney International. 2005;68(4): 1834–1839.
71. Ginevri F, Azzi A, Hirsch HH, et al. Prospective monitoring of polyomavirus BK replication and impact of pre-emptive intervention in pediatric kidney recipients. American Journal of Transplantation. 2007;7(12):2727–2735.
72. Hardinger KL, Koch MJ, Bohl DJ, et al. BK-Virus and the impact of pre-emptive immunosuppression reduction: 5-year results. American Journal of Transplantation. 2010;10(2):407–415.
73. Almeras C, Foulongne V, Garrigue V, et al. Does reduction in immunosuppression in viremic patients prevent BK virus nephropathy in de novo renal transplant recipients? A prospective study. Transplantation. 2008;85(8):1099–1104.
74. Saad ER, Bresnahan BA, Cohen EP, et al. Successful treatment of BK viremia using reduction in immunosuppression without antiviral therapy. Transplantation. 2008;85(6):850–854.
75. Wu SW, Chang HR, Hsieh MC, et al. Early diagnosis of polyomavirus type BK infection in tailoring immunosuppression for kidney transplant patients: screening with urine qualitative polymerase chain reaction assay. Transplantation Proceedings. 2008;40(7):2389–2391.
76. Giraldi C, Noto A, Tenuta R, et al. Prospective study of BKV nephropathy in 117 renal transplant recipients. New Microbiologica. 2007;30(2):127–130.
77. Ahya VN, Douglas LP, Andreadis C, et al. Association between elevated whole blood Epstein–Barr Virus (EBV)-encoded RNA EBV polymerase chain reaction and reduced incidence of acute lung allograft rejection. Journal of Heart and Lung

Transplantation. 2007;26(8):839–844.
78. Doesch AO, Konstandin M, Celik S, et al. Epstein-Barr virus load in whole blood is associated with immunosuppression, but not with post-transplant lymphoproliferative disease in stable adult heart transplant patients. Transplant International. 2008;21(10):963–971.
79. Schubert S, Renner C, Hammer M, et al. Relationship of immunosuppression to Epstein–Barr viral load and lymphoproliferative disease in pediatric heart transplant patients. Journal of Heart and Lung Transplantation. 2008;27(1): 100–105.
80. Bakker NA, Verschuuren EA, Erasmus ME, et al. Epstein-Barr virus-DNA load monitoring late after lung transplantation: a surrogate marker of the degree of immunosuppression and a safe guide to reduce immunosuppression. Transplantation. 2007;83(4):433–438.
81. Hayden RT, Yan X, Wick MT, et al. Factors contributing to variability of quantitative viral PCR results in proficiency testing samples: a multivariate analysis. Journal of Clinical Microbiology. 2012;50(2):337–345.
82. Pang XL, Fox JD, Fenton JM, et al. Interlaboratory comparison of cytomegalovirus viral load assays. American Journal of Transplantation. 2009;9(2):258–268.
83. Preiksaitis JK, Pang XL, Fox JD, et al. Interlaboratory comparison of Epstein-Barr virus viral load assays. American Journal of Transplantation. 2009;9(2): 269–279.
84. Humar A, Mazzulli T, Moussa G, et al. Clinical utility of cytomegalovirus (CMV) serology testing in high-risk CMV D+/R– transplant recipients. American Journal of Transplantation. 2005;5(5):1065–1070.
85. Emery VC, Asher K, Sanjuan C. Importance of the cytomegalovirus seropositive recipient as a contributor to disease burden after solid organ transplantation. Journal of Clinical Virology. 2012;54(2):125–129.
86. Salomon B, Bluestone JA. Complexities of CD28/B7: CTLA-4 costimulatory pathways in autoimmunity and transplantation. Annual Review of Immunology. 2001;19:225–252.
87. Klenerman P, Cerundolo V, Dunbar PR. Tracking T cells with tetramers: new tales from new tools. Nature Reviews. Immunology. 2002;2(4):263–272.
88. Waldrop SL, Pitcher CJ, Peterson DM, et al. Determination of antigen-specific memory/effector CD4+ T cell frequencies by flow cytometry: evidence for a novel, antigen-specific homeostatic mechanism in HIV-associated immunodeficiency. Journal of Clinical Investigation. 1997;99(7):1739–1750.
89. Anthony DD, Milkovich KA, Zhang W, et al. Dissecting the T cell response: proliferation assays vs. cytokine signatures by ELISPOT. Cells. 2012;1(2): 127–140.
90. Egli A, Humar A, Kumar D. State-of-the-art monitoring of cytomegalovirus-specific cell-mediated immunity after organ transplant: a primer for the clinician. Clinical Infectious Diseases. 2012.
91. Engstrand M, Tournay C, Peyrat MA, et al. Characterization of CMVpp65-specific CD8+ T lymphocytes using MHC tetramers in kidney transplant patients and healthy participants. Transplantation. 2000;69(11):2243–2250.
92. Hassan-Walker AF, Vargas Cuero AL, Mattes FM, et al. CD8+ cytotoxic lymphocyte responses against cytomegalovirus after liver transplantation: correlation with time from transplant to receipt of tacrolimus. Journal of Infectious Diseases. 2001;183(6):835–843.
93. Radha R, Jordan S, Puliyanda D, et al. Cellular immune responses to cytomegalovirus in renal transplant recipients. American Journal of Transplantation. 2005;5(1):110–117.
94. Bunde T, Kirchner A, Hoffmeister B, et al. Protection from cytomegalovirus after transplantation is correlated with immediate early 1–specific CD8 T cells. Journal of Experimental Medicine. 2005;201(7):1031–1036.
95. Egli A, Binet I, Binggeli S, et al. Cytomegalovirus-specific T-cell responses and viral replication in kidney transplant recipients. Journal of Translational Medicine. 2008;6:29.
96. Binggeli S, Egli A, Schaub S, et al. Polyomavirus BK-specific cellular immune response to VP1 and large T-antigen in kidney transplant recipients. American Journal of Transplantation. 2007;7(5):1131–1139.
97. Hammer MH, Brestrich G, Andree H, et al. HLA type-independent method to monitor polyoma BK virus-specific CD4+ and CD8+ T-Cell immunity. American Journal of Transplantation. 2006;6(3):625–631.
98. Guppy AE, Rawlings E, Madrigal JA, et al. A quantitative assay for Epstein-Barr Virus-specific immunity shows interferon-[gamma] producing CD8+ T cells increase during immunosuppression reduction to treat posttransplant lymphoproliferative disease. Transplantation. 2007;84(11):1534–1539.
99. La Rosa C, Limaye AP, Krishnan A, et al. Longitudinal assessment of cytomegalovirus (CMV)—specific immune responses in liver transplant recipients at high risk for late CMV disease. Journal of Infectious Diseases. 2007;195(5): 633–644.
100. Sester U, Gärtner BC, Wilkens H, et al. Differences in CMV-specific T-cell levels and long-term susceptibility to CMV infection after kidney, heart and lung transplantation. American Journal of Transplantation. 2005;5(6):1483–1489.
101. Walker S, Fazou C, Crough T, et al. Ex vivo monitoring of human cytomegalovirus-specific CD8+ T-cell responses using QuantiFERON-CMV. Transplant Infectious Disease. 2007;9(2):165–170.
102. Westall GP, Mifsud NA, Kotsimbos T. Linking CMV serostatus to episodes of CMV reactivation following lung transplantation by measuring CMV-specific CD8+ T-cell immunity. American Journal of Transplantation. 2008;8(8): 1749–1754.
103. Kumar D, Chernenko S, Moussa G, et al. Cell-mediated immunity to predict cytomegalovirus disease in high-risk solid organ transplant recipients. American Journal of Transplantation. 2009;9(5):1214–1222.
104. Lisboa LF, Kumar D, Wilson LE, et al. Clinical utility of cytomegalovirus cell-mediated immunity in transplant recipients with cytomegalovirus viremia. Transplantation. 2012;93(2):195–200.
105. Dharnidharka VR, Stablein DM, Harmon WE. Post-transplant infections now exceed acute rejection as cause for hospitalization: a report of the NAPRTCS1. American Journal of Transplantation. 2004;4(3):384–389.
106. Ozaki KS, Camara NOS, Galante NZ, et al. Decreased Cytomegalovirus infection after antilymphocyte therapy in sirolimus-treated renal transplant patients. International Immunopharmacology. 2005;5(1):103–106.
107. Haririan A, Morawski K, West MS, et al. Sirolimus exposure during the early post-transplant period reduces the risk of CMV infection relative to tacrolimus in renal allograft recipients. Clinical Transplantation. 2007;21(4):466–471.
108. Viganò M, Dengler T, Mattei MF, et al. Lower incidence of cytomegalovirus infection with everolimus versus mycophenolate mofetil in de novo cardiac transplant recipients: a randomized, multicenter study. Transplant Infectious Disease. 2010;12(1):23–30.
109. Demopoulos L, Polinsky M, Steele G, et al. Reduced risk of cytomegalovirus infection in solid organ transplant recipients treated with sirolimus: a pooled analysis of clinical trials. Transplantation Proceedings. 2008;40(5):1407–1410.
110. Grinyo J, Charpentier B, Pestana JM, et al. An integrated safety profile analysis of belatacept in kidney transplant recipients. Transplantation. 2010;90(12): 1521–1527.

第 92 章 器官移植供体来源感染

Marissa B. Wilck, Emily A. Blumberg

引言

众所周知，移植受体存在发生各种感染性疾病的风险（见第 93 章和第 94 章）。这种风险除了与移植术后免疫抑制治疗和潜在器官衰竭造成的免疫损伤有关之外，还与移植器官本身密不可分。事实上，移植器官在破坏机体本身机械屏障的同时，带入的主要组织相容性分子扰乱了原有免疫状态。本章将概述供体来源感染性疾病的诊断、治疗和预防。

一般认知

供体来源的感染性疾病是实体器官移植预后不佳的重要因素。这些感染性疾病的发生率很难准确统计，主要原因在于来源多样性，未能及时识别和(或)上报意料之外的供体来源事件。美国器官捐献与移植网络(OPTN)数据显示，仅有不到 1%的移植发生了供体来源的感染性疾病[1,2]。由于大部分数据来源于死亡供体，因此无法得知这是否能同时准确反映活体供体移植的感染性疾病发病率。值得注意的是，现有数据并不包含一些常见的潜在感染性疾病，如巨细胞病毒(CMV)或 Epstein-Barr 病毒(EBV)感染。如果把它们也统计在内，供体来源感染性疾病的发生率将进一步增加。

供体来源感染已经得到越来越多重视，在明确供体感染的情况下，一般会采取预防策略来减轻病原传播造成的危害。而一些难以预料的供体感染性疾病，如真菌感染和结核感染，则会由于没有及时采用预防策略而在移植术后表现出临床症状。最近的研究报道也已逐渐聚焦于那些很难诊断或者缺乏有效预防/治疗措施的感染性疾病。

供体来源感染的病原体形式多样，细菌、病毒、真菌、原生动物、寄生虫和朊病毒均被报道可以通过器官移植进行传播[1-4]。供体来源感染的类型与供体所在地区也有关联(表 92.1)。考虑到供体人群的地区差异性和日益放宽的捐献标准(见第 53 章)，具有地域人群特征的感染性疾病发生率也存在日益增加的风险[5]。

影响供体来源感染性疾病预后的重要因素，除供体人群特征之外，还包括免疫抑制剂选择、疾病筛查与诊断手段的改进、预防性抗菌药物的开发。移植受体感染性疾病的临床表现存在个体差异性[1,3]，主要原因在于病原体、供体器官、受体免疫状态、免疫抑制剂和抗菌药物使用等诸多方面存在不同。

供体来源感染性疾病的发生、发展与病原体、抗菌药物和免疫抑制剂密切相关(见第 94 章)。细菌感染通常发生在移植后第 1 个月，其他病原体则会更晚一些[4]。预防措施可能会延迟某些感染性疾病临床症状的出现，比如 CMV 感染。

有很多线索可以提示受体感染性疾病是否来源于供体，比如移植术后短时间内发生感染，又或者受体感染很难用其他原因解释，使用同一供器官来源的多名受体都发生同样类型的感染。此外，不管供体在去世前还是去世后发现了感染存在，都应该警惕其对受体传播感染性疾病的风险。

筛选

供体筛选应包含病史、社会史和常见感染性疾病检测的实验室检查[7](表 92.2)。因为供器官常常来源于远程医院，所以受体的主治医生应该能够很娴熟地从

表 92.1　常见的供体来源感染病原体*

病原体	分布	简介
细菌		
生脓原(如金黄色葡萄球菌、铜绿假单胞菌)	全球	
苍白密螺旋体	全球	
结核分枝杆菌	全球	最常见于非洲、东南亚、印度、巴基斯坦、阿富汗和俄罗斯；或供体存在监禁史、无家可归、酒精滥用、结核病未规范治疗或结核病接触史等情况
真菌		
白色念珠菌	全球	腹腔穿孔
组织胞浆菌	美国俄亥俄州和密西西比州河谷地区；南美洲、亚洲和非洲	
球孢菌	美国西南部、墨西哥中北部和南美洲	
曲霉菌	全球	与受体免疫抑制有关
隐球菌	全球	与受体免疫抑制、肝硬化有关
寄生虫/原生动物		
弓形体	全球	常见于拉丁美洲、撒哈拉以南的非洲、欧洲部分地区
克氏锥虫	拉丁美洲	
类圆线虫	全球	常见于热带、亚热带和暖温带地区
病毒		
巨细胞病毒	全球	
EB 病毒	全球	
乙型肝炎病毒	全球	常见于东南亚和非洲
丙型肝炎病毒	全球	常见于注射吸毒者、性工作者、高风险的性行为，或 1994 年之前的输血史
人类免疫缺陷病毒(HIV)	全球	
人类 T 细胞淋巴细胞病毒 1	全球	亚洲、加勒比海地区、南美洲、大洋洲和西非
西尼罗河病毒	全球	与季节性蚊虫有关

*供体来源感染的病原体还包括其他细菌(布鲁杆菌、巴氏杆菌、非结核分枝杆菌)；真菌(足放线病菌、原壁菌)、寄生虫/原生动物(疟原虫、阿米巴)、病毒(其他疱疹病毒、细小病毒、狂犬病病毒、淋巴细胞性脉络丛脑膜炎病毒)和朊病毒。

捐献协调中心获取上述信息并加以评判供体传播感染性疾病的风险。由于潜伏性或活动性感染性疾病都可以造成传播，因此这两种类型都应该被充分评估。美国 OPTN 已经制定了供体筛选相关标准，包括人类免疫缺陷病毒(HIV)、乙型和丙型肝炎病毒(HBV 和 HCV)、梅毒、CMV、EBV 的血清学检测，以及血液培养和尿液培养[8]。弓形体抗体(特别是对于心脏供体)、单纯疱疹病毒和水痘病毒抗体、人类 T 细胞嗜淋巴病毒 1 和 2 (HTLV 1 和 HTLV 2)抗体则被列为可选检测项目[7]。供体的地域、既往史和社会史等信息可能提供潜在感染性疾病的重要线索，以便后续选择合适的实验室检查(表 92.2)。这些评估结果有时会因为疾病传播风险而将供体排除在捐献队列之外，有时则可以帮助受体采取预防性干预措施。

不管是什么检测手段，都必须考虑血液稀释造成的实验误差[7,8]。因为供器官可能被大量血液制品、胶体或晶体进行灌注，从而造成检测结果假阴性。因此要尽量使用预灌注之前的血清样本用于供体筛查[7-9]。如果唯一可用于检测的是灌注后样本，那么应该根据美国食品和药品监督局(FDA)的指南来计算以消除血液稀释影响[10]。

供体感染的筛查平台取决于病原体类型和现存检测手段。值得注意的是，虽然器官捐献包含组织捐献，但受制于检测方法，器官捐献和组织捐献的检测应加以区分。在美国，供器官筛选检测方法必须经 FDA 批准[8]。血清学检测是明确既往感染病史的最有效筛查手

表 92.2 供体主要感染病原体筛查

疾病	首选筛查手段*	辅助筛查手段	死亡供体	活体供体
巨细胞病毒	巨细胞病毒 IgG*		需要	需要
人类免疫缺陷病毒	抗 HIV 1 和 HIV 2*	NAT 检测(不能替代血清学)	需要,存在高危因素时进行 NAT	需要,存在高危因素时进行 NAT
乙型肝炎病毒	HBsAg,抗 HBcAb*	HBV DNA(不能替代血清学)	需要,存在高危因素时进行 NAT	需要,存在高危因素时进行 NAT
丙型肝炎病毒	抗 HCV*	NAT 检测(不能替代血清学)	需要,存在高危因素时进行 NAT	需要,存在高危因素时进行 NAT
梅毒	RPR 或 VDRL*		需要	需要
EB 病毒	EB 病毒抗体检测*		需要	需要
细菌	血培养、尿培养*	呼吸道分泌物培养	需要	不需要
HTLV 1 和 HIV 2	血清学	NAT		
西尼罗河病毒	血清学	NAT		
弓形体	血清学		心脏供体	
克氏锥虫	血清学(EIA、IFA)	外周血涂片、NAT		
类圆线虫	血清学	粪便寄生虫卵		
利什曼原虫	血清学			
疟原虫	外周血涂片	抗原检测		
血吸虫	尿液或粪便寄生虫卵	血清学	肾脏供体	肾脏供体
结核分枝杆菌	PPD 实验	干扰素-γ 释放测定	不需要	需要
球孢菌	血清学(免疫扩散、补体结合)	抗原检测		
组织胞浆菌	血清学(免疫扩散、补体结合)	尿或血清抗原		

*美国国家器官获取和移植网络科学登记系统要求的检测项目。

NAT,核酸扩增检测;HBsAg,乙型肝炎表面抗原;HBcAb,乙型肝炎核心抗体;HBsAb,乙型肝炎表面抗体;EIA,酶联免疫测定;IFA,间接免疫荧光测定;RPR,快速血浆反应;VRDL,病毒和立克次体性疾病实验室。

段，恰恰有些既往感染非常容易在移植后重燃,如 CMV 感染。核酸扩增试验(NAT)则多用于鉴定 HIV、HCV 和 HBV，因为 NAT 可以在机体发生抗体应答之前就检测到这些病原体。感染窗口期因病原体和检测手段不同而各有差异。研究表明,利用 NAT 可以检测出组织供体 7 天内发生的 HIV 和 HCV 感染,而抗体检测阳性则需感染发生 22 天和 70 天后[11](表 92.3)。最新的抗原抗体检测可以在 3~5 天之内就鉴定出 HIV 感染,但该类检测方法在美国目前还没有被批准用于器官捐献筛查[12]。供体来源感染性疾病的窗口期感染(指利用现有实验室检测方法未能检出的已实际发生的感染)比较少见。NAT 检测是尽早发现 HCV 窗口期感染的有效手段[13,14]。由于 NAT 存在假阳性从而造成供器官丢失,而且不是所有器官捐献组织(OPO)都可以

表 92.3 供体 HIV 与 HCV 窗口期感染对筛查检测的影响

		窗口期*血清学	窗口期*感染未被血清学检出的风险	窗口期*核酸实验	窗口期*感染未被核酸实验检出的风险
HIV	正常人群	22	1.72(0.63~4.40)	7	0.55(0.2~1.3)
	高危人群	22	8.54(1.52~23.99)	7	2.72(0.49~7.44)
HCV	正常人群	70	3.65(1.69~8.30)	7	1.16(0.53~2.61)
	高危人群(定义依据[19])	70	19.91(10.75~31.93)	7	1.99(1.09~3.23)

Adapted from Ellingson et al.[13], with permission from John Wiley & Sons Ltd.

*窗口期:病毒达到可传播水平至其可通过标准实验室检测(血清学或 NAT)被检测出的时间间隔。

进行 NAT，所以是否将 NAT 纳入供体 HIV、HBV 和 HCV 的筛查标准还存在争议。2009 年的一项会议共识指出，当供体有 HIV、HCV 和 HBV 感染可能时，推荐进行 NAT 检测[15]。

受体评估

由于移植后感染有可能来源于受体潜在感染再燃，也可能来源于供体，因此供体来源感染性疾病的鉴别诊断关键在于移植前受体评估。一些已知感染病史的供器官可能更适于分配给之前有相同感染病史的受体，如 HCV。移植前受体评估还可以帮助提前预防以降低移植后感染性疾病的发生风险，比如 HBV，这在一定程度上也扩大了供器官来源。美国 OPTN 强制要求受体进行 HIV、HBV 和 HCV 检测[16]。其他一些备选项目则包括 CMV 抗体、HTLV 1 和 HTLV 2 抗体，VDRL 或快速血浆反应素(RPR)(筛选梅毒)、EBV 抗体(病毒衣壳抗原或 EBNA)以及弓形体病抗体检测[17]。具有地域暴露特征的受体应进行寄生虫/原生动物(如锥虫和类圆线虫)或真菌(如粗球孢子菌和组织胞浆菌)的血清学检测，并可能因此而受益[17]。

明确供体来源感染的瓶颈难题

尽管供体来源的感染性疾病越来越被重视，但准确识别还存在很多瓶颈难题[18]。供体评估包括既往病史和社会史调查，对于死亡供体而言，很多时候并不能得到全面信息，这些不全面的信息会影响后续实验筛查手段的选择。实验室筛查手段也是瓶颈难题之一，如血清学检测要求合适取样时间点，NAT 检测方法并不适用于所有病原体。血清学检测和 NAT 检测存在假阳性与假阴性问题，血液稀释对检测结果也会有所影响。对于一些特定病原体而言，目前还缺乏标准检测手段。特别是对于那些有不明病因精神状态改变的供体应该进行仔细评估，如果其死亡原因中包含未被诊断出的感染性疾病，那么应该被排除在捐献人群之外(表 92.4)。

表 92.4　供体存在可疑脑膜脑炎和(或)异常精神状态时的主要感染病原体*

- 病毒
  - 淋巴细胞性脉络丛脑膜炎病毒
  - 西尼罗河病毒
  - 狂犬病病毒
- 细菌
  - 结核分枝杆菌
- 真菌
  - 球孢菌
  - 隐球菌
  - 曲霉菌
- 寄生虫/原生动物
  - 阿米巴

* 如果常规筛选结果阳性，应将供体排除。

知情同意问题

器官移植存在感染性疾病传播的巨大风险，受体应该在术前对此有充分认知。因此，OPTN 政策规定如果供体存在传播感染性疾病可能时，受体必须被充分告知[16]。根据美国公共卫生系统指南，如果供体有HIV、HBV 或 HCV 感染的医疗或社会高危因素，或者进行上述感染性疾病筛查时使用了稀释后血清样本，受体必须被充分告知其可能感染 HIV、HBV 或 HCV 的风险[19]。受体也应该认识到，供体筛查很难一应俱全，现有实验室检测还存在很多缺陷。很多时候，移植完成之后供体感染才被确诊，这种情况同样应该详细告知受体。

供体来源感染性疾病的相关报道

供体来源感染性疾病的相关报道日益增多。在美国，所有潜在的或已被证实的疾病传播都必须上报 OPTN 患者安全系统。疾病传播调查委员会将对这些病例进行分析，以明确供体传播风险[2,16]。这有助于移植中心对其他存在潜在感染风险的受体采取预防性措施。世界卫生组织倡议供体来源感染性疾病的规范化上报，以便建立数据库从而实现供器官的最大有效利用[18]。

特异病原体感染

细菌感染

供体来源的细菌感染并不常见，但会导致受体死亡率升高，特别是当它们诱发血管内疾病、吻合部位感染或弥漫性感染时。供体细菌培养如果为阳性,则可以同时反映其定殖部位,且转移至受体的风险最小[20]。大约有15%的供体会出现细菌培养阳性[20,21]。受体感染可能来源于供体血液、供体器官或污染的器官保存液。死亡供体通常在捐献前就存在多种细菌感染风险,如气管插管、静脉留置针、导尿管及重症监护室的长期滞留[22-24]。

细菌培养是否阳性取决于取材部位。有时候很难区分污染与真正的感染。比如,血培养分离出凝固酶阴性葡萄球菌、棒杆菌属、短棒菌苗属或芽孢杆菌属时,通常提示污染。但多份标本培养出同一病原体(即便是上述常见污染源),则可提示供体存在感染。

供体来源的细菌感染通常发生在移植后7~14天,也可能由于抗生素使用或其他治疗措施而延迟发生。另外,常见的院内或社区病原体并非来自供体。供体来源感染的确认需要从分子层面证实供体和受体存在相同菌株。在多位受体中找到与供体一致的微生物可以帮助确诊供体来源的感染性疾病[2]。

许多回顾性分析试图量化受体使用感染供器官时发生供体来源感染性疾病的风险[20,25,26]。一项研究回顾性分析了3322名供体,其中8.8%被确诊为“感染”[20]。感染主要见于肺脏,其次为血液、尿道、中枢神经系统、腹部伤口和保存液。虽然供体感染的发生率很高,但只有1.71%的受体发生了供体来源的细菌感染性疾病。大部分发生术后感染的受体,其供体细菌培养一般为阴性[20]。研究认为,如果在移植后给受体制订合理标准的抗菌方案,那么供体的细菌感染将不会传播给受体[25,26]。而且使用细菌感染的供器官不会影响受体和供器官的存活率[20,22,23,25-28]。因此,如果在移植术后7~14天给予受体规范敏感的抗生素治疗方案,即便使用存在细菌感染的供器官也是安全的。

患有细菌性脑膜炎的供体也可以被考虑允许捐献。一些研究表明,受体在接受携带有链球菌肺炎、脑膜炎奈瑟菌和流感嗜血杆菌的供体器官后,预后良好且并未发现传播证据[28-30]。而那些携带转移风险较高菌种,如李斯特菌、沙门菌、结核杆菌、金黄色葡萄球菌和铜绿假单胞菌的脑膜炎供体,是否可以安全使用尚未见报道。但一般认为这些供体发生细菌传播的概率很高,因此不建议使用[31]。

肺脏是一个特殊器官,因为易于被细菌定殖,在器官获取过程也非常容易被感染[32]。细菌可以通过供体肺脏传播给受体,但供体革兰染色阳性并不代表受体术后早期会发生肺炎[33]。一项回顾性分析表明,尽管超过50%的供体发现肺部感染或者细菌定殖,但发生细菌感染传播的供体比例仅为15%[34]。

由于现有报道太少,对于那些特定供体来源细菌感染的预后信息还很少。金黄色葡萄球菌和铜绿假单胞菌是造成吻合口感染和受体术后死亡最常见的菌种。也有报道指出供体金黄色葡萄球菌菌血症并不容易传播给受体[20,25]。铜绿假单胞菌更容易发生传播,还有一些病例报道指出铜绿假单胞菌感染可以导致受体死亡,并与造成移植物失功的血管并发症有关[35-38]。可能这些报道存在一定偏倚,但对于存在铜绿假单胞菌感染的供体应非常警觉,并对受体进行相应的早期抗菌治疗[6]。供体感染菌种如果存在多重耐药,则可能导致预防性感染措施失败,因为标准抗菌治疗无法完全覆盖这些菌种。当发生多重耐药细菌传播时,受体预后往往不佳,但目前并没有建议剔除这类供体[39-41]。

结核病

结核分枝杆菌已被越来越多地认为是供体来源感染的重要原因。结核感染主要发生在器官移植例数较少的发展中国家。但随着移民、全球化及器官移植在结核高发地区的推广,受体被潜伏结核或未被确诊的活动性结核影响的可能性也越来越大。美国和欧洲一些早期研究表明,移植受体发生结核病的概率为0.35%~6.5%,而其中供体来源的比例仅占其中的4%,这个数据可能有些被低估[42]。2005—2009年,美国OPTN报道了22例器官移植发生结核的病例,其中10例受体发生结核感染,2例受体死亡,均被证实与供体来源感染有关[1,2]。肺脏移植受体发生受体来源结核病的概率最高,而对于浸润性肺结核,所有移植器官类型都会受累[43,44]。

受体来源结核病是否来源于供体很难判断,因为结核可能存在肺外播散,供体筛查也很困难[44,45]。报道中常见的供体结核高危因素包括结核高发地区居留史、社会因素(无家可归或监禁史)、可疑病史(持续且无法解释的复发性肺炎),如有类似情况,需对供体进行更仔细的筛查[43,44]。供体不明原因的脑膜炎也可能与结核杆菌有关[44]。即便高度怀疑供体存在结核感染,明确诊断也相当困难。供体结核筛查依赖于感染暴露史和危险因素评估,但器官捐献时这些信息可能还很不详尽。体格检查和影像学检查(如胸片、CT)会有一定帮助。也可以在移植后进行痰液或组织 AFB 涂片检查，但因为不是常规评价手段，因此只有在特殊情况下才会实施。确诊感染一般需要 6~8 周甚至更长时间。如果想缩短确诊时间，必要时可以利用生物学方法进行结核杆菌培养和鉴定。

美国移植学会和加拿大移植学会已经形成会议共识并制定了结核筛查指南[46]。指南提及，由于全球结核病流行地区差异而很难进行标准筛查。即便不考虑地区因素，那些存在活动性结核杆菌感染的供体也应该被排除在外，因为其会导致受体预后不佳[17,45]。对于那些有结核杆菌潜伏感染的供体应用尚缺乏共识。目前还没有供体自动排除体系，因此必须认真权衡该类移植的风险和益处[17]。如何筛查和管理结核潜伏感染的供体，特别是在结核高发地区，目前还存在很大争议。死亡供体的结核筛查非常困难，目前还没有相应检测手段。在结核低发地区，应该充分利用病史采集、实验室检查、结核菌素皮肤试验或干扰素 γ 释放测定来评估活体供体的结核潜在感染风险[17,45]。如果供体之前有未治疗的潜伏性结核病，那么既往无感染史的受体应通过化学药物来预防供受体之间的传播。由于利福霉素会与免疫抑制剂相互作用，应避免使用[47]。在捐献前 1~2 个月内有活动性结核病病史的供体结核复发风险和传播给受体的风险均较高。使用该类供器官之前，应该充分评估移植的受益和风险，并且强烈推荐药物预防[17]。如果在移植后发现了供体活动性结核病，则应为受体制订相应治疗方案。

梅毒

所有实体器官移植都应进行梅毒血清学检查。因为存在比较成熟的治疗方案，血清学阳性或者既往病毒病史都不属于捐献禁忌。现有报道供体来源梅毒感染率为 0.15%[48]。受体免疫抑制状态可能会滞后梅毒血清学反应且不能用来诊断受体疾病。对供受体进行早期治疗可以阻止其临床进展[49-52]。未治疗供体来源梅毒的长期预后尚不清楚，但可导致疾病增加。那些接受活动性或潜伏性梅毒感染供器官的受体，应该根据指南进行治疗，并监测其对治疗的临床和血清学反应[7,53]。

病毒感染

病毒感染很容易从供体传播给受体。很多可以预见的感染，如 CMV 和 EBV，并不包含在这一章节中。关于这些感染将在第 94 章进行介绍，本章节主要关注那些容易被忽略的供体来源病毒感染。

供体来源的病毒感染存在独特挑战，因为在器官移植前很难明确诊断。很多情况下，病毒感染可能是无症状的，或者被当成其他类型感染，供体捐献前病毒感染有可能通过血液传播途径获得。因此，目前常规诊断方法不足以识别移植前病毒感染。即便在移植前后确诊了病毒感染，也面临着治疗措施不足的尴尬。

当供体存在没有明确病因的发热时，应怀疑病毒感染。特别是当供体存在精神状态改变时，应该怀疑是否存在病毒性脑膜炎和(或)脑炎。淋巴细胞性脉络丛脑膜炎病毒、西尼罗河病毒(WNV)和狂犬病病毒都可以通过供体传播给受体[54-56]。当高度怀疑上述病毒感染时，应进行详尽的病史采集(啮齿动物和昆虫接触史)、体格检查、脑部和腰椎的 CT 扫描或磁共振成像(MRI)。在明确诊断并且制订合适的治疗方案之前，应尽可能推迟器官捐献[17]。

因为很多供体病毒感染为潜伏感染，标准筛查方法很难检测。一般供体病毒筛查包括 HIV、HBV、HCV 和 EBV[17]。是否所有供体应该接受 HTLV 或 WNV 筛查还存在争议。一些情况下，WNV 的 NAT 假阳性结果可能会导致一些不必要的供体资源浪费[57]。因此，尽管组织样本库已经常规筛查 WNV，但供体器官评估的标准流程并不包含 WNV 筛查。在美国，由于 HTLV 感染率较低，HTLV 1 和 HTLV 2 也不是供体器官评估的强制检测项目。FDA 也已经不再批准这两种病毒的常规临床筛查[58]。

人类免疫缺陷病毒

虽然供体来源的人类免疫缺陷病毒(HIV)感染发生率很低，但 HIV 仍是最可怕的供体来源感染之一。在美国，HIV 感染的供体被排除在捐献系统之外，而且 HIV 在 1985 年便已被列为供体筛查的强制检测项目[59]。这很大程度上减少了供体传播感染的发生，但美国和欧洲仍有关于死亡或者活体供体来源 HIV 感染的零星报道[60-66]。受体感染的预后差异很大，随着获得性免疫缺陷综合征(AIDS)进展，受体很早便会发生移植物失功和死亡。在一定程度上，预后不佳也受双重感染(如 HCV)、有限治疗方式和术后免疫抑制的影响。在南非，经过严格筛选匹配，HIV 感染供肾已成功使用于 HIV 感染的受体[67]。

最近发生的HIV意外感染事件使得大众又重新关注讨论更合适的供体HIV筛选方案。死亡供体的HIV筛查应该包含详细的病史调查和严格的实验室检查，而实验室检查主要指血清学检测[8]。如前所述，NAT可以帮助检测新近发生的HIV感染，从而减少窗口期感染的干扰[11](表92.3)。因为最近的两个HIV传播事件正好发生于感染窗口期，因此NAT正被考虑列为强制性检测项目[63,64]。2008年，美国OPO的一项调查显示供体HIV筛查几乎都包含NAT检测[68]。但NAT不能完全替代血清学检测，因为那些接受HAART治疗的患者很难通过NAT检测到病毒存在。如果不联合血清学检测，很容易出现假阴性。

活体捐献相对而言更容易进行充分的风险评估，并且可以通过重复的血清学检测来规避窗口期感染。如果检测时间与捐献时间间隔很长，建议在器官捐献前重新评估检测。

供体未被检测到的潜在HIV感染发生率很难估计。从献血者的数据推断，一般风险的供体人群HIV发生率为0.10%，而高风险供体人群的HIV发生率为0.50%[13]。血清学检测既应该考虑如何最大程度降低HIV传播风险，又应该避免因为自身假阳性造成的供器官资源浪费。美国OPTN要求充分告知受体，移植过程中所有可能的HIV传播风险[8]。指南也建议对于高危供体进行NAT检测，并对受体在移植术后1、3和12个月进行HIV病毒检测，以排除供体来源HIV传播[15]。

乙型肝炎病毒

尽管传播风险很大，但携带HBV的捐献者仍被认为是供体的重要来源，特别是在HBV发病率比美国更高的东南亚和欧洲部分地区[7,69,70]。大多数情况下，供体来源的HBV感染风险评估基于血清学测试。在任何器官移植中，HBV表面抗原和(或)HBV-DNA阳性的供体传播风险最高，核心抗体阳性的供体也可能传播HBV[71,72]。影响HBV传播风险与预后的因素包括移植器官种类、受体免疫状态、预防措施和免疫抑制剂[7,72-78]。

器官捐献者的HBV检测内容一般包括乙型肝炎表面抗原、表面抗体和核心抗体[17]。有时也会进行乙型肝炎核心IgM抗体和HBV-DNA测定，这些检测可以帮助筛查乙型肝炎窗口期感染，特别是对于那些高危供体而言更有意义[17]。供体血清学检测表明核心抗体阳性人群的HBV-DNA检出率为1.6%[79,80]。值得注意的是HBV-DNA水平通常较低，有研究表明仅有36%的表面抗原阳性个体可以同时检测到HBV-DNA。因此仅仅通过DNA检测筛查并不能完全识别出供体HBV感染[79-81]。目前为止，只有1例病例报道HBV抗体阴性和DNA复制水平低下状态下造成了移植后感染，1例多器官供体在5例非免疫状态受体中造成了3例感染HBV[82]。目前没有对乙肝病毒核心蛋白δ的检测要求，也不清楚其表达阳性的HBV供体是否存在更高的传播风险。

目前，由于传播风险极高，乙型肝炎表面抗原、核心IgM和(或)HBV-DNA阳性的供体被建议排除在捐献之外，除非受体存在危及生命情况[7]。而表面抗体和(或)核心抗体阳性的供体在某些情况下则可以被使用[7]。

肝脏移植受体接受HBV核心抗体阳性供肝发生乙型肝炎的风险极大，在没有预防措施的情况下其发生率可以高达33%~100%[72]。而对于其他种类的器官移植，如果供体核心抗体阳性，受体的HBV感染率很低，且长期预后和移植物存活率也很好[70,73,83-88]。预先免疫可以减少感染传播的发生。受体的感染病史(表面和核心抗体均阳性)可能比疫苗具有更大的保护作用[73,76,87]。但HBV疫苗仍然是一种重要的预防措施，特别是在供体核心抗体阳性的情况下[7]。抗体水平会影响感染传播效率，抗体水平减小至200mIU/mL以下时应加强剂量[75,78]。

抗病毒药物和免疫球蛋白在防治核心抗体阳性供体的HBV传播中同样发挥重要作用，尤其是肝脏移植患者，传染病和有症状疾病发生率急剧下降时[72,74,76,77,89]。目前还没有最优预防策略，很多中心采用早期联合乙型肝炎免疫球蛋白与抗肝炎药物(拉米夫定)的策略[90]。对于非肝脏移植的受体则没有具体建议。

识别供体来源的乙型肝炎可能很困难，特别是感染可能在移植后60个月之后才会发生[72]。新发感染一定程度上可以反映受体免疫状态。没有乙型肝炎病史的受体发生新发感染的平均时间为14.7个月；而对于表面抗体和核心抗体阳性的受体，发生新发感染的平均时间为23.7个月[76]。正因为如此，建议潜在的移植感染受体，特别是肝脏移植患者，在术后5年内每3个月进行乙型肝炎表面抗原、表面抗体、核心抗体和HBV-DNA检测[72]。

丙型肝炎病毒

HCV在供受体间的传播已经被充分认知多年[91-93]。与HBV不同，受体的HCV感染率为50%~93%[92,94-97]。

许多因素会影响 HCV 传播，特别是对于非肝脏移植受体。这些因素主要包括供体是否存在病毒血症及其严重程度[97]。并不是所有抗体阳性的供体都存在病毒血症，如果移植器官不是肝脏，供体又没有病毒血症，那么传播 HCV 的概率非常低[98]。器官保存方式也会影响病毒感染，脉冲式灌注被报道可以减少 HCV 病毒载量，从而减少肾移植时发生传播的风险[99]。

接受 HCV 阳性供器官的受体会发生很多术后并发症，而且其预后随 HCV 状态和移植器官不同而不同。发生 HCV 感染的肝脏移植受体预后一般较佳。一些情况下，供体存活时间与其是否存在 HCV 感染无关[100-104]。HCV 感染供器官与受体 HCV 早期复发相关，而 HCV 早期复发是影响移植受体长期存活与移植物失功的重要因素[103]。美国肾脏数据系统和 OPTN 数据库的回顾性分析表明 HCV 阳性供肾存活时间更短，与受体年龄无关；而且由肝病和感染造成的死亡在 HCV 阳性供器官中更为常见[105,106]。当受体是 HCV 阳性时，无论供体是 HCV 阳性或者阴性，受体预后相差无几[107,108]。因为使用 HCV 阳性供肾可以减少移植等待时间，这也提高了一些透析患者的生存率[106,109]。几项研究表明，与接受 HCV 阴性供心相比，接受 HCV 阳性供心的移植受体长期存活率较低，而与受体年龄及 HCV状态无关[110,111]。接受 HCV 阳性供心的受体易发生血管病变和晚期肝病。因此，HCV 阳性供器官（尤其是肾脏和肝脏）一般被用于 HCV 阳性或者生命垂危的受体[112]。

HCV 常规筛查包括抗体检测。NAT 也可以显著增加窗口期感染的检出率，应该常规用于 HCV 高危供体筛查[15]。NAT 最常用于有静脉注射吸毒史、性工作者和一些有高危性行为的供体[14]。一般不进行供体 HCV 基因型检测，对于供受体 HCV 基因型是否需要匹配也没有相应的指南规范。移植后哪种基因型更占优势往往取决于基因型本身，而与 HCV 数量无关。基因型 1 一般会占优势地位[71,90,113]。

西尼罗河病毒

近年来，人们越来越关注西尼罗河病毒（WNV）感染。这反映了 WNV 在供体人群中越来越高的发病率，以及其作为受体潜在感染源的进一步认识。实际上，供体来源 WNV 感染报道很少。真实的传播率也不得而知，因为供体 WNV 感染通常无症状，受体也通常不做 WNV 筛查。虽然大部分接受了感染供器官的受体会表现出临床症状，但是对于那些没有临床症状或者非典型临床症状的受体感染很难诊断。

不管供体是否存在典型临床症状，都可能导致感染传播[56,114,115]。血制品也是 WNV 传播的重要途径，有时正是由于供体使用了受感染的血制品后发生 WNV 感染，这也造成了识别供体来源感染的困难[116,117]。供体来源 WNV 感染造成的最严重后果包括神经系统症状和死亡，也可以不表现出临床症状[56,114,116,117]。也有供体 WNV 感染未传播给受体的报道。影响传播的危险因素还不明了。单个器官发生 WNV 感染的概率很低。受体的免疫移植状态对 WNV 感染预后有很大影响，有研究报道表明，对高危受体进行免疫球蛋白预处理可以改善预后[56,115]。

是否所有供体都应该进行 WNV 筛选还存在争议。尽管在美国，血液和组织捐献时常规进行 WNV 检测，但在器官捐献中并不常规检测。一些欧洲移植中心要求常规筛选 WNV[118]。检测方法主要包括血清学检测和 NAT。单一检测手段可能存在很大不足，因为不管是血清学检测还是 NAT 检测都无法完全识别潜在的受体感染[114]。地理因素和季节变化造成的干扰都会增加筛查困难。这时常规筛选会看上去意义不大。2003—2005 年，一项在加拿大艾伯塔省进行的大规模筛选没有发现 1 例确诊患者[119]。此外，基于 2002 年医疗决策分析的流行调查数据显示，假阳性造成了 452 例不必要的受体死亡[57]。所以没有足够证据支持需要对所有供体进行筛查。在 WNV 流行率较高的地区，容易获得抗体或者 NAT 阳性的结果。因为 WNV 感染与神经系统症状相关，因此那些伴有精神症状或者四肢无力、发热原因也没有明确诊断的潜在捐献者都应该被排除。

如果供体被发现存在感染，一些学者主张使用免疫球蛋白对受体进行预防[56]。但也没有足够的循证医学证据来支持上述措施。所以供体的合适筛选以及受体围术期管理都需要进行更详细的研究。

沙粒病毒：淋巴细胞脉络丛脑膜炎病毒

器官移植供体来源的沙粒病毒感染非常罕见，但其死亡率非常高[55,120,121]。淋巴细胞性脉络丛脑膜炎病毒是报道最多的一种，供体来源感染中至少有 1 例为新发沙粒病毒。因为大多数供体没有表现出临床症状，因此在移植术前筛查出感染供体非常困难，只有 1 例供体被报道有发热症状[120-122]。供体沙粒病毒感染也不被常规筛查。

受体感染最早可以在移植术后3~4天就发生肝细胞坏死、血细胞减少和脑炎等症状，而大多数受体基本在移植术后2~3周才会出现上述症状。一般会在移植后2个月内发生死亡[120-122]。有病例报道指出，症状出现后早期使用利巴韦林可以改善预后[120]。目前没有足够证据来常规推荐利巴韦林用于疑似获得供体来源沙粒病毒感染的受体。

人类嗜淋巴细胞病毒1和2

尽管流行病学有所不同，但由于相同的检测方法，HTLV 1和HTLV 2这两种逆转录病毒经常被同时进行检测。HTLV 1主要发生在亚洲、加勒比海地区、南美洲、西非和大洋洲部分地区，在北美和欧洲流行率较低。它会导致急性T细胞白血病和淋巴瘤、HTLV 1相关性脊髓病（HAM）和热带痉挛性截瘫（TSP）。HTLV 2主要流行于美国印第安人地区和非洲中西部，常见于静脉吸毒者和性工作者。它不会导致某种特殊疾病类型。即便在HTLV 1和HTLV 2流行国家，确诊的供体来源感染也非常罕见。可能这种感染传播大多数情况下并没有引起临床症状，或者没有影响预后[58,123-127]。当发生临床症状时，受体一般会在移植后2年内表现出神经系统症状（TSP/HAM）[125]。

是否对上述两种存在地理区域特征的病毒进行供体筛查也存在争议[58,128]。这一定程度上反映了现有检测手段的不足[58]。HTLV 1和HTLV 2的标准血清学检测方法为酶联免疫吸附测定（ELISA），但无法区分两种病毒。尽管这种方法灵敏度很高，但特异度很差，所以经常造成假阳性。一般也不会用蛋白印迹或NAT进行验证。每年由于假阳性大概会造成167~227个潜在供器官丢失[58]。2010年，美国FDA停止授权供体HTLV筛查。结合极低流行病学数据、对受体不良预后的微弱影响和不会造成供器官失功，OPTN在2010年也停止了受体HTLV筛查。在西班牙，HTLV筛查仅限于来自流行地区的供体[128]。

供体来源的真菌感染

真菌感染是移植后受体死亡的重要原因之一，但供体传播的真菌感染非常罕见。供体来源的真菌感染发生后可以导致器官失功与受体死亡[1]。供体传播的真菌感染可能与供体潜在感染、器官捐献过程中发生的血液污染或保存液污染有关。证明供体来源的某些真菌感染尤为困难，因为受体可能与供体存在同样的地理暴露因素。

念珠菌病

供体来源的念珠菌感染虽然不常见，但很重要，因为其可以造成移植物失功和受体死亡。腹部器官和肾移植受体的发生风险最高，这可能与念珠菌肠道定殖从而容易播散至移植物有关[129]。这些感染的实际发生率仍然未知；法国的一项多中心研究表明肾移植受体真菌感染发生率为1/1000[129]。

念珠菌感染的来源非常多样，包括血液、尿道、供器官保存液污染、腹部损伤或者肠破裂污液[20,129-132]。由于念珠菌常在十二指肠定居，胰腺非常容易受到直接感染[133,134]。供体来源的念珠菌感染较少常见于心肺移植[135]。念珠菌常定居于口咽部，供体的呼吸道分泌物可以培养出念珠菌，但其临床意义还不确定。供体培养阳性时吻合口念珠菌感染发生率不高，这可能与两性霉素B的常规给药有关，但吻合口念珠菌感染不应被忽略[34,135]。心脏移植中供体来源的念珠菌感染尚未见报道。

明确器官保存液中是否存在念珠菌感染非常困难，而且由其导致的感染发生率也很难估计。当器官保存液培养阴性时，发生感染的概率非常低，至少在肾移植中如此[136,137]。在肾移植受体中，器官移植保存液检出污染的比例为5%~23%，2%~10%归因于真菌[133]。大概4%的肝脏移植器官保护液可以培养出念珠菌[22,138,139]。

供体来源的念珠菌感染在肾移植受体中具有显著临床特征，而且一般在移植后第1个月便会出现症状[129]。其感染并发症非常多样，主要包括移植受体肾周集合感染、尿道瘤、肾盂肾炎、念珠菌病、手术部位感染以及血管受累等[129-131,140]。其他腹部移植器官最重要的并发症为血管并发症，可能导致吻合口破裂、动脉炎和真菌感染性动脉瘤，最终导致灾难性出血并伴随移植物失功或受体死亡[129,130,134]。

为了防止供体来源念珠菌感染带来的不良后果，对于那些接受念珠菌感染供器官的受体采取预防措施尤为重要，特别是肾移植受体。当在器官保存液中检测到念珠菌感染或有粘性穿孔时，专家建议进行为期2周的抗真菌治疗，并在治疗开始和治疗7天后进行影像学评估。如果没有真菌感染的表现，抗真菌治疗可在2周后停药[141]。存在临床症状或者培养阳性的受体，应该延长真菌治疗时间并重复影像学评估。因为肝脏、胰腺和小肠特别容易受到肠道菌群污染，一些移植中心推荐在器官捐献过程中将两性霉素 B 滴注到供体十二指肠[134]。其他移植中心可能会预防性使用抗真菌治疗。考虑到动脉炎和移植物失功，当胰腺移植供体培养阳性时，应该考虑对胰腺进行影像学评估。心脏移植很少进行供体保存液培养。因为肺脏非常容易发生真菌感染，因此抗真菌治疗是肺脏移植的常规措施。当肺脏移植供体念珠菌培养阳性时，受体需要进行系统性抗真菌治疗[34,135]。抗真菌治疗疗程取决于吻合口情况。如果心脏供体保存液中培养出念珠菌，因其与受体感染相关性不大，并不是进行抗真菌治疗的指征[142]。

尽管一些存在念珠菌感染的供器官被成功使用，但是基于一些潜在不良后果，存在未经治疗念珠菌血症和肾盂肾炎的供体不应被使用[20,25,143]。当供体有念珠菌尿时，发生传播的风险未知，其传播给非肾移植受体的概率应该非常低。

如果供体被怀疑存在念珠菌感染，那么应该尽可能进行基于药物敏感性实验的抗真菌治疗。氟康唑通常是抗真菌首选，因为它能被很好吸收并在尿液中达到高水平。另外，唑类不能在尿中达到高水平，因此当存在尿道感染时应尽量避免使用。因为棘白菌素代谢广泛，而且不容易渗透至尿道，因此应该被用于非白色假丝酵母菌感染（可能对氟康唑存在耐药）、肾外和肾实质疾病[144]。两性霉素 B 脱氧胆酸盐对大部分念珠菌感染都有作用，但是由于其潜在的肾毒性和不能在尿液中达到高水平，使之成为次选，特别是对于肾移植受体感染。肾切除患者可采取手术治疗或保守治疗，全面的抗真菌治疗和密切监测应尽早进行[130,131,145]。一般来说，必要时需进行肾囊肿穿刺引流，或当有动脉炎或动脉瘤时应尽快进行肾切除术评估。

隐球菌感染

隐球菌是一种普遍存在的荚膜酵母，但其造成的供体来源感染非常罕见。感染的主要传播途径为吸入传播。它在正常宿主中通常无症状并且主要在肺脏中潜伏，因此可以造成没有症状的供体来源感染[146]。

绝大多数移植受体的隐球菌感染并非供体来源，而是其自身潜伏感染的激活[147,148]。尽管不太常见，但受体来源的隐球菌感染在 1971 年就有被报道[149,150]。区分是受体来源还是供体来源的念珠菌感染非常困难，但是如果供体存在未确诊的神经系统疾病或脑膜脑炎，感染应怀疑为供体来源[150]。如果供体存在免疫抑制状态，如激素使用史、器官衰竭病史（终末期肾病、终末期肝病）、肉瘤状病、风湿病等，感染念珠菌的概率会非常高，供体应进行仔细筛查，特别是存在诊断不明的神经系统症状和肉芽肿肺病时。虽然大部分念珠菌感染来源于死亡供体，但是活体供体也有传播念珠菌感染的相关报道[151]。

供体的念珠菌感染非常难以识别，而且很难在器官捐献前诊断。当供体存在神经症状时，检测血清和脑脊液样本中的念珠菌抗原会有所帮助。供体血清念珠菌抗原阳性可帮助诊断，但如果为阴性也不能排除诊断。这时就需要进一步对供体组织和体液进行微生物学和组织生物学检测以明确诊断。当活体供体肺部具有肉芽肿影像学表现时，应该在术前进行详细的念珠菌感染排查[151]。一般来说，移植后第 1 个月发生的念珠菌感染通常是供体来源，但也应该认识到一些特殊类型器官移植，特别是肝脏移植，受体本身在术前就容易感染念珠菌。这在某种程度上会混淆感染来源。

如果供体被怀疑或者确诊念珠菌感染，则不被鼓励进行器官捐献，因为其可能增加受体发生严重疾病的风险。如果供体只有肺部感染，那么非肺脏受体感染的风险未知，因为供体肺部的感染可能还很局限而没有发生全身播散。如果在移植后才确诊供体感染，那么应该对受体进行抗真菌治疗。有 1 例移植病例报道，受体在移植术后进行了为期 3 个月成功的抗真菌治疗，没有表现出肺部症状，但这种治疗期限目前缺乏大规模临床证据支持[151]。供体来源念珠菌感染治疗应遵循指南和感染病专家意见[152]。

曲霉菌病

曲霉菌在日常环境中并不常见。它是移植后第二常见的真菌感染，但并不常见于供体来源感染[153]。供体来源的曲霉菌感染主要见于肺脏移植受体，最大问题在于缝合处感染与血管侵入。一项包含 197 例肺脏移植的研究表明在 5 例供体存在曲霉菌感染的前提下，即便进行了两性霉素 B 的雾化吸入预防，仍有 3 例受体发生了供体来源曲霉菌感染。其中 2 例为支气管肺炎，1 例为致命性纵隔炎[34]。

因为极少会考虑到曲霉菌感染，因此捐献前确诊曲霉菌感染很困难。但是当评估那些因为免疫抑制而处于曲霉菌高感染风险的供体时，还是应该将其纳入考虑。当潜在供体死于病因不清的神经系统疾病时，这一点更为重要。有2例关于供体来源曲霉菌感染的病例报道，2例供体本身也是实体器官移植受体，均死于脑出血[154,155]。因为预后不佳且容易造成移植物失供，因此当供体被确诊或者怀疑存在曲霉菌感染时，应被排除在捐献之外。

当捐献后供体才被怀疑或者发现曲霉菌病时，应该对受体采取预防性干预措施，比如唑类药物、伏利康唑、棘白菌素、两性霉素等。目前没有抗真菌治疗的规范指南。很多肺脏移植中心在移植后很长时间内采取预防性抗真菌治疗，直到受体呼吸道分泌物培养阴性证实没有曲霉菌感染定殖。这种预防性策略可以避免很多潜在的供体来源感染。

球孢子菌病

球孢子菌病在美国西南部、墨西哥北部和中南美洲的部分地区比较常见。一般通过吸入导致肺部感染，通常无症状，孢子通过血行播散[156]。大部分球孢菌病源于潜伏感染的重燃[157,158]。供体来源的球孢菌病发病率未明，一般认为其发生率很低。不管有没有表现出临床症状，活体或者死亡供体都可以造成受体球孢菌感染[159-162]。供体球孢菌病的发生率与其在流行病区的暴露有关。在一个位于流行区的移植中心，活体供体球孢菌血清学阳性率为2.1%[163]。

供体来源的球孢菌病会导致受体高死亡率，主要死因包括播散性感染、重度低氧血症以及在50%受体中都会发生的中枢神经系统感染[162]。球孢菌病感染可以发生在很多器官移植中，而肺脏移植患者感染球孢菌病的概率最高，预后与T细胞功能受损以及抗真菌治疗时长有关[161,164]。供体来源感染一般会在移植后第1个月发生，特别是当供体存在未被识别的活动性感染时。当存在免疫抑制不足和(或)抗真菌治疗时，发病时间也会延后。对受体使用伏利康唑或者伊曲康唑可以延缓受体感染进展[163]。

由于早期抗菌感染有助于预后，因此受体感染的早期确诊非常关键。如果死亡供体之前在流行病区长期停留，同时有诊断不明的神经症状、肺部感染或结节时，应该高度警惕供体来源球孢菌感染[160,162]。不幸的是，由于大多数人没有临床症状或者缺乏详细的流行病区暴露史，因此在捐献前很难明确球孢菌病诊断。不同血清学检测方法的灵敏度和特异度不同，培养物分离困难也加大了诊断难度。目前有很多可以用于球孢菌抗体检测的血清学方法，包括补体结合、酶联免疫、管沉淀和免疫扩散等。抗原检测、PCR和真菌培养可以检测活动性感染，但在供体中不太适用。因为每种方法灵敏度和特异度不同，所以抗体筛查应该联合多种方法[163]。血清学可以帮助检测死亡供体和活体供体的既往感染，但是对诊断急性感染存在不足，因为机体出现反应性抗体需要一段时间，特别是在使用免疫抑制剂的情况下[163,165,166]。当血清学检测阴性时，抗原检测可能发挥一点作用[165]。有时候也会要求进行组织病原学检测以诊断活动性感染。

尽管存在活动性感染的供体应排除在外，但球孢菌的既往感染史并不是绝对的排除指征，而且既往存在感染病史且目前没有活动性感染的供体已被成功用于肾脏与肝脏移植[163]。那些接受存在静息感染供器官的受体应该接受预防性伏利康唑和伊曲康唑治疗。如果已经在接受预防其他真菌感染的唑类药物治疗，则一般不需要再同时使用伏利康唑[167]。而对于静息感染受体，预防性抗真菌治疗的剂量与疗程还不清楚。一般至少使用1个月的100mg伏利康唑进行治疗，也有专家推荐加大伏利康唑剂量，并最少使用6~12个月[157,163]。因为疾病进展受供体感染程度、移植器官类型和免疫抑制程度影响，因此受体治疗方案应体现个体差异性，并向感染病专家咨询。

组织胞浆菌病

器官移植中组织胞浆菌病可见于各种地区，主要包括美国、亚洲和非洲。在美国，主要分布于俄亥俄州密西西比河沿岸地区。在流行病区，大约75%的居民会发生感染，但绝大多数都没有临床症状[168]。流行地区移植受体组织胞浆菌病的发生率为0.1%~0.5%，大部分被认为是既往感染重燃或新发感染，在移植后第1个月内发生的感染被认为是供体来源[168-170]。

供体来源的组织胞浆菌病发生率不得而知，即便在流行病地区也不会太高[171]。有推测认为流行地区的供体来源组织胞浆菌病感染率为万分之一[172]。当供体存在组织胞浆菌病时，不是所有受体都会受到影响，最可能受影响的是肾移植受体。一项流行地区的回顾性研究表明，大约0.1%的肺脏移植受体发生组织胞浆菌病[170]。但没有发现供体来源的感染病例，可能是由于术后常规抗真菌药物的使用。

目前关于供体来源组织胞浆菌病感染的报道也很少[173-177]。大部分受体会在移植后 2~3 周表现出供体来源感染，但也有术后 36 周才发生感染的报道。临床表现主要包括非特异性发热、移植物失功、全血细胞减少和体重下降。

考虑到供体来源组织胞浆菌病发生率很低，以及较高的人群暴露率，供体的常规筛查并不推荐；但应该明确存在活动性感染的供体，因为他们发生传播的概率很高[141]。供体组织胞菌病诊断需要多重手段，包括尿液和血清抗原检测、抗体检测（免疫扩散与补体结合实验）、相关组织的培养与组织学检测。为排除活动性感染，来自流行地区并且有不明原因肺炎的供体，应进行详细排查。因为感染播散主要累及肝脾，这些器官也应该包含在组织学评估中。流行地区活体供体的评估应该包括既往感染病史和不明原因的肺炎史调查、影像学检查和血清抗原检测。专家建议在器官捐献前对活动性感染进行至少 6 周的治疗[141]。因为抗体反应可能在 3 个月之后才出现，而且在免疫抑制的状态下可能延迟出现，因此在免疫抑制和早期感染的状态下进行抗原检测更为合适[178]。

对于疑似或者确诊的受体感染如何治疗，目前没有大规模的实验数据支持。专家认为如果通过培养或者抗原检测明确了供体感染，那么应该对受体进行 1 年的治疗[141]。如果组织学证据存在，或者供体抗体结合滴度大于 1:32，或者 H/M 沉淀素存在，那应该给予受体 3~6 个月的伊曲康唑治疗[141]。抗体滴度较低的那些没有明确感染的受体，术后进行血清与尿液抗原的监测有利于早期发现感染[179]。

寄生虫病

除弓形体病之外，大部分供体来源的寄生虫感染可能与地理区域和（或）供体风险有关。即便是在流行地区，这种感染传播也不太常见。很多时候很难将受体移植后的感染归因于供体，因为供体和受体可能存在同样的流行暴露史。对于那些来自非流行地区的供体，目前有零星的关于死亡供体或活体供体来源的寄生虫感染报道，包括供体锥形虫、类圆形虫、血吸虫、疟疾、丝虫病和华支睾吸虫[180-189]。因为不同病原体存在不同的器官嗜好，因此传播风险各有不同。比如血吸虫和华支睾吸虫大多发生在肝脏移植，而克氏锥虫大多发生在心脏移植[180,181,188]。通过对肝脏移植供体进行血清学筛查、外周血涂片、大便、尿液或组织中寄生虫卵检查，然后通过器官捐献前治疗可以避免感染发生[180,189,190]。因为很多检测手段不适用，对于死亡供体而言很难在器官捐献前确诊。应该留意供体的疫区旅行居留史，对于那些来自疫区的供体，必要时可以进行外周血涂片或组织穿刺活检。如果供体嗜酸细胞比例偏高，应该进行寄生虫血清学检测和预防性治疗措施来避免供体感染重燃（见表 92.2）。如果供体没有明确既往感染史，那么不建议仅仅依靠死亡供体高危暴露史便将其排除在捐献之外。

弓形体病

弓形体病主要由弓形虫引起，在世界范围内可见。主要流行于拉丁美洲与亚撒哈拉地区，法国也是高发区，发病率高达 90%[191]。美国为 10%~20%[192,193]。在美国，感染主要病因包括食用生肉或者未熟的肉、接触土壤和猫的粪便[194]。移植后急性期感染可能是供体来源的，可能是潜伏感染再燃，也可能是极少见的新发感染。

尽管有其他类型的移植传播，但是由于弓形虫对心肌的偏好性，心脏移植受体感染供体来源弓形体病的风险最高[195]。如果不加预防，血清学阴性的受体接受血清学阳性供器官后，发生感染并表现出临床症状的概率为 50%~75%[196,197]。受体血清学阴性是获得供体来源感染的最主要原因。在所有的心脏移植中，供体来源感染占所有感染的 60%左右[198]。

实体器官移植后弓形体病可能会导致严重疾病，常暴发性发作。没有预防治疗的前提下，一般会在移植后 3 个月内发生，没有特异性临床表现[195,199]。心肌炎、肺炎、脑脓肿、脑膜炎、脉络膜视网膜炎、肝炎、淋巴结炎和播散感染都有可能发生[195,198,199]。

供体感染一般都是潜伏感染，很容易通过标准血清学方法明确。由于美国流行率极低，即便是心脏移植受体也不建议血清学检测。加拿大的一项研究也支持这种举措。他们发现供体和受体的感染率都很低，由于标准预防措施的采用，新发感染率也很低[200]。因此在那些高流行地区进行筛查可能会更有效。

可以通过使用甲氧苄啶（TMP）和磺胺甲噁唑（SMX）、乙胺嘧预防感染发生，特别是那些高危受体（血清学阴性受体接受阳性供器官）[192,199,201]。TMP-SMX 的最佳剂量和疗程仍不明确。大多数研究每周使用三次 160mg TMP 和 800mg SMX [201,202]。目前指南推荐每天使用 TMP-SMX [192,203]。对于那些不能耐受 TMP-SMX 的受体，可以使用乙胺嘧啶、阿托伐琨和氨苯。在预防性治疗结束以后，很少会发生有临床症状的感染[199,203]。

可以在移植后 7.5+2 周左右，通过血清学明确供体来源感染的诊断，但单纯血清学转阴也并不能排除新发感染可能[198]。活动性感染可以表现为心脏受体的心肌感染和脑部环行强化损伤。相关的组织病理学检测、脑脊液中弓形虫抗体阳性、脑脊液或支气管肺泡灌洗液 DNA 阳性都可以帮助诊断[192]。磺胺嘧啶是一线治疗，也可以被克拉霉素、阿奇霉素或阿托伐醌替代[192]。

克氏锥虫(Chagas 病)

克氏锥虫是 Chagas 病的主要病原体，最常见于拉丁美洲。潜伏期通常较长，在潜伏期内通过输血和器官移植传播。在美国，大概有 300 000 例患者发生输入性锥形虫感染，主要发生于佛罗里达和加利福尼亚[204]。由于从拉丁美洲播散，其在欧洲、日本和其他国家也正成为潜在问题[205]。因为供体的病因学信息不足或当地流行率偏低，在克氏锥虫低流行地区很难诊断。

供体来源感染最常见于心脏移植受体，也可以见于肾移植并造成移植后受体死亡[206-208]。供体来源的克氏锥虫病一般会有非特异性发热和全身乏力。急性期感染与移植排斥症状类似，特别是在心脏移植[206-208]。

供体感染筛查主要通过抗体检测，大多数通过 EIA、间接免疫荧光抗体检测，有时也会用放射免疫沉淀方法[209]。由于单一方法灵敏度和特异度不高，一般会建议联合两种方法进行检测[209,210]。对于流行率低的地区不推荐进行实体器官供体克氏锥虫的筛选[209,211]。在美国，鼓励对来自拉丁美洲的供体进行筛查[209]。

因为供体感染发生锥形虫传播的概率很低，非心脏移植的供器官都可以被使用[209,211]。即便供体存在 Chagas 病，考虑到传染概率、花费和药物副作用，一般不推荐进行预防性治疗，但是推荐血清学监测和 Giemsa 染色 [209]。因为心脏移植传播率高，应尽量避免使用来自感染供体的供心。如果移植后需要强力免疫抑制时，其他器官移植类型也建议避免使用感染供器官[209]。如果怀疑锥形虫感染，应该及时联系 CDC，进行确诊实验并采取必要治疗措施[209]。

总结

虽然供体来源的感染经常不能被提前诊断或避免使用，但仔细的供体评估、相应干预措施都能将其可能带来的危害降至最低。移植中心和 OPO 应该意识到供体来源感染的潜在发生风险。如果怀疑供体来源感染那么应该及时联系 OPO 或移植中心，以便对接受同一供体供器官的其他受体采取干预措施，避免不可逆的损害。

(魏绪勇 译　徐骁 校)

参考文献

1. Ison MG, Hager J, Blumberg E, et al. Donor-derived disease transmission events in the United States: data reviewed by the OPTN/UNOS Disease Transmission Advisory Committee. American Journal of Transplantation. 2009;9(8): 1929–1935.
2. Ison MG, Nalesnik MA. An update on donor-derived disease transmission in organ transplantation. American Journal of Transplantation. 2011;11(6): 1123–1130.
3. Blumberg ECS, Taranto S, Taylor K, et al. Donor derived transmission events in 2010: a report of the OPTN Ad Hoc Diseases Transmission Advisory Committee (DTAC). American Journal of Transplantation. 2011;11(Suppl S2):458.
4. Fishman JA. Infection in solid-organ transplant recipients. New England Journal of Medicine. 2007;357(25):2601–2614.
5. Tuttle-Newhall JE, Krishnan SM, Levy MF, et al. Organ donation and utilization in the United States: 1998-2007. American Journal of Transplantation. 2009;9(4 Pt 2):879–893.
6. Humar A, Snydman D. Cytomegalovirus in solid organ transplant recipients. American Journal of Transplantation. 2009;9(Suppl 4):S78–S86.
7. Grossi PA, Fishman JA. Donor-derived infections in solid organ transplant recipients. American Journal of Transplantation. 2009;9(Suppl 4):S19–S26.
8. Network OPaT. Minimum Procurement Standards for an Organ Procurement Organization (Policy 2.0). [cited 2011 December 28]; Available from: http://optn.transplant.hrsa.gov/PoliciesandBylaws2/policies/pdfs/policy_2.pdf.
9. Eastlund T. Hemodilution due to blood loss and transfusion and reliability of cadaver tissue donor infectious disease testing. Cell and Tissue Banking. 2000;1(2):121–127.
10. US Department of Health and Human Services Food and Drug Administration CfBEaR. Guidance for Industry. Eligibility Determination for Donors of Human Cells, Tissues, and Cellular and Tissue-Based Products (HCT/Ps). 2007 [cited 2011 December 28]; Available from: http://www.fda.gov/downloads/BiologicsBloodVaccines/GuidanceComplianceRegulatoryInformation/Guidances/Tissue/ucm091345.pdf.
11. Zou S, Dodd RY, Stramer SL, et al. Probability of viremia with HBV, HCV, HIV, and HTLV among tissue donors in the United States. New England Journal of Medicine. 2004;351(8):751–759.
12. Sickinger E, Jonas G, Yem AW, et al. Performance evaluation of the new fully automated human immunodeficiency virus antigen-antibody combination assay designed for blood screening. Transfusion. 2008;48(4):584–593.
13. Ellingson K, Seem D, Nowicki M, et al. Estimated risk of human immunodeficiency virus and hepatitis C virus infection among potential organ donors from 17 organ procurement organizations in the United States. American Journal of Transplantation. 2011;11(6):1201–1208.
14. Kucirka LM, Sarathy H, Govindan P, et al. Risk of window period hepatitis-C infection in high infectious risk donors: systematic review and meta-analysis. American Journal of Transplantation. 2011;11(6):1188–1200.
15. Humar A, Morris M, Blumberg E, et al. Nucleic acid testing (NAT) of organ donors: is the 'best' test the right test? A consensus conference report. American Journal of Transplantation. 2010 Apr;10(4):889–899.
16. Allander T, de Lamballerie X, Simmonds P. A new arenavirus in transplantation. New England Journal of Medicine. 2008;358(24):2638, author reply 359.
17. Fischer SA, Avery RK. Screening of donor and recipient prior to solid organ transplantation. American Journal of Transplantation. 2009;9(Suppl 4):S7–S18.
18. Garzoni C, Ison MG. Uniform definitions for donor-derived infectious disease transmissions in solid organ transplantation. Transplantation. 2011;92(12): 1297–1300.
19. Guidelines for preventing transmission of human immunodeficiency virus

through transplantation of human tissue and organs. Centers for Disease Control and Prevention. MMWR. Recommendations and Reports: Morbidity and Mortality Weekly Report. Recommendations and Reports. 1994; 43(RR-8):1-17.
20. Len O, Gavalda J, Blanes M, et al. Donor infection and transmission to the recipient of a solid allograft. American Journal of Transplantation. 2008;8(11): 2420-2425.
21. Paredes D, Gambra MP, Cervera C, et al. Characterization of the organ donor with bacteremia. Transplantation Proceedings. 2007;39(7):2083-2085.
22. Cerutti E, Stratta C, Romagnoli R, et al. Bacterial- and fungal-positive cultures in organ donors: clinical impact in liver transplantation. Liver Transplantation. 2006;12(8):1253-1259.
23. Gonzalez-Segura C, Pascual M, Garcia Huete L, et al. Donors with positive blood culture: could they transmit infections to the recipients? Transplantation Proceedings. 2005;37(9):3664-3666.
24. Askarian M, Gooran NR. National nosocomial infection surveillance system-based study in Iran: additional hospital stay attributable to nosocomial infections. American Journal of Infection Control. 2003;31(8):465-468.
25. Freeman RB, Giatras I, Falagas ME, et al. Outcome of transplantation of organs procured from bacteremic donors. Transplantation. 1999;68(8):1107-1111.
26. Lumbreras C, Sanz F, Gonzalez A, et al. Clinical significance of donor-unrecognized bacteremia in the outcome of solid-organ transplant recipients. Clinical Infectious Diseases. 2001;33(5):722-726.
27. Battaglia M, Ditonno P, Selvaggio O, et al. Kidney transplants from infected donors: our experience. Transplantation Proceedings. 2004;36(3):491-492.
28. Kubak BM, Gregson AL, Pegues DA, et al. Use of hearts transplanted from donors with severe sepsis and infectious deaths. Journal of Heart and Lung Transplantation. 2009;28(3):260-265.
29. Little DM, Farrell JG, Cunningham PM, et al. Donor sepsis is not a contraindication to cadaveric organ donation. QJM. 1997;90(10):641-642.
30. Satoi S, Bramhall SR, Solomon M, et al. The use of liver grafts from donors with bacterial meningitis. Transplantation. 2001;72(6):1108-1113.
31. Issa NC, Patel R. Potential for expansion of the donor pool using liver allografts from donors with bacterial meningitis. Liver Transplantation. 2002;8(10): 977-979.
32. Low DE, Kaiser LR, Haydock DA, et al. The donor lung: infectious and pathologic factors affecting outcome in lung transplantation. Journal of Thoracic and Cardiovascular Surgery. 1993;106(4):614-621.
33. Weill D, Dey GC, Hicks RA, et al. A positive donor gram stain does not predict outcome following lung transplantation. Journal of Heart and Lung Transplantation. 2002;21(5):555-558.
34. Ruiz I, Gavalda J, Monforte V, et al. Donor-to-host transmission of bacterial and fungal infections in lung transplantation. American Journal of Transplantation. 2006;6(1):178-182.
35. Simkins J, Muggia V. Favorable outcome in a renal transplant recipient with donor-derived infection due to multidrug-resistant Pseudomonas aeruginosa. Transplant Infectious Disease. 2012;14(3):292-295.
36. Kumar D, Cattral MS, Robicsek A, et al. Outbreak of pseudomonas aeruginosa by multiple organ transplantation from a common donor. Transplantation. 2003;75(7):1053-1055.
37. Orlando G, Di Cocco P, Gravante G, et al. Fatal hemorrhage in two renal graft recipients with multi-drug resistant Pseudomonas aeruginosa infection. Transplant Infectious Disease. 2009;11(5):442-447.
38. Nelson PW, Delmonico FL, Tolkoff-Rubin NE, et al. Unsuspected donor pseudomonas infection causing arterial disruption after renal transplantation. Transplantation. 1984;37(3):313-314.
39. Martins N, Martins IS, de Freitas WV, et al. Severe infection in a lung transplant recipient caused by donor-transmitted carbapenem-resistant *Acinetobacter baumannii*. Transplant Infectious Disease. 2012;14(3):316-320.
40. Transmission of multidrug-resistant Escherichia coli through kidney transplantation — California and Texas, 2009. MMWR. Morbidity and Mortality Weekly Report. 2010;59(50):1642-1646.
41. Goldberg E, Bishara J, Lev S, et al. Organ transplantation from a donor colonized with a multidrug-resistant organism: a case report. Transplant Infectious Disease. 2012;14(3):296-299.
42. Singh N, Paterson DL. *Mycobacterium tuberculosis* infection in solid-organ transplant recipients: impact and implications for management. Clinical Infectious Diseases. 1998;27(5):1266-1277.
43. Winthrop KL, Kubak BM, Pegues DA, et al. Transmission of *Mycobacterium tuberculosis* via lung transplantation. American Journal of Transplantation. 2004;4(9):1529-1533.
44. Transplantation-transmitted tuberculosis-Oklahoma and Texas, 2007. MMWR. Morbidity and Mortality Weekly Report. 2008;57(13):333-336.
45. Subramanian A, Dorman S, Practice ASTIDCo. *Mycobacterium tuberculosis* in solid organ transplant recipients. American Journal of Transplantation. 2009;9(Suppl 4):S57-S62.
46. Morris MI, Daly JS, Blumberg E, et al. Diagnosis and management of tuberculosis in transplant donors: a donor-derived infections consensus conference report. American Journal of Transplantation. 2012;12(9):2288-2300. Erratum 2013;13(2): 528.
47. American Thoracic Society, Centers for Disease Control and Prevention, et al. American Thoracic Society/Centers for Disease Control and Prevention/ Infectious Diseases Society of America: controlling tuberculosis in the United States. American Journal of Respiratory and Critical Care Medicine. 2005;172(9):1169-1227.
48. Gibel LJ, Sterling W, Hoy W, et al. Is serological evidence of infection with syphilis a contraindication to kidney donation? Case report and review of the literature. Journal of Urology. 1987;138(5):1226-1227.
49. Caballero F, Domingo P, Rabella N, et al. Successful transplantation of organs retrieved from a donor with syphilis. Transplantation. 1998;65(4):598-599.
50. Cortes NJ, Afzali B, MacLean D, et al. Transmission of syphilis by solid organ transplantation. American Journal of Transplantation. 2006;6(10): 2497-2499.
51. Ko WJ, Chu SH, Lee YH, et al. Successful prevention of syphilis transmission from a multiple organ donor with serological evidence of syphilis. Transplantation Proceedings. 1998;30(7):3667-3668.
52. Steinmann J, Marggraf G, Buer J, et al. Syphilis-specific immunoglobulin G seroconversion after double-lung transplantation. Journal of Heart and Lung Transplantation. 2009;28(8):857-859.
53. Workowski KA, Berman S, Centers for Disease Control and Prevention. Sexually transmitted diseases treatment guidelines, 2010. MMWR. Recommendations and Reports: Morbidity and Mortality Weekly Report. Recommendations and Reports. 2010;59(RR-12):1-110.
54. Srinivasan A, Burton EC, Kuehnert MJ, et al. Transmission of rabies virus from an organ donor to four transplant recipients. New England Journal of Medicine. 2005;352(11):1103-1111.
55. Brief report: lymphocytic choriomeningitis virus transmitted through solid organ transplantation-Massachusetts, 2008. MMWR. Morbidity and Mortality Weekly Report. 2008;57(29):799-801.
56. Morelli MC, Sambri V, Grazi GL, et al. Absence of neuroinvasive disease in a liver transplant recipient who acquired West Nile virus (WNV) infection from the organ donor and who received WNV antibodies prophylactically. Clinical Infectious Diseases. 2010;51(4):e34-e37.
57. Kiberd BA, Forward K. Screening for West Nile virus in organ transplantation: a medical decision analysis. American Journal of Transplantation. 2004;4(8): 1296-1301.
58. Kaul DR, Taranto S, Alexander C, et al. Donor screening for human T-cell lymphotrophic virus 1/2: changing paradigms for changing testing capacity. American Journal of Transplantation. 2010;10(2):207-213.
59. Turkowski-Duhem A, Kamar N, Cointault O, et al. Predictive factors of postrenal transplant anemia. Transplantation Proceedings. 2005;37(2): 1009-1011.
60. Human immunodeficiency virus infection transmitted from an organ donor screened for HIV antibody-North Carolina. MMWR. Morbidity and Mortality Weekly Report. 1987;36(20):306-308.
61. Simonds RJ, Holmberg SD, Hurwitz RL, et al. Transmission of human immunodeficiency virus type 1 from a seronegative organ and tissue donor. New England Journal of Medicine. 1992;326(11):726-732.
62. Quarto M, Germinario C, Fontana A, et al. HIV transmission through kidney transplantation from a living related donor. New England Journal of Medicine. 1989;320(26):1754.
63. Ison MG, Llata E, Conover CS, et al. Transmission of human immunodeficiency virus and hepatitis C virus from an organ donor to four transplant recipients. American Journal of Transplantation. 2011;11(6):1218-1225.
64. HIV transmitted from a living organ donor-New York City, 2009. MMWR. Morbidity and Mortality Weekly Report. 2011;60(10):297-301.
65. Kumar P, Pearson JE, Martin DH, et al. Transmission of human immunodeficiency virus by transplantation of a renal allograft, with development of the acquired immunodeficiency syndrome. Annals of Internal Medicine. 1987; 106(2):244-245.
66. Prompt CA, Reis MM, Grillo FM, et al. Transmission of AIDS virus at renal transplantation. Lancet. 1985;2(8456):672.
67. Muller E, Kahn D, Mendelson M. Renal transplantation between HIV-positive donors and recipients. New England Journal of Medicine. 2010;362(24): 2336-2337.
68. Kucirka LM, Alexander C, Namuyinga R, et al. Viral nucleic acid testing (NAT) and OPO-level disposition of high-risk donor organs. American Journal of Transplantation. 2009;9(3):620-628.
69. Rosengard BR, Feng S, Alfrey EJ, et al. Report of the Crystal City meeting to maximize the use of organs recovered from the cadaver donor. American Journal

of Transplantation. 2002;2(8):701–711.
70. Salvadori M, Rosso G, Carta P, et al. Donors positive for hepatitis B core antibodies in nonliver transplantations. Transplantation Proceedings. 2011;43(1): 277–279.
71. Natov SN. Transmission of viral hepatitis by kidney transplantation: donor evaluation and transplant policies (Part 1: hepatitis B virus). Transplant Infectious Disease. 2002;4(3):124–131.
72. Avelino-Silva VI, D'Albuquerque LA, Bonazzi PR, et al. Liver transplant from Anti-HBc-positive, HBsAg-negative donor into HBsAg-negative recipient: is it safe? A systematic review of the literature. Clinical Transplantation. 2010;24(6): 735–746.
73. Mawhorter SD, Avery RK. Can donors with prior hepatitis be safely used for heart transplantation? Journal of Heart and Lung Transplantation. 2006; 25(7):805–813.
74. Cholongitas E, Papatheodoridis GV, Burroughs AK. Liver grafts from anti-hepatitis B core positive donors: a systematic review. Journal of Hepatology. 2010;52(2):272–279.
75. Lin CC, Chen CL, Concejero A, et al. Active immunization to prevent de novo hepatitis B virus infection in pediatric live donor liver recipients. American Journal of Transplantation. 2007;7(1):195–200.
76. Skagen CL, Jou JH, Said A. Risk of de novo hepatitis in liver recipients from hepatitis-B core antibody-positive grafts – a systematic analysis. Clinical Transplantation. 2011;25(3):E243–E249.
77. Nery JR, Nery-Avila C, Reddy KR, et al. Use of liver grafts from donors positive for antihepatitis B-core antibody (anti-HBc) in the era of prophylaxis with hepatitis-B immunoglobulin and lamivudine. Transplantation. 2003;75(8): 1179–1186.
78. Su WJ, Ho MC, Ni YH, et al. High-titer antibody to hepatitis B surface antigen before liver transplantation can prevent de novo hepatitis B infection. Journal of Pediatric Gastroenterology and Nutrition. 2009;48(2):203–208.
79. Hennig H, Puchta I, Luhm J, et al. Frequency and load of hepatitis B virus DNA in first-time blood donors with antibodies to hepatitis B core antigen. Blood. 2002;100(7):2637–2641.
80. Stramer SL, Wend U, Candotti D, et al. Nucleic acid testing to detect HBV infection in blood donors. New England Journal of Medicine. 2011;364(3):236–247.
81. Kuhns MC, Kleinman SH, McNamara AL, et al. Lack of correlation between HBsAg and HBV DNA levels in blood donors who test positive for HBsAg and anti-HBc: implications for future HBV screening policy. Transfusion. 2004; 44(9):1332–1339.
82. Centers for Disease Control and Prevention. Notes from the field: transplant-transmitted hepatitis B virus - United States, 2010. MMWR. Morbidity and Mortality Weekly Report. 2011;60(32):1087.
83. Madayag RM, Johnson LB, Bartlett ST, et al. Use of renal allografts from donors positive for hepatitis B core antibody confers minimal risk for subsequent development of clinical hepatitis B virus disease. Transplantation. 1997;64(12): 1781–1786.
84. Fong TL, Bunnapradist S, Jordan SC, et al. Impact of hepatitis B core antibody status on outcomes of cadaveric renal transplantation: analysis of United Network of Organ Sharing database between 1994 and 1999. Transplantation. 2002; 73(1):85–89.
85. Dhillon GS, Levitt J, Mallidi H, et al. Impact of hepatitis B core antibody positive donors in lung and heart-lung transplantation: an analysis of the United Network for Organ Sharing Database. Transplantation. 2009;88(6):842–846.
86. Pinney SP, Cheema FH, Hammond K, et al. Acceptable recipient outcomes with the use of hearts from donors with hepatitis-B core antibodies. Journal of Heart and Lung Transplantation. 2005;24(1):34–37.
87. De Feo TM, Poli F, Mozzi F, et al. Risk of transmission of hepatitis B virus from anti-HBC positive cadaveric organ donors: a collaborative study. Transplantation Proceedings. 2005;37(2):1238–1239.
88. Lai Q, Molinaro A, Spoletini G, et al. Impact of anti-hepatitis B core-positive donors in liver transplantation: a survival analysis. Transplantation Proceedings. 2011;43(1):274–276.
89. Satterthwaite R, Ozgu I, Shidban H, et al. Risks of transplanting kidneys from hepatitis B surface antigen-negative, hepatitis B core antibody-positive donors. Transplantation. 1997;64(3):432–435.
90. Gallegos-Orozco JF, Vargas HE. Should antihepatitis B virus core positive or antihepatitis C virus core positive subjects be accepted as organ donors for liver transplantation? Journal of Clinical Gastroenterology. 2007;41(1):66–74.
91. Pereira BJ, Milford EL, Kirkman RL, et al. Prevalence of hepatitis C virus RNA in organ donors positive for hepatitis C antibody and in the recipients of their organs. New England Journal of Medicine. 1992;327(13):910–915.
92. Tesi RJ, Waller K, Morgan CJ, et al. Transmission of hepatitis C by kidney transplantation–the risks. Transplantation. 1994;57(6):826–831.
93. Ong JP, Barnes DS, Younossi ZM, et al. Outcome of de novo hepatitis C virus infection in heart transplant recipients. Hepatology. 1999;30(5): 1293–1298.
94. Tugwell BD, Patel PR, Williams IT, et al. Transmission of hepatitis C virus to several organ and tissue recipients from an antibody-negative donor. Annals of Internal Medicine. 2005;143(9):648–654.
95. Wreghitt TG, Gray JJ, Allain JP, et al. Transmission of hepatitis C virus by organ transplantation in the United Kingdom. Journal of Hepatology. 1994;20(6): 768–772.
96. Pfau PR, Rho R, DeNofrio D, et al. Hepatitis C transmission and infection by orthotopic heart transplantation. Journal of Heart and Lung Transplantation. 2000;19(4):350–354.
97. Fabrizi F, Messa P, Martin P. Current status of renal transplantation from HCV-positive donors. International Journal of Artificial Organs. 2009; 32(5):251–261.
98. Aswad S, Khan NS, Comanor L, et al. Role of nucleic acid testing in cadaver organ donor screening: detection of hepatitis C virus RNA in seropositive and seronegative donors. Journal of Viral Hepatitis. 2005;12(6):627–634.
99. Zucker K, Cirocco R, Roth D, et al. Depletion of hepatitis C virus from procured kidneys using pulsatile perfusion preservation. Transplantation. 1994;57(6): 832–840.
100. Vargas HE, Laskus T, Wang LF, et al. Outcome of liver transplantation in hepatitis C virus-infected patients who received hepatitis C virus-infected grafts. Gastroenterology. 1999;117(1):149–153.
101. Marroquin CE, Marino G, Kuo PC, et al. Transplantation of hepatitis C-positive livers in hepatitis C-positive patients is equivalent to transplanting hepatitis C-negative livers. Liver Transplantation. 2001;7(9):762–768.
102. Velidedeoglu E, Desai NM, Campos L, et al. The outcome of liver grafts procured from hepatitis C-positive donors. Transplantation. 2002;73(4):582–587.
103. Ghobrial RM, Steadman R, Gornbein J, et al. A 10-year experience of liver transplantation for hepatitis C: analysis of factors determining outcome in over 500 patients. Annals of Surgery. 2001;234(3):384–393, discussion 93–94.
104. Burr AT, Li Y, Tseng JF, et al. Survival after liver transplantation using hepatitis C virus-positive donor allografts: case-controlled analysis of the UNOS database. World Journal of Surgery. 2011;35(7):1590–1595.
105. Bucci JR, Matsumoto CS, Swanson SJ, et al. Donor hepatitis C seropositivity: clinical correlates and effect on early graft and patient survival in adult cadaveric kidney transplantation. Journal of the American Society of Nephrology. 2002;13(12):2974–2982.
106. Maluf DG, Archer KJ, Mas VR. Kidney grafts from HCV-positive donors: advantages and disadvantages. Transplantation Proceedings. 2010;42(7):2436–2446.
107. Morales JM, Campistol JM, Dominguez-Gil B, et al. Long-term experience with kidney transplantation from hepatitis C-positive donors into hepatitis C-positive recipients. American Journal of Transplantation. 2010;10(11):2453–2462.
108. Ali MK, Light JA, Barhyte DY, et al. Donor hepatitis C virus status does not adversely affect short-term outcomes in HCV+ recipients in renal transplantation. Transplantation. 1998;66(12):1694–1697.
109. Abbott KC, Lentine KL, Bucci JR, et al. The impact of transplantation with deceased donor hepatitis c-positive kidneys on survival in wait-listed long-term dialysis patients. American Journal of Transplantation. 2004;4(12): 2032–2037.
110. Haji SA, Starling RC, Avery RK, et al. Donor hepatitis-C seropositivity is an independent risk factor for the development of accelerated coronary vasculopathy and predicts outcome after cardiac transplantation. Journal of Heart and Lung Transplantation. 2004;23(3):277–283.
111. Gasink LB, Blumberg EA, Localio AR, et al. Hepatitis C virus seropositivity in organ donors and survival in heart transplant recipients. JAMA. 2006; 296(15):1843–1850.
112. Levitsky J, Doucette K. Practice ASTIDCo. Viral hepatitis in solid organ transplant recipients. American Journal of Transplantation. 2009;9(Suppl 4): S116–S130.
113. Schussler T, Staffeld-Coit C, Eason J, et al. Severe hepatitis C infection in a renal transplant recipient following hepatitis C genotype mismatch transplant. American Journal of Transplantation. 2004;4(8):1375–1378.
114. Rhee C, Eaton EF, Concepcion W, et al. West Nile virus encephalitis acquired via liver transplantation and clinical response to intravenous immunoglobulin: case report and review of the literature. Transplant Infectious Disease. 2011; 13(3):312–317.
115. Centers for Disease Control and Prevention. West Nile virus infections in organ transplant recipients–New York and Pennsylvania, August-September, 2005. MMWR. Morbidity and Mortality Weekly Report. 2005;54(40):1021–1023.
116. Iwamoto M, Jernigan DB, Guasch A, et al. Transmission of West Nile virus from an organ donor to four transplant recipients. New England Journal of Medicine. 2003;348(22):2196–2203.
117. Centers for Disease Control and Prevention. West Nile virus transmission via organ transplantation and blood transfusion - Louisiana, 2008. MMWR. Morbidity and Mortality Weekly Report. 2009;58(45):1263–1267.

118. Capobianchi MR, Sambri V, Castilletti C, et al. Retrospective screening of solid organ donors in Italy, 2009, reveals unpredicted circulation of West Nile virus. Euro Surveillance. 2010 15(34): pii: 19648.
119. Tilley PA, Fox JD, Lee B, et al. Screening of organ and tissue donors for West Nile virus by nucleic acid amplification–a three year experience in Alberta. American Journal of Transplantation. 2008;8(10):2119–2125.
120. Fischer SA, Graham MB, Kuehnert MJ, et al. Transmission of lymphocytic choriomeningitis virus by organ transplantation. New England Journal of Medicine. 2006;354(21):2235–2249.
121. Palacios G, Druce J, Du L, et al. A new arenavirus in a cluster of fatal transplant-associated diseases. New England Journal of Medicine. 2008; 358(10):991–998.
122. Centers for Disease Control and Prevention. Brief report: lymphocytic choriomeningitis virus transmitted through solid organ transplantation–Massachusetts, 2008. MMWR. Morbidity and Mortality Weekly Report. 2008;57(29):799–801.
123. Nakamura N, Arakaki Y, Sunagawa H, et al. Influence of immunosuppression in HTLV-1-positive renal transplant recipients. Transplantation Proceedings. 1998;30(4):1324–1326.
124. Nakatsuji Y, Sugai F, Watanabe S, et al. HTLV-I-associated myelopathy manifested after renal transplantation. Journal of the Neurological Sciences. 2000; 177(2):154–156.
125. Toro C, Rodes B, Poveda E, et al. Rapid development of subacute myelopathy in three organ transplant recipients after transmission of human T-cell lymphotropic virus type I from a single donor. Transplantation. 2003;75(1):102–104.
126. Marvin MR, Brock GN, Kwarteng K, et al. Increasing utilization of human T-cell lymphotropic virus (+) donors in liver transplantation: is it safe? Transplantation. 2009;87(8):1180–1190.
127. Shames BD, D'Alessandro AM, Sollinger HW, et al. Cell lymphotrophic virus infection in organ donors: a need to reassess policy? American Journal of Transplantation. 2002;2(7):658–663.
128. Toro C, Benito R, Aguilera A, et al. Infection with human T lymphotropic virus type I in organ transplant donors and recipients in Spain. Journal of Medical Virology. 2005;76(2):268–270.
129. Albano L, Bretagne S, Mamzer-Bruneel MF, et al. Evidence that graft-site candidiasis after kidney transplantation is acquired during organ recovery: a multicenter study in France. Clinical Infectious Diseases. 2009;48(2): 194–202.
130. Mai H, Champion L, Ouali N, et al. Candida albicans arteritis transmitted by conservative liquid after renal transplantation: a report of four cases and review of the literature. Transplantation. 2006;82(9):1163–1167.
131. Matignon M, Botterel F, Audard V, et al. Outcome of renal transplantation in eight patients with Candida sp. contamination of preservation fluid. American Journal of Transplantation. 2008;8(3):697–700.
132. Veroux M, Corona D, Scriffignano V, et al. Contamination of preservation fluid in kidney transplantation: single-center analysis. Transplantation Proceedings. 2010;42(4):1043–1045.
133. Gottesdiener KM. Transplanted infections: donor-to-host transmission with the allograft. Annals of Internal Medicine. 1989;110(12):1001–1016.
134. Ciancio G, Burke GW, Viciana AL, et al. Destructive allograft fungal arteritis following simultaneous pancreas-kidney transplantation. Transplantation. 1996;61(8):1172–1175.
135. Kanj SS, Welty-Wolf K, Madden J, et al. Fungal infections in lung and heart-lung transplant recipients. Report of 9 cases and review of the literature. Medicine. 1996;75(3):142–156.
136. Spees EK, Light JA, Oakes DD, et al. Experiences with cadaver renal allograft contamination before transplantation. British Journal of Surgery. 1982; 69(8):482–485.
137. Veroux M, Corona D, Giuffrida G, et al. Acute renal failure due to ureteral obstruction in a kidney transplant recipient with *Candida albicans* contamination of preservation fluid. Transplant Infectious Disease. 2009;11(3):266–268.
138. Audet M, Piardi T, Panaro F, et al. Incidence and clinical significance of bacterial and fungal contamination of the preservation solution in liver transplantation. Transplant Infectious Disease. 2011;13(1):84–88.
139. Janny S, Bert F, Dondero F, et al. Microbiological findings of culture-positive preservation fluid in liver transplantation. Transplant Infectious Disease. 2011;13(1):9–14.
140. Laouad I, Buchler M, Noel C, et al. Renal artery aneurysm secondary to *Candida albicans* in four kidney allograft recipients. Transplantation Proceedings. 2005;37(6):2834–2836.
141. Singh N, Huprikar S, Burdette S, et al. Donor-derived fungal infections in organ transplant recipients: guidelines of the American Society of Transplantation, infectious diseases community of practice. American Journal of Transplantation. 2012;12(9):2414–2428.
142. Mossad SB, Avery RK, Goormastic M, et al. Significance of positive cultures from donor left atrium and postpreservation fluid in heart transplantation. Transplantation. 1997;64(8):1209–1210.
143. Zibari GB, Lipka J, Zizzi H, et al. The use of contaminated donor organs in transplantation. Clinical Transplantation. 2000;14(4 Pt 2):397–400.
144. Fisher JF, Sobel JD, Kauffman CA, et al. Candida urinary tract infections–treatment. Clinical Infectious Diseases. 2011;52(Suppl 6):S457–S466.
145. Canaud G, Timsit MO, Zuber J, et al. Early conservative intervention for candida contamination of preservative fluid without allograft nephrectomy. Nephrology, Dialysis, Transplantation. 2009;24(4):1325–1327.
146. Goldman DL, Khine H, Abadi J, et al. Serologic evidence for *Cryptococcus neoformans* infection in early childhood. Pediatrics. 2001;107(5):E66.
147. Husain S, Wagener MM, Singh N. *Cryptococcus neoformans* infection in organ transplant recipients: variables influencing clinical characteristics and outcome. Emerging Infectious Diseases. 2001;7(3):375–381.
148. Pappas PG, Alexander BD, Andes DR, et al. Invasive fungal infections among organ transplant recipients: results of the Transplant-Associated Infection Surveillance Network (TRANSNET). Clinical Infectious Diseases. 2010;50(8): 1101–1111.
149. Ooi BS, Chen BT, Lim CH, et al. Survival of a patient transplanted with a kidney infected with *Cryptococcus neoformans*. Transplantation. 1971;11(4): 428–429.
150. Baddley JW, Schain DC, Gupte AA, et al. Transmission of *Cryptococcus neoformans* by Organ Transplantation. Clinical Infectious Diseases. 2011;52(4): e94–e98.
151. Matsumoto M, Kita Y, Gocho T, et al. Successful liver transplantation from a living donor with asymptomatic pulmonary cryptococcosis. Liver Transplantation. 2011;17(3):351–353.
152. Perfect JR, Dismukes WE, Dromer F, et al. Clinical practice guidelines for the management of cryptococcal disease: 2010 update by the Infectious Diseases Society of America. Clinical Infectious Diseases. 2010;50(3): 291–322.
153. Minari A, Husni R, Avery RK, et al. The incidence of invasive aspergillosis among solid organ transplant recipients and implications for prophylaxis in lung transplants. Transplant Infectious Disease. 2002;4(4):195–200.
154. Keating MR, Guerrero MA, Daly RC, et al. Transmission of invasive aspergillosis from a subclinically infected donor to three different organ transplant recipients. Chest. 1996;109(4):1119–1124.
155. Mueller NJ, Weisser M, Fehr T, et al. Donor-derived aspergillosis from use of a solid organ recipient as a multiorgan donor. Transplant Infectious Disease. 2010;12(1):54–59.
156. Einstein HE, Johnson RH. Coccidioidomycosis: new aspects of epidemiology and therapy. Clinical Infectious Diseases. 1993;16(3):349–354.
157. Blair JE, Logan JL. Coccidioidomycosis in solid organ transplantation. Clinical Infectious Diseases. 2001;33(9):1536–1544.
158. Holt CD, Winston DJ, Kubak B, et al. Coccidioidomycosis in liver transplant patients. Clinical Infectious Diseases. 1997;24(2):216–221.
159. Tripathy U, Yung GL, Kriett JM, et al. Donor transfer of pulmonary coccidioidomycosis in lung transplantation. Annals of Thoracic Surgery. 2002; 73(1):306–308.
160. Wright PW, Pappagianis D, Wilson M, et al. Donor-related coccidioidomycosis in organ transplant recipients. Clinical Infectious Diseases. 2003;37(9): 1265–1269.
161. Brugiere O, Forget E, Biondi G, et al. Coccidioidomycosis in a lung transplant recipient acquired from the donor graft in France. Transplantation. 2009; 88(11):1319–1320.
162. Blodget E, Geiseler PJ, Larsen RA, et al. Donor-derived *Coccidioides immitis fungemia* in solid organ transplant recipients. Transplant Infectious Disease. 2012;14:305–310.
163. Blair JE, Mulligan DC. Coccidioidomycosis in healthy persons evaluated for liver or kidney donation. Transplant Infectious Disease. 2007;9(1):78–82.
164. Dierberg KL, Marr KA, Subramanian A, et al. Donor-derived organ transplant transmission of coccidioidomycosis. Transplant Infectious Disease. 2012;14(3): 300–304.
165. Durkin M, Connolly P, Kuberski T, et al. Diagnosis of coccidioidomycosis with use of the Coccidioides antigen enzyme immunoassay. Clinical Infectious Diseases. 2008;47(8):e69–e73.
166. Pappagianis D, Zimmer BL. Serology of coccidioidomycosis. Clinical Microbiology Reviews. 1990;3(3):247–268.
167. Keckich DW, Blair JE, Vikram HR, et al. Reactivation of coccidioidomycosis despite antifungal prophylaxis in solid organ transplant recipients. Transplantation. 2011;92(1):88–93.
168. Wheat LJ. Histoplasmosis in Indianapolis. Clinical Infectious Diseases. 1992;14(Suppl 1):S91–S99.
169. Freifeld AG, Iwen PC, Lesiak BL, et al. Histoplasmosis in solid organ transplant recipients at a large Midwestern university transplant center. Transplant Infectious Disease. 2005;7(3–4):109–115.

170. Cuellar-Rodriguez J, Avery RK, Lard M, et al. Histoplasmosis in solid organ transplant recipients: 10 years of experience at a large transplant center in an endemic area. Clinical Infectious Diseases. 2009;49(5):710–716.
171. Vail GM, Young RS, Wheat LJ, et al. Incidence of histoplasmosis following allogeneic bone marrow transplant or solid organ transplant in a hyperendemic area. Transplant Infectious Disease. 2002;4(3):148–151.
172. Assi M, Martin S, Wheat LJ, et al. Histoplasmosis after solid organ transplant. Clinical Infectious Diseases. 2013;57(11):1542–1549..
173. Davies SF, Sarosi GA, Peterson PK, et al. Disseminated histoplasmosis in renal transplant recipients. American Journal of Surgery. 1979;137(5):686–691.
174. Limaye AP, Connolly PA, Sagar M, et al. Transmission of *Histoplasma capsulatum* by organ transplantation. New England Journal of Medicine. 2000;343(16): 1163–1166.
175. Hood AB, Inglis FG, Lowenstein L, et al. Histoplasmosis and thrombocytopenic purpura: transmission by renal homotransplantation. Canadian Medical Association Journal. 1965;93(11):587–592.
176. Wong SY, Allen DM. Transmission of disseminated histoplasmosis via cadaveric renal transplantation: case report. Clinical Infectious Diseases. 1992;14(1): 232–234.
177. Botterel F, Romand S, Saliba F, et al. A case of disseminated histoplasmosis likely due to infection from a liver allograft. European Journal of Clinical Microbiology & Infectious Diseases. 1999;18(9):662–664.
178. Hage CA, Ribes JA, Wengenack NL, et al. A multicenter evaluation of tests for diagnosis of histoplasmosis. Clinical Infectious Diseases. 2011;53(5):448–454.
179. Wheat LJ, Freifeld AG, Kleiman MB, et al. Clinical practice guidelines for the management of patients with histoplasmosis: 2007 update by the Infectious Diseases Society of America. Clinical Infectious Diseases. 2007;45(7):807–825.
180. Martin-Davila P, Fortun J, Lopez-Velez R, et al. Transmission of tropical and geographically restricted infections during solid-organ transplantation. Clinical Microbiology Reviews. 2008;21(1):60–96.
181. Vincenzi R, Neto JS, Fonseca EA, et al. *Schistosoma mansoni* infection in the liver graft: The impact on donor and recipient outcomes after transplantation. Liver Transplantation. 2011;17(11):1299–1303.
182. Rodriguez-Hernandez MJ, Ruiz-Perez-Pipaon M, Canas E, et al. *Strongyloides stercoralis* hyperinfection transmitted by liver allograft in a transplant recipient. American Journal of Transplantation. 2009;9(11):2637–2640.
183. Hamilton KW, Abt PL, Rosenbach MA, et al. Donor-derived *Strongyloides stercoralis* infections in renal transplant recipients. Transplantation. 2011;91(9): 1019–1024.
184. Chiche L, Lesage A, Duhamel C, et al. Posttransplant malaria: first case of transmission of Plasmodium falciparum from a white multiorgan donor to four recipients. Transplantation. 2003;75(1):166–168.
185. Fischer L, Sterneck M, Claus M, et al. Transmission of malaria tertiana by multi-organ donation. Clinical Transplantation. 1999;13(6):491–495.
186. Menichetti F, Bindi ML, Tascini C, et al. Fever, mental impairment, acute anemia, and renal failure in patient undergoing orthotopic liver transplantation: post-transplantation malaria. Liver Transplantation. 2006;12(4):674–676.
187. Gupta RK, Jain M. Renal transplantation: potential source of microfilarial transmission. Transplantation Proceedings. 1998;30(8):4320–4321.
188. Ho JK, Lau WY, Liu K, et al. Liver infested with *Clonorchis sinensis* in orthotopic liver transplantation: a case report. Transplantation Proceedings. 1994;26(4): 2269–2271.
189. Lee KW, Joh JW, Kim SJ, et al. Living donor liver transplantation using graft infested with clonorchis sinensis: two cases. Transplantation Proceedings. 2003;35(1):66–67.
190. Sobh MA, el Sharkawy SE, Shokeir AA, et al. Effects of schistosomiasis on living kidney donors. Scandinavian Journal of Urology and Nephrology. 1992; 26(4):409–412.
191. Desmonts G, Couvreur J. Congenital toxoplasmosis: a prospective study of 378 pregnancies. New England Journal of Medicine. 1974;290(20): 1110–1116.
192. Kotton CN, Lattes R. Practice ASTIDCo. Parasitic infections in solid organ transplant recipients. American Journal of Transplantation. 2009;9(Suppl 4): S234–S251.
193. Jones JL, Kruszon-Moran D, Wilson M, et al. *Toxoplasma gondii* infection in the United States: seroprevalence and risk factors. American Journal of Epidemiology. 2001;154(4):357–365.
194. Jones JL, Dargelas V, Roberts J, et al. Risk factors for *Toxoplasma gondii* infection in the United States. Clinical Infectious Diseases. 2009;49(6):878–884.
195. Campbell AL, Goldberg CL, Magid MS, et al. First case of toxoplasmosis following small bowel transplantation and systematic review of tissue-invasive toxoplasmosis following noncardiac solid organ transplantation. Transplantation. 2006;81(3):408–417.
196. Ryning FW, McLeod R, Maddox JC, et al. Probable transmission of *Toxoplasma gondii* by organ transplantation. Annals of Internal Medicine. 1979; 90(1):47–49.
197. Fishman JA. *Pneumocystis carinii* and parasitic infections in transplantation. Infectious Disease Clinics of North America. 1995;9(4):1005–1044.
198. Gallino A, Maggiorini M, Kiowski W, et al. Toxoplasmosis in heart transplant recipients. European Journal of Clinical Microbiology & Infectious Diseases. 1996;15(5):389–393.
199. Fernandez-Sabe N, Cervera C, Farinas MC, et al. Risk factors, clinical features, and outcomes of toxoplasmosis in solid-organ transplant recipients: a matched case-control study. Clinical Infectious Diseases. 2012;54(3):355–361.
200. Gourishankar S, Doucette K, Fenton J, et al. The use of donor and recipient screening for toxoplasma in the era of universal trimethoprim sulfamethoxazole prophylaxis. Transplantation. 2008;85(7):980–985.
201. Baden LR, Katz JT, Franck L, et al. Successful toxoplasmosis prophylaxis after orthotopic cardiac transplantation with trimethoprim-sulfamethoxazole. Transplantation. 2003;75(3):339–343.
202. Munoz P, Arencibia J, Rodriguez C, et al. Trimethoprim-sulfamethoxazole as toxoplasmosis prophylaxis for heart transplant recipients. Clinical Infectious Diseases. 2003;36(7):932–933, author reply 933.
203. Keogh A, Macdonald P, Richens D, et al. Mini-dose trimethoprim with sulphamethoxazole prevents pneumocystis and toxoplasmosis infections after heart transplantation. Transplantation Proceedings. 1992;24(5):2263.
204. Bern C, Montgomery SP. An estimate of the burden of Chagas disease in the United States. Clinical Infectious Diseases. 2009;49(5):e52–e54.
205. Gascon J, Bern C, Pinazo MJ. Chagas disease in Spain, the United States and other non-endemic countries. Acta Tropica. 2010;115(1–2):22–27.
206. Centers for Disease Control and Prevention. Chagas disease after organ transplantation–United States, 2001. MMWR. Morbidity and Mortality Weekly Report. 2002;51(10):210–212.
207. Centers for Disease Control and Prevention. Chagas disease after organ transplantation–Los Angeles, California, 2006. MMWR. Morbidity and Mortality Weekly Report. 2006;55(29):798–800.
208. Kun H, Moore A, Mascola L, et al. Transmission of *Trypanosoma cruzi* by heart transplantation. Clinical Infectious Diseases. 2009;48(11):1534–1540.
209. Chin-Hong PV, Schwartz BS, Bern C, et al. Screening and treatment of Chagas disease in organ transplant recipients in the United States: recommendations from the Chagas in transplant working group. American Journal of Transplantation. 2011;11(4):672–680.
210. Bern C, Montgomery SP, Katz L, et al. Chagas disease and the US blood supply. Current Opinion in Infectious Diseases. 2008;21(5):476–482.
211. Riarte A, Luna C, Sabatiello R, et al. Chagas' disease in patients with kidney transplants: 7 years of experience 1989-1996. Clinical Infectious Diseases. 1999;29(3):561–567.

第 93 章
器官移植围术期感染

Daniel Kaul, Michael Green

引言

感染并发症是实体器官移植(SOT)受体死亡的重要原因。并不受限于移植器官类型,一些特异性感染的发生时间是可以预测的,临床上大部分重要感染都发生在移植后 180 天内。移植后不同时间点的病原体感染及其症状有一定规律可循(图 94.1)。但某些特殊病原体(如 CMV)的临床表现可能会受预防策略、免疫抑制状态和二次手术等因素影响。根据发生时间,我们将移植后感染并发症分为三类:①早期感染综合征(移植后 0~30 天)、②中期(31~180 天)、③晚期(>180 天)。对于某些感染,如导管相关菌血症,只要其风险因素存在,就可以在移植后持续发生。尽管也存在其他特例,但这种分类方法可以有效指导 SOT 受体潜在感染的鉴别诊断。本章将重点介绍移植术后 30 天内发生的感染。我们还会讨论在这一时期常用的预防策略。关于其他感染并发症的具体介绍详见第 92 章和第 94 章。

我们将移植后围术期感染定义为发生在 SOT 后 30 天内的感染。在这段时间内发生的感染经常与受体原有状态、移植手术本身或手术并发症相关。此外,一些感染可能来源于供体(见第 92 章)。一般来说,细菌或酵母是该时期最常见的病原体[1,2]。50%或者更多比例的细菌感染发在移植术后早期[1,2]。这一阶段最常见的感染综合征为浅表或深部手术部位感染。对大部分器官移植而言,吻合口狭窄或渗漏是术后 1 个月内侵入性感染发生最主要的风险因素之一。鉴于大多数早期感染与手术部位密切相关,供器官是感染最常发生的部位[3]。胸部、腹部和尿道是胸部器官、肝脏、肾脏移植后最常见的感染部位。这些部位的特异性感染可以归因于局部缺血性损伤和出血,或手术过程中造成的污染[4]。

诱发因素

器官移植后早期感染的主要诱发因素可以分为两大类:一类来源于移植前供体,一类来源于移植术中和术后。

移植前因素

潜在疾病造成的供器官衰竭是 SOT 后早期感染的重要危险因素。如囊性纤维化病史可能使受体在肺脏移植术后早期感染假单胞菌和真菌;这类人群还很容易出现艰难梭菌定殖,继而使移植受体发生相应感染[5]。糖尿病是移植后泌尿系统感染(UTI)的危险因素[6]。移植术前姑息性手术病史可能增加移植难度,也会相应增加移植后感染风险[7]。移植时疾病的严重程度与术后发病率和死亡率相关[8]。例如,MELD 评分高的肝脏移植受体,其发生术后感染的概率也很高[9]。同样,围术期长期营养不良也会增加术后感染机会。当肠外营养纠正营养不良降低感染风险时,也会相应增加围术期导管相关的感染风险。等待器官移植时,入住重症监护室(ICU)和机械通气都会增加院内获得性病原体定殖与感染的风险,这些病原体很多都具备多重耐药能力,其造成的感染病程可能会超过 1 个月。

年龄是影响移植后特殊病原体易感性和感染程度的重要因素。那些年龄因素造成的病原体感染表现差异可能在移植后第 1 个月内并不显著。与大龄儿童或者成人相比,接受器官移植的幼儿在感染特定病毒时,如呼吸道合胞体病毒(RSV)或副流感病毒,其临床症状更为严重[10,11]。当术后早期受体还处于高度免疫抑制并且没有从器官移植中恢复时,情况更是如此[10,11]。较小的腰大肌是老年人体弱的标志,并与肝脏移植受体死亡率相关,而且术前体弱意味着更容易在术后早期发生细菌和真菌感染[12]。心脏移植中老年受体的年龄会增加早期感染发生风险[13]。

移植受体还存在从供体获取病原的风险，因为在器官捐献时供体可能存在活动或潜伏性感染。很多供体来源感染，包括细菌相关的供体全身感染[14]、西尼罗河病毒、类芽孢杆菌和新型隐球菌等，容易在移植术后早期出现。对于供体来源感染的讨论详见第92章。

术中因素

器官移植造成术后感染的术中因素各有不同。如肝脏移植中胆道重建方式会影响术后感染发生[15]。同样，胰腺移植术后不同引流方式与不同感染风险相关[16,17]。术中操作也会影响感染风险。术中膈肌、迷走神经和喉返神经损伤会影响痰液排出，从而增加肺脏移植受体发生肺炎的概率[18]。移植过程中移植物缺血过程会影响器官活力，增加感染风险。其他因素，包括较长手术时间、手术部位污染、邻近部位出血都会增加术后感染风险。不同器官移植外科手术的具体内容详见第55~64章。

移植后因素

围术期感染并发症最重要的风险因素是手术技术水平。肝脏移植后肝动脉易于形成血栓，并造成囊肿和血行感染(BSI)[19]；肾移植后膀胱输尿管反流易于发生肾盂肾炎[20,21]；胸部移植需要重新探查的纵隔出血易于发生纵隔炎和BSI[2]。

留置管道长期使用也是移植后感染的重大风险因素。中央静脉导管易于诱发BSI，导尿管易于诱发尿路感染，胆道引流不畅易于诱发胆管炎，气管插管时间延长易于诱发肺炎。留置管道的使用与移植术后感染在任意时间段都密切相关，但其在移植术后早期使用最多。因此，它是围术期感染的重要原因。

院内暴露也是移植后感染危险的重要因素。所有移植受体都存在感染输血相关病原体的风险，虽然这些感染都具有较长潜伏期，在表现出临床症状时已超过移植后1个月。儿童和部分成年人在冬季进行移植时可能暴露于常见季节流行性社区获得性病毒，如呼吸道合胞病毒(RSV)和流行性感冒。移植后早期感染已被证实可增加受体术后死亡率，特别是儿童移植受体[10,11]。医院重污染区的致病真菌如曲霉属菌种，会增加受体发生侵袭性真菌疾病的风险。多重耐药细菌的院内播散也极易诱发感染。

移植术后感染的风险因素还包括免疫抑制。虽然免疫抑制在移植术后早期不太重要，但依然是主要危险因素。免疫抑制方案总是期望能够在对免疫功能损伤最小的前提下控制排斥。然而，所有免疫抑制方案都会干扰宿主防御。排斥反应的治疗加剧了感染风险，使用抗淋巴细胞制剂或其他生物制剂会增加感染风险[15,22,23]。随着新型免疫抑制剂(特别是日益多样化的新型生物制剂)的不断引入，临床医生必须意识到SOT受体术后感染可能发生的变化[24,25]。

早期术后感染

移植术后早期感染并发症一般可分为两大类：SOT受体共有感染、某些器官移植特有感染(表93.1)。

大多数器官移植的常见感染

绝大多数器官移植早期术后感染来自细菌、念珠菌和病毒[26]。术后早期感染并发症一般表现为全身性败血症、血行播散或受累部位的局部症状，伴或不伴发热。早期感染通常与手术操作有关，因此也可以分类为浅表感染与深部感染。浅表感染可以发生在任何SOT受体中，主要影响手术部位的皮肤和(或)筋膜，很难与术后发生的伤口感染相鉴别。因此，这种感染的治疗与普通手术造成的手术切口感染类似。深部感染通常发生在靠近移植器官的部位，通常与吻合或其他使得移植复杂化的手术技术有关。因为移植器官部位不同、技术难题不同，因此深部感染与移植器官类型有关(见下文)。在本节中，我们更强调围术期感染发生的细节，而不关注移植类型。

医用导管相关感染

导管相关感染类型最主要是细菌感染，其次是真菌感染，可在围术期影响所有SOT受体。中心静脉导管(CVC)与中心导管相关血液感染(CLABSI)发生相关。只要中心静脉导管没有拔除，CLABSI的风险就会一直存在。大多数SOT受体只需要在术后1~2周使用中心静脉导管，但一部分患者因为营养需求、透析、有限的替代性血管通路或病情不稳定而需要长期使用。尽管目前存在一些可以长期使用的中心静脉导管，比如Broviac，或输液港植入以降低CLABSI的风险，但这

表93.1 不同器官移植早期感染的危险因素和预防策略

	危险因素	特异性感染	预防策略
肾脏	导尿管/尿路支架	UTI	避免使用导尿管/缩短支架使用时间
	糖尿病[6]		
	膀胱输尿管反流[20,21]		抗菌预防
	女性[57]		尿道囊肿造口术
胰腺	十二指肠残端	腹腔内感染±BSI	
	吻合口漏	UTI	肠道引流
	胆漏[16,17]		
肝脏	吻合口漏	胆汁瘤感染	T管引流可能增加风险(晚期感染)
	肝动脉血栓形成[19]	肝脓肿/胆管炎±BSI	超声和早期干预
	肾衰竭/手术时长/假丝酵母定殖/输血需求/胆总管吻合[74,75]	念珠菌病	抗真菌预防
	移植物功能障碍/入住ICU[15,78,79,112]	曲霉病	模式激活预防
肺脏	囊性纤维化/手术性神经损伤/长时间机械通气	肺炎	
	缺血	真菌吻合部位感染	抗真菌感染
	供体或受体病原体定殖[112]	曲霉病	模式激活感染
心脏	长期机械通风	肺炎	
	术后循环支持	BSI	
	再手术/出血/VAD[2,89]	纵隔炎	
小肠	使用mesh	腹腔内感染	
	二次手术	感染	
	黏膜屏障破坏(损伤或排斥)	BSI	

UTI,尿路感染;BSI,血流感染;VAD,心室辅助装置。

些患者仍存在较高感染发生风险,直到中心静脉导管被移除。一般来说,SOT受体CLABSI的治疗方式与非移植患者类似。美国感染病学会指南提供了一些基于病原体与患者临床表现的适当建议(包括未移除中心静脉导管时的治疗持续时间与可能效果)[27,28]。

艰难梭菌结肠炎

艰难梭菌结肠炎(CDAD)是一种可以影响所有SOT受体的潜在并发症。艰难梭菌是成人SOT后腹泻最常见的感染性病因。一般来说,SOT受体发生CDAD的比例比其他住院人群要高[29]。最新研究表明由于NAP1菌株的出现,该种并发症在过去十年发病率显著增加了大约5%[29-35]。当局限于儿童SOT受体时,器官移植后发生CDAD的比例为5%~13%[5,36]。大多数情况下,发生CDAD的中位时间小于30天[29,32,34,37],当然移植术后晚期也可以发生。移植早期CDAD常见风险因素包括抗生素使用、住院和抑酸治疗。在肝脏移植受体,再移植、高MELD评分、腹腔内感染并发症以及其他全身感染均与CDAD有关[29]。囊性纤维化患者更易于艰难梭菌定殖,也易于在肺脏或肝脏移植后发生感染[5]。CDAD一般不会造成SOT受体死亡或严重疾病,死亡发生率小于5%[35,37-39]。早期诊断和治疗可能会改善预后。CDAD诊断性检测一般用于移植术后早期发生不明原因腹泻时因为CDAD早期治疗可改善预后,并且免疫抑制患者的临床表现如腹痛、发热、白细胞增多可能是非特异性的。随着高度敏感的聚合酶链反应(PCR)和抗原测试发展,CDAD诊断测试方法也在迅速发展。相对之前的酶免疫测定(EIA),目前的检测方法可以提高检测效率。但是,即便检测结果阴性,还是应该对那些具有高度提示性的病例进行经验性治疗。

SOT受体的CDAD治疗与非移植患者没有差异,而且有可以遵照的指南作为参考[40,41]。如果可能的话,应该停用其他抗生素。在紧急情况下,可以在获得检测结果之前便开始经验性治疗[40,41],初始治疗和复发治疗方案均有相应推荐[40,41]。CDAD预防依赖于限制抗生素使用(用于治疗和预防)和感染控制措施,如洗手(使用肥皂、乙醇类消毒剂不能杀死孢子)和室内清洁中使用漂白剂溶液[41]。

多药耐药细菌感染

在过去十年中,住院患者多重耐药(MDR)感染发生显著增加[42-45],SOT受体也受到这种趋势的影响[46-48]。万古霉素耐药肠球菌(VRE)是一个主要问题,但对于大多数VRE感染患者目前有很多有效的抗菌药物。MDR(耐受两类或两类以上广谱抗菌药)和极耐药(XDR,对除了替加环素和黏菌素之外的药物均耐药)革兰阴性病原菌的出现是临床新问题,新的耐药抵抗机制不断涌现。因此,临床医生必须了解所在移植中心的耐药情况,并为移植后危重患者选择合适的经验性治疗方案。肝脏移植受体腹部感染和囊性纤维化患者术后肺炎发生MDR和XDR感染的概率很高。在一些情况下,存在MDR/XDR革兰阴性菌感染的移植患者死亡率可以高达90%,远远高于对药物敏感细菌感染的对照组[46,47,49,50]。对于XDR微生物而言,治疗非常困难而且经常存在肾毒性。可以采用联合治疗和早期研发的抗生素(如黏菌素)[48,49,51]。

与移植过程相关的围术期感染并发症

肾移植

肾移植后第1个月常见的致命性败血症感染大多数源于泌尿道下、呼吸道或移植伤口[21,52]。UTI,特别是肾盂肾炎,是最常见的感染并发症,大概占50%[53,54]。在移植术后早期,UTI比例大概为23%~45%[55-57]。常见风险因素包括女性(特别是对于后期UTI)、糖尿病(虽然最近的两项研究认为其不是危险因素)、高龄、反流病、急性排斥反应、输尿管支架使用、死亡供体供器官和泌尿系统先天畸形[6,57-59]。移植后1个月内长期使用导尿管是特别重要的风险因素[60]。大肠杆菌是最常见的病原体,肠球菌属和其他革兰阴性细菌也有相关报道。真菌病原体则主要是念珠菌,但不足所有感染的5%。耐药细菌(例如绿脓杆菌)和产广谱β-内酰胺酶(ESBL)的病原体通常见于移植后早期,可能与院内更容易接触耐药病原体及围术期抗生素使用有关[56,59,61]。每个移植中心的耐药细菌谱各不相同;对于移植术后早期UTI选择合适的经验性治疗取决于移植中心的抗生素耐药模式。UTI会导致额外抗生素治疗,住院时间延长,急性肾盂肾炎败血症等,但其对移植器官功能长期预后和移植受体死亡率的影响存在争议[6,57-59,62]。通过输尿管囊肿切除术和每日预防性使用甲氧苄啶/磺胺甲噁唑(TMP-SMX)可能会减少肾移植受体UTI的发生率(参见下文"肾移植受体UTI预防")[20,63,64]。

肝脏移植

肝脏移植常见细菌和真菌感染[65-68]。腹腔感染或中心静脉导管的存在易于发生BSI。肠道革兰阴性病原(通常是MDR)占感染一半以上。涉及腹部或手术伤口的细菌感染特别常见。移植后胆道并发症及其所致的感染也是主要问题,其中吻合口漏和肝动脉血栓形成是最重要的影响因素,胆道狭窄则主要发生于移植术后后期。研究报道胆漏率为4.9%~18%,晚期胆漏通常与T管拔除有关[69-72]。在许多情况下吻合口胆漏通过保守治疗可以好转,也不会发生感染。但还是有部分患者会发展为胆汁瘤感染,并且需要长期重复的抗生素治疗与引流。在这种情况下,MDR感染比较常见。肝动脉血栓形成可能导致胆漏、肝坏死并产生脓肿,但其发生率低于2%[72]。在一些移植中心,移植后早期应用多普勒监测血栓形成,并结合血栓切除术和溶栓治疗,可以有效消除肝动脉血栓形成和移植物感染。

由念珠菌之外病原体造成的真菌感染在肝脏移植后第1个月并不常见[26,73]。最近一项研究表明,成年肝脏移植受体7%的真菌感染源于隐球菌且术后45未发生感染[73]。可能受体在移植前就存在亚临床感染或感染源于供体。相反,念珠菌感染(典型的念珠菌病,伴或不伴有传播)更易在术后早期发生。研究表明,成人肝脏移植受体感染念珠菌的风险非常高[74,75]。危险因素包括肾衰竭、手术时长、再移植或手术并发症、念珠菌定殖、高输血需求以及胆总管空肠吻合[74,75]。基于这些风险因素,大多数移植中心对高风险成人患者制订了抗真菌预防措施,通常为1个月或直到危险因素解决(详见下文"抗真菌预防")[75,76]。

肝脏移植后侵袭性曲霉病罕见,受体发生率低于2%[77-79]。其多会发生在移植后早期。这些患者一般移植术后病情不平稳。早期曲霉病风险因素包括再移植、透析、移植物功能障碍和持续的ICU护理需求。侵袭性曲霉病之前较多发生在接受肝脏移植的囊性纤维化儿童[67]。发生侵袭性曲霉病的肝脏移植受体预后往往很差[78,79]。

小肠移植

成人和儿童患者小肠移植例数不断增加,许多病例为肝肠联合移植或多脏器移植。细菌感染经常发生在小肠移植患者,特别在移植后第1个月[1,80,81]。BSI

比较常见，可能归因于损伤或排斥造成的黏膜屏障破坏[80,81]。凝固酶阴性葡萄球菌、肠球菌和革兰阴性菌肠道杆菌占大多数，偶尔出现 MDR 菌株。小肠移植受体在所有 SOT 受体中真菌感染风险最高[26]。这些患者在移植后的第 1 个月经常发生腹腔感染。因为关闭腹腔时移植器官太大，或移植时不能完全闭合伤口而使用网状物会增加感染风险。腹腔感染风险还与潜在性剖腹探查术有关。腹腔感染的治疗类似于免疫低下患者腹腔感染所使用的治疗措施。如果条件允许，建议收集排泄物和脓肿（术中或通过介入放射学）。经验性抗生素治疗应涵盖肠道革兰阴性杆菌和肠球菌。既往 MDR 感染或定殖史提示应尽可能保证使用涵盖这些病原体的敏感药物。特别是在患者存在脓毒性休克表现或病情波动时。因此，小肠移植人群经常使用的抗生素为碳青霉烯（抗革兰阴性杆菌）或利奈唑胺（用于抗万古霉素肠球菌）。然而，一旦得到培养结果和药敏数据，应尽量缩窄抗菌谱。

心脏移植

感染是心脏移植术后围术期死亡的重要原因。据报道，此期间感染发生率高达 22%[82]，其他研究结果则表明感染造成的心脏移植术后早期死亡占 11%~18%[82-86]。早期感染常见部位包括肺脏、血液、胸骨和尿道[13,82,83]。术后循环支持，如体外膜氧合、主动脉内球囊泵、左心室辅助设备（LVAD）等，都会增加导管或设备相关感染风险[87]。在大多数心脏移植受体，下呼吸道感染（包括肺炎和肺脓肿）发生率非常高[13,83,88]。纵隔炎是心脏移植术后早期比较重要的感染类型，其发病率和死亡率均很高。心脏移植受体纵隔炎的发病率据报道为 2.4%~3.8%[83,89]。与纵隔炎最相关的病原体是金黄色葡萄球菌和革兰阴性肠杆菌。最近研究表明心脏移植受体接受 mTOR 受体抑制剂时，易于发生胸骨伤口感染和纵隔炎[82,89]。除了非移植人群的风险因素以外，还包括胸部重新探查、移植年龄、机械通气持续时间和移植前使用心室辅助装置[89]。非移植胸腔手术患者发生纵隔炎会表现为发热、白细胞增多和局部发红，而在移植受体中纵隔炎诊断相对困难。与胸骨切开术不成比例的疼痛是一条重要诊断线索。CT 扫描发现纵隔空气或液体可以进一步支持诊断，抽液或手术探查可以明确诊断。一旦确诊，应进行手术引流和清创术，并切除坏死组织。同时适当提供抗菌治疗。

接受心脏移植的低龄儿童发生侵袭性肺炎链球菌感染的风险比较高[90]。接受心脏移植的婴儿为另一种特殊人群，其发生细菌或真菌感染的风险也非常高。Backer 等报道超过 20% 的心脏移植婴儿存在严重的细菌感染[91]。与此类似，在匹兹堡接受心脏移植的小于 6 个月的婴儿中也观察到非常高的细菌或真菌感染率。此外，成年患者也可发生术后早期侵入性霉菌感染（常常为播散性），如曲霉菌病[83,92]。

作为移植桥梁的心室辅助装置，其使用频率不断增加[84]，与术后感染相关[13]。这些设备可能在术前就存在感染，利用抗生素慢性抑制这些感染可能导致 MDR 菌发生。此外，设备移除后仍可能残存定殖菌株，导致难以治疗的深部感染。

肺脏移植与心肺联合移植

成人和儿童肺脏移植和心肺联合移植术后 30 天内的供体死亡原因，感染占 10%~20%[93]。肺脏移植受体发生呼吸道细菌感染的风险非常高。肺炎是最重要的感染并发症，但却很难区分慢性定殖和呼吸道感染。革兰阴性病原体（通常为 MDR 菌）和金黄色葡萄球菌可以在表现或不表现临床症状的情况下被发现。影像学异常几乎普遍存在于肺炎或移植排斥患者[94-96]。因此，经常需要利用支气管肺泡灌洗（BAL）或支气管活检进行鉴别诊断。

由于囊性纤维化而进行肺脏移植的患者具有较高感染并发症发生率。他们通常存在假单胞菌或曲霉菌定殖。伯克霍尔德菌的定殖与受体高死亡率有关[97-99]。在囊性纤维化肺脏移植患者中，由于移植术前存在的病原体造成 BSI 非常常见[100,101]。因为这些细菌并发症治疗的重要性和困难性，大多数移植中心移植术前会进行供体微生物菌群评估。包括抗生素协同作用测试和实验室伯克霍尔德菌分离。

发生在术后早期的真菌感染常常使肺脏移植患者病情复杂化，偶尔也会在晚期发生于气道吻合部位[102,103]。所有 SOT 受体中，肺脏移植受体发生侵袭性曲霉菌的风险最高，而且是唯一一类曲霉菌感染比念珠菌感染更常见的 SOT 受体[26]。尽管如此，包括念珠菌病、深部手术部位感染和吻合口感染的早期念珠菌感染也会发生。早期真菌感染更可能发生在因为囊性纤维化而接受肺脏移植的患者，因为这些患者先前就存在曲霉菌定殖。早期真菌感染也可能是由于供体肺中存在的隐性或潜伏性真菌病。对于地方性真菌病尤其如此,如组织胞浆菌病和球孢子菌病。早期真菌病相对较高的发生率和临床预后不佳促使许多移植中心进行包含抗曲霉菌试剂的真菌预防[104]。

胰腺移植

胰腺移植主要适用于糖尿病控制不佳的成人患者,因此,一个风险感染已经存在。对于终末期肾病患者,还必须同时进行或顺序进行肾移植。胰腺移植或胰肾联合移植术后早期感染率比单纯肾移植要高,这可能与污染的供体十二指肠残端以及移植导致的坏死、感染、血栓形成、吻合口漏、免疫抑制需求增加和高排斥率相关。报道表明移植后45天内发生血行感染败血症的比例为16%,也是腹腔感染最常见来源[105]。改进手术技术并减慢血栓形成速率会降低腹腔感染发生率[106]。1.2%~1.4%的胰腺移植受体死于感染,使感染成为仅次于心血管疾病的第二位死亡原因[107]。胰腺引流可能通过供体十二指肠残端或内引流至膀胱。膀胱引流患者的UTI发生率也非常高[16,17]。胰腺移植受体发生真菌感染的风险比肾脏移植受体要高,可能与肠漏和UTI相关,比例分别为4%和1.3%[26]。

术后早期感染预防

术后早期存在多种预防策略。其中一些集中于预防围术期和早期感染性并发症,另外一些则旨在防治晚期感染性并发症。在高危器官受体中,如何进行一般预防或针对特殊病原体进行靶向预防都会详细讨论(表93.2)。

围术期抗菌预防

器官移植尽管已有40多年临床经验,但却有很少数据可以用来指导制订移植受体合适的围术期抗菌方案。围术期预防的一般原则是标准手术方案与特殊风险环境因素相结合。欧洲一项包含61家肝脏移植中心的调查结果表明,大多数移植中心赞成延长预防时间(中位时间3天),但在选择何种抗菌预防策略方面存在极大差异[76]。预防策略涵盖从相对较窄的β-内酰胺抗菌药物到联合新一代β-内酰胺抗菌药物(例如第三代或第四代头孢菌素或哌拉西林/他唑巴坦)与万古霉素治疗。虽然目前还缺乏临床数据支持,围术期预防方案还应该覆盖皮肤微生物(所有器官移植类型)和肝脏、胰腺和肠移植手术的肠革兰阴性厌氧菌和肠球菌。如果预先知道存在耐甲氧西林葡萄球菌、金黄色葡萄球菌(MRSA)、VRE和MDR革兰阴性菌定殖,制订围术期预防方案应体现个体化。

某些特殊情况应采用长期特异性预防。许多移植中心会在心脏移植受体覆盖呼吸道病原体,而且如果术前明确LVAD定殖或术后LVAD管道培养阳性,移植后一般给予1~2周治疗。对肺移植受体,如果供体BAL培养发现细菌或真菌病原体,那么应根据病原体药敏实验进行为期2周的抗菌治疗。当供体存在菌血症,或移植物或中枢神经系统存在感染的特殊情况下,应该改变预防药物或者延长预防时间。

肾移植受体泌尿系统感染预防

许多中心使用抗菌药物来预防移植后1~12个月内的UTI。最近一项荟萃分析发现20世纪80年代至90年代,抗生素预防可以降低败血症、菌血症和菌尿发生率,但对移植物长期预后无影响[64]。在一定程度上,超过80%的美国移植中心在移植后3~6个月使用TMP-SMX预防性治疗肺孢子虫病[108]。最近证据表明微生物耐药性(特别是尿液分离物中的TMP-SMX)限制了药物功效[61],并且降低了通过延长疗程进行UTI预防的意愿。增大抗菌谱,如加用氟喹诺酮,会产生一些严重并发症,如更严重的耐药性、没有可用的口服药物治疗UTI,以及其他不良事件和超级感染。

抗真菌预防

如上所述,SOT后侵袭性真菌感染风险因素相对明确,并且由于这些感染的严重并发症,很多移植中心会对高危人群进行抗真菌预防治疗。没有证据表明预防治疗会降低死亡率,药物相互作用和耐药性反而可能会限制抗真菌预防的受益。肺脏移植受体和高危肝脏移植受体最常应用靶向抗真菌预防策略。

肝脏移植

具有危险因素(见上文)的成年肝脏移植受体术后早期感染念珠菌的风险很高[74,75]。一些使用不同剂量氟康唑或伊曲康唑的随机研究已证实其可以减少真菌感染,但不能降低总体死亡率[109-111]。由于与CNI相关作用较少且药物递送率高,氟康唑一般优于伊曲康唑。氟康

表 93.2 器官类型相关非病毒感染的预防策略

	伤口感染	UTI 预防	抗真菌预防	PCP 预防[8]	弓形体病
肾脏	皮肤菌群[1]	大多数中心移植术后使用 TMP-SMX 1~3 个月	无	4~12 个月,如果有高危事件再延长 2~3 个月[2]	无
胰肾联合/单独胰腺	皮肤菌群[1] 肠道菌群[3]	对于单独胰腺移植不需要	无	4~12 个月,如果有高危事件再延长 2~3 个月[2]	无
肝脏	皮肤菌群[1]	无	高危成人受体[4]使用 1 个月氟康唑直到危险因素撤除	4~12 个月,如果有高危事件再延长 2~3 个月[2]	无
	肠道菌群[3]		超高危受体激活模式预防[5]		
肺脏	皮肤菌群[1] 呼吸道菌群[6] 供体来源或者受体自身病原体治疗超过 14 天	无	大多数中心使用模式预防[7]	最少 12 个月;或终身预防	无
心脏	皮肤菌群[1](一些中心包括受体定殖的 MRSA) 呼吸道菌群[6] LVAD 定殖	无	无	4~12 个月,如果有高危事件再延长 2~3 个月[2]	供体+/受体-IgG 血清学[9]
小肠	皮肤菌群[1] 肠道菌群[3]	无	无	最少 12 个月;或终身预防	无

[1] 用于皮肤菌群预防的抗生素主要包括头孢唑林和克林霉素。
[2] 巨细胞病毒,抗排斥的细胞耗竭治疗,高剂量皮质类固醇使用延长。
[3] 覆盖肠道微生物(革兰阴性+厌氧菌)的抗生素包括哌拉西林/他唑巴坦、氨苄西林/他唑巴坦和头孢西丁,这些也可以预防皮肤菌群。
[4] 肾衰,手术时间、非计划二次手术、假丝酵母菌定殖、高输血需求和胆总管造口术。
[5] 以上风险因素合并移植物衰竭、血液透析、长期 ICU 治疗。
[6] 涵盖呼吸道病原体的抗生素包括头孢吡肟和哌拉西林/他唑巴坦,这些也可预防皮肤菌群。
[7] 对霉菌具有活性的试剂包括棘白菌素、伏立康唑和泊沙康唑。
[8] 有些专家建议终生 PCP 预防。
[9] 单独使用 TMP-SMX,或联合氨苯砜、阿托伐醌、乙胺嘧啶、甲酰四氢叶酸组合。
UTI,尿路感染;PCP,肺囊虫;TMP-SMX,甲氧苄 -磺胺甲恶唑;MRSA,耐甲氧西林金黄色葡萄球菌;LVAD,左心室辅助装置。

唑每日 400mg 的剂量可能会有些高,许多中心采用较低剂量(每日 100mg)也可以取得令人满意的疗效。氟康唑预防应用增加了氟康唑耐药菌株比率[73]。肝脏移植后大约 50%的念珠菌属为非白色念珠菌[26,73]。由于非白色种类更可能为唑类抗性,因此需要使用棘白菌素治疗非白色念珠菌,高危患者的临床实验还在进行中。尽管存在药物相互作用、肝毒性、药物输送问题或其他不良事件可能会限制伏立康唑或泊沙康唑等药物在移植术后早期使用,专家仍建议对侵入性曲霉菌病发生风险较高的重症患者(二次移植、长期 ICU 滞留、移植物功能障碍、血液透析)进行早期预防[75,112]。值得注意的是,抗真菌预防并不适用于儿童肝脏移植受体。这可能是由于念珠菌感染在儿童肝脏移植中的发生率和预后有所不同。

肺脏移植

对于 SOT 受体,肺脏移植受体是侵袭性真菌感染发生风险最高的群体;侵袭性肺曲霉病(IPA)是这些患者最常见真菌感染类型[26]。因为IPA高发且后果严重，大多数移植中心都会对其进行预防[104]。但目前缺乏随机安慰剂对照数据来确认预防疗效。报道的结果也各不相同，因此没有成熟的推荐方案[112-115]。预防性治疗选择包括吸入性两性霉素、伊曲康唑或伏立康唑[112]。许多移植中心选择治疗3~6个月或持续至支气管镜下获得的真菌培养为阴性[104]。一些中心报道了伏立康唑延长使用后肝毒性发生率会有所升高[113,115]，以及其他不良事件如疼痛性骨膜炎[116]和皮肤癌的风险增加。考虑到唑类和CNI药物之间的相互作用，吸入使用两性霉素获得越来越多关注。其他移植中心试图对具有IPA额外危险因素的患者进行预防，如曲霉菌定居、细胞耗竭诱导治疗、CMV感染[112,113]。目前亟须多中心随机研究明确高危人群的最佳抗真菌预防方案。

肺囊虫预防

在常规进行预防之前，SOT受体肺囊虫肺炎(PCP)的发生率被报道为1%~88%，特别是胸部器官移植受体术后第1年[117]。因此，美国和欧洲指南都建议SOT后4~12个月进行PCP预防[118,119]。然而，一些专家也建议对于非免疫抑制的患者不进行预防。但考虑到肺脏移植和小肠移植受体的高风险，许多移植中心对这两类人群会进行终身预防。鉴于多达85%的美国移植中心目前在移植后进行至少3个月PCP预防[108]，免疫抑制状态下PCP发生率很难确定。然而，最近一些报道表明进行有限预防或不进行预防，低危人群(如肾移植受体)的PCP发生率比预期低，这也提出了新的问题，是否需要进行普遍预防[120-125]。有趣的是，一些报道指出人传人的PCP爆发在经过一段时间之后，发生率变得很低[121-125]。一种可能性是正好在PCP爆发期间观测到较高发生率。当存在PCP高风险因素时，如CMV感染、排斥治疗、细胞耗竭剂、高剂量的皮质类固醇，大多数移植中心会重新启动(或继续)2~3个月的预防。包含TMP-SMX的PCP预防非常有效。大多数试验未发现已治疗患者存在PCP[126]。每日两片或每周3次。儿童SOT受体的剂量为5mg/(kg·d)(甲氧苄啶组分)。一些移植中心倾向于每天使用单片片剂，并根据肾功能调整药物用量。TMP-SMX还可以同时预防虽然罕见但非常重要的其他潜在感染，如诺卡菌病和弓形体病。不能耐受TMP-SMX的患者可以每日50~100mg氨苯砜，1500mg阿托伐醌或者每月吸入300mg喷他脒。儿童SOT受体则建议根据体重计算药物用量。每周给予1次氨苯砜，剂量为2mg/kg(最大剂量100mg/d)或4mg/kg(最大剂量200mg)。对于阿托伐醌，剂量则需因年龄而异。4~24个月的儿童应接受45mg/(kg·d)，每天一次(最大剂量1500mg/d)，而年龄>24个月的患者应每天用30mg/(kg·d)治疗(最大剂量1500mg/d)。儿童吸入喷他脒的给药频率为每3~4周1次，小于5岁的儿童每次接受150mg的剂量，而大于5岁的儿童每次接受成人剂量300mg。

弓形体病预防

弓形虫通常潜伏感染在10%~20%的北美原生动物，其在世界其他地区的流行率也很高。最重要问题在于当血清阳性心脏供体移植到血清阴性受体时，SOT受体心肌中的潜伏感染会被激活。因此，所有心脏供体和受体都应该接受血清学检测，以确定是否存在高风险(供体阳性，受体阴性)。常规筛查对于非心脏供体和受体则不是必需的。PCP部分提及的TMP-SMX剂量同样可以有效防治弓形体病，但是一些移植中心倾向于给高风险受体每日给药[127,128]。不能耐受TMP-SMX的患者可以用氨苯砜或阿托伐醌，也可以与乙胺嘧啶或亚叶酸联用；一些移植中心则单独使用阿托伐醌。任何治疗方案都将同时提供PCP预防。预防时间未知很多移植中心预防治疗6个月至1年，但有些中心终身维持预防。

抗病毒预防

虽然由CMV、EBV、BK病毒(BKV)、乙型肝炎(HBV)和丙型肝炎病毒(HCV)导致的临床疾病直到SOT后期才表现出典型临床症状，但针对这些病毒病原体感染的预防策略在围术期就已存在。以下分别进行讨论。

巨细胞病毒

CMV的预防策略主要包括两种。普遍化学预防指在特定时间段对所有"有风险"的移植受体提供更昔洛韦或缬更昔洛韦的抗病毒治疗。目前的建议倾向于口服3~6个月的缬更昔洛韦，虽然有些移植中心选择更长疗程，特别是肺脏移植受体[129-131]。先行治疗是基于血液中检测到的病毒载量，在其处于亚临床感染时便启动预防性抗病毒治疗。建议移植后特定时间段(例如6个月)内每周进行病毒载量测定[129,131]。一旦启动，抗病毒治疗通常持续到CMV负荷检测阴性。先行治疗主要用于那些已明确诊断的亚临床感染，采取更昔洛韦或缬更昔洛韦治疗。但 SOT 受体每周监测血清病毒载量可能会增加经济负担。但这种策略对于 CMV 高风险患者可能无效(供体阳性而受体阴性胸部器官移植受体)。第三种策略,被称为“混合策略”,特别适用于儿童移植中心,因为可供儿童口服的缬更昔洛韦刚上市不久[131]。混合策略先对 CMV 感染高风险的患者进行短期抗病毒化学预防治疗(通常 2~4 周),然后在指定时间段监测病毒载量。每种治疗方法的优缺点详见第 94 章。

Epstein–Barr 病毒

尽管付出了越来越多努力,EBV 感染和移植后淋巴增殖性疾病(PTLD)预防工作还远远不够。除了少数前瞻性、随机试验,支持 EBV 预防策略的回顾性临床研究质量参差不齐。阿昔洛韦或更昔洛韦的化学预防效力仍不清楚。支持这种方法的回顾性研究缺乏适当控制,并被随时间变化的免疫抑制方案所混淆。一项多中心随机临床研究评估了静脉注射免疫球蛋白的效用,虽看似存在受益趋势,但在两组之间无统计学差异[132]。大部分专家推荐的现有预防策略是监测外周血 EBV 载量,然后相应减弱免疫抑制[132]。当 EBV 负荷上升时,支持优先使用利妥昔单抗[133]。评价方法有效性的研究一般受到回顾性研究设计限制。一般来说,仅推荐移植术前 EBV 血清阴性患者进行病毒监测,因为移植术前 EBV 血清阳性的受体术后很少发生 EBV 感染。但这不适用于小肠移植受体，因为其 EBV 血清阳性(至少在儿童受体中)并不发挥保护性作用。关于 EBV 和 PTLD 预防的细节详见第 96 章。

BK 病毒

对于肾移植受体 BKV 相关肾病(BKVAN)的预防也已经付出了很多努力。一般来说,通过监测 BKV 载量评估 BKVAN 风险适用于肾脏移植受体[134]。尿液中 BKV 检测为无创手段,应用比较广泛。但尿液中 BKV 负荷增加并不能预判 BKVAN 进展。因此,先行治疗干预需要检测血液中 BKV 负荷。目前一致赞成当病毒载荷持续增高时应减弱免疫抑制[134]。目前对于西多福韦、来氟米特、静脉免疫球蛋白和环丙沙星治疗亚临床或临床 BKV 感染的潜在作用还缺乏相关研究。大多数专家目前认为这些治疗措施可能无效。

乙肝与丙肝病毒

如果没有预防策略,HBV 感染在肝脏移植受体极易复发,并且在免疫抑制状态下进展迅速。因为之前缺乏有效预防策略,HBV 复发导致 HBV 相关肝脏移植受体存活率远远低于其他移植指征的群体[135]。移植术前，存在活动性乙型肝炎的受体应按指南进行抗病毒治疗以保证移植时较低病毒载量,这样可降低 HBV 复发风险[136,137]。移植后结合乙型肝炎免疫球蛋白(HBIg)和抗病毒治疗可以有效预防乙型肝炎复发并且优于单独使用 HBIg 或单独使用拉米夫定[137-141]。虽然大多数研究使用拉米夫定作为抗病毒药物，耐药也随之发生,因此优先使用组合疗法或不易产生耐药的抗病毒药物[137]。未来研究需更好地定义各种抗病毒制剂或抗病毒组合功效。大多数移植中心采用终身抗病毒药物预防；对移植时病毒无法检测或无耐药史的肝脏移植受体可短期应用 HBIg(1~6 个月)[137,142]。对于防治 HBV 阳性供体到 HBV 阴性受体的传播,预防策略相似。从围术期角度而言，应该对血清阴性受体进行主动免疫以减少他们在移植时获得 HBV 的风险。供体来源的 HBV 感染详见第 92 章。

HCV 易于在大多数感染的肝脏移植受体中复发,且目前没有被广泛接受的预防策略[137]。未来更为有效的 HCV 治疗方法将会对其防治具有积极的作用。

总结

移植受体在围术期易于感染多种疾病。这与受体在移植时的状态和移植器官类型密切相关。非移植手术中一些不太常见的感染类型表现会非常典型。但移植固有的免疫抑制状态和供器官暴露使得受体易于发生机会性感染,这些感染需要快速诊断和治疗。

(魏绪勇 译　徐骁 校)

参考文献

1. Al-Hasan MN, Razonable RR, Eckel-Passow JE, et al. Incidence rate and outcome of Gram-negative bloodstream infection in solid organ transplant recipients. American Journal of Transplantation. 2009;9(4):835–843.
2. Green M, Wald ER, Fricker FJ, et al. Infections in pediatric orthotopic heart transplant recipients. Pediatric Infectious Disease Journal. 1989;8(2):87–93.
3. Dummer JS, Hardy A, Poorsattar A, et al. Early infections in kidney, heart,

and liver transplant recipients on cyclosporine. Transplantation. 1983;36(3): 259-267.

4. Ho M, Dummer JS. Risk factors and approaches to infection in transplant recipients. In: Mandell GL, Douglas RJ, Bennett JE, editors. Principles and Practice of Infectious Disease. New York, NY: Churchill Livingstone; 1990: 2294-2300.
5. Rosen JB, Schecter MG, Heinle JS, et al. Clostridium difficile colitis in children following lung transplantation. Pediatric Transplantation. 2010;14(5):651-656.
6. Abbott KC, Swanson SJ, Richter ER, et al. Late urinary tract infection after renal transplantation in the United States. American Journal of Kidney Diseases. 2004;44(2):353-362.
7. Cuervas-Mons V, Rimola A, Van Thiel DH, et al. Does previous abdominal surgery alter the outcome of pediatric patients subjected to orthotopic liver transplantation? Gastroenterology. 1986;90(4):853-857.
8. Hsu J, Griffith BP, Dowling RD, et al. Infections in mortally ill cardiac transplant recipients. Journal of Thoracic and Cardiovascular Surgery. 1989;98(4): 506-509.
9. Sun HY, Cacciarelli TV, Singh N. Identifying a targeted population at high risk for infections after liver transplantation in the MELD era. Clinical Transplantation. 2011;25(3):420-425.
10. Apalsch AM, Green M, Ledesma-Medina J, et al. Parainfluenza and influenza virus infections in pediatric organ transplant recipients. Clinical Infectious Diseases. 1995;20(2):394-399.
11. Pohl C, Green M, Wald ER, et al. Respiratory syncytial virus infections in pediatric liver transplant recipients. Journal of Infectious Diseases. 1992;165(1): 166-169.
12. Englesbe MJ, Patel SP, He K, et al. Sarcopenia and mortality after liver transplantation. Journal of the American College of Surgeons. 2010;211(2):271-278.
13. Smart FW, Naftel DC, Costanzo MR, et al. Risk factors for early, cumulative, and fatal infections after heart transplantation: a multiinstitutional study. Journal of Heart and Lung Transplantation. 1996;15(4):329-341.
14. Ison MG, Hager J, Blumberg E, et al. Donor-derived disease transmission events in the United States: data reviewed by the OPTN/UNOS Disease Transmission Advisory Committee. American Journal of Transplantation. 2009;9(8):1929-1935.
15. Kusne S, Dummer JS, Singh N, et al. Infections after liver transplantation. An analysis of 101 consecutive cases. Medicine. 1988;67(2):132-143.
16. Jiménez-Romero C, Manrique A, Meneu JC, et al. Comparative study of bladder versus enteric drainage in pancreas transplantation. Transplantation Proceedings. 2009;41(6):2466-2468.
17. Pirsch JD, Odorico JS, D'Alessandro AM, et al. Posttransplant infection in enteric versus bladder-drained simultaneous pancreas-kidney transplant recipients. Transplantation. 1998;66(12):1746-1750.
18. Dummer JS. Infectious complications. In: Cooper DK, Novitzky D, editors. The Transplantation and Replacement of Thoracic Organs. Norwell, MA: Kluwer Academic Publishers; 1990.
19. Schroter GP, Hoelscher M, Putnam CW, et al. Infections complicating orthotopic liver transplantation: a study emphasizing graft-related septicemia. Archives of Surgery. 1976;111(12):1337-1347.
20. Hanevold CD, Kaiser BA, Palmer J, et al. Vesicoureteral reflux and urinary tract infections in renal transplant recipients. American Journal of Diseases of Children. 1987;141(9):982-984.
21. Zaontz MR, Hatch DA, Firlit CF. Urological complications in pediatric renal transplantation: management and prevention. Journal of Urology. 1988;140(5 Pt 2):1123-1128.
22. Bowman JS, Green M, Scantlebury VP. OKT3 and viral disease in pediatric liver transplant recipients. Clinical Transplantation. 1991;5:294-300.
23. Koo S, Marty FM, Baden LR. Infectious complications associated with immunomodulating biologic agents. Infectious Disease Clinics of North America. 2010;24(2):285-306.
24. Grinyo J, Charpentier B, Pestana JM, et al. An integrated safety profile analysis of belatacept in kidney transplant recipients. Transplantation. 2010;90(12): 1521-1527.
25. Humar A, Michaels M. American Society of Transplantation recommendations for screening, monitoring and reporting of infectious complications in immunosuppression trials in recipients of organ transplantation. American Journal of Transplantation. 2006;6(2):262-274.
26. Pappas PG, Alexander BD, Andes DR, et al. Invasive fungal infections among organ transplant recipients: results of the Transplant-Associated Infection Surveillance Network (TRANSNET). Clinical Infectious Diseases. 2010;50(8): 1101-1111.
27. Mermel LA, Allon M, Bouza E, et al. Clinical practice guidelines for the diagnosis and management of intravascular catheter-related infection: 2009 Update by the Infectious Diseases Society of America. Clinical Infectious Diseases. 2009;49(1):1-45.
28. O'Grady NP, Alexander M, Burns LA, et al. Guidelines for the prevention of intravascular catheter-related infections. Clinical Infectious Diseases. 2011; 52(9):e162-e193.
29. Albright JB, Bonatti H, Mendez J, et al. Early and late onset *Clostridium difficile*-associated colitis following liver transplantation. Transplant International. 2007;20(10):856-866.
30. Apaydin S, Altiparmak MR, Saribas S, et al. Prevalence of *Clostridium difficile* toxin in kidney transplant recipients. Scandinavian Journal of Infectious Diseases. 1998;30(5):542.
31. Collini PJ, Bauer M, Kuijper EJ, et al. *Clostridium difficile* infection in HIV-seropositive individuals and transplant recipients. Journal of Infection. 2012;64(2):131-147.
32. Hashimoto M, Sugawara Y, Tamura S, et al. *Clostridium difficile*-associated diarrhea after living donor liver transplantation. World Journal of Gastroenterology. 2007;13(14):2072-2076.
33. Mochon M, Kaiser BA, Dunn S, et al. Urinary tract infections in children with posterior urethral valves after kidney transplantation. Journal of Urology. 1992;148(6):1874-1876.
34. Munoz P, Giannella M, Alcala L, et al. *Clostridium difficile*-associated diarrhea in heart transplant recipients: is hypogammaglobulinemia the answer? Journal of Heart and Lung Transplantation. 2007;26(9):907-914.
35. Stelzmueller I, Goegele H, Biebl M, et al. *Clostridium difficile* colitis in solid organ transplantation-a single-center experience. Digestive Diseases and Sciences. 2007;52(11):3231-3236.
36. Stelzmueller I, Wiesmayr S, Eller M, et al. Enterocolitis due to simultaneous infection with rotavirus and *Clostridium difficile* in adult and pediatric solid organ transplantation. Journal of Gastrointestinal Surgery. 2007;11(7):911-917.
37. Keven K, Basu A, Re L, et al. *Clostridium difficile* colitis in patients after kidney and pancreas-kidney transplantation. Transplant Infectious Disease. 2004;6(1): 10-14.
38. Gellad ZF, Alexander BD, Liu JK, et al. Severity of *Clostridium difficile*-associated diarrhea in solid organ transplant patients. Transplant Infectious Disease. 2007;9(4):276-280.
39. Mitu-Pretorian OM, Forgacs B, Qumruddin A, et al. Outcomes of patients who develop symptomatic *Clostridium difficile* infection after solid organ transplantation. Transplantation Proceedings. 2010;42(7):2631-2633.
40. Cohen SH, Gerding DN, Johnson S, et al. Clinical practice guidelines for *Clostridium difficile* infection in adults: 2010 update by the society for healthcare epidemiology of America (SHEA) and the infectious diseases society of America (IDSA). Infection Control and Hospital Epidemiology. 2010;31(5):431-455.
41. Dubberke ER, Riddle DJ. *Clostridium difficile* in solid organ transplant recipients. American Journal of Transplantation. 2009;9(Suppl 4):S35-S40.
42. National Nosocomial Infections Surveillance (NNIS) System Report, data summary from January 1992 through June 2004, issued October 2004. American Journal of Infection Control. 2004;32(8):470-485.
43. Fournier PE, Richet H. The epidemiology and control of *Acinetobacter baumannii* in health care facilities. Clinical Infectious Diseases. 2006;42(5):692-699.
44. McDonald LC. Trends in antimicrobial resistance in health care-associated pathogens and effect on treatment. Clinical Infectious Diseases. 2006;42(Suppl 2):S65-S71.
45. Pop-Vicas AE, D'Agata EM. The rising influx of multidrug-resistant Gram-negative bacilli into a tertiary care hospital. Clinical Infectious Diseases. 2005;40(12):1792-1798.
46. Reddy P, Zembower TR, Ison MG, et al. Carbapenem-resistant *Acinetobacter baumannii* infections after organ transplantation. Transplant Infectious Disease. 2010;12(1):87-93.
47. Shi SH, Kong HS, Jia CK, et al. Risk factors for pneumonia caused by multidrug-resistant Gram-negative bacilli among liver recipients. Clinical Transplantation. 2010;24(6):758-765.
48. van Delden C, Blumberg EA. Multidrug resistant gram-negative bacteria in solid organ transplant recipients. American Journal of Transplantation. 2009;9(Suppl 4):S27-S34.
49. Shields RK, Kwak EJ, Potoski BA, et al. High mortality rates among solid organ transplant recipients infected with extensively drug-resistant *Acinetobacter baumannii*: using in vitro antibiotic combination testing to identify the combination of a carbapenem and colistin as an effective treatment regimen. Diagnostic Microbiology and Infectious Disease. 2011;70(2):246-252.
50. Linares L, Cervera C, Hoyo I, et al. *Klebsiella pneumoniae* infection in solid organ transplant recipients: epidemiology and antibiotic resistance. Transplantation Proceedings. 2010;42(8):2941-2943.
51. Sun HY, Shields RK, Cacciarelli TV, et al. A novel combination regimen for the treatment of refractory bacteremia due to multidrug-resistant *Pseudomonas aeruginosa* in a liver transplant recipient. Transplant Infectious Disease. 2010; 12(6):555-560.
52. Fox BC, Sollinger HW, Belzer FO, et al. A prospective, randomized, double-blind study of trimethoprim-sulfamethoxazole for prophylaxis of infection in renal

transplantation: clinical efficacy, absorption of trimethoprim-sulfamethoxazole, effects on the microflora, and the cost-benefit of prophylaxis. American Journal of Medicine. 1990;89(3):255-274.
53. Krieger JN, Brem AS, Kaplan MR. Urinary tract infection in pediatric renal transplantation. Urology. 1980;15(4):362-369.
54. Martin-Pena A, Cordero E, Fijo J, et al. Prospective study of infectious complications in a cohort of pediatric renal transplant recipients. Pediatric Transplantation. 2009;13(4):457-463.
55. Di Cocco P, Orlando G, Mazzotta C, et al. Incidence of urinary tract infections caused by germs resistant to antibiotics commonly used after renal transplantation. Transplantation Proceedings. 2008;40(6):1881-1884.
56. Kawecki D, Kwiatkowski A, Michalak G, et al. Urinary tract infections in the early posttransplant period after simultaneous pancreas-kidney transplantation. Transplantation Proceedings. 2009;41(8):3148-3150.
57. Chuang P, Parikh CR, Langone A. Urinary tract infections after renal transplantation: a retrospective review at two US transplant centers. Clinical Transplantation. 2005;19(2):230-235.
58. Kamath NS, John GT, Neelakantan N, et al. Acute graft pyelonephritis following renal transplantation. Transplant Infectious Disease. 2006;8(3):140-147.
59. Pellé G, Vimont S, Levy PP, et al. Acute pyelonephritis represents a risk factor impairing long-term kidney graft function. American Journal of Transplantation. 2007;7(4):899-907.
60. Rabkin DG, Stifelman MD, Birkhoff J, et al. Early catheter removal decreases incidence of urinary tract infections in renal transplant recipients. Transplantation Proceedings. 1998;30(8):4314-4316.
61. Valera B, Gentil MA, Cabello V, et al. Epidemiology of urinary infections in renal transplant recipients. Transplantation Proceedings. 2006;38(8):2414-2415.
62. Muller V, Becker G, Delfs M, et al. Do urinary tract infections trigger chronic kidney transplant rejection in man? Journal of Urology. 1998;159(6): 1826-1829.
63. Casale P, Grady RW, Mitchell ME, et al. Recurrent urinary tract infection in the post-transplant reflux nephropathy patient: is reflux in the native ureter the culprit? Pediatric Transplantation. 2005;9(3):324-327.
64. Green H, Rahamimov R, Gafter U, et al. Antibiotic prophylaxis for urinary tract infections in renal transplant recipients: a systematic review and meta-analysis. Transplant Infectious Disease. 2011;13(5):441-447.
65. Colonna JO, Winston DJ, Brill JE, et al. Infectious complications in liver transplantation. Archives of Surgery. 1988;123(3):360-364.
66. Hollenbeak CS, Alfrey EJ, Sheridan K, et al. Surgical site infections following pediatric liver transplantation: risks and costs. Transplant Infectious Disease. 2003;5(2):72-78.
67. Verma A, Wade JJ, Cheeseman P, et al. Risk factors for fungal infection in paediatric liver transplant recipients. Pediatric Transplantation. 2005;9(2):220-225.
68. Zitelli BJ, Gartner JC, Malatack JJ, et al. Pediatric liver transplantation: patient evaluation and selection, infectious complications, and life-style after transplantation. Transplantation Proceedings. 1987;19(4):3309-3316.
69. Qian YB, Liu CL, Lo CM, et al. Risk factors for biliary complications after liver transplantation. Archives of Surgery. 2004;139(10):1101-1105.
70. Sundaram V, Jones DT, Shah NH, et al. Posttransplant biliary complications in the pre- and post-model for end-stage liver disease era. Liver Transplantation. 2011;17(4):428-435.
71. Verdonk RC, Buis CI, Porte RJ, et al. Biliary complications after liver transplantation: a review. Scandinavian Journal of Gastroenterology. 2006;243 (Suppl): 89-101.
72. Welling TH, Heidt DG, Englesbe MJ, et al. Biliary complications following liver transplantation in the model for end-stage liver disease era: effect of donor, recipient, and technical factors. Liver Transplantation. 2008;14(1):73-80.
73. Neofytos D, Fishman JA, Horn D, et al. Epidemiology and outcome of invasive fungal infections in solid organ transplant recipients. Transplant Infectious Disease. 2010;12(3):220-229.
74. Collins LA, Samore MH, Roberts MS, et al. Risk factors for invasive fungal infections complicating orthotopic liver transplantation. Journal of Infectious Diseases. 1994;170(3):644-652.
75. Pappas PG, Silveira FP. Candida in solid organ transplant recipients. American Journal of Transplantation. 2009;9(Suppl 4):S173-S179.
76. Vandecasteele E, De Waele J, Vandijck D, et al. Antimicrobial prophylaxis in liver transplant patients–a multicenter survey endorsed by the European Liver and Intestine Transplant Association. Transplant International. 2010;23(2): 182-190.
77. Kusne S, Torre-Cisneros J, Manez R, et al. Factors associated with invasive lung aspergillosis and the significance of positive Aspergillus culture after liver transplantation. Journal of Infectious Diseases. 1992;166(6):1379-1383.
78. Singh N, Arnow PM, Bonham A, et al. Invasive aspergillosis in liver transplant recipients in the 1990s. Transplantation. 1997;64(5):716-720.
79. Singh N, Avery RK, Munoz P, et al. Trends in risk profiles for and mortality associated with invasive aspergillosis among liver transplant recipients. Clinical Infectious Diseases. 2003;36(1):46-52.
80. Green M, Bueno J, Sigurdsson L. Unique aspects of infectious complications of intestinal transplantation. Current Opinion in Organ Transplantation. 1999;4: 361-367.
81. Sigurdsson L, Reyes J, Kocoshis SA, et al. Bacteremia after intestinal transplantation in children correlates temporally with rejection or gastrointestinal lymphoproliferative disease. Transplantation. 2000;70(2):302-305.
82. van de Beek D, Kremers WK, Del Pozo JL, et al. Effect of infectious diseases on outcome after heart transplant. Mayo Clinic Proceedings.. 2008;83(3): 304-308.
83. Montoya JG, Giraldo LF, Efron B, et al. Infectious complications among 620 consecutive heart transplant patients at Stanford University Medical Center. Clinical Infectious Diseases. 2001;33(5):629-640.
84. Almenar L. Spanish registry on heart transplantation. 22nd official report of the Spanish Society of Cardiology Working Group on Heart Failure and Heart Transplantation (1984-2010). Revista Española de Cardiologia. 2011;64(12): 1138-1146.
85. Stehlik J, Edwards LB, Kucheryavaya AY, et al. The Registry of the International Society for Heart and Lung Transplantation: twenty-seventh official adult heart transplant report-2010. Journal of Heart and Lung Transplantation. 2010; 29(10):1089-1103.
86. Kirk R, Edwards LB, Kucheryavaya AY, et al. The Registry of the International Society for Heart and Lung Transplantation: thirteenth official pediatric heart transplantation report—2010. Journal of Heart and Lung Transplantation. 2010;29(10):1119-1128.
87. Mihaljevic T, Jarrett CM, Gonzalez-Stawinski G, et al. Mechanical circulatory support after heart transplantation. European Journal of Cardio-Thoracic Surgery. 2012;41(1):200-206.
88. Cisneros JM, Munoz P, Torre-Cisneros J, et al. Pneumonia after heart transplantation: a multi-institutional study. Spanish Transplantation Infection Study Group. Clinical Infectious Diseases. 1998;27(2):324-331.
89. Zuckermann A, Barten MJ. Surgical wound complications after heart transplantation. Transplant International. 2011;24(7):627-636.
90. Stovall SH, Ainley KA, Mason EO, et al. Invasive pneumococcal infections in pediatric cardiac transplant patients. Pediatric Infectious Disease Journal. 2001;20(10):946-950.
91. Backer CL, Zales VR, Harrison HL, et al. Intermediate term results of infant orthotopic cardiac transplantation from two centers. Journal of Thoracic and Cardiovascular Surgery. 1991;101(5):826-832.
92. Hofflin JM, Potasman I, Baldwin JC, et al. Infectious complications in heart transplant recipients receiving cyclosporine and corticosteroids. Annals of Internal Medicine. 1987;106(2):209-216.
93. Hertz MI, Aurora P, Benden C, et al. Scientific registry of the international society for heart and lung transplantation: introduction to The 2011 Annual Reports. Journal of Heart and Lung Transplantation. 2011;30(10):1071-1077.
94. Millet B, Higenbottam TW, Flower CD, et al. The radiographic appearances of infection and acute rejection of the lung after heart-lung transplantation. American Review of Respiratory Disease. 1989;140(1):62-67.
95. Scott JP, Higenbottam TW, Smyth RL, et al. Transbronchial biopsies in children after heart-lung transplantation. Pediatrics. 1990;86(5):698-702.
96. Starnes VA, Theodore J, Oyer PE, et al. Pulmonary infiltrates after heart-lung transplantation: evaluation by serial transbronchial biopsies. Journal of Thoracic and Cardiovascular Surgery. 1989;98(5 Pt 2):945-950.
97. Aris RM, Routh JC, LiPuma JJ, et al. Lung transplantation for cystic fibrosis patients with Burkholderia cepacia complex. Survival linked to genomovar type. American Journal of Respiratory and Critical Care Medicine. 2001;164(11): 2102-2106.
98. De Soyza A, McDowell A, Archer L, et al. *Burkholderia cepacia complex genomovars* and pulmonary transplantation outcomes in patients with cystic fibrosis. Lancet. 2001;358(9295):1780-1781.
99. Lipuma JJ. Update on the *Burkholderia cepacia* complex. Current Opinion in Pulmonary Medicine. 2005;11(6):528-533.
100. Noyes BE, Michaels MG, Kurland G, et al. *Pseudomonas cepacia* empyema necessitatis after lung transplantation in two patients with cystic fibrosis. Chest. 1994;105(6):1888-1891.
101. Palmer SM, Alexander BD, Sanders LL, et al. Significance of blood stream infection after lung transplantation: analysis in 176 consecutive patients. Transplantation. 2000;69(11):2360-2366.
102. Sims KD, Blumberg EA. Common infections in the lung transplant recipient. Clinics in Chest Medicine. 2011;32(2):327-341.
103. Puchalski J, Lee HJ, Sterman DH. Airway complications following lung transplantation. Clinics in Chest Medicine. 2011;32(2):357-366.
104. Husain S, Zaldonis D, Kusne S, et al. Variation in antifungal prophylaxis strategies

in lung transplantation. Transplant Infectious Disease. 2006;8(4):213–218.
105. Berger N, Guggenbichler S, Steurer W, et al. Bloodstream infection following 217 consecutive systemic-enteric drained pancreas transplants. BMC Infectious Diseases. 2006;6:127.
106. Humar A, Kandaswamy R, Granger D, et al. Decreased surgical risks of pancreas transplantation in the modern era. Annals of Surgery. 2000;231(2):269–275.
107. Gruessner AC, Sutherland DE. Pancreas transplant outcomes for United States (US) and non-US cases as reported to the United Network for Organ Sharing (UNOS) and the International Pancreas Transplant Registry (IPTR) as of October 2002. Clinical Transplants. 2002:41–77.
108. Batiuk TD, Bodziak KA, Goldman M. Infectious disease prophylaxis in renal transplant patients: a survey of US transplant centers. Clinical Transplantation. 2002;16(1):1–8.
109. Lumbreras C, Cuervas-Mons V, Jara P, et al. Randomized trial of fluconazole versus nystatin for the prophylaxis of Candida infection following liver transplantation. Journal of Infectious Diseases. 1996;174(3):583–588.
110. Sharpe MD, Ghent C, Grant D, et al. Efficacy and safety of itraconazole prophylaxis for fungal infections after orthotopic liver transplantation: a prospective, randomized, double-blind study. Transplantation. 2003;76(6):977–983.
111. Winston DJ, Pakrasi A, Busuttil RW. Prophylactic fluconazole in liver transplant recipients. A randomized, double-blind, placebo-controlled trial. Annals of Internal Medicine. 1999;131(10):729–737.
112. Singh N, Husain S. Invasive aspergillosis in solid organ transplant recipients. American Journal of Transplantation. 2009;9(Suppl 4):S180–S191.
113. Husain S, Paterson DL, Studer S, et al. Voriconazole prophylaxis in lung transplant recipients. American Journal of Transplantation. 2006;6(12): 3008–3016.
114. Drew RH, Dodds Ashley E, Benjamin DK, et al. Comparative safety of amphotericin B lipid complex and amphotericin B deoxycholate as aerosolized antifungal prophylaxis in lung-transplant recipients. Transplantation. 2004;77(2): 232–237.
115. Cadena J, Levine DJ, Angel LF, et al. Antifungal prophylaxis with voriconazole or itraconazole in lung transplant recipients: hepatotoxicity and effectiveness. American Journal of Transplantation. 2009;9(9):2085–2091.
116. Wang TF, Wang T, Altman R, et al. Periostitis secondary to prolonged voriconazole therapy in lung transplant recipients. American Journal of Transplantation. 2009;9(12):2845–2850.
117. Gordon SM, LaRosa SP, Kalmadi S, et al. Should prophylaxis for *Pneumocystis carinii* pneumonia in solid organ transplant recipients ever be discontinued? Clinical Infectious Diseases. 1999;28(2):240–246.
118. EBPG Expert Group on Renal Transplantation. European best practice guidelines for renal transplantation. Section IV: long-term management of the transplant recipient. IV.7.1 Late infections. *Pneumocystis carinii* pneumonia. Nephrology, Dialysis, Transplantation. 2002;17(Suppl 4):36–39.
119. Martin SI, Fishman JA. *Pneumocystis pneumonia* in solid organ transplant recipients. American Journal of Transplantation. 2009;9(Suppl 4):S227–S233.
120. Anand S, Samaniego M, Kaul DR. *Pneumocystis jirovecii* pneumonia is rare in renal transplant recipients receiving only one month of prophylaxis. Transplant Infectious Disease. 2011;13(6):570–574.
121. de Boer MG, Bruijnesteijn van Coppenraet LE, Gaasbeek A, et al. An outbreak of *Pneumocystis jiroveci* pneumonia with 1 predominant genotype among renal transplant recipients: interhuman transmission or a common environmental source? Clinical Infectious Diseases. 2007;44(9):1143–1149.
122. Gianella S, Haeberli L, Joos B, et al. Molecular evidence of interhuman transmission in an outbreak of *Pneumocystis jirovecii* pneumonia among renal transplant recipients. Transplant Infectious Disease. 2010;12(1):1–10.
123. Rabodonirina M, Vanhems P, Couray-Targe S, et al. Molecular evidence of interhuman transmission of *Pneumocystis pneumonia* among renal transplant recipients hospitalized with HIV-infected patients. Emerging Infectious Diseases. 2004;10(10):1766–1773.
124. Schmoldt S, Schuhegger R, Wendler T, et al. Molecular evidence of nosocomial *Pneumocystis jirovecii* transmission among 16 patients after kidney transplantation. Journal of Clinical Microbiology. 2008;46(3):966–971.
125. Yazaki H, Goto N, Uchida K, et al. Outbreak of Pneumocystis jiroveci pneumonia in renal transplant recipients: *P. jiroveci* is contagious to the susceptible host. Transplantation. 2009;88(3):380–385.
126. Green H, Paul M, Vidal L, et al. Prophylaxis of *Pneumocystis pneumonia* in immunocompromised non-HIV-infected patients: systematic review and meta-analysis of randomized controlled trials. Mayo Clinic Proceedings. 2007;82(9):1052–1059.
127. Baran DA, Alwarshetty MM, Alvi S, et al. Is toxoplasmosis prophylaxis necessary in cardiac transplantation? Long-term follow-up at two transplant centers. Journal of Heart and Lung Transplantation. 2006;25(11):1380–1382.
128. Kotton CN, Lattes R. Parasitic infections in solid organ transplant recipients. American Journal of Transplantation. 2009;9(Suppl 4):S234–S251.
129. Humar A, Snydman D. Cytomegalovirus in solid organ transplant recipients. American Journal of Transplantation. 2009;9(Suppl 4):S78–S86.
130. Palmer SM, Limaye AP, Banks M, et al. Extended valganciclovir prophylaxis to prevent cytomegalovirus after lung transplantation: a randomized, controlled trial. Annals of Internal Medicine. 2010;152(12):761–769.
131. Kotton CN, Kumar D, Caliendo AM, et al. International consensus guidelines on the management of cytomegalovirus in solid organ transplantation. Transplantation. 2010;89(7):779–795.
132. Allen U, Preiksaitis J. Epstein-Barr virus and posttransplant lymphoproliferative disorder in solid organ transplant recipients. American Journal of Transplantation. 2009;9(Suppl 4):S87–S96.
133. Martin SI, Dodson B, Wheeler C, et al. Monitoring infection with Epstein-Barr virus among seromismatch adult renal transplant recipients. American Journal of Transplantation. 2011;11(5):1058–1063.
134. Hirsch HH, Randhawa P. BK virus in solid organ transplant recipients. American Journal of Transplantation. 2009;9(Suppl 4):S136–S146.
135. Kim WR, Poterucha JJ, Kremers WK, et al. Outcome of liver transplantation for hepatitis B in the United States. Liver Transplantation. 2004;10(8):968–974.
136. Lok AS, McMahon BJ. Chronic hepatitis B. Hepatology. 2007;45(2):507–539.
137. Levitsky J, Doucette K. Viral hepatitis in solid organ transplant recipients. American Journal of Transplantation. 2009;9(Suppl 4):S116–S130.
138. Seehofer D, Berg T. Prevention of hepatitis B recurrence after liver transplantation. Transplantation. 2005;80(1 Suppl):S120–S124.
139. Perrillo RP, Lai CL, Liaw YF, et al. Predictors of HBeAg loss after lamivudine treatment for chronic hepatitis B. Hepatology. 2002;36(1):186–194.
140. Samuel D, Muller R, Alexander G, et al. Liver transplantation in European patients with the hepatitis B surface antigen. New England Journal of Medicine. 1993;329(25):1842–1847.
141. Zheng S, Chen Y, Liang T, et al. Prevention of hepatitis B recurrence after liver transplantation using lamivudine or lamivudine combined with hepatitis B Immunoglobulin prophylaxis. Liver Transplantation. 2006;12(2):253–258.
142. Buti M, Mas A, Prieto M, et al. A randomized study comparing lamivudine monotherapy after a short course of hepatitis B immune globulin (HBIg) and lamivudine with long-term lamivudine plus HBIg in the prevention of hepatitis B virus recurrence after liver transplantation. Journal of Hepatology. 2003;38(6):811–817.

第 94 章
器官移植后晚期感染性疾病

Jay A. Fishman, Robin K. Avery

引言

实体器官移植(SOT)后感染风险随着新型免疫抑制剂的应用、同种异体移植物和受体存活期延长不断增大。因此,移植相关感染治疗不仅需要有效抗微生物药物,还需要考虑预防移植排斥时免疫抑制剂的使用。本章节将阐述免疫抑制强度与新型预防策略之间的动态关联,同时介绍抗菌药物最新进展,以便为移植临床医生防治大多数机会性感染提供参考。

对于大多数移植患者,一些重要概念对于评估移植后感染风险非常有用:

1.与具有正常免疫功能的个体相比,移植受体感染性疾病较难识别,因为后者临床症状大多不明显,非感染性发热、移植排斥和药物毒性都会增加鉴别难度。

2.潜在感染病原体范围广泛,有时还会存在多重感染,如病毒和霉菌。不断改进的微生物测定方法有助于指导治疗常见病原体[3]。

3.感染风险与预防移植物排斥的免疫抑制强度有关[1,2]。

4.受体因为免疫受损,如果发生感染性疾病,进展会非常迅速。因此感染性疾病预防非常重要。

5.快速准确的诊断可帮助指导抗生素应用,以避免药物相互作用和毒性。有时需采取有创性诊断程序。

免疫抑制方案应在指导药物最佳剂量或组合预防移植排斥的同时,尽量避免感染性疾病发生。但目前缺乏精准的个体化免疫治疗方案。移植后临床管理和定期随访对降低移植受体感染风险至关重要。

感染的风险和时间表

移植受体感染风险很大程度上取决于两个关键因素:

1.受体和供体的流行病学暴露,包括受体未及时识别的既往暴露史(表 94.1)[2,4]。

2.受体的"免疫抑制状态",包括所有可能造成感染风险的因素(表 94.2)[2]。

这些因素会随着时间推移而演变。因此,可以通过公式计算曲线下面积来评估感染风险,这个公式会考虑受体的流行病学和免疫功能:当免疫功能长时间处于抑制状态时,即便是较低水平的"暴露"也会导致感染风险增加。当免疫抑制处于较低水平时,感染性疾病和药物不良反应发生率下降,但移植排斥风险增加。特异性免疫移植方案会使受体易于感染某些特定类型生物体,如 T 淋巴细胞消耗会激活潜在巨细胞病毒(CMV),并允许病毒复制,而皮质类固醇使用则更易于发生肺囊虫感染[5]。成功的预防策略(预防或先行治疗)在减少病原体感染风险的同时,还能够达到最佳免疫抑制状态。因此预防策略的制订不仅需要考虑免疫因素,还需要考虑其他可能导致感染的危险因素。关于感染性疾病预防策略详见第 99 章。

流行病学暴露

流行病学暴露可以分为四种类别:供体来源(见第 92 章)、预先存在的受体来源感染、社区或社区衍生的暴露。这些在前面章节中已有详细讨论。本章节将强调一些突出特点。在免疫抑制之前,移植受体中任何未被根除的感染性疾病都可能在后期病程中再现。

受体和供体来源的感染

供体和受体筛查(见第 92 章)对移植术后感染防治策略的制订具有重要意义[6,7]。预防策略因人而异,如对乙型肝炎病毒(HBV)感染的患者应尽量避免使用激素,对潜在的结核感染患者应利用异烟肼进行预处理,

表 94.1 移植相关的重大流行病学暴露

- 供体来源
- 病毒：
  - 疱疹组(巨细胞病毒,EBV,人类疱疹病毒6、7和8,单纯疱疹,水痘带状疱疹病毒)
  - 肝炎病毒(特别是HBV和HCV)
  - 逆转录病毒(人类免疫缺陷病毒,人类T淋巴细胞病毒1和2)
  - 其他：西尼罗河病毒,淋巴细胞性脉络丛脑膜炎病毒,狂犬病
- 细菌：
  - 革兰阳性菌和革兰阴性菌(葡萄球菌属,假单胞菌属,肠杆菌科)
  - 分枝杆菌(结核和非结核)
  - 诺卡菌种
- 真菌：
  - 假丝酵母属
  - 曲霉菌种
  - 地方性真菌
  - 地理性真菌,副球形菌
- 寄生虫：
  - 弓形虫
  - 克氏锥虫
  - 类圆线虫
  - 利什曼原虫
  - 阿米巴
- 医院暴露：
  - 耐甲氧西林葡萄球菌
  - 万古霉素抗性肠球菌(也是利奈唑胺和奎奴普丁-达福普汀抗性)
  - 多药耐药革兰阴性杆菌
  - 曲霉菌种
  - 假丝酵母非白色念珠菌菌株
- 社区风险：
  - 食物和水传播(单核细胞增多性李斯特菌,沙门菌,隐孢子虫属,甲型肝炎病毒,弯曲杆菌属)
  - 呼吸道病毒(呼吸道合胞病毒,流感,副流感,腺病毒,间质肺病毒)
  - 常见病毒,通常暴露于儿童(柯萨奇病毒,细小病毒)
  - 其他病毒(多瘤病毒,乳头瘤病毒)
  - 基孔肯雅病毒
  - 非典型呼吸道病原体(军团杆菌属,支原体属,衣原体)
  - 地理真菌和隐球菌,杰氏肺囊虫
- 寄生虫(通常遥远)：
  - 类圆线虫
  - 利什曼原虫
  - 弓形虫
  - 克氏锥虫
  - 纳氏虫属

表 94.2 “净免疫抑制状态”相关因素

- 免疫抑制治疗：类型,时间序列,强度
- 既往治疗措施(化疗或抗菌)
- 黏膜屏障完整性(导管)
- 中性粒细胞减少,淋巴细胞减少(常常是药物诱导)
- 基础免疫缺陷(例如蛋白尿导致的低丙种球蛋白血症,系统性红斑狼疮,补体缺陷)
- 代谢状况：尿毒症,营养不良,糖尿病,酒精中毒/肝硬化
- 病毒感染(巨细胞病毒,乙型和丙型肝炎,呼吸道合胞病毒)

对来自地衣昆虫地区的患者应使用伊维菌素预防；对水痘带状疱疹病毒(VZV)血清学阴性的患者进行主动免疫；对接受念珠菌感染供器官的受体进行经验性抗真菌治疗。对于巨细胞病毒(CMV)或Epstein-Barr病毒(EBV)治疗策略则需要根据血清学检测对移植受体进行个体化评估(下文讨论)。

一些供体来源感染,如结核杆菌或组织胞浆菌,在围术期可能表现不明显。同样的情况,定殖在供体肺部的伯克霍尔德菌、曲霉属或隐球菌属,或定殖在受体尿道或胆道的万古霉素抗性肠球菌(VRE),可能仅在某些特殊情况下发生感染,如抗排斥或抗病毒细菌感染的免疫治疗。受体来源暴露也在一定程度上反映近期可能的感染或者在免疫抑制和(或)技术问题情况下可能出现的定殖激活。那些有未完全治愈的慢性肺炎或者慢性腹膜炎患者可能在停止抗菌治疗后出现复发。

社区暴露风险

近期或者久远之前的流行病学暴露都有可能在移植后被重新激活。旅行、新爱好、儿童或者工作都有可能会暴露于污染的食物或水(李斯特菌、隐孢子虫)、土壤(曲霉属或诺卡菌属)、鸟类(隐球菌属)和地理限制性系统性真菌病(皮炎芽生菌、粗球孢子菌、副球虫属、荚膜组织胞浆菌),甚至是呼吸道病毒感染,或合并细菌真菌感染。

院内暴露风险

院内感染在移植受体中越来越重要(见第93章)。在一定程度上,这反映了医学移植中心耐药菌株的数量。受体等待移植时间越长,就越不可避免增加了抗感染治疗和暴露于耐药菌株的概率。最常见的病原体包括VRE、甲氧西林抗性金黄色葡萄球菌(MRSA)、氟康

唑耐药假丝酵母属、曲霉属和高度抗性的革兰阴性细菌[8]。呼吸道病毒感染有可能通过医务人员获得，这一点应该被考虑在免疫功能低下受体发烧和呼吸代偿障碍的原因中。

净免疫抑制状态

净免疫抑制状态评估量表包含了所有可能造成受体感染的风险因素（表 94.2）[2]。主要风险因素包括：

• 特异性免疫抑制治疗，包括剂量、持续时间和免疫抑制剂服用次序。

• 移植手术的技术问题：导致的渗漏（血液、淋巴、尿液）和积液、组织损伤、伤口愈合不良以及术后引流。

• 长期气管插管。

• 广谱抗生素使用。

• 移植后肾、肝、肺或心脏功能障碍或糖尿病。

• 长期使用导尿管、血管通路、透析导管或其他造成皮肤或黏膜损伤的有创操作。

• 免疫调节性病毒感染，包括 CMV、EBV、HBV、丙型肝炎病毒（HCV）或人类免疫缺陷病毒（HIV）。注意大多数病毒，包括社区获得性呼吸道病毒，可能会发展为超级感染。

• 营养不良。

• 药物造成的中性粒细胞减少，如霉酚酸莫非替克（MMF）、硫唑嘌呤、更昔洛韦和缬更昔洛韦。

不同免疫移植剂组合对于特定个体免疫功能的影响不可预测。对特定病原体的“免疫”能力测定，如细胞免疫功能或针对特异微生物的血清抗体水平，是一种新兴技术。血清学测定可以帮助确定既往对各种病原体的可能暴露，但无法在免疫抑制受体中评估其对特定病原体的免疫应答功效。全身免疫功能评估技术仍不成熟[9]。某些药物与特定感染的风险增加有关（表 94.3）[5]；药剂组合可能会增加这种风险或造成毒性，如肾毒性。目前对于特殊状态下的免疫重建数据还很缺乏，如 T 或 B 淋巴细胞严重消耗、抗体肿瘤坏死因子应用或共刺激阻断等。器官功能障碍（如肝硬化和肾功能障碍）对全身免疫功能的影响也有待确定。

其中比较重要的免疫缺陷包括皮肤破损与天然固有免疫损害。同时也应注意皮肤定殖的黏性生物，如 VRE 或金黄色葡萄球菌，皮下留置导管会增加菌血症风险。这些影响又被那些可以造成中性粒细胞减少的药物放大[更昔洛韦、MMF、硫唑嘌呤、别嘌呤醇、甲氧苄啶-磺胺甲噁唑（TMP-SMX）等]。外科性、侵入性放射学、胃肠道手术会造成并发症，如胆漏、胆道/尿道狭窄、细菌远处播散的风险增加，并且会导致局部脓肿形成和移植物缺血。

表 94.3　免疫抑制和感染常见关联

- 抗淋巴细胞球蛋白（溶解消减）和同种免疫反应：
  - T 淋巴细胞：潜伏（疱疹）病毒的活化，发热，细胞因子
  - B 淋巴细胞：细菌
- 血浆置换：细菌
- 共刺激阻滞：可能增加 EBV/移植后淋巴增生性疾病的风险
- 皮质类固醇：细菌，肺囊虫（以前的卡里尼）肺炎，乙型肝炎，丙型肝炎
- 硫唑嘌呤：中性粒细胞减少症，乳头瘤病毒
- 霉酚酸酯（MMF）：早期细菌感染，B 细胞，晚期巨细胞病毒
- 钙依赖磷酸酶抑制剂：增强的病毒复制（无免疫力），牙龈感染，细胞内病原体
- mTOR 抑制剂：
  - 伤口愈合不良
  - 与其他药剂组合的过度感染
  - 特发性间质性肺炎

感染时间表

随着免疫抑制方案的标准化，移植后大部分感染性疾病可以在不同时间点提前预见（图 94.1）。这反映了随着时间变化，不同风险因素的变化情况：手术/住院、免疫抑制、急性和慢性排斥、潜在感染出现和新型社区感染暴露[1]。感染模式随多种因素而改变，如免疫抑制方案（副作用、避免移植排斥的强化）、并发病毒感染、中性粒细胞减少（药物毒性）、移植物功能障碍或显著的流行病学暴露（旅行或食物）。同样也包括预防性抗菌治疗，当推迟有效抗菌治疗时，感染出现会比平时更晚一些。这些现象表明随着时间推移，免疫抑制的净状态是可以达到的。这样即便在抗菌治疗停止以后，也不太会发生感染[10,11]。

时间表反映了感染风险的三个重叠期：① 围术期，移植后 0~30 天（见第 93 章）；② 移植后 1~6 个月（取决于免疫抑制强度、类型、剂量、抗淋巴细胞效应）；③ 移植后 6~12 个月。这些时间段反映了与感染相关的不断变化的主要风险因素：① 手术技术并发症；② 强力免疫抑制导致的病毒激活；③ 回归正常生活后的社区获得性暴露。

这条时间线可以用于多个方面：① 对怀疑感染的

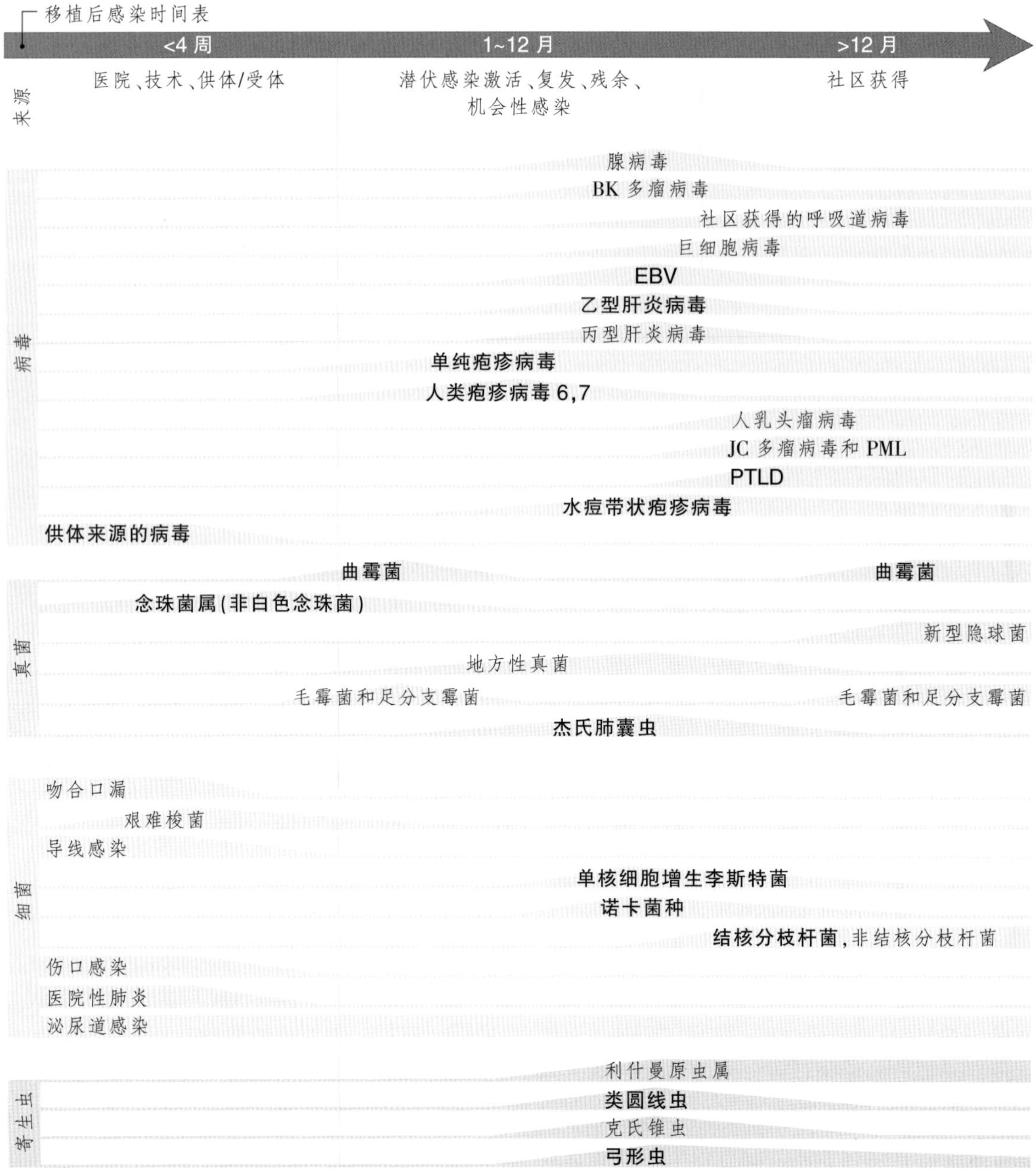

图 94.1 器官移植后感染时间表。器官移植后的感染风险在与免疫抑制的净状态和流行病学暴露有关。可以被预防措施(包括疫苗接种和抗微生物剂)影响感染风险的潜在病原体用粗体表示。个体感染风险则会被抗排斥或恶性肿瘤所影响。线条粗细表示相对风险大小。可预防的感染也被用粗体表示。可能会延迟直到预防停止。(Modified from Fishman [1] and Fisham and Rubin [2].)
PML,进行性多灶性脑白质病;PTLD,移植后淋巴增生性疾病。

移植患者进行鉴别诊断;② 作为个人在医院或社区的环境危害评估线索;③ 指导预防性抗菌药物使用。在常见时间点之外发生的异常严重感染常常提示过多的流行病学危险或过度免疫抑制[1]。感染预防一定要与移植后不同时间段感染的各种风险因素相联系。马萨诸塞州总医院的常规预防策略在表 94.4 和表 94.5 中概述。需要注意的是,这些预防策略在面对过多流行病学压力时只能推迟感染发生。使用抗生素预防、疫苗或者改变生活习惯,如洗手或未戴口罩在花园工作,也仅仅是把感染拖回到相应的时间点,除非减低免疫抑制强度或者增强免疫才有可能避免感染。

移植后第一阶段(0~30 天)

移植后第 1 个月的常见感染类型已在第 93 章中

表 94.4 杰氏肺囊虫肺炎(PCP)的预防

背景

低剂量甲氧苄啶-磺胺甲噁唑(TMP-SMX)预防(成人:每天口服一片单强度片剂)可以很好地耐受,并且基本上能够根除这个群体的肺囊虫感染。低剂量(3 天/周)可以预防 PCP,但不能预防其他感染,如尿道感染,包括易感性诺卡菌和李斯特菌、弓形体病以及各种胃肠道和肺部感染。

治疗方案

一片单强度 TMP-SMX 片剂 (含有 80mg 甲氧苄啶,400mg 磺胺甲噁唑)移植后口服至少 4~6 个月。巨细胞病毒感染、慢性排斥、复发性感染以及大多数肺、肝和心脏受体建议终身预防。

替代方案

对于那些不耐受 TMP-SMX 的患者,替代方案包括:

- 每天饭中口服阿托伐醌 1500mg,加用每日一次 250mg 左氧氟沙星(或等量氟喹诺酮)
- 戊脒(每 3~4 周静脉注射或吸入 300mg)
- 氨苯砜(每天或一周两次,每次 100mg),可选择联用乙胺嘧啶

每一种药物都具有自身副作用,如葡萄糖-6-磷酸缺陷宿主使用氨苯砜会发生溶血。没有任何一种替代治疗可以达到 TMP-SMX 的治疗效果。

概述。这些感染通常是移植手术并发症、移植前已存在的受体或供体感染或院内感染。除非这些感染被根除,否则会在患者病程中造成很多麻烦。复发性感染主要与技术问题有关(狭窄、渗漏、移植损伤),非常难解决。如果术后早期拔除引流管、停用不必要的药物包括抗生素、细致的切口护理,那么患者感染的风险会大大降低。值得注意的是,移植后的第 1 个月机会性感染不太常见,即便在这期间每天的免疫抑制剂用量很大。这说明免疫抑制剂需要持续管理以保证避免那些小的天然毒力生物体可以引起侵袭性疾病。因此,移植受体如果在术前没有预防性抗菌治疗,那么应用皮质类固醇后可能会发生肺孢子虫肺炎。术后早期霉菌感染大多是因为术前定殖或医院过多环境暴露,如在废气处理管道处或人口密集区域。供体来源和围术期感染的治疗措施详见第 92 章和第 93 章。

移植后第二阶段(1~6 个月)

在移植后 1~6 个月,有很多原因可以造成受体发热综合征。常规使用的抗 CMV 治疗和 TMP-SMX 预防已经改变了这一阶段的感染模式。每天给予 TMP-SMX 可以消除肺囊虫肺炎(PCP),降低尿道感染(UTI)、单核细胞增多性李斯特菌脑膜炎,尿毒症、诺卡菌感染和弓形虫感染的发生率[12]。值得注意的是,在磺胺类过敏患者中使用 TMP-SMX 的替代药物可能不会带来上述益处。有效的抗 CMV 药物应该在治疗期间可以阻止大部分 CMV 感染(大部分由疱疹病毒引起)。因此,这一阶段的主要感染性综合征包括:

- 移植排斥,特别是钙调神经磷酸酶抑制剂(CNI)-休眠免疫抑制方案。
- 围术期感染,包括复发性艰难梭菌结肠炎、未充分治疗的肺炎或与手术技术相关的感染,如胸膜渗出、尿漏、由于胆道缺血引起的胆管炎、淋巴囊肿感染性血肿、气道坏死和肺脏移植受体气道开裂等。
- 住院期间留下的院内感染。
- 病毒感染,包括 CMV、单纯疱疹病毒(HSV)、带状疱疹(VZV 造成的局部或弥散性带状疱疹)、人类疱疹病毒(HHV)6 或 7、BK 多瘤病毒、EBV、复发性肝炎(HBV 和 HCV),以及社区获得性呼吸病毒[腺病毒、流感、副流感、呼吸道合胞体病毒(RSV)和间质肺病毒]。相对于正常个体,移植受体中病毒感染通常更持久,更具侵入性。
- 机会性感染,由耶氏肺孢子菌、李斯特菌、T.弓形虫、诺卡菌属、曲霉属等造成的感染。机会性感染可以反映免疫抑制强度,或免疫调节性病毒感染的有无。

疱疹病毒特别常见,它产生的感染血清标志物终生阳性。疱疹病毒在移植中比较突出是因为 T 细胞免疫可以控制这些感染和来自血清阳性供体的传播效率。与其他慢性病毒感染类似,疱疹病毒一方面可以产生全身性免疫抑制,一方面又会通过细胞因子产生和其他机制诱导免疫排斥[13,14]。

在这个阶段,还包含另外一组亚群,主要指那些需要更高免疫抑制维持器官功能,或者存在未被治疗的病毒感染和机会性感染的人群(在第三个阶段进行讨论)[2]。这些个体可能需要更长的预防治疗[抗菌和(或)抗病毒]、仔细的临床和实验室监测来避免危及生命的感染。

移植后第三阶段(6~12 个月)

移植术后 6 个月以上的受体根据感染风险可以分为三类。首先,那些手术顺利、移植物功能良好而可以进行免疫抑制剂减量的受体发生潜伏感染再燃的风险

表 94.5 疱疹病毒预防*

背景

人疱疹病毒是移植受体感染性疾病发病率和死亡率的最重要原因之一。预防方案根据临床风险制订，其主要决定因素是供体既往感染史、受体是否携带病毒（移植前循环抗体是否阳性）和免疫抑制治疗方案。

通用 CMV 病毒预防策略

巨细胞病毒（CMV）血清学状态±抗淋巴细胞球蛋白诱导治疗（ALG）	预防	监测（抗原血症）
D+/R-，不进行 ALG	静脉注射更昔洛韦 5mg/kg（负荷剂量），然后口服 3 个月的缬更昔洛韦（900mg/d，根据肾功能调整剂量）或更昔洛韦（3g/d）†	终止治疗后 6 个月内每月检查一次*
D+或 R+，联合 ALG	静脉注射更昔洛韦 5mg/kg（首剂量），然后根据肾功能终止治疗或者继续口服 6 个月的缬更昔洛韦（900mg/d，根据肾功能调整剂量）或更昔洛韦（3g/d）†	终止治疗后 6 个月内每月检查一次*
D-/R+，不进行 ALG	口服 3 个月的缬更昔洛韦（900mg/d，根据肾功能调整剂量）	症状
D-/R-	口服 3~4 个月的泛昔洛韦，500mg/d（或者 500mg 伐昔洛韦，每天两次；400mg 阿昔洛韦，每天三次）	症状、发热/中性粒细胞减少
	使用 CMV 阴性或白细胞过滤的血液	如上
感染状态未知，联合 ALG	静脉注射更昔洛韦 5mg/kg（首剂量），然后每天口服，并根据肾功能调整剂量，直到血清学转阴	

中性粒细胞减少症：一般来说，抗病毒治疗的剂量不会引起中性粒细胞减少。

* ALG：抗淋巴细胞抗体包括任何裂解或者消耗淋巴细胞的抗体制剂。

† 伐昔洛韦在肾移植受体中作为替代药物时的剂量为 8g/d。

先行治疗

优先治疗需要患者良好的依从性与详细的治疗监测程序，CMV 病毒载量试验或 pp65 抗原血症实验都可以用于治疗监视。在移植后的 12~24 个月应每周监测一次。如果监测结果阳性，则应该口服缬更昔洛韦（900mg，每天两次）或静脉注射更昔洛韦（5mg/kg，每天两次）。根据肾功能的结果调整剂量。治疗应持续至血清病毒转阴。

混合预防

许多中心对最高风险的受体（D+/R-或 R+，合并淋巴细胞消耗）采用普遍预防，其他受体则采用先行治疗。

背景

人疱疹病毒是移植受体感染性疾病发病率和死亡率的最重要原因之一。预防方案根据临床风险制订，其主要决定因素是供体既往感染史、受体是否携带病毒（移植前循环抗体是否阳性）和免疫抑制治疗方案。

CMV 通用抗病毒预防

很低。社区获得性呼吸病毒感染是其主要风险，还可能同时引发更严重的机会性感染。这些患者还有可能发生社会获得性原发 CMV 感染，或现有疾病造成的感染，如糖尿病皮肤感染。

第二类指那些发生复发病毒感染的受体，其预后取决于抗微生物治疗的有效性。这些患者的主要危险包括 CMV、EBV、BK 多瘤病毒感染、肝脏移植受体的 HCV、乳头瘤病毒（皮肤疣）。在没有有效治疗手段时期，这类患者还受到 HBV 和 HIV 的潜在威胁。不断出现的 HCV 药物可能会改变疾病预后。这些感染造成的主要危害包括：

- 器官晚期损害：BK 多瘤病毒肾病、冷蛋白血症、HCV 造成的肝硬化。
- 恶性肿瘤：EBV 造成的移植后淋巴细胞增生性疾病、乳头状病毒造成的皮肤和阴部恶性肿瘤。
- 器官排斥可能由感染造成，也有可能与治疗感染而减弱的免疫抑制有关。

第三组受体预后极差则是因为移植技术不佳、供器官质量不良或者慢性器官排斥（细胞或体液）。很多受体还会因为慢性 CNI 副作用而造成肾功能不全。他们也会遭受上述病毒的慢性感染。因此，这些受体一般免疫抑制使用量较大，其移植器官功能往往不佳。这些受体很容易区分,因为他们在移植后功能恢复不佳、发生各种并发症(出血、渗漏、药物相互作用、重症监护需求)或疾病复发。这类移植受体还特别容易发生机会性感染,最常见的病原体包括耶氏肺孢子菌、李斯特菌、星状诺卡菌、曲霉属和新型隐球菌[2]。还有一些造成 AIDS 免疫受损状态的病原体(巴氏杆菌属、红球菌属、隐孢子虫属和小孢子菌属)和侵袭性真菌病原体(丝孢菌属、接合菌和暗色孢菌)。非常细小的临床症状可以帮助进行这些高危群体的评估。受体或许会受益于长期的 TMP-SMX 预防或者抗真菌治疗。

移植后选择性感染

一般情况

免疫受损个体的感染谱很广。考虑到抗微生物药物潜在毒性和早期干预的需要,感染的早期诊断非常必要。不断发展的影像学技术和分子微生物学技术都极大地促进了诊断水平的提高。但是一般不太使用侵入性诊断方法。这些方法如果无法明确诊断和有效指导治疗,反而会带来一些风险。一般都是先采取经验性治疗,尽可能覆盖多的病原体,然后再根据数据逐渐缩窄抗菌谱。

当受体表现出感染症状时,最核心的考虑是是否需要降低免疫抑制强度,承担移植排斥或免疫重建综合征(IRIS)风险[15]。治疗感染时,如果移植排斥已经存在,那么有可能会加速感染发生。感染与排斥密切关联,有时很难区分。例如,HCV 感染复发会增加移植肝脏排斥的风险。误吸、社区获得性呼吸道病毒、CMV、细菌性感染造成的肺炎会增加肺脏移植受体闭塞性气管炎的发生风险[16-18]。CMV 还与心脏和肾脏移植物排斥有关[19,20]。实际情况中,当面对特殊感染时,经常会降低免疫抑制强度;但是,确实也可能发生排斥。如何调整免疫抑制方案取决于分离到的病原体。一些免疫缺陷(中性粒细胞减少症和丙种球蛋白减少症)可以通过辅助治疗(集落刺激因子或抗体)来逆转[21]。合并 CMV 感染时也需要考虑附加治疗手段。

巨细胞病毒

尽管已经有很成熟的抗病毒措施,巨细胞病毒仍然是移植受体非常重要的病原体[22,23]。由于感染部位和宿主反应不同,CMV 感染可以表现出不同的症状。潜伏感染一般存在于单核细胞,但病毒复制可以在多种细胞中进行,如成纤维细胞、上皮细胞、内皮细胞和其他实质细胞。

CMV 感染的表现传统上分为直接和间接效应[13]。更准确的表述应该是“病毒血症/细胞病变性”效应和“细胞/免疫性”效应。最常见的直接效应和临床综合征包括:

- CMV 综合征:发热和中性粒细胞减少综合征,伴或不伴有单核细胞增多症,包括肝炎、肾炎、淋巴结炎、白细胞减少症和(或)血小板减少症。
- 肺炎。
- 胃肠道疾病,食管炎、结肠炎、胃炎、溃疡、出血或穿孔。
- 肝炎、胰腺炎、心肌炎、脉络膜视网膜炎。
- 脑膜脑炎。
- 溶血性尿毒症综合征或者微血管栓塞。

如果没有预防措施,除了脉络膜视网膜炎之外,CMV 感染的直接临床反应一般在移植后 1~6 个月内发生。在有效的抗病毒治疗下,很少会发生病毒血症和症状性感染[24],也会在治疗中断或移植排斥下增强免疫抑制后发生[25]。脉络膜视网膜炎一般在病毒复制水平很低的情况下也可以发生,而且发生的时间通常较晚。移植受体发生率很低,AIDS 患者合并 CMV 感染时非常容易发生视网膜炎[26]。

CMV 感染的细胞性免疫性临床表现(下文讨论)主要是由于宿主防御屏障的损害,从而易感于继发性疾病,主要病原体包括耶氏肺孢子虫、念珠菌、曲霉属以及其他细菌等。CMV 感染还会增加移植排斥风险,PTLD、HHV6 和 HHV7 感染,受体死亡率。

传播方式

移植受体 CMV 传播包含三种方式:原发性感染、重新激活感染和超级感染。

原发性感染

原发性 CMV 感染是风险最大的感染类型,常发生于血清学阴性受体接受潜伏感染或者血清学阳性供器官时[供体血清学阳性,受体血清学阴性(D+/R-)],移植后会发生病毒的再激活与感染全身播散[17,27]。在没有预防措施前提下,超过 50%的受体会发生病毒血症,可以没有临床症状。同样,在抗病毒预防措施停止之后,超过 50%的受体会发生病毒血症,25%~35%会表现出临床症状。血清学阴性个体可以通过输血和性接触获得原发性CMV感染。这种疾病可能会非常严重。最大的病毒负荷被认为是供体器官，特别是在D+/R-组合中。供器官被认为是病毒复制的特殊位点，因为MHC限制性，当供体与受体的MHC不匹配时，病毒特异性细胞毒性T细胞不能有效清除病毒感染细胞。

再激活感染

在再激活感染中，移植后血清学阳性个体重新激活内源性病毒 [供体血清学阳性或血清学阴性(D+或D-)，受体血清学阳性(R+)]。当使用常规免疫抑制治疗(无抗淋巴细胞抗体的“诱导”治疗)时，10%~15%的受体直接会产生疾病感染临床症状，而应用包含抗淋巴细胞抗体的“诱导”治疗防治移植排斥时，发生率会更高。高达50%的个体会产生经常无症状的病毒血症。

超感染

来自供体的病毒还可能在特定情况下被激活，如血清学阳性的供器官移植给血清学阳性受体(D+ R+)。即便是去除白细胞之后进行输血，CMV感染也有4%的传播率。一些移植中心给血清学阴性受体使用抗体阳性血清，而其他一些移植中心则使用白细胞过滤后的血制品。这一现象提醒我们应注意围术期管理以避免CMV感染传播。

感染发病机制

CMV感染激活受多种因素影响，包括免疫抑制强度，特别是脉冲剂量的皮质类固醇应用；移植物中病毒量；裂解性T细胞消耗疗法；特别是伴随炎症和发热的HHV6和HHV7共感染[通过包括肿瘤坏死因子(TNF-α)在内的促炎细胞因子]；移植排斥(可能通过炎症或对感染内皮细胞的损伤)。病毒的激活风险因素包括联合强化免疫抑制与抗淋巴细胞治疗免疫排斥。促炎细胞因子和趋化因子相关的免疫反应通常靶向发生在移植物，也是病毒载量最大的部位。当CMV激活增加移植排斥风险时，移植排斥也在增加病毒复制的风险。因此，Reinke等的研究表明，21例患者中有17例活检提示“晚期急性排斥反应”的受体对抗病毒治疗有反应[28]。而且，Lowance等证明了预防CMV感染的预防也可以降低移植排斥发病率[20]。

细胞和免疫效应

血清转换是宿主免疫系统进展和良好细胞免疫应答存在的标志。CMV感染的控制主要通过MHC限制性、病毒特异性、细胞毒性T淋巴细胞反应(CD8$^+$细胞)进行[29-32]。CD4$^+$淋巴细胞在维持细胞免疫反应中起重要作用，并可以直接杀伤人类CMV(HCMV)感染的细胞[33]。γδT细胞的作用则有待明确[34,35]。抗体中和反应在临床中非常重要[36]。HCMV糖蛋白B(gB)与细胞附着和CMV穿透作用有关，也是抗体中和反应的主要靶标和HCMV疫苗的主要成分[37]。HCMV与Toll样受体(TLR9和TLR3)相互作用，激活炎症细胞因子通路和共刺激通路[38]。巨噬细胞、树突状细胞和自然杀伤(NK)细胞都参与对CMV的先天免疫反应。

CMV的细胞和免疫效应(间接效应)与侵入性病毒感染一样，对于免疫受损宿主很重要[30,39]。这些效应的机制非常复杂，并且与病毒逃避宿主抗病毒反应有关，后者通过HCMV感染的抗原呈递细胞(APC)进行传播[39-41]。HCMV感染阻断单核细胞前体分化为APC，损害APC迁移，并减弱抗原呈递。HCMV基因产物UL18，通过MHCⅠ类分子抑制NK细胞活化，并抑制细胞毒性的信号激活[42,43]。HCMV干扰正常的CD8$^+$ T淋巴细胞MHCⅠ类呈递与识别。人类基因的多个同源产物(跨膜G蛋白偶联、趋化因子受体、TNF受体、补体)会抑制炎症细胞募集和感染细胞杀伤。CMV编码的抗细胞凋亡基因产物可延迟感染细胞凋亡[44]。HCMV编码的Fc-γ受体通过掩盖病毒抗原来保护受感染的细胞免受抗体介导的细胞毒性[45]。这些特征改变了先天和适应性免疫应答的许多方面，因此当联合外源性免疫抑制防治移植排斥时容易发生机会性感染[30]。

CMV感染或疾病与移植物排斥损伤之间的双向联系已在多种临床试验中被观察到，包括心脏、肺、肝和肾移植患者[19,20,39,46]。有症状的疾病和无症状的感染都会刺激同种免疫应答，正如在CMV感染防治临床实验中所证明的那样。最清楚的关联之一是在发热或排斥中TNF-α的作用[47]，它可以激活细胞内NF-κB。NF-κB易位至细胞核并控制早期（IE）启动子/增强子。CMV *IE*基因编码对于病毒复制非常重要[48]。TNF-α和其他炎症细胞因子在细胞移植排斥中发挥重要作用。CMV还有促进移植物纤维化，增加纤维化和血管生长因子的作用，如肿瘤生长因子(TGF)-β、血小板衍生的生长因子(PDGF)、结缔组织生长因子(CTGF)、血管内皮生长因子以及黏附分子[包括细胞间黏附分子(ICAM-1)和血管细胞黏附分子(VCAM-1)][49-57]。CMV感染的促纤维化作用放大了伴随同种异体移植排斥的免疫与炎症损伤[58,59]。内皮损伤使得血小板黏附于基底膜，同时伴随 PDGF 释放、基质金属蛋白酶(MMP)-2 活性增加和基质基因表达降低，最终导致平滑肌细胞迁移，促进血管新生内膜增生[60-62]。CMV 介导的细胞凋亡抑制因子减少了 CMV 感染平滑肌细胞凋亡。白介素 IL-8 的产生则增加全身炎症与中性粒细胞、巨噬细胞和内皮细胞的激活。

诊断

由于近 20 年 CMV 感染敏感定量诊断方法以及治疗措施的不断进步，CMV 的临床管理取得了长足进步[63-65]。血清学测试在移植之前的风险预测中非常重要，但是在移植后定义临床疾病的价值很小[包括抗 CMV 免疫球蛋白 M(IgM)水平检测]。如果受体血清检测到 CMV 抗体，可以证明其既往暴露于 CMV 并已具备一定的免疫力[66]。但是，移植受体的血清反应化一般很迟出现，因此诊断意义不大。过去，CMV 细胞培养常与免疫荧光结合检测，虽然有用但相对太慢，而且不敏感，临床应用价值小[64]。此外，免疫受损宿主的呼吸分泌物或者尿液 CMV 培养物(或小瓶培养物)阳性也具有很小的诊断价值，因为许多患者可以在没有侵袭性疾病的情况下分泌 CMV。组织学中 CMV 包涵体存在或者免疫染色阳性是诊断组织浸润性 CMV 疾病的金标准[23,67]。活检证实的免疫组织学诊断对于可能的胃肠道疾病也至关重要。在移植受体出现溃疡性结肠病、胃部病变、弥漫性红斑或出血时，必须考虑 CMV。这些受体经常具有低至检测不出的病毒血症[23,68]，组织学检测也不太容易发现细胞内包涵体。

CMV 感染强度与移植感染受体风险相联系。因此，移植后 CMV 感染管理的金标准已经发展为定量测定。目前已开发了两种类型的定量测定方法：病毒 DNA 或 RNA 分子测定、抗原测定。任意一种方法都适用。抗原检测方法是一种基于劳动密集型、半定量荧光或免疫过氧化物酶的测定方法，它将循环中性粒细胞的 CMV 早期抗原(pp65)染色，然后被用来非特异性评估机体病毒总负荷量[64,69,70]。分子生物学方法[直接定量 DNA 聚合酶链反应(PCR)、杂交捕获、扩增测定]对于探测病毒血症具有高度特异性和敏感性[63,64]。检测方法通常包括基于血浆的 PCR 测试和全血杂交捕获测定，基于全血和血浆的测定结果不能直接比较，因为全血测定通常会产生较高的病毒载量[64,65,71,72]。世界卫生组织(WHO)已经制订了 CMV 实验室检测标准[65]。CMV 感染时病毒载量差异很大。最高的病毒载量通常与组织浸润性疾病相关，而最低的病毒载量与胃肠或中枢神经系统(CNS)疾病相关[23,73,74]。在这种情况下，CMV 检测方法通常为阴性，因此需要必要的侵入性(活检)诊断。

病毒测定在 CMV 预防和治疗中发挥重要作用(表 94.5)。筛选时间表与感染风险相关。因此，对于高危患者(D+/R-或 R+，联合抗胸腺细胞球蛋白治疗)，在预防完成后的 3~6 个月中应每两周或每月进行筛查以确保没有感染[23,75]。这种防治措施非常常见，但是在实际情况中因移植中心和患者群体不同而差别很大。虽然共识指南已经出版，但目前还缺乏可以指导实践的具体数据[23,75]。在治疗 CMV 感染患者时，测定方法可以提示什么时间开始预防，什么时间终止治疗。

预防

CMV 感染的预防应根据免疫抑制方案和患者而个体化。两种策略比较常见：① 普遍预防；② 抢先治疗[23,76]。普遍预防指给予所有处于风险中的患者在移植时或移植后马上进行一定时间的抗病毒治疗。抢先治疗则是指通过定量方法进行检测，早期诊断以便尽早治疗。阳性测定需要进行治疗。这种策略需要额外的监控和患者出院后配合，但也同时降低药物成本及药物毒性[77]。普遍预防不仅可以预防 CMV 感染，同时还可以减少 HSV、VZV、HHV6、HHV7 和 EBV 感染[27]。此外，CMV 感染造成的移植排斥、机会性感染和死亡率也可以通过常规、普遍预防所降低[27]。任何一种策略都不够完美。在两种策略的实际应用中都发现了控制不良的疾病和更昔洛韦抗性[78-80]。普遍预防完成后会观察到“后期”疾病[81,82]。在 D+/R-受体中“后期”疾病的发生率为 17%~37%。IMPACT 研究证实 D+/R-肾受体 200 天(相比于 100 天)的预防治疗更有效[11]。

鉴于有侵入性感染风险，对于原发性感染风险的心脏、肝脏、胰腺和肾移植患者(CMV D+/R-)应在移植后给予 3~6 个月的预防性治疗(表 94.5)[23,75]。很多移植中心对于接受抗淋巴细胞抗体的 CMV D+/R-或 R+受体进行 6 个月的预防治疗[11]。最近一项肺脏移植后关于缬更昔洛韦 3 个月与 12 个月对比使用的随机试验表明，肺脏移植受体可能更会受益于更长的预防治疗

(12 个月)[10]。如果有适当的监测系统,而且受体依从性良好,抢先治疗则会更合适[23,75]。在一些心脏移植与肺脏移植中,CMV 超免疫球蛋白也被常规使用[23,75,83,84]。

治疗

CMV 的标准治疗通常为 3 周静脉注射更昔洛韦(5mg/kg,每日两次,肾功能不良者可进行剂量调整)或者缬更昔洛韦(900mg 口服,每日两次肾功能不良者可进行剂量调整)[23,75]。在最近的一项临床试验中,对于携带中等病毒载量的轻至中度 CMV 感染患者,口服缬更昔洛韦不逊于静脉注射更昔洛韦治疗[85]。这项实验排除了那些高病毒载量和侵入性胃肠道疾病的患者。两组 21 天内清除病毒血症的比例大约为 50%[85]。对于那些治疗反应不佳或者血清学阴性的患者,一些移植中心对血清学阴性的个体使用 3 个月 CMV 超免疫球蛋白(150mg/kg,每月静脉注射)。低丙种球蛋白血症应该在治疗期间进行纠正[86]。复发主要发生在那些由于定量阴性而没有接受治疗[85]或对一些胃肠道疾病仅仅采取了口服药物治疗的受体。实际应用中,应该一开始就启动更昔洛韦静脉注射治疗,并每周进行检测直到监测阴性。当静脉用药完成后,口服 2~4 个月缬更昔洛韦(每日 900mg,基于肌酐清除率)可以作为二线方案[87,88]。这种方法极少发生复发和病毒抗性的出现。测定肌酸酐清除率非常必要,可以确保合适的药物剂量。

更昔洛韦的抗性一般不太常见,可能在肺脏移植中比例高一些[78]。D+/R-受体发生耐药的风险最大,特别当存在高病毒载量、预防性或治疗性更昔洛韦的剂量不足,更强的免疫抑制包括抗淋巴细胞抗体诱导,和长期抗病毒预防[78,79]。临床上,患者的病毒载量或临床症状有时对适当的治疗反应欠佳。遗传抗性测试可用于 CMV 感染抗药性管理;病毒 UL97(胸苷激酶)或 UL54(DNA 聚合酶)基因突变可以产生更昔洛韦耐药[89]。另外一些常见的 UL97 基因突变对高剂量的更昔洛韦静脉注射更敏感[90]。联合突变(UL97 和 UL54)会导致更高的更昔洛韦抗性。替代疗法仅存在静脉用药形式。包括膦甲酸和西多福韦[78]。膦甲酸对许多对更昔洛韦耐药的 CMV 有效,尽管它可以造成镁钾丢失、癫痫(特别是联合 CNI 治疗时)和一些肾毒性。西多福韦常常引起显著的肾毒性和眼毒性。加入超免疫球蛋白的联合治疗(更昔洛韦和膦甲酸)可能会更有效[91]。大多数移植中心试图减少治疗过程中的免疫抑制程度。UL54 突变可能导致膦甲酸和西多福韦抗性,这取决于突变性质[89]。耐药的巨细胞病毒感染可能需要多疗程的抗病毒治疗来治愈。鉴于可用药物的毒性,一些正在研究中的药物可能在将来改变耐药 CMV 的治疗[92-94]。

移植后淋巴增生性疾病和 Epstein-Barr 病毒

PTLD 的特征为良性多克隆淋巴细胞增殖到恶性单克隆淋巴瘤[95-98]。大部分 PTLD 与 EBV 感染有关,并且以 B 淋巴细胞为主目标。在免疫抑制的移植受体,原发性 EBV 感染 (和没有抗病毒免疫情况下的复发)会引起单核细胞增多型综合征,通常表现为 B 细胞淋巴细胞增多症,伴或不伴淋巴结病或咽炎。有时还可以观察到脑膜炎,肝炎和胰腺炎。原因缓解-复发性 EBV 感染在儿童中很常见,可能反映了抗病毒免疫进化与免疫抑制之间的相互作用。这种综合征提示免疫抑制过度。PTLD 最明确的危险因素是原发性 EBV 感染,其将 PTLD 风险增加 10~76 倍[95]。然而,在没有 EBV 感染或血清学阳性患者中,PTLD 也可能发生。

移植后非霍奇金淋巴瘤(NHL)是常见的实体器官移植并发症。淋巴瘤占所有成人受体肿瘤的 15%(儿童受体的 51%),死亡率为 40%~60%。与一般人群相比,PTLD 具有增加的淋巴结外侵犯,常规治疗反应差和预后不良。疾病谱范围从良性多克隆 B 细胞感染性单核细胞增多症到恶性单克隆淋巴瘤。大多数是 B 细胞来源。T 细胞、NK 细胞和无效细胞肿瘤在成人中发生率为 37%,经常是单细胞性的,预后极差。其他预后不良指证包括 CNS 疾病、多发性部位疾病、EBV 阴性 PTLD、疾病受体来源,以及原癌基因和肿瘤抑制基因突变[95,99-101]。

PTLD 诊断由于 EBV 阴性 PTLD 和同种异体移植物 T 细胞 PTLD 的存在而复杂化,很容易与移植物排斥或其他病毒感染相混淆。EBV 阴性 PTLD 在成人移植中更是经常在晚期发生(>1~2 年)[95]。

除原发性 EBV 感染外,PTLD 的风险因素包括 CMV 供体-受体血清失配、T 细胞耗竭治疗、低龄儿童、高龄、免疫抑制总体强度[95]。PTLD 可以发生在移植后任何时候,如果是原发性 EBV 感染引起,一般在移植后 12 周内就会发生。一些风险与移植器官种类相关,虽然这可能反映病毒负荷、共感染的存在和免疫抑制强度。因此,儿童肠移植 PTLD 的发生率为 32%,而心、肺、肝和胰腺移植的PTLD发生率较低(3%~12%),肾移植PTLD发生率甚至更低(1%~2%)[95]。

EBV相关PTLD的临床表现包括:

- 不明原因发热(未知来源的发热)。
- 单核细胞增多型综合征,伴有发热和不适,伴或不伴咽炎或扁桃体炎(经常通过扁桃体切除标本偶然诊断)。通常没有淋巴结病。
- 胃肠道出血、阻塞和穿孔。
- 腹部肿块(最常见于腹部移植)。
- 同种异体移植物浸润性疾病。
- 肝细胞或胰腺功能障碍。
- 孤立的中枢神经系统疾病或脑膜炎。
- 肺浸润性病变。

诊断

血清学检查对急性EBV感染或PTLD诊断作用有限。但血清学阴性受体接受阳性供器官时(EBV D+/R-),应监测EBV感染相关临床症状。任何排斥表现都应该通过组织穿刺来明确是否存在PTLD。EBV病毒载量定量对于EBV阳性PTLD的诊断和治疗都非常有帮助[102-104]。这些方法的灵敏度很高,但是特异度不强。一些移植中心喜欢使用全血而不是血浆样品用于EBV病毒载量监测[105]。系列方法测定比单一病毒载量测定更有用[102]。因为这些测定方法都不是标准化的,不能直接相互比较[105]。WHO实验室检测标准可以用于能力验证。一般来说,组织诊断对PTLD的诊断和管理是必须的。这些组织应请病理学专家进行评估以便避免与其他病变混淆[100]。使用RNA原位杂交测定组织或循环淋巴细胞中EBV编码的小核RNA(EBER),相对于杂交靶向病毒DNA更为灵敏[106]。通常利用免疫组化进行补充检测EBV潜伏抗原EBNA-1、EBNA-2和LMP-1[107,108]。淋巴细胞抗体克隆、癌基因、肿瘤抑制基因或染色体、治疗靶标记(CD20的表达、细胞毒性T细胞表位)都可以通过供体和受体研究进行很好的补充。

治疗

临床管理取决于疾病阶段。在多克隆形式,特别是在儿童中,通过减少免疫抑制重建免疫功能可能就足以使PTLD消退[95]。在这个阶段,考虑到病毒血症和EBV作为免疫抑制病原,抗病毒治疗可能会有一定的作用[103,109]。CMV是PTLD的共同因子,因此有必要对EBV病毒血症个体使用更昔洛韦或缬更昔洛韦进行预防性治疗。关于这种治疗功效的确切数据非常有限。随着疾病进展到淋巴结外和单克隆恶性形式,减少免疫抑制可能有用,但通常需要替代疗法。目前一般会联合抗B细胞治疗(抗CD20、利妥昔单抗)、组合化疗(CHOP)和(或)采用经刺激T细胞的过继性免疫治疗[95,110,111]。但是反应持续时间往往令人失望。在移植中,免疫抑制消退不明显可能表明需要牺牲同种异体移植患者生存期。在活动性病毒血症时,移植排斥非常罕见,但是一些受体死亡也确实与撤除免疫抑制治疗恶性肿瘤期间的移植物失功有关[96]。CNS PTLD一般需要放射治疗[111]。如果没有神经系统外的疾病表现,一般需要活检明确诊断。

多瘤病毒

多瘤病毒在一些移植受体中被确认存在,如肾病和输尿管梗阻(BK病毒),类似于艾滋病的脑脱髓鞘疾病(JC病毒)[112]。成人血清学阳性率为65%~90%。BK病毒潜伏在肾小管上皮细胞。JC病毒也已从肾组织中分离,但是似乎对神经组织更具有嗜好性。重新激活的发生与免疫缺陷、免疫抑制和组织损伤有关,如缺血再灌注。

BK多瘤病毒感染

BK病毒尿症和病毒(BKV)与免疫受损宿主一系列临床综合征相关:病毒血症、输尿管溃疡和狭窄以及出血性膀胱炎[112,113]。肾移植活动性感染与一些个体移植物功能的进行性丧失相关,被称为“BK肾病”或多瘤病毒相关性肾病(PyVAN或PVAN)。尽管存在病毒复制和病毒尿症,在非肾脏器官的受体中PVAN很少被识别,说明肾损伤如缺血再灌注或者其他肾移植相关的操作会引起肾病。不常见的是,BKV还可能引起肺炎、血噬细胞综合征、脑炎或多瘤病毒相关多灶性白细胞性脑病(PVML,最常见于JC病毒)[114,115]。

疾病临床表现通常包括在没有血细菌或真菌感染的前提下,尿液细胞检测提示肾小管和输尿管上皮细胞脱落。这些含有病毒壳并通过尿检检测得到的细胞被称作“诱饵细胞”[116,117]。在大多数情况下,并不进行这些细胞检测,而受体会表现出移植物功能减弱,或较不常见的输尿管狭窄和梗阻。在这种患者中,肾功能下降的病因必须仔细评价,如机械阻塞、药物毒性、肾盂肾炎、排斥、血栓形成和复发性疾病。必须在增加免疫抑制治疗疑似移植物排斥或减少免疫抑制以允许免疫系统来控制感染之间做出抉择。BK肾病患者增大免疫抑制强度时容易发生移植物功能损害[112,118]。减少免疫抑制可以稳定肾同种异体移植物功能[119],但又会存在移植物排斥风险。以组织学表现和肾功能障碍为特征多瘤相关肾病在移植患者中的比例为1%~8%[112]。

30%~50%具有高病毒水平的肾脏受体可以进展到PVAN。风险因素包括缺血再灌注损伤、BKV特异性免疫缺乏、他克莫司为基础的免疫抑制过强、HLA不匹配、急性排斥包括脉冲剂量类固醇使用和用于治疗排斥的T细胞耗竭[112]。特异性免疫抑制剂的作用目前还没有确认[120]。

筛查、预防与诊断

BKV感染通常是无症状的。管状上皮细胞损伤及炎症反映在缓慢上升的血清肌酐，这也是PVAN的第一个临床征兆。大多数移植中心已经发展筛选程序记录早期疾病[118,120,121]。利用尿液细胞学检测是否存在感染的诱饵细胞,其BKV感染的敏感性可以达到100%,但预后判断价值较差(29%)。诱饵细胞可用于筛查,但不能用于明确诊断[117]。尿液中的BKV可以通过电子显微镜检测;当尿液BKV(DNA)含量>7log gEq/mL或BKV VP1 mRNA>6log拷贝/ng时对诊断很有帮助。Hirsch等的研究表明与没有BK肾病的患者相比,BK肾病患者血液病毒载量偏高(>7700BKV拷贝/mL血浆;$P<0.001$;50%阳性预测率,100%阴性预测率)，并且具有统计学意义[122]。当血清病毒负荷高合并血清肌酐高时,应该调整免疫抑制强度，但是明确诊断依赖于移植肾脏BKV细胞病变表现、BKV蛋白的免疫组化检测或穿刺标本的BKV核酸原位杂交[112]。PVAN的特征在于管状上皮和(或)肾小球细胞中核内多瘤病毒包涵体。肾脏活检通常会证实上皮细胞病变，并评估细胞浸润的逐渐演变与间质性肾炎的诊断。纤维化经常发生,偶尔伴有钙化。免疫组化中可利用的抗体包括猿猴病毒40大T抗原交叉反应抗体、BKV VP1或抗原蛋白抗体[117]。PVAN病灶通常比较局限,易造成活检假阴性,因此有些病例需要重复穿刺。PVAN可能与移植排斥并存,从而使得前者诊断变得困难。目前有针对PVAN组织学变化的半定量评分系统[117]。

关于筛选BKV感染的建议目前存在异议,但一般建议在移植后两年内每3个月检查一次，第2~5年每年至少检查1次[112,118]。BKV的尿液检测(诱饵细胞的尿液细胞学检查或BKV病毒载荷>7log gEq/mL）适用于筛查。如果结果阴性,那么发生PVAN的风险极低。尿液BKV阳性的患者应继续测定血浆BKV DNA载量[118]。一些移植中心直接使用血浆BKV DNA负荷进行筛查。当患者血清病毒负荷在2~3周之内重复检测均大于4log 10gEq/mL时,可以确诊PVAN并减轻免疫抑制程度(见下文)。如果使用血清学方法进行筛查,那么在移植后应至少每6个月测定一次。这提示在永久性肾损伤之前,病毒血症患者的尿液中也已出现病毒。对血清肌酐升高并且BKV筛查阳性的受体应进行肾活检[112]。

治疗

除降低免疫抑制强度外，没有PVAN的特效治疗方式[112,119,123]。可以用血浆病毒载量监测治疗反应。尽管存在争议，当监测血清BKV病毒负荷时应逐步减少CNI和抗代谢物的药物剂量。鉴于CNI的毒性管状细胞、BKV激活造成损伤、抗BK T细胞活性需要等,这些药物应该在一开始就进行减量。减药目标为:他克莫司谷浓度水平<6ng/mL,环孢菌素谷浓度<150ng/mL,西罗莫司谷浓度<6ng/mL,和(或)MMF日剂量当量≤1000mg。不管使用哪种方法,肾功能(每周至少1~2次)、药物水平和病毒载量(每两周1次)应该在减药期间规律监测[112]。如果反应不佳则有必要进行重复穿刺。

使用辅助抗病毒治疗仍有争议。一些中心主张在BK肾病使用低剂量西多福韦[124](每2周0.25~1mg/kg)。值得注意的是,使用该药物可以造成肾功能损害,特别是联合使用CNI时。一些数据支持在认真筛选的受体中使用交替治疗方法。包括来氟米特(一种同时具有抗BKV病毒活性的免疫抑制剂)、免疫球蛋白静脉注射和氟喹诺酮抗微生物剂[125,126]。前瞻性临床试验数据和FDA并没有批准这些疗法。最好在移植感染专家的指导下使用上述治疗方法。

当PVAN患者移植物失功时可以进行再次移植，可能需要免疫抑制减弱之后免疫能力再建[127,128]。大部分移植中心在撤除免疫抑制剂一段时间后(6个月),血液和尿液中均不能检测到BKV时再次进行移植。未来,撤除免疫抑制后BKV细胞免疫的特殊检测方法可以帮助决定合适的再移植时机[129]。供器官的外科切除并不能保证未来不感染 BKV 或不发生 PVAN,但是在免疫抑制无法撤除(双移植、同种致敏作用)和(或)病毒载量持续升高时,也不得不进行外科切除。

JC 病毒

JC 多瘤病毒造成的 CNS 感染和其导致的进行性多灶性脑白质病(PML)在移植受体中并不常见[130]。这种感染可能伴随局灶性神经功能缺陷或癫痫发作、缓慢进行性神经病变，并可能进展为广泛脱髓鞘然后致死。PML 可能与钙调磷酸酶神经毒性相混淆,因为两者都对减低药物水平有反应。基于 AIDS 患者 PML 的免疫重建，一般在移植后 PML 发生时减弱免疫抑制强度,但目前仍然缺乏已经被证实有效的治疗手段。

真菌感染

移植受体可能会感染各种真菌，主要类型包括念珠菌属、曲霉属、新型隐球酵母和地方性真菌病及地理真菌[131-134]。随着受体长期存活和流行病学暴露,其他种类的真菌感染也越来越多地被报道[135]。

念珠菌

移植受体最常见的侵入性真菌病原体为假丝酵母菌属、白色念珠菌、热带假丝酵母和光滑假丝酵母,约占该类感染的 90%[134]。念珠菌定殖部位明确,而且各移植中心氟康唑耐药的发生率也各有不同，移植受体中非白色念珠菌感染的比例正在不断提高。黏膜念珠菌感染,如鹅口疮、食管感染、睫毛间皮肤感染、念珠菌性阴道炎等，特别容易发生在免疫抑制下糖尿病控制不佳、口腔卫生差以及接受广谱抗菌治疗的受体。这些感染可以通过纠正潜在的代谢异常、局部应用克霉唑和制备菌素进行治疗。念珠菌病对于肾移植受体比较特殊,因为通常无症状[136,137]。特别是在膀胱功能差的个体,可以在肾盂输尿管连接处形成真菌球,进而导致阻塞性疾病、肾盂肾炎及全身性传播。

念珠菌血症是移植术后最常见的院内感染类型，与血管通路导管、外科导管、膀胱导管、抗微生物使用、外周静脉营养和糖尿病有关[134,138]。但对于存在胆道吻合问题的肝脏移植受体，念珠菌血症可在持续性胆管炎抗菌治疗之后发生。胆肠吻合的肝脏移植受体其念珠菌发生率高于胆管-胆管吻合。胆漏和出血会导致念珠菌再次感染。胰腺移植受体感染发生率很高,一般使用氟康唑进行预防[139]。长期肠道引流感染发生侵入性念珠菌病的概率比膀胱引流大得多。与念珠菌血症相关的其他因素包括肾和肝脏移植物功能障碍、重症监护病房(ICU)停留、大量输血、腹部移植后再次手术、移植物胰腺炎、胃肠外高营养、定殖和广谱抗微生物治疗[134]。感染诊断基于血清培养。血培养阳性的受体应及时治疗,并应去除外界异物,如血管通路导管等。治疗延迟与死亡率显著相关。所有分离物都应该检测抗生素药敏实验以确保治疗有效，因为氟康唑耐药菌种如光滑念珠菌和克鲁斯念珠菌越来越普遍[140]。还应进行视网膜检查排除视网膜炎。应该注意的是肺念珠菌病非常罕见,其通常定殖于咽部。一种例外情况是肺脏移植后受体存在气道吻合并暴露在外[141]。念珠菌属还可以与 HSV 或 CMV 一起多重感染食管。血管吻合感染可导致有破裂风险的真菌性动脉瘤。在一些研究中，念珠菌感染与器官保存液污染有关[142];区别器官保存液污染和捐献过程中的外科操作污染非常困难。

曲霉菌种

侵入性曲霉病是移植受体的一种紧急情况。大部分通过肺和鼻窦侵入。非常容易转移至 CNS 并决定临床表现。在移植后早期,累及 CNS 的真菌感染主要为曲霉菌;而移植一年以后则主要以其他真菌(接合菌、暗色丝孢真菌)为主[143,144]。侵入性曲霉病发病率为 1%~15%,取决于移植器官类型[145]。一般风险因素包括定殖、CMV 感染、中性粒细胞减少、移植排斥、ICU 停留、肾功能不全和透析[133]。此外,器官特异性风险因素包括重新探查(肝和肺)、HCV 感染、再移植(肝)、气管缺血和获得性低丙种球蛋白血症(肺)[146]。应该特别注意肺脏移植气管吻合感染中是否存在曲霉菌[141],以及造血干细胞或实体器官移植患者出现病毒感染和药物毒性造成的中性粒细胞减少时。

早期诊断对于预后至关重要,通常需要活检。在气道分泌物中检测到曲霉菌,常提示心脏、肺和肝脏受体发生侵入性感染的风险较高。半乳甘露聚糖测试对侵入性曲霉病早期诊断效用不如中性粒细胞[147]。半乳甘露聚糖测定法进行移植受体侵入性曲霉病诊断最适用于气管肺泡灌洗样本[148]。曲霉菌的组织或培养诊断非常必要,因为对不同抗真菌药物的敏感性不同,可能还会存在其他感染。每种有效的抗真菌剂都有自身局限性。脂质体两性霉素与 CNI 联合使用时会增加肾毒性风险；伏立康唑和其他唑类具有增加 CNI 血清水平和西罗莫司的显著作用;棘白菌素具有肝毒性,并且对接合菌的活性和隐球菌属没有效果。

中枢神经系统感染和新型隐球菌

移植受体CNS感染是医疗紧急情况。致病生物范围广泛，预后通常与治疗及时性有关。许多转移到CNS的感染来自于肺。因此，转移来源是CNS病情评价的组成部分，包括病因来源曲霉属、隐球菌属、诺卡菌属等。病毒感染主要包括CMV（结节性血管炎）、单纯疱疹脑膜脑炎、JC病毒（PML）和VZV。常见的细菌感染包括单核细胞增生李斯特菌、分枝杆菌、诺卡菌属，偶尔还会有沙门菌属。脑脓肿和硬膜外脓肿中可以观察到MRSA、青霉素抵抗肺炎链球菌和喹诺酮抗性链球菌，这些治疗都很困难。转移性真菌包括曲霉属和隐球菌属，但也会来源于鼻窦（毛霉菌）、皮肤（暗色孢科）和血液（组织胞浆菌和假杆菌/镰刀菌）。寄生虫包括刚地弓形虫和类圆线虫。

鉴于病因谱广泛，精确诊断必不可少。特别是当等待腰穿、血培养和放射性数据时，经验治疗必须“覆盖”李斯特菌（氨苄西林）、隐球菌（氟康唑或两性霉素）和HSV（阿昔洛韦或更昔洛韦），以及常见的细菌性脑膜炎（肺炎球菌、流感嗜血杆菌）和已知的肺定殖病原体。非感染性病因的鉴别诊断包括CNI毒性、淋巴瘤以及转移性癌症。确诊通常需要通过活检。

新型隐球菌

隐球菌感染比较常见，但移植术后6个月内的感染很少，一般感染发生在16个月之后[132]。移植受体的隐球菌感染最常见的临床表现为无症状的肺结节，常常伴有病原体存在。在其他患者中可能出现脑膜炎、肺炎、组织损伤部位（导管）皮肤感染、蜂窝织炎、结节性或者丘疹性病变。当移植受体在移植1年以后出现不明原因头痛（特别是伴有发热时）、意识冷漠、发育不良、肺炎或不明原因局灶性皮肤病（需要穿刺活检培养和病理学评估）时，应考虑隐球菌感染[132]。风险因素包括暴露于鸟类和蝙蝠排泄物、供体来源感染性感染和T细胞耗竭。肝脏受体在所有移植受体中感染风险最大。

一般通过隐球菌血清抗原检测来诊断，但这些患者需同时进行腰椎穿刺以用于细胞计数和培养、脑脊液（CSF）压力测量和隐球菌抗原测定。最初使用脂质两性霉素和5-氟胞嘧啶，然后联合高剂量氟康唑直到血液和CSF中无法检测到隐球菌抗原。长期治疗建议使用氟康唑。IRIS或瘢痕形成可能会造成CSF压力升高和脑积水[15]。

类圆线虫

在免疫治疗情况下，类原虫感染可以在初次接触的30年内再次被激活。这种再激活会导致腹泻、寄生虫迁移伴过度感染综合征（特征为出血性小肠结肠炎或出血性肺炎，或两者均有）、弥漫性感染伴革兰阴性菌血症或脑膜炎[149,150]。热带地区和美国东南部的患者应在移植前进行类圆线虫血清IgG筛选，如果血清学阳性，则应提前利用伊维菌素治疗[6]。

发热、肺炎和肺囊虫感染

肺脏移植潜在病原体非常广泛。一些基本概念值得考虑。对于所有移植感染而言，侵入性技术诊断肺炎经常是必需的。免疫功能低下的移植受体对于感染免疫反应滞后可能会改变或延迟通过放射学发现肺脏损伤。因此，在评估早期或者胸片没有特异性发现时应尽早行CT检查，还可以指导诊断性穿刺，如支气管镜、细针穿刺活检或术中活检。CT对于明确疾病严重程度以及发展可能也很有帮助。胸部急性发作的局灶性或多灶性X线征象很可能是由细菌感染引起的。进展较慢的多灶性病变可能继发于真菌、结核病或诺卡菌感染。大结节通常是真菌、诺卡菌或PTLD的感染迹象，特别是当呈现亚急性或慢性发作时。亚急性疾病伴随弥漫性异常，如支气管血管区域或粟粒微结节，通常由病毒（特别是CMV）或耶氏肺孢子菌造成。肺部病变的空洞也可以提供一些线索，空洞一般提示真菌（曲霉属或毛霉科）、诺卡菌属、葡萄球菌属和某些革兰阴性杆菌感染，最常见的是肺炎克雷白杆菌和铜绿假单胞菌。

肺囊虫性肺炎

PCP的感染风险在移植后6个月和免疫抑制增加期间最大[151]。与其他受体相比，肺脏移植受体存在终身感染肺囊虫的风险[152]。考虑到PCP常规预防的应用，肺囊虫肺炎可能发生在预防治疗期之外，特别是当供体存在与胸部检查不符的显著低氧血症时。其感染来源尚未知晓。动物实验和临床实验已经证明，PCP可以通过气体传播，特别是在HIV感染者和移植受体人群中[153]。病因主要是在免疫抑制的受体中发生了潜在感染激活。在实体器官移植受体中，包括皮质类固醇在内的慢性免疫抑制与肺囊炎密切相关。皮质类固醇、环孢素、CMV或其他社区获得性呼吸道病毒合并感染都会增加肺炎杆菌肺炎发病风险。

大多数移植中心报道移植后 6 个月内，在不接受 TMP-SMX(或替代药物)预防的受体中，耶氏肺孢子菌肺炎的发生率为 10%[151]。在三个相互重叠的移植受体群体中存在继续感染的风险：① 由于移植物功能较差或慢性排斥而长时间需要高于正常水平的免疫抑制；② 合并慢性 CMV 感染；③ 接受造成免疫受损的治疗措施，如癌症化疗或由于药物毒性引起的中性粒细胞减少。与其他免疫缺陷的宿主相比，环孢菌素患者中肺孢子虫肺炎的死亡率较高。耶氏肺孢子菌感染的标志是明显的低氧血症、呼吸困难和咳嗽，而缺乏阳性体征与影像学表现。在移植受体，肺孢子虫肺炎一般由急性转归为亚急性。非典型肺囊虫感染（影像学或临床）一般发生在受体存在其他肺部感染或者接受二线药物治疗(喷他脒和阿托伐醌)时。发生在非高危感染期的 PCP 可能会与心力衰竭相混淆。这类患者一般需要侵入性诊断手段进行确诊[151]。

西罗莫司毒性可能有助于弥漫性间质肺炎发展[154]；不清楚这种效应是由西罗莫司本身引起，还是 RSV、PCP 和(或)CMV 的共感染引起。

诊断

PCP 特征性低氧血症会使肺泡-动脉间梯度明显。大多数肺囊虫肺炎患者血清乳酸脱氢酶(LDH)水平会升高(>300IU/mL)。但是，其他一些弥漫性肺病也会增加血清 LDH 水平。与许多“非典型”肺炎(肺部感染，无痰产生)一样，肺囊虫肺炎的常规胸部 X 线片不会有特殊表现。胸片可以完全正常，也可以表现为间质性肺炎经典的“磨玻璃”影。也可以表现为微小囊肿、结节、小渗出、淋巴结病及不对称性的线性带。相对于常规的影像学检查，胸部 CT 扫描可能对于间质弥漫性病变和结节更为敏感。PCP 的临床和放射学表现与 CMV 几乎相同。事实上，确定两种病原体是否同时存在一直是临床难题。移植受体不太发生明显的肺外疾病[151]。

在免疫功能低下的患者中确诊耶氏肺孢子菌为特异性病原体对于治疗是否有效尤为关键。AIDS 患者和非 AIDS 患者的肺炎球菌感染诊断应加以区分。相比其他免疫受损宿主，AIDS 患者一般会存在更多微生物病原体，而且非侵入性诊断方法(痰培养)即可以明确诊断。一般来说，应采用非侵入性方法进行初步诊断，但在临床可行时应使用侵入性技术。耶氏肺孢子菌感染的诊断随着痰培养、免疫荧光单克隆抗体检测以及分子诊断技术的进步得到了很大提高。抗体可以结合囊壁和滋养体。囊壁可以通过各种染色技术显示；其中青霉胺类——硝酸银方法(将微生物染成褐色或黑色)是最可靠的，即使它容易受到伪像的影响。荧光增白剂也常用于检测肺囊虫。孢子和滋养体可以被多色染料染色，特别是 Giemsa 染色，但对于非专家而言，不太容易观察到病原体。

治疗

早期治疗一般采用 TMP-SMX，几乎没有移植患者能够耐受长期的全剂量 TMP-SMX。当需要使用比预防剂量更多的药物时，推荐给药浓度[15~20mg/(kg·/d)甲氧苄啶组分]没有在肾功能不全的成人中很好地进行过研究。毒性表现为甲氧苄啶和磺胺药物对移植肾损伤造成的肌酐升高。水化和逐步增加给药浓度可能有所帮助。替代治疗有成功应用案例，但疗效仍无法令人满意，包括静脉注射戊脒、阿托伐醌和克林霉素及伯氨喹或乙胺嘧啶。减弱免疫抑制强度一般被认为是移植受体抗感染的重要部分，渐近性的辅助性类固醇短期应用对于移植受体和 AIDS 患者有效[151]。

肺囊虫感染预防的重要性无须过分强调。在没有具体数据证明过敏或者导致间质性肾炎的前提下，应使用耐受性良好的低剂量 TMP-SMX。替代性预防策略，包括氨苯砜、阿托伐醌、吸入或静脉内应用戊脒，相比 TMP-SMX 效果较差，但是在磺胺药物过敏的患者中非常有效。TMP-SMX 是最有效的 PCP 预防药物。TMP-SMX 的优点在于疗效明确、花费低、可口服，而且对其他一些病原体也有预防作用，如刚地弓形虫、环孢子囊菌以及常见的泌尿、呼吸和胃肠道细菌病原体。替代性预防策略则没有这些优点[151]。

总结

基于敏感分子诊断技术的防治策略和早期治疗是移植感染性疾病领域的重要内容。与早期移植相比，在 CMV 感染和其他机会性病原体的预防方面有了长足进步，但感染仍然是受体面临的重要问题。在未来，移植受体会在特异性病原体免疫测定方法、供受体微生物筛查、基于免疫调节元件和受体遗传多态性宿主感染风险评估、移植免疫抑制个体化治疗等方面取得长足发展。

（魏绪勇　译　徐骁　校）

参考文献

1. Fishman JA. Infection in solid-organ transplant recipients. New England Journal of Medicine. 2007;357(25):2601–2614.
2. Fishman JA, Rubin RH. Infection in organ-transplant recipients. New England Journal of Medicine. 1998;338(24):1741–1751.
3. Fishman JA. Transplantation microbiology: an evolving pillar of transplant care. American Journal of Transplantation. 2009;9(2):249–250.
4. Rubin RH. The compromised host as sentinel chicken. New England Journal of Medicine. 1987;317(18):1151–1153.
5. Issa NC, Fishman JA. Infectious complications of antilymphocyte therapies in solid organ transplantation. Clinical Infectious Diseases. 2009;48(6):772–786.
6. Fischer SA, Avery RK. Screening of donor and recipient prior to solid organ transplantation. American Journal of Transplantation. 2009;9(Suppl 4):S7–S18.
7. Grossi PA, Fishman JA. Donor-derived infections in solid organ transplant recipients. American Journal of Transplantation. 2009;9(Suppl 4):S19–S26.
8. van Delden C, Blumberg EA. Multidrug resistant gram-negative bacteria in solid organ transplant recipients. American Journal of Transplantation. 2009;9(Suppl 4):S27–S34.
9. Husain S, Raza K, Pilewski JM, et al. Experience with immune monitoring in lung transplant recipients: correlation of low immune function with infection. Transplantation. 2009;87(12):1852–1857.
10. Palmer SM, Limaye AP, Banks M, et al. Extended valganciclovir prophylaxis to prevent cytomegalovirus after lung transplantation: a randomized, controlled trial. Annals of Internal Medicine. 2010;152(12):761–769.
11. Humar A, Lebranchu Y, Vincenti F, et al. The efficacy and safety of 200 days valganciclovir cytomegalovirus prophylaxis in high-risk kidney transplant recipients. American Journal of Transplantation. 2010;10(5):1228–1237.
12. Hibberd PL, Tolkoff-Rubin NE, Doran M, et al. Trimethoprim-sulfamethoxazole compared with ciprofloxacin for the prevention of urinary tract infection in renal transplant recipients. A double-blind, randomized controlled trial. Online Journal of Current Clinical Trials. 1992;Doc No 15.
13. Rubin RH. The indirect effects of cytomegalovirus infection on the outcome of organ transplantation. JAMA. 1989;261(24):3607–3609.
14. Rubin RH. The pathogenesis and clinical management of cytomegalovirus infection in the organ transplant recipient: the end of the 'silo hypothesis'. Current Opinion in Infectious Diseases. 2007;20(4):399–407.
15. Singh N, Lortholary O, Alexander BD, et al. An immune reconstitution syndrome-like illness associated with Cryptococcus neoformans infection in organ transplant recipients. Clinical Infectious Diseases. 2005;40(12):1756–1761.
16. Avery RK. Infections after lung transplantation. Seminars in Respiratory and Critical Care Medicine. 2006;27(5):544–551.
17. Bando K, Paradis IL, Komatsu K, et al. Analysis of time-dependent risks for infection, rejection, and death after pulmonary transplantation. Journal of Thoracic and Cardiovascular Surgery. 1995;109(1):49–57, discussion 57–59.
18. Kroshus TJ, Kshettry VR, Savik K, et al. Risk factors for the development of bronchiolitis obliterans syndrome after lung transplantation. Journal of Thoracic and Cardiovascular Surgery. 1997;114(2):195–202.
19. Potena L, Valantine HA. Cytomegalovirus-associated allograft rejection in heart transplant patients. Current Opinion in Infectious Diseases. 2007;20(4):425–431.
20. Lowance D, Neumayer HH, Legendre CM, et al. Valacyclovir for the prevention of cytomegalovirus disease after renal transplantation. International Valacyclovir Cytomegalovirus Prophylaxis Transplantation Study Group. New England Journal of Medicine. 1999;340(19):1462–1470.
21. Yamani MH, Avery RK, Mawhorter SD, et al. Hypogammaglobulinemia following cardiac transplantation: a link between rejection and infection. Journal of Heart and Lung Transplantation. 2001;20(4):425–430.
22. Snydman DR, Limaye AP, Potena L, et al. Update and review: state-of-the-art management of cytomegalovirus infection and disease following thoracic organ transplantation. Transplantation Proceedings. 2011;43(3 Suppl):S1–S17.
23. Humar A, Snydman D. Cytomegalovirus in solid organ transplant recipients. American Journal of Transplantation. 2009;9(Suppl 4):S78–S86.
24. Paya C, Humar A, Dominguez E, et al. Efficacy and safety of valganciclovir vs. oral ganciclovir for prevention of cytomegalovirus disease in solid organ transplant recipients. American Journal of Transplantation. 2004;4(4):611–620.
25. Freeman RB, Paya C, Pescovitz MD, et al. Risk factors for cytomegalovirus viremia and disease developing after prophylaxis in high-risk solid-organ transplant recipients. Transplantation. 2004;78(12):1765–1773.
26. Eid AJ, Bakri SJ, Kijpittayarit S, et al. Clinical features and outcomes of cytomegalovirus retinitis after transplantation. Transplant Infectious Disease. 2008;10(1):13–18.
27. Snydman DR. The case for cytomegalovirus prophylaxis in solid organ transplantation. Reviews in Medical Virology. 2006;16(5):289–295.
28. Reinke P, Fietze E, Ode-Hakim S, et al. Late-acute renal allograft rejection and symptomless cytomegalovirus infection. Lancet. 1994;344(8939–8940):1737–1738.
29. Gerna G, Lilleri D, Rognoni V, et al. Preemptive therapy for systemic and pulmonary human cytomegalovirus infection in lung transplant recipients. American Journal of Transplantation. 2009;9(5):1142–1150.
30. Emery VC. Cytomegalovirus: recent progress in understanding pathogenesis and control. QJM. 2012;105(5):401–405.
31. Cummins NW, Deziel PJ, Abraham RS, et al. Deficiency of cytomegalovirus (CMV)-specific CD8+ T cells in patients presenting with late-onset CMV disease several years after transplantation. Transplant Infectious Disease. 2009;11(1):20–27.
32. Chiereghin A, Gabrielli L, Zanfi C, et al. Monitoring cytomegalovirus T-cell immunity in small bowel/multivisceral transplant recipients. Transplantation Proceedings. 2010;42(1):69–73.
33. Sund F, Lidehall AK, Claesson K, et al. CMV-specific T-cell immunity, viral load, and clinical outcome in seropositive renal transplant recipients: a pilot study. Clinical Transplantation. 2010;24(3):401–409.
34. Couzi L, Lafarge X, Pitard V, et al. Gamma-delta T cell expansion is closely associated with cytomegalovirus infection in all solid organ transplant recipients. Transplant International. 2011;24(5):e40–e42.
35. Pitard V, Roumanes D, Lafarge X, et al. Long-term expansion of effector/memory Vdelta2-gammadelta T cells is a specific blood signature of CMV infection. Blood. 2008;112(4):1317–1324.
36. Couzi L, Pitard V, Sicard X, et al. Antibody-dependent anti-cytomegalovirus activity of human gammadelta T cells expressing CD16 (FcgammaRIIIa). Blood. 2012;119(6):1418–1427.
37. Griffiths PD, Stanton A, McCarrell E, et al. Cytomegalovirus glycoprotein-B vaccine with MF59 adjuvant in transplant recipients: a phase 2 randomised placebo-controlled trial. Lancet. 2011;377(9773):1256–1263.
38. Razonable RR. Cytomegalovirus infection after liver transplantation: current concepts and challenges. World Journal of Gastroenterology. 2008;14(31):4849–4860.
39. Nickel P, Bold G, Presber F, et al. High levels of CMV-IE-1-specific memory T cells are associated with less alloimmunity and improved renal allograft function. Transplant Immunology. 2009;20(4):238–242.
40. Varani S, Frascaroli G, Landini MP, et al. Human cytomegalovirus targets different subsets of antigen-presenting cells with pathological consequences for host immunity: implications for immunosuppression, chronic inflammation and autoimmunity. Reviews in Medical Virology. 2009;19(3):131–145.
41. Jackson SE, Mason GM, Wills MR. Human cytomegalovirus immunity and immune evasion. Virus Research. 2011;157(2):151–160.
42. Wilkinson GW, Tomasec P, Stanton RJ, et al. Modulation of natural killer cells by human cytomegalovirus. Journal of Clinical Virology. 2008;41(3):206–212.
43. Wills MR, Ashiru O, Reeves MB, et al. Human cytomegalovirus encodes an MHC class I-like molecule (UL142) that functions to inhibit NK cell lysis. Journal of Immunology. 2005;175(11):7457–7465.
44. Skaletskaya A, Bartle LM, Chittenden T, et al. A cytomegalovirus-encoded inhibitor of apoptosis that suppresses caspase-8 activation. Proceedings of the National Academy of Sciences of the United States of America. 2001;98(14):7829–7834.
45. Namboodiri AM, Pandey JP. The human cytomegalovirus TRL11/IRL11-encoded FcgammaR binds differentially to allelic variants of immunoglobulin G1. Archives of Virology. 2011;156(5):907–910.
46. Smith JM, Corey L, Bittner R, et al. Subclinical viremia increases risk for chronic allograft injury in pediatric renal transplantation. Journal of the American Society of Nephrology. 2010;21(9):1579–1586.
47. Zhang H, Fu S, Busch A, et al. Identification of TNF-alpha-sensitive sites in HCMVie1 promoter. Experimental and Molecular Pathology. 2001;71(2):106–114.
48. Hummel M, Abecassis MM. A model for reactivation of CMV from latency. Journal of Clinical Virology. 2002;25(Suppl 2):S123–S136.
49. Burns LJ, Pooley JC, Walsh DJ, et al. Intercellular adhesion molecule-1 expression in endothelial cells is activated by cytomegalovirus immediate early proteins. Transplantation. 1999;67(1):137–144.
50. Inkinen K, Soots A, Krogerus L, et al. Cytomegalovirus enhance expression of growth factors during the development of chronic allograft nephropathy in rats. Transplant International. 2005;18(6):743–749.
51. Shahgasempour S, Woodroffe SB, Garnett HM. Alterations in the expression of ELAM-1, ICAM-1 and VCAM-1 after in vitro infection of endothelial cells with a clinical isolate of human cytomegalovirus. Microbiology and Immunology. 1997;41(2):121–129.

52. Lebranchu Y, al Najjar A, Kapahi P, et al. The association of increased soluble VCAM-1 levels with CMV disease in human kidney allograft recipients. Transplantation Proceedings. 1995;27(1):960.
53. Lautenschlager I, Hockerstedt K, Taskinen E, et al. Expression of adhesion molecules and their ligands in liver allografts during cytomegalovirus (CMV) infection and acute rejection. Transplant International. 1996;9(Suppl 1): S213–S215.
54. Steinhoff G, You XM, Steinmuller C, et al. Enhancement of cytomegalovirus infection and acute rejection after allogeneic lung transplantation in the rat. Transplantation. 1996;61(8):1250–1260.
55. Allen MD, King C, MacDonald TO, et al. VCAM-1 and E-selectin expression during cytomegalovirus infection in post-transplant myocardial biopsies. Clinical Transplantation. 1996;10(6 Pt 1):528–537.
56. Martelius T, Krogerus L, Hockerstedt K, et al. Cytomegalovirus infection is associated with increased inflammation and severe bile duct damage in rat liver allografts. Hepatology. 1998;27(4):996–1002.
57. Nordoy I, Muller F, Nordal KP, et al. Chemokines and soluble adhesion molecules in renal transplant recipients with cytomegalovirus infection. Clinical and Experimental Immunology. 2000;120(2):333–337.
58. Inkinen K, Soots A, Krogerus L, et al. Cytomegalovirus increases collagen synthesis in chronic rejection in the rat. Nephrology, Dialysis, Transplantation. 2002;17(5):772–779.
59. Reischig T, Jindra P, Hes O, et al. Effect of cytomegalovirus viremia on subclinical rejection or interstitial fibrosis and tubular atrophy in protocol biopsy at 3 months in renal allograft recipients managed by preemptive therapy or antiviral prophylaxis. Transplantation. 2009;87(3):436–444.
60. Prochnau D, Lehmann M, Straube E, et al. Human cytomegalovirus induces MMP-1 and MMP-3 expression in aortic smooth muscle cells. Acta Microbiologica et Immunologica Hungarica. 2011;58(4):303–317.
61. Reinhardt B, Winkler M, Schaarschmidt P, et al. Human cytomegalovirus-induced reduction of extracellular matrix proteins in vascular smooth muscle cell cultures: a pathomechanism in vasculopathies? Journal of General Virology. 2006;87(Pt 10):2849–2858.
62. Straat K, de Klark R, Gredmark-Russ S, et al. Infection with human cytomegalovirus alters the MMP-9/TIMP-1 balance in human macrophages. Journal of Virology. 2009;83(2):830–835.
63. Caliendo AM, St George K, Kao SY, et al. Comparison of quantitative cytomegalovirus (CMV) PCR in plasma and CMV antigenemia assay: clinical utility of the prototype AMPLICOR CMV MONITOR test in transplant recipients. Journal of Clinical Microbiology. 2000;38(6):2122–2127.
64. Mazzulli T, Drew LW, Yen-Lieberman B, et al. Multicenter comparison of the digene hybrid capture CMV DNA assay (version 2.0), the pp65 antigenemia assay, and cell culture for detection of cytomegalovirus viremia. Journal of Clinical Microbiology. 1999;37(4):958–963.
65. Pang XL, Fox JD, Fenton JM, et al. Interlaboratory comparison of cytomegalovirus viral load assays. American Journal of Transplantation. 2009; 9(2):258–268.
66. Humar A, Mazzulli T, Moussa G, et al. Clinical utility of cytomegalovirus (CMV) serology testing in high-risk CMV D+/R- transplant recipients. American Journal of Transplantation. 2005;5(5):1065–1070.
67. Ljungman P, Griffiths P, Paya C. Definitions of cytomegalovirus infection and disease in transplant recipients. Clinical Infectious Diseases. 2002;34(8): 1094–1097.
68. Eid AJ, Arthurs SK, Deziel PJ, et al. Clinical predictors of relapse after treatment of primary gastrointestinal cytomegalovirus disease in solid organ transplant recipients. American Journal of Transplantation. 2010;10(1):157–161.
69. Tanabe K, Tokumoto T, Ishikawa N, et al. Comparative study of cytomegalovirus (CMV) antigenemia assay, polymerase chain reaction, serology, and shell vial assay in the early diagnosis and monitoring of CMV infection after renal transplantation. Transplantation. 1997;64(12):1721–1725.
70. van den Berg AP, van der Bij W, van Son WJ, et al. Cytomegalovirus antigenemia as a useful marker of symptomatic cytomegalovirus infection after renal transplantation – a report of 130 consecutive patients. Transplantation. 1989; 48(6):991–995.
71. Caliendo AM, Shahbazian MD, Schaper C, et al. A commutable cytomegalovirus calibrator is required to improve the agreement of viral load values between laboratories. Clinical Chemistry. 2009;55(9):1701–1710.
72. Razonable RR, Brown RA, Wilson J, et al. The clinical use of various blood compartments for cytomegalovirus (CMV) DNA quantitation in transplant recipients with CMV disease. Transplantation. 2002;73(6):968–973.
73. Sia IG, Wilson JA, Groettum CM, et al. Cytomegalovirus (CMV) DNA load predicts relapsing CMV infection after solid organ transplantation. Journal of Infectious Diseases. 2000;181(2):717–720.
74. Mendez J, Espy M, Smith TF, et al. Clinical significance of viral load in the diagnosis of cytomegalovirus disease after liver transplantation. Transplantation. 1998;65(11):1477–1481.
75. Kotton CN, Kumar D, Caliendo AM, et al. International consensus guidelines on the management of cytomegalovirus in solid organ transplantation. Transplantation. 2010;89(7):779–795.
76. Kalil AC, Levitsky J, Lyden E, et al. Meta-analysis: the efficacy of strategies to prevent organ disease by cytomegalovirus in solid organ transplant recipients. Annals of Internal Medicine. 2005;143(12):870–880.
77. Singh N, Wannstedt C, Keyes L, et al. Efficacy of valganciclovir administered as preemptive therapy for cytomegalovirus disease in liver transplant recipients: impact on viral load and late-onset cytomegalovirus disease. Transplantation. 2005;79(1):85–90.
78. Limaye AP. Ganciclovir-resistant cytomegalovirus in organ transplant recipients. Clinical Infectious Diseases. 2002;35(7):866–872.
79. Limaye AP, Corey L, Koelle DM, et al. Emergence of ganciclovir-resistant cytomegalovirus disease among recipients of solid-organ transplants. Lancet. 2000; 356(9230):645–649.
80. Limaye AP, Raghu G, Koelle DM, et al. High incidence of ganciclovir-resistant cytomegalovirus infection among lung transplant recipients receiving preemptive therapy. Journal of Infectious Diseases. 2002;185(1):20–27.
81. Singh N. Late-onset cytomegalovirus disease as a significant complication in solid organ transplant recipients receiving antiviral prophylaxis: a call to heed the mounting evidence. Clinical Infectious Diseases. 2005;40(5):704–708.
82. Limaye AP, Bakthavatsalam R, Kim HW, et al. Late-onset cytomegalovirus disease in liver transplant recipients despite antiviral prophylaxis. Transplantation. 2004;78(9):1390–1396.
83. Valantine HA. Prevention and treatment of cytomegalovirus disease in thoracic organ transplant patients: evidence for a beneficial effect of hyperimmune globulin. Transplantation Proceedings. 1995;27(5 Suppl 1):49–57.
84. Valantine HA, Luikart H, Doyle R, et al. Impact of cytomegalovirus hyperimmune globulin on outcome after cardiothoracic transplantation: a comparative study of combined prophylaxis with CMV hyperimmune globulin plus ganciclovir versus ganciclovir alone. Transplantation. 2001;72(10):1647–1652.
85. Asberg A, Humar A, Rollag H, et al. Oral valganciclovir is noninferior to intravenous ganciclovir for the treatment of cytomegalovirus disease in solid organ transplant recipients. American Journal of Transplantation. 2007;7(9): 2106–2113.
86. Carbone J, Sarmiento E, Palomo J, et al. The potential impact of substitutive therapy with intravenous immunoglobulin on the outcome of heart transplant recipients with infections. Transplantation Proceedings. 2007;39(7):2385–2388.
87. Turgeon N, Fishman JA, Doran M, et al. Prevention of recurrent cytomegalovirus disease in renal and liver transplant recipients: effect of oral ganciclovir. Transplant Infectious Disease. 2000;2(1):2–10.
88. Helantera I, Lautenschlager I, Koskinen P. The risk of cytomegalovirus recurrence after kidney transplantation. Transplant International. 2011;24(12): 1170–1178.
89. Lurain NS, Bhorade SM, Pursell KJ, et al. Analysis and characterization of antiviral drug-resistant cytomegalovirus isolates from solid organ transplant recipients. Journal of Infectious Diseases. 2002;186(6):760–768.
90. West P, Schmiedeskamp M, Neeley H, et al. Use of high-dose ganciclovir for a resistant cytomegalovirus infection due to UL97 mutation. Transplant Infectious Disease. 2008;10(2):129–132.
91. Mylonakis E, Kallas WM, Fishman JA. Combination antiviral therapy for ganciclovir-resistant cytomegalovirus infection in solid-organ transplant recipients. Clinical Infectious Diseases. 2002;34(10):1337–1341.
92. Avery RK, Mossad SB, Poggio E, et al. Utility of leflunomide in the treatment of complex cytomegalovirus syndromes. Transplantation. 2010;90(4):419–426.
93. Avery RK, Marty FM, Strasfeld L, et al. Oral maribavir for treatment of refractory or resistant cytomegalovirus infections in transplant recipients. Transplant Infectious Disease. 2010;12(6):489–496.
94. Painter W, Robertson A, Trost LC, et al. First pharmacokinetic and safety study in humans of the novel lipid antiviral conjugate CMX001, a broad-spectrum oral drug active against double-stranded DNA viruses. Antimicrobial Agents and Chemotherapy. 2012;56(5):2726–2734.
95. Allen U, Preiksaitis J. Epstein-barr virus and posttransplant lymphoproliferative disorder in solid organ transplant recipients. American Journal of Transplantation. 2009;9(Suppl 4):S87–S96.
96. Kasiske BL, Kukla A, Thomas D, et al. Lymphoproliferative disorders after adult kidney transplant: epidemiology and comparison of registry report with claims-based diagnoses. American Journal of Kidney Diseases. 2011;58(6):971–980.
97. Dharnidharka VR, Araya CE. Post-transplant lymphoproliferative disease. Pediatric Nephrology. 2009;24(4):731–736.
98. Nalesnik MA. Clinicopathologic characteristics of post-transplant lymphoproliferative disorders. Recent Results in Cancer Research.. 2002;159:9–18.
99. Craig FE, Johnson LR, Harvey SA, et al. Gene expression profiling of Epstein-

Barr virus-positive and -negative monomorphic B-cell posttransplant lymphoproliferative disorders. Diagnostic Molecular Pathology, Part B. 2007;16(3): 158–168.
100. Nalesnik MA. The diverse pathology of post-transplant lymphoproliferative disorders: the importance of a standardized approach. Transplant Infectious Disease. 2001;3(2):88–96.
101. Nelson BP, Nalesnik MA, Bahler DW, et al. Epstein-Barr virus-negative posttransplant lymphoproliferative disorders: a distinct entity? American Journal of Surgical Pathology. 2000;24(3):375–385.
102. Green M, Cacciarelli TV, Mazariegos GV, et al. Serial measurement of Epstein-Barr viral load in peripheral blood in pediatric liver transplant recipients during treatment for posttransplant lymphoproliferative disease. Transplantation. 1998;66(12):1641–1644.
103. McDiarmid SV, Jordan S, Kim GS, et al. Prevention and preemptive therapy of postransplant lymphoproliferative disease in pediatric liver recipients. Transplantation. 1998;66(12):1604–1611.
104. Tsai DE, Douglas L, Andreadis C, et al. EBV PCR in the diagnosis and monitoring of posttransplant lymphoproliferative disorder: results of a two-arm prospective trial. American Journal of Transplantation. 2008;8(5):1016–1024.
105. Preiksaitis JK, Pang XL, Fox JD, et al. Interlaboratory comparison of epstein-barr virus viral load assays. American Journal of Transplantation. 2009;9(2): 269–279.
106. Randhawa PS, Jaffe R, Demetris AJ, et al. Expression of Epstein-Barr virus-encoded small RNA (by the EBER-1 gene) in liver specimens from transplant recipients with post-transplantation lymphoproliferative disease. New England Journal of Medicine. 1992;327(24):1710–1714.
107. Lones MA, Shintaku IP, Weiss LM, et al. Posttransplant lymphoproliferative disorder in liver allograft biopsies: a comparison of three methods for the demonstration of Epstein-Barr virus. Human Pathology. 1997;28(5):533–539.
108. Niedobitek G, Mutimer DJ, Williams A, et al. Epstein-Barr virus infection and malignant lymphomas in liver transplant recipients. International Journal of Cancer. 1997;73(4):514–520.
109. Funch DP, Walker AM, Schneider G, et al. Ganciclovir and acyclovir reduce the risk of post-transplant lymphoproliferative disorder in renal transplant recipients. American Journal of Transplantation. 2005;5(12):2894–2900.
110. Jagadeesh D, Woda BA, Draper J, et al. Post transplant lymphoproliferative disorders: risk, classification, and therapeutic recommendations. Current Treatment Options in Oncology. 2012;13(1):122–136.
111. Buell JF, Gross TG, Hanaway MJ, et al. Posttransplant lymphoproliferative disorder: significance of central nervous system involvement. Transplantation Proceedings. 2005;37(2):954–955.
112. Hirsch HH, Randhawa P. BK virus in solid organ transplant recipients. American Journal of Transplantation. 2009;9(Suppl 4):S136–S146.
113. Mylonakis E, Goes N, Rubin RH, et al. BK virus in solid organ transplant recipients: an emerging syndrome. Transplantation. 2001;72(10):1587–1592.
114. Lopes da Silva R, Ferreira I, Teixeira G, et al. BK virus encephalitis with thrombotic microangiopathy in an allogeneic hematopoietic stem cell transplant recipient. Transplant Infectious Disease. 2011;13(2):161–167.
115. Bratt G, Hammarin AL, Grandien M, et al. BK virus as the cause of meningoencephalitis, retinitis and nephritis in a patient with AIDS. AIDS. 1999;13(9): 1071–1075.
116. Singh HK, Bubendorf L, Mihatsch MJ, et al. Urine cytology findings of polyomavirus infections. Advances in Experimental Medicine and Biology. 2006;577: 201–212.
117. Drachenberg CB, Papadimitriou JC. Polyomavirus-associated nephropathy: update in diagnosis. Transplant Infectious Disease. 2006;8(2):68–75.
118. Hirsch HH, Brennan DC, Drachenberg CB, et al. Polyomavirus-associated nephropathy in renal transplantation: interdisciplinary analyses and recommendations. Transplantation. 2005;79(10):1277–1286.
119. Schaub S, Hirsch HH, Dickenmann M, et al. Reducing immunosuppression preserves allograft function in presumptive and definitive polyomavirus-associated nephropathy. American Journal of Transplantation. 2010;10(12): 2615–2623.
120. Suwelack B, Malyar V, Koch M, et al. The influence of immunosuppressive agents on BK virus risk following kidney transplantation, and implications for choice of regimen. Transplantation Reviews. 2012;26(3):201–2011.
121. Smith F, Panek R, Kiberd BA. Screening to prevent polyoma virus nephropathy in kidney transplantation: a cost analysis. American Journal of Transplantation. 2009;9(9):2177–2179.
122. Hirsch HH, Knowles W, Dickenmann M, et al. Prospective study of polyomavirus type BK replication and nephropathy in renal-transplant recipients. New England Journal of Medicine. 2002;347(7):488–496.
123. Ginevri F, Azzi A, Hirsch HH, et al. Prospective monitoring of polyomavirus BK replication and impact of pre-emptive intervention in pediatric kidney recipients. American Journal of Transplantation. 2007;7(12):2727–2735.
124. Araya CE, Lew JF, Fennell RS, et al. Intermediate dose cidofovir does not cause additive nephrotoxicity in BK virus allograft nephropathy. Pediatric Transplantation. 2008;12(7):790–795.
125. Josephson MA, Williams JW, Chandraker A, et al. Polyomavirus-associated nephropathy: update on antiviral strategies. Transplant Infectious Disease. 2006;8(2):95–101.
126. Josephson MA, Gillen D, Javaid B, et al. Treatment of renal allograft polyoma BK virus infection with leflunomide. Transplantation. 2006;81(5):704–710.
127. Ramos E, Vincenti F, Lu WX, et al. Retransplantation in patients with graft loss caused by polyoma virus nephropathy. Transplantation. 2004;77(1): 131–133.
128. Hirsch HH, Ramos E. Retransplantation after polyomavirus-associated nephropathy: just do it? American Journal of Transplantation. 2006;6(1): 7–9.
129. Comoli P, Hirsch HH, Ginevri F. Cellular immune responses to BK virus. Current Opinion in Organ Transplantation. 2008;13(6):569–574.
130. Mateen FJ, Muralidharan R, Carone M, et al. Progressive multifocal leukoencephalopathy in transplant recipients. Annals of Neurology. 2011;70(2): 305–322.
131. Proia L, Miller R. Endemic fungal infections in solid organ transplant recipients. American Journal of Transplantation. 2009;9(Suppl 4):S199–S207.
132. Singh N, Forrest G. Cryptococcosis in solid organ transplant recipients. American Journal of Transplantation. 2009;9(Suppl 4):S192–S198.
133. Singh N, Husain S. Invasive aspergillosis in solid organ transplant recipients. American Journal of Transplantation. 2009;9(Suppl 4):S180–S191.
134. Pappas PG, Silveira FP. Candida in solid organ transplant recipients. American Journal of Transplantation. 2009;9(Suppl 4):S173–S179.
135. Kubak BM, Huprikar SS. Emerging & rare fungal infections in solid organ transplant recipients. American Journal of Transplantation. 2009;9(Suppl 4): S208–S226.
136. Delgado J, Calvo N, Gomis A, et al. Candiduria in renal transplant recipients: incidence, clinical repercussion, and treatment indication. Transplantation Proceedings. 2010;42(8):2944–2946.
137. Safdar N, Slattery WR, Knasinski V, et al. Predictors and outcomes of candiduria in renal transplant recipients. Clinical Infectious Diseases. 2005;40(10): 1413–1421.
138. Pappas PG, Andes D, Schuster M, et al. Invasive fungal infections in low-risk liver transplant recipients: a multi-center prospective observational study. American Journal of Transplantation. 2006;6(2):386–391.
139. Benedetti E, Gruessner AC, Troppmann C, et al. Intra-abdominal fungal infections after pancreatic transplantation: incidence, treatment, and outcome. Journal of the American College of Surgeons. 1996;183(4):307–316.
140. Silveira FP, Husain S. Fungal infections in solid organ transplantation. Medical Mycology. 2007;45(4):305–320.
141. Hadjiliadis D, Howell DN, Davis RD, et al. Anastomotic infections in lung transplant recipients. Annals of Transplantation. 2000;5(3):13–19.
142. Mai H, Champion L, Ouali N, et al. *Candida albicans* arteritis transmitted by conservative liquid after renal transplantation: a report of four cases and review of the literature. Transplantation. 2006;82(9):1163–1167.
143. Singh N, Aguado JM, Bonatti H, et al. Zygomycosis in solid organ transplant recipients: a prospective, matched case-control study to assess risks for disease and outcome. Journal of Infectious Diseases. 2009;200(6):1002–1011.
144. Husain S, Alexander BD, Munoz P, et al. Opportunistic mycelial fungal infections in organ transplant recipients: emerging importance of non-Aspergillus mycelial fungi. Clinical Infectious Diseases. 2003;37(2):221–229.
145. Minari A, Husni R, Avery RK, et al. The incidence of invasive aspergillosis among solid organ transplant recipients and implications for prophylaxis in lung transplants. Transplant Infectious Disease. 2002;4(4):195–200.
146. Goldfarb NS, Avery RK, Goormastic M, et al. Hypogammaglobulinemia in lung transplant recipients. Transplantation. 2001;71(2):242–246.
147. Husain S, Kwak EJ, Obman A, et al. Prospective assessment of Platelia Aspergillus galactomannan antigen for the diagnosis of invasive aspergillosis in lung transplant recipients. American Journal of Transplantation. 2004;4(5):796–802.
148. Husain S, Paterson DL, Studer SM, et al. Aspergillus galactomannan antigen in the bronchoalveolar lavage fluid for the diagnosis of invasive aspergillosis in lung transplant recipients. Transplantation. 2007;83(10):1330–1336.
149. Schaeffer MW, Buell JF, Gupta M, et al. Strongyloides hyperinfection syndrome after heart transplantation: case report and review of the literature. Journal of Heart and Lung Transplantation. 2004;23(7):905–911.
150. Kotton CN, Ryan ET, Fishman JA. Prevention of infection in adult travelers after solid organ transplantation. American Journal of Transplantation. 2005; 5(1):8–14.
151. Martin SI, Fishman JA. Pneumocystis pneumonia in solid organ transplant recipients. American Journal of Transplantation. 2009;9(Suppl 4):S227–S233.
152. Gordon SM, LaRosa SP, Kalmadi S, et al. Should prophylaxis for Pneumocystis

carinii pneumonia in solid organ transplant recipients ever be discontinued? Clinical Infectious Diseases. 1999;28(2):240–246.

153. Sassi M, Ripamonti C, Mueller NJ, et al. Outbreaks of pneumocystis pneumonia in 2 renal transplant centers linked to a single strain of pneumocystis: implications for transmission and virulence. Clinical Infectious Diseases. 2012; 54(10):1437–1444.

154. Morelon E, Stern M, Israel-Biet D, et al. Characteristics of sirolimus-associated interstitial pneumonitis in renal transplant patients. Transplantation. 2001; 72(5):787–790.

第 95 章 器官移植术后常见恶性肿瘤

Oriol Bestard, Josep M. Cruzado, Josep M. Grinyó

引言

实体器官移植(SOT)可以延长各种原因所致的不可逆的慢性器官衰竭患者的预期寿命。由于新的免疫抑制剂的出现及更多有效的免疫抑制剂的联合使用，在过去几十年里，同种异体移植物的短期转归取得了显著改善，但是移植物与患者的长期存活还有待进一步改善。长期应用免疫抑制剂引起的并发症被认为会降低移植物和受体的长期存活率。除了机会性感染和心血管事件外，新生的恶性肿瘤是实体器官移植术后的主要不良结果[1,2]。

许多研究已表明移植受体罹患癌症风险较一般人群增加 2~500 倍,其变化程度取决于移植类型和恶性肿瘤的具体类型。然而,因为研究方法和患者纳入标准的不同，这些数据可能并不能精确反映实际情况。甚至不同文献报道之间也存在显著的差异[3-11]。值得注意的是,恶性肿瘤的组织学类型和发生率因地理区域、人群和所使用的免疫抑制剂的不同而有所不同。虽然存在上述提到的许多差异,但是主流的文献报道数据都明确显示移植受体恶性肿瘤发生风险显著增加。

一旦癌症发生,移植受体的生存将受到严重影响,并且其治疗选择会受到移植、维持移植物功能的免疫抑制剂及并发症的限制。因此,更为重要的是要了解导致癌症发生的主要危险因素以及在移植人群发生率增高的那些癌症的特征。这将有助于患者移植后进行系统、合理的筛检与监测。为此,科学家正在努力研究可能影响实体器官移植后新生恶性肿瘤的主要危险因素、致癌机制和抗肿瘤免疫应答。

流行病学

器官移植后新发恶性肿瘤风险显著增加与患者长期免疫抑制状态有关这一观点已被人们广泛接受。来自不同区域移植人群的癌症注册处的数据使我们可以更好地了解器官移植受体的癌症患病率、发病率、预后以及识别更多的潜在危险因素。

单中心、小样本的数据很难精确地确定大多数肿瘤的发病率或将其发病率与一般人群进行比较。目前移植注册处报道癌症发病率的数据不多[1-5]。最近一项英国注册处的研究通过比较不同类型移植器官的受体与一般人群的恶性肿瘤的发病率,发现移植术后 10 年移植受体恶性肿瘤的总体发病率为 90/1000[4]。由于注册处记录的癌症患者往往存在信息丢失情况，因此很难确定其低估癌症真实发生率的程度[12-16]。除了免疫抑制外，许多队列研究明确了癌症风险变化还取决于受体年龄和性别；移植受体的年龄是影响恶性肿瘤发病率的明显混杂因素。具体来说,与年龄匹配的一般人群相比,65 岁的移植受体发展肿瘤的风险只增加 2 倍,而年轻移植受体风险却增加了 15~30 倍。

大样本的移植注册处的研究显示移植受体中不同癌症风险的广泛变化。一些恶性肿瘤的发生可能与免疫抑制后致癌病毒感染相关,但是其他恶性肿瘤的发生与已知的病毒感染无关。除此之外,一些癌症常见的危险因素还包括慢性免疫紊乱或炎症、潜在的疾病或药物毒性等。与病毒感染相关的恶性肿瘤，例如，Epstein-Barr 病毒(EBV)相关的非霍奇金淋巴瘤[NHL，移植后淋巴增生性疾病(PTLD)]、人疱疹病毒 8(HHV 8)相关的卡波西肉瘤,还有其他一些特殊的恶性肿瘤,如非黑色素瘤皮肤癌(NMSC,包括基底细胞癌和鳞状细胞癌)以及唇部和肛门癌症,这些恶性肿瘤在 SOT 受体中较一般人群显著增加[6]。一般人群中常见的癌症发病率在移植受体也升高(如结肠癌、肺癌或肝癌);而其他恶性肿瘤,如乳腺癌或前列腺癌的发病率与一般人群类似(表 95.1)。来自澳大利亚的研究发现,癌症随着观察时间的延长而逐渐增加。在暴露于阳光下的皮肤癌高危人群中,皮肤癌的累积发病率从使用免疫抑制 1 年后的 7%逐渐增加至 11 年后的 45%,20 年后的 70%[17]。

不同器官移植后的恶性肿瘤类型

值得注意的是，不同器官移植后的恶性肿瘤类型及其发病率不同(表 95.1)。不考虑器官移植类型的情况下,NMSC、PTLD、唇和肛门癌是 SOT 术后最常见的恶性肿瘤,其标准化发病风险(SIR)较一般人群高 7.5~61.4;其他恶性肿瘤在肺、肝和肾移植受体亚组中的风险显著增加[4,18]。

来自肾移植注册处的数据显示,与一般人群相比,移植术后发生各种恶性肿瘤的 SIR 显著增加。移植受体发生恶性肿瘤的总体 SIR 为 3.27(95%CI 3.09~3.46);与之相比,透析期间(SIR 1.35,95%CI 1.27~1.45)和肾脏替代治疗前(1.16,95%CI 1.08~1.25),患癌症的增加程度明显降低。其中,NHL 和 NMSC 是最常见的恶性肿瘤,结直肠癌和肾细胞癌(RCC)是最常见的实体器官肿瘤[6,19]。

表 95.1　器官移植术后受体(美国、英国、澳大利亚、新西兰)各种新发恶性肿瘤的标准化发生率比值,按发生率从高到低排列

恶性肿瘤	USRTR[18] 175732 名患者 (1987–2008)	UKRA[4] 25104 名患者 (1980–2007)	ANZDATA[1,14] 12623 名患者 (1980–2002)	
			男	女
所有恶性肿瘤*	2.1	2.4	2.5	3.1
非黑色素皮肤癌	13.8	16.6	60	90
卡波西肉瘤	64.4	17.1	17.4	62
非霍奇金淋巴瘤	7.5	12.5	6.9	29.1
肾癌	4.6	7.9	14.1	14.6
膀胱癌	1.5	2.4	1.6	3.6
黑色素瘤	2.3	2.6	6.9	5.2
宫颈癌	1.0	2.3	4.3	5.7
肝癌	1.1	2.4	4.2	4.5
食管癌	1.5	1.8	2.4	2.8
结直肠癌	1.2	1.8	1.6	2.8
肺癌	1.4	1.4	2.3	3.6
前列腺癌	0.9	1.1	1.6	–
乳腺癌	0.8	1.0	–	1.1

* 不包括非黑色素皮肤癌。

USRTR，美国器官移植受体登记;UKRA，英国器官移植登记审计;ANZDATA,澳大利亚和新西兰器官透析和移植登记。

肝移植受体中，新发实体器官恶性肿瘤的 SIR 为 2.7,与一般人群相比,结肠癌、口咽癌、肝癌和 RCC 的风险增加。癌症相关死亡率从 0.6%到 8%不等[20]。值得注意的是,35~50 岁的肝移植患者术后第 1 年 NHL 的 SIR 高于肾移植受体[21]。

心脏移植受体在移植术后比其他实体器官移植受体有相对较高的恶性肿瘤发生率,其原因可能是心脏移植受体接受了相对高水平的免疫抑制[22,23]。实体器官肿瘤是心脏移植受体中最常见的恶性肿瘤,一些研究报道在心脏移植受体常见的实体肿瘤中肺癌发生率较高[24,25],然而另一项包括 572 例患者的研究未证明这一点[26]。

肺移植受体中高达 10%~15%的死亡原因是随访期间发生恶性肿瘤[27]。

据报道,在小肠或多脏器移植受体中,新发恶性肿瘤的发病率为 15%，其中 PTLD 占 13%，非淋巴瘤占 3.2%。儿童 PTLD 的风险显著增高,而成年人更容易受到非淋巴瘤的影响[28]。在这些移植人群中,PTLD 似乎与 EBV 感染和移植物抗宿主病有很强的相关性。

病因和危险因素

明确 SOT 受体中恶性肿瘤发生的危险因素有助于理解免疫系统、感染和其他因素在恶性肿瘤发生发展中的作用,并且有助于提高移植手术的安全性。目前很难精确定义移植术后癌症的发病机制。虽然某些恶性肿瘤与特定的危险因素有关，但其他恶性肿瘤大多与多个危险因素的累积作用有关。无论如何,人们普遍认为:在移植术后新发恶性肿瘤的危险因素中,长期的免疫抑制起到重要作用。这些癌症的类型与在感染人类免疫缺陷病毒(HIV)的患者中所观察到的类型相似[11]。虽然 HIV 相关研究表明同种异体移植受体恶性肿瘤的发生率增加主要由免疫抑制引起，但这并不能解释为什么与一般人群相比，移植受体患不同类型的肿瘤风险不同。因此,除免疫抑制外,其他危险因素如导致患

者需要器官移植的原发疾病相关的危险因素可能也起一定作用。

在一般人群中，恶性肿瘤的发生与包括遗传易感性和致癌因素在内的许多因素有关，如吸烟、饮酒及紫外线的过度暴露。除此之外，移植受体发生特定类型的恶性肿瘤可能还与一些慢性或潜伏性的病毒感染有关，如 NHL(EBV)、卡波西肉瘤(HHV 8)、肛门癌(人乳头瘤病毒 HPV)及肝癌(丙型和乙型肝炎病毒)。在这些患者中，癌症风险增加一方面是由于免疫抑制导致病毒失控；另一方面也与病毒的直接作用有关。此外，目前常用免疫抑制剂(如环孢菌素、他克莫司或硫唑嘌呤)可引起 DNA 损伤，或干扰正常 DNA 修复机制、诱导和促进促癌因子[如转化生长因子-β(TGF-β)和血管内皮生长因子(VEGF)]或在 DNA 水平抑制剪接和引发密码子误读引起 DNA 损伤，从而引起癌症风险增加。最后，移植受体接受长期免疫抑制治疗导致体机内可有效预防恶性肿瘤生长和发展的免疫监视功能的损伤，同样引起癌症风险增加(图 95.1)[29,30]。

常见危险因素及区域危险因素

通常情况下，一般人群中已知的癌症危险因素也适用于移植受体。其中，高龄、烟酒、某些饮食和镇痛剂滥用都是移植术后恶性肿瘤发生的危险因素[31,32]。

分析移植术后恶性肿瘤的危险因素时，另一个要考虑的是地域差异。众所周知，在日本，移植后恶性肿瘤最常见的是胃肠道恶性肿瘤(主要是肝、胃、结肠、直肠)，这与该国一般人群中胃肠道癌的高发生率相一致。因此，地方性风险与移植带来的风险存在叠加效应。与之类似，在澳大利亚和新西兰，器官受体中皮肤癌，特别是棘细胞癌发生的风险非常高。最可能的解释就是浅肤色的白种人对于紫外线的过度暴露[33]。在欧洲和美国，最常见的移植后恶性肿瘤是 NMSC、NHL、RCC、消化系统肿瘤和卡波西肉瘤[10,34]。而在沙特阿拉伯和一些地中海国家中，HHV 8 的感染比在北欧更常见[35]，因此最常见的恶性肿瘤是卡波西肉瘤、感染性淋巴瘤(特别是在儿童中)、皮肤恶性肿瘤(黑色素瘤在儿

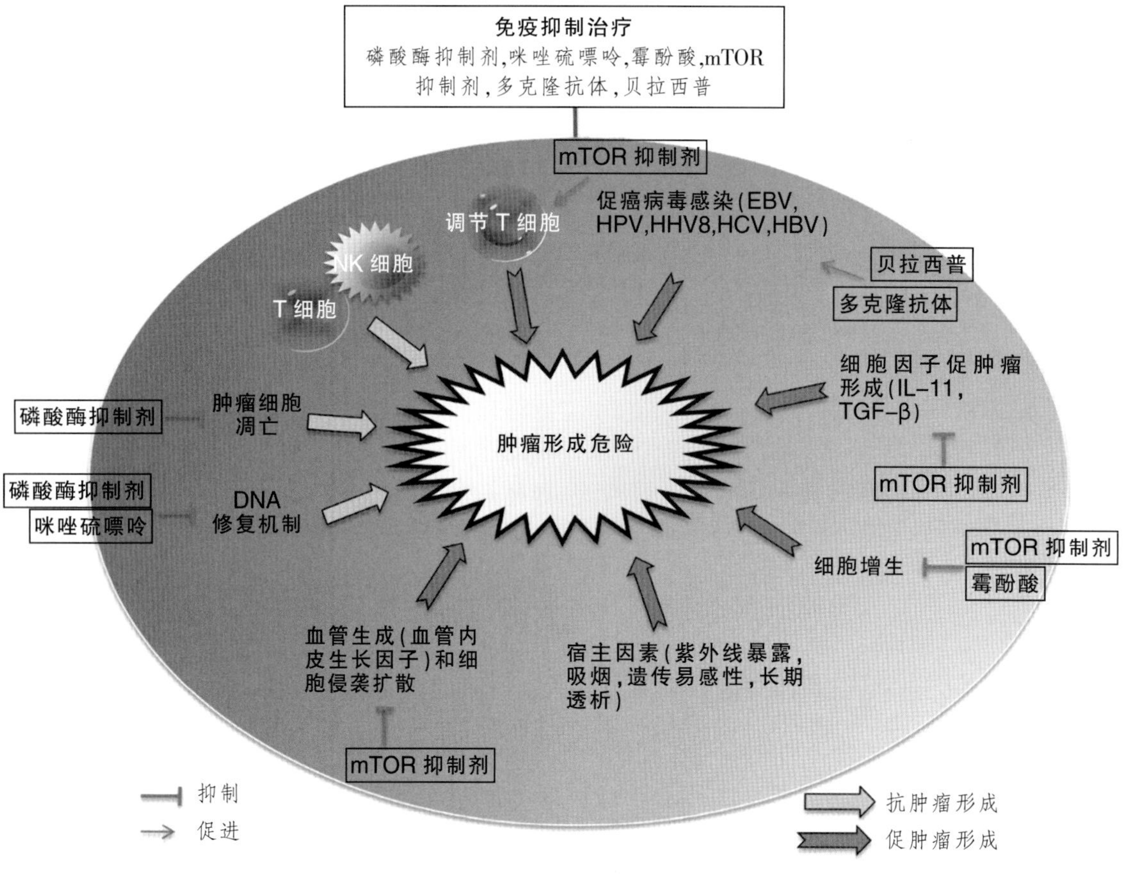

图 95.1 移植后新生恶性肿瘤发病机制。

童中较成人更常见)和肛门癌[36]。在乙型和丙型肝炎高发的东南亚,肾移植后的肝癌发生率也相当高[37]。

遗传因素

在一般人群中,遗传因素可促进恶性肿瘤的发生发展。事实上,也存在一些已知的疾病,例如 Von Hippel-Lindau 病,与侵袭性 RCC 的发生密切相关。这些患者接受同种异体肾移植后,RCC 的发生率进一步增加[38]。移植术后癌症发生的风险显著增加,这种现象在 Wiskott-Aldrich 综合征或 Drash 综合征的患者中也可以观察到。在这些罕见疾病的移植受体中,发生淋巴瘤和 Wilms 肿瘤的病例也有报道[39,40]。因此,有假说提出器官移植术后恶性肿瘤的发生有遗传学倾向,并与最初器官衰竭的病因有关,而恶性肿瘤患者移植术后常发生不止一种类型的肿瘤的事实也支持这一假说[39]。在同时患有两种恶性肿瘤的患者中,最常见的继发性恶性肿瘤是皮肤癌[34]。

致癌病毒

已经明确某些病毒的慢性感染可以促使移植患者发生特定类型的恶性肿瘤(表 95.2)。病毒感染可以通过多种机制促使细胞增殖失控,包括病毒介导的细胞周期和分裂进程的失控、通过肿瘤细胞表面上携带的病毒衍生颗粒介导的免疫监视逃逸以及抑制宿主细胞凋亡[41,42]。抑制细胞凋亡是非常重要的因素,因为它被认为是被致癌病毒转化后宿主细胞不断生长的必需条件。FLIP(FADD 1 样白介素 1B 转化酶样蛋白酶抑制蛋白)一类蛋白可能通过作用于具有共同信号通路的凋亡抑制受体(包括 CD95、TNF-R1、TRAMP/DR3 和 TRAIL-R1),从而干扰细胞凋亡的启动[43,44]。某些疱疹病毒如 Saimiri 疱疹病毒(HVS)或 HHV 8 可编码 FLIP 蛋白。所有编码 vFLIP 的病毒都可以在体外转化细胞,它可导致易感宿主肿瘤的发生。HVS 可在易感灵长类动物中引起淋巴瘤和白血病,并可在体外诱导人类 T 细胞的稳定转化生长。病毒诱导恶性肿瘤的另一个重要途径是干扰抑癌基因 p53,p53 可在 DNA 损伤时诱导细胞周期停滞或细胞凋亡[45]。小 DNA 病毒通过直接与 p53 结合、抑制 p53 介导的转录激活或通过泛素途径促使 p53 降解等多种方式来对抗 p53。HPV E6 和 E7 蛋白抑制 p53 基因而参与了恶性肿瘤的诱导。此外,皮肤组织暴露于紫外线(UV)后形成胸腺嘧啶二聚体引起了 DNA 突变,导致 p53 基因的失活。细胞无法修复此类突变造成恶性增殖。

表 95.2　器官移植后病毒感染与相关的恶性肿瘤

病毒	恶性肿瘤(靶器官)
乙型肝炎病毒(HBV)	肝细胞肝癌(肝脏)
丙型肝炎病毒(HCV)	肝细胞肝癌(肝脏)
EB 病毒(EBV)	鼻咽癌、霍奇金及非霍奇金淋巴瘤
人类疱疹病毒 8(HHV8)	卡波西肉瘤(脉管)
人乳头状瘤病毒(HPV)	宫颈,阴茎,外阴癌
人乳头状瘤病毒 58(HPV58)	鲍恩病
人乳头状瘤病毒 8,9(HPV8,9)	非黑色素皮肤癌
人乳头状瘤病毒 16,20(HPV16,20)	皮肤、扁桃体癌

在接受单克隆或多克隆抗体作为免疫抑制诱导或接受类固醇抵抗的挽救治疗的受体中[48],EBV 通常与淋巴瘤(霍奇金和非霍奇金淋巴瘤)密切相关,HHV 8 则与卡波西肉瘤关系密切[46,47]。多种 HPV 与皮肤、宫颈、阴茎或肛门生殖器癌相关[49]。此外,多瘤 BK 病毒——在肾移植受体中可诱导急性间质性肾炎的双链 DNA 病毒,通过中等 T 抗原的活动来转化细胞从而增加致瘤能力[51,52]。

免疫抑制的作用

如上所述,器官移植后发生恶性肿瘤的风险显著增加,这表明免疫抑制治疗在此过程中起关键作用。临床医生通常在恶性肿瘤治愈后等待 2~5 年再进行移植。该措施主要考虑到免疫抑制将加速残余瘤的生长。表 95.3 中提供了一些临床指南,但支持这些指南的数据并不是特别强有力。基于恶性肿瘤风险的免疫抑制维持的内容在第 66 章中讨论。澳大利亚[6]的一项非常具有说服力的基于群体的队列研究支持这一观点:在末期肾脏疾病的患者中,移植使癌症发生的风险增加了 3 倍多,而在移植前并未观察到这种易感性。同样,自身免疫性疾病如类风湿性关节炎、系统性红斑狼疮或皮肌炎的患者接受免疫抑制治疗后发生肿瘤,这也支持了免疫抑制药物是移植受体肿瘤发病率增加的部分原因[53-55]。直观上看,免疫抑制药物的总量是移植后恶性肿瘤风险的相关因素[56]:如之前提到的,接受相对较高的免疫抑制用量的心脏移植受体在移植后比其他实体器官受体(接受的免疫抑制用量较低)的恶性肿瘤

表 95.3 原发性肿瘤发生后实体器官移植建议的等待时间

恶性肿瘤	移植前建议等待时间(年)
肺	2
结肠	
Ⅰ期	2
Ⅱ期或以上	5
乳腺	
原位癌	2
非原位癌	5
前列腺	2
肝脏	不建议(除非在肝转移患者)
膀胱	
非浸润型	2
浸润型	5
原位黑色素瘤	5
非黑色素皮肤癌	
鳞状细胞癌	2
基底细胞癌	不等待
多发性骨髓瘤	不建议(骨髓移植,肾脏移植)
白血病	2
生殖系肿瘤	
睾丸	2
宫颈/子宫	2

发病率更高[22]。然而,由于缺乏对治疗的随机分配造成的选择偏倚、大多数研究中药物暴露的记录有限以及缺乏肿瘤预后的相关信息,目前对具体的免疫抑制剂或联合应用的相对致癌性仍知之甚少。所有这些问题阻碍了我们对混杂变量的评估[2,6,57]。但目前已经有研究报道了不同免疫抑制剂和肿瘤易感性之间的相关联系。

使用多克隆或单克隆淋巴细胞消耗性抗体用于免疫抑制或补救诱导可明确增加PTLD的发生率(见第96章)。这在肾脏和心脏移植受体中已被观察到[58,59],但并不是在所有恶性肿瘤中使用所有药物都存在这种关系[60]。

糖皮质激素已经广泛用于SOT。它们已被证实对不同肿瘤类型的癌细胞具有抗细胞凋亡和促进增殖作用[61,62]。目前已有的证据表明其在仅接受糖皮质激素的非移植患者(主要为NMSC)中发挥促癌作用[63],几乎没有流行病学数据显示其在SOT后具有潜在的致癌作用。

钙调神经磷酸酶抑制剂 (CNI), 包括环孢菌素A(CyA)和他克莫司(TAC),除了抑制钙调磷酸酶复合物作用外,还可促进TGF-β和VEGF的表达,特别是较高剂量使用时作用更强。这些行为均可促进肿瘤侵袭、扩散和肿瘤血管生成[64-66]。初步研究表明,与仅接受硫唑嘌呤(AZA)的移植受体相比,CyA使肿瘤发病率更高[67-69],特别是接受CyA、AZA和皮质类固醇的三联免疫抑制方案及维持高剂量CyA的移植受体[22,68,70-73]。尽管如此,在Gallagher等人[74]最近的一项研究中,489例首次尸体肾移植受体分别接受AZA联合皮质类固醇治疗,或CyA单一疗法3个月后换为AZA联合皮质类固醇治疗[74]。中位随访20.6年,比较了各组移植后恶性肿瘤(非皮肤癌及皮肤癌)的发病率。有趣的是,在多因素分析中,免疫抑制方案与两种恶性肿瘤的发生无关;相反,年龄的增加、既往吸烟史、非褐色眼睛和浅肤色等一般癌症发生的危险因素也是肾移植后新发肿瘤的独立危险因素。CyA和TAC之间的比较表明,TAC治疗的患者中PTLD的累积发病率略高,但其他实体肿瘤的发生率较CyA治疗的患者相比较低[75-80]。

一项大型的、随访3年的观察性队列研究比较了来自两个大型注册系统(OPTN/UNOS和CTS)的接受或未接受霉酚酸酯 (MMF) 免疫抑制治疗的肾移植患者,结果表明接受MMF免疫抑制的患者发生恶性肿瘤的风险较低[81]。这种潜在的抑癌作用可能是由于MMF能够抑制肌苷一磷酸脱氢酶, 这种酶在多种恶性肿瘤中显著升高[82,83]。

除了免疫抑制作用, 哺乳动物西罗莫司靶标(mTOR)抑制剂[mTORi;西罗莫司(SRL)和依维莫司(EVL)]也具有抗增殖的特性。这是由于它们可以干扰细胞周期和某些生长过程,如信号翻译、核糖体生物发生和编码不同代谢及生物合成通路的基因转录过程[84]。尽管mTOR复合物Ⅱ对SRL/EVL部分不敏感,但也可被这类药物部分阻断, 从而导致PI3K/Akt/mTOR信号通路的抑制。在多种人类恶性肿瘤中,mTOR的上下游信号传导组分, 包括PI3K/Akt/mTOR通路的异常活化和(或)细胞周期过程的调节改变十分常见。此外,与CNI药物相比,体外和体内实验均表明mTORi可通过干扰VEGF信号通路发挥抗血管生成作用,从而消除肿瘤生长甚至转移[86,87]。总而言之,这些免疫抑制剂的多种生物学效应使得移植界对评估免疫制剂在实体器官移植术后抑制恶性肿瘤发生的潜能上产生了强烈的兴趣[88]。

几项短期随访回顾性研究(移植后2~3年)比较了

肾移植受体术后接受 CyA 或 SRL 治疗的恶性肿瘤发病率：在 SRL 治疗组中，恶性肿瘤特别是 NMSC 的发病率略低[89]。OPTN/UNOS 数据库[90]的一项回顾性研究比较了接受仅 mTORi、mTORi 联合 CNI 或基于 CNI 治疗的肾移植受体的恶性肿瘤发病率，截尾随访时间为 963 天，治疗组之间具有可比较性：无论何种恶性肿瘤，相比单独应用 CNI 的恶性肿瘤发病率为 1.81%，单独应用 SRL、EVL 或 SRL/EVL 加上 CNI 均可使其发病率显著降低(0.60%)。SRL 或 EVL 治疗组的新发实体恶性肿瘤的发病率为 0%，SRL/EVL 联合 CNI 治疗组为 0.47%，单独 CNI 治疗组为 1.0%。多因素分析表明 mTORi 维持免疫抑制可降低 60%的恶性肿瘤发生风险和 55%的实体恶性肿瘤发生风险。近期一项随访 24 个月的研究纳入从 CNI 方案（TAC 或 CyA）转化为 mTORi 或接受 mTORi 方案(SRL)的肾移植受体，两组都有使用 AZA/MMF 及皮质类固醇，转为 SRL 的患者发生非皮肤癌的风险有所降低[91,92]。另一项最近 4 年的欧洲前瞻性研究报道显示，肾移植术后 3 个月，从 CyA 转化为 SRL 治疗的患者新发恶性肿瘤更少(3:9)[93]。然而，其他试验或荟萃分析报道了相反的观察结果，显示 mTORi 并没有明确减少移植后恶性肿瘤的发病率[94,95]。

尽管已有报道显示接受 mTORi 免疫抑制治疗的患者一般有恶性肿瘤发病率降低的总趋势，但是缺乏长期随访的前瞻性随机研究来证实其可以预防移植后恶性肿瘤的作用。一项有趣的病例报道了一例肝移植受体的免疫抑制方案从 CyA 和 AZA 转换为 SRL 和 MMF 后，肝细胞癌的三个肺转移灶完全消退[96]。

值得注意的是，在接受 SRL 治疗的患者中，NMSC 及卡波西肉瘤的发生率显著低于非 SRL 治疗的患者。此外，也有报道称患者从 CNI 转换为 mTORi 治疗后，卡波西肉瘤成功消退[97-99]。

在长期随访的前瞻性随机研究提供更强有力的结论前，许多移植专家们建议恶性肿瘤患者移植前应接受 mTORi 治疗或在肿瘤发展时转换为 mTORi 治疗。尽管如此，大家也普遍认为转换至 mTORi 治疗对较大的、侵袭性的、转移的恶性肿瘤作用有限[100]。

新型免疫抑制剂仍被不断地开发以期改善移植物及患者的长期存活。通常认为具有更特异性位点的药物的促癌风险较低。贝拉西普——最具潜力的新型试剂，是一种共刺激阻断融合蛋白，可与抗原提呈细胞上的 B7 家族成员 CD80/86 结合，最近已经用于肾移植患者。到目前为止，有三个使用两种不同剂量的贝拉西普的前瞻性研究，均以接受 CyA 治疗的患者作为对照组。在一项中位随访时间为 2.4 年的研究中，贝拉西普组中 PTLD [特别位于中枢神经系统(CNS)]的风险更高，特别是 EBV 血清学阴性且使用高剂量药物的患者[101]。研究未显示贝拉西普明显增加实体器官肿瘤的风险，但仍需要更长的随访时间来证明。

恶性肿瘤的免疫监测

免疫系统不仅可以识别自身与病原体或自身与非自身，而且可以识别自身和自身转化之间的细微差别。这种现象解释了恶性肿瘤免疫监视的假说，其中包括肿瘤中免疫的两种相反的功能：宿主保护与肿瘤诱发。这些功能形成目前肿瘤免疫编辑的概念基础。在这一概念中，免疫系统能够阻断肿瘤生长、发展及存活，或通过改变肿瘤免疫原性及抑制宿主保护性的抗肿瘤反应来促进肿瘤生长[102-105]。固有免疫及适应性免疫系统能识别并消除肿瘤细胞。有趣的是，恶性肿瘤的局部免疫环境被认为发挥关键作用。Galon 等人研究发现，在结直肠癌中，与常用的基于肿瘤大小和扩散的分期标准相比，T 细胞及其产物的存在、位置和密度能更好地预测患者的生存[106]。由 T 细胞识别的来自黑色素瘤和其他癌症的肿瘤抗原，有助于发展更有效的抗原特异性抗癌免疫疗法以及多种黑色素瘤抗原来源的抗原肽或树突细胞(DC)联合抗原肽的疫苗。这些进展在恶性肿瘤的治疗中具有极大的潜力[107-109]。此外，调节 T 细胞(Treg)作为预测肿瘤预后的潜在标志物将在未来的研究中备受关注。一般癌症人群中，肿瘤及外周循环中 Treg 数目增加与不良预后相关[110-113]。值得注意的是，在鼠肿瘤模型中阻断 Treg 的功能可导致细胞抗肿瘤免疫应答增强，甚至完全破坏肿瘤[114-118]，这表明 Treg 在肿瘤免疫中起到关键作用。此外，自然杀伤细胞(NK)也在宿主防御恶性肿瘤中发挥重要作用：无论体外或体内的研究均显示其控制或抑制癌症出现的作用[119-121]。

因此，很显然，在免疫抑制条件下，移植受体中的抗肿瘤免疫应答将受到阻碍，从而有利于恶性肿瘤的发生和进展。事实上，研究者们已经尝试通过测量淋巴细胞亚群来筛选移植后癌症风险增加的那些患者。两项研究提示低 CD4 计数预示移植后癌症 [包括鳞状细胞癌(SCC)]发生的风险[122,123]。然而，尽管具有预测性，CD4 T 细胞计数在这类人群中的临床应用有限。类似地，最近研究提示，在患有SCC的肾移植受体中，高的外周Foxp3⁺ Treg及低的外周NK细胞与新发SCC的风险显著相关。此外，肿瘤中CD8/Foxp3的表达比例新发的皮肤SCC相关[124]。这些结果表明，对免疫系统的监测有助于预测癌症的发生。

供体肿瘤传播

来自供体的隐匿性的恶性肿瘤的传播相对罕见，特别是活体供体在器官捐献前被彻底地评估过；然而，对于死亡供体可能性则较大，移植后的恶性肿瘤的鉴别诊断中应该考虑到这一点。移植术后，在免疫抑制条件下，来自供体的（微小）恶性肿瘤或转移灶均易发生播散。根据OPTN/UNOS的数据，在总共108 062例的移植受体中，0.2%的恶性肿瘤与供体相关[125]。

部分恶性肿瘤比其他种类的恶性肿瘤播散风险更高，如黑色素瘤和绒毛膜癌；而局限在肾囊内没有血管浸润的RCC及CNS肿瘤的播散风险非常低。另一种情况是病毒感染导致恶性肿瘤：如EBV感染的供体将病毒传递到血清学阴性受体可能导致移植后继发性PTLD，特别是接受特异性免疫抑制剂如多克隆抗体或贝拉西普治疗的受体。

在一项报道中，50%接受患有癌症的供体器官的同种异体移植受体发生了恶性肿瘤，其中一半为转移癌[81]。在一些患者中，消除免疫抑制治疗可导致对供体来源的恶性肿瘤的排斥反应，而不需要进一步的治疗。然而，在大多数供体传播恶性肿瘤的患者中，除了减少免疫抑制，特异性的抗癌治疗也是必要的。供体相关恶性肿瘤的总死亡率为38%，其中46%来自供体传播肿瘤，33%来自新生肿瘤。总体而言，死亡供体相关肿瘤死亡率为0.007%（108 062例受体中有8例）[125]。

肿瘤类型

非恶性及恶性皮肤病变

NMSC，包括基底细胞癌（BCC）和SCC，是SOT后最常见的恶性肿瘤[126]，它占皮肤癌的大多数，发生率比一般人群高10~200倍[127]。此外，一般人群中两种肿瘤类型的比例与移植受体中相反（SCC/BCC，4:1）[128]。虽然其他皮肤恶性病变的发生率低于NMSC，但它们在SOT患者中较一般人群仍显示增加的趋势：如黑色素瘤（风险高3.6倍）、Merkel细胞癌（10倍）和卡波西肉瘤（80倍）[129-131]。移植术后NMSC的发生率随时间的延长而增加。在美国和欧洲，肾移植后2年、10年和20年NMSC的发生率分别为5%、10%~27%和40%~60%[10,132,133]。这些皮肤病变也可以在年轻个体中出现，虽然普遍认为它们不如其他实体恶性肿瘤严重，但相比一般群体，它们在移植受体中的侵袭性更高，生长更快，切除后局部复发及转移能力更强[134]。

NMSC的发展与以下几种情况有关：例如，具有直接致癌特性的高强度免疫抑制、强烈的日光照射、已存在的角化病皮肤损伤、免疫监视降低以及一些致癌病毒的作用。累积的日光暴露是重要的致癌因子，因为这些病损主要发生在皮肤暴露于阳光的区域，并且在强光照的国家发病率明显增高。年龄是皮肤癌的另一个重要危险因素。与年轻受体相比，年龄高于55岁的患者发生皮肤癌的风险显著增加[135]。

此外，抑癌基因p53的突变在皮肤癌中很常见。这些突变有助于皮肤斑块的形成，而这也可能是SCC的危险因素[44]。

如前所述，HPV感染与皮肤癌风险增加相关[136,137]。免疫抑制剂如CNI（特别是维持标准剂量的CyA）[55]，由于其产生某些促进血管生成的细胞因子，可促进肿瘤生长甚至转移。类似地，由于可使皮肤细胞对UVA诱导的皮肤损伤更加敏感，AZA也与皮肤癌的发展相关[138]。与之相反，已有报道称，一开始即接受SRL/EVL或从其他免疫抑制剂（基本上为CNI）转换到SRL/EVL治疗的肾移植受体，其恶性肿瘤特别是NMSC的发病率较低[93]。尽管如此，目前仍然缺乏临床对照试验数据支持转换为基于mTORi的免疫抑制方案能够特异性诱导肿瘤消退这一论断。其中卡波西肉瘤也许是个例外，有报道显示从CNI转换到SRL可增强其消退[98,99]。尚不清楚卡波西肉瘤的消退是由于CNI的消除，还是SRL的特异性作用或两者二者协同作用兼有之。之所以有这样的争论，是因为在另一项报道中，通过减少/停止免疫抑制药物治疗，24例卡波西肉瘤患者中有8例患者产生了完整的肿瘤应答[139]。

SOT患者中，恶性黑色素瘤的发生风险仅略有增加。然而，黑色素瘤的死亡率非常高。此外，与非移植人群相比，移植受体中的黑色素瘤具有更差的预后。尽管相关报道的数据稀缺，但从已有信息来看，似乎病灶的厚度决定预后：恶性黑色素瘤<0.76mm的受体与一般

人群的预后相似，而> 0.76mm 的受体死亡率高，预后更差[140]。

实体癌

肾细胞癌和其他泌尿系统恶性肿瘤

泌尿系统恶性肿瘤是移植受体第二大常见的肿瘤。在不同报告中，RCC 的发生风险较同年龄和性别的一般人群高 5~100 倍[141-143]。大多数 RCC 发生在自身肾脏而不是移植肾，特别在多囊肾患者中发生风险明显增高。

目前没有用于在肾移植人群中筛选肾癌的统一建议。美国移植肾脏疾病改善协会（KDIGO）肾移植受体临床实践管理指南认为，目前并无证据支持对肾移植受体常规筛查肾癌，并且对一般风险的肾移植受体不推荐应用超声筛查[144,145]，但欧洲泌尿外科协会指南建议对高危受体的自身肾及移植肾应每年进行超声检查[146]。由于对于风险患者没有明确的定义，肾移植受体进行常规筛查的成本效益值得商榷[147]。尽管如此，仍推荐对移植受体的自身肾脏每年进行超声监测，而且患有 Bosniak Ⅰ或Ⅱ型囊肿伴或不伴有成年多囊肾病（APKD）的患者应接受每年两次肾脏超声检查[148]。

与 RCC 类似，其他泌尿系统肿瘤的发生率也所有增加，其中前列腺癌显著增加[149]。美国肾脏数据系统显示前列腺癌的 3 年累积发病率为 3.1%，RCC 为 2.2%，膀胱癌为 0.7%，睾丸癌为 0.1%。此外，因镇痛剂引起肾病接受肾移植的患者发生了上尿路移行性细胞癌的风险较高[150,151]。虽然尚未证实对前列腺癌筛查存在生存优势，甚至对微小恶性肿瘤存在过度诊断的风险，肿瘤筛查指南仍建议对前列腺癌进行筛查。

结直肠恶性肿瘤

肾移植受体中结直肠恶性肿瘤的发病率是否增加目前尚存在争议。部分研究报道，与一般人群中的男性和女性相比，其发病率均有所增加[10]，但是这些结果却受到其他研究团队的质疑[152,153]。然而，对于接受肝移植的原发性硬化性胆管炎且患有炎性肠病史的患者，其结直肠恶性肿瘤发生风险明显增加[154]。

肛门生殖器恶性肿瘤

所有移植受体的肛门癌发病率明显增加。妇科恶性肿瘤如宫颈原位癌、外阴、卵巢和宫颈癌也在移植后显著增加。所有这些恶性肿瘤都与 HPV 16 或 HPV 18 感染相关，占移植术后总癌症发病的 2%~3%[155,156]。然而，HPV 疫苗的作用还存在争议。移植后接种疫苗可能对 HPV 阴性患者无效，因为与一般人群相比，这些患者可能次级反应更低，抗体衰亡更快[157]。这些肿瘤往往是广泛的或多发的，特别是女性，30%合并有宫颈癌。因此，移植术后应该每年进行妇科检查。

肺癌及乳腺癌

在 SOT 受体中，肺癌和乳腺癌的发病率增加了两倍。在两项纳入大量接受 SOT 患者的研究中，高达 0.3%的患者发展为肺癌。与一般人群相反，非吸烟者的肺癌发生率高于吸烟者。此外，未进行肿瘤切除的患者中，肿瘤进展迅速[158,159]。Jimenez 等人[160]的一项研究表明，因酒精性肝硬化行肝移植的患者肺癌发生率显著高于因其他原因行移植的患者（4.3%对 0.7%）。但是这一结果有混杂影响因素：饮酒的患者吸烟风险更高，在该研究中，73.3%的新发肺癌患者是重度饮酒者同时也是中重度吸烟者。

在女性 SOT 受体中，乳腺癌的发病率存在一定的争议。一项研究中显示，与一般人群相比，女性心脏移植受体的乳腺癌发病率降低[161]；另一项研究显示，接受肝移植的女性乳腺癌发病率增加[162]。然而，与一般人群相比，移植受体中乳腺癌的生物学侵袭性更高[163]。对于乳腺癌，针对一般群体建立的常规筛查指南也适合于移植受体。

实体器官移植患者中的恶性肿瘤筛查

随着对 SOT 后恶性肿瘤发生风险增加的认识，国际移植协会对 SOT 患者行常规肿瘤筛查进行了相关研究[144,155,164-166]。然而，移植受体肿瘤筛查的主要指南是从一般人群的数据中推断而来。一般人群和移植受体之间的差异、诊断检测的差异及其他原因（例如心血管疾病）导致的死亡而造成总体预期寿命的降低都使 SOT 人群中应用这些指南的有效性遭到质疑。在 SOT 人群中应用为一般人群制订的指南需要评估其适用性，权衡筛查的成本效益及对个体的潜在危害[167]。有关移植受体预防性医疗筛查的其他信息，请参见第 88 章。

一些国际移植协会对不同类型SOT的肿瘤筛查发布了相应的指南或建议。一般来说,尽可能地避免过度免疫抑制治疗、避免与消耗性抗淋巴细胞抗体反复接触、筛查供体和受体的恶性肿瘤以及避免致癌因素(如持续的强日照)都是预防新生恶性肿瘤的措施。此外,移植受体年龄的增加以及等待移植时间的延长都增加了恶性肿瘤检测逃脱的风险,因此原本就存在肿瘤的受体应优先接受移植。

在预防皮肤癌方面,除了避免强烈的日晒、穿防晒服和涂防晒霜外,另外重要的是对皮肤肿瘤的筛查。强烈建议每个月进行皮肤自检及每6~12个月由专科医生和皮肤科医生进行一次全身的皮肤检查。高风险患者,如之前被诊断为SCC的患者,需要更频繁的检查。

对于没有进行子宫切除的女性患者,强烈建议每年行妇科检查和经阴道超声检查以排除外阴、会阴和子宫的恶性肿瘤。由于宫颈癌是病毒相关的肿瘤,而且它在免疫功能低下的患者中更具侵袭性,因而欧洲和美国移植学会建议所有成年女性肾移植受体每年通过宫颈刮片和盆腔检查进行宫颈癌筛查[145,165]。

慢性肾病患者的自体多囊肾是众所周知的癌前病变。虽然没有RCC高风险患者的精确定义,但是应该每年对移植受体的肾脏进行超声检查,特别是有Bosniak Ⅰ型或Ⅱ型囊肿的患者。

对于出现镜下血尿的有镇痛剂肾病史及接受环磷酰胺治疗(特别是累积剂量超过20g)的患者,应进行泌尿系统检查[168]。一些研究者还建议对使用AZA超过10年的患者进行泌尿系统检查[169]。

由于移植术后结直肠癌的发生频率较高,应定期检测粪便潜血。然而,对于乙状结肠镜检查的建议并不明确;目前建议从50岁开始每5年检查一次。肝移植后的结直肠癌右侧多发并更具侵袭性,而且转移率更高。此外,患有原发性硬化性胆管炎和炎性肠病的肝移植受体在肝移植术后发生结肠癌的风险增加,需要更频繁的筛查/监测,建议每年结肠镜检查随访并行随机结直肠黏膜活检来早期检测[170]。

对于其他实体器官(如前列腺和乳腺)的恶性肿瘤,移植受体应当严格遵守用于一般群体的筛查和预防实体器官恶性肿瘤的指南。对于乳腺癌,美国和欧洲移植学会建议对所有50~69岁的女性移植受体每隔12~24个月进行一次筛查[171-173]。40~49岁的女性可以每1~2年检查一次钼靶X线,但目前没有证据支持或反对该年龄组患者筛查[145,165]。对一般人群和SOT受体的前列腺癌筛查目前尚无统一意见。但美国和欧洲移植学会均鼓励所有男性肾移植受体(年龄大于50岁,预期寿命至少10年)每年进行数字直肠检查(DRE)及前列腺特异性抗原(PSA)检测[145,165]。

实体器官移植后新生恶性肿瘤的治疗

移植患者新发恶性肿瘤的治疗非常具有挑战性,并根据肿瘤的类型、分期及治疗目的(治愈性或姑息性)而有所不同。然而,移植受体也应该接受与一般人群相同的预防性建议。这包括改变生活方式,如健康饮食、定期运动和戒烟。然后,根据特定肿瘤类型酌情使用手术摘除、放射治疗或化疗等特定的治疗策略[174]。

除了癌症特定治疗措施,建议对免疫应答性肿瘤减少或撤除免疫抑制要非常谨慎,需要考虑到器官衰竭和恶性肿瘤进展的风险。对于维持生命的重要器官(如心脏、肺或肝脏),特别是对于不能被免疫抑制诱导的恶性肿瘤,不推荐完全撤除免疫抑制。但是,对于有些免疫应答性恶性肿瘤(如EBV相关的淋巴瘤)或肾移植患者可以根据情况撤除。也可以考虑转换至基于mTORi的免疫抑制方案。然而,转换为具有抗增殖活性的免疫抑制剂对治疗的整体成功仍然未知。因为肝脏急性排斥在移植后并不常见,而且通常是轻度并容易逆转的,所以肝移植受体可以维持在最小剂量的泼尼松龙和AZA/MMF或转换为mTORi。在肾移植受体中,CNI浓度应降至最低,而且可以被SRL/EVL所替代[175,176]。在其他SOT受体(例如心、肺或肠移植受体),仍需要考虑到重要器官排斥的后果,免疫抑制的管理可遵循相同的建议。

转换为具有抗增殖作用的免疫抑制方案(如MMF,特别是mTORi)可能有助于降低移植排斥反应的发生率,甚至可以消除恶性肿瘤。该策略应特别适用于NHL、皮肤癌、卡波西肉瘤或供体来源的恶性肿瘤患者[177-179]。虽然越来越多的证据表明,在移植后恶性肿瘤的早期阶段,mTORi对肿瘤消退和患者存活有益[175],但是它们的作用需要长期前瞻性临床研究进一步确定。

当患者患有严重的恶性肿瘤,特别是HLA完全匹配的患者,应该考虑最小化甚至完全停止使用免疫抑制剂。虽然在严重恶性肿瘤中免疫反应似乎相对受损[180],

短期内移植监测(特别在移植后的早期阶段)仍是必要的,否则爆发性排斥常因诊断过晚而导致移植物失功。移植物的失功程度首先根据恶性肿瘤的分期及免疫应答程度而变化;终末情况下,移植物失功的程度与生活质量受损程度直接相关。在供体来源的恶性肿瘤中,一定程度的移植排斥反应可能有利于恶性肿瘤的消除。

有趣的是,一些恶性肿瘤如黑色素瘤[181]、结直肠癌[182]和 RCC[183]的免疫治疗研究目前正在非移植患者中进行。这些治疗方式在器官移植患者中是否有效需要进一步研究。

总结

总之,恶性肿瘤在移植受体中非常常见,所有实体器官移植的受体均应考虑到这一点。相关的危险因素或肿瘤的发展应受到关注并进行系统的监测。此外,肿瘤的快速检测有助于进行有效治疗。鉴于移植物衰竭和肿瘤转移性进展的多种竞争性危险因素,以及各自的相关发病率和死亡率,移植后恶性肿瘤患者的管理应涉及多学科协作诊治。鉴于处理移植后恶性肿瘤的复杂性,预防应该是移植医生的主要目标。

(刘治坤 译 徐骁 校)

参考文献

1. McDonald S, Excell L, Livingston B, editors. ANZDATA Registry Report 2010. Australia and New Zealand Dialysis and Transplant Registry. Adelaide, South Australia, Australia. 2010. Available from: http://www.anzdata.org.au/.
2. Vajdic CM, van Leeuwen MT. Cancer incidence and risk factors after solid organ transplantation. International Journal of Cancer. 2009;125:1747–1754.
3. Birkeland SA, Storm HH, Lamm LU, et al. Cancer risk after renal transplantation in the Nordic countries, 1964–1986. International Journal of Cancer. 1995;60: 183–189.
4. Collett D, Mumford L, Banner NR, et al. Comparison of the incidence of malignancy in recipients of different types of organ: a UK Registry audit. American Journal of Transplantation. 2010;10:1889–1896.
5. Villeneuve PJ, Schaubel DE, Fenton SS, et al. Cancer incidence among Canadian kidney transplant recipients. American Journal of Transplantation. 2007;7: 941–948.
6. Vajdic CM, McDonald SP, McCredie MR, et al. Cancer incidence before and after kidney transplantation. JAMA. 2006;296:2823–2831.
7. Adami J, Gäbel H, Lindelö B, et al. Cancer risk following organ transplantation: a nationwide cohort study in Sweden. British Journal of Cancer. 2003;89: 1221–1227.
8. Kyllönen L, Salmela K, Pukkala E. Cancer incidence in a kidney-transplanted population. Transplant International. 2000;13(Suppl 1):S394–S398.
9. Serraino D, Piselli P, Angeletti C, et al. Risk of Kaposi's sarcoma and of other cancers in Italian renal transplant patients. British Journal of Cancer. 2005;92: 572–575.
10. Kasiske BL, Snyder JJ, Gilbertson DT, et al. Cancer after kidney transplantation in the United States. American Journal of Transplantation. 2004;4: 905–913.
11. Grulich AE, van Leeuwen MT, Falster MO, et al. Incidence of cancers in people with HIV/AIDS compared with immunosuppressed transplant recipients: a meta-analysis. Lancet. 2007;370:59–67.
12. Brunner FP, Landais P, Selwood NH. Malignancies after renal transplantation: the EDTA-ERA registry experience. European dialysis and transplantation association–European Renal Association. Nephrology Dialysis Transplantation. 1995;10:74–80.
13. Stewart T, Tsai S-CJ, Grayson H, et al. Incidence of de-novo breast cancer in women chronically immunosuppressed after organ transplantation. Lancet. 1995;346:796–798.
14. Stewart JH, Vajdic CM, van Leeuwen MT, et al. The pattern of excess cancer in dialysis and transplantation. Nephrology Dialysis Transplantation. 2009;24: 3225–3231.
15. Birkeland SA, Lokkegaard H, Storm HH. Cancer risk in patients on dialysis and after renal transplantation. Lancet. 2000;355:1886–1887.
16. Adami J, Gabel H, Lindelof B, et al. Cancer risk following organ transplantation: a nationwide cohort study in Sweden. British Journal of Cancer. 2003;89: 1221–1227.
17. Bouwes Bavinck JN, Hardie DR, Green A, et al. The risk of skin cancer in renal transplant recipients in Queensland, Australia: a follow-up study. Transplantation. 1996;61:715–721.
18. Engels EA, Pfeiffer RM, Fraumeni JF Jr, et al. Spectrum of cancer risk among US solid organ transplant recipients. JAMA. 2011;306:1891–1901.
19. Wong G, Howard K, Craig J, et al. 29th report —Australia and New Zealand Dialysis and Transplant Registry— 2006. McDonald S, Chang S, Excell L, eds. 2006: 138–142.
20. Sanchez W, Talwalkar JA, Gores GJ. Will all liver transplantation patients eventually die from cancer? Journal of Hepatology. 2006;44:13–18.
21. Jiang Y, Villeneuve PJ, Fenton SS, et al. Liver transplantation and subsequent risk of cancer: findings from a Canadian cohort study. Liver Transplantation. 2008;14:1588–1597.
22. Shapiro R, Nalesnik M, McCauley J, et al. Posttransplant lymphoproliferative disorders in adult and pediatric renal transplant patients receiving tacrolimus-based immunosuppression. Transplantation. 1999;68:1851–1854.
23. Ippoliti G, Rinaldi M, Pellegrini C, et al. Incidence of cancer after immunosuppressive treatment for heart transplantation. Critical Reviews in Oncology. 2005;56:101–113.
24. Rinaldi M, Pellegrini C, D'Armini AM, et al. Neoplastic disease after heart transplantation: single center experience. European Journal of Cardio-Thoracic Surgery. 2001;19:696–701.
25. Goldstein DJ, Williams DL, Oz MC, et al. De novo solid malignancies after cardiac transplantation. Annals of Thoracic Surgery. 1995;60:1783–1789.
26. Potaris K, Radovancevic B, Thomas CD, et al. Lung cancer after heart transplantation: a 17-year experience. Annals of Thoracic Surgery. 2005;79:980–983.
27. Pierson RN 3rd. Lung transplantation: current status and challenges. Transplantation. 2006;81:1609–1615.
28. Abu-Elmagd KM, Mazariegos G, Costa G, et al. Lymphoproliferative disorders and de novo malignancies in intestinal and multivisceral recipients: improved outcomes with new outlooks. Transplantation. 2009;88:926–934.
29. Ajithkumar T, Parkinson C, Butler A. Management of solid tumours in organ-transplant Recipients. Lancet Oncology. 2007;8:921–932.
30. Morath C, Mueller M, Goldschmidt H, et al. Malignancy in renal transplantation. Journal of the American Society of Nephrology. 2004;15:1582–1588.
31. Danpanich E, Kasiske BL. Risk factors for cancer in renal transplant recipients. Transplantation. 1999;68:1859–1864.
32. Pommer W, Bronder E, Klimpel A, et al. Urothelial cancer at different tumour sites: role of smoking and habitual intake of analgesics and laxatives. Results of the Berlin Urothelial Cancer Study. Nephrology Dialysis Transplantation. 1999;14:2892–2897.
33. Kimlin MG, Parisi AV, Wong JC. Quantification of personal solar UV exposure of outdoor workers, indoor workers and adolescents at two locations in Southeast Queensland. Photodermatology, Photoimmunology and Photomedicine. 1998;14:7–11.
34. London NJ, Farmery SM, Will EJ, et al. Risk of neoplasia in renal transplant patients. Lancet. 1995;346:403–406.
35. Pietrosi G, Vizzini G, Pipitone L, et al. Primary and reactivated HHV8 infection and disease after liver transplantation: a prospective study. American Journal of Transplantation. 2011;11:2715–2723.
36. Al-Sulaiman MH, al-Khader AA. Kaposi's sarcoma in renal transplant recipients. Transplantation Science. 1994;4:46–60.
37. Luengrojanakul P, Vareesangthip K, Chainuvati T, et al. Hepatitis C virus infection in patients with chronic liver disease or chronic renal failure and blood donors in Thailand. Journal of Medical Virology. 1994;44:287–292.
38. Goldfarb DA, Neumann HP, Penn I, et al. Results of renal transplantation in patients with renal cell carcinoma and von Hippel-Lindau disease. Transplantation. 1997;64:1726–1729.

39. Cleper R, Davidovitz M, Krause I, et al. Unexpected Wilms' tumor in a pediatric renal transplant recipient: suspected Denys-Drash syndrome. Transplantation Proceedings. 1999;31:1907–1909.
40. Fischer A, Binet I, Oertli D, et al. Fatal outcome of renal transplantation in a patient with the Wiskott-Aldrich syndrome. Nephrology Dialysis Transplantation. 1996;11:2077–2079.
41. Thomson BJ. Viruses and apoptosis. International Journal of Experimental Pathology. 2001;82:65–76.
42. Hay S, Kannourakis G. A time to kill: viral manipulation of the cell death program. Journal of General Virology. 2002;83:1547–1564.
43. Scaffidi C, Schmitz I, Krammer PH, et al. The role of c-FLIP in modulation of CD95-induced apoptosis. Journal of Biological Chemistry. 1999;274: 1541–1548.
44. Muller M, Wilder S, Bannasch D, et al. p53 activates the CD95 (APO-1/Fas) gene in response to DNA damage by anticancer drugs. Journal of Experimental Medicine. 1998;188:2033–2045.
45. Hanahan D, Weinberg RA. The hallmarks of cancer. Cell. 2000;100:57–70.
46. Lye WC. Successful treatment of Epstein-Barr virus-associated T-cell cutaneous lymphoma in a renal allograft recipient: case report and review of the literature. Transplantation Proceedings. 2000;32:1988–1989.
47. Schmidtko J, Wang R, Wu CL, et al. Posttransplant lymphoproliferative disorder associated with an Epstein-Barr-related virus in cynomolgus monkeys. Transplantation. 2002;73:1431–1439.
48. Cathomas G, Tamm M, McGandy CE, et al. Transplantation-associated malignancies: restriction of human herpes virus 8 to Kaposi's sarcoma. Transplantation. 1997;64:175–178.
49. Harwood CA, Surentheran T, McGregor JM, et al. Human papillomavirus infection and non-melanoma skin cancer in immunosuppressed and immunocompetent individuals. Journal of Medical Virology. 2000;61:289–297.
50. Nickeleit V, Klimkait T, Binet IF, et al. Testing for polyomavirus type BK DNA in plasma to identify renal-allograft recipients with viral nephropathy. New England Journal of Medicine. 2000;342:1309–1315.
51. Ichaso N, Dilworth SM. Cell transformation by the middle Tantigen of polyoma virus. Oncogene. 2001;20:7908–7916.
52. Benjamin TL. Polyoma virus: old findings and new challenges. Virology. 2001;289:167–173.
53. Beauparlant P, Papp K, Haraoui B. The incidence of cancer associated with the treatment of rheumatoid arthritis. Seminars in Arthritis and Rheumatism. 1999;29:148–158.
54. Kamel OW, van de Rijn M, LeBrun DP, et al. Lymphoid neoplasms in patients with rheumatoid arthritis and dermatomyositis: frequency of Epstein-Barr virus and other features associated with immunosuppression. Human Pathology. 1994;25:638–643.
55. Arellano F, Krupp P. Malignancies in rheumatoid arthritis patients treated with cyclosporin A. British Journal of Rheumatology. 1993;32(Suppl 1):72–75.
56. Dantal J, Hourmant M, Cantarovich D, et al. Effect of long-term immunosuppression in kidney-graft recipients on cancer incidence: randomized comparison of two cyclosporine regimens. Lancet. 1998;351:623–628.
57. Webster AC, Craig JC, Simpson JM, et al. Identifying high risk groups and quantifying absolute risk of cancer after kidney transplantation: a cohort study of 15,183 recipients. American Journal of Transplantation. 2007;7:2140–2151.
58. Opelz G, Henderson R. Incidence of non-Hodgkin lymphoma in kidney and heart transplant recipients. Lancet. 1993;342:1514–1516.
59. Cherikh WS, Kauffman HM, McBride MA, et al. Association of the type of induction immunosuppression with posttransplant lymphoproliferative disorder, graft survival, and patient survival after primary kidney transplantation. Transplantation. 2003;76:1289–1293.
60. Kirk AD, Cherikh WS, Ring R, et al. Dissociation of depletional induction and post transplant lymphoproliferative disease in kidney recipients treated with alemtuzumab. American Journal of Transplantation. 2007;7:2619–2625.
61. Rutz HP. Effects of corticosteroid use on treatment of solid tumours. Lancet. 2002;360:1969–1970.
62. Herr I, Ucur E, Herzer K, et al. Glucocorticoid cotreatment induces apoptosis resistance toward cancer therapy in carcinomas. Cancer Research. 2003;63: 3112–3120.
63. Cidlowski JA, king KL, Evans-Storms RB, et al. The biochemistry and molecular biology of glucocorticoid-induced apoptosis in the immune system. Recent Progress in Hormone Research. 1996;51:457–490.
64. Li B, Sehajpal PK, Khanna A, et al. Differential regulation of transforming growth factor beta and interleukin 2 genes in human T cells: demonstration by usage of novel competitor DNA constructs in the quantitative polymerase chain reaction. Journal of Experimental Medicine. 1991;174:1259–1265.
65. Shihab FS, Andoh TF, Tanner AM, et al. Role of transforming growth factor-beta 1 in experimental chronic cyclosporine nephropathy. Kidney International. 1996;49:1141–1151.
66. Maluccio M, Sharma V, Lagman M, et al. Tacrolimus enhances transforming growth factor-beta1 expression and promotes tumor progression. Transplantation. 2003;76:597–602.
67. Vogt P, Frei U, Repp H, et al. Malignant tumours in renal transplant recipients receiving cyclosporin: survey of 598 first-kidney transplantations. Nephrology Dialysis Transplantation. 1990;5:282–288.
68. Shuttleworth D, Marks R, Griffin PJ, et al. Epidermal dysplasia and cyclosporine therapy in renal transplant patients: a comparison with azathioprine. British Journal of Dermatology. 1989;120:551–554.
69. Penn I, First MR. Development and incidence of cancer following cyclosporine therapy. Transplantation Proceedings. 1986;18:210–215.
70. McGeown MG, Douglas JF, Middleton D. One thousand renal transplants at Belfast City Hospital: post-graft neoplasia 1968–1999, comparing azathioprine only with cyclosporin-based regimes in a single centre. Clinical Transplants. 2000;193–202.
71. Hiesse C, Rieu P, Kriaa F, et al. Malignancy after renal transplantation: analysis of incidence and risk factors in 1700 patients followed during a 25-year period. Transplantation Proceedings. 1997;29:831–833.
72. Kyllönen L, Salmela K, Pukkala E. Cancer incidence in a kidney-transplanted population. Transplant International. 2000;13(Suppl 1):S394–S398.
73. Marcén R, Pascual J, Tato AM, et al. Influence of immunosuppression on the prevalence of cancer after kidney transplantation. Transplantation Proceedings. 2003;35:1714–1716.
74. Gallagher M, Kelly P, Jardine M, et al. Long-term cancer risk of immunosuppressive regimens after kidney transplantation. Journal of the American Society of Nephrology. 2010;21:852–858.
75. Caillard S, Dharnidharka V, Agodoa L, et al. Posttransplant lymphoproliferative disorders after renal transplantation in the United States in era of modern immunosuppression. Transplantation. 2005;80:1233–1243.
76. Webster A, Woodroffe RC, Taylor RS, et al. Tacrolimus versus cyclosporin as primary immunosuppression for kidney transplant recipients. Cochrane Database of Systematic Reviews. 2005;(4):CD003961.
77. Bustami RT, Ojo AO, Wolfe RA, et al. Immunosuppression and the risk of post-transplant malignancy among cadaveric first kidney transplant recipients. American Journal of Transplantation. 2004;4:87–93.
78. Baumeister S, Kleist C, Döhler B, et al. Risks of allogeneic hand transplantation. Microsurgery. 2004;24:98–103.
79. Wiesner RH. A long-term comparison of tacrolimus (FK506) versus cyclosporine in liver transplantation: a report of the United States FK506 Study Group. Transplantation. 1998;66:493–499.
80. Johnson SR, Cherikh WS, Kauffman HM, et al. Retransplantation after post-transplant lymphoproliferative disorders: an OPTN/UNOS database analysis. American Journal of Transplantation. 2006;6:2743–2749.
81. Robson R, Cecka JM, Opelz G, et al. Prospective registry-based observational cohort study of the long-term risk of malignancies in renal transplant patients treated with mycophenolate mofetil. American Journal of Transplantation. 2005;5:2954–2960.
82. Buell JF, Gross TG, Woodle ES. Malignancy after transplantation. Transplantation. 2005;80:s254–s264.
83. Engl T, Makarević J, Relja B, et al. Mycophenolate mofetil modulates adhesion receptors of the beta1 integrin family on tumor cells: impact on tumor recurrence and malignancy. BMC Cancer. 2005;5:4.
84. Wullschleger S, Loewith R, Hall MN. TOR signaling in growth and metabolism. Cell. 2006;124:471–484.
85. Vignot S, Faivre S, Aguirre D, et al. mTOR-targeted therapy of cancer with rapamycin derivates. Annals of Oncology. 2005;16:525–537.
86. Guba M, Yezhelyev M, Eichhorn ME, et al. Rapamycin induces tumor-specific thrombosis via tissue factor in the presence of VEGF. Blood. 2005;105: 4463–4469.
87. Luan FL, Ding R, Sharma VK, et al. Rapamycin is an effective inhibitor of human renal cancer metastasis. Kidney International. 2003;63:917–926.
88. Campistol JM, Eris J, Oberbauer R, et al. Sirolimus therapy after early cyclosporine withdrawal reduces the risk for cancer in adult renal transplantation. Journal of the American Society of Nephrology. 2006;17:581–589.
89. Mathew T, Kreis H, Friend P. Two-year incidence of malignancy in sirolimus-treated renal transplant recipients: results from five multicenter studies. Clinical Transplantation. 2004;18:446–449.
90. Kauffman HM, Cherikh WS, Cheng Y, et al. Maintenance immunosuppression with TOR inhibitors is associated with a reduced incidence of de novo malignancies. Transplantation. 2005;80:883–889.
91. Schena FP, Pascoe MD, Alberu J, et al. Conversion from calcineurin inhibitors to sirolimus maintenance therapy in renal allograft recipients: 24-Month efficacy and safety results from the CONVERT trial. Transplantation. 2009;87:233–242.
92. Alberú J, Pascoe MD, Campistol JM, et al. Sirolimus CONVERT Trial Study Group. Lower malignancy rates in renal allograft recipients converted to

sirolimus-based, calcineurin inhibitor-free immunotherapy: 24-month results from the CONVERT trial. Transplantation. 2011;92:303–310.
93. Lebranchu Y, Thierry A, Thervet E, et al. Efficacy and safety of early cyclosporine conversion to sirolimus with continuous MMF-four-year results of the Postconcept study. American Journal of Transplantation. 2001;11:1665–1675.
94. Ekberg H, Bernasconi C, Tedesco-Silva H, et al. Calcineurin inhibitor minimization in the SYMPHONY study: observational results 3 years after transplantation. American Journal of Transplantation. 2009;9:1876–1885.
95. Webster AC, Lee VW, Chapman JR, et al. Target of rapamycin inhibitors (TOR-I; sirolimus and everolimus) for primary immunosuppression in kidney transplant recipients. Cochrane Database of Systematic Reviews. 2006;(2):CD004290.
96. Zhou J, Fan J, Wang Z, et al. Conversion to sirolimus immunosuppression in liver transplantation recipients with hepatocellular carcinoma: report of an initial experience. World Journal of Gastroenterology. 2006;12:3114–3118.
97. Campistol JM, Gutierrez-Dalmau A, Torregrosa JV. Conversion to sirolimus: a successful treatment for posttransplantation Kaposi's sarcoma. Transplantation. 2004;77:760–762.
98. Stallone G, Schena A, Infante B, et al. Sirolimus for Kaposi's sarcoma in renal-transplant recipients. New England Journal of Medicine. 2005;352: 1317–1323.
99. Zmonarski SC, Boratynska M, Rabczynski J, et al. Regression of Kaposi's sarcoma in renal graft recipients after conversion to sirolimus treatment. Transplantation Proceedings. 2005;37:964–966.
100. Monaco AP. The role of mTOR inhibitors in the management of posttransplant malignancy. Transplantation. 2009;87:157–163.
101. Grinyó J, Charpentier B, Pestana JM, et al. An integrated safety profile analysis of belatacept in kidney transplant recipients. Transplantation. 2010;90: 1521–1527.
102. Schreiber RD. Cancer immunoediting: from immunosurveillance to tumor escape. Nature Immunology. 2002;3:991–998.
103. Dunn GP, Old LJ, Schreiber RD. The three Es of cancer immunoediting. Annual Review of Immunology. 2004;22:329–360.
104. Dunn GP, Old LJ, Schreiber RD. The immunobiology of cancer immunosurveillance and immunoediting. Immunity. 2004;21:137–148.
105. Shankaran V, Turner DM, Williams DM, et al. IFNγ and lymphocytes prevent primary tumour development and shape tumour immunogenicity. Nature. 2001;410:1107–1111.
106. Galon J, Costes A, Sanchez-Cabo F, et al. Type, density, and location of immune cells within human colorectal tumors predict clinical outcome. Science. 2006;313:1960–1964.
107. Wang RF, Rosenberg SA. Human tumor antigens for cancer vaccine development. Immunological Reviews. 1999;170:85–100.
108. Houghton AN, Gold JS, Blachere NE. Immunity against cancer: lessons learned from melanoma. Current Opinion in Immunology. 2001;13:134–140.
109. Rosenberg SA. Progress in human tumour immunology and immunotherapy. Nature. 2001;411:380–384.
110. Fenoglio D, Ferrera F, Fravega M, et al. Advancements on phenotypic and functional characterization of non-antigen-specific CD8CD28 regulatory T cells. Human Immunology. 2008;69:745–750.
111. Filaci G, Fenoglio D, Fravega M, et al. CD8CD28 T regulatory lymphocytes inhibiting T cell proliferative and cytotoxic functions infiltrate human cancers. Journal of Immunology. 2007;179:4323–4334.
112. Viguier M, Lemaitre F, Verola O, et al. Foxp3 expressing CD4CD25(high) regulatory T cells are overrepresented in human metastatic melanoma lymph nodes and inhibit the function of infiltrating T cells. Journal of Immunology. 2004;173:1444–1453.
113. Bates GJ, Fox SB, Han C, et al. Quantification of regulatory T cells enables the identification of high risk breast cancer patients and those at risk of late relapse. Journal of Clinical Oncology. 2006;24:5373–5380.
114. Yu P, Lee Y, Liu W, et al. Intratumor depletion of CD4+ cells unmasks tumor immunogenicity leading to the rejection of late-stage tumors. Journal of Experimental Medicine. 2005;201:779–791.
115. Imai H, Saio M, Nonaka K, et al. Depletion of CD4+CD25+ regulatory T cells enhances interleukin-2-induced antitumor immunity in a mouse model of colon adenocarcinoma. Cancer Science. 2007;98:416–423.
116. Viehl CT, Moore TT, Liyanage UK, et al. Depletion of CD4+CD25+ regulatory T cells promotes a tumor-specific immune response in pancreas cancer-bearing mice. Annals of Surgical Oncology. 2006;13:1252–1258.
117. Comes A, Rosso O, Orengo AM, et al. CD25+ regulatory T cell depletion augments immunotherapy of micrometastases by an IL-21-secreting cellular vaccine. Journal of Immunology. 2006;176:1750–1758.
118. Nagai H, Horikawa T, Hara I, et al. In vivo elimination of CD25+ regulatory T cells leads to tumor rejection of B16F10 melanoma, when combined with interleukin-12 gene transfer. Experimental Dermatology. 2004;13:613–620.
119. Farag SS, VanDeusen JB, Fehniger TA, et al. Biology and clinical impact of human natural killer cells. International Journal of Hematology. 2003;78:7–17.
120. Seaman WE, Sleisenger M, Eriksson E, et al. Depletion of natural killer cells in mice by monoclonal antibody to NK-1.1. Reduction in host defense against malignancy without loss of cellular or humoral immunity. Journal of Immunology. 1987;138:4539–4544.
121. Rushfeldt C, Sveinbjornsson B, Seljelid R, et al. Early events of hepatic metastasis formation in mice: role of Kupffer and NK-cells in natural and interferon-gamma-stimulated defense. Journal of Surgical Research. 1999;82:209–215.
122. Thibaudin D, Alamartine E, Mariat C, et al. Long-term kinetic of T-lymphocyte subsets in kidney-transplant recipients: influence of anti-T-cell antibodies and association with posttransplant malignancies. Transplantation. 2005; 80:1514–1517.
123. Ducloux D, Carron PL, Rebibou JM, et al. CD4 lymphocytopenia as a risk factor for skin cancers in renal transplant recipients. Transplantation. 1998;65: 1270–1272.
124. Carroll R, San Segundo D, Hollowood K, et al. Immune phenotype predicts risk for posttransplantation squamous cell carcinoma. Journal of the American Society of Nephrology. 2010;21:713–722.
125. Myron Kauffman H, McBride MA, Cherikh WS, et al. Transplant tumor registry: donor related malignancies. Transplantation. 2002;74:358–362.
126. Euvrard S, Kanitakis J, Claudy A. Skin cancers after organ transplantation. New England Journal of Medicine. 2003;348:1681–1691.
127. Ramsay HM, Fryer AA, Hawley CM, et al. Factors associated with nonmelanoma skin cancer following renal transplantation in Queensland, Australia. Journal of the American Academy of Dermatology. 2003;49:397–406.
128. Ulrich C, Kanitakis J, Stockfleth E, et al. Skin cancer in organ transplant recipients–where do we stand today? American Journal of Transplantation. 2008;11:2192–2198.
129. Berg D, Otley CC. Skin cancer in organ transplant recipients: epidemiology, pathogenesis, and management. Journal of the American Academy of Dermatology. 2002;47:1–17.
130. Moosa MR. Kaposi's sarcoma in kidney transplant recipients: a 23-year experience. QJM. 2005;98:205–214.
131. Buell JF, Trofe J, Hanaway MJ, et al. Immunosuppression and merkel cell cancer. Transplantation Proceedings. 2002;34:1780–1781.
132. Ramsay HM, Reece SM, Fryer AA, et al. Seven-year prospective study of non-melanoma skin cancer incidence in U.K. renal transplant recipients. Transplantation. 2007;84:437–439.
133. Bordea C, Wojnarowska F, Millard PR, et al. Skin cancers in renal-transplant recipients occur more frequently than previously recognized in a temperate climate. Transplantation. 2004;77:574–579.
134. Harwood CA, Proby CM, McGregor JM, et al. Clinicopathologic features of skin cancer in organ transplant recipients: a retrospective case-control series. Journal of the American Academy of Dermatology. 2006;54:290–300.
135. Birkeland SA, Storm HH. Risk for tumor and other disease transmission by transplantation: a population-based study of unrecognized malignancies and other diseases in organ donors. Transplantation. 2002;74:1409–1413.
136. Harwood CA, Surentheran T, McGregor JM, et al. Human papillomavirus infection and non-melanoma skin cancer in immunosuppressed and immunocompetent individuals. Journal of Medical Virology. 2000;61:289–297.
137. Euvrard S, Chardonnet Y, Pouteil-Noble C, et al. Association of skin malignancies with various and multiple carcinogenic and noncarcinogenic human papillomaviruses in renal transplantat recipients. Cancer. 1993;72:2198–2206.
138. O'Donovan P, Perrett CM, Zhang X, et al. Azathioprine and UVA light generate mutagenic oxidative DNA damage. Science. 2005;309:1871–1874.
139. El-Agroudy AE, El-Baz MA, Ismail AM, et al. Clinical features and course of Kaposi's sarcoma in Egyptian kidney transplant recipients. American Journal of Transplantation. 2003;3:1595–1599.
140. Zwald FO, Christenson LJ, Billingsley EM, et al. Melanoma in solid organ transplant recipients. American Journal of Transplantation. 2010;10:1297–1304.
141. Australian and New Zealand Dialysis and Transplant Registry. The 30th Annual Report. 2007. 11-1-0007.
142. Bosniak MA. The use of the Bosniak classification system for renal cysts and cystic tumors. Journal of Urology. 1997;157:1852–1853.
143. Denton MD, Magee CC, Ovuworie C, et al. Prevalence of renal cell carcinoma in patients with ESRD pre-transplantation: a pathologic analysis. Kidney International. 2002;61:2201–2209.
144. Members of the KDIGO Working Group. KDIGO clinical practice guidelines for the care of kidney transplant recipients. American Journal of Transplantation. 2009;9:S1–S155.
145. Kasiske BL, Vazquez MA, Harmon WE, et al. Recommendations for the outpatient surveillance of renal transplant recipients. Journal of the American Society of Nephrology. 2000;11:1910–1917.

146. Kälble T, Lucan M, Nicita G, et al. ; European Association of Urology Guidelines on renal transplantation. Wiesel MEuropean Urology. 2005;47:156–166.
147. Wong G, Howard K, Webster AC, et al. Screening for renal cancer in recipients of kidney transplants. Nephrology Dialysis Transplantation. 2011;26:1729–1739.
148. Israel GM, Bosniak MA. An update of the Bosniak renal cyst classification system. Urology. 2005;66:484–488.
149. Muruve NA, Shoskes DA. Genitourinary malignancies in solid organ transplant recipients. Transplantation. 2005;80:709–716.
150. US Renal Data System. USRDS 2003 annual data report: atlas of end-stage renal disease in United States. Bethesda MD: National Institutes of Health, National Institute of Diabetes and Digestive and Kidney Diseases, 2003.
151. Swindle P, Falk M, Rigby R, et al. Transitional cell carcinoma in renal transplant recipients: the influence of compound analgesics. British Journal of Urology. 1998;81:229–233.
152. Aigner F, Boeckle E, Albright J, et al. Malignancies of the colorectum and anus after solid organ recipients. Transplant International. 2007;20:497–504.
153. Saidi RF, Dudrick PS, Goldman MH. Colorectal cancer after renal transplantation. Transplantation Proceedings. 2003;35:1410–1412.
154. Vera A, Gunson BK, Ussatoff V, et al. Colorectal cancer in patients with inflammatory bowel disease after liver transplantation for primary sclerosing cholangitis. Transplantation. 2003;75:1983–1988.
155. Adami J, Gabel H, Lindelof B, et al. Cancer risk following organ transplantation: a nationwide cohort study in Sweden. British Journal of Cancer. 2003;89: 1221–1227.
156. Euvrard S, Kanitakis J, Chardonnet Y, et al. External anogenital lesions in organ transplant recipients. A clinicopathologic and virologic assessment. Archives of Dermatology. 1997;133:175–178.
157. Webster AC, Wong G, Craig JC, et al. Managing cancer risk and decision making after kidney transplantation. American Journal of Transplantation. 2008;8: 2185–2191.
158. Ahmed Z, Marshall MB, Kucharczuk JC, et al. Lung cancer in transplant recipients: a single-institution experience. Archives of Surgery. 2004;139: 902–906.
159. de Perrot M, Fischer S, Waddell TK, et al. Management of lung transplant recipients with bronchogenic carcinoma in the native lung. Journal of Heart and Lung Transplantation. 2003;22:87–89.
160. Jimenez C, Manrique A, Marques E, et al. Incidence and risk factors for the development of lung tumors after liver transplantation. Transplant International. 2007;20:57–63.
161. Stewart T, Tsai SC, Grayson H, et al. Incidence of de-novo breast cancer in women chronically immunosuppressed after organ transplantation. Lancet. 1995;346: 796–798.
162. Oruc MT, Soran A, Jain AK, et al. De novo breast cancer in patients with liver transplantation: University of Pittsburgh's experience and review of the literature. Liver Transplantation. 2004;10:1–6.
163. Buell JF, Hanaway MJ, Trofe J, et al. De novo breast cancer in renal transplant recipients. Transplantation Proceedings. 2002;34:1778–1779.
164. EBPG Expert Group on Renal Transplantation. European best practice guidelines for renal transplantation. Section IV: Long-term management of the transplant recipient. IV. 6.1. Cancer risk after renal transplantation. Post-transplant lymphoproliferative disease (PTLD): prevention and treatment. Nephrology Dialysis Transplantation. 2002;17(Suppl 4):31–33, 35–36.
165. EBPG Expert Group on Renal Transplantation. European best practice guidelines for renal transplantation. Section IV: Long-term management of the transplant recipient. IV. 6.3. Cancer risk after renal transplantation. Solid organ cancers: prevention and treatment. Nephrology Dialysis Transplantation. 2002;17(Suppl 4):32, 34–36.
166. EBPG Expert Group on Renal Transplantation. European best practice guidelines for renal transplantation. Section IV: Long-term management of the transplant recipient. IV. 6.2. Cancer risk after renal transplantation. Skin cancers: prevention and treatment. Nephrology Dialysis Transplantation. 2002; 17(Suppl 4):31–36.
167. Wong G, Chapman JR, Craig JC. Cancer screening in renal transplant recipients: what is the evidence? Clinical Journal of the American Society of Nephrology. 2008;3:S87–S100.
168. Matzkies FK, Tombach B, Dietrich M, et al. MVAC-therapy for advanced urothelial carcinoma in an anuric renal transplant recipient. Nephrology Dialysis Transplantation. 2000;15:110–112.
169. Whang M, Geffner S, Khachikian Z, et al. Renal transplantation and prostate cancer: guidelines for screening and treatment. Transplantation Proceedings. 2002;34:3196–3199.
170. Nishihori T, Strazzabosco M, Wasif Saif M. Incidence and Management of Colorectal Cancer in Liver Transplant Recipients. Clinical Colorectal Cancer. 2008;7:260–266.
171. American Cancer Society. American Cancer Society issues redefined breast cancer screening guidelines. Iowa Medicine. 2003;93:27.
172. ACOG. ACOG practice bulletin. Breast cancer screening. International Journal of Gynaecology and Obstetrics. 2003;81:313–323.
173. US Preventive Services Task Force. Screening for breast cancer: recommendations and rationale. American Family Physician. 2002;65:2537–2544.
174. Rama I, Grinyó JM. Malignancy after renal transplantation: the role of immunosuppression. Nature Reviews Nephrology. 2010;6:511–519.
175. Gomez-Camarero J, Salcedo M, Rincon D, et al. Use of everolimus as a rescue immunosuppressive therapy in liver transplant patients with neoplasms. Transplantation. 2007;84:786–791.
176. Sanchez-Fructuoso A, Conesa J, Perez Flores I, et al. Conversion to sirolimus in renal transplant patients with tumors. Transplantation Proceedings. 2006;38: 2451–2452.
177. Duman S, Töz H, Aşçi G, et al. Successful treatment of posttransplant Kaposi's sarcoma by reduction of immunosuppression. Nephrology Dialysis Transplantation. 2002;17:892–896.
178. Campistol JM. Minimizing the risk of posttransplant malignancy. Transplantation. 2009;87(Suppl):S19–S22.
179. Penn I. Incidence and treatment of neoplasia after transplantation. Journal of Heart and Lung Transplantation. 1993;12:S328–S336.
180. Camus M, Galon J. Memory T-cell responses and survival in human cancer: remember to stay alive. Advances in Experimental Medicine and Biology. 2010;684:166–177.
181. Weber JS, Aparicio A. Novel immunologic approaches to the management of malignant melanoma. Current Opinion in Oncology. 2001;13:124–128.
182. Safa MM, Foon KA. Adjuvant immunotherapy for melanoma and colorectal cancers. Seminars in Oncology. 2001;28:68–92.
183. Rosenberg SA. Progress in human tumour immunology and immunotherapy. Nature. 2001;411:380–384.

第 96 章
移植术后淋巴增生性疾病

Michael Green, Steven A. Webber

引言

实体器官移植(SOT)作为对心脏、肾脏、肺、肝脏、肠等器官终末期疾病的治疗方法已逐渐被广泛接受。SOT 取得长足发展和显著成果的同时，我们也应该认识到移植后淋巴增生性疾病(PTLD)的重要性。尤其对儿童器官移植受体来说，因为儿童在器官移植时 EB 病毒(EBV)阴性可能性大；成人 PTLD 也是增加术后并发症和死亡率的重要原因[1]。尽管大多数 PTLD 与 EBV 感染有关，但是 EBV 阴性的 PTLD 也有发生[2,3]。虽然 PTLD 的病理学研究日益清楚，但仍有大量问题尚待解决，并且在 SOT 受体中 PTLD 的最佳治疗方式也存在争议。本章节将回顾 PTLD 生物学、病理学、流行病学、临床表现、诊断、治疗方面的研究，并讨论关于 SOT 受体 PTLD 的可行性预防方案。第 95 章节对移植术后恶性肿瘤的情况进行了总述，本章节将在 PTLD 方面进行补充和完善。

历史回顾

1968 年首次发现移植术后淋巴瘤与免疫抑制治疗有关[4]。随着外科和免疫抑制方案的发展，器官移植术后恶性淋巴瘤的发生率逐渐升高。尽管此疾病一直被人们所关注，但是直到 20 世纪 80 年代早期才由明尼苏达州大学发现 EBV 在 PTLD 中具有重要作用[5,6]。随着更有效的抗 T 细胞免疫抑制的引入，PTLD 的问题变得越来越明显，促使人们越来越重视该疾病的病因和可能的治疗方案。后来的研究证实 EBV 是导致大部分器官移植患者 PTLD 的主要病原体。然而，随着 EBV 分子探针的应用，我们发现存在一个 PTLD 亚型，在这个亚型中大量病例（特别是成年人或移植后长期存活的儿童)与 EBV 感染无关[2,3]。无论是否与 EBV 感染相关，移植受体都应该强调免疫监视在预防肿瘤中的重要性，特别是被病毒感染的患者。

EBV 相关的 PTLD 涵盖病毒感染到恶性肿瘤发生的全过程[1]。SOT 受体发生 EBV 感染可表现为非特异性发热到 PTLD 的连续的临床及组织病理过程，包括多种与淋巴瘤相关的基因改变[1,7]。通过 30 年来对 EBV 相关疾病严重性和预后影响因素的研究，人们发现适当的宿主免疫反应和外源性免疫抑制水平是其决定性因素。Starzl 等人初步研究发现减少免疫抑制有助于 PTLD 的逆转[8]。由于 EBV 在大多数 PTLD 中发挥关键作用，因此抗病毒可能在 PTLD 中发挥治疗作用。20 世纪 80 年代，Hanto 等人提供了阿昔洛韦在治疗 PTLD 的初步证据[5]。随后，更有效的抗病毒药物受到许多临床医生的青睐，使用这种药剂治疗 EBV 相关性疾病和 PTLD[9]。然而，对 EBV 相关 PTLD 发病机制的认识，特别是其与病毒潜伏期相关(参见下文)而不是与其进展中的溶解性感染相关，以及缺乏支持抗病毒治疗与预防 PTLD 的确切数据，引起了人们对 PTLD 抗病毒治疗的质疑。

20 世纪 80 年代后期的研究确定了外周血中 EBV 载量的升高与移植受体 EBV 相关疾病之间存在相关性[10]。越来越多的 EBV 载量测定方法已被广泛采用，但 20 年来的经验突显了它们的前景和局限性[11]。EBV 载量的升高可鉴别大多数 EBV 阴性受体新发感染处于 EBV 相关性疾病的风险中或已发展 EBV 相关性疾病。然而，部分患者不表现 EBV 载量升高，而其他 EBV 载量升高的患者也可能不表现或不会发展为 EBV 相关性疾病。尽管如此，由于 EBV 载量在疾病发展前几周转为阳性或上升至高水平，人们可以通过连续动态测量 EBV 载量来指导移植时 EBV 血清学阴性的受体预防 EBV 相关性疾病的发生[1,11]。EBV 载量对于在移植时

EBV 血清学阳性受体 PTLD 的预测价值不清楚。

EBV 相关 PTLD 的生物学

EBV 是 γ 家族的双链 DNA 病毒[12]。病毒主要通过唾液传播，尽管它可能也会通过过继白细胞从供体传递到受体。无论是通过唾液还是白细胞，EBV 主要是感染 B 淋巴细胞。B 淋巴细胞的感染分为两个阶段。在溶解期，EBV 在 B 细胞内主动复制，随后产生和释放感染性病毒体，其可扩散并感染未感染的 B 细胞。第二期或潜伏期更为复杂[12,13]。EBV 相关的潜伏期涉及几个不同的阶段。其中一种称为潜伏期Ⅲ型，其特征为受感染的 B 细胞被激活并自主增殖。被感染的 B 细胞类似于免疫功能正常的抗原活化的 B 淋巴母细胞，其中 EBV 特异性细胞毒性 T 淋巴细胞(CTL)最终可控制溶解性感染和 EBV 激活的淋巴母细胞的生长。在正常宿主中，Ⅲ型潜伏期首先发展为Ⅱ型潜伏期(发生在次级淋巴组织的 B 细胞滤泡中)，然后在记忆 B 细胞中发展为Ⅰ型感染潜伏期[13]。这种进展部分由 EBV 特异性 T 细胞免疫介导的，涉及感染的 B 细胞迁移到次级淋巴组织和不同基因的序贯性表达，最终导致在潜伏期Ⅰ型感染的记忆 B 细胞。实际上，EBV 的潜伏基因序列与人免疫系统相互作用，通常不导致慢性或严重疾病，最终导致终生潜伏感染。然而，在移植受体中，免疫抑制破坏了足够的宿主免疫应答，就可能导致潜伏期Ⅲ型中的 B 细胞持续扩增，并因此导致 EBV 相关疾病，如 PTLD[12-14]。

在初次感染免疫状态正常的个体中，潜伏期Ⅲ型淋巴母细胞主要由 EBV 特异性 $CD8^+$ CTL 控制其增殖[13]。随后，血清学阳性的免疫功能正常的个体长期从 T 细胞库释放高比例的对裂解和潜在期发挥作用的 EBV 特异性 T 细胞来控制 EBV。关于 $CD4^+$ T 细胞对 EBV 的应答知之甚少，体液应答在器官移植受体中防止 PTLD 的作用也不清楚。虽然从感染到 PTLD 的确切机制仍不清楚，但缺乏充足的免疫反应抑制 EBV 显然是 EBV 相关 PTLD 发展的关键。

EBV 阴性的 PTLD

虽然大多数 PTLD 损伤与 EBV 感染相关，但人们发现越来越多的 PTLD 没有 EBV 的证据[2,3]。多达 21%~34%的组织学诊断 PTLD 是 EBV 阴性[2,3]，这个数字可能还在增加。并且一些病变为 T 细胞来源的 PTLD[7,15]。EBV 阴性病例通常晚于 EBV 阳性病例发病，且通常是 T 细胞来源的；并且如果 B 细胞正常的话，通常表现出单形态组织学。这类疾病也倾向于较差的预后[3]。

目前发现许多因素是 EBV 阴性 PTLD 的潜在原因。可能存在未知的感染因子刺激淋巴细胞增生。Vilchez 等在 16 例 PTLD 中找到 2 例有 SV40 肿瘤抗原序列的证据，包括 1 例 EBV 阴性 T 细胞疾病[16]。个别病例与人类疱疹病毒 8(HHV 8)感染有关[17]。不论其病因是什么，目前已明确 EBV 阴性 PTLD 似乎代表一类不同的亚群，其生物学行为、治疗反应性和预后都存在差异[2,3]。

病理学

PTLD 是在移植术后发生的淋巴和浆细胞增殖的一类疾病。如上所述，它们大部分与 EBV 感染相关，但也有少部分与 EBV 感染无关。SOT 患者中的大多数 PTLD 是宿主来源的，但在骨髓/干细胞移植受体中它们也可以来源于供体。这些疾病的分类在过去二十年中几经演变，并且有时也使得临床医生和病理学家困惑。世界卫生组织(WHO)制订了分类标准，目前在大多数中心使用[7]。在 2008 年世界卫生组织修订的分类中，确定了四个主要类别(表 96.1)。应当注意，同一患者可以显示不同类型的 PTLD，有时是与克隆无关的，或甚至是来源于不同细胞。这些可以同时发生或在不同时间发生。复发可能会从多形态性病变进展为 B 细胞或 T 细胞单形态性 PTLD 或霍奇金淋巴瘤[15,18]。

要诊断 PTLD，必须要排除其他淋巴或浆细胞炎症病变的可能性。在同种异体移植中，必须与排斥反应鉴

表 96.1 WHO 移植后淋巴增殖异常分类

- 早期损害
  - 浆细胞增生
  - 感染性单核细胞样
- 多形性 PTLD
- 单形性 PTLD(B,T/NK 细胞型)*
- 典型霍奇金淋巴瘤样 PTLD

*根据淋巴瘤特征进一步分型。

PTLD，移植后淋巴增生性疾病；NK，自然杀伤细胞。

别。在极少数情况下，PTLD 和排斥反应可同时发生。PTLD 仍然是一种病理诊断，并且当可疑诊断时，应进行活检；需要进行切除活检或穿刺活检（通常是 CT 或超声引导）而不是细胞学检查。组织的处理应当与免疫功能正常的宿主中淋巴瘤的处理方式相同，并且应该由病理学家参与给出该诊断。进一步的评估应包括组织学切片、免疫表型研究、新鲜/冰冻组织的基因型研究。经典的细胞遗传学研究在某些情况下可能也是有价值的[7]。

早期病变

非破坏性淋巴浆细胞增生可分为两个亚组：浆细胞增生和感染性单核细胞样 PTLD。部分病变不属于上述任何一类，归于滤泡增生，例如舌扁桃体。这些病变可引起显著的症状，包括气道阻塞，但传统上尚未被归类为 PTLD；这仍然存在争议。早期病变可能类似于在免疫功能正常的宿主的淋巴组织中发生的反应性变化。一般来说，这些病变是非克隆的，缺乏细胞遗传学异常。

多形性 PTLD

多形性 PTLD 是儿童移植受体最常见的类型，免疫组织化学提示病变为潜伏 EBV 阳性，即表达非编码 EBV RNA（EBER）或 EBV 核抗原（EBNA）（图 96.1A，B）。这些也是破坏性病变，但不符合非移植人群中的任何经典淋巴瘤的标准。传染性单核细胞样的 PTLD 或单形性 PTLD 的鉴别诊断有时是非常困难。这些病变包括各种类型、大小和形状、各个阶段的淋巴细胞，以及成熟的浆细胞。通常存在各种大小的 B 细胞和异质性 T 细胞的混合物。转化的 B 细胞/免疫母细胞倾向于少数并且可能类似于 R-S 细胞。这些病变并不满足典型恶性淋巴瘤的标准。尽管如此，B 细胞/浆细胞克隆通常通过分子研究来鉴定。在一些多形性 PTLD 中发现了 Bcl-6 的突变，但是肿瘤抑癌基因和原癌基因通常是正常的[19]。

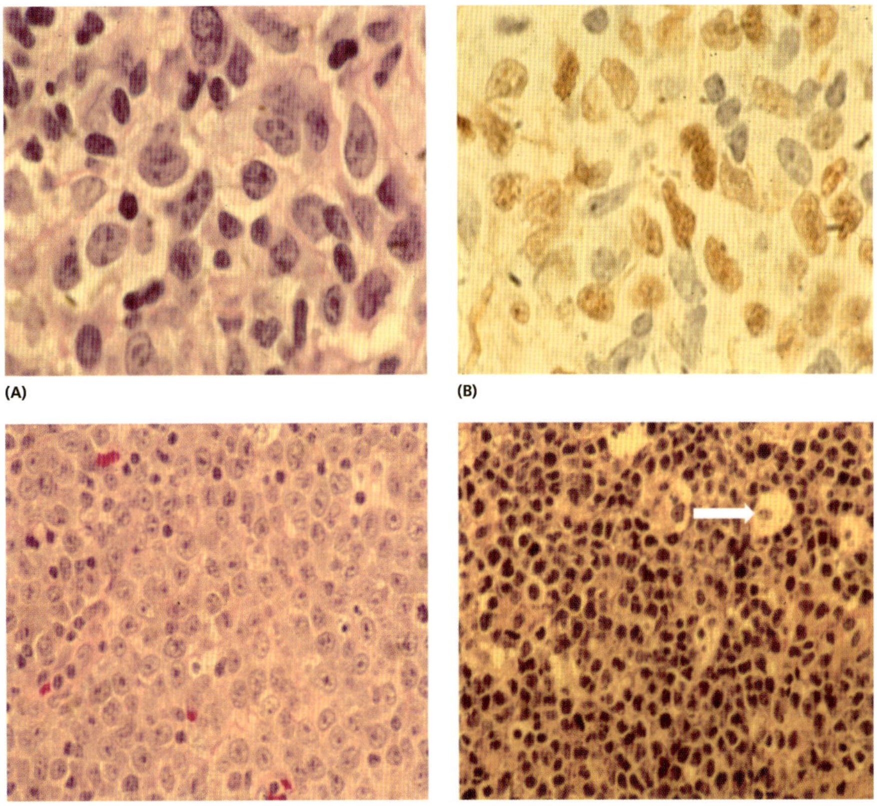

图 96.1　移植后淋巴增生性疾病组织学特征。（A，B）多形性 PTLD。（A）多形性病变和大量异常转化细胞。（B）非编码 EB 病毒 RNA 的免疫组化，A 图中可见细胞中潜伏 EB 病毒（棕黑色）。（C）单形性 PTLD，大量的细胞一致性（D）具有伯基特淋巴瘤特征的单形性 PTLD，巨噬细胞吞噬死亡细胞（箭头）形成的满天星图像。

单形性 PTLD

单形性 PTLD 通常满足弥漫性大 B 细胞淋巴瘤(DLBCL)的标准(图 96.1C);还观察到伯基特淋巴瘤(图 96.1D)、浆细胞瘤和 T /天然杀伤(NK)细胞淋巴瘤。它们是基于在非移植人群中最相似的淋巴瘤的类型来分类。目前,小 B 细胞淋巴瘤不被认为是 PTLD,尽管在移植受体中观察到 MALT 淋巴瘤。

B 细胞单形性 PTLD 在成熟阶段主要由许多转化的淋巴样细胞组成,即单形性。然而,通常存在一定程度的细胞多形性。这些病变通常是单克隆。EBV 阴性病例最多见单形性 PTLD。DLBCL 是 CD20 阳性;伯基特淋巴瘤通常具有 $CD20^+$、$CD10^+$、$Bcl\text{-}6^+$、$Bcl\text{-}2^-$表型。浆细胞肿瘤通常缺乏 B 细胞标记物,但是 $CD138^+$通常表现出轻链类型限制。单形性 B 细胞 PTLD 通常显示肿瘤抑制基因(例如 TP53)、癌基因(N-RAS)和 Bcl-6 的突变。易位,如 MYC,是伯基特淋巴瘤的典型特征[7]。其他细胞遗传学异常也相对比较常见。

单形性 T 细胞 PTLD 满足 T 细胞肿瘤之一的 WHO 标准,与 DLBCL 相反,通常不由单形性大的转化细胞组成。通常,它们类似于外周 T 细胞淋巴瘤。T 细胞 PTLD 的组织病理学差异较大, 如在免疫功能正常的宿主中 T 细胞淋巴瘤中所看到的一样。因为许多 T 细胞淋巴瘤异质性很大,与反应性病变和多形性 PTLD 融合时有发生。免疫表型研究是诊断的关键。分子研究有助于识别克隆 T 细胞群。偶尔,也可以看到 NK 细胞来源的淋巴瘤。

经典霍奇金淋巴瘤

移植人群中罕见的经典霍奇金淋巴瘤。这些病变符合免疫功能正常宿主中经典霍奇金淋巴瘤的诊断标准。大多数情况下, 移植受体符合混合细胞型的标准的,大多数是 EBV 阳性。如前所述,类似于 R-S 的细胞可见于许多不同类型的 PTLD,包括多形性病变。虽然一些病变描述了“霍奇金样”PTLD[20],但这些不包括在 WHO 分类中的经典霍奇金型 PTLD[7]。

流行病学

PTLD 的流行病学最近已由 Dharnidharka 等人综述[21]。本节重点介绍 PTLD 的发病率/患病率及其发病的危险因素。

发病率

移植术后第 1 年 PTLD 的发病风险最高, 但患者在医源性免疫抑制下发病风险持续存在[22]。PTLD 的发病时间随着年龄、移植的器官和供体/受体 EBV 状态等因素而变化。较早发病的受体多见于强有效的免疫抑制方案以及儿童移植受体,特别是那些 EBV 阴性的受体接受 EBV 阳性的器官[22]。早发性疾病更可能是多态性的、B 细胞来源的以及 EBV 阳性, 这种情况多见于儿童[23]。

任何类型疾病的发生率取决于术后生存和随访时间,以及疾病定义。移植后很快死亡的患者处于“危险”状态的时间也很短。因此,有些报道是包含了存活 30 天受体的发病率。大多数报道似乎排除所谓的“早期病变”并且仅报道破坏性的疾病类型。在移植后 5 年,儿童移植受体的“发病率”为:肾脏 3%,心脏 5%,肝脏 6%和肺 11%[21]。在成年受体中,5 年累积发病率近 1%[24],但肝和肺(2%~4%)似乎略高一点[21]。

对于随着随访时间可变的相关事件发生率,更合适的分析方法包括发生密度或“存活分析”方法。后者在疾病发展的风险不断变化时尤其适用。最近的一项研究评估了 1993—2009 年间进行的 3170 例原发性心脏儿童移植受体 PTLD 的发生率和危险度[22](图 96.2)。PTLD 的整体风险在最近的 9 年里(2001—2009)下降。这与许多儿科移植医生的印象相一致,病毒载量监测和其他预防策略一定程度上减少早期 PTLD 发生。然而,儿童心脏移植研究(PHTS)数据集显示了一个令人担忧的现象[22];在长期的随访中,迟发性 PTLD 的危险性增加(图 96.2)。这些晚期 PTLD 在本质上更可能是单形性的,并包括强侵袭性的病变,例如伯基特病[25,26]。

危险因素

PTLD 的许多危险因素已经明确[21],包括感染相关因素(特别是受体和供体 EBV 血清学状态)、宿主相关因素(如年龄)、原发性疾病相关因素以及免疫抑制的强度和类型。EBV 血清学状态可能是单个最强的危险因素,并且在儿童移植中影响最大(移植时这些受体中大多数未接触过 EBV 病毒)。供体 EBV 血清学阳性是 PHTS 中血清学阴性受体中 PTLD 非常强的危险因

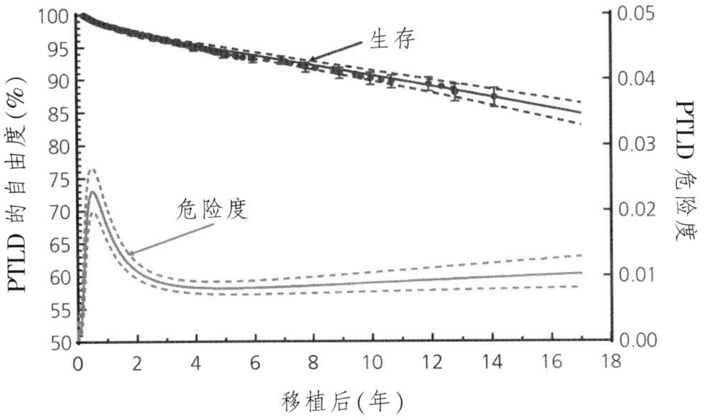

图 96.2 儿童心脏移植研究(1993–2009)中 PTLD 的自由度。第一年疾病危险度高,后期危险度缓慢上升。(Modified from Chinnock et al. [22], with permission from John Wiley & Sons.)

素[22],但危险的大小取决于移植时受体的年龄。当供体 EBV 血清学阳性时,近 25%的 EBV 阴性、年龄在 4~7 岁的受体发生 PTLD。巨细胞病毒(CMV)共感染也是一个危险因素[27]。除了年龄,Dharnidharka 等从美国器官共享联合网(UNOS)和全美器官获取和移植网(OPTN)以及北美儿科肾脏试验和协作研究(NAPRTCS)注册处的数据中发现儿童肾移植中男性和白种人也是风险因素[28]。

许多研究关注各种免疫抑制剂对 PTLD 的影响。这些研究很少是随机对照试验,很难确定特定的药物对 PTLD 的影响,也很难确定风险是否与总体免疫抑制强度有关,特别是靶向 T 细胞免疫的免疫抑制剂(监测 EBV 感染 B 细胞的主要机制;参见上文)。PTLD 最初是在使用硫唑嘌呤类固醇的受体中发现,当引入环孢菌素后,报道的数量有所增加。20 世纪 80 年代末,Swinnen 等人报道 OKT3 是 PTLD 的危险因素[29]。一项近期的随机研究发现在儿童肾移植后撤除类固醇,改用巴利昔单抗诱导、钙调神经磷酸酶抑制剂(CNI)、西罗莫司和皮质类固醇,PTLD 的发生率高达 6.9%[30]。这些数据不支持特定免疫抑制剂在 PTLD 中的作用,但提示我们在该群体中的总体免疫抑制程度过高。自从 Swinnen 等人[29]的报道发表以来,有人担心 T 细胞耗竭抗体可能与 PTLD 的发病率增加相关。对移植受体科学注册处(SRTR)的分析,Kirk 等人检查了在肾移植受体中使用 IL-2 缺失诱导,与没有诱导治疗的患者相比,发现 OKT3 和多克隆兔抗胸腺细胞球蛋白都有增加 PTLD 的风险,而白介素-2(IL-2)受体特异性免疫抑制剂的非消耗诱导并没有增加[31]。有趣的是,消耗性的阿仑单抗与 PTLD 的风险增加无关,可能与该药实际维持在较低水平有关,类似于不用类固醇和较低的 CNI 水平,或者阿仑单抗减少 T 和 B 细胞的同时可以消除一些潜伏期的 EBV。最后,应该指出的是,贝伐珠单抗的使用与肾移植后成人 EBV 血清学阴性中 PTLD 发生率增加有关[32]。需要长期随访和人群的研究来了解这些观察性结果的相关机制。

EBV 相关 PTLD 的预防

EBV 感染在 PTLD 发展中具有重要作用,引起预防 EBV 相关疾病的兴趣。预防 EBV 疾病的潜在方法可以大致分类为免疫预防、化学预防和先发制人治疗策略。

免疫预防

免疫预防可分为主动或被动预防。主动免疫预防是通过使用 EBV 疫苗来实现。在移植前用有效疫苗免疫所有 EBV 血清学阴性受体,可能显著降低移植后 EBV 相关性疾病和 PTLD 的风险。可惜的是,EBV 疫苗的开发进展缓慢,短时间内不可能获得有效的疫苗[33-35]。被动免疫预防是通过静脉输注免疫球蛋白(IVIG)提供抗 EBV 抗体来实现的。在严重的联合免疫缺陷(SCID)小鼠模型中证明了 IVIG 对 EBV 疾病的预防作用[36,37]。这些实验数据支持在 EBV 血清学阴性儿童肝移植受体中开始多中心、随机对照试验[38]。虽然没有观察到统计学显著性差异,但研究表明,与接受安慰剂的受体相比,接受 CMV-IVIG 的患者 EBV 感染率和 PTLD 发生率有降低趋势。该研究中 CMV-IVIG 疗效缺乏显著性差异可能是由于小样本的限制,药物的功效缺乏或由于本研究的后几年引入聚合酶链反应(PCR)测定后的 EBV 载量从而采用预防减少免疫抑制等的混杂效应的存在。最后,使用 EBV 特异性细胞毒性 T 淋巴细胞作为过继性免疫治疗可能成为第三种潜在的免疫预防策略。然而,虽然这种方法已被证明在干细胞移植受体中有效,但是其在 SOT 受体中预防 EBV 疾病和 PTLD 目前还没实现[39]。

化学预防

使用抗病毒剂如阿昔洛韦和更昔洛韦进行的化学预防是另一种预防 EBV 疾病和 PTLD 的方法。阿昔洛韦和更昔洛韦都在体外有效抑制溶解性 EBV 复制,但是这两种药物都不对潜伏状态 EBV 及 EBV 转化的 B 细胞增殖具有任何作用。因此,如果 EBV 疾病进展依赖于 EBV 转化的 B 细胞扩增而不是溶解期的 EBV 复制,则更昔洛韦或阿昔洛韦的使用不可能有效地预防 EBV 疾病的发展。然而,目前缺乏临床数据来明确抗病毒治疗在预防人类 EBV/PTLD 的效果。支持抗病毒药物效果的研究大部分是回顾性的或缺乏适当的对照组[40,41]。也有其他的研究试图通过分析临床注册处数据来解决抗病毒治疗在预防 EBV 疾病中的效果[42,43]。但是这两项研究结果也不一致:Funch 等人结论是抗病毒治疗可以预防 EBV 疾病[42],而 Opelz 等人发现抗病毒治疗不具有相关的保护性作用[43]。

截至目前,只有一项随机对照试验评估抗病毒药物在预防 EBV/PTLD 中的作用[44]。在儿童肝移植受体中,这项随机试验比较了静脉注射更昔洛韦单药 2 周与更昔洛韦治疗 2 周后接受 50 周高剂量口服阿昔洛韦治疗,两组之间没有观察到 EBV/PTLD 显著性差异。这表明延长使用阿昔洛韦并不能防止 EBV/PTLD。然而,值得注意的是,在长期接受静脉注射更昔洛韦治疗的患者中仍然可观察到 PTLD 的发生[45]。

病毒载量监测和预防策略

与历史对照相比,监测 EBV 载量来指导预防性减少免疫抑制可使 EBV 疾病和 PTLD 的发生率降低。McDiarmid 等人报道注射 EBV 病毒载量监测来指导联合减少免疫抑制和静脉使用更昔洛韦,可以使儿童肝移植受体的 PTLD 发生率从 10%降低至 5%[41]。Lee 等人发现 EBV 载量升高后,单独减少免疫抑制,儿童肝移植受体 PTLD 的发生率从 16%下降到 2%[46]。Ganschow 等人也发现降低免疫抑制应对病毒载量升高,儿童肾移植受体 PTLD 发生率为 0.9%[47]。

最近,Martin 等人探讨了 EBV 载量检测指导使用抗 CD20 单克隆抗体,即利妥昔单抗在 EBV 供体阳性/受体阴性成人肾移植且持续性 EBV 病毒血症受体中的作用[48]。尽管作者提出了该方法的有效作用,由于样本量小,在使用利妥昔单抗之前观察时间相对较短且伴随免疫抑制减少,需要另外的研究来证实这些结果。目前还没有随机试验来明确利妥昔单抗对 PTLD 的预防作用。

临床表现和诊断

在器官移植受体中,EBV 感染表现出一系列临床症状[1]。临床上表现为从非特异性病毒感染综合征到移植后 PTLD。值得注意的是,感染 EBV 的患者不同发展阶段存在明显的重叠,而与随后是否发展成 PTLD 无关。此外,EBV 阴性的 PTLD 患者表现出的临床症状与 EBV 相关 PTLD 亦难以区分。

PTLD 与 EBV 相关疾病的诊断主要基于病史和体格检查以及实验室检查结果(表 96.2)。做出该诊断时最重要的始终是结合临床上高度可疑的相关因素。与早期 PTLD 的诊疗相比,提高的诊断意识和改进的诊断工具使那些 PTLD 危重患者大大减少。要实现早期诊断,必须注意到更细微的症状,如昏睡乏力、萎靡不振、体重减轻和发热,这些都是 PTLD 常见的表现。此外呕吐和(或)腹泻病史(可能粪便检查阳性),提示胃肠道受累(被越来越多地认为是该疾病常见的累及部位)。这在肠移植受体中尤其如此,几乎所有肠移植受体都表现出受累,可以是同种异体移植肠,也可以是自身原有的肠道受累。肠道出血、梗阻和穿孔也可以在累及肠道的 PTLD 患者中见到。令人惊讶的是,穿孔的最高风险可能是由于治疗期间透壁性损伤发展引起的坏疽所致。

其他受累部位因所接受的器官移植的类型而不同。肺部受累在心脏移植受体中非常常见,而在肺部移

表 96.2 疑似 PTLD 患者的诊断性评估

常规	进一步检查患者
全血细胞计数、血小板、白细胞及分类	胃肠道内镜
血电解质、钙、尿素氮、肌酐	骨扫描
肝功能检查	骨穿活检
尿酸	脑部 CT/MRI
乳酸脱氢酶	腰椎穿刺
免疫球蛋白定量	联合病变感染筛查
血清蛋白电泳	PET 扫描
EB 病毒血清学	
定量 PCR 的 EB 病毒负荷	
大便隐血	
胸片(前后位、侧位)	
胸/腹/骨盆 CT	
病变穿刺或切除活检	

植受体中几乎普遍出现。接受同种异体肺移植的受体，肺部表现从常规胸片检查时发现的无症状结节到危及生命的肺部功能障碍。后者可能类似于在胸片上的肺排斥反应，具有弥散的肺实变但又没有明显确定的大块病变。这种误判可能导致免疫抑制的增加，而免疫抑制又会引起严重后果[49]。累及肝脏的 EBV 疾病和 PTLD 在肝移植受体中最常见，可能表现为弥漫性肝炎或肝脏的结节性损害。有趣的是，心脏是同种异体器官移植中唯一没有被该类疾病影响的器官。在大多数 SOT 中，同种异体移植物功能障碍可能是 PTLD 的表现，并可能与急慢性排斥反应相似。

其他表现包括持续的咽喉疼痛、淋巴结肿大和皮肤结节，以及癫痫、头痛和伴有中枢神经系统(CNS)疾病的局灶性神经病变。PTLD 有时是在儿童实行选择性摘除肿大的扁桃体和淋巴结肿大时被发现。因此，对于移植受体来说，所有手术摘除的淋巴组织和扁桃体组织应该接受常规病理检查。

虽然体格检查可能没有特异的发现，但常常可以发现脸色苍白、体重减轻、周围性淋巴结肿大或肝脾肿大的证据。全身体格检查是必要的，还应包括彻底的神经系统检查。对全身皮肤和体表淋巴结的检查以及口咽部的仔细检查也是必要的。

对于诊断 PTLD 所需的检验室检查的总结见表 96.2。初步检测应包括白细胞分型和血小板在内的全血细胞计数。白细胞减少症常与非典型淋巴细胞增多症有关，血小板减少症也比较常见。另外，可常常表现出贫血，一般是正常细胞性贫血，而当存在隐匿性胃肠道出血时则表现为缺铁性。很少发现溶血性贫血。大便隐血应常规检测。终末器官功能(肝肾)应进行评估。尿酸和乳酸脱氢酶升高很常见，应该在生化检查中进行检测。免疫球蛋白水平可能升高，特别是 IgE，可能是由于 PLTD 患者存在以 Th2 占主要优势的细胞因子环境所引起的。一些医学中心还常规进行血清蛋白电泳检测以查找单克隆丙种球蛋白病的证据。虽然很多患者并不显示单克隆或寡克隆丙种球蛋白病，但是如果存在相关证据，这就提供了另一种跟踪患者的治疗反应的方法。

多种成像检查有助于评估移植受体是否患有 PTLD。胸片常能显示肺部结节病和(或)纵隔淋巴结肿大的证据。最有价值的诊断性研究通常是检查评估胸部、腹部和盆部的增强 CT，结节或结节外疾病的证据常能在 CT 上的一个或多个部位上明显显示。胸部，普通胸片上显示正常的，增强 CT 则可以显示出小的肺部结节或增大的纵隔淋巴结。腹部，疾病可在包括胃肠道上的正常淋巴结上或结节外的部位被发现，如肝脾肾。有些中心会常规进行脑部 CT 或 MRI，因此如果有任何关于中枢神经系统疾病方面的临床提示，应该需要进行上述检查。

在诊断和评估 PTLD 的治疗临床反应方面，PET 和 FDG 的潜在作用正受到越来越多的关注[50]。与常规 CT 相比，PET 的潜在优势包括在诊断阶段对病变损伤部位具有更强大的检测灵敏性，以及在随后的治疗期间或治疗后，能潜在地区分活性肿瘤灶与坏死的或纤维化的病灶。常规使用 PET 扫描能否改善临床预后还需要进一步研究。

根据临床发现选择了一些特定患者进行研究，具体见表 96.2。当出现胃肠道症状或隐匿性胃肠道出血时，应进行上/下消化道的内镜检查。当有中枢神经系统疾病的证据时，应进行腰椎穿刺。当出现骨髓衰竭的证据和存在单形态细胞疾病时，应在开始治疗前进行骨髓穿刺检测。但目前并不太清楚是否需要在具有早期病变或多形性疾病的患者(主要是儿童患者)中进行这些检测。

使用 PCR 技术测量外周血中 EBV 的载量作为诊断工具已用于评估包括 PTLD 在内的有症状的 EBV 患者病情[10,11,48,51,52]。越来越多的研究表明，升高的 EBV 载量将会出现在绝大多数与 EBV 相关的 PTLD 儿童患者中，对成年患者来说也是如此。当接受移植时，EBV 血清学阴性的受体中 EBV 相关 PTLD 的这一现象最为明显。需要着重指出的是，EBV 载量的高浓度在 EBV 相关的病毒综合征和 PTLD 的患者中通常是相当的。此外，病毒载量可以在没有活动性疾病的情况下升高，于是一些患者在无症状的 EBV 感染后变成了慢性高浓度病毒的携带者[25]。因此，尽管对可疑 EBV 患者进行 EBV 载量的测量是一个十分有用的筛选方法，但由于该检测缺乏特异性，并不能代替组织学检查，而后者是对涉及的可疑部位进行诊断 PTLD 所必需的。最后，临床医生不应该依赖血清学试验来做出 PTLD 的诊断，因为很多患者基于血液制品(或婴儿接受了母体来源)导致的被动免疫，以及其他患者可能因为血清转化出现了 EBV 滴度阳性，但并没有表现出任何临床症状。此外，在移植受体中应用免疫抑制剂，可能会导致某些患者出现假阴性血清学结果。

治疗

尽管对PTLD的病理生理学认知日益增长，但其最佳治疗方案仍然存在争议。对于临床医生来说，治疗手段越来越多，但是如何、何时使用或联合使用这些治疗方法并不清楚。值得注意的是，还没有对任何治疗手段进行过重要的随机试验验证。治疗方式的选择是随意的，例如，机构偏好等，但也可以受预测因素（客观真实的或主观的）影响，例如病理性结果、发病年龄、移植物、发病阶段、EBV的存在与否、并发症的情况以及先前排斥反应史。

PTLD最佳治疗方案应是能快速根除疾病，不增加同种异体移植排斥（急性或慢性的）的风险，并且给药方式简单方便、成本低且不良事件少。很显然，并没有单一的治疗手段满足上述这些标准。此外，治疗还需个体化，例如对于接受肺部移植并在移植早期就有严重排斥反应的受体，与那些接受肾脏移植但有较轻排斥的移植晚期受体相比，治疗严重的PTLD所需的最佳治疗很可能明显不同。涉及具有临床异质性的罕见疾病时，设计临床试验时将会面临巨大的挑战。临床反应也可能取决于肿瘤的固有特性，例如有丝分裂的速度、原癌基因、EBV的存在与否，以及重建T细胞免疫监视的控制能力。不幸的是，目前很难预测肿瘤行为，即便是在完成了广泛的病理评价之后。

减少免疫抑制

1984年，Starzl等人报道了接受环孢素治疗的患者通过减少免疫抑制成功逆转PTLD[8]。这种策略仍然是大多数医学中心初始的治疗手段，以此治疗大多具有早期病变或多态性细胞病变的数患者。对单形态病变而言，虽然更多地使用现代疗法，包括辅助治疗，如自诊断之时起采用抗B细胞单克隆抗体治疗，但减少免疫抑制也被作为一些特殊群体（尤其是儿童）的一线治疗。无论如何，免疫抑制减少应该是对PTLD治疗的关键部分。减少（或停止）免疫抑制的目的是为了允许宿主恢复天然免疫监视，以及随后获得对潜伏EBV感染的B细胞增殖的控制。免疫监视的恢复也可能助于EBV阴性PTLD的缓解，尽管似乎缓解率较低[53]。儿童（特别是多态性细胞病变）中的大多数PTLD将对免疫抑制的减少有反应，尽管具有显著的急性细胞排斥的可能性（随器官不同而不同）[23,54]。在成年人中，PTLD对减少免疫抑制的反应率差异较大，一些报道低风险患者取得了不错的效果，而另一报道其效果非常差[56,57]。这些不同的结果可能反映了不同的参照模式和患者的特征及病理，例如，多形态和单形态病变的比例，以及可能在使用辅助治疗（如抗病毒剂）方面的差异。与儿童一样，免疫抑制减少后成年人的排斥率显著增高，且是一个重要的死亡原因，尤其是对那些在接受心脏移植后为了治疗PTLD而减少免疫抑制的患者[56]。

一般来说，减少免疫抑制后，大多数患者在2–4周内出现临床反应的证据，虽然某些患者几个月后才观察到延迟反应。对弥散性大B细胞性淋巴瘤（DLBCL），移植后霍奇金病和其他更罕见PTLD（T细胞淋巴瘤）患者而言，通过减少免疫抑制来实现完全缓解是不可能的，如果真的发生了，也是不完全或者不持久的[53,57]。因此，越来越少使用减少免疫抑制这一方法作为唯一初始治疗手段。

减少免疫抑制的方法有很多，差异也很大。许多中心最初使用CNI和辅助抗增殖剂，并维持受体可接受的皮质类固醇。因为肝脏代谢受损，他克莫司和环孢菌素的水平在起始阶段可能是高的。随后的用法变化也很大。在肝移植方案中，存在一种长期甚至无限期撤销CNI的可能[54]。这在心肺和肠道移植中是不大可能的。用西罗莫司靶蛋白（mTOR）抑制剂代替CNI引起了广泛的兴趣。西罗莫司已经常用于这种情况。在PTLD中使用这些药物的好处，已经部分反映了它们的抗肿瘤特性，包括抑制EBV相关B细胞淋巴瘤。然而，mTOR抑制剂也是有效的T细胞抑制剂，因此会损害T细胞免疫监视作用。在临床中，很难知道使用mTOR抑制剂是否有益，因为它们可能足以防止移植物排斥（不需要重新引入CNI），也不清楚这些药物在体内是否真正表现出抗PTLD的作用。值得注意的是，使用mTOR抑制剂而非CNI的免疫抑制方案的受体，仍然可能发展成PTLD[58]。

手术和放射治疗

切除活检，一般用作诊断目的，也可以治愈孤立性的PTLD病变，但通常与减少免疫抑制相结合。几乎所有患者都需要接受系统的治疗，因此，PTLD被认为可能是系统性过程。手术也可能有助于局部并发症的处理，例如胃肠道出血、肠梗阻或穿孔。

虽然很多病变会对放射治疗起反应，但是其在 PTLD 治疗中的作用有限。当需要局部快速治疗反应时，如肿瘤肿块压迫气道引起阻塞或者其他关键性结构受到压迫，这时可用放射治疗。它还可以在一些中枢神经系统的 PTLD 病例中起作用(参见下文)。

抗病毒治疗

起初用抗病毒治疗 PTLD 的兴趣发生在 1982 年，Hanto 等人描述了 1 例 EBV 相关的 PTLD 患者，其病变的消退似乎与阿昔洛韦的治疗相关[5]。阿昔洛韦和更昔洛韦都能抑制溶解期 EBV DNA 在体外的复制，可能在治疗 EBV 感染的溶解期有价值。然而，对于潜伏感染与无限增殖 B 细胞没有明显作用；因此，它们用于治疗 PTLD 的合理性还不清楚。然而，许多医学中心已经常规性使用这些药剂治疗 PTLD。

治疗严重的人类孢疹病毒(HHV)及 EBV 感染的抗病毒药物制剂已经取得了诸多进展[59,60]。不依赖于病毒酶靶标、胸苷激酶而发挥作用的药物或许对 PTLD 有效。西多福韦在这方面发挥作用，但其具有重大的毒性。研究表明，西多福韦和环状西多福韦的脂质类似物可能比母体药物具有更大的抗 EBV 活性，可能是用于Ⅰ期临床试验的合适药物[60]。

另一种抗病毒方法是在 EBV 感染的肿瘤中诱导 EBV 胸苷激酶，从而使得肿瘤对核苷型抗病毒药物如更昔洛韦敏感。可实现这一目标的药物是丁酸精氨酸。在 15 例难治性 EBV 阳性的成人淋巴瘤患者的Ⅰ/Ⅱ临床试验中，连续输注丁酸精氨酸以及标准剂量的更昔洛韦，2/3 的患者出现了显著的抗肿瘤反应[61]。最近已经证明短期、不连续暴露于丁酸精氨酸中(与连续输注相比)，足以引起溶解期 EBV 基因表达和胸苷激酶诱导[62]。这种疗法为 EBV 相关 PTLD 患者带来了希望。

干扰素和其他细胞因子

已有研究表明干扰素(IFN)可作为治疗 PTLD 的一个选择[63,64]。干扰素既是一种促炎症细胞因子，也是一种天然抗病毒剂，并呈现出一种能控制 EBV 感染 B 细胞增殖的能力。由于它是一种非特异性免疫刺激剂，因此经常可以看到抗供体反应，并且在治疗期间引起严重的排斥反应。在一些对免疫抑制减少无反应的成人 PTLD 患者中，13 例使用 IFN-α2b 的病例中仅有 1 例(7%)达到了持久的完全缓解[57]。目前，大多中心并没有常规使用 IFN 治疗 PTLD。

白介素-6(IL-6)被认为是 EBV 感染 B 细胞的生长因子。为此，已经在Ⅰ/Ⅱ期临床试验中评估抗 IL-6 单克隆抗体的疗效[65]。抗 IL-6 单克隆抗体具有良好的耐受性，大约 40%的患者中观察到了完全应答，而这些患者都是对短暂的减少免疫抑制没有反应。但目前，它并未在临床中常规运用。

随着进一步认识 EBV-PTLD 的生物学特征[12]，更多干预的靶标将会被发现。

静脉注射免疫球蛋白

静脉注射免疫球蛋白(IVIG)已被建议作为一种潜在治疗 PTLD 的方法。几项报道发现在 EBV 感染器官移植受体中，至少一种 EBV 核抗原(EBNA)抗体的减少或缺失与随后 PTLD 的发展有关联[66]。此外，已经证明了升高的抗 EBNA 抗体(包括通过输血输入的)水平与 EBV 载量的减少之间存在关联。总之，这些研究提示在预防和(或)治疗 EBV 疾病和 PTLD 中考虑使用抗体，虽然控制 EBV 感染的主要机制似乎是细胞毒性 T 细胞介导的免疫反应。IVIG 单独使用或与 IFN-α 组合使用治疗 PTLD[64]。IVIG 和 CMV-IVIG 已经用于治疗部分 PTLD 患者。在治疗 PTLD 上，与使用抗病毒剂和 IFN 一样，并没有比较试验来评价 IVIG 的疗效，尤其是 CMV-IVIG 的疗效。

抗 B 细胞抗体

大多数 PTLD 是 B 细胞来源的，并且大多数表达 CD20。抗 CD20 人/鼠嵌合单克隆抗体利妥昔单抗(Genentech Inc. and IDEC Pharmaceuticals)，用于治疗成人非移植受体中 $CD20^+$的 B 细胞非霍奇金淋巴瘤，目前已商业上市。2000 年，法国临床研究人员发表了一项 32 例 PTLD 患者使用利妥昔单抗的回顾性分析[67]。在所有实体器官移植受体中总体反应率为 65%，其中大多数获得长期缓解。然而，大约 20%的应答者在完成利妥昔单抗治疗后中位随访时间为 7 个月时 PTLD 复发。后续几项研究来自单中心[53,68-70]和多中心Ⅱ期试验[71,72]。成年人的总体反应率差异显著，当利妥昔单抗被用作免疫抑制失败的二线治疗时，完全缓解率为 28%~59%[68,71,72]。然而，一组 60 例患者的长期随访显示，57%的患者在完成治疗后 1 年出现疾病进展期，而无进展生存期的中位时间仅为6个月[73]。尽管利妥昔单抗在PTLD的成人患者中疗效欠佳，但它具有良好的耐受性，大量患者将获得持久的完全应答而不需要化疗，并且那些进展性疾病或者复发的患者仍然可以进行化疗[53]。有趣的是,利妥昔单抗在一些先前接受过化疗但无效或者复发的患者中也可能有效[74]。

利妥昔单抗的疗效可能在儿童中更具优越，尽管只有很少的数据支持这一观点。在一项小型的前瞻性多中心Ⅱ期试验中,80%的难治性PTLD儿童患者在4次或8次剂量治疗后出现了完全应答，但有25%的复发率[75]。

关于在移植中使用利妥昔单抗有几个重要问题：

• 长期消除B细胞是否会导致额外的机会性感染或其他并发症？

• 是否将利妥昔单抗应用在所有确诊的患者,或仅仅适用于那些减少免疫抑制初始治疗失败的患者？

• 如果在使用利妥昔单抗后复发，该如何继续治疗？

• 每6个月进行维持治疗是否合理？

• 利妥昔单抗治疗后PTLD的高复发率是否与应用在那些高风险患者，即那些有难治性疾病或旧病复发高危因素有关？

• 当确诊后使用利妥昔单抗时，临床医生的免疫抑制减少程度会降低吗？

似乎我们可以认为，除非实现EBV-细胞毒性T淋巴细胞(EBV-CTL)反应的重建,否则持久的缓解不能实现[76]。最后,值得注意的是关于较新的抗B细胞抗体的放射偶联物(所谓的放射免疫疗法)的经验很少。这些药物是否提供了优于利妥昔单抗的好处，以及是否安全？希望正在进行中的和未来的研究将回答这些重要问题。

化疗

化疗通常用于侵袭性的移植后淋巴瘤如伯基特病(图96.3)或T细胞淋巴瘤的一线治疗,并且也适用于移植后经典霍奇金病的大多数病例。如前所述,尚不清楚在组织学上呈现弥漫性大B细胞淋巴瘤(DLBCL)的单形态疾病患者是否该接受使用免疫抑制减少或连用利妥昔单抗治疗，也不清楚他们是否该接受化疗作为一线治疗。这是目前PTLD治疗管理中最具争议的问题之一。

难治性多态性PTLD儿童患者对使用环磷酰胺和泼尼松的“低剂量”化疗有相当高的初始反应率,尽管2年无进展期生存率在58%左右[77]。最近还研究了在该方案中加入利妥昔单抗[78]。目前并不清楚化疗在完成利妥昔单抗试验之前是否起作用,因为单独使用利妥昔单抗在儿童难治性疾病中给出了令人鼓舞的结果[75]。在减少免疫抑制治疗的儿童患者中，目前还没有低剂量化疗直接与利妥昔单抗进行比较研究。化疗应该给予那些使用利妥昔单抗治疗进展性疾病的儿童，并且化

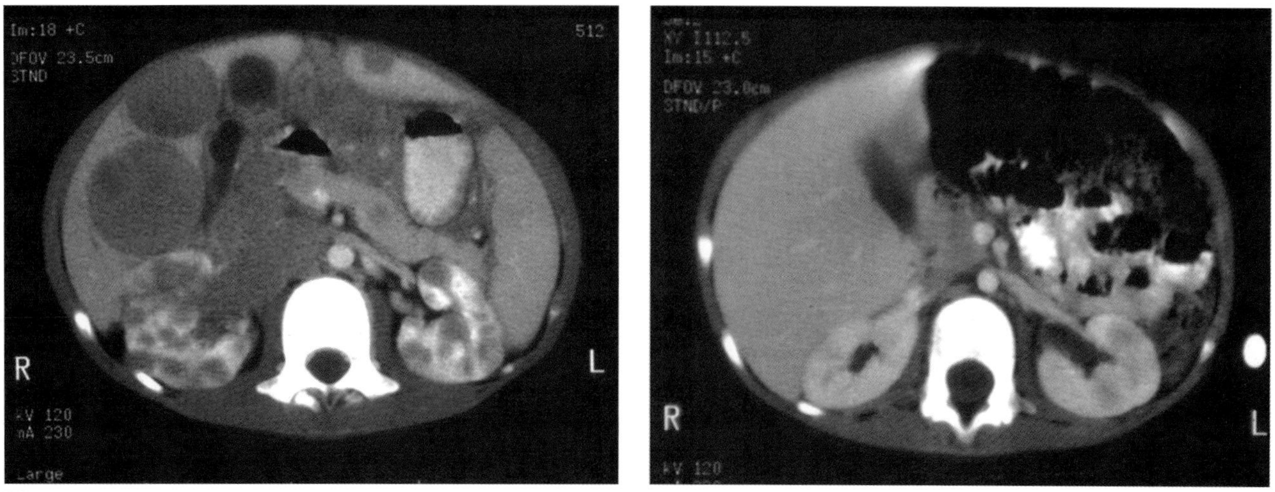

图96.3 儿童心脏移植后伯基特淋巴瘤。(A)腹部广泛病变存在,下颌及眼眶也受侵犯。(B)化疗2个疗程后,病变明显好转,达到持续完全反应。[Reproduced from Dharnidharka V, Green M, Webber SA (2010). Post-transplant lymphoproliferative disorders (figure 9.2), with kind permission from Springer Science+Business Media B.V. Copyright 2010, Springer-Verlag.]

疗对那些罕见的伴有同种异体移植排斥的活动性PTLD也是有用的。儿童和成年人中的伯基特病对多种药物化疗方案(使用或不使用利妥昔单抗;图 96.3)也有良好的反应,但最佳方案仍有待确定[26,79,80]。我们并不建议在这种情况下单用利妥昔单抗。

成年人化疗的适应证与儿童大致类似。医疗中心关于 DLBCL(成年人中最常见的病理类型)是否应该用化疗作为主要治疗手段,还是仅仅在未能对减少的免疫抑制和利妥昔单抗起反应后再使用化疗方面分成了两派。化疗通常会保护移植物免受排斥反应和移植物功能受损[81],但是与在非移植人群中使用的类似方案相比,有更高的感染发病率和死亡率[53]。目前存在多种不同的化疗方案,包括环磷酰胺-泼尼松(用或不用利妥昔单抗)、"CHOP""CHOP-利妥昔单抗""ACVBP"和"ProMACE-CytaBOM"[53,57,77-86]。目前缺乏各种方案之间的直接比较研究。总体反应率为 65%~80%,尽管长期死亡率非常高[87]。

细胞免疫治疗

虽然可能存在其他机制,EBV 特异性 T 细胞反应不足是 EBV 相关 PTLD 发展中重要或关键的病理性步骤。EBV 特异性 CTL 的输注已经被用于治疗和预防骨髓/干细胞移植中的 PTLD[88]。这种情况下,PTLD 通常是供体来源的,并且供体通常可用于为受体提供 CTL 来源。这种过继性免疫治疗在干细胞受体中的成功激起了将这种方法用到 SOT 受体的 PTLD 治疗研究中[89]。理论上,这是一种合理的治疗方案,因为其针对 PTLD,并且应该减少抗供者反应,即排斥反应。然而,PTLD 病变内的 EBV 感染的细胞通常是受体来源,这一事实限制了实体器官受体中使用 CTL 输注。理想情况下,EBV 特异性 CTL 应是 HLA 单倍体相同。因此,自体 CTL 是用于实体器官移植受体的 EBV 特异性 CTL 输注的理想来源。然而,来自器官受体的 EBV 特异性 CTL 的发展具有挑战性,因为大多数处于 EBV-PTLD 风险的患者在移植时是 EBV 阴性的,免疫抑制造成 CTL 的产生受损,并且当 PTLD 发展时 T 细胞应答进一步严重抑制。因此,用于实体器官移植受体中 EBV 相关 PTLD 的过继性免疫治疗的技术主要集中于开发体外"免疫"和刺激器官受体自身的 T 细胞来抗衡 EBV 的策略,随后当患者发展为难治性 EBV 感染/PTLD 时,将这些 EBV 特异性 CTL 输注回受体[39,89,90]。这种方法也可用于预防,当 EBV 病毒载量开始在原发性移植后 EBV 感染后上升时进行输注[39]。理想情况下,用于培养的细胞应当在移植前获得,并且在高危受体(移植时 EBV 血清学阴性)中开始免疫抑制。但这种方法代价较大,因为大多数受体将可能不需要 CTL 治疗。此外,使用自体 CTL 过继性免疫在实体器官移植受体中的效果与在骨髓/干细胞移植后观察到的并不一致。另一种方法已经取得一些成功,其使用来自 EBV 阳性血液供体的同种异体 T 细胞输注,其尽可能与接受体的 HLA 类型匹配。使用这种方法的Ⅱ期临床试验中观察到约 50%的患者有效[91]。尽管过继性免疫治疗作为实体器官移植后 PTLD 治疗的进步,但它仍然处于研究阶段,仅有非常少的中心提供基于细胞的免疫治疗。目前的研究集中在用于开发针对 EBV 感染的靶细胞的高细胞毒性的离体培养细胞。刺激细胞的特性,如淋巴母细胞样细胞系或装载有 EBV 抗原的树突细胞和细胞因子环境,如添加 IL-7 和 IL-12,可能是离体产生用于临床输注的 CTL 成功的关键因素[92,93]。

联合治疗

由于缺乏相关的大型随机对照试验,使用联合治疗证据不足。然而,与其他疾病一样,联合使用通过不同机制起作用的治疗方案可能也是合理的。联合疗法也使得鉴定治疗方案的有效组分非常具有挑战性。例如,自体 EBV 特异性 CTL 在多次化疗后立即与利妥昔单抗联合使用[90]。由于在该疾病中开展随机对照试验是非常有挑战性的,联合疗法仍然是基于经验性的。

中枢神经系统疾病

CNS 疾病可能是原发的[94,95],或者可能同时合并有颅外疾病[94]。疾病通常是多灶的,并且可发生在任何部位,尽管在脑半球最常见[96]。几乎所有的病变显示增强。鉴别诊断包括其他恶性肿瘤和感染,特别是真菌。必要时需要通过活检来确诊,预后一般非常差[94,95]。CNS 通常是受保护的,其中正常的免疫监测难以控制其疾病发生发展。尽管如此,正常的免疫监测可能足以控制罕见的疾病(图 96.4)。然而,其发生频率较低,不足以证明减少免疫抑制是唯一的治疗。在肾移植患者中,完全停止免疫抑制治疗似乎是合理的,直到根除疾病。通常给予辅助治疗,尽管其疗效难以确定。这些包括全身或鞘内利妥昔单抗、化疗(特别是使用高剂量甲

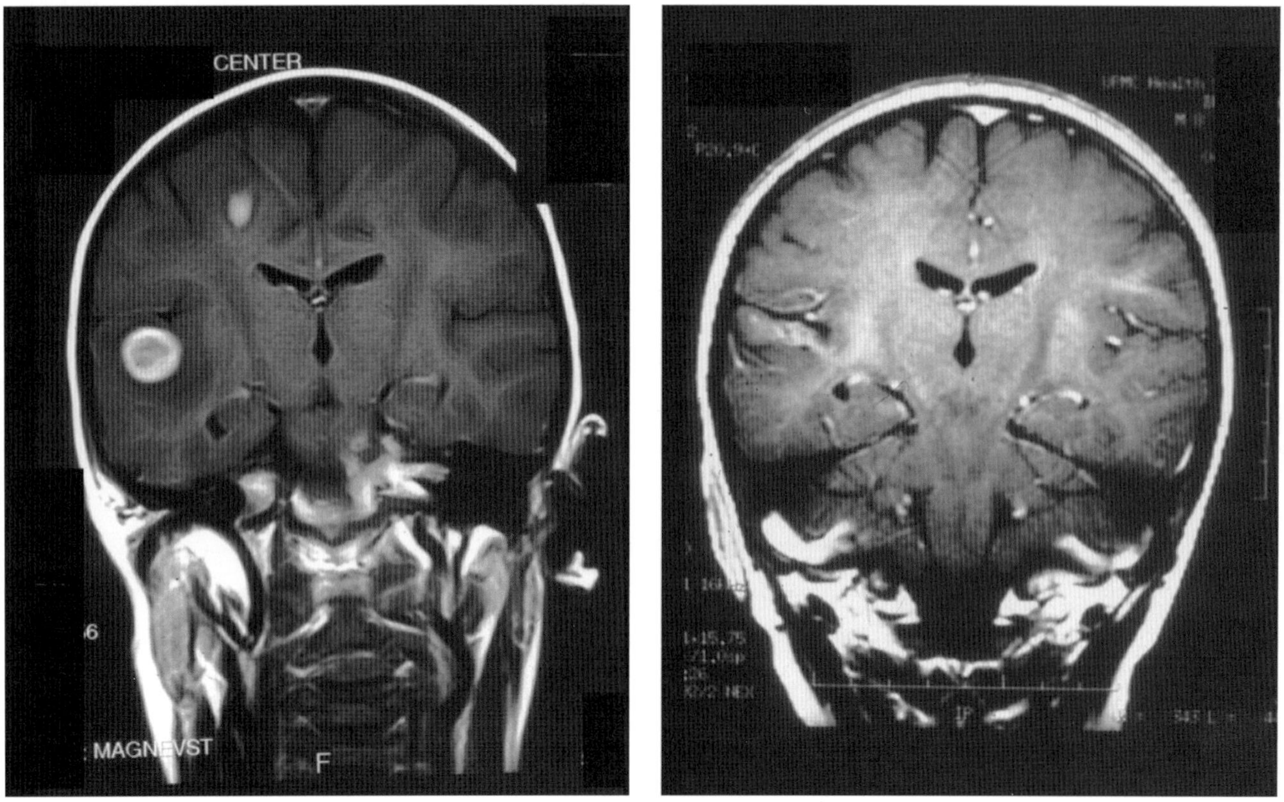

(A) (B)

图 96.4 (A)中枢神经系统单形性 PTLD 伴有第六神经麻痹多发强化占位病变(A 图)。(B)暂时去除免疫抑制剂后病变完全缓解。[Reproduced from Dharnidharka V, Green M, Webber SA (2010). Post-transplant lymphoproliferative disorders (figure 9.3), with kind permission from Springer Science+Business Media B.V. Copyright 2010, Springer-Verlag.]

氨蝶呤)和放疗。

预后和结果

PTLD 的预后差异较大,跨年龄组(例如儿童与成人)及跨器官移植类型的移植物和患者存活率能够提供给医生指导个体化治疗的有用信息很少。当研究特定人群时,PTLD 确实对移植物和患者的长期预后具有显著的负面影响[23]。此外,PTLD 确诊后,急性和慢性排斥而不是疾病进展是预后的重要决定因素[23]。因此,治疗策略必须是在减少的免疫抑制期间保护移植物以及有效地治疗 PTLD [81]。

最近一篇综述报道了预后因素[97],也是另几项研究的主要内容[98-100]。在许多研究中,不良预后因素与非移植人群的传统非霍奇金淋巴瘤类似,包括差的体能状态、多灶性疾病、骨髓受累和年龄增加[97,100]。T 细胞来源的 PTLD 和 CNS 的 PTLD 在大多数研究中显示预后不良,尽管最近的数据表明积极治疗可以使一些 CNS 疾病患者获得持续缓解[96]。有关单形性组织学、缺乏 EBV 或迟发性疾病是不利的预后因素也存在不一致的看法。在未来,有可能对 PTLD 的生物学和分子病理学有更详细的了解,这将提高我们对疾病行为的理解并进行个体化治疗[101]。这个目标的中心是理解 PTLD 是一组异质性疾病,因此一个最佳治疗不可能适合于所有 PTLD 的患者。令人鼓舞的是,最近的数据表明,新的治疗方法可能会改善疾病预后,提高患者生存率[98]。

总结

PTLD 仍然是器官移植受体中重要的潜在致命性疾病。其与 EBV 生物学的相关性提供了关于免疫抑制对病毒相关恶性肿瘤影响的重要作用,并有助于对其临床风险因素的认识和治疗方案的发展。PTLD 的分类已达到共识,并且用于指导临床治疗。PTLD 的早期诊断和治疗已经有所改善,但 PTLD 继续影响移植术后的并发症和死亡率,特别是在儿童移植受体,以及 EBV

阴性受体接受 EBV 血清学阳性的器官。因此，了解移植受体 EBV 血清学状态是非常重要的，并且应该纳入移植临床医生诊疗常规中。

（刘治坤 译　徐骁 校）

参考文献

1. Allen U, Preiksaitis J, AST Infectious Disease Community of Practice. Epstein-Barr virus and posttransplant lymphoproliferative disorder in solid organ transplant recipients. American Journal of Transplantation. 2009;9(Suppl 4): S87–S96.
2. Leblond V, Davi F, Charlotte F, et al. Posttransplant lymphoproliferative disorders not associated with Epstein-Barr virus: a distinct entity? Journal of Clinical Oncology. 1998;16:2052–2059.
3. Nelson BP, Nalesnik MA, Bahler DW, et al. Epstein-Barr virus-negative post-transplant lymphoproliferative disorders - A distinct entity? American Journal of Surgical Pathology. 2000;24:375–385.
4. Murray JE, Wilson RE, Tilney NL, et al. Five years' experience in renal transplantation with immunosuppressive drugs: survival, function, complications, and the role of lymphocyte depletion by thoracic duct fistula. Annals of Surgery. 1968; 168:416–435.
5. Hanto DW, Frizzera G, Gajl-Peczalska KJ, et al. Epstein-Barr virus-induced B-cell lymphoma after renal transplantation. New England Journal of Medicine. 1982;306:913–918.
6. Hanto DW, Frizzera G, Gajl-Peczalska KJ, et al. Epstein-Barr virus, immunodeficiency, and B cell lymphoproliferation. Transplantation. 1985;39:461–472.
7. Swerdlow SH, Webber SA, Chadburn A, et al. Post-transplant lymphoproliferative disorders. In: Swerdlow SH, Campo E, Harris NL, et al., editors. WHO Classification of Tumours of Haematopoietic and Lymphoid Tissues. Lyon: IARC; 2008.
8. Starzl TE, Nalesnik MA, Porter KA, et al. Reversibility of lymphomas and lymphoproliferative lesions developing under cyclosporin-steroid therapy. Lancet. 1984;1:583–587.
9. Lin JC, Smith MC, Pagano JS. Prolonged inhibitory effect of 9-(1,3-dihydroxy-2-propoxymethyl) guanine against replication of Epstein-Barr virus. Journal of Virology. 1984;50:50–55.
10. Green M, Webber SA. EBV viral load monitoring: unanswered questions. American Journal of Transplantation. 2002;2:894–895.
11. Green M, Reyes J, Webber S, et al. The role of Epstein-Barr viral load in the diagnosis, management and possible prevention of EBV-associated post-transplant lymphoproliferative disease following solid organ transplantation. Current Opinion in Organ Transplantation. 1999;4:292–296.
12. Martinez O. The biology of Epstein-Barr virus and posttransplant lymphoproliferative disease. In: Dharnidharka VR, Green M, Webber SA, editors. Post-Transplant Lymphoproliferative Disorders. Berlin: Springer Verlag; 2010: 29–43.
13. Thorley-Lawson DA. Epstein-Barr virus: exploiting the immune system. Nature Reviews. Immunology. 2001;1:75–82.
14. Snow AL, Martinez OM. Epstein-Barr virus: evasive maneuvers in the development of PTLD. American Journal of Transplantation. 2007;7:271–277.
15. Swerdlow SH. T-cell and NK-cell posttransplantation lymphoproliferative disorders. American Journal of Clinical Pathology. 2007;127:887–895.
16. Vilchez RA, Jauregui MP, Hsi ED, et al. Simian virus 40 in posttransplant lymphoproliferative disorders. Human Pathology. 2006;37:1130–1136.
17. Kapelushnik J, Ariad S, Benharroch D, et al. Post renal transplantation human herpesvirus 8-associated lymphoproliferative disorder and Kaposi's sarcoma. British Journal of Haematology. 2001;113:425–428.
18. Wu TT, Swerdlow SH, Locker J, et al. Recurrent Epstein-Barr virus-associated lesions in organ transplant recipients. Human Pathology. 1996; 27:157–164.
19. Cesarman E, Chadburn A, Liu YF, et al. BCL-6 gene mutations in posttransplantation lymphoproliferative disorders predict response to therapy and clinical outcome. Blood. 1998;92:2294–2302.
20. Ranganathan S, Webber S, Ahuja S, et al. Hodgkin-like posttransplant lymphoproliferative disorder in children: does it differ from posttransplant Hodgkin lymphoma? Pediatric and Developmental Pathology. 2004;7:348–360.
21. Dharnidharka VR. Epidemiology of PTLD. In: Dharnidharka VR, Green M, Webber SA, editors. Post-Transplant Lymphoproliferative Disorders. Berlin: Springer Verlag; 2010: 17–28.
22. Chinnock R, Webber SA, Dipchand AI, et al., Pediatric Heart Transplant Study. A 16-year multi-institutional study of the role of age and EBV status on PTLD incidence among pediatric heart transplant recipients. American Journal of Transplantation. 2012;12:3061–3068.
23. Webber SA, Naftel DC, Fricker FJ, et al. Lymphoproliferative disorders after paediatric heart transplantation: a multi-institutional study. Lancet. 2006;367: 233–239.
24. Caillard S, Lamy FX, Quelen C, et al., French Transplant Centers. Epidemiology of posttransplant lymphoproliferative disorders in adult kidney and kidney pancreas recipients: report of the French registry and analysis of subgroups of lymphomas. American Journal of Transplantation. 2012;12: 682–693.
25. Bingler MA, Feingold B, Miller SA, et al. Chronic high Epstein-Barr viral load state and risk for late-onset posttransplant lymphoproliferative disease/lymphoma in children. American Journal of Transplantation. 2008;8:442–445.
26. Picarsic J, Jaffe R, Mazariegos G, et al. Post-transplant Burkitt lymphoma is a more aggressive and distinct form of post-transplant lymphoproliferative disorder. Cancer. 2011;117:4540–4550.
27. Manez R, Breinig MC, Linden P, et al. Posttransplant lymphoproliferative disease in primary Epstein-Barr virus infection after liver transplantation: the role of cytomegalovirus disease. Journal of Infectious Diseases. 1997;176: 1462–1467.
28. Dharnidharka VR, Tejani AH, Ho PL, et al. Post-transplant lymphoproliferative disorder in the United States: young Caucasian males are at highest risk. American Journal of Transplantation. 2002;2:993–998.
29. Swinnen LJ, Costanzo-Nordin MR, Fisher SG, et al. Increased incidence of lymphoproliferative disorder after immunosuppression with the monoclonal antibody OKT3 in cardiac- transplant recipients. New England Journal of Medicine. 1990;323:1723–1728.
30. McDonald RA, Smith JM, Ho M, et al., CCTPT Study Group. Incidence of PTLD in pediatric renal transplant recipients receiving basiliximab, calcineurin inhibitor, sirolimus and steroids. American Journal of Transplantation. 2008;8:984–989.
31. Kirk AD, Cherikh WS, Ring R, et al. Dissociation of depletional induction and post transplant lymphoproliferative disease in kidney recipients treated with alemtuzumab. American Journal of Transplantation. 2007;7:2619–2625.
32. Pestana JO, Grinyo JM, Vanrenterghem Y, et al. Three-year outcomes from BENEFIT-EXT: a phase III study of belatacept versus cyclosporine in recipients of extended criteria donor kidneys. American Journal of Transplantation. 2012;12:630–639.
33. Elliott SL, Suhrbier A, Miles JJ, et al. Phase I trial of a CD8+ T-cell peptide epitope-based vaccine for infectious mononucleosis. Journal of Virology. 2008;82:1448–1457.
34. Moutschen M, Leonard P, Sokal EM, et al. Phase I/II studies to evaluate safety and immunogenicity of a recombinant gp350 Epstein-Barr virus vaccine in healthy adults. Vaccine. 2007;25:4697–4705.
35. Sokal EM, Hoppenbrouwers K, Vandermeulen C, et al. Recombinant gp350 vaccine for infectious mononucleosis: a phase 2, randomized, double-blind, placebo-controlled trial to evaluate the safety, immunogenicity, and efficacy of an Epstein-Barr virus vaccine in healthy young adults. Journal of Infectious Diseases. 2007;196:1749–1753.
36. Nadal D, Guzman J, Frohlich S, et al. Human immunoglobulin preparations suppress the occurrence of Epstein-Barr virus-associated lymphoproliferation. Experimental Hematology. 1997;25:223–231.
37. Abedi MR, Linde A, Christensson B, et al. Preventive effect of IgG from EBV-seropositive donors on the development of human lympho-proliferative disease in SCID mice. International Journal of Cancer. 1997;71:624–629.
38. Green M, Michaels MG, Katz BZ, et al. CMV-IVIG for prevention of Epstein Barr virus disease and posttransplant lymphoproliferative disease in pediatric liver transplant recipients. American Journal of Transplantation. 2006;6:1906–1912.
39. Savoldo B, Goss JA, Hammer MM, et al. Treatment of solid organ transplant recipients with autologous Epstein Barr virus-specific cytotoxic T lymphocytes (CTLs). Blood. 2006;108:2942–2949.
40. Malouf MA, Chhajed PN, Hopkins P, et al. Anti-viral prophylaxis reduces the incidence of lymphoproliferative disease in lung transplant recipients. Journal of Heart and Lung Transplantation. 2002;21:547–554.
41. McDiarmid SV, Jordan S, Kim GS, et al. Prevention and preemptive therapy of postransplant lymphoproliferative disease in pediatric liver recipients. Transplantation. 1998;66:1604–1611.
42. Funch DP, Walker AM, Schneider G, et al. Ganciclovir and acyclovir reduce the risk of post-transplant lymphoproliferative disorder in renal transplant recipients. American Journal of Transplantation. 2005;5:2894–2900.

43. Opelz G, Daniel V, Naujokat C, et al. Effect of cytomegalovirus prophylaxis with immunoglobulin or with antiviral drugs on post-transplant non-Hodgkin lymphoma: a multicentre retrospective analysis. Lancet Oncology. 2007;8:212–218.
44. Green M, Kaufmann M, Wilson J, et al. Comparison of intravenous ganciclovir followed by oral acyclovir with intravenous ganciclovir alone for prevention of cytomegalovirus and Epstein-Barr virus disease after liver transplantation in children. Clinical Infectious Diseases. 1997;25:1344–1349.
45. Kuo PC, Dafoe DC, Alfrey EJ, et al. Post-transplant lymphoproliferative disorders and Epstein-Barr virus prophylaxis. Transplantation. 1995;59:135–138.
46. Lee TC, Savoldo B, Rooney CM. Quantitative EBV viral loads and immunosuppression alterations can decrease PTLD incidence in pediatric liver transplant recipients. American Journal of Transplantation. 2005;5:2222–2228.
47. Ganschow R, Schulz T, Meyer T, et al. Low-dose immunosuppression reduces the incidence of post-transplant lymphoproliferative disease in pediatric liver graft recipients. Journal of Pediatric Gastroenterology and Nutrition. 2004;38:198–203.
48. Martin SI, Dodson B, Wheeler C, et al. Monitoring infection with Epstein-Barr virus among seromismatch adult renal transplant recipients. American Journal of Transplantation. 2011;11:1058–1063.
49. Sweet SC, Spray TL, Huddleston CB. Pediatric lung transplantation at St. Louis Children's Hospital, 1990-1995. American Journal of Respiratory and Critical Care Medicine. 1997;155:1027–1035.
50. Blaes AH, Cioc AM, Froelich JW, et al. Positron emission tomography scanning in the setting of post-transplant lymphoproliferative disorders. Clinical Transplantation. 2009;23:794–799.
51. Tsai DE, Douglas L, Andreadis C, et al. EBV PCR in the diagnosis and monitoring of posttransplant lymphoproliferative disorder: results of a two-arm prospective trial. American Journal of Transplantation. 2008;8:1016–1024.
52. Rowe DT, Qu L, Reyes J, et al. Use of quantitative competitive PCR to measure Epstein-Barr virus genome load in the peripheral blood of pediatric transplant patients with lymphoproliferative disorders. Journal of Clinical Microbiology. 1997;35:1612–1615.
53. Elstrom RL, Andreadis C, Aqui NA, et al. Treatment of PTLD with rituximab or chemotherapy. American Journal of Transplantation. 2006;6:569–576.
54. Hurwitz M, Desai DM, Cox KL, et al. Complete immunosuppression withdrawal as a uniform approach to post-transplant lymphoproliferative disease in pediatric liver transplantation. Pediatric Transplantation. 2004;8:267–272.
55. Tsai DE, Hardy CL, Tomaszewski JE, et al. Reduction in immunosuppression as initial therapy for posttransplant lymphoproliferative disorder: analysis of prognostic variables and long-term follow-up of 42 adult patients. Transplantation. 2001;71:1076–1088.
56. Aull MJ, Buell JF, Trofe J, et al. Experience with 274 cardiac transplant recipients with posttransplant lymphoproliferative disorder: a report from the Israel Penn International Transplant Tumor Registry. Transplantation. 2004;78:1676–1682.
57. Swinnen LJ, LeBlanc M, Grogan TM, et al. Prospective study of sequential reduction in immunosuppression, interferon alpha-2B and chemotherapy for posttransplant lymphoproliferative disorder. Transplantation. 2008;86:215–222.
58. Traum AZ, Rodig NM, Pilichowska ME, et al. Central nervous system lymphoproliferative disorder in pediatric kidney transplant recipients. Pediatric Transplantation. 2006;10:505–512.
59. Prichard MN, Hartline CB, Harden EA, et al. Inhibition of herpes virus replication by hexadecyloxypropyl esters of purine- and pyramidine-based phosphonomethoxyethyl nucleoside phosphonates. Antimicrobial Agents and Chemotherapy. 2008;52:4326–4330.
60. Williams-Aziz SL, Hartline CB, Harden EA, et al. Comparative activities of lipid esters of cidofovir and cyclic cidofovir against replication of herpes viruses in vitro. Antimicrobial Agents and Chemotherapy. 2005;49:3724–3733.
61. Perrine SP, Hermine O, Small T, et al. A phase I/II trial of arginine butyrate and ganciclovir in patients with Epstein-Barr virus associated lymphoid malignancies. Blood. 2007;109:2571–2578.
62. Ghosh SK, Forman LW, Akinsheye I, et al. Short discontinuous exposure to butyrate effectively sensitizes latently EBV-infected cells to nucleoside analogue antiviral agents. Blood Cells, Molecules and Diseases. 2007;38:57–65.
63. Davis CL, Wood BL, Sabath DE, et al. Interferon-alpha treatment of posttransplant lymphoproliferative disorder in recipients of solid organ transplants. Transplantation. 1998;66:1770–1779.
64. Shapiro RS, Chauvenet A, McGuire W, et al. Treatment of B-cell lymphoproliferative disorders with interferon alfa and intravenous gamma globulin [letter]. New England Journal of Medicine. 1988;318:1334.
65. Haddad E, Paczesny S, Leblond V, et al. Treatment of B-lymphoproliferative disorder with a monoclonal anti-interleukin-6 antibody in 12 patients: a multicenter phase 1-2 clinical trial. Blood. 2001;97:1590–1597.
66. Riddler SA, Breinig MC, McKnight JLC. Increased levels of circulating Epstein-Barr virus-infected lymphocytes and decreased EBV nuclear antigen antibody responses are associated with the development of posttransplant lymphoproliferative disease in solid-organ transplant recipients. Blood. 1994;84:972–984.
67. Milpied N, Vasseur B, Parquet N, et al. Humanized anti-CD20 monoclonal antibody (rituximab) in post transplant B-lymphoproliferative disorder: a retrospective analysis on 32 patients. Annals of Oncology. 2000;11(Suppl 1):113–116.
68. Blaes AH, Peterson BA, Bartlett N, et al. Rituximab therapy is effective for posttransplant lymphoproliferative disorders after solid organ transplantation: results of a phase II trial. Cancer. 2005;104:1661–1667.
69. Jain AB, Marcos A, Pokharna R, et al. Rituximab (chemeric anti-CD20 antibody) for post-transplant lymphoproliferative disorder after solid organ transplantation in adults: long-term experience from a single center. Transplantation. 2005;80:1692–1698.
70. Knoop C, Kentos A, Remmelink M, et al. Post-transplant lymphoproliferative disorders after lung transplantation: first-line treatment with rituximab may induce complete remission. Clinical Transplantation. 2006;20:179–187.
71. Choquet S, Leblond V, Herbrecht R, et al. Efficacy and safety of rituximab in B-cell post-transplantation lymphoproliferative disorders: results of a prospective multicenter phase 2 study. Blood. 2006;107:3053–3057.
72. Oertel SH, Verschuuren E, Reinke P, et al. Effect of anti-CD20 antibody rituximab in patients with post-transplant lymphoproliferative disorder (PTLD). American Journal of Transplantation. 2005;5:2901–2906.
73. Choquet S, Oertel S, Leblond V, et al. Rituximab in the management of post-transplantation lymphoproliferative disorder after solid organ transplantation: proceed with caution. Annals of Hematology. 2007;86:599–607.
74. Trappe RU, Choquet S, Reinke P, et al. Salvage therapy for relapsed posttransplant lymphoproliferative disorders (PTLD) with a second progression of PTLD after upfront chemotherapy: the role of single agent rituximab. Transplantation. 2007;84:1708–1712.
75. Webber S, Harmon W, Faro A, et al. Anti-CD20 monoclonal antibody (rituximab) for refractory PTLD after pediatric solid organ transplantation: multicenter experience from a registry and from a prospective clinical trial. Blood. 2004;104-1:213a.
76. Salvado B, Rooney CM, Quiros-Tejeira RE, et al. Cellular immunity to Epstein-Barr virus in liver transplant recipients treated with rituximab for post-transplant lymphoproliferative disease. American Journal of Transplantation. 2005;5:566–572.
77. Gross TG, Bucuvalas JC, Park JR, et al. Low-dose chemotherapy for Epstein-Barr virus-positive post-transplantation lymphoproliferative disease in children after solid organ transplantation. Journal of Clinical Oncology. 2005;23:6481–6488.
78. Gross TG, Orjuela MA, Perkins SL, et al. Low-dose chemotherapy and rituximab for posttransplant lymphoproliferative disease (PTLD): a Children's Oncology Group Report. American Journal of Transplantation. 2012;12:3069–3075.
79. Windebank K, Walwyn T, Kirk R, et al. Post cardiac transplantation lymphoproliferative disorder presenting as t(8;14) Burkitt leukaemia/lymphoma treated with low intensity chemotherapy and rituximab. Pediatric Blood and Cancer. 2009;53:392–396.
80. Zimmermann H, Reinke P, Neuhaus R, et al. Burkitt post-transplantation lymphoma in adult solid organ transplant recipients: sequential immunochemotherapy with rituximab (R) followed by cyclophosphamide, doxorubicin, vincristine, and prednisone (CHOP) or R-CHOP is safe and effective in an analysis of 8 patients. Cancer. 2012;118:4715–4724.
81. Trappe R, Hinrichs C, Appel U, et al. Treatment of PTLD with rituximab and CHOP reduces the risk of renal graft impairment after reduction of immunosuppression. American Journal of Transplantation. 2009;9:2331–2337.
82. Trappe R, Oertel S, Leblond V, et al., German PTLD Study Group; European PTLD Network. Sequential treatment with rituximab followed by CHOP chemotherapy in adult B-cell post-transplant lymphoproliferative disorder (PTLD): the prospective international multicentre phase 2 PTLD-1 trial. Lancet Oncology. 2012;13:196–206.
83. Choquet S, Trappe R, Leblond V, et al. CHOP-21 for the treatment of post-transplant lymphoproliferative disorders (PTLD) following solid organ transplantation. Haematologica. 2007;92:273–274.
84. Fohrer C, Caillard S, Koumarianou A, et al. Long-term survival in post-transplant lymphoproliferative disorders with a dose-adjusted ACVBP regimen. British Journal of Haematology. 2006;134:602–612.
85. Swinnen LJ, Mullen GM, Carr TJ, et al. Aggressive treatment for postcardiac transplant lymphoproliferation. Blood. 1995;86:3333–3340.
86. Trappe R, Riess H, Babel N, et al. Salvage chemotherapy for refractory and relapsed posttransplant lymphoproliferative disorders (PTLD) after treatment with single-agent rituximab. Transplantation. 2007;83:912–918.
87. Buell JF, Gross TG, Hanaway MJ, et al. Chemotherapy for post-transplant lym-

phoproliferative disorder: the Israel Penn International Transplant Tumor Registry. Transplantation Proceedings. 2005;37:956–957.

88. Rooney CM, Smith CA, Ng CYC, et al. Use of gene-modified virus-specific T lymphocytes to control Epstein-Barr virus related lymphoproliferation. Lancet. 1995;345:9–13.
89. Swinnen LJ. Immune-cell treatment of Epstein-Barr-virus-associated lymphoproliferative disorders. Best Practice and Research. Clinical Haematology. 2006;19:839–847.
90. Comoli P, Maccario R, Locatelli F, et al. Treatment of EBV-related postrenal transplant lymphoproliferative disease with a tailored regimen including EBV-specific T cells. American Journal of Transplantation. 2005;5:1415–1422.
91. Haque T, Wilkie GM, Jones MM, et al. Allogeneic cytotoxic T cell therapy for EBV-positive posttransplant lymphoproliferative disease: results of a phase 2 multicenter clinical trial. Blood. 2007;110:1123–1131.
92. Comoli P, Ginevri F, Maccario R, et al. Successful in vitro priming of EBV-specific CD8+ T cells endowed with strong cytotoxic function from T cells of EBV seronegative children. American Journal of Transplantation. 2006;6:2169–2176.
93. Metes D, Storkus W, Zeevi A, et al. *Ex vivo* generation of effective Epstein-Barr Virus (EBV)-specific CD8+ cytotoxic T cells from peripheral blood of immunocompetent EBV-seronegative individuals. Transplantation. 2000;70: 1507–1515.
94. Buell JF, Gross TG, Hanaway MJ, et al. Post-transplant lymphoproliferative disorder: significance of central nervous system involvement. Transplantation Proceedings. 2005;37:954–955.
95. Castellano-Sanchez AA, Li S, Qian J, et al. Primary central nervous system posttransplant lymphoproliferative disorders. American Journal of Clinical Pathology. 2004;121:246–253.
96. Cavaliere R, Petroni G, Lopes MB, et al., International Primary Central Nervous System Lymphoma Collaborative Group. Primary central nervous system posttransplantation lymphoproliferative disorder: an international primary central nervous system lymphoma collaborative group report. Cancer. 2010;116: 863–870.
97. Maniar T, Tsai D. Dharnidharka VR, Green M, Webber SA, editors. Prognostic factors for PTLD. In: Post-Transplant Lymphoproliferative Disorders. Berlin: Springer Verlag; 2010: 105–116.
98. Dharnidharka VR, Martz KL, Stablein DM, et al. Improved survival with recent Post-Transplant Lymphoproliferative Disorder (PTLD) in children with kidney transplants. American Journal of Transplantation. 2011;11:751–758.
99. Maecker B, Jack T, Zimmermann M, et al. CNS or bone marrow involvement as risk factors for poor survival in post-transplantation lymphoproliferative disorders in children after solid organ transplantation. Journal of Clinical Oncology. 2007;25:4902–4908.
100. Reshef R, Vardhanabhuti S, Luskin MR, et al. Reduction of immunosuppression as initial therapy for posttransplantation lymphoproliferative disorder. American Journal of Transplantation. 2011;11:336–347.
101. Hatton O, Martinez OM, Esquivel CO. Emerging therapeutic strategies for Epstein-Barr virus+ post-transplant lymphoproliferative disorder. Pediatric Transplantation. 2012;16:220–229.
102. Webber SA. Treatment of PTLD. In: Dharnidharka VR, Green M, Webber SA, editors. Post-Transplant Lymphoproliferative Disorders. Berlin: Springer Verlag; 2010.

第 97 章 移植术后的妊娠和避孕

Serban Constantinescu, Veronica Gomez-Lobo, John M. Davison, Michael J. Moritz, Vincent T. Armenti

引言

移植是许多终末期器官衰竭患者的首选治疗方法。人类第一例成功的肾移植完成于 1954 年 12 月[1]。然而,直到 20 世纪 60 年代免疫抑制的出现及 20 世纪 80 年代环孢素的使用,才使得术后移植物可长期存活,进而提高受者的生存率(见第 1 章)。随着器官功能的恢复,患者的健康得到整体改善,性冲动与生育能力也得以恢复。移植受者希望与正常人一样有为人父母的机会是移植手术成功之后的自然结果,事实上,移植手术成功最明确的指标之一,就是使患者拥有基本生活的能力。首次移植术后的妊娠发生在 1958 年 3 月并于 1963 年被报道[2]。该患者在接受了她同卵双胞胎姐妹的肾脏后,通过剖宫产产下一个健康的男婴。

随着移植技术的改善,各种器官移植术后的患者均有妊娠的报道,这其中绝大多数是接受肾脏移植的患者[3-10]。成功妊娠是可能的,但相比正常人的低风险妊娠,器官移植患者的妊娠仍有巨大的不同。诸如母体移植物的功能、母体的健康状况、妊娠对移植物功能的短期及长期影响,以及药物和移植物功能对胎儿发育的影响都是必须考虑的问题。还有一个问题,即使出生时一切正常,移植带来的细微及长期影响是否会影响受体后代的生长发育[11,12]。

在本章中,我们将回顾目前对移植受者避孕的建议、孕前和产前指南,以及可获得的实体器官移植受者的妊娠结局数据。

移植受者的避孕

女性移植受者如果想要妊娠的话,应使用安全、有效的避孕方法并有计划地妊娠。虽然存在妊娠风险,许多移植受者并未被告知避孕或节育的必要性[13,14]。最近对肾移植受者的两份问卷调查显示,29.1%(伊朗)和88.2%(中国)的移植受者妊娠是意外妊娠[15,16]。值得注意的是,中国的研究显示 94%未妊娠的女性采取了避孕措施,而只有 56%的妊娠者采取了避孕措施。在这项研究中,大多数不使用避孕方法的女性不知道自己的生育能力在移植术后得到恢复[16]。在西方国家,显示避孕失败的相关数据相当少见。

美国目前有很多避孕方法:含雌激素的贴剂、环和药丸;孕激素药片;植入物和宫内节育器(IUD);紧急避孕;各种屏障避孕方法及绝育术。这些方法中有许多并不能避孕反而有其他风险及副作用。

2010 年,美国疾病控制和预防中心(CDC)颁布了第一个具有美国医疗资格标准的避孕方案,其中“实体器官移植”是推荐实行避孕的指征之一。这种情况进一步细分为“复杂:移植失败(急性或慢性),排斥,心脏移植物血管病变”和“非复杂”。每种分类都分为:1=使用此种方法不受限制;2=使用此方法的优点超过理论或已证实的风险;3=理论或已证明的风险超过使用该方法的优势;4=该方法对健康存在不可接受的风险[17]。风险评估基于充分的文献回顾以及专家意见。其他并发症的风险,如高血压和凝血紊乱也被纳入其中。总结见表 97.1。

表 97.1　移植受者不同避孕方法的获益与风险

方法	获益	问题	移植相关问题	CDC 分类非复杂*	CDC 分类复杂*
铜 T 形宫内节育器	绝大多数有效，持续时间长	月经增多	大多数免疫抑制剂不会影响巨噬细胞介导的反应	2	3(起始期) 2(持续期)
含黄体酮的宫内节育器	绝大多数有效，持续时间长，减少贫血的发生	不规则流血		2	3(起始期) 2(持续期)
长效醋酸甲羟孕酮(DMPA)	有效率高，减少贫血的发生	骨密度降低，不规则流血	可能引起胆汁阻塞	2	2
孕激素植入物	绝大多数有效，持续时间长，不降低骨密度	不规则流血		2	2
复合口服避孕药	减少贫血的发生，调节月经		经过肝的首过效应；体内浓度受免疫抑制剂影响 在不能控制的高血压、活动性肝病及有心衰、中风、深静脉血栓病史的人群中禁忌使用 免疫抑制剂导致的胃肠功能紊乱降低吸收功能 免疫抑制剂可能引起高钾血症，从而阻碍含有黄体酮成分的药物作用	2(不能用于有布加综合征病史的妇女)	4
避孕贴	不经过肝的首过效应	血液循环中雌激素水平升高较大	在不能控制的高血压、活动性肝病及有心衰、卒中、深静脉血栓病史的人群中禁忌使用 如果器官功能稳定且无禁忌，可以试用	2(不能用于有布加综合征病史的妇女)	4
阴道环	血液循环中雌激素水平升高不大 不经过肝的首过效应		在不能控制的高血压、活动性肝病及有心衰、卒中、深静脉血栓病史的人群中禁忌使用 如果器官功能稳定且无禁忌，可以试用	2(不能用于有布加综合征病史的妇女)	4
孕激素药丸		没有 COCS 有效	经过肝的首过效应	2	2
避孕套	预防性传播疾病 无药物间相互作用	有效性稍差		1	1
宫颈帽/膈	无药物间相互作用	有效性稍差		1	1
紧急避孕	性接触后有效	没有上述方法有效		1	1
体外排精	无药物间相互作用	有效性最差		N/A	N/A

* CDC 分类：1，使用不受限制；2，优点超过风险；3，风险超过优点；4，有非常严重的风险。

含雌激素的避孕措施

含雌激素的避孕药包括口服复合避孕药(OC)、避孕贴，由于阴道环可能引起血栓形成及肝毒性，因此移植受者通常避免使用。这些药物的好处是减少月经出血、贫血、痛经、痤疮、多毛症以及卵巢和子宫内膜肿瘤的发生[18]。主要风险是血栓形成和血压升高。

目前美国的 OC 在雌激素和黄体酮的配比上不尽

相同,但绝大多数含有“低剂量”的激素。避孕贴可致血液雌二醇水平升高,因此相比OC具有更高的静脉血栓栓塞(VTE)风险[19]。即便这样,这种风险仍低于妊娠期间静脉血栓栓塞的发生风险。相比其他避孕措施,避孕环升高血液循环中雌激素的水平较弱,且可以避开肝脏的首过效应,因此,原则上它导致静脉血栓栓塞的风险亦较低,但这仍需进一步的临床研究证实[19]。

移植受者中应用含雌激素的避孕药的研究目前仅限于小样本的病例研究和少量病例报道。在当前可检索到的研究中,有两个关于肾移植受者接受低剂量OC(26名女性)或避孕贴(10名女性)的前瞻性队列研究[20]。其中应用OC的一位受者在用药18个月后出现血栓性静脉炎,另一位在移植术后10年时发生了排斥相关的肝功能恶化。避孕措施应用18个月时,受者的肝酶、胆固醇、血清肌酐和葡萄糖并未发生显著变化。但在6个月时,葡萄糖和肌酐从1.31mg/dL增加到1.47mg/dL($P<0.01$)。在研究过程中,一些受者需要调整她们的抗高血压方案,以控制血压[20]。在参与研究的受者中,OC和避孕贴都使受者的血细胞比容明显增加。一个纳入15名肝移植受者的回顾性研究发现OC未导致肝功能、葡萄糖代谢、血压或体重指数(BMI)的显著改变[21]。在一篇病例报告中,一位接受高剂量避孕药治疗月经过多的移植受者发生了胆汁淤积,病情在停药后得以改善[22]。在最近来自中国的问卷调查中,在34名使用OC的移植受者,其中4人意外妊娠[16]。

基于这些小型研究的数据以及专家意见,CDC指南在“复杂”的实体器官移植(SOT)中对使用联合激素避孕的风险设定为第4类(即这些患者使用联合激素避孕的风险非常严重)[17]。对于“非复杂”实体器官移植,风险为第2类(即获益超过理论或已证实的风险)[17]。因此,在具有稳定的器官功能和血压控制良好的移植受者中(除非其对于含雌激素的化合物存在禁忌),医务人员可以为其提供含雌激素的避孕措施。

与其他全身给药一样,避孕药理论上可能影响免疫抑制剂的作用,反之亦然。雌激素在肝脏中代谢,免疫抑制剂可以激活细胞色素P450 3A4系统。因此,免疫抑制剂在理论上会减少避孕药在血液中的含量而影响其疗效。然而,现有数据表明二者间相互影响较小,OC在移植受者中仍然有效[19]。此外,避孕药也可能会影响免疫抑制剂的作用水平,但目前尚无相关研究[23]。因此,实体器官移植的女性接受含雌激素的避孕药时必须密切监测血压、相关副作用及免疫抑制水平的变化。

孕激素避孕

对于雌激素避孕禁忌的患者,可以选择含黄体酮成分的避孕方法,如长效醋酸甲羟孕酮(DMPA),依托孕烯植入剂和孕激素药丸。这些产品含有不同类型和剂量的黄体酮。孕激素药丸需每天服用,相比OC失败率较高,并且在肝脏中存在首过效应。DMPA可以每12周皮下或肌内注射。它在肝脏中代谢,故患有活动性肝病的女性应避免使用,但DMPA代谢不受其他药物的影响[19]。有研究显示DMPA可导致可逆性的骨密度降低,移植受者中骨质疏松患病率的增加提示监测患者骨矿物质密度的必要性(见第100章)。此外,DMPA可延迟生育力的恢复,因此可作为没有妊娠计划女性的最佳避孕方法。依托孕烯植入物是最有效的避孕方法之一,它的优点与DMPA类似。此外,依托孕烯植入物不会降低骨密度[19]。

到目前为止,尚没有评估黄体酮避孕在移植受者中的作用。CDC指南在“复杂”及“非复杂”的实体器官移植将黄体酮避孕药设定为第2类[17]。因此,这种避孕方法对移植受者是相对安全的。

宫内节育器

目前在美国,有两种宫内节育器(IUD)可用:铜IUD和含黄体酮的IUD(LNG-IUD)。铜宫内节育器可能会增加月经出血量,不能用于Wilson病患者。研究证明LNG-IUD可明显减少月经出血量,增加血红蛋白量[24]。一名患有子宫肌瘤和月经过多的肾移植受体在使用LNG-IUD 1年后,痛经和月经过多均得到显著改善[25]。

宫内节育器是最有效的节育方法之一,但在一个肾移植受者的研究中,只有5.2%的患者在移植术后推荐使用宫内节育器[14]。1981年,两名肾移植受者使用铜宫内节育器后发生妊娠,研究者推测可能是免疫抑制剂降低了宫内节育器的效能。但有证据表明巨噬细胞在卵子破坏中发挥最重要的作用,而目前的免疫抑制剂对巨噬细胞的功能影响非常小[19,26]。此外,在最近中国的问卷调查中,使用宫内节育器的178名女性中无一例妊娠,但在研究中使用的宫内节育器的类型没有说明[16]。在另一项研究中,12名移植受者接受LNG-IUD植入1年后均未发生妊娠[27]。

关于宫内节育器使用的另一个问题是感染的风

险。没有研究评估移植受者中使用宫内节育器发生感染的情况，但对患有人类免疫缺陷病毒(HIV)/自身免疫性免疫缺陷综合征(AIDS)女性的研究显示，应用宫内节育器发生盆腔炎的风险较低[28]。

CDC 指南对于使用宫内节育器的初试期和持续期进行区分。对于行“非复杂”实体器官移植的女性，两种宫内节育器的风险为第 2 类（即宫内节育器的获益通常超过风险）[17]。对于“复杂”的实体器官移植女性，如果宫内节育器为持续使用，风险亦为第 2 类(例如，如果受体发生排斥、器官衰竭或心血管病变，无需移除宫内节育器)[17]。对于“复杂”实体器官移植的受者，无论哪种宫内节育器的初始使用都被评价为第 3 类（即理论或已证明的风险超过获益)[17]。

紧急避孕

紧急避孕的方法包括：黄体酮药、抗黄体酮药、复合避孕药以及植入铜 IUD 宫内节育器。需要强调的是，在紧急避孕时，OC 和黄体酮药丸的风险在 CDC 指南中被划分类为 1 类。在实体器官移植受者中不应该对这两种方法进行使用限制[17]。由于在移植受者中有关紧急避孕尚无相关报道，该条属专家建议。

屏障法、体外排精及节育术

屏障法和输卵管结扎是肾脏和肝脏移植受者中最常用的避孕方法[14,16,29]。需要注意的是，避孕套失败率较高，但却是预防性传播疾病的唯一方法。部分患者经常选择体外排精避孕，但来自伊朗的研究表明，92%的意外妊娠是由体外排精引起的。在中国的研究中，使用安全期避孕法、避孕套和体外排精与意外妊娠关系密切[16]。

女性绝育术可以通过腹腔镜或宫腔镜进行。后者可以按规范化程序执行，因此可以作为移植受者的选择之一。

总之，移植受者有意外妊娠的风险。移植受者应在移植术前，特别是在手术评估过程中，向医生咨询避孕方案。这些患者可以有很多选择。当选择避孕方法时，必须考虑避孕和不避孕的好处和风险以及可能的药物相互作用(表 97.1)。长效避孕措施，如宫内节育器和黄体酮植入物是最有效的避孕方法[17]。这些方法具有可逆性，专家推荐它们可能是有意外妊娠风险的行实体器官移植的女性的最佳选择[17]。

移植术后妊娠

如上文所提，第一名妊娠的移植受者——伊迪丝·赫尔姆在 1958 年 3 月妊娠[2]。妊娠过程安全无事，正常的排泄性尿路造影解除了大家对于妊娠会对移植物产生压迫的担忧。重约 3300g 的正常男婴通过剖宫产分娩，理论上避免了顺产时胎儿沿产道下降时对移植肾造成创伤的可能。妊娠对移植功能亦未造成影响。1960 年，该受者第二次妊娠，并通过剖宫产分娩了一个健康的女婴。她妊娠期间的排泄性尿路造影显示排泄迅速，但值得注意的是，相比生理条件下肾盂扩张要少。因此可以得出结论，移植到骨盆中的孤立肾可以维持妊娠，并且没有压迫问题。事实上，伊迪丝·赫尔姆活到了 76 岁，她姐姐的肾在移植后维持了 53 年。

1967 年，Hume 等报道了使用免疫抑制(硫唑嘌呤和泼尼松)的肾移植术后第一次成功的妊娠[30]。1976 年，其中一位作者(JMD)和他在英国的同事发表了一篇对肾移植受者在妊娠期间密切随访的报告[31]。通过这次经验及对现有文献的分析，作者制订了指导女性肾移植受者妊娠的指南。这些指导建议多年来只有略微改动。修订版本已被美国移植学会纳入共识指南[32]（见下文），另外还有较早的欧洲最佳实践指南[33]。

鉴于需要为移植群体提供更多更有用的信息，1991 年，国家移植妊娠登记中心(NTPR)在托马斯杰斐逊大学成立，其目标是维持一个可更新的数据库，以评估女性及男性移植受者孕育后代的安全性[3,9]。所有报告的妊娠结局将被分析，包括活产、自然流产、治疗性流产、死胎和异位妊娠。数据包括父母和后代的随访，以确定移植后妊娠对受者、移植物和后代的长期影响。

表 97.2 和表 97.3 显示截至 2011 年 12 月，在 NTPR 1247 名女性受者中有 2054 次生育，830 名男性受者有 1257 次生育。21 岁以前接受移植的受者妊娠数目列于表 97.4。

英国移植妊娠登记中心(TPR)成立于 1997 年，但于 2002 年中止，最近的一份关于英国移植受者妊娠的报告于 2007 年出版[34,35]。英国报告的数据与来自美国 NTPR 的结果相似[3,35](表 97.5)。

移植受者生育相关的几个问题

大多数移植术后生育的结局都较为乐观，但由于

表 97.2 NTPR:女性移植受者的生育情况[3]

器官	受者	生育	结局 *
肾	922	1490	1525
肝	179	319	325
肝-肾联合	5	7	8
肠	2	2	2
胰-肾联合	50	90	95
胰	2	5	6
心	60	105	109
心-肺联合	5	5	5
肺	22	31	33
总计	1247	2054	2108

* 包括双胞胎、三胞胎及四胞胎。

NTPR,国家移植妊娠登记中心,截至 2011 年 12 月。

表 97.3 NTPR:男性移植受者的生育情况[3]

器官	受者	生育	结局 *
肾	605	925	941
肝	69	109	115
肝-肾联合	3	7	7
肝-心-肾联合	1	1	1
肝-肠-肾联合	1	2	2
肠	1	1	1
肠-胃-胰联合	2	2	2
胰-肾联合	34	43	45
心	108	158	162
心-肺联合	1	2	2
心-肺-肾联合	1	3	3
肺	4	4	4
总计	830	1257	1285

* 包括双胞胎、三胞胎及四胞胎。

NTPR,国家移植妊娠登记中心,截至 2011 年 12 月。

表 97.4 NTPR:21 岁以前接受移植的女性的生育情况

器官	受者	生育	结局 *
肾	299	499	511
肝	76	150	153
肝-肾联合	2	4	5
肠	1	1	1
胰-肾联合	0	0	0
胰	0	0	0
心	24	45	45
心-肺联合	0	0	0
肺	1	1	1
总计	403	700	716

* 包括双胞胎、三胞胎及四胞胎。

NTPR,国家移植妊娠登记中心,截至 2011 年 12 月。

表 97.5 肾移植受者的生育结局

	NTPR[3]	英国 TPR[35]
受者	335	176
生育	515	193
结局 *	527	188
治疗性流产(%)	8.4	6
自发性流产(%)	12	11
异位妊娠(%)	0.6	1
死产(%)	3	2
活产(%)	76	79
活产	401	121**
胎龄(周)	35.8±3.4	35.6±0.3
早产(<37 周)(%)	53%	50%
平均出生体重(g)	2490±756	2316±80
低体重(<2500g)(%)	46	54
剖宫产(%)	54%	72%
新生儿复杂情况(%)	41	NR
新生儿死亡(生后 30 天)[数目(%)]	4(1)	NR

* 包括双胞胎及三胞胎。

** 报道数据。

NR,未报道;NTPR,国家移植妊娠登记中心。

移植后情况相对复杂,以下问题必须考虑:

(1)母体:母体长期健康及为人母亲的能力和(或)生存的风险。

(2)移植物:妊娠导致移植物功能障碍和(或)丧失的风险,妊娠期间潜在的药物代谢变化可能增加排斥的风险。

(3)胎儿/新生儿:免疫抑制剂及其他药物相关的潜在致畸风险,不仅可以表现为形体缺陷,还可表现为微小的发育改变,可能直到儿童期才显现,或对后代产生影响。

其他要考虑的长期问题包括移植术后的父母在抚养子女期间应对疾病和(或)移植物功能障碍的能力,以及移植术后的父母生病或死亡对其子女的影响。

免疫抑制剂及致畸作用

美国食品药品监督管理局(FDA)对免疫抑制药物的妊娠安全分类见表 97.6。这些药物的作用机制见第 98 至第 102 章。

表 97.6 FDA 对移植术后常规免疫抑制剂的妊娠安全分类[3]

药物	FDA 妊娠安全分类 *
皮质激素(泼尼松,泼尼松龙,甲基泼尼松龙)	B/C
硫唑嘌呤(Imuran®)	D
环孢素(Sandimmune®)	C
改良环孢素(Neoral®)	C
他克莫斯(Prograf®)	C
麦考酚酸吗乙酯(Cellcept®)	D
肠溶麦考酚酸吗乙酯(Myfortic®)	D
西罗莫司(Rapamune®)	C
贝拉西普(Nulojix®)	C
抗胸腺细胞球蛋白(Atgam®,ATG)	C
抗胸腺细胞球蛋白(Thymoglobulin®)	C
莫罗单抗-CD3(OKT3®)	C
巴利昔单抗(Simulect®)	B
达利珠单抗(Zenapax®)	C

* FDA 分类:B,对胎儿无风险,无对照研究;C,胎儿风险不能排除;D,已证实的胎儿风险。

糖皮质激素

在动物研究中,糖皮质激素可引起腭裂,但在人类中尚未见报道[36,37]。临床上,这些药物可能引起未足月胎膜早破及新生儿肾上腺功能不全[38]。泼尼松在移植术后的维持治疗及临床上其他领域(如风湿类疾病)治疗中的应用已超过 45 年。

硫唑嘌呤(Imuran®)

在环孢素出现之前,高剂量硫唑嘌呤与泼尼松联合的免疫抑制方案应用广泛且有相当多的临床经验。临床数据并不支持早期关于其致畸性的担忧,也没有确定其导致的主要结构畸形。文献报道了极少数可能与其相关的新生儿问题,包括胸腺萎缩、白细胞减少、贫血、血小板减少、短暂染色体畸变、败血症和免疫球蛋白水平降低[39-41]。虽然硫唑嘌呤在妊娠期应用的安全性归为 D 类(对胎儿毒性),其在维持免疫抑制的辅助治疗中的剂量对于致畸来说是相对安全的。

环孢素(Sandimmune®,Neoral®,Gengraf®及其他)

第一代钙调神经磷酸酶抑制剂(CNI)——环孢素,是 20 世纪 80 年代初应用的主要免疫抑制剂。环孢素的妊娠安全类别是 C(胎儿风险不能排除)。在动物研究中报道了环孢素的胎儿毒性和致畸性,但其发生剂量远高于临床使用的剂量[42-44]。早期研究认为该药使胎儿生长受限的风险较大,但这一作用在后来的研究中并不明显[7]。致畸风险似乎很少,目前没有关于新生儿畸形的报告。在应用环孢素治疗的肾脏受者后代中的结构畸形的最大分析报告中,NTPR 登记的 479 名接受肾移植的女性在接受环孢素维持治疗,共生产 362(76%)个活胎[45],其中 18 个具有先天缺陷,占活胎数目的 5%,与一般人群报告的 3%~5%相似[46]。

他克莫司(Prograf®及其他)

自 1995 年推出以来,他克莫司作为肾移植的维持性 CNI 治疗在美国已取代环孢素。在动物研究中,胎儿吸收药物的发生剂量远高于临床使用剂量[47]。由于该药可使母体糖尿病的发病率升高,目前已有该药导致短暂性新生儿高钾血症的报道[48]。与环孢素类似,尚未发现孕期应用他克莫司与畸形有关。根据 NTPR 的数据,使用 CNI 治疗而未联合霉酚酸制剂的肾移植受者的后代发生缺陷的概率与一般人群相似[49]。

霉酚酸制剂(麦考酚酸吗乙酯,CellCept®及其他;肠溶麦考酚酸吗乙酯,Myfortic®)

FDA 在 1994 年批准霉酚酸制剂(MMF)取代硫唑嘌呤作为 CNI 的辅助治疗。在有关生殖毒性的动物研究中,相比 CNI,MMF 的致畸风险似乎更大。大鼠和兔的发育毒性包括畸形和子宫内生长受限。基于体表面积计算的推荐临床使用剂量也可导致死胎的发生[50,51]。NTPR 数据显示,该药物导致新生儿畸形的发生率增加,此外,暴露于 MMF 的新生儿还有其他问题[52-60]。从 2007 年开始,CellCept®和 Myfortic®的包装说明已经将 FDA 安全类别从 C 改为 D[29,30],并强调了服用 MMF 的育龄女性必须避孕,因为服药后流产及先天性畸形的可能性增加。欧洲最佳实践指南也提出类似建议[33]。结合 NTPR 数据,罗氏公司收集 1995—2007 年药品上市后的数据,发现 77 名接受 MMF 治疗的女性,其中 25 人发生自然流产,14 人有畸形的婴儿或胎儿(其中 6 例有耳畸形)。

西罗莫司(Rapamune®)

西罗莫司是 mTOR 抑制剂,自从 2000 年被批准用于CNI的辅助治疗，该药在孕期的使用已经开始得到关注。在动物研究中没有发现其致畸作用，但有报道该药可导致胎儿体重降低及骨化延迟[61]。在妊娠动物模型中，当与环孢素联合应用时，胎儿流产率增加，表明该药物存在一定毒性。然而，尚缺乏临床妊娠结果数据[52,62-66]。

男性服用西罗莫司后精子数量和运动性显著降低，进而影响生育率[67]。因此，服用西罗莫司的男性受者应该被告知这种潜在的副作用。

其他制剂

用于诱导或抗排斥的其他制剂在妊娠中的作用较小。在一个病例观察中，作者报道了少量患者应用莫罗单抗-CD3（OKT3®）[68]、皮质类固醇和抗胸腺细胞球蛋白（Thymoglobulin®）在妊娠期间进行治疗。利妥昔单抗用于移植排斥的治疗，但目前尚无孕期使用的报告。

最近批准的贝拉西普（Nulojix®）是用于维持免疫抑制的选择性T细胞共刺激阻断剂。目前NTPR尚无该药物的妊娠结局数据。

器官移植群体

肾移植受者

在20世纪七八十年代硫唑嘌呤应用的时代，文献报告了数千名移植后成功妊娠的肾移植受者。在其中，自然流产率约为14%，治疗性流产率约为20%。前3个月妊娠期安全渡过者，90%以上可成功妊娠。其中约15%的女性发生肾损伤，约30%发生高血压。早产较为常见，可影响45%~60%的妊娠女性，胎儿生长受限的发生率约为20%[69,70]。

有关妊娠期使用环孢素的数据显示胎儿生长受限和高血压的发生率增高，这可能与20世纪80年代初使用较高的药物剂量有关[43]。有学者提出，环孢素可能不是妊娠期使用的最佳选择。由于硫唑嘌呤的使用经验更为丰富，这部分受者被换回基于硫唑嘌呤的治疗方案。随着环孢素的使用经验增加，不论是个例报告还是移植中心，或注册的数据报告了越来越多的成功妊娠案例，但该药物对母亲和新生儿的潜在风险是不可忽视的[71]。NTPR上报告的应用CNI的肾脏受者的妊娠结局见表97.7[3]。

母体预后

总体而言，与一般人群相比，女性移植受者在妊娠期间患高血压和先兆子痫的风险更大。据NTPR报告，53%~64%应用CNI的肾移植受者在妊娠期间患有需药物干预的高血压。肾脏受者更有可能在妊娠前已患有高血压，单这一条就是妊娠结局不佳（包括低出生体重）的危险因素[72]。先兆子痫在普通人群的发病率为7%~10%，但在移植受者中则为该数量的3倍。许多移植受者在妊娠前已经患有高血压，这更增加了先兆子痫的诊断难度[70]。

根据NTPR的报告，12%使用CNI的肾移植受者需要在妊娠期使用胰岛素。在妊娠的前3个月，严格控制血糖非常关键，因为在此期间妊娠期糖尿病与子代缺陷之间的关系密切[73]。在这一数据中，对于不需要胰岛素治疗的轻度妊娠期糖尿病并未进行评估，因此妊娠期糖尿病的实际发生率可能比NTPR报道的还要高。

NTPR中妊娠期最常见的感染性并发症是尿路感染。这通常可以通过合适的抗生素治愈。

移植功能

临床研究及非移植的动物模型均显示，如果妊娠前的肾功能稳定，其长期功能将不受妊娠影响[74]。类似地，在移植人群中，通过严谨的病例对照研究已经证实，如果妊娠前移植物功能稳定，妊娠将不会导致移植物功能的恶化[75-79]。然而，Sturgiss和Davison报道了一项病例对照研究[76]，该研究的最新进展表明，妊娠可能对移植肾的功能有微小的影响，但在统计学上差异并不显著[77]。

排斥反应

妊娠期间移植排斥的发生率较低，并未高于未妊娠的移植人群。类似地，分娩2年内移植物失功的发生率也并未受妊娠的影响。在受者中，妊娠期前即存在移植物功能损害与不可逆和不可预测的移植物事件更加相关。

根据NTPR的数据，2%的肾脏受者在妊娠期伴有活检证实的急性排斥反应。对症治疗包括激素冲击、淋巴细胞消耗剂和（或）免疫抑制剂的基线调整，经过合理治疗，仍可能继续妊娠。妊娠期的移植排斥会影响新生儿和移植物的预后[80]。妊娠期或产后马上发生排斥

表 97.7　NTPR：女性肾移植受者妊娠期间应用 CNI 的妊娠结局[3]

	环孢素（336 位受者，517 次妊娠）	改良环孢素（150 位受者，241 次妊娠）	他克莫司（170 位受者，278 次妊娠）
产妇因素（妊娠数量）	517	241	278
移植术后至受孕的平均时间（年）	3.6±2.8	6.2±4	4.4±3
妊娠期高血压(%)	62	64	53
妊娠期糖尿病(%)	12	5	10
妊娠期感染(%)	23	18	21
子痫前期(%)	30	32	32
妊娠期排斥 *(%)	1	2	2
平均血肌酐(mg/dL)			
妊娠前	1.4±0.5	1.3±0.4	1.2±0.3
妊娠中	1.4±0.7	1.3±0.5	1.3±0.8
妊娠后	1.6±0.97	1.4±0.5	1.4±0.7
分娩 2 年内移植物失功(%)	9	6	6
结局 †	529	254	283
治疗性流产(%)	8	1	1
自发性流产(%)	12	20	25
异位妊娠(%)	0.6	1	0.4
死产	3	2	2
活产(%)	76	77	71
活产	402	196	200
胎龄（周）	35.9±3.4	35.8±3.4	35.3±3.5
早产(<37 周)(%)	52	52	53
平均出生体重(g)	2490±755	2501±748	2494±844
低体重(<2500g)(%)	46	43	43
剖宫产	54	43	57
新生儿复杂情况	41%	44%	49%
新生儿死亡（生后 30 天）[数目(%)]	4(1)	4(2)‡	4(2)

* 活检证实发生急性排斥反应。

† 包括双胞胎、三胞胎及四胞胎。

‡ 妊娠 24 周的四胞胎，全部死亡。

反应是妊娠后 5 年内移植肾失功的重要危险因素[81]。

NTPR 的一份报告对接受活体肾移植和尸体肾移植的妊娠女性进行研究，发现受者及新生儿的状况并没有明显不同[82]。

多胎妊娠及连续妊娠

许多移植受者成功连续妊娠，也有一些受者成功行多胎妊娠及试管婴儿[82-87]。在 478 例移植受者首次妊娠后，189 例在此后有 1~4 次妊娠。在各组之间，活产的比例并无统计学差异。对于连续妊娠者，有妊娠年龄增加的趋势，导致了低或极低体重早产新生儿的数量显著减少。各组间移植排斥率相似[82]。连续妊娠与胎儿结局及母体移植物失功无关。因此，具有良好移植肾功能的受者可以多次妊娠。

不良事件的预测因素

移植受者妊娠成功是指移植肾在妊娠中或产后功能良好并保持稳定，受者和新生儿情况正常。具体指活产、产妇及胎儿并发症发生率低以及移植肾功能稳定，这些与妊娠期间血肌酐的水平稳定密切相关[88]（表 97.8）。

如果女性开始妊娠时移植肾功能较差，如血清肌酐>1.5mg/dL(>133μmol/L)，则在妊娠期和产后发生移植肾功能障碍的可能性较大[89]。此外，妊娠期血清肌酐

表 97.8 妊娠期间肾移植受者肌酐水平与生育结局的关系

血肌酐[mg/dL (μmol/L)]	胎儿生长受限(%)	早产(%)	子痫前期(%)	围生期死亡(%)	失去>25%的肾功能		
					妊娠期(%)	产后(%)	1年内发展为终末期肾疾病(%)
<1.4(<125)	30	35	24	3	15	4	—
1.4~1.85(125~160)	50	70	45	7	20	7	10
>1.85(>160)	60	90	60	12	45	35	70

参考文献自1991—2007年，所有妊娠至少24周胎龄。

Adapted from Armenti et al[88], with permission from Elsevier.

的升高与移植不良反应及新生儿结局较差相关[88]。因此在妊娠期血清肌酐的上升不该简单地归因于妊娠，此时需要明确原因。由于血清肌酐通常在妊娠期间随着肾小球滤过率增加而减少，因此妊娠期间血清肌酐的轻度增加即可能是妊娠期间移植物排斥的重要信号。

NTPR中1个研究对服用他克莫司维持治疗的133名肾移植女性受者进行观察，结果发现妊娠前较高的血清肌酐和妊娠期或产后立即发生排斥反应是产后5年内移植肾失功的重要危险因素。若妊娠前血清肌酐水平>1.3mg/dL(>115μmol/L)，则产后5年内移植物失功的相对风险为3.3(P=0.005)；若妊娠前肌酐>1.6mg/dL(>140μmol/L)，则妊娠后5年内移植物失功的相对风险为7.4(P=0.00001)[81]。

Deshpande等对25个国家的50项研究进行了系统评价和荟萃分析[90]。总体上讲，肾移植术后妊娠的预后较好，这在全世界的趋势是一致的。如前所述，不良生育结局的相关因素包括妊娠期高血压、血清肌酐水平增高及蛋白尿。

新生儿结局

肾移植受者平均早产1个月，早产(<37周)的发生率为50%，平均新生儿出生体重为约2500g。关于两种CNI，目前有两个对比环孢素和他克莫司导致新生儿畸形的流行病学研究。一项接受环孢素治疗的受者的荟萃分析中，后代畸形率为4.1%(339例中有14例)[91]。NTPR数据显示，在接受环孢素治疗的肾移植受者的362例活产婴儿中，5%为畸形[45]。畸形的种类在不同系统中不尽相同，并无主要类型。妊娠期接受他克莫司治疗的受者(84名女性，100次妊娠)，71名活产婴儿中有4名(5.6%)为畸形，但没有特异的畸形类型[92]。

在肾移植子代中，妊娠期应用MMF的受体子代畸形发生率较高[52]。来自NTPR的数据和病例报告均提及了一类畸形模式。其表型包括影响口腔(唇裂和腭裂)、耳朵(小耳畸形)和眼异常(眼间距过宽)的颅面畸形[3,52-60]。一些胎儿畸形可在产前超声检测到[93]。

在评估新生儿的发育风险时，必须考虑遗传因素，特别当这些因素造成母体器官衰竭时。此外值得关注的是潜在的更细微的影响，在出生时不明显，但可能会对长期的生长发育及对下一代造成影响。

后代的长期结局

有临床报告提出，T细胞亚群的变化可能会影响预防接种或长期免疫，但目前实体器官移植受者的后代发育良好[11,12,94,95]。NTPR的一个关于175个接受环孢素治疗的肾移植受者新生儿的研究表明，并未观察到预想中的新生儿生长发育延迟发生率的增加[11]。与之相似，相比于未暴露的儿童，在子宫内有环孢素暴露的3~15岁儿童的神经发育没有显著性差异及IQ或行为异常[12]。此外，考虑到肾移植受者的早产率和低出生体重率，药物对受者子代的长期神经认知发展的影响可以不用太担心。

胰肾联合移植受者

目前已有数篇关于胰肾联合移植术后妊娠的文献报道[4,96-101]。与单纯肾移植受者相比，胰肾联合移植受者中所需关注的问题是需评估胰腺移植物失去功能和血糖控制，更高的高血压发生率和更低的新生儿出生体重，以及移植物存活是否受到更不利的影响。但在这一群体中，目前的临床数据非常有限。

NTPR中报告的50例胰肾联合移植受者中共发生89次妊娠，生产94例（包括双胞胎和三胞胎，见表97.9)。在89例妊娠中，88例应用CNI进行免疫抑制治

表 97.9　NTPR：胰肾联合移植受者妊娠期间应用 CNI 的妊娠结局[3]

	环孢素（17 位受者，23 次妊娠）	改良环孢素（14 位受者，23 次妊娠）	他克莫司（22 位受者，42 次妊娠）
产妇因素（妊娠数量）	23	23	42
移植术后至妊娠的平均时间（年）	3.4±2.3	5.5±3.5	3.9±2.2
妊娠期高血压（%）	95	78	41
妊娠期糖尿病（%）	0	4	5
妊娠期感染（%）	62	55	21
子痫前期（%）	22	31	32
妊娠期排斥（%）	14	0	5
分娩 2 年内移植物失功（%）	13	17	10
结局 *	24	24	45
治疗性流产（%）	8	4	2
自发性流产（%）	8	25	31
异位妊娠（%）	4	0	2
死产（%）	0	0	0
活产（%）	79	71	64
活产	19	17	29
胎龄（周）	34±3	34.8±2.5	33.7±3.6
早产（<37 周）（%）	84	65	76
平均出生体重（g）	1436±647	2195±624	2096±797
低体重（<2500g）（%）	68	65	59
剖宫产（%）	61	69	65
新生儿复杂情况（%）	44	53	52
新生儿死亡（生后 30 天）[数目（%）]	1(5)	0	0

有些受者服用不同种类的 CNI 制剂后妊娠多次，对于服用其他药物或药物不能明确的受者未列入表格结果。

* 包括双胞胎。

疗（其中 8 例联合应用霉酚酸制剂），1 例应用 MMF 行免疫抑制治疗[3]。3 名受者（妊娠前具有良好的胰腺功能）在妊娠期使用了胰岛素。11 名受者发生了 5 个胰腺和 4 个肾脏失功；2 名受者在产后 2 年内胰肾同时失功；5 名受者在妊娠期间发生了移植后排斥。65 例活产儿的平均胎龄为（34.1±3.2）周；75%为早产（<37 周）。平均出生体重为（2075±709）g；63%是低出生体重（<2500g）。有一例 26 周胎龄的新生儿因败血症而死亡。在这些儿童的最后一次随访中[平均年龄为（8.5±5.6）岁]，所有 64 例儿童均报告身体健康且发育良好。有一些持续的问题报道：一个孩子患有注意缺陷多动障碍（ADHD），一个有胰岛素依赖性糖尿病（IDDM），一个同时患有 ADHD 和 IDDM，还有一个患有 ADHD 及癫痫。母亲的随访[平均（11.2±5.3）年]显示，30 名（60%）受者的胰腺和肾功能良好；7 名受者死亡，13 名受体患有不同程度的移植物功能障碍/损失。

NTPR 中也有胰肾联合移植后成功妊娠的妇女在妊娠期间少量使用胰岛素的报道。这组受者的后代中早产和低出生体重的发生率很高，因此这类妊娠的风险较高，需要跨学科管理。此外，妊娠对胰肾联合移植受者移植物存活的长期影响需要继续观察。

必须强调的是针对肾脏受体所概述的许多管理方法同样也适用于其他移植。以下部分将回顾非肾器官受者特有的问题。

肝移植受者

在慢性肝病的女性中，高达 50%患有闭经或伴有生育力下降的月经异常[102-113]。移植成功后由于促性腺功能恢复，几乎均可使月经周期和生殖功能迅速恢复至正常。这是生育年龄的受者社会康复的重要部分[104,109,110]，在世界范围内报道的肝移植后妊娠数量也逐渐增加[5,48,102-113]。

母体和新生儿的结局

与肾脏受者相反，肝脏受者的妊娠特点是妊娠期高血压和先兆子痫的发生率低，足月产的比例高。目前在 NTPR 上登记的肝受者的妊娠结局见表 97.10[3]。

在 21 岁前接受肝移植的受者中，75%的妊娠为活产。如果移植受者是未成年人，那么受者的妊娠、受者和新生儿的潜在风险及受者的长期生存情况应与受者和受者的父母等相关因素进行分析[108]。

移植功能

受体妊娠期通常会发生皮肤瘙痒和胆汁淤积。肝移植术后约 35%的“正常”妊娠中会有碱性磷酸酶升高。此时需要排除移植排斥，并与其他情况进行鉴别。目前也有关于移植受体妊娠期发生溶血、低血小板综合征和贫血的报道[104]。

排斥反应

活检证实急性排斥反应的发生率为 2%~8%[3,9,105]。当考虑急性排斥反应时，建议在超声引导下行经皮肝穿刺活检，以降低并发症的发生风险。移植物功能不全的评估可行肝脏多普勒超声，以排除解剖源性的移植物功能不全。通常移植排斥可以通过调整免疫抑制药物成功治疗。对于严重的排斥反应，可使用类固醇激素治疗。有报道称，母亲在妊娠期发生排斥反应，会导致新生儿低体重和早产的发生[105]。

应特别注意移植患者的肝动脉血流。有篇文献报道了 1 例妊娠子宫的压迫导致移植物血栓形成最后致使受者死亡的病例[111]。

多胎妊娠和连续妊娠

NTPR 数据报道了肝移植受者多胎妊娠的结果。在

表 97.10 NTPR：肝移植受者妊娠期间应用 CNI 的妊娠结局[3]

	环孢素(62 位受者，100 次妊娠)	改良环孢素(35 位受者，64 次妊娠)	他克莫司(85 位受者，140 次妊娠)
产妇因素(妊娠数量)	100	64	140
移植术后至妊娠的平均时间(年)	3.6±3.1	8.8±5.5	5.9±4.9
妊娠期高血压(%)	40	39	17
妊娠期糖尿病(%)	3	2	13
妊娠期感染(%)	31	31	19
子痫前期(%)	24	20	20
妊娠期排斥(%)	11	2	5
分娩 2 年内移植物失功(%)	8	3	5
结局 *	101	66	143
治疗性流产(%)	10	0	1
自发性流产(%)	15	17	20
异位妊娠(%)	0	2	1
死产(%)	3	0	1
活产(%)	72	82	76
活产	73	54	109
胎龄(周)	36.4±3.9	37.3±2.7	36±3.7
早产(<37 周)(%)	40	30	48
平均出生体重(g)	2619±803	2757±669	2747±875
低体重(<2500g)(%)	36	31	30
剖宫产(%)	44	29	45
新生儿复杂情况(%)	27	37	40
新生儿死亡(生后 30 天)[数目(%)]	1(1)	0	1(1)

有些受者服用不同种类的 CNI 制剂后妊娠多次，对于服用其他药物或药物不能明确的受者未列入表格结果。

* 包括双胞胎及三胞胎。

125 例有过首次妊娠史的肝移植受者中，有 61 例随后又有 1~4 次的妊娠。共 213 次妊娠，217 个产儿（含双胞胎）。在这些案例中，新生儿结局、妊娠期排斥反应和妊娠后 2 年内的移植物失功没有显著差异。因此，对于没有明显疾病复发或慢性移植排斥，肝功能良好者可以进行多次妊娠[49]。

不良事件的预测因素

NTPR 一项纳入 161 名女性肝移植受者的分析，在分娩后的 5 年内，移植物失功的最强危险因素为妊娠期排斥反应，其次是低龄妊娠[112]。在最终模型中，病毒性肝炎的影响并不显著，但它 5 年内移植物失功的相关因素中仅有肝病因素。

Coffin 等对美国住院患者数据库中 1993—2005 年的患者进行了调查研究[113]。他们将产科住院患者中肝移植受者（n = 206）和对照组（n = 4060）进行了分析比较，其中肝移植受者中的大多数妊娠结局良好。相比正常人群，肝移植受者有较高的胎儿死亡率、产前入院、母亲和胎儿并发症。这项研究提示肝移植受者妊娠有一定的风险。

肝病的病因

肝病复发，特别是病毒性肝炎，给母体和子代带来了风险。在无免疫预防的情况下，10%~20%HBsAg 阳性 HBeAg 阴性的非移植母体可发生乙型肝炎病毒（HBV）的垂直传播。为了防止垂直传播，HBsAg 阳性的女性产出的新生儿应在出生后 12h 内接受乙型肝炎免疫球蛋白（HBIg）和 HB 疫苗，这样可预防 90%以上的新生儿 HBV 感染[114]。丙型肝炎（HCV）RNA 阳性妇女的垂直传播率为 3%~5%（在没有其他病毒共感染的情况下）[115]。移植后高病毒载量的患者应特别注意，因为它是 HCV 垂直传播的重要危险因素。

自身免疫性肝炎（AIH）的肝移植受者通常需要比其他原因肝移植受者更多的免疫抑制。NTPR 分析了患有 AIH 女性的妊娠结果[3]。AIH 肝移植受者在接受移植手术及妊娠时平均年龄偏大，移植术后到妊娠的间隔时间较短，但 AIH 和非 AIH 肝移植受体在母体、妊娠和新生儿情况这些方面没有显著差异。

心脏移植受者

近年来，有大量复杂先天性心脏病的年轻患者进行了心脏移植，因此有必要来评估这一人群的生育能力[116]。

心脏移植受体在计划妊娠时，应进行一系列检测，包括心电图（ECG）和超声心动图，必要时应行冠状动脉造影。如果有临床指征的话，还可以选择右心导管检测和心内膜活检（EMB）[117]。当发生移植物失功或心脏移植物血管病变时，心脏移植受者应避免妊娠。

与肾移植受体相反，心脏移植受体的妊娠通常足月产较多，先兆子痫及妊娠 2 年内移植物失功的发生率较低。然而，孕妇的生存率独立于妊娠相关事件，应在妊娠前充分考虑。表 97.11 显示了服用 CNI 的心脏移植受体的妊娠结局[3]。

移植功能

妊娠对移植心脏的影响包括增加心脏负荷、心排血量和母体耗氧量[118,119]。当移植功能稳定时，移植心脏可以适应这些变化[120,121]。

排斥反应

确定心脏移植受者排斥反应需要 EMB。NTPR 报道了 57 名心脏受体，在她们的 103 次妊娠中，妊娠期移植排斥反应的发生率达 11%，这其中很多是轻度反应，并没有严重临床后果[3]。治疗排斥包括使用皮质类固醇，增加环孢素的剂量，如果排斥反应非常轻微，也可以继续观察[122]。有一例报道称心脏移植受体产后发生的排斥由抗体介导，所以在妊娠期间或之后发生排斥的心脏受体，应评估抗 HLA 抗体水平[123]。

他汀类药物

他汀类药物在心脏移植受者中经常用到，但由于其潜在的致畸作用，不建议在妊娠期间使用。来自 Motherisk 的一项研究表明妊娠期间服用他汀类药物的风险并不大，所以如果妊娠期服用了他汀类药物并不一定要终止妊娠[124]。如果可以的话，建议避免使用这些药物，以降低胎儿的风险。在一项 NTPR 的研究中，评估了服用他汀类药物的心脏移植受体的 10 例妊娠，这些新生儿有 6 例存活，没有畸形儿[125]。

分娩

类似于其他实体器官移植受体，阴道分娩是心脏移植受者推荐的分娩方式[32]。剖宫产应遵循产科指征。

表 97.11 NTPR：胰肾联合移植受者妊娠期间应用 CNI 的妊娠结局[3]

	环孢素(23位受者，43次妊娠)	改良环孢素(16位受者，25次妊娠)	他克莫司(20位受者，35次妊娠)
产妇因素(妊娠数量)	43	25	35
移植术后至妊娠的平均时间(年)	4.4±3.6	5.9±4.1	8.5±5.4
妊娠期高血压(%)	51	28	31
妊娠期糖尿病(%)	2	4	0
妊娠期感染(%)	12	8	23
子痫前期(%)	10	10	25
妊娠期排斥(%)	21	4	3
分娩2年内移植物失功(%)	0	4	3
结局 *	43	25	35
治疗性流产(%)	9	4	0
自发性流产(%)	19	44	36
异位妊娠(%)	2	0	3
死产(%)	0	4	0
活产(%)	70	48	62
活产	3	12	24
胎龄(周)	36.9±3.0	37.8±1.4	36.1±2.5
早产(<37周)(%)	37	8	54
平均出生体重(g)	2658±590	2690±540	2483±570
低体重(<2500g)(%)	37	33	46
剖宫产(%)	30	42	57
新生儿复杂情况(%)	24	25	46
新生儿死亡(生后30天)[数目(%)]	0	0	0

有些受者服用不同种类的 CNI 制剂后妊娠多次，服用其他药物或药物不能明确的受者未列入表格结果。

* 包括双胞胎。

在 NTPR 报告的心脏移植受体妊娠中，40%经剖宫产分娩。在分娩期间，由于心律失常的风险增加，必须进行 ECG 监测。但没有必要行更多的侵入性心血管监测。硬膜外麻醉可减少疼痛诱导的交感反应，并减少分娩期间的急性血压波动[13]。医务人员需要注意的是心脏受者可能对血管活性药物有不可预测的反应，同时，去神经支配的心脏对血管舒张药(阿托品)无反应。

母体预后

大多数心脏移植受者在妊娠后可维持良好的移植物功能。在 NTPR 报道的 57 名心脏移植受者中，40 名受者产后维持了良好的移植物功能(70%)。2 名受体在妊娠 2 年内有移植物失功，其中 1 名在移植后 17 年死亡，另 1 名发生在分娩后 9 个月，需要重新移植手术。后者目前身体情况良好，且移植物功能正常[3]。16 例产妇死亡，均发生在妊娠 2 年后。死亡原因包括血管病变、动脉粥样硬化、急性排斥、肺炎和败血症。如前所述，妊娠前必须考虑到心脏移植受者的寿命可能有限。

肺移植受者

与心脏移植受者相比，肺移植受者发生排斥反应、围生期移植物失功及新生儿低体重的概率更高[8,126]。由于他们的总体风险较高，妊娠者较少，目前尚无相关指南。

NTPR 报告了 22 例女性肺移植受者的 31 例妊娠(33 例新生儿)(包括一例三胞胎)[3](表 97.12)。免疫抑制方案包括：环孢素(8 例)，改良的环孢素(2 例)和他克莫司(21 例)。所有发生排斥反应的受者都是在 1996 年之前接受的肺移植手术，她们采用的是基于环孢素的免疫抑制方案。在 22 名受者中，11 例因肺囊性纤维化行肺移植，她们共有 13 次妊娠(8 例活产，3 例自发流产，2 例治疗性流产)。3 名囊性纤维化受者在妊娠期

表 97.12　NTPR：22 例肺移植受者的妊娠结局[3]

器官	肺
产妇因素(妊娠数量)	31
移植术后至妊娠的平均时间(年)	3.6±3.2
妊娠期高血压(%)	52
妊娠期糖尿病(%)	26
妊娠期感染(%)	21
妊娠期排斥(%)	16
子痫前期(%)	5
分娩 2 年内移植物失功(%)	14
结局 *	33
治疗性流产(%)	15
自发性流产(%)	27
异位妊娠(%)	0
死产(%)	0
活产(%)	58
活产	19
胎龄(周)	33.9±5.0
早产(<37 周)(%)	63
平均出生体重(g)	2206±936
低体重(<2500g)(%)	61
剖宫产(%)	32
新生儿复杂情况(%)	63
新生儿死亡(生后 30 天)[数目(%)]	2(11)†

* 包括三胞胎。

† 三胞胎：1 个在 14 周自发性流产，2 个在 22 周生产并在 24 小时内死亡。

间发生排斥反应。在最近的一次随访中，14 例移植物功能良好，1 例功能降低，5 例已经死亡(2 例囊性纤维化)，1 例移植物失功。19 名活产儿的平均孕龄为(33.9±5.0)周，平均出生体重为(2206±936)g。有 1 例三胞胎中的两胎在 22 周生产时死亡（另一个在 14 周自发性流产）。在最后一次随访时，17 名存活的儿童均健康且发育良好。

肺移植受者(包括肺囊性纤维化者)有可能成功妊娠。1996 年前，移植受者妊娠期间发生排斥反应的较多。目前尚需要更多数据来分析明确肺移植后妊娠的情况。此外，妊娠对母体长期生存的影响还需要进一步研究。

小肠移植受者

小肠移植术后的妊娠在 NTPR 中有过报道[3,6,127]，但缺乏相关的预后数据。有 2 例肠移植受者发生妊娠。2 例受者产下健康足月儿，且在妊娠期间及产后未出现移植并发症。

其他器官组

目前相关的报道有限，但女性肝肾联合及心肺联合移植受者也有成功妊娠的报道[3]。

哺乳

女性移植受者母乳喂养目前仍存在争议[3,32,128–132]。NTPR 收集了使用多种免疫抑制方案的移植受者进行母乳喂养的数据，包括 64 例肾移植受者母乳喂养的 80 个婴儿，21 例肝移植受者母乳喂养的 28 个婴儿，1 例肝肾受者母乳喂养的 3.5 个月的婴儿，3 例胰肾移植受者母乳喂养的 4 个婴儿[3]，2 例肺移植受者母乳喂养的婴儿：一个 10 周，另一个 3 个月，6 例心脏移植受者母乳喂养的 10 个孩子(年龄从出生几天到 2 岁)。在最后一次随访中，没有关于这些儿童与母乳喂养有关问题的报道。

因此，任何免疫抑制药物暴露于婴儿都可能超过安全阈值，但相对少的暴露给婴儿的药物剂量、尚无不良反应的记录以及母乳喂养的益处均可能超过这种暴露的理论风险。此外，母乳喂养的婴儿应该检查其血液中免疫抑制剂的水平——能检测出免疫抑制剂是停止母乳喂养的标志。在移植受者母乳喂养方面需要进一步研究，特别是免疫抑制药物暴露对婴儿发育的影响。

移植受者的管理

移植受者妊娠的管理建议已有详细的公布[3,32,133–140]。管理指南的摘要见表 97.13。

妊娠前咨询

移植术后可恢复生育能力，因此移植受者应在移植前和移植后早期咨询避孕的相关问题。对于所有移植受者，移植术后最好在移植物功能稳定建立的同时将免疫抑制剂减量到维持水平后再妊娠。NTPR 数据显示，接受环孢素治疗的肾移植受者，移植至妊娠间隔<6 个月的，妊娠终止和围生期排斥的发生率较时间间隔更长的移植受者高。从移植到妊娠的最短安全间隔尚未明确，但建议至少在移植术后 1 年，以使移

表 97.13 移植术后妊娠管理建议

妊娠
• 移植受者应通过合理避孕至少在器官移植1年后妊娠
• 评估移植物功能(器官特异性)
○ 活检
○ 蛋白尿
○ 乙型肝炎或丙型肝炎的病情
○ 巨细胞病毒,弓形虫病,单纯疱疹的病情
• 维持免疫抑制治疗建议
○ 硫唑嘌呤
○ 环孢素
○ 他克莫司
○ 糖皮质激素
○ 麦考酚酸吗乙酯
○ 肠溶麦考酚酸吗乙酯
○ 西罗莫司
○ 依维莫司
○ 贝拉西普
• 同治病的影响:如是否有糖尿病及高血压,如果有,应优化治疗方案。非肾移植受者应评估她们的肾功能基线
• 如需要,予以疫苗预防疾病,如风疹疫苗
• 寻找病因,考虑基因相关因素
• 考虑子宫内生长受限、早产和低出生体重儿的风险
产前
• 妊娠的早期诊断
• 对移植器官功能及免疫移植水平进行临床及实验室监测:
○ 32周前每月一次
○ 36周前每两周一次
○ 36周后每周一次直至妊娠结束
• 每月进行尿培养
• 如果考虑发生排斥反应,进行组织活检
• 对细菌或病毒等病原体的检测,如巨细胞病毒、弓形虫和疱疹
• 胎儿监测
• 高血压及肾脏疾病的管理
• 子痫前期的监测
• 妊娠糖尿病的监测
分娩
• 推荐经阴道分娩,有产科指征时剖宫产
• 对于心脏移植/心肺联合移植/肺移植受者
○ 警惕咳嗽反射的缺乏,需要气道保护
○ 对于血管活性药物的反应不可预计
○ 正确的静脉用药
产后
• 产后至少1个月的免疫抑制药物监测,尤其对于妊娠期药物剂量增加者
• 如果考虑发生排斥反应,予以活检
• 合理避孕

Adapted from Armenti et al[88], with permission from Elsevier.

植物功能充分稳定,并将免疫抑制剂用量减至维持水平[32,141,142]。

免疫抑制药物

霉酚酸类免疫抑制剂应用时要兼顾到抗排斥反应与潜在的胎儿致畸作用。目前没有关于更换为其他低妊娠风险的替代免疫方案的数据，也没有关于排斥反应预防的可靠研究结果。因此,每名计划妊娠的移植受者，特别是在器官功能会直接影响生育力及妊娠安全的情况下,必须进行个体评估,来判断更换免疫抑制剂给移植器官带来的风险。妊娠前必须权衡继续使用具有潜在危害胎儿的免疫抑制方案的风险。此时,最终的决定最好是在患者、患者伴侣和移植团队的共同参与下进行决策。对于意外妊娠,只能根据具体情况最后做出决定。

抗高血压药物

许多移植受者患有原发性高血压，且可能正在接受降压药物的联合治疗。血管紧张素转换酶抑制剂和血管紧张素Ⅱ受体拮抗剂在妊娠期间禁用，目前对于该类药物暴露的时间风险仍存在一些争议[32,143]。如果需要对降压方案进行调整,应在妊娠前进行。

母体伴发疾病

除了高血压和先兆子痫，还应注意可能发生的其他与母亲有关的疾病,包括感染和妊娠糖尿病。妊娠期间的感染性疾病最常见的是尿路感染，妊娠期间应每月进行尿培养。其他包括酵母菌感染、肺炎、败血症或不明确的病毒感染均可使妊娠复杂化。巨细胞病毒(CMV)感染通常是无症状的,但可以通过血清学、抗原或病毒学方法检测。CMV急性感染是移植术后第1年最常见的感染类型，这在早期妊娠中尤其危险。CMV感染可造成先天性畸形(小头症、脑性麻痹、感音神经性聋)或先天性肝病。10%~15%感染了CMV的妊娠可出现这种畸形。更昔洛韦和缬更昔洛韦用于预防和治疗CMV感染,这些抗病毒药物在妊娠中的安全性尚不确定[105]。

非移植人群中HCV的垂直传播率为5%[144]。HBV感染的移植受者也可以将病原体传播给子代[114]。如前所述，出生后几小时内给新生儿应用HBIg和HBV疫苗通常可防止疾病传播。急性弓形虫感染的发生率为

0.2%~1%,且大多数病例未确诊且无症状。先天性弓形虫病可能有严重后果,可通过培养、直接抗原检测或血清学测试帮助诊断[145]。

高血压和先兆子痫的检查是必需的,尽管血清尿酸水平和尿蛋白排泄受药物肾毒性的干扰使先兆子痫的诊断比较困难。其他潜在并发症包括 HELLP 综合征、输尿管梗阻和剖宫产分娩的相关并发症。如果血清肌酐升高,需进行围生期超声检查,以排除尿梗阻。

排斥反应

除非发生免疫抑制剂毒性或排斥反应,一般情况下最好维持妊娠前免疫抑制剂量和血药水平。妊娠期间血药浓度可能会降低,原因包括母体体液增加以及药物在胎儿中的代谢。有时,由于担心药物对胎儿有影响,移植受者可能会私自在妊娠期间停服药物,这是不允许的。NTPR 的报告显示,大多数受者在妊娠期间免疫抑制剂用量保持不变或有所增加。无论妊娠期间药物剂量是多少,围生期机体发生的变化要求产后免疫抑制剂剂量调整最好通过血药浓度来管理。

妊娠期间的排斥反应并不常见,但在移植物功能障碍时必须考虑是否发生了排斥反应。通常血清肌酐水平在妊娠早期轻微下降,并于产后回到基线。在肾移植受者中,妊娠期和产后血清肌酐≥15%时必须进行评估。对于所有 SOT 受者,考虑移植物功能恶化时均应进行活检,如果确诊为急性排斥反应,则需要合适的抗排斥治疗。考虑到排斥和先兆子痫的风险,从妊娠中期起,血压、移植物功能和免疫抑制药物水平应进行常规监测。

分娩

对于移植受者的分娩,目前报道剖宫产比例高达 29%~69%(表 97.7,表 97.9 至表 97.12)。然而,建议只有符合产科指征时才行剖宫产。免疫抑制剂不能在分娩期间中断,并建议预防性使用抗生素。

产后护理

大多数口服免疫抑制剂很容易吸收,免疫抑制治疗可以在剖宫产后不久恢复。当不能恢复口服药物治疗时,大多数药物有对应的静脉制剂。应监测免疫抑制剂的水平,并适当调节剂量,注意对血压、肾功能的影响及药物毒性。必须意识到移植受者可能伴有产后抑郁症,药物可能因此被遗忘或漏服。所以在产后几个月需要密切监测用药情况。

如前所述,母乳喂养仍然存在争议。新生儿暴露于任何免疫抑制药物都可能是有害的,但目前认为母乳中存在的药量很小。母乳喂养的好处可能超过其带来的风险。

活体捐献后妊娠

活体肾捐献后的妊娠首次由 Murray 等于 1963 年报道[2]。早期研究的结论认为供体肾切除术不会对产前或妊娠结局带来风险[146-148]。然而,最近的两项研究提高了我们的认识,并使活体捐献后妊娠得到了高度关注[149,150]。

Reisæter 等基于挪威出生注册处的数据,描述了 326 名女性肾捐献者,捐献前有 620 次妊娠,捐献后有 106 次妊娠,并且使用来自该处的随机样本作为对照[149]。在肾捐赠者和一般人群之间,除了捐献后先兆子痫的发生率更高(5.7%对 2.6%),母体和新生儿的结局没有差异。由于数量过少,因此应谨慎解释该结果。最重要的是,捐献后的妊娠结局类似于非捐献者。

Ibrahim 等调查了美国单一大规模移植中心 1589 名女性捐献者的捐献前后妊娠结果,该研究包括 1085 名捐献者的 3213 次妊娠[150]。肾捐献后的胎儿和母体结果与一般人群的相似。然而,捐献后妊娠与捐献前妊娠进行比较时,显而易见,捐献后妊娠的不良事件可能性更高,例如更低比例的足月婴儿,更高的胎儿流产、妊娠糖尿病、妊娠高血压、蛋白尿和先兆子痫发生率。值得注意的是,捐献前不良反应的发生率非常低,提示可能存在选择偏倚,且有妊娠糖尿病、高血压或先兆子痫病史的妇女不太可能成为肾脏供体。

现有数据认为与一般人群相比,肾捐献后妊娠的母体和胎儿不良事件的发生率并未增加。然而,对肾捐献者的妊娠期血压、尿蛋白排泄和胎儿超声应进行严密监测[151]。

目前,肾脏捐献后与妊娠的时间间隔尚未确定。有共识建议肾捐献术后至少 2 个月后再评估妊娠前的肾脏代偿能力[152]。也有人认为肾捐献术后 1 年才可以让女性从捐肾的情绪中恢复过来并适应新的肾功能水平[151]。捐献后妊娠及其潜在问题应与所有育龄的捐献者及其受体共同讨论[151,153,154]。

有趣的是,Soyama等报道了一位右肝脏捐献后6个月内妊娠的女性并结局成功的病例[155]。

男性受体

表97.14显示了NTPR中男性移植受者生育的活产儿和新生儿结局,其中包括多器官移植受者。总体而言,男性移植受者的生育结局与一般人群相似。NTPR还在继续收集SOT后男性受者生育的数据。与男性移植受者生育有关的问题还需要进一步的研究。

总结

移植后妊娠的要点见表97.15。

随着移植医学中免疫抑制剂的不断发展和改进,临床医生应为所有移植前和移植后的育龄受者提供妊娠咨询。由各个中心的医生一起积累的这些治疗经验,无论对于阳性和阴性妊娠结果的报道都至关重要。今后还需要制订更好和更具体的器官特异性的妊娠管理指南。随着新的免疫抑制剂的不断出现,专家间持续的密切合作将有助于更好地识别移植受者群体的潜在妊娠风险。

表97.14 NTPR:男性移植受者生育后代情况[3]

	肾	肝	胰肾联合	心
受者数量	594	69	34	106
生育	915	109	43	157
结局 *	930	115	45	160
活产(%)	93	89	91	88
平均胎龄(周)	39.1±2.2	39.1±1.9	38.7±2.4	38.9±2.3
平均出生体重(g)	3329	3296	3321	3440
新生儿复杂情况(%)	16	19	15	19

* 包括双胞胎及三胞胎。

表97.15 要点

- 推荐通过以下建议优化妊娠结局:
  - 移植后身体状况良好≥1年
  - 稳定的移植物功能[血肌酐<1.5mg/mL(<130μmol/L)],目前无免疫排斥证据
  - 高血压稳定控制或无高血压
  - 微量或无蛋白尿(<1g/24h)
  - 稳定的免疫抑制治疗方案
- 潜在的母体及新生儿并发症包括子痫前期,早产,胎儿生长受限及低出生体重
- 妊娠过程本身不影响稳定的移植物功能
- 其他并发疾病的影响,如糖尿病及高血压,应优化治疗方案
- 推荐维持妊娠期免疫抑制治疗,除非像霉酚酸酯类有胎儿风险的药物应考虑是否需要更换

致谢

感谢Lisa A. Coscia,RN,BSN在编写方面提供了诚挚的帮助。

NTPR感谢北美超过250个中心的移植受者和工作人员的合作,感谢他们向注册机构提供信息及付出的时间。NTPR得到了诺华制药公司、Astellas Pharma公司、Genentech公司、Pfizer公司、Teva美国制药公司、Sandoz公司和Bristol-Myers Squibb公司的资助。要联系NTPR,请发送电子邮件至:NTPR@giftoflifeinstitute.org(http://www.NTPRegistry.org)。

(刘治坤 译 徐骁 校)

参考文献

1. Merrill JP, Murray JE, Harrison JH, et al. Successful homotransplantation of the human kidney between identical twins. JAMA. 1956;160:277–282.
2. Murray JE, Reid DE, Harrison JH, et al. Successful pregnancies after human renal transplantation. New England Journal of Medicine. 1963;269:341.
3. National Transplantation Pregnancy Registry. 2011 Annual Report. Thomas Jefferson University: June 2012. 2012. Available from: http://www.jefferson.edu/ntpr.
4. Castro LA, Baltzer U, Hillebrand G, et al. Pregnancy in juvenile diabetes mellitus under cyclosporine treatment after combined kidney and pancreas transplantation. Transplantation Proceedings. 1986;18(6):1780.
5. Walcott WO, Derick DE, Jolley JJ, et al. Successful pregnancy in a liver transplant patient. American Journal of Obstetrics and Gynecology. 1978;132:340–341.
6. Kosmach-Park B, Doshi B, Seward L, et al. Successful pregnancy following intestine transplant in a long-term survivor. Transplantation. 2006;82(S2):855.
7. Lowenstein BR, Vain NW, Perrone SV, et al. Successful pregnancy and vaginal delivery after heart transplantation. American Journal of Obstetrics and Gynecology. 1988;73:667–683.
8. Donaldson S, Novotny D, Paradowski L, et al. Acute and chronic lung allograft rejection during pregnancy. Chest. 1996;110(1):293–296.
9. Armenti VT, Constantinescu S, Moritz MJ, et al. Pregnancy after transplantation. Transplantation Reviews. 2008;22:223–240.
10. Scott JR, Branch DW, Holman J. Autoimmune and pregnancy complications in the daughter of a kidney transplant patient. Transplantation. 2002;73:815.
11. Stanley CW, Gottlieb R, Zager R, et al. Developmental well-being in offspring of women receiving cyclosporine post-renal transplant. Transplantation Proceedings. 1999;31:241–242.
12. Nulman I, Sgro M, Barrera M, et al. Long-term neurodevelopment of children exposed in utero to ciclosporin after maternal renal transplant. Pediatric Drugs. 2010;12(2):113–122.
13. Mastrobatista JM, Gomez-Lobo V. Pregnancy after solid organ transplantation. Obstetrics and Gynecology. 2008;112(4):919–931.
14. Guazzelli CA, Torlini MR, Sanches TF, et al. Contraceptive counseling and

use among 197 female kidney transplant recipients. Transplant. 2008;86(5): 669–672.
15. Ghazizadeh S, Lessan-Pezeshki M, Khatami M, et al. Unwanted pregnancy among kidney transplant recipients in Iran. Transplantation Proceedings. 2005; 37(7):3085–3086.
16. Xu L, Yang Y, Shi JG, et al. Unwanted pregnancy among Chinese renal transplant recipients. European Journal of Contraception and Reproductive Health Care. 2011;16(4):270–276.
17. Curtis K. U.S medical eligibility for contraceptive use. MMWR. Morbidity and Mortality Weekly Report. 2010;56 (early release):1–6;; [February 6, 2012] Available from: http://www.cdc.gov/mmwr/preview/mmwrhtml/rr59e0528a1.htm.
18. Maguire K, Westhoff C. The state of hormonal contraception today: established and emerging noncontraceptive health benefits. American Journal of Obstetrics and Gynecology. 2011;205(4 Suppl):s4–s8.
19. Estes C, Westhoff C. Contraception for the transplant patient. Seminars in Perinatology. 2007;31:372–377.
20. Pietrzak B, Bobrowska K, Jabiry-Zieniewicz Z, et al. Oral and transdermal hormonal contraception in women after kidney transplantation. Transplantation Proceedings. 2007;39(9):2759–2762.
21. Jabiry-Zieniewicz Z, Bobrowska K, Kamiski P, et al. Low-dose hormonal contraception after liver transplantation. Transplantation Proceedings. 2007;39(5): 1530–1532.
22. Fedorkow DM, Corenblum B, Shaffer EA. Cholestasis induced by oestrogen after liver transplantation. BMJ (Clinical Research Edition). 1989;299: 1080–1081.
23. Sucato GS, Murray PJ. Developmental and reproductive health issues in adolescent solid organ transplant recipients. Seminars in Pediatric Surgery. 2006; 15(3):170–178.
24. Hubacher D, Grimes DA. Noncontraceptive health benefits of intrauterine devices: a systematic review. Obstetrical and Gynecological Survey. 2002; 57(2):120–128.
25. Fong YF, Singh K. Effects of the levonorgestrel-releasing intrauterine system on uterine myomas in a renal transplant patient. Contraception. 1999;60: 51–53.
26. Zerner J, Doil KL, Drewry J, et al. Intrauterine contraceptive device failures in renal transplant patients. Journal of Reproductive Medicine. 1981;26(2): 99–102.
27. Bahamondes MV, Hidalgo MM, Bahamondes L, et al. Ease of insertion and clinical performance of the levonorsgestrel-releasing intrauterine device in nulligravidas. Contraception. 2011;84(5):e11–e16.
28. Stringer EM, Kaseba C, Levy J, et al. A randomized trial of the intrauterine contraceptive device vs hormonal contraception in women who are infected with the human immunodeficiency virus. American Journal of Obstetrics and Gynecology. 2007;197(2):144, e 1–8.
29. Kosola S, Lampela H, Lauronen J, et al. General health, health related quality of life and sexual health after pediatric liver transplantation: a nationwide study. American Journal of Transplantation. 2012;12(2):420–427.
30. Board JA, Lee HM, Draper DA, et al. Pregnancy following kidney homotransplantation from a non-twin. Report of a case with concurrent administration of azathioprine and prednisone. Obstetrics and Gynecology. 1967;29(3): 318–323.
31. Davison JM, Lind T, Uldall PR. Planned pregnancy in a renal transplant recipient. British Journal of Obstetrics and Gynaecology. 1976;83:518–527.
32. McKay DB, Josephson MA, Armenti VT, et al., Women's Health Committee of the American Society of Transplantation. Reproduction and transplantation: report on the AST consensus conference on reproductive issues and transplantation. American Journal of Transplantation. 2005;5(7):1592–1599.
33. EBPG Expert Group on Renal Transplantation. European best practice guidelines for renal transplantation. Pregnancy in renal transplant recipients. Nephrology, Dialysis, Transplantation. 2002;17(S4):50–55.
34. Davison JM, Redman CWG. Pregnancy post-transplant: the establishment of a UK registry. British Journal of Obstetrics and Gynaecology. 1997;104: 1106–1107.
35. Sibanda N, Briggs JD, Davison JM, et al. Pregnancy after organ transplantation: a report from the UK transplant pregnancy registry. Transplantation. 2007; 83(10):1301–1307.
36. Fraser FC, Fainstat TD. Production of congenital defects in the off-spring of pregnant mice treated with cortisone; progress report. Pediatrics. 1951;8(4): 527–533.
37. Fraser FC, Sajoo A. Teratogenic potential of corticosteroids in humans. Teratology. 1995;51(1):45–46.
38. Hou S. Pregnancy in chronic renal disease insufficiency and end-stage renal disease. American Journal of Kidney Diseases. 1999;33:235–252.
39. Leb DE, Weisskopf B, Kanovitz BS. Chromosome aberrations in the child of a kidney transplant recipient. Archives of Internal Medicine. 1971;128(3): 441–444.
40. Davison JM. Dialysis, transplantation, and pregnancy. American Journal of Kidney Diseases. 1991;17(2):127–132.
41. Cleary BJ, Källén B. Early pregnancy azathioprine use and pregnancy outcomes. Birth Defects Research. Part A, Clinical and Molecular Teratology. 2009;85(7): 647–654.
42. Fein A, Vechoropoulos M, Nebel L. Cyclosporin-induced embryotoxicity in mice. Biologia Neonatorum. Neo-Natal Studies. 1989;56:165–173.
43. Pickrell MD, Sawers R, Michael J. Pregnancy after renal transplantation: severe intrauterine growth retardation during treatment with cyclosporin A. British Medical Journal. 1988;296:825.
44. Mason RJ, Thomson AW, Whiting PH, et al. Cyclosporine-induced feto-toxicity in the rat. Transplantation. 1985;39(1):9–12.
45. Armenti VT, Radomski JS, Moritz MJ, et al. Report from the National Transplantation Pregnancy Registry (NTPR): outcomes of pregnancy after transplantation. In: Cecka JM, Terasaki PI, editors. Clinical Transplants 2001. Los Angeles, CA: Terasaki Foundation Laboratory; 2002: 97–105.
46. Finnell RH. Teratology: general considerations and principles. Journal of Allergy and Clinical Immunology. 1999;103:S 337–S 342.
47. Farley DE, Shelby J, Alexander D, et al. The effect of two new immunosuppressive agents, FK506 and didemnin B, in murine pregnancy. Transplantation. 1991;52(1):106–110.
48. Jain A, Venkataramanan R, Fung JJ, et al. Pregnancy after liver transplantation under tacrolimus. Transplantation. 1997;64(4):559–565.
49. Coscia LA, Constantinescu S, Moritz MJ, et al. Report from the National Transplantation Pregnancy Registry (NTPR): outcomes of pregnancy after transplantation. In: Cecka JM, Terasaki PI, editors. Clinical Transplants 2007. Los Angeles, CA: Terasaki Foundation Laboratory; 2008: 29–42.
50. Mycophenolate mofetil package insert. Nutley, NJ, Roche Laboratories, 2009.
51. Mycophenolic acid package insert. East Hanover, NJ, Novartis Pharmaceuticals, 2009.
52. Sifontis NM, Coscia LA, Constantinescu S, et al. Pregnancy outcomes in solid organ transplant recipients with exposure to mycophenolate mofetil or sirolimus. Transplantation. 2006;82:1698–1702.
53. Le Ray C, Coulomb A, Elefant E, et al. Mycophenolate mofetil in pregnancy after renal transplantation: a case of major fetal malformations. Obstetrics and Gynecology. 2004;103:1091–1094.
54. Pérgola PE, Kancharla A, Riley DJ. Kidney transplantation during the first trimester of pregnancy: immunosuppression with mycophenolate mofetil, tacrolimus and prednisone. Transplantation. 2001;71:994–997.
55. Tjeertes IFA, Bastiaans DET, van Ganzewinkel CJLM, et al. Neonatal anemia and hydrops fetalis after maternal mycophenolate mofetil use. Journal of Perinatology. 2007;27:62–64.
56. Perez-Aytes A, Ledo A, Boso V, et al. In utero exposure to mycophenolate mofetil: a characteristic phenotype? American Journal of Medical Genetics Part A. 2008;146:1–7.
57. El Sebaaly Z, Charpentier B, Snanoudj R. Fetal malformations associated with mycophenolate mofetil for lupus nephritis. Nephrology, Dialysis, Transplantation. 2007;22:2722.
58. Velinov M, Zellers N. The mycophenolate mofetil syndrome. Clinical Dysmorphology. 2008;17:77–78.
59. Jackson P, Paquette L, Watiker V, et al. Intrauterine exposure to mycophenolate mofetil and multiple congenital anomalies in a newborn: possible teratogenic effect. American Journal of Medical Genetics Part A. 2009;149A:1231–1236.
60. Lin AE, Singh KE, Strauss A, et al. An additional patient with mycophenolate mofetil embryopathy: cardiac and facial analyses. American Journal of Medical Genetics Part A. 2011;155A(4):748–756.
61. Sirolimus package insert. Philadelphia, Wyeth Laboratories, 2008.
62. Jankowska I, Oldakowska-Jednyak U, Jabiry-Zieniewicz Z, et al. Absence of teratogenicity of sirolimus used during early pregnancy. Transplantation Proceedings. 2004;36:3232–3233.
63. Guardia O, del Rial MC, Casadei D. Pregnancy under sirolimus-based immunosuppression. Transplantation. 2006;81:636.
64. Chu SH, Liu KL, Chiang YJ, et al. Sirolimus used during pregnancy in a living related renal transplant recipient: a case report. Transplantation Proceedings. 2008;40:2446–2448.
65. Veroux M, Corona D, Veroux P. Pregnancy under everolimus-based immunosuppression. Transplant International. 2011;24(12):e115–e117.
66. Framarino dei Malatesta M, Corona LE, et al. Successful pregnancy in a living-related kidney transplant recipient who received sirolimus throughout the whole gestation. Transplantation. 2011;91(9):e69.
67. Zuber J, Anglicheau D, Elie C, et al. Sirolimus may reduce fertility in male renal transplant recipients. American Journal of Transplantation. 2008;8(7):1471–1479.

68. Armenti VT, Moritz MJ, Davison JM. Drug safety issues in pregnancy following transplantation and immunosuppression. Drug Safety. 1998;19(3):219–232.
69. Davison JM. Renal disorders in pregnancy. Current Opinion in Obstetrics & Gynecology. 2001;13(2):109–114.
70. Davison JM. Pregnancy in renal allograft recipients. Problems, prognosis and practicalities. In: Lindheimer MD, Davison JM, editors. Ballière's Clinical Obstetrics and Gynaecology. 1994: 501–525.
71. Armenti VT, Ahlswede KM, Ahlswede BA, et al. National Transplantation Pregnancy Registry: outcomes of 154 pregnancies in cyclosporine-treated female kidney transplant recipients. Transplantation. 1994;57(4):502–506.
72. Barron WM. Hypertension. In: Barron WM, Lindheimer MD, editors. Medical Disorders During Pregnancy. St. Louis, MO: Mosby; 2000: 1–38.
73. Correa A, Gilboa SM, Besser LM, et al. Diabetes mellitus and birth defects. American Journal of Obstetrics and Gynecology. 2008;199(3):237, e1–9.
74. Baylis C. Glomerular filtration and volume regulation in gravid animal models. In: Lindheimer MD, Davison JM (eds): Ballière's Clinical Obstetrics & Gynaecology 1994;8(2):235–264.
75. First MR, Combs CA, Weiskittel P, et al. Lack of effect of pregnancy on renal allograft survival or function. Transplantation. 1995;59(4):472–476.
76. Sturgiss SN, Davison JM. Effect of pregnancy on long-term function renal allografts. American Journal of Kidney Diseases. 1992;19(2):167–172.
77. Sturgiss SN, Davison JM. Effect of pregnancy on the long-term function of renal allografts: an update. American Journal of Kidney Diseases. 1995; 26(1):54–56.
78. Rahamimov R, Ben-Haroush A, Wittenberg C, et al. Pregnancy in renal transplant recipients: long-term effect on patient and graft survival. A single-center experience. Transplantation. 2006;81:660–664.
79. Fischer T, Neumayer HH, Fischer R, et al. Effect of pregnancy on long-term kidney function in renal transplant recipients treated with cyclosporine and with azathioprine. American Journal of Transplantation. 2005;5: 2732–2739.
80. Armenti VT, Radomski JS, Moritz MJ, et al. Report from the National Transplantation Pregnancy Registry (NTPR): outcomes of pregnancy after transplantation. In: Cecka JM, Terasaki PI, editors. Clinical Transplants 2002. Los Angeles, CA: Terasaki Foundation Laboratory; 2003: 121–130.
81. Constantinescu S, Axelrod P, Coscia LA, et al. Risk factors for graft loss within 5 years post pregnancy in female kidney recipients. American Journal of Transplantation. 2011;11(S 2):205, A591.
82. Coscia LA, Constantinescu S, Moritz MJ, et al. Report from the National Transplantation Pregnancy Registry: outcomes of pregnancy after transplantation. In: Cecka JM, Terasaki PI, editors. Clinical Transplants 2009. Los Angeles, CA: Terasaki Foundation Laboratory; 2010: 103–122.
83. Case AM, Weissman A, Sermer M, et al. Successful twin pregnancy in a dual-transplant couple resulting from in-vitro fertilization and intracytoplasmic sperm injection. Human Reproduction. 2000;15(3):626–628.
84. Jimenez E, Gonzalea-Carabello Z, Morales-Otero L, et al. Triplets born to a kidney transplant recipient. Transplantation. 1995;59:435–436.
85. Coscia LA, Cardonick EH, Moritz MJ, et al. Multiple gestations in female kidney transplant recipients maintained on calcineurin inhibitors. American Journal of Transplantation. 2003;5:A1603.
86. Fichez A, Labrousse C, Fromajoux C, et al. Successful pregnancy outcome after in vitro fertilization in a pancreas-kidney recipient. Fertility and Sterility. 2008;90(3):849, e1–3.
87. Termini SM, Coscia LA, Potti S, et al. National Transplantation Pregnancy Registry (NTPR): in vitro fertilization outcomes in female transplant recipients. American Journal of Obstetrics and Gynecology. 2011;204(S1): S322.
88. Armenti VT, Moritz MJ, Davison JM. Pregnancy following transplantation. In: James DK, Steer PJ, Weiner CP, et al., editors. High Risk Pregnancy: Management Options. 4th ed. Philadelphia, PA: Elsevier Science; 2011: 961–972.
89. Armenti VT, Ahlswede KM, Ahlswede BA, et al. Variables affecting birthweight and graft survival in 197 pregnancies in cyclosporine-treated female kidney transplant recipients. Transplantation. 1995;59(4):476–479.
90. Deshpande NA, James NT, Kucirka LM, et al. Pregnancy outcomes in kidney transplant recipients: a systematic review and meta-analysis. American Journal of Transplantation. 2011;11(11):2388–2404.
91. Oz BB, Hackman R, Einarson T, et al. Pregnancy outcome after cyclosporine therapy during pregnancy: a meta-analysis. Transplantation. 2001;71(8): 1051–1055.
92. Kainz A, Harabacz I, Cowlrick IS, et al. Review of the course and outcome of 100 pregnancies in 84 women treated with tacrolimus. Transplantation. 2000; 70(12):1718–1721.
93. Huang SY, Chueh HY, Shaw SW, et al. Sonographic diagnosis of fetal malformations associated with mycophenolate mofetil exposure in utero. American Journal of Obstetrics and Gynecology. 2008;199(2):e6–e8.
94. Pilarski LM, Yacyshyn BR, Lavarovits AI. Analysis of peripheral blood lymphocyte populations and immune function from children exposed to cyclosporine or azathioprine in utero. Transplantation. 1994;57:133–144.
95. Di Paolo S, Schena A, Morrone L, et al. Immunologic evaluation during the first year of life of infants born to cyclosporine-treated kidney transplant recipients: analysis of lymphocyte subpopulation and immunoglobulin serum levels. Transplantation. 2000;69:2049–2054.
96. Barrou BM, Gruessner AC, Sutherland DER, et al. Pregnancy after pancreas transplantation in the cyclosporine era. Transplantation. 1998;65:524–527.
97. Wilson GA, Coscia LA, McGrory CH, et al. National Transplantation Pregnancy Registry: postpregnancy graft loss among female pancreas-kidney recipients. Transplantation Proceedings. 2001;33:1667–1668.
98. Jain AB, Shapiro R, Scantlebury VP, et al. Pregnancy after kidney and kidney-pancreas transplantation under tacrolimus: a single center's experience. Transplantation. 2004;77(6):897–902.
99. McGrory CH, Groshek MA, Sollinger HW, et al. Pregnancy outcomes in female pancreas-kidney recipients. Transplantation Proceedings. 1999;31:652–653.
100. Bramham K, Lightstone L, Taylor J, et al. Pregnancy in pancreas-kidney recipients: report of three cases and review of the literature. Obstetric Medicine. 2010;3:73–77.
101. Koyama S, Tomimatsu T, Kanagawa T, et al. Successful pregnancy after simultaneous pancreas-kidney transplantation from a brain-dead donor: the first case report in Japan. Journal of Obstetrics and Gynaecology Research. 2011;37(11): 1711–1716.
102. Laifer SA, Darby MJ, Scantlebury VP, et al. Pregnancy and liver transplantation. Obstetrics and Gynecology. 1990;76(6):1083–1088.
103. Jabiry-Zieniewicz Z, Cyganek A, Luterek K, et al. Pregnancy and delivery after liver transplantation. Transplantation Proceedings. 2005;37(2):1197–1200.
104. Nagy S, Bush MC, Berkowitz R, et al. Pregnancy outcome in liver transplant recipients. Obstetrics and Gynecology. 2003;102(1):121–128.
105. Armenti VT, Herrine SK, Radomski JS, et al. Pregnancy after liver transplantation. Liver Transplantation. 2000;6(6):671–685.
106. Christopher V, Al-Chalabi T, Richardson PD, et al. Pregnancy outcome after liver transplantation: a single-center experience of 71 pregnancies in 45 recipients. Liver Transplantation. 2006;12:1138–1143.
107. Heneghan MA, Selzner M, Yoshida EM, et al. Pregnancy and sexual function in liver transplantation. Journal of Hepatology. 2008;49(4):507–519.
108. Ramirez CB, Maley WR, Doria C, et al. Pregnancy outcomes in female liver recipients transplanted under the age of 21. American Journal of Transplantation. 2010;10(4):459.
109. Bonanno C, Dove L. Pregnancy after liver transplantation. Seminars in Perinatology. 2007;31:348–353.
110. Cundy TF, O'Grady JG, Williams R. Recovery of menstruation and pregnancy after liver transplantation. Gut. 1990;31(3):337–338.
111. Jain AB, Reyes J, Marcos A, et al. Pregnancy after liver transplantation with tacrolimus immunosuppression: a single center's experience update at 13 years. Transplantation. 2003;76(5):827–832.
112. Coscia LA, Constantinescu S, Moritz MJ, et al. Report from the National Transplantation Pregnancy Registry (NTPR): outcomes of pregnancy after transplantation. In: Terasaki PI, Cecka JM, editors. Clinical Transplants 2010. Los Angeles, CA: Terasaki Foundation Laboratory; 2011: 65–85.
113. Coffin CS, Shaheen AA, Burak KW, et al. Pregnancy outcomes among liver transplant recipients in the United States: a nationwide case-control analysis. Liver Transplantation. 2010;16(1):56–63.
114. Lai CL, Ratziu V, Yuen MF, et al. Viral hepatitis B. Lancet. 2003;362: 2089–2094.
115. Ferrero S, Lungaro P, Bruzzone BM, et al. Prospective study of mother-to-infant transmission of hepatitis C virus: a 10-year survey (1990–2000). Acta Obstetricia et Gynecologica Scandinavica. 2003;82(3):229–234.
116. Hunt SA, Haddad F. The changing face of heart transplantation. Journal of the American College of Cardiology. 2008;52(8):587–598.
117. Wu DW, Wilt J, Restaino S. Pregnancy after thoracic organ transplantation. Seminars in Perinatology. 2007;31:354.
118. Wagoner LE, Taylor DO, Olsen SL, et al. Immunosuppressive therapy, management and outcome of heart transplant recipients during pregnancy. Journal of Heart and Lung Transplantation. 1993;12:993–1000.
119. Metcalfe J, McAnulty JH, Ueland K. Cardiovascular physiology. Clinical Obstetrics and Gynecology. 1981;24:693–695.
120. Hunt S, Burch M, Bhat G, et al. The international society of heart and lung transplantation guidelines for the care of heart transplant recipients Task force 3: Long-term care of heart transplant recipients. Journal of Heart and Lung Transplantation. 2010;29(8):914–956.
121. Hunt SA. Pregnancy in heart transplant recipients: a good idea? Journal of Heart and Lung Transplantation. 1991;10:499–503.

122. Cowan SW, Coscia LA, Philips LZ, et al. Pregnancy outcomes in female heart and heart-lung transplant recipients. Transplantation Proceedings. 2002;34: 1855–1856.
123. O'Boyle PJ, Smith JD, Danskine AJ, et al. De Novo HLA sensitization and antibody mediated rejection following pregnancy in a heart transplant recipient. American Journal of Transplantation. 2010;10:180–183.
124. Kazmin A, Garcia-Bournissen F, Koren G. Risks of statin use during pregnancy: a systematic review. Journal d'Obstetrique et Gynecologie du Canada. 2007; 29(11):906–908.
125. Sifontis NM, Constantinescu S, Coscia LA, et al. Long-term survival in female heart transplant recipients following pregnancy. American Journal of Transplantation. 2009;S2:198A.
126. Gyi KM, Hodson ME, Yacoub MY. Pregnancy in cystic fibrosis lung transplant recipients: case series and review. Journal of Cystic Fibrosis. 2006;5: 171–175.
127. Guerra J, Kozlowski S, Matsumoto C, et al. Male and female fertility after intestinal transplantation. 2011. Presented at the XII International Intestinal Transplant Symposium, Washington, D.C.
128. Thiagarajan KD, Easterling T, Davis C, et al. Breast-feeding by a cyclosporine-treated mother. Obstetrics and Gynecology. 2001;97(5):816–818.
129. French AE, Soldin SJ, Soldin OP, et al. Milk transfer and neonatal safety of tacrolimus. Annals of Pharmacotherapy. 2003;37:815–818.
130. Gardiner SJ, Begg EJ. Breastfeeding during tacrolimus therapy. Obstetrics and Gynecology. 2006;107:453–455.
131. Morton A. Cyclosporine and lactation. Correspondence in Nephrology. 2011;16:249–250.
132. Bramham K, Chusney G, Lee J, et al. Tacrolimus and breastfeeding: how safe is it? Journal of the American Society of Nephrology. 2011;22:206A.
133. Armenti VT, Moritz MJ, Cardonick EH, et al. Immunosuppression in pregnancy. Choices for infant and maternal health. Drugs. 2002;62(16):2361–2375.
134. McKay DB, Josephson MA. Pregnancy in recipients of solid organs-effects on mother and child. New England Journal of Medicine. 2006;354:1281–1293.
135. Rudolph JE, Schweizer RT, Bartus SA. Pregnancy in renal transplant patients. Transplantation. 1979;27(1):26–29.
136. Kozlowska-Boszko B, Lao M, Gaciong Z, et al. Chronic rejection as a risk factor for deterioration of renal allograft function following pregnancy. Transplantation Proceedings. 1997;29:1522–1523.
137. Toma H, Tanabe K, Tokumoto T, et al. Pregnancy in women receiving renal dialysis or transplantation in Japan: a nationwide survey. Nephrology, Dialysis, Transplantation. 1999;14:1511–1516.
138. Källén B, Westgren M, Aberg A, et al. Pregnancy outcome after maternal organ transplantation in Sweden. BJOG. 2005;112(7):904–909.
139. Lindheimer MD, Katz AI. Gestation in women with kidney disease: prognosis and management. In: Lindheimer MD, Davison JM (eds): Bailliere's Clinical Obstetrics and Gynaecology. 1994;8(2):387–404.
140. Armenti VT, Jarrell BE, Radomski JS, et al. National Transplantation Pregnancy Registry (NTPR): cyclosporine dosing and pregnancy outcome in female renal transplant recipients. Transplantation Proceedings. 1996;28:2111–2112.
141. Gaughan WJ, Coscia LA, Dunn SR, et al. National Transplantation Pregnancy Registry: relationship of transplant to conception interval to pregnancy outcome in cyclosporine-treated female kidney recipients. American Journal of Transplantation. 2001;1:S377.
142. Kim HW, Seok HJ, Kim TH, et al. The experience of pregnancy after renal transplantation: pregnancies even within postoperative 1 year may be tolerable. Transplantation. 2008;85:1412–1419.
143. Cooper WO, Hernandez-Diaz S, Arbogast PG, et al. Major congenital malformations after first-trimester exposure to ACE inhibitors. New England Journal of Medicine. 2006;354:2443–2451.
144. Conte D, Fraquelli M, Prati D, et al. Prevalence and clinical course of chronic hepatitis C virus (HCV) infection and rate of HCV vertical transmission in a cohort of 15,250 pregnant women. Hepatology. 2000;31(3):751–755.
145. Wong SY, Remington JS. Toxoplasmosis in pregnancy. Clinical Infectious Diseases. 1994;18:853–862.
146. Buszta C, Steinmuller DR, Novick AC, et al. Pregnancy after donor nephrectomy. Transplantation. 1985;40:651.
147. Jones JW, Acton RD, Elick B, et al. Pregnancy following kidney donation. Transplantation Proceedings. 1993;25:3082.
148. Wrenshall LE, McHugh L, Felton P, et al. Pregnancy after donor nephrectomy. Transplantation. 1996;62:1934–1936.
149. Reisæter VA, Roiselien J, Henriksen T, et al. Pregnancy and birth after kidney donation: the Norwegian experience. American Journal of Transplantation. 2008;9:820–824.
150. Ibrahim HN, Akkina SK, Leister E, et al. Pregnancy outcomes after kidney donation. American Journal of Transplantation. 2009;9(4):825–834.
151. Nevis IF, Garg AX. Donor Nephrectomy Outcomes Research (DONOR) maternal and fetal outcomes after living kidney donation. Network. American Journal of Transplantation. 2009;9(4):661–668.
152. DelMonico F, et al. A report of the Amsterdam forum on the care of the live kidney donor: data and medical guidelines. Transplantation. 2005;79:S53–S66.
153. Josephson MA. Transplantation: pregnancy after kidney donation: more questions than answers. Nature Reviews Nephrology. 2009;5(9):495–497.
154. Nayak-Rao S. Pregnancy after kidney donation—placing things in perspective. Saudi Journal of Kidney Diseases and Transplantation. 2011;22(3):552–553.
155. Soyama A, Eguchi S, Takatsuki M, et al. Pregnancy and delivery after partial liver donation for living-donor liver transplantation. Transplantation. 2007;84(2):283.

第 98 章 特批用于移植的药物

Winston A. Ally, Avinash Agarwal

引言

美国食品药品监督管理局(FDA)参与调控了超过1万亿美金的产品,包括80%的食品供应到医疗产品、电子产品、生物制剂以及化妆品等的调控。在这些受调控的产品中,食品占4660亿,药品占2750亿,化妆品占600亿[1]。美国FDA通过严格有力的审批监控制度来保护其公民免受伤害,并期望以快速、高效的方式完成审批,同时又能够兼顾发现潜在的安全以及未知不良事件。由于科技的进步,要求这一组织以及它的法规构架需要不停地更新改进,以应对日新月异的需求。

本章将简述FDA的工作模式以及药物审批过程,并以免疫抑制药物的复杂性作为一个突出例子。每个国家都有其独有的规定,以便管理审批过程,但其中的主体部分在大部分国家中还是相似的。本部分将针对那些从FDA获得一项或多项移植适应证的产品做一个简要总结,并根据每种被批准的药物列出建议。但这实际上并不是普通药物转化至临床应用的常规流程。事实上,临床应用中的药物疗法是许多药物的混合制剂,而一些"脱标"的药物实际上并未经过审批。基于药物机制提出的可能的药物疗效其实非常重要,但目标人群以及特殊用途的受限就需要对药物的临床实际效应做一定的筛查。本章以及涵盖脱标药物的第101章,其中所列的药物机制在第17章中也有提及,同时有关的临床实践的应用在许多器官术后管理和治疗专题的章节中均有提及。FDA审批过程中的临床相关研究往往是首先需要考虑的问题,因此第135章中的临床研究设计也应与本章结合起来一起探讨。

FDA 的革新

1902年以前,美国政府在注册药物管理中的作用非常小。当时缺乏针对临床疗效的法律,没有管理制度,也没有任何标准。1820年美国药典发布,这是首个官方认证的有关药品管理的制度。美国药典为医生和药剂师们制订了药物剂量和纯度等方面的标准。针对美军在墨西哥受劣质奎宁影响的事件,1848年,美国首个药品监督管理法《进口药品法案》颁布。该法案明确要求未达标的药物产品必须经由实验室严格检测,并对其进行销毁。

FDA的起源通常可以追溯到美国农业化学部[2]。1883年,在当时部门首席化学家Harvey W. Wiley的领导下,该部门开始对国家的食品和药品进行研究调查。通过规范化的人体临床研究,他证实了当时的美国有大量的药物质量不合格以及产品标签缺失。在Wiley博士的努力下,特别是Upton Sinclair编写的《丛林》(描写腐朽的肉类产业)的出版,美国开始意识到现有食品工业的危害性。1902年,在圣路易斯的一个小研究室里,一头名叫Jim的退休奶牛被用于开发并生产白喉抗毒素,然而很不幸,它感染了破伤风被人道毁灭。与此同时,通过它生产开发的白喉抗毒素却并未经过破伤风检测,而药品的使用直接导致十多名学龄期儿童因使用感染血清而死亡。这一事件直接促成了《病毒、血清、毒素法案》(《生物制剂控制法案》)的通过。

1906年,国会通过了罗斯福总统签署的第一份食品药物监管法律《美国纯食品和药品法》(USPDA,也称为Wiley法)。Wiley法案禁止销售被污染的食品或错配的药物，而依据则来自产品标签。随后，在 1927 年，USDA 下的化学工业部门重组，命名为食品药品杀虫剂组织，也就是 FDA 的前身[3]。但遗憾的是，根据相关的司法规定，FDA 只能对那些明显违反说明书生产的产品进行质量管理，对于产品虚假广告却无能为力。1937 年，一场悲剧改变了现代医疗的命运[4]。在危及生命的感染治疗方面，磺胺类被视为一种奇迹药物。遗憾的是它的口味实在不怎么样。Bristol TN 的 S.E. Massingill 有限公司开发出了一种名为“磺胺类长生不老药”的覆盆子饮品。但它用到了二甘醇来溶解磺胺类，超过 100 人死于这种药品。

这一事件导致美国医疗卫生相关法律中最为全面的法律条款中的一条诞生——《联邦食品、药品和化妆品法案》(FDCA)。这项法案要求所有新药在进入市场前都必须经过政府有关部门的测试并通过新药审批(NDA)。FDCA 至今为止仍是 FDA 的工作基础。1962 年，Kefauver-Harris 法案起草完成[5]。这项法案的关键在于所有的新药审批中都必须证明新药的疗效，同时也必须提供新药安全性方面的数据。此外，在进行人体试验之前，都必须取得患者的知情同意。这一新法案的实施直接导致新药的研发周期延长。1984 年，国会又讨论通过了《价格竞争及专利保护法案》，也称为 Waxman-Hatch 法案[6]。这项法案主要包括两方面的内容。第一个方面是鼓励研发新型药，只要新型药物的主要成分、药效以及剂量等方面与传统药物没有明显差异，便可以较快地通过审批进入市场。第二个方面则是通过延长专利时间，来弥补药物在审批过程中所消耗的时间，从而鼓励新药的研发工作。

获得性免疫缺陷综合征(AIDS)的流行使得新药审批过程过长的现象得到了足够的重视[7]。来自 AIDS 的压力是促使相关法案改革的动力。1992 年，美国国会起草通过了《处方药使用收费标准》(PDUFA)，允许 FDA 从中扣取一定的金额用于完善相关的审批流程[8]。为了能够保证持续有效地收取该项费用，FDA 相应地对审核过程中的某些环节做了一定的加速调整。对那些主要开发针对“孤儿病”的药物或者是非公众需求药物的小型药物研发企业，该项法案予以了一定的豁免权。1997 年，为了进一步发展以满足不断增长的公民需求，国会通过了《FDA 现代化法案》，提高了 FDA 的权威性及其管理范围[8]。

目前，FDA 有权启动加速审批和快速跟踪程序，以加快急救药物的上市。快速发展项目是 FDA 推出的针对那些承诺能有效解决一些尚没有较好治疗方案、严重影响生命健康的医学难题的药物研发的特殊快速程序。现状使得 FDA 经常开会讨论新药的研发，以达到快速审批以及患者的参与。FDA 可以允许试用一种药物，但会事先合理地定义临床上的直接或间接终点事件。一个较常用的方法就是先确立一个生物标记分子，然后去研究药物对该项生物标记分子的实际作用。例如在肿瘤治疗方面，其中一种就是比较肿瘤大小以及肿瘤标志物，如前列腺特异性抗原(PSA)的变化情况。相比较传统的如患者生存率这样需要大样本长期随访的临床终点指标，这种监测指标截然不同。

FDA 的架构

正如上文所介绍的，FDA 成立于 1906 年，是美国人类健康服务机构(HHS)下的一个子机构。其他子机构则包括有 CDC、NIH 以及医疗保险和医疗补助服务中心(CMS)。FDA 由多个办事中心组成，并由一名由总统任命的经参议院审核通过的专员领导。图 98.1 展示了其办公组成以及职责。FDA 的总部位于马里兰州的西尔弗斯普林斯，它的大部分办事机构也在那里。FDA 目前有六大中心：药物研究审计中心(CDER)、生物制剂审计中心(CBER)、放射医疗及设备中心(CDRH)、食品安全与应用营养中心(CFSAN)、烟草制品中心和兽医中心。还有一些其他的办公室，它们都承担着各自唯一的药物研发工作，如特殊程序和产业联合办公室、监察专员办公室、孤儿产品发展办公室，还有法律事务办公室，用以建立并维护组织的标准和规程。所有这些组织机构都有它特定的角色定义。然而，随着科技的快速发展，这些组织机构中很可能存在一定的管辖重叠，这也是正常情况。药品作为小分子产品归属 CDER 的管辖，但其他机构的参与管理也是必需的。生物制剂的生产来源于生物本身的一些成分物质，如抗毒素、血清、血液制品、重组蛋白和细胞疗法。生物制剂生产商必须持有 CDER 颁布的许可令。CBER 负责多克隆抗体制剂和血液/组织衍生产品，如丙种球蛋白或疫苗。如果某个药物中的一部分被认定为需要一种设备，那么它也需要受到 CDRH 的监管。

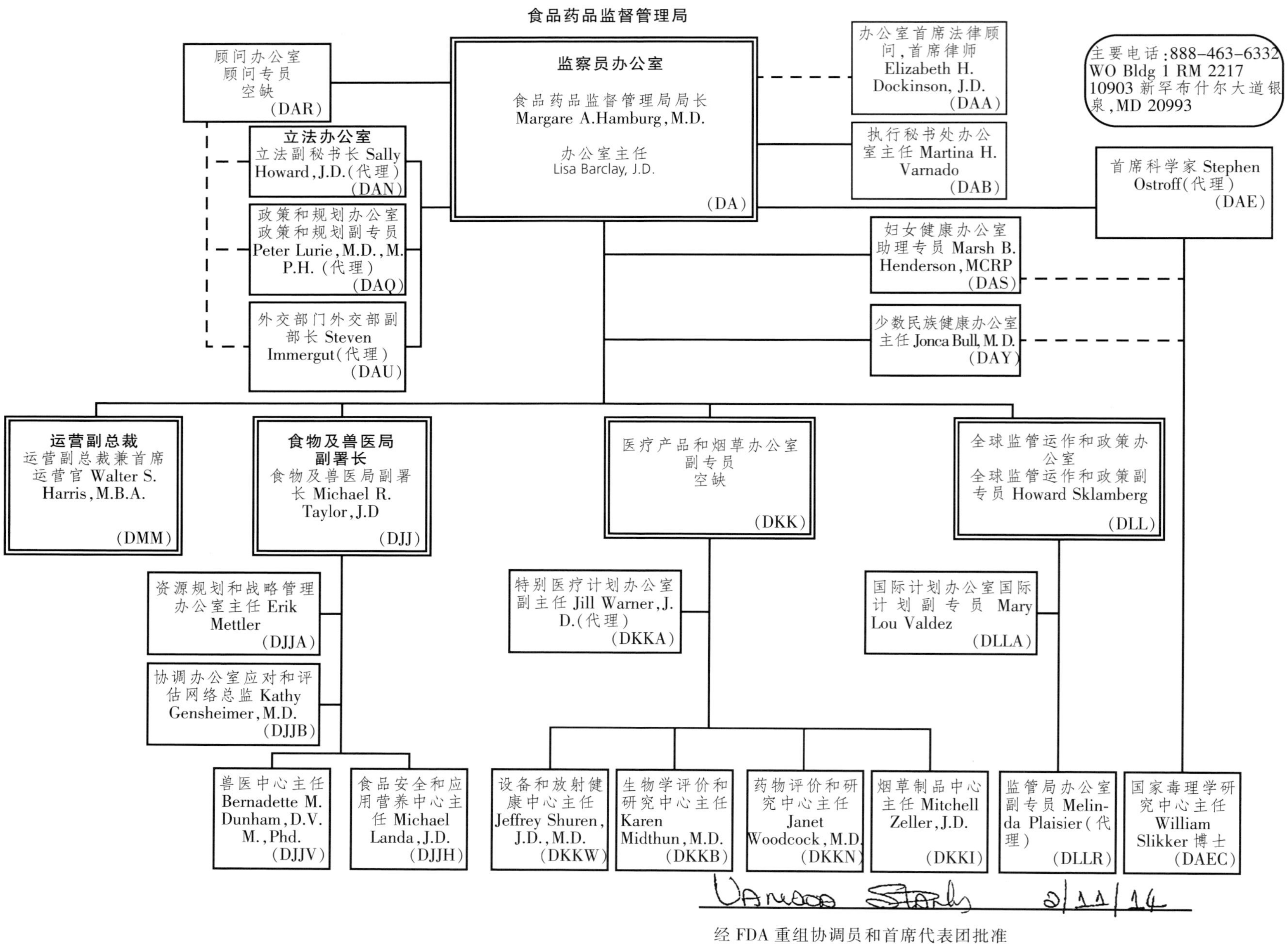

图 98.1 FDA 组织图。(Reproduced from http://www.fda.gov/downloads/AboutFDA/CentersOffices/OrganizationCharts/UCM291886.pdf.)

新药的研发过程

FDA 认为只要是有药效的物质,不论是为了诊断、治疗还是预防,它都属于“新”药的范畴[9]。关键在于预期用途或反映其基本组成以及必要的安全性及有效性研究证明的产品说明。一种“新”药的定义同样也适用于那些已经通过 FDA 审批的药品，只要它有新的用途、新的给药方式,或者一些其他的有意义的临床应用[10]。在这样的情况下,新产品必须经过适当的物质检验以及 FDA 的审批。致力于临床药物开发的项目其新药申请都需要经历临床前研究(如毒理、动物实验等)。简单地说,程序起始于非临床研究,包括体外研究和动物实验。这些都要在三期的临床研究前完成。美国联邦法规(CFR)中的相关法规规定了其基本的充分控制性研究,包括有详细的目的、终点事件、变量、合理的数据分析以及合格标准。法规同样包括随机实验以及盲法实验的重要性。尤其重要的是,FDA 通过 CFR 和 FDA 指南明确了特殊定量数据对效果的证明(然而安全性和危险因素的测定往往依赖于定性研究或半定量研究)。FDA 将回顾所有这些数据,以判断是否予以通过审核。药物同样要经过四期检验,也被称为上市后监测,这就可能包括后期教育以及患者监护等。

非临床研究

如果某个药物分子的临床安全性尚未得到证实，那么就需要进行临床前的动物体内及体外实验研究，这也是新药研发过程中重要的第一步。其主要目的在于针对药物的安全性以及早期人体相关研究的重要数据做一个收集[11]。最开始是药物的发现阶段,也就是对混合药物中可能有药理作用的药物做一个筛选。然后大量的体外实验用以阐明该药物的药理作用以及它的药效学等。而药代动力学研究则需要在多种物种中进行研究,从而为药物的半衰期等提供一定的数据基础。这些大量实验主要是为了阐明药物的吸收、分布、代谢过程和排泄时间等(ADME 描述)。毒理学研究对药物的长短期生理影响有很重要的研究意义。半数致死率(代表能导致半数实验动物死亡的剂量)已经逐渐被增加剂量的单剂量法所替代。其目的是为了明确其没有明显不良反应的剂量范围(NOAEL)或者是在产生必要的药理学作用的前提下而又没有明显不良反应的用量。FDA 对非临床研究没有做明确的规范要求。但为了保证数据质量，所有实验室都必须遵从实验室管理规范(GLP)。管理规范对组织、个人、维护以及设备操作流程都做了明确的规定[12]。FDA 将通过实地考察的办法来监管管理规范的执行情况。

试验性临床新药申请

FDA 对临床研究的监控非常小心，以保证人用产品的安全,同时也保证了最高质量的研究数据。一旦临床前研究数据已经积攒了足够多的新药药理资料,同时证明它在人体试验中相对比较安全时，那么将进入试验性新药申请(IND)阶段。IND 是申请 FDA 开展临床研究调查的一项流程。从技术上来说,IND 就是为了获得联邦食品药品化妆品法案(FD&C)对新药贸易的豁免权。简单来说,IND 是将一种未经批准的药物合法化的交易。IND 申请需要向 FDA 提供一些必需的数据,以便说明目前设计的实验安全性是否合理。如果你想对一种尚未经过审批的新药进行相应的临床研究(如新的适应证、新剂型以及其他药物的联用)，那么 IND 就显得必不可少了[13]。如果符合以下条件,根据规章制度就能豁免申请药物的研究[14]。

(1)产品的标签广告没有改变或不是为了新的适应证。

(2)不涉及新的给药途径或剂量水平或患者人群。

(3)研究严格遵照 IRB 和知情同意。

开发商需向 FDA 提供的 IND 相关材料主要包括:介绍性说明、基本研究方案、综合性条款、研究手册(临床前研究,如动物药理毒理学研究、药理作用和药代动力学研究)、产业信息化和研究人员信息。提交材料后,申请者必须等待 30 天后才能开始进行临床研究。FDA 实际上并不会特意去批准一项 IND，但一旦有任何异议提出，将会组织一个临床会议。在每个人体研究之前，必须先制订一份相应的条款并送机构审查委员会(IRB)审查。IRB 是医学以及伦理研究委员会,主要审查临床研究并被委托建立有效的标准，以保证人身安全。一旦 IRB 审核并通过了包括知情同意书在内的必需文件和研究流程协议,人体试验便可正式开始。临床研究一般情况下根据其目的的不同分为三期。

Ⅰ期临床研究——首次应用于人的研究，主要被设计用于明确临床前研究的数据结果是否适用于人体。它的目的在于明确该药物在健康人体的药代动力学以及药物安全的给药管理。这项研究将关注是否有预想的药理作用，尽管它的统计学设计往往没有明确这一点。Ⅱ期临床研究则将药物应用于疾病或相关疾病状态的人群。这也表明了工作的中心从安全性转向了有效性。研究有时会涉及上百人的受试群体。这一期研究的目的主要在于明确新药是否有预期的对疾病的治疗效果。比较典型的做法就是将多种治疗方案与安慰剂进行比较。同样的，此项研究的结果将用于分析并制订下一步的研究方案。Ⅱ期临床研究中有一个关键部分就是观察治疗效果的观察量级，这将用于决定Ⅲ期临床研究的样本量大小。在Ⅱ期临床研究的最后，FDA 和申请者将进行会谈，讨论已有的结果并计划下一步的研究内容。

最后，最关键的Ⅲ期临床研究将对比开发的新药和已有的 FDA 审核通过的药物。此项临床研究是为了开发者编写适应人群以及临床方案相关标签。这些研究往往非常巨大，并且需要成百上千的受试者。大量的受试者使得研究者能够从中发现可能的新的治疗方向。在此项研究结束时，研究者必须提供大量证据或者有严格的质量管理证据，使得专家们能够足够公正地得出药物对相关疾病有实际作用的结论。除少数例外情况，针对某种药物，至少有两项研究必须通过 FDA 的审核，从而得到科学的重现。然而，这两项研究的方案设计不能相同，它们将在不同疾病严重程度的人群中重现，或者说在不同类型供体的移植病例中。一旦对所有研究数据都进行了汇总分析，且受试药物达到了既定的Ⅲ期临床研究目的，开发者就能够向 FDA 申请批准该药上市。

明确药物疗效的 FDA 标准指南

鉴于一份药物审批文件的重要组成部分是关于其药效的描述，实验设计的重点关注部分以及前瞻点都应该聚焦在这一点上。法律法规以及规章制度能够大体上描述预期要求，但对其中词汇的解读也同样非常重要。出于对管理实施的负责，FDA 需要经常对所制订的法规以及管理制度进行检验。在某些情况下，FDA 会发行指南文件来阐明它目前的思想理念。指导并没有法律强制性，也并不意味着 FDA 会相应地坚持某些方针，但可以提供一些重要的视野，这对一些利益相关者挑选兴趣方向有很大帮助。

迄今为止，没有指南特别指明了器官移植临床研究的设计。但 FDA 出台了一些有关临床证据的指南性文章。如 1998 年发表的《产业指南：为临床药物生物制剂提供临床证据》阐述了证据质量问题对支持效果的重要性，其中就包括常见的两种不同实验结果佐证，当然只用一种实验方案有时也是适用的[15]。另外还有三个指南，《人用药品注册技术要求国际协调会议》(ICH)中值得一提的 ICH E8(临床研究共识)，它由美、欧、日本三方共同协定，还包括 ICH E9(临床研究数据准则)和 ICH E10(临床研究对照组选择及相关问题)，它们分别在 1997 年、1998 年和 2000 年发表[15]。这三份 ICH 文件为 FDA 审核多样的研究提供了可行的关注点，包括对非劣质并发症控制的讨论。

优势及非劣效性研究

对药效的说明可以通过优势或非劣效性研究来证明。在预定的初期临床或替代终点的优势性实验中，要想说明产品的有效性需要利用统计学差异，通常用的是 95%置信区间。对此类实验设计的说明非常简单：如果终点事件能达到，那么我们就可以相对自信地认为研究表明产品有一定的作用效果。非劣效性实验（在 FDA 中更多地被称为等效性实验)，换句话说就是通过说明产品和有已知效果的产品比较，效果并没有大幅度下降，从而证明它的有效性。非劣效性研究旨在说明两种治疗方案之间的差异事实上非常小，从而证明新药的有效性。一项成功的优势性试验要求它的结果能够直接说明自身的有效性。非劣效性研究则建立于假设新药本身是有效果的基础上，而这些往往需要外部数据或历史信息的支持。

新药的申请

自从具有里程碑意义的 1983 年起，新药申请(NDA)已经成为美国药物发展的重要方式。开发商将提交数千页的文件内容，包括临床前和临床数据及分析、药物手册，以及其他许多不同领域的信息。当开发商准备上市药物之前，这其中的信息将成为其说明标签上内容的基础。一个高度专业化的专家小组将审核 NDA 并决定是否予以通过。审核流程差不多，但对生物制剂而言，生物制剂生产许可证(BLA)才更关键。对于一份 NDA 所必须包含的内容，食品药品化妆品法案和美国联邦法规(CFR)第 21 条已经有了概述。所有申请书都必须提供足够明确的证据，以便审核人员能够判断药物是否安全，是否针对其开发目的而言有明确的作用效果，药物的优势是否大于其劣势，药物标签的合理性，药物开发商的胜任能力等。此外，FDA 制订了大量的指导文件，用以说明目前在 NDA 审核过程中的关注方向等[15]。正如前文提到的，《处方药使用收费标准》(PDUFA) 要求快速更有据可循的同时能够建立一个时间表，以对开发商提出一定的反馈。

时间表起始于 NDA 送达文档管理室，而 FDA 有 60 天的时间决定是否对该项 NDA 进行审核。为建立一个 NDA 档案并开始审批流程，开发商支付相应的处方药费用，目前而言（2013 年），针对需要临床数据的申请要支付 1 958 800 美元，不需要临床数据支持的申请则需要 979 400 美元[15]。每项 NDA 都将指派一名项目负责人，对项目申请做一个初步审核，以保证所有重要的材料都已经提供，没有缺失。接下来，项目负责人会将该 NDA 材料转发给不同的审查小组成员，其中可能包括临床医生、药剂师、毒理学家、统计学家和化学家，由他们来进行第二次评审，来决定是否对其进行正式审查（通常在收到 NDA 后 45 天内完成）。最后，该 NDA 将受到正式的审查，包括检查药品生产站点和潜在的临床试验地点。所有小组成员都将提交一份手写的评价材料来声明他对申请的态度。“批准”代表该药物已经可以准备上市了。“可批准”代表开发商需要在上市前解决一些问题。最后审查小组可以给出“不批准”，但需要予以说明理由。

对 FDA 下的 CDER 和 CBER 而言，开发商递交的 NDA 和 BLA 复申请有较高的优先级。FDA 中的资源系统能够对资源进行有效分配。为了对生产和组织负责，开发商将对那些对 NDA 或 BLA 有利的数据负责。该系统依靠经济压力促使开发商进行重要的实验研究，并提供相关数据以供审核。就 FDA 而言，此系统的一个重要结果就是申请决定了是否能被批准（包括很多其他修改标签的）。在 FDA 看来，对实体器官移植相关审核的批准最重要的一点就是开发商提供的申请。

可能公众会认为 FDA 批准一项产品可能基于它自身对该产品安全性和有效性的重复性研究。如果没有 FDA 对说明的批准，则说明申请没有提交完全或申请没有充分地阐明产品的安全性和有效性。在特殊情况下，FDA 可以要求开发商在处方药的标签和文字叙述部位予以黑框警示。这是 FDA 要求的最强烈警告，表示医学研究表明该药物具有严重甚至是危及生命的不良反应及重大风险[16]。

上市后监控

在过去十年中，许多药物在批准后出现了一系列安全问题，包括罗非考昔、罗格列酮和那他珠单抗。即使在 NDA 批准通过后，申请人必须对安全性和新报告的不良事件进行上市后监测。由于药物是基于良好对照的临床试验批准的，上市后监测可以进一步定义药物在被引入具有各种各样的医学状况的一般人群之后的安全性。2007 年，国会通过了 2007 年 FDA 现代化法案（FDAAA）的立法，其中包含新战略和安全计划，专门评估和最小化新药的风险。大会介绍了风险评估、缓解策略（REMS）和营销后要求（PMR）的概念，为 FDA 强制执行风险规避策略提供了更大的权限。

根据《联邦食品、药品和化妆品法案》第 505-1 部分，第Ⅸ条，第 A 款，第 901 节，FDA 有权要求一家公司在新药申请期间或在批准后的任何时间提交 REMS，以确保药物的好处大于其风险[17]。REMS 被定义为管理与使用药物相关的已知或潜在严重风险的策略。所有 REMS 必须有特定的目标，元素构成实现目标的工具。REMS 的元素可以包括以下中的一个或多个：药物指南和（或）患者档案插页（PPI）、医疗保健提供者的通信计划和确保安全使用的元素（ETASU）。药物指南旨在为潜在患者提供有关产品安全使用的信息。指南的目的是通过潜在地影响患者使用或继续使用药物的决定，或者当具体说明可以帮助改善患者的依从性时来防止严重不良事件的发生。PPI 旨在指导患者安全使用药物产品。每次分配产品时，必须向患者提供药物指导，而不是 PPI[18]。通信计划旨在通过各种通信手段，包括给提供者的信函或材料，教育医疗保健提供者适当和安全地使用产品。最后，当患者对具有已知风险的产品的安全问题不清楚时，可利用 ETASU。ETASU 可能包括医疗保健提供者的特殊认证，其规定药品或药物的特别认证，或产品分发的限制(限于登记在注册表中的患者或在特定治疗设置中)。作为 REMS 的一部分，开发商必须展示一个上市后计划，以监测潜在风险，并向 FDA 提供评估频率不低于批准后 18 个月、3 年和 7 年这样的频次。本报告应评论 REMS 要素在实现其目标方面的成功。在 2008—2011 年期间，大约 35%的

NDA需要REMS,虽然大多数只需要一个药物指南。在178个REMS中，有48个REMS需要一个通信计划，只有21个具有ETASU[15]。在需要REMS的仿制药的设置中，创新药和通用药物将共享相同的REMS，包括ETASU所需的系统。

孤儿药

和上述大多数方法相比，批准孤儿药的过程具有一些显著差异。孤儿药物是用于治疗在美国折磨少于200 000名患者的“罕见”疾病的药物。重要的是,器官移植被认为是标准的孤儿药适应证,因此,该政策与为移植适应证开发的每种药物相关。此外，对于药企来说,新药研发的收益往往有限,很难填补由于新药开发的超高成本。1993年的《孤儿药法案》为赞助者提供财政奖励,以促进这些必要的新药发展,如用于临床研究的联邦赠款、用于发展的税收抵免,以及获得联邦批准的赞助商的7年市场独占性。

缩短新药申请周期

FDA通过简化新药申请(ANDA)途径批准仿制药。制造商能够提交此缩略申请，以便一旦原始产品的专利过期,批准将立即生效。与NDA的申请不同,ANDA的申请不需要包括临床试验数据来确立安全性和有效性。相反,FDA基于建立仿制药与被批准的创新产品的生物等效性和药物等效性的数据批准ANDA的应用。重要的是要注意，等价被定义为没有统计学上的显著差异。FDA已经设置为药代动力学数据的范围为新产品PK是传统产品的80%~125%。移植领域最近进入了一个时代,其中主要药剂,如霉酚酸酯(MMF)和他克莫司的使用已经变得普遍。

实体器官移植特有的药物开发挑战

在移植免疫抑制维持试验中考虑疗效终点

自环孢素出现以来，批准为初始或维持免疫抑制剂的产品通常使用急性排斥反应、移植物损失和死亡的组合终点作为主要功效终点。在移植文献中,这种组合终点有时被称为“传统的FDA联合终点”。这样的分析已经用于确立更新的试剂的有效性，但值得注意的是,FDA不认为这样的分析代表“FDA”终点或“组合”终点。相反,在那些审查期间,FDA支持急性排斥用于调节免疫应答治疗失败的显著临床事件。从FDA的角度来看,这些试验的终点是急性排斥反应。缺失数据的患者,无论是由于死亡、移植物丢失或随访丢失,都被认定为有急性排斥反应。

在移植免疫抑制剂研究中，将急性排斥反应作为终点事件在公共认可方面有着一定的局限性。终点不对临床上重要的元素,如排斥发作的严重性进行权衡。目前已经提出使用替代终点，如基于肾小球滤过率(GFR)和活检,可以增强对免疫抑制方案的移植试验中患者结果的评价。事实上,例如在审查贝拉西普和依维莫司期间,GFR有被考虑作为终点事件。

FDA开放审查替代终点，既用于预防急性排斥反应,也用于更新的适应证。然而应该基于充分良好控制的调查建立疗效任务，与临床医生使用随机对照试验确定最佳治疗方案。主要功效终点的最重要功能是提供研究药物的有效性的定量证据。它应该能够清楚地证明测试产品的贡献。不论临床重要性,不是所有的结果测量在所有情况下都非常适合于此目的。急性排斥终点仍然是有相关性的，因为来自过去试验的丰富经验和数据告诉我们使用这些终点可用于新试验的设计和解释。

通过基于急性排斥的终点测量，为目前可用的免疫抑制维持方案提供了相当有效的功效。但在所有药物中,它们与已知的毒性(包括对GFR的可逆和不可逆减少以及在组织病理学上显而易见的一些特定肾毒性)相关。考虑到市售产品的效力,更新产品有效性通常使用旨在确定非劣效性而不是测试产品优越性的试验来建立。非劣效性试验用以验证新产品不比阳性对照差太多。

为了执行一个有意义的非劣效性分析，必须知道该试验产品所期望达到的与阳性对照相对应的贡献效果。为了确定这种贡献,必须获得历史试验,通过比较接受阳性对照的患者和接受安慰剂的患者的结果来研究期望的终点。使用基于急性排斥的终点确定移植试验的非劣效性是有挑战性的,但有时是可能的,因为许多历史试验存在为这些终点捕获提供的可靠数据。使用新的终点事件建立非劣效性研究通常是不可能的,因为必要的历史数据往往不存在或不可用。

鉴于相关历史试验数据的缺乏，更新的终点通常必须依赖于设计用于测试研究剂相对于阳性对照更优异的试验。由于当前可用的治疗是有效的,证明实验产品比市售产品更有效具有挑战性。由于市售产品具有已知的毒性,这限制了它们的有用性,可以通过证明不存在相关毒性，使用新产品具有更好的研究结果。然而,在设计这些试验时必须小心:没有毒性本身不能构成试验产品的功效。如果某项结果与阳性对照的已知毒性混淆,结果可能不适合作为主要终点事件,以支持产品批准。

GFR 和 CAN 作为肾移植维持免疫抑制相关适应证功效终点的经验

肾移植试验中的 GFR 研究说明它不总是适合用作重要临床结果的终点事件。作为肾功能的量度,GFR 似乎代表了免疫抑制剂在肾移植中功效的合理量度:在没有有效免疫抑制的情况下，免疫介导的肾损伤将导致肾衰竭和 GFR 降低。事实上,FDA 认同这样的终点在安慰剂对照试验的设置中是可行的。然而,它通常用于临床试验中代替阳性对照中的钙调神经磷酸酶抑制剂。理论上,可以追求非劣效性试验设计,但需要可靠的安慰剂相关 GFR 数据结果。相反,开发商通常提出使用试验设计通过研究 GFR，以确立较新产品的优越性。但钙调神经磷酸酶抑制剂(特别是环孢素)会引起传入肾动脉的血管收缩,导致继发于血流动力学(非免疫抑制)作用的 GFR 的生理性降低。在随机分配的患者中观察到统计学上的 GFR 不一定能证明测试产品具有更大(或甚至相等)的功效。先前的试验设计的缺陷在于不排除在维持免疫抑制试验的情况下使用 GFR 作为主要功效终点；这样的试验应该依赖于能确保终点不被混淆的设计。

同种异体移植活检方案也被提议在维持免疫抑制方面作为替代疗效终点,但同样面临类似的挑战。开发商建议比较组织病理学诊断，如慢性同种异体移植肾病(CAN)。CAN 是一种非特异性改变,用于描述肾脏组织学的各种变化，认为它往往继发于免疫学和非免疫学损伤。部分历史试验数据已经提交和审查,使得非劣效性边界能通过规范的活检进行判定。此外，将 CAN 用于测试产品的优越性评判的试验设计的主要终点是有问题的,原因有两个:①钙调神经磷酸酶抑制剂毒性是肾脏非免疫学损伤的潜在来源之一；②CAN 诊断的临床意义是不确定的。如果 CAN 的发生率在某些情况下可归因于暴露于阳性对照组,则 CAN 的不存在不能证明测试试剂的功效。在免疫维持的临床试验中,应基于组织活检来制订药物的效益终点，这需要富有经验的临床组织病理学诊断,同时避免误解和混淆。

FDA 批准用于实体器官移植的产品

免疫抑制剂

本节的目的是简要回顾具有 FDA 批准适应证且目前在美国使用的免疫抑制剂。简而言之,除了介绍导致各自药物批准的临床试验的结果之外，还将回顾该药物处方信息的关键特征。读者将快速地注意到,大多数药物的批准指示明显比移植中药物的常见使用范围更有限。此外,对任何移植从业者来说显而易见的是,机构给药指南通常偏离批准的给药方式，事实上即使在移植中最适用且常见的适应证，也没有给出明确的方案。此外,在批准的标签中对随时间改变而改变给药量方面并没有明确指导，例如目前适用这些药物的患者,几年后通常减少给药,并没有任何明确的监管来批准这种操作。这些药物作用机制的综合评价以及关于和其他药物的“脱标”使用的更多细节将分别在第 17 章和第 101 章中讨论。关于器官移植后的管理在特定章节中描述了实际使用情况。有几种 FDA 批准的器官移植药物不予讨论，因为它们不再用于实体器官移植受体。这些药物包括马抗胸腺细胞球蛋白、达珠单抗和莫罗单抗-CD3。

硫唑嘌呤(Imuran)

硫唑嘌呤和类固醇被认为是器官移植自 20 世纪 60 年代初到 20 世纪 80 年代初免疫抑制的主要药物。基于 1968 年 3 月 Prometheus 实验室提交的 NDA 文件,FDA 批准了硫唑嘌呤的适用[19]。目前,通过已提交 ANDA 的几家公司硫唑嘌呤可作为通用药物。硫唑嘌呤是用于预防肾移植排斥的辅助治疗选择。根据处方信息,“超过 16 000 例移植的经验显示患者 5 年存活率为 35%~55%”[20]。这基于以下几个因素,包括供体、HLA 抗原的匹配、抗供体或抗 B 细胞同种抗原抗体以及在对照试验中未测试的其他变量。硫唑嘌呤被认为能够抑制细胞介导的超敏反应，并且导致抗体产生的改变,对建立的移植物排斥或次级反应几乎没有影响。硫唑嘌呤在儿科患者中的安全性和有效性尚未确定。

处方信息中建议给药从移植时开始每日 3~5mg/kg 作为初始剂量。血浆水平监测预测价值较小,因为硫唑嘌呤的代谢广泛,转化为 6-巯基嘌呤,并随后转化为硫嘌呤核苷酸。硫嘌呤 S-甲基转移酶(TPMT)水平降低的患者可能有严重威胁生命的风险，需要降低硫唑嘌呤的剂量。同时对所有患者进行全血细胞计数监测及 TPMT 基因分型或表型,可以用于识别患者风险。最后,导致 FDA 批准的用于肾移植的指示数据不一定反映当前移植药物情况的原因是因为处方信息不包含关于硫唑嘌呤与其他维持免疫抑制剂联合使用的信息[20]。

环孢素(Sandimmune/Neoral/Gengraf)

环孢素是一种强大的免疫抑制药物，在器官移植中作为第一个钙调神经磷酸酶抑制剂。使用环孢素的影响不仅发生在肾移植中，也发生于心脏和肝移植中。环孢素于 1983 年 11 月获得 FDA 批准生产口服和注射溶液,然而,由于其生物利用度差,在 1990 年和 1995 年分别开发和批准了新的制剂。环孢素的胶囊制剂在 1990 年由诺华公司(巴塞尔,瑞士)获得专利批准[21]。1995 年 FDA 批准诺华公司以 Neoral 为品牌名生产改进后的环孢素[22]。

环孢素和改良环孢素都用于预防肾脏、肝脏和心脏同种异体移植中的器官排斥。然而,在环孢素和修改后环孢素的适应证之间存在轻微的变化。环孢素的处方信息表明它总是与肾上腺皮质类固醇一起使用,并且可用于治疗先前用其他免疫抑制剂治疗的患者慢性排斥反应[23]。修改后的环孢素的处方信息表明它已经与硫唑嘌呤和皮质类固醇联合使用[24]。处方信息的差异也反映在两种药剂的临床药理学中。环孢素的临床药理学基于以下陈述：环孢素的确切作用机制未知，但“实验证据表明环孢素的有效性是由于细胞的 G0 或 G1 期中免疫活性淋巴细胞的特异性和可逆抑制周期”[23]。

环孢素和修改后环孢素的给药建议反映了制剂药代动力学性质的差异,并且可以肯定地说,在现代临床实践中很少遵循批准的给药方式。推荐在移植前 4~12h 施用 15mg/kg 初始口服剂量的环孢素,该单次日剂量应持续长达 2 周,随后是将每日剂量减少 5%,直至 3mg/(kg·d)[23]。修改后的环孢素可以在移植前或手术后 4~13h 给予,剂量范围为 7~9mg/(kg·d),以两个等分的剂量给予。应调整后续剂量,以获得目标环孢素血药浓度。尽管与环孢素相比,患者在任何给定的靶范围修饰后环孢素的作用更强，二者的波谷水平目标范围是相同的，因此修改后环孢素可利用较低靶标槽提供足够的免疫抑制。此外,使用 1:1 比例将患者从修改后的环孢素转化为环孢素可导致较低的环孢素血药浓度[24]。两种制剂的处方信息还包括肾上腺皮质类固醇的辅助治疗剂量建议,其有 2 个月的锥形化策略。虽然没有进行充分和良好控制的儿科研究，年龄为 6 个月的患者已经接受该药物,没有“不寻常的”不良反应。儿童给药建议基于药代动力学类似的成人剂量[23,24]。

环孢素的多重 ANDA 应用已被批准，利用环孢素和修改后环孢素作为参考产品。为了区分所有可用的产品,以下是用于每种制剂的完全通用名称。环孢素胶囊,USP 和环孢素口服溶液,USP 是指脂溶性的产品 Sandimmune®，而环孢素胶囊,USP 修饰和环孢素口服溶液,USP 修饰是指微乳液产品 Neoral®。品牌通用修改后环孢素可以商品名 Gengraf 获得,具有以下通用药物名称:环孢素胶囊,USP 修饰。

他克莫司

他克莫司是一种免疫抑制剂，在肝和肾移植中能显著改善临床结果。与其他药物不同，他克莫司在 1994 年首次获得 FDA 批准用于肝脏而不是肾脏同种异体移植受者[25]。1997 年,他克莫司的适应证收入肾移植同种异体移植受者。最后,2006 年,心脏同种异体移植也加入他克莫司的适应证中——这是他克莫司最新的适应证。自 2009 年以来,FDA 已批准了多种 ANDA 应用于他克莫司的仿制版本[26]。

FDA 批准他克莫司用于预防肾脏、肝脏和心脏移植中的器官排斥。他克莫司推荐与硫唑嘌呤或 MMF 和肾上腺皮质类固醇联合用于肾脏和心脏移植。对于肝移植患者，建议同时使用他克莫司与肾上腺皮质类固醇[27]。如处方信息中所述,他克莫司通过结合细胞内蛋白 FKBP12 抑制 T 淋巴细胞活化。然后该复合物与钙、钙调蛋白和钙调磷酸酶结合,以防止淋巴因子的形成,防止 T 淋巴细胞活化[27]。与环孢素一样,他克莫司的实际使用和其说明有一定偏差。

由于药代动力学个体间的显著性差异，他克莫司需要个体化给药,以达到最佳治疗效果。他克莫司的吸收程度与食物存在相关性。在使用他克莫司的小药代动力学研究中，发现给药后 10~12h 的血液水平或 Cmin 水平与 AUC 相关。他克莫司 99%与血浆蛋白结合,并通过肝脏细胞色素 P-450 系统,特别是 CYP3A4

进行代谢。一项对健康志愿者的小型研究使用放射性标记他克莫司,证明他克莫司 92.6%由粪便排除。他克莫司在儿童移植人群中的药代动力学研究有限，但在处方信息中包括了儿童肝移植给药建议。

FDA 批准的他克莫司给药建议对象包括成年心脏、肝和肾移植患者以及儿童肝移植患者,见表 98.1。所有剂量基于 mg/kg 体重，作为两个分开的剂量,每 12h 时间隔使用。处方信息包括起始剂量的他克莫司与个体化剂量滴定的目标全血浓度。此外,处方信息表明，非洲裔美国人和小儿肝移植患者可能需要更高剂量的他克莫司,以达到目标水平[27]。

如前所述，促成 1994 年最初 FDA 批准他克莫司的临床试验首先在肝移植中进行。两项前瞻性随机非盲法Ⅲ期多中心试验评估他克莫司方案的安全性和有效性。研究评估 12 个月的患者和移植物存活率,比较由他克莫司和肾上腺皮质类固醇组成的方案与环孢素、硫唑嘌呤和肾上腺皮质类固醇组成的方案。首次研究在美国进行(n=529)[28],其他的在欧洲进行(n=545)[29]。两项研究报道了治疗组之间类似的一年患者和移植物存活率。两个研究之间的总体结果在患者和移植物存活方面也相似。该研究报告了移植后 1 年内的血药浓度,其范围为 9.8~19.4ng/mL。因此在这些研究中,他克莫司方案被发现效果相当于环孢素方案,并获得 FDA 批准用于肝移植。

表 98.1 初始口服剂量建议和全血浓度终点

患者人群	推荐的初始口服剂量[a]	全血浓度
成人肾移植患者		
与硫唑嘌呤联用	0.2mg/(kg·d)	1~3 个月:7~20ng/mL 4~12 个月:5~15ng/mL
与 MMF/IL-2 受体拮抗剂联用[b]	0.1mg/(kg·d)	1~12 个月:4~11ng/mL
成人肝移植患者	0.10~0.15mg/(kg·d)	1~12 个月:5~20ng/mL
儿科肝移植患者	0.15~0.20mg/(kg·d)	1~12 个月:5~20ng/mL
成人心脏移植患者	0.075mg/(kg·d)	1~3 个月:10~20ng/mL ≥4 个月:5~15ng/mL

[a] 注:两次分剂量,ql21h。

[b] 在第二个较小的研究中,他克莫司的初始剂量为 0.15~0.2mg/(kg·d),在第 1~3 个月期间,他克莫司浓度为 6~16ng/mL,在第 4~12 个月期间为 5~12ng/mL(参见临床研究)。

Reproduced from [27] with permission.

随后试验在肾移植中使用他克莫司,1997 年,FDA 批准添加肾移植作为他克莫司的适应证。在Ⅲ期随机多中心非盲性前瞻性研究中，首次评估他克莫司与硫唑嘌呤和皮质类固醇联用的效果[30]。所有患者(n=412)接受由抗淋巴细胞抗体制剂、皮质类固醇和硫唑嘌呤组成的诱导免疫抑制治疗。将患者随机分成他克莫司(n=205)或环孢素(n=207),一旦血清肌酐低于 4mg/dL,开始第一次给药。一年后,比较他克莫司和环孢素组患者或移植物存活没有显著差异。患者存活率分别为 95.6%和 96.6%，而移植物存活率分别为 91.2%和 87.9%。然而,他克莫司治疗组中活检证实的急性排斥显著减少(30.7%对 46.4%,P=0.001)。作者得出结论是与环孢素相比,他克莫司在减少急性排斥反应方面更有效,同时减少了所需的抗淋巴细胞抗体制剂的量[30]。本研究使得 FDA 批准他克莫司与肾脏肾上腺皮质类固醇在肝或肾移植患者中联合使用。

最近,两项Ⅲ期研究评估他克莫司与 MMF 联用于肾移植患者。ELITE-Symphony 研究涉及 1589 名肾移植患者,其被随机分成由他克莫司(C 组,n=401)、西罗莫司(D 组,n=399)或两种环孢素方案(标准剂量,n=390)和 B 组(低剂量,n=399)[31]。除了 MMF 和皮质类固醇外，除 A 组外的所有组都接受达克珠单抗的诱导免疫抑制治疗。研究使用肌酐清除率(由 Cockcroft-Gault 计算)比较 12 个月时的肾功能。接受他克莫司的患者在 12 个月时肾功能显著改善,与其他治疗组相比有更高的肌酐清除率(表 98.2)。

在次要结果方面，治疗失败被定义为活检证实的急性排斥、移植物丢失、死亡和(或)随访失去的患者。接受他克莫司(C 组)的患者表现出较少的治疗失败案例,C 组和每个治疗组之间的差异有统计学意义。值得注意的是,接受他克莫司与 MMF 的患者更有可能出现腹泻和糖尿病[31]。

第二项研究是在美国、加拿大和巴西进行的Ⅲ期随机(1:1:1)开放标记多中心非劣效性研究[32]。本研究比较了与肾移植患者相关的缓释他克莫司(n=214)、标准他克莫司(n=212)和环孢素(n=212)联用 MMF、皮质类固醇和巴利昔单抗诱导的三种方案。本研究的主要终点是 1 年时的联合功能衰竭,包括活检证实的急性排斥、排除死亡的移植物损失、死亡率和随访失败。缓释他克莫司目前不是 FDA 批准的，因此处方信息仅报告这项研究关于标准他克莫司治疗组的结果(表

表 98.2 肾移植患者第 12 个月的肌酐清除率

分组	第 12 个月的肌酐清除率 [a] N	MEAN	SD	MEDIAN	与 C 组治疗差异(99.2%CI[b])
(A)CsA/MMF/CS	390	56.5	25.8	56.9	−8.6(−13.7, −3.7)
(B)CsA/MMF/CS/达利珠单抗	399	58.9	25.6	60.9	−6.2(−11.2, −1.2)
(C)Tac/MMF/CS/达利珠单抗	401	65.1	27.4	66.2	−
(D)SRL/MMF/CS/达利珠单抗	399	56.2	27.4	57.3	−8.9(−14.1, −3.9)
合计	1589	59.2	26.8	60.5	

[a] 所有死亡/移植物损失(组 A、B、C 和 D 中的 n=41、27、23 和 42)和最后记录的肌酐值在第 3 个月访视之前的患者(组 A、B、C 和 D 中的 n=10、9、7 和 9)分别以 10mL/min 的肾小球滤过率(GFR)输入;在第 12 个月(对于组 A、B、C 和 D,分别为 n=11、12、15 和 19)中,将受试者从第 3 个月最后观察到的肌酐值用于剩余的具有缺失肌酐的受试者。如果缺失,重量也计算在估计的 GFR 中。

[b] 使用 Bonferroni 校正对多个[6]成对比较进行调整。

Reproduced from [69] Pestana et al. with permission from John Wiley and Sons.

98.3),尽管根据主要结果,他克莫司组对环孢素具有非劣效性。虽然死亡率的差异没有统计学意义,标准他克莫司组(4.2%)相对于环孢素(2.4%)死亡率更高。虽然在他克莫司组中认定了归因于败血症等的三种死亡方式,而在环孢素组中没有发现该趋势。作为本研究的结果,以及 ELITE-Symphony 研究,与 MMF 联用于肾

表 98.3 肾移植患者随访 12 个月的 BPAR、移植物丢失或死亡的发生率

	他克莫司/MMF (n=212)	环孢素/MMF (n=212)
总体失败率	32(15.1%)	36(17.0%)
衰竭因素		
BPAR	16(7.5%)	29(13.7%)
移植物损失	6(2.8%)	4(1.9%)
死亡	9(4.2%)	5(2.4%)
失去随访	4(1.9%)	1(0.5%)
与 Prograf/MMF 组(95% CI[a])相比的功效衰竭差异	−	1.9%(−5.2%, 9.0%)

[a] 使用 Fisher 精确检验计算 95%置信区间。

移植成为他克莫司的适应证[32]。

由于两项Ⅲ期研究比较了他克莫司和基于环孢素方案的安全性和有效性,他克莫司在 2006 年获得 FDA 批准用于心脏移植。第一项研究在欧洲(n=314)进行,并将患者分别用他克莫司或改良环孢素联合皮质类固醇和硫唑嘌呤诱导治疗 18 个月[33]。第二项研究(n=331)在美国进行,并由以下三组方案治疗一年:皮质类固醇加他克莫司和西罗莫司,他克莫司加 MMF 或环孢霉素改性加 MMF[34]。在每项研究中,在 18 个月(91.7%他克莫司对 89.2%环孢素)或 1 年(91.7%他克莫司对86.1%环孢素)的治疗终点时,患者/移植物存活没有显著差异。美国进行研究的西罗莫司组确实发现伤口愈合并发症和胰岛素依赖性移植后的糖尿病的风险增加,因此不推荐使用该组[34]。

霉酚酸酯(Cellcept)

霉酚酸酯是一种强大的抗代谢物,于 1995 年被首次批准用于肾移植[35]。2000 年,随后的研究增加心脏和肝脏移植作为适应证。自 2009 年以来,FDA 批准了若干针对 MMF 使用的 ANDA 申请[36]。目前 FDA 批准的 MMF 指征是预防接受同种异体肾脏、心脏和肝脏移植患者的器官排斥[37]。处方信息还指出 MMF 将与环孢素和皮质类固醇联合使用。霉酚酸酯是麦考酚酸的前药,是一种活性代谢物。霉酚酸是一种有选择性并能有效抑制合成嘌呤所需的肌苷一磷酸脱氢酶的非竞争性可逆抑制剂。由于 T 淋巴细胞和 B 淋巴细胞缺乏嘌呤合成的补救途径,霉酚酸能够预防淋巴细胞增殖[37]。

MMF 的药代动力学性质已有详细描述。它在口服给药后被快速吸收并水解形成霉酚酸。口服相对静脉内 MMF 的生物利用度为 94%。有证据表明霉酚酸经历肠肝再循环,有助于维持血浆浓度水平。由于其致畸作用,MMF 属于妊娠 D 类药。在妊娠期与妊娠前期使用 MMF 会增加流产或先天性畸形的风险。这来源于国家移植妊娠登记(NTPR)的生殖毒理学研究数据[38]。该风险自 2012 年 11 月起,由 FDA 以所有含有霉酚酸酯的化合物的风险评估和减轻策略计划的形式解决[38]。

基于三个随机双盲多中心前瞻性试验,霉酚酸酯被批准用于肾移植。三个研究均比较两个剂量(1g 和 1.5g)MMF 每天两次与硫唑嘌呤(2 项研究)或安慰剂(1 项研究)联用的效果差异。所有研究都联合环孢素和皮质类固醇治疗,一项研究利用马抗胸腺细胞球蛋白。第一项研究在美国进行(n=499;表 98.4),第二项研

究在欧洲进行(n=503),最后一项研究在欧洲、加拿大和澳大利亚进行(n=491)[39-41]。三个研究的主要终点是前六个月内的治疗失败、定义为活检证实的急性排斥、死亡、移植物损失和来自研究的早期终止。接受 MMF 的患者在移植后的前 6 个月内治疗失败的发生率有统计学意义上的降低。很多接受 MMF 的患者停止治疗,但相比对照组没有明显增多的急性排斥反应、死亡或移植物丢失。当 MMF 的剂量为 3g/d 时,患者停药率最高,这可能是由于在较高剂量下药物不耐受性增加。与对照相比,MMF 在一年患者或移植物存活方面没有明显优势[37]。

2000 年,基于双盲随机平行组多中心研究结果,心脏移植成为 MMF 的适应证,其结果总结在表 98.5[42]。该多中心研究在原发性心脏移植受者中进行,患者接受每日两次 MMF1.5g(n=289)或联合环孢素和皮质类固醇的硫唑嘌呤(n=289)。两个主要终点是心内膜活检证实的排斥反应、在前 6 个月内有血流动力学损害和移植物衰竭或死亡、前 12 个月死亡或重新移植。组织活检证实的排斥或患者存活的发生率在治疗组之间没有差异。基于这项研究,显示 MMF 在排斥和存活方面至少与硫唑嘌呤同样有效[42]。

基于对原发性肝移植患者进行双盲随机比较平行组的多国多中心研究结果,肝移植最终在 2000 年由FDA 批准成为 MMF 的适应证[43]。患者(n=565)接受改良的环孢素和皮质类固醇与 MMF1g 组合每天两次,每日两次静脉内给药 14 天,随后 MMF1.5g 每日两次或硫唑嘌呤静脉内给药,再转为口服硫唑嘌呤。两个主要终点如下:活检证实患者在前 6 个月内发生排斥反应、死亡或再移植的比例,以及在前 12 个月内由于死亡或再移植而导致的移植物损失的患者比例。当死亡或再

表 98.5 心脏移植患者 6 个月时的排斥反应,1 年后死亡率或再移植

	所有患者		治疗患者	
	AZA (N=323)	MMF (N=327)	AZA (N=289)	MMF (N=289)
活检证实 6 个月时血流动力学损伤的排斥反应[a]	121(38%)	120(37%)	100(35%)	92(32%)
1 年后死亡或二次移植	49(15.2%)	42(12.8%)	33(11.4%)	18(6.2%)

[a] 如果满足以下任一标准,则出现血流动力学损害:肺毛细血管楔压≥20mm 或增加 25%;心脏指数<2.0L/min/m² 或降低 25%;射血分数≤30%;肺动脉血氧饱和度≤60%或降低 24%;存在新的 S3 加速;分数缩短≤20%或降低 25%;控制临床症状需要正性肌力支持。

表 98.4 移植后 6 个月内肾移植患者治疗失败的发生率

美国的研究[a](N=499)	MMF 2g/d(n=167)	MMF 3g/d(n=166)	硫唑嘌呤 1~2mg/(kg·d)(n=166)
总体失败率	31.1%	31.3%	47.6%
早期终止,无急性排斥[b]	9.6%	12.7%	6.0%
活检证实排斥反应	19.8%	17.5%	38.0%
欧洲/加拿大/澳大利亚的研究[c](N=505)	**MMF 2g/d(n=173)**	**MMF 3g/d(n=164)**	**硫唑嘌呤 100~150mg/d(n=166)**
总体失败率	38.2%	34.8%	50.0%
早期终止,无急性排斥[b]	13.9%	15.2%	10.2
活检证实排斥反应	19.7%	15.9%	35.5%
欧洲的研究[d](N=491)	**MMF 2g/d(n=165)**	**MMF 3g/d(n=160)**	**安慰剂(n=166)**
总体失败率	30.3%	38.8%	56.0%
早期终止,无急性排斥[b]	11.5%	22.5%	7.2%
活检证实排斥反应	17.0%	13.8%	46.4%

[a] 抗胸腺细胞球蛋白诱导/MMF 对硫唑嘌呤/环孢素/皮质类固醇。
[b] 不包括死亡和功能丧失作为提前终止的理由。
[c] MMF 或硫唑嘌呤/环孢素/皮质类固醇。
[d] MMF 或安慰剂/环孢素/皮质类固醇。

移植作为主要终点的一部分时，研究（总结在表98.6中）发现，使用MMF的患者在6个月时的急性排斥率显著降低。

当排斥反应这一主要终点用于检验死亡或再移植造成的移植物损失时，MMF和硫唑嘌呤之间的差异没有统计学意义。关于患者一年存活率，在治疗组之间移植物损失没有明显差异[43]。

霉酚酸钠肠溶片（Myfortic）

霉酚酸钠缓释剂是直接递送霉酚酸活性部分的肠溶衣制剂。霉酚酸钠肠溶片（EC-MPS）于2004年被批准与环孢素和皮质类固醇联用于预防同种异体肾移植受者的器官排斥[44]。由于具有相同的活性代谢物，霉酚酸钠具有与MMF相同的作用机制。EC-MPS是肌苷一磷酸脱氢酶的可逆性非竞争抑制剂，其抑制从嘌呤合成开始，并因此抑制缺乏嘌呤补救途径的B淋巴细胞和T淋巴细胞的增殖[45]。

由于其肠溶包衣制剂，霉酚酸钠具有独特的药代动力学性质。预期缓释霉酚酸浓度的升高范围为0.25~1.25h，中值时间至最大浓度范围为1.5~2.75h。相比之下，MMF最大浓度的中值时间为0.5~1.0h。EC-MPS的绝对生物利用度为72%。就等摩尔剂量而言，在单剂量和多剂量交叉试验中，用麦考酚酸钠720mg和MMF 1000mg均每日两次给药的剂量测定的AUC测定的平均系统霉酚酸浓度是相似的。与MMF类似，EC-MPS是妊娠期D类药物[45]。在妊娠期间使用EC-MPS与妊娠前期流产和先天性畸形的风险增加有关。这是基于动物生殖毒理学研究和国家移植妊娠登记（NTPR）的数据。该风险自2012年11月起，由FDA以所有含有霉酚酸酯的化合物的风险评估和减轻策略计划的形式解决[38]。EC-MPS在儿科肾移植患者中的安全性和有效性尚未确立。在稳定的儿科肾移植患者（5~16岁）中，安全性和有效性来自控制合理的成人研究的支持，然而由此得出的药代动力学数据有限[45]。

EC-MPS的处方信息包括成人和儿科患者的给药建议。EC-MPS推荐的成人剂量为空腹、食物摄取前1h或后2h，口服720mg，每日两次。缓释片在摄入之前不应被咀嚼、碾碎或切割。EC-MPS的推荐儿科剂量为400mg/m^2，每日两次，最大剂量为720mg，每日两次，四舍五入为最接近的整个180mg片剂。儿科患者体表面积<1.19m^{2}者[2]不应接受EC-MPS，因为该剂量不能用目前可用的片剂制剂精确地给药[45]。

基于两个Ⅲ期多中心随机试验从肾移植开始到维持阶段的研究，霉酚酸钠获得FDA批准用于肾移植患者。两项研究都将1.44g/d剂量的EC-MPS与每日2g MMF进行比较。该研究是一项多国研究，患者在移植后48h内随机分为MMF（n=213）或EC-MPS（n=210），与改良的环孢素和皮质类固醇比较[46]。值得注意的是，不控制抗体诱导使用的前提下仅有41%的患者接受抗体诱导。研究的主要终点是治疗失败，定义为活检证实的急性排斥、移植物丢失、死亡或在6个月后失访。这项研究的结果如表98.7所示，表明在EC-MPS和MMF之间，6个月或12个月治疗失败的发生率没有明显差异。

维持研究在移植后至少6个月的322名患者中进行，这些患者正在使用MMF和改良环孢素合用或不合用皮质类固醇[47]。患者被随机分配至霉酚酸钠或MMF，主要终点为治疗失败，如活检证实的急性排斥、移植物丢失、死亡或在6个月或12个月失访。再次，在任一时间点处理组之间的主要终点没有观察到明显差异（表98.8）。

西罗莫司

西罗莫司是抑制哺乳动物雷帕霉素靶标（mTOR）的相对新型免疫抑制剂的原始成员。西罗莫司在1999年被FDA批准用于肾移植[48]。西罗莫司结合FK506结合蛋白-12形成抑制mTOR的免疫抑制复合物。通过抑制mTOR，西罗莫司阻止蛋白质合成以及细胞周期从G1到S的进展，最终抑制T淋巴细胞增殖[49]。

西罗莫司可用于预防13岁以上肾移植患者的器官排斥。基于初次移植后的免疫风险，建议与环孢素和皮质类固醇联合治疗。建议低或中度免疫风险的患者在移植后2~4个月内停止环孢素治疗。对于高免疫风险的患者，建议在移植后第一年继续使用西罗莫司、环孢素和皮质类固醇的三联疗法。高免疫风险定义为黑色受体、高反应性抗体的患者（峰值PRA>80%）或由于免疫学原因而失去先前肾脏同种异体移植的二次移植

表98.6 肝移植患者6个月时的排斥反应，1年后死亡率或再移植

	AZA N=287	CellCept N=278
6个月活检证实排斥（包括死亡或再移植）	137（47.7%）	107（38.5%）
1年后死亡或二次移植	42（14.6%）	41（14.7%）

表 98.7 6 个月和 12 个月环孢素 * 和皮质类固醇联合治疗肾移植患者的失败案例

	EC-MPS 1.44g/d(n=213)	霉酚酸酯 2g/d(n=210)
6 个月	n(%)	n(%)
治疗失败 #	55(25.8)	55(26.2)
病理证实急性排斥	46(21.6)	48(22.9)
移植物丢失	7(3.3)	9(4.3)
死亡	1(0.5)	2(1.0)
失访 **	3(1.4)	0
12 个月	n(%)	n(%)
移植物丢失或死亡或失访 ***	20(9.4)	18(8.6)
治疗失败	61(28.6)	59(28.1)
病理证实急性排斥	48(22.5)	51(24.3)
移植物丢失	9(4.2)	9(4.3)
死亡	2(0.9)	5(2.4)
失访 **	5(2.3)	0

* USP(修改后)。

** 失访后表明，在没有事先活检的情况下失去随访的患者证实为急性排斥、移植物丢失或死亡。

*** 失访后表示失去随访而无先前移植物丢失或死亡的患者(9 名顽固性患者和 4 名霉酚酸酯患者)。

\# 6 个月治疗失败的差异(霉菌素)的 95%置信区间为(-8.7%, 8.0%)。

表 98.8 6 个月和 12 个月环孢素 * 和皮质类固醇联合治疗转换移植患者的失败案例

	EC-MPS 1.44g/d(n=159)	霉酚酸酯 2g/d(n=163)
6 个月	n(%)	n(%)
治疗失败 #	7(4.4)	11(6.7)
病理证实急性排斥	2(1.3)	2(1.2)
移植物丢失	0	1(0.6)
死亡	0	1(0.6)
失访 **	5(3.1)	7(4.3)
12 个月	n(%)	n(%)
移植物丢失或死亡或失访 ***	10(6.3)	17(10.4)
治疗失败	12(7.5)	20(12.3)
病理证实急性排斥	2(1.3)	5(3.1)
移植物丢失	0	1(0.6)
死亡	2(1.3)	4(2.5)
失访 **	8(5.0)	10(6.1)

* USP(修改后)。

** 失访后表明，在没有事先活检的情况下失去随访的患者证实为急性排斥、移植物丢失或死亡。

*** 失访后表示失去随访而无先前移植物丢失或死亡的患者(8 名顽固性患者和 12 名霉酚酸酯患者)。

\# 6 个月治疗失败的差异(霉菌素)的 95%置信区间为(-7.4%, 2.7%)。

患者[49]。重要的是应该注意到经验显示与环孢素联用后相关的肾毒性显著加剧,因此在现代实践中,在标签上指示西罗莫司与环孢素联用相对来说是不常见的。

西罗莫司的处方信息包括针对 13 岁以上患者的给药建议。应采用相当于维持剂量 3 倍(即 6mg 负荷剂量,随后为每日 2mg)的西罗莫司作为初始负荷剂量。推荐初始维持剂量为 2mg，尽管在临床研究中有报道为每天 5mg。年龄在 13 岁以上,体重在 40kg 以下的患者应根据体表面积(负荷剂量为 3mg/m^2,维持剂量为 1mg/m^2)给药。随机多中心对照试验发现西罗莫司口服溶液和片剂在临床预防肾移植后器官排斥的作用等同。由于西罗莫司的长半衰期为 62h,频繁剂量调整可导致过量给药或剂量不足。因此,新的维持剂量应在基于谷水平调节之前持续至少 7 天。在处方信息中描述了若干目标血药浓度，高免疫风险患者合用环孢素治疗的剂量为 10~15ng/mL,已经撤回环孢素治疗的低至中等风险患者为 16~24ng/mL。在现实中,这些目标水平远远高于实践中使用的水平。重要的是注意由于用不同的测定方法测量西罗莫司水平[49],因此每个组的用法不能通用。

西罗莫司是少数具有两种不同“黑盒”警告的免疫抑制剂之一。根据处方信息,西罗莫司在肝或肺移植患者中的安全性和有效性尚未确定,因此不推荐。对于肝移植，该警告是特异性针对首次肝移植患者的过量死亡率、移植物丢失和肝动脉血栓形成。对于肺移植,由于潜在致命的支气管吻合开裂的风险，西罗莫司不推荐用于首次肺移植患者[49]。

涉及西罗莫司在初次肝移植患者（使用他克莫司或与环孢素组合)中使用的两项研究证明过量死亡率、移植物丢失和肝动脉血栓形成的发生率增加。在第一项研究中，发现西罗莫司与他克莫司死亡率和移植物损失约为 22%对 9%[50]。两项研究接受西罗莫司的患者中肝动脉血栓形成的研究显示，使用西罗莫司为 7%，对照组为 2%。大多数移植物丢失或死亡病例发生在移植后 30 天内[49]。此外,在从基于钙调神经磷酸酶抑制剂的方案转化为西罗莫司的稳定肝移植患者的 2:1 随机、多中心控制的临床研究中，与未转化的那些相比，在西罗莫司队列中观察到死亡数增加（3.8%对1.4%，*P*=NS）[51]。西罗莫司不推荐用于首次肺移植，因为有许多支气管吻合开裂的病例，其中大多数是致命的[49]。

在两项Ⅲ期随机双盲多中心对照试验中评估西罗莫司口服溶液预防肾同种异体移植排斥的安全性和有效性。第一项研究（表98.9a）比较了西罗莫司每天2mg（n=284），西罗莫司每天5mg（n=274）和硫唑嘌呤（n=161），所有这些与环孢素和皮质类固醇联用[52]。第二项研究（表98.9b）比较了西罗莫司每天2mg（n=227），西罗莫司每天5mg（n=219）和硫唑嘌呤（n=130），所有这些与环孢素和皮质类固醇联用[53]。在两项研究中，禁止抗淋巴细胞抗体诱导。主要终点是功效衰竭，定义为活检证实的急性排斥反应、移植物损失或6个月时的患者死亡。在两项研究中，与硫唑嘌呤或安慰剂相比，任一剂量（2mg或5mg）的西罗莫司可显著降低失功率。患者和移植物存活在第一次研究的1年和2年以及第二次研究的1年和3年的治疗组之间是类似的。发现在两个研究中接受西罗莫司的患者在较晚时间点的平均肾小球滤过率较低。当第一个研究中的患者通过种族分层时，与黑人患者中的硫唑嘌呤相比，每日5mg的西罗莫司具有降低失功率的作用。然而，在黑人患者中使用较高剂量的西罗莫司时必须细致权衡，因为观察到的剂量依赖性不良事件的风险增加[52]。

在Ⅲ期随机多中心对照研究中评价了钙调神经磷酸酶抑制剂与西罗莫司联用戒断策略（表98.10）[54,55]。所有患者被随机分为持续的环孢素（n=215）或戒断环孢素（n=215）组，且前3个月接受西罗莫司、环孢素和皮质类固醇。主要终点是移植后12个月的移植物存活。移植后1年、2年或3年患者或移植物存活没有差异。接受具有4个或更多HLA错配的肾同种异体移植（15.3%环孢素戒断对3.0%环孢素）的患者，其活检证实的急性排斥的发生显著增加。对于接受具有3个或更少HLA错配的同种异体移植物的患者，组之间的排斥率没有差异。在移植后1年、2年和3年，接受环孢素戒断的患者的平均肾小球滤过率显著高于连续给予环孢素的患者[54,55]。

在肾移植中尚未建立没有钙调神经磷酸酶抑制剂的西罗莫司的使用。在新生肾移植患者中进行的Ⅲ期研究比较了西罗莫司与环孢素联合IL-2受体拮抗剂、MMF和类固醇。西罗莫司组具有显著更高的急性排斥

表98.9a 6个月和24个月研究[1][a,b]失效的发生率(%)

参数	西罗莫司口服溶液2mg/d (n=284)	西罗莫司口服溶液5mg/d (n=274)	硫唑嘌呤2~3mg/(kg·d) (n=161)
6个月失效[c]	18.7	16.8	32.3
功能衰竭的原因			
病理证明急性排斥	16.5	11.3	29.2
移植物丢失	1.1	2.9	2.5
死亡	0.7	1.8	0
失访	0.4	0.7	0.6
24个月失效	32.8	25.9	36.0
功能衰竭的原因			
病理证明急性排斥	23.6	17.5	32.3
移植物丢失	3.9	4.7	3.1
死亡	4.2	3.3	0
失访	1.1	0.4	0.6

[a] 患者接受环孢素和皮质类固醇。
[b] 包括过早停止治疗的患者。
[c] 主要终点。

表98.9b 6个月和36个月研究[2][a,b]失效的发生率(%)

参数	西罗莫司口服溶液2mg/d (n=227)	西罗莫司口服溶液5mg/d (n=219)	硫唑嘌呤 (n=130)
6个月失效[c]	30.0	25.6	47.7
功能衰竭的原因			
病理证明急性排斥	24.7	19.2	41.5
移植物丢失	3.1	3.7	3.9
死亡	2.2	2.7	2.3
失访	0	0	0
36个月失效	44.4	41.6	54.6
功能衰竭的原因			
病理证明急性排斥	32.2	27.4	43.9
移植物丢失	6.2	7.3	4.6
死亡	5.7	5.9	5.4
失访	0	0.9	0.8

[a] 患者接受环孢素和皮质类固醇。
[b] 包括过早停止治疗的患者。
[c] 主要终点。

表 98.10 研究 [3][a,b,c] 在 12 个月、24 个月和 36 个月时通过 Nankivell 方程计算移植后肾小球滤过率(mL/min)

参数	西罗莫司与环孢素治疗	环孢素戒断后西罗莫司
12 个月	53.2±1.5(n=208)	59.3±1.5(n=203)
24 个月	48.4±1.7(n=203)	58.4±1.6(n=201)
36 个月	47.0±1.8(n=196)	58.5±1.9(n=199)

[a] 包括过早停止治疗的患者。

[b] 有移植物损失的患者在分析中其 GFR 设置为 0.0。

[c] 所有患者接受皮质类固醇。

率和更高的死亡率[49]。最后,在稳定的肾移植患者中至少 6 个月后评价从钙调神经磷酸酶抑制剂(CNI)到西罗莫司的转化。这项研究是一项随机多中心全球性研究,涉及 111 个中心和 830 例患者[56]。该研究旨在证明肾功能将通过从钙调神经磷酸酶抑制剂转化为西罗莫司而得到改善。然而,在转化为西罗莫司的患者中,蛋白尿的发生率没有得到与转化相关的益处。此外,由于严重不良事件的发生率较高,肾小球滤过率<49 的患者不入组。

依维莫司(Zortress)

依维莫司是 mTOR 抑制剂类免疫抑制剂的第二名成员。依维莫司在美国获得 FDA 批准,在 2010 年以商标名 Zortress®用于移植[57]。依维莫司也可在美国以商品名 Afinitor®用于肿瘤学。此外,值得注意的是,自 2003 年以来,依维莫司已在美国以外的 70 多个国家以商品名 Certican®用于器官移植[58]。

依维莫司用于预防接受肾移植的低-中度免疫风险的成年患者的器官排斥[59]。依维莫司应与巴利昔单抗和低剂量的环孢素和皮质类固醇一起使用。这种较低剂量的推荐反映了从西罗莫司收集的数据经验,其中标准剂量的环孢素被发现是有毒性的。处方信息还包括对依维莫司使用的几个限制。如前所述,依维莫司是一种预防 T 淋巴细胞和 B 淋巴细胞增殖的 mTOR 抑制剂。依维莫司结合 FK506 结合蛋白-12 以形成抑制 mTOR 的免疫抑制复合物,从而防止蛋白质合成和细胞增殖。依维莫司的处方信息特别警告移植后 30 天,肾动脉和静脉血栓形成的风险增加,从而导致移植物损失。此外,处方信息包括在首次心脏移植患者的临床试验中增加死亡率的警告。因此,在心脏移植中不推荐使用依维莫司。目前已确定依维莫司在儿科患者中的安全性和有效性。

FDA 批准的依维莫司的推荐剂量是:使用剂量减少的环孢素的成年患者的初始剂量为 0.75mg,每天两次。应调整剂量至推荐的 3~8ng/mL 的全血浓度水平。降低的靶水平与西罗莫司给药的实际迁移相互协同到更低的目标水平。由于长达 30h 的消除半衰期,建议以 4~5 天的间隔进行剂量调整,以达到治疗范围。处方信息包括针对降低环孢素用量的全血浓度的建议,移植后第一个月的目标范围从 100~200ng/mL 开始,在移植后 6~12 个月之间降至 25~50ng/mL[59]。

肾移植后 24 个月多国家开放标签的随机试验中评价浓度控制的依维莫司给药的安全性和功效,结果见表 98.11[60]。这是一项三臂研究,比较了两种不同的依维莫司剂量与巴利昔单抗、减量环孢素和皮质类固醇的联用,与接受巴利昔单抗、标准剂量环孢素、霉酚酸和皮质类固醇联用的对照组(n=277)。两个依维莫司剂量分别为 1.5mg/d,目标波谷水平为 3~8ng/mL (n=277)和 3mg/d,目标波谷水平为 6~12ng/mL(n=279)。研究人群包括接受第一次肾移植的患者,他们处于低到中度的免疫风险(ABO 兼容移植,Ⅰ类 PRA<20%,和阴性 T 细胞交叉匹配)。研究的主要终点是 12 个月时的功效衰竭,为活检证实的急性排斥反应、死亡、移植物丢失或

表 98.11 治疗组(ITT 人群)在 12 个月的功能衰竭

疗效终点 [3]	依维莫司 1.5mg/d,减少 CsA 剂量 N=277 n(%)	霉酚酸 1.44mg/d 与标准剂量 CsA N=277 n(%)
主要功能衰竭终点 [1]	70(25.3)	67(24.2)
活检证实急性排斥	45(16.2)	47(17.0)
死亡	7(2.5)	6(2.2)
移植物丢失	12(4.3)	9(3.2)
失访	12(4.3)	9(3.2)
移植物丢失或死亡或失访 [2]	32(11.6)	26(9.4)
移植物丢失或死亡失访 [2]	18(6.5)	15(5.4)
	14(5.1)	11(4.0)

[1] 包括治疗的 BPAR、移植物丢失、死亡或到第 12 个月失访,其中失访表示未经历治疗的 BPAR、移植物丢失或死亡的患者,并且其最后的联系日期是在 12 个月访问之前。

[2] 包括治疗的 BPAR、移植物丢失、死亡或失访,在第 12 个月,其中失访表示未经历治疗的 BPAR、移植物丢失或死亡的患者。

[3] 失访(移植物丢失、死亡或随访失败)表示未经历死亡或移植物丢失且在 12 个月访问之前失去联系的患者。

失去随访的患者。发现每天以 1.5mg 给药的依维莫司与对照组相比在 12 个月(25.3%依维莫司每天 1.5mg 对 24.2%对照)的功效衰竭方面是相当的。此外,通过计算肾小球滤过率,12 个月时的肾功能分别为每日 1.5mg [54.6mL/(min·1.73m²)]和对照组[52.3mL/(min·1.73m²)]。停用更高剂量(3mg/d)依维莫司率为 34%,其中 20%是由于不良事件,因此不予推荐。

两项针对首次肾移植患者的多中心双盲随机试验评价了未进行治疗药物监测的依维莫司的固定剂量[61,62]。两项研究比较了两种不同固定剂量的依维莫司(每天 1.5mg 和每天 3mg) 与标准环孢素和类固醇联用, 与用环孢素、MMF 和皮质类固醇治疗的患者对照。与对照组相比,利用肾小球滤过率的 12 个月肾功能分析显示两种依维莫司组中肾损伤的情况。这些研究的结果显示,应进行治疗药物监测,以维持 3~8ng/mL的依维莫司波谷水平。此外,当与依维莫司一起使用时,应减少环孢素的剂量,以避免肾功能障碍[59]。

贝拉西普

贝拉西普属于针对特定共刺激分子和途径的新型免疫抑制剂。2011 年,FDA 批准贝拉西普用于肾移植[63]。贝拉西普用于预防成人肾移植患者的器官排斥,这些患者都是 EB 病毒(EBV)血清阳性[64]。它与巴利昔单抗、霉酚酸酯和皮质类固醇联合使用。

贝拉西普用于预防肾脏以外的移植器官排斥的用途尚未确定。贝拉西普是一种新型免疫抑制剂,提供选择性 T 淋巴细胞协同刺激阻断。它是融合蛋白,结合抗原呈递细胞上的 CD80 和 CD86, 从而阻断 CD28 介导的 T 淋巴细胞共刺激, 这能防止 T 淋巴细胞信号 2 的活化,从而抑制细胞增殖和细胞因子白细胞介素-2、干扰素-γ、白细胞介素-4 和 TNF-α 的产生。贝拉西普 10mg/kg 剂量的消除半衰期为 9.8 天,5mg/kg 剂量的消除半衰期为 8.2 天。FDA 批准贝拉西普的给药方案是在第 1 天和第 5 天, 第 2 周和第 4 周结束时静脉内输注 10mg/kg;然后每 4 周输注直至移植后第 12 周。从第 16 周开始,应每 4 周静脉内输注贝拉西普 5mg/kg。剂量应根据移植时患者的实际体重计算, 并且在治疗过程中不应修改,除非患者的体重变化大于 10%。所有剂量的贝拉西普应在 30min 内输注完[64]。

贝拉西普的处方信息包含移植后淋巴增殖性疾病(PTLD)、感染和其他恶性肿瘤的黑框警告。与基于环孢素的方案相比, 接受贝拉西普的患者具有增加累及中枢神经系统(CNS)的 PTLD 的风险。此外,与 FDA 批准的给药方案相比, 在接受贝拉西普较高累积和较高频率给药方案的患者中,CNSPTLD、PML 和其他 CNS 感染的发生更频繁。在这种治疗方案中,8 例 PTLD 中的 6 例伴有 CNS 参与。因此,不推荐服用这种更高剂量的方案。总体而言,在用贝拉西普治疗的患者中,与 EBV 血清阳性(5/810)相比,EBV 血清阴性或未知血清阳性(8/139)的 PTLD 的发生率高出 9 倍。因此,贝拉西普不应用于 EBV 血清阴性或未知血清的患者,因为在没有 EBV 免疫的患者中,PTLD 的风险会增加。由于这些安全问题, 制造商需要在产品批准中纳入风险评估和减缓战略计划[64]。

此外,贝拉西普带有黑色警告,由于移植物丢失和死亡的风险增加,建议不要在肝移植中使用。这种黑盒警告是基于Ⅲ期试验的结果[64]。在与肾移植中研究的给药方案相比,在与 MMF 和皮质类固醇联合的给药方案中贝拉西普给药更频繁。与他克莫司治疗组相比,贝拉西普治疗与较高的移植物损失和死亡率相关。此外,有两例 PTLD 涉及肝脏同种异体移植(一例死亡)和一例致命性 PML[64]。

在两个开放标签随机多中心试验中评价贝拉西普在新生肾移植中的安全性和功效[65,66]。将贝拉西普的两种不同给药方案与基于环孢素的方案进行比较,所有患者都接受巴利昔单抗、MMF 和皮质类固醇。两种贝拉西普方案是目前推荐的具有更高累积和更频繁给药的方案。所有治疗组接受 MMF、皮质类固醇和巴利昔单抗联用。两项研究排除了高免疫风险的患者,定义为具有>50%的面板反应性抗体(PRA)、PRA>30%的再移植、HIV、丙型肝炎、活动性 TB 或活动性乙型肝炎。一年功能衰竭被定义为活检证实的急性排斥、移植物丢失、死亡或失访的患者。

第一项研究(BENEFIT)仅包括具有活体供体和标准供体的肾移植受体[65,67]。与环孢素相比,两个贝拉西普组中一年和三年活检证实的急性排斥率更高 (表 98.12)。在贝拉西普组经历急性排斥反应的患者中,70%的患者在第三个月经历排斥反应,84%的患者在移植后 6 个月经历排斥反应。此外,接受贝拉西普的患者比对照患者(6%贝拉西普对 2%对照)更频繁地经历活检证实的急性排斥,分类为 Banff Ⅱb 级或更高。然而,在移植后一年和三年患者和移植物存活没有差异。通过肾小球滤过率测量一年和两年的肾功能, 并且在移植后一年、两年和三年使用肾脏疾病方案中的饮食修改计算。与所有时间点的环孢素相比，接受贝拉西普的患者的测量和计算的肾小球滤过率更高(表 98.13)。在解释本研究中肾功能的终点时，FDA 利用肾小球滤过数据来评估贝拉西普对肾功能的安全性，而不是作为疗效测量[68]。

第二项研究(BENEFIT-EXT)包括具有延长标准的肾移植受者死亡的供体，并且是在 ECD 群体中特异性寻求指征的试验[66,69]。本研究发现，在移植后 1 年和 3 年，活检证实的急性排斥反应率没有差异。活组织检查证实的急性排斥比例为 Banff Ⅱb 级或更高，在治疗组之间也是可比的(贝拉西普为 5%，环孢素治疗组为 4%)。在移植后 1 年和 3 年，患者和移植物存活没有差异。此外，与贝拉西普治疗的患者相比，用环孢素治疗的患者的测量和计算的肾小球滤过率更高(图98.2)。与第一项研究类似，FDA 将这些肾小球滤过率结果解释为贝拉西普对肾功能的安全性评估，而不是作为疗效测量[68]。

免抗人胸腺细胞球蛋白(Thymoglobulin)

免抗人胸腺细胞球蛋白(Thymoglobulin®，RATG)是一种有效的免疫抑制剂，最初于 1998 年 12 月获得 FDA 批准，成为市场上可获得的第二种抗胸腺细胞球蛋白[70]。第一种抗胸腺细胞球蛋白制剂(ATGAM)是来源于马的，并且最初在 1981 年得到 FDA 批准。然而在美国，大多数移植中心的抗胸腺细胞剂的选择中它已经被 RATG 替代[71]。

重要的是要注意，尽管其用于预防实体器官移植患者中的器官排斥，经 FDA 批准的唯一作用是治疗成年肾移植急性排斥以及伴随的免疫抑制。RATG 是通

表 98.12　第 1 年和第 3 年的结果：存活受体和供体肾脏标准

参数	贝拉西普推荐方案 N=226 n(%)	环孢素(CSA) N=221 n(%)	贝拉西普–CSA (97.3%CI)
死亡	4(1.8)	7(3.2)	
失访	0	1(0.5)	
第 3 年功能衰竭	58(25.7)	57(25.8)	–0.1(–9.3,9)
功能衰竭的原因 *			
病理证实急性排斥	50(22.1)	31(14)	
移植物丢失	9(4)	10(4.5)	
死亡	10(4.4)	15(6.8)	
失访	2(0.9)	5(2.3)	
患者和移植物存活率⁺			
1 年	218(96.5)	206(93.2)	
3 年	206(91.2)	192(86.9)	4.3(–2.2,10.8)

* 患者可能不止一项临床事件。

⁺ 已知的存活的移植器官正常的患者。

表 98.13　测量和计算 GFR：受益人生活标准和标准死亡供体肾脏

参数	贝拉西普推荐方案 N=226	环孢素(CSA) N=221	贝拉西普–CSA (97.3%CI)
测量的 GFR*mL/(min·1.73m²)(SD)			
1 年	63.4(27.7)(n=206)	50.4(18.7)(n=199)	13.0(7.3,18.7)
2 年⁺	67.9(29.9)(n=199)	50.5(20.5)(n=185)	17.4(11.5,23.4)
测量的 GFR‡ mL/min/1.73m²(SD)			
1 年	65.4(22.9)(n=200)	50.1(21.1)(n=199)	15.3(10.3,20.3)
2 年	65.4(25.2)(n=201)	47.9(23)(n=182)	17.5(12,23.1)
3 年	65.8(27)(n=190)	44.4(23.6)(n=171)	21.4(15.4,27.4)

* 使用冷的碘他酸盐方法测量 GFR。

⁺ 在第 3 年没有评估测量的 GFR。

‡ 使用 MDRD 公式计算 GFR。

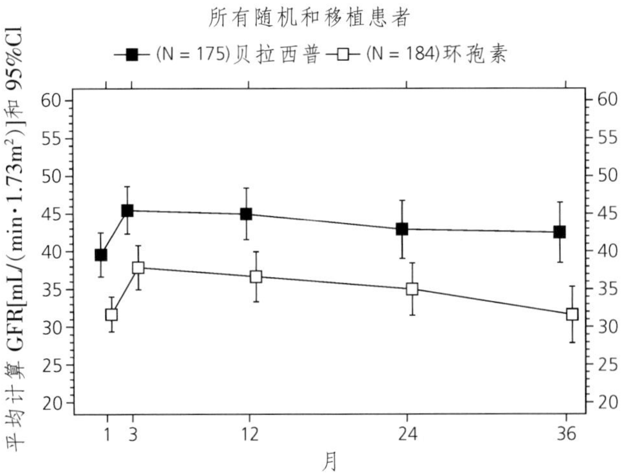

图 98.2　计算(MDRD)GFR 到第 36 个月；研究 2：延长标准供体肾脏的受者。

过用兔抗人胸腺细胞免疫获得的多克隆抗淋巴细胞制剂。它是γ免疫球蛋白产物,其由针对T淋巴细胞抗原的多克隆细胞毒性抗体组成。RATG诱导免疫抑制的作用机制尚未完全了解,但可能涉及T细胞清除、活化调节、归巢和细胞毒性活性。RATG是兔过敏以及免疫抑制导致急性或慢性感染的患者的禁忌[71]。

针对RATG治疗急性排斥的批准剂量和给药建议为每天每千克体重1.5mg,通过静脉内给药7~14天。它应该通过0.22μm过滤器输注,第一次输注最少6h,后续输注至少4h。淋巴细胞的裂解,与第一次或第二次输注的发生与细胞因子释放综合征一致的输注反应相关。细胞因子释放综合征的体征和症状包括:发热、寒战、严重呼吸困难、低血压、高血压、恶心、呕吐和腹泻、不适、皮疹或头痛。输注速率的降低,以及用对乙酰氨基酚、皮质类固醇和抗组胺药的预处理已经显示能降低输注反应的发生率。据报道,血清病的症状包括发热、皮疹、关节痛和肌痛,治疗后5~15天出现症状。与RATG相关的显著不良事件包括白细胞减少、血小板减少症、感染和恶性肿瘤。

处方信息参考了在美国进行的导致RATG批准的一项Ⅲ期研究[72]。这项双盲多中心平行组随机的非劣效性试验比较接受RATG和ATGAM的急性移植物排斥肾移植患者。如果患者在他们的第一次或第二次肾移植中具有活检证实的Banff Ⅱ级、Ⅲ级或类固醇抗性Ⅰ级急性细胞排斥,则将其包括在研究中。用1.5mg/(kg·d)的RATG(n=82)或15mg/(kg·d)的ATGAM(n=81)给予抗排斥治疗7~14天。这项研究的主要终点是急性排斥反应的逆转,定义为在排斥诊断后14天内血清肌酐水平恢复到基线。发现RATG具有比ATGAM更高的抗排斥效果(88%对76%,P=0.027),在用RATG治疗的患者中,治疗后90天发生的排斥复发较少(17%对36%,P=0.011)。不良事件、一年患者和移植物存活在治疗组之间相当。在研究的后半期,两个治疗组都因他克莫司和霉酚酸的使用而关闭方案,但对总体结果没有影响。总体加权治疗差异为11.1%(RATG-ATGAM),置信区间为0.07%(表98.14)。结果,发现RATG在逆转肾移植患者的急性移植排斥中至少与ATGAM同样有效[72]。

巴利昔单抗(Simulect)

巴利昔单抗是一种非淋巴细胞消耗性诱导免疫抑制剂,于1998年5月获得FDA批准[73]。巴利昔单抗属于白细胞介素2受体拮抗剂[74]。这种药物类别的另一个成员是达利珠单抗(Zenapax®),于1997年获得FDA批准[75]。2010年,由于市场对药物的需求减少,制造商停止生产达利珠单抗。结果,巴利昔单抗是美国唯一可用的白细胞介素2受体拮抗剂。

表98.14 研究治疗的排斥反应严重程度和半研究应答

	总体		前半段		后半段	
成功/n	RATG	ATGAM	RATG	ATGAM	RATG	ATGAM
危险因素:排斥严重性基线						
轻度	9/10 (90.0%)	5/8 (62.5%)	5/5 (100%)	1/3 (33.3%)	4/5 (80.0%)	4/5 (80.0%)
中等	44/58 (75.5%)	41/58 (70.7%)	22/28 (84.8%)	22/32 (68.8%)	22/32 (68.8%)	18/26 (73.1%)
严重	11/14 (71.6%)	8/14 (57.1%)	6/8 (75.0%)	3/8 (37.5%)	5/8 (83.3%)	5/8 (83.3%)
总体	64/82 (78.0%)	54/80 (87.5%)	33/39 (84.8%)	26/43 (60.5%)	31/43 (72.1%)	28/37 (75.7%)
加权差分		11.1%[a]		19.3%		-3.2%
较低的单侧95%置信界限		0.07%		4.6%		-19.7%
P值[b]		0.061[c]		0.008[d]		0.625[d]

[a] 跨越排斥严重性和半研究。

[b] 在无假设的等效试验中(Codhran-Mantel-Haenszel检验)。

[c] 单方面排斥严重性和半研究。

[d] 单方面排斥严重性。

巴利昔单抗用于预防肾移植患者中的急性器官排斥反应，作为由改良环孢素和皮质类固醇组成的免疫抑制方案的一部分[74]。它是设计用于抑制 T 细胞活化信号 3 的嵌合(鼠/人)单克隆抗体。这是由于在活化的 T 淋巴细胞表面上的巴利昔单抗对白细胞介素 2 受体 α(也称为 CD25 抗原)的高亲和力。当与改良环孢素和皮质类固醇联合使用时，成人和儿科患者中白细胞介素 2 受体 α 饱和的持续时间为 36 天，而当与改良环孢素、皮质类固醇和硫唑嘌呤或 MMF 联合使用时，持续时间分别为 50 天和 59 天。巴利昔单抗通常耐受良好，大多数报道的不良事件由胃肠道疾病(恶心、呕吐、便秘、腹痛、消化不良和腹泻)组成。

处方信息包含成人和儿科患者的给药建议。对于成人，推荐的给药方案由两个剂量的静脉巴利昔单抗 20mg 组成。第一剂量应在手术前 2h 施用，第二剂应在移植后 4 天施用。根据与成人给药相同的时间表，基于体重将儿科给药方案分层，其中体重在 35kg 以下的患者接受两次 10mg 剂量，35kg 以上的接受两次 20mg 剂量。

四个成年随机双盲安慰剂对照临床试验和儿科药代动力学安全性研究，使 FDA 批准巴利昔单抗用于肾移植[74]。最初的研究利用了巴利昔单抗与改良环孢素和皮质类固醇的组合。第一项研究在欧洲和加拿大进行，而第二项研究在美国进行[76,77]。这两项研究都在接受死亡供体肾移植的患者中进行，但美国的研究也包括活体供体肾移植。将患者分为巴利昔单抗或安慰剂治疗。两个研究的主要终点是在移植后 6 个月期间死亡、移植物损失或急性排斥发作的发生率。次要终点包括 6 个月和 12 个月时活检证实的排斥反应，所有主要终点在 12 个月时评估 1 年患者和移植物存活。在比较接受巴利昔单抗(n=190)与安慰剂(n=186)的欧洲和加拿大研究的患者中，接受巴利昔单抗的患者的主要终点的发生率降低有统计学意义(42%对 57%，P=0.003)[76]。在比较接受巴利昔单抗(n=173)与安慰剂(n=173)的美国研究的患者中，接受巴利昔单抗的患者的主要终点的发生率有统计学意义的降低(38%对 55%，P=0.002)[51,77]。就两项研究的次要终点而言，主要终点在 12 个月，以及在 6 个月和 12 个月时排斥发作的发生率显著降低。两个研究的 12 个月的患者和移植物存活率在组之间是相当的。欧洲/加拿大研究评价了 71%的患者移植物和患者存活，美国研究评估了 58%的患者。两个研究中移植物存活没有差异。美国研究的患者存活在组之间是可比的；然而对于欧洲/加拿大的研究，存在数值上较低的患者存活率(87%的巴利昔单抗对 95%的安慰剂)。处方信息指出，这种差异的原因是未知的，没有指出恶性肿瘤或感染的增加[74]。

在两个双盲随机安慰剂对照研究中评价了基于三联疗法的维持免疫抑制方案中的巴利昔单抗的使用。两项研究均在死亡或活体供体成人第一次或第二次肾移植患者中进行。两个研究的主要终点是移植后 6 个月的急性排斥反应。第一项研究比较了采用(n=168)或未采用(n=172)巴利昔单抗联合环孢素、皮质类固醇和硫唑嘌呤治疗的患者[78]。对于主要终点，用巴利昔单抗(21%巴利昔单抗对 35%安慰剂，P=0.005)治疗的患者的急性排斥发作显著减少。第二项研究比较了用 (n=59)或不用(n=64)巴利昔单抗联合环孢素、皮质类固醇和 MMF 治疗的患者[79]。对于本研究的主要终点，6个月时活检证实的急性排斥反应没有显著差异 (15%的巴利昔单抗对 27%的安慰剂，P>0.05)。两个研究的患者和移植物存活在 12 个月时相当。

在 41 名中位年龄为 8.1 岁[1~11 岁(n=27)]和 12~16 岁(n=14)的儿科患者中进行安全性和药代动力学研究[80]。除了用改良环孢素、硫唑嘌呤、MMF 和(或)皮质类固醇的标准免疫抑制外，这些患者还用巴利昔单抗治疗。发现 6 个月的急性排斥率与接受基于三重疗法的免疫抑制的成年患者相当，具有相当的不良事件概况。报告最常见的不良事件是发热、多发性高血压、高血压、鼻炎和尿路感染[74]。

抗病毒药

所有移植患者均应接受一系列药物，以预防所使用的免疫抑制剂的不良作用。第 94 章深入讨论了移植前和移植后感染预防的管理，但大多数所使用的药物并未特别批准用于移植。以下药剂已经正式批准用于实体器官移植。

更昔洛韦钠(Cytovene-IV)

更昔洛韦钠是对抗巨细胞病毒(CMV)的合成鸟嘌呤衍生物，最初被 FDA 于 1989 年批准用于治疗获得性免疫缺陷综合征(AIDS)患者中的 CMV 视网膜炎[81]。1992 年，更昔洛韦在 CMV 疾病风险的移植受者中获得了预防 CMV 疾病的扩展指征[82]。最初，更昔洛韦仅以更昔洛韦钠的形式在静脉内使用，然而在1994年，口服更昔洛韦制剂被引入市场[81]。口服更昔洛韦用于预防CMV疾病风险的患者中的CMV疾病，包括实体器官移植受者和患有AIDS的患者。最近，口服更昔洛韦在长期药物短缺后退出了市场。

静脉内和口服更昔洛韦的药代动力学性质已经得到很好地描述。在吸收方面，与静脉内更昔洛韦相比，口服更昔洛韦的生物利用度较低，据报道绝对生物利用度为8.53%[83]。更昔洛韦的主要消除途径是以药物原形经肾脏排泄。因此，当给予更昔洛韦时，需要注意肾损伤。对于儿科患者，其药代动力学性质与在成人中观察到的相似。然而，由于更昔洛韦不适用于儿科患者，在处方信息中不包括给药建议。最后，由于更昔洛韦的致突变性和致畸潜力，育龄妇女建议适当避孕[82]。

FDA批准更昔洛韦用于预防移植接受者中的CMV疾病，肾功能正常患者的剂量为每12h 5mg/kg，7~14天，然后5mg/kg每天一次（每周7天）或6mg/kg每天一次（每周5天）。治疗的持续时间取决于免疫抑制的程度，处方没有明确建议。

更昔洛韦给药应根据肌酐清除率调整肾损伤，如表98.15所述[82]。

三个预防器官移植患者CMV疾病的随机对照试验对更昔洛韦进行了评价。第一项Ⅲ期研究在149名有CMV疾病风险的心脏移植患者中进行，CMV疾病风险定义为CMV受体血清阳性或供体血清阳性和受体血清阴性[84]。患者随机接受更昔洛韦（n=76）或安慰剂（n=73），共28天。在移植后120天期间观察，与安慰剂（31/73或43%）相比，更昔洛韦治疗的患者（12/76或16%）CMV疾病的总发病率在统计学上显著降低。第二项研究是一项随机双盲安慰剂对照的72例无症状CMV感染（尿液、唾液或血液CMV培养阳性）骨髓移植患者的试验[85]。患者分组接受安慰剂或更昔洛韦，共100天。在第100天和第180天接受更昔洛韦的患者中，CMV疾病的发病率在统计学上显著降低。此外，更昔洛韦治疗的患者在第100天和第180天的总存活率也显著更高。第三个随机开放标记研究评估了40个同种异体骨髓移植受者的CMV疾病风险[86]。患者在移植后第35天进行支气管镜检查和支气管肺泡灌洗。有肺部CMV感染的组织学或病毒学证据的患者随后被随机分组接受更昔洛韦治疗。在更昔洛韦治疗的患者中，CMV疾病的发病率显著降低，在用更昔洛韦治疗的20名患者中有4名（20%）患者，20名对照患者中有14名（70%）发展为间质性肺炎。这些结果被发现与前面提到的骨髓移植受者的研究一致。

表98.15 肾功能损害患者的剂量

肌酐清除率*(mL/min)	更昔洛韦IV诱导剂量(mg/kg)	加药间隔(h)	更昔洛韦IV维持剂量(mg/kg)	加药间隔(h)
≥70	5.0	12	5.0	24
50–69	2.5	12	2.5	24
25–49	2.5	24	1.25	24
10–24	1.25	24	0.625	24
<10	1.25	血透后每周三次	0.625	血透后每周三次

*根据Cookcroft-gault方程确定肌酐清除率。

缬更昔洛韦（Valcyte）

缬更昔洛韦是更昔洛韦的前药，其最初被FDA于2001年批准用于治疗AIDS患者中的CMV视网膜炎[87]。2003年，FDA扩大了缬更昔洛韦的适应证，包括在特定类型的实体器官移植中预防CMV疾病，对于CMV高风险的成人和儿科患者，定义为CMV IgG供体阳性和受体阴性的患者。FDA批准的缬更昔洛韦的适应证是预防CMV高风险的肾脏、心脏或肾脏–胰腺成人移植患者中的CMV疾病和CMV高风险的小儿（年龄在4个月至16岁）心脏或肾脏移植患者[88]。重要的是注意到缬更昔洛韦不适用于成人或小儿肝移植患者。

缬更昔洛韦是更昔洛韦的L–缬氨酸酯，其通过肠或肝酯酶迅速转化为更昔洛韦。与更昔洛韦相比，在实体器官移植患者中评价了缬更昔洛韦的药代动力学。与1000mg的更昔洛韦相比，900mg的缬更昔洛韦的平均全身暴露为更昔洛韦1.7倍[88]。获得的全身暴露在肾、心脏和肝移植中是相当的。与成人患者相比，缬更昔洛韦的药代动力学在儿科器官移植受者中相似。由于其活性代谢物是更昔洛韦，缬更昔洛韦应被认为是潜在的致癌物。

缬更昔洛韦的给药建议包括对于CMV高风险患者的成人和儿科给药建议。对于成年心脏或肾脏胰脏移植患者，推荐剂量为900mg，在移植后10天内每天一次开始，持续至后续第100天。对于成人肾移植患者，推荐剂量为900mg口服，应注意所有成人剂量的缬更昔洛韦应基于通过 Cockcroft-Gault 方程计算的肌酐清除率调整肾功能。在心脏或肾脏儿科移植患者中，缬更昔洛韦的每日剂量应在移植后 10 天开始，并根据以下方程式给药：

儿科剂量(mg)=7×体表面积×CrCl(使用改进的施瓦茨公式计算，不超过 $150mL/min/1.73m^2$)。

$$体表面积(m^2)=\sqrt{\frac{身高(cm)\times体重(kg)}{3600}}$$

Schwartz 式肌酐清除率$[mL/(min\cdot1.73m^2)]$=

$$\frac{k\times身高(cm)}{血清肌酐浓度(mg/dL)}$$

K=

0.45　　4 个月~<1 岁

0.45　　1 岁~<2 岁

0.55　　男孩 2~<13 岁，女孩 2~16 岁

0.7　　男孩 13~16 岁

关于器官移植的指征，有三个主要临床试验在处方信息中提及。第一个是在被认为对 CMV(供体 CMV 血清阳性和受体 CMV 血清阴性）高风险的 372 个肝脏、肾脏、心脏和肾脏胰腺移植受体中进行的双盲双模拟活性比较研究[89]。患者从移植后 10~100 天以 2:1 被随机分为缬更昔洛韦 900mg(n=239)或口服更昔洛韦 1000mg，每天 3 次(n=125)。在移植后的前六个月期间发生 CMV 疾病的患者的比例在缬更昔洛韦(12.1%)和更昔洛韦(15.2%)之间是相当的。作者得出结论，每日三次口服缬更昔洛韦和更昔洛韦在高危实体器官移植患者同样有效且耐良好受。然而重要的是注意到，当根据器官类型分组时，与更昔洛韦组相比，接受缬更昔洛韦的肝移植患者组织浸润性 CMV 疾病的发生率显著增高(见表 98.16)[89]。

第二项研究旨在评估将 CMV 预防从 100 天延长至 200 天的安全性和有效性[90]。这是一项在 326 名CMV 高危肾移植患者中进行的双盲安慰剂对照研究，他们被随机分配每天接受缬更昔洛韦 900mg 200 天或 100 天后改用 100 天安慰剂。使用缬更昔洛韦的延长的 CMV 预防方案在移植后的前 12 个月内在预防 CMV 疾病中是相对有效的(见表 98.17)。然而，移植后 24 个月，CMV 疾病率在治疗组之间是相似的。

最后，第三项研究是在年龄 4 个月至 16 岁的儿科移植患者中进行的，以评估缬更昔洛韦预防 CMV 的安全性和有效性[91]。共有 63 名患有 CMV 疾病风险的儿科实体器官移植患者被纳入口服缬更昔洛韦的开放标签安全性药代动力学研究。儿童患者包括 33 名肾脏、17 名肝脏、12 名心脏和 1 名肾脏肝脏移植患者。基于体表面积和肌酐清除率计算缬更昔洛韦的日剂量。器官移植类型中更昔洛韦的药代动力学相似。平均每日更昔洛韦暴露与每天接受 900mg 的成人受试者相当。重要的是要注意，由于缬更昔洛韦不被批准用于成人肝移植，它也不推荐用于儿科肝移植患者。

静脉用巨细胞病毒免疫球蛋白(CytoGam)

静脉用巨细胞病毒(CMV)免疫球蛋白(CMV–I-GIV)是由含有标准化量的对巨细胞病毒特异性抗体的

表 98.16　CMV 患者类型，组织侵袭性 CMV 疾病或 CMV 综合征的患者的百分比：以 6 个月 ITT 群体为终点

器官	CMV 病[1]		组织浸润性 CMV 疾病		CMV 综合征[2]	
	VGCV(N=239)	GCV(N=125)	VGCV(N=239)	GCV(N=125)	VGCV(N=239)	GCV(N=125)
肝脏	19%	12%	14%	3%	5%	9%
(n=177)	(22/118)	(7/59)	(16/118)	(2/59)	(6/118)	(5/59)
肾脏	6%	23%	1%	5%	5%	18%
(n=120)	(5/81)	(9/39)	(1/81)	(2/39)	(4/81)	(7/39)
心脏	6%	10%	0%	5%	6%	5%
(n=56)	(2/35)	(2/21)	(0/35)	(1/21)	(2/35)	(1/21)
胰肾联合	0%	17%	0%	17%	0%	0%
(n=11)	(0/5)	(1/6)	(0/5)	(1/6)	(0/5)	(0/6)

GCV=口服更昔洛韦；VGCV=缬更昔洛韦。

[1] 患有 CMV 疾病的患者数目=具有组织浸润性 CMV 疾病或 CMV 综合征的患者数目。

[2] CMV 综合征被定义为在 7 天内间隔至少 24h 的两次或更多次的发热≥38℃的 CMV 病毒血症的证据，以及伴随以下一种或多种：不适、白细胞减少、非典型淋巴细胞增多症、血小板减少症和肝转氨酶升高。

表 98.17 具有 CMV 疾病,组织侵袭性 CMV 疾病或 CMV 综合征的肾移植患者的百分比,12 个月 ITT 群体

	CMV 病 [1]		组织浸润性 CMV 疾病		CMV 综合征 [2]	
	100 天 VGCV (*N*=163)	200 天 VGCV (*N*=155)	100 天 VGCV (*N*=163)	200 天 VGCV (*N*=155)	100 天 VGCV (*N*=163)	200 天 VGCV (*N*=155)
病例数	36.8% (60/163)	16.8% (26/155)	1.8% (3/163)[3]	0.6% (1/155)	35.0% (57/163)	16.1% (25/155)

VGCV=缬更昔洛韦。

[1] 患有 CMV 疾病的患者数目=具有组织浸润性 CMV 疾病或 CMV 综合征的患者数目。

[2] CMV 综合征被定义为伴有以下至少一种 CMV 病毒血症的证据:发热≥38℃、严重不适、白细胞减少、非典型淋巴细胞增多、血小板减少和肝转氨酶升高。

[3] 100 天组中的两名患者具有组织浸润性 CMV 疾病和 CMV 综合征,然而,这些患者被认为仅具有组织侵袭性 CMV 疾病。

免疫球蛋白 G(IgG)组成的血浆产品。CMV-IGIV 最初于 1991 年被批准用于 CMV 感染高风险的肾转移患者中减弱原发性 CMV 疾病，定义为 CMV IgG 供体阳性和受体阴性的患者[92]。该适应证在 1998 年扩大,包括其他移植器官。目前 FDA 批准 CMV-IGIV 用于预防与肾、肺、肝、胰腺和心脏移植相关的 CMV 疾病。对于 CMV 感染高风险的移植患者,除了接受肾移植的患者外,应考虑与更昔洛韦联合应用 CMV-IGIV[92]。

CMV-IGIV 衍生自高 CMV 抗体滴度的成年人血浆池。结果,球蛋白含有相对高浓度的针对 CMV 的抗体。施用时,其可以将 CMV 抗体提高到足以减轻或降低严重 CMV 疾病发生率的水平。由于 CMV-IGIV 是从人血浆中获得，理论上它有用于血源性病毒试剂传输以及克雅病病原体传输的可能性。此外，由于 CMV-IGIV 是基于免疫球蛋白的产品,其具有其他免疫球蛋白产物相关的不良事件的风险[92]。无菌性脑膜炎综合征通常在治疗后数小时至数天内开始，并且与严重的头痛、颈部僵硬、嗜睡、发热和畏光有关。非心源性肺水肿据报道已经出现在接受 IGIV 治疗后 1~6h 的患者中,并且与严重的呼吸窘迫、肺水肿、正常的左心室功能、发热和低氧血症相关。肾脏功能障碍、血栓形成和溶血也很少报道与 IGIV 有关。FDA 批准的每次输注 CMV-IGIV 的推荐总剂量为 150mg/kg。基于移植后时间的完全给药建议见表 98.18。

基于 1987 年和 1991 年发表的两项临床试验，CMV-IGIV 对于肾移植患者中的 CMV 预防是有效的。第一项随机试验表明,CMV 综合征的发生率从对照患者(n=35)的 60%显著降低至 21%,在 CMV-IGIV 治疗的患者中(n=24)[93]。在接受 CMV-IGIV 的患者中,严重

表 98.18 静脉用巨细胞病毒免疫球蛋白(CytoGam)

	移植形式	
	肾脏	肝、胰、肺、心
移植后 72h 内	150mg/kg	150mg/kg
2 周后	100mg/kg	150mg/kg
4 周后	100mg/kg	150mg/kg
6 周后	100mg/kg	150mg/kg
8 周后	100mg/kg	150mg/kg
12 周后	50mg/kg	100mg/kg
16 周后	50mg/kg	100mg/kg

CMV 疾病的发生率从 46%降低至 13%。在第二项非随机试验中,36 名肾移植患者接受 CMV-IGIV 治疗,发现 CMV 相关综合征的发生率为 36%[94]。此外,与第一次研究的对照组相比，两项研究中严重的 CMV 疾病,伴随的真菌和寄生性超感染的比率也较低。

根据在其他移植器官中使用 CMV-IGIV 的研究,FDA 在 1998 年批准 CMV-IGIV 用于包括肝、肺、心、脏和胰腺的移植。在分为 CMV-IGIV(n=69)和对照(n=72）的肝移植患者的随机双盲安慰剂对照研究中，CMV-IGIV 治疗组的严重 CMV 疾病的发生率从 27%显著降低至 12%[95]。值得注意的是,在 CMV 高风险的肝移植患者中,严重 CMV 疾病的减少小于其他供体和受体血清学状态的移植。在肝移植患者的随访研究中,将对照患者与接受 CMV-IGIVI 的患者进行比较,一年存活率分别为 72%和 86%(*P*=0.03)[96]。

另外的研究表明，与 CMV-IGIV 和更昔洛韦组合的 CMV 预防可降低 CMV 疾病高风险患者的严重 CMV 相关疾病的发生率，低于单独一种药物所预期

的。与以前的单药预防经验相比，在实体器官移植患者（包括 14 例高危 CMV 肾-胰腺移植患者）中进行的一项研究报道，联合治疗可降低严重 CMV 疾病的发生率[92]。另一项心胸移植的研究比较了 CMV-IGIV 联合静脉更昔洛韦与单用更昔洛韦的预防效果[97]。在 CMV 高危心脏移植患者中，CMV 疾病的发病率从更昔洛韦组（n=16）的 55%降至联合治疗组（n=16）的 46%。此外，患者存活率为 61%~94%，有统计学意义的增加（$P \leq 0.001$）。在 CMV 高风险的心肺或肺单独移植患者中，CMV 疾病的发病率从单用更昔洛韦的 85%降低到联合治疗的 36%。生存率分别从 60%提高到 80%（$P \leq 0.01$）。作为这些研究的结果，CMV-IGIV 接受适应证扩大，包括肾、胰腺、肝、肺和心脏移植受体。

总结

药物批准在大多数国家是一个复杂和高度管制的过程，并且批准过程的知识是必要的，这不仅是为了促进药物试验设计，而且对于特定药物建立剂量推荐的方式有一定的实际认识。已经正式批准用于移植的这些药物具有相对安全性和有效性的明确证据，其在药物批准时达到了相应的标准。虽然这些药物构成了移植受者现代免疫管理的基础，随着时间的推移和新兴知识的发展，额外的辅助疗法和临床医生的经验都会使之不断发展。可以合理地说，所有移植患者在其移植后都需要接受标准化的治疗。本章和第 101 章将帮助读者了解现代免疫管理的良好基础，同时了解临床实践差异。

（沈恬 译　沈恬 校）

参考文献

1. New York Times. [accessed February 12, 2014]; Available from: http://www.nytimes.com/2008/11/02/magazine/02fda-t.html.
2. Food and Drug Administration [accessed February 12, 2014]; Available from: http://www.fda.gov/AboutFDA/WhatWeDo/History/Origin/ucm054819.htm.
3. Food and Drug Administration [accessed February 12, 2014], Available from: http://www.fda.gov/AboutFDA/WhatWeDo/History/Milestones/ucm128305.htm.
4. Independent Policy Report [accessed February 12, 2014]; Available from: http://www.independent.org/pdf/policy_reports/2010-02-10-fda.pdf.
5. Temple R. Policy developments in regulatory approval. Statistics in Medicine. 2002;21(19):2939–2948.
6. Karki L. Review of FDA law related to pharmaceuticals: the Hatch-Waxman Act, regulatory amendments and impications for drug patent enforcement. Journal of the Patent and Trademark Office Society. 2005;87:602–620.
7. Orlando VI. The FDA's accelerated approval process: does the pharmaceutical industry have adequate incentives for self-regulation? American Journal of Law & Medicine. 1999;25(4):543–568.
8. Prescription Drug User Fee Act (PDUFA) CRSRR, by Susan Thaul, Congressional Research Services, 12 July 2007.
9. 21 USC Sec. 321(g)(1).
10. Pisano DJ, Mantus DS. FDA Regulatory Affairs. 2nd ed. New York, NY: Informa Healthcare USA, Inc; 2008.
11. Mathieu M. New Drug Development: A Regulatory Overview. 8th ed. Waltham, MA: Parexel International Corporation; 2008.
12. 21 CFR Part 58.
13. Federal Food, Drug & Cosmetic Act Chapter II Section 201 (g)(1).
14. Code of Federal Regulations Title 21 Section 312.2.
15. Food and Drug Administration [accessed February 12, 2014]; Available from: http://www.fda.gov/cder/guidance/index.htm.
16. Food and Drug Administration [accessed February 12, 2014]; Available from: http://www.fda.gov/downloads/Drugs/GuidanceComplianceRegulatoryInformation/Guidances/ucm075096.pdf.
17. Gabardi S, Halloran PF, Friedewald J. Managing risk in developing transplant immunosuppressive agents: the new regulatory environment. American Journal of Transplantation. 2011;11(9):1803–1809.
18. Food and Drug Administration Guidance for Industry: Format and Content of Proposed Risk Evaluation and Mitigation Strategies (REMS), REMS Assessment, and Proposed REMS Modifications. 2009.
19. Food and Drug Administration [accessed February 12, 2014]; Available from: http://www.accessdata.fda.gov/scripts/cder/drugsatfda/index.cfm?fuseaction=Search.Set_Current_Drug&ApplNo=016324&DrugName=IMURAN&ActiveIngred=AZATHIOPRINE&SponsorApplicant=PROMETHEUS%20LABS&ProductMktStatus=1&goto=Search.DrugDetails.
20. DailyMed [accessed February 12, 2014]; Available from: http://dailymed.nlm.nih.gov/dailymed/drugInfo.cfm?id=46199.
21. Food and Drug Administration [accessed February 12, 2014]; Available from: http://www.accessdata.fda.gov/scripts/cder/drugsatfda/index.cfm?fuseaction=Search.Set_Current_Drug&ApplNo=050625&DrugName=SANDIMMUNE&ActiveIngred=CYCLOSPORINE&SponsorApplicant=NOVARTIS&ProductMktStatus=1&goto=Search.DrugDetails.
22. Food and Drug Administration [accessed February 12, 2014]; Available from: http://www.accessdata.fda.gov/scripts/cder/drugsatfda/index.cfm?fuseaction=Search.Set_Current_Drug&ApplNo=050715&DrugName=NEORAL&ActiveIngred=CYCLOSPORINE&SponsorApplicant=NOVARTIS&ProductMktStatus=1&goto=Search.DrugDetails.
23. DailyMed [accessed February 12, 2014]; Available from: http://dailymed.nlm.nih.gov/dailymed/lookup.cfm?setid=5e5926a7-1de0-4b54-a5c0-286b6200ff82.
24. DailyMed [accessed February 12, 2014]; Available from: http://dailymed.nlm.nih.gov/dailymed/lookup.cfm?setid=94461af3-11f1-4670-95d4-2965b9538ae3.
25. Food and Drug Administration [accessed February 12, 2014]; Available from: http://www.accessdata.fda.gov/scripts/cder/drugsatfda/index.cfm?fuseaction=Search.Set_Current_Drug&ApplNo=050708&DrugName=PROGRAF&ActiveIngred=TACROLIMUS&SponsorApplicant=ASTELLAS&ProductMktStatus=1&goto=Search.DrugDetails.
26. Food and Drug Administration [accessed February 12, 2014]; Available from: http://www.accessdata.fda.gov/scripts/cder/drugsatfda/index.cfm?fuseaction=Search.Overview&DrugName=TACROLIMUS.
27. DailyMed [accessed February 12, 2014]; Available from: http://dailymed.nlm.nih.gov/dailymed/lookup.cfm?setid=7f667de1-9dfa-4bd6-8ba0-15ee2d78873b.
28. A comparison of tacrolimus (FK 506) and cyclosporine for immunosuppression in liver transplantation. The U.S. Multicenter FK506 Liver Study Group. The New England Journal of Medicine. 1994;331(17):1110–1115.
29. Otto G, Bleyl J, Neuhaus P, et al. Corticosteroids and concomitant medication in the European multicentre study of FK 506 and cyclosporin in primary liver transplantation. Transplant International. 1994;7(Suppl 1):S7–S10.
30. Pirsch JD, Miller J, Deierhoi MH, et al. A comparison of tacrolimus (FK506) and cyclosporine for immunosuppression after cadaveric renal transplantation. FK506 Kidney Transplant Study Group. Transplantation. 1997;63(7):977–983.
31. Ekberg H, Tedesco-Silva H, Demirbas A, et al. Reduced exposure to calcineurin inhibitors in renal transplantation. The New England Journal of Medicine. 2007;357(25):2562–2575.
32. Silva HT Jr, Yang HC, Abouljoud M, et al. One-year results with extended-release tacrolimus/MMF, tacrolimus/MMF and cyclosporine/MMF in de novo kidney transplant recipients. American Journal of Transplantation. 2007;7(3):595–608.
33. Grimm M, Rinaldi M, Yonan NA, et al. Superior prevention of acute rejection by tacrolimus vs. cyclosporine in heart transplant recipients–a large European trial. American Journal of Transplantation. 2006;6(6):1387–1397.
34. Kobashigawa JA, Miller LW, Russell SD, et al. Tacrolimus with mycophenolate mofetil (MMF) or sirolimus vs. cyclosporine with MMF in cardiac transplant patients: 1-year report. American Journal of Transplantation. 2006;6(6):1377–1386.

35. Food and Drug Administration [accessed February 12, 2014]; Available from: http://www.accessdata.fda.gov/scripts/cder/drugsatfda/index.cfm?fuseaction=Search.Set_Current_Drug&ApplNo=050722&DrugName=CELLCEPT&ActiveIngred=MYCOPHENOLATE%20MOFETIL&SponsorApplicant=ROCHE%20PALO&ProductMktStatus=1&goto=Search.DrugDetails.
36. Food and Drug Administration [accessed February 12, 2014]; Available from: http://www.accessdata.fda.gov/scripts/cder/drugsatfda/index.cfm?fuseaction=Search.Overview&DrugName=MYCOPHENOLATE%20MOFETIL.
37. DailyMed [accessed February 12, 2014]; Available from: http://dailymed.nlm.nih.gov/dailymed/lookup.cfm?setid=37241e87-4af4-4dc3-a1aa-ea6f20d8dc40.
38. Mycophenolate REMS (Risk Evaluation and Mitigation Strategy) [access February 24th, 2014]; Available from: https://www.mycophenolaterems.com.
39. Sollinger HW. Mycophenolate mofetil for the prevention of acute rejection in primary cadaveric renal allograft recipients. U.S. Renal Transplant Mycophenolate Mofetil Study Group. Transplantation. 1995;60(3):225–232.
40. A blinded, randomized clinical trial of mycophenolate mofetil for the prevention of acute rejection in cadaveric renal transplantation. The Tricontinental Mycophenolate Mofetil Renal Transplantation Study Group. Transplantation. 1996;61(7):1029–1037.
41. Placebo-controlled study of mycophenolate mofetil combined with cyclosporin and corticosteroids for prevention of acute rejection. European Mycophenolate Mofetil Cooperative Study Group. Lancet. 1995;345(8961):1321–1325.
42. Kobashigawa J, Miller L, Renlund D, et al. A randomized active-controlled trial of mycophenolate mofetil in heart transplant recipients. Mycophenolate Mofetil Investigators. Transplantation. 1998;66(4):507–515.
43. Wiesner R, Rabkin J, Klintmalm G, et al. A randomized double-blind comparative study of mycophenolate mofetil and azathioprine in combination with cyclosporine and corticosteroids in primary liver transplant recipients. Liver Transplantation. 2001;7(5):442–450.
44. Food and Drug Administration [accessed February 12, 2014]; Available from: http://www.accessdata.fda.gov/scripts/cder/drugsatfda/index.cfm?fuseaction=Search.Set_Current_Drug&ApplNo=050791&DrugName=MYFORTIC&ActiveIngred=MYCOPHENOLIC%20ACID&SponsorApplicant=NOVARTIS&ProductMktStatus=1&goto=Search.DrugDetails.
45. DailyMed [accessed February 12, 2014]; Available from: http://dailymed.nlm.nih.gov/dailymed/lookup.cfm?setid=eed26501-890d-4ff6-88e7-6dbea4726e53.
46. Salvadori M, Holzer H, de Mattos A, et al. Enteric-coated mycophenolate sodium is therapeutically equivalent to mycophenolate mofetil in de novo renal transplant patients. American Journal of Transplantation. 2004;4(2):231–236.
47. Budde K, Glander P, Diekmann F, et al. Enteric-coated mycophenolate sodium: safe conversion from mycophenolate mofetil in maintenance renal transplant recipients. Transplantation Proceedings. 2004;36(2 Suppl):524S–527S.
48. Food and Drug Administration [accessed February 12, 2014]; Available from: http://www.accessdata.fda.gov/scripts/cder/drugsatfda/index.cfm?fuseaction=Search.Set_Current_Drug&ApplNo=021083&DrugName=RAPAMUNE&ActiveIngred=SIROLIMUS&SponsorApplicant=WYETH%20PHARMS%20INC&ProductMktStatus=1&goto=Search.DrugDetails.
49. DailyMed [accessed February 12, 2014]; Available from: http://dailymed.nlm.nih.gov/dailymed/lookup.cfm?setid=3275b824-3f82-4151-2ab2-0036a9ba0acc.
50. Neff GW, Montalbano M, Tzakis AG. Ten years of sirolimus therapy in orthotopic liver transplant recipients. Transplantation Proceedings. 2003;35(3 Suppl):209S–216S.
51. Abdelmalek MF, Humar A, Stickel F, et al. Sirolimus conversion regimen versus continued calcineurin inhibitors in liver allograft recipients: a randomized trial. American Journal of Transplantation. 2012;12(3):694–705.
52. Kahan BD. Efficacy of sirolimus compared with azathioprine for reduction of acute renal allograft rejection: a randomised multicentre study. The Rapamune US Study Group. Lancet. 2000;356(9225):194–202.
53. MacDonald AS. A worldwide, phase III, randomized, controlled, safety and efficacy study of a sirolimus/cyclosporine regimen for prevention of acute rejection in recipients of primary mismatched renal allografts. Transplantation. 2001;71(2):271–280.
54. Johnson RW, Kreis H, Oberbauer R, et al. Sirolimus allows early cyclosporine withdrawal in renal transplantation resulting in improved renal function and lower blood pressure. Transplantation. 2001;72(5):777–786.
55. Oberbauer R, Kreis H, Johnson RW, et al. Long-term improvement in renal function with sirolimus after early cyclosporine withdrawal in renal transplant recipients: 2-year results of the Rapamune Maintenance Regimen Study. Transplantation. 2003;76(2):364–370.
56. Schena FP, Pascoe MD, Alberu J, et al. Conversion from calcineurin inhibitors to sirolimus maintenance therapy in renal allograft recipients: 24-month efficacy and safety results from the CONVERT trial. Transplantation. 2009;87(2):233–242.
57. Food and Drug Administration [accessed February 12, 2014]; Available from: http://www.accessdata.fda.gov/scripts/cder/drugsatfda/index.cfm?fuseaction=Search.Set_Current_Drug&ApplNo=021560&DrugName=ZORTRESS&ActiveIngred=EVEROLIMUS&SponsorApplicant=NOVARTIS&ProductMktStatus=1&goto=Search.DrugDetails.
58. Insciences [accessed February 12, 2014]; Available from: http://insciences.org/article.php?article_id=8804.
59. DailyMed [accessed February 12, 2014]; Available from: http://dailymed.nlm.nih.gov/dailymed/lookup.cfm?setid=e082a024-7850-400b-a5c2-2a140612562a.
60. Tedesco Silva H Jr, Cibrik D, Johnston T, et al. Everolimus plus reduced-exposure CsA versus mycophenolic acid plus standard-exposure CsA in renal-transplant recipients. American Journal of Transplantation. 2010;10(6):1401–1413.
61. Lorber MI, Mulgaonkar S, Butt KM, et al. Everolimus versus mycophenolate mofetil in the prevention of rejection in de novo renal transplant recipients: a 3-year randomized, multicenter, phase III study. Transplantation. 2005;80(2):244–252.
62. Vitko S, Margreiter R, Weimar W, et al. Everolimus (Certican) 12-month safety and efficacy versus mycophenolate mofetil in de novo renal transplant recipients. Transplantation. 2004;78(10):1532–1540.
63. Food and Drug Administration [accessed February 12, 2014]; Available from: http://www.accessdata.fda.gov/scripts/cder/drugsatfda/index.cfm?fuseaction=Search.Set_Current_Drug&ApplNo=125288&DrugName=NULOJIX&ActiveIngred=BELATACEPT&SponsorApplicant=BRISTOL%20MYERS%20SQUIBB&ProductMktStatus=1&goto=Search.DrugDetails.
64. DailyMed [accessed February 12, 2014]; Available from: http://dailymed.nlm.nih.gov/dailymed/lookup.cfm?setid=c16ac648-d5d2-9f7d-8637-e2328572754e.
65. Vincenti F, Charpentier B, Vanrenterghem Y, et al. A phase III study of belatacept-based immunosuppression regimens versus cyclosporine in renal transplant recipients (BENEFIT study). American Journal of Transplantation. 2010;10(3):535–546.
66. Durrbach A, Pestana JM, Pearson T, et al. A phase III study of belatacept versus cyclosporine in kidney transplants from extended criteria donors (BENEFIT-EXT study). American Journal of Transplantation. 2010;10(3):547–557.
67. Vincenti F, Larsen CP, Alberu J, et al. Three-year outcomes from BENEFIT, a randomized, active-controlled, parallel-group study in adult kidney transplant recipients. American Journal of Transplantation. 2012;12(1):210–217.
68. Archdeacon P, Dixon C, Belen O, et al. Summary of the US FDA approval of belatacept. American Journal of Transplantation. 2012;12(3):554–562.
69. Pestana JO, Grinyo JM, Vanrenterghem Y, et al. Three-year outcomes from BENEFIT-EXT: a phase III study of belatacept versus cyclosporine in recipients of extended criteria donor kidneys. American Journal of Transplantation. 2012;12(3):630–639.
70. Food and Drug Administration [accessed February 12, 2014]; Available from: http://www.fda.gov/BiologicsBloodVaccines/BloodBloodProducts/ApprovedProducts/default.htm.
71. DailyMed [accessed February 12, 2014]; Available from: http://dailymed.nlm.nih.gov/dailymed/lookup.cfm?setid=bbd8ab99-552e-4b81-aca4-6b0c7af8b9ae.
72. Gaber AO, First MR, Tesi RJ, et al. Results of the double-blind, randomized, multicenter, phase III clinical trial of Thymoglobulin versus Atgam in the treatment of acute graft rejection episodes after renal transplantation. Transplantation. 1998;66(1):29–37.
73. Food and Drug Administration [accessed February 12, 2014]; Available from: http://www.accessdata.fda.gov/scripts/cder/drugsatfda/index.cfm?fuseaction=Search.Set_Current_Drug&ApplNo=103764&DrugName=SIMULECT&ActiveIngred=BASILIXIMAB&SponsorApplicant=NOVARTIS&ProductMktStatus=1&goto=Search.DrugDetails.
74. DailyMed [accessed February 12, 2014]; Available from: http://dailymed.nlm.nih.gov/dailymed/lookup.cfm?setid=1af01887-b69d-444b-91ed-ebfe12784440.
75. Food and Drug Administration [accessed February 12, 2014]; Available from: http://www.accessdata.fda.gov/scripts/cder/drugsatfda/index.cfm?fuseaction=Search.Set_Current_Drug&ApplNo=103749&DrugName=ZENAPAX&ActiveIngred=DACLIZUMAB&SponsorApplicant=HOFFMAN%2DLA%20ROCHE&ProductMktStatus=1&goto=Search.DrugDetails.
76. Nashan B, Moore R, Amlot P, et al. Randomised trial of basiliximab versus placebo for control of acute cellular rejection in renal allograft recipients. CHIB 201 International Study Group. Lancet. 1997;350(9086):1193–1198.
77. Kahan BD, Rajagopalan PR, Hall M. Reduction of the occurrence of acute cellular rejection among renal allograft recipients treated with basiliximab, a chimeric anti-interleukin-2-receptor monoclonal antibody. United States Simulect Renal Study Group. Transplantation. 1999;67(2):276–284.
78. Ponticelli C, Yussim A, Cambi V, et al. A randomized, double-blind trial of basiliximab immunoprophylaxis plus triple therapy in kidney transplant recipients. Transplantation. 2001;72(7):1261–1267.
79. Lawen JG, Davies EA, Mourad G, et al. Randomized double-blind study of immunoprophylaxis with basiliximab, a chimeric anti-interleukin-2 receptor monoclonal antibody, in combination with mycophenolate mofetil-containing triple therapy in renal transplantation. Transplantation. 2003;75(1):37–43.
80. Offner G, Broyer M, Niaudet P, et al. A multicenter, open-label, pharmacokinetic/pharmacodynamic safety, and tolerability study of basiliximab (Simulect) in pedi-

atric de novo renal transplant recipients. Transplantation. 2002;74(7):961–966.
81. Food and Drug Administration [accessed February 12, 2014]; Available from: http://www.accessdata.fda.gov/scripts/cder/drugsatfda/index.cfm?fuseaction=Search.Set_Current_Drug&ApplNo=019661&DrugName=CYTOVENE&ActiveIngred=GANCICLOVIR%20SODIUM&SponsorApplicant=ROCHE%20PALO&ProductMktStatus=1&goto=Search.DrugDetails.
82. DailyMed [accessed February 12, 2014]; Available from: http://dailymed.nlm.nih.gov/dailymed/lookup.cfm?setid=38e8f819-985c-4d20-aafd-3ba953af26ca.
83. Anderson RD, Griffy KG, Jung D, et al. Ganciclovir absolute bioavailability and steady-state pharmacokinetics after oral administration of two 3000-mg/d dosing regimens in human immunodeficiency virus- and cytomegalovirus-seropositive patients. Clinical Therapeutics. 1995;17(3):425–432.
84. Merigan TC, Renlund DG, Keay S, et al. A controlled trial of ganciclovir to prevent cytomegalovirus disease after heart transplantation. The New England Journal of Medicine. 1992;326(18):1182–1186.
85. Goodrich JM, Mori M, Gleaves CA, et al. Early treatment with ganciclovir to prevent cytomegalovirus disease after allogeneic bone marrow transplantation. The New England Journal of Medicine. 1991;325(23):1601–1607.
86. Schmidt GM, Horak DA, Niland JC, et al. A randomized, controlled trial of prophylactic ganciclovir for cytomegalovirus pulmonary infection in recipients of allogeneic bone marrow transplants; The City of Hope-Stanford-Syntex CMV Study Group. The New England Journal of Medicine. 1991;324(15):1005–1011.
87. Food and Drug Administration [accessed February 12, 2014]; Available from: http://www.accessdata.fda.gov/scripts/cder/drugsatfda/index.cfm?fuseaction=Search.Set_Current_Drug&ApplNo=021304&DrugName=VALCYTE&ActiveIngred=VALGANCICLOVIR%20HYDROCHLORIDE&SponsorApplicant=HOFFMANN%20LA%20ROCHE&ProductMktStatus=1&goto=Search.DrugDetails.
88. DailyMed [accessed February 12, 2014]; Available from: http://dailymed.nlm.nih.gov/dailymed/lookup.cfm?setid=dc548ff9-e8ea-4d6e-b9b4-e31f53ac4078.
89. Paya C, Humar A, Dominguez E, et al. Efficacy and safety of valganciclovir vs. oral ganciclovir for prevention of cytomegalovirus disease in solid organ transplant recipients. American Journal of Transplantation. 2004;4(4):611–620.
90. Humar A, Lebranchu Y, Vincenti F, et al. The efficacy and safety of 200 days valganciclovir cytomegalovirus prophylaxis in high-risk kidney transplant recipients. American Journal of Transplantation. 2010;10(5):1228–1237.
91. Vaudry W, Ettenger R, Jara P, et al. Valganciclovir dosing according to body surface area and renal function in pediatric solid organ transplant recipients. American Journal of Transplantation. 2009;9(3):636–643.
92. DailyMed [accessed February 12, 2014]; Available from: http://dailymed.nlm.nih.gov/dailymed/lookup.cfm?setid=d72d56e3-1f27-4ec1-a49d-7c0f8f5bc512.
93. Snydman DR, Werner BG, Heinze-Lacey B, et al. Use of cytomegalovirus immune globulin to prevent cytomegalovirus disease in renal-transplant recipients. The New England Journal of Medicine. 1987;317(17):1049–1054.
94. Snydman DR, Werner BG, Tilney NL, et al. Final analysis of primary cytomegalovirus disease prevention in renal transplant recipients with a cytomegalovirus-immune globulin: comparison of the randomized and open-label trials. Transplantation Proceedings. 1991;23(1 Pt 2):1357–1360.
95. Snydman DR, Werner BG, Dougherty NN, et al. Cytomegalovirus immune globulin prophylaxis in liver transplantation. A randomized, double-blind, placebo-controlled trial. Annals of Internal Medicine. 1993;119(10):984–991.
96. Snydman DR, Werner BG, Dougherty NN, et al. A further analysis of the use of cytomegalovirus immune globulin in orthotopic liver transplant patients at risk for primary infection. Boston Center for Liver Transplantation CMVIG-Study Group. Transplantation Proceedings. 1994;26(5 Suppl 1):23–27.
97. Valantine HA, Luikart H, Doyle R, et al. Impact of cytomegalovirus hyperimmune globulin on outcome after cardiothoracic transplantation: a comparative study of combined prophylaxis with CMV hyperimmune globulin plus ganciclovir versus ganciclovir alone. Transplantation. 2001;72(10):1647–1652.

第 99 章
器官移植后感染性疾病的预防

G. Marshall Lyon, III

引言

“一盎司的预防值一磅的治疗。”这句话常归功于本杰明·富兰克林。然而,这句话的起源比富兰克林要早得多。第一个书面记载可追溯到 13 世纪 Henry de Bracton 的手稿。不论其起源如何,都很适用于移植。预防感染通常比尝试和治愈感染更容易。对于移植患者和供者,这种预防可以采取多种形式——药物治疗、免疫接种或通过卫生或避免患者接触来防止疾病。

移植受体的预防措施不可能完全避免疾病或感染。它们可以减轻疾病,使感染性发作程度减轻。它们也可以延迟疾病的发作,直到移植后期。延迟感染的发生可能有好处。目前更常使用更有效的免疫抑制诱导,延迟感染发作直到免疫系统恢复。类似地,移植前疫苗接种可能不能完全防止移植后的疾病,但可以减轻疾病的严重性并缩短持续时间。这似乎也是实验性巨细胞病毒(CMV)疫苗的情况,其中与安慰剂受体相比,疫苗受体需要的抗病毒治疗天数更少。当考虑实体器官移植中的感染时,机会性感染通常存在 1~6 个月(见第 94 章中的图 94.1)。然而,在使用有效预防性药物的情况下,该时间框架可以转移到 6~12 个月。

在本章中,我们将讨论实体器官移植中针对感染性疾病所使用的有效预防措施。本章补充了关于供体来源、围术期和术后感染疾病诊断和管理的内容(第 92 章至第 94 章)。

肾、胰腺和肾/胰腺移植中的预防

表 99.1 总结了肾、胰腺和肾/胰腺受体推荐的抗微生物治疗的剂量和持续时间。

细菌预防

手术预防

一般认为即使是膀胱被定植,肾移植手术产生的也是干净的外科切口。在任意情况下,手术部位感染(SSI)均为低风险(通常<2%)。通常引起 SSI 的细菌是葡萄球菌属(Staphylococcus sp)。肾移植是典型的清洁手术。因此,外科预防应使用具有抗葡萄球菌活性的抗生素,包括抗葡萄球菌青霉素和第一代头孢菌素。优选在皮肤切割前 30min 内预防性给予抗生素[1]。抗生素可以在术后持续使用长达 24h,但延长持续时间未显示能降低 SSI 的发生率。对于对青霉素过敏的患者,主要的选择是万古霉素[1]。由于通常会被定义为起效时间轻慢的药物,万古霉素应在皮肤切开前 60min 开始使用。万古霉素也可用于具有耐甲氧西林金黄色葡萄球菌(MRSA)定植记录的患者。第二代头孢菌素也可用于没有青霉素或头孢菌素过敏的患者。

胰腺移植被认为是清洁-污染伤口。这是因为十二指肠在手术过程中被打开过(详见前面的章节)。因此,除葡萄球菌外,通常胰腺移植相关的 SSI 还与定居在十二指肠的微生物有关,包括肠球菌属、克雷白菌属、大肠杆菌、肠杆菌属、厌氧革兰阴性杆菌和假丝酵母属。尽管在胰腺移植中引起手术部位感染的微生物的种类较多,头孢唑林仍然是有效的预防剂。这是因为大多数需氧革兰阴性杆菌对它高度敏感。肾移植中如果患者有青霉素或头孢菌素过敏,那么可以使用万古霉素[1]。然而,它应该与庆大霉素或左氧氟沙星结合,以防止革兰阴性菌感染。虽然没有强大的数据支持,一些中心选择加入氟康唑,以预防念珠菌[2]。如果使用,氟康唑通常在移植后持续 5~14 天。许多中心培养腹部器官的灌注液,并针对可能生长的任何潜在病原体进行靶向

表 99.1 肾脏或肾脏/胰腺移植受体的一般预防措施建议

	优选预防措施	替代预防措施
手术预防	头孢唑啉 1g iv 皮肤切口前 0~30min	万古霉素 1g iv 皮肤切开前 60min
CMV	缬更昔洛韦、阿昔洛韦和伐昔洛韦，需要对肾功能不全进行剂量调整	
D+/R-*	缬更昔洛韦每天 450~900mg，3~6 个月	抢先监控
R+[†]	缬更昔洛韦每天 450~900mg，3 个月	抢先监控
D-R-[‡]		阿昔洛韦 400~800mg TID[§]或伐昔洛韦 500mg BID 3~6 个月
真菌		
念珠菌	氟康唑每日 200mg，最多 14 天	阿托伐醌每天 1500mg
PCP**	Smx/tmp 1DS[‖] 每周三次	氨苯砜每日 100mg
		吸入戊脒氯林可霉素+乙胺嘧啶

* 供体血清阳性/受体血清阴性；[†]受体血清阳性；[‡]供体血清阴性/受体血清阴性；[§]每天三次（每 8 小时），每天两次（每 12 小时）；** 肺炎；[‖]双重强度（磺胺甲恶唑 800mg-甲氧苄啶 160mg）。

治疗。

牙科预防

几乎没有数据支持在进行牙科手术之前对移植受者使用常规抗生素预防。然而，无论是否是侵入手术，大多数中心建议患者在牙科手术前服用抗生素[3]。如果使用，大多数移植中心使用美国心脏协会心内膜炎预防指南推荐的方案[3,4]。

治疗无症状菌尿

美国传染病学会（IDSA）指南建议对无症状菌尿进行治疗[5]。然而，这些指南为刚刚接受泌尿生殖外科手术的患者提供了例外。许多中心在输血移植后约 90 天内留下输尿管支架。如果在支架保留在适当位置时检测到无症状的细菌尿，则大多数中心将进行治疗。这是因为更严重的感染，如败血症或肾盂肾炎，与移植后早期的无症状菌尿有关[6]。抗微生物剂的选择应通过敏感性试验来指导，尽管没有明确定义，持续时间可能为 7~10 天。

在美国，结核分枝杆菌的感染相对不常见。然而，参与透析的患者与一般人群相比，潜伏感染结核分枝杆菌的风险是 30 倍[7]。建议所有潜在的移植受体在移植前筛查潜伏性结核病（TB）[8]。然而，潜伏性 TB 感染的治疗时间可以在移植之前或之后立即进行。韩国研究评估了在移植时进行干扰素-γ 释放测定（IGRA）对潜伏性 TB 感染的作用[9]。所有四个最终发展为结核的移植后患者均为 IGRA 阳性。此外，所有皮肤测试为潜伏性结核感染阳性的患者在移植后接受 9 个月的异烟肼（INH）治疗[9]。这些患者中没有一个（n=24）发展为活动性 TB[9]。这项研究表明，即使潜在结核病的所有治疗均在移植后给予，仍能有效降低活动性 TB 的风险。然而，移植后 IGRA 测试的灵敏度尚未评估。因此，重要的是在移植前进行某种形式的潜伏性 TB 筛选。

真菌预防

除了上面关于胰腺移植所提到的，特异性抗真菌预防通常不是肾、胰腺或肾/胰腺移植的保证。肾脏和胰腺移植受体在移植后有发展为隐球菌病的风险。目前 IDSA 指南推荐至少 6 个月的氟康唑维持，然后停用氟康唑后检测血清隐球菌抗原（CrAg）[10]。如果血清 CrAg 在治疗停止后上升，并且没有活动性疾病的迹象，大多数移植感染病专家将重新开始使用氟康唑且无限期使用。

耶式肺孢子虫以前被称为卡氏肺囊虫（P.carinii），已经从寄生虫重新归类为真菌。所有移植受体接受针对肺孢子虫肺炎（PCP）的某种预防。磺胺甲恶唑/甲氧苄啶（smx/tmp）是防止 PCP 的优选试剂。许多患者对 smx/tmp 有过敏反应。smx/tmp 在预防 PCP 方面明显优于二线药物，所以应该查明患者有什么样的不良反应。许多人在使用 smx/tmp 时有光敏反应，这可以通过限制阳光暴露来避免。PCP 预防的持续时间通常为移植后 6 个月。然而，如果患者接受抗淋巴细胞抗体来治疗排斥反应，则应继续给予 smx/tmp 3~6 个月。此外，一些使用抗胸腺细胞免疫球蛋白诱导免疫抑制的中心将 PCP 预防的时间延长至至少两年，有些甚至为终生预防。

smx/tmp 的替代品包括氨苯砜、阿托伐醌、吸入喷他脒和克林霉素+乙胺嘧啶[11]。氨苯砜具有磺胺成分。因此,对磺胺过敏的患者不应给予氨苯砜。氨苯砜也与肺移植患者的溶血性贫血有关[12]。氨苯砜通过肾脏清除,但没有关于调节肾功能的具体建议。在研究肺受体对发生溶血性贫血的氨苯砜的研究中,肌酐的峰值与血液性贫血的最终发展之间存在联系[12]。这表明移植后肾功能降低的患者(如延迟移植功能)应降低氨苯砜剂量或使用阿托伐醌用于 PCP 预防。阿托伐醌从医学角度来说通常耐受良好。阿托伐醌是一种液体,可以与任何液体混合。然而,许多患者不喜欢阿托伐醌的味道,也不喜欢喝大量的液体来掩饰味道。

寄生虫预防

在美国,寄生虫感染通常不是大多数移植受体的主要问题。此外,用于 PCP 预防的 smx/tmp、氨苯砜和阿托伐醌也具有抗弓形虫的活性,弓形虫是移植受体中最常见的寄生虫感染。弓形虫病不是移植人群中的一个主要问题,但仍建议患者不要清理猫便盆或吃未煮熟的生肉。

随着来自拉丁美洲移民的捐赠者和受体人口比例越来越大,克氏锥虫越来越受到关注。最近在美国进行的监测显示血清阳性率为 0.026%。然而,在墨西哥出生的捐献者中,患病率为 0.3%,在中美洲出生的患者为 0.5%[13]。由于目前美国没有 FDA 批准的治疗查加斯病(美国锥虫病)的药物,因此该病值得关注。心脏移植已经成功地解决了查加斯心脏病,但结果不太有利,因为早期死亡率为 18%[14]。查加斯病在来自两个查加斯阳性供体的非心脏器官中没有发生,但使用来自克氏锥虫血清反应阳性供体的肾脏或胰腺移植只应在挽救生命的情况下才进行。如果潜在的移植受体术前的查加斯病检测为阳性,则在移植前治疗较为明智。苯并咪唑或硝苯呋醇都具有一些抗克氏锥虫的活性,然而通常不可能治愈。如果使用来自克氏锥虫血清阳性供体的器官,则应考虑治疗受体。治疗使用苄硝唑,持续时间应为 30~60 天[15]。

病毒预防

除 CMV,呼吸道病毒(流感、副流感、呼吸道合胞病毒等)是移植受体中最常见的病毒感染源。目前,年度流感疫苗是减少呼吸道病毒感染的最佳措施。推荐的疫苗将在本章后面讨论。虽然有流感免疫诱发同种抗体的关注[16-18],似乎常规的流感疫苗是安全的。在 2000—2006 年间的一项大型研究中,Hurst 等发现流感疫苗在移植术后第一年与急性排斥反应无关[19]。然而,流感疫苗接种与移植物流失风险降低 [校正风险比(HR)=0.77:95%置信区间 (CI);0.69~0.85,P<0.001]和死亡(HR=0.82:95%CI;0.76~0.89,P<0.001)有关[19]。由于数据细节的限制,作者无法将免疫的时间与排斥发作相关联。他们也未能够评估流感病毒的排除时间[19]。多个其他研究已经研究了针对神经氨酸酶和血凝素的中和抗体的替代终点以及不良反应(发热、注射部位的疼痛、肌酐的变化)。所有这些研究的结论是,流感免疫似乎能安全、有效地使肾移植受体产生抗体[20-23]。

CMV 已经是与移植最相关的病毒感染。CMV 能够感染许多器官系统,包括胃肠道、肝脏、骨髓、中枢神经系统和眼睛。未治疗的 CMV 疾病可具有灾难性后果,包括永久性脑损伤、失明和死亡。1989 年,Balfour 及其同事评估了阿昔洛韦在肾移植后预防 CMV 疾病方面的用途。患者随机服用阿昔洛韦或安慰剂 12 周。有症状的 CMV 疾病的发生率在阿昔洛韦组为 7.5%,而安慰剂组为 29%,P=0.002[24]。因此,许多中心采用阿昔洛韦用于初步预防高风险患者中的 CMV 疾病,如供体阳性和 CMV 受体阴性(D+/R-)。然而,CMV 对体外阿昔洛韦敏感性差。更昔洛韦被开发为针对 CMV 的抗病毒剂。Flechner 等以随机化方式评价 3 个月的口服更昔洛韦或口服阿昔洛韦。除 CMV 疾病,他们对 CMV 进行了常规血培养。移植后 6 个月,CMV 病毒血症发生在 2.5%的更昔洛韦治疗的患者和 36%的阿昔洛韦治疗的患者中,P=0.0001。在 D+/R-患者中观察到更昔洛韦比阿昔洛韦的效果更好,为 54%对 0%(P=0.0008)。因此,许多中心转为使用更昔洛韦常规预防移植受体中的 CMV 感染。

然而,随着诊断技术的进步和更昔洛韦相关毒性的出现,许多移植中心寻求用抗病毒药物进行普遍预防的替代方案,先发制人地治疗巨细胞病毒感染。改进的诊断技术意味着可以在症状发展之前很好地检测 CMV。这些测定包括 pp65 检测和 CMV 核酸检测。pp65 测定使用针对 pp65(CMV 上的表面蛋白)的直接荧光抗体。该测试可以在症状发作前 1 周检出阳性。核酸扩增测定通常更敏感,并且可以在症状之前 7~14 天在血清或血浆中检测 CMV 的存在。先发制人依赖于非常灵敏的测定和频繁的监测。提前制订方法的益处是减少抗病毒药物剂量暴露,从而使毒性降低,潜在地降低更昔洛韦的抗性以及患者成本。缺点是移植中心的成本较高以及潜在的更严重的疾病，特别是如果患者对频繁的测试方案不依从或移植中心工作人员错过阳性结果时。当直接比较时,普遍预防和先发制人的方法在预防 CMV 疾病方面似乎是相同的。

更昔洛韦的前药缬更昔洛韦,于 2000 年初由 FDA 开发并批准。缬更昔洛韦的生物利用度更高,能保证与静脉内更昔洛韦相当的血浆水平。一项大型随机临床研究评估口服缬更昔洛韦的剂量为 900mg/d,相对于口服更昔洛韦 1000mg,每日 3 次,用于预防 D+/R−移植受体的 CMV 疾病[25]。本研究纳入所有器官移植患者。在 364 名可评估的患者中,120 名（33%）是肾移植患者。患者在移植后 3 个月内接受研究药物。在移植后 6 个月和 12 个月时，对于 CMV 治疗的患者数量在组之间相当,缬更昔洛韦分别为 23%和 30.5%,口服更昔洛韦为 21.6%和 28.0%[25]。该研究符合非劣效标准,缬更昔洛韦被大多数中心迅速采用作为预防 CMV 的优选药物。然而,当 FDA 批准缬更昔洛韦时,在肝移植受体中没有 CMV 预防的指征。这一决定是基于在接受缬更昔洛韦的肝移植受体发生了更多的组织侵入性疾病(更多细节参见下一部分关于肝移植的预防)。

随后关于在肾移植受体中使用缬更昔洛韦预防的研究进一步改进了其作用。最初发表的研究表明,在肾移植患者中每天口服 450mg 导致血液水平足以预防 CMV。然后,Humar 等的一项研究显示,延长缬更昔洛韦 900mg/d 预防从 100~200 天导致移植后 2 年 CMV 疾病显著减少,为 38.7%对 21.3%,$P<0.001$[26]。移植物排斥或患者存活没有差异[26]。Humar 等的研究之前公布的共有指南[27]建议在 D+/R−患者中使用 900mg/d 的缬更昔洛韦 3~6 个月,在 R+患者中使用 3 个月。对于 CMV 为 D−R−的患者，应进行单纯疱疹和水痘带状疱疹病毒的预防[27]。

主要是由于缺乏有效的抗病毒药物，除一些非常具体的情况外,不推荐对其他病毒的常规预防。大多数患有终末期肾病(ESRD)的患者应接种乙型肝炎病毒(HBV)疫苗。然而,如果受体没有对疫苗接种产生有效的抗体反应，并且他们最终从 HBV 感染的供体(HBV cAb+,HBV sAg+或 HBV DNA+)接受肾脏,则受体应尽可能接受 HBV 免疫球蛋白和(或)开始抗病毒预防。对 HBV 有活性的抗病毒药物包括拉米夫定、替诺福韦、恩曲他滨和恩替卡韦。除抗病毒药物,患者应对 HBV 感染进行监测。这包括在移植后第 1、第 3、第 6 和第 12 个月对 HBV sAg 和 HBV DNA 进行检测。如果其中任一种变为阳性,则患者应保持抗病毒治疗,直到患者形成可检测的 HBVsAb。如果患者接受来自急性流感感染供体的器官，则考虑在移植后给予受体奥司他韦 5~10 天。当然这是一个非硬性的推荐,因为没有流感通过肾移植传播的记录。

肝移植中的预防

肝移植中推荐的预防策略概述见表 99.2。

细菌预防

肝移植术后细菌感染常见。根据 CDC 监测,手术部位感染在肝移植手术高达 20%[28]。这些感染范围从表面伤口感染到深部器官感染。正如在任何外科手术中一样，表面和深部伤口感染通常与典型的皮肤生物体有关。然而,深部器官感染通常与胆道或肠的菌群有关,这取决于所进行的外科手术。在作者的培训期间, Robert H. Rubin 被认为是移植感染病的早期领导者之一,其曾经说过“移植中的感染风险与外科医生的技能直接相关”。更准确的说法是越复杂的手术越有可能感染并发症。通过 Mayo Jacksonville 的经验,作者在 2 年内分析了 370 例肝移植[29],多变量分析后,只有 2 个因素与感染风险显著相关,即手术时间(>6h)和低肝移植物重量与受体 BMI 比率(<0.01)[29]。此外,在这项研究中，手术部位感染与移植物丢失或死亡的风险增加显著相关。手术部位感染患者的 12 个月累积移植物丢失或死亡率超过 20%，而没有手术部位感染的患者约为 8%[29]。因此,重要的是选择用于外科预防的抗生素,且应对十二指肠和胆道的菌群具有良好的作用。

西班牙移植组涵盖了西班牙的所有移植中心,在 2 年内回顾了他们的肝移植队列，以了解抗生素的选择是否影响手术感染的发生率。在队列中有 1222 个肝移植病例。累计 12 个月手术部位感染率为 8.8%。其中大多数(42%)为切口感染,仅 26%为深部脓肿[30]。在单变量分析中，头孢唑林的使用与手术部位感染的风险增加相关。然而,由于在某个中心头孢唑啉使用率非常高,这种关联在多变量分析上退出。多因素分析后,发生手术部位感染的几个危险因素包括：胆总管空肠造

表 99.2 肝移植一般预防措施建议

	优选预防措施	替代预防措施
手术预防	氨苄西林或万古霉素	氨苄西林/舒巴坦与哌拉西林/他唑巴坦或碳青霉烯
	第三代头孢菌素或碳青霉烯或	
	氟喹诺酮或氨基糖苷	
	氟康唑(仅高危患者)	
CMV	缬更昔洛韦、阿昔洛韦和伐昔洛韦,需要对肾功能障碍进行剂量调整	
D+/R-*	抢先监控	缬更昔洛韦 900mg/d,3 个月
R+†	抢先监控	缬更昔洛韦 900mg/d,3 个月
D-R-‡		阿昔洛韦 400~800mg TID§或
		伐昔洛韦 500mg BID 3~6 个月
真菌	氟康唑每日 200mg,最多 70 天	
念珠菌	Smz/tmp 1DS‖ 每周 3 次	
PCP**		阿托伐醌每日 1500mg,氨苯砜每日 100mg,吸入戊脒氯林可霉素+乙胺嘧啶
乙肝	拉米夫定+乙型肝炎免疫球蛋白	拉米夫定+恩替卡韦或
		恩曲他滨+替诺福韦或
		拉米夫定+替诺福韦

* 供体血清阳性/受体血清阴性;† 受体血清阳性;‡供体血清阴性/受体血清阴性;§每天 3 次(每 8h),每天 2 次(每 12h);** 肺炎;‖ 双重强度(磺胺甲恶唑 800mg-甲氧苄啶 160amg)。

口术(OR=4.2:95%CI;1.6~10.7,P=0.003),先前的肝或肾移植(OR=2.6:95%CI;1.1~6.3,P=0.029),红细胞输注>4U(OR=2.0:95%CI;1.1~3.4)[30]。值得注意的是,大量输血也被发现会增加念珠菌感染的风险[31]。所有这些研究结果都加强了 Rubin 博士指出的原则的合理性,即如果手术由于任何原因而复杂,那么感染的风险就会增加。

然而,这些研究如何帮助选择手术抗生素预防的方案?西班牙研究发现,肠球菌属菌种对其队列中的所有感染负责。因此,重要的是选择具有抗肠球菌活性的抗生素方案。西班牙研究的学者认为,含或不含氨苄西林的第二代或第三代头孢菌素可能是足够的。他们的数据表明糖肽类药物加上氟喹诺酮也是可接受的选择(OR=1.2:95%CI;0.01~13.4,单变量分析)[30]。这在具有所述青霉素/头孢菌素过敏的患者中或在已知患有 MRSA 的患者中也是可接受的方案。这些方案得到目前正在进行修订的指南的支持[1]。尽管选择了抗生素,重要的是,一般建议初始或最后一次给药后 6h,或存在大体积失血时重新给予抗生素,并继续使用抗生素 48h[1],复杂手术后抗生素通常持续更长时间。

除手术预防外,通常无需常规的抗生素预防。目前显然认为如果在术后从体液收集物中分离出细菌,然后使用抗生素是治疗而不是预防。

真菌预防

念珠菌感染是肝移植后最常见的真菌感染[32]。氟康唑在移植后 70 天的常规应用能降低肝移植中念珠菌感染的发生率[33]。然而,这项随机安慰剂对照研究的氟康唑组念珠菌感染率高于大多数中心所遇到的[32,33]。因此,许多中心在发生真菌感染的高风险患者中使用氟康唑。用于确定高风险的标准是:已知的念珠菌定植(尿道、伤口或呼吸道)、胆总管吻合术、再移植、术中施用>40U 的细胞血液制品(红细胞或血小板)、术前肌酐≥2.0mg/dL,或返回手术室修复黏性渗漏或出血并发症[34]。如果患者具有这些标准中的两个或更多个,则认为他处于真菌感染的高风险中,应在围术期进行抗真菌预防[34,35]。然而,小于两个上述标准的患者无需常规抗真菌预防[36]。

在移植后的前 6~12 个月,推荐对所有移植受体进行肺孢子虫预防(包括肝移植)[11]。抗生素的选择与肾移植受体相同,包括磺胺甲恶唑/甲氧苄啶、氨苯砜、阿托伐醌、吸入喷他脒和克林霉素+吡甲胺[11]。对于磺胺过敏患者,阿托伐醌或喷他脒是可接受的替代品。戊脒具有每月给药的方便性。然而,喷他脒气溶胶需要专门的设备和有经验的人员进行有效的给药[11]。

曲霉菌病和隐球菌病在肝移植中通常是低频晚

期感染，且常规抗真菌预防不是必需的，但由于某些特定情况下可能在供体中检测到疾病，预防疾病传播是需要的。

寄生虫预防

对于肾移植受者，用于 PCP 预防的一些药剂对弓形虫有效。然而，肝移植中通常无需预防弓形体感染。有时与肾移植类似的，拉丁美洲农村地区出生的肝移植受者应考虑查加斯病。如果发现且时间允许，应在移植前对患者进行治疗或治疗移植后复发的受体。

病毒预防

CMV

像肾移植一样，CMV 是肝移植后最容易感染的病毒，然而不推荐使用用于肾移植受者的常规 CMV 化学预防。在 D+/R–受体中，缬更昔洛韦在预防 CMV 疾病方面不逊色于口服更昔洛韦。然而，当 FDA 分析数据时，他们发现与口服更昔洛韦相比，接受缬更昔洛韦的肝移植受体组织浸润性 CMV 疾病发病率更高[37]。因此，预防肝移植中 CMV 疾病不是缬更昔洛韦的适应证。与每天 450mg 口服相比，每天 900mg 口服的研究和批准的剂量似乎与增加的毒性风险相关。在一个尚未发表的摘要中，Kalil 等发现高剂量的缬更昔洛韦与白细胞减少的风险相关（OR=5.24；95%CI：2.09~13.15，$P<0.001$）[38]。

如果不进行 CMV 预防，则应考虑使用伐昔洛韦或阿昔洛韦预防单纯疱疹病毒（HSV）和水痘带状疱疹病毒感染[39,40]。HSV 通常发生在移植后的第一个月。

乙型肝炎

在移植前未接受乙型肝炎免疫的患者应接受免疫接种。如果需要，可以加速注射免疫进度。接受肝移植的慢性乙型肝炎患者应在移植前进行治疗。治疗通常由联合治疗组成，因为拉米夫定单药治疗失败率高[41]。拉米夫定耐受性良好，具有极好的安全性。它通常与替诺福韦或阿德福韦组合。拉米夫定联合乙型肝炎免疫球蛋白也能有效预防移植后复发[42]。

丙型肝炎

至今还没有用于预防移植后丙型肝炎复发的特异性药物。然而，许多中心使用不同方法来最小化移植后丙型肝炎复发的风险。这是通过：类固醇的快速减量，通过缓慢慢速类固醇减量降低排斥反应的风险或避免 CMV[43]。

呼吸道病毒

常规季节性流感免疫是预防肝移植中流感的最有效手段[44,45]。感染流感后移植的受体可以接受奥司他韦治疗 10 天[46,47]。

肺移植中的预防

肺移植中的一般预防建议见表 99.3。

细菌和真菌预防

肺移植与其他外科手术类似，因为患者浅表性伤口感染的风险最可能来自皮肤菌群。然而，与其他外科

表 99.3 肺移植建议的一般预防措施

	优选预防措施	替代预防措施
手术预防	氨苄西林或万古霉素和第三代头孢菌素或碳代青霉烯或氟喹诺酮	哌拉西林/他唑巴坦或碳青霉烯或克林霉素+头孢他啶或氟喹诺酮
CMV	缬更昔洛韦、阿昔洛韦和伐昔洛韦，需要对肾功能障碍进行剂量调整	
D+/R–*	缬更昔洛韦每日 900mg，12 个月	提前监控
R+†	缬更昔洛韦每日 900mg，12 个月	提前监控
D–R–‡		阿昔洛韦 400~800mg TID§或伐昔洛韦 500mg BID 3~6 个月
真菌		
霉菌	伏立康唑 200mg，每日 2 次，≥4 个月	伊曲康唑 200~400mg，每 2 两次
PCP**	Smx/tmp 1DS‖ 每周 3 次	阿托伐醌每天 1500mg，氨苯砜每天 100mg，吸入戊脒氯林可霉素+乙胺嘧啶

* 供体血清阳性/受体血清阴性；† 受体血清阳性；‡供体血清阴性/受体血清阴性；§每天 3 次（每 8h），每天 2 次（每 12h）；** 肺炎；‖ 双重强度（磺胺甲恶唑 800mg–甲氧苄啶 160mg）。

手术不同，肺移植涉及切入气管树。因此，手术预防的选择还必须考虑可能存在于该身体部位中的细菌。这包括捐助者和受体的气道。许多中心和器官采购组织经常带有气道菌群，然后选择针对任何生物生长的抗生素。这种做法主要基于观察性研究，显示肺炎是肺移植后最常见的感染[48]。美国健康系统药剂师协会的指南建议头孢唑林、头孢呋辛或万古霉素用于青霉素过敏患者。然而，这些指南没有实际数据支持，因此默认为是用于非移植心胸外科手术的预防性方案[1]。这些指南表明，治疗应根据供体培养的结果进行调整。对于经验性围术期预防，许多中心选择可能涵盖呼吸系统相关或吸入性肺炎的抗生素。在我们中心，经验方案是万古霉素和头孢他啶，可覆盖口腔菌群、可能的 MRSA 和假单胞菌。然而，碳青霉烯、抗假单胞菌青霉素或抗假单胞菌头孢菌素+/-氨苄西林或万古霉素也有合理的覆盖范围。对于脓毒性肺病患者、囊性纤维化或支气管扩张，围术期方案通常基于受体最近的情况来设计。该方案应包括对革兰阳性口腔菌群有活性的抗微生物剂。或者如果 MRSA 是本地的流行病问题，万古霉素也应该包括在抗生素方案中。当然，抗生素管理的时间安排应遵循卫生保健控制实践咨询委员会[49]的现行指南。最近的数据表明，万古霉素和氟喹诺酮类药物除外，其应在切皮前 1h 内服用，抗生素应在皮肤切口之前 0~30min 给予[50]。

肺炎是一种重要的移植后并发症，但支气管吻合口是感染的关键部位。由于支气管吻合口需要 6~12 周的时间愈合，它容易感染病原性和腐生生物。对于已经显示假丝酵母和青霉菌导致吻合口感染可能导致吻合破裂的真菌尤其如此[51]。此外，除小肠移植，肺移植受体在侵袭性真菌感染，特别是曲霉病中的风险最高。移植后 12 个月，8.6%的肺移植患者将发生侵袭性真菌感染，其中 64%是曲霉病或不明的感染[32]。因此，防止真菌感染可能对肺移植非常有利。然而，还未明确最有效的抗真菌剂。大多数中心使用伏立康唑，联用或不联用吸入两性霉素 B[52]。然而，一些中心仅使用吸入的两性霉素 B 产品，并且脂质复合物两性霉素 B 已被证明仅在间歇给药时(2 周后每周一次)可耐受[53]。Drew 等研究在吸入性两性霉素 B 组中有 14.3%的预防失败，在吸入性脂质复合物两性霉素 B 组中有 11.8%的失败[53]。这些比率优于匹兹堡大学使用氟康唑普遍预防 3 个月的回顾性分析。如果发现患者感染曲霉菌，则使用系统性的氟康唑与吸入的两性霉素 B 的靶向干预[54]。采用这种方法，他们在一年内经历了 23%的侵袭性曲霉菌。然而，在切换到使用伏立康唑 200mg 每日 2 次，移植后最少持续 4 个月的普遍预防方法后，他们将侵入性曲霉菌率减少至 1.5%[54]。因此，普遍吸入两性霉素 B——脱氧胆酸盐或脂质复合物比氟康唑更好，但伏立康唑的普遍预防似乎优于吸入性两性霉素 B，分别为 1.5%对 11%~15%。虽然这些数据从来没有被好好地比较过。遗憾的是，伏立康唑还是存在问题。研究已表明伏立康唑用于肺移植受体会增加皮肤癌的发生率[55-57]。虽然存在这一问题，这种风险必须与发生侵袭性曲霉病的高风险和高相关死亡率相比较。幸运的是，泊沙康唑、伊曲康唑或目前正在研究的药物伊沙康唑可能成为另一种选择。其中，目前只有伊曲康唑显示有效[58]。然而，伊曲康唑的生物利用度较差，并且许多中心遵循血液浓度以确保水平足够高。泊沙康唑可有效预防急性骨髓性白血病或骨髓增生异常综合征患者的真菌感染[59,60]。因此，目前只能假定泊沙康唑在肺转移预防中有效是合理的，但这还没有得到证实。

肺移植受体的 PCP 风险增加。然而，不像其他移植受体，这种风险可能随着生存提高。因此，目前的指南推荐继续使用 PCP 预防终生[11]。与其他器官移植受体一样，smx/tmp 是优选试剂。替代药物包括氨苯砜、阿托伐醌、吸入喷他脒和克林霉素加乙胺嘧啶。然而，在肺移植受体中应谨慎使用氨苯砜，因为葡萄糖-6 磷酸酶缺乏(G6PD)的溶血性贫血的风险可能增加，特别是伴随肾衰竭时[12]。

寄生虫预防

和肾移植受体一样，一些用于 PCP 预防的药剂对弓形虫有效。然而肝移植中通常不需要弓形体预防。与肾移植类似的，肝移植中拉丁美洲农村地区出生的受体应考虑查加斯病的可能。如果发现且时间允许，应在移植前对患者进行治疗或治疗移植后复发的受体。

病毒预防

移植前对乙型肝炎病毒的免疫可能有助于减少乙型肝炎与器官传播的机会。然而，如果肺部已知是从活跃感染的捐赠者获得或最近感染的(例如 HBV cAb IgM 阳性)，则应考虑使用拉米夫定与 HBIG 预防感染。如果肺移植受体确实发展成慢性/活动性 HBV 感染，则需要使用抗病毒剂联合治疗。

针对季节性流感的疫苗接种在肺移植受体中诱导免疫应答是有效的[61-63]。而且在一般群体中,中和抗体与针对季节性流感的保护相关。因此,建议肺移植受体每年免疫,优选在疫苗可用时立即免疫。

CMV 是移植后发病的主要原因。CMV 与闭塞性支气管炎综合征(BOS)的发病相关[64,65]。在 Paya 等[25]的关键研究中没有足够数量的肺移植受体加入使得 FDA 给予缬更昔洛韦作为这些患者的 CMV 预防的适应证。然而,一项随访研究检查了肺移植术后 12 个月和 3 个月时缬更昔洛韦每日 900mg(对于肾功能障碍调整)哪个更好[66]。随机分组患者在标准的 3 个月预防期后接受额外 9 个月的药物治疗或安慰剂。移植后一年,延长预防期的患者在统计学和临床上 CMV 疾病的发病情况都显著降低,为 3.6%对 35%[66]。这种益处在研究戒断或更昔洛韦抗性时,显示其毒性增加并不明显。因此,建议供体或受体血清 CMV 呈阳性的肺移植受体应在移植后 12 个月内接受缬更昔洛韦。建议在预防时采取某种形式的 CMV 病毒血症监测,以确保没有发病。

如果不使用 CMV 预防,则应考虑使用伐昔洛韦或阿昔洛韦预防单纯疱疹和水痘(HSV)带状疱疹[39,40]。HSV 通常发生在移植后的第一个月。

心脏移植预防

心脏移植中的一般预防建议见表 99.4。

细菌预防

心脏移植后的手术部位感染率不高于冠状动脉旁路移植术[28]。因此,可以接受使用类似的围术期预防性抗生素。目前的指南[1]推荐头孢唑啉或头孢呋辛预防。对于青霉素或头孢菌素过敏的患者,万古霉素是可接受的替代品。头孢菌素应理想地在皮肤切口之前 30min 给予,万古霉素输注应在皮肤输注前 30~60min 开始[49]。

真菌预防

与其他移植受体一样,所有心脏移植受体应接受 PCP 预防。Smx/tmp 是预防 PCP 的首选药物[11]。此外,如果患者接受抗淋巴细胞抗体以治疗排斥反应,应考虑重建 smx/tmp 3~6 个月。许多患者对 smx/tmp 有过敏反应。smx/tmp 的替代品包括氨苯砜、阿托伐醌、吸入喷他脒和克林霉素加乙胺嘧啶[11]。氨苯砜具有磺胺成分。因此,有磺胺过敏的患者不应给予氨苯砜。如前所述,氨苯砜也与肺移植患者的溶血性贫血有关[12]。因此,在患有贫血的心脏移植受体中应考虑溶血性贫血。即使没有 G6PD 也会发生这种情况。

心脏移植受体在移植后发生真菌感染的风险相对较低[32]。因此,未指明常规抗真菌预防(除 PCP 外)。

寄生虫预防

心脏移植受体具有刚地弓形虫显著发病率的最高风险。心脏移植受体也具有从供体获得弓形体的最高风险。在从血清反应阳性供体接受心脏的血清阴性受体中弓形体病的风险最高。幸运的是,所有心脏移植受体接受 PCP 预防和 smx/tmp,阿托伐醌和氨苯砜都是有效预防弓形虫的。高危患者(D+/R−)应继续预防,因为在停止预防后会复发[67]。除化学预防外,心脏移植受

表 99.4 心脏移植中的一般预防措施建议

	优选预防措施	替代预防措施
手术预防	头孢唑啉 1g iv 皮肤切口前 0~30min	万古霉素 1g iv 皮肤切口前 60min
CMV	缬更昔洛韦、阿昔洛韦和伐昔洛韦,需要对肾功能障碍进行剂量调整	
D+/R−*	缬更昔洛韦每日 900mg,3 个月	提前监控
R+†	缬更昔洛韦每日 900mg,3 个月	提前监控
D−R−‡		阿昔洛韦 400~800mg TID§或伐昔洛韦 500mg BID 3~6 个月
真菌		
PCP**	Smx/tmp 1DS‖ 每周 3 次	阿托伐醌每天 1500mg,氨苯砜每天 100mg,吸入戊脒氯林可霉素+乙胺嘧啶

* 供体血清阳性/受体血清阴性;† 受体血清阳性;‡供体血清阴性/受体血清阴性;§每天 3 次(每 8h),每天 2 次(每 12h);** 肺炎;
‖ 双重强度(磺胺甲恶唑 800mg-甲氧苄啶 160amg)。

体应避免在移植后获得弓形虫。这意味着避免吃未煮熟的肉和动物粪便，特别是猫或其他食肉动物。应提醒患者动物粪便可污染土壤。所以，应注意保证猫不使用花园或在花坛排便。

查加斯心肌病是巴西心脏移植的主要原因[14]，但早期死亡率高(18%)。建议对移植前的Chagas阳性患者使用苯并咪唑治疗。治疗的持续时间应为30~60天，使用苯并咪唑或硝苯呋酮[15]。虽然苯并咪唑和硝苯莫司在美国未经FDA批准，可以通过CDC的寄生虫病和疟疾司(404-718-4745；电子邮件chagas@cdc.gov)或在正常营业时间之外呼叫CDC紧急行动中心(770-488-7100)，并联系寄生虫疾病管理专家。如果在移植前无法进行治疗，则应密切监测移植后症状的发展，如果出现症状则应对其进行治疗。

病毒预防

CMV感染与心脏移植受体的移植后血管病变有关[68,69]。基于Paya等的研究，CMV D+/R-的心脏移植受体在移植后3个月接受缬更昔洛韦预防对患者有益[25]。本研究中有56名心脏受者。到12个月为止，与口服更昔洛韦28.0%的比率相比，缬更昔洛韦组患者30.5%有CMV疾病[25]。由于口服更昔洛韦在美国不再可用，口服缬更昔洛韦或高剂量的伐昔洛韦是唯一可用的预防药物。许多中心选择在心脏移植受体中使用CMV预防性治疗方法。这可能使更多数量的患者接受CMV治疗。然而，缬更昔洛韦可能能减少CMV疾病且毒性小。虽然研究表明CMV预防可减少内膜增厚和可能的移植后血管病变[70]。

如果不使用CMV预防，则应考虑使用伐昔洛韦或阿昔洛韦预防HSV[39,40]。HSV通常发生在移植后的第一个月。

与其他器官一样，心脏移植受体应接受年度流感免疫接种，因为它减少了症状性流感样疾病[71]。流感免疫在心脏移植后也是安全的。正在等待心脏移植的患者也应该接受流感疫苗接种。流感注射已被证明可以减少心血管事件的发生和潜在的总死亡率[72,73]。这对于缺血性心肌病患者尤其如此。如果移植后患者确实暴露于有流感的人，则可以考虑用奥司他韦进行第二次预防。通常的剂量和持续时间为75mg，每日1次，持续10天。

如果死者的心脏捐赠者最近或有活跃的HBV(如HBV cAb IgM阳性或阳性HBV sAg)证据，则应考虑使用拉米夫定与HBIG预防感染。如果心脏移植受体确实发展为慢性/活动性HBV感染，则需要用抗病毒剂联合治疗。

小肠和复合血管同种异体移植(CVA)的预防

小肠和CVA移植中预防策略的数据积累很少。尽管如此，上述原则可以经验地应用于这两种移植情况。像肝脏移植一样，小肠移植涉及切入肠。因此，手术抗菌预防应包括对小肠菌群有活性的药物，包括氨苄西林与第三代头孢菌素或β-内酰胺与β-内酰胺酶抑制剂（氨苄西林加舒巴坦或哌拉西林加他唑巴坦)的组合。大量失血或手术时间延长应加大抗生素使用强度。像其他非黏性外科手术一样，头孢唑林或万古霉素应该对CVA肢体手术有足够的预防作用。然而，如果CVA外科手术涉及面部，则应在万古霉素之外加用覆盖革兰阴性菌的药物，如氟喹诺酮、氨基糖苷或氨曲南。

根据观察性报告，小肠和CVA移植的CMV疾病率更高。大多数专家建议在这两个患者群体中使用缬更昔洛韦进行抗病毒预防。移植后3个月应该是最短的。然而，可能需要更长的疗程。

实体器官移植中的免疫预防

移植中的疫苗接种建议见表99.5。

一般来说，移植患者应与相同年龄的成年或儿科患者进行类似免疫。CDC的免疫实践咨询委员会为儿童和成人免疫方案定期更新[74]。然而，对于实体器官移植受者有一个重要的警告：不应向接受免疫抑制的移植后受者施用活疫苗。有最小免疫抑制的失败同种异体移植物的受者可接受活疫苗。此外，如果感觉到接受活疫苗的益处超过了用疫苗毒株发展慢性感染的风险，则需要接受活疫苗接种。移植受者不应接受轮状病毒疫苗或口服脊髓灰质炎疫苗。此外，家庭接触者应在更换尿布后彻底清洗他们的手，以防止疫苗株的传播。值得注意的是，在美国不再进行口服脊髓灰质炎疫苗接种。然而，外国出生的婴儿可能已经接受口服脊髓灰质炎疫苗接种。除了这两种情况，移植受者通常不需要避免与活病毒疫苗受体接触。需要注意的是，如果水痘

表 99.5　移植受体(成人)推荐疫苗

疫苗	说明
流感-三价,灭活	每年尽快提供
破伤风+白喉+无细胞百日咳(Tdap)	给予一次,如果从未接受
破伤风+白喉(Td)	10 年一次
人乳头瘤病毒(HPV)	如果潜在受体<26 岁且未接种疫苗,请考虑给予移植。疫苗因性别而异
甲肝	如果未接种和非免疫,移植前或移植后均可
乙肝	给予如果未接种和非免疫,移植前或移植后均可,移植前优先
肺炎球菌	每五年一次
脑膜炎球菌	如果觉得有风险每五年一次
活病毒疫苗,不应在移植后给予	
水痘	如果没有免疫,给予预移植
水痘带状疱疹	如果潜在受体>50 岁,考虑移植
麻疹+腮腺炎+风疹	如果疫苗接种史是有问题的,考虑检查风疹滴度和免疫移植
活减毒流感疫苗(鼻内)	目前(2012 年)不推荐移植受体或家庭联系人,或照顾移植受体的医护人员

疫苗接种者出现皮疹，那么移植受体应避免直接接触皮疹[74]。

总结

目前移植领域已经在采用有效措施预防感染方面取得了进展，同时大量经过数据验证的化学预防措施也已经在移植过程中被使用。这要求移植施行者们要全面掌握微生物知识，并结合防治疾病的有力规章制度，考虑感染性疾病的风险，从而改善移植预后。然而除了采取各种预防措施以外，为了正确预期感染性疾病并在必要时有效应对，还需要良好的临床监测并对感染保持高度怀疑的态度，此外还需要和临床移植团队与感染性疾病服务中心协同合作。

（沈恬 译　沈恬 校）

参考文献

1. American Society of Health-System Pharmacists. ASHP therapeutic guidelines on antimicrobial prophylaxis in surgery. American Journal of Health-System Pharmacy. 1999;56:1839–1888.
2. Singh N. Antifungal prophylaxis for solid organ transplant recipients: seeking clarity amongst controversy. Clinical Infectious Diseases. 2000;31(2):545–553.
3. Guggenheimer J, Eghtesad B, Stock DJ. Dental management of the (solid) organ transplant patient. Oral Surgery, Oral Medicine, Oral Pathology, Oral Radiology, and Endodontics. 2003;95(4):383–389.
4. Wilson W, Taubert KA, Gewitz M, et al. Prevention of infective endocarditis: uidelines from the American Heart Association: a guideline from the American Heart Association Rheumatic Fever, Endocarditis and Kawasaki Disease Committee, Council on Cardiovascular Disease in the Young, and Council on Clinical Cardiology, Council on Cardioivascular Surgery and Anesthesia, and the Quality of Care and Outcomes Research Interdisciplinary Working Group. Circulation. 1997;116:1736–1754.
5. Nicolle LE, Bradley S, Colgan R, et al. Infectious Diseases Society of America Guidelines for the diagnosis and treatment of asymptomatic bacteriuria in adults. Clinical Infectious Diseases. 2005;40(5):643–654.
6. Schmaldienst S, Dittrich E, Horl WH. Urinary tract infections after renal transplantation. Current Opinion in Urology. 2002;12:125–130.
7. American Thoracic Society, Centers for Disease Control and Prevention, Infectious Diseases Society of America. Americal Thoracic Society/Centers for Disease Control and Prevention/Infectious Diseases Society of Ameica: controlling tuberculosis in the United States. American Journal of Respiratory and Critical Care Medicine. 2005;172:1169–1227.
8. Fischer SA, Avery RK. Screening of donor and recipient prior to solid organ transplantation. American Journal of Transplantation. 2009;9(Suppl 4):S7–S18.
9. Kim SH, Lee SO, Park JB, et al. A prospective longitudinal study evaluating the usefullness of a T-cell-based assay for latent tuberculosis infection in kidney transplant recipients. American Journal of Transplantation. 2011;11:1927–1935.
10. Perfect J, Dismukes WE, Dromer F, et al. Clinical practice uidelines for the management of cryptococcal disease: 2010 update by teh Infectious Diseases Society of America. Clinical Infectious Diseases. 2010;50:291–322.
11. Martin SI, Fishman JA. Pneumocystis pneumonia in solid organ transplant recipients. American Journal of Transplantation: Official Journal of the American Society of Transplantation and the American Society of Transplant Surgeons. 2009;9(Suppl 4):S227–S233.
12. Naik PM, Lyon GM, Ramirez A, et al. Dapsone-induced hemolytic anemia in lung alloraft recipients. Journal of Heart and Lung Transplantation. 2008;27:1198–1202.
13. Custer B, Agapova M, Bruhn R, et al. Epidemiologic and laboratory findings from 3 years of testing United States blood donors for Trypanosoma cruzi. Transfusion. 2012;52:1901–1911.
14. Fiorelli AI, Santos RHB, Oliveira JL, et al. Heart Transplantation in 107 cases of Chagas' Disease. Transplantation Proceedings. 2011;43(1):220–224.
15. Lattes R. Chagas disease (American trypanosomiasis) in transplant recipients. 2012 [cited 2012 May 25, 2012]; Available from: http://www.antimicrobe.org.
16. Katerinis I, Hadaya K, Duquesnoy R, et al. De novo anti-HLA antibody after pandemic H1N1 and seasonal influenza immunization in kidney transplant recipients. American Journal of Transplantation. 2011;11(8):1727–1733.
17. Kumar D, Campbell P, Humar A. Donor-specific alloantibody upregulation after influenza vaccination in transplant recipients. American Journal of Transplantation. 2011;11(11):2538, author's reply 9–40.
18. Danziger-Isakov L, Cherkassky L, Siegel H, et al. Effects of influenza immunization on humoral and cellular alloreactivity in humans. Transplantation. 2010;89(7):838–844.
19. Hurst FP, Lee JJ, Jindal RM, et al. Outcomes associated with influenza vaccination in the first year after kidney transplantation. Clinical Journal of the American Society of Nephrology. 2011;6(5):1192–1197.
20. Scharpe J, Evenepoel P, Maes B, et al. Influenza vaccination is efficacious and safe in renal transplant recipients. American Journal of Transplantation. 2008;8(2):332–337.
21. Wyzgal J, Brydak LB, Zygier D, et al. Grochowiecki T. Study on efficacy of influenza vaccination in renal allograft recipients. Transplantation Proceedings. 2002;34(2):572–575.
22. Esposito S, Meregalli E, Daleno C, et al. An open-label, randomized clinical trial assessing immunogenicity, safety and tolerability of pandemic influenza A/H1N1 MF59-adjuvanted vaccine administered sequentially or simultaneously with seasonal virosomal-adjuvanted influenza vaccine to paediatric kidney transplant recipients. Nephrology, Dialysis, Transplantation. 2011;26(6):2018–2024.
23. Miraglia JL, Abdala E, Hoff PM, et al. Immunogenicity and reactogenicity of 2009

influenza A (H1N1) inactivated monovalent non-adjuvanted vaccine in elderly and immunocompromised patients. PLoS ONE. 2011;6(11):e27214.
24. Balfour HH Jr, Chace BA, Stapleton JT, et al. A randomized, plaebo-controlled trial of oral acyclovir for the prevention of cytomegalovirus disease in recipients of renal allografts. New England Journal of Medicine. 1989;320:1381-1387.
25. Paya C, Humar A, Dominguez E, et al. Efficacy and safety of valganciclovir vs. oral ganciclovir for prevention of cytomegalovirus disease in solid organ transplant recipients. American Journal of Transplantation: Official Journal of the American Society of Transplantation and the American Society of Transplant Surgeons. 2004;4(4):611-620.
26. Humar A, Limaye AP, Blumberg EA, et al. Extended valganciclovir prophylaxis in D+/R- kidney transplant recipients is associated with a long-term reduction in cytomegalovirus disease: two-year results of IMPACT study. Transplant Infectious Disease. 2010;90(12):1427-1431.
27. Kotton CN, Kumar D, Caliendo AM, et al. International consensus guidelines on the management of cytomegalovirus in solid organ transplantation. Transplantation. 2010;89(7):779-795.
28. Edwards JR, Peterson KD, Mu Y, et al. National Healthcare Safety Network (NHSN) report: data summary for 2006 through 2008, issued December 2009. American Journal of Infection Control. 2009;37:783-805.
29. Hellinger WC, Crook JE, Heckman MG, et al. Surgical site infection after liver transplantation: risk factors and association with graft loss or death. Transplantation. 2009;87:1387-1393.
30. Asensio A, Ramos A, Cuervas-Mons V, et al. Effect of antibiotic prophylaxis on the risk of surgical site infection in orthotopic liver transplant. Liver Transplantation. 2008;14(6):799-805.
31. Collins LA, Samore MH, Roberts MS, et al. Risk factors for invasive fungal infections complicating orthotopic liver transplantation. Journal of Infectious Diseases. 1994;170:644-652.
32. Pappas PG, Alexander BD, Andes DR, et al. Invasive fungal infections among transplant recipients: results of the transplant-associated infection surveillance network (TRANSNET). Clinical Infectious Diseases. 2010;50:1101-1111.
33. Winston DJ, Pakrasi A. Busuttil RWCINAIMM, Pmid. Prophylactic fluconazole in liver transplant recipients. A randomized, double-blind, placebo-controlled trial. Annals of Internal Medicine. 1999;131(10):729-737.
34. Hadley S, Huckabee C, Pappas PG, et al. Outcomes of antifungal prophylaxis in high-risk liver transplant recipients. Transplant Infectious Disease. 2009; 11(1):40-48.
35. Playford EG, Webster AC, Sorell TC, et al. Antifungal agents for preventing fungal infections in solid organ transplant recipients. Cochrane Database of Systematic Reviews (Online). 2004(3):CD004291.
36. Pappas PG, Andes D, Schuster M, et al. Invasive fungal infections in low-risk liver transplant recipients: a multi-center prospective obersvational study. American Journal of Transplantation. 2006;6:386-391.
37. Marcus KA, FDA. Cross-discipline team leader review [valganciclovir oral solution]. 2009 [cited 2011]; Available from: http://www.accessdata.fda.gov/drugsatfda_docs/nda/2009/022257Original-1_021304s007sumr.pdf.
38. Kalil AC, Mindru C, Florescu DF Valganicloivr 900mg versus 450mg daily for cytomegalovirus prophylaxis in solid organ transplantation: direct and indirect comparison meta-analysis. IDSA 48th Annual Meeting, October 22, 2010; Vancouver2010.
39. Zuckermann A, Wald A. Herpes simplex virus infections in solid organ transplant recipients. American Journal of Transplantation. 2009;9(Suppl 4):S104-S107.
40. Pergam SA, Limaye AP. Varicella zoster virus (VZV) in solid organ transplant recipients. American Journal of Transplantation: Official Journal of the American Society of Transplantation and the American Society of Transplant Surgeons. 2009;9(Suppl 4):S108-S115.
41. Perrillo RP, Wright T, Rakela J, et al. A multicenter United States-Canadian trial to assess lamivudine monotherapy before and after liver transplantation for chronic hepatitis B. Hepatology (Baltimore, Md.). 2001;33:424-432.
42. Zheng S, Chen Y, Liang T, et al. Prevention of hepatitis B recurrence after liver transplantation using lamivudine or lamivudine combined wiht hepatitis B immunoglobulin prophylaxis. Liver Transplantation. 2006;12:253-258.
43. Levitsky J, Doucette K. Viral hepatitis in solid organ transplant recipients. American Journal of Transplantation. 2009;9(Suppl 4):S116-S130.
44. Gaeta GB, Pariani E, Amendola A, et al. Influenza vaccination in patients with cirrhosis and in liver transplant recipients. Vaccine. 2009;27(25):3373-3375.
45. Lawal A, Basler C, Branch A, et al. Influenza vaccination in orthotopic liver transplant recipients: absence of post administration ALT elevation. American Journal of Transplantation. 2004;4(11):1805-1809.
46. Kute V, Goplani KR, Godara SM, et al. Post-exposure prophylaxis for H1N1 with oseltamivir in renal allograft recipient-safe and effective without any immunosuppresive drug interaction. Journal of the Association of Physicians of India. 2011;59:49-51.
47. Marfo K, Chapochnick-Friedmann J, Akalin E, et al. Postexposure prophylaxis of H1N1 with oseltamivir in a newly transplanted kidney recipient receiving intense immunosuppressive therapy. Transplantation Proceedings. 2009;41(10): 4411-4413.
48. Maurer JR, Tullis DE, Grossman RF, et al. Infectious complications following isolated lung transplantation. Chest. 1992;101:1056-1059.
49. Mangram AJ, Horan TC, Pearson ML, et al. Guideline for prevention of surical site infection, 1999. Infection Control and Hospital Epidemiology. 1999;20(4): 247-278.
50. Steinberg JP, Braun BI, Hellinger WC, et al. Timing of antimicrobial prophylaxis and the risk of surgical site infections: results from the Trial to Reduce Antimicrobial Prophylaxis Errors. Annals of Surgery. 2009;250(1):10-16.
51. Nunley DR, Gal AA, Vega JD, et al. Saprophytic fungal infections and complications involving the bronchial anastamosis following human lung transplantation. Chest. 2002;112(4):1185-1191.
52. Neoh CF, Snell GI, Kotsimbos T, et al. Antifungal prophylaxis in lung transplantation-a world-wide survey. American Journal of Transplantation. 2011; 11(2):361-366.
53. Drew RH, Dodds Ashley E, Benjamin DK Jr, et al. Comparative safety of amphotericin B lipid complex and amphotericin B deoxycholate as aerosolized antifungal prophylaxis in lung-transplant recipients. Transplantation. 2004;77(2): 232-237.
54. Husain S, Paterson DL, Studer S, et al. Voriconazole prophylaxis in lung transplant recipients. American Journal of Transplantation: Official Journal of the American Society of Transplantation and the American Society of Transplant Surgeons. 2006;6(12):3008-3016.
55. Vadnerkar A, Nguyen MH, Mitsani D, et al. Voriconazole exposure and geographic location are independent risk factors for squamous cell carcinoma of the skin among lung transplant recipients. Journal of Heart and Lung Transplantation: The Official Publication of the International Society for Heart Transplantation. 2010;29(11):1240-1244.
56. Zwald FO, Spratt M, Lemos BD, et al. Duration of voriconazole exposure: an independent risk factor for skin cancer after lung transplantation. Dermatologic Surgery. 2012;38(8):1369-1374.
57. Epaulard O, Saint-Raymond C, Villier C, et al. Multiple aggressive squamous cell carcinomas associated with prolonged voriconazole therapy in four immunocompromised patients. Clinical Microbiology and Infection. 2010;16(9):1362-1364.
58. Cadena J, Levine DJ, Angel LF, et al. Antifungal prophylaxis with voriconazole or itraconazole in lung transplant recipients: hepatotoxicity and effectiveness. American Journal of Transplantation. 2009;9(9):2085-2091.
59. Cornely OA, Maertens J, Winston DJ, et al. Posaconazole vs. fluconazole or itraconazole prophylaxis in patients with neutropenia. New England Journal of Medicine. 2007;356(4):348-359.
60. Ullmann AJ, Lipton JH, Vesole DH, et al. Posaconazole or fluconazole for prophylaxis in severe graft-versus-host disease. New England Journal of Medicine. 2007;356(4):335-347.
61. Hayney MS, Moran J, Wiegert NA, et al. Lung transplant patients' T cell responses to influenza vaccine viruses between seasons. Vaccine. 2008;26(21):2596-2600.
62. Hayney MS, Welter DL, Francois M, et al. Influenza vaccine antibody responses in lung transplant recipients. Progress in Transplantation (Aliso Viejo, Calif.). 2004;14(4):346-351.
63. Mazzone PJ, Mossad SB, Mawhorter SD, et al. The humoral immune response to influenza vaccination in lung transplant patients. European Respiratory Journal: Official Journal of the European Society for Clinical Respiratory Physiology. 2001;18(6):971-976.
64. Westall GP, Michaelides A, Williams TJ, et al. Human cytomegalovirus load in plasma and bronchoalveolar lavage fluid: a longitudinal study of lung transplant recipients. Journal of Infectious Diseases. 2004;190(6):1076-1083.
65. Westall GP, Michaelides A, Williams TJ, et al. Bronchiolitis obliterans syndrome and early human cytomegalovirus DNAaemia dynamics after lung transplantation. Transplantation. 2003;75(12):2064-2068.
66. Palmer SM, Limaye AP, Banks M, et al. Extended valganciclovir prophylaxis to prevent cytomegalovirus after lung transplantation: a randomized, controlled trial. Annals of Internal Medicine. 2010;152(12):761-769.
67. Keogh A, Macdonald P, Richens D, et al. Mini-dose trimethoprim with sulphamethoxazole prevents pneumocystis and toxoplasmosis infections after heart transplantation. Transplantation Proceedings. 1992;24(5):2263.
68. Fateh-Moghadam S, Bocksch W, Wessely R, et al. Cytomegalovirus infection status predicts progression of heart-transplant vasculopathy. Transplantation. 2003; 76(10):1470-1474.
69. Kocher AA, Bonaros N, Dunkler D, et al. Long-term results of CMV hyperimmune globulin prophylaxis in 377 heart transplant recipients. Journal of Heart and Lung Transplantation. 2003;22(3):250-257.
70. Potena L, Grigioni F, Magnani G, et al. Prophylaxis versus preemptive therapy for prevention of the consequences of cytomegalovirus infection in transplant recipients: a still unresolved issue. Transplantation. 2009;87(2):305-306, author reply 6-7.
71. Magnani G, Falchetti E, Pollini G, et al. Safety and efficacy of two types of influenza

vaccination in heart transplant recipients: a prospective randomised controlled study. Journal of Heart and Lung Transplantation. 2005;24(5):588–592.

72. Ciszewski A, Bilinska ZT, Brydak LB, et al. Influenza vaccination in secondary prevention from coronary ischaemic events in coronary artery disease: FLUCAD study. European Heart Journal. 2008;29(11):1350–1358.

73. Gurfinkel EP, Leon de la Fuente R, Mendiz O, et al. Flu vaccination in acute coronary syndromes and planned percutaneous coronary interventions (FLUVACS) Study. European Heart Journal. 2004;25(1):25–31.

74. Kroger AT, Sumaya CV, Pickering LK, et al. General recommendations on immunizations: recommendations of the ADvisory Committee on Immunization Practices (ACIP). MMWR. Morbidity and Mortality Weekly Report. 2011; 60(RR-2):1–61.

第 100 章 器官移植受体的代谢和内分泌管理

Naim Issa, Scott A. Reule, Aleksandra Kukla

引言

移植实体器官受体可能产生多种代谢和内分泌相关疾病。在已存并发症的背景下，这些疾病的产生由移植器官相关的生理变化、移植后生活方式的变化、免疫抑制药物和遗传易感性之间的复杂相互作用引起。

移植后，患者需要实时密切监测多种电解质的浓度变化。这些与手术过程有关，但很快这些将发展为由器官功能变化和改变电解质的免疫抑制剂带来的病症。通常需要特异性处理的有高钾血症、高钙血症、低镁血症和低磷血症。急性高血糖症并不罕见，可在多达 87%的没有糖尿病史的肾移植受者中观察到[1]。从长期来看，由糖尿病、高血压和血脂异常组成的代谢综合征的患病率在肝脏和肾脏移植中可能至少达到 40%~50%[2,3]。代谢综合征与心脏移植受者的同种异体移植物血管病变的发展相关，且会导致肾移植受体心血管疾病风险的增加[3,4]。移植后的新发糖尿病（NODAT）与肝肾移植后的移植物衰竭和死亡率[5,6]相关[7]。

实体器官移植后内分泌和代谢疾病的成功管理需要仔细考虑并发症、肾功能受损和药物的相互作用。有一些证据表明移植相关治疗的毒性有遗传易感性。单核苷酸多态性（SNP）已与免疫抑制剂的特定副作用相关[8-10]。遗传因素的鉴定可帮助我们对疾病代谢兴奋和其他并发症病因的理解，并为未来的个体化免疫抑制创造机会。移植肾病科医生、内分泌专家和初级保健医生之间密切合作并积极管理移植后并发症非常必要，以达到优化并发症并使药物相关毒性的风险最小化的目标。读者可参考第 88 章关于代谢问题的长期管理的其他信息，因为它们与移植后的心血管疾病有关。

实体器官移植后的高血糖和糖尿病

高血糖的移植后管理根据血糖水平升高的时间和预期持续时间的不同而变化（图 100.1）。在移植后，高糖可因手术压力和免疫抑制而发生。值得注意的是，移植后的急性高血糖与 NODAT 的发生率呈 4 倍相关[11]。胰岛素是围术期的优选疗法，因为急性高血糖通常对口服药物有抗性，且免疫抑制剂（特别是皮质类固醇）每日剂量的变化导致不可预测的血糖水平。

从长远来看，NODAT 的发生率在所有移植器官中可能高达 30%，特别是在成年实体器官移植受者中（表 100.1）。虽然传统的危险因素（年龄、肥胖、种族）是公认的诱因，肝炎 C 感染和免疫抑制也增加了风险（图 100.2）[3,6,12-18]。NODAT 的病理生理学是复杂的，围绕两个重要途径：对胰腺 β 细胞的直接毒性和增加的胰岛素抵抗（图 100.2）。此外，肾脏在循环胰岛素的清除和降解中起着重要作用，因此肾功能的恢复可能“预防”先前存在的糖尿病[19]。对个体药物致敏作用背后的病因理解可指导临床医生选择靶向治疗。

所有非糖尿病实体器官移植受者应筛选 NODAT。肾病：改善全球肾脏病预后组织（KDIGO）移植工作组建议每周测量空腹血糖、口服葡萄糖耐量试验和（或）评估 HbA1C，前四周每周一次，每 3 个月 1 次持续一年，之后每年一次[20]。许多患者可能会发生与胰岛素抵抗相关的餐后高血糖，由于缺乏敏感性，空腹血糖的检测作用受到限制，并且作为筛选可能诊断不到 25%的患者的 NODAT[21]。HbA1C 可用于筛选，但可能会由于尿毒症、输血、红细胞生成素施用和溶血（在移植后不常见的早期）而混杂。此外，当在移植后早期测量时，HbA1C 可反映瞬时高血糖。

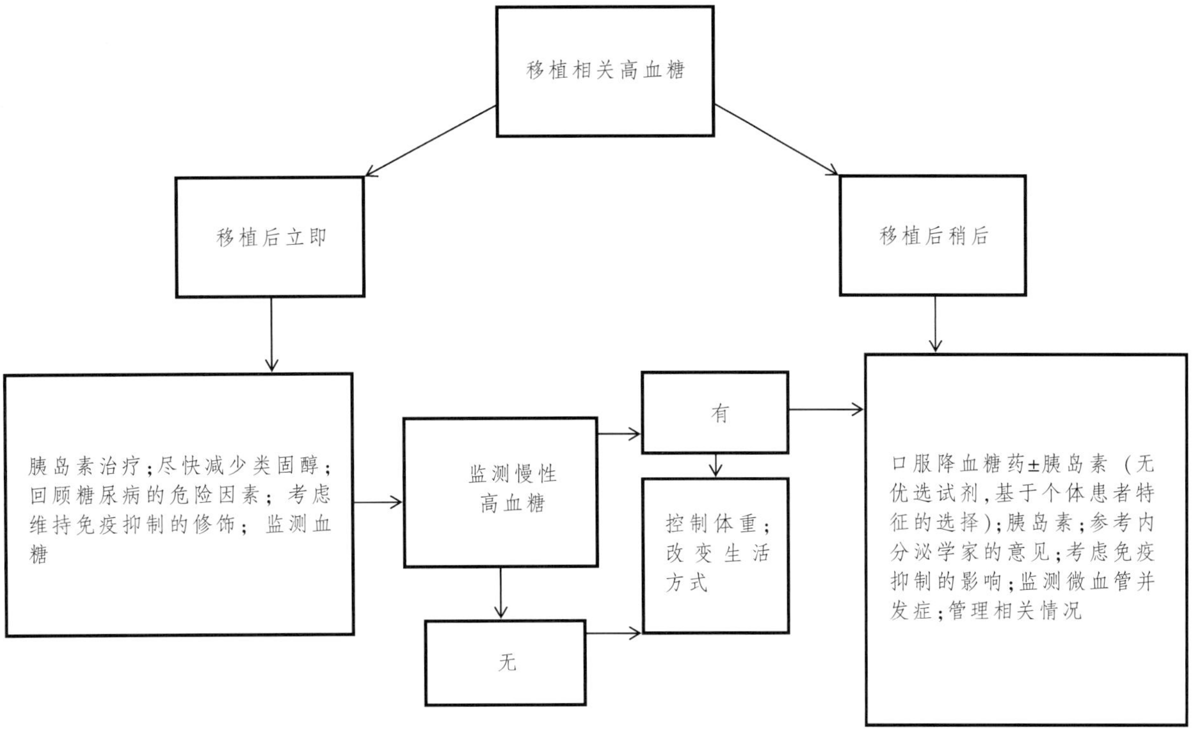

图 100.1　移植相关的高血糖。

胰腺移植后葡萄糖障碍的管理与其他器官移植葡萄糖障碍的管理不同，这已经在第 77 章中进行了讨论。

免疫抑制剂的作用

糖皮质激素

糖皮质激素主要通过增加胰岛素抵抗来诱导 NODAT，其由肝脏糖异生和体重的增加以及肌肉中糖原合成和葡萄糖摄取减少引起。糖皮质激素也对 β 细胞的功能产生直接的负面影响。皮质类固醇的累积剂量和持续时间似乎影响 NODAT 的风险[22]。为了避免不利的代谢并发症而开发的类固醇节约方案越来越常见[23]。这些方案已与 NODAT 发病率的降低相关，并可能减少其他心血管危险因素，包括高甘油三酯血症和体重增加[24-27]。关于类固醇节食方案在其他器官移植受者中的益处的现有文献较为有限。

钙调神经磷酸酶抑制剂

两种钙调神经磷酸酶抑制剂（CNI），环孢素和他克莫司，是器官移植后维持免疫抑制的主要药物。使用这些药物，特别是他克莫司，有助于 NODAT 的发展[28-30]。CNI 通过破坏活化 T 细胞（NFAT）途径的核因子的钙调神经磷酸酶/转录因子抑制胰岛素的转录和合成，NFAT 途径是 β 细胞功能的必需调节物[31]。

雷帕霉素靶蛋白抑制剂

雷帕霉素靶蛋白抑制剂（mTOR 抑制剂）曾经被认为是发生 NODAT 的服用 CNI 的患者的替代药物。然而，研究未能证明经历了从 CNI 到西罗莫司的转化的肾移植受者中的葡萄糖代谢有所改善。相反，转化与葡萄糖耐量降低的发生率增加有 30%的相关性[32]。西罗莫司的抗糖尿病作用可能与胰岛素介导的抑制肝葡萄糖产生、胰岛素抵抗和直接 β 细胞毒性有关[33-35]。

共刺激阻滞剂

贝拉西普是一线的生物制剂，通过作用于共刺激途径选择性抑制 T 细胞活化。贝拉西普被设计为是 CNI 的替代药物，希望通过避免 CNI 相关毒性并使代谢并发症最小化延长肾同种异体移植物的存活时间。两项前瞻性试验比较了肾移植受者随机分到环孢素或贝拉西普的代谢性并发症发生率。在预先指定的合并分析中，贝拉西普的使用与 12 个月时 NODAT 的发生率较低有关[36]。更长的随访非常必要，以描述这种新型药物的真正代谢益处。

其他免疫抑制剂

硫唑嘌呤和霉酚酸酯未显示出独立的致糖尿病作用,事实上,在一个分析中显示具有“保护”效应[6]。这种关系需要谨慎解释,因为没有好的解释存在。

免疫抑制剂的调整

鉴于免疫抑制剂在NODAT发展中的重要作用,在个体患者中进行风险评估可指导临床医生对于维持免疫抑制的选择。某些危险因素在所有实体移植器官中是一致的(表100.1)。他克莫司已反复显示出比环孢素更有可能导致糖尿病的发生[37]。老年患者、非裔美国人、丙型肝炎感染患者和肥胖移植受者易患NODAT,这些患者可能最好服用环孢素,而不是他克莫司。类似地,先前的研究显示,具有NODAT的受者在维持他克莫司时可以从转化为环孢素时受益[38-40]。贝拉西普可能是代谢并发症高风险人群的一个很好的选择,但更长的随访需要充分评估其长期安全性。皮质类固醇-最小化方案如果被认为安全,应考虑用于有NODAT风险的患者。对于维持类固醇的受体,剂量降低至5mg/d可使葡萄糖代谢改善[41]。

用口服降血糖药治疗移植后糖尿病:安全性和副作用(表100.2)

胰岛素敏化剂

二甲双胍被推荐作为非移植2型糖尿病患者的一线治疗。它对体重稳定性或体重减轻以及有限的副作用分布(主要是胃肠道不耐受)具有有利的影响。二甲双胍单药治疗可将HbA1C水平降低1.5%,并且通常不会引起低血糖[42]。二甲双胍的使用在肾病患者中受到限制,因为其存在乳酸性酸中毒的风险,然而,它被证明在慢性肾脏疾病(CKD)1-3期的患者中是安全的,没有严重的并发症[43,44]。二甲双胍患者的乳酸性酸中毒发生率非常低(4.3例/100 000名患者/年),与非二甲双胍治疗患者相当(5.4例/100 000名患者/年)[45]。乳酸性酸中毒的风险随着严重的并发症,如肝功能障碍、肾衰竭、心力衰竭和缺氧而增加。尽管数据有限,二甲双胍已被证明是肾脏移植受者肾脏功能保护的安全选择[46]。在非移植人群中,二甲双胍可以降低代谢综合征的风险,改善心血管[44,47]。这一发现需要更多的研究来确认实体器官移植受者存在这些好处。

胰岛素促分泌素

磺胺类和格列奈类直接刺激胰岛素分泌并可能对CNI诱导的胰岛素分泌不足患者特别有利。磺胺类和瑞格列奈使血红蛋白A1C降低1.5%,而那格列奈作为单一治疗时效果较差[42]。这些药物的主要副作用是长期低血糖,其在老年患者中更常见。

格列本脲及其活性代谢物在肾脏清除,因此在肾功能不全患者中积累,导致频繁和长期的低血糖发作[48]。在动物研究中,格列本脲的降血糖作用被环孢素抑制[49]。相比之下,格列吡嗪在肝脏中广泛代谢为无活性代谢物。格列吡嗪不与环孢素相互作用,并且较少引起低血糖[48,50]。肝病患者中格列吡嗪的清除延长,因此在有显著肝损伤的患者应避免使用。瑞格列奈和那格列奈也是肝代谢的,在患有肝衰竭的患者中应避免,但无需对肾功能障碍进行剂量调整。虽然瑞格列奈被证明是肾移植受者的一个安全且有效的选择[51],它通过肝细胞色素p450同工酶CYP 3A4代谢。这种同工酶被CNI抑制,因此钙调神经磷酸酶抑制剂的患者可能有低血糖的危险[52]。

噻唑烷二酮

噻唑烷二酮(TZD)可增加肌肉、脂肪组织和肝对内源和外源胰岛素的敏感性。单用TZD可使HbA1C降低0.5%~1.4%,但与磺胺类药物相比,它们的作用更持久[53]。它们通常需要3~6周的治疗来显示效果。主要副作用是体重增加和外周水肿,它们的使用也与心力衰竭的风险成倍增加相关[54]。TZD对脂质分布发挥积极作用,但它们对心血管事件发生率的影响仍有争议[55]。还有证据表明,TZD患者的骨质流失加快,骨折风险增高,这可能是由于过氧化物酶体增殖物激活受体γ(PPARγ),抑制骨形成并增强骨吸收[56]。TZD在肾移植受体中的使用显示出良好的耐受性,与短期内免疫抑制药物没有显著的相互作用[57]。尽管如此,在移植受体中应谨慎使用TZD,因为其中许多受试者易患骨折。此外,缺乏对心血管结果的积极影响使得这类药物在实体器官移植受体中不太需要。

胰高血糖素样肽-1类似物

小肠产生的肠促胰岛素,是响应于碳水化合物摄

表 100.1 实体器官移植受者新发糖尿病的发病率

研究项目	器官	数据库	N	移植后时间(月)	发生率(累计)(%)	风险增加	风险不增加	风险降低
Israni 等[3]	肾	PORT	1840*	12~60	13	移植后 6~12 个月 年龄较大(每 10 年) 非洲裔美国人 GFR(每 10) BMI>30kg/m²	–	–
Shah 等[17]	肾	OPTN/UNOS	15 309	主要 306 天	10	老年高血压之前移植 非洲裔美国人 BMI>30kg/m² HCV Tac	扩展标准捐助者 活体捐赠者 HLA-A,-B 错配的数量	阿仑单抗
Kasiske 等[6]	肾	USRDS	11 659	3, 12, 36	9.1 16 24	年龄>45 对 18~44 岁 非洲裔美国人 西班牙种族男性供者 HCV 感染	–	年龄<17 岁对 18~44 岁 MMF AZA ESRD 继发于 GN
Kuo 等[18]	儿科肾	OPTN/UNOS	2726	中位 693 天	4.6	年龄>10 岁 BMI<5% 和 > 85% 出院时使用类固醇	性别;高血压;非白种族诱导 mTOR 抑制剂 Tac MMF	活体供体器官
Ye 等[15]	肺	OPTN/UNOS	3540	中位 670 天	33.4	性别(男) 年龄(>50 岁) 非洲裔美国人 BMI≥25kg/m² 囊性纤维化(作为肺病的病因)出院时的 Tac	HCV 免疫抑制(MMF、mTOR 抑制剂,类固醇)	CMV 阴性(供体/受体);BMI<18kg/m²
Kuo 等[14]	肝	OPTN/UNOS	15 463	中位 685 天	26.4	年龄(>50 岁) 非洲裔美国人 BMI≥25kg/m² HCV 肝硬化 捐献者年龄>60 岁 Tac 类固醇	受者为男性 1A 身份 冷缺血时间	活体捐献者诱导
Kuo 等[13]	儿科肝	OPTN/UNOS	1161	中位 770 天	10.1	年龄>13 岁 非洲裔美国人 继发于 AHN、肝硬化、PSC 或囊性纤维化的 ESLD 血清胆红素>3mg/dL AR 类固醇治疗	性别 捐助者性别 捐助者年龄 捐献者类型(活体对尸体) HCV 肥胖 移植因素[冷缺血时间、免疫抑制(CNI、MMF、mTOR 抑制剂、类固醇)];1 年维持类固醇	–

(待续)

表 100.1(续) 实体器官移植受者新发糖尿病的发病率

研究项目	器官	数据库	N	移植后时间(月)	发生率(累计)(%)	风险增加	风险不增加	风险降低
Ye 等[16]	成人心脏	OPTN/UNOS	3763	中位 713 天	28.6	年龄增加(> 50 岁) 非白种族 BMI≥25kg/m² 缺血性心脏病 CMV 阳性(受体) 烟草使用 出院时使用类固醇	受体性别 HCV 出院时 mTOR 出院时的 MMF	–

* 移植后 1 年内的移植后新发糖尿病受者被排除;Tac,他克莫司;MMF,吗替麦考酚酯;AZA,硫唑嘌呤;GFR,肾小球滤过率;ESLD,终末期肝病;AHN,急性肝坏死;PSC,原发性硬化性胆管炎;HCV,丙型肝炎病毒;AR,急性排斥反应;CNI,钙调磷酸酶抑制剂。

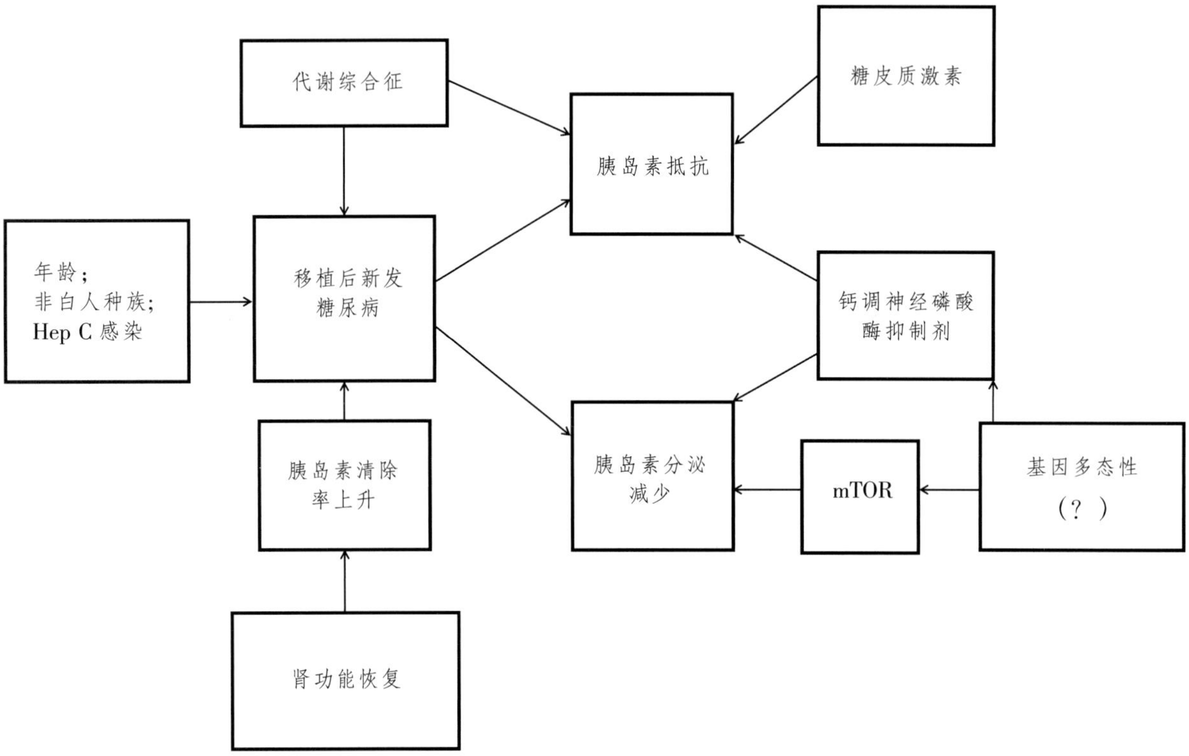

图 100.2 移植后新发糖尿病的危险因素。

入而分泌的天然激素，其可加强葡萄糖刺激的胰岛素分泌。基于胰岛素激素的治疗,包括胰高血糖素样肽 1 (GLP-1)激动剂和二肽肽酶Ⅳ(DDP-4)抑制剂,对于患有 2 型糖尿病的患者是新的治疗选择。GLP-1 激动剂与 GLP-1 受体结合并增加 GLP-1 活性,导致葡萄糖依赖性胰岛素分泌，减少葡萄糖分泌和肝脏葡萄糖产生。艾塞那肽主要通过降低餐后葡萄糖水平使 HbA1C 降低 0.5%~1%。主要副作用包括胃肠道紊乱,如恶心、呕吐和腹泻。艾塞那肽通过诱导饱腹感和减慢胃动力促进体重减轻,因此不推荐用于严重胃轻瘫患者。艾塞那肽不应用于 GFR<30mL/min 的患者。类似地,严重肾功能不全的患者应避免使用利拉鲁肽[42,58]。

DPP-4 抑制剂防止内源性 GLP-1 和胃抑制性多肽酶失活,导致生理水平的内源性 GLP-1 增加的可用性。它们将 HbA1C 降低 0.5%~0.8%。与 GLP-1 激动剂类似,DPP-4 抑制剂对体重减轻发挥积极作用，并且不引起低血糖。剂量调整对于肾功能障碍是必需的。总体而言,由于缺乏关于安全性和有效性的数据以及潜在的药

表 100.2　口服降血糖药物

药物	作用	代谢/消除	优点	风险、预防措施和禁忌证
胰岛素敏化剂				
二甲双胍、丁福明、苯乙双胍	减少葡萄糖产生，增加骨骼肌的葡萄糖摄取	主要：肾小管分泌	血糖风险低 体重减轻	GI 不耐受 禁用于有肾脏疾病和肝脏疾病的患者 伴有肾脏和肝脏疾病的乳酸性酸中毒的风险增加
胰岛素促分泌素				
磺胺类药物格列吡嗪、格列本脲、格列美脲	增加胰腺胰岛素分泌	主要：肝糖尿病肾脏排泄	快速开始血糖效应	低血糖(格列本脲最高风险) 体重增加调整剂量或避免肾病或肝衰竭患者
美格列奈、瑞格列奈、那格列奈		主要：CYP2C8 和 3A4	快速开始血糖效应	低血糖 体重增加 肝衰竭患者中调整剂量或避免免疫抑制药物相互作用
其他有不同的药物				
噻唑烷二酮衍生物吡格列酮、罗格列酮	结合过氧化物酶体增殖物激活受体(PPARs)并刺激胰岛素敏感基因	主要：CYP2C8 次要：CYP3A4	低血糖风险降低 改善血脂谱 肾脏疾病无需调整	体重增加 外周水肿 心力衰竭 骨折 在 NYHA Ⅲ级和Ⅳ级心衰的患者中禁忌 避免 肝病患者
胰高血糖素样肽-1 类似物艾塞那肽，利拉鲁肽;	增加胰腺胰岛素分泌	主要：肾脏	低血糖风险低 体重减轻	GI 不耐受 不推荐用于胰腺癌患者 在晚期肾脏疾病患者中不要使用(艾塞那肽)或谨慎使用(利拉鲁肽)
二肽基肽酶-4 抑制剂西他列汀，沙格列汀	增加内源性肠促胰岛素	主要：肾脏 次要：CYP3A42C8	低血糖风险低 可能改善脂质分布	减少中度或重度肾脏疾病的剂量，观察免疫抑制药物的相互作用

物相互作用，在移植受体中应谨慎使用这类药物[42,58]。

移植后糖尿病的管理

目标 HbA1C 尚未在实体器官移植受者中建立，但目标<7%通常可从一般人群中治疗 2 型糖尿病的指南推断[42]。类似于非移植人群，生活方式和饮食的改变在 NODAT 的管理中发挥重要作用，但有持续性高血糖的患者需要药理学治疗。

文献缺乏足够的研究，以解决口服降糖药与胰岛素在移植后长期糖尿病治疗中的安全性和有效性。尽管增加了对 NODAT 病理生理学的理解，在临床实践中，胰岛素抵抗与胰岛素分泌减少的全面评估并不常规进行。

尽管不优选单一的口服降血糖药，应仔细检查每种药物的风险和益处，以确定其与实体器官移植受者中免疫抑制剂的潜在相互作用。二甲双胍似乎是胰岛素抵抗和肾功能稳定患者的良好选择。如果患者经历急性肾功能变化和急性疾病，如胃肠道紊乱和严重感染，或可导致缺氧(包括心脏或呼吸衰竭)的情况，二甲双胍应停止使用。二甲双胍应谨慎用于肾移植受者，特别是在移植后的前六个月，在排斥反应、移植物功能障碍发生率最大时。

胰岛素促分泌素可用于移植人群，特别是如果主要机制被怀疑是胰岛素分泌降低时。然而，特定的降血糖剂应基于个体患者并发症背景下的药代动力学来选择。应谨慎使用 TZD，因为它们有引起水肿、心力衰竭和骨折的倾向。肠促胰岛素疗法是一种新的、有希望的药物疗法，但其在移植患者中的安全性和功效尚未得到充分研究。基于高血糖的严重性和对治疗的初始反应，可能需要来自不同类别的口服降血糖药的组合疗法。

实体器官移植后的高脂血症

高脂血症在实体器官移植中很常见，可能影响一半以上的肝、肾和心脏移植受者[59-61]。作用因素包括遗传倾向、肥胖、肾病综合征、甲状腺功能减退、糖尿病和药物使用，包括免疫抑制剂。

免疫抑制剂的作用

皮质类固醇

皮质类固醇对胆固醇代谢有许多有害作用。之前研究已经描述了高胆固醇水平和皮质类固醇的累积剂量之间的相关性。它们的长期使用诱导胰岛素抵抗和高胰岛素血症，从而导致甘油三酯(TG)、总胆固醇(TC)和极低密度脂蛋白(VLDL)水平的增加，以及高密度脂蛋白(HDL)水平的降低。其他脂肪生成机制包括乙酰辅酶A羧化酶和游离脂肪酸合成酶的活性的上调、HMG-CoA还原酶活性的增加、脂蛋白脂肪酶的抑制和LDL受体活性的下调[62-65]。

CNI

环孢素诱导的高脂血症的机制包括通过抑制26-羟化酶和下调LDL受体从胆固醇合成胆汁酸[66]。这种效果不依赖于皮质类固醇的同时使用，提取皮质类固醇对血脂异常有影响[67]。在肾移植受者中使用霉酚酸酯和皮质类固醇治疗的晚期环孢素减少试验显示脂质水平的剂量反应性降低[68]。使用他克莫司治疗的肾和肝移植受者的血脂异常发生率低于用环孢素治疗的患者[69,70]。一些研究表明，从头使用和从环孢素转化为他克莫司对血脂异常有积极影响[71,72]。

mTOR抑制剂

使用mTOR抑制剂以剂量依赖性模式可显著增加胆固醇和TG水平。西罗莫司的不良脂质效应的机制是未知的，并且可以是多因素的，包括阻断胰岛素刺激的脂蛋白脂肪酶、增加的肝脏产生的TG和脂蛋白，降低的血浆清除率和细胞转运，以及降低的apoB100脂蛋白的分解代谢[73-78]。从CNI到西罗莫司的转化与高甘油三酯血症和高胆固醇血症的高发病率相关[79]。西罗莫司与CNI的联合治疗与总胆固醇和TG水平的显著增加相关[80-82]。

其他免疫抑制剂

没有数据表明硫唑嘌呤或霉酚酸酯导致血脂异常。使用共刺激阻断剂贝拉西普与非环磷酰胺和总胆固醇相比，环磷酰胺减少25%~50%，与移植后TG浓度降低相关[36,83]。

用抗高血脂药物治疗：安全性和副作用(表100.3)

用于临床使用的降血脂药包括他汀类药物、依泽替米贝、烟酸、贝特类和鱼油。他汀类药物是最常用的处方药，有有效降低LDL的作用、优异的耐受性和已证实的降低心血管事件的能力[84]。实体器官移植受者与一般人群血脂异常的治疗的主要区别源于免疫抑制剂和降脂药物之间的药物相互作用。

他汀类药物

他汀类药物是HMG-CoA还原酶抑制剂（胆固醇生物合成中的限速步骤）和降低低密度脂蛋白胆固醇的最有效药物，可降低20%~60%[85-87]。它们还表现出多效性，包括抑制炎症活性和细胞因子活化、减弱内皮功能障碍、减轻血管高凝状态并增加其心血管益处[88-91]。随机临床试验表明，普伐他汀和辛伐他汀可改善心脏移植受者的生存，并降低急性排斥反应和移植血管病变的发生率[92-94]。在ALERT试验中检查了氟伐他汀对肾移植受者心血管结局的影响[95]。实际上，该试验在第134章中作为临床试验设计的示例性标本。尽管初始结果未显示出显著性差异，试验后期显示使用氟伐他汀使主要心血管事件减少21%[96]。

他汀的效价、代谢和药物相互作用不同(表100.3)。阿托伐他汀和罗苏伐他汀是最有效的，分别在80mg/d和40mg/d的剂量下将LDL-胆固醇水平降低约60%[97]。阿托伐他汀和罗苏伐他汀的另一个作用是改善甘油三酯水平并适度升高HDL-胆固醇水平[98,99]。

大多数他汀类药物，包括洛伐他汀、辛伐他汀和阿托伐他汀，被肝同工酶CYP3A4代谢。当与CNI共同使用时，由于其对CYP3A4或CYP2C9同工酶的抑制作

表 100.3 降脂药物的药物治疗

	一般人群常用日剂量	给药说明	代谢	选择性药物相互作用	副作用
HMG CoA 还原酶抑制剂(他汀类药物)					
普伐他汀	10~80mg/d	睡前	50%肾脏清除未改变的药物。较小的量通过胆汁排泄清除或经历非 CYP 和 CYP3A4 肝转化	环孢素：由于添加剂毒性和 CYP 3A4 的竞争性抑制，他汀类药物血清水平升高而增加肌病的风险。普伐他汀和氟伐他汀不太可能比其他他汀类药物与环孢素相互作用显著 mTOR 抑制剂(西罗莫司、依维莫司)：与阿托伐他汀组合的增加的西罗莫司和依维莫司的血清水平 FDA 建议在接受氨氯地平的患者中避免使用高于 20mg 剂量的辛伐他汀	转氨酶，GI 不耐受，CPK 升高，肌肉毒性，横纹肌溶解（罕见）转氨酶的密切监测可提供他汀类药物水平和毒性升高的早期证据
氟伐他汀	20~80mg/d	睡前	75%由 CYP2C9 进行肝转化，20%由CYP3A4进行		FDA 警告用高剂量辛伐他汀（80mg/d）会增加肌病风险
阿托伐他汀	10~80mg/d	全天	接受广泛的 CYP3A4 转化为活性代谢物		
瑞舒伐他汀	5~40mg/d	全天	清除为未更改的药物。10%经历 CYP2C9 转化为部分活性代谢物		
辛伐他汀	10~80mg/d(FDA 警告剂量>40mg /d)	睡前	接受广泛的 CYP3A4 转化为活性和非活性代谢物		
胆固醇吸收抑制剂					
依泽替米贝	10mg，每日 1 次	全天	在肝脏和小肠中接受葡萄糖醛酸苷共轭，形成活性代谢物。通过肠肝循环和粪便排泄清除	他汀类药物：如果不耐受他汀类药物，与他汀类药物联合或作为单一药物联合使用降低 LDL 环孢素：升高依泽替米贝的血清水平并可能改变环孢素水平。50%剂量减少至 5mg 依泽替米贝联合环孢素	增加转氨酶与他汀类药物的组合

（待续）

表 100.3 降脂药物的药物治疗(续)

	一般人群常用日剂量	给药说明	代谢	选择性药物相互作用	副作用
贝特类药物 吉非贝齐	600mg,每日2次	餐前30~60min	通过葡萄糖苷酸共轭与少量的CYP 3A4转化进行非CYP转化。吉非贝齐抑制其他药物由CYP 2C8,2C9和2C19代谢	环孢素:在环孢素治疗的患者中潜在的肾毒性 他汀类药物:肝毒性、肌病和横纹肌溶解的风险增加 避免将吉非贝齐与他汀类药物联用 他汀类药物:肌病和横纹肌溶解的风险增加	皮疹、胃肠不耐症(腹胀、痉挛、恶心)、胆石症、肌痛、肌肉毒性、横纹肌溶解
非诺贝特	剂量根据制剂而变化	不推荐肾功能不全(特别是GFR <30mL/min)的患者使用	通过血浆和组织酯酶代谢为活性中间体。不接受葡萄糖醛酸苷共轭的CYP代谢	环孢素:肾毒性的附加风险	
胆汁酸螯合剂					
考来烯胺 考来维仑 考来替泊	4~24g/d 3.75g/d 5~30g/d	饭后30min内 用餐时 应在饭后30min内服用	没有很好地吸收从肠道进入血液。因此,胆汁酸多价螯合剂连同与药物结合的任何胆汁酸在通过GI道后通过粪便排泄	影响其他药物的吸收,结合和减少脂溶性维生素,如维生素A、维生素D、维生素E和维生素K、地高辛、华法林、甲状腺素和苯巴比妥的吸收	恶心、腹胀、腹部绞痛、便秘、转氨酶异常
杂项					
烟酸	1~2g/d(避免高剂量)	应与每日膳食一起服用。从低剂量开始	未从肠道吸收到血液中	胆汁酸螯合剂:可能降低烟酸的吸收	皮肤潮红、头痛、温热感和瘙痒、恶心、呕吐、腹泻、心绞痛和肌炎
ω-3-酸乙酯(鱼油)	1~2g,每天2次	全天	未明	他汀类药物:烟酸可能增强其毒性作用,特别是每天1g或更高剂量的烟酸 基于体外数据,没有CYP介导的与免疫抑制剂、他汀类、贝特类或依泽替米贝的相互作用	消化不良、呕吐、鱼腥味味觉、LDL适度增加、出血时间适度增加

用,他汀类药物的系统暴露可以增加3~20倍。这在服用环孢素的患者中尤其明显[100-103]。环孢素还抑制其他转运蛋白,如P-糖蛋白有机阴离子转运多肽(OATP1B1),这能解释非CYP3A4依赖性他汀类药物,如普伐他汀、氟伐他汀和瑞舒伐他汀的升高[104]。

更大的他汀类药物暴露增加了他汀类药物引起肌病的风险,从肌肉疼痛和无力,到潜在的致命并发症,横纹肌溶解。在对美国肾脏数据系统(USRDS)数据库中的20 366名肾移植受体的回顾性分析中,横纹肌溶解的发生率为1.4/1000/年(95%CI,1.1~1.8),且环孢素相比他克莫司或西罗莫司更易发[105]。发现他汀诱导的肌病在非移植人群中是剂量依赖性的[106],导致美国食品药品监督管理局（FDA）对高剂量辛伐他汀(80mg/d)的使用提出了警告。

在 CNI 的移植受者中，由细胞色素 P450 代谢的他汀类药物的最大剂量应降低至一般群体最大剂量的 50%。应避免或管理抑制肝细胞色素 P450 酶的药物的共同给药[107]。这种相互作用的一个实例涉及使用氨氯地平，其通常用于高血压，并且需要进一步降低他汀类药物剂量，因为氨氯地平是 CYP3A4 同工酶的弱抑制剂[108]。对于具有相同代谢途径的其他药剂，也存在类似的关注必要(表 100.4)。

他汀的使用与高达 3%的治疗患者的肝转氨酶升高相关。这以剂量依赖的方式发生，在大多数情况下发生自发性消退。他汀类药物很少导致严重的药物性肝损伤、慢性肝病或急性肝衰竭。在启动他汀类药物和任何剂量增加后，应立即监测肝功能。如果肝转氨酶高于正常值上限的 3 倍，应停用或减少他汀类药物的使用。

依泽麦布

依泽麦布是一种选择性胆固醇吸收抑制剂，可有效阻止饮食和胆汁中胆固醇的肠道吸收。在肾移植受者中，依泽麦布可以有效降低总胆固醇和 TG 水平，具有良好的安全性[109,110]。非移植人群中可用的随机试验的综述表明，将依泽麦布加入他汀类药物治疗并不会增加肌痛、肌酸激酶水平升高、溶骨性溶解、转氨酶升高、胃肠道不良事件或戒断等不良事件的发生[111]，因此，可以考虑在实体器官移植受者中使用依泽麦布，以避免他汀类药物剂量递增。然而，没有令人信服的证据表明其添加改善了单独使用他汀类药物治疗后的临床结果。

表 100.4　增强 HMG-CoA 还原酶抑制剂水平的细胞色素 P450 同工酶抑制剂 *

药物	P450 同工酶
环孢素	3A4
大环内酯类(红霉素、克拉霉素)	3A4
唑杀真菌剂(酮康唑、氟康唑、伊曲康唑、伏立康唑)	主要是 3A4 和 2C9
非二氢吡啶类钙阻滞剂(地尔硫卓、维拉帕米)	3A4
氨氯地平	3A4(主要与高剂量辛伐他汀)
吉非贝齐	3A4
胺碘酮	3A4 和 2C9
奥美拉唑	2C9
甲氧苄啶/磺胺甲恶唑	2C9
蛋白酶抑制剂	3A4

*这些药物通常可以导致他汀类药物血浆深度曲线下面积增加 2 倍以上。

烟酸

烟酸可降低甘油三酯和低密度 LDL 颗粒的水平，并提高 HDL 的水平。烟酸与他汀类药物联合已被证明能有效降低患有冠状动脉疾病风险的高甘油三酯血症患者的动脉粥样硬化的进展[112]。可能的副作用包括潮红、头晕和恶心，这常常限制了该试剂在临床实践中的使用。

贝特

贝特类是过氧化物酶体增殖物激活受体 α(PPA-Rα)激动剂，并且可有效降低 TG 水平。在肾脏功能障碍的患者中，与他汀类药物联合使用时，贝特类诱发的肌炎和横纹肌溶解的风险更高，尤其是吉非贝齐。非诺贝特与肾移植受者的肾功能下降相关，并且剂量调整对于肾功能障碍是必要的[113-115]。在控制糖尿病(ACCORD)心血管风险的试验中，用非诺贝特联合治疗的 2 型糖尿病患者，与单独接受辛伐他汀患者的致命性心血管事件、非致命性心肌梗死或非致命性卒中的比率没有显著差异[116]。鉴于其未经证实的益处和药物相互作用的潜力，应避免在实体器官移植受者中使用贝特类。

鱼油

鱼油的优点包括良好的耐受性、轻微的不良反应和无药物相互作用。

来自肾移植受者随机对照试验数据的荟萃分析显示，在鱼油治疗的患者中，甘油三酯水平降低，HDL 水平升高，但对患者存活、移植物存活、急性排斥和 CNI 毒性没有影响[117]。它可以用作他汀类药物的辅助治疗。

血脂异常的管理

KDIGO 移植工作组建议在移植后 2~3 个月测量空腹血清、总胆固醇、低密度脂蛋白、高密度脂蛋白和 TG，改变其他已知导致血脂异常的条件，并每年都进行一次[20]。

推荐生活方式的改变，如减肥、低脂肪饮食和增加体育活动来治疗糖尿病，但通常需要药理治疗来达到

LDL目标(表100.5)。当前移植受体的目标脂质水平已经相对一般群体扩展。在肾移植受者,LDL水平>100mg/dL(>2.6mmol/L)应被治疗到更小的推荐目标,即<100mg/dL(<2.6mmol/L)。一些专家目前降低一般人群二级冠心病预防的目标为低于70mg/dL(1.8mmol/L)。这些更具挑战性的指南也可适用于实体器官移植受者,因为这些患者被认为是高风险的。然而,更积极治疗的风险可能超过益处,这些建议未被2009年KDIGO指南采纳。在肝、心脏和肺移植受者,高脂血症的治疗是类似的,没有正式的指导方针。

甘油三酯水平>500mg/dL

在TG水平>500mg/dL的患者中,建议将生活方式改变作为一线治疗,除非存在严重的高甘油三酯血症。如果2~3个月后水平不足,可以开始用烟酸治疗[112]。鱼油几乎没有副作用,应被认为是一种替代药剂。

LDL ≥100mg/dL

在LDL≥100mg/dL的患者中,建议为他汀类药物治疗联合生活方式改变。在心脏移植受者中,他汀类药物的益处超越了胆固醇治疗,应该使用而不考虑胆固醇水平[93]。最安全的他汀类药物是氟伐他汀和普伐他汀,因为它们不会被细胞色素P450 3A4代谢,并且几乎没有肌肉毒性。然而,这些他汀类药物的效力低于其他药物,因此应用于有轻度LDL升高的患者。在大多数实体器官移植受者中,考虑到与他克莫司联合能减少一般人群的心血管事件且耐受性良好,他汀类药物,如阿托伐他汀可能是一个更合适的选择[104]。

如果单独的他汀类不能充分降低LDL-胆固醇水平,伊泽麦布可以是另外的选择。如果使用他汀类药物产生不良反应,可以考虑减少剂量或切换到不同的他汀类药物。单独的伊泽麦布或烟酸可用于不能耐受他汀类药物的患者。在药物治疗难以治愈的严重失血性

表100.5 移植受者血脂异常的管理(改编自KDIGO 2009指南[11])

风险类别	目标	一线治疗	优选试剂	额外治疗	备选*	特殊考虑
空腹TG≥500mg/dL	TG<500mg/dL	生活方式改变+/-烟酸	烟酸	他汀类	贝特类(优选吉非贝齐)	TG≥500mg/dL会增加急性胰腺炎的风险 肾衰竭患者通常不推荐使用贝特类药物,特别是GFR<15mL/min/1.73m²;GFR<60mL/min/1.73m²的患者剂量减少50%
LDL 100~129mg/dL	LDL<100mg/dL	生活方式改变+/-他汀类	阿托伐他汀(更有效) 氟伐他汀或普伐他汀	他汀类	单用烟酸	在用环孢素治疗的患者中,他汀类药物剂量需减少约50%,也可能与他克莫司相比
LDL≥130mg/dL	LDL<100mg/dL	生活方式改变+他汀类	阿托伐他汀(更有效) 氟伐他汀或普伐他汀	依泽麦布	单用烟酸	药物治疗难治的病例可能需要减少免疫抑制剂的剂量或停止,并转换到另一种免疫抑制剂
LDL<100mg/dL,空腹TG≥200mg/dL,非HDL-C≥130mg/dL	非HDL-C<130mg/dL	生活方式改变+他汀类	阿托伐他汀(更有效) 氟伐他汀或普伐他汀	依泽麦布	单用烟酸	相对较少的具有正常或低LDL,增加的TG和高的非HDL-C患者被认为具有高水平的致动脉粥样硬化脂蛋白残余物。这些患者的治疗类似于具有高LDL患者的治疗

TG,甘油三酯;LDL,低密度脂蛋白;HDL,高密度脂蛋白;非HDL-C,非高密度脂蛋白胆固醇;GFR,肾小球滤过率。*替代疗法:在一线治疗不耐受的情况下。

贫血病例中，可能需要降低患者当前免疫抑制剂的剂量或停止使用,并切换到另一种。这种调整应始终在移植专家的指导下进行。

实体器官移植后的骨和矿物质疾病

骨和矿物质疾病在实体器官移植受者中常见。促成因素包括高龄、预先存在的骨营养不良、导致终末期器官衰竭的潜在疾病、维生素 D 缺乏、吸烟、糖尿病和移植特异性治疗,特别是免疫抑制剂[118]。

在实体器官移植后的前 6~12 个月内,骨丢失尤其迅速,0~24%在脊柱,2%~11%在髋部[119]。在移植后期,骨丢失率降低，这可能是由于较低剂量的免疫抑制剂以及代谢和内分泌异常改善，并且可能有一些骨矿物质密度(BMD)的恢复,特别是在脊柱处可以观察到[120]。用于治疗排斥或其他原因的糖皮质激素剂量的增加可能导致骨丢失的加速。因此,骨折的频率在肾移植受者中为 6%~45%，在心脏、肺和肝移植受体中为 22%~42%[119-125]。

肾移植受体在具有预先存在的慢性肾脏疾病(CKD)中是独特的,其影响矿物质代谢的许多方面,包括磷酸盐保留、低钙血症和降低的维生素 D 活化。这些效应刺激甲状旁腺,导致继发性甲状旁腺功能亢进。如果不适当治疗，这些代谢紊乱可导致甲状旁腺细胞增生和三级甲状旁腺功能亢进。成功的肾移植逆转了矿物质和骨代谢中的许多这些异常,然而,改善程度常常不完全[126-131]。持续高钙血症可对肾同种异体移植物(包括移植物微钙化和功能障碍，来自传入小动脉血管收缩的肾衰竭、骨脱矿质和损失、软组织和血管钙化,以及增加的断裂率)有不利影响[132-136]。

持续性甲状旁腺功能亢进和高钙血症

肾移植后持续性甲状旁腺功能亢进的发生率可高达 50%[132,137-144]。移植后甲状旁腺功能亢进和肾功能的严重程度决定了移植后长期的甲状旁腺功能[133]。虽然甲状旁腺在移植后逐渐恢复，这一过程需要几个月到几年才能完成[129,130,137,138]。

在移植后的前 3 个月内，高达 41%的受体会发生短暂的高钙血症[145]。第一年后,高达 20%的患者会出现持续性高钙血症和甲状旁腺激素(PTH)水平升高[146,147]。高钙血症的发展与移植前透析的持续时间、甲状旁腺增生的程度和腺体大小相关,因此,1 年后高钙血症的自发性消退不常见[139]。持续性甲状旁腺功能亢进是肾脏后移植高钙血症的主要原因，但其他因素可能有助于在新的肾脏同种异体移植物中提高肾小管钙重吸收和骨化三醇生产的正常化，这提高了对骨的 PTH 效应,也增加了肠钙吸收[132,148]。

三级甲状旁腺功能亢进的治疗考虑

对于三级甲状旁腺功能亢进的适应证，治疗方案没有普遍的建议。维生素 D 类似物通常对甲状旁腺具有负的生物反馈效应,但其在高钙血症患者中的使用可能受到限制。钙化可能是那些持续性甲状旁腺功能亢进和高钙血症的有希望的治疗,因为它们的使用可有效降低钙水平，但 PTH 水平的降低一直未得到证实[149-154]。肾移植受者中描述了西那卡塞和他克莫司之间的相互作用，导致他克莫司全身暴露的中度显著减少,而环孢素和霉酚酸酯的药代动力学不受影响[155]。在用西那卡塞治疗 12 个月的少数肾移植受者中显示出 BMD 的改善，但需要进一步的研究和更长的随访,以更好地阐明拟钙剂的功效和安全性特征，特别是对于长期骨组织学和肾脏结果[156]。

甲状旁腺切除术被认为是肾移植后三级甲状旁腺功能亢进的确定性治疗。一些研究已经证明甲状旁腺切除术后,高钙血症改善,骨矿物质密度增加,血压改善,脂质得到控制[157-161]。在肾移植患者中有甲状旁腺切除术的两个主要适应证:严重的症状性高钙血症,通常发生在移植后早期,以及持续的、明显的高钙血症,药物治疗无效。没有关于甲状旁腺切除术的最佳时机的共识。由于缺乏基于证据的指南,一个保守的方法是等待至少 12 个月,然后考虑甲状旁腺切除术患者的三级甲状旁腺功能亢进。西那卡塞的使用以及仔细监测他克莫司、钾离子水平和钙水平可以是甲状旁腺切除术的替代方案，尽管它未被 FDA 批准用于肾移植受者。需要进一步的研究来确定肾移植术后三级甲状旁腺功能亢进手术治疗的相对危险度和获益。

维生素 D 缺乏是慢性肾脏疾病患者 PTH 升高的重要原因,甚至在肾移植后仍然存在[162,163]。没有关于移植受者维生素 D 替代的指南,因此,在没有高钙血症的情况下，建议根据国家肾脏基金会在非移植人群中的建议,保持 25-OH-维生素 D 浓度>30ng/mL。用维生素 D 治疗需要每日最少 1000~2000 IU 的维生素 D_3[164]。

低磷酸盐血症

低磷酸血症可在肾移植后的最初几个月内发展到高达93%的患者[165],并且很少在其他实体器官移植后发生。该病症通常在移植后1~3个月内消退,但可持续长达10年[165]。一般来说,鼓励恢复富含磷的食物是较好的治疗措施。

持续低磷血症主要是由甲状旁腺功能亢进、相对钙三醇缺乏以及使用糖皮质激素和其他免疫抑制剂(mTor抑制剂和环孢素比他克莫司更多)引起的肾脏磷酸盐消耗引起的[165-169]。在移植后早期,主要是由于在CKD患者中积累的磷酸化成纤维细胞生长因子-23(FGF-23)[165,170-173]。然而,持续性甲状旁腺功能亢进,而不伴随FGF-23增加,似乎是持续超过一年的磷酸盐消耗的基础[143]。

大多数低磷水平的患者是无症状的。血浆磷酸盐水平<1.5mg/dL可引起全身肌肉无力。严重低磷血症虽然移植后通常罕见,可以与急性呼吸衰竭、肌肉无力、溶血性贫血、横纹肌溶解和改变的精神状态有关。低磷血症对骨密度和骨折风险的净效应尚不清楚;然而,长期和严重的低磷血症可导致骨软化和立克次体。

大多数移植后低磷血症会自发解决。如果没有预测持续性或症状性低磷血症的因素,尚不清楚哪些患者可能从药理学治疗中受益。一些研究支持磷酸盐补充[静脉和(或)口服][174],但担心磷酸盐替代可能产生高磷水平的爆发,从而触发更多的PTH产生,进而延迟继发性甲状旁腺功能亢进的解决。其他人主张磷替代不可能比观察等待和恢复正常饮食有更显著的影响。更合理的方法可能是补充骨化三醇,增加管状Na^+/磷酸盐共转运蛋白活性,从而增强磷酸盐的重吸收[175]。如前所述,通过治疗三级甲状旁腺功能亢进(无论是医学还是手术)降低PTH水平也将有助于通过抑制PTH诱导的磷酸盐肾脏消瘦来治疗低磷血症。

免疫抑制剂的作用(表100.6)

对早期移植后骨丢失的最大影响似乎是皮质类固醇的使用。类固醇通过直接的成骨细胞毒性和增加的破骨细胞活性而损伤骨形成,并且促进负钙平衡(通过减少胃肠吸收和增加尿排泄)。它们还减少性腺激素和胰岛素样生长因子-1的产生,降低对PTH的敏感性,增加NF-κβ配体的受体激活剂,并增加破骨细胞发生[176,177]。

表100.6 免疫抑制药物和骨病

免疫抑制剂	骨矿物质密度损失的机制
皮质类固醇	通过直接毒性损害成骨细胞骨形成
	减少钙胃肠道吸收
	增加钙尿排泄
	降低性腺激素的产生(雌激素、睾酮肾上腺雄激素)
	减少胰岛素样生长因子-1生产降低对PTH的敏感性
	增加NF-κβ配体的受体激活剂
	增加破骨细胞形成
环孢素	冲突的报告
	? 增加破骨细胞数量和骨转换
	? 抑制成骨细胞
	? 降低矿物质附着和骨形成速率
他克莫司	? 与环孢素类似,但毒性较小
霉酚酸	没有不良骨质影响的证据
硫唑嘌呤	没有不良骨质影响的证据
西罗莫司	至今没有人类数据;动物数据:干扰成骨细胞的增殖和分化
依维莫司	至今没有人类数据;动物数据:减少破骨细胞介导的骨吸收

类固醇剂量与骨丢失量正相关。即使小剂量的类固醇也可导致明显的骨损失[178]。

关于环孢素对骨密度丢失的影响的研究结果尚不明确。有部分报道在无激素免疫抑制方案中使用环孢素并不会显著增加骨密度减少风险[179,180]。但也有研究表明,环孢素可能会增加骨钙蛋白表达,从而增加破骨细胞数量并加速骨转换,最终导致骨密度丢失[181,182]。总的来看,环孢素似乎比他克莫司对骨密度有更多的负面影响[180,183,184]。

流行病学研究无法建立CNI与骨折风险之间的关联[125,185]。没有关于霉酚酸酯和硫唑嘌呤对骨的影响的可用数据。最近的体外研究表明,西罗莫司可能干扰小鼠中成骨细胞的增殖和分化[186],而卵巢切除的大鼠的研究发现,依维莫司可通过减少破骨细胞介导的骨吸收来减少小梁骨损失[187]。

用抗再吸收剂治疗:安全性和副作用(表100.7)

钙和维生素D类似物

在非高钙血症患者中应考虑每日至少1000mg的

表 100.7 用于治疗实体器官移植受者的矿物和骨疾病的药理学试剂

药物家族(品牌)	对血清钙和磷的影响	对血清 PTH 的影响	注释/证据
二磷酸盐			
阿仑膦酸钠(福善美)	减少	减少	增加骨矿物质密度,特别是在腰椎
帕米膦酸(APD、阿可达)	减少	减少	可能导致骨转换减少
唑来膦酸(择泰、密固达)	减少	减少	不清楚它们是否真的降低了骨折的风险
利塞膦酸盐	减少	减少	不推荐均匀使用
伊班膦酸钠	减少	减少	当 GFR<30mL/min 时指示
依替膦酸钠	减少	减少	
氯膦酸盐	减少	减少	
维生素 D.			
胆固醇(德利斯多)	增加	减少	改善骨矿物质密度
胆钙化醇(骨化二醇、维生素 D_3)	增加	减少	可能导致高钙血症
25(OH)D(骨化二醇、骨化)	增加	减少	
维生素 D 受体激活剂			
1 – 阿法骨化醇(1-α)	增加	减少	改善骨矿物质密度
度骨化醇	增加	减少	可能导致高钙血症
骨化三醇(溉纯、罗盖全)	增加	减少	
维生素 D 模拟物			
帕立骨化醇	无改变或增加	减少	改善骨矿物质密度
拟钙剂			
西那卡塞	减少	减少	未经 FDA 批准用于肾移植受者二级/三级甲状旁腺功能亢进 可能改善骨矿物质密度 可能与他克莫司联用(他克莫司水平应仔细监测)
其他药物			
特立帕肽	钙:增加,磷:减少	增加	在移植患者中未证明有效,不推荐移植后使用
降钙素	减少	减少	在移植患者中未证明有效

钙补充,因为糖皮质激素治疗会降低肠钙吸收。在移植人群中,维生素 D 缺乏症的发生率高,并且与未治疗相比,用 25-羟基-和 1,25-羟基-维生素 D 治疗与改善的骨矿物质密度相关[188-190]。在维生素 D 治疗的受体中需仔细监测高钙血症。

二磷酸盐

在非移植人群中,二磷酸盐用于预防骨量减少并治疗骨质疏松症。几项临床介入试验证实二磷酸盐在肝、心、肺和肾移植受体移植后预防和治疗骨丢失的功效[191-196]。值得注意的是,大多数研究无法使用足够的统计学力量来检测治疗和未治疗患者的骨折差异。在移植后的前 12 个月,涉及在肾、肝、心脏或肺移植患者中用二磷酸盐或活性维生素 D 类似物治疗的试验的荟萃分析结果表明,用二磷酸盐或维生素 D 治疗可改善患者的骨矿物质密度、骨折和椎骨骨折[197]。当分别分析二磷酸盐试验时,有骨折的受试者的数量减少,但椎骨骨折没有改善。

在某些人群中应谨慎使用二磷酸盐。用二磷酸盐治疗的肾移植受者由于预先存在肾性骨营养不良,可能处于骨转移低风险,尽管骨活检研究显示出有争议的结果[193,198]。

类似地,在患有晚期 CKD(4~5 期)的患者中应避免二磷酸盐,因为肾排泄是唯一的消除途径。二磷酸盐在骨中积累,半衰期超过 10 年,并逐渐释放回循环并再次吸收或排泄[199]。长期使用二磷酸盐可能导致骨形成的过度抑制,因此在 CKD 患者中,应考虑骨活检,以在开始治疗之前排除低骨转换疾病。

特立帕肽

特立帕肽是具有完全生理活性的氨基末端甲状旁腺激素。它可增加骨矿物质的密度，降低绝经后妇女和类固醇治疗患者的骨折风险[200,201]。在移植受者中，迄今为止没有证明特立帕肽的使用益处[202]。直到进行进一步的研究，不建议移植后使用特立帕肽。

降钙素和其他治疗

另一种潜在治疗剂是降钙素，但它对肾移植后患者的死亡率、移植物损失和骨折风险没有影响[203,204]。常规运动和激素替代治疗显示可降低肺损伤和骨髓移植受体的骨折风险，但它们尚未在肾移植受者中证实[205,206]。早期阶段的骨坏死通常保守或伴随骨移植的减压。

骨病的治疗

实体器官移植受者骨病的预防和管理应注意纠正任何可能影响骨代谢的因素和生活方式，以改善身体活动代谢水平。骨疾病预防和治疗的正式指南只适用于肾移植受者。国家肾脏基金会疾病预后质量倡议(KDOQI)指南建议移植后及移植后1~2年时行DEXA(双能X射线吸收测定法)扫描。如果在移植或随后的评估时T值≤-2，则应考虑用双磷酸盐治疗[207]。KDIGO指南建议，对低骨矿物质密度和GFR>约30mL/min/1.73mm^{2}的患者，应考虑使用维生素D、骨化三醇或双磷酸盐治疗[208]。这些试剂的选择由异常的钙、磷酸盐、PTH、碱性磷酸盐和25-羟基维生素D水平决定。在非肾实体器官移植受者中，来自临床试验的数据表明，双磷酸盐和维生素D类似物是用于预防和治疗移植后骨质疏松症和骨折的安全且有效的药物[119,197]。

骨矿物质密度低和GFR<30mL/min/1.72mm^{2}的实体器官移植受者应在饮食中限制磷酸盐并替换维生素D储备。患有晚期CKD的患者应谨慎使用二磷酸盐，并且在开始治疗之前尽量进行骨活检[209]。

研究已经开发了类固醇戒断或避免免疫抑制方案，并且发现与使用标准类固醇免疫抑制方案相比，骨矿物质密度更高。最大的差异见于腰椎。然而，随机对照试验显示晚期类固醇戒断(移植后数周至数月完成)与肾移植中急性排斥的风险增加相关[210,211]。因此，目前的KDIGO指南不建议采取类固醇戒断，同时避免单纯地治疗骨疾病。

实体器官移植后的高尿酸血症和痛风

高尿酸血症在实体器官移植后常见。其病因是复杂的，并与降低的GFR、移植低龄、肥胖症、代谢综合征、前移植物高尿酸血症的存在以及利尿剂和免疫抑制剂使用相关的尿酸排泄相关。肾移植受者高尿酸血症的患病率可高达80%，特别是在接受环孢素的受者中，肝移植受者中则接近50%[212,213]。但痛风的发生率则相对低得多(6%~7%)[213,214]。

在一般人群中，血清尿酸水平升高与心血管和全因死亡率的风险增加相关[215]。高尿酸血症也与胰岛素抵抗和代谢综合征的发展相关[216]。尿酸是否在疾病的发展中起致病作用或仅仅作为伴随疾病的问题仍不清楚。

无症状高尿酸血症对实体器官移植受者的发病率和死亡率的影响未知。类似地，关于高尿酸血症对肾移植患者中同种异体移植物功能的影响的数据是矛盾的。一项研究表明，高尿酸血症与405名肾移植受体在3年内同种异体移植功能降低有关[217]，而多数前瞻性试验的结果未发现关联[212]。

免疫抑制剂的作用

钙调神经磷酸酶抑制剂

环孢素诱导GFR的减少和过滤后尿酸盐肾小管吸收的净增加，导致高尿酸血症[218,219]。他克莫司具有许多与环孢素相同的血流动力学和毒性作用，但高尿酸血症的发生率在基于他克莫司的方案中似乎较低[220]。已经采用CNI剂量减少的策略作为免疫抑制管理的一部分，以解决高尿酸血症和痛风。一个报告记录了从环孢素转化为他克莫司后尿酸减少，但数据有限[221]。

其他免疫抑制剂

长期使用糖皮质激素与胰岛素抵抗和代谢综合征的发展相关。高尿酸血症也与代谢综合征相关，尽管没有确定的研究将糖皮质激素的使用与高尿酸血症联系起来[216,222]。

硫唑嘌呤、霉酚酸吗啉乙酯和西罗莫司未显示能显著影响尿酸。

利尿剂的作用

带环和噻嗪类利尿剂治疗导致痛风和高尿酸血症的风险增加。利尿治疗与血清尿酸的增加具有剂量依赖性关系。这是由于诱导的相对血容量不足，导致肾小管尿酸盐重吸收增加和尿酸盐排泄减少[223]。

高尿酸血症和痛风的治疗考虑

非甾体抗炎药

非甾体抗炎药(NSAID)通过非选择性抑制环氧化酶起作用，导致前列腺素和各种炎症介质的合成减少。非甾体抗炎药在非移植人群中治疗急性痛风发作有效，但在移植人群中肾功能下降的高流行性和 CNI 中则限制了它们的使用。NSAID 的短期治疗可用于肾功能正常的移植患者。

糖皮质激素

糖皮质激素的抗炎作用通过减少白细胞进入炎症区域的外周迁移来介导。在随机对照试验中的急性痛风发作期间，在 120 名非移植患者中比较系统性口服皮质类固醇(35mg 口服泼尼松龙，5 天)与萘普生的疗效。泼尼松龙的安全性和有效性与萘普生相当[224]。虽然没有进行移植受者的类似研究，短期的皮质类固醇被认为是有效的。关节内制备可能是治疗单关节疾病的合理选择。

秋水仙碱

秋水仙碱通常用于非移植人群急性痛风的发生和预防。其可快速缓解疼痛(48h 内)，但其显著的副作用可能限制其在移植受体中的使用。秋水仙碱诱导的肌病尤其会在肾功能损伤的背景下发生，因此，应考虑慢性肾脏疾病阶段 3~5 的替代治疗[225]。在肾脏和心脏移植受者中报道了与秋水仙碱有关的神经毒性[226,227]。环孢素共同给药通过双重机制增加秋水仙碱毒性：环孢素抑制 P–糖蛋白，这导致增加的细胞内秋水仙素浓度和减少的药物和环孢素的肝和肾排泄与 CYP3A4 相互作用，其减少秋水仙碱在肝中的消除[228,229]。伴随的他汀类药物使用会增加肌肉损伤的风险。骨髓抑制在肾转移受体中并不罕见，也可由秋水仙碱引起。

别嘌呤醇

别嘌呤醇是嘌呤类似物和酶黄嘌呤氧化酶的抑制剂，它是生产尿酸所必需的[228]。别嘌呤醇常常是长期治疗高尿酸血症和痛风的首选治疗方法。与硫唑嘌呤的共同给药可能由于其活性代谢物巯基嘌呤的代谢抑制而导致严重的骨髓抑制，因此，应考虑替代治疗。如果不可能，那么硫唑嘌呤的剂量应减少 50%~75%，应使用剂量减少的别嘌呤醇[230]。尽管剂量调整，在数月或甚至数年的治疗后可以看到全血细胞减少[231]。CKD 需要调整剂量。

非布索坦

非布索坦是非嘌呤抑制剂的黄嘌呤氧化酶，在临床试验中显示可比别嘌呤醇更有效地减少尿酸[232]。CKD 3 期的患者无需减少剂量，但对于晚期肾脏疾病患者的研究数据不足[225]。联合给予硫唑嘌呤可增加骨髓抑制的风险。

尿酸剂

丙磺舒通过增加肾排泄降低尿酸。它在肾功能降低的患者中是无效的。此外，其可导致肾脏中尿酸晶体的沉积，导致尿酸肾病和(或)尿酸结石。一种更有效的尿毒症药苯唑酮在肾脏疾病患者中有效，并且已被证明在肾移植受者中有效，但肝毒性是一个重要的关注点[230,233]。

氯沙坦显示具有适度的尿酸排泄作用及抗高血压活性，其效果未被其他血管紧张素受体阻断剂证实[234]。

普瑞凯希

普瑞凯希，哺乳动物的重组尿酸氧化酶，使得尿酸代谢为其胺囊代谢物尿囊素，并可有效降低不能耐受嘌呤醇或难治痛风患者的尿酸[235]。它尚未在慢性肾脏疾病和实体器官移植受者的研究中进行深入研究。

痛风的治疗

渐进性高尿酸血症患者治疗目标的证据是矛盾的，由于数据不足和副作用风险，一般不推荐在移植受者中使用。然而，对于症状性高尿酸血症，如痛风和尿酸结石，治疗是必要的。治疗策略针对与爆发相关的急性炎症反应和高尿酸血症。饮食改变，如减少饮酒、海鲜和红肉，是重要生活方式的组成部分。应注意含有果糖的食品,因为它们的消耗促使血清尿酸迅速增加[222]。

抗痛风治疗剂的风险和益处需要在其他疾病治疗的背景下仔细检查。高血压和高脂血症在移植人群中常见,并且它们的治疗剂可影响尿酸水平或加强毒性。如果可能,应避免使用利尿剂,并且可能需要使用替代治疗剂来治疗高血压。

对于急性痛风的发生,可以使用短期皮质类固醇。NSAID的短期治疗也可用于肾功能正常的患者。eGFR<60mL/(min·1.73m^2)的患者应避免长期使用秋水仙碱。如果绝对必要,秋水仙碱可以在eGFR>10mL/(min·1.73m^2)且无需透析的患者中以减少的剂量使用<1周[20]。

长期、低剂量的尿酸可能需要开始治疗。通常使用别嘌呤醇,但可能需要调整免疫抑制,并且需要在肾脏疾病中减少剂量。较新的低尿酸剂,如非布索坦或聚乙二醇重组尿酸酶,被证明可能在移植受体中有用,但需要更多的研究。

实体器官移植后的电解质紊乱

高钾血症

高钾血症是实体器官移植后最常见的电解质紊乱,特别是在最初几周。其原因几乎总是多因素的,包括饮食摄入增加、再分配和肾排泄减少。常用于移植受者的药物,如甲氧苄啶和CNI,会增加高钾血症的风险。甲氧苄啶通过抑制远端肾单位中的钾清除而诱导高钾血症,并且这种效应在肾功能受损的患者中尤其常见[236]。CNIs减少醛固酮的产生,减弱肾脏对醛固酮的反应,并抑制集合管中的钾分泌[237,238]。

实体器官移植受体中高钾血症的急性治疗遵循非移植人群中的一般治疗。选择包括静脉葡萄糖酸钙和葡萄糖,随后胰岛素注射,碳酸氢钠,甚至血液透析(当其他治疗失败时)。治疗由肾功能的程度、EKG变化的存在或不存在以及钾的绝对水平决定。更换某些药物,如甲氧苄啶可能是必要的,在大多数情况下足以降低血清钾水平。高钾血症的慢性处理包括优化肾功能,使用钾消耗剂,如树脂黏合剂和盐皮质激素(如氟氢可的松),以及在严重的情况下最小化或撤除钙调神经磷酸酶抑制剂。

低镁血症

低镁血症在用CNI治疗的实体器官移植受体中非常常见。其通常发生在前几个星期,并可能因使用CNI而慢性持续。大约80%的血清镁在肾小球中自由过滤,超过95%的血清镁在小管中被重吸收。CNI具有直接镁质管状效应,它们减少镁的再吸收,增加尿镁消耗,从而引起低镁血症[239]。

在用环孢素治疗的肾移植受者中,血清镁水平与肾脏同种异体移植物功能的下降速度和移植物丢失率增加相关[239]。严重的低镁血症可能与心律失常和癫痫发作有关。低镁血症也是肾移植受者新发移植后糖尿病的独立预测因素[240]。当膳食补充剂无法维持镁水平时,尤其是在用CNI治疗的患者中,可能需要长期补充氧化镁。

代谢性酸中毒

实体器官移植后的代谢性酸中毒可由肾功能和CNI减少引起。在动物研究中,通过在近端小管和远端肾脏中主要酸碱转运蛋白的调节,CNI诱导代谢性酸中毒[241]。使用CNI的移植后受体可能由于收集管中钾分泌的抑制存在高钾血症代谢性酸中毒(Ⅳ型肾小管性酸中毒)[237]。应及时开始治疗,以纠正酸中毒和高钾血症。有胰腺膀胱排尿的胰腺移植受体可能由于来自胰腺分泌物的尿液中的碳酸氢盐损失而呈现代谢性酸中毒。由于胰腺膀胱引流的这种主要副作用,伴随着慢性体积耗竭,肠道排泄的胰腺移植已经获得普及。此外,大多数情况下肠道排水转化可以纠正代谢性酸中毒[242]。已经证明口服碳酸氢钠补充剂可以在非移植性慢性肾脏疾病患者中保持肾功能,但缺乏关于移植后肾脏结果的数据[243]。

总结

在实体器官移植受体中,代谢病和电解质紊乱常见。术后早期会经常遇到电解质异常,如高钾血症、高钙血症、低镁血症和低磷血症。从长期来看,受体需要密切监测并管理糖尿病、高脂血症、骨病和痛风等并发症。由于与移植药物的潜在相互作用以及肾脏和肝脏功能的变化,治疗尤其具有挑战性。在本章中,我们回顾了可用于治疗移植后代谢和电解质疾病的治疗选择,应特别关注常用药物的潜在副作用和药物的相互作用。

(沈恬 译 沈恬 校)

参考文献

1. Chakkera HA, Weil EJ, Castro J, et al. Hyperglycemia during the immediate period after kidney transplantation. Clinical Journal of the American Society of Nephrology. 2009;4(4):853-859.
2. Perito ER, Laul A, Rhee S, et al. Post-transplant metabolic syndrome in children and adolescents after liver transplant: a systematic review. Liver Transplantation. 2012;18(9):1009-1028.
3. Israni AK, Snyder JJ, Skeans MA, et al. for the PORT Investigators. Clinical diagnosis of metabolic syndrome: predicting new-onset diabetes, coronary heart disease, and allograft failure late after kidney transplant. Transplant International. 2012;25(7):748-757.
4. Sanchez-Gomez JM, Martinez-Dolz L, Sanchez-Lazaro I, et al. Influence of metabolic syndrome on development of cardiac allograft vasculopathy in the transplanted heart. Transplantation. 2012;93(1):106-111.
5. Dong M, Parsaik AK, Eberhardt NL, et al. Cellular and physiological mechanisms of new-onset diabetes mellitus after solid organ transplantation. Diabetic Medicine. 2012;29(7):e1-12.
6. Kasiske BL, Snyder JJ, Gilbertson D, et al. Diabetes mellitus after kidney transplantation in the United States. American Journal of Transplantation. 2003; 3(2):178-185.
7. Parekh J, Corley DA, Feng S. Diabetes, hypertension and hyperlipidemia: prevalence over time and impact on long-term survival after liver transplantation. American Journal of Transplantation. 2012;12(8):2181-2187.
8. Jacobson PA, Schladt D, Israni A, et al. Genetic and clinical determinants of early, acute calcineurin inhibitor-related nephrotoxicity: results from a kidney transplant consortium. Transplantation. 2012;93(6):624-631.
9. Jacobson PA, Schladt D, Oetting WS, et al. Genetic determinants of mycophenolate-related anemia and leukopenia after transplantation. Transplantation. 2011;91(3):309-316.
10. Tavira B, Coto E, Diaz-Corte C, et al. KCNQ1 gene variants and risk of new-onset diabetes in tacrolimus-treated renal-transplanted patients. Clinical Transplantation. 2011;25(3):E284-E291.
11. Chakkera HA, Knowler WC, Devarapalli Y, et al. Relationship between inpatient hyperglycemia and insulin treatment after kidney transplantation and future new onset diabetes mellitus. Clinical Journal of the American Society of Nephrology. 2010;5(9):1669-1675.
12. Claes K, Meier-Kriesche HU, Schold JD, et al. Effect of different immunosuppressive regimens on the evolution of distinct metabolic parameters: evidence from the Symphony study. Nephrology, Dialysis, Transplantation. 2012;27(2): 850-857.
13. Kuo HT, Lau C, Sampaio MS, et al. Pretransplant risk factors for new-onset diabetes mellitus after transplant in pediatric liver transplant recipients. Liver Transplantation. 2010;16(11):1249-1256.
14. Kuo HT, Sampaio MS, Ye X, et al. Risk factors for new-onset diabetes mellitus in adult liver transplant recipients, an analysis of the Organ Procurement and Transplant Network/United Network for Organ Sharing database. Transplantation. 2010;89(9):1134-1140.
15. Ye X, Kuo HT, Sampaio MS, et al. Risk factors for development of new-onset diabetes mellitus after transplant in adult lung transplant recipients. Clinical Transplantation. 2011;25(6):885-891.
16. Ye X, Kuo HT, Sampaio MS, et al. Risk factors for development of new-onset diabetes mellitus in adult heart transplant recipients. Transplantation. 2010;89(12):1526-1532.
17. Shah T, Kasravi A, Huang E, et al. Risk factors for development of new-onset diabetes mellitus after kidney transplantation. Transplantation. 2006;82(12): 1673-1676.
18. Kuo HT, Poommipanit N, Sampaio M, et al. Risk factors for development of new-onset diabetes mellitus in pediatric renal transplant recipients: an analysis of the OPTN/UNOS database. Transplantation. 2010;89(4):434-439.
19. Rabkin R, Ryan MP, Duckworth WC. The renal metabolism of insulin. Diabetologia. 1984;27(3):351-357.
20. Kidney Disease: Improving Global Outcomes (KDIGO) Transplant Work Group. KDIGO clinical practice guideline for the care of kidney transplant recipients. American Journal of Transplantation. 2009;9(Suppl 3):S1-155.
21. Caillard S, Eprinchard L, Perrin P, et al. Incidence and risk factors of glucose metabolism disorders in kidney transplant recipients: role of systematic screening by oral glucose tolerance test. Transplantation. 2011;91(7):757-764.
22. van Raalte DH, Nofrate V, Bunck MC, et al. Acute and 2-week exposure to prednisolone impair different aspects of beta-cell function in healthy men. European Journal of Endocrinology. 2010;162(4):729-735.
23. Meier-Kriesche HU, Li S, Gruessner RW, et al. Immunosuppression: evolution in practice and trends, 1994-2004. American Journal of Transplantation. 2006;6(5 Pt 2):1111-1131.
24. Luan FL, Steffick DE, Ojo AO. New-onset diabetes mellitus in kidney transplant recipients discharged on steroid-free immunosuppression. Transplantation. 2011;91(3):334-341.
25. Rizzari MD, Suszynski TM, Gillingham KJ, et al. Ten-year outcome after rapid discontinuation of prednisone in adult primary kidney transplantation. Clinical Journal of the American Society of Nephrology. 2012;7(3):494-503.
26. Knight SR, Morris PJ. Steroid sparing protocols following nonrenal transplants; the evidence is not there. A systematic review and meta-analysis. Transplant International. 2011;24(12):1198-1207.
27. Woodle ES, First MR, Pirsch J, et al. A prospective, randomized, double-blind, placebo-controlled multicenter trial comparing early (7 day) corticosteroid cessation versus long-term, low-dose corticosteroid therapy. Annals of Surgery. 2008;248(4):564-577.
28. Vincenti F, Friman S, Scheuermann E, et al. Results of an international, randomized trial comparing glucose metabolism disorders and outcome with cyclosporine versus tacrolimus. American Journal of Transplantation. 2007;7(6):1506-1514.
29. Flechner SM, Glyda M, Cockfield S, et al. The ORION study: comparison of two sirolimus-based regimens versus tacrolimus and mycophenolate mofetil in renal allograft recipients. American Journal of Transplantation. 2011;11(8): 1633-1644.
30. Ekberg H, Bernasconi C, Noldeke J, et al. Cyclosporine, tacrolimus and sirolimus retain their distinct toxicity profiles despite low doses in the Symphony study. Nephrology, Dialysis, Transplantation. 2010;25(6):2004-2010.
31. Heit JJ. Calcineurin/NFAT signaling in the beta-cell: from diabetes to new therapeutics. Bioessays. 2007;29(10):1011-1021.
32. Teutonico A, Schena PF, Di Paolo S. Glucose metabolism in renal transplant recipients: effect of calcineurin inhibitor withdrawal and conversion to sirolimus. Journal of the American Society of Nephrology. 2005;16(10):3128-3135.
33. Gyurus E, Kaposztas Z, Kahan BD. Sirolimus therapy predisposes to new-onset diabetes mellitus after renal transplantation: a long-term analysis of various treatment regimens. Transplantation Proceedings. 2011;43(5):1583-1592.
34. Johnston O, Rose CL, Webster AC, et al. Sirolimus is associated with new-onset diabetes in kidney transplant recipients. Journal of the American Society of Nephrology. 2008;19(7):1411-1418.
35. Bussiere CT, Lakey JR, Shapiro AM, et al. The impact of the mTOR inhibitor sirolimus on the proliferation and function of pancreatic islets and ductal cells. Diabetologia. 2006;49(10):2341-2349.
36. Vanrenterghem Y, Bresnahan B, Campistol J, et al. Belatacept-based regimens are associated with improved cardiovascular and metabolic risk factors compared with cyclosporine in kidney transplant recipients (BENEFIT and BENEFIT-EXT studies). Transplantation. 2011;91(9):976-983.
37. Heisel O, Heisel R, Balshaw R, et al. New onset diabetes mellitus in patients receiving calcineurin inhibitors: a systematic review and meta-analysis. American Journal of Transplantation. 2004;4(4):583-595.
38. van Duijnhoven EM, Boots JM, Christiaans MH, et al. Metabolic aspects of tacrolimus in renal transplantation. Consequences for the choice of an immunosuppressive regimen and for the management of post-transplant diabetes mellitus. Minerva Urologica e Nefrologica. 2003;55(1):33-42.
39. Emre S, Genyk Y, Schluger LK, et al. Treatment of tacrolimus-related adverse effects by conversion to cyclosporine in liver transplant recipients. Transplant International. 2000;13(1):73-78.
40. Mor E, Sheiner PA, Schwartz ME, et al. Reversal of severe FK506 side effects by conversion to cyclosporine-based immunosuppression. Transplantation. 1994;58(3):380-382.
41. Hjelmesaeth J, Hartmann A, Kofstad J, et al. Glucose intolerance after renal transplantation depends upon prednisolone dose and recipient age. Transplantation. 1997;64(7):979-983.
42. Nathan DM, Buse JB, Davidson MB, et al. Medical management of hyperglycemia in type 2 diabetes: a consensus algorithm for the initiation and adjustment of therapy: a consensus statement of the American Diabetes Association and the European Association for the Study of Diabetes. Diabetes Care. 2009;32(1): 193-203.
43. Shaw JS, Wilmot RL, Kilpatrick ES. Establishing pragmatic estimated GFR thresholds to guide metformin prescribing. Diabetic Medicine. 2007;24(10): 1160-1163.
44. Pilmore HL. Review: metformin: potential benefits and use in chronic kidney disease. Nephrology (Carlton). 2010;15(4):412-418.
45. Salpeter SR, Greyber E, Pasternak GA, et al. Risk of fatal and nonfatal lactic acidosis with metformin use in type 2 diabetes mellitus. Cochrane Database of Systematic Reviews. 2010;(4):CD002967.
46. Kurian B, Joshi R, Helmuth A. Effectiveness and long-term safety of thiazolidinediones and metformin in renal transplant recipients. Endocrine Practice.

2008;14(8):979–984.
47. Holman RR, Paul SK, Bethel MA, et al. 10-year follow-up of intensive glucose control in type 2 diabetes. New England Journal of Medicine. 2008;359(15): 1577–1589.
48. Harrower AD. Pharmacokinetics of oral antihyperglycaemic agents in patients with renal insufficiency. Clinical Pharmacokinetics. 1996;31(2):111–119.
49. Pollock SH, Reichbaum MI, Collier BH, et al. Inhibitory effect of cyclosporine A on the activity of oral hypoglycemic agents in rats. Journal of Pharmacology and Experimental Therapeutics. 1991;258(1):8–12.
50. Yates CJ, Fourlanos S, Hjelmesaeth J, et al. New-onset diabetes after kidney transplantation-changes and challenges. American Journal of Transplantation. 2012;12(4):820–828.
51. Turk T, Pietruck F, Dolff S, et al. Repaglinide in the management of new-onset diabetes mellitus after renal transplantation. American Journal of Transplantation. 2006;6(4):842–846.
52. Jindal RM, Hjelmesaeth J. Impact and management of posttransplant diabetes mellitus. Transplantation. 2000;70(11 Suppl):SS58–SS63.
53. Kahn SE, Haffner SM, Heise MA, et al. Glycemic durability of rosiglitazone, metformin, or glyburide monotherapy. New England Journal of Medicine. 2006;355(23):2427–2443.
54. Komajda M, McMurray JJ, Beck-Nielsen H, et al. Heart failure events with rosiglitazone in type 2 diabetes: data from the RECORD clinical trial. European Heart Journal. 2010;31(7):824–831.
55. Hamnvik OP, McMahon GT. Balancing risk and benefit with oral hypoglycemic drugs. Mount Sinai Journal of Medicine. 2009;76(3):234–243.
56. Wei W, Wan Y. Thiazolidinediones on PPAR gamma: the roles in bone remodeling. PPAR Research. 2011;2011:867180.
57. Voytovich MH, Simonsen C, Jenssen T, et al. Short-term treatment with rosiglitazone improves glucose tolerance, insulin sensitivity and endothelial function in renal transplant recipients. Nephrology, Dialysis, Transplantation. 2005;20(2): 413–418.
58. Goldman-Levine JD. Beyond metformin: initiating combination therapy in patients with type 2 diabetes mellitus. Pharmacotherapy. 2011;31(12 Suppl): 44S–53S.
59. Watt KD. Metabolic syndrome: is immunosuppression to blame? Liver Transplantation. 2011;17(Suppl 3):S38–S42.
60. Sanchez-Lazaro IJ, Sanchez-Gomez JM, Almenar-Bonet L, et al. Long-term prognostic implications of metabolic syndrome in heart transplant recipients. Transplantation Proceedings. 2011;43(6):2257–2259.
61. Ramezani M, Einollahi B, Ahmadzad-Asl M, et al. Hyperlipidemia after renal transplantation and its relation to graft and patient survival. Transplantation Proceedings. 2007;39(4):1044–1047.
62. Watson KE, Horowitz BN, Matson G. Lipid abnormalities in insulin resistant states. Reviews in Cardiovascular Medicine. 2003;4(4):228–236.
63. Borggreve SE, De Vries R, Dullaart RP. Alterations in high-density lipoprotein metabolism and reverse cholesterol transport in insulin resistance and type 2 diabetes mellitus: role of lipolytic enzymes, lecithin:cholesterol acyltransferase and lipid transfer proteins. European Journal of Clinical Investigation. 2003;33(12):1051–1069.
64. Kobashigawa JA, Kasiske BL. Hyperlipidemia in solid organ transplantation. Transplantation. 1997;63(3):331–338.
65. Perry CG, Spiers A, Cleland SJ, et al. Glucocorticoids and insulin sensitivity: dissociation of insulin's metabolic and vascular actions. Journal of Clinical Endocrinology and Metabolism. 2003;88(12):6008–6014.
66. de Groen PC. Cyclosporine, low-density lipoprotein, and cholesterol. Mayo Clinic Proceedings. Mayo Clinic. 1988;63(10):1012–1021.
67. Hricik DE, Mayes JT, Schulak JA. Independent effects of cyclosporine and prednisone on posttransplant hypercholesterolemia. American Journal of Kidney Diseases. 1991;18(3):353–358.
68. Pascual M, Curtis J, Delmonico FL, et al. A prospective, randomized clinical trial of cyclosporine reduction in stable patients greater than 12 months after renal transplantation. Transplantation. 2003;75(9):1501–1505.
69. Ekberg H, Bernasconi C, Tedesco-Silva H, et al. Calcineurin inhibitor minimization in the Symphony study: observational results 3 years after transplantation. American Journal of Transplantation. 2009;9(8):1876–1885.
70. Canzanello VJ, Schwartz L, Taler SJ, et al. Evolution of cardiovascular risk after liver transplantation: a comparison of cyclosporine A and tacrolimus (FK506). Liver Transplantation and Surgery. 1997;3(1):1–9.
71. Artz MA, Boots JM, Ligtenberg G, et al. Improved cardiovascular risk profile and renal function in renal transplant patients after randomized conversion from cyclosporine to tacrolimus. Journal of the American Society of Nephrology. 2003;14(7):1880–1888.
72. Kohnle M, Zimmermann U, Lutkes P, et al. Conversion from cyclosporine A to tacrolimus after kidney transplantation due to hyperlipidemia. Transplant International. 2000;13(Suppl 1):S345–S348.
73. Kasiske BL, de Mattos A, Flechner SM, et al. Mammalian target of rapamycin inhibitor dyslipidemia in kidney transplant recipients. American Journal of Transplantation. 2008;8(7):1384–1392.
74. Massy ZA, De Bandt JP, Morelon E, et al. Hyperlipidaemia and post-heparin lipase activities in renal transplant recipients treated with sirolimus or cyclosporin A. Nephrology, Dialysis, Transplantation. 2000;15(6):928.
75. Kraemer FB, Takeda D, Natu V, et al. Insulin regulates lipoprotein lipase activity in rat adipose cells via wortmannin- and rapamycin-sensitive pathways. Metabolism. 1998;47(5):555–559.
76. Hoogeveen RC, Ballantyne CM, Pownall HJ, et al. Effect of sirolimus on the metabolism of apoB100- containing lipoproteins in renal transplant patients. Transplantation. 2001;72(7):1244–1250.
77. Groth CG, Backman L, Morales JM, et al. Sirolimus (rapamycin)-based therapy in human renal transplantation: similar efficacy and different toxicity compared with cyclosporine. Sirolimus European Renal Transplant Study Group. Transplantation. 1999;67(7):1036–1042.
78. Kreis H, Cisterne JM, Land W, et al. Sirolimus in association with mycophenolate mofetil induction for the prevention of acute graft rejection in renal allograft recipients. Transplantation. 2000;69(7):1252–1260.
79. Schena FP, Pascoe MD, Alberu J, et al. Conversion from calcineurin inhibitors to sirolimus maintenance therapy in renal allograft recipients: 24-month efficacy and safety results from the CONVERT trial. Transplantation. 2009;87(2): 233–242.
80. Kahan BD, Podbielski J, Napoli KL, et al. Immunosuppressive effects and safety of a sirolimus/cyclosporine combination regimen for renal transplantation. Transplantation. 1998;66(8):1040–1046.
81. Chueh SC, Kahan BD. Dyslipidemia in renal transplant recipients treated with a sirolimus and cyclosporine-based immunosuppressive regimen: incidence, risk factors, progression, and prognosis. Transplantation. 2003;76(2):375–382.
82. McAlister VC, Gao Z, Peltekian K, et al. Sirolimus-tacrolimus combination immunosuppression. Lancet. 2000;355(9201):376–377.
83. Larsen CP, Grinyo J, Medina-Pestana J, et al. Belatacept-based regimens versus a cyclosporine A-based regimen in kidney transplant recipients: 2-year results from the BENEFIT and BENEFIT-EXT studies. Transplantation. 2010;90(12): 1528–1535.
84. Baigent C, Landray MJ, Reith C, et al. The effects of lowering LDL cholesterol with simvastatin plus ezetimibe in patients with chronic kidney disease (Study of Heart and Renal Protection): a randomised placebo-controlled trial. Lancet. 2011;377(9784):2181–2192.
85. Larsen ML, Illingworth DR. Drug treatment of dyslipoproteinemia. Medical Clinics of North America. 1994;78(1):225–245.
86. Levy RI, Troendle AJ, Fattu JM. A quarter century of drug treatment of dyslipoproteinemia, with a focus on the new HMG-CoA reductase inhibitor fluvastatin. Circulation. 1993;87(4 Suppl):III45–53.
87. Illingworth DR, Stein EA, Mitchel YB, et al. Comparative effects of lovastatin and niacin in primary hypercholesterolemia. A prospective trial. Archives of Internal Medicine. 1994;154(14):1586–1595.
88. Kwak B, Mulhaupt F, Myit S, et al. Statins as a newly recognized type of immunomodulator. Nature Medicine. 2000;6(12):1399–1402.
89. Holschermann H, Hilgendorff A, Kemkes-Matthes B, et al. Simvastatin attenuates vascular hypercoagulability in cardiac transplant recipients. Transplantation. 2000;69(9):1830–1836.
90. Blum A, Shamburek R. The pleiotropic effects of statins on endothelial function, vascular inflammation, immunomodulation and thrombogenesis. Atherosclerosis. 2009;203(2):325–330.
91. Weis M, Pehlivanli S, Meiser BM, et al. Simvastatin treatment is associated with improvement in coronary endothelial function and decreased cytokine activation in patients after heart transplantation. Journal of the American College of Cardiology. 2001;38(3):814–818.
92. Wenke K, Meiser B, Thiery J, et al. Simvastatin reduces graft vessel disease and mortality after heart transplantation: a four-year randomized trial. Circulation. 1997;96(5):1398–1402.
93. Wenke K, Meiser B, Thiery J, et al. Simvastatin initiated early after heart transplantation: 8-year prospective experience. Circulation. 2003;107(1):93–97.
94. Kobashigawa JA, Katznelson S, Laks H, et al. Effect of pravastatin on outcomes after cardiac transplantation. New England Journal of Medicine. 1995;333(10): 621–627.
95. Holdaas H, Fellstrom B, Jardine AG, et al. Effect of fluvastatin on cardiac outcomes in renal transplant recipients: a multicentre, randomised, placebo-controlled trial. Lancet. 2003;361(9374):2024–2031.
96. Holdaas H, Fellstrom B, Cole E, et al. Long-term cardiac outcomes in renal transplant recipients receiving fluvastatin: the ALERT extension study. American Journal of Transplantation. 2005;5(12):2929–2936.
97. Jones P, Kafonek S, Laurora I, et al. Comparative dose efficacy study of atorvas-

tatin versus simvastatin, pravastatin, lovastatin, and fluvastatin in patients with hypercholesterolemia (the CURVES study). American Journal of Cardiology. 1998;81(5):582–587.
98. Bakker-Arkema RG, Davidson MH, Goldstein RJ, et al. Efficacy and safety of a new HMG-CoA reductase inhibitor, atorvastatin, in patients with hypertriglyceridemia. Journal of the American Medical Association. 1996;275(2):128–133.
99. Davidson M, McKenney J, Stein E, et al. Comparison of one-year efficacy and safety of atorvastatin versus lovastatin in primary hypercholesterolemia. Atorvastatin Study Group I. American Journal of Cardiology. 1997;79(11):1475–1481.
100. Dunn CJ, Wagstaff AJ, Perry CM, et al. Cyclosporin: an updated review of the pharmacokinetic properties, clinical efficacy and tolerability of a microemulsion-based formulation (neoral)1 in organ transplantation. Drugs. 2001;61(13):1957–2016.
101. Asberg A. Interactions between cyclosporin and lipid-lowering drugs: implications for organ transplant recipients. Drugs. 2003;63(4):367–378.
102. Fehrenbach T, Cui Y, Faulstich H, et al. Characterization of the transport of the bicyclic peptide phalloidin by human hepatic transport proteins. Naunyn-Schmiedeberg's Archives of Pharmacology. 2003;368(5):415–420.
103. Kasiske B, Cosio FG, Beto J, et al. Clinical practice guidelines for managing dyslipidemias in kidney transplant patients: a report from the Managing Dyslipidemias in Chronic Kidney Disease Work Group of the National Kidney Foundation Kidney Disease Outcomes Quality Initiative. American Journal of Transplantation. 2004;4(Suppl 7):13–53.
104. Lemahieu WP, Hermann M, Asberg A, et al. Combined therapy with atorvastatin and calcineurin inhibitors: no interactions with tacrolimus. American Journal of Transplantation. 2005;5(9):2236–2243.
105. Hurst FP, Neff RT, Jindal RM, et al. Incidence, predictors and associated outcomes of rhabdomyolysis after kidney transplantation. Nephrology, Dialysis, Transplantation. 2009;24(12):3861–3866.
106. Study of the Effectiveness of Additional Reductions in Cholesterol and Homocysteine (SEARCH) Collaborative Group, Armitage J, Bowman L, et al. Intensive lowering of LDL cholesterol with 80 mg versus 20 mg simvastatin daily in 12,064 survivors of myocardial infarction: a double-blind randomised trial. Lancet. 2010;376(9753):1658–1669.
107. Riella LV, Gabardi S, Chandraker A. Dyslipidemia and its therapeutic challenges in renal transplantation. American Journal of Transplantation. 2012;12(8):1975–1982.
108. Nishio S, Watanabe H, Kosuge K, et al. Interaction between amlodipine and simvastatin in patients with hypercholesterolemia and hypertension. Hypertension Research. 2005;28(3):223–227.
109. Kohnle M, Pietruck F, Kribben A, et al. Ezetimibe for the treatment of uncontrolled hypercholesterolemia in patients with high-dose statin therapy after renal transplantation. American Journal of Transplantation. 2006;6(1):205–208.
110. Buchanan C, Smith L, Corbett J, et al. A retrospective analysis of ezetimibe treatment in renal transplant recipients. American Journal of Transplantation. 2006;6(4):770–774.
111. Kashani A, Sallam T, Bheemreddy S, et al. Review of side-effect profile of combination ezetimibe and statin therapy in randomized clinical trials. American Journal of Cardiology. 2008;101(11):1606–1613.
112. Brunzell JD. Clinical practice. Hypertriglyceridemia. The New England Journal of Medicine. 2007;357(10):1009–1017.
113. Angeles C, Lane BP, Miller F, et al. Fenofibrate-associated reversible acute allograft dysfunction in 3 renal transplant recipients: biopsy evidence of tubular toxicity. American Journal of Kidney Diseases. 2004;44(3):543–550.
114. McQuade CR, Griego J, Anderson J, et al. Elevated serum creatinine levels associated with fenofibrate therapy. American Journal of Health-System Pharmacy. 2008;65(2):138–141.
115. Hottelart C, El Esper N, Rose F, et al. Fenofibrate increases creatininemia by increasing metabolic production of creatinine. Nephron. 2002;92(3):536–541.
116. ACCORD Study Group, Ginsberg HN, Elam MB, et al. Effects of combination lipid therapy in type 2 diabetes mellitus. New England Journal of Medicine. 2010;362(17):1563–1574.
117. Lim AK, Manley KJ, Roberts MA, et al. Fish oil treatment for kidney transplant recipients: a meta-analysis of randomized controlled trials. Transplantation. 2007;83(7):831–838.
118. Chauhan V, Ranganna KM, Chauhan N, et al. Bone disease in organ transplant patients: pathogenesis and management. Postgraduate Medicine. 2012;124(3):80–90.
119. Cohen A, Sambrook P, Shane E. Management of bone loss after organ transplantation. Journal of Bone and Mineral Research. 2004;19(12):1919–1932.
120. Leidig-Bruckner G, Hosch S, Dodidou P, et al. Frequency and predictors of osteoporotic fractures after cardiac or liver transplantation: a follow-up study. Lancet. 2001;357(9253):342–347.
121. Ball AM, Gillen DL, Sherrard D, et al. Risk of hip fracture among dialysis and renal transplant recipients. Journal of the American Medical Association. 2002;288(23):3014–3018.
122. Grotz WH, Mundinger FA, Gugel B, et al. Bone fracture and osteodensitometry with dual energy X-ray absorptiometry in kidney transplant recipients. Transplantation. 1994;58(8):912–915.
123. Shane E, Papadopoulos A, Staron RB, et al. Bone loss and fracture after lung transplantation. Transplantation. 1999;68(2):220–227.
124. Sprague SM, Josephson MA. Bone disease after kidney transplantation. Seminars in Nephrology. 2004;24(1):82–90.
125. Vautour LM, Melton LJ 3rd, Clarke BL, et al. Long-term fracture risk following renal transplantation: a population-based study. Osteoporosis International. 2004;15(2):160–167.
126. Heaf JG. Bone disease after renal transplantation. Transplantation. 2003;75(3):315–325.
127. Parfitt AM. The hyperparathyroidism of chronic renal failure: a disorder of growth. Kidney International. 1997;52(1):3–9.
128. Julian BA, Benfield M, Quarles LD. Bone loss after organ transplantation. Transplantation Reviews. 1993;7:82.
129. Julian BA, Quarles LD, Niemann KM. Musculoskeletal complications after renal transplantation: pathogenesis and treatment. American Journal of Kidney Diseases. 1992;19(2):99–120.
130. Cundy T, Kanis JA, Heynen G, et al. Calcium metabolism and hyperparathyroidism after renal transplantation. The Quarterly Journal of Medicine. 1983;52(205):67–78.
131. Bonarek H, Merville P, Bonarek M, et al. Reduced parathyroid functional mass after successful kidney transplantation. Kidney International. 1999;56(2):642–649.
132. Borchhardt K, Sulzbacher I, Benesch T, et al. Low-turnover bone disease in hypercalcemic hyperparathyroidism after kidney transplantation. American Journal of Transplantation. 2007;7(11):2515–2521.
133. Torres A, Rodriguez AP, Concepcion MT, et al. Parathyroid function in long-term renal transplant patients: importance of pre-transplant PTH concentrations. Nephrology, Dialysis, Transplantation. 1998;13(Suppl 3):94–97.
134. Carlini RG, Rojas E, Weisinger JR, et al. Bone disease in patients with long-term renal transplantation and normal renal function. American Journal of Kidney Diseases. 2000;36(1):160–166.
135. Hernandez D, Rufino M, Bartolomei S, et al. Clinical impact of preexisting vascular calcifications on mortality after renal transplantation. Kidney International. 2005;67(5):2015–2020.
136. Gwinner W, Suppa S, Mengel M, et al. Early calcification of renal allografts detected by protocol biopsies: causes and clinical implications. American Journal of Transplantation. 2005;5(8):1934–1941.
137. D'Alessandro AM, Melzer JS, Pirsch JD, et al. Tertiary hyperparathyroidism after renal transplantation: operative indications. Surgery. 1989;106(6):1049–1055, discussion 1055–1056.
138. David DS, Sakai S, Brennan BL, et al. Hypercalcemia after renal transplantation. Long-term follow-up data. The New England Journal of Medicine. 1973;289(8):398–401.
139. Garvin PJ, Castaneda M, Linderer R, et al. Management of hypercalcemic hyperparathyroidism after renal transplantation. Archives of Surgery. 1985;120(5):578–583.
140. Parfitt AM. Hypercalcemic hyperparathyroidism following renal transplantation: differential diagnosis, management, and implications for cell population control in the parathyroid gland. Mineral and Electrolyte Metabolism. 1982;8(2):92–112.
141. Messa P, Sindici C, Cannella G, et al. Persistent secondary hyperparathyroidism after renal transplantation. Kidney International. 1998;54(5):1704–1713.
142. Torres A, Lorenzo V, Salido E. Calcium metabolism and skeletal problems after transplantation. Journal of the American Society of Nephrology. 2002;13(2):551–558.
143. Sirilak S, Chatsrisak K, Ingsathit A, et al. Renal phosphate loss in long-term kidney transplantation. Clinical Journal of the American Society of Nephrology. 2012;7(2):323–331.
144. Heaf J, Tvedegaard E, Kanstrup IL, et al. Hyperparathyroidism and long-term bone loss after renal transplantation. Clinical Transplantation. 2003;17(3):268–274.
145. Evenepoel P, Van Den Bergh B, Naesens M, et al. Calcium metabolism in the early posttransplantation period. Clinical Journal of the American Society of Nephrology. 2009;4(3):665–672.
146. Ansell D, Udayaraj UP, Steenkamp R, et al. Chronic renal failure in kidney transplant recipients. Do they receive optimum care?: data from the UK renal registry. American Journal of Transplantation. 2007;7(5):1167–1176.
147. Marcen R, Ponte B, Rodriguez-Mendiola N, et al. Secondary hyperparathyroidism after kidney transplantation: a cross-sectional study. Transplantation

Proceedings. 2009;41(6):2391-2393.
148. Bonnin MR, Gonzalez MT, Huguet J, et al. 1,25-Dihydroxycholecalciferol as measured by a radioreceptor assay in normal subjects and patients after kidney transplantation. Clinical Chemistry. 1990;36(2):389-390.
149. Serra AL, Schwarz AA, Wick FH, et al. Successful treatment of hypercalcemia with cinacalcet in renal transplant recipients with persistent hyperparathyroidism. Nephrology, Dialysis, Transplantation. 2005;20(7):1315-1319.
150. Szwarc I, Argiles A, Garrigue V, et al. Cinacalcet chloride is efficient and safe in renal transplant recipients with posttransplant hyperparathyroidism. Transplantation. 2006;82(5):675-680.
151. Kruse AE, Eisenberger U, Frey FJ, et al. The calcimimetic cinacalcet normalizes serum calcium in renal transplant patients with persistent hyperparathyroidism. Nephrology, Dialysis, Transplantation. 2005;20(7):1311-1314.
152. Leca N, Laftavi M, Gundroo A, et al. Early and severe hyperparathyroidism associated with hypercalcemia after renal transplant treated with cinacalcet. American Journal of Transplantation. 2006;6(10):2391-2395.
153. El-Amm JM, Doshi MD, Singh A, et al. Preliminary experience with cinacalcet use in persistent secondary hyperparathyroidism after kidney transplantation. Transplantation. 2007;83(5):546-549.
154. Srinivas TR, Schold JD, Womer KL, et al. Improvement in hypercalcemia with cinacalcet after kidney transplantation. Clinical Journal of the American Society of Nephrology. 2006;1(2):323-326.
155. Falck P, Vethe NT, Asberg A, et al. Cinacalcet's effect on the pharmacokinetics of tacrolimus, cyclosporine and mycophenolate in renal transplant recipients. Nephrology, Dialysis, Transplantation. 2008;23(3):1048-1053.
156. Bergua C, Torregrosa JV, Fuster D, et al. Effect of cinacalcet on hypercalcemia and bone mineral density in renal transplanted patients with secondary hyperparathyroidism. Transplantation. 2008;86(3):413-417.
157. Triponez F, Clark OH, Vanrenthergem Y, et al. Surgical treatment of persistent hyperparathyroidism after renal transplantation. Annals of Surgery. 2008; 248(1):18-30.
158. Collaud S, Staub-Zahner T, Trombetti A, et al. Increase in bone mineral density after successful parathyroidectomy for tertiary hyperparathyroidism after renal transplantation. World Journal of Surgery. 2008;32(8):1795-1801.
159. Rostaing L, Moreau-Gaudry X, Baron E, et al. Changes in blood pressure and renal function following subtotal parathyroidectomy in renal transplant patients presenting with persistent hypercalcemic hyperparathyroidism. Clinical Nephrology. 1997;47(4):248-255.
160. Evenepoel P, Claes K, Kuypers D, et al. Impact of parathyroidectomy on renal graft function, blood pressure and serum lipids in kidney transplant recipients: a single centre study. Nephrology, Dialysis, Transplantation. 2005;20(8): 1714-1720.
161. Milas M, Weber CJ. Near-total parathyroidectomy is beneficial for patients with secondary and tertiary hyperparathyroidism. Surgery. 2004;136(6):1252-1260.
162. Chandra P, Binongo JN, Ziegler TR, et al. Cholecalciferol (vitamin D3) therapy and vitamin D insufficiency in patients with chronic kidney disease: a randomized controlled pilot study. Endocrine Practice. 2008;14(1):10-17.
163. Wolf M, Shah A, Gutierrez O, et al. Vitamin D levels and early mortality among incident hemodialysis patients. Kidney International. 2007;72(8):1004-1013.
164. Marcen R, Ponte B, Rodriguez-Mendiola N, et al. Vitamin D deficiency in kidney transplant recipients: risk factors and effects of vitamin D3 supplements. Transplantation Proceedings. 2009;41(6):2388-2390.
165. Bhan I, Shah A, Holmes J, et al. Post-transplant hypophosphatemia: tertiary 'hyper-phosphatoninism'? Kidney International. 2006;70(8):1486-1494.
166. Rosenbaum RW, Hruska KA, Korkor A, et al. Decreased phosphate reabsorption after renal transplantation: evidence for a mechanism independent of calcium and parathyroid hormone. Kidney International. 1981;19(4):568-578.
167. Loffing J, Lotscher M, Kaissling B, et al. Renal Na/H exchanger NHE-3 and Na-PO4 cotransporter NaPi-2 protein expression in glucocorticoid excess and deficient states. Journal of the American Society of Nephrology. 1998;9(9): 1560-1567.
168. Falkiewicz K, Nahaczewska W, Boratynska M, et al. Tacrolimus decreases tubular phosphate wasting in renal allograft recipients. Transplantation Proceedings. 2003;35(6):2213-2215.
169. Tataranni T, Biondi G, Cariello M, et al. Rapamycin-induced hypophosphatemia and insulin resistance are associated with mTORC2 activation and Klotho expression. American Journal of Transplantation. 2011;11(8):1656-1664.
170. Pande S, Ritter CS, Rothstein M, et al. FGF-23 and sFRP-4 in chronic kidney disease and post-renal transplantation. Nephron Physiology. 2006;104(1): p23-32.
171. Ghanekar H, Welch BJ, Moe OW, et al. Post-renal transplantation hypophosphatemia: a review and novel insights. Current Opinion in Nephrology and Hypertension. 2006;15(2):97-104.
172. Evenepoel P, Naesens M, Claes K, et al. Tertiary 'hyperphosphatoninism' accentuates hypophosphatemia and suppresses calcitriol levels in renal transplant recipients. American Journal of Transplantation. 2007;7(5):1193-1200.
173. Trombetti A, Richert L, Hadaya K, et al. Early post-transplantation hypophosphatemia is associated with elevated FGF-23 levels. European Journal of Endocrinology. 2011;164(5):839-847.
174. Ambuhl PM, Meier D, Wolf B, et al. Metabolic aspects of phosphate replacement therapy for hypophosphatemia after renal transplantation: impact on muscular phosphate content, mineral metabolism, and acid/base homeostasis. American Journal of Kidney Diseases. 1999;34(5):875-883.
175. Steiner RW, Ziegler M, Halasz NA, et al. Effect of daily oral vitamin D and calcium therapy, hypophosphatemia, and endogenous 1-25 dihydroxycholecalciferol on parathyroid hormone and phosphate wasting in renal transplant recipients. Transplantation. 1993;56(4):843-846.
176. Weinstein RS, Jilka RL, Parfitt AM, et al. Inhibition of osteoblastogenesis and promotion of apoptosis of osteoblasts and osteocytes by glucocorticoids. Potential mechanisms of their deleterious effects on bone. Journal of Clinical Investigation. 1998;102(2):274-282.
177. Lukert BP, Raisz LG. Glucocorticoid-induced osteoporosis: pathogenesis and management. Annals of Internal Medicine. 1990;112(5):352-364.
178. Van Staa TP, Leufkens HG, Abenhaim L, et al. Use of oral corticosteroids and risk of fractures. Journal of Bone and Mineral Research. 2000;15(6):993-1000.
179. Cunningham J. Posttransplantation bone disease. Transplantation. 2005;79(6): 629-634.
180. Goffin E, Devogelaer JP, Lalaoui A, et al. Tacrolimus and low-dose steroid immunosuppression preserves bone mass after renal transplantation. Transplant International. 2002;15(2-3):73-80.
181. Cayco AV, Wysolmerski J, Simpson C, et al. Posttransplant bone disease: evidence for a high bone resorption state. Transplantation. 2000;70(12):1722-1728.
182. Movsowitz C, Epstein S, Fallon M, et al. Cyclosporin-A in vivo produces severe osteopenia in the rat: effect of dose and duration of administration. Endocrinology. 1988;123(5):2571-2577.
183. Albano L, Casez JP, Bekri S, et al. Effects of tacrolimus vs cyclosporin-A on bone metabolism after kidney transplantation: a cross-sectional study in 28 patients. Nephrologie and Therapeutique. 2005;1(2):115-120.
184. Monegal A, Navasa M, Guanabens N, et al. Bone mass and mineral metabolism in liver transplant patients treated with FK506 or cyclosporine A. Calcified Tissue International. 2001;68(2):83-86.
185. Patel S, Kwan JT, McCloskey E, et al. Prevalence and causes of low bone density and fractures in kidney transplant patients. Journal of Bone and Mineral Research. 2001;16(10):1863-1870.
186. Singha UK, Jiang Y, Yu S, et al. Rapamycin inhibits osteoblast proliferation and differentiation in MC3T3-E1 cells and primary mouse bone marrow stromal cells. Journal of Cellular Biochemistry. 2008;103(2):434-446.
187. Kneissel M, Luong-Nguyen NH, Baptist M, et al. Everolimus suppresses cancellous bone loss, bone resorption, and cathepsin K expression by osteoclasts. Bone. 2004;35(5):1144-1156.
188. Palmer SC, Strippoli GF, McGregor DO. Interventions for preventing bone disease in kidney transplant recipients: a systematic review of randomized controlled trials. American Journal of Kidney Diseases. 2005;45(4):638-649.
189. Cueto-Manzano AM, Konel S, Freemont AJ, et al. Effect of 1,25-dihydroxyvitamin D3 and calcium carbonate on bone loss associated with long-term renal transplantation. American Journal of Kidney Diseases. 2000;35(2):227-236.
190. El-Agroudy AE, El-Husseini AA, El-Sayed M, et al. Preventing bone loss in renal transplant recipients with vitamin D. Journal of the American Society of Nephrology. 2003;14(11):2975-2979.
191. Kaemmerer D, Schmidt B, Lehmann G, et al. Monthly ibandronate for the prevention of bone loss in patients after liver transplantation. Transplantation Proceedings. 2012;44(5):1362-1367.
192. Shane E, Addesso V, Namerow PB, et al. Alendronate versus calcitriol for the prevention of bone loss after cardiac transplantation. New England Journal of Medicine. 2004;350(8):767-776.
193. Coco M, Glicklich D, Faugere MC, et al. Prevention of bone loss in renal transplant recipients: a prospective, randomized trial of intravenous pamidronate. Journal of the American Society of Nephrology. 2003;14(10):2669-2676.
194. Crawford BA, Kam C, Pavlovic J, et al. Zoledronic acid prevents bone loss after liver transplantation: a randomized, double-blind, placebo-controlled trial. Annals of Internal Medicine. 2006;144(4):239-248.
195. Aris RM, Lester GE, Caminiti M, et al. Efficacy of alendronate in adults with cystic fibrosis with low bone density. American Journal of Respiratory and Critical Care Medicine. 2004;169(1):77-82.
196. Fan SL, Kumar S, Cunningham J. Long-term effects on bone mineral density of pamidronate given at the time of renal transplantation. Kidney International. 2003;63(6):2275-2279.
197. Stein EM, Ortiz D, Jin Z, et al. Prevention of fractures after solid organ transplantation: a meta-analysis. The Journal of Clinical Endocrinology and Metabolism. 2011;96(11):3457-3465.

198. Haas M, Leko-Mohr Z, Roschger P, et al. Zoledronic acid to prevent bone loss in the first 6 months after renal transplantation. Kidney International. 2003;63(3): 1130–1136.
199. Lin JH. Bisphosphonates: a review of their pharmacokinetic properties. Bone. 1996;18(2):75–85.
200. Saag KG, Shane E, Boonen S, et al. Teriparatide or alendronate in glucocorticoid-induced osteoporosis. The New England Journal of Medicine. 2007;357(20): 2028–2039.
201. Neer RM, Arnaud CD, Zanchetta JR, et al. Effect of parathyroid hormone (1–34) on fractures and bone mineral density in postmenopausal women with osteoporosis. The New England Journal of Medicine. 2001;344(19):1434–1441.
202. Cejka D, Benesch T, Krestan C, et al. Effect of teriparatide on early bone loss after kidney transplantation. American Journal of Transplantation. 2008;8(9): 1864–1870.
203. El-Husseini AA, El-Agroudy AE, El-Sayed MF, et al. Treatment of osteopenia and osteoporosis in renal transplant children and adolescents. Pediatric Transplantation. 2004;8(4):357–361.
204. Grotz WH, Rump LC, Niessen A, et al. Treatment of osteopenia and osteoporosis after kidney transplantation. Transplantation. 1998;66(8):1004–1008.
205. Braith RW, Magyari PM, Fulton MN, et al. Resistance exercise training and alendronate reverse glucocorticoid-induced osteoporosis in heart transplant recipients. Journal of Heart and Lung Transplantation. 2003;22(10):1082–1090.
206. Mitchell MJ, Baz MA, Fulton MN, et al. Resistance training prevents vertebral osteoporosis in lung transplant recipients. Transplantation. 2003;76(3):557–562.
207. National Kidney Foundation. K/DOQI clinical practice guidelines for bone metabolism and disease in chronic kidney disease. American Journal of Kidney Diseases. 2003;42(4 Suppl 3):S1–S201.
208. Kidney Disease: Improving Global Outcomes (KDIGO) CKD-MBD Work Group. KDIGO clinical practice guideline for the diagnosis, evaluation, prevention, and treatment of Chronic Kidney Disease-Mineral and Bone Disorder (CKD-MBD). Kidney International. Supplement. 2009;113:S1–S130.
209. Gordon PL, Frassetto LA. Management of osteoporosis in CKD Stages 3 to 5. American Journal of Kidney Diseases. 2010;55(5):941–956.
210. Kasiske BL, Chakkera HA, Louis TA, et al. A meta-analysis of immunosuppression withdrawal trials in renal transplantation. Journal of the American Society of Nephrology. 2000;11(10):1910–1917.
211. Pascual J, Quereda C, Zamora J, et al. Steroid withdrawal in renal transplant patients on triple therapy with a calcineurin inhibitor and mycophenolate mofetil: a meta-analysis of randomized, controlled trials. Transplantation. 2004;78(10):1548–1556.
212. Meier-Kriesche HU, Schold JD, Vanrenterghem Y, et al. Uric acid levels have no significant effect on renal function in adult renal transplant recipients: evidence from the symphony study. Clinical Journal of the American Society of Nephrology. 2009;4(10):1655–1660.
213. Neal DA, Tom BD, Gimson AE, et al. Hyperuricemia, gout, and renal function after liver transplantation. Transplantation. 2001;72(10):1689–1691.
214. Abbott KC, Kimmel PL, Dharnidharka V, et al. New-onset gout after kidney transplantation: incidence, risk factors and implications. Transplantation. 2005;80(10):1383–1391.
215. Niskanen LK, Laaksonen DE, Nyyssonen K, et al. Uric acid level as a risk factor for cardiovascular and all-cause mortality in middle-aged men: a prospective cohort study. Archives of Internal Medicine. 2004;164(14):1546–1551.
216. Nakagawa T, Tuttle KR, Short RA, et al. Hypothesis: fructose-induced hyperuricemia as a causal mechanism for the epidemic of the metabolic syndrome. Nature Clinical Practice Nephrology. 2005;1(2):80–86.
217. Bandukwala F, Huang M, Zaltzman JS, et al. Association of uric acid with inflammation, progressive renal allograft dysfunction and post-transplant cardiovascular risk. American Journal of Cardiology. 2009;103(6):867–871.
218. Marcen R, Gallego N, Orofino L, et al. Impairment of tubular secretion of urate in renal transplant patients on cyclosporine. Nephron. 1995;70(3): 307–313.
219. Zurcher RM, Bock HA, Thiel G. Hyperuricaemia in cyclosporin-treated patients: GFR-related effect. Nephrology, Dialysis, Transplantation. 1996;11(1): 153–158.
220. Claes K, Meier-Kriesche HU, Schold JD, et al. Effect of different immunosuppressive regimens on the evolution of distinct metabolic parameters: evidence from the Symphony study. Nephrology, Dialysis, Transplantation. 2012;27(2): 850–857.
221. Urbizu JM, Zarraga S, Gomez-Ullate P, et al. Safety and efficacy of tacrolimus rescue therapy in 55 kidney transplant patients treated with cyclosporine. Transplantation Proceedings. 2003;35(5):1704–1705.
222. Mazali FC, Mazzali M. Uric acid and transplantation. Seminars in Nephrology. 2011;31(5):466–471.
223. Noordzij TC, Leunissen KM, Van Hooff JP. Renal handling of urate and the incidence of gouty arthritis during cyclosporine and diuretic use. Transplantation. 1991;52(1):64–67.
224. Janssens HJ, Janssen M, van de Lisdonk EH, et al. Use of oral prednisolone or naproxen for the treatment of gout arthritis: a double-blind, randomised equivalence trial. Lancet. 2008;371(9627):1854–1860.
225. Curiel RV, Guzman NJ. Challenges associated with the management of gouty arthritis in patients with chronic kidney disease: a systematic review. Seminars in Arthritis and Rheumatism. 2012;42(2):166–178.
226. Rieger EH, Halasz NA, Wahlstrom HE. Colchicine neuromyopathy after renal transplantation. Transplantation. 1990;49(6):1196–1198.
227. Rana SS, Giuliani MJ, Oddis CV, et al. Acute onset of colchicine myoneuropathy in cardiac transplant recipients: case studies of three patients. Clinical Neurology and Neurosurgery. 1997;99(4):266–270.
228. Stamp LK, Chapman PT. Gout and organ transplantation. Current Rheumatology Reports. 2012;14(2):165–172.
229. Eleftheriou G, Bacis G, Fiocchi R, et al. Colchicine-induced toxicity in a heart transplant patient with chronic renal failure. Clinical Toxicology. 2008; 46(9):827–830.
230. Stamp L, Searle M, O'Donnell J, et al. Gout in solid organ transplantation: a challenging clinical problem. Drugs. 2005;65(18):2593–2611.
231. Cummins D, Sekar M, Halil O, et al. Myelosuppression associated with azathioprine-allopurinol interaction after heart and lung transplantation. Transplantation. 1996;61(11):1661–1662.
232. Becker MA, Schumacher HR, Espinoza LR, et al. The urate-lowering efficacy and safety of febuxostat in the treatment of the hyperuricemia of gout: the CONFIRMS trial. Arthritis Research and Therapy. 2010;12(2):R63.
233. Zurcher RM, Bock HA, Thiel G. Excellent uricosuric efficacy of benzbromarone in cyclosporin-A-treated renal transplant patients: a prospective study. Nephrology, Dialysis, Transplantation. 1994;9(5):548–551.
234. Kamper AL, Nielsen AH. Uricosuric effect of losartan in patients with renal transplants. Transplantation. 2001;72(4):671–674.
235. Sundy JS, Baraf HS, Yood RA, et al. Efficacy and tolerability of pegloticase for the treatment of chronic gout in patients refractory to conventional treatment: two randomized controlled trials. Journal of the American Medical Association. 2011;306(7):711–720.
236. Ho JM, Juurlink DN. Considerations when prescribing trimethoprim-sulfamethoxazole. Canadian Medical Association Journal. 2011;183(16): 1851–1858.
237. Riveiro-Barciela M, Campos-Varela I, Tovar JL, et al. Hyperkalemic distal renal tubular acidosis caused by immunosuppressant treatment with tacrolimus in a liver transplant patient: case report. Transplantation Proceedings. 2011;43(10): 4016–4018.
238. Heering PJ, Kurschat C, Vo DT, et al. Aldosterone resistance in kidney transplantation is in part induced by a down-regulation of mineralocorticoid receptor expression. Clinical Transplantation. 2004;18(2):186–192.
239. Mazzola BL, Vannini SD, Truttmann AC, et al. Long-term calcineurin inhibition and magnesium balance after renal transplantation. Transplant International. 2003;16(2):76–81.
240. Van Laecke S, Van Biesen W, Verbeke F, et al. Posttransplantation hypomagnesemia and its relation with immunosuppression as predictors of new-onset diabetes after transplantation. American Journal of Transplantation. 2009;9(9): 2140–2149.
241. Mohebbi N, Mihailova M, Wagner CA. The calcineurin inhibitor FK506 (tacrolimus) is associated with transient metabolic acidosis and altered expression of renal acid-base transport proteins. American Journal of Physiology Renal Physiology. 2009;297(2):F499–509.
242. Kleespies A, Mikhailov M, Khalil PN, et al. Enteric conversion after pancreatic transplantation: resolution of symptoms and long-term results. Clinical Transplantation. 2011;25(4):549–560.
243. de Brito-Ashurst I, Varagunam M, Raftery MJ, et al. Bicarbonate supplementation slows progression of CKD and improves nutritional status. Journal of the American Society of Nephrology. 2009;20(9):2075–2084.

第 101 章
实体器官移植中免疫抑制剂的非标签使用

Jill C. Krisl, Rita R. Alloway, E. Steve Woodle

引言

美国食品药品监督管理局(FDA)通过法规负责维护食品和药物的公共安全，通过严格的药物审批程序确保这一点。为了使药物被 FDA 批准，申办者必须提供关于药物在特定患者群体中安全性和有效性，以及确定的临床状况的满意证据。药品审批流程的关键是产品标签的创建和定义，包括剂量、管理、预期患者人群和临床状况。在标签的这些方面之外使用药物通常被认为是脱标使用。理论上，FDA 有关于制造商标签外药物使用和促销的规定，但在实践中，这种规定是有限的[1]。

在美国，医生选择在限定标签之外使用 FDA 批准的药物是合法且常见的做法[2,3]。脱标使用不同于以下一或多种方面的标签使用，包括临床适应证、患者群体、剂量或给药途径。FDA 已经认识到这些未标记的用途可能是适当的，并且得到医学期刊中的证据支持[4]。"标签外"一词来自美国 FDA，但药物使用超出特定药物适应证的概念在世界范围内是常见的，因此本章的适用性远超出国界。实际上，在实体器官移植中，标签外使用已经变得非常常见，它被认为是大多数免疫抑制方案的"标准治疗"，并且有许多随机试验提供的大量证据支持(表 101.1)。本章将讨论标签外药物使用的概念和实践，并作为对第 98 章的补充，该章涉及正式表明用于移植的药物。有关本章中列出的许多药物的详细信息，请参见第 17 章和第 18 章。

在移植中使用非标签方案给药

现代医学中的标签外药物使用效果是显著的，并且在移植实践中尤其常见。据估计，在美国，每年标签外药物使用占 7.5 亿处方的 20%[2]。在移植和肿瘤学两门医学专业中，标签外药物使用已成为惯例。据估计，肿瘤学中使用的 50%或更多的药物是标签外的[5,6]。其主要原因是大量的癌症患者，而抗癌药物最初通常被批准用于特定癌症。肿瘤学分子谱的出现导致在大量癌症中共有基因突变的识别。因此，靶向特异性基因突变的药物在具有相似基因突变的其他癌症类型中可以享有大量的标签外使用。

在移植中，标签外使用范围在各药物和各种器官类型之间有显著差异。移植中标签外使用的一个显著案例是联合运用他克莫司和麦考酚酯预防肾移植患者的排斥反应。他克莫司于 1994 年获得批准，在 FDA 批准麦考酚酯之前不久。他克莫司和麦考酚酯的研究同时进行但各自独立，因此并未对两种药物联合使用进行分析。首次批准时，吗替麦考酚酯(MMF)被标记用于与环孢素一起使用，没有关于其与他克莫联用的安全性和疗效的数据。在 MMF 获得批准后几乎立即开始了评估他克莫司/ MMF 组合的研究，因为许多中心认为他克莫司是比环孢素更优选的钙调神经磷酸酶抑制剂(CNI)。他克莫司被广泛认为是一种更有效的免疫抑制剂，并与更好的肾功能相关[7]。采用他克莫司/MMF 联合进行大型多中心随机试验证实了该方案的有效性和安全性[8,9]。如今，他克莫司是肾移植中最常用的CNI，约 80%的肾移植受者出院时携带他克莫司。同样地，他克莫司/ MMF 组合是最常规的方案，超过 70%的肾移植受者在出院时接受该方案[7,10]。

数年来，他克莫司/ MMF 组合是肾移植受者最常用的免疫抑制方案，但其在 2009 年之前一直被认为是标签外的[11]。2006 年，安斯泰来[品牌为 Prograf™(他克莫司)]提交了补充的新药申请(sNDA)，以寻求 FDA 批准他克莫司/MMF 方案用于肾移植的排斥预防。在实体器官移植领域的新型调节作用中，FDA 批准了基于大

表 101.1 FDA 批准的和非标签的免疫抑制的临床使用。Adapted from:Micromedex [Internet database]

药物	FDA 批准的适应证	标签外临床用于移植和药物推荐				
				DrugDex©		
			AHFS-DI	总体	证据	效果
他克莫司	心脏:预防排斥	心脏:排斥反应的治疗	NN	无	无	无
	肝脏:预防排斥	肝脏:排斥反应的治疗	NN	Ⅱb	B	满意,Ⅱa
	肾脏:预防排斥	肾脏:排斥反应的治疗	支持	Ⅱa	B	满意,Ⅱa
		肺移植	NN	Ⅱb	C	满意,Ⅱa
		肾/胰腺:预防排斥	NN	Ⅱa	C	满意,Ⅱa
		胰腺:排斥反应的治疗	NN	Ⅱa	B	满意,Ⅱa
环孢素	心脏:预防排斥	肺:预防排斥	NN	Ⅱa	B	满意,Ⅱa
	心脏:治疗排斥	肺:治疗排斥	NN	Ⅱa	B	满意,Ⅱa
	肝脏:预防排斥	胰腺:预防排斥	NN	无	无	无
	肝脏:治疗排斥	胰腺:治疗排斥	NN	无	无	无
	肾脏:预防排斥					
	肾脏:治疗排斥					
西罗莫司	肾脏:预防排斥(低、中、高免疫风险)	心脏:预防排斥	NN	Ⅲ	B	满意,Ⅱa
		肾脏:治疗排斥	NN	Ⅱb	B	满意,Ⅱa
		肝脏:预防排斥	无支持	Ⅲ	B	不确定
依维莫司	肾脏:预防排斥	心脏:预防排斥	NN	Ⅲ	B	满意,Ⅱa
		肾脏:治疗排斥	NN	无	无	无
贝拉西普	肾脏:当与EBV血清阳性受者中的巴利昔单抗诱导联合使用时预防排斥	肾脏:当与抗胸腺细胞联合使用时预防排斥	NN	无	无	无
霉酚酸酯	心脏:预防排斥	肾脏:治疗排斥	NN	Ⅱb	B	满意,Ⅱa
	肝脏:预防排斥	肾脏:替代疗法	NN	Ⅱb	B	满意,Ⅱa
	肾脏:预防排斥					
霉酚酸	肾脏:预防排斥	肾脏:治疗排斥	NN	无	无	无
硫唑嘌呤	肾脏:用于预防排斥的辅助治疗	肝脏:预防排斥	NN	Ⅱb	B	满意,Ⅱa
		胰腺:预防排斥	NN	Ⅱb	B	满意,Ⅱa
巴利昔单抗	肾脏:与环孢素和皮质类固醇联合预防排斥反应	肝脏:预防排斥	NN	Ⅱb	B	满意,Ⅱa
兔抗胸腺细胞球蛋白	肾脏:排斥的治疗,伴随免疫抑制	心脏:预防排斥	NN	Ⅱb	B	满意,Ⅱa
		心脏:治疗排斥	NN	Ⅱb	B	满意,Ⅱa
		肝脏:预防排斥	NN	Ⅱb	C	满意,Ⅱa
		肾脏:预防排斥	支持	Ⅲ	B	满意,Ⅱa
		肺:预防排斥	NN	Ⅱb	C	满意,Ⅱa
		胰腺:预防排斥	NN	Ⅱb	B	满意,Ⅱa
		胰腺:治疗排斥	NN	Ⅱb	B	满意,Ⅱa
马抗胸腺细胞球蛋白	肾脏:预防排斥	非肾脏器官中兔抗胸腺球蛋白的替代品	支持	无	无	无
	肾脏:治疗排斥					
阿仑单抗	B细胞慢性淋巴细胞白血病	肾脏:预防排斥	NN	Ⅱb	B	满意,Ⅱa
利妥昔单抗	类风湿性关节炎(中至重度)	治疗 PTLD	NN	Ⅱb	B	满意,Ⅱa
	CD20 阳性慢性淋巴细胞白血病	脱敏方案	NN	无	无	无
	CD20 阳性非霍奇金淋巴瘤	抗体介导的排斥反应的治疗	NN	无	无	无
硼替佐米	多发性骨髓瘤	脱敏方案与血浆置换组合	NN	无	无	无
	套细胞淋巴瘤	抗体介导的排斥反应的治疗	NN	无	无	无

型多中心随机试验的他克莫司/ MMF 组合，这些试验证明了该组合的有效性和安全性，代替了预期进行的3期注册试验。FDA 接受来自非注册随机试验的大量证据基础作为批准依据，这一行动在移植领域树立了先例。

FDA 传统上要求使用 FDA 批准的免疫抑制药物组合作为对照试验中的对照组。在批准他克莫司/MMF 组合之前,该策略需要由作为维持诱导治疗的白细胞介素-2 受体拮抗剂(IL-2RA)和环孢素,MMF 和类固醇形成的对照组[7]。这种以环孢素为基础的治疗方案作为对照组的劣势在注册试验中大幅地限制了患者注册,从而给开发商带来了相当大的负担。因此,FDA 的政策导致了开发商避免开发移植领域的药物，导致了免疫抑制药物在自身免疫疾病而不是移植中开发的转变。这种趋势一直持续到目前，导致移植患者的弱势。

同时,历史上认为 FDA 可接受的端点和由开发商在药物开发方面的实用性正在经历重大变化。随着患者和移植物存活率由于免疫抑制的进展而改善，实现统计功效所需的患者数量超过了开发商的预算限制。类似地,由于需要大量患者实现统计功效,与发病率显著相关并且被认为是注册试验传统终点的活检证实的急性排斥(BPAR)已经降低到这样低的比例,它也变成不可行的终点[12,13]。因此,复合或替代终点(如肾功能的变化)允许更合理的样本大小,并且最近被 FDA 接受用于登记试验。临床研究人员在很大程度上认为 FDA 批准他克莫司/ MMF 方案在创建使用该方案作为对照组对将来的注册试验至关重要。

临床上需要以 FDA 标记的方案作为对照组,使兔抗人胸腺细胞球蛋白(rATG,Thymoglobulin™,赛诺菲)在肾移植中的注册试验变得复杂化。目前,rATG 仅被 FDA 批准用于肾移植排斥的治疗，大量的移植术后的诱导治疗并不是 FDA 批准的。与其他可用于肾移植诱导治疗的药物相比,rATG 是最常用的药物，在大多数移植项目中,对于高免疫风险、移植功能延迟恢复和需避免或最低剂量应用皮质类固醇的患者,rATG 被认为是首选的诱导因子。这些使得肾移植的诱导试验不可行,因为对照组中没有 rATG。已经建议类似于他克莫司/ MMF 组合的方法用于与 rATG 相比,将其作为肾移植诱导剂注册试验的对照组。在移植领域中具有实际药物开发经验的研究者已经发出这样的声明：

我认为对移植专业人员(通过他们的社会)来说,重要的是让 FDA 参与关于标签使用的药物的监管事项，不论是由于专利期满还是移植团体不具有安慰剂组，例如当有足够的临床数据时批准高免疫风险患者使用抗体类药物。如在 TAC-MMF 组合的情况下,批准高风险患者使用兔抗人胸腺细胞球蛋白。我们已经证明,一个恭敬而坚定的倡导可以产生结果。[个人通信,Flavio Vincenti,MD] [14]。

FDA 新药批准的监管程序

为了获得 FDA 的批准,药品公司必须提交新药申请(NDA)或生物许可申请(BLA),提供来自注册试验的支持药物有效性和安全性的数据[15]。当公司想扩大药物的适应证(如他克莫司/麦考酚酯组合被批准的过程)时,提交 sNDA。当一家公司希望获得新临床指征的批准时,应提交一份研究性新药(IND)申请[15]。

孤儿药提供了在特定条件下 FDA 批准的替代方法。孤儿药用于治疗、预防或诊断罕见病或在美国影响不到 20 万人的疾病[15]。孤儿药也可用于罕见疾病中影响 20 万人以上的药物,但市场永远不会帮助恢复发展成本。2009 年,美国进行了大约 16 000 例肾移植,其他实体器官的移植更少,所有移植均符合稀有条件[10]。

标签外药物的医疗保险报销批准过程

在过去几年中，付款人报销已成为标签外使用免疫抑制剂(ISA)的最大障碍。在 FDA 批准的适应证外使用时，私人健康保险运营商和健康管理提供者越来越难以偿还药物(特别是昂贵的药物)费用。这一问题经常使标签外药物不能作为免疫抑制剂使用。

卫生和公共服务部(HHS)的监察长办公室(OIG)发布关于处方药物覆盖率的年度政策声明，为医疗保险和医疗补助服务中心(CMS),医疗保健 ISA 制订了移植受者的保险范围。这为其他保险付款人制订保险政策提供了基础。2012 财年的 OIG 政策指出：

……联邦法律通常要求根据医学上的适应证,例如由 FDA 批准的或由 HHS 秘书鉴定的一个或多个权威药物支持的那些[16]。

该政策规定，如果药物概要报告了足够的证据表明药物对于该临床疾病或病症是安全且有效的，则药物的标签外使用被覆盖。

历史上，“社会保障法”[第 1861(t)(2)(B)(ii)(Ⅰ)条]认可三个纲要作为可接受的标签外药物使用来源。这三个纲要包括医学协会药物评价(AMA-DE)、美国药典信息(USP-DI)或其后续出版物[在 DRA 的第 6001(f)(1)节中修订]和美国医院处方服务-药物信息(AFHS-DI)。目前医疗保险认可的药典包括美国医院处方药服务药物信息(AHFS-DI)、临床药理学和药物索引[16]。对于抗癌药物，则利用国家综合癌症网络(NCCN)药物和生物制剂纲要。其他保险公司可以使用相同或不同的概略。

Thomson Reuters 维护着 DrugDex compendia(一个大型 Micromedex 资源中的数据库)，长期以来一直致力于涵盖关于标签外药物使用的信息[17]。通过对初级文献和有影响力的药物信息来源的持续评估，如 FDA、国家卫生研究所(NIH)和疾病控制和预防中心(CDC)，监测非标记适应证。此外，数据库接受添加标签外适应证的请求。对于每种药物，所有 FDA 批准的适应证以及各种标签外的适应证都包括在内。每个指征同样评估功效强度、证据强度和推荐强度(表 101.2)[17]。根据是否有证据支持疗效，给予Ⅰ、Ⅱa、Ⅱb 或Ⅲ的等级。Ⅰ类被认为是最高的有效性水平。证据强度为 A、B、C 类或“无证据”。A 类证据基于荟萃分析和(或)随机对照试验。推荐的总体强度考虑到效力和证据评级。Ⅰ类、Ⅱa 或Ⅱb 被认为可以接受使用，不推荐Ⅲ类[17]。

AHFS-DI，另一个 HHS 公认的药物简编，是一个旨在基于现有证据提供药物安全性和有效性信息的资源。药物资源任务的一个重要部分是评估药物标签外使用的证据。通过支持性叙述，AHFS-DI 提供了标签外药物的使用建议。AHFS-DI 数据也可通过 Lexicomp 药物资源获得[18]。

医疗保险福利政策规定，如果在 AHFS-DI 或临床药理学中提供支持性文本，或在 DrugDex 中给出Ⅰ、Ⅱa 或Ⅱb 类推荐，则可以涵盖非标签药物使用[19]。然而，覆盖决策过程由于各种药物资源在其支持和不合标签 ISA 使用的证据方面的不一致而变得复杂。AHFS-DI 对非标签药物使用的支持基于是否讨论使用以及叙述

表 101.2 药物概略中推荐和分级定义

药物代码			
AHFS-DI	叙述性文本是支持的——被认为是可接受的标签外药物使用		
	叙述性文本不支持——被认为是不可接受的非标签药物使用		
	支持性文本中没有叙述(NN)		
DrugDex	可接受的标签外药物使用	Ⅰ类	推荐。已证明治疗有效且应该施用
		Ⅱa 类	推荐，在大多数情况下。治疗通常被认为是有效的，并且在大多数情况下表明
		Ⅱb 类	推荐，在某些情况下。治疗可能是有效的，并且在一些但不是大多数情况下指示
	不可接受的非标签药物使用	Ⅲ类	不建议。治疗无效，应避免
	证据强度	A 类	证据是基于以下数据得出的：具有同质性的随机对照试验的荟萃分析关于个别研究之间的结果的方向和程度。多次，完成的随机临床试验涉及大量患者
		B 类	证据来源于：对各个研究之间的结果方向和程度具有冲突结论的随机对照试验的荟萃分析。涉及少量患者或具有显著方法缺陷(如偏倚、辍学率、有缺陷的分析等)的随机对照试验。非随机研究(如队列研究、病例对照研究和观察性研究)
		C 类	证据基于以下数据：专家意见或共识、病例报告或病例系列
		无证据	
	效果	Ⅰ类	有效。证据和(或)专家意见表明，针对特定适应证的给定药物治疗是有效的
		Ⅱa 类	证据有利于功效。证据和(或)专家意见对于特定指征的给定药物治疗是否有效是相互矛盾的，但证据的重量和(或)专家意见有利于效力
		Ⅱb 类	证据和(或)专家意见对于特定适应证的给定药物治疗是否有效相互矛盾，但证据的重量和(或)专家意见反对效力
		Ⅲ类	证据和(或)专家意见表明，对于特定药物的给定药物治疗是无效的

性内容是支持性还是不支持性(表 101.2)。然而,这种叙述的程度非常有限。表 101.1 中列出的 ISA 的大部分在 AHFS-DI 中没有关于标签外使用的叙述,因此不支持其使用。相比之下,DrugDex 提供了标签外使用是否可接受的评级。该汇编继续提供证据强度和效力的评级。

AHFS-DI 和 DrugDex compendia 之间存在差异,使得关于标签外使用的 ISA 的覆盖决定变得复杂。例如,使用西罗莫司预防心脏移植排斥反应被评为Ⅲ(非标签使用不可接受),但有证据表明其有利于疗效。鉴于这些事实,评级不可接受的基础不清楚。有趣的是,AHFS-DI 没有提供同样的非标签使用的叙述。

在标记适应证外支持使用 rATG 治疗肾移植排斥反应(目前 FDA 批准的适应证)方面,AHFS-DI 和 DrugDex 之间存在显著差异。在 AHFS-DI,用于移植的非标签使用仅用于预防肾移植排斥反应。具体来说,AHFS-DI 没有提到使用 rATG 治疗或预防心脏或胰腺移植排斥反应,并且不包括叙述文支持此应用。相比之下,DrugDex 支持使用 rATG 治疗和预防心脏移植受者的排斥反应,并被指定Ⅱb 类推荐,这被认为是 OIG 批准非标签使用。

用于测定 ISA 覆盖度的药典的缺点可以由用于肾移植中用作诱导治疗的 rATG 的 DrugDex 指定最好地表示。尽管提供了证据效力和强度的支持评级,DrugDex 将 rATG 分为Ⅲ类(即不推荐),用于预防肾同种异体移植排斥反应。

由于临床现状和现有的证据基础,很难证明在肾移植中缺乏对 rATG 的标签外使用。根据移植受者科学登记(SRTR),rATG 是 2009 年最常用的诱导剂,近 48%的肾移植受者接受 rATG,并且该试剂在很大程度上被认为是美国移植中心的标准治疗[10]。此外,科学文献广泛支持这种标签外使用 rATG 诱导治疗[20-24]。药物纲要、临床实践和现有科学证据之间的这种差异提供了对当前状态重新合理评估有力的理由。这个问题给移植提供者为他们的患者提供最佳护理上带来了相当大的挑战。一种处理问题的方法是,主要的专业移植学会(美国移植外科医师协会和美国移植学会)参与开发并提供用于开发的科学证据分类和叙述。

标签外 ISA 的额外报销选项在同行评议的期刊文章中提供了治疗效果的源文档。如果通过了权威医学文献或护理标准的验证,则使用非标签药物是可以接受的。对于抗癌药物和生物制剂的标签外使用,OIG 和 Medicare 提供了如何评估和接受医学文献的具体细节[19]。本政策提供了可接受的文献资料来源清单,专门用于抗癌药物的研究。在移植生物制剂方面,主要的实体器官移植学术期刊不包括在批准的医学文献列表中,从而严重地使得用于非标签 ISA 使用的医疗保险覆盖的问题复杂化。这种情况为移植领域的主要专业学会提供了参与和影响既定方法的机会。

肿瘤患者人群中的标签外药物使用已经得到 OIG 政策的充分认可和解决。然而,OIG 对移植中脱标药物的使用没有 ISA 中那么严格。由于在移植中存在更大的时间限制,移植中缺乏关于标签外药物使用的 OIG 政策使得问题进一步复杂化——移植通常在紧急情况下进行,急性排斥治疗必须在紧急情况下进行。这些观察结果提供了有力的理由说明在联邦政策制订和政策法规应用方面需更集中的努力。

免疫抑制药物在移植中的标签外使用

在过去的几年中,三种具有 FDA 肿瘤适应证的药物已被作为免疫抑制剂在移植中进行标签外使用:阿仑单抗、利妥昔单抗和硼替佐米。以下部分详细介绍了这些肿瘤药物在移植中的已公布的临床应用,以及它们如何成为许多移植中心的实践标准。

阿仑单抗

阿仑单抗(Campath-1H)是在 T 和 B 淋巴细胞、单核细胞、巨噬细胞和嗜酸性粒细胞上表达的 CD52 抗原的特异性单克隆抗体[25,26]。阿仑单抗最初被 FDA 批准用于治疗 B 细胞慢性淋巴细胞白血病(CLL)。这种引起快速和持续的淋巴细胞消耗的细胞溶解剂已经在实体器官移植中作为诱导疗法被广泛研究。阿仑单抗在 2001 年被美国批准用于 CLL,之前一直在美国之外使用。1998 年,英国的一项研究调查了使用阿仑单抗作为诱导治疗的 13 名肾脏移植受者[26]。2005 年发表了一项具有较大患者群的 5 年随访研究[27]。与标准治疗相比,阿仑单抗联合低剂量环孢素对于患者和移植物存活是安全且有效的[27]。在亚洲三个中心进行的另一项研究表明,阿仑单抗是无类固醇方案中的有效诱导剂[28]。

将阿仑单抗与 rATG 和 IL-2RA(达利珠单抗或巴利昔单抗)进行比较的随机研究提供了实质性证据,支持在肾移植中将阿仑单抗作为诱导治疗的非标记使用。Cianco 等发表相关研究将患者随机分为阿仑单抗、rATG 或达利珠单抗组,15 个月的研究表明急性排斥反应率、肾功能或患者或移植物存活率没有差异[29]。支持阿仑单抗在移植中的标签外使用的最佳证据源自多中心随机 INTAC 试验,其中将阿仑单抗与巴利昔单抗(在低免疫风险患者中) 或 rATG (在高免疫风险患者中)进行比较。在这项研究中,发现阿仑单抗具有与 rATG 类似的功效,并且在低风险患者中具有比巴利昔单抗更潜在的优势[24]。此外,还有其他几个非随机的阿仑单抗试验。阿仑单抗被用作诱导疗法, 但 Genzyme-Sanofi 尚未寻求 FDA 批准阿仑单抗在肾移植中的使用。

2009 年,约 13%的移植中心在肾移植受者中使用阿仑单抗[10]。阿仑单抗主要在肾移植中使用,但阿仑单抗已经用于其他实体器官移植受体。移植受者 SRTR 显示,阿仑单抗被用于 12%的肠移植,8%的肺移植和 11%~12.6%的胰腺移植(胰肾、肾后胰腺和单独胰腺)[10]。阿仑单抗也已在更有限的方面用作肝移植和儿科移植受者的诱导疗法。

遗憾的是, 阿仑单抗似乎不太可能获得 FDA 的批准用于移植。2012 年 9 月,宣布将不再通过常规药物分配机制提供阿仑单抗(以 Campath 为专有名称),并且只能通过美国 Campath 分销计划提供[30]。人们普遍认为, 这一举动是赛诺菲努力获得 FDA 批准阿仑单抗在多发性硬化中使用的准备。赛诺菲的这一决定可能基于市场潜力考虑,因为炎症和自身免疫性疾病具有更大的市场潜力,因此具有更大的利润率。尽管通过美国 Campath 分布计划提供了用于多发性硬化外指征的阿仑单抗,这种方案的长期可持续性是个问题。阿仑单抗是移植领域在药物开发方面所面临的问题的典型案例。与自身免疫性疾病和肿瘤学适应证相比,由移植代表的相对较小的市场规模提供了较小的潜在经济利润率。这些考虑导致药物开发的转变,使得新的免疫抑制剂远离移植,转向肿瘤学或自身免疫性疾病。

利妥昔单抗

利妥昔单抗是针对 B 淋巴细胞上的 CD20 抗原特异性的单克隆抗体。利妥昔单抗的确切机制是复杂的。然而,B 细胞消耗是最显著的作用,其消耗通过几种潜在的途径,包括补体依赖性细胞毒性作用、抗体依赖性细胞毒性作用和凋亡介导[31]。利妥昔单抗被 FDA 批准用于治疗:对肿瘤坏死因子(TNF)拮抗剂缺乏反应的成年患者的 CD20 阳性非霍奇金淋巴瘤、CD20 阳性 CLL、中至重度活动性类风湿性关节炎(与甲氨蝶呤组合)、韦格纳肉芽肿和微血管多发性血管炎。在实体器官移植中,利妥昔单抗已经开发出了几种标签外使用,包括移植后淋巴增殖性疾病(PTLD)、排斥反应的预防、ABO 不相容移植、排斥反应的治疗和 HLA 敏化患者的脱敏[31]。最大的成功领域是利妥昔单抗用于PTLD,然而本节将重点关注利妥昔单抗用于治疗排斥反应和脱敏。

利妥昔单抗用于治疗难治性排斥反应目前限于小型和非随机性研究。基于这样的观察结果:难治性排斥反应的患者在肾同种异体移植活检中显示出显著数量的 $CD20^+$染色 B 细胞[31]。Becker 及其同事描述了接受利妥昔单抗治疗的 27 例患者的病例系列,这些患者具有激素抵抗型或抗体介导的排斥反应(AMR)。几乎所有这些患者还接受类固醇(24/27)、血浆置换术及 rATG (22/27)。只有 3 名患者经历了与患者死亡无关的移植物损失。这个病例系列太小从而无法评估结果,但它的确表明利妥昔单抗是一种有效的治疗患者耐药性排斥反应的疗法[32]。另一个关于 4 例慢性 AMR 患者的病例系列描述了利妥昔单抗联合静脉注射免疫球蛋白(IVIg)的使用。这些患者在治疗后 3 个月和 6 个月显示肾同种异体移植功能改善,2 名患者供体特异性抗体(DSA)减少[33]。其他研究表明,当与血浆置换联合使用时,利妥昔单抗对 AMR 有效[34]。

Tydén 及其同事进行了一项利妥昔单抗诱导治疗的前瞻性、随机双盲研究,与他克莫司、霉酚酸酯和类固醇相组合。在血运重建的 24h 内,将 140 名患者随机分配接受一剂量的利妥昔单抗 (375 mg/m^2 体表面积)或一剂安慰剂[35]。在接受利妥昔单抗的 68 名患者中,观察到 CD19/CD20 细胞的显著消耗。在利妥昔单抗组中观察到在 6 个月时排斥反应更少的趋势, 然而这没有统计学的显著性差异。相比之下,在一项比较利妥昔单抗和达利珠单抗诱导的开放性随机研究中, 移植后 3 个月在利妥昔单抗组中, 由于 83%的急性细胞排斥率,仅招募 13 名患者后,这项研究被迫终止[36]。

利妥昔单抗也已用于HLA高度致敏患者的脱敏方案中。在一项拥有20名患者的研究中,16名患者在服用两剂1g利妥昔单抗(第7和第22天)和两剂2g/kg IVIg(第0和第30天)[37]后接受移植。

总之,利妥昔单抗的证据基础通常不如阿仑单抗的强。然而,来自非控制性临床试验的数据表明,利妥昔单抗在脱敏方案和抗体介导排斥反应治疗方面可能有疗效。

硼替佐米

硼替佐米是一种小分子第一类蛋白酶体抑制剂,被FDA批准用于治疗多发性骨髓瘤和套细胞淋巴瘤[38]。硼替佐米的作用机制复杂,并且对细胞信号传导途径具有多种作用。然而,这些作用被认为很少有助于其在多发性骨髓瘤中的功效。目前认为,多发性骨髓瘤中的主要机制来源于内质网(ER)应激的诱导,以及最终导致细胞凋亡的末端未折叠蛋白质应答[39]。硼替佐米还是已知的有效导致细胞凋亡的细胞周期抑制剂和核因子κB(NFκB)介导的抗性抑制剂。

硼替佐米在移植中的首次报道是用于治疗难治性抗体介导的排斥反应(AMR)[40]。在这项研究中,用硼替佐米治疗6名有记录的难治性AMR患者。在标准AMR治疗失败的每名患者中,这种脱标使用硼替佐米导致AMR逆转。初始适应证外的支付覆盖范围是可变的,付款人覆盖范围的持续不一致使得硼替佐米疗法研究的扩展变得复杂。根据这一经验,治疗成功的文件和提供科学出版物已经大大有助于获得付款人覆盖范围。根据我们的经验,硼替佐米的使用由医院药房检测和监测,并且由于其成本相当高(在11天周期内4次剂量约5000美元),硼替佐米的标签外使用引起了相当大的关注。然而,潜在的同种异体移植节省效应有助于抵制医院药房和处方委员会的反对。

在同行评审的科学文献中发表的经验成为硼替佐米非标记使用治疗肾移植受者难治性AMR的最有效策略。然而,如果硼替佐米治疗不如原始系列那样有效,这种方法可能失败。

硼替佐米的脱标使用说明了未来移植中非标签药物使用需要重点考虑。一般来说,关于注册试验的决定基于几个因素,包括已知的机制,以及潜在市场的规模。一种药物可能适用于几种潜在疾病,能够进一步开发,但临床注册试验的高昂费用将研究限于单一适应证。对单一适应证的限制导致标签外药物开发是其他大多数潜在治疗适应证的唯一可行选择。积极的第四阶段发展计划可以为新治疗领域的非标记评价提供实质性支持。然而,当这些资金不可用时,标签外使用变得具有挑战性。就硼替佐米而言,在辛辛那提大学,作者幸运地拥有三个临床试验的相关资金,包括两个小型随机试验,一个有关诱导治疗,另一个有关肾移植急性混合性排斥反应。第三个试验作为高敏感肾移植受体中的脱敏试验进行。

在初步报告硼替佐米治疗难治性AMR后出现了许多报告。遗憾的是,这些发表的报告的结果成功率各不相同。然而,硼替佐米在心脏和肺受体以及儿科移植受体中显示出逆转AMR的潜在功效[41,42]。一项大规模的合作研究证实了难治性AMR肾移植受者的原始观察结果[43]。最近,大型脱敏研究证实了硼替佐米对高度敏感的肾移植候选物的影响,从而为基于IVIG的方案提供了潜在的替代方案。

总之,硼替佐米的适应证外开发受到成本高、支付者覆盖范围、医院药房和处方委员会的成本控制限制,以及赞助商对Ⅳ期研究的有限资助的影响。临床结果的科学出版、预防难治性AMR患者移植物损失的功效,以及缺乏替代性的FDA批准的AMR疗法,有助于提高硼替佐米的非标签使用的覆盖率。

法国再定义非标签药物使用的法律框架

最近通过的法国法律和相关的“法令”已经建立了一个调节批准药物的非标签使用的过程。这个新的规章框架旨在为新批准药物的脱标使用提供支持和评估,同时确保公共安全[44]。该项法律的主要影响是要求赞助商(即药品制造公司)监督非标签使用,并确定是否必须采取以下行动:

(1)告知国家监管机构(国家安全局)药品和保健产品(ANSM)的非传统处方。

(2)采取措施教育医疗保健专业人员并防止非标签使用。

该法令[“临时使用建议”(TRU)]规定,对一种药物的一次性TRU指定授权,如果没有其他药物可用于指定用途,则需要由付款人报销。监管机构(ANSM)可以通过具有既得利益的若干组中的任何一组(如国家卫生部、国家癌症研究所或患者宣传组)通知 TRU 的需要。然后,ANSM 可以决定采用正在考虑的 TRU 的建议,由此它将对发起人或从已发表的文献提交的数据进行考虑[44]。

对于授予 TRU, 必须没有其他经批准的药物用于此适应证。在批准 TRU 时要考虑的因素包括:

- 支持提议的 TRU 的证据基础的质量;
- 药物的安全性;
- 疾病的预后;
- 疾病/病症的发病率。

法国的监管框架可能加强安全,但一些因素引起了相当大的关注。最受关注的是,每一种药物只能给予一次 TRU。因此,如果药物具有几种潜在的脱标用途(如几种不同的癌症类型),则赞助者需决定哪种适应证应得到 TRU 应用。如果药物有两种(或更多种)潜在的标签外使用, 这两种都是潜在致命的条件呢?做出这种决定的伦理框架是什么? 显然,在美国医疗界和美国公众可以接受此类系统之前, 需要额外考虑。

非标签使用、标准治疗和药物的研究性使用

药物的非标签使用已在本章前面定义。然而,标签外使用可以根据标准治疗进一步限定, 或者可以构成研究用途。如前所述,非标签使用可能成为这样的常见实践,即它成为标准治疗(如他克莫司/MMF 方案用于预防肾移植的排斥反应),但非标签使用与标准治疗的转变点很难定义。类似地,非标签使用可以是或不是研究性的, 并且该定义引起了人们对人类受试者的保护和管理问题的关注。因此, 在药物非标签使用的背景下,考虑提供标准治疗和研究使用的定义非常重要。

从法律角度来看,标准治疗已被很好地定义。法律词典将"治疗标准"定义为"在某种情况下合理的人会警惕、注意、谨慎和审慎地行使"[45]。在不当行为中,治疗标准的定义至关重要, 因为原告在特定医学专业或全科医学执业中必须建立治疗标准。

相比之下,治疗标准没有明确确定的医学定义。此外, 医疗从业者的治疗标准可能因医生的执业地点而异。即使在美国,在治疗标准方面也可能存在明显的区域性甚至局部差异。例如,在俄亥俄州内,六个成年人肾移植项目之间存在显著差异。即使在同一城市内的个别项目之间,尽管地域临近,标准的免疫抑制治疗方案也有显著差异。美国许多大型城市有多个移植项目,然而免疫抑制疗法与同一城市的其他项目有很大不同。

鉴于这些差异, 了解一个项目如何制订其治疗标准很重要。CMS 以及器官采购和移植网络(OPTN)通过计划认证和建立认证标准来规范移植领域。这些标准需要针对团队的操作方案, 并且还需要开发用于免疫抑制和预防感染的标准。CMS 和 OPTN 不规定哪些药物用于免疫抑制或感染预防, 只是由经认证的移植医生和外科医生的多学科小组开发出这些药物的标准。在本地, 特定的医生共识的项目在决定免疫抑制方案时必须考虑证据基础、先前经验、持续经验、财务成本、付款人覆盖范围和个体患者群体。

最常见的免疫抑制剂和免疫抑制方案的电子处方数据很容易获得, 其可以代表定义治疗标准的替代方法。如果给定的方案代表最常规的处方,这样的数据可以表示代表治疗标准的特定组合的强论据。然而,对于较小的患者群体,如高风险人群,处方用于定义治疗标准比较困难, 除非这样的高风险群体可以由处方数据库可靠地定义。

另一方面,在国家、区域和地方范围内从电子处方数据库对当前美国最常见规定的免疫抑制方案进行追踪。有些情况下,当地的治疗标准可能与全国范围内定义的标准大不相同。在这些情况下,地方方案应能够证明当地选择的治疗标准的基础。

循证医学和患者护理指南代表定义护理标准的另一种方法。然而,由国家肾脏基金会 KDIGO 小组建立的肾病:改善全球预后(KDIGO)指南列举了建立实践指南所固有的困难。KDIGO 中的免疫抑制建议备受争议,因为一些医生认为他们没有达到适度的客观性,并带有责任作者(Dr. E. Steve Woodle,未发表的观察)的过度偏倚。因此,在没有多中心双盲试验明确优势方法的情况下,治疗标准的定义在本质上是主观的。

当机构审查委员会(IRB)赞助协议生效时,更容易定义当标签外使用构成调查性使用时的问题。然而,在没有 IRB 批准方案的情况下研究非标记使用可以论证。例如,执业医师或一组执业医师可以选择标签外使用药物治疗患者并收集数据,以用于评估治疗效果。当这些数据发布时,它开始接近研究使用。这方面的示例

可参考我们使用硼替佐米治疗难治性抗体介导的反应(AMR)的初期经历中所遇到的问题和经验[40]。在治疗已知治疗剂难以治疗的AMR患者 [包括IVIG和利妥昔单抗(有意义的,也用于标签外治疗AMR)]之前,应由肾脏科医师、移植外科医生和移植药剂师进行内部程序性讨论,对IVIG和利妥昔单抗失败的AMR患者应当被允许取消同种异体移植(并且返回透析),而非额外尝试逆转排斥反应。因为肾脏同种异体移植的透析和损失的恢复与患者预期寿命的显著降低有关,在此情况下,我们选择考虑使用硼替佐米。在使用硼替佐米之前,应从科学文献中仔细研究其作用和毒性以及安全性,我们还聘用了肿瘤学家和经过肿瘤学专业培训的药剂师。在考虑治疗的患者群体中,安全性和毒性需要明确。移植小组讨论了这些结果并做出决定,以治疗下一个合适的难治性AMR患者,此患者被判定具有肾同种异体移植物丢失的高风险,对其脱标使用硼替佐米作为挽救疗法。当确定患者时,并未与患者讨论进一步治疗的预后,但讨论了缺乏替代选择,硼替佐米的潜在脱标使用,包括潜在成本、安全性和毒性等问题。前6位接受治疗的患者都证实了硼替佐米具有实质性疗效,并且经历了AMR逆转[40]。在治疗了2名患者后,我们与当地IRB的负责人讨论了这种标签外使用,特别针对这种治疗是否代表研究应该在IRB批准方案指导下进行。会议同意,在某些时候,首选方法是进行IRB资助的试验,然而很明显,这种非标签使用显然是主治医师的特权。迄今为止,我们已经提交了研究硼替佐米AMR治疗的研究建议,但还未获得这项试验的资金。在移植史上,只有少数抗菌药物耐药性研究被资助。迄今为止,硼替佐米治疗AMR的集体经验提供了类似于IVIG曾经所获得的结果[43]。

在一个完美的世界,资金将可用于所有研究,无论多么罕见,可为标签外药物治疗提供适当的证据基础。然而,现代医学的现实是许多新药物相当昂贵,进行这些临床试验的成本越来越高。这些在很大程度上阻碍了行业资助这些试验的潜力,使得NIH和其他实体成为这些研究的唯一可能的替代选择。

总结

标签外药物使用在实体器官移植领域是众所周知的,部分是由于该领域新型药物的开发水平和程度不如其他领域(如自身免疫疾病和肿瘤学)。标签外的ISA使用和药物开发由于保险公司拒绝提供报销而变得复杂,这可能导致患者在完成治疗前需花费数千美元。尽管备受阻碍,标签外药物使用和发展已经持续到现在。然而,未来似乎并不乐观,并且随着新药的成本增加,地方和联邦可能会增强对标签外药物使用的审查和限制。历史上,非标签药物使用已逐渐成为移植受体的治疗标准。然而,这种做法可能在未来改变。法定限制,如在法国设立的限制,正在重新界定这一药物开发领域,其他国家也可能很快就会出台相关规定。

(沈恬 译 沈恬 校)

参考文献

1. Ventola CL. Off-label drug information: regualtion, distribution, evaluation, and related controversies. Pharmacy and Therapeutics. 2009;34(8):428–449.
2. Stafford RS. Regulating off-label drug use – rethinking the role of the FDA. New England Journal of Medicine. 2008;358(14):1427–1429.
3. Nightingale S. Off-label use of prescription drugs. American Family Physician. 2003;68(3):425–427.
4. American Society of Health-Systems Pharmacist. ASHP statement on the use of medications for unlabeled uses. American Journal of Hospital Pharmacy. 1992;49:2006–2008.
5. European Society of Medical Oncology (ESMO). The off-label use of drugs in oncology: a position paper by the European Society for Medical Oncology. Annals of Oncology. 2007;18:1923–1925.
6. American Society of Clinical Oncology. Reimbursement for cancer treatment: coverage of off-label drug indications. Journal of Clinical Oncology. 2006;24(19):3206–3208.
7. Vincenti F, Klintmalm G, Halloran PF. Open letter to the FDA: new drug trials must be relevant. American Journal of Transplantation. 2008;8:733–734.
8. Ahsan N, Johnson C, Gonwa T, et al. Randomized trial of tacrolimus plus mycophenolate mofetil or azathioprine versus cyclosporine oral solution (modified) plus mycophenolate mofetil after cadaveric kidney transplantation: results at 2 years. Transplantation. 2001;72(2):245–250.
9. Miller J, Mendez R, Pirsch JD, et al. Safety and efficacy of tacrolimus in combination with mycophenolate mofetil (MMF) in cadaveric renal transplant recipients. FK506/MMF Dose-Ranging Kidney Transplant Study Group. Transplantation. 2000;69(5):875–880.
10. Organ Procurment and Transplantation Network (OPTN) and Scientific Registry of Transplant Recipients(SRTR). OPTN/SRTR 2010 Annual Data Report. 2009.
11. PRNewswire. Astellas Receives FDA Approval for Use of Prograf (tacrolimus) in Conjuction with Mycophenolate Mofetil (MMF) in Kidney Transplant Recipients. PRNewswire. 2009.
12. Albrecht R. Introduction. FDA Workshop on Endpoint in Clinical Trials of Kidney Transplantation. 2012 September 10; Silver Spring, MD.
13. Cavaille-Coll M. Past and current regulatory approaches to endpoints in kidney transplantation. FDA Workshop: Endpoints in Clinical Trials of Kidney Transplantation. 2012 September 10; Silver Spring, MD.
14. Vincenti F. [Personal Communication]. 2012.
15. U.S. Food and Drug Administration. How Drugs are Developed and Approved. 2010 [updated April 23, 2012; cited 2012 September 29, 2012]; Available from: http://www.fda.gov/Drugs/DevelopmentApprovalProcess/HowDrugsareDevelopedandApproved/default.htm.
16. Office of Inspector General. Office of Inspector General Work Plan. In: U.S. Department of Health and Human Services. 2012.
17. DrugDex® System [Internet database] Greenwood Village, Colo. Thomson Reuters (Healthcare) Inc. Updated periodically..
18. AHFS-DI. [Internet database]. Hudson, Ohio. LexiComp Inc. Udpated periodically.
19. Center for Medicaid and Medicare Services. Medicare Benefit Policy Manual [Online Policy Manual]. 2012 [cited 2012 October 10, 2012]; Available from: http://www.cms.gov/Regulations-and-Guidance/Guidance/Manuals/Internet-

Only-Manuals-IOMs-Items/CMS012673.
20. Brennan DC, Daller JA, Lake KD, et al. Rabbit antithymocyte globulin versus basiliximab in renal transplantation. New England Journal of Medicine. 2006; 355(19):1967–1977.
21. Cole EH, Cattran DC, Farewell VT, et al. A comparison of rabbit coantithymocyte serum and OKT3 as prophylaxis against renal allograft rejection. Transplantation. 1994;57(1):60–67.
22. Buchler M, Hurault de Ligny B, Madec C, et al. Induction therapy by anti-thymocyte globulin (rabbit) in renal transplantation: a 1-yr follow-up of safety and efficacy. Clinical Transplantation. 2003;17(6):539–545.
23. Hardinger KL. Rabbit antithymocyte globulin induction therapy in adult renal transplantation. Pharmacotherapy. 2006;26(12):1771–1783.
24. Hanaway MJ, Woodle ES, Mulgaonkar S, et al. Alemtuzumab induction in renal transplantation. New England Journal of Medicine. 2011;364(20):1909–1919.
25. Hale G. The CD52 antigen and development of the CAMPATH antibodies. Cytotherapy. 2001;3:137–143.
26. Morris PJ, Russell NK. Alemtuzumab (Campath-1H): a systematic review in organ transplantation. Transplantation. 2006;81:1361–1367.
27. Watson CJE, Bradley JA, Friend PJ, et al. Alemtuzumab (CAMPATH-1H) induction therapy in cadaveric kidney transplantation – efficacy and safety at five years. American Journal of Transplantation. 2005;5:1347–1533.
28. Vathsala A, Ona ET, Tan S, et al. Randomized trial of alemtuzumab for prevention of graft rejection and preservation of renal function after kidney transplantation. Transplantation. 2005;80:765–774.
29. Ciancio G, Burke GW, Gaynor JJ, et al. A randomizied trial of three renal transplant induction antibodies: early comparison of tacrolimus, mycophenolate, and steroid dosing, and newer immune-monitoring. Transplantation. 2005;80: 457–465.
30. Genzyme-Sanofi. US Campath Distribution Program [press release]. 2012.
31. Pescovitz MD. Rituximab, an anti-CD20 monoclonal antibody: history and mechanism of action. American Journal of Transplantation. 2006;6:859–866.
32. Becker Y, Becker BN, Pirsch JD, et al. Rituximab as treatment for refractory kidney transplant rejection. American Journal of Transplantation. 2004;4:996–1001.
33. Fehr T, Rusi B, Flescher A, et al. Rituximab and intravenous immunoglobulin treatment of chronic antibody-mediated kidney allograft rejection. Transplantation. 2009;87:1837–1841.
34. Faguer S, Kamar N, Guilbeaud-Frugier C, et al. Rituximab therapy for acute humoral rejection after kidney transplantation. Transplantation. 2007;83:1277–1280.
35. Tydén G, Genberg H, Tollemar J, et al. A randomized, doubleblind, placebo-controlled, study of single-dose rituximab as induction in renal transplantation. Transplantation. 2009;87:1325–1329.
36. Clatworthy MR, Watson CJE, Plotnek G, et al. B-cell depleting induction therapy and acute cellular rejection. New England Journal of Medicine. 2009;360(25): 2683–2684.
37. Vo AA, Lubovksy M, Toyoda M, et al. Rituximab and intravenous immune globulin for desensitization during renal transplantation. New England Journal of Medicine. 2008;359:242–251.
38. Woodle ES, Alloway RR, Girnita AL. Proteasome-inhibitor treatment of antibody-mediated allograft rejection. Current Opinion in Organ Transplantation. 2011; 16(4):434–438.
39. Walsh RC, Alloway RR, Girnita AL, et al. Proteasome inhibitor-based therapy for antibody-mediated rejection. Kidney International. 2012;81(11):1067–1074.
40. Everly MJ, Everly JJ, Susskind B, et al. Bortezomib provides effective therapy for antibody- and cell-mediated acute rejection. Transplantation. 2008;86: 1754–1761.
41. Morrow WR, Frazier EA, Mahle WT, et al. Rapid reduction in donor-specific anti-human leukocyte antigen antiibodies and reversal of antibody-mediated rejection with bortezomib in pediatric heart transplant patients. Transplantation. 2012;93:319–324.
42. Neumann J, Tarrasconi H, Bortolotto A, et al. Acute humoral rejection in a lung recipient: reversion with bortezomib. Transplantation. 2010;89(1): 125–126.
43. Walsh RC, Braily P, Girinta A, et al. Early and late acute antibody-mediated rejection differ immunologically and in response to proteasome inhibition. Transplantation. 2011;91:1218–1226.
44. Emmerich J, Dumarcet N, Lorence A. France's new framework for regulating off-label drug use. New England Journal of Medicine. 2012;367(14):1279–1281.
45. Hill GN, Hill KT. Legal-Dictionary. The Free Dictionary. [cited 2012 October 14, 2012]; Available from: http://legal-dictionary.thefreedictionary.com/standard+of+care.

第 102 章
器官移植中的药物相互作用

William D. Simmons, Pamala A. Jacobson, Karen L. Hardinger

引言

药物之间的相互作用是指一种药物在另一种药物的作用下发生改变或干扰而出现非目的效应。药物的相互作用对移植受体来说可能会危及他们的生命，因为他们具有发生药物相互作用的危险因素，包括患有多种伴随疾病及使用治疗区间狭窄的药物。这些有害作用的概率随着年龄的增长也会增加。移植受体中的药物间相互作用的发生率并不明确，但在一般人群中，该作用在急诊、住院及复诊中的发生率为 0~7.6%[1]。住院期间急性药物相互作用的发生率为 5.3%~14.3%[1]。而移植患者发生率较高的原因显然是在移植时给予大量药物，标签外用药时药物分布不同，对药物代谢至关重要的器官功能快速变化，尤其是在肝和肾移植方面。药物相互作用可以大致分为两类：药代动力型及药效型。

药代动力学

药代动力学是研究药物吸收、分布、代谢及在体内外排泄的学科。药代动力学的药物相互作用发生在一种药物影响另一种药物的吸收、分布、代谢及排泄时。表 102.1 列出了部分药物间相互作用的例子。

药效动力学

药效动力学是研究药物剂量与靶组织效应或临床结果关系的学科。药代动力学型的药物-药物相互作用可能引起叠加、协同或相反的药效学效应。每一类型的药物间作用都可以对患者造成不良效果。现在越来越多的证据表明，基因多样性或药理遗传学可能影响药物间相互作用。

本章的目的在于专注于免疫抑制剂，描述药代动力学和药效动力学的药物-药物作用，探索药物间作用对移植受体药理基因组学的影响，以及提出处理药物间作用的方法。在 17 章中可看到一篇关于移植免疫抑制剂的通用机制的概论。对于在移植中常用的药物的详细描述可以在第 98 至第 101 章中找到。

药代动力学型药物间相互作用

药代动力型相互作用可导致药物的药代动力学参数改变，如时间对浓度曲线下的面积(AUC)、半衰期($t_{1/2}$)、血药浓度达到峰值的时间(T_{max})、最大血药浓度(C_{max})或最小血药浓度(C_{min})。

吸收

药物吸收是指药物进入循环系统的过程。药物被消化后，首先是剂型溶解或破裂，然后才是吸收。吸收过程取决于某些因素，包括药物配方、食物或胆汁对吸收的影响、伴随药物、消化道物理环境及转运蛋白。

是否进食、进食时机以及食物的组分可能会影响许多免疫抑制剂的吸收[2-9](表 102.2)。由于给药时禁食并不常用于临床实践，许多临床医生推荐患者服药应坚持一贯性，不管有无进食，依照一种习惯服药。

另一个影响移植药物吸收的因素是同时常规应用二价阳离子。在健康志愿者中进行的交叉实验显示，单剂量下联用他克莫司和镁/铝氢氧化物与单用他克莫司相比，联用时他克莫司的 AUC 均值增加 21%，C_{max} 均值减少 10%[2]。在一项临床研究中，他克莫司与镁/铝氢氧化物联用的患者并不需要调整他克莫司剂量[10]。在霉酚酸酯（MMF）试验中，铝/镁氢氧化物使麦考酚酸(MPA)的 AUC 降低了 17%，C_{max} 降低了 33%[4,9]。当给予肠溶型麦考酚酸钠(EC-MPS)时，铝/镁氢氧化物使 MPA 的 AUC 降低了 25%，C_{max} 降低了 37%[4](药品说明

表 102.1 选择的药物与免疫抑制剂的相互作用

免疫抑制剂	交互剂	研究条件(如已报道)	结果	参考文献
硫唑嘌呤	别嘌呤醇	未报道	需要硫唑嘌呤剂量减少约为通常剂量的 1/3 至 1/4	[6]
环孢素	乙酰唑胺	3 名男性在共同施用乙酰唑胺前及 72h 后进行研究	增加环孢素的平均谷值水平，170ng/mL(范围 54~270ng/mL)至 1130ng/mL（范围 517~1827ng/mL)	[76]
环孢素	阿利吉仑	14 名健康受试者，开放性实验，单序列，平行组，单剂量研究。阿利吉仑 75mg 口服(1 期)，随后阿利吉仑 75mg+环孢素 200mg(2 期)，在 7 天的清除期后，阿利吉仑 75mg+环孢素 600mg(3 期)(14 天清除期)	使阿利吉仑的 AUC 增加 4~5 倍，C_{max} 增加 2.5 倍，将平均 t1/2 从 25h 增加到 45h。但未改变环孢素的药代动力学	[77]
环孢素	安倍生坦	28 名健康受试者每日接受安立生坦单药 5mg 或与环孢素 100~150mg，2 次/天联用，其他 24 名受试者接受单药环孢素或与安立生坦联用	安倍生坦 C_{max} 增加 1.5 倍，AUC 增加 2 倍；环孢素（CsA)的 C_{max} 和 AUC 仅轻微增加(906ng/mL 对 1014ng/mL 和 3.05μgh/mL 对 3.37μgh/mL)。安倍生坦若与 CsA 联用，推荐的最大剂量是 5mg	[42]
环孢素	氟康唑	在 16 例稳定肾移植受者中行随机双盲安慰剂对照研究，患者接受环孢素的剂量恒定，加用氟康唑每日 200mg 或安慰剂，共 14 天	在两周的治疗中，环孢素浓度增加缓慢，其谷浓度大约增加 2 倍	[78]
环孢素	氟康唑	比较开始口服氟康唑后第 2、4、7 天时的药代动力学，氟康唑剂量为 200mg/d	CsA 的 AUC 从第 0 天的 2887+/−1729ngh/mL 增加至第 2 天的 3842+/−1975ngh/mL ($P<0.05$)，第 4 天的 4750+/−1718ngh/mL ($P< 0.01$)，随后在第 7 天时降至 4052+/−1687ngh/mL ($P<0.01$)	[79]
环孢素	茚地那韦和奈非那韦	同时服用环孢素、茚地那韦和奈非那韦的肾移植患者	需要环孢素的剂量减少 85%	[80]
环孢素	酮康唑	未报道	环孢素的 AUC 增加几乎 3 倍，需要减少高达 80% 的环孢素剂量	[81]
环孢素	洛匹那韦/利托那韦	接受环孢素及洛匹那韦/利托那韦治疗的肝移植患者	需要减少 5%~20% 的环孢素剂量	[82]
环孢素	甲氨蝶呤	20 例类风湿关节炎患者	甲氨蝶呤的 AUC 增加约 30%，环孢素的浓度无明显改变	[7]
环孢素	甲氧氯普胺	14 例肾功能稳定的肾移植患者，甲氧氯普胺的总剂量为 20mg	环孢素的 AUC 增加 29%	[22]
环孢素	奈法唑酮	维持环孢素并开始使用奈法唑酮的心脏移植受者的病例报告	环孢素谷浓度在开始使用奈法唑酮后增加 10 倍	[83]
环孢素	泊沙康唑	3 例心脏移植受者已服用环孢素 3 次/天，持续 6 周或更长，加用泊沙康唑 200mg/d，持续 10 天	环孢素暴露增加和必要剂量减少 14%~29%	[84]

（待续）

表 102.1(续) 选择的药物与免疫抑制剂的相互作用

免疫抑制剂	交互剂	研究条件(如已报道)	结果	参考文献
环孢素	奎奴普丁/达福普汀	同时使用环孢素奎奴普丁/达福普汀	在2~3天内环孢素的谷浓度增加2.5倍以上，AUC增加1.6倍，C_{max}增加1.3倍	[85]
环孢素	瑞格列奈	12名健康男性接受2剂100mg环孢素胶囊，每剂间隔12h口服，单剂瑞格列奈0.25mg在环孢素初始剂量13h后口服	瑞格列奈平均C_{max}增加1.8倍（范围:0.6~3.7倍），AUC增加2.4倍（范围1.2~5.3倍）	[7]
环孢素	利福平	单剂量利福平	环孢素浓度降低73%	[86]
环孢素	利福平	肾移植患者在接受利福平治疗前或后接受环孢素治疗	环孢素的剂量需要增加2.5~3倍来维持最理想的浓度	[87]
环孢素	特拉匹韦	10名健康志愿者单独服用CsA作为单次100mg的口服剂量，随后是一个最短8天的清洗期，以及随后单一10mg口服剂量的环孢素联合单剂量的特拉匹韦750mg或稳态特拉匹韦750mg/8h	环孢素的剂量归一化，AUC大约增长4.6倍，环孢素的末端消除t 1/2从平均值[标准偏差(SD)从]12(1.67)h增加到42.1(11.3)h	[88]
环孢素	伏立康唑	7例肾移植受体在CsA基础上加用伏立康唑，随机双盲交叉研究	CsA的平均AUC增加1.7倍	[89]
依维莫司	阿托伐他汀	24名健康受试者给予单次口服剂量的阿托伐他汀20mg和依维莫司2mg	依维莫司的AUC降低5%，C_{max}降低9%。没有阿托伐他汀AUC的变化，因此没有剂量需要调整	[90]
依维莫司	环孢素	健康受试者中的单剂量研究，环孢素175mg与依维莫司2mg联用和单用依维莫司比较	依维莫司AUC增加2.7倍(168%，范围46%~365%)，C_{max}增加82%(范围25%~158%)	[91]
依维莫司	红霉素	16名健康受试者给予红霉素500mg 3次/天，共9天，单次2mg剂量的依维莫司在第5天加用	依维莫司的AUC增加4.4倍(90%CI，3.5~5.4)，从116+/-37ngh/mL降至524+/-225ngh/mL。依维莫司t1/2延长39%，从32+/-6h至44+/-6h	[92]
依维莫司	伊曲康唑	肾移植受体病例报告	伊曲康唑清除率降低74%	[93]
依维莫司	酮康唑	12名健康志愿者给予酮康唑200mg，2次/天，共8天，单次2mg剂量的依维莫司在酮康唑治疗第4天共同给药	依维莫司的AUC增加15倍(90%CI，13.6~16.6)，C_{max}增加3.9倍(90%CI，3.4~4.6)，t 1/2延长1.9倍；依维莫司不改变酮康唑浓度	[94]
依维莫司	泊沙康唑	接受泊沙康唑与依维莫司联合治疗的肾移植受者病例报告	依维莫司血液谷浓度增加3.8倍	[95]
依维莫司	普伐他汀	24名健康受试者给予单一口服剂量的普伐他汀20mg和依维莫司2mg	依维莫司C_{max}降低10%，AUC降低6%，普伐他汀AUC降低5%，因此无需剂量调整	[90]
依维莫司	利福平	12名健康受试者给予利福平600mg，每日一次，持续8天，随后为单剂量4mg依维莫司	依维莫司清除率增加172%，AUC降低63%，$t_{1/2}$从32h降低至24h	[96]

（待续）

表 102.1(续)　选择的药物与免疫抑制剂的相互作用

免疫抑制剂	交互剂	研究条件(如已报道)	结果	参考文献
依维莫司	异搏定	16 名健康志愿者给予维拉帕米 80mg,3 次/天,持续 5 天,第二天单次给予 2mg 依维莫司	依维莫司 C_{max} 增加 2.3 倍,AUX 增加 3.5 倍	[97]
依维莫司	伏立康唑	接受伏立康唑和依维莫司联合治疗的肾移植患者病例报告	依维莫司血谷浓度增加 7.5 倍	[95]
麦考酚酯	环丙沙星或阿莫西林+克拉维酸	已在使用 MMF 的肾移植受者同时口服环丙沙星 500mg bid 或阿莫西林加克拉维酸 375mg 3 次/天,持续 7~14 天	在 3 天内 MPA 的中值波峰浓度减少约 50%	[3]
麦考酚酯	左炔诺孕酮	18 名患有牛皮癣的妇女连续 3 次月经周期联用 MMF (1g bid)、炔雌醇 (0.02mg~0.04mg)和左炔诺孕酮(0.05mg~0.20mg),去氧孕烯(0.15mg)或孕二烯酮的组合口服避孕药(0.05mg~0.10mg)	平均左炔诺孕酮 AUC(0~24h)降低约 15%,乙炔雌二醇和 3-酮去氧孕烯的平均 AUC(0-24h)相似	[3]
麦考酚酯	镁铝悬浮液	10 例类风湿关节炎患者给予单剂量 MMF (2g),同时使用 TC 10mL ,4 次/天	MPA C_{max} 降低 37%,AUC (0~24h)降低 15%	[3]
麦考酚酯	诺氟沙星和甲硝唑	11 名健康志愿者在诺氟沙星和甲硝唑组合的 5 天疗程的第 4 天施用单剂量 MMF(1g)	平均 MPA AUC 0-48 和单独施用 MMF 相比降低 33%	[9]
麦考酚酯	泮托拉唑	36 例自身免疫性疾病患者接受稳定的 MMF 维持治疗,其中 23 例患者同时使用泮托拉唑,另 13 名患者未接受 PPI 或抗酸药的治疗	在泮托拉唑治疗的患者中 MPA AUC 降低 37%(P<0.01),MPA 暴露与 IMPDH 活性的抑制相关,并且泮托拉唑治疗的患者中酶活性曲线的面积高 42%(P<0.01)	[28]
麦考酚酯	丙磺舒	猴子	血浆 MPA AUC 增加 3 倍,血浆 MPA AUC 增加 2 倍	[3]
麦考酚酯	利福平	心肺移植受体病例报告	减少 MPA 暴露的 AUC(0-12)67%	[3]
麦考酚酯	利福平	心肺移植受体病例报告	MMF 暴露降低超过 2 倍	[73]
麦考酚酯	司维拉姆	成人和儿科患者	平均 MPA C_{max} 降低 36%,AUC (0~12h)减少 26%	[3]
麦考酚酯	司维拉姆	单独和重复同时服用司维拉姆和 MMF 的肾移植受者	MPA 平均降低 25%	[20]
麦考酚酯/麦考酚酸钠	奥美拉唑	12 名健康志愿者(6 名男性/ 6 名女性)接受单次口服剂量的 MMF 1000mg 或等摩尔剂量的 EC-MPS 720mg,禁食,给或不给予奥美拉唑 20mg 2 次/天	MPA AUC 减少 20%,峰浓度在用 MMF 时减半,但用 EC MPS 时没有变化	[29]
麦考酚酸吗啉/麦考酚酸钠	泮托拉唑	12 名健康志愿者(6 名男性/ 6 名女性)接受单次口服剂量的 MMF 1000mg 或等摩尔剂量的 EC-MPS 720mg,禁食,给或不给予泮托拉唑 40mg 2 次/天	MPA AUC(0~12)降低 27%,C_{max} 降低 57%,但泮托拉唑不改变肠溶衣的麦考酚酸钠的药代动力学	[25]
麦考酚酸钠	镁铝悬浮液	12 例病情稳定的肾移植患者服用含镁铝的抗酸药 30mL 和 MMF	MPA 平均降低最大 25%,AUC 降低 37%	[4]
麦考酚酸钠	泮托拉唑	21 例心脏或肺移植受者使用泮托拉唑 40mg,每日一次,和平均剂量为 960mg 的 EC-MPS,2 次/天	MPA AUC、C_{max}、T_{max} 或 IMPDH 活性的 AUC 都没有显著变化	[98]

(待续)

表 102.1(续) 选择的药物与免疫抑制剂的相互作用

免疫抑制剂	交互剂	研究条件(如已报道)	结果	参考文献
西罗莫司	环孢素	24名健康志愿者在单剂量研究中同时或在一剂量的新山地明300mg后4h给予西罗莫司片剂10mg	同时使用与单独使用西罗莫司相比,西罗莫司平均 C_{max} 增加512%,AUC为148%。使用CsA后4h:与单独的西罗莫司相比,西罗莫司 C_{max} 和AUC增加33%	[5]
西罗莫司	环孢素	24名健康志愿者在单剂量研究中同时或在一剂量的新山地明300mg后4h给予西罗莫司片剂10mg	同时给药与单独的西罗莫司相比,西罗莫司平均 C_{max} 增加116%,AUC增加230%。给CsA后4h与单独西罗莫司相比,西罗莫司 C_{max} 增加37%,AUC减少80%	[5]
西罗莫司	环孢素	33名健康志愿者在单剂量交叉研究中接受单剂新山地明300mg的2h前和2h后接受西罗莫司口服溶液5mg	在使用CsA前2h给药,西罗莫司 C_{max} 和AUC与单独施用西罗莫司相当。在使用CsA后2h:与单独使用西罗莫司相比,增加西罗莫司平均 C_{max} 126%,AUC增加141%	[5]
西罗莫司	地尔硫卓	18名健康志愿者同时口服西罗莫司口服溶液10mg和地尔硫120mg	西罗莫司 C_{max} 显著增加1.4倍,T_{max} 增加1.3倍,AUC增加1.6倍,西罗莫司不影响地尔硫的药代动力学	[5]
西罗莫司	红霉素	24名健康志愿者在稳定状态下每日口服西罗莫司溶液2mg和每8h口服红霉素乙基琥珀酸片剂800mg	西罗莫司 C_{max} 增加4.4倍,AUC增加4.2倍,T_{max} 增加0.4h,红霉素 C_{max} 增加1.6倍,AUC增加1.7倍,并且 T_{max} 增加0.3h	[5]
西罗莫司	酮康唑	酮康唑多剂量给药同时服用西罗莫司口服溶液	西罗莫司 C_{max} 增加4.3倍,T_{max} 增加38%,AUC增加10.9倍。西罗莫司的最终 $t_{1/2}$ 没有改变;单剂量西罗莫司不影响酮康唑稳态12h血浆浓度	[5]
西罗莫司	利福平	14名健康志愿者每天服用利福平600mg,给药14天,然后给予单剂量西罗莫司口服溶液20mg	西罗莫司AUC降低82%,C_{max} 降低71%	[5]
西罗莫司	异搏定	26名健康志愿者在稳态下每日给予西罗莫司口服溶液2mg,同时每12h给予维拉帕米180mg	西罗莫司 C_{max} 增加2.3倍,AUC增加2.2倍,T_{max} 没有实质变化	[5]
西罗莫司	伏立康唑	健康男性每12h给口服伏立康唑400mg,1天,然后改为每12h给200mg,8天和单剂量西罗莫司2mg	西罗莫司 C_{max} 增加7倍,AUC增加11倍	[99]
他克莫司	地瑞那韦	肾移植受体病例报告	他克莫司谷浓度增加,需要剂量减少相当于通常剂量的3.5%	[100]

(待续)

表 102.1(续)　选择的药物与免疫抑制剂的相互作用

免疫抑制剂	交互剂	研究条件(如已报道)	结果	参考文献
他克莫司	洛匹那韦/利托那韦	3 例肝移植受者病例报告共同给予洛匹那韦/利托那韦和他克莫司	他克莫司暴露,$t_{1/2}$ 增加约 10 倍	[101]
他克莫司	奈法唑酮	2 例稳定服用他克莫司并加用奈法唑酮的肾移植受者病例报告	他克莫司谷浓度增加>3~5 倍	[102,103]
他克莫司	奈非那韦	5 例与历史对照相比较的肝移植受者和在基于他克莫司的方案中添加奈非那韦之后进行肝移植的病例报告患者	需要他克莫司剂量降低 38~70 倍,以保持相似的谷浓度	[104,105]
他克莫司	奥美拉唑和艾美拉唑,而非兰索拉唑	具有稳定的血液浓度的肾移植受体保持在 5~8ng/mL 之间,而对兰索拉唑(30mg/d)转换为艾美拉唑(40mg/d)	一个月后,他克莫司血液浓度升至 27.4ng/mL。患者切换回兰索拉唑并且他克莫司浓缩归一化至 5~8ng/mL 的目标范围	[106]
他克莫司	泊沙康唑	36 名健康志愿者接受他克莫司 0.05mg/kg/d,以及泊沙康唑 400mg,2 次/天。	他克莫司 C_{max} 增加 121%,AUC 增加 358%,未影响泊沙康唑的药代动力学	[84]
他克莫司	特拉匹韦	单次他克莫司 2mg 口服剂量, 随后为最少 14 天的清除期,随后共同施用单剂 0.5mg 的他克莫司与稳态特拉匹韦 750mg/8h	他克莫司 AUC 增加 70 倍,$t_{1/2}$ 从 40.7(5.85)h 的平均(SD)增加达到 196(159)h	[88]
他克莫司	伏立康唑	原发性肾同种异体移植受者病例报告	他克莫司谷浓度增加≥5 倍,3 天后为 10 倍,5~7 天后为 10 倍	[107]
他克莫司	伏立康唑	健康志愿者每 12h 重复给予口服伏立康唑 400mg×1 天,然后每 12h 予 200mg×6 天和他克莫司 0.1mg/kg 单剂量	他克莫司的 AUC 增加 3 倍(90% CI,2.7~3.8),C_{max} 平均增加 2 倍(90%CI,1.9~2.5)	[99]

MMF,霉酚酸酯;CsA-环孢素;AUC,时间对浓度曲线下的面积;C_{max},最大血药浓度;C_{min},最小血药浓度或低谷;EC-MPS,肠溶型麦考酚酸钠;$t_{1/2}$,半衰期;T_{max},血药浓度达到峰值的时间。

书)。钙离子对 MPA 吸收的影响已有相关研究。在一项以 6 名健康男性志愿者为对象的研究中,使用了 MMF 和聚卡波非钙的受试者的 MPA 暴露降低了 50%[11]。这可能是由于在胃肠道中 MMF 和钙离子之间有螯合作用[11]。研究表明,MMF 与铁离子之间也有类似的相互作用。对 7 名健康志愿者使用 MMF 的同时给予硫酸亚铁缓释片,MPA 暴露降低了 90%[12]。尽管如此,别的研究并没有在肾移植受体中发现 MPA 的吸收减少[13-16],所以这种相互作用的重要性仍然存在争议。当 MPA 和钙依赖磷酸酶抑制剂(CNI)与二价阳离子联用时,建议检测 MPA 和 CNI 的浓度并合理调整剂量。为了使这些潜在的相互作用最小化,包含镁和铝成分的制剂与他克莫司或霉酚酯制剂的服用时间应间隔至少 2h。

考来烯胺也会抑制许多药物的吸收[17]。虽然在移植受体中的数据很少,考来烯胺一般会作为治疗血脂异常的最后选择[18,19]。镧、司维拉姆等一些药物还可能抑制免疫抑制剂的吸收。司维拉姆会降低 MPA 的 C_{max} 和 AUC,必要时应使两种药的给药时间间隔至少 2h[3,20]。镧有可能结合阳离子解酸剂形成复合物[21],因此有可能也会与 MPA 结合。

胃肠道的变化可能会影响免疫抑制剂的吸收。来自胃肠道的影响因素包括蠕动缓慢(常见于腹内手术之后)、排空障碍(常见于Ⅰ型糖尿病相关的胃轻瘫)、pH 值的变化、低血流量以及表面积减少,这些因素都会阻碍吸收。泻药会通过加快药物通过肠道的速度来减少药物的吸收,而减少肠蠕动的药物(如麻醉药、阿托品)会延长药物通过肠道的时间以增加吸收时间。液体摄入,如 250mL 水,可以通过增加溶解度来提高药物的吸收。同样的,促胃肠运动的药品,如甲氧氯普胺[22]和红霉素可以通过促进胃肠道蠕动和胃排空,促进药物在小肠的吸收来增加血药浓度。

这种相互作用可能是由胃肠道中的运载体和酶介导的。西罗莫司和环孢素之间的强相互作用就被认为是通过这种机制介导的。环孢素和西罗莫司都是

表 102.2 常见的免疫抑制剂和食物相互作用及其常见的代谢和转运途径[3-8]

药物分类	药物	食物对吸收的影响	代谢和运输	
			对 CYP P450 3A4/5 的影响	对 P-糖蛋白的影响
皮质类固醇	泼尼松	无影响	底物	底物
钙调神经磷酸酶抑制剂	环孢素	多变	底物,抑制剂	底物,抑制剂
	他克莫司	高脂肪餐:C_{max} 减少 77%,AUC 减少 37%;高碳水化合物餐:C_{max} 减少 65%,AUC 减少 28%	底物,抑制剂	无
mTOR 抑制剂	西罗莫司	高脂肪餐:AUC 减少 23%~35%	底物	底物
	依维莫司	高脂肪餐:C_{max} 减少 60%,AUC 减少 16%	底物	底物
增殖抑制	硫唑嘌呤	无影响	无	无
	麦考酚酯	C_{max} 减少 40%,AUC 无变化	无	无
	肠溶包衣麦考酚酸钠	高脂肪餐:C_{max} 减少 33%,AUC 无变化	无	无
抗 T 细胞治疗	马抗胸腺细胞球蛋白	无影响	无	无
	兔抗胸腺细胞球蛋白	无影响	无	无
IL-2 受体阻断剂	巴利昔单抗	无影响	无	无
协同刺激信号阻断	贝拉西普	无影响	无	无

AUC,时间对浓度曲线下的面积;C_{max},最大血药浓度或峰值。

CYP3A4 和磷酸化的糖蛋白的基质。环孢素还是 CYP3A4 和磷酸化的糖蛋白的强效抑制剂(见表 102.3)[23,24]。当同时摄入环孢素和西罗莫司时,环孢素被认为抑制了西罗莫司在内脏中的代谢,从而增强西罗莫司的生物利用度。环孢素对磷酸化的糖蛋白的抑制作用也减少了西罗莫司从消化道排泄,从而使西罗莫司的生物利用率增高。这两种机制的联合作用使西罗莫司和环孢素联用时,西罗莫司的 C_{max} 和 AUC 大幅提升。当西罗莫司和环孢素的给药时间间隔在 4h 时,这种相互作用的强度会降低,但仍有较大意义(表 102.4)。有趣的是,这种作用对环孢素的血药浓度影响不大。要提醒患者注意这种作用,并且不要随意改变服药习惯。临床医生需要密切监控西罗莫司的使用,因为环孢素剂量要求和血药浓度会随时间减少。

药物相互作用也可以发生在联用质子泵抑制(PPI)和 MPA 时。质子泵抑制剂抑制胃酸分泌并增加胃 pH 值。研究表明,MMF 与泮托拉唑、兰索拉唑、雷贝拉唑和奥美拉唑联用会使 MMF 在胃 pH 值较高时的溶解度减少,导致其生物利用度降低和全身性 MPA 暴露降低[25-31]。质子泵抑制剂联合用药会减少服用 MMF 的心脏移植受者的 MPA 暴露[26,27]。然而,回顾性研究没有证据表明当 MMF 与 PPI 一起使用时 MPA 的 AUC 会降低[32]。因此,PPI 治疗对 MMF 吸收的影响仍然存在争议。尽管在临床实践中这是一种令人苦恼的非典型现象,接受这种联合治疗的患者仍应该能够达到 MPA 血浆浓度。肠溶剂型的 MPA、EC-MPS 可以通过胃里的酸性环境并在到达小肠的中性环境中溶解[33]。因此,当 PPI 与 EC-MPS 联用时,会对 MPA 的生物利用率和系统暴露的影响有限制作用。这在泮托拉唑和奥美拉唑中得到证实[25,29]。

分布

分布是药物从血管内向血管外空间转移的过程,两个隔室在移植后处于动态通量中。许多过程可影响药物的分布,包括药物结合血浆蛋白的能力、药物转运蛋白、脂质溶解度、组织渗透性和血流量。然而,许多药物的相互作用通过蛋白质或药物诱导的运输变化影响分布机制而发生。

许多药物与蛋白质结合,然而蛋白质结合的程度变化很大。一般来说,高蛋白质的药物存在通过结合变

表 102.3　通过药物类别诱导、抑制或作为 CYP3A4/5 底物的药物[3-8,43,74,75]

药物类别	CYP450 3A4/5 的底物
抗惊厥药	卡马西平、乙琥胺
抗感染药	克拉霉素、氨苯砜、红霉素、酮康唑
抗反转录病毒	依曲韦林、茚地那韦、洛匹那韦、奈非那韦、利托那韦、沙奎那韦、特拉匹韦
抗肿瘤剂	克唑替尼、多西他赛、依托泊苷、氟他胺、伊马替尼、伊立替康、索拉非尼、舒尼替尼、他莫昔芬、紫杉醇、长春新碱
心血管药物	胺碘酮、氨氯地平、阿托伐他汀、地尔硫卓、决奈达隆、依普利酮、非洛地平、伊拉地平、洛伐他汀、尼卡地平、硝苯地平、尼莫地平、尼索地平、奎尼丁、辛伐他汀、维拉帕米
免疫抑制剂	环孢素、依维莫司、地塞米松、泼尼松、西罗莫司、他克莫司
镇痛类药物	芬太尼、美沙酮
精神类药物	舍曲林
其他	阿普匹坦、阿莫达夫尼、布地奈德、溴隐亭、大麻素、西沙必利、康尼伐坦、达沙替尼、地塞米松、炔雌醇、非索非那定、氢化可的松、伊马替尼、兰索拉唑、莫达非尼、昂丹司琼、孕酮、利福布汀、唑吡坦
药物类别	**CYP450 3A4/5 的诱导剂**
抗感染药	异烟肼、萘夫西林、利福平、利福喷丁、利福布汀
抗惊厥药	卡马西平、磷苯妥英、奥卡西平、苯巴比妥、苯妥英、扑米酮
抗反转录病毒	依法韦仑*、依曲韦林、奈韦拉平
免疫抑制剂	地塞米松、泼尼松、泼尼松龙
其他	阿莫沙芬、波生坦、溴隐亭、地拉罗司、灰黄霉素、莫达非尼、奥曲肽#、吡格列酮、圣约翰草
药物类别	**CYP450 3A4/5 抑制剂**
抗生素	氯霉素、环丙沙星、诺氟沙星(仅报道了环孢素)、喹诺酮
止吐药	阿瑞匹坦
抗肿瘤药	克里唑蒂尼、达沙替尼、依托泊苷、伊马替尼、尼罗替尼、舒尼替尼、他莫昔芬、维莫司尼
抗反转录病毒	安定奈韦、阿扎那韦、波普瑞韦、地瑞那韦、地拉夫定、依法韦仑*、福沙那韦、茚地那韦(强效)、奈非那韦(强效)、利托那韦、沙奎那韦(强效)、特拉匹韦、替拉那韦
唑类抗真菌剂	克霉唑、氟康唑、伊曲康唑(强效)、酮康唑(强效)、咪康唑、泊沙康唑、伏立康唑
钙通道阻滞剂	地尔硫卓、非洛地平、尼卡地平、维拉帕米
心血管药物	胺碘酮、决奈达隆
免疫抑制剂	环孢素(仅限 3A4 抑制剂)、依维莫司、他克莫司
大环内酯类	克拉霉素(强效)、红霉素、泰利霉素(强效)
精神类药物	氟西汀、氟伏沙明、奈法唑酮(强效)、舍曲林
其他	溴隐亭、西咪替丁、西沙必利、考尼伐坦、达那唑、乙炔雌二醇、葡萄柚汁、格列本脲、甲基泼尼松龙、莫达非尼、匹莫齐特、异丙酚、奎宁、杨桃、扎鲁司特

* 可能诱导或抑制。

奥曲肽抑制生长激素分泌，这可能减少由 CYP3A4 代谢的药物的代谢清除。

化介导的潜在药物相互作用的风险。蛋白质，如 α-1-酸性糖蛋白、脂蛋白或白蛋白可以结合血液或组织中的药物，并降低到达靶点的药物的速率和(或)量。只有未结合的药物具有药理活性，因此蛋白质结合率的变化对于与一种或多种蛋白高度结合的药物十分重要。许多药物与蛋白质结合，然而，作为蛋白质结合的结果仅有少数药物相互作用与临床相关。使用高蛋白结合的药物可以从它们的共同蛋白质中置换，从而增加未结合的药物部分。弱酸主要结合白蛋白，碱性药物结合 α-酸糖蛋白。参与药物结合最重要的蛋白质是白蛋白。因此，某些与白蛋白高度结合的酸性药物(如 MPA、呋塞米、非甾体抗炎药、青霉素、苯妥英、水杨酸盐和磺胺类药物)与另一种与白蛋白结合的药物联用时可能导致游离药物浓度增加。同样，与 α-1-酸性糖蛋白结合的碱性药物(如利多卡因、吩噻嗪、普萘洛尔、喹那啶和三环抗抑郁药)与另一种与 α-1-酸性糖蛋白结合的药物联用时也会使游离药物浓度增加。

麦考酚酸及其主要代谢产物麦考酚酸葡萄糖醛酸

表 102.4 钙调神经磷酸酶抑制剂、mTOR 抑制剂和麦考酚酸的相互作用[2,3,5,8,23,24]

西罗莫司			依维莫司	麦考酚酸
环孢素	同时服用 西罗莫司溶液：西罗莫司 C_{max} 增加 116%，AUC 增加 230%，波谷升高，T_{max} 下降 西罗莫司片剂：西罗莫司 C_{max} 升高 512%，AUC 升高 148% 对 CSA 浓度没有显著影响	间隔 4h 服用 西罗莫司溶液：西罗莫司 C_{max} 升高 37%，AUC 升高80%，波谷升高，T_{max} 降低 西罗莫司片：西罗莫司 C_{max} 增加，AUC 升高 33%	依维莫司 C_{max} 增加 82%，AUC 增加 168% 依维莫司随着时间的推移可能轻微增加 CsA 浓度	MPA 浓度降低 30%~50%，由于抑制肠肝再循环，CsA 浓度未受显著影响
他克莫司	他克莫司水平降低，对西罗莫司浓度没有显著影响		对他克莫司或依维莫司的浓度没有显著影响	对他克莫司或 MPA 浓度无显著影响

C_{max}，最大血药浓度；CsA，环孢素，MPA，麦考酚酸。

苷(MPAG)可与白蛋白[3]高度结合(分别> 98%和82%)。随着 MPAG 的累积(与肾功能不良的个体一样)，其可以从白蛋白结合位点置换 MPA，导致 MPA 游离增加并具有更大潜在的药理作用[34]。麦考酚酸盐和苯妥英或茶碱结合治疗可导致茶碱的蛋白质结合从 53%降低至 45%，苯妥英从 90%降至 87%[3]。因此，在需要严格控制苯妥英或茶碱浓度的患者中，当与麦考酚酸盐一起使用时，可能需要额外监测(游离苯妥英，如果有的话)。这些类型的相互作用难以检测，并且仅可通过测量游离药物浓度来注意。具有这些相互作用风险的患者应密切监测不良反应和过度免疫抑制。

活性药物转运蛋白

活性药物转运蛋白控制药物在细胞内外的移动，并可影响生物利用度、靶组织的药物浓度和许多药物的消除。常见的活性药物转运系统包括 P-糖蛋白和人类有机阴离子转运多肽(OATP)。这些转运系统受遗传因素调节，但也可受食物和药物的影响。药物可以上调或下调这些蛋白质，从而改变肠吸收、近端肾小管排泄或胆汁排泄。药物-药物相互作用可以通过转运蛋白介导，尽管临床上难以检测。如果一种药物是抑制剂而另一种是相同转运蛋白的底物，则这种类型的药物相互作用更有可能发生。许多影响 CYP450 的药物和食物也影响活性药物传输系统，大大混淆了这些相互作用发生的基本机制[35]。

P-糖蛋白

P-糖蛋白是分布或表达在许多细胞(包括肠上皮、肝细胞、肾近端肾小管细胞、肾上腺和血脑屏障)中的流出转运蛋白的家族的一部分。P-糖蛋白也被称为多药耐药蛋白 1(MDR1)或 ATP 结合亚家族 B 成员 1(ABCB1)蛋白。P-糖蛋白是涉及底物穿过细胞膜运动的外排转运蛋白，并且在许多临床上重要的治疗物质的分布和消除中起重要作用。药物、食物和体内代谢物质可以作为这些转运蛋白的抑制剂和(或)诱导物。环孢素、依维莫司、西罗莫司和泼尼松是 P-糖蛋白的底物(表 102.2)。体外数据表明，他克莫司既不是 P-糖蛋白的底物也不是抑制剂[36]。环孢素是 P-糖蛋白的抑制剂[37,38]。在这种类型的相互作用的实例中，环孢素可通过抑制 P-糖蛋白和减少药物从肿瘤细胞外排而增强柔红霉素、多西他赛、多柔比星、表柔比星、依托泊苷、米托蒽醌、紫杉醇和长春花生物碱的功效。卡维地洛抑制 P-糖蛋白，因此可增加环孢素的血液浓度[39]。

有机阴离子转运多肽

有机阴离子转运多肽也在药物-药物相互作用中起作用。例如，环孢素抑制瑞格列奈的代谢[40,41]。环孢素似乎通过抑制 OATP1B1 (其是活性肝摄取转运蛋白)而减少瑞格列奈的肝脏摄取。在一项对健康志愿者的随机交叉研究中，与安慰剂相比，环孢素使瑞格列奈的血浆浓度提高 175%，AUC 提高 244%[40]。可以发生涉及 CYP450、P-糖蛋白和 OATP 的复杂药物相互作用。例如，环孢素是 CYP3A4、P-糖蛋白和 OATP 的抑制剂。安立生坦是 ET(A)选择性内皮素受体拮抗剂，是 CYP3A4、OATPs 和 P-糖蛋白的潜在底物。28 名健康受试者单独使用安利生坦 5mg 每日一次或环孢素 100~150mg 每日两次，另外 24 名受试者在安利生坦稳定状态下单独接受环孢素[42]。环孢素和安立生坦联用的组合，安立生坦 C_{max} 增加 1.5 倍，AUC 增加 2 倍。环孢素 C_{max} 和 AUC 仅轻微增加(分别为 906ng/mL 对 1014ng/mL 和 3.05μgh/mL 对 3.37μgh/mL)。因此，如果与环孢素联合给药，安立生坦推荐的最大剂量为 5mg。

代谢

即使当药物吸收和分布正在进行时，药物消除也会开始。在达到全身循环之前，口服给药的药物通过门静脉循环通过肝脏。胃肠道和肝脏含有可以在某些药物到达全身循环之前代谢它们的酶。大多数药物被这些酶代谢为无活性或活性较低的代谢物。在移植受者中，最常见类型的药代动力学药物相互作用涉及细胞色素 P450 酶系统。通过 CYP3A 酶代谢的免疫抑制剂的概述见表 102.2。

虽然有许多代谢位点，肝脏是药物氧化、还原、水解和结合的最重要位点。许多亲脂性药物经历生物转化为待排泄的亲水性化合物。药物生物转化反应由主要在肝脏中发生的阶段Ⅰ(如氧化、还原)或阶段 2(如缀合)反应组成。CYP450 酶系统是参与药物代谢的氧化生物转化反应的关键途径。CYP450 是可以分为家族、亚家族和(或)单一酶的血蛋白超家族。CYP450 酶由字母 CYP(代表 CYP)指定，后面是表示家族的阿拉伯数字、表示亚家族的字母(当存在 2 个或更多个字母时)和表示个体基因的另一个阿拉伯数字亚家族(如 CYP2D6)。在 CYP450 的不同同种型中，CYP3A4 和 5 在人类中普遍存在，并且对移植药物的药物代谢非常重要。

药物可以是一种或多种 CYP450 酶的底物和(或)也是相同或不同酶的抑制剂或诱导剂(表 102.3)[43]。在人类中，这些通常包括 CYP450 3A4、3A5、2C9、2C19、2D6、2A6、2E1 和 1A2。根据定义，底物是作用于或受酶影响的药物。抑制剂降低酶的代谢能力，因此可以降低特定底物的代谢，通常导致药物效应增加。相反，诱导剂可以增加特定底物的代谢，通常导致药物效应降低。如果一种药物是抑制剂或诱导剂而另一种是相同酶的底物，则这种类型的药物相互作用更有可能发生。许多药物是 CYP 抑制剂和诱导剂，但它们的效力变化很大。抑制剂或诱导剂的效力极大地影响这些相互作用的临床相关性。依维莫司、西罗莫司、环孢素和他克莫司是 CYP3A4/5 的底物。泼尼松和泼尼松龙的活性代谢物也是 CYP3A4 的底物，尽管临床上很少发生显著的相互作用。环孢素是 CYP3A4/5 的抑制剂和底物，依维莫司是 CYP3A4/5 的竞争性抑制剂和 CYP2D6 的混合抑制剂。

CYP3A4/5 的抑制剂和诱导剂列于表 102.3。如果患者已使用 CYP3A4/5 底物，则应避免使用这些药物。如果患者不能避免使用 CYP3A4/5 的强抑制剂或诱导剂，则必须密切监测药物浓度和毒性。当抑制剂与环孢素和他克莫司共同给药时，可获得有关精确剂量调整的有限数据。当接受他克莫司治疗的患者开始接受伏立康唑或泊沙康唑治疗时，他克莫司剂量最初应减少到当前剂量的 1/3，随后的剂量应根据他克莫司全血浓度进行调整[2]。

虽然大多数代谢相互作用通过 CYP450 发生，特别是在使用 CNI 和哺乳动物类雷帕霉素靶蛋白(mTOR)抑制剂的情况下，其他类型的相互作用发生于使用非 CYP450 酶系统代谢的免疫抑制剂时。别嘌呤醇抑制黄嘌呤氧化酶，导致硫唑嘌呤代谢减少和严重的骨髓抑制和全血细胞减少[44]。这种组合具有潜在的严重的相互作用，应当避免。如果不可能，这种组合可用于硫唑嘌呤剂量显著减少 67%~75%[6]以及密切监测的情况下。

麦考酚酸被尿苷-二磷酸葡糖醛酸转移酶(UGT)酶广泛代谢。然而，临床上尚未明确与 MPA 相关的相互作用。

排泄

排泄是涉及药代动力学的最后一个过程，指药物从体内消除的过程。肾脏是水溶性药物的主要排泄位置。尿液 pH 值可能影响药物的重吸收和排泄。尿液酸化使弱酸类重吸收增加排泄减少并使弱碱类重吸收减少。尿液碱化具有相反的效果。

对于一些药物，肾小管中的活性分泌物是重要的消除途径。药物也可以通过肾小球滤过，分子的被动转运过程由肾脏排泄。当药物浓度高时，分泌转运变得饱和。霉酚酸和抗病毒药包括阿昔洛韦、更昔洛韦和伐昔洛韦，缬更昔洛韦经肾小管分泌。伴随使用 MPA 和这些抗病毒剂可导致管状分泌的竞争和 MPA 和(或)抗病毒暴露的增加。12 名健康志愿者使用霉酚酸酯(1g)和阿昔洛韦(800mg)显示 MPA AUC 和 C_{max} 没有显著变化。然而，MPAG 和阿昔洛韦血浆 AUC 分别增加了 10.6%和 21.9%[3]。单剂量给予 12 名稳定的肾移植患者

MMF(1.5g)和静脉注射更昔洛韦(5mg/kg)后,在两者之间未观察到药代动力学相互作用。在肾损伤的存在下,MPAG和更昔洛韦在肾小管竞争分泌,但两者的血浆浓度都增加了。在肾损伤患者中共同使用MPA和更昔洛韦、缬更昔洛韦、阿昔洛韦或伐昔洛韦时,必须仔细监测血液毒性和过度免疫抑制的迹象[3]。

其他次要的排泄部位是胆道系统、唾液、汗液和肺。高分子量的极性亲脂性药物通过活性分泌转运在胆汁中排泄。麦考酚酸和MPAG的胆汁排泄、远端吸收和再吸收可利用几种运输机制,包括OATP和多药耐药相关蛋白(MRP-2)[45]。

麦考酚酯经历肠肝再循环,并且一些MPA药物相互作用通过干扰该过程介导。在肠肝再循环中,在胆汁中分泌的药物从肠道重吸收到循环中(图102.1)。就麦考酚酸而言,MPA在肠和肝中通过UGT酶进行葡萄糖醛酸化,以形成主要葡萄糖醛酸苷代谢物MPAG,其被排泄到胆汁中。在那里,MPAG解偶联回到MPA并在胃肠道中被再吸收到体循环中,从而增加MPA的血浆浓度。胆汁酸螯合剂,如考来烯胺,通过抑制肠肝再循环减少MPA AUC,导致MPA AUC降低约40%[3]。环孢素还通过抑制MRP-2转运蛋白来中断MPA的肠肝再循环,从而减少排泄到胆汁中的MPAG的量,并且不太可转化为MPA和重吸收。当与环孢素同时给予时,与单独给予或与他克莫司或西罗莫司共同给药相比,麦考酚酸血浆浓度下降30%~40%[13]。在肾移植患者中,与MMF和环孢素共同给药相比,单独给予MMF时平均MPA $AUC_{0\text{-}12}$增加30%~50%[3,33]。

抗生素也可能与麦考酚酸相互作用。麦考酚酸葡糖苷酸在胃肠道中通过葡糖醛酸糖苷酶转化为MPA。葡糖醛酸酶由细菌产生,并且在抗生素存在下,可获得较少的葡糖醛酸糖苷酶。在患者和健康志愿者中使用减少胃肠道菌群的抗生素,可减少MPA的解偶联和MPA的肠肝再循环[46,47]。

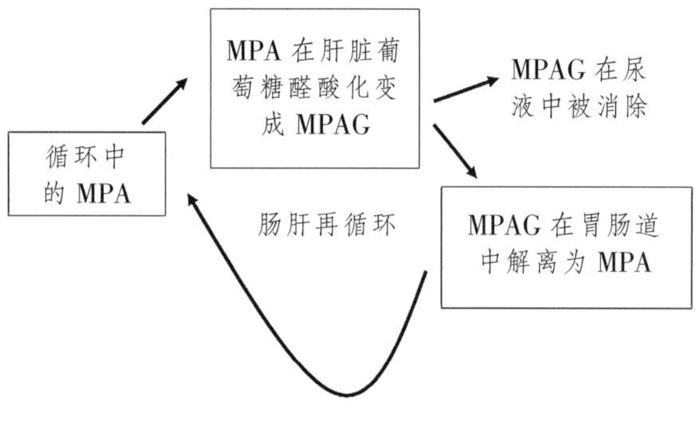

图102.1 麦考酚酯肠肝再循环。麦考酚酯经历肠肝再循环,并且这种机制介导了一些MPA药物的相互作用。在肠肝再循环中,分泌在胆汁中的药物从肠中再吸收到循环中。MPA,麦考酚酸;MPAG,麦考酚酸酸葡糖苷酸。

药效学相互作用

药效学研究药物暴露与药理作用或临床反应(疗效或毒性)之间的关系。

药效学影响因素包括药物与其受体之间的关系、年龄、耐受性和生理因素。几个术语被用来描述药物与其受体之间的相互作用。协同药物效应指两种或多种药物联用时产生的效应大于它们各自效应的总和。例如,呋塞米和美托拉宗联用时,可产生比单独给药时更强的利尿作用。当两种药物结合形成总效应时,就会产生加性药物效应。在移植受者中,药效动力学药物相互作用通常导致毒性增强或功效变化。

药物之间的相互作用——CNI

CNI的常见副作用包括神经毒性、肾毒性、高血压、糖尿病、血脂异常和电解质紊乱。如有可能,应避免在移植受体中也使用引起相同副作用的药物。高钾血症在移植后常见,因此当联用与高钾血症相关的药物(如保钾利尿剂、ACE抑制剂、血管紧张素Ⅱ受体阻断剂、阿米洛利、螺内酯和氨苯蝶啶)和CNI时,应密切监测。与环孢素和安慰剂或硫唑嘌呤对照相比,用环孢素和西罗莫司治疗的移植受者具有更高的血清肌酐水平和更低的肾小球滤过率[5]。依维莫司与标准剂量环孢素联用增加了肾毒性的风险,导致较低的肾小球滤过率。为了减少肾功能障碍,环孢素与依维莫司联用时需减少剂量[8]。

药物相互作用——抗代谢物

骨髓抑制(包括贫血、白细胞减少和血小板减少症)是与麦考酚酸盐和硫唑嘌呤治疗相关的常见不良反应。鉴于硫唑嘌呤和麦考酚酸均抑制嘌呤代谢,不推荐联合使用[3,4]。

当给予抗代谢物时,应密切监测增加出血风险的药物(如抗凝血剂、血小板抑制剂和血栓形成剂)。当抗代谢物与抗病毒剂,如阿昔洛韦、更昔洛韦、伐昔洛韦和缬更昔洛韦一起给予时，可能发生骨髓抑制[3,4,48–50]。因此，当这些药物联合给药时，应更频繁地获得全血细胞计数。减少麦考酚酯剂量或使用粒细胞集落刺激因子是治疗麦考酚酯和抗病毒药物所致骨髓抑制的选择。

硫唑嘌呤和来氟米特都与肝毒性有关。当这些药物一起给予时，需定期监测肝功能。使用硫唑嘌呤和血管紧张素转化酶(ACE)抑制剂可导致贫血的风险增加。

药物–器官相互作用

表 102.5 提供了与移植相关的潜在药效学相互作用的列表。两种或多种肾毒性药物联用是导致加重肾毒性的药效学相互作用的实例。例如，应避免联合使用氨基糖苷和利尿剂，特别是在具有潜在的肾功能减退并正在接受 CNI 治疗的肾移植受者。根据移植的器官，某些药物–器官的相互作用可能相当显著。表 102.6 给出了因对移植物具有高度毒性而应避免或最小化的药物–器官相互作用。草药或天然产物有时不被认为是药物，但可对肝脏具有显著的毒性作用，特别是当与其他肝毒性药物联用时。表 102.7 是肝移植受者应避免的肝毒素的列表。同样，胰腺、心脏或肺移植受者应避免可能增加胰腺炎、高血糖或损害心脏或肺功能的药物。

药物–疾病相互作用

已知引起高血糖的 CNI 与已经存在糖尿病的患者高血糖症的恶化或新发糖尿病的发展相关，特别是在非洲血统的受试者中[51–53]。为了使这种药效学相互作用最小化，应定期监测移植后患者的血糖和体重。

一般来说，移植受体不应接受活的病毒疫苗，因为他们的免疫反应能力受损，因此病毒复制的风险很高。移植受者可能需要更高剂量或更频繁的灭活疫苗的加强剂。同样，在移植受者中应仔细考虑共同给予可能危及免疫系统的任何药物的风险和益处，如抗肿瘤药、自身免疫性疾病治疗和具有免疫抑制性质的天然产物(即紫锥菊)[54]。

许多其他药物–疾病状态相互作用也可能发生。与 CNI 和 mTOR 抑制剂相关的罕见不良反应是血栓性微血管病变。这些免疫抑制剂联用与血栓性微血管病变风险增加相关[55]。他克莫司和奎尼丁，决奈达隆

表 102.5 药效学相互作用

免疫抑制剂	相互作用的药物	效果
所有免疫抑制	疫苗	疫苗效果降低
所有免疫抑制	抗肿瘤药、自身免疫性疾病治疗	免疫抑制和骨髓抑制加强
钙调神经磷酸酶抑制剂	保钾利尿剂、阿米洛利、螺内酯、氨苯蝶啶、TMP/SMZ	高钾血症增加
钙调神经磷酸酶抑制剂	西罗莫司/依维莫司	血栓性微血管病/溶血性风险增加，尿毒症综合征/血栓性血小板减少性紫癜
钙调神经磷酸酶抑制剂	降糖药/抗糖尿病药	直接 β 细胞毒性–高血糖
钙调神经磷酸酶抑制剂	有关肾毒素的列表，见表 102.6	肾毒性风险增加
他克莫司	奎尼丁、决奈达隆、胺碘酮、阿夫唑嗪、蒿甲醚/本芴醇、氯喹、环丙沙星、克唑替尼、尼罗替尼、喹硫平、奎宁、丁苯那嗪、硫利达嗪、凡德他尼、托瑞米芬、齐拉西酮、雷诺嗪、西沙必利、达沙替尼	增加 QT 间期延长和室速
环孢素	米诺地尔	附加性多毛症
环孢素	雄激素	肝毒性增加
麦考酚酯	硫唑嘌呤	骨髓移植增加
麦考酚酯	抗凝剂、血小板抑制剂、血栓形成剂	出血风险增加
麦考酚酯	抗生素	可能改变 GI 菌群和肠肝再循环
麦考酚酯	阿昔洛韦、更昔洛韦、伐昔洛韦、缬更昔洛韦、TMP–SMX	增加中性粒细胞减少的风险
硫唑嘌呤	来氟米特	增加肝毒性的风险
硫唑嘌呤	ACEi	增加贫血的风险
西罗莫司/依维莫司	ARB/ACEi、头孢菌素、NSAID/水杨酸盐、青霉素	增加血管性水肿的风险
泼尼松	安非他酮	增加癫痫发作的风险

ARB，血管紧张素受体阻断剂；ACEi，血管紧张素转换酶抑制剂；GI，胃肠道；TMP–SMZ，甲氧苄啶/磺胺甲恶唑。

表 102.6 可能损害或对抗移植器官的有益效果的选择性药物

肾脏(肾毒性)	肝脏(肝毒性)	肺(肺毒性)	胰腺(胰腺炎)	心脏(心脏毒性)
阿昔洛韦	对乙酰氨基酚	胺碘酮	硫唑嘌呤	多柔比星
阿德福韦	阿莫西林-克拉维酸	β阻断剂	雌激素	曲妥珠单抗
氨基糖苷类	硫唑嘌呤	博来霉素	呋塞米	
两性霉素 B	卡托普利	白消安	甲硝唑	
ARB/ACEi	卡马西平	环磷酰胺	戊脒	
卡铂	红霉素	甲氨蝶呤	水杨酸盐	
西多福韦	HMG-CoA 还原酶抑制剂	米诺地尔	柳氮磺吡啶	
顺铂	异烟肼	丝裂霉素-C	四环素	
环孢素和他克莫司	萘夫西林	亚硝基脲	噻嗪利尿剂	
膦甲酸	呋喃妥英	普鲁卡因胺		
更昔洛韦	苯妥英	奎尼丁		
免疫球蛋白 IV	罗格列酮			
戊脒 IV	四环素			
甲氨蝶呤	甲氧苄啶-磺胺甲恶唑			
NSAIDS				
帕米膦酸盐				
多黏菌素				
甲氧苄啶-磺胺甲恶唑				
万古霉素				
唑来膦酸				

ARB,血管紧张素受体阻断剂; ACEi,血管紧张素转换酶抑制剂; IV,血管内。

或胺碘酮的联用与QT间期和尖端扭转型室间隔的延长有关[56-58]。如需联用,则应使用EKG进行闭合监测。西罗莫司和依维莫司与ACE抑制剂、非甾体抗炎药、水杨酸盐、头孢菌素或青霉素的给药可能增加血管性水肿的风险[5,8,59]。泼尼松和安非他酮的组合可能增加癫痫的发作风险[60]。

胆固醇药物和药物相互作用

血脂异常在移植受者中常见,并且常需要治疗,因此,降低胆固醇药物和免疫抑制剂之间的相互作用可能性很高。许多HMG-CoA还原酶抑制剂(他汀类药物)是CYP3A4的底物,并与横纹肌溶解症和肌炎有关。抑制CYP3A4的药物,如环孢素,可能与他汀有显著的相互作用,增加他汀类药物浓度并增加肌肉毒性的风险。为了避免或使这些相互作用最小化,当与环孢素联用时,推荐使用较低剂量的他汀类(表102.8)[61,62]。匹伐他汀(一种HMG-CoA还原酶抑制剂)禁止与环孢素联用。环孢素也是OATP转运蛋白的已知抑制剂,并且匹伐他汀主要通过OATP1B1进入人肝细胞。这种相互作用可导致匹伐他汀浓度增加。罗苏伐他汀、普伐他汀、氟伐他汀与其他HMG-CoA还原酶抑制剂相比,不太可能与环孢素有显著的相互作用,因为它们是CYP3A4的不良底物。

血脂异常的其他治疗选择包括纤维酸衍生物、依泽替米贝和胆甾酮。对于高甘油三酯血症通常选择的

表 102.7 作为潜在肝毒素的草药产品[54]

• African remedy	• 石蚕属植物	• 薄荷油
• Black colash	• 戈多洛洛茶	• 锯棕榈
• 八角莲	• 金不换	• 檫树
• 小槲树	• 生命根	• 美黄芩
• 小槲树叶	• 卡瓦	• 小柴胡汤
• CHM	• 康普茶菇	• 如松萝酸
• 中国凉茶	• 马黛茶	• 缬草
• 紫草	• Mediterranean remedy	• Venencapsan
• 七叶树	• 楝油	• Zulu remedy
• European remedy	• 槲寄生	

表 102.8 当给予环孢素时,HMG-CoA 还原酶抑制剂剂量[7,61,62]

药物	代谢途径	通常起始剂量 *	与环孢素合用的剂量
罗苏伐他汀	CYP2C9	10mg/d	5mg/d
洛伐他汀	CYP3A4	10~20mg/d	10mg/d
匹伐他汀	由 CYP2C9 次要	2mg/d	禁用于服用环孢素的患者
普伐他汀	无已知的 CYP 代谢	40mg/d	环孢素 10mg 每天一次
氟伐他汀	CYP2C9	20~40mg/d	不变
阿托伐他汀	CYP3A4	10~20mg/d	10mg/d
辛伐他汀 *	CYP3A4	10~20mg/d	禁用于服用环孢素的患者^

HMG,3-羟基-3-甲基-戊二酰基;CoA, 辅酶 A;* 服用氨氯地平和雷诺嗪的患者不超过 20mg;胺碘酮、维拉帕米和地尔硫卓的患者不超过 10mg;由于横纹肌炎的风险,患者的初始剂量不要大于 80mg。

治疗是纤维酸衍生物。然而, 吉非贝齐和环孢素联用时,存在肾功能障碍的附加风险。环孢素也可增加依泽替米贝血清浓度,依泽替米贝也可增加环孢素的浓度。接受这种药物组合的患者应监测依泽替米贝的不良反应。考来烯胺通过与药物结合而减少许多药物的吸收,包括免疫抑制药物。因此,在移植受者中,考来烯胺通常保留作为治疗血脂异常的最后一步。

草药产品、葡萄柚和药物相互作用

草药产品可能与免疫抑制剂具有显著的药效学相互作用,导致不利的免疫结果和不良反应,如出血。遗憾的是,草药产品在移植患者中的疗效研究不足。圣约翰草是与免疫抑制剂相互作用的草药产品的实例。圣约翰草产生 CYP3A4 和 P-糖蛋白。因此,肾脏、胰腺、肝脏和心脏移植受者中报道了圣约翰草与免疫抑制剂联用而产生了排斥反应[63]。紫锥菊是一种草药产品,也可能对免疫系统产生不良影响。体外研究表明,它激活吞噬细胞、T 淋巴细胞增殖和细胞因子的产生[64]。天然草药可能危害肝脏或移植肝脏,列于表 102.7[54]。几种草药产品也可能增加出血的风险。建议在移植手术前至少 2~3 周停用草药产品。临床医生应仔细考虑天然产品对免疫系统的影响、与移植药物相互作用的可能性以及对移植器官造成伤害的风险。如果有同样有效和安全的处方药物可用,则一般应避免草药。

葡萄柚是维生素和植物化学品的优良来源, 但葡萄柚与许多重要的药物有相互作用。葡萄柚中的一组活性化合物,称为呋喃香豆素,是 CYP3A4 酶的有效抑制剂。基于 CYP3A4 酶在肠中的抑制机制,通过呋喃香豆素,导致酶的完全失活[63]。这导致对 CYP3A4 底物肠清除的抑制作用延长, 需要重新恢复同工酶以恢复正常的代谢功能。许多口服药剂需经 CYP3A4 的首关代谢,酶抑制作用十分显著,导致作为 CYP3A4(特别是环孢素)底物的药物全身暴露的增加。应指导教育患者葡萄柚汁与免疫抑制剂之间的相互作用非常重要。频繁地监测血液 CNI 浓度在经常食用葡萄柚的患者中可能是必需的。杨桃也可能具有类似作用。

药物基因组学和药物相互作用

遗传变异对药物的药代动力学和药效学有重要影响。然而,相对于其他治疗领域,除他克莫司外,移植方面的药物基因组数据有限,其中,CYP3A5 酶变异对其药代动力学有良好的影响[65-68]。增加的数据表明,通过抑制 CYP3A、2D6、2C9 和 2C8 酶(通常具有有限的临床相关性)产生的药物相互作用可能在具有潜在遗传变异的个体中变得高度显著[69-71]。

联用 MMF 和他克莫司、用或不用 PPI 的 61 名肾移植受者被分型为 CYP2C19 *1、*2、*3 和多药耐药性(MDR)1 C3435T 等位基因 [31]。相对于没有兰索拉唑和相同基因型的个体, 具有 CYP2C19 *1/*2 或 *1/*3 或 MDR1 CC 基因型的个体使用兰索拉唑 30mg 治疗后的 MPA AUC 降低了 25%~30%。这些数据表明,具有这些基因型的需抑酸治疗的个体可以用替代的抑酸剂或更高剂量的 MMF。

将唑类抗真菌剂加入他克莫司治疗通常需要显著减少他克莫司剂量,以维持类似的血液暴露。接受他克莫司和酮康唑 100mg/d 的肾脏受体(n=79)基因分型为 CYP3A5, 基因型为 CYP3A5 *3/*1 或 *3/*3 的个体在开始酮康唑治疗后他克莫司的浓度增加 79%~112%,而基因型为 *1/*1 的个体在剂量标准化后浓度仅增加 30%[72]。在 29 名肾移植受体中,他克莫司和氟康唑之间的相互作用也提示了基因型效应[73]。相对于氟康唑治疗之前, 在添加氟康唑后立即出现的剂量标准化的他克莫司浓度在具有 CYP3A5 *3/*3 基因型的那些中增加73%,在具有*1/*3基因型的那些中增加45%。具有*3/*3基因型而不是*1/*3基因型(73.9%对16.6%)的更多受试者在开始氟康唑后谷氨酸浓度> 25ng/mL。这些数据表明,通过CYP3A介导的他克莫司药物相互作用的效力部分是基础基因型的功能。用CYP3A5基因型的相关信息可以更优先准确地确定减少的剂量。

总结

在对移植受者用药时,必须仔细考虑药代动力学、药效学和药物基因组学,并且基本上对所有患者都应预期药物的相互作用。应考虑采取预防或尽量减少药物相互作用的方法。首先,使患者接受的药物数量最小化是一般的最佳方法。应在每次移植随访中构建完整的用药史,包括处方、非处方、违禁药品和草药等。注意在移植方案中添加或移除相互作用的药物。通常,当添加或中断CYP3A抑制剂或诱导剂时,CNI和mTOR抑制剂的剂量需要调整。对于与吸收相关的相互作用,可能需要调整药物使用的时间,以使相互作用最小化。在药效学相互作用的情况下,应仔细监测患者的药物毒性、感染或排斥的早期迹象。对于所有类型的药物相互作用,可能需要更积极地监测药物浓度和化学性质。

(沈恬 译 沈恬 校)

参考文献

1. Magro L, Moretti U, Leone R, et al. Epidemiology and characteristics of adverse drug reactions caused by drug-drug interactions. Expert Opinion on Drug Safety. 2012;11(1):83–94.
2. Prograf [Prescription Information] Deerfield, IL: Astellas; Sept 2011.
3. Cellcept [Prescription Information] San Francisco, CA: Genentech USA; Feb 2010.
4. Myfortic [Prescription Information] East Hanover, NJ: Novartis Pharmaceutical Corp; Oct 2010.
5. Rapamune [Prescription Information] Philadelphia, PA: Pfizer Inc; Nov 2010.
6. Imuran [Prescription Information] Hunt Valley, MD: Prometheus Lab Inc; Apr 2009.
7. Neoral [Prescription Information] East Hanover, NJ: Novartis Pharmaceutical Corp; Oct 2009.
8. Zortress [Prescription Information] East Hanover, NJ: Novartis Pharmaceutical Corp; March 2010.
9. Bullingham R, Shah J, Goldblum R, et al. Effects of food and antacid on the pharmacokinetics of single doses of mycophenolic mofetil in rheumatoid arthritis patients. British Journal of Clinical Pharmacology. 1996;41(6):513–516.
10. Chisholm MA, Mulloy LL, Jagadeesan M, et al. Coadministration of tacrolimus with anti-acid drugs. Transplantation. 2003;76(4):665–666.
11. Kato R, Ooi K, Ikura-Mori M, et al. Impairment of mycophenolate mofetil absorption by calcium polycarbophil. Journal of Clinical Pharmacology. 2002;42(11):1275–1280.
12. Morii M, Ueno K, Ogawa A, et al. Impairment of mycophenolate mofetil absorption by iron ion. Clinical Pharmacology and Therapeutics. 2000; 68(6):613–616.
13. Staatz CE, Tett SE. Clinical pharmacokinetics and pharmacodynamics of mycophenolate in solid organ transplant recipients. Clinical Pharmacokinetics. 2007;46(1):13–58.
14. Mudge DW, Atcheson B, Taylor PJ, et al. The effect of oral iron administration on mycophenolate mofetil absorption in renal transplant recipients: a randomized, controlled trial. Transplantation. 2004;77(2):206–209.
15. Gelone DK, Park JM, Lake KD. Lack of an effect of oral iron administration on mycophenolic acid pharmacokinetics in stable renal transplant recipients. Pharmacotherapy. 2007;27(9):1272–1278.
16. Lorenz M, Wolzt M, Weigel G, et al. Ferrous sulfate does not affect mycophenolic acid pharmacokinetics in kidney transplant patients. American Journal of Kidney Diseases. 2004;43(6):1098–1103.
17. Bays HE, Dujovne CA. Drug interactions of lipid-altering drugs. Drug Safety. 1998;19(5):355–371.
18. Keogh A, Day R, Critchley L, et al. The effect of food and cholestyramine on the absorption of cyclosporine in cardiac transplant recipients. Transplantation Proceedings. 1988;20(1):27–30.
19. Jensen RA, Lal SM, Diaz-Arias A, et al. Does cholestyramine interfere with cyclosporine absorption? A prospective study in renal transplant patients. American Society for Artificial Internal Organs Journal. 1995;41(3):M704–M706.
20. Pieper AK, Buhle F, Bauer S, et al. The effect of sevelamer on the pharmacokinetics of cyclosporin A and mycophenolate mofetil after renal transplantation. Nephrology, Dialysis, Transplantation. 2004;19(10):2630–2633.
21. Fosrenal [Prescription Information] Shire US INC, Wayne, PA: Aug 2011.
22. Wadhwa NK, Schroeder TJ, O'Flaherty E, et al. The effect of oral metoclopramide on the absorption of cyclosporine. Transplantation Proceedings. 1987;19(1 Pt 2):1730–1733.
23. Zimmerman JJ, Harper D, Getsy J, et al. Pharmacokinetic interactions between sirolimus and microemulsion cyclosporine when orally administered jointly and 4 hours apart in healthy volunteers. Journal of Clinical Pharmacology. 2003;43(10):1168–1176.
24. Kaplan B, Meier-Kriesche HU, Napoli KL, et al. The effects of relative timing of sirolimus and cyclosporine microemulsion formulation coadministration on the pharmacokinetics of each agent. Clinical Pharmacology and Therapeutics. 1998;63(1):48–53.
25. Rupprecht K, Schmidt C, Raspé A, et al. Bioavailability of mycophenolate mofetil and enteric-coated mycophenolate sodium is differentially affected by pantoprazole in healthy volunteers. Journal of Clinical Pharmacology. 2009;49: 1196–1201.
26. Kofler S, Shvets N, Bigdeli AK, et al. Proton pump inhibitors reduce mycophenolate exposure in heart transplant recipients-a prospective case-controlled study. American Journal of Transplantation. 2009;9:1650–1656.
27. Kofler S, Deutsch M, Bigdeli AK, et al. Proton pump inhibitor co-medication reduces mycophenolate acid drug exposure in heart transplant recipients. Journal of Heart and Lung Transplantation. 2009;28:605–611.
28. Schaier M, Scholl C, Scharpf D, et al. Proton pump inhibitors interfere with the immunosuppressive potency of mycophenolate mofetil. Rheumatology (Oxford, England). 2010;49:2061–2067.
29. Kees MG, Steinke T, Moritz S, et al. Omeprazole impairs the absorption of mycophenolate mofetil but not of enteric-coated mycophenolate sodium in healthy volunteers. Journal of Clinical Pharmacology. 2011;52(8):1265–1272.
30. Doesch AO. Proton pump inhibitor co-medication reduces MPA exposure in heart transplant recipients receiving mycophenolate mofetil. Transplantation Proceedings. 2010;42(10):4243–4246.
31. Miura M, Satoh S, Inoue K, et al. Influence of lansoprazole and rabeprazole on mycophenolic acid pharmacokinetics one year after renal transplantation. Therapeutic Drug Monitoring. 2008;30:46–51.
32. Kiberd BA, Wrobel M, Dandavino R, et al. The role of proton pump inhibitors on early mycophenolic acid exposure in kidney transplantation: evidence from the CLEAR study. Therapeutic Drug Monitoring. 2011;33(1):120–123.
33. Arns W, Breuer S, Choudhury S, et al. Enteric-coated mycophenolate sodium delivers bioequivalent MPA exposure compared with mycophenolate mofetil. Clinical Transplantation. 2005;19:199–206.
34. Shaw LM, Nawrocki A, Korecka M, et al. Using established immunosuppressant therapy effectively: lessons from the measurement of mycophenolic acid plasma concentrations. Therapeutic Drug Monitoring. 2004;26(4):347–351.
35. Dubuske LM. The role of P-glycoprotein and organic anion-transporting polypeptides in drug interactions. Drug Safety. 2005;28(9):789–801.
36. Saitoh H, Saikachi Y, Kobayashi M, et al. Limited interaction between tacrolimus and P-glycoprotein in the rat small intestine. European Journal of Pharmaceutical Sciences. 2006;28(1–2):34–42.
37. Staatz CE, Goodman LK, Tett SE. Effect of CYP3A and ABCB1 single nucleotide polymorphisms on the pharmacokinetics and pharmacodynamics of calcineurin

inhibitors: Part I. Clinical Pharmacokinetics. 2010;49(3):141–175.
38. Ejendal KF, Hrycyna CA. Differential sensitivities of the human ATP-binding cassette transporters ABCG2 and P-glycoprotein to cyclosporin A. Molecular Pharmacology. 2005;67(3):902–911.
39. Amioka K, Kuzuya T, Kushihara H, et al. Carvedilol increases ciclosporin bioavailability by inhibiting P-glycoprotein-mediated transport. Journal of Pharmacy and Pharmacology. 2007;59(10):1383–1387.
40. Türk T, Witzke O. Pharmacological interaction between cyclosporine and repaglinide. Is it clinically relevant? American Journal of Transplantation. 2006;6(9):2223.
41. Kajosaari LI, Niemi M, Neuvonen M, et al. Cyclosporine markedly raises the plasma concentrations of repaglinide. Clinical Pharmacology and Therapeutics. 2005;78(4):388–399.
42. Spence R, Mandagere A, Richards DB, et al. Potential for pharmacokinetic interactions between ambrisentan and cyclosporine. Clinical Pharmacology and Therapeutics. 2010;88(4):513–520.
43. Flockhart DA Drug Interactions: Cytochrome P450 Drug Interaction Table. Indiana University School of Medicine (2007). 2007 [cited January 4, 2012]; Avaiable from: http://medicine.iupui.edu/clinpharm/ddis/table.aspx.
44. Kennedy DT, Hayney MS, Lake KD. Azathioprine and allopurinol: the price of an avoidable drug. Annals of Pharmacotherapy. 1996;30(9):951–954.
45. Kuypers DR, Naesens M, Vermeire S, et al. The impact of uridine diphosphate -glucuronosyltransferase 1A9 (UGT1A9) gene promoter region single-nucleotide polymorphisms T-275A and C-2152T on early mycophenolic acid dose-interval exposure in de novo renal allograft recipients. Clinical Pharmacology and Therapeutics. 2005;78(4):351–361.
46. Naderer OJ, Dupuis RE, Heinzen EL, et al. The influence of norfloxacin and metronidazole on the disposition of mycophenolate mofetil. Journal of Clinical Pharmacology. 2005;45:219–226.
47. Borrows R, Chusney G, Loucaidou M, et al. The magnitude and time course of changes in mycophenolic acid 12-hour predoses during antibiotic therapy in mycophenolate mofetil-based renal transplantation. Therapeutic Drug Monitoring. 2007;29:122–126.
48. Izquierdo MJ, Rodrigo E, de Cos MA, et al. Leukopenia in kidney transplantation resulting from the interaction between mycophenolate mofetil and valganciclovir. Nefrologia. 2007;27(2):232–233.
49. Gimenez F, Foeillet E, Bourdon O, et al. Evaluation of pharmacokinetic interactions after oral administration of mycophenolate mofetil and valaciclovir or aciclovir to healthy subjects. Clinical Pharmacokinetics. 2004;43(10):685–692.
50. Royer B, Zanetta G, Bérard M, et al. A neutropenia suggesting an interaction between valacyclovir and mycophenolate mofetil. Clinical Transplantation. 2003;17(2):158–161.
51. Heisel O, Heisel R, Balshaw R, et al. New onset diabetes mellitus in patients receiving calcineurin inhibitors: a systematic review and meta-analysis. American Journal of Transplantation. 2004;4(4):583–595.
52. Vincenti F, Friman S, Scheuermann E, et al. DIRECT (Diabetes Incidence after Renal Transplantation: neoral C monitoring versus tacrolimus) investigators. Results of an international, randomized trial comparing glucose metabolism disorders and outcome with cyclosporine versus tacrolimus. American Journal of Transplantation. 2007;7(6):1506–1514.
53. Ekberg H, Tedesco-Silva H, Demirbas A, et al. ELITE-Symphony Study. Reduced exposure to calcineurin inhibitors in renal transplantation. New England Journal of Medicine. 2007;357(25):2562–2575.
54. Natural Standards. 2011 [cited October 5, 2011]; Available from: http://www.naturalstandard.com/.
55. Fortin MC, Raymond MA, Madore F, et al. Increased risk of thrombotic microangiopathy in patients receiving a cyclosporin-sirolimus combination. American Journal of Transplantation. 2004;4(6):946–952.
56. Johnson MC, So S, Marsh JW, et al. QT prolongation and Torsades de Pointes after administration of FK506. Transplantation. 1992;53(4):929–930.
57. Multag [Prescription Information] Bridgewater, NJ: Sanofi-Aventis; June 2011.
58. Li EC, Esterly JS, Pohl S, et al. Drug-induced QT-interval prolongation: considerations for clinicians. Pharmacotherapy. 2010;30(7):684–701.
59. Hoover T, Lippmann M, Grouzmann E, et al. Herscu P. Angiotensin converting enzyme inhibitor induced angio-oedema: a review of the pathophysiology and risk factors. Clinical and Experimental Allergy. 2010;40(1):50–61.
60. Wellbutrin XL [Prescription Information] Research Triangle Park, NC: GlaxoSmithKline; Aug 2011.
61. US Food and Drug Administration. FDA drug safety communication: new restriction, contraindications, and dose limitations for Zocor (simvastatin) to reduce the risk of muscle injury. 2011. [cited August 8, 2011]; Available from: http://www.fda.gov/Drugs/DrugSafety/ucm256581.htm.
62. U.S. prescribing information for simvastatin revised to include new limits on the use of the highest dose -80 mg—and updated drug interaction information [press release]. Whitehouse Station, NJ: Merck & Co., Inc.; June 8, 2011.
63. Ernst E. St John's Wort supplements endanger the success of organ transplantation. Archives of Surgery. 2002;137(3):316–319.
64. Melchart D, Linde K, Worku F, et al. Results of five randomized studies on the immunomodulatory activity of preparations of Echinacea. Journal of Alternative and Complementary Medicine. 1995;1(2):145–160.
65. Jacobson PA, Oetting WS, Brearley AM, et al. Novel polymorphisms associated with tacrolimus trough concentrations: results from a multicenter kidney transplant consortium. Transplantation. 2011;91(3):300–308.
66. Kuypers DR. Pharmacogenetic vs. concentration-controlled optimization of tacrolimus dosing in renal allograft recipients. Clinical Pharmacology and Therapeutics. 2010;88(5):595–596.
67. Tavira B, Coto E, Díaz-Corte C, et al. Pharmacogenetics of tacrolimus after renal transplantation: analysis of polymorphisms in genes encoding 16 drug metabolizing enzymes. Clinical Chemistry and Laboratory Medicine. 2011;49(5):825–833.
68. Ware N, MacPhee IA. Current progress in pharmacogenetics and individualized immunosuppressive drug dosing in organ transplantation. Current Opinion in Molecular Therapeutics. 2010;12(3):270–283.
69. Samer CF, Daali Y, Wagner M, et al. The effects of CYP2D6 and CYP3A activities on the pharmacokinetics of immediate release oxycodone. British Journal of Pharmacology. 2010;160(4):907–918.
70. Zi J, Liu D, Ma P, et al. Effects of CYP2C9*3 and CYP2C9*13 on Diclofenac metabolism and inhibition-based drug-drug interactions. Drug Metabolism and Pharmacokinetics. 2010;25(4):343–350.
71. Gao Y, Liu D, Wang H, et al. Functional characterization of five CYP2C8 variants and prediction of CYP2C8 genotype-dependent effects on in vitro and in vivo drug-drug interactions. Xenobiotica. 2010;40(7):467–475.
72. Chandel N, Aggarwal PK, Minz M, et al. CYP3A5*1/*3 genotype influences the blood concentration of tacrolimus in response to metabolic inhibition by ketoconazole. Pharmacogenetics and Genomics. 2009;19(6):458–463.
73. Kuypers DR, de Jonge H, Naesens M, et al. Effects of CYP3A5 and MDR1 single nucleotide polymorphisms on drug interactions between tacrolimus and fluconazole in renal allograft recipients. Pharmacogenetics and Genomics. 2008;18(10):861–868.
74. Clinical Pharmacology. 2012 [cited January 10, 2012]; Available from: www.clinicalpharmacology.com.
75. Lexi-Comp. 2012 [cited January 10, 2012]; Available from: www.lexi.com.
76. Tabbara KF, Al-Faisal Z, Al-Rashed W. Interaction between acetazolamine and cyclosporine. Arch Ophthalmol. 1998;116:832–833.
77. Rebello S, Compain S, Feng A, et al. Effect of cyclosporine on the pharmacokinetics of aliskiren in healthy subjects. J Clin Pharmacol. 2011; 51:1549–1560.
78. Canafax DM, Graves NM, Hilligoss DM, et al: Interaction between cyclosporine and fluconazole in renal allograft recipients. Transplantation. 1991;51(5):1014–1018.
79. Sud K, Singh B, Krishna VS, et al. Unpredictable cyclosporin-fluconazole interaction in renal transplant recipients. Nephrology Dialysis Transplantation. 1999; 14:1698–1703.
80. Frassetto LA, Baluom M, Jacobsen W, et al. Cyclosporine pharmacokinetics and dosing modifications in human immunodeficiency virus-infected liver and kidney transplant recipients.Transplantation. 2005; 80:13–17.
81. Abraham MA, Thomas PP, John GT, et al. Efficacy and safety of low-dose ketoconazole (50 mg) to reduce the cost of cyclosporine in renal allograft recipients. Transplant Proceedings. 2003; 35: 215–216.
82. Vogel M, Voigt E, Michaelis HC, et al. Management of drug-to- drug interactions between cyclosporine A and the protease- inhibitor lopinavir/ritonavir in liver-transplanted HIV-infected patients. Liver Transplant. 2004;10:939–944.
83. Wright DH, Lake KD, Bruhn PS, Emery Jr. RW. Nefazodone and cyclosporine drug-drug interaction. Journal of Heart and Lung Transplantation. 1999;18:913–915.
84. Sansone-Parsons A, Krishna G, Martinho M, et al. Effect of oral posaconazole on the pharmacokinetics of cyclosporine and tacrolimus. Pharmacotherapy. 2007;27:825–834.
85. Stamatakis MK, Richards JG. Interaction between quinupristin/dalfopristin and cyclosporine. Annals of Pharmacotherapy. 1997;31:576–578.
86. Wandel C, Böhrer H, Böcker R, et al. Rifampicin and cyclosporine dosing in heart transplant recipients. J Cardiothorac Vasc Anesth 1995; 9:621–622.
87. Kim YH, Yoon YR, Kim YW et al. Effects of rifampin on cyclosporine disposition in kidney recipients with tuberculosis. Transplantation Proceedings. 1998; 30: 3570–3572.
88. Garg V, van Heeswijk R, Lee JE, et al. The effect of telaprevir on the pharmacokinetics of cyclosporine and tacrolimus. Hepatology. 2011: 54: 20–27.
89. Romero AJ, Pogamp PL, Nilsson LG, Wood N. Effect of voriconazole on the pharmacokinetics of cyclosporine in renal transplant patients. Clinical Pharmacology and Therapeutics. 2002; 71: 226–234.
90. Kovarik JM, Hartmann S, Hubert M, et al. Pharmacokinetic and pharmacodynamic assessments of HMG-CoA reductase inhibitors when coadministered with everolimus. Journal of Clinical Pharmacology. 2002; 42: 222–228.

91. Kovarik JM, Kalbag J, Figueiredo J, et al. Differential influence of two cyclosporine formulations on everolimus pharmacokinetics: a clinically relevant pharmacokinetic drug interaction. Journal of Clinical Pharmacology. 2002; 42: 95–99.
92. Kovarik JM, Beyer D, Bizot MN, et al. Effect of multiple-dose erythromycin on everolimus pharmacokinetics. European Journal of Clinical Pharmacology. 2005;61(1):35–38.
93. Kovarik JM, Hsu CH, McMahon L, et al. Population pharmacokinetics of everolimus in de novo renal transplant patients: impact of ethnicity and comedications. Clinical Pharmacology and Therapeutics. 2001; 70:247–254.
94. Kovarik JM, Beyer D, Bizot MN, et al. Blood concentrations of everolimus are markedly increased by ketoconazole. Journal of Clinical Pharmacology. 2005; 45(5):514–518.
95. Billaud EM, Antoine C, Berge M, et al. Management of metabolic cytochrome P450 3A4 drug-drug interaction between everolimus and azole antifungals in a renal transplant patient. Clinical Drug Investigation. 2009; 29(7):481–416.
96. Kovarik JM, Hartmann S, Figueiredo J, et al. Effect of rifampin on apparent clearance of everolimus. Annals of Pharmacotherapy. 2002; 36:981–985.
97. Kovarik JM, Beyer D, Bizot MN, et al. Pharmacokinetic interaction between verapamil and everolimus in healthy subjects. British Journal of Clinical Pharmacology. 2005; 60(4):434–437.
98. Kofler S, Wolf C, Shvets N, et al. The proton pump inhibitor pantoprazole and its interaction with enteric-coated mycophenolate sodium in transplant recipients. Journal of Heart Lung Transplant. 2011; 30:565–571.
99. Vfend [Prescription Information] VFEND® (voriconazole) Tablets, Oral Suspension, and I.V. Initial U.S. Approval: 2002.
100. Mertz D, Battegay M, Marzolini C, Mayr M. Drug-drug interaction in a kidney transplant recipient receiving HIV salvage therapy and tacrolimus. American Journal of Kidney Diseases. 2009; 54(1):e1–4.
101. Jain AB, Venkataramanan R, Eghtesad B. Effect of coadministered lopinavir and ritonavir (Kaletra) on tacrolimus blood concentration in liver transplantation patients. Liver Transplantation. 2003; 9:954–960.
102. Campo JV, Smith C, Perel JM. Tacrolimus toxic reaction associated with the use of nefazodone: paroxetine as an alternative agent. Archives of General Psychiatry. 1998; 55:1050–1052.
103. Olyaei AJ, deMattos AM, Norman DJ, Bennett WM. Interaction between tacrolimus and nefazodone in a stable renal transplant recipient. Pharmacotherapy. 1998; 18:1356–1359.
104. Jain A, Venkataramanan R, Shapiro R, et al. The interaction between antiretroviral agents and tacrolimus in liver and kidney transplant patients. Liver Transplant. 2002; 8:841–845.
105. Schvarcz R, Rudbeck G, Söderdahl G, Ståhle L. Interaction between nelfinavir and tacrolimus after orthoptic liver transplantation in a patient coinfected with HIV and hepatitis C virus (HCV). Transplantation. 2000; 69:2194–2195.
106. Maguire M, Franz T, Hains DS. A clinically significant interaction between tacrolimus and multiple proton pump inhibitors in a kidney transplant recipient. Pediatric Transplantation. 2011; 16(6):e217–220.
107. Kuypers DR, Claes K, Evenepoel P, Vanrenterghem Y. Clinically relevant drug interaction between voriconazole and tacrolimus in a primary renal allograft recipient. Transplantation. 2006; 81:1750–1752.

第 7 篇

移植长期预后

第 103 章
肾移植长期预后

Sundus A. Lodhi, Neema Stephens

引言

肾移植在过去三十多年里取得了重大进步，目前已成为终末期肾病的常规治疗方法。随着肾移植的成功推广，门诊有越来越多的肾移植受者前来随访，相比短期存活情况，他们的长期预后也越来越受重视。影响长期预后的因素与影响短期预后的因素有很大不同，相关数据还在不断积累中。本章内容包括肾移植受体长期预后、影响患者及移植肾存活的供受体相关危险因素、远期患者死亡及移植肾失功的原因等。

肾移植受体的长期预后

评价肾移植成功与否的临床指标包括经典终点，如急性排斥率、移植肾和患者存活率。目前大多数临床试验仅关注短期存活率。事实上，最终可以指导临床实践的大部分重要研究和临床试验的主要终点都是 1 年排斥率和 1 年存活率。对长期预后进行准确评估的主要困难在于：

- 随访时间需要足够长
- 在长时间的随访过程中数据要准确

解决这些问题的方法之一是从大型移植登记系统中获取数据，通过 Kaplan-Meier 法进行观察性或回顾性分析。一项合并了美国肾脏数据系统(USRDS)和科学肾移植登记系统(SRTR)数据的研究表明，尸体肾移植长期预后优于维持性血透。这种优越性与性别、年龄和种族无关。这些发现再次激起对肾移植的研究关注。目前，肾移植仍被视为是优于透析的 ESRD 患者的治疗选择[1,2]。

随着移植术后更长时间的随访数据越来越多，评估患者及移植肾存活情况越来越准确。以往基于短期随访的预测现在被长期随访的实际数据所替代。这不但可以计算实际存活率，还使得更精确的预测成为可能。我们对长期移植肾存活的认识，从开始时过于乐观的状态逐渐转变，慢慢意识到提高患者及移植物存活情况主要依赖于提高第一年存活率[3]。

免疫抑制处理的进步不断改善了总体排斥率，手术技术的发展提高了移植物质量。因此，未调整的 1 年移植物存活率从 1987 年的 76%提高到了 2008 年的 93%(OPTN/SRTR2010 年年报)。即使是在早年间(1975—1990 年)，1 年移植物存活率有显著提高，然而 1 年后移植物存活情况(如移植物半衰期)并没有相应改善[4]。

最新的肾移植长期预后分析表明，大部分进步使得第一年存活情况大幅改善，但长期存活率改善较小[5]。

过去 20 年里，急性排斥率有了显著下降，但长期移植肾寿命并没有相应改变。这种不一致原因部分可能由于即使是发生了排斥，但只要能回到基线肾功能水平，6 年移植肾存活率和未发生排斥的情况类似。然而，排斥后不能回到基线肾功能水平时，移植肾存活率将下降(6 年移植肾存活率为 50.2%对 72.7%)[6]。

当接受患者移植前咨询时，移植物半衰期可以作为一个有效的提供给患者的合理预期存活率的临床指标。移植物年丢失率能够帮助评估早期及远期移植后存活情况。

基于 Kaplan-Meier 分析 1989—2005 年累积半衰期时，我们发现尸体肾移植的实际半衰期从 1989 年的 6.6 年提高到了 2000 年的 8.2 年，预测 2005 年可达到 8.8 年。尸体肾移植中，标准供肾的半衰期从 1989 年的 6.7 年提高到了 2000 年的 8.8 年，预测 2005 年可达到 9.5 年。更加显著的改善是扩大标准供肾的半衰期从 1989 年的 3 年提高到了 2000 年的 5.6 年，预测 2005 年可达到 6.4 年。活体肾移植更佳，但随着时间的提升空间较小，1989 年是 11.4 年，预测 2005 年为 11.9 年。

许多研究中认为存在种族差异，黑人作为受体时移植物存活率较低[7,8]。当比较黑人和非黑人的移植物半衰期时，同样有类似的改善趋势（黑人 4.1 年提高到 7.4 年，非黑人 7.8 年提高到 10.9 年），但种族间差异并没有显著缩小（图 103.1）。

影响长期移植肾存活的因素与影响短期存活的因素不同。移植物特异性的因素包括慢性排斥、感染和与长期免疫抑制有关的危险因素，如移植后淋巴增殖性疾病。随着某个个体移植肾和患者寿命延长，更多、更复杂的因素，像心血管疾病、体重增加和是否得到妥善照顾等会变得越来越重要。事实上我们也确实开始关注老年肾移植受体的相关问题，因为这些问题使得带功死亡率上升。

临床医生试图寻找导致移植物失功的慢性移植物损伤的最佳解读方式。慢性排斥这个词曾用于描述功能不全的移植肾的病理改变。这个词被过度简化，因为排斥并不是导致移植物失功的慢性损伤的唯一因素。20 世纪 90 年代初，慢性移植肾肾病（chronic allograft nephropathy，CAN）这个词开始用于强调进行性移植肾功能不全的多方面病因。CAN 的特征性病理表现包括小管萎缩、间质纤维化、小球硬化和小动脉透明变性。2005 年，第 8 版 Banff 标准弃用了 CAN 这个概念，改为慢性移植物损伤。这个词包括一系列导致慢性移植物功能不全的过程。高血压、糖尿病、感染（如 BK 病毒）、钙调磷酸酶抑制剂（calcineurin inhibitor，CNI）中毒、肾小球疾病复发或新发、慢性排斥均可引起慢性移植物损伤，最终导致移植肾失功。

器官质量和供体因素

器官类型和大小

移植物失功的危险因素因肾移植类型的不同而不同。器官质量对预后有非常重要的影响[9]。活体肾移植冷缺血时间短，预后佳，表现为较低的急性排斥率、较低的延迟复功率和较长的移植物寿命。尸体肾移植在不考虑 HLA 错配的前提下，长期预后总体劣于活体肾移植。要更好地理解这一问题，我们可以比较 HLA 全错配的活体肾移植和 HLA 全相合的尸体肾移植，前者移植肾存活仍然优于后者。

移植肾功能性肾单位的数量对其功能和存活状态

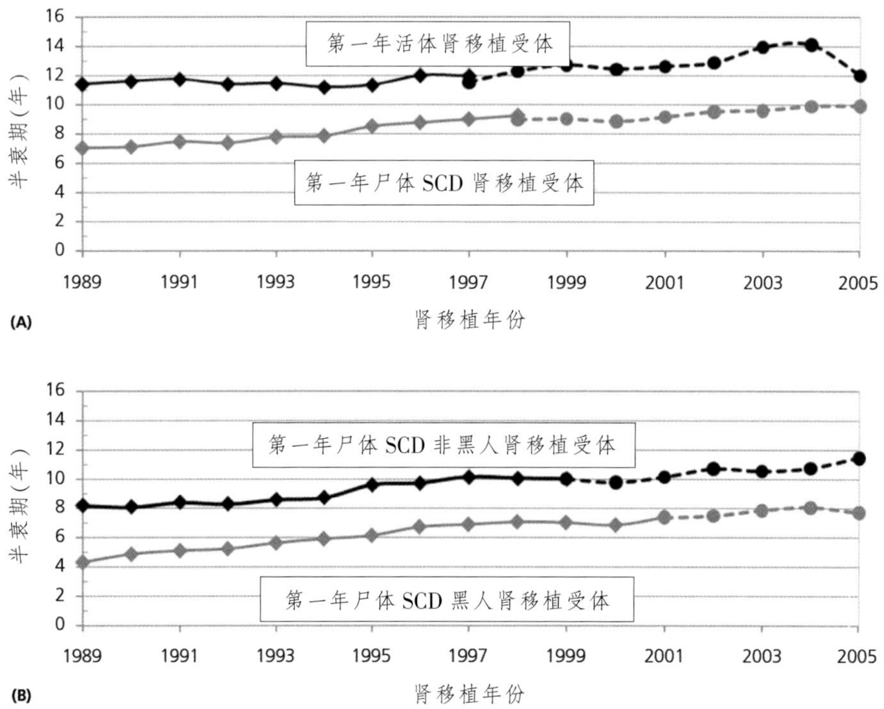

图 103.1 实际（方点，实线）和预测（圆点，虚线）累积半衰期。(A)第一年活体肾移植对尸体肾移植。(B)第一年尸体肾移植非黑人受体对黑人受体。（Reproduced from [5] Lamb et al. Am J Transplant. 2011, with permission from Wiley-Blackwell.）

起着重要作用。一项首次移植的多中心研究表明,移植肾重/受体体重低于 2.3g/kg 是 2 年随访移植肾失功的独立危险因素[10]。这一观点被衍伸到幼龄及老龄供肾,因为这两种情况下功能性肾单位相对不足。

供体危险指数

肾脏供体危险指数是设计用于帮助临床医生进行尸体器官评估决策的实用工具。该工具将影响移植物存活的供体因素纳入考虑:供体年龄、身高、体重、种族、糖尿病、高血压、中风、DCD、末次肌酐、HCV[11]。这种计算方法将移植肾失功的风险与“平均”40 岁的 SCD 供肾相关联。这一评分有助于评价一个供肾移植后的表现,但它并不能反映影响长期移植肾存活的其他因素,也未经过确切检验。

当研究预测预后的因素时,应将危险因素(例如,糖尿病是移植肾失功的危险因素)与预后因素区别开来,因为预后因素应当是可靠的、能够预测每一个预后的。肾脏供体危险指数(KDRI)将供体分为高风险和低风险是合理的,但它不足以区分大部分“中距”供肾的预后。能够可靠地预测长期移植物存活并被前瞻性验证的危险指数尚不存在。

受体因素

移植时机

移植前透析时间是已知的不利于移植物存活的因素。抢先肾移植(移植前未开始透析或透析时间<6 个月)被认为具有更好的患者及移植肾存活率[12]。不论是活体还是尸体肾移植,抢先肾移植最突出的是可以显著降低患者死亡风险(RR 0.84 和 0.69)和移植肾失功风险(RR 0.75 和 0.73)。然而,抢先肾移植中受体大多比较年轻,医保完善,受教育水平较高[13]。这些相关研究又大多是回顾性的,不可避免地存在选择偏倚。尽管如此,通过统计学方法校正供体因素及选择偏倚后,结果仍然显示,较早移植有利于改善长期预后。虽然原因尚未被完全厘清,尽早移植能够减少透析相关感染及心血管发病率,可以改善预后。

带功死亡

尽管移植的存活优势和净寿命获益均高于透析,肾移植受体的预期寿命仍低于总体人群。心血管疾病是肾移植受体带功死亡的主要原因(图 103.2)。

每年心血管事件导致的死亡率估计为 5%。终末期肾病患者移植前即有很高的心血管疾病风险,术后将影响预后。肾移植受体往往同时具有经典及非经典心血管疾病危险因素。经典 Framingham 危险因素包括高血压、高血脂、糖尿病、吸烟、肥胖和缺乏锻炼。非经典危险因素有免疫抑制药物不良反应。管理受体心血管疾病危险因素具有极为重要的作用,因为心血管疾病是导致带功死亡的首要原因。本节将详细回顾每一项危险因素。

高血压

高血压是远期移植肾失功的独立危险因素。移植后 1 年的血压可预测移植肾存活情况。收缩压、舒张压、平均动脉压每增加 10mmHg,移植肾存活都会显著降低[14]。虽然缺乏前瞻性随机对照试验研究降压方案及目标范围,KDIGO 指南推荐将血压控制在<130/80mmHg。

高血压定义为血压高于 140/90mmHg,这在肾移植受体中极为常见。它可能是既往高血压、肥胖或其他移植相关因素的结果。导致移植肾功能不全的急慢性原因也会导致高血压。

免疫抑制剂治疗本身可以直接引起高血压。糖皮质激素从移植早期开始使用,可通过水钠潴留引起高

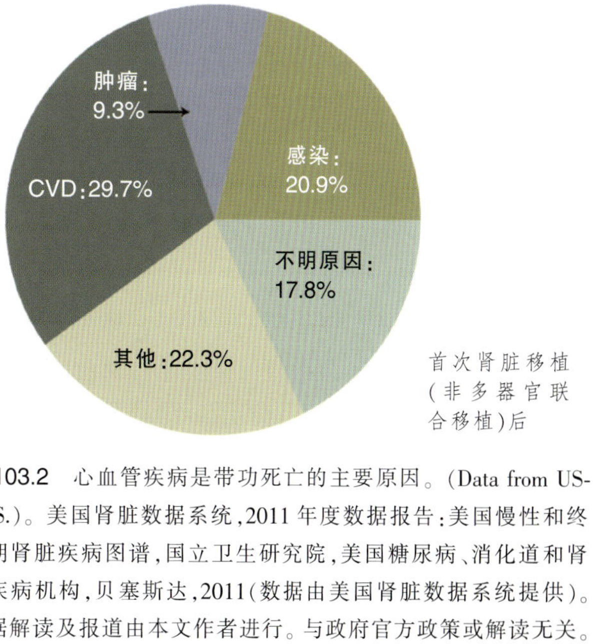

图 103.2 心血管疾病是带功死亡的主要原因。(Data from USRDS.)。美国肾脏数据系统,2011 年度数据报告:美国慢性和终末期肾脏疾病图谱,国立卫生研究院,美国糖尿病、消化道和肾脏疾病机构,贝塞斯达,2011(数据由美国肾脏数据系统提供)。数据解读及报道由本文作者进行。与政府官方政策或解读无关。

血压。在20世纪80年代,50%~60%的肾移植受体患有高血压。在应用CNI后,这一比例升至75%~90%[15]。许多移植研究为避免这项不良反应,尝试采用减少激素及避免CNI的方案。

高血脂

在移植后第一年,至少一半的患者会有血脂异常。高血脂,特别是LDL升高,是心血管疾病的独立危险因素。KDIGO指南推荐术后3个月内复查血脂谱,其后每年复查。某些免疫抑制药物,如糖皮质激素、CNI和mTOR可加重或引发高血脂。因此,可考虑调整免疫抑制方案来帮助改善血脂谱。西罗莫司可能同时升高总胆固醇和甘油三酯水平。在CNI中,环孢素对总胆固醇和LDL的影响最大。ALERT试验是一个前瞻性随机对照研究,关注他汀治疗对肾移植受体心血管预后的影响。2000多例患者随机分为氟伐他汀组和安慰剂组。他汀组的次要终点(非致死性心梗和心源性死亡)有明显降低,心脏事件发生率也有减少趋势(虽然无统计学差异)[16]。基于此,他汀被推荐为治疗肾移植受体高脂血症的一线用药。生活方式的改变可能有帮助,但大部分患者还是需要药物治疗。当选择他汀治疗时,应注意与CNI的药物相互作用。由于两类药物都是通过细胞色素P450系统代谢,某些他汀在与CNI同时使用时需要减量。总体来说,氟伐他汀、阿托伐他汀和普伐他汀在移植患者中具有较好的安全性。由于移植受体具有较高的心血管疾病风险,KDIGO指南推荐LDL目标值<100mg/dL。对于糖尿病或已有心血管疾病史的受体,一些临床医生倾向于选择<70mg/dL。

吸烟

多达1/3的肾移植受体经常吸烟。移植时未戒烟是全因死亡、缺血性心脏病、卒中、充血性心力衰竭和外周血管疾病的独立危险因素。一项单中心研究表明,吸烟者的心血管死亡风险升高2倍。此外,来自USRDS的数据表明,吸烟将增加带功死亡和总体患者死亡的风险。这独立于移植前肺病[17]。患者因移植入院后会有所节制,因此这是戒烟的好时机。戒烟咨询应包括以下“5A”:

(1)询问烟草使用情况;

(2)劝说戒烟;

(3)评估戒烟意愿;

(4)帮助戒烟;

(5)安排随访和帮助。

戒烟有一系列药物选择,包括尼古丁替代口香糖、糖果、贴片、尼古丁受体部分激动剂和抗抑郁药。

糖尿病

作为美国ESRD的首要原因,移植时有1/5的患者有糖尿病。在移植前没有糖尿病的患者中,24%会在移植后3年内有新发糖尿病。若原发病是糖尿病肾病,可能影响移植肾功能,尽管较少独立导致移植肾失功。USRDS回顾性研究表明,移植后新发糖尿病(newonset diabetes after transplantation,NODAT)与移植肾失功和患者死亡相关。研究阐述了一系列NODAT的关键危险因素,包括年龄、非洲裔美国人、西班牙裔、肥胖和丙肝[18]。移植医生可通过美国糖尿病协会提供的标准,识别空腹血糖受损和糖尿病患者。空腹血糖受损是指无糖尿病,但空腹血糖为100~125mg/dL,这同样会增加心血管事件的发生率。改变生活方式,特别是对肥胖患者很必要。根据KDIGO指南,药物治疗目标是控制HbA1c在7%~7.5%。在所有患有糖尿病的受体中,建议服用低剂量阿司匹林,以预防心血管疾病。

免疫抑制治疗同样可以引起NODAT。CNI,尤其是他克莫司,可减少胰岛素分泌,糖皮质激素可引起胰岛素抵抗。因此,应根据实际情况调整方案。

肥胖

很多肾移植受体和普通人群一样,受到肥胖的困扰。事实上,UNOS回顾性研究表明,约一半受体处于肥胖状态。肥胖定义为BMI>30,肥胖症定义为BMI>35。肥胖症是延迟复功和低移植肾存活率的独立危险因素[19]。除了对移植肾预后的影响,肥胖还与胰岛素抵抗、糖尿病和动脉粥样硬化性心脏病有关。因为移植后胃纳增加,移植患者应进行锻炼和营养咨询。这可以与定期随访相结合。

心血管疾病

心血管疾病包括缺血性心脏病、充血性心衰、外周血管疾病和卒中。这都是引起带功死亡的重要临床终点。临床医生应极为警觉。血管重建,如经皮血管成形术和冠状动脉搭桥等均可用于肾移植患者,其2年患者存活率约为80%[20]。手术过程存在AKI的风险,但移植肾失功率有所下降。

CNI 肾毒性

CNI 包括环孢素和他克莫司，是目前免疫抑制治疗的基石。它们是移植后短期移植物存活率改善的药物之一。它们的弱点在于肾毒性。血栓性微血管病、小动脉透明变性和空泡形成的小管损伤是 CNI 相关肾毒性的病理表现。肾毒性可表现为急性的氮质血症，也可在长期使用中表现为缓慢的慢性损伤。二氢吡啶类钙通道阻滞剂对于 CNI 的血管收缩作用有保护效应。在一项纳入 107 例环孢素治疗患者的前瞻性研究中，服用硝苯地平的患者延迟复功率低、GFR 高、术后 1 年活检间质纤维化发生率低[21]。人们提出假说，钙通道阻滞剂不仅使入球小动脉扩张，而且阻断钙离子内流，减轻缺血再灌注损伤。如前所述，CNI 除了对入球小动脉的直接收缩作用，还会显著增加心血管风险。

目前较少证据支持 CNI 减量方案被认为能够改善长期预后。但贝拉西普治疗在术后 3 年仍能维持较好的移植肾功能[22]。并且患者的代谢异常风险和高血压发生率都较低[23]。虽然缺乏长期随访数据，贝拉西普相对环孢素的优势仍有较大前景。

肾小球疾病复发或新发

原发疾病为 FSGS、膜增生性肾小球肾炎、IgA 肾病的患者术后复发导致移植物失功风险较高。狼疮性肾炎、GBM 疾病复发后失功风险较小。30%~50%的特发性 FSGS 患者术后会复发。确诊 3 年内快速进展至终末期肾病、首次移植因 FSGS 复发失败是疾病复发的强有力预测因子。

一项回顾性研究比较了 167 例复发或新发肾小球疾病的肾移植受体和 4746 例无肾小球疾病的受体。

前者移植肾存活中位时间为 1360 天，后者为 3382 天（$P<0.0001$）。前者 5 年存活率为 39.8%，后者为 67.6%[24]。疾病复发已在第 77 章详细阐述。

免疫损伤

肾移植受体移植时 PRA 较高则长期预后不佳。对 4000 例 HLA 相合亲属肾移植受体进行回顾性研究发现，术前 PRA 为 0 的受体 10 年存活率为 72.4%，而 PRA 1%~50%的受体 10 年存活率为 63.3%[25]。一些研究还认为，低剂量免疫抑制治疗的受体慢性移植肾肾病发生率较高。这表明慢性和亚临床免疫损伤在长期移植物存活中扮演重要角色。非 HLA 免疫仍然是改善慢性移植物损伤的重要挑战。

致敏与 DSA

致敏患者是术前可检测出 HLA 抗体的患者。妊娠、输血、既往移植史都是致敏事件，可导致 HLA 抗体产生。当产生到足够的量，这些 DSA 会引起阳性的交叉配型。美国的一些移植中心报道了脱敏治疗后阳性交叉配型的移植成功案例。脱敏治疗方案包括移植前血浆置换联合静脉免疫球蛋白输注。移植时 DSA 的存在与移植后早期抗体介导排斥以及较短的移植物半衰期相关。关于 DSA 及其检测的更多内容见第 77 章。

非致敏患者在新生 DSA 的介导下也会发生抗体介导排斥。一项多中心前瞻性研究认为，20%的带功患者有 HLA 抗体[26]。在检测出这些抗体 1 年后，移植物失功发生率增加。这种关系适用于移植时致敏及移植后新产生 DSA 的患者。在移植物功能不全之前的几个月甚至几年，DSA 即可出现。对 300 例移植时 HLA 抗体阴性的首次肾移植受体进行前瞻性研究，发现 15%的患者在术后 6 个月内产生了 DSA。新生 DSA 的两个预测指标包括 HLA-DR 错配和用药依从性差。在 10 年随访中，新生 DSA 患者移植肾存活率为 57%，无新生 DSA 的患者移植肾存活率为 96%[27]。另一项单中心研究随访 347 例患者 3 年后，18%的患者产生了 DSA，DQ 抗体最多见[28]。DQ 抗体和其他抗体都有的患者 3 年移植肾存活率（52%）低于只有 DQ 抗体、只有其他抗体、无 DSA 的患者（92%~94%）。这与普遍认为 HLA Ⅱ类抗体对远期移植肾存活影响较大的观点一致。图 103.3 表示了新生 DSA 的过程和影响。

抗体介导损伤

HLA 抗体是 AMR 的主要因子。AMR 传统上范围包括超急性排斥、急性排斥、慢性排斥以及最后导致的移植肾肾小球病。迟发型急性 AMR 不论能不能检测到 DSA，都是用药依从性差的表现。

目前有很多有效的 AMR 治疗方法，如血浆置换、免疫吸附、IVIG、利妥昔单抗、硼替佐米和依库里单抗。这些方法在本书其他章节详细阐述。

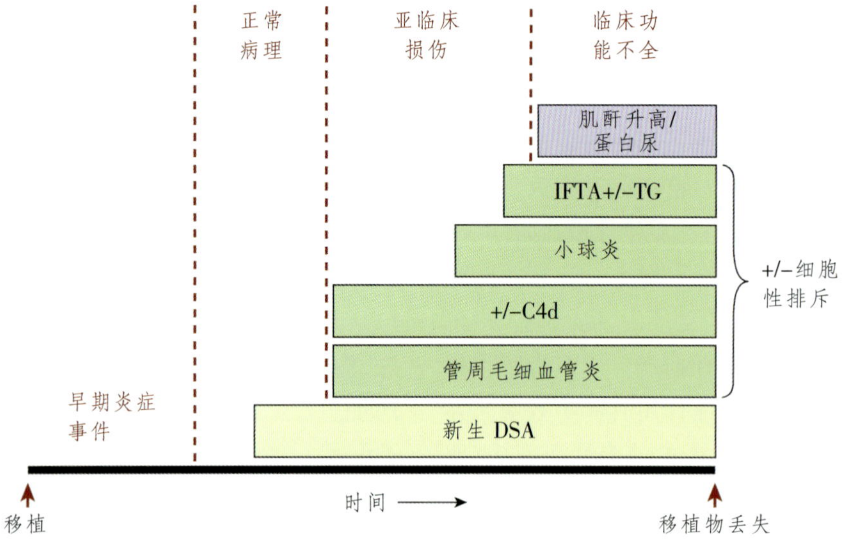

图 103.3 新生 DSA 的过程及其对移植肾的影响。(Adapted from [27] Wiebe et al. Am J Transplant. 2012, with permission from Wiley-Blackwell.)

针对性治疗往往能够逆转急性 AMR,改善移植肾功能,但 AMR 的发生对长期预后仍有消极影响。即使临床指标好转,AMR 患者仍有可能发生移植肾小球病。移植肾小球病被认为是免疫介导内皮损伤所致,与移植肾预后不佳相关。

慢性 AMR 是远期移植肾失功的主要原因。慢性 AMR 与移植肾小球病、管周毛细血管炎等表现有关。慢性 AMR 常伴有明显小管间质纤维化和小管萎缩,以及微血管改变。因为抗体的作用开始于黏附微血管内皮。虽然有有效的免疫抑制及一系列抗急性体液排斥方案,慢性 AMR 仍无有效治疗。临床上,慢性 AMR 可表现为亚急性、进行性肾功能不全和蛋白尿。患者也可能有外周水肿和高血压。移植前 DSA、高敏状态和移植后 DSA 形成都与慢性 AMR 的发生有关。依从性差也是一个重要原因,可从患者的血药浓度得到依据。

感染及移植后肿瘤

移植一直以来都受到感染和肿瘤的影响。更详细的内容在第 94 章和第 95 章介绍。在此仅概括这些并发症的主要特点。

CMV 感染

CMV 错配(供体阳性/受体阴性)与移植物存活率低和患者死亡率高相关。CMV 病在 HLA-DR 零错配患者中多见[29]。单中心回顾 470 例受体发现,CMV 病和 HLA-DR 零错配的移植肾存活率下降。较早的移植肾失功部分是由于 CMV 感染所致,也有部分是由于减少免疫抑制药物。虽然尽量同时兼顾 CMV 血清学状态及 HLA 匹配情况,目前的器官短缺导致前者受到限制。因此大多数中心选择术后进行 6~9 个月的预防性用药来减少 CMV 病的发生。

BK 多瘤病毒

肾移植受体的免疫抑制治疗可能会引起 BK 感染活动,导致小管间质性肾炎、输尿管狭窄和膀胱炎。诊断大多是通过筛查得出, 大部分患者在术后 1 年发生感染,也可延后。一线治疗包括减少免疫抑制药物,对于移植肾的不良反应在于:

- 由于病毒的直接损伤将导致肾实质和输尿管并发症
- 减少免疫抑制药物可导致慢性免疫损伤
- 炎症和纤维化后肾功能快速下降

由于 BK 肾病相关的移植物失功数据较少, 且局限于小型研究,免疫抑制调整方案多变,使得 BK 感染的长期影响难以估计。在一项 41 例 BK 肾炎的研究中,3 年和 5 年存活率从无 BK 感染的 83%和 76%降至 58%和 47%。46%的 BK 感染受体会发生移植肾失功。BK 感染后恢复的患者达到肾功能稳定需要 112 天[30]。BK 病毒性肾病对短期和长期预后都是重大威胁。

EB 病毒和移植后淋巴增殖性疾病

移植后淋巴增殖性疾病(PTLD,在第 96 章详述)仅发生于约 1%的移植患者,但其死亡风险很高。PTLD 与 EB 病毒诱导 B 细胞增殖有关,但也有 EBV 阴性的 PTLD 报道。除非黑色素瘤皮肤癌外,这是最常见的肾移植术后肿瘤。移植时 EBV 血清学阴性及移植后免疫抑制是 PTLD 的高危因素。CLTA-4 抑制剂贝拉西普治疗的 EBV 阴性患者中 PTLD 高发,表明其与 T 细胞抑制相关[22]。

大多数 PTLD 是在术后 18 个月内诊断的,10 年发生率约为 1%。虽然发生率低,一旦发生,患者存活率将降至 51%(1 年)和 39%(5 年)[31]。OPTN 数据分析认为,诊断为 PTLD 后,带功死亡的风险增加 17.5 倍,移植肾失功风险增加 5.5 倍[32]。

社会和种族因素

近来对移植受者长期结果的社会经济因素的关注越来越多。

黑人受体移植肾和患者存活率都较低。生物学影响因素包括 HLA 多态性、免疫抑制治疗需求和药代动力学变异引起较高的排斥率和影响移植物的生存[7,33]。随着免疫抑制剂的进步，某些生物学因素逐渐让位于社会经济学因素。低移植肾存活率与低收入、低教育水平、低保险报销比例和较差的看护有关。当收入和教育水平接近,移植肾存活的种族差异也会缩小。许多社会经济因素的影响在黑人受体中尤为突出。

研究长期预后时，移植肾年损耗率是区别早期和远期的有效工具。黑人受体的移植肾年损耗率更高(图 103.4)。不仅仅是在早期损耗明显,在远期也可以看到较缓慢但仍可识别的损耗。

慢性移植肾失功的多因素性质是目前肾移植的重大挑战。控制免疫反应改善了短期存活率,但干预措施会增加长期损耗。最终，心血管疾病、感染并发症和 PTLD 成为移植肾和患者存活的突出威胁因素。

慢性疾病状态与社会经济负担一起使得准确干预较为困难。当前改善长期预后需要在个体水平长时间随访。干预危险因素及术前开始预防性健康保健将成为必需。随着肾移植受体寿命的延长,短期预后的提升空间较小，我们应当开始关注慢性疾病的防治和减轻社会经济压力。

总结

肾移植依然是较为满意的替代透析治疗的方法。然而，长期应用免疫抑制药物对患者及移植肾长期存活具有不良影响。短期预后的改善为调整免疫抑制剂治疗和防治慢性并发症提供了机会。临床医生需要对这些问题有较为透彻的理解，以期未来获得更好的肾移植效果。

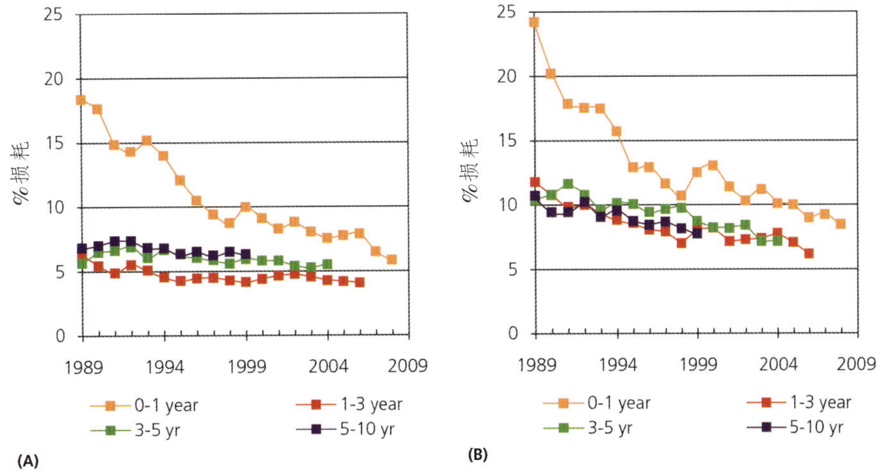

图 103.4 首次肾移植受体累积年损耗率。(A)非黑种人尸体 SCD 供体;(B)黑种人尸体 SCD 供体。(Reproduced from [5] Lamb et al. Am J Transplant. 2011, with permission from Wiley-Blackwell.)

(吴建永 译 吴建永 校)

参考文献

1. Port FK, Wolfe RA, Mauger EA, et al. Comparison of survival probabilities for dialysis patients vs cadaveric renal transplant recipients. Journal of the American Medical Association. 1993;270(11):1339–1343.
2. Wolfe RA, Ashby VB, Milford EL, et al. Comparison of mortality in all patients on dialysis, patients on dialysis awaiting transplantation, and recipients of a first cadaveric transplant. New England Journal of Medicine. 1999;341(23): 1725–1730.
3. Meier-Kriesche HU, Schold JD, Kaplan B. Long-term renal allograft survival: have we made significant progress or is it time to rethink our analytic and therapeutic strategies? American Journal of Transplantation. 2004;4(8):1289–1295.
4. Gjertson DW. Survival trends in long-term first cadaver-donor kidney transplants. Clinical Transplants. 1991;225–235.
5. Lamb KE, Lodhi S, Meier-Kriesche HU. Long-term renal allograft survival in the United States: a critical reappraisal. American Journal of Transplantation. 2011;11(3):450–462.
6. Meier-Kriesche HU, Schold JD, Srinivas TR, et al. Lack of improvement in renal allograft survival despite a marked decrease in acute rejection rates over the most recent era. American Journal of Transplantation. 2004;4(3):378–383.
7. Butkus DE, Meydrech EF, Raju SS. Racial differences in the survival of cadaveric renal allografts. Overriding effects of HLA matching and socioeconomic factors. New England Journal of Medicine. 1992;327(12):840–845.
8. Isaacs RB, Nock SL, Spencer CE, et al. Racial disparities in renal transplant outcomes. American Journal of Kidney Diseases. 1999;34(4):706–712.
9. Matas AJ, Gillingham KJ, Humar A, et al. Immunologic and nonimmunologic factors: different risks for cadaver and living donor transplantation. Transplantation. 2000;69(1):54–58.
10. Giral M, Foucher Y, Karam G, et al. Kidney and recipient weight incompatibility reduces long-term graft survival. Journal of the American Society of Nephrology. 2010;21(6):1022–1029.
11. Rao PS, Schaubel DE, Guidinger MK, et al. A comprehensive risk quantification score for deceased donor kidneys: the kidney donor risk index. Transplantation. 2009;88(2):231–236.
12. Meier-Kriesche HU, Kaplan B. Waiting time on dialysis as the strongest modifiable risk factor for renal transplant outcomes: a paired donor kidney analysis. Transplantation. 2002;74(10):1377–1381.
13. Kasiske BL, Snyder JJ, Matas AJ, et al. Preemptive kidney transplantation: the advantage and the advantaged. Journal of the American Society of Nephrology. 2002;13(5):1358–1364.
14. Kasiske BL, Anjum S, Shah R, et al. Hypertension after kidney transplantation. American Journal of Kidney Diseases. 2004;43(6):1071–1081.
15. Ojo AO. Cardiovascular complications after renal transplantation and their prevention. Transplantation. 2006;82(5):603–611.
16. Holdaas H, Fellstrom B, Jardine AG, et al. Effect of fluvastatin on cardiac outcomes in renal transplant recipients: a multicentre, randomised, placebo-controlled trial. Lancet. 2003;361(9374):2024–2031.
17. Hurst FP, Altieri M, Patel PP, et al. Effect of smoking on kidney transplant outcomes: analysis of the United States Renal Data System. Transplantation. 2011;92(10):1101–1107.
18. Kasiske BL, Snyder JJ, Gilbertson D, et al. Diabetes mellitus after kidney transplantation in the United States. American Journal of Transplantation. 2003;3(2): 178–185.
19. Gore JL, Pham PT, Danovitch GM, et al. Obesity and outcome following renal transplantation. American Journal of Transplantation. 2006;6(2):357–363.
20. Herzog CA, Ma JZ, Collins AJ. Long-term outcome of renal transplant recipients in the United States after coronary revascularization procedures. Circulation. 2004;109(23):2866–2871.
21. McCulloch TA, Harper SJ, Donnelly PK, et al. Influence of nifedipine on interstitial fibrosis in renal transplant allografts treated with cyclosporin A. Journal of Clinical Pathology. 1994;47(9):839–842.
22. Vincenti F, Larsen CP, Alberu J, et al. Three-year outcomes from BENEFIT, a randomized, active-controlled, parallel-group study in adult kidney transplant recipients. American Journal of Transplantation. 2012;12(1):210–217.
23. Vanrenterghem Y, Bresnahan B, Campistol J, et al. Belatacept-based regimens are associated with improved cardiovascular and metabolic risk factors compared with cyclosporine in kidney transplant recipients (BENEFIT and BENEFIT-EXT studies). Transplantation. 2011;91(9):976–983.
24. Hariharan S, Adams MB, Brennan DC, et al. Recurrent and de novo glomerular disease after renal transplantation: a report from Renal Allograft Disease Registry (RADR). Transplantation. 1999;68(5):635–641.
25. Opelz G. Non-HLA transplantation immunity revealed by lymphocytotoxic antibodies. Lancet. 2005;365(9470):1570–1576.
26. Terasaki PI, Ozawa M. Predicting kidney graft failure by HLA antibodies: a prospective trial. American Journal of Transplantation. 2004;4(3):438–443.
27. Wiebe C, Gibson IW, Blydt-Hansen TD, et al. Evolution and clinical pathologic correlations of de novo donor-specific HLA antibody post kidney transplant. American Journal of Transplantation. 2012;12(5):1157–1167.
28. Devos JM, Gaber AO, Knight RJ, et al. Donor-specific HLA-DQ antibodies may contribute to poor graft outcome after renal transplantation. Kidney International. 2012;82(5):598–604.
29. Schnitzler MA, Lowell JA, Hmiel SP, et al. Cytomegalovirus disease after prophylaxis with oral ganciclovir in renal transplantation: the importance of HLA-DR matching. Journal of the American Society of Nephrology. 2003;14(3):780–785.
30. Vasudev B, Hariharan S, Hussain SA, et al. BK virus nephritis: risk factors, timing, and outcome in renal transplant recipients. Kidney International. 2005;68(4): 1834–1839.
31. Faull RJ, Hollett P, McDonald SP. Lymphoproliferative disease after renal transplantation in Australia and New Zealand. Transplantation. 2005;80(2):193–197.
32. Hricik DE. Posttransplant lymphoproliferative disorders: a continued threat for kidney transplant recipients. American Journal of Kidney Diseases. 2011;58(6): 870–871.
33. Kerman RH, Kimball PM, Van Buren CT, et al. Possible contribution of pretransplant immune responder status to renal allograft survival differences of black versus white recipients. Transplantation. 1991;51(2):338–342.

第 104 章
肝移植长期预后

Heidi Yeh, Paulo Martins, James F. Markmann

引言

目前，肝移植是终末期肝病的标准治疗方式及唯一可能治愈的方法。50 年前，人类肝移植刚刚起步，3 例患者接受移植手术，第 1 例受者术中死亡，第 2 例受者术后 3 周死亡，最后一例受者移植后一周死亡[1]。到 1980 年，受者移植后一年生存率不到 40%[2]。2009 年 SRTR 年度报告表明，移植物一年生存率为 86%，5 年生存率为 70%，10 年生存率为 53%，同时，受者一年生存率为 90%，5 年生存率为 75%，10 年生存率为 60%[3]。

虽然供肝数量不足，移植物及受者长期生存期逐渐延长，主要的进展发生在 1980—1995 年之间的 15 年(图 104.1)。过去 30 年肝移植的实践，手术方式、免疫抑制治疗和器官保存技术的改进，促成了这些进展。具体内容可见第 56 章、第 66 章和第 21 章。1988 年，人类发明氩气凝血器，20 世纪 90 年代，术中血液回收装置(细胞保存器)的使用完全改变了术中出血的重要性。20 世纪 90 年代初，免疫治疗方案转变为应用他克莫司，减少了高剂量皮质醇的使用及 T 细胞清除的副作用，降低了排斥的发生率，极大地提高了长期生存时间。20 世纪 80 年代晚期，威斯康星大学保存液(Viaspan)最初用于胰腺保存，它能够改善远期预后，很快取代了欧洲柯林液，成为肝脏的标准保存液，一直沿用至今。重症监护的发展对于肝移植术后死亡率的降低也意义重大，相关内容已在 43 章详细阐述。20 世纪 90 年代，每年的活体肝移植数量基本少于 100 例，移植物及受者长期生存统计数据并不稳定，1999 年以后，每年开展的活体肝移植超过 200 例，自此之后，移植物及受者长期生存率并没有明显提高(图 104.2，也可见第 24 章和第 57 章)。

有趣的是，不同时期移植后生存曲线的变化趋势在 3 个月的节点之后十分相似，移植后 90 天内受者死亡率下降趋势最大(图 104.3)。因此，肝移植后短期预后改善能够显著改善远期预后。虽然我们尽力去控制影响围术期死亡率的因素，由于患者已存在的基础疾病及长期免疫抑制治疗产生的副作用，肝移植长期预后并没有明显改善。本章讨论导致受者死亡和移植肝失功的晚期因素、肝移植后远期转归影响因素和肝移植晚期并发症。

移植后晚期死亡及供肝失活的原因

超过一半的肝移植受者在移植肝具有功能时死亡。北美大量单中心及多中心研究报道，移植肝失功造成 9%~43%的晚期死亡(移植后 1~3 年)[4-9]。对比之下，移植后早期死亡（移植后 3 个月内）的主要原因是感染、移植肝功能不全及手术相关并发症。

原病复发与慢性排斥反应

原病复发是导致移植肝失功的主要原因，其次是慢性排斥反应。原病复发包括丙肝复发，小部分为酒精性肝炎。在英国，各种原因导致的移植肝失功占移植后死亡原因的 10%[10]。值得注意的是，1996 年英国因丙肝开展的肝移植占 10%，2008 年这一数字上升到 21%[11]。预计再经过差不多长的时间，因丙肝开展的肝移植将从 21%上升到超过 40%[12]。第 78 章详细阐述了移植后复发疾病的治疗原则及方法。

肿瘤与感染

除原病复发和慢性排斥外，肿瘤与感染是移植后死亡的主要原因。尽管肿瘤和感染不能表明移植肝失功，作为免疫抑制的并发症，两者确实与移植物相关。新发肿瘤导致 9%~24%的移植后死亡率，原肿瘤复发

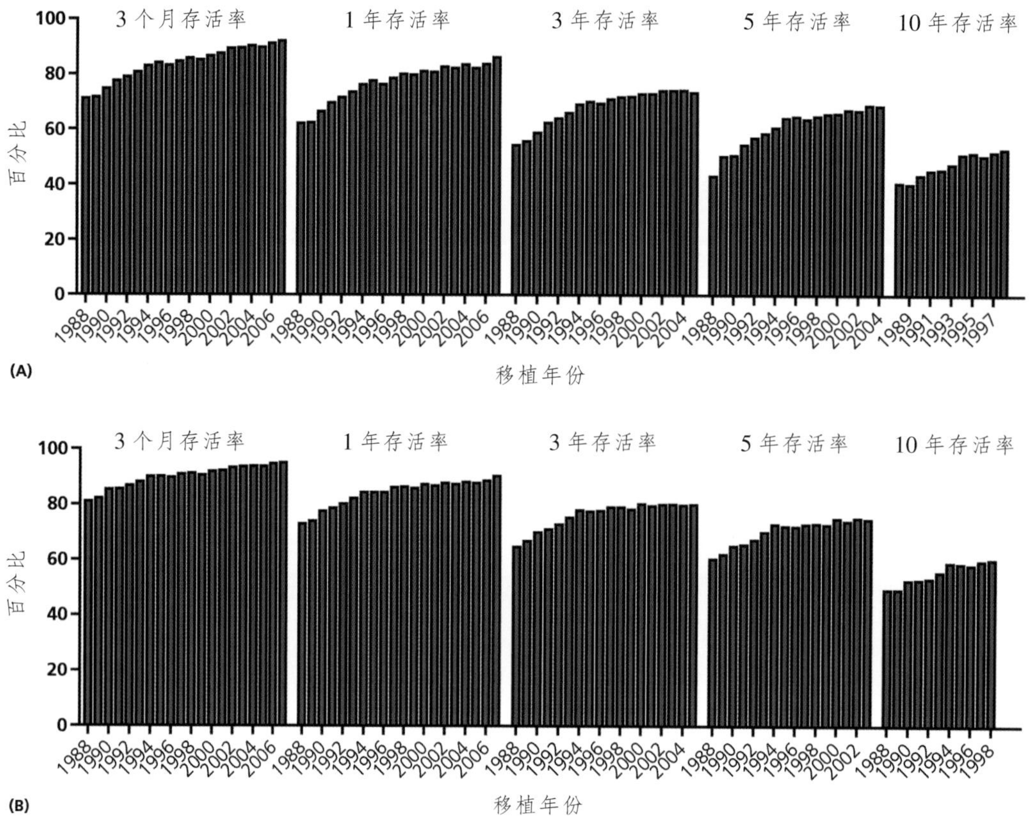

图 104.1 (A)尸体供肝肝移植调整后移植物存活率。(B)尸体供肝肝移植调整后患者生存率。

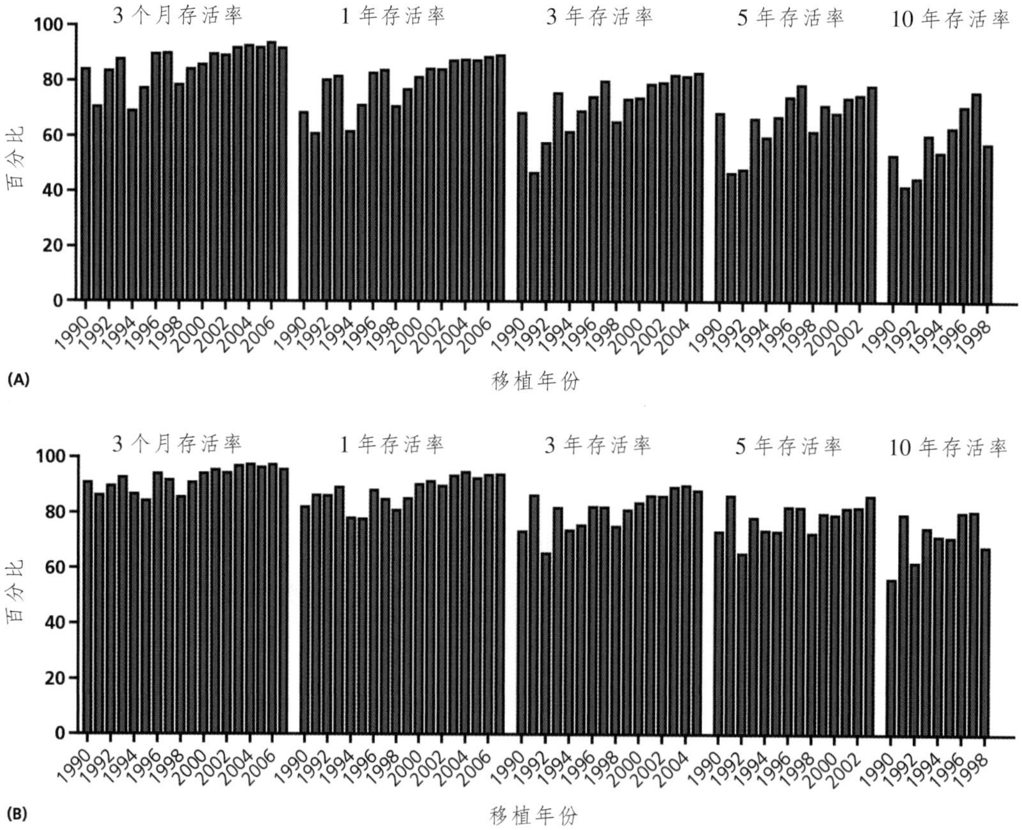

图 104.2 (A)活体供肝肝移植调整后移植物存活率。(B)活体供肝肝移植调整后患者生存率。

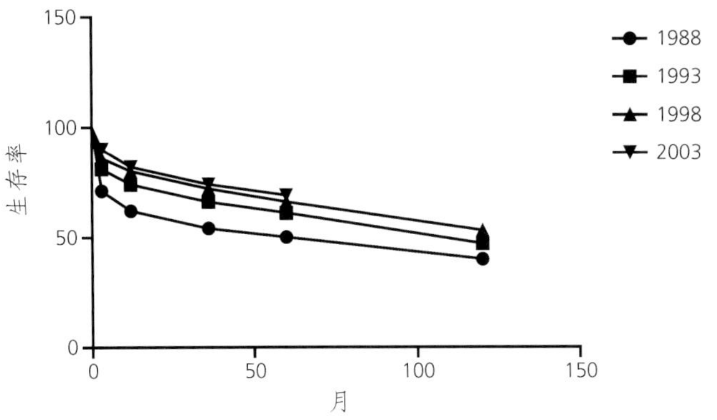

图 104.3　三组存活率:生存率。

所导致的死亡率与新发肿瘤相同。因此,肿瘤是导致肝移植受者远期死亡的主要原因[4,6,7,9,10]。移植后淋巴组织增生性疾病的 15 年累计发生率仅占移植后死亡原因的 4.7%,该种疾病将死亡风险增加了 10%~15%[13]。第 95 章和第 96 章分别详细阐述了上述疾病的治疗原则及方法。

感染,作为免疫抑制治疗最显著的副作用,尽管仅 10%的“多系统器官衰竭”和感染相关,但感染占移植后死亡原因的 8%~20%[4,5,8,9]。由于感染引起的死亡率较高,由于慢性排斥反应引起的死亡率较低,反之亦然。感染已在第 94 章进行了详细阐述。

心血管疾病

非移植物相关的主要死亡原因为心血管疾病(也可见第 98 章),约占移植后远期死亡原因的 20%[4-9,14]。使用皮质醇和钙调磷酸酶抑制剂会增加发生心血管疾病(高血压、糖尿病、高脂血症)的风险,因此心血管疾病有时被认为是皮质醇和钙调磷酸酶抑制剂治疗方案的副作用。研究表明,死于心血管疾病的患者在移植前存在冠心病高危因素或已存在冠心病[4]。加拿大的一项研究表明,心血管疾病发生率和匹配年龄人群之间不存在统计学意义[5]。

随着非酒精性脂肪肝病肝移植逐渐增加,心血管疾病很有可能成为肝移植后死亡的主要原因。未来 5~10 年,非酒精性脂肪肝病(NAFLD)可能是进行肝移植的首要指征[15],引起 NAFLD 的危险因素与心血管疾病的危险因素一致,包括糖尿病、高脂血症、高血压以及肥胖。事实上,因非酒精性脂肪肝病导致的肝移植与因原发性胆汁淤积性肝硬化、原发性硬化性胆管炎、酒精性肝病或丙肝相关肝移植相比,心血管事件所致死亡率更高[16]。

影响患者长期预后的受者因素

原发疾病

由于肝移植术后主要的死亡原因之一为恶性肿瘤的复发,作为肝移植首要指征,恶性肿瘤所致死亡率最高并不令人惊讶。相关研究估计,肝癌肝移植的死亡率约为非肝癌肝移植死亡率的 2 倍[17]。根据 SRTR 报道,与其他原因导致的移植相比,恶性肿瘤移植后 3 个月及 1 年生存率相近甚至更好,但 5 年和 10 年生存率分别降低约 10%和 20%。一项单中心研究表明,在该中心,两者 1 年生存率相差 10%,5 年及 5 年以上生存率相差超过 40%[18]。恶性肿瘤移植后 5 年和 10 年生存率分别只有 67%和 50%[3]。

暴发性肝衰竭所致肝移植与慢性非恶性肿瘤肝病所致肝移植相比,移植后死亡风险更高,其 5 年和 10 年生存率分别为 71%和 58%[3]。恶性疾病移植后 3 个月生存率明显较低,3 个月后,其生存率下降趋势与慢性非恶性疾病所致肝移植的受者相近[3]。这和术后高发的脓毒病/多器官衰竭及神经并发症所致的移植后死亡率一致[19]。移植前肾衰竭是移植后死亡率的最强预测因素[19]。

尽管最早认为丙肝所致移植的预后与其他移植适应证相似[20],将 20 世纪 80 年代初和 20 世纪 90 年代进行的移植例数包括在内,统计分析所得出的肝移植后 1 年生存率仅为 70%。同时,非丙肝相关肝移植受者生存期已逐渐延长,但丙肝相关肝移植受者生存期并未明显延长[21-23]。最近,越来越多的研究表明丙肝患者与非丙肝患者相比,其死亡风险提高约 23%,移植肝衰竭发生风险提高约 30%[24]。肝癌肝移植和丙肝肝移植与其他移植适应证相比,长期预后均较差。肝癌肝移植和丙肝肝移植数量增加,移植物远期预后和短期预后均有改善。

另一方面,胆道闭锁和代谢疾病所致肝移植远期预后是最好的。尽管两者是儿童肝移植的主要适应证,两者在全美肝移植总量中不足 1%。第 114 章详细阐述了儿童肝移植的内容。相比其他更常见的肝移植适应证,胆汁淤积性疾病(包括原发性胆道硬化和原发性硬化性胆管炎)远期预后最好[3,18]。

肝肺综合征和门静脉高压

肝肺综合征源于肺内扩张和分流,未经氧合的血液直接回到左心房，导致血氧不足。有 8%~32%的终末期肝病患者会发生肝肺综合征[25,26]，其唯一的治疗手段为肝移植。但与氧合正常的移植患者相比，肝肺综合征患者术后恢复差[26,27]，尽管部分患者与非肝肺综合征患者术后恢复情况相近[27]，大部分患者 90 天死亡率接近 30%[26]。无论患者氧分压是否低于 60mmHg，术后死亡主要是因为分流量的增加[26]。移植后分流的恢复需要数周至数月。

相比之下，肝移植并非门脉性肺动脉高压的标准治疗方法，并非因为存在其他可替代的治疗手段，而是因为严重门静脉高压移植后预后极差。4%~16%的肝纤维化患者会发生门脉性肺动脉高压，并发有严重腹水的肝硬化患者发生率更高[28]，其机制尚未研究明了。肺血管高压的产生主要是由于终末期肝病血管调控失衡，血管收缩增加，内皮损伤，血管重塑导致高压，最终血管平滑肌增殖，微血管栓塞，右心房衰竭[28]。依据血管重塑的程度，移植后肺血管高压可能改善，也可能无法逆转。

门脉性肺动脉高压背景下的肝移植，移植开始时的总体死亡率接近 40%，术中总体死亡率约为移植开始死亡率的 3 倍[27]。依据平均肺动脉压力，相关研究将受者分层，证明如果平均肺动脉压力在 25~35mmHg，门脉性肺动脉高压患者与非门脉性肺动脉高压患者围术期死亡率相近。若平均肺动脉压力在 35~50mmHg，围术期死亡率超过 50%[29]。若平均肺动脉压力>50mmHg，死亡率为 100%。对于初始平均肺动脉压力>50mmHg 的患者，服用环前列腺素将肺动脉压力降至 35mmHg 以下，其远期预后能明显改善[30]。能够通过血管舒张剂将平均肺动脉压力降低是可逆转性肺动脉高压及良好预后的指标。

年龄、性别和人种

某些研究团体曾报道，年龄>60 岁的受者与年龄<60 岁的受者相比，其预后较差[31-37]。事实上，中位生存率在 60 岁并没有突然的转变。总体而言，年轻受者，尤其是青春期前儿童，其移植后一年生存期与老年患者相比更好，而各年龄组术后 3 个月生存期没有明显差异(图 104.4)。

最近针对老年群体的研究表明，70 岁以上受者与 60 岁以下受者的术后生存期没有明显差异。但老年患者的 MELD(终末期肝病模型)评分更低，肌酸酐水平更高，术后重症监护室停留时期更长，白蛋白浓度更高[38,39]，这项研究表明，年老移植受者的选择标准应更加严格，这对保证移植后良好的远期预后有重要意义。两项研究均表明，70 岁以上人群移植后发生心血管并发症的风险更高，提示在老年人群中筛查心血管风险因素非常重要。

男性接受肝移植的数量为女性的 2 倍，但性别似

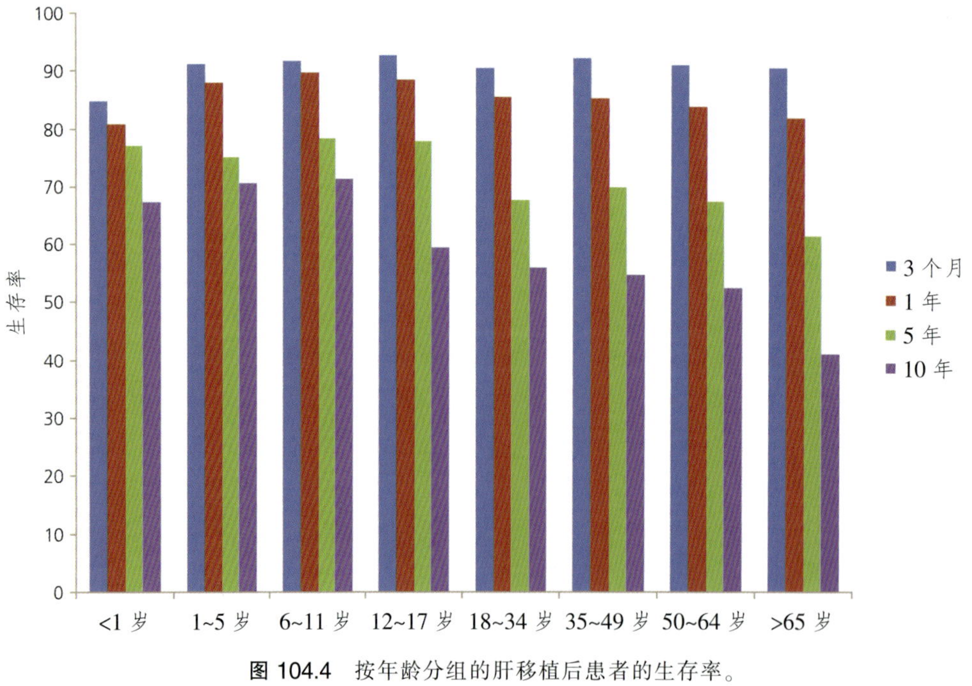

图 104.4 按年龄分组的肝移植后患者的生存率。

乎并不会影响移植后总体生存[3,40]。值得注意的是，女性患者作为移植人群组成部分之一，若为丙肝患者，与男性丙肝患者相比，其 1 年、5 年和 10 年移植后死亡的风险增高 14%~15%[40]。

较早的研究表明，相比白种人与西班牙裔，亚洲裔美国人与非洲裔美国人的预后较差[41]。几十年来，亚洲裔美国人移植后预后不断改善，截至目前，亚洲裔美国人移植后预后是最好的[3,42]。乙肝相关肝硬化而非丙肝是亚洲裔美国人进行肝移植的主要适应证，而乙肝相关肝硬化的治疗取得较大进展，这可能是导致这一现象的部分原因[42]。最初，乙肝所致肝移植的预后非常差，甚至被认为是肝移植的禁忌证。随着乙肝抗体和核苷类似物拉米夫定、替诺福韦及恩替卡韦的研发，乙肝复发能够被避免，未复发的乙肝患者移植后生存能够明显改善[43-46]。

但非洲裔美国人移植后生存依然较差。非洲裔美国人的慢性排斥发生率更高[47]。同时，丙肝更易复发且治疗不敏感[48]，也更易发生移植后糖尿病，增加并发症，提高死亡率[49]。

体重指数

约 3%的肝移植受者的体重指数(BMI)>35kg/m^2[50]。有关肥胖受者(BMI 27~32kg/m^2)、严重肥胖受者(BMI >32kg/m^2)和正常体重受者的单中心研究并没有发现三者的远期移植后生存有明显差异，但肥胖受者术后呼吸衰竭发生率更高，住院时间更长，医疗花费更高[51]。严重肥胖受者容易增加手术难度，使热缺血时间延长，这可能是导致他们更易发生移植物功能不全的原因[52]。大样本研究表明，BMI>35~40kg/m^2 死亡率提高 40%，主要原因是移植后第一年发生的心血管意外事件[50,52]。

大样本研究与小样本研究的差异主要是统计差异。小样本研究不足以发现生存期差异。但一些研究者认为如果将腹水因素考虑其中，修正 BMI 后，不同 BMI 群体生存期不存在统计学意义差异。约 20%的患者修正 BMI 后，归入轻度肥胖群体。这些研究者指出每升腹水约提高 7%的死亡率[53]。肥胖本身可能并不是移植术后死亡率的强力预测指标，但病态肥胖群体并发症更多见，这些并发症对死亡风险影响较大[54]。

移植后生存时间是移植价值的一项评估指标，但一些关注生存获益的研究认为，如果移植后生存时间与未移植生存时间相同，那么移植后生存时间是没有意义的。综合考虑移植后死亡风险率和未移植死亡风险率，以 5kg/m^2 为分层间隔，不同 BMI 群体生存获益不存在差异[55]。

BMI<18.5kg/m^2(体重过低)的受者约占移植人群的 2%[50]。尽管他们也被认为是移植高危人群，关于该人群移植后预后的相关研究鲜有出版。仅有的一些研究指出，该人群移植后容易发生术后出血和脑血管并发症，移植后死亡率较正常人群提高 55%~60%[50,51]。同样的，该人群移植后死亡时间大多发生在移植后第一年[50]。相比其他 BMI 人群，该人群移植后生存获益略低(0.14 对 0.14~0.17)，但该差异并不存在统计学意义[55]。

终末期肝病的多器官移植

在目前开展的多器官复合移植中，肝肾联合移植是最常见的，在 2005 年之后，每年开展的肝肾联合移植超过 300 例，有些年份甚至超过 400 例[56]。在美国，肾衰竭能够明显增加肝移植受者的 MELD 评分，器官分配政策也相应做出调整。肝肾联合移植的适应证不在本章详细阐述，相关研究表明肝肾联合移植与单独肝移植相比，受者术后生存不存在差异[57,58]。事实上，虽然不同研究对于肾衰竭严重程度及透析时间长短的定义不同，一部分肾功能下降的终末期肝病患者接受了肝肾联合移植后，其预后比单独进行肝移植要好[58-60]。同时，大量研究已经证明，移植前肾衰竭会增加移植后死亡率[61,62]，提示肝肾联合移植能够逆转肾衰竭对于肝移植后的不利影响。值得注意的是，虽然肾脏的体液性排斥的保护机制尚未研究清楚[66]，可能是由于清除了供者特异性抗体[63-65]，与单独肝移植相比，肝肾联合移植后移植肾存活期比未移植更长[63]。

除了肝肾联合移植，其他腹腔脏器联合肝移植的预后均比单独肝移植要差得多，但其预后相比未移植要好一些。美国每年进行的肝肠联合移植约为 100 例(包括联合胰腺或肾脏的几例)，近十年来，尽管肠移植的预后生存极大改善，肝肠联合移植后 1 年患者、移植物生存率仅为 70%，远比单独肝移植或单独肠移植低[67]。3 年、5 年患者、移植物生存率分别为约 60%和不到 60%，10 年患者生存率不足 50%[67]。每年进行的肝胰腺联合移植(联合或不联合肾移植)仅仅开展数例[56]，其 3 年、5 年生存率分别为 71%和 64%[68]。肝肠移植和多内脏移植的预后在 109 章详细阐述。

肝-胸腔器官联合移植同样少之又少。2009 年，共开展了11例肝心联合移植(包括1例肝-肺-心联合移植)和10例肝肺联合移植(包括1例肝-肺-心联合移植)[56]。尽管开展例数极少,肝心联合移植预后仅比单独肝移植稍差,与单独心移植相同,其1年、3年和5年生存率分别为85%、77%和75%[69,70]。这可能是由于肝心联合移植的主要适应证是遗传性淀粉样变性,这些患者除了甲胎蛋白异常,术前无肝功能紊乱[69-71]。此外,2007年统计报道,所有肝心联合移植患者的平均年龄仅为46岁[69]。和肝肾联合移植相同,相比单独心脏移植,肝心联合移植似乎也能够减轻抗排斥反应[70]。

肝肺联合移植主要针对囊状纤维化并发α1抗胰蛋白酶病的患者开展[72]。2008年统计的患者1年生存率不到70%[72,73],目前,尤其是针对囊性纤维化患者,肝-肺联合移植手术时机的选择以及是否应该进行双器官移植仍存在众多争议[73-75]。目前报道的肝肺心三器官联合移植1年生存率为50%,5年生存率为37.5%[74]。

再次移植

首次移植如果失败,唯一可行的治疗方法为再次移植。近20年,用于再次移植的器官占比下降,再次移植后预后生存极大改善,但目前超过15%的肝移植是为了替代前次移植后衰竭的移植肝,再次肝移植后生存预后较首次移植低。最近的移植受者科学登记报告处报道的再次移植患者1年生存率为71%~77%[76-79],远低于首次移植患者的1年生存率(90%)[3]。配备长期随访的单中心研究表明,再次移植患者5年生存率为48%~62%[80-82]。有文献记录的德国单中心进行的再次移植后最佳1年生存率、最佳5年生存率分别为70%和67%[83]。但是其他欧洲研究表明再次移植后1年生存率最高不超过65%[81,84]。第3次、4次、5次移植相比第2次移植,死亡率更高[78]。再次移植1年移植物生存期仅为66%[76,79]。

MELD评分较高、需要呼吸机维持呼吸、肾功能下降、需要ICU监护等都是再次移植后预后的不良因素[80,83-86]。大部分大样本研究指出,丙肝血清阳性会提高移植物失功率和患者死亡率[79,85,87,88],当再次移植时MELD评分增高,丙肝血清阳性的这一作用会被放大。SRTR的一项分析研究表明,MELD评分>30、丙肝阳性患者移植后1年生存率仅为42%(丙肝阴性患者为55%),移植后5年生存率仅为21%(丙肝阴性患者为47%)[85]。相反,原发性移植肝失功导致的再次移植对于预后没有影响[81],或能改善预后[88]。相比首次移植后7天内或数月(年)后移植物失功的患者,首次移植后7~30天再次进行移植的患者预后要差得多[80,84]。高龄供者[44-54]、心死亡供者与移植预后负相关[80,83,89]。已存在的抗供体HLA-1抗体会降低约20%的生存率,有趣的是,这一现象仅存在于成人受者,儿童受者不存在此现象[90]。该项研究并未表明抗体阳性受者发生移植物失功(患者死亡)是由排斥反应造成的。

ABO血型与HLA配对

最初,人们认为ABO血型不配对会在移植术后30天造成约50%的移植物功能不全、受者死亡或再次移植[91]。移植物功能不全是抗体导致的肝内弥散性血管内凝血[91]、动脉血栓形成、胆管病以及排斥反应引起的[92,93]。血型不配对所致的再次肝移植以及O型血受者的预后非常差,相应的死亡风险分别为首次肝移植和ABO血型不符但非O型血受体的2.46倍和3.43倍[92,94]。

随着抗体调节机制相关临床经验的积累,血浆置换方法的多样组合、IV抗体、血浆除去法、利妥昔单抗、脾切、环磷酰胺以及T细胞去除法用于治疗ABO血型不合肝移植,这些方法主要是针对抗A、B抗体滴度较低的新生儿[95]。这些方法也用于治疗年龄稍大一些的儿童及成年人,小样本(6~14例)的移植物和患者生存预后时间接近ABO血型配对肝移植[96-99]。尽管不同研究的排斥反应及胆管病变发生率不同,总体而言,皮质醇反应是导致排斥反应发生的主要原因,强化免疫抑制、去除抗体的治疗方案可极大地降低胆道损伤的发生率[96-99]。移植后即时(两周)抗体滴度和排斥反应并不相关,细胞或抗体可能调控移植后即时抗体滴度,一些患者即使接受抗体清除疗法,其抗体滴度依然很高,另一些患者在中断抗体清除治疗后的数月,抗体滴度极低甚至无法检测到[96]。

小样本组(6~10例/组)研究结果表明,未应用抗体清除法直接移植A2亚型供体来源器官到O型血受者的预后和应用抗体清除法的预后相近[100,101]。这是由于A2亚型转移酶不同于A1亚型转移酶,不能高效地将抗原前体(H)转化为A抗原,导致A2亚型供体来源器官缺少细胞表面 A 抗原[102]。因此在移植器官分配时,O 型受者的中位等待时间约为 A 型和 AB 型受者的 2 倍,是 AB 型受者的约 5 倍[103]。

近 10 年,ABO 血型不配对移植占儿童移植的 2%~4%,在成人移植中不到 1%[104]。新生儿及儿童进行 ABO 血型不配对移植后,移植物存活时间与 ABO 血型配对移植相等[104,105],但成人 ABO 血型不配对移植后,移植物 1 年、3 年及 5 年存活率下降约 10%, 移植物 10 年存活时间与与 ABO 血型配对移植相等[104]。事实上,对于移植物存活 3 个月以上的受者,ABO 血型符合和 ABO 血型不合对受者的长期存活时间是一样的[104]。

HLA 配对对于肝移植后移植物存活和患者预后生存并没有影响[106,107]。在儿童活体相关移植中,HLA 配对导致移植后 6 周的低排斥率[108],当排斥反应发生时,可以检测到抗 HLA 抗体和 C4d 沉积[109,110],但这对于远期生存预后并没有影响。但相关报道生存,T 细胞交叉实验阳性容易导致急性排斥反应[111],使移植物 1 年、3 年、5 年存活率降低约 10%[112]。在美国,移植前 HLA 配对并非常规检查项目, 但回顾性交叉实验可用于指导排斥及移植物失功高风险患者的免疫抑制治疗管理。

供者影响受者及移植物存活预后的因素

供者短期风险因素

供者因素主要在移植后 90 天内影响移植物及受者存活预后,导致移植物长期功能紊乱和原发性失功。供者年龄是最重要的影响因素之一,70 岁以下的供者,每增加 10 岁,移植物失功率会增加 15%~20%。70 岁以上供者的移植物失功率是 40 岁以下供者的 1.65 倍[113]。冷缺血时间每增加 1h 仅提高 1%的移植物失功率[113],但冷缺血时间超过 12h 合并 45 岁以上的供者年龄会增加肝衰竭的发生[114],在丙肝患者中,年龄因素作用尤为明显。有趣的是,地区共享会增加约 11%的衰竭发生率,国内共享会增加约 28%的衰竭发生率[113]。卒中所致死亡的供体器官与缺氧或创伤所致死亡的供体器官相比会提高约 16%的移植物失功率[113]。非洲裔美国人来源的供肝相比白人供肝, 供肝衰竭发生率会提高 1.2 倍[113]。劈裂肝和部分肝移植相比全肝肝移植,失功率会提高 50%[113]。

脂肪变性是否能相反地影响移植肝功能、脂肪沉积是否直接引起毒性反应或是增强缺血-再灌注损伤均尚不清楚, 脂肪变性提示近期发生或正在发生的肝细胞损伤。不同程度的微血管脂肪变性并不会导致移植物失功和预后变差[114],但大血管脂肪变性超过 25%会导致 62%的功能失调、12%的原发性失功以及患者预后生存期缩短[114]。其他研究表明,脂肪变性超过 30%的移植肝 AST/ALT 和 INR 升高,肝功能紊乱,但 5 年移植物存活率改变不存在统计学意义[115,116]。一项研究表明,无脂肪变性的移植肝 1 年存活率为 82%,0~10%脂肪变性的移植肝为 73%,11%~30%脂肪变性的移植肝为 74%,31%~60%脂肪变性的移植肝为 62%。几乎没有一家中心供肝的脂肪变性超过 60%。值得注意的是,丙肝阳性受者如果接受脂肪变性超过 30%的供肝,丙肝的复发会更早、更频繁[117]。脂肪变性在移植后能够被逆转[118],大量研究正在研究移植前逆转供肝的脂肪变性[119]。

活体供肝移植

活体肾移植比尸体供体移植受者状况相对较好,移植物存活期更长[120],而肝移植与此不同,在活体肝移植中,供者处在死亡和并发症高风险状态,相比尸体供体移植并没有明显优势。在美国,活体肝移植相比尸体供体肝移植,移植后生存并没有优势。即使活体肝移植受者在接受移植时更年轻,MELD 评分更低[121,122]。活体供肝移植的移植后 10 年生存率稍高于尸体供体肝移植,但两者的差异不存在统计学意义[122]。事实上,丙肝阳性受者进行活体肝移植后, 其术后 1~3 年的生存率反而可能降低 12%~15%[122]。急性排斥反应常见于尸体供体肝移植[122],但活体肝移植移植物失功率更高[123]。

相对于尸体供体肝移植, 活体肝移植更易发生手术并发症。在移植后 90 天,主要的手术并发症是胆漏,其发生率比尸体供体肝移植高 3 倍(10%~32%对 8%~12%)[124,125]。90 天之后容易发生胆道梗阻,其发生率比尸体供体肝移植高 2~3 倍(28%~32%对 5%~15%)[125-127]。活体肝移植肝动脉栓塞发生率比尸体供体肝移植高 3 倍(6.5%对 2.3%),门静脉栓塞发生率为 3%,而这些在尸体供体肝移植中很少见[126]。手术中心的临床经验对于减少活体肝移植后手术并发症非常重要[124]。

然而,基于治愈目的的患者生存研究表明,活体肝移植受者相比等待尸体供体的受者,死亡率降低一半[128-130]。对于 MELD 评分<15,但死亡风险很高的供体等待者而言,活体肝移植的优势更加突出[130]。这一现象的原因是等待供体的受者最终因为无法得到供肝而死亡[128-130]。总之,尽管会提高发生并发症或是再次肝移植的风险,活体肝移植能够给那些最终无法等到供体的受者提供重要的生存获益。因此,在那些供体等待时间更长、死亡风险更高的国家,活体肝移植会更广泛地开展[131]。

心死亡(DCD)器官捐献

心死亡(DCD)器官捐献的数量在近 15 年中增长超过 10 倍[132,133]。虽然 DCD 器官增加了供体数量,DCD 器官的使用也存在风险。尽管 DCD 器官大多来源于较年轻的供者,冷缺血时间较短,相比脑死亡(DBD)器官,DCD 器官移植后移植物失功率远高于脑死亡来源供器官,为 50%~85%[132,134],相对应的 3 年移植物存活率比脑死亡来源供器官低 10%~15%[132,133,135,136]。在低风险受者中,不同来源的移植物生存率差异较小。年龄、是否为首次移植、正常的肾脏功能和良好的医疗条件等因素[133,136]影响低风险受者移植物生存率,这说明受者的选择标准对于 DCD 供体移植的预后至关重要。DCD 供肝移植受者生存率较低[133,137],热缺血时间少于 30min、冷缺血时间小于 10h 的 DCD 供肝有较好的移植预后[136]。

尽管脑死亡供肝胆管损伤发生率与冷缺血时间相关[141],DCD 供肝比 DBD 供肝更易发生不同缺血类型的胆管损伤(20%~40%对 5%)[138-140]。不同于吻合口狭窄,这些胆管狭窄不能通过内镜或手术治疗,高达一半的患者需要进行再次肝移植[142]。而吻合口狭窄的患者只有 1%~2%需要再次肝移植[143]。

乙肝阳性和丙肝阳性供者

在美国,15%的供体乙肝核心抗体阳性[144],但表面抗体阴性,提示病毒滴度未知的乙肝感染。在无预防的情况下,源自乙肝阳性供体的受体乙肝感染率为 25%~95%,这会导致严重的肝炎以及移植肝失功[145]。但通过乙肝抗体、拉米夫定、阿德福韦酯和(或)恩替卡韦的联合应用,乙肝病毒阳性的肝脏可以用于乙肝表面抗体阴性的受者,感染风险可以被控制在 5%以下[145-147],同时,1 年、3 年、5 年移植物及受者存活率和乙肝病毒阴性供体移植相近[144,145]。

同样地,大量研究表明,只要供肝功能正常,丙肝阳性受者接受丙肝阳性或阴性供肝移植[148-152],其移植肝及受者预后并没有明显差异。但老年供者(年龄≥50 岁)来源的供器官和年轻供者(年龄<50 岁)来源的供器官相比,受者发生移植肝功能不全和死亡的概率提高了 6 倍,供者年龄的影响远大于乙肝阴性供者,这主要是因为丙肝病毒引起的肝纤维化[152]。50 岁及以上供者来源的供器官中,丙肝阳性供者来源供器官发生供肝功能不全的可能性提高了 3 倍,这一现象不存在于年轻供者来源的供肝中。即使发生再次肝移植,受者预后相近[152]。

肝移植的远期并发症

肾衰竭

肝移植后 1 年、3 年、5 年及 10 年,Ⅳ型和Ⅴ型慢性肾脏病(GFR<29L/min)的发生率分别为 8%、14%、18%及 25%[153]。导致肝移植后终末期肾病的最常见原因是神经钙调蛋白抑制剂的毒性作用。其他原因包括糖尿病性肾病、血栓性微血管病、急性肾小管坏死、部分肾小球硬化症以及原先未治愈的肝肾综合征[154,155]。

年龄增加、糖尿病、高血压、急性肾损伤以及神经钙调蛋白抑制剂的使用增加慢性肾脏疾病的发生可能,其中,移植前就存在的肾脏疾病是移植后慢性肾脏疾病的提示因素[153,155]。丙肝感染也是慢性肾脏疾病发生的一个危险因素,这可能是由于丙肝与免疫复合体型肾小球体性肾炎[156]和糖尿病[157,158]之间存在某种联系。用西罗莫司代替神经钙调蛋白抑制剂,有时能够提高肾小球滤过率[159-162]。

在所有非肾脏移植患者中,终末期肾脏疾病将死亡风险提高了将近 5 倍[153]。在一项肝移植患者系列研究中,患有终末期肾脏疾病的肝移植患者移植后第 13 年生存率只有 28%,而这一数字在无肾脏疾病的患者群体中为 55%[154]。在其他非肾移植患者中[155],肾脏移植受者发生终末期肾脏疾病后,移植后第 6 年生存率只有 71%,而依赖肾脏替代治疗方案的患者,第 6 年生存率只有 27%[154]。

移植后糖尿病

根据相关报道,肝移植后新发糖尿病(包括 1 型和 2 型)的发生率为 5%~27%[163-166]。当接受大剂量类固醇治疗时,很多患者需要短暂的胰岛素治疗。45 岁以上受者发生移植后糖尿病的风险提高了 2 倍[163]，丙肝阳性受者这一风险提高了 2~6 倍[163,164,166,167]。即使在非移植患者中，丙肝感染相比乙肝感染更易引起糖尿病[164]，这可能是由于感染后反应性产生的细胞因子和病毒本身导致的胰岛素敏感性改变[168]。病毒血症的严重程度正相关影响胰岛素抵抗程度[168,169]，其部分原因是丙肝病毒核心蛋白引导的胰岛素信号蛋白（胰岛素受体亚基-1）的降解[170,171]以及胰岛素生长因子结合蛋白表达量的减少[170]。他克莫司具有 β 细胞毒性，直接减少胰岛素的分泌[172]，使用他克莫司而不是环孢素以维持免疫抑制状态，使糖尿病的发生概率提高了 3 倍[163,164]。有趣的是，如果移植肝活检存在 10%以上的脂肪变性，那么移植后发生糖尿病的概率也会增高 3 倍[163]。

感染、肾衰竭、神经及心血管并发症常见于移植后新发糖尿病的患者[173,174]。一些研究者发现，移植后新发糖尿病的患者和未新发糖尿病的患者其移植物存活率和患者存活率相近[163,165]。另外一些研究者发现移植后新发糖尿病患者的死亡率提高了将近 3 倍[167]。造成这种差异的部分原因可能是研究人群中囊括了 1 型和 2 型糖尿病患者，但移植后新发 1 型糖尿病患者移植物和患者存活率均降低了 40%，移植后新发 2 型糖尿病患者移植物存活率和移植后未发生糖尿病的患者相同[175]。

新发恶性肿瘤

在不同的系列研究中，肝移植后患者新发恶性肿瘤的发生率为 3%~55%[173,174]。根据肿瘤类型的不同，某些肿瘤发生率（非黑色素皮肤肿瘤）比总人群高了约 70 倍[173]，乳腺癌和泌尿生殖道肿瘤发生率和总人群相似或更低[176]。和免疫健全的个体相比，免疫抑制状态的个体发生恶性疾病的概率要高得多，无论这种恶性疾病是遗传相关、药物相关还是感染相关。这可能是由于 T 细胞、巨噬细胞以及清除蛋白质异常表达的肿瘤病毒或是恶性细胞的自然杀伤细胞功能丧失造成的。包括神经钙调蛋白抑制剂和抗代谢药物在内的许多免疫抑制药物也被认为可以直接导致肿瘤的产生[174]。

在非移植患者中，吸烟和长期饮酒会增加癌症，尤其是口咽肿瘤的发生概率[176,177]，而这一概率在肝移植患者中提高了 7 倍[173]。在众多原发性疾病中，原发性硬化性胆管炎最易导致非皮肤恶性肿瘤，虽然溃疡性结肠炎在原发性硬化性胆管炎患者中的发生率尚不清楚，原发性硬化性胆管炎最易导致结直肠癌[174,176]。值得注意的是，在非移植患者中，与单独患有溃疡性结肠炎相比，原发性硬化性胆管炎和溃疡性结肠炎并存会增加结直肠癌的发生率[178]，而原发性硬化性胆管炎患者发生结直肠癌的风险尚未研究清楚。总体而言，在肝移植后患者和非移植患者的配对研究中，结直肠癌的发生风险提高了 12 倍。

与普通人群相比，肝移植受者群体不仅患癌症的风险提高，也更易患恶性疾病。关于实质器官移植受者的研究表明，移植受者确诊结直肠癌后 5 年生存率仅为相匹配的同期结直肠癌患者的不到一半[179,180]。肝移植受者移植后 5 年因诊断非皮肤恶性肿瘤后的死亡概率不到 50%[176]。如此糟糕的预后究竟是由于移植患者患有更多不同肿瘤生物学特性的强侵袭性疾病，还是仅仅是由于免疫抑制状态造成的肿瘤防御机制减弱，目前众说纷纭。无论由于何种机制，肝移植受者移植后应严格监测皮肤损伤情况，一些研究者认为即使肝移植患者年龄低于 50 岁[180]，也必须每 3 年进行一次结直肠镜检查，对于原发性硬化性胆管炎的患者，每年都必须进行结直肠镜检查[181]。

操作性耐受

肝移植受者免疫耐受指的是外源免疫抑制下，移植物功能保持正常。这一报道最早见于 5 名依从性差的患者，他们在移植后一年左右停止服用免疫抑制剂，但他们的肝功能仍能保持正常，停止服药 13 年后各项临床指标及实验室检查仍然正常[182]。随后的一些研究在受者移植数年后探索性地停止服用免疫抑制剂，发生的副作用包括感染、恶性肿瘤以及较少见的肾衰竭，这些研究报道的耐受成功率在停止服用免疫抑制剂 10 年后高达 23%[183–185]。大体上，发生肝功能异常和(或)穿刺确认排斥反应发生的患者，重新应用神经钙调蛋白抑制剂或是应用低剂量类固醇，肝功能以及组织学结果均能够恢复正常。对于复发丙型肝炎的受者而言，停用免疫抑制反而能够改善组织疾病，或使组织疾病病情保持稳定[186]。对于原先存在自身免疫性肝脏疾病的受者，不建议撤除免疫抑制剂。

但据相关报道，部分患者在停止使用免疫抑制剂后数年发生慢性排斥反应[183,187]，但这些现象在早期发现，重新应用神经钙调蛋白抑制剂也能够逆转这些排斥反应[187]，这意味着肝功能正常的移植患者在停止使用免疫抑制剂后，每隔数年进行1次活检作为监测手段是有益的，因此，一些学者甚至建议未停用免疫抑制药物的患者也接受同样的检查[188]。对未停用免疫抑制药物的移植受者，增强免疫抑制是否能够影响慢性排斥反应的出现仍不清楚。

在一项研究中，早期（移植后6个月）指导下停用免疫抑制剂耐受率极低，许多严重排斥的患者最终失败，需要采用高剂量类固醇和T细胞去除治疗方案[189]。一项免疫抑制剂撤除临床研究，其研究对象为接受父母活体供肝移植的儿童受者，该研究发现，那些撤除免疫抑制剂后没有不良反应的受者（占总人数的60%），他们从移植完成到撤除药物的时间比那些出现不良反应的要更长（100个月对73个月）[190]。

为了找到新的免疫耐受的预测指标，大量的回顾性研究报道成功耐受的患者Th1细胞因子含量更低[191]，而$CD4^+CD25^+$T细胞、伽马-δT细胞[192,193]、B细胞[192]频数较高。基因表达分析表明，与正常人群和耐受失败的患者相比，成功耐受的受者应激及炎症反应基因表达下调，DNA修复以及细胞周期调控基因表达上调[193,194]。最近一项前瞻性研究，在停止使用免疫抑制剂前进行移植物组织测序，发现耐受与HAMP mRNA含量相关[195]，当铁离子沉积时，它在肝细胞中表达上调。HAMP在中性粒细胞和巨噬细胞中也有表达，在固有免疫中承担重要作用。TFRC mRNA主要负责肝细胞摄取转铁蛋白结合铁，在成功耐受患者的肝细胞中低表达[195]，在抗原激活时，它在T细胞和B细胞中高表达。这些发现令人欣喜雀跃，但耐受和不耐受患者中这些指标的表达水平存在交叉现象[195]，意味着mRNA水平检测还不适用于临床。

总结

当前，对于终末期肝病患者，肝移植毫无疑问是最佳的长期治疗手段。然而，多种因素限制了患者的长期生存，包括肝移植原发适应证相关因素和免疫抑制剂相关因素。相比其他器官移植受者，肝移植受者的预后相对理想，但与正常人群相比还存在许多问题。手术流程、免疫抑制剂使用方法的完善，以及抗病毒、抗肿瘤治疗方案的改进，都是提高远期预后所必须解决的问题。

（徐骁 杨帆 译 徐骁 校）

参考文献

1. Starzl TE, Marchioro TL, Von Kaulla MD, et al. Homotransplantation of the liver in humans. Surgery, Gynecology and Obstetrics. 1963;117:659–676.
2. Starzl TE, Goran B, Lintmalm G, et al. Liver transplantation with use of cyclosporin A and prednisone. New England Journal of Medicine. 1981;305: 266–269.
3. Organ Procurement and Transplantation Network (OPTN) and Scientific Registry of Transplant Recipients (SRTR). OPTN/SRTR 2009 Annual Data Report. Rockville, MD: Department of Health and Human Services, Health Resources and Services Administration, HealthCare Systems Bureau, Division of Transplantation. American Journal of Transplantation. 2012;12(Suppl 1).
4. Pruthi J, Medkiff KA, Esrason KT, et al. Analysis of causes of death in liver transplant recipients who survived more than 3 years. Liver Transplantation. 2001;9:811–815.
5. Asfar S, Metrakos P, Fryer J, et al. An analysis of late deaths after liver transplantation. Transplantation. 1996;61(9):1377–1381.
6. Ashok J, Reyes J, Randeep K, et al. Long-term survival after liver transplantation in 4,000 consecutive patients at a single center. Annals of Surgery. 2000; 232(4):490–500.
7. Vogt DP, Henderson JM, Carey WD, et al. The long-term survival and causes of death in patients who survive at least 1 year after liver transplantation. Surgery. 2002;132(4):775–780, discussion 780.
8. Watt KD, Pedersen RA, Kremers WK, et al. Evolution of causes and risk factors for mortality post-liver transplant: results of the NIDDK long-term follow-up study. American Journal of Transplantation. 2010;10(6):1420–1427.
9. Abbasoglu O, Levy MF, Brkic BB, et al. Ten years of liver transplantation: an evolving understanding of late graft loss. Transplantation. 1997;64(12): 1801–1807.
10. Gelson W, Hoare M, Dawwas MF, et al. The pattern of late mortality in liver transplant recipients in the United Kingdom. Transplantation. 2011;91(11): 1240–1244.
11. Health Protection Agency. Hepatitis C in the UK. [accessed February 7, 2012]; Available from: http://www.hpa.org.uk/webc/HPAwebFile/HPAweb_C/1259152221464.
12. Schiano TD, Martin P. Management of HCV infection and liver transplantation. International Journal of Medical Sciences. 2006;3(2):79–83. doi: 10.7150/ijms.3.79.
13. Kremers WK, Devabhavi HC, Wiesner RH, et al. Post-transplant lymphoproliferative disorders following liver transplantation: incidence, risk factors and survival. American Journal of Transplantation. 2006;6:1017–1024.
14. Fouad TR, Abdel-Razek WM, Burak KW, et al. Prediction of cardiac complications after liver transplantation. Transplantation. 2009;87(5):763–770.
15. Charlton, M. Nonalcoholic fatty liver disease: a review of current understanding and future impact. Clinical Gastroenterology and Hepatology. 2004;2(12): 1048–1058.
16. Malik SM, deVera ME, Fontes P, et al. Outcome after liver transplantation for NASH cirrhosis. American Journal of Transplantation. 2009;9:782–793.
17. Mailey B, Buchberg B, Prendergast DO, et al. A disease-based comparison of liver transplantation outcomes. American Surgeon. 2009;75:901–908.
18. Busuttil RW, Farmer DG, Yersiz H, et al. Analysis of long-term outcomes of 3200 liver transplantations over two decades. Annals of Surgery. 2005;241(6): 905–918.
19. Farmer DG, Anselmo DM, Ghobrial R, et al. Liver transplantation for fulminant hepatic failure: experience with more than 200 patients over a 17-year period. Annals of Surgery. 2003;237(5):666–676.
20. Gane EJ, Portmann BC, Naoumov NV, et al. Long-term outcome of hepatitis C infection after liver transplantation. New England Journal of Medicine. 1996;334(13):815–820.
21. Belli LS, Burroughs AK, Burra P, et al. Liver transplantation for HCV cirrhosis: improved survival in recent years and incerased severity of recurrent disease in female recipients: results of a long-term retrospective study. Liver Transplantation. 2007;13:733–740.
22. Thuluvath PJ, Krok KL, Segev DL, et al. Trends in post-liver transplant survival in patients with hepatitis C between 1991 and 2001 in the United States. Liver Transplantation. 2007;13:719–724.
23. Berenguer M. Recurrent hepatitis C: worse outcomes established, interventions still inadequate. Liver Transplantation. 2007;13:641–643.
24. Forman L, Lewis JD, Berlin JA, et al. The association between hepatitis C infection and survival after orthotopic liver transplantation. Gastroenterology. 2002;122(4):889–896.

25. Fallon MB, Krowka MJ, Brown RS, et al. Pulmonary vascular complications of liver disease study group. Impact of hepatopulmonary syndrome on quality of life and survival in liver transplant candidates. Gastroenterology. 2008;135(4): 1168–1175.
26. Arguedas MR, Abrams GA, Krowka MB. Prospective evaluation of outcomes and predictors of mortality in patients with hepatopulmonary syndrome undergoing liver transplantation. Hepatology (Baltimore, Md.). 2003;37(1):192–197.
27. Krowka MJ, Mandell MS, Ramsay MA, et al. Hepatopulmonary syndrome and portopulmonary hypertension: a report of the multicenter liver transplant database. Liver Transplantation. 2004;10(2):174–182.
28. Swanson KL, Korowka MJ. Screen for portopulmonary hypertension, especially in liver transplant candidates. Cleveland Clinic Journal of Medicine. 2008; 75(2):121–136.
29. Krowda M, Plevak DJ, Findlay JY, et al. Pulmonary hemodynamics and perioperative cardiopulmonary related mortality in patients with portopulmonary hypertension undergoing liver transplant. Liver Transplantation. 2000;6: 443–450.
30. Bandara M, Gordon FD, Sarwar A, et al. Successful outcomes following liver donor liver transplantation for portopulmonary hypertension. Liver Transplantation. 2010;16(8):983–989.
31. Collins BH, Pirsch JD, Becker YT, et al. Long-term results of liver transplantation in older patients 60 years of age and older. Transplantation. 2000;70(5): 780–783.
32. Bromley PN, Hilmi I, Tan KC, et al. Orthotopic liver transplantation in patients over 60 years old. Transplantation. 1994;58(7):800–803.
33. Emre S, Mor E, Schwartz ME, et al. Liver transplantation in patients beyond age 60. Transplantation Proceedings. 1993;25(1 Pt 2):1075–1076.
34. Garcia CE, Garcia RF, Mayer AD, et al. Liver transplantation in patients over sixty years of age. Transplantation. 2001;72(4):679–684.
35. Prisch JD, Kalayoglu M, D'Alessandro AM, et al. Orthotopic liver transplantation in patients 60 years of age and older. Transplantation. 1991;51(2):431–433.
36. Stieber AC, Gordon RD, Todo S, et al. Liver transplantation in patients over sixty years of age. Transplantation. 1991;51(1):271–273.
37. Zetterman RK, Belle SH, Hoofnagle JH, et al. Age and liver transplantation: a report of the liver transplantation database. Transplantation. 1998;66(4): 500–506.
38. Lipshutz GS, Hiatt J, Ghobrial RM, et al. Outcome of liver transplantation in septuagenarians: a single-center experience. Archives of Surgery (Chicago, Ill.: 1960). 2007;142(8):775–781.
39. Aduen JF, Sujay B, Dickson RC, et al. Outcomes after liver transplant in patients aged 70 years or older compared with those younger than 60 years. Mayo Clinic Proceedings. Mayo Clinic. 2009;84(11):973–978.
40. Thuluvarth PJ, Guidinger MK, Fung JJ, et al. Liver transplantation in the United States, 1999–2008. American Journal of Transplantation. 2010;10(4):1003–1019.
41. Hong JC, Kosari K, Benjamin E, et al. Does race influence outcomes after primary liver transplantation? A 23-year experience with 2,700 patients. Journal of the American College of Surgeons. 2008;206(5):1009–1016.
42. Kemmer NM, Neff GW. Liver transplantation trends and survival in the Asian population. Transplantation. 2009;88(3):392–394.
43. Schreibman IR, Schiff ER. Prevention and treatment of recurrent hepatitis B after liver transplantation: the current role of nucleoside and nucleotide analogues. Annals of Clinical Microbiology and Antimicrobials. 2006;5:8.
44. Paptheodoridis GV, Sevastianos V, Burroughs AK. Prevention of and treatment for hepatitis B virus infection after liver transplantation in the nucleoside analogues era. American Journal of Transplantation. 2003;3(3):250–258.
45. Fung J, Cheung C, Chan SC, et al. Entecavir monotherapy is effective in suppressing hepatitis B virus after liver transplantation. Gastroenterology. 2011;141(4): 1212–1219.
46. Karlas T, Hartmann J, Weiman A, et al. Prevention of lamivudine-resistant hepatitis B recurrence after liver transplantation with entecavir plus tenofovir combination therapy and perioperative hepatitis B immunoglobulin only. Transplant Infectious Disease. 2011;13(3):299–302. doi: 10.1111/j.1399-3062.2010.00591.x.
47. Nair S, Eustace J, Thuluvath PJ, et al. Effect of race outcome of orthotopic liver transplantation: a cohort study. Lancet. 2002;359(9303):287–293.
48. Smallwood GA, Coffey G, Davis L, et al. Hepatits C treatment outcomes of African Americans following liver transplantation. Transplantation Proceedings. 2002;34:3317–3318.
49. Nguyen GC, Thuluvath PJ. Racial disparity in liver disease: biological, cultural, or socioeconomic factors. Hepatology (Baltimore, Md.). 2008;47(3):1058–1066.
50. Dick AAS, Spitzer AL, Seifert CF, et al. Liver transplantation at the extremes of the body mass index. Liver Transplantation. 2009;15(8):968–977.
51. Nair S, Cohen DB, Cohen MP, et al. Postoperative morbidity, mortality, costs and long-term survival in severely obese patients undergoing orthotopic liver transplantation. The American Journal of Gastroenterology. 2001;96(3):842–845.
52. Nair S, Verma S, Thuluvath PJ, et al. Obesity and its effect on survival in patients undergoing orthotopic liver transplantation in the United States. Hepatology (Baltimore, Md.). 2002;35(1):105–109.
53. Leonard J, Heimbach JK, Malinchoc M, et al. The impact of obesity on long-term outcomes in liver transplant recipients-results of the NIDDK liver transplant database. American Journal of Transplantation. 2008;8(3):667–672.
54. Thuluvath PJ. Morbid obesity with one or more other serious comorbidities should be a contraindication for liver transplantation. Liver Transplantation. 2007;12:1627–1629.
55. Pelletier SJ, Schaubel DE, Wei G, et al. Effectof body mass index on the survival benefit of liver transplantation. Liver Transplantation. 2007;12:1678–1683.
56. Organ Procurement and Transplantation Network (OPTN) and Scientific Registry of Transplant Recipients (SRTR). OPTN/SRTR 2009 Annual Data Report. Rockville, MD: Department of Health and Human Services, Health Resrouces and Services Administration, HealthCare Systems Bureau, Division of Transplantation. 2011.
57. Martin EF, Huang J, Xiang Q, et al. Recipient and graft survival are not diminished by simultaneous liver-kidney transplantation: an analysis of the UNOS database. Liver Transplantation. 2012;18(8):914–929. doi: 10.1002/lt.23440; Abstract.
58. Schmitt TM, Kumer SC, Al-Osaimi A, et al. Combined liver-kidney and liver transplantation in patients with renal failure outcomes in the MELD era. Transplant International. 2009;22:876–883.
59. Locke JE, Warren DS, Singer AL, et al. Declining outcomes in simultaneous liver-kidney transplantation in the MELD era: ineffective usage of renal allografts. Transplantation. 2008;85(7):935–942.
60. Eason JD, Gonwa TA, Davis CL, et al. Proceedings of consensus conference on simultaneous liver kidney transplantation (SLK). American Journal of Transplantation. 2008;8:2243.
61. Nair S, Verma S, Thuluvath PJ. Pretransplant renal function predicts survival in patients undergoing orthotopic liver transplantation. Hepatology (Baltimore, Md.). 2002;35:1179.
62. Markmann JF, Markmann JW, Markmann DA, et al. Preoperative factors associated with outcome and their impact on resource use in 1148 consecutive primary liver transplants. Transplantation. 2001;72:1113.
63. Simpson N, Cho YW, Cicciarelli JC, et al. Comparison of renal allograft outcomes in combined liver-kidney transplantation verus subsequent kidney transplantation in liver transplant recipients: analysis of UNOS database. Transplantation. 2006;82(10):1298–1303.
64. Askar M, Schold JD, Eghtesad B, et al. Combined liver-kidney transplants: allosensitization and recipient outcomes. Transplantation. 2011;91(11): 1286–1292.
65. Dar W, Agarwal A, Watkins C, et al. Donor-directed MHC class I antibody is preferentially cleared from sensitized recipients of combined liver/kidney transplants. American Journal of Transplantation. 2011;11:841–847. doi: 10.111/j. 1600-6143.2011.03467.x.
66. Barth RN, Campos L, Kukuruga DL, et al. Clinical Transplantation. 2010;24:685–690. doi: 10.111/j.1399-0012.2009.01161.x.
67. Mazariegos GV, Steffick DE, Horslen S, et al. Intestine transplantation in the United States, 1999–2008. American Journal of Transplantation. 2010;10(Pt 2):1020–1034. doi: 10.1111/j.1600-6143.2010.03044.x.
68. Kornberg A, Kupper B, Barthel E, et al. Combined en-bloc liver-pancreas transplantation in patients with liver cirrhosis and insulin-dependent type 2 diabetes mellitus. Transplantation. 2009;87(4):542–545.
69. Te HS, Anderson AS, Millis JM, et al. Current state of combined heart-liver transplantation in the United States. Journal of Heart and Lung Transplantation. 2008;27(7):753–759.
70. Raichlin E, Daly RC, Rosen CB, et al. Combined heart and liver transplantation: a single-center experience. Transplantation. 2009;88(2):219–225.
71. Rauchfuss F, Breuer M, Dittmar Y, et al. Implantation of the liver during reperfusion of the heart in combined heart-liver transplantation: own experience and review of the literature. Transplantation Proceedings. 2011;43:2707–2713.
72. Grannas G, Neipp M, Hoeper MM, et al. Indications for and outcomes after combined lung and liver transplantation: a single-center experience on 13 consecutive cases. Transplantation. 2008;85(4):524–531.
73. Mendizabal M, Rajender Reddy K, Cassuto J, et al. Liver transplantation in patients cystic fibrosis: analysis of united network for organ sharing data. Liver Transplantation. 2011;17:243–250.
74. Nash KL, Collier JD, French J, et al. Cystic fibrosis liver disease: to transplant or not to transplant? American Journal of Transplantation. 2008;8:162–169. doi: 10.1111/j.1600-6143.2007.02028.x.
75. Noble-Jamieson G, Barnes N, Jamieson N, et al. Liver transplantation for hepatic cirrhosis in cystic fibrosis. Journal of the Royal Society of Medicine. 1996;89(Suppl 27):31–37.
76. Reese PP, Yeh H, Thomasson AM, et al. Transplant center volume and outcomes after liver retransplantation. American Journal of Transplantation. 2009;

9(2):309–317.
77. Thuluvath PJ, Guidinger MK, Fung JJ, et al. Liver transplantation in the United States, 1999–2008. American Journal of Transplantation. 2010;10(Pt 2): 1003–1019.
78. Akpinar E, Selvaggi G, Levi D, et al. Liver retransplantation of more than two grafts for recurrent failure. Transplantation. 2009;88(7):884–890.
79. Ghabril M, Dickson R, Wiesner R. Improving outcomes of liver retransplantation: an analysis of trends and the impact of hepatitis C infection. American Journal of Transplantation. 2008;8:404–411.
80. Hong JC, Kaldas FM, Kositamongkol P, et al. Predictive index for long-term survival after retransplantation of the liver in adult recipients. Annals of Surgery. 2011;254(3):444–449.
81. Marudanayagam R, Shanmugam V, Gunson BK, et al. Liver retransplantation in adults: a single-centre, 25-year experience. HPB: Official Journal of the International Hepato Pancreato Biliary Association. 2010;12:217–224.
82. Yao FY, Saab S, Bass NM, et al. Prediction of survival after liver retransplantation for late graft failure based on preoperative prognostic scores. Hepatology (Baltimore, Md.). 2004;39(1):230–238.
83. Pfitzmann R, Benscheidt B, Langrehr JM, et al. Trends and experiences in liver retransplantation over 15 years. Liver Transplantation. 2007;13:248–257.
84. Linhares MM, Azoulay D, Matos D, et al. Liver retransplantation: a model for determining long-term survival. Transplantation. 2006;81(7):1016–1021.
85. Watt KDS, Lyden ER, McCashland TM. Poor survival after liver retransplantation: is hepatitis C to blame? Liver Transplantation. 2003;9(10):1019–1024.
86. Andes A, Gerstel E, Combescure C, et al. A score predicting survival after liver retransplantation for hepatitis C virus cirrhosis. Transplantation. 2012;93(7): 717–722.
87. Pelletier SJ, Schaubel DE, Punch JD, et al. Hepatitis C is a risk factor for death after liver retransplantation. Liver Transplantation. 2005;11(4):434–440.
88. Yoo HY, Maheshwar A, Thuluvath PJ. Retransplantation of liver: primary graft nonfunction and hepatitis C virus are associated with worse outcome. Liver Transplantation. 2003;9(9):897–904.
89. Perry DK, Willingham DL, Sibulesky L, et al. Should donation after cardiac death liver grafts be used for retransplantation. Annals of Hepatology. 2011;10(4): 482–485.
90. Goh A, Scalamogna M, DeFeo T, et al. Human leukocyte antigen crossmatch testing is important for liver retransplantation. Liver Transplantation. 2010; 16:308–313.
91. Demetris AJ, Jaffe R, Tzakis A, et al. Antibody-mediated rejection of human orthotopic liver allografts. A study of liver transplantation across ABO blood group barriers. American Journal of Pathology. 1988;132(3):489–502.
92. Gugenheim J, Samuel D, Reynes M, et al. Liver transplantation across ABO blood group barriers. Lancet. 1990;336:519–523.
93. Sanchez-Urdazpal L, Batts KP, Gores GJ, et al. Increased bile duct complications in liver transplantation across the ABO barrier. Annals of Surgery. 1993;218: 152–158.
94. Lo C, Shaked A, Busuttil RW. Risk factors for liver transplantation across the ABO barrier. Transplantation. 1994;58:548–547.
95. Fong SW, Qaqundah BY, Taylor WF. Developmental patterns of ABO isoagglutinins in normal children correlated with the effects of age, sex, and maternal isoagglutinins. Transfusion. 1974;14:551–559.
96. Urbani L, Mazzoni A, Bianco I, et al. The role of immunomodulation in ABO-incompatible adult liver transplant recipients. Journal of Clinical Apheresis. 2008;23(2):55–62.
97. Hanto DW, Fecteau AH, Alonso MH, et al. ABO-incompatible liver transplantation with no immunological graft losses using total plasmaexchange, splenectomy, and quadruple immunosuppression: evidence of accommodation. Liver Transplantation. 2003;9(1):22–30.
98. Heffron T, Welch D, Pillen T, et al. Successful ABO-incompatible pediatric liver transplantation utilizing standard immunosuppression with selective postoperative plasmapheresis. Liver Transplantation. 2006;12(6):972–978.
99. Yamada Y, Hoshino K, Morikawa Y, et al. Successful liver transplantation across the ABO incompatibility barrier in 6 cases of biliary atresia. Journal of Pediatric Surgery. 2006;41(12):1976–1979.
100. Fishbein T, Emre S, Guy S, et al. Safe transplantation of blood type A2 livers to blood type O recipients. Transplantation. 1999;67:1071–1073.
101. Skogsberg U, Breimer ME, Friman S, et al. Successful ABO-incompatible liver transplantation using A2 donors. Transplantation Proceedings. 2006;38(8): 2667–2670.
102. Sorensen JB, Grant WJ, Belnap LP, et al. Transplantation of ABO group A^2 kidneys from living donors into group O and B recipients. American Journal of Transplantation. 2001;1(3):296–299.
103. Organ Procurement and Transplantation Network (OPTN). [cited March 25, 2012]; Available from: http://optn.transplant.hrsa.gov/latestData/rptStrat.asp.
104. Stewart ZA, Locke JE, Montgomery RA, et al. ABO-incompatible decreased donor liver transplantation in the United States: a national registry analysis. Liver Transplantation. 2009;15(8):883–893.
105. Wu J, Ye S, Xu X, et al. Recipient outcomes after ABO-incompatible liver transplantation: a systemic review and meta-analysis. PLoS ONE. 2011;6(1):e16521.
106. Navarro V, Herrine S, Katopes C, et al. The effect of HLA class I (A and B) and class II (DR) compatibility on liver transplantation outcomes: an analysis of the OPTN database. Liver Transplantation. 2006;12(4):652–658.
107. Castillo-Rama M, Castro MJ, Bernardo I, et al. Preformed antibodies detected by cytotoxic assay or multibead array decrease liver allograft survival: role of human leukocyte antigen compatibility. Liver Transplantation. 2008;14:554–562.
108. Sugawara Y, Mizuta K, Kawarasaki H, et al. Risk factors for acute rejection in pediatric living related liver transplantation: the impact of HLA matching. Liver Transplantation. 2001;9:769–773.
109. Fontana M, Moradpour D, Aubert V, et al. Prevalence of anti-HLA antibodies after liver transplantation. Transplant International. 2010;8:858–859.
110. Sakashita H, Haga H, Ashihara E, et al. Significance of C4d staining in ABO-identical/compatible liver transplantation. Modern Pathology. 2007;6:676–684.
111. Takakura K, Kiuchi T, Kashara M, et al. Clinical implications of flow cytometry corssmatch with T or B cells in living donor liver transplantation. Clinical Transplantation. 2001;15:309–316.
112. Castillo-Rama M, Castro MJ, Bernardo I, et al. Preformed antibodies detected by cytotoxic assay or multibead array decrease liver allograft survival: role of human leukocyte antigen compatibility. Liver Transplantation. 2008;14: 554–562.
113. Feng S, Goodrich NP, Bragg-Gresham JL, et al. Characteristics associated with liver graft failure: the concept of a donor risk index. American Journal of Transplantation. 2006;6(4):783–790.
114. Reese PP, Sonawane SB, Thomasson A, et al. Donor age and cold ischemia interact to produce inferior 90-day liver allograft survival. Transplantation. 2008;85(12): 1737–1744.
115. Angele MK, Rentsch M, Hartl WH, et al. Effect of graft stenosis on liver function and organ survival after liver transplantation. American Journal of Surgery. 2008;195(2):214–220.
116. Fiorentino M, Vasuri F, Ravaioli L, et al. Predictive value of frozen-section analysis in the histological assessment of steatosis before liver transplantation. Liver Transplantation. 2009;15(12):1821–1825.
117. Briceno J, Ciria R, Pleguezuelo M, et al. Impact of donor graft steatosis on overall outcome and viral recurrence after liver transplantation for hepatitis C virus cirrhosis. Liver Transplantation. 2009;15(1):37–48.
118. Li J, Liu B, Yan LN, et al. Reversal of graft steatosis after liver transplantation: prospective study. Transplantation Proceedings. 2009;41(9):3560–3563.
119. Nagrath D, Xu H, Tanimura Y. Metabolic preconditioning of donor organs: defatting fatty livers by normothermic perfusion ex vivo. Metabolic Engineering. 2009;11(4–5):274–283.
120. Davis C, Delmonico F. Living-donor kidney transplantation: a review of the current practices for the live donor. Journal of the American Society of Nephrology. 2005;16(7):2098–2110.
121. Olthoff KM, Merion RM, Ghobrial RM, et al. Outcomes of 385 adult-to-adult living donorr liver transplant recipients: a report from the A2ALL consortium. Annals of Surgery. 2005;242:314–323.
122. Fisher RA, Cotterell AH, Maluf DG, et al. Adult living donor versus deceased donor liver transplantation: a 10-year prospective single center experience. Annals of Hepatology. 2009;8(4):298–307.
123. Abt PL, Mange KC, Olthoff KM, et al. Allograft survival following adult-to-adult living donor liver transplantation. American Journal of Transplantation. 2004;4(8):1302–1307.
124. Freise CE, Gillespie BW, Koffron AJ, et al. Recipient morbidity after living and deceased donor liver transplantation: findings from the A2ALL Retrospective Cohort Study. American Journal of Transplantation. 2008;8: 2569–2579.
125. Akamatsu N, Sugawara Y, Hashimoto D. Biliary reconstruction, its complications and management of biliary complications after adult liver transplantation: a systemic review of the incidence, risk factors and outcome. Transplant International. 2011;24(4):379–392.
126. Ryu CH, Lee SK. Biliary strictures after liver transplantation. Gut and Liver. 2011;5(2):133–142.
127. Sharma S, Gurakar A, Jabbour N. Biliary strictures following liver transplantation: past, present and preventive strategies. Liver Transplantation. 2008;14(6): 759–769.
128. Russo MW, LaPointe-Rudow D, Kinkhabwala M, et al. Impact of adult living donor liver transplantation on waiting time survival in candidates listed for liver transplantation. American Journal of Transplantation. 2004;4(3):427–431.
129. Berg CL, Gillepsie BW, Merion RM, et al. Improvement in survival associated with adult-to-adult living donor liver transplantation. Gastroenterology. 2007; 133(6):1806–1813.

130. Berg CL, Merion RM, Shearon TH, et al. Liver transplant recipient survival benefit with living donation in the model for endstage liver disease allocation era. Hepatology (Baltimore, Md.). 2011;54(4):1314–1321.
131. Yeh H, Smoot E, Schoenfeld D, et al. Geographic inequity in access to livers for transplantation. Transplantation. 2011;91(4):479–486.
132. DeVera ME, Lopez-Solis R, Dvorchik I, et al. Liver transplantation using donation after cardiac death donors: long-term follow-up from a single center. American Journal of Transplantation. 2009;9(4):773–781.
133. Saidi RF, Bradley J, Greer D, et al. Changing pattern of organ donation at a single center: are potential brain dead donors being lost to donation after cardiac death? American Journal of Transplantation. 2010;10(11):2536–2540.
134. Abt PL, Desai NM, Crawford MD, et al. Survival following liver transplantation from non-heart beating donors. Annals of Surgery. 2004;239(1):87–92.
135. Grewal HP, Willingham DL, Nguyen WR, et al. Liver transplantation using controlled donation after cardiac death donors: an analysis of a large single-center experience. Liver Transplantation. 2009;15(9):1028–1035.
136. Mateo R, Cho Y, Singh G, et al. Risk factors for graft survival after liver transplantation from donation after cardiac death donors: an analysis of OPTN/UNOS data. American Journal of Transplantation. 2006;6:791–796.
137. Doshi MD, Hunsicker LG. Short- and long-term outcomes with the use of kidneys and livers donated after cardiac death. American Journal of Transplantation. 2007;7:122–129.
138. Jay CL, Lyukemburg V, Ladner DP, et al. Ischemic cholangiopathy after conrolled donation after cardiac death liver transplantation: a meta-analysis. Annals of Surgery. 2011;253(2):259–264.
139. Skaro A, Jay CL, Baker TB, et al. The impact of ischemic cholangiopathy in liver transplantation using donors after cardiac death: the untold story. Surgery. 2009;146(4):543–552.
140. Cameron AM, Busuttil RW. Ischemic cholangiopathy after liver transplantation. Hepatobiliary and Pancreatic Diseases International. 2005;4(4):495–501.
141. Sanchez-Urdazpal L, Gores GJ, Ward EM, et al. Ischemic-type biliary complications after orthotopic liver transplantation. Hepatology (Baltimore, Md.). 1992;16:49–53.
142. Verdonk RC, Buis CL, Porte RJ, et al. Biliary complications after liver transplantation: a review. Scandinavian Journal of Gastroenterology. Supplement. 2006; 243:89.
143. Akamatsu N, Sugawara Y, Hashimoto D. Biliary reconstruction, its complications and management of biliary complications after adult liver transplantation: a systemic review of the incidence, risk factors and outcome. Transplant International. 2011;24(4):379–392.
144. MacConmara MP, Vachharajani N, Wellen JR, et al. Utilization of hepatitis B core antibody-positive donor liver grafts. HPB: Official Journal of the International Hepato Pancreato Biliary Association. 2011;14.
145. Saab S, Waterman B, Chi AC, et al. Comparison of different immunoprophylaxis regimens after liver transplantation with hepatitis B core antibody-positive donors: a systemic review. Liver Transplantation. 2010;16(3):300–307.
146. Holt D, Thomas R, Van Thiel D, et al. Use of hepatitis B core antibody-positive donors in orthotopic liver transplantation. Archives of Surgery (Chicago, Ill.: 1960). 2002;137(5):572–575.
147. Celebi Kobak A, Karasu Z, Kilic M, et al. Living donor liver transplantation from hepatitis B core antibody positive donors. Transplantation Proceedings. 2007; 39(5):1488–1490.
148. Northup PG, Argo CK, Nguyen DT, et al. Liver allografts from hepatitis C positive donors can offer good outcomes in hepatitis C positive recipients: a US National Transplant Registry analysis. Transplant International. 2010; 23(10):1038–1044.
149. Burr AT, YouFu L, Tseng JF, et al. Survival after liver transplantation using hepatitis C virus-positive donor allografts: case-controlled analysis of the UNOS database. World Journal of Surgery. 2011;35(7):1590–1595. doi: 10.1007/s00268-011-1019-5.
150. Marroquin CE, Marino G, Kuo PC, et al. Transplantation of hepatitis C-positive livers in hepatitis C-positive patients is equivalent to transplanting hepatitis C-negative livers. Liver Transplantation. 2001;7(9):762–768.
151. Velidedeoglu E, Desai NM, Campos L, et al. The outcome of liver grafts procured from hepatitis C-positive donors. Transplantation. 2002;73(4):582–587.
152. Khapra AP, Agarwal K, Kontorinis N, et al. Impact of donor age on survival and fibrosis progression in patients with hepatitis C undergoing liver transplantation using HCV+ allografts. Liver Transplantation. 2006;12(10):1496–1503.
153. Ojo AO, Held PJ, Port FK, et al. Chronic renal failure after transplantation of a nonrenal organ. New England Journal of Medicine. 2003;349:931–939.
154. Gonwa TA, Mai ML, Melton LB, et al. Renal replacement therapy and orthotopic liver transplantation: the role of continuous venovenous hemodialysis. Transplantation. 2001;71:1424–1428.
155. Bahirwani R, Reddy KR. Outcomes after liver transplantation: chronic kidney disease. Liver Transplantation. 2009;15(Suppl 2):S70–S74.
156. McGuire BM, Julian BA, Bynon JS Jr, et al. Brief communication: glomerulonephritis in patients with hepatitis C cirrhosis undergoing liver transplantation. Annals of Internal Medicine. 2006;144:735–741.
157. Khalili M, Lim JW, Bass N, et al. New onset diabetes mellitus after liver transplantation: the critical role of hepatitis C infection. Liver Transplantation. 2004;10:349–355.
158. Delgado-Borrego A, Liu YS, Jordan SH, et al. Prospective study of liver transplant recipients with HCV infection: evidence for a causal relationship between HCV and insulin resistance. Liver Transplantation. 2008;14:193.
159. Campbell MS, Rai J, Kozin E, et al. Effects of sirolimus vs. Calcineurin inhibitors on renal dysfunction after orthotopic liver transplantation. Clinical Transplants. 2007;21(3):377–384.
160. Fairbanks KD, Eustace JA, Fine D, et al. Renal function improves in liver transplant recipients when switched from a calcineurin inhibitor to sirolimus. Liver Transplantation. 2003;9(10):1079–1085.
161. Sanchez EQ, Martin AP, Ikegami T, et al. Sirolimus conversion after liver transplantation: improvement in measured glomerular filtration rate after 2 years. Transplantation Proceedings. 2005;37(10):4416–4423.
162. Asrani MD, Leise CP, West CP, et al. Use of sirolimus in liver transplant recipients with renal insufficiency: a systemic review and meta-analysis. Hepatology (Baltimore, Md.). 2010;52(4):1360–1370.
163. Mirabella S, Brunati A, Ricchiuti A, et al. New-onset diabetes after liver transplantation. Transplantation Proceedings. 2005;37(6):2636–2637.
164. Khalili M, Lim JW, Bass N, et al. New onset diabetes mellitus after liver transplantation: the critical role of hepatitis C infection. Liver Transplantation. 2004;10(3):349–355.
165. John PR, Thuluvath PJ. Outcome of patients with new-onset diabetes mellitus after liver transplantation compared with those without diabetes mellitus. Liver Transplantation. 2002;8(8):708–713.
166. AlDosary AA, Ramji AS, Elliott TG, et al. Post-liver transplantation diabetes mellitus: an association with hepatitis C. Liver Transplantation. 2002;8(4): 356–361.
167. Khalili M, Lim JW, Bass N, et al. New onset diabetes mellitus after liver transplantation: the critical role of hepatitis C infection. Liver Transplantation. 2004;10(3):349–355.
168. Parvaiz F, Manzoor S, Tariq H, et al. Hepatitis C virus infection: molecular pathways to insulin resistance. Virology Journal. 2011;8:474.
169. Delgado-Borrego A, Jordan SH, Negre B, et al. Reduction of insulin resistance with effective clearance of hepatitis C infection: results from the HALT-C trial. Clinical Gastroenterology and Hepatology. 2010;8(5):458–462.
170. Alberstein M, Zornitzki T, Zick Y, et al. Hepatitis C core protein impairs insulin downstream signalling and regulatory role of IGFBP-1 expression. Journal of Viral Hepatitis. 2012;19(1):65–71.
171. Pazienza V, Clement S, Pugnale P, et al. The hepatitis C virus core protein of genotypes 3a and 1b downregulates insulin receptor substrate 1 through genotype-specific mechanisms. Hepatology (Baltimore, Md.). 2007;45(5):1164–1171.
172. Drachenberg CB, Klassen DK, Weir MR, et al. Islet cell damage associated with tacrolimus and cyclosporine: morphological features in pancreas allograft biopsies and clinical correlation. Transplantation. 1999;68(3):396–402.
173. Haagsma EB, Hagens VE, Schaapveld M, et al. Increased cancer risk after liver transplantataion: a population-based study. Journal of Hepatology. 2001;34(1): 84–91.
174. Chak E, Saab S. Risk factors and incidence of de novo malignancy in liver recipients: a systemic review. Liver International. 2010;30(9):1247–1258.
175. Yoo HY, Thuluvath PJ. The effect of insulin-dependent diabetes mellitus on outcome of liver transplantation. Transplantation. 2002;74(7):1007–1012.
176. Watt KD, Pedersen RA, Kremers WK, et al. Long-term probability of and mortality from de novo malignancy after liver transplantation. Gastroenterology. 2009;137(6):2010–2017.
177. Jain AB, Yee LD, Nalesnik MA, et al. Comparative incidence of de novo nonlymphnoid malignancies after liver transplantation under tacrolimus using surveillance epidemiologic end result data. Transplantation. 1998;66(9): 1193–1200.
178. Shetty K, Rybicki L, Brzezinski A, et al. The risk of cancer or dysplasia in ulcerative colitis patients with primary sclerosing cholangitis. American Journal of Gastroenterology. 1999;94:1643–1649.
179. Buell JF, Papaconstantinou HT, Skalow B, et al. De novo colorectal cancer: five-year survival is markedly lower in transplant recipients compared with the general population. Transplantation Proceedings. 2005;37(2):960–961.
180. Johnson EE, Leverson GE, Pirsch JD, et al. A 30-year analysis of colorectal adenocarcinoma in transplant recipients and proposal for altered screening. Journal of Gastrointestinal Surgery. 2007;11(3):272–279.
181. Saint Nicholaas J, De Jonge V, Steyerberg E, et al. Risk of colorectal carcinoma in post-liver transplant patients: a systemic review and Meta-analysis. American Journal of Transplantation. 2010;10(4):868–876.

182. Starzl TE, Demetris AJ, Trucco M, et al. Cell mighration and chimerism after whole-organ transplantation: the basis of graft acceptance. Hepatology (Baltimore, Md.). 1993;17:1127–1152.
183. Manez R, Kusne S, Linden P, et al. Temporary withdrawal of immunosuppression for life-threatening infections after liver transplantation. Transplantation. 1994;57:149–151.
184. Hurwitz M, Desai DM, Cox KL, et al. Complete immunosuppressive withdrawal as a uniform approach to post-transplant lymphoproliferative disease in pediatric liver transplantation. Pediatric Transplantation. 2004;8:267–272.
185. Devlin J, Doherty D, Thomson L, et al. Defining the outcome of immunosuppression withdrawal after liver transplantation. Hepatology (Baltimore, Md.). 1998; 27:926–933.
186. Takatsuki M, Uemoto S, Inomata Y, et al. Weaning of immunosuppression in living donor liver transplant recipients. Transplantation. 2001;72:449–454.
187. Lerut J, Sanchez-Fueyo A. An appraisal of tolerance in liver transplantation. American Journal of Transplantation. 2006;6:1774–1780.
188. Sebagh M, Rifai K, Feray C, et al. All liver recipients benefit from the protocol 10-year liver biopsies. Hepatology (Baltimore, Md.). 2003;37:1293–1301.
189. Eason JD, Cohen AJ, Nair S, et al. Tolerance: is it worth the risk? Transplantation. 2005;79:1157–1159.
190. Feng S, Ekong UD, Lobritto SJ, et al. Complete immunosuppression withdrawal and subsequent allograft function among pediatric recipients of parental living donor liver transplants. JAMA: Journal of the American Medical Association. 2012;307(3):283–293.
191. Mazariegos GV, Zahorchak AF, Reyes J, et al. Dendritic cell subset ratio in peripheral blood correlates with successful withdrawal of immunosuppression in liver transplant patients. American Journal of Transplantation. 2003;3:689–696.
192. Takatsuki M, Uemoto S, Inomata Y, et al. Analysis of alloreactivity and intragraft cytokine profiles in living donor liver transplant recipients with graft acceptance. Transplant Immunology. 2001;8:279–286.
193. Martinez-Llordella M, Lozano JJ, Puig-Pey I, et al. Using transcriptional profiling ato develop a diagnostic test of operational tolerance in liver transplant recipients. Journal of Clinical Investigation. 2008;118(8):2845–2857.
194. Martinez-Llordella M, Puig-Pey I, Orlando G, et al. Multiparameter immune profiling of operational tolerance in liver transplantation. American Journal of Transplantation. 2007;7:309–319.
195. Bohne F, Martinez-Llordella M, Lozano JJ, et al. Intra-graft expression of genes involved in iron homeostasis predicts the development of operational tolerance in human liver transplantation. Journal of Clinical Investigation. 2012; 122(1):368–382.

第 105 章
心脏移植长期预后

Michelle M. Kittleson, Jon A. Kobashigawa

引言

尽管近年来慢性心力衰竭的治疗药物和仪器设备均有了长远进步，但仍有很大一部分患者进展为终末期心力衰竭，其长期死亡率和并发症发生率仍处于较高水平。有症状心衰患者的 5 年死亡率接近 50%，而对于终末期心衰患者，其 1 年死亡率可能接近 80%[1]。在过去的 40 年内，心脏移植已成为部分终末期心力衰竭患者更适宜的治疗手段。在美国，每年大约要开展 2400 例心脏移植手术。根据国际心肺移植协会(ISHLT)的统计，对于术后 1 年存活的患者，其中位生存时间可以达到 10~13 年[2](图 105.1)，这相比于单纯药物治疗的心衰患者，生存时间有显著延长。

免疫抑制治疗方案的不断优化对于心脏移植术后存活来说至关重要。免疫抑制、供体心脏获取、手术技术及术后监护等方案的发展对于移植患者术后生存率的提升有长足的促进作用。尽管如此，这些方面仍有许多问题存在，本章将就当前心脏移植术后长期并发症的发生进行阐述。

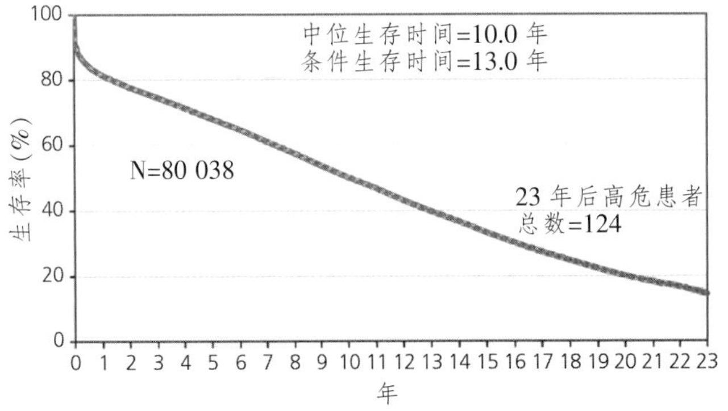

图 105.1 1982 年 1 月至 2009 年 6 月，成人心脏移植生存率曲线。在一篇超过 80 000 病例的国际报告中表明，心脏移植术后 1 年存活的患者，其中位生存时间为 10~13 年。(Reproduced from [2] Stehlik et al., J Heart Lung Transplant 2010;29:1089–1103. Copyright © 2010, with permission from Elsevier.)

本章将综述心脏移植术后导致死亡和并发症发生的主要原因。术后死亡的主要病因包括排斥、感染、癌变及移植相关的冠状动脉疾病。由于移植相关冠状动脉疾病的重要性和危险性，该主题将在另一章(第 79 章)进行重点阐述。主要并发症的发病原因包括肾功能不全、高血压、糖尿病、血脂异常、痛风和骨质疏松。

心脏移植术后长期疗效

生存率

近 30 年来，心脏移植术后生存率已得到了显著提升。在 20 世纪 80 年代，心脏移植术后 1 年生存率为 70%，条件下半数存活时间，即在所有术后 1 年存活的患者中，有 50%的患者可以生存到至少术后 9.4 年。最近由 ISHLT 发表的一篇报告指出[2]，移植术后患者 1年生存率已达到 90%，条件下半数存活时间也已达到 14 年。值得注意的是，移植术后死亡率尽管在 1992 年时较之前有所降低，近 20 年来，移植术后患者的死亡率并未明显降低。术后患者平均每年的死亡率为 3%~4%，这一数字比普通人群要高得多。这种现象的存在可能同部分影响远期死亡率的因素有关，这些因素包括移植心脏血管病变及癌变，这为临床监测和治疗带来了挑战。因此，未来对于移植术后生存的提升将重点着眼于移植心脏血管病变和癌变的监测及治疗等方面。

ISHLT 研究对术后 1 年、5 年、10 年、15 年和 20 年生存的影响因子进行了逐层分析[2]。研究表明，术后 1 年死亡最重要的危险因素为技术因素，包括临时机械灌注支持、移植前机械通气治疗、透析，以及移植术前的根本病因，包括先天性心肌病、非缺血性心肌病和移植史等。这些因素能够使术后1年死亡率提高50%甚至更高。影响术后5年和10年的因素，则更多地同免疫相关因素、免疫抑制不良反应，包括透析、术后感染、术后第一年排斥反应以及非正规免疫抑制治疗（正规免疫抑制移植应包括以下至少两项治疗：细胞周期抑制剂、钙调神经磷酸酶抑制剂、增殖信号抑制剂）等相关。

不同时代进行心脏移植的患者，其术后20年生存率有明显差异。1990年进行心脏移植的患者，其术后20年生存率优于1985年进行心脏移植的患者。其他影响20年生存率的因素包括移植病因、性别、年龄、心肌缺血时间以及中心容量。进行再移植，或是因缺血性心肌病或瓣膜病进行移植的患者，其相比于因非缺血性心肌病而移植的患者，20年生存率明显降低。而其机制目前仍不清楚，其具体原因可能同致病疾病进展、缺血性心肌病或瓣膜病受体患者年龄较高等原因有关。女性患者相比于男性患者，移植术后死亡风险相对较高。低供体年龄、低受体年龄、短移植缺血时间、高中心容量同术后生存率提高有关，有关这些方面的研究在不同国家都有类似的结果。

生存质量

心脏移植术后患者不仅生存时间延长，生活治疗也得以提高。ISHLT数据显示，心脏移植术后1年中，约75%的受体患者表示已回归正常的、健康的日常生活，或仅有少量症状。有15%的患者已可以进行正常的活动，仅有少许活动障碍。仅有不到10%的患者表现出了生存质量降低[2]。

一个小样本的心脏移植术后患者的逐层分析研究表明，心脏移植术后最常见的长期症状，占50%~65%，为疲劳、心功能减退、记忆障碍、淤青和痉挛[3]。而这些症状在已婚患者和高学历患者中较少见。

基于ISHLT的研究数据，许多患者术后均能回归正常工作。在25~55岁的受体患者中，约50%的患者在术后5年即被雇用[2]。综上所述，心脏移植术后患者可以从事正常工作。然而在美国，由于健康保险等情况的存在，可能会在一定程度上制约心脏移植术后患者回归正常岗位。

排斥反应

诊断

排斥反应仍是目前移植术后死亡的主要原因之一[2]。移植排斥反应在术后1个月时发生率最高，之后逐步减低。急性排斥反应是移植患者术后死亡率和发病率升高的重要原因之一，通常需要严密监测并进行临床干预。由于移植排斥反应的临床表现通常不明显，对无症状患者进行常规检查已成为目前的标准策略。同肾移植或肝移植不同，心脏移植术后排斥反应目前仍缺乏有效的实验室检查手段。心内膜心肌活检是目前对移植排斥反应进行监测的标准手段。心内膜心肌活检一般在造影引导下从右颈内静脉入路。该方法一般发生并发症的风险较低，可在门诊进行操作。最严重的并发症（发生率约为0.5%）包括三尖瓣损伤及心脏穿孔，易导致心包填塞[4,5]。在不同的医疗中心，进行心内膜心肌活检的时间窗各有差异，但总体上，心脏移植术后早期应较多地进行心内膜心肌活检，随着时间的推移，频率可以逐渐降低。在我中心，我们一般在术后第1个月要求患者每周2次门诊复查随访，并在第1个月内每周进行一次心内膜心肌活检。接下来，患者在第2个月内每周门诊复查1次，每两周进行1次活检。在术后第3~6个月，患者每月进行一次活检，到了术后8~12个月，患者每两月进行一次活检（表105.1）。因此，患者总计要在术后第1年内进行13次活检。在我中心，术后1年之后排斥风险相对较低，因此1年之后并不进行常规的定期活检。1年之后，仅在患者表现出排斥反应的症状或体征时进行心内膜心肌活检。尽管如此，我们对每位患者每6个月进行一次心超检查，每年进行一次血管造影，以评估移植心脏血管病变情况（在第79章有详细描述）。

心内膜心肌活检的目的主要在于评估细胞或抗体介导排斥反应下的心脏损伤情况。根据ISHLT分级，可以对细胞排斥进行诊断并分级。该分级标准于2005年发表，并对之前1990年的分级标准进行了简化[6,7]。活检结果分级如下：

- 0R级——无排斥（同1990年版相同）；
- 1R级——轻度排斥（1990年版的1A、1B和2级）；

表 105.1　移植术后监测

	门诊	抗 HLA 抗体检测	心超	心内膜心肌活检	血管造影
第 1 周	XX		X	X	
第 2 周	XX		X	X	
第 3 周	XX		X	X	
第 4 周	XX	X	X	X	
第 5 周	X				
第 6 周	X		X	X	
第 7 周	X				
第 8 周	X		X	X	
第 3 个月	X	X	X	X	
第 4 个月	X		X	X	
第 5 个月	X		X	X	
第 6 个月	X	X	X	X	
第 8 个月	X		X	X	
第 10 个月	X		X	X	
第 12 个月	X	X	X	X	
半年	X		X		
每年	X	X	X		X

• 2R 级——中度排斥(1990 年版的 3A 级)；

• 3R 级——重度排斥(1990 年版的 3B 级和 4 级)。

其中,2R 及以上等级的活检结果有临床意义,应给予相应治疗,在下文中进行详细阐述(也可见第 83 章)。

抗体介导排斥反应的诊断相对不够直观，但在 2010 年的会议后取得了更一致的诊断分级标准[8]。根据该标准，将心内膜心肌活检的结果根据组织学和免疫学表现进行分级。组织学表现包括内皮血管内巨噬细胞活化及毛细血管损伤。免疫学表现包括补体和 HLA 沉积。活检的分级标准如下：

• 无组织学或免疫学证据(阴性,0 级抗体介导排斥反应)；

• 有组织学或免疫学之一证据(可疑,1 级抗体介导排斥反应)；

• 同时有组织学和免疫学证据(阳性,2 级抗体介导排斥反应)；

• 重度心肌损伤表现(3 级抗体介导排斥反应)。

分级的明确化有助于临床上对抗体介导排斥反应的诊断,从而促进对心脏移植自然病程的研究,并指导对罕见情况的治疗。

虽然对于抗体介导排斥反应的诊断并无要求,我们中心依然对所有心脏移植术后患者的抗 HLA 抗体进行了监测。我们对患者在术后 1 个月、3 个月、6 个月及 12 个月进行抗体水平检测,之后每年检测 1 次(表 105.1)。检测发现高水平的抗体特异性抗 HLA 抗体通常具有细胞毒性,可能会对治疗造成影响,这点在之后进行进一步讨论。

进行心内膜心肌活检比较直接，但该侵入性操作仍有一定的危险性，目前也正在对其他排斥诊断方法进行开发。目前已研究并应用许多非侵入性的诊断指标,包括心电图、心超或磁共振的改变,以及 B 型钠尿肽等实验室指标。然而,并没有哪个指标能够提供足够的准确性和有效性。但在 Allomap,一个从外周血单个核细胞中提取的 11 个基因组成的基因表达特征可能对预测细胞排斥反应有显著的效果[9]。根据某临床试验结果,Allomap 基因表达谱对于细胞排斥的诊断效果并不亚于心内膜心肌活检[10]。然而,由于临床试验和其一般用于等方面的限制,Allomap 目前在临床上并未得到广泛应用[11,12]。

具有标志性意义的随机对照试验——IMAGE 研究,在心脏移植术后 6 个月至 5 年的患者中比较了 Allomap 基因表达谱同心内膜心肌活检的诊断效果,这批患者中有 85%都成功生存至术后 1 年之后。许多中心因心脏移植术后 1 年之后抗体介导排斥反应的发生率较低，因此没有在1年后对患者进行心肌活检，导致Allomap对于这批患者的适用性并没有得到很好的检验[12,13]。进一步地，Allomap因此并没有检测到抗体介导的排斥反应，且也不能用于30天内接受过血液制品输注或影响白细胞的造血细胞生长因子(如粒细胞刺激因子)输注的患者[9]。因此，Allomap在国际范围内的应用受到了阻碍，需要进一步的临床随机对照研究或广泛的临床研究经验，以证明其相比于心内膜心肌活检的优越性。

危险因素

移植排斥反应的危险因素根据移植术后的时间有所不同。移植术后早期，即移植术后一年以内的危险因素包括年龄低、女性供体、女性受体、巨细胞病毒血清学阳性、感染史以及OKT3诱导治疗[2]。相对地，术后远期的危险因素包括术后第一年多次移植排斥反应发作及巨细胞感染史[2]。

虽然移植术后远期排斥反应的发生较少见，根据部分中心对患者随访的心内膜心肌活检结果，部分术后患者远期依然存在移植排斥反应。远期排斥通常同患者免疫抑制药物治疗依从性不强、使用导致免疫抑制水平下降的干扰药物(如利福平)、停用一些已经在维持水平的药物(地尔硫卓、氮唑类抗真菌药或大环内酯类抗生素)或感染事件等相关[14]。抗体介导的排斥反应在术后远期更常见[15]，其可能是移植相关冠状动脉疾病[16]及死亡[17,18]的危险因素。

治疗

排斥反应的治疗应根据活检结果以及患者的临床表现循序渐进(表105.2)。移植排斥反应在移植术后早期最常发生，不同发生时间下治疗方法均类似。1R级细胞排斥反应，或疑似抗体介导排斥反应，即AMR1级，若无明显临床或血流动力学上的改变，一般无需特殊干预。对于AMR1级的治疗上目前还存在争议，在一些中心，更高级别的排斥反应一般才需要治疗干预，具体阐述见下文。

活检所发现的更严重的排斥反应，包括2R级及以上细胞排斥反应或AMR2级及以上抗体介导排斥反应，需要治疗干预。具体治疗方案应根据患者的临床表现决定。若患者无明显的心衰症状且左室射血分数正常，应给予口服或静脉冲击量激素治疗，并给予更高级

表105.2 抗排斥治疗力度主要依据患者的临床评估结果及活检结果确定，对于临床表现较不稳定的患者，可以考虑采用更积极的抗排斥治疗策略

	无症状	EF下降	心力衰竭/休克
细胞排斥	• 维持更高的CNI水平 • 口服激素冲击治疗 • 西罗莫司	• 口服激素冲击治疗 或 • 静脉激素冲击治疗	• 静脉激素冲击治疗 • 溶细胞治疗(ATG) • 血浆置换 • 静脉免疫球蛋白
抗体介导排斥反应	• 不治疗 或 • 口服激素冲击治疗	• 口服激素冲击治疗 或 • 静脉激素冲击治疗 ± • 静脉免疫球蛋白	• 肌力疗法 • IABP或ECMO支持

EF，左室射血分数；CNI，钙离子通道拮抗剂；ATG，抗胸腺细胞球蛋白；IABP，主动脉球囊反搏；ECMO，体外膜肺氧合。

别的免疫抑制药物，如将环孢素改为他克莫司[19,20]，或将霉酚酸酯改为增殖信号抑制剂等[21-23]。若静脉或口服皮质激素对无症状细胞排斥反应的治疗效果明显[24]，对于这部分患者，一线治疗方案为门诊予口服皮质激素治疗。无症状的抗体介导排斥反应则相对不易处理。近期部分研究表明，无症状抗体介导排斥反应可能预示不良预后[16-18]，并且治疗对于预后的改善效果目前也不太确切。在Cedars-Sinai心脏研究中心，对于这部分患者，给予口服皮质激素治疗，并根据情况给予静脉免疫球蛋白治疗，以及供体特异性HLA抗体的严密监测。

对于心超发现射血分数降低的患者，应予以更积极的治疗。若心脏射血分数降低，但无明显活检证据时，可静脉予皮质激素及抗胸腺细胞球蛋白，并根据上述方案更改免疫抑制治疗。如有AMR2或更高级别的证据，对于这部分患者，应同时给予静脉免疫球蛋白治疗。如果患者在AMR或射血分数降低的同时，存在供体特异性抗HLA抗体阳性证据，应在给予口服激素的同时，加用更积极的治疗，如静脉免疫球蛋白、利妥昔单抗或硼替佐米。

最后，若患者表现为心源性休克，那么不论活检结果如何，均应给予激进的治疗方案，包括静脉皮质激

素、溶细胞治疗、血浆置换、静脉免疫球蛋白、静脉肝素(尸检常发现患者存在心脏微血管栓塞现象)[25,26]以及经主动脉球囊反搏甚至给予体外膜肺氧合 (ECMO)治疗,以提供血流动力学支持[27]。

不同移植中心对于移植排斥的治疗策略不同,并且目前对于这些治疗策略还没有临床对照研究验证其优劣。然而，由于目前国际范围内移植样本量依然不大,其发生此类排斥反应病例较少,相关的临床随机对照研究较难开展。因此,临床医生必须依靠临床经验,以采取对患者预后最佳、不良反应最小的治疗方案。

长期治疗

细胞排斥反应通常可以通过糖皮质激素以及溶细胞治疗达到心衰的缓解及心脏射血分数的恢复[28],但抗体介导排斥反应的治疗相对较复杂。患者常出现持续性射血分数降低、心衰症状反复发作及移植相关冠状动脉疾病加速进展等情况[28]。

此类射血分数持续下降的患者,对于其有症状排斥反应的后续治疗方案,目前还没有明确的报道。在 Cedars-Sinai 心脏研究所，我们常依赖于降低供体特异性抗 HLA 抗体水平的治疗手段,包括利妥昔单抗、硼替佐米以及长期体外光分离疗法来调节 T 细胞功能。对于小部分患者,这些治疗手段可以起到明显的疗效[29,30],而对于大部分患者,可能仍需要进行再次移植手术治疗。

感染

概述

由于采用了免疫抑制治疗,心脏移植受体患者常处于感染高危状态,且感染的发生一般可以预测[31](见第 94 章,图 94.1)。葡糖球菌和链球菌等细菌感染常在术后早期即出现,并常累及手术切口造成切口感染。机会性感染通常在移植术后几周后才有可能出现。机会感染的病原常包括真菌(念珠菌、曲霉菌)、寄生虫(肺囊虫、弓形虫)以及病毒(巨细胞病毒)等。

对于常见机会性感染病原体的预防对于降低特定感染至关重要,这些感染包括口腔念珠菌病、肺孢子菌肺炎、弓形虫病以及巨细胞病毒感染等,但即使采取预防性治疗策略,这些感染还是有发生的可能。此外,由于免疫反应被抑制，移植患者术后部分活动性感染的临床表现可能会被掩盖从而难以发现。对于实质脏器移植术后患者的感染的诊断必须要果断，因为在免疫抑制的患者个体中,感染可能会迅速进展。此外,对于实质脏器移植术后感染,早期应给予广谱治疗,并且,熟悉移植术后感染的感染病学专家的诊断和治疗意见对于这部分患者而言至关重要。

感染风险

对于急性排斥反应，如何监测免疫状态和感染风险依然是一个难题。目前有许多针对移植后免疫监测方法的相关研究,然而均未得到明确验证,因此,目前临床上对于移植患者术后感染还没有明确的诊断和评估方法。然而,目前有一种新的淋巴细胞活性检测方法(ImmuKnow;Cylex,Columbia,MD),该方法利用外周血检测激活的淋巴细胞中 ATP 的释放,可能对重度免疫抑制患者的诊断给予有效的帮助[32,33]。一项目前为止最大样本量的研究显示,利用免疫监测评分对患者进行评估，那些评估后一月内出血感染表现的患者,其评分值要显著低于一般状况平稳的患者[34]。免疫评分<200ngATP/mL 的患者,其感染可能性较高。

在我们中心，对于免疫评分<200ngATP/mL 的,尤其是有多次复发感染的患者，我们可能考虑降低其钙调神经磷酸酶抑制剂低谷水平，或是减少霉酚酸酯剂量。然而,这种检测方法也存在一定局限。对于非重度免疫抑制的患者,其对于治疗的指导意义相对较小,而反复感染或重度感染本身就是重度或过度免疫抑制的最确切的诊断依据。进一步地,患者根据免疫评分调整免疫抑制治疗后的治疗效果，目前还没有明确的研究证据。

供体传播或受体再激活感染

供体传播的或是受体再激活的感染，虽然比较少见,但一旦发生,对于器官移植来说可能是灾难性的并发症。尽管利用各种手段对供体可能传播的疾病或受体可能再激活的疾病进行检测，这些感染性疾病依然有可能发生，主要发生在移植术后早期和免疫抑制最强的阶段。

供体传播感染可能通过移植组织中的潜伏感染或是菌血症造成。潜伏感染包括巨细胞病毒(这就是为什么供体暴露状态是决定受体预防性治疗疗程的关键因素)、结核和克氏锥虫(查加斯病)。病毒血症和菌血症在器官获取时很可能不易被察觉。较少见的供体传播性感染包括西尼罗河病毒、狂犬病、HIV 和淋巴细胞性脉络丛脑膜炎等。这些之前未被检测发现的病毒之所以会发病，是因为血清学病原检测的准确率并不是100%,在急性排斥反应阶段,病毒可能不表现出血清阳性表现,且并不是所有可能的病原都被检测了。在未来，分子诊断学的应用可能有助于提高供体检测的准确率,针对特定地区(例如对于得克萨斯州和美国西南部进行查加斯病的检测）扩大检测范围也可能有助于检测到潜在的可能传播的感染。一旦发现此类感染,相应地给予强力的预防和治疗措施，将有助于有效遏制该疾病在受体体内的进一步进展。

受体的感染再激活也是目前的关注重点之一,有活跃感染证据的受体患者一般应被排除于实体器官移植候选人之外。然而,移植术后远期也可能出现短暂性感染现象,可能为类圆线虫病或查加斯病等寄生虫。在南加利福尼亚州的 Cedars-Sinai 心脏研究所，查加斯病高发地区的患者一般在移植术前进行查加斯病的检测，移植术后也利用 PCR 技术进行该病原的严密监测,以防再激活的发生。克氏锥虫病原 PCR 检测阳性的患者,一般在移植传染病学家的指导下,给予苯并咪唑预防治疗。

真菌感染

所有移植受体患者都应预防性给予口服抗生素以防鹅口疮的发生。在 Cedars-Sinai 心脏研究所,这种预防治疗一般每 3 个月给予一次，与糖皮质激素降至泼尼松 10mg 每天的剂量以下的过程基本同步。预防治疗的选择包括复方磺胺甲恶唑(喉糖)或制霉菌素口服制剂。对于表现为系统性真菌感染的患者,如来自球孢子菌病高发的患者，可以预防性给予氟康唑或伊曲康唑治疗。唑类抗菌药的使用会使钙调神经磷酸酶抑制剂和增殖信号抑制剂类药物的浓度提高，因此在开始唑类抗生素疗程时,应将环孢素、他克莫司、西罗莫司和依维莫司的药物剂量减少到 50%，并对血药浓度进行严密监测。

寄生虫

移植受体患者按标准应给予一年的复方磺胺甲恶唑(TPM-SMX),以预防肺孢子虫病。TMP-SMX 几乎能够完全根除心脏移植受体患者体内的肺囊虫，并能预防诺卡氏菌和弓形虫感染。对于有磺胺类药物过敏的患者,只要患者没有 G6PD 缺陷相关证据,可给予氨苯砜或阿托伐醌治疗。

病毒感染

对于巨细胞病毒感染高危,即巨细胞病毒 IgG 滴度较低的患者,应给予巨细胞病毒预防性治疗。巨细胞病毒 IgG 滴度阴性(即未曾感染巨细胞病毒)的患者,且将要接受来自巨细胞病毒 IgG 阳性患者供心的,其移植术后感染巨细胞病毒的风险最大。在 Cedars-Sinai 心脏研究所,对于这些患者,一般给予一年的缬更昔洛韦治疗。对于供体和受体患者均为巨细胞病毒 IgG 阴性的,这些患者发生巨细胞病毒感染的可能性最低,对于这部分患者,可以给予 3 个月的缬更昔洛韦或阿昔洛韦(巨细胞病毒感染防治效果稍弱,但价格较便宜)治疗。其他患者应给予 6 个月的缬更昔洛韦治疗。当然,利用大剂量激素或溶细胞疗法对急性排斥治疗之后,患者应进行 3 个月的缬更昔洛韦联合 TMP-SMX 预防治疗。

疫苗

对于心脏移植受体患者进行疫苗注射目前还存在争议。由于这部分患者处于免疫抑制状态,活疫苗是严格禁止的。但即便是灭活疫苗,由于其可能通过促进免疫系统活化导致排斥反应的发生,也存在一定风险。在 Cedars-Sinai 心脏研究所,我们推荐仅对移植术后 6 个月以上，且前 6 个月没有排斥发作史的患者采用灭活死疫苗,如流感或肺炎球菌疫苗等。

恶变

发生率

除移植心脏血管病变外，移植心脏恶变是心脏移植术后致死的第二常见原因[2]。心脏移植术后恶变的发生率是肾移植术后发生率的 2~4 倍[35-38]。ISHLT 注册项目研究显示，移植心脏术后 8 年的累及恶变概率大约为 26%,其中 18%是由于皮肤癌转移[2]。心脏移植术后患者癌症发病率升高的原因可能同心脏移植术后大剂量免疫抑制治疗有关，而心脏移植术后需要大剂量免疫抑制的可能原因有两个：一是同移植心脏本身免疫要求有关，二是因为缺乏肝移植术后的转氨酶或肾移植术后的血清肌酐这样的无创排斥监测指标[39]。

恶变的发生可能同免疫抑制治疗下机体缺乏对肿瘤的免疫监视作用有关。除糖皮质激素外，所有种类的免疫抑制剂都有加速恶变的可能。有文献报道，对于卡波西肉瘤，利用西罗莫司可以起到使肿瘤完全缓解的效果[40]。也有其他实质性器官移植受体相关报道表明，利用增殖信号抑制剂，如西罗莫司和依维莫司，能够有效降低恶变的发生和进展[41-43]。

临床表现

实质脏器移植受体中癌症通常发生在移植术后3~5年。皮肤恶性肿瘤是心脏移植术后最常见的类型，主要包括鳞状细胞癌和基底细胞癌[44]。同普通人群相比，器官移植受体发生鳞状细胞癌的概率要升高65~250倍，发生基底细胞癌的概率升高10~16倍[45,46]。发生皮肤恶性肿瘤的危险因素包括白皙皮肤、皮肤癌症史、病变位置（容易阳光照射处）以及免疫移植治疗的完整性等[47,48]。

移植术后淋巴增生性疾病（PTLD），最常见的为同EB病毒感染相关的B细胞淋巴瘤，可能在移植术后发生。术后免疫抑制高负荷是淋巴瘤发生的危险因素，因此由于移植术后1年内免疫抑制的强度最高，PTLD在这一时间段内的发生率相对较高[49,50]。50%以上的PTLD患者均可表现出淋巴结外肿块，可累及消化道、肺、皮肤、肝脏、中央神经系统以及移植器官本身。PTLD发病的危险因素包括主要同溶细胞诱导治疗等高水平的免疫抑制有关[50]以及EB病毒血清学检测结果有关（EB病毒阴性受体及EB病毒阳性供体组合者风险最高）[51]。

最后，一般人群中高发的肿瘤，在心脏移植术后也常发生，包括乳腺、肺和前列腺肿瘤。心脏移植患者发生肺癌的概率要高于其他实质脏器移植患者，其原因可能同吸烟史有关，吸烟史既是肺癌的高危因素，也是需要进行移植治疗的终末期心脏和肺部疾病发生的高危因素[52]。

治疗

对于移植术后癌变的发生来说，最重要的治疗手段便是预防。在我们中心，我们鼓励所有心脏移植患者在他们的全科医师处进行常规的健康筛查，项目包括乳腺钼靶摄片、宫颈涂片、前列腺检查以及结肠镜等非移植患者一般体检项目。此外，我们鼓励患者进行防日照保护，并在皮肤科医生处进行常规的皮肤检查。尽管每年胸部X线片对于肺癌的早期监测目前尚未纳入常规流程，我们曾在部分患者中利用X线片检测到早期肺癌，因此，我们对我们中心的患者推荐每年进行胸部X线片摄影。

对于癌变的控制来说，第一步应该是减少免疫抑制力度，并且，对于部分PTLD患者来说，这可能是唯一的治疗策略。在我们中心，我们会考虑将新诊断为癌变患者的免疫抑制治疗中的钙调磷酸酶抑制剂或霉酚酸酯调整为增殖信号抑制剂，如西罗莫司或依维莫司，这两种药物对于癌变可能有一定的保护作用。相比于以钙调磷酸酶抑制剂为基础的治疗策略，利用雷帕霉素靶蛋白（mTOR）类免疫抑制剂，如西罗莫司和依维莫司可能可以减少癌变的发生，如减少实质脏器移植后患者非黑色素皮肤癌的发生[41-43]。利用免疫监测方法，如前文提到的淋巴细胞活性检测，可能可以对患者的全局免疫抑制状态进行了解[32-34]，从而为癌变患者降低免疫抑制剂剂量提供着手点。

除降低免疫抑制剂剂量，以及将钙调磷酸酶抑制剂类或霉酚酸酯类免疫抑制剂调整为增殖信号抑制剂两种方法外，其余方法建议咨询相关专家的意见。皮肤病学可能常需要进行广泛的肿瘤切除术，以治疗鳞状细胞癌或基底细胞癌。PTLD可能还需要化疗药物的治疗，最常见的为利妥昔单抗联合环磷酰胺、多柔比星、长春新碱及糖皮质激素（一般称为R-CHOP方案）。

一般治疗

对于所有心脏移植患者，都应该有相应的内科医师进行全程常规医疗指导。心脏移植患者应同一般患者一样给予常规检查和治疗，如根据患者年龄进行常见肿瘤的筛查，包括宫颈、乳腺、结肠和前列腺肿瘤等。此外，由于心脏移植患者好发皮肤恶性肿瘤，对于心脏移植患者，尤其是肤色白皙或有皮肤肿瘤既往史的移植患者，应配备一名内科医师或皮肤科医师每年进行皮肤检查。并且，内科医师还需对患者心脏移植术后长期慢性并发症进行管理，具体包括肾功能不全、高血压、血脂异常、糖尿病骨质疏松和痛风等。但也必须告诫患者，若内科医师针对一般慢性疾病开具了新的处方时，在用药之前需及时通知心脏移植中心，以确保药物之间没有明显的交叉作用。

肾功能不全

肾功能不全是钙调磷酸酶抑制剂的一种常见不良反应，且常随时间而逐渐加重，大约 8%的心脏移植患者在术后 5 年或更长时间发展为终末期肾病[2,53,54]。对于这部分患者，常需要给予不影响肾功能的免疫抑制方案，如降低钙调磷酸酶抑制剂剂量或用西罗莫司替代进行治疗等[55]。为了成功达到预期疗效，用药时间至关重要。若血肌酐过高，超过 2.5mg/dL 时，肾功能的损伤可能是不可逆的。如果利用西罗莫司代替钙调磷酸酶抑制剂治疗，那么该过程的关键步骤在于，在 2~4 周的时间内将钙调磷酸酶抑制剂缓慢撤药并同时等待西罗莫司药物水平逐渐上升，并在钙调磷酸酶抑制剂完全停药后 1 个月对患者进行心超和活检随访[56]。尽管目前仍无随机对照研究证实这种不影响肾功能的治疗方案的有效性，我们中心已发现，按照上述方法进行时，这种不影响肾功能的治疗方法是有效的、安全的且对部分患者有显著的改善作用。

高血压

心脏移植术后高血压主要同钙调磷酸酶抑制剂的应用有关，大约 80%的患者会出现移植术后高血压的情况[2]。移植术后高血压通常控制起来比较困难，往往需要多种降血压药物联合应用才能达到满意的效果[57,58]。目前，还没有临床研究证实[59-61]哪个降血压药物对于肾脏或心脏移植患者[62]的疗效要优于其他降压药物。但对于心脏移植患者，一般不推荐使用 β 受体阻滞剂，这是因为当机体运动时，去神经支配的移植心脏往往需要依靠循环中的儿茶酚胺以维持正常的心脏功能，而应用 β 受体阻滞剂的心脏移植患者常感到疲劳乏力感。部分移植患者由于术后肾功能不全和高血钾等情况的存在，往往也无法耐受血管紧张素转化酶抑制剂(ACEI)及血管紧张素受体阻断剂(ARB)。二氢吡啶类钙通道阻滞剂，如氨氯地平和硝苯地平，一般疗效显著，但可能会导致难治性水肿，且可能会增加钙调磷酸酶抑制剂的血药浓度，因此在初始使用时应予以严密监测。

血脂异常

由于皮质激素、钙调磷酸酶抑制剂和增殖信号抑制剂的使用，心脏移植术后脂质水平异常比较常见[63]。3-羟基-3-甲基戊二酰辅酶 A 还原酶抑制剂(他汀类)对于心脏移植患者术后的总胆固醇和低密度脂蛋白胆固醇的降低有明显效果。值得一提的是，心脏移植术后 2 周内开始应用他汀类，可以降低移植排斥反应中血流动力学的改变，并可有效提升术后 1 年生存率[64]。这些药物除了降脂作用外，可能存在免疫抑制作用。由于血脂异常在心脏移植术后较常见，所有移植患者都应常规接受他汀治疗。普伐他汀是他汀中的首选药物，其可以通过细胞色素 3A4 系统进行代谢，从而降低同钙调磷酸酶抑制剂之间的相互作用[14]。

糖尿病

糖尿病是导致终末期心脏疾病发生的重要心血管危险因素，同样地，糖尿病在心脏移植术前的患者中也较多见。并且，利用糖皮质激素及他克莫司进行移植术后免疫抑制可能会导致或加重糖尿病的发生。有数据显示，心脏移植患者在术后 5 年时，糖尿病的发生率高达 32%[2]。虽然糖尿病同远期生存率的降低有明显关系[64]，目前依然缺乏足够的临床数据，以指导这部分患者的治疗。总体来看，心脏移植术后肾功能不全的发生率较高，因此在治疗糖尿病时应尽量避免用二甲双胍类药物。此外，噻唑烷二酮类由于易导致液体潴留，也不推荐试用。短效磺酰脲类可能是大多数心脏移植术后患者首选的降糖药物[14]。

骨质疏松症

骨质疏松症导致的椎体压缩性骨折在心脏移植术后较多见，将进一步导致机体功能下降，并且激素类药物的使用会使骨质疏松进一步进展。在我们中心，我们推荐患者每年至内科医师处进行一次骨密度检测。为了预防骨质疏松的发生，患者应摄入足量的钙和维生素 D，并保持一定负荷量的运动，并根据初级保健医师的意见摄入适量的二磷酸盐。

痛风

心脏移植术后痛风发生的原因包括钙调磷酸酶抑制剂、利尿剂的应用以及肾功能不全的发生等。非甾体消炎药(NSAID)由于具有潜在的加速肾功能不全进展的作用，心脏移植术患者应尽量避免服用。对于痛风急性发作的患者，可用秋水仙碱治疗，但由于秋水仙碱同钙调磷酸酶抑制剂之间有相互作用，有造成神经病变的可能。因此，对于急性发作，通常首选静脉或关节内激素注射作为首选治疗。别嘌呤醇是有效的抑制方案，但由于其同硫唑嘌呤联合应用时可导致严重的骨髓抑制，在应用别嘌呤醇时应避免同硫唑嘌呤联合使用。鉴于不同药物之间的相互作用可能导致不良反应，对于心脏移植患者，在应用这些药物之前应咨询风湿病学家。

总结

目前，在免疫抑制、供体器官获取、手术技术和术后监护等方面的进步已大大提高了心脏移植患者的术后生存率。但当下依然存在许多难点问题，包括排斥反应、感染、恶变、移植冠脉疾病、肾功能不全、高血压、糖尿病、血脂异常、骨质疏松和痛风等。针对这些并发症防治策略的研究目前正在展开，未来在非有创监测手段上的进步将有助于我们更好地对排斥反应和免疫应答进行评估。本章使临床医师们能够根据每名心脏移植患者的具体情况更好地调整治疗方案，从而将治疗疗效最大化，并将治疗相关不良反应降到最低。

（赵海格 倪一鸣 郑骏楠 译 倪一鸣 校）

参考文献

1. Hunt SA, Abraham WT, Chin MH, et al. 2009 focused update incorporated into the ACC/AHA 2005 Guidelines for the Diagnosis and Management of Heart Failure in Adults: a report of the American College of Cardiology Foundation/American Heart Association Task Force on Practice Guidelines: developed in collaboration with the International Society for Heart and Lung Transplantation. Circulation. 2009;119:e391–479.
2. Stehlik J, Edwards LB, Kucheryavaya AY, et al. The Registry of the International Society for Heart and Lung Transplantation: twenty-seventh official adult heart transplant report-2010. Journal of Heart and Lung Transplantation. 2010;29:1089–1103.
3. Grady KL, Wang E, Higgins R, et al. Symptom frequency and distress from 5 to 10 years after heart transplantation. Journal of Heart and Lung Transplantation. 2009;28:759–768.
4. Saraiva F, Matos V, Goncalves L, et al. Complications of endomyocardial biopsy in heart transplant patients: a retrospective study of 2117 consecutive procedures. Transplantation Proceedings. 2011;43:1908–1912.
5. Baraldi-Junkins C, Levin HR, Kasper EK, et al. Complications of endomyocardial biopsy in heart transplant patients. Journal of Heart and Lung Transplantation. 1993;12:63–67.
6. Stewart S, Winters GL, Fishbein MC, et al. Revision of the 1990 working formulation for the standardization of nomenclature in the diagnosis of heart rejection. Journal of Heart and Lung Transplantation. 2005;24:1710–1720.
7. Billingham ME, Cary NR, Hammond ME, et al. A working formulation for the standardization of nomenclature in the diagnosis of heart and lung rejection: Heart Rejection Study Group. The International Society for Heart Transplantation. Journal of Heart Transplantation. 1990;9:587–593.
8. Kobashigawa J, Crespo-Leiro MG, Ensminger SM, et al. Report from a consensus conference on antibody-mediated rejection in heart transplantation. Journal of Heart and Lung Transplantation. 2011;30:252–269.
9. Deng MC, Eisen HJ, Mehra MR, et al. Noninvasive discrimination of rejection in cardiac allograft recipients using gene expression profiling. American Journal of Transplantation. 2006;6:150–160.
10. Pham MX, Teuteberg JJ, Kfoury AG, et al. Gene-expression profiling for rejection surveillance after cardiac transplantation. New England Journal of Medicine. 2010;362:1890–1900.
11. Jarcho JA. Fear of rejection–monitoring the heart-transplant recipient. New England Journal of Medicine. 2010;362:1932–1933.
12. Mehra MR, Parameshwar J. Gene expression profiling and cardiac allograft rejection monitoring: is IMAGE just a mirage? Journal of Heart and Lung Transplantation. 2010;29:599–602.
13. Patel JK, Kobashigawa JA. Should we be doing routine biopsy after heart transplantation in a new era of anti-rejection? Current Opinion in Cardiology. 2006;21:127–131.
14. Page RL 2nd, Miller GG, Lindenfeld J. Drug therapy in the heart transplant recipient: part IV: drug-drug interactions. Circulation. 2005;111:230–239.
15. Michaels PJ, Espejo ML, Kobashigawa J, et al. Humoral rejection in cardiac transplantation: risk factors, hemodynamic consequences and relationship to transplant coronary artery disease. Journal of Heart and Lung Transplantation. 2003;22:58–69.
16. Wu GW, Kobashigawa JA, Fishbein MC, et al. Asymptomatic antibody-mediated rejection after heart transplantation predicts poor outcomes. Journal of Heart and Lung Transplantation. 2009;28:417–422.
17. Kfoury AG, Hammond ME, Snow GL, et al. Cardiovascular mortality among heart transplant recipients with asymptomatic antibody-mediated or stable mixed cellular and antibody-mediated rejection. Journal of Heart and Lung Transplantation. 2009;28:781–784.
18. Kfoury AG, Stehlik J, Renlund DG, et al. Impact of repetitive episodes of antibody-mediated or cellular rejection on cardiovascular mortality in cardiac transplant recipients: defining rejection patterns. Journal of Heart and Lung Transplantation. 2006;25:1277–1282.
19. Kobashigawa JA, Miller LW, Russell SD, et al. Tacrolimus with mycophenolate mofetil (MMF) or sirolimus vs. cyclosporine with MMF in cardiac transplant patients: 1-year report. American Journal of Transplantation. 2006;6:1377–1386.
20. Kobashigawa JA, Patel J, Furukawa H, et al. Five-year results of a randomized, single-center study of tacrolimus vs microemulsion cyclosporine in heart transplant patients. Journal of Heart and Lung Transplantation. 2006;25:434–439.
21. Keogh A, Richardson M, Ruygrok P, et al. Sirolimus in de novo heart transplant recipients reduces acute rejection and prevents coronary artery disease at 2 years: a randomized clinical trial. Circulation. 2004;110:2694–2700.
22. Eisen HJ, Tuzcu EM, Dorent R, et al. Everolimus for the prevention of allograft rejection and vasculopathy in cardiac-transplant recipients. New England Journal of Medicine. 2003;349:847–858.
23. Mancini D, Pinney S, Burkhoff D, et al. Use of rapamycin slows progression of cardiac transplantation vasculopathy. Circulation. 2003;108:48–53.
24. Kobashigawa JA, Stevenson LW, Moriguchi JD, et al. Is intravenous glucocorticoid therapy better than an oral regimen for asymptomatic cardiac rejection? A randomized trial. Journal of the American College of Cardiology. 1993;21:1142–1144.
25. Arbustini E, Roberts WC. Morphological observations in the epicardial coronary arteries and their surroundings late after cardiac transplantation (allograft vascular disease). American Journal of Cardiology. 1996;78:814–820.
26. Fishbein MC, Kobashigawa J. Biopsy-negative cardiac transplant rejection: etiology, diagnosis, and therapy. Current Opinion in Cardiology. 2004;19:166–169.
27. Kittleson MM, Patel JK, Moriguchi JD, et al. Heart transplant recipients supported with extracorporeal membrane oxygenation: outcomes from a single-center experience. Journal of Heart and Lung Transplantation. 2011;30:1250–1256.
28. Patel JK, Kittleson M, Kobashigawa JA. Cardiac allograft rejection. The Surgeon: Journal of the Royal Colleges of Surgeons of Edinburgh and Ireland. 2011;9:160–167.
29. Patel J, Everly M, Chang D, et al. Reduction of alloantibodies via proteosome inhibition in cardiac transplantation. Journal of Heart and Lung Transplantation. 2011;30:1320–1326.
30. Kirklin JK, Brown RN, Huang ST, et al. Rejection with hemodynamic compromise: objective evidence for efficacy of photopheresis. Journal of Heart and Lung Transplantation. 2006;25:283–288.
31. Fishman JA. Infection in solid-organ transplant recipients. New England Journal of Medicine. 2007;357:2601–2614.
32. Kowalski R, Post D, Schneider MC, et al. Immune cell function testing: an adjunct to therapeutic drug monitoring in transplant patient management. Clinical Transplantation. 2003;17:77–88.
33. Kowalski RJ, Post DR, Mannon RB, et al. Assessing relative risks of infection and rejection: a meta-analysis using an immune function assay. Transplantation. 2006;82:663–668.
34. Kobashigawa JA, Kiyosaki KK, Patel JK, et al. Benefit of immune monitoring in heart transplant patients using ATP production in activated lymphocytes. Journal of Heart and Lung Transplantation. 2011;29:504–508.

35. Penn I. Incidence and treatment of neoplasia after transplantation. Journal of Heart and Lung Transplantation. 1993;12:S328–S336.
36. Mihalov ML, Gattuso P, Abraham K, et al. Incidence of post-transplant malignancy among 674 solid-organ-transplant recipients at a single center. Clinical Transplantation. 1996;10:248–255.
37. Fortina AB, Caforio AL, Piaserico S, et al. Skin cancer in heart transplant recipients: frequency and risk factor analysis. Journal of Heart and Lung Transplantation. 2000;19:249–255.
38. Jensen P, Hansen S, Moller B, et al. Skin cancer in kidney and heart transplant recipients and different long-term immunosuppressive therapy regimens. Journal of the American Academy of Dermatology. 1999;40:177–186.
39. Dantal J, Soulillou JP. Immunosuppressive drugs and the risk of cancer after organ transplantation. New England Journal of Medicine. 2005;352:1371–1373.
40. Campistol JM, Gutierrez-Dalmau A, Torregrosa JV. Conversion to sirolimus: a successful treatment for posttransplantation Kaposi's sarcoma. Transplantation. 2004;77:760–762.
41. Mathew T, Kreis H, Friend P. Two-year incidence of malignancy in sirolimus-treated renal transplant recipients: results from five multicenter studies*. Clinical Transplantation. 2004;18:446–449.
42. Campistol JM, Eris J, Oberbauer R, et al. Sirolimus therapy after early cyclosporine withdrawal reduces the risk for cancer in adult renal transplantation. American Journal of Nephrology. 2006;17(2):581–589.
43. Salgo R, Gossmann J, Schöfer H, et al. Switch to a sirolimus-based immunosuppression in long-term renal transplant recipients: reduced rate of (pre-) malignancies and nonmelanoma skin cancer in a prospective, randomized, assessor-blinded, controlled clinical trial. American Journal of Transplantation. 2010;10:1385–1393.
44. Vajdic CM, van Leeuwen MT. Cancer incidence and risk factors after solid organ transplantation. International Journal of Cancer. 2009;125:1747–1754.
45. Greenberg JN, Zwald FO. Management of skin cancer in solid-organ transplant recipients: a multidisciplinary approach. Dermatologic Clinics. 2011;29:231–241.
46. Moloney FJ, Comber H, O'Lorcain P, et al. A population-based study of skin cancer incidence and prevalence in renal transplant recipients. British Journal of Dermatology. 2006;154:498–504.
47. Caforio ALP, Fortina AB, Piaserico S, et al. Skin cancer in heart transplant recipients: risk factor analysis and relevance of immunosuppressive therapy. Circulation. 2000;102(19 Suppl 3):III-222–III-227.
48. Ramsay HM, Fryer AA, Hawley CM, et al. Factors associated with nonmelanoma skin cancer following renal transplantation in Queensland, Australia. Journal of the American Academy of Dermatology. 2003;49:397–406.
49. Opelz G, Henderson R. Incidence of non-Hodgkin lymphoma in kidney and heart transplant recipients. Lancet. 1993;342:1514–1516.
50. Swinnen LJ, Costanzo-Nordin MR, Fisher SG, et al. Increased incidence of lymphoproliferative disorder after immunosuppression with the monoclonal antibody OKT3 in cardiac-transplant recipients. New England Journal of Medicine. 1990;323:1723–1728.
51. Walker RC, Marshall WF, Strickler JG, et al. Pretransplantation assessment of the risk of lymphoproliferative disorder. Clinic of Infectious Diseases. 1995;20(5):1346–1353.
52. Rinaldi M, Pellegrini C, D'Armini AM, et al. Neoplastic disease after heart transplantation: single center experience. European Journal of Cardio-Thoracic Surgery. 2001;19:696–701.
53. Goldstein DJ, Zuech N, Sehgal V, et al. Cyclosporine-associated end-stage nephropathy after cardiac transplantation: incidence and progression. Transplantation. 1997;63:664–668.
54. Zietse R, Balk AH, vd Dorpel MA, et al. Time course of the decline in renal function in cyclosporine-treated heart transplant recipients. American Journal of Nephrology. 1994;14:1–5.
55. Gustafsson F, Ross HJ. Renal-sparing strategies in cardiac transplantation. Current Opinion in Cardiology. 2009;14(5):566–570.
56. Flechner SM, Kobashigawa J, Klintmalm G. Calcineurin inhibitor-sparing regimens in solid organ transplantation: focus on improving renal function and nephrotoxicity. Clinical Transplantation. 2008;22:1–15.
57. Frohlich ED, Ventura HO, Ochsner JL. Arterial hypertension after orthotopic cardiac transplantation. Journal of the American College of Cardiology. 1990;15:1102–1103.
58. Starling RC, Cody RJ. Cardiac transplant hypertension. American Journal of Cardiology. 1990;65:106–111.
59. Midtvedt K, Hartmann A, Holdaas H, et al. Efficacy of nifedipine or lisinopril in the treatment of hypertension after renal transplantation: a double-blind randomised comparative trial. Clinical Transplantation. 2001;15:426–431.
60. Sennesael J, Lamote J, Violet I, et al. Comparison of perindopril and amlodipine in cyclosporine-treated renal allograft recipients. Hypertension. 1995;26(3):436–444.
61. Hausberg M, Barenbrock M, Hohage H, et al. ACE inhibitor versus beta-blocker for the treatment of hypertension in renal allograft recipients. Hypertension. 1999;33(3):862–868.
62. Brozena SC, Johnson MR, Ventura H, et al. Effectiveness and safety of diltiazem or lisinopril in treatment of hypertension after heart transplantation. Results of a prospective, randomized multicenter trail. Journal of the American College of Cardiology. 1996;27(7):1707–1712.
63. Lindenfeld J, Page RL 2nd, Zolty R, et al. Drug therapy in the heart transplant recipient: part III: common medical problems. Circulation. 2005;111:113–117.
64. Kobashigawa JA, Starling RC, Mehra MR, et al. Multicenter retrospective analysis of cardiovascular risk factors affecting long-term outcome of de novo cardiac transplant recipients. Journal of Heart and Lung Transplantation. 2006;25:1063–1069.

第 106 章 肺移植和心肺联合移植的长期预后

Toshihiro Okamoto, David Wheeler, Kenneth R. McCurry

引言

终末期肺衰竭仍然是美国和全世界都很常见的发病和死亡原因。对于许多患者,肺移植提供了延长生命的唯一希望。自 1983 年第一例肺移植成功以来,提供肺移植的机构和移植量都稳步增加。特别是在过去 10 年,每年美国和全世界进行的肺移植量

都在显著增长。仅在美国,每年进行 1700~1800 例肺移植,全球每年进行超过 3500 例肺移植[1,2](图 106.1)。

随着移植量的增加,我们已经看到了患者预后正随着时间的推移和各移植中心后续护理的稳步改善而逐渐改善[1-3]。肺移植成功数量增加的关键在于多年来一直不断地努力完善免疫抑制疗法,以减少糖皮质激素对支气管愈合的不良反应和其他并发症,以及评估技术的改善和肺移植手术的进展,还有移植后的保护和管理的进展。这些都已在第 26 章、第 59 章和第 72 章进行了特别阐述,覆盖了器官的复苏和保存、外科技术和围术期免疫管理。这些努力已经改善了生存,特别是短期生存,但肺移植 5 年中位生存率仍令人失望[1]。晚期(即移植后 1 年以上)移植失败和死亡通常是由于闭塞性细支气管炎综合征(BOS)和感染,在过去的 20 年里未见改观。除了这些往往致命的并发症,肾功能不全、高血压、糖尿病或骨质疏松症也较为常见。

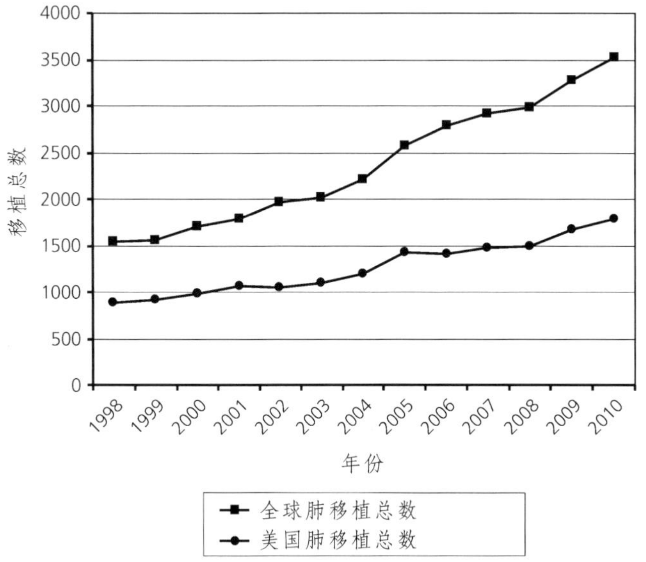

图 106.1 1998—2010 年期间,在全球和美国进行的年度肺移植手术数量。国际心肺移植协会(ISHLT)登记处报告,2010 年是迄今为止年手术量最多的一年,全球共进行了 3519 例肺移植(2599 例双肺移植和 920 例单肺移植)。在美国,根据器官获取和移植网络(OPTN)的年度报告,2010 年美国进行了 1785 例肺移植(1246 例双肺移植和 539 例单肺移植)。图根据 2011 年 ISHLT 登记处和 OPTN 报告的数据生成。

肺移植后的短期结果在第 72 章和第 80 章进行了讨论。本章将回顾成人肺移植的长期预后,包括主要的发病和死亡原因。心肺联合移植较孤立肺移植少,长期结果更接近于肺移植患者而非心脏移植患者。由于这个原因,心肺联合移植的长期预后也将在此讨论。小儿肺移植的讨论见第 116 章。

长期预后

生存

肺移植术后生存率在过去的 20 年里稳步提高。在 20 世纪 80 年代和 20 世纪 90 年代初,1 年生存率约为 70%,中位生存时间约 3.9 年,第一年存活的患者,7 年存活率为 50%[2](图 106.2)。在一份国际心肺移植协会(ISHLT)登记处的报告中,2004 年到 2010 年 6 月,1 年生存率已经提高到 81%,中位生存时间增加到 5.9 年[2](图 106.2)。这个随时间改善的生存时间同样反映在美国的数据里[1]。长期生存的改善在很大程度上是早期生存的增加,第一年以后移植失败率一直是相对稳定的

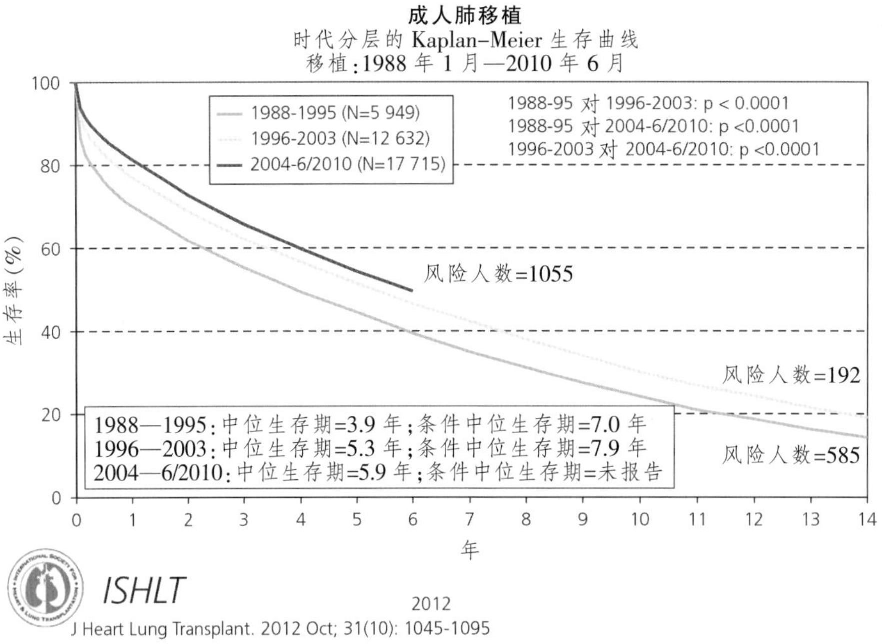

图 106.2 使用 Kaplan-Meier 方法计算的成人肺移植生存曲线。包含可以提供任何随访信息的移植患者的数据。由于许多患者仍然存活并且部分已失访,不是所有患者的死亡时间是明确已知的,因此这里的存活率只是估计值。使用对数秩检验比较存活率。多重比较未进行校整。(Source: International Society for Heart and Lung Transplantation, accessible from http://www.ishlt.org/registries/slides.asp?slides=heartLungRegistry)

(图 106.2)。尽管有这些改善,肺移植受者的生存数据相比其他实体器官移植,如心脏、肾脏和肝移植受者的中位生存时间都相对要低。

影响生存的因素

在之前已经提到,从 ISHLT 注册处的最新报告显示,双肺移植(DLT)受者较单肺移植(SLT)受者具有更大的生存优势[2]。这些数据应被谨慎解读,然而,由于生存率的差异,移植方式的选择还需要考虑其他临床因素(如患者年龄、并发症、诊断以及捐赠者的问题)。许多研究者检查了移植类型生存率与受者疾病诊断之间的相关性[4-9]。Meyer 等发现,接受双肺移植治疗慢性阻塞性肺疾病(COPD)较单肺移植有较高的中位生存时间(6.7 年对 4.6 年),虽然没有统计学显著差异,60 岁以上受者获益更多[10]。此外,有人认为移植类型可能影响 BOS 的风险。Hadjiliadis 等报道,COPD 受者接受 DLT 的 3 年内 BOS 风险较 SLT 要小(57.4%对 50.7%),移植后 5 年分别是 44.5%和 17.9%[5]。猜测可能是 DLT 受者有更多的肺储备。

在肺间质纤维化(IPF)患者接受肺移的植人群中,2011 年 ISHLT 注册报告显示,肺移植术后 3 年或更长时间,未调整的生存率方面 DLT 优于 SLT[6]。然而,在 UNOS 注册报告中,包含 3327 例 IPF 患者,DLT 和 SLT 之间调整受者和供者的基线特征后并没有显著不同的生存率[7]。Weiss 等分析了美国高危 IPF 患者在引入肺分配评分(LAS)的生存情况。DLT[8] 1 年死亡率下降至 14.4%,这表明 DLT 较 SLT 有利。对于肺动脉高压(PAH),许多报道表明 DLT 是有利的选择[9]。

在过去 10 年中,65 岁及以上患者进行肺移植的数量急剧增加。2001 年在美国,3.4%的肺移植受者为 65 岁及以上,而在 2011 年,这已增加至 26.6%[1]。这一趋势在 ISHLT 注册中也可以看到[2]。注意到这一人口数据的改变,也很清楚地表明肺移植后的生存率受患者年龄的影响。特别是在 65 岁及以上受者,中位生存期是 3.6 年,而在 35~49 岁受者是 6.5 年[2]。预后差异的主要原因似乎是后期事件导致 1 年长期生存率更差[2]。

疾病特异性生存差异明显,但可能受疾病严重性、不同的并发症以及人群疾病平均年龄的影响。此外,某些诊断带来手术并发症和移植物失功的风险更大。在至少生存 1 年以上的受者中,囊性纤维化(CF)的中位生存时间为 10.4 年,PAH 为 10 年,而结节病是 8.4 年,α_1-抗胰蛋白酶缺乏是 8.6 年,COPD 和 IPF 是 6.8 年[2]。

COPD 肺移植患者 1 年生存率最高，PAH 具有最低的一年生存率。IPF 肺移植受者比其他疾病的 1 年和 10 年生存率都低。

需要注意的是，美国大多数已公布的生存数据是基于之前的器官分配体系，等待时间长的受者优先。2005 年 5 月，新的肺分配评分(LAS)系统启动，将患者的死亡风险(紧迫度)和移植后 1 年生存率纳入考量[11]。这个 LAS 系统部分基于疾病严重程度，这可能对患者的选择以及生存预后产生影响[12]。很快在 LAS 启动后，等待时间和等待名单的死亡人数出现轻度但有差异的下降。随着时间的推移，移植受者的平均得分增加[13]，而有争议的是，一些数据表明，更高的 LAS 评分与增加的发病率和肺移植后死亡率相关[14,15]。在美国，这将如何影响预后和器官分配目前尚不清楚。作为 LAS 系统的一部分，等待名单死亡和移植后生存将被持续监控，仍迫切需要对 LAS 系统进行修订。LAS 对等待名单管理的影响在第 40 章阐述。

最近 ISHLT 注册报告对肺移植术后死亡率的风险因素进行了深入分析(在之前讨论的那些因素之外)[2]。5 年死亡率的最强分类危险因素包括受者静脉注射强心药物[相对危险(RR)为 2.13]和透析(RR 为 1.79)。5 年死亡率的持续危险因素，通过生存超过 1 年调整，包括受体低或高年龄和移植中心规模小。

心肺联合移植

每年进行的成人心肺联合移植数量与世界范围内的肺移植相比明显少，自 2003 年以来每年为 86~114 例[2]。主要适应证仍然是先天性心脏病和肺动脉高压，以及逐渐减少的 CF。心肺联合移植的存活率与肺移植存活率有所不同，其早期死亡率相对较高。心肺联合移植受者的 1 年生存率为 63%，但存活一年后的生存率较好，1 年后中位生存时间为 10 年。与肺移植相比，心肺联合移植术后存活率在 1982—2010 年间每十年均有显著提高。心肺联合移植患者移植前的诊断也与生存相关。艾森门格综合征整体生存时间最佳，而术前诊断为 PAH 等先天性心脏病则相对较差[2]。

生活质量

肺移植的目的不仅是延长那些患有终末期肺病患者的生存期，也要提高与健康相关的生活质量(HRQL)。移植后生存分析和肺功能分析较常见，但深度分析肺移植后 HRQL 相对较少。ISHLT 注册处有登记移植后的状态，尽管由于报告不完整而资料有限，数据显示，85%以上的存活患者在 1 年、3 年和 5 年没有活动受限，在移植 5 年后，35%的存活患者从事兼职或全职工作，46%不工作，19%退休[2]。在最近发表的研究中，专题分析了肺移植患者的 HRQL。Singer 等发表了一些重要见解[16]。首先，他们分析发现，支持肺移植改善 HRQL 的结果体现在身体健康和功能上的改善。第二，他们发现肺移植受者可能得到比其他实体器官移植更大的 HRQL 获益。第三，肺移植受者在 HRQL 方面明显改善归属于等待肺移植的患者 HRQL 极差。最后，他们的数据支持，肺移植术后 HRQL 仍然是一个需要充分研究的领域。虽然他们确定了在 1983 年 1 月 1 日和 2011 年 12 月 31 日之间 73 项已发表的关于肺移植 HRQL 的研究，心脏移植在同时期有 1131 篇文章发表，肝移植有 1291 篇，肾移植有 1689 篇。这一领域在未来无疑会有更多的调查。

急性排斥反应

尽管新的免疫抑制药物应用于肺移植，急性和慢性排斥反应仍然很常见。事实上，在肺移植中，排斥反应给受者带来的负担可能较其他器官移植更大，小肠移植受者除外。肺暴露于外部环境(包括感染)且有丰富的免疫背景是重要的影响因素(这可能也适用于小肠移植)。从历史上看，急性细胞排斥反应(ACR)被认为是肺移植急性排斥反应的主要形式，然而，抗体介导排斥反应(AMR)目前也被认为起重要作用，像在其他实体器官移植中那样。移植后第一年的死亡主要原因是 BOS，也是长期生存的主要障碍。这些问题在以下各节中将讨论。相关的肺移植受者与心肺联合移植受者之间的差异将进行讨论。

急性细胞排斥反应

ACR 的临床和病理特点在第 72 章和第 84 章已经全部讨论。然而，ACR 是预后的一个重要因素，因此在这里介绍。肺移植患者出现 ACR 可无症状或有广泛的症状和表现。非特异性症状包括咳嗽、呼吸困难和痰，而非特异性症状可包括低氧血症、发热和异常呼吸音，很难从症状和体征上与感染相鉴别[17]。同样，影像学研究和肺功能研究(PFT)的结果不敏感或不够特异性而无法区别于感染[18,19]。因此,经支气管肺活检(TBBx)仍然是ACR诊断的金标准。TBBx的风险包括出血和气胸,已促使许多研究人员试图通过纤维支气管镜支气管肺泡灌洗(BAL)液内相关蛋白或细胞标记确立ACR的诊断[20]。然而,迄今为止,尽管有一些希望,没有外周血相应的细胞或分子标记被证明具有足够的敏感性和特异性可以取代TBBx在ACR诊断中的地位。

ACR病理分级分为急性细胞血管性排斥反应(A级ACR)和急性细胞气道排斥反应(B级ACR),每个类别又分不同程度[21](表106.1)。ACR是常见的肺移植并发症,至少1/3的肺移植受者在移植后第一年经历ACR。移植第一年之后,ACR的频率明显下降。肺移植受者的管理,尽管有争议,包括在许多肺移植中心常规使用监测性支气管镜检查及TBBxs[22]。而一些肺移植方案进行TBBxs取决于临床环境[23],许多人认为,监测性TBBxs(至少对于移植后前18~24个月)可提供有价值的信息,以允许适当免疫抑制方案的微调来治疗无症状性排斥反应[24]。然而没有数据能证实监测性TBBxs对BOS或生存的影响。

尽管严重的ACR可以致命,但ACR通常是可以治愈的,且在肺移植的死亡原因中占不到2%[2]。ACR是肺移植后的一大焦点,然而是BOS发生的最重要危险因素。研究表明,高级别的ACR、更加频繁的ACR、反复高级别ACR和B级ACR(淋巴细胞性细支气管炎)是BOS的危险因素,而A级排斥反应则不是[25-27]。此外,由于存在有大气道炎症[29],最小的A1级ACR在一些研究中已被确定为是BOS的风险因素。

ACR的风险因素已在第72章进行了详细介绍,但这里还是简要介绍一下ACR、BOS和长期预后之间的联系。有报告的ACR的危险因素包括供受者HLA差异、免疫抑制的类型、受者因素及感染。几个大型研究分析HLA差异与ACR风险的相关性,虽然确切的关系需要进一步研究确定,似乎表明越来越多的HLA差异将恶化肺移植的结果,并与ACR风险增加相关[30,31]。关于免疫抑制,未调整ISHLT注册数据表明,基于他克莫司的维持方案上给予白介素-2受体拮抗剂导致移植后第一年ACR的发生率明显降低[2]。几个随机比较环孢素与他克莫司为基础的试验,虽然有不同的结果,最新和最大的随机试验发现,他克莫司与较低的BOS累积发病率相关,尽管与ACR发病无关[32]。受者与ACR风险相关的因素包括:与免疫减少或提高有关的基因型[20],增强针对移植肺自身免疫反应的胃食管反流病[33,34]。最后,各种病毒和细菌感染被证实与ACR加重和(或)BOS恶化风险相关,导致长期预后受影响[35]。

虽然大多数肺移植受者需终身使用三联免疫抑制方案,包括钙调磷酸酶抑制剂(CI)、抗代谢药物和糖

表106.1 肺同种异体移植物排斥反应的修订分类和分级

排斥类别	分级	程度	组织学发现
A级	0	无	正常肺
急性细胞性血管排斥	1	轻微	散在,不常见的血管周围单核细胞浸润
	2	轻度	较低的放大倍数下可见更频繁的血管周围浸润,可有嗜酸性粒细胞
	3	中度	容易识别,密集的血管周围浸润,延伸到支气管周围隔膜和气腔,通常与内皮炎相关,可见嗜酸性粒细胞和嗜中性粒细胞
	4	重度	弥漫性血管周围、间质和气腔浸润,显著的肺细胞损伤和内皮炎
B级	0	无	无细支气管炎证据
急性细胞性气道排斥	1R	低级别	不常见和分散的淋巴细胞(或形成圆带),没有上皮损伤或上皮内浸润
	2R	高级别	细支气管黏膜下层有较大并活化的淋巴细胞,嗜酸性粒细胞和浆细胞样细胞较多,上皮内淋巴细胞浸润与上皮损伤有关
	X	无法定级	组织无法定级
C级	0	无	无闭塞性细支气管炎
慢性气道排斥	1	有	有闭塞性细支气管炎
D级			加速性移植物血管硬化
慢性血管排斥			

R表示修订等级,以避免与1996年的分类混淆。

基于2007年修订的标准化命名工作分类(21)。

皮质激素,但关于最佳方案缺乏共识,用药剂量差异很大[2,36]。同样,在各治疗中心之间没有标准化的方法应对 ACR,且缺乏随机试验数据支持药物选择。然而一般认为,2 级 ACR 或更高级别需要治疗。初始治疗通常为糖皮质激素冲击式治疗 (每天 500~1000mg)3~5 天,随后给予口服糖皮质激素和(或)增加其他免疫抑制药物[36]。高级别急性排斥反应可导致移植肺功能不全,一些中心选择利用多克隆或单克隆抗淋巴细胞药物。持续性或反复 ACR 一般是重复使用糖皮质激素,可在维持免疫抑制剂(例如,在 CI 或增加一种 mTOR 抑制剂)和(或)多克隆或单克隆抗淋巴细胞药物上做调整[36]。其他报告的方法包括使用阿仑单抗[37]、吸入环孢素[38]、全淋巴照射[39]和体外照光[40]。虽然如上所述,A1 级和 B 级(淋巴细胞性细支气管炎)急性排斥反应伴随 BOS 的发展,不同方案在是否治疗之间有争议,且是否治疗改变了 BOS 的风险。在最近美国的一项调查中,80%的受访者表示会治疗 A1 级排斥反应,而只有 35%的受访者表示会治疗无症状的 A1 级排斥反应。此外,12%的受访者表示,他们不会治疗淋巴细胞性细支气管炎[22]。进一步将问题复杂化,淋巴细胞性细支气管炎的分级也有很大差异。

抗体介导的排斥反应(AMR)

抗 HLA 抗体的排斥反应在肾移植和心脏移植方面已经被确认,而且在第 6 章进行了机制探讨,在第 89 章进行了临床探讨。其在肺移植中的重要性,除外超急性排斥反应,在过去的 10~15 年有越来越多的证据证明了肺移植后 AMR 的存在,肺 AMR 的后果包括持续性和难治性 ACR 和 BOS[41]。基于最近发布的 ISHLT 病理共识[41],诊断的典型要素包括:

(1)临床证实移植肺功能不全

(2)循环供者特异性抗体(DSA),和

(3)病理结果[41]

学者强调了组织病理学,这在第 84 章已经描述,各种疾病 AMR 具有损伤的非特异性,并指出,毛细血管 C4d 阳性和循环 DSA 常见于 AMR,也可以没有。他们还强调,基于目前的定义和大多数移植病理学家的经验,AMR 是一种相对罕见的发现,诊断 AMR 要依靠病理学家、免疫学家和临床医生的配合。他们还鼓励中心设计方案定期评估 DSA,并结合临床随访或监测性支气管镜检查。

目前没有随机对照试验评价肺移植后 AMR 的治疗,在肾移植也一样。治疗方面现有数据大多来自单中心报告。血浆置换术(清除循环抗体)、免疫球蛋白(IVIG-导致 B 细胞凋亡,阻断供者反应性抗体和抑制补体激活)和利妥昔单抗(抗 CD20 抗体)是常见的治疗方法,可单独或联合使用[20]。一些中心现在正在使用的两种新药物包括硼替佐米 (26s 蛋白酶体抑制剂,导致浆细胞凋亡)和依库珠单抗(补体 C5 的抗体,封锁终端补体激活)[20]。辅助治疗通常包括多克隆抗淋巴细胞药物和霉酚酸酯抗 B 细胞增殖。关于治疗药物的构成还有许多悬而未决的问题,包括治疗时间和对临床预后的影响(包括 BOS 的风险)。

问题也依然存在,如患者在 AMR 的经典诊断方面的不一致和如何管理这些患者。例如,许多患者已被发现有循环 DSA,但缺乏明显的组织病理学改变或 C4d 染色,有或无移植肺功能不全。这是否是免疫抑制不足,导致 T 淋巴细胞和早期的同种抗体产生或别的细胞活化,目前还不清楚在。此外,针对自身上皮抗原 Kα-1 微管蛋白体液自身免疫与 BOS 发生相关,至少有一项研究表明,在抗 Kα-1 微管蛋白抗体 DSA 的发生表明,DSA 介导损伤可能增强[42,43]。更多的工作有待澄清这些复杂的相互作用、临床结局和潜在治疗疗效。

慢性移植肺功能不全

从历史上看,肺慢性排斥反应被认为是细胞免疫反应导致纤维增生,引起狭窄小气道阻塞,进一步导致移植肺功能不全。由于经纤维支气管镜活检诊断慢性排斥反应的病变特征的效率低[44],而临床阻塞性分级量表利用 1s 用力呼气量(FEV1)与最佳术后值至少 20%的差异可识别 BOS。BOS 被认为是一种阻塞性、不可逆的细支气管纤维化阻塞导致的肺功能不全。最近研究表明,不是所有 FEV1 下降都是 BOS,长期慢性移植肺功能不全(CLAD)已被提议作为一个总体名称,包含了 BOS 作为一种表型。其他两个新的表型包括中性粒细胞可逆性肺功能不全(NRAD)和限制性移植肺综合征(RAS),随后提出了不同的临床表现和治疗反应率。本节对此做一个概述。

BOS

CLAD 最常见的形式是 BOS,也是移植一年后死亡的主要原因。在肺移植后1~3年和3~5年,BOS作为主要死亡原因占到了26%和29.2%[2]。BOS也导致显著的致病率,减少HRQOL,导致肺移植费用增加。ISHLT注册报道,在移植后5年和10年,BOS发生率分别是48%和76%,而BOS在移植后第一年是9.6%[2]。

BOS被定义为一个持续的(>3周)从最佳基线FEV1下降,而没有其他可以解释的原因(如感染、急性排斥反应和气道狭窄、吻合口狭窄等)[45]。最佳基线被定义为移植后最少每3周一次检测两个最好的FEV1值的平均值。从基线下降至少20%定义为BOS,BOS渐进阶段定义为功能逐渐丧失(表106.2)。BOS的典型病理表现,如果有的话,包括:

• 黏膜下淋巴细胞性炎症和小气道上皮细胞的早期阶段破坏;

• 黏液样肉芽组织长入气道管腔,导致部分或完全梗阻,以及;

• 肉芽组织瘢痕性模式和由此产生的纤维化,最终阻塞气道管腔。

典型症状是非特异性的,包括呼吸困难、咳嗽、痰和运动能力受限。胸部CT显示支气管扩张,伴支气管周围增厚和空气潴留。RAS患者胸部CT通常表现为间质模糊、肺上叶纤维化、磨玻璃影和蜂窝肺。BOS最常见于移植后1.5~4年之间[46]。病程高度可变,可在起病和进展中不明显,渐进肺功能不全持续数月或数年下降,或可能导致突然而严重的下降,在几周之内[47]。最初的恶化和随后稳定在较低的水平也常有描述[47]。早发BOS和高级别BOS[2,3]起病往往提示生存不佳[46]。

BOS的发病机制复杂,涉及同种免疫与非免疫性机制,独立或联合。一般来说,BOS是同种免疫介导的移植物损伤。支持这篇定论的,之前已经讨论,是ACR与BOS的相关性。同样,如前面所讨论的,针对HLA的体液同种免疫与BOS发生也相关。过去十年中的许多工作也集中在自体免疫的作用而非同种免疫[42,48]。数据显示,在肺损伤过程中V型胶原抗原表位的暴露(如随着移植时的缺血再灌注损伤)和K-α1微管蛋白可导致自身免疫,进而导致移植肺损伤和BOS。许多正在进行的工作都集中在这一领域和潜在的干预措施。

大量证据证明BOS的其他危险因素似乎与非同种异体免疫相关,包括原发移植肺功能不全、胃食管反流病和各种感染,如巨细胞病毒(CMV)感染和社区获得性病毒感染(CARV)以及其他。而导致BOS发生的机制尚不明确,有认为这些事件导致高炎症状态,进而导致移植物损伤,而其他人认为有其他途径,包括损伤后异常愈合[49,50]。

原发性移植物功能不全(PGD)是BOS的一个风险因素,不同于急性排斥反应、淋巴细胞性支气管炎和社区获得性呼吸道病毒感染,并且这种风险因素直接关系到原发移植肺功能不全的严重程度[51]。Whitson等进行了回顾性分析,指出双肺移植受者出现3级PGD后长期生存较差,BOS的发生率较高,会发生更严重的肺功能受损[52]。PGD和BOS之间的联系被认为是氧化应激,减少一氧化氮的产生,而在缺血再灌注损伤上调了HLA Ⅱ类抗原。

某单中心研究表明胃食管反流病(GERD)在肺移植受者中的发生率高达73%[53]。大量证据表明,GERD与BOS的发病相关。早期手术(胃底折叠术)对肺移植后GERD可以免于发生BOS,比患者接受药物治疗要有优势[53,54]。很多工作仍希望进行一项随机临床试验。

巨细胞病毒感染一直被认为是BOS发生的一个危险因素[55]。虽然某个单中心研究[56]没有证实这一结

表106.2 闭塞性细支气管炎综合征的分类

	1993年的原始分类		2001年的目前分类
BOS 0	FEV_1>基线的80%	BOS 0	FEV_1>基线的90%且FEF_{25-75}>基线的75%
		BOS 0-p	FEV_1>基线的81%~90%和(或)FEF_{25-75}≤基线的75%
BOS 1	FEV_1>基线的66%~80%	BOS 1	FEV_1>基线的66%~80%
BOS 2	FEV_1>基线的51%~65%	BOS 2	FEV_1>基线的51%~65%
BOS 3	FEV_1<基线的50%	BOS 3	FEV_1<基线的50%

BOS,闭塞性细支气管炎综合征;FEF_{25-75},呼气中期流速;FEV_1,用力1s呼气量。

Modified from Estenne M, Maurer JR, Boehler A, et al. Bronchiolitis obliterans syndrome 2001: an update of the diagnostic criteria. J Heart Lung Transplant 2002; 21:297.

果,另一个单中心队列研究表明,移植后前 6 个月内发生巨细胞病毒性肺炎,明显增加了 BOS 的风险[57]。同样,在一个单中心报道中,CARV[58]、人类疱疹病毒 6 型[59]和肺炎衣原体[60]感染与 BOS 相关。在一项包含 161 例病例的单中心研究中,Valentine 等发现肺炎和革兰阳性菌、革兰阴性菌和真菌致病菌气道定植是慢性移植肺功能不全的独立决定因素[61]。此外,Weigt 等报道称,曲霉菌定植与 BOS 和 BOS 相关死亡率显著相关[62]。

到目前为止,BOS 没有行之有效的治疗方法。从历史上看,许多单中心研究中的药物和治疗方法进行了评估,但这些研究的结果由于样本量小,缺乏合适的对照组,将 FEV1 的稳定、FEV1 下降的速率降低(而不是改进)作为终点而被质疑,因为这些情况可以发生在 BOS 的自然病程中。治疗方法包括将环孢素替换为他克莫司的免疫抑制维持治疗,以及从硫唑嘌呤改为霉酚酸酯[63,64]。利用抗淋巴细胞药物、抗胸腺细胞药物或阿仑单抗(人源化 CD52 抗体)作为细胞治疗也被报道在部分患者有效[65,66]。

也许最有证据证明的方法是阿奇霉素、体外光照(ECP)和外科手术治疗 GERD 的患者。2003 年的一个小规模研究首次报道在 BOS 患者给予阿奇霉素治疗(250mg,每周 3 次)[67]。在这项研究中,6 例患者中有 5 例表现出显著的 FEV1 改善。大多数后续研究也提出一部分 BOS 患者对阿奇霉素有效,FEV1 得到改善,许多研究也表明,有效的患者支气管肺泡灌洗液(BALF)中存在中性粒细胞增多[68]。这导致了许多研究者认为,该群 BALF 中性粒细胞增多的患者是一种独特的 CLAD 表型,因此他们把这叫作中性粒细胞增多性可逆性移植肺功能不全(NRAD)。

ECP 是通过一个封闭静脉循环系统进行的,采集大约 700mL 的患者血液,并分离白细胞,随后加入 8-甲氧沙林(8-MOP)并给予紫外线照射[69]。8-MOP 结合于 DNA 碱基诱导淋巴细胞凋亡。ECP 是安全的,于 1998 年被美国食品药品监督局批准用于治疗皮肤 T 细胞淋巴瘤、急性和慢性移植物抗宿主病和各种其他疾病,包括心脏移植受者急性细胞性排斥反应[70,71]。确切的作用机制尚不明确,但已经表明,ECP 引起的免疫调节作用,可能是通过诱导调节性 T 淋巴细胞而发挥的[72]。第一例 ECP 成功用于肺移植后急性排斥反应的报告见于 1995 年[73]。从那时起,一些研究表明,ECP 在肺移植受者的难治性急性排斥反应或 BOS 均有疗效。然而,由于样本量小、没有与免疫抑制治疗的对照研究、随访时间短、费用和依赖静脉注射的原因,对于 ECP 的使用热情有限。近来,Greer 等发表了一系列 BOS 患者的回顾性研究,65 例患者中有 64 例尽管给予了阿奇霉素治疗依然恶化。中位随访时间为 503 天,这项研究表明,ECP 治疗对 54%的患者有效,并确定了三个亚组的 CLAD(限制性移植综合征、急进性和非中性粒细胞增多),这些亚组对 ECP 可能不太敏感[69]。这项研究有可能引发 ECP 作为新的治疗手段的热情。

最后,再次肝移植可以挽救 BOS 患者的生命,然而,再移植仍存在争议,因为供肺数量有限,生存率一般较低且移植后 BOS 发展更快[74]。

预防 BOS 的策略(以及其他形式的 CLAD)之前已经部分讨论过。鉴于急性排斥反应和 BOS 密切相关,监控策略包括使用监测性支气管镜和 TBBx,许多中心都采取这些措施,希望能预防并积极治疗急性排斥反应。目前没有明确的证据能表明监测性活检 TBBxs 对 BOS 的生存能产生影响。问题在于 TBBx 的采样误差[75]以及病理学家之间对 ACR 分级的认定[76]缺乏一致性,这导致急性排斥不能被明确诊断。在 ISHLT 注册处,诱导治疗的使用与更长的生存期相关,但数据未调整[2]。临床数据有限且不确定,需要进一步的多中心研究。ISHLT 数据[2]也表明,他克莫司的使用较环孢素在相关生存率方面有优势,之前讨论的随机研究数据也支持发生 BOS 或 ACR 的机会更小[32]。2011 年,Vos 等发表了肺移植患者出院后阿奇霉素预防治疗的随机试验[77]。2年后,阿奇霉素组的 BOS 发生率明显较安慰剂组低(12.5%对 44.2%,P=0.0017)。阿奇霉素组也表现出了更好的 FEV1,并降低 BALF 中性粒细胞。

中性粒细胞增多可逆性移植肺功能不全和限制性移植肺综合征

随着 Gerhardt 等[67]首次发表的 BOS 接受阿奇霉素治疗,大量研究证实了这一发现,虽然有些没有。一些患者没有治疗反应的原因在于最初并不清楚后来所发现的 BALF 中性粒细胞增多和 IL-8 水平高相关研究与阿奇霉素治疗之间的关系[69,78]。研究者总结对阿奇霉素有反应的病例的特点是 BALF 中中性粒细胞百分比高(>15%),CLAD(阻塞性生理特征)移植后早期发生,他们在阿奇霉素治疗 3~6 个月后至少有 10%的 FEV1

改善。这组似乎预示阿奇霉素治疗的良好预后。

限制性移植肺综合征被多伦多肺移植计划定义为肺移植受者FEV1持续下降(与最佳术后基线相比>20%)和限制性肺动力学模式[定义为总的肺容量比基线水平(TLC)下降大于10%][79]。这种模式在肺移植受者发生CLAD中有25%~30%可以观察到。BOS或NRAD患者的诊断是依靠肺功能检查和高分辨率胸部CT显示肺间质模糊、肺上叶纤维化、磨玻璃影和蜂窝肺[79]。RAS患者诊断后生存率低,来自比利时的一个研究表明中位生存期为8个月,多伦多的一个研究中位生存期为16个月(阻塞性BOS患者分别为35个月和46个月)[79,80]。迄今为止,RAS患者对阿奇霉素不应答则没有任何治疗方法被确认是有效的。一些研究者发现,一些患者首先表现为经典的阻塞性BOS表现(没有TLC改变),然后发展为RAS(TLC下降>10%)。需要进一步的研究来明确这种情况,包括更好地了解病理生理学。

感染

与所有实体器官移植受者一样,在第92章至第94章已经描述,肺移植受者由于免疫抑制治疗引起感染的风险增加。然而,普遍认为肺移植受者比大多数其他实体器官移植更容易感染。

因此,在这里具体提出肺移植受者感染的治疗方案。加剧感染风险的因素包括:需要较高水平的免疫抑制治疗、局部防御机制受损(淋巴引流受损、黏膜纤毛功能受损、咳嗽减少)和持续环境暴露,以及微生物经气管吸入。因此,感染仍然是肺移植术后发病和死亡的常见原因。的确,非巨细胞病毒感染(20%人死亡)是第一年报告死亡原因中仅次于移植肺衰竭的原因,是移植第一年之后死亡的常见原因,仅次于BOS[2]。细菌和病毒在肺移植术后感染中占主导地位,然而,真菌和分枝杆菌感染也有增加。机会性感染的预防,如巨细胞病毒、真菌、卡氏肺囊虫在临床实践中常见,预防可减少这些微生物感染的危险但仍有可能发生。

肺移植术后肺部感染的诊断有时相当棘手。症状和体征包括发热、呼吸急促、咳痰和低氧血症,难以区分急性排斥反应。同时痰培养和BAL培养阳性,活检不提示ACR,可高度提示或明确感染,很少有其他确定性检验和检查结果,综合考虑各项检查发现对指导治疗非常必要。Cylex免疫细胞功能测定方法(Immuno-Know;Cylex公司,哥伦比亚市,MD)的研发,可以全面评估实体器官受者的免疫功能,并有助于诊断感染或排斥反应。这一检测方法检测外周血T细胞受刺激后产生的ATP,与感染和肾、肝、心、小肠移植受者的排斥反应均有相关性[81]。非常低的ATP水平与感染相关,非常高的ATP水平和ACR相关,但这一测定方法仍不足以诊断感染或ACR并指导治疗[82,83]。

细菌感染

细菌感染,尤其是革兰阴性菌是肺移植术后肺部感染的最常见原因[84]。常见的革兰阴性细菌有绿脓杆菌、不动杆菌属、肠杆菌科、嗜麦芽窄食属和洋葱克雷白杆菌。移植前的气道定植需重视,尤其是囊性纤维化患者,因为它可能会导致术后并发症,如肺炎。关于定植细菌和洋葱伯克霍尔德菌的多药耐药性,需要高度警觉。洋葱伯克霍尔德菌以前被称为洋葱假单胞菌,包括9种不同的菌株。最近的研究表明,一种特异性的洋葱伯克霍尔德菌、基因型Ⅲ型洋葱伯克霍尔德菌,与移植后死亡率增加相关[85]。因此,许多肺移植方案将不会提供移植机会给洋葱伯克霍尔德菌定植的患者(最常见的是囊性纤维化)。绿脓杆菌在移植前期多重耐药不认为是死亡的危险因素[86]。但移植后假单胞菌的定植与BOS的高发病率相关,与无BOS生存也相关[87]。

病毒感染

巨细胞病毒感染在肺移植受者是最主要的病毒感染,并且是仅次于细菌感染的第二常见感染[88]。因此,肺移植方案中将预防巨细胞病毒作为一种常规。肺移植受者在病毒负荷高时巨细胞病毒感染风险增加,比其他器官移植更明显。缺乏积极的预防,据估计,肺移植受者巨细胞病毒发病率为38%~75%[89]。

CMV感染的危险因素包括供者和受者的感染状况,血清学阳性供者和阴性受者这种组合风险最高。根据Zuk等发表的研究,94.9%的中心对供者阳性和受者阴性的移植受者使用预防巨细胞病毒的措施[90]。关于预防的持续时间,2010年,国际移植协会的国际CMV共识小组指南建议CMV D+/R−的受者至少接受6个月的预防,CMV D+/R +以及D−/R+的受者接受3~6个月的预防[91]。在最近的一项多中心随机试验中,在巨细胞病毒感染的高风险肺移植患者扩展巨细胞病毒预防(12个月),巨细胞病毒发病率较预防3个月的患者显著降低[92]。

CMV 感染在移植 1 年以后死亡中占不到 1%，然而如先前所讨论的，巨细胞病毒感染似乎是 BOS 发病的一个危险因素[57]，进而可能导致 BOS 受者死亡率的增加。

除巨细胞病毒，许多其他病毒也越来越多地被确认，对肺移植受者的短期和长期预后有潜在的重要影响。我们之前讨论的社区获得性呼吸道病毒感染在肺移植受者中常见，并已被证明是一种常见的引起急性排斥反应和(或)BOS 的病原体[93]。移植前带状疱疹病毒暴露也很常见，潜伏病毒再激活引起带状疱疹，但很少有广泛皮肤或内脏受累。人类疱疹病毒 6 型(HHV-6)和人类疱疹病毒(HHV-7)的血清学阳性，在成人很常见，实体器官移植后病毒再激活也很常见[94]。肝移植受者 HHV-6 与急性和慢性排斥反应相关[95]。迄今为止的研究认为，在肺移植受者已经发现了 HHV-6 和间质性肺炎有相关性，却没有显示与急性排斥反应或 BOS 有关联[96,97]。

真菌感染

虽然细菌和病毒感染比较常见，真菌感染发生在 15%~35%的肺移植受者，与死亡率增高相关[98]。曲霉菌和念珠菌是肺移植术后真菌感染的主要原因，其中，念珠菌感染的发病率在下降。其他不常见的导致移植受者肺部感染的真菌病原体包括镰刀菌属、放线菌属和接合菌属。这些病原体的侵袭性感染，即使接受抗真菌治疗，依然导致 34%~78%的死亡率[99]。

肺移植受者 44%的侵袭性真菌感染是由于曲霉菌，肺移植受者在所有实体器官移植中发生侵袭性曲霉病(IA)的机会最高[100]。这也许是由于曲霉菌在环境中是普遍存在的，并通过呼吸道吸入。因此，许多注意力都集中在肺移植受者的曲霉菌感染。从气管支气管树分离到的曲霉菌在气管支气管炎合并气道吻合口感染、侵袭性或播散性肺疾病(如 IA)都可能是一种定植(不致病)。曲霉菌性气管支气管炎较以前已变得不太常见，通常平均在移植后 50 天发生[99,101]。并发症包括气道狭窄、吻合口裂开和出血。曲霉菌支气管炎的死亡率为 20%，如没有抗真菌治疗，进展到 IA 并导致死亡的风险很大。

IA 发生的平均时间比以前要更长，一般发生在移植后 500 天左右[102]。这种时间上的转变可能是由于移植后真菌预防的应用。侵袭性曲霉菌感染的危险因素包括移植前或后定植、单肺移植、巨细胞病毒感染、低丙种球蛋白血症、环境暴露、慢性排斥反应和免疫抑制状态[99]。IA 的治疗包括减少免疫抑制，以及根据 IDSA 2008 年曲霉菌治疗指南给予抗真菌治疗(伏立康唑是一线治疗)[102]。由于治疗的进步，IA 的死亡率已从以前的 81%下降到目前的 38%[98]。尽管缺乏证据，真菌感染预防是普遍实行的。在最近的一次世界范围的调查中，59%的肺移植方案认为，在移植后前 6 个月通常使用广谱抗真菌药物预防，这些药物 97%能靶向治疗曲霉菌。所使用的药物差异较大，有伏立康唑单药或联合吸入两性霉素。普遍认为需要制订抗真菌预防指南[103]。

恶性肿瘤

实体器官移植是恶性肿瘤的重要危险因素，在第 95 章已经讨论。发生恶性肿瘤的机制被认为是移植后慢性免疫抑制降低了免疫监视功能。恶性肿瘤在移植后第一年死亡率中占很小一部分，在移植第一年后，9.1%~15.9%的死亡是由于癌症的发生[2]。非黑色素瘤的皮肤癌症是最常见的恶性肿瘤，但移植后淋巴组织增生性疾病(PTLD)位居第二，是肺移植和心肺联合移植存活一年以后最常见的恶性肿瘤。

移植后淋巴组织增生性疾病

移植后淋巴组织增生性疾病(PTLD)被定义为实体器官移植与异基因造血干细胞移植后淋巴和(或)浆细胞增殖。PTLD 的发生是 Epstein Barr 病毒(EBV)介导的。由于对 T 细胞反应抑制的减少，EBV 诱导 B 细胞增殖，从而导致单纯的淋巴组织增生或非霍奇金淋巴瘤等侵袭性病变。PTLD 的一般特征已在 96 章描述。

发展 PTLD 的风险因素包括 T 细胞免疫抑制剂的强化、受者血清 EBV 的状况、原发巨细胞病毒感染、男性和老年受者[104]。根据 Kremer 等的一项单中心研究表明，PTLD 的发病率是 4.8%，且最近有下降[105]。作者认为 2000 年之前早期使用抗胸腺细胞球蛋白(ATG)可能与 PTLD 的发病率相关。

手术后第一年 PTLD 往往发生在移植物或纵隔淋巴结。晚期 PTLD 往往在胸腺以外，多有肠道受累。诊断 PTLD 多在肺移植后 22.5~40 个月[105-107]。

预防 PTLD 的重要因素包括识别高危 EB 病毒感染患者、对血清 EBV 转阳性或 EBV 负荷增高的患者常规监测 EBV 病毒量、抗病毒预防和减少免疫抑制。PTLD 的治疗包括减少免疫抑制、抗病毒、抗 CD20(利妥昔单抗),有时需联合化疗,如CHOP方案(环磷酰胺、阿霉素、长春新碱、泼尼松)。大肿块或腹部梗阻的患者,外科手术可以是一种治疗选择。抗CD20的报道在肺移植受者发生PTLD后,有66%的有效率[108]。据报道,抗CD20治疗具有类似的效果[109]。对于扩散性疾病,利妥者单抗治疗后临床进展以及非B细胞的PTLD患者,应选择CHOP方案进行化疗。利妥昔单抗联合化疗治疗PTLD的临床试验证明实体器官受者可以获得60%的临床缓解率,延长生存至平均6.6年[110]。

皮肤癌

皮肤癌约占器官移植受者发生恶性肿瘤的40%[111,112]。移植受者最常见的皮肤癌症为鳞状细胞癌、基底细胞癌、黑色素瘤和卡波西肉瘤。鳞状细胞癌和基底细胞癌的危险因素包括免疫抑制治疗的强度和持续时间、老年移植患者以及紫外线暴露和地理位置。虽然目前还不清楚某个特定的免疫抑制药物是否会促使受者发生恶性肿瘤,最近有研究表明,霉酚酸酯比硫唑嘌呤可能更少诱发皮肤癌发病[113]。在一项前瞻性随机对照试验[114]发现,西罗莫司可降低肾移植受者恶性肿瘤与非黑色素瘤皮肤癌的风险,而一些研究表明,环孢素和硫唑嘌呤在实体器官移植中使用有导致皮肤癌发生的倾向[115,116]。这些药物具有一定的致癌作用[117,118]。对于肺移植受者经常使用的其他药物,长时间使用伏立康唑已报道与肾移植和肺移植受者的非黑色素瘤皮肤癌发病有关[119,120]。移植受者皮肤癌的预防需要患者教育,并建议减少太阳照射。维A酸的预防作用一直没有定论。

其他医疗并发症

免疫抑制药物对其他脏器的毒性导致发病,在肺移植患者和其他实体器官移植患者中一样常见。常见的并发症包括高血压、肾功能不全、高脂血症、糖尿病和骨质疏松症。许多并发症在移植后第一年内发病,尽管随着时间的推移逐渐减少免疫抑制药物的使用,但累积患病率继续上升。ISHLT的数据表明,高血压的发病率在移植后第一年为52%,移植后存活5年以上的受者中上升到83%[2]。同样,糖尿病的发病率由移植后1年的26%增加到5年后的41%,高脂血症在移植后1年发病率为25%,5年后上升到58%。重要的是要管理这些医疗问题,这三个都是心血管疾病的主要危险因素。

肾功能不全可能是肺移植术后很棘手的问题,由于慢性肾脏疾病会对生活质量产生严重的负面影响,导致死亡率急剧上升[121]。根据ISHLT的数据,严重肾功能不全的发生率在移植5年后不高,需要透析或接受肾移植的在这一群体中占4%,15.5%的患者肌酐高于2.5mg/dL[2]。在移植后10年,存活的患者需要透析或肾移植的比例上升到14.4%[2]。一般来说,肺移植计划中试图采取肾脏保护措施,如增加钙拮抗剂和(或)转换为西罗莫司为主的免疫抑制方案。同样,移植后免疫抑制药物相关的骨质疏松症至少一部分相关,可导致骨折并影响生活质量[122]。

总结

受者和供者的选择、外科手术技术、免疫抑制方案和移植后护理的日益改善,使许多肺移植患者的生存和HRQOL获益。尽管有进步,显著的困难和挑战仍然存在。生存目前已经得到了极大改善,很大程度是依赖于移植后1年生存率的改善。后期患者死亡在很大程度上是由于慢性排斥反应和感染。此外,免疫抑制剂的使用导致感染、恶性肿瘤、高血压、高脂血症、肾功能不全、糖尿病和骨质疏松症很常见。更好地理解导致慢性肺移植损伤的机制,有更好的和更多的非侵入性方法来指导免疫抑制治疗,可以改善患者预后。

(韩威力 译 韩威力 校)

参考文献

1. Valapour M, Paulson K, Smith JM, et al. OPTN/SRTR 2011 Annual Data Report. American Journal of Transplantation. 2013;13(s1):149–177.
2. Christie JD, Edwards LB, Kucheryavaya AY, et al. The Registry of the International Society for Heart and Lung Transplantation: 29th adult lung and heart-lung transplant report-2012. Journal of Heart and Lung Transplantation. 2012; 31(10):1073–1086.
3. Thabut G, Christie JD, Kremers WK, et al. Survival differences following lung transplantation among US transplant centers. JAMA: Journal of the American Medical Association. 2010;304(1):53–60.
4. Meyer DM, Bennett LE, Novick RJ, et al. Single vs bilateral, sequential lung transplantation for end-stage emphysema: influence of recipient age on survival and secondary end-points. Journal of Heart and Lung Transplantation. 2001; 20(9):935–941.
5. Hadjiliadis D, Chaparro C, Gutierrez C, et al. Impact of lung transplant operation on bronchiolitis obliterans syndrome in patients with chronic obstructive pulmonary disease. American Journal of Transplantation. 2006;6(1):183–189.
6. Christie JD, Edwards LB, Kucheryavaya AY, et al. The Registry of the International Society for Heart and Lung Transplantation: twenty-eighth adult lung and heart-lung transplant report-2011. Journal of Heart and Lung Transplantation. 2011;30(10):1104–1122.
7. Thabut G, Christie JD, Ravaud P, et al. Survival after bilateral versus single-lung

transplantation for idiopathic pulmonary fibrosis. Annals of Internal Medicine. 2009;151(11):767–774.
8. Weiss ES, Allen JG, Merlo CA, et al. Survival after single versus bilateral lung transplantation for high-risk patients with pulmonary fibrosis. Annals of Thoracic Surgery. 2009;88(5):1616–1625, discussion 1625–1626.
9. Doyle RL, McCrory D, Channick RN, et al. Surgical treatments/interventions for pulmonary arterial hypertension: ACCP evidence-based clinical practice guidelines. Chest. 2004;126(1 Suppl):63S–71S.
10. Thabut G, Christie JD, Ravaud P, et al. Survival after bilateral versus single lung transplantation for patients with chronic obstructive pulmonary disease: a retrospective analysis of registry data. Lancet. 2008;371(9614):744–751.
11. Egan TM, Murray S, Bustami RT, et al. Development of the new lung allocation system in the United States. American Journal of Transplantation. 2006;6(5 Pt 2):1212–1227.
12. Orens JB, Estenne M, Arcasoy S, et al. International guidelines for the selection of lung transplant candidates: 2006 update-a consensus report from the Pulmonary Scientific Council of the International Society for Heart and Lung Transplantation. Journal of Heart and Lung Transplantation. 2006;25(7):745–755.
13. Iribarne A, Russo MJ, Davies RR, et al. Despite decreased wait-list times for lung transplantation, lung allocation scores continue to increase. Chest. 2009;135(4): 923–928.
14. Russo MJ, Iribarne A, Hong KN, et al. High lung allocation score is associated with increased morbidity and mortality following transplantation. Chest. 2010;137(3):651–657.
15. Liu V, Zamora MR, Dhillon GS, et al. Increasing lung allocation scores predict worsened survival among lung transplant recipients. American Journal of Transplantation. 2010;10(4):915–920.
16. Singer JP, Chen J, Blanc PD, et al. A thematic analysis of quality of life in lung transplant: the existing evidence and implications for future directions. American Journal of Transplantation. 2013;13:839–850.
17. DeVito Dabbs A, Hoffman LA, Iacono AT, et al. Are symptom reports useful for differentiating acute rejection and pulmonary infection after lung transplantation? Heart and Lung: Journal of Critical Care. 2004;33(6):372–380.
18. Ng YL, Paul N, Patsios D, et al. Imaging of lung transplantation: review. AJR. American Journal of Roentgenology. 2009;193(3):S1–S13.
19. Van Muylem A, Melot C, Antoine M, et al. Role of pulmonary function in the detection of allograft dysfunction after heart-lung transplantation. Thorax. 1997;52(7):643–647.
20. McManigle W, Pavlisko EN, Martinu T, et al. Acute cellular and antibody-mediated allograft rejection. Seminars in Respiratory and Critical Care Medicine. 2013;34:320–335.
21. Stewart S, Fishbein MC, Snell GI, et al. Revision of the 1996 working formulation for the standardization of nomenclature in the diagnosis of lung rejection. Journal of Heart and Lung Transplantation. 2007;26(12):1229–1242.
22. Gordon IO, Bhorade S, Vigneswaran WT, et al. SaLUTaRy: survey of lung transplant rejection. Journal of Heart and Lung Transplantation. 2012;31(9): 972–979.
23. Valentine VG, Taylor DE, Dhillon GS, et al. Success of lung transplant without surveillance bronchoscopy. Journal of Heart and Lung Transplantation. 2002; 21(3):319–326.
24. Glanville AR. Bronchoscopic monitoring after lung transplantation. Seminars in Respiratory and Critical Care Medicine. 2010;31(2):208–221.
25. Bando K, Paradis IL, Similo S, et al. Obliterative bronchiolitis after lung and heart-lung transplantation. An analysis of risk factors and management. Journal of Thoracic and Cardiovascular Surgery. 1995;110(1):4–13.
26. Sharples LD, McNeil K, Stewart S, et al. Risk factors for bronchiolitis obliterans: a systematic review of recent publications. Journal of Heart and Lung Transplantation. 2002;21(2):271–281.
27. Glanville AR, Aboyoun CL, Havryk A, et al. Severity of lymphocytic bronchiolitis predicts long-term outcome after lung transplantation. American Journal of Respiratory and Critical Care Medicine. 2008;177(9):1033–1040.
28. Hachem RR, Khalifah AP, Chakinala MM, et al. The significance of a single episode of minimal acute rejection after lung transplantation. Transplantation. 2005;80(10):1406–1413.
29. Greenland JR, Jones KD, Hays SR, et al. Association of large-airway lymphocytic bronchitis with bronchiolitis obliterans syndrome. American Journal of Respiratory and Critical Care Medicine. 2013;187(4):417–423.
30. Pelz M, Edwards LB, Jessen ME, et al. HLA mismatches influence lung transplant recipient survival, bronchiolitis obliterans and rejection: implications for donor lung allocation. Journal of Heart and Lung Transplantation. 2011;30(4): 426–434.
31. Opelz G, Susal C, Ruhenstroth A, et al. Impact of HLA compatibility on lung transplant survival and evidence for an HLA restriction phenomenon: a collaborative transplant study report. Transplantation. 2010;90(8):912–917.
32. Treede H, Glanville AR, Kleptko W, et al. European and Auatralian investigators in lung transplantation. Tacrolimus and cyclosporine have differential effects on the risk of development of bronchiolitis obliterans syndrome: results of a prospective, randomized international trial in lung transplantation. Journal of Heart and Lung Transplantation. 2012;31(8):797–804.
33. Hartwig MG, Appel JZ, Li B, et al. Chronis aspiration of gastric fluid accelerates pulmonary allograft dysfunction in a rat model of lung transplantation. Journal of Thoracic and Cardiovascular Surgery. 2006;131(1):209–217.
34. Fisichella PM, Davis CS, Lundberg PW, et al. The protective role of laproscopic antireflux surgery against aspiration of pepsin after lung transplantation. Surgery. 2011;150(4):598–606.
35. Lease ED, Zaas DW. Update in infectious complications following lung transplantation. Current Opinion in Pulmonary Medicine. 2011;17(3): 20609.
36. Korom S, Boehler A, Weder W. Immunosuppressive therapy in lung transplantation: state of the art. European Journal of Cardio-Thoracic Surgery. 2009;35(6): 1045–1055.
37. Reams BD, Musselwhite LW, Zaas DW, et al. Alemtuzumab in the treatment of refractory acute rejection and bronchiolitis obliterans syndrome after human lung transplantation. American Journal of Transplantation. 2007;7(12): 2802–2808.
38. Keenan RJ, Iacono A, Dauber JH, et al. Treatment of refractory acute allograft rejection with aerosolized cyclosporine in lung transplant recipients. Journal of Thoracic and Cardiovascular Surgery. 1997;113(2):335–340.
39. Valentine VG, Robbins RG, Wehner JH, et al. Total lymphoid irradiation for refractory acute rejection in heart-lung and lung allografts. Chest. 1996; 109(5):1184–1189.
40. Dall'Amico R, Murer L. Extracorporeal photochemotherapy: a new therapeutic approach for allograft rejection. Transfusion and Apheresis Science. 2002; 26(3):197–204.
41. Berry G, Burke M, Andersen C, et al. Pathology of pulmonary antibody-mediated rejection:2012 update from the Pathology Council of the ISHLT. Journal of Heart and Lung Transplantation. 2013;32(1):14–21.
42. Goers TA, Ramachandran S, Aloush A. De novo production of K-alpha1 tubulin-specific antibodies: role in chronic lung allograft rejection. Journal of Immunology. 2009;180(7):4487–4494.
43. Saini D, Weber J, Ramachandran S, et al. Alloimmunity-induced autoimmunity as a potential mechanism in the pathogenesis of chronic rejection of human lung allografts. Journal of Heart and Lung Transplantation. 2011;30(6):624–631.
44. Chamberlain D, Maurer JR, Chaparro C, et al. Evaluation of transbronchial biopsy specimens in the diagnosis of bronchiolitis obliterans after lung transplantation. Journal of Heart and Lung Transplantation. 1994;13(6):963–971.
45. Estenne M, Maurer JR, Boehler A, et al. Bronchiolitis obliterans syndrome 2001: an update of the diagnostic criteria. Journal of Heart and Lung Transplantation. 2002;21(3):297–310.
46. Finlen Copeland CA, Snyder LD, Zaas DW, et al. Survival after bronchiolitis obliterans syndrome among bilateral lung transplant recipients. American Journal of Respiratory and Critical Care Medicine. 2010;182(6):784–789.
47. Lama VN, Murray N, Lonigro RJ, et al. Course of FEV(1) after onset of bronchiolitis obliterans syndrome in lung transplant recipients. American Journal of Respiratory and Critical Care Medicine. 2007;175(11):1192–1198.
48. Sumpter TL, Wilkes DS. Role of autoimmunity in organ allograft rejection: a focus on immunity to type V collagen in the pathogenesis of lung transplant rejection. American Journal of Physiology. Lung Cellular and Molecular Physiology. 2004;286(6):L1129–L1139.
49. Shilling RA, Wilkes DS. Immunobiology of chronic lung allograft dysfunction: new insights from the bench and beyond. American Journal of Transplantation. 2009;9(8):1714–1718.
50. Snell GI, Westall GP. The contribution of airway ischemia and vascular remodelling to the pathophysiology of bronchiolitis obliterans syndrome and chronic lung allograft dysfunction. Current Opinion in Organ Transplantation. 2010; 15(5):558–562.
51. Daud SA, Yusen RD, Meyers BF, et al. Impact of immediate primary lung allograft dysfunction on bronchiolitis obliterans syndrome. American Journal of Respiratory and Critical Care Medicine. 2007;175(5):507–513.
52. Whitson BA, Prekker ME, Herrington CS, et al. Primary graft dysfunction and long-term pulmonary function after lung transplantation. Journal of Heart and Lung Transplantation. 2007;26(10):1004–1011.
53. Davis RD Jr, Lau CL, Eubanks S, et al. Improved lung allograft function after fundoplication in patients with gastroesophageal reflux disease undergoing lung transplantation. Journal of Thoracic and Cardiovascular Surgery. 2003;125(3): 533–542.
54. Bobadilla JL, Jankowska-Gan E, Xu Q, et al. Reflux-induced collagen type v sensitization: potential mediator of bronchiolitis obliterans syndrome. Chest. 2010;138(2):363–370.
55. Smith MA, Sundaresan S, Mohanakumar T, et al. Effect of development of anti-

bodies to HLA and cytomegalovirus mismatch on lung transplantation survival and development of bronchiolitis obliterans syndrome. Journal of Thoracic and Cardiovascular Surgery. 1998;116(5):812–820.
56. Tamm M, Aboyoun CL, Chhajed PN, et al. Treated cytomegalovirus pneumonia is not associated with bronchiolitis obliterans syndrome. American Journal of Respiratory and Critical Care Medicine. 2004;170(10):1120–1123.
57. Snyder LD, Finlen-Copeland CA, Turbyfill WJ, et al. Cytomegalovirus pneumonitis is a risk for bronchiolitis obliterans syndrome in lung transplantation. American Journal of Respiratory and Critical Care Medicine. 2010;181(12): 1391–1396.
58. Kumar D, Husain S, Chen MH, et al. A prospective molecular surveillance study evaluation the clinical impact of community-acquired respiratory viruses in lung transplant recipients. Transplantation. 2010;89(8):1028–1033.
59. Neurohr C, Huppman P, Leuchte H, et al. Human herpes 6 in bronchoalveolar lavage fluid after lung transplantation: a risk factor for bronchiolitis obliterans syndrome? American Journal of Transplantation. 2005;5(12):2982–2991.
60. Kotsimbos TC, Snell GI, Levvey B, et al. Chlamydia pneumonia serology in donors and recipients and the risk of bronchiolitis obliterans syndrome after lung transplantation. Transplantation. 2005;79(3):269–275.
61. Valentine VG, Gupta MR, Walker JE Jr, et al. Effect of etiology and timing of respiratory tract infections on development of bronchiolitis obliterans syndrome. Journal of Heart and Lung Transplantation. 2009;28(2):163–169.
62. Weigt SS, Elashoff RM, Huang C, et al. Aspergillus colonization of the lung allograft is a risk factor for bronchiolitis obliterans syndrome. American Journal of Transplantation. 2009;9(8):1903–1911.
63. Kesten S, Chaparro C, Scavuzzo M, et al. Tacrolimus as rescue therapy for bronchiolitis obliterans syndrome. Journal of Heart and Lung Transplantation. 1997;16(9):905–912.
64. Hayes D Jr. A review of bronchiolitis obliterans syndrome and therapeutic strategies. Journal of Cardiothoracic Surgery. 2011;6:92.
65. Kesten S, Rajagopalan N, Maurer J. Cytolytic therapy for treatment of bronchiolitis obliterans syndrome following lung transplantation. Transplantation. 1996;61(3):427–430.
66. Reams BD, Musselwhite LW, Zaas DW, et al. Alemtuzumab in the treatment of refractory acute rejection and bronchiolitis obliterans after human lung transplantation. American Journal of Transplantation. 2007;7(12):2802–2808.
67. Gerhardt SG, McDyer JF, Girgis RE, et al. Maintenance azithromycin therapy for bronchiolitis obliterans syndrome: results of a pilot study. American Journal of Respiratory and Critical Care Medicine. 2003;168(1):121–125.
68. Gottlieb J, Szangolies J, Koehnlein T, et al. Long-term azithromycin for bronchiolitis obliterans syndrome after lung transplantation. Transplantation. 2008; 85(1):36–41.
69. Greer M, Dierich M, De Wall C, et al. Phenotyping established chronic lung allograft dysfunction predicts extracorporeal photopheresis response in lung transplant patients. American Journal of Transplantation. 2013;13:911–918.
70. Rook AH, Cohen J. Therapeutic applications of photopheresis. Dermatologic Clinics. 1993;11(2):339.
71. Barr ML, Meiser BM, Eisen HJ, et al. Photopheresis for the prevention of rejection in cardiac transplantation. New England Journal of Medicine. 1998;339(24): 1744–1751.
72. George JF, Gooden CW, Guo L, et al. Role for CD4+CD25+ T cells in inhibition of graft rejection by extracorporeal photopheresis. Journal of Heart and Lung Transplantation. 2008;27(6):616–622.
73. Andreu G, Achkar A, Couetil J. Extracorporeal photochemotherapy treatment for acute lung rejection episode. Journal of Heart and Lung Transplantation. 1995;14(4):793–796.
74. Kawut SM, Lederer DJ, Keshavjee S, et al. Outcomes after lung retransplantation in the modern era. American Journal of Respiratory and Critical Care Medicine. 2008;177(1):114–120.
75. Scott JP, Smyth RL, Higenbottam T, et al. Transbronchial biopsy after lung transplantation. Journal of Thoracic and Cardiovascular Surgery. 1991;101(5): 935–937.
76. Arcasoy SM, Berry G, Marboe CC, et al. Pathologic interpretation of transbronchial biopsy for acute rejection of lung allograft is highly variable. American Journal of Transplantation. 2011;11(2):320–328.
77. Vos R, Vanaudenaerde BM, Verleden SE, et al. A randomised controlled trial of azithromycin to prevent chronic rejection after lung transplantation. The European Respiratory Journal. 2011;37(1):164–172.
78. Verleden GM, Vanaudenaerde BM, Dupont LJ, et al. Azithromycin reduces airway neutrophilia and interleukin-8 in patients with bronchiolitis obliterans syndrome. American Journal of Respiratory and Critical Care Medicine. 2006;174(5):566–570.
79. Sato M, Waddell TK, Wagnetz U, et al. Restrictive allograft syndrome (RAS): a novel form of chronic lung allograft dysfunction. Journal of Heart and Lung Transplantation. 2011;30(7):735–742.
80. Verleden GM, Vos R, Verleden SE, et al. Survival determinants in lung transplant patients with chronic allograft dysfunction. Transplantation. 2011;92(6): 703–708.
81. Kowalski RJ, Post DR, Mannon DR, et al. Assessing relative risks of infection and rejection: a meta-analysis using an immune function assay. Transplantation. 2006;82(5):663–668.
82. Husain S, Raza K, Pilewski JM, et al. Experience with immune monitoring in lung transplant recipients: correlation of low immune function with infection. Transplantation. 2009;87(12):1852–1857.
83. Shino MY, Weigt SS, Saggar R, et al. Usefulness of immune monitoring in lung transplantation using adenosine triphosphate production in activated lymphocytes. Journal of Heart and Lung Transplantation. 2012;31(9):996–1002.
84. Aguilar-Guisado M, Givalda J, Ussetti P, et al. Pneumonia after lung transplantation in the RESITRA Cohort: a multicenter prospective study. American Journal of Transplantation. 2007;7(8):1989–1996.
85. Alexander BD, Petzold EW, Reller LB, et al. Survival after lung transplantation of cystic fibrosis patients infected with Burkholderia cepacia complex. American Journal of Transplantation. 2008;8(5):1025–1030.
86. Aris RM, Gilligan PH, Neuringer IP, et al. The effects of panresistant bacteria in cystic fibrosis patients on lung transplant outcome. American Journal of Respiratory and Critical Care Medicine. 1997;155(5):1699–1704.
87. Botha P, Archer L, Anderson RL, et al. Pseudomonas aeruginosa colonization of the allograft after lung transplantation and the risk of bronchiolitis obliterans syndrome. Transplantation. 2008;85(5):771–774.
88. Zamora MR. Cytomegalovirus and lung transplantation. American Journal of Transplantation. 2004;4(8):1219–1226.
89. Alexander BD, Tapson VF. Infectious complications of lung transplantation. Transplant Infectious Disease. 2001;3(3):128–137.
90. Zuk DM, Humar A, Weinkauf JG, et al. An international survey of cytomegalovirus management practices in lung transplantation. Transplantation. 2010; 90(6):672–676.
91. Kotton CN, Kumar D, Caliendo AM, et al. International consensus guidelines on the management of cytomegalovirus in solid organ transplantation. Transplantation. 2010;89(7):779–795.
92. Palmer SM, Limaye AP, Banks M, et al. Extended valganciclovir prophylaxis to prevent cytomegalovirus after lung transplantation: a randomized, controlled trial. Annals of Internal Medicine. 2010;152(12):761–769.
93. Kumar D, Husain S, Chen MH, et al. A prospective molecular surveillance study evaluating the clinical impact of community-acquired respiratory viruses in lung transplant recipients. Transplantation. 2010;89(8):1028–1033.
94. Humar A, Asberg A, Kumar D, et al. An assessment of herpesvirus co-infections in patients with CMV disease: correlation with clinical and virologic outcomes. American Journal of Transplantation. 2009;9(2):374–381.
95. Humar A, Kumar D, Caliendo AM, et al. Clinical impact of human herpesvirus 6 infection after liver transplantation. Transplantation. 2002;73(4):599–604.
96. Costa C, Curtoni A, Bergallo M, et al. Quantitative detection of HHV-6 and HHV-7 in transbronchial biopsies from lung transplant recipients. New Microbiologica. 2011;34(3):275–280.
97. Manuel O, Kumar D, Moussa G, et al. Lack of association between betaherpesvirus infection and bronchiolitis obliterans syndrome in lung transplant recipients in the era of antiviral prophylaxis. Transplantation. 2009;87(5): 719–725.
98. Sole A, Salavert M. Fungal infections after lung transplantation. Current Opinion in Pulmonary Medicine. 2009;15(3):243–253.
99. Bhaskaran A, Hosseini-Moghaddam SM, Rotstein C, et al. Mold Infections in Lung Transplant Recipients. Seminars in Respiratory and Critical Care Medicine. 2013;34(3):371–379.
100. Pappas PG, Alexander BD, Andes DR, et al. Invasive fungal infections among organ transplant recipients: results of the Transplant-Associated Infection Surveillance Network (TRANSNET). Clinical Infectious Diseases. 2010;50(8): 1101–1111.
101. Singh N, Husain S. Aspergillus infections after lung transplantation: clinical differences in type of transplant and implications for management. Journal of Heart and Lung Transplantation. 2003;22(3):258–266.
102. Walsh TJ, Anaissie EJ, Denning DW, et al. Treatment of aspergillosis: clinical practice guidelines of the Infectious Diseases Society of America. Clinical Infectious Diseases : an Official Publication of the Infectious Diseases Society of America. 2008;46(3):327–360.
103. Neoh CF, Snell GI, Kotsimbos T, et al. Antifungal prophylaxis in lung transplantation—a world-wide survey. American Journal of Transplantation. 2011;11(2): 361–366.
104. Allen U, Preiksaitis J. Epstein-barr virus and posttransplant lymphoproliferative disorder in solid organ transplant recipients. American Journal of Transplantation. 2009;9(Suppl 4):S87–S96.
105. Kremer BE, Reshef R, Misleh JG, et al. Post-transplant lymphoproliferative dis-

order after lung transplantation: a review of 35 cases. Journal of Heart and Lung Transplantation. 2012;31(3):296–304.
106. Wudhikarn K, Holman CJ, Linan M, et al. Post-transplant lymphoproliferative disorders in lung transplant recipients: 20-yr experience at the University of Minnesota. Clinical Transplantation. 2011;25(5):705–713.
107. Baldanti F, Rognoni V, Cascina A, et al. Post-transplant lymphoproliferative disorders and Epstein-Barr virus DNAemia in a cohort of lung transplant recipients. Virology Journal. 2011;8:421.
108. Cook RC, Connors JM, Gascoyne RD, et al. Treatment of post-transplant lymphoproliferative disease with rituximab monoclonal antibody after lung transplantation. Lancet. 1999;354(9191):1698–1699.
109. Elstrom RL, Andreadis C, Aqui NA, et al. Treatment of PTLD with rituximab or chemotherapy. American Journal of Transplantation. 2006;6(3):569–576.
110. Trappe R, Oertel S, Leblond V, et al. Sequential treatment with rituximab followed by CHOP chemotherapy in adult B-cell post-transplant lymphoproliferative disorder (PTLD): the prospective international multicentre phase 2 PTLD-1 trial. Lancet Oncology. 2012;13(2):196–206.
111. Euvrard S, Kanitakis J, Claudy A. Skin cancers after organ transplantation. New England Journal of Medicine. 2003;348(17):1681–1691.
112. Greenberg JN, Zwald FO. Management of skin cancer in solid-organ transplant recipients: a multidisciplinary approach. Dermatologic Clinics. 2011;29(2): 231–241, ix.
113. Einollahi B, Nemati E, Lessan-Pezeshki M, et al. Skin cancer after renal transplantation: results of a multicenter study in Iran. Annals of Transplantation: Quarterly of the Polish Transplantation Society. 2010;15(3):44–50.
114. Salgo R, Gossmann J, Schofer H, et al. Switch to a sirolimus-based immunosuppression in long-term renal transplant recipients: reduced rate of (pre-)malignancies and nonmelanoma skin cancer in a prospective, randomized, assessor-blinded, controlled clinical trial. American Journal of Transplantation. 2010;10(6): 1385–1393.
115. Dantal J, Hourmant M, Cantarovich D, et al. Effect of long-term immunosuppression in kidney-graft recipients on cancer incidence: randomised comparison of two cyclosporin regimens. Lancet. 1998;351(9103):623–628.
116. Wisgerhof HC, Edelbroek JR, de Fijter JW, et al. Subsequent squamous- and basal-cell carcinomas in kidney-transplant recipients after the first skin cancer: cumulative incidence and risk factors. Transplantation. 2010;89(10):1231–1238.
117. O'Donovan P, Perrett CM, Zhang X, et al. Azathioprine and UVA light generate mutagenic oxidative DNA damage. Science. 2005;309(5742):1871–1874.
118. Wu X, Nguyen BC, Dziunycz P, et al. Opposing roles for calcineurin and ATF3 in squamous skin cancer. Nature. 2010;465(7296):368–372.
119. Vanacker A, Fabre G, Van Dorpe J, et al. Aggressive cutaneous squamous cell carcinoma associated with prolonged voriconazole therapy in a renal transplant patient. American Journal of Transplantation. 2008;8(4):877–880.
120. Zwald FO, Spratt M, Lemos BD, et al. Duration of voriconazole exposure: an independent risk factor for skin cancer after lung transplantation. Dermatologic Surgery. 2012;38(8):1369–1374.
121. Wehbe E, Brock R, Budev M, et al. Short-term and long-term outcomes of acute kidney injury after lung transplantation. Journal of Heart and Lung Transplantation. 2012;31(3):244–251.
122. Kulak CA, Cochenski BV, Kulak J, et al. Osteoporosis after solid organ transplantation. Minerva Endocrinologica. 2012;37(3):221–231.

第 107 章
胰腺移植长期预后

Philip Y. Wai, Hans W. Sollinger

引言

胰腺移植主要用于治疗那些未用外源性胰岛素仍有能力维持正常血糖的Ⅰ型糖尿病(T1D)患者。对于伴有晚期肾病的Ⅰ型糖尿病患者，胰肾联合移植(SPK)是最佳的长远治疗方法。成功的SPK术可使患者免于透析并能够重新维持血糖的正常调节。SPK术两个明显的缺点是手术并发症以及长期免疫抑制的副作用，这也大大限制了SPK术的潜在候选人数量。在过去的40多年里,胰腺移植术后早期和长期疗效都有显著改善[1-4]。手术技术的改良、免疫抑制的进展、术后临床护理的进步都有助于移植后疗效的改善和患者存活率的提高。

合适的资源分配对受者来说仍然是个挑战，因为必须考虑到个人的区域等待时间以及在患者需要同时移植肾脏和胰腺时，衡量纠正尿毒症和纠正糖尿病的利弊。活体肾脏捐赠带来了一个关键问题:有些患者是否最好先进行活体供肾移植(LDK),然后再行胰腺移植(PAK)。最近的研究对接受SPK术患者的病史数据进行了分析,这些长期的疗效分析提示,SPK术是糖尿病伴有尿毒症患者的最佳治疗方式。

在本章，我们描述了胰腺移植手术技术的演变，讨论分析了胰腺移植术远期疗效的数据、相关并发症、胰腺移植对继发性糖尿病并发症的影响,以及扩大捐赠库的新方法。手术技术我们在第60章已有详细的描述。最后,本章将为优化胰腺供体并提高患者生存给出目前的建议。关于识别和治疗胰腺排斥反应的附加信息,我们在第73章中有描述,关于胰腺移植候选人的标准和选择,以及胰岛移植,我们在第32章中有描述。

胰腺移植手术技术的演变

对胰腺移植术后长期疗效的充分论述必须要提到外科技术的演进。同种异体胰腺移植患者生存率的提高不仅得益于免疫抑制的改进，而且与手术者改良手术技术有关。1966年12月17日,Kelly等运用胰管节段移植方法为一名28岁的青年做了首例胰肾联合移植术[5]。继这次里程碑事件后,一系列胰腺移植方法得以开展,如全胰十二指肠伴或不伴脾脏移植、胰岛注射方法和十二指肠肠袢将外分泌胰液引流至泌尿系。这些移植方法都由于技术过于复杂或免疫排斥，未能提供长期良好的疗效或提高患者的生存率。胰腺移植术后1年,据报道移植物生存率为21%,1年患者死亡率为39%(国际胰腺移植登记处;1980)。

之前已描述过如何准备胰十二指肠异体移植物和手术移植的步骤[6-9]。在威斯康星大学,胰腺和肝脏在供体的分离基本上是由移植团队完成的(详见第21章和第22章腹部器官恢复过程的详细描述)。在这一技术过程中，胰腺与肝脏和异体移植物的分离是在低温的UW溶液中完成的连续过程 (ViaSpan,Bristol Myers Squibb,Garden City,NY)。当多个器官恢复团队在共同操作时，一般不会整体移除器官，而是在原位分离器官。胰腺的脉管和实质都很容易被损坏,所以必须保护好。在胰腺移植技术过程中,移植物的准备仍然是最关键的步骤。应仔细检查胰腺的脂肪含量、纤维化、胰腺实质的质地、胰腺血管的大小和质量,以及移植的供体血管是否有异常解剖[6,9]。脾切除术是通过分离胰尾和脾并选择性结扎远端的脾动脉远端和临近的脾静脉完成。十二指肠段缝合近端和远端切缘。应仔细分离肠系膜上动脉(SMA)和脾动脉周围的区域神经和淋巴组织。

小静脉分支的结扎可使门静脉延长，动脉的重建一般用髂血管 Y 形血管完成[6]。对于胰腺移植物和肠道异体移植物分开获取的情况，则需要保留近端 SMA 和肠系膜上静脉(SMV)向胰腺移植物胰头和十二指肠的分支和血供[9]。

胰腺经常植入右侧腹部，静脉与远端下腔静脉或髂总静脉吻合(图 107.1)。最近的报告不断证实，无论是门静脉或全身静脉回流技术，都无明显的生存优势[2,10]。不常规运用静脉延长移植，移植物的十二指肠部通常是向头侧。动脉的吻合也通常在近端右髂总动脉进行。膀胱引流技术在威斯康星大学得到了发展，但仍然只在某些中心进行。通常优先使用胰肠引流技术，距十二指肠悬韧带 20~60cm 处，将供者十二指肠段缝合至受者的空肠，采用双层手工缝制吻合技术。通过吻合左髂静脉和髂动脉，将肾脏移植到左髂窝。虽然作者的移植中心中，胰腺首先移植并没有增加血栓形成的概率，其他中心则报道了当需要多个手术团队参与及多个手术部位暴露时，首先行肾移植能够使胰腺血栓的风险降低[11]。对目前最大的胰腺移植库的分析显示，目前美国大多数中心从膀胱引流改为肠道引流，供者门静脉通常与受者体静脉吻合[2]。这些方法使过去的某些技术又得到了重新使用，如活体胰腺移植中的分段移植物使用[12]和门胃(供者空肠与受体胃的吻合)吻合[13]，这些技术一直在探索，但在美国中心不常规开展。

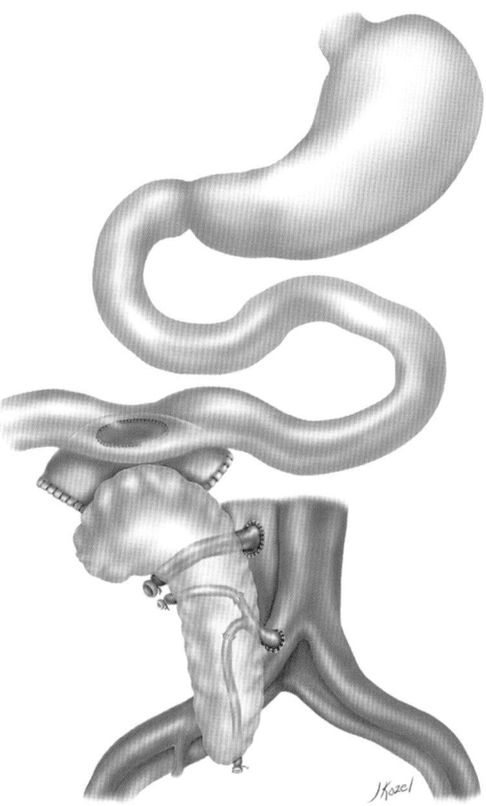

图 107.1 胰腺移植的肠引流技术。[Reprinted from [4] Sollinger HW, Odorico JS, Becker YT, D'Alessandro AM, Pirsch JD. One thousand simultaneous pancreas-kidney transplants at a single center with 22-year follow-up. Ann Surg 2009, 250 (4):618–630, with permission from Wolters Kluwer Health.]

胰腺移植后的远期疗效

10 多年前，Ojo 等就证明与单独肾移植或透析相比，胰腺移植能提高 I 型糖尿病患者及糖尿病肾病患者的生存率[14]。最近来自一些综合报道的数据描述了患者胰腺移植后目前的远期疗效(表 107.1)。

登记处和大型多中心数据

国际胰腺和胰岛移植登记处(IPITR)成立于 1980 年，位于明尼苏达大学，由 David E.R. Sutherland 教授指导，拥有所有关于胰腺移植在世界范围内最全面的数据库的报道(www.iptr.umn.edu)。对 18 159 例胰腺移植从 1978 年 7 月 25 日到 2005 年 12 月 31 日进行跨时代分析，证明过去 30 年里患者的短期和长期疗效有了很大改进。在美国，胰腺移植的数量从 1966—2005 年持续增长，自 2005 年后，数量就开始下降，最明显的是胰肾联合移植术 [1-3](图 107.2 和图 107.3)。最近 5 年、10 年和 20 年的胰肾移植物功能率分别为 80%、68%和 45%，肾移植后胰腺移植分别为 62%、46%和 16%，单独胰腺移植为 59%、39%和 12%[1-3](图 107.4 和图 107.5)。胰肾联合移植、肾移植后胰腺移植和单独胰腺移植移植后 5 年存活率分别是 87%、83%和 89%[2]。截至 2010 年 12 月，国际胰腺移植登记处共登记了 37 000 多例胰腺移植(25 000 例在美国，12 000 例在其他国家)[2]。分析过去 30 年的趋势，可以发现膀胱引流向肠道引流转换，免疫抑制治疗方案从环孢素/硫唑嘌呤方案向在接受的抗体 T 细胞诱导的基础上的他克莫司/霉酚酸酯方案转换。在胰腺的三个类别中，胰腺移植受体的年龄范围有了很大提高，应注重使用更年轻的捐赠者及缺血保存时间较短的器官，避免因早期技术操作问题及免疫抑制问题降低移植成功率[2]。

其他国家的胰腺移植案例并没有强制要求要去国

表 107.1 描述胰腺移植后的长期疗效的分析研究,来源于大型单中心分析、区域协作和注册表的数据

来源[参考文献]	来自国际胰腺移植登记处的最新数据分析[2]	18 159 例国际胰腺移植登记处胰腺移植的数据分析[1]	欧洲登记处[20,21]	全球最大系列的胰肾移植患者[4]	年度更新(www.srtr.org)器官获取和移植网	美国以外的其他国家的最全面的数据分析[15]	13个选中的欧洲国家的数据分析[19]	拉丁美洲最大的系列报道(巴西)[16]	欧洲最大系列报道的生存率结果(葡萄牙)[17]	欧洲最大系列报道的生存率结果(瑞典)[18]
登记处/合作单位/单中心	国际胰腺移植登记处(IPTR)	国际胰腺移植登记处	登记处	单中心(威斯康星大学)	器官获取和移植网络	登记处/合作单位	登记处/合作单位	合作单位	单中心	单中心

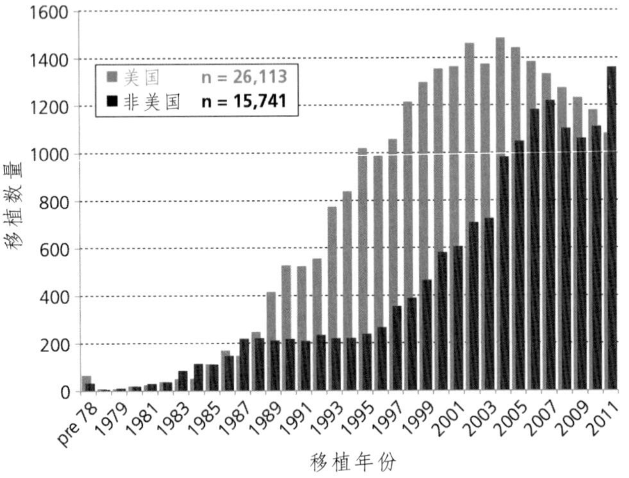

图 107.2 据 UNOS/IPTR 报道,美国和世界其他国家胰腺移植的年数据,1966 年—2013 年 6 月。(Reproduced with permission of Professor Angelika Gruessner.)

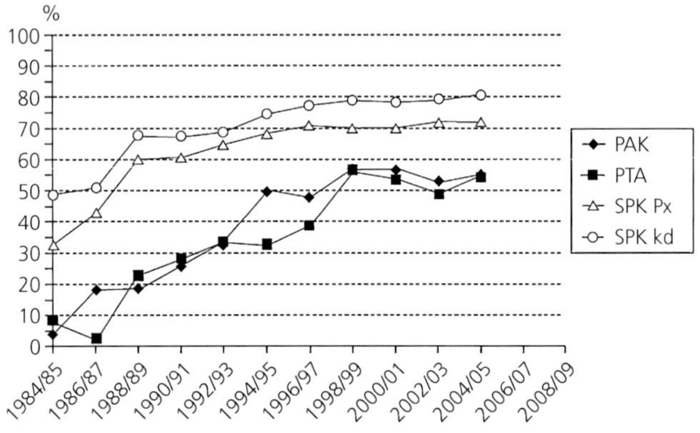

图 107.4 1985 年 1 月 1 日至 2005 年 12 月 31 日,胰腺和胰肾联合移植术后 5 年移植物功能研究。[Reprinted from [1] Gruessner AC, Sutherland DE, Gruessner RW: Long-term outcome after pancreas transplantation. Curr Opin Organ Transplant 2012, 17(1):100–105, with permission from Wolters Kluwer Health.]

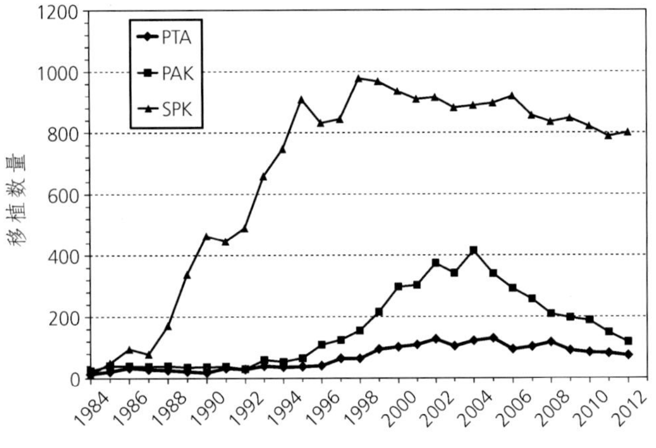

图 107.3 年度美国胰腺移植的主要接受者类别数量,1988—2012 年。(Reproduced with permission of Professor Angelika Gruessner.)

际胰腺移植登记处(IPTR)汇报,因此,IPTR 中其他国家胰腺移植的数据也往往不完整。其他国家的胰腺移植案例主要在多个公共系统和登记处有记录[2,15-18]。Perosa 及其同事全面地研究了美国以外的胰腺移植的案例。这 10 108 例移植大部分在欧洲进行(n=6766),其次是拉丁美洲(n=1945)、加拿大(n=671)、大洋洲(n=499)、亚洲(n=222)和非洲(n=5)[15](图 107.6)。这项研究还表明,之前国际胰腺移植登记处分析低估了美国以外的国家的胰腺移植数量[3],认为美国以外的胰腺移植的数量每年约 1100 例,而事实是在美国以外已有 10 000 多例胰腺移植[15]。有趣的是,Perosa 的研究时间段是美国以外的国家进行胰肾联合移植比例较高的时期,达到了 85%(与之前的 67%相比)[15,19]。在比较分析

13 个选中的欧洲国家和美国的胰腺移植数据后，发现胰腺移植率与尸体捐赠的概率不相关[19]。Perosa 等把这一现象用共同数据库来解释。这些登记处不会把移植物信息和患者的生存率情况详细记录。例如，欧洲国家器官储运组织负责奥地利、比利时、克罗地亚、德国、卢森堡、荷兰和斯洛文尼亚的器官分配[20]。这种国际性的合作包括所有的移植医院、组织分型实验室和捐赠者捐赠器官的医院。欧洲国家器官储运组织的有效数据包括胰腺移植的捐赠者名单、胰腺移植的类型和等待列表信息，但长期疗效及器官移植的结果未被报道。同样，位于法国斯特拉斯堡的欧洲委员会也有不同的关注点，如维护人权、保持社会公正和文化认同，它们也收集和发布年度时事通讯，其中包含在欧盟(EU)完成的胰腺移植数量。2010 年，在欧盟(27 个国家)报道了 769 例胰腺移植，同期有 9206 名尸体供者[21]。相比之下，欧洲的一家中心分析它们的长期疗效数据，发表了 10 年胰肾联合移植术后，患者、肾脏和胰腺异体移植物的生存率分别为 94%、62%和 69%，这与国际胰腺移植登记处的记录相似[17,18]。

在拉丁美洲，最近有一项对 500 例胰腺移植的研究，这也是来自这个洲的最大的系列报道。胰肾联合移植、肾移植后的胰腺移植和单独胰腺移植的患者一年生存率分别为 82%、93%和 95%。移植后的胰腺移植物 1 年生存率分别为 70%、86%和 77%[16]。有趣的是，胰肾联合移植术后的患者生存率更低。这些学者认为，这一趋势反映了社会经济贫困地区的受者的生存率，因为在这些地区，为了更多的开展移植，领导和中心会扩大捐助者和受者的选择标准[16]。

胰肾联合移植(SPK)

对于那些 1 型糖尿病和终末期肾病的患者，其治疗选择包括透析、尸体捐献肾移植、活体捐献肾移植、胰肾联合移植，以及在尸体或活体供体肾移植后再胰腺移植。若患者没有进行肾移植而仅凭透析维持，其死亡率会很高，10 年生存率仅为 9.6%~11.2%(数据来自 USRDS，10 年生存率：血液透析患者)。

长期随访的累积研究显示，SPK 移植对于 1 型糖尿病和糖尿病性肾病的患者，相比较尸体捐献肾移植和活体捐献肾移植，可提高其生存率，是最佳的治疗方法[2-4]。根据 IPTR 2010 年的数据，在美国，SPK 移植的例数占所有胰腺移植的 72%[2]。分析显示，PTA 等待时间的中位数是 110 天，而 SPK 等待时间是 243 天[2]。SPK 移植患者中肠道引流占 91%。此外，在术后第 1 年，胰腺移植物功能从 1987—1993 年的 77.2%提高至 2006—2010 年的 85.5%。SPK 移植术后，5 年移植胰腺和肾移植物存活率分别为 72%和 80%，这些数据自 1996 年以来未再有明显提高[1]。SPK 受者 5 年存活率可达到 87%[2,4]。

在威斯康星大学，从 1985 年开始，我们就致力于研究 SPK 移植。最近我们报道了 1000 名 SPK 患者移植术后 22 年的随访记录[4]。在这份目前全球最大的SPK 研究数据中，我们发现 SPK 移植患者的 5 年、10 年和 20 年生存率分别为 89%、80%和 58%[2]。而且我们观察到，SPK 移植患者的生存率比接受活体捐献肾移植的糖尿病尿毒症患者(图 107.7)的生存率还高，这与以前报道中的一些数据不符。在 Young 等的一篇研究中[22]，接受活体捐献肾移植的患者 1 年生存率比 SPK 要高(97%对 95%)，然而 6 年的生存率，仍是 SPK 高(85%对 80%)[23-25]。其他研究也显示 SPK 在生存率上有优势，且对于控制血糖是更为持久而有效的治疗方法。胰腺移植对于移植肾和患者都能发挥一个好的保护作用，这一概念并不新颖，Kleinclaus 等早前就证明 PAK 患者的肾功能比单独做活体捐献肾移植的要好[26]。总之，这些数据显示改善代谢可能带来一种纠正尿毒症的生存优势。然而，诸多研究的累积数据证明，其对于糖尿病性视网膜病变、心脏恶化和 SPK 后血管疾病等次要并发症进展的作用是有限的[27-29]。因此，这些观察结果背后的潜在致病因素仍未确定。

SPK 移植带来的生存优势依赖于技术上成功的胰腺移植。由于早期移植物衰竭与患者和移植肾的存活率相关，因此移植物 1 年内功能保留率是一个重要的因素[24,30]。仔细选择适当的接受者和匹配捐献器官对于 SPK 仍然至关重要。此外，影响患者和胰腺生存率的因素包括捐献者肥胖[31]、接受者肥胖(BMI>30kg/m^2)[32]、年老的捐献者(>45 岁)[33]以及年老的接受者(>50 岁)[34,35]。然而，最近的研究表明，如果在明智而审慎地考虑后选择年老的接受者、肥胖的捐献者和肥胖的接受者，其结果还是可以接受的[36-39]。

移植物和患者生存率的提高也导致了肾脏移植物或胰腺移植物功能衰竭的病例数增加。近期的一项分析检测了初期 SPK 后再次肾移植患者的移植胰腺的存活率[40]。其结果是，在 1 年、5 年和 10 年时胰腺的存活

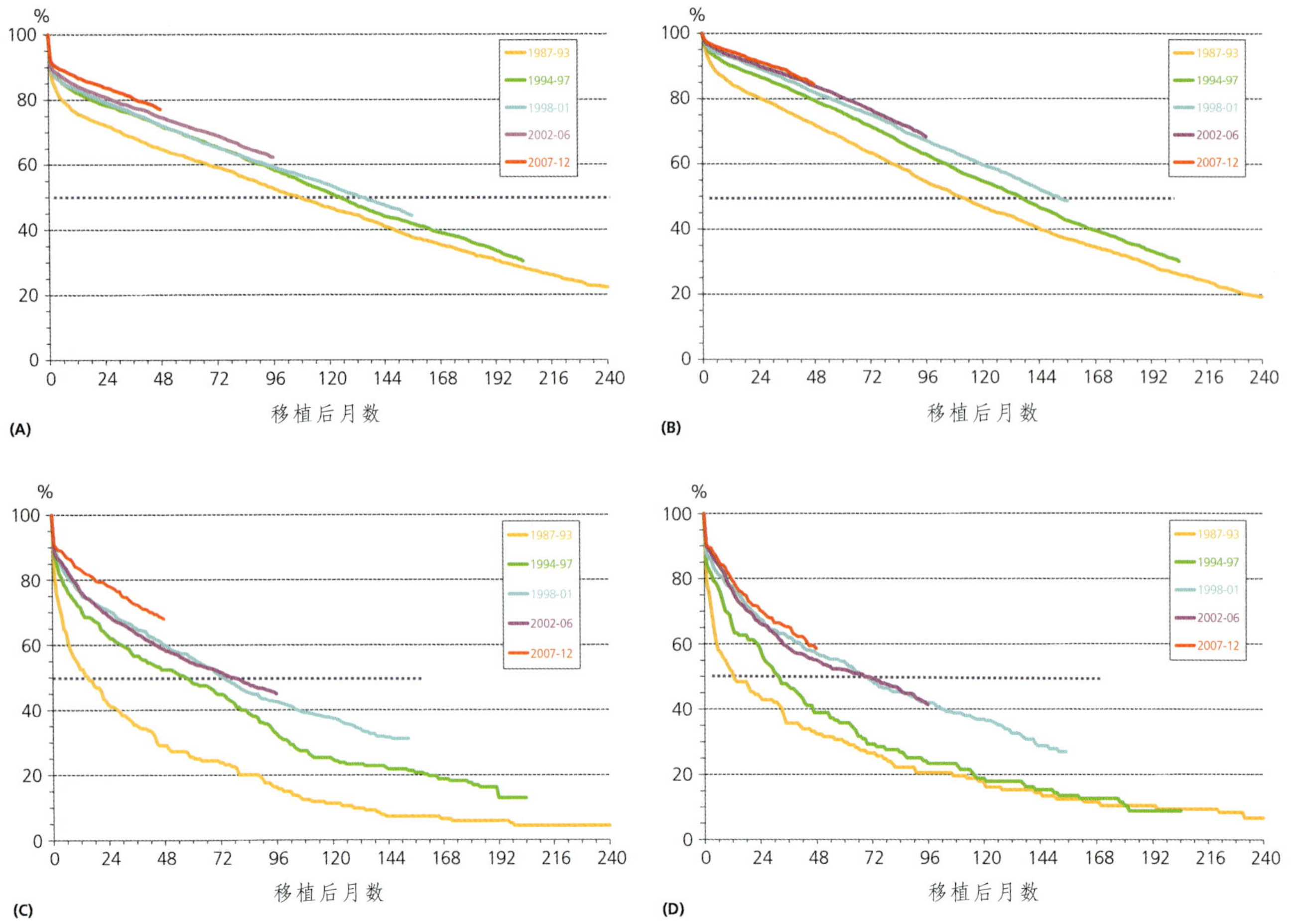

图 107.5 在 5 个阶段中，主要为尸体捐献移植物功能。胰肾联合移植（SPK）的胰腺移植物（A）；SPK 肾移植物（B）；肾移植后胰腺（PAK）移植物（C）；和单独胰腺移植（PTA）的胰腺移植物（D）。

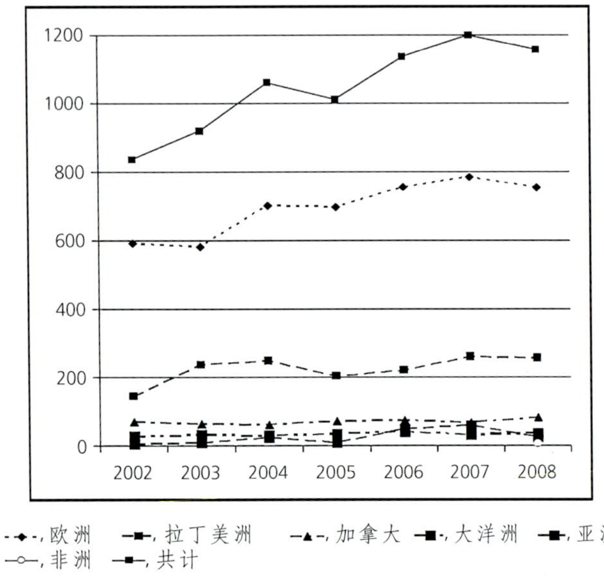

图 107.6 1 型糖尿病患者生存率。[Reprinted from [4] Sollinger HW, Odorico JS, Becker YT, D'Alessandro AM, Pirsch JD. One thousand simultaneous pancreas-kidney transplants at a single center with 22-year follow-up. Ann Surg 2009, 250 (4):618-630, with permission from Wolters Kluwer Health.]

率分别为 78%、49%和 40%。这意味着尽管移植胰腺存在一定风险（20%~25%的患者可能会有移植胰腺衰竭），考虑到再次透析的风险和再次肾移植的成功，应建议合适的患者再次移植。初次 SPK 后再次 SPK 的概念已经被提出了[41]。在再次移植之前或移植时，大部分患者采取了肾切除（89%）或胰切除（78%）[41]。

肾移植后胰腺移植

那些接受活体供肾的糖尿病终末期肾病患者将可能减少或避免透析。从务实的角度讲，这些活体器官移植也减少了对尸体供肾的需求。分配规则和地理原因导致时间等待，也限制了 SPK 移植，使得活体供肾移植后胰腺移植成为部分患者的首要选择[42]。分配到可用的移植胰腺和肾脏概率的差异，对于考虑患者是等待 SPK 还是 PAK 至关重要。具体关于器官分配策略的讨论见第 137 章。此外，另一个重要的考虑点是 PAK 和 SPK 移植的移植胰腺在长期存活率上的差异。尽管差

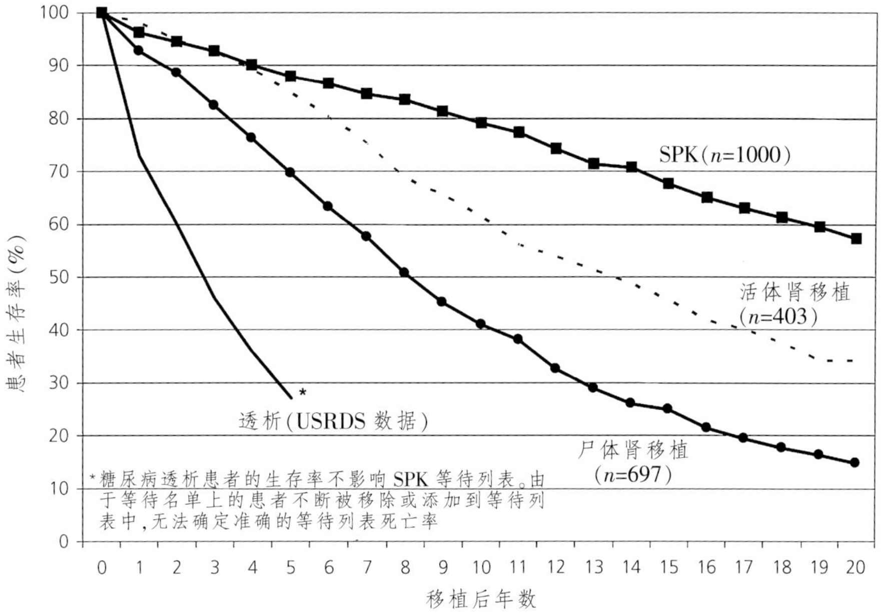

图 107.7 非美国地区每年胰腺移植数目。(Reprinted from[15] Perosa M, Boggi U, Cantarovich D, Robertson P: Pancreas transplantation outside the USA: an update. Curr Opin Organ Transplant 2011, with permission from Wolters Kluwer Health.)

距在缩小,PAK 的移植胰腺存活率仍不如 SPK 的移植物存活率(80%对 86%)[2,25,34,43]。结果的差异可部分归因于较高的排斥率和免疫因素增加的移植物 3 年失功率,PAK 与 SPK 的移植物失功率分别为 14%和 5%[34]。

肾移植受者考虑后续胰腺移植往往是个极具挑战性的决定,许多文献也关注到了后续胰腺移植对肾脏移植物的影响。累积证据表明,PAK 时的心血管危险分层和仔细评估肾移植功能,对于合适的候选人的 PAK 移植成功是两项重要的考虑。PAK 后移植肾结果不佳,可能与外科手术风险、接受者并发症的发生、免疫事件和药物引起的肾毒性等有关[44]。通过对前瞻性、随机化和控制方法的严格分析并考虑了固有的选择性偏差后,比较了 PAK 患者的移植肾结果和仅做肾移植的糖尿病患者的移植肾结果,发现它们并不一样,并不是所有的肾移植患者都适合 PAK。因此,许多现有研究并没有提供一个"公平"的评估结果。然而,Browne 等最近根据 PAK 倾向得分并利用多变量模型中的时间依赖和时间变量[42],通过调整他们的分析而不是如先前的研究那般仅局限于对 PAK 等待列表上的患者的分析[43,45,46]。他们的结果表明,相比于仅做肾移植的患者,PAK 接受者的移植肾衰竭风险在前 2 周内更高,在 143 天时相等,在 366 天后则相反,PAK 接受者在长期肾存活率上有更显著的提高[42]。这些发现证实了如之前报道的那样,胰腺移植术后围术期死亡的风险增加[47],也强调了选择合适 PAK 患者的重要性。更重要的是,Browne 等也证明 69%的 10 年期移植肾存活率,以及肾功能可被长期保留。他们认为,PAK 代表了一种安全、可行的方法。这份报告的结论,结合之前的关于 126 名 PAK 患者的研究,警示那些肾小球滤过率(GFR) <45mL/min,肾移植后再胰腺移植的时间间隔大于 1 年,PAK 前有肾脏排斥和蛋白尿的患者,不适合做肾移植后胰腺移植[44]。这两项研究都显示,PAK 患者降低的 GFR 值[<40mL/(min·1.73m^2)或<45mL/(min·1.73m^2)]与其移植肾之后的衰竭有关。尽管在 Browne 的研究中,这种效应在胰腺移植 3 年后才突显出来。想要准确地分析移植结果,需要足够的长期随访数据,虽然这是一项回顾性研究,在已报道的文献中,我们近 20 年的随访分析数据是独一无二的。Poommipanit 等报道的最近研究结果表明,活体肾移植后胰腺移植(PALK)相比 SPK,可提高患者生存率[43]。数据中的生存率都是移植后 5 年的随访记录分析结果。作者认为,主要差异在于移植早期的 3 个月和 12 个月生存率分别为 2.3%和 3.7%。在那些 12 个月时仍有肾功能的 PALK 和 SPK 患者中,研究未发现在后续 4 年中他们有显著的生存率上的区别。若以胰腺移植时间为开始日期,PALK 和 SPK 患者的生存率也无区别[43]。报道的 1 年内生存率差异很小(PALK 对 SPK 为 99.24%对 95.55%),这在很大程度上反映了 LDK 赋予的早期优势。在我们的研究

中，也发现对于1型糖尿病而言，SPK与LDK的生存率在移植早期也是有小的差异的[4]。然而，主要区别在移植后5年才体现出来，10年后生存率差异超过20%(图107.7)。20年的纵向随访系列提供了重要的长期分析，弥补了短期随访研究上的不足。PAK后肾脏或胰腺的排斥增加了肾脏和胰腺同种异体移植物的衰竭和患者的死亡[44]。有趣的是，肾脏和胰腺移植的间隔之间的关系和其后的肾移植物衰竭[44]在其他研究中并未被观察到[42,48]。总之，这些数据表明，对于不适合SPK的患者或已在做透析的患者，PAK移植手术的死亡率和随后的肾移植失败的风险在当前的时代可能相对较小，这也使活体肾移植后胰腺移植成为一个安全的替代考虑(表107.2)[49]。如果SPK可用作初步的治疗方式且患者还未开始透析，患有肾病的1型糖尿病患者适合的治疗选择则是SPK移植。

PTA

对于PTA是否可提高未发现糖尿病性肾病的1型糖尿病患者长期生存率和改善继发性并发症，这一观点仍有争议。成功的PTA在很大程度上可改善生活质量，但大量研究并未证实它能否提高生存率。PTA的应用局限于部分患者：

(1)有较长的严重的代谢并发症病史(低血糖未察觉、高血糖、酮症酸中毒)，需要就医；

(2)常规胰岛素治疗不佳[50]。

从免疫学的角度看，在三种胰腺移植类别中，PTA风险最高，其移植物1年衰竭率为6.0%，而PAK和SPK分别为3.7%和1.8%[2]。在最近的研究报告中，PTA后患者5年生存率为90%~98%[51]，移植物5年存活率为73%~89%[1,52]，半数移植物存活时间为9年[53]。与等待名单上的患者相比[46,47,54]，PTA患者并没有明确的生存优势，且糖尿病微血管并发症的改善也并不是基于前瞻性随机研究[55]。有趣的是，Boggi及其同事最近报告，PTA移植前后糖化血红蛋白和脂质水平明显降低了[52]。然而，由于没有未移植仅胰岛素治疗组的患者和未纳入PTA候选人组的患者[52]，所以没有适当的对照。更重要的是，钙调磷酸酶抑制剂(CI)和其他肾毒性药物可能潜在地有害影响PTA带来的血糖控制。不同的研究结果显示接受PTA治疗后，GFR降低值≥40mL/(min·1.73m^2)的患者中有32%表现出了肾毒性，高达9.9%的患者需要肾移植[56]。一群患者接受单独胰腺移植(PTA和PAK两种)，移植后肾衰竭需要透析或肾移植的速率为8%[45]。常规活检的数据也证实了他克莫司和环孢素对肾脏的副作用[57,58]。

胰腺移植后的并发症

胰腺移植后的早期技术障碍

IPTR对技术性并发症的定义包括移植物血栓形成、胰腺炎、吻合部泄漏、感染和出血[3]。在胰腺移植后前6个月内的移植失败事件中，技术性并发症的原因占了约50%[59]。在最近一份关于6282名SPK接受者的分析中，早期胰腺移植失败与随后的肾移植和患者生存率降低有关[60]。预防早期移植失败涉及受体选择的标准化和术后药物预防方案[61]。SPKT后总体并发症的发生率很高(图107.8)[4]，但多年来由于免疫抑制的改善和移植后管理的改进，已经极大地减少了总体并发

表107.2 糖尿病性肾病移植选择的利弊

	优点	缺点
活体供体单独肾移植(LDKA)	1.大大减少透析等待时间	1.血糖不能控制到正常范围
	2.降低早期并发症发生率和死亡率	2.生存率不如SPK患者
SPK	1.血糖可正常调节	1.早期并发症发生率和死亡率比肾移植的高
	2.质量高，减少了供体肾移植次数	2.早期胰腺衰竭(<1年)，预后比LDKA差
活体供体肾移植后胰腺移植	1.血糖可正常调节	1.要两次手术，胰腺移植后术后并发症发生率增加
		2.肾移植存在潜在风险

(Adapted from [49] Wiseman AC: Pancreas transplant options for patients with type 1 diabetes mellitus and chronic kidney disease: simultaneous pancreas kidney or pancreas after kidney? Curr Opin Organ Transplant 2012, 17 (1):80-86 with permission from Wolters Kluwer Health)

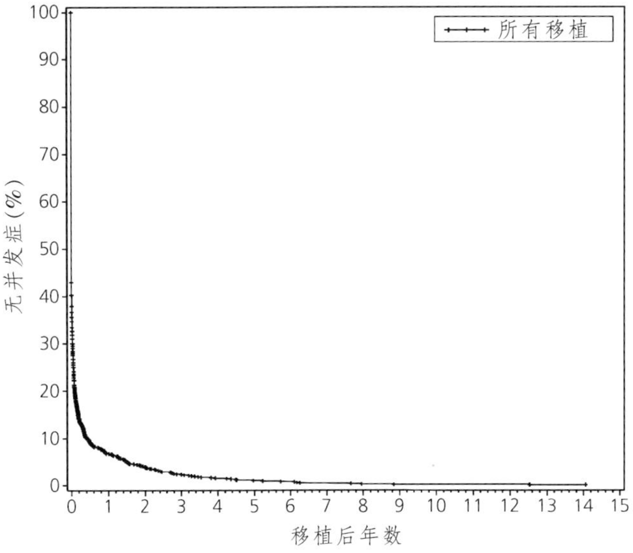

图 107.8 1985—2007 年 SPK 移植后总体并发症情况。(Reprinted from [4] Sollinger HW, Odorico JS, Becker YT, D'Alessandro AM, Pirsch JD. One thousand simultaneous pancreas-kidney transplants at a single center with 22-year follow-up. Ann Surg 2009, 250 (4):618-630, with permission from Wolters Kluwer Health.)

症。给予患者细致的护理以避免早期并发症是获得长期移植生存的关键，避免早期再手术也与改良预后直接相关[62]。早期技术性并发症的患者仍可行胰腺再移植。这些患者的胰腺移植生存、长期生存、急性排斥反应率和初次 SPK 患者也无差异[63]。

出血

移植后再次手术最常见的原因是术后出血。与移植物血栓形成不同，术后出血通常并不导致胰腺移植的移植物衰竭(< 0.3%)[3]。胰腺移植后，出血可发生在腹腔内、胃肠道或膀胱引流患者的膀胱内。围术期抗凝和腹腔出血关系密切[64]。腹腔血肿的临床处理包括停止抗凝治疗，纠正任何潜在的或持续的凝血障碍，如果血流动力学不稳定或有血肿继发感染的潜在来源，则是再次开腹的指征。胰腺移植后早期消化道出血往往源于十二指肠-空肠吻合术[64,65]。晚期出血往往是由于胃炎、胃或十二指肠溃疡、结肠炎、主动脉-肠瘘和细菌性动脉瘤[64,66]。晚期出血通常需要干预，它代表了一个重要的疾病事件。主动脉-肠瘘或假动脉瘤的发生可能会成为影响移植可行性和患者生存的一个潜在危险因素，往往高度提示可能需要介入或手术干预[66]。

血栓形成

胰腺移植后可能会发生动脉和静脉血栓形成，且静脉血栓更为常见，为动脉的 2 倍[67]。血栓事件可分为早期或晚期，部分或完全。早期溶栓可抢救移植物，但完全的静脉或动脉闭塞往往会导致同种异体移植物衰竭，常需要胰腺切除[66]。许多中心移植后使用了某种形式的抗凝，如阿司匹林、普通肝素或低分子肝素等，但华法林应用较少[66,67]。对于胰腺移植后血栓形成，通过避免使用肝素或右旋糖酐来系统性抗凝，可使那些出血量大、需要再次手术的风险比率维持在较低值(< 1%)[68]。因此我们研究中的血栓形成率比其他研究报道(10%~20%)都低[69-71]。根据来自 IPTR 的数据，在过去的几十年里，胰腺移植后血栓形成的发病率似乎相当一致(4%~8%)[1]。这些注册表数据也表明，相比 PAK 或 PTA，SPK 接受者胰腺移植后血栓形成较少[3]。这可能部分是由于 SPK 患者尿毒症的抗凝效果和较低的免疫排斥率[67]。其他组织，包括 Troppmann 等，曾发现血栓形成的危险因素，包括供者年龄、供者心脑血管方面的死亡原因、使用主动脉 Carrel 补片、使用脾动脉吻合肠系膜上动脉做胰腺移植后动脉重建、在脾动脉和肠系膜上动脉间架桥、门静脉延长架桥、移植到受者腹腔左侧以及移植物胰腺炎[69]。最近的数据也表明，组氨酸-色氨酸-酮戊二酸(HTK)液的使用与血栓形成率增加有关，特别是在冷保存超过 12h[72]。移植后早期血管血栓形成的原因是多因素的，但超出两周后血栓形成主要是由于炎症和急性排斥反应[67]。门静脉血栓是否有症状也很关键，意外发现的局部血栓形成也可以采用系统性抗凝[73]。成功的非手术治疗的共同因素包括无症状和侧支回流的存在[74]。我们在研究中也认为不使用静脉移植来延长门静脉对于降低胰腺移植血栓的形成风险至关重要，其他中心研究也支持这一做法[69]。根据长期的经验，移植物血栓形成而导致移植物衰竭非常罕见。在各项研究中，只有不到 3.6%的胰腺移植接受者的移植物衰竭是由血栓引起的[75]。这一发生率已经低于其他报道(3%~17%)[3,71,76]。当然，一旦发生血栓形成，移植物衰竭的发生风险就会很高。尽管早期的开腹手术探查可能是阴性的(43%)，但及时的手术探查可以抢救 45%的血栓形成患者[77]。

吻合口瘘

吻合口瘘仅占导致移植物失败事件原因的不足0.5%[1,3]。相比肠内引流的SPK患者(ED-SPK)(胰肠吻合术,5.7%)[4],膀胱引流的SPK患者(BD-SPK)吻合口瘘的发生率更高(胰腺膀胱引流,22.8%)。ED胰腺移植后出现吻合口漏的患者会有肠内容物流出及腹膜炎的潜在危险,而BD引流吻合口漏常常风险较小。血清淀粉酶和脂肪酶水平的升高,多因腹膜吸收肠液所致,可作为提示肠瘘的早期指标。鉴于免疫抑制药物的影响,虽然肠内容物流入腹部,腹膜反应可能不明显。对于ED-SPK患者,采用Roux-en-Y形吻合的手术方式较多,且这种手术修补方式也更容易成功。在BD-SPK患者中,手术修补却不那么容易,而且有时引流也会导致瘘口阻塞。如果脓毒症持续存在,则要考虑胰切除。

心血管并发症

SPK患者死亡的主要原因是心血管事件(7.2%)[4]。这些事件,包括心肌梗死,可通过尸体解剖、临床表现和实验室检查来诊断。因此,在威斯康星大学实施的研究中,我们制订了更严格的术前检查标准。严格的SPK患者选择标准(见第32章)也使得我们的观察研究结果和其他中心有所不同。心血管事件死亡率是患者预后的一个重要指标。在这一系列研究中,术前心血管的干预比率很低,这也意味着这些患者的总体心血管风险很低,反过来说,这组患者的生存率会较高。除心血管事件外,其他导致死亡的原因有感染(3.4%)、卒中(1.8%)、肾衰竭(1.5%)、恶性肿瘤(1.3%)和出血(0.8%)[4]。还有一些死亡事件(n=57)由于解剖被拒绝或不确定而不能准确诊断。

肠内引流、膀胱引流和肠内引流转换

在做了390位膀胱引流的SPK患者后,我们中心(威斯康星大学)开始采用肠内引流的方式做胰腺移植[6]。我们分析了ED-SPK和BD-SPK患者的移植肾存活率和移植胰腺存活率情况。有趣的是,在这两组患者之间,我们未发现其移植肾脏或胰腺的存活率有显著差异(图107.9和图107.10)。这个结果让我们出乎意料,因为BD患者有较高的排斥反应和感染并发症发生率,而EB患者则经常使用霉酚酸酯和他克莫司,从而有着更好的免疫抑制。

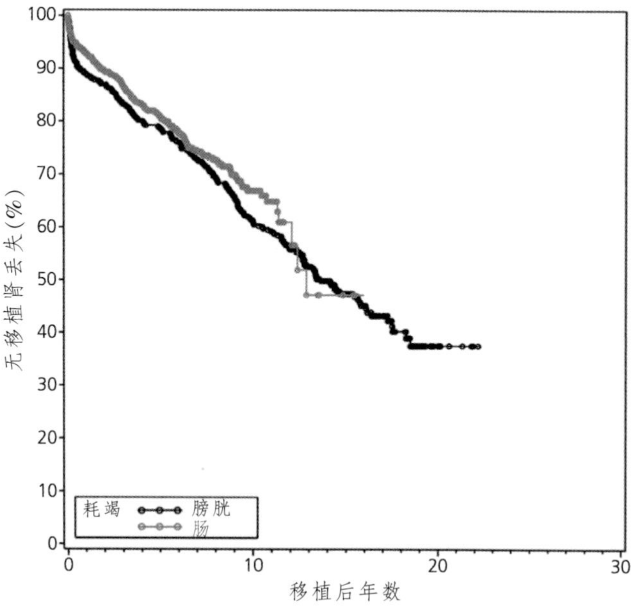

图107.9 1985—2007年肾胰移植患者膀胱引流与肠内引流对移植肾存活率的影响。(Reprinted from [4] Sollinger HW, Odorico JS, Becker YT, D'Alessandro AM, Pirsch JD. One thousand simultaneous pancreas-kidney transplants at a single center with 22-year follow-up. Ann Surg 2009, 250 (4):618-630, with permission from Wolters Kluwer Health.)

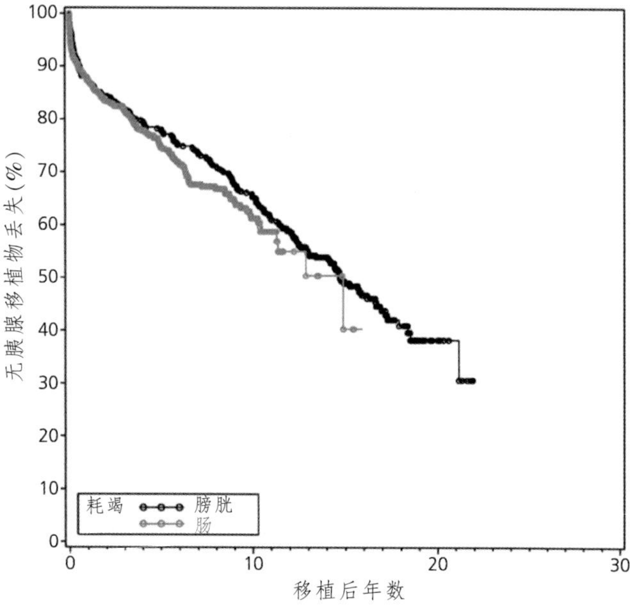

图107.10 1985—2007年肾胰移植患者膀胱引流与肠内引流对移植胰腺存活率的影响。(Reprinted from [4] Sollinger HW, Odorico JS, Becker YT, D'Alessandro AM, Pirsch JD. One thousand simultaneous pancreas-kidney transplants at a single center with 22-year follow-up. Ann Surg 2009, 250 (4):618-630, with permission from Wolters Kluwer Health.)

ED-SPK 和 BD-SPK 患者在移植物存活率上没有差异，我们研究发现 ED 患者移植后生活质量提高，优于 BD 患者。BD 患者的并发症包括代谢性酸中毒、较高的尿路感染发生率、血尿、尿道炎、尿道中断和排尿困难。在我们中心存活的 BD 患者中，超过一半通过转换为肠内引流来纠正严重的尿路感染和代谢性酸中毒。在移植后的 15 年内，大约 50%的患者转换做了肠内引流[4]。根据我们的经验，移植后再转换为肠内引流的话，由于十二指肠段易碎性增加，引起吻合口瘘并发症的风险更高。在最近的一份研究中报道了 EC 和初次 ED-SPK 患者在 1 年、5 年和 10 年的移植胰腺和患者生存率[78]，但我们仍应注意到，EC 后早期并发症的发生率很高(手术并发症：31.1%，再次手术概率：25%，早期移植失败：6.3%)。对于这些患者，应该明智地选择肠内引流转换，并在转换后期采用 Roux-en-Y 形吻合。这是当前我们处理早期移植 ED 患者的经验。

BD 的支持者认为，测量尿淀粉酶水平为早期排斥反应判断提供一个检测方法。但我们自己中心(威斯康星大学)所做的 ED 单独胰腺移植(SP-ED)的患者结果并不支持这一观点。在这项研究中，通过胰腺活检来诊断急性排斥反应，再比较 SP-ED 接受者和 SPK 接受者的排斥发生率和移植物存活率[79]。我们假设，如果 BD 在胰腺移植中至关重要，那么在 SP-ED 患者排斥由于无法监测尿淀粉酶导致了急性排斥反应时抢救的概率很低。在 SPK 患者中，移植肾的功能会增强排斥反应的检测，与之相比，我们发现在单独和联合胰腺移植之前，其急性排斥反应后抢救概率是没有差异的[79]。这些数据证实，SPK 患者移植后排斥反应的诊断和治疗与是否采用 BD 无显著关系。相比 BD 患者，ED 患者在移植后早期阶段由于并发症而再次手术的概率/情况更多。有 24%的 ED-SPK 患者在移植后 30 天内发生了并发症，而 BD-SPK 患者仅为 15%。然而，BD-SPK 患者中需要再次手术的大部分并发症(76%)发生在后期(>1 年)，且许多是需要做肠内引流转换的[4]。

移植后 1 型糖尿病(T1D)复发

Sutherland 博士在明尼苏达大学通过研究一批 HLA 相同的接受胰腺移植的患者，第一次描述了移植后 1 型糖尿病复发[80-83]。在未采用免疫抑制的情况下，移植后 4~8 周可能发生 T1D 复发，表现为单核细胞浸润和选择性 β-细胞破坏，但未发生胰腺排斥[83]。根据这些初步研究和其他的观察，他认为采用加倍的免疫抑制剂可对非 HLA 相同患者的排斥反应和胰腺炎后的自身免疫起到抑制效果。然而，随着该领域知识的拓展，在有足够免疫抑制来防止排斥反应的患者身上发生 T1D 复发被认为是一件临床上确实会发生的事件[84,85]。复发性疾病的基本特性包括高血糖的临床症状、活检证实的伴选择性 β-细胞损失的胰腺炎、自身抗体的持续存在或再现(GAD，IA2)、保留的外分泌功能和循环中自身反应性 T 细胞的存在[83]。这些特性很重要，移植后高血糖可能发生[86]，但并不意味着自身免疫性 T1D 也会复发。另一个关键发现是，自体抗原转换而不是持久或消耗与复发性糖尿病的高风险相关。迈阿密大学的一项研究发现，复发性疾病的发生率等于慢性排斥反应的发生率，约为 5%。慢性移植排斥反应导致的移植后高血糖可能与复发性 T1D 难以区分。在 Pugilese 等所做的研究中，他们的胰腺移植受者是采用了膀胱引流，从而观察到了外分泌功能。肠内引流已成为美国的主流术式，而且测量这些患者的尿淀粉酶是不可能的[2]。在这一临床过程中需要提高诊断、预防和治疗。其他关于胰腺移植后复发病的讨论见第 77 章。

胰腺移植对继发性糖尿病并发症的影响

恢复内源性胰岛素分泌和肾功能已证明可以缓解继发性糖尿病的并发症，而且证据表明移植可延长 T1D 患者的寿命。然而，关于这一问题的多项研究并非是前瞻性的，没有充分平衡控制病例选择和变量控制，其对照组往往是那些非移植患者或移植失败的患者。此外，测量参数经常使用替代标记物来评估复杂的继发性糖尿病并发症，在某些情况下，这些检测指标是否相关或是否临床相关仍有争议。

肾病

糖尿病肾病的病理生理特点是基底膜增厚、系膜基质积累、肾小球动脉透明变性和肾小球硬化[55,87]。Bohman 等所做的研究表明，成功的胰腺移植可防止糖尿病性肾小球肾病发生[88,89]。糖尿病性肾小球肾病的标准包括肾小球基底膜宽度，总系膜和系膜基质总量在 5 年内持平但 10 年内明显减少意味着糖尿病性肾小球和管状病变是可逆的。最近的一些研究也表明,如果单独胰腺移植的患者没有尿毒症,那么其糖尿病性肾病的病变是可逆的[58,90,91]。然而,PAK患者人群的各种病变是相关的,长期免疫抑制带来的肾毒性使患者体内的平衡更加复杂化。此外,糖尿病性肾病的长期形态学变化已经被改善或稳定下来,但以GFR降低评估肾功能,无论是否按仔细的、设计的和可控的分析做出来的,它都是有争议的。另外的关于糖尿病性肾病复发的讨论见第77章。

视网膜病

大多数对视网膜病变的研究进展都不大。Ramsay等报道,在成功的胰腺移植后情况平稳的前三年内,多达30%的患者发生了视网膜病变[92]。而且移植失败的患者也会发生视网膜事件。最近的研究证实了这些数据[27,93]。Giannarelli等分析了33名接受胰腺移植的患者,并比较了他们与36名未移植的T1D患者,在30个月的随访中发现,91%的移植患者发生了视网膜病变,而非移植患者仅为43%[93]。相比而言,平行观察提示移植后有10%~35%的不稳定眼疾患者发生了视网膜恶化[55],且类固醇和钙调磷酸酶的使用可能恶化白内障和青光眼[94]。

神经病变

几项研究已经证明了胰腺移植受者的外周肾病改善。Solders等报道,胰腺移植后患者的神经病变也改善了,而未移植或移植失败的患者神经病变依然进展。Kennedy等通过与接受强化胰岛素治疗的患者比较,评估了胰腺移植患者的糖尿病自主神经和感觉运动神经病变进展[95]。两组比较了移植后12个月、24个月和42个月时的情况,还记录了胰岛素治疗患者的感觉运动和自主神经病变情况,发现移植后神经病变有改善。最近,Martinenghi等比较了胰肾联合移植患者和胰腺移植失败患者的神经传导速度,发现移植后神经传导速度提高了,证实了上述发现[96]。这些研究的缺点是神经进展测量困难。不管神经传导速度增加是否有临床相关性,但部分症状往往是主观的,是难以量化的。

周围性血管疾病

总的来说,糖尿病患者下肢截肢的风险高出非糖尿病患者15倍多[97]。患者血糖降到正常理论上可以降低周围性血管疾病的发生风险。然而,仍有一小部分分析发现胰腺移植后有周围性血管疾病的发生风险[98-100]。Morrissey等表明,与仅做肾移植(KTA)的糖尿病患者相比,SPK患者移植后早期的周围性血管疾病发生率(定义为截肢、需要治疗的缺血性溃疡和下肢搭桥手术或血管成形术)似乎增加了[101]。周围性血管并发症在移植前后的差异在各组间无差异(P=0.94),但18/39的SPK患者中有35个新血管并发症事件,在20/65的KTA患者中,有32个事件(P=0.005)。由于患者数量少,且KTA患者在胰腺移植前未完全筛选入选资格、相关疾病、肾功能和高血糖程度,所以这些数据也有局限性。Biesenbach等最近的研究也指出,SPK患者的周围性血管疾病发生率比KTA患者的低[99]。然而,其研究中只有12名SPK患者和10名KTA的糖尿病患者,且其关于心肌梗死(16%对50%)、卒中(16%对40%)和截肢(16%对30%)结果上的差异使其结论说服力不足。

疾病控制中心发布的分析中,年龄调整后的每千人糖尿病患者腿部和足部截肢率从1996年的1.12%降至2008年的0.39%[102]。胰腺移植后的T1D患者需要截肢的发生率据报道为8%~9.5%[100,103,104]。相比之下,2型DM患者的截肢率为6.1%~19%[105-107]。近年来,T1D患者累积的非创伤性下肢截肢率女性为11.0%,男性为20.7%[108]。许多研究利用截肢率来代替周围性血管疾病或作为结果的主要衡量方法。然而,截肢是多因素的结果,其中包括神经病变和反复的足部受伤,其次是伤口愈合受损、细菌感染引起的免疫反应以及内膜的血管病变。单独的截肢率不能充分衡量这些患者的周围性血管疾病。在接受胰腺移植的T1D患者中,代谢调节改善和血糖恢复正常带来的疗效需综合下列因素来分析研究,其中包括年龄相关性血管病变的生理过程、预先存在的疾病和免疫抑制药物对主动脉的副作用等多个因素。

扩大供体池

心脏死亡后捐献和胰腺移植

在威斯康星大学,我们经常接到心脏死亡后的捐助者(DCD)来用于SPK和单独胰腺移植[109]。我们用惯例标准来评估捐赠胰腺是否适合移植,并控制缺血时间在30~45min。在我们的研究中,8.6%的SPK患者通过接受 DCD 捐赠的器官而康复[4]。

DBD 和 DCD 用于 SPK 移植后，其移植患者的 10 年生存率相近(分别为 80%和 84%;P=0.97)[4]。其胰腺移植物存活率也无明显差异(5 年:76%对 75%,10 年:64%对 60%;P=0.57)。以 GFR 和肌酸酐作为评估移植肾脏功能的标志,发现 DBD 和 DCD-SPK 患者相似(分别为 P=0.89,P=0.78),尽管 DCD 肾脏有较高的移植物功能延迟恢复发生率。这些数据与其他研究传统供体同边缘性供体胰腺移植效果的文献报道相一致[110]。

活体供体肾移植

许多中心的活体供体胰腺移植很少。如果有活体供体肾移植的话，那将可以缩短移植患者的尸体供体等待时间,而且一些对 HLA 抗原过敏的患者也可以采用活体移植治疗。在最近的一份报道中,明尼苏达大学发表了 Sutherland 等的研究。他们发现活体供体肾移植比尸体供体肾移植的移植失败风险更低，并预测这将使更多的胰腺移植接受者可以添加到等待名单中来[12]。目前,活体供体肾移植要求候选人去指定的中心,而且手术并发症和相关风险,以及捐献后供体糖尿病风险限制了潜在的手术患者数量。

供者和受者特异性对结果的影响

目前，移植的更大挑战在于匹配供者与适当的受者。Feng 等在肝移植文献中提出了供者风险指数的概念。在胰腺移植方面,有报道提出了供者特异性和受者特异性因素,这可能有助于指导器官分配及移植后影响[111]。Axelrod 等最近公布了胰腺供体风险指数(PDRI)[112]。PDRI 增加就意味着胰腺移植后 1 年内的存活率降低。这一风险指数可根据不同区域和中心的情况来具体使用,作者认为这仍是一个进展中的工作。大多数胰腺移植中心更倾向于用自己获得的捐赠移植器官，但使用区域外的胰腺移植物仍被认为是一条安全、可行的途径[113]。有效运用这些器官需要对冷冻缺血时间进行密切监测，要注意适合的供者与受者的风险因素。在单独的研究中,Luan 等提出了其他风险因素,包括受者种族,因为他们最近发现非裔美国人 SPK 受者有高达 38%的肾移植失败和 47%胰腺移植失败风险，且非裔美国人排斥后移植物丧失的风险比其他种族高 2 倍[114]。

免疫抑制药物

最初，我们中心在胰腺移植后给予的常规免疫抑制剂是环孢素联合硫唑嘌呤和泼尼松。1995 年,霉酚酸酯、他克莫司取代了硫唑嘌呤。我们目前的方案包括他克莫司、霉酚酸和低剂量泼尼松。诱导治疗从抗胸腺细胞球蛋白、莫罗单抗、达利珠单抗、阿来组单抗到巴利昔单抗。一般诱导和维持免疫抑制疗法的讨论可分别见第 65 章和第 66 章。

MMF 的引入对我们威斯康星大学而言是一个范例式的转变，其大大降低了肾脏和胰腺的急性排斥反应发生率（肾脏:34%对 75%,P=0.001；胰腺:7%对 24%,P=0.003)，同时也降低了需要抗淋巴细胞急救治疗的固醇类难治性排斥发作事件的发生率（15%对 52%,P=0.01)[6]。其他人也发表了类似结果，抗胸腺细胞球蛋白诱导有副作用(相比达利珠单抗),而他克莫司联合 MMF 治疗,相比于他克莫司联合西莫莫司或环孢素联合 MMF,其并发症发生率要低得多[111]。

我们最近经验性地使用阿仑单抗后,发现其与 IL-2 受体抗体诱导相比并没有更好地改善生存率[115]。此外统计显示，阿仑单抗治疗组有更高的巨细胞病毒感染和病毒血症发生率。因此,我们认为阿仑单抗没有显著的疗效，目前对于初次移植患者采用巴利昔单抗诱导的方法。

总结

为肾衰竭的 T1D 患者选择合适的治疗方式,是否需要胰腺移植是一个至关重要的决策。治疗方式包括透析、DDK、LDK、SPK 和 PAK。我们中心(威斯康星大学)的原则和指导方针是由 SPK 移植的受益要超过术后并发症风险以及终身免疫抑制治疗的风险。文献累积的证据表明,相比肾单独移植,SPK 患者糖尿病导致的代谢紊乱,在纠正后其生存率可提高。适当的选择应基于每个地区中不同器官接受者的发病率和不同的等待时间。上述结果的总结和我们对于临床实践的建议如下:

(1)SPK、PAK 和 PTA 患者移植后 5 年内胰腺移植物功能存活率分别为 80%、62%和 59%。其 5 年患者生存率则分别为87%、83%和89%。对于有糖尿病性肾病且未开始透析的T1D患者,应首先考虑SPK,它可以提高移植器官存活率和患者生存率。对于开始透析的T1D患者,如果SPK治疗等待时间过长的话,可以选择活体供肾移植。细致的手术技术,特别是移植器官准备,有利于长期的良好预后和移植物存活。对于PAK患者,相比胰腺移植,在选择其他治疗方式时更应注意避免对移植肾功能的影响,要充分考虑两个重要的术前指标:心血管情况和移植肾的功能。

(2)胰腺移植后早期技术失败会导致移植肾存活率和患者生存率下降。

(3)移植物血栓形成和心血管事件是移植后最严重的并发症。不同的中心常规使用的系统性抗凝剂各有不同,也没有哪种抗凝剂被证明有较好疗效,手术技术和捐献肾质量仍然是影响移植物血栓形成的重要因素。

(4)肠内引流是胰腺移植时外分泌引流的推荐方法,也是目前最广泛应用的选择。当患者症状明显、代谢紊乱以及生活质量改变时,应考虑将膀胱引流改为肠内引流,谨慎的选择和决策至关重要。

(5)胰腺移植后,糖尿病的一些次级并发症也会有所改善,但这方面的研究数据由于前瞻性设计不足和对照组不够等原因而缺乏准确性。

(6)如果谨慎而明智地进行捐献者-接受者匹配,那么利用心脏死亡后捐献的器官或引进的同种异体移植物来做移植是可行的。

感谢

作者认为,威斯康星大学胰腺移植部门在本研究项目的进展过程中发挥了关键作用。包括Marilyn Groshek、Elaine Snyder、Michael Armbrust、Munci Kalayoglu、Stuart Knectle和L.Tomas Chin。我们的移植患者,Barbara Voss、Glen Leverson、Judy Kozminski和Janet Fox。本报告没有任何利益冲突,也不披露任何利益关系。

(刘原兴 译 刘原兴 校)

参考文献

1. Gruessner AC, Sutherland DE, Gruessner RW. Long-term outcome after pancreas transplantation. Current Opinion in Organ Transplantation. 2012;17(1):100–105.
2. Gruessner AC. 2011 update on pancreas transplantation: comprehensive trend analysis of 25,000 cases followed up over the course of twenty-four years at the International Pancreas Transplant Registry (IPTR). Review of Diabetic Studies. 2011;8(1):6–16.
3. Gruessner AC, Sutherland DE. Pancreas transplant outcomes for United States (US) cases as reported to the United Network for Organ Sharing (UNOS) and the International Pancreas Transplant Registry (IPTR). Clinical Transplants. 2008;45–56.
4. Sollinger HW, Odorico JS, Becker YT, et al. One thousand simultaneous pancreas-kidney transplants at a single center with 22-year follow-up. Annals of Surgery. 2009;250(4):618–630.
5. Kelly WD, Lillehei RC, Merkel FK, et al. Allotransplantation of the pancreas and duodenum along with the kidney in diabetic nephropathy. Surgery. 1967;61(6):827–837.
6. Sollinger HW, Odorico JS, Knechtle SJ, et al. Experience with 500 simultaneous pancreas-kidney transplants. Annals of Surgery. 1998;228(3):284–296.
7. Gill IS, Sindhi R, Jerius JT, et al. Bench reconstruction of pancreas for transplantation: experience with 192 cases. Clinical Transplantation. 1997;11(2):104–109.
8. Bunzendahl H, Ringe B, Meyer HJ, et al. Combination harvesting procedure for liver and whole pancreas. Transplant International. 1988;1(2):99–102.
9. Fridell JA, Powelson JA, Sanders CE, et al. Preparation of the pancreas allograft for transplantation. Clinical Transplantation. 2011;25(2):E103–E112.
10. Bazerbachi F, Selzner M, Marquez MA, et al. Portal venous versus systemic venous drainage of pancreas grafts: impact on long-term results. American Journal of Transplantation. 2012;12(1):226–232.
11. Salzedas-Netto A, Linhares M, Lopes-Filho G, et al. Simultaneous pancreas-kidney transplantation: which organ should be transplanted first? Transplantation Proceedings. 2010;42(7):2647–2649.
12. Sutherland DE, Radosevich D, Gruessner R, et al. Pushing the envelope: living donor pancreas transplantation. Current Opinion in Organ Transplantation. 2012;17(1):106–115.
13. Shokouh-Amiri H, Zakhary JM, Zibari GB. A novel technique of portal-endocrine and gastric-exocrine drainage in pancreatic transplantation. Journal of the American College of Surgeons. 2011;212(4):730–738, discussion 738–739.
14. Ojo AO, Meier-Kriesche HU, Hanson JA, et al. The impact of simultaneous pancreas-kidney transplantation on long-term patient survival. Transplantation. 2001;71(1):82–90.
15. Perosa M, Boggi U, Cantarovich D, et al. Pancreas transplantation outside the USA: an update. Current Opinion in Organ Transplantation. 2011;16(1):135–141.
16. Perosa M, Crescentini F, Noujaim H, et al. Over 500 pancreas transplants by a single team in Sao Paulo, Brazil. Clinical Transplantation. 2011;25(4):E422–E429.
17. Martins L, Henriques AC, Dias L, et al. One hundred eleven simultaneous pancreas-kidney transplantations: 10-year experience from a single center in Portugal. Transplantation Proceedings. 2011;43(1):205–208.
18. Yamamoto S, Tufveson G, Wahlberg J, et al. Factors influencing outcome of simultaneous kidney and pancreas transplantation: a 23-year single-center clinical experience. Transplantation Proceedings. 2010;42(10):4197–4201.
19. Manuel Gonzalez-Posada J, Marrero D, Hernandez D, et al. Pancreas transplantation: differences in activity between Europe and the United States. Nephrology, Dialysis, Transplantation. 2010;25(3):952–959.
20. Eurotransplant website [cited February 15, 2012]; Available from: http://eurotransplant.org/cms/.
21. Council of Europe website [cited February 23, 2012]; Available from: http://www.coe.int/lportal/web/coe-portal/22-october-european-day-for-organ-donation.
22. Young BY, Gill J, Huang E, et al. Living donor kidney versus simultaneous pancreas-kidney transplant in type I diabetics: an analysis of the OPTN/UNOS database. Clinical Journal of the American Society of Nephrology : CJASN. 2009;4(4):845–852.
23. Morath C, Zeier M, Dohler B, et al. Metabolic control improves long-term renal allograft and patient survival in type 1 diabetes. Journal of the American Society of Nephrology. 2008;19(8):1557–1563.

24. Weiss AS, Smits G, Wiseman AC. Twelve-month pancreas graft function significantly influences survival following simultaneous pancreas-kidney transplantation. Clinical Journal of the American Society of Nephrology : CJASN. 2009; 4(5):988–995.
25. Lodhi SA, Lamb KE, Meier-Kriesche HU. Solid organ allograft survival improvement in the United States: the long-term does not mirror the dramatic short-term success. American Journal of Transplantation. 2011;11(6):1226–1235.
26. Kleinclauss F, Fauda M, Sutherland DE, et al. Pancreas after living donor kidney transplants in diabetic patients: impact on long-term kidney graft function. Clinical Transplantation. 2009;23(4):437–446.
27. Wang Q, Klein R, Moss SE, et al. The influence of combined kidney-pancreas transplantation on the progression of diabetic retinopathy. A case series. Ophthalmology. 1994;101(6):1071–1076.
28. Gaber AO, el-Gebely S, Sugathan P, et al. Early improvement in cardiac function occurs for pancreas-kidney but not diabetic kidney-alone transplant recipients. Transplantation. 1995;59(8):1105–1112.
29. Solders G, Tyden G, Tibell A, et al. Improvement in nerve conduction 8 years after combined pancreatic and renal transplantation. Transplantation Proceedings. 1995;27(6):3091.
30. Hill M, Garcia R, Dunn T, et al. What happens to the kidney in an SPK transplant when the pancreas fails due to a technical complication? Clinical Transplantation. 2008;22(4):456–461.
31. Stegall MD, Dean PG, Sung R, et al. The rationale for the new deceased donor pancreas allocation schema. Transplantation. 2007;83(9):1156–1161.
32. Sampaio MS, Reddy PN, Kuo HT, et al. Obesity was associated with inferior outcomes in simultaneous pancreas kidney transplant. Transplantation. 2010;89(9):1117–1125.
33. Salvalaggio PR, Schnitzler MA, Abbott KC, et al. Patient and graft survival implications of simultaneous pancreas kidney transplantation from old donors. American Journal of Transplantation. 2007;7(6):1561–1571.
34. Gruessner RW. Pancreas transplantation. Current Opinion in Organ Transplantation. 2010;15(1):92.
35. Gruessner AC, Sutherland DE, Gruessner RW. Pancreas transplantation in the United States: a review. Current Opinion in Organ Transplantation. 2010; 15(1):93–101.
36. Gruessner AC, Sutherland DE. Access to pancreas transplantation should not be restricted because of age: invited commentary on Schenker et al. Transplant International. 2011;24(2):134–135.
37. Schenker P, Vonend O, Kruger B, et al. Long-term results of pancreas transplantation in patients older than 50 years. Transplant International. 2011;24(2): 136–142.
38. Fridell JA, Mangus RS, Taber TE, et al. Growth of a nation part I: impact of organ donor obesity on whole-organ pancreas transplantation. Clinical Transplantation. 2011;25(3):E225–E232.
39. Fridell JA, Mangus RS, Taber TE, et al. Growth of a nation part II: impact of recipient obesity on whole-organ pancreas transplantation. Clinical Transplantation. 2011;25(4):E366–E374.
40. Lamattina J, Sollinger H, Becker Y, et al. Long-term pancreatic allograft survival after renal retransplantation in prior simultaneous pancreas-kidney recipients. American Journal of Transplantation. 2012.
41. Lamattina JC, Sollinger HW, Becker YT, et al. Simultaneous pancreas and kidney (SPK) retransplantation in prior SPK recipients. Clinical Transplantation. 2011; 26(3):495–501.
42. Browne S, Gill J, Dong J, et al. The impact of pancreas transplantation on kidney allograft survival. American Journal of Transplantation. 2011;11(9): 1951–1958.
43. Poommipanit N, Sampaio MS, Cho Y, et al. Pancreas after living donor kidney versus simultaneous pancreas-kidney transplant: an analysis of the organ procurement transplant network/united network of organ sharing database. Transplantation. 2010;89(12):1496–1503.
44. Pavlakis M, Khwaja K, Mandelbrot D, et al. Renal allograft failure predictors after PAK transplantation: results from the New England Collaborative Association of Pancreas Programs. Transplantation. 2010;89(11):1347–1353.
45. Odorico JS, Voss B, Munoz Del Rio A, et al. Kidney function after solitary pancreas transplantation. Transplantation Proceedings. 2008;40(2):513–515.
46. Venstrom JM, McBride MA, Rother KI, et al. Survival after pancreas transplantation in patients with diabetes and preserved kidney function. JAMA: Journal of the American Medical Association. 2003;290(21):2817–2823.
47. Gruessner RW, Sutherland DE, Gruessner AC. Mortality assessment for pancreas transplants. American Journal of Transplantation. 2004;4(12): 2018–2026.
48. Humar A, Sutherland DE, Ramcharan T, et al. Optimal timing for a pancreas transplant after a successful kidney transplant. Transplantation. 2000;70(8): 1247–1250.
49. Wiseman AC. Pancreas transplant options for patients with type 1 diabetes mellitus and chronic kidney disease: simultaneous pancreas kidney or pancreas after kidney? Current Opinion in Organ Transplantation. 2012; 17(1):80–86.
50. Anand SG, Mehta SD, Adams WG. Diabetes mellitus screening in pediatric primary care. Pediatrics. 2006;118(5):1888–1895.
51. Gruessner RW, Sutherland DE, Kandaswamy R, et al. Over 500 solitary pancreas transplants in nonuremic patients with brittle diabetes mellitus. Transplantation. 2008;85(1):42–47.
52. Boggi U, Vistoli F, Amorese G, et al. Long-term (5 years) efficacy and safety of pancreas transplantation alone in type 1 diabetic patients. Transplantation. 2012;93(8):842–846.
53. Sutherland DE, Gruessner AC. Long-term results after pancreas transplantation. Transplantation Proceedings. 2007;39(7):2323–2325.
54. Gruessner RW, Sutherland DE, Gruessner AC. Survival after pancreas transplantation. JAMA: Journal of the American Medical Association. 2005;293(6):675, author reply 675–676.
55. Gremizzi C, Vergani A, Paloschi V, et al. Impact of pancreas transplantation on type 1 diabetes-related complications. Current Opinion in Organ Transplantation. 2010;15(1):119–123.
56. Scalea JR, Butler CC, Munivenkatappa RB, et al. Pancreas transplant alone as an independent risk factor for the development of renal failure: a retrospective study. Transplantation. 2008;86(12):1789–1794.
57. Fioretto P, Najafian B, Sutherland DE, et al. Tacrolimus and cyclosporine nephrotoxicity in native kidneys of pancreas transplant recipients. Clinical Journal of the American Society of Nephrology : CJASN. 2011;6(1):101–106.
58. Fioretto P, Mauer M. Effects of pancreas transplantation on the prevention and reversal of diabetic nephropathy. Contributions to Nephrology. 2011;170: 237–246.
59. Humar A, Ramcharan T, Kandaswamy R, et al. Technical failures after pancreas transplants: why grafts fail and the risk factors-a multivariate analysis. Transplantation. 2004;78(8):1188–1192.
60. Norman SP, Kommareddi M, Ojo AO, et al. Early pancreas graft failure is associated with inferior late clinical outcomes after simultaneous kidney-pancreas transplantation. Transplantation. 2011;92(7):796–801.
61. Schnickel GT, Busuttil RW, Lipshutz GS. Improvement in short-term pancreas transplant outcome by targeted antimicrobial therapy and refined donor selection. American Surgeon. 2011;77(10):1407–1411.
62. Perez-Saez MJ, Toledo K, Navarro MD, et al. Long-term survival of simultaneous pancreas-kidney transplantation: influence of early posttransplantation complications. Transplantation Proceedings. 2011;43(6):2160–2164.
63. Wang SN, Sturdevant M, Kandaswamy R, et al. Technical failure of the pancreas after SPK transplant: are these patients good candidates for later pancreas retransplant? Clinical Transplantation. 2008;22(1):50–54.
64. Troppmann C. Complications after pancreas transplantation. Current Opinion in Organ Transplantation. 2010;15(1):112–118.
65. Orsenigo E, Fiorina P, Dell'Antonio G, et al. Gastrointestinal bleeding from enterically drained transplanted pancreas. Transplant International. 2005;18(3): 296–302.
66. Fridell JA, Johnson MS, Goggins WC, et al. Vascular catastrophes following pancreas transplantation: an evolution in strategy at a single center. Clinical Transplantation. 2012;26(1):164–172.
67. Farney AC, Rogers J, Stratta RJ. Pancreas graft thrombosis: causes, prevention, diagnosis, and intervention. Current Opinion in Organ Transplantation. 2012;17(1):87–92.
68. Sollinger HW. Pancreatic transplantation and vascular graft thrombosis. Journal of the American College of Surgeons. 1996;182(4):362–363.
69. Troppmann C, Gruessner AC, Benedetti E, et al. Vascular graft thrombosis after pancreatic transplantation: univariate and multivariate operative and nonoperative risk factor analysis. Journal of the American College of Surgeons. 1996;182(4):285–316.
70. Ionescu C, Wolf P, Ellero B, et al. The venous thrombosis of the pancreatic graft. Journal of Gastrointestinal and Liver Diseases. 2007;16(3):287–292.
71. Schenker P, Vonend O, Ertas N, et al. Incidence of pancreas graft thrombosis using low-molecular-weight heparin. Clinical Transplantation. 2009;23(3): 407–414.
72. Stewart ZA, Cameron AM, Singer AL, et al. Histidine-tryptophan-ketoglutarate (HTK) is associated with reduced graft survival in pancreas transplantation. American Journal of Transplantation. 2009;9(1):217–221.
73. Troppmann C. Complications after pancreas transplantation. Current Opinion in Organ Transplantation. 2010;15(1):112–118.
74. Garcia-Roca R, Samame J, Garcia-Criado MA, et al. Preservation of pancreas graft function after complete venous thrombosis: report of four cases treated conservatively. Transplantation. 2012;93(2):214–218.

75. Sollinger HW, Odorico JS, Becker YT, et al. One thousand simultaneous pancreas-kidney transplants at a single center with 22-year follow-up. Annals of Surgery. 2009;250(4):618–630.
76. Martins L, Henriques AC, Dias L, et al. Pancreas-kidney transplantation: complications and readmissions in 9-years of follow-up. Transplantation Proceedings. 2010;42(2):552–554.
77. Fridell JA, Mangus RS, Mull AB, et al. Early reexploration for suspected thrombosis after pancreas transplantation. Transplantation. 2011;91(8):902–907.
78. Kleespies A, Mikhailov M, Khalil PN, et al. Enteric conversion after pancreatic transplantation: resolution of symptoms and long-term results. Clinical Transplantation. 2011;25(4):549–560.
79. Odorico JS, Pirsch JD, Becker YT, et al. Results of solitary pancreas transplantation with enteric drainage: is there a benefit from monitoring urinary amylase levels? Transplantation Proceedings. 2001;33(1–2):1700.
80. Sutherland DE, Sibley R, Xu XZ, et al. Twin-to-twin pancreas transplantation: reversal and reenactment of the pathogenesis of type I diabetes. Transactions of the Association of American Physicians. 1984;97:80–87.
81. Sibley RK, Sutherland DE, Goetz F, et al. Recurrent diabetes mellitus in the pancreas iso- and allograft. A light and electron microscopic and immunohistochemical analysis of four cases. Laboratory Investigation; a Journal of Technical Methods and Pathology. 1985;53(2):132–144.
82. Sutherland DE, Goetz FC, Sibley RK. Recurrence of disease in pancreas transplants. Diabetes. 1989;38(Suppl 1):85–87.
83. Pugliese A, Reijonen HK, Nepom J, et al. Recurrence of autoimmunity in pancreas transplant patients: research update. Diabetes Management (London, England). 2011;1(2):229–238.
84. Vendrame F, Pileggi A, Laughlin E, et al. Recurrence of type 1 diabetes after simultaneous pancreas-kidney transplantation, despite immunosuppression, is associated with autoantibodies and pathogenic autoreactive CD4 T-cells. Diabetes. 2010;59(4):947–957.
85. Laughlin E, Burke G, Pugliese A, et al. Recurrence of autoreactive antigen-specific CD4+ T cells in autoimmune diabetes after pancreas transplantation. Clinical Immunology (Orlando, Fla.). 2008;128(1):23–30.
86. Neidlinger N, Singh N, Klein C, et al. Incidence of and risk factors for posttransplant diabetes mellitus after pancreas transplantation. American Journal of Transplantation. 2010;10(2):398–406.
87. Mauer SM, Steffes MW, Ellis EN, et al. Structural-functional relationships in diabetic nephropathy. Journal of Clinical Investigation. 1984;74(4):1143–1155.
88. Bohman SO, Tyden G, Wilczek H, et al. Prevention of kidney graft diabetic nephropathy by pancreas transplantation in man. Diabetes. 1985;34(3): 306–308.
89. Bohman SO, Wilczek H, Tyden G, et al. Recurrent diabetic nephropathy in renal allografts placed in diabetic patients and protective effect of simultaneous pancreatic transplantation. Transplantation Proceedings. 1987;19(1 Pt 3): 2290–2293.
90. Fioretto P, Mauer M. Reversal of diabetic nephropathy: lessons from pancreas transplantation. Journal of Nephrology. 2012;25(1):13–18.
91. Fioretto P, Sutherland DE, Najafian B, et al. Remodeling of renal interstitial and tubular lesions in pancreas transplant recipients. Kidney International. 2006;69(5):907–912.
92. Ramsay RC, Goetz FC, Sutherland DE, et al. Progression of diabetic retinopathy after pancreas transplantation for insulin-dependent diabetes mellitus. New England Journal of Medicine. 1988;318(4):208–214.
93. Giannarelli R, Coppelli A, Sartini M, et al. Effects of pancreas-kidney transplantation on diabetic retinopathy. Transplant International. 2005;18(5):619–622.
94. Chow VC, Pai RP, Chapman JR, et al. Diabetic retinopathy after combined kidney-pancreas transplantation. Clinical Transplantation. 1999;13(4):356–362.
95. Kennedy WR, Navarro X, Goetz FC, et al. Effects of pancreatic transplantation on diabetic neuropathy. New England Journal of Medicine. 1990;322(15): 1031–1037.
96. Martinenghi S, Comi G, Galardi G, et al. Amelioration of nerve conduction velocity following simultaneous kidney/pancreas transplantation is due to the glycaemic control provided by the pancreas. Diabetologia. 1997;40(9): 1110–1112.
97. Most RS, Sinnock P. The epidemiology of lower extremity amputations in diabetic individuals. Diabetes Care. 1983;6(1):87–91.
98. Morrissey PE, Shaffer D, Monaco AP, et al. Peripheral vascular disease after kidney-pancreas transplantation in diabetic patients with end-stage renal disease. Archives of Surgery (Chicago, Ill: 1960). 1997;132(4):358–361, discussion 361–352.
99. Biesenbach G, Konigsrainer A, Gross C, et al. Progression of macrovascular diseases is reduced in type 1 diabetic patients after more than 5 years successful combined pancreas-kidney transplantation in comparison to kidney transplantation alone. Transplant International. 2005;18(9):1054–1060.
100. Kalker AJ, Pirsch JD, Heisey D, et al. Foot problems in the diabetic transplant recipient. Clinical Transplantation. 1996;10(6 Pt 1):503–510.
101. Morrissey PE, Shaffer D, Madras PN, et al. Progression of peripheral vascular disease after combined kidney-pancreas transplantation in diabetic patients with end-stage renal failure. Transplantation Proceedings. 1997;29(1–2):662–663.
102. Li Y, Burrows NR, Gregg EW, et al. Declining rates of hospitalization for nontraumatic lower-extremity amputation in the diabetic population aged 40 years or older: U.S., 1988-2008. Diabetes Care. 2012;35(2):273–277.
103. Woeste G, Wullstein C, Pridohl O, et al. Incidence of minor and major amputations after pancreas/kidney transplantation. Transplant International. 2003;16(2): 128–132.
104. Knight RJ, Zela S, Schoenberg L, et al. The effect of pancreas transplantation on peripheral vascular disease complications. Transplantation Proceedings. 2004;36(4):1069–1071.
105. O'Hare AM, Bacchetti P, Segal M, et al. Factors associated with future amputation among patients undergoing hemodialysis: results from the Dialysis Morbidity and Mortality Study Waves 3 and 4. American Journal of Kidney Diseases. 2003;41(1):162–170.
106. Ramsey SD, Newton K, Blough D, et al. Incidence, outcomes, and cost of foot ulcers in patients with diabetes. Diabetes Care. 1999;22(3):382–387.
107. Moulik PK, Mtonga R, Gill GV. Amputation and mortality in new-onset diabetic foot ulcers stratified by etiology. Diabetes Care. 2003;26(2):491–494.
108. Jonasson JM, Ye W, Sparen P, et al. Risks of nontraumatic lower-extremity amputations in patients with type 1 diabetes: a population-based cohort study in Sweden. Diabetes Care. 2008;31(8):1536–1540.
109. Bellingham JM, Santhanakrishnan C, Neidlinger N, et al. Donation after cardiac death: a 29-year experience. Surgery. 2011;150(4):692–702.
110. Singh RP, Rogers J, Farney AC, et al. Outcomes of extended donors in pancreatic transplantation with portal-enteric drainage. Transplantation Proceedings. 2008;40(2):502–505.
111. Fellmer PT, Pascher A, Kahl A, et al. Influence of donor- and recipient-specific factors on the postoperative course after combined pancreas-kidney transplantation. Langenbeck's Archives of Surgery. 2010;395(1):19–25.
112. Axelrod DA, Sung RS, Meyer KH, et al. Systematic evaluation of pancreas allograft quality, outcomes and geographic variation in utilization. American Journal of Transplantation. 2010;10(4):837–845.
113. Fridell JA, Mangus RS, Hollinger EF, et al. No difference in transplant outcomes for local and import pancreas allografts. Transplantation. 2009;88(5):723–728.
114. Luan FL, Kommareddi M, Cibrik DM, et al. Influence of recipient race on the outcome of simultaneous pancreas and kidney transplantation. American Journal of Transplantation. 2010;10(9):2074–2081.
115. Pascual J, Pirsch JD, Odorico JS, et al. Alemtuzumab induction and antibody-mediated kidney rejection after simultaneous pancreas-kidney transplantation. Transplantation. 2009;87(1):125–132.

第 108 章 胰岛移植长期预后

A.M. James Shapiro, Camillo Ricordi

引言

胰岛移植的开展以及预后在过去 12 年里取得了显著进展[1-6]。这一明确的微创治疗方法为不能用其他方式替代治疗的 1 型糖尿病患者提供了可靠、有效的血糖控制可能。约 40 个国际网站登记结果显示，目前已有超过 1000 名患者接受了胰岛移植(协同胰岛移植注册系统已登记了 752 例同种异体胰岛移植和 333 例自体胰岛移植)[5,7]。有趣的是，相比于实体器官移植，获取死亡供体的胰腺并不是限制胰腺移植的唯一阻碍因素。临床胰岛细胞分离设备(cGMP)限制和必需的临床良好生产规范的超净环境、加工胰岛的技能和专业知识、从可用器官获取胰岛普遍效率偏低，以及明显有限的临床研究经费都是开展胰岛移植的限制因素。在美国，胰岛移植目前正计划获得美国食品药品监督管理局(FDA)的生物应用许可，这意味着医疗补助、医疗保险和其他第三方报销对胰岛移植的发展会产生巨大影响。

从长远来看，胰岛供应有限和需要强化免疫抑制被视为两个缺点，限制了胰岛移植在 T1DM 中更广泛的应用[3,7]。糖尿病控制不良和免疫抑制的风险是明确的。许多糖尿病社区往往过于担心移植和免疫抑制治疗的风险，而那些每天照顾胰岛移植患者的人反而认识到糖尿病并发症带来的更大风险。随着胰岛移植变得更为常规且免疫抑制管理更加精简，很可能移植和终身免疫抑制的风险与这些最稳定的胰岛素控制的糖尿病患者取得平衡。这将扩大程序化适应证，并开放这一疗法在小儿科的应用[8]。越早成功地在糖尿病发生过程中应用胰岛移植，防止继发性并发症的潜在保护效应就会越大。但同时，终身免疫抑制持续时间越长、恶性肿瘤、感染和肾损伤的累积风险就越大[9-12]。只有同时采用严格设计的 T1DM 患者接受胰岛素或移植治疗的随机对照试验和意向性治疗基础上的终身随访才能明确这样的平衡何时能达到。

同时，由于目前移植耐受仍无法实现，一些基金组织已经投资探索干细胞来源和异种移植的胰岛作为常规临床稳定血糖控制的替代方式，包括采用高科技的闭环传感器胰岛素泵作为过渡或终身疗法，甚至可以完全避免移植[13]。我们往往先入为主地认为持续正常血糖无法通过外源性胰岛素皮下持久释放达到，即使是最好的胰岛素泵和传感器也达不到自身胰腺胰岛或足够体积的移植胰岛提供的精确的即时血糖控制。本章讨论了目前胰岛移植的临床预后，以及为进一步进行随机对照试验将要面临的挑战。

糖尿病和替代干预策略的风险

T1DM 是一个变化无常的和普遍的疾病，同时影响儿童和成人，目前无法预防，发病率逐渐增加。此外，胰岛素治疗只能拯救生命，不能治愈。T1DM 发病率介于 17~40/10 万人口，发病率最高的是芬兰和撒丁岛，且仍在迅速增加[14]。15 岁以下的 T1DM 儿童患者估计有 490 100 例[15]，而死亡率在第一和第三世界国家之间相差很大。即使是在富裕国家，T1DM 儿童和成人的死亡率至少是年龄相仿的未患患者群的 2 倍[16,17]。在美国，糖尿病是第七大死因，是肾衰竭、非创伤性截肢和成人失明新发病例的主要原因，消耗了超过 1740 亿美元的医疗成本[17,18]。而糖尿病控制和并发症试验(DCCT)清楚地表明，通过强化胰岛素改善血糖控制可大幅降低继发性并发症的风险，并降低糖化血红蛋白(HbA1C)水平，使低血糖的风险显著增加[19-21]。

低血糖早已被确认为是过量胰岛素治疗的并发症，事实上一个单位的胰岛素量是指诱发一只兔子发生致命性低血糖的剂量[22]。用于血糖监测和药物持久释放的皮下位点是有缺陷的方法，响应滞后必然不能提供完整的生理血糖控制。尤其是在部分易感个体中，纠正糖化血红蛋白并进一步降低继发性并发症的风险的措施会加剧低血糖的风险[21,23,24]。欧美国家患有T1DM的汽车司机发生车祸的次数是他们的非糖尿病配偶的2倍，在某种程度上与神经性低血糖、视网膜病变和周围神经病变有关[25-27]。

“死在床上”综合征仍是胰岛素治疗的T1DM患者发生低血糖症的最可怕的并发症之一，患者通常被发现死在清晨，占不明原因死亡病例的4.7%~7.3%，也占年龄在40岁以下的T1DM患者整体死亡率的6%[27-30]。图108.1表明了两名患者携带连续皮下葡萄糖监测系

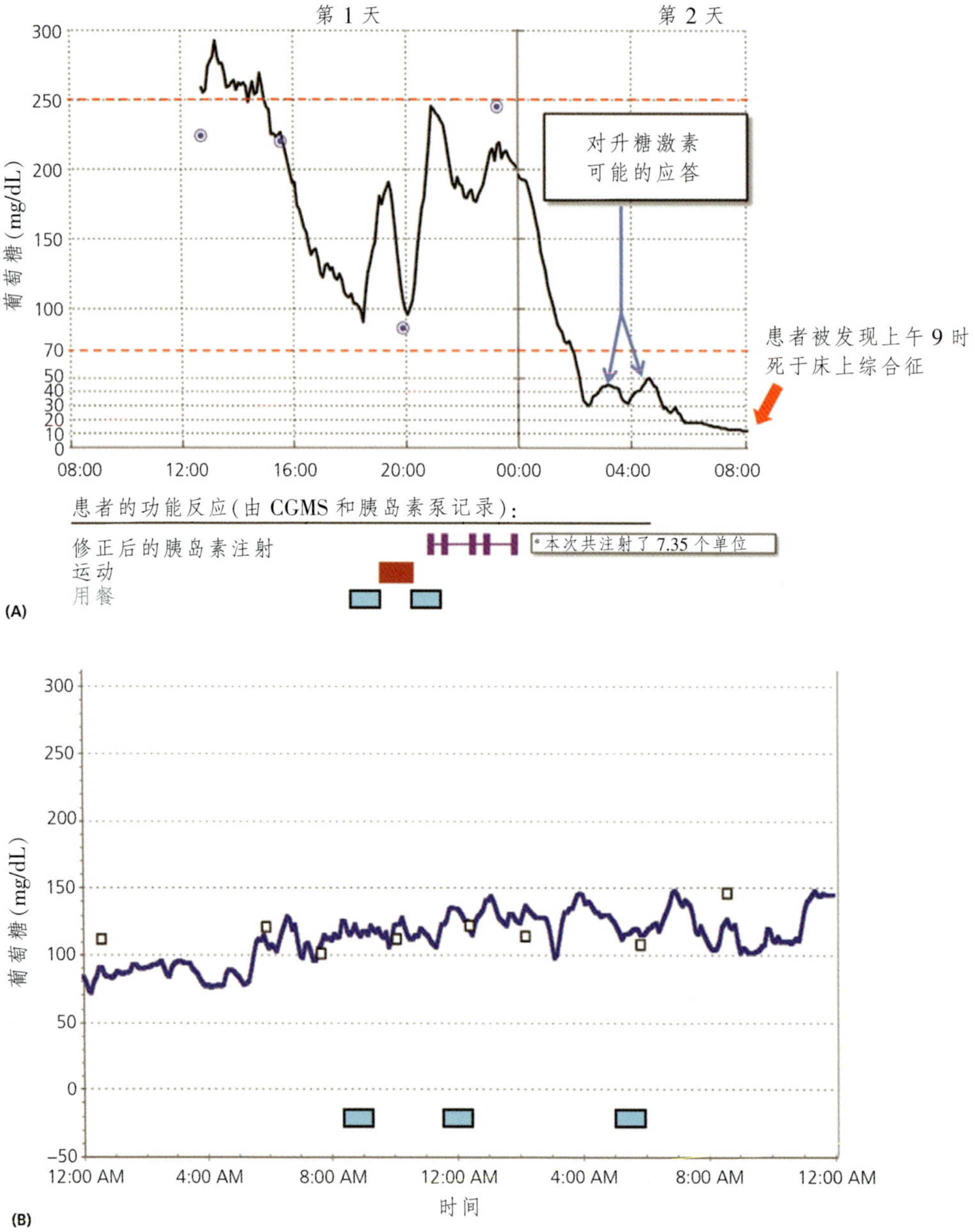

图108.1 连续皮下葡萄糖监测系统(CGMS)记录:(A)一名23岁的T1DM患者使用胰岛素泵，并发严重低血糖，被母亲发现有痉挛后送往急诊，服用了橙汁。第二天早晨，他的家人在上午9时发现其没有反应和脉搏。CGMS记录和尸体解剖证实其因低血糖而死亡(死于床综合征)。(B)一名44岁的女性，曾经在阿尔伯塔大学接受过T1DM治疗，接受了两次胰岛移植，CGMS证实持续出现血糖异常，HbA1C为5.5%，不需要胰岛素3年。[Figure 1A modified from the original published in reference [31], and generously provided by Professor R.J. Tanenberg with kind permission. Reprinted from Endocrine Practice, Vol 16, Confirmation of hypoglycemia in the “dead-in-bed” syndrome, as captured by a retrospective continuous glucose monitoring system, p.246, Copyright (2010), with permission from the American Association of Clinical Endocrinologists.]

统(CGMS)的葡萄糖参数,在(A)图(CGMS)记录显示一名23岁男子使用胰岛素泵,HbA1C为6.4%,但仍出现低血糖,死于床上综合征[31],(B)图显示了一名44岁的老年女性的血糖,她既往有严重的低血糖发作史且依赖外源性胰岛素维持血糖,胰岛移植后HbA1C为5.5%。

改善的胰岛素传递算法的精确技术的进步和葡萄糖传感技术为预防低血糖而纠正HbA1C提供了可能,从而扩大了胰岛素耐受的治疗窗[32,33]。然而,目前电流传感器的滞后现象、皮下位点注入胰岛素的输送和吸收仍然是这一技术的持续局限性。胰岛素泵上自动化的低葡萄糖暂停(LGS)胰岛素截流阀与闭环传感器相连接是缓解严重低血糖风险的重大进步[34,37]。该技术的现有局限性包括理想精度、可靠性和长时间连续葡萄糖监测的可持续性和与皮下胰岛素输送相关的时间间隔延迟。单用胰岛素,没有额外的反向调控的胰高血糖素,也被视为这一方法的另一个不足之处。

短期和长效胰岛素制剂的进步改善了血糖控制。最初的从牛和猪胰岛素转变到重组合成人类胰岛素时,人们担心反向调节反应降低会导致低血糖和昏迷的增加[38-40]。最近引入的长效基础微晶体胰岛素类似物,甘精(赛诺菲-安万特公司,巴黎,法国)具有更长的18~26h作用时效,相比于中性鱼精蛋白胰岛素,一般发生严重低血糖的风险较低,但仍不能解决易感患者严重的复发性低血糖症[41-44]。最初促进吸入型胰岛素的发展被视为一种很有前途的和创新的方法,因为其血管吸收更加迅速,而且看起来有吸引力,因为它不需要重复注射。在实践中,对照试验未能证明该方法的优势,2007年,辉瑞退出了Exuberta的生产,其他公司相继退出,只有MannKind公司仍在接受FDA审查。由于存在可能会轻微增加肺癌的风险、缺乏优势以及相当大的和不合理的费用等问题,这些都会阻碍这一方法的进一步发展[45,46]。

尽管在自身免疫性糖尿病小鼠模型中得出的数据表现出巨大的前景,旨在预防和早期干预T1DM的努力仍令人失望。在非肥胖糖尿病(NOD)小鼠模型中,超过463例/次介入治疗已证明其能够不同程度地预防或逆转自身免疫性糖尿病[47]。尽管投资巨大并在最近开展了一系列大规模的临床试验,致力于转化从老鼠到T1DM患者的几个最有前途的方法仍然受挫[48]。这带来人类疾病小鼠模型的效用问题[49]。一些初步临床试验数据是令人鼓舞的,包括非Fc段结合的CD3抗体[50-53]、霉酚酸酯(MMF)+达利珠单抗[54]、美罗华B淋巴细胞消耗[55,56]、可溶性NBI-6024修饰的胰岛素多肽配体[57]、维生素D_3[58]、烟酰胺[59]、肠胃外胰岛素、口服胰岛素、鼻喷剂胰岛素、消婴儿牛奶喂养可能减轻糖尿病发病,以及延长内源性C-肽代谢维持蜜月期[48,59-61]。到目前为止,当进行足够有力的随机对照试验时,这些方法都无法显示出强有益的效力。Voltarelli等首先报道,也许目前最有前途的方法是在粒细胞集落刺激因子动员后使用静脉内非脊髓抑制的自体造血干细胞移植,并使用抗胸腺细胞球蛋白和环磷酰胺调节[62-67]。这种“免疫重置”方法旨在消除自身免疫和非自身免疫淋巴细胞克隆以及后续的免疫重建。更新报告显示,20名新发病T1DM患者实现胰岛素自主分泌,其中12人保持这一状态平均31个月,2例发生医院获得性肺炎,9例出现精子减少,无死亡病例[63,68,69]。这种方法的机制可能是恢复凋亡相关基因的失调所导致免疫耐受障碍和T1DM[70]。这一有趣方法的风险收益和可持续性仍需持续的试验进一步明确。

因此,对于大多数T1DM患者,标准或强化胰岛素治疗方案目前仍然是金标准,同时清楚地了解到更严格的血糖控制可降低继发性糖尿病并发症的风险,但大大增加了麻烦的、偶尔危及生命的低血糖症的风险。胰岛素泵、动态血糖监测系统和胰岛素晶体结构设计的改进相当大地改善了许多T1DM患者的病情。然而,对于少数患者,日常中经常性低血糖或继发性并发症则是难以承受的负担。对这些人来说,胰岛移植是一个越来越有吸引力的选择。全胰腺移植提供了恢复血糖的可能,并且通常比胰岛移植可以抵制更大的代谢压力储备。两种方法都需要类似水平的免疫抑制,但胰岛移植代表一个更简便的解决方案(图108.2)。没有外分泌组件的内分泌替代的胰岛移植很容易通过非手术和极低风险的方法完成。相比之下,全胰腺移植的风险和预后在过去的四分之一个世纪有了很大改进,目前国际上已有30 000多人接受了这一治疗方法[71-74]。从患者的角度来看,避免胰腺移植过程中潜在的剖腹手术、胰腺炎、移植物血栓形成、手术部位感染和偶尔的死亡风险使得胰岛移植成为更有吸引力的选择,能够随着时间的推移,提供类似的代谢作用[75-78]。

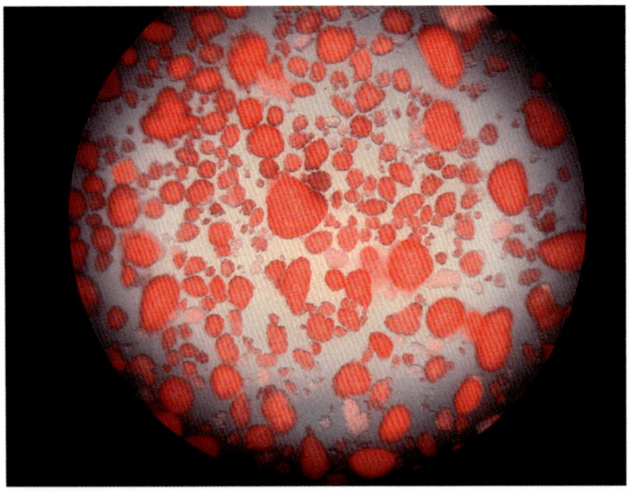

图 108.2 制备完成的提纯人胰岛细胞，用二硫腙染色进行定量。胰岛的大小在 50~500μm 之间，采用胰岛等同物(IEQ)来评估最终的胰岛质量，通常制备>5000 IEQ/kg 受体体重的胰岛可足够用于移植。

胰岛移植的患者选择和程序性适应证

临床胰岛移植患者的选择基于表 108.1 总结的适应证。患者选择的额外讨论，等待胰岛或胰腺移植患者的管理见第 33 章和第 41 章。

胰岛移植

胰岛移植的适应证(ITA)需要 T1DM 的证据(C-肽阴性)，有足够的时间(> 5 年)来证明，已经由一个独立的糖尿病专家或内分泌学家通过所有合理的替代尝试来纠正和稳定血糖，包括优化强化胰岛素或胰岛素泵治疗联合频繁的血糖监测[79]。一系列客观评分的应用，包括详细的患者调查问卷(克拉克分数)[80]，并严格审查详细的血糖记录，以允许计算低血糖得分和不稳定性指数(LI)[81]。表 108.1 总结的阈值代表目前大多数中心或 CIT 联合实验中心可接受的胰岛移植的适应证[79]。选择 T1DM > 5 年的患者，以确保足够的机会选择提供的最佳医疗方案。年龄>18 岁的限制反映了普遍的共识，即在儿科人群应避免终身免疫抑制，除了在极其罕见的情况下，替代手段不能避免低血糖造成的死亡风险或不可逆脑损伤[8]。避免受者体重> 90kg 与每日胰岛素需求>1.0U/kg 的目的是避免存在显著的胰岛素抵抗时的无效移植(表 108.1A)。

表 108.1 胰岛移植的适应证

A.胰岛移植(ITA)
1 型糖尿病，持续时间>5 年
年龄>18 岁，体重<90kg，胰岛素用量<1.0U/kg/d
无恶性肿瘤或未受控制的感染
依从性较好
难治性低血糖血症或血糖不稳定，尽管：
1.合理监控的最优的强化胰岛素或胰岛素泵
2.在内分泌专家的指导下用药
3.有明显的低血糖风险迹象：
Ⅰ.克拉克评分≥4
Ⅱ.HYPO 评分≥1000
Ⅲ.不稳定指数(LI)≥400
Ⅳ.同时 HYPO 指数≥400 和 LI 指数≥300
B.肾移植后胰岛移植
成功的肾移植术后发生 1 型糖尿病
免疫抑制剂耐受
肾上腺皮质激素≤5mg/d
无 BK 病毒感染或其他活跃的机会性感染
PRA<20%

For Clarke Score, see ref [80].

For HYPO Score and Lability Index, see ref [81].

肾移植后胰岛移植

在肾移植后胰岛移植的情况下，胰岛移植的适应证更加明确，因为患者已经承受免疫抑制的慢性风险(表 108.1b)。在 IAK 移植情况，患者必须首先有一个功能良好的移植肾，并能够耐受标准的免疫抑制治疗。一些中心使用糖皮质激素用于肾移植后维持治疗，尽管有人担心强的松的胰岛素抵抗和胰岛毒性，如果剂量为每天≤5mg，副作用是可以忽略的，事实上胰岛移植排斥可通过加用类固醇治疗成功逆转[82-85]。肾移植比其他器官更容易受到 BK 病毒感染，在 1971 年从第一例肾移植患者尿液中分离出这种多瘤病毒并以患者的姓名首字母命名[86]。BK 肾病的恶化会带来问题，而且在消耗疗法过程中有加重可能。因此在潜在 IAK 受者中应筛查 BK 病毒，以避免额外风险[87]。最后，避免广泛 HLA 致敏状态的受者和之前肾移植排斥高反应性抗体(PRA)、输血或妊娠可能对胰岛移植的成功有重要帮助[88,89]。此外，应认识到肾移植仅有 8~15 年的有限半生期[90,91]，二次肾移植可能很快会成为肾移植的最常见适应证(肾移植名单上 20%的患者是由于首次移植失败)，进一步额外的胰岛致敏增加的 PRA 问题在这类人群中格外突出[92–94]。因此,初始 PRA<20%可能是 IAK 移植的合理界限。

胰岛移植的风险

程序性风险

胰岛移植这种细胞疗法尤其有吸引力，因为这种细胞疗法可以通过一个简单的经皮经肝方法安全地输送入肝内门静脉系统,避免了手术。事实上,在经验丰富的高容量胰岛移植中心，目前这一过程比其他任何实体器官移植更安全。尽管如此,门静脉内输注方法仍存在潜在风险,包括腹腔出血和门静脉血栓形成,但通过针道消融等细节措施和门静脉内治疗性肝素化密切结合则可以避免这些并发症[95]。胰岛移植的技术细节在第 61 章深入讨论。

最常见的并发症是轻微疼痛或导管插入位点的不适,或右肩牵涉性疼痛,是短暂的,多达 50%的患者会发生,其很容易通过标准的镇痛药物控制,通常在 24~48h 之内完全缓解。

出血

尽管使用肝素抗凝治疗（70U/kg 受者体重门脉内灌注，然后以每小时 3U/kg 静脉输液调整至 60~80s的即按即通），现在我们的病例中需要外科干预的大量出血仍然极其罕见,比率<1%(3/342 例,阿尔伯塔大学)[95,96]。使用 4F 或 5F 的导管在肝实质留下较窄的穿刺道,且这种带有胶原糊或 D–STAT 的穿刺道轨道长度至少为 4cm,可有效防止腹腔出血[97–99]。使用这种方法,最近在埃德蒙顿的 150 次操作中,我们无需输血、腹腔镜或手术治疗腹腔出血[95,96]。在一个特殊病例中,我们遇到了右胸腔内出血，出血很快就被发现并通过血管造影消融肋间动脉及随后的胸引流管插入得以控制。针道消融技术不能控制这种伤害。使用超声引导帮助进入门静脉,避免肋下或肋骨边缘穿刺,可能有助于避免这种伤害[100–102]。

门静脉血栓形成

完全性门静脉系统血栓形成是门脉内胰岛移植最可怕的并发症[103–105]。然而,在当前低内毒素胶原酶,连续梯度净化,常规胰岛培养,门脉压力监测,治疗性肝素化,控制胰岛组织块体积≤5cc 的时代[106–115],完整的血栓形成伴慢性门静脉高血压后遗症已是罕见的并发症。在阿尔伯塔大学 164 名患者的 342 次经皮门静脉内输注，我们现在还没有遇到胰岛移植后完全性门静脉主干血栓形成(发生率为 0%)。此外,13 年的随访中没有一名患者表现出门静脉高压的迹象[95,96]。

我们偶尔观察到门静脉分支闭塞这种完全良性的情况。这往往不会波及门脉主干，也不会引起门脉高压。门静脉分支闭塞在之前的病例中发病率为 3.7%，但自从引入治疗性肝素化后，过去 5 年的发生率明显降低[95,116]。肝素治疗后常使用维生素 K 拮抗剂(华法林)治疗 3 个月,但这可能是没有必要的,因为刺激因素(胰岛沉积)是短暂的过程。患者存在潜在的血栓形成倾向,包括蛋白质 C、S 和抗凝血酶 3 缺乏,V 因子莱顿突变可能增加这一并发症的风险，筛查患者之前血栓形成病史可能会降低这种风险[117]。

胆囊穿刺损伤和偶然胆道穿刺损伤

经皮经肝方法可能会导致无意的胆囊刺穿损伤，但如果常规应用超声指导可以完全避免这一并发症[97,99,100]。肝实质内胆管造影术预计使用 22 gauge 导引穿刺针,一般不会导致胆漏[118]。

短暂肝功能指标上升和肝脏脂肪变性

在前面已描述过门脉内胰岛移植后肝脏转氨酶短暂轻微的升高，可见于一半的病例,27%可能升高到5倍。往往在没有干预的情况下,一个月内可完全恢复正常[119]。有趣的是,采用常规胰岛培养步骤,如改善的胶原酶、治疗性肝素化并使用抗炎剂(英夫利昔单抗、依那西普、阿那白滞素,阿司匹林),根据我们最近的经验,转氨酶升高的发生率和严重性已经明显降低。

超声波、磁共振成像(MRI)和肝活检可观察到在胰岛移植和自体移植受者中肝脂肪变性多达 20%[120–124]。脂肪沉积通常呈泡状,处于中央部位,可能反映了局部功能胰岛的高胰岛素释放。胰岛发生免疫排斥时这些变化是可逆的[120,122]。这些变化与胰岛受者非酒精性脂肪肝(NASH)无关,但它们的长期影响仍需进一步随访来明确。

肝癌风险

之前有人担忧当胰岛栓塞肝脏会有潜在的肝细胞

转化为肝细胞癌(HCC)的可能。Dombrowski 等最先描述链脲佐菌素诱导的糖尿病大鼠在接受胰岛移植后组织块出现肝腺瘤和肝细胞肝癌的发生率增加，随后在自发糖尿病 BB/Pfd 的老鼠模型中观察到类似的变化，肝内移植胰岛局部释放一系列营养因子增加了这一风险[125,126]。这一观测似乎只局限于大鼠。自 1977 年来，已有超过 1500 人接受临床胰岛自体或同种异体移植，目前仍没有关于这一并发症的个案报告，因此推测临床胰岛移植引起肝脏恶变的风险可以忽略[7,127-129]。

传播感染和受污染的胰岛准备

在实体器官移植中已经很好地描述了供体来源的严重感染风险(细菌、真菌、病毒或朊病毒相关)。典型的例子包括来自供体宠物仓鼠的丙型肝炎的传播、人类免疫缺陷病毒(HIV)和淋巴细胞性脉络丛脑膜炎导致 3 名器官受者死亡，1 名供者被蝙蝠咬伤而感染狂犬病毒，导致 4 名肾脏、肝脏和一个动脉节段移植的受者死亡。幸运的是，供体来源的传染性感染在胰岛移植受者中已很少见[130-133]。在一名 45 岁女性西尼罗河病毒性脑炎的致命病例中，患者既往三年曾接受 2 次胰岛移植[134]。但在这个病例，受体有在马厩被蚊子咬的病史，感染显然不是供体来源[134]。仔细筛选供体、避免高风险供体用于非抢救移植、胰岛培养期间对供体组织长期的附加测试可以进一步降低供体来源的感染风险。供体选择提倡艾滋病毒、乙肝和丙肝的核酸检测(NAT)，供体感染高风险病例缩短检测窗口。我们推迟了几个高风险供体来源的胰岛移植，直到 NAT 测试已经发布且结果为阴性[135]。第 92 章对供体来源的传染性风险进行了更全面的叙述。

当胰岛分离和培养储存时，在准备工作过程中可能发生细菌污染。在培养基中添加抗生素可以降低这种风险。最终胰岛产品的革兰染色必须是阴性的，内毒素含量要低(<5EU/kg 受者体重)，必须留出一份没有暴露于抗生素的胰岛产品样本用于后来的特殊细菌和真菌培养。在 1998 年之前使用内毒素含量高的污染胶原酶可能是导致受者胰岛功能不佳的原因[136,137]。目前胶原酶混合物内毒素含量低。

因此，建议所有病例的胰岛移植受者预防性使用广谱抗生素治疗。然而，尽管在极少数情况下无意输注了污染的胰岛产品，也未观察到肝内脓肿或系统性感染后遗症，这无疑是让人放心的[138]。这种较低的感染风险可能与肝血流量高和肝脏内皮系统有着活跃的可吞噬细菌的枯否细胞有关。

免疫抑制挑战

胰岛毒性控制自身免疫和排斥

广义免疫抑制需要抑制同种异体移植物反应，这与许多特征明显的风险和副作用相关，最明显的是机会性感染和恶性肿瘤的风险增加。免疫抑制剂的类型、剂量和联合使用，决定了这些风险的发生频率增加。在临床胰岛移植，必须抑制强有力的复发性 T1DM 自身免疫反应和同种异体免疫反应。此外，与实体器官肝脏或肾脏移植早期就可检测到移植物失功相比，出现进展性高血糖内分泌失调往往已是胰岛排斥晚期和不可逆的标志[3,83,139]。临床上很难通过皮质类固醇治疗逆转胰岛排斥[84]，因此从一开始进行充分和持续的预防被认为是成功的关键因素[1]。尽管使用强有力的联合免疫抑制疗法，全胰腺移植后自身免疫性 T1DM 仍有复发，这可能是胰腺移植后 50%的胰岛素自主分泌维持 5 年的根本原因[140-143]。临床胰岛移植后复发性自身免疫伴选择性 β 细胞破坏也被肝活检标本明确[144]，这是经典的埃德蒙德方案系随访 5 年后不可逆的失去胰岛素自主分泌最可能的解释[145-147]。Roep 及其同事已经设计出一系列体外实验，用于检测胰岛移植后自身免疫反应，最近应用 HLA 量子点纳米技术更精确地定义胰岛肽段对前胰岛素原、胰岛抗原 2、谷氨酸脱羧酶 65、胰岛淀粉样多肽和其他靶标的反应[148-152]。这些和其他研究表明，有效控制自身免疫反应和同种异体免疫反应对 T1DM 胰岛移植的长期功能性生存至关重要[153-155]。

然而应用强有力的免疫抑制的同时，越来越多的研究发现，许多关键性免疫抑制剂对 β 细胞有特异毒性[156]。这无疑增加了胰岛移植的挑战，因为我们不能假定最佳实体器官移植免疫抑制策略同样适用于胰岛移植[82]。使用谱系追踪技术，Nir 等证明了他克莫司和西罗莫司(用于埃德蒙顿方案)明显抑制了小鼠 β 细胞再生[157]。Ricordi 等在免疫缺陷小鼠中强调了他克莫司对人类胰岛功能有早期直接毒性，Rostambeigi 等最近的研究也观察到胰岛素分泌和线粒体密度的降低[158,159]。我们知道，特别是在移植后早期，胰岛暴露于门静脉局部高浓度免疫抑制药物中[160,161]。有趣的是，西罗莫司被证明能够改善体内外的胰岛素分泌，而且其抗炎作用可能改善胰岛细胞培养的生存[162,163]。相反，Zhang 等在边缘质量小鼠胰岛移植模型观察到胰岛移植存活率下降和 β 细胞功能受损[164]。Merani 等发现在人类胰岛小鼠模型长效 GLP-1 类似物可保护性拮抗他克莫司和西罗莫司的免疫抑制毒性[165]。新型免疫抑制剂，如 sphingosine-1 磷酸酶受体调节剂 FTY720 缺乏 β 细胞毒性，在小鼠和灵长类动物的边缘组织块胰岛移植模型中看起来是有前景的，但其缺陷是被证明在早期临床试验中加速黄斑变性，这对 T1DM 伴预先存在的视网膜病变患者是一个不幸的副作用[166-171]。综上所述，尚无理想的用于胰岛移植的免疫抑制药物。目前只能使用可以提供可靠保护防止自身免疫和同种异体免疫，同时又不过分损害胰岛功能的折中方案。

胰岛移植免疫抑制的实用方法

第 65 章至第 67 章提供了一个诱导、维持和恢复免疫抑制管理策略的综述。我们这里关注当前临床胰岛移植免疫抑制的实用方法。

诱导疗法——达利珠单抗、巴利昔单抗、抗胸腺细胞球蛋白和阿仑单抗，以及巨细胞病毒、乙脑病毒及淋巴组织增生性疾病的风险

抗 IL2R 单克隆抗体达利珠单抗和巴利昔单抗自 2000 年以来已被广泛用于胰岛移植[1,2]。其授权的公司基于财政考虑决定达利珠单抗不再进行商业销售。尽管耐受性良好没有副作用，这些制剂对免疫抑制方案添加效力不大，并对 T1DM 自身免疫的影响很小。事实上，大规模的临床介入试验使用达利珠单抗和霉酚酸酯未能保护 β 细胞功能或扩展新发 T1DM 的蜜月期[54]。所以我们推荐 Hering 等提出的在临床胰岛移植使用淋巴细胞耗竭的方法，尤其是在初次胰岛移植时[4,172-174]。大量临床研究表明，在自身免疫调节和耐受方面，淋巴细胞耗竭是一个强有力的辅助策略[151,152,175-177]。Bellin 等最近分析了国际胰岛移植注册中心和明尼苏达州的数据，证明不考虑维护免疫抑制方案，特别是结合肿瘤坏死因子-α(TNF-α)阻滞，初次耗竭治疗对 5 年胰岛素非依赖预后产生深远影响(图 108.3)[172]。抗胸腺细胞球蛋白给出的累积剂量为 6mg/kg 的外周静脉输液超过 2~3 天，目标是胰岛被注入前至少 2mg/kg 同时保持胰岛细胞培养，以避免在耗竭细胞因子风暴期间移植[178]。在埃德蒙顿方案中，我们一直习惯用超过 3h 外周静脉注入 30mg 阿仑单抗进行淋巴细胞耗竭，是基于效能、耐受性、持续效果和成本。初始剂量阿仑单抗包括对乙酰氨基酚 650mg 口服，静脉注射苯海拉明 50mg 和甲泼尼龙 250mg。Calne 等首次开发阿仑单抗用于临床器官移植诱导与可耐受的方法结合低剂量环孢素[179-181]。我们在 2002 年开始将阿仑单抗用于胰岛移植，最初结合西罗莫司单一疗法，但观察到排斥率高，这和肾移植早期经验相类似[182-185]。在转换到他克莫司(目标槽前 3 个月 ≥10ng/mL)后，随后剂量是 8~10ng/mL，霉酚酸酯根据耐受情况每日最高 2g 的个体化剂量，我们发现这种方法是患者最耐受，且有着最优患者的 5 年胰岛素自主分泌(2012 年 Shapiro 个人观察)。Tan 等在中国福州的 7 名 IAK 受者使用阿仑单抗诱导结合西罗莫司和他克莫司维持，4/7 的患者获得 1 年胰岛素自主分泌[186]。迈阿密的 Froud 等使用阿仑单抗诱导结合短期钙调磷酸酶抑制，使用他克莫司和西罗莫司 3 个月，随后使用西罗莫司和霉酚酸酯，3 名患者中的 2 名获得胰岛素自主分泌[187]。尽管会导致严重而持续的淋巴细胞耗竭，目前仍有超过 2000 名实体器官移植患者接受阿仑单抗诱导，表明这种方法是安全的[74,188-204]。目前在阿尔伯塔大学和其他地方正在探索阿仑单抗在控制胰岛移植受者自身免疫中的作用。我们报道了胰岛移植受者运用抗胸腺细胞球蛋白或阿仑单抗耗竭疗法，尤其是在最初的巨细胞病毒预防时期后的应用，会伴有巨细胞病毒传播和激活的比例增加[205-207]。幸运的是这些事件很大程度上是亚临床的，只是通过 PCR 检测到，并没有导致相关的特定器官疾病，而且可很容易地通过静脉注射更昔洛韦或口服缬更昔洛韦治疗[205]。

OKT3 和 ATGAM 之前已证明与 EBV 相关的移植后淋巴组织增生失调(PTLD)发生率增加相关，而抗胸腺细胞球蛋白和阿仑单抗风险较低[208,209]。2246 例肾脏和心脏移植受者接受抗胸腺细胞球蛋白治疗的荟萃分析发现 5 年 PTLD 的发病率为 0.98%，显著低于缬更昔洛韦抗病毒预防的患者(0.63%)[210,211]。Kirk 等回顾了美

国大型数据库中 59 560 例肾移植受者的 PTLD 发病率,发现阿仑单抗(0.37%)发生 PTLD 的风险显著低于抗胸腺细胞球蛋白组(0.67%)[212]。分析中 mTOR 抑制剂的使用总体与 PTLD 强烈相关,作者认为,淋巴细胞耗竭本身不是 PTLD 的一个独立危险因素,而整体强度的免疫抑制是更相关的度量标准[212]。有趣的是,阿仑单抗已经有效用于治疗骨髓移植和血液恶性肿瘤的 PTLD[213,214]。在淋巴耗竭后骨髓和干细胞移植的情况下,尽管在这些高危人群有 EBV 激活,使用阿仑单抗与 PTLD 发生率极低有关(<1%)[215]。在实体器官移植阿仑单抗诱导后,PTLD 的报道很少。目前在任何主要临床试验中,即使诱导和维持方案不同,均无胰岛移植后 PTLD 的报道。尽管 Cure 等报道在 3 名接受他克莫司和西罗莫司的 IAK 受者中发现 EBV 迟发激活,但没有人转化为 PTLD[1,2,101,118,146,216,217]。

维持免疫抑制

选择普遍耐受的协同维持免疫抑制在胰岛移植中非常具有挑战性。希望使用"对胰岛有益的"对 β-细胞无毒的药物往往与提供强有力的持续性自身免疫和同种异体免疫的保护无法两全[7,156]。埃德蒙顿方案提倡高剂量西罗莫司(最初 3 个月维持 12~15μg/L 水平,然后减少至 10~12μg/L)结合低剂量他克莫司(4~6μg/L)作为一种手段,用以减少明显的或隐蔽性 T1DM 肾病的患者暴露于钙调磷酸酶抑制剂[1,218]。尽管这种方法在三大胰岛移植中心导致了前所未有的高比例的 1 年期胰岛素自主分泌[219],但当延伸到国际多中心试验时,这样的组合很难精确掌握[2,220]。高剂量西罗莫司在这一方案中被认为是主要原因[221],伴有无法忍受的口腔溃疡[105,118]、卵巢囊肿和女性闭经[222~224]、疲劳、腹泻、偶发严重的小肠溃疡[225]、肺炎[226]、外周和腹膜后水肿[123,227],以及西罗莫司导致的蛋白尿增加,这些副作用停药后是可逆的[228,229]。尽管西罗莫司在美国临床胰岛移植注册试验中仍是不可或缺的组成部分,由于上述副作用,阿尔伯塔大学放弃了在胰岛移植中常规使用这一制剂。更标准的移植免疫抑制方案中他克莫司加霉酚酸酯有着较好的耐受性,同时在副作用和依从性方面有很大优势。淋巴耗竭诱导和高剂量他克莫司和霉酚酸酯维持治疗可以使 5 年胰岛素自主分泌率大幅增加,表明理论上其胰岛毒性备受关注,但在实践中,这种组合可以有效地预防排斥和自身免疫复发。这种方法的缺点是需要在开始时排除潜在的糖尿病肾功能损害患者。目前一般建议治疗开始前需要肾功能储备充足的证据,估计基线为肾小球滤过率> 60mL/(min·1.73m²),白蛋白排泄率<300mg/g 肌酐。

胰腺移植中钙调磷酸酶抑制剂的避免

由于糖尿病是肾移植中最常见的并发症,因此在该领域中常优先考虑可以提供等效的无副作用,同时避免钙调磷酸酶抑制剂(CNI)的方案。虽然西罗莫司和霉酚酸酯可以提供有效的短期预防,在胰腺移植中只有结合淋巴耗竭诱导时才具有一定疗效,目前尚不清楚完全撤除 CNI 是否将影响 5 年胰岛素自主分泌率[172,187]。Posselt 等已经探索了两种不同的可能实现这些目标的策略[230]。他们发现胸腺细胞球蛋白诱导淋巴耗竭,联合贝拉西普的融合稳定共刺激通路可以保证只需西罗莫司或霉酚酸酯的无 CNI 方案[230]。此外,他们测试了通过抗白细胞功能性抗原 1 型抗体来阻断共刺激通路[230]。虽然非常令人鼓舞,这些早期观察目前仅限于每组的 5 个病例。而且由于其在治疗银屑病患者中出现了进行性多灶性白质脑病(在超过 46 000 名患者中,3 名确诊,1 名疑似),抗 LFA1 抗体非常不幸地退出了市场[231~233]。目前关于贝拉西普结合淋巴耗竭治疗的临床试验的许可也许会被进一步限制,此外,移植后贝拉西普疗法的药品市场监测,可能需要百时美施贵宝公司一个低风险的容忍度。因此,目前一个完美的在胰腺移植中消除 CNI 的方法尚不存在,仍需更长期广泛的测试。

辅助性围移植期预防性用药处理

预防性抗细菌、抗真菌和抗病毒管理一般遵循当地的实践指南,与移植传染病专家观点一致,通常我们建议在胰腺移植前服用广谱抗生素进行预防处理。

抗凝治疗

抗凝治疗已在第 61 章详细描述。总的说来,肝素(70U/kg)和胰岛一起门脉输注,启始肝素注入每小时 3U/kg,然后滴定保持 PTT 在 60~80s,并持续到移植后 48h。这种方法,结合强化胰岛素治疗,改善了我们的单供体胰岛移植预后[116]。此后,如果多普勒超声检查未发现出血或血栓形成,我们继续使用低分子量肝素(肝素 30mg,2 次/日)7 天,移植后 14 天内服用阿司匹林肠溶片 81mg。

抗炎药物

伴随药物治疗可能包括应用维生素 E(800iU 移植前和移植后 7 天口服),用依那西普进行抗 TNF-α 阻断(50mg 静脉移植前, 然后移植后第 3、第 7 和第 10 天 25mg 皮下注射,Hering 等的方案。)[4,174]。Farney 等最初在老鼠身上描述这种方法[234]。当联合使用依那西普、抗 IL1β 受体抗体和阿那白滞素时,McCall 等最近在免疫缺陷小鼠临界组织块人类胰岛移植中发现显著的作用[235]。Matsumoto 等的初步临床数据表明,这种组合可能在小部分胰岛受者中是有益的[236]。Bellin 等令人鼓舞的数据表明,进行胰岛移植时用依那西普或英夫利昔单抗强力抗炎、抗 TNFα 策略可能对 5 年胰岛素自主分泌率具有持久的积极影响,特别是当结合淋巴耗竭诱导疗法时(图 108.3)[172]。我们通常在移植后 7 天给予己酮可可碱 400mg 口服,之后采用经典的吉森方案[237]。

巨细胞病毒的预防

建议所有接受耗竭疗法的受试者使用缬更昔洛韦预防巨细胞病毒和 EBV, 无论供体和受体巨细胞病毒状态如何,开始 450mg 每日一次,移植后持续 14 天,然后增加到 900mg 每日一次,维持 12 周[205]。我们进一步推荐磺胺甲噁唑 400mg-甲氧苄啶 80mg 每日一次,维持 6 个月,预防移植后肺孢子虫。如果对磺胺过敏,可用喷他脒 300mg 吸入取代,但应避免使用氨苯砜,因为它会干扰糖化血红蛋白测定[238]。

胰岛移植患者其他长期风险

死亡

胰岛移植后死亡风险极其少见。现在在阿尔伯塔大学,13 年随访后我们精确的生存概率是 96%(158/164 例)。就我们所知,没有由于直接或非直接的免疫抑制原因死亡的病例。在 6 例死亡病例中,4 例是由于潜在的心脏微血管病、冠脉阻塞或是心律失常,1 例是由于胰岛移植失败及免疫抑制剂延长使用导致的致死性低血糖,1 例是由于严重的眼痛使用了过量的美沙酮,患者之前是逐步增加美沙酮剂量,然后停止服用。两年后突然重新服用之前的剂量导致死亡。

最近来自 CIT 国际注册中心的数据显示当前共有 18 例死亡患者(包括之前 6 例在埃德蒙顿死亡的),总计 1.3%,其中 15 例患者是在 1999—2003 年间行胰岛移植的[239]。对于这些病例来说,1 例明确是和胰岛移植或免疫抑制剂使用相关的,3 例可能是相关的。但并没有收集合适的非胰岛移植病例数据作为对照, 在与胰岛移植等待列表里的病例头对头研究中, 越来越多的证据显示因严重低血糖导致死亡的病例, 与在胰岛移植和优化胰岛素的药物治疗中的比例类似。

肿瘤

按照肿瘤来看, 在 CITR 有 16 例皮肤基底癌或鳞

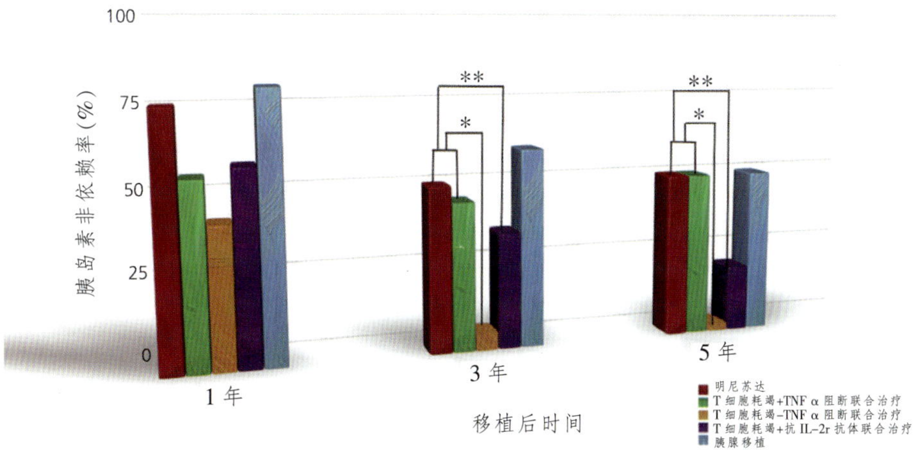

图 108.3 胰腺单独移植(PTA)与临床胰岛移植中不同诱导和抗炎策略的 5 年胰岛素非依赖性的比较。来自美国移植杂志的数据(reproduced from [172] Bellin et al. 2012, with kind permission from Wiley)显示,当 T 细胞耗竭+TNF-α 阻断联合应用时,5 年胰岛素非依赖率为 50%。这些结果等同于国际胰腺移植登记资料中 5 年间观察到的 PTA 的 50%胰岛素非依赖率。*$P<0.01$;**$P\leqslant 0.05$。

状细胞癌发生，总比例为2.3%[239]。大多数被认为和免疫抑制有关，都进行了完全切除治疗。此外，CITR中还发生2例乳腺癌、2例肺癌和2例甲状腺癌(0.35%的发生率)[239]。越来越多的证据表明西罗莫司可能在减少移植患者恶性肿瘤的发生中扮演保护角色[240-249]。

HLA致敏作用

HLA的致敏风险已经被高度关注，这是因为患者接受来自超过1个供体的胰岛以及不合适的免疫抑制方案会由于排斥变得高致敏。这可能阻止他们未来成功地接受胰岛、胰腺或肾脏移植。来自埃德蒙顿的Campbell等证明HLA抗体的存在与更差的胰岛移植预后有关，强调更详细的高分辨率和标准化的HLA抗体筛查和移植术前的交叉配血是必要的[88]。我们曾报道广泛HLA致敏率较高的高反应组抗体（PRA）与C肽阴性胰岛移植病例的失败有关，但这种分组仅代表受检总数的一小部分，占整体风险的16%[89]。完全撤除免疫抑制是一个激进的因素，是否有可能用预防性低剂量持续单一疗法预防致敏依旧是个问题。有趣的是，更强力的阿仑单抗、他克莫司和骁悉方案被认为与低的PRA致敏有关(未发表的数据，Shapiro Edmonton)，Geneva-GRAGIL network已经报道在IAK患者中低HLA致敏(10.8%的风险)，虽然用了多个供体，在比例上相当于单独肾移植[250]。回顾CITR数据库HLA Ⅰ级致敏风险表明，移植后PRA≥20%会使器官衰竭风险增加3.6倍[251]。Rickels等已经明确建议使致敏风险最小化，包括避免使用多个胰岛移植，在移植前用高分辨率手段等待阴性的细胞毒交叉配型，避免供受体在移植前出现可识别的抗原不和[252]。

长期结局

现在CIT注册中心积累了最近的570名患者，一系列最近来自胰岛移植中心的数据表明，5年胰岛素非依赖比例正在逐年升高[172,239]。原始的埃德蒙顿系列报道术后5年胰岛素非依赖率不可避免地降低了，只有15%的患者仍然完全不需要胰岛素(图108.4A)[2,7,145,146]。虽然长期结果对于埃德蒙顿来说低于他们的预期，随访10年后73%的病例血糖控制稳定，完全避免了低血糖症的复发，校正HbA1C少于6.5%。相似的结果在CITR数据库中也有反映[253]。除非使用胰岛素泵或CGMS管理器，这种血糖控制稳定很少见，但要求终身免疫抑制治疗，对比仍有不同的观点[254-259]。胰岛素储备退化的解释多种多样，但明显是多因素作用的结果。自身免疫复发、排斥反应和胰岛B细胞增殖能力受抑制可能是显性因素，对一个受伤的、发炎的、低剂量的最初的胰岛植入物会增加额外的压力(图108.4B)[124,260-264]。对边缘胰岛移植物进行代谢过度刺激会引起内质网相关胰岛细胞凋亡和对胰岛功能有害的淀粉蛋白沉积[265-268]。现在注册在ClinicalTrials.gov的超过80个临床研究有很多机会，以完全的生理的无损伤无发言状态的最初胰岛移植物作为初步目标，从而研究未来避免终身使用

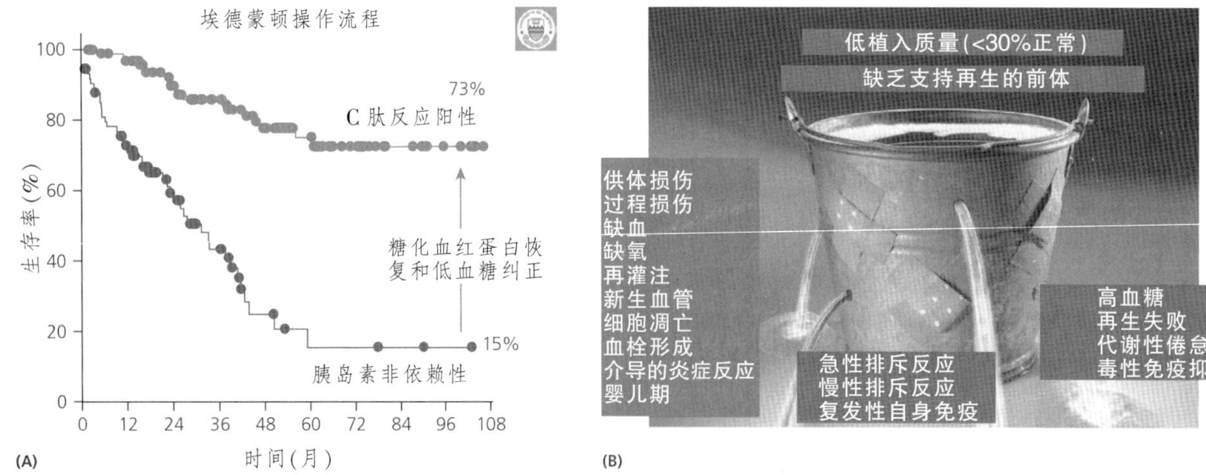

图108.4 (A)根据原始埃德蒙顿操作流程，胰岛素非依赖性在5年内必然损失，但在规律的C肽分泌维持下，73%的病例能够有糖化血红蛋白的校正并预防低血糖发作。(Data from [2,7,145,146].)(B)对这些患者逐渐丧失胰岛素独立性的可能多因素解释。有限的初始胰岛移植质量和再生失败，特别是复发性自身免疫是未来胰岛移植试验中必须克服的主要挑战。背景图：www.tsamedien.de。

免疫抑制的耐受实验。

现在，至少 5 个独立胰岛移植中心报道术后 5 年有 50%~70%的胰岛素非依赖患者应用不同的诱导和维持方案[4,172-174,269,270]。胰岛单独移植在这方面的结果表现出持续上升的趋势，而且根据 IPTR 的数据在 5 年内结果已经接近全胰腺移植[71,172]。这种等效性结果带来的影响需要一段时间才能在患者和移植界中有所反应。一项经皮下的胰岛细胞移植受到了新的追捧，操作容易，同时可以避免大型手术的创伤和与之伴随的严重并发症。但目前这项细胞移植需要多名胰岛供者，同时有 50%的失败率，且仅具有 cGMP 胰岛分离技术的少数几个中心具有该项资质，所以仍然有待提升。值得一提的是，目前这项技术并没有广泛的医保覆盖(美国)。最近一组令人印象深刻的来自旧金山的研究数据显示，在 45 个来自 50 岁以下供体的胰腺组织有 82%的成功率，供体平均 BMI 为 34，同时分离出来胰岛物平均有 630 000IEQ。如果这一水平的胰岛分离技术能够传播到其他中心，这将会对胰岛的分配模式和选择更年轻的最佳捐献者产生重大影响。

CIT 联盟实验和其他政府资助

CIT 联盟是一个在 2004 年由过敏传染疾病国家研究所(NIAID)和美国国立卫生研究院(NIH)下糖尿病和消化及肾脏疾病国家研究所(NIDDK)最初以 750 万设计促进临床胰岛移植的机构[5,271]。共 10 个胰岛制造点和 12 个临床中心是积极参与者，包括美国、加拿大和瑞典的中心。这一联盟的主要目标是发起两个Ⅲ期临床试验(CIT-07、islet alone IAT 和 CIT-06，IAK)，将被 FDA 用于生物执照申请(BLA)和以后的第三方美国胰岛移植的医疗补助和医疗保险的报销[5]。BLA 需要向 FDA 提交详细的、标准的胰岛制造方案，还要综合评述这一生物产品的医疗效果。最后，CIT 联合组织形成了标准的胰岛生产工艺、临床患者的护理、严格的终点判定，以及两种不同的 ITA 和 IAK 人群的风险因素[5]。可预计的是，CIT-07 项目将会在 2013 年底完成 HbA1C 对低血糖血症保护作用的相关性研究，最终在 2014—2015 年间公布最终研究结果。这份最终研究报告会形成 BLA 的基础。

其他 CIT 中心Ⅰ/Ⅱ期试验目前正在研究接近于通过抑制瞬时的血液介导的炎症反应提升胰岛移植，更安全，通过贝拉西普或脱氧精胍菌素进行共刺激封锁的不使用 CNI 的免疫抑制方案，或者联合使用 B 细胞和 T 细胞消耗治疗，或者艾塞那肽(GLP-1)治疗[5]。

数个其他国家已经成功得到了政府支持，特别是在加拿大(通过阿尔伯塔政府的省级资助)、英国(促进健康和临床国家研究所——NICE)、瑞士和澳大利亚，澳大利亚政府联合青少年糖尿病研究基金会(表 108.2)。

单独胰岛和胰岛后肾移植比较——类似的结局

与全胰腺移植只有 18%最终成为 PTA 相反，过去 10 年中，84%的胰岛移植为 ITA，只有 16%为 IAK[71,73,239]。这反映了一个普遍的观点，就是伴随终末期肾病的 T1DM 是最适合外科联合或连续实体器官移植的，而拥有良好肾功能及控制能力的 TIDM 患者适合胰岛移植，和 SPK 移植相比，PTA 风险更高且结果也略差[71,77,272]。同时胰岛-肾移植(SIK)已经在有限的病例中被证实是成功的，但要在同一尸体供者中实施可行仍有一些细节问题，而且在 50%的胰岛分离失败的可能性下并不适合广泛应用[186,273,274]。

更进一步考虑 IAK 移植似乎是恰当的，由于先行肾移植可带来免疫抑制的风险收益平衡。IAK 移植现在是在 CIT-06 与 CIT 联盟 BLA 试验中主要的平行试验[5]。在早些时候，有个担忧就是胰岛移植可能通过供体致敏作用增加移植肾的免疫风险，但至今为止没有这种病例发生，并且有功能的胰岛存在确实能对肾脏起到保护作用[250,273,275-278]。

表 108.2 国家报销胰岛移植

国家	机构	年度
加拿大	省级报销	2001 年
	阿尔伯塔省政府	
英国	国立临床卓越研究所(NICE)	2008 年
澳大利亚	澳大利亚政府	2011 年
	青少年糖尿病研究基金会(联合资金)	
瑞士	瑞士政府 GRAGIL 联盟	2000 年
北欧网络	瑞典政府	2008 年
美国	FDA	
	生物许可证申请(BLA)	2014—2015 年

胰岛移植和对继发糖尿病并发症的影响

全胰腺移植积累的令人瞩目的数据清晰地证明接近完美的血糖控制的主要保护获益在于稳定和反转冠脉疾病、颈动脉内膜的增厚、糖尿病肾病、神经病变、视网膜病变和其他继发的T1DM并发症，并且能降低心血管疾病的死亡率[279-291]。临床胰岛移植中也有同样引人注目的数据，在稳定正常的血糖和逆转次要的糖尿病并发症中有保护效果。米兰小组已经证实临床胰岛移植伴随C肽阳性能稳定T1DM的大血管和微血管病变,而与独立的胰岛素水平无关[263,277,292-296]。来自温哥华小组的Thompson等设计了一个前瞻性队列交叉研究来比较胰岛移植介入的最佳药物治疗[297]。在胰岛移植组视网膜病变进展减少了，神经传导速度有改善的趋势[298]。此外,虽然CNI免疫抑制剂增加,在胰岛移植组相比较药物治疗组肾小球滤过率有下降[297]。尚需要更多的随机对照研究来更深入地证实这一阳性结果,但有可能在资金和实施方面存在困难。

单供体胰岛移植

2000年,埃德蒙顿方案使用多个(平均2个,2~4个)胰岛供体进行胰岛移植提供了一个足量的胰岛数量来维持短期的(1~3年)胰岛素非依赖,但也有人对这一方法的实用性和潜在的HLA致敏作用带来的风险有顾虑[1,88,89]。目前的观念是单个胰腺能够提供足够的胰岛来治疗多个受体，这第一次由Payne等在兔子中证实,随后,Griffin等在犬中也证实了[299,300]。这种做法会主要影响胰岛支持并影响T1DM的治疗范围,但它尚未在临床上证明。也许最接近成功的一个例子是日本活体胰岛自移植,母亲移植到女儿身上。T1DM受体仅用了50%的远端胰腺就获得了胰岛素非依赖[301]。

因此,明尼苏达州系列病例有着明显的优点,它们通过非Fc结合抗CD3抗体用于诱导，同时与胰岛优化净化梯度一起，使用Optiprep在胰岛素样生长因子Ⅰ存在下进行胰岛培养，应用依那西普抗TNFα阻断和移植前的胰岛素和肝素，最终能够保持较高的单供体移植比例[4]。供体和受体潜在的选择偏倚因素可能有利于高胰岛素效力、产量、胰岛素需要量和受体抵抗，从而影响了阐明单供体一致的成功的机制，但很明显这是一个理想的结果[302]。数个其他中心和方法报道了不同的单供体移植成功率(表108.3)。Markmann等在7名患者中的5名患者里应用类似埃德蒙顿的方案,应用高BMI供体获得了类似的单供体胰岛移植成功[303]。我们确信使用Hering的方法联合术前加强胰岛素和肝素作为调节移植物提升方案，发现使用这一方案单供体胰岛素的非依赖比率从10%上升到40%，是IBMIR效果令人鼓舞的临床示范[116,304,305]。埃默里和旧金山小组都描述了在单供体胰岛移植中依法丽珠单抗在无CNI方案中的高比例使用,但不再在临床使用(早些讨论)[230,306,307]。当精准的胰岛效力测定实验普及到应用实验的各方面时，我们就可以明确哪个方案的特点部分有助于单供体细胞植入[308-310]。

GLP-1类似物的临床试验

使用短活力的GLP-1类似物艾塞那肽已经被迈阿密、温哥华和伊利诺伊大学组广泛应用作为促进单供体和补充的胰岛移植物的一种手段[311-317]。虽然艾塞那肽明显对胰岛功能有积极的直接和间接影响，仍需要持续治疗,以维持边缘移植物功能。高达30%的患者不能耐受因艾塞那肽产生的严重恶心。长效GLP-1类似物利拉鲁肽作为代替物，已经有更低的恶心反应和临床不耐受发生率。Merani等发现,利拉鲁肽在小鼠中

表108.3 单供体胰岛方案

作者	中心	方法	年[参考文献]
Hering等	明尼苏达	抗-CD3+依那西普	2005[4,172]
Markmann等	宾夕法尼亚	埃德蒙顿类似	2003[303]
Turgeon等	埃默里	依法珠单抗+霉酚酸酯	2010[306]
Posselt等	旧金山	ATG+依法利珠单抗+西罗莫司/霉酚酸酯	2010[230]
Posselt等	旧金山	ATG+贝拉西普+西罗莫司/霉酚酸酯	2010[230]
Koh等	埃德蒙顿	围移植期胰岛素+肝素	2010[116]
Matsumoto等	京都	活体胰岛移植	2005[301]
Matsumoto等	贝勒	ATG+阿那白滞素+依那西普	2011[236]
Ghofaili等	温哥华	艾塞那肽	2007[316]
Faradji等	迈阿密	艾塞那肽	2009[311]
Gangemi等	UIC芝加哥	艾塞那肽	2008[317]

能提升人边缘数量的胰岛移植物，在体内和体外减少免疫抑制剂对 β 细胞的毒性作用[165]。当在一个快速增长的大型动物猪胰岛自体移植模型中测试时，利拉鲁肽的应用有助于帮助抵抗代谢移植物失功[318]。当加入胰岛培养基，利拉鲁肽在小鼠中明显增加了人胰岛细胞边缘数量移植物的存活,减少了凋亡[319]。基于这些数据,Novo Nordisk 在 16 处主要的国际试验点,对利拉鲁肽在临床胰岛移植中的作用做随机对照研究[320]。

目前临床试验中的不同策略

IBMIR 控制

瑞士研究小组一直对在门脉内胰岛移植后数分钟内发生的,通过增加组织因子表达、血小板聚集、炎症反应导致的内源性 IBMIR 胰岛损伤感兴趣[304,321],从死亡胰岛释放的凝血酶-抗凝血酶复合物和 C 肽的高循环水平证实这是一个明确的临床实体，通过正电子发射断层扫描成像在经门脉内胰岛移植的患者中标记的人胰岛可以检测出的丧失也证实这是在围移植期的胰岛保护的一个主要因素[322,323]。外源性胰岛素和肝素可以部分影响该反应并提高单个供体的移植率[116]。在猪胰岛移植模型中，肝素与胰岛的表面结合测试是一种有效方法,有待临床进一步评估[305]。此外,如同肝素一样，将血管内皮生长因子锚定在胰岛表面可以潜在地刺激胰岛血管生成[324]。临床上可能进一步测试几种策略,包括低分子量葡聚糖、直接凝血酶抑制剂(如水蛭素、去唾液酸、美拉曲坦、达比加群)和其他外在凝血途径的高特异性抑制剂。这些方法对于胰岛存活平衡,同时避免过度出血的风险将至关重要。

控制凋亡

我们的基础实验关注于胰岛凋亡临时抑制，这是因为我们最初的实验证明这条通路对人胰岛具有损伤作用。Emamaullee 等证明,病毒转染体外胰岛细胞与 x 连锁抑制剂细胞凋亡蛋白(XIAP)可以改善边缘数量胰岛移植物的存活[325-327]。一个 Fluoromethylketone(FMK)代替物 ZVAD-FMK 也很高效,但由于其毒性太大而限制了其临床应用[328]。Nakano 等证明 FMK 来源的 caspase-3 抑制剂在体外能保护人胰岛细胞,但缺乏蛋白酶(pan-caspase)抑制作用可能降低这一效果[329]。我们进一步探索一种有效的被称为 EP1013 的泛蛋白酶抑制剂，发现只需要 10%~30%的边缘数量小鼠或人胰岛移植物就可以扭转小鼠糖尿病,此外这也是一个促进高效共刺激封锁诱导免疫耐受诱导小鼠的方法[330,331]。由于 EP1013 失去专利和地位,不再可用于试验。因此,我们首先用人胰岛在小鼠中测试了类似的泛蛋白酶 (IDN-6556,科莱特斯制药公司,圣地亚哥)抑制剂,并随后在大型动物猪边缘数量胰岛自体移植模型进行测试,都得到类似的令人信服的数据[332]。这一机构目前正在进行临床前 Ⅰ/Ⅱ 期实验并进行埃德蒙顿的有效的胰岛移植患者的临床研究。虽然当细胞凋亡受抑制,尤其是与强的免疫抑制相组合有导致恶性肿瘤发生的相关理论问题,短期(2 周)临时治疗应该有希望抵消这种风险。

免疫耐受

通过消除在 T1DM 中活跃的自身反应性 T 细胞克隆以及永久消除同种异体反应，完全恢复自我耐受性是胰岛移植从治疗状态达到治愈的关键变革步骤。尽管这种耐受性可在小鼠中常规获得，偶尔在大型动物非自身免疫性灵长类动物移植模型中也可以实现对这些有区别但又相互关联的攻击途径的双重耐受[3]。第 11 章和第 76 章详细论述了与临床有关的耐受和应用的具体细节,在此不再赘述。共刺激阻断是诱导小鼠外周耐受诱导的有前途的方法,但由于不同的成熟度、暴露情况、结合亲和力、受体表达和异源免疫的混杂效应，共刺激(使用 CTLA4-Ig 或 belatacept)不能作为单一策略来诱导临床耐受[333-340]。抗 CD40L(Hu5c8)在灵长动物肾移植中结果良好，但在临床应用中未能产生类似的结果,且会进一步导致患者致命性血栓栓塞事件[341]。一种替代的嵌合抗人 CD40 抗体血栓栓塞风险较小,并具有强大的免疫抑制特性[342]。Adams 等在食蟹猴胰岛同种异体移植模型中证明了抗 CD40 与贝伐他汀的显著协同作用,这种方法可能有临床转化的潜力[343]。

共刺激阻滞目前尚未显示出对临床耐受性的影响,但具有 HLA 匹配的同种异体骨髓输注的清髓性和非清髓性调理方法在血液恶性肿瘤患者的肾脏和骨髓移植联合中具有一定诱导耐受性前景，同时也给出了策略(通常涉及总淋巴样照射)[344-350]。随着时间的推移，通过对骨髓富集、剂量和调理的进一步了解,胰岛移植也可能将借鉴相似策略。来自 The Cure Alliance(www.thecurealliance.org)和糖尿病研究所(DRI)联合会的福州和迈阿密组织最近的一项合作研究已经评估了自体间充质干细胞(MSC)用于临床活体肾移植诱导策略的潜力[351]。159 例患者随机接受以(1~2)×10^6/kg 给药的自体 MSC,采用标准或低剂量 CNI 维持,与接受标准抗 IL2R 加 CNI 的对照者进行比较。发现前者排斥风险明显降低,并降低了机会性感染的风险,改善了肾移植生存[351]。类似通过和 T 细胞耗竭相结合的方法,已经证明了在胰岛素非依赖的新发 T1DM 中具有明显的再生潜力(见上文),并且如果与该方法结合,可以提供消除自身反应性并控制同种异体免疫的缺失环节。单独或与 MSC 组合的调节性 T 细胞的外周输注可进一步促进这种方法。

此外,最近芝加哥的路易斯维尔的 Ildstad 小组和 Leventhal 小组的一个联合研究报道称使用非清髓性调整的受体成功建立了持久嵌合体和供体特异性耐受的肾移植受体[352]。如果这种方法被证实在自身免疫性疾病可行,那么它不仅对实体器官和胰岛细胞移植,而且对 T1D 患者中自身免疫耐受恢复也将起到作用。

总结

本章回顾了目前的 T1DM 的风险和状态, 目前正在开发的替代策略能进一步改善血糖控制, 胰岛移植能够提供恢复正常血糖的潜力、外源性胰岛素无法做到的完全防治低血糖,且比胰腺移植风险低。自 2000 年埃德蒙顿方案开始后胰岛移植出现了明显进步,目前在 40 多个国际中心, 超过 1000 例患者已经接受了胰岛自体或异体移植。最初 5 年的结果显示胰岛素非依赖的大幅减少但仍有持续保护性, 最近来自 5 个独立的胰岛中心的报告,包括 CITR 中心和最值得注意的 Minnesota 胰岛中心,都报告了胰岛素非依赖比例超过 50%,可与全胰腺移植相媲美。单供体胰岛移植已经逐渐出现, 并可能会加速一系列的临床试验。目前尚在 CIT 联盟内的研究表明一种胰岛制备的 BLA 将在 2014—2015 年对美国的中心产生重大影响。平行临床试验旨在恢复自身耐受,调节性 T 细胞或 MSC 输注试验将分步实现精准稳健地治疗 T1DM。

(刘原兴 译 刘原兴 校)

参考文献

1. Shapiro AM, Lakey JR, Ryan EA, et al. Islet transplantation in seven patients with type 1 diabetes mellitus using a glucocorticoid-free immunosuppressive regimen. The New England Journal of Medicine. 2000;343(4):230–238.
2. Shapiro AM, Ricordi C, Hering BJ, et al. International trial of the Edmonton protocol for islet transplantation. The New England Journal of Medicine. 2006;355(13):1318–1330.
3. Ricordi C, Strom TB. Clinical islet transplantation: advances and immunological challenges. Nature Reviews Immunology. 2004;4(4):259–268.
4. Hering BJ, Kandaswamy R, Ansite JD, et al. Single-donor, marginal-dose islet transplantation in patients with type 1 diabetes. JAMA: Journal of the American Medical Association. 2005;293(7):830–835.
5. Consortium CIT. 2012. Available from: http://www.citisletstudy.org/.
6. Ricordi C. Islet transplantation: a brave new world. Diabetes. 2003;52(7): 1595–1603.
7. Shapiro AM. State of the art of clinical islet transplantation and novel protocols of immunosuppression. Current Diabetes Reports. 2011;11(5):345–354.
8. Hathout E, Lakey J, Shapiro J. Islet transplant: an option for childhood diabetes? Archives of Disease in Childhood. 2003;88(7):591–594.
9. Bustami RT, Ojo AO, Wolfe RA, et al. Immunosuppression and the risk of post-transplant malignancy among cadaveric first kidney transplant recipients. American Journal of Transplantation. 2004;4(1):87–93.
10. Colegio OR, Billingsley EM. Skin cancer in transplant recipients, out of the woods. Scientific retreat of the ITSCC and SCOPE. American Journal of Transplantation. 2011;11(8):1584–1591.
11. Kuschal C, Thoms KM, Schubert S, et al. Skin cancer in organ transplant recipients: effects of immunosuppressive medications on DNA repair. Experimental Dermatology. 2012;21(1):2–6.
12. Ojo AO, Held PJ, Port FK, et al. Chronic renal failure after transplantation of a nonrenal organ. New England Journal of Medicine. 2003;349(10): 931–940.
13. McCall MD, Toso C, Baetge EE, et al. Are stem cells a cure for diabetes? Clinical Science (London, England: 1979). 2010;118(2):87–97.
14. Harjutsalo V, Sjoberg L, Tuomilehto J. Time trends in the incidence of type 1 diabetes in Finnish children: a cohort study. Lancet. 2008;371(9626): 1777–1782.
15. International Diabetes Federation. Diabetes Atlas. 2011, IDF, editor. Brussels.
16. Guariguata L. Estimating the worldwide burden of type 1 diabetes. Diabetes Voice. 2011;56(Special Issue 2):6–8.
17. National Diabetes Information Clearinghouse (NDIC). National Diabetes Statistics. 2012 Available from: http://diabetes.niddk.nih.gov/dm/pubs/statistics/.
18. Nathan DM. Long-term complications of diabetes mellitus. New England Journal of Medicine. 1993;328(23):1676–1685.
19. The Diabetes Control and Complications Trial Research Group. The effect of intensive treatment of diabetes on the development and progression of long-term complications in insulin-dependent diabetes mellitus. New England Journal of Medicine. 1993;329(14):977–986.
20. Pedersen-Bjergaard U, Pramming S, Heller SR, et al. Severe hypoglycaemia in 1076 adult patients with type 1 diabetes: influence of risk markers and selection. Diabetes/Metabolism Research and Reviews. 2004;20(6):479–486.
21. Cryer PE. Elimination of hypoglycemia from the lives of people affected by diabetes. Diabetes. 2011;60(1):24–27.
22. Sahyun M, Blatherwick N. The physiological response of rabbits to insulin. Journal of Biological Chemistry. 1928;79(2):443–460.
23. Cryer PE. Hypoglycemia in diabetes: pathophysiological mechanisms and diurnal variation. Progress in Brain Research. 2006;153:361–365.
24. Cryer PE. Minireview: glucagon in the pathogenesis of hypoglycemia and hyperglycemia in diabetes. Endocrinology. 2012;153(3):1039–1048.
25. Songer T. Low blood sugar and motor vehicle crashes in persons with type 1 diabetes. Annual Proceedings / Association for the Advancement of Automotive Medicine Association for the Advancement of Automotive Medicine. 2002; 46:424–427.
26. Cox DJ, Ford D, Gonder-Frederick L, et al. Driving mishaps among individuals with type 1 diabetes: a prospective study. Diabetes Care. 2009;32(12): 2177–2180.
27. Campbell LK, Gonder-Frederick LA, Broshek DK, et al. Neurocognitive differences between drivers with type 1 diabetes with and without a recent history of recurrent driving mishaps. International Journal of Diabetes Mellitus. 2010; 2(2):73–77.
28. O'Reilly M, O'Sullivan EP, Davenport C, et al. "Dead in bed": a tragic complication of type 1 diabetes mellitus. Irish Journal of Medical Science. 2010;179(4):

585–587.
29. Koltin D, Daneman D. Dead-in-bed syndrome - a diabetes nightmare. Pediatric Diabetes. 2008;9(5):504–507.
30. Hanas R. Dead-in-bed syndrome in diabetes mellitus and hypoglycaemic unawareness. Lancet. 1997;350(9076):492–493.
31. Tanenberg RJ, Newton CA, Drake AJ. Confirmation of hypoglycemia in the "dead-in-bed" syndrome, as captured by a retrospective continuous glucose monitoring system. Endocrine Practice. 2010;16(2):244–248.
32. Cengiz E. Putting brakes on insulin pump infusion to prevent hypoglycemia. Journal of Diabetes Science and Technology. 2011;5(5):1142–1143.
33. Nathan DM, Dunn FL, Bruch J, et al. Postprandial insulin profiles with implantable pump therapy may explain decreased frequency of severe hypoglycemia, compared with intensive subcutaneous regimens, in insulin-dependent diabetes mellitus patients. American Journal of Medicine. 1996;100(4):412–417.
34. Danne T, Kordonouri O, Holder M, et al. Prevention of hypoglycemia by using low glucose suspend function in sensor-augmented pump therapy. Diabetes Technology & Therapeutics. 2011;13(11):1129–1134.
35. Tamborlane WV. Closed-loop insulin delivery: we're "virtually" there. Diabetes Technology & Therapeutics. 2012;14(3):203–204.
36. Kumareswaran K, Evans ML, Hovorka R. Closed-loop insulin delivery: towards improved diabetes care. Discovery Medicine. 2012;13(69):159–170.
37. Pickup JC. Semi-closed-loop insulin delivery systems: early experience with low-glucose insulin suspend pumps. Diabetes Technology & Therapeutics. 2011; 13(7):695–698.
38. Teuscher A, Berger WG. Hypoglycaemia unawareness in diabetics transferred from beef/porcine insulin to human insulin. Lancet. 1987;2(8555):382–385.
39. Wolff SP. Trying times for human insulin. Nature. 1992;356(6368):375–376.
40. Amiel SA. Human insulin in hypoglycemia. A new arena? Diabetes. 1995; 44(3):257–260.
41. Deiss D, Kordonouri O, Hartmann R, et al. Treatment with insulin glargine reduces asymptomatic hypoglycemia detected by continuous subcutaneous glucose monitoring in children and adolescents with type 1 diabetes. Pediatric Diabetes. 2007;8(3):157–162.
42. Dailey G, Strange P. Lower severe hypoglycemia risk: insulin glargine versus NPH insulin in type 2 diabetes. American Journal of Managed Care. 2008;14(1): 25–30.
43. Brunetti P, Muggeo M, Cattin L, et al. Incidence of severe nocturnal hypoglycemia in patients with type 1 diabetes treated with insulin lispro or regular human insulin in addition to basal insulin glargine. Nutrition, Metabolism, and Cardiovascular Diseases: NMCD. 2010;20(7):519–526.
44. Singh SR, Ahmad F, Lal A, et al. Efficacy and safety of insulin analogues for the management of diabetes mellitus: a meta-analysis. CMAJ: Canadian Medical Association Journal = Journal de l'Association Medicale Canadienne. 2009; 180(4):385–397.
45. Kling J. Dreamboat sinks prospects for fast approval of inhaled insulin. Nature Biotechnology. 2011;29(3):175–176.
46. Mitri J, Pittas AG. Inhaled insulin–what went wrong. Nature Clinical Practice Endocrinology and Metabolism. 2009;5(1):24–25.
47. Shoda LK, Young DL, Ramanujan S, et al. A comprehensive review of interventions in the NOD mouse and implications for translation. Immunity. 2005; 23(2):115–126.
48. Herold KC, Bluestone JA. Type 1 diabetes immunotherapy: is the glass half empty or half full? Science Translational Medicine. 2011;3(95):95fs1.
49. Roep BO, Atkinson M, von Herrath M. Satisfaction (not) guaranteed: re-evaluating the use of animal models of type 1 diabetes. Nature Reviews Immunology. 2004;4(12):989–997.
50. Sherry N, Hagopian W, Ludvigsson J, et al. Teplizumab for treatment of type 1 diabetes (Protege study): 1-year results from a randomised, placebo-controlled trial. Lancet. 2011;378(9790):487–497.
51. Herold KC, Gitelman S, Greenbaum C, et al. Treatment of patients with new onset Type 1 diabetes with a single course of anti-CD3 mAb Teplizumab preserves insulin production for up to 5 years. Clinical Immunology (Orlando, Fla.). 2009;132(2):166–173.
52. Herold KC, Hagopian W, Auger JA, et al. Anti-CD3 monoclonal antibody in new-onset type 1 diabetes mellitus. New England Journal of Medicine. 2002; 346(22):1692–1698.
53. Chatenoud L. Immune therapy for type 1 diabetes mellitus-what is unique about anti-CD3 antibodies? Nature Reviews Endocrinology. 2010;6(3):149–157.
54. Gottlieb PA, Quinlan S, Krause-Steinrauf H, et al. Failure to preserve beta-cell function with mycophenolate mofetil and daclizumab combined therapy in patients with new- onset type 1 diabetes. Diabetes Care. 2010;33(4):826–832.
55. Herold KC, Pescovitz MD, McGee P, et al. Increased T cell proliferative responses to islet antigens identify clinical responders to anti-CD20 monoclonal antibody (rituximab) therapy in type 1 diabetes. Journal of Immunology. 2011;187(4): 1998–2005.
56. Pescovitz MD, Greenbaum CJ, Krause-Steinrauf H, et al. Rituximab, B-lymphocyte depletion, and preservation of beta-cell function. New England Journal of Medicine. 2009;361(22):2143–2152.
57. Walter M, Philotheou A, Bonnici F, et al. No effect of the altered peptide ligand NBI-6024 on beta-cell residual function and insulin needs in new-onset type 1 diabetes. Diabetes Care. 2009;32(11):2036–2040.
58. Walter M, Kaupper T, Adler K, et al. No effect of the 1alpha,25-dihydroxyvitamin D3 on beta-cell residual function and insulin requirement in adults with new-onset type 1 diabetes. Diabetes Care. 2010;33(7):1443–1448.
59. Bingley PJ, Mahon JL, Gale EA. Insulin resistance and progression to type 1 diabetes in the European Nicotinamide Diabetes Intervention Trial (ENDIT). Diabetes Care. 2008;31(1):146–150.
60. Skyler JS. Update on worldwide efforts to prevent type 1 diabetes. Annals of the New York Academy of Sciences. 2008;1150:190–196.
61. Skyler JS. Immune intervention for type 1 diabetes mellitus. International Journal of Clinical Practice Supplement. 2011;170:61–70.
62. Voltarelli JC, Couri CE, Rodrigues MC, et al. Stem cell therapies for type 1 diabetes mellitus. Indian Journal of Experimental Biology. 2011;49(6): 395–400.
63. Voltarelli JC, Couri CE. Stem cell transplantation for type 1 diabetes mellitus. Diabetology and Metabolic Syndrome. 2009;1(1):4.
64. Couri CE, Oliveira MC, Stracieri AB, et al. C-peptide levels and insulin independence following autologous nonmyeloablative hematopoietic stem cell transplantation in newly diagnosed type 1 diabetes mellitus. JAMA: Journal of the American Medical Association. 2009;301(15):1573–1579.
65. Voltarelli JC, Couri CE, Stracieri AB, et al. Autologous hematopoietic stem cell transplantation for type 1 diabetes. Annals of the New York Academy of Sciences. 2008;1150:220–229.
66. Couri CE, Voltarelli JC. Autologous stem cell transplantation for early type 1 diabetes mellitus. Autoimmunity. 2008;41(8):666–672.
67. Voltarelli JC, Couri CE, Stracieri AB, et al. Autologous nonmyeloablative hematopoietic stem cell transplantation in newly diagnosed type 1 diabetes mellitus. JAMA: Journal of the American Medical Association. 2007;297(14): 1568–1576.
68. Fiorina P, Voltarelli J, Zavazava N. Immunological applications of stem cells in type 1 diabetes. Endocrine Reviews. 2011;32(6):725–754.
69. De Santis GC, de Pina Almeida Prado B Jr, de Lima Prata K, et al. Mobilization and harvesting of PBPC in newly diagnosed type 1 diabetes mellitus. Bone Marrow Transplantation. 2011;47:993–994.
70. de Oliveira GL, Malmegrim KC, Ferreira AF, et al. Up-regulation of fas and fasL pro-apoptotic genes expression in type 1 diabetes patients after autologous haematopoietic stem cell transplantation. Clinical and Experimental Immunology. 2012;168(3):291–302.
71. Gruessner AC. 2011 update on pancreas transplantation: comprehensive trend analysis of 25,000 cases followed up over the course of twenty-four years at the International Pancreas Transplant Registry (IPTR). Review of Diabetic Studies: RDS. 2011;8(1):6–16.
72. Gruessner AC, Sutherland DE, Gruessner RW. Pancreas transplantation in the United States: a review. Current Opinion in Organ Transplantation. 2010;15(1): 93–101.
73. Sutherland DE, Gruessner AC, Radosevich DM. Transplantation: kidney or kidney-pancreas transplant for the uremic diabetic? Nature Reviews Nephrology. 2009;5(10):554–556.
74. Muthusamy AS, Vaidya AC, Sinha S, et al. Alemtuzumab induction and steroid-free maintenance immunosuppression in pancreas transplantation. American Journal of Transplantation. 2008;8(10):2126–2131.
75. Wang SN, Sturdevant M, Kandaswamy R, et al. Technical failure of the pancreas after SPK transplant: are these patients good candidates for later pancreas retransplant? Clinical Transplantation. 2008;22(1):50–54.
76. Muthusamy AS, Giangrande PL, Friend PJ. Pancreas allograft thrombosis. Transplantation. 2010;90(7):705–707.
77. Venstrom JM, McBride MA, Rother KI, et al. Survival after pancreas transplantation in patients with diabetes and preserved kidney function. JAMA: Journal of the American Medical Association. 2003;290(21):2817–2823.
78. Dy EC, Harlan DM, Rother KI. Assessment of islet function following islet and pancreas transplantation. Current Diabetes Reports. 2006;6(4):316–322.
79. Ryan EA, Bigam D, Shapiro AM. Current indications for pancreas or islet transplant. Diabetes, Obesity & Metabolism. 2006;8(1):1–7.
80. Clarke WL, Cox DJ, Gonder-Frederick LA, et al. Reduced awareness of hypoglycemia in adults with IDDM. A prospective study of hypoglycemic frequency and associated symptoms. Diabetes Care. 1995;18(4):517–522.
81. Ryan EA, Shandro T, Green K, et al. Assessment of the severity of hypoglycemia and glycemic lability in type 1 diabetic subjects undergoing islet transplantation. Diabetes. 2004;53(4):955–962.
82. Shapiro AM, Geng Hao E, Lakey JR, et al. Defining optimal immunosuppression

for islet transplantation based on reduced diabetogenicity in canine islet autografts. Transplantation. 2002;74(11):1522–1528.
83. Nanji SA, Shapiro AM. Islet transplantation in patients with diabetes mellitus: choice of immunosuppression. Biodrugs: Clinical Immunotherapeutics, Biopharmaceuticals and Gene Therapy. 2004;18(5):315–328.
84. Moreau F, Toti F, Bayle F, et al. Rescue of a pancreatic islet graft after steroid therapy. Transplantation. 2012;93(3):e10–e11.
85. Toso C, Baertschiger R, Morel P, et al. Sequential kidney/islet transplantation: efficacy and safety assessment of a steroid-free immunosuppression protocol. American Journal of Transplantation. 2006;6(5 Pt 1):1049–1058.
86. Gardner SD, Field AM, Coleman DV, et al. New human papovavirus (B.K.) isolated from urine after renal transplantation. Lancet. 1971;1(7712):1253–1257.
87. Mujtaba M, Fridell J, Sharfuddin A, et al. BK virus nephropathy in simultaneous pancreas kidney transplant: a potentially preventable cause of kidney allograft loss. Clinical Transplantation. 2012;26(2):E87–E93.
88. Campbell PM, Salam A, Ryan EA, et al. Pretransplant HLA antibodies are associated with reduced graft survival after clinical islet transplantation. American Journal of Transplantation. 2007;7(5):1242–1248.
89. Campbell PM, Senior PA, Salam A, et al. High risk of sensitization after failed islet transplantation. American Journal of Transplantation. 2007;7(10): 2311–2317.
90. Schroppel B, Heeger PS. Gazing into a crystal ball to predict kidney transplant outcome. Journal of Clinical Investigation. 2010;120(6):1803–1806.
91. Meier-Kriesche HU, Schold JD, Kaplan B. Long-term renal allograft survival: have we made significant progress or is it time to rethink our analytic and therapeutic strategies? American Journal of Transplantation. 2004;4(8): 1289–1295.
92. Rao PS, Schaubel DE, Wei G, et al. Evaluating the survival benefit of kidney retransplantation. Transplantation. 2006;82(5):669–674.
93. Barba Abad J, Robles Garcia JE, Saiz Sansi A, et al. Impact of renal retransplantation on graft and recipient survival. Archivos Espanoles de Urologia. 2011;64(4): 363–370.
94. Koch MJ. Considerations in retransplantation of the failed renal allograft recipient. Advances in Chronic Kidney Disease. 2006;13(1):18–28.
95. Kawahara T, Kin T, Kashkoush S, et al. Portal vein thrombosis is a potentially preventable complication in clinical islet transplantation. American Journal of Transplantation. 2011;11(12):2700–2707.
96. Kawahara T, Kin T, Shapiro AM. A comparison of islet autotransplantation with allotransplantation and factors elevating acute portal pressure in clinical islet transplantation. Journal of Hepato-Biliary-Pancreatic Sciences. 2012;19(3): 281–288.
97. Owen RJ, Ryan EA, O'Kelly K, et al. Percutaneous transhepatic pancreatic islet cell transplantation in type 1 diabetes mellitus: radiologic aspects. Radiology. 2003;229(1):165–170.
98. Villiger P, Ryan EA, Owen R, et al. Prevention of bleeding after islet transplantation: lessons learned from a multivariate analysis of 132 cases at a single institution. American Journal of Transplantation. 2005;5(12):2992–2998.
99. Froud T, Yrizarry JM, Alejandro R, et al. Use of D-STAT to prevent bleeding following percutaneous transhepatic intraportal islet transplantation. Cell Transplantation. 2004;13(1):55–59.
100. Venturini M, Angeli E, Maffi P, et al. Technique, complications, and therapeutic efficacy of percutaneous transplantation of human pancreatic islet cells in type 1 diabetes: the role of US. Radiology. 2005;234(2):617–624.
101. Hafiz MM, Faradji RN, Froud T, et al. Immunosuppression and procedure-related complications in 26 patients with type 1 diabetes mellitus receiving allogeneic islet cell transplantation. Transplantation. 2005;80(12):1718–1728.
102. Neeman Z, Hirshberg B, Harlan D, et al. Radiologic aspects of islet cell transplantation. Current Diabetes Reports. 2006;6(4):310–315.
103. Walsh TJ, Eggleston JC, Cameron JL. Portal hypertension, hepatic infarction, and liver failure complicating pancreatic islet autotransplantation. Surgery. 1982; 91(4):485–487.
104. Shapiro AM, Lakey JR, Rajotte RV, et al. Portal vein thrombosis after transplantation of partially purified pancreatic islets in a combined human liver/islet allograft. Transplantation. 1995;59(7):1060–1063.
105. Hirshberg B, Rother KI, Digon BJ 3rd, et al. Benefits and risks of solitary islet transplantation for type 1 diabetes using steroid-sparing immunosuppression: the National Institutes of Health experience. Diabetes Care. 2003;26(12): 3288–3295.
106. Casey JJ, Lakey JR, Ryan EA, et al. Portal venous pressure changes after sequential clinical islet transplantation. Transplantation. 2002;74(7):913–915.
107. Froud T, Ricordi C, Baidal DA, et al. Islet transplantation in type 1 diabetes mellitus using cultured islets and steroid-free immunosuppression: Miami experience. American Journal of Transplantation. 2005;5(8):2037–2046.
108. Noguchi H, Naziruddin B, Jackson A, et al. Low-temperature preservation of isolated islets is superior to conventional islet culture before islet transplantation. Transplantation. 2010;89(1):47–54.
109. Murdoch TB, McGhee-Wilson D, Shapiro AM, et al. Methods of human islet culture for transplantation. Cell Transplantation. 2004;13(6):605–617.
110. Kin T, Senior P, O'Gorman D, et al. Risk factors for islet loss during culture prior to transplantation. Transplant International: Official Journal of the European Society for Organ Transplantation. 2008;21(11):1029–1035.
111. Kerr-Conte J, Vandewalle B, Moerman E, et al. Upgrading pretransplant human islet culture technology requires human serum combined with media renewal. Transplantation. 2010;89(9):1154–1160.
112. Fraker C, Montelongo J, Szust J, et al. The use of multiparametric monitoring during islet cell isolation and culture: a potential tool for in-process corrections of critical physiological factors. Cell Transplantation. 2004;13(5):497–502.
113. Berney T. Islet culture and counter-culture. Commentary on: effect of short-term culture on functional and stress-related parameters in isolated human islets by Ihm. Transplant International: Official Journal of the European Society for Organ Transplantation. 2009;22(5):531–533.
114. O'Gorman D, Kin T, Imes S, et al. Comparison of human islet isolation outcomes using a new mammalian tissue-free enzyme versus collagenase NB-1. Transplantation. 2010;90(3):255–259.
115. Misawa R, Ricordi C, Miki A, et al. Evaluation of viable beta-cell mass is useful for selecting collagenase for human islet isolation: comparison of collagenase NB1 and liberase HI. Cell Transplantation. 2012;21(1):39–47.
116. Koh A, Senior P, Salam A, et al. Insulin-heparin infusions peritransplant substantially improve single-donor clinical islet transplant success. Transplantation. 2010;89(4):465–471.
117. Brennan DC, Shannon MB, Koch MJ, et al. Portal vein thrombosis complicating islet transplantation in a recipient with the Factor V Leiden mutation. Transplantation. 2004;78(1):172–173.
118. Ryan EA, Paty BW, Senior PA, et al. Risks and side effects of islet transplantation. Current Diabetes Reports. 2004;4(4):304–309.
119. Rafael E, Ryan EA, Paty BW, et al. Changes in liver enzymes after clinical islet transplantation. Transplantation. 2003;76(9):1280–1284.
120. Bhargava R, Senior PA, Ackerman TE, et al. Prevalence of hepatic steatosis after islet transplantation and its relation to graft function. Diabetes. 2004;53(5): 1311–1317.
121. Maffi P, Angeli E, Bertuzzi F, et al. Minimal focal steatosis of liver after islet transplantation in humans: a long-term study. Cell Transplantation. 2005;14(10): 727–733.
122. Markmann JF, Rosen M, Siegelman ES, et al. Magnetic resonance-defined periportal steatosis following intraportal islet transplantation: a functional footprint of islet graft survival? Diabetes. 2003;52(7):1591–1594.
123. Low G, Hussein N, Owen RJ, et al. Role of imaging in clinical islet transplantation. Radiographics: A Review Publication of the Radiological Society of North America, Inc. 2010;30(2):353–366.
124. Toso C, Isse K, Demetris AJ, et al. Histologic graft assessment after clinical islet transplantation. Transplantation. 2009;88(11):1286–1293.
125. Dombrowski F, Bannasch P, Pfeifer U. Hepatocellular neoplasms induced by low-number pancreatic islet transplants in streptozotocin diabetic rats. American Journal of Pathology. 1997;150(3):1071–1087.
126. Dombrowski F, Mathieu C, Evert M. Hepatocellular neoplasms induced by low-number pancreatic islet transplants in autoimmune diabetic BB/Pfd rats. Cancer Research. 2006;66(3):1833–1843.
127. Najarian JS, Sutherland DE, Matas AJ, et al. Human islet autotransplantation following pancreatectomy. Transplantation Proceedings. 1979;11(1): 336–340.
128. Najarian JS, Sutherland DE, Matas AJ, et al. Human islet transplantation: a preliminary report. Transplantation Proceedings. 1977;9(1):233–236.
129. Sutherland DE, Matas AJ, Najarian JS. Pancreas and islet transplantation. World Journal of Surgery. 1977;2(1):185–195.
130. Humar A, Fishman JA. Donor-derived infection: old problem, new solutions? American Journal of Transplantation. 2008;8(6):1087–1088.
131. Len O, Gavalda J, Blanes M, et al. Donor infection and transmission to the recipient of a solid allograft. American Journal of Transplantation. 2008;8(11): 2420–2425.
132. Srinivasan A, Burton EC, Kuehnert MJ, et al. Transmission of rabies virus from an organ donor to four transplant recipients. New England Journal of Medicine. 2005;352(11):1103–1111.
133. Morris MI, Fischer SA, Ison MG. Infections transmitted by transplantation. Infectious Disease Clinics of North America. 2010;24(2):497–514.
134. Barshes NR, Agee EE, Zgabay T, et al. West Nile Virus encephalopathy following pancreatic islet transplantation. American Journal of Transplantation. 2006; 6(12):3037.
135. Humar A, Morris M, Blumberg E, et al. Nucleic acid testing (NAT) of organ donors: is the 'best' test the right test? A consensus conference report. American Journal of Transplantation. 2010;10(4):889–899.

136. Vargas F, Vives-Pi M, Somoza N, et al. Endotoxin contamination may be responsible for the unexplained failure of human pancreatic islet transplantation. Transplantation. 1998;65(5):722–727.
137. Bucher P, Oberholzer J, Bosco D, et al. Microbial surveillance during human pancreatic islet isolation. Transplant International: Official Journal of the European Society for Organ Transplantation. 2005;18(5):584–589.
138. Kin T, Rosichuk S, Shapiro AM, et al. Detection of microbial contamination during human islet isolation. Cell Transplantation. 2007;16(1):9–13.
139. Shapiro AM, Hao EG, Lakey JR, et al. Novel approaches toward early diagnosis of islet allograft rejection. Transplantation. 2001;71(12):1709–1718.
140. Burke GW 3rd, Vendrame F, Pileggi A, et al. Recurrence of autoimmunity following pancreas transplantation. Current Diabetes Reports. 2011;11(5): 413–419.
141. Laughlin E, Burke G, Pugliese A, et al. Recurrence of autoreactive antigen-specific CD4+ T cells in autoimmune diabetes after pancreas transplantation. Clinical Immunology (Orlando, Fla.). 2008;128(1):23–30.
142. Pugliese A, Reijonen HK, Nepom J, et al. Recurrence of autoimmunity in pancreas transplant patients: research update. Diabetes Manag (Lond). 2011;1(2): 229–238.
143. Vendrame F, Pileggi A, Laughlin E, et al. Recurrence of type 1 diabetes after simultaneous pancreas-kidney transplantation, despite immunosuppression, is associated with autoantibodies and pathogenic autoreactive CD4 T-cells. Diabetes. 2010;59(4):947–957.
144. Rossini AA. Autoimmunity after islet-cell allotransplantation. New England Journal of Medicine. 2006;355(13):1397–1399.
145. Ryan EA, Paty BW, Senior PA, et al. Beta-score: an assessment of beta-cell function after islet transplantation. Diabetes Care. 2005;28(2):343–347.
146. Ryan EA, Paty BW, Senior PA, et al. Five-year follow-up after clinical islet transplantation. Diabetes. 2005;54(7):2060–2069.
147. Jaeger C, Brendel MD, Hering BJ, et al. Progressive islet graft failure occurs significantly earlier in autoantibody-positive than in autoantibody-negative IDDM recipients of intrahepatic islet allografts. Diabetes. 1997;46(11):1907–1910.
148. Harlan DM, Kenyon NS, Korsgren O, et al. Current advances and travails in islet transplantation. Diabetes. 2009;58(10):2175–2184.
149. Huurman VA, Velthuis JH, Hilbrands R, et al. Allograft-specific cytokine profiles associate with clinical outcome after islet cell transplantation. American Journal of Transplantation. 2009;9(2):382–388.
150. Roep BO, Stobbe I, Duinkerken G, et al. Auto- and alloimmune reactivity to human islet allografts transplanted into type 1 diabetic patients. Diabetes. 1999;48(3):484–490.
151. Roep BO, Peakman M. Antigen targets of type 1 diabetes autoimmunity. Cold Spring Harbor Perspectives in Medicine. 2012;2(4):a007781.
152. Roep BO, Buckner J, Sawcer S, et al. The problems and promises of research into human immunology and autoimmune disease. Nature Medicine. 2012;18(1): 48–53.
153. Shi Q, Lees JR, Scott DW, et al. Endogenous expansion of regulatory T cells leads to long-term islet graft survival in diabetic NOD mice. American Journal of Transplantation. 2012;12(5):1124–1132.
154. Bartlett ST, Schweitzer EJ, Kuo PC, et al. Prevention of autoimmune islet allograft destruction by engraftment of donor T cells. Transplantation. 1997; 63(2):299–303.
155. Bartlett ST, Chin T, Dirden B, et al. Inclusion of peripancreatic lymph node cells prevents recurrent autoimmune destruction of islet transplants: evidence of donor chimerism. Surgery. 1995;118(2):392–397, discussion 7–8.
156. Chatenoud L. Chemical immunosuppression in islet transplantation–friend or foe? New England Journal of Medicine. 2008;358(11):1192–1193.
157. Nir T, Melton DA, Dor Y. Recovery from diabetes in mice by beta cell regeneration. Journal of Clinical Investigation. 2007;117(9):2553–2561.
158. Ricordi C, Zeng YJ, Alejandro R, et al. In vivo effect of FK506 on human pancreatic islets. Transplantation. 1991;52(3):519–522.
159. Rostambeigi N, Lanza IR, Dzeja PP, et al. Unique cellular and mitochondrial defects mediate FK506-induced islet beta-cell dysfunction. Transplantation. 2011;91(6):615–623.
160. Shapiro AM, Gallant HL, Hao EG, et al. The portal immunosuppressive storm: relevance to islet transplantation? Therapeutic Drug Monitoring. 2005;27(1): 35–37.
161. Desai NM, Goss JA, Deng S, et al. Elevated portal vein drug levels of sirolimus and tacrolimus in islet transplant recipients: local immunosuppression or islet toxicity? Transplantation. 2003;76(11):1623–1625.
162. Kneteman NM, Lakey JR, Wagner T, et al. The metabolic impact of rapamycin (sirolimus) in chronic canine islet graft recipients. Transplantation. 1996;61(8): 1206–1210.
163. Mita A, Ricordi C, Miki A, et al. Anti-proinflammatory effects of sirolimus on human islet preparations. Transplantation. 2008;86(1):46–53.
164. Zhang N, Su D, Qu S, et al. Sirolimus is associated with reduced islet engraftment and impaired beta-cell function. Diabetes. 2006;55(9):2429–2436.
165. Merani S, Truong W, Emamaullee JA, et al. Liraglutide, a long-acting human glucagon-like peptide 1 analog, improves glucose homeostasis in marginal mass islet transplantation in mice. Endocrinology. 2008;149(9):4322–4328.
166. Fu F, Hu S, Deleo J, et al. Long-term islet graft survival in streptozotocin- and autoimmune-induced diabetes models by immunosuppressive and potential insulinotropic agent FTY720. Transplantation. 2002;73(9):1425–1430.
167. Truong W, Emamaullee JA, Merani S, et al. Human islet function is not impaired by the sphingosine-1-phosphate receptor modulator FTY720. American Journal of Transplantation. 2007;7(8):2031–2038.
168. Wijkstrom M, Kenyon NS, Kirchhof N, et al. Islet allograft survival in nonhuman primates immunosuppressed with basiliximab, RAD, and FTY720. Transplantation. 2004;77(6):827–835.
169. Yamasaki T, Inoue K, Hayashi H, et al. Effect of a new immunosuppressive agent, FTY720, on survival of islet allografts. Cell Transplantation. 1998; 7(4):403–406.
170. Ontaneda D, Cohen JA. Potential mechanisms of efficacy and adverse effects in the use of fingolimod (FTY720). Expert Review of Clinical Pharmacology. 2011;4(5):567–570.
171. Salvadori M, Budde K, Charpentier B, et al. FTY720 versus MMF with cyclosporine in de novo renal transplantation: a 1-year, randomized controlled trial in Europe and Australasia. American Journal of Transplantation. 2006; 6(12):2912–2921.
172. Bellin MD, Barton FB, Heitman A, et al. Potent induction immunotherapy promotes long-term insulin independence after islet transplantation in type 1 diabetes. American Journal of Transplantation. 2012;12(6):1576–1583.
173. Bellin MD, Kandaswamy R, Parkey J, et al. Prolonged insulin independence after islet allotransplants in recipients with type 1 diabetes. American Journal of Transplantation. 2008;8(11):2463–2470.
174. Hering BJ. Achieving and maintaining insulin independence in human islet transplant recipients. Transplantation. 2005;79(10):1296–1297.
175. Parker MJ, Xue S, Alexander JJ, et al. Immune depletion with cellular mobilization imparts immunoregulation and reverses autoimmune diabetes in nonobese diabetic mice. Diabetes. 2009;58(10):2277–2284.
176. Ildstad ST, Chilton PM, Xu H, et al. Preconditioning of NOD mice with anti-CD8 mAb and costimulatory blockade enhances chimerism and tolerance and prevents diabetes, while depletion of alpha beta-TCR+ and CD4+ cells negates the effect. Blood. 2005;105(6):2577–2584.
177. Glandt M, Herold KC. Treatment of type 1 diabetes with anti-T-cell agents: from T-cell depletion to T-cell regulation. Current Diabetes Reports. 2004;4(4): 291–297.
178. Rabinovitch A, Sumoski W, Rajotte RV, et al. Cytotoxic effects of cytokines on human pancreatic islet cells in monolayer culture. Journal of Clinical Endocrinology and Metabolism. 1990;71(1):152–156.
179. Clatworthy MR, Friend PJ, Calne RY, et al. Alemtuzumab (CAMPATH-1H) for the treatment of acute rejection in kidney transplant recipients: long-term follow-up. Transplantation. 2009;87(7):1092–1095.
180. Watson CJ, Bradley JA, Friend PJ, et al. Alemtuzumab (CAMPATH 1H) induction therapy in cadaveric kidney transplantation–efficacy and safety at five years. American Journal of Transplantation. 2005;5(6):1347–1353.
181. Calne R, Friend P, Moffatt S, et al. Prope tolerance, perioperative campath 1H, and low-dose cyclosporin monotherapy in renal allograft recipients. Lancet. 1998;351(9117):1701–1702.
182. Newell KA, Cendales LC, Kirk AD. Finding the right job for the tool: alemtuzumab and its role in renal transplantation. American Journal of Transplantation. 2008;8(7):1363–1364.
183. Kirk AD, Hale DA, Mannon RB, et al. Results from a human renal allograft tolerance trial evaluating the humanized CD52-specific monoclonal antibody alemtuzumab (CAMPATH-1H). Transplantation. 2003;76(1):120–129.
184. Knechtle SJ, Pirsch JD, H Fechner JJ, et al. Campath-1H induction plus rapamycin monotherapy for renal transplantation: results of a pilot study. American Journal of Transplantation. 2003;3(6):722–730.
185. Knechtle SJ, Fernandez LA, Pirsch JD, et al. Campath-1H in renal transplantation: the university of Wisconsin experience. Surgery. 2004;136(4):754–760.
186. Tan J, Yang S, Cai J, et al. Simultaneous islet and kidney transplantation in seven patients with type 1 diabetes and end-stage renal disease using a glucocorticoid-free immunosuppressive regimen with alemtuzumab induction. Diabetes. 2008; 57(10):2666–2671.
187. Froud T, Baidal DA, Faradji R, et al. Islet transplantation with alemtuzumab induction and calcineurin-free maintenance immunosuppression results in improved short- and long-term outcomes. Transplantation. 2008;86(12): 1695–1701.
188. LaMattina JC, Mezrich JD, Hofmann RM, et al. Alemtuzumab as compared to alternative contemporary induction regimens. Transplant International: Official Journal of the European Society for Organ Transplantation. 2012;25(5):

518–526.
189. Macedo C, Walters JT, Orkis EA, et al. Long-term effects of alemtuzumab on regulatory and memory T-cell subsets in kidney transplantation. Transplantation. 2012;93(8):813–821.
190. Gallon L, Chhabra D, Skaro AI. T-cell-depleting agents in kidney transplantation: is there a place for alemtuzumab? American Journal of Kidney Diseases: The Official Journal of the National Kidney Foundation. 2012; 59(1):15–18.
191. Haynes R, Friend P. Alemtuzumab: right drug, right dose? Transplant International: Official Journal of the European Society for Organ Transplantation. 2011;24(11):1051–1052.
192. Uemura T, Ramprasad V, Matsushima K, et al. Single dose of alemtuzumab induction with steroid-free maintenance immunosuppression in pancreas transplantation. Transplantation. 2011;92(6):678–685.
193. Myrvang H. Transplantation: alemtuzumab induction is safe for renal transplant recipients. Nature Reviews Nephrology. 2011;7(7):362.
194. Markmann JF, Fishman JA. Alemtuzumab in kidney-transplant recipients. New England Journal of Medicine. 2011;364(20):1968–1969.
195. Hanaway MJ, Woodle ES, Mulgaonkar S, et al. Alemtuzumab induction in renal transplantation. New England Journal of Medicine. 2011;364(20): 1909–1919.
196. Levitsky J, Thudi K, Ison MG, et al. Alemtuzumab induction in non-hepatitis C positive liver transplant recipients. Liver Transplantation: Official Publication of the American Association for the Study of Liver Diseases and the International Liver Transplantation Society. 2011;17(1):32–37.
197. Scarsi M, Bossini N, Malacarne F, et al. The number of circulating recent thymic emigrants is severely reduced 1 year after a single dose of alemtuzumab in renal transplant recipients. Transplant International: Official Journal of the European Society for Organ Transplantation. 2010;23(8):786–795.
198. Safdar N, Smith J, Knasinski V, et al. Infections after the use of alemtuzumab in solid organ transplant recipients: a comparative study. Diagnostic Microbiology and Infectious Disease. 2010;66(1):7–15.
199. Teuteberg JJ, Shullo MA, Zomak R, et al. Alemtuzumab induction prior to cardiac transplantation with lower intensity maintenance immunosuppression: one-year outcomes. American Journal of Transplantation. 2010;10(2):382–388.
200. Dhesi S, Boland B, Colquhoun S. Alemtuzumab and liver transplantation: a review. Current Opinion in Organ Transplantation. 2009;14(3):245–249.
201. Pascual J, Pirsch JD, Odorico JS, et al. Alemtuzumab induction and antibody-mediated kidney rejection after simultaneous pancreas-kidney transplantation. Transplantation. 2009;87(1):125–132.
202. Tan HP, Donaldson J, Basu A, et al. Two hundred living donor kidney transplantations under alemtuzumab induction and tacrolimus monotherapy: 3-year follow-up. American Journal of Transplantation. 2009;9(2):355–366.
203. Margreiter R, Klempnauer J, Neuhaus P, et al. Alemtuzumab (Campath-1H) and tacrolimus monotherapy after renal transplantation: results of a prospective randomized trial. American Journal of Transplantation. 2008;8(7):1480–1485.
204. Farney A, Sundberg A, Moore P, et al. A randomized trial of alemtuzumab vs. anti-thymocyte globulin induction in renal and pancreas transplantation. Clinical Transplantation. 2008;22(1):41–49.
205. Gala-Lopez BL, Senior PA, Koh A, et al. Late cytomegalovirus transmission and impact of T-depletion in clinical islet transplantation. American Journal of Transplantation. 2011;11(12):2708–2714.
206. Toso C, Edgar R, Pawlick R, et al. Effect of different induction strategies on effector, regulatory and memory lymphocyte sub-populations in clinical islet transplantation. Transplant International: Official Journal of the European Society for Organ Transplantation. 2009;22(2):182–191.
207. Hafiz MM, Poggioli R, Caulfield A, et al. Cytomegalovirus prevalence and transmission after islet allograft transplant in patients with type 1 diabetes mellitus. American Journal of Transplantation. 2004;4(10):1697–1702.
208. Hardinger KL, Schnitzler MA, Miller B, et al. Five-year follow up of thymoglobulin versus ATGAM induction in adult renal transplantation. Transplantation. 2004;78(1):136–141.
209. Hardinger KL, Rhee S, Buchanan P, et al. A prospective, randomized, double-blinded comparison of thymoglobulin versus Atgam for induction immunosuppressive therapy: 10-year results. Transplantation. 2008;86(7): 947–952.
210. Schenker P, Ozturk A, Vonend O, et al. Single-dose thymoglobulin induction in living-donor renal transplantation. Annals of Transplantation: Quarterly of the Polish Transplantation Society. 2011;16(2):50–58.
211. Marks WH, Ilsley JN, Dharnidharka VR. Posttransplantation lymphoproliferative disorder in kidney and heart transplant recipients receiving thymoglobulin: a systematic review. Transplantation Proceedings. 2011;43(5):1395–1404.
212. Kirk AD, Cherikh WS, Ring M, et al. Dissociation of depletional induction and posttransplant lymphoproliferative disease in kidney recipients treated with alemtuzumab. American Journal of Transplantation. 2007;7(11): 2619–2625.
213. Vallejo C, Rios E, de la Serna J, et al. Incidence of cytomegalovirus infection and disease in patients with lymphoproliferative disorders treated with alemtuzumab. Expert Review of Hematology. 2011;4(1):9–16.
214. Bartakke S, Abla O, Weitzman S. Successful use of alemtuzumab in a child with refractory peripheral T-cell posttransplant lymphoproliferative disorder. Journal of Pediatric Hematology/Oncology: Official Journal of the American Society of Pediatric Hematology/Oncology. 2008;30(10):787–788.
215. Carpenter B, Haque T, Dimopoulou M, et al. Incidence and dynamics of Epstein-Barr virus reactivation after alemtuzumab-based conditioning for allogeneic hematopoietic stem-cell transplantation. Transplantation. 2010;90(5):564–570.
216. Muzaffar M, Taj A, Ratnam S. Aggressive posttransplant lymphoproliferative disease in a renal transplant patient treated with alemtuzumab. American Journal of Therapeutics. 2010;17(6):e230–e233.
217. Cure P, Froud T, Leitao CB, et al. Late Epstein Barr virus reactivation in islet after kidney transplantation. Transplantation. 2008;86(9):1324–1325.
218. Leitao CB, Cure P, Messinger S, et al. Stable renal function after islet transplantation: importance of patient selection and aggressive clinical management. Transplantation. 2009;87(5):681–688.
219. Shapiro AM, Lakey JR, Paty BW, et al. Strategic opportunities in clinical islet transplantation. Transplantation. 2005;79(10):1304–1307.
220. Shapiro AM, Ricordi C, Hering B. Edmonton's islet success has indeed been replicated elsewhere. Lancet. 2003;362(9391):1242.
221. Berney T, Secchi A. Rapamycin in islet transplantation: friend or foe? Transplant International: Official Journal of the European Society for Organ Transplantation. 2009;22(2):153–161.
222. Alfadhli E, Koh A, Albaker W, et al. High prevalence of ovarian cysts in premenopausal women receiving sirolimus and tacrolimus after clinical islet transplantation. Transplant International: Official Journal of the European Society for Organ Transplantation. 2009;22(6):622–625.
223. Del Olmo Garcia MI, Lauriola V, Gomez Aracena A, et al. Alterations of the female reproductive system in islet recipient receiving immunosuppression. Cell Transplantation. 2011;20(10):1649–1651.
224. Cure P, Pileggi A, Froud T, et al. Alterations of the female reproductive system in recipients of islet grafts. Transplantation. 2004;78(11):1576–1581.
225. Molinari M, Al-Saif F, Ryan EA, et al. Sirolimus-induced ulceration of the small bowel in islet transplant recipients: report of two cases. American Journal of Transplantation. 2005;5(11):2799–2804.
226. Digon BJ 3rd, Rother KI, Hirshberg B, et al. Sirolimus-induced interstitial pneumonitis in an islet transplant recipient. Diabetes Care. 2003;26(11): 3191.
227. Senior PA, Shapiro AM, Ackerman TE, et al. Magnetic resonance-defined perinephric edema after clinical islet transplantation: a benign finding associated with mild renal impairment. Transplantation. 2004;78(6):945–948.
228. Leitao CB, Froud T, Cure P, et al. Nonalbumin proteinuria in islet transplant recipients. Cell Transplantation. 2010;19(1):119–125.
229. Senior PA, Paty BW, Cockfield SM, et al. Proteinuria developing after clinical islet transplantation resolves with sirolimus withdrawal and increased tacrolimus dosing. American Journal of Transplantation. 2005;5(9):2318–2323.
230. Posselt AM, Szot GL, Frassetto LA, et al. Islet transplantation in type 1 diabetic patients using calcineurin inhibitor-free immunosuppressive protocols based on T-cell adhesion or costimulation blockade. Transplantation. 2010; 90(12):1595–1601.
231. Kothary N, Diak IL, Brinker A, et al. Progressive multifocal leukoencephalopathy associated with efalizumab use in psoriasis patients. Journal of the American Academy of Dermatology. 2011;65(3):546–551.
232. Gadzia J, Turner J. Progressive multifocal leukoencephalopathy in two psoriasis patients treated with efalizumab. Journal of Drugs in Dermatology: JDD. 2010;9(8):1005–1009.
233. Carson KR, Focosi D, Major EO, et al. Monoclonal antibody-associated progressive multifocal leucoencephalopathy in patients treated with rituximab, natalizumab, and efalizumab: a review from the research on adverse drug events and reports (RADAR) project. Lancet Oncology. 2009;10(8):816–824.
234. Farney AC, Xenos E, Sutherland DE, et al. Inhibition of pancreatic islet beta cell function by tumor necrosis factor is blocked by a soluble tumor necrosis factor receptor. Transplantation Proceedings. 1993;25(1 Pt 2):865–866.
235. McCall M, Pawlick R, Kin T, et al. Anakinra potentiates the protective effects of etanercept in transplantation of marginal mass human islets in immunodeficient mice. American Journal of Transplantation. 2012;12(2):322–329.
236. Matsumoto S, Takita M, Chaussabel D, et al. Improving efficacy of clinical islet transplantation with iodixanol based islet purification, thymoglobulin induction and blockage of IL-1-beta and TNF-alpha. Cell Transplantation. 2011;20(10):1641–1647.

237. Bretzel RG, Brandhorst D, Brandhorst H, et al. Improved survival of intraportal pancreatic islet cell allografts in patients with type-1 diabetes mellitus by refined peritransplant management. Journal of Molecular Medicine (Berlin, Germany). 1999;77(1):140–143.
238. Froud T, Faradji RN, Gorn L, et al. Dapsone-induced artifactual a1c reduction in islet transplant recipients. Transplantation. 2007;83(6):824–825.
239. CITR. The Collaborative Islet Transplant Registry Seventh Annual Report. 2011 Bethesda, MD 2011 December 30.
240. Alberu J, Pascoe MD, Campistol JM, et al. Lower malignancy rates in renal allograft recipients converted to sirolimus-based, calcineurin inhibitor-free immunotherapy: 24-month results from the CONVERT trial. Transplantation. 2011;92(3):303–310.
241. Kahan BD, Yakupoglu YK, Schoenberg L, et al. Low incidence of malignancy among sirolimus/cyclosporine-treated renal transplant recipients. Transplantation. 2005;80(6):749–758.
242. Geissler EK, Schlitt HJ. The potential benefits of rapamycin on renal function, tolerance, fibrosis, and malignancy following transplantation. Kidney International. 2010;78(11):1075–1079.
243. Manuelli M, De Luca L, Iaria G, et al. Conversion to rapamycin immunosuppression for malignancy after kidney transplantation. Transplantation Proceedings. 2010;42(4):1314–1316.
244. Feldmeyer L, Hofbauer GF, Boni T, et al. Mammalian target of rapamycin (mTOR) inhibitors slow skin carcinogenesis, but impair wound healing. British Journal of Dermatology. 2012;166(2):422–424.
245. Campbell SB, Walker R, Tai SS, et al. Randomized controlled trial of sirolimus for renal transplant recipients at high risk for nonmelanoma skin cancer. American Journal of Transplantation. 2012;12(5):1146–1156.
246. Geissler EK, Schlitt HJ. Transplantation: can sirolimus prevent skin cancer in transplant recipients? Nature Reviews Nephrology. 2010;6(11):639–641.
247. Decaens T, Luciani A, Itti E, et al. Phase II study of sirolimus in treatment-naive patients with advanced hepatocellular carcinoma. Digestive and Liver Disease: Official Journal of the Italian Society of Gastroenterology and the Italian Association for the Study of the Liver. 2012;44(7):610–616.
248. Liang W, Wang D, Ling X, et al. Sirolimus-based immunosuppression in liver transplantation for hepatocellular carcinoma: a meta-analysis. Liver Transplantation: Official Publication of the American Association for the Study of Liver Diseases and the International Liver Transplantation Society. 2012;18(1):62–69.
249. Toso C, Merani S, Bigam DL, et al. Sirolimus-based immunosuppression is associated with increased survival after liver transplantation for hepatocellular carcinoma. Hepatology (Baltimore, Md.). 2010;51(4):1237–1243.
250. Ferrari-Lacraz S, Berney T, Morel P, et al. Low risk of anti-human leukocyte antigen antibody sensitization after combined kidney and islet transplantation. Transplantation. 2008;86(2):357–359.
251. Naziruddin B, Wease S, Stablein D, et al. HLA class I sensitization in islet transplant recipients - report from the collaborative islet transplant registry. Cell Transplantation. 2011;21(5):901–908.
252. Rickels MR, Kearns J, Markmann E, et al. HLA sensitization in islet transplantation. Clinical Transplants. 2006; 413–420.
253. Tiwari JL, Schneider B, Barton F, et al. Islet cell transplantation in type 1 diabetes: an analysis of efficacy outcomes and considerations for trial designs. American Journal of Transplantation. 2012;12(7):1898–1907.
254. Robertson RP. Islet transplantation a decade later and strategies for filling a half-full glass. Diabetes. 2010;59(6):1285–1291.
255. Morris PJ, Monaco AP. Pancreatic islet transplantation: is the glass half-empty or half-full? Transplantation. 2005;79(10):1287–1288.
256. Bromberg JS, Kaplan B, Halloran PF, et al. The islet transplant experiment: time for a reassessment. American Journal of Transplantation. 2007;7(10):2217–2218.
257. Ruggenenti P, Remuzzi A, Remuzzi G. Decision time for pancreatic islet-cell transplantation. Lancet. 2008;371(9616):883–884.
258. Shapiro AM. Islet transplantation–the imperative need for continued clinical trials. Nature Clinical Practice Nephrology. 2008;4(12):662–663.
259. Witkowski P, Zakai SB, Rana A, et al. Pancreatic islet transplantation, what has been achieved since Edmonton break-through. Annals of Transplantation: Quarterly of the Polish Transplantation Society. 2006;11(2):5–13, discussion 32–43.
260. Gadi VK, Nelson JL, Guthrie KA, et al. Soluble donor DNA and islet injury after transplantation. Transplantation. 2011;92(5):607–611.
261. Lacotte S, Berney T, Shapiro AJ, et al. Immune monitoring of pancreatic islet graft: towards a better understanding, detection and treatment of harmful events. Expert Opinion on Biological Therapy. 2011;11(1):55–66.
262. Koh A, Imes S, Kin T, et al. Supplemental islet infusions restore insulin independence after graft dysfunction in islet transplant recipients. Transplantation. 2010;89(3):361–365.
263. Fiorina P, Shapiro AM, Ricordi C, et al. The clinical impact of islet transplantation. American Journal of Transplantation. 2008;8(10):1990–1997.
264. Smith RN, Kent SC, Nagle J, et al. Pathology of an islet transplant 2 years after transplantation: evidence for a nonimmunological loss. Transplantation. 2008;86(1):54–62.
265. Sjolander J, Westermark GT, Renstrom E, et al. Islet amyloid polypeptide triggers limited complement activation and binds complement inhibitor C4b-binding protein, which enhances fibril formation. Journal of Biological Chemistry. 2012;287(14):10824–10833.
266. Westermark GT, Davalli AM, Secchi A, et al. Further evidence for amyloid deposition in clinical pancreatic islet grafts. Transplantation. 2012;93(2):219–223.
267. Westermark P, Andersson A, Westermark GT. Islet amyloid polypeptide, islet amyloid, and diabetes mellitus. Physiological Reviews. 2011;91(3):795–826.
268. Prentki M, Madiraju SR. Glycerolipid/free fatty acid cycle and islet beta-cell function in health, obesity and diabetes. Molecular and Cellular Endocrinology. 2012;353(1–2):88–100.
269. Berney T, Ferrari-Lacraz S, Buhler L, et al. Long-term insulin-independence after allogeneic islet transplantation for type 1 diabetes: over the 10-year mark. American Journal of Transplantation. 2009;9(2):419–423.
270. Gibly RF, Graham JG, Luo X, et al. Advancing islet transplantation: from engraftment to the immune response. Diabetologia. 2011;54(10):2494–2505.
271. NIH. NIH News. NIH Funds Centers to Study Islet Transplantation. 2004 [cited May 23, 2012]; Available from: http://www.nih.gov/news/pr/oct2004/niddk-04.htm.
272. Hirshberg B. Benefits of simultaneous islet-kidney transplantation versus simultaneous pancreas-kidney transplantation. Current Diabetes Reports. 2008;8(4):307–309.
273. Lehmann R, Weber M, Berthold P, et al. Successful simultaneous islet-kidney transplantation using a steroid-free immunosuppression: two-year follow-up. American Journal of Transplantation. 2004;4(7):1117–1123.
274. Gerber PA, Pavlicek V, Demartines N, et al. Simultaneous islet-kidney vs pancreas-kidney transplantation in type 1 diabetes mellitus: a 5 year single centre follow-up. Diabetologia. 2008;51(1):110–119.
275. Carroll PB, Ricordi C, Shapiro R, et al. Frequency of kidney rejection in diabetic patients undergoing simultaneous kidney and pancreatic islet cell transplantation. Transplantation. 1993;55(4):761–764, discussion 4–5.
276. Kaufman DB, Baker MS, Chen X, et al. Sequential kidney/islet transplantation using prednisone-free immunosuppression. American Journal of Transplantation. 2002;2(7):674–677.
277. Fiorina P, Folli F, Zerbini G, et al. Islet transplantation is associated with improvement of renal function among uremic patients with type I diabetes mellitus and kidney transplants. Journal of the American Society of Nephrology: JASN. 2003;14(8):2150–2158.
278. Shapiro AM. Islet transplants and impact on secondary diabetic complications: does C-Peptide protect the kidney? Journal of the American Society of Nephrology: JASN. 2003;14(8):2214–2216.
279. Gremizzi C, Vergani A, Paloschi V, et al. Impact of pancreas transplantation on type 1 diabetes-related complications. Current Opinion in Organ Transplantation. 2010;15(1):119–123.
280. Lee TC, Barshes NR, Agee EE, et al. The effect of whole organ pancreas transplantation and PIT on diabetic complications. Current Diabetes Reports. 2006;6(4):323–327.
281. Luzi L. Pancreas transplantation and diabetic complications. New England Journal of Medicine. 1998;339(2):115–117.
282. Becker BN, Brazy PC, Becker YT, et al. Simultaneous pancreas-kidney transplantation reduces excess mortality in type 1 diabetic patients with end-stage renal disease. Kidney International. 2000;57(5):2129–2135.
283. Smets YF, Westendorp RG, van der Pijl JW, et al. Effect of simultaneous pancreas-kidney transplantation on mortality of patients with type-1 diabetes mellitus and end-stage renal failure. Lancet. 1999;353(9168):1915–1919.
284. Tyden G, Bolinder J, Solders G, et al. Improved survival in patients with insulin-dependent diabetes mellitus and end-stage diabetic nephropathy 10 years after combined pancreas and kidney transplantation. Transplantation. 1999;67(5):645–648.
285. Giannarelli R, Coppelli A, Sartini MS, et al. Pancreas transplant alone has beneficial effects on retinopathy in type 1 diabetic patients. Diabetologia. 2006;49(12):2977–2982.
286. Koznarova R, Saudek F, Sosna T, et al. Beneficial effect of pancreas and kidney transplantation on advanced diabetic retinopathy. Cell Transplantation. 2000;9(6):903–908.
287. Fioretto P, Mauer M. Reversal of diabetic nephropathy: lessons from pancreas transplantation. Journal of Nephrology. 2012;25(1):13–18.
288. Fioretto P, Steffes MW, Sutherland DE, et al. Reversal of lesions of diabetic nephropathy after pancreas transplantation. New England Journal of Medicine. 1998;339(2):69–75.

289. Kendall DM, Rooney DP, Smets YF, et al. Pancreas transplantation restores epinephrine response and symptom recognition during hypoglycemia in patients with long-standing type I diabetes and autonomic neuropathy. Diabetes. 1997;46(2):249–257.
290. Larsen JL, Ratanasuwan T, Burkman T, et al. Carotid intima media thickness decreases after pancreas transplantation. Transplantation. 2002;73(6):936–940.
291. Ojo AO, Meier-Kriesche HU, Hanson JA, et al. The impact of simultaneous pancreas-kidney transplantation on long-term patient survival. Transplantation. 2001;71(1):82–90.
292. Del Carro U, Fiorina P, Amadio S, et al. Evaluation of polyneuropathy markers in type 1 diabetic kidney transplant patients and effects of islet transplantation: neurophysiological and skin biopsy longitudinal analysis. Diabetes Care. 2007;30(12):3063–3069.
293. Venturini M, Fiorina P, Maffi P, et al. Early increase of retinal arterial and venous blood flow velocities at color Doppler imaging in brittle type 1 diabetes after islet transplant alone. Transplantation. 2006;81(9):1274–1277.
294. Fiorina P, Gremizzi C, Maffi P, et al. Islet transplantation is associated with an improvement of cardiovascular function in type 1 diabetic kidney transplant patients. Diabetes Care. 2005;28(6):1358–1365.
295. Fiorina P, Folli F, Maffi P, et al. Islet transplantation improves vascular diabetic complications in patients with diabetes who underwent kidney transplantation: a comparison between kidney-pancreas and kidney-alone transplantation. Transplantation. 2003;75(8):1296–1301.
296. Fiorina P, Folli F, Bertuzzi F, et al. Long-term beneficial effect of islet transplantation on diabetic macro-/microangiopathy in type 1 diabetic kidney-transplanted patients. Diabetes Care. 2003;26(4):1129–1136.
297. Thompson DM, Meloche M, Ao Z, et al. Reduced progression of diabetic microvascular complications with islet cell transplantation compared with intensive medical therapy. Transplantation. 2011;91(3):373–378.
298. Warnock GL, Thompson DM, Meloche RM, et al. A multi-year analysis of islet transplantation compared with intensive medical therapy on progression of complications in type 1 diabetes. Transplantation. 2008;86(12):1762–1766.
299. Payne WD, Sutherland DE, Matas AJ, et al. Amelioration of diabetes in rats by transplantation of islet tissue from a single donor to multiple recipients. Surgical Forum. 1977;28:301–304.
300. Griffin SM, Alderson D, Farndon JR. Comparison of harvesting methods for islet transplantation. British Journal of Surgery. 1986;73(9):712–715.
301. Matsumoto S, Okitsu T, Iwanaga Y, et al. Insulin independence after living-donor distal pancreatectomy and islet allotransplantation. Lancet. 2005;365(9471):1642–1644.
302. Shapiro AM, Ricordi C. Unraveling the secrets of single donor success in islet transplantation. American Journal of Transplantation. 2004;4(3):295–298.
303. Markmann JF, Deng S, Huang X, et al. Insulin independence following isolated islet transplantation and single islet infusions. Annals of Surgery. 2003;237(6):741–749, discussion 9–50.
304. Nilsson B, Ekdahl KN, Korsgren O. Control of instant blood-mediated inflammatory reaction to improve islets of Langerhans engraftment. Current Opinion in Organ Transplantation. 2011;16(6):620–626.
305. Cabric S, Sanchez J, Lundgren T, et al. Islet surface heparinization prevents the instant blood-mediated inflammatory reaction in islet transplantation. Diabetes. 2007;56(8):2008–2015.
306. Turgeon NA, Avila JG, Cano JA, et al. Experience with a novel efalizumab-based immunosuppressive regimen to facilitate single donor islet cell transplantation. American Journal of Transplantation. 2010;10(9):2082–2091.
307. Oberholzer J, Kinzer K, Fiorina P. The anti-LFA-1 trial in islet transplantation. American Journal of Transplantation. 2010;10(8):1725–1726.
308. Ichii H, Miki A, Yamamoto T, et al. Characterization of pancreatic ductal cells in human islet preparations. Laboratory Investigation; a Journal of Technical Methods and Pathology. 2008;88(11):1167–1177.
309. Sweet IR, Gilbert M, Scott S, et al. Glucose-stimulated increment in oxygen consumption rate as a standardized test of human islet quality. American Journal of Transplantation. 2008;8(1):183–192.
310. Papas KK, Colton CK, Nelson RA, et al. Human islet oxygen consumption rate and DNA measurements predict diabetes reversal in nude mice. American Journal of Transplantation. 2007;7(3):707–713.
311. Faradji RN, Froud T, Messinger S, et al. Long-term metabolic and hormonal effects of exenatide on islet transplant recipients with allograft dysfunction. Cell Transplantation. 2009;18(10):1247–1259.
312. Froud T, Ricordi C, Alejandro R. Exenatide Use in Islet Transplantation - Reasons to Remain Optimistic. Transplantation. 2009;87(1):154.
313. Rickels MR, Naji A. Exenatide use in islet transplantation: words of caution. Transplantation. 2009;87(1):153, author reply 4.
314. Faradji RN, Tharavanij T, Messinger S, et al. Long-term insulin independence and improvement in insulin secretion after supplemental islet infusion under exenatide and etanercept. Transplantation. 2008;86(12):1658–1665.
315. Froud T, Faradji RN, Pileggi A, et al. The use of exenatide in islet transplant recipients with chronic allograft dysfunction: safety, efficacy, and metabolic effects. Transplantation. 2008;86(1):36–45.
316. Ghofaili KA, Fung M, Ao Z, et al. Effect of exenatide on beta cell function after islet transplantation in type 1 diabetes. Transplantation. 2007;83(1):24–28.
317. Gangemi A, Salehi P, Hatipoglu B, et al. Islet transplantation for brittle type 1 diabetes: the UIC protocol. American Journal of Transplantation. 2008; 8(6):1250–1261.
318. Emamaullee JA, Merani S, Toso C, et al. Porcine marginal mass islet autografts resist metabolic failure over time and are enhanced by early treatment with liraglutide. Endocrinology. 2009;150(5):2145–2152.
319. Toso C, McCall M, Emamaullee J, et al. Liraglutide, a long-acting human glucagon-like peptide 1 analogue, improves human islet survival in culture. Transplant International: Official Journal of the European Society for Organ Transplantation. 2010;23(3):259–265.
320. Berney T. Liraglutide in islet transplantation: from bench to bedside. Transplant International: Official Journal of the European Society for Organ Transplantation. 2010;23(3):257–258.
321. Moberg L, Johansson H, Lukinius A, et al. Production of tissue factor by pancreatic islet cells as a trigger of detrimental thrombotic reactions in clinical islet transplantation. Lancet. 2002;360(9350):2039–2045.
322. Eriksson O, Eich T, Sundin A, et al. Positron emission tomography in clinical islet transplantation. American Journal of Transplantation. 2009;9(12):2816–2824.
323. Eich T, Eriksson O, Lundgren T. Visualization of early engraftment in clinical islet transplantation by positron-emission tomography. New England Journal of Medicine. 2007;356(26):2754–2755.
324. Cabric S, Sanchez J, Johansson U, et al. Anchoring of vascular endothelial growth factor to surface-immobilized heparin on pancreatic islets: implications for stimulating islet angiogenesis. Tissue Engineering Part A. 2010;16(3):961–970.
325. Emamaullee JA, Shapiro AM. Interventional strategies to prevent beta-cell apoptosis in islet transplantation. Diabetes. 2006;55(7):1907–1914.
326. Emamaullee JA, Rajotte RV, Liston P, et al. XIAP overexpression in human islets prevents early posttransplant apoptosis and reduces the islet mass needed to treat diabetes. Diabetes. 2005;54(9):2541–2548.
327. Emamaullee J, Liston P, Korneluk RG, et al. XIAP overexpression in islet beta-cells enhances engraftment and minimizes hypoxia-reperfusion injury. American Journal of Transplantation. 2005;5(6):1297–1305.
328. Emamaullee JA, Stanton L, Schur C, et al. Caspase inhibitor therapy enhances marginal mass islet graft survival and preserves long-term function in islet transplantation. Diabetes. 2007;56(5):1289–1298.
329. Nakano M, Matsumoto I, Sawada T, et al. Caspase-3 inhibitor prevents apoptosis of human islets immediately after isolation and improves islet graft function. Pancreas. 2004;29(2):104–109.
330. Emamaullee JA, Davis J, Pawlick R, et al. The caspase selective inhibitor EP1013 augments human islet graft function and longevity in marginal mass islet transplantation in mice. Diabetes. 2008;57(6):1556–1566.
331. Emamaullee JA, Davis J, Pawlick R, et al. Caspase inhibitor therapy synergizes with costimulation blockade to promote indefinite islet allograft survival. Diabetes. 2010;59(6):1469–1477.
332. McCall M, Toso C, Emamaullee J, et al. The caspase inhibitor IDN-6556 (PF3491390) improves marginal mass engraftment after islet transplantation in mice. Surgery. 2011;150(1):48–55.
333. Arora S, Tangirala B, Osadchuk L, et al. Belatacept: a new biological agent for maintenance immunosuppression in kidney transplantation. Expert Opinion on Biological Therapy. 2012;12(7):965–979.
334. Parameswaran S, Swaminathan RP. Belatacept: good, but not good enough? Journal of Pharmacology and Pharmacotherapeutics. 2012;3(1):82–83.
335. Vincenti F. Beyond belatacept: praise and progress for the FDA. American Journal of Transplantation. 2012;12(3):513–514.
336. Wekerle T, Grinyo JM. Belatacept: from rational design to clinical application. Transplant International: Official Journal of the European Society for Organ Transplantation. 2012;25(2):139–150.
337. Larsen CP, Grinyo J, Medina-Pestana J, et al. Belatacept-based regimens versus a cyclosporine A-based regimen in kidney transplant recipients: 2-year results from the BENEFIT and BENEFIT-EXT studies. Transplantation. 2010;90(12):1528–1535.
338. Vincenti F, Blancho G, Durrbach A, et al. Five-year safety and efficacy of belatacept in renal transplantation. Journal of the American Society of Nephrology: JASN. 2010;21(9):1587–1596.
339. Kaplan B. Belatacept: the promises and challenges of belatacept and costimulatory blockade. American Journal of Transplantation. 2010;10(3):441–442.
340. Larsen CP, Pearson TC, Adams AB, et al. Rational development of LEA29Y (belatacept), a high-affinity variant of CTLA4-Ig with potent immunosuppressive

properties. American Journal of Transplantation. 2005;5(3):443–453.
341. Kirk AD, Harlan DM, Armstrong NN, et al. CTLA4-Ig and anti-CD40 ligand prevent renal allograft rejection in primates. Proceedings of the National Academy of Sciences of the United States of America. 1997;94(16): 8789–8794.
342. Pearson TC, Trambley J, Odom K, et al. Anti-CD40 therapy extends renal allograft survival in rhesus macaques. Transplantation. 2002;74(7):933–940.
343. Adams AB, Shirasugi N, Jones TR, et al. Development of a chimeric anti-CD40 monoclonal antibody that synergizes with LEA29Y to prolong islet allograft survival. Journal of Immunology. 2005;174(1):542–550.
344. Sykes M. Hematopoietic cell transplantation for tolerance induction: animal models to clinical trials. Transplantation. 2009;87(3):309–316.
345. Spitzer TR, Delmonico F, Tolkoff-Rubin N, et al. Combined histocompatibility leukocyte antigen-matched donor bone marrow and renal transplantation for multiple myeloma with end stage renal disease: the induction of allograft tolerance through mixed lymphohematopoietic chimerism. Transplantation. 1999;68(4):480–484.
346. Strober S, Spitzer TR, Lowsky R, et al. Translational studies in hematopoietic cell transplantation: treatment of hematologic malignancies as a stepping stone to tolerance induction. Seminars in Immunology. 2011;23(4):273–281.
347. Spitzer TR, Sykes M, Tolkoff-Rubin N, et al. Long-term follow-up of recipients of combined human leukocyte antigen-matched bone marrow and kidney transplantation for multiple myeloma with end-stage renal disease. Transplantation. 2011;91(6):672–676.
348. Sachs DH, Sykes M, Kawai T, et al. Immuno-intervention for the induction of transplantation tolerance through mixed chimerism. Seminars in Immunology. 2011;23(3):165–173.
349. Kawai T, Cosimi AB, Sachs DH. Preclinical and clinical studies on the induction of renal allograft tolerance through transient mixed chimerism. Current Opinion in Organ Transplantation. 2011;16(4):366–371.
350. Scandling JD, Busque S, Shizuru JA, et al. Induced immune tolerance for kidney transplantation. The New England Journal of Medicine. 2011;365(14): 1359–1360.
351. Tan J, Wu W, Xu X, et al. Induction therapy with autologous mesenchymal stem cells in living-related kidney transplants: a randomized controlled trial. JAMA: The Journal of the American Medical Association. 2012;307(11):1169–1177.
352. Leventhal J, Abecassis M, Miller J, et al. Chimerism and tolerance without GVHD or engraftment syndrome in HLA-mismatched combined kidney and hematopoietic stem cell transplantation. Science Translational Medicine. 2012;4(124):124ra28.

第 109 章 小肠和多器官联合移植的长期预后

Jennifer Garcia, Gennaro Selvaggi, Akin Tekin, Phillip Ruiz, Andreas Tzakis

引言

小肠移植是复杂小肠坏死患者的救命措施。尽管预后落后于其他大多数实质性器官的移植，个别小肠移植患者存活超过 20 年且能独立进食，恢复健康和社会生活表明其有长期成功的可能性。影响小肠移植后预后最主要的问题为由于排斥、疾病复发或感染导致的移植器官失功或死亡。这些可能与肠道屏障和供体器官对受体的同种免疫功能间的复杂相互关系相关。包含肝移植和其他多器官联合移植能在某种程度上减小免疫障碍，小肠同种移植对于患者和医生而言仍然存在免疫障碍。本章将回顾小肠移植的长期预后和影响预后的因素。

长期移植及患者预后

尽管小肠移植领域持续取得进展，预后也在改善，其长期预后仍然落后于肾脏、肝脏及心脏移植，其预后与肺移植相当。根据第 12 届国际小肠移植讨论会的小肠移植登记(2011)，全世界范围已经进行了 2611 例小肠移植，超过一半(55%)为儿童患者(详见第 117 章)。患者的 5 年生存率仅约 50%，2000 年后的移植患者预后有所改善。随着时间进展，生存率持续下降：35%的患者于第 10 年时存活，这在儿童及成人间没有区别。联合移植(多脏器和肝脏-小肠联合移植)的远期预后好于单纯移植（移植 5 年后生存率分别为 55%及 65%对 45%)。危险因素包括移植时年龄<1 岁、免疫抑制的诱导和患者移植时的状态，患者在医院的病房，特别是重症监护室，为预示因子。移植时在家或大型中心的患者移植预后可见改善。包括肝移植的联合移植与良好预后显著相关，相对危险度为 0.68(P=0)[1,2]。

当分析我们中心的小肠移植术后生存超过 5 年的成人患者的预后可以发现相似的结果[3]。从 1994—2010 年，115 名成人患者接受了 126 次移植，其中 79 例患者于 1994—2005 年间接受移植。36 名(42%)患者生存超过 5 年。中位随访时间为(9.2±3.2)年，全部患者均脱离肠外营养。长期生存和未长期生存患者的免疫移植诱导、供体年龄、供体/受体人类白细胞抗原匹配(位点数量)或交叉配对(阴性/阳性)间无显著差异。但接受包括肝脏移植(肝脏-小肠或多器官移植)的患者的 5 年生存率显著好于接受不包括肝脏移植(改良多器官移植或单纯小肠移植)(图 109.1)的患者。此外，移植前状态间有显著性差异：52%的长期生存患者和 78%的未长期生存患者接受移植时处于家中(P=0.015)(图 109.2)[3]。这表明移植前状态不仅影响短期预后，也影响远期预后。

在最近美国外科医师学会的介绍中，来自时间最悠久及世界最大的中心，匹兹堡大学的研究者报道了

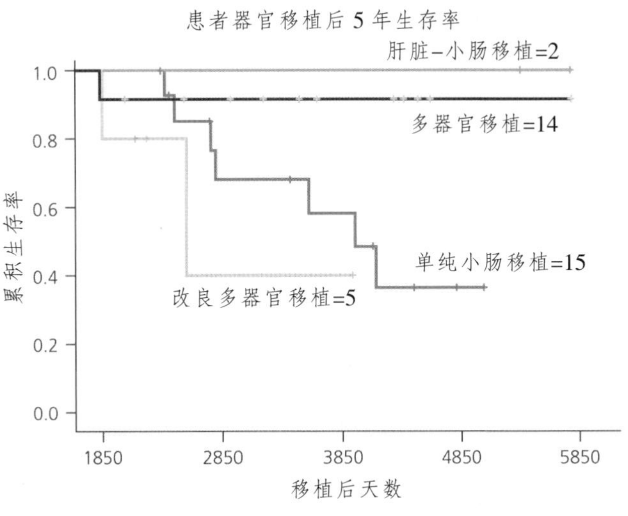

图 109.1 迈阿密大学米勒医学院至少 5 年的长期生存患者，图示为肝脏-小肠移植、多器官移植、单纯小肠移植和改良多器官移植患者的预后。

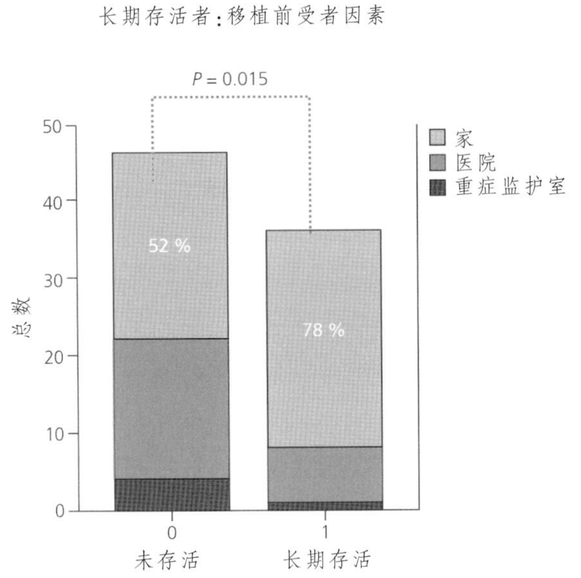

图 109.2　小肠移植后长期生存患者的特点分层。长期生存与患者移植时能健康地待在家里有关。

患者和移植器官 5 年生存率分别为 60%及 50%。生存超过 5 年的患者 10 年及 15 年的生存率分别为 75%和 61%。相应的移植物存活率分别为 59%和 50%[4]。导致死亡的原因有排斥、感染和肾衰竭。相较于儿童，肾衰竭在成人中更常见。导致移植物失功的原因为排斥。

这个研究证实以前的观察结果：

- 大部分长期生存患者(92%)能摄入日常饮食，实现营养独立。
- 大部分长期生存患者(92%)的移植器官有正常的可量化的功能。
- 接受小肠移植的患者的生活质量显著好于依赖肠外营养的患者。
- 长期神经精神障碍行为发生率高(儿童中更高)，如抑郁、焦虑和认知功能障碍。
- 尽管这些疾病发生率高，这些患者有超乎寻常的社会调节力。大部分儿童能上学，大部分成人能保有家庭和工作。

这个研究第一次表明长期生存的最重要危险因素为缺乏社会支持，应严谨处理这一过程及相关资料显示的各类并发症。移植物(不包括肝脏)为影响长期生存的第二重要危险因素。其他预后因素包括早期排斥、受体的年龄及性别、免疫抑制的类型、脾切除和人类白细胞抗原不匹配。

慢性肾衰竭是小肠移植后的常见并发症，报道的 5 年发生率约为 21.3%。据报道，5%~9%的长期生存患者需要肾脏替代治疗。肾衰竭可为小肠移植后的致命并发症，因为缺乏静脉通路对于透析乃至肾移植都是禁忌。类似的，恶性肿瘤的发生率升高，主要是淋巴来源的移植后淋巴组织增生性疾病。其他恶性肿瘤（皮肤、结肠等)更常见于其他实质性器官移植。

排斥，作为导致长期生存患者死亡的主要原因，应被预防或治疗。其诊断往往基于出现排斥的临床表现(腹胀、腹泻或肠梗阻、肠出血)后的活检(见第 86 章)。临床表现和小肠排斥管理的详细细节见第 74 章。大部分这些患者生活于远离移植中心的地方。当吻合口闭合时，不容易进行内镜检查。

我们证实血清瓜氨酸的减少有助于诊断。其水平在移植 3 个月后稳定下来。排除严重感染情况后，下降超过基线的 25%或绝对值<13~15m/L 为排斥的重要指标[5]。我们中心或其他中心正在开展排斥的非侵入性指标的研究。

有越来越多的证据表明反应性抗体和疾病易感抗原水平与急性排斥的进展、严重度和对治疗的反应相关[6]。它们在远期预后中的作用仍未知，也是现在监视的目标。

儿童生长和发育

接受小肠移植的儿童脱离了肠外营养，但在移植后最初的 2~5 年内为了生长，仍然需要肠内营养支持[7-10]。这很有可能是由于部分患者存在长期厌食。

一位来自法国研究者的报道显示，在 31 名不依赖肠外营养的儿童患者中，84%的儿童始终不需要肠外营养，而 45%的儿童需要肠内营养[10]。持续的脂肪吸收不良促使需要更多的营养摄入，通过必需的肠内营养摄入，以确保正常生长[10]。

比推荐值(根据年龄)多 20%~30%卡路里的营养支持是正常生长的关键[11]。

患者生活质量和移植器官功能的丧失

在小肠移植中，排斥是导致移植小肠功能丧失的最常见原因。早期发现，排斥需要正确的实现筛查方案，包括内镜和一些可行的非特异性的生物质指标(瓜氨酸、钙卫蛋白)。

急性排斥

小肠移植后,生存患者仍需注意迟发性急性排斥。一项大中心的综述报道,包括36名小肠移植术后生存超过5年的成年患者的迟发急性排斥发生率为14%。这些患者都为单纯小肠移植，且都接受了胸腺免疫球蛋白治疗[3]。

迟发急性排斥常与不遵医嘱相关，或跟随胃肠炎发作[12,13]。迟发排斥罕见,但其往往很严重,导致移植器官功能丧失。

慢性排斥

早期、复发和(或)严重急性排斥使患者易发生慢性排斥。此外,单纯小肠移植的受体相对于接受包含肝移植的患者更易发生慢性排斥。准确诊断慢性排斥需要全层组织活检,其临床诊断往往基于临床表现,诊断被证实于再次移植时肠切除或尸检。据许多中心报道，慢性排斥的发生率约为15%[12-14]。目前除再次移植外，无其他措施可以治疗慢性排斥。

再次移植

移植器官功能丧失,即需要移除移植器官,常需要再次移植。小肠移植登记处的报道[1,2]显示早期接受小肠再移植的患者预后非常糟糕。最近,一项研究报道了更好的预后,患者的生存率为71%[15]。一项包含500名成人和儿童受体的研究报道了相似的结果[16]。

感染

感染为小肠移植受体最常见的并发症和导致死亡的原因[1]。感染在移植后早期更常见,50%的感染发生于最初的3个月,25%发生于3~12个月，仅25%发生于移植后12个月[17]。然而,即使过了移植后早期阶段，感染导致的死亡仍占总数的60%[1]。当发生迟发性感染性肠炎时,肠管吻合口往往闭合,急诊内镜检查往往不可行,所以其为一困难的挑战。感染性肠炎能引起排斥的进展,使其变得更致命[18-20]。

肿瘤疾病

显著数量的小肠移植患者可见新发肿瘤，报道发生率约为15%[21]。这当中,13%为移植后淋巴组织增生性疾病,仅有3.2%为非淋巴癌。移植后淋巴组织增生性疾病的详细描述见第96章。考虑到需要高强度的免疫抑制使移植小肠免于出现排斥，以及相较于其他实质性脏器移植,移植小肠内出现大量淋巴组织,移植后淋巴组织增生性疾病在小肠移植受体中的出现风险最高。绝大部分移植后淋巴组织增生性疾病为EB病毒促使的异常B淋巴细胞增生而非T淋巴细胞,Burkitt淋巴瘤和EB病毒阴性亚型也被报道过[22]。最常见的移植后淋巴组织增生性疾病涉及小肠移植物。总共累计风险为移植后6个月8%,1年11%,5年16%和10年27%[21]。免疫抑制、受体年龄、脾切除和排斥治疗为移植后淋巴组织增生性疾病的危险因素。即使最近的研究报道移植后淋巴组织增生性疾病的发生率已经降低到7%,儿童受体发生移植后淋巴组织增生性疾病的风险更高是因为绝大部分儿童在接受移植时无EBV免疫力[21]。移植后淋巴组织增生性疾病的管理也有改善,这归因于通过血液EBV定量PCR分析的早期检测及利妥昔单抗的使用[23]。

更常见于成人的非淋巴癌症的累计风险为5年4%及10年10%。非淋巴癌症最常见的包括非黑色素皮肤癌。其他癌症包括肺癌,睾丸、子宫、结直肠、外阴和前列腺癌。最后,小肠移植后Gradner综合征、纤维瘤复发很可能与免疫抑制相关。

移植物抗宿主病

相较于其他实质脏器移植,小肠移植受体中移植物受体疾病的发生率更高。据报道,小肠移植患者的发生率为5%~10%,其他实质性脏器移植受体的发生率为1%~2%[24,25]。发生移植物受体疾病的死亡率相当高,尤其当患者最初未接受激素治疗时[26]。大多数患者死亡是由于持续的感染和多器官衰竭。积极主动地监测肠道受者外周血供体嵌合水平,可以在症状出现时更早地诊断,并被证明是决定治疗成功的重要纵向工具。

肾功能障碍

一些研究已经表明小肠移植患者相对于其他实质性脏器移植受体发生慢性肾衰竭的风险更高。Ojo等[27]第一个发现这一情况，报道了移植后5年的风险为21.3%。这些患者在移植前和移植后经历了长期的脱水，钙调磷酸酶抑制剂和长期脱水共同造成了肾毒性的进展和恶化。肾功能障碍的预测因子包括术前肾小球滤过率<75%、术前处于 ICU 和高剂量的 FK 免疫抑制剂。移植后肾小球滤过率<75%为预后不佳的预测因子[28]。来自匹兹堡的 Thomas E. Starzl 研究所的研究者报道了 9%的移植后长期生存超过 5 年的患者需要肾移植[4]。

总结

小肠移植仍是一项富有挑战性的治疗，其结果仍落后于其他脏器移植。而同种特性新免疫和保护性免疫并发症的种类与其余实质性脏器移植中的种类相似，它们的程度及频率仍很高，且持续发生。合适的患者选择，尤其需注意家庭社会支持和患者对风险的认知是取得良好预后的关键。尽管存在这些挑战，小肠移植仍是特定条件下的最好选择。

（周舒扬 杨梦凡 译 周舒扬 校）

参考文献

1. Intestinal Transplant Registry. [accessed February 8, 2014] Available at: http://www.intestinaltransplant.org.
2. Grant D, Abu-Elmagd K, Reyes J, et al. 2003 report of the intestinal transplant registry: a new era has dawned. Annals of Surgery. 2005;241(4):607–613.
3. Uchida K, Nishida S, Levi D, et al. Current Status of Long Term Survivors after Intestinal and Multivisceral Transplantation in Adults. Oral Presentation, ISBTS. 2011.
4. Abu-Elmagd K, Costa G, Kosmach-Park B, et al. Long term survival, nutritional autonomy, and quality of life after intestinal and multivisceral transplantation. Annals of Surgery. 2012;256(3):494.
5. David AI, Selvaggi G, Ruiz P, et al. Blood citrulline level is an exclusionary marker for significant acute rejection after intestinal transplantation. Transplantation. 2007;84(9):1077–1081.
6. Gonzalez-Pinto IM, Tzakis AG, Tsai HL, Chang JW, et al. Association between panel reactive antibodies and acute small bowel rejection: analysis of a series of 324 intestinal transplants. Transplantation Proceedings. 2010;42(10):4269–4271.
7. Iyer K, Horslen S, Iverson A, et al. Nutritional outcome and growth of children after intestinal transplantation. Journal of Pediatric Surgery. 2002;37:464.
8. Nucci AM, Barksdale EM Jr, Beserock N, et al. Long-term nutritional outcomes after pediatric intestinal transplantation. Journal of Pediatric Surgery. 2002;37:460.
9. Venick RS, Farmer DG, Saikali D, et al. Nutritional outcome following intestinal transplantation. Transplantation Proceedings. 2008;38:1718.
10. Lacaille F, Vass N, Sauvat F, et al. Long term outcome, growth and digestive function in children 2 to 18 years of age after intestinal transplantation. Gut. 2008;57:455–461.
11. Ueno T, Kato T, Revas K, et al. Growth after intestinal transplant in children. Transplantation Proceedings. 2006;38:1702.
12. Gupte G, Sharif K, Muiesan P, et al. Small Bowel Transplant Programme- 1993-2011; Strategies for Improvement in Medium and Long Term Survival. Oral Presentation, ISBTS. 2011. Available at: https://www.tts.org/index.php?option=com_tts&view=presentations&meeting=27&Itemid=312&limitstart=100 [accessed April 21, 2014].
13. Chandrashekhar K, Mangus R, Tector J, et al. Intestinal/Multivisceral Transplantation: Indiana University Experience. Oral Presentation, ISBTS. 2011. Available at: https://www.tts.org/index.php?option=com_tts&view=presentations&meeting=27&Itemid=312&limitstart=100 [accessed April 21, 2014].
14. Lacaille F, Chardot C, Goulet O, et al. Intestinal Transplantation 17 Years Down the Road: Lessons and Future. Oral Presentation, ISBTS. 2011. Available at: https://www.tts.org/index.php?option=com_tts&view=presentations&meeting=27&Itemid=312&limitstart=100 [accessed April 21, 2014].
15. Mazariegos GV, Soltys K, Bond G, et al. Pediatric intestinal retransplantation: techniques, management, and outcomes. Transplantation. 2008;86:1777–1782.
16. Abu-Elmagd KM, Costa G, Bond GJ, et al. Five hundred intestinal and multivisceral transplantations at a single center: major advances with new challenges. Annals of Surgery. 2009;250:567–579.
17. Kato T, Tzakis AG, Selvaggi G, et al. Intestinal and multivisceral transplantation in children. Annals of Surgery. 2006;243:756.
18. Farmer D. Infectious Complications. Oral Presentation, ISBTS. 2011. Available at: https://www.tts.org/index.php?option=com_tts&view=presentations&meeting=27&Itemid=312&limitstart=100 [accessed April 21, 2014].
19. Eisengart LJ, Chou PM, Iyer K, et al. Rotavirus infection in small bowel transplant: a histological comparison with acute cellular rejection. Pediatric and Developmental Pathology. 2009;12:85.
20. Parizhskaya M, Walpush J, Mazariegos G, et al. Enteric adenovirus infection in pediatric small bowel transplant recipients. Pediatric and Developmental Pathology. 2001;4:122.
21. Abu-Elmagd KM, Mazariegos G, Costa G, et al. Lymphoproliferative disorders and denovo malignancies in intestinal and multivisceral recipients: improved outcomes with new outlooks. Transplantation. 2009;88(7):926–934.
22. Debray D, Baudouin V, Lacaille F, et al. De novo malignancy after solid organ transplantation in children. Transplantation Proceedings. 2009;41:674–675.
23. Berney T, Delis S, Kato T, et al. Successful treatment of posttransplant lymphoproliferative disease with prolonged rituximab in intestinal transplant recipients. Transplantation. 2002;74:1000–1006.
24. Mazariegos GV, Abu-Elmagd K, Bond JR, et al. Graft versus host disease in intestinal transplantation. American Journal of Transplantation. 2004;4(9):1459–1465.
25. Andres AM, Santamaria ML, Ramos F, et al. Graft-vs-host disease after small bowel transplantation in children. Journal of Pediatric Surgery. 2010;45:330–336.
26. Shin CR, Nathan J, Alonso M, et al. Incidence of acute and chronic acute and chronic graft-versus-host disease and donor T cell chimerism after small bowel or combined organ transplantation. Journal of Pediatric Surgery. 2011;46:1732–1738.
27. Ojo AO, Held P, Port FK, et al. Chronic renal failure and transplantation of a nonrenal origin. New England Journal of Medicine. 2003;349:931–940.
28. Watson MJ, Venick RS, Kaldas F, et al. Renal function impacts outcomes after intestinal transplantation. Transplantation. 2008;88(1):117–122.

第 110 章 同种异体复合组织移植的长期预后

Alessandrina M. Freitas, Linda C. Cendales

引言

同种异体复合组织移植(VCA)为多组织缺陷重建的发展领域,可改善自体组织。迄今为止,这类移植已被用于全世界超过 90 名患者。据报道,最常见的同种异体复合组织移植部位包括手和(或)手指(54 名患者)、喉部(16 名患者)、腹壁(9 名患者)和脸部(7 名患者)。其他移植,包括膝盖、子宫、股骨干和下肢也被报道过[1]。

同种异体复合组织移植在目前可能是由于显微手术和移植的进展。这些同种异体复合组织移植技术为组织转移,技术已经被扩展用于重建手术数十年。环孢素后免疫抑制的进展已经被用于同种异体复合组织移植。然而,大部分患者目前仍然使用多种药物方案,典型的方案包括他克莫司、霉酚酸酯和激素。考虑到同种异体复合组织移植为一项关乎生命质量的移植,其得到更广泛应用的一个障碍为传统免疫抑制制剂相关的副反应和毒性。

同种异体复合组织移植中的急性和慢性排斥

在书写本章时,85%的同种异体复合组织移植受体在第一年内可观察到急性排斥[2]。一些理论解释了为什么其排斥反应的发生率高于实质性脏器移植。首先,真皮和上皮富含树突状细胞,这赋予了皮肤高度的免疫原性。其次,诊断出的急性排斥反应的次数可能部分反映了这样一个事实,即我们能够不断观察移植的皮肤,这可能导致检测到排斥事件,而在实体器官移植中,这种情况可能会注意不到。第三,同种异体复合组织移植中耐受试验的数量可能会影响免疫抑制的亚治疗水平。最后,同种异体复合组织移植物与环境不断接触,皮肤会因环境暴露(温度、阳光照射、过敏原)而出现变化,这可能被严重误认为是排斥反应。

2005 年,为了使报告标准化,促进执行同种异体复合组织移植的各个中心之间的前瞻性数据收集和协作,并促进对同种异体复合组织移植病理学的理解,一个国际共识小组成立了 Banff 工作组。这于 2007 年的含有复合同种异体皮肤病理学的工作分类上被报道[3],目前作为同种异体复合组织移植中排斥反应相关组织学基础被持续报道。

慢性排斥和抗体调节排斥已经被报道存在于同种异体复合组织移植,且其数量随着病例数和移植生存时间的累积持续上升。Banff 2007 共识提出的同种异体复合组织移植中慢性损害的可能特征包括血管狭窄、附件损失、皮肤和肌肉萎缩性改变、深层组织纤维化、指甲改变和肌内膜增生[3]。至今在西方国家中,仅有一例报道同种异体复合组织移植可能存在慢性排斥。这名患者在路易斯维尔接受移植,且免疫抑制方案为阿仑单抗诱导及霉酚酸酯/他克莫司维持治疗,在经历了严重移植器官缺血 9 个月后,其移植手需要截肢。检查发现引起供体动脉缺血的原因是供体动脉内膜增生严重。当移植器官失功时,尽管深部组织有细胞浸润,表面活检不会显示存在组织排斥。以前未检测到的 Ⅰ 和 Ⅱ 类供体特异性抗体在免疫抑制终止及移植器官切除后变成阳性[4]。关于同种异体复合组织移植排斥的临床特征的额外信息见第 75 章,对排斥组织的病理学表现的更深理解见第 85 章。

同种异体复合组织移植的并发症

免疫抑制并发症

与免疫抑制相关的并发症包括代谢障碍、恶性肿瘤和机会感染[5]。本书的其他章节回顾了各种实质性器官移植的免疫抑制并发症。同种异体复合组织移植受体中常见免疫抑制相关的和社会心理的并发症，本章将回顾这些并发症。同种异体复合组织移植被认为是生命质量移植，因此，与挽救生命的移植相比，风险-效益比(潜在风险:生命质量改善)使其需要仔细检查其他因素。

本章着眼于同种异体复合组织移植的长期预后，其至今仍未被定义。我们定义长期为移植后超过一年。与大多数新兴领域一样，对同种异体复合组织移植预后的量化面临着挑战，因为迄今为止进行的移植手术相对较少，可供长期随访的患者也很少。此外，移植中心的随访方法差异很大，这进一步加大了收集统一数据的难度。我们必须根据实质性脏器移植的经验来指导监测远期预后，并收集能够用来比较各中心目标的数据。肾移植患者常通过血清肌酐来检测，移植肾功能障碍意味着需要再次透析。相似的，移植心脏和肺的功能随访根据射血分数和肺功能测试。随着这一领域的前进，有必要将客观的、功能上重要的成果措施标准化。由于移植组织的具体风险和随访方法差异很大，我们目前重点关注一些特定类型的同种异体复合组织移植，以便对哪些移植(至少在功能上)是广泛可变的进行更具体的讨论。

手移植

背景

手移植在技术上是可行的，其手术技术和并发症(如动脉栓塞、静脉堵塞等)与自体肢体的显微再植相似，其详细记录见第 64 章。据我们所知，在书写本章时，西方国家有 45 名患者接受了手移植(23 名单侧及 22 名双侧)。然而，仅有 21 名单侧和 18 名双侧手移植患者被国际注册处报道[1]。并且，仅有 13 名单侧和 14 名双侧患者的细节被发表。

患者选择

合适的患者选择、筛选和多规则评估至关重要。它们的重要性怎么强调也不过分。由于这项治疗较新奇，候选者可能会表现出渴望接受风险，但他们可能并不适合这项治疗。候选者可能医学上合适，但缺乏耐受、社会支持和承诺随访方面的证据。患者招募应包括教育、关于国际预后的信息、包括假体和自体组织外科重建在内的护理选择标准、免疫抑制、康复、并发症和整个移植过程[6]。

将潜在候选人限制为双侧截肢者的理由包括，即使使用假肢，双侧手丧失后的生活质量也很差，且双侧截肢者可能更倾向于遵循康复计划[7]。患者有很高的不满倾向是因为他们会比较移植手和自己的手的功能[5]。然而，根据患者满意度调查报告的文献，这一假设不被支持。此外，再植文献通常支持单侧上肢再植，表明单侧再植的患者比那些接受手术截肢和使用假肢的患者更有可能获得“优秀”或“良好”的长期结果(通过 Carroll 评分)[8]。

Louisville 分析了各种同种异体复合组织移植个体能接受的风险度[9,10]。结果显示，健康对照组和肾脏移植受体对接受双手移植和肾脏移植的风险水平相等。此外，单侧手移植风险的接受程度显著高于脚移植[9]。

手移植的预后

患者死亡率

已经有双侧手和脸部联合移植术后 2 月患者死亡的报道，导致患者死亡的原因有移植手部和脸部的假单胞菌感染，最后导致心搏骤停和气道阻塞所致的缺氧损伤[11]。第二例死亡发生于双手移植后第 1 周内。在那时没有可用的更进一步的数据。这使移植受体的死亡率变为 4.5%。

移植器官存活

迄今为止，4 名患者的移植手失功并需要在移植后一年内截肢。第 1 例为由于动脉栓塞导致的围术期单侧移植手失功[12]。第 2 例为移植 9 个月后由于严重内膜增生导致移植手缺氧[4]。虽然没有被学术文献报道，已经被手术队伍和媒体所证实，第 3 例和第 4 例患者失去了移植手(其中一例联合脸部移植)[13]。因此，移植手第一年内失功的概率为 8.9%。

在西方国家 41 名移植手存活超过 1 年的患者中，1 名于 1998 年接受移植的患者最后移植手失功。其原因为患者不能耐受免疫抑制方案，导致移植排斥，最后患者要求于移植后 29 个月截去移植手[14]。因此，目前移植手一年后发生移植失功的概率为 2.4%。

移植手的功能预后

感觉运动功能

手移植后的感觉运动恢复涉及多种因素。神经再生至关重要，与再植相比，同种异体移植的神经再生似乎加快了，这是由于钙调神经磷酸酶抑制剂他克莫司的使用，已证明他克莫司可促进轴突再生[7]。肌肉再神经支配所需的时间是预期功能结果可能与移植水平相关的原因之一，有些病例表明，更多的远端移植可以更快、更完全地恢复功能[15]。这在一定程度上可能是由于手部固有肌肉保持失神经状态的时间过长，导致移植后出现一定程度的肌肉萎缩。随着远端截肢次数的增加，恢复有效控制的可能性增加[8,16,17]。然而，手部一定程度的损伤（手指Ⅱ区）后再植功能恢复较差[18]。

此外，功能恢复无可置疑与所有手移植受者所需的损伤机制、外科重建和治疗方案有关，一些学者认为，正式的康复和患者依从性是决定肢体移植成功与否的两个最重要因素[19]。同样，上肢再植文献支持患者的康复依从性和心理社会倾向作为功能预后的重要指标[17]。对于肢体移植来说，开始时间、强度、用夹板固定、方式（如电刺激、超声波）和康复时间尚未确定。目前，每个中心已经根据自己的重建步骤经验采用相应的复原计划。

我们经历了重建的过程。手移植患者的长期功能评估富有挑战性，目前，这一队伍使用多种方法来完成这一过程。大多肢体/手功能的测量用于量化评估上肢残疾。一些测量工具现被用于评估手移植患者。

Carroll 测试为上肢评分方法之一，被用于手移植的功能恢复随访。文献中证实报道仅有 3 例单侧和 1 例双侧手移植患者（全部移植中心）有 Carrol 评分。除了仅仅做功能评价，如 Carroll 测试，一些工具用于评估手功能对患者生命的影响。例如，一些手移植中心使用 Chen 评分，常规用于评估再移植后手的功能。将功能分为 4 个等级，Chen 评分考虑活动范围、肌力、感觉恢复和独立工作的能力。Chen 评分的变化可用于比较移植前后的功能水平。然而，Chen 评分的有效性、敏感性和可靠性未被验证过。在任意给定的时间，患者可能无法归入单一的分类[20]。Tamai 和 Ipsen 评分与 Chen 评分系统相类似[21]。有文献报道，5 名手移植患者的移植后 Chen 评分都为Ⅱ级[15,20,22]。

DASH（肢体、肩膀和手残疾）评分是经过验证的 30 项报告上肢残疾的评分，评分越高，反映残疾水平越高（图 110.1）。它要求患者在 5 分量表上对他们执行各种任务的能力、上肢活动造成的限制、疼痛程度，以及对自我形象和社交活动的干扰进行评分[23]。DASH 评分的一个优势是它可以综合比较移植前和移植后的情况。

国际手部和复合组织移植登记处于 2007 年提出了手部移植评分系统（HTSS）（图 110.2）。这一评分系统提出了一项用于报道各中心移植结果的工具，但其仍未被验证。HTSS 提出了更高的评分（最高 100 分），用于评估手部功能的 6 个方面，包括：运动、感觉、外

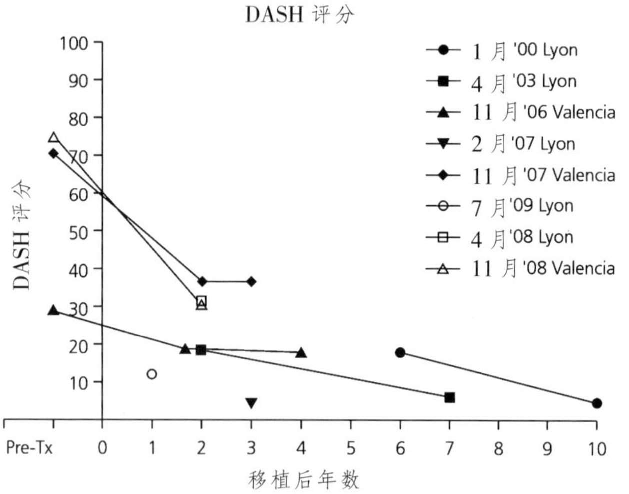

[13, 19]

图 110.1 报道的手部移植的 DASH 评分。

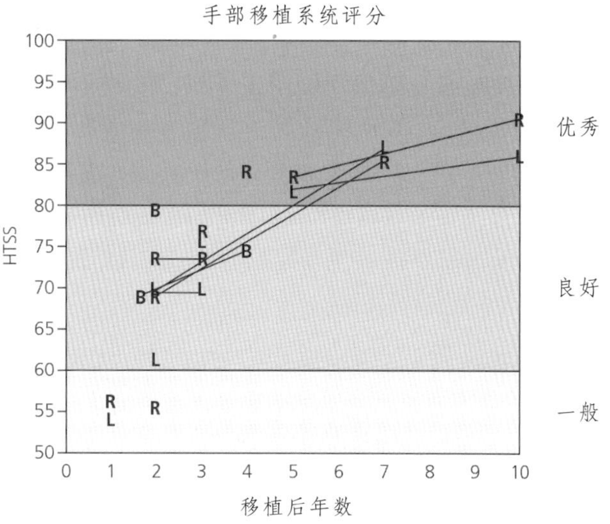

[13, 14, 19, 21, 29]

图 110.2 报道的手部移植的 HTSS 评分。

观、心理和社会接受度、日常活动和工作状态、患者满意度和幸福感[2]。HTSS 的一项限制为其仅能评估移植后的功能，因此临床医生不能直接将其与移植前相比较。一个队伍报道了 9 名患者和他们的 HTSS 评分，随访时间最长的患者其 HTSS 评分处于“良好”的范围内[14,20,22]（表 110.1）。

社会心理预后

考虑到手移植的最主要目标为改善受体的生命质量，患者对移植肢体的满意度是最重要的预后。尽管如此，少数移植中心已经报道了正式的生命质量[12]。然而，在学术文献中报道的移植手患者（13 名单侧和 14 名双侧），超过 51%在移植后已经能够独立完成日常活动和（或）重返工作。

除了发生不能耐受药物后患者要求截肢外，迄今只有 1 例文献报道患者对功能恢复结果不满，这名患者的移植肢体被烧伤，导致右肘僵硬[14]。

手移植后的皮质重组

同种异体复合组织移植的皮质可塑性，尤其是手移植，是一个令人感兴趣的领域且被许多小组所研究。最主要的运动皮质（M1）包含一个躯体感觉的“地图”或个体躯体分割方向中央沟[24]。非侵入性模式用于探究皮质变化，包括功能磁共振。大脑是一直在进化的结果。在上肢截肢后的 24h 内，皮质开始变化[25]。手移植提供了一个机会，来研究这些皮质变化的可逆性（有时在截肢后数年）、移植肢体与受体运动皮质结合的程度，以及由此信息得出的潜在预后、康复或功能影响。在有限数量的患者中已经证明，在手移植后，截肢过程中发生的皮质重组可以逆转，并且新移植的内在肌肉能够获得受者运动皮质内的表现[26,27]。

报道的手移植的并发症

免疫抑制并发症

报道的手移植的最常见代谢并发症为肾功能异常、高糖血症和血脂异常（表 110.2）。病毒感染导致至少有 5 名患者发生巨细胞病毒感染，至少各 1 名患者发生单纯Ⅰ型疱疹病毒、EB 病毒和水痘带状疱疹病毒感染[4,5,12,14,20,28]。移植器官的细菌感染已经被报道过[11,13,14]。有 1 例皮肤真菌感染的报道[20]。有 2 例发生肿瘤并发症的报道，为鼻子的基底细胞癌和周围区域淋巴瘤[4,20]。

社会心理并发症

在书写本章时，不能耐受免疫抑制已经被报道为导致一例单侧移植手失功的原因[14]。一例患者发生人为疾病，表现为急性失明，使对患者的照顾变得复杂[29]。

面部移植

背景

第一例免疫移植开展于 2005 年，至今全世界实施了 18 例面部移植[1,30,31]。然而，其中仅有 7 例被国际注册处[1]报道，且仅有 11 例移植（代表 8 个移植小组）已经在学术文章中发表了它们的结果。数量稀少的面部同种异体移植的报道表明，该手术在技术上是可行的，并且有可能恢复传统重建无法达到的功能和美学特性。然而，其潜在风险包括死亡。

一些已经开展的研究探究了人们为了能够进行面部移植能接受的相关风险。研究表明，健康个体和已经接受了肾脏移植的患者（易感免疫抑制风险）为了面部移植，能接受比肾移植更高的风险[9]。相较于其他 5 种提到的同种异体复合组织移植和肾移植，风险最高的为全脸移植[9]。77%的毁容患者在被告知 20 种潜在的免疫抑制副作用后会接受面部移植，假如在第一年发生排斥的概率为 50%，71%的患者会接受面部移植[10]。

面部移植的预后

患者死亡率

已经有 2 例面部移植的受体死亡，造成死亡率高于 11%。第一例死亡是移植 27 个月后由于不能耐受免疫抑制和多器官衰竭造成的[32]。第二例发生在面部和单侧上肢移植后 2 个月。这例死亡是由于气管造口闭塞，缺氧性心搏骤停，导致不可逆的大脑损伤[11,31]。然而，导致这一系列致命并发症的病理学原因为移植器官的严重假单胞菌感染。

移植器官存活

在书写本章时，没有移植面部失功的病例。考虑到

表 110.1 手移植评分系统

外观(最高 15 分)		
皮肤颜色和血管化	正常	3 分
	不正常	0 分
皮肤纹理	正常	3 分
	不正常	0 分
头发生长	正常	3 分
	不正常	0 分
指甲生长	正常	3 分
	不正常	0 分
与对侧的手匹配(单边移植:大小、颜色、纹理)	优秀	3 分
	良好	2 分
	一般	0.5 分
	较差	0 分
与上肢/身体匹配(双侧移植)	优秀	3 分
	良好	2 分
	一般	0.5 分
	较差	0 分
移动(最高 20 分)		
关节活动度		
前臂(包括旋前旋后)		
	>150	2 分
	>120	1 分
	>90	0.5 分
腕关节(包括伸展)		
	>90	2 分
	>45	1 分
	>25	0.5 分
拇指和长手指(对侧或正常手的总关节活动-度%)		
	>50	2 分
	>25	1 分
	>10	0.5 分
力量(Jamar 测力计)		
握	>10kg	2 分
	>5kg	1 分
	>2.5kg	0.5 分
捏	>2kg	2 分
	>1kg	1 分
	>0.5kg	0.5 分
内在肌肉活动		
	临床上有用	6 分
	肌电图检测	3 分
	无	0 分
手皮质再整合		
	是	4 分
	否	0 分

(待续)

表 110.1(续)　手移植评分系统

心理和社会接受度(最高 15 分)		
社交行为(每个行为 1 分)		
握/握手		
在团体中感觉良好		
克服尴尬感		
被人接受的感觉		
建立新关系的能力		
能够克服障碍		
获得全球社会的认可		
情感(每个方面 1 分)		
爱抚		
拥抱		
触摸		
与伴侣的亲密感		
令人满意的全球情感		
身体图像(每个方面 1 分)		
拥有完整身体的感觉		
个人外表上的自信		
使用手头珠宝(手表等)		
灵敏度(最高 20 分)		
触觉感受(Semmes-Weinstein 单纤维测试)		
正中神经	绿色(1.65~2.83)	3 分
	蓝色(3.22~3.61)	3 分
	紫色(3.84~4.31)	2 分
	红色(4.56)	1 分
	红色(6.65)	0 分
尺神经	绿色(1.65~2.83)	3 分
	蓝色(3.22~3.61)	3 分
	紫色(3.84~4.31)	2 分
	红色(4.56)	1 分
	红色(6.65)	0 分
保护性感觉(热-冷-痛)		
是(尺-正中)		5 分
是(正中)		2 分
是(尺)		1 分
否		0 分
桡神经		1 分
辨别性感觉		
正中神经	S2PD 等级 S4	3 分
	S2PD 等级 S3+(7~12mm)	2.5 分
	S2PD 等级 S3(>15mm)	1.5 分
	S2PD 等级 2(无)	0 分
尺神经	S2PD 等级 S4(2~6mm)	3 分
	S2PD 等级 S3+(7~12mm)	2.5 分
	S2PD 等级 S3(>15mm)	1.5 分
	S2PD 等级 2(无)	0 分

(待续)

表 110.1(续) 手移植评分系统

出汗	正常	2分
	不正常	0分
日常活动和工作状态(最高15分)		
日常活动(每项1分)		
驾驶/骑自行车		
梳头/个人卫生/剃须		
抓握玻璃		
从瓶子里倒水		
使用餐具/筷子		
刷牙		
牵手		
写作		
手的对称使用		
工作状态		
	被雇佣	6分
	未被雇佣	0分
患者满意度和总体幸福感(最高15分)		
患者满意度	非常满意	5分
	满意	3分
	不满意	0分
幸福感	身心健康	5分
	药物治疗的副作用	0分
	药物的永久性副作用/病变	–5分
生活质量	改善很多	5分
	改善	3分
	相同	0分
	恶化	–3分
	恶化很多	–5分

重建方法的有限选择,移植面部失功的后果深远。移植器官失功会发生于部分受体移植后的某些时间点,移植面部失功的管理对于决定这一过程的风险–收益比至关重要。

面部移植的功能预后

感觉运动功能

面部移植的目标有功能和美容。从功能的观点来说,最好的结果为通过面部表情实现感情表达,通过咀嚼实现正常的进食、更好的发言、控制口腔分泌、经鼻呼吸及保护眼睛。全部功能独立于移植器官神经功能的再生。一些侵入性及非侵入性的方法已经被用于面部移植后运动和感觉等恢复水平的评估。然而,目前没有标准的检测来评估面部移植后的功能,这使得跨中心结果的客观比较非常困难(表110.3)。

社会心理并发症

拥有一张审美上可以接受的脸的社会重要性不应该被低估。其目的是获得一种优于传统重建技术的结果。严重毁损的面部对人与社会的交互能力、自尊和生活质量有负面影响[30]。严重面部毁损可与其他严重医学情况一样对生活质量产生影响,如艾滋病、I型糖尿病和需要透析的终末期肾病[33]。一群普通人群的样本显示,若他们被告知有严重面部畸形,他们会愿意接受34%的死亡风险和交换12年生命来行面部移植[33]。面部移植后,大多数生活质量评定为定性的[11,34,35]。目前,关于面部移植术后生活质量的定量研究还很少。

表 110.2　手移植受者的并发症报告

移植时间和地点	单侧手移植受者并发症报告			参考文献
	代谢类	感染类	其他	
1998 年 9 月，法国里昂	高血糖、肌酐升高	单纯疱疹病毒	不遵医嘱导致 29 个月时移植物丢失	[14,15,65]
1999 年 1 月，美国路易斯维尔	未报道	巨细胞病毒	未报道	[4,66]
2001 年 2 月，美国路易斯维尔	糖尿病	未报道	骨坏死(双侧髋部)，不遵医嘱导致排斥反应发作	[4,66]
2006 年 4 月，波兰弗罗茨瓦夫	短暂性高血糖	未报道	未报道	[12,22]
2006 年 11 月，美国路易斯维尔	高脂血症	巨细胞病毒(结肠炎)	严重中性粒细胞减少、前臂血肿需要清创和植皮、边缘区淋巴瘤(血液中不常见的 B 和 T 细胞克隆)	[4,66]
2008 年 1 月，波兰弗罗茨瓦夫	未报道	未报道	动脉血栓形成导致围术期移植物丢失	[12]
2008 年 7 月，美国路易斯维尔	未报道	未报道	9 个月移植物丢失(内膜增生)	[4]
2008 年 9 月，波兰弗罗茨瓦夫	高血糖	未报道	未报道	[12]
2008 年 11 月，美国路易斯维尔	未报道	未报道	未报道	[4]
2009 年 10 月，波兰弗罗茨瓦夫	未报道	巨细胞病毒	未报道	[12]
2000 年 1 月，法国里昂	高血糖	未报道	血清病	[14,15]
2000 年 3 月，奥地利因斯布鲁克	肌酐升高、血脂异常、糖尿病	巨细胞病毒	胸腺球蛋白、房室积液引起支气管痉挛/动静脉瘘管(需要结扎)	[5,67–69]
2003 年 2 月，奥地利因斯布鲁克	未报道	巨细胞病毒	未报道	[28,67]
2003 年 4 月，法国里昂	未报道	骨髓炎(左尺骨)	围术期左尺动脉血栓形成	[14,15]
2006 年 11 月，西班牙瓦伦西亚	高血压、糖尿病、血脂异常	带状疱疹病毒再发	精神性人为障碍，表现为急性视力丧失、口腔溃疡和基底细胞癌(鼻)	[20,29,70,71]
2007 年 2 月，法国里昂	未报道	EB 病毒	未报道	[14]
2007 年 11 月，西班牙瓦伦西亚	肌酐升高、高血压	混合性/真菌性皮肤感染	阿仑单抗引起的细胞因子释放综合征(皮疹、低血压、对机械通气的抵抗)、口腔溃疡	[20,72]
2008 年 11 月，西班牙瓦伦西亚	肌酐升高、高血压、糖尿病、血脂异常加重	无	贫血、头痛	[20,73,74]
2009 年 7 月，法国里昂	高血糖	无	中性粒细胞减少相关的口腔蜂窝织炎、术后第 5 天右桡动脉和左尺动脉血栓形成	[14]
2009 年 4 月，法国巴黎*	未报道	同种异体移植物的假单胞菌感染	心搏骤停，死亡	[11]
2010 年 8 月，美国路易斯维尔	未报道	未报道	围术期动脉血栓形成、缺血性坏死需要经拇指指间关节切除拇指和经远端指间关节切除小指	[4]
2010 年 6 月，波兰弗罗茨瓦夫	肾功能正常的多尿	未报道	围术期左末节指骨动脉血栓形成、表皮松解和坏死，需要截肢	[12]
2011 年 5 月，美国波士顿 *	未报道	肺炎	围术期双侧同种异体手移植物丢失	[13]

* 同时异体面部移植。

表 110.3 面部移植的感觉运动恢复情况

移植时间和地点	运动恢复	感觉恢复	参考文献
2005 年 11 月,法国亚棉	1 周:能吃/喝 6 个月:完全唇接触 18 个月:对称微笑	6 个月:正常温度、浅触觉	[34]
2006 年,中国西安	2 年:能吃、能喝、能说话,但面神经功能不全 无对称性微笑,患者于 27 个月死亡	3 个月:区分性感觉恢复 8 个月:温度感觉恢复	[32,38]
2007 年 1 月,法国巴黎	术后 10 天:能说话/吃东西 肌电图: 3 个月:面神经刺激引起的轻微运动反应(左眼轮匝肌) 6 个月:左眼轮匝肌和双侧口轮匝肌自主收缩 9 个月:自发模仿 12 个月:面三叉神经运动再支配(对神经刺激和不自主眨眼的运动反应)	3 个月:机械和温度感觉存在	[11,39]
2008 年 12 月,美国克利夫兰	可以吃、喝、闻、噘起嘴唇	未报道	[32]
2009 年 3 月,法国巴黎	术后 24 天:易懂的语言 8 个月:完全闭嘴	深部压力敏感性恢复	[11]
2009 年 4 月,法国巴黎	不适用–2 个月后患者死亡	不适用–2 个月后患者死亡	[11]
2009 年 4 月,美国波士顿	即时语言改善	6 个月:轻触感,刺痛,寒冷;两点分辨实验=15mm	[41]
	术后 3 天:经口摄入 1 年:经鼻呼吸,能闻,对称微笑		
2009 年 8 月,西班牙瓦伦西亚	16 个月:能够吞咽(移植包括舌)	未报道	[75]
2009 年 8 月,法国巴黎	术后 20 天:易懂的语言 8~12 个月:完全闭嘴	未报道	[11]
2010 年 1 月,西班牙塞维利亚	语言能力提高,能吃东西 6 个月:提唇肌和颊肌的运动恢复	3 个月:感觉开始恢复 6 个月: 对疼痛和体温的几乎完全感觉	[35]
2010 年 3 月,西班牙巴塞罗那	10 周:软性饮食	4 个月:前额、眼睑、脸颊和口腔黏膜的感觉恢复。嘴唇没有感觉	[40]
	120 天:肌电图显示肌肉活动的初步迹象		

外貌的预后

面部移植的一个伦理关注点为供体的外貌会被转到受体。已经在尸体模型上开展了表皮下肌腱膜系统面部移植的研究,其结果显示,相较于供体,移植的面部与受体更相似,其基于一些测量工具(头颅宽度和颅面高度)[36]。其他方面(眼间距)在供体和受体的外貌相似[37]。面部移植的尸体研究与供体面部相似[30]。

没有正式的用来测量面部移植后外貌改善的工具,但已经有外貌得到改善的报道。在书写本章时,没有患者对外貌不满意的报道,且有许多患者满意外貌,恢复正常的社会生活,返回工作岗位的报道(图 110.3)[11,34,35,38-41]。

面部移植的并发症

免疫抑制并发症

在 11 名患者报道的结果中,2 名移植后发生肾功能异常,2 名新发糖尿病[34,35,38,41]。6 名患者有感染的并发症[11,34,38,42]。2 名患者感染巨细胞病毒,2 名患者感染Ⅰ型疱疹病毒,1 名患者感染痘病毒[11,34,42,43]。已经有移植面部感染、肺感染和胃肠道感染的报道[11,41,43]。1 名患者被报道发生口腔念珠菌病[44]。1 名患者于移植后 50

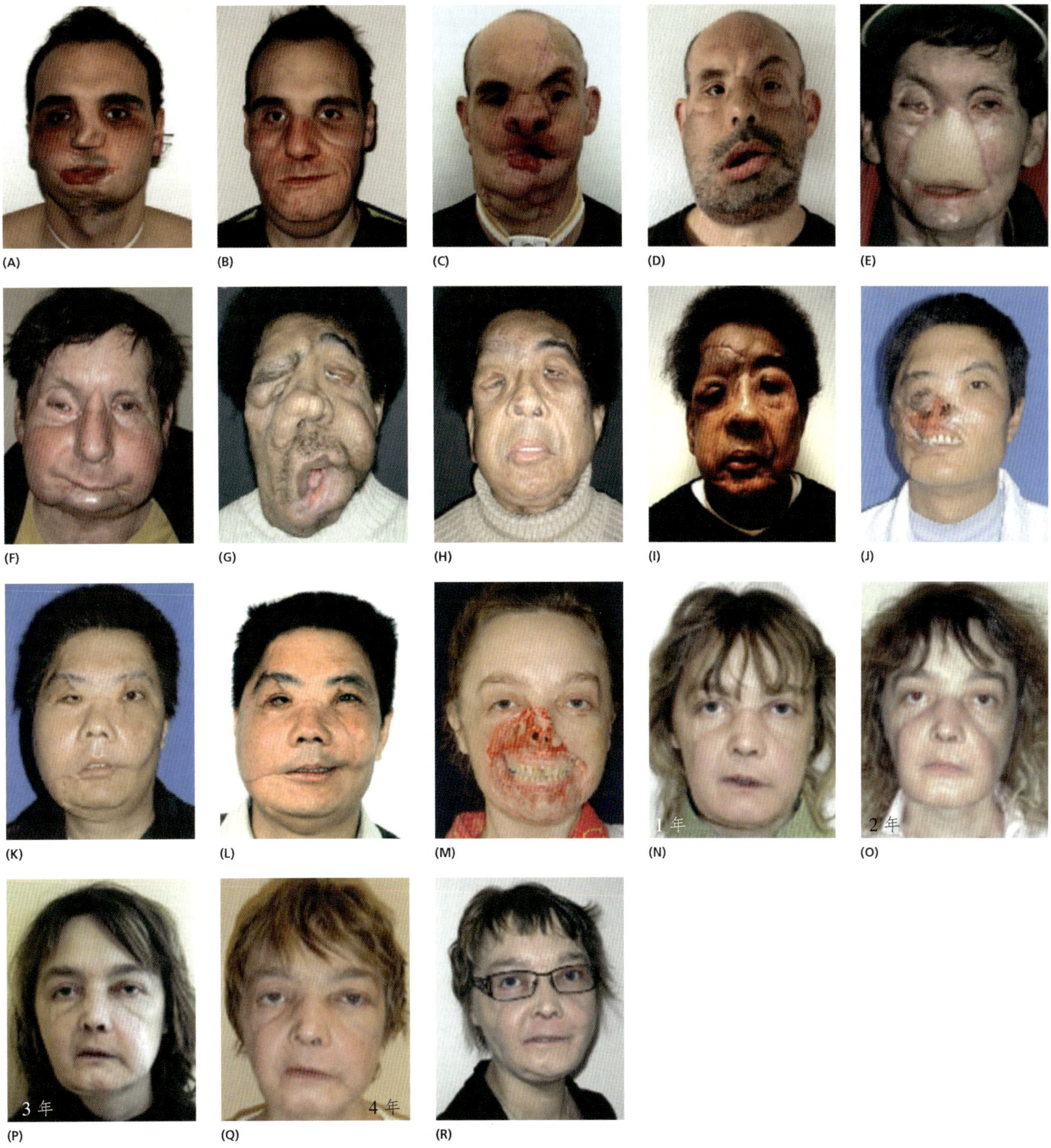

图 110.3　面部移植的美学效果。(A)术前。(B)11 个月随访。(C)术前。(D)1 年随访。(E)术前。(F)1 年随访。(G)术前。(H)1 年随访。(I)3 年随访。(J)术前。(K)20 个月随访。(L)2 年随访。(M)术前。(N)1 年随访。(O)2 年随访。(P)3 年随访。(Q)4 年随访。(R)5 年随访。[(A–D, I) Reproduced from [11] Lantieri L et al. with permission from John Wiley and Sons. (E,F) Reproduced from [41] Pomahac et al. with permission from John Wiley and Sons. (G,H) Reproduced from [39] The Lancet ,Vol 372. Lantieri L, Meningaud JP, Grimbert P et al. Repair of the lower and middle parts of the face by composite tissue allotransplantation in a patient with massive plexiform neurofibroma: a 1-year follow-up study. Lancet, 2008;639–645. Copyright 2008 with permission from Elsevier. (J,K,L) Reproduced from [38] The Lancet, Vol 372. Guo S, Han Y, Zhang X et al. Human facial allotransplantation: a 2-year follow-up study. Lancet 2008;631–638, Copyright 2008 with permission from Elsevier. (M) Reproduced from [44] The Lancet, Vol 368. Devauchelle B, Badet L, Lengelé B et al. First human face allograft: early report. Lancet, 2006;368:203–209, Copyright © 2006 with permission from Elsevier. (N–R) Reproduced from [43] Petruzzo P, Testelin S, Kanitakis J et al. First human face transplantation: 5 years outcomes. Transplantation, 2012;93:236–240, with permission from Wolters Kluwer Health.]

个月发生原位宫颈癌[43]。

社会心理并发症

不能耐受免疫抑制已经导致1名面部移植患者死亡(表110.4)[32]。

腹壁移植

背景

由于多次手术，肠外瘘和肿瘤导致腹壁缺失或腹壁严重损坏的患者可同时进行腹壁移植与小肠或多脏器联合移植。腹壁移植的最终目标为多器官联合移植后能关腹，覆盖和支持下面的器官。由于原来的移植已经需要长期的免疫抑制，所以，腹壁移植有独特的免疫方面的考虑和随访。

腹壁同种异体移植的预后

在书写本章时，文献报道共有14名患者进行了15次腹壁移植，其中仅有9次正式报道于国际注册处[1,45]。在这14名患者中，4名为儿童受体。全部患者包括9名小肠移植，4名多脏器移植和2名不含肝的多脏器移植。2名患者在腹腔脏器移植后接受腹壁移植二次手术。全部患者接受阿仑单抗(抗CD52)的免疫抑制诱导和他克莫司单药维持治疗，除1名儿童接受达克珠单抗诱导及他克莫司维持治疗[45]。

在15例腹壁移植中，2例由于移植后1周内血管血栓形成而失败(1名患者接受再次移植)，致使围术期移植物失功率为13%[45]。

在14名术后移植腹部存活的患者中，9名患者已经由于脓毒症和多器官衰竭而死亡，1例由于淋巴细胞增生性疾病而死亡。没有患者因为移植腹壁而死亡。在5名生存的患者中，1名移植的腹壁失去功能，腹壁移植的最长随访时间为7.1年(图110.4)[45]。

也有一例肝脏和双肾移植的儿童为了能关腹而移植带血管的腹直肌鞘后筋膜的报道。在这一病例中，10cm×20cm大小的腹直肌鞘后筋连同镰状韧带被获

表110.4 面部移植并发症报告

移植时间和地点	面部移植受者的并发症报告			参考文献
	代谢类	感染类	其他	
2005年11月，法国亚棉	血栓性微血管病（血小板减少、溶血性贫血、急性肾衰竭、高血压)、肾功能不全、高血压、血脂异常	单纯疱疹病毒Ⅰ(嘴唇)、传染性软疣(面颊)、念珠菌性口炎	宫颈原位癌、胆管炎	[34,43,44]
2006年，中国西安	糖尿病	无	不遵医嘱，死亡	[32,38]
2007年1月，法国巴黎	无	巨细胞病毒病毒血症	短暂性类固醇性精神错乱	[11,39]
2008年12月，美国克利夫兰	无	巨细胞病毒病毒血症、艰难梭菌和气单胞菌性腹泻	中性粒细胞减少	[42]
2009年3月，法国巴黎	无	假单胞菌肺炎	无	[11]
2009年4月，法国巴黎	无	同种异体移植物的假单胞菌感染	心搏骤停、死亡	[11]
2009年4月，美国波士顿	糖尿病	无	从捐赠者处转移的红斑痤疮	[41]
2009年8月，西班牙瓦伦西亚	无	无	良性假肉瘤梭形细胞术后结节(舌)	[75]
2009年8月，法国巴黎	无	单纯疱疹病毒Ⅰ(嘴唇)	无	[11]
2010年1月，西班牙塞维利亚	肾功能不全	无	无	[35]
2010年3月，西班牙巴塞罗那	无	无	急性口腔皮肤瘘	[40]

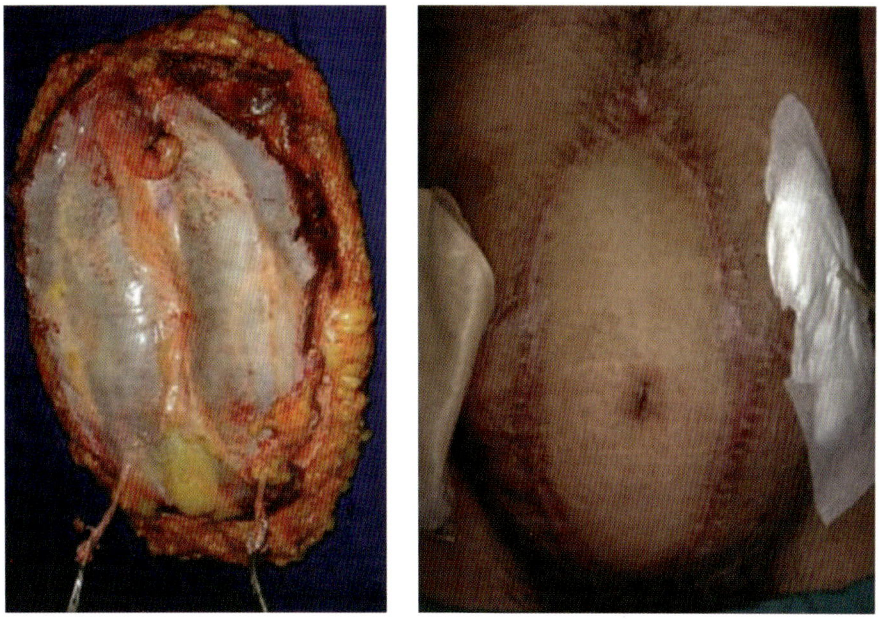

(A)　(B)

图 110.4　腹壁移植。(A)带 2 个蒂的上腹壁移植。(B)腹壁移植后 3 个月。(Reproduced from [64] with permission from John Wiley and Sons.)

取，并从原位肝移植的吻合的肝动脉获取血供。免疫抑制方案为激素诱导、激素、他克莫司及达克珠单抗维持。组织活检未发现排斥迹象。然而，患者可能由于呼吸系统来源的真菌性败血症于移植后 51 天死亡[76]。

喉部移植

背景

由于外伤或肿瘤原因而丧失的喉部功能的常规恢复方法效果不理想[47]。说话能力丧失，不能保护上呼吸道及预防支气管感染，味觉及嗅觉丧失。与其他影响生命质量的移植相似，关于这些功能是否值得冒手术及免疫抑制的风险仍存在争议。

已有一些研究探讨了喉部移植的生命质量[48-50]。20 名健康的志愿者，假如发生喉癌，会选择放射性治疗而不是手术以保留自然的发音，即使这一选择会使 3 年生存率下降 20%~30%[50]。在一项喉部切除患者的研究中，在理想条件下，75%的患者会接受喉部移植。当需要气管切开或更长的住院时间时，这一数字并没有显著降低。并且，一半的喉切除患者会接受移植，即使这并不会使其声音恢复正常，但有不到 20%的患者愿意冒生命危险来做移植[48]。喉切除患者愿意接受的风险比肾移植患者及健康人对照组低[49]。尽管有这些风险，告知免疫抑制的副作用后仍然有超过一半的患者对喉部移植感兴趣，即使有 50%的排斥可能性，超过 1/3 的患者仍愿意接受移植[49]。绝大多数患者由于癌症而切除喉部。肿瘤患者的合适移植免疫抑制仍有争议，尤其在生命质量相关的移植患者中。

国际注册处已经报道了 16 例喉部移植，第一例实施于 1998 年俄亥俄州的克里夫兰[1]。

然而，仅有 1 例患者的预后被正式报道[51,52]。这一移植受体为一名 40 岁男性，由于摩托车事故造成喉部急性损伤失声 20 年。移植包括喉部、气管、咽、甲状腺及甲状旁腺。免疫抑制方案为环孢素、霉酚酸酯和甲强龙。他克莫司 15 个月后替换环孢素。此外，患者移植后第一周内接受莫罗单抗-CD3。没有进一步随访的报道。

喉部移植的预后

第一名患者于术后第 3 天第一次发声。4 个月后，右侧声带恢复到中线位置，到第 6 个月时，左侧声带恢复到近中线位置。通过肌电图确认了双侧声带的神经再生和环咽肌。第 36 个月后，全部发音均为正常范围。未发现甲状腺异常。14 周后嗅觉和味觉恢复。患者的生命质量得到改善且成为了一名励志演说家[51]。

喉部移植的并发症

免疫抑制并发症

口服降压药和环孢素减量导致高血压及肌酐升高。感染并发症包括口咽鹅口疮、气管支气管炎和囊虫肺炎[51]。

社会心理并发症

患者不能耐受一段时间的排斥预防方案导致上述的肺炎[51]。

膝关节移植

背景

膝关节异体移植用于重建有功能的因暴力外伤或感染而损伤的关节。国际注册处记录了6例实施于德国穆尔瑙一个单中心的膝关节移植[1]。这些受体都因为关节和感染[53]导致骨和韧带缺失。未报道手术并发症，冷缺血时间为18到25h[53]。5例患者接受胸腺细胞球蛋白、环孢素、硫唑嘌呤和激素的诱导及环孢素和硫唑嘌呤两药维持的免疫抑制治疗。6例关节移植患者接受了胸腺细胞球蛋白、霉酚酸酯、他克莫司和激素的诱导及霉酚酸酯、他克莫司维持的免疫抑制治疗[53,54]。

膝关节移植的预后

没有带血管的膝关节移植的死亡病例报道。1例膝关节移植由于术后第5周手术部位感染而失败。剩余的5例移植由于术后第14个月、15个月、24个月、36个月和56个月发生排斥相关的并发症而失败[53,54]。特别的是第36个月器官功能丧失的患者是由于不能耐受免疫抑制[54]。排斥的临床表现包括关节不稳、活动范围减小和水肿[54]。4名患者最终移植膝关节被去除，剩下的2名患者进行了关节固定术[53,54]。

最初的5例膝关节患者遇到的一个重要问题是无法监测移植关节的免疫状态，这是由于没有可视的特定的生物指标。移植队伍使用局部炎症表现来预示排斥，但这可能导致未诊断出的排斥[55]。为了更好地检测移植关节，第6名患者接受了用于免疫监测的带血管的皮瓣。这个团队的经验的重要贡献为在一些患者中观察到的血管变化。第一例患者在15个月后发生血管堵塞，其被认为与排斥相关，并连同血管周围淋巴细胞浸润[56]。最后一名患者也由于血管堵塞而发生移植器官功能丧失。表面皮肤坏死预示着移植器官的滑膜组织和软组织出现血管周围浸润、内膜增生及同心性闭塞和血管堵塞。这些血管改变导致器官坏死、深层感染及最终功能丧失。移植队伍认为，肌内膜增生为感染的后遗症[54]。

没有免疫移植的代谢或肿瘤的副反应被报道过。然而，100%的膝关节移植受体有感染的并发症[53-55]。考虑到全部患者最终都由于移植膝关节失功而需要再次截去移植膝关节，因此对急性、抗体介导和慢性同种异体免疫损伤的研究正在进行中(表110.5和图110.5)。

股骨干移植

背景

国际注册处记录了3例实施于德国穆尔瑙单中心的股骨干移植[1]。骨缺陷范围从12~33cm，其中2例是由于骨髓炎，1例由于5年无病生存的软骨肉瘤。没有手术并发症的报道，冷缺血时间为16~25h。免疫抑制方案为环孢素、硫唑嘌呤、抗T细胞球蛋白和泼尼松龙联合诱导，1周后由环孢素和硫唑嘌呤维持[57]。

股骨干移植的预后

没有膝关节移植后患者死亡的报道。2名患者实现了骨愈合[56]。第3名患者需要移除移植的股骨干，这是由于18个月时深部感染复发且接受了同种骨重建[55]。据报道，这三名患者都是完全负重的，膝关节和髋关节的屈曲不受阻碍[57]。

其他同种异体复合组织移植

下肢移植

有1例坐骨联胎双胞胎中的1名由于心脏畸形无法存活而将下肢移植给双胞胎中的另一名的病例。2003年，在一名3周岁的患者实施了这项移植。现在这名患者已经随访超过6年。到移植后30个月，可以观察到捐献的腿部运动和感觉。除了脚部背屈和跖屈

表 110.5　膝关节移植的预后

移植时间	功能实现	并发症	移植物/肢体预后	参考文献
1996 年 4 月	6 个月:完全骨整合 12 个月:完全关节活动度	血管蒂闭塞、全膝关节置换术后植入物感染	15 个月后排斥 全膝关节置换术 膝上截肢	[53]
1996 年 11 月	12 个月:关节稳定,能走路,能参加运动,能复工	不遵守免疫抑制方案导致移植物丢失,全膝关节置换术后种植体感染	36 个月后排斥 全膝关节置换术 膝上截肢	[53]
1996 年 12 月	不适合	手术部位感染	5 周后移植物摘除 关节固定术	[53]
1997 年 7 月	关节稳定,能走路,能复工(全膝关节置换术后)	2 年疲劳性骨折,全膝关节置换术后植入物感染	24 个月后排斥 全膝关节置换术 膝上截肢	[53]
1998 年 2 月	全膝关节置换术后完全关节活动度	14 个月时疲劳性骨折, 全膝关节置换术后再损伤后感染	14 个月后排斥 全膝关节置换术 关节固定术	[53]
2002 年 4 月	8 周:部分承重 6 个月:回归工作 1.5 年:良好的关节活动度,完全承重 4 年:完全承重,满意的关节活动度	排斥反应引起的血管改变引起的坏死/缺血引起的感染	56 个月后排斥 膝上截肢	[53,54]

外,各种运动肌力逐渐得到改善。膝跳反射和足底反射未引出。移植的腿比原始腿短导致骨盆倾斜和 Trendelenberg 步态。然而,这名儿童能跑短距离路,参加运动,可以上学且没有显著的心理问题(图 110.6)[58]。

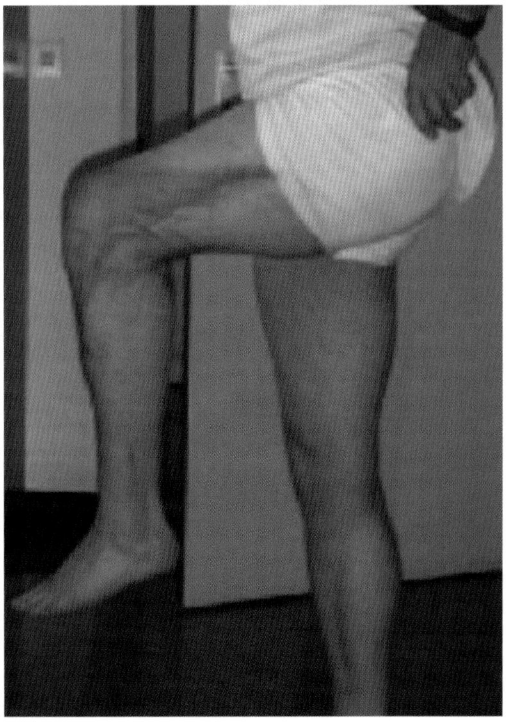

图 110.5　膝关节移植后 1.5 年的活动范围。(Reproduced from [53] with permission from John Wiley and Sons.)

尽管并没有被学术文献所报道, 来自西班牙的瓦伦西亚的手术队伍通过发布会确认他们已经于 2011 年 7 月完成了双侧膝盖以上腿部的移植[59]。现在评价患者的恢复效果还太早。

带血管的腓骨移植

1988 年, 一个日本小组从活着的母亲体内移植了带血管的腓骨给其 2 岁的儿子,以重建由于先天性假关节和神经纤维瘤导致的巨大胫骨损伤。带蒂血管包括供体的腓骨动静脉,这些血管汇入受体的胫前动静脉。免疫抑制方案包括环孢素和 2 周的激素。移植后第 1 天的骨扫描显示适量的示踪剂摄入。然而,移植后 2 周,环孢素水平低于目标范围,导致排斥反应。移植后 3 周的反复骨扫描显示示踪剂摄取减少,3 个月的动脉造影显示血管阻塞。只有远端实现了骨质愈合。为了实现近端愈合,移植 1 年后进行了带血管的腓骨自体移植[60]。

子宫移植

子宫移植被认为可能用于治疗先天性子宫缺如或已手术切除子宫的情况。2000 年,在沙特阿拉伯进行

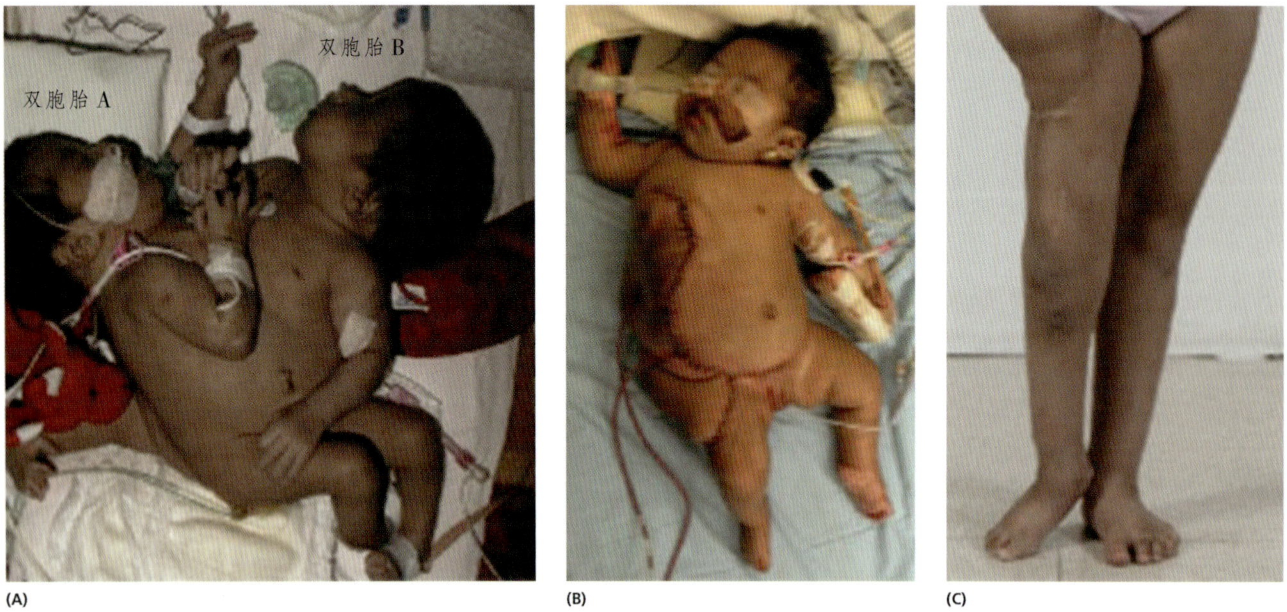

图 110.6 下肢移植。(A)坐骨联体儿的术前外观。(A)双胞胎中的一名儿时由于有致命心脏畸形为供体,另一名儿时为受体。(B)双生儿分开后的下肢移植术后外观。(C)移植腿比原生腿短 6.5cm。(Reproduced from [58] with permission from John Wiley and Sons.)

了 1 例人类子宫移植。6 年前由于产后出血而切除子宫的 26 岁的女性患者，活体原位移植了一不相关的 46 岁的供体的子宫。免疫抑制方案为环孢素、硫唑嘌呤和激素。有一例 9 天后发生急性排斥并用抗胸腺细胞球蛋白治疗的报道。排斥最初有如阴道流液、腹痛、发热和不适的系统症状。多普勒超声显示子宫肌层水肿。外周血流式细胞检测分析显示 CD4/CD8 比率颠倒。未进行组织活检来确认发生排斥。激素治疗后子宫内膜增生和两次停搏止血证实了最初的功能成功。然而,由于急性血管栓塞，导致子宫梗死 99 天后移植后的子宫被切除。血管栓塞归因于缺乏子宫支持,其导致血管扭结[61]。然而,抗体介导的反应不能被排除参与移植子宫失功。在书写本章时,没有其他人类子宫移植的报道。

舌头移植

2003 年,在奥地利维也纳开展了舌头移植。42 岁的受体由于舌鳞状细胞癌失去了说话、吃和吞咽能力。肿瘤根治性切除后立即进行了移植。免疫抑制由抗胸腺细胞球蛋白和激素诱导,由他克莫司、霉酚酸酯和激素维持。没有围术期并发症和排斥的报道。10 个月后,

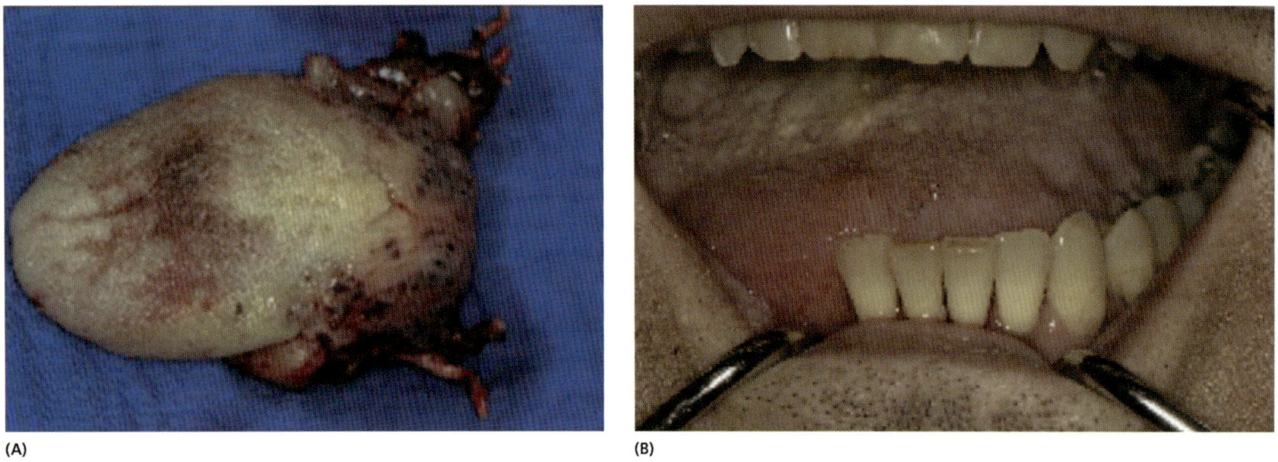

图 110.7 (A)舌头移植。(B)舌头移植术后的外观。(Reproduced from [62] Kermer C, Watzinger F, Oeckher M. Tongue transplantation: 10-month follow-up. Transplantation, 2008;85:654-655 with permission from Wolters Kluwer Health.)

患者能够讲话，吞咽唾液和小量的食物，并且舌头具有部分味觉。舌头的运动能力从未恢复。移植后 1 年，肿瘤于患者颈部复发，患者可能由于肺栓塞于移植后 13 个月死亡(图 110.7)[46,62]。

前臂放射状筋膜皮瓣移植用于半脸重建

2008 年，一个埃及的队伍移植了活体母亲的前臂筋膜皮瓣到她的被着色性皮肤干燥症折磨的孩子上。着色性皮肤干燥症由 DNA 缺陷导致许多皮肤癌暴露于紫外线。患者基本于 20 岁前死亡。在这一独特的病例中，外科医师将同种异体复合组织移植作为预防措施，用不携带着色性皮肤干燥症缺陷的供体皮肤替换患者自己的皮肤。对受体的半脸皮肤进行全厚度切除，并用同种异体移植的筋膜皮肤桡侧前臂代替。免疫抑制包括类固醇、霉酚酸酯、莫非特和环孢素。最初的愈合是正常的。移植 6 周后，在同种异体皮肤上发现了一个孤立的皮肤变色区域，但这在没有干预的情况下得以解决。然而，在移植后 5 个月内，连续 3 次随访失败，出现低于目标的免疫抑制水平后，同种异体移植经历了不可逆的排斥反应，需要完全切除。伤口随后因第二次计划而愈合。值得注意的是，移植的皮肤上未发生癌症，尽管未移植的对侧仍有新的癌症发生[63]。

总结

纵观历史，临床移植的发展与研究密切相关。同种异体复合组织移植已经在过去 10 年内取得了显著发展。然而，与其他移植相似，同种异体复合组织移植也面临一些挑战，一些为同种异体移植共同的挑战，其他为同种异体复合组织移植特有的。尽管这些移植在技术上是可行的，这些挑战仍然存在，包括决定最好的候选者，平衡免疫抑制负担和生命质量，决定移植的适宜时间，及时获取学术群体报道的预后，决定免疫学特点。这些内容在本章的范围外，这些挑战必然成为研究的前沿。

从最初，同种异体复合组织移植项目就应该以跨学科的方法为目标。目前，至少有来自 17 个国家的团体已经开展了这些复杂移植。目前，少于 10 名同种异体复合组织移植患者的生存超过 10 年。已有报道在手、脸部、喉部和膝关节移植受体出现不耐受免疫移植或预防方案的情况，且其与一名移植手失功和一名面部移植受体死亡相关[14,32]。即使处于最佳的免疫移植和复原的过程，这些移植受体的经历仍然未知。慢性排斥和抗体介导的过程在同种异体复合组织移植中的作用仍然未知。研究的关键范围为：皮质可塑性，缺血–再灌注损伤对功能的影响，存在先天性或儿童缺陷的潜在的同种异体复合组织移植申请者，组织供体的接受度和公众教育。现在，移植仍为免疫学和移植相关应用的独特领域，作为移植的一部分，不管在现在还是将来，同种异体复合组织移植应着重于保持同种异体复合组织移植受体最好的预后。

(周舒扬　杨梦凡　译　周舒扬　校)

参考文献

1. International Registry of Hand and Composite Tissue Transplantation. World Experience. 2011 [cited 2011 17 August; 2012]; Available from: http://www.handregistry.com.
2. Lanzetta M, Petruzzo P, Dubernard JM, et al. Second report (1998-2006) of the international registry of hand and composite tissue transplantation. Transplant Immunology. 2007;18:1–6.
3. Cendales LC, Kanitakis J, Schneeberger S, et al. The Banff 2007 working classification of skin-containing composite tissue allograft pathology. American Journal of Transplantation. 2008;8:1396–1400.
4. Kaufman CL, Breidenbach W. World experience after more than a decade of clinical hand transplantation: update from the Louisville hand transplant program. Hand Clinics. 2011;27:417–421.
5. Margreiter R, Brandacher G, Ninkovic M, et al. A double hand transplant can be worth the effort! Transplantation. 2002;74:85–90.
6. Cendales L, Granger D, Henry M, et al. Implementation of vascularized composite allografts in the United States: recommendations from the ASTS VCA Ad Hoc Committee and the Executive Committee. American Journal of Transplantation. 2011;11:13–17.
7. Dubernard JM, Owen ER, Lanzetta M, et al. What is happening with hand transplants? Lancet. 2001;357:1711–1712.
8. Graham B, Adkins P, Tsai TM, et al. Major replantation versus revision amputation and prosthetic fitting in the upper extremity: a late functional outcomes study. Journal of Hand Surgery. 1998;23A:783–791.
9. Brouha P, Naidu D, Cunningham M, et al. Risk acceptance in composite-tissue allotransplantion reconstructive procedures. Microsurgery. 2006;26:144–150.
10. Barker JH, Furr A, Cunningham M, et al. Investigation of risk acceptance in facial transplantation. Plastic and Reconstructive Surgery. 2006;118:663–670.
11. Lantieri L, Hivelin M, Audard V, et al. Feasibility, reproducibility, risks, and benefits of face transplantation: a prospective study of outcomes. American Journal of Transplantation. 2011;11:367–378.
12. Jablecki J. World experience after more than a decade of clinical hand transplantation: update on the polish program. Hand Clinics. 2011;27:433–442.
13. Brigham and Women's Hospital. Press Conference: Charla Nash. 2011 [cited 2011 14 December; 2011]; Available from: http://bwhedtech.media.partners.org/programs/publicaffairs/20110610/index.htm#.
14. Petruzzo P, Dubernard JM. World experience after more than a decade of clinical hand transplantation: update on the French program. Hand Clinics. 2011;27:411–416.
15. Petruzzo P, Badet L, Gazarian A, et al. Bilateral hand transplantation: six years after the first case. American Journal of Transplantation. 2006;6:1718–1724.
16. Chung KC, Alderman AK. Replantation of the upper extremity: indications and outcomes. Journal of the American Society for Surgery of the Hand. 2002;2:78–94.
17. Medling BD, Bueno RA, Russell RC, et al. Replantation outcomes. Clinics in Plastic Surgery. 2007;34:177–185.
18. Wilhelmi B, Lee WP, Pagensteert GI, et al. Replantation in the mutilated hand. Hand Clinics. 2003;19:89–120.
19. Siemionow MZ, Zor F, Gordon CR. Face, upper extremity, and concomitant transplantation: potential concerns and challenges ahead. Plastic and Reconstructive Surgery. 2010;226:308–315.
20. Cavadas PC, Landin L, Thione A, et al. The Spanish experience with hand, forearm,

and arm transplantation. Hand Clinics. 2011;27:443–453.
21. Herzberg G, Parmentier H, Erhard L. Assessment of functional outcome in hand transplantation patients. Hand Clinics. 2003;19:505–509.
22. Jablecki J, Kaczmarzyk L, Domanasiewicz A, et al. First Polish forearm transplantation—final report (outcome after 4 years). Annals of Transplantation: Quarterly of the Polish Transplantation Society. 2010;15:61–67.
23. The Institute for Work and Health. The DASH Outcome Measure. 2011 [cited 2011 14 December; 2011]; Available from: http://www.dash.iwh.on.ca/score.htm.
24. Sirigu A, Vargas C, Dubernard JM. Novel hand representations in the human motor cortex after hand allograft. Proceedings of the American Philosophical Society. 2011;155:29–40.
25. Borsook D, Becerra L, Fishman S, et al. Acute plasticity in the human somatosensory cortex following amputation. Neuroreport. 1998;9:1013–1017.
26. Vargas CD, Aballea A, Rodrigues EC, et al. Re-emergence of hand muscle representation in human motor cortex after hand allograft. Proceedings of the National Academy of Sciences USA. 2009;10617:7197–7202.
27. Giraux P, Sirigu A, Schneider F, et al. Cortical reorganization in motor cortex after graft of both hands. Nature Neuroscience. 2001;4:691–692.
28. Schneeberger S, Kreczy A, Brandacher G, et al. Steroid and ATG resistant rejection after double forearm transplantation responds to Campath-1H. American Journal of Transplantation. 2004;4:1372–1374.
29. Cavadas PC, Landin L, Ibanez J. Bilateral hand transplantation: result at 20 months. Journal of Hand Surgery European. 2009;34:434–443.
30. Pomahac B, Nowinski D, Diaz-Siso JR, et al. Face transplantation. Current Problems in Surgery. 2011;48:293–357.
31. Shanmugarajah K, Hettiaratchy S, Clarke A, et al. Clinical outcomes of facial transplantation: a review. International Journal of Surgery. 2011;9: 600–607.
32. Hui-Chou HG, Nam AJ, Rodriguez ED. Clinical facial composite tissue allotransplantation: a review of the first four global experiences and future implications. Plastic and Reconstructive Surgery. 2010;125:538–546.
33. Sinno HH, Thibaudeau S, Duggal A, et al. Utility scores for facial disfigurement requiring facial transplantation [outcomes article]. Plastic and Reconstructive Surgery. 2010;126:443–449.
34. Dubernard JM, Lengelé B, Morelon E, et al. Outcomes 18 months after the first human partial face transplant. New England Journal of Medicine. 2007; 357:2451–2460.
35. Sicilia-Castro D, Gomez-Cia T, Infante-Cossio P, et al. Reconstruction of a severe facial defect by allotransplantation in neurofibromatosis type I: a case report. Transplantation Proceedings. 2011;43:2831–2837.
36. Baccarani A, Follmar KE, Das RR, et al. A pilot study in Sub-SMAS face transplantation: defining donor compatibility and assessing outcomes in a cadaver model. Plastic and Reconstructive Surgery. 2006;119:121–129.
37. Follmar KE, Baccarani A, Das RR, et al. Osteocutaneous face transplantation. Plastic and Reconstructive Surgery. 2008;61:518–524.
38. Guo S, Han Y, Zhang X, et al. Human facial allotransplantation: a 2-year follow-up study. Lancet. 2008;372:631–638.
39. Lantieri L, Meningaud JP, Grimbert P, et al. Repair of the lower and middle parts of the face by composite tissue allotransplantation in a patient with massive plexiform neurofibroma: a 1-year follow-up study. Lancet. 2008;372: 639–645.
40. Barret JP, Gavaldà J, Bueno J, et al. Full Face Transplant: the first case report. Annals of Surgery. 2011;254:252–256.
41. Pomahac B, Pribaz J, Eriksson E, et al. Restoration of facial form and function after severe disfigurement from burn injury by a composite facial allograft. American Journal of Transplantation. 2011;11:386–393.
42. Gordon CR, Avery RK, Abouhassan W, et al. Cytomegalovirus and other infectious issues related to face transplantation: specific considerations, lessons learned, and future recommendations. Plastic and Reconstructive Surgery. 2011;127: 1515–1523.
43. Petruzzo P, Testelin S, Kanitakis J, et al. First human face transplantation: 5 years outcomes. Transplantation. 2012;93:236–240.
44. Devauchelle B, Badet L, Lengelé B, et al. First human face allograft: early report. Lancet. 2006;368:203–209.
45. Selvaggi G, Levi DM, Cipriani R, et al. Abdominal wall transplantation: surgical and immunologic aspects. Transplantation Proceedings. 2009;41:521–522.
46. CDS Review. Recipient of first tongue transplant recovering. Chicago Dental Society (CDS) Review. 2003;96:44.
47. Birchall MA, Lorenz RR, Berke GS, et al. Laryngeal transplantation in 2005: a review. American Journal of Transplantation. 2006;6:20–26.
48. Potter CS, Birchall MA. Laryngectomees' views on laryngeal transplantation. Transplant International. 1998;11:433–438.
49. Reynolds CC, Martinez SA, Furr A, et al. Risk acceptance in laryngeal transplantation. Laryngoscope. 2006;116:1770–1775.
50. McNeil BJ, Weichselbaum R, Pauker SG. Speech and survival: tradeoffs between quality and quantity of life in laryngeal cancer. New England Journal of Medicine. 1981;305:982–987.
51. Strome M, Stein J, Esclamado R, et al. Laryngeal transplantation and 40-month follow-up. New England Journal of Medicine. 2001;344:1676–1679.
52. Lorenz RR, Hicks DM, Shields RW Jr, et al. Laryngeal nerve function after total laryngeal transplantation. Otolaryngology and Head and Neck Surgery. 2004; 131:1016–1018.
53. Diefenbeck M, Wagner F, Kirschner MH, et al. Outcome of allogeneic vascularized knee transplants. Transplant International. 2007;20:410–418.
54. Diefenbeck M, Nerlich A, Schneeberger S, et al. Allograft vasculopathy after allogeneic vascularized knee transplantation. Transplant International. 2011;24:e1–e5. doi: 10.1111/j.1432-2277.2010.01178.
55. Hofmann GO, Kirschner MH. Clinical experience in allogenic vascularized bone and joint allografting. Microsurgery. 2000;20:375–383.
56. Kirschner MH, Brauns L, Gonschorek O, et al. Vascularized knee joint transplantation in man: the first two years experience. European Journal of Surgery. 2000;166:320–327.
57. Hofmann GO, Kirschner MH, Wagner FD, et al. Allogeneic vascularized transplantation of human femoral diaphysis and total knee joints – first clinical experiences. Transplantation Proceedings. 1998;30:2754–2761.
58. Fattah A, Cypel T, Donner EJ, et al. The first successful lower extremity transplantation: 6-year follow-up and implications for cortical plasticity. American Journal of Transplantation. 2011;11:2762–2767.
59. The Spokesman – Review. Doctors in Spain perform double-leg transplant. 2011 [cited 2011 14 December; 2011]; Available from: http://m.spokesman.com/stories/2011/jul/12/doctors-spain-perform-double-leg-transplant/.
60. Doi K, Akino T, Shigetomi M, et al. Vascularized allografts: review of current concepts. Microsurgery. 1994;15:831–841.
61. Fageeh W, Raffa H, Jabbad H, et al. Transplantation of the human uterus. International Journal of Gynaecology and Obstetrics. 2002;76:245–251.
62. Kermer C, Watzinger F, Oeckher M. Tongue transplantation: 10-month follow-up. Transplantation. 2008;85:654–655.
63. Amin A, Bassiouny M, Sallam K, et al. Living related hemi-face skin transplant using radial forearm free flap for a xeroderma pigmentosa patient: early outcome. Head and Neck Oncology. 2010;2:18.
64. Cipriani R, Contedini F, Santoli M, et al. Abdominal wall transplantation with microsurgical technique. American Journal of Transplantation. 2007;7: 1304–1307.
65. Dubernard JM, Owen E, Herzberg G, et al. Human hand allograft: report on first 6 months. Lancet. 1999;353:1315–1320.
66. Ravindra KV, Buell JF, Kaufman CL, et al. Hand transplantation in the United States: experience with 3 patients. Surgery. 2008;144:638–643.
67. Ninkovic M, Weissenbacher A, Gabl M, et al. Functional outcome after hand transplantation: what can be achieved? Hand Clinics. 2011;27:455–465.
68. Schneeberger S, Ninkovic M, Piza-Katzer H, et al. Status 5 years after bilateral hand transplantation. American Journal of Transplantation. 2006;6:834–841.
69. Piza-Katzer H, Ninkovic M, Pechlaner S, et al. Doucle hand transplantation: functional outcome after 18 months. Journal of Hand Surgery (Edinburgh, Lothian). 2002;4:385–390.
70. Landin L, Cavadas PC, Rodriguez-Perez JC. Improvement in renal function after late conversion to sirolimus-based immunosuppression in composite tissue allotransplantation. Transplantation. 2010;90:691–692.
71. Landin L, Cavadas PC, Ibanez J, et al. CD3+ mediated rejection and C4d deposition in two composite tissue (bilateral hand) allograft recipients after induction with alemtuzumab. Transplantation. 2009;87:776–781.
72. Landin L, Cavadas PC, Garcia-Cosmas P, et al. Perioperative ischemic injury and fibrotic degeneration of muscle in a forearm allograft: functional follow-up at 32 months post transplantation. Annals of Plastic Surgery. 2011;66:202–209.
73. Landin L, Cavadas PC, Nthumba P, et al. Preliminary results of bilateral arm transplantation. Transplantation. 2009;88:749–751.
74. Cavadas PC, Ibáñez J, Thione A, et al. Bilateral Trans-humeral arm transplantation: result at 2 years. American Journal of Transplantation. 2011;11:1085–1090.
75. Cavadas PC, Ibáñez J, Thione A, Surgical aspects of a lower face, mandible, and tongue allotransplantation. Journal of Reconstructive Microsurgery. 2011;10: 43–48.
76. Agarwal S, Dorafshar AH, Harland RC, et al. Liver and vascularized posterior rectus sheath fascia composite tissue allotransplantation. American Journal of Transplantation. 2010;10:2712–2716.

第 8 篇

儿童移植

第 111 章 儿童器官移植简介

Steven A. Webber, Allan D. Kirk

本章主要介绍儿童移植。虽然儿童移植在许多方面与成人移植相似,但依然有其特殊性。本章内容旨在阐述两者之间的差异,并补充前文未提及的内容。

由于儿童护理及自身的特点,儿科需要专门的执业医生。同样,与成人移植不同之处在于,儿童移植不仅在手术技术上有差异,在免疫生物学、病理学、药理学,心理学和保护性免疫等方面都有独特的表现。研究者和临床医生必须认识到上述问题是接受器官移植的患儿首先需要考虑的。

在第一部分,Urschel 和 West 对免疫系统的发育成熟以及在不同年龄组免疫系统与器官移植相关性进行了详细描述。通常认为,免疫系统在人出生时基本已经发育成熟,但是新生儿专科医生或儿科专家并不完全认同这种观点。虽然人体抗原受体库是在出生时建立的,但是免疫功能是随着免疫反应逐渐完善的。对此的一种解释是儿童和成人的免疫系统有诸多不同,包括免疫系统内各组织细胞和生物分子均存在差异。这些发现有助于解释同种免疫应答与年龄相关的差异和移植急性排斥反应以及慢性移植物功能障碍在人出生早期发生率低的原因。上述情况在心脏移植的新生儿和婴儿早期受体中表现最为显著,因为该年龄组的其他器官移植很罕见。这被视为一种"免疫豁免"时期,虽然这种优势免疫的精确时间窗并不完全清楚。但相对来说,这些年幼的移植受体感染率高,并且淋巴增生性疾病的发病率最高。

接下来的章节将主要围绕肾脏、肝脏、心脏,肺和小肠移植进行阐述。这些章节提醒我们儿童器官移植在器官移植史上发挥着重要作用。儿童器官移植是与成人器官移植平行发展的,而非后者成功的结果。鲜有人知,世界上首例儿童肾脏移植是在 1952 年巴黎的平安夜完成的。移植完成后,移植肾马上就开始发挥功能,但在移植后的第 21 天,可能因为排斥反应导致该少年患者的死亡。尽管如此,移植手术的可行性已被证明。第一例儿童心脏移植手术计划于 1966 年施行,早于 Christian Barnard 在 1967 年 12 月完成的首例成人心脏移植手术。但因器官捐献者病情恶化,移植并未完成。新的受体是于 1967 年确认的,移植手术的时间比 Barnard 的手术时间仅晚了 3 天。人类历史上第 2 例原位心脏移植患者是一位患有致死性先天性心脏病的 3 周大的婴儿。供者是一位先天性无脑畸形的新生儿,出生就被送往器官捐献中心[2]。心脏跳动了约 6 小时。婴幼儿还具有悠久的肝移植的历史。早在 1963 年 3 月,Starzl 完成了首例肝移植手术,不幸的是,受体的器官移植未能完成,主要原因是"虽然我们尽全力止血,但这个 3 岁的患儿仍然失血过多而死"[3]。虽然大多数早期移植手术没有取得成功,但这些观察性资料仍然使这些儿童和他们的家庭成为器官移植领域的开拓者,并使人们积累了最早期的经验教训。

儿童特定器官移植章节重点讲述儿童与成人移植方式的区别。最显著的区别也许是导致儿童终末期器官功能衰竭的原因明显不同。这就需要专注于诊治儿童终末期器官功能衰竭的团队进行移植前的评估。一些特殊情况需要专门的外科技术,例如先天性尿路畸形或先天性心脏病的儿童。这些差异会使移植手术在技术上很有挑战性,需要手术团队在这些先天性异常的重建方面有着丰富的经验。先天性异常的重建失败常导致早期移植失败。

移植后的管理策略也受到年龄和移植前诊断的影响。免疫功能成熟可能影响免疫抑制策略,而患者的体型和解剖变异可能影响到移植后进行移植物的活检。皮质类固醇药物已率先在儿童移植人群中停止使用。该药物对于成人移植中的使用尚在探索中。传染因素(尤其是人类疱疹病毒)的接触提示我们发生感染和淋巴增殖性疾病的风险,并影响移植后病毒预防和检测的策略。

在特定器官移植章节之后，我们主要介绍儿童移植受体和他们家庭的几个至关重要的问题。器官移植的目标是尽可能长的延长受体的生存期，使受体恢复最佳的健康状态，以提高生活质量，并使儿童回归正常的生活，和与年龄相应的活动。实现这些目标仍有许多障碍。药物有很多副作用，生理发育和青春期可能会延误受体的治疗。类固醇皮质激素的影响以及生长激素的治疗性使用对于人体细胞生长的影响，在儿童器官受体中进行了广泛的研究。认知发展受损和精神疾病也是常见的问题。对免疫抑制药物的依从性差可能是对于儿童移植团队最具挑战性的问题，同时依从性差也是现在许多研究共同面临的重要难题。提高依从性研究的新的干预措施也在本章进行了说明。对于儿童和成人移植团队成员都非常重要的一个问题，在本章进行了总结，即“护理过渡期”。受体在这个十分脆弱的时期中，移植排斥反应和坏死的风险增加。本章将总结一些制订有效过渡方案的具体建议。

综上所述，本节的重点是儿童器官移植。本章可以单独作为儿童移植的专著。但最好与本书的其他章节一起阅读，因为这些章节也是与儿童移植领域相关的。其他章节的一些参考文献主要是为了突出成人和儿童器官移植之间存在的一些共同点。

（柯庆宏 译　柯庆宏 校）

参考文献

1. Michon L, Hamburger J, Oeconomos N, et al. Une tentative de transplantation renale chez l'homme: aspects medicaux et biologique. La Presse Medicale. 1953; 61:1419–1923.
2. Kantrowitz A, Haller JD, Joos H, et al. Transplantation of the heart in an infant and an adult. American Journal of Cardiology. 1968;22:782–790.
3. Starzl TE. Memoirs of a Transplant Surgeon: The Puzzle People. Pittsburgh University Press; Pittsburgh, PA: 1992.

第 112 章
免疫系统发育：从出生到成人

Simon Urschel，Lori J. West

引言

免疫系统的个体发育过程是在各种外界因素的综合作用下逐步完善，在其连续发展过程中具有“关键窗口期”[1,2]。这些窗口期中的抗原暴露或治疗干预可能具有长期甚至永久性的后果，部分是不利的，部分是有利的（表 112.1）。与那些在妊娠末期解剖和功能就完全发育的器官系统相比，免疫系统没有完全发育成熟，在整个童年和青年时期发生重大的变化。在出生时免疫系统的不成熟与缺乏抗原接触有关，同时和其出生后需继续发育的固有特征有关。了解免疫发育的各个方面及其儿童移植医学中的最佳决策的影响需要整合从各个领域收集的知识的医学研究和临床实践，包括传染病、自身免疫、免疫缺陷和内分泌等。至少，从一些动物试验及近半个世纪试验工作的研究成果中有助于我们理解在免疫发育过程中发生的复杂变化。在本章中，我们将阐述一些与移植医学相关的发育免疫学的概念。在第 2 章中，还会对生理机体免疫功能进行更广泛的讨论。

表 112.1　人体发育的主要阶段

1	孕前期，即卵母细胞和精子发育，尤其对卵母细胞发育特别重要，因为其可在受精前多年受到影响
2	妊娠期：胚胎到妊娠中期，胎儿晚期（器官发生、细胞迁移、生长教育）
3	围生期：产后早期（哺乳期）
4	婴儿期：儿童早期 – 传染性暴露
5	童年期–胸腺退化
6	青少年期–激素影响
7	“性成熟期”
8	衰老期

Reproduced from [1] West LJ (2002). Defining critical windows in the development of the human immune system. Human and Experimental Toxicology, 21(9–10): 499–505, copyright ⓒ 2002 by Sage Publications. Reprinted by Permission of SAGE.

免疫系统的自然发展与童年的成熟

在讨论新生儿的免疫反应时，重要的是，尽管有从试验系统尤其是小鼠模型中得到的大量关于免疫系统发育的信息，但这些信息却不能精确分析完整的人类新生儿体内发生的复杂的相互作用。尽管如此，从 20 世纪 50 年代 Peter Medawar 和他的同事开展的试验开始[3,4]，新生小鼠由于出生时免疫系统极不成熟以及易于操作，被作为研究免疫发育的理想物种。出生的事件，并不意味着任何特定程度的免疫成熟，而是标志着胎儿离开宫内环境的时刻。免疫发育在出生时达到的程度以及出生后的成熟率，随物种而异；新生小鼠的免疫成熟度不及人类出生时达到的程度（小鼠和人类的发育阶段粗略估算在表 112.2 中列出）[5]。

新生儿和婴儿的免疫系统

虽然新生儿的严格定义为出生后 1~28 天的儿童，但是免疫系统的变化是不固定的，并且具有较大的个体差异。目前最小的出生和存活的新生儿的孕龄为 23 周，提前 17 周从保护性母体环境中出生。除了其他器官的发育不全，早产儿也面临免疫系统发育不成熟的挑战，从而增加感染的风险。然而，所有的新生儿易发生一些致病菌引发的严重的全身性感染。有报道，引起新生儿免疫功能低下的原因包括获得性及固有免疫系统中的定量和定性的因素，这些因素在鼠模型以及在人类中进行了描述。这些总结在表 112.3 和下面的章节中详细讨论。

新生儿和婴儿的固有免疫反应

如第 7 章所描述的，固有免疫系统包括的各种细

表 112.2 人类与小鼠 T 细胞发育比较

功能	小鼠	人
妊娠期	21 天	40 周
淋巴造血细胞定殖于原始胸腺	11~12 天	第 9 周
胸腺组织分化出皮质和髓质	13~14 天	第 11~14 周
γδTCR 和 αβTCR 的表达	14~16 天	第 11~13 周
MLR 发育	16~18 天	第 12 周(胸腺) 第 19 周(脾) (直到第 23 周)
有丝分裂原反应	第 18 天(胸腺)(部分有丝分裂原直到出生后)	第 13~14 周(胸腺) 第 16~18 周(脾,外周血)
细胞毒反应(CML)	产后 7 天开始变强	从第 20~23 周开始(胸腺)

Reprinted from [5] West LJ. Developmental aspects of immunomodulation: exploiting the immature immune system for organ transplantation. Transplant Immunology, 2002: 9(2-4): 149-153. Copyright (2002), with permission from Elsevier.

表 112.3 未成熟的免疫成分在新生儿或婴儿和成人中的差异

固有免疫系统
• 吞噬细胞:低反应性模式识别受体
• 树突状细胞和单核细胞:低表达 MHC Ⅱ和共刺激分子
• 多形核嗜中性白细胞:小库和受损的趋化性
• 补体系统: 少量 C9,显著的替代激活途径
• 自然杀伤细胞: 数量较少且功能不全
适应性免疫系统
• 出生时淋巴细胞减少,出生后第一年淋巴细胞增多
• T 细胞:表型和功能不成熟;缺乏免疫记忆;大量新生的非复制的 T 细胞;Th2 细胞在特异性免疫反应中差异较大
• 调节性 T 细胞:未成熟细胞大量存在,活化细胞极少
• B 淋巴细胞:出生时数量较少,出生后第一年主要为淋巴细胞;缺乏记忆细胞和边缘区 B 细胞;未成熟细胞为主;过渡性 B 细胞比例增加
• 抗体: 母体 IgG 在出生后约 6 个月达最低点;内源性 IgG、IgA、IgM 从出生开始产生并在十岁左右达到成年人的浓度;IgG2 产生减弱
• 脾和淋巴结: 组织结构(如生发中心)发育;3~6 个月后边缘区发育

胞和酶,它们对病原体、非人生物体、或改变的人类细胞起作用,可以概括为一种非特异性的第一道防线。顾名思义,固有免疫反应是在出生时起作用,很可能开始于妊娠早期,并且是不依赖暴露于特定抗原或免疫记忆。然而,词语“先天”往往会被误认为不需要发育成熟;实际上,固有免疫反应的不成熟在不同的临床和试验研究中得到了阐述。举个例子,每 1000 个发育成熟的新生儿中约有 2 个发生早期败血症;约 41%的病原体是 B 群链球菌,新生儿对它具有有限的抵抗力,这些细菌无害定植于母体产道中[6]。新生儿吞噬细胞通过模式识别受体(PRR)包括 Toll 样受体(TLR)对各种病原相关分子模式(PAMP)和损伤相关分子模式(DAMP)的刺激下,其反应较成人下降[7,8]。新生儿的树突状细胞和单核细胞的抗原呈递细胞降低表达与反应相关的重要的分子表明结构,包括Ⅱ型主要组织相容性复合体(MHC)[9,10]以及共刺激分子,例如 CD40、CD80 和 CD86 [11]。细菌感染和败血症期间,骨髓中的中性粒细胞增殖和释放在新生儿期比以后更易耗尽[12],导致败血症期间中性粒细胞减少及更高的死亡率[13,14]。新生儿的中性粒细胞的自发迁移能力和对趋化因子的反应下降[15],在败血症期间尤为明显[16]。补体因子 C9,作为细菌感染时的膜攻击复合物的一个重要组成部分,其数量在新生儿期明显降低[17]。可能与缺乏发育良好的适应性免疫和相应的特异性抗体有关,在细菌感染时新生儿不能检测到经典途径的补体活化,而是通过旁路途径响应,通过血浆中 C3a 和 C5a 水平增加而加以鉴定[18]。

这些总结只是一些当前最为认可和熟悉的限制新生儿和婴儿的固有免疫反应的相关因素。在移植中对同种异体免疫应答的影响大多数仍然未知,尽管越来越多的证据表明,固有免疫和适应性免疫之间的相互作用被大大低估了。认识到通过固有免疫应答增强抗原特异性适应性免疫和潜在的增加长期移植物损伤是至关重要的。这将不仅可以更好地了解早期和长期移植接受的个体间差异,而且可能揭示在器官移植时最终改善移植物存活可能的治疗靶标。

动物和人类从产前到幼儿期 T 细胞和 B 细胞的反应发展

婴儿对各种传染性病原体的易感性不仅与前面所述的尚未完全发育成熟的固有免疫有关,而且还与缺乏先前存在的免疫记忆和外周淋巴器官中的淋巴细胞及其他适应性免疫成分有关(表 112.3)。对于淋巴细胞

(包括 T 细胞和 B 细胞)的缺陷已进行了描述。免疫细胞亚群的数量在发展过程中出现差异,并且在表型和功能上与成人来源的细胞存在差异(综述[19,20])。T 细胞和 B 细胞在表型和功能上都是不成熟的,通常缺乏具有记忆细胞的表型和功能。自然杀伤(NK)细胞在出生时出现频率低、功能也并不成熟。有文献报道,在出生时淋巴细胞相对减少,外周 T 细胞数量最低,此后随着功能尚不成熟的外周淋巴器官的发育,其数量逐渐增加[21,22]。

近几十年来的报道,新生小鼠 T 细胞在数量和功能上均存在缺陷。不过,最近较多研究报道新生小鼠 T 细胞在各种体外和体内模型均可发挥效应[23-25]。此外,新生小鼠辅助 T 细胞在向 Th2 细胞分化上被认为并非完全反应"缺陷"[26,27],至少部分由产生 IL-12 的树突状细胞亚群延迟成熟引起[28]。主要涉及 Th1 和 Th2 功能的 T 辅助应答在某些情况下无效但在其他情况下有效[29-31],这种情况在人类是否正确还并不明确。胎儿起源的 $CD4^+T$ 细胞在新生儿期持续存在,影响向 Th2 分化的早期反应,而 Th2 分化在子宫内已比较明显[32,33]。此外,关于新生儿的 $CD4^+T$ 细胞功能有效性和 T 辅助应答存在广泛的多样性,在不同报道之间存在矛盾。虽然新生儿 $CD8^+T$ 细胞在某些情形下(包括先天性获得性感染中)能逐渐进化成熟的细胞溶解功能[34-36],但是它们在正常的健康新生儿中功能与成年人相比仍然较不完善[37]。此外,新生儿的淋巴细胞相对减少症可能引起稳态增殖的上升,这在小鼠中已得到充分研究,但在人类中尚未得到证实,这可能影响到新兴的 T 细胞库。在早期阶段,因为 T 细胞不断离开胸腺,外周血细胞数量增加,导致相对于成人,新生儿在脾和淋巴结内具有较高的外周循环的胸腺细胞比例[38,39]。在细胞因子的产生和增殖反应方面,这些细胞表型和功能在定量和定性方面,新生儿与成年人均存在差异。这可能有助于新生儿不同的 T 辅助应答。近期一些研究通过分析 TCR 重排剪切环(TREC)作为外周循环的胸腺细胞的分子标志物,发现人类脐带血 T 细胞对 IL-7 刺激后的增殖数量高于成年人的不成熟的 $CD4^+$细胞,提示在人类也存在功能差异[39,40]。

新生儿比儿童时期具有更高的循环 B 细胞比例。但是,新生儿 B 细胞表型尚不成熟[41],与成年人细胞具有不同的表型转换模式。这些因素和新生儿 $CD4^+$ T 细胞对 B 细胞功能的"帮助"不足一起导致新生儿抗体反应普遍存在缺陷:生成时间晚、持续时间较短、抗体水平低,抗体的亲和力和亲合力较低。边缘区 B 细胞在生命的前几个月基本上是缺失的[42];循环浆细胞也很罕见。在早期新生儿中淋巴器官发生是持续的,淋巴结和脾结构尚在发育(生发中心,边缘区)。因此,"T 细胞依赖"和"T 细胞非依赖"性的抗体反应较后期的效应低[43]。特别是 T 细胞非依赖的反应出现明显受损[44];据报道,下面所述的许多因素导致受损发生。

抗原呈递能力不足导致新生儿有限的免疫反应。树突状细胞数量很少,且报道提示其功能不足,共刺激分子的表达低。在临床器官移植中,年龄较大的个体这种"不成熟"的表型重演是试图通过使用药物或生物阻断共刺激途径等免疫抑制策略予以实现。

越来越多地被认识到,调节性细胞群是免疫成熟的重要参与者,同时也是婴儿时期"免疫抑制"的重要原因,起着预防自身免疫性疾病的作用。文献报道 $CD4^+$ 调节性 T 细胞在幼儿中比年长的个体具有更高的比例,但是已探究的功能相对并不完善。新生儿主要是不成熟的调节性 T 细胞,这被认为对自我耐受有利,在试验模型中,则对非自体抗原反应有利[45,46]。对于最近描述调节 B 细胞[47],证据显示婴幼儿[48]比[49]年长个体具有更高的发生率,但影响仍有待进一步明确。此外,抑制途径(如 PD-1[50])在儿童移植免疫中的作用还有待探索。

儿童早期固有免疫和适应性免疫系统的相互作用

固有免疫和适应性免疫在很多方面可相互作用、激活和调节。在移植的文中所提及的"T 细胞非依赖性"对于多糖结构的反应主要是指非自体 ABO 血型抗原的免疫应答。与其他多糖类似,一般认为 ABO 抗原不通过 MHC Ⅱ 复合物呈递导致 T 细胞介导的 B 细胞激活的经典途径,而是通过固有免疫分子相互作用激活 B 细胞。如果抗原与补体片段体 C3d 组成复合物,相较于无补体状态,B 细胞受体(BCR)的活化仅需要低于 100~1000 倍抗原浓度。这种效应是通过 C3d 与其受体 CD21 结合完成的,效应 B 细胞共受体复合物将介导 BCR 通过 CD19 发挥效应[51]。补体介导共信号在对自身抗原的免疫耐受中发挥重要作用[52,53],并可能对同种抗原发挥至关重要的作用。婴儿中这种相互作用的功能受损在临床上多表现为多糖荚膜细菌[44]感染发生率和严重性增加。分析外周血 ABO 血型不相容与 ABO 血型相容的儿童发现,心脏移植(下面将详细描述)没有显示出明确的C3d水平与年龄依赖性；然而，心脏移植ABO血型不匹配的婴儿受者相较于ABO血型匹配的婴儿受者血浆中C3d的水平显著降低[54]。在新生儿和婴幼儿中B细胞CD21的存在比例较后期并未发现显著差异[54]，通过信号通路的改变[55]或由于进一步机制的作用，由补体结合所诱导的效应似乎受到损害。补体在成人宿主长期ABO血型不相容肾移植物的作用如前所述[56]。

依靠母体免疫球蛋白的被动免疫

早在胎龄13周时，免疫球蛋白G(IgG抗体)开始从母体通过胎盘转移到胎儿血液中[57,58]。32周妊娠后此效应将大幅提高，在约36周时几乎能完全反映母体的血清状况。实际上足月新生儿将超出产妇特异性IgG抗体浓度20%~30%[57]。这种转移是主动转运过程，因为高分子量结构无法被动通过胎盘屏障。产妇的IgG与胎儿侧胎盘的IgG受体的结晶部分（Fcγ）相结合(‘新生儿Fcγ受体’，FcRn)[59]。这些I类MHC样受体是pH值敏感的，相较于母体生理血液pH值7.4时，当pH值为6.0时对于Fcγ具有高出100°的亲和力。目前假说认为母体的IgG通过低pH值的内涵体的体液相进行内吞捕获从而免受溶酶体酶的降解。内涵体是通过细胞胞饮作用并与朝向胎儿血管的细胞膜融合，在胎儿血较高的生理pH值下，此处IgG将再次从FcRn释放[60]。

母体的IgG可在一定程度上对新生儿先前由母体适应性免疫或免疫接种的感染物质进行保护。母体IgG的存在表明既往已与抗原进行接触；母源抗体的强度部分反映了与抗原接触的时间间隔。在可通过胎盘传播感染到胎儿的感染中，母体血清学阳性的儿童感染高于母体血清学阴性的儿童，只作为以前母体感染的替代[61]。然而，针对特定病原体，更高母体抗体水平已被发现可降低此病原体所致的感染风险。例如，B组链球菌所致的新生儿败血症的风险与在母体和脐带血中针对这些细菌的抗原滴度呈负相关[62]。然而，被动输入的IgG只能提供部分保护，特别是针对细胞内病原体，并且各种IgG亚型的转移不相同，IgG2是转移效率最低的亚型[63]。对现有的一般抗体的分析表明，胎盘转移的比例变化取决于抗原的性质。针对蛋白质的抗体(如破伤风类毒素)，婴儿血中的比例相较于母体血浆中比例高(平均165%)，而抗多糖抗体(如抗流感嗜血杆菌和大肠杆菌脂多糖)比母亲略低[57]。此现象的发现对婴儿移植是非常重要的，因为特定ABO血型的血型抗原就是表面多糖，而IgG2是针对多糖抗原产生效应的主要抗体亚类[64]。由此推测，这有助于保护O型血的母亲孕有A型或B型血胎儿，或AB血型胎儿及其他血型的母亲避免发生溶血反应。胎盘免疫球蛋白的转移将在后面的章节进一步讨论。

哺乳

与其他动物比较而言，人类不表达在肠中的FcRn，由此似乎没有从肠腔未消化的免疫球蛋白的主动吸收[65]。因此，健康婴儿的IgG水平将经历生理性下降，大约6个月的时候达到低值，在随后青春期早期逐步升高[66]，(达到成人正常水平的中位值年龄在9岁左右)。母乳喂养与配方奶喂养的婴幼儿血浆中的抗体IgG(和IgM)水平不同[67]。IgM和IgA由儿童时期产生，但不通过胎盘也不经由肠道的吸收传送，从出生到17、18岁的年龄显示出一个稳定增加[66]。然而，基于对IgA的表达的B细胞中的乳腺腺泡的选择性富集，人母初乳中含有高浓度的IgA的水平(分泌超过5000mg/d)和中等浓度的母体的IgG和IgM水平(第一周超过70mg /d，产后3~4周降至10mg/d)[68,69]。尽管缺乏肠道吸收，但可通过腔内结合和抗原毒素中和为新生儿和婴儿提供保护[70]。有趣的发现是，母乳喂养的儿童血浆IgA水平较配方奶喂养者高，这可能是由于儿童自身适应或保存IgA的能力[67]。

母体免疫系统的要素也通过白细胞转移到胎儿的胃肠道。而在转移的白细胞中，巨噬细胞比例高达85%[71]，与明显的吞噬作用和失活有害物质相关[72]，记忆T细胞和B细胞的存在表明，一种功能完善的适应性免疫反应的产妇细胞可能在胎儿肠道内发生[68]。母乳中的附加免疫活性的底物包括乳铁蛋白，有文献报道可损伤细菌对黏膜的黏附能力[73]。溶酶体与细菌腔内裂解有关[74]。各种母乳原发性非免疫组分在婴儿的免疫系统发育过程中担任重要的免疫角色，细菌对黏膜表面的细菌黏附受体结构竞争非消化性寡糖[73]，可减少细菌与侵入婴儿内环境的细菌[75]。肠腔内母源性的免疫成分发挥的免疫效应与母乳喂养婴儿的低过敏发生率相关[76]，也和母乳喂养的早产儿坏死性结肠炎的低发生率相关[77]。目前认为，免疫系统可能的“吸收”的效应，可用来鉴别消化道营养或其他基本成分等“良性”外来物质与靶向损伤免疫系统的有害物质。机制包括与致病物质减少物理相互作用，通过分泌细胞因子及与腔内母体淋巴细胞的互动改变免疫环境[68]。

尽管专家之间意见尚不一致，在母乳中各种特异性和非特异性免疫成分可在某种程度上对婴儿有害物质起保护作用[78],很少有临床对照试验可证明这一假设。绝大多数公开的临床试验都在发展中国家,这反映了等待器官移植的新生儿所面临的威胁与“发达”国家的新生儿不同。几项 Cochrane 回顾得出的结论是,现有科学数据均强烈支持母乳喂养是新生儿最好的选择这一观点,特别是在发展中国家,以致近期世界卫生组织的指南推荐尽可能纯母乳喂养 6 个月[78]。

母乳喂养对新生儿移植方案的选择和诊断的影响需要深入考虑。

幼儿和学龄儿童:成熟和经验

婴儿和年老者,具有更高的感染易感性和预后不良,主要是因为各自的免疫不成熟和衰老,与之相比,童年中间阶段往往具有有力的免疫应答。研究提示,与健康的年轻人相比,诸多传染类疾病在 4~13 岁的年龄阶段,死亡率较低,病程也较缓和[79,80]。研究发现,这种强大的免疫力的儿童与其他年龄组相比,对流感和结核感染的易感性降低,此外当儿童感染病毒如水痘、麻疹、腮腺炎和 EB 病毒(EBV)后,疾病的临床表现的严重程度下降。这与记忆 B 细胞可在体内维持多年,并能够迅速地激活而产生保护性抗体有关。产生的抗体可以通过终末分化的长寿命浆细胞在血浆中维持多年[81-86]。记忆 $CD4^+$和 $CD8^+T$ 细胞也有助于针对病原体的保护性免疫,部分原因是它们效应功能的发展速度。除了免疫记忆和保护性抗体,免疫应答的保护于儿童和年长儿童的致病性方面存在差异,最终利于现有的或广泛破坏后病原体去除后的组织修复和再生[87]。

在移植实践中,这些正常发育过程对临床结果的影响还没有从婴儿时期接受移植的儿童的这一角度进行探讨。但是,儿童在童年中期进行(心脏)移植效果没有在出生后第一年接受移植的长期效果好[105]。

青春期

青春期是人类发展的关键时期。独立于移植后的时间和其他危险分层，器官移植的移植物损失率最高的时期是 15~25 岁年龄组[88-90]。有多方面的因素可以解释这一结果,这里将进行综述。同时在第 120 章将进行深入探讨。

行为影响

最重要的是,青少年这个发育阶段发生的巨大的精神和心理的变化将对移植效果产生不利影响。随着儿童长大成人,他们经历着身份和责任的转变。其中包括越来越希望掌控自己的生活，而大多数患者仍无法恰当地处理多方面的挑战，如移植后护理相关的医疗方案。家长和医务人员等遭到质疑和挑战,偏激、冒险和自毁倾向伴随着不成熟的处理问题的方式以及情绪敏感。显然,坚持医疗和日常生活的约束在这个年龄组经常表现较差[90,91]。对日常免疫抑制药物及消遣物限制的建议虽然与其他组显示并无不同，但往往与个人意愿相左。鉴于对免疫抑制药物的依从性欠佳,可以部分解释在青少年中急性排斥反应发生率较高、供体特异性的人类白细胞抗原(HLA)的抗体产生频率较高和移植失败率较高的原因[92]。不过,这些解释仍有较大的局限性,其忽略了青春期主要代谢和与免疫相关变化。

内分泌和代谢改变对免疫系统的影响

神经内分泌因子、性激素和类固醇以及生长激素对免疫系统的各个方面产生重大影响。在青春期这些激素在数量和分泌模式上发生巨大变化。在过去数十年,两性之间免疫系统的差异已在临床证实,并进行相关科学探究;但在许多方面尚不明确。与许多其他的动物类似,女性的自身免疫性疾病比男性的发病率更高[93]。已有研究证实，月经周期和怀孕期间性激素定量差异与自身免疫性疾病的发病具有相关性。同样,已经发现持续感染所致的反复发生的症状(如单纯疱疹)已被证实与月经周期和免疫组分以及细胞因子/趋化因子的变化有关[94]。一些病症(如多发性硬化[95]和类风湿性关节炎[96])在怀孕期间表现出活性显著下降。与此相反，对于其他疾病(如系统性红斑狼疮)导致炎症活动的加重和减轻均有报道,妊娠末期激素变化已被发现可触发疾病[97]。这种效果并不仅仅受到激素影响,而且还涉及暴露于胎儿的 HLA 分子,并且对免疫反应调节的程度不一样[98]。皮质类固醇,不论是由肾上腺产生或者药物来源,均可对固有免疫和适应性免疫产生重大影响。类固醇治疗因其调节免疫作用而用于治疗各种自体免疫和过敏性疾病，同时也可用于移植后减少同种异体免疫反应。雄激素和雌激素本质上具有糖皮质激素作用，高剂量性激素的使用显示对免疫系统有类似的作用[99]。进一步发现高剂量的睾酮导致肿瘤坏死因子 α (TNF-α)的释放和 $CD4^{+}CD8^{+}$“双阳性”不成熟的胸腺细胞的凋亡[100]。

胸腺退化被发现与性类固醇和它们调节激素的分泌增加强烈相关[101]，且可通过外科去势或化学去势逆转[102]。此外，已有报道，固有和适应性免疫系统的许多细胞受生长激素[103]和性激素[104]的影响，但是在生理功能和临床相关性上仍有待确定。这些激素在青春期达到高峰；这种激素“混乱”的相互作用对人体发育的影响可能远远超出单个内分泌信使的效果。这表明，对免疫成熟、免疫反应和免疫耐受以及其他治疗后果的影响目前被低估，并需要进一步探索。

免疫成熟程度对移植的影响

幼儿期的“允许性”的环境

如果在生命早期进行器官移植，此时免疫发生巨大变化，在这个过程中对两个固有的主要因素仍然知之甚少：外来抗原和化学免疫抑制大量而持续的侵入，在瞬息万变的发育过程中既无法设定也无法检测。在心脏（和肺）移植中，新生胸腺切除对免疫功能的潜在影响使情况变得更为复杂。临床器官移植的免疫后果不限于增加感染并发症（例如与其他生命阶段相比，对更广泛的感染性致病体具有更高的易感性，常见的病毒导致移植后感染病程也存在差异）。但与此同时，其对移植结果也会提供一个有利的环境。免疫系统发育易受到耐受诱导，并具有一定程度的可塑性，随着时间的推移，它表现出对移植的器官的存在发生的慢性“适应性”的免疫抑制影响下降。因此，不成熟的状态为非常年轻但如安全血型（ABO）不符的患者的器官移植（见下文）提供了特殊的机会，而后来，随着青春期的神经内分泌发生显著变化同时伴有心理和行为问题，为临床小组诊疗移植患儿带了巨大挑战。

卓越的长期预后

根据国际心脏和肺移植学会（ISHLT）的数据[105]，多个研究组发现，虽然早期移植死亡率较高，但是一岁以下的儿童接受心脏移植与其他年龄组相比长期生存率最好[106,107]。相比于移植前年龄较大的儿童，接受心脏移植的婴幼儿经常处于一个比较紧急的临床状态，其中约 12%患者需要在体外膜肺氧合（ECMO）的形式的机械循环支持，并且越来越多的患者需接受心室辅助装置（VAD）。尽管预期的早期移植后的死亡率较高，婴儿移植受者的实际存活率曲线与那些年龄较大的儿童和成人相比，有更好的移植物中位存活时间，目前达到 19.7 年。根据过去 21 年的文献报道，移植后第一年存活的儿童（图 112.1），其生存优势变得尤为明显，虽然目前还没有达到 50%的移植物存活率。

儿童肝移植后，有近 20%的儿童实现手术耐受，表现为移植物功能正常以及在无须维护免疫抑制药物治疗下无排斥反应[108,109]，其比例高于成人。同样的“免疫特权”也适用于非常年轻的肾和肺的移植受者，但是这些接受移植的患儿数量太少以致很难证明免疫系统未发育成熟的优势。

在移植受者中，调节性 T 细胞在抗供体免疫反应的控制中的作用尚不清楚。在儿科移植胸腺切除患者中，诱导治疗和慢性免疫抑制对调节性 T 细胞的发育和功能的影响，还有待深入研究。T 细胞亚群和 T 细胞库明显受胸腺切除影响，其通常伴随胸骨切开术[110,111]。初步数据表明，外周血调节性 T 细胞的数量在心脏移植受者中显著低于胸腺切除非移植患者组（不接受 T 细胞耗竭和维持免疫抑制的患者）以及健康年龄匹配对照组中的细胞数[112,113]。此外，幼稚 T 细胞与效应调节性 T 细胞的比例在移植患者中较健康对照组低[114]。在异体抗原持续存在和免疫抑制作用下引起调节性 T 细胞亚群的多样性改变促进稳定供体的调节性 T 细胞的发展和移植物更好地存活，这点还有待进一步阐明。

总之，婴儿因其免疫系统的不成熟，较成年个体有更高的感染率。疫苗的发展旨在帮助婴儿促进免疫系统成熟并在较早的年龄增加免疫应答。这些发育的差异同样可有助于解释婴儿移植受者的较好疗效，并且可以借此进一步解决其他问题。虽然文献报道很少，但是儿童移植医生普遍认为年龄小的儿童接受移植手术后较年长的儿童需要更少的免疫抑制治疗[115]。许多研究治疗中心在婴儿中不使用诱导治疗，幼儿仅早期用类固醇治疗（或不用），且在年龄较大的儿童较年轻儿童中具有较低的钙调磷酸酶目标水平。在最近的我们组牵头多中心研究发现，只有在年长阶段移植的儿童

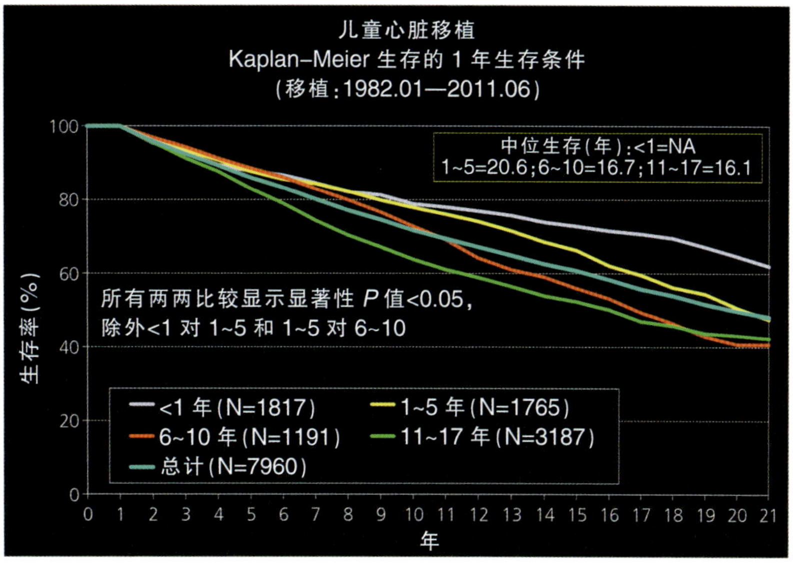

图 112.1 根据移植的年龄分层后，儿童心脏移植受者术后一年生存率。Source: International Society for Heart and Lung Transplantation，accessible from http://www.ishlt.org/downloadables/slides/2013/heart_pediatric.pptx.

出现供体特异性 HLA 抗体[116]。此外，抗Ⅱ类敏感 HLA 抗体在 6 岁以下的患者中没有发现。移植物血管病变、复发的慢性排斥反应，在新生儿和婴儿移植中发生率最低，而该发生率在 1~10 岁的患儿中增加，10 岁以上患者的发病率和成人相似[105]。

显然这种效果不能仅由未成熟的免疫系统来解释，还要考虑幼儿中和成人相比较低的其他危险因素，如高血压、血浆脂质异常、心脏动脉粥样硬化、糖尿病和慢性肾衰竭等[117]。但是，毫无疑问，年轻移植受者的免疫系统的发育增加了移植物长期耐受的可能性。

ABO 血型不符移植

婴儿期后植入 ABO 血型不符的移植物，由于存在高浓度的预成形同型血球凝集素，会引起高风险的超急性抗体介导的排斥反应。在成年人肾移植中，预先存在的抗体可在移植时通过各种手段减少、克服供者和受者 ABO 血型不符的问题[118-123]，从而扩大潜在的捐赠者库。对于需要心脏移植的婴幼儿，由于其自然缺乏超急性免疫介质排斥以及等待 ABO 血型相符的供体期间的高死亡风险，ABO 血型不符最初被设想为一个合理的安全选择[124]。过去的十年中，从我们第一组 ABO

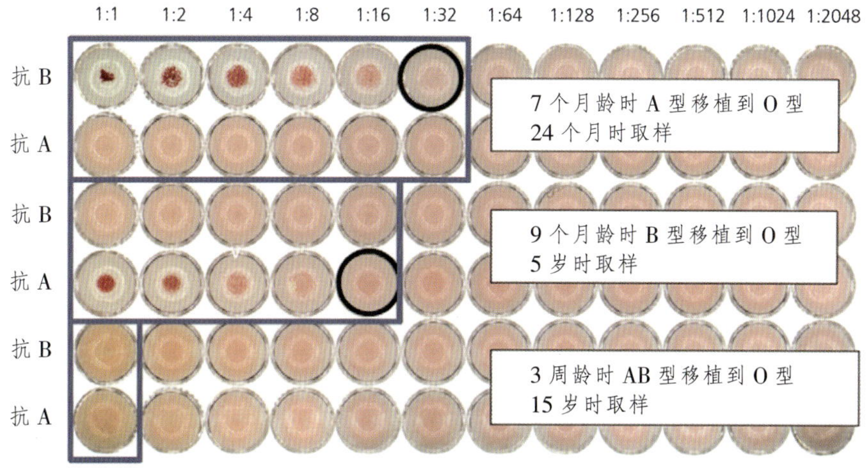

图 112.2 ABO 血型不符的移植心脏的微量凝集试验评估的同族血凝素滴度的例子。Source: [138] West LJ.(2011). ABO-incompatible hearts for infant transplantation. Curr Opin Organ Transplant 16:548 - 554 with permission of Wolters Kluwer Health.

血型不符心脏移植研究开始,已经证明幼儿ABO血型不符的心脏移植死亡率或发病率与ABO血型相符相同,是扩大现有婴幼儿供体库的有效策略[125-127]。事实上,在一些国家的小儿心脏移植中心现在经常列出很年幼患者进行移植,而不需要捐赠者血型相符[128,129],虽然安全的限制有待最后确定[130]。值得注意的是,与加拿大和英国相比,UNOS法规在美国不断削弱实现这种策略的全部好处[130-132]。基于数十年来形成的器官分配规则,供体器官必须首先被分配到ABO血型相同或者相符的受者,之后才被考虑分配给ABO血型不符的受者,尽管这一政策对婴幼儿心脏移植没有科学依据或相关性。

几十年前,人们在成人ABO血型不相符的肾移植中注意到,当针对供者血型的抗体重新积累,移植物经常能耐受抗体介导的损伤。Platt和同事们描述了这种现象,称为"耐受"[56,133];HLA和ABO抗体的移植物耐受机制仍是目前研究的重点,并将在本书的第4章、第6章和第36章中详细讨论。相比之下,ABO血型不符的年轻心脏移植受者,移植前普遍缺乏足够的血球凝集素,通常随时间的推移,在产生针对其他非自身抗原的抗体的同时,缺乏针对血型的抗体(图112.2),这一模式与移植物耐受相比,和B细胞的耐受性更一致[134-138]。此外,当受到各种具体的体内外非特异性刺激,ABO血型不符的移植受者的外周血细胞不产生针对供者血型的抗体,表明成熟B细胞在早期长期接触A/B抗原导致类似自我耐受的过程的发生。

当考虑ABO抗体及其在ABO血型不符的移植中的潜在重要性,了解目前同型血球凝集素临床检测方法的固有缺陷至关重要[140]。连续稀释的血清样品中的抗体凝集红细胞被读出并称为"抗体滴度"。众所周知,该方法有很大的局限性,包括凝集度的主观评价以及不同中心缺乏标准的方法[141]。另一个潜在的混杂因素是ABO碳水化合物亚结构在不同红细胞和组织表达中存在差异。红细胞具有A和B抗原的六个糖链的子类型,而一般没有组织[142,143]。只在红细胞上拥有,而组织中不存在的A和B抗原凝集的抗体可能和ABO血型不相符移植没有关系。因此,对ABO血型凝集试验的解读必须谨慎。不凝集能可靠地指示没有ABO抗体,A或B的红细胞凝集表明可能存在供体非特异性的抗体。

胎盘免疫和母乳喂养对移植的影响

新生儿和婴儿的感染性疾病诊断

新生儿的血清学检测反映的是母体的情况,因此不能作为婴幼儿感染性疾病诊断的可靠依据。然而,对于弓形虫、巨细胞病毒(CMV)等可以通过母婴垂直传播的感染,诊断有很大挑战[144,145]。区分被动获得性抗体和婴儿自身感染的区别在于血清中IgM抗体的出现。IgM五聚体因分子体积大和不能通过FcRn介导的跨细胞转运而不能穿过胎盘。因此,除非接受输血,IgM抗体由婴儿免疫系统自身产生,可明确自身感染。不过,IgM抗体被认为是适应性免疫的第一线反应,并且很快转换成IgG抗体,通常只存在于感染后的几周内。因此在婴儿血清中出现IgG抗体而不出现IgM抗体,并不能排除孕期感染,因为IgM抗体可能已消退。直接检测感染可能有帮助但不能保证绝对的正确。在部分疑似感染的病例中,唯一可靠的方法就是遵循感染治疗,直到总体和抗原特异性的IgG抗体同步消退[146]。

在新生儿和婴儿移植中,特别需要关注的感染包括CMV、EB病毒、弓形虫病和疱疹单纯形(HSV),其中前两个病毒对小儿移植长期预后有重要影响。在CMV IgG抗体血清抗体阳性的情况下,尿和咽拭子病毒培养能有效区分未感染的儿童。对于EB病毒,检测病毒衣壳抗原(VCA)特异性抗体能较好地表明近期感染;IgM抗体的出现表明婴幼儿期感染,而高滴度并与产妇血清学无关的IgG能起到一定提示作用[147]。核酸检测聚合酶链反应(PCR)阳性对于感染的诊断具有很高的特异性[148]。

由于母乳中的抗体不被吸收,母乳喂养并不改变通过产后的血清学测试诊断的相关传染病。然而,由于母乳中存在的产妇白细胞有携带传染性疾病母婴传播的风险,尤其在移植后的免疫抑制状态宿主防御功能受损的状态下。因此,当母亲发生临床感染的症状时,母乳喂养需要谨慎。母亲如果感染具有通过母乳垂直传播风险的人类免疫缺陷病毒(HIV)、新感染或者重新激活的CMV或EB病毒时,应禁止母乳喂养[149]。有一种特殊的情况,如果出现一个CMV血清学阳性母亲的孩子通过培养被认定为CMV阴性,并且移植了CMV阴性的捐献者的器官。在这些患者中,尽管发生率很低,但仍有通过母乳传染的风险,不推荐移植后母乳喂养。

新生儿、婴儿 HLA 和 ABO 诊断

报道显示,高达 60%有手术或者输血史的健康成人体内存在可以用高敏感的方法检测到的 HLA 抗体[150]。和其他 IgG 抗体一样,那些针对 HLA 表位的抗体可以穿过胎盘,导致胎儿被动获得这类抗体[57],其浓度逐渐降低但持续存在至 18 个月龄[151,152]。因此,评估新生儿过敏是很困难的,只能通过记录过程和产妇的抗体相对于婴儿的自然下降来确认。即使是新生儿也能够产生针对外源性 HLA 分子的特异性抗体,例如,早期心脏手术需要涉及血小板输血和其他血液制品以及体外循环,特别是血管重建需人类同种异体组织的植入。事实上,在不使用免疫抑制的情况下,由于持续暴露于外源性组织抗原,血管移植的婴儿通常产生明显和广泛的抗体反应[153-155]。对于那些后续需要移植的患者,这显然会产生很高的免疫风险。我们团队此前研究发现,只要简单的在术中用戊乙醛浸泡就可以在不损害供器官完整性的前提下,预防过敏的发生[156]。婴儿 HLA 致敏目前在我们中心已经很少发生,这对于需要做心脏手术的患者而言是巨大优势。

活性 HLA 致敏与被动获得抗体对于制订围术期和术后计划至关重要。对于被动获得的抗体,在移植时去除抗体能有效避免儿童受者发生抗体介导的排斥,而对于产生免疫记忆人群则需要在移植时给予更强的脱敏治疗,包括抗体去除、B 细胞耗竭(利妥昔单抗)和浆细胞减少(硼替佐米)治疗以及用 IVIG 的免疫调节。如果有被受者 HLA 针对的合适供体,这些患者将被排除接受移植;如果跨越 HLA 不符,他们将面临早期发生的抗体介导的损伤的高风险。因致敏产生供体特异性抗体和免疫记忆的人群与被动获得抗体的人群相比,长期抗 HLA 抗体负担更重。这些移植受者有重新激活免疫应答的高风险,导致抗体介导移植损伤。这可能不局限于急性抗体介导的排斥反应,也可能包括加快的慢性排斥过程,如心脏移植中的快速发生的移植物血管病变。

在 ABO 不相符的心脏移植新生儿中,通常较少发现被动获得的抗 A 和抗 B 抗体并且具有比其他抗体更低的滴度(比如针对 CMV 或 EBV 的抗体),胎盘转移 IgG 亚类的差异和特异性可能部分解释我们的观察结果。另外,根据我们的经验和来自其他组的观察,母亲血型特异性抗体倾向于在几个星期内迅速下降或消失,而其他母亲血清学标志持续存在,直到 9~12 个月龄,有时长达 18 个月。

如本章前面详述,母体 IgG 或 IgM 抗体不能通过完整的肠屏障吸收,因此,对于等待移植或移植后的婴儿,母亲 HLA 或 ABO 抗体的存在不应排除母乳喂养。

成长期:免疫系统发育完善

儿童只占移植受者的小部分;然而,发育不成熟导致儿童受者与成年受者相比可更好地接受供器官的机制和要素,对所有年龄的移植用药均有作用。在骨髓移植准备过程中,受体自身的淋巴系统通过辐射和白细胞耗竭剂消除。我们可以推测,这表示免疫系统实际上被“重置”,进而形成更容易接受供体的免疫环境。分析免疫系统恢复后可以发现,这种情况下各种成分恢复经历的阶段和新生儿免疫系统发育相近[157-159]。但是,与婴儿或幼儿相比,成人免疫系统的重构取决于很多附加因素[160]。这包括上述讨论的一些方面,例如缺少胸腺、性激素和生长激素的差异,以及可能在移植组织本身完成生长发育和与多个细胞周期复制相关结构变化的差异。在骨髓移植中,目前甚至多次延长的致死剂量的辐射和额外的治疗仍无法去除每一种免疫细胞[161]。特别是在休息或蛰伏期的细胞阶段可以持续存在并且在恢复期间被重新激活。因此,恢复中的成人免疫系统不能像发育中的婴幼儿的免疫系统那样接受外来抗原。正如第 76 章描述的那样,通过淋巴细胞去除、部分去除骨髓细胞和降低剂量的辐射诱导免疫耐受,虽然成功率在逐渐提高,但仍非常受限。因此,为了发展成人和年龄较大的儿童的靶向治疗方法,精确识别未成熟的免疫系统信号通路和相互作用的表征变得更加重要。在这一点上,B 细胞可能的关键作用正在显现。骨髓去除后,新产生的 B 细胞经历产前和早期婴儿期类似的发育阶段。特别是过渡期的不同阶段 B 细胞有很高的出现率。这些细胞表面表达 CD5 和 CD10,在第一阶段,表达低密度 CD21[162]。在成熟期间,因 BTK 遗传重组,过渡性 B 细胞表达 CD21 以及 CD23、CD44、Bcl-2、BAFF-R 和 IgD 逐渐增加[162]。在鼠胰岛移植模型中,通过阻断 B 细胞成熟信号或受体,成功诱导这种未成熟细胞[163,164],并导致体液同种异体移植耐受[165]。当在第一例成功操作性耐受的肾移植病例中分析 B 细胞间隔室重组观察到了类似的结果,其 HLA 不匹配供器官的长

期生存和功能通过部分去除骨髓和输入肾移植供者的干细胞实现，详见第76章[166]。在成功诱导耐受的患者中，过渡性B细胞和B细胞激活因子(BAFF)的血浆水平较高[167]。

在用利妥昔单抗去除B细胞的成人中，能否观察到接受ABO不相符心脏婴儿的供体特异性耐受的状态(见上述)仍未明确。在大样本的成人ABO不相符的肾移植中，大多数受者最终重新积累到一定程度的针对供体血液的抗体，尽管比移植前滴度更低，并且通常没有临床排斥。但是，部分人群观察到持续缺少的对供体血液的抗体，而少数出现不可控制的高滴度和移植物丢失[120,122]。因此，只有少数的成人在B细胞去除后出现婴儿类似的免疫系统重建，而大多数并不是这种模式。

总结

总之，理解免疫系统的不成熟和发展，不仅有助于个性化的临床移植，也有助于理解自体耐受和同种异体耐受机制。探索自然发生的免疫系统不成熟对移植物和受体生存的益处必将是移植研究的重要部分。

(柯庆宏 译 柯庆宏 校)

参考文献

1. West LJ. Defining critical windows in the development of the human immune system. Human and Experimental Toxicology. 2002;21(9-10):499-505.
2. Spencer SJ, Martin S, Mouihate A, et al. Early-life immune challenge: defining a critical window for effects on adult responses to immune challenge. Neuropsychopharmacology. 2006;31(9):1910-1918.
3. Billingham RE, Brent L, Medawar PB. Actively acquired tolerance of foreign cells. Nature. 1953;172(4379):603-606.
4. Streilein JW. Neonatal tolerance of H-2 alloantigens. Procuring graft acceptance the "old-fashioned" way. Transplantation. 1991;52(1):1-10.
5. West LJ. Developmental aspects of immunomodulation: exploiting the immature immune system for organ transplantation. Transplant Immunology. 2002;9(2-4):149-153.
6. Benitz WE, Gould JB, Druzin ML. Risk factors for early-onset group B streptococcal sepsis: estimation of odds ratios by critical literature review. Pediatrics. 1999;103(6):e77.
7. Corbett NP, Blimkie D, Ho KC, et al. Ontogeny of Toll-like receptor mediated cytokine responses of human blood mononuclear cells. PLoS ONE. 2010;5(11): e15041.
8. Yan SR, Qing G, Byers DM, et al. Role of MyD88 in diminished tumor necrosis factor alpha production by newborn mononuclear cells in response to lipopolysaccharide. Infection and Immunity. 2004;72(3):1223-1229.
9. Hunt DW, Huppertz HI, Jiang HJ, et al. Studies of human cord blood dendritic cells: evidence for functional immaturity. Blood. 1994;84(12):4333-4343.
10. Hoeman C, Dhakal M, Zaghouani H. Overcoming dendritic cell tardiness to triumph over IL-13 receptor: a strategy for the development of effective pediatric vaccines. Discovery Medicine. 2010;9(49):554-559.
11. Velilla PA, Rugeles MT, Chougnet CA. Defective antigen-presenting cell function in human neonates. Clinical Immunology. 2006;121(3):251-259.
12. Christensen RD, Rothstein G. Exhaustion of mature marrow neutrophils in neonates with sepsis. Journal of Pediatrics. 1980;96(2):316-318.
13. Squire E, Favara B, Todd J. Diagnosis of neonatal bacterial infection: hematologic and pathologic findings in fatal and nonfatal cases. Pediatrics. 1979;64(1): 60-64.
14. Doron MW, Makhlouf RA, Katz VL, et al. Increased incidence of sepsis at birth in neutropenic infants of mothers with preeclampsia. Journal of Pediatrics. 1994;125(3):452-458.
15. Turkmen M, Satar M, Atici A. Neutrophil chemotaxis and random migration in preterm and term infants with sepsis. American Journal of Perinatology. 2000;17(2):107-112.
16. Merry C, Puri P, Reen DJ. Defective neutrophil actin polymerisation and chemotaxis in stressed newborns. Journal of Pediatric Surgery. 1996;31(4): 481-485.
17. Lassiter HA, Watson SW, Seifring ML, et al. Complement factor 9 deficiency in serum of human neonates. Journal of Infectious Diseases. 1992;166(1):53-57.
18. Zilow EP, Hauck W, Linderkamp O, et al. Alternative pathway activation of the complement system in preterm infants with early onset infection. Pediatric Research. 1997;41(3):334-339.
19. Adkins B, Leclerc C, Marshall-Clarke S. Neonatal adaptive immunity comes of age. Nature Reviews. Immunology. 2004;4(7):553-564.
20. Zaghouani H, Hoeman CM, Adkins B. Neonatal immunity: faulty T-helpers and the shortcomings of dendritic cells. Trends in Immunology. 2009;30(12): 585-591.
21. Helbert M, Breuer J. Monitoring patients with HIV disease. Journal of Clinical Pathology. 2000;53(4):266-272.
22. Schatorje EJ, Gemen EF, Driessen GJ, et al. Pediatric reference values for the peripheral T-cell compartment. Scandinavian Journal of Immunology. 2011;3(4):e28.
23. Ridge JP, Fuchs EJ, Matzinger P. Neonatal tolerance revisited: turning on newborn T cells with dendritic cells. Science. 1996;271(5256):1723-1726.
24. Sarzotti M. Response: immunological tolerance. Science. 1996;272(5267):1408a.
25. Forsthuber T, Yip HC, Lehmann PV. Induction of TH1 and TH2 immunity in neonatal mice. Science. 1996;271(5256):1728-1730.
26. Adkins B, Bu Y, Vincek V, et al. The primary responses of murine neonatal lymph node CD4+ cells are Th2-skewed and are sufficient for the development of Th2-biased memory. Clinical and Developmental Immunology. 2003; 10(1):43-51.
27. Adkins B, Bu Y, Guevara P. The generation of Th memory in neonates versus adults: prolonged primary Th2 effector function and impaired development of Th1 memory effector function in murine neonates. Journal of Immunology. 2001;166(2):918-925.
28. Lee HH, Hoeman CM, Hardaway JC, et al. Delayed maturation of an IL-12-producing dendritic cell subset explains the early Th2 bias in neonatal immunity. Journal of Experimental Medicine. 2008;205(10):2269-2280.
29. Hussey GD, Watkins ML, Goddard EA, et al. Neonatal mycobacterial specific cytotoxic T-lymphocyte and cytokine profiles in response to distinct BCG vaccination strategies. Immunology. 2002;105(3):314-324.
30. Vekemans J, Amedei A, Ota MO, et al. Neonatal bacillus Calmette-Guerin vaccination induces adult-like IFN-gamma production by CD4+ T lymphocytes. European Journal of Immunology. 2001;31(5):1531-1535.
31. Xainli J, Baisor M, Kastens W, et al. Age-dependent cellular immune responses to Plasmodium vivax Duffy binding protein in humans. Journal of Immunology. 2002;169(6):3200-3207.
32. Adkins B. Peripheral CD4+ lymphocytes derived from fetal versus adult thymic precursors differ phenotypically and functionally. Journal of Immunology. 2003;171(10):5157-5164.
33. Prescott SL, Macaubas C, Holt BJ, et al. Transplacental priming of the human immune system to environmental allergens: universal skewing of initial T cell responses toward the Th2 cytokine profile. Journal of Immunology. 1998; 160(10):4730-4737.
34. Opiela SJ, Levy RB, Adkins B. Murine neonates develop vigorous in vivo cytotoxic and Th1/Th2 responses upon exposure to low doses of NIMA-like alloantigens. Blood. 2008;112(4):1530-1538.
35. Marchant A, Appay V, Van Der Sande M, et al. Mature CD8(+) T lymphocyte response to viral infection during fetal life. Journal of Clinical Investigation. 2003;111(11):1747-1755.
36. Hermann E, Truyens C, Alonso-Vega C, et al. Human fetuses are able to mount an adultlike CD8 T-cell response. Blood. 2002;100(6):2153-2158.
37. Ruckwardt TJ, Malloy AM, Gostick E, et al. Neonatal CD8 T-cell hierarchy is distinct from adults and is influenced by intrinsic T cell properties in respiratory syncytial virus infected mice. PLoS Pathogens. 2011;7(12):e1002377.
38. Fink PJ, Hendricks DW. Post-transplant-thymic maturation: young T cells assert their individuality. Nature Reviews. Immunology. 2011;11(8):544-549.
39. Hendricks DW, Fink PJ. Recent thymic emigrants are biased against the T-helper type 1 and toward the T-helper type 2 effector lineage. Blood. 2011; 117(4):1239-1249.

40. Opiela SJ, Koru-Sengul T, Adkins B. Murine neonatal recent thymic emigrants are phenotypically and functionally distinct from adult recent thymic emigrants. Blood. 2009;113(22):5635–5643.
41. Schatorje EJ, Gemen EF, Driessen GJ, et al. Age-matched reference values for B-lymphocyte subpopulations and CVID classifications in children. Scandinavian Journal of Immunology. 2011;74(5):502–510.
42. Timens W, Boes A, Rozeboom-Uiterwijk T, et al. Immaturity of the human splenic marginal zone in infancy. Possible contribution to the deficient infant immune response. Journal of Immunology. 1989;143(10):3200–3206.
43. Rijkers GT, Dollekamp EG, Zegers BJM. The invitro B-cell response to pneumococcal polysaccharides in adults and neonates. Scandinavian Journal of Immunology. 1987;25(5):447–452.
44. Rijkers GT, Sanders EAM, Breukels MA, et al. Infant B-cell response to polysaccharide determinants. Vaccine. 1998;16(14–15):1396–1400.
45. Miyara M, Yoshioka Y, Kitoh A, et al. Functional delineation and differentiation dynamics of human CD4+ T cells expressing the FoxP3 transcription factor. Immunity. 2009;30(6):899–911.
46. van Gent R, van Tilburg CM, Nibbelke EE, et al. Refined characterization and reference values of the pediatric T- and B-cell compartments. Clinical Immunology. 2009;133(1):95–107.
47. Yanaba K, Bouaziz JD, Haas KM, et al. A regulatory B cell subset with a unique CD1dhiCD5+ phenotype controls T cell-dependent inflammatory responses. Immunity. 2008;28(5):639–650.
48. Ling Y, Dijke E, West LJ, et al. Impact of CD1d+CD5+ B Cells on T dependent and T independent immune response in early childhood. Journal of Heart and Lung Transplantation. 2012;31(4):S146
49. Urschel S, Larsen IM, Rebeyka IM, et al. High prevalence of B-10 B-cells in human infants: Regulatory impact on immune response following heart transplantation? Transplantation. 2010;90(S2):403.
50. Riella LV, Paterson AM, Sharpe AH, Chandraker A. Role of the PD-1 pathway in the immune response. American Journal of Transplantation. 2012;12(10): 2575–2587.
51. Boackle SA, Holers VM, Karp DR. CD21 augments antigen presentation in immune individuals. European Journal of Immunology. 1997;27(1):122–129.
52. Prodeus AP, Goerg S, Shen L-M, et al. A critical role for complement in maintenance of self-tolerance. Immunity. 1998;9(5):721–731.
53. Rickert RC. Regulation of B lymphocyte activation by complement C3 and the B cell coreceptor complex. Current Opinion in Immunology. 2005;17(3): 237–243.
54. Urschel S, Larsen IM, Derkatz K, et al. Linking innate and adaptive immunity: C3d plasma levels and CD21 expressing B-cells in ABO-incompatible infant heart transplantation. Transplantation. 2010;90(10(S1)):405(S1).
55. Ryan LA, West LJ, Urschel S. Determining Developmental Immaturity in B-Cell Receptor Signaling. 32nd Annual Meeting of the International Society of Heart and Lung Transplantation. 2012.
56. Platt JL. C4d and the fate of organ allografts. Journal of the American Society of Nephrology. 2002;13(9):2417–2419.
57. Palmeira P, Quinello C, Silveira-Lessa AL, et al. IgG placental transfer in healthy and pathological pregnancies. Clinical and Developmental Immunology. 2012;2012:985646.
58. Saji F, Samejima Y, Kamiura S, et al. Dynamics of immunoglobulins at the feto-maternal interface. Reviews of Reproduction. 1999;4(2):81–89.
59. Leach J, Sedmak D, Osborne J, et al. Isolation from human placenta of the IgG transporter, FcRn, and localization to the syncytiotrophoblast: implications for maternal-fetal antibody transport. Journal of Immunology. 1996;157(8): 3317–3322.
60. Firan M, Bawdon R, Radu C, et al. The MHC class I-related receptor, FcRn, plays an essential role in the maternofetal transfer of gamma-globulin in humans. International Immunology. 2001;13(8):993–1002.
61. de Moraes-Pinto MI, Almeida AC, Kenj G, et al. Placental transfer and maternally acquired neonatal IgG immunity in human immunodeficiency virus infection. Journal of Infectious Diseases. 1996;173(5):1077–1084.
62. Lin FY, Weisman LE, Azimi PH, et al. Level of maternal IgG anti-group B streptococcus type III antibody correlated with protection of neonates against early-onset disease caused by this pathogen. Journal of Infectious Diseases. 2004;190(5):928–934.
63. Nagao AT, Martinez CC, Vieira VS, et al. Placental transfer of IgG and IgG subclass antibodies anti-purified Escherichia coli LPS O16, O6 and O111. Scandinavian Journal of Immunology. 1998;47(6):609–614.
64. Jefferis R, Kumararatne DS. Selective IgG subclass deficiency: quantification and clinical relevance. Clinical and Experimental Immunology. 1990;81(3): 357–367.
65. Baker K, Qiao SW, Kuo T, et al. Immune and non-immune functions of the (not so) neonatal Fc receptor, FcRn. Seminars in Immunopathology. 2009;31(2): 223–236.
66. Belldegrin A, Shoenfeld Y, Pick AI, et al. Age related distribution of serum immunoglobulin concentration in 1003 healthy children and adults. Biomedicine / [Publiee Pour L'A.A.I.C.I.G.]. 1980;33(1):8–12.
67. Kanariou M, Petridou E, Liatsis M, et al. Age patterns of immunoglobulins G, A & M in healthy children and the influence of breast feeding and vaccination status. Pediatric Allergy and Immunology. 1995;6(1):24–29.
68. Lepage P, Van de Perre P. The immune system of breast milk: antimicrobial and anti-inflammatory properties. Advances in Experimental Medicine and Biology. 2012;743:121–137.
69. Ogra SS, Ogra PL. Immunologic aspects of human colostrum and milk. I. Distribution characteristics and concentrations of immunoglobulins at different times after the onset of lactation. The Journal of Pediatrics. 1978;92(4): 546–549.
70. Glass RI, Svennerholm AM, Stoll BJ, et al. Protection against cholera in breast-fed children by antibodies in breast milk. New England Journal of Medicine. 1983;308(23):1389–1392.
71. Crago SS, Prince SJ, Pretlow TG, et al. Human colostral cells. I. Separation and characterization. Clinical and Experimental Immunology. 1979;38(3): 585–597.
72. Pitt J. The milk mononuclear phagocyte. Pediatrics. 1979;64(5 Pt 2 Suppl): 745–749.
73. Lonnerdal B. Nutritional and physiologic significance of human milk proteins. American Journal of Clinical Nutrition. 2003;77(6):1537S–43S.
74. Ellison RT 3rd, Giehl TJ. Killing of gram-negative bacteria by lactoferrin and lysozyme. Journal of Clinical Investigation. 1991;88(4):1080–1091.
75. Shah NP. Effects of milk-derived bioactives: an overview. British Journal of Nutrition. 2000;84(Suppl 1):S3–S10.
76. Mihrshahi S, Ampon R, Webb K, et al. The association between infant feeding practices and subsequent atopy among children with a family history of asthma. Clinical and Experimental Allergy. 2007;37(5):671–679.
77. Quigley MA, Henderson G, Anthony MY, et al. Formula milk versus donor breast milk for feeding preterm or low birth weight infants. Cochrane Database of Systematic Reviews. 2007;(4):CD002971.
78. World Health Organization (WHO). Exclusive Breastfeeding for Six Months Best for Babies Everywhere. 2011; Available from: http://www.who.int/maternal_child_adolescent/documents/infant_feeding/en/index.html.
79. Ahmed R, Oldstone MB, Palese P. Protective immunity and susceptibility to infectious diseases: lessons from the 1918 influenza pandemic. Nature Immunology. 2007;8(11):1188–1193.
80. Feigin RD, Cherry J, Demmler GJ, et al. Textbook of Pediatric Infectious Diseases, 5th ed. Philadelphia, PA: W.B. Saunders; 2004.
81. Amanna IJ, Slifka MK, Crotty S. Immunity and immunological memory following smallpox vaccination. Immunological Reviews. 2006;211:320–337.
82. Bernasconi NL, Traggiai E, Lanzavecchia A. Maintenance of serological memory by polyclonal activation of human memory B cells. Science. 2002; 298(5601):2199–2202.
83. Manz RA, Thiel A, Radbruch A. Lifetime of plasma cells in the bone marrow. Nature. 1997;388(6638):133–134.
84. Slifka MK, Antia R, Whitmire JK, et al. Humoral immunity due to long-lived plasma cells. Immunity. 1998;8(3):363–372.
85. Kalia V, Sarkar S, Gourley TS, et al. Differentiation of memory B and T cells. Current Opinion in Immunology. 2006;18(3):255–264.
86. Crotty S, Felgner P, Davies H, et al. Cutting edge: long-term B cell memory in humans after smallpox vaccination. Journal of Immunology. 2003;171(10): 4969–4973.
87. Swain SL, Agrewala JN, Brown DM, et al. CD4+ T-cell memory: generation and multi-faceted roles for CD4+ T cells in protective immunity to influenza. Immunological Reviews. 2006;211:8–22.
88. Foster BJ, Dahhou M, Zhang X, et al. Association between age and graft failure rates in young kidney transplant recipients. Transplantation. 2011;92(11): 1237–1243.
89. LaRosa C, Baluarte HJ, Meyers KE. Outcomes in pediatric solid-organ transplantation. Pediatric Transplantation. 2011;15(2):128–141.
90. Burra P, Germani G, Gnoato F, et al. Adherence in liver transplant recipients. Liver Transplantation. 2011;17(7):760–770.
91. Dew MA, Dabbs AD, Myaskovsky L, et al. Meta-analysis of medical regimen adherence outcomes in pediatric solid organ transplantation. Transplantation. 2009;88(5):736–746.
92. Hsiau M, Fernandez HE, Gjertson D, et al. Monitoring nonadherence and acute rejection with variation in blood immunosuppressant levels in pediatric renal transplantation. Transplantation. 2011;92(8):918–922.
93. Jacobson DL, Gange SJ, Rose NR, et al. Epidemiology and estimated population burden of selected autoimmune diseases in the United States. Clinical Immunology and Immunopathology. 1997;84(3):223–243.

94. Mysliwska J, Trzonkowski P, Bryl E, et al. Lower interleukin-2 and higher serum tumor necrosis factor-a levels are associated with perimenstrual, recurrent, facial Herpes simplex infection in young women. European Cytokine Network. 2000;11(3):397–406.
95. Voskuhl RR, Gold SM. Sex-related factors in multiple sclerosis susceptibility and progression. Nature Reviews. Neurology. 2012;8(5):255–263.
96. Ostensen M, Brucato A, Carp H, et al. Pregnancy and reproduction in autoimmune rheumatic diseases. Rheumatology. 2011;50(4):657–664.
97. Baer AN, Witter FR, Petri M. Lupus and pregnancy. Obstetrical and Gynecological Survey. 2011;66(10):639–653.
98. Zrour SH, Boumiza R, Sakly N, et al. The impact of pregnancy on rheumatoid arthritis outcome: the role of maternofetal HLA class II disparity. Joint, Bone, Spine: Revue Du Rhumatisme. 2010;77(1):36–40.
99. Butts CL, Sternberg EM. Neuroendocrine factors alter host defense by modulating immune function. Cellular Immunology. 2008;252(1–2):7–15.
100. Guevara Patino JA, Marino MW, Ivanov VN, et al. Sex steroids induce apoptosis of CD8+CD4+ double-positive thymocytes via TNF-alpha. European Journal of Immunology. 2000;30(9):2586–2592.
101. Hince M, Sakkal S, Vlahos K, et al. The role of sex steroids and gonadectomy in the control of thymic involution. Cellular Immunology. 2008;252(1–2): 122–138.
102. Pejcic-Karapetrovic B, Kosec D, Leposavic G. Differential effects of male and female gonadal hormones on the intrathymic T cell maturation. Developmental Immunology. 2001;8(3–4):305–317.
103. Meazza C, Pagani S, Travaglino P, et al. Effect of growth hormone (GH) on the immune system. Pediatric Endocrinology Reviews. 2004;1(Suppl 3):490–495.
104. Wunderlich F, Benten WP, Lieberherr M, et al. Testosterone signaling in T cells and macrophages. Steroids. 2002;67(6):535–538.
105. Dipchand AI, Kirk R, Edwards LB, et al. The Registry of the International Society for Heart and Lung Transplantation: sixteenth official pediatric heart transplantation report 2013; focus theme: age. Journal of Heart and Lung Transplantation. 2013;32(10):979–988.
106. Pahl E, Naftel DC, Canter CE, et al. Death after rejection with severe hemodynamic compromise in pediatric heart transplant recipients: a multi-institutional study. Journal of Heart and Lung Transplantation. 2001;20(3):279–287.
107. Canter C, Naftel D, Caldwell R, et al. Survival and risk factors for death after cardiac transplantation in infants. A multi-institutional study. The Pediatric Heart Transplant Study. Circulation. 1997;96(1):227–231.
108. Williams R. Forty years of liver transplantation in the United kingdom-reflections on challenges and achievements. Transplantation. 2009;87(9):1268–1272.
109. Ng VL, Fecteau A, Shepherd R, et al. Outcomes of 5-year survivors of pediatric liver transplantation: report on 461 children from a north american multicenter registry. Pediatrics. 2008;122(6):e1128–e1135.
110. Sauce D, Larsen M, Fastenackels S. Evidence of premature immune aging in patients thymectomized during early childhood. Journal of Clinical Investigation. 2009;119(10):3070–3078.
111. Ogle BM, West LJ, Driscoll DJ, et al. Effacing of the T cell compartment by cardiac transplantation in infancy. Journal of Immunology. 2006;176(3):1962–1967.
112. Derkatz K, Dijke E, West L. High Expression of the B-Cell Inhibitory Molecule CD22 on Memory B-Cells in Early Life May Contribute to Better Transplant Outcomes. Journal of Heart and Lung Transplantation. 2012;31(4):S31–S.
113. Dijke E, Urschel S, Larsen I, et al. Altered naive and effector FOXP3+T-cell frequencies after thymectomy and heart transplantation (HTx) in infants. Journal of Heart and Lung Transplantation. 2012;31(4):S103–S.
114. Dijke E, Urschel S, Larsen I, et al. CD4(+)FOXP3(+) regulatory T-cell diversity is altered after infant heart transplantation. American Journal of Transplantation. 2011;11:521–522.
115. Urschel S, Altamirano-Diaz LA, West LJ. Immunosuppression armamentarium in 2010: mechanistic and clinical considerations. Pediatric Clinics of North America. 2011;57(2):433–457, table of contents.
116. Urschel S, Campbell PM, Meyer SR, et al. Absence of donor-specific anti-HLA antibodies after ABO-incompatible heart transplantation in infancy: altered immunity or age? American Journal of Transplantation. 2010;10(1):149–156.
117. Chinnock RE, Bailey LL. Heart transplantation for congenital heart disease in the first year of life. Current Cardiology Reviews. 2011;7(2):72–84.
118. Stegall MD, Dean PG, Gloor JM. ABO-incompatible kidney transplantation. Transplantation. 2004;78(5):635–640.
119. Takagi T, Ishida H, Shirakawa H, et al. Evaluation of low-dose rituximab induction therapy in living related kidney transplantation. Transplantation. 2010; 89(12):1466–1470.
120. Tanabe K. Japanese experience of ABO-incompatible living kidney transplantation. Transplantation. 2007;84(12 Suppl):S4–S7.
121. Tanabe K, Ishida H, Shimizu T, et al. Evaluation of two different preconditioning regimens for ABO-incompatible living kidney donor transplantation. A comparison of splenectomy vs. rituximab-treated non-splenectomy preconditioning regimens. Contributions to Nephrology. 2009;162:61–74.
122. Toki D, Ishida H, Horita S, et al. Impact of low-dose rituximab on splenic B cells in ABO-incompatible renal transplant recipients. Transplant International. 2009;22(4):447–454.
123. Shirakawa H, Ishida H, Shimizu T, et al. The low dose of rituximab in ABO-incompatible kidney transplantation without a splenectomy: a single-center experience. Clinical Transplantation. 2011;25(6):878–884.
124. West LJ, Pollock-Barziv SM, Dipchand AI, et al. ABO-incompatible heart transplantation in infants. New England Journal of Medicine. 2001;344(11): 793–800.
125. Dipchand AI, Pollock BarZiv SM, Manlhiot C, et al. Equivalent outcomes for pediatric heart transplantation recipients: ABO-blood group incompatible versus ABO-compatible. American Journal of Transplantation. 2011;10(2):389–397.
126. Roche SL, Burch M, O'Sullivan J, et al. Multicenter experience of ABO-incompatible pediatric cardiac transplantation. American Journal of Transplantation. 2008;8(1):208–215.
127. West LJ, Karamlou T, Dipchand AI, et al. Impact on outcomes after listing and transplantation, of a strategy to accept ABO blood group-incompatible donor hearts for neonates and infants. Journal of Thoracic and Cardiovascular Surgery. 2006;131(2):455–461.
128. Urschel S, Larsen IM, Kirk R, et al. ABO-incompatible heart transplantation in early childhood: an international multicenter study of clinical experiences and limits. Journal of Heart and Lung Transplantation. 2013;32(3):285–292.
129. Everitt MD, Donaldson AE, Casper TC, et al. Effect of ABO-incompatible listing on infant heart transplant waitlist outcomes: analysis of the United Network for Organ Sharing (UNOS) database. Journal of Heart and Lung Transplantation. 2009;28(12):1254–1260.
130. West LJ. Lost in regulation: why do U.S. policies for ABO-incompatible transplantation for infants lag behind? Journal of Heart and Lung Transplantation. 2009;28(12):1246–1248.
131. West LJ, Platt JL. And justice for all: consideration of ABO compatibility in allocation of hearts for infant transplantation. Circulation. 2010;121(17): 1884–1886.
132. Almond CS, Gauvreau K, Thiagarajan RR, et al. Impact of ABO-incompatible listing on wait-list outcomes among infants listed for heart transplantation in the United States: a propensity analysis. Circulation. 2010;121(17):1926–1933.
133. Chopek MW, Simmons RL, Platt JL. ABO-incompatible kidney transplantation: initial immunopathologic evaluation. Transplantation Proceedings. [Case Reports Research Support, Non-U.S. Gov't Research Support, U.S. Gov't, P.H.S.]. 1987;19(6):4553–4557.
134. Fan XH, Ang A, BarZiv SMP, et al. Donor-specific B-cell tolerance after ABO-incompatible infant heart transplantation. Nature Medicine. 2004;10(11): 1227–1233.
135. Obhrai JS, Lakkis FG. Transplantation tolerance: babies take the first step. Nature Medicine. 2004;10(11):1165–1166.
136. West LJ. Targeting antibody-mediated rejection in the setting of ABO-incompatible infant heart transplantation: graft accommodation vs. B cell tolerance. Current Drug Targets. Cardiovascular and Haematological Disorders. 2005;5(3):223–232.
137. West LJ. Antibodies and ABO-incompatibility in pediatric transplantation. Pediatric Transplantation. 2011;15(8):778–783.
138. West LJ. ABO-incompatible hearts for infant transplantation. Current Opinion in Organ Transplantation. 2011;16(5):548–554.
139. West LJ. B-cell tolerance following ABO-incompatible infant heart transplantation. Transplantation. 2006;81(3):301–307.
140. Jeyakanthan M, West LJ. Donor-specific isohemagglutinins: measuring the unknown. American Journal of Transplantation. 2012;12(4):803–805.
141. Kobayashi T, Saito K. A series of surveys on assay for anti-A/B antibody by Japanese ABO-incompatible Transplantation Committee. Xenotransplantation. 2006;13(2):136–140.
142. Ravn V, Dabelsteen E. Tissue distribution of histo-blood group antigens. APMIS: Acta Pathologica, Microbiologica, et Immunologica Scandinavica. 2000;108(1): 1–28.
143. Clausen H, Hakomori S. ABH and related histo-blood group antigens; immunochemical differences in carrier isotypes and their distribution. Vox Sanguinis. 1989;56(1):1–20.
144. Lazzarotto T, Guerra B, Lanari M, et al. New advances in the diagnosis of congenital cytomegalovirus infection. Journal of Clinical Virology. 2008;41(3): 192–197.
145. Sensini A. Toxoplasma gondii infection in pregnancy: opportunities and pitfalls of serological diagnosis. Clinical Microbiology and Infection. 2006;12(6): 504–512.
146. Gross U, Luder CG, Hendgen V, et al. Comparative immunoglobulin G antibody profiles between mother and child (CGMC test) for early diagnosis of congenital toxoplasmosis. Journal of Clinical Microbiology. 2000;38(10):3619–3622.

147. Odumade OA, Hogquist KA, Balfour HH Jr. Progress and problems in understanding and managing primary Epstein-Barr virus infections. Clinical Microbiology Reviews. 2011;24(1):193–209.
148. de Vries JJ, van der Eijk AA, Wolthers KC, et al. Real-time PCR versus viral culture on urine as a gold standard in the diagnosis of congenital cytomegalovirus infection. Journal of Clinical Virology. 2012;53(2):167–170.
149. Nijman J, de Vries LS, Koopman-Esseboom C, et al. Post-transplantnatally acquired cytomegalovirus infection in preterm infants: a prospective study on risk factors and cranial ultrasound findings. Archives of Disease in Childhood. Fetal and Neonatal Edition. 2012;97(4):F259–63.
150. Morales-Buenrostro LE, Terasaki PI, Marino-Vazquez LA, et al. "Natural" human leukocyte antigen antibodies found in nonalloimmunized healthy males. Transplantation. 2008;86(8):1111–1115.
151. Holmlund E, Nohynek H, Quiambao B, et al. Mother-infant vaccination with pneumococcal polysaccharide vaccine: persistence of maternal antibodies and responses of infants to vaccination. Vaccine. 2011;29(28):4565–4575.
152. Saffar MJ, Ajami A, Khalilian AR, et al. The impact of maternal measles-rubella immunization on the 12-month-old infant's immune response to measles-mumps-rubella vaccine immunogenicity. European Journal of Clinical Microbiology and Infectious Diseases. 2009;28(7):845–847.
153. Shaddy RE, Hunter DD, Osborn KA, et al. Prospective analysis of HLA immunogenicity of cryopreserved valved allografts used in pediatric heart surgery. Circulation. 1996;94(5):1063–1067.
154. Shaddy RE, Thompson DD, Osborne KA, et al. Persistence of human leukocyte antigen (HLA) antibodies after one year in children receiving cryopreserved valved allografts. American Journal of Cardiology. 1997;80(3):358–359.
155. Meyer SR, Campbell PM, Rutledge JM, et al. Use of an allograft patch in repair of hypoplastic left heart syndrome may complicate future transplantation. European Journal of Cardio-Thoracic Surgery. 2005;27(4):554–560.
156. Laing BJ, Ross DB, Meyer SR, et al. Glutaraldehyde treatment of allograft tissue decreases allosensitization after the Norwood procedure. Journal of Thoracic and Cardiovascular Surgery. 2010;139(6):1402–1408.
157. Farnault L, Chambost H, Zandotti C, et al. Early recovery of immunity after cord-blood transplantation in children: qualitative features and impact of cytomegalovirus infection. Acta Haematologica. 2012;128(1):7–16.
158. Moretta A, Maccario R, Fagioli F, et al. Analysis of immune reconstitution in children undergoing cord blood transplantation. Experimental Hematology. 2001;29(3):371–379.
159. Inoue H, Yasuda Y, Hattori K, et al. The kinetics of immune reconstitution after cord blood transplantation and selected CD34+ stem cell transplantation in children: comparison with bone marrow transplantation. International Journal of Hematology. 2003;77(4):399–407.
160. Fallen PR, McGreavey L, Madrigal JA, et al. Factors affecting reconstitution of the T cell compartment in allogeneic haematopoietic cell transplant recipients. Bone Marrow Transplantation. 2003;32(10):1001–1014.
161. Morecki S, Gelfand Y, Nagler A, et al. Immune reconstitution following allogeneic stem cell transplantation in recipients conditioned by low intensity vs myeloablative regimen. Bone Marrow Transplantation. 2001;28(3):243–249.
162. Suryani S, Fulcher DA, Santner-Nanan B, et al. Differential expression of CD21 identifies developmentally and functionally distinct subsets of human transitional B cells. Blood. 2010;115(3):519–529.
163. Parsons RF, Redfield RR 3rd, Rodriguez E, et al. Primary B cell repertoire remodeling to achieve humoral transplantation tolerance. Seminars in Immunology. 2012;24(2):109–114.
164. Parsons RF, Vivek K, Redfield RR 3rd, et al. B-lymphocyte homeostasis and BLyS-directed immunotherapy in transplantation. Transplantation Reviews. 2010;24(4):207–221.
165. Parsons RF, Vivek K, Rostami SY, et al. Acquisition of humoral transplantation tolerance upon de novo emergence of B lymphocytes. Journal of Immunology. 2011;186(1):614–620.
166. Kawai T, Cosimi AB, Spitzer TR, et al. HLA-mismatched renal transplantation without maintenance immunosuppression. New England Journal of Medicine. 2008;358(4):353–361.
167. Porcheray F, Wong W, Saidman SL, et al. B-cell immunity in the context of T-cell tolerance after combined kidney and bone marrow transplantation in humans. American Journal of Transplantation. 2009;9(9):2126–2135.

第 113 章 儿童肾移植

William Harmon

引言

在儿童和成人中，肾移植均是大多数终末期肾病的首选治疗方式，尤其是对体重超过 10kg 的患者。然而，儿童肝移植的适应证和并发症与成人不同。此外，儿童人群面临独特的技术挑战（特别是泌尿科），与先天异常、社会支持问题和不遵从性问题相关，以及免疫、身体和情感成熟的细微差别和成人移植存在显著不同。本章补充成人肾移植开展和患者管理的内容。

移植在儿童中的作用

慢性透析和肾移植是治疗终末期肾脏疾病（ESRD）的有效方式。大多数 ESRD 成年人接受透析而不是接受肾脏移植。寻求肾移植的成年人数正在上升，但每年完成移植的数量受到捐助者数量的限制[1]。几乎在所有候选人中，移植都具有生存的优势。近三十年前，肾移植被认为是治疗儿童 ESRD 的更好的方式[2]，并已被多次证明为儿童提供了生存获益[3,4]。

腹膜透析，作为持续不卧床或循环腹膜透析（CAPD 或 CCPD），和血液透析均表现出更差的生活质量和不令人满意的生长速率以及持续并发症。来自北美儿科肾脏试验和协作研究（NAPRTCS）注册表[5]透析部分的数据显示，在透析开始 24 个月后，总体身高从低于平均值的–1.8 个标准差降低到–2.16 个标准差。另外，透析儿童会失去自信和产生情感失调，因而难以接受依赖透析[6]。认知成就测试也可能随着透析时间延长而下降[7]。相比之下，肾移植的便捷性和不受饮食限制能使儿童过上接近正常的生活。尽管肾移植儿童还不能像正常儿童那样的成长，但其中的很多人能在短期内明显的增高，成年后的身高也得到改善[8-12]。重要的是，成功移植可以使儿童正常学习和发展，移植后学校功能测试显著改善[13,14]。在所有年龄组中，幼儿的长期移植效果最好，证明移植在这个年龄组的作用[15,16]。由于这些原因，成功的肾移植仍然是治疗ESRD 儿童的主要目标[3,17]。儿童受者的肾移植具有活体捐献者的最高百分比；并且他们在死亡供体（DD）中大量获益[18]，从而缩短等待时间。因此，ESRD 的儿童患者应尽快安排接受移植，尽管快速得到肾脏移植的目标尚未普遍实现[19]。

儿童肾移植的发生率和频率

2008—2012 年，美国每年开展约 16 500 例肾移植，其中约 800 例是年龄小于 18 岁的儿童[19]（图113.1），提示儿童患者约占所有移植受者中的 5%。虽然每年进行的儿童移植的数量变化通常不超过 10%，但捐赠者来源发生了重大变化。移植受者科学登记注册（SRTR）数据显示活体肾脏捐赠大量增加，活体供体（LD）肾移植在 2001 年首次超过了死亡供体的数量[20]。然而，活体捐赠的数量在 2004 年前逐渐增加到顶峰并从那之后开始下降；而死亡供体的数量保持稳定[21]。活体捐赠目前占美国所有肾移植的 36%。在 1987 年，所有儿童移植中，只有 40%来自活体捐献；到 1991 年，这一数字已上升到 53%，直到 2005 年活体捐赠成为儿童肾移植捐赠的主要来源。等待移植儿童优先分配死亡供体的改变使死亡供体肾移植急剧增加，并占据优势（图 113.1）。虽然这种改变会导致这些儿童更快地接受移植，但也可能导致平均移植存活率下降[22]。

父母是大多数活体捐赠来源。大多数家长捐赠者是母亲；父亲占 46%。与女孩相比有更多的男孩接受肾移植，64%父亲捐给儿子，60%母亲捐给儿子。父亲或者母亲捐赠对移植结果没有影响，除了一岁以下婴儿对母亲捐献器官的排斥更少[23,24]。由于孩子的兄弟姐妹往往太年轻不能捐赠（小于 18 岁），很少有兄弟姐妹之间

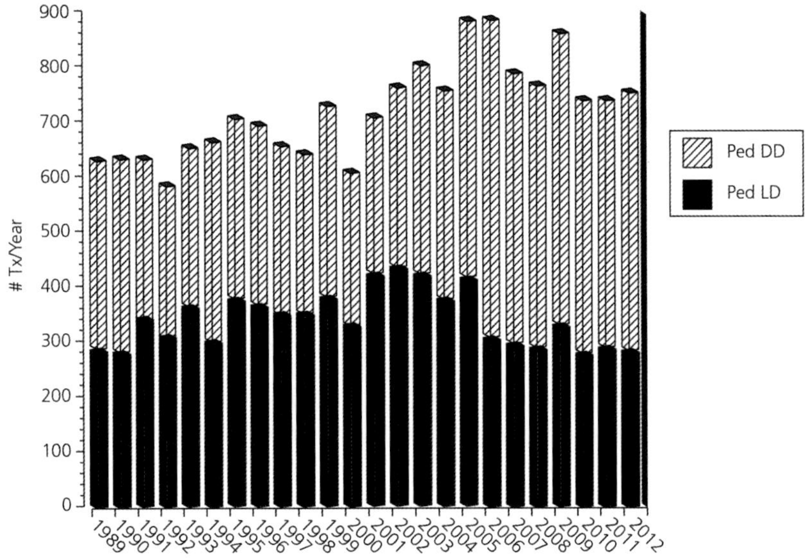

图 113.1 1989—2010 年年龄 18 岁以下的儿童中活体及死亡供体肾移植的数量。adapted from UNOS data: www.optn.org.

的移植。NAPRTCS 已经鉴定了 150 个移植物来自 21 岁以下的捐赠者。NAPRTCS 登记册确定只有 12 名 18 岁以下的活体捐赠者,其中 11 个是兄弟姐妹之间的移植,1 个是来自婴儿的父母。很明显,大多数的项目不倾向于用年龄小的捐赠者[25,26]。但是,UNOS 数据显示,1987—2000 年,在美国约 40 000 活体供体中,60 例来自 18 岁以下的捐赠者[27]。受者中 24 例为儿童,36 例为成人;只有 7 例移植在同卵双胞胎之间进行。近年来,非亲属供体捐赠是成人移植研究的热点,因为移植的结果已经显示比死亡供体肾脏好[28]。NAPRTCS 确定 1987—2001 年非亲属供体捐赠 123 例,对前 38 例受者进行初步分析,23 例(61%)为男性,30 例(79%)为白种人,8 例为 6 岁以下儿童,20 例为 12 岁以上儿童[29]。在 38 个捐赠者中,22 例是非生物学父母,10 例来自家庭朋友。2008 年,UNOS 记录了 293 例儿童活体肾移植:189 例(68%)来自父母,24 例来自兄弟姐妹,30 例来自其他生物学相关的供体。83%的儿童活体肾移植来自生物相关活体捐赠者。

大多数儿童的死亡供体肾脏来源于成人。在 20 世纪 80 年代开始倾向于婴幼儿来源的供体优先给予婴幼儿受者[30]。这些数据的广泛传播[31,32]也引起临床实践的显著变化。1987—1990 年,10 岁以上死亡供体的比例为 59%~68%。1991—1994 年,比例为 78%~88%并继续上升至 90%以上。1991 年前,两岁以下儿童供者占死亡供者的 3.2%。1991 年,没有儿童移植受者的供体来源于小于两岁的供者;在 1995 年和 1996 年,没有这样的肾脏在儿童中使用[33]。来源于年轻捐赠者的肾脏分配的早期变化导致移植物存活改善[30]。使用年轻捐赠者器官的肾移植的预后在近些年来得到改善[17,34,35],但在许多移植手术中,移植物从非常年轻的捐赠者移植给年长的受者[36,37]。

患者的选择和移植指征

儿童 ESRD 病因学

一般来说,儿童 ESRD 是由于先天性或遗传性疾病造成。在审查 NAPRTCS 数据库中的 10 632 例移植时,最常见的先天性疾病是阻塞性的肾病和肾脏再生障碍/发育不全/发育不良,每一类均占约 16%的患者 [3](表 113.1)。在肾小球疾病中,局灶性节段性肾小球硬化(FSGS)最常见,1987—2011 年,1246 名儿童因 FSGS 接受肾移植。不同种族受者的主要诊断也不同。总体而言,在 NAPRTCS 登记册中,白种人儿童占所有受者的 64%。然而,白种人儿童占 FSGS 移植儿童的 50%以下。FSGS 导致 ESRD 可以通过透析患者的观察更好地体现,其中两个最常见的诊断是 FSGS 和肾脏再生障碍/发育不良,每个占 14%。因 FSGS 透析的 733 个儿童中,白种人儿童只占 34%,非裔美国儿童和西班牙裔儿童占患者的 62%。24%的非洲裔美国儿童透析患者,以及 30%的 12 岁以上的儿童有 FSGS。主要诊断的信息对移植物存活和原发病复发的预测至关重要,将在下文详细讨论。

表 113.1 根据主要诊断儿童肾脏移植性别与种族分布

	数量	%	% 男性	% 白种人	% 活检
总数	10 632	100	59	64	56
诊断					
肾脏发育不全	1681	15.8	62	67	30
梗阻性肾病	1630	16.5	85	67	30
局灶性节段性肾小球硬化	1246	12.6	58	48	94
反流性肾病	549	5.5	44	78	35
慢性肾小球肾炎	340	3.4	44	50	75
多囊性疾病	323	3.2	51	78	52
髓质囊性疾病	287	2.9	50	87	66
先天性肾病综合征	277	2.8	52	68	87
溶血性尿毒症综合征	273	2.7	57	82	52
梨状腹综合征	268	2.7	98	63	38
家族性肾炎	241	2.4	81	60	72
膀胱炎	221	2.2	53	90	45
Ⅰ型膜增生性肾小球肾炎	187	1.8	45	60	96
肾盂/间质性肾炎	186	1.8	47	74	77
特发性新月体肾小球肾炎	181	1.8	34	56	95
SLE 肾炎	159	1.6	17	27	95
肾梗死	140	1.4	48	82	37
伯杰(IgA)肾炎	135	1.3	54	72	94
过敏性紫癜性肾炎	113	1.1	40	75	85
Ⅱ型膜增生性肾小球肾炎	85	0.8	49	78	96
韦格纳肉芽肿	66	0.6	44	68	91
威尔姆斯肿瘤	56	0.5	55	75	93
Drash 综合征	55	0.5	56	70	91
草酸中毒	55	0.5	51	92	75
膜肾病	47	0.4	64	51	94
其他全身免疫疾病	34	0.3	12	61	94
镰状细胞肾病	13	0.1	56	0	75
糖尿病肾小球肾炎	11	0.1	36	36	64
其他	1110	11.2	53	63	64
未知	663	6.7	53	34	34

Adapted from Smith et al.[3].

儿童肾移植指征

在过去数十年中，儿童肾移植的长期预后取得了显著的进展[3,38-40]。以前,幼儿被认为短期和长期移植生存更差,其中一个原因是增强的免疫应答,特别是在婴儿中[41,42]。最近的注册信息已经清楚地表明,婴儿和年轻患者和肾移植物存活出现了显著逆转[16,21,38,39,43]。事实上，已经有几个分析发现非常年轻的接受者在所有年龄段受者中具有最好的预后[16,23,38,44](图 113.2)。因此,儿童是所有年龄段中最优秀的移植受者。儿童慢性肾病(CKD)发展到 4~5 期的时候应开始规划,并开始移植前准备工作。儿童肾移植的禁忌证很少。可能只有两个情况存活时间短,例如转移性 Wilms'瘤和严重神经损害。约 75%的儿童在之前用慢性透析治疗,但除非有特殊移植前准备需要,否则移植前透析没有优势。早期肾移植确实有生存优势[45-49]。

移植时受者年龄

小于 6 个月,或在受者体重小于 6kg 是例外情况。自 1987 年以来,UNOS 记录了 111 例 12 个月龄以下儿童和 3500 例 1~5 岁儿童。其中,3~5 个月龄儿童 7 例,6~8 个月龄儿童 22 例,9~11 个月龄儿童 63 例。自 2000 年以来只报道了 31 例婴儿。因为婴幼儿和青少年受者,受者和移植物具有不同的危险因素,儿童常被分为五个年龄组:0~1 岁,2~5 岁,6~12 岁,13~17 岁和 18~21 岁。在 1987 年,开展 1~5 岁的儿童肾移植 119 例,而在 2012 年同一年龄组接受了 187 例移植。早期,在少数中心,儿童受者取得了很好的预后[44,50],但年轻受者免疫反应增强的概念表明他们是一个高风险组[51-53]。与儿童移植相关的特殊问题可能是感染、技术和药代动力学的差异[23,54-58],而不是他们的免疫反应。

在过去数十年中,儿童肾移植的长期预后取得了显著的进展[38-40]。之前,幼儿被认为短期和长期移植生存更差,其中一个原因是增强的免疫应答,特别是在婴儿中[41,42]。最近的注册信息已经清楚地表明结果发生了惊人的逆转。手术技术改善[59-63]、供体选择[64]、免疫抑制方法[65-69]、专业化儿科移植团队[70],以及发展多中心研究联盟都促成了儿童肾移植患者和肾移植物存活的显著改善[38,39,43]。事实上,一些分析已经确定了这些非常年轻的接受者,是所有年龄组中长期存活最好的[16,23,38,44,71]。事实上,接受成年人供器官并且供器官具有功能的年轻受者,具有最长的移植物半衰期,甚至超过那些成人受体的 2-单倍型匹配活体供体(LD)移植[72]。

11 岁以下的接受活体肾移植的儿童受者,移植物 3 年存活率和其他人群一样或更好(年龄为 0~5 岁的儿童为 93%,年龄为 6~10 岁的儿童为 92%)[16]。死亡供体的年轻受者的肾移植结果类似于成人,1~5 岁和 6~10 岁的受者,3 年移植存活率为 82%[16]。不幸的是,这个很好的结果在青少年[73,74]中没有出现,其 3 年移植物存活率差于所有其他年龄组,无论对于活体移植(85%)还是死亡供体移植(76%)(图 113.2)。

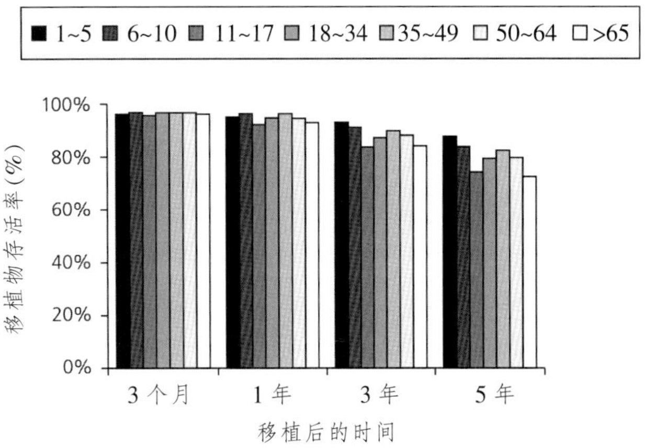

图 113.2 活体肾移植根据受体在移植时的年龄的存活率。Reprinted from Magee JC, Krishnan SM, Benfield MR, et al. Pediatric transplantation in the United States, 1997-2006. American Journal of Transplantation. 2008;8(4 Pt 2):935-945.

移植受者管理

移植准备

在儿童可以进行肾移植之前,如果可能的话,必须解决慢性肾功能不全(CRI)引起的问题。那些由于泌尿系统畸形引起的 ESRD 的情况,应在移植前先进行矫正重建手术,特别是下尿路。CRI 的两个主要后果是贫血和生长延迟,这两者都应该在移植之前解决。最近研究表明,移植后到最终成年身高的改善和移植前身高不足有关,而不是移植后净增加身高[10,12,75]。尿毒症也导致消耗和儿童营养不良,这可能会影响移植的成功。例如,预防性肾切除术和蛋白质消耗、营养不良的逆转改善了先天性肾病综合征儿童移植的结果[76-78]。仔细的移植前准备在儿童移植中特别重要。因为活病毒疫苗通常在慢性免疫抑制患者中不推荐使用或无效,儿童应在移植前接受所有适当的疫苗接种。有很多关于移植前免疫方法的报道[79-82]。

泌尿系统准备

因泌尿系统原因引起 ESRD 的儿童需要进行彻底的移植前泌尿系统评估,他们经常需要移植前重建[83-86]。在 NAPRTCS 报道中,7651 例儿童肾移植中 1865(25%)有下尿路异常[43]。对这样的患者,在发展成 ESRD 之前的排尿模式的病史是最有帮助的。初步调查包括测量尿流率和超声估计移植后排尿量。尿流率应该至少 15mL/s[87],残余尿量应该小于 30mL。进一步的检查包括在疑似尿路狭窄的患者中的尿路镜检查,膀胱压力容积测定术对于评估膀胱功能是必须的[88]。这可以提供膀胱的容量、压力升高和排空效率等信息。还有更多信息可以通过结合尿动力学研究和放射性同位素成像获得。年龄较大的患者若没有相关的泌尿系统相关症状，不常规行排尿膀胱尿路造影[89]。

非常小容量的膀胱可能不适宜用于功能移植。偶尔会在长期少尿患者中发现小容量的膀胱。但是如果膀胱是可扩张的并且膀胱壁有顺应性，那么膀胱可安全地用于肾移植。可用的膀胱的其他标准是灌注压力小于30cm H_2O 和良好的流速。在流量差的患者中，如果尿路和膀胱出口阻塞被排除，问题可能是由于逼尿肌功能障碍[87]。当膀胱不能完全排空，感染和阻塞是潜在的并发症，这可能缩短移植物存活。清洁间歇自我导尿术广泛应用于泌尿科实践，可以安全应用于那些当原发疾病未完全根治或者逼尿肌功能障碍的移植后患者。大多数儿童患者的膀胱能适应新的肾脏。虽然膀胱可能不一定具有足够的容量，特别是移植前长期透析的患者，但也会随着使用逐渐扩张[90]。然而，在真正低容量或高压的患者中，在移植之前增大膀胱可能是必需的[91-94]。

现代重建儿科泌尿学的目标是有一个足够的低压尿储存空间，可通过排空或通过间歇性导尿得以实现。增强膀胱成形术包括向膀胱中加入肠或胃壁，而替代性膀胱成形术是在进行膀胱切除后大多数时候用肠替代。增强膀胱成形术中使用胃壁组织比较流行，但他们可能导致尿中过多的酸丢失，导致不适和代谢性碱中毒。用生物工程材料重建膀胱的早期尝试正在进行。有很多有潜力的“生物工程”膀胱材料，虽然这些还没有在移植受者中使用过[95-97]。泌尿系统重建，包括增加膀胱成形术，通常用在移植之前[85,86,93,94,98-102]，虽然有些报道移植后成功重建[84]。在已经进行增强膀胱成形术的那些患者中，长期抗生素治疗和间歇性导尿术是必须的，以防止尿潴留和感染的发生。一般来说，尿路感染及其他并发症的发生率在这些受者中较高，他们的预后不比没有泌尿系统异常的儿童受者差[94]。如果ESRD患儿的原发性肾脏引起高血压、慢性感染或蛋白质、尿液或其他物质的过量丢失，应该考虑在移植前或移植时行肾脏切除术[103]。约有25%的儿童在移植前进行肾切除术[104]。

供体准备

供体选择

在移植过程中，合适的受者选择是不可或缺的重要组成部分，对每个肾移植儿童来说，都是一个影响长期预后的重要限制因素。在儿童移植中，活体供体的应用比成人移植中更加常见[3,16,32,33,38,43,104,105]。平均而言，活体供体的移植物存活时间是死亡供体的两倍[22,38,104,105]。使用活体移植物有很多限制，比如供者情况稳定、血型相符、年龄等。因此，并非每个儿童都可以有合适的活体供体。使用活体移植需要注意的是，早期移植物失功和原发病复发这样的重大风险[106,107]。当死亡供体用于儿童时，低危供体被仔细筛选，因此儿童肾移植的死亡率很低，并且这些移植物将会被长期使用。

活体供体

首例成功的肾移植使用活体供体，从那时起活体供体成为儿童肾移植的主流。重要的是，随着供体缺乏越来越严重，供体安全问题越来越凸显[111]。目前，移植学界已经关注这个问题，并且在活体供体合理使用、评估过程、合理的随访以及对供者关怀等方面达成共识[1,112]。供者不得因受者利益而受到生理、情感以及心理上的风险。原则包括，年龄在18岁以下者不得成为活体供者，尽管这点尚未受到普遍重视[27,113]。基因无相关供者扩大了活体供体范围，活体供者最初只包括配偶，后来扩大到无基因相关的其他家庭成员、朋友甚至是非定向的供者。重要的是，这些无基因相关的供者与基因相关的供者相比，移植预后不相上下[114,121]。甚至有人提出建议，对非定向供者的捐赠进行补偿，形成商业化的捐助系统，扩大捐助范围[122,123]。尽管商业化的器官捐助已经存在于世界上很多地方，很多国家都已经宣布这样的做法是非法的，移植学界也对这种做法进行谴责[124,125]。非定向活体供体的使用，通过供者信息交流的做法，在扩大捐助范围的过程中发挥了重要作用。这种程序允许活体供者捐助给不相关的受者，以换取受者已有的抗原不相容供者，捐赠给前者的家人[126-128]。这种程序包括两种简单的交换，多人多米诺骨牌式交换以及死亡供体等待名单的交换[129,139]。在第138章中可以找到活体捐赠的伦理深度分析，在第27章中有对交换捐赠队列的具体描述。

供者收入的工作在第23章中详细描述。总体来说，所有的活体供者与潜在的移植受者都进行检测，包括ABO血型检测、人白细胞抗原(HLA)组织相容性检测，以及一些交叉配型。家长作为儿童肾移植的主要活体供者，约占80%。无亲属关系的供者、兄弟姐妹以及偶然的非定向供者弥补了剩余的不足[105]。因此，儿童肾移植的供者大多数为 HLA-Ⅰ型匹配供者，很少为 HLA-Ⅱ型。尽管缺乏 HLA-B 配型会有一定的不利[105]，儿童受者总体上缺乏 HLA 配型，特别是婴儿，不过这似乎并不影响长期预后。

如上所述，所有供者都应被仔细评估，确保所有供者都没有商业交易、胁迫或者在捐献过程中受到任何伤害。合适供者的评估部分已被报道[140,141]。很多评估是用于确认供者安全，但这也用于确保供者没有将感染或其他疾病传给受者，以及供者器官能够为受者提供足够的功能。总体来说，以下情况的供者会被排除：太年轻（≤18 岁），或者太老[个人年龄、肾小球滤过率（GFR）低、潜在的癌症、心血管及其他疾病概率增加]，或存在因捐赠手术加重的医疗问题，以及单肾生活供者[112]。存在如高血压、糖尿病以及转移性癌症患者会被排除。并且，慢性感染如 HIV、乙肝、丙肝者也被排除，因为他们存在传播的可能。尽管巨细胞病毒（CMV）、人乳头瘤病毒（HPV）以及 EB 病毒也可能被传播，但是这些可以在受者体内被治愈，所以并不被排除。

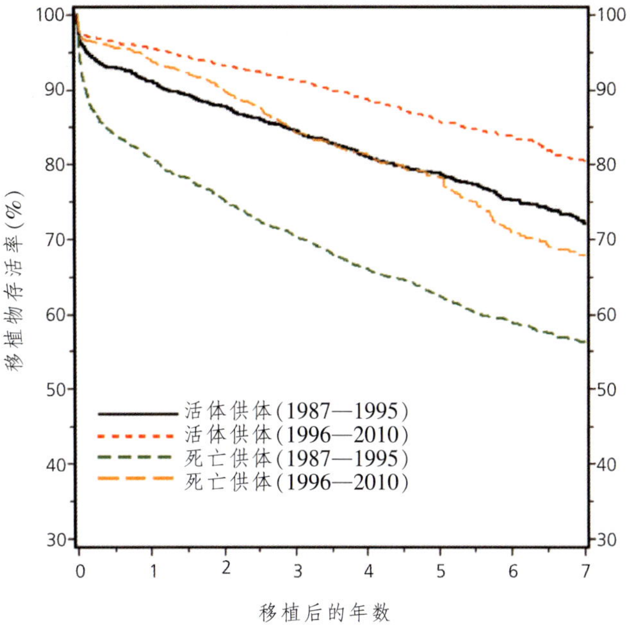

图 113.3 两个时代活体供肾移植供者七年存活率。Reproduced from NAPRTCS 2010 Annual Report: www.naprtcs.org. https://web.emmes.com/study/ped/annlrept/2010_Report.pdf. [December 19, 2013].

死亡供体

目前大多数肾移植都来自死亡供体。而在过去，儿童移植中活体供体更常见，2006 年以来，美国的分配政策导致儿童移植中死亡供体移植成为主流（图 113.1）[4,16,18]。这种变化的结果在几年中也许并不显著，但是儿童活体肾移植的长期预后显著优于死亡供体移植（图 113.3）[3,16,18,104,105]，这说明快速获取死亡供体的短期收益可能被移植物存活时间缩短抵消。

多年来，有一种用婴儿和年幼儿童的肾脏移植给年轻受者的趋势[30]。早期研究显示，25%的儿童死亡供体移植来自 10 岁以下的儿童[41]。一项关于 NAPRTCS 的研究[64]，证明了优先将小肾脏植入婴儿和年幼儿童体内会为移植物存活带来灾难性的后果，这也被后来更大规模的研究所证实[142]。因此，儿童移植死亡供体分配政策的变化改善了预后[30]。最新研究显示这种做法引起了实质性的变化[43]。1991 年以来，儿童受者不到 1%的死亡供体肾脏来自 2 岁以下的供者。同一时期，来自 10 岁以上供者肾脏的百分比从 78%上升到 88%。重要的是，年轻供者的肾脏并没有被放弃，而是通过整块技术移植用于成人受者[36,142,143]。单中心报道年轻供者来源器官，按照精细的操作流程取得更高的成功率[34,35]。年长的供者与移植物存活时间缩短相关，并且应该避免用于年轻的受者[64,146,147]。

配型对移植预后的影响是巨大的，但从免疫抑制发展以来，配型的影响减少了很多[148-151]。儿童死亡供体肾移植预后很少被供者组织相容配型影响[18,104,105]。ABO 血型相容以及交叉配型仍然是必要的。总体来说，已经存在抗体或者在移植后产生抗体的移植候选者发生早期排斥的风险更高，应该加强免疫抑制[152-156]。

死亡供体通常需要检测确定移植物能够为受者提供足够的功能，并且供者无传染病或转移性肿瘤。在过去，决定供者资格的标准是脑死亡（DBD）。努力扩大供体供应，最新的研究进展发现，心脏死亡基础上确定的供体也能使用，即所谓的心脏死亡捐献（DCD）。儿童正在更加频繁地接受移植（图 113.4）。尽管使用这样的供体发生移植物肾功能延迟恢复的可能性更高，DCD 供者的移植肾与 DBD 移植肾短期疗效相当[118,128,157,158]，但是存在晚期移植物失功的风险[159]。

大多数国家的国家器官分配系统提供了一些儿童死亡供体移植候选者的优先选择。在美国器官获取和移植网络（OPTN）有一个最新变化，该系统为 18 岁以下儿童按照时间顺序列出名单，优先于其他大多数候选者，等待时间比成人候选者更短[18]。使用年长或扩展条件供体（ECD）与不良预后持续相关[119,128,145,160]。儿童

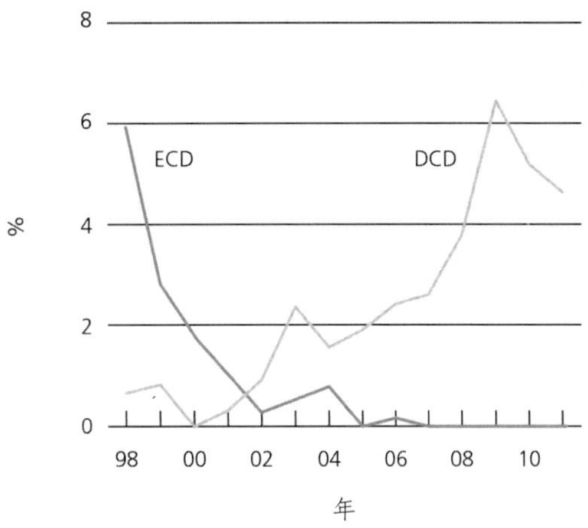

图 113.4 扩展条件供体(ECD)和捐赠者心脏死亡后(DCD)为源的死亡供体儿童肾移植频率（1998—2010 年）。SRTR 2012 Annual Report: http://www.srtr.org/ [accessed December 19, 2013].

很少接受年长死亡供体或者扩展条件供者的器官(图 113.4)[104]。

移植过程

移植的技术问题

按照不同体重的儿童选择手术方式。对于较小的儿童,体重低于 15kg,移植通常用中线切口,较大的血管用于吻合供体肾[90]。在盲肠和右结肠之后,主动脉前壁和下腔静脉暴露并解剖分离[161]。主动脉从肠系膜上动脉的上方移到右侧髂外动脉。结扎后,分离腰支、髂动脉及肠系膜下动脉。接下来将下腔静脉从左肾静脉转到髂静脉上。结扎腰静脉后,环扎髂静脉,供体肾静脉以末端吻合技术吻合到受者腔静脉上[162]。供者肾动脉以末端吻合技术吻合到受者主动脉上。需要特别注意夹紧和松开主要血管时,受者的血流动力学反应,松开夹子前需要保持 15~18cmH_2O 的中心静脉压[90,161]。

移植肾的灌注比较缓慢可能是由于成人的肾脏较大,会占用很多正常儿童的血容量。血流动力学研究发现,要充分灌注成人肾脏,婴儿的心输出量必须加倍[163]。因此容量替换是十分重要的(图 113.5)。通过供者输尿管进入受者膀胱完成输尿管吻合术，应用 Ledbetter-Politano 法或者非回流法。然而,大多数外科医生更喜欢使用非回流法而不是经膀胱的输尿管膀胱吻合术(见第 55 章),因为这种方法更快。不需要行单独的膀胱切开术,但是需要缩短输尿管长度,来保证远端输尿管血供。

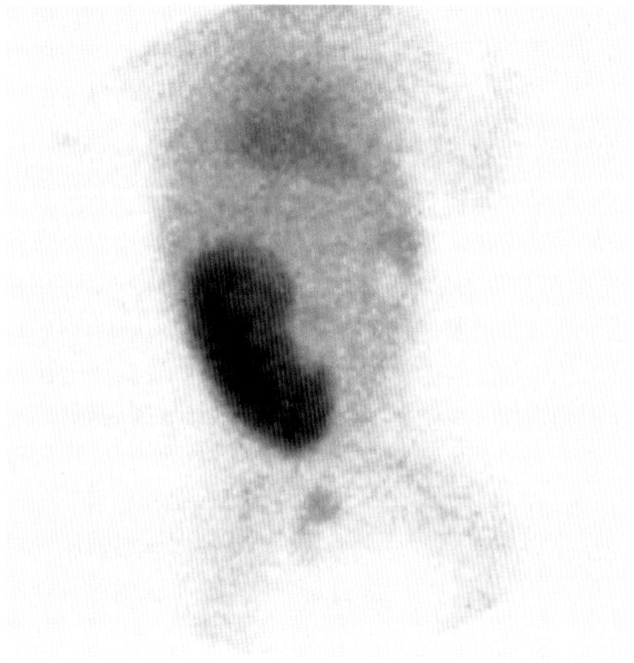

图 113.5 ^{99M}Tc-MAG3 核素肾扫描 1 名 9 个月龄的婴儿接受活体(从他的父亲)肾移植。移植物在腹腔内,占据腹膜右侧的大部分空间。注意移植物和心脏的相对大小。Reprinted from [315] Harmon WE. Pediatric kidney transplantation (Chapter 75). In: Avner ED, Harmon WE, Niaudet P, et al., editors. Pediatric Nephrology, 6th ed. Springer; 2009: Oxford University, UK:1867-1901.

对于体重超过 20kg 的儿童,移植技术与成人移植技术类似,这在第 55 章中有描述。与年幼儿童经腹膜路径不同,这种移植是通过腹膜外路径,将肾静脉吻合到髂总静脉或者髂外静脉上[161]。动脉吻合到髂总动脉或者是髂内动脉。膀胱输尿管吻合使用上述描述的技术。

目前,用腔镜技术来移除活体供体肾脏十分流行,因为这可以缩短供者的住院和康复时间。这个过程需要的手术时间更长,延迟移植物功能的概率也较高。尽管大多数研究都说明这个过程是安全的,10 000 例活体器官捐献的综述发现 3 例死亡或者严重并发症;3 例都是腔镜术后。尽管一些儿童受者研究中出现了严重并发症[168,169],大多数报道都证实了腔镜肾切除术的良好预后。

移植物失功的评估

完成血管吻合并松开夹子时的移植肾功能可以通过产生的尿量来判断。很多原因影响初始肾功能,即时肾功能评估以及这种情况下的鉴别诊断对肾移植医生十分重要。

延迟移植物功能(DGF)

一个功能良好的移植肾应该在 2~3 天达到正常肾功能。缺乏正常肾功能,如血清肌酐水平下降到正常水平,被称为延迟移植物功能(DGF)。目前对 DGF 的定义尚未达成共识[176]。在一些研究中,DGF 仅用于判断移植后透析患者,这是最严格但最常用的定义。急性肾小管坏死(ATN)是最常见的早期移植物无功能的原因。早期 ATN 的风险与以下因素相关,如有移植史、延迟冷缺血、缺乏预防性抗体治疗,移植前使用超过 5 种血液灌注。如果移植物功能恢复延迟,其他诊断性检查无法区分 ATN 与排斥、原发病的突然复发,就需要进行移植物活检[177-179]。重要的是,早期急性排斥类似 ATN 或能与 ATN 共存[180]。移植后出现 ATN 预示不良预后,特别是死亡供体移植物的受者,合并 ATN 者常常出现移植物衰竭和死亡[181,182]。DGF 是移植物失功和死亡的单独风险因素。重要的是,尽管 DGF 的发生率在 DCD 供者移植病例中很高,但是 DGF 对于长期移植预后的不利影响,在活体捐献或脑死亡移植术后并不显著[157,158,176]。

移植物血栓

移植物血栓是儿童移植的独立并发症。虽然这是早期移植物失功的主要原因,但也会在后来的病程中出现,并且记录到移植后 15 天。移植物血栓是儿童肾移植中第三个常见的移植物衰竭原因,约占 10%的移植物失功[3,43]。这在大多数病例中是不可逆的,并需要去除移植物。病例中出现少尿或者无尿就应该怀疑移植物血栓。通过二乙三胺五乙酸(DTPA)或 MAG3 放射性核素扫描来诊断[186],显示了没有被移植肾吸收的光子减少缺陷(图 113.6)。

由于移植物血栓的预后普遍较差,大量研究尝试理解和预测这种并发症。移植物血栓的病因是多方面的,这种并发症常见于年轻受者[110]。一项 2060 例活体供体和 2334 例死亡供体的研究中[187],NAPRTCS 发现有移植病史会增加风险,而受者年龄较大则对活体供体肾有保护作用。预防性使用抗淋巴细胞抗体也有保护作用,这很可能是因为 IL2r 单抗的作用[188]。死亡供体肾脏,冷缺血超过 24 小时会增加血栓形成的风险。使用抗体诱导治疗,捐献者年龄大于 5 岁、受者年龄增加都能降低血栓形成的风险。高度的血栓状态也会产生影响[186,189,190]。一项研究显示,较少进行儿童移植的中心移植物血栓的发生率更高[70]。其他研究提示移植前使用腹膜透析会增加血栓的风险[191,192],但是之后的研究认为这种联系是有争议的。有的中心对移植物血栓高风险的儿童受者常规应用抗凝剂,但是目前还没有临床研究证实其有效性,这种做法也并非没有并发症[193]。

梗阻、漏尿、泌尿系统并发症

早期移植物失功的罕见但可控制的原因是泌尿系统梗阻,表现为尿量减少以及肾积水。超声与核素扫描用呋塞米冲刷有助于临床医生诊断。梗阻可能是因为输尿管扭曲,在输尿管连接部位出现水肿阻塞或形成淋巴囊肿。尿外渗进入盆腔或腹腔是非常痛苦,并且建立放射性核素扫描(图 113.7)。腹腔内阴囊、外阴的示踪剂的出现,或腹股沟区修补和立即手术矫正的诊断是必要的。

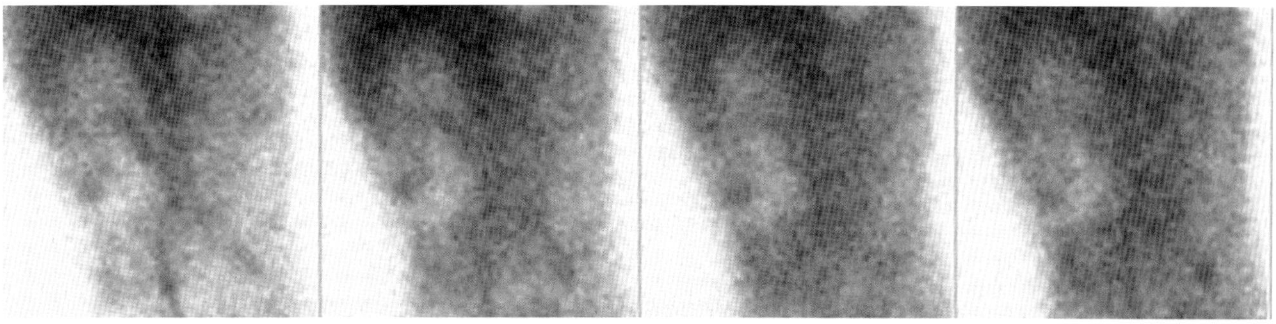

图 113.6　^{99M}Tc-MAG3 放射性核素肾扫描 1 名 6 岁女孩,有局灶性肾小球硬化(FSGS),接受活体(LD)肾移植手术,手术进行 16 小时。注意右腹部的放射缺损区,说明无灌注移植血栓形成。Reprinted from[315] Harmon WE. Pediatric kidney transplantation(Chapter 75). In: Avner ED, Harmon WE, Niaudet P, et al., editors. Pediatric Nephrology, 6th ed. Springer; 2009: Oxford University, UK:1867-1901.

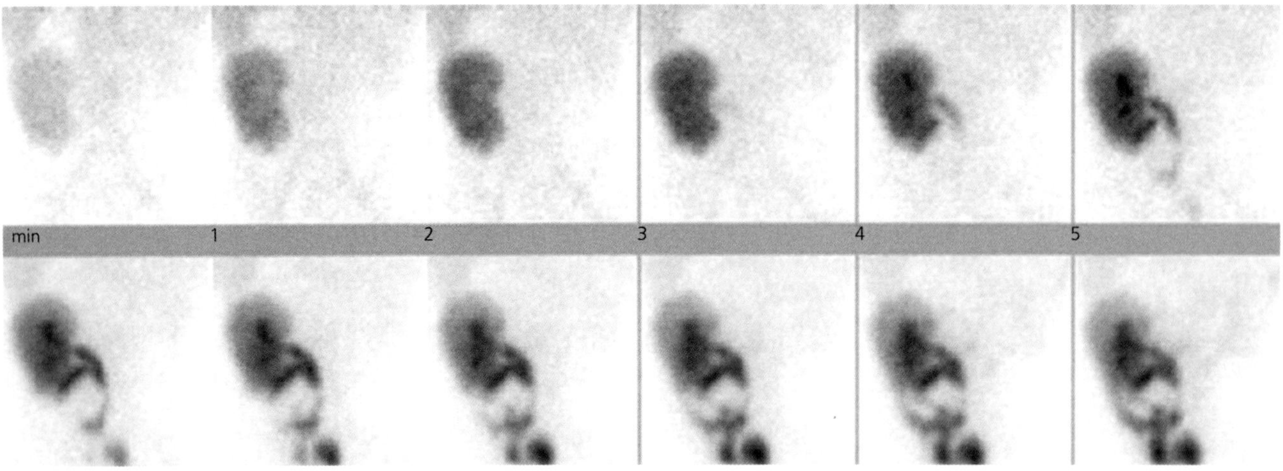

图 113.7　^{99M}Tc-MAG3 放射性核素肾扫描在 1 名 8 岁的女孩，接受了死亡供体的肾移植，术后 12 小时。值得注意的是，移植肾的良好灌注、快速浓缩和排泄。示踪物迅速积聚在右下象限，在膀胱外。调查显示创伤性膀胱破裂。Reprinted from [315] Harmon WE. Pediatric kidney transplantation(Chapter 75). In: Avner ED, Harmon WE, Niaudet P, et al., editors. Pediatric Nephrology, 6th ed. Springer; 2009: Oxford University, UK:1867-1901.

免疫抑制策略

免疫抑制策略与文中描述的成人情况一致。一半的儿童肾移植受者移植后接受抗体诱导治疗，其中约一半的受者接受抗淋巴细胞药物[3,194-198]。移植后 30 天，大部分儿童接受三联免疫抑制剂维持治疗(他克莫司、霉酚酸酯、类固醇)[3,108]，越来越多的患者不再使用类固醇激素。就像 NAPRTCS 年度报道中所述，传统免疫抑制疗法在过去 20 年中被频繁修改(图 113.8)。然而，儿童接受一种联合用药后就会应用这种疗法。目前很多多中心研究致力于研究减少慢性免疫抑制剂的使用种类，包括类固醇激素以及钙调磷酸酶抑制剂等常用靶向药物都被移除[199]。很多单中心[175,199-201]和多中心[202-204]临床试验报道已成功停用类固醇激素，尽管这些报道中也存在部分副作用[202,205,206]。也有一些报道在儿童中避免使用钙调磷酸酶抑制剂来预防神经毒性。至少有一项临床试验发现了良好的长期移植物功能，但是存在高概率的早期急性排斥[207]。随后的临床试验中加强抗体诱导可能得到更好的短期预后[195]。

移植后管理

超急性排斥反应

超急性排斥反应是反复的抗宿主 HLA、ABO 或其他抗原抗体的特异性排斥[208]。不可逆转的移植物快速破坏，组织学上有肾小球的血栓形成、纤维素样坏死和多形核白细胞浸润。移植早期，HLA 配对技术还未成熟，超急性排斥反应更加普遍。目前，在大多数中心，超急性排斥反应已经非常罕见。最近 NAPRTCS 数据显示过去 24 年中只有 19 例[3]。唯一的治疗方法是外科手术移除同种异体移植物。

急性排斥反应

发生率的信息以及儿童肾移植中急性排斥的预后很难被标准化，因为目前有很多不同的定义。常见的排斥定义是基于患者接受抗排斥反应治疗的情况，尽管活检确诊越来越常见。目前对儿童肾移植的回顾发现，活检确诊率为 95%，一年累计急性排斥反应报道为 15%[3]。在过去 20 年中(表 113.2)，急性排斥反应发生率显著降低。死亡供体的危险因素包括：缺少预防性使用 T 细胞抗体治疗、供者年龄小于 5 岁、黑种人，以及无 Dr 匹配。活体移植的危险因素是：缺乏使用 T 细胞抗体、1~2 种 Dr 错配、黑种人以及急性肾小管坏死。婴儿和儿童间是否有强烈的免疫反应及急性排斥，这方面数据存在争议[42]。而且 UNOS 注册中心的数据证明，不论活体供体还是死亡供体移植，年幼儿童具有更高的急性排斥反应发生率[23]。另一方面，移植后活检数据提示所有分组中排斥反应发生率相同[52]。大型儿科移植试验证明婴儿比儿童有更好的临床预后[54]。SRTR 报

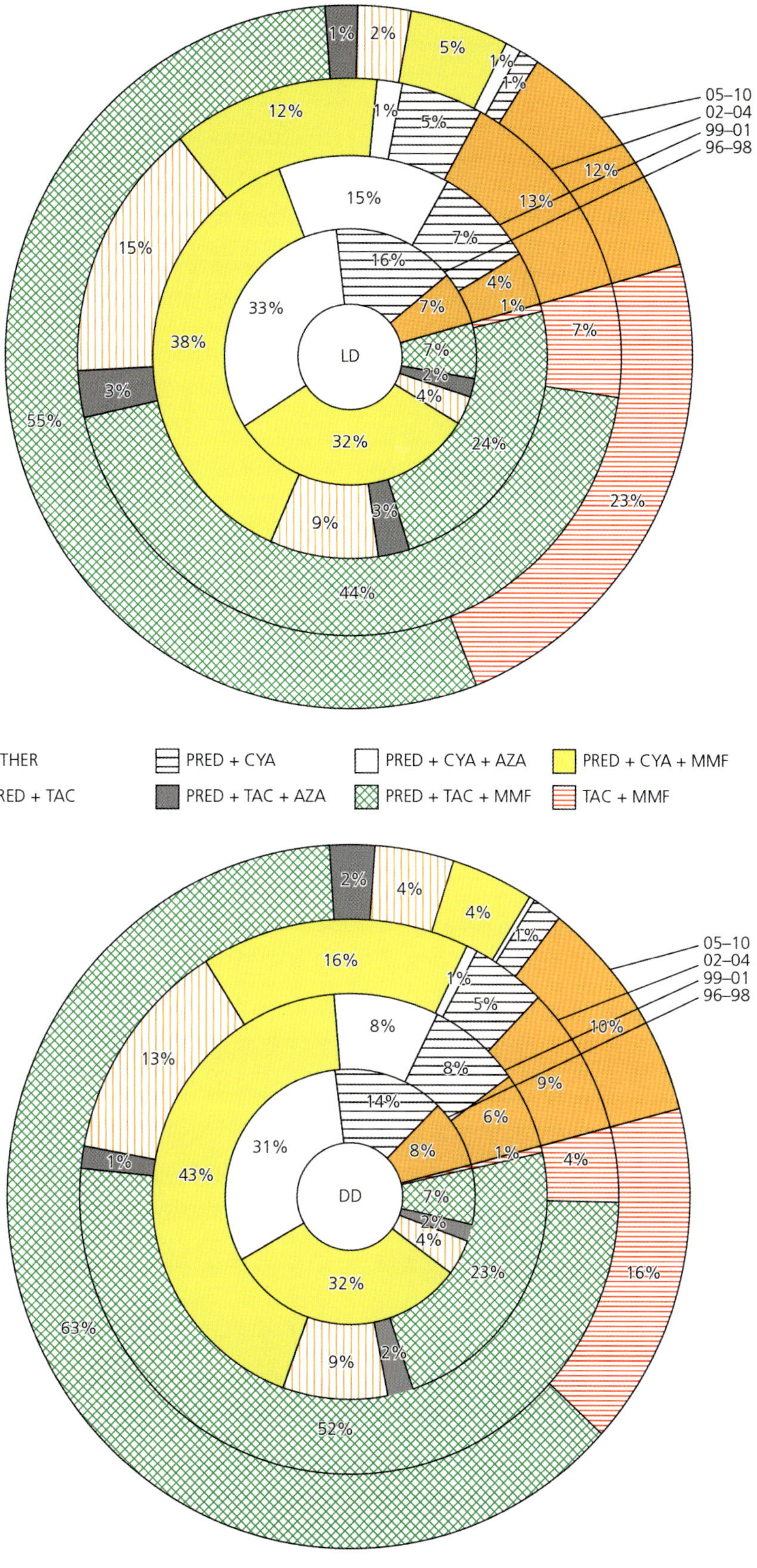

图 113.8 在移植后 30 天小儿活体（LD）和死亡供体肾移植受者（DD）三年组（1997—2010 年）维持免疫抑制。adapted from NAPRTCS 2010 Annual Report: www.naprtcs.org. https://web.emmes.com/study/ped/annlrept/2010_Report.pdf. [December 19, 2013].

表 113.2 按移植年份分列的 12 个月首次排斥反应概率(%)

	活体供体		死亡供体	
移植年份	%	SE	%	SE
1987–1990	54.2	1.7	68.9	1.5
1991–1994	44.9	1.5	60.3	1.6
1995–1998	33.0	1.4	40.5	1.7
1999–2002	21.9	1.3	26.6	1.8
2003–2007	12.8	1.3	17.1	1.5
2007–2010	8.6	1.8	16.6	2.1

Adapted from Smith et al.[3].

道证明了婴儿和儿童在所有年龄分组中的预后是最好的[15]。因此,不管是通过加强免疫抑制克服免疫反应,还是引起之前提到的不良预后都与其他因素相关。

急性排斥反应的诊断

当出现尿量减少以及血肌酐增加时应考虑排斥反应。在过去,急性排斥反应的临床标志包括发热和移植物柔软。在钙调磷酸酶抑制剂和预防性抗体疗法下,这些标志越来越罕见;因此早期出现移植物功能紊乱甚至没有其他标志,也应该引起关注。鉴别诊断包括:输尿管梗阻、肾血管狭窄、尿瘘和急性感染。当怀疑发生排斥时,验尿和尿培养应该用于确认是否有感染。验尿出现蛋白尿、尿沉出现白细胞或其他细胞,也有助于确认移植物内炎症和免疫反应。超声用于排除梗阻。肾周液体收集可以引起梗阻、大囊状淋巴管瘤、血肿,罕见的也出现脓肿。超声可以提供移植物血流和压力信息[177]。放射性核素肾扫描,使用MAG3示踪剂,对诊断很有帮助(图113.6和图113.7)[209]。肾脏快速摄取示踪剂但出现延迟的排泄被认为存在排斥。遗憾的是,放射性核素扫描无法鉴别不同原因的移植物功能紊乱,如排斥、环孢素毒性和急性肾小管坏死。因此排斥的明确诊断需要进行移植物活检。

儿童肾移植活检

肾移植活检是在意识清醒的情况下,按照超声指导进行,非常安全简单。通过超过150例儿童肾移植活检的数据分析,包括腹膜内肾和移植后第一周检查,发现风险非常低[178]。降低移植术后活检出血的重要因素是使用自动穿刺针,使用小型号(18号)而不是标准型针(15号)。无论什么时候怀疑存在排斥,都应该进行活检。

急性排斥反应的治疗

急性排斥反应的标准治疗是静脉内给予甲强龙,10~20mg/kg(最大剂量为0.5Gm),连续3天。大多数Ⅰ、Ⅱ型排斥反应需要类固醇疗法。类固醇抵抗排斥反应需要T细胞抗体治疗,比如多克隆抗胸腺细胞球蛋白抗体。球蛋白予以1.5~2mg/kg,10~14天。建议在细胞治疗期间监控$CD3^+$细胞,限制给药频率,特别是计数超过20个细胞/mm^3。所有抗体都有一些副作用。预防与多克隆抗体相关的潜在的过敏反应,用500mg甲强龙,并给予抗体及抗组胺药(如苯海拉明),提前1.5小时给药。

慢性同种异体移植物肾病

从急性到慢性排斥反应的过程是逐渐发生的;但很多活检都能看出两者特征,慢性排斥的一些特征性血管改变可以在移植后10天被发现[211]。临床表现为肾功能逐渐下降合并不同程度的血尿和高血压[212]。这种临床情况被称为移植肾小球疾病、慢性排斥、慢性同种异体移植物功能紊乱(CAD)、慢性同种异体移植物肾病(CAN)或间质纤维化以及肾小管萎缩(IFTA)[213]。逐渐形成的名称反映了缺乏明确病因,这个过程在这一章中被称为慢性同种异体移植物肾病,是儿童肾移植后移植物功能缺失的主要原因。

一个关于慢性排斥反应的持续争论是,是否存在于高免疫介导的、感染激发反应、缺血性或由于高滤过率导致的非免疫性损伤中[214–217]。儿童数据清楚地显示急性排斥反应是慢性排斥的一个预测因子[40]。1699例活体供体和1795例死亡供体的受者研究中,NAPRTCS提出急性排斥是慢性排斥的一个相对危险因素(RR=3.1),多种急性排斥将RR提高到4.3。晚期急性排斥也是慢性排斥临床相关的[218]。甚至急性排斥是最重要的慢性排斥反应原因,其他免疫机制可能介导其进程,比如抗体介导的抗宿主反应、MICA、内皮细胞和B淋巴细胞[156,219]。CAN患者的移植物活检中,基因表达谱显示纤维化和生长因子上调[220]。

复发性肾病

在第77章中有详细描述,一些疾病会在移植肾中复发,复发疾病可能会导致移植物功能缺失,就像患者原来的肾一样。原发疾病复发占儿童肾移植功能缺失的 7%[3]。5 年 FSGS 儿童移植物生存率是 71%，肾小球肾炎儿童则是 77%；对比其他所有引发 ESRD 的原因，其 5 年移植物生存率高达 83%。在死亡供体组，5 年 FSGS、肾小球肾炎和先天性肾病综合征儿童移植物生存率都低于 64%。溶血性尿毒症综合征(HUS)和家族性肾炎生存率为 66%；其他原因生存率为 70%。很多出版物回顾了儿童肾移植中疾病复发的过程[106,221,222]。在某些病例中，某些疾病复发的特点并没有影响到移植物生存。不幸的是，儿童移植物中疾病复发情况几乎没有好转，尽管在过去 20 年中免疫抑制药物得到了极大的发展[3,223]。

局灶节段性肾小球硬化是激素耐药型肾病综合征导致终末期肾病的最常见原因，也是儿童 ESRD 最常见的获得性原因。复发性 FSGS 的报道，介于 15%~50% 和大约 50%的复发导致移植物功能缺失[221-223]。遗传性疾病似乎并没有在移植物中复发。复发的危险因素包括：早期尿毒症、快速进展到 ESRD、对治疗抵抗、白种人或亚洲人种、前次移植复发，以及可能出现“肾小球通透因子存在”[179,223]。复发可以立即出现在移植后，并且导致大量蛋白尿、急性肾小管坏死，甚至是小管栓塞引起的移植物衰竭[179]。总体来说，活跃期肾病综合征的儿童不宜优先移植，因为可能发生很严重的蛋白尿和随后发生的移植物栓塞，以及复发延迟诊断[221]。很多治疗过程会行肾切除术，并对儿童维持一段时间透析，确保改善营养状态以及维持正常的人血白蛋白水平。对于 FSGS 的儿童进行活体移植并没有好处，尽管由于排斥引起的移植物功能缺失在活体受者中发生率更低，但是复发引起的移植物功能缺失率更高，导致活体与死亡供体移植物类似的生存率[179,224]。去除血浆常在移植前或移植后用于预防和治疗 FSGS 的复发[225-228]，在一些报道中，使用这种方法使完全缓解率达 60%。尽管没有特异性的免疫移植方法证明治疗或预防 FSGS 复发是明确有效的，有一些证据显示，大剂量环孢素可能在这方面有效[227,228]。是否需要大剂量来抵消高血清水平的低密度脂蛋白，这种蛋白不结合游离环孢素，这种原因是否由于直接作用于足细胞引起尚不明确[106,229]。利妥昔单抗被用于治疗儿童复发 FSGS[230-233]。

MPGN 的类型可在移植物中复发，频率为 30%~60%[106]。2 型显得更加严重，不管哪种都不是复发后可治愈的[240]。

原发性草酸过多几乎在所有肾移植后立刻复发，被认为是肾移植禁忌证，不过治疗前和移植后透析能降低体内草酸负荷，肝肾联合移植能有更好的预后结果[241-246]。如果考虑肝移植，就必须认真考虑决定儿童是否对终身吡哆醇治疗敏感，而不是肝移植[106]。肾移植可以改善部分的甲基丙二酸血症，但是完整的治疗需要肝移植[106]。ESRD 是胱氨酸贮积症儿童中最早出现的器官衰竭，常常是这种疾病死亡的主要原因。用半胱氨酸减少胱氨酸疗法以及肾移植延长了患者 50 年寿命[247-250]。虽然胱氨酸可能在肾移植物小管间隙中累积，但是这并不能引起移植物衰竭。持续的胱氨酸累积也会导致非肾脏原因发病率死亡率增加[249,251]。

预后和危险因素

为了取得更好的人口组合，代表性别、年龄和人种多样性，多中心注册结果(如 SRTR 和 NAPRTCS 年度报告)准确地报道肾移植预后[3,16,21]。

NAPRTCS 记录了 1987—2010 年间 11 603 例肾移植数据中 10 632 例儿童受者。2920 例移植物衰竭中，约 9%出现移植物死亡，13%是因为急性排斥，36%是因为慢性排斥。血管栓塞仍然是衰竭的主要病因，13.5%是由于原发性无功能、血管栓塞、或各种技术原因。这些数据显示这些问题在所有儿童移植患者的 4%儿童移植中出现[70,110,187,189,191,192,252]。原发病复发是移植物衰竭的原因之一，占移植物衰竭的 7%。特异性疾病包括局灶性阶段性肾小球肾炎，占移植物功能缺失的 44%，膜性增生性肾小球肾炎 2 型占 9%，HUS 占 9%，草酸过多症占 5%，慢性肾小球肾炎占 4%，其他占 28%。

图 113.2 显示的是受者年龄相关的 10 年活体移植物生存曲线，图 113.3 显示的是供者来源和年代相关的 7 年移植物生存率。在过去十年内，活体供体移植物 1、3、5 年生存率分别是 97%、92%、84%，死亡供体移植物存活率分别是 95%、84%、78%[3,21]。在短期和中期的移植物存活率方面，有一个持续的改善，主要是由于早期移植存活率显著改善。这可能与急性排斥反应发生率下降的频率和急性排斥反应的发病率下降、移植物功能缺失的原因相关。不过需要注意的是，如图 113.3 所示，在过去的 20 年中，移植物的存活曲线的斜率没有显著改变。在过去的 10 年中，儿童活体和死亡

供体肾移植中移植物存活率提高的趋势结果常常被报道[3,15,21,32,105]。

表113.3显示了活体和死亡供体移植中移植失败的相对危险因素。移植失败的相对风险,采用Cox比例风险回归模型。对于移植的受者,对移植物存活的最重要的预后变量是种族(非裔美国人对非非裔美国人),以前的移植缺乏诱导抗体治疗和移植年份。死亡供体受者的重要预后因素包括:非裔美国人、移植病史、年龄超过2岁和移植年份。透析史、缺乏HLA-B和DR匹配以及延长冷藏时间可能会有轻微的相对风险。在活体和死亡供体移植中,男性受者与女性受者相比似乎风险较低。同样对于活体和死亡供体移植,超过5次输血的历史似乎与较差的存活率有关,但这一发现在现代的意义还不明确。此外,诱导抗体治疗往往被促使使用这种治疗方法的因素妨碍了,这些偏倚的大小和方向不能被量化,这些因素能否用于评价还不明确。更重要的是,在活体供体受者中,非常年轻的受者移植物存活率的改善是最强的,这个年龄组的整体改善可能与他们所使用的高比例的活体供体有关。

移植后生长

成人受者与儿童受者的主要区别是儿童需要生长。在移植的时候,通常观察到的儿童生长障碍是多因素的,但是最重要的原因是许多机制引起的对内源性生长激素反应减少[253]。许多年来,研究一直认为一个功能的移植将使儿童能够实现追赶生长[9]。不幸的是,从注册表研究的长期数据显示了一个更令人失望的结果。

NAPRTCS数据显示,移植时的平均身高是-1.75,男性(-1.78),更年轻的患者在移植时有更大的生长赤字[43]。这个赤字一直在稳步上升,且平均赤字从1987年的-2.43提高到2009年的-1.23[3]。移植时小于5岁的年幼儿童通常表现出早期的追赶生长[3,9],2年后Z值全反转达0.60。年龄较大的儿童可能以正常的速度生长,但很少表现出追赶生长。终末期肾病儿童的成年身高在不断地改善,但所有的改善都是在治疗CKD中获得而不是移植后[10,12]。近期移植的患儿的成人身高比以前移植的患儿的成人身高有所改善。在儿童移植中,1987—1991年移植患儿的最终身高Z值为-1.93,而1997—2001年为-1.08。

表113.3 儿童肾移植失败的相对危险性分析

	活体供体		死亡供体	
	RH	*P*值	RH	*P*值
受体年龄(>2)	1.23	NS	0.67	0.0040
先前移植	1.50	<0.0001	1.45	0.0001
诱导抗体	0.84	0.0050	0.92	NS
>5次输血	1.22	0.0160	1.25	0.0006
非HLA-B不匹配	1.32	0.0183	1.15	0.0170
非HLA-DR不匹配	0.82	NS	1.13	0.0333
黑人种族	1.94	<0.0001	1.58	<0.0001
先前透析	1.16	0.0375	0.0375	0.0326
冷保存时间>24小时	–	–	1.15	0.0200
移植年份(1987-2010)	0.95	<0.0001	0.94	<0.0001

Adapted from Smith et al.[3].

坚持慢性免疫抑制治疗

不坚持往往被认为是儿童肾移植受者长期移植物功能缺失的重要原因,尤其是青少年[254]。这在第120章中进行了深度描述。依从性差的主要原因是由于免疫抑制药物引起的外观改变,包括库兴面容及长期皮质类固醇使用引起的生长迟缓、多毛症、环孢素相关的牙龈肥大等。然而,不能坚持治疗的发病率是未知的。有报道,不坚持率为22%[255]、43%[256]和高达64%[257]。不坚持率升高与年轻、青春期、社会经济状况不佳以及家庭压力有关[255,257-259]。重要的是,医护人员不能够识别的非依从患者占很大比例[260]。教育计划[256]和家庭为基础的治疗[261]等措施并没有得到广泛的成功[254]。改善非依从性的另一个建议是改变免疫抑制药物的类型或使用频率,使受者不必坚持严格的时间表,但这些建议目前只是假设[175,262]。

住院治疗

再住院率在2000—2010年间已大幅下降。活体移植受者的再住院率已经从49%下降到39%,而住院时间已从8天下降到6天。对于死亡供体受者而言,再住院率已经从57%下降到42%,而住院时间已从10天下降到6天[3]。住院的最常见原因曾经是排斥反应。但是,最新的文献表明病毒和细菌感染是住院的下一个最常见的原因[3,263]。头 6 个月内治疗高血压住院的受者占 5%~8%，移植后 5 年降至约 1%[33]。

移植后淋巴组织增生性疾病和恶性肿瘤(PTLD)

多年前 PTLD 已被报道为儿童器官移植并发症[264]，目前文献报道越来越多[265]。目前尚不清楚这个潜在的致命并发症的发生率是正在增加，或者仅仅是更多地被识别。如果发生率正在增加，这可能是“改进”免疫抑制的不幸后果[266]。综述报道，UNOS 数据(<18 岁)表明，白种人和男性是显著的发病的危险因素[267]。目前儿童肾移植 PTLD 的发生率为 1%~2%，有些报道高于此数值[206]。

这种并发症在第 96 章中已有明确表述。PTLD 常出现在淋巴结内，但它也可以发生在淋巴结外。PTLD 经常在胃肠道内[268]发生，接近或在移植物内[269]或远离移植物[270]。中枢神经系统中的 PTLD 往往是破坏性的，并迅速致命。PTLD 通常被认为由 EBV 感染而来[268,271,272]。因此，移植前供者和受者的 EBV 感染状态可能是一个重要的决定因素，这也解释了 PTLD 为什么在儿童中的发生率比成人高[273,274]。在几个报道中，PTLD 的发病率在 EBV 阴性的受者中比 EBV 抗体阳性高[275-277]。在大多数情况下，其是来源于供者[278]。然而，EBV 阳性受者可能引起其他致命的疾病[279]。初次感染巨细胞病毒的受者可增加 PTLD 发生 5 倍的风险[275]。免疫抑制的强度也与儿童受者 PTLD 发生相关[277,280]。治疗用抗淋巴细胞抗体(如 OKT3)，无论是诱导或抗排斥治疗，都可能会增加 PTLD 的发生风险[275,276,279,281]。在环孢素和他克莫司治疗这两种免疫抑制方案中，他克莫司方案 PTLD 发生率较高[266,273,282]。然而，最近有一份注册报道显示麦考酚酯或他克莫司都不是 PTLD 发生的危险因素；当然，免疫抑制的强度很重要[267]。

PTLD 的诊断必须依靠病理结果。EBV DNA 检测技术的进步[283-287]和转化淋巴细胞生长[288-290]使 PTLD 高危患者检测成为可能。建议进行血液监测和免疫抑制剂调整，但目前仍没有被普遍接受的方案[291]。类似的测试也被用于指导治疗[283]，但其效果仍待评估。

PTLD 的治疗首先是减少或停止免疫抑制剂的使用[278,292,293]。有趣的是，停止或减少免疫抑制药物的使用，移植物并未发生排斥。干扰素-α 和静脉内 γ 球蛋白[294,295]、更昔洛韦[296,297]甚至化疗被用于治疗，但功效存在差异。高危患者的预防可能是有用的[298]。用单克隆抗体利妥昔单抗治疗已显示出有希望的结果[299-303]。

其他感染

免疫抑制使成人和儿童受者更易受多种病毒和细菌感染。这些在第 92 章至第 94 章中被提及。感染是儿童肾移植后的最主要并发症。预防性治疗感染在肾移植中更常见。

免疫缺陷受者移植后的巨细胞病毒感染可能导致致命的疾病，特别是当受体血清阴性并且供体血清是阳性时。预防性口服缬更昔洛韦 3~12 个月在儿童肾移植中已成为常规[297,304,305]。类似地，也可预防性使用甲氧苄啶-磺胺、喷他脒、氨苯砜或阿托瓦宗。

水痘在免疫功能低下时可能引起非常严重或甚至致命的结果[306,307]。儿童应在移植前接种水痘疫苗[308,309]，必要时应该重复以确保在慢性免疫抑制使用前血清阴性[81]。移植后接种水痘疫苗的报道为数不多[309]，但它可能是安全的，虽然不一定成功。BK 病毒性肾病是一种日益被认可的并发症，其在儿童和成人肾移植中的发生率相近[310-313]。正如 EBV 那样，典型的方法是预防、仔细筛选病毒血症和选择性减少免疫抑制剂。一些患者可以从来氟米特治疗中受益[314]。

死亡率

接受肾移植的儿童死亡率显著降低。活体和死亡供体受者存活率都有所增高(图 113.9)[3]，目前的 5 年患者生存率分别是 97%和 96%。婴儿的存活，特别是那

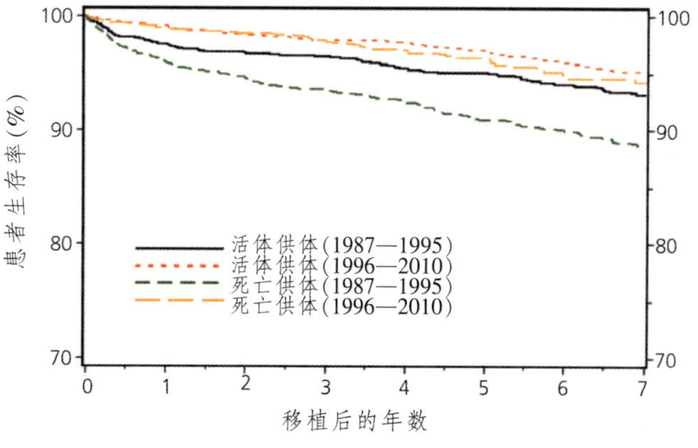

图 113.9 儿童活体和死亡供体肾移植 7 年患者生存率。adapted from NAPRTCS 2010 Annual Report: www.naprtcs.org. https://web.emmes.com/study/ped/annlrept/2010_Report.pdf. [December 19, 2013].

些接受死亡供体移植物的，不如年龄大的儿童好。儿童死亡的主要原因是感染，其次是心肺问题、恶性和透析相关问题。约50%的死亡发生与功能移植相关[3]。

总结

一般来说，儿童肾移植的效果因为成人移植的成熟而提高，然而儿童肾移植仍需改进。和儿童体形相关的手术技术和先天性异常在这个人群中非常常见。结果令人欣喜，明显优于通过透析获得的收益，尽管这在青少年中效果仍然不是最佳的。免疫治疗类似于成人移植受者，虽然这主要是药物发展中的产物，少数儿童受到制药公司的一些注意。该领域的未来机遇包括使用特殊的免疫抑制方案，应考虑到动态的、发展中的儿童免疫系统（见第112章），并仅仅用于儿童患者的需要。

（柯庆宏 译 柯庆宏 校）

参考文献

1. Gaston RS, Danovitch GM, Adams PL, et al. The report of a national conference on the wait list for kidney transplantation. American Journal of Transplantation. 2003;3(7):775–785.
2. Fine RN. Renal transplantation for children-the only realistic choice. Kidney International. Supplement. 1985;17(7):S15–S17.
3. Smith JM, Martz K, Blydt-Hansen TD. Pediatric kidney transplant practice patterns and outcome benchmarks, 1987-2010: a report of the North American Pediatric Renal Trials and Collaborative Studies. Pediatric Transplantation. 2013;17(2):149–157.
4. Gillen DL, Stehman-Breen CO, Smith JM, et al. Survival advantage of pediatric recipients of a first kidney transplant among children awaiting kidney transplantation. American Journal of Transplantation. 2008;8(12):2600–2606.
5. Warady BA, Hebert D, Sullivan EK, et al. Renal transplantation, chronic dialysis, and chronic renal insufficiency in children and adolescents. The 1995 Annual Report of the North American Pediatric Renal Transplant Co-operative Study. Pediatric Nephrology (Berlin, Germany). 1997;11(1):49–64.
6. Trachtman H, Hackney P, Tejani A. Pediatric hemodialysis: a decade's (1974-1984) perspective. Kidney International. Supplement. 1986;19(22):S15–S22.
7. Brouhard BH, Donaldson LA, Lawry KW, et al. Cognitive functioning in children on dialysis and post-transplant-transplantation. Pediatric Transplantation. 2000;4(4):261–267.
8. Sarwal MM, Yorgin PD, Alexander S, et al. Promising early outcomes with a novel, complete steroid avoidance immunosuppression protocol in pediatric renal transplantation. Transplantation. 2001;72(1):13–21.
9. Ingelfinger JR, Grupe WE, Harmon WE, et al. Growth acceleration following renal transplantation in children less than 7 years of age. Pediatrics. 1981;68(2):255–259.
10. Fine RN, Ho M, Tejani A, et al. The contribution of renal transplantation to final adult height: a report of the North American Pediatric Renal Transplant Co-operative Study (NAPRTCS). Pediatric Nephrology (Berlin, Germany). 2001;16(12):951–956.
11. Fine RN, Stablein D, Cohen AH, et al. Recombinant human growth hormone post-transplant-renal transplantation in children: a randomized controlled study of the NAPRTCS. Kidney International. 2002;62(2):688–696.
12. Fine RN, Martz K, Stablein D. What have 20 years of data from the North American Pediatric Renal Transplant Co-operative Study taught us about growth following renal transplantation in infants, children, and adolescents with end-stage renal disease? Pediatric Nephrology (Berlin, Germany). 2010;25(4):739–746.
13. Mendley SR, Zelko FA. Improvement in specific aspects of neurocognitive performance in children after renal transplantation. Kidney International. 1999;56(1):318–323.
14. Fennell EB, Fennell RS, Mings E, et al. The effects of various modes of therapy for end stage renal disease on cognitive performance in a pediatric population–a preliminary report. International Journal of Pediatric Nephrology. 1986;7(2):107–112.
15. Colombani PM, Dunn SP, Harmon WE, et al. Pediatric transplantation. American Journal of Transplantation. 2003;3(Suppl 4):53–63.
16. Magee JC, Krishnan SM, Benfield MR, et al. Pediatric transplantation in the United States, 1997-2006. American Journal of Transplantation. 2008;8(4 Pt 2):935–945.
17. Moudgil A, Martz K, Stablein DM, et al. Good outcome of kidney transplants in recipients of young donors: a NAPRTCS data analysis. Pediatric Transplantation. 2011;15(2):167–171.
18. Gritsch HA, Veale JL, Leichtman AB, et al. Should pediatric patients wait for HLA-DR-matched renal transplants? American Journal of Transplantation. 2008;8(10):2056–2061.
19. Nguyen S, Martz K, Stablein D, et al. Wait list status of pediatric dialysis patients in North America. Pediatric Transplantation. 2011;15(4):376–383.
20. Gaston RS, Alveranga DY, Becker BN, et al. Kidney and pancreas transplantation. American Journal of Transplantation. 2003;3(Suppl 4):64–77.
21. Matas AJ, Smith JM, Skeans MA, et al. OPTN/SRTR 2011 annual data report: kidney. American Journal of Transplantation. 2013;13(Suppl 1):11–46.
22. Dale-Shall AW, Smith JM, McBride MA, et al. The relationship of donor source and age on short- and long-term allograft survival in pediatric renal transplantation. Pediatric Transplantation. 2009;13(6):711–718.
23. Cecka JM, Gjertson DW, Terasaki PI. Pediatric renal transplantation: a review of the UNOS data. Pediatric Transplantation. 1997;1(1):55–64.
24. Neu AM, Stablein DM, Zachary A, et al. Effect of parental donor sex on rejection in pediatric renal transplantation: a report of the North American Pediatric Renal Transplant Co-operative Study. Pediatric Transplantation. 1998;2(4):309–312.
25. Spital A. Should children ever donate kidneys? Views of U.S. transplant centers. Transplantation. 1997;64(2):232–236.
26. Price DP. Minors as living donors: ethics and law. Transplantation Proceedings. 1996;28(6):3607–3608.
27. Delmonico FL, Harmon WE. The use of a minor as a live kidney donor.[see comment]. American Journal of Transplantation. 2002;2(4):333–336.
28. Terasaki PI, Cecka JM, Gjertson DW, et al. High survival rates of kidney transplants from spousal and living unrelated donors [see comments]. New England Journal of Medicine. 1995;333(6):333–336.
29. Al-Uzri A, Sullivan EK, Fine RN, et al. Living-unrelated renal transplantation in children: a report of the North American Pediatric Renal Transplant Co-operative Study (NAPRTCS)[see comment]. Pediatric Transplantation. 1998;2(2):139–144.
30. Davies DB, Breen TJ, Guo T, et al. Waiting times to pediatric transplantation: an assessment of the August 1990 change in renal allocation policy. Transplantation Proceedings. 1994;26(1):30–31.
31. McEnery PT, Alexander SR, Sullivan K, et al. Renal transplantation in children and adolescents: the 1992 annual report of the North American Pediatric Renal Transplant Co-operative Study. Pediatric Nephrology (Berlin, Germany). 1993;7(6):711–720.
32. Tejani A, Sullivan EK, Fine RN, et al. Steady improvement in renal allograft survival among North American children: a five year appraisal by the North American Pediatric Renal Transplant Co-operative Study. Kidney International. 1995;48(2):551–553.
33. Feld LG, Stablein D, Fivush B, et al. Renal transplantation in children from 1987-1996: the 1996 Annual Report of the North American Pediatric Renal Transplant Co-operative Study. Pediatric Transplantation. 1997;1(2):146–162.
34. Filler G, Lindeke A, Bohme K, et al. Renal transplantation from donors aged <6 years into children yields equal graft survival when compared to older donors. Pediatric Transplantation. 1997;1:119–123.
35. Butani L, Troppmann C, Perez RV. Outcomes of children receiving en bloc renal transplants from small pediatric donors. Pediatric Transplantation. 2013;17(1):55–58.
36. Hiramoto JS, Freise CE, Randall HR, et al. Successful long-term outcomes using pediatric en bloc kidneys for transplantation. American Journal of Transplantation. 2002;2(4):337–342.
37. Kayler LK, Zendejas I, Gregg A, et al. Kidney transplantation from small pediatric donors: does recipient body mass index matter? Transplantation. 2012;93(4):430–436.
38. Harmon WE, McDonald RA, Reyes JD, et al. Pediatric transplantation, 1994-2003. American Journal of Transplantation. 2005;5(4 Pt 2):887–903.
39. Tejani A, Stablein DM, Donaldson L, et al. Steady improvement in short-term graft survival of pediatric renal transplants: the NAPRTCS experience. Clinical Transplants. 1999:95–110.
40. Tejani A, Ho PL, Emmett L, et al. Reduction in acute rejections decreases chronic

rejection graft failure in children: a report of the North American Pediatric Renal Transplant Co-operative Study (NAPRTCS). American Journal of Transplantation. 2002;2(2):142–147.

41. McEnery PT, Stablein DM, Arbus G, et al. Renal transplantation in children. A report of the North American Pediatric Renal Transplant Co-operative Study. New England Journal of Medicine. 1992;326(26):1727–1732.
42. Ettenger RB, Blifeld C, Prince H, et al. The pediatric nephrologist's dilemma: growth after renal transplantation and its interaction with age as a possible immunologic variable. Journal of Pediatrics. 1987;111(6 Pt 2):1022–1025.
43. Seikaly M, Ho PL, Emmett L, et al. The 12th Annual Report of the North American Pediatric Renal Transplant Co-operative Study: renal transplantation from 1987 through 1998 (updated at http://www.naprtcs.org). Pediatric Transplantation. 2001;5(3):215–231.
44. Briscoe DM, Kim MS, Lillehei C, et al. Outcome of renal transplantation in children less than two years of age. Kidney International. 1992;42(3):657–662.
45. Fine RN, Tejani A, Sullivan EK. Pre-emptive renal transplantation in children: report of the North American Pediatric Renal Transplant Co-operative Study (NAPRTCS). Clinical Transplantation. 1994;8(5):474–478.
46. Butani L, Perez RV. Effect of pretransplant dialysis modality and duration on long-term outcomes of children receiving renal transplants. Transplantation. 2011;91(4):447–451.
47. Liem YS, Weimar W. Early living-donor kidney transplantation: a review of the associated survival benefit. Transplantation. 2009;87(3):317–318.
48. Ellis EN, Martz K, Talley L, et al. Factors related to long-term renal transplant function in children. Pediatric Nephrology (Berlin, Germany). 2008;23(7): 1149–1155.
49. Kasiske BL, Snyder JJ, Matas AJ, et al. Preemptive kidney transplantation: the advantage and the advantaged. Journal of the American Society of Nephrology. 2002;13(5):1358–1364.
50. Najarian JS, Frey DJ, Matas AJ, et al. Renal transplantation in infants. Annals of Surgery. 1990;212(3):353–365.
51. Ingulli E, Matas AJ, Nevins TE, et al. Impact of age on renal graft survival in children after the first rejection episode. Pediatric Nephrology (Berlin, Germany). 1996;10(4):474–478.
52. Strehlau J, Sharma VK, Pavalakis M, et al., editors Do children have a heightened immune response to acute allograft rejection? A preliminary comparative study of intragraft gene transcripts of immune activation markers in adult and peditric graft rejection. 16th Annual Meeting of the American Society of Transplant Physicians; 1997; Chicago: Abstract.
53. Scomik JC, Cecka M. Clinical parameters of immune responsiveness in children and African American transplant patients. 16th Annual Meeting of the American Society of Transplant Physicians; 1997; Chicago: Abs.
54. Chavers BM, Gillingham KJ, Matas AJ. Complications by age in primary pediatric renal transplant recipients. Pediatric Nephrology (Berlin, Germany). 1997; 11(4):399–403.
55. Schachter AD, Benfield MR, Wyatt RJ, et al. Sirolimus pharmacokinetics in pediatric renal transplant recipients receiving calcineurin inhibitor co-therapy. Pediatric Transplantation. 2006;10(8):914–919.
56. Schachter AD, Meyers KE, Spaneas LD, et al. Short sirolimus half-life in pediatric renal transplant recipients on a calcineurin inhibitor-free protocol. Pediatric Transplantation. 2004;8(2):171–177.
57. Lemire J, Capparelli EV, Benador N, et al. Neoral pharmacokinetics in Latino and Caucasian pediatric renal transplant recipients. Pediatric Nephrology (Berlin, Germany). 2001;16(4):311–314.
58. Hoppu K, Koskimies O, Holmberg C, et al. Pharmacokinetically determined cyclosporine dosage in young children. Pediatric Nephrology (Berlin, Germany). 1991;5(1):1–4.
59. Adams J, Gudemann C, Tonshoff B, et al. Renal transplantation in small children– a comparison between surgical procedures. European Urology. 2001;40(5): 552–556.
60. Humar A, Arrazola L, Mauer M, et al. Kidney transplantation in young children: should there be a minimum age? Pediatric Nephrology (Berlin, Germany). 2001;16(12):941–945.
61. Matas AJ, Payne WD, Sutherland DE, et al. 2,500 living donor kidney transplants: a single-center experience. Annals of Surgery. 2001;234(2):149–164.
62. Millan MT, Sarwal MM, Lemley KV, et al. A 100% 2-year graft survival can be attained in high-risk 15-kg or smaller infant recipients of kidney allografts. Archives of Surgery. 2000;135(9):1063–1068, discussion 8–9.
63. Salvatierra O Jr, Sarwal M. Renal perfusion in infant recipients of adult-sized kidneys is a critical risk factor. Transplantation. 2000;70(3):412–413.
64. Harmon WE, Alexander SR, Tejani A, et al. The effect of donor age on graft survival in pediatric cadaver renal transplant recipients–a report of the North American Pediatric Renal Transplant Co-operative Study. Transplantation. 1992;54(2):232–237.
65. Elshihabi I, Chavers B, Donaldson L, et al. Continuing improvement in cadaver donor graft survival in North American children: the 1998 annual report of the North American Pediatric Renal Transplant Co-operative Study (NAPRTCS). Pediatric Transplantation. 2000;4(3):235–246.
66. McDonald R, Donaldson L, Emmett L, et al. A decade of living donor transplantation in North American children: the 1998 annual report of the North American Pediatric Renal Transplant Co-operative Study (NAPRTCS). Pediatric Transplantation. 2000;4(3):221–234.
67. Trompeter R, Filler G, Webb NJ, et al. Randomized trial of tacrolimus versus cyclosporin microemulsion in renal transplantation. Pediatric Nephrology (Berlin, Germany). 2002;17(3):141–149.
68. Weber LT, Shipkova M, Armstrong VW, et al. The pharmacokinetic-pharmacodynamic relationship for total and free mycophenolic Acid in pediatric renal transplant recipients: a report of the german study group on mycophenolate mofetil therapy. Journal of the American Society of Nephrology. 2002; 13(3):759–768.
69. Benfield MR, Symons JM, Bynon S, et al. Mycophenolate mofetil in pediatric renal transplantation. Pediatric Transplantation. 1999;3(1):33–37.
70. Schurman SJ, Stablein DM, Perlman SA, et al. Center volume effects in pediatric renal transplantation. A report of the North American Pediatric Renal Transplant Co-operative Study. Pediatric Nephrology (Berlin, Germany). 1999;13(5): 373–378.
71. Sweet SC, Wong HH, Webber SA, et al. Pediatric transplantation in the United States, 1995-2004. American Journal of Transplantation. 2006;6(5 Pt 2): 1132–1152.
72. Sarwal MM, Cecka JM, Millan MT, et al. Adult-size kidneys without acute tubular necrosis provide exceedingly superior long-term graft outcomes for infants and small children: a single center and UNOS analysis. Transplantation. 2000;70(12):1728–1736. United Network for Organ Sharing.
73. Van Arendonk KJ, James NT, Boyarsky BJ, et al. Age at graft loss after pediatric kidney transplantation: exploring the high-risk age window. Clinical Journal of the American Society of Nephrology. 2013;8(6):1019–1026.
74. Levine MH, Reese PP, Wood A, et al. Inferior allograft outcomes in adolescent recipients of renal transplants from ideal deceased donors. Annals of Surgery. 2012;255(3):556–564.
75. Fine RN. Growth following solid-organ transplantation. Pediatric Transplantation. 2002;6(1):47–52.
76. Kim MS, Primack W, Harmon WE. Congenital nephrotic syndrome: preemptive bilateral nephrectomy and dialysis before renal transplantation. Journal of the American Society of Nephrology. 1992;3(2):260–263.
77. Fasola CG, Gillingham KJ, Troppmann C, et al. Kidney transplant or retransplant can effectively treat congenital nephrotic syndrome: a single-center experience. Transplantation Proceedings. 1994;26(1):9.
78. Holmberg C, Jalanko H, Koskimies O, et al. Renal transplantation in small children with congenital nephrotic syndrome of the Finnish type. Transplantation Proceedings. 1991;23(1 Pt 2):1378–1379.
79. Chaves TS, Pereira LM, De Santos SS, et al. Evaluation of the vaccination status in pediatric renal transplant recipients. Pediatric Transplantation. 2008;12(4): 432–435.
80. Laube GF, Berger C, Goetschel P, et al. Immunization in children with chronic renal failure. Pediatric Nephrology (Berlin, Germany). 2002;17(8):638–642.
81. Furth SL, Fivush BA. Varicella vaccination in pediatric kidney transplant candidates. Pediatric Transplantation. 2002;6(2):97–100.
82. Olson AD, Shope TC, Flynn JT. Pretransplant varicella vaccination is cost-effective in pediatric renal transplantation. Pediatric Transplantation. 2001;5(1): 44–50.
83. Routh JC, Yu RN, Kozinn SI, et al. Urological complications and vesicoureteral reflux following pediatric kidney transplantation. Journal of Urology. 2013;189(3):1071–1076.
84. Basiri A, Otookesh H, Hosseini R, et al. Kidney transplantation before or after augmentation cystoplasty in children with high-pressure neurogenic bladder. BJU International. 2009;103(1):86–88, discussion 8.
85. Djakovic N, Wagener N, Adams J, et al. Intestinal reconstruction of the lower urinary tract as a prerequisite for renal transplantation. BJU International. 2009;103(11):1555–1560.
86. Alam S, Sheldon C. Urological issues in pediatric renal transplantation. Current Opinion in Urology. 2008;18(4):413–418.
87. Rudge CJ. Transplantation and the abnormal bladder. In: Morris PJ, editor. Kidney Transplantation: Principles and Practice, 4th ed. Philadelphia, PA: WB Saunders; 1994: 138–148.
88. Lopez Pereira P, Jaureguizar E, Martinez Urrutia MJ, et al. Does treatment of bladder dysfunction prior to renal transplant improve outcome in patients with post-transplanterior urethral valves? Pediatric Transplantation. 2000;4(2): 118–122.
89. Ramirez SP, Lebowitz RL, Harmon WE, et al. Predictors for abnormal voiding cystourethrography in pediatric patients undergoing renal transplant evaluation.

[see comment]. Pediatric Transplantation. 2001;5(2):99–104.
90. Salvatierra O, Tanney D, Mak R, et al. Pediatric renal transplantation and its challenges. Transplantation Reviews. 1997;11:51–69.
91. Koo HP, Bunchman TE, Flynn JT, et al. Renal transplantation in children with severe lower urinary tract dysfunction.[comment]. Journal of Urology. 1999;161(1):240–245.
92. Power RE, O'Malley KJ, Khan MS, et al. Renal transplantation in patients with an augmentation cystoplasty. BJU International. 2000;86(1):28–31.
93. Nahas WC, Mazzucchi E, Arap MA, et al. Augmentation cystoplasty in renal transplantation: a good and safe option–experience with 25 cases. Urology. 2002;60(5):770–774.
94. Pereira DA, Barroso U Jr, Machado P, et al. Effects of urinary tract infection in patients with bladder augmentation and kidney transplantation. Journal of Urology. 2008;180(6):2607–2610, discussion 10.
95. Atala A. Bladder regeneration by tissue engineering. BJU International. 2001;88(7):765–770.
96. Atala A. Future trends in bladder reconstructive surgery. Seminars in Pediatric Surgery. 2002;11(2):134–142.
97. Horst M, Madduri S, Gobet R, et al. Engineering functional bladder tissues. Journal of Tissue Engineering and Regenerative Medicine. 2013;7(7):515–522.
98. Otukesh H, Basiri A, Simfroosh N, et al. Kidney transplantation in children with post-transplanterior urethral valves. Pediatric Transplantation. 2008;12(5): 516–519.
99. Franc-Guimond J, Gonzalez R. Renal transplantation in children with reconstructed bladders. Transplantation. 2004;77(7):1116–1120.
100. Capizzi A, Zanon GF, Zacchello G, et al. Kidney transplantation in children with reconstructed bladder. Transplantation. 2004;77(7):1113–1116.
101. DeFoor W, Tackett L, Minevich E, et al. Successful renal transplantation in children with post-transplanterior urethral valves. Journal of Urology. 2003;170(6 Pt 1):2402–2404.
102. DeFoor W, Minevich E, McEnery P, et al. Lower urinary tract reconstruction is safe and effective in children with end stage renal disease. Journal of Urology. 2003;170(4 Pt 2):1497–1500, discussion 500.
103. Broyer M. What are the indications for nephrectomy, either bilateral or unilateral, prior to transplantation in children? Pediatric Nephrology (Berlin, Germany). 1991;5(1):11.
104. NAPRTCS. 2008 Annual Report. 2008 [accessed May 1, 2007]; Available from: http://www.naprtcs.org.
105. Smith JM, Stablein DM, Munoz R, et al. Contributions of the transplant registry: the 2006 annual report of the North American Pediatric Renal Trials and Collaborative Studies (NAPRTCS). Pediatric Transplantation. 2007;11(4):366–373.
106. Cochat P, Fargue S, Mestrallet G, et al. Disease recurrence in paediatric renal transplantation. Pediatric Nephrology (Berlin, Germany). 2009;24(11): 2097–2108.
107. Loirat C, Fremeaux-Bacchi V. Hemolytic uremic syndrome recurrence after renal transplantation. Pediatric Transplantation. 2008;12(6):619–629.
108. Horslen S, Barr ML, Christensen LL, et al. Pediatric transplantation in the United States, 1996-2005. American Journal of Transplantation: Official Journal of the American Society of Transplantation and the American Society of Transplant Surgeons. 2007;7(Suppl 1):1339–1358.
109. Delmonico FL, Harmon WE. Pediatric kidney transplantation in the United States: the current realities. American Journal of Transplantation. 2008;8(12): 2487–2488.
110. Harmon WE, Stablein D, Alexander SR, et al. Graft thrombosis in pediatric renal transplant recipients. A report of the North American Pediatric Renal Transplant Co-operative Study. Transplantation. 1991;51(2):406–412.
111. Ibrahim HN, Foley R, Tan L, et al. Long-term consequences of kidney donation. New England Journal of Medicine. 2009;360(5):459–469.
112. Delmonico F, Council of the Transplantation S. A report of the Amsterdam forum on the care of the live kidney donor: data and medical guidelines. Transplantation. 2005;79(6 Suppl):S53–S66.
113. Joseph JW, Thistlethwaite JR Jr, Josephson MA, et al. An empirical investigation of physicians' attitudes toward intrasibling kidney donation by minor twins. Transplantation. 2008;85(9):1235–1239.
114. Gheith O, Sabry A, El-Baset SA, et al. Study of the effect of donor source on graft and patient survival in pediatric renal transplant recipients. Pediatric Nephrology (Berlin, Germany). 2008;23(11):2075–2079.
115. Ahmad N, Ahmed K, Khan MS, et al. Living-unrelated donor renal transplantation: an alternative to living-related donor transplantation? Annals of the Royal College of Surgeons of England. 2008;90(3):247–250.
116. Kaneku HK, Terasaki PI. Thirty year trend in kidney transplants: UCLA and UNOS Renal Transplant Registry. Clinical Transplants. 2006:1–27.
117. Spital A. Increasing the pool of transplantable kidneys through unrelated living donors and living donor paired exchanges. Seminars in Dialysis. 2005;18(6):469–473.
118. O'Connor KJ, Delmonico FL. Increasing the supply of kidneys for transplantation. Seminars in Dialysis. 2005;18(6):460–462.
119. Cecka JM. The OPTN/UNOS renal transplant registry. Clinical Transplants. 2005:1–16.
120. Morrissey PE, Dube C, Gohh R, et al. Good samaritan kidney donation. Transplantation. 2005;80(10):1369–1373.
121. Jacobs CL, Roman D, Garvey C, et al. Twenty-two nondirected kidney donors: an update on a single center's experience. American Journal of Transplantation. 2004;4(7):1110–1116.
122. Matas AJ, Hippen B, Satel S. In defense of a regulated system of compensation for living donation. Current Opinion in Organ Transplantation. 2008;13(4): 379–385.
123. Matas AJ. Should we pay donors to increase the supply of organs for transplantation? Yes. BMJ (Clinical Research Ed.). 2008;336(7657):1342.
124. Steering Committee of the Istanbul S. Organ trafficking and transplant tourism and commercialism: the Declaration of Istanbul. Lancet. 2008;372(9632): 5–6.
125. International Summit on Transplant T, Organ T. The declaration of Istanbul on organ trafficking and transplant tourism. Clinical Journal of the American Society of Nephrology. 2008;3(5):1227–1231.
126. Gentry SE, Segev DL, Simmerling M, et al. Expanding kidney paired donation through participation by compatible pairs. American Journal of Transplantation. 2007;7(10):2361–2370.
127. Delmonico FL, Morrissey PE, Lipkowitz GS, et al. Donor kidney exchange for incompatible donors. American Journal of Transplantation. 2003;3(Suppl 5):550.
128. Marks WH, Wagner D, Pearson TC, et al. Organ donation and utilization, 1995-2004: entering the collaborative era. American Journal of Transplantation. 2006;6(5 Pt 2):1101–1110.
129. Huh KH, Kim MS, Ju MK, et al. Exchange living-donor kidney transplantation: merits and limitations. Transplantation. 2008;86(3):430–435.
130. Hanto RL, Reitsma W, Delmonico FL. The development of a successful multiregional kidney paired donation program. Transplantation. 2008;86(12): 1744–1748.
131. den Hartogh G. Trading with the waiting-list: the justice of living donor list exchange. Bioethics. 2010;24(4):190–198.
132. de Klerk M, Witvliet MD, Haase-Kromwijk BJ, et al. Hurdles, barriers, and successes of a national living donor kidney exchange program. Transplantation. 2008;86(12):1749–1753.
133. de Klerk M, Weimar W. Ingredients for a successful living donor kidney exchange program. Transplantation. 2008;86(4):511–512.
134. Kim BS, Kim YS, Kim SI, et al. Outcome of multipair donor kidney exchange by a web-based algorithm. Journal of the American Society of Nephrology. 2007;18(3):1000–1006.
135. Waterman AD, Schenk EA, Barrett AC, et al. Incompatible kidney donor candidates' willingness to participate in donor-exchange and non-directed donation. American Journal of Transplantation. 2006;6(7):1631–1638.
136. de Klerk M, Witvliet MD, Haase-Kromwijk BJ, et al. A highly efficient living donor kidney exchange program for both blood type and crossmatch incompatible donor-recipient combinations. Transplantation. 2006;82(12):1616–1620.
137. Tuncer M, Tekin S, Yucetin L, et al. Comparison of paired exchange kidney transplantations with living related kidney transplantations. Transplantation Proceedings. 2012;44(6):1626–1627.
138. Bohmig GA. Impact of live-donor exchange on transplant waiting time. Transplant International: Official Journal of the European Society for Organ Transplantation. 2012;25(10):1024–1025.
139. Montgomery RA, Lonze BE, Jackson AM. Using donor exchange paradigms with desensitization to enhance transplant rates among highly sensitized patients. Current Opinion in Organ Transplantation. 2011;16(4):439–443.
140. Davis CL. Evaluation of the living kidney donor: current perspectives. American Journal of Kidney Diseases. 2004;43(3):508–530.
141. Bia MJ, Ramos EL, Danovitch GM, et al. Evaluation of living renal donors. The current practice of US transplant centers. Transplantation. 1995;60(4): 322–327.
142. Bresnahan BA, McBride MA, Cherikh WS, et al. Risk factors for renal allograft survival from pediatric cadaver donors: an analysis of united network for organ sharing data. Transplantation. 2001;72(2):256–261.
143. Ruff T, Reddy KS, Johnston TD, et al. Transplantation of pediatric en bloc cadaver kidneys into adult recipients: a single-center experience. American Surgeon. 2002;68(10):857–859.
144. Takemoto S, Terasaki PI. Donor age and recipient age. Clinical Transplants. 1988:345–356.
145. Terasaki PI, Gjertson DW, Cecka JM, et al. Significance of the donor age effect on kidney transplants. Clinical Transplantation. 1997;11(5 Pt 1):366–372.

146. Tejani A, Stablein DM, Sullivan EK, et al. The impact of donor source, preoperative immunotherapy and prophylactic antibody therapy on first rejection episodes in children. Pediatric Transplantation. 1998;2(4):318–324,
147. Toma H, Tanabe K, Tokumoto T, et al. Time-dependent risk factors influencing the long-term outcome in living renal allografts: donor age is a crucial risk factor for long-term graft survival more than 5 years after transplantation. Transplantation. 2001;72(5):940–947.
148. Cecka JM. The UNOS scientific renal transplant registry-ten years of kidney transplants. Clinical Transplants. 1997:1–14
149. Terasaki PI, Cho Y, Takemoto S, et al. Twenty-year follow-up on the effect of HLA matching on kidney transplant survival and prediction of future twenty-year survival. Transplantation Proceedings. 1996;28(3):1144–1145.
150. Cho YW, Cecka JM, Terasaki PI. HLA matching effect: better survival rates and graft quality. Clinical Transplants. 1994;435–449.
151. Takamoto S, Terasaki PI, Cecka JM, et al. Survival of nationally matched kidney transplants from cadaveric donors. New England Journal of Medicine. 1992;327:834–839.
152. Haas M, Montgomery RA, Segev DL, et al. Subclinical acute antibody-mediated rejection in positive crossmatch renal allografts. American Journal of Transplantation. 2007;7(3):576–585.
153. Takemoto SK, Zeevi A, Feng S, et al. National conference to assess antibody-mediated rejection in solid organ transplantation. American Journal of Transplantation: Official Journal of the American Society of Transplantation and the American Society of Transplant Surgeons. 2004;4(7):1033.
154. Terasaki PI. Humoral theory of transplantation. American Journal of Transplantation. 2003;3(6):665–673.
155. Terasaki PI, Ozawa M, Castro R. Four-year follow-up of a prospective trial of HLA and MICA antibodies on kidney graft survival. American Journal of Transplantation. 2007;7(2):408–415.
156. Ozawa M, Terasaki PI, Lee JH, et al. 14th International HLA and Immunogenetics Workshop: report on the Prospective Chronic Rejection Project. Tissue Antigens. 2007;69(Suppl 1):174–179.
157. Farney AC, Singh RP, Hines MH, et al. Experience in renal and extrarenal transplantation with donation after cardiac death donors with selective use of extracorporeal support. Journal of the American College of Surgeons. 2008; 206(5):1028–1037, discussion 37.
158. Locke JE, Segev DL, Warren DS, et al. Outcomes of kidneys from donors after cardiac death: implications for allocation and preservation. American Journal of Transplantation. 2007;7(7):1797–1807.
159. Van Arendonk KJ, James NT, Locke JE, et al. Late graft loss among pediatric recipients of DCD kidneys. Clinical Journal of the American Society of Nephrology. 2011;6(11):2705–2711.
160. Sumrani N, Delaney V, Ding ZK, et al. Renal transplantation from elderly living donors. Transplantation. 1991;51(2):305–309.
161. Jones JW, Matas AJ, Najarian JS. Surgical technique. In: Tejani AH, Fine RN, editors. Pediatric Renal Transplantation. New York, NY: Wiley-Liss; 1994: 187–200.
162. Lee HM. Surgical techniques of renal transplantation. In: Morris PJ, editor. Kidney Transplantation: Principles and Practice, 4th ed. Philadelphia, PA: WB Saunders; 1994: 127–137.
163. Salvatierra O, Singh T, Shifrin R, et al. Successful transplantation of adult-sized kidneys into infants requires maintenance of high aortic blood flow. Transplantation. 1998; 66(7):819–823.
164. French CG, Acott PD, Crocker JF, et al. Extravesical ureteroneocystostomy with and without internalized ureteric stents in pediatric renal transplantation. Pediatric Transplantation. 2001;5(1):21–26.
165. Zaontz MR, Maizels M, Sugar EC, et al. Detrusorrhaphy: extravesical ureteral advancement to correct vesicoureteral reflux in children. Journal of Urology. 1987;138(4 Pt 2):947–949.
166. Wacksman J, Gilbert A, Sheldon CA. Results of the renewed extravesical reimplant for surgical correction of vesicoureteral reflux. Journal of Urology. 1992;148(2 Pt 1):359–361.
167. Matas AJ, Bartlett ST, Leichtman AB, et al. Morbidity and mortality after living kidney donation, 1999-2001: survey of United States transplant centers. American Journal of Transplantation. 2003;3(7):830–834.
168. Magee JC. Does laparoscopic donor nephrectomy put pediatric recipients at risk? Pediatric Transplantation. 2008;12(5):503–505.
169. Troppmann C, McBride MA, Baker TJ, et al. Laparoscopic live donor nephrectomy: a risk factor for delayed function and rejection in pediatric kidney recipients? A UNOS analysis.[see comment]. American Journal of Transplantation. 2005;5(1):175–182.
170. Hsu TH, Su LM, Trock BJ, et al. Laparoscopic adult donor nephrectomy for pediatric renal transplantation. Urology. 2003;61(2):320–322.
171. Troppmann C, Pierce JL, Wiesmann KM, et al. Early and late recipient graft function and donor outcome after laparoscopic vs open adult live donor nephrectomy for pediatric renal transplantation. Archives of Surgery. 2002;137(8):908–915, discussion 15–6.
172. Basiri A, Simforoosh N, Heidari M, et al. Laparoscopic v open donor nephrectomy for pediatric kidney recipients: preliminary report of a randomized controlled trial. Journal of Endourology. 2007;21(9):1033–1036.
173. Chandak P, Kessaris N, Durkan A, et al. Is laparoscopic donation safe for paediatric recipients?–a study of 85 paediatric recipients comparing open and laparoscopic donor nephrectomy. Nephrology, Dialysis, Transplantation. 2012;27(2):845–849.
174. Mamode N, Johnson RJ, Hadjianastassiou VG. Laparoscopic donor nephrectomy does not compromise outcomes for pediatric transplant recipients. Transplantation. 2011;91(9):1005–1009.
175. Tan HP, Donaldson J, Ellis D, et al. Pediatric living donor kidney transplantation under alemtuzumab pretreatment and tacrolimus monotherapy: 4-year experience. Transplantation. 2008;86(12):1725–1731.
176. Yarlagadda SG, Coca SG, Garg AX, et al. Marked variation in the definition and diagnosis of delayed graft function: a systematic review. Nephrology, Dialysis, Transplantation. 2008;23(9):2995–3003.
177. Briscoe DM, Hoffer FA, Tu N, et al. allografts in children: correlation between renal blood flow and clinical findings. Pediatric Radiology. 1993;23(5): 365–368.
178. Benfield MR, Herrin J, Feld L, et al. Safety of kidney biopsy in pediatric transplantation: a report of the Controlled Clinical Trials in Pediatric Transplantation Trial of Induction Therapy Study Group. Transplantation. 1999; 67(4):544–547.
179. Baum MA. Outcomes after renal transplantation for FSGS in children. Pediatric Transplantation. 2004;8(4):329–333.
180. Aquino-Dias EC, Joelsons G, da Silva DM, et al. Non-invasive diagnosis of acute rejection in kidney transplants with delayed graft function. Kidney International. 2008;73(7):877–884.
181. Tejani A, Sullivan EK, Alexander S, et al. Post-transplanttransplant deaths and factors that influence the mortality rate in North American children. Transplantation. 1994;57(4):547–553.
182. Gjertson DW. Impact of delayed graft function and acute rejection on kidney graft survival. Clinical Transplants. 2000:467–480.
183. Patel SJ, Duhart BT Jr, Krauss AG, et al. Risk factors and consequences of delayed graft function in deceased donor renal transplant patients receiving antithymocyte globulin induction. Transplantation. 2008;86(2):313–320.
184. Yarlagadda SG, Coca SG, Formica RN Jr, et al. Association between delayed graft function and allograft and patient survival: a systematic review and meta-analysis. Nephrology, Dialysis, Transplantation. 2009;24(3):1039–1047.
185. Yarlagadda SG, Klein CL, Jani A. Long-term renal outcomes after delayed graft function. Advances in Chronic Kidney Disease. 2008;15(3):248–256.
186. Balachandra S, Tejani A. Recurrent vascular thrombosis in an adolescent transplant recipient. [Review] [20 refs]. Journal of the American Society of Nephrology. 1997;8(9):1477–1481.
187. Singh A, Stablein D, Tejani A. Risk factors for vascular thrombosis in pediatric renal transplantation: a special report of the North American Pediatric Renal Transplant Co-operative Study. Transplantation. 1997; 63(9):1263–1267.
188. Smith JM, Stablein D, Singh A, et al. Decreased risk of renal allograft thrombosis associated with interleukin-2 receptor antagonists: a report of the NAPRTCS. American Journal of Transplantation: Official Journal of the American Society of Transplantation and the American Society of Transplant Surgeons. 2006;6(3):585–588.
189. Wheeler MA, Taylor CM, Williams M, et al. Factor V Leiden: a risk factor for renal vein thrombosis in renal transplantation. Pediatric Nephrology (Berlin, Germany). 2000;14(6):525–526.
190. Kim MS, Stablein D, Harmon WE. Renal transplantation in children with congenital nephrotic syndrome: a report of the North American Pediatric Renal Transplant Co-operative Study (NAPRTCS). Pediatric Transplantation. 1998;2(4):305–308.
191. Vats AN, Donaldson L, Fine RN, et al. Pretransplant dialysis status and outcome of renal transplantation in North American children: a NAPRTCS Study. North American Pediatric Renal Transplant Co-operative Study. Transplantation. 2000;69(7):1414–1419.
192. McDonald RA, Smith JM, Stablein D, et al. Pretransplant peritoneal dialysis and graft thrombosis following pediatric kidney transplantation: A NAPRTCS report. Pediatric Transplantation. 2003;7(3):204–208.
193. Lundin C, Bersztel A, Wahlberg J, et al. Low molecular weight heparin prophylaxis increases the incidence of lymphocele after kidney transplantation. Upsala Journal of Medical Sciences. 2002;107(1):9–15.
194. Ona ET, Danguilan RA, Africa J, et al. Use of alemtuzumab (Campath-1H) as induction therapy in pediatric kidney transplantation. Transplantation Proceedings. 2008;40(7):2226–2229.

195. McDonald R, Smith J, Meyers K, et al. A phase II exploratory study to evaluate the safety of induction therapy with Campath-1H, combined with chronic immunosuppression with MMF and sirolimus: a study of the co-operative clinical trials in pediatric transplantation (abs). American Journal of Transplantation: Official Journal of the American Society of Transplantation and the American Society of Transplant Surgeons. 2008;8(s-2):192.
196. Tan HP, Kaczorowski D, Basu A, et al. Steroid-free tacrolimus monotherapy after pretransplantation thymoglobulin or campath and laparoscopy in living donor renal transplantation. Transplantation Proceedings. 2005;37(10):4235.
197. Shapiro R, Basu A, Tan H, et al. Kidney transplantation under minimal immunosuppression after pretransplant lymphoid depletion with Thymoglobulin or Campath. Journal of the American College of Surgeons. 2005;200(4):505.
198. Kaabak MM, Babenko NN, Samsonov DV, et al. Alemtuzumab induction in pediatric kidney transplantation. Pediatric Transplantation. 2013;17(2):168–178.
199. Sarwal MM. Out with the old, in with the new: immunosuppression minimization in children. Current Opinion in Organ Transplantation. 2008;13(5):513–521.
200. Barletta GM, Kirk E, Gardner JJ, et al. Rapid discontinuation of corticosteroids in pediatric renal transplantation. Pediatric Transplantation. 2009;13(5):571–578.
201. Chavers BM, Chang YC, Gillingham KJ, et al. Pediatric kidney transplantation using a novel protocol of rapid (6-day) discontinuation of prednisone: 2-year results. Transplantation. 2009;88(2):237–241.
202. Benfield MR, Bartosh S, Ikle D, et al. A randomized double-blind, placebo controlled trial of steroid withdrawal after pediatric renal transplantation. American Journal of Transplantation. 2010;10(1):81–88.
203. Sarwal M, Benfield MR, Ettenger RB, et al. One year results of a prospectie, randomized, multicenter trial of steroid avoidance in pediatric renal transplantation (abs). American Journal of Transplantation: Official Journal of the American Society of Transplantation and the American Society of Transplant Surgeons. 2008;8(s-2):192.
204. Hocker B, Weber LT, Feneberg R, et al. Prospective, randomized trial on late steroid withdrawal in pediatric renal transplant recipients under cyclosporine microemulsion and mycophenolate mofetil. Transplantation. 2009;87(6):934–941.
205. Hymes LC, Warshaw BL. Sirolimus in pediatric patients: results in the first 6 months post-transplant-renal transplant. Pediatric Transplantation. 2005;9(4):520–522.
206. McDonald RA, Smith JM, Ho M, et al. Incidence of PTLD in pediatric renal transplant recipients receiving basiliximab, calcineurin inhibitor, sirolimus and steroids. American Journal of Transplantation. 2008;8(5):984–989.
207. Harmon W, Meyers K, Ingelfinger J, et al. Safety and efficacy of a calcineurin inhibitor avoidance regimen in pediatric renal transplantation. Journal of the American Society of Nephrology: JASN. 2006;17(6):1735–1745.
208. Tilney NL. Early course of a patient. In: Morris PJ, editor. Kidney Transplantation: Principles and Practice. Philadelphia, PA: WB Saunders; 1988: 278–283.
209. Treves ST, Majd M, Kuruc A, et al. Kidneys. In: Treves WT, editor. Pediatric Nuclear Medicine, 2nd ed. New York, NY: Springer-Verlag; 1995: 339–399.
210. Peddi VR, Bryant M, Roy-Chaudhury P, et al. Safety, efficacy, and cost analysis of thymoglobulin induction therapy with intermittent dosing based on CD3+ lymphocyte counts in kidney and kidney-pancreas transplant recipients. Transplantation. 2002;73(9):1514–1518.
211. Dunnill MS. Histopathology of renal allograft rejection. In: Morris PJ, editor. Kidney Transplantation: Principles and Practice, 4th ed. Philadelphia, PA: WB Saunders; 1994: 266–285.
212. Nankivell BJ, Borrows RJ, Fung CL, et al. The natural history of chronic allograft nephropathy. The New England Journal of Medicine. 2003;349(24):2326–2333.
213. Solez K, Colvin RB, Racusen LC, et al. Banff '05 meeting report: differential diagnosis of chronic allograft injury and elimination of chronic allograft nephropathy ('CAN'). American Journal of Transplantation. 2007;7(3):518–526.
214. Feehally J, Harris KP, Bennett SE, et al. Is chronic renal transplant rejection a non-immunological phenomenon? Lancet. 1986;2(8505):486–488.
215. Tilney NL, Guttmann RD. Effects of initial ischemia/reperfusion injury on the transplanted kidney. [Review] [23 refs]. Transplantation. 1997;64(7):945–947.
216. Ishii Y, Sawada T, Kubota K, et al. Injury and progressive loss of peritubular capillaries in the development of chronic allograft nephropathy. Kidney International. 2005;67(1):321–332.
217. Streblow DN, Kreklywich C, Yin Q, et al. Cytomegalovirus-mediated upregulation of chemokine expression correlates with the acceleration of chronic rejection in rat heart transplants. Journal of Virology. 2003;77(3):2182–2194.
218. Tejani A, Cortes L, Stablein D. Clinical correlates of chronic rejection in pediatric renal transplantation. A report of the North American Pediatric Renal Transplant Co-operative Study. Transplantation. 1996;61(7):1054–1058.
219. Mizutani K, Terasaki P, Bignon JD, et al. Association of kidney transplant failure and antibodies against MICA. Human Immunology. 2006;67(9):683–691.
220. Hotchkiss H, Chu TT, Hancock WW, et al. Differential expression of profibrotic and growth factors in chronic allograft nephropathy. Transplantation. 2006;81(3):342–349.
221. Baqi N, Tejani A. Recurrence of the original disease in pediatric renal transplantation. Journal of Nephrology. 1997;10(2):85–92.
222. Seikaly MG. Recurrence of primary disease in children after renal transplantation: an evidence-based update. Pediatric Transplantation. 2004;8(2):113–119.
223. Hariharan S, Savin VJ. Recurrent and de novo disease after renal transplantation: a report from the Renal Allograft Disease Registry. Pediatric Transplantation. 2004;8(4):349–350.
224. Baum MA, Stablein DM, Panzarino VM, et al. Loss of living donor renal allograft survival advantage in children with focal segmental glomerulosclerosis. Kidney International. 2001;59(1):328–333.
225. Cochat P, Kassir A, Colon S, et al. Recurrent nephrotic syndrome after transplantation: early treatment with plasmaphaeresis and cyclophosphamide. Pediatric Nephrology (Berlin, Germany). 1993;7(1):50–54.
226. Dantal J, Bigot E, Bogers W, et al. Effect of plasma protein adsorption on protein excretion in kidney-transplant recipients with recurrent nephrotic syndrome. New England Journal of Medicine. 1994;330(1):7–14.
227. Cochat P, Schell M, Ranchin B, et al. Management of recurrent nephrotic syndrome after kidney transplantation in children. Clinical Nephrology. 1996;46(1):17–20.
228. Nathanson S, Cochat P, Andre JL, et al. Recurrence of nephrotic syndrome after renal transplantation: influence of increased immunosuppression. Pediatric Nephrology (Berlin, Germany). 2005;20(12):1801–1804.
229. Faul C, Donnelly M, Merscher-Gomez S, et al. The actin cytoskeleton of kidney podocytes is a direct target of the antiproteinuric effect of cyclosporine A. Nature Medicine. 2008;14(9):931–938.
230. Bayrakci US, Baskin E, Sakalli H, et al. Rituximab for post-transplant-transplant recurrences of FSGS. Pediatric Transplantation. 2009;13(2):240–243.
231. Marks SD, McGraw M. Does rituximab treat recurrent focal segmental glomerulosclerosis post-transplant-renal transplantation? Pediatric Nephrology (Berlin, Germany). 2007;22(1):158–160.
232. Nozu K, Iijima K, Fujisawa M, et al. Rituximab treatment for post-transplanttransplant lymphoproliferative disorder (PTLD) induces complete remission of recurrent nephrotic syndrome. Pediatric Nephrology (Berlin, Germany). 2005;20(11):1660–1663.
233. Yabu JM, Ho B, Scandling JD, et al. Rituximab failed to improve nephrotic syndrome in renal transplant patients with recurrent focal segmental glomerulosclerosis. American Journal of Transplantation. 2008;8(1):222–227.
234. Ferraris JR, Ramirez JA, Ruiz S, et al. Shiga toxin-associated hemolytic uremic syndrome: absence of recurrence after renal transplantation. Pediatric Nephrology (Berlin, Germany). 2002;17(10):809–814.
235. Loirat C, Niaudet P. The risk of recurrence of hemolytic uremic syndrome after renal transplantation in children. Pediatric Nephrology (Berlin, Germany). 2003;18(11):1095–1101.
236. Quan A, Sullivan EK, Alexander SR. Recurrence of hemolytic uremic syndrome after renal transplantation in children: a report of the North American Pediatric Renal Transplant Co-operative Study. Transplantation. 2001;72(4):742–745.
237. Krid S, Roumenina LT, Beury D, et al. Renal transplantation under prophylactic eculizumab in atypical hemolytic uremic syndrome with CFH/CFHR1 hybrid protein. American Journal of Transplantation. 2012;12(7):1938–1944.
238. Dorresteijn EM, van de Kar NC, Cransberg K. Eculizumab as rescue therapy for atypical hemolytic uremic syndrome with normal platelet count. Pediatric Nephrology (Berlin, Germany). 2012;27(7):1193–1195.
239. Nester C, Stewart Z, Myers D, et al. Pre-emptive eculizumab and plasmapheresis for renal transplant in atypical hemolytic uremic syndrome. Clinical Journal of the American Society of Nephrology. 2011;6(6):1488–1494.
240. Braun MC, Stablein DM, Hamiwka LA, et al. Recurrence of membranoproliferative glomerulonephritis type II in renal allografts: The North American Pediatric Renal Transplant Co-operative Study experience. Journal of the American Society of Nephrology. 2005;16(7):2225–2233.
241. Cochat P, Liutkus A, Fargue S, et al. Primary hyperoxaluria type 1: still challenging! Pediatric Nephrology (Berlin, Germany). 2006;21(8):1075–1081.
242. Ellis SR, Hulton SA, McKiernan PJ, et al. Combined liver-kidney transplantation for primary hyperoxaluria type 1 in young children.[comment]. Nephrology, Dialysis, Transplantation. 2001;16(2):348–354.
243. Gagnadoux MF, Lacaille F, Niaudet P, et al. Long term results of liver-kidney transplantation in children with primary hyperoxaluria. Pediatric Nephrology (Berlin, Germany). 2001;16(12):946–950.
244. Hoppe B, Langman CB. A United States survey on diagnosis, treatment, and outcome of primary hyperoxaluria. Pediatric Nephrology (Berlin, Germany). 2003;18(10):986–991.
245. Jamieson NV, European PHITSG. A 20-year experience of combined liver/kidney

transplantation for primary hyperoxaluria (PH1): the European PH1 transplant registry experience 1984-2004. American Journal of Nephrology. 2005;25(3): 282–289.
246. Harambat J, van Stralen KJ, Espinosa L, et al. Characteristics and outcomes of children with primary oxalosis requiring renal replacement therapy. Clinical Journal of the American Society of Nephrology. 2012;7(3):458–465.
247. Kashtan CE, McEnery PT, Tejani A, et al. Renal allograft survival according to primary diagnosis: a report of the North American Pediatric Renal Transplant Co-operative Study. Pediatric Nephrology (Berlin, Germany). 1995;9(6): 679–684.
248. Langlois V, Geary D, Murray L, et al. Polyuria and proteinuria in cystinosis have no impact on renal transplantation. A report of the North American Pediatric Renal Transplant Co-operative Study.[erratum appears in Pediatr Nephrol 2001 Feb;16(2):201]. Pediatric Nephrology (Berlin, Germany). 2000;15(1–2):7–10.
249. Nesterova G, Gahl W. Nephropathic cystinosis: late complications of a multisystemic disease. Pediatric Nephrology (Berlin, Germany). 2008;23(6):863–878.
250. Wuhl E, Haffner D, Offner G, et al. Long-term treatment with growth hormone in short children with nephropathic cystinosis. Journal of Pediatrics. 2001; 138(6):880–887.
251. Ueda M, O'Brien K, Rosing DR, et al. Coronary artery and other vascular calcifications in patients with cystinosis after kidney transplantation. Clinical Journal of the American Society of Nephrology. 2006;1(3):555–562.
252. van Lieburg AF, de Jong MC, Hoitsma AJ, et al. Renal transplant thrombosis in children. Journal of Pediatric Surgery. 1995;30(4):615–619.
253. Fine RN, Kohaut EC, Brown D, et al. Growth after recombinant human growth hormone treatment in children with chronic renal failure: report of a multicenter randomized double-blind placebo-controlled study. Genentech Co-operative Study Group. Journal of Pediatrics. 1994;124(3):374–382.
254. Fine RN, Becker Y, De Geest S, et al. Nonadherence consensus conference summary report. American Journal of Transplantation. 2009;9(1):35–41.
255. Meyers KE, Weiland H, Thomson PD. Paediatric renal transplantation non-compliance. Pediatric Nephrology (Berlin, Germany). 1995;9(2):189–192.
256. Beck DE, Fennell RS, Yost RL, et al. Evaluation of an educational program on compliance with medication regimens in pediatric patients with renal transplants. Journal of Pediatrics. 1980;96(6):1094–1097.
257. Ettenger RB, Rosenthal JT, Marik JL, et al. Improved cadaveric renal transplant outcome in children. Pediatric Nephrology (Berlin, Germany). 1991;5(1): 137–142.
258. Foulkes LM, Boggs SR, Fennell RS, et al. Social support, family variables, and compliance in renal transplant children. Pediatric Nephrology (Berlin, Germany). 1993;7(2):185–188.
259. Bell F. Post-transplant-renal transplant compliance. Journal of Child Health Care. 2000;4(1):5–9.
260. Blowey DL, Hebert D, Arbus GS, et al. Compliance with cyclosporine in adolescent renal transplant recipients. Pediatric Nephrology (Berlin, Germany). 1997;11(5):547–551.
261. Fennell RS, Foulkes LM, Boggs SR. Family-based program to promote medication compliance in renal transplant children. Transplantation Proceedings. 1994;26(1):102–103.
262. Traum AZ, Ko DS, Kawai T. The potential for tolerance in pediatric renal transplantation. Current Opinion in Organ Transplantation. 2008;13(5):489–494.
263. Dharnidharka V, Stablein D, Harmon W. Risk of hospitalization due to infection now exceeds risk due to acute rejection at early and late time oints in pediatric renal transplantation. American Journal of Transplantation. 2003;3(Suppl 5): 319.
264. Hanto DW, Frizzera G, Purtilo DT, et al. Clinical spectrum of lymphoproliferative disorders in renal transplant recipients and evidence for the role of Epstein-Barr virus. Cancer Research. 1981;41(11 Pt 1):4253–4261.
265. Nocera A, Ghio L, Dall'Amico R, et al. De novo cancers in paediatric renal transplant recipients: a multicentre analysis within the North Italy Transplant programme (NITp), Italy. European Journal of Cancer. 2000;36(1):80–86.
266. Ciancio G, Siquijor AP, Burke GW, et al. Post-transplant-transplant lymphoproliferative disease in kidney transplant patients in the new immunosuppressive era. Clinical Transplantation. 1997;11(3):243–249.
267. Dharnidharka VR, Tejani AH, Ho PL, et al. Post-transplant-transplant lymphoproliferative disorder in the United States: young Caucasian males are at highest risk. American Journal of Transplantation. 2002;2(10):993–998.
268. Chang H, Wu JD, Cheng KK, et al. Epstein-Barr virus-associated lymphoproliferative disorders in oral cavity after heart transplantation: report of a case. Journal of the Formosan Medical Association. 1994;93(4):332–336.
269. Renoult E, Aymard B, Gregoire MJ, et al. Epstein-Barr virus lymphoproliferative disease of donor origin after kidney transplantation: a case report. American Journal of Kidney Diseases. 1995;26(1):84–87.
270. Gonthier DM, Hartman G, Holley JL. Post-transplanttransplant lymphoproliferative disorder presenting as an isolated skin lesion. American Journal of Kidney Diseases. 1992;19(6):600–603.
271. Cen H, Williams PA, McWilliams HP, et al. Evidence for restricted Epstein-Barr virus latent gene expression and anti-EBNA antibody response in solid organ transplant recipients with post-transplanttransplant lymphoproliferative disorders. Blood. 1993;81(5):1393–1403.
272. Delecluse HJ, Kremmer E, Rouault JP, et al. The expression of Epstein-Barr virus latent proteins is related to the pathological features of post-transplant-transplant lymphoproliferative disorders. American Journal of Pathology. 1995;146(5): 1113–1120.
273. Cox KL, Lawrence-Miyasaki LS, Garcia-Kennedy R, et al. An increased incidence of Epstein-Barr virus infection and lymphoproliferative disorder in young children on FK506 after liver transplantation. Transplantation. 1995;59(4):524–529.
274. Andrews W, Sommerauer J, Roden J, et al. 10 years of pediatric liver transplantation. Journal of Pediatric Surgery. 1996;31(5):619–624.
275. Walker RC, Marshall WF, Strickler JG, et al. Pretransplantation assessment of the risk of lymphoproliferative disorder. Clinical Infectious Diseases : an Official Publication of the Infectious Diseases Society of America. 1995;20(5): 1346–1353.
276. Cockfield SM, Preiksaitis JK, Jewell LD, et al. Post-transplant-transplant lymphoproliferative disorder in renal allograft recipients. Clinical experience and risk factor analysis in a single center. Transplantation. 1993;56(1):88–96.
277. McDonald RA, McIntosh M, Stablein D, et al. Increased Incidence of PTLD in pediatric renal transplant recipients enrolled in a randomized controlled trial of steroid withdrawal: a study of the CCTPT (abs). American Journal of Transplantation. 2005;5(S11):418.
278. Sokal EM, Caragiozoglou T, Lamy M, et al. Epstein-Barr virus serology and Epstein-Barr virus-associated lymphoproliferative disorders in pediatric liver transplant recipients [see comments]. Transplantation. 1993;56(6): 1394–1398.
279. Cleper R, Ben Shalom E, Landau D, et al. Post-transplant-transplantation lymphoproliferative disorder in pediatric kidney-transplant recipients - a national study. Pediatric Transplantation. 2012;16(6):619–626.
280. Srivastava T, Zwick DL, Rothberg PG, et al. Post-transplanttransplant lymphoproliferative disorder in pediatric renal transplantation. Pediatric Nephrology (Berlin, Germany). 1999;13(9):748–754.
281. Swinnen LJ, Costanzo-Nordin MR, Fisher SG, et al. Increased incidence of lymphoproliferative disorder after immunosuppression with the monoclonal antibody OKT3 in cardiac-transplant recipients [see comments]. New England Journal of Medicine. 1990;323(25):1723–1728.
282. Ellis D, Shapiro R, Jordan ML, et al. Comparison of FK-506 and cyclosporine regimens in pediatric renal transplantation. Pediatric Nephrology (Berlin, Germany). 1994;8(2):193–200.
283. Kenagy DN, Schlesinger Y, Weck K, et al. Epstein-Barr virus DNA in peripheral blood leukocytes of patients with post-transplanttransplant lymphoproliferative disease. Transplantation. 1995;60(6):547–554.
284. Campe H, Jaeger G, Abou-Ajram C, et al. Serial detection of Epstein-Barr virus DNA in sera and peripheral blood leukocyte samples of pediatric renal allograft recipients with persistent mononucleosis-like symptoms defines patients at risk to develop post-transplant-transplant lymphoproliferative disease. Pediatric Transplantation. 2003;7(1):46–52.
285. Gupta M, Filler G, Kovesi T, et al. Quantitative tissue polymerase chain reaction for Epstein-Barr virus in pediatric solid organ recipients. American Journal of Kidney Diseases. 2003;41(1):212–219.
286. Wagner HJ, Wessel M, Jabs W, et al. Patients at risk for development of post-transplanttransplant lymphoproliferative disorder: plasma versus peripheral blood mononuclear cells as material for quantification of Epstein-Barr viral load by using real-time quantitative polymerase chain reaction. Transplantation. 2001;72(6):1012–1019.
287. Sato T, Fujieda M, Maeda A, et al. Monitoring of Epstein-Barr virus load and killer T cells in pediatric renal transplant recipients. Clinical Nephrology. 2008;70(5):393–403.
288. Rooney CM, Loftin SK, Holladay MS, et al. Early identification of Epstein-Barr virus-associated post-transplant-transplantation lymphoproliferative disease. British Journal of Haematology. 1995;89(1):98–103.
289. Falco DA, Nepomuceno RR, Krams SM, et al. Identification of Epstein-Barr virus-specific CD8+ T lymphocytes in the circulation of pediatric transplant recipients. Transplantation. 2002;74(4):501–510.
290. Tanaka E, Sato T, Ishihara M, et al. Asymptomatic high Epstein-Barr viral load carriage in pediatric renal transplant recipients. Pediatric Transplantation. 2011;15(3):306–313.
291. Shroff R, Trompeter R, Cubitt D, et al. Epstein-Barr virus monitoring in paediatric renal transplant recipients. Pediatric Nephrology (Berlin, Germany). 2002;17(9):770–775.
292. Harris KM, Schwartz ML, Slasky BS, et al. Post-transplanttransplantation cyclosporine-induced lymphoproliferative disorders: clinical and radiologic

manifestations. Radiology. 1987;162(3):697–700.
293. Chen JM, Barr ML, Chadburn A, et al. Management of lymphoproliferative disorders after cardiac transplantation. Annals of Thoracic Surgery. 1993;56(3): 527–538.
294. Taguchi Y, Purtilo DT, Okano M. The effect of intravenous immunoglobulin and interferon-alpha on Epstein-Barr virus-induced lymphoproliferative disorder in a liver transplant recipient. Transplantation. 1994;57(12):1813–1815.
295. Shapiro RS, Chauvenet A, McGuire W, et al. Treatment of B-cell lymphoproliferative disorders with interferon alfa and intravenous gamma globulin [letter]. New England Journal of Medicine. 1988;318(20):1334.
296. Pirsch JD, Stratta RJ, Sollinger HW, et al. Treatment of severe Epstein-Barr virus-induced lymphoproliferative syndrome with ganciclovir: two cases after solid organ transplantation. American Journal of Medicine. 1989;86(2):241–244.
297. Hocker B, Bohm S, Fickenscher H, et al. (Val-)Ganciclovir prophylaxis reduces Epstein-Barr virus primary infection in pediatric renal transplantation. Transplant International: Official Journal of the European Society for Organ Transplantation. 2012;25(7):723–731.
298. Davis CL, Harrison KL, McVicar JP, et al. Antiviral prophylaxis and the Epstein Barr virus-related post-transplant-transplant lymphoproliferative disorder. Clinical Transplantation. 1995;9(1):53–59.
299. Herman J, Vandenberghe P, van den Heuvel I, et al. Successful treatment with rituximab of lymphoproliferative disorder in a child after cardiac transplantation. Journal of Heart and Lung Transplantation. 2002;21(12):1304–1309.
300. Berney T, Delis S, Kato T, et al. Successful treatment of post-transplanttransplant lymphoproliferative disease with prolonged rituximab treatment in intestinal transplant recipients. Transplantation. 2002;74(7):1000–1006.
301. McGhee W, Mazariegos GV, Sindhi R, et al. Rituximab in the treatment of pediatric small bowel transplant patients with post-transplanttransplant lymphoproliferative disorder unresponsive to standard treatment. Transplantation Proceedings. 2002;34(3):955–956.
302. Serinet MO, Jacquemin E, Habes D, et al. Anti-CD20 monoclonal antibody (Rituximab) treatment for Epstein-Barr virus-associated, B-cell lymphoproliferative disease in pediatric liver transplant recipients.[comment]. Journal of Pediatric Gastroenterology and Nutrition. 2002;34(4):389–393.
303. Dotti G, Rambaldi A, Fiocchi R, et al. Anti-CD20 antibody (rituximab) administration in patients with late occurring lymphomas after solid organ transplant. Haematologica. 2001;86(6):618–623.
304. Zhao W, Fakhoury M, Fila M, et al. Individualization of valganciclovir prophylaxis for cytomegalovirus infection in pediatric kidney transplant patients. Therapeutic Drug Monitoring. 2012;34(3):326–330.
305. Paya C, Humar A, Dominguez E, et al. Efficacy and safety of valganciclovir vs. oral ganciclovir for prevention of cytomegalovirus disease in solid organ transplant recipients. American Journal of Transplantation. 2004;4(4): 611–620.
306. Lynfield R, Herrin JT, Rubin RH. Varicella in pediatric renal transplant recipients. Pediatrics. 1992;90(2 Pt 1):216–220.
307. Harmon WE. Opportunistic infections in children following renal transplantation. [Review] [80 refs]. Pediatric Nephrology (Berlin, Germany). 1991;5(1): 118–125.
308. Broyer M, Tete MJ, Guest G, et al. Varicella and zoster in children after kidney transplantation: long-term results of vaccination. Pediatrics. 1997; 99(1):35–39.
309. Zamora I, Simon JM, Da Silva ME, et al. Attenuated varicella virus vaccine in children with renal transplants. Pediatric Nephrology (Berlin, Germany). 1994;8(2):190–192.
310. Dharnidharka VR, Abdulnour HA, Araya CE. The BK virus in renal transplant recipients-review of pathogenesis, diagnosis, and treatment. Pediatric Nephrology (Berlin, Germany). 2011;26(10):1763–1774.
311. Smith JM, Davis CL. Screening for BK virus in pediatric renal transplant recipients. Pediatric Transplantation. 2010;14(5):559–560.
312. Smith JM, Dharnidharka VR, Talley L, et al. BK virus nephropathy in pediatric renal transplant recipients: an analysis of the North American Pediatric Renal Trials and Collaborative Studies (NAPRTCS) registry. Clinical Journal of the American Society of Nephrology. 2007;2(5):1037–1042.
313. Alexander RT, Langlois V, Tellier R, et al. The prevalence of BK viremia and urinary viral shedding in a pediatric renal transplant population: a single-center retrospective analysis. Pediatric Transplantation. 2006;10(5):586–592.
314. Araya CE, Garin EH, Neiberger RE, et al. Leflunomide therapy for BK virus allograft nephropathy in pediatric and young adult kidney transplant recipients. Pediatric Transplantation. 2010;14(1):145–150.
315. Harmon WE. Pediatric kidney transplantation (Chapter 75). In: Avner ED, Harmon WE, Niaudet P, et al., editors. Pediatric Nephrology, 6th ed. Springer; 2009: Oxford University, UK: 1867–1901.

第 114 章
儿童肝移植

John C. Bucuvalas, Sandy Feng

引言

对于儿童和成人肝移植,虽然在基本原则上对急性或者慢性肝脏疾病肝移植评估和选择是一样的,但候选人群显然是不同的。儿童受者和成人受者的区别,不仅是年龄不同,而且在肝脏的疾病谱、技术性变异移植物的渗透增加、疾病复发的风险减少、长期暴露于免疫抑制药物和生命活力的显著增加方面都是不同的[1]。

死亡供体器官分配

将死亡供体(DD)供肝分配给儿童候选人的方案是基于 2000 年建立监管框架并由美国卫生部在 2002 年实施。儿童终末期肝病(PELD)和梅奥终末期肝病(MELD)评分系统使用客观措施来估计疾病严重性和医疗紧急性。器官分配中涉及的伦理可在第 137 章中找到,国家分配政策在第 128 章被提及。PELD 评分包括年龄、人血白蛋白水平、总血清胆红素水平、国际标准化比率(INR)以及存在或不存在的发育延缓[2]。而 MELD 评分由血清胆红素水平、INR 和血清肌酐计算所得[3]。器官被分配给 12 岁以下的儿童根据 PELD 评分,而分配给 12~18 岁的青少年根据 MELD 评分。供肝提供方可以请求额外的 PELD / MELD 评估,因为单从一个区域审查委员会如果计算 PELD/MELD 评分被认为不足以反映患者疾病的严重程度[4-6]。

儿童肝移植指征

这里描述的数据是从研究中检索的儿童肝移植(SPLIT)注册表和在北美进行的 2000 多例儿童肝移植中获得。胆道闭锁是最常见的肝移植指征,约占全部病例的 37%。急性肝衰竭、再移植和原发性肝脏肿瘤(包括肝母细胞瘤)分别占 13.5%、10%和 9%。约 21.5%的儿童肝移植是因遗传基因缺陷而进行的移植:①胆汁淤积性疾病(4.5%);②药物治疗难治性的代谢疾病(无肝硬化)(6%);③代谢紊乱导致结构性肝损伤与肝硬化(11%)。剩余的情况包括:隐源性肝硬化、自身免疫性肝炎、硬化性胆管炎和线粒体肝病。原发病复发比较罕见,仅在因自身免疫性疾病或胆汁淤积性疾病而接受肝移植的受者中可能发生[7]。肝病分布在儿童和成年人之间存在差异,最明显是成人主要为丙型肝炎肝硬化、酒精和非酒精脂肪性肝炎和肝细胞癌。

胆道闭锁

对于胆道闭锁的儿童而言,肝移植可以改善生存。所有胆道闭锁的患者未经治疗,两岁以内均会死亡;超过 70%需要做肝移植[8-10]。移植是肝门肠吻合术失败患者唯一的选择。免疫抑制剂和手术技术的进步,使得胆道闭锁的受者活体肝移植 5 年生存率为 92.3%,死亡供体肝移植 5 年生存率为 85.8%(2009 年 OPTN / SRTR 1999—2008 年度报告。HHS / HRSA / HSB / DOT;UNOS;Arbor 研究协作健康)。对于年长患者做决定是复杂的,其在行肝门肠吻合术后可能出现并发症(门静脉高

表 114.1 儿童肝移植的适应证。来自 SPLIT 注册表(2005 年 6 月 1 日至 2009 年 5 月 31 日首次移植的患者)

主要诊断	原发性移植(%)
胆道闭锁	41.2%
Alagille 综合征	3.1%
急性肝衰竭	14.5%
肝肿瘤	5.2%
无肝硬化的代谢性肝病	11.2%
其他	15.8%

压症),生存收益不明确[9,11-14]。

急性肝衰竭

急性肝衰竭(ALF)由于疾病的特征(复杂且临床变化快),使得对儿童肝移植的决策更难。此外,移植后早期和晚期死亡率增高的风险损害了生存获益[15-17]。病因不确定的ALF与那些明确病因的ALF相比,需要肝移植的可能性增加1.5倍。后者包括儿童急性对乙酰氨基酚中毒、单纯疱疹和血细胞淋巴组织细胞增多症[16,18-21]。现有急性肝衰竭评分系统包括国王大学医院标准(KCH)[22]、Clichy评分[23,24]、MELD / PELD[24-26],但也不能可靠地区分那些能够生存的患者和需要移植的患者[16,21]。管理ALF儿童时面临紧迫的临床问题是:

1.儿童是否有可以治疗的病症?

2.每个连续的恶化或改善的风险是什么?

3.患者生存需要移植吗?

4.不移植可能完全恢复吗?

5.相关的疾病是否可以恢复或不可逆转?

肝脏肿瘤

肝母细胞瘤是儿童中最常见的原发性肝肿瘤,约占因恶性肿瘤肝移植的70%以及所有儿童肝移植的5%。根治性切除术后有良好的生存预后,>90%可无瘤生存。不幸的是,只有1/3的患者可行根治性切除术。其余可行新辅助化疗。即使对于在化疗后被认为不可切除的儿童,肝移植也是长期生存所必需的[27-29]。临床结果的主要预测因素是存在或不存在转移性疾病、组织学和肿瘤可切除性,由PRETEXT分期[27,30-32]确定。当前美国拨款政策规定的供肝分配状况表1B。

代谢性疾病

移植可以纠正由肝脏产生的变异蛋白和其他任意的结构损伤[33](表114.2)。对于具有结构性肝损伤的代谢性疾病亚组,进行移植的决定是基于生存收益和医疗紧急程度,由PELD /MELD评分确定。然而,对于没有结构性肝病的亚组,肝移植的目的不仅是为了纠正基因缺陷,而且为了防止由基因缺陷引起肝外器官的损伤。因此,紧急情况反映了不可逆转的中枢神经系统或肾脏损害风险,而不是死亡的风险。移植决策必须平衡风险,预防可能的肝外疾病进展需要多学科方法和相关专家共同参与。

表114.2 代谢性疾病儿童肝移植的适应证。来自SPLIT注册表(2005年6月1日至2009年5月31日首次移植的患者)

主要诊断	例数
α1-抗胰蛋白酶缺乏症	71
威尔森病	28
酪氨酸血症	24
原发性高草酸血症	6
囊性纤维化	37
尿素循环缺陷	58
Crigler-Najjar症	15
糖原贮积病	18
新生血液色素沉着病	13
先天性胆酸合成障碍	2

再移植

再移植的主要适应证是原发性无功能、肝动脉血栓形成、慢性排斥和晚期血管或胆汁并发症。原发性无功能和早期肝动脉血栓形成在医学上是急症,通常发生在移植后数天内。再移植后受者和移植物的存活率低于初次移植[34]。供者年龄小于1岁、使用技术性变异移植物和重新植入时的INR是生存的独立预测因子;INR可能作为肝衰竭的替代指标。

移植评估

一个儿童应该从被确定为不可逆的或潜在危及生命的肝脏疾病开始评估肝移植。评估的时间取决于儿童的临床状态以及对原发性疾病进展过程的理解。例如,一个无症状的6个月龄的胆道闭锁、血清胆红素8mg/dL的儿童需要在2岁前行肝移植,以确保生存。相比之下,6个月龄的有Alagille综合征的儿童在没有心脏病的情况下可能不需要移植。评估过程旨在:①估计移植提供的生存获益[35];②识别进行性和不可逆的非肝病是否存在移植的收益;③确定心理社会支持是否足以优化结果。

肝移植对生活质量的影响仍然很重要,需与患者和家属进行评估和讨论。然而,由于有限的生活质量数据、有限的肝移植时间及死亡供体短缺,生活数量替代了生活质量[4,36]。跨学科移植团队由外科医生、肝病专家、协调员、心理学家组成,社会工作者、财务顾问和其他相关顾问应参加候选人的评估。术前移植候选人的一般评估可以在第 29 章中找到。

生存获益

在许多情况下,没有足够的数据来提供关于肝移植对儿童的获益证据。和成人相比,短期生存获益受到肝病严重程度强烈影响。对于 PELD 评分为 17~27 的儿童,肝移植 1 个月后产生生存获益。相反,对于 PELD 评分为 7~16 的患者,生存获益没有累积直到移植后 10 个月[37]。

肝移植的一般禁忌是不可逆的多系统衰竭、肝外恶性肿瘤、肝胆外活动性感染系统或进行性和(或)不可逆的心肺或中枢神经系统疾病。但也有例外,单个可手术切除的肝母细胞瘤转移后不排除移植[27,28]。通常,对不可逆肝外疾病定义是模糊的。可以说,肝移植如果可能无用,就不应该考虑。但是,对无用的定义是难以确定的,因为它取决于复杂的相互作用的因素包括原发性诊断、移植中心技能和器官的可用性和质量。此外,定义对儿童的无用性可能不同于成年人,应更多考虑潜在的生存获益和较低的医疗负担。我们社会愿意接受儿童有更好的生存获益而带来增高的风险吗?SRTR 数据分析描绘了儿童肝移植后的第一年生存获益[38]。使用 PELD 评分作为疾病严重性的评估,无效阈值无法确定。由于缺乏一个定义阈值,所以一个有效的跨学科团队对于促进良好决策至关重要。

是否有心理社会支持足以优化结果?心理社会评估不仅关注于候选人,而且确定和减轻心理社会风险可能会优化移植后的效果[39]。结构化评估应旨在确定是否存在:①有儿童受虐的证据;②儿童或父母是抑郁症或有创伤后应激的证据;③家庭可以支持孩子移植过程。这些因素不应认为是移植的禁忌证,但需要由肝移植团队解决这些挑战。

移植前治疗

移植前的时间是具有显著风险的时间。对于不到 1 岁的儿童,急性肝衰竭的儿童在移植列表中是死亡率最高的[21,37](表 114.3)。移植的结果反映了多个过程的相互作用:①原发性疾病;②移植前护理;③器官分配;④供体/移植物质量;⑤手术和全身移植护理[40];这也在第 20 章和第 38 章中介绍过。

移植前期的护理影响早期患者和移植物存活。为了让儿童候选人在移植时达到医学和心理最佳优化状态,移植团队必须进行以下流程:①进行患儿和其家属的教育;②最大限度地得到合适的器官(活体或死亡供体);③优化营养状况;④预防感染;⑤预防和(或)治疗门静脉高压的并发症。

表 114.3 儿童肝移植以特定症状为主要指标的患病率。源自 SPLIT 注册表(2005 年 6 月 1 日至 2009 年 5 月 31 日的首次移植患者)

移植的主要指标	N	%
未成熟	255	26.6
腹水	308	32.1
自发性细菌性腹膜炎	31	3.2
肝性脑病	130	13.6
门静脉高血压出血	80	8.3
难治性瘙痒	99	10.3
其他	56	5.8
总计	959	100.0

肝肺综合征

肝肺综合征(HPS)是指在没有原发的心肺疾病情况下,出现严重肝脏疾病、室内空气下的低氧血症、肺内血管扩张[41,42]。HPS 是肝硬化受者不良预后的危险因素[43]。不过,HPS 在肝移植以后是可逆的,尤其是在发生严重低氧血症之前进行移植[44,45]。虽然儿童数据有限,肝移植对于成人 HPS 已显示能改善生存[45]。因此,当前的分配策略将 HPS 设定为移植的特殊指征。符合设定标准的成人的 MELD 评分相当于 3 个月 15%死亡率。MELD 评分每 3 个月增加 10%的死亡率。还没有为 HPS 儿童建立标准。

静脉曲张出血

肝移植预防静脉曲张的效果在成人中被认可,但在儿童中未知。急性静脉曲张出血的治疗应该与成人患者相同,从稳定血流动力学开始,接着进行诊断和治疗性内镜检查。

营养不良

充分营养的维持是一个挑战,慢性肝病影响营养摄入和内分泌功能,后者包括对生长激素的反应减弱[46]。基于来自 SPLIT 注册表的数据,40%的 2 岁以上移植候选者的体重和身高比标准低出一个或以上的标准差,甚至在移植时低于标准的两个标准差。看起来更大的比例患儿存在轻度的营养缺乏。优化具有中度或重度肝脏疾病严重性儿童的营养状况(MELD / PELD 评分> 15),需每月进行彻底的连续评估。深入地评估饮食史、身体测量和生长、审查药物和维生素/矿物质补充、测定能量、蛋白质、大量营养素和(或)微量营养素摄入量和流体要求。等待名单上营养充足的儿童在遭受感染可能性更小,而感染可以延迟移植或使移植复杂化。移植后,良好的营养状况可减少感染、改善伤口愈合以及降低顽固性腹水的风险[12,47]。

腹水和自发性腹膜炎

腹水管理应针对维持患者血容量、血清钠大于 130meq/L 以及足够的营养和呼吸状况。腹水突然明显增加可能反映门静脉血栓形成,应使用多普勒超声检查。成人的指导原则和管理策略也适用于儿童[48,49]。

自发性细菌性腹膜炎(SBP)定义为细菌性腹水感染但不能找到特定的感染源。注册表数据表明,SBP 发生在 10%的等待肝移植的儿童患者中。发热、脑病恶化、腹痛以及有腹水的患者的任何临床症状改变,应行诊断性腹水穿刺检查。SBP 最常由腹水中性粒细胞增多(> 250 细胞/mm^3)予以诊断,有或没有阳性培养。广谱抗生素治疗应在发现腹水中性粒细胞计数增多时开始。头孢噻肟是研究最广泛的抗生素,并涵盖三种最常见的分离细菌株:埃希氏菌属大肠杆菌,肺炎克雷伯氏菌和肺炎链球菌[48,49]。不需要重复穿刺,除非症状持续或对治疗的反应不典型。关于儿童患者的研究有限。即使如此,初级和二级预防可能改善儿童与肝硬化和腹水结果。当然,这通常是规定。

移植和手术技术

从历史上看,儿童肝移植在最初的肝移植和随后移植创新中起到了重要的作用。1963 年第一次尝试肝移植[50]和 1967 年第一次 3 个成功的肝移植都涉及幼儿[51]。后来,在 20 世纪 80 年代末,儿童肝移植在等待名单中的死亡率为 25%~46%(成人为 8%),由于缺乏大小匹配器官,这就需要创新[52-54]。肝脏的节段性解剖学启发外科医生移植部分移植物给合适的特定候选人[55,56]。最初,整个肝脏通过减体积到右叶、左叶或左外叶侧移植给 1 个儿童[53,57,58]。此后不久,创新性的将整个肝脏分成两个可移植的移植物完成 2 个儿童或 1 个成人和 1 个儿童的移植[58-60](图 114.1)。最初,劈裂式移植的并发症发生率高于全肝移植或减体积移植[59]。这些问题很快被克服,为最终的活体移植创新铺平道路[61,62]。随着移植技术的快速发展,等候名单死亡率急剧下降[54,63],从而使儿童肝脏移植的领域逐渐成熟。全肝移植手术的技术细节可以在第 56 章中找到。活体肝移植手术从 1989 年的两例(0.4%)稳步增加到 2000 年的 120 例(20.4%)(图 114.2)。随着 2002 年 2 月死亡供体器官分配政策的巨大变化,活体供体目前占所有儿童肝脏移植的 9%~12%。图 114.3 显示活体移植的比例因候选人年龄而异。活体供体移植一贯占婴儿移植最大比例(<1 岁),其次是幼儿(1~5 岁)。然而,有趣的是,在过去几年中年长儿童(6~17 岁)活体移植占较大比例,也许是成人至成人活体肝移植技术成熟的结果。

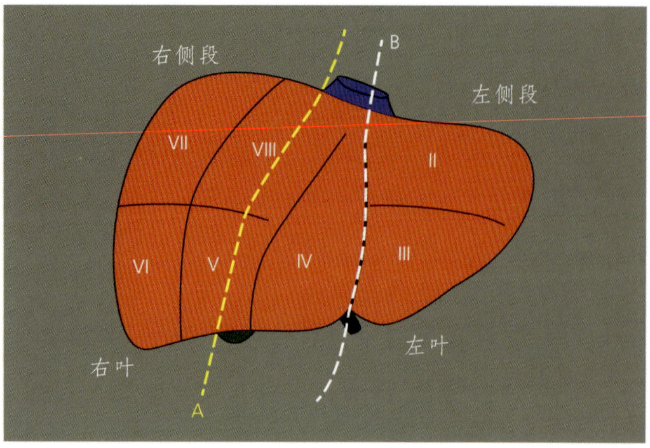

图 114.1 劈裂式肝移植。移植给一个儿童和一个成人,肝脏通常分为两个移植物,由白色虚线“B”表示:(A)左侧段(Couinaud 的 Ⅱ 和 Ⅲ 段)占肝脏质量的 20%~25%,和(B)右侧段(Couinaud 的 Ⅰ、Ⅳ~Ⅷ段)占肝脏质量的 75%~80%。左侧段通常伴有左肝静脉、左门静脉、腹腔轴与 Carrel 主动脉瓣和左肝管。右侧段的移植通常伴有下腔静脉、门静脉主段、右肝动脉和胆总管。另一种劈离方法是将肝脏分成右叶 (Couinaud 的 Ⅴ~Ⅷ段) 和左叶 (Couinaud 的 Ⅰ~Ⅳ段),如黄色虚线“A”所示。Reproduced from Renz JF, Yersiz H, Reichert PR, Hisatake GM, Farmer DG, Emond JC et al. Split-liver transplantation: a review. Am J Transplant 2003;3 (11):1323-1335, with permission from John Wiley and Sons.

移植后早期并发症

血管并发症

儿童肝移植的实质性技术挑战反映在移植后早期观察到的手术并发症发生率。肝动脉血栓形成(HAT)

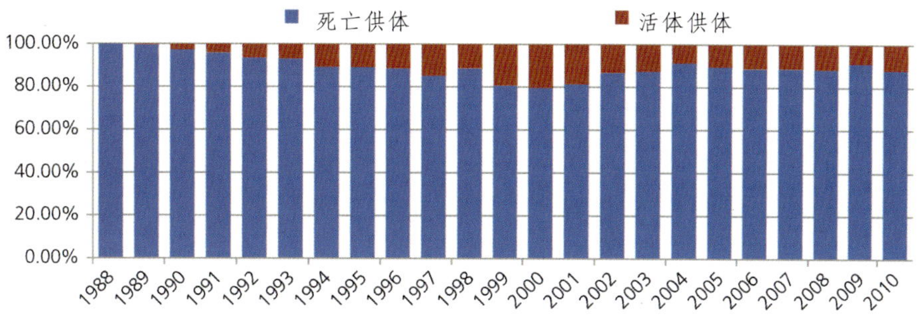

图 114.2 儿童(<18 岁)中死亡供体与活体肝移植的比例。自从第一例儿童活体供体肝移植在 1989 年实施以来,活体供体的比例在 1990 年后稳步上升。然而,2001 年 2 月根据 MELD/PELD 来进行肝脏分配的政策实施以来,全国活体供体肝移植数量下降,目前占儿童肝移植的 10%左右。基于 2012 年 1 月 12 日的 OPTN 数据。

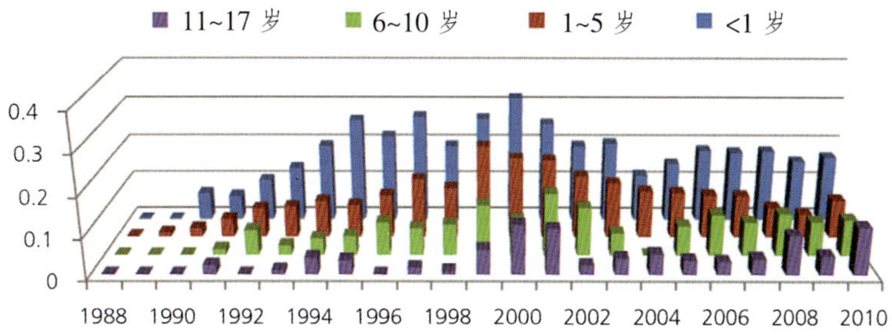

图 114.3 根据受者年龄划分的活体供体移植比例。活体供体移植的比例与供者年龄和移植年份有显著差异。虽然活体供体移植主要服务于婴儿和幼儿(0~5 岁),儿童肝移植的百分比似乎有相对增加。基于 2012 年 1 月 12 日的 OPTN 数据。

作为一种严重的潜在的威胁生命的儿童肝移植并发症。虽然 HAT 可以在临床上无症状,也可以导致急性的移植失败伴随大量的肝脏坏死或亚急性问题(如肝内脓肿形成或缺血性胆管并发症,如胆漏或胆道狭窄)。历史上,肝动脉血栓形成率高达 38%。但最近,许多中心发生率低于 10%[64-70]。类似于门静脉并发症,年龄小于 3 岁(体重小于 15kg)、使用整个移植物需和多个动脉重建和(或)单独的吻合时 HAT 的危险因素[67,68,70-72]。

由于血栓形成导致了对手术技术和额外的药物治疗方案的探索。早期,在死亡供体的全肝或部分肝移植中,动脉血管直接重建或通过移植物重建,间断缝合技术被作为先进技术[67,68,70,73]。然而,随着活体移植的出现,使用微血管手术技术与高放大倍数(大于 10×)大大降低肝动脉血栓发生率[66,74-77]。最近,许多报道建议高功率放大镜放大率(3.5 至 6×)可能就足够了[64,65,78]。抗凝策略减少 HAT 的风险。阿司匹林、肝素和(或)低分子量葡聚糖经常被使用,但疗效未得到证实[65,71,79,80]。

考虑到 HAT 干预的成功取决于早期诊断,许多儿童移植中心在肝移植后一或两周每日甚至每日两次进行多普勒超声检查[65]。可疑结果通常通过血管造影证实,尽管一些中心建议立即探查[72,81,82]。在手术室行取栓术进行或不进行溶栓治疗,同时需要重新评估原吻合口,并在必要时进行修改。也可进行完全抗凝。

发生 HAT 后,患者和移植物的预后是不一致的。许多报道表明,HAT 不影响移植后患者的存活[69,72,81]。然而,60%~75%的 HAT 发生后移植物存活明显受到损害,需要再移植[69,82,83]。急性血管重建的成功率为 30%~50%[69,82]。然而,即使成功进行血管重建后,许多 HAT 儿童仍患胆管并发症[69,72,84]。

门静脉并发症,最常见的是狭窄或血栓形成,是儿童肝移植后第二常见的血管并发症。据报发生率为 4%~16%。虽然早期观察到发生率较高,高于 35% [85-94]。门静脉并发症的潜在危险因素包括受者人口统计变量、解剖学和功能特征以及吻合技术。人口统计特征包括年龄≤1 岁和体重<10kg,门静脉并发症主要和门静脉直径较小有关[86,87,92,94]。此外,儿童胆道闭锁共存结构异常使门静脉重建复杂化。这些异常包括内脏异构(左异构)、脾异常(通常为多脾综合征)、十二指肠前门静脉、门静脉发育不全、无门静脉、无下腔静脉或先天性肠旋转不良[95-99]。最后,不利的功能特性因素包括低门静脉流量或非入肝性(波动、缺失或离肝),血流也与移植相关门静脉并发症增加有关[86,87,94]。

最常用的方法是供者和受者门静脉的端对端吻合。但是,如果受者门静脉不适宜,必须采用更复杂的策略。一个选择是完全切除门静脉在脾静脉和肠系膜静脉的汇合处端对端吻合,或与肠系膜上静脉进行端对侧吻合。其次可以进行门静脉成形术或使用静脉补片进行重建。相应地,使用导管或插入移植物增加了门静脉相关并发症[87,90,91]。

门静脉早期并发症使用手术取栓以及改进门静脉吻合、反射介入溶栓及支架治疗或联合治疗[97,100-102]。根据文献报道,一些小样本的单中心数据表明,治疗后门静脉有较好的长期通畅率。

第三种类型的儿童肝移植后血管并发症是静脉流出道梗阻。就像在成人中一样,经典原位移植比背驼式的静脉流出道并发症低。因此,特别是在儿童的部分肝移植的早期,流出道梗阻的发生率为17%~28%[62,103]。后期,发生率有所下降,为4.5%~10.5%[103-106]。人们普遍认为,一个简单的端对端吻合方法是移植物扭转的危险因素,可引起流出道梗阻,导致移植物功能障碍、液体潴留和腹水,甚至发生急性移植物衰竭。几个提出替代的吻合方法的重点是创造一个宽而短的流出道。包括用肝静脉汇合处剪开到下腔静脉进行三角吻合、或直接吻合到下腔静脉[62,103,107,108]。

临床上,静脉流出道问题在临床上早期表现为急性移植物衰竭。常见的表现为腹水进展和(或)外周水肿,有或没有移植物功能障碍的生化证据。建议用多普勒超声进行诊断,显示无典型的肝静脉多普勒频谱波形,并经颈静脉造影证实。在围移植期,若出现急性症状,外科干预通常应立即进行。另外,静脉流出道阻塞时,用经皮血管腔内治疗解决压力梯度[103,104,109,110]。首先尝试气囊扩张,初始的成功率和复发率都很高。压力梯度持续存在或复发应考虑行支架置入。对于临床症状的改善和移植物功能的保存的长期疗效良好。

胆道并发症

对于儿童肝移植来说,供肝和受体的胆管小,因此Roux-en-Y胆管空肠吻合术较胆总管端对端吻合术有明显的优势,是最佳吻合手术策略。血管并发症的发生率儿童高于成人,与此不同的是,胆道并发症发生率儿童与成人无明显差距,均为10%~33%[111-116]。胆道并发症主要是胆漏和胆道狭窄,其中胆漏更常见。尽管吻合彻底,胆漏也可能发生在移植物的切缘。胆道狭窄可发生在移植术后早期或晚期。类似的,吻合口狭窄较弥漫性肝内胆管狭窄更常见。儿童肝移植术后胆道并发症的危险因素有:肝动脉血栓导致胆道缺血,多胆管,ABO血型不相符肝移植[112-114,116]。移植类型(全肝移植或半肝移植)和供体来源(死亡供体或活体供体)与胆道并发症无相关性。最近,多项报道提到了胆总管端对端吻合术联合外支架的吻合手术策略[117-120]。从并发症的角度来说,转换成Roux-en-Y术式常常是必要的,特别是婴儿受者。

尽管非侵入检查手段(如超声影像、核素影像等)可以提示胆道并发症的发生,但经皮肝穿刺胆道造影仍是诊断金标准。当诊断确立时,优先评估肝动脉对于胆道并发症的治疗十分重要。在围移植期,通常立刻进行手术治疗,而在移植后期,更常使用经皮穿刺或胆道内镜治疗[121-125]。尽管胆道并发症发生率高,但其并不会影响移植物及受者的生存率。

早期移植术后管理注意事项

免疫抑制策略

在早期,移植术后免疫抑制仅仅依靠糖皮质激素和硫唑嘌呤,甚至当环孢素出现后,诱导免疫抑制还常常被用于成人及儿童肝移植。随着对如霉酚酸酯、他克莫司等更多更有效的免疫抑制因子的深入研究和探索,诱导免疫抑制被逐渐抛弃。然而,在儿童肝移植领域,随着糖皮质激素和钙调磷酸酶抑制剂毒性研究进展,诱导免疫抑制刮起了复兴之风。现在的观点是:与其通过诱导增加整体免疫抑制,减少急性排斥反应发生率,不如在诱导免疫抑制的辅助下,以不改变急性排斥反应的发生率、移植物和患者生存率为前提,尽量少用甚至完全不用糖皮质激素和(或)钙调磷酸酶抑制剂[117,126-132]。如今,儿童肝移植免疫抑制诱导率是31%。一线诱导免疫抑制剂为抗白介素2(IL-2)受体抗体及抗胸腺球蛋白抗体。历史上曾出现过两种抗IL-2受体抗体——巴利昔单抗和达克珠单抗,但后者现已不再使用。总体来说,抗IL-2受体抗体具有良好的安全性,不增加包括移植后淋巴组织增生性疾病在内的血液动力、代谢、肾脏、神经、感染等系统的恶性不良事件发生率[127-130,132]。

过去的20年里,免疫抑制维持疗法得到长足发展(详述于第66章)。众所周知,钙调磷酸酶抑制剂与环孢素将移植带入了新纪元,但其早已经被他克莫司取代。在随机对照试验中,与环孢素相比,他克莫司显著降低急性和慢性排斥反应，但不增加患者及移植物生存率[134-136]。与环孢素相比，他克莫司的毒性较复杂，其与糖尿病和移植后淋巴组织增生性疾病(PTLD)关系更加密切，但与多毛症及牙龈增生关系不大[137-141]。随着时间的推移，他克莫司的渗透率稳步提升，如今超过 90%的儿童肝移植受者因为他克莫司不用再住院治疗[142]。

与他克莫司和环孢素相似，霉酚酸酯作为抗代谢药已全面取代咪唑硫嘌呤，成为维持免疫抑制的一线药物。关于霉酚酸酯的研究最早出现于 1999 年，其联合微乳化环孢素和糖皮质激素的新疗法，与一项关于咪唑硫嘌呤的历史队列研究比较，作者认为在维持免疫抑制时更加安全有效，患者更易耐受且避免了静脉诱导免疫抑制[143]。有研究报道，使用霉酚酸酯可以通过减少钙调磷酸酶抑制剂的暴露从而提升肾功能[144-150]，且能作为难治性排斥反应的拯救疗法[148,151-153]。如今，40%的儿童肝移植受者使用霉酚酸酯维持免疫抑制。

随着他克莫司与霉酚酸酯的广泛应用，少用甚至避免使用糖皮质激素成为研究热点。第一个相关的研究是由 20 名受者组成的前瞻性队列，他们接受巴利昔单抗和他克莫司的治疗，并与一个同样由 20 名接受糖皮质激素和他克莫司治疗的受者组成的回顾性队列进行比较[131]。免类固醇方案(steroid free regimen)的受者术后第一年无排斥生存率更高，且随着时间的推移该差别更明显。随后更多研究证明，巴利昔单抗可以有效减少糖皮质激素的使用，且显著降低急性排斥反应、感染，特别是病毒感染的发生率。不使用糖皮质激素还能减少血压下降并增加补偿性生长。如今在美国，20%的儿童肝移植术后完全不使用糖皮质激素。尽管大部分患儿依然在肝移植时使用糖皮质激素，但为了更好地(补偿性)生长，减少糖皮质激素的使用是不可避免的趋势。移植一年后，大约仅有 40%的儿童肝移植受者仍使用糖皮质激素。

急性细胞性排斥的诊断和处理

儿童肝移植早期细胞排斥反应(术后 6 个月内)的诊断与治疗与成人差别不大，在第 70 章中已经涉及。鉴于儿童肝移植技术难度更高，手术并发症更多，超声和多普勒检查成为十分重要的评估移植物功能障碍的首选检查手段。如果没有明显的证据证明肝动脉、门静脉及胆道并发症的存在，则需要加做肝活检。最常用的肝活检手段是超声引导经皮肝穿刺活检。由放射科医生实施的颈静脉内穿刺使用也较广泛，因为出血都被限制在血管内[161,162]。

急性排斥反应的诊断和分级都基于 Banff 分类[163]，在第 82 章中已经涉及。在围移植期，主要的移植物功能障碍的原因有急性细胞性排斥反应、缺血再灌注损伤、移植物保存损伤和胆管周围炎症导致胆管狭窄等。如今，早期急性细胞性排斥反应的发生率为 40%~45%，且绝大多数发生在移植后 6 周内(如图 114.4)。对 SPLIT 数据库中数据的分析显示，与急性排斥反应独立负相关的因素有：移植时年龄在 0~5 个月与其他年龄相比；胆汁淤积、代谢及其他造成肝脏疾病的病因和胆道闭锁相比；ABO 血型不符与 ABO 血型相符相比；他克莫司与环孢素为主的其他免疫抑制剂相比；2002 年以后的移植[164]。

儿童肝移植术后早期急性细胞性排斥反应的治疗主要是静脉注射糖皮质激素。后续的组织活检可以有效评估疗效，特别是如果怀疑对激素不敏感时。当急性细胞性排斥反应不能被静脉注射糖皮质激素解决时，常常需要加用单克隆或多克隆抗体治疗。为了治疗急性排斥反应，除了诱导免疫抑制的剂量，还需加大剂量以维持免疫抑制。方案包括强化(增加剂量)、转化[137](单药到多药联合，特别是同一类型的)或添加(增加药物)[153,165-168]。在某些特定情况下，这些方案本身可能代表了不同的治疗方法[169]。尽管最温和且有效的治疗方案是最优选择，但应该避免因为治疗不充分而导致的慢性排斥反应，这是一个更难以处理和逆转的状况。

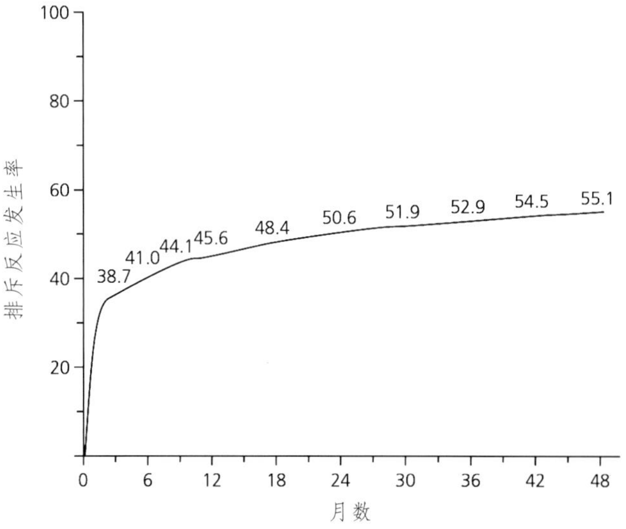

图 114.4 排斥反应发生可能性与移植后时间的关系。Kaplan-Meier 生存分析显示，1995—2006 年，2291 名在 SPLIT 数据库登记的儿童肝移植受者排斥发生可能性随着时间变化的规律。Reproduced from [164] Shepherd et al. with permission from John Wiley and Sons.

移植术后感染的处理

随着手术技术的进步和免疫抑制药物的研究深入，毫无疑问，全科医学已经和儿童肝移植密不可分，术后感染的预防、检测和治疗技术的进展对提高移植术后患者生存率有极大的改善。当免疫抑制治疗的强度和效率增加时，患者的耐受性也会随之降低，因此对感染的控制显得尤为重要。由于大多数儿童肝移植的受者是婴幼儿，他们缺乏对许多病原体的免疫力，因此儿童肝移植术后感染更常见。慢性肝病及营养不良，会削弱细胞免疫防御机制，从而诱发特定的感染，如自发性细菌性腹膜炎和胆源性脓毒症[170-172]。并且，移植时需抑制免疫，同样会增加感染的风险。因此，尽管试验研究已经取得进展，但是儿童肝移植术后感染依然是制约生活质量的重要因素之一[17,164,173-175]。

感染与移植术后时间的关系

虽然许多患儿准备接受移植手术时没有明显的感染，部分可能近期有感染或者目前感染已被控制，以及容易被忽视的情况（如留置导管），但是众所周知，未控制的感染是移植的禁忌证。像每一位经历了大手术的患者一样，儿童接受肝移植容易发生感染，涉及手术部位，尤其是当有不利的解剖或技术因素以及相关的留置装置，例如导尿管、血管导管和（或）气管内插管。移植后的第一个月内最常见的病原体是细菌，包括革兰阳性菌和革兰阴性菌以及念珠菌[164,175-178]。尽管抗细菌及抗真菌药物对于治疗十分重要，感染的治愈需要解决所有出现的解剖或技术问题，否则感染会复发，并且可能涉及用抗感染剂之前的抗药性微生物。SPLIT 来源的数据表明，38%的儿童肝移植受者在术后第一个月内有培养确诊的细菌或真菌感染[164]。

在移植术后的1~6个月内，假设可能出现的解剖及技术问题均被解决，机会性感染与社区获得性感染可能发生在免疫抑制治疗后[174,175]。针对念珠菌和肺孢子虫的预防措施已经有了预期的效果。尽管病毒感染或感染复发已经是一个重要的问题，但是其已经可以被预防用药和（或）预防治疗所控制，具体内容将在本章中详述。随着移植术后时间的推移，感染发生的可能性逐渐降低，特别是那些移植物功能良好且免疫抑制维持合理的患者。例外的情况有：接受针对排斥反应激进治疗的患儿、本身有慢性（常常是病毒）感染和移植物功能不理想。

重要的病毒感染：巨细胞病毒

巨细胞病毒（CMV）属于疱疹病毒家族，是一类DNA病毒，在肝移植术后免疫抑制状态下易感染。其临床症状包括无症状感染、自限性发热和严重的组织浸润性疾病（肺、肝、胃肠道，以及很少见的中枢神经系统）[174,175,178-181]。根据病毒复制状态，刚感染时可能没有症状，当产生临床症状时才成为感染性疾病。接受儿童肝移植的受者往往是婴幼儿，他们不曾感染 CMV，因此缺乏针对 CMV 的免疫力，这正是 CMV 感染和（或）感染性疾病最重要的危险因素。接触曾经感染过 CMV 的供体移植物和血液制品还会增加这一风险。原发感染被广泛认为是比继发感染毒性更强的感染状态。第二个重要的危险因素是在移植准备阶段接受了如兔抗胸腺细胞球蛋白或 OKT3 等抗体治疗[178,180,182,183]。在儿童肝移植中，这些药物常规应用于对糖皮质激素不耐受的患者，因此，这种状况比较少见。

为了提高 CMV 感染患者的生存率，降低死亡率，针对移植患者的免疫抑制主要有两种策略。许多中心根据风险预测，给予移植受者预防剂量抗病毒药物时，持续时间往往不同[184-189]。更昔洛韦在住院期间往往通过静脉注射，当出院后则按照预订的计划改成口服给药。这种做法简单易行，但是长期服用抗病毒药物会有副作用。数据显示，感染和感染性疾病常常出现于停用预防剂量药物后[181]，导致用药时间延长从而进一步增加毒性。另一种方法是在 CMV DNA 复制数量超过预警值之前即开始治疗[185-187]。该方案可有效减少药物剂量，但需要个体化治疗方案，因此需要耗费更多资源。因此，许多移植中心制订了多种混合策略，包括针对高危受者的预防性治疗和针对低危受者的早期治疗或在一段时间的监控后再行预防治疗。

CMV 感染和感染性疾病的诊断在过去几十年内发展迅速。如今，循环 CMV DNA 的检测是最重要的手段，早已经取代了 pp65 血抗原检测和血、尿或其他分泌物中的病毒培养[190-192]。病毒 DNA 阳性的患者必须根据临床情况做出相应处理。CMV DNA 可以在临床症状没有出现之前即可检测到。根据 DNA 浓度不同，可以考虑开始治疗或者后续检查。需要说明的是，CMV DNA 在组织浸润性疾病中可能无法被检测到，这种状况多见于胃肠道浸润性疾病。此时，当临床症状提示有感染时需要行组织活检以确诊。

最重要的治疗CMV感染和感染性疾病的药物是静脉内注射更昔洛韦,这是一种核苷类药物,其主要毒副作用是骨髓抑制。口服更昔洛韦或缬更昔洛韦(可提高生物利用度的前体药物)更常用于预防性或早期治疗,而后者现在正在研究用于常规治疗方案[181,182,184,186-189,193]。替代药物包括作为辅助治疗的CMV高效免疫球蛋白和膦甲酸钠,或拥有较少副作用的二线药物(如西多福韦等)。最后,应考虑针对严重CMV感染患者减少免疫抑制的程度。

重要的病毒感染

Epstein-Barr 病毒,包括移植后淋巴增生性疾病

Epstein-Barr病毒(EBV)是淋巴细胞疱疹病毒。EBV感染是许多疾病的病因,包括感染与恶性疾病,是导致儿童肝移植术后死亡的重要原因之一[178,194-198]。关于器官移植后淋巴增殖紊乱性疾病(PTLD)的内容参见第96章。与CMV一样,初次感染会导致更加严重的临床症状。婴幼儿往往在接受移植手术时,免疫系统尚不成熟且没有暴露于一些病原体,因此他们特别脆弱。初次感染发生于围移植期,通过移植物本身和(或)输血的血液制品传播,后者可以通过常规去除白细胞从而降低感染风险。急性感染可以完全没有症状,或者仅仅有通过血清学证实的轻微的非特异性病毒感染表现。同时,急性感染也可以产生一系列全身症状,如发热、全身乏力、厌食和肌痛。还可以有器官炎症的症状或体征,包括咽炎、淋巴结肿大、脾肿大、肝炎、肺炎和肠胃炎。EBV导致的炎症信号可以使淋巴细胞增生[主要(>85%)是B细胞],这也被认为是移植后淋巴增殖紊乱性疾病(PTLD)。除了免疫系统对EBV没有成熟的免疫力以外,全身免疫抑制是另一个众所周知的产生PTLD的危险因素[195,199-203]。

CMV和EBV感染和感染性疾病的处理有显著的相似之处,特别是两者的抗病毒药物结构是一致的[184]。一些中心使用预防治疗,或者是给所有受者,或者是给高危受者——不曾感染EBV且供体器官来自曾感染过的供者。另一些中心根据外周血EBV浓度使用早期治疗策略。因为PTLD的进展与“高”EBV DNA复制数量有关,因此减少免疫抑制从而增加抗病毒能力是治疗的重要组成部分。一些研究证实这一策略可有效减少PTLD的发生率[204-213]。PTLD的发病率已经从历史上的20%降低到如今的不到5%[199,200,207,214-216]。

通过临床、实验室和影像学检查需要精确评估疾病的预后及风险。PTLD的精准诊断需要进行组织活检。病理学分级是根据世界卫生组织制订的标准来划分。在儿童中,大部分PTLD是EBV感染所致,且组织分型多样。完整的病理学分型、临床表现及治疗方法的细节详见第96章。针对不同的器官,由活检确诊的PTLD的治疗需遵循一定的顺序,形成一个层次化结构性的治疗方案。在治疗金字塔的底部是减少免疫抑制,那些发生“早期病变”或者多形性疾病的患者身上,免疫抑制往往是过量的,在某些患有单形性疾病的儿童亦是如此。一些中心主张完全终止免疫抑制[217]。手术或放射治疗也可用于减轻症状或局限病灶。另一个现代医学治疗手段是利妥昔单抗,这是一种针对CD20的单克隆抗体,CD20在大部分PTLD患者中存在,是表达于B细胞表面的一类抗原。自从2002年,第一例用于PTLD儿童患者身上被报道以来,后续不断有研究证实其在CD20阳性PTLD患者治疗中所起的重要作用[218-221]。在治疗金字塔的顶端是标准化疗方案,该化疗方案是针对非移植诊断患有淋巴瘤的患者。许多研究报道,这一治疗方案明显降低PTLD的发病率与死亡率,从而可以制订较温和的治疗措施,进而减少药物的毒性以达到更好的治疗效果[222,223]。

儿童肝移植PTLD患者的结局表明,健康的受者和优质的供体器官之间的微妙平衡十分重要。PTLD确诊后最重要的死亡原因,既不是PTLD本身,也不是因为治疗PTLD所带来的毒副作用(感染、脓毒血症、多器官功能障碍或严重移植物功能障碍)。其中严重移植物失功是损失移植器官的重要原因之一,通常由免疫抑制减少导致的急性和继发性慢性排斥反应所引起[207,209,217]。过去10~20年间的研究报道,其死亡率从12%到60%。

晚期移植术后的挑战

在儿童肝移植中,晚期死亡与移植物失功并不常见。晚期死亡主要是由于免疫抑制的并发症,如感染(脓毒血症或多器官功能障碍)或恶性疾病(PTLD或肝母细胞瘤复发)[17,226]。而晚期移植物失功的原因主要是免疫抑制不足导致的慢性排斥反应或技术性并发症,如肝动脉血栓和(或)胆道狭窄。晚期死亡与移植物失功的高危因素有肝癌肝移植以及移植术后一年内入院次数超过5次。其他晚期死亡的独立危险因素有:重型肝衰竭的肝移植、受者体重过轻的肝移植和肝动脉血栓。其他晚期移植物失功的独立危险因素有:早期再次

手术和糖皮质激素抵抗急性细胞性排斥反应[17]。儿童在移植术后会面临更大的死亡和无免疫并发症风险,因其潜在寿命更长,有更多暴露于危险因素的机会。当前的免疫抑制治疗手段会增加糖尿病、高脂血症、高血压、肥胖和代谢综合征的风险。除了这些风险外,慢性免疫抑制还会影响患儿生长和器官功能恢复,进而决定健康相关生活质量,相关内容将在第118章中详述。如今,仅有1/3的超过10年生存期的患儿,在接受免疫抑制治疗的同时,拥有稳定的移植物功能、正常的生长发育以及没有发生免疫抑制导致的并发症。

晚期手术并发症

血管和胆道并发症在移植术后一年内常常被忽视,因此有着极大的发病率和潜在的移植物失功风险[17,226]。晚期肝动脉血栓可能没有任何临床症状,故其发病率未知。即使偶然诊断出患有肝动脉血栓,但是没有肝功能损害或临床症状的情况下,可以考虑不使用干预措施。晚期肝动脉血栓可能是难治性胆道并发症的诱因,而后者则需要再次移植。晚期胆道并发症在儿童肝移植中的发病率为13%,其中主要是胆道狭窄[111,116,228]。肝功能可以由一些常见的症状和体征来进行评估,特别是病情有起伏时或者胆道有炎症时。在制订治疗计划时,必须保证肝动脉的通畅。经皮导管或内镜介入是首选的治疗胆道狭窄的措施,特别是同时存在肝动脉血栓时,可以最大限度保存侧支循环[111,115,123]。发生反复胆源性败血症和(或)继发性胆汁性肝硬化时,再次移植不可避免。15%~20%的移植物失功归因于胆道并发症[17,226,229,230]。

晚期血管并发症发生率远低于胆道并发症[85,89,231]。门静脉狭窄或血栓的典型症状主要表现为门静脉高压,包括消化道出血、腹水和(或)肝脾肿大[85]。流出道狭窄常伴随腹水,伴或不伴有周围水肿。门静脉或肝静脉狭窄的首选治疗措施是球囊扩张。首次成功率高,但是易复发,因此需要频繁的扩张和支架置入[89,104,105,110,231]。门静脉血栓时必须规范处理由门静脉高压引起的各类并发症。

晚期移植物失功

移植物排斥

晚期移植物失功是指在移植术90天后发生的急性细胞性排斥反应,在临床上并不常见。仅发生于10%的儿童肝移植受者中,发生时间在术后3~12个月,再往后的发生率非常低(见图114.4)[164]。移植物排斥与免疫抑制治疗密切相关,无论是否严格遵守预定的治疗计划[232-234]。不遵从治疗计划引起的移植物排斥在儿童肝移植中常见,详细内容参见第120章。通过钙调磷酸酶抑制剂的变化来检测血药浓度,从而判断患者是否严格遵循治疗计划[235,236]。临床上,急性排斥反应常常没有明显症状,一般由肝功能检查异常疑诊,组织活检确诊。移植物组织活检是急性和(或)慢性排斥反应诊断和分级的金标准。活检应根据Banff全球评估标准做出解释[163](参见第82章)。当活检发现没有排斥反应时,其他可能导致肝功能异常的原因应全面考虑。

急性排斥反应的治疗策略应充分考虑临床和组织学特点,应排除可以证明不遵从治疗的证据和潜在的先前存在可能导致恶化的疾病,如肾功能不全或糖尿病。轻度或中度急性排斥反应(排斥活动指数小于6)可以强化治疗(增加剂量、用药频率或加用钙调磷酸酶抑制剂)、换更有效的药物、增加一种新药或以上几种方法的联合使用来进行治疗。如果肝功能没有在2周内稳定或改善,应使用糖皮质激素。中度到重度急性排斥反应应使用糖皮质激素,无论静脉注射、口服或者两者兼有。如果肝功能正常或回到基准值,可以考虑排斥反应消失。肝功能迟迟不恢复时,应考虑再行组织活检以确认排斥反应程度,判断是否为糖皮质激素不敏感型,进而考虑使用抗体药物,如兔抗胸腺细胞球蛋白或OKT3。慢性排斥反应不常见,在儿童肝移植受体中发生率低于2%[17]。尽管如此,慢性排斥反应导致40%的晚期移植物失功[17]。与使用环孢素为主的免疫抑制治疗相比,接受他克莫司治疗的受者慢性排斥反应发生率更低[136,237]。根据Banff标准,慢性排斥反应的诊断主要依靠肝组织学检查[136,238]。患儿在早期被确诊为慢性排斥反应,其病程进展尚可能被逆转,此时应加强免疫抑制。然而,除了一些早期从环孢素改为他克莫司的研究以外[137,239],尚未发现比再移植更有效的处理办法。

慢性肝炎与肝纤维化

儿童肝移植受者(甚至转氨酶正常)移植超过5年后发生慢性炎症和纤维化非常普遍[240,243]。不同严重程度的纤维化在移植术后10年内的发生率为75%。慢性肝炎和纤维化的病理学尚不明确,可能受不同移植技术引起的晚期并发症、典型排斥反应、慢性病毒性肝炎或新发自身免疫性肝炎的影响。对于临床、血清学和组织学可确诊的新发自身免疫性肝炎，硫唑嘌呤、糖皮质激素和(或)西罗莫司可能有效[244,245]。

免疫抑制药物引起的非免疫并发症

移植后肾病

儿童肝移植受体中，慢性肾功能不全的发生率为24%~70%[246-248]。患有先天性代谢异常、Alagille综合征、先天性肝纤维化的受体和那些在手术前接触对肾脏有害因素(化疗药物、氨基糖苷类药物)的患者，其术后慢性肾功能不全发生率增加[246,247,249]。有间接证据证明，围移植期急性肾损伤可导致术后慢性肾功能不全[250,251]。在这关键时期，对肾功能的保护措施有：密切监视血清肌酐值、维持足够的血容量、避免使用肾毒性药物和早期诊断与缓解急性肾损伤[252]。免疫抑制治疗可有效降低肾功能不全发生的风险，特别是针对那些曾患有肾脏疾病的患者和(或)在移植时肾小球滤过率(GFR)降低的受者。针对肾小球滤过率在移植术后降低，移植后一年以上的成人和儿童的观察与对照研究证实，减少钙调磷酸酶抑制剂剂量25%~50%和加用霉酚酸酯可有效提高肾功能[147]。

糖尿病

移植后新发糖尿病在儿童肝移植中发生率为10%~15%，较成人低[253-255]。移植后糖尿病平均持续时间为75天，推测可能是在围移植期使用大剂量糖皮质激素导致的[203]。危险因素有西班牙裔、青春期、肝囊性纤维化、糖皮质激素和他克莫司的使用[141,254]。与成人肝移植患者类似，早期减少或停用糖皮质激素可以有效控制血糖水平，特别是针对移植前就有糖尿病或有高危因素的患者。

新发恶性肿瘤

在成人中已经证实，实质器官移植受体在术后新发恶性肿瘤的可能性增加，而在儿童中相关数据尚未被报道[226,256-258]。一项有趣的试验证明，皮肤癌在儿童肝移植受者术后10~15年更罕见[259,260]，在一项瑞典的研究中，收集国家癌症注册中心1970—2007年所有的儿童实质性器官移植患者病例(536例)，仅有2例发生非黑色素瘤皮肤癌[261]。但是考虑到儿童潜在生存期长，对皮肤癌的预防措施仍是必要的。其他的癌症也有报道，但是与常规人群比较的相对危险度并无定论。危险因素、筛选标准和最优治疗方案在儿童肝移植受者中尚未建立。

健康相关生活质量

健康相关生活质量(HRQOL)涉及与健康直接相关的生活质量和潜在被健康护理系统影响的方面。世界健康组织定义组成健康相关生活质量的5个方面：①躯体健康；②心理健康；③社会功能；④角色功能；⑤通常健康观念[262-264]。一个北美的大型横断面多中心儿童肝移植研究表明，儿童肝移植受者较正常群体而言，包括学校功能在内的健康相关生活质量的各方面均下降，但最大的影响是在学校功能方面[265]。一个更细节的研究显示，肝移植受者与正常群体相比，平均智商至少在移植后的两年内是下降的[266](参见第119章)。在同样的队列里，肝移植受者较正常群体而言更经常出现学习障碍和执行功能的下降[265]。这个观察结果对教育策略的选择和受者不遵守的管理有明显的启示意义，并过渡到成人护理。

成人护理的过渡

儿童移植受者转换到成人导向的护理模式是一个复杂的问题，在第121章中有详细讲解。为了成功过渡到成人护理系统，青少年和年轻的成人必须知道他(她)的器官衰竭和需要移植的原因。患者应该意识到不同的行为，包括遵从医学指示的行为会促进好的结果，同时避免冒险行为，并且积累健康护理系统的知识[233,267-271]。医学遵从在过渡过程中被认为是一个非常重要的因素，而且在转换到成人护理后可能会减少医学遵从。为了确保一个安全的转换护理，将父母的责任转换到青少年和年轻的成人的策略应该在真正的转换护理前几年就开始实施。

总结

儿童肝移植已经是儿童终末期肝病的首选治疗，在实施过程中发展出许多与成人肝移植不同的做法。临床医生必须理解这些(包括技术、药理及社会等方面)的细微差别，才能投入到这个高度复杂却非常有意义的临床实践中。

(柯庆宏 译　柯庆宏 校)

参考文献

1. Bucuvalas JC, Campbell KM, Cole CR, et al. Outcomes after liver transplantation: keep the end in mind. Journal of Pediatric Gastroenterology and Nutrition. 2006;43(Suppl 1):S41-S48.
2. McDiarmid SV, Anand R, Lindblad AS. Development of a pediatric end-stage liver disease score to predict poor outcome in children awaiting liver transplantation. Transplantation. 2002;74(2):173-181.
3. Kamath PS, Wiesner RH, Malinchoc M, et al. A model to predict survival in patients with end-stage liver disease. Hepatology (Baltimore, Md.). 2001;33(2): 464-470.
4. Freeman RB. Mortality risk versus other endpoints: who should come first on the liver transplant waiting list? Liver Transplantation. 2004;10(5):675-677.
5. Olthoff KM, Brown RS Jr, Delmonico FL, et al. Summary report of a national conference: evolving concepts in liver allocation in the MELD and PELD era. Liver Transplantation. 2004;10(10 Suppl 2):A6-A22.
6. Voigt MD, Zimmerman B, Katz DA, et al. New national liver transplant allocation policy: is the regional review board process fair? Liver Transplantation. 2004;10(5):666-674.
7. Jara P, Hierro L, Martinez-Fernandez P, et al. Recurrence of bile salt export pump deficiency after liver transplantation. New England Journal of Medicine. 2009;361(14):1359-1367.
8. Utterson EC, Shepherd RW, Sokol RJ, et al. Biliary atresia: clinical profiles, risk factors, and outcomes of 755 patients listed for liver transplantation. Journal of Pediatrics. 2005;147(2):180-185.
9. Shneider BL, Brown MB, Haber B, et al. A multicenter study of the outcome of biliary atresia in the United States, 1997 to 2000. Journal of Pediatrics. 2006;148(4):467-474.
10. Shneider BL, Mazariegos GV. Biliary atresia: a transplant perspective. Liver Transplantation. 2007;13(11):1482-1495.
11. Barshes NR, Lee TC, Balkrishnan R, et al. Orthotopic liver transplantation for biliary atresia: the U.S. experience. Liver Transplantation. 2005;11(10): 1193-1200.
12. DeRusso PA, Ye W, Shepherd R, et al. Growth failure and outcomes in infants with biliary atresia: a report from the Biliary Atresia Research Consortium. Hepatology (Baltimore, Md.). 2007;46(5):1632-1638.
13. Karrer FM, Price MR, Bensard DD, et al. Long-term results with the Kasai operation for biliary atresia. Archives of Surgery (Chicago, Ill.: 1960). 1996; 131(5):493-496.
14. Sokol RJ, Mack CL. Optimizing outcomes and bridging biliary atresia into adulthood. Hepatology (Baltimore, Md.). 2005;41(2):231-233.
15. Baliga P, Alvarez S, Lindblad A, et al. Post-transplant survival in pediatric fulminant hepatic failure: the SPLIT experience. Liver Transplantation. 2004; 10(11):1364-1371.
16. Squires RH Jr, Shneider BL, Bucuvalas J, et al. Acute liver failure in children: the first 348 patients in the pediatric acute liver failure study group. Journal of Pediatrics. 2006;148(5):652-658.
17. Soltys KA, Mazariegos GV, Squires RH, et al. Late graft loss or death in pediatric liver transplantation: an analysis of the SPLIT database. American Journal of Transplantation. 2007;7(9):2165-2171.
18. Bucuvalas J, Yazigi N, Squires RH Jr. Acute liver failure in children. Clinics in Liver Disease. 2006;10(1):149-168, vii.
19. Filipovich AH. Life-threatening hemophagocytic syndromes: current outcomes with hematopoietic stem cell transplantation. Pediatric Transplantation. 2005;9(Suppl 7):87-91.
20. Filipovich AH. Hemophagocytic lymphohistiocytosis (HLH) and related disorders. Hematology / the Education Program of the American Society of Hematology. American Society of Hematology. Education Program. 2009;1: 127-131.
21. Squires RH Jr. Acute liver failure in children. Seminars in Liver Disease. 2008;28(2):153-166.
22. McPhail MJ, Wendon JA, Bernal W. Meta-analysis of performance of Kings's College Hospital Criteria in prediction of outcome in non-paracetamol-induced acute liver failure. Journal of Hepatology. 2010;53(3):492-499.
23. Blei AT. Selection for acute liver failure: have we got it right? Liver Transplantation. 2005;(11 Suppl 2):S30-S34.
24. Yantorno SE, Kremers WK, Ruf AE, et al. MELD is superior to King's college and Clichy's criteria to assess prognosis in fulminant hepatic failure. Liver Transplantation. 2007;13(6):822-828.
25. Rhee C, Narsinh K, Venick RS, et al. Predictors of clinical outcome in children undergoing orthotopic liver transplantation for acute and chronic liver disease. Liver Transplantation. 2006;12(9):1347-1356.
26. Sindhi R, Soltys K, Bond G, et al. PELD allocation and acute liver/graft failure. Liver Transplantation. 2007;13(5):776-777.
27. Faraj W, Dar F, Marangoni G, et al. Liver transplantation for hepatoblastoma. Liver Transplantation. 2008;14(11):1614-1619.
28. Otte JB, Pritchard J, Aronson DC, et al. Liver transplantation for hepatoblastoma: results from the International Society of Pediatric Oncology (SIOP) study SIOPEL-1 and review of the world experience. Pediatric Blood and Cancer. 2004;42(1):74-83.
29. Tiao GM, Bobey N, Allen S, et al. The current management of hepatoblastoma: a combination of chemotherapy, conventional resection, and liver transplantation. Journal of Pediatrics. 2005;146(2):204-211.
30. Aronson DC, Schnater JM, Staalman CR, et al. Predictive value of the pretreatment extent of disease system in hepatoblastoma: results from the International Society of Pediatric Oncology Liver Tumor Study Group SIOPEL-1 study. Journal of Clinical Oncology. 2005;23(6):1245-1252.
31. Perilongo G, Shafford E, Plaschkes J. SIOPEL trials using preoperative chemotherapy in hepatoblastoma. The Lancet Oncology. 2000;1:94-100.
32. Roebuck DJ, Aronson D, Clapuyt P, et al. 2005 PRETEXT: a revised staging system for primary malignant liver tumours of childhood developed by the SIOPEL group. Pediatric Radiology. 2007;37(2):123-132, quiz 249-150.
33. Hansen K, Horslen S. Metabolic liver disease in children. Liver Transplantation. 2008;14(5):713-733.
34. Ng V, Anand R, Martz K, et al. Liver retransplantation in children: a SPLIT database analysis of outcome and predictive factors for survival. American Journal of Transplantation. 2008;8(2):386-395.
35. Merion RM, Schaubel DE, Dykstra DM, et al. The survival benefit of liver transplantation. American Journal of Transplantation. 2005;5(2):307-313.
36. Freeman RB. MELD and the quality of life. Liver Transplantation. 2005; 11(2):134-136.
37. Magee JC, Krishnan SM, Benfield MR, et al. Pediatric transplantation in the United States, 1997-2006. American Journal of Transplantation. 2008;8(4 Pt 2):935-945.
38. Barshes NR, Lee TC, Udell IW, et al. The pediatric end-stage liver disease (PELD) model as a predictor of survival benefit and post-transplant survival in pediatric liver transplant recipients. Liver Transplantation. 2006;12(3):475-480.
39. Shemesh E. Assessment and management of psychosocial challenges in pediatric liver transplantation. Liver Transplantation. 2008;14(9):1229-1236.
40. Feng S, Goodrich NP, Bragg-Gresham JL, et al. Characteristics associated with liver graft failure: the concept of a donor risk index. American Journal of Transplantation. 2006;6(4):783-790.
41. Sarkar P, Basu AK, Mandal SK, et al. Hepatopulmonory syndrome-an uncommon and severe complication of certain liver diseases. Journal of the Indian Medical Association. 2005;103(9):469-470, 472.
42. Schenk P, Schoniger-Hekele M, Fuhrmann V, et al. Prognostic significance of the hepatopulmonary syndrome in patients with cirrhosis. Gastroenterology. 2003;125(4):1042-1052.
43. Arguedas MR, Abrams GA, Krowka MJ, et al. Prospective evaluation of outcomes and predictors of mortality in patients with hepatopulmonary syndrome undergoing liver transplantation. Hepatology (Baltimore, Md.). 2003;37(1):192-197.
44. Yi HM, Wang GS, Yi SH, et al. Prospective evaluation of postoperative outcome after liver transplantation in hepatopulmonary syndrome patients. Chinese Medical Journal. 2009;122(21):2598-2602.
45. Al-Hussaini A, Taylor RM, Samyn M, et al. Long-term outcome and management of hepatopulmonary syndrome in children. Pediatric Transplantation. 2010;14(2):276-282.
46. Bucuvalas JC, Cutfield W, Horn J, et al. Resistance to the growth-promoting and metabolic effects of growth hormone in children with chronic liver disease. Journal of Pediatrics. 1990;117(3):397-402.
47. Nightingale S, Ng VL. Optimizing nutritional management in children with chronic liver disease. Pediatric Clinics of North America. 2009;56(5): 1161-1183.
48. Runyon BA. Management of adult patients with ascites due to cirrhosis. Hepatology (Baltimore, Md.). 2004;39(3):841-856.
49. Runyon BA. Management of adult patients with ascites due to cirrhosis: an update. Hepatology (Baltimore, Md.). 2009;49(6):2087-2107.
50. Starzl TE, Marchioro TL, Vonkaulla KN, et al. Homotransplantation of the Liver in Humans. Surgery, Gynecology & Obstetrics. 1963;117:659-676.
51. Starzl TE, Groth CG, Brettschneider L, et al. Extended survival in 3 cases of orthotopic homotransplantation of the human liver. Surgery. 1968;63(4): 549-563.
52. Esquivel CO, Koneru B, Karrer F, et al. Liver transplantation before 1 year of age. Journal of Pediatrics. 1987;110(4):545-548.
53. Broelsch CE, Emond JC, Thistlethwaite JR, et al. Liver transplantation, including the concept of reduced-size liver transplants in children. Annals of Surgery.

1988;208(4):410-420.
54. de Ville de Goyet J, Hausleithner V, Reding R, et al. Impact of innovative techniques on the waiting list and results in pediatric liver transplantation. Transplantation. 1993;56(5):1130-1136.
55. Couinaud C. [Contribution of anatomical research to liver surgery]. France Medecine. 1956;19(5):5-12.
56. Couinaud C. [Surgical anatomy of the liver. Several new aspects]. Chirurgie; Memoires de l'Academie de Chirurgie. 1986;112(5):337-342.
57. Otte JB, Yandza T, de Ville de Goyet J, et al. Pediatric liver transplantation: report on 52 patients with a 2-year survival of 86%. Journal of Pediatric Surgery. 1988;23(3):250-253.
58. Ringe B, Burdelski M, Rodeck B, et al. Experience with partial liver transplantation in Hannover. Clinical Transplants. 1990;135-144.
59. Broelsch CE, Emond JC, Whitington PF, et al. Application of reduced-size liver transplants as split grafts, auxiliary orthotopic grafts, and living related segmental transplants. Annals of Surgery. 1990;212(3):368-375, discussion 375-367.
60. Otte JB, de Ville de Goyet J, Alberti D, et al. The concept and technique of the split liver in clinical transplantation. Surgery. 1990;107(6):605-612.
61. Broelsch CE, Whitington PF, Emond JC, et al. Liver transplantation in children from living related donors. Annals of Surgery. 1991;214(4):428-437, discussion 437-429. Surgical techniques and results.
62. Emond JC, Heffron TG, Whitington PF, et al. Reconstruction of the hepatic vein in reduced size hepatic transplantation. Surgery, Gynecology & Obstetrics. 1993;176(1):11-17.
63. Otte JB, de Ville de Goyet J, Sokal E, et al. Size reduction of the donor liver is a safe way to alleviate the shortage of size-matched organs in pediatric liver transplantation. Annals of Surgery. 1990;211(2):146-157.
64. Guarrera JV, Sinha P, Lobritto SJ, et al. Microvascular hepatic artery anastomosis in pediatric segmental liver transplantation: microscope vs loupe. Transplant International. 2004;17(10):585-588.
65. Heffron TG, Welch D, Pillen T, et al. Low incidence of hepatic artery thrombosis after pediatric liver transplantation without the use of intraoperative microscope or parenteral anticoagulation. Pediatric Transplantation. 2005; 9(4):486-490.
66. Inomoto T, Nishizawa F, Sasaki H, et al. Experiences of 120 microsurgical reconstructions of hepatic artery in living related liver transplantation. Surgery. 1996;119(1):20-26.
67. Rela M, Muiesan P, Bhatnagar V, et al. Hepatic artery thrombosis after liver transplantation in children under 5 years of age. Transplantation. 1996;61(9): 1355-1357.
68. Stevens LH, Emond JC, Piper JB, et al. Hepatic artery thrombosis in infants. A comparison of whole livers, reduced-size grafts, and grafts from living-related donors. Transplantation. 1992;53(2):396-399.
69. Stringer MD, Marshall MM, Muiesan P, et al. Survival and outcome after hepatic artery thrombosis complicating pediatric liver transplantation. Journal of Pediatric Surgery. 2001;36(6):888-891.
70. Tan KC, Yandza T, de Hemptinne B, et al. Hepatic artery thrombosis in pediatric liver transplantation. Journal of Pediatric Surgery. 1988;23(10):927-930.
71. Mazzaferro V, Esquivel CO, Makowka L, et al. Hepatic artery thrombosis after pediatric liver transplantation-a medical or surgical event? Transplantation. 1989;47(6):971-977.
72. Uchida Y, Sakamoto S, Egawa H, et al. The impact of meticulous management for hepatic artery thrombosis on long-term outcome after pediatric living donor liver transplantation. Clinical Transplantation. 2009;23(3):392-399.
73. Busuttil RW, Seu P, Millis JM, et al. Liver transplantation in children. Annals of Surgery. 1991;213(1):48-57.
74. Mori K, Nagata I, Yamagata S, et al. The introduction of microvascular surgery to hepatic artery reconstruction in living-donor liver transplantation-its surgical advantages compared with conventional procedures. Transplantation. 1992;54(2):263-268.
75. Tanaka K, Uemoto S, Tokunaga Y, et al. Surgical techniques and innovations in living related liver transplantation. Annals of Surgery. 1993;217(1):82-91.
76. Bade SA, Bayley GJ, Coren RA, et al. Microsurgical hepatic artery reconstruction in paediatric liver transplantation. Hepato-Gastroenterology. 2009;56(94-95): 1414-1416.
77. Panossian A, Diamond I, Fecteau A, et al. Hepatic artery microvascular anastomosis in pediatric living donor liver transplantation: a review of 35 consecutive cases by a single microvascular surgeon. Journal of Reconstructive Microsurgery. 2009;25(7):439-443.
78. Enne M, Pacheco-Moreira L, Balbi E, et al. Hepatic artery reconstruction in pediatric living donor liver transplantation under 10 kg, without microscope use. Pediatric Transplantation. 2010;14(1):48-51.
79. Hashikura Y, Kawasaki S, Okumura N, et al. Prevention of hepatic artery thrombosis in pediatric liver transplantation. Transplantation. 1995;60(10): 1109-1112.
80. Wolf DC, Freni MA, Boccagni P, et al. Low-dose aspirin therapy is associated with few side effects but does not prevent hepatic artery thrombosis in liver transplant recipients. Liver Transplantation and Surgery: Official Publication of the American Association for the Study of Liver Diseases and the International Liver Transplantation Society. 1997;3(6):598-603.
81. Nishida S, Kato T, Levi D, et al. Effect of protocol Doppler ultrasonography and urgent revascularization on early hepatic artery thrombosis after pediatric liver transplantation. Archives of Surgery (Chicago, Ill.: 1960). 2002;137(11): 1279-1283.
82. Warnaar N, Polak WG, de Jong KP, et al. Long-term results of urgent revascularization for hepatic artery thrombosis after pediatric liver transplantation. Liver Transplantation. 2010;16(7):847-855.
83. Martin SR, Atkison P, Anand R, et al. Studies of pediatric liver transplantation 2002: patient and graft survival and rejection in pediatric recipients of a first liver transplant in the United States and Canada. Pediatric Transplantation. 2004;8(3):273-283.
84. Garcia-Gallont R, Bar-Nathan N, Shaharabani E, et al. Hepatic artery thrombosis in pediatric liver transplantation: graft salvage after thrombectomy. Pediatric Transplantation. 1999;3(1):74-78.
85. Buell JF, Funaki B, Cronin DC, et al. Long-term venous complications after full-size and segmental pediatric liver transplantation. Annals of Surgery. 2002;236(5):658-666.
86. Cheng YF, Chen CL, Huang TL, et al. Risk factors for intraoperative portal vein thrombosis in pediatric living donor liver transplantation. Clinical Transplantation. 2004;18(4):390-394.
87. de Magnee C, Bourdeaux C, De Dobbeleer F, et al. Impact of pretransplant liver hemodynamics and portal reconstruction techniques on post-transplant portal vein complications in pediatric liver transplantation: a retrospective analysis in 197 recipients. Annals of Surgery. 2011;254(1):55-61.
88. Jean-Bernard O. Approach to avoid and to manage vascular thrombosis and stenosis in pediatric liver transplantation. Pediatric Transplantation. 2007; 11(2):124-126.
89. Kawano Y, Mizuta K, Sugawara Y, et al. Diagnosis and treatment of pediatric patients with late-onset portal vein stenosis after living donor liver transplantation. Transplant International: Official Journal of the European Society for Organ Transplantation. 2009;22(12):1151-1158.
90. Millis JM, Seaman DS, Piper JB, et al. Portal vein thrombosis and stenosis in pediatric liver transplantation. Transplantation. 1996;62(6):748-754.
91. Saad S, Tanaka K, Inomata Y, et al. Portal vein reconstruction in pediatric liver transplantation from living donors. Annals of Surgery. 1998;227(2):275-281.
92. Suzuki L, de Oliveira IR, Widman A, et al. Real-time and Doppler US after pediatric segmental liver transplantation: I. Portal vein stenosis. Pediatric Radiology. 2008;38(4):403-408.
93. Yilmaz A, Arikan C, Tumgor G, et al. Vascular complications in living-related and deceased donation pediatric liver transplantation: single center's experience from Turkey. Pediatric Transplantation. 2007;11(2):160-164.
94. Ou HY, Concejero AM, Huang TL, et al. Portal vein thrombosis in biliary atresia patients after living donor liver transplantation. Surgery. 2011;149(1):40-47.
95. Andreani P, Srinivasan P, Ball CS, et al. Congenital absence of the portal vein in liver transplantation for biliary atresia. International Journal of Surgical Investigation. 2000;2(1):81-84.
96. Falchetti D, de Carvalho FB, Clapuyt P, et al. Liver transplantation in children with biliary atresia and polysplenia syndrome. Journal of Pediatric Surgery. 1991;26(5):528-531.
97. Funaki B, Rosenblum JD, Leef JA, et al. Angioplasty treatment of portal vein stenosis in children with segmental liver transplants: mid-term results. AJR. American Journal of Roentgenology. 1997;169(2):551-554.
98. Karrer FM, Hall RJ, Lilly JR. Biliary atresia and the polysplenia syndrome. Journal of Pediatric Surgery. 1991;26(5):524-527.
99. Tanano H, Hasegawa T, Kawahara H, et al. Biliary atresia associated with congenital structural anomalies. Journal of Pediatric Surgery. 1999;34(11): 1687-1690.
100. Bueno J, Perez-Lafuente M, Venturi C, et al. No-touch hepatic hilum technique to treat early portal vein thrombosis after pediatric liver transplantation. American Journal of Transplantation. 2010;10(9):2148-2153.
101. Cheng YF, Ou HY, Tsang LL, et al. Vascular stents in the management of portal venous complications in living donor liver transplantation. American Journal of Transplantation. 2010;10(5):1276-1283.
102. Wei BJ, Zhai RY, Wang JF, et al. Percutaneous portal venoplasty and stenting for anastomotic stenosis after liver transplantation. World Journal of Gastroenterology. 2009;15(15):1880-1885.
103. Tannuri U, Mello ES, Carnevale FC, et al. Hepatic venous reconstruction in pediatric living-related donor liver transplantation-experience of a single center. Pediatric Transplantation. 2005;9(3):293-298.
104. Cheng YF, Chen CL, Huang TL, et al. Angioplasty treatment of hepatic vein

stenosis in pediatric liver transplants: long-term results. Transplant International: Official Journal of the European Society for Organ Transplantation. 2005;18(5): 556–561.
105. Krishna Kumar G, Sharif K, Mayer D, et al. Hepatic venous outflow obstruction in paediatric liver transplantation. Pediatric Surgery International. 2010; 26(4):423–425.
106. Sakamoto S, Egawa H, Kanazawa H, et al. Hepatic venous outflow obstruction in pediatric living donor liver transplantation using left-sided lobe grafts: Kyoto University experience. Liver Transplantation. 2010;16(10):1207–1214.
107. Ringe B, Pichlmayr R, Burdelski M. A new technique of hepatic vein reconstruction in partial liver transplantation. Transplant International. 1988;1(1):30–35.
108. Tannuri U, Santos MM, Tannuri AC, et al. Which is the best technique for hepatic venous reconstruction in pediatric living-donor liver transplantation? Experience from a single center. Journal of Pediatric Surgery. 2011;46(7): 1379–1384.
109. Sakamoto S, Ogura Y, Shibata T, et al. Successful stent placement for hepatic venous outflow obstruction in pediatric living donor liver transplantation, including a case series review. Pediatric Transplantation. 2009;13(4):507–511.
110. Carnevale FC, Machado AT, Moreira AM, et al. Midterm and long-term results of percutaneous endovascular treatment of venous outflow obstruction after pediatric liver transplantation. Journal of Vascular and Interventional Radiology. 2008;19(10):1439–1448.
111. Anderson CD, Turmelle YP, Darcy M, et al. Biliary strictures in pediatric liver transplant recipients - early diagnosis and treatment results in excellent graft outcomes. Pediatric Transplantation. 2010;14(3):358–363.
112. Bhatnagar V, Dhawan A, Chaer H, et al. The incidence and management of biliary complications following liver transplantation in children. Transplant International. 1995;8(5):388–391.
113. Egawa H, Uemoto S, Inomata Y, et al. Biliary complications in pediatric living related liver transplantation. Surgery. 1998;124(5):901–910.
114. Heffron TG, Emond JC, Whitington PF, et al. Biliary complications in pediatric liver transplantation. A comparison of reduced-size and whole grafts. Transplantation. 1992;53(2):391–395.
115. Kling K, Lau H, Colombani P. Biliary complications of living related pediatric liver transplant patients. Pediatric Transplantation. 2004;8(2):178–184.
116. Salvalaggio PR, Whitington PF, Alonso EM, et al. Presence of multiple bile ducts in the liver graft increases the incidence of biliary complications in pediatric liver transplantation. Liver Transplantation. 2005;11(2):161–166.
117. Ando H, Kaneko K, Ono Y, et al. Biliary reconstruction with wide-interval interrupted suture to prevent biliary complications in pediatric living-donor liver transplantation. Journal of Hepato-Biliary-Pancreatic Sciences. 2011;18(1): 26–31.
118. Liu C, Loong CC, Hsia CY, et al. Duct-to-duct biliary reconstruction in selected cases in pediatric living-donor left-lobe liver transplantation. Pediatric Transplantation. 2009;13(6):693–696.
119. Sakamoto S, Egawa H, Ogawa K, et al. The technical pitfalls of duct-to-duct biliary reconstruction in pediatric living-donor left-lobe liver transplantation: the impact of stent placement. Pediatric Transplantation. 2008;12(6):661–665.
120. Tanaka H, Fukuda A, Shigeta T, et al. Biliary reconstruction in pediatric live donor liver transplantation: duct-to-duct or Roux-en-Y hepaticojejunostomy. Journal of Pediatric Surgery. 2010;45(8):1668–1675.
121. Funaki B, Zaleski GX, Straus CA, et al. Percutaneous biliary drainage in patients with nondilated intrahepatic bile ducts. AJR. American Journal of Roentgenology. 1999;173(6):1541–1544.
122. Belenky A, Mor E, Bartal G, et al. Transhepatic balloon dilatation of early biliary strictures in pediatric liver transplantation: successful initial and mid-term outcome. Cardiovascular and Interventional Radiology. 2004;27(5):491–494.
123. Lorenz JM, Denison G, Funaki B, et al. Balloon dilatation of biliary-enteric strictures in children. AJR. American Journal of Roentgenology. 2005;184(1): 151–155.
124. Sunku B, Salvalaggio PR, Donaldson JS, et al. Outcomes and risk factors for failure of radiologic treatment of biliary strictures in pediatric liver transplantation recipients. Liver Transplantation. 2006;12(5):821–826.
125. Miraglia R, Maruzzelli L, Caruso S, et al. Interventional radiology procedures in pediatric patients with complications after liver transplantation. Radiographics: A Review Publication of the Radiological Society of North America, Inc. 2009;29(2):567–584.
126. Dell-Olio D, Kelly DA. Calcineurin inhibitor minimization in pediatric liver allograft recipients. Pediatric Transplantation. 2009;13(6):670–681.
127. Ganschow R, Broering DC, Stuerenburg I, et al. First experience with basiliximab in pediatric liver graft recipients. Pediatric Transplantation. 2001;5(5):353–358.
128. Ganschow R, Grabhorn E, Schulz A, et al. Long-term results of basiliximab induction immunosuppression in pediatric liver transplant recipients. Pediatric Transplantation. 2005;9(6):741–745.
129. Gras JM, Gerkens S, Beguin C, et al. Steroid-free, tacrolimus-basiliximab immunosuppression in pediatric liver transplantation: clinical and pharmacoeconomic study in 50 children. Liver Transplantation. 2008;14(4):469–477.
130. Heffron TG, Pillen T, Smallwood GA, et al. Pediatric liver transplantation with daclizumab induction. Transplantation. 2003;75(12):2040–2043.
131. Reding R, Gras J, Sokal E, et al. Steroid-free liver transplantation in children. Lancet. 2003;362(9401):2068–2070.
132. Spada M, Petz W, Bertani A, et al. Randomized trial of basiliximab induction versus steroid therapy in pediatric liver allograft recipients under tacrolimus immunosuppression. American Journal of Transplantation. 2006;6(8):1913–1921.
133. Di Filippo S. Anti-IL-2 receptor antibody vs. polyclonal anti-lymphocyte antibody as induction therapy in pediatric transplantation. Pediatric Transplantation. 2005;9(3):373–380.
134. McDiarmid SV, Farmer DA, Goldstein LI, et al. A randomized prospective trial of steroid withdrawal after liver transplantation. Transplantation. 1995;60(12): 1443–1450.
135. Kelly D, Jara P, Rodeck B, et al. Tacrolimus and steroids versus ciclosporin microemulsion, steroids, and azathioprine in children undergoing liver transplantation: randomised European multicentre trial. Lancet. 2004;364(9439): 1054–1061.
136. Jain A, Mazariegos G, Pokharna R, et al. The absence of chronic rejection in pediatric primary liver transplant patients who are maintained on tacrolimus-based immunosuppression: a long-term analysis. Transplantation. 2003; 75(7):1020–1025.
137. Reding R, Wallemacq PE, Lamy ME, et al. Conversion from cyclosporine to FK506 for salvage of immunocompromised pediatric liver allografts. Efficacy, toxicity, and dose regimen in 23 children. Transplantation. 1994;57(1):93–100.
138. McDiarmid SV, Busuttil RW, Ascher NL, et al. FK506 (tacrolimus) compared with cyclosporine for primary immunosuppression after pediatric liver transplantation. Results from the U.S. Multicenter Trial. Transplantation. 1995;59(4): 530–536.
139. Cacciarelli TV, Esquivel CO, Cox KL, et al. Oral tacrolimus (FK506) induction therapy in pediatric orthotopic liver transplantation. Transplantation. 1996; 61(8):1188–1192.
140. Jain A, Mazariegos G, Kashyap R, et al. Comparative long-term evaluation of tacrolimus and cyclosporine in pediatric liver transplantation. Transplantation. 2000;70(4):617–625.
141. Hathout E, Alonso E, Anand R, et al. Post-transplant diabetes mellitus in pediatric liver transplantation. Pediatric Transplantation. 2009;13(5):599–605.
142. Organ procurement and transplantation network and scientific registry of transplant recipients 2010 data report. American Journal of Transplantation. 2012;12(Suppl 1):1–156.
143. Renz JF, Lightdale J, Mudge C, et al. Mycophenolate mofetil, microemulsion cyclosporine, and prednisone as primary immunosuppression for pediatric liver transplant recipients. Liver Transplantation and Surgery: Official Publication of the American Association for the Study of Liver Diseases and the International Liver Transplantation Society. 1999;5(2):136–143.
144. Aw MM, Samaroo B, Baker AJ, et al. Calcineurin-inhibitor related nephrotoxicity-reversibility in paediatric liver transplant recipients. Transplantation. 2001;72(4):746–749.
145. Nobili V, Comparcola D, Sartorelli MR, et al. Mycophenolate mofetil in pediatric liver transplant patients with renal dysfunction: preliminary data. Pediatric Transplantation. 2003;7(6):454–457.
146. Ferraris JR, Duca P, Prigoshin N, et al. Mycophenolate mofetil and reduced doses of cyclosporine in pediatric liver transplantation with chronic renal dysfunction: changes in the immune responses. Pediatric Transplantation. 2004;8(5): 454–459.
147. Evans HM, McKiernan PJ, Kelly DA. Mycophenolate mofetil for renal dysfunction after pediatric liver transplantation. Transplantation. 2005;79(11):1575–1580.
148. Klupp J, Pfitzmann R, Langrehr JM, et al. Indications of mycophenolate mofetil in liver transplantation. Transplantation. 2005;80(1 Suppl):S142–S146.
149. Mention K, Lahoche-Manucci A, Bonnevalle M, et al. Renal function outcome in pediatric liver transplant recipients. Pediatric Transplantation. 2005;9(2): 201–207.
150. Tannuri U, Gibelli NE, Maksoud-Filho JG, et al. Mycophenolate mofetil promotes prolonged improvement of renal dysfunction after pediatric liver transplantation: experience of a single center. Pediatric Transplantation. 2007;11(1):82–86.
151. Chardot C, Nicoluzzi JE, Janssen M, et al. Use of mycophenolate mofetil as rescue therapy after pediatric liver transplantation. Transplantation. 2001;71(2): 224–229.
152. Aw MM, Taylor RM, Verma A, et al. Basiliximab (simulect) for the treatment of steroid-resistant rejection in pediatric liver transpland recipients: a preliminary experience. Transplantation. 2003;75(6):796–799.
153. Aw MM, Verma A, Rela M, et al. Long-term outcome of mycophenolate mofetil

rescue therapy for resistant acute allograft rejection in pediatric liver transplant recipients. Liver Transplantation. 2008;14(9):1303–1308.
154. Agarwal A, Pescovitz MD. Immunosuppression in pediatric solid organ transplantation. Seminars in Pediatric Surgery. 2006;15(3):142–152.
155. Alonso EM, Shepherd R, Martz KL, et al. Linear growth patterns in prepubertal children following liver transplantation. American Journal of Transplantation. 2009;9(6):1389–1397.
156. Al-Sinani S, Dhawan A. Corticosteroids usage in pediatric liver transplantation: to be or not to be! Pediatric Transplantation. 2009;13(2):160–170.
157. Diem HV, Sokal EM, Janssen M, et al. Steroid withdrawal after pediatric liver transplantation: a long-term follow-up study in 109 recipients. Transplantation. 2003;75(10):1664–1670.
158. Lopez-Espinosa J, Yeste D, Iglesias J, et al. Analysis of growth during prepubertal years in long-term survivors after pediatric orthotopic liver transplantation. Journal of Pediatric Endocrinology & Metabolism: JPEM. 2004;17(9): 1221–1229.
159. Reding R. Steroid withdrawal in liver transplantation: benefits, risks, and unanswered questions. Transplantation. 2000;70(3):405–410.
160. Saito T, Mizuta K, Hishikawa S, et al. Growth curves of pediatric patients with biliary atresia following living donor liver transplantation: factors that influence post-transplantation growth. Pediatric Transplantation. 2007;11(7): 764–770.
161. Miraglia R, Maruzzelli L, Spada M, et al. Transjugular liver biopsy in pediatric patients with left split liver transplantation and severe coagulation impairment. Pediatric Transplantation. 2012;16(1):58–62.
162. Smith TP, Presson TL, Heneghan MA, et al. Transjugular biopsy of the liver in pediatric and adult patients using an 18-gauge automated core biopsy needle: a retrospective review of 410 consecutive procedures. AJR. American Journal of Roentgenology. 2003;180(1):167–172.
163. Demetris A, Adams D, Bellamy C, et al. Update of the International Banff Schema for Liver Allograft Rejection: working recommendations for the histopathologic staging and reporting of chronic rejection. An International Panel. Hepatology (Baltimore, Md.). 2000;31(3):792–799.
164. Shepherd RW, Turmelle Y, Nadler M, et al. Risk factors for rejection and infection in pediatric liver transplantation. American Journal of Transplantation. 2008;8(2):396–403.
165. Jara P, Robledo MJ, Frauca E, et al. Tacrolimus for steroid-resistant liver rejection in children. Transplant International. 1998;11(Suppl 1):S275–S277.
166. Reggiani P, Gridelli B, Colledan M, et al. Rescue FK506 early conversion for refractory rejection after pediatric liver transplantation: experience in 20 children. Transplant International. 1998;11(Suppl 1):S272–S274.
167. Reyes J, Jain A, Mazariegos G, et al. Long-term results after conversion from cyclosporine to tacrolimus in pediatric liver transplantation for acute and chronic rejection. Transplantation. 2000;69(12):2573–2580.
168. Basso MS, Subramaniam P, Tredger M, et al. Sirolimus as renal and immunological rescue agent in pediatric liver transplant recipients. Pediatric Transplantation. 2011;15(7):722–727.
169. Feng S, Ekong UD, Lobritto SJ, et al. Complete immunosuppression withdrawal and subsequent allograft function among pediatric recipients of parental living donor liver transplants. JAMA: Journal of the American Medical Association. 2012;307(3):283–293.
170. Maggiore G, De Giacomo C, Marconi M, et al. Defective neutrophil motility in children with chronic liver disease. American Journal of Diseases of Children. 1983;137(8):768–770.
171. Kaido T, Mori A, Oike F, et al. Impact of pretransplant nutritional status in patients undergoing liver transplantation. Hepato-Gastroenterology. 2010; 57(104):1489–1492.
172. Cakir M, Arikan C, Akman SA, et al. Infectious complications in pediatric liver transplantation candidates. Pediatric Transplantation. 2010;14(1):82–86.
173. Fridell JA, Jain A, Reyes J, et al. Causes of mortality beyond 1 year after primary pediatric liver transplant under tacrolimus. Transplantation. 2002;74(12): 1721–1724.
174. Fonseca-Aten M, Michaels MG. Infections in pediatric solid organ transplant recipients. Seminars in Pediatric Surgery. 2006;15(3):153–161.
175. Allen U, Green M. Prevention and treatment of infectious complications after solid organ transplantation in children. Pediatric Clinics of North America. 2010;57(2):459–479.
176. George DL, Arnow PM, Fox A, et al. Patterns of infection after pediatric liver transplantation. American Journal of Diseases of Children. 1992;146(8): 924–929.
177. Gladdy RA, Richardson SE, Davies HD, et al. Candida infection in pediatric liver transplant recipients. Liver Transplantation and Surgery: Official Publication of the American Association for the Study of Liver Diseases and the International Liver Transplantation Society. 1999;5(1):16–24.
178. Saint-Vil D, Luks FI, Lebel P, et al. Infectious complications of pediatric liver transplantation. Journal of Pediatric Surgery. 1991;26(8):908–913.
179. Breinig MK, Zitelli B, Starzl TE, et al. Epstein-Barr virus, cytomegalovirus, and other viral infections in children after liver transplantation. Journal of Infectious Diseases. 1987;156(2):273–279.
180. Pehlivanoglu E, Ament ME, Spolidoro JV, et al. Severe cytomegalovirus infection and immunosuppressive therapy in pediatric liver transplantation. The Turkish Journal of Pediatrics. 1990;32(1):3–11.
181. Bedel AN, Hemmelgarn TS, Kohli R. Retrospective review of the incidence of cytomegalovirus infection and disease post liver transplantation in pediatric patients: comparison of prophylactic oral ganciclovir versus oral valganciclovir. Liver Transplantation. 2012;18(3):347–354.
182. Dussaix E, Wood C. Cytomegalovirus infection in pediatric liver recipients. A virological survey and prophylaxis with CMV immune globulin and early DHPG treatment. Transplantation. 1989;48(2):272–274.
183. King SM, Petric M, Superina R, et al. Cytomegalovirus infections in pediatric liver transplantation. American Journal of Diseases of Children. 1990; 144(12):1307–1310.
184. Green M, Kaufmann M, Wilson J, et al. Comparison of intravenous ganciclovir followed by oral acyclovir with intravenous ganciclovir alone for prevention of cytomegalovirus and Epstein-Barr virus disease after liver transplantation in children. Clinical Infectious Diseases: An Official Publication of the Infectious Diseases Society of America. 1997;25(6):1344–1349.
185. Campbell AL, Herold BC. Strategies for the prevention of cytomegalovirus infection and disease in pediatric liver transplantation recipients. Pediatric Transplantation. 2004;8(6):619–627.
186. Gerna G, Lilleri D, Callegaro A, et al. Prophylaxis followed by preemptive therapy versus preemptive therapy for prevention of human cytomegalovirus disease in pediatric patients undergoing liver transplantation. Transplantation. 2008;86(1): 163–166.
187. Madan RP, Campbell AL, Shust GF, et al. A hybrid strategy for the prevention of cytomegalovirus-related complications in pediatric liver transplantation recipients. Transplantation. 2009;87(9):1318–1324.
188. Lapidus-Krol E, Shapiro R, Amir J, et al. The efficacy and safety of valganciclovir vs. oral ganciclovir in the prevention of symptomatic CMV infection in children after solid organ transplantation. Pediatric Transplantation. 2010;14(6):753–760.
189. Bueno J, Ramil C, Green M. Current management strategies for the prevention and treatment of cytomegalovirus infection in pediatric transplant recipients. Paediatric Drugs. 2002;4(5):279–290.
190. Macartney M, Gane EJ, Portmann B, et al. Comparison of a new quantitative cytomegalovirus DNA assay with other detection methods. Transplantation. 1997;63(12):1803–1807.
191. Aw MM, Murugasu B, Tan AW, et al. Quantitation of peripheral blood cytomegalovirus DNA for monitoring recurrent cytomegalovirus retinitis in pediatric solid organ transplant recipients. Pediatric Transplantation. 2000;4(2):100–106.
192. Kullberg-Lindh C, Ascher H, Krantz M, et al. Quantitative analysis of CMV DNA in children the first year after liver transplantation. Pediatric Transplantation. 2003;7(4):296–301.
193. Megison SM, Andrews WS. Combination therapy with ganciclovir and intravenous IgG for cytomegalovirus infections in pediatric liver transplant recipients. Transplantation. 1991;52(1):151–154.
194. Lamy ME, Favart AM, Cornu C, et al. Epstein-Barr virus infection in 59 orthotopic liver transplant patients. Medical Microbiology and Immunology. 1990;179(3):137–144.
195. Cox KL, Lawrence-Miyasaki LS, Garcia-Kennedy R, et al. An increased incidence of Epstein-Barr virus infection and lymphoproliferative disorder in young children on FK506 after liver transplantation. Transplantation. 1995;59(4):524–529.
196. Martinez OM, Villanueva JC, Lawrence-Miyasaki L, et al. Viral and immunologic aspects of Epstein-Barr virus infection in pediatric liver transplant recipients. Transplantation. 1995;59(4):519–524.
197. Bodeus M, Smets F, Reding R, et al. Epstein-Barr virus infection in sixty pediatric liver graft recipients: diagnosis of primary infection and virologic follow-up. The Pediatric Infectious Disease Journal. 1999;18(8):698–702.
198. Smets F, Bodeus M, Goubau P, et al. Characteristics of Epstein-Barr virus primary infection in pediatric liver transplant recipients. Journal of Hepatology. 2000; 32(1):100–104.
199. Newell KA, Alonso EM, Whitington PF, et al. Post-transplant lymphoproliferative disease in pediatric liver transplantation. Interplay between primary Epstein-Barr virus infection and immunosuppression. Transplantation. 1996;62(3):370–375.
200. Sokal EM, Antunes H, Beguin C, et al. Early signs and risk factors for the increased incidence of Epstein-Barr virus-related post-transplant lymphoproliferative diseases in pediatric liver transplant recipients treated with tacrolimus. Transplantation. 1997;64(10):1438–1442.
201. Cao S, Cox KL, Berquist W, et al. Long-term outcomes in pediatric liver recipients: comparison between cyclosporin a and tacrolimus. Pediatric Transplanta-

tion. 1999;3(1):22-26.
202. Younes BS, McDiarmid SV, Martin MG, et al. The effect of immunosuppression on post-transplant lymphoproliferative disease in pediatric liver transplant patients. Transplantation. 2000;70(1):94-99.
203. Cacciarelli TV, Reyes J, Jaffe R, et al. Primary tacrolimus (FK506) therapy and the long-term risk of post-transplant lymphoproliferative disease in pediatric liver transplant recipients. Pediatric Transplantation. 2001;5(5):359-364.
204. Rogers BB, Conlin C, Timmons CF, et al. Epstein-Barr virus PCR correlated with viral histology and serology in pediatric liver transplant patients. Pediatric Pathology and Laboratory Medicine: Journal of the Society for Pediatric Pathology, Affiliated With the International Paediatric Pathology Association. 1997;17(3):391-400.
205. Rowe DT, Qu L, Reyes J, et al. Use of quantitative competitive PCR to measure Epstein-Barr virus genome load in the peripheral blood of pediatric transplant patients with lymphoproliferative disorders. Journal of Clinical Microbiology. 1997;35(6):1612-1615.
206. Green M, Cacciarelli TV, Mazariegos GV, et al. Serial measurement of Epstein-Barr viral load in peripheral blood in pediatric liver transplant recipients during treatment for post-transplant lymphoproliferative disease. Transplantation. 1998;66(12):1641-1644.
207. McDiarmid SV, Jordan S, Kim GS, et al. Prevention and preemptive therapy of postransplant lymphoproliferative disease in pediatric liver recipients. Transplantation. 1998;66(12):1604-1611.
208. Kogan DL, Burroughs M, Emre S, et al. Prospective longitudinal analysis of quantitative Epstein-Barr virus polymerase chain reaction in pediatric liver transplant recipients. Transplantation. 1999;67(7):1068-1070.
209. Gridelli B, Spada M, Riva S, et al. Circulating Epstein-Barr virus DNA to monitor lymphoproliferative disease following pediatric liver transplantation. Transplant International. 2000;13(Suppl 1):S399-S401.
210. Kogan-Liberman D, Burroughs M, Emre S, et al. The role of quantitative Epstein-Barr virus polymerase chain reaction and preemptive immunosuppression reduction in pediatric liver transplantation: a preliminary experience. Journal of Pediatric Gastroenterology and Nutrition. 2001;33(4):445-449.
211. Holmes RD, Orban-Eller K, Karrer FR, et al. Response of elevated Epstein-Barr virus DNA levels to therapeutic changes in pediatric liver transplant patients: 56-month follow up and outcome. Transplantation. 2002;74(3):367-372.
212. Scheenstra R, Verschuuren EA, de Haan A, et al. The value of prospective monitoring of Epstein-Barr virus DNA in blood samples of pediatric liver transplant recipients. Transplant Infectious Disease. 2004;6(1):15-22.
213. Lee TC, Savoldo B, Rooney CM, et al. Quantitative EBV viral loads and immunosuppression alterations can decrease PTLD incidence in pediatric liver transplant recipients. American Journal of Transplantation. 2005;5(9):2222-2228.
214. Cao S, Cox KL. Epstein-Barr virus lymphoproliferative disorders after liver transplantation. Clinics in Liver Disease. 1997;1(2):453-469, x-xi.
215. Cacciarelli TV, Green M, Jaffe R, et al. Management of post-transplant lymphoproliferative disease in pediatric liver transplant recipients receiving primary tacrolimus (FK506) therapy. Transplantation. 1998;66(8):1047-1052.
216. Fernandez MC, Bes D, De Davila M, et al. Post-transplant lymphoproliferative disorder after pediatric liver transplantation: characteristics and outcome. Pediatric Transplantation. 2009;13(3):307-310.
217. Hurwitz M, Desai DM, Cox KL, et al. Complete immunosuppressive withdrawal as a uniform approach to post-transplant lymphoproliferative disease in pediatric liver transplantation. Pediatric Transplantation. 2004;8(3):267-272.
218. Serinet MO, Jacquemin E, Habes D, et al. Anti-CD20 monoclonal antibody (Rituximab) treatment for Epstein-Barr virus-associated, B-cell lymphoproliferative disease in pediatric liver transplant recipients. Journal of Pediatric Gastroenterology and Nutrition. 2002;34(4):389-393.
219. Al-Akash SI, Al Makadma AS, Al Omari MG. Rapid response to rituximab in a pediatric liver transplant recipient with post-transplant lymphoproliferative disease and maintenance with sirolimus monotherapy. Pediatric Transplantation. 2005;9(2):249-253.
220. Savoldo B, Rooney CM, Quiros-Tejeira RE, et al. Cellular immunity to Epstein-Barr virus in liver transplant recipients treated with rituximab for post-transplant lymphoproliferative disease. American Journal of Transplantation. 2005;5(3):566-572.
221. Hayashida M, Ogita K, Matsuura T, et al. Successful prolonged rituximab treatment for post-transplant lymphoproliferative disorder following living donor liver transplantation in a child. Pediatric Transplantation. 2007;11(6):671-675.
222. Gross TG, Bucuvalas JC, Park JR, et al. Low-dose chemotherapy for Epstein-Barr virus-positive post-transplantation lymphoproliferative disease in children after solid organ transplantation. Journal of Clinical Oncology. 2005;23(27):6481-6488.
223. Gross TG, Hinrichs SH, Winner J, et al. Treatment of post-transplant lymphoproliferative disease (PTLD) following solid organ transplantation with low-dose chemotherapy. Annals of Oncology. 1998;9(3):339-340.
224. Malatack JF, Gartner JC Jr, Urbach AH, et al. Orthotopic liver transplantation, Epstein-Barr virus, cyclosporine, and lymphoproliferative disease: a growing concern. Journal of Pediatrics. 1991;118(5):667-675.
225. Molmenti EP, Nagata DE, Roden JS, et al. Post-transplant lymphoproliferative syndrome in the pediatric liver transplant population. American Journal of Transplantation. 2001;1(4):356-359.
226. Wallot MA, Mathot M, Janssen M, et al. Long-term survival and late graft loss in pediatric liver transplant recipients-a 15-year single-center experience. Liver Transplantation. 2002;8(7):615-622.
227. Ng VL, Alonso EM, Bucuvalas JC, et al. Health status of children alive 10 years after pediatric liver transplantation performed in the US and Canada: report of the studies of pediatric liver transplantation experience. Journal of Pediatrics. 2012;160(5):820-826.
228. Lopez-Santamaria M, Martinez L, Hierro L, et al. Late biliary complications in pediatric liver transplantation. Journal of Pediatric Surgery. 1999;34(2):316-320.
229. Bucuvalas J. Long-term outcomes in pediatric liver transplantation. Liver Transplantation. 2009;15(Suppl 2):S6-S11.
230. Sieders E, Peeters PM, TenVergert EM, et al. Graft loss after pediatric liver transplantation. Annals of Surgery. 2002;235(1):125-132.
231. Heffron TG, Pillen T, Smallwood G, et al. Incidence, impact, and treatment of portal and hepatic venous complications following pediatric liver transplantation: a single-center 12 year experience. Pediatric Transplantation. 2010;14(6):722-729.
232. Shemesh E, Shneider BL, Emre S. Adherence to medical recommendations in pediatric transplant recipients: time for action. Pediatric Transplantation. 2008;12(3):281-283.
233. Shemesh E, Shneider BL, Savitzky JK, et al. Medication adherence in pediatric and adolescent liver transplant recipients. Pediatrics. 2004;113(4):825-832.
234. Venkat VL, Nick TG, Wang Y, et al. An objective measure to identify pediatric liver transplant recipients at risk for late allograft rejection related to non-adherence. Pediatric Transplantation. 2008;12(1):67-72.
235. Shemesh E, Fine RN. Is calculating the standard deviation of tacrolimus blood levels the new gold standard for evaluating non-adherence to medications in transplant recipients? Pediatric Transplantation. 2010;14(8):940-943.
236. Stuber ML, Shemesh E, Seacord D, et al. Evaluating non-adherence to immunosuppressant medications in pediatric liver transplant recipients. Pediatric Transplantation. 2008;12(3):284-288.
237. Jain A, Reyes J, Kashyap R, et al. Long-term survival after liver transplantation in 4,000 consecutive patients at a single center [In process citation]. Annals of Surgery. 2000;232(4):490-500.
238. Banff schema for grading liver allograft rejection: an international consensus document. Hepatology (Baltimore, Md.). 1997;25(3):658-663.
239. Moreno M, Manzanares C, Castellano F, et al. Monitoring of tacrolimus as rescue therapy in pediatric liver transplantation. Therapeutic Drug Monitoring. 1998;20(4):376-379.
240. Ekong UD, Melin-Aldana H, Seshadri R, et al. Graft histology characteristics in long-term survivors of pediatric liver transplantation. Liver Transplantation. 2008;14(11):1582-1587.
241. Evans HM, Kelly DA, McKiernan PJ, et al. Progressive histological damage in liver allografts following pediatric liver transplantation. Hepatology (Baltimore, Md.). 2006;43(5):1109-1117.
242. Herzog D, Soglio DB, Fournet JC, et al. Interface hepatitis is associated with a high incidence of late graft fibrosis in a group of tightly monitored pediatric orthotopic liver transplantation patients. Liver Transplantation. 2008;14(7):946-955.
243. Scheenstra R, Peeters PM, Verkade HJ, et al. Graft fibrosis after pediatric liver transplantation: ten years of follow-up. Hepatology (Baltimore, Md.). 2009;49(3):880-886.
244. Guido M, Burra P. De novo autoimmune hepatitis after liver transplantation. Seminars in Liver Disease. 2011;31(1):71-81.
245. Kerkar N, Dugan C, Rumbo C, et al. Rapamycin successfully treats post-transplant autoimmune hepatitis. American Journal of Transplantation. 2005;5(5):1085-1089.
246. Campbell KM, Bucuvalas JC. Renal function in the long term after pediatric liver transplantation: is there a need for protocol kidney biopsies? Current Opinion in Organ Transplantation. 2010;15(5):608-613.
247. Campbell KM, Yazigi N, Ryckman FC, et al. High prevalence of renal dysfunction in long-term survivors after pediatric liver transplantation. Journal of Pediatrics. 2006;148(4):475-480.
248. Kivela JM, Raisanen-Sokolowski A, Pakarinen MP, et al. Long-term renal function in children after liver transplantation. Transplantation. 2011;91(1):115-120.

249. Campbell K, Ng V, Martin S, et al. Glomerular filtration rate following pediatric liver transplantation–the SPLIT experience. American Journal of Transplantation. 2010;10(12):2673–2682.
250. Goldstein SL, Devarajan P. Progression from acute kidney injury to chronic kidney disease: a pediatric perspective. Advances in Chronic Kidney Disease. 2008;15(3):278–283.
251. Goldstein SL, Devarajan P. Pediatrics: acute kidney injury leads to pediatric patient mortality. Nature Reviews Nephrology. 2010;6(7):393–394.
252. Goldstein SL. Advances in pediatric renal replacement therapy for acute kidney injury. Seminars in Dialysis. 2011;24(2):187–191.
253. Hathout E, Alonso E, Anand R, et al. Post-transplant diabetes mellitus in pediatric liver transplantation. Pediatric Transplantation. 2009;13(5):599–605.
254. Kuo HT, Lau C, Sampaio MS, et al. Pretransplant risk factors for new-onset diabetes mellitus after transplant in pediatric liver transplant recipients. Liver Transplantation. 2010;16(11):1249–1256.
255. Kuo HT, Sampaio MS, Ye X, et al. Risk factors for new-onset diabetes mellitus in adult liver transplant recipients, an analysis of the Organ Procurement and Transplant Network/United Network for Organ Sharing database. Transplantation. 2010;89(9):1134–1140.
256. Penn I. Cancers complicating organ transplantation. The New England Journal of Medicine. 1990;323(25):1767–1769.
257. Penn I. Occurrence of cancers in immunosuppressed organ transplant recipients. Clinical Transplants. 1998;147–158.
258. Penn I. Post-transplant malignancy: the role of immunosuppression. Drug Safety: An International Journal of Medical Toxicology and Drug Experience. 2000; 23(2):101–113.
259. Euvrard S, Kanitakis J, Cochat P, et al. Skin cancers following pediatric organ transplantation. Dermatologic Surgery. 2004;30(4 Pt 2):616–621.
260. Thomson MA, Suggett NR, Nightingale PG, et al. Skin surveillance of a U.K. paediatric transplant population. The British Journal of Dermatology. 2007; 156(1):45–50.
261. Simard JF, Baecklund E, Kinch A, et al. Pediatric organ transplantation and risk of premalignant and malignant tumors in Sweden. American Journal of Transplantation. 2011;11(1):146–151.
262. Bucuvalas JC, Britto M. Health-related quality of life after liver transplantation: it's not all about the liver. Journal of Pediatric Gastroenterology and Nutrition. 2003;37(2):106–108.
263. Bucuvalas JC, Britto M, Krug S, et al. Health-related quality of life in pediatric liver transplant recipients: a single-center study. Liver Transplantation. 2003; 9(1):62–71.
264. Varni JW, Seid M, Rode CA. The PedsQL: measurement model for the pediatric quality of life inventory. Medical Care. 1999;37(2):126–139.
265. Alonso EM, Limbers CA, Neighbors K, et al. Cross-sectional analysis of health-related quality of life in pediatric liver transplant recipients. Journal of Pediatrics. 2010;156(2):270–276 e271.
266. Sorensen LG, Neighbors K, Martz K, et al. Cognitive and academic outcomes after pediatric liver transplantation: Functional Outcomes Group (FOG) results. American Journal of Transplantation. 2011;11(2):303–311.
267. Fredericks EM. Nonadherence and the transition to adulthood. Liver Transplantation. 2009;15(Suppl 2):S63–S69.
268. Fredericks EM, DoreStites D, Lopez MJ, et al. Transition of pediatric liver transplant recipients to adult care: patient and parent perspectives. Pediatric Transplantation. 2011;15(4):414–424.
269. Fredericks EM, DoreStites D, Well A, et al. Assessment of transition readiness skills and adherence in pediatric liver transplant recipients. Pediatric Transplantation. 2010;14(8):944–953.
270. Fredericks EM, Lopez MJ, Magee JC, et al. Psychological functioning, nonadherence and health outcomes after pediatric liver transplantation. American Journal of Transplantation. 2007;7(8):1974–1983.
271. Shemesh E, Lurie S, Stuber ML, et al. A pilot study of posttraumatic stress and nonadherence in pediatric liver transplant recipients. Pediatrics. 2000;105(2):E29.

第 115 章 儿童心脏移植

Steven A. Webber

引言

自从心脏移植开展以来，儿童心脏移植一直是其重要组成部分。儿童心脏移植在其发展过程中，不仅关注心脏移植的技术问题，而且关注移植免疫与耐受问题。目前，心脏移植已成为儿童心脏结构性或功能性疾病的治疗选择之一。本章主要讲述儿童心脏移植的发展过程，并概述了儿童心脏移植的指征、准备、实施、随访过程，重点阐述儿童的特殊之处，而成人相关内容在本书其他章节进行描述。

发展历史

1967 年 12 月 3 日，世界第一例异体心脏移植手术由 Christian Barnard 在南非开普敦格罗特·舒尔医院开展[1]。在 3 年后的 12 月 6 日，第一例儿童心脏移植由 Kantrowitz 及其同事在纽约布鲁克林的迈蒙尼德医学中心开展[2]。该医疗小组曾于 1966 年 6 月尝试进行婴儿心脏移植，但最后还是终止了。新的受者最初被诊断为三尖瓣闭锁，但最终确定为严重房室间隔缺损和功能性肺动脉闭锁。在出生后的第 3 天，该婴儿接受了体肺分流术，但疾病最终还是进展为心力衰竭与肺水肿。11 月 24 日，医疗团队给患者提供了原位心脏移植的机会，移植心脏来源于一位无脑儿患者。在 Barnard 开展第一次心脏移植前一周，家属签署了手术知情同意书。供者与受者均为 A 型血，且“组织配型显示无免疫不相容迹象”。在 12 月 6 日，一位无脑儿患者被确定为潜在的合适供体，两位儿童被带入手术室，并通过泡入冰水来进行外部冷却(图 115.1)。供体心脏在 27℃时停止跳动，医疗团队便进行了相应的移植操作(先于脑死亡诊断标准确立时进行)。虽然手术是在循环停止下进行，但是移植过程还是利用了 Lower 和 Shumway 技术(图 115.2)。最初受者表现良好并能自主活动四肢，但数小时后即发生代谢性和呼吸性酸中毒，并于移植后约 6 小时发生心搏骤停而复苏抢救失败。尸检结果显示手术结果良好且缝线止血合适，然而肺主动脉分流未完全关闭。纽约和南非的首次心脏移植是在多次动物异位或原位移植试验后开展的。在这些首批移植后面，成为心脏移植第一人是背后的部分驱动力，而 20 世纪 60 年代末这些外科先驱者确信儿童和成人进行成功的心脏移植是可行的。

1968 年，在 Barnard 和 Kantrowitz 之后有一大批外科医生尝试心脏移植。到该年年末，17 个国家开展了

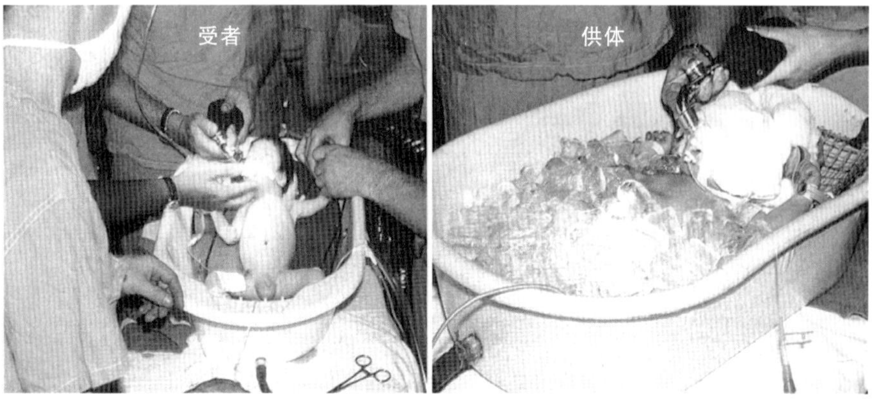

图 115.1 第一次儿童心脏移植在 1967 年 12 月 6 日进行。通过将无脑儿供体(右图)和受体(左图)置于冰水浴中诱导低温。当供体心脏跳动停止时，进行移植程序。

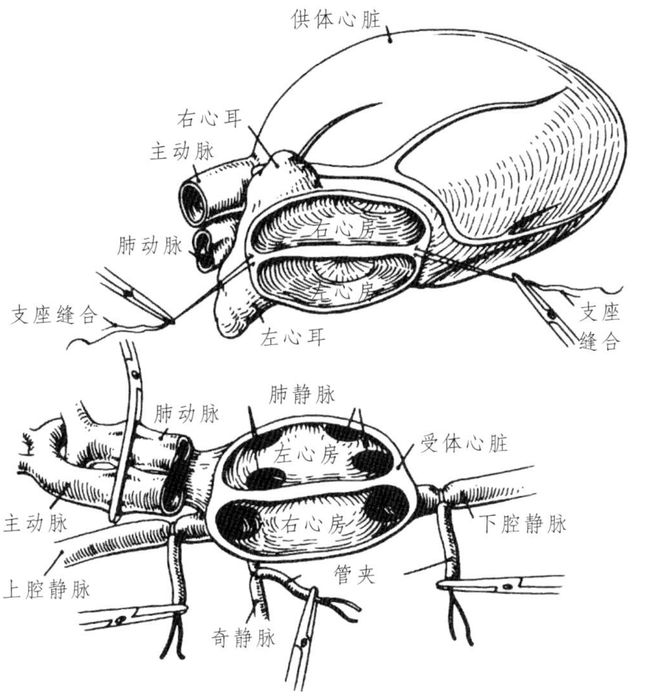

图 115.2 首次儿童心脏移植手术的技术图解(术后不久绘制)。Reproduced from [87] Fine R, Webber SA, Harmon W, et al. (2007). Pediatric Solid Organ Transplantation, Second Edition, with permission from John Wiley and Sons.

102 例手术,平均生存期仅为 29 天[3]。接下去的 10 年内,因为针对异体排斥反应的医疗手段相对匮乏而不利于患者移植后生存,世界范围对人类心脏移植的热情骤然下降[4]。一部分中心,尤其是斯坦福大学的外科医生,选择性地对成人开展心脏移植。此外,斯坦福大学的团队也开展了青少年心脏移植,1974—1980 年间共进行了 8 例手术。尽管只能应用皮质激素和硫唑嘌呤进行免疫抑制,仍有 4 名患者移植后存活了 10 年以上[5]。此外,脑死亡被广泛接受后,供者器官存活率也得到了提升[6,7]。

环孢素对于心脏移植受者存活的提升作用相当显著[8,9],并重新引起了斯坦福、匹兹堡大学(1982)及随后世界其他地区的多个医疗中心对儿童心脏移植的兴趣。最早的受者都是大龄儿童或是青少年,但不久后婴幼儿也成了心脏移植受者。Bailey 及其同事在大量动物试验基础上提出新生儿或能成为良好的实体器官受体[10,11]。他们第一次为新生儿移植是在一位患有主动脉瓣和二尖瓣闭锁的 12 日龄的 2.2kg 新生儿身上的狒狒–人体异种移植[12]。该婴儿仅仅存活了 20 天,但左心发育不全综合征(HLHS)的心脏移植手术可行性已经得到了验证。原位新生儿心脏移植于 1985 年 11 月在罗马琳达开展[13]。第一个受者是患有 HLHS 的 4 岁婴儿,尽管有 Norwood 的姑息性手术,但其状态在当时被认为是十分危重的[14]。在 20 世纪 90 年代,儿童心脏移植中 HLHS 的移植是发展得最迅速的。最近,HLHS 的阶段性姑息手术治疗效果的提升及受者的器官等待时间的增加也导致许多医疗中心放弃将心脏移植作为 HLHS 患儿的第一治疗选择。

在过去的 15 年间,儿童心脏移植领域克服了许多挑战,有多个发展的里程碑。早期结果显示,对曾接受姑息手术的复杂性先天性心脏病患者进行心脏移植的结果并不尽如人意[15]。然而,患者选择的优化与手术经验的增加,使心脏移植手术现能在多个医疗中心开展[16]。

供者器官的短缺依旧是一个严峻的问题,等候捐献的婴幼儿,尤其是那些接受 ECMO 机械循环支持的供体的死亡率依旧维持在一个较高的水平[17]。因为婴儿期后阶段开始就不产生主要血型抗原(在第 112 章有深入的讨论),新生儿与婴儿的 ABO 不相符的移植最近也得到了多伦多医疗小组的支持[18]。该方法或能改善等候捐献的婴幼儿的生存情况[19]。在异种器官移植能够安全有效实施并被广泛接受之前,供者器官短缺问题就不能得到很好的解决。

移植指征与候选者评估

儿童移植指征

当患者预计生存时间少于 2 年,或生活质量极低时,可以考虑做心脏移植。心肌病(主要是扩张型心肌病)和复杂性先天性心脏病依然是主要的手术指征,约占儿童心脏移植的 90%[20]。因为供者器官的短缺,移植手术数量在过去 10 年内一直保持稳定。移植候选的诊断是基于年龄考虑的,超过 50%的先天性心脏病的移植是在婴儿身上完成的,而有将近 2/3 的心肌病的心脏移植受者是青少年[20]。值得注意的是,接受心脏移植的确诊为先天性心脏病(CHD)的婴儿比例在北美要显著高于世界其他地区[20]。

合理的儿童心脏移植指征于 1999 年由美国移植学会儿科委员会总结得出[21]。最近,美国心脏协会的一个共识小组也得出了同样结论[22]。总体上就移植指征而言,儿童心脏委员会有着一致的共识。心脏移植指征的争议之处在于新生儿 HLHS 和相关病理。在有经验的医疗中心中,HLHS 患者 Norwood 重建或心脏移植每年生存率超过 80%。在美国,新生儿心脏移植受者的中位等待时间约为 2 个月(在部分国家则更久),这导致了移植前护理的高费用支出与移植前的高死亡率,其中,等候名单中患者的死亡率高达 30%[23]。基于这些观察结果,绝大部分医疗中心减少了患有 HLHS 新生儿的心脏移植,而更倾向于阶段性重建。这增加了不适于行姑息性手术治疗的心脏病患儿的心脏移植率。

心脏移植的相对或绝对禁忌证包括:乙肝病毒、丙肝病毒或人类免疫缺陷病毒(HIV)感染的慢性感染,先前对治疗的不依从,现阶段或最近的肿瘤治疗且无足够随访能够确定治愈,活动性急性病毒、真菌或细菌感染,过度且恒定的肺血管阻力(10IU 以上),肺实质血管床不足,弥漫性肺血管狭窄,以及心脏移植难以治愈的严重心外疾病(如严重全身肌病)。当然,部分医疗中心认为的绝对禁忌证可能被其他中心认为是相对禁忌证。而心脏移植的最终决策是在医疗小组、家庭医生和转诊医生一起讨论后做出的。

候选者评估

儿童心脏移植的评估流程大致基于成人心脏移植候选者的评估原则(见第 30 章)。评估流程包括无移植预计生存时间、目前生活质量、其他手术或治疗方法,以及移植手术内在风险的估计。

解剖结构和血流动力学考察

只要肺血管充分发育且肺血管阻力适合,复杂的解剖结构也能完成心脏移植。外科医生最关注的解剖学要点包括:心脏或其他脏器异位情况(尤其是全身或肺静脉回流异常),肺动脉主干及其分支的位置和解剖学情况(包括狭窄、变形和不汇合),而心内解剖相对不重要,因为心脏大部分会被移植物取代。大动脉位置的畸形常会引发一系列问题。譬如右心室肺动脉连接管道、胸骨后的巨大右心房(Fontan 手术后)等关键部位之间的关系应当引起足够的重视。CT 或磁共振成像能够很好地勾画出心脏解剖结构,心脏导管常用于移植术前的肺血管阻力的测定。过度的恒定阻力可能会导致供体器官的急性心室衰竭,最终使受者难以脱离体外循环。

总体而言,肺血管阻力系数(PVRI)≤9IU 的儿童发生供体器官右心衰竭和早逝的风险较低。PVRI 大于 9 时风险较高[24],只有在有效的肺血管舒张治疗后才能进行移植。PVRI 在临界值附近时,因为 PVRI 常会发生显著下降,所以应在应用数日的肌力药物和血管舒张剂的治疗后进行重新评估。然而肺部阻力的迅速下降可能导致左心房压的急剧上升,进而导致左心房功能不全,甚至引发肺水肿。心室辅助装置(VAD)能否降低左心室压并进一步减少 PVRI 从而为儿童原位心脏移植做准备,在目前看来尚不明确,但是最近病例报道显示,在部分病例中短暂的 VAD 支持能够显著降低 PVRI,并成功地进行了心脏移植。

实验室研究

血型鉴定是确定移植器官 ABO 相容性的必要手段,但缺少或有较低水平的抗 A 或抗 B 同种红细胞凝集素的婴幼儿能够绕过传统 ABO 屏障而安全完成移植。因为 West 及其同事在多伦多发现抗血型抗原的同种红细胞凝集素在婴儿期晚期才能正常生成[18,19]。抗 A 和抗 B 同种红细胞凝集素正常产生前的跨血型移植在最终治疗结果上与 ABO 相容性移植相近[25,26]。此外,在长期随访过程中,绝大部分移植的婴儿并不会形成抗移植器官的抗体[27],这可能是由于 B 细胞耐受性的产生[28]。有报道表明,即使相关抗体产生,最终结果也良好[27]。移植前后的血液制品需要小心应用,以防输血中包含抗 A 或抗 B 抗体。血库与临床需要充分沟通,以提供合适的血液制品,相关输血信息也应在患者出院前就充分告知患者家属。

对于抗 HLA 抗体的形成(“致敏作用”)的评估,传统上是利用群体反应性抗体(PRA)测试进行的。而现在绝大部分医疗中心是利用固相分析,尤其是 Luminex 平台(可伴有基于细胞的 PRA 试验)。固相分析平台敏感性很高,且有未发表的儿童器官移植临床试验(CTOT-C)的数据显示,约 50%儿童心脏移植候选者有形成抗 HLA 抗体,但其中许多人的抗体滴度较低,即使是针对供者而言,该项研究的意义仍需进一步探讨。许多医疗中心将 HLA 分子分型作为评估的流程之一,若要在致敏的候选者身上进行交叉配对试验,那么该步骤是十分必要的(在第 89 章有深入的探讨)。

传染病评估包括对巨细胞病毒(CMV)、EB 病毒(EBV)、水痘、单纯疱疹病毒、弓形虫、艾滋病毒、麻疹病毒和甲、乙、丙、丁肝炎病毒的血清学测试,有助于移植后发热的预防与评估。在极少数情况下,这会导致儿童移植候选者的排除。传染病评估也应包括预防接种史的回顾。非紧急的移植候选者应当进行最新且合适的预防接种。此外,年幼患者移植评估后在其移植之时应当再次进行传染病抗体的检测,因为这可能影响巨细胞病毒的预防以及移植后淋巴组织增生性疾病(PTLD)的风险评估。

应诊

一个包括心脏移植医生、外科医生、社工、移植协调员和传染病专家在内的多学科团队会对每个移植候选者进行评估。对儿童及其家庭进行精神病学和心理学的筛查也是十分有益的。这个评估的主要目标在于鉴定等候移植和移植后儿童及其家庭的不良心理社会结果的风险。对于治疗依从性较差的既往史的评估也是十分关键的,此外也可与血液肿瘤学(若有肿瘤病史)、儿童发育学、基因学、神经学、营养学等专家进行额外的咨询。而接受过 Fontan 手术的患者需要评估肝硬化的情况,或需要接受正式的肝脏病学咨询。

等候名单的管理与结局

一旦进入移植等候名单,患者及其家属就会关注患者存活的概率。但是,移植前死亡率、等候名单中死亡率以及移植最佳时间依旧很少得到关注。过早的移植会增加受者的移植风险,并使受者长期处于免疫抑制状态。但等候过久而未移植可能会引起患者死亡或是患者的病态从而增加移植难度。这些病态包括进展性的终末期器官功能不全(尤其是肾脏)、严重心力衰竭相关的营养不良和肺血管阻力的增加。

美国移植受者科学登记系统(SRTR)的数据显示,所有年龄组的儿童的心脏移植等候时间均要小于成人,但儿童等候者死亡风险要高于成人(www.ustransplant.org)。其中,小于 1 岁的婴儿的死亡率最高,而且诊断为先天性心脏病的患者的死亡率更是显著增加。ABO 血型不符的心脏移植可能会降低婴儿心脏移植候选者在等候名单时的死亡率[19]。

儿童心脏移植研究(从 1993 年开始的世界范围内 40 余个医疗中心开展的关于移植等候名单和移植后结局的研究)的多个分析集中于进入移植等候名单后的危险因素和最佳移植时间的选择。处于低风险状态(在美国为 UNOS 等级 2)而进入等候名单的儿童中,病因是扩张性心肌病者猝死风险最低。与此相反,患有缺血性疾病的成人移植候选者的猝死风险最高。这些数据表明自动植入型心律转复除颤器(AICD)不必在等候名单的儿童中进行常规应用,即使其中某些亚群会有一定的受益[29]。除此之外,有一项研究表明,UNOS 等级 2 的移植候选者至少有 4 年以上的生存时间[30]。

对进入等候名单的心肌病患儿结局的详细分析已经通过儿童心脏移植研究(PHTS)数据库进行[31-33]。对于扩张性心肌病而言,每年等候名单死亡率是 10%,另外 74%接受了移植,而 16%则仍在等待[31],这与儿童移植最常见的适应证相矛盾。等候名单死亡的危险因素包括了机械通气史、体外膜氧合器(ECMO)和心律失常。

相比之下,等候名单中先天性心脏病患儿则相当之少,尤其是那些 UNOS 等级 1A 和婴儿期就进入等候名单者。婴儿等候名单中某些确诊的亚群死亡率甚至高至 30%[23],这或许反映了现有医疗和外科治疗条件对某些等待移植患者而言也是无能为力的。虽然 VAD 支持的患儿在过去 15 年间显著增加,但与心肌病相比,CHD 患者的最终结局仍是相当不佳[34]。几乎所有的儿童都是接受了辅助泵的支持,而且 30kg 以下的患儿(接近成人设备的限制)通过柏林心脏辅助装置成功地完成了移植[35,36],但最终结局仍是令人失望的。尽管如此,婴儿中最常用的机械辅助装置还是 ECMO,该装置的应用与移植前后的高死亡率有关[17,36]。因为绝大多数医疗中心的中位等待时间均超出了儿童利用 ECMO 所能支持的最长时间,而且急需机械支持的情况下利用 VAD 也增加移植后的死亡率[35]。但是,对于绝大部分CHD 患儿,解剖因素严重地限制了该技术的成功应用[34]。

供者评估,手术技术与移植后早期管理

本部分的重点是儿童心脏移植供者的评估,手术技术(主要是针对 CHD 患者)和集中护理及首次入院期间的早期移植后管理。手术技术部分主要是儿童常见疾病相关的,且与第 58 章中的心脏移植一般技术相一致。

儿童受者的心脏供体评估

供体心脏评估的第一步就是对病史的仔细回顾,包括了供者的年龄、性别、体型、死因、是否有胸部创

伤、是否需要心肺复苏、复苏时间的长短、血流动力学状态的评估(包括血压、心率及中心静脉压)。此外,还包括了正性肌力支持量及其应用趋势等数据。对受者而言,供者接受心肺复苏的病史是一项禁忌证[37,38],因为脑死亡会导致供者动态性的生理紊乱,包括了体温的不稳定及体温过低、循环血容量改变(主要是减少)和神经内分泌紊乱,还有全身甲状腺素、糖皮质激素、胰岛素、血管升压素、抗利尿激素(ADH)的消耗。

为了排除心脏结构异常及评估心功能,完整的超声心动图检查是必要的。绝大部分医疗中心避免使用那些经正性肌力药物或甲状腺激素治疗后收缩功能仅高于轻微受损心脏的供体心脏(比如短轴缩短率小于26%,射血分数低于50%等)。某些程度的二尖瓣或三尖瓣反流多见于脑死亡供者,而轻度的反流则不是器官捐献的禁忌证。心包积液则可能预示心肌损伤。轻度非特异性的ST段和T段改变较为常见,常反映了中枢神经系统的影响、电解质紊乱或体温过低,这些并非器官捐献的禁忌证。在广泛创伤的情况下,对心肌酶结果进行解释可能会变得困难。供者血清中心肌肌钙蛋白I的水平或可作为儿童心脏移植后失败的预测因子[39]。不过,最近的一项SRTR数据库的研究表明,移植手术前肌钙蛋白I的升高与移植失败或移植受者住院时间无关[40]。

在成人移植中,通过选择性冠状动脉造影对成人供者冠状动脉疾病的评估是十分普遍的。儿童心脏移植使用成年供体心脏(供者为35岁以上),则与移植后冠心病和较低的长期生存率有关[41]。因此这样的供者被排除在儿童心脏移植之外,因此供者通常不需要进行冠脉造影。

器官大小匹配是选择潜在供者的关键问题。大多数医疗中心避免选择低于受者体重的75%~80%的供者。低于这个范围,供者的心输出量可能并不能满足受者的要求。但是最近来自SRTR数据库的一份报道显示低于受者器官大小60%的供受者不匹配与较差的移植结局无关[42]。这项回顾性分析并不能明确供者器官大小、冷缺血时间、术前供者器官功能之间的复杂联系。因此,这并不能断定尺寸严重过小的器官能够在移植常规基础上安全使用。

使用过大的器官在儿童移植中是十分常见的,因为很少有能与受者尺寸完全相符的供者器官。大多数患有心肌病的候选者有明显的心肥大,这为过大的供体心脏提供了足够的胸腔空间。供受者体重比2.5:1在儿童心脏移植中是比较常见的,3:1及以上的比例也有成功的先例[43],特别是在新生儿和婴儿身上。明显过大的移植心脏体积会导致胸骨闭合延迟,而在婴儿受者中,供受者体重比大于2时会导致呼吸机使用时间延长和原发性移植物功能不全的风险增高[44]。过大的供体心脏也会导致术后综合征的产生,其特征有与全身性高血压、高颅内压甚至精神状态改变相关的高输出状态。虽然受到广泛推荐,但在显著肺动脉高压的受者身上,较大的供体心脏能否改善治疗结果是不明确的。绝大部分医疗机构认可在受者患有肺动脉高压的情况下应当避免明显过小尺寸的移植器官。

所有的供者应该进行CMV、EBV、HIV 1和2、人嗜淋巴病毒1和2(HTLV-1,HTLV-2)和甲、乙、丙型肝炎的筛查。此外,供者也应进行梅毒和弓形虫抗体的筛查。CMV、EBV或弓形虫抗体的存在并非移植的禁忌证,但有助于移植后治疗及监测方案的制订。供者受逆转录病毒感染(HIV或HTLV)的证据则被认为是心脏移植的一种绝对禁忌证。而供者乙型肝炎表面抗原阳性也常被视为绝对禁忌证。而对于丙型肝炎阳性供者的心脏的使用仍存在争议。

移植物植入的手术技术

对手术技术的详细描述超出了本书的范围,而且最近也有文章进行了综述[45]。1960年,Lower和Shumway列举了原位心脏移植的基本外科原理,最初他们在狗身上试验,数年后则是在人身上研究[46]。他们开创性的工作也带来了心脏移植中双心房吻合技术的应用。这项技术已在数千位各种年龄段的患者身上成功应用。

尽管双心房吻合术取得了巨大成功,但这在解剖学上仍有缺陷,会形成巨大的房腔。由此产生的异常心房可能会增加三尖瓣功能障碍。此外,手术创伤或缺血也可能引起窦房结功能障碍。基于这些原因,许多医疗中心在原位心脏移植中选用了双腔吻合。某些特定的先天性心脏病患者选用双腔吻合术较为合适,比如曾接受过Mustard后Senning手术的患者,或者是那些曾经接受Glenn吻合手术者。双腔吻合术可能与上腔静脉狭窄有关,尤其是对婴儿而言[47]。当手术伤口完全愈合后的最初数周,该狭窄可经心导管介入术成功治疗[47]。

先天性心脏病的移植通常在多个姑息性手术后进

行，对移植手术而言这可能存在巨大挑战。从解剖学上来说，挑战主要分为全身静脉回流的异常、肺静脉回流的异常以及包括 HLHS 在内的大血管异常。对于这些解剖学改变而言，双房吻合术和双腔吻合术的改进是必要的。总体而言，大动脉位置的异常带来的困难相对较少，而全身静脉回流的异常则是最大的挑战。对左位下腔静脉的患者(例如右位心或是内脏异位综合征)进行心脏移植时需要特殊的考虑，有多个手术技巧能够克服这些解剖学改变带来的困难(图 115.3)[16,45]。其中最关键的步骤是取得包括无名静脉在内的供者的腔静脉。当存在没有连接静脉的双侧上腔静脉时，供者的无名静脉可以用于受者左心室的端对端吻合。当受者脏器完全呈镜像排列时(右位心和内脏左右转位)，可以利用房室瓣作为通道，改变上腔静脉和下腔静脉的流向。

通常，先前的心脏手术涉及的肺动脉包括全身至肺的分流和腔肺吻合术等等。在任何情况下，都应该尽可能多地收集供者的肺动脉。最常见的是，在双向 Glenn 或 Fontan 手术中，将腔肺吻合端取下，对肺动脉进行修补，再进行双腔吻合术。牛的心包、同种移植物、受者或供者的组织均可以用于手术中的修复。而修复最好是在受者心脏部分切除术后和器官移植前进行。在肺动脉不连续的情况下，供体器官应有完整的肺动脉与肺静脉(图 115.4)。之后就可直接进行左肺动脉与右肺动脉的吻合。或者在心脏植入前利用供者的主动脉连接左肺动脉与右肺动脉。当单肺缺血或严重的肺动脉发育不全时，单肺的移植也是可行的[48]，但这只能在主要的肺动脉发育良好且肺血管阻力极低的情况下进行。否则供体心脏发生急性右心衰竭的风险会大大增加。

目前很少有医疗中心会为 HLHS 进行原位移植，因为广泛的动脉弓发育不全，供者的外科医生必须连带整个横向和近端降主动脉获得供体心脏。而动脉弓的手术重建也应在低温停循环的条件下进行。

术后管理与早期并发症

儿童患者心脏移植后早期术后管理的许多基本原则与其他心肺旁路手术较为相似。本部分重点介绍移植受者的护理内容。

心血管因素

低心排血量

当供体心脏发生缺血或缺氧时，心肌功能的异常是不可避免的。收缩功能的恢复通常较快，而舒张功能异常可能持续数周。尽管需要 2~3 天，但大多数受者在移植后的短期内应用小剂量的正性肌力药物是能够获益的。正性肌力药物的选择取决于用药医生的偏好及心率、肺血管阻力、血压等血流动力学因素，小剂量的多巴酚丁胺和异丙肾上腺素是比较常用的选择，其中，

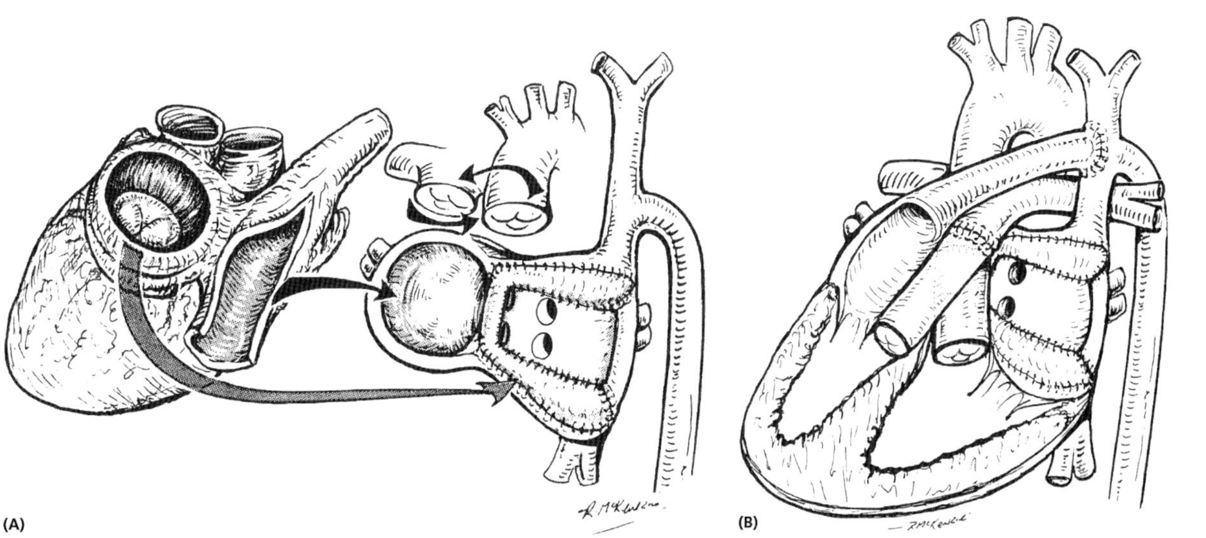

图 115.3　在 Mustard 术后(心房挡板)，对已修复的大血管进行移植与镜像器官的操作(内脏转位)。(A)保存 Mustard 挡板以将左侧全身静脉回流引导至供体右心房。(B)由于上腔静脉的狭窄，供体上腔静脉吻合到靠近挡板的受体上腔静脉。

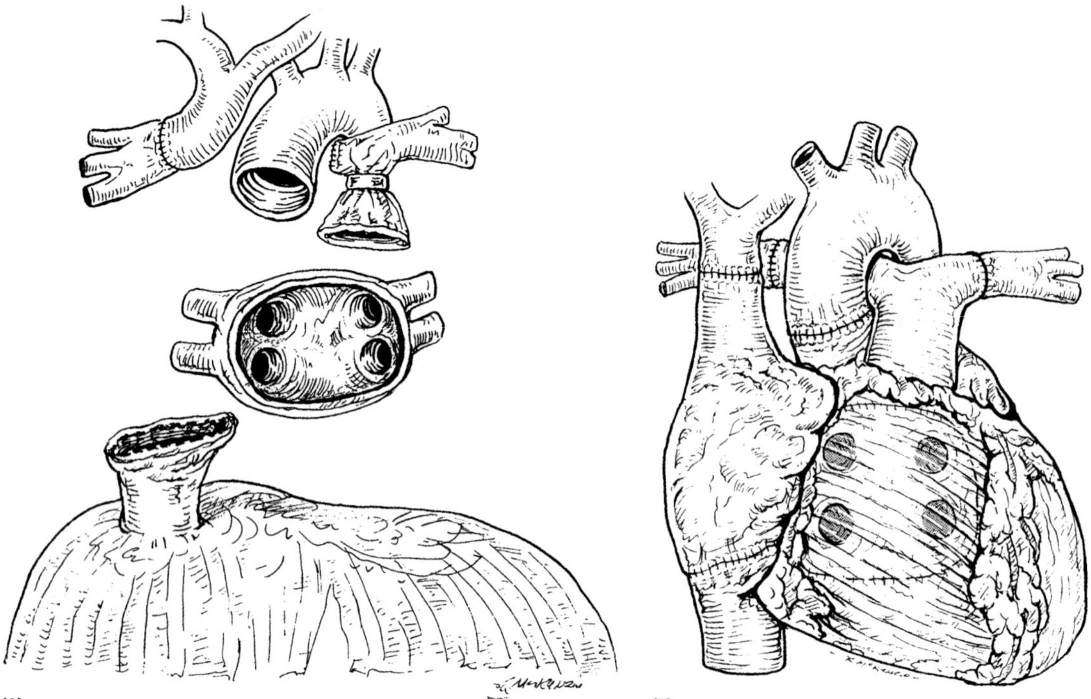

图 115.4 一位肺动脉不连续的患儿,先进行右侧经典 Glenn 分流和肺动脉束缩,后进行 Bicaval 心脏移植。(A)在切除受者心脏后,制备下腔静脉套和左心房扣,并取消经典 Glenn 分流。(B)供体器官采用两个肺动脉的分支和上部静脉的延伸段,并进行肺和吻合口吻合术。

异丙肾上腺素因其变时作用、正性肌力作用和肺血管收缩作用而得到了更多的应用。当存在低心排血量和高全身血管阻力的证据时,加用如米力农等血管扩张剂和(或)正性肌力药物是合理的。当供体心脏过大时, 改善心功能最简单的方法是在移植结束时开胸。在术后 24 小时内, 偶有体外循环脱离失败或术后原发性移植物衰竭。这种原发性移植物衰竭是与术后高死亡率密切相关的并发症。原发性移植物衰竭主要是由于急性左心室或双心室衰竭, 而非肺血管阻力过高。较差的供者选择、心肌缺血时间延长、较差的保存技术及超急性排斥反应应当得到全面的考虑。当发生原发性移植失败时(非超急性排斥导致),若循环能够得到支持则通常可以恢复,这通常是通过体外膜氧合器(ECMO)实现的[49]。原发性移植物衰竭后的再移植通常与较差的预后有关[50],许多人将其视为再移植的禁忌证[51]。

系统性高血压

与非移植的心脏外科患者相比, 系统性高血压是十分常见的。有多种因素导致系统性高血压,包括超大供体器官和高剂量皮质激素引起的心血管动力过强。在成功的移植手术后 24 小时内观察到相当严重的收缩期高血压是不寻常的。如果超声心动图证实心室功能良好,则应立刻撤除正性肌力药物的应用。当全身性血管阻力较高时,静脉内血管扩张剂是合理的选择。也有人主张在超大供体心脏的病例中应用 β-肾上腺素受体阻断剂。

肺动脉高压

前文已经讨论了肺血管阻力作为急性供体右心室衰竭的危险因素重要性。若有心肺血管阻力升高的风险,则应在术前评估的基础上采取额外的预防措施。一氧化氮从手术室开始应用,并用于中断体外循环。酸中毒应当避免,并提供高浓度的吸入氧。在术后早期进行过度通气和足量药物镇静。右心可能需要正性肌力药物支持,此外,尽管对肺血管阻力可能产生潜在的不良效应,但在米力农和多巴酚丁胺之外,有时也需要应用肾上腺素。若存在右心室功能障碍伴心排血量不足,在相应支持之外也应提供机械辅助支持。如果肺血管阻力在移植前有轻微升高 (或在低血管阻力儿童接受心肺旁路手术后发生的急性血管阻力升高),24~48 小时的机械支持常常能使右心室恢复到满足血液循环的要求,尽管这会导致肺动脉压的升高。如果候选者选择的问题导致了供体右心急性衰竭（比如血管扩张剂使用后肺动脉阻力指数大于 9IU),那么右心功能是通常难以恢复的。

心率与心律

在心脏移植后的儿童中观察到术后快速性和缓慢性心律失常。除窦性心动过速之外最常见的节律异常是窦房结功能障碍，并会导致有或没有心房或节段性逸搏心率的窦性心动过缓。去神经支配的窦房结适当地响应于外源性的变时性药物，异丙肾上腺素就有这样的作用。有一种简单的方法是心房起搏,所有移植受者都应当在术中放置临时起搏线。窦房结功能障碍反映缺血性和(或)创伤性损伤,但这通常在几天内恢复。室性异位和非持续性室性心动过速在移植后的第一周或两周也相当常见。这些可能与缺血再灌注损伤有关,且很少需要治疗。新的心脏同种异体移植物具有有限的增加心搏量的能力，因此建立起足够的心率对于维持心排血量是十分重要的。而心房起搏则最常用于控制心率。

呼吸支持

呼吸支持的原则与其他儿科开放性心脏手术的原则相同,早期拔管应该是治疗目标。需要长期术前机械通气的患者在术后通常需要更长时间，因为他们往往需要重新训练呼吸肌。长期心脏肥大的婴儿常常具有显著的支气管软化症，而持续性或复发性肺动脉狭窄并不常见,尤其是在左下叶。

肾功能

慢性心力衰竭联合心肺旁路应用和环孢素或他克莫司的使用,会增加移植术后肾功能障碍。如果术后有低心排血量状态,则肾功能障碍会加剧,少尿则是常见的症状。但儿童发生急性肾衰竭很少,因而很少需要透析。当发生持续性少尿时,可用袢利尿剂和低剂量多巴胺[例如 3~5μg/(kg·min)]治疗。前述的正性肌力药物可用于治疗心排血量过低,连续输注呋塞米[最多 6mg/(kg·d)]也可能有效。以上这些治疗通常能够成功地刺激足够尿量的产生[>1mL/(kg·h)]。当尿输出持续减低时,可能需要停用钙调磷酸酶抑制剂(他克莫司或环孢素)数天,静脉诱导剂使用作为早期免疫抑制方案的一部分可能有帮助(参见本章中的更多内容)。

胃肠道因素

胃肠道并发症在儿童心脏移植术后是十分常见的[52]。所有患者应接受静脉内 H_2 拮抗剂治疗,并随后口服 H_2 拮抗剂，以降低手术后早期应激性溃疡的风险。该治疗通常要持续到皮质类固醇减至低剂量乃至撤药为止。一旦患者拔管能够口服食物与药物,就移除鼻胃管。注意食物应提供最佳的热量而非过量,因为大多数患者在术后早期倾向于体液潴留。胰腺炎在移植后并非罕见,当有腹痛或不明原因的喂食不耐受时,应考虑胰腺炎。避免使用硫唑嘌呤和皮质类固醇的免疫抑制方案可以减少这种并发症。儿童使用免疫抑制药物，特别是使用皮质类固醇时，可能会导致胃肠道穿孔。许多慢性心力衰竭儿童患有胃食管反流病,此类疾病应当积极管理,但是免疫抑制剂和包括抗酸药、抗组胺药和促胃动力药物在内的用于胃食管反流疾病的药物之间有许多药物相互作用。

感染预防

感染是儿童心脏移植后首年死亡的主要原因[20],最严重的感染通常发生在最初的住院期间。移植后的第一周内,应尽快移除埋线和插管。给予患者短疗程的抗生素(例如 72 小时)用于预防纵隔和伤口感染,通常第一代头孢菌素效果就符合要求。如果患者的 ICU 时间延长并且具有长期存在的缝线,则应给予覆盖更多葡萄球菌的抗生素(即万古霉素),长期存在的缝线通常在手术室中更换。感染 MRSA 的患者也应用万古霉素治疗。在 ICU 中，如果受体或供体的血清中 CMV 为阳性,那么应当同时口服制霉菌素与更昔洛韦。对于真菌感染高风险的患者（例如移植前接受 ECMO 的患者)常常用氟康唑进行预防。应当注意的是,所有“唑类”抗真菌药对钙调磷酸酶抑制剂通过细胞色素 P450 系统对其代谢具有很大的影响。同时使用唑类抗真菌剂时,需要明显减少(50%~90%)他克莫司或环孢素给药剂量。此外,在邻近出院之时可以开始预防肺囊虫。

免疫抑制和早期急性排斥反应

高剂量静脉内甲基泼尼松龙(例如 15~20mg/kg)常在手术过程中应用。大多数医疗中心通常在术后 1~2

周在对患者进行维持性皮质类固醇治疗过程中，给予患者逐步减量的皮质类固醇治疗[2]。如果排斥过程不危及生命,某些医疗中心会使患者停用类固醇[53]。然而在儿童治疗过程中，非类固醇免疫抑制方案的使用越来越多[54],这可能需要诱导治疗才能成功。一旦确定患者尿量正常时，环孢素或他克莫司在术后24~48小时内就可通过静脉或肠内给药。如果使用抗T细胞诱导治疗(最常见的是兔多克隆抗胸腺细胞球蛋白,而白细胞介素-2受体拮抗剂使用相对较少)，在第一次治疗过程中不必立即使用(最初1~2天)钙调磷酸酶抑制剂(CNI):环孢素或他克莫司是通过口服途径而非静脉给药。当尿量少或肾功能恶化时,这些药物在诱导治疗的覆盖范围内延迟数天应用或有很好的效果。在过去10年中,诱导治疗的应用在2010年达到了70%[20],但这种趋势并没有反映在成年人群中。这可能表明在低免疫风险病例中应避免应用皮质类固醇，并延迟对儿童受者行侵入性心内膜活检(EMB)。

虽然除了致敏患者外,在术后7~10天之前罕有严重免疫排斥反应，但对于免疫排斥仍应进行仔细的日常评估。诱导治疗的应用通常会延迟免疫排斥反应。婴儿和幼儿的急性排斥反应比青少年更少。皮肤苍白、心动过速、腹痛、奔马律和少尿都反映了严重的排斥反应，在这些体征出现之前最好能通过超声心动图和(或)检测性活检确定排斥反应的存在,心电图可能显示缩心前电压的减少。在移植后早期,排斥反应的进展可能相当迅速，任何术后初期患者状况的恶化都必须严肃对待。若有明确证据表明有移植物功能障碍的迹象,应该立刻进行经验性治疗(通常包括静脉内注射皮质类固醇)或EMB。活检通常显示淋巴细胞浸润(主要是T细胞),且伴有不同程度的水肿和肌细胞损伤。心内膜活检的分级应当根据ISHLT创立的国际认可的分类系统进行[55]。

移植后管理和移植的长期并发症

儿童心脏移植受者长期管理的主要目标是使长期生存率最大化,尽量减少免疫抑制治疗的并发症,并提高生活质量。关于心脏移植术后发生的所有并发症的详细讨论超出了本章的范围，而在本书的其他章节中有叙述。本章重点讨论儿童心脏移植受体的特定并发症,以及预防和治疗这些并发症的策略。

免疫抑制治疗的维持

免疫抑制治疗目的在于防止或最小化宿主对供体器官的有害免疫应答，同时避免治疗性免疫抑制的并发症。抑制的免疫并发症分为两大类:①同种异体移植排斥和急、慢移植物功能障碍,这反映了免疫抑制的不足以及包括感染和恶性肿瘤在内的非特异性免疫抑制的表现;②免疫抑制治疗的非免疫副作用(即组织和器官毒性),这是儿童心脏移植后发病及偶然死亡的重要原因。

如前所述，目前大多数儿童在围术期接受了某种方式的诱导治疗,最常见的是兔抗胸腺细胞球蛋白。与成年人一样,几乎所有的儿童都接受了含有抗代谢剂和(或)抗增殖剂的CNI。目前,他克莫司和霉酚酸酯是最常用的药物组合,在移植后一年,他克莫司使用率约为66%,而霉酚酸酯(MMF)或霉酚酸(MPA)则为70%[20]。5年内,MMF/MPA的使用已经减少了一半[20],这可能是因为MMF/MPA在儿童中不耐受的情况较多[56]。皮质类固醇的使用并非必须，尽管在国际上有64%的儿童仍然接受皮质类固醇的治疗，在移植1年后则下降到39%[20]。正如之前讨论的那样,许多医疗中心在非致敏儿童的心脏移植后的最初几天内避免使用类固醇激素[54],这为儿童移植受者提供了许多明显的优势。总体而言，需要进一步的研究来确定哪些患者不适合使用类固醇激素。

急性排斥反应

尽管移植后排斥反应的风险会随着时间而减少,但患者仍将一直存在急性排斥的风险。目前并没有证据表明心脏移植受者能够真正耐受同种异体移植物。当检查心脏移植后的死亡原因时，急性排斥反应就变得相当重要。来自ISHLT的数据显示,急性排斥反应是心脏移植后30天至3年之间死亡的最常见原因[20]。在此期间,20%的死亡是由于急性排斥反应,另外31%则归因于“移植物衰竭”。首次排斥的最大风险或即时风险发生在移植后的1~2个月。移植术后1年,约64%的儿童心脏移植受者无急性排斥反应[23](图115.5)。发生在移植后第一年之后的晚期急性排斥反应常有着较差的预后,特别是该排斥反应与移植物功能障碍有关时[57,58]。当发生任何程度的急性排斥伴收缩功能障碍

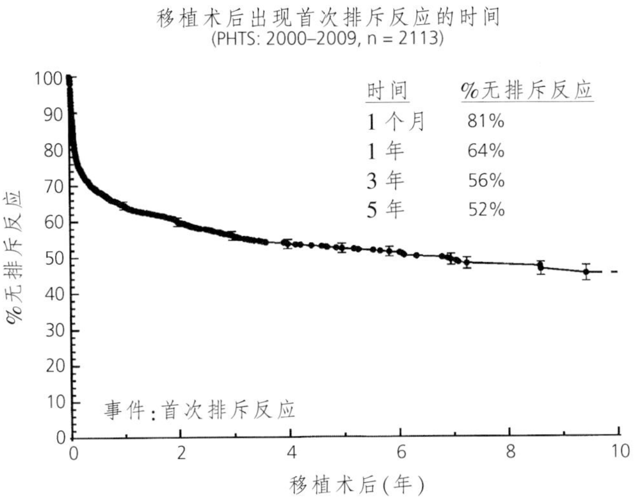

图 115.5 2000 年 1 月至 2009 年 12 月间，在儿童心脏移植研究(PHTS)数据库中移植患者的无急性排斥反应事件时间。Published with permission of PHTS.

时,即使患者状况良好且无心力衰竭,病情也很容易快速恶化。因此,应当谨慎地将所有急性移植物衰竭的患者纳入重症监护室治疗。如果发生超过轻度以上的收缩性衰竭时,应该静脉注射米力农,并且应该监测患者的心律失常情况。除非移植物衰竭是由于冠状动脉疾病,否则发生急性排斥和(或)移植物功能障碍时应该立刻开始静脉注射甲泼尼龙 10~15mg/kg (最大剂量为 1g),共 3~5 天。除非患者状态不稳定,否则 EMB 是最佳选择，因为在组织学上急性移植物功能障碍可能与"无细胞排斥"(预后较差)或抗体介导的排斥(AMR)有关。有时这可能需要额外的治疗,如紧急血浆置换等。需要指出的是，严重急性排斥反应的治疗不应该在等待 EMB 执行或获得结果时被延迟。急性排斥伴血流动力学改变可以迅速导致移植物衰竭。因为这种情况通常是可逆的,所以除非有特定的禁忌证,这些患者应该得到全面的动态支持,包括使用机械支持等,其中 ECMO 是最常用的装置 [59]。在发生活动性急性排斥反应时,应避免再移植,因为其预后通常不佳[51]。

PHTS 的三个最近的研究分析了急性排斥反应的年代效应[58,60,61]。从 1993 年开始到现在,移植后急性排斥反应事件显著减少[60],晚期排斥反应的首发和复发事件也明显减少[57,58]。已经有研究发现晚期排斥反应与随后发展的中重度移植物血管病变、死亡和重新移植的高风险因素相关[57,58]。特别值得注意的是,尽管所有急性排斥反应事件的总体频率下降,PHTS 内急性排斥反应与严重血流动力学改变的发生率并没有随时间而改变[61]。此外,与排斥事件后 1 年和 5 年时严重血流动力学改变相关的急性排斥反应的生存率 (1 年后为 63%,5 年后为 49%)没有随着时间改变而改善[61]。

急性排斥反应的危险因素也已经在 PHTS 中开展了广泛研究。首次排斥的风险与年代较早的移植、高龄和阳性的供体特异性的交叉配型相关[60]。值得注意的是,在近些年的急性排斥反应中,种族并非危险因素,但它仍是晚期排斥反应和伴严重血流动力学改变的排斥反应的危险因素[58,61]。

正如在成人一样，在儿童心脏移植后也观察了到抗体介导的排斥反应。大多数排斥反应发生在阳性的供体特异性细胞毒性交叉配型的患者中[62,63]。由于过去手术的频率高，先前用于修复先天性心脏缺陷的主动脉和肺同源移植物的使用率较高，致敏作用在儿童中是十分常见的。这些冷冻保存的同种异体移植物具有巨大的致敏作用[64]。某些儿童就有这样广泛的敏感性,但由于无法找到与 HLA 相符的供体,患者的移植等待时间非常长[65]。在该群体中,移植前脱敏方案并没有效果。在 100%PRA 等情况下,并不能找到可用的供体。一些医疗中心在已知供体特异性交叉配型阳性的情况下,尝试了对这些患者开展移植手术。典型的手术方案包括:手术中血浆置换、移植后短期血浆置换、T 细胞耗竭抗体诱导治疗、三重药物免疫抑制(他克莫司、MMF、类固醇激素)和静脉内免疫球蛋白的连续输注等。目前有一项进行中的试验正在评估这种策略的效果[66]。利妥昔单抗、硼替佐米和其他试验药物在这种情况下的作用是未知的。虽然没有进行前瞻性随机试验,但这些药物已被用于治疗已确立 AMR 的儿童心脏移植者[67]。

慢性排斥反应和同种异体移植心脏的血管病变

慢性排斥反应和同种异体移植心脏的血管病变(CAV)通常被用作同义词。移植后的冠状动脉疾病是一种加速性血管病变，它是儿童心脏移植晚期存活者死亡的主要原因[20,41]。它占到了移植后三年内死亡人数的 25%以上[20]。CAV 的病理生理的细节将在本书其他部分进行描述。可以这样说:儿童受体并不对这种并发症免疫，虽然在移植后任意时间点上儿童受体在 CAV 上优于成年受体[41]。最近发布的一项有趣的数据显示,通过聚合酶链反应检测心脏活组织样本中的各种病毒(尤其是腺病毒)的病毒基因组的持续性,预测了儿童的冠状动脉疾病进展和晚期的移植物失功。高龄供体的使用、晚期急性排斥反应的发作和更大的受体年龄都是儿童发生移植后CAD的危险因素[41]。儿童CAV中的巨细胞病毒血清状况和感染的作用还不完全清楚,相比于成人,儿童的研究较少[69]。

即使进行心脏的去神经支配操作,虽然有些儿童会经历腹部疼痛和(或)胸痛的发作,但局部缺血的症状往往缺乏[70]。晕厥和猝死也是儿童CAV的常见症状。如今最常在选择性冠状动脉造影中得出诊断。血管内超声在此诊断上有着更强的灵敏度,虽然它在儿童中的经验要比成人有限得多[71,72]。评估儿童的冠脉血流储备也是可行的,但由于涉及的技术性挑战和对结果解释说明的不确定性几乎很少被使用[73]。

不幸的是,对已有的冠状动脉疾病还没有根治性疗法。舒张功能障碍往往发生于早期并可被观测到,即使此时还几乎没有心外膜冠状动脉狭窄的证据[74]。这可能是许多患者的一种弥漫性小血管疾病的反映。一旦明显的心脏收缩随之而来,其生存率会很低,应考虑再次移植。再次移植的晚期结果(初次移植超过6个月)与初次移植类似[50]。缺血导致晕厥的儿童如果在等待再次移植的过程中要出院,应接受自动植入型心律转复除颤器(AICD)。如果不处于晚期的心力衰竭,则为了抗局部缺血作用可给予β受体阻滞剂,而且不需要β受体激动剂。支架植入术和搭桥手术在桥接再次移植发挥的作用有限,而且受到CAV的扩散性质的限制。在一年内的经皮血管重建术的过程中,52%的儿童被报道有移植物失功,表明了这些干预措施的作用有限[75]。

感染

对于儿童群体整体来说,各种形式的感染的患病率有所增加。大多数感染是由病原体引起的,它也导致非免疫抑制宿主的感染。常见的例子包括呼吸道病毒、肺炎链球菌和水痘病毒。非免疫抑制的心脏移植受者发生的所有感染可引起更严重的疾病。在这方面特别值得注意的是,由于巨细胞病毒(CMV)和EB病毒(EBV)导致的感染,它们几乎不在具有免疫能力的宿主中导致严重的疾病。更罕见的是,可见如因卡氏肺孢子虫(原卡氏肺孢子虫)导致的机会性感染[76]。虽然大多数感染都能被很好地耐受,在移植后的第一个月,感染是导致移植失败的第二大原因,并且它依然是患者移植后第一年的一个重要死亡原因[20]。

任何心脏移植后出现败血症的儿童都需要使用广谱抗生素,直到确定病原体。肺炎链球菌感染的发生频率增加,并且抗生素的选择必须覆盖这种病原体。当有肺炎的临床和影像学证据和恶化的临床状态时,应该有一个进行支气管肺泡灌洗的下限阈值,以获得病毒、真菌和细菌的深度培养。当有缺氧和特征性胸部X线改变时,应排除卡氏肺囊虫[76]。当心脏移植受者有严重呼吸道感染的证据时,应该寻找呼吸道病毒病原菌(如呼吸道合胞病毒、流感病毒、副流感病毒、腺病毒)。在年龄较大和移植后很久的儿童中,病毒性呼吸系统疾病往往能被很好地耐受,在移植后的最初几个星期获得这些呼吸系统病毒的其中一种有时会导致毁灭性的疾病,特别是婴儿。侵袭性真菌感染在严重移植后感染的儿童中约占7%,最常见的是念珠菌和曲霉属真菌感染[77]。主要是在移植后的六个月内,这些都与侵入性移植前操作(例如,ECMO、手术前、VAD)的数量增加相关,并与高死亡率相关[77]。

在心脏移植患者中原发性巨细胞病毒感染的问题比肺移植受者要小,但仍能引起严重的发病率和偶尔的病死率。心脏移植受者中肺炎是相当罕见的,而这是一个肺和心肺移植受体移植后发生原发性感染的发病部位。相比之下,病毒性肝炎、肝炎和骨髓抑制是比较常见的现象。通过对外周血的PCR或抗原检测(pp65)来进行诊断。巨细胞病毒病的诊断仍是一个组织诊断。当确诊较早时,静脉注射更昔洛韦和(或)口服缬更昔洛韦治疗通常是非常有效的。预防策略一般与成年人相同(见第94章)。

免疫功能低下的EBV感染儿童可无症状,或可能导致非特异性病毒综合征、单核细胞增多症、暴发性病毒感染或移植后淋巴组织增生性疾病(PTLD)。发展为PTLD最危险的因素是移植后发生EBV原发感染,虽然那些在移植的时候EBV血清阳性的儿童并不完全能够防止发生该并发症。两项针对PHTS数据库的分析提供了儿童心脏移植人群PTLD的最全面的分析。1993—2009年35个机构的3170位初次心脏移植患者中的147位被诊断为PTLD,移植10年后免于发生PTLD的概率为90%。在治疗PTLD过程中的排斥反应反跳仍然是主要的问题,并且移植失败(对比PTLD疾病进展)占了诊断为 PTLD 后约 50%的死亡人数[78]。PTLD 的病理学、流行病学、治疗及预后的进一步细节在第 96 章中进行描述。

非免疫性并发症

对于免疫抑制过强或者不足的后果来说，移植受者受到大量免疫抑制治疗的非免疫毒性影响。儿童免疫抑制药物的毒性先前已有总结[80,81]。与成人相比,生长障碍是儿童的一个独特问题，并导致许多儿科移植中心的类固醇最小化和避免方案的愿望。特别值得关注的一个并发症是由于钙调磷酸酶抑制剂导致的进行性肾功能障碍。这越来越成为问题,因为越来越多的儿童心脏移植后长期生存。一些已经发展到终末期肾衰竭需要肾移植[82]。应该指出的是,在这一人群中肌酐清除率的估计和直接测量会过高估计肾小球滤过率(GFR),并且肾脏疾病的严重程度一般大于感觉[82]。在最近一次关于 PHTS 患者中的肾衰竭的分析中，晚期肾衰竭被发现与更早期肾移植、黑种人、第一年有血流动力学相关排斥反应和移植一年后最低 25%的肾小球滤过率评估值相关[83]。另一项最近的儿童多机构研究,无法证实先前关于常见的遗传变异可能影响 CNI 为基础的免疫抑制状态下的移植后肾功能的报道[84]。值得注意的是，从移植时间来避免 CNI 的临床试验还没有在儿童心脏移植人群中进行。

移植后生存率与危险因素

从 ISHLT 的注册数据来看[20],SRTR 和儿童心脏移植的研究[23]都显示出在过去的 20 年中移植后生存率的重要的趋势。重要的是,最近几年的结果有了显著的改善；在婴儿组和较小规模中心的生存率的提升是最明显的。值得注意的是,在 21 世纪第一个 10 年的前 5 年与后 5 年之间的结果都有了明显的提升(图 115.6)。大多数的改善显示是由于早期死亡率的减少。在许多医疗中心一年生存率现在约为 90%，在接下来的 1~4 年只有一个相对较小的下降。PHTS 和 ISHLT 数据库继续显示婴儿受者稍高的围术期和早期死亡率，但有趣的是这些最年轻的患者有一个中位生存时间，现在接近 20 年,婴儿存活一年的条件中位生存时间优于其他年龄组。相比之下,青少年患者的中位生存时间只有

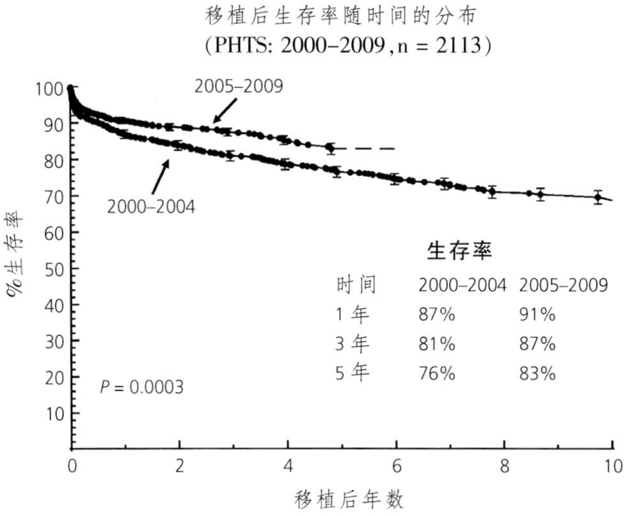

图 115.6 2000 年 1 月至 2009 年 12 月儿童心脏移植的研究(PHTS) 数据库的患者移植后总体生存率随时间的分布。Published with permission of PHTS.

11.9 年[20]。这可能反映了在非常年轻受者的一个较低的移植后冠状动脉疾病的发病率和一定程度的免疫豁免特权。在更为年长的儿童中较高的移植物失功和死亡率可能反映(至少部分反映),这个年龄组的低依从性。利用诱导治疗、初始 CNI 选择(环孢素或他克莫司)和在手术后一年使用他克莫司或环孢素与儿童心脏移植后的生存率没有相关性[20]。

先天性心脏病的移植结果仍然落后于心肌病的移植结果;这种差异是由于较高的围术期死亡率造成的。这种差异在婴儿受者中最显著,在青少年中最不明显。ISHLT 报道患有心肌病的婴儿 10 年生存率相较于冠心病有 12%的优势;差异完全是由于早期死亡率增加。青少年组的差异无统计学意义。

重要的是，仍然有证据表明黑人儿童的存活率与其他种族群体相比较低。这种差异主要是由于移植后的第一年移植物失功的增加。社会经济地位较低也与第一年移植物失功的增加有关[86]。

在 ISHLT 登记信息的最新分析中，第一年的移植死亡危险因素包括:ECMO、再次移植、先天性疾病、透析、机械通气、前胸骨切开术、供体年龄、术前肌酐水平及总缺血时间[20]。供者的死亡原因和脑血管事件也被认为是一个危险因素,第一年死亡率相比于头部外伤,缺氧保护相比于头部外伤有着更高第一年死亡率的相对风险。后者的观察结果的意义尚不清楚,因为最近一个 PHTS 数据库分析(3122 例)并没有揭示传统危险因

素影响供体移植后的结果，包括供者的死亡原因，供者心肺复苏和正性肌力应用(移植物获取前)。在不到6个月龄的婴儿中，没有影响移植后生存率的供者相关因素。较长的缺血时间和较大的供受者年龄差异确实影响了10岁以上的受者的生存率。

总结

儿童心脏移植术后现在已经取得了优异的结果，5年生存率超过80%。提升的结果似乎很有限，而且主要是早期的术后阶段，并且这种改善在婴儿和患有先天性心脏病的患者中最明显。第一年存活的婴儿有着最好的长期结果，移植物中位生存时间超过20年。移植等候名单的死亡率似乎也有改善，可能反映了包括对危重者更好的医疗保障、作为与儿童移植桥梁的VAD支持的延长和分配政策的变化等多种因素。尽管取得了这些进展，心脏移植仍然是权宜之计，所有移植受者都暴露在非特异性免疫抑制的副作用的风险中，包括感染、淋巴组织增生性疾病和非淋巴恶性肿瘤。此外，目前的免疫抑制剂有着狭窄的治疗窗，并表现出广泛的器官毒性。这对必须忍受终身免疫抑制的年轻患者带来了特殊的挑战。新的免疫抑制方案降低了急性排斥反应率（但没有排斥反应伴随严重的血流动力学障碍），而对CAV的发病率的影响相对较小，它是后期移植物失功的主要原因。

（柯庆宏 译 柯庆宏 校）

参考文献

1. Bernard CN. The operation. A human cardiac transplant: an interim report of a successful operation performed at Groote Schuur Hospital, Cape Town. South African Medical Journal. 1967;41:1271–1274.
2. Kantrowitz A, Haller JD, Joos H, et al. Transplantation of the heart in an infant and an adult. American Journal of Cardiology. 1968;22:782–790.
3. Cooley DA, Bloodwell RD, Hallman GL, et al. Organ transplantation for advanced cardiopulmonary disease. Annals of Thoracic Surgery. 1969;8:30–46.
4. Griepp RB. A decade of human heart transplantation. Transplantation Proceedings. 1979;11:285.
5. Baum D, Kaye MP, Miller WW. Pediatric heart, heart-lung, and lung transplantation: historical perspective. Progress in Pediatric Cardiology. 1993;2:1–3.
6. Report of the Ad Hoc Committee of the Harvard Medical School to examine the definition of brain death: a definition of irreversible coma. JAMA: Journal of the American Medical Association. 1968;205:337–340.
7. Black PM. Brain death. New England Journal of Medicine. 1978;299:338.
8. Oyer PE, Stinson EB, Jamieson SW, et al. Cyclosporine in cardiac transplantation: a 2 1/2 year follow up. Transplantation Proceedings. 1983;15:2546–2552.
9. Grattan MT, Moreno-Cobral CE, Starnes VA, et al. Eight-year results of cyclosporine-treated patients with cardiac transplants. Journal of Thoracic and Cardiovascular Surgery. 1990;90:500–509.
10. Bailey LL, Li Z, Lacour-Gayet F, et al. Orthotopic cardiac xenotransplantation in the cyclosporine-treated neonate. Transplantation Proceedings. 1983;15(Suppl 1):2956–2959.
11. Bailey LL, Jang J, Johnson W, et al. Orthotopic cardiac xenografting in the newborn goat. Journal of Thoracic and Cardiovascular Surgery. 1985;89:242–247.
12. Bailey LL, Nehlsen-Cannarella SL, Conception W, et al. Baboon to human cardiac xenotransplantation in a neonate. JAMA: Journal of the American Medical Association. 1985;254:3321–3329.
13. Bailey LL, Nehlsen-Cannarella SL, Doroshow RW,et al. Cardiac allotransplantation in newborns as therapy for hypoplastic left heart syndrome. New England Journal of Medicine. 1986;315:949–951.
14. Noorwood WI, Lang P, Hansen D. Physiologic repair of aortic atresia-hypoplastic left heart syndrome. New England Journal of Medicine. 1983;308:23–26.
15. Trento A, Griffith BP, Fricker FJ, et al. Lessons learned in pediatric heart transplantation. Annals of Thoracic Surgery. 1989;48:617–623.
16. Webber SA, Fricker FJ, Michael M, et al. Orthotopic heart transplantation in children with congenital heart disease. Annals of Thoracic Surgery. 1994;58:1664–1669.
17. Dipchand AI, Mahle W, Tresler M, et al. Extracorporeal membrane oxygenation as a bridge to pediatric heart transplantation: impact on post-listing and post-transplantation outcomes (abstract). Circulation. 2011;124(21 Suppl 1):A16269.
18. West LJ, Pollock-Barziv SM, Dipchand AI, et al. ABO-incompatible heart transplantation in infants. New England Journal of Medicine. 2001;344:793–800.
19. West LJ, Karamlou T, Dipchand AI, et al. Impact on outcomes after listing and transplantation, of a strategy to accept ABO blood group-incompatible donor hearts for neonates and infants. Journal of Thoracic and Cardiovascular Surgery. 2006;131:455–461.
20. Kirk R, Dipchand AI, Edwards LB, et al. The registry of the International Society for Heart and Lung Transplantation: fifteenth pediatric heart transplantation report–2012. Journal of Heart and Lung Transplantation. 2012;31:1065-72.
21. Fricker FJ, Addonizio L, Bernstein D, et al. Heart transplantation in children: indications. Pediatric Transplantation. 1999;3:333–342.
22. Canter CE, Shaddy RE, Bernstein D, et al. Indications for heart transplantation in pediatric heart disease: a scientific statement from the American Heart Association Council on Cardiovascular Disease in the Young; the Councils on Clinical Cardiology, Cardiovascular Nursing, and Cardiovascular Surgery and Anesthesia; and the Quality of Care and Outcomes Research Interdisciplinary Working Group. Circulation. 2007;115:658–676.
23. Dipchand AI, Kirk R, Mahle WT, et al. Ten years of pediatric heart transplantation: a report from the Pediatric Heart Transplant Study. Pediatric Transplantation. 2013;17:99–111.
24. Chiu P, Russo MJ, Davies RR, et al. What is high risk? Redefining elevated pulmonary vascular resistance index in pediatric heart transplantation. Journal of Heart and Lung Transplantation. 2012;31:61–66.
25. Henderson HT, Canter CE, Mahle WT, et al. ABO-incompatible heart transplantation: analysis of the Pediatric Heart Transplant Study (PHTS) database. Journal of Heart and Lung Transplantation. 2012;31:173–179.
26. Urschel S, Larsen IM, Kirk R, et al. ABO-incompatible heart transplantation in early childhood: an international multicenter study of clinical experiences and limits. Journal of Heart and Lung Transplantation. 2013;32:285–292.
27. Conway J, Manlhiot C, Allain-Rooney T, et al. Development of donor-specific isohemagglutinins following pediatric ABO-incompatible heart transplantation. American Journal of Transplantation. 2012;12:888–895.
28. Fan X, Ang A, Pollock-Barziv SM, et al. Donor-specific B-cell tolerance after ABO-incompatible infant heart transplantation. Nature Medicine. 2004;10:1227–1233.
29. Rhee EK, Canter CE, Basile S, et al. Sudden death prior to pediatric heart transplantation: would implantable defibrillators improve outcome? Journal of Heart and Lung Transplantation. 2007;26:447–452.
30. Kirklin JK, Naftel DC, Caldwell RL, et al. Should status II patients be removed from the pediatric heart transplant waiting list? A multi-institutional study. Journal of Heart and Lung Transplantation. 2006;25:271–275.
31. Dipchand AI, Naftel DC, Feingold B, et al. Outcomes of children with cardiomyopathy listed for transplant: a multi-institutional study. Journal of Heart and Lung Transplantation. 2009;28:1312–1321.
32. Kirk R, Naftel D, Hoffman TM, et al. Outcome of pediatric patients with dilated cardiomyopathy listed for transplant: a multi-institutional study. Journal of Heart and Lung Transplantation. 2009;28:1322–1328.
33. Zangwill SD, Naftel D, L'Ecuyer T, et al. Outcomes of children with restrictive cardiomyopathy listed for heart transplant: a multi-institutional study. Journal of Heart and Lung Transplantation. 2009;28:1335–1340.
34. Blume ED, Naftel DC, Bastardi HJ, et al. Outcomes of children bridged to heart transplantation with ventricular assist devices: a multi-institutional study. Circula-

tion. 2006;113:2313–2319.
35. Morales DL, Almond CS, Jaquiss RD, et al. Bridging children of all sizes to cardiac transplantation: the initial multicenter North American experience with the Berlin Heart EXCOR ventricular assist device. Journal of Heart and Lung Transplantation. 2011;30:1–8.
36. Fraser CD Jr, Jaquiss RD, Rosenthal DN, et al. Berlin Heart Study Investigators. Prospective trial of a pediatric ventricular assist device. New England Journal of Medicine. 2012;367:532–541.
37. Conway J, Chin C, Kemma M, et al. Donor characteristics and impact on outcomes in pediatric heart transplant recipients. Journal of Heart and Lung Transplantation. 2011;30(4 Suppl 1):S133.
38. L'Ecuyer T, Sloan K, Tang L. Impact of donor cardiopulmonary resuscitation on pediatric heart transplant outcome. Pediatric Transplantation. 2011;15: 742–745.
39. Grant JW, Canter CE, Spray TL, et al. Elevated donor cardiac troponin I. A marker of acute graft failure in infant heart recipients. Circulation. 1994;90(6): 2618–2621.
40. Lin KY, Sullivan P, Salam A, et al. Troponin I levels from donors accepted for pediatric heart transplantation do not predict recipient graft survival. Journal of Heart and Lung Transplantation. 2011;30:920–927.
41. Pahl E, Naftel DC, Kuhn MA, et al. The impact and outcome of transplant coronary artery disease in a pediatric population: a 9-year multi-institutional study. Journal of Heart and Lung Transplantation. 2005;24:645–651.
42. Tang L, Du W, Delius RE, et al. Low donor-to-recipient weight ratio does not negatively impact survival of pediatric heart transplant patients. Pediatric Transplantation. 2010;14:741–745.
43. Kanani M, Hoskote A, Carter C, et al. Increasing donor-recipient weight mismatch in pediatric orthotopic heart transplantation does not adversely affect outcome. European Journal of Cardio-Thoracic Surgery. 2012;41:427–434.
44. Huang J, Trinkaus K, Huddleston CB, et al. Risk factors for primary graft failure after pediatric cardiac transplantation: importance of recipient and donor characteristics. Journal of Heart and Lung Transplantation. 2004;23: 716–722.
45. Pigula FA, Webber SA. Donor evaluation, surgical technique and perioperative management. Chapter 33, Section 5, Heart Transplantation. In: Fine R, Webber SA, Harmon W, et al., editors. Pediatric Solid Organ Transplantation. Oxford: Blackwell Publishing; 2007.
46. Lower RR, Shumway NE. Studies on orthotopic homotransplantation of the canine heart. Surgical Forum. 1960;11:18–25.
47. Sachdeva R, Seib PM, Burns SA, et al. Stenting for superior vena cava obstruction in pediatric heart transplant recipients. Catheterization and Cardiovascular Interventions. 2007;70:888–892.
48. Lamour JM, Hsu DT, Quaegebeur JM, et al. Heart transplantation to a physiologic single lung in patients with congenital heart disease. Journal of Heart and Lung Transplantation. 2004;23:948–953.
49. Fenton KN, Webber SA, Danford DA, et al. Long-term survival after pediatric cardiac transplantation and postoperative ECMO support. Annals of Thoracic Surgery. 2003;76:843–846.
50. Chin C, Naftel D, Pahl E, et al. Cardiac retransplantation in pediatrics: a multi-institutional study. Journal of Heart and Lung Transplantation. 2006;25: 1420–1424.
51. Johnson MR, Aaronson KD, Canter CE, et al. Heart retransplantation. American Journal of Transplantation. 2007;7:2075–2081.
52. Rakhit A, Nurko S, Gauvreau K, et al. Gastrointestinal complications after pediatric cardiac transplantation. Journal of Heart and Lung Transplantation. 2002;21: 751–759.
53. Canter CE, Moorhead S, Saffitz JE, et al. Steroid withdrawal in the pediatric heart transplant recipient initially treated with triple immunosuppression. Journal of Heart and Lung Transplantation. 1994;13(1 Pt 1):74–79.
54. Singh TP, Faber C, Blume ED, et al. Safety and early outcomes using a corticosteroid-avoidance immunosuppression protocol in pediatric heart transplant recipients. Journal of Heart and Lung Transplantation. 2010;29:517–522.
55. Stewart S, Winters GL, Fishbein MC, et al. Revision of the 1990 working formulation for the standardization of nomenclature in the diagnosis of heart rejection. Journal of Heart and Lung Transplantation. 2005;24:1710–1720.
56. Ohmann EL, Burckart GJ, Brooks MM, et al. Genetic polymorphisms influence mycophenolate mofetil-related adverse events in pediatric heart transplant patients. Journal of Heart and Lung Transplantation. 2010;29:509–516.
57. Webber SA, Naftel DC, Parker J, et al. Late rejection episodes greater than 1 year after pediatric heart transplantation: risk factors and outcomes. Journal of Heart and Lung Transplantation. 2003;22:869–875.
58. Ameduri RK, Zheng J, Schechtman KB, et al. Has late rejection decreased in pediatric heart transplantation in the current era? A multi-institutional study. Journal of Heart and Lung Transplantation. 2012;31:980–986.
59. Chen JM, Richmond ME, Charette K, et al. A decade of pediatric mechanical circulatory support before and after cardiac transplantation. Journal of Thoracic and Cardiovascular Surgery. 2012;143(2):344–351.
60. Gossett JG, Canter CE, Zheng J, et al. Decline in rejection in the first year after pediatric cardiac transplantation: a multi-institutional study. Journal of Heart and Lung Transplantation. 2010;29:625–632.
61. Everitt MD, Pahl E, Schechtman KB, et al. Rejection with hemodynamic compromise in the current era of pediatric heart transplantation: a multi-institutional study. Journal of Heart and Lung Transplantation. 2010;30:282–288.
62. Holt DB, Lublin DM, Phelan DL, et al. Mortality and morbidity in pre-sensitized pediatric heart transplant recipients with a positive donor crossmatch utilizing peri-operative plasmapheresis and cytolytic therapy. Journal of Heart and Lung Transplantation. 2007;26:876–882.
63. Pollock-BarZiv SM, den Hollander N, Ngan BY, et al. Pediatric heart transplantation in human leukocyte antigen sensitized patients: evolving management and assessment of intermediate-term outcomes in a high-risk population. Circulation. 2007;116(11 Suppl):I172–I178.
64. Shaddy RE, Hunter DD, Osborn KA, et al. Prospective analysis of HLA immunogenicity of cryopreserved valved allografts used in pediatric heart surgery. Circulation. 1996;94:1063–1067.
65. Feingold B, Bowman P, Zeevi A, et al. Survival in allosensitized children after listing for cardiac transplantation. Journal of Heart and Lung Transplantation. 2007;26:565–571.
66. CTOT-C04 Study Protocol. [assessed December 23, 2013]; Available at: https://www.ctotc.org/Approved_Studies.htm.
67. Morrow WR, Frazier EA, Mahle WT, et al. Rapid reduction in donor-specific anti-human leukocyte antigen antibodies and reversal of antibody-mediated rejection with bortezomib in pediatric heart transplant patients. Transplantation. 2012;93:319–324.
68. Shirali GS, Ni J, Chinnock RE, et al. Association of viral genome with graft loss in children after cardiac transplantation. New England Journal of Medicine. 2001;344:1498–1503.
69. Hussain T, Burch M, Fenton MJ, et al. Positive pretransplantation cytomegalovirus serology is a risk factor for cardiac allograft vasculopathy in children. Circulation. 2007;115:1798–1805.
70. Price JF, Towbin JA, Dreyer WJ, et al. Symptom complex is associated with transplant coronary artery disease and sudden death/resuscitated sudden death in pediatric heart transplant recipients. Journal of Heart and Lung Transplantation. 2005;24:1798–1803.
71. Nicolas RT, Kort HW, Balzer DT, et al. Surveillance for transplant coronary artery disease in infant, child and adolescent heart transplant recipients: an intravascular ultrasound study. Journal of Heart and Lung Transplantation. 2006;25(8): 921–927.
72. Costello JM, Wax DF, Binns HJ, et al. A comparison of intravascular ultrasound with coronary angiography for evaluation of transplant coronary disease in pediatric heart transplant recipients. Journal of Heart and Lung Transplantation. 2003;22(1):44–49.
73. Schubert S, Abdul-Khaliq H, Wellnhofer E, et al. Coronary flow reserve measurement detects transplant coronary artery disease in pediatric heart transplant patients. Journal of Heart and Lung Transplantation. 2008;27(5):514–521.
74. Law Y, Boyle G, Miller S, et al. Restrictive hemodynamics are present at the time of diagnosis of allograft coronary artery disease in children. Pediatric Transplantation. 2006;10:948–952.
75. Jeewa A, Chin C, Pahl E, et al. Outcomes after percutaneous coronary artery revascularization procedures for allograft vasculopathy in pediatric heart transplant recipients: a multi-institutional experience. Journal of Heart and Lung Transplantation. 2011;30(4S):S133.
76. Ng B, Dipchand A, Naftel D, et al. Outcomes of Pneumocystis jiroveci pneumonia infections in pediatric heart transplant recipients. Pediatric Transplantation. 2011;15:844–848.
77. Zaoutis TE, Webber S, Naftel DC, et al. Invasive fungal infections in pediatric heart transplant recipients: incidence, risk factors, and outcomes. Pediatric Transplantation. 2011;15:465–469.
78. Webber SA, Naftel DC, Fricker FJ, et al. Lymphoproliferative disorders after pediatric heart transplantation: a multi-institutional study. Lancet. 2006;367: 233–239.
79. Chinnock R, Webber SA, Dipchand AI, et al. A 16-year multi-institutional study of the role of age and EBV status on PTLD incidence among pediatric heart transplant recipients. American Journal of Transplantation. 2012;12: 3061–3068.
80. Smith JM, Nemeth TL, McDonald RA. Current immunosuppressive agents: efficacy, side effects, and utilization. Pediatric Clinics of North America. 2003; 50:1283–1300.
81. Russo L, Webber SA. Pediatric heart transplantation: immunosuppression and its complications. Current Opinion in Cardiology. 2004;19:104–109.
82. English RF, Pophal SA, Bacanu S, et al. Long-term comparison of tacrolimus and cyclosporine induced nephrotoxicity in pediatric heart transplant recipients. American Journal of Transplantation. 2002;2:769–773.

83. Feingold B, Zheng J, Law YM, et al. Risk factors for late renal dysfunction after pediatric heart transplantation: a multi-institutional study. Pediatric Transplantation. 2011;15:699–705.
84. Feingold B, Brooks MM, Zeevi A, et al. Renal function and genetic polymorphisms in pediatric heart transplant recipients. Journal of Heart and Lung Transplantation. 2012;31:1003–1008.
85. Mahle WT, Kanter KR, Vincent RN. Disparities in outcome for black patients after pediatric heart transplantation. Journal of Pediatrics. 2005;147:739–743.
86. Singh TP, Naftel DC, Addonizio L, et al. Association of race and socioeconomic position with outcomes in pediatric heart transplant recipients. American Journal of Transplantation. 2010;10:2116–2123.
87. Fine R, Webber SA, Harmon W, et al. Pediatric Solid Organ Transplantation, 2nd ed. Oxford: John Wiley and Sons; 2007.

第 116 章
儿童肺移植

Albert Faro, Stuart C. Sweet

引言

1963 年 Hardy 博士对一名终身监禁的罪犯进行了第一次成功的人类肺移植。免疫抑制包括:硫唑嘌呤、泼尼松和放射治疗。患者 18 天后死于肾功能不全。尽管 ABO 血型不匹配,尸检没有发现排斥反应。1968 年,库勒博士和他的团队对一个 12 个月大的完全性房室管缺损和肺动脉高压婴儿进行了第一次人类心肺移植。患者只存活了 14 个小时[1]。这种肺移植主要是在实验室实施,直到手术技术、保存液和免疫抑制方案提升或者可用。20 世纪 80 年代初成年人成功的心肺和肺移植报道,允许这个流程扩展和应用到儿科人群[2,3]。1986 年和 2010 年 6 月间,在小于 18 岁的患者中,国际心肺移植协会(ISHLT)报道了 1664 例肺移植和 653 例心肺移植(ISHLT)[4]。

为儿童进行移植的决定带来了独特的挑战。在成人肺移植领域获得的所有经验、适应证、方法、并发症、免疫抑制剂的药代动力学和监测对儿童来说往往是非常不同的。因此,儿童群体的肺移植必须被视为一个独特的领域,并单独研究。本章将试图突出儿童肺移植的一些独特特性。第 31 章、第 45 章、第 59 章、第 72 章、第 80 章、第 84 章和第 106 章囊括了成人肺移植的总体和特性方面的内容。儿童特殊事项涉及儿童的体型和生长、气道吻合口并发症、在幼儿园或学校感染的暴露增加、免疫抑制的非依从性,过渡到成人医疗供应和移植相关监测的障碍。

移植患者的选择和适应证

肺移植应考虑在特定的患有终末期或进行性肺疾病或没有其他治疗可选择的肺血管疾病的儿童中进行。到肺移植中心进行评估儿童的诊断通常与成人的诊断不同(第 31 章)。慢性阻塞性肺疾病(COPD)、肺气肿、特发性肺纤维化是最常见的三项成人移植前诊断。在过去的 20 年中,儿童肺移植的适应证已经经历了相当大的变化,即使是婴儿肺移植的经验也已经提高[5,6]。图 116.1 根据移植时的年龄列出了儿童移植时最常见的诊断。在 1 岁以下的儿童中,最常见的适应证是肺动脉高压,通常与先天性心脏病、其他肺血管疾病、原发

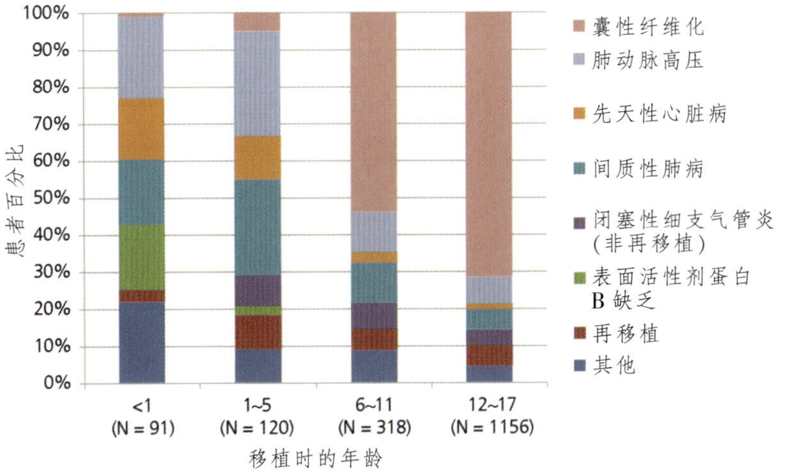

图 116.1 儿童肺移植的年龄和适应证分布。Data adapted from [4] with permission.

性肺静脉狭窄和罕见的肺泡毛细血管发育不良有关。表面活性剂的代谢紊乱包括:表面活性蛋白 B(SPB)和 C (SPC) 的不足,ATP 结合盒转运体 A3 (ABCA3)与 NKX2.1 的突变[6-9]。较不常见的适应证包括:间质性肺疾病、支气管肺发育不良、肺发育不全[10]。在 1~5 岁年龄组,导致肺动脉高压的疾病仍然是一个常见的适应证。在 6~11 岁的患者中,囊性纤维化(CF)成为最常见的适应证。原发性肺动脉高压导致的肺移植儿童的相对百分比在过去的 10 年中显著减少,在很大程度上是因为有效的药物治疗包括:前列腺素(依前列醇)、磷酸二酯酶抑制剂(如西地那非)和内皮素受体拮抗剂(如波生坦)[4]。在青少年中,囊性纤维化几乎占到肺移植人数的 3/4。换言之,与成年候选者相比,儿童候选者可出现脓毒症的肺部疾病,病原菌在肺移植后可继续定植于上呼吸道。

从历史上看,寻求肺移植治疗的时机是根据预测的死亡率与预期等待供肺的时间决定的。在安排肺移植之前,考虑到并不完美的疾病具体标准,大多数儿童医疗中心仔细考虑肺功能之外的多种因素,包括潜在的疾病进展、生长和营养状况、住院次数、心理社会因素和潜在的整体生活质量(QOL)的改进等。

儿童和成人患者的绝对禁忌证类似,包括:明显会给儿童造成移植后不良预后的风险的情况,包括全身性疾病(如恶性肿瘤或多器官功能衰竭)。相对禁忌证增加移植风险,但应根据具体情况进行权衡。一般禁忌证不是静态的,并且可以随着时间出现新的信息、治疗方法或技术而变化。禁忌证同时也基于医疗中心个体经验而有中心特异性。例如,许多医疗中心不会考虑给予患者静脉-动脉体外支持(VA-ECMO)。

一个具有挑战性的所有的儿童移植必须解决的问题是不遵守医疗管理。与成人相比,这对儿童是更大的问题,因为提供儿童治疗或带他们到诊所预约的责任属于父母,而不是儿童。在第 120 章中,可以找到详细的讨论。在这些情况下,咨询中心和移植中心必须与家庭合作分担责任,以解决治疗中的障碍。这可能需要制订一个咨询医生和家庭之间的契约,强调需要严格遵守移植前可能超过 6 个月的治疗计划。总的来说,在一些移植中心当非依从性问题难以干预时,它就成为一个绝对的禁忌证。虽然在一些医疗中心可以依据法律效力把孩子寄养,但许多医疗中心将临时安置在寄养家庭作为移植的绝对禁忌证。

移植评估本身包括一些实验室和影像学研究,以及与多个项目的咨询(表 116.1)。该评估是多学科的性质,涉及医疗和社会心理等因素。

疾病特异性评价

囊性纤维化

囊性纤维化(CF)是一种高度可变的疾病,是终末期肺部疾病最常见的死亡原因。治疗技术的提高进一步提高了中位生存时间,但仍有患囊性纤维化的儿童

表 116.1 儿童肺和心脏肺候选的推荐评价

血液检查
血型(ABO)
全血细胞计数
凝血试验(PT、INR、PTT)
全血生化包括电解质和肝肾功能测试
血脂分析
血清学包括:巨细胞病毒、EB 病毒、人类免疫缺陷病毒、乙肝和丙肝病毒、麻疹、水痘、单纯疱疹、刚地弓形虫
抗 HLA 抗体筛选
动脉血气分析
自身免疫筛选(ANA、ANCA、类风湿因子、定量免疫球蛋白)
甲状腺功能
肺功能测试
6 分钟步行试验
痰或喉深部培养和敏感性测试
结核杆菌测试
心电图
心导管(特定患者)
影像
胸片
胸部 CT
鼻窦 CT(CF 或免疫缺陷患者)
超声心动图
骨密度测定
会诊
心胸外科
心脏内科(特定患者)
感染科
社会服务
心理科
营养科
物理治疗
儿童生活

进展到呼吸功能不全。Liou 等使用比例风险模型来评估肺移植是否为囊性纤维化儿童提供了生存上的改善，并得出没有改善的结论[11]。然而他们的模型有几个缺陷[12]。它的数据来自移植等候名单，并且不是移植的时间。他们的研究完成于 2005 年，那时美国依据在等候名单上等待的时间来分配肺，而不是由肺分配系统（在本章进一步阐述）进行器官分配。患者通常在让他们继续生存下去的实际移植前等待 2~3 年。医生会考虑到名单上的日期将不是移植的日期，承认如果患者能够存活到移植的时候，他们将累积名单上的时间。这个缺陷，它本身影响了计算该方案的生存获益。其他研究发现[13]，肺移植仍然是囊性纤维化和终末期肺部疾病患者的有延长寿命可能性的唯一可用的治疗选择[14]。

特殊适应证

囊性纤维化的早期研究建议，一旦预测一秒钟用力呼气容积（FEV_1）下降到 30%以下[15]，即要接受肺移植治疗。虽然更多的近期研究试图添加到这些标准[16]，但没有一项显著改善了预测等候名单的死亡率。即使在最好的模型中，阳性预测值也是小于 50%[17]。

特殊禁忌证

个别移植中心有特定的移植微生物相关禁忌证；最常见 Burkholderia cenocepacia 的慢性感染。病例报告表明慢性脓肿分枝杆菌感染的患者预后可能更糟[18]，但其他研究人员已经证明这些患者的成功结果[19]。严重肝疾病在一些医疗中心可能是一个禁忌证，但可能在其他医疗中心是联合肺肝移植的适应证。胸膜固定术不是移植的绝对禁忌证，但可能因为手术期间较多的出血而延长缺血时间。

表面活性剂过程异常

表面活性物质缺陷的患者通常表现为出生后不久的呼吸衰竭。SPC 缺陷的儿童，ABCA3 转运蛋白突变，或 NK2.1x 突变可以有不同的表现[20]。肺活检可显示弥漫性肺泡Ⅱ型上皮细胞增生、肺泡间隔增厚和肺泡蛋白沉积症。遗传分析进一步证实了诊断。

特殊适应证

一旦决定进行移植，表面活性物质缺陷患者应该尽可能快地转移到移植中心，因为许多患者最终需要高频振荡通气或 ECMO。对于其他的表面活性剂过程异常的肺移植表明难治性呼吸衰竭或进行性呼吸功能不全对医疗干预反应迟钝。

特殊禁忌证

正如上面所提到的，许多移植中心 VA-ECMO 依赖是移植的绝对禁忌证。明显的脑出血或其他严重的带有显著延迟发育可能的神经损伤也是一个禁忌证。

肺血管疾病

儿童的肺血管疾病有多种潜在病因，包括肺动脉高压（IPH）、先天性心脏病和肺静脉异常。这些必须进行仔细区分，以进行适当的管理。治疗的进展已经大大提高肺动脉高压患儿的预后，并且他们应该只在药物治疗失败时接受移植。确定何时给予艾森门格综合征患者移植仍然是具有挑战性的。这些患者中很多在诊断后也可以活很多年。

特殊适应证

心脏指数降低小于 2L/(min·m^2)、肺血管阻力升高、右心房压力大于 7.4mmHg 和右室舒张压超过 10.4mmHg 预示着较差的生存时间，是肺移植的适应证。其他可能与生存相关的因素包括：血管性血友病因子水平超过 240%、血尿酸水平升高与血浆脑钠肽（BNP）大于 180pg/mL。

艾森门格综合征和进行性疾病患者，包括严重的缺氧、晕厥或非常有限的生活质量，心肺移植必须被考虑。简单的心脏病变的患者可以是双侧肺移植时进行心脏修复的候选人[21,22]。

对于表面活性剂缺陷患者，一旦肺泡毛细血管发育不良（ACD）、肺静脉闭塞性疾病或肺静脉狭窄的患者决定进行肺移植，应该尽可能快地实施，因为这些疾病对药物或手术干预的反应很差。

特殊禁忌证

在这一人群中，广泛的主动脉-肺动脉侧支循环的存在（见于小或无中心肺动脉的肺动脉闭锁），和已多次开胸手术与预后不良有联系[23,24]。此外，曾经历多次外科手术或有同种瓣膜或血管植入患者，有同种致敏可能和随后的同种异体移植物抗移植物损伤风险增加的可能。这些危险因素是许多医疗中心的相对禁忌证。

等候名单的管理

在美国，处理等候名单的做法是，>12 岁的儿童和成人由器官获取和移植网络（OPTN）[25]（见第 31 章）按照 2005 年被采用的“肺分配系统”（LAS）来分配。为了最大限度地提高一年移植存活率，LAS依据等候名单死亡率和移植后生存模型来分配供肺。模型中的因素包括诊断、年龄、身高体重比、需要氧气支持、肺动脉压、6分钟步行距离和肺功能等。在美国等候时间和等待名单的死亡率下降与LAS的采用有关[26]。然而，等候名单死亡率对LAS（LAS=移植后存活-2×等候名单生存率，归一化到0~100尺度）的双重贡献作用已增加重症患者接受移植的数量，并且高LAS评分的移植患者有着更差的总体生存率（主要是那些需要机械通气的患者）[27]。LAS的一个重要方面是，能从肺移植患者名单中连续收集数据，对模型进行细化并产生优先级得分；在2012年初发布了一个LAS升级版本，用于公共评价。虽然没有足够的数据来创建一个年龄小于12岁的儿童LAS分型系统，但从2010年，该人群的肺分配已基于两个紧急层和更广泛的地理共享（表116.2）[28]。

术前管理的目标是保持患者的健康状态，使移植后达到最佳预后，并解决在评估过程中发现的不足之处。因此无论什么诊断，在这段时间内的许多干预措施是相同的。策略包括：最大限度地提高儿童的营养状况；让儿童参加物理和康复治疗，以减少肌肉松弛；尽量减少感染的暴露；提供适当的预防接种；如果有关于依从性问题，和家庭一起建立能够适应移植后续复杂生活的方案。

其他具体的术前管理将因疾病状态而改变。在囊性纤维化患者中，继续积极地进行气道清理、营养支持、抗菌治疗和身体康复是至关重要的。特殊病因的肺血管疾病的患者中，使用肺血管扩张剂治疗、利尿剂、抗凝剂、氧气支持、和（或）心脏房隔造口术可能延长生命。患有间质性肺疾病的儿童中，类固醇激素的使用可能有利。

表116.2 美国12岁以下等待肺移植高优先级儿童

呼吸衰竭表现为
• 需要持续机械通气，或
• 需要任何方式提高 FiO_2 大于50%，氧饱和度大于90%，或
• 存在动脉或毛细血管 PCO_2 大于50mmHg，静脉 PCO_2 大于56mmHg
肺动脉高压表现为
• 3个或以上肺静脉狭窄，或
• 在药物治疗下仍出现晕厥、咯血、心指数小于2L/(min·m²)，心电图或心导管提示的肺动脉高压

值得注意的是，虽然机械通气在成年肺移植受者中是一个不良预后的危险因素，但这对于婴儿和幼儿却不是。与非通气的患者相比，3岁以下的机械通气儿童1~3年的移植物存活率并没有不同[29]。

在长时间难以管理机械通气的患者中，介入肺辅助装置（Novalung®iLA），一种无泵转膜机，已被证明是一种有效的二氧化碳去除装置和可能用于移植的有用装置。在第50章中可找到附加的关于人工肺细节[30]。该装置已成功地用于一个2岁的儿童[31]。在我们医疗中心，我们也在使用Maquet® quadrox ID膜式氧合器在避免肌肉松弛的时候试图提供足够的气体交换。这些装置有ECMO抗凝相关并发症的类似风险；因此他们的长期支持作用仍不明确。

移植程序和外科技术

潜在的儿童供体肺用一种与成年患者类似的方式进行评估。对比成人肺移植（第59章），儿童的大多数流程在体外循环打开时进行。手术方法仍然采用双前外侧经胸骨（“翻盖”）切口，来提供双侧胸腔的最佳入路和视野。大多数程序涉及端对端连续性双肺移植而不是可伸缩的支气管对支气管吻合来降低狭窄的可能性[32]。为了给吻合口提供最佳的血液供应，降低感染从气道向邻近血管结构扩散的风险，吻合口一般覆盖供体或受体来源的心包或支气管周围淋巴组织[32,33]。在囊性纤维化患者中，在移植前对受者气管及支气管残端用抗生素溶液用力冲洗可减少气道微生物向供体移植物传播的可能性。

在儿科心肺移植是一个相对罕见的事件[4]。虽然在过去，肺动脉高压伴显著的右心室功能障碍被认为是心肺移植的适应证，甚至可以在成功的双侧肺移植中看到显著的右心室肥大和功能障碍[34,35]。当临床中先天性心脏缺损需要修复时，心内修复可以在双侧肺切除时或切除后，并在供体肺移植前进行，从而避免心肺移植[22]。由于儿童的肺疾病的高患病率，以及考虑到肺的生长，单肺移植很少在儿童中使用[4]。

自从LAS使用以来，在美国活体供肺移植已经几乎消失了。不过，被植入受体的一个右下叶来自一个健康的供者，左下叶来自另一个供者（一般是家庭成员）的手术仍然在日本使用，那里得到适合儿童的供体器官受到很多限制。其他在儿童中使用的外科技术包括用线性吻合器进行供体裁剪或者叶切除术和肺叶移植[37]。这些通常用于增加婴儿和年幼儿童移植器官的可获取范围。

移植后管理

我们将突出儿童移植后管理不同于成人方案中的几个重要的方面。关于成人管理的具体细节可以在第80章找到。一些移植后管理内容在儿童和成人肺移植受者中是相同的，如原发性移植物功能障碍或排斥反应的处理，这里将简要提及而不进行进一步细述。

免疫抑制方案

在儿童移植中，医生在考虑免疫抑制方案疗效的同时，也要考虑到该方案的副作用是否会影响患儿正常生长发育，或引起患者对免疫抑制方案的不依从性。在移植后1年中，80%的儿童肺移植受者使用他克莫司，65%使用MMF，因为肺移植受者与其他器官移植受者相比，具有更高的排斥风险，更强的免疫抑制方案已经问世。例如，他克莫司最低剂量的初始目标通常为10~20ng/mL。泼尼松的初始给药量通常为0.5~1.0mg/(kg·d)，移植后3~4个月的目标量为0.25~0.5mg/(kg·d)。在移植后5年，很少有患者停用泼尼松[4]。免疫诱导治疗在大多数儿科肺移植中心使用；最近数据显示，超过60%的患者接受多克隆抗体(抗淋巴细胞或抗胸腺细胞球蛋白)或IL-2受体拮抗剂(巴利昔单抗)治疗[4]。

儿童中类固醇的使用值得注意，因为它可能对儿童的生长发育产生不利影响。有其他儿科器官受体的数据显示，避免用类固醇激素策略可以有良好的免疫抑制效果，但对儿童肺移植受者没有系统性研究[38]。这方面的进一步研究是必要的。

抗微生物方案

大多数患者在肺移植之前和之后接受预防性静脉内抗生素治疗，以覆盖常见的气道病原体以及已知在其气道中定植的微生物。抗微生物方案可以基于供体培养结果进行修改。无囊性纤维化患者使用单一广谱抗革兰阳性和革兰阴性抗生素，囊性纤维化患者术前痰培养结果可以指导抗微生物治疗。一般需要覆盖革兰阴性菌，例如铜绿假单胞菌和偶然的无色杆菌属。近期在患有囊性纤维化和晚期肺部疾病的儿童中流行的耐甲氧西林金黄色葡萄球菌（MRSA），用万古霉素覆盖。对移植前检测出烟曲霉菌的患者，大部分医疗中心用伏立康唑或阿尼芬净预防。在某些情况下，雾化吸入的两性霉素，口服伊曲康唑或口服伏立康唑也在使用[39]；对于移植后不久出现的肺囊虫，使用甲氧苄啶和(或)磺胺甲恶唑(TMP /SMX)1周3次。预防念珠菌病可口服制霉菌素。

虽然肺移植受者中更昔洛韦预防显著降低了CMV肺炎的发病率，但CMV(巨细胞病毒)仍然是患者死亡的重大潜在风险[40,41]。在儿童肺移植受体中，CMV的预防方法在移植中心之间差别很大。一般来说，当受体和供体都是CMV血清阴性时，不给予预防[42]。当供体或受体CMV血清阳性时，用4~12周更昔洛韦或缬更昔洛韦。最近，研究表明预防(使用更昔洛韦或口服缬更昔洛韦）的持续时间延长至6个月或更长有益于预后[43,44]。虽然基于成人经验，一些儿科中心除了使用更昔洛韦外还使用CMV超免疫球蛋白（CMVIg)[45]，但CMVIg的益处仍不清楚[46]。

对移植物的监测

儿童肺功能的测量更具挑战性，特别是对于6岁以下的儿童，因为肺活量测量通常在该年龄组是不可用或不可靠的。对于较大的儿童和成人一样，肺活量测量是临床诊断闭塞性细支气管炎综合征(BOS)所必需的。对于婴儿，使用胸腹压缩技术，肺功能测试可以识别气流阻塞的存在，但需要专门的设备和经验，且仅限于体长小于90cm的儿童[47,48]。此外，因为测试需要在安静环境下进行，所以婴儿肺功能测试不能像常规肺活量测定法那样频繁进行。而且最新的BOS诊断标准中并不包含婴儿肺功能测试[49]。因此，一些儿科移植中心常规开展胸部HRCT以及通气和(或)灌注扫描，以帮助早期识别闭塞性细支气管炎。

脉冲震荡(IOS)是一种有效的技术，以评估2岁以下儿童是否存在气流阻塞[50,51]。该技术要求受试者在短时间内正常地呼吸到吹口（或者是针对那些不能在吹口周围闭合嘴唇的幼儿的特殊面罩)。它不需要患者积极配合，值得在学龄前儿童术后人群中进一步研究。

在婴儿和幼儿中获得活检也颇具难点。虽然匹配儿科支气管镜的更小的支气管活检钳已经在临床应用了一段时间，但是该技术每次获取的活检组织相应地也更小了。因此，如何获得足够的组织以可靠地判断婴儿是否出现排斥反应现在仍是难题[52]。

预后及危险因素

生存率

1990年1月至2009年6月进行的儿童肺移植后生存与成人的生存相当(图116.2)。参见第106章关于肺移植结果的额外讨论。总体而言,儿童受者的中位生存期为4.5年,与成人的结果无统计学差异。儿童受体的一年生存率显著改善,从1988—1994年的67%,到近期(2002—2009年)的83%(图116.3)。但是5年生存率没有显著改善,这表明早期死亡率改善的主要原因是时间效应。Kaplan-Meier生存分析还显示,1~11岁移植的儿童同12~17岁的移植相比,存活率更高(图116.4a和116.4b)。在最近的ISHLT报道中,移植后第一年内的最常见的两种死亡原因是感染和移植物衰竭。移植后1~3年,闭塞性细支气管炎成为死亡的主要原因,占死亡率的近40%。感染和移植物衰竭在整个随访期间仍然是死亡的重要原因。

值得注意的是,尽管与首次移植相比,再移植(总体37%的5年生存率)结果仍然较差,但现在再次移

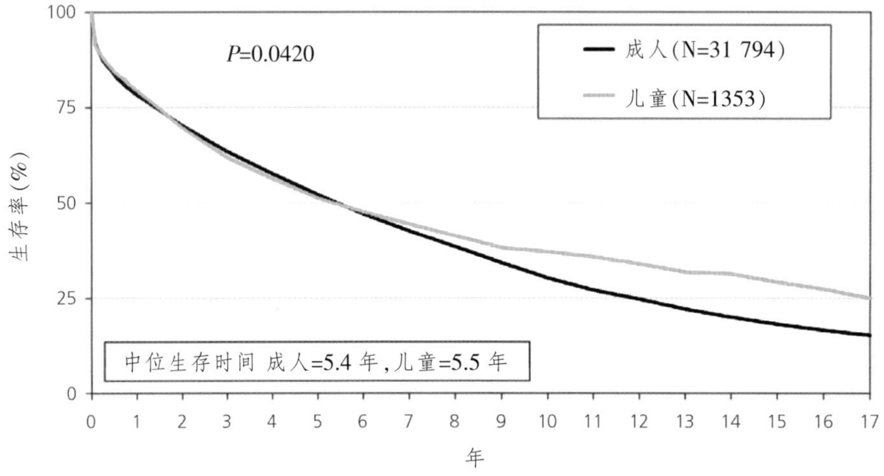

图116.2 成人与儿童肺移植存活率比较。(Reprinted from [4] Benden C, Aurora P, Edwards LB, Kucheryavaya AY, Christie JD, Dobbels F, et al. The Registry of the International Society for Heart and Lung Transplantation: Fourteenth Pediatric Lung and Heart-Lung Transplantation Report (2011). J Heart Lung Transplant. 2011 Oct;30(10):1123–1132. Copyright © 2011, with permission from Elsevier.)

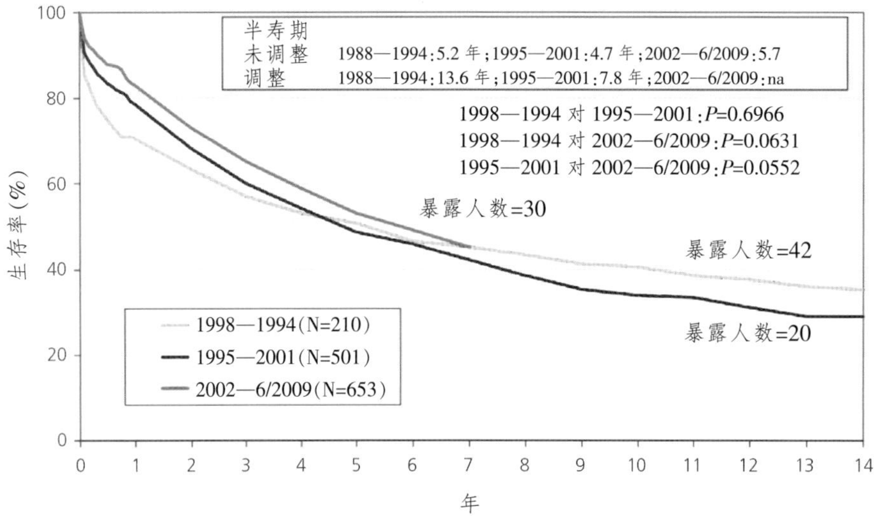

图116.3 不同时期儿童肺移植存活率。Reprinted from [4] Benden C, Aurora P, Edwards LB, Kucheryavaya AY, Christie JD, Dobbels F, et al. The Registry of the International Society for Heart and Lung Transplantation: Fourteenth Pediatric Lung and Heart-Lung Transplantation Report (2011). J Heart Lung Transplant. 2011 Oct;30(10):1123–1132. Copyright © 2011, with permission from Elsevier.

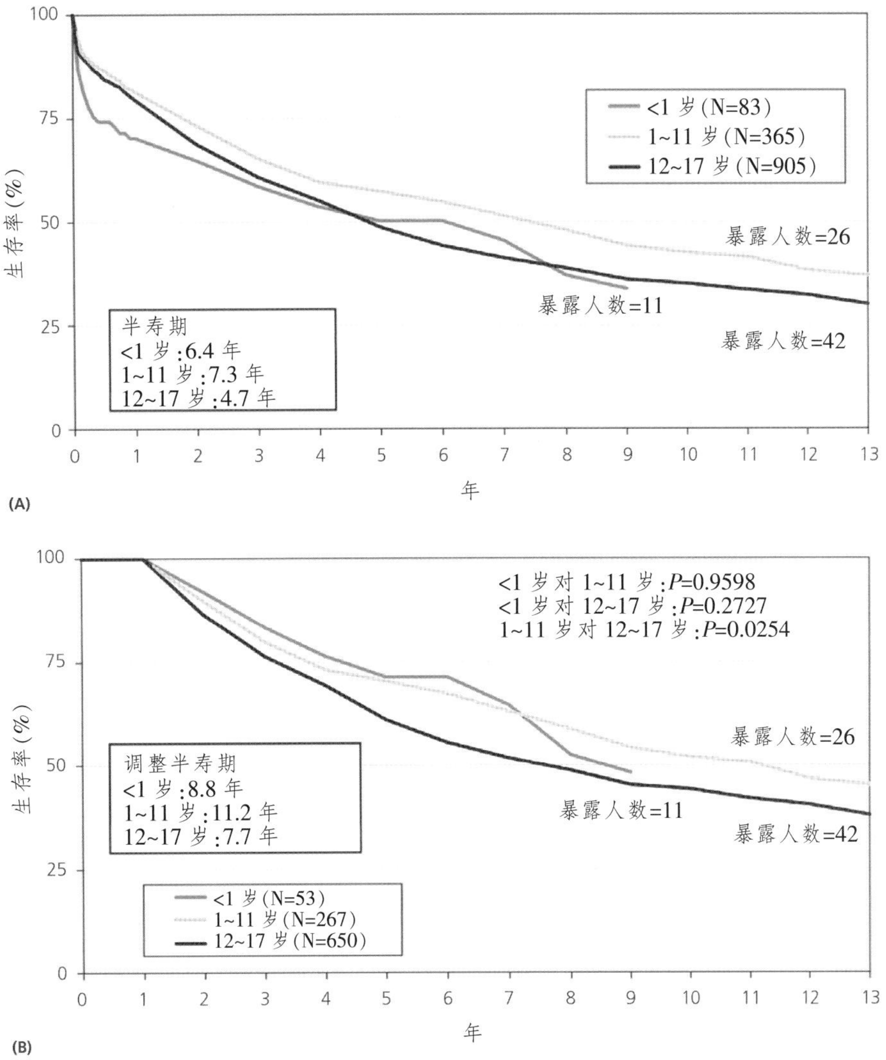

图 116.4 (A)不同年龄组儿童肺移植生存率。(B)不同年龄组儿童肺移植一年条件生存率。Reprinted from [4] Benden C, Aurora P, Edwards LB, Kucheryavaya AY, Christie JD, Dobbels F, et al. The Registry of the International Society for Heart and Lung Transplantation: Fourteenth Pediatric Lung and Heart-Lung Transplantation Report (2011). J Heart Lung Transplant. 2011 Oct;30(10):1123-1132. Copyright ⓒ 2011, with permission from Elsevier.

植[4,26]已很普遍,可能是因为 LAS 为 12 岁及以上儿童提供了更多的机会[53]。选择合适的再次肺移植受者因优先考虑。

并发症

气道并发症

血管或支气管吻合口瘘是一种罕见的并发症,需要再次手术。大多数移植中心在移植后的第一个 24~48 小时期间通过软支气管镜检查气道吻合口的完整性,并获取下呼吸道的培养物。用血管化组织覆盖吻合口的技术显著降低了这种并发症的发生率[3,33,54]。同时令人惊讶的是,儿童肺移植后纤维化狭窄、过度肉芽组织或吻合口气道塌陷发生率与成人类似[55,56]。当临床表现严重时,气道狭窄可通过经支气管镜球囊扩张术缓解。

大多数医疗中心避免放置可膨胀金属支架,因为它们并没有能扩张到适应儿童气道最大生长所需程度的能力,需要最终去除。不幸的是,移除这些支架可能引起致命并发症[57]。此外,肉芽组织的形成可能导致严重的气道阻塞。在我们的机构,硅橡胶支架用于 12 例支气管吻合中,4 例发生并发症,包括移位或阻塞[56]。新的生物可降解支架具有缓解狭窄的潜力,还能允许气道之后的生长发育[58],值得进一步研究。

血管并发症

由于大多数儿童肺移植手术在心肺旁路手术中进行，出血（特别是在胸膜腔或血管吻合部位的出血）并不少见，尤其是在既往有开胸手术中的患者中[10]。血管吻合并发症通常与低血压和造影异常有关。肺静脉或左心房吻合缝合线的血栓形成可能发生在术后早期[59]。灌注扫描和超声心动图应用于评估吻合口。

免疫学并发症

在婴幼儿群体中发生急性细胞排斥和BOS的风险似乎较低[29]。免疫学并发症的诊断和治疗方法与成年移植受者相同。抗体介导的排斥是最近认识到的肺移植免疫学并发症，并且以类似的方式影响儿童和成人。尽管有关治疗的具体标准尚未定论，在同种异体移植物功能障碍的情况下，循环供体特异性抗体（使用固相流式细胞术鉴定），肺泡毛细血管补体（C4d）沉积和毛细血管炎的鉴定通常被认为是足够的证据[60]。在儿科移植中心中，体液排斥的治疗也是各不相同。大多数移植中心使用类固醇、血浆置换、静脉注射免疫球蛋白和B细胞减少（环磷酰胺或利妥昔单抗）等组合治疗[61]。较新的药物（如硼替佐米，靶向浆细胞的蛋白体抑制剂）或补体抑制剂（如依库珠单抗）越来越多地被使用[62,63]。

免疫抑制的重要并发症是恶性肿瘤。在移植后1年和5年，肺移植后的恶性肿瘤发生率分别为5.9%和13.1%。移植后淋巴增生性疾病（PTLD）是迄今为止最常见的恶性肿瘤[4]。在免疫抑制的儿童患者中，PTLD通常是EB病毒介导的，B细胞淋巴增殖在组织学上可变很多[64,65]。同成人患者相比，儿童患者与囊性纤维化患者作为肺移植受体（同其他实体器官受体相比）时更易发生PTLD。这可以用移植前血清EB病毒抗体阴性和免疫抑制的强度解释。PTLD经常表现为无其他症状，胸部成像意外的发现单一或多个圆形或卵圆形肺结节[67]。肺外PTLD的发生率在移植第一年后增加。部位包括胃肠道、皮肤、鼻咽、淋巴结和其他淋巴组织[68,69]。大多数移植中心通过PCR监测EBV的定量测量，PCR是PTLD的一种敏感且特异性的标志物[70]。正电子发射断层扫描（PET）是敏感的检查手段[71]。PTLD的组织学诊断对预后至关重要，因为CD20阳性肿瘤可能更适合于抗体治疗，单形PTLD具有较差的预后[72]。

虽然一些成人医疗中心在发现升高的EBV PCR后，随之减少免疫抑制[73]。最近的一项研究表明，在儿童中使用这种方法需谨慎[74]。虽然它可以在一些患者中取得成功，但减少的免疫抑制带来急性排斥的风险显著提高。在许多情况下，需要另外的治疗来诱导缓解。许多医疗中心现在遵循儿童肿瘤小组的方案，使用ANHL 0221（利妥昔单抗，低剂量环磷酰胺和泼尼松有效），并证实了在儿童实体器官移植受者发生PTLD时有效[75]。

社区获得性呼吸道病毒

由于上幼儿园、学校或兄弟姐妹的存在，儿童往往更容易暴露于呼吸道病毒感染。这些感染在移植后特别容易引起并发症。腺病毒[76]和副黏病毒包括副流感和呼吸道合胞病毒（RSV）可引起显著的肺损伤或死亡[77,78]。许多医疗中心分别用西多福韦和利巴韦林分别治疗这些病毒[78-80]。呼吸道病毒感染也与闭塞性细支气管炎综合征（BOS）的晚期发展有关[81]。

移植获益，功能预后和生活质量

尽管成年肺移植受者的生存质量（QOL）和生存率优于仍在等候名单上的患者[82-84]，推广应用至儿童和青少年时仍应保持谨慎。虽然登记报告数据表明，超过80%的肺移植幸存者移植后的1年、3年和5年没有活动受限的报道[4]，但是关于儿童肺移植生存质量的高质量研究还很有限。一项小型研究显示肺移植受者的健康质量提高24%[85]。在另一项研究中，一组47名胸部器官受者（6名肺移植受者）报道的健康状况低于正常人群，但与哮喘、青少年类风湿性关节炎和顽固性癫痫患儿的健康状况相似[86]。需要注意的是，生活质量的评估可能受到移植前儿童的生存质量和移植后预期的影响[85]。此外，儿童的生长发育水平也必须包括在生活质量研究中。对儿科移植术后系统评估和发展影响的未来纵向研究，对儿童受者的生存质量很重要。

肺的生长发育

在婴儿和幼儿中成功的肺移植引起了行业内对肺同种异体移植物是否会随着儿童生长这一问题的关注。在动物模型中，同种异体肺移植的肺容量和气道大小随着年龄的增加而增加[88]。肺活量和肺体积测量在婴儿[89]和较大的儿童[24]中是正常的。然而，这些测量反映的是增加的肺泡容积和气体交换的表面积，而不是肺泡数量。Ro 和同事连续 CT 扫描数据支持胸腔内气道随时间而生长[90]。然而，一家医疗中心研究表明死亡供体和活体供体移植的儿童受者中一氧化碳扩散能力(DLCO)并没有出现随生长而升高的表现[91]。尽管 DLCO 能更好地估计气体交换表面积，但是在婴儿中不容易测量。有待进一步研究以证明婴儿和幼儿肺移植受者的肺生长的程度。

儿童的发展

神经认知结果难以预测。婴儿具有一定程度的神经认知可塑性，使他们能够更好地面对环境改变、循环系统损害、感染、营养异常和生长状态。接受实体器官移植的婴儿有发展成学习障碍、视觉和空间缺陷以及运动迟缓的风险[92]。头围、运动技能和认知功能的测量都显示移植后有改善，大多数儿童正常或接近正常[92]。至关重要的是，婴儿移植体系中需要有一个方案，对儿童的神经发育进行评估，以便在必要时实施早期干预。这一领域值得进一步研究，以更好地定义与发展迟缓相关的危险因素。

青少年移植

青少年移植受者值得特别提及。青春期是一个情感脆弱的生活阶段，个体与自我同一性、认知发展和自我自主性进行斗争。青少年移植受者有冒险行为的可能性增加，会表现为不依从治疗。他们感觉很好，低估免疫抑制治疗的重要性，可能导致晚期急性排斥发生率的增加，较差的结果如移植失败甚至死亡[93,94]。

毫无疑问，移植团队要和青少年的移植人群建立与其他人群相比更稳健的关系，以提供正规的教育、鼓励和开放的沟通。这一时期的医疗结果可能很差[95]，这并不奇怪。过渡需要协调一致地改善儿童和成人医疗中心之间的沟通，特别是提供者之间的沟通[96,97]。如何更好地处理过渡的过程是一个需要积极研究的领域，随着我们能更好地管理儿童肺移植受者[98,99]，这一挑战会越来越大。

总结

儿童肺移植有很多独特的挑战和机会。显然，肺移植可以在具有终末期肺实质和血管疾病的婴儿和儿童中成功地进行，能够延长存活时间及改善生活质量。然而，许多人的长期结果远远低于我们的预期。闭塞性细支气管炎缺乏有效疗法，供体短缺等问题和成人移植一样。在儿科领域也能遇到的一些特有的问题和解决方法。

(柯庆宏 译 柯庆宏 校)

参考文献

1. Cooley DA, Bloodwell RD, Hallman GL, et al. Organ transplantation for advanced cardiopulmonary disease. Annals of Thoracic Surgery. 1969;8(1):30–46.
2. Reitz BA, Wallwork JL, Hunt SA, et al. Heart-lung transplantation: successful therapy for patients with pulmonary vascular disease. New England Journal of Medicine. 1982;306(10):557–564.
3. Grossman RF, Frost A, Zamel N, et al. Results of single-lung transplantation for bilateral pulmonary fibrosis. The Toronto Lung Transplant Group. New England Journal of Medicine. [10.1056/NEJM199003153221104 doi]. 1990;322(11):727–733.
4. Benden C, Aurora P, Edwards LB, et al. The registry of the international society for heart and lung transplantation: fourteenth pediatric lung and heart-lung transplantation report–2011. Journal of Heart and Lung Transplantation. 2011; 30(10):1123–1132.
5. Bridges ND, Mallory GB, Huddleston CB, et al. Lung transplantation in infancy and early childhood. Journal of Heart and Lung Transplantation. 1996;15(9): 895–902.
6. Hamvas A, Nogee LM, Mallory GB Jr, et al. Lung transplantation for treatment of infants with surfactant protein B deficiency. Journal of Pediatrics. 1997;130(2): 231–239.
7. Nogee LM, Dunbar AE III, Wert SE, et al. A mutation in the surfactant protein C gene associated with familial interstitial lung disease. New EnglandJournal of Medicine. 2001;344(8):573–579.
8. Shulenin S, Nogee LM, Annilo T, et al. ABCA3 gene mutations in newborns with fatal surfactant deficiency. [see comment]. New EnglandJournal of Medicine. 2004;350(13):1296–1303.
9. Maquet E, Costagliola S, Parma J, et al. Lethal respiratory failure and mild primary hypothyroidism in a term girl with a de novo heterozygous mutation in the TITF1/NKX2.1 gene. Journal of Clinical Endocrinology and Metabolism. [Case Reports Research Support, Non-U.S. Gov't]. 2009;94(1):197–203.
10. Sweet SC. Pediatric lung transplantation: update 2003. [Review] [98 refs]. Pediatric Clinics of North America. 2003;50(6):1393–1417.
11. Liou TG, Adler FR, Cox DR, et al. Lung transplantation and survival in children with cystic fibrosis. New England Journal of Medicine. 2007;357(21):2143–2152.
12. Sweet SC, Aurora P, Benden C, et al. Lung transplantation and survival in children with cystic fibrosis: solid statistics–flawed interpretation. [see comment]. Pediatric Transplantation. 2008;12(2):129–136.
13. Aurora P, Whitehead B, Wade A, et al. Lung transplantation and life extension in children with cystic fibrosis. Lancet. 1999;354(9190):1591–1593.
14. Adler FR, Aurora P, Barker DH, et al. Lung transplantation for cystic fibrosis. Proceedings of the American Thoracic Society. 2009;6(8):619–633.
15. Kerem E, Reisman J, Corey M, et al. Prediction of mortality in patients with cystic fibrosis. New England Journal of Medicine. 1992;326(18):1187–1191.
16. Belkin RA, Henig NR, Singer LG, et al. Risk factors for death of patients with cystic fibrosis awaiting lung transplantation. American Journal of Respiratory and Critical Care Medicine. 2006;173(6):659–666.
17. Mayer-Hamblett N, Rosenfeld M, Emerson J, et al. Developing cystic fibrosis lung transplant referral criteria using predictors of 2-year mortality. [comment]. American Journal of Respiratory and Critical Care Medicine. 2002;166(12 Pt 1): 1550–1555.
18. Taylor JL, Palmer SM. Mycobacterium abscessus chest wall and pulmonary infection in a cystic fibrosis lung transplant recipient. Journal of Heart and Lung Transplantation. [Case Reports]. 2006;25(8):985–988.
19. Gilljam M, Schersten H, Silverborn M, et al. Lung transplantation in patients with cystic fibrosis and Mycobacterium abscessus infection. Journal of Cystic Fibrosis. [Case Reports Research Support, Non-U.S. Gov't]. 2010;9(4):272–276.
20. Faro A, Hamvas A. Lung transplantation for inherited disorders of surfactant metabolism. NeoReviews. 2008;9(10):e468–e476.
21. Choong CK, Sweet SC, Guthrie TJ, et al. Repair of congenital heart lesions combined with lung transplantation for the treatment of severe pulmonary hypertension: a 13-year experience. Journal of Thoracic and Cardiovascular Surgery.

2005;129(3):661–669.
22. Mendeloff EN, Huddleston CB. Lung transplantation and repair of complex congenital heart lesions in patients with pulmonary hypertension. Seminars in Thoracic and Cardiovascular Surgery. 1998;10(2):144–151.
23. Grady RM, Gandhi S, Sweet SC, et al. Dismal lung transplant outcomes in children with tetralogy of Fallot with pulmonary atresia compared to Eisenmenger syndrome or pulmonary vein stenosis. Journal of Heart and Lung Transplantation. 2009;28(11):1221–1225.
24. Sweet SC, Spray TL, Huddleston CB, et al. Pediatric lung transplantation at St. Louis Children's Hospital, 1990-1995. American Journal of Respiratory and Critical Care Medicine. 1997;155(3):1027–1035.
25. Egan TM, Murray S, Bustami RT, et al. Development of the new lung allocation system in the United States. American Journal of Transplantation. 2006;6(5 Pt 2):1212–1227.
26. Yusen RD, Shearon TH, Qian Y, et al. Lung transplantation in the United States, 1999-2008. American Journal of Transplantation. 2010;10(4 Pt 2):1047-68.
27. Sweet SC. Improving the lung allocation system: statistical significance does not guarantee predictive value. Journal of Heart and Lung Transplantation. [Comment Editorial]. 2010;29(7):756–758.
28. Organ Distribution: Allocation of Thoracic Organs. 2012 [updated May 23, 2012]; Available from: http://optn.transplant.hrsa.gov/PoliciesandBylaws2/policies/pdfs/policy_9.pdf.
29. Elizur A, Faro A, Huddleston CB, et al. Lung transplantation in infants and toddlers from 1990 to 2004 at St. Louis Children's Hospital. American Journal of Transplantation. 2009;9(4):719–726.
30. de Perrot M, Granton JT, McRae K, et al. Impact of extracorporeal life support on outcome in patients with idiopathic pulmonary arterial hypertension awaiting lung transplantation. Journal of Heart and Lung Transplantation. [Comparative Study]. 2011;30(9):997–1002.
31. Gazit AZ, Sweet SC, Grady RM, et al. First experience with a paracorporeal artificial lung in a small child with pulmonary hypertension. Journal of Thoracic and Cardiovascular Surgery. [Case Reports]. 2011;141(6):e48–e50.
32. Huddleston CB. Airway complications in children following lung transplantation. In: Cooper DKC, Miller LW, Patterson GA, editors. The Transplantation and Replacement of Thoracic Organs. Dordrecht: Springer Netherlands; 1996: 581–588.
33. Pasque MK, Cooper JD, Kaiser LR, et al. Improved technique for bilateral lung transplantation: rationale and initial clinical experience. Annals of Thoracic Surgery. 1990;49(5):785–791.
34. Carere R, Patterson GA, Liu P, et al. Right and left ventricular performance after single and double lung transplantation. The Toronto Lung Transplant Group. Journal of Thoracic and Cardiovascular Surgery. 1991;102(1):115–122.
35. Katz WE, Gasior TA, Quinlan JJ, et al. Immediate effects of lung transplantation on right ventricular morphology and function in patients with variable degrees of pulmonary hypertension. Journal of the American College of Cardiology. [0735-1097(95)00502-1 pii]. 1996;27(2):384–391.
36. Starnes VA, Barr ML, Cohen RG. Lobar transplantation. Indications, technique, and outcome. Journal of Thoracic and Cardiovascular Surgery. 1994;108(3):403–410.
37. Benden C, Inci I, Weder W, et al. Size-reduced lung transplantation in children–an option worth to consider! Pediatric Transplantation. [PTR1267 pii; 10.1111/j.1399-3046.2009.01267.x doi]. 2010;14(4):529–533.
38. Vidhun JR, Sarwal MM. Corticosteroid avoidance in pediatric renal transplantation. Pediatric Nephrology. 2005;20(3):418–426.
39. Mallory GB, Spray TL. Paediatric lung transplantation. European Respiratory Journal. [24/5/839 pii;10.1183/09031936.04.00064804 doi]. 2004;24(5):839–845.
40. Danziger-Isakov LA, DelaMorena M, Hayashi RJ, et al. Cytomegalovirus viremia associated with death or retransplantation in pediatric lung-transplant recipients. Transplantation. 2003;75(9):1538–1543.
41. Danziger-Isakov LA, Worley S, Michaels MG, et al. The risk, prevention, and outcome of cytomegalovirus after pediatric lung transplantation. Transplantation. 2009;87(10):1541–1548.
42. Danziger-Isakov LA, Faro A, Sweet S, et al. Variability in standard care for cytomegalovirus prevention and detection in pediatric lung transplantation: survey of eight pediatric lung transplant programs. Pediatric Transplantation. 2003;7(6):469–473.
43. Valentine VG, Weill D, Gupta MR, et al. Ganciclovir for cytomegalovirus: a call for indefinite prophylaxis in lung transplantation. Journal of Heart and Lung Transplantation. 2008;27(8):875–881.
44. Jaksch P, Zweytick B, Kerschner H, et al. Cytomegalovirus prevention in high-risk lung transplant recipients: comparison of 3- vs 12-month valganciclovir therapy. Journal of Heart and Lung Transplantation. 2009;28(7):670–675.
45. Valantine HA, Luikart H, Doyle R, et al. Impact of cytomegalovirus hyperimmune globulin on outcome after cardiothoracic transplantation: a comparative study of combined prophylaxis with CMV hyperimmune globulin plus ganciclovir versus ganciclovir alone. Transplantation. 2001;72(10):1647–1652.
46. Ranganathan K, Worley S, Michaels MG, et al. Cytomegalovirus immunoglobulin decreases the risk of cytomegalovirus infection but not disease after pediatric lung transplantation. Journal of Heart and Lung Transplantation. 2009;28(10):1050–1056.
47. Tepper RS, Reister T. Forced expiratory flows and lung volumes in normal infants. Pediatric Pulmonology. 1993;15(6):357–361.
48. Castile R, Filbrun D, Flucke R, et al. Adult-type pulmonary function tests in infants without respiratory disease. Pediatric Pulmonology. 2000;30(3):215–227.
49. Estenne M, Maurer JR, Boehler A, et al. Bronchiolitis obliterans syndrome 2001: an update of the diagnostic criteria. Journal of Heart and Lung Transplantation. 2002;21(3):297–310.
50. Klug B, Bisgaard H. Measurement of lung function in awake 2-4-year-old asthmatic children during methacholine challenge and acute asthma: a comparison of the impulse oscillation technique, the interrupter technique, and transcutaneous measurement of oxygen versus whole-body plethysmography. Pediatric Pulmonology. [Comparative Study Research Support, Non-U.S. Gov't]. 1996;21(5):290–300.
51. Nielsen KG, Bisgaard H. Discriminative capacity of bronchodilator response measured with three different lung function techniques in asthmatic and healthy children aged 2 to 5 years. American Journal of Respiratory and Critical Care Medicine. [Clinical Trial Comparative Study Randomized Controlled Trial Validation Studies]. 2001;164(4):554–559.
52. Visner GA, Faro A, Zander DS. Role of transbronchial biopsies in pediatric lung diseases. Chest. 2004;126(1):273–280.
53. Scully BB, Zafar F, Schecter MG, et al. Lung retransplantation in children: appropriate when selectively applied. Annals of Thoracic Surgery. 2011;91(2):574–579.
54. Mendeloff EN. Donor selection, organ preservation, surgical technique and perioperative management. In: Tejani AH, Harmon WE, Fine RN, editors. Pediatric Solid Organ Transplantation. Copenhagen: Munksgaard; 2000: 471–481.
55. Kaditis AG, Gondor M, Nixon PA, et al. Airway complications following pediatric lung and heart-lung transplantation. AmericanJournal of Respiratory and Critical Care Medicine. 2000;162(1):301–309.
56. Choong CK, Sweet SC, Zoole JB, et al. Bronchial airway anastomotic complications after pediatric lung transplantation: incidence, cause, management, and outcome. Journal of Thoracic and Cardiovascular Surgery. 2006;131(1):198–203.
57. Vinograd I, Keidar S, Weinberg M, et al. Treatment of airway obstruction by metallic stents in infants and children. Journal of Thoracic and Cardiovascular Surgery. 2005;130(1):146–150.
58. Vondrys D, Elliott MJ, McLaren CA, et al. First experience with biodegradable airway stents in children. Annals of Thoracic Surgery. [Case Reports]. 2011; 92(5):1870–1874.
59. Schulman LL, Anandarangam T, Leibowitz DW, et al. Four-year prospective study of pulmonary venous thrombosis after lung transplantation. Journal of the American Society of Echocardiography. 2001;14(8):806–812.
60. Takemoto SK, Zeevi A, Feng S, et al. National conference to assess antibody-mediated rejection in solid organ transplantation. American Journal of Transplantation. [10.1111/j.1600-6143.2004.00500.x doi; AJT500 pii]. 2004;4(7):1033–1041.
61. Martinu T, Chen DF, Palmer SM. Acute rejection and humoral sensitization in lung transplant recipients. [Review] [107 refs]. Proceedings of the American Thoracic Society. 2009;6(1):54–65.
62. Everly MJ. A summary of bortezomib use in transplantation across 29 centers. Clinical Transplants. 2009;323–337.
63. Stegall MD, Gloor JM. Deciphering antibody-mediated rejection: new insights into mechanisms and treatment. Current Opinion in Organ Transplantation. [10.1097/MOT.0b013e3283342712 doi]. 2010;15(1):8–10.
64. Purtilo DT, Strobach RS, Okano M, et al. Epstein-Barr virus-associated lymphoproliferative disorders. Laboratory Investigation; a Journal of Technical Methods and Pathology. 1992;67(1):5–23.
65. Boyle GJ, Michaels MG, Webber SA, et al. Posttransplantation lymphoproliferative disorders in pediatric thoracic organ recipients. Journal of Pediatrics. 1997;131(2):309–313.
66. Cohen AH, Sweet SC, Mendeloff E, et al. High incidence of posttransplant lymphoproliferative disease in pediatric patients with cystic fibrosis. American Journal of Respiratory and Critical Care Medicine. 2000;161(4 Pt 1):1252–1255.
67. Lim GY, Newman B, Kurland G, et al. Posttransplantation lymphoproliferative disorder: manifestations in pediatric thoracic organ recipients. Radiology. 2002;222(3):699–708.
68. Herrmann BW, Sweet SC, Molter DW. Sinonasal posttransplant lymphoproliferative disorder in pediatric lung transplant patients. Otolaryngology–Head and Neck Surgery. 2005;133(1):38–41.
69. Herrmann BW, Sweet SC, Hayashi RJ, et al. Otolaryngological manifestations of posttransplant lymphoproliferative disorder in pediatric thoracic transplant patients. International Journal of Pediatric Otorhinolaryngology. 2006;70(2):303–310.
70. Wheless SA, Gulley ML, Raab-Traub N, et al. Post-transplantation lymphoproliferative disease: Epstein-Barr virus DNA levels, HLA-A3, and survival. American Journal of Respiratory and Critical Care Medicine. 2008;178(10):1060–1065.
71. Blaes AH, Cioc AM, Froelich JW, et al. Positron emission tomography scanning

in the setting of post-transplant lymphoproliferative disorders. Clinical Transplantation. [CTR938 pii; 10.1111/j.1399-0012.2008.00938.x doi]. 2009;23(6):794–799.

72. Chadburn A, Chen JM, Hsu DT, et al. The morphologic and molecular genetic categories of posttransplantation lymphoproliferative disorders are clinically relevant. Cancer. [Clinical Trial Controlled Clinical Trial]. 1998;82(10):1978–1987.
73. Bakker NA, Verschuuren EA, Erasmus ME, et al. Epstein-Barr virus-DNA load monitoring late after lung transplantation: a surrogate marker of the degree of immunosuppression and a safe guide to reduce immunosuppression. Transplantation. 2007;83(4):433–438.
74. Benden C, Aurora P, Burch M, et al. Monitoring of Epstein-Barr viral load in pediatric heart and lung transplant recipients by real-time polymerase chain reaction. Journal of Heart and Lung Transplantation. 2005;24(12):2103–2108.
75. Gupta S, Fricker FJ, Gonzalez-Peralta RP, et al. Post-transplant lymphoproliferative disorder in children: recent outcomes and response to dual rituximab/low-dose chemotherapy combination. Pediatric Transplantation. 2010;14(7):896–902. [PTR1370 pii; 10.1111/j.1399-3046.2010.01370.x doi].
76. Bridges ND, Spray TL, Collins MH, et al. Adenovirus infection in the lung results in graft failure after lung transplantation. Journal of Thoracic and Cardiovascular Surgery. 1998;116(4):617–623.
77. Wendt CH, Fox JM, Hertz MI. Paramyxovirus infection in lung transplant recipients. Journal of Heart and Lung Transplantation. 1995;14(3):479–485.
78. McCurdy LH, Milstone A, Dummer S. Clinical features and outcomes of paramyxoviral infection in lung transplant recipients treated with ribavirin. Journal of Heart and Lung Transplantation. 2003;22(7):745–753.
79. Doan ML, Mallory GB, Kaplan SL, et al. Treatment of adenovirus pneumonia with cidofovir in pediatric lung transplant recipients. Journal of Heart and Lung Transplantation. [S1053-2498(07)00511-6 pii; 10.1016/j.healun.2007.06.009 doi]. 2007;26(9):883–889.
80. Glanville AR, Scott AI, Morton JM, et al. Intravenous ribavirin is a safe and cost-effective treatment for respiratory syncytial virus infection after lung transplantation. Journal of Heart and Lung Transplantation. 2005;24(12):2114–2119.
81. Khalifah AP, Hachem RR, Chakinala MM, et al. Respiratory viral infections are a distinct risk for bronchiolitis obliterans syndrome and death. American Journal of Respiratory and Critical Care Medicine. [Research Support, Non-U.S. Gov't Research Support, U.S. Gov't, P.H.S.]. 2004;170(2):181–187.
82. Yacoub MH, Gyi K, Khaghani A, et al. Analysis of 10-year experience with heart-lung transplantation for cystic fibrosis. Transplantation Proceedings. [S0041-1345(96)00368-5 pii]. 1997;29(1–2):632.
83. Smeritschnig B, Jaksch P, Kocher A, et al. Quality of life after lung transplantation: a cross-sectional study. Journal of Heart and Lung Transplantation. 2005; 24(4):474–480.
84. Kugler C, Fischer S, Gottlieb J, et al. Health-related quality of life in two hundred-eighty lung transplant recipients. Journal of Heart and Lung Transplantation. 2005;24(12):2262–2268.
85. Nixon PA, Morris KA. Quality of life in pediatric heart, heart-lung, and lung transplant recipients. [Review] [21 refs]. International Journal of Sports Medicine. 2000;21:S109–S111.
86. Hirshfeld AB, Kahle AL, Clark BJ III, et al. Parent-reported health status after pediatric thoracic organ transplant. Journal of Heart and Lung Transplantation. [10.1016/j.healun.2003.08.016 doi; S105324980300411X pii]. 2004;23(9):1111–1118.
87. Noyes BE, Kurland G, Orenstein DM, et al. Experience with pediatric lung transplantation. Journal of Pediatrics. 1994;124(2):261–268.
88. Hislop AA, Rinaldi M, Lee R, et al. Growth of immature lung transplanted into an adult recipient. The American Journal of Physiology. 1993;264(1 Pt 1):L60–L65.
89. Cohen AH, Mallory GB Jr, Ross K, et al. Growth of lungs after transplantation in infants and in children younger than 3 years of age. American Journal of Respiratory and Critical Care Medicine. 1999;159(6):1747–1751.
90. Ro PS, Bush DM, Kramer SS, et al. Airway growth after pediatric lung transplantation. Journal of Heart and Lung Transplantation. 2001;20(6):619–624.
91. Sritippayawan S, Keens TG, Horn MV, et al. Does lung growth occur when mature lobes are transplanted into children? Pediatric Transplantation. 2002;6(6):500–504.
92. Baum M, Freier MC, Chinnock RE. Neurodevelopmental outcome of solid organ transplantation in children. Pediatric Clinics of North America. [Review]. 2003;50(6):1493–1503, x.
93. Ringewald JM, Gidding SS, Crawford SE, et al. Nonadherence is associated with late rejection in pediatric heart transplant recipients. Journal of Pediatrics. 2001;139(1):75–78.
94. Gaston RS. Maintenance immunosuppression in the renal transplant recipient: an overview. [erratum appears in Am J Kidney Dis 2002 Apr;39(4):898]. [Review] [69 refs]. American Journal of Kidney Diseases. 2001;38(6 Suppl 6):S25–S35.
95. Annunziato RA, Emre S, Shneider B, et al. Adherence and medical outcomes in pediatric liver transplant recipients who transition to adult services. [see comment]. Pediatric Transplantation. 2007;11(6):608–614.
96. Reiss JG, Gibson RW, Walker LR. Health care transition: youth, family, and provider perspectives. Pediatrics. [Research Support, U.S. Gov't, Non-P.H.S.]. 2005;115(1):112–120.
97. Stabile L, Rosser L, Porterfield KM, et al. Transfer versus transition: success in pediatric transplantation brings the welcome challenge of transition. Progress in Transplantation. 2005;15(4):363–370.
98. McDonagh JE, Kelly DA. The challenges and opportunities for transitional care research. Pediatric Transplantation. [Review]. 2010;14(6):688–700.
99. Bell LE, Bartosh SM, Davis CL, et al. Adolescent transition to adult care in solid organ transplantation: a consensus conference report. American Journal of Transplantation. [Congresses]. 2008;8(11):2230–2242.

第 117 章
儿童小肠和多脏器移植

Douglas G. Farmer

引言

肠移植的起源与儿童的肠道和肝脏疾病密切相关。正是这些疾病促进了早期移植的开展。几个重要的里程碑值得铭记。1967 年，由 Tomas Starzl [1]成功实施一例儿童肝移植，同时几例肠移植没有成功[2]。随着 20 世纪 60 年代后期肠外营养的临床引入[3]，之后近 20 年没有其他肠移植病例的报道。20 世纪 80 年代中期，成人肠移植的成功实施的报道[4–6]，再次激发了儿童肠移植的实施[7]。生存最长的受者于 1988 年在法国巴黎接受了肠移植[8]。随后，系列病例也逐渐被报道[9]，从而开启了儿童肠移植的新时代。

适应证和患者选择

肠移植的主要指征是不可逆的肠衰竭：胃肠道不能维持患者的体液和(或)电解质、热量、大量和微量营养素需要的临床状况。较不常见的指征通常是技术问题，例如不可切除的肿瘤、不适于标准外科治疗的涉及肠系膜根部或胰–门静脉–肠系膜平面静脉血栓形成。这一主题的其他治疗见第 33 章。肠衰竭大致分为三类：手术、功能或黏膜(见表 117.1)。三者的表现和诊断可以相互重叠。

表 117.1 常见儿童肠移植原因分类

手术	功能	黏膜
腹裂	假性梗阻	微绒毛包涵体病
空肠闭锁	希尔施普戈病	先天性簇绒肠病
肠扭转	–	神经内分泌疾病
坏死性肠炎	–	–

发生肠衰竭的儿童通过肠外营养管理来稳定。一般来说，最初的目标是肠内适应，尽量避免移植。这些患者在肠衰竭/康复的这个阶段的特异性管理超出了本章的范围，相关内容可以阅读其他信息[10,11]。与肠衰竭的不可逆性相比，有几个预后因素被评估可能与适应有关。这些因素(表 117.2)已经在大型研究中显示能够预测适应，尽管没有一个是绝对的[12]。

表 117.2 与不可逆性肠衰竭相比，可能适应的预后因素评估

预后因素	有利影响	不利影响
年龄	年轻	老年
残余肠管	长	短
回盲瓣	有	无
结肠	有	无
肠癌	无	有
发病时间	短	长
发病期肠病	无	有
小肠部位	空肠	回肠

预后不良和(或)没有表现出早期肠道适应证据的患者应转诊至移植中心进行评估。其他能够辅助适应的内外科手段都应加以考虑。移植手术指征，是存在不可逆的肠衰竭和一种或多种威胁生命的肠胃外营养相关并发症。并发症通常包括如下。

1.中心静脉通路中断。

2.多中心静脉导管的病史。

3.多发性血液感染史。

4.存在肠衰竭相关肝病。

5.与肠衰竭相关的慢性疼痛综合征。

6.体液、电解质、营养难以管理。

对适应预后极差的患者亚群，在常见的肠外营养相关并发症发作之前应该考虑移植。该标准在 2001 年由美国移植学会出版的文件中阐述[13]，现在仍在使用。

等候名单

等候名单中死亡率是儿童肠移植的主要障碍。这一问题在 1993—2001 年在 UNOS 数据库的一项研究中首次暴露[14],该研究表明肝-肠或多器官移植儿童的等候名单死亡率远远超过肝移植的儿童的等候名单死亡率。回顾性研究表明,这一发现并不出人意料,因为肝-肠和多器官移植等候者基本上是等待脏器大小匹配的儿童供者,而肝移植等候者可有多种选择,包括大小匹配的儿童供者、成人死亡供体劈离移植物、活体移植物。

此外,回顾性研究发现,终末期肝病和儿童末期肝病(MELD/PELD)评分系统不能准确预测肠衰竭相关患者的 3 个月生存率。因此,美国肠道分配系统进行了重大改革,包括为等待肝脏或器官簇移植的儿童增加 23 个 PELD/MELD 点,在更广泛的地理区域分配儿童器官给儿童受者,使等候名单死亡率急剧下降[15]。

移植选择与手术技术

要根据患者的疾病情况来选择肠移植的类型。一般常见的类型有:单独的肠移植,肝肠联合移植,多器官移植和多器官改进移植。这些操作的技术细节见第 62 和第 63 章。

1.单独肠移植:将部分或全部供体空肠移植到受体中。适用于无上消化道(胃、十二指肠、胰腺)疾病、无或处于早期肝病、不可逆肠衰竭患者,血供通常从肾下动脉或肠系膜上动脉建立,静脉回流肠系膜静脉或下腔静脉。

2.肝肠联合移植:移植部分或全部肝、胰、空肠。此处应注意,供体胰腺现在通常包括在移植器官复合体中,简化供体和受体手术步骤[17]。受者肝和残留空回肠切除,胰十二指肠保留原位。肝肠联合移植适用于无上消化道病变、有不可逆性肝病和不可逆性肠衰竭患者。血供来自主动脉来源的血管,经移植肝回流至上下腔静脉。

3.多器官移植:移植部分或全部肝、胰、空肠,包括或不包括胃。适用于有上消化道疾病、不可逆性肝病和不可逆性肠衰竭患者。多器官移植和肝肠联合移植间主要区别在于受者的胃也一并切除,两者的血供类似。

4.多器官改进移植:移植部分或全部胰、空肠、包括或不包括胃。注意肝并不在移植范围内。适用于有上消化道疾病、不可逆性肠衰竭患者。血供来自主动脉来源的血管,经门静脉回流。

免疫移植与排斥反应

促进肠移植发展的主要因素之一是免疫抑制剂。肠道是唯一一个依靠自身吸收药物以防止自身免疫介导破坏的器官。因此,吸收性好和强效的免疫抑制剂和(或)免疫抑制剂的静脉制剂的开发极大地推动了这一领域的发展。第一个重大突破就是来自他克莫司的发现[18]和临床应用[19]。在临床使用这种药剂之前,肠移植的成功是极其罕见的。这一领域的下一个重大突破是使用诱导免疫治疗。在常规使用之前,肠移植后的短期存活率通常为 25%~50%[20]。在 1999—2000 年,大多数医疗中心开始使用诱导疗法与白介素-2 受体拮抗剂(达珠单抗或巴利昔单抗),兔抗人胸腺细胞免疫球蛋白(即复宁)。最近,阿仑单抗也已用于诱导治疗,效果良好。所有试剂使短期存活率显著增加高达 75%~90%[21-24]。

预后

生存率

肠移植后的一般预后在第 109 章详细讨论。为了评价肠移植后的预后,有几个不同的数据来源。标准的多中心数据来自肠移植登记网[25]。目前这一数据已经收集了自 1985 年以来在世界各地开展的几乎所有肠移植。其他可用的数据来自器官共享/器官获取和移植网络(UNOS/OPTN),通过移植受者科学登记系统(SRTR)进行报道[26]。对于所有注册登记的数据存在一定的局限,如对于每位患者收集的数据点的数量、输入的数据点的完整性以及来自不同医疗中心的输入数据的解释的可变性等。预后数据的另一个主要来源是单中心报道。很少报道单纯来源于儿童。这里综述的一些经验见表 117.3[20,21,22,24-31]。

UNOS/OPTN 数据库表明,在 1988—2011 年间,美国进行了 2138 例肠移植,56%实施于儿童中[26]。在移植后 3 年和 5 年,患者存活率分别为 51%~79%和 33%~76%,而相应的移植物存活率分别为 44%~64%和 30%~

表 117.3 大型登记处和单中心出版物的肠移植经验总结

来源/参考文献	年份	数量	患者生存率	移植物生存率	死亡原因	移植物失功原因	排斥	移植后淋巴组织增生性疾病	巨细胞病毒
ITR[25]	2011	1351C	72 MO:50% 6+47% 2000+42% 1995+33% 1990+19% 1985+	72 MO:40% 2006+45% 2000+35% 1995+20% 1990+0% 1985+	NR	NR	NR	NR	NR
ITR[20]	2009	1151C	60 MO:NR% 2005+70% 2000+68% 1995+58% 1990+65% 1985+	NR	脓毒症 46% 多器官功能衰竭 35%	NR	NR	NR	NR
UNOS/OPTN[26]	2011	1198C	72 MO:51%~79% 60 MO:33%~76%	72 MO:44%~64% 60 MO:30%~69%	NR	NR	NR	NR	NR
PITTSBURGH[24]	2011	213C	72 MO:73% 60 MO:68%	72 MO:66% 60 MO:55%	NR	NR	82%无 79%CPP/L2RA 68%RATG 36%CAMPATH	23% CPP/L2RA 11%RATG	26%CPP/L2RA 13%RATG+CAMPATH
PITTSBURGH[21]	2009	500T 184C	60 MO:70% C 61% T	60MO:50% T	NR	排斥 20% T 感染 11% T	90D rate 50%~75%T	41/184(22%)	16%T
PITTSBURGH[27]	2002	84C	72 MO:59% 60 MO:56%	72 MO:53% 60 MO:47%	13/39(33%)感染 7/39(18%)排斥	NR	345E/89G(377%) 73G/89G(82%)	15/34(44%)ERA1 12/51(24%)ERA2	22%
MIAMI[29]	2006	123C 141TX	72 MO:32% 1994+38% 1998+60% 2001+(IL2RA)44% 2001+(CAMPATH)	NR	20/67(30%)排斥 22/67(33%)感染	NR	191/141(135%)	14/123(11%)	NR

（待续）

表 117.3(续)

来源/参考文献	年份	数量	患者生存率	移植物生存率	死亡原因	移植物失功原因	排斥	移植后淋巴组织增生性疾病	巨细胞病毒
MIAMI[28]	2005	108C	60 MO:41%	NR	19/55(35%)排斥 19/55(35%)感染	NR	21/108(19%) 严重	NR	NR
UCLA[22]	2010	88T 63C	72 MO:70% 60 MO:65%	72 MO:68% 60 MO:64%	感染 58% 神经 16%	排斥 33% 感染 10%	NR	NR	NR
PARIS[30]	2005	52C	72 MO:72%	72 MO:53%	技术性 3/15(20%) 感染 10/15(67%) PTLD 2/15(13%)	27/52(52%) 患者死亡	25/52(48%)T	12/52(23%)	11/52(21%)
MT SINAI MC[31]	2002	31T 18C	NR	12 MO:58% 对 92% RAPA	感染 4/6(66%) PTLD 2/6(33%)	NR	30D:72%对 17% RAPA	NR	NR

C,儿童;CMV,巨细胞病毒;COD,死因;COGL,移植物失功原因;CPP,环磷酰胺;E,发作;G,移植物;IL2RA,白细胞介素-2 受体拮抗剂;ITR,肠移植登记;MO,月;n,数量;NR,未报道;PTLD,移植后淋巴增生性疾病;RAPA,雷帕霉素;rATG,兔抗胸腺细胞球蛋白;T,患者总数;TX,移植;UCLA,加州大学洛杉矶分校;MC,医学中心;UNOS/OPTN,器官共享/器官获取和移植网络。

69%。2009年ITR关于儿童肠移植的报道表明，在全世界，1151例患者接受了1236次移植[32]。5年生存率不断提高，在2000年以后，出现了70%患者存活率的报道。患者死亡的最常见原因是败血症(46%)和多器官衰竭(35%)。

3年生存率(56%~72%)和移植物存活率(53%~92%)，并随着时代进步不断提高。最常见导致移植物失功和死亡的原因是感染、排斥和移植后淋巴增生性疾病(PTLD)。移植中心报道见表117.3。

急性排斥反应

急性排异反应是肠移植成功的最大障碍。历史上，排斥在肠移植后几乎普遍发生，并且是移植物失功的主要原因。可惜并没有一个统一的关于排斥发生时间、有无排斥发生及排斥发生率的系统报道。单中心报道仍然是评估排斥率的最佳来源。这些报道中，排斥率最低的是联合阿仑单抗诱导治疗与西罗莫司的维持治疗(分别为36%和17%)的方案。

关于这个问题的最详细的报道之一由迈阿密大学发布[33]。在研究间隔期间，299名患者(包括128名儿童)接受肠移植。32%无排斥发生，而其余的发生290次，平均每名患者2次。首次排斥的中位时间为18天。统计数据表明，2001年以前，缺乏阿仑单抗诱导、供体不含脾及较长的冷缺血时间是最强预测排斥的因素。

这些数据表明，虽然排斥反应仍然是肠移植的主要障碍，排斥速率和严重程度随时间改善。严格的内镜监测方案已在大多数医疗中心实施，有助于排斥反应的早期发现。任何种类的诱导免疫治疗似乎有助于减少排斥的发生率。需要开发预测排斥的非侵入性检查方法来帮助解决这个问题。

巨细胞病毒病

组织侵袭性巨细胞病毒(CMV)疾病是肠移植后的一个问题。这种病毒在免疫缺陷患者的肠道内极易生长。2000年早期的报道显示，这一比例高达26%[34]。不过，最近的报道表明这种感染减少为11%~24%，见表117.3。最近在加州大学洛杉矶分校的综述表明CMV疾病的总体比例降低到5%[35]。而这些成果的获得归结于针对该病毒的预防性治疗方案的进展。UCLA方案包括每周血液监测病毒DNA以及用静脉注射更昔洛韦进行预防性治疗[36]。

移植后淋巴增生性疾病

与CMV病毒相似，可引起感染及与肿瘤相关的EB病毒(EBV)是肠移植后的另一个主要问题。EB病毒在免疫不全的患者中发展迅速。文献中关于EBV感染的实际发病率还不清楚。相比之下，PTLD的发病率有明确报道。然而，并非所有PTLD都是EB病毒相关和(或)驱动的，因此在文献中缺乏一致性。从单中心报道来看，PTLD(与EB病毒相关或不相关)的历史发病率为23%~44%(见表117.3)。在最近的研究中，这些比率从24%降至11%。在UCLA中，PTLD的发生率为8%[35]。尽管因果关系难以确定，PTLD的发病率的改善似乎在很大程度上与针对CMV使用相同的预防策略有关。PTLD的讨论详见第96章。

肾衰竭

在OPTN/SRTR的报道中首次阐明了肠移植后肾功能问题的严重性。其中228名受者5年内慢性肾衰竭的发生率为21%±3.4%[37]，这一发现刺激了几个医疗中心对这一问题的研究。在一项对44名儿童肠移植的研究中，Ueno及其同事发现，移植前估计肾小球滤过率(eGFR)为138±42mL/(min·m²)，移植后24个月，相应的eGFR降至基线的81%[38]。eGFR降低与术后前12个月他克莫司的高谷浓度相关。UCLA对45名儿童和23名成人进行肠移植后的数据进行分析，以多个时间点测量的eGFR/正常GFR的量化数值来评估术后肾功能[39]。移植前，eGFR为正常值的83%~91%。移植后，eGFR范围为正常值的64%~95%。研究发现移植前低eGFR、ICU状态、移植前TPN长时间段、高剂量他克莫司和年龄> 18岁，可以作为eGFR <75%正常值的预测因素。从这些研究中我们可以得出结论，肾功能障碍或衰竭是肠移植后的主要问题，高他克莫司水平是引起该问题的主要原因。

营养

肠移植的最终目标是自主肠内营养。可是对这一问题的研究很少。为了解决这个问题，Venick和同事对33例儿童肠移植后的营养结果进行了详细评估[40]。肠内营养开始的中位时间是移植后8天，并且在移植后31天中止了胃肠外营养。血清白蛋白和前白蛋白(白蛋白：2.7~3.7g/dL；前白蛋白：15~25.1mg/dL）得到了改善。但微量营养元素缺乏常见为铁和锌。这项研究为肠同种异体移植可以在移植术后长期支持自主营养提供了具体的证据。

总结

肠移植后的结果在过去 10 年有显著改善，这无疑是多种因素促进了这些进步。手术技术、各移植中心独特的经验、诱导免疫治疗和抗感染药物的进展均发挥了巨大作用。肠移植成功可以实现自主营养。然而，排斥反应、病毒感染和肾功能恶化等影响移植的障碍仍然存在，有待一一解决。尽管存在种种问题，肠移植患者的预后和其他实体器官移植的预后几乎没有区别。

（柯庆宏 译 柯庆宏 校）

参考文献

1. Starzl TE, Groth CG, Brettschneider L, et al. Extended survival in 3 cases of orthotopic homotransplantation of the human liver. Surgery. 1968;63(4):549-563.
2. Watson AJ, Lear PA. Current status of intestinal transplantation. Gut. 1989; 30(12):1771-1782.
3. Dudrick SJ, Wilmore DW, Vars HM, et al. Long-term total parenteral nutrition with growth, development, and positive nitrogen balance. Surgery. 1968;64(1): 134-142.
4. Grant D, Wall W, Mimeault R, et al. Successful small-bowel/liver transplantation. Lancet. 1990;335(8683):181-184.
5. Deltz E, Schroeder P, Gebhardt H, et al. [First successful clinical small intestine transplantation. Tactics and surgical technic]. Der Chirurg; Zeitschrift fur Alle Gebiete Der Operativen Medizen. 1989;60(4):235-239. German.
6. Deltz E, Schroeder P, Gundlach M, et al. Successful clinical small-bowel transplantation. Transplantation Proceedings. 1990;22(6):2501.
7. Starzl TE, Rowe MI, Todo S, et al. Transplantation of multiple abdominal viscera. JAMA: The Journal of the American Medical Association. 1989;261(10): 1449-1457.
8. Goulet O, Revillon Y, Brousse N, et al. Successful small bowel transplantation in an infant. Transplantation. 1992;53(4):940-943.
9. Todo S, Tzakis AG, Abu-Elmagd K, et al. Cadaveric small bowel and small bowel-liver transplantation in humans. Transplantation. 1992;53(2):369-376.
10. Mazariegos GV, Superina R, Rudolph J, et al. Current status of pediatric intestinal failure, rehabilitation, and transplantation: summary of a colloquium. Transplantation. 2011;92(11):1173-1180.
11. Sigalet D, Boctor D, Brindle M, et al. Elements of successful intestinal rehabilitation. Journal of Pediatric Surgery. 2011;46(1):150-156.
12. Quirós-Tejeira RE, Ament ME, Reyen L, et al. Long-term parenteral nutritional support and intestinal adaptation in children with short bowel syndrome: a 25-year experience. The Journal of Pediatrics. 2004;145(2):157-163.
13. Kaufman SS, Atkinson JB, Bianchi A, et al. Indications for pediatric intestinal transplantation: a position paper of the American Society of Transplantation. Pediatric Transplantation. 2001;5(2):80-87.
14. Fryer J, Pellar S, Ormond D, et al. Mortality in candidates waiting for combined liver-intestine transplants exceeds that for other candidates waiting for liver transplants. Liver Transplantation. 2003;9(7):748-753.
15. Mazariegos GV, Steffick DE, Horslen S, et al. Intestine transplantation in the United States, 1999-2008. American Journal of Transplantation. 2010;10(4 Pt 2): 1020-1034.
16. Abu-Elmagd KM. The small bowel contained allografts: existing and proposed nomenclature. American Journal of Transplantation. 2011;11(1):184-185.
17. Sudan DL, Iyer KR, Deroover A, et al. A new technique for combined liver/small intestinal transplantation. Transplantation. 2001;72(11):1846-1848.
18. Kino T, Hatanaka H, Hashimoto M, et al. FK-506, a novel immunosuppressant isolated from a Streptomyces. I. Fermentation, isolation, and physico-chemical and biological characteristics. The Journal of Antibiotics. 1987;40(9): 1249-1255.
19. Starzl TE, Todo S, Fung J, et al. FK 506 for liver, kidney, and pancreas transplantation. Lancet. 1989;2(8670):1000-1004.
20. Grant D. Intestinal transplantation: 1997 report of the international registry. Intestinal Transplant Registry. Transplantation. 1999;67(7):1061-1064.
21. Abu-Elmagd KM, Costa G, Bond GJ, et al. Five hundred intestinal and multivisceral transplantations at a single center: major advances with new challenges. Annals of Surgery. 2009;250(4):567-581.
22. Farmer DG, Venick RS, Colangelo J, et al. Pretransplant predictors of survival after intestinal transplantation: analysis of a single-center experience of more than 100 transplants. Transplantation. 2010;90(12):1574-1580.
23. Farmer DG. Clinical Immunosuppression for intestinal transplantation. Current Opinion in Organ Transplantation. 2004;9:214-291.
24. Nayyar NS, McGhee W, Martin D, et al. Intestinal transplantation in children: a review of immunotherapy regimens. Paediatric Drugs. 2011;13(3):149-159.
25. Intestine Transplant Registry Report. [assessed December 27, 2013]; Available from: http://www.tts.org/images/stories/ITA/curren_update_worldwide_experience.pdf.
26. Scientific Registry of Transplant Recipients. [assessed December 27, 2013]; Available from: http://optn.transplant.hrsa.gov/data; based on OPTN data 12/14/2011.
27. Reyes J, Mazariegos GV, Bond GM, et al. Pediatric intestinal transplantation: historical notes, principles and controversies. Pediatric Transplantation. 2002;6(3): 193-207.
28. Kato T, Gaynor JJ, Selvaggi G, et al. Intestinal transplantation in children: a summary of clinical outcomes and prognostic factors in 108 patients from a single center. Journal of Gastrointestinal Surgery. 2005;9(1):75-89.
29. Kato T, Tzakis AG, Selvaggi G, et al. Intestinal and multivisceral transplantation in children. Annals of Surgery. 2006;243(6):756-764.
30. Goulet O, Sauvat F, Ruemmele F, et al. Results of the Paris program: ten years of pediatric intestinal transplantation. Transplantation Proceedings. 2005;37(4): 1667-1670.
31. Fishbein TM, Florman S, Gondolesi G, et al. Intestinal transplantation before and after the introduction of sirolimus. Transplantation. 2002;73(10):1538-1542.
32. EIR, 2009 Biannual Report. In D. Grant (Ed), Intestinal Transplant Registry. Toronto, ON: Intestinal Transplant Association.
33. Selvaggi G, Gaynor JJ, Moon J, et al. Analysis of acute cellular rejection episodes in recipients of primary intestinal transplantation: a single center, 11-year experience. American Journal of Transplantation. 2007;7(5):1249-1257.
34. Abu-Elmagd KM, Reyes J, Bond GJ, et al. Clinical intestinal transplantion: A decade of experience at a single center. Annals of Surgery. 2001;234(3): 404-417.
35. Farmer DG, Venick RS, Woznak L, et al. The liver, spleen, and preformed antibodies are important predictors of survival after intestinal transplantation. Abstract #238, XIIth International Small Bowel Transplant Symposium, Washington, DC, September, 17th, 2011.
36. Farmer DG, McDiarmid SV, Winston D, et al. Effectiveness of aggressive prophylatic and preemptive therapies targeted against cytomegaloviral and Epstein-Barr viral disease after human intestinal transplantation. Transplantation Proceedings. 2002;34(3):948-949.
37. Ojo AO, Held PJ, Port FK, et al. Chronic renal failure after transplantation of a nonrenal organ. The New England Journal of Medicine. 2003;349(10): 931-940.
38. Ueno T, Kato T, Gaynor J, et al. Renal function after pediatric intestinal transplant. Transplantation Proceedings. 2006;38(6):1759-1761.
39. Watson MJ, Venick RS, Kaldas F, et al. Renal function impacts outcomes after intestinal transplantation. Transplantation. 2008;86(1):117-122.
40. Venick RS, Wozniak LJ, Colangelo J, et al. Long-term nutrition and predictors of growth and weight gain following pediatric intestinal transplantation. Transplantation. 2011;92(9):1058-1062.

第 118 章 器官移植术后生长和发育

Franz Schaefer

引言

对患者生长发育的基因潜能认知是器官移植儿童和青少年的一个关键目标。原则上,器官功能的完全恢复应达到青春期正常的生长和发育。然而,器官移植术后患者的生长发育恢复往往是受影响的。到目前为止,大部分在童年期间接受器官移植的患者其最后的成年身高往往低于正常水平。本章将详细阐述影响实质性器官移植术后生长发育的各种因素和改善器官移植术后生长发育的最新策略。第 119 章和第 121 章将提供额外的关于认知发育的相关内容,以及影响从儿童到成人的转变的问题。

慢性器官衰竭过程中的生长发育迟缓

慢性器官衰竭会影响儿童患者的生长和成熟。因此,生长发育迟缓在儿童实质性器官移植受体中非常常见。一般骨骼成熟和青春期发育的迟缓往往跟生长的迟缓相符。

许多登记中心和大型单中心调查研究提供了实质性器官移植受体的平均生长发育迟缓信息。终末期肾病(ESRD)儿童的自然生长历史特点为婴儿期和童年中期渐进的每年约 0.2~0.5 的标准差评分(SDS),在青春期前的末期其生长发育明显减慢,青春期的成长将推迟 1.5~2 年,低于正常的程度和持续时间,导致了低于健康儿童 50%的累积发育[1]。幸运的是,发育失败在慢性肾功能不全和终末期肾病的患者中是可以通过加强营养管理及重组人生长激素(rhGH)治疗来预防和治疗的。对生长失败的强烈关注会导致在移植前生长模式的改进。北美儿童肾移植登记表(NAPRTCS)的信息显示,肾移植儿童的平均标准身高从 1987 年第一例肾移植的-2.4 SDS 到 1999 年的-1.5 SDS,而 1999—2009 年间仅有轻微的进一步改善(0.25 SDS)[2](图 118.1)。

由于儿童肝脏疾病最常发生于婴儿期,因此严重的营养不良和快速生长失败是肝衰竭的常见后遗症。事实上,生长失败已被认为是患有胆道闭锁或 Alagille 综合征等患者的肝移植适应证。SPLIT 登记的 569 名

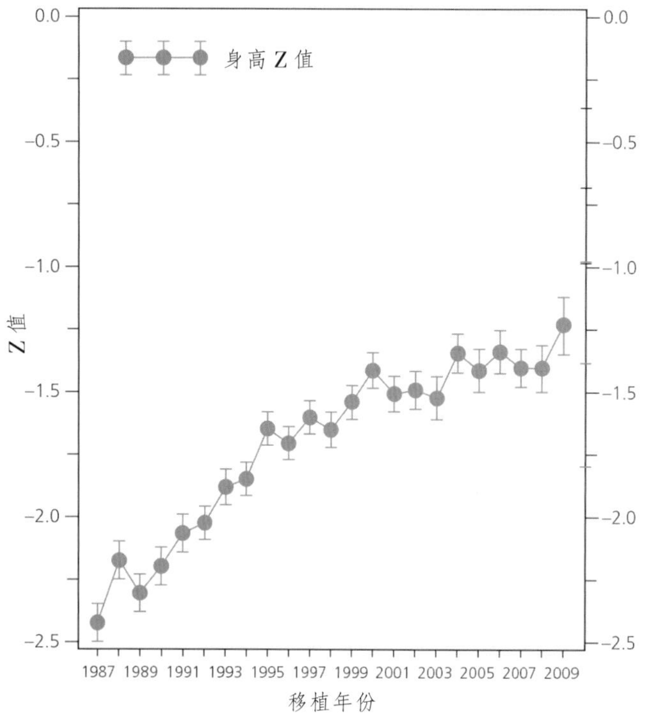

图 118.1 1997—2009 年,接受肾移植的北美儿童移植时平均标准化身高的改善状况。Adapted from [2], with permission from North American Pediatric Renal Trials and Collaborative Studies.

患者的移植前平均高度 SDS 为-1.3[3]。由来自加州大学洛杉矶分校[4]、芝加哥大学[5],以及英国[6]的包含 236 294 名儿童和 107 名儿童受体的单中心研究显示，其报道的基线高度 SDS 分别为-1.7,-1.6 和-1.2。

终末期肝病儿童的生长迟缓通常与年龄负相关，这一结论论证了肝衰竭对于婴儿期营养依赖生长阶段患者更为关键的论点。营养的重要地位也在大多数需要单独小肠移植或肝-小肠联合移植的短肠综合征患儿中得到强调[7]。相比之下,在婴儿期之后获得终末期肝病的患者行拯救性肝移植,通常是由于急性的(如暴发性肝炎或中毒等)原因所致,多不伴有之前的生长失败。第三组肝衰竭患者则由伴有肝脏参与的综合征组成。在这些儿童中,慢性肝衰竭可能是导致严重生长迟缓的因素之一。Alagille 综合征或 Byler 综合征可导致矮小身材的基因倾向；宫内生长迟缓发生在 50%的受这些疾病影响或移植肝功能正常化后并未引起生长追赶的患者中[8-10]。

生长发育在因严重心脏疾病等待移植的患者中也是次优的。受损的组织氧化作用会导致肠道蠕动受损和营养吸收不良、酸中毒、能量消耗增加,甚至下丘脑-垂体轴缺血性损伤导致一个或多个内分泌系统分泌促进生长发育的激素不足[11]。其总体的生长失败一般为中等程度。在最新的大规模的单中心报道中,UCLA 的 46 名青春期前儿童在移植时平均身高 SDS 为-0.7,多伦多的 130 名儿童为-1.3[12,13]。

影响移植术后生长发育的因素

肾移植

器官移植术后生长发育在肾移植受体中进行了系统性的研究。个别医疗中心报道了肾移植术后从进行性生长失败到完全生长追赶的多种生长模式经验[14-28],大多数结论都支持器官移植术后生长状况为主要影响因素。其包括接受移植时的年龄和疾病对生长的妨碍程度[17,18,28-31],移植肾的功能状况和糖皮质激素治疗模式。

器官移植术后生长追赶的潜力似乎与移植时的年龄呈负相关。良好的生长追赶通常出现在婴儿期的移植受体[17,29-32]。从 2~12 年的不同的研究[17,27,29-31,33]表明，关键年龄超过婴儿期的儿童患者,其身高标准差改善将不会发生。青春期生长从肾移植获益最少。在进行透析的尿毒症患者中,其移植后在青春期开始以及青春期的生长均会延迟大约 2年。即使有明显的生长加速,由于青春期高速生长时间的缩短其身高仍会低于正常[34]。目前已观察到青春期身高增长速度的峰值与累积的糖皮质激素之间的反比关系[34,35]。

除了年龄的影响，肾移植术后标准化身高的变化与移植时的身高密切相关[32,36]。因此,要求的生长追赶的一般原则为：一个有机体去除生长抑制状态后恢复到一个预定的生长通道的趋势，这也适用于肾移植受体。

移植术后的生长发育对于移植器官的功能状况非常的敏感。当肾小球滤过率(GFR)持续下降到低于 30mL/(min·1.73m^2)时,原生肾功能只影响线性生长，任何 GFR 低于 60mL/(min·1.73m^2)均会显著降低移植术后的生长速度[2,16,29]。多因素分析证实,移植肾功能不佳导致的生长抑制与糖皮质激素剂量无关[24,27]。

鉴于糖皮质激素对于生长抑制内分泌和代谢的深刻影响(见后续章节),毫无疑问这种免疫抑制药物对移植术后的生长发育有重要的影响。改良的类固醇药物临床试验的结果显示，完全性无类固醇药物或者甚至主要无类固醇方案证实了糖皮质激素对肾移植受体生长追赶的影响。另一方面,令人惊讶的是,很少有研究证实类固醇的剂量和移植术后标准化身高变化之间的关系[14,35]。糖皮质激素的剂量和移植术后生长之间一致性关系的缺乏,或者可以一个非线性的“阈值”关系以及糖皮质激素吸收和药代动力学个体差异来解释。事实上,血清甲泼尼龙浓度曲线以下区域在预测移植术后生长速度上优于给予的糖皮质激素剂量[37]。

目前已有关于 mTOR 抑制剂可能抑制生长的矛盾结果的报道。在细胞水平,这类免疫抑制剂有通过干扰关键合成代谢信号通路而产生抗增殖的特性[38]。试验研究显示雷帕霉素通过在生长板抗血管生成作用诱导生长迟缓[39,40]。在首个临床病例报告提示西罗莫司导致生长障碍后[41],一项回顾性分析比较了 34 名由于钙调磷酸酶抑制剂(CNI)毒性、急性或慢性排斥反应或肿瘤而从 CNI 转换为西罗莫司的儿童,与 34 名年龄、性别、肾功能和类固醇剂量相匹配的配对儿童之间的生长状况[42]。其生长追赶随着时间的推移逐渐出现在 CNI 组的儿童中,但西罗莫司组并未观察到。在一个有良好肾小球滤过率和低类固醇剂量的青春期前儿童分组中，接受西罗莫司治疗组的平均身高两年改变SDS为-0.22，而CNI治疗组为+0.77，差异更为显著。相反，在一个比较25名接受西罗莫司、MMF和泼尼松治疗的儿童和配对的23名接受他克莫司、MMF和泼尼松治疗的儿童的单中心研究中，从接受移植时开始的前2年内未发现西罗莫司对于生长速度有任何不利的影响，两组的平均身高SDS均无改变[43]。

经过30年以上的儿童肾移植发展，全世界有数千名患者获得了"最终成人身高"。这提供了评估移植术后生长追赶的最终完整性，及分析上述影响纵向生长终点的调节因子的机会。最终身高在单中心研究和各个登记报道中进行了评估[2,34,36,44,45]。在所有儿童期间发展为终末期肾病并接受肾移植治疗的患者中，25%~41%的患者表现为较矮的成人身高。最终平均身高随着时间的推移大幅增加；NAPRTCS登记中心显示1987—1991年、1992—1996年、1997—2001年，以及2002以后的成人身高平均SDS分别为-1.93、-1.51、-1.05和-0.94[2]。然而，该数据的增加几乎完全与移植前生长管理的改善相关。NAPRTCS登记中心报道的于12岁以下接受移植的237名患者中，其平均最终身高SDS与移植时的标准化身高完全相同，这表明儿童肾移植人群作为一个整体缺乏生长追赶[45]。据上述提到的早期移植术后生长研究显示，最后身高与移植年龄呈负相关；青春期前的患者其有显著的生长追赶受限。生长发育不良最严重的患者表现出最明显的移植术后生长改善，移植肾的功能是最终身高的一个独立预测因素。此外，平均泼尼松剂量超过0.15mg/(kg·d)与延缓的最终身高独立相关[45]。

肝移植

肝移植术后生长追赶可在40%~50%肝移植受体中观察到[5,8,46]。如在肾移植中，年龄和在移植时的生长迟缓程度是移植术后生长追赶的重要预测因素[5,46]，较小的婴儿通常表现出最快速和最完全的生长追赶[4,5,46,47]。

不同的"原发肝脏疾病"也可能影响移植术后的生长潜力。McDiarmid等报道，胆道闭锁患者行肝移植术后5年的身高SDS分数为+0.7，而在那些暴发性肝衰竭的患者中为-1.0，原发性疾病为肿瘤的患者则为-0.9[47]。生长追赶缺乏还见于Alagille综合征和家族性肝硬化的受体[6,47]。这一变化也可能是由于肝移植术后生长状况的持续性差异或终末期肝病发生时患者年龄差异的简单反应。

长期观察到的生长发育结果似乎有利于肝移植受体。McDiarmid等发现236名儿童移植术后标准化身高从-1.7SDS的基线到-1.4SDS的改善，Viner等发现107名受体的移植术后7年标准化身高从-1.2SDS增加到了-0.8SDS，Fouquet等发现80名胆道闭锁患者移植10年后的标准化身高从-1.4SDS增加到-0.5SDS[4,6,47]。北美SPILT登记中心的121名儿童移植术后10年平均身高SDS为-0.5[48]。因此，大部分儿童肝同种异体移植受体的身高能达到正常的范围。

肝移植受体的长期生长状况关键取决于激素的使用状况(具体见本章后续内容)和移植肝的功能状况[4,5,49,50]。在免疫方面低风险的同时有良好的肝功能可以完全脱离激素的患者，其完整的生长追赶很常见[4,51,52]。这些发现已被日本一项分析237名随访15年的肝移植受体的研究所证实[53]。移植术后第一年平均标准化身高从-1.70SDS增加到-0.64SDS，随后有一个稳定期，到术后10年其生长追赶至-0.33SDS。在2岁之前接受移植的患者在移植术后10年后其表现为迟发性的生长退化，这主要与移植物功能不良有关，平均身高SDS在15年为-0.47。长期的生长失败主要与激素治疗密切相关；在移植术后10年，仍然接受激素治疗的患者中43%的高度低于平均身高10个百分点，而无激素治疗患者中仅为11%。

心脏移植

在心脏移植受体中存在多种不同的生长模式。在以激素为基础的免疫抑制方案的患者样本中，其移植6年后的标准身高无明显改变或为轻度的降低[12,13 54-57]。

无激素免疫治疗方案在心脏移植中的早期传播已证实糖皮质激素的持续治疗对于接受心脏移植的儿童患者的长期生长状况有着至关重要的影响。

英国纽卡斯尔市的一项无激素维持治疗并随访时间超过1年的小样本心脏移植研究显示标准化身高SDS从平均-2.15的基线增加到-1.15[58]。同样的，一项包含77名在年龄小于6月时接受移植并维持无激素方案的婴儿的研究中发现这些患者在移植术后第一年普遍发现明显的生长追赶[59]。可预测接受无激素免疫抑制方案的患者，其移植术后5年低于正常身高的因素包括：术后第一年内长期住院，频繁的迟发性排斥，以及低于平均水平的父母身高。

肺移植

迄今为止,全球尽管已有超过 1500 名儿童接受肺移植，但其中有限的长期生存患者导致了移植术后生长模式分析的困难[60]。由于营养不良、感染以及激素治疗的高发生率,这些儿童多有术前即存在的生长迟缓。如果患者术后接受包含激素的免疫抑制治疗，其生长追赶状况往往不明显，而激素的撤除仅可能出现在极少的患者中。目前为止,仅有一篇 1997 年的文章报道了 88 例儿童肺移植受体的身高状况[61]。其接受移植时的平均身高为正常人的 72%，最后观察到的平均身高仅为正常人的 64%。

小肠移植

两份研究描述了接受小肠移植(伴或不伴肝移植)儿童的移植术后生长状况[7,62]。在 46 名儿童中,其中 35 名在术后平均 3 年中保留有功能的移植小肠的同时没有任何额外肠外营养需求[7],其免疫抑制维持包括他克莫司和泼尼松。尽管这些患者接受移植时的年龄更小(平均 3.7 岁),但其并未发现明显的生长追赶。其移植术后 2 年内的中位身高 SDS 稳定在–1.8 左右。一项随访 31 名接受移植时年龄为 2~15 岁的患者，发现平均身高 SDS 为–1.2。即使其中 5 名儿童生长速度受损,仍有 25 名儿童患者的身高 SDS 保持稳定,仅有 1 名术前有严重的生长失败的儿童其术后有明显的生长追赶。

糖皮质激素诱导生长失败的内分泌机制

在婴儿后期，纵向生长的主要驱动因素为促进生长的激素,青春期则主要为促性腺激素轴的作用。这些内分泌系统在儿童移植受体中受到了糖皮质激素免疫抑制剂很大的影响。

在接受肾移植的儿童中，生长板会回应生长轴通过所显示生长激素(GH)脉冲振幅与身高增长速度之间的正相关作用产生的刺激[63]。然而,垂体生长激素的分泌易减少，其多由于糖皮质激素治疗对下丘脑生长激素抑制素合成和释放的慢性刺激效应[64]。因此,一些在移植术后接受糖皮质激素药物治疗的儿童可出现部分生长激素缺乏现象。在正常的青春期,增强的脉冲式促性腺激素的分泌可刺激性激素分泌。循环性激素浓度的增加会同时通过对生长板的直接作用和刺激性激素脉冲式分泌来诱发发育期生长的陡增。在肾移植受体中,青春期促性腺激素分泌的激增往往完好,但至少在男孩中性激素水平上升是不够的[64]。这是由于生长激素脉冲增加的迟缓和低于正常的发育期升高获得有关[20,64]。最近一份芬兰的报道显示,一组平均年龄为 5 岁的移植患者有更多的青春期正常性类固醇模式,这表明低剂量类固醇的使用以及在童年早期接受移植可保持青春期正常的内分泌状况[65]。

除了抑制生长激素分泌,试验和临床证据表明,糖皮质激素的使用还可能抑制目标器官的生长激素水平。在大鼠中肝生长激素受体表达随着甲泼尼龙治疗的生长抑制剂量的增加而减少[66,67],循环中的生长激素结合蛋白，反应性肝生长激素受体含量等在儿童肾移植受体中的水平较低[20,68,69]。激素介导的生长激素分泌改变和作用意味着生长激素主要下游介质 IGF–1 有效性的降低。的确,降低的 IGF–1 基因转录已在糖皮质激素治疗的动物中被证实[67,70]。然而,令人惊讶的是,在糖皮质激素治疗的肾移植受体血浆中 IGF–1 水平在正常范围内[20,68,69]。这种差异可以用额外的激素诱导的 IGF–1 的 mRNA 稳定性的改变、转录后的处理和 IGF–1 的分泌肽或 IGF–1 结合蛋白组成物半衰期的改变来解释[70]。与正常的免疫反应性的 IGF–1 血浆浓度相比，IGF 的生物活性在糖皮质激素治疗的患者中被显著抑制[68,71]。有证据显示糖皮质激素可能引起 IGF 抑制剂的产生[71]。这些假定的 IGF 抑制剂分子量为 12~20 kD，但至今没有进一步发现。

除了这些内分泌作用外，糖皮质激素还通过多个机制干预生长和生长板内软骨细胞水平的软骨内成骨。其可抑制增殖,抑制 IGF–1 的自分泌和(或)旁分泌合成,下调软骨细胞生长激素和 IGF–1 受体的表达,干扰骺软骨基质的硫酸盐化和矿化作用[72,73]。

促进移植术后最佳生长的模式

糖皮质激素治疗对同种异体移植儿童受体的内分泌功能和生长,及身体组成,脂类代谢,骨矿化和血压调节等在内的多个其他系统有深远影响。激素影响长期健康和生活质量的副作用越来越促使人们寻找在儿童器官移植受体中日常用甲泼尼龙治疗的替代方法[74]。

激素治疗的修正

临床试验的登记结果和证据表明，相同的糖皮质激素总量进行隔日给药相较于每日给药可以改善纵向生长且不产生对移植物长期功能的影响[22,27]。NAPRTCS登记显示，完全的激素总量通过隔日给药(17%的移植受体)证实在移植术后的前2年对其身高SDS有积极改善。在这两项研究中,相较于每日给药组无变化的标准化身高SDS，隔日给药均可观察到标准化身高0.5SDS的增加。一项对接受激素隔日给药的30名年轻肾移植受体长期随访(5~7年的随访)结果的分析表明，在接受移植时年龄为2~5岁的儿童中身高从-1.9DS增加到-0.4SDS,获得了的几乎完全的生长追赶,在2岁以内的移植受体获得了稳定的生长(接受移植时和移植术后7年身高SDS为-1.1)[32]。由于其已证实的良好的安全性，激素的隔日给药方式已成为许多有经验的中心的首选模式。在2010年NAPRTCS登记中心的年度报告中,34%的同种异体移植受体在移植术后4年内接受激素的隔日给药治疗[2]。

激素的撤除

在儿童肾移植受体的第一个二十年中，由于基于环孢素(CsA)和硫唑嘌呤单独的无激素免疫抑制方案,导致了至少50%的儿童的肾功能恶化，完全的激素撤除仍存在问题[21,75]。尽管如此,一些不受控制的小范围研究表明,该方案如果成功,完全的激素撤除可导致显著的生长追赶[76,77]。随着过去15年里更强大的免疫抑制剂的引入,尤其是他克莫司对CsA和霉酚酸吗啉乙酯对硫唑嘌呤的接近完全的替换,增加了肾移植受体的激素撤除的治疗窗[78]。北美儿童肾移植登记中心(NAPRTCS)的最新年度报告显示,1996—2009年的患者移植术后3年内无激素治疗的比例为:死亡供体移植为17%,活体移植为25%[2]。移植术后1个月接受激素治疗的患者比例从20世纪90年代的95%下降到了2009年的49%。

在过去的10年里,对早期及晚期的激素撤除方案均进行了相应的评估:

"晚期激素撤除"方案在至少70%接受他克莫司治疗的儿童同种异体移植受体中是可行的。Höcker等对52个儿童移植受体采用基于CsA和MMF的免疫抑制方案,在移植术后6个月撤除激素,其3年后的平均身高SDS从-2.41增加到-1.31[79]。由于严重的激素副作用,在移植术后第2年成功停止糖皮质激素的20名筛选后患者中，均维持了稳定的移植肾功能和不超过一次前述的排斥[80]。经过4年的随访,相比于标准化身高SDS无变化的持续每日甲泼尼龙治疗的配对控制组,其身高SDS从-1.6增加到-1.0。生长追赶仅限于6名青春期前儿童,其身高SDS从-2.24增加到-0.77,而青春期患者的生长并没有从激素撤除治疗中受益。激素治疗(如肥胖和高血压等)的后遗症也从激素撤除中得到了明显的改善。

早期的激素撤除方案对生长的促进效果已在随机对照试验TWIST中进行了评估,该试验中196名患者均采用了他克莫司及MMF,激素使用随机分为每日给药或达克珠单抗诱导治疗，并在移植术后第5天撤除激素。6个月观察到在激素撤除组的标准化身高有了显著的改善(0.16 SDS对0.03 SDS,P=0.005),并且在代谢和血压控制方面也有了明显的改善。在6个月的随访中，移植物生存和排斥发生率两组间并无明显差异[82]。该试验的扩展结果至今并未发表。一些更小的研究发现早期激素撤除并行单克隆或多克隆抗体诱导治疗的病史控制组在随访1~2年也获得了相似的结果,同时其也具有了良好的安全性[82-85]。然而,生长状况从早期激素撤除中的获益似乎随着时间逐渐减少。在一个前瞻性的对照研究中比较了95名基于他克莫司和MMF的免疫治疗方案行激素早期撤除的疗效,激素治疗组和无激素治疗组平均身高SDS分别从移植时的-2.4增加到了1年后的-1.5、-2.2,2年后的-1.3、-1.9,5年后的-1.0、-1.2[85]。

激素仍然是许多儿童肝移植免疫抑制剂中的基石。一些非对照研究[86]和一个对照研究[87]评估了儿童肝移植受体的激素撤除概念。5个非对照研究尝试在移植术后3~58个月同时行CsA治疗时撤除激素,其急性排斥发生率为7%~27%,慢性排斥为4%~13%,移植物失功及受体死亡率为3%~13%。相比较,McDiarmid等采用严格的筛选标准对23名患者在术后平均3.5年撤除了激素,其急性排斥发生率仅为6%,无相应导致的慢性排斥、移植物失功或患者死亡。不幸的是,在激素撤除组和激素持续治疗组之间在纵向生长上并未发现显著的差异。在3个尝试在移植术后一年内使用他克莫司治疗的同时撤除激素的试验中，急性排斥的发生率为14%~29%[86]。Reding等比较了接受CsA或他克莫司治疗的受体撤除激素后的纵向生长状况[86]。在激素撤除后的 12 个月内,相较于他克莫司组(-0.2~+0.3),CsA 组的标准化身高改善效果欠佳(-0.2~-0.4)。该差异可能是由于他克莫司组更短的激素暴露（平均术后 1.2 年),而 CsA 组为术后平均 5~6 年。

在许多儿童心脏移植中激素多在移植术后早期撤除;多于 50%的心脏受体在移植术后 12 个月内维持无激素方案[88]。在一项包括接受心脏移植时年龄小于 3 个月的 25 名婴儿的研究中，比较了 18 名在移植术后 7 个月撤除激素和 8 名持续激素治疗患者之间的生长状况[89],随访期间两组之间的标准化身高并无明显差异。然而,心脏移植受体组的移植术后总体生长状况相当差。其平均标准化身高从移植时的-1.08 下降到移植术后 4 年的-1.8。

激素的避免

随着新的强有力的和选择性免疫抑制剂的增加，完全无激素方案开始成为儿童器官移植中的一个可实现的选择。除了可以避开激素开始治疗时的副作用,动物试验数据还显示无激素治疗模式甚至可诱导对同种异体器官的免疫耐受。

无激素方案目前已在心脏移植中倡导。生长追赶在儿童心脏移植受体中几乎是普遍的。在一项大型研究中，仅 12%的受体移植术后 5 年的身高低于标准的 5%[59]。

在肾移植方面,斯坦福组第一次报道了在 50 名接受联合他克莫司和 MMF 或西罗莫司治疗同时行补偿性 IL-2 受体阻断治疗儿童中,术后 6 个月内采用完全无激素方案的有利结果[90,91]。经过 22 个月的随访,相较于接受基于激素治疗的病史配对对照组的 32%，其急性排斥发生率仅为 8%。无激素组的生长状况更优。这在年龄小于 5 岁的儿童中最为明显，相较于激素治疗组无改善的平均标准化身高，其在移植术后第一年的生长追赶为 1.7±0.8SDS。该初步经验促使了一项持续 3 年包括 130 名儿童的多中心研究，肾移植儿童在接受他克莫司和 MMF 治疗的同时,随机再分为无激素同时行标准剂量达克珠单抗诱导和基于激素同时行超剂量达克珠单抗诱导的免疫抑制治疗[92]。

令人失望的是，那些在接受移植时仍有生长潜能的患者，其移植 3 年后的纵向生长在无激素组身高 SDS 改变为-0.92±2.29,而激素治疗组为-0.9±1.16(P=0.732),并无明显的差异。只有 5 岁以下接受无激素免疫抑制方案的儿童的身高 SDS 有显著改善的趋势,但是该效果在移植术后 1 年和 3 年失去了效果。其在 3 年随访中的经穿刺证实的急性排斥发生率（16.7%对 17.1%;P=0.94）和移植物生存率无明显差异没有差异(95%对 90%)。无激素组表现为更低的收缩压和胆固醇水平。

无激素免疫抑制方案第一次是在比利时布鲁塞尔的儿童肝移植项目中进行了应用。其比较了 20 名同时接受他克莫司和巴利昔单抗的儿童与 20 名病史配对的同时接受他克莫司和激素治疗的儿童。他克莫司和巴利昔单抗组拥有更高的无排斥生存期以及移植术后 1 年更为显著的生长改善。无激素组患者在移植时的轻度生长迟缓(-0.57SDS)在移植术后 6 个月内就得到了完全的生长追赶，然而激素治疗组儿童表现为更慢的生长恢复节奏[93]。在获得积极的初步经验后,相同的方案分别在包括 72 名和 84 名儿童肝移植的前瞻性研究中进行了比较[94,95]。两个研究结果在患者和移植物生存率上基本相似,但他克莫司和巴利昔单抗组有更长的无排斥间隔、更低的感染发生率,以及更少的抗高血压治疗需求。3 年内,无激素组患者出现了完全的标准化身高正常化(平均基准为-1.16SDS,3 年后为 0.21SDS),而激素治疗组的生长追赶是不完全的（平均基准为-1.15SDS,3 年后为-0.42SDS,P<0.001)[95]。

生长激素治疗

重组人生长激素的慢性管理已证实在慢性肾功能不全伴有生长失败的儿童中有明显的效果,在过去 15 年中其促使儿童肾移植受体产生了稳定的身高 SDS 增长。因此,重组人生长激素已被认为是移植术后未表现出生长追赶的生长迟缓肾移植受体调整或撤除激素治疗的替代方案。

动物试验结果显示重组人生长激素治疗能通过调节激活循环中或局部的 IGF-1 合成[97-99]弥补糖皮质激素治疗的生长抑制效应[96]。

大量的非对照试验认为长达 3 年的重组人生长激素治疗对于肾移植受体儿童有明显的生长促进作用[68,69,100-106],其标准化身高每年增加的中位数在术后的第一个 2 年可达到 0.5SDS。4 个随机对照试验证实了肾移植受体应用重组人生长激素的短期效果[107-110];在两项更大型的试验中，相较于控制组一年生长速度的

4.2~4.6cm，其生长速度增加到每年7.7~9.0cm。一项NAPRTCS登记中心评估了513名移植术后儿童患者和2263名无生长激素治疗患者的结果显示重组人生长激素组获得了更多的累积身高增长和更好的最终身高(−1.83±0.14SDS对−2.63±0.05SDS)。

重组人生长激素的成功生长激活同时在7名接受氢化可的松的肝移植患者中获得了证实。在治疗的第一年，每年生长速度从3.9cm增加到8.2cm，中位身高SDS从−2.7增加到−2.1[111]。

重组人生长激素被认为不仅可以对抗生长抑制，还包括糖皮质激素的免疫抑制效果。两项大型对照试验和对儿童肾移植受体的登记分析已实行来评估重组人生长激素治疗期间在排斥和移植物衰竭方面的任何改变。然而没有一项研究发现有排斥或肾功能损害发生率的增加，前瞻性研究发现，在那些治疗前就有一次以上排斥病史的患者中，其随后的排斥发生率有所增加。

总结

总之，实体器官移植患者的生长和青春期发育表现非常多样，但仍有许多儿童移植受体成年后较为矮小。移植术后生长和发育的主要决定因素为接受移植时的年龄和生长不足、长期的移植物功能状况、潜在的代谢紊乱和免疫抑制治疗的选择。完全的激素撤除或一开始即采用的无激素免疫治疗方案在大部分的实体器官移植儿童中成为了可能。然而，早期生长促进效果和最小激素暴露的免疫安全仍然需要长期试验的证实。生长激素治疗在高免疫风险的患者中可作为激素撤除的替代方案。这些方法在日常临床实践中的转换应使移植受体获得改善的生长追赶和最终正常的成年身高，即使不是大多数。

(柯庆宏 译 柯庆宏 校)

参考文献

1. Schaefer F. Endocrine and growth disorders in chronic renal failure. In: Avner ED, Niaudet P, Harmon W, editors. Pediatric Nephrology. 6th ed. Berlin and Heidelberg: Springer-Verlag; 2009: 1714–1753.
2. North American Pediatric Renal Trials and Collaborative Studies (NAPRTCS). 2010 Annual Transplant Report. 2010. [assessed December 28, 2013]; Available from: https://web.emmes.com/study/ped/annlrept/2010_Report.pdf.
3. Studies of Pediatric Liver Transplantation (SPLIT). Annual Report, 2000. Rockville, MD, EMMES Corporation, 2000.
4. McDiarmid S, Gornbein J, DeSilva P, et al. Factors affecting growth after pediatric liver transplantation. Transplantation. 1999;67:404–411.
5. Bartosh SM, Thomas SE, Sutton MM, et al. Linear growth after pediatric liver transplantation. Journal of Pediatrics. 1999;135:624–631.
6. Viner RM, Forton JTM, Cole TJ, et al. Growth of long-term survivors of liver transplantation. Archives of Disease in Childhood. 1999;80:235–240.
7. Iyer K, Horslen S, Iverson A, et al. Nutritional outcome and growth of children after intestinal transplantation. Journal of Pediatric Surgery. 2002;37: 464–466.
8. Burdelski M, Nolkemper D, Ganschow R, et al. Liver transplantation in children: longterm outcome and quality of life. European Journal of Pediatrics. 1999;158:S34–S42.
9. Quiros-Tejeira RE, Ament ME, Heyman MB, et al. Does liver transplantation affect growth pattern in Alagille syndrome? Liver Transplantation. 2000;6: 582–587.
10. Arvay JL, Zemel BS, Gallagher PR, et al. Body composition of children aged 1 to 12 years with biliary atresia or Alagille syndrome. Journal of Pediatric Gastroenterology and Nutrition. 2005;40:146–150.
11. Hathout EH, Chinnock RE. Growth after heart transplantation. Pediatric Transplantation. 2004;8:97–100.
12. Peterson RE, Perens GS, Alejos JC, et al. Growth and weight gain of prepubertal children after cardiac transplantation. Pediatric Transplantation. 2008;12:436–441.
13. Bannister L, Manlhiot C, Pollock-BarZiv S, et al. Anthropometric growth and utilization of enteral feeding support in pediatric heart transplant recipients. Pediatric Transplantation. 2010;14:879–886.
14. DeShazo CV, Simmons RL, Berstein SM, et al. Results of renal transplantation in 100 children. Surgery. 1974;76:461–463.
15. Potter DE, Holliday MA, Wilson SJ, et al. Alternate day steroids in children after renal transplantation. Transplantation Proceedings. 1975;7:79.
16. Pennisi AJ, Costin G, Phillips LS, et al. Linear growth in long-term renal allograft recipients. Clinical Nephrology. 1977;8:415–421.
17. Ingelfinger JR, Grupe WE, Harmon WE, et al. Growth acceleration following renal transplantation in children less than 7 years of age. Pediatrics. 1981;68:255–259.
18. Bosque M, Munian A, Bewick M, et al. Growth after renal transplants. Archives of Disease in Childhood. 1983;58:110–114.
19. Offner G, Hoyer PF, Jüppner H, et al. Somatic growth after kidney transplantation. American Journal of Diseases of Children. 1987;141:541–546.
20. Rees L, Greene SA, Adlard P, et al. Growth and endocrine function after renal transplantation. Archives of Disease in Childhood. 1988;63:1326–1332.
21. Reisman L, Lieberman KV, Burrows L, et al. Follow-up of cyclosporine-treated pediatric renal allograft recipients after cessation of prednisone. Transplantation. 1990;49:76–80.
22. Broyer M, Guest G, Gagnadoux M-F. Growth rate in children receiving alternate-day corticosteroid treatment after kidney transplantation. Journal of Pediatrics. 1992;120:721–725.
23. Kaiser BA, Polinsky MS, Palmer JA, et al. Growth after conversion to alternate-day corticosteroids in children with renal transplants: a single-center study. Pediatric Nephrology (Berlin, Germany). 1994;8:320–325.
24. Hokken-Koelega AC, Van Zaal MA, de Ridder MA, et al. Growth after renal transplantation in prepubertal children: impact of various treatment modalities. Pediatric Research. 1994;35:367–371.
25. Chao SM, Jones CL, Powell HR, et al. Triple immunosuppression with subsequent prednisolone withdrawal: 6 years′ experience in paediatric renal allograft recipients. Pediatric Nephrology (Berlin, Germany). 1994;8:62–69.
26. Ellis D. Clinical use of tacrolimus (FK-506) in infants and children with renal transplants. Pediatric Nephrology (Berlin, Germany). 1995;9:487–494.
27. Jabs K, Sullivan EK, Avner ED, et al. Alternate-day steroid dosing improves growth without affecting graft survival or long-term graft function. A report of the North American Pediatric Renal Transplant Cooperative Study. Transplantation. 1996;61:31–36.
28. Tejani A, Cortes L, Sullivan EK. A longitudinal study of the natural history of growth post- transplantation. Kidney International. 1996;53:103–108.
29. Tejani A, Fine R, Alexander S, et al. Factors predictive of sustained growth in children after renal transplantation. The North American Pediatric Renal Transplant Cooperative Study. Journal of Pediatrics. 1993;122:397–402.
30. Helling TS, Nelson PW, Reed L, et al. A seven year experience with kidney transplantation for pediatric end stage renal disease. Missouri Medicine. 1994;91:33–37.
31. Kohaut EC, Tejani A. The 1994 annual report of the North American Pediatric Renal Transplant Cooperative Study. Pediatric Nephrology (Berlin, Germany). 1996;10:422–434.
32. Qvist E, Marttinen E, Rönnhom K, et al. Growth after renal transplantation in infancy or early childhood. Pediatric Nephrology (Berlin, Germany). 2002;17: 438–443.

33. Fine RN, Stablein D. Long-term use of recombinant human growth hormone in pediatric allograft recipients: a report of the NAPRTCS Transplant Registry. Pediatric Nephrology (Berlin, Germany). 2005;20:404–408.
34. Nissel R, Brazda I, Feneberg R, et al. Effect of renal transplantation in childhood on longitudinal growth and adult height. Kidney International. 2004;66: 792–800.
35. Schaefer F, Seidel C, Binding A, et al. Pubertal growth in chronic renal failure. Pediatric Research. 1990;28:5–10.
36. Englund MS, Tyden G, Wikstad I, et al. Growth impairment at renal transplantation – a determinant of growth and final height. Pediatric Transplantation. 2003;7:192–199.
37. Sarna S, Hoppu K, Neuvonen PJ, et al. Methylprednisolone exposure, rather than dose, predicts adrenal suppression and growth inhibition in children with liver and renal transplantation. Journal of Clinical Endocrinology and Metabolism. 1997;82:75–77.
38. Hay N, Sonenberg N. Upstream and downstream of mTOR. Genes and Development.2004:18:1926–1945.
39. Alvarez-Garcia O, Carbajo-Pérez E, Garcia E, et al. Rapamycin retards growth and causes marked alterations in the growth plate of young rats. Pediatric Nephrology (Berlin, Germany). 2007;22:954–961.
40. Alvarez-García O, García-López E, Loredo V, et al. Rapamycin induces growth retardation by disrupting angiogenesis in the growth plate. Kidney International. 2010;78:561–568.
41. Rangel GA, Ariceta G. Growth failure associated with sirolimus: case report. Pediatric Nephrology (Berlin, Germany). 2009;24:2047–2050.
42. González D, García CD, Azócar M, et al. Growth of kidney-transplanted pediatric patients treated with sirolimus. Pediatric Nephrology (Berlin, Germany). 2011;26:961–966.
43. Hymes LC, Warshaw BL. Linear growth in pediatric renal transplant recipients receiving sirolimus. Pediatric Transplantation. 2011;15:570–572.
44. Rodriguez-Soriano J, Vallo A, Quintela MJ, et al. Predictors of final adult heigth after renal transplantation during childhood: a single-center study. Nephron. 2000;86:266–273.
45. Fine RN, Ho M, Tejani A. The contribution of renal transplantation to final adult height: a report of the North American Pediatric Renal Transplant Cooperative Study (NAPRTCS). Pediatric Nephrology (Berlin, Germany). 2001;16:951–956.
46. Renz JF, de Roos M, Rosenthal P, et al. Posttransplantation growth in pediatric liver recipients. Liver Transplantation. 2001;7:1040–1055.
47. Fouquet V, Alves A, Branchereau S, et al. Long-term outcome of pediatric liver transplantation for biliary atresia: a 10-year follow-up in a single center. Liver Transplantation. 2005;11:152–160.
48. Ng VL, Alonso EM, Bucuvalas JC, et al.; Studies of Pediatric Liver Transplantation (SPLIT) Research Group. Health status of children alive 10 years after pediatric liver transplantation performed in the US and Canada: report of the studies of pediatric liver transplantation experience. Journal of Pediatrics. 2012;160:820–826.
49. Lopez-Espinosa J, Yeste D, Iglesias J, et al. Analysis of growth during prepubertal years in long-term survivors after pediatric orthotopic liver transplantation. Journal of Pediatric Endocrinology and Metabolism. 2004;17:1221–1229.
50. Superina R, Zangari A. Acal L: growth in children following liver transplantation. Pediatric Transplantation. 1998;2:70–75.
51. Kelly D. Nutritional factors affecting growth before and after liver transplantation. Pediatric Transplantation. 1997;1:80–84.
52. Orii T, Ohkohchi N, Koyamada N, et al. Growth of pediatric patients with biliary atresia after liver transplantation: influence of age at transplantation and steroid administration. Transplantation Proceedings. 2000;32:2210–2212.
53. El Moghazy WM, Ogura Y, Harada K, et al. Can children catch up in growth after living donor liver transplantation? Liver Transplantation. 2010;16:453–460.
54. Cohen A, Addonizio LJ, Softness B, et al. Growth and skeletal maturation after pediatric cardiac transplantation. Pediatric Transplantation. 2004;8:126–135.
55. De Broux E, Huot CH, Chartrand S, et al. Growth and pubertal development following pediatric heart transplantation: a 15-year experience at Ste-Justine Hospital. Journal of Heart and Lung Transplantation. 2000;19:825–833.
56. Baum MF, Cutler DC, Fricker FJ, et al. Session VII: physiologic and psychological growth and development in pediatric heart transplant recipients. Journal of Heart and Lung Transplantation. 1991;10:848–855.
57. Lebidois J, Kachaner J, Vouhe P, et al. Heart transplantation in children: mid-term results and quality of life. European Journal of Pediatrics. 1992;151:S59–S64.
58. Au J, Gregory JW, Colquhoun IW, et al. Paediatric cardiac transplantation with steroid-sparing maintenance imunosuppression. Archives of Disease in Childhood. 1992;67:1262–1266.
59. Chinnock R, Baum M. Somatic growth in infant heart transplant recipients. Pediatric Transplantation. 1998;2:30.
60. Benden C. Specific aspects of children and adolescents undergoing lung transplantation. Current Opinion in Organ Transplantation. 2012;17:509–514.
61. Sweet SC, Spray T, Huddleston CB. Pediatric lung transplantation at St. Louis Children's Hospital, 1990–95. American Journal of Respiratory and Critical Care Medicine. 1997;155:1027–1035.
62. Lacaille F, Vass N, Sauvat F, et al. Long-term outcome, growth and digestive function in children 2 to 18 years after intestinal transplantation. Gut. 2008;57:455–461.
63. Schaefer F, Hamill G, Stanhope R, et al. Cooperative Study on Pubertal Development In Chronic Renal Failure: pulsatile growth hormone secretion in peripubertal patients with chronic renal failure. Journal of Pediatrics. 1991; 119:568–577.
64. Wehrenberg WB, Janowski BA, Piering AW. Glucocorticoids: potent inhibitors and stimulators of growth hormone secretion. Endocrinology. 1990;126: 3200–3203.
65. Tainio J, Qvist E, Vehmas R, et al. Pubertal development is normal in adolescents after renal transplantation in childhood. Transplantation. 2011;92:404–409.
66. Tönshoff B, Eden S, Weiser E, et al. Reduced hepatic growth hormone (GH) receptor gene expression and increase in plasma GH binding protein in experimental uremia. Kidney International. 1994;45:1085–1092.
67. Gabrielsson BG, Carmignac DF, Flavell DM, et al. Steroid regulation of growth hormone (GH) receptor and GH binding protein messenger ribonucleic acids in the rat. Endocrinology. 1995;133:2445–2452.
68. Tönshoff B, Haffner D, Mehls O, et al. German Study Group for Growth Hormone Treatment in Chronic Renal Failure: efficacy and safety of growth hormone treatment in short children with renal allografts: three year experience. Kidney International. 1993;44:199–207.
69. van Dop C, Jabs KL, Donohue PA, et al. Accelerated growth rates in children treated with growth hormone after renal transplantation. Journal of Pediatrics. 1992;120:244–250.
70. Luo J, Murphy LJ. Dexamethasone inhibits growth hormone induction of insulin-like growth factor-I (IGF-I) messenger ribonucleic acid (mRNA) in hypophysectomized rats and reduces IGF-I mRNA abundance in the intact rat. Endocrinology. 1989;125:165–171.
71. Unterman TG, Phillips LS. Glucocorticoid effects on somatomedins and somatomedin inhibitors. Journal of Clinical Endocrinology and Metabolism. 1985;61:618–626.
72. Silbermann M, Maor G. Mechanisms of glucocorticoid-induced growth retardation: impairment of cartilage mineralization. Acta Anatomica. 1978;101: 140–149.
73. Jux C, Leiber K, Hügel U, et al. Dexamethasone inhibits growth hormone (GH)-stimulated growth by suppression of local insulin-like growth factor (IGF)-I production and expression of GH- and IGF-I receptor in cultured rat chondrocytes. Endocrinology. 1998;139:3296–3305.
74. Reding R, Webber SA, Fine R. Getting rid of steroids in pediatric solid-organ transplantation? Pediatric Transplantation. 2004;8:526–530.
75. Ingulli E, Sharma V, Singh A, et al. Steroid withdrawal, rejection and the mixed lymphocyte reaction in children after renal transplantation. Kidney International. Supplement. 1993;43:S36–S39.
76. Chakrabati P, Wong HY, Scantlebury VP, et al. Outcome after steroid withdrawal in pediatric renal transplant patients receiving tacrolimus-based immunosuppression. Transplantation. 2000;15:5–760.
77. Klare B, Montoya CR, Fischer DC, et al. Normal adult height after steroid-withdrawal within 6 months of pediatric kidney transplantation: a 20 years single center experience. Transplant International. 2012;25:276–278.
78. Pascual J, Zamora J, Galeano C, et al. Steroid avoidance or withdrawal for kidney transplant recipients. Cochrane Database of Systematic Reviews. 2009;(1): CD005632.
79. Ellis D. Growth and renal function after steroid-free tacrolimus-based immunosuppression in children with renal transplants. Pediatric Nephrology (Berlin, Germany). 2000;14:689–694.
80. Höcker B, John U, Plank C, et al. Successful withdrawal of steroids in pediatric renal transplant recipients receiving cyclosporine A and mycophenolate mofetil treatment: results after four years. Transplantation. 2004;78:228–234.
81. Grenda R, Watson A, Trompeter R, et al. A randomized trial to assess the impact of early steroid withdrawal on growth in pediatric renal transplantation: the TWIST Study. American Journal of Transplantation. 2010;10:828–836.
82. Birkeland SA, Larsen KE, Rohr N. Pediatric renal transplantation without steroids. Pediatric Nephrology (Berlin, Germany). 1998;12:87–92.
83. Oberholzer J, John E, Lumpaopong A, et al. Early discontinuation of steroids is safe and effective in pediatric kidney transplant recipients. Pediatric Transplantation. 2005;9:456–463.
84. Chavers BM, Chang YC, Gillingham KJ, et al. Pediatric kidney transplantation using a novel protocol of rapid (6-day) discontinuation of prednisone: 2-year results. Transplantation. 2009;88:237–241.
85. Delucchi A, Valenzuela M, Lillo AM, et al. Early steroid withdrawal in pediatric

renal transplant: five years of follow-up. Pediatric Nephrology (Berlin, Germany). 2011;26:2235–2244.
86. Reding S. Steroid withdrawal in liver transplantation. Transplantation. 2000;70: 405–410.
87. McDiarmid S, Farmer DA, Goldstein LI, et al. A randomized prospective trial of steroid withdrawal after liver transplantation. Transplantation. 1995;60:1443.
88. Boucek MM, Edwards LB, Keck BM, et al. The registry of the International Society of Heart and Lung Transplantation: fifth official pediatric report - 2001 to 2002. Journal of Heart and Lung Transplantation. 2002;21:827–840.
89. Hirsch R, Huddleston CB, Mendeloff EN, et al. Infant and donor organ growth after heart transplantation in neonates with hypoplastic left heart syndrome. Journal of Heart and Lung Transplantation. 1996;15:1093–1100.
90. Sarwal MM, Yorgin PD, Alexander S, et al. Promising early outcomes with a novel, complete steroid avoidance immunosuppression protocol in pediatric renal transplantation. Transplantation. 2001;72:13–21.
91. Sarwal MM, Vidhun JR, Alexander SR, et al. Continued superior outcomes with modification and lengthened follow-up of a steroid-avoidance pilot with extended daclizumab induction in pediatric renal transplantation. Transplantation. 2003;76:1331–1339.
92. Sarwal MM, Ettenger RB, Dharnidharka V, et al. Complete steroid avoidance is effective and safe in children with renal transplants: a multicenter randomized trial with three-year follow-up. American Journal of Transplantation. 2012;12:2719–2729.
93. Reding R, Gras J, Sokal E, et al. Steroid-free liver transplantation in children. Lancet. 2003;362:2068–2070.
94. Spada M, Petz W, Bertani A, et al. Randomized trial of basiliximab induction versus steroid therapy in pediatric liver allograft recipients under tacrolimus immunosuppression. American Journal of Transplantation. 2006;6:1913–1921.
95. Gras JM, Gerkens S, Beguin C, et al. Steroid-free, tacrolimus-basiliximab immunosuppression in pediatric liver transplantation: clinical and pharmacoeconomic study in 50 children. Liver Transplantation. 2008;14:469–477.
96. Kovàcs G, Fine RN, Worgall S, et al. Recombinant human growth hormone prevents catabolic effects of methylprednisolone in the healthy and uremic organism. Kidney International. 1991;40:1032–1040.
97. Tomas FM, Knowles SE, Owens PC. Insulin-like growth factor I (IGF-I) variants are anabolic in dexamethasone treated rats. Biochemical Journal. 1992; 282:91–97.
98. Mehls O, Tönshoff B, Kovacs G, et al. Interaction between glucocorticoids and growth hormone. Acta Paediatrica. Supplementum. 1993;388:77–82.
99. Kovacs GT, Oh J, Kovacs J, et al. Growth promoting effects of growth hormone and IGF-I are additive in experimental uremia. Kidney International. 1996;49:1413–1421.
100. Johannson G, Janssens F, Proesmans W. Treatment with Genotropin in short children with chronic renal failure, either before active replacement therapy or with functioning renal transplants. An interim report on five European studies. Acta Paediatrica Scandinavica. 1990;370:36–42.
101. Fine RN, Yadin O, Nelson PA, et al. Recombinant human growth hormone treatment of children following renal transplantation. Pediatric Nephrology (Berlin, Germany). 1991;5:147–151.
102. van Es A. Growth hormone treatment in short children with chronic renal failure and after renal transplantation: combined data from European clinical trials. Acta Paediatrica Scandinavica. 1991;379:42–48.
103. Hokken-Koelega AC, Stijnen T, de Jong RC, et al. A placebo-controlled, double-blind trial of growth hormone treatment in prepubertal children after renal transplant. Kidney International. Supplement. 1996;53:S128–S134.
104. Rees L, Rigden SPA, Ward G, et al. Treatment of short stature in renal disease with recombinant human growth hormone. Archives of Disease in Childhood. 1990;65:856–860.
105. Hokken-Koelega AC, de Jong RC, Donckerwolcke RA, et al. Use of recombinant human growth hormone (rhGH) in pubertal patients with CRI/dialysis/post-transplant: dutch data. Dutch Study Group on Growth in Children with Chronic Renal Disease. British Journal of Clinical Practice. Symposium Supplement. 1996;85:5–6.
106. Hokken-Koelega AC, Stijnen T, de Ridder MA, et al. Growth hormone treatment in growth-retarded adolescents after renal transplant. Lancet. 1994;343:1313–1317.
107. Hokken-Koelega ACS, Stijnen T, de Jong RC, et al. A placebo-controlled double-blind trial of growth hormone treatment in prepubertal children with renal allografts. Kidney International. 1996;49(Suppl):S128–S134.
108. Maxwell H, Rees L, for the British Association for Paediatric Nephrology. Randomised controlled trial of recombinant human growth hormone in prepubertal and pubertal renal transplant recipients. Archives of Disease in Childhood. 1998;79:481–487.
109. Guest G, Berard E, Crosnier H, et al. Effects of growth hormone in short children after renal transplantation. Pediatric Nephrology (Berlin, Germany). 1998;12:437–446.
110. Fine RN, Stablein D, Cohen AH, et al. Recombinant human growth hormone post-renal transplantation in children: a randomized controlled study of the NAPRTCS. Kidney International. 2002;62:688–696.
111. Rodeck B, Kardoff R, Melter M, et al. Improvement of growth after growth hormone treatment in children who undergo liver transplantation. Journal of Pediatric Gastroenterology and Nutrition. 2000;31:286–290.

第 119 章 器官移植术后的认知发展和功能结果

Estella M. Alonso, Saeed Mohammad, Lisa G. Sorensen

引言

实体器官移植的期望不仅仅是延长生命和恢复器官衰竭终末期的严重后果，还包括得到能明显改善移植前状况的希望和维持良好的健康状况。考虑到儿童健康的各个方面，医生需要检查的不仅仅是生理状况还需要检查心理状况，包括认知发展和学习功能。然而，在儿童心脏、肾、肝和肠移植中，这个领域的研究仍存在相当大的差距。在本章中，我们将复习最新的关于实体器官移植儿童受体认知功能检查的文献并以目前的知识来讨论他们的发现。

由于需要根据年龄相适应的方法来评估认知的发展，所以还需要研究新兴的评估方法。那些从非常规治疗（如器官移植）中生存下来的儿童组，其结果样本往往偏小同时包括不同年龄的异质性。因此，有些研究者利用不同的工具对年龄进行分组来打散研究结果，尝试去发现有意义的结论。针对这一点，许多针对接受实体器官移植治疗儿童的认知发展研究多局限于一个医疗中心以及相对较小的样本。然而，在过去的几年里，一些重要的研究已经发表，可以帮助我们扩展对于这些患者发展结果和康复的认识。

认知功能

认知发展的结果可以根据年龄，并通过数种方式来检测。对于婴儿的评估主要集中于自主功能、社会和环境反应，以及语言发展和适应技能，年龄较大儿童则可根据智力、学习成绩、行为和更多的特异性认知领域（如注意力、执行能力、语言、视觉空间的处理、学习和记忆等）来检测。在儿童晚期出现的异常更有可能预示其可能会持续到成人期。许多儿童时期的慢性疾病对于认知发展有不利的影响。由于在神经系统快速成熟期经历了疾病的暴发，在婴儿期经历了实体器官功能衰竭的儿童对于认知延迟有特别的风险。目前，对于移植前和移植术后神经发展损失的影响仍无仔细的研究。同样的，对于实体器官移植术后神经认知结果和发展康复的研究仍然有限。

经过多器官受体组神经认知的研究包含了一些相同的方法。最常见的研究领域为智力，其多数通过智商（IQ）来评估。IQ 最常用 Wechsler 评分法来评估。当前对于儿童评估的版本为 Wechsler 学前儿童和初级智力评分第 3 版（WPPSI-Ⅲ），和 Wechsler 儿童智力评分第 4 版（WPPSI-Ⅳ），其标准为 100 分及 15 分的偏差[1,2]。认知发展延迟分为：轻到中度，典型的“全量表智商”（FSIQ）71~85 分，重度，FSIQ≤70 分，其低于正常人群 2 个标准差。严重迟缓的患者的 IQ 多预示着精神迟缓，而那些轻到中度迟缓患者的智力多处于平均水平的下缘[3]。学习障碍同样也是研究较多的方面，但是学习障碍的定义随着时间不停地变化。在一些研究中，学习障碍的定义为通过 IQ 和阅读和（或）数学竞赛测试的智力水平低于 15 分或更多[3]。已明确诊断的患者学习障碍也可通过父母的报告来评估，特别是那些在学校期间已接受过特殊教育服务测试的父母，其被认为更加准确。

肾移植受体

慢性肾衰竭已被证实对于神经认知的发育有不利的影响，该影响可通过肾移植的改善来减轻。肾移植受体儿童的智力水平常常在正常水平的下缘，一项研究报道显示肾移植术后儿童的智力平均 FSIQ 为 87 分（正常平均为 100 分，标准差为 15 分），另一项更新的研究显示，27 名受体的中位 FSIQ 为 97 分，仅有 22% 的FSIQ<85 分[5]。研究显示肾移植受体语言功能相较于

非语言功能受到更严重损害，注意力的集中时间更短，记忆困难，特别是那些一出生就有肾脏疾病的患者[4]。对于那些接受移植时年龄更大的儿童，其操作 IQ 会明显受损害，其测定智力能力多不依靠一个人的知识量、词汇和基础知识，而更多的借助于流体智力[5]。肾移植受体的运动功能与正常人相比也会出现显著迟缓，其表现在多个功能领域包括：纯运动任务 $P<0.001$，自适应的精细运动任务 $P=0.01$，自适应粗大运动任务 $P<0.001$，以及静态平衡 $P=0.001$[5]。运动技能在同伴关系和学习任务（如画画、书法）中发挥着关键的作用。

很少有评估移植术前及术后认知功能的纵向研究。最近的一项研究评估了 6 名慢性肾脏病（CKD）儿童移植前和移植术后的认知功能，并与 28 名中重度肾病儿童以及 23 名对照儿童进行了比较[6]。肾移植受体组的 FSIQ 有平均 12 分的改善，即使这是在移植术后第一年（平均移植术后 6 个月）这个相对早期的时间评估的。无论肾病组还是健康组均无这种趋势。

尽管样本量小，许多肾移植受体研究仍然尝试对导致认知功能差的危险因素进行了分析。肾病发病早、长期透析治疗、术前病态（如癫痫）[4]，和较低的社会经济状况被认为对认知功能发展有显著的影响[7-9]。然而，也有其他研究[5]认为医疗因素和认知结果之间并无关系。但是，目前普遍认为避免长期的透析可部分改善认知的损害。假定持续的如高血压和尿毒症等肾病终末期并发症对于神经髓鞘形成突触的发展有不利的影响。事实上，婴儿在移植术后 1 年，早期移植显示可改善头部循环，SDS 从 −1.4 增长到 −0.9（$P=0.02$），粗大运动显著改善，社会和语言发展（$P=0.02-0.0006$）[10]。

在肾移植术后，大约 70% 的患者接受常规的教室学习，而剩下的多需要特殊的教育或有严重的神经系统疾病（如癫痫）[4,7]。有许多长期研究发现，这些患者的最终受教育水平多低于全国平均水平[11,12]。而其他研究也显示，其教育水平与一般人群或其民族人群相似。

肝移植受体

即使获得资质最早的儿童肝移植医生对于肝移植受体的神经认知结果也特别感兴趣。大量研究表示移植术后儿童的智力水平往往显著低于健康儿童[14-18]。婴儿期的肝病被认为会增加神经认知发育迟缓的风险，其甚至可持续到成功的肝移植以后。儿童肝移植受体一些独特的方面理论上可被认为是认知损害的危险因素。由于大约一半的儿童肝移植受体接受移植时的年龄小于 2 岁，因此研究该婴儿人群的神经认知功能非常的重要。慢性肝病患者导致门静脉高压可出现慢性肝性脑病的临床症状。包括血氨等的神经抑制物质血浆浓度不仅仅改变心理过程，还可能造成成功移植术后的认知功能的不可逆的损害。最终，钙调神经磷酸酶抑制剂可造成严重的神经毒性，儿童肝移植受体相对于其他的实体器官移植受体该并发症发生率更高[19-21]。

得克萨斯大学一系列对于肝移植早期经验的研究评估了终末期肝病和胆道闭锁患者，发现这些患者的 IQ 和发展功能基本位于正常水平以下。早期发病，肝功能和生长参数（特别是年龄更小的儿童）与智力缺陷的相关性进行了强调。较小的患者（0.5~5 岁）恐怕更糟；其总体认知功能在 Bayley 或 Stanford-Binet 的边缘范围，并伴有极低的运动技能。婴儿的精神和运动发育与生长参数相关，而较大儿童则与肝功能的关系更为密切[22]。一项最近的针对胆道闭锁婴儿小型研究（n=15，平均年龄 4~20 个月）证实了这些发现，其显示这部分患者存在严重的发育迟缓特别是非常小的患者[23]。在这项研究中，Mullen 测试的所有尺度均低于正常，伴有粗大运动和语言表达能力中最弱的执行能力。肝功能，生长参数与年龄在 Kassai 手术中有一定的关系。值得注意的是，有接近一半的患者母语为西班牙语，测试过程中需要翻译者，所以语言结果的解释需要仔细点。

得克萨斯大学也进行了两项评估对比儿童肝移植受体与囊性纤维化控制组的神经心理发育状况的小型研究。这两项研究强调并进一步扩展了终末期肝病患者的移植前认知损害是不可逆的[24,25]。

从历史观点来说，极少有研究成功评估移植前后的认知功能状况。其中在最重要的一项关于胆道闭锁婴儿的纵向研究中，患者在等待移植过程中其心理和运动发展评分均位于较低的平均水平[26]。移植术后的检测显示这些评估分数在移植早期进一步降低，仅在移植术后 12 个月才恢复到术前水平。这个结果显示婴儿受体直到移植术后第 2 年才会出现认知的追赶。该研究同样提示长期住院的婴儿以及那些移植时有生长损害的婴儿会有显著的迟缓现象。

最新的评估肝移植受体认知功能的研究更强调了早期发现。IQ 几乎普遍下降至正常水平以下[15,27,28]。儿童肝移植患者 IQ 明显有一个下降趋势，其平均 IQ 为 85 分~90 分，以及 70 分以下发病率的增加（27% 相比于预计的 2%)[14,16,28,29]。值得注意的是,唯一一项针对儿童肝移植患者 IQ 的多中心研究和最大样本的研究(n=144,年龄 5~6 岁)发现,虽然 FSIQ、VIQ 以及 PIO 均显著低于正常(FSIQ=94.7±13.5;VIQ=95.0±13.8;PIQ=94.9±13.5)以及预期 2 倍的患者有轻到中度的 IQ 迟缓(71~85 分)[28],FSIQ 低于 70 分的比例仍是最小的(4%)。初步分析表明,后续这些患者在 2 年内智商并不能显著提高。

学习障碍和学校表现同样在肝移植受体中进行了评估。一项针对 3~9 岁移植受体的长期研究显示,根据学习障碍的定义约不到 20%的患者 IQ 低于 70 分,26%的患者在 IQ 和学术成就上有差别[30]。在那个研究中许多 IQ 低和学习障碍儿童的学习状况并未得到评估。一项儿童肝移植(SPLIT)网络针对学习调查显示 40%的患者需要一些特殊类型的教育支持,8%有学习障碍以及 5%的儿童 IQ 低于 70[31]。失学的时间也可能是缺失的学校功能所致。SPLIT 的数据显示,30%~40%的患者在长期随访中每年的未上学时间超过 10 天,其中青少年的缺课率最高[31]。

心脏及肺移植受体

针对有发绀的心脏病儿童的研究显示,慢性发绀与进行性的认知损害相关,越早期的发绀纠正可以获得越好的认知结果[32-34]。其他因素包括循环骤停,心肺转流以及栓塞事件也会导致认知发展低于预期[32-38]。心脏移植儿童主要是婴儿的认知发展状况,在 Chinnock 等的研究中进行了详细的综述[39]。一般来说,那些描述心脏移植儿童发展状况的报道提示,相较于那些手术纠正的先天性心脏病患者,这些移植患者中的大多数智力位于正常水平的下缘。然而,有显著的一部分(可能高达 40%)患者,其智力分数在正常的低缘(FSIQ<85),高达 10%可能有严重的神经损伤,其多有频繁的缺血性时间并被排除测试。Freier 等在 2004 年报道了利用 Bayley 评分评估了 39 名小婴儿(移植时平均年龄 53 天)的纵向神经发展状况的研究[40]。这些患者在移植术后 4~6 周及其后 6~12 个月接受了测试,其平均智力发育指数在正常范围内,平均精神运动发育指数则有轻度的延迟。Wray 等在 2006 年一项研究中评估了 34 名年龄为 1.3~15.3 岁的心肺移植患者[41],认知功能和学习成就在移植术后 1 年和 3 年进行了评估,除了较小的儿童的算术有下降外,其他人的智力和学习成就平均分数均在正常范围内,并在测试期间保持稳定。一些研究评估了低认知结果的危险因素,发现循环骤停、出生时的头围、长时间住院、心肺转流、栓塞事件、等待移植时间和移植前诊断都是影响这些患者认知发展变化的潜在因素[35-39,41]。评估初步诊断影响的研究显示,因心肌病接受心脏移植的患者评分要高于有发绀病史的先天性心脏病患者。一份最新的包含 18 名年龄为 6~16.5 岁患者的研究显示,平均 FSIQ,言语 IQ(VIQ)及执行智商(PIQ)均显著低于精神发育迟滞 26%的范围标准(<70 分)[42]。如果患者按照神经损伤病史进行分组(比如移植前神经影像学提示),显然这种高风险组导致了平均的差异,而其他患者均在正常范围内。在该研究中发现,脑部影像学异常与移植前心脏手术次数及先天性心脏病相关。

另外一项关于平均年龄 2.5 岁(14 个月~10 岁)的 21 名心脏移植受体的研究发现,这些患者不仅是全面的智力较低,还包括语言表达(P=0.01,46% 的人低于正常 1SD 以上)、适应能力(P<0.005)、视觉运动(P=0.01),和精细运动技能(P<0.005)。作者认为,适应性行为的某些方面会受到语言表达能力延迟及运动合作等的影响[43]。

尽管这些评估患者智力的研究结果较为积极,心脏移植受体的学校表现往往较正常差,且行为问题随着移植术后的时间逐渐增加[44]。Ikle 等利用 Vineland 评分研究了因左心室发育不全接受心脏移植的 26 名受者。其结果发现其中许多日常生活技能评分低于平均水平超过 1SD(39%)、社会化(29%)、交流技能(48%)以及总体适应性行为(52%)[45]。这些发现认为,针对改善这些技能领域的治疗介入能改善包括学校状况等在内的功能预后。

肺移植受体的研究并没有如心脏移植受体这么广泛。一项针对 18 名婴儿和 11 名幼童的研究显示,40%~50%的婴儿和 20%~30%的幼童有严重的发育迟缓。值得注意的是,有 2 名存在严重发育迟缓的儿童伴有听力障碍。这些患者的测试多在其移植术后的相对早期,超过 50%在移植术后一年内[46]。

如上所述,Wray 等报道了智力及学习成就上的正常范围[41]。同样这些作者研究了一组连续登记 99 名 3~17 岁的心、肺或心肺/移植的患者,比较不同诊断组之间的认知延迟状况。这项研究包括 56 名先天性心脏病患者 (CHD,34%登记为心/肺),10 名心肌病(CM),15

名囊性纤维化(CF,100%等待肺移植)和9名原发性肺高压(PPH,100%等待肺移植)。这组患者智力和学习成就的各个方面平均分数均显著低于正常水平。10%的患者 (8名先天性心脏病,1名心肌病)IQ低于70分,所有组中23%的患者的学习成就低于正常2个标准差。低成就或学习障碍定义为IQ低于一个标准差的学习成就标准化分数,其出现在23%的患者中(22%为数学,14%为阅读)。一般来说,心肌病和原发性肺高压患者的表现较先天性心脏病和囊性纤维化患者好。双变量研究显示诊断,出生后的累积住院时间和评估IQ时的年龄之间存在关系。然而,在多因素分析中,仅有住院时间能解释在IQ和学习成就上的显著比例差异(13%)。这些发现进一步强调了慢性疾病持续时间对于将接受移植治疗儿童的认知的影响。这效应可能无法在成功的器官移植术后完全恢复。

肠移植受体

据报道,肠移植受体有更高比例的认知迟缓[47-49],同时患者在移植术后的第1个2个月内有更差的发展延迟,这与肝移植受体的报道结果相似。在肠衰竭的儿童患者中,研究最多的是伴有坏死性小肠结肠炎(NEC)的早产儿。一些研究发现,NEC患者的神经发育损害(NDI)较其他儿童发病率更高,即使各组之间有相似的妊娠时间和出生体重。更严重的NEC患者(Bell3期)以及需要手术的NEC患者发现,其发生NDI的风险较无NEC或NEC可通过药物控制的患者高。然而,这种联系是否能反映疾病的严重程度或影响手术和并发症的因素并不清楚(比如促炎症细胞因子、稳定的血压改变、更严重的营养不良和更多的败血症发病)。多脏器移植受体的婴儿的发育也较单肝脏移植受体晚。这些患者往往比接受肝、心或肾移植的患者恢复得更慢,并有更多的额外手术过程。一些患者有肠造口,其需要后续手术来关闭。当移植的肠适应新环境时,许多患者需要后续的肠外营养支持。因此,相对于其他的实体器官移植受体,肠移植患者有相对高的慢性病影响,这可能是由于其发育复原的更慢。终末期肝病患者婴儿的主要危险因素包括慢性营养不良以及长期住院和早产。

认知功能概要

目前评估实体器官移植儿童受体神经发展结果的文献越来越多。利用不同的评分来评估可以获得的以小样本配对的不同年龄组认知的需求来得到可理解的结论较为困难。考虑到发绀型先天性心脏病更早期的研究,相较于预期,接受心脏移植的儿童受体可能有更好的认知结果。肝和肾移植受体的认知结果也获得了改善,但是许多仍然要求特殊的教育支持。要求行肠移植或肝肠联合移植的婴儿认知延迟的风险可能最高,但是仍缺少可证实这些迟缓无法恢复的纵向研究。在所有病例中神经合并症会增加延缓的风险。尽管有最新的进展,仍有较多的部分肝和心脏受体患者有严重的发育迟缓和(或)神经损伤。发育迟缓的危险因素仍在检测中,但是限制无支持脏器功能衰竭时间的策略和慢性营养不良,特别是在婴儿期间被认为有明显的影响。

实体器官移植受体显示了广泛的发育结果状况,包括正常结果以及那些有显著延迟的患者,见表119.1。导致这些延迟的准确机制仍未被完全阐明,例如长期住院、移植前慢性营养不良,以及手术并发症病史等因素都有影响,见图119.1。初级保健医生在帮助早期的发育迟缓诊断和促进合适的评估以及社区的治疗介入有重要作用。早期介入身体及职业上的治疗能减轻身体残疾。对认知发育迟缓和学校功能异常的最佳认识可以在教育开始早期帮助固定特殊的教育资源。再次,设定家庭和学校系统关于认知结果的期望值是他们预期健康保健的一个重要方面。

功能结果

那些通过器官移植存活的儿童在恢复期间需要面对许多的障碍,甚至当移植的过程完全恢复时,相较于那些健康同龄人,他们的健康状况常常类似于那些患有慢性疾病的儿童。这些患者往往需要与包括身体和发育缺陷在内的合并症斗争。当这些儿童时期接受移植的患者长大成年并努力独立生活,在社会中寻找自身位置时,这些缺陷会显得越发明显。

评估功能结果包括健康相关生活质量(HRQOL)的评估和日常生活技能的特殊评估。指导患者测试物理技能和认知状况也可并入功能结果评估。很少有实体器官儿童受体有明显的身体残疾,除非其有终末期的移植物衰竭或移植期间有严重的神经损伤。但如上所述,许多患者有明显的认知损伤。指导患者测试,比

表 119.1　实体器官移植儿童患者的智力测试

参考文献	样本数	年龄	智力(IQ)	较低或临界 IQ
肾				
Qvist 等[76]	33	7~12 岁	平均 言语 IQ 87.5±13.4 非言语 IQ 87.5±14.9	9% IQ<70 42% 70≤IQ<90
Falger 等[5]	27	6~17 岁	中位数(范围) 全量表智商(FSIQ)97(49~133) 言语 IQ 104(50~146)	4% IQ<70 19% 70≤IQ<85
肝				
Adeback 等[14]	21	4~16 岁	平均 总体 IQ 86.6 言语 IQ 90.6 非言语 IQ 84.5	15% FSIQ<70 35% 70≤FSIQ<85
Sorensen 等[28]	134	5~7 岁	平均 FSIQ 94.7±13.5 言语 IQ 95.0±13.8 执行 IQ 94.9±13.5	4% FSIQ≤70 26% 70≤FSIQ≤85
心/肺				
Wray 等[41]	22 心和心-肺	平均年龄 7.88±5.1 岁	平均 总体 IQ 103.7±13.3(移植术后 12 个月) 总体 IQ 100.2±12.9(移植术后 3 年)	100% IQ≥85
Haavisto 等[42]	18 心和心-肺	6~16 岁	平均 FSIQ 85.6±18.8 言语 IQ 89.8±22.7 执行 IQ 82.2±18.9	26% IQ<70 16% 70≤IQ<85
Uzark 等[43]	21 心	1~10 岁	平均 总体 IQ 86.7 言语 IQ 88.4 非言语 IQ 87.5	43% 总体 IQ<85

所有测试标准化为 100 分，标准差为 15 分。正常人群预期 14%，70<IQ≤85，4% IQ<70。

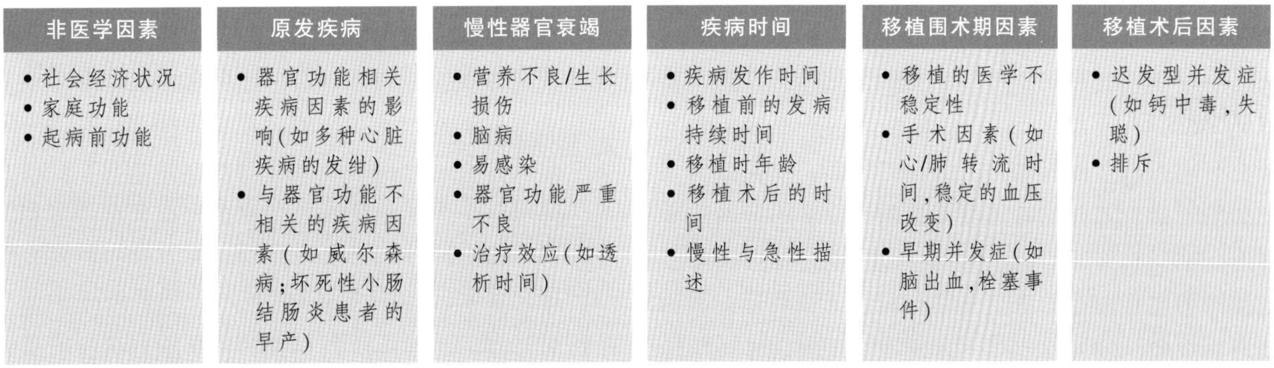

图 119.1　影响实体器官移植受体认知功能的因素。

如神经认知测试或运动/力量测试,可以让调查者获得有关患者生理和心理HRQOL的功能技能的特殊信息。这些信息对于指定合适的恢复计划和评估患者是否符合合适的年龄预期是不可或缺的。移植术后的恢复应主要关注于身体和认知功能,且不间断的结果评估应对这两者的改变敏感。对于这个范围内的损害的理解在儿童期随后的教育预期指导和其成年后的工作定位中非常关键。

与QOL相关的健康定义为一个个体对于其自身疾病主观的经历和疾病及其治疗对于个体功能的影响。移植多可改善身体健康状况。然而,药物治疗、住院、临床随访和侵入步骤的影响,以及移植物生存的不确定和长期健康状况都可能影响个体的HRQOL。QOL相关健康状况可通过一般和疾病特殊的角度来评估。其同样可通过父母或儿童的角度来评估,工具必须敏感,同时有与年龄适应的版本。对于HRQOL的评估有助于患者结果的评估,为儿童和家庭对于实体器官移植经历和治疗提供了更全面的理解。

一般HRQOL的调查包括普通问题如:“你在举重物时有困难吗?”或者“你的孩子有低能量状况吗?”这些问题与任何儿童都相关,无论其健康状况。从这个一般角度评估HRQOL会让我们比较移植受体跟健康儿童及那些慢性病儿童的状况。但是,这些问题可能无法触及一些移植受体儿童的真实状况,因为其许多问题是独特的。疾病特殊HRQOL评估可以帮助我们理解这些健康状况随着时间微妙的改变,并且对于治疗和移植物功能的变化更为敏感。大多数针对实体器官移植HRQOL的研究只利用一般工具,但是现在随着新的疾病特殊工具是可以获得的[50],疾病相关的特异HRQOL数据正在完善。

为评估幼儿的HRQOL必须以委托人的方式来报告儿童的状况。然而,年龄稍大的儿童(5岁或以上),或许有能力自行准确地评估自身的状态。在青春期父母和孩子报告之间的相关性是合理的,除了那些主要为内在症状相关的区域,比如疼痛或焦虑。父母对于学校功能和同伴关系的报告多具有良好的相关性,因为这些患者较大可能会与其家庭频繁地讨论相关问题。来自父母和儿童角度的评估是相互补充的,同时包括两个报告可对儿童的结果有一个更完全的评估。同样的,一般和特殊的疾病评估提供了互相补充的信息,并且两个同时可以获得更佳的效果。

我们将简短地回顾所有实体器官移植组的功能结果评估状况,但是需要注意,这些受体经历是非常相似的。集中组讨论和对于受体及其父母的个体采访能一致地认同相关药物和治疗是非常重要的[51,52]。如同经过年龄分组和同时来自儿童和父母的角度,疾病特殊HRQOL的评估可区分治疗焦虑、反复的疼痛和不适,以及对药物副作用的担心[50]。免疫抑制剂管理策略逐步进化减少了药物相关的身体副作用,比如肥胖和矮小。HRQOL的这些方面对如何随着治疗不同而改变的评估已经进行了管理。同样的,对低HRQOL的预测分析已经进行了限制,且其无法持续地确定干预目标。然而,人口统计可变量(比如社会经济状态等)也是关键决定因素。

肾移植受体

一般来说,儿童肾移植对于生理和心理HRQOL是有利的,并远远好于那些仍持续行透析治疗的患者。从中等效应量来看,相比于持续血液透析或腹膜透析的患者儿童肾移植患者有更高的HRQOL[53-56]。然而,一些研究比较了肾移植受体和健康对照显示患者的HRQOL更低[53,56-58]。患者被其身体的形象和身体的症状、与同伴和家庭交流的困难,学校的破坏显著困扰[59]。初级看护者报告了由于儿童健康导致的情感状态和家庭活动限制的不利影响[558,59]。由于父母倾向报告更低的生理和心理功能,儿童和父母的HRQOL报告存在显著的不一致部分[53,58]。虽然大多数成年的儿童肾移植受者对于其QOL感到满意,并报道了成功的私人关系,但高达83%的患者伴有焦虑、绝望或两者均有[13]。与一般人相比,他们有更大的失业概率,更小的独立生活可能[11-13]。最终成人身高和功能结果之间的关系很有意思,包括教育水平、参与的活动、婚姻生活和独立生活[11]。

肝移植受体

通过肝移植存活的儿童受到多种潜在的影响短期和长期HRQOL的生理和心理的损害。最初研究报道的肝移植术后儿童的HRQOL显示存活者有很少的身体限制,一般QOL良好[62-64]。然而,在随后使用经过验证的工具的研究中显示儿童肝移植受体的HRQOL水平显著低于健康儿童,更多的与儿童慢性疾病患者群持平[65-67]。儿童肝移植前后HRQOL改变的较少研究中的其中一个,Cple等对在移植术后第一个6个月内变化最大、所有功能得到显著改善的 5 岁以下儿童进行了纵向评估。一项多中心研究检查了 102 名儿童移植术后 2 年的时间点，将其分为 2 组：年幼组小于 5 岁（n=7）和年长组大于 5 岁（n=35）[65]。结果根据年龄区分，根据父母报告显示年长儿童的 HRQOL 显著低于正常组和 2~5 岁的年幼组。这些年幼患者的生理和心理 HRQOL 与平行对照组的结果相似。分量表的单因素分析确定人口统计学，但是在所有年龄组中临床变量并不是显著的 HRQOL 预测因素。

SPLIT 功能结果组（FOG）最近有一项包括 2~18 岁的 873 名儿童（363 名自我报告）肝移植受体平均从移植到调查随访 3.1 年的一般 HRQOL 的大型横向分析研究[69]。其结果与根据年龄、性别、种族和（或）人种划分随机配对的健康儿童进行了比较。肝移植受体的生理和心理功能相较于其他慢性儿童疾病更为良好，见图 119.2，但是并不同于健康组。效应量在小（情感功能）到中等（学习功能）范围内，PelsQL™4.0 一般核心量表的总量表分数和分量表均显著低于健康儿童。考虑到评估学校功能的调查问题，那些与失学相关的问题在这个领域内对分数有最大的影响。

人口统计学及医学变量可预测人群 HRQOL 的水平[67,68]。研究分析了 SPILT/FOG 的横向数据来检查年龄对于父母的 HRQOL 报告测试的影响，其结果显示年龄确实对于 HRQOL 有重要的影响，更年幼的儿童有最高的分数，更年轻的青少年有最低的分数。事实上，年龄对于测试的影响似乎比移植的介入治疗更有意义。评估多因素对于 SPILT/FOG 中患者 HRQOL 影响的多因素分析最初结果显示单亲家庭、移植术后最初住院时间、较大的年龄、癫痫病史，移植时 Z 评分更低和最近随访的住院天数均为消极预测因素。

患者的 HRQOL 与家庭动态之间的关系需要进一步的考虑。包含了评估儿童健康状况对父母影响的研究显示其对父母情感状况和家庭生活有许多的负面影响[14,58,65]。然而，当家庭功能在移植术后 2 年正式测定时，其家庭功能与那些报道的参考人群相当[65]。这些初步结果显示支持父母处理儿童健康状态的服务将改善儿童的 HRQOL。由于患者 HRQOL 水平与依赖行为相关并很可能长期维持移植物功能，因此该策略尤为重

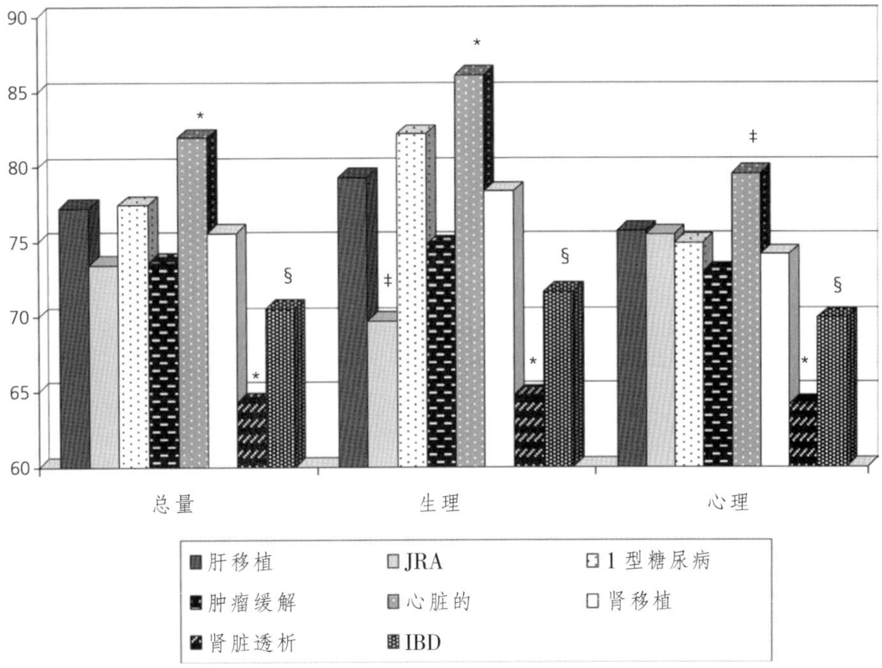

* $P \leqslant 0.001$
‡ $P \leqslant 0.01$
§ $P \leqslant 0.05$

图 119.2　父母、委托人报道的肝移植受体组和慢性疾病组 PedsQL 评分。Reproduced from Limbers et al. Health-related quality of life in pediatric liver transplant recipients compared with other chronic disease groups. Pediatric Transplant. 2011;15(3):245－253, with permission from Wiley.

要[70]。

心脏和肺移植受体

虽然根据报道大部分患者在移植术后调整良好，但HRQOL并没有系统性的进行研究。一项包含了儿童时接受心脏移植的23名成年患者的研究显示利用SF-36(质量标准)测定的生理和精神健康分数与普通的美国人群相似[71]。其中70%患者与父母或家庭成员一起居住，拥有私人医疗保险并完成了高中学习。在肺移植受体中，其表现为很大一部分患者出现了家中的行为问题及与其同伴的社会能力减少，其中大部分为男性患者。报道的抑郁症发病率为1年后的23%和3年后的13%[41,72]。

肠移植受体

肠移植术后的QOL评估受到小样本量和喂养及持续胃肠道症状等问题的限制。肠外营养支持患者的QOL评分随着时间逐渐退化，特别是肝脏疾病等并发症。相反的，有报道显示，肠移植术后患者的QOL随时间逐渐改善[73]。经过最初的术后阶段，肠外营养依赖患者和肠移植患者的QOL分数大致相似。在纵向的随访中，肠移植患者在焦虑、睡眠、冲动和控制方面获得了显著的改善，这反映了移植术后进行性的调整适应[73]。肠移植受体父母报告了疾病对其孩子在生理和心理健康上的明显限制，而患者本身认为相对于其他正常的儿童，其对大多数领域的影响均较小[74]。这些作者总结认为，尽管这些儿童与其同伴之间有区别，但并不认为这些不同会影响他们的功能。

功能结果概要

接受实体器官移植儿童的HRQOL和功能结果多低于正常人群，其与那些慢性疾病的儿童最具可比性。儿童实体器官移植受体的父母经历了孩子疾病相关的压力，其报告的功能结果较儿童自身报告的结果要差。测试时的年龄会影响HRQOL的结果，年幼儿童的父母报告的功能结果更为良好。看来人口统计学因素对于HRQOL有显著的影响，对实体器官移植受体家庭看护和教育提供支持的介入可改善这些儿童的结果。

QOL相关健康是对患者感觉如何、他们怎么看待自身与其他人的关系和其在所处环境中的功能问题的全面评估。尽管实体器官移植的长期状况和移植物生存较好，仍有许多受体在与减退的HRQOL、次佳或不完全的恢复斗争。关于这些儿童器官移植受体的长期HRQOL数据仍缺乏，最好有进一步多医疗中心的研究。初级保健提供者通过他们与家庭及其他兄弟姐妹的良好关系在恢复的一些需求或社会支持上提供帮助。通过促进社区的评价和试验监测，初级保健提供者可帮助减少学校的缺课和家庭活动的缺席。初级保健提供者也可帮助家庭使其在那些其他慢性疾病的儿童家长范围内，并分享那些改善其他更常见疾病儿童功能结果的干预策略，比如哮喘或糖尿病。

长期随访的概要和影响

当我们回顾实体器官移植受体发育结果的各个方面，一些常见的问题出现了。虽然许多受体有完全的认知功能并在学校表现良好，仍有不成比例的患者存在低于平均智力、学习困难和在课堂上预期的问题。如精细运动技能和高频听力损伤等微妙生理损害会导致这些患者很难跟上其同伴。随着学习任务越来越复杂及儿童成长进入青春期，处理区分这些相关的压力显著增加了。慢性疾病的持续时间和严重程度，无论是透析、门静脉高压或先天性心衰竭均明显影响结果。社会经济和环境因素同样也有影响，那些限制家庭确保其孩子特殊资源的能力可混合医学危险因素的影响。对于大多数移植家庭，他们与医疗系统联系最多的多是经过他们的移植团队。然而，尽管引入专业的移植社会服务，移植团队可能也不会经常在移植术后随访期间引出认知迟缓或学习任务的病史。移植医生和初级保健提供者需在随访期间特别关注医学病史的这些方面。

由于发育测试昂贵并需要许多人力，因此很难对所有的受体进行。然而，通过系统的筛查项目进入常规移植术后保健，患者将受益于确定损害的更严格测试。一些筛选方法的建议和合适推荐可见表119.2。如果找到问题，已推荐来自合适医生更全面的评价。

关于生理和社会发育里程碑的问题和语言获得应常规包含4岁以下儿童的随访评估。年龄更大的儿童(5岁或以上)，应根据学习的困难和缺课频率来评估。对于肝移植受体（5~7岁），“PedsQL 4.0 认知功能量表”调查问卷与执行功能有更广泛的相关性，并能在诊

表 119.2　每年根据年龄评估发育迟缓的筛查方法的建议

年龄	功能领域	筛查方法 工具	管理模式	推荐 ***
1~5 岁	适应性行为：社会化，运动，交流，日常生活技能	适应性行为评估系统，第二版(ABAS-Ⅱ)[77]* 或 Vineland 适应性行为量表，第二版(Vineland-Ⅱ)[78]*	父母完成调查(15~20 分钟)	发育评估(心理学家)
	发育的里程碑：社会，运动，语言	Denver-Ⅱ[79]	诊所内筛查(10~20 分钟)	发育评估(心理学家)
	语言	学前语言量表，第五版(PLS-5) 家庭沟通问卷[80]	父母完成调查(10~20 分钟)	发育评估(心理学家)和说话和(或)语言评估
	听力	听力筛查 **		全面的听力评估
6~13 岁	一般生理和心理功能	PedsQL-4.0 一般核心量表[81]*	父母和孩子完成调查(5~10 分钟)	心理诊断评估(儿科医学心理学家)
	执行功能	PedsQL-CF 量表[75]*	父母和孩子完成调查(5 分钟)	神经心理评估(神经心理学家)
		执行功能的行为评定量表(BRIEF)[82]	父母和老师完成调查；儿童完成调查(11 岁以上)(10~15 分钟)	
	注意力	ADHD 评定量表Ⅳ[83]*	父母和老师完成调查(10~15 分钟)	
	学校表现	医学临床医生和(或)社会服务支持团队应该评估学校的问题如下 父母有无报告学习延误 孩子是否有接受特殊教育服务，如个性化的教育计划(IEP)或 504 计划 孩子的成绩低于平均水平，高度变量或较以前变差 相较于同龄人做作业是否需要更多的努力，帮助或时间 孩子对学业感到过度沮丧吗?孩子逃避和(或)抵制作业和(或)对上学感到痛苦吗 由于疾病或医疗访问有多少天未去学校		
	听力	1~5 岁及以上		
14~18 岁	一般生理和心理功能 执行功能 注意力 学校表现	6~13 岁及以上		
	过渡计划	医学临床医生和(或)社会服务支持团队应该在认知功能和学校表现历史范围内讨论先进教育或就业上的计划。认知功能，尤其是智力和执行功能在发展计划中应考虑为自身管理或医疗保健、自我保健	父母和(或)患者访谈(10~15 分钟)	自我医疗保健、自我管理保健的过渡计划：心理诊断评价(儿科医学心理学家)。继续教育或职业发展的过渡计划：学校

* 可通过英语和西班牙语获得。

** 移植术后至少推荐一次的听力筛查。如果问题是在筛选，可参考全面的听力学评估。除非临床怀疑和(或)之前的听力学测试显示有问题，否则没有进一步筛查的必要。

*** 全面的神经心理学、发育、言语和(或)语言，和心理诊断评估不需要每年进行。如果儿童已经完成了一项评估，请咨询相关专家有关后续随访的建议，如果最初的评估后新的担忧出现或担忧增加，请重新评估。

所里进行简单的管理[75]。如需要进行更为全面的执行功能评估,可以使用BRIEF。因为认知功能在个体化的治疗计划转换中非常关键,那些在小学阶段需要特殊教育支持的青少年会与许多需要自我管理的任务作斗争。儿童受体的最终目标就是使他们成长为健康和有生育能力的成人。那些帮助这些儿童规避认知缺陷的干预期望能改善成年时的功能状态。同样的,区分特殊问题(比如临界智力或减退的执行技能)能帮助患者和他们的家庭设置职业选择和长期功能结果的现实期望。

(奚斌 译 徐骁 校)

参考文献

1. Wechsler D. Wechsler Preschool and Primary Scale of Intelligence-Third Edition. San Antonio, TX: The Psychological Corporation; 2002.
2. Weschler D, editor. Weschler Intelligence Scale for Children-Fourth Edition. San Antonio, TX: The Psychological Corporation; 2003.
3. Association D-IAP. Diagnostic and Statistical Manual of Mental Disorders. 4th ed. (DSM-IVTM). Washington, DC: American Psychiatric Association; 1994.
4. Qvist E, Marttinen E, Ronnholm K, et al. Growth after renal transplantation in infancy or early childhood. Pediatric Nephrology (Berlin, Germany). 2002; 17(6):438-443.
5. Falger J, Latal B, Landolt MA, et al. Outcome after renal transplantation. Part I: intellectual and motor performance. Pediatric Nephrology. 2008;23(8): 1339-1345.
6. Icard P, Hooper SR, Gipson DS, et al. Cognitive improvement in children with CKD after transplant. Pediatric Transplantation. 2010;14(7):887-890.
7. Brouhard BH, Donaldson LA, Lawry KW, et al. Cognitive functioning in children on dialysis and post-transplantation. Pediatric Transplantation. 2000;4(4): 261-267.
8. Warady BA. Neurodevelopment of infants with end-stage renal disease: is it improving? Pediatric Transplantation. 2002;6(1):5-7.
9. Warady BA, Belden B, Kohaut E. Neurodevelopmental outcome of children initiating peritoneal dialysis in early infancy. Pediatric Nephrology (Berlin, Germany). 1999;13(9):759-765.
10. Motoyama O, Kawamura T, Aikawa A, et al. Head circumference and development in young children after renal transplantation. Pediatrics International. 2009; 51(1):71-74.
11. Broyer M, Le Bihan C, Charbit M, et al. Long-term social outcome of children after kidney transplantation. Transplantation. 2004;77(7):1033-1037.
12. Groothoff JW, Cransberg K, Offringa M, et al. Long-term follow-up of renal transplantation in children: a Dutch cohort study. Transplantation. 2004;78(3): 453-460.
13. Karrfelt HME, Berg UB. Long-term psychosocial outcome after renal transplantation during childhood. Pediatric Transplantation. 2008;12(5):557-562.
14. Adeback P, Nemeth A, Fischler B. Cognitive and emotional outcome after pediatric liver transplantation. Pediatr Transplantation. 2003;7:385-389.
15. Kaller T, Schulz K, Sander K, et al. Cognitive abilities in children after liver transplantation. Transplantation. 2005;79:1252-1256.
16. Krull K, Fuchs C, Yurk H, et al. Neurocognitive outcome in pediatric liver transplant recipients. Pediatric Transplantation. 2003;7(2):111-118.
17. Stewart S, Campbell R, McCallon D, et al. Cognitive patterns in school-age children with end-stage liver disease. Journal of Developmental and Behavioral Pediatrics. 1992;13:331-338.
18. Stewart S, Kennard B, Waller D, et al. Cognitive function in children who receive organ transplantation. Health Psychology. 1994;13:3-13.
19. Bronster DJ, Emre S, Boccagni P, et al. Central nervous system complications in liver transplant recipients-incidence, timing, and long-term follow-up. Clinical Transplantation. 2000;14(1):1-7.
20. Guarino M, Stracciari A, Pazzaglia P, et al. Neurological complications of liver transplantation. Journal of Neurology. 1996;243(2):137-142.
21. Wijdicks EF, Plevak DJ, Wiesner RH, et al. Causes and outcome of seizures in liver transplant recipients. Neurology. 1996;47(6):1523-1525.
22. Stewart S, Uauy R, Waller D, et al. Mental and motor development correlates in patients with end-stage biliary atresia awaiting liver transplantation. Pediatrics. 1987;79:882-888.
23. Caudle SE, Katzenstein JM, Karpen SJ, et al. Language and motor skills are impaired in infants with biliary atresia before transplantation. Journal of Pediatrics. 2010;156(6):936-940.
24. Stewart SM, Hiltebeitel C, Nici J, et al. Neuropsychological outcome of pediatric liver transplantation. Pediatrics. 1991;87(3):367-376.
25. Stewart SM, Silver CH, Nici J, et al. Neuropsychological function in young children who have undergone liver transplantation. Journal of Pediatric Psychology. 1991;16(5):569-583.
26. Wayman K, Cox K, Esquivel C. Neurodevelopmental outcome of young children with extrahepatic biliary atresia 1 year after liver transplantation. Journal of Pediatrics. 1997;131:894-898.
27. Kaller T, Boeck A, Sander K, et al. Cognitive abilities, behaviour and quality of life in children after liver transplantation. Pediatric Transplantation. 2010;14(4): 496-503.
28. Sorensen L, Neighbors K, Martz K, et al. Cognitive and academic outcomes after pediatric liver transplatation: functional outcomes group (FOG) results. American Journal of Transplantation. 2011;11:303-311.
29. Gilmour S, Adkins R, Liddell GA, et al. Assessment of psychoeducational outcomes after pediatric liver transplant. American Journal of Transplantation. 2009;9(2):294-300.
30. Kennard B, Stewart S, Phelan-McAuliffe D, et al. Academic outcome in long-term survivors of pediatric liver transplantation. Journal of Developmental and Behavioral Pediatrics. 1999;20:17-23.
31. Gilmour S, Sorenson L, Anand R, et al. School outcomes in children registered in the studies of pediatric liver transplantation (SPLIT) consortium. Liver Transplantation. 2010;16(9):1041-1048.
32. Newburger JW, Silbert AR, Buckley LP, et al. Cognitive function and age at repair of transposition of the great arteries in children. New England Journal of Medicine. 1984;310(23):1495-1499.
33. O'Dougherty M, Wright FS, Loewenson RB, et al. Cerebral dysfunction after chronic hypoxia in children. Neurology. 1985;35(1):42-46.
34. Wright M, Nolan T. Impact of cyanotic heart disease on school performance. Archives of Disease in Childhood. 1994;71(1):64-70.
35. Bellinger DC, Jonas RA, Rappaport LA, et al. Developmental and neurologic status of children after heart surgery with hypothermic circulatory arrest or low-flow cardiopulmonary bypass. New England Journal of Medicine. 1995;332(9): 549-555.
36. Bellinger DC, Wypij D, Kuban KC, et al. Developmental and neurological status of children at 4 years of age after heart surgery with hypothermic circulatory arrest or low-flow cardiopulmonary bypass. Circulation. 1999;100(5):526-532.
37. Miller G, Mamourian AC, Tesman JR, et al. Long-term MRI changes in brain after pediatric open heart surgery. Journal of Child Neurology. 1994;9(4): 390-397.
38. Miller G, Tesman JR, Ramer JC, et al. Outcome after open-heart surgery in infants and children. Journal of Child Neurology. 1996;11(1):49-53.
39. Chinnock RE, Freier MC, Ashwal S, et al. Developmental outcomes after pediatric heart transplantation. Journal of Heart and Lung Transplantation. 2008; 27(10):1079-1084.
40. Freier MC, Babikian T, Pivonka J, et al. A longitudinal perspective on neurodevelopmental outcome after infant cardiac transplantation. Journal of Heart and Lung Transplantation. 2004;23(7):857-864.
41. Wray J, Radley-Smith R. Longitudinal assessment of psychological functioning in children after heart or heart-lung transplantation. Journal of Heart and Lung Transplantation. 2006;25(3):345-352.
42. Haavisto A, Korkman M, Jalanko H, et al. Neurocognitive function of pediatric heart transplant recipients. Journal of Heart and Lung Transplantation. [Research Support, Non-U.S. Gov't]. 2010;29(7):764-770.
43. Uzark K, Spicer R, Beebe DW. Neurodevelopmental outcomes in pediatric heart transplant recipients. Journal of Heart and Lung Transplantation. [Comparative Study]. 2009;28(12):1306-1311.
44. Nixon PA, Morris KA. Quality of life in pediatric heart, heart-lung, and lung transplant recipients. International Journal of Sports Medicine. 2000;21(Suppl 2):S109-S111, discussion S12.
45. Ikle L, Hale K, Fashaw L, et al. Developmental outcome of patients with hypoplastic left heart syndrome treated with heart transplantation. Journal of Pediatrics. 2003;142(1):20-25.
46. Elizur A, Faro A, Huddleston CB, et al. Lung transplantation in infants and toddlers from 1990 to 2004 at St. Louis Children's Hospital. American Journal of Transplantation. 2009;9(4):719-726.
47. Thevenin DM, Baker A, Kato T, et al. Neurodevelopmental outcomes of infant multivisceral transplant recipients: a longitudinal study. Transplantation Proceedings. 2006;38(6):1694-1695.

48. Thevenin DM, Baker A, Kato T, et al. Neuodevelopmental outcomes for children transplanted under the age of 3 years. Transplantation Proceedings. 2006;38(6): 1692–1693.
49. Thevenin DM, Mittal N, Kato T, et al. Neurodevelopmental outcomes of infant intestinal transplant recipients. Transplantation Proceedings. 2004;36(2):319–320.
50. Weissberg-Benchell J, Zielinski T, Rodgers S, et al. Health-related quality of life: feasibility, reliability and validity of the PedsQL™ transplant module. American Journal of Transplantation. 2010;10:1686–1694.
51. Anthony SJ, Hebert D, Todd L, et al. Child and parental perspectives of multidimensional quality of life outcomes after kidney transplantation. Pediatric Transplantation. 2010;14(2):249–256.
52. Nicholas DB, Otley AR, Taylor R, et al. Experiences and barriers to health-related quality of life following liver transplantation: a qualitative analysis of the perspectives of pediatric patients and their parents. Health and Quality of Life Outcomes. 2010;8:150.
53. Goldstein SL, Graham N, Burwinkle T, et al. Health-related quality of life in pediatric patients with ESRD. Pediatric Nephrology. 2006;21(6):846–850.
54. Goldstein SL, Graham N, Warady BA, et al. Measuring health-related quality of life in children with ESRD: performance of the generic and ESRD-specific instrument of the pediatric quality of life inventory (PedsQL). American Journal of Kidney Diseases. 2008;51(2):285–297.
55. Goldstein SL, Rosburg NM, Warady BA, et al. Pediatric end stage renal disease health-related quality of life differs by modality: a PedsQL ESRD analysis. Pediatric Nephrology. 2009;24(8):1553–1560.
56. Riano-Galan I, Malaga S, Rajmil L, et al. Quality of life of adolescents with end-stage renal disease and kidney transplant. Pediatric Nephrology. 2009;24(8): 1561–1568.
57. Qvist E, Narhi V, Apajasalo M, et al. Psychosocial adjustment and quality of life after renal transplantation in early childhood. Pediatric Transplantation. 2004;8(2):120–125.
58. Sundaram SS, Landgraf JM, Neighbors K, et al. Adolescent health-related quality of life following liver and kidney transplantation. American Journal of Transplantation. 2007;7(4):982–989.
59. Anthony SJ, Hebert D, Todd L, et al. Child and parental perspectives of multidimensional quality of life outcomes after kidney transplantation. Pediatric Transplantation. 2010;14(2):249–256.
60. Rees L. Long-term outcome after renal transplantation in childhood. Pediatric Nephrology (Berlin, Germany). 2009;24(3):475–484.
61. Rosenkranz J, Reichwald-Klugger E, Oh J, et al. Psychosocial rehabilitation and satisfaction with life in adults with childhood-onset of end-stage renal disease. Pediatric Nephrology (Berlin, Germany). 2005;20(9):1288–1294.
62. Asonuma K, Inomata Y, Uemoto S, et al. Growth and quality of life after living-related liver transplantation in children. Pediatric Transplantation. 1998;2(1):64–69.
63. Burdelski M, Nolkemper D, Ganschow R, et al. Liver transplantation in children: long-term outcome and quality of life. European Journal of Pediatrics. 1999;158(Suppl 2):S34–S42.
64. Sokal EM. Quality of life after orthotopic liver transplantation in children. An overview of physical, psychological and social outcome. European Journal of Pediatrics. 1995;154(3):171–175.
65. Alonso EM, Neighbors K, Barton FB, et al. Health-related quality of life and family function following pediatric liver transplantation. [see comment]. Liver Transplantation. 2008;14(4):460–468.
66. Alonso EM, Neighbors K, Mattson C, et al. Functional outcomes of pediatric liver transplantation. Journal of Pediatric Gastroenterology and Nutrition. 2003;37(2): 155–160.
67. Bucuvalas JC, Britto M, Krug S, et al. Health-related quality of life in pediatric liver transplant recipients: a single-center study. Liver Transplantation. 2003;9(1): 62–71.
68. Cole CR, Bucuvalas JC, Hornung RW, et al. Impact of liver transplantation on HRQOL in children less than 5 years old. Pediatric Transplantation. 2004;8(3): 222–227.
69. Alonso EM, Limbers C, Neighbors K, et al. Cross-sectional analysis of health-related quality of life in pediatric liver transplant recipients. Journal of Pediatrics. 2010;156:270–276.
70. Fredericks EM, Magee JC, Opipari-Arrigan L, et al. Adherence and health-related quality of life in adolescent liver transplant recipients. Pediatric Transplantation. 2008;12(3):289–299.
71. Petroski RA, Grady KL, Rodgers S, et al. Quality of life in adult survivors greater than 10 years after pediatric heart transplantation. Journal of Heart and Lung Transplantation. 2009;28(7):661–666.
72. Wray J, Radley-Smith R. Beyond the first year after pediatric heart or heart-lung transplantation: changes in cognitive function and behaviour. Pediatric Transplantation. 2005;9(2):170–177.
73. Rovera GM, DiMartini A, Schoen RE, et al. Quality of life of patients after intestinal transplantation. Transplantation. 1998;66(9):1141–1145.
74. Sudan D, Iyer K, Horslen S, et al. Assessment of quality of life after pediatric intestinal transplantation by parents and pediatric recipients using the child health questionnaire. Transplantation Proceedings. 2002;34(3):963–964.
75. Varni J, Limbers C, Sorensen L, et al. PedsQL™ cognitive functioning scale in pediatric liver transplant recipients: feasibility, reliability and validity. Quality of Life Research. 2011;20:913–921.
76. Qvist E, Pihko H, Fagerudd P, et al. Neurodevelopmental outcome in high-risk patients after renal transplantation in early childhood. Pediatric Transplantation. 2002;6(1):53–62.
77. Harrison P, Oakland T. Adaptive Behavior Assessment System (ABAS-II). 2th ed. San Antonio, TX: Psychcorp; 2003.
78. Sparrow S, Cicchetti D, Balla D. Vineland Adaptive Behavior Scales (Vineland II). 2th ed. San Antonio, TX: Psychcorp; 2005.
79. Frankenburg WK, Dodds J, Archer P, et al. The Denver II: a major revision and restandardization of the Denver Developmental Screening Test. Pediatrics. 1992;89(1):91–97.
80. Zimmerman I, Steiner V, Pond R. Preschool Language Scales (PLS-5). 5th ed. San Antonio, TX: Psychcorp; 2011.
81. Varni JW, Burwinkle TM, Seid M, et al. The PedsQL™ 4.0 as a pediatric population health measure: feasibility, reliability, and validity. Ambulatory Pediatrics. 2003;3:329–341.
82. Gioia G, Isquith P, Guy S, et al. Behavior Rating Inventory of Executive Function. Odessa, FL: Psychological Assessment Services, Inc.; 2000.
83. DuPaul G, Power T, Anastopoulos A, et al., editors. ADHD Rating Scale-IV. New York, NY: The Guilford Press; 1998.

第 120 章
不依从、心理适应及其在儿童移植中的影响

Robert Ettenger, Margaret L. Stuber

引言

世界卫生组织定义药物依从性为“一个人的行为在多大程度上[服药、推荐的饮食和(或)生活方式变化的执行]符合约定的医疗服务提供者的建议[1]”。正如这个定义所暗示的那样，有很多的建议慢性病移植患者预计遵守，包括出席医疗预约、执行血液测试、避免饮酒或使用非法药物。在这个章节中，我们专注于免疫抑制药物的不依从性，如果一个家庭或受体不遵守推荐保健计划的其他方面，这对受体的健康和幸福也有不利的影响。更明显的是不依从仍然是迟发性移植物失功和患者死亡的主要原因，因此其仍然是新知识获得和增强依从性干预的关键目标。

移植受体健康中药物不依从的责任

一项 Cochrane 回顾显示，“增强药物依从性的干预”得出结论，改善药物服用相对于任何谨慎的治疗改善对临床结果有更深远的影响[2]。由于目前确实没有实用、可重复的方法来确保没有免疫抑制药物进行的移植，药物治疗依从性是成功的实体器官移植的原因。事实上，在绝大多数的成年器官移植受体中，药物依从性已被证明是预防同种异体移植物排斥反应的关键[3,4]。

现代移植的成功在很大程度上是得益于更有潜力的抑制排斥的免疫抑制剂。然而，这些免疫抑制剂的进步也付出了代价。目前所有可获得的维持药物均为口服的，需要一生持续维持同种异体移植物。对于维持生活的器官(比如心脏)，移植受体放弃服用药物，甚至即使是几天，就有发生急性排斥和移植物失功的风险，使得患者进入透析的困难生活[5-8]或死亡。

除了人力成本，药物不依从还有巨大的经济成本。据估计实体器官移植不依从导致的代价为每年 1500 万到 1 亿美元[9]。每年维持肾移植良好功能的花费中位数约为 8500 美元，失败移植的代价约为 51 000 美元[9]。此外，基于平均成本，它大约需要两年半的移植的成本来抵消避免透析的成本[10]。欧洲的相似分析也获得了本质上相同的结论[11]。更持久的移植功能是医疗保健系统的一项巨大经济收益。在这个时候关注医疗保健财务状况，药物依从性的改善可对医疗保健支持有巨大的影响。

发病率的忽视和不依从的影响

实体器官移植受体的药物不依从的发病率和影响经常被忽略。根据美国器官共享网络(UNOS)的数据显示，在儿童肝移植受体组中仅有 2%的不依从发生率[12]。然而，一项回顾性报道显示，35%的移植物失功是由于不依从所致[12]。还有缺少药物不依从认识的其他例子[9]，然而对依从性改善的重视仍然不够[13,14]。甚至儿童肾移植社区对药物依从性影响的接受已经晚了。儿童肾试验和协作研究(NAPRTCS)的 2010 年度报道中，几乎 50%的移植物衰竭是由于排斥。然而，由于患者未持续服药导致的移植物失功仅占移植物失功的 4.5%[15]。

独特的儿童影响

实体器官移植作为儿童和青少年终末期器官衰竭的治疗选择已被广泛接受。比如，肾移植在健康和认知功能上的收益远远超过了任何形式的透析[16,17]。美国肾数据系统(USRDS)数据显示肾移植受体存活时间远远长于透析的患者，这种效应在儿童患者中更加明显，预期生命时间为 20~30 年[18]。成功移植的获益包括生长

的改善和性发育[19,20]以及采用“健康”人的角色来代替慢性疾病个体的能力。在儿科，这种变化为谈判的机会和享受角色及成熟的责任[21-23]。

尽管有这些积极的结果，据估计药物不依从发生率在儿童肾移植受体中仍然很高，特别是青少年[24]。对于所有年龄大于 1 岁的儿童移植肾生存超过一年是极好的，那些青少年时接受移植或存活到青少年的患者，移植肾功能下降更大以及比年轻接受体同种异体移植物生存期少 3~5 年。在移植术后 5 年，那些在青少年时接受移植的患者在所有年龄段中的移植物失功发生率最高，包括所有成人组[17]。青少年移植受体移植物失功发生率增加的大部分原因是药物不依从。

不依从的定义

之前提到的 WHO 关于依从性的定义未能明确不按照规定服用药物带来的问题。对于部分患者来说，不依从不应仅仅视为一种任性的无视或粗心的行为。相反，不依从代表了医疗保健交付的限制。这可能是药物提供者和患者在最初对于处方未完全达成一致导致的结果，或者代表了缺乏识别和提供教育、情感、或患者需要的经济支持[25]。因此，微妙的药物依从性不仅强调患者的责任，而且要看护理人员的方法。

服从

要求患者遵循医学团队的决定且不需要研究这些决定的原因。这就是青少年移植受体发现自身的状况。

依从性

依从性描述了一个状况，患者理解医学团队的决定并参与遵循这些决定的执行。在儿童和青少年实体器官移植中，这往往能获得的最佳状况。

一致性

这是依从性理论上的目标。患者的欲望和动机和医学团队的是一致的。因此，结论就是患者想要做那些医学团队相信能使他(她)获益的事情。

器官移植中不依从的操作型定义

围绕实体器官移植受体药物依从或服从的问题往往很难让患者及其家庭领会。另一方面，这些问题对于医疗团队来说更加明显。Chapman 提供了以下的有用定义：“不依从是服用规定的同种异体抗排斥药物的失败，这会潜在地导致移植物组织学或功能损害[26]。”该定义有两个重要临床特点：①不依从一定是隐蔽的，在青少年不依从的大部分病例中，满足此条件。偶尔情况下，青少年公开表示不满来拒绝接受规定药物。通常，当患者不依从时儿童移植医生和医疗团队不能准确识别；②不依从应有一个对移植物临床结果的行为不符的可衡量效果[26]。

有一些问题使儿童移植不依从很难以文字来解释。Matas 和 Nevins[8]提出了相关问题：关于药物不服从(不依从)权威的、临床有用的定义是什么？多少服从是足够的？给药延迟呢[8]？真的存在阈值效应，超过这个标准移植物就会出现损伤？由于免疫反应、器官免疫原性、组织相容性匹配、药物代谢和无数的其他因素(许多是未明确的)的个体差异，有时候很难应用固定的定义。

打个比方，考虑到同行评审文章关于“药物不依从”的定量方面的多种定义，Greenstein 和 Siegal 定义不服从为漏过、忘记，改变或推迟服药每月至少 1 次(2%的给药预计每天 2 次)[27]。Nevins 等定义不服从为遗漏至少 10%的服药，也就是说每月 6 次[28]。Chisholm 等和 Blowey 等定义不服从为遗漏至少 20%的给药，或者每月 12 次[29,30]。服药过晚定义为不依从，合适时间的截止是什么时候[31]？为了识别这个难题，一项最新的共识会议定义器官移植的不依从为“相对于规定服药可足够导致严重影响治疗方案预期效果的任何偏差”[9]。毫无疑问，所有临床医生都努力争取 100%的服从。做不到这点，临床医生必须回到器官病理学作为不依从的真正标志和随后的免疫抑制导致急性或慢性排斥的操作性定义。

儿童移植患者免疫抑制剂不依从的发病率

根据最新的 meta 分析[32]，大约 50%关于儿童移植不依从的研究都是关于肾移植受体的。这些研究中 30%是关于儿童肝脏同种异体移植的，13%的报道是心脏移植受体。因此，肾移植的研究是至今最为频繁的。在所有移植类型中，免疫抑制剂不依从发生率为每年

100名患者中6名。免疫抑制药物不依从在不同的器官移植类型中的发生率无显著差异[32]。

很难比较成人和儿童之间免疫抑制药物不依从的发病率和(或)患病率,其中涉及各个研究之间的关于不依从的不同定义。所以,这导致了包括文献综述和所有研究的meta分析往往会得出不同的结论。例如,上面提到的,Dew等[32]发现儿童免疫抑制剂不依从发生率仅为100人中6例/年,在成人中,其发生率为100人中19~25例/年[33]。其他的meta分析也得出了不同的结论[24,34,35]。各个研究之间的发病率差别巨大,为5%~80%[36],反映了研究质量、方法、不依从定义及其他因素的多样性。在儿童肾移植中,16项研究关于免疫抑制剂不依从的加权平均发病率为30.7%[34]。同一作者的之前一项研究比较了不同实体器官移植类型之间的药物不依从加权发病率,该研究报道了儿童肾移植受体32%的加权平均发病率,肝移植受体为30.8%,心脏受体为15.9%[24]。

大量的研究认为青少年期是不依从的高发时期。Dobell等的系统分析认为儿童移植中青少年期是药物不依从的最令人担忧的阶段。其加权发病率在青少年和儿童中有明显差异,分别为43.2%和22.4%[24,32,34]。在其综述中青少年期定义为除了其他指定的原因外,年龄≥10岁。其他的分析也显示较年长的儿童移植受体(青少年)的药物不依从发生率更高[37]。在其他(如哮喘、HIV感染、类风湿性关节炎和糖尿病等)要求慢性药物治疗的状态中,报道也显示青少年的药物不依从发生率也很高[38,39]。

超过50%的儿童肾移植是在青少年期进行的,特别是当其低于10岁[15,40]。在大多数研究中,患者多数根据他们接受肾移植的年龄来区分[15]。因此,当患者在青少年期接受移植,无法预料在哪个特殊年龄会出现药物不依从导致的医学并发症。

目前已有新的数据阐述了该原理。Foster等[41]用更精确的年龄划分来评估那些经历移植物失功的青少年。利用USRDS数据库,在他们的分析中控制移植术后的时间,作者发现约在9岁开始,青少年患者的移植物失功发生率随着年龄增大而增加,直到19~20岁到达高峰。他们同样发现在小于12岁的儿童中,移植物失功发生率在移植术后晚期戏剧性的增加,即患者到青少年末期的时候。移植物失功发生的最高峰为17~24岁的患者。Foster等发现那些在年幼的时候接受移植的儿童,移植物失功发生的最高时间为移植术后13~17年,而那些在青少年期接受移植的患者在移植术后几年内的发生率更高。综合来看,这些数据有力显示,在此期间青少年本身即是移植物失功的特殊危险因素。由于儿童移植的移植物失功过程非常复杂,这些发现的潜在原因并不能简单的明确。Foster等发现的最明显的解释是药物不依从。其他免疫生物学过程,包括更年长儿童时期增强的同种异体反应与环境致病菌导致的感染,特别是病毒[42-45],也可能在移植物排斥和失功中扮演了重要角色。

儿童和青少年移植受体的心理和发育适应

移植受体术后药物不依从的问题随着年龄和发育状况而变化[32]。为了理解如何更好地促进依从性,移植团队必须不仅仅考虑移植受体的认知发育状况,还要考虑各年龄组的发育任务。

童年早期

一般来说,7岁以下儿童的不依从问题往往被认为是父母或社会因素所致,而较少考虑的是儿童的理解水平或合作问题[32]。3岁以下的儿童多生活在当下,他们多表达正在经历的身体感受的愉快或不愉快。他们不理解为什么需要看医生或服药,且不会非常抵抗。大部分父母让婴儿或蹒跚学步的幼儿服药是比较舒适的,并且许多父母擅长做这件事。但是,如果他们经历了他们依赖的成年人情绪失控、经常生气,或者任何理由的身体难以忍受的不适,即使实际上是为他们好,这些非常年幼的儿童也会受到创伤[46,47]。安全感(可预测未来情感稳定性)依靠于可预测的、反应敏捷的成人。不安全感显示晚期依从性差,这将后续进一步讨论。

3~7岁的儿童是Piaget称为认知发育前的运算阶段[48]。虽然他们现在可以理解相对复杂的语言,但他们并没有对理由和效应的良好感觉,且并不能理解对药物的需求。他们正在发展他们的自主意识和以后学校期间将会用到的交往技能。那些非常焦虑的学龄前儿童父母会认为移植受体等同为“脆弱”,并过度保护和警惕[49]。依据服药依从性、焦虑甚至创伤后应激障碍(PTSD)对一部分父母来说可能是(至少暂时)有益的[50]。然而,那些保持这种依赖角色的儿童,当他们在医学或发育上不再合适时,其在将来照顾上的参与能力更弱。他们可能会在不依从行为上故意尝试来证实独立能力。

学龄期

7~11 岁的儿童可以更有逻辑的思考并理解服药的原因[51]。这个阶段 Piaget 称为“具体操作性思维”。因为学龄期儿童不理解解剖，会从字面上认识和解释并视指南为规则，所以临床医生和父母在解释事情时必须小心[52]。学龄期儿童会听从说明,但是并没有非常好的独立判断,且普遍没有良好的组织或责任感。评估学龄期儿童在移植术后角色的研究发现,11 岁以下的儿童普遍开始对服药有一定的责任感，但是这经常会受限并需要监督[53,54]。这种监督是非常恰当的。

青少年期

青少年的移植预后最差，这要将很大一部分原因归于不依从[41]。这很有意思,因为从单纯的认知发育角度来讲,年龄大于 11 岁的受体被期待的依从性是最好的。他们被 Piaget 称为正式操作阶段,他们能理解事情的多个原因并能抽象性的理解[55]。然而,青少年行为的 3 个最突出特点是冒险的增加、感觉寻找的增加和想要离开父母寻求更好的同伴关系[56]。这些行为导致的移植术后行为问题阶段我们称为“不依从”。

基于累计的青少年发育大脑神经影像学研究,出现了 3 大主题[57]。第一个,由于大脑的多个区域越来越集成相关认知活动出现了增加[58]。第二个结构性主题有一个普遍特点是儿童时到高峰(比如突触增殖)随后在青少年期下降(称为修剪)。因此大脑得到了修正[57]。第三个,可能是我们讨论的最重要的一点,即不同认知的竞争神经元网络和情感系统成熟之间的不同速度导致的平衡改变[57]。这导致了包括了注意力、反应抑制、情绪调节、组织与远期规划等在内的一系列广泛能力的增加。这些功能位于前额叶并且成熟相对较晚[57]。随着时间的推移,对于一定数量的认知任务,与边缘系统活动相反的比例正在增加[59]。

导致不依从的一个额外因素是青少年的分离和个性化的主要发育任务[60]。青少年比学龄期儿童更适应那些能被他们同龄人接受的事情。他们会试验性地看待父母的价值观和期望哪些是他们想保留,哪些是他们要拒绝的。权威的人(如医生和教师)也会被作为青少年相信的东西同时也会质疑[61]。一个质疑日常药物必要性的青少年可能尝试如果他们跳过一次服药会发生什么问题。他们发现停止用药物,无论是故意的或因为他们“遗忘”导致的,并没有直接的负面影响。而当出现排斥的时候往往太晚了。

年轻成人

年轻成人的发育任务也会表现出对依从性的挑战[62]。这个年龄的年轻人决定追求更先进的教育、职业、生活伴侣、住房和教养。这些领域的限制,感知的或真实的,均会让年轻人感到毁灭感。有一些建议基于从儿童时期癌症生存下来的无症状的 PTSD 患者，因为儿童或青少年也会成长为这样的年轻成人，他们也会碰到这样的发育任务[63]。不依从反映了对与疾病和移植相关的每件事终止的欲望，从而能使他们返回到如果他们健康时能拥有的生活。

与儿童患者药物不依从相关的因素

有许多关于那些与免疫抑制剂不依从相关的因素的研究[24,34,64]。许多因素已经得到了确认(表 120.1)。然而，很重要的一点是要意识到那些研究中用来明确影响因素的方法是非常多变的。因此证实这些因素的有效性或比较预测能力具有挑战性。根据一般规则,临床医生(与药物依从性领域研究者相反)利用这些因素作为大致的指南来发现不依从和确认和(或)接触那些可能被修改的依从性的障碍。表 120.1 包含了一系列与药物不依从相关的危险因素。其中的许多儿童和(或)青少年患者的因素是与那些在成人中观察到的相重叠的。在文献中有最大一致性的因素将在后续进一步讨论。

WHO 确定了 5 个不同类别的药物不依从危险因素[1]。其包括社会经济因素、患者相关因素、状况相关因素、治疗相关因素,医疗保健系统和团队相关的因素。其中的一定数量的因素分布到多个不同的类别中。

社会经济因素

进入这个类别的患者遇到了药物负担[65]、低社会经济状况[65-67]、非洲裔美国人[68]、家庭不稳定、来自父母较差的社会支持[30,66,69],和单亲家庭[66,67]等问题。其他的因素在表 120.1 中具体描述。

在一般情况下,青少年生活在稳定的、有支持的环境下相比于那些生长在家庭冲突且缺少家庭凝聚力的氛围患者会有更好的药物治疗依从性[24,67,69-74]。还有重要的是要意识到患者的社会支持网络会随着时间而改变。医学团队同患者自身要持续的评估其社会支持网络。照顾者"筋疲力尽"时会进入更差的药物依从性阶段[75,76]。

患者相关因素

这些因素包括那些会导致青少年放弃药物管理的行为因素。其中的一些在表120.1中列出。Greenstein和Siegal[27]证实了一项有用的患者相关因素分类。他们确定了至少3项不依从特点：意外的不依从意味着遗忘[30]；固执己见的特点[30,65]，这在青少年中较为普遍；决定性不依从的特点涉及冒险行为[24,77-79]。在成人中，似乎肾移植受体的不依从更多是由于遗忘而不是故意行为[80]。

其他的患者相关特点与移植的经历相关，如创伤事件或由于PTSD症状导致的事件[81]。对于这些移植受体，每日服药如同他们所有负面经历的创伤提醒。避免药物带来的一些来自住院记忆、疾病、没有朋友和血液测试的刺激。这可以帮助他们感到"正常"，这个愿望在青少年移植受体研究中经常被引用[82]。对创伤后应激的干预可能会改善这些状况的不依从[67]。有趣的是，父母由于对孩子幸福的焦虑也会经历PTSD[24,66]。疾病和必要治疗的应激也会导致临床显著的焦虑和抑郁[66,71,78]，特别是那些移植前就已经沮丧的受体。受体可能有较低的自尊感[65,71]，这可能与不依从，特别是如果治疗会导致身体形象的改变这点有关。另一方面，对于儿童和成年患者的依从性有很大希望得到改善。

让儿童移植受体逐渐能控制自己的医疗保健是很重要的。然而，假设儿童移植受体为其自身的服药负责，而减少父母在管理药物中的作用，其观察到依从性有所下降[37,85,86]。相似的是，移植受体在儿童医疗保健系统过渡到成人保健系统的过程中也观察到依从性的下降[87,88]。

一个相信健康结果是偶然而不是通过他们自身行为(外部的轨迹控制)获得的个体更有可能放弃药物[89]。另一方面，其清楚地表明，如果青少年知道他们服用的药物名称，这些药物的作用，他们会有更好的依从性[90]。

表120.1 与药物不依从相关的因素(Data from Wolff [64], Dobells [24, 34], Butler [123], Denhaerynck [3], Bunzel 和 Laedrach-Hofmann [211])

社会经济因素
儿童
贫穷或差的社会经济状态
种族和(或)文化背景(往往是一个低社会经济地位的替代)
药物代价和(或)不完全的医疗保健覆盖
家庭动力学
Ⅰ.家庭不稳定和(或)家庭凝聚力差
Ⅱ.单亲家庭
Ⅲ.缺乏父母监督和(或)社会支持
Ⅳ.缺少家庭成员间交流
Ⅴ.父母焦虑、过度保护，或社会孤立后的创伤后应激障碍
成人
更年轻的年龄
种族和(或)文化背景(通常是一个低社会经济地位的替代品)
较低的教育背景
婚姻问题和(或)离婚
缺乏社会支持
患者相关的因素
儿童
对以下知识的缺乏
Ⅰ.药物名称和剂量和(或)时间
Ⅱ.药物作用
Ⅲ.不适当的健康理念
低自尊
Ⅰ.身体形象差
Ⅱ.不喜欢随身携带药物
健忘
Ⅰ.忙碌的生活方式
发育延迟
年龄
Ⅰ.移植时
Ⅱ.患者最近随访时
心理
Ⅰ.以前的不依从[222]
Ⅱ.抑郁和(或)焦虑
Ⅲ.创伤后应激障碍
Ⅳ.愤怒
Ⅴ.辍学
Ⅵ.儿童时虐待史
Ⅶ.拒绝
Ⅷ.物质滥用
Ⅸ.应对机制差
a.感觉移植问题不堪重负

(待续)

表 120.1(续)

社会
- Ⅰ.社会技能差
- Ⅱ.社会调整问题
- Ⅲ.缺乏社会支持
- Ⅳ.不愿承认接受移植的患者为朋友

心理发展阶段
- Ⅰ.风险行为
- Ⅱ.走向独立的过程
  - a.解决依赖父母与对自主性的需要的困难

成人
- 对自己医疗保健知识的缺乏
- 与医疗团队健康理念的不同
  - Ⅰ.外部控制源
  - Ⅱ.自觉缺乏自主性
- 健忘
  - Ⅰ.组织能力差
  - Ⅱ.生活方式和(或)工作的干扰
- 移植前的不依从
- 缺乏动机
  - Ⅰ.低自我效能感
  - Ⅱ.自我保健困难
  - Ⅲ.物质滥用

疾病相关的条件

儿童
- 时间
  - Ⅰ.疾病的持续时间
  - Ⅱ.移植术后时间较长
- 良好健康的感觉
  - Ⅰ.脆弱性的低感知
- 从未接受过透析

成人
- 抑郁
- 移植术后时间较长
- 良好健康的感觉
- 继发于感染或排斥的物理限制

治疗相关的因素

儿童
- 化妆品的副作用
- 药物治疗方案的复杂性
  - Ⅰ.药物和(或)药片的总数
  - Ⅱ.白天更高的给药剂量(如每天 3 次和每天 2 次)
- 药物的其他属性
  - Ⅰ.口味
  - Ⅱ.药丸大小和吞咽困难程度

成人
- 关注药物的严重不良影响

(待续)

表 120.1(续)

- 使用非处方药
- 增加给药的频率
- 增加给药的数量
- 晚上给药

医疗保健系统和团队相关因素

儿童
- 父母和医疗保健团队之间的沟通
- 医疗保健团队的选择性归因
  - Ⅰ.医疗工作者认为不依从患者“坏”
  - Ⅱ.医疗保健团队不知道他们的哪些态度可以影响患者和(或)家长坚持方案的愿望

成人
- 缺少保险
- 无力支付汽车费用
- 不良的医患关系
- 从儿童到成人护理的过渡

疾病状况相关因素

当移植术后状况良好 1 年或多年以后不依从的可能性更高[91]。这是一个普遍点即医生感觉他们不需要频繁地关注移植受体。不幸的是,这种下降的医学团队干预与青少年依从性的下降相关[92]。当不依从在移植术后早期证实,随着时间的流逝服药的紧迫性会降低,药物的依从性也会降低[93-95]。具有讽刺意味的是,成功移植导致的良好健康感觉对于青少年的药物依从性的发生是鼓励而不是阻止。因为当一次服药被遗忘时并没有直接的副作用,这导致了青少年简单地认为不服药也没有严重的后果。

治疗相关因素

治疗相关因素包括管理的药物的特点和治疗方案的复杂性。对于儿童,口味差[86]、难以下咽的药物,或者会导致严重副作用的药物[85]都可能与不依从相关。治疗方案的复杂性也与移植术后的不依从高度相关[96]。这同时包括给药频率和需要服用药片的数量。

医疗系统和团队相关因素

医疗团队的方式也是不依从的一个重要因素。Wolff 等[64]强调医疗团队需要避免选择性的将所有导致不依从的问题归咎于患者[34]。医疗团队给出的信息必须是清楚明确的。比如一个有问题的干预方式[34],一项研究发现调度测试或一次随访发出适得其反的消息会干扰药物的管理[97]。一些支持团队作用的证据显示各个移植中心的不依从发生率有区别[34,98]。医疗团队怎样与受体和父母联系在决定药物不依从的出现和严重程度中扮演了关键的角色。

医疗保健系统因素(如保险覆盖到的药物费用)明显对于社会经济因素有影响。然而,还有一些其他的医疗保健系统因素导致不依从的例子。这些例子包括在一个特别的年龄强制性地让患者从儿童转到成人状况,当她(他)到21岁时失去了保险的覆盖(或者几岁被认为是过渡年龄)[99,100]。无论患者是否准备好,经常都有一个强制性过渡的系统。当一个已计划或未计划的过渡出现时药物不依从会增加[53,87,88],提供一个能识别在关键时刻增加不依从的危险因素的组织好的过渡计划是符合患者和医疗保健系统最佳利益的。这个计划同时必须包括财务咨询[100]。

依从的障碍

上面讨论的与不依从相关的因素为那些在评估特定的人口统计学因素、治疗和依从性特定评估的系统变量之间的相关性研究中受到关注的。"是什么导致不依从的另一个理解方式是问移植受体和他们的父母哪些方面他们认为是依从的障碍。"其中一个用来评估依从障碍最频繁的方法是由Simon等发现的[85]。作者使用标准化的确定依从障碍重要范畴维度的开放式问题查询了80名青少年移植受体和他们的父母,并将他们按照4个类别来描述[101]。

可感知到的障碍总数在医学依从评估(MAM)[86,101]中确定为不依从的那些移植受体中更大。此外,研究中那些经历了排斥事件的患者有更多的障碍数目。表120.2显示这个研究中主要的两个障碍类型为遗忘、分心和差的计划和安排[101]。当青少年而不是父母管理药物及早上给药而不是晚上(因为他们上学要迟到)时,不依从的发生率更高。这些结果与那些描述包括认知障碍[102-104]、这些药物的问题特点[103,105]和对服药的自主抵抗[104]等在内的显著障碍的其他研究一致。

Simons和Blount使用两张有效的基于这项工作的调查问卷使药物依从性的测试正式化。父母药物障碍分数(PMBS)和青少年药物障碍分数(AMBS)[101]。PMBS包含16项Cronbach's alpha为0.87,预示强烈的内部一致性。有4个因素分析的派生分量表:"疾病挫折和(或)青少年问题"伴有7项(α=0.84),"方案适应和(或)认知"有5项(α=0.82),"摄入问题"有3项(α=0.69),和"父母提醒"1项。AMBS包含17项Cronbach's alpha为0.86,预示强烈的内部一致性。其有3项因素分析派生分量表:"疾病挫折和(或)青少年问题"伴有项(α=0.84),"摄入问题"有5项(α=0.70),"方案适应和(或)认知"有4项(α=0.76)。每一项额定一个5分的Likert分数从"强烈不同意"到"强烈同意"。

在一项上述讨论的感知到的障碍研究的一个重要随访中,Simons等[106]在2010年发现这些感知到的障碍并没有随着时间而改变。更重要的是,"疾病挫折和(或)青少年问题"的青少年感知障碍和"方案适应和(或)认知"的父母感知障碍与随访期间药物更差的依从性是相关的。医学并发症和死亡率同时与父母和青少年感知的"摄入问题"障碍显著相关。

其他研究也研究了儿童移植受体依从性障碍的出现和药物不依从性的发生率。基于依从性的电子监测,Gerson等[107]发现增加的父母压力、无效的父母和孩子之间的沟通,和儿童行为问题等水平与更差的药物依从性相关。他们同样发现了支持对形象的主观不满和

表120.2 依从的各种障碍[102]

障碍类型	例子	父母报告障碍/数量/%	青少年报告障碍/数量/%
障碍总数		76	73
忘记或分心	"没注意还剩下多少","没有了";"完全忘记了","做别的事情"	13/17.1	21/28.8
差的计划和规划问题	"保持24小时围着药丸转是困难的";"周末,睡觉"	52/68.4	42/57.5
身体障碍或药物问题	"太累""早上恶心"	4/5.3	7/9.6
自主抵抗或尝试变得正常	"当我看到朋友不需要服药,我也不想吃""少年生活方式""不做"	7/9.2	3/4.1

更差的药物依从性之间关系的证据。

Tielen 等提出了一个通过对不依从患者对移植术后生活方式态度的调查来确定青少年不依从行为风险的替代方法[108]。他们利用了一项结合了定性和定量测量的强大混合技术。这项技术允许对主体性、信念、感情和意见的系统性学习[109]。Q 方法的这一类型已被用来研究他们的健康生活方式态度[110]。其对年轻成人受体确定了 4 种不同的健康生活方式态度：①关注和控制；②外表表现；③固执己见和独立的；④随和和顺从的[108]。这些态度类型的自我分类可用来预测不依从性。当态度①~③与依从性积极相关，其显示②和③类型的态度需要更紧密的专业医学监测。Bullington 等[110]利用 Q 方法并发现 3 个因素：药物问题(口味、药片大小、服药频率和时间表)；“麻烦”的青少年(差的家庭生活、压性的医疗状况、抑郁)和故意的不依从(注意力关注者、可靠的态度) 可帮助确定那些有不依从风险和通知管理办法的患者。Pai 报道了治疗责任分配(ATR)量表的效应，这是一个通过肾移植儿童的家庭成员对治疗任务分配的简单测定。在这最初的报道中，这个标准化和有效的测量可修改的家庭流程工具允许发展针对性的干预措施[54]。

免疫抑制剂的费用作为依从的障碍在儿童和成人移植受体中都很常见。在美国，门诊患者缺少连续的免疫抑制药物的保险覆盖是成功药物管理的一个明显障碍。在 2010 年，一项包括美国移植协会(AST)，美国器官分配网络(UNOS)和 NAPRTCS 在内的合作项目开展了一项对移植项目描述性的研究来证实这个问题的范围和大小[112]。所有项目中超过 70%的报道显示至少 20%的患者在支付免疫抑制剂上碰到了困难。超过 43%的项目报道有至少 10%的患者由于费用问题未规范服药。这个问题在成人中尤其尖锐，由于成人受体的医疗费用主要来源为医疗保险，而医疗保险仅仅只覆盖移植术后免疫抑制剂的前 3 年。这个问题在儿童移植受体中相对不那么尖锐，因为在许多国家都有相应的援助项目。由于免疫抑制剂的覆盖在经济上是划算的，所以是否应该无限延伸的医疗保险已经在讨论[113,114]。

药物不依从的后果

药物不依从的后果非常严重。对于儿童肾移植受体来说，压倒性的数据显示药物不依从是迟发性移植物预后差的主要原因[5,6]。大多数研究证实了药物不依从与包括排斥和移植物失功的灾难性临床后果之间的关系[6,32,115]。一项最新的文献回顾发现，14%的肾移植物失功均因免疫抑制剂不依从所致[24]。在其他的实体器官移植受体中，约 16%的肝移植儿童受体和 35%的心脏受体的移植物失功是由药物不依从所致[24]。另外，移植物失功在青少年中占优势[5]。在那些仅关注青少年的研究中，不依从导致了约 32%的移植物失功；在其他评估混合了儿童和(或)青少年人群的研究中，发生率为 14.1%。免疫抑制剂依从性是儿童肾移植结果的重要预测因子[115]。研究加强了药物不依从是移植的一个巨大损失的结论，无论是临床结果还是经济花费。两项研究利用了大型数据库并计算了“药物状况比率”，该数据定义为一年内的药物提供天数。这个指标利用药房数据比较了药物提供的天数和假如依从性完美时需要提供的天数[116]。Pinsky 等发现根据该指标在 19~24 岁之间的患者的不依从水平最低[117]。令人惊奇的是，Chisholm-Burn 等利用同样的指标发现青少年的依从性比更年幼的患者要好[115]。两个研究都证实了伴有药物不依从的患者其不良的临床预后和高昂的经济代价。在 Chisholm-Burns 构建的模型中，10%的药物状况比率改善会减少儿童中 8%的移植物衰竭[115]。

迟发性急性排斥多是药物不依从的结果[4]。在青少年中，23%的迟发性急性排斥是由于不依从，这同时高度预示慢性移植物衰竭[24]。33%的儿童肝移植受体迟发性急性排斥[118-120]和超过 70%的儿童心脏移植受体的迟发性排斥[121]与药物不依从相关。儿童肝[79]和肾[122]移植的前瞻性研究证实了这些结果。在成人受体研究中也发现了相似的结果[3,123]。有良好依从性的儿童肾移植受体相对于成人有明显更好的长期预后[115]。在成人受体中，免疫抑制剂不依从与进行性的肾功能恶化[14]及迟发性急性排斥[124]显著相关。甚至即使没有明显的急性排斥，肾功能也可能随着时间持续恶化[125]。

不依从的另一个后果也开始显现。在肾移植中，抗 HLA 抗体指导着对供体抗原的对抗，所以被称为供体特异抗体(DSA)，其与抗体介导排斥[126,127]和差的移植物结果[128]有强烈的联系。抗体介导排斥，随着间质纤维化、肾小管萎缩和细胞介导排斥，反过来与药物不依从显著相关[125,128]。因此，这可能显示同时发生的 DSA 发展是药物不依从的良好指示因子[129]。这个建议在我们的儿童肾移植受体工作[130]和其他最新出版的研究[128,131]中都有出现。

评估不依从

对于怎样的不依从会导致严重临床后果的定义目前仍没有共识。对于药物不依从造成的损害的评估被临床上有意义的不依从的定义和记录所混淆。同样目前仍没有精确评估不依从后果的共识。移植专家需要"实时"即在允许出现移植物不可逆损害前进行干预的时间发现不依从[9]。

Shemesh 和 Fine 已推荐可提供现实和有用的依从性评估特性[132]。这些推荐的特性包括：①可被集成到临床实践中；②对患者没有额外的负担；③可直接评估药物的摄入；④依靠尽可能简单的过程；⑤需与一项严重后果有关，比如排斥；⑥有提高患者行为有效关注的歧视性能力；⑦实时（或事后）提供证据，故可及时进行干预。

不依从的两大类监测方法：直接和间接方法[133]

直接方法

这些包括直接观察到的治疗（DOT），对于药物在血或尿中的代谢产物浓度进行测定，或对药物配方增加生物或电子标志物的发现。作为一般规则，药物依从性的直接措施烦琐、昂贵，其增加的医疗保健团队负担和可能导致的耐药性会受到患者的抵抗[133]。无需置疑，DOT 是评估依从性最精确的方法。父母常常可作为儿童患者的观察者，但是当儿童成长为青少年，其提交给 DOT 的意愿会减少。除了其一般的不切实际，DOT 会使儿童"无礼对待"药物然后丢弃药片。儿童患者会变得擅长这个行为，这样他们就可以逃避服药，即使在医院的直接观察下。

免疫抑制药物浓度测定的利用成为了标准做法。钙调磷酸酶抑制剂（CNI）药物水平在临床复查时常规检查，但是使用单独的水平来精确评估依从性仍具有挑战性[133]。利用单独的异常水平来进行临床判断是不可取的。这在评估 12 小时低谷期水平时尤其真实。患者可能调整服药时间，这使得药物水平异常的高或低。或许更重要的是，不依从的患者可能会通过临床复查或血液测试的前一个晚上大剂量的服药来掩盖他们的不依从。所有这些行为都被称为"白外套服从"[134]。

因此，评估药物随着时间的波动水平比评估依从性更有逻辑。这已在许多儿童肝移植中心进行了测试[67,132,135-137]。具体地说，这些移植中心确定了他克莫司随着时间变化的标准差，发现设定阈值 1 个 SD 以上的水平与迟发性排斥显著相关[132,137]。这个方法与电子监测（见后文）的结果良好相关[138]。Pollack-BarZiv 等把这个 SD 方法扩展到了其他实体器官移植儿童受体中，发现其对于迟发性排斥之间的相似结果[139]。

我们利用这个 SD 技术来评估其在 46 名肾移植受体中的应用。我们发现排斥患者的平均 SD 为 5.3，未经历排斥患者为 3.5（P=NS）。然后我们利用变异系数（CV，CV%=SD/平均增加到 100）作为他克莫司水平的可变性标志[122]。在 46 名青少年受体中，有排斥患者的他克莫司 CV% 中位数（53.4）比无排斥患者更高（30%）（P=0.005）。没有重叠的差别值。重要的是，当研究霉酚酸水平时，我们未发现任何相似的关系，所以这项技术似乎只针对他克莫司[122]。随后的仅针对青少年的研究使该方法行之有效并证实 CV%≥ 31%与迟发性排斥有显著相关[140]。

或许是最直接的方法，诊断临床上显著不依从的最侵入性和最不实际的方法是肾活检。在标准化时间的计划性活检可以发现"亚临床"排斥[141,142]，这可能是药物不依从的第一手证据。肾移植的计划性活检有用性不在我们的讨论范围内[143]，活检证实急性排斥（BPAR）是测定移植物损伤必不可少的部分，因此其是确定临床免疫抑制剂显著不依从的一个直接形式[26,144]。计划性穿刺的使用同样是许多心脏移植中心的照顾标准[145]。

目前有一项新技术承诺可以直接测量依从性[146]。其可提取的事件标志（IEM）是微小的，由吞咽后由胃激活的食物成分组成的可消化的传感器。IEM 是用硅在"晶体规模"制造，所以其生产费用极度的便宜，在大量生产时费用仅为每个几美分。一旦被激活，通过一个微电子记录配置像一个绷带风格的皮肤补丁，IEM 产生超低功耗、私人的数字信号。这个探测器根据时间标记，解码并记录信息。这些信息随后可以上传到患者的手机。从那里，这些信息可进一步上传到一个"云"系统，可供调查者下载。这项技术最近被应用于临床试验,并已被欧盟和FDA批准。在撰写时,关于这项技术的信息仅提供摘要形式[146]。移植的临床试验已经在进行,第一个出版物已经急切的等待出版。

间接方法

这些药物依从性评估一般被推荐用来更好的识别(满足)不依从的出现[31,147,148]。目前,使用多维的"工具箱"可能并不完全实际或有证据基础[149],但是公平地说这是一个与文献一致的研究和监测药物依从性的有效方法[31,150,151]。

患者(与父母)自我报告量表

这可能是测量药物不依从最容易和最简洁的方法了[152]。其优点包括:①简单;②低成本;③易于管理;④在临床情况下实用;⑤患者自我报告很可能是真实的;⑥自我报告可以洞察导致不依从的社会、情境和这一行为模式[31,53-157]。缺点包括:①自我报告高估了依从性;②由于回忆偏倚,社会和医学愿望导致的错误("告诉医生他们想听的");③问题的表述会令人困惑;④依从性回忆的时间表会影响精度;⑤需要一个无偏倚的方法[153,154,156-158]。自我报告的固有困难,总的来说是患者或父母可能无法准确地反馈他们的经历[152]。在比较的方法中,相对于其他测定方法,自我报告倾向于低估了不依从的实际发生率[151]。

文献报道了许多依从性自我报告量表,但没有哪个单一量表被认为最有用。正如所预期的那样,有更多的文献是关于成人的。一项详尽的meta分析确定了3个自我报告工具来实现成人的可靠性、有效性和反应性,可推荐进入临床移植实践[31]。这些测试包括Basel免疫抑制剂依从性评估量表(BAASIS)[31,159,160,161]、简短的抗逆转录依从性指数[162-164],药物依从性自我报告清单(MASRI)[165,166]。后两个已通过艾滋病的验证,接下来将在移植中进行验证。这些被认为是最适合移植的临床保健是因为[31]:

1.这些工具同时考虑了药物的服用和规律性。

2.其使用简单并容易评分,适用于忙碌的临床工作。

3.所有工具都经过验证,并显示了良好的心理属性。

因为BAASIS是针对移植设计的,所以其特别适合在儿童移植受体中应用。该量表可在约5分钟内完成,使其具有良好的可操作性。有意思的是,这工具在儿童肾移植中也使用得很成功[167]。

特别针对儿童移植自我报告的可靠工具发展缓慢。上面提到的MAM,通过广泛的健康行为和障碍来评估依从性[168]。由于其聚焦于药物的时间管理和药物服用本身,据报道其特别有用[134]。基本医疗问卷(BMQ)也能评估自我效能,这使其在移植术后临床中很有用[169,170]。它直接提出谁对药物管理负责[患者、父母和(或)监护人,还是共同责任],此问卷从中收集关于药物管理(或缺乏的)和免疫抑制剂不依从的可能原因信息。

药片数量

虽然看似简单,但药片数量评估依从性是出了名的不可靠[152]。丢弃药物并反馈空的药瓶是很简单的,这会错误地得出良好的免疫抑制药物依从性[171]。当通过电子监测设备测定时,已证明通过药物数量的评估低估了不依从程度[172]。在某些低资源领域,药物数量和药房记录(见后文)已在HIV的治疗中使用,但是其已表明这些措施必须使用直接的依从性测量措施来补充才会有效[173]。

处方补充率

一个可获得的大数据会使依从性的研究有更加强大的工具[115,117]。这对个体患者同样有用[174],特别是有封闭的药物系统和(或)使用邮件来订购处方或补充[175]。在一个地方,患者可以使用补充率多达四个不同的药店[176]。然而,在多个管理保健组织的环境下,物流可能会受到挑战。这可以通过更广泛的使用电子医疗记录系统与另一个系统相互沟通来改变。关于青少年的一个更大的问题在于,缺少一颗药片并不能直接反映药物的摄入。

电子监测

电子监控系统已经被吹捧为衡量药物不依从性的"金标准",并被公认是发现不依从最好的间接方法[97,122,146]。一个附加在药物容器帽的连续微处理器,记录容器的每一次打开为一个假定的剂量,并根据日期来记录给药的时间和频率[28]。记录的数据可以检索,基于假设这些药物事件对应于药物服用,没有打开相对应错过了药物可以进行依从性评估[28,94,152]。许多电子监控系统目前正在使用,引用最多的通常为药物事件监测系统（MEMS，Aardex Ltd）中儿童不依从的文献。MEMS利用在线传递每个临床复诊的用药历史到受保护的服务器。数据根据一些设定和已验证的算法进行处理。依从性信息报告在门户网站显示(如日程图、年表图)。在研究的最后会生成一个可供统计学家分析的报告。

电子监测已经在肾移植受体研究中进行了使用[28,94,152,177]。这些数据成功确定了早期的不依从特点，其将延续至移植术后晚期[94]。这种方法被认为提供了最精确的发现不依从的方法[123,177,178]，在正确使用的情况下，药物服用的动力学将清楚地被记录下来。这种方法已被成功地用于儿童患者，来测量依从性[107]。不幸的是，这种方法价格比较昂贵，在临床实践中很难实现(见后文)。它最大的使用是在临床试验研究中检查可能的在临床实践中可实行的对于药物不依从的干预。

最近的一项研究详细地检查了可能危及成人移植受体电子监测有效性的一些因素[179]。第一个因素是要求设备功能正常。早期的肾移植受体研究不允许对无功能帽的准确数量的评估[98]。在Denhaerynck等的研究中，系统功能是可靠的，故障率≤0.5%[179]。

电子监测可靠性的第二个因素是假设每次患者旋开EM瓶子帽他(她)也立即服用了处方的剂量。但是可能并非如此，也有可能没有服用，药物服用晚点或不服用，从而低估了不依从性[178]。也可能患者能够从MEMS瓶以外的地方正确地服用药物，或从之前MEMS瓶拿出的药物获得提供（可能因为不切实际或尴尬)，导致过高的估计不依从性[98,180,181]。这可以通过询问那些不依从的患者来保留每日可能的差异，在某种程度上得到改善[4,181]，特别是青少年，很可能继续[182]或故意混淆这一过程。Denhaerynck等使用电子监控系统来评估这个方法，发现准确记录日志的成年人，其依从性的确定超过了96%的准确给药天数[179]。

评估MEMS可靠性考虑的第三个因素是“霍桑”效应[183,184]。这是患者对于意识到他(她)在被研究的反应性行为改变的趋势。观察到的评估不能被认为反映了患者在没有被研究时的行为。药物依从性可能由于研究参与而得到增强[181]。然而，因为患者每日使用药盒被MEMS盒子所约束，所以这也有可能阻碍药物治疗的依从性[185]。Denhaerynck及其他人以前的关于MEMS对于依从性影响的调查并没有得出确定性的结果[179,186]。

关于电子监测有效性的最后一个担忧是选择偏差。MEMS的使用需要承诺，因为，只有增加依从性激发的患者才会参加或保留在MEMS研究。因此，对于人群的精确采样是不可能的[182,185]。Denhaerynck等无法证实或否认这样选择偏差的存在[179]。

总的来说，可以认为MEMS系统是一个潜在的强大的工具，但有几个因素会影响设备的实用性[185]和有效性。因此，重要的是认识到依从性测量“金标准”的局限性[187]。MEMS帽通常不适合接受液体药物治疗的年轻患者。在Shellmer和Zelikovsky的研究中[187]，41%的患者报告认为将他们的药物放到指定的药瓶子是烦琐的，27%的觉得携带药瓶是一种负担，22%的患者认为它改变了他们的习惯，10%担心它会导致错过服用药物[185,187]。这使51%的患者拒绝参与MEMS的研究。然而，27位利用MEMS技术的人中只有1位认为这可能增加药物不依从的可能性。一项使用MEMS作为依从性测量措施的研究遇到了困难，40%的青少年根本未返还瓶帽及其中的记忆芯片[84]。Shellmer和Zelikovsky描述了实现MEMS更大接受性的策略[187]。

一些评估不依从的研究调查使用多个措施来优化其准确性[147,148,151]。结合不依从的自我报告或至少一个临床医生对于不依从的评估报告对于代替治疗血液水平的敏感性为72%，特异性为43%[151]。在未来的前瞻性研究中利用和验证直接和间接测量如DSA、IEM、抗HLA抗体和肾活检，单独或一起来确定最准确的措施。

阻止或改善不依从的干预

在医学、心理、行为和护理文献中有大量的关于干预措施以避免或改善慢性病患者（包括儿童和成人)的服药依从性的描述。许多类型的干预在移植人群中已被应用。作为一般规则，这些干预措施是针对确定那些与不依从及影响药物治疗依从性的障碍相关因素制订的。干预措施包括但并不限于:教育方法[53,69,188,189]；包括合同化的[191]行为方法[39,190]；消除购买免疫抑制药物的经济障碍[192]；多个利用电子和数字技术的研究[187,193-196]。

令人失望的是，只有很少的证据证明可在移植受体中成功识别干预措施预防或纠正免疫抑制药物不依从[34,197,198]。在成人移植受体中，发表了一些药物缺乏依从性方法论上的声音和随机对照研究设计的文章[24,198,199]。这显示有许多可用的且已被使用来解决其他类型药物或治疗不依从的干预措施。但即使到目前为止,还是缺乏严格的证据基础。

在移植中缺乏以证据为基础的方法已通过考虑KDIGO(肾脏疾病改善全球结果)移植受体保健指南得到了说明[200]。专家小组甚至不能对药物不依从的管理推荐的证据进行质量分级[201]。许多在 KDIGO 指南或其他地方描述的干预措施代表"常识",与证据基础相反的是,其是基于对那些与不依从相关的因素的识别[202]。

当评估服药不依从的干预措施是否成功时,有两种基本类型的结果测定。其可关注医疗小组的指令的真正的依从性行为的评价。但是,如果主要的问题是临床上显著的不依从,生物学结果将会是最有用的测量[203]。这是儿童艾滋病毒研究中一个常见的过程[204,205],其依从性能通过改善 $CD4^+$ T 细胞计数或减少病毒载量来推定。肾移植依从性的成功干预措施可使用晚期排斥频率、同种异体移植物生存、或活检结果来评估。

作为指导的第一原则,应该清楚药物不依从性的不同模式,从偶尔的误时药物,到严重违规时机;通过偶尔错过剂量,到频繁严重的时机违规行为;直接拒绝采取任何形式的服药[28,206]。因此,应该明确,许多类型的不依从活动、很多行为"预测",以及各种各样的依从障碍,"一刀切"的做法是不切合实际并注定要失败的。干预措施也必须根据受体的发展阶段个体化制订[207,208]。随着青少年努力成为一名独立的决策者,缺乏错过了一次服药直接的后果和免疫反应个体差异的了解,导致青少年质疑他们父母和医疗团队指示的倾向[209]。青少年有一种强烈的倾向关注"此时、此刻、此地"[206]。他们在抽象的长期思考上有困难。特别是,错过一次服用免疫抑制药物并没有立即的疼痛或痛苦。因为个体的免疫反应不同[208],所以到目前为止没有可以给出可靠的即时反馈的生物测试。在肾移植中,医疗团队仍然依赖于血清肌酐水平,其同时具有敏感性和特异性。缺乏可靠的即时反馈阻碍了支持及时发现免疫抑制药物依从性和提示干预的措施。

即使是在青春期,干预措施的制订必须考虑患者的特定发展阶段[205]。不管患者实际年龄如何,不同的青少年可能会沿着不同的发展谱发展。青少年努力成为独立的决策者,但他们经常出现尝试成为独立于他们看护者和(或)父母的独立决策者的负面行为[209]。问题可能会进一步发展,因为不同的医疗团队成员在其评估一个青少年是否能胜任一个建设性和积极自主的决定制订者上有所不同[209,210]。因此现任的医疗保健团队需要仔细的制订不依从干预措施——它应该有理论基础并能具体解决所有这些挑战。记住这些告诫,我们将接下来阐述一系列文献中讨论的干预措施的分类和其在临床实践中的实用性。

移植前评估和行为矫正

直观看来,移植前药物不依从以及其他行为和心理问题,或可预测移植术后的不依从[211]。令人惊讶的是,这是一个缺乏数据的主题[212]。在这个主题上似乎有相互矛盾的意见[212]。一份检查术前不依从预测价值的报告由于其回顾性质和定义术前不依从的弱标准而受到了限制[213]。另一方面,理论模型旨在解释健康行为,过去的行为可以是预测未来行为(如药物不依从)的强大工具[212,214]。移植前评估是测定药物不依从的第一个临床机会。即使根据移植前行为预测,移植前临床干预措施能否显著改善移植术后不依从行为仍不完全明确[215-219]。

另一方面,Dobbel 等最近的一项前瞻性研究[220]表明移植前药物治疗依从性、差的药物服用社会支持、低分的性格特征"责任心",和高等教育水平可预测移植术后不依从和差的移植物预后。关于高等教育水平预测移植术后不依从的发现是令人惊讶的,由于其他研究显示低的教育水平与不依从相关[221]。最值得注意的是,移植前不依从是晚期急性排斥反应的重要预测因素[220]。

关于肾移植的 KDIGO 指南[200]推荐不依从的预防干预措施,包括提供"教育、预防和治疗措施使免疫抑制剂服用不依从最小化和筛选那些有不依从风险增加的患者"[215]。然而,这些一般移植前干预实施的特别方法并没有详细的描述。关于 KDIGO 指南移植前干预的 KDOQI 评论了确定暗示移植术后不依从的因素。然而,他们指出,KDIGO 除了申明在提供适当干预时采用多个学科很重要外,其提供了很少的证据[216]。现已提出了成人肾移植的移植前评估应该考虑透析计划和药物服用的不依从,并应推迟移植直到达到了合适的依从性[14]。然而,在一个领域的不依从不能保证另一个领域的不依从。例如,在肝移植领域的研究已经发现移植前药物滥用(视为不依从活动)并不一定预示药物不依从的发生[217,218]。

明尼苏达大学的移植项目报道了他们一项结果可能揭示移植前评估和干预措施草案的经验。该草案描述了那些第一次移植由于不依从而失败而必须考虑第二次肾移植的患者的阶段。这个草案第一次是在1995年提出，在2009年进行更新[218,219]。虽然这些报道不是来源于一个临床试验，他们利用一个历史对照组和代表了唯一的大型出版的临床经验。114位由于药物不依从失去了第一次移植肾的患者，根据自我报告记录，接受了完整的重新评估，其中包括一个教育类和一个完整的移植团队的访问。具体评估组成是:①一个候选人和移植协调员，肾脏专科医生和外科医生之间个体化的讨论，处理之前的不依从性原因以及如何预防后续不依从；②社会工作者和神经心理学家的评估的移植以找到更多的可能导致不依从性因素；③逐点与候选人讨论移植前必须满足的条件[219]。明尼苏达草案需要完全满足的主要标准包括: ①至少6个月的完整透析，药物和(或)实验室和其他测试、诊所访问在内的完整的依从性；②完成社会工作者和神经心理学家的所有建议；③改善这些被确认为导致之前不依从的因素；④当有一个活体供体的计划时，需充分讨论这个未来供者的所有草案。最后一个咨询是安排时间使医疗小组能确保其候选人充分理解和计划来实现移植的要求和条件。这整个移植前干预和许多移植中心具体实施的不同。

114位患者中的75位(66%)启动了移植前筛查和干预草案。这75位中的48位能够圆满地完成评估和(或)干预草案，48位中的37位在这个报道时接受了肾移植。作者发现这些患者与历史对照组患者之间的患者生存率、除去死亡后的移植物生存、或慢性无排斥生存之间并无显著性差异，虽然有建议提示在后面几类之间出现差异的趋势。在那些第一次移植中出现不依从的患者中急性排斥发生有显著的增加。然而，药物不依从的一个特点，晚期急性排斥发生率并没有显著增加。这似乎与其他的报道结果相反[220]。不幸的是，尽管移植前行干预措施，但不依从行为似乎有一些重要的耐久性。之前不依从的患者组，14%由于不依从导致移植失败，而仅2%的对照再次移植的移植物失功是由于不依从[219]。此外，57%的最初不依从的再移植受体表现出了不依从行为。

本研究提出了什么程度移植前干预可以有效的一些重要问题。一方面，令人失望的是不依从行为仍持续出现在那些之前不依从的二次移植术后患者身上[222]。另一方面，我们没有从明尼苏达研究中得到足够的信息(如抗HLA DSA的存在)，同时研究并没有真正足够的说服力，也没有重组的控制来完全回答他们的移植前干预是否有效的问题。事实上，如果不追求最优的话，该临床结果是可以接受的。

综上所述，使用移植前干预措施来阻止不依从可以得出什么结论？它似乎合理地得出一个移植前评估的必要部分是候选人依从性状态的调查。每个移植前候选人应考虑不依从的风险[222]。在移植前，患者的依从性应该反复评估，最好是由擅长识别不依从和利用可获得的时间(如患者透析时)的人来进行。评估者应该探索患者问题行为的潜在原因。移植前团队(特别是社会工作者、心理学家、移植协调员)应该利用之前列出的因素实现对那些能够确定的潜在问题制订干预措施[222](见表120.1)。

对于儿童和(或)青少年候选人，适当的移植前干预措施(尽管没有一个严格的基于证据的评估)应该包括:

- 指导青少年和照顾者关于移植术后医学问题和一致的、长期的依从性的教育干预措施；
- 弥补技能缺陷的干预措施(例如组织策略、公共交通使用，温度计读数和实验室值的解释)；
- 确定的情感和(或)行为问题的治疗；
- 改善供者、患者关系和沟通的干预措施；
- 增加和(或)优化青少年社会、情感支持的干预措施。

移植前的教育干预措施也应该遵循以下指南:

- 信息应该由几个不同的教育者提供；
- 具有确定药物知识、副作用和时机等的特殊问题；
- 强调患者、父母和健康提供者之间健康理念的调解；
- 以一种理解的方式建议患者。

我们使用承认有时依从性是困难的(“当你和朋友一起或在学校时我知道你一定觉得记住服药是困难的”)，与他(她)一起承认困难，所以他们容易接受。

Siegal和Greenstein在以上描述中已经确定了3种模式的药物不依从[223]。以下关于干预类型的建议是针对解决这些特定模式或情况。

意外

这些人往往有强烈的信念相信免疫抑制药物是有

效的并理解药物的管理不应该错过或延误。他们倾向于认为,免疫抑制剂的作用方式问题是限制为 12 个小时。这些患者需要干预工作来提醒患者服药。每周补充一次的每日药盒是有帮助,可以使用暗示方式。他们还需要咨询集成他们的药物与他们的生活方式。

不易接受的

这些患者往往更年轻的,缺少良好的教育,相比于其他组他们的肾移植时间更短。他们有更高的趋势不相信药物的效果或定时服药的要求。教育干预需要明确药物不依从的长期后果。

果断的不坚持者

这些患者往往平均受过更高等教育, 或者如果是成年人,多为白领。他们习惯于独立决策和理解免疫抑制药物的需求, 但相信药物治疗的效果持续> 24 小时并进一步认为,偶尔延迟或错过服药没有大的影响。这些个人的干预措施需要考虑他们独立决定的习惯。

心理压力

许多患者可能不属于这些类别中的任何一种,但是相反可能受到(如对他们疾病的抑郁或创伤后应激障碍等)心理问题的困扰[67]。如果可能,这些问题需要在移植前识别和处理。照顾者,如亲密的家庭成员,也可能出现类似的障碍并需要护理[50]。

围移植期和移植术后干预

与移植前干预一样, 每一个器官移植受体都应该被假定存在药物不依从的风险[92,222]。因此,利用每一个移植术后诊所访问来加强依从行为是很重要的, 包括药物管理和他们的健康活动、临床复查和健康生活方式选择。因为在谨慎干预后的短期内其结果更加的明显, 所以医疗团队必须不断地教育或接受他们的措施来使依从性最大化[39]。随着时间的推移,一个独立的干预结果随时间减少。这当然与干预特别是心理治疗效果往往随着时间的推移而削弱的发现相符合[224]。一些预防干预的总体指南见下面。

1.干预包括医疗团队与患者和(或)家属的沟通:

• 采用一种“相互作用的模式”,而不是“我们/他们”的方法;倾听患者/家属意见。

• 采用非主观判断的方法。

• 避免选择性归因(“是患者的错”)[64]。

• 强调“团队”的方法——父母是帮助 “指导”(提醒)团队的一部分,而不是控制;医疗保健专业人士是团队的一部分。

• 有不同的团队成员针对特定的患者开发 “个人特点”。这些连接应该在医务人员和患者特别是青少年患者之间的相互作用培养。

2.移植术后的干预措施尝试预先阻止不依从:

• 每一次访问都持续教育。

• 修改随着时间的推移而修改的书面指示。

• 识别和解决患者和家长心理和社会问题(抑郁、焦虑、保险的变化、学校咨询)。

• 讨论要点:

a.药物有效时间只有 12~24 小时。

b.延迟或推迟服药不会有立即的后果,但有长远影响。伤害不是立即明显,但它是慢慢累积的。

对于干预措施的研究文献的描述经常不完整[225-227]。在 De Bleser 等最近的一次回顾中[198],有 12 篇确定是处理移植术后受体不依从干预措施的研究。研究发现,处理研究干预措施导致的移植受体。这些研究中绝大多数只有弱或中度的等级[198]。下面我们将回顾这些移植特异的干预措施。只有同行评议的出版物将被列出。干预分为:①教育和(或)认知:传递信息;②咨询和(或)行为:让患者参与他们的保健和发展新的自理技能的行为的改变;③心理和(或)情绪:处理感情、情绪或社会关系的策略;④利用这些组合的混合干预措施[188,197]。

教育和(或)认知干预

关于儿童患者慢性疾病(不是移植)服药不依从的文献,一篇最新的 meta 分析发现教育干预是每次依从性增强干预的重要组成部分[228]。一项包括 21 位儿童移植受体的研究,其中 17 人是青少年,其结果并不积极[72]。21 位患者和(或)父母在每一次诊所访问都被劝告,平均每 2 个月左右 1 次。提供了纸质的包括药物日志、日程安排和小册子的劝告。作者得出的结论是,医学教育项目改善了患者和父母对于药物的了解, 但是没有显著提高依从。然而,由于本研究只包含一个小样本量,在方法上使用了有缺陷的药物依从性措施,所以本报告不应作为教育是一种改善依从性工具的结论。

Annunziato 等[53]评价了一个目的为从父母照顾到

自理过渡的教育干预。22名儿童肝移植受体都报名参加了1~2个会议教育研究。其中10名是由于从照顾者到父母过渡中有困难而纳入,11名患者没有任何的纳入标准。根据他克莫司浓度的标准差分数的改进,教育干预显著改善了那些被预知有从父母照顾到自理过渡困难的患者的依从性。然而,在进入研究时没有任何过渡过程困难的患者组,依从性没有明显改善。虽然这项研究样本小,没有对照组,但是针对那些存在责任从父母过渡到青少年困难的父母和家庭,报告显示教育干预有潜在的价值。在另一项研究中,照顾者对服药的语言提示和验证均与更高的依从性相关[229]。Klein 等[188]在先前的研究的基础上,评估了教育策略,其建议临床药学服务可以对肾移植和其他医学领域[230]的药物依从性产生积极的影响[224]。在一个前瞻性随机对照试验中,作者通过研究比较了20名肝移植患者和21名对照患者12个月的随访来确定药物依从性的计划。干预组患者在移植前的每周和移植术后的每1~3个月会收到关于免疫抑制药物的教育咨询。通过电子监测(MEMS)来测定不依从、"免疫抑制剂药物浓度"、药片数量、Morisky调查表[231]和自我报告。干预组显示了所有措施在依从性统计学上的显著改善,特别是电子监测组。患者的样本量小,由于MEMS的麻烦有的患者放弃了。此外,作者不可能纠正霍桑效应。然而,与之前的一项研究一致[224],这些发现强烈建议药剂师可以在一个教育依从性干预中发挥重要的作用。

相比之下,Dean 等发现,在儿童和青少年中,单独的教育干预本身不足以促进或维持最佳的依从性[232]。这结果得到了 Kahana 等分析的证实[39]。另外,慢性疾病依从性的 meta 分析认为单独教育项目无法改善依从性或对结果产生积极的影响[233]。这可得出结论认为教育干预是成功的必要组成部分,但并不足以阻止药物不依从性[234-236]。

咨询和(或)行为干预

Hardstaff 等[190]研究了75名手术1年以后的肾移植受体的行为和(或)咨询干预的影响。所有的患者均使用MEMS系统。患者被随机分配为接受他们第一次复查MEMS结果的反馈或者无反馈。两组均不接受任何剩下12个月试验中的进一步反馈。一个会议的反馈导致并没有改善药物治疗的依从性。这可能是因为干预太短暂,或者没有针对性。其他一些负面结论的研究显示更多的研究是必要的[231,236-238]。然而,儿童艾滋病毒文献强烈表明,行为部分可成功地改善结果[39,237]。从文献显示持续评估和对患者反馈行为干预有最高的成功可能[233],这些策略应该在混合干预时强烈推荐。在成人慢性疾病的文献中,有使用财务强化原则的操作性条件的成功干预[238]。换句话说,患者为了依从而付费。一个类似的概念试图在青少年中应用,即奖励是颁发给那些可取的行为。这证明是有效的[239]。其认为这种正面强化可能是青少年依从性干预成功的一部分,只要选择合适的强化部分。它已经证明青少年的慢性疾病患者疾病和治疗的个人意义以及个人动机的程度,明显影响依从性[240]。

心理和(或)情绪干预

尽管试点研究建议针对PSTD的干预成功改善了儿童肝移植受体的依从性[65],目前还没有任何证实仅仅利用心理和(或)情绪干预的儿童移植受体获得重大成功的研究[196]。

联合干预

在考察慢性病依从性管理的干预中,多组分和行为干预对依从行为产生了特别明显的影响[39,241]。最常见的联合干预措施包括教育和行为干预措施,另有小部分使用有教育或行为因素的社会支持策略[233]。因此,可以合理地期待联合干预措施在移植中取得了成功。De Blesser 等的评论[198]确定了5项采用联合了教育/认知、辅导/行为和情感/心理方法的干预措施的研究[198]。

De Geest 等[150]引导了这5项研究的最高质量。他们在那些确定了不依从的成人肾移植受体中确定了低自我效能感[242]和抑郁[243]作为随机对照研究的目标。患者被随机分为"增强的常规护理组"和干预组。使用MEMS电子监测了随访期6个月的3个月干预/控制期。作者使用了结构化的面试技术[4]来评估MEMS的有效性和可靠性。对于每一名患者(可获取的所有家庭成员)都进行了一个全面的家访来评估可针对的特定依从性障碍。"干预护士"讨论并开始一系列包括行为因素的干预措施来增强自我效能感(如动机性访谈[244]),和提醒患者服药的其他行为干预,加强患者依从性知识的定制教育模块,并帮助组织药物治疗的社会支持。18名不依从患者被选入参与了这个试验。6名在干预组,12名在对照组。两组患者的药物治疗依从性都得到了提高,并似乎在干预组有更明显的改善,虽然效果没有达到显著的统计学意义。该随机对照试验结果不够权威。此外,干预的多个元素非常费时和费力的。作者认为虽然他们的模型在日常临床是不切实际的,但进行心理和行为元素的设置可用于持续的护理模型或慢性疾病管理模型[245,246]。这个方法在许多儿童移植诊所进行了应用,在诊所中许多患者和家人不仅接受了医疗,而且包括心理和行为等多学科的处理。

第一个针对儿童肾移植的联合干预研究同时使用了教育和行为结合的方法[70,247],并涉及整个家庭,是适合儿童的干预。除了教育材料,干预还涉及家长每周给予的依从性行为的奖励。利用多参数测量系统,试验组中的受体对于移植更为了解。此外,试验组硫唑嘌呤和泼尼松的依从性提高了约60%,而对照组只提高了33%。

Shemesh等[248]明确了儿童肝移植受体的不依从性,并使用方法增加诊所访问的频率,并提供针对患者和家庭的对于依从性重要性的教育计划。他们使用他克莫司浓度的标准差的同时增加访问次数。干预后,谷丙转氨酶高的患者数量的水平从干预前的8位明显减少到之后的4位。其他包括排斥发生数量和他克莫司的依从性等结果也得到了改善,但是仍没有达到统计学意义[248]。因为这种类型的干预在临床实践中是可行的[192],进行随机和更权威的试验很重要,可能需要增加更正式的行为模块(如通过电子监测检查依从性措施)。

另一个小型的研究利用联合干预方法包含了12名患者[236]。临床药师工作每月进行教育咨询和药物调解,通过电话直接反馈和行为动机咨询。通过配药和免疫抑制药物的血浓度来评估依从性,接受临床药师干预的组相对于12名控制组在统计学上有显著的改善。这项研究样本量小,同时依从性评估的方法是薄弱的。然而,这种联合干预支持了针对特殊患者的多种干预措施是有价值的概念。一个使用网络基础的与健康保健团队的4个月电子沟通使那些最积极参与的患者的药物依从获得了改善,但对于整个组并没有统计学意义[194]。

应该承认,这些报道中的大部分有足够的弱点来要求更多基于不依从干预的证据。尽管如此,看起来多维干预措施,不仅涉及教育,还包括行为修改、自我保健的鼓励、稳定的社会支持发展和适当的(如抑郁等)心理问题的治疗,可以在防止或改善药物不依从性的建设中发挥重要作用。

改善药物不依从的其他干预

简化药物疗法

简化药物疗法能显著改善慢性疾病患者的药物依从性[134,233,249,250-253]。Eisen等证明随着药物剂量的频率减少依从性改善递增[254]。这种效应中也在成人肾移植受体中得到了证实[98]。由于移植受体药物方案经常很复杂,简化有明显的优势。例如,最近使用新的每天1次缓释配方的他克莫司[255]的研究,其对药物依从性有积极的影响[248,256],虽然这种测量依从性的方法不权威。这种方法并不是没有问题[257]。单一的药代动力学(在本例中为他克莫司)可能与每天2次剂量是不等价的,会迫使剂量变化[258,259]。此外,如果患者不依从,错过了他(她)每天1次的剂量,可能增加临床影响[257]。尽管如此,对依从性的适当监测,简化免疫抑制药物是理性的,虽然简化细节的明确数据需要适当研究证实的有效性。

避免药物的毒副作用

不可接受的某些免疫抑制药物副作用可能会导致药物不依从,尤其是青少年。一个典型的例子是移植术后免疫抑制使用糖皮质激素。类固醇激素对身体形象[261,262]和生长[260](在其他副作用中)的有害副作用是患者对这些药物不依从的重要原因[263]。无激素方案的使用已经被证明是成功的[19,264,265]。通过减少或完全避免用糖皮质激素,可以认为至少有一个依从性的重要障碍已经克服。

额外可能的药物修改

临床耐受性

根据定义,免疫耐受状态指的是在没有额外的免疫抑制情况下有能力维持一个运转良好的同种异体移植物和针对第三方侵略者良好的免疫系统[266]。虽然这可能不修改青少年的移植受体的其他冒险行为特征,免疫耐受状况将代表药物不依从性的答案[267-269]。不幸的是,它不可能在人类临床中产生可靠的耐受性,尤其在儿科[270]。自发或人为的耐受可偶尔在当一个器官面临免疫抑制剂撤除后可存活的状况下观察到,要么在医学监督下或由于缺乏依从性。如果生物标志物可以识别人为的耐受，理论上一些移植患者可以退出免疫抑制药物[271]。这可能对青少年有些好处,尤其可能在肝移植受体中特别常见[271]。在这方面有趣的是,在儿科患者中，行肝肾移植的受体移植肾存活率相比只接收肾移植的患者高[272]。

长期肠外免疫抑制药物

使用安全、长效的免疫抑制药物在药物不依从的环境中是有吸引力的，这种药物的管理是简单和可以直接观察到的[133]。这种策略促使我们检查 Figolimod (FTY 720)的使用,其可以降低外周淋巴细胞持续一个星期[273]。有来自药物医务人员对于这种肠外管理药物的更大的理论呼吁。在儿童肾移植中,达克珠单抗,一种人源化单克隆抗 CD25 抗体已被成功地应用超过 6 个月并获得成功的结果[265]。在非传染性的眼部炎症疾病,达克珠单抗成功使用超过了 3 年[274]。很长时间内,皮下注射用于管理达克珠单抗目前在评估复发缓和多发性硬化中的使用[275],但现在并没有对用于肾移植的评估。

目前使用贝拉西普的策略已经吸引了研究领域相当大的兴趣。为了完全激活 T 细胞,信号必须通过 T 细胞受体和共刺激分子或分子来传导。中断这个共刺激表现了 T 淋巴细胞的无能。有很多二分体(抗原呈递细胞上的一个分子切断 T 淋巴细胞上的一个抗原),这些细节在本书的其他章节会详细讨论。这些共刺激通路中第一个报道并最突出的是 CD 28/B7 (如 CD80 和 CD86)连接。在 T 细胞上 CD28 通过抗原呈递细胞表面的 B7 进行衔接,通过 MHC 抗原激活的 T 细胞受体信号使标记的 T 细胞活化和增殖。CTLA-4,另一个 T 细胞表面受体,热切结合 B7 抗原 100 倍,从而阻止 CD28 共刺激信号。贝拉西普包含 CTLA-4 的一个融合蛋白。这导致强烈的 B7 结合和阻断 CD28 信号[276]。这个讨论重要的是,贝拉西普可以每月不经肠道给药,拥有优秀和可能的免疫抑制安全性。这个项目目前正在进行三期试验研究,持续管理时间将会为3~5 年[277,278]。至该书编写的时候还没有开始正式的临床试验。如果青少年患者可稳定地获得至少一个有效的免疫抑制剂量则可以持谨慎的乐观态度,这可能会导致一些药物不依从影响的改进[279]。两点必须谨慎的注意:贝拉西普只建议在 EBV 血清反应阳性的患者中使用，防止生成 PTLD[280];因此贝拉西普可能并不适合每一位青少年。此外，贝拉西普的成功管理可能并不伴随其他口服免疫抑制药物的良好依从性。

解决潜在的心理问题

成人慢性疾病患者[281,282]特别是终末期肾脏疾病患者,经常会出现抑郁症状。在一项研究中,开始慢性血液透析的成人开始接受心理分析，其中 44%的患者显示有明显的抑郁[283]。心理压力似乎持续存在,虽然肾移植之后稍有一定程度的下降[284]。儿童患者也是如此。相比于健康的儿童，患有慢性疾病的儿童出现心理和行为问题发生率是其两倍[285]。接受透析和移植的儿童显示有抑郁、学校问题和情绪困扰[279,286,287]。后来的研究使用更复杂的工具证实了这些观察[77]。当有希望减轻抑郁症状时[84],疾病相关的不确定性似乎在其中扮演了重要的角色[84,288]。

在如抑郁、焦虑等情绪问题和药物不依从性之间似乎有一个强大的联系[289,290]。这发生在大量的慢性疾病患者身上,包括肾和肝移植受体[291-295]。同样,在患有慢性疾病的青少年中，依从性差和情感问题之间也有相关性[83,296-298]。Penkower 等[77]研究了 22 名青少年移植受体,发现不依从性与愤怒之间有显著的关系,而并不是抑郁或焦虑。其他研究显示在儿童移植受体中,妥协的情感功能和不依从之间存在相关性[72,299]。强烈建议疾病相关不确定性可以调节抑郁,同时期可以反过来调解药物的不依从[84]。另一方面,希望的存在、缓解抑郁,似乎与免疫抑制相关药物治疗良好的依从性相关[84]。有趣的是，似乎移植术后焦虑的发展并不预示着药物不依从水平的增加，但实际上可能与更稳定的依从性模式有关[300]。最后,创伤后应激障碍的发展,正如这一章前面详细所说,与医学不依从的困难相关。

总结

这不是夸大代表实体器官移植中最重要的未满足需求之一的药物依从性的问题。与药物不依从性有关的问题仍在鉴别中,不管是儿童还是成人。这一领域的研究饱受无正式定义、检测技术、相关障碍的协议和诱发因素、行之有效的干预措施等的困扰。长期移植的结果,尤其是肾移植,并没有随着时间的推移发生翻天覆地的变化,虽然在短期上有了一些改进。很有可能部分或大部分改善移植物结果的障碍随着更体贴和共同的努力改善免疫抑制药物治疗的依从性来实现。

（奚斌　译　徐骁　校）

参考文献

1. Sabate E. Adherence to Long-Term Therapies: Evidence for Action. Geneva, Switzerland: World Health Organization; 2003.
2. Haynes RB, et al. Interventions for enhancing medication adherence. Cochrane Database of Systematic Reviews. 2008;(2):CD000011.
3. Denhaerynck K, et al. Prevalence, consequences, and determinants of non-adherence in adult renal transplant patients: a literature review. Transplant International. 2005;18(10):1121–1133.
4. De Geest S, et al. Late acute rejection and subclinical non-compliance with cyclosporine therapy in heart transplant recipients. Journal of Heart and Lung Transplantation. 1998;17(9):854–863.
5. Rianthavorn P, et al. Non-compliance with immunosuppressive medications in pediatric and adolescent patients receiving solid-organ transplants. Transplantation. 2004;77(5):778–782.
6. Rianthavorn P, Ettenger RB. Medication non-adherence in the adolescent renal transplant recipient: a clinician's viewpoint. Pediatric Transplantation. 2005; 9(3):398–407.
7. De Geest S, Vanhaecke J. Methodological issues in transplant compliance research. Transplantation Proceedings. 1999;31(4A):81S–83S.
8. Nevins TE, Matas AJ. Medication non-compliance: another iceberg's tip. Transplantation. 2004;77(5):776–778.
9. Fine RN, et al. Non-adherence consensus conference summary report. American Journal of Transplantation. 2009;9(1):35–41.
10. Loubeau PR, Loubeau JM, Jantzen R. The economics of kidney transplantation versus hemodialysis. Progress in Transplantation (Aliso Viejo, Calif.). 2001; 11(4):291–297.
11. Rocha MJ, Ferreira S, Martins LS, et al. Cost analysis of renal replacement therapy by transplant in a system of bundled payment of dialysis. Clinical Transplantation. 2012;4:529–531.
12. Sudan DL, Shaw BW Jr, Langnas AN. Causes of late mortality in pediatric liver transplant recipients. Annals of Surgery. 1998;227(2):289–295.
13. Pascual M, et al. Strategies to improve long-term outcomes after renal transplantation. The New England Journal of Medicine. 2002;346(8):580–590.
14. Prendergast MB, Gaston RS. Optimizing medication adherence: an ongoing opportunity to improve outcomes after kidney transplantation. Clinical Journal of the American Society of Nephrology. 2010;5(7):1305–1311.
15. *Annual Report of the North American Pediatric Renal Trials and Collaborative Studies (NAPRTCS)*. 2006.
16. Tsai EW, et al. Kidney transplantation in children. In: Danovitch GM, editor. Handbook of Kidney Transplantation. Philadelphia, PA: Wolters Kluwer / Lippincott Williams & Wilkins; 2010: 355–388.
17. Horslen S, et al. Pediatric transplantation in the United States, 1996–2005. American Journal of Transplantation. 2007;7(5 Pt 2):1339–1358.
18. Atlas of chronic kidney disease and end-stage renal disease in the United States. In: United States Renal Data System Annual Data Report. National Institute of Diabetes and Digestive and Kidney Diseases; 2009.
19. Grenda R, Watson A, Trompeter R, et al. A randomized trial to assess the impact of early steroid withdrawal on growth in pediatric renal transplantation: the TWIST study. American Journal of Transplantation. 2010;10(4):828–836.
20. Rees L, et al. Growth and endocrine function after renal transplantation. Archives of Disease in Childhood. 1988;63(11):1326–1332.
21. Bucuvalas JC, et al. Improving long-term outcomes after liver transplantation in children. American Journal of Transplantation. 2008;8(12):2506–2513.
22. DeBolt AJ, et al. A survey of psychosocial adaptation in long-term survivors of pediatric liver transplants. Children's Healthcare: Journal of the Association for the Care of Children's Health. 1995;24(2):79–96.
23. Neu AM. Special issues in pediatric kidney transplantation. Advances in Chronic Kidney Disease. 2006;13(1):62–69.
24. Dobbels F, et al. Growing pains: non-adherence with the immunosuppressive regimen in adolescent transplant recipients. Pediatric Transplantation. 2005; 9(3):381–390.
25. Nunes V, N.J., O'Flynn N, Calvert N, et al. Practitioners RCOG, editor. Clinical Guidelines and Evidence Review for Medicines Adherence: involving patients in decisions about prescribed medicines and supporting adherence. Hyde Park, London: National Collaborating Centre for Primary Care and Royal College of General Practitioners. 2009.
26. Chapman JR. Compliance: the patient, the doctor, and the medication? Transplantation. 2004;77(5):782–786.
27. Greenstein S, Siegal B. Compliance and non-compliance in patients with a functioning renal transplant: a multicenter study. Transplantation. 1998;66(12): 1718–1726.
28. Nevins TE, et al. The natural history of azathioprine compliance after renal transplantation. Kidney International. 2001;60(4):1565–1570.
29. Chisholm MA, et al. Renal transplant patient compliance with free immunosuppressive medications. Transplantation. 2000;70(8):1240–1244.
30. Blowey DL, et al. Compliance with cyclosporine in adolescent renal transplant recipients. Pediatric Nephrology (Berlin, Germany). 1997;11(5):547–551.
31. Dobbels F, Berben L, De Geest S, et al. The psychometric properties and practicability of self-report instruments to identify medication non-adherence in adult transplant patients: a systematic review. Transplantation. 2010;90(2): 205–219.
32. Dew MA, et al. Meta-analysis of medical regimen adherence outcomes in pediatric solid organ transplantation. Transplantation. 2009;88(5):736–746.
33. Dew MA, et al. Rates and risk factors for non-adherence to the medical regimen after adult solid organ transplantation. Transplantation. 2007;83(7): 858–873.
34. Dobbels F, Ruppar T, De Geest S, et al. Adherence to the immunosuppressive regimen in pediatric kidney transplant recipients: a systematic review. Pediatric Transplantation. 2010;14(5):603–613.
35. Shellmer DA, Dabbs AD, Dew MA. Medical adherence in pediatric organ transplantation: what are the next steps? Current Opinion in Organ Transplantation. 2011;16(5):509–514.
36. Fredericks EM, Dore-Stites D. Adherence to immunosuppressants: how can it be improved in adolescent organ transplant recipients? Current Opinion in Organ Transplantation. 2010;15(5):614–620.
37. Kahana SY, Frazier TW, Drotar D. Preliminary quantitative investigation of predictors of treatment non-adherence in pediatric transplantation: a brief report. Pediatric Transplantation. 2008;12(6):656–660.
38. Lemanek KL, Kamps J, Chung NB. Empirically supported treatments in pediatric psychology: regimen adherence. Journal of Pediatric Psychology. 2001;26(5): 253–275.
39. Kahana S, Drotar D, Frazier T. Meta-analysis of psychological interventions to promote adherence to treatment in pediatric chronic health conditions. Journal of Pediatric Psychology. 2008;33(6):590–611.
40. *United States Renal Data System 2009 Annual Data Report Atlas of Chronic Kidney Disease and End Stage Renal Disease in the United States*. 2009.
41. Foster BJ, Dahhou M, Zhang X, et al. Association between age and graft failure rates in young kidney transplant recipients. Transplantation. 2010;92(11): 1237–1243.
42. Welsh RM, Selin LK. No one is naive: the significance of heterologous T-cell immunity. Nature Reviews. Immunology. 2002;2(6):417–426.
43. Adams AB, Pearson TC, Larsen CP. Heterologous immunity: an overlooked barrier to tolerance. Immunological Reviews. 2003;196:147–160.
44. Welsh RM, et al. The privacy of T cell memory to viruses. Current Topics in Microbiology and Immunology. 2006;311:117–153.
45. Koelle DM, et al. Herpes simplex virus type 2-specific CD8 cytotoxic T lymphocyte cross-reactivity against prevalent HLA class I alleles. Blood. 2002; 99(10):3844–3847.
46. Stuber ML. Psychiatric issues in pediatric organ transplantation. Child and Adolescent Psychiatric Clinics of North America. 2010;19(2):285–300, viii–ix.
47. Stuber ML. Psychiatric issues in pediatric organ transplantation. Pediatric Clinics of North America. 2011;58(4):887–901, x.
48. Zetlin AG. Problem solving in pre-operational youngsters. Journal of Mental Deficiency Research. 1981;25(Pt 2):127–132.
49. Chambers PL, Mahabee-Gittens EM, Leonard AC. Vulnerable child syndrome, parental perception of child vulnerability, and emergency department usage. Pediatric Emergency Care. 2011;27(11):1009–1013.
50. Young GS, et al. Symptoms of posttraumatic stress disorder in parents of transplant recipients: incidence, severity, and related factors. Pediatrics. 2003;111(6 Pt 1):e725–e731.
51. Berry SL, et al. Conceptions of illness by children with juvenile rheumatoid arthritis: a cognitive developmental approach. Journal of Pediatric Psychology. 1993;18(1):83–97.
52. Borzekowski DL. Considering children and health literacy: a theoretical approach. Pediatrics. 2009;124(Suppl 3):S282–S288.
53. Annunziato RA, et al. Transitioning healthcare responsibility from caregivers to patient: a pilot study aiming to facilitate medication adherence during this process. Pediatric Transplantation. 2008;12(3):309–315.
54. Pai AL, Gray E, Kurivial K, et al. The Allocation of Treatment Responsibility scale:

a novel tool for assessing patient and caregiver management of pediatric medical treatment regimens. Pediatric Transplantation. 2010;14(8):993–999.
55. Gordon DE. Formal operational thinking: the role of cognitive-developmental processes in adolescent decision-making about pregnancy and contraception. American Journal of Orthopsychiatry. 1990;60(3):346–356.
56. Giedd JN. The digital revolution and adolescent brain evolution. Journal of Adolescent Health. 2012;51(2):101–105.
57. Giedd JN. The teen brain: insights from neuroimaging. Journal of Adolescent Health. 2008;42(4):335–343.
58. Paus T. Mapping brain maturation and cognitive development during adolescence. Trends in Cognitive Sciences. 2005;9(2):60–68.
59. Rubia K, et al. Progressive increase of frontostriatal brain activation from childhood to adulthood during event-related tasks of cognitive control. Human Brain Mapping. 2006;27(12):973–993.
60. Daniels JA. Adolescent separation-individuation and family transitions. Adolescence. 1990;25(97):105–116.
61. Tong A, et al. Adolescent experiences following organ transplantation: a systematic review of qualitative studies. The Journal of Pediatrics. 2009;155(4):542–549.
62. Fredericks EM. Non-adherence and the transition to adulthood. Liver Transplantation. 2009;15(Suppl 2):S63–S69.
63. Stuber ML, Meeske KA, Krull KR, et al. Prevalence and predictors of posttraumatic stress disorder in adult survivors of childhood cancer. Pediatrics. 2010;125(5):e1124–e1134.
64. Wolff G, et al. Non-compliance following renal transplantation in children and adolescents. Pediatric Nephrology (Berlin, Germany). 1998;12(9):703–708.
65. Bunchman TE. Compliance in pediatric transplant. Pediatric Transplantation. 2000;4(3):165–169.
66. Warady BA, et al. Transplant allograft loss in the adolescent patient. Advances in Renal Replacement Therapy. 1996;3(2):154–165.
67. Shemesh E, et al. A pilot study of posttraumatic stress and non-adherence in pediatric liver transplant recipients. Pediatrics. 2000;105(2):E29.
68. Tucker CM, et al. Associations with medication adherence among ethnically different pediatric patients with renal transplants. Pediatric Nephrology (Berlin, Germany). 2002;17(4):251–256.
69. Beck DE, et al. Evaluation of an educational program on compliance with medication regimens in pediatric patients with renal transplants. Journal of Pediatrics. 1980;96(6):1094–1097.
70. Foulkes LM, et al. Social support, family variables, and compliance in renal transplant children. Pediatric Nephrology (Berlin, Germany). 1993;7(2):185–188.
71. Korsch BM, Fine RN, Negrete VF. Non-compliance in children with renal transplants. Pediatrics. 1978;61(6):872–876.
72. Shaw RJ, et al. A typology of non-adherence in pediatric renal transplant recipients. Pediatric Transplantation. 2003;7(6):489–493.
73. Falkenstein K, et al. Non-compliance in children post-liver transplant. Who are the culprits? Pediatric Transplantation. 2004;8(3):233–236.
74. Serrano-Ikkos E, et al. Heart or heart-lung transplantation: psychosocial outcome. Pediatric Transplantation. 1999;3(4):301–308.
75. Cohen M, Katz D, Baruch Y. Stress among the family caregivers of liver transplant recipients. Progress in Transplantation (Aliso Viejo, Calif.). 2007;17(1):48–53.
76. Rodrigue JR, Dimitri N, Reed A, et al. Quality of life and psychosocial functioning of spouse/partner caregivers before and after liver transplantation. Clinical Transplantation. 2011;25(2):239–247.
77. Penkower L, et al. Psychological distress and adherence to the medical regimen among adolescent renal transplant recipients. American Journal of Transplantation. 2003;3(11):1418–1425.
78. Griffin KJ, Elkin TD. Non-adherence in pediatric transplantation: a review of the existing literature. Pediatric Transplantation. 2001;5(4):246–249.
79. Shemesh E, et al. Medication adherence in pediatric and adolescent liver transplant recipients. Pediatrics. 2004;113(4):825–832.
80. Griva K, Davenport A, Harrison M, Newman SP. Non-adherence to immunosuppressive medications in kidney transplantation: intent vs. forgetfulness and clinical markers of medication intake. Annals of Behavioral Medicine: A Publication of the Society of Behavioral Medicine. 2012;44(1):85–93.
81. Mintzer LL, et al. Traumatic stress symptoms in adolescent organ transplant recipients. Pediatrics. 2005;115(6):1640–1644.
82. Tong A, Morton R, Howard K, et al. "When I had my transplant, I became normal." Adolescent perspectives on life after kidney transplantation. Pediatric Transplantation. 2011;15(3):285–293.
83. van Servellen G, et al. Individual and system level factors associated with treatment non-adherence in human immunodeficiency virus-infected men and women. AIDS Patient Care and STDS. 2002;16(6):269–281.
84. Maikranz JM, et al. The relationship of hope and illness-related uncertainty to emotional adjustment and adherence among pediatric renal and liver transplant recipients. Journal of Pediatric Psychology. 2007;32(5):571–581.
85. Simons LE, et al. Parent and patient perspectives on barriers to medication adherence in adolescent transplant recipients. Pediatric Transplantation. 2009;13(3):338–347.
86. Zelikovsky N, et al. Perceived barriers to adherence among adolescent renal transplant candidates. Pediatric Transplantation. 2008;12(3):300–308.
87. Annunziato RA, et al. Adherence and medical outcomes in pediatric liver transplant recipients who transition to adult services. Pediatric Transplantation. 2007;11(6):608–614.
88. Kennedy A, Sawyer S. Transition from pediatric to adult services: are we getting it right? Current Opinion in Pediatrics. 2008;20(4):403–409.
89. Raiz LR, et al. Medication compliance following renal transplantation. Transplantation. 1999;68(1):51–55.
90. Meyers KE, Thomson PD, Weiland H. Non-compliance in children and adolescents after renal transplantation. Transplantation. 1996;62(2):186–189.
91. Germani G, Lazzaro S, Gnoato F, et al. Non-adherent behaviors after solid organ transplantation. Transplantation Proceedings. 2011;43(1):318–323.
92. Ettenger RB, Tsai EW, Fine RN. A paradigm shift and a few modest suggestions in the care of adolescent transplant recipients. Transplantation. 2011;92(11):1191–1193.
93. Cramer J, et al. Medication compliance feedback and monitoring in a clinical trial: predictors and outcomes. Value in Health. 2003;6(5):566–573.
94. Nevins TE, Thomas W. Quantitative patterns of azathioprine adherence after renal transplantation. Transplantation. 2009;87(5):711–718.
95. Haynes RB, McDonald HP, Garg AX. Helping patients follow prescribed treatment: clinical applications. JAMA: The Journal of the American Medical Association. 2002;288(22):2880–2883.
96. Hansen R, Seifeldin R, Noe L. Medication adherence in chronic disease: issues in posttransplant immunosuppression. Transplantation Proceedings. 2007;39(5):1287–1300.
97. Gordon EJ, et al. Adherence to immunosuppression: a prospective diary study. Transplantation Proceedings. 2007;39(10):3081–3085.
98. Weng FL, et al. Race and electronically measured adherence to immunosuppressive medications after deceased donor renal transplantation. Journal of the American Society of Nephrology. 2005;16(6):1839–1848.
99. Bell LE, Sawyer SM. Transition of care to adult services for pediatric solid-organ transplant recipients. Pediatric Clinics of North America. 2010;57(2):593–610, table of contents.
100. Bell LE, et al. Adolescent transition to adult care in solid organ Transplantation: a consensus conference report. American Journal of Transplantation. 2008;8(11):2230–2242.
101. Logan D, et al. The Illness Management Survey: identifying adolescents' perceptions of barriers to adherence. Journal of Pediatric Psychology. 2003;28(6):383–392.
102. Simons LE, Blount RL. Identifying barriers to medication adherence in adolescent transplant recipients. Journal of Pediatric Psychology. 2007;32(7):831–844.
103. Marhefka SL, et al. Clinical assessment of medication adherence among HIV-infected children: examination of the Treatment Interview Protocol (TIP). AIDS Care. 2004;16(3):323–338.
104. Penza-Clyve SM, Mansell C, McQuaid EL. Why don't children take their asthma medications? A qualitative analysis of children's perspectives on adherence. The Journal of Asthma. 2004;41(2):189–197.
105. Chisholm MA. Identification of medication-adherence barriers and strategies to increase adherence in recipients of renal transplants. Managed Care Interface. 2004;17(9):44–48.
106. Simons LE, McCormick ML, Devine K, Blount RL. Medication barriers predict adolescent transplant recipients′ adherence and clinical outcomes at 18-month follow-up. Journal of Pediatric Psychology. 2010;35(9):1038–1048.
107. Gerson AC, et al. Assessing associations between medication adherence and potentially modifiable psychosocial variables in pediatric kidney transplant recipients and their families. Pediatric Transplantation. 2004;8(6):543–550.
108. Tielen M, et al. Q-methodology to identify young adult renal transplant recipients at risk for non-adherence. Transplantation. 2008;85(5):700–706.
109. Cross RM. Exploring attitudes: the case for Q methodology. Health Education Research. 2005;20(2):206–213.
110. van Exel J, de Graaf G, Brouwer W. Give me a break! Informal caregiver attitudes towards respite care. Health Policy. 2008;88(1):73–87.
111. Bullington P, et al. Identification of medication non-adherence factors in adolescent transplant patients: the patient's viewpoint. Pediatric Transplantation. 2007;11(8):914–921.
112. Evans RW, Applegate WH, Briscoe DM, et al. Cost-related immunosuppressive medication non-adherence among kidney transplant recipients. Clinical Journal of the American Society of Nephrology. 2010;5(12):2323–2328.

113. Page TF, Woodward RS. Cost-effectiveness of Medicare's coverage of immunosuppression medications for kidney transplant recipients. Expert Review of Pharmacoeconomics & Outcomes Research. 2009;9(5):435–444.
114. Kasiske BL, et al. Payment for immunosuppression after organ transplantation. American Society of Transplantation. JAMA: Journal of the American Medical Association. 2000;283(18):2445–2450.
115. Chisholm-Burns MA, et al. Immunosuppressant therapy adherence and graft failure among pediatric renal transplant recipients. American Journal of Transplantation. 2009;9(11):2497–2504.
116. De Geest S, Dobbels F. Transplantation: increasing adherence to immunosuppression: a clinical priority. Nature Reviews Nephrology. 2010;6(3):139–140.
117. Pinsky BW, et al. Transplant outcomes and economic costs associated with patient non-compliance to immunosuppression. American Journal of Transplantation. 2009;9(11):2597–2606.
118. D'Antiga L, et al. Late cellular rejection in paediatric liver transplantation: aetiology and outcome. Transplantation. 2002;73(1):80–84.
119. Jain A, et al. Reasons why some children receiving tacrolimus therapy require steroids more than 5 years post liver transplantation. Pediatric Transplantation. 2001;5(2):93–98.
120. Sellers M, et al. Incidence of late acute rejection and progression to chronic rejection in pediatric liver recipients. Transplantation Proceedings. 1997;29(1–2):428–429.
121. Ringewald JM, et al. Non-adherence is associated with late rejection in pediatric heart transplant recipients. The Journal of Pediatrics. 2001;139(1):75–78.
122. Hsiau M, Fernandez HE, Gjertson D, et al. Monitoring non-adherence and acute rejection with variation in blood immunosuppressant levels in pediatric renal transplantation. Transplantation. 2011;92(8):918–922.
123. Butler JA, et al. Frequency and impact of non-adherence to immunosuppressants after renal transplantation: a systematic review. Transplantation. 2004;77(5):769–776.
124. Vlaminck H, et al. Prospective study on late consequences of subclinical non-compliance with immunosuppressive therapy in renal transplant patients. American Journal of Transplantation. 2004;4(9):1509–1513.
125. Lerut E, et al. Acute rejection in non-compliant renal allograft recipients: a distinct morphology. Clinical Transplantation. 2007;21(3):344–351.
126. Sis B, Mengel M, Haas M, et al. Banff '09 meeting report: antibody mediated graft deterioration and implementation of Banff working groups. American Journal of Transplantation.2010;10(3):464–471.
127. Solez K, et al. Banff 07 classification of renal allograft pathology: updates and future directions. American Journal of Transplantation. 2008;8(4):753–760.
128. Sellares J, de Freitas DG, Mengel M, et al. Understanding the causes of kidney transplant failure: the dominant role of antibody-mediated rejection and non-adherence. American Journal of Transplantation. 2012;12(2):388–399.
129. Terasaki PI, Ozawa M, Castro R. Four-year follow-up of a prospective trial of HLA and MICA antibodies on kidney graft survival. American Journal of Transplantation. 2007;7(2):408–415.
130. Tzeng J, Reed EF, et al. The presence of de novo donor specific anti-HLA antibody is associated with medication non-adherence and allograft loss in pediatric renal transplant recipients. American Journal of Transplantation. 2012;12(Suppl 3):310.
131. Wiebe C, et al. Evolution and clinical pathologic correlations of de novo donor-specific HLA antibody post kidney transplant. American Journal of Transplantation. 2012;12(5):1157–1167.
132. Shemesh E, Fine RN. Is calculating the standard deviation of tacrolimus blood levels the new gold standard for evaluating non-adherence to medications in transplant recipients? Pediatric Transplantation. 2010;14(8):940–943.
133. Osterberg L, Blaschke T. Adherence to medication. New England Journal of Medicine. 2005;353(5):487–497.
134. Claxton AJ, Cramer J, Pierce C. A systematic review of the associations between dose regimens and medication compliance. Clinical Therapeutics. 2001;23(8):1296–1310.
135. Venkat VL, et al. An objective measure to identify pediatric liver transplant recipients at risk for late allograft rejection related to non-adherence. Pediatric Transplantation. 2008;12(1):67–72.
136. Bucuvalas JC, et al. A novel approach to managing variation: outpatient therapeutic monitoring of calcineurin inhibitor blood levels in liver transplant recipients. Journal of Pediatrics. 2005;146(6):744–750.
137. Stuber ML, et al. Evaluating non-adherence to immunosuppressant medications in pediatric liver transplant recipients. Pediatric Transplantation. 2008;12(3):284–288.
138. Kerkar N, et al. Prospective analysis of non-adherence in autoimmune hepatitis: a common problem. Journal of Pediatric Gastroenterology and Nutrition. 2006;43(5):629–634.
139. Pollock-Barziv SM, Finkelstein Y, Manlhiot C, et al. Variability in tacrolimus blood levels increases the risk of late rejection and graft loss after solid organ transplantation in older children. Pediatric Transplantation. 2010;14(8):968–975.
140. Fernandez HE, Ettenger RB. TsaiEW, tacrolimus percent coefficient of variation as a superior marker ofLate acute rejection associated with non-adherence in adolescent renal transplant recipients. Journal of the American Society of Nephrology: JASN. 2011;22:841A. (Abstract).
141. Buchmann TN, Wolff T, Bachmann A, et al. Repeat true surveillance biopsies in kidney transplantation. Transplantation. 2012;93(9):908–913.
142. Seron D, Moreso F. Protocol biopsies in renal transplantation: prognostic value of structural monitoring. Kidney International. 2007;72(6):690–697.
143. Wilkinson A. Protocol transplant biopsies: are they really needed? Clinical Journal of the American Society of Nephrology. 2006;1(1):130–137.
144. Birk PE, et al. Surveillance biopsies are superior to functional studies for the diagnosis of acute and chronic renal allograft pathology in children. Pediatric Transplantation. 2004;8(1):29–38.
145. Orrego CM, et al. Usefulness of routine surveillance endomyocardial biopsy 6 months after heart transplantation. The Journal of Heart and Lung Transplantation. 2012;31(8):845–9.
146. Wütrich RP, Eisenberger U, Bock A, et al. *Towards a Gold Standard for Adherence Assessment in Transplantation: High Accuracy of the Proteus Raisin System (PRS) Combined with Enteric-Coated Mycophenolate Sodium (ECMPS) in Stable Kidney Transplant Recipients*, in *24th International Congress of The Transplantation Society*. 2012: Berlin, Germany. (Abstract).
147. Simons LE, et al. Multidimensional adherence classification system: initial development with adolescent transplant recipients. Pediatric Transplantation. 2009;13(5):590–598.
148. Pai AL, Rausch J, Tackett A, et al. System for integrated adherence monitoring: real-time non-adherence risk assessment in pediatric kidney transplantation. Pediatric Transplantation. 2012;16(4):329–334.
149. Shemesh E. Measuring adherence to medications: are complex methods superior to simple ones? Pediatric Transplantation. 2012;16(4):315–317.
150. De Geest S, et al. Supporting medication adherence in renal transplantation (SMART): a pilot RCT to improve adherence to immunosuppressive regimens. Clinical Transplantation. 2006;20(3):359–368.
151. Schafer-Keller P, et al. Diagnostic accuracy of measurement methods to assess non-adherence to immunosuppressive drugs in kidney transplant recipients. American Journal of Transplantation. 2008;8(3):616–626.
152. Butler JA, et al. Measuring compliance with drug regimens after renal transplantation: comparison of self-report and clinician rating with electronic monitoring. Transplantation. 2004;77(5):786–789.
153. Paterson DL, Potoski B, Capitano B. Measurement of adherence to antiretroviral medications. Journal of Acquired Immune Deficiency Syndromes. 2002;31(Suppl 3):S103–S106.
154. Miller LG, Hays RD. Measuring adherence to antiretroviral medications in clinical trials. HIV Clinical Trials. 2000;1(1):36–46.
155. Bender B, Milgrom H, Rand C. Non-adherence in asthmatic patients: is there a solution to the problem? Annals of Allergy, Asthma and Immunology. 1997;79(3):177–185, quiz 185–6.
156. Farmer KC. Methods for measuring and monitoring medication regimen adherence in clinical trials and clinical practice. Clinical Therapeutics. 1999;21(6):1074–1090, discussion 1073.
157. Hecht FM. Measuring HIV treatment adherence in clinical practice. AIDS Clinical Care. 1998;10(8):57–59.
158. Turner BJ. Adherence to antiretroviral therapy by human immunodeficiency virus-infected patients. The Journal of Infectious Diseases. 2002;185(Suppl 2):S143–S151.
159. Siegal BR. Postrenal transplant compliance: report of 519 responses to a self-report questionnaire. Transplantation Proceedings. 1993;25(4):2502.
160. Deschamps AE, et al. Diagnostic value of different adherence measures using electronic monitoring and virologic failure as reference standards. AIDS Patient Care and Stds. 2008;22(9):735–743.
161. Lennerling A, Forsberg A. Self-reported non-adherence and beliefs about medication in a Swedish kidney transplant population. Open Nursing Journal. 2012;6:41–46.
162. Chesney MA, et al. Self-reported adherence to antiretroviral medications among participants in HIV clinical trials: the AACTG adherence instruments. Patient Care Committee & Adherence Working Group of the Outcomes Committee of the Adult AIDS Clinical Trials Group (AACTG). AIDS Care. 2000;12(3):255–266.
163. Reynolds NR, et al. Optimizing measurement of self-reported adherence with the ACTG Adherence Questionnaire: a cross-protocol analysis. Journal of Acquired Immune Deficiency Syndromes. 2007;46(4):402–409.
164. Mathews WC, et al. Predictive validity of a brief antiretroviral adherence index: retrospective cohort analysis under conditions of repetitive administration. AIDS

Research and Therapy. 2008;5:20.
165. Walsh JC, Mandalia S, Gazzard BG. Responses to a 1 month self-report on adherence to antiretroviral therapy are consistent with electronic data and virological treatment outcome. AIDS (London, England). 2002;16(2):269–277.
166. Koneru S, et al. Effectively measuring adherence to medications for systemic lupus erythematosus in a clinical setting. Arthritis and Rheumatism. 2007; 57(6):1000–1006.
167. Pape L, Heidotting N, Ahlenstiel T. Once-daily tacrolimus extended-release formulation: 1 year after conversion in stable pediatric kidney transplant recipients. International Journal of Nephrology. 2011;126251.
168. Zelikovsky N, Schast AP. Eliciting accurate reports of adherence in a clinical interview: development of the Medical Adherence Measure. Pediatric Nursing. 2008;34(2):141–146.
169. Lavsa SM, Holzworth A, Ansani NT. Selection of a validated scale for measuring medication adherence. Journal of the American Pharmaceutical Association. 2011;51(1):90–94.
170. Svarstad BL, et al. The Brief Medication Questionnaire: a tool for screening patient adherence and barriers to adherence. Patient Education and Counseling. 1999;37(2):113–124.
171. Rudd P, et al. The natural history of medication compliance in a drug trial: limitations of pill counts. Clinical Pharmacology and Therapeutics. 1989;46(2): 169–176.
172. Lee JY, et al. Assessing medication adherence by pill count and electronic monitoring in the African American Study of Kidney Disease and Hypertension (AASK) Pilot Study. American Journal of Hypertension. 1996;9(8):719–725.
173. Ndubuka NO, Ehlers VJ. Adult patients' adherence to anti-retroviral treatment: a survey correlating pharmacy refill records and pill counts with immunological and virological indices. International Journal of Nursing Studies. 2011; 48(11):1323–1329.
174. Grossberg R, Zhang Y, Gross R. A time-to-prescription-refill measure of antiretroviral adherence predicted changes in viral load in HIV. Journal of Clinical Epidemiology. 2004;57(10):1107–1110.
175. Gross R, Zhang Y, Grossberg R. Medication refill logistics and refill adherence in HIV. Pharmacoepidemiology and Drug Safety. 2005;14(11):789–793.
176. de Boer IM, Prins JM, Sprangers MA, Nieuwkerk PT. Using different calculations of pharmacy refill adherence to predict virological failure among HIV-infected patients. Journal of Acquired Immune Deficiency Syndromes. 2010;55(5):635–640.
177. Hardstaff R, Green K, Talbot D. Non-compliance postrenal transplantation: measuring the extent of the problem using electronic surveillance and nurse practitioner interviews. Transplantation Proceedings. 2002;34(5):1608.
178. Liu H, et al. A comparison study of multiple measures of adherence to HIV protease inhibitors. Annals of Internal Medicine. 2001;134(10):968–977.
179. Denhaerynck K, et al. Examining assumptions regarding valid electronic monitoring of medication therapy: development of a validation framework and its application on a European sample of kidney transplant patients. BMC Medical Research Methodology. 2008;8:5.
180. Bova CA, et al. Use of electronic monitoring devices to measure antiretroviral adherence: practical considerations. AIDS and Behavior. 2005;9(1): 103–110.
181. Deschamps AE, et al. Prevalence and correlates of non-adherence to antiretroviral therapy in a population of HIV patients using Medication Event Monitoring System. AIDS Patient Care and Stds. 2004;18(11):644–657.
182. Matsui D, et al. Critical comparison of novel and existing methods of compliance assessment during a clinical trial of an oral iron chelator. Journal of Clinical Pharmacology. 1994;34(9):944–949.
183. Fernald DH, Coombs L, DeAlleaume L, et al. An assessment of the Hawthorne Effect in practice-based research. Journal of the American Board of Family Medicine. 2012;25(1):83–86.
184. McCarney R, et al. The Hawthorne Effect: a randomised, controlled trial. BMC Medical Research Methodology. 2007;7:30.
185. Wendel CS, et al. Barriers to use of electronic adherence monitoring in an HIV clinic. The Annals of Pharmacotherapy. 2001;35(9):1010–1015.
186. Wagner GJ. Does discontinuing the use of pill boxes to facilitate electronic monitoring impede adherence? International Journal of STD and AIDS. 2003; 14(1):64–65.
187. Shellmer DA, Zelikovsky N. The challenges of using medication event monitoring technology with pediatric transplant patients. Pediatric Transplantation. 2007;11(4):422–428.
188. Klein A, Otto G, Kramer I. Impact of a pharmaceutical care program on liver transplant patients' compliance with immunosuppressive medication: a prospective, randomized, controlled trial using electronic monitoring. Transplantation. 2009;87(6):839–847.
189. Cifani L, Vargo R. Teaching strategies for the transplant recipient: a review and future directions. Focus on Critical Care. 1990;17(6):476–479.
190. Hardstaff R, Green K, Talbot D. Measurement of compliance posttransplantation–the results of a 12-month study using electronic monitoring. Transplantation Proceedings. 2003;35(2):796–797.
191. Cupples SA, Steslow B. Use of behavioral contingency contracting with heart transplant candidates. Progress in Transplantation (Aliso Viejo, Calif.). 2001;11(2):137–144.
192. Chisholm MA. Enhancing transplant patients' adherence to medication therapy. Clinical Transplantation. 2002;16(1):30–38.
193. De Bleser L, Vincke B, Dobbels F, et al. A new electronic monitoring device to measure medication adherence: usability of the Helping Hand. Sensors (Basel). 2010;10(3):1535–1552.
194. Pangarakis SJ, et al. Electronic feedback messages for home spirometry lung transplant recipients. Heart and Lung: Journal of Critical Care. 2008;37(4): 299–307.
195. Miloh T, et al. Improved adherence and outcomes for pediatric liver transplant recipients by using text messaging. Pediatrics. 2009;124(5):e844–e850.
196. Dew MA, et al. An internet-based intervention to improve psychosocial outcomes in heart transplant recipients and family caregivers: development and evaluation. Journal of Heart and Lung Transplantation. 2004;23(6): 745–758.
197. van Dulmen S, et al. Patient adherence to medical treatment: a review of reviews. BMC Health Services Research. 2007;7:55.
198. De Bleser L, et al. Interventions to improve medication-adherence after transplantation: a systematic review. Transplant International. 2009;22(8): 780–797.
199. DeVito Dabbs A, et al. Evaluation of a hand-held, computer-based intervention to promote early self-care behaviors after lung transplant. Clinical Transplantation. 2009;23(4):537–545.
200. Kasiske BL. KDIGO clinical practice guideline for the care of kidney transplant recipients. American Journal of Transplantation. 2009;9(Suppl 3):S1–S155.
201. Kasiske BL, Zeier MG, Chapman JR, et al. KDIGO clinical practice guideline for the care of kidney transplant recipients: a summary. Kidney International. 2010;77(4):299–311.
202. Knoll GA, Blydt-Hansen TD, Campbell P, et al. Canadian Society of Transplantation and Canadian Society of Nephrology commentary on the 2009 KDIGO clinical practice guideline for the care of kidney transplant recipients. American Journal of Kidney Diseases. 2010;56(2):219–246.
203. Bain-Brickley D, Butler LM, Kennedy GE, Rutherford GW. Interventions to improve adherence to antiretroviral therapy in children with HIV infection. Cochrane Database of Systematic Reviews. 2010;(12):CD009513.
204. Funck-Brentano I, et al. Evaluation of a peer support group therapy for HIV-infected adolescents. AIDS (London, England). 2005;19(14):1501–1508.
205. Muller AD, Myer L, Jaspan H. Virological suppression achieved with suboptimal adherence levels among South African children receiving boosted protease inhibitor-based antiretroviral therapy. Clinical Infectious Diseases : an Official Publication of the Infectious Diseases Society of America. 2009;48(1):e3–e5.
206. Urquhart J. The odds of the three nons when an aptly prescribed medicine isn't working: non-compliance, non-absorption, non-response. British Journal of Clinical Pharmacology. 2002;54(2):212–220.
207. Yeo M, Sawyer S. Chronic illness and disability. BMJ (Clinical Research Ed.). 2005;330(7493):721–723.
208. Christie D, Viner R. Adolescent development. BMJ (Clinical Research Ed.). 2005;330(7486):301–304.
209. Byczkowski TL, Kollar LM, Britto MT. Family experiences with outpatient care: do adolescents and parents have the same perceptions? Journal of Adolescent Health. 2010;47(1):92–98.
210. Butner J, et al. Parent-adolescent discrepancies in adolescents' competence and the balance of adolescent autonomy and adolescent and parent well-being in the context of Type 1 diabetes. Developmental Psychology. 2009;45(3):835–849.
211. Bunzel B, Laederach-Hofmann K. Solid organ transplantation: are there predictors for posttransplant non-compliance? A literature overview. Transplantation. 2000;70(5):711–716.
212. Rhodes F, et al. Using theory to understand how interventions work: project RESPECT, condom use, and the Integrative Model. AIDS and Behavior. 2007;11(3):393–407.
213. Douglas S, Blixen C, Bartucci MR. Relationship between pretransplant noncompliance and posttransplant outcomes in renal transplant recipients. Journal of Transplant Coordination. 1996;6(2):53–58.
214. Chisholm MA, et al. Predicting adherence to immunosuppressant therapy: a prospective analysis of the theory of planned behaviour. Nephrology, Dialysis, Transplantation. 2007;22(8):2339–2348.
215. KDIGO clinical practice guideline for the care of kidney transplant recipients. American Journal of Transplantation. 2009;9(Suppl 3):S1–S155.
216. Bia M, Adey DB, Bloom RD, et al. KDOQI US commentary on the 2009 KDIGO clinical practice guideline for the care of kidney transplant recipients. American

Journal of Kidney Diseases. 2010;56(2):189–218.
217. Dew MA, et al. Meta-analysis of risk for relapse to substance use after transplantation of the liver or other solid organs. Liver Transplantation. 2008;14(2):159–172.
218. Troppmann C, et al. Retransplantation after renal allograft loss due to non-compliance. Indications, outcome, and ethical concerns. Transplantation. 1995;59(4):467–471.
219. Dunn TB, et al. Selective retransplant after graft loss to non-adherence: success with a second chance. American Journal of Transplantation. 2009;9(6):1337–1346.
220. Dobbels F, et al. Pretransplant predictors of posttransplant adherence and clinical outcome: an evidence base for pretransplant psychosocial screening. Transplantation. 2009;87(10):1497–1504.
221. DiMatteo MR. Variations in patients' adherence to medical recommendations: a quantitative review of 50 years of research. Medical Care. 2004;42(3):200–209.
222. Dobbels F, Hames A, Aujoulat I, et al. Should we retransplant a patient who is non-adherent? A literature review and critical reflection. Pediatric Transplantation. 2012;16(1):4–11.
223. Siegal B, Greenstein SM. Profiles of non-compliance in patients with a functioning renal transplant: a multicenter study. Compliance Study Group. Transplantation Proceedings. 1999;31(1-2):1326–1327.
224. Chisholm MA, et al. Impact of clinical pharmacy services on renal transplant patients' compliance with immunosuppressive medications. Clinical Transplantation. 2001;15(5):330–336.
225. Conn VS, et al. Searching for the intervention in intervention research reports. Journal of Nursing Scholarship. 2008;40(1):52–59.
226. Pignone MP, et al. Counseling to promote a healthy diet in adults: a summary of the evidence for the U.S. Preventive Services Task Force. American Journal of Preventive Medicine. 2003;24(1):75–92.
227. Haynes RB, et al. Interventions to enhance medication adherence. Cochrane Database of Systematic Reviews. 2005;(4):CD000011.
228. Salema NE, Elliott RA, Glazebrook C. A systematic review of adherence-enhancing interventions in adolescents taking long-term medicines. Journal of Adolescent Health. 2011;49(5):455–466.
229. Ingerski L, Perrazo L, Goebel J, Pai AL. Family strategies for achieving medication adherence in pediatric kidney transplantation. Nursing Research. 2011; 60(3):190–196.
230. Schulz M, et al. Pharmaceutical care services for asthma patients: a controlled intervention study. Journal of Clinical Pharmacology. 2001;41(6):668–676.
231. Morisky DE, et al. Predictive validity of a medication adherence measure in an outpatient setting. Journal of Clinical Hypertension (Greenwich, Conn.). 2008;10(5):348–354.
232. Dean AJ, Walters J, Hall A. A systematic review of interventions to enhance medication adherence in children and adolescents with chronic illness. Archives of Disease in Childhood. 2010;95(9):717–723.
233. Kripalani S, Yao X, Haynes RB. Interventions to enhance medication adherence in chronic medical conditions: a systematic review. Archives of Internal Medicine. 2007;167(6):540–550.
234. Roter DL, et al. Effectiveness of interventions to improve patient compliance: a meta-analysis. Medical Care. 1998;36(8):1138–1161.
235. Peterson AM, Takiya L, Finley R. Meta-analysis of trials of interventions to improve medication adherence. American Journal of Health-System Pharmacy. 2003;60(7):657–665.
236. Haynes RB, et al. Interventions for helping patients to follow prescriptions for medications. Cochrane Database of Systematic Reviews. 2002;(2):CD000011.
237. Rapoff MA, et al. Prevention of non-adherence to nonsteroidal anti-inflammatory medications for newly diagnosed patients with juvenile rheumatoid arthritis. Health Psychology. 2002;21(6):620–623.
238. Petry NM, Rash CJ, Byrne S, et al. Financial reinforcers for improving medication adherence: findings from a meta-analysis. American Journal of Medicine. 2012;125(9):889–896.
239. Godley SH, et al. Contingent reinforcement of personal goal activities for adolescents with substance use disorders during post-residential continuing care. American Journal on Addictions. 2008;17(4):278–286.
240. KyngAs HA, Kroll T, Duffy ME. Compliance in adolescents with chronic diseases: a review. Journal of Adolescent Health. 2000;26(6):379–388.
241. DiMatteo MR. Social support and patient adherence to medical treatment: a meta-analysis. Health Psychology. 2004;23(2):207–218.
242. De Geest S, et al. Development of the long-term medication behaviour self-efficacy scale: qualitative study for item development. Journal of Advanced Nursing. 1994;19(2):233–238.
243. DiMatteo MR, Lepper HS, Croghan TW. Depression is a risk factor for non-compliance with medical treatment: meta-analysis of the effects of anxiety and depression on patient adherence. Archives of Internal Medicine. 2000;160(14):2101–2107.
244. Krummenacher I, Cavassini M, Bugnon O, Schneider MP. An interdisciplinary HIV-adherence program combining motivational interviewing and electronic antiretroviral drug monitoring. AIDS Care. 2011;23(5):550–561.
245. Bodenheimer T, et al. Patient self-management of chronic disease in primary care. JAMA: Journal of the American Medical Association. 2002;288(19):2469–2475.
246. Gordon EJ, et al. Can focusing on self-care reduce disparities in kidney transplantation outcomes? American Journal of Kidney Diseases. 2005;45(5):935–940.
247. Fennell RS, Foulkes LM, Boggs SR. Family-based program to promote medication compliance in renal transplant children. Transplantation Proceedings. 1994;26(1):102–103.
248. Doesch AO, Mueller S, Konstandin M, et al. Increased adherence after switch from twice daily calcineurin inhibitor based treatment to once daily modified released tacrolimus in heart transplantation: a pre-experimental study. Transplantation Proceedings. 2010;42(10):4238–4242.
249. Saini SD, et al. Effect of medication dosing frequency on adherence in chronic diseases. American Journal of Managed Care. 2009;15(6):e22–e33.
250. Baird MG, et al. A study of efficacy, tolerance and compliance of once-daily versus twice-daily metoprolol (Betaloc) in hypertension. Betaloc Compliance Canadian Cooperative Study Group. Clinical and Investigative Medicine. Medecine Clinique et Experimentale. 1984;7(2):95–102.
251. Becker LA, et al. A randomized trial of special packaging of antihypertensive medications. Journal of Family Practice. 1986;22(4):357–361.
252. Brown BG, et al. Moderate dose, three-drug therapy with niacin, lovastatin, and colestipol to reduce low-density lipoprotein cholesterol <100 mg/dl in patients with hyperlipidemia and coronary artery disease. American Journal of Cardiology. 1997;80(2):111–115.
253. Girvin B, McDermott BJ, Johnston GD. A comparison of enalapril 20 mg once daily versus 10 mg twice daily in terms of blood pressure lowering and patient compliance. Journal of Hypertension. 1999;17(11):1627–1631.
254. Eisen SA, et al. The effect of prescribed daily dose frequency on patient medication compliance. Archives of Internal Medicine. 1990;150(9):1881–1884.
255. First MR. First clinical experience with the new once-daily formulation of tacrolimus. Therapeutic Drug Monitoring. 2008;30(2):159–166.
256. Guirado L, et al. Efficacy and safety of conversion from twice-daily to once-daily tacrolimus in a large cohort of stable kidney transplant recipients. American Journal of Transplantation. 1965;11(9):71.
257. Hougardy JM, de Jonge H, Kuypers D, Abramowicz D. The once-daily formulation of tacrolimus: a step forward in kidney transplantation? Transplantation.2012;93(3):241–243.
258. de Jonge H, Kuypers DR, Verbeke K, et al. Reduced C0 concentrations and increased dose requirements in renal allograft recipients converted to the novel once-daily tacrolimus formulation. Transplantation.2010;90(5):523–529.
259. Hougardy JM, Broeders N, Kianda M, et al. Conversion from Prograf to Advagraf among kidney transplant recipients results in sustained decrease in tacrolimus exposure. Transplantation. 2011;91(5):566–569.
260. Shield CF 3rd, McGrath MM, Goss TF. Assessment of health-related quality of life in kidney transplant patients receiving tacrolimus (FK506)-based versus cyclosporine-based immunosuppression. FK506 Kidney Transplant Study Group. Transplantation. 1997;64(12):1738–1743.
261. Fine RN, Martz K, Stablein D. What have 20 years of data from the North American Pediatric Renal Transplant Cooperative Study taught us about growth following renal transplantation in infants, children, and adolescents with end-stage renal disease? Pediatric Nephrology (Berlin, Germany).2010;25(4):739–746.
262. Sarwal MM, Yorgin PD, Alexander S, et al. Promising early outcomes with a novel, complete steroid avoidance immunosuppression protocol in pediatric renal transplantation. Transplantation. 2001;72(1):13–21.
263. Filler G, Huang SH. Progress in pediatric kidney transplantation. Therapeutic Drug Monitoring. 2010;32(3):250–252.
264. Srinivas TR, Meier-Kriesche HU. Minimizing immunosuppression, an alternative approach to reducing side effects: objectives and interim result. Clinical Journal of the American Society of Nephrology. 2008;3(Suppl 2):S101–S116.

第 121 章 器官移植受者从儿童过渡到成人的健康管理

Sandra Amaral, Lorraine E. Bell

引言

在二十世纪六七十年代是儿童移植的初始阶段。儿童移植很少且死亡率高[1]。受体成功地成长为成人的数量少，所以他们到成人的临床结果很少得到关注。从二十世纪八十年代以来，儿童移植随着医学、药物和外科手术的明显进步，一些器官受体的 10 年生存率达到了 95%[1,2]。儿童移植的全部数量和在婴儿及儿童早期接受移植的儿童比例有明显增加，且儿童受体成长为成人的数量持续增加。儿童看护者在帮助儿童慢性疾病的复杂医学问题、疾病知识和技能上过渡到成人健康保健系统的过程中存在较大挑战。本章将讨论成功过渡的促进因素和障碍，并回顾增强过渡患者保健质量的最佳实践的推荐。其他关于该话题依从性问题的讨论参见第 120 章。

背景

将过渡期和转移作为两个独立的整体很关键。前者是过程，后者是事件。过渡最佳的定义为“慢性生理和医学状况的青少年和年轻成年有目的、有计划地从儿童为中心转移为成人为中心的健康保健系统的过程”[3]。这个定义综合了包括心理、生理和青少年期间发育改变的广泛因素。过渡期保健的提供是会随着转移为医疗保健分离点出现并持续很长一段时间的过程。过渡青年的定义与儿童器官移植并无特异之处。事实上，许多最新的关于青少年和年轻成年最佳保健的实践推荐和指南是从那些有广泛的慢性疾病的患者研究中得出的[3,4]。

解决青少年和年轻成年移植受体的过渡需求并不仅包括其移植物功能，还包括他们的生存，这些都很关键。一些大型研究在转移为成人保健的时间框架和年龄范围中观察到了更高的移植物衰竭发生率。Samuel 等利用一个加拿大的登记数据，评估了转移适应期间移植物失功是否有所增加[5]。他们采用“适应时间”为第一次记录的成人访问前 6 个月到访问后 2.5 年之间。与之前的时期相比，适应时间为 2.24 (95%CI:1.19~4.20)。当他们缩小适应时间到转移前 6 个月到转移后 6 个月，调整的移植物失功危险比甚至更高，为 5.42 (95%CI:2.83~10.39)。相似的，美国审计办公室的一项政府报告评估了不同年龄组的肾移植失败率，儿童对比“过渡期”对比成人[6]。该研究确定那些儿童期接受移植并在随后 7 年内到 18 岁的移植受体为“过渡期”。到移植术后 5 年，过渡期受体的移植失败率为 33%，两倍于儿童受体的 16%，轻度高于成人受体的 28%。其假定该过渡组在随访期间转移了医学保健。相反，加拿大的一项 115 例肾移植受体的单医疗中心研究发现过渡期的移植物衰竭无明显增加，新西兰的胰腺研究显示转移为成人保健期间的患者(平均年龄为 18 岁)急性排斥发生率并无增加[7,8]。因此，转移并不是必定会导致排斥或移植物失功。需要进一步的研究来弄清楚哪些患者和医疗保健系统因素可在过渡期间保护或预示移植物功能不良或丢失。

年龄也被认为是青少年和年轻的成年人过渡期间同种异体移植物失功风险增加的一个独立的危险因素。Smith 和他的同事们报道了相比于北美儿童肾移植协会(NAPRTCS)的更年轻的肾移植受体，美国 13~17 岁的青少年肾移植受体的移植物失功，晚期急性排斥和不完全排斥的风险更高[9]。使用一个更大的数据库，美国肾脏数据系统(USRDS)，Foster 等发现转移时年龄小于 21 岁的患者年龄标准化移植失败率是每 100 人 12.9，相比于那些转移时年龄≥21 岁的患者为每 100 人 8.7[10]。在加拿大，Kiberd 在两个不同的年龄范围:18~24 岁和 25~35 岁，比较了< 18 岁时在儿童医院接受移

植和在成人医院接受移植的年轻成人之间的移植物生存率[11]。25~35 岁之间的患者相较于儿童和年轻患者(18~24 岁)组(HR 0.45;95%CI 为 0.25~0.82)有明显更好的移植物生存率。然而,移植生存率在儿童和 18~24 岁的年轻患者中无明显差异,无论护理是否转移。在最近的一次非常重要的 USRDS 研究中,Foster 等研究了移植时年龄和当前年龄作为同种异体移植物失功的危险因素的状况[12]。在第一次肾移植时小于 40 岁的患者中,相比于更年轻和更年长的年龄组,无论移植时年龄和移植术后时间,年龄较大的青少年和年轻患者(17~24 岁)移植失败的风险最高。

青春期和年轻成人的正常的发育过程可能导致这个时期观察到的移植物失功的增加(表 121.1)[13-17]。“情感”大脑和“执行”大脑有不同的发展轨迹,且执行功能是成熟最慢的[18]。良好的神经成像研究表明,大脑直到 20 几岁的中晚期才会完全成熟[19-22]。风险通常在成年早期达到顶峰;这在复杂的神经心理学试验和发病率-死亡率统计中都能看到[18,23]。年轻人(18~25 岁)意外死亡,药物滥用和性风险的概率最高[23]。这个风险最高时正值青年转到成人保健的时间。它通常是其他压力事件可能发生的时期,如要离开家,搬到另一个城市工作或接受教育,以及强烈的情感或浪漫的关系。所有这些因素的融合,在一个年轻人慢性疾病的药物不依从性和错过医疗预约中发挥了作用。

无论是年龄或转移哪个更重要,一个过渡的年轻成人移植受体防止同种异体移植物失功的需求不仅对于患者个体同时对于社会也至关重要。每一个潜在的由于发生的转移或过渡问题出现的可预防的器官失功增加了世界上本有限的器官供应的需求。此外,患者失去一个同种异体移植物并回到透析治疗增加了大量经济负担。透析状态患者相比于一个移植患者工作的可能性更少,并且透析的医疗成本远远高于移植患者[6]。

虽然认为不依从会导致同种异体移植物在过渡期间失功,依从性在本书中有专门章节进行介绍;当前章

表 121.1　青少年和年轻成人的发育阶段和相应临床方法建议

	青少年早期(10~13 岁)	青少年中期(14~16 岁)	青少年晚期(17~21 岁)
认知、情感和道德	• 具体思维 • 一些抽象思维的开始 • 不能把握决定的长期结果 • 提高情感唤起能力 • 感觉寻求 • 以奖励为导向	• 抽象思维的增加 • 紧张情况下的具体思维 • 可能开始考虑行动的未来后果,但决策时不采用 • 冒险行为的高度脆弱性 • 调节影响和行为时会有困难	• 复杂的抽象思维 • 更面向未来的:制订长期计划,延迟满足,设定限制 • 更好的情绪稳定性 • 理想主义但有时专制主义,对反对意见的不宽容
自我概念和(或)身份的形成	• 幻想和面向现实 • 对形象的自我意识	• 自省的增加 • 可能有强烈的内心躁动感 • 关注自身吸引力	• 个人认识的发展 • 更稳定的身体形象;吸引力可能仍然很重要
家人和同事	• 来自父母的情感分离的开始 • 隐私的需求 • 强烈的认同感和归属感的开始	• 从父母和家庭情感的进一步分离 • 在自治中斗争和冲突 • 强烈的同伴的认同和参与	• 从情感和身体上与家庭分离 • 同龄群体和(或)同行的重要性降低 • 稳定关系的形成
社会关系	• 对中学和(或)高中早期的适应	• 技能和机会的评估 • 早期职业计划 • 现实角色模型至关重要	• 职业决策中心 • 职业能力和经济独立的发展
在诊所访问探讨和讨论的建议主题	• 对患者和父母介绍私人秘密访问的概念 • 简单指导患者的互动问题 • 简单互动咨询	• 朋友、空闲时间活动、家庭生活、学校的询问 • 以无威胁的、中立的方式询问任何关于毒品、酒精、性行为或其他法律上有麻烦的尝试 • 讨论健康生活	• 讨论健康生活习惯和改善整体健康的个人干预措施 • 识别不健康的生活习惯及其后果 • 讨论个人、教育和职业目标 • 建立早期年龄段的相关问题(见左侧)

节将更关注于与过渡性照顾提供相关的系统性问题。

过渡青少年和成年移植受体保健提供的推荐和指南

有很多文献提供了过渡期保健的推荐建议，但很少有数据支持的特定的循证指南[17,24-29]。Bell 等报道了多个移植协会的国际合作中对实体器官移植受体过渡期的保健建议[17]。这份报道反映了来自各种儿童和成人移植的医生和护士、心理学家、社会工作者，以及管理员的专家意见。Webb 等之后在英国进行了一次类似的会议，同时包括了患者和父母[30]。一般来说，不同的专家小组推荐了几个主要的主题和关键的过渡因素，其与由青少年医学协会推进的过渡保健措施的基本原则和基本步骤是一致的(表 121.2)的[3]。这些建议中的很多仅受到了来自不同过渡期患者的观点的小的定性研究支持。这里我们将讨论这些至关重要的因素。至关重要的是，记住"过渡的最优目标是提供不间断的、协调发展的、相适应的、心理的需求和全面的医疗保健"[3]。

早期开始

大多数共识指南和推荐建议过渡的准备应在青春期早期开始，一般年龄为 12~14 岁[31-33]；之前的一些建议是为了促进社会和医学上的进行性独立[17,25,34]，没有一个年龄、时间和方法是最适合用来介绍转移概念的。早期的介绍可能意味着简单地承认有一天患者会成年并需要转移。父母意识到医生希望自己的孩子长大成人，尽管他们患有疾病，他们需要为他(她)的未来制订计划。早期引入过渡的概念可以帮助父母建立年龄和发展适当的任务和他们慢性疾病孩子应负的职责，并增强孩子定期上学和参加社会活动的需求。表 121.3 说明了父母和他们的孩子如何分享医疗任务以及从父母到孩子逐渐转变的主要责任[17,35,36]。这些是帮助一个孩子发展自我负责和自主权的关键因素。

表 121.2 对提供青少年和年轻成人移植受体过渡保健的关键因素

1.在青春期早期开始讨论过渡问题
2.过渡期保健必须灵活、个体化和适当发展。保健必须解决青少年常见地对健康和生活方式担忧问题
3.必须针对提高患者的自主权、增加患者的个人责任感和促进自力更生与患者潜在的独立
4.必须有一个指定的医疗专业人士负责过渡的过程。每位患者和家庭应该有一个过渡保健协调员和倡导者
5.应该有一个详细的书面过渡计划，并根据每一位年轻人和他(她)的家庭来更新
6.必须有一个方便患者和接受医疗服务提供者的简洁、便携式医学总结
7.必须关注支持移植受体在过渡和过渡期间连续健康保险覆盖
8.在转移保健之前、期间和之后的时间里，儿童和成人卫生保健提供者之间必须有沟通
9.转移不应该发生在危机时刻，应该由家庭成员、患者和儿童以及成人提供者共同商定
10.监护和法律能力问题应该在成人之前澄清

在医学访问中，儿科护士和医生应该花一部分的时间直接与儿童沟通，鼓励他(她)回答一些病史的问题和了解治疗方案。这可以帮助患者感觉自己是团队的一员，增强他(她)在治疗过程中的积极作用。

此外，甚至在青春期的早期，儿科医生需在部分访问中单独访问患者。医疗访问期间私人一对一的医疗访问在年轻人感知到的保健质量中扮演重要的角色，并被美国儿科学会推荐作为青少年的医疗质量的一个组成部分[37]。在青春期的早期，这种独立访问可能是非常具体的，访问者会问"你在学校最喜欢的科目是什么?你喜欢做什么?"内容不重要，重要的是访问者和患者之间开始构建的关系和信任。这个私人访问(照顾者没有表现的）提供了患者一个磨炼对成人健康自我管理至关重要的沟通技巧和提供患者交流可能仍未揭露的私密信息的机会。患者报告中说被认为独立是让他们准备转移的重要的部分[38,39]。一些医疗中心在候诊室张贴了海报，这些海报会解释隐私权，并提醒患者和家庭：和家庭初级卫生保健提供者之间发生主要关系的是患者而不是其父母。医疗服务提供者知道并理解国家、省和(或)联邦法律对未成年人管理隐私和知情同意的问题很重要，因为这些会由于不同的管辖而有所不同。

灵活的、个性化的、发展的适当关心

器官移植受体可能有神经认知和成熟的延迟，有时这些都不是显而易见的[40-43]。因此过渡保健的策略需要灵活性。根据患者神经认知功能的状况制订一个过渡计划很重要。这可能需要一个心理学家来参与正式评估患者医疗自我管理和独立的潜能，以及避免不切

表 121.3 儿童和青少年的领导和(或)自我管理技能发展的建议方法

阶段/年龄	形成管理技能基础的儿童能力、行动	父母的领导力行为支持孩子增加能力
婴幼儿(1~3 岁)父母作为执行者	• 配合常规治疗作用有限 • 理解受到父母的限制 • 帮助管理设备和用品(如口服药物分配器、肠内喂养用品)	• 治疗仪式:孩子知道会发生什么,可以通过重复学习 • 与孩子分享识别可能的治疗作用 • 强调卫生预防感染(如洗手、牙齿清洁、安全处理宠物)
学前期(4~5 岁)儿童开始学习基本自我保健	• 进一步参与自我保健(如帮助收集药物或治疗用品) • 医疗中的扮演:如通过护士或医生包、玩偶,来经历患者相似的治疗(如静脉穿刺、腹膜透析、营养管等) • 开始识别身体部位对他(她)的健康状况很重要 • 学习健康状况的名称(如心脏、肾脏、肝移植手术等) • 学习移植相关问题和药物副作用的名词(如感觉不适、恶心、尿痛、皮肤病变)	• 在诊所和(或)医院访问时用简单具体的名词来解释 • 设置公平且适当的限制(例如按时服药、刷牙、饮食和液体要求,感染预防战略) • 允许选择(适当的时候),如哪种药先吃 • 接受管理例程和限制 • 当治疗引起不适(如注射、抽血)时,安慰他(她)而不是责备或惩罚
学龄期早期 (6~9 岁) 儿童能提供一些自我保健	• 识别一个或两个主要的身体内部问题的线索(例如发热、腹痛、移植物疼痛、排尿困难、肿胀) • 积极参与具体的保健和监测状况 (如口腔卫生、液体摄入量、在个人药物记录本上记录药物) • 增加对健康状况的理解,原发器官衰竭原因,治疗要求的具体水平	• 与孩子的"规则"谈判来合作完成所有治疗(如在父母面前按时服药) • 鼓励健康生活(有规律的锻炼,健康的食物选择) • 支持规范活动(体育、其他组织的活动)来鼓励健身,团队合作,获得成就感 • 讨论和规范方法告诉老师、朋友,对教练分享关于健康状况和细节
青少年早期 (10~13 岁)父母成为"管理者"对比"执行者"青少年表现越来越多的自我保健和一些自我管理	• 增加对移植条件和对日常生活影响的理解 • 学习移植器官排斥的症状和(或)体征 • 开始直接与卫生保健提供者进行交流,最初在父母的面前 • 独立完成一些医学自我管理任务 (如药物的警示,预约和测试的行程,学习药物名称、剂量和时间,以及过敏情况) • 在家长的监督下准备药物剂量盒子 • 学习如何应对来自同辈的压力,但仍然照顾自己	• 提供工具让孩子自己管理[如记录治疗和服药的笔记本和(或)议事日程] • 密切观察过程,提供及时的纠正性反馈 • 保持现状和参与保健、决策和监控 • 有新的症状,治疗和紧急情况的变化 • 确保孩子已告知重要他人(如朋友、老师、教练)关于他(她)的移植情况,如果需要他们可以提供哪些帮助 • 进一步鼓励上述的健康生活和规范的活动
青少年中期 (14~16 岁)父母成为"监督人"青少年成为日常常规保健的主要"管理者"	• 获得治疗要求、并发症预防和移植器官排斥的更多抽象知识 • 发展策略来完成日常管理任务,比如按时服药(警示、日常常规提示) • 学习药物的作用,不规则服药的副作用 • 参加预约过程 • 在复杂情况下有效地要求援助 • 阅读更多关于移植和他(她)的潜在条件	• 谈判和协商谁做什么 • 讨论新问题(如:性、毒品、酒精),相关的同龄群体活动、压力和任何对移植条件的影响 • 开始讨论职业教育目标和保险问题 • 鼓励社区参与(如俱乐部、志愿工作、课外活动组) • 考虑青少年参与兼职工作或暑期就业
青少年晚期、父母成为青少年的"顾问"	• 实现作为胜任的移植状况管理者的自我意识 • 整合他(她)移植保健的现实和相关风险 • 尽管约束管理还能感受移植的好处 • 继续发展更加独立的过渡到成人基础服务的健康和社区支持网络 • 承诺终身治疗	• 采用灵活的沟通方式与青少年保持知情但不干预 • 保持现在的支持并解决问题 • 提供青年从儿童过渡到成人保健服务的鼓励和指导 • 鼓励职业学院或大学培训和(或)融入劳动力

实际的过高或过低的期望。过渡保健的目的包括帮助患者设定目标、自我宣传、医疗自我管理和解决问题。患者、家庭和医疗团队的期望必须考虑患者的能力和潜力。

提供发展的适当保健同样适用于青少年为中心的保健。提供者需要解决常见青少年和年轻人的健康和生活方式的问题,如生殖健康、消极的健康行为(喝酒、吸烟、无保护措施的性行为),以及积极的健康行为(健康饮食、锻炼)和情绪障碍筛查。在美国,据估13%以上的高中青少年有严重的自杀倾向,47%有性行为史,其中12.9%没有使用避孕措施[44]。暴力也在美国高中青少年中流行,32.8%的报告存在身体对抗和8%报告性虐待[44]。一个广泛的包括性历史的社会心理访谈对于男女同样重要。最近的研究表明,男性青少年的性和生殖健康需求往往得不到关注[45]。一个常见的青少年社会心理访谈是HEEAADSSS(家,教育和就业,饮食,活动,情感,毒品,性,自杀和抑郁,安全)[13]。虽然移植专科医生可能觉得这些青少年问题对于一般儿童看护者最好延迟,通常青少年的初级保健使用率很低[46,47]。因此,青少年移植受体可能没有一个与他们建立起信任和融洽关系的保健提供者。此外,他们可能受益于讨论和他们移植相关的心理问题和医疗方案,并有需要更多关注的特殊领域,比如优化疫苗接种、健康相关旅游风险、性、生育期的遗传咨询。

另一个全面、个性化保健的部分是职业和教育的评估、指导和支持。教育是健康相关行为、自主权、就业、社会经济地位和医疗保险的一个重要决定因素[48,49]。优化儿童移植受体的潜力教育可以促进他们的长期健康和幸福以及他们在成年生活中的适应。社会工作者是来帮助解决这些问题的多学科过渡服务中的重要团队成员。

有时,患者可能在门诊预约时带来同伴或者重要的人。这些都是评估和参与患者的支持系统的良好机会。患者的支持系统中包括概念化的同伴,是很重要的。患者也表达了渴望有相似经历的"伙伴"帮助过渡[50]。在英国,青年工人作为同行和榜样已经纳入一个过渡诊所模型[51]。同伴支持的可能性包括鼓励青少年和年轻成人移植受体在诊所访问中互相参与和促进为他们定期安排医疗以外的社交活动[51]。

增强患者自主权

年轻成人移植受体往往在转移之前表达让自己能作为成年人对待的偏好[33,38]。医疗服务提供者与患者及其家庭合作来识别那些责任增加的特定患者的特殊任务,这是必不可少的。例如,患者可能听父母的话联系药房补充药物,然后在他(她)父母监督下完成这件事,最后独立做这件事。医疗保健预约是另一个需要的学习技能。患者可以听父母的建议通过电话或一次临床访问后亲自预约。患者可以与父母一起完成几次,然后独立完成。类似于一个青少年学习如何开车。家长或监护人可能先做然后孩子学习,让他们熟悉刹车和油门,如何启动,如何加速等。然后青少年在父母陪伴的情况下驾驶,并提供反馈。最后,经过实践后,青少年足以获得驾照和独立驾驶。虽然驾驶不等同于医疗自我管理,但所涉及的学开车步骤与许多的独立的健康倡导是相同的。这些基于任务的成就需要时间、实践和监督,家长或监护人应在这过程中积极参与。自主权的进一步增强建议可见表121.1和表121.3。

指定的专业健康保健

指南建议应该有一个促进保健成果的过渡"领导者"[17,31]。一般来说,在成人或儿童医疗中心这一责任将由医生承担。还有每位患者都有过渡倡导或协调员的需求,通常有直接服务者,比如移植协调员、护士、社会工作者或病例管理员。在一些中心,他(她)可能是一位青年工人[51],主要接触评估患者的过渡进程,帮助患者在过渡期间掌握医疗系统保健。理想的网站资源包括移植医生、外科医生、指定移植护士、护士协调员、社会工作者、心理学家和指定的转移联络人;在成人医疗中心可能还包括生殖专家和泌尿科医生[17,51]。此外,强烈推荐患者有一个可提供连续性一般护理的初级保健提供者。

书面的过渡计划

重要的是,提供者、患者和家庭成员共同努力构建一个特定的过渡计划。一个医疗中心可能首先是对所有患者提供一般的计划并根据患者和家人的反馈以及患者的发展阶段和潜在的独立性来调整。一份书面计划鼓励拥有可以清楚设置和系统评估的期望和目标。同时应该基于患者进展和挑战定期检查和更新。一些项目每年都进行正式的过渡评估。其间期可能取决于所需的患者和项目的资源,但至少应该是每年评估。

便携式医疗总结

儿科医疗服务提供者应该制订一个综合患者和接受的医疗服务提供者的简洁但全面的医疗总结,以便于在患者转移和紧急情况时传播知识。至少应该包括主要诊断、移植日期、移植重大事件(如活检、排斥、药物治疗变化、感染等)、一个更新的药物清单、药物过敏和禁忌、心理状况、医疗保险状态、最近的实验室研究和可以使健康提供者联系到患者和(或)照顾者的全面联系信息。以患者为导向的便携式医疗总结的一个很好的例子是来自加拿大多伦多儿童医院的"我的健康护照"[52]。它可在互联网存取,包括特定的移植模型,患者可以在医疗服务提供者的帮助下完成。输入的数据将转换为可打印、钱包大小的医疗总结。其也可以根据电子健康记录产生一个简明医学总结。轻便、简洁的总结可以有许多形式,包括图片、音频、视频或存储于 USB 驱动器。美国儿科学会通过信息技术的使用加强了医疗卫生信息在医疗提供者和多个健康保健设定之间的传播,也改善了患者过渡保健的质量[53]。

健康保险覆盖

转移到成人保健应适当考虑青少年和(或)年轻成人的经济因素。如果一个患者有即将失去医疗保险的风险,应考虑延迟转移。相比于其他年龄组,年轻成人的医疗保险覆盖率最低[54]。2000—2010 年,18~64 岁之间的美国成年人的私人健康保险覆盖百分比有明显下降,没有保险的人群明显增加[54]。在美国有广泛的宣传来扩大肾移植受体的免疫抑制药物覆盖，以避免由于保险缺口导致的移植物失功。据估计,免疫抑制药物覆盖的延伸会产生显著的节约成本[55]。虽然没有保险是一个大问题,不足额保险就显得没有那么严重了。许多青少年由于所需的服务覆盖不足而承受不良的健康结果,包括预防、生殖和行为健康[47,56,57]。无论国家医疗系统如何,在过渡期间及之后,确保过渡年轻人可以使用并负担继续接受促进移植物和患者的生存的必要的药物和治疗是至关重要。

成人和儿童提供者之间的沟通

在一些移植中心，儿童和成人提供者共同参与随访患者,交替访问或同时访问。在其他中心,过渡的努力分别集中在儿童或成人中心。过渡护理模型的实施在很大程度上取决于可获得的资源和医疗系统的结构。目前没有一个已知的模型优于另一个。无论什么样的保健模型,儿童医疗提供者和成人提供者互相沟通来确保患者保健的最佳连续性是至关重要的。患者对于不足的儿童和成人医疗提供者之间的沟通表示失望[33]。沟通应该贯穿转移发生的之前、期间和之后,并应通过多种形式出现,如书面交流以及电话或生活会议等。交流也应该专注针对相关的医学和心理问题提供一个简洁但全面的总结。

儿科医疗团队成员在典型的诊所时间做一个成人移植中心的网站访问是非常有帮助的，这样过渡的患者可以被告知更准确的期望。这可能包括医生和护士互动、预约时间、血液测试如何安排、候诊室的样子、通常等待多长时间、哪里停车等等。许多患者对于儿童和成人医疗中心之间的差异是缺乏了解的[50]。成人的一些医疗中心在首次正式访问前可以参观设施，这获得了患者良好的反馈[38,50]。

沟通的另一个重要方面是治疗方案信息的分享。成人和儿童移植专家互相熟悉对方的方法是很重要的。任何理想的免疫抑制修改方案应该发生在转移之前，并允许患者在更改之前的一段时间内维持药物水平稳定。转移后早期的药物治疗修正会导致混乱、计量混乱,有时会导致缺乏信任。

避免在危急时转移

理想情况下,转移的时机应该预先获得患者、家庭成员和提供者的同意[17,30,50]。虽然许多卫生保健系统授权特定年龄界限,目前仍没有理想的转移年龄。然而,如果一个患者是在一个不稳定的或转移要求年龄时不断出问题的医疗情况(比如出现严重的并发症,如排斥或移植术后恶性肿瘤)下,应尽一切努力推迟转移直到达到一个合理稳定的状态。在治疗不断变化的情况下或者当患者的病情恶化时转移患者，可能会破坏患者和家庭成员对新的治疗团队的信心。同样心理危机期间应避免转移。在某些情况下,一些意外事件可能导致需要紧急或意外转移;例如,一些儿科中心会迫使怀孕女性转移到其他有可以帮助患者随后的分娩之前及之后高位风险的青少年医学服务的中心。当需要紧急转移时，最好的方法是儿童和成人提供者之间的良好的沟通，儿童和成人团队，患者和家庭之间有一个透明的转移计划。这将有助于避免“退回”的问题。如果有了计划，关键是要增强家庭关于成人团队将接管后续医疗的意识。在这种情况下，患者应该被劝阻避免那些反复的事情，因为这会导致保健不连续的问题和增加无意的负面健康的风险。

监护，同意和保密问题

转移之前和成年之前，一个提供者应该与患者和他（她）的家庭讨论患者的合法权益，以及任何年龄相关的保密和知情权利。在某些司法领域，未成年人18岁之前可以提供定义过程或有条件的知情同意。医疗服务提供者意识到国家，省级和（或）联邦法律管理与年龄相关的保密性和同意问题是很重要的，因为这些是根据不同的管辖权变化的[58-62]。一些患者可能会因为自我同意的责任感到不知所措，一些家长由于他们控制的突然中断会觉得自己被忽视了。先行咨询可以帮助避免发生混乱、焦虑和不满。

当存在认知限制时，监护问题尤为重要；在过渡计划中考虑个人的发展阶段和患者个体的独立能力是至关重要的。神经认知评估可能是必要的。这将在本章进一步讨论。

智力障碍的患者

认知延迟的患者面临的医疗差距和增加的健康风险超过健康的移植青少年[63-65]。与他们的过渡计划和准备相关的挑战包括对于转移的高度焦虑、常规改变的适应性、独立生活的能力、性、职业问题、沟通方式、决策和知情同意、监护和替代决策。

这些患者的转移文档的关键组成部分是他们的自我管理和医疗决策的总结[64]。日常生活活动的知识能力和执行能力不是同义的实体。尽管智商低于70传统上被认为是认知推迟，智商测试只是独立功能评估的一部分，测试结果可能会误导，尤其是当学习障碍或抑郁并发症存在时。以受教育层次、发育年龄和智商来标记青少年的能力可能无法反映他（她）执行自我保健或听从指导的能力。适应性行为如日常生活活动，沟通和社交技巧的评估等是至关重要的。一个临床实用的方法是让父母或照顾者来描述他们的孩子典型的一天，尤其询问关于他（她）做了哪些自我保健、他（她）如何沟通，以及他（她）如何解决问题[64]。临床观察本身可能具有欺骗性和潜在的高估或低估他们的能力。青少年在临床设置中表现的行为可能不同，有限的时间可能限制观察到的适应性行为范围。此外，除非一个人进行深入观察，不然可能很难确定一个年轻人并没有完全理解面临的问题或给予的指示。

不同类型的过程和治疗及是否需要替换决策的知情同意问题可能很复杂，并和部分过程类型相关（如静脉开始注射抗生素和复杂的选择性外科手术），与理解好处和风险及医疗或手术的紧迫性的理解水平的需求相关。最好在患者成人之前评估和计划这些突发事件。成人提供者如何与智力障碍年轻人沟通也非常重要。必须评估一个人表达和理解能力，并定制相适应的方法。通过冷静清楚的对话是必要的。访问中一般应包括护理人员，并提供时间与患者单独交流。

职业和教育问题对于认知挑战青年来说是主要的问题，且其选择可能受到更多的限制。不过，工作可以提供结构、稳定和保险覆盖。在青春期早期，过渡团队应该询问患者如何准备目前的职业。一位社会工作者可以作为教育系统的一个优秀联络员以确保修改的教育计划在早期获得实施[66]。让患者与另一个已经获得工作的认知障碍个体会面是有帮助的。此外，形成社交网络对患者是具有挑战性的，但可能有可以帮助患者学习社会技能和以安全、监督方式参与社会的社区组织。

与其他青少年患者一样，适当的性教育对这些患者发展是非常重要的。不能假设认为认知障碍患者不会参与危险行为或不会有性活跃；同样不应该认为性行为是非双方自愿的。另一个要考虑的因素是生活安排。父母可能认为患者会永远与他们或与另一个照顾者一起，不会充分理解患者独立生活的能力或渴望。

因为认知推迟的青少年通常结构化的日常做得很好，他们的依从性可能比正常智力者更好。然而他们可能不太能适应非常规的变化，比如当不在家时如何服药或者因病错过服药时如何处理。在过渡过程中以及转移可以使用特定的组织能力解决，以及到位的应急支持。

给智力障碍患者在他们保健中承担更多责任的机会和在他们能力范围内尽可能地允许他们发展更多的

自主权是有价值的。这可能需要较长的过渡期和更多的社区支持。适当的认知延迟评估对于帮助家庭获得潜在的社会和经济资源也很重要。这些都是在整个过渡过程中需要考虑到的问题。

平稳过渡和评估过渡准备的障碍

有许多潜在的年轻人平稳过渡的障碍。要克服障碍必须首先确定并理解它们的含义。考虑三种可能障碍来源是有用的:提供者和(或)医疗保健系统,家长和(或)照顾者,以及患者自己。

医疗服务提供者和医疗系统相关的障碍

儿科医生经常会与患者和他们的家庭确定长期的关系,并经历使他们放弃保健的困难。这可能导致患者被留在儿科医疗系统的时间比必要的时间长。它也可能导致儿科医生感受到患者和家庭的依赖感。儿科提供者可能在无意的交流中表现出对成人患者医疗环境的不信任。提高成人和儿童提供者之间的沟通有助于克服儿科医生在转移其患者时的犹豫。

目前没有正式的“过渡保健”能力存在的成人或儿童提供者，处理通常在对方的领域的问题时可能会觉得经验不足。成人提供者已经表示了在先天和儿童状况下更好的培训需求，以及对青少年和年轻的成年患者的心理问题和成熟的担忧[67]。儿科医生可以帮助提供特别遗传的状况，先天性泌尿道异常和其他需要谨慎随访或考虑其他器官相关的症状。相反,成人提供者可能传授对他们的实践的先行指导有用的信息，以及更多对生殖医疗、癌症预防和筛查、心血管疾病和其他移植晚期并发症的关注。

通过改善成人和儿童提供者之间的沟通，他们将获得互相学习的机会。儿童和成人提供者可以通过参与讨论过渡患者相互受益，无论是非正式讨论或安排会议。共同回顾患者的情况可以帮助减轻一些障碍而获得平稳过渡。例如,成人社会工作者进行早期介入来阻止保健获得的妨碍,如保险缺口等。有严重认知延迟的患者，共同讨论可以帮助由成人医疗团队根据患者可以独立从事医疗他(她)自我管理的程度来设定现实的预期。

改善那些照顾有慢性疾病的青少年患者的卫生保健专业人员的培训是非常必要的。在英国,国民健康服务(NHS)赞助了一个医疗保健专业人士电子学习模块的青少年健康计划，来支持青少年和年轻的成年人的保健质量[68]。这些模块涵盖了广泛的青少年健康问题,其没有特定疾病要求,包括了知情同意和保密性问题。他们还为参与者提供反馈，并有资格提供继续教育学分。这种创新的程序可能在青少年医疗保健交付中作为一个创建质量指标的模型。

医疗体系障碍是一个需要解决的关键领域，包括医疗服务提供者的时间和资源不足以及卫生保健系统经常低下的效率。年轻的成年患者可能需要更长时间访问以确保全面,而保健提供者可能觉得时间受限[67]。由于更高容量的患者导致的更长的时间延迟，过渡患者在一个成人医院获得预约设置可能是具有挑战性的。此外,那些有较少辅助支持的患者容易错过预约或实验室检测。上述每个对于年轻的成年患者在新的医疗环境不能舒适的独立管理因素都可能导致后续失访。此外,即使儿童和成人保健是在相同的医疗保健系统内，不相容或缺乏电子医疗记录系统可以损害转移或医疗信息。一个固定的转移年龄,没有对健康危机或空间需求的适应性空间,也可以成为成功的主要障碍。

在美国历史上，转移时间和移植免疫抑制剂药物治疗公共保险终止的时间往往同时，导致年轻患者容易受到保险缺口的伤害。最近的医疗改革措施可能减轻这一特定障碍,但需要更进一步的研究。

平稳过渡的父母和(或)照顾者的障碍

移植受体的父母可能经历放弃他们的青少年医疗保健责任控制的困难，如果排除在医疗咨询成人中心之外他们会感到受伤害和愤怒,特别是如果他们既往参与了每一次的儿科访问。在文献中,关于父母是否应该被排除在成人中心的咨询以外并没有明确的共识[30,31]。

据报道肝移植受体的父母意识到了过渡保健的重要性,但对于过程的了解仍然匮乏[69]。儿科医生需要鼓励家长逐步促进孩子从小的独立和自我责任(表121.3)。这包括随着逐渐增加的责任和技能在年龄合适水平对医疗保健例程的监督参与。在青少年的早期到中期,这可能包括父母给患者增加的打电话处方的责任，也可以从那些非必需的药物开始。父母可以转向另一个特定的任务,如预约医疗访问。同时,应鼓励孩子参与与其正常年龄相关的活动和任务，由此一个年龄对应的自立感觉可以得到发展。如果父母不愿与他们的青少

年分享健康责任，对医疗保健预期和其他适龄的生活预期做一个平行比较会有所帮助，比如独立做作业和学习开车。作为青少年学习新任务，家长应该保持监控和支持他们。父母积极健康行为的模范作用也需要强调。

平稳过渡的患者障碍

许多过渡过程的患者障碍多来自青春期和新兴成年的正常发展阶段，或者从小有复杂的慢性疾病的后果。此外，转移到成人保健通常发生成人初期(18~25岁)，这正是危险行为发生的高峰期[70]。

青少年和(或)成人初期是一个探索、身份形成、边界测试、冒险、激烈情感和创造力的时期[70]。青春的想象力、精力和理想主义导致了在许多领域的重要进展。然而，慢性疾病的负担可以毁坏潜在的无忧无虑的生活时间。青少年对感知现在行动的未来后果的困难加剧了这一点，使他们很难理解当前的限制与未来健康的相关性[71,72]。青少年和新兴成人移植受体模仿同龄人更随意的生活方式的尝试可能导致治疗不依从，从而导致移植失败。依从性被认为是青少年和成人初期，以及过渡到成人保健过程中高移植物失功率的主要因素[5,12,73]。

儿童时的慢性疾病经验会导致认知、情感和社会的挑战，这是成功过渡到成人保健潜在的重要障碍[63-76]。Berney-Martinet 和他的同事最近的一次研究使用半结构化精神病学诊断访谈和问卷(青年自我报告)，来检查40名青少年肾移植受体(平均年龄15.2岁)和经过年龄、性别、社会经济地位和种族背景配对的40名健康青少年控制的心理和精神资料。患者的父母也接受了采访，两组患者的父母均填写了调查问卷(儿童行为检查表)。该研究发现上学延迟或教育问题是惊人的。60%的移植受体至少重复读了一个年级（控制组为12.5%，$P<0.001$)。学习障碍的患病率为30%(控制组7.5%，P为0.03)，其与肾脏疾病诊断时年龄小、血液透析治疗，以及较低的社会经济阶层有关。由于行为问题和(或)残疾(27.5%对比控制组2.5%，P为0.005)，几乎所有那些在研究中学习困难的人被分到一个特殊的班级中。精神疾病伴随发病率高，65%的受体达到了生活精神障碍的DSM-Ⅳ标准，50%的人有两个或以上并发的精神疾病诊断。包括有抑郁症(35%)、注意缺陷多动障碍(ADHD)(23%)和恐惧症(20%)。接受移植的青少年相比于他们的同龄人有显著的孤独和社会孤立。另一份涉及定性研究的系统回顾包括了300多名青少年移植受体，发现他们存在自尊低、感知到来自同龄人的负面反应、失去归属感、对他们预期寿命的不确定性[77]。这两个研究都说明了积极评价儿童移植受体心理健康的重要性。

教育是健康和后期生活成功的一个重要的社会决定因素[48,49,78]。作为一个群体，儿童器官移植受体相比于同龄人有更多的学业成绩挑战与成人时更高的失业率[70,79]。尽管他们中的许多人希望建立长期的学术和职业目标，但广泛的学校缺勤率可能会导致落后，从而对于如何达到满意成绩不知所措[77]。重复或延长的学校缺席不仅错失了掌握核心技能的机会，同时还会使年轻人失去回到学校的信心和对社会的适应，因为他们需要经历重建友谊的挑战[70]。儿科卫生专业人员需要保持警惕，经常检查移植受体的教育和在社会上的困难，并指导他们的父母获得适当的支持和介入资源。优化移植受体教育和职业的潜能方法包括教育干预计划，对于有长时间的缺席的儿童的重新整合计划，以及医院和学校之间更好地协调[80]。适时的干预很关键，因为在青少年初期即表现出低水平的青少年更容易辍学[81]。Wolf Branigin 等开发了一个创新的计划来帮助整合残疾青少年进入到成年。它包含课后活动、工作“新兵训练营”、夏季就业准备、自我宣传技能发展、六周的工作经验“夏季研究所”和课堂活动、每月工作室、父母支持课程、青年领袖论坛和重点关注高中的强化个性化教育项目[82]。参与者的年龄为12~20岁，平均年龄为14.8岁。通过儿童生活质量量表4.0的评估，两年计划期间的身体健康状况、学校功能和总功能得到了改善。职业成熟量表-态度量表(CMI-AS)被用来评估就业准备，其显示仅有那些最小的年龄和(或)年级组获得了超过2年的平均改善，其预示了在青春期早期干预的必要性。

额外的转换障碍可能是由于青少年缺乏参与和缺乏转移过程中的知识。该发现结合了青少年和年轻成人如何看待过渡保健的重要性。Anthony 和他的同事们进行了14名青少年心脏移植受体(11.7~17.8岁、平均年龄为15.7岁)观点和信念的定性研究[83]。他们发现青少年对于过渡过程是不感兴趣和冷漠的，与他们父母的恐惧和焦虑形成鲜明对比。没有青少年对于他们保健表现出更多地参与或自主兴趣。作者推测看护者的过度保护可能会鼓励青少年脱离过渡的过程。Freder-

icks 等利用全面的问卷研究了青少年和(或)新兴成人肝移植受体转换的视角[69]。该队列研究由 31 名 12~17 岁和 15 名 18~21 岁的肝移植受体组成,还包括了较年轻组的父母。这些研究者发现了对于转变前期思考和过渡过程的知识的水平很低，只对其学习存在适度的兴趣。当患者按照年龄分组时,那些在 16 岁以上的患者对于学习转换的知识有更多的兴趣。这两项研究证实了关于从小开始讨论过渡和对父母宣传促进孩子的参与他(她)的保健的并在监督下自我责任感逐渐增强的重要性的推荐[17,25,31–34]。一些人表达了对于青少年承担他们药物责任程度的担忧。Simons 等检查了青少年肾移植受体药物依从性的障碍。其发现当青少年负责他们的药物而不是他们父母负责时的不依从性发生率更高；但他们没有报告药物责任从父母过渡到青少年是如何发生的[84]。研究也表明,医疗责任从父母到青少年的突然转变可能会导致两者都感到痛苦。不依从与较低的家庭凝聚力和父母的痛苦感相关,家庭冲突会对青少年移植受体的心理健康产生负面的影响[85–87]。医疗保健从业者需要对这些风险保持敏感并对患者和他们的家属在整个医疗责任的过渡中提供建议和支持。

总之，患者克服成功转移障碍包括青春期和成年初期患者正常的神经认知发育过程、依从性问题、学习困难、错过的教育机会、减少的社会和工作经验、精神疾病和缺乏综合患者准备。增强集成青少年移植受体转为成人保健和优化他们成年后的生活质量需要及时、主动、多层次跨学科的过程。

过渡的准备

实现成功转型的一个重大的挑战是识别正确的转移时间。一些医疗中心有转移必须发生的特定时间。然而相似年龄患者的发展可能是非常不同的，一些人可能比别人更早地准备转移。过渡过程不仅包括医疗保健的过渡,也包括医疗保健责任转移(从父母到患者的转移)。许多共识建议和指南建议转移应在患者、护理人员、儿童和成人医疗团队都认为患者已经做好准备时进行[17,31]。然而,如何提供最好的评估患者的过渡准备？这需要真正理解需要如何优化年轻人参与成人医疗体系，评估转变准备的标准化工具和指标需要进一步开发和研究。这是一个生机勃勃的领域,一些最近开发的工具有望为临床和研究使用提供帮助。评估器官移植受体过渡准备状况的工具体现四个主要原则:

1.评估应该包括多个方面,包括患者和家庭两方面的信息。几项研究显示患者和家长之间的报告不整合[69,88,89]。一般来说,患者倾向于比他们的照顾者报告更多的医疗独立[69]。

2.评估的过渡准备应该从理论上知情、可靠和有效。实现过渡的准备需要部分患者、照顾者和提供者进步的行为变化。使用行为理论和模型通知评估工具会促使对于行为干预的成功或失败有更好的理解[90]。

3.评估应基于整个过渡过程重复进行。理想的过渡准备措施评估应对变化敏感并可以纵向应用。

4.除了疾病相关技能和知识外,评估还应该包括自我保健、医疗保健决策和维护自己的权利的精通[91]。过渡准备的里程碑在各种文献回顾和共识声明中进行了建议[17,92](表 121.4)。

从儿童过渡到成人保健计划协调的目标是“优化健康和促进每个人的最大健康成就潜力。”[93] Sawicki 等建立了过渡准备评估问卷(TRAQ)来识别那些有特殊健康保健的成年初期患者，需要额外的准备来达到医疗保健自我管理的领域[94]。它是基于“改变的阶段”需要评估一个人的准备阶段来采用特定的行为的模型。TRAQ 是 33 项需要患者完成来衡量成功转变所需的健康、教育、工作和日常生活等技能的问卷。据报道这个等级分类，着重于两个领域——自我管理和自主权利。自我管理问题包括管理药物、医疗预约和健康保险等项目。自主权利问题包括与健康提供者之间的沟通,以及在教育和就业上的自主权利维护。此问卷不包括照顾者或提供者的视角。这在有各种各样的特殊的医

表 121.4 过渡的里程碑

1.理解并能够描述器官衰竭的病因
2.注意移植对于整体健康的长期和短期并发症
3.了解疾病对性和生殖健康的影响
4.对自己的医疗保健有责任感。这包括电话续药,药物知识,准备药盒子,坚持医疗方案和管理医疗预约
5.显示提供大部分自我保健的能力
6.表示已准备好进入成年
7.形式简洁的医疗信息总结
8.成为一个知识渊博的健康消费者。能够传递个人病史。了解医疗保险覆盖。知道如何寻求紧急援助。知道如何独立的与提供者沟通健康问题

疗保健需求的16~26岁患者中得到了验证。它还没有经过作为一个纵向测量预测效度的测试。

另一个疾病的问卷,基于发育的技能清单,被用来评估肝移植受体的医疗保健自我管理技能。它由22个关于了解身体状况、与提供者的沟通、管理药物和预约,以及健康的生活方式问题组成。患者需对每一个特殊行为回应“永不,有时或经常”[95]。在肝移植受体中,发现了一些领域显著的基线损害,如预约和理解保险。然而,是否与过渡准备或医学或行为的结果有关仍未知,并作为一个纵向测量使用。像TRAQ是患者关注测量并没有平行的看护者评估。

Pai等创建了治疗责任分配量表(ATR)来评估青少年和成人初期移植受体和他们的照顾者的健康保健责任[89]。这18项指标包含3个分量表:口服药物治疗,诊所出勤和实验室检查。它是由患者和照顾者单独完成,来评估谁是主要负责在家里治疗相关任务的人。这在39名7~18岁儿童肾移植受体和他们的照顾者中得到了验证。总体患者责任在患者和照顾者报告之间的差异与更明显的不依从相关。ATR可能成为医疗保健自我管理潜在的指标,但尚未被证明能够反映过渡准备状况。

Fredericks等开发了一种评估11~20岁儿童肝移植患者过渡准备的工具[96]。它由38项和4个医疗服务提供者管理的问题组成。反应为Likert量表(问题)自我报告或直接演示的技能。4个领域包括:自我管理,药物知识,技能和心理调整。另有针对护理人员的单独的36项调查。作者将71名患者的过渡准备分数与年龄、服药依从性、诊所出勤和肝功能进行了比较。转变准备与依从性,诊所出席或健康状况之间没有明显的关联。但年长患者报告了更高的自我管理技能,如能够描述一个人的药物疗程,但是他们的知觉不等同于能更好地演示这些技能。此外,青少年或成人初期更大的医疗保健自我管理会增加不依从性,这提示家长参与下降与患者更多的药物失检相关。这个发现也在儿童肾移植受体的研究中得到了支持,其显示当有管理他们药物的主要责任时患者不依从的可能性更大[84]。这些数据强调了提供者帮助患者和父母通过系统的方式而不是让父母突然放弃全部责任,或者相反,对成熟青少年保持完全控制的过渡医疗保健责任。

在另一项15~21岁肾移植受体研究中,Gilleland等测试了过渡准备问卷(RTQ),包含了22项分别调查患者和护理人员:①医疗自我管理行为中患者的责任和②这些行为中父母的参与[88]。此外,患者和医护人员分别报告患者的准备:①承担医疗的全部责任和②转移到成人保健。患者和家长对整体转移准备的报告与他们报告的患者责任积极相关,但与父母的参与状况相反。因此,患者准备转变时已增加了其医疗责任并减少了父母的参与。这些患者也报道了更多的药物知识,更有可能自己续药和与父母的关系更好。报告中增加的过渡准备与更少的药物障碍相关,但令人惊讶的是与服药依从性无关。RTQ在多个角度的评估中很有效,其是基于理论和有效的,同时考虑了医疗技能和知识以及个人健康宣传。然而,这一方法,像以上提及的其他方法一样,尚未经过纵向测试。

因此,尽管上述同行评审发表的过渡准备和医疗责任措施目前正在使用,但没有一个是完美的。他们还没有经过纵向测试或已证明其对改变的敏感。此外,他们是自我和(或)照顾者报告但不包括医疗服务提供者。卫生保健提供者的输入也是转换过程的一部分,他们的目标评估需要结合患者和家长的报告。也有几个额外的基于网络的工具,读者可以参考但没有一个严格经过了可靠性、有效性和持续的预测值的评估[97-99]。

实施转移准备评估的一个理论模型为青少年和年轻成年人转移准备的社会生态模型(SMART),见图121.1[91]。这个模型包含了患者、家庭和提供者、社会人口统计学状态和健康经历间复杂的相互作用。一些因素可能不容易受干预影响,如年龄、种族、民族、家庭结构以及潜在的转换障碍,如受损的医疗访问和神经认知障碍。另一个组成关注于患者的发育成熟、健康知识、医疗保健管理技能、转移信念、目标、关系和心理社会功能。这个模型在癌症生存患者中进行了测试,但其也可以为移植受体未来发展的过渡准备的工具提供一个全面的评估基础。它通过提供考虑了医疗保健系统和患者医疗以外的个人生活中提供者,患者和家庭伙伴关系的一项全面的理论模型增加了当前的措施。这个模型显示了通知、构建和测试未来的过渡准备工具和干预措施的承诺。

虽然建立过渡准备的指标仍然是具有挑战性的,在过去的十年里已经取得了很大进展,目前的研究工作将继续推进科学的过渡。

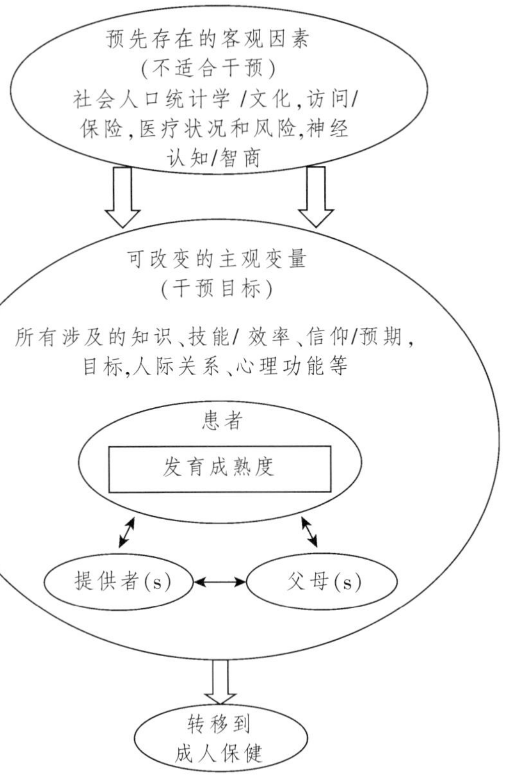

图 121.1　青少年和年轻成年人转移准备的社会生态模型。Reproduced from [91] Schwartz et al. with permission from Wiley.

过渡的结果和研究的需要

青少年过渡到成人保健的整体目标，最初出版于 2002 年,并在许多期刊文章中进行了重申,是因为“通过高质量,以患者为中心的、灵活的、协调的、响应、全面发展适当的不间断的医疗保健服务来最大化终身功能和潜能”[100]。在本节中,我们将讨论上述目标的过渡效果和研究需要。

两个出版的大型数据库研究清楚地表明，青少年和(或)成人初期年龄段的移植受体移植物失功的风险非常高,该事件段围绕着向成人保健转移的过渡事件,尤其是第一年,与移植的显著高失败相关[5,12]。这两个报道提供了特别警惕 17~24 岁年龄范围的受体和改善过渡和转移的过程的医疗的需求。他们是重要的研究,而之前过渡作为一个风险的证据主要是基于小的单医疗中心研究。

该如何继续改善过渡的过程并评价干预措施的效果?定义可靠措施的结果,测量什么和如何测量它具有优先级和挑战性。为了评估“最大化终生功能和潜能”的转移目标,我们需要看看广泛的因素,包括移植物功能、移植物和患者生存、整体身心健康和心理因素。然而许多转型研究的目的中移植物和患者的生存可能是不足的。明确严格的终止点需要敏感性(如移植物功能而不是移植物失功的生物标志,如代谢组学、蛋白质组学和基因组学领域)还有特异性,需要明确界定正常和异常的范围。我们需要在重大损害发生之前早期辨别移植物功能的变化。转移后移植物功能变化评估的一个综合因素是,对于大多数器官移植而言,正常的功能也会随着时间有小的改变，所以当前使用措施的敏感性和特异性仍不够。

评估在整个过渡时期和进入成人初期健康和保险充足率和覆盖率的连续性是评估“不间断保健”的关键因素,可能会被认为是有良好结果的措施。然而,“不间断的医疗服务”需要准确的评估过渡患者及转移到成人保健之前及之后其移植相关的数据库。目前国家数据库的主要限制是其没有定义转移到成人保健的点,使得很难大规模评估过渡和转移的影响。需要学习的重要因素包括患者在转移之后是否保持随访,定义了移植和初级保健可获得的卫生保健提供者和参加预期的临床和实验室预约。住院和急诊访问也可以检查,但是实践和住院及急诊室政策的变化可能在儿童和成人医疗中心不同,使得患者难以作为他(她)自己的控制者。

健康相关生活质量(HRQOL)是最大化患者潜力的核心,是评估在过渡过程中患者的一个重要的因素。在评估转移之前患者需记住,父母、照顾者和患者报告可能有所不同是非常重要的，患者的评估将随着时间继续[87,101]。有助于 HRQOL 的因素包括健康营养、体育锻炼和调节,社会整合可以积极纳入过渡计划和评估。还需要注意优化教育的潜能、健康的主要决定因素、令人满意的工作准备,对于长期的生活质量是很重要的。因此,教育和职业培训结果至关重要。目前缺乏一个可以纵向应用和解释从童年成熟到成年的 HRQOL 应用的措施。一种独特的随着时间的推移可以通过条件和年龄范围来测量 HRQOL 的工具是美国健康患者报告结果测量信息系统(PROMIS),这是一个可靠的、有效的、精确的和响应性的测量患者报告的健康状况的评估工具[102]。然而这个工具不具有疾病特异性。

一旦定义了结果,报道也必须加以考虑。一个转移成功或失败的结果评估重要组成部分必须包括促使最佳的移植物功能和患者生存的治疗因素，如药物治疗依从性(在本文分别讨论)和治疗后遗症(如恶性肿瘤、糖尿病、高脂血症、改变的免疫力)。

在考虑不同的研究设计，定性和定量研究都有价值,但研究设计和目标必须清晰和可重复的。定性研究评估元素,比如"与发展相适应的、灵活的和响应的"护理是很重要的。患者可以用更丰富的经历仔细和深入分析进行定性描述研究，随后可以用一个更广泛的量化方式来帮助定义这些问题。此外,患者的经历可以在项目水平获得质量保证[17]。

过渡研究必须协作。在一个机构水平,研究应该多学科努力来纳入转变的各种生物心理社会方面。而单中心研究在报告可行性和设计各种方法上很重要,多中心的合作确保足够的权威和普遍性是很必要的。到目前为止,很少有出版的过渡过程结果,且大多数的结果是小型的描述性分析,通常为单中心,且有时候是历史控制[7,51,103]。尽管结果是鼓舞人心的,历史控制的研究一般不能解释治疗方案上微妙但重大的调整、医疗人员或疾病特征的变化，特别是儿童移植中较小的患者数目。

过渡的研究应该是纵向的。一个纵向数据收集的挑战是确保患者同意长期随访[17]。有建议国家登记收集更细致的数据来更好地评估患者的长期结果[104]。

除了患者的结果，未来的过渡研究工作应该检查过渡保健的卫生保健专业人员促进服务交付全面和系统的教育和培训。在英国,已经提出建立一套管理过渡服务的性能标准,以使项目可以进行评估[30]。1993年,Blum等报道,"虽然我们可以定义过渡的概念和目标,但对于过程有太多不知道的东西"[3]。当时,Blum等缺乏关于哪个护理模式是最有效的，对谁及健康状况是否需要根据正式转移计划变化的有关知识。这些知识的缺陷在20年后仍然存在。如果提供的过渡保健是系统的和理论的，临床干预和解释理解观察到的结果会更容易。系统的质量保证与改进研究及成本效益分析支持研究方法是至关重要的。

总结

• 过渡与许多利益相关者一样是一个动态的过程。护理必须是有计划的、可理解的、协调的、持续及心理和发展合适的。思考患者的过渡保健应从10~12岁甚至更早开始。

• 考虑各种来源的平稳过渡的障碍,包括患者、护理提供者和医疗保健系统。一旦识别障碍,需要与患者和家属一起来研究有针对性的促进成功过渡的方法。

• 评估"高质量、发展适当的、不间断的以患者为中心、灵活的、协调的、响应性的和全面性的医疗服务",有众多因素需要研究,其中一些比其他的更容易。一个主要领域是帮助患者和家人准备过渡和转移。我们需要通过患者准备的明确定义工具、过程的纵向评估和转移准备的指标来衡量。干预设计中使用行为理论是很重要的，最有效的努力可能来源于临床医生、心理学家、社会工作者、教育工作者和行为理论家的合作。

结论

青少年和成人初期移植受体转移项目的目标是提高长期的健康状况,包括移植物生存和心理因素,如有利的就业和健康相关的生活质量。防止过渡期间移植受体同种异体移植物损失的需求不仅对于个别患者而且对于社会也是至关重要的。由于有问题的过渡或转移导致的每一个潜在的，可预防的器官丢失增加了对于有限器官更多的需求。尽管多学科治疗可能需要大量的资源,但潜在的好处也是巨大的。

当提供者、患者和家属早期参与医疗自我管理的过程时,基于一个正在进行的基础,平稳过渡需求并不仍然是一个难以捉摸的概念。推进转移改进的一个重要组成是教育和医疗保健专业人员来促进系统化且有效的服务。研究评价干预措施的效果是至关重要的,未来的研究工作应该是多学科、全面和纵向的。

(奚斌 译　徐骁 校)

参考文献

1. McDonald SP, Craig JC, Australian and New Zealand Paediatric Nephrology Association. Long-term survival of children with end-stage renal disease. New England Journal of Medicine. 2004;350:54–62.
2. Organ Procurement and Transplantation Network (OPTN) and Scientific Registry of Transplant Recipients (SRTR). OPTN/SRTR 2010 Annual Data Report. 2011 Rockville, MD: Department of Health and Human Services, Health Resources and Services Administration, Healthcare Systems Bureau, Division of Transplantation.
3. Blum RW, Garell D, Hodgman CH, et al. Transition from child-centered to health-care systems for adolescents with chronic conditions. a position paper of the Society for Adolescent Medicine. Journal of Adolescent Health. 1993;14:570–576.
4. Reiss JG, Gibson RW, Walker LR. Health care transition: youth, family and provider perspectives. Pediatrics. 2005;115:112–120.
5. Samuel SM, Nettel-Aguirre A, Hemmelgarn BR, et al. Graft failure and adaptation

period to adult healthcare centers in pediatric renal transplant patients. Transplantation. 2011;91:1380–1385.
6. United States Government Accountability Office. End-Stage Renal Disease: Characteristics of Kidney Transplant Recipients, Frequency of Transplant Failures, and Cost to Medicare. 2007 [cited September 3, 2012]. GAO-07-1117. Available from: http://www.gao.gov/.
7. Koshy SM, Hebert D, Lam K, et al. Renal allograft loss during transition to adult healthcare services among pediatric renal transplant patients. Transplantation. 2009;87:1733–1736.
8. van den Heuvel ME, van der Lee JH, Cornelissen EA, et al. Transition to the adult nephrologist does not induce acute renal transplant rejection. Nephrology, Dialysis, Transplantation. 2010;25:1662–1667.
9. Smith JM, Ho PL, McDonald RA. Renal transplant outcomes in adolescents: a report of the North American Pediatric Renal Transplant Co-operative Study. Pediatric Transplantation. 2002;6:493–499.
10. Foster BJ, Platt RW, Dahhou M, et al. The impact of age at transfer from pediatric to adult-oriented care on renal allograft survival. Pediatric Transplantation. 2011;15:750–759.
11. Kiberd JA, Acott P, Kiberd BA. Kidney transplant survival in pediatric and young adults. BMC Nephrology. 2011;12:54–59.
12. Foster BJ, Dahhou M, Zhang X, et al. Association between age and graft failure rates in young kidney transplant recipients. Transplantation. 2011;92: 1237–1243.
13. Christie D, Viner R. Adolescent development. British Medical Journal (Clinical Research Ed.). 2005;330:301–304.
14. Marcell AV. Adolescence. In: Kliegman RM, Behrman RE, Jensen HB, et al., editors. Nelson Textbook of Pediatrics. Philadelphia, PA: Saunders Elsevier; 2007.
15. Steinberg L. Cognitive and affective development in adolescence. Trends in Cognitive Sciences. 2005;9:69–74.
16. Gutgesell ME, Payne N. Issues of adolescent psychological development in the 21st century. Pediatrics in Review. 2004;25:79–85.
17. Bell LE, Bartosh SM, Davis CL, et al. Adolescent transition to adult care in solid organ transplantation: a consensus conference report. American Journal of Transplantation. 2008;8:2230–2242.
18. Steinberg L. A social neuroscience perspective on adolescent risk-taking. Developmental Review. 2008;28:78–106.
19. Lebel C, Beaulieu C. Longitudinal development of human brain wiring continues from childhood to adulthood. Journal of Neuroscience. 2011;31:10937–10947.
20. Giorgio A, Watkins KE, Douaud G, et al. Changes in white matter microstructure during adolescence. Neuroimage. 2008;39:52–61.
21. Westlye LT, Walhovd KB, Dale AM, et al. Life-span changes of the human brain white matter: diffusion tensor imaging (DTI) and volumetry. Cerebral Cortex (New York, N.Y.: 1991). 2010;20:2055–2068.
22. Giedd JN, Rapoport JL. Structural MRI of pediatric brain development: what have we learned and where are we going. Neuron. 2010;67:728–734.
23. Mulye TP, Park MJ, Nelson CD, et al. Trends in adolescent and young adult health in the United States. Journal of Adolescent Health. 2009;45:8–24.
24. LaRosa C, Glah C, Baluarte HJ, et al. Solid-organ transplantation in childhood: transitioning to adult health care. Pediatrics. 2011;127:742–753.
25. Alpay H. Transition of the adolescent patient to the adult clinic. Peritoneal Dialysis International: Journal of the International Society for Peritoneal Dialysis. 2009;S2:S180–S182.
26. Icard PF, Hower SJ, Kuchenreuther AR, et al. The transition from childhood to adulthood with ESRD: educational and social challenges. Clinical Nephrology. 2008;69:1–7.
27. McDonagh JE, Southwood TR, Shaw KL. The impact of a coordinated transitional care programme on adolescents with juvenile idiopathic arthritis. Rheumatology. 2007;46:161–168.
28. American Academy of Pediatrics, American Academy of Family Physicians, American College of Physicians, et al. Supporting the health care transition from adolescence to adulthood in the medical home. Pediatrics. 2011;128: 182–200.
29. Health Networks Branch, Department of Health, Western Australia. Paediatric Chronic Diseases Transition Framework. Perth, 2009. Available at www .healthnetworks.health.wa.gov.au/modelsofcare/docs/ [accessed Dec 14, 2013].
30. Webb N, Harden P, Lewis C, et al. Building consensus on transition of transplant patients from paediatric to adult healthcare. Archives of Disease in Childhood. 2010;95:606–611.
31. Watson AR, Harden P, Ferris M, et al. Transition from pediatric to adult renal services: a consensus statement by the International Society of Nephrology (ISN) and the International Pediatric Nephrology Association (IPNA). Pediatric Nephrology (Berlin, Germany). 2011;26:1753–1757.
32. McDonagh JE, Kaufman M. Transition from pediatric to adult care after solid organ transplantation. Current Opinion Organ Transplantation. 2009;14:526–532.
33. Stabile L, Rosser L, Porterfield KM, et al. Transfer versus transition: success in pediatric transplantation brings the welcome challenge of transition. Progress in Transplantation (Aliso Viejo, Calif.). 2005;15:363–370.
34. van Staa AL, Jedeloo S, van Meeteren J, et al. Crossing the transition chasm: experiences and recommendations for improving transitional care of young adults, parents and providers. Child: Care, Health and Development. 2011;37: 821–832.
35. Kieckhefer GM, Trahms CM. Supporting development of children with chronic conditions: from compliance toward shared management. Pediatric Nursing. 2000;26:354–363.
36. Reiss J, Gibson R, Institute for Childhood Health Policy at University of Florida. Health Care Transition Workbooks for Ages 12-14, 15-17 and 18 and up. Available from: http://hctransitions.ichp.ufl.edu/hct-promo/ [accessedSeptember 4, 2012].
37. Committee on Adolescence. Achieving quality health services for adolescents. Pediatrics. 2008; 121:1263–1270.
38. Belair C, Gilleland J, Amaral S. Assessing the satisfaction of teens with kidney transplants who have attended an adolescent transition clinic. International Journal of Child and Adolescent Health. 2011;4:00–00.
39. van Staa AL, van der Stege HA, Jedeloo S, et al. Readiness to transfer to adult care of adolescents with chronic conditions: exploration of associated factors. Journal of Adolescent Health. 2011;48:295–302.
40. Baum M, Freier MC, Chinnock RE. Neurodevelopmental outcome of solid organ transplantation in children. Pediatric Clinics of North America. 2003;50: 1493–1503.
41. Duquette PJ, Hooper SR, Wetherington CE, et al. Brief report: intellectual and academic functioning in pediatric chronic kidney disease. Journal of Pediatric Psychology. 2007;8:1011–1017.
42. Gipson DS, Hooper SR, Duquette PJ, et al. Memory and executive functions in pediatric chronic kidney disease. Child Neuropsychology. 2006;12:391–405.
43. Mohammad S, Alonso EM. Approach to optimizing growth, rehabilitation, and neurodevelopmental outcomes in children after solid-organ transplantation. Pediatric Clinics of North America. 2010;57:539–557.
44. Office of Surveillance, Epidemiology and Laboratory Services, Centers for Disease Control and Prevention (CDC), et al. Youth risk behavior surveillance-United States 2011. Morbidity and Mortality Weekly Report. 2012;61:1–168.
45. Marcell AV, Wibbelsman C, Seigel WM, et al. Male adolescent sexual and reproductive health care. Pediatrics. 2011;128:e1658–e1676.
46. Klein JD, Wilson KM, NcNulty M, et al. Access to medical care for adolescents: results from the 1997 Commonwealth Fund Survey of the Health of Adolescent Girls. Journal of Adolescent Health. 1999;25:120–130.
47. Lotstein DS, Inkelas M, Hays RD, et al. Access to care for youth with special health care needs in the transition to adulthood. Journal of Adolescent Health. 2008;43:23–29.
48. Feinstein L. Quantitative Estimates of the Social Benefits of Learning. *2: Health (Depression and Obesity)*. London, England: Centre for Research on the Wider Benefits of Learning; 2002. [cited August 29, 2012] Available at:: http://citeseerx .ist.psu.edu/viewdoc/download?doi=10.1.1.107.6227&rep=rep1&type=pdf.
49. Low BJ, Low DM. Education and education policy as social determinants of health. Virtual Mentor. 2006;8:756–761.
50. Chaturvedi S, Jones CL, Walker RG, et al. The transition of kidney transplant recipients: a work in progress. Pediatric Nephrology (Berlin, Germany). 2009;24:1055–1060.
51. Harden PN, Walsh G, Bandler N, et al. Bridging the gap: an integrated paediatric to adult clinical service for young adults with kidney failure. British Medical Journal (Clinical Research Ed.). 2012;344:e3718.
52. The Hospital for Sick Children, Toronto, Canada. MyHealth Passport. Available from: https://www.sickkids.ca/MyHealthPassport/[accessed September 3, 2012].
53. Council on Clinical Information Technology. Health Information Technology and the Medical Home. Pediatrics. 2011;127:978–982.
54. Centers for Disease Control/National Center for Health Statistics. Health, United States, 2011. Data from the National Health Interview Survey. Figure 15. Health insurance coverage among adults 18-64 years of age, by age and type of coverage: United States, 2000-2010.
55. Gill JS, Tonelli M. Penny wise, pound foolish? Coverage limits on immunosuppression after kidney transplantation. New England Journal of Medicine. 2012;366:586–589.
56. Committee on Adolescence and Committee on Child Health Financing. Underinsurance of adolescents: recommendations for improved coverage of preventive, reproductive and behavioral health care services. Pediatrics. 2009;123:191–196.
57. Committee on Child Health Financing. Scope of health care benefits for children from birth through age 26. Pediatrics. 2012;129:185–189.
58. Berlan ED, Bravender T. Confidentiality, consent, and caring for the adolescent patient. Current Opinion in Pediatrics. 2009;21:450–456.
59. The Canadian Association for Adolescent Health (CAAH). Parents-

Communication. [cited August 30, 2012]; http://www.youngandhealthy.ca/caah/Informations/Parents/t429c436s4360x415/Communication.aspx.
60. Evans KG. Consent – A Guide for Canadian Physicians, 4th ed. Ottawa, Canada: Canadian Medical Protective Association; 2006 [accessed August 31, 2012]; Available from: http://cmpa.org/cmpapd04/docs/resource_files/ml_guides/consent_guide/pdf/com_consent-e.pdf.
61. National Center for Youth Law. Teen health law- Minor Consent –California. [accessed August 30, 2012]; Available from: http://www.teenhealthlaw.org/minorconsent/.
62. National Center for Youth Law. Teen Health law- Resources for US States other than California. [accessed 2012 August 30, 2012]; Available from: http://www.teenhealthlaw.org/resources_for_other_us_states/.
63. Horowitz S, Kerker B, Owens P, et al. The Health Status and Needs of Individuals with Mental Retardation. New Haven, : Yale University School of Medicine: Special Olympics, Inc; 2001.
64. Kaufman M. Transition of cognitively delayed adolescent organ transplant recipients to adult care. Pediatric Transplantation. 2006;10:413–417.
65. National Institutes of Health. Eunice Kennedy Shriver National Institute of Child Health and Human Development. Appendix D: Health Disparities and Mental Retardation: Programs and Creative Strategies to Close the Gap. [accessed January 3, 2012]; Available from: http://www.nichd.nih.gov/publications/pubs/closingthegap/sub18.cfm.
66. National Dissemination Center for Children with Disabilities. Transition to Adulthood. [accessed September 3, 2012]; Available from: http://nichcy.org/schoolage/transitionadult.
67. Peter NG, Forke CM, Ginsburg KR, et al. Transition from pediatric to adult care: internists' perspectives. Pediatrics. 2009;123:417–423.
68. Royal College of Pediatrics and Child Health. E-learning resources: Adolescent Health Programme. [accessed September 3, 2012]; Available from: http://www.rcpch.ac.uk/.
69. Fredericks EM, Dore-Stites D, Lopez MJ, et al. Transition of pediatric liver transplant recipients to adult care: patient and parent perspectives. Pediatric Transplantation. 2011;15:414–424.
70. Bell LE, Sawyer SM. Transition of care to adult services for pediatric solid-organ transplant recipients. Pediatric Clinics of North America. 2010;57:593–610.
71. Nurmi JE. Development of orientation to the future during early adolescence: a four-year longitudinal study and two cross-sectional comparisons. International Journal of Psychology. Journal International de Psychologie. 1989;24:195.
72. Nurmi JE. How do adolescents see their future? A review of the development of future orientation and planning. Developmental Review. 1991;11:1–59.
73. Ettenger RB, Tsai EW, Fine RN. A paradigm shift and a few modest suggestions in the care of adolescent transplant recipients. Transplantation. 2011;92:1191–1193.
74. Mongeau JG, Clermont MJ, Robitaille P, et al. Study of psychosocial parameters related to the survival rate of transplantation in children. Pediatric Nephrology (Berlin, Germany). 1997;11:542–546.
75. Gerson AC, Furth SL, Neu AM, et al. Assessing associations between medication adherence and potentially modifiable psychosocial variables in pediatric kidney transplant recipients and their families. Pediatric Transplantation. 2004;8:543–550.
76. Maikranz JM, Steele RG, Dreyer ML, et al. The relationship of hope and illness-related uncertainty to emotional adjustment and adherence among pediatric renal and liver transplant recipients. Journal of Pediatric Psychology. 2007;32:571–581.
77. Tong A, Morton R, Howard K, et al. Adolescent experiences following organ transplantation: a systematic review of qualitative studies. Journal of Pediatrics. 2009;155:542–549.
78. Bynner J. Childhood risks and protective factors in social exclusion. Child Society. 2001;15:285–301.
79. Groothoff JW, Grootenhuis MA, Offringa M, et al. Social consequences in adult life of end-stage renal disease in childhood. Journal of Pediatrics. 2005;146:512–517.
80. Martinez YJ, Ercikan K. Chronic illnesses in Canadian children: what is the effect of illness on academic achievement, and anxiety and emotional disorders? Child: Care, Health & Development. 2009;35:391–401.
81. Janosz M, Archambault I, Morizot J, et al. School engagement trajectories and their differential predictive relations to dropout. Journal of Social Issues. 2008;64:21–40.
82. Wolf-Branigin M, Schuyler V, White P. Improving quality of life and career attitudes of youth with disabilities: experiences from the Adolescent Employment Readiness Center. Research on Social Work Practice. 2007;17:324–333.
83. Anthony SJ, Martin K, Drabble A, et al. Perceptions of transitional care needs and experiences in pediatric heart transplant recipients. American Journal of Transplantation. 2009;9:614–619.
84. Simons LE, McCormick ML, Mee LL, et al. Parent and patient perspectives on barriers to medication adherence in adolescent transplant recipients. Pediatric Transplant. 2009;13:338–347.
85. Dew MA, Dabbs AD, Myaskovsky L, et al. Meta-analysis of medical regimen adherence outcomes in pediatric solid organ transplantation. Transplantation. 2009;88:736–746.
86. Simons LE, Anglin G, Warshaw BL, et al. Understanding the pathway between the transplant experience and health-related quality of life outcomes in adolescents. Pediatric Transplantation. 2008;12:187–193.
87. Devine KA, Reed-Knight B, Loiselle KA, et al. Predictors of long-term health realted quality of life in adolescent solid organ transplant recipients. Journal of Pediatric Psychology. 2011;36:891–901.
88. Gilleland J, Amaral S, Mee L, et al. Getting ready to leave: transition readiness in adolescent kidney transplant recipients. Journal of Pediatric Psychology. 2012;37:85–96.
89. Pai AH, Gray E, Kurivial K, et al. The Allocation of Treatment Resonsibility scale: a novel tool for assessing patient and caregiver management of pediatric medical treatment regimens. Pediatric Transplantation. 2010;14:993–999.
90. Glanz K, Rimer BK, Viswanath K. Theory, research and practice in health behavior and health education, Chapter 2. In: Glanz K, Rimer BK, Viswanath K, editors. Health Behavior and Health Education: Theory, Research, and Practice, 4th ed. San Francisco, CA: Jossey-Bass; 2008: 23–38.
91. Schwartz LA, Tuchman LK, Hobbie WL, et al. A social-ecological model of readiness for transition to adult-oriented care for adolescents and young adults with chronic health conditions. Child: Care, Health and Development. 2011;37:883–895.
92. Shemesh E, Annunziato RA, Arnon R, et al. Adherence to medical recommendations and transition to adult services in pediatric transplant recipients. Current Opinion Organ Transplantation. 2010;15:288–292.
93. Rosen DS, Blum RW, Britto M, et al. Transition to adult health care for adolescents and young adults with chronic conditions. Position paper of the Society for Adolescent Medicine. Journal of Adolescent Health. 2003;33:309–311.
94. Sawicki GS, Lukens-Bull K, Yin X, et al. Measuring the transition readiness of youth with special healthcare needs: validation of the TRAQ-Transition Readiness Assessment Questionnaire. Journal of Pediatric Psychology. 2011;36:160–171.
95. Annunziato RA, Parkar S, Dugan CA, et al. Brief report: deficits in health care management skills among adolescent and young adult liver transplant recipients transitioning to adult care settings. Journal of Pediatric Psychology. 2011;36:155–159.
96. Fredericks EM, Dore-Stites D, Well A, et al. Assessment of transition readiness skills and adherence in pediatric liver transplant recipients. Pediatric Transplantation. 2010;14:944–953.
97. GotTransition Transition Preparation-Transition Readiness Assessment (youth and family versions)[accessed September 23, 2012]; Available from: http://www.gottransition.org/6-core-Elements-Table; http://www.gottransition.org/UploadedFiles/Files/NHCTC_ReadinessYouthTool_06_Oct_2011.pdf; http://www.gottransition.org/UploadedFiles/Files/NHCTC_ReadinessFamilyTool_06Oct2011.pdf.
98. Good2Go Transition Readiness Checklists: Teen and parent versions. [cited September 23, 2012]; Available from: http://www.sickkids.ca/Good2Go/Transition-Interventions-Tools/Readiness-checklists/index.html.
99. UNC STARx Transition Scale Assessment and Transition Readiness Survey. [cited 2012 September 23, 2012] Available from: http://www.unckidneycenter.org/hcprofessionals/toolsfortransition.html.
100. American Academy of Pediatrics, American Academy of Family Physicians, American College of Physicians-American Society of Internal Medicine. A consensus statement on healthcare transitions for young adults with special healthcare needs. Pediatrics. 2002;110:1304–1306.
101. Devine KA, Reed-Knight B, Simons LE, et al. Prospective comparison of parent and adolescent report of health-related quality of life in adolescent solid organ transplant recipients. Pediatric Transplantation. 2010;14:1000–1006.
102. National Institutes of Health. PROMIS Overview. [cited September 4, 2012]; Available from: http://www.nihpromis.org/about/overview.
103. Prestidge C, Romann A, Djurdjev O, et al. Utility and cost of a renal transplant transition clinic. Pediatric Nephrology. 2012;27:295–302.
104. Bartosh SM, Ryckman FC, Shaddy R, et al. A national conference to determine research priorities in pediatric solid organ transplantation. Pediatric Transplantation. 2008;12:153–166.

第 9 篇

移植管理

第 122 章
移植协调

Dianne LaPointe Rudow

引言

移植患者成功管理的部分原因是多学科团队在移植术前、术中和术后护理。移植协调员是移植多学科团队的必要成员，在所有大型移植中心他们在移植护理过程中的必要性已被确定。移植协调员的作用有很多，但总的来说包括帮助患者度过复杂的移植护理并协助医生确定所必需的监测和护理。这章内容着重阐述移植协调员作为移植团队重要成员的转变过程，详细描述他们多种作用及责任，总结现有的培训认证模式。另外分别在第 124 章和第 125 章详细探讨协调员在住院患者及出院患者的服务方式中的作用。

移植协调员的历史及产生过程

移植协调目前是护理的作用，其发展是由于早些时候对于器官捐献及移植过程各个方面“协调”的必要。早期协调员来自许多专业人员包括：护理、外科技术和实验室人员。他们涉及器官复苏、储存和术后移植患者管理。

移植协调员已经从护理角色发展成为具有执业范围、技能及能力认证的专业人员。协调员通常有两种类型：获取协调员管理器官捐献的过程；临床移植协调员护理移植患者。临床移植协调员的作用进一步细化到器官特别的作用包括术前和术后。新兴的使用高级护理人员作为移植协调员，专门护理活体器官供者。

移植协调员最初的作用

早在移植的先驱者努力通过外科技术及免疫学方法使器官移植成为可能时，许许多多的幕后工作人员努力完成任务支持他们的工作。这些任务包括了捐献器官的复苏、储存和再灌注，选择和评估移植受者，协助发展器官分配方案等。本质上来讲包括了所有非医生的必要工作。“移植协调员”可能是移植外科医生创造的，为了寻找能完成多种任务的且具有多学科技能人员，以协调正在进行的工作。

美国的第一位移植协调员早在 20 世纪 60 年代，欧洲早在 20 世纪 70 年代，亚洲最早在 20 世纪 80 年代。最初的移植协调作为“能做各种事的人”，随着多种类型的移植协调员参与成功的器官移植，它逐渐转变成为一个职业并且是一种非常专业的职业。早期协调员主要宣传促进许多家庭理解器官捐献观念并促进捐献者同意捐献，同时协助外科医生获取器官、储存和灌注器官并将器官，安全地送到目的地。

第一批临床协调员常常是负责透析的护士，他们是从负责采购转变到负责管理移植等候名单，协助患者进行术前评估，在外科医生手术时管理移植术后问题，如术后并发症和移植免疫管理。事实上，移植协调员和内外科医生工作时可能是第一种模式，多学科团队合作对于移植的成功是至关重要的。

1979 年国家级协会北美移植协调员组织(NATCO)被创立，在这个协会中确立了移植协调员作为一个职业所需的教育背景、实践能力。这个早期的协调员组织也需要协作解决许多分配、法律、医学、社会、经济和宗教方面的问题，以促进移植的成功进行。

在美国器官共享网络(UNOS)和器官获取和移植网络(OPTN)创建之前，早期肾脏是由东南获取基金组织(SEOPF)完成分配的。但是大部分人没有意识到这些是移植协调员通过 NATCO 的“24 小时警惕系统”分配肾脏以外的器官。最初作为一个电话应答机，最后由计算机系统每周 7 天 24 小时分配器官。这些早期的移植先驱带着坚持、对移植成功的热情和动力定义了我们现在移植协调员的适用范围和实践能力。

移植认证

随着移植领域的发展，更多的人选择移植协调作为职业，这个职业由国家认证，并严格执行行业标准以护理器官供体和受体。假定为移植协调员的多个移植专业人员组成的特别小组，对其他健康组织进行职业分析、资格审查，并与其他涉及器官捐献和移植的专业人员进行讨论。1988年，一个独立非营利性组织——美国移植委员会认证组织(ABTC)被创立。起初这个组织提供获取和临床移植认证，现在ABTC作为四种移植认证代理：获取协调员认证(CPTC)、临床移植协调员认证(CCTC)、临床移植护士认证(CCTN)和移植保存员认证(CTP)。这些认证考试在器官移植领域是自愿的。它们的目标如下。

- 为移植专业建立教育和能力标准。
- 作为专业定义移植协调、移植护理和器官保存。
- 移植专业人员凭证。
- 维护从业人人员名单。
- 通过教育和认证促进从业人员的持续职业发展。

目前，移植协调员在考试之前必须工作至少一年，而且满足继续教育学分要求。在2010年，美国有超过2100名被认证的移植协调员。

获取协调员

如今获取协调员必须具有许多能力，而且可能承担一个或多个以下的器官获取代理机构的任务。

- 促进医院发展和职业教育。
- 评估器官和组织供者。
- 与家庭商谈器官捐献问题并获得知情同意。
- 通过访问家庭和可利用的资源得到广泛的医疗和社会背景。
- 确保器官捐献和恢复的所有医学和法律要求被优先满足。
- 帮助器官供者管理以维持器官功能良好。
- 确保器官分配的高效及时并按照UNOS政策进行。
- 协助外科团队进行器官恢复和组织储存。
- 维护供体记录。
- 与捐献家庭沟通并可以支持。
- 与捐赠医院的工作人员沟通合作并支持他们的工作。

临床移植协调员

正如获取协调员的作用随着时间的推移发生了变化一样，临床移植协调员也在变化。这个原因是多方面的：首先，患者变得更加复杂，许多患者和老年人同时患有多种合并症，有更多的管理要求和更多的移植手术要进行，药物治疗更加个性化，每个器官有其特有的程序。此外UNOS/OPTN和美国医疗保险都要求专业人员能胜任临床移植协调员并完成任务。

OPTN描述临床移植协调员在移植团队中负责协调候选人临床护理的各个方面。这些工作包括整个移植前后对患者及其家属进行登记随访。移植协调员必须是注册护士或别的许可的执行医疗保健工作的临床医生。

美国医疗保险(COP)要求临床移植协调员在患者和活体供体移植前、移植中、移植后恢复阶段提供持续的护理照顾。这包括认定和评估治疗方案、教育患者、活体捐献者和家庭治疗选择、术后护理和治疗、医疗监测、外科和心理状态，以及为其他团队成员提供反馈。肾移植协调员必须能证明其与透析设备厂家保持沟通。此外，所有协调员必须是注册医生或护士，而且在该州具有行医资格，并且具有捐献及移植相关知识及经验。

此外，美国医疗保险要求对护理及临床移植协调员进行培训，培训内容包括完全的职前培训计划、工作准则与工作规程学习、组织继续教育、评估协调员培训需求等。

如果同一人或不同人完成术前、术中或术后的多个任务都不符合管理部门的规定。每个个体的移植方案及所需任务都不相同。移植协调员具有术前、术后移植模式，另外在整个过程中都使用相同护理任务。另外一些方案只使用注册护士，而另外一些则具有多位健康管理专业人员协同工作完成多种任务。护理模式的案例显示在表122.1以及临床移植协调员的核心能力在表122.2中列出。

表 122.1 移植计划中使用的移植协调员护理模式

成员
• 移植协调员的注册护士
• 高级实践护士(APN)和(或)医生助理被聘为执行传统的移植协调员角色但没有自主权
• 组合高级实践护士 APN / RN 注册护士模型
• 只有高级实践护士模式
护理模式
• 用职责区分移植前和移植后协调员
• 连续性护理模型:移植前和移植后相同的协调者
• 电话服务模式
• 单器官团队和多器官团队
• 成人和儿科联合或分开

表 122.2 临床移植协调员(CTC)的能力

移植前
移植推荐及评估
• CTC 必须理解其目的是帮助协调移植评估
• CTC 必须遵守 UNOS/OPTN 规定登记候选人
等待期
• CTC 必须有知识和能力去监督和协调护理等待移植患者
• CTC 必须知道 CMS 和 UNOS/OPTN 要求
• CTC 必须维护和保留移植前教育和记录文件
围术期
• 当一个器官对等待的候选人适合时,CTC 具有促进移植完成的知识和能力
• CTC 必须遵守 UNOS/OPTN 分配原则
移植后
住院时
• CTC 具有移植术后管理相应的药物、并发症及干预知识
• CTC 参与出院计划
• CTC 与多学科团队有效的合作
门诊时
• CTC 具有协调门诊受体护理的知识
• CTC 促进受体能够具有最佳的体能、社交能力和良好情绪
专业实践
• CTC 能精通和不断扩充其移植知识
• CTC 对正确的判断力和管理受体、供体及他们家庭优质的护理负责

Adapted from the NATCO Core Competencies for the Clinical Transplant Coordinator [7].

移植前

评估

移植评估是通过确定适合的候选人治疗终末期器官衰竭最初的步骤。临床移植协调员必须理解术前评估的目的并协助其完成。这些包括:医学、心理学、实验室、放射学、营养学和经济评估。他们必须与多学科团队合作去确定血型、免疫学组织相容性、有无感染性疾病、扫描癌症证据、鉴别其他可能增加移植风险或阻碍移植成功的疾病,并将这些作为候选人评估项目[5-7]。

候选人的心理、精神和经济状况必须被评估,而且临床移植协调员必须与团队合作确定候选人的教育水平、文化背景、依从性和支持移植成功的充分证据。此外,他们必须和咨询医生、咨询公司合作评估患者的候选资格。

临床移植协调员必须理解和遵守所有 UNOS/OPTN 和 CMS 登记候选人的规定[5,6]。最后也是最重要的,临床移植协调员必须教育患者、患者家庭和支持团队所有移植相关的事物并做好医学记录。对移植患者教育的关键点见表 122.3。

等待期

临床移植协调员确定并管理等候名单对大型的腹腔移植尤为重要,由于器官获取时间长,要求评估测试的结果为最新的,因此,当一个器官被分配时要确定候选人已为移植做好了准备。根据年龄、疾病和器官需要,再次评估测试的类型及频率。临床协调员必须理解管理等候名单的工作准则和工作规程,熟悉国家对于重新检测以确保持续候选资格的建议。他们必须有知识和能力去监督和协调等待移植患者的护理,维持和患者的联系并与当地医生及透析中心保持广泛合作[7]。根据法律规定,移植前全部的病案资料、检测结果、患者教育与知情同意、任何患者与相关团队的通信都应以文档的形式被保留和维护。

围术期

当有器官被提供时,临床移植协调员需与器官获取机构(OPO)外科团队和患者密切合作。当一个器官对等待患者有用时,他们必须有相关知识及能力去促进移植的过程[7]。这些包括但不限于理解什么使器官适

表 122.3 教育及知情同意的关键点

- 移植评估过程
- 移植选择
  - 活体供体
  - 标准死亡供体
  - 扩大标准死亡供体
- 替代移植
- 器官分配
- OPTN 规定
- 移植等待
- 需要时重新评估
- 整个过程所需支持
- 选择多个队列移植
- 移植过程
- 移植风险及收益
- CDC 高风险因素
- 疾病复发风险
- 医学中心特殊患者和移植生存率与国家生存率比较
- 移植的经济因素
- 术后过程
  - 监测生命体征
  - 饮食及活动
  - 药物治疗目的、计量和副作用
  - 必要的活检和实验室检查
  - 健康保健及遵守治疗方案
- 怎样和移植团队交流
- 频繁随访的必要性
- 获得社会心理服务及当地医学护理的方法
- 怎样鉴别并发症
  - 排斥
  - 感染

Data from UNOS/OPTN Policy, CMS conditions of participation and NATCO Core com-petencies [5-7].

合移植，与移植团队和 OPO 交流关于器官的适合性、转运和政策，遵守器官分配政策，教育告知候选人器官分配的详细政策及过程。其他任务包括：协调运输，获取交叉配血结果，等候名单管理，核查供受体的重要数据，安排手术前程序(如透析等)，手术过程文档记录可能也需要临床移植协调员完成。临床移植协调员在围术期坚持目前的 UNOS/OPTN 分配策略是非常重要的。

移植后

住院期间

在移植时，患者和其支持系统都会忙于接受新生命依赖于供体的器官。不论是恢复顺利还是出现并发症，临床移植协调员都和多学科团队一起工作去护理患者度过过渡期。临床移植协调员必须对患者移植后的管理(包括药物治疗、并发症及干预措施)熟悉。多学科团队需要和咨询医生、咨询公司和付款人保持联系。移植协调员应促进这些联系和交流。另外，协调员必须参与出院计划制订，以预料患者出院后可能需要的医学心理学和经济需求[7]。对患者的教育是最重要的，必须以文明和适当的方法进行。

门诊服务期

临床协调员在受体出院后对受体进行照顾，必须能够熟悉和配合器官移植护理。这些患者情况都是非常复杂并且有出现并发症、药物副作用和意外的风险。移植协调员必须通过电话或亲自监护患者，能够了解患者的需要并干预患者并发症的危险因素。他们必须不断加强对患者的教育并确保患者充分理解。另外，他们必须评估许多可能影响器官功能的证据，这些证据可能并不相关。这些监护可能包括回顾器官功能相关的检测数据，评估药物的治疗范围以及识别并发症。协调员经常依据移植后指南，根据患者实验室检测结果调整患者的药物。他们必须协调团队中的外科和内科医生对患者的治疗方案做出调整。他们也参与患者联系会诊医生和病情随访，同样和其他学科人员一起促进患者身体、心理和情绪达到最佳状态[7]。

专业实习

临床移植协调员是移植过程中必不可少的角色，随着这个领域的发展，移植协调员依然是必须的。他们必须精通并不断地学习移植知识。为了不断学习，他们可以完成移植协调员认证并参加现在的继续教育研讨会。此外，他们必须阅读移植杂志的专业文献并将其与患者的护理工作相结合。移植协调员常常被要求参加移植相关的科研工作，并适当地发表他们的发现。

为了确保持续高质量的护理，有经验的移植协调员必须指导新成员专业技能的发展。坚持专业规定、分配原则、专业管理和正确的判断力是为供体、受体提供高质量的护理的必要条件。

活体供体协调员

随着对移植项目法律要求的增加，活体器官捐赠者护理的要求也增加了。活体捐献的移植项目必须有不同于受体的单独团队来护理活体供体。每一个供体必须分配一个独立的律师，而且活体供体移植协调员参与多学科过程去协调护理移植捐献前后的护理[6,8]。

活体供体协调员与临床移植协调员的职能相似，但是随之活体捐献领域的不断发展，活体器官提供的要求变得非常专业，从而成为移植的亚专科[9]。协调员护理活体供体需要一些特别的能力以提供高质量的护理。这些能力可见表 122.4。对移植、相关法规和规程理解并具有应用知识对活体供体协调员是非常重要的，因为潜在的供体需要理解器官接受过程、捐献风险、生存概率，并依靠一个经验和知识丰富的供体团队为捐献做出准备。他们必须确定合适的活体供体候选人并协调对活体供体的评估过程。供体安全是非常重要的而且是优先考虑的，那些具有禁忌证的人员在这个过程的早期将被排除[10]。协调员必须具有丰富的经验以评估供体的动机，理解风险的能力，以及成为捐献者的愿望。协调员常常参与到对患者、患者家庭及大众的教育中，这些教育包括：移植过程、危险、获益和随访的需要。协调员与多学科团队合作参与供体的护理和决定供体的适用性。如果供体不合适或供体决定不捐献，协调员需要确保供体对结果满意并对他们的需要提供支持。协调员为患者提供直接护理、支持和移植后捐献教育，这些贯穿于围术期和术后长期随访。最后，活体供体协调员为捐献前、捐献后，或者选择不再捐献的供体提供护理和倡议。

表 122.4 活体供体协调员的职责

• 保持对移植的理解和具有移植相关政策和程序的应用知识。
• 明确 OPTN/UNOS 的政策和要求
• 识别合适的活体供体候选人
• 协调活体供体的评估过程
• 对患者、家属及公众进行活体捐献、捐献流程、相关风险、收益及随访要求的教育
• 评估供体是否适合
• 与多学科团队合作参与供体护理和活体捐献的倡议
• 为患者提供直接护理、支持和移植后捐献的相关教育，这些贯穿于围术期和术后长期随访
• 为捐献前、捐献后，或者选择不再捐献的供体提供护理和倡议

协调员在教育中的作用

临床移植协调员很可能最重要的角色是作为教育者[11]。尽管比过去更为常见，但仍然只有有限的数量的医生能够护理移植如此复杂的患者群体。不管他们进行哪种器官移植工作或护理哪些方面，移植协调员必须对他们的患者及患者家庭进行宣教。这些主题在之前已经被讨论过了。另外对其他护士、顾问、咨询医生、住院医生、医学生、移植研究人员的教育也是必要的。除医疗小组以外，临床移植协调员还需要对付款人、监管机构、财务协调员、药师和大众进行教育，告知他们不同移植之间的差别以更好的支持患者。因此，了解移植的各个方面对协调员是非常重要的。

高级实践护士(APN)作为协调员的作用

临床移植协调员的传统作用具有明显的自主性。因此，许多移植项目使用临床专业实践护士照顾移植患者。原因包括如下。

• APN 接受过身体评估和诊断测试的培训，同时受过独立管理复杂疾病过程的训练。

• APN 的自主练习是经过授权的。

• APN 在大多数州具有处方权。

• APN 能够要求医疗保险、医疗援助及私人付款人为服务付款。

• 大量患者需要健康照顾，移植中心已经不堪重负，并且移植领域住院医生和内科医生较为缺乏，APN 能填补这些空白。

APN 作为临床移植协调员的任务包括：移植前教育和评估，等候名单管理，与咨询医生协调，在手术室协助外科医生，移植前及移植后住院患者管理，移植后出院患者免疫抑制及并发症管理，移植受者长期管理，护理活体器官供体，护理儿童移植受者，推广门诊管理，移植前后的心理照顾，专业发展和领导力[9,12-17]。

APN 补充了现有人员的配置模式。利用 APN 的护理模式多种多样，但是对护理能力的补充依赖于经济激励[18]。他们可以减轻医疗团队过重的负担，为患者提供优质的护理和教育。图 122.1 示出 APN 如何并入当前移植小组的例子。他们可以和内外科医生合作，与移

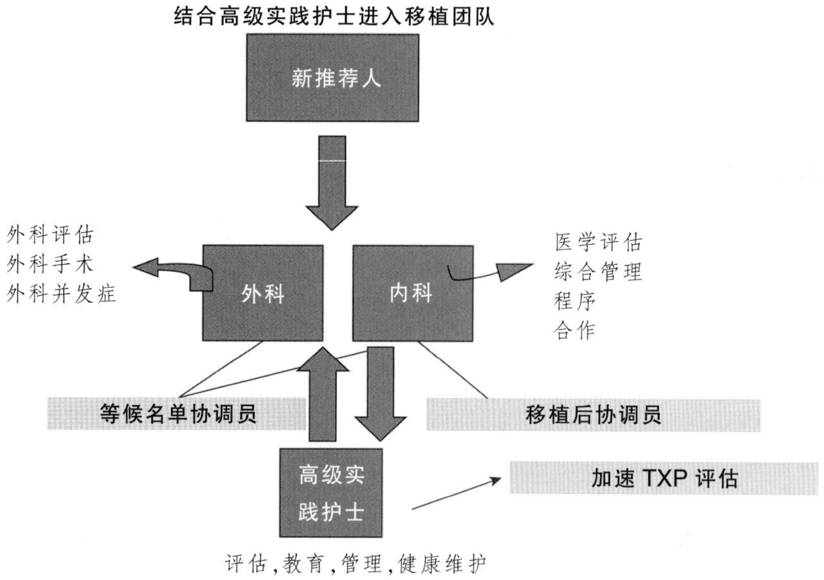

图 122.1 使用高级实践护士的护理模式。

植协调员一起工作或者代替他们照顾移植前后的患者。我们需要用广泛成本分析和成功使用的数据,了解能对移植前和移植后的患者真正受益的方案。

总结

不管移植协调员在器官捐献或移植的哪个方面的工作,他们都是患者支持、临床管理、教育、协调移植团队的其他人员以取得成功的关键组成部分。传统上的协调员是一个有多方面知识和经验的注册护士,现在有许多的专业人员来做协调员,其中包括了高级实践护士。随着移植领域医疗改革的不断深入,移植协调员的作用也在发生着转变,以适应患者的需求。

(郭海军 译 徐骁 校)

参考文献

1. Shafer T. History of the transplant coordinator. In: LaPointe Rudow D, Ohler L, Schaefer T, editors. A Clinicians Guide to Organ Donation and Transplantation. Lenexa, KS: Applied Measurements Professionals; 2006: 25–78.
2. American Board of Transplant Certification Handbook. [assessed January 3, 2012]; Available from: http://abtc.net/documents/ABTChandbookDec2010.pdf.
3. American Board of Transplant Certifications. [assessed January 3, 2012]; Available from: http://abtc.net/.
4. Core Competencies for the Procurement Transplant Coordinator. [assessed January 3, 2012]; Available from: http://www.natco1.org/prof_development/documents/CPTCCompetencies_May09.pdf.
5. OPTN Evaluation Plan, section IV, Membership Criteria. [assessed January, 2012]; Available from: http://optn.transplant.hrsa.gov/ContentDocuments/Evaluation_Plan_123111.pdf.
6. Medicare Conditions of Participation for organ transplant programs. [assessed January 3, 2012]; Available from: http://www.cms.gov/CertificationandComplianc/20_Transplant.asp.
7. Core Competencies for the Clinical Transplant Coordinator. [assessed January 3. 2012]; Available from: http://www.natco1.org/prof_development/documents/CCTCCompetencies_May09.pdf.
8. Organ Procurement and Transplant Network (OPTN) policies about live donation. [assessed January 7, 2012]; Available from: http://optn.transplant.hrsa.gov/PoliciesandBylaws2/policies/pdfs/policy_172.pdf.
9. LaPointe Rudow D. Development of the Center for Living Donation: incorporating the role of the nurse practitioner as director. Progress in Transplantation. 2011;21(4):312–317.
10. Garvey G. Living kidney donors. In: LaPointe Rudow D, Ohler L, Schaefer T, editors. A Clinicians Guide to Organ Donation and Transplantation. Lenexa, KS: Applied Measurements Professionals; 2006: 527–535.
11. Charlton M, Ventura K. Education and the transplant patient. In: LaPointe Rudow D, Ohler L, Schaefer T, editors. A Clinicians Guide to Organ Donation and Transplantation. Lenexa, KS: Applied Measurements Professionals; 2006: 549–559.
12. Core Competencies for the Advanced Practice Transplant Professional. [assessed January 3, 2012]; Available from: http://natco1.org/prof_development/documents/NATCOAPTPCoreCompetencies_FinalWeb.pdf.
13. Martin RK. The role of the transplant advanced practice nurse: a professional and personal evolution. Critical Care Nursing Quarterly. 1999;21(4):69–76.
14. Tedesco J. Acute care nurse practitioners in transplantation: adding value to your program. Progress in Transplantation. 2011;21(4):278–284.
15. Lerret SM, Stendahl G. Working together as a team: adolescent transplant recipients and nurse practitioner. Progress in Transplantation. 2011;21(4):288–294.
16. Hoy H, Alexander S, Payne J, et al. The role of advanced practice nurses in transplant center staffing. Progress in Transplantation. 2011;21(4):294–299.
17. Brennan J, McEnhill M. Use of nurse practitioners in pediatric kidney transplant: a model for providing comprehensive care to children and families. Progress in Transplantation. 2011;21(4):306–312.
18. Hoch DA, Maynard E, Whiting J. Billing and reimbursement for advanced practice in solid organ transplantation. Progress in Transplantation. 2011;21(4):274–278.

第 123 章
移植药学服务

Christin C. Rogers, Nicole A. Pilch, Eric M. Tichy, Lonnie D. Smith, David J. Taber, Rita R. Alloway

引言

移植的成功主要依赖在其他因素的作用下一系列药物的适当使用。事实上,管理免疫移植药物、抗感染药物,常常需要移植团队付出大量努力处理疾病状况的药物清单,常常需要考虑关键药物间的相互作用和不相容性。因此,药剂师已经成为大部分移植团队的重要成员,移植药剂师已经被列入编制。本章将介绍移植药剂师作为多学科移植服务的一部分的作用,为读者提供成为移植药剂师必要培训的一般理解,以及其能改善患者的治疗效果和护理的方式。移植的药理学的具体内容在第 98~第 102 章中介绍。

移植药剂师的发展

药剂师作为多学科移植医疗团队的一部分已有近半个世纪。1976 年,俄亥俄州立大学 John Mitchell 首次详细介绍了药剂师在移植团队中的作用[1]。Mitchell 在 20 世纪 70 年代描述的药剂师的作用和今天执业药剂师的作用非常相似。2007 年,Gilbert Burckart 博士发表了对过去 30 年移植药学的反思[2]。在这本著作中,他将功劳归功于匹兹堡大学的 Thomas Starzl 博士和美国明尼苏达大学的 John Najarian 博士,因为他们最先将药剂师看作移植团队的成员并认识到他们药物治疗的专长。1986 年,Burckart 和同事 Venkataramanan 及 Ptachcinski 在临床实践中改进了环孢素的治疗药物监测,并出版了环孢素详细的药代动力学著作[3]。自 20 世纪 80 年代中期以来,药剂师在移植药代动力学著作的发表上不断做出显著的贡献,除了免疫抑制剂治疗的药物基因组学外,还将重点放在临床移植疗效的相关著作[4-10]。移植药剂师对患者的治疗效果的直接影响已被论文证明,这篇论文表明移植药学服务改善用药的依从性和血压管理[11-13]。

对于今天的移植医生而言,移植团队内的药剂师已经完成了从新奇到期望的转变。最值得注意的是,第一次描述药剂师作为移植多学科团队成员的作用的论文发表在 2011 年的美国移植杂志[14]。这篇文章概述了药剂师在住院患者、门诊和研究环境时的各种作用,并介绍了胜任这些任务所需要的培训。

除了对论文的贡献,移植药剂师已经越来越受到各专业药店和医疗社会认可。在过去的 5 年里这个专业的成员已经成倍的增长。自 1994 年成立以来,美国大学临床药学院(ACCP)的免疫学移植实践和研究网络已经从 75 名成员发展到 330 名成员,最引人注目的是 2004—2011 年的成员从 170 增长到 332 名[15]。这些增长主要与对于移植药剂师的需求的增加以及美国医疗保险和医疗补助服务中心(CMS)的规定有关,这将在本章的后面进行讨论。

ACCP 和美国药师协会(ASHP)现在确定移植药剂师是一个值得肯定的专业,为特殊的患者人群服务。ASHP 现已有对移植药剂师的认定标准为参加 2 年制的移植住院医师培训(PGY2),在全国实施移植药师住院医生培训计划[16]。这对于移植药剂师的培训非常重要,它确保了移植药剂师住院医生必须达到特定的标准,并且接受高质量的培训。PGY2 移植住院医生培训计划的数量也在过去十年急剧增加,从不到 6 个增长到 2012 年 20 多个,其中大部分是 ASHP 认证的。这些使移植药剂师行业持续发展,并保持提供给所有移植的供者和受者卓越的高标准的药学服务。

2008 年,美国移植学会(AST)主任委员将移植药剂师加入实践团队模式(CoP)。CoP 是 2009 年启动的,至 2011 年 11 月已有超过 160 名成员,其中包括主席、主席当选人、前任主席及四名成员。自从一名移植药剂师被美国移植杂志正式任命为编委会成员开始，移植药剂师发展成为美国移植协会的正式组织成员，移植药剂师对于整个移植的成功非常重要，并且在持续教育高危患者药物治疗方面做出杰出贡献。

管理部门对移植药剂师的支持

1984年，根据国家器官移植法(NOTA)，美国国会建立了同意的移植网络被誉为器官获取和移植网络(OPTN)。法律要求移植网络为私人经营，基于联邦协议是一个非营利组织。OPTN的两个主要目的是：①增加器官共享的效果和效率，增加器官分配的公平性；②增加移植器官的供给。OPTN是连接所有参与捐献和移植体系专业人士独特的机构。OPTN是由器官共享网络执行，主要依据与美国卫生人类服务部分的健康资源与服务管理局签订的协议[17]。

由UNOS制订的一系列章程确定了每个移植过程的确切标准，这些章程是为了使所有移植过程都符合标准。这些规章在2004年进行了修订，为了确定药剂师作为移植小组的重要成员的作用和责任。具体而言，这些章程强制要求"所有的移植方案应该确定一个以上药剂师为固体器官移植受者提供药学服务"[18]。移植药剂师是团队中的特定成员，发挥团队中药物信息专家的关键作用，并有责任遵守制度，筛选和预测药物相互作用，教育患者和看护人员，具体在本章的后面部分论述。CMS为可以接受服务收费的移植项目提供认证。CMS每3~4年实地考察所有被其认可的移植中心，以确保这些移植中心符合确立的条件。2007年3月30日，CMS出版了审批和重新审批移植中心执行器官移植医疗的医学需求。该文概述了CMS认证的特殊要求。至于药剂师在移植团队中的作用，该文件指出"一个移植中心必须确定一个多学科移植小组(由医学、护理、营养、社会服务、移植协调、药理学成员组成)，并描述了团队的每一个成员的责任。该文献没有特别指出药剂师必须加入具有药理学知识的团队。然而，在CMS一个开放性评论中提到UNOS章程详细描述了药剂师对移植小组的特别作用[19]。指南说明的更新版本在2008年6月出版[20]。文中列出了的重要更新，包括需要多学科团队的所有成员在病历中记录所有活动，以及需要多学科团队全程参与照顾在捐献和移植的过程中各个不同的阶段的供体和受体。这些阶段包括了等待移植阶段、围术期、移植后住院期间以及出院后。

除了更新指南说明，2008年9月CMS发表了一系列文件协助对医学中心的调查计划[21]。文件规定了在CMS访问住院期间要会见移植药剂师。这个文件提供了药剂师将被问及的典型问题。还会审查药剂师的人事档案，以评估药剂师的移植专业培训、目前的能力和与移植继续教育。

移植药剂师的教育和培训

移植药剂师有多种水平的训练和教育。最近ACCP移植和免疫学的实践与研究网络(PRN)的一项调查显示，大多数执业移植药剂师都接受过先进的训练，这些已经超出了他们的药学博士学位。66%的移植药剂师完成了1年的PGY培训，另外45%完成了高级移植培训和(或)收到奖学金。尽管多数移植药剂师都接受高级培训，但是移植药剂师的最低要求每个移植中心均不相同。37%调查回应者表示，他们的人员要求最少为药学博士学位。另外35%的要求至少1年PGY1培训，29%的表示至少5年移植经验或者毕业后2年PGY2培训，26%要求移植PGY2培训。

从历史看，一个注册药剂师要求4年的理学学士学位。然而在20世纪90年代，学位要求转变为博士学位。目前，大部分药学院都同意四年的药学博士计划，随后完成前提条件，或者完成4年的理学学士，随后完成2年的药学博士。最后一年博士课程主要由一系列患者护理为主的临床轮转组成。取得药学博士学位以后，所有人必须通过国家和州法律规定的考试，并且在药房作为药剂师完成特定的实践时间，才能得到药剂师注册执照。

正规研究生培养之前的移植药剂师实践

许多现有的移植药剂学学者没有正规的住院医师培训就进入了实践阶段。这些药剂师对新药剂师的发展原则、现有教育标准和认可的培训项目负责。

毕业后的住院医生培训

复杂的移植学和在药学博士课程中有限的接触，需要药学博士接受正式的毕业后临床培训。研究生培养的第一阶段往往是PGY1药学住院医生培训项目完成。这个住院医生是ASHP认证的。完成PGY1住院医生培训，就可以通过各种临床护理培训，例如：内科、外科、重症监护，专科如移植、感染科、心内科、卧床护理等等。除了临床轮转，PGY1 住院医生还参与管理实践，教学活动，并通过临床研究增加他们的相关经验。这篇介绍可以作为技能和能力发展的基础，以在多个实践过程中提供药学服务。

紧随着 PGY1 住院医生培训，移植药剂师应该完成 PGY2 在移植的专科培训。大多数 PGY2 培训项目是 ASHP 认证的。PGY2 药剂住院医生器官移植培训的目的、目标和教育成绩的设计都是为了使 PGY1 住院医生从全科实践转变到器官移植的专科实践，并注重器官移植、活体器官移植受体的护理。毕业生准备好参加跨学科团队，这些团队患者医学相关护理负责，包括了住院及出院患者的教育和研究。

移植研究员培训

尽管非常少的移植药剂师经历专科团队培训。适合此类培训项目的数目是有限的。这些项目需要两年而且要求完成 PGY1 或者 PGY2 住院医生培训。不同于 PGY2 移植专科住院医生培训，PGY2 强调的是患者护理，移植研究员培训重点是移植领域的基础和（或）临床研究。研究员的目的是训练药剂师成为移植领域独立的研究者。

附加的正规教育

理学硕士临床研究（MCR）项目已面向全国，目的是为临床医生提供必要的多学科技能和教育，促进他们作为独立的或者合作者进入临床研究。这些项目增加了新移植药剂师在试验设计、流行病学和生物统计方面的研究潜能。另外，一些移植药剂师参加了其他类型的附加正式教育，包括理学硕士的公众健康或商业管理。

患者护理团队的角色和职责的描述

住院患者移植药剂师的职责与责任

临床移植药剂师结合几个亚专科原理，将会是多学科住院移植患者护理团队的有效成员（可见第 124 章）。这些包括患者从重症监护室到出院整个护理过程的药物优化治疗，这些患者包括成人、儿童受体和活体供体。有关于药物输送系统、药物经济学、药品信息和药物文献评估、统计、免疫学、药代动力学、药理学、药物基因组学、生理学、药物、药物安全、监管标准，和用药安全的知识是必要的。移植药剂师需要具有大量的专业知识，在新型与传统免疫管理中，并将其与其他二级专科相结合，例如传染病、心脏病学、肝脏病学、肾病学、肺病学、内分泌科、血液学、儿科学和特级护理学，为了管理有多种合并疾病的患者。

当移植药剂师为住院临床团队服务时，他们在移植围术期及移植后有许多责任。这些包括：通过安全和有效的参数主动持续监测药物治疗处方的恰当运用以及治疗结果。移植药剂师每日的主要任务包括：移植药物监测、药代动力学及药效评估、药物（药物与食物间）相互作用管理、药物最优化管理、药物输送及消耗。此外，移植药剂师还担任与护士协调员、执业医生、社会工作者及患者护理团队的其他成员对住院及出院药物的协调工作。

移植药剂师通常还参与移植用药指南的编写，并确保在移植过程中使用指南，主动监测指南相关的预后，收集相关数据用于之后指南的修改。涉及评估指南效果的数据搜集常常和移植中心的研究任务一同进行，移植药剂师在医疗质量的改善上逐渐发挥重要作用[22]。

这些指南要求和移植医生达成一致并得到医疗机构内的药物使用监督委员会批准，这些委员会如药学治疗学会。在这种情况下，移植药剂师需要确保指南与机构指导方针一致，为了确保医疗安全指南要求监督委员会批准。这些指南将与实践协议一起执行。

医生和药剂师之间的合作协议存在于一个或多个药剂师和一个或多个医生在任何环境下的药物治疗协议中，在这些环境中药剂师和患者的关系已经成立[23]。一个治疗合作协议提供了药剂师在治疗的范围内管理药物的权力。在移植时，这样的协议授权药剂师根据患者的个体需求提供护理服务，这些服务包括但是不限于随访：

- 提供处理配药服务外的医患关系。
- 执行评估和面谈，以获得完整的用药、医疗、社会以及其他相关的患者信息评估。
- 通过获取和评估有效性和（或）耐受性的客观和主观指标监测药物治疗。
- 启动、修改和终止药物治疗。

• 对患者和照顾者开展药物培训，包括用药条件、相关的非药物干扰、健康促进因素。

• 患者健康档案中记录与交流。

移植药师的另一个重要任务是对患者和护理人员的教育。对患者及家属教育的一个重要部分就是在移植后住院期间接受相关药物。药剂师提供或者协助大部分此类的教育并评估患者和家属独立管理出院后药物的能力。移植药物及时与多学科团队的其他护理成员一起协助，在协助药物治疗方面起着重要的作用，因为他们随访患者贯穿其整个治疗过程。

另外在教育患者及其护理者移植后药物的适当管理时，患者对免疫抑制剂的副作用及危险因素的教育需求很大。这种风险意识的提升源于新的食品药品管理局(FDA)关于风险评估和缓解策略条例(REM)。如果确定了REM是必要的以确保药物的益处大于风险，在2008年3月美国FDA被授权要求药品生产企业提交药品推荐的REM作为审批过程的一部分[24]。REM组成部分的变化是基于风险的严重性。REM要求任何或所有以下情况：①用药向导及药品包装；②交流计划；③确保安全使用的元素(ETASO)。

REM项目都需要接受制造商和FDA定期评估。这些评估最少要在批准后的18个月、3年、7年进行。移植供体必须留在不断变化的REM要求内，保证患者接受他们药物治疗风险的适当的教育。mTOR受体抑制剂(依维莫司)是经FDA的REM项目批准的第一个免疫抑制剂。原来的REM计划包括交流计划和用药指导，一年半后用药指南被批准从REM移除。(用药指南）加入西罗莫司的REM项目10多年，在它被FDA批准后，在6个月前才被移除[25]。贝拉西普是在2011年6月贝拉西普FDA批准的第一个生物类免疫抑制剂。贝拉西普被批准时要求有REM项目，该项目要求使用药物向导和交流计划。通常药物指南被零售药房和最初的处方及所有后来的再填充一起分发。贝拉西普是第一个静脉内维持的免疫抑制药物。鉴于贝拉西普的给药方式及移植围术期首次计量，出现了一些争议，在必要时为患者提供用药指南。2011年11月，FDA公布了为住院患者提供用药指南的规定。该文件指出，药物治疗指南应该包括如下。

• 患者或护理者可在任何时候要求药物指南。

• 如果药物受限于一个因素，为了确保安全需使用REM，REM要求提供和审查用药指南。

• 药物第一次在诊所或者输液室被医务人员用于患者时。

• 药物用药指南发生大的修改后第一次在诊所或者输液室被医务人员用于患者时。

• 任何时候，药物在院外被直接发到患者及其照料者时。

Gabardi和他的同事在2011年出版了评论REM系统的细节和REM在移植影响。这些评论应该被查阅，以了解REM在移植概述中更多的细节[27,28]。

移植药剂师发明一些工具、个性化策略和系统以改进药物的依从性。这些范围中的一些来自教育技术使用的提醒工具，帮助确认复杂药物治疗方案的依从性。

例子包括：教育材料的发展材料，视频或其他视觉辅助；规定和指导使用药丸或其他存储设备；电子方法如自动短信或电子邮件提醒;实现基于Web的药物名单和组织方案；患者管理新药的自动药物程序；在移植团队直接管理药物时，建立信赖及承担管理药物的责任。

除了教育患者及其家庭成员外，移植药剂师也对别的移植护理提供者及医学中心的其他药剂师负有教育责任，这些药剂师可能管理移植受者的药物治疗。在住院部设置的移植药剂师交流和记录所有行为在病历上，保证各个水平从业者理解护理移植药物的治疗计划。此外，移植药剂师对患者、患者家人和护理者解释清楚药物变化的关键问题和治疗计划是很有必要的。在此，药剂师在创造一个平稳安全的护理过渡中做出重大贡献[14]。

移植药剂师参与日间护理设定

实现移植药学服务进入门诊并添加到各种影响患者预后的服务中。移植药剂师提供了广泛的临床和手术服务，补充了门诊移植服务的处理任务(见第125章)。一些研究已经评估了移植药剂师在门诊设定中的影响。Chisholm和他的同事评估了肾移植门诊临床药剂师主导的辅助计划的成本节约情况[29]。共有61例患者入选，通过行业赞助援助计划应用免费免疫抑制剂，在计划的第一年节约了124 793美元的成本。药剂师的时间成本估计有16 650美元。2008年，Chisholm和他的同事随后的研究评估了临床药学服务对移植预后和依从性的影响。这项研究调查了两组肾移植受者。干预组(n=12)提供了旨在促进服从性、依从性、药物教育和获得药物治疗的强烈的临床药学服务，而对照组（n=12）接受标准护理。结果表明，在干预组有较高的药物依从性坚持率（96.1%±4.7%），而对照组为（81.6%±11.5%，$P<0.001$）。在这些患者中最终成为不依从的患者，干预组比对照组坚持服药持续时间长（平均 11 个月而对照组为 9 个月，$P<0.05$）[30]。

实施专门药剂师服务的移植服务的投资回报包括：改善患者及移植的预后，通过促进适当的编码和计费程序增加特殊治疗的费用报销（例如，巴利昔单抗、抗胸腺细胞球蛋白、静脉注射免疫球蛋白）。此外，移植药剂师在诊所能更好地识别患者不服从引发的继发财务问题的高危风险。药剂师可以参考这些个体的患者援助项目或修改他们的方案使成本效益最大化。

多个移植中心也实现了门诊药房移植药学服务以提高门诊药房的收入，通过开发更多的疾病状态管理服务（例如，药剂师协助糖尿病、抗凝、高血压、或丙型肝炎治疗）改善患者的预后，这些服务允许快速、简洁的指导产生直接结果或利用药剂师为患者提供的建议回到门诊药房补充超出了他们的免疫抑制剂的处方[31]。一些门诊移植药剂师模式的存在，可以帮助患者从住院到出院持续改善患者的护理。具体而言，当药剂师在住院和门诊服务之间转换时，专业的门诊药剂师可以为门诊患者提供住院后的药物辅导。此外，利用提供者均可进入的电子信息系统可以促进患者问题的交流，如患者需要问询、依从性障碍、或可能引起感染或免疫排斥的病情变化。

最近，从监管的角度来看，移植药剂师被医疗保险和医疗服务中心（CMS）要求在移植前对患者进行评估。这是一个额外的机会让移植团队利用移植药剂师调整移植之前的药物情况，识别移植后服药依从性的阻碍，必要时为围术期药物的选择提供建议。

综合住院和药学服务程序在移植后药物依从性的影响发表在 2009 年[32]。这项研究是一项前瞻性的随机对照试验，旨在评估 50 位肝移植受者 12 个月的药学护理服务项目对移植后依从性的影响。这项研究中用以评估依从性的方法包括：药物事件监测系统（MEM）、免疫抑制剂浓度、药片数量、自我报告和 Morisky 问卷。除了常规的临床护理，患者随机分配到干预组，在干预组患者将受到一个专门的医院药剂师提供的医药监护服务。药剂师在患者出院前大约一个星期开始会见患者，在这次会见中，他们会讨论药物剂量、可能的副作用、药物监测和出院后药物指导。这样的会面通常在出院前发生 3~4 次。此外，在出院时，这些患者将被给予药物、出院计划和记录生命体征和试验的书面指导。在第一年，移植后患者按季度会见药剂师，主要讨论药物更改、实验室和药物相关问题。结果表明，被随机分配接受医药监护的患者比对照组依从率更高（90.2%±6.2%比 80.8%±12.4%，$P=0.015$），这个数据是电子依从性检测系统评估的 [(# 正确的开启瓶子天数/# 监控天数)×100]。根据药片计数评测依从性的结果显示，在患者内部存在很大的差异，尤其是控制组。然而，在接受药学监护的患者中坚持服药率仍然明显高于对照组。血清免疫抑制剂水平在接受药物监护的患者中与对照组相比有显著较高比例（78%对 51%，$P<0.001$）[32]。

尽管在住院及出院患者中药学服务都是需要的，但近期的一项调查结果显示 43%的移植药剂师更关注患者的住院期间的服务。36%移植药剂师能够将他们的时间分配给住院和门诊患者，另有 3%的药剂师将时间分配到在院、门诊、研究和移植管理。大部分的努力都集中在肾肝脏和胰腺移植受者中。越来越多的药剂师也对心脏（34%）、肺（29%）移植受者提供药物服务。由于复合组织异体移植方案变得越来越普遍，回应调查的 5%的药剂师表示他们已经成为这种多学科团队的一部分。

确定药剂师与理想患者的比例仍然是一个挑战。这项调查获得了每个站点药剂师的数量和年移植率，并允许计算在研究的医疗中心现有药剂师与患者的比率（图 123.1）。每年超过 200 例移植患者的移植中心中有（78%）的中心雇佣超过 2 位药剂师，他们覆盖了所有器官移植及提供所有住院及门诊患者的服务。

药剂师在临床研究中的作用

理解药剂师作为专业临床专家的潜能

临床和转化研究不是一个单一的活动而是一个连续的过程。由于其跨学科性质，药剂学与这种连续性结合得非常好[33]。特别是在移植中，许多移植药剂师作为住院和门诊医疗团队之间的联络人[14]。移植药剂师的先进观点使他们发展很好，并通过临床和转化研究促进和分析移植相关的预后。

药剂师在免疫抑制药物研究中存在一些独特的挑

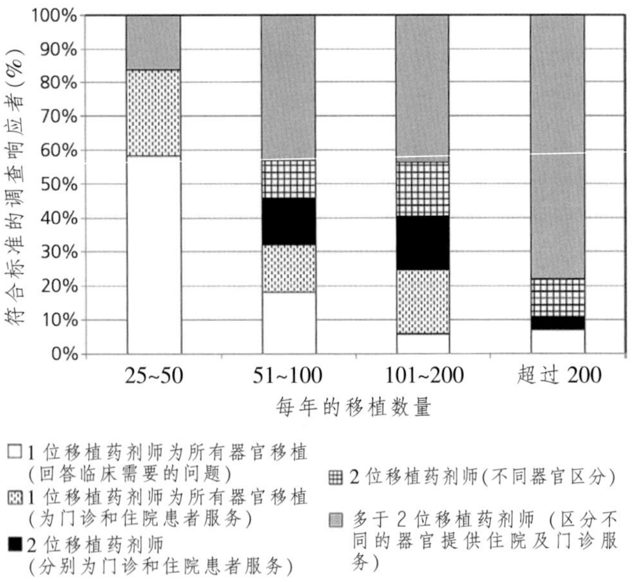

图 123.1 移植药剂师与移植数量的比例。

战。他们越来越需要了解药物开发流程，最佳临床实践，联邦法规和准则，和临床研究指南的发展、实施和监督。另外，编写临床研究指南是需要广泛的训练和经验，任何临床研究指南都包括背景、原理和方法部分。药剂师在剂型技术、药物化学、药理学和对药物开发和商业化过程中的关键的治疗学上有强力的技术背景，而且是临床免疫抑制药物治疗研究的有效研究者。在发现和转化研究的领域，受过特别培训的药剂师可以提供临床前研究，这些研究能评估新技术和新方法是否适用于药物基因组学，而且他们能够设计方法开发临床上有用的生物标志物。他们还可以监督和规划临床发展战略；设计研究；书写研究方案；监督研究实施；分析数据、作者报告和出版物；审查信息资料的科学内涵。受过药代动力学和药物代谢学专门训练的药剂师通常被要求设计和分析从各种移植研究获得的数据。移植药剂师牵涉了研究的这些领域，聚集于Ⅱ和Ⅲ阶段研究的安全性和有效性，或第Ⅳ阶段上市后研究，以解决新型免疫抑制剂的组合和优化治疗策略[34]。

很少在移植中进行大型研究，以恰当地评估各种器官移植的类型或方案组合使用的所有药物。随着从研究到实践这样一个快速过渡，药剂师是唯一受过将自己治疗的知识与临床移植的知识相结合这种教育，来审慎评估这种疗法的疗效和毒性。虽然这不应取代良好对照的临床试验，但这种做法在移植中是不可避免的。药剂师独特的定位使其谨慎地评估小试点的经验，并慎重地将其应用于实践中，但是必须遵从无伤害原则。

随着引进比较效益研究，一个新的研究终点被开发注重于整体医疗成本控制。虽然许多药物治疗的成本效益存在争论，但是药物治疗花费被看成医疗费用中包含的最简单的部分。药剂师对药物花费的整体影响有独特的理解，这些观点可能与药物花费与整体医疗成本管理独立的观点相距较远。这在移植尤其重要，因为药物费用关系到终生免疫抑制治疗的成本。

药剂师在连续的临床研究中的作用

研究领域的成功通常需要与医生或多学科研究者的团队有效的合作。在移植多学科的团队中已经建立了很好的合作，最近这个团队中药剂师的作用加强了。药剂师的作用可能采用多种形式体现，主要是有关个人的知识基础和个人能力，再结合体制的需求。同样地，药剂师的角色和责任在研究中也可以发生变化。作为一名临床研究人员，药剂师参与临床试验中Ⅰ~Ⅳ期的所有阶段。在各种研究中，药剂师的主要角色包括：首席研究员，合作研究者，副研究员，协调员，研究性的药剂师，研究协调员，研究助理等。作为主要研究者的药剂师，是最终对研究设计、实施、报告和监测的负责者。药剂师作为副研究员或共同参与者与医生协同工作开展，以确保符合这些日益复杂的研究所需的监管和报告要求。作为共同研究者的药剂师必须有应用免疫抑制药物知识的能力，用于针对纳入试验的不同患者，在整个移植过程中跟上他们的进展。药剂师日常参与病房巡视及门诊，协助临床医生和研究人员试验程序，以及提供药物治疗管理的专业知识。

移植与研究药剂学之间的界限

首席调查员负责计划，以控制试验用药物。例如，它如何存储、控制和分散，因此只有合格的研究员和参与者可以使用研究药物。很多时候这个责任委托给研究药物的药剂师。研究性药学服务在实体器官移植的研究中可能非常复杂，因为大部分移植没有预定的时间表，因此要求大部分移植研究需要实时服务和长期研究药物来评估长期的预后。实体器官移植中有经验的专业研究药学服务能促进各方面的进行。在许多移植研究中，研究产品的随机化和(或)管理必须在移植前或移植过程中发生。以保证此项服务及移植产品能够及时交付,避免移植程序被延迟,这是非常重要的。这需要研究性药剂师与临床研究团队密切合作与沟通。促进慢性药物长期、及时并遵守相关规定标准的发放对于临床试用产品是一个挑战。这必须在有准备的复杂移植后药物治疗情况下进行。了解各个研究的复杂性和研究性药物服务(IDS)可以使有效的沟通最大化。在每个阶段进行有效的沟通是效果最佳的。表 123.1 概述了必要的沟通阶段以保证最佳的效果。

随着大量使用了适应证外药物,移植的基本挑战之一是你的研究是否包括研究药物。要确定你的研究是否符合研究药物的定义,你可能会问"在人类研究中使用的药物的主要目的是为了积累科学知识?"如果是这样的话,你的研究可考虑使用研究药物。是否研究药物服务的必要性,可由图 123.2 来了解。决策图包括了基本的问题,但是,对具体的问题要求必须量身制订。研究药物服务的使用并不一定需要由药房发药。

药剂师作为临床研究的指挥者

一些药剂师已经成为临床研究的指挥者。在此期间,药剂师结合行政和临床知识,以促进一个给定机构内移植临床研究的整体进行。当许多高校倾向于对美国卫生研究院(NIH)资助的研究提供基础设施时,很多高校却不为正在进行的临床研究方案提供所需的基础设施。不同于科学研究,成功的临床研究项目要求有补充领域,如监管、实验室、临床技能、财务、行政的专业知识、并且和几个部门合作,如麻醉科、外科、肾内科、病理科等。增强在这些领域的能力和专业知识对促进临床研究的整体成功同等重要。在当今的经济环境下,产业需要中心很快招收大量患者并提供优质的数据。同样,大学再也不能在财政上支持那些经济上不可行的临床研究团队。不仅科学和患者护理不可能没有一个重点,而且在商业和金融也同样。

表 123.1 临床研究性药学协调阶段

阶段	状态
Ⅰ计划	研究者和(或)指定者意识到管理临床药物试验的潜在研究的时间。在此阶段,活动可包括确定个别药物服务(IDS)工作范围,确定所需的 IDS 服务,为 IDS 服务建立准确的预算,为后续研究阶段确定时间表,与现场评估访问的研究监测员会面等。在这时,研究方案可以是或不是最终确定。如果研究者的意图是以任何物质的储存、库存控制和分发管理作为研究一部分,调查员或指定人员必须提交此过程的适当文档以供审核
Ⅱ起始	该计划是在物质储存和分配的其他制度规定的背景下研究者和(或)指定者认为研究很可能开始的时间。在此阶段,活动可包括 IRB 提交、合同复核、授予通知书等
Ⅲ开始入组	在 IRB、合同和机构批准的时间完成。研究药物可在现场和随时可用
Ⅳ关闭入组	当入组已完成,患者还在随访时
Ⅴ研究结束	最后一个患者最后一次访问后,所有研究文件完成和更正后

临床药学服务的经济原因

临床药学服务集合

这是公认的临床药剂师是医院和卫生系统患者护理团队的重要组成部分。医院及卫生系统需要门诊药剂师和临床药剂师,他们的共同作用是为患者提供一步到位的监护,这些包括出院时门诊处方的设定及出院后持续的药物监护。除了提高监护质量,门诊药剂师需要具有开出 Medicare B 部分(医疗保险)的账单,专业的药学服务允许医院和卫生系统获取额外收益,目前正在寻找途径来降低成本,并最大限度地提高收入。通过获取这种门诊收入及相关患者转健康的药学项目,药剂师资源的费用可以被抵扣,这就允许有关各方得到一个双赢的局面。在移植中心和医院领导的支持下,一个受过培训的药学工作人员愿意接受通过移植的专业药学服务线的机会,可以实现显著的收入。当机构发展了移植专科药学服务线,并能够在自己系统内维持患者,他们便有机会利用这些收入进一步支持临床药学服务。移植药剂师提高自己收入的另一个潜在机会是为自己的服务定出价格。虽然正在实现这种思路的移植药剂师数量有限,但 Maldonado 和他的同事证明,在一年(208 次热线)中,药剂师门诊收入提高近 10 000 美元或约 100 美元/次的费用。其他因素增加的收入被用来证明临床药学服务的情况[35]。在目前的医疗环境下,任何抵消和(或)调整资源的机会必须被评估。新健康技术、电子病历、电子处方和药物治疗管理将继续允许药剂师扩大自己的作用,并确保患者的用药需求在住院和门诊治疗的各个阶段得到适当的解决。

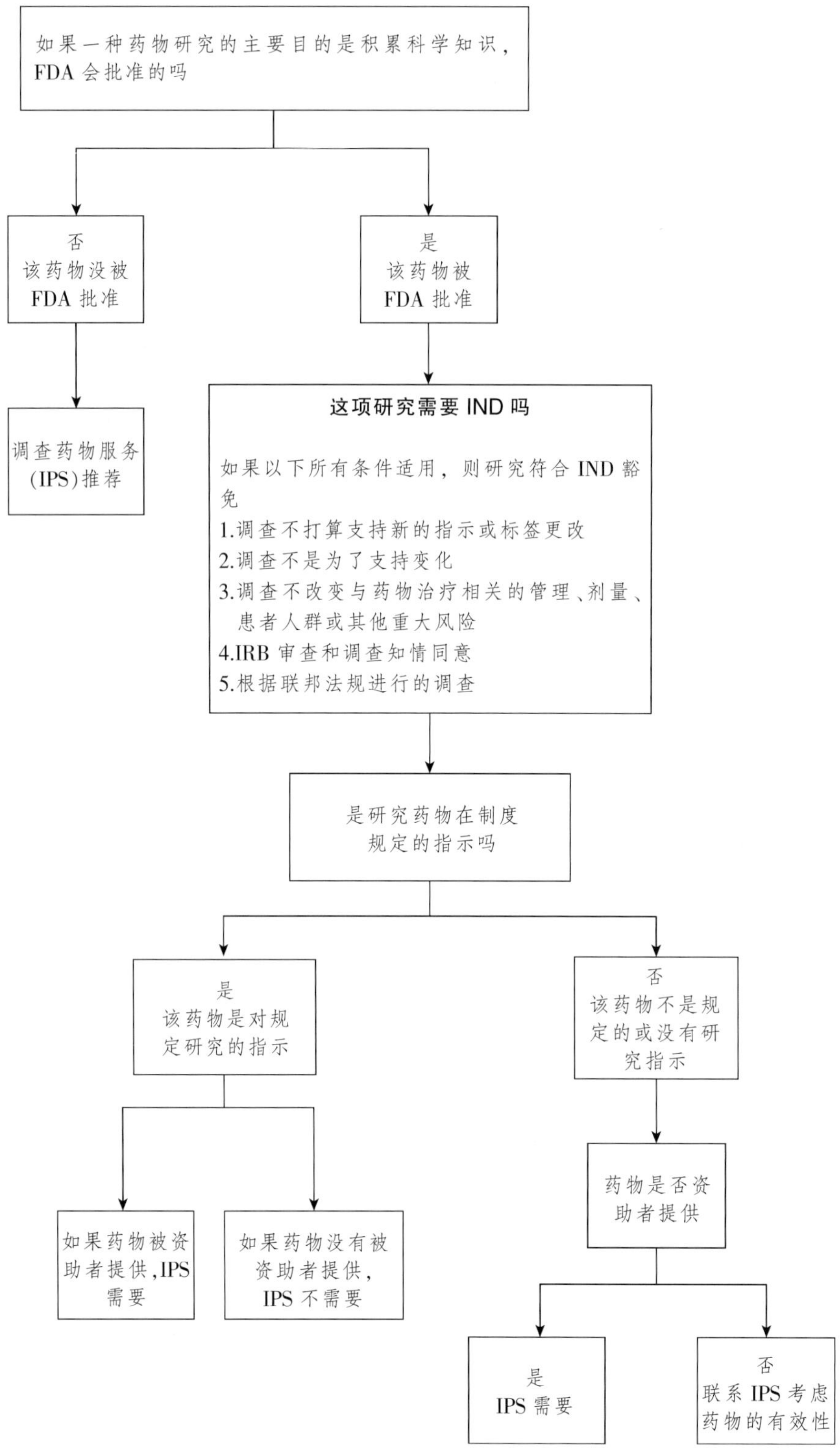

图 123.2 评估调查药物服务的需要。

建立邮购移植药学服务-340B药物定价方案的影响

340B药物定价计划的建立是为了响应美国公法102-585的340B部分，即1992年退伍军人医疗保健法案。这个法案的340B部分限制了某些联邦机构和其他被识别的实体的接受者的药物花费。该计划是由药房事务卫生资源(OPA)和服务管理办公室(HRSA)管理,在美国联邦政府的卫生和人类服务(HHS)部下属。联邦 340B 药物价格计划减少价格处方药超过 16 869 美元(截止到 2011 年 9 月 30 日),由 HHS 认证的医疗设施卫生与公众服务部为“实体”覆盖。这些诊所、医院和移植中心轮番为在 50 个州中为十几万的患者提供服务。

最大化参与 340b 定价在联邦公共卫生法案下允许储备增长和扩大各州及诊所获得处方药。这表明了移植项目获取收益的重要机会,340B 价格是比平均医疗补助“最佳价格”网低 19%,比平均保险报销低 39%,低于平均批发价格(AWP)51%。最大化节省成本的策略是为药店最昂贵的项目,或者最昂贵的患者群体和(或)疾病状态,如心理健康、移植、血友病、艾滋病和其他类别昂贵的慢性疾病的患者。追求建立门诊药学系统并维护他们的患者在他们的移植机构,将有机会产生显著经济收益,并再次证明移植药剂师的薪水合法化的收入。

专业药房建立

药物的成本高以及药店结算和报销的复杂性使许多独立和小型零售药店对参加医保 B 部分和“专业”的市场望而却步,零售巨头和邮购药店获准的业务范围更大且更“复杂”。在过去的 30 年中,“专业”药房已经从一个概念到一个行业,每年接近一千亿美元收入,已经成为医疗质量和创新的重要力量[36]。

专业药店为供应商和保险公司提供服务,以简化交付流程和调整医疗保健交付中的挑战。许多专业药店注重具有极高的购买成本的医药和生物产品,从患者护理和报销的角度很难管理。患者的处方药福利计划往往需要患者从邮购药店获得,这些邮购药店加入了保险公司的专业药物网络。药物监管和使用说明在某些注射药物中被要求提供,许多药物被认为是“耐用医疗设备”。其结果是,许多药物可以被药房或医疗福利覆盖,对于护理提供者、患者和药店职工的护理更加复杂。

当成本高的治疗药物被药店和(或)主要医疗福利覆盖时,了解如何识别和正确列出这些药物是非常重要的。药疗保险包括但不限于注射和输液的治疗药物,以及需要复杂护理的疾病如癌症、艾滋病、器官移植、丙型肝炎和类风湿性关节炎。药店设施与现有的移植和肿瘤患者群体必须制订工作流程计划和进程,以便为患者提供无缝的服务级个性化用药管理。创建一个强大的邮购药店以满足药房邻近区域以外的地区,并让患者在系统保留长期用药的需求,这些增加了大量的利润给医院和(或)设施,从而再次提供了机会抵消与移植药剂师相关昂贵的费用及其他急需资源。

医疗保险覆盖面的影响

每年有成千上万有医保的人通过医保终末期肾病(ESRD)计划完成肾移植。肾衰竭或者终末期肾病是唯一可以享用医疗保险福利的疾病,包括提供透析、移植和免疫抑制药物以及其他服务。如果 ESRD 患者或他们的配偶或父母已经支付社保至少十年,将可以自动获得医疗保险。

自 1993 年医保确定免疫抑制药物的福利后,移植后免疫抑制药物花费的范围不断增加。2000 年医保福利改进及保护法案去除了之前医保年龄 36 个月及移植时符合医保的残疾人受者的限制。现在如果患者只符合 ESRD,医保覆盖至移植后 36 个月。然而,一位肾移植受者为医保 ESRD 状态而且 36 个月的期限已满,如果他们后来再次基于年龄及残疾的原因获得医保,他们的免疫抑制药物医保覆盖将恢复。立法废除免疫抑制药物 36 个月的限制已经被反复提交至国会商议。通过这一立法是由于财政和医学的双重原因。

对于门诊处方药物,医疗保险有两种截然不同的程序,每一种都有大量复杂的政策。药房供应商广告的、耐用品医疗器械管理的药品能被医保 B 部分支付,如一些被药品供应商广告的和被患者自我管理的药品、免疫抑制药物和抗癌药物。对于医保 B 部分覆盖的药物,这些药物必须提供批准文件给医生。这通常意味着该药物是凭医生处方分配的或遵医嘱给予的。医保 B 部分药物覆盖通常限于通过注射和输注施用的药物或生物制品,除非注射是自动进行的。医保是实行本地和国家医保组合决定的,如果 CMS 国家医保覆盖缺失,当地医保由供应商决定。医疗保险 B 部分定义了几种作为耐用医疗器械的带回家药物,包括喷雾溶液、免疫抑制药物、糖尿病药物、某些口服抗癌药物[37-39]。

医保费用报告和器官获取讨论

如今美国器官移植的最主要支付者是医保。移植必须对所有适用于医保成本的直接及间接的费用负责,以获得医保补偿,在报销持续缩减的市场中,获得所有容许的医疗费用是成功的关键。医保报销医院是经过医保认证的移植中心，涉及器官获取相关费用的福利。医保要求费用是合理地使用适当的分配和支持的。医保容许作为器官获取的费用包括器官供者和受者入院手术前的费用，及供者住院后的费用。每年年末时，各个医院上交一份费用报告，这份报告被医保审核以确定所有的费用是符合医疗法规和政策规定的。医保要求移植医院只拨出部分器官获取行动的时间费用，这些器官获取费用在医保费用报告上。移植中心被要求用合理的依据来分配移植前、移植后、非移植相关行为的费用。对于所有移植中心，获取移植前相关的个人工资是非常重要的。所有移植中心都能非常熟悉地使用工具，如时间研究、获得移植协调员时间、社会工作者、金融协调和管理人员在移植前阶段的工作。这些移植前的工资费用是医保允许的，应该被获取通过成本报表部分报销。由于医疗保险和UNOS现在都需要在移植前阶段移植药剂师的参与，移植中心含有移植药剂师的时间研究是很重要的。当移植中心在移植前记录并获得适合的移植药剂师，可以将这些列入成本报告，因此药剂师的大部分的工资可以抵消。报销的数目由每个中心器官的百分比及移植前参与药剂师的数量决定[40-42]。

总结

CMS及UNOS意识到移植药剂师的作用已经从多学科团队的移植新成员变成必需成员。移植药剂师作为住院、门诊、研究和移植管理团队成员的价值越来越明显。移植药剂师在住院部、门诊和研究中心进行的各种活动见表123.2。基本活动被定义为预期的活动，以确保安全和有效的药学服务，并使移植受体获得药物治疗。基本活动不应该被认为是移植药剂师工作的最低标准。期望中的活动包括结合增强的移植相关药物的责任和移植相关研究的基本活动。最佳活动包括基本活动和期望的活动，包含了移植药剂师作为移植相关药物研究和教育领导者的角色和责任。他们还结合专业技术的最高水平，以优化患者和移植的预后。移植药剂师应该成为他们所在团队的药物治疗专家，在实践中优化药物治疗方案，除此之外还有许多其他的责任。这些药剂师活动列表并不能包含所有活动，而是随着医学和药学的实践不断发展。

表123.2 移植药剂师的活动

基本活动
1.药剂师的时间都奉献给移植患者，几乎没有为其他患者服务
2.药剂师一直致力于小时门诊和住院移植服务
3.药剂师作为多学科移植团队的一员定期进行巡视，为所有的移植患者提供药物治疗管理
4.药剂师协调药物治疗指南和(或)移植途径的发展和实践，使药物治疗发挥最大的益处
5.药剂师前瞻性评估了所有的药物治疗相应的适应证、剂量、药物相互作用，以及药物过敏;监测患者药物治疗方案的有效性、药物不良反应事件和干预需要
6.药剂师需要确保医院诊所之间在移植中心的用药记录的协调
7.结合临床营养学、药剂师建议修改的营养方案
8.药剂师识别并帮助他们管理和预防药物不良事件，改进开发过程以减少用药错误及防止不良事件
9.药剂师用病历作为一种手段与其他医护专业人员进行沟通并记录具体的药物治疗建议
10.必要时，药剂师需提供免疫抑制药物和其他药物的药代动力学监测
11.药剂师为移植团队提供药物信息
12.药剂师参与对药学学生、住院医生及通过轮转的研究人员的培训
13.药剂师维护移植指南并做适当引用
14.药剂师为移植团队人员提供药物相关治疗的教育
15.药剂师参与报告药物不良事件给本机构的质量保证委员会和美国FDA的MedWatch计划
16.药剂师提供的内容更新和对有REM要求的免疫抑制治疗移植小组的教育
17.药剂师提供和记录对所有移植的用药教育，证明患者有能力管理自己的药物，协调移植后家庭药物目录

（待续）

表 123.2(续) 移植药剂师的活动

18.药剂师回顾患者用药史,以确定移植后应该继续用哪些药物
(a)药剂师弄清先前的有效剂量,给药方案和在移植后需要时提供药物剂量调整的建议
(b)药剂师确保对药物–药物的相互作用进行适当的管理
(c)对于所有可疑药物相关的住院,药剂师评估历史用药的因果关系并在病历中记录可能影响患者管理的任何发现
19.药剂师保证患者出院时可优先获得所有需要的移植的药物
20.药剂师记录的临床活动包括,但不限于:疾病状态管理、一般药物治疗监测、药代动力学监测、药物不良事件、教育和其他患者护理活动
21.药剂师作为药学、护理学、以及医务人员的联络人,教育健康专业人员药物有关的程序、政策、指导方针
22.药剂师贡献了医院简报和有关药物移植利用率相关药物内容
23.药剂师执行和维护安全有效使用移植药物相关的政策和法规
24.药剂师与护理、医务人员和医院管理人员合作,为联合委员会(TJC)、医疗保险和医疗补助服务中心(CMS)和联合器官共享网络(UNOS)的调查和响应做准备,以发现任何的缺陷
25.当进行移植的药物治疗问题审查时,药剂师为医院提供咨询,比如药物和治疗
26.药剂师需要识别如何通过适当使用移植药物和通过实施成本控制使药物花费最小化
27.药剂师应确保一般治疗药物的安全使用
28.药剂师参与加强药学服务的质量保障过程
29.药剂师参与非患者护理活动,包括多学科医学评审及在职教育
令人满意的活动
1.药剂师在移植门诊定期与患者会面,以提供后续教育确保正确遵守规定的药物治疗方案
2.药剂师维持目前的主要移植药物相关文献知识
3.药剂师为医学学生提供移植药理学和治疗学的知识
4.药剂师使用文档程序,这个程序既有临床意义又有临床干预措施的经济价值
5.药剂师积极参与移植药物的研究,可以作为研究的协调者和联系人,通过帮助筛选入组患者参与研究
6.药剂师参与研究设计和数据分析
7.药剂师贡献医学文献,例如病例报告,给编辑的信和治疗、药代动力学、药物经济学报告
8.药剂师促进对器官捐赠重要性的认识
最佳活动
1.药剂师协助医生与患者和(或)家庭成员讨论治疗方案,并做出决策
2.药剂师提供正式被认可的教育时间,如面对医务人员、学生和住院医生的大查房
3.药剂师在移植药学实践中发展住院医生和(或)奖学金
4.药剂师认同和教育社会团体以及医务人员关于药剂师作为多学科移植团队的一部分的作用
5.药剂师独立地调查或与其他移植参与者合作来评估,用于移植的药物给药和终末期器官疾病相关的疾病状态的管理指南的影响
6.药剂师使用药物经济学分析,为了前瞻性评估现有的或新的药学服务以及移植药物治疗新药的位置
7.药剂师积极设计,优先推进新医药方案和移植患者服务
8.药剂师寻求资金进行研究
9.药剂师在地区或国家会议中向药学医学学会报告临床研究和药物经济学分析结果
10.药剂师发表在同行评审的药学和医疗文献,作为下列任何活动的结果
(a)定量或定性评估药物治疗和药学服务的临床研究或其他的原创性研究
(b)研究者发起的赠款和合同
(c)药物经济学与结果研究

(郭海军 译 徐骁 校)

参考文献

1. Mitchell JF. Pharmacist involvement as a member of a renal transplant team. American Journal of Hospital Pharmacy. 1976;33(1):55–58.
2. Burckart GJ. Transplant pharmacy: 30 years of improving patient care. Annals of Pharmacotherapy. 2007;41(7):1261–1263.
3. Ptachcinski RJ, Venkataramanan R, Burckart GJ. Clinical pharmacokinetics of cyclosporin. Clinical Pharmacokinetics. 1986;11(2):107–132.
4. Jacobson PA, Schladt D, Oetting WS, et al. Genetic determinants of mycophenolate-related anemia and leukopenia after transplantation. Transplantation. 2011;91(3):

309–316.
5. Tichy EM, Medwid AJ, Mills EA, et al. Significant sirolimus and dronedarone interaction in a kidney transplant recipient. Annals of Pharmacotherapy. 2010;44(7–8):1338–1341.
6. Everly MJ, Everly JJ, Susskind B, et al. Bortezomib provides effective therapy for antibody- and cell-mediated acute rejection. Transplantation. 2008;86(12): 1754–1761.
7. van Gelder T, Silva HT, de Fijter H, et al. How delayed graft function impacts exposure to mycophenolic acid in patients after renal transplantation. Therapeutic Drug Monitoring. 2011;33(2):155–164.
8. Thielke JJ, West-Thielke PM, Herren HL, et al. Living donor kidney transplantation across positive crossmatch: the University of Illinois at Chicago experience. Transplantation. 2009;87(2):268–273.
9. Alloway R, Steinberg S, Khalil K, et al. Two years post-conversion from a prograf-based regimen to a once-daily tacrolimus extended-release formulation in stable kidney transplant recipients. Transplantation. 2007;83(12):1648–1651.
10. Park JM, Lake KD, Cibrik DM. Impact of changing from cyclosporine to tacrolimus on pharmacokinetics of mycophenolic acid in renal transplant recipients with diabetes. Therapeutic Drug Monitoring. 2008;30(5):591–596.
11. Chisholm MA, Mulloy LL, Jagadeesan M, et al. Impact of clinical pharmacy services on renal transplant patients' compliance with immunosuppressive medications. Clinical Transplantation. 2001;15(5):330–336.
12. Chisholm MA, Mulloy LL, Jagadeesan M, et al. Effect of clinical pharmacy services on the blood pressure of African-American renal transplant patients. Ethnicity and Disease. 2002;12(3):392–397.
13. Wang HY, Chan AL, Chen MT, et al. Effects of pharmaceutical care intervention by clinical pharmacists in renal transplant clinics. Transplantation Proceedings. 2008;40(7):2319–2323.
14. Alloway RR, Dupuis R, Gabardi S, et al. Evolution of the role of the transplant pharmacist on the multidisciplinary transplant team. American Journal of Transplantation. 2011;11(8):1576–1583.
15. American College of Clinical Pharmacy. Immunology/Transplantation Practice and Research Network (PRN) history report. 2009 [accessedaccessed December 1, 2011]; Available from: http://www.accp.com/prns/history.aspx.
16. American Society of Health-System Pharmacists Required Educational Outcomes and Objectives for Postgraduate Year Two (PGY2) Pharmacy Residencies in Solid Organ Transplant. Bethesda, MD. 2008 [accessed November 23, 2011]; Available from: http://www.ashp.org/menu/Accreditation/ResidencyAccreditation.aspx.
17. Title 42 of the Public Health Service Act. Part 121-Organ Procurement and Transplantation Network. Washington, D.C. Sections 215, 371-376 of the Public Heath Service Act (42 U.S.C. 216, 273-274d); sections 1102,1106,1138 and 1871 of the Social Secutiry Act 942 U.S.C. 1302,,1306, 1320b-8 and 1395hh); and section 301 of the National Organ Transplant Act, as amended (42 U.S.C. 274e).
18. (UNOS) United Network or Organ Sharing Bylaws. Attachment 1 to Appendix B of the UNOS Bylaws; Designated Transplant Program Criteria. UNOS-Appendix B- Attachment I-XII-1-91.[accessed December 14, 2013]; Available from: http://www.unos.org/docs/Appendix_B_AttachI_XIII.pdf.
19. Anonymous, Department of Health and Human Services, Centers for Medicare and Medicaid Services. 42 CFR Parts 405,482,488, and 498. Medicare program; hospital conditions of participation: requirements for approval and re-approval of transplant centers to perform organ transplants; final rule. Federal Register. 2007;72(61):15197–15279.
20. Department of Health and Human Services Centers for Medicare and Medicaid Services. Advance Copy – Organ Transplant Program Intrepretive Guidelines. 2008 [accessed December 1, 2011]; Available from: https://www.cms.gov/SurveyCertificationGenInfo/downloads/SCLetter08-25.pdf.
21. Department of Health and Human Services Centers for Medicare and Medicaid Services. Advance Copy – Organ Transplant Program State Operations Manual (SOM) and Survey Protocol. 2008 [accessed December 1, 2011]; Available from: https://www.cms.gov/SurveyCertificationGenInfo/downloads/SCLetter09-09.pdf.
22. McDevitt-Potter LM, Sadaka B, Tichy EM, et al. A multicenter experience with generic tacrolimus conversion. Transplantation. 2011;92(6):653–657.
23. Hammond RW, Schwartz AH, Campbell MJ, et al. Collaborative drug therapy management by pharmacists–2003. Pharmacotherapy. 2003;23(9): 1210–1225.
24. Anonymous, Department of Health and Huma Services. Identification of drug and biological products deemed to have risk evaluation and mitigation strategies for purposes of the food and drug administration amendments act of 2007. Federal Register. 2008;73(60):16313–16314.
25. United States Food and Drug Administration. Approved Risk Evaluation and Mitigation Strategies (REMS). [accessed January 5, 2012]; Available from: http://www.fda.gov/Drugs/DrugSafety/PostmarketDrugSafetyInformationforPatientsandProviders/ucm111350.htm.
26. U.S. Department of Health and Human Services Food and Drug Administration. Guidance-Medication Guides-Distribution Requirements and Inclusion in Risk Evaluation and Mitigation Strategies (REMS). [accessed January 5, 2012]; Available from: http://www.fda.gov/downloads/Drugs/GuidanceComplianceRegulatoryInformation/Guidances/UCM244570.pdf.
27. Gabardi S, Halloran PF, Friedewald J. Managing risk in developing transplant immunosuppressive agents: the new regulatory environment. American Journal of Transplantation. 2011;11(9):1803–1809.
28. Gabardi S. Understanding risk evaluation and mitigation strategies in organ transplantation. Pharmacotherapy. 2011;31(7):714–722.
29. Chisholm MA, Vollenweider LJ, Mulloy LL, et al. Cost-benefit analysis of a clinical pharmacist-managed medication assistance program in a renal transplant clinic. Clinical Transplantation. 2000;14(4 Pt 1):304–307.
30. Chisholm-Burns MA, Spivey CA, Garrett C, et al. Impact of clinical pharmacy services on renal transplant recipients' adherence and outcomes. Patient Preference and Adherence. 2008;2:287–292.
31. Schuh MJ, Crumb DJ, Dubois J. Building a pharmacist-managed pharmacotherapy medication therapy management practice. The Consultant Pharmacist. Journal of the American Society of Consultant Pharmacists. 2011;26(6):404–413.
32. Klein A, Otto G, Krämer I. Impact of a pharmaceutical care program on liver transplant patients' compliance with immunosuppressive medication: a prospective, randomized, controlled trial using electronic monitoring. Transplantation. 2009;87(6):839–847.
33. Blouin RA, Pollack GM. Training clinical pharmaceutical scientists in today's highly competitive times: it's time to commit to change. Pharmacotherapy. 2009;29(2):134–136, discussion 6-7.
34. Dowling TC, Murphy JE, Kalus JS, et al. Recommended education for pharmacists as competitive clinical scientists. Pharmacotherapy. 2009;29(2):236–244.
35. Maldonado AQ, Seiger TC, Urann CL, et al. Billing for outpatient transplant pharmacy services. American Journal of Health-System Pharmacy. 2012;69(2): 144–147.
36. Suchanek D. The rise and role of specialty pharmacy. Biotechnology Healthcare. 2005;2(5):31–35.
37. Center for Medicare and Medicaid Services. Medicare Coverage of Kidney Dialysis and Kidney Transplant Services. [accessed January 1, 2012]; Available from: http://www.medicare.gov/publications/pubs/pdf/10128.pdf.
38. Yen EF, Hardinger K, Brennan DC, et al. Cost-effectiveness of extending Medicare coverage of immunosuppressive medications to the life of a kidney transplant. American Journal of Transplantation. 2004;4(10):1703–1708.
39. Woodward RS, Schnitzler MA, Lowell JA, et al. Effect of extended coverage of immunosuppressive medications by medicare on the survival of cadaveric renal transplants. American Journal of Transplantation. 2001;1(1):69–73.
40. Abecassis M. Organ acquisition cost centers Part I: medicare regulations–truth or consequence. American Journal of Transplantation. 2006;6(12):2830–2835.
41. United States Department of Health and Human Services. Office of the Inspector General. [accessed December 23, 2011]; Available from: http://oig.hhs.gov.
42. Center for Medicaid and Medicare Services. Title 42–Public Health Chapter IV–Title 42–Public Health Chapter IV– Part 412—Prospective Payment Systemsn for Inpatient Hospital Services 42 CFR 412.100-Special treatment: Renal transplantation centers. [accessed December 23, 2011]; Available from: http://edocket.access.gpo.gov/cfr_2004/octqtr/pdf/42cfr412.100.pdf.

第 124 章
移植住院病房管理

Linda Ohler, Margaret Schaeffer, Kelly Carter, Donna George

引言

对实体器官移植受者的护理要求移植中心成员具有专业技能和高水平的能力。这个患者群体监护的复杂性要求通过多学科的日常查房计划来指导。由外科医生、内科医生、护士、移植协调员、执业护士、药剂师、社会工作者、营养师组成的多学科团队,通过合作和规划每位移植受者或活体供体个性化的治疗。床旁的护士实施护理计划,评估结果,并将结果与移植团队成员进行交流,教育患者和家属。一位执业护士在移植住院病房的作用已随着时间不断地演变并随着移植项目的不同而不同。在病房有 3 个或更多的执业护士变得非常普遍,在移植病房及重症监护室这些护士的作用等同于住院医生[1]。一些护士管理着移植病房。

心脏移植或肝移植候选人常常在重症监护病房或专门的高级监护病房被护理,以等待合适的器官移植。在过去十年里,机械循环支持设备的使用急剧上升,这些设备(如左心室辅助装置或人工心脏)被视为心脏移植的桥梁。这些设备需要高度专业化和较高能力的人员来确保安全高效的照顾患者。鉴于移植后受者护理的复杂性,许多移植中心已指定移植后受者护理的专业病房。大部分病房进一步专门为胸部或腹部移植受者使用。外科手术后,肝、肺或心脏受者被带到为他们专设的重症监护病房。许多医院在高级监护病房照顾肾移植和活体供肾者,而不是在 ICU 环境。然而,一些外科医生倾向于让所有肾移植受者在重症监护病房中监护至少最初的 24 小时。本章主要介绍胸部、腹部移植病房中的管理和人员配置,以及他们相关的候选人和受者护理。门诊管理和移植护理协调员的作用将在第 122 章和第 125 章中分别介绍。

物理环境和资源(感染控制)

少数人能有幸经历从头开始入住移植病房,享受全新的环境。我们中的大多数人继承了我们活动的空间。我们最大的移植愿望是为每一位患者提供私人房间。当只有一个半私人房间配置可用时,最大限度地控制感染对患者安置非常重要。对于刚刚接受了实体器官移植的患者,以及新免疫抑制患者,私人房间里的情况似乎是显而易见的。对一位移植前患者来说私人房间同样是非常重要的,因为任何感染都可能使患者暂时无法接受器官,延长在等候名单的时间。可以考虑申请重症监护室、高级病房或一般病房。在那里有多个半私人房间,往往需要进行阻断而变成双人房,以创建私人房间的环境。当整个设施的费用偏高时,获得医院管理者的支持就变成了一项挑战。讨论和规划这一潜在的情况应先于实际实行。医院流行病学的专家对这样的看法很支持。

另一个在任何移植病房都需考虑的感染控制问题是空气质量。如果病房的通风系统不是恒定状态,高效微粒空气流(HEPA)应该是容易获得的。正压通气(PPV)是指在密闭房间中具有极高的空气交换率,长期以来其优点一直争论不休,但从来没有被科学证明[2]。曲霉菌病在移植病房内爆发可能是致命的。这是 PPV 优劣的讨论中最常听到的。预防是最好的干预。频繁地评估在物理环境中的潜在问题是避免问题的关键。例如,在一个移植病房中透析是很常见的,因为并非所有的患者都能够前往中央透析区。透析的过程需要水,而且需要大量的水。机器需要安全地连接到水源和一个排出水的地方。差的连接可导致不断潮湿的地区,这是导致发霉和产生曲霉菌病的条件。比透析不太常见的是,一个大雨长期泄漏的窗户,但是湿气建立的一个来源。聪明的移植病房管理者发明了一种永远的警惕状态,促进床旁护士和辅助人员(环境服务等)保持警惕。

人力资源(人员)

胸部移植和(或)机械辅助装置病房是由心脏病医生、心胸外科医生、执业护士、高级护士、注册护士(RN)、护理的合作伙伴、营养师、物理治疗师、职业治疗师、药剂师、社会工作者和护理协调员(评审/出院计划)的多学科团队组成的,这个病房的操作主要由护理人员执行。护理安排由临床护士、护理的合作伙伴、病房秘书、临床协调员、临床护理专家和护士管理者组成。护理管理者为所有病房工作人员编配预算,并倡导为复杂的心胸外科患者提供安全的护理所需的必要的资源。

要为住院部编制手术预算,护士管理者必须熟悉金融结构和组织的目标。护理管理者必须对该组织的工作重点有很深地理解,使病房的计划与组织的战略方向一致。预算是一年的计划,为使组织能准备活动和控制成本。

护士和护理管理者是成本控制的关键,更重要的是,他们对维护患者安全和确保患者预后良好有较大帮助。在各类不同组织中护理管理者的培训和知识水平也不同。行政主管护士对护理预算的发展和管理费用给付最终责任。一线管理人员必须具备规划预算和控制成本的技能,并能对资源配置做出有效的决策[3]。预算确定了组织的服务水平,工作量决定了个人和非个人的资源要求[4]。护理人员预算是医疗机构的人工费用的很大一部分。成功经营移植住院病房的关键是领导者管理和分配这些资源的能力。

传统监护护士人员的方式有两种:一种按每位患者每天小时制;另一种是护士与患者的比例。住院移植病房护士人员配备是组织通过每个患者一天(HPPD)护理时间确定的。这项评估方法(HPPD),是由美国护理协会护理质量指标(NDNQI)的国家数据库开发的[5]。护理HPPD是指相对于护理工作量需要护理的小时数。该HPPD值是由医院直接护理时间和单位普查数据确定的,普查数据是基于历史普查数据的、单位个性化的。护理工作量在重症监护病房要比急性监护病房更大。急性护理病房可能是中级或高级护理或手术遥测病房。由于护理工作量增加,护士对患者的比例必须下降。每年人员预算是根据历史日均普查(住院日)决定。患者住院日预测在今年的基础上,基于历史普查数据。配置移植护理病房的人员是非常重要的,管理者必须能够提供足够的资源来照顾复杂的患者。每位患者一天的工作时间和人力资源配置近年来已经在被研究,以评估工作人员人数和患者预后之间的关系[6,7]。这些研究示出工作人员和患者的治疗效果之间的关系不同的结果。研究表明护理时间和患者的治疗效果之间的相关性[6-8]。增加护士人力资源是非常昂贵的,护理的预算已经占医院预算的很大一部分。然而,减少不良事件和改善护士敏感指标被证明是有益的组织成本。护理人员水平的增加显示可以改善患者预后,研究将继续评估这项措施工作量的有效性和可靠性[6-8]。

一旦病房的预算确立,有效地管理这些资源是护士长的职责。必须认真考虑工作人员技能的混合以及对患者敏感性的护理。在作者的工作机构,人员编制指南是基于HPPD和护士患者比确定的,已提供一线职工中多少护士应该工作的指导,基于目前总的单位普查。

劳动管理学院是一个咨询、教育和研究机构,为人力资源管理和运营领域提供服务。他们对45个国家的360家医院的进行年度调查,关于患者天、小时和护士患者比例。据劳动管理协会2009年度调查结果显示,中级监护病房(降低)HPPD和每位患者一天总时间,平均为9.6~11.1(总HPPD)。每位患者一天直接小时平均为9.3~10.8。教学医院护士患者的比例为1:3.6~1:3.8[9]。

一旦配备了精心设计的人力资源计划,对于领导者来说分配护理资源去保证复杂心脏手术患者安全和专业的护理就是一项挑战,可以开发一个表格作为确定所需工作人员数量的指导,这个表格是根据当前患者普查结果来制作的。这个工具对维护框架内费用很有帮助。当人口普查浮动时,工作人员可被分配在组织内需要的地方。

胸部移植病房

在胸部移植/机械循环辅助装置(MCSD)病房,分三个阶段来确定能力:雇佣期,方向确定期,持续的基础。在雇佣期,注册护士(RN)能力通过验证执照、注册、认证、行为面试,及以往的经验进行评估。初始能力阶段侧重于就业第一年必要的技能和照顾患者的能力[10]。

在方向确定期，对胸部移植/MCSD 病房 RN 工作人员培训各种经验，为独立照顾移植和 MCSD 患者做准备。初始的方向期是 12 周，包括课堂教育、体验各种 MCSD 设备和观察经验。RN 被分配给初级的指导医生，指导他们在病房里照护患者。他们将被立即分配给需要 MCSD 护理的患者，包括左心室辅助装置的患者（LVAD）和全人工心脏（TAH）的患者，在导师的监督下。他们的方向的培训部分通常在定位结束时提供。他们的导师在课堂培训之前亲自审查和培训，以更好地理解课堂内容。在培训结束之前，培训者亲自完成能力评定，包括紧急措施更换电池、对警报的反应、一些需要转换设置的情况（全人工心脏与便携式 HAT-t）（表 124.1）[11]。病房的工作人员需要完成移植能力测试及 MCSD 能力测试。

该教学内容包括，左心室辅助装置适应证，设备的组成部分，患者术后管理，报警管理，水泵故障，驱动线护理（伤口护理），更换电池和充电，并发症和设备管理。完成在病房环境中使用每一台设备的能力清单。新员工必须观察并且在导师的监督下完成切口护理和驱动线护理。必须细心和保持无菌，二氧化碳麻醉槽必须被放置，以确保驱动线在出口位置移动幅度最小。

其他移植护理/MCSD 患者重要的概念包括术后心外科患者护理。一旦患者转出重症监护室，护理的重点包括药物管理、防止肺部并发症、患者运动发展、伤口护理、疼痛管理，并且照顾 MCSD 患者的心理。

对于一些小的项目，当规程简单时，保持胜任力是一项挑战。护理的领导者可能会为了保持竞争胜任力，考虑限制员工的数量来适应 MCSD 和移植患者的护理。对于其他的项目，那些需要机械循环辅助设备和胸部移植的项目更是平常。所有护理的人员都应该接受培训和年度能力评估。能力评估应包括新的规程、技术、政策或措施、或措施的变化、程序、政策。高风险的责任可能导致伤害、死亡或法律诉讼也应列入正在进行的能力评估[10]。应该使用各种能力评估方法来评估工作技能的各个方面，包括技术、批判性思维和人际关系。有很多方法可以用来展示能力，包括后测试、范例、技能观察、案例研究、同行评审、模拟事件[10]。

表 124.1 机械循环辅助装置(MCSD)能力测试(Reprinted from [11] Savage L, Murphy J, Joyce K. Developing and maintaining competency with circulatory assist devices: How to meet the challenge. Progress in Transplantation 2010;20:125–128 with permission from InnoVision Communications, Inc)

主题	审核（日期）	实施（日期）	日期/签名/方法 S =模拟 C =认知 D =证明
1.TAH-t/LVAD 植入			
A.术前教学			
B.所需设备			
a.OR 需要什么			
b.备份支持			
c.如何获得额外的设备			
C. 设置 PBU /系统监控			
2.患者护理			
A.现场护理			
B.系统检查/数据卡			
C.电池			
D.手动装置			
E.文档			
F.HAT-t 特殊实验室			
3.故障排除			
A.低流量状态(病因和行为)			
B.更换系统控制器			
C.警报			
D.黄色扳手			
E.红色心脏			
F.除颤/心脏复律			
G.空气罐			
4.LVAD 退出计划			
5.LVAD / TAH-t 多元活动			
6.资源			
A.TAH-t Syncardia			
B.VAD 协调员			
C.Heartline 24/7			

腹部移植病房

腹部移植病房为肾、肾-胰联合、胰腺、肝脏、肠和（或）多内脏器官移植患者群体提供服务。这些患者大多数都有多系统复杂的疾病过程，几乎没有单限于一个器官。在一些情况下，患者正在接受两种或更多种腹部器官联合移植。维持一个成功的腹部移植住院病房所需的资源包括：适当的物理环境，有知识、有技能以及专业的患者护理工作人员。

住院病房小的 10 张床，大的 80 张床。如果小的移植病房,可能只提供术后即刻照顾,有时也被称为新鲜移植的患者。大的移植病房为患者提供持续护理,包括移植评估阶段、等待期、围术期或者移植术后入院。在较大的移植病房,许多患者可能会在其慢性、急性和恢复期中出入院多次。这些反复住院的患者,可以为患者和护理人员创造一个非常个性化的环境,特别是护理和辅助治疗的工作人员。这是在移植护理中获益的一个部分。

腹部移植病房特殊的患者可能是肾或者肝段的活体供者。我们知道,有些项目经常把相关的和不相关的、已知的和机密的捐助者与接受者放在同一单位。一个相关或者不相关的供体,如果其身份信息受者是已知的,通常不会安排在同一个房间或一个连通的房间。物理的隔离是为了保护隐私,同时也是保护患者减少其心理压力。在我们工作的病房中,受体与供体隔离时,当他们互相知道彼此时,常常会成为一方首先走出病房探访另一方的原动力。这些探访常常为患者及全体员工带来欣喜和满足。

在保密捐赠时,众所周知的心地善良或者无私的供者,供者和受者置于同一个房间是可能的。但是,必须小心地保护两位患者的身份。病房大小和物理环境的设计,以及员工的数量决定了如何完成保密。例如,同一名护士照顾供体和受体是不明智的。在一些项目中,所有的供者或只是保密供者被置于隔离的外科病房,为了保密。

腹部病房人员

与胸部移植病房相似,腹部移植团队由肾病学家、移植外科医生、移植专业药剂师、移植协调员、执业护士、注册护士、营养师和社会工作者、无证辅助和办事人员组成。物理治疗和职业治疗的辅助服务也参与护理的日常规划。人员配置的责任落在了病房管理人员身上,包括直接护理的注册护士和无证助理人员。

工作人员人数的配置就像前面提到的,是任何医院住院病房员工配置的核心。全职人员(FTS)的数量(包括有执照和无执照的协助人员),每年被确定并形成人员结构,这些是由病房管理者负责的。随着时间的变化,人员是不断变化的,部分是由于腹部移植病房普查和敏感度的变化,这些都是常态。

外科移植在很大程度上是个不确定的事件。如果是活体肾或肝捐献,外科手术床及工作人员需要提前安排。然而,死亡供体的有效性不能预测。移植中心等待患者的数量、等待名单上患者的人口学统计资料(ABO血型、疾病等严重程度)、供体池的大小和质量,地理区域内移植中心的数量都会对器官移植的数量和频率产生影响。员工必须精通基线数据并随着普查改变上下浮动计划。

一个有20张床的移植病房,有位刚从ICU转入的肝移植患者,有位需要血管活性药物新肾移植受体,10位处于不同干预阶段的患者,这个病房需要护士患者比要高于具有20张病床且10张床近期无其他移植患者的病房。这种人员配置的变化是一种潜在的再分配,通常涉及流动的员工到其他病房,当他们不需要在家或强迫使用他们的带薪假期。这些措施都不利于床边护理者,并可能导致不满、轮转和员工空缺。所有这些结果都会导致患者预后不佳[12]。

维护全面和稳定的普查结果在病房中的策略是确定移植服务患者在无感染监控及员工能力欠佳的病房中状态良好。我们熟悉的病房能够安全地接受神经病和心脏病领域的转移患者,和一些个性化的外科手术,例如甲状腺次全切术。这个策略的关键是在接受他们进入的移植病房之前快速筛选所有患者感染的迹象。安置这些患者到移植病房对组织的需求有利,而且能稳定普查的波动和腹部移植病房的员工。

员工的培训、教育,和能力认证

护理人员选择在腹部移植病房工作的人员,包括新手和有经验的护士。雇佣时的基本能力是由执业资格、行为面试、核心护理技能认证决定的。通过广泛的适应(12~14周培训和亲自工作),基础能力得到不断发展。每位注册护士被分配给一个初级和第二级导师。这些导师都已经成功地完成了训练他们的一般导师课程。导师首要的工作是在整个训练期间指导他们。在我们特殊病房中,这个过程是被护理医生监督的,护理医生是一种高级实践护士。在腹部移植病房,初始能力是从临床知识和实践的角度观察。护士完成腹部移植病房定位之前那些掌握的具体的核心竞争力包括如下。

- 管理免疫抑制药物,静脉内(IV)和口服。
- 监测治疗水平的实验室值。
- 监测患者对这些药物的反应并快速识别不良反

应。

• 识别排斥和感染症状。

• 管理血管活性药物，实现严密控制血压。

• 早期识别体液平衡的需要，调整液体摄入量，能根据需要精确的置换体液，利用已确立的指南。

• 监测出血症状，在手术部位、引流液和血流动力学稳定方面。

• 监测中心静脉压(CVP)；能够解读并确定变化的原因。

• 监测、解释，并完成 12 导联心电图(ECG)。

• 识别心脏监测电解质水平。

• 护理导管，包括外周插入中心导管(PICC)和透析导管。

• 监控代谢紊乱的迹象，如糖尿病。

在所有包含的行为中演示出更加宽广和综合的竞争力。这些能力已经被国际移植护理协会认证并且被概括为 15 个领域[13]。表 124.2 概括了这些领域，并且总结了一些典型的活动。

表 124.2 移植护理人员的能力

分类	能力	证明能力的活动
评估	系统全面地收集记录特定患者的资料，包括过去和现在的病史	识别当前历史条件下的影响
		标识系统对患者和潜在预后的影响
	评估和记录家人和照顾者的支持系统的各个方面（任务、压力等）	确定危险因素，识别患者、家庭等教育的需要
	评估过去和现在的治疗建议	
护理敏感诊断	根据评估做出护理诊断。基于新的数据持续地提炼和修改诊断	对于移植人群区分正常及非正常指标
	记录并与患者、家属，其他照料者的诊断和多学科小组的成员讨论诊断	
预后识别	识别预期的结果，是患者确定并与病情发展相适应的，以证据为基础，可在持续评估的基础上修改预期	确保患者和医护人员双方都能接受的预期结果。用可测量的目标记录预后
计划	开发护理的个性化方案，与患者人口统计学指标一致，利用策略和备选方案，以满足预期的结果	与患者、护理人员，以及团队的成员合作发展计划并设定优先顺序。考虑患者经济对计划的影响
	定义计划，以反映移植护理实践的现行法规和标准	记录计划，采用标准化的术语和技术
履行	使用安全及时的鉴别工具	与跨学科的团队实现合作
	使用基于证据的干预措施，特别是对诊断	记录执行和任何修改或改变
	采取策略，以促进健康和安全环境	记录明确的协调
		创建学习和提供健康教育的环境
评估	对患者预后进行系统的持续的基于标准的评估	评估计划策略的有效性
专业实践评估	在目前的监管环境下，评估自己相关的护理实践专业标准和指南	从同行、患者和同事中获得反馈。采取行动以实现在评估过程中确定的目标
讨论	有助于同行和同事们的专业发展	与同行和同事共享知识和技能，包括反馈、指导其他人
伦理	在实践中遵从道德原则	保持耐心和保守捐助者保密
	通过参加跨专业团队及伦理委员会等有助于道德问题的解决	通知患者医疗保健方案的风险、效益、替代品和潜在的效果
研究	综合研究成果转化为实践	在实践中使用最好的证据;积极参与科研活动
资源利用	考虑计划和服务提供的有关安全性、有效性、成本的影响因素	协助患者和家属，理解对护理方案、成本、风险和关怀的益处
领导	提供护理实践和护理专业指导	在从事团队工作作为一个团队成员和一个团队建设者
	对别人的固有尊严和价值的尊重	
		心甘情愿地接受自己和他人的失误，并用它们作为学习的机会

认证

认证是确认一个护士在特别定义的工作领域的资格证书和专业知识的过程[14]。其中授予认证的组织是非政府组织,授予是基于一组预定标准[15]。护士资格证是基于最基本的职业要求。认证表示公认的高标准的知识和实践。而要求根据特定护理专业而变化,所有认证包括实践板块、已知身体所需知识,和一个测试规划[16]。

对于在移植方面工作的护士，这里有许多认证选项：

- 逐行护理认证护士(PCCN)。
- 重症监护注册护士(CCRN)。
- 认证的临床移植护士(CCTN)。
- 认证的临床移植协调员(CCTC)。

为什么移植护士需要通过认证？护理专业的美国委员会(ABNS)在2006年发表了护理认证的白皮书,其中指出,认证被护士和公众认为是有责任感的,专业素养和专业知识证[17]。该文件指出,护士感到更大的个人成就、专业挑战和专业信誉。

为什么一个护士管理者、护士领导者,在病房促进和鼓励移植专业认证？有强有力的证据表明护理专业认证会对组织作为一个整体、对护理专业、并对护理满意度和忠诚产生积极的影响[16]。

出院计划

为患者准备出院是从入院开始，需要大量的个性化的规划。在出院时计划过程中分散的护理会导致再住院[17]。患者出院时多学科规划要求互相沟通,以确保筹备最高质量的准备工作。从医院控制过渡到在家中不良事件和错误用药和自我保健的可能性[18]。据医学研究报道,“是人都会犯错”,多数医疗差错是系统性问题的结果[19]。由于出院计划是一个系统性的过程,错误可能发生。随着多学科的方法,规划患者出院必须有据可查,以保持工作人员连续性的关怀和沟通。多学科查房必须证明团队的每个成员签署的护理计划，以指出协调护理。出院计划应该是精心策划和协调的,以防止错误。

结构化、个性化的出院计划已被证明可以减少住院时间和再住院率[20]。一些移植中心使用多学科团队的出院通路[21]。每个学科签署了分配给他们教育患者出院准备的部分。其他中心也用出院通路,在病历中记录他们对患者的教育。在多学科患者查房的进展会被讨论,以迅速决定是否有出院障碍。

对患者和其家庭进行教育是移植协调员、执业护士和护理人员在患者准备出院时最重要的任务之一。患者教育实际开始在移植前阶段,并持续在整个入院、出院、门诊和后续随访中。对患者和家属最复杂的过程可能是掌握移植后必需的药物。教育患者,并要求他们展示自我服药在繁忙的医院环境中是一项挑战。患者开始自我服药的过程后，为错误的药物治疗提供了许多机会。在剂量和次数频繁变化时(有时每天变化),更增加了其复杂性。当药物的剂量个性化时,并不经常改变免疫抑制剂,从而增加了混淆。即使患者已经了解,他们将被要求服下的移植后的许多药物，当他们出院时依然可能出现真实的情况。

许多移植项目使用名为MedActionPlan在线出院药物的规划方案[22]。当患者回到家中,或在患者住院治疗和门诊护理期间，患者或其医生可访问该程序。这是临床医生的优秀资源和患者教育工具。药物可以每天进行更新，并打印为可在钱包或在笔记本中携带的格式。大多数药物的图片都可以指导患者，通过每一个新的药物的复杂的学习过程。访问也可用于iPhone和Android设备通过电子邮件或短信提醒被推送给患者[22]。

案例管理人员和社会工作者经常协助出院计划过程,通过教育患者和家属对社区资源的利用,帮助患者过渡到家庭护理环境。过渡到门诊护理往往使一些人害怕，尤其是那些使用机械辅助循环装置正在出院的患者。患者和家属在出院前接受个性化教育,一旦他们在家里关注许多疑问和回答。所有的移植设置程序有一个呼叫系统，患者及家属可以打电话提问并寻求指导。出院规划过程的一个重要部分是为患者提供呼叫的号码，其中一个医生或护士每天24小时提供回应。书面指南和指导提供护理人员呼叫应对患者的问题,并且有医生为更复杂的情况做出回应。这个呼叫系统帮助患者从住院到门诊医疗过渡。电话的工作人员还必须具有针对每个器官系统和机械循环辅助设备了解的能力。

质量评估和性能改进

直到 2007 年，大部分移植中心在内部审查其结果。很少有质量改进计划。如今,移植项目必须向调查员和保险公司证明,他们正在监测结果,并与医院质量保证和绩效改进项目(QAPI)共享他们的数据。监管环境导致许多移植项目开发了一个任务为移植 QAPI 大项目的质量改进进行协调。医疗保险和医疗补助(CMS) 的中心已经提供了指引移植界和调查员初始 CMS 调查审查质量计划工作表。2007—2010 年在最初的 CMS 调查中，调查员评估他们遵守政策和程序程度。在移植中心的第二次调查中,重点显然是 QAPI。项目被要求提供质量小组会议、QAPI 会议,并展示医院质量计划。当调查员审核中心的质量计划时,除了审查计划中遇到的不良事件，他们还要求正在进行或已完成的过程改进项目的证据。

建立绩效评估,这样可以反映移植过程,移植前、移植后随访的工作,对每一个移植计划都很关键。虽然项目利用从科学登记为移植受者的报道，这一数据代表最多 5 年的结果来确定 3 年预后[23]。为了紧密联系当前项目的成果,实时数据必须保持在关键领域,如等候名单中死亡、移植物失功、患者死亡。虽然大多数移植程序 QAPI 要求门诊随访，这是明确的移植受者和候选人护理的住院病房所需要的。护理人员、重症监护和手术室(OR)工作人员应是 QAPI 小组的成员。QAPI 季度报告结果应提交给每一位病房的工作人员以及 OR 工作人员。

沟通是为 QAPI 计划获取数据的关键组成部分。要求对不良事件报告与住院部和门诊医疗诊所进行交流。从护理移植候选人及受者的 QAPI 团队获取成员有助于保证数据完整。移植程序必须坚持不良事件监测系统。各病房应坚持记录不良事件日志。发病率和死亡率会议应包括不良事件的审查。委员会会议纪要包括每个 QAPI 会议。议程项目都是基于病房事件和随访计划以及对以往各次会议问题。

流程改进是基于每个项目的需求而开发的。患者满意度评分、患者安全问题或增加的移植物失功是可以由移植项目进行选择改进的。这些项目也应与医院的目标保持一致。举例来说,在这个时候患者的安全是医院的一大关注点。工作人员被邀请参与的项目,以改善在各自的领域的工作。在项目中共同工作人员可以有机会在移植小组中发挥领导作用。领导者被选出并在工作人员会议和器官特别质量小组会议中提供更新内容。

监管问题

2007 年 3 月 30 日,CMS 确立了器官移植项目的参与条件(COP),有效日期至 2007 年 6 月 28 日[24]。随着新的 CMS 移植 COP 的出现,一个新的移植项目监管运动在进行,这些将决定移植的未来。由 CMS 确定的移植项目作为移植医院的组成部分，提供了一个独特器官类型的移植。所有的器官移植项目必须在具有医疗提供者达成协议的医院中。除了满足移植 COP,移植项目还必须遵守医院的医疗 COP,特别是第 42 号联邦法规 482.1 至 482.57 条,这与移植 COP 是不同文件[25]。

在 2007 年 6 月 28 日之前的医保批准的移植项目,被要求在 2007 年 12 月 26 日前申请继续参与 CMS[24]。有些 COP 的关键点包括移植程序的显著变化通知 CMS、评估符合医疗保险的需求,并要求在 CMS 决定医保认证的器官移植中心考虑移植因素[24]。

移植项目有显著改变时被要求 7 天内通知 CMS,否则可能影响医疗符合保险第 42 号联邦法规 482.74 条的要求。内容包括:关键职工的变化(如主要特别项目的外科医生和内科医生),移植管理者变化,移植项目数量和预后明显减少，终止医院和器官获取组织的协议,移植项目关闭[24]。

随着移植中心 COP 方案的实施,成果是由监管机构通过每个项目的移植数据上传,并通过 SRTR 分析[23]。数据通过电子方式将每个候选人和受者的数据上传到器官获取和移植网络(OPTN)。以确保 95%中心的数据在到期日(COP482.8)90 天前提交。未能及时提交数据可能会导致研究员访问失败[23]。

候选人在 OPTN 注册用于获取新的器官的计算机排队系统。一旦移植完成,第一年随访的表格将会定期递交,然后受者每年的生活定期递交。移植物和患者的预后是基于表格提交到 OPTN,最后科学注册移植受者(SRTR)分析的[23]。这些成果都是每半年公开报道,并提供第 30 天、1 年和 3 年移植物和患者生存率的结果。CMS、保险公司及 OPTN 监测所有这些结果。如移植中心没有达到预期成果,将会收到 CMS 发布的系统改进协议(SIA)的改进要求。该文件要求移植项目在为期一年的试用期内改进他们的业绩。如果项目没有改善,它可能会失去移植医疗保险和医疗保险覆盖。

在要求考虑抑制因素的CMS决定器官移植中心保险批准过程中，有三种大体的领域将被评估决定是否获得批准,主要基于以下的抑制因素。

- 预后测量达到或超越的程度。
- 医保中心批准的抑制中心在区域内的有效性;
- 可以减轻劣处的程度以满足COP要求。

在审查结果的措施失败时,CMS评估程度和措施失败的性质以及在结果调整过程将远离标准。重要的趋势评估正在改善，由于长期低于标准状态会变得更糟。一个由CMS测量的关键因素是风险调整异常。CMS评估证据，以确定其性能受到移植风险不利影响的程度,这些危险因素不包括在SRTR风险调整方法中。试验的指南也将列入审查。其他因素包括:访问护理的证据和对护理问题的特殊访问、患者人群、器官类型以及一些不受医院控制的因素、自然灾害等其他因素。

移植项目在一个医院的住院部和门诊医疗都发挥作用。平均每三年CMS会暗访调查,但CMS可以提前调查移植项目,如果患者和移植物的预后始终在变差。调查员用绘图的方法来评估是否符合文件要求，并确定从业者是否遵循他们的政策和指南。这个过程涉及住院和门诊医疗病例。在调查中,将每天住进医院患者的信息提供给现场调查员。他们可能会在这段时间调查一下患者关于他们护理的问题。在现场审查期间,调查员还可以要求门诊医疗就诊的所有患者的名字。从审查部分患者和门诊患者的记录可咨询他们的照护问题[26]。

OPTN还进行现场调查,然而,他们提供自己计划访问移植项目的日期,同时也给移植中心一份他们1~3天的调查将会去访问的患者名单[27]。2011年,OPTN开始分别调查活体器官移植项目和死亡供体器官移植。因此，进行活体和死亡供体肾移植的中心可能一年内有三次调查:一个CMS网站的调查,以及两个独立的OPTN现场调查。虽然移植的监管方面已经创造了移植的项目规范的结构,监管人员要求增加监督数据管理、质量和法规遵从问题。住院和门诊医疗正在进行更紧密的合作,以确保安全、有质量的项目认识以及数量和预后都被监督,并捆绑支付。

除了CMS法规和OPTN政策,联合委员会进行特定疾病的认证调查,如美国心室辅助装置(VAD)与心脏移植项目相关[28]。机械循环辅助设备,如各种VAD已经成为大多数心脏移植项目的重要组成部分，无论是作为心脏移植桥梁或目标治疗[29]。调查由联合委员会每两年进行一次，以保持该验证程序已符合联合委员会建立的安全和质量标准认证[28]。负责在重症监护和高级护理病房照顾使用机械循环辅助设备患者的护士是通过面试来评估他们的患者护理方面的知识,并讨论他们的服务方向。工作人员能力的审查往往与员工的继续教育一起被要求。

联合委员会调查人员对患者从急诊室到门诊护理的机械循环辅助设备的设置进行调查。一旦出院,通过移植前的工作人员随访患者在门诊护理就诊情况,包括心脏病专家、外科医生、注册护士和执业护理师。护士和工作人员在门诊护理也由联合委员会调查员审查他们更新案例情况的能力。调查员要求护士掌握治疗定向文档和继续教育文件，以确保具有目标护理人群的知识和专业技能。

一些心脏移植项目也植入全人工心脏(TAH)。在重症监护室和高级护理病房照顾这类患者的护理人员,在护理TAH患者时联合委员会调查人员会审查他们的知识、专业知识和能力。2011年便携式TAH(研究的设备),让TAH患者可以出院。

当患者被植入服务时,VAD的特殊疾病认证要求项目改进质量指示指标以便随访。该QAPI项目必须包括针对预后和过程的至少四个绩效指标。这时的绩效指标不是联合委员会规定的，可以根据每个项目临床实践指南确定。一旦分析所有的认证项目的数据,联合委员会计划使用统一的绩效指标。数据每个季度提交给联合委员会。凡是通过认证的VAD项目都必须参加名为INTERMACS国家数据库注册。无论是住院患者还是门诊治疗的患者，只要他们应用一个VAD项目,这些数据将被收集并提交给INTERMACS。基于该数据库的预后报告,每年进行公布[29]。

总结

移植由于其高成本和高风险，是一个高度管制医疗领域。在这个监管环境下移植项目变得更加标准化和关注预后结果。很多移植项目拓展员工包括质量和专业能力以及额外的数据协调员实时监控结果。CMS、

OPTN 和联合委员监管调查的频率会带来了额外的人力需求,以准备那些未提前告知的调查。在大型移植项目中,候选人和受者往往被在专业病房进行照顾,要求护士熟悉技能的复杂性以便有能力照顾这些患者和其家属。在较小的移植程序中,患者可能与非移植的患者同住。在这种情况下,一个专门的核心组护士为移植候选人和受者提供护理。对护理人员能力测试可能是半年或一年进行 1 次。认证是强烈推荐给护士工作人员以及移植协调员的,是为了进一步确保他们在其专业领域保持目前最新的知识。多学科小组从不同角度照顾这些复杂的患者人群的做法是非常有效的,每个团队成员的不同的意见最终能满足全面护理这些患者的需要。

(郭海军 译 徐骁 校)

参考文献

1. Landsperger JS, Williams KJ, Hellervik SM, et al. Implementation of a medical intensive care unit acute-care nurse practitioner service. Hospital Practice. 2011;39(2):32–39.
2. Humphreys H. Positive pressure ventilation and the prevention of invasive aspergillosis. What is the evidence? Journal of Hospital Infection. 2004;56: 93–100.
3. Finkler SA, Kovner CT, Jones CB. Financial management for nurse managers and executives. 3rd ed. St. Louis, MO: Saunders; 2007. ISBN# 978-1-4160-3342-4.
4. Finkler SA, McHugh ML. Budgeting concepts for nurse managers. St. Louis, MO: Saunders; 2008. ISBN# 978-1-4160-3341-7.
5. Montalvo I. The National Database on Nursing Quality Indicators. Online Journal of Issues in Nursing. 2007;12(3): [accessed December 14, 2013] http://www.nursingworld.org/MainMenuCategories/Policy-Advocacy/State/Legislative-Agenda-Reports/State-StaffingPlansRatios
6. Twigg D, Duffield C, Brumner A, et al. Impact of skill mix variations on patient outcomes following implementation of nursing hours per day staffing: a retrospective study. Journal of Advanced Nursing. 2012;68(12): 2710–2718.
7. Unruh LY, Zhang NJ. Nurse staffing and patient safety in hospitals: new variable and longitudinal approaches. Nursing Research. 2012;61(1):3–12.
8. Aiken LH, Clarke SP, Sloane DM, et al. Hospital nurse staffing and patient mortality, nurse burnout and job dissatisfaction. Journal of the American Medical Association. 2002;288:1987–1993.
9. Labor Management Institute. Annual Survey of Hours Report. [accessed March 25, 2012]; Available from: http://www.lminstitute.com/1864/1948.html.
10. Wright D. The Ultimate Guide to Competency Assessment in Health Care. 3rd ed. Minneapolis, MN: Creative Healthcare Management; 2005.
11. Savage L, Murphy J, Joyce K. Developing and maintaining competency with circulatory assist devices: how to meet the challenge. Progress in Transplantation. 2010;20:125–128.
12. Hayes B, Bonner A, Pryor J. Factors contributing to nurse satisfaction in the acute hospital setting: a review of recent literature. Journal of Nursing Management. 2010;18:804–814.
13. Transplant Nursing Competency Task Force. Introduction to Transplant Nursing Core Competencies. Pittsburgh, PA: International Transplant Nurses Society; 2011.
14. Sechrist KR, Valentine W, Berlin LE. Perceived value of certification among certified, noncertified, and administrative perioperative nurses. Journal of Professional Nursing. 2006;22(4):242–247.
15. Altman M. Let's get certified, best practices for nurse leaders to create a culture of certification. AACN Advanced Critical Care. 2011;22(1):68–75.
16. American Board of Nursing Specialties Specialty Nursing Certification: Nurses Perceptions, Values and Behaviors. [accessed March 31, 2012]; Available from: http://www.nursingcertification.org/resources-position.html.
17. Anthony D, Chetty VK, Kartha A, et al. Re-engineering the hospital discharge: an example of a multifaceted process evaluation. In: Henriksen K, Battles JB, Marks ES, et al., editors. Advances in Patient Safety: From Research to Implementation, Vol. 2, Concepts and Methodology. Rockville, MD: AHRQ; 2005.
18. Forster AJ, Murff HJ, Peterson JF, et al. The incidence and severity of adverse events affecting patients after discharge from the hospital. Annals of Internal Medicine. 2003;138:161–167.
19. Kohn LT, Corrigan JM, Donaldson MS, editors. To Err is Human: Building a Safer Health System, A report from the Committee on Quality of Health Care in America. Institute of Medicine, Washington, DC: National Academy Press; 1999.
20. Shepard S, McClaran J, Phillips CO, et al. Discharge Planning from hospital to home. Cochrane Database of Systemic Reviews. 2010; [accessed April 8, 2012] http://summaries.cochrane.org/CD000313/discharge-planning-from-hospital-to-home.
21. Frank-Bader M, Beltran K, Dojlidko D. Improving discharge education using a structured teaching approach. Progress in Transplantation. 2011;11(4):332–339.
22. MedActionPlan. [accessed January 3, 2012]; Available from: http://www.medactionplan.com/.
23. Scientific Registry for Transplant Recipients. [accessed April 8, 2012]; Available from: http://www.srtr.org.
24. Centers for Medicare and Medicaid. Final Rule for Transplant Conditions of Participation. Federal Register, Friday, March 30, 2007 [accessed March 25, 2012]; Available from: http://www.gpo.gov/fdsys/pkg/FR-2007-03-30/content-detail.htm.
25. Conditions for Coverage and Conditions of Participation for Healthcare Organizations. [accessed April 8, 2012]; Available from: http://www.cms.gov/Regulations-and-Guidance/Legislation/CFCsAndCoPs/index.html?redirect=/CFCsandCOPs/06_Hospitals.asp.
26. CMS Transplant Conditions of Participation Interpretive Guidelines. [accessed January 10, 2012]; Available from: https://www.cms.gov/Medicare/Provider-Enrollment-and-Certification/SurveyCertificationGenInfo/downloads//SCLetter08-25.pdf.
27. About OPTN. [accessed March 17, 2012]; Available from: http://optn.transplant.hrsa.gov/optn/.
28. The Joint Commission Disease Specific Certification for VADS. [accessed March 25, 2012]; Available from: http://www.jointcommission.org/certification/ventricular_assist_device.aspx.
29. Kirklin JK, Naftel DC, Kormos RL, et al. The Fourth INTERMACS annual report: 4,000 implants and counting. Journal of Heart and Lung Transplantation. 2012; 31(2):117–126.

第 125 章
移植门诊管理

Elizabeth A. Kallenborn, Chris Shay-Downer, Kathy Schwab, Shelley Zomak

引言

移植领域已经远远超出传说中的 13 世纪 Saints Cosmos 和 Damien 手术室，成为目前复杂的多项目移植中心。除了手术技能和医疗进步，随着时间的推移，很明显需要额外的临床资源对日益复杂的患者提供长期护理。临床专家组成门诊诊所移植已经发展到移植受者、接受者和活体供者提供全面的、具有成本效益的服务。今天面对移植项目的主要挑战包括：面临着越来越长的等待时间，老化移植接受者的人群面临着许多慢性疾病的问题，和移植前短期住院和移植后长期住院。

文献中关于开发或进化早期的门诊患者移植诊所只有很少的信息，但护理组织的价值得到了普遍的认可。有序组织的护理工作改善保健和控制慢性病的临床质量，提高患者满意度，并减少住院、急诊、处方药费用[1]。开创性的移植努力在很大程度上是一个“团队”，通常由外科医生、内科医生和移植协调员组成。从外科医生的角度写关于早期移植协调的文章很多，但是很少有出版物关注早期移植诊所的作用[2]。因此，本章的目的是描述当前门诊移植诊所管理运营策略。这个概述适用于移植的各个阶段：评估，候选和（或）等候名单管理，以及受体和（或）活体长期护理管理。

在美国，移植深受联邦政府监管。本章讨论的操作策略通常是基于这些规则，这将在某种程度上影响诊所管理。在 128 章中可以找到更详细的政府监管治疗细节。在 124 章可以找到详细的住院治疗病房设计和管理。

监管机构的角色

器官供应移植网络/器官共享联合网络（OPTN/UNOS）

直到 20 世纪 80 年代，只有相对较少的医疗中心是本地管理移植和器官分配。随着移植预后的改善，提高了现有的移植项目的数量，并且更多的患者成为移植候选者，联邦政府认识到需要一个集中的、全国器官分配系统确保所有患者有平等的机会获得供体器官。随着 1984 年全国器官移植法案（NOTA）的颁布，国家器官供应移植网络（OPTN）被要求建立一个公平分配捐赠器官的系统，增加可用捐赠器官移植的供应是在联邦合同的约束下进行、由私人运营的非营利组织。器官共享联合网络（UNOS）目前持有 OPTN 运营合同。UNOS 的使命是推动器官移植可用性以及团结和支持移植社区，通过教育、技术和政策的发展造福患者[3]。同时，为移植受者的全国科学登记（SRTR）旨在汇编和分析所有移植者数据对潜在的改进进行鉴定，以提高移植患者的生命[4]。

2000 年 3 月 16 日，OPTN 规则开始实施，对整个美国的实体器官移植环境有很大影响。最终规则为 OPTN 建立了一个监管框架。有几个因素影响器官移植，其中最深刻的是供体器官的全国性紧缺。由于这个短缺，需要建立透明的授权评估移植供应程序，以及捐献器官的分配、管理部门。器官供应移植网络（OPTN）是一个私人、非营利性组织，专门进行器官供应移植器官分配，职责是维护一个公平的分配系统，维持潜在受者的等候名单,匹配潜在受者的器官捐赠者,根据既定标准列出和删除移植患者。OPTN 还收集、分析和发布关于移植前后的事件数据来推进器官移植、器官获取、器官保存和免疫遗传学领域的发展。这些数据是通过一个被称为 UNet 的在线数据库系统管理的。自 1987 年 10 月 1 日,UNet 记录了每一个关于捐赠和移植数据事件。OPTN 针对美国官方政策开发、捐赠器官的分配和移植数据的收集建立了政策和规章制度。OPTN 由 22 个国家委员会,23 个地区和国家审查委员会和众多董事会制定政策。OPTN /UNOS 定义 11 个区域服务领域;每个区域被细分为器官组织(OPO)捐赠服务领域(DSA)支持公平合理分配捐献器官[5](图 125.1)。

OPTN 进行持续的定期调查和评估每一个 OPO 和移植的医院是否符合 OPTN 规则和政策。为了合规监控,OPTN 定义的流程和协议、申请项目成员和关键人员、具体要求通知内容、现场绩效审计,全部由 OPTN 承担者按照联邦规定开发。OPTN 力求通过整改计划,实施制裁包括:必要的及时纠正措施和匿名的同行评审,使会员遵守专业标准委员会(MPSC)。这个过程鼓励参与质量改进;使用以下纪律制裁的警告(机密同行评审),试用期(公告),和宣告"会员未达到好的标准"(公告)[7,8]。

医疗保险和医疗补助服务中心(CMS)

器官移植计划的参与条件(CoP)成立于 2007 年。最终规则提出了由医疗保险参与设施提供安全、优质的服务移植预期。监管的领域包括遵守联邦、州和地方法律,和法律相关的患者护理计划,患者的权利、利用率、服务需求和合理和必要的覆盖全国的决定。

2004 年监察长办公室(OIG),这似乎是当前 CoP 最初的步骤,建议 CMS 应该开发受体数量和存活率标准,制订指导方针和程序处理移植项目不符合数量和存活率标准,并监督改进数据,收集移植受者的生存相关数据。

随着时间的推移,其他程序的质量和服务的具体问题以及投诉,证明了自我报告的重大变化并不足以确保高质量和安全移植服务。另外,认证标准没有被 OIG 确定。其结果是,最终规定和随后的 CoP 建立了最初的审批和医疗保险的重新审批医疗保险认证医院的核定要求,这些医院对成人和儿童患者和活体捐献提供移植服务。

2007 年 3 月,美国卫生与公众服务部 (HHS),与 CMS 作为负责的联邦机构,推出了移植方案审批和重新审批申请程序。CMS 调查认证过程初始评估移植程

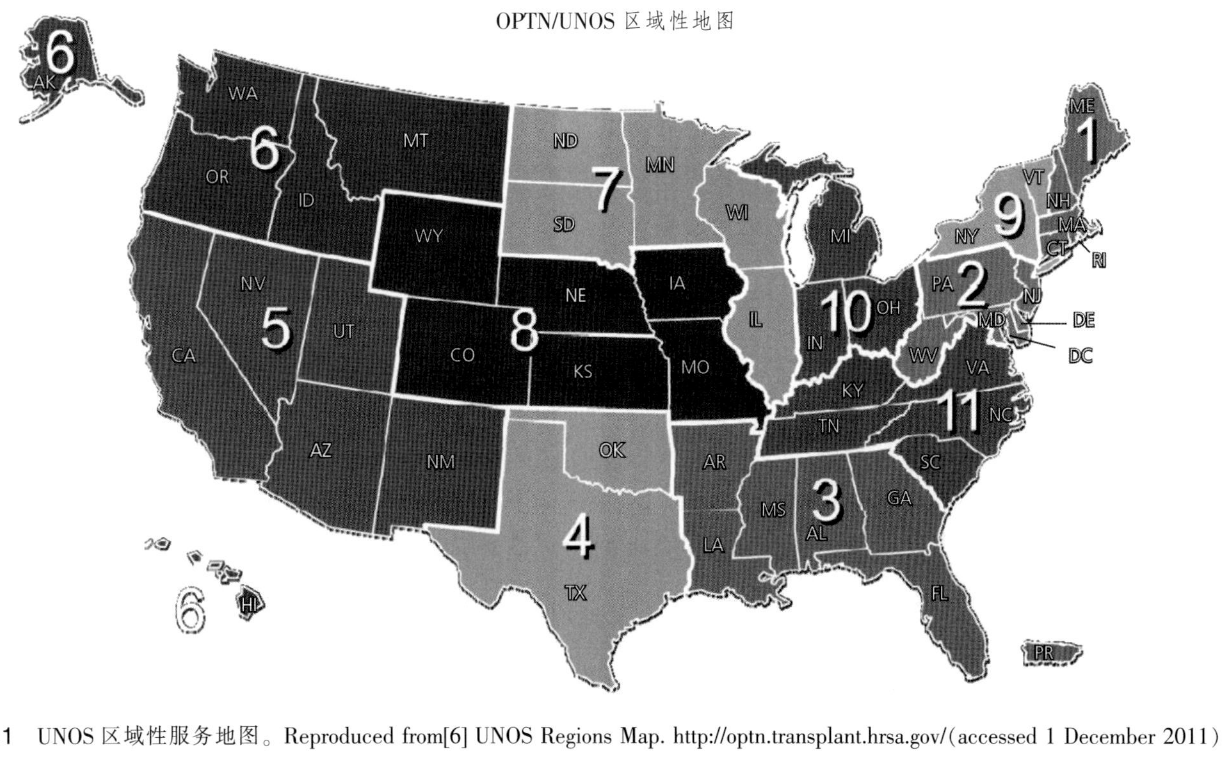

图 125.1　UNOS 区域性服务地图。Reproduced from[6] UNOS Regions Map. http://optn.transplant.hrsa.gov/(accessed 1 December 2011)

序和持续评估是否符合 CoP。移植医院预计被要求提供通知到 CMS，移植方案的变化其中包括关键人员的变动、在临床经验和成果的变化、器官获取组织（OPO）协议终止和（或）失活移植程序的任何显著变化。自我报告后，当移植中心不符合 CoP 要求时，必须申请“考虑缓和因素”[9]。

其他机构

美国卫生和公众服务部咨询委员会的器官移植（ACOT）的成立，通过卫生资源和服务管理局（HRSA）扮演了一个咨询委员会代理的角色，由卫生部长指导关于器官捐赠、采购、分配和移植问题。该委员会的任务是审查 OPTN 政策提议，对提交的各种移植相关的问题进行审批。

在 HRSA 的指导下，于 2003 年捐赠与移植实践委员会通过提高死亡供体捐献者的数量，减少移植等候名单的死亡，增加捐赠可供移植器官的数量，并创建最佳实践指南。这些协作努力继续扩大到捐献和移植的各个方面。2007 年，HRSA 移植中心增长和协同管理最佳实践最终报告被颁布。这份报告提供了从选择高性能的移植中心的最佳实践观察，这些中心器官移植率和器官恢复的使用效率高，同时保持预期或高于预期的患者和移植器官的生存结果[10]。

移植门诊诊所的设计和（或）布局

目标和目的

门诊诊所的范围可以从一个简单的医疗机构提供初级保健，到以高度专业化、复杂的工具或者说是没有住院床位的医院。移植门诊诊所的目标纳入各个中心的任务说明，但通常范围很广，维护共同的愿景和保证候选人、受者活体供体和他们的家庭的健康和幸福。诊所的宗旨是为移植候选人和活体供体提供评估，并优化移植候选人和受体的医学管理，包括处方、监测和免疫调节的医疗管理；诊断和管理移植的急性和长期并发症和活体的随访。为了确保最佳的患者护理和连续性的照顾，移植团队需要有一种协作方式。

操作

移植诊所操作和设计可以变化。大多数是基于需要、面积和在其移植中心的患者数量。所有这些都作为较大的医疗中心的一部分而存在，成为患者从住院到门诊护理的延续，因此成为患者的移植相关保健服务的主要中心。

为了满足不断扩大的患者需求，提高接入移植相关服务，乡村诊所也被用于促进患者护理。卫星诊所已经成为综合医疗体系的一部分，综合医疗体系包括大型学术中心、社区中心，以及为便于患者护理的乡村中心。这是一个机会，利用乡村外科手术中心，对移植前后患者进行随访护理，这些包含在较大的医疗系统内。这些诊所减少患者的治疗路费和经济负担，最终可能促进他们遵守规定的移植护理计划。乡村诊所也可以帮助增加推荐，使移植中心最终扩大移植计划。这些诊所都配备有在实验室、放射学和程序方面指定的人员；而多学科的团队有能力在这个系统中搜索、查看这些地方的移植患者，如同在移植中心一样[11]。

监管移植诊所可以属于医院门诊部管理或门诊诊所管理。操作规程和偿还时间根据临床管理类型和国家认证机构的不同而有所不同。简单地说，医院为基础的诊所作用相当于医生的办公室从而为患者提供具体服务；他们在医院的许可下运行，并对联邦政府和监管机构负责，即医疗组织的联合认证委员会（JCAHO）。必须注意，不同类型的诊所被当地、州和联邦监管机构以及国家认证机构按照各自的需求调查。

设计

针对移植临床操作，一个专门的移植结构化诊所是最优的。移植结构化诊所背后的概念是受过专门移植训练的人员在一个空间提供综合移植服务，这个空间设计是为了照顾移植候选人、受体和活体供体。这种类型的诊所的作用范围从一个广泛的协调候选人或活体供体，到评估移植受者的长期随访和生活。

医院和移植管理，与医生领导者一同，提供任何诊所发展的基础、设计和管理。在设计诊所空间时必须考虑结构支持和限制。提供不同规模和类型的服务是移植门诊诊所的共同属性。移植患者来到医疗中心以解决棘手的问题，这类患者常有多个家庭成员陪伴并带医疗设备如氧气瓶、步行器、轮椅。为了提高工作环境的功能，诊所设计团队应该包括政府、医疗建设人员、移植团队人员，以便在给定的空间内提供服务。一般认为是在构建门诊诊所的主要关注内容包括:①以成本有效的方式提供服务的能力;②灵活性和可扩展性,以满足当前和未来的需求计划;③环境质量和安全;④可视性和可访问性,包括美国残疾人法案规定;⑤为患者治疗安全的环境;⑥可持续性;⑦健康保险流通与隐私的责任法案和安全(HIPAA)合规[12]。

在理想情况下,设备管理将充分支持移植项目的需要。临床上,足够数量的诊所咨询和评估的房间可以为医疗团队提供专门工作区检查记录和完成文档。诊所房间的需求数量取决于项目的规模和年度诊所容量。

配备有熟悉移植血液检查人员的专业移植实验室,也应该在诊所或其附近提供。设施,如:为患者检查和申报登记区;私人咨询室;患者教育设施,为个人或小组教学设施;患者库;宽敞的等候室,都需要在移植诊所的物理设计和布局中考虑。

诊所调度模型

模型

各种类型的临床调度模型可用于移植诊所作为其标准开发的基础。无论将哪种模型作为诊所结构的基础, 以患者和家庭为中心的方法提供任何所需的移植服务的能力以及持续的质量结果是所有移植计划的共同目标。基本上有两种类型的患者服务交付模式:医生驱动或诊所/服务专线驱动的方法。传统的医生驱动诊所每次调度是根据门诊时间。在一间诊所/服务专线带动诊疗模式,按患者通常的到达时间安排,根据器官类型和移植状态(移植前/等候名单/移植后/活体),没有指定的直接提供者。

无论采用哪个诊疗模式, 诊所人员模式可以相差很大。一个工作人员模式是有充分专门的诊所工作人员。这种类型的人员配置将包括:辅助人员、抽血人员、医疗助理和移植诊所的护士, 专门的诊所护士长和护理人员都是以患者在诊所中治疗护理为目的。另一种模式工作人员是其中的诊所空间为服务专线, 包括移植协调员和支持人员。无论如何选择人员结构,必须维持高效优质的医护服务, 以及监测合规性和持续的患者满意度。

就诊者的类型:移植前和移植后

移植前就诊

通常情况下, 首先遇到的潜在候选人或活体供体将在移植中心评估用于移植或捐赠的时间。移植候选人评估的目的是确定医疗需要器官移植治疗终末期器官功能衰竭时,传统的医学已经无计可施。潜在的移植候选者将根据终末期器官功能衰竭的各个阶段置于移植中心。在实际移植的评估之前,病历是由多学科小组成员审核,以安排确定评估的适当水平。一旦患者被医生批准以及经济授权到位,正式安排移植评估计划。在最初的移植评估过程中,终末期疾病的原因、移植的适应证和禁忌证将被确定。必须进一步处理和管理共存疾病管理以便完成评估。一个专门的移植诊所要有安排协调全面的测试的能力。通常,每个候选人的评估将针对其医疗需求,以及器官特异性特点。一个专门的移植诊所和人员提供了潜在的移植候选者的多学科综合评估的场所。临床移植团队成员必须与转诊医生合作,让他(她)掌握患者的整个评估进展。这是开始转诊点,并成为患者终身的护理团队相互合作的基础(图 125.2)。

从患者的角度来看, 预约诊疗在实际访问之前启动。提示信息包发送给患者即将进行的访问概述。这个信息包通常包括:行车路线,当地的住房信息,医疗中心的方向,患者的评估时间表,具体的测试编制说明(如果有器官特异性教育材料), 规范性文件 (例如,UNOS材料、知情同意)和其他医疗中心的具体项目。候选人的评估即将推出的确认也应传达给转诊医生。对调度的项目要关注包括获得患者及住宿地点的替代电话号码。调度还应提前 24~48 小时确认预约。由于移植候选人的医疗条件的复杂性, 频繁住院治疗的情况并不少见, 但贡献较高的失约率。这也延长了转诊和移植时间,最终可能会影响患者整体的治疗效果。

从移植小组的角度来看, 诊所预约安排在任何一天的数目由可用的门诊室、提供者的可用性、会面类型和时间长短来决定。辅助科室之间的测试和磋商协调是访问效果和成功的关键。

在患者到来之前, 通过系统停车和导航的辅助功能确认。设施,如在指定的患者落客区或代客泊车配有残疾人专用的无障碍标志帮助第一次来的患者减少焦

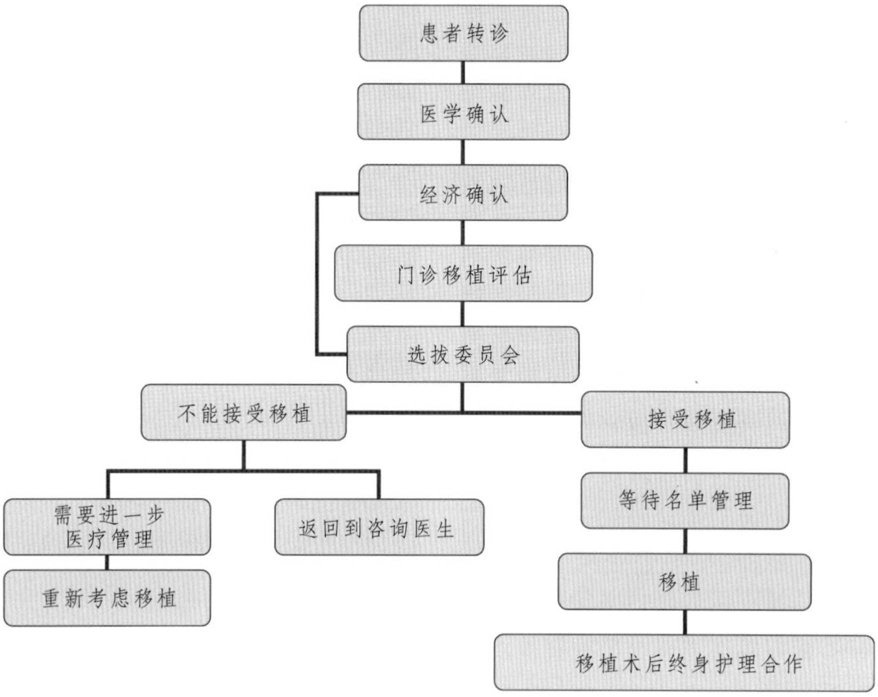

图 125.2 移植过程图。

虑。轮椅和(或)踏板车应在患者抵达时随时可供患者使用,另外还配有医院的服务人员和交通专家。医院标牌必须是最新的,易于寻找。

一旦患者到达移植诊所,就需要办理入住手续和登记。由于移植评价的程度,预期这些患者将在诊所停留些时间,可能会停留数天。评估的时长是可变的,取决于每个移植中心的器官特异性的选择标准要求和患者的整体健康状态。诊所团队将通过评估过程指导患者。这将包括服务(如抽血、医疗评估、药物使用、协商、耐心教育),还需测试移植候选人的医疗状态和病史。该工作人员完成任务概述可能每个都有差异:医疗助理(MA),注册护士(RN),移植协调员(TC),先进的执业护士(APN),医生助理(PA),或移植的医生。在每次访谈的最后,应提前与患者及家属安排即将到来的评估。

移植评估过程中一定要坚持 UNOS 和 CMS 法规。CMS 参与条件确定需要参与候选人和活体捐赠者评估的移植专业人员。在多学科团队中包括:医生(移植外科医生和移植医生),护理,社会服务,临床移植协调员,营养和药理学。具体到活体供体的评估是独立的活体倡导的评估。多学科移植小组的其他成员可能包括:行政支持人员,调度,负责病历人员,UNOS 的数据协调,移植协调员资金方面和科研人员。每一个确定的团队成员拥有全面提供终身护理,对于整个移植过程患者需要独特的技能和专业知识。CMS 法规要求的机构发展自己的移植中心[13]中指定的多学科评估小组成员个人了解政策,以及他们的学历,证书和作用。

医生(移植医生和外科医生)

移植的医生和外科医生是负责监督直接移植手术和医疗服务的。若有可供移植的供体器官,必须配有一位可靠的医生。初级医生和外科医生必须由 OPTN[13]的批准。

护理

护士向移植患者提供移植期间所有时间点的护理。从医生办公室,到门诊移植诊所,手术中,重症监护病房,一般护理单位,康复服务单位,长期护理设施,专业护理设施,家庭护理护士,研究团队,护理教育,护理管理人员都是不同的参与护理移植患者的护士。护理教育范围为执业的/高职(LPN/LVN)、注册护士(RN)、或高级执业护士(APN)。在移植专业认证可移植护士的移植具体护理经验[13,14]至少一年。

社会服务

社会服务是移植小组的固有重要组成部分,整个过程中为患者提供的连续服务。他们的重点是传达给他们不单单是经历移植过程的患者，而且是作为团队成员。移植社工提供支持、教育和咨询服务，以帮助减少进行移植的压力。执行评估的评估是通过目标 CMS 任务确保患者和团队必须实现患者和程序都具有潜在取得圆满成功所需的所有信息。在社会服务的评估涉及的主要方面包括：

- 移植获益和风险须知；
- 遵守评估；
- 心理健康史，包括药物和酒精使用和(或)滥用；
- 可用的应对能力进行评估；
- 经济能力，资源评估；
- 适当的社会、交通、住宿评估[13]。

临床移植协调员

移植协调员(TC)是必须注册的具备移植方面的知识和经验并经国家许可实践的护士或医生。移植协调员确保护理的连续性和协调整个移植和(或)捐赠的所有阶段的临床护理候选人、受者/捐助者，也作为与患者的护理[14,15]的多学科团队的所有成员的联络人。移植协调已演变成基本上所有的移植团队的重要组成部分，是覆盖在深入第 122 章。

营养

营养评估和饮食咨询必须在评估阶段由专业营养师提供给所有移植患者，候选人和活体捐献移植中心。教育是提供给患者针对他们的个性化需求。营养师提供医学营养治疗。营养服务也提供给受者和供者术后营养关键和问题(即体重增加、体重下降、电解质失衡、药物原因的饮食限制)。单个移植中心的政策必须明确营养服务，包括营养评估、饮食咨询、或营养干预[15]。

药理学

移植药剂师帮助管理移植患者的日常护理。他们评估和建议是根据个人情况而不仅仅是特定的移植器官护理计划。他们提供了宝贵的关于免疫管理和拒绝治疗的见解。纵观连续移植，移植药剂师专门监督规定药物相互作用和药物治疗水平。必须考虑到在处方药和患者补充药物，要使用好。移植药剂师往往是移植研究团队[15,16]的成员。移植药剂师的作用在第 123 章进行了详细讨论。

活体供体倡导者

执行活体移植的移植中心必须是一个独立的活体供体倡导者，以确保准活体供者的权益保护。这个人应该从移植小组[15]中独立运作。

UNOS 的数据协调员

一些大型的、多程序移植中心的多学科小组有 UNOS 的数据协调员。UNOS 的数据协调员是管理 UNOS/UNet 相关数据录入者。移植求职登记(TCR)，移植受者登记(TRR)，移植患者随访表单(TRF)，激活，在激活完成后，上传和清除任务 UNOS 的数据协调员执行的例子。这些协调员也都是质量改进委员会(QAPI)的重要成员，并参与质量控制审核。

移植财务协调员

一个移植小组一个符合条件的新患者首先接触的是移植财务协调员(TFC)。此人充当辅导患者以及为其提供保险的联络员和(或)协调员。在深入审查和保险福利验证后，咨询预约评估期间安排与患者审查所有符合条件的保险覆盖面的优点和局限性。TFC 解释了高成本移植相关业务的财务影响，并指导是给那些因覆盖范围和福利限制而需要额外援助的人，TFC 也作为医疗管理部门的联络员，提醒团队限制覆盖范围，以及何时需要进行服务授权[17]。

移植后门诊随访

移植后的随访往往很短，但在促进患者长期成功的治疗效果也同样重要。这种类型访问的目标包括：免疫抑制，监测与移植有关的急性和慢性并发症的诊断优化管理，以及促进整体健康。这些访问可能包括或不包括实验室指标，但需要包括患者评估、药物作用、咨询、教育和移植具体的测试。值得注意的是，由于护士和医生对患者和家庭的再教育水平，可以预期移植后的初始随访将更深入、更长久。

单独移植诊所不能提供所有的服务移植患者需要。服务的协调必须在医疗中心系统内使用。护理与多学科的移植团队，包括但不限于病理科、放射科、感染性疾病、肾病、肝病、心脏病、肺、麻醉、内分泌、药物学、精神病学和姑息治疗联合对于患者长期预后十分重要。协议或方式可通过移植小组进行开发，与查明的特色相结合,以促进执行患者护理。

一个专门的移植门诊手术单位对于治疗这种复杂的患者群很关键。这种类型的病房提供器官特异性移植前和移植后的服务和治疗，以及独特的需要比门诊更密集的医疗管理可以提供移植人口其他侵入性操作的中间水平。包括干预和治疗,不需要住院,但确实需要耐心的监督,以确保患者的安全。典型的护士与患者的比例是一名护士与三名或四名移植患者。门诊及门诊手术室可以提供的服务包括出院后的日常监测、静脉切开术、活组织检查、血液制品管理、用药管理、侵入性放射学检测和血浆置换。这种类型的服务相关的节约成本的好处包括:促进早期放电,预防再入院,护理的中间级不能在家庭中设置的输送。

在某个时间点，照顾移植受者可能会转移到移植小组对长期医疗服务以外的医疗服务提供者，如初级护理医生(主治医生)或其他非移植相关的专家。移植小组和多学科团队的其他成员之间的关怀协调必须通过开诚布公的沟通和协作完成为这种复杂的患者群体提供相应的服务。长期移植随访必须通过移植办公室进行协调,以确保符合监管报告要求。

人员编制

CMS参保条件规定多学科小组成员必须参加移植患者的护理。CoP明确规定,每位患者必须处于一个多学科小组照顾。这个团队在整个移植阶段是由移植医生必须参与患者护理的各个环节，包括协调评估和常规随访护理[13]。然而,个别移植中心如何集成这些角色计划之间差别很大。对于多学科小组必须解决团队成员、角色、资格的组成和支持文档中心的具体政策。移植候选人、受者或生活再加上需要专门的医疗管理供体的复合物,慢性的进一步增加了工作人员的困境。其他限制因素包括：检查室提供的门诊每年人口增加的数量、检查室数量、供体数量和支持人员的水平。

一般工作人员的做法包括两种类型:“医学模式”和“护理模式”。“医学模式”中的传统提供者(医生,PA),医疗助理(MA)和支持人员运行诊所。这种类型的经营的诊所拥有更低的运营成本，但因此提供服务的范围有限。在“护理模式”下的诊所,这样的环境会增加护士经济管理和支持人员的提供者(医生,PA)的利用率。这种类型的护士引领的诊所通过增强为患者提供服务和教育的范围,提高患者的治疗效果[18]支持专科护理门诊环境的敏锐度。

为了应对工作人员的困境,2003年UNOS制定了移植管理员、调查人员配备通过UNet,以帮助确定给出的移植方案的方式和特点水平最佳。本次调查确定多学科移植小组成员的角色。移植管理员委员会人事调查检查每一个移植项目的规模和范围。人员类型方面,它还确定以及许多在每个角色如何执行在中心工作、交互式报表允许移植中心在保密的基础上的人员配置水平,与其他类似规模的移植中心进行比较。同样,这个工具是目前没有可衡量的,被用作工作人员指导。报道这一调查数据只适用于已参加调查[19]移植中心。

能力

移植的专业人士为候选者、受者、家庭成员、活体供者提供高度专业化的服务。随着技术、手术、药物和继续进步，移植的专业人士必须不断更新自己的知识基础,并展示在自己的领域的专业知识,以照顾日益复杂的患者群。所有的医疗服务提供者需具备一定程度的能力。“能力”是用来得到性能广泛的因素的一个包容各方的流程。能力包括行为评估,技能,技术知识和在医疗系统的熟练程度,具体的部门和监管水平。年度医疗保健体系能力培训可以通过电子全球竞争力完成，并在组织核心竞争力的交付和确保一致性中提供便利。具体部门能力和监管能力为另外进行的个性化的规章和医疗服务提供者提供服务。移植协调员将预期参与它们所提供照顾的特殊患者群体，以及监管特定移植相关的能力。UNOS的数据协调员或其他辅助人员将有望参加与文书和行政工作相关的任务。这可能包括UNet和监管的具体移植相关的任务。

2009年,国际护士移植学会(ITNS)与美国护士协会(ANA)合作开发了移植护理范围和执业标准。这些标准的实践和专业性能作用，提供可以由护理人员用来测量专业性能[20]具体的衡量因素。他们部门内建立移植具体的年度能力评估时,移植中心可参照此文件。

电子病历

在过去的20年里一直是电子病历(EMR)不断增

长的推动力。随着更严格的联邦政府监督和正在进行的医疗改革，大多数移植中心将电子病历集成到实践中。电子病历是通过在任何护理服务设置一个或多个生成的患者健康信息的纵向电子记录。电子病历提供由授权患者记录的即时访问、增强质量、安全和患者护理[21]的效率。

根据美国卫生信息管理协会(AHIMA)EMR 的主要功能是在实时医疗点捕获数据的能力，整合来自多个内部和外部数据源的数据，并支持临床决策。核心要素/任何电子病历的功能包括：健康信息和数据存储，高效的结果管理，订单录入管理，临床决策支持，沟通和连接加强对所有提供者之间的持续护理，患者的支持并获得他们的受保护的健康记录，并直接参与监管报告[22]。

有许多商业电子病历可用于医疗保健系统。电子病历必须生成一个完整的病历，以及直接或间接地支持通过接口其他保健相关活动的能力。包括以证据为基础的决策支持活动，质量管理和结果报告。提供者需要选择最适合的方案需求的系统。移植特定的程序可以同时支持日常运营、研究数据收集和监管报告的集成。

患者教育和(或)知情同意书

移植患者的教育已被公认为是移植成功的一个因素。综合患者和家庭教育开始在移植转诊时间。移植是压倒性的，需要患者和移植团队之间的开放和信任的关系，以确保成功。移植涉及重大生活方式的变化，移植中心成为患者和家庭教育的主要来源。从患者被告知需要进行移植手术开始，多学科团队的所有成员都参与教育过程。整个移植过程持续的教育是必要的，能让患者及家属成功管理健康做出决策。

知情同意

CMS 参保条件提供了所有移植教育计划的基础。参保条件清楚地勾勒出患者和活体供体的权利，包括获得知情同意和患者教育文档的过程。被列入知情同意书内容包括：评估过程，外科手术，替代疗法，医疗或心理风险，临床结局，供体的风险因素，拒绝权，以及通过移植中心无医保进行移植的局限性。在评估阶段实验室和诊断测试结果、选择标准、社会心理问题可能影响移植、财务问题，以及移植后严格遵守医疗制度的必要性等问题进行了详细的讨论。必须讨论移植前手术方式，必须先考虑很多方面，如手术的麻醉风险与使用血液制品风险，移植后恢复，以及相关的风险和益处，同时对患者的限制，必须在电子病历记录。选择用于替代的疗法要根据每个器官的类型和患者的整体健康状况，必须提前列出潜在候选人。讨论医疗风险需要包括术后并发症，特别是伤口感染、肺炎、血栓、排斥、需要再次移植、需要终身免疫抑制、多器官功能衰竭，甚至死亡。社会心理风险的讨论必须包括与抑郁症、创伤后应激障碍(PTSD)、和焦虑相关的问题。CMS 参保条件需要将最近 SRTR 报告国家和特定移植中心的成果提供给所有潜在候选人。内容包括移植中心的观察值与预期一年期患者和移植物存活率，全国一年期患者和移植物存活率，并通知不是由移植中心满足所有医疗成果的要求。更新成果报告必须提供给所有在评估的候选人，并且等待名单的阶段每半年更新一次。可能影响移植物功能的成功的器官捐献者的危险因素的讨论需要包括：医疗/社会史，年龄，器官状态，感染 HIV 的风险，乙型肝炎病毒，丙型肝炎病毒，或癌症。候选者需要被告知在过程[23]中，有随时拒绝的权利。

对活体捐献必须包括上述所有，并专门解决相关的捐赠将来的健康问题可能不考虑在捐赠者的健康保险内，捐助者可能获得健康、残疾，或可能会永久影响人寿保险能力，讨论概述了捐赠者的在捐赠过程[23]随时退出捐赠的权利[23]。

在 CMS 调查中，审计人员要求查看提供给患者的所有教育材料的复印件作为移植中心的概述知情同意过程的一部分，以及提供给患者及家庭配套的教育材料和患者的病历记录。移植中心必须制订具体的器官知情同意书及关于谁负责与患者沟通知情同意过程，谁负责获得知情同意的政策和方法，以及每个 CMS 指导患者教育[23](图 125.3)。

多重列表

在最初的评估潜在的移植候选者时必须告知为“多重列表”的选项。根据目前的 OPTN/ UNOS 的政策 3.2 器官分布：UNOS 患者 2011 年等候名单，患者可能被列为在多中心移植的候选人。多重列表是增加接收机构报价机会的一种方式。患者一定要意识到这个选项，以及一些相关的责任和成本。要求通知患者每项

教育文件工具样本

门诊跨学科患者/家庭教育记录

患者：__________

协调员：__________

移植前：器官

移植前

新患者一起发送 __________（发送日期）
- 包括教材
- 多重列表及等待移植时间(UNOS)手册
- 知情同意

初步评估诊所预约 ________（日期）
- 医学咨询 ________（日期）
- 手术咨询 ________（日期）
- 社会服务咨询 ________（日期）
- 营养咨询 ________（日期）
- 药理学咨询 ________（日期）
- 移植财务协调员咨询 ________（日期）
- 活体供体协调员咨询 ________（日期）
- 移植协调员咨询 _______（日期）
  - 移植协调员的作用
  - 所需评估测试教育
  - 移植过程概述
  - 器官特异性分配系统概述
  - 患者在等待期间的责任
  - 要求移植时期望什么
  - 外科手术概述
  - 住院概况和移植后随访
  - 免疫抑制药物
  - 移植后并发症：排斥，感染，恶性肿瘤

集体教学班 ________（日期安排/参加）
额外的个人教学课程 ________（根据需要，中心具体举措）
何时呼叫移植中心
移植中心电话号码 ____________

我了解提交的材料，并有持续的机会，让移植团队回答有关我作为____________移植候选人的任何问题。
患者签名：____________ 日期：____________
教育者签名：____________ 日期：____________

A

教育文件工具样本

门诊跨学科患者/家庭教育记录

患者：__________

协调员：__________

移植后：器官

移植后

初次移植后诊所预约 ________（日期）
- 医生咨询 ________（日期）
- 移植协调员咨询 ________（日期）
  - 移植团队的作用
  - 给予移植手册的副本 ________（日期）
  - 参加移植教育班 ________（日期）
    - 认识护理人员
    - 药物检查
    - 实验室检查
    - 伤口护理
    - 饮食和运动
    - 生活质量问题
    - 长期随访要求
    - 排斥反应，感染，恶性肿瘤的监测
    - 短期和长期并发症检查
    - 当地医生的作用
    - 监管报告要求 UNOS
    - 患者的责任
- 何时呼叫移植中心
- 移植中心电话号码 ____________

我了解提交的材料，并有持续的机会，让移植团队回答有关我____________移植的任何问题。
患者签名：____________ 日期：____________
教育者签名：____________ 日期：____________

B

图 125.3 移植前和移植后教育的教育文件工具样本。

OPTN 政策，并通知该患者已在多个移植中心的列表选项的文档审计[24]。

继续教育

如前所述，对移植患者的教育是一个持续的过程，在很多层面上必须进行。对于大多数的患者和家属，移植是一个高度紧张和改变生活的过程。患者和家庭教育的重点是维持最佳健康状态，虽然经历移植评估和等待器官，以及一个健康的器官移植后的维护。与患者每次会面应被看作是一个教学机会。在每位患者就诊时给予一致性的清晰、简洁的教育，确保患者理解目前的保健治疗方案和患者的责任。所有患者学习情况不同。压力和情绪状态、身体状况、学习风格、愿意学习、不确定的学习障碍，都必须纳入个性化教育计划。由于所有学习者学习方式不同，应该采取一个多感官的做法。书面材料应符合阅读水平并且通俗易懂，使那些读者能够领悟其中内容。在教育方面，商定为六年级的教育水平。材料还需要外语口译或必须提供翻译。加强书面材料的直观教具（如图片和海报），应纳入教学计划。基于计算机的教育工具应提供给团体或个人观看。结构化群体教育课程可内置候选人评估和术后至出院。在就诊期间以任何形式与患者沟通的过程中出现个别教育巩固。每天 24 小时，1 周 7 天的手机操作服务移植中心必须提供。此服务必须提供解答患者的有关治疗方案及相关并发症的问题。

移植候选人的教育是终身移植学习的过程。包括候选者按要求参与器官移植。患者必须学会通过坚持治疗计划、按照饮食指南、正确服药、并知道何时向移植中心呼救，以管理自己的健康。这些可以成为对患者主要的生活方式改变，他们期待着移植中心作为教育的一个主要来源。在转诊点开始患者教育是非常重要的。这包括移植和移植后的生活过程中器官特异性教育。必要时必须对关键信息进行审查，以促进患者和家属记忆。与每个患者的互动，提供清晰、一致和持续教育，确保患者及家属了解他们的角色和责任[25]（表 125.1）。

表 125.1 患者教育表[13,26,27]

主题	移植前	出院	移植后
概述	X	–	–
疾病进程	X	–	–
移植过程	X	–	–
移植团队的作用	X	–	X
评估过程	X	–	–
诊断测试	X	–	–
血液工作	X	–	–
结果	X	–	–
知情同意	X	–	–
保持健康	–	–	–
等候	X	–	–
饮食和运动	X	X	X
什么时候打电话	X	X	X
器官分配	X	–	–
外科手术	X	–	–
术后恢复	X	–	–
停留时间	X	–	–
伤口护理	–	X	X
药物	–	–	–
免疫抑制	X	X	X
副作用	X	X	X
非处方药	X	X	X
草药	X	X	X
术后并发症	–	–	–
排斥	X	X	X
感染	X	X	X
恶变	X	X	X
长期			X
心理问题	X	X	X
随访	X	X	X
随访次数	X	X	X
必要的实验室工作	X	X	X
经济问题	X	X	X
生活质量	X	X	X
返回工作	–	X	X
牙齿保健	–	X	X
性问题	–	X	X
旅行	–	X	X
预防接种	–	X	X
宠物	–	X	X
持续健康	–	–	X

结果衡量报告

移植领域（包括活体捐献），深受 OPTN/UNOS、HRSA 和 CMS 管理。CMS 参保条件清楚地识别结果的报告要求。移植结果衡量包括：在整个移植连续报道，移植失败或患者死亡开始在移植名单上激活。

从移植中心 OPTN/UNOS 的数据提交直接创建 SRTR 方案的具体报告。方案的具体报告包括患者和家属，支付方，移植中心，以及联邦政府。这些方案的具体报告包括移植方案很多方面：

- 等候名单活动–添加和去除原因。
- 等候名单患者的特征。
- 等候名单患者的移植和死亡率。
- 等候时间。
- 进行移植的数量。
- 受者，捐助者和移植手术的特点。
- 移植物和患者存活率报道 1 个月内、1 年、3 年结果与 2.5 年队列的患者预期利率相比。

这些报告在 1 月和 7 月每半年发表有关美国每个移植计划的修正数据。该结果被调整，以反映特定中心的供者、受者和实践。风险调整允许个人中心将其报告的结果与国家成果比较，找出全国各地移植方案之间的类似患者。调整了受者和供者的特点，确保移植中心不处罚很难接受治疗的患者，并积极使用扩展的供者。移植中心需要积极主动地学习管理自己的数据的准确性，找出失败的风险，并制订质量成果的最佳做法。准确和及时的个别方案，以独立地监控他们的成果以及证明符合监管报告提交要求[28]“移植候选人登记”“移植受者注册”和“移植受者跟进”形式的意见是必要的。监测方案的最佳实践的成功和发展的所有数据是非常重要的；三年移植物和患者生存率的数据最能反映目前的门诊管理。

患者满意度的标准

一个相当新的方法来衡量为患者提供护理质量水平的新方法是要求患者就他们的经验来反馈[29]。开发满意度较强的医患关系是一个具有挑战性的、但现实的目标。患者和提供者相互信任，理解个体患者的需求能促进患者护理质量。政府需要讨论患者的满意度时，应对考虑以下问题：什么是衡量患者满意度的效用；它是如何最适合衡量特定患者人群；什么是最终的结果？临床医生、医疗中心和纳税人都在衡量患者满意度为了实用、专业和道德上的原因。衡量患者的满意度是不明确的，而是患者医疗保健体验的看法的定性指标。

有可用来监测患者满意度的众多有偿服务机构。其中最流行的是 Press Ganey 公司。Press Ganey 公司一直在帮助提供者改进医疗服务，交付业务已超过 25 年。Press Ganey 公司理念是，患者有一个有价值的观点向需要者提供关于他们接受护理工作质量，确保患者由医疗机构寻找方法来评估和提高护理质量。通过使用专门的工具、服务、咨询和数据分析，Press Ganey 公司向医疗保健机构提供它们的效果如何，以及如何提高其性能[30]。

2010 年，Press Ganey 公司与 UNOS 移植管理委员会（TAC）联合开发了一个专门的住院和门诊移植调查。具体到门诊移植调查项目包括：移植通用背景问题，器官移植以及临床上的等待时间。注册、移植设施相关的非移植的具体问题得到解决。移植的具体照顾和教育项目包括：药物，饮食，伤口护理，血液工作，何时调用移植小组，如何与移植小组沟通，相关的成本，以及多学科团队成员的患者评级。移植中心可以利用这些成果来提高患者的满意度[31]（图 125.4）。

移植经济方面的考虑

移植被认为是一种选择性的挽救生命的手术，有时是终末期器官疾病患者的唯一治疗方法。移植机构需要在竞争激烈的市场中保持财政实力。该计划的资金实力、报销、性能、监测、成果、协助合同谈判和维护移植中心的整体财政实力。移植中心需要有效地竞争力提供服务，保持盈利。由于移植的复杂性和长期性，对服务的相关成本可能是一个天文数字，而且时间长。经济限制可能会影响患者的移植服务。在患者的利益彻底的评估之前启动任何移植服务，必须由专门的经济移植协调员确定。

对大多数患者有四种基本类型覆盖：医疗/医疗援助（MA），医疗保险（MC），商业付款人和私人/自己负担。CMS 包括 MA/MC 计划，是美国最大的单一付款人。大多数商业纳税人遵循 CMS 有关报销规定。移植中心必须制订明确的政策，概述移植相关服务的覆盖面和补偿的可接受的水平。以下是在移植中的常见保险的简要概述。有患者援助基金会药理援助，基金会帮助患者筹款和慈善关怀选项。

医疗有偿服务

大多数州要求 MA 受者在居住地所在州获得医疗服务。所有护理提供者，包括医院和治疗患者的每个医生，必须在指定（登记）的状态下报销。国家资金是有限

CLIENT LOGO

出院患者移植服务问卷

首先非常感谢您能够完成这些问题，当填写完该问卷后，请回复我们。

背景问题

1. 您是否已经进行了移植手术？ ○是 ○否

2. 从您的预约时间开始到您被告知做问卷等待了多少分钟？ □□□

3. 从您的预约时间开始到您开始做问卷等待了多少分钟？ □□□

4. 您最近一次随访是在周几？
○周一 ○周二 ○周三
○周四 ○周五 ○周六
○周日

5. 您最近一次随访是在一天中的什么时候？
○6:00-8:00 ○8:00-10:00
○10:00-12:00 ○12:00-14:00
○14:00-16:00 ○16:00-18:00
○18:00-20:00 ○20:00-22:00

请您对我们移植团队的出院患者移植服务做出评价：数字 1~5 分别代表非常差到非常好的 5 个等级，请选择出最符合您的经历的选项，如果某一问题不适合，请跳过，回答下一个问题。

登记	非常差 1	差 2	一般 3	好 4	非常好 5
1. 为您登记的人员是否提供了足够的帮助	○	○	○	○	○
2. 登记过程的舒心程度	○	○	○	○	○
3. 登记的等待过程	○	○	○	○	○
4. 如果您是通过电话和移植中心的人员交谈，获得了什么程度的帮助	○	○	○	○	○
5. 当您被告知延期时，会有什么样的感受	○	○	○	○	○

评价（描述好或不好的经历）：________

设施	非常差 1	差 2	一般 3	好 4	非常好 5
1. 等待区域的舒适程度	○	○	○	○	○
2. 容易找到的程度	○	○	○	○	○
3. 设施的清洁程度	○	○	○	○	○

评价（描述好或不好的经历）：________

检查或治疗	非常差 1	差 2	一般 3	好 4	非常好 5
1. 为您提供服务人员的友好及礼貌程度	○	○	○	○	○
2. 是否为您详细解释了检查或治疗过程中可能出现的情况	○	○	○	○	○
3. 您对在检查或治疗过程中可能出现的风险了解多少	○	○	○	○	○
4. 您对该检查或治疗的替代方法了解多少	○	○	○	○	○
5. 您对自己有权拒绝该检查或治疗的了解程度	○	○	○	○	○
6. 为您提供服务的人员的技能水平	○	○	○	○	○
7. 相关人员对您是否足够放松舒适的关注程度	○	○	○	○	○
8. 相关人员对您的问题和担忧的关注程度	○	○	○	○	○

评价（描述好或不好的经历）：________

15179385

待续

图 125.4 出院患者移植服务问卷。Reproduced from [32] with permission from Press Ganey Associates, Inc.

移植护理及教育	非常差 1	差 2	一般 3	好 4	非常好 5
仅需要回答您经历过的情况					
1. 关于下列几项措施,您受到什么程度的教育					
a.药物	○	○	○	○	○
b.饮食	○	○	○	○	○
c.切口护理	○	○	○	○	○
d.血液检测	○	○	○	○	○
e.何时去联系移植团队	○	○	○	○	○
f.怎样联系移植团队	○	○	○	○	○
g.移植护理所需要的费用(例如,房间、交通、药物)	○	○	○	○	○
2. 移植团队在多大程度上致力于解决您的需求	○	○	○	○	○

评价(描述好或不好的经历):______

个人问题	非常差 1	差 2	一般 3	好 4	非常好 5
1. 我们对您隐私的关注程度	○	○	○	○	○
2. 我们对您的需求的敏感程度	○	○	○	○	○
3. 我们的员工在您本次随访过程中的关心或不满所表现出的关注度	○	○	○	○	○
4. 工作人员佩戴身份识别徽章的程度	○	○	○	○	○
5. 工作人员向您做自我介绍的程度	○	○	○	○	○
6. 当您进入房间时,工作人员双手的清洁程度	○	○	○	○	○
7. 您对自己接受的护理所做决定的参与度	○	○	○	○	○
8. 您的家人对您接受的护理所做决定的参与度	○	○	○	○	○

评价(描述好或不好的经历):______

整体评估	非常差 1	差 2	一般 3	好 4	非常好 5
1. 在本次随访中,您对我们工作人员所提供服务的整体评价如何	○	○	○	○	○
2. 您在本次随访中所接受的服务的等级	○	○	○	○	○
3. 您有多大可能把这些设施介绍给其他人	○	○	○	○	○

评价(描述好或不好的经历):______

等级

请您用 0~10 这 11 个数字对我们门诊移植团队的服务做出评价,0 代表最差的体验,10 代表最好的服务体验:

最差 0	1	2	3	4	5	6	7	8	9	最好 10
○	○	○	○	○	○	○	○	○	○	○

患者签名:______

电话号码:______

15179385

PRESS GANEY™

这项调查在印刷和发放时是最新的。如果您想确认它是否仍是最新版本,请联系您的负责人。

图 125.4(续)

的；这就影响了现有支付移植相关的医疗费用金额。根据MA报销进度，提供者可能会遇到收入的净损失。移植协调员必须审查移植状态，移植患者是否在所在州治疗，是否满足保险范围。MA按服务收费计划受到严格监督，不与其他福利共享。

托管医疗机构

管理医疗组织（MMO）产品类似MA产品。MMO的可能不要求供者在州内注册报销，但受者需接受协调所有的初级护理医生（主治医生）的管理。这将创建为获得转诊和移植后的服务不是由PCP下令授权的挑战。如果患者被认为和（或）网络脱离状态，移植提供者可以与MMO服务洽谈可接受的报销比例。

传统医疗保险

传统的医疗保险（MC）可以被认为是普遍的，因为有在地理上确定没有分配网络或州和报销率的情况。几乎所有的提供者都纳入MC，不需要转介。患者可通过年龄、残疾、或终末期肾病（ESRD）拥有MC资格。然而，一个人必须有资格得到MC的益处。资格是基于工作经历；因此，TFC必须进行个人检查。

医保组成

MC有四个组成部分：部分A、B、C、D，获得MA资格的个体被自动免费归入MC A部分。MC A部分涵盖了住院医院护理；但是，扣除额和共同保险由住院时间的长短来决定。个人必须选择并支付每月保费为MC B部分，它涵盖了医院门诊和专业费用的80%。除了MC A/B部分，应劝告个人购买MC D部分，涵盖处方药。共同支付适用于大多数处方。

正如上文指出的MC不提供全覆盖，暴露个人潜在的经济困难。应建议MC受者购买“补充医疗保险”。它可以补充MC支付给个人将被视为完全程度覆盖，消除了免赔额和共同保险人的责任。

管理医疗/医疗优势

许多公司在健康维护组织（HMO）或优先提供者组织（PPO）提供托管医疗/医疗优势（MC类C部分）的，但个人必须在MC A部分和MC B部分。MC C部分的缺点是有分配网络，个人不能选择在哪里就医。就像MMO，需要请示。在某些情况下，MC C公司将与提供者合作，谈判同意报销其中还包括免收会员更高的资金责任[33]。

商业保险

个人可以通过雇主团体或通过单独购买获得商业保险。在这两种情况下并非所有计划都相同，即使覆盖率是通过相同的公司。当购买个人保险，免赔额成员和（或）共同保险责任金额由溢价支付的金额确定。更高的溢价意味着较低资金成员的责任；同样较低的保费意味着更高资金成员的责任。在大多数情况下，通过覆盖雇主团体提供了最好的覆盖面。

无论是以个人或团体基础得到了保险，患者一定要注意覆盖范围的差异，必须非常小心，并了解他们选择的保险级别。当考虑商业保险时，还有赔偿计划、优先提供者组织（PPO）计划和健康维护组织（HMO）计划的选择。保险公司可以提供的部分或所有的计划，所以再次不能假定同一家公司的所有成员覆盖一样。赔偿计划是商用的限制最少的计划。PPO计划，同时拥有在网络内和网络外的好处。如果成员应用网络内提供者发生金融负债的数额会少些。

在某些情况下，保险公司和提供者可能考虑通常被称为单例协议（SCA）代表个人的协议。当有必要寻求一个网络外提供者治疗，这种类型的协议被使用。该SCA提供指定的报销；因此，如果护理是在网络内提供，上面的约定速率和实际收费余额以相同的方式被放弃。

HMO计划是限制最严格的选择，因为成员仅限于看到网络内提供者，因此这种类型的计划具有最低的保费和成员责任。如果成员必须使用网络外提供者，该公司必须给予授权和SCA谈判。

自费/个人支持

没有保险的患者是最有挑战性的。TFC中应该考虑，患者是否有资格获得公共援助计划，或者是否有低成本的保险计划。也有适用于符合条件的移植患者的众多受资助的援助方案。资格规则根据个人的计划、以及提供的援助金额而有所不同。应大力鼓励没有医疗保险的患者联系援助方案。移植项目必须有资格获得移植服务、专门为没有医疗人群的保险财务政策。

外国患者

UNOS的政策6.0非居民外国人移植允许外国患者在美国寻求移植服务。当前UNOS的政策6.0 2005

年允许每年外籍患者的个别移植项目移植占整体体量的5%[34]。单个移植中心必须制订有关外籍患者的管理政策。卫生系统内部设立一个专门的国际部安排便利服务,包括文化需求、在整个移植过程中这个独特群体的后勤工作。这些服务可能包括抵达前援助,提供获得签证和患者所需的其他旅行证件及随行家属正在进行的援助;安排住宿再接受评估,移植名单上等待时间,移植后的护理;协助患者在整个移植过程1天24小时,1周7天口译服务;门诊的协调与多学科移植小组访问;住院患者/住院时间;从患者祖国过渡;并促进患者的祖国纵向护理监测援助。通过这些为患者提供的个性化服务,并减少在国外医疗保健系统应用困难,可以帮助消除一些在移植过程中遇到的障碍。

对这个人群移植患者的一些特殊挑战,包括有关移植过程,以及患者和家属的期望受限。当期望与患者的满意服务不符,由于缺乏对器官分配系统的理解,并延长等待时间,这可以是特别困难的。患者不愿回家,当医疗出院,出院后家庭护理的协调可能是特别具有挑战性的,尤其是当移植的服务在患者国家中受限。根据现有的资金和移植的赞助,返回移植中心进行后续治疗的能力也可能受到限制。谈判必须明确移植方案服务的覆盖范围,并商定费用、患者和赞助商,但不包括并发症。移植患者教育和知情同意过程的所有方面都必须提前用患者的母语提供。

住宿费

移植患者可来自世界各地。对患者及家属来说与移植相关的住宿的经济成本可能是毁灭性的。由于这个空白,全国范围内出现了招待所。"全国医院招待所协会(NAHHH)由近200家独特的、非营利性组织组成,为很远的接受治疗的患者、家庭和亲人提供住宿和配套服务,是全国性专业协会"[35]。这些房子从只能容纳几个人,到可容纳近200居民设施。在美国任何特定的房子中,目前居民20%~25%为移植相关的患者。目前美国的设施,可根据是儿童还是成人而不同;然后患者可以留在该处,或者仅仅是患者住院治疗的家。自1981年第一家这样的住所在费城开设,这不仅仅是为患者和家属提供睡觉的地方。

这些房子是严格的住宅设施和酒店业的一部分,因此它们也按照酒店的规定和标准,不提供直接的医疗服务,不保持医院的规定。它们已成为医疗服务的患者远离家乡的一个组成部分。就像如果患者从医院移植后出院或等待移植回自己的家,他们遇到任何医疗紧急情况需要拨打911。家庭健康工作人员访问提供家庭治疗的设施,提供耐用医疗设备所需的支持,允许用辅助设备。感染控制标准,一般从医院到返回家中之前,成为患者和家人的一个学习工具。他们得到如何安全清洁的训练,以及如何与他人生活,为他们过渡到自己的家中做准备。

这些房子为患者及其家人不断发展的"正常"恢复提供了一个社区环境。在任何时候,房子的目前居住者成为一个支持小组,因为他们学会一起应用医疗制度。像这些设施能够提供一个全面的方法来安排活动,而减少家庭经济和精神压力。住房成本的降低,如果需要,从符合501(c)的财政支持(3)募捐可用以补充哪些家庭可以负担。这些家庭都是有偿服务,涵盖的费用约为65%,其余的收入来自捐赠和募捐。

通常情况下,房子内的活动随着探视时间而在晚上回升。在公共场所家庭聚集来分享食物,谈论他们的一天,学习如何从别人已经经历了一个较长的时间段类似的经历中预期。某些设施利用志愿者帮助提供整个月(活动或餐)体验,同时使试图维持正常的生活方式成为可能。医疗住房在不断地发展,以满足客人的需求,以及发展长寿命的精神和力量。

总结

随着移植领域的不断发展,移植候选人、受者和活体供体的临床管理还需加强。通过扩展的多学科团队得到更多护理,门诊移植诊所提供。每个移植中心的功能不同,但必须以同样的联邦法规为政策依据承担责任。移植中心必须有一个指导他们的实践证明,同时监管合规,透明和可衡量质量的患者治疗效果的愿景和使命宣言。本章中包含的主题并不意味着囊括一切,但可作为一个参考指南,以纳入门诊的临床实践的发展。

(郭海军 译 徐骁 校)

参考文献

1. McCarthy D. Integrative models & performance. In: Kovner A, Knickman J, editors. Jonas & Kovnec's Healthcare Delivery in the United States. 10th ed. New York, NY: Springer Publishing Co., LLC; 2011: 224.
2. Shafer T, et al. The history of the transplant coordinator: the advent of modern

organ transplantation. In: Rudow D, editor. A Clinician's Guide to Donation and Transplantation. 1st ed. Lenexa, KS: Applied Measurement Professionals, Inc; 2006: 17.
3. UNOS. [accessed 2011 December 27, 2011]; Available from: http://www.unos.org/.
4. National Organ Transplant Act, 42 United States Code, Section 273 et seq. 1987 [accessed 2011 December 1, 2011]; Available from: http://optn.transplant.hrsa.gov/policesAndBylaws/nota.asp/.
5. Department of Health and Human Services. Organ Procurement and Transplantation Network: Final Rule. 42 Code of Federal Regulations, Section 121.1(b)(2), 2005 [accessed 2011 December 1, 2011]; Available from: http://optn.transplant.hrsa.gov/policiesAndBylaws/final_rule.asp/.
6. UNOS Regions Map. [accessed 2011 December 1, 2011]; Available from: http://optn.transplant.hrsa.gov/members/regions.asp/.
7. OPTN Website. [accessed 2011 December 1, 2011]; Available from: http://optn.transplant.hrsa.gov/policiesAndBylaws/charterAndBylaws.asp/.
8. Centers for Medicare and Medicaid Services (Formerly Healthcare Financing Administration). Medicare and medicaid programs. Organ procurement and transplantation network rules and membership actions. Federal Register. 54:51802.
9. Centers for Medicare and Medicaid Services. Medicare program. Conditions of participation: requirements for approval and re-approval of transplant centers to perform organ transplants; final rule. Federal Register. 2007;72:15198-15209.
10. Department of Health & Humans Services USA. HRSA Transplant Center Growth and Management Collaborative: Best Practices Evaluation Final Report. US Department of Health and Human Services, Health Resources & Services Administration. Healthcare Systems Bureau: Division of Transplantation. September 2007.
11. Department of Health & Humans Services USA. HRSA Transplant Center Growth and Management Collaborative: Best Practices Evaluation Final Report. US Department of Health and Human Services, Health Resources & Services Administration. Healthcare Systems Bureau: Division of Transplantation. September 2007: 53.
12. National Institute of Building Sciences. Whole Building Design Guide. Carr, R. Outpatient Clinic. Updated 21 April 2011 [accessed 2011 December 1, 2011]; Available from: http://www.wbdg.org/design/outpatient.php/.
13. Centers for Medicare and Medicaid Services. Conditions of Participation: Requirements for Approval and Re-Approval of Transplant Centers to Perform Organ Transplants; Final Rule. S482.94 Condition of Participation: Patient and Living Donor Management. March 30, 2007.
14. McNatt G. Nursing and transplant coordination: a call for clarity. Progress in Transplantation. 2008;18:208-215.
15. Centers for Medicare and Medicaid Services. Conditions of Participation: Requirements for Approval and Re-Approval of Transplant Centers to Perform Organ Transplants; Final Rule. S482.98 Condition of Participation: Human Resources. March 30, 2007.
16. Alloway R, et al. Evolution of the role of the transplant pharmacist on the multidisciplinary transplant team. American Journal of Transplantation. 2011;11: 1576-1583.
17. Transplant Financial Coordinators Association. [accessed 2011 December 1, 2011]; Available from: http://www.tfcassociation.org/.
18. American Academy of Ambulatory Care Nursing. [accessed 2011 December 1, 2011]; Available from: http://www.aaacn.org/.
19. Transplant Administrators Staffing Survey. [accessed 2011 December 1, 2011]; Available from: https://www.portal.unos.org/.
20. International Transplant Nurses Society. Transplant Nursing: Scope and Standards of Practice. Silver Spring, MD: American Nurses Association; 2009: 23.
21. Kropf R. Health information technology. In: Kovner A, Knickman J, editors. Jonas & Kovnec's Healthcare Delivery in the United States. 10th ed. New York, NY: Springer Publishing Co. LLC.; 2011: 332-346.
22. American Health Information Management Association. [accessed 2011 December 1, 2011]; Available from: http://www.ahima.org/.
23. Centers for Medicare and Medicaid Services. Conditions of Participation: Requirements for Approval and Re-Approval of Transplant Centers to Perform Organ Transplants; Final Rule. S482.102 Condition of Participation: Patient and Living Donor Rights. March 30, 2007.
24. Multiple Listing and Waiting Time Transfer. [accessed 2011 December 1, 2011]; Available from: http://optn.transplant.hrsa.gov/policiesAndBylaws/policies.asp/.
25. Department of Health & Humans Services USA. HRSA Transplant Center Growth and Management Collaborative: Best Practices Evaluation Final Report. US Department of Health and Human Services, Health Resources & Services Administration. Healthcare Systems Bureau: Division of Transplantation. September 2007: 58-59.
26. Ohler L. Patient education. In: Cupples S, Ohler L, editors. Transplantation Nursing Secrets. 1st ed. Philadelphia, PA: Elsevier Publishing; 2003: 305-312.
27. Ford E, John E. Patient education for the transplant recipient. In: Ohler L, Cupples S, editors. Core Curriculum for Transplant Nurses, 1st ed. Philadelphia, PA: Elsevier Publishing; 2008: 51-88.
28. Scientific Registry of Transplant Recipients. [accessed 2011 December 1, 2011]; Available from: http://www.srtr.org/.
29. Clancy C, Lloyd R. High quality healthcare. In: Kovner A, Knickman J, editors. Jonas & Kovnec's Healthcare Delivery in the United States. 10th ed. New York, NY: Springer Publishing Co., LLC; 2011: 236.
30. Press Ganey. [accessed 2011 December 1, 2011]; Available from: http://www.pressganey.com/.
31. Patient Satisfaction Survey. [accessed 2011 December 1, 2011]; Available from: https://www.portal.unos.org/.
32. Press Ganey Transplant Survey. [accessed 2011 December 1, 2011]; Available from: http://www.pressganey.com.
33. Medicare Basics. [accessed 2011 December 28, 2011]; Available from: http://www.medicare.gov/navigation/medicare-basics/medicare-basics-overview.aspx/.
34. Transplantation of Non-Resident Aliens. [accessed 2011 December 1, 2011]; Available from: http://optn.transplant.hrsa.gov/policiesAndBylaws/policies.asp/.
35. National Association of Hospital Hospitality Houses. [accessed 2011 December 1, 2011]; Available from: http://www.nahhh.org/.

第 126 章
移植中心管理和领导:内部企业架构范例

Luke Preczewski, Gwen McNatt, Michael Abecassis

引言

企业家是利用金融和商业智慧将创新转化为经济产品的个体。这种行为可能需要组建一个新的组织,或者给现有组织提供一个振兴的机会。尽管该术语在传统意义上是指业务计划,但它已被广泛应用。社会、政治以及最近的知识企业家精神已经出现。关于企业家精神的研究可以追溯到 17 世纪和 18 世纪后期的 Richard Cantillon 和 Adam Smith,但是在过去的几十年中,人们对商业和经济学动态的兴趣再次兴起,使我们重新关注了企业家的重要性。创业是一个将新思想或新发明转化为成功且通常有利可图的创新的过程。在这种情况下,创新更有可能代表渐进式改进,而不是量子发现。企业家可能会冒风险,以一个想法将财务安全或职业放在首位,在面对不确定性时表现出主动性。

创新和企业家精神在移植中的作用源于这样的事实,即没有其他可行的替代方法可治疗晚期器官衰竭,尤其是肾衰竭。首次成功的肾脏移植手术是在传统透析无效的时候进行的。也许是因为针对移植技术挑战的外科解决方案在有效的免疫抑制之前已经进行了数十年,所以外科医生被认为是移植的最初创新者,而免疫学家和科学家则同时定义了移植免疫学的本质。通过外科手术先驱的进取精神和毅力,逐渐说服了主要的学术机构(医学院和合作医院)成为这些空前实验的实验室。外科医生为了实现创新想法而冒着个人职业风险,而机构也承担了声誉和财务安全风险。越来越清楚的是,移植是终末期器官衰竭的可行治疗选择,越来越多的机构加入了现有移植计划的行列,这表明在减少不确定性的情况下对移植计划的承诺。随着移植的发展,标志着其诞生和成长的企业家精神仍然是移植文化的重要方面,使移植中心继续成为医疗中心创新的重点,将新思想转化为治疗方法。特别是在过去的三十年中,见证了移植程序从试验和研究活动过渡到经过验证的治疗干预措施。

随着移植计划的发展,支持它们的行政结构也越来越复杂。起初,移植团队通常由一名或两名外科医生、协作医生和一名或两名护士协调员组成,他们分配给中低级医院管理员,并由医院领导进行不同程度的监督。在这个创业阶段,主要是与患者直接护理密切相关的人们充满了热情,而清晰的愿景则激发了热情,通常由外科手术负责人传达。医疗中心其他人的态度通常是支持的,但可能支持程度不同。在这个早期阶段,团队通常会得到手术室主任的大力支持(很可能招募了首席外科医生),并得到了医院主任不同程度的支持。随着移植中心的成功发展以及移植试验的成功,管理机构也不断发展以适应计划的需求。这与需要进一步投入资源和人员同时发生,引起了医院管理者的更高关注。在典型情况下,外科团队会继续推动议程,招募更多的协作医生,将一些移植前和移植后的护理归于各自的专业,而团队的非医生组成部分也将扩大以满足患者的需求。越来越多的患者被评估、列出和移植。同样,外科团队领导了这些工作,但逐渐失去了医院管理员的行政和领导职能,放弃了有关运营和预算问题的一些决策点。尽管该计划的医生组成部分的增长可能需要对部门(医学院)和实践计划层次结构进行一些结构和组织上的更改,例如在外科部门内创建移植手术部门,但非医生组成部分的增长可能与医院行政和管理结构的重大变化相关,例如固有的和必不可少的规则和操作程序。

总之,组织结构的这些变化将不可避免地引入公司文化和纪律要素,尤其是随着移植计划越来越受到机构领导者的关注。尽管大家更关注计划的成功，但他们也有各自的议程，因为他们通常负责更广泛的预算和合规性问题。随着该计划的发展，其主要监督将从医学院和医生实践逐步转移到医院，由医院承担该计划的法规遵从性责任。直接的结果是，与该计划的增长相吻合的是，该计划的需求适应更加公司化的组织结构，其中充满了管理孤岛，每个孤岛都有自己的一套流程和规则。这种演进发展的意外结果是，从负责项目成功的企业家精神过渡到更严格的公司纪律，充斥着不可避免的阻碍创新自由的局限性障碍。因此，机构对遵守明确的组织结构图和报告线、政策和程序手册，对机构和监管要求的遵守以及针对财政责任的纪律的要求最终可能会扼杀持续创新所需的精力和激情。随着该计划的重心从企业家精神向企业文化过渡，医生不可避免地要遵循与非医生同事相同的企业规范和标准。在完全集成的医疗保健提供系统中，一组通用规则支配该计划的所有组成，而这些规则几乎总是向公司倾斜。在集成程度较低的系统中，医学院校和实践计划都必须遵守日益增长的监管环境并对此做出响应，以使学术领导者可能会欢迎医院领导者施加的行政管理措施。因此，不可避免的是，随着程序的发展和成熟，从某种意义上说，他们会因自身的成功而“受害”，牺牲了其敏捷性，并限制了其对某些更新颖的方法应对移植挑战的能力。

企业文化所决定的行政结构对于实现高可靠性、提高效率、实现财务目标以及保持完全的法规遵从性至关重要，但与此同时，其固有的以流程为导向和规避风险的文化可以阻碍企业家精神和革新。因此，对于移植领导者来说，挑战包括维持“团队精神”和创新精神，这首先激励了团队，同时实现了与公司文化和结构相关的收益。成功的移植企业将适应企业文化的要求，同时利用两者的优势以确保高度可靠、高效且合规的中心仍然是创新的引擎。在本章中，我们将进一步讨论移植中心的演变，概述领导和管理已建立的移植服务线的关键要素，并探索在其他领域证明的机制，移植领导者可以使用这些机制来建立和捍卫这一重要的中间立场。

移植中心文化的演变

移植的早期是“顽强男子气概的文化”的一个明显例子，其特点是冒险和快速的反馈与奖励[1]。在 Deal 和 Kennedy 模型中，组织文化由两个轴定义：风险容忍度和反馈即时性。Starzl 在光谱的两端阐述了这一点，他强调了《人物拼图》[2]中“外科医生对官僚的争论性冲突”。随着移植已从研究领域发展成为一种被广泛接受的疗法，移植中心发现自己正在向较少的冒险以及较少的即时反馈和回报过渡。Deal 和 Kennedy 框架定义的这种“过程文化”以官僚、安全和企业文化为标志。考虑到财务和声誉方面的责任，大型医疗机构对自我保护的亲和力是明智的。企业责任和问责制的现实预示着创新的诱惑。结果，旨在遏制风险并提高可预测性的机构、政策和程序，可能击败任何企业家承担风险的愿望，尤其是在极有可能发生高调失败案例的情况下。

最近对移植中心法规和公共政策的关注加剧了医院避免风险的趋势。《国家器官移植法》(NOTA)首先在联邦一级规范了死者捐献器官作为公共物品的分配[3]，并建立了器官采购和移植网络(OPTN)以及移植受者科学注册（SRTR）合同，对卫生资源和服务管理局(HRSA)的移植进行监管。NOTA 的规定包括要求公开披露特定中心的患者结果[4]。此外，终末期肾脏疾病(ESRD)的权利还通过拒绝报销[5]赋予了医疗保险和医疗补助中心(CMS)监管移植中心的更多权限。在 21 世纪初期，许多受到广泛关注的事件引起了政府的关注。这些事件包括纽约一个中心的活体肝供体死亡[6]，北卡罗来纳州一种血型不相符的心脏移植导致儿童患者死亡[7]以及 Charles 的一系列文章和《洛杉矶时报》的Ornstein 详细介绍了加利福尼亚几个移植中心的问题。Ornstein 强调了器官共享联合网络(CMS)和 CMS 在检测和解决这些问题方面的失败[8]。这些事件导致监察长办公室（OIG）进行了调查和国会听证会，发现 CMS 缺乏监督责任。结果创建和发布了专门针对移植的医疗保险参与条件[9]。这些法规创建了规定性要求，要求移植医院制订特定于移植的政策和程序，并满足一定的数量和结果要求。CMS 对移植中心实施了三年一次的合规性审核，以执行这些要求。作为回应，移植中心已将法规遵从问题提高到医院机构内部的最高领导水平。HRSA 以类似的方式通过 OPTN 承包商加强了监督。随着 2000 年对 NOTA 的修订以及 2005 年《最终规则》的修订，OPTN 的范围和权限得到了显著增强。其包括但不限于患者教育、员工资格、活体供体的评估和选择以及预防疾病传播。OPTN 通过监管绩效和结果以及对政策遵守情况进行现场调查来行使监管职责。外部调查和合规性审核的常年周期使日常移植临床操作变得复杂。

在过去十年中，法规对创新的威胁成倍增长。HRSA和CMS都具有改善移植患者和活体供体成果的值得称赞的目标[4,10],但是政策和法规的严格执行以及政府机构和负责强制执行这些规定的测量员可能过度解释这种无意识的依从性，实际上降低了移植计划的可靠性和适应性,扼杀了创新和创造力,并在临床实践中浪费了资源。在CMS调查的第一轮中,由于数量少或结果差[8,11],有几个中心自愿或被迫退出了医疗保险的参与和报销，而其他移植中心报告为了避免相似的命运改变了做法[12]。过度监管比任何医院的公司机构都更具压迫性,威胁了移植的整体生命力。计划和国家两级移植领导力的挑战将是与政府领导人一起倡导，以保持监管者的适当作用：促进客观的外部审查者[10]促进良好的自治,并提供同行审评指南[4];不会造成不可持续的行政负担。医院管理者越来越意识到必须遵守这些法规,尤其是结果要求。因此,移植中心向公司结构的演进和政府法规的迅速部署以及可能采取的惩罚性措施，在规避风险方面掀起了一场完美风暴。结果，移植计划见证了官僚机构的既定目标与监督目标之间的重大融合。

实施以证据为基础的最佳实践、流程标准化、企业组织和法规共同支持的成果非常有价值，因为标准化流程是提高可靠性和降低风险的关键要素。在1999年和2001年,实施高可靠性原则[13]在医学研究所的具有里程碑意义的报告的推动下提高医疗质量的计划已变得尤为重要[14]。这些原则不仅包括结构化的过程和角色,还包括“对失败的关注”,并将其定义为对错误和事故源的持续警惕以及对成功管理意外事件的操作敏感性。高度可靠的组织(HRO)文化要求安全、一致地提供既定的疗法,并努力降低个人失败的风险。为预防临床错误而制订的这些原则也可以成功地减轻财务和法律风险。事实证明,HRO原则有助于管理已证明的程序向高度可靠的服务线的演进，并且要求熟悉业务原则的专业人员进行行政监督,这些原则使大型组织可靠、高效、适应性强,并且具有许多复杂性以及移植实践、业务运营和合规性的细微差别。结果,这种文化在移植中心变得越来越普遍,并被移植中心所接受。因此,不再容忍普遍的冒险行为，这种冒险行为通常发生在那些移植初期绝望患者中，几乎没有可行的治疗方案。“从不发生事件”的文化在有关医疗保健服务的讨论中占主导地位，并可能导致移植领导者更具创新精神和规避风险的公司行政领导者之间的文化冲突。尽管每个人都希望避免风险，但是大多数移植临床医生都会同意，永远不会发生重大并发症的唯一方法是永远不要进行移植。无论具体的问题是活体供体死亡、供体传染性疾病的传播,还是免疫耐受的新方法,最佳实践和过程的实施都不能保证完全避免潜在的严重并发症。而且,如果在解决并发症时几乎没有缓解的余地,那么所产生的风险规避可能就不允许潜在并发症涉及如此复杂的程序。因此,在整个HRO原则的应用中,移植中心不得让自己盲目地采用规避风险的文化。移植中心领导需要保持警惕,以设定期望值并减轻潜在风险,然后抓住机会从失败和成功中吸取经验。对失败的关注不应被误用于扼杀企业家精神,相反,应通过更加严格地探索新的护理方法来增强创新能力。所有参与者都应充分理解和接受创新的风险，应尽最大可能减少创新的风险,虽然有一些不可避免的挫折,但仍应支持这些努力。为此,必须部署严格的知情同意程序。

创业精神—在企业家精神和企业文化之间取得平衡

移植领导者面临的挑战是，在保持企业家精神的同时成功利用企业文化的优势。必须尽可能确保安全、可靠和高效地进行服务。这些流程受益于标准化、可重复性和透明性。同时,新思想的开发和新程序的创建将需要使移植成为创新引擎的企业家文化。Collins和Hansen提出,最成功的公司(10Xers)将创造力和纪律相结合:“伟大的任务(很少实现)是将创造力与纪律相结合,以扩大创造力而不是破坏创造力。当您将卓越运营与创新相结合时,您就可以将创造力的价值相乘”[15]。许多企业解决了在企业文化中保持企业家精神的问题,这种企业文化被称为“企业内创业精神”,这些模式可能对移植中心具有指导意义。企业家内创业和企业家精神最早是由Gifford和Pinchot[16]在1970年代后期描述的,并在1982年由Macrae[17]推广使用。1985年,《时代》杂志在一篇名为“企业家来了”的文章中[18]首次使用了这些术语,同年,苹果公司董事长Steve Jobs在《新闻周刊》中引用了这些术语[19]。1992年,《美国传统词典》承认“创业”一词[20]。鼓励内部企业家在大型组织的资源、能力和安全性背景下以企业家的身份行事，这可以实现企业家精神的动态和活力，同时提供针对通常与企业家失败相关的风险和责任的保护[21]。因此，企业内创业精神结合了个人通过果断的冒险和创新将想法转变为可盈利产品的能力，以及大公司的保护和支持，允许在“小型公司”内应用公司管理实践。

与企业内创业概念的发展同时，波士顿咨询集团(BCG)开发了增长份额矩阵(图 126.1)，以评估针对投资或收购目标的组织内的产品线。作者使用该矩阵表示，随着市场份额的增加，产生的现金也随之增加，并且随着增长率的增加，一个周期[其中一个新想法(以问号表示)]消耗了大量资源而没有产生太多收入。这些“问号”代表着冒险的目标，但是如果它们通过成功建立竞争而成功地进入了较高的市场份额，它们将成为“明星类”，需要继续投资，但也会产生收入和利润来抵消投资。由于该产品被认为是有利可图的，因此对该产品的进一步创新的投资减少了，并且该产品成为“金牛类”，继续产生收入而几乎不需要成本。虽然从财务角度来看，这似乎是最佳的产品位置，但是随着将这些

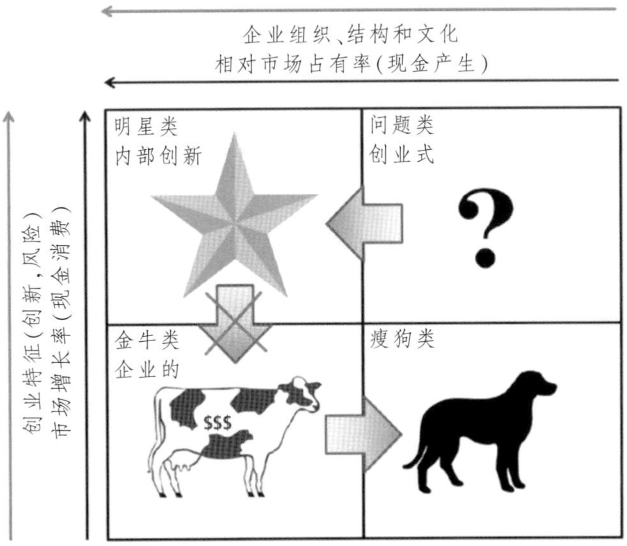

改编自波士顿咨询集团增长矩阵(1984)

图 126.1　波士顿咨询集团(BCG)的成长份额矩阵适用于移植文化。要建立持久的移植计划，必须建立高度可靠的公司组织，以在产品增长过程中保持市场份额，并利用企业家文化的力量来确保差异化创新和持续增长，以及在新产品线的基础上引入新的产品线。自己成为“明星类”，避免成为注定要商品化的“金牛类”，同时最大化强大的公司组织和积极创新是企业内创业的标志。

产品与竞争对手区分开来并从消费者处获得溢价并产生良好的利润逐渐消失，这种产品系列不可避免地成为商品。竞争对手复制并成功竞争，产品线很快就变成了“瘦狗类”，在饱和的市场上争夺较小的市场份额，现在更多地取决于谁可以最便宜地生产产品。我们认为，企业文化是与市场份额在同一轴线上的积极力量，可以有效地增加销量。另一方面，企业文化是沿着增长轴的积极力量，使产品线得以继续发展。因此，在此类推中，就像应该通过创新投资来继续使产品保持差异化一样，要尽一切努力使产品线保持在“明星”类别中(并避免其自然地成为“金牛类”)，旨在保持企业家精神和创新精神的活力，同时利用公司组织的益处。如图 126.1 所示，可以按以下两种方式之一推向 2×2 网格的特定象限。显然，“问号”可以成为“明星类”(毕竟是自然周期)，或者可以通过对创新进行再投资并通过将企业家精神保留在公司结构中来避免向“金牛类”过渡。两者都是企业内创业的例子。

创业精神可以通过两种模式来实现。首先，它是广泛文化变革的一部分。3M 就是一个例子，它使工程师能够将多达 15%的时间统一用于自己的项目[22]。该倡议导致了诸如便利贴等创新的发展。类似的环境产生了 Sony PlayStation 和 JAVA 编程语言。第二种模式包括在较大的企业文化中建立一个小的企业家团体。该团队有权采用创新文化，摆脱了大型企业文化的诸多限制，但仍能够利用其资源和能力。该模型的经典示例是 Lockheed Martin 公司的 Skunk Works™，它的成立是为了快速设计新飞机。在一位名叫 Kelly Johnson 的年轻工程师的带领下，该小组的任务是在第二次世界大战期间设计一种全新的飞机。他们在 143 天内这样做了。Lockheed Martin 公司将此归因于 Johnson 的自主权，以真正创造出一种不同的文化。“凯利如此高效地运营 Skunk Works™ 的原因是他非常规的组织方法。他打破了规则，挑战了当前阻碍创新的体系”[23]。正是这种内部创业模式，使团队能够在公司环境中作为企业家团体发挥作用，我们认为这与移植最相关。

Govindarajan 和 Trimble 通过记录各种组织(例如，纽约时报公司、康宁、孩之宝、思科、柯达、强生、汤姆森公司)的计划，研究了这种特定的企业内部模型，以他们的“管理战略试验”总结最佳实践，被定义为高风险、潜在高回报的创新，需要独特的管理方法。他们确定了三个关键策略：

1."遗忘",脱离核心业务,即使在对核心业务成功至关重要的领域也是如此;

2."借用",充分利用核心业务的经验和资产,使企业内计划明显胜过独立的企业家竞争者;

3."学习",可以按需要借鉴经验,但不能照搬[24]。

我们认为,这三种策略与在移植中心采用内部培养有关。这些作者还描述了跨行业实施此模型时所犯的错误,我们认为这对于希望采用此模型的移植领导者应作为重要的警告注意事项。他们观察到,核心业务通常将其工作方式(从组织结构到流程管理)投射到新企业上。这导致缺乏适应性,因为新举措需要更大的自由更改权,并且需要对新信息做出更灵活的反应。使大型组织成功和高效的相同业务标准扼杀了新企业。同时,许多新企业未能充分利用成为大型组织机构的优势。他们以纽约时报数字集团为例,该团队努力使自己独立于原始组织,未能利用原本的内容和广告商基础。作为学习的失败案例,作者研究了孩之宝公司,其领导者太专注于成长和远见,他们失去了自省,未能从错误中吸取教训。领导人运用了错误的指标并设定了不切实际的目标,最终导致了他们的失败[24]。

移植中心的领导者如果听取这些倡议的经验,将是成功的。成功的中心将在遗忘、借用和学习之间取得平衡。一方面,他们将利用资产、经验、数据、计划、人力、流程改进等资源,这些资源可以作为大型、成功的医疗保健组织的一部分提供给他们。另一方面,他们将保持创新精神和企业家精神、快速变革的能力以及愿意承担风险的意愿,这些风险使他们的计划在发展和增长阶段获得成功。

移植中心管理:构建企业内部

我们大多数人都听说过:"您见过一个移植中心,而您已经看到了一个移植中心"。该声明暗示着管理移植计划的组织结构在各个机构之间有很大差异。这主要有两个原因。首先,通常包含移植程序的学术医学中心本身在结构上有很大差异。实际上,甚至有少数移植程序不在学术机构中。在学术机构内部,有许多类型,包括医院、医学院和医生[25]。其次,即使在两个几乎完全相同的学术医学中心内,移植计划的发展也可能随着时间的推移而有所不同,因此其结构可能会有很大差异。例如,有些可能是复杂的部门结构,通常是外科部门,而另一些可能已经演变为中心或研究所[26]。即使在中心或研究所之间,由这些结构支配的职能也可能存在重大差异。本部分的目的不是列出所有可能的组合和排列,也不是建议某一种结构,而是建议在研究潜在的结构框架时拥护创业精神的宗旨,因为它们适用于移植。

医疗主管和管理人员必须共同努力,领导和管理移植计划中复杂多样的组成部分,同时他们分别抵御内部压力和外部压力,以在 Deal 和 Kennedy 系列的任何一端开展业务。HRO 专家 Karl Wieck(1987)将其描述为"必不可少的品种",并建议运用复杂性,并抵制公司过度简化和集中化的趋势[27]。移植中心内的不同功能需要专门的技能和知识来实现(表 126.1)。在移植计划发展的早期,外科团队主要专注于移植服务的临床交付,管理技能和过程关注较少。随着计划的发展以及监管和财务影响更加显著,行政和管理变得更重要,并且移植领导者必须抵御公司集中职能的趋势,并且必须成为移植特定利益和资源的拥护者,特别是保持创新的自由。

随着操作复杂性的增加,尤其是在高度监管的医疗保健专业领域,向上述形式化的 HRO 过渡至关重要。但是,该计划的医生经常会为正式流程的最终附件以及决策,成长和变更的批准层层挣扎。尽管医院往往具有定义明确的组织结构图,某些区域要向特定的副总裁报告,这些副总裁分别专注于运营、财务、人力资源、法规遵从等,但是医生通常会嵌入学术部门,并且在实践计划中可能不能处理移植的复杂性,特别是其跨学科性质。因此,随着移植计划的发展,其管理重心转向更好的组织结构并采用其固有的组织行为和文化并不少见。医院为此组织提供了良好的住所,并且设备齐全,可支持包括移植在内的大型复杂服务线。相反,医师基础设施往往不那么僵化,更灵活。不幸的是,学术部门和医师团体通常无法提供大量资源。移植医生的实践通常需要其医院的支持,因为代表该计划完成的大量工作无法通过标准相对价值单位(RVU)机制进行计费,因此,在医学院校和实践计划计算医生生产率时不会被认可。对于医生雇主来说,很难证明其医生和外科医生的薪水支持是合理的。特别是医学部门,通常需要为其移植医生提供支持。结果是医院在合同基础上启动了一项服务转让协议,该协议符合 Stark 和其他反回扣法律。不可避免的结果是医生的某些控制权转

表126.1 移植中心的行政职能

职能	专业知识要求	内容
财务		
支付账户	是	成本报告
收入账单	是	管理移植护理阶段/医疗保险二次支付
收入:收集	否	低容量/高费用
收入:价格	是	管理护理合同/标准器官收费(SAC)
成本报告准备	是	
预算准备和管理	是	收购成本中心
签订合同	是	管理移植护理阶段
分析	是	成本报销报告
患者咨询	是	管理式医疗,ESRD医疗保险,OPTN/ENOS要求
市场营销拓展	是	专业产品知识
人力资源		
福利及工资	否	
行政管理		
薪酬结构	是	通话补偿,外展营销补偿
招聘(非医生)	否	需要针对性的广告
员工管理(医生和非医生)	是	临床知识评估,必要的CMS、OPTN知识
非医生职工护理人员、社会工作者、中等水平提供者、餐饮服务人员	是	按照CMS、OPTN要求,专业知识及专业培训
质量保证/绩效改进/法规遵从	是 是	必须具备CMS、OPTN法规和报告的知识
数据管理	是	移植特殊数据管理
整体项目管理	是	管理整个程序所需的复杂性

移到了医院。医院既要履行对监管者的责任,又要履行其治理职责,因此需要对与该计划有关的医生活动进行某种形式的监督。在高度集成的医疗保健提供系统中,尤其是那些医院雇用医生的系统中,这些情况不利于移植的创业起源。例如,医院可能难以量化和激励诸如创新研究之类的学术努力。研究通常由院外拨款机构提供的资金不足,尤其是对于外科医生和其他专家,他们的市场化工资超过了联邦将其纳入美国国家卫生研究院(NIH)和其他联邦拨款机构的上限,这威胁了学术移植医生的财务可行性实践。既定的补偿计划将奖励研究活动以外的临床活动,从而激励移植外科医生在报酬丰厚的普通外科手术病例中填补临床移植职责所未占的任何时间,并阻碍参加研究和教学活动。不管支撑医疗服务的结构如何,随着移植计划的数量和收入的增长,它们冒着采用倾向于促进临床生产力和对创新与研究进行成本控制的企业文化的风险。该结构严格遵循临床企业的规范,使用最简单的公式在整个临床企业中运作,分配资源的方式与分配开销的方式一样多。而且由于移植的复杂性和微妙性,最初意外的后果之一就是丧失了创新精神,而创新精神首先使该计划取得了成功。另外,移植外科医生通常在移植中心内被分配管理角色,这导致他们不可避免地采用公司文化。鉴于这些外科医生/管理人员通常是该机构高级领导的一部分,尽管他们从根本上不同意对真正的创新计划施加的限制,但他们仍然经常需要接受这种文化。

内科医生和外科医生及其受训者通常居住在医学院内的部门中。Braunwald的综合论文[28]提供了中心和研究所发展的历史观点,以及中心和研究所发展的强大理由。在本文中,作者还支持矩阵组织的价值。但是在总结中,他们提醒我们,组织的管理细节,特别是学术医疗保健,只是达到目的的一种手段,特别是执行教育,研究和患者护理的三方使命的手段。尽管如此,作者强调了围绕共同主题激发不同专业的重要性,在移植中心的背景下,该主题或任务是为了满足移植患者的需求。Mallon在另一项研究中警告读者注意中心和研究所的风险,并建议,尽管利用中心和研究所的优势很重要,但在建立合作伙伴关系时奖励那些拥护协作观点的领导人也很重要。他的主要论点是必须在学术机构中保持自己的位置[29]。尽管有这些论点,但很明显,移植体现的多专业计划要求组织和行政结构超越学术环境中部门结构的传统孤岛。Braunwald了解了心脏外科手术前后心脏中心的演变。这个例子和移植之间有很多相似之处。当然,与心血管疾病相比,其参与提供者的移植多样性明显更高。重要的是,所使用的任何结构均应用于促进移植的发展,并且不要成为个人对独立和建立帝国的渴望所驱动的官僚主义障碍。阐明中心的目标(表126.2)可以作为一组指导原则,以防止原始意图的退化。移植中心的此类指导原则应包括以下内容:

1.促进跨学科成员之间的相互依存,以履行三方使命;

表 126.2 在高度可靠的移植中心实现企业内创业的两套独特但互补的指导原则

移植中心的学术任务指导原则	移植中心的临床任务指导原则
• 促进跨学科成员之间的相互依存(以履行三方使命)	• 提供高质量的护理,以达到出色的临床结果
• 增强,促进和消除跨学科合作的障碍	• 尽可能高效(经济高效地)运营
• 克服潜在的限制性组织结构,以便有效访问必要的资源以支持进度	• 保持完全合规性
• 围绕移植调整部门间目标	• 确保以团队为基础的多学科护理,重点放在沟通上
• 提供支持移植计划学术任务的财政结构	• 以患者为中心
• 培养企业的自豪感,并在从事移植的各个学科之间分享责任感和命运感	• 争取最大的本地市场份额

2.加强,促进和消除阻碍跨学科合作的因素;

3.克服潜在的限制性组织结构,从而可以有效地获取必要的资源以支持进度;

4.围绕移植确定部门间目标;

5.提供支持移植计划学术任务的财政结构;

6.促进企业的自豪感,并在从事移植的各个专业中分担责任和命运。

此外,移植中心不应该:

1.与现有机构的现有能力重复;

2.与其他中心不公平地竞争可用资源;

3.使部门过时。

如果遵循这些原则, 中心和研究所应被部门视为积极的发展, 而不是威胁竞争对手的权力和资源。为此, 应从一开始就明确中心或研究所的利益相关者包括部门主席,例如外科和医学部门。最后,应该理解的是,如果可以在不需要结构的情况下实现最初的目标,那么它将在短期内"落日",或者,中心或研究所提供的任何职能可以归还给部门 更有意义。在这些原则下运作的中心或研究所的明显好处之一是能够将所需的教职人员集中在共同感兴趣的领域。

尽管围绕三方任务的研究和教育组成部分建立中心或研究所相对容易, 但调和其临床组成部分变得更加困难。这个问题主要围绕医生补偿。不同的部门可能使用不同的量表来衡量医生的工作效率, 由于上一节中所述的原因,在移植设置中可能难以评估。因此,随着医院在支持基础设施方面的作用随着移植计划的发展和壮大而增加,这些问题不再是金钱上的问题,而更多地是关于权限和控制上的问题, 这些问题可能引起巨大的摩擦,并且已知会导致非常活跃的内爆。当个人变得不高兴并离开他们所偏爱的位置时, 他们就会成为中心。该机构的领导者还应建立一套指导原则(表126.2),该原则可用于调节资金流向和资源分配。以这种身份,移植中心的临床任务应被视为提供:

1.高质量(临床结果);

2.高价值(具有成本效益);

3.法规符合性;

4.团队合作,协调一致;

5.以患者为中心的护理。

6.此外,护理服务应努力争取在本地市场中占据较高的市场份额。

根据交付系统的集成程度, 医生可能会被医院雇用,或者从根本上充当移植服务的承包商。因此,实际的合同协议可能会有所不同,但是最终,目标仍然是相同的。读者应该注意的是,上一个列表中没有"创新",尽管人们可能会认为它在其他一些术语上是间接暗示的,包括高质量和市场份额,因为如果没有通过创新实现增长的计划可能就没有竞争力。。但是,移植计划可能是创新产品系列的先行者或后期采用者。现实情况是,大多数大型学术医院并没有将重点放在先行者上,而只是在有一定余地的情况下才是晚采用者。取而代之的是,这些机构对医疗的更多公司要素更加感兴趣,这在上一清单中已明确阐明。这是更多的学术伙伴(即医生)必须在其中提供平衡。我们认为,这两套指导原则都不能孤立地使用。相反,我们建议将内置的移植程序纳入两者的要素。

尽管很明显, 移植中心内许多已建立的程序可以根据 HRO 的原理运行,在行之有效的治疗和过程中达到效率,质量和一致性,以及克服失败的韧性,但要求移植中心保持肾内神经身份能够进行研究并建立新程序。以前的作者提出了令人信服的案例,说明了跨越公司界限并授权进行移植的临床科学家的中心和研究所[26]。在这个想法的基础上,我们建议各机构应建立移植中心和研究所，以开展前沿研究并建立以先前讨论的脑内群体为模型的新计划。在 Lockhed Martin 公司成立 Skunk 工厂时,Kelly Johnson 提出了 14 项“规则和做法”，他认为这对于集团的成功至关重要[30]。“Kelly 的 14 条规则”已成为成功的脑内组织的指南。尽管这些规则是特定于国防承包商的，并且更容易推广到工程学,但我们根据原始清单开发了一组新规则。遵循这些规则将确保移植中心(或研究所)的研究和新程序开发组件能够蓬勃发展(表 126.3)。这些规则旨在确保最高程度的灵活性和责任感，以使肾内移植中心可以在公司环境中进行创新和领导，从而确保程序一旦启动并运行就具有高度的可靠性。该规则还与先前所述[24]的新企业的经验教训以及先前尝试建立综合医疗中心的经验[31]相一致。

最后，成功的移植中心的一个基本要素是强大的领导力。这对于整个领导团队至关重要:医生领导,管理员,医疗主管以及经理和团队负责人。真正出色的移植中心始终只有一名有远见的医生领导，通常是外科医生。从优秀到优秀:为什么有些公司实现飞跃,而其他人则没有,Collins 指出,每家从单纯的好公司跃升为优秀的公司的公司都被他称为“5 级高管”的领导。他指出,许多有名望的企业领导者,例如 Lee Iacocca,都是“四级有效领导者”,他形容为“催化并致力于并追求清晰而引人注目的愿景,以刺激更高的绩效标准”。毫无疑问，这种描述对任何关注大多数移植巨头的人以及当今许多大型移植中心的领导人都是正确的。成功的移植中心可能需要拥有 4 级领导者。但是,在确定 5 级高管时,Collins 描述了一种真正的变革型领导者模

表 126.3 基于 Lockhed Martin 公司 Skunk 工厂 Kelly14 个规则的西北大学 14 个内部移植中心(右栏)规则。Reproduced from [30]

Kelly 的 14 个规则	西北大学 14 个规则
1.团队管理必须被完全授权控制团队的各个方面,再向董事长报告	1.中心领导者必须在各方面完全控制自己的方案。他应该向医院的院长和医院的首席执行官报告
2.强大但小型的项目办公室必须由军事和工业提供	2.该机构必须提供少而强大的核心行政人员,以确保中心灵活性
3.与项目有任何联系的人的数量必须以一种近乎苛刻的方式加以限制。使用少量的好人(所谓的正常的系统的 10%~25%)	3.中心成员应限于积极从事移植研究和新举措者,由中心领导掌握具体目标
4.必须提供非常简单的流程系统,具有很大进行更改的灵活性	4.项目计划应该是直接、高层次的,具有很大的灵活性
5.必须用最少数量的报告,但必须彻底记录重要的工作	5.必须有最少数量的报告,但项目应具有明确的绩效指标
6.必须每月进行一次费用审查,不仅涵盖了所花费和已付出的费用,而且涵盖了计划结束时预计的费用	6.必须定期进行成本和绩效审查,涵盖项目预计程序的状态和所需的任何变化
7.承包商必须被委派,必须承担超过正常责任,以获得良好的供应商投标项目的分包合同。商业招标程序通常比军事程序更好	7.该中心必须得到授权并有望发展与其他专业人士合作,创建项目不同学科的交叉点
8.目前由空军和海军批准的 Skunk 工程使用的检查系统符合现有军事要求的意图。将更多的基本检查责任推回给分包商和供应商。不要做这么多重复的检查	8.机构领导者必须承诺促进而不是阻碍研究项目和新举措
9.承包商必须被授权在飞行中测试其最终产品。他可以而且必须在初始阶段进行测试。如果不这样做,他就迅速失去了设计其他车辆的资格	9.中心必须得到支持,努力快速而安全地将研究发现转化为新的临床计划
10.适用于硬件的规格必须在订约前事先达成一致。Skunk 公司的做法有一个规范部分，明确说明哪些重要的军事规格项目不会被遵守及原因,因此被强烈要求	10.任何项目的成功和失败的指标必须被提前同意,并且不能立即修复这些指标或者终止项目,还有未支出的资金回报
11.资助计划必须及时,以至承包商不必继续向银行支付政府项目支持	11.为新计划提供资金必须完全可用,直到方案达到自我维持目标或由于无法实现目标而终止
12.军事项目组织和承包商之间必须有相互信任、日常密切的合作和联络。这将误解和通信减少到绝对最小值	12.移植中心、医学院和医院之间必须相互信任,对财务、目标和战略的变化具有充分的透明度
13.外部人员对项目及其人员的接触必须通过适当的安全措施严格控制	13.中心的成员必须能够在预算范围内管理项目,免除外部审查和批准的计划
14.由于只有少数人在工程和大多数其他领域被使用,所以必须提供奖励良好表现的方式	14.由于中心教师将努力实现超出医生普遍生产力指标的目标,所以补偿计划必须允许中心成员获得实现这些目标的奖励

型，能够使组织取得最高成就。在描述组织领导力的级别和模型时，Collins 指出，“第四级领导者”通常是“拥有一千个助手的天才”，具有远见卓识的意志坚强的领导者和无数可互换的经理人可以执行一个人的计划。相反，最好的公司有一个5级执行团队，在团队中，一个意志坚强的领导者会与最好的人围绕在一起，并与他们一起寻找开发和推进愿景的最佳方法。Collins 将这些5级领导者定性为不愿主动承担信用的人，而是将信用授予他们的团队成员，同时又将错误归咎于自己。他进一步描绘他们采取安静而镇定的态度，树立鼓舞人心的标准，将他们的组织摆在自己面前[32]。寻找移植负责人的组织不仅要确定有远见的医生将领导他们的计划推向新的高度，而且要使第5级领导者与众不同，这是非常罕见的无私领导。

总结

逐步实施《平价医疗法案》(ACA)的规定无疑将产生基于证据，基于团队、协调、纵向、负责和价值驱动的护理。正在进行的有关未来交付和付款改革的讨论和辩论强调了当前移植中交付和付款模式的许多特征和关键成功因素。美国其他医疗机构似乎正在采取的方向模仿了过去几十年来的移植成果。但是，一直没有强调创新。其重点似乎主要集中在监管、价值激励和奖励对患者进行协调和综合护理的护理模式上。尽管这些都是值得称赞的目标，但最大的，也是大多数人被忽视的很可能是创新和研究，而培训和教育却排在第二位。谁来为创新付费，我们将如何确保通过用质量代替数量来弯曲成本曲线的顽强决心不会减轻法规和对新颖疗法的追求？医疗改革可能预示着企业家精神的消亡，这进一步加剧了移植领导者的挑战以及在组织框架内需要开展企业内行动的挑战。

(郭海军 译 徐骁 校)

参考文献

1. Deal TE, Kennedy AA. Corporate Cultures: The Rites and Rituals of Corporate Life. Harmondsworth: Penguin Books; 1982.
2. Starzl TE. The Puzzle People: Memoirs of a Transplant Surgeon. Pittsburgh, PA: University of Pittsburgh Press; 1992.
3. Department of Health and Human Services. Public Law 98-507, STST 2339 National Organ Transplantation Act. 1984 [accessed January 26, 2012]; Available from: http://history.nih.gov/research/downloads/PL98-507.pdf.
4. McDiamid SV, Pruett TL, Graham WK. The oversight of solid organ transplantation in the United States. American Journal of Transplantation. 2008;8: 739–744.
5. Rettig RA. Special treatment – the story of Medicare's ESRD entitlement. New England Journal of Medicine. 2011;364:596–598.
6. Gorman C, Bjerklie D. The ultimate sacrifice. *Time Magazine*. 2002; Jan 28.
7. Campion EW. A death at Duke. New England Journal of Medicine. 2003; 348:1083–1084.
8. Weber T, Ornstein C. Transplant centers penalized. *Los Angeles Times*. 2006; Nov 29.
9. Centers for Medicare and Medicaid Services. 42 CFR Parts 405, 482, 488, and 498 Medicare Program; Hospital Conditions of Participation: Requirements for Approval and Re-Approval of Transplant Centers to Perform Organ Transplants; Final Rule. [accessed January 13, 2012]; Available from: http://www.cms.hhs.gov/CertificatonandComplianc/downloads/Transplantfinal.pdf.
10. Hamilton TE. Improving organ transplantation in the United States – A regulatory perspective. American Journal of Transplantation. 2008;8:2503–2505.
11. Hamilton TE. Accountability in health care – Transplant community offers leadership. American Journal of Transplantation. 2009;9:1287–1293.
12. Schold JD, Arrington CJ, Levine G. Significant alterations in reported clinical practice associated with increased oversight of organ transplant centers performance. Progress in Transplantation. 2010;20:279–287.
13. Weick KE, Sutcliffe KM. Managing the Unexpected. Assuring High Performance in an Age of Complexity. 1st ed. San Francisco, CA: Jossey-Bass; 2001.
14. Dixon MM, Shofer M. Struggling to invent high-reliability organizations in health care settings: insights from the field. Health Services Research. 2006;41: 1618–1632.
15. Collins J, Hansen M. Great by Choice. New York, NY: HarperCollins; 2011.
16. Intra-corporate Entrepreneuring. [accessed 2012 January 13, 2012]; Available from: http://www.intrapreneur.com/MainPages/History/IntraCorp.html.
17. Macrae N. Intrapreneurial now. *Economist*. 1982; April 17.
18. DeMott JS, Byrne R. Here come the Intrapreneurs. *Time Magazine*. 1985; Feb 4.
19. Lubenow GC, Rogers M. The onetime whiz kid professes no bitterness toward Apple, but he is plainly hurt by his abrupt ouster. *Newsweek*. 2008; September 29.
20. Editors of the American Heritage Dictionary. The American Heritage Dictionary of the English Language. 3rd ed. Boston, MA: Houghton; 1992.
21. Kotler P. Marketing Management: Analysis, Planning and Control. 13th ed. Englewood Cliffs, NJ: Prentice-Hall; 2009.
22. Nayak PR, Ketteringham J. 3M's post-it notes: a managed or accidental innovation? In: Katz R, editor. The Human Side of Managing Technological Innovation: A Collection of Readings. Oxford: Oxford University Press; 1997: 367–377.
23. Peters TJ. Creating innovative climates: a skunkworks tale. In: Katz R, editor. The Human Side of Managing Technological Innovation: A Collection of Readings. Oxford: Oxford University Press; 1997: 347–355.
24. Govindarajan V, Trimble C. Building breakthrough business within established organizations. Harvard Business Review. 2005;83:58–68.
25. Levin S, Maddrey G, Bagnall A. Achieving Optimal Alignment in Academic Health Centers. The Chartis Group, May 2010 [accessed January 26, 2012]; Available from: http://www.chartis.com/files/pdfs/chartis-achieving-alignment-health-care-consulting.pdf.
26. Howard KJ, Kaplan B. The time is now: formation of true transplant centers. [Personal Viewpoint]. American Journal of Transplantation. 2008;8:2225–2229.
27. Weick KE. Organizational culture as a source of high reliability. California Management Review. Winter. 1987;29:112–127.
28. Braunwald E. Departments, divisions, and centers in the evolution of medical schools. The American Journal of Medicine. 2006;119:457–462.
29. Mallon WT. The benefits and challenges of research centers and institutions in academic medicine: findings from six universities and their medical schools. Academic Medicine. 2006;81:502–512.
30. Lockheed Martins. Kelly's 14 Rules. [accessed January 14, 2012]; Available from: http://www.lockheedmartin.com/aeronautics/skunkworks/14rules.html.
31. Levin SA, Saxton JW, Johns MME. Developing integrated clinical programs. It's what academic health centers should do better than anyone. So why don't they? Academic Medicine. 2008;83:59–65.
32. Collins J. Good to Great. New York, NY: HarperCollins; 2001.

第 127 章 移植质量项目

Christian Morath, Peter Schemmer, and Martin G. Zeier

引言

通过第 103 章~第 110 章的基本介绍，我们发现过去几十年里几乎所有实体器官移植整体的水平都在不断提高。根据国际和国家移植网站登记的统计数据显示，过去几十年中，世界范围内至少已经开展了 50 万例肾移植和超过 10 万例肝移植和心脏移植[1]。对于肾移植受体而言，尽管随着受体年龄的增大，终末期肾病的并发症有所增加，但总体患者的生存质量和移植物的存活时间在不断提高[2]。同时，在非肾移植的其他器官移植领域中我们也发现了类似的结果[3]，过去几十年中，我们虽然降低了肝移植受体的基础情况标准，提高了心脏移植的供体年龄标准，肝移植和心脏移植总体的预后还是得到了显著的提高[4]。根据国际心脏和肝脏移植协会(ISHLT)1982—2009 年的心脏移植数据表明，心脏移植患者术后的中位生存时间为 11 年，目前每年至少有 3700 例患者接受心脏移植[5]。随着器官移植在世界范围的大规模推广，移植术后的治疗方式(如免疫抑制剂的使用、手术方式的选择等)呈现出多样化的态势，同时，移植患者的预后管理以及术后质量评估标准的规范要求也愈发迫在眉睫。

本章列出了大量临床需要特别关注的主要指标以便于进行临床的前瞻性研究，这些临床数据的采集及解读将通过统计学及信息技术的方式进行统一分析，具体详见第 132 章。本章则着重于针对不同的器官移植及移植术后不同时期影响预后的主要临床参数及指标作统一的归纳。

移植预后质量：移植登记注册的作用

移植协会会定期检查临床预后，以确保有限的供体器官的最佳利用[5]。器官移植在不断变化的外部和内在因素的影响下持续发展。这些因素包括外科手术技术、围术期护理、移植后的随访、新的免疫抑制药物和免疫抑制药物的组合。在高质量的治疗方式下，没有移植注册系统分析随访数据则无法评估移植的质量标准。来自大型移植登记系统的结果会影响器官移植的质量及将来的发展。虽然移植登记系统是回顾性分析，但巨大的患者人数和高比例的随访能够得出有效的结论(亦可见第 133 章，注册表数据使用)。有许多国家和国际移植登记系统可以计算患者和移植物的累积存活率。一个大型国际移植登记中心是一项全球协作移植研究，该研究涉及全球超过 35 万个肾脏、6 万个肝脏、11 000 个胰腺和 5 万个心脏移植受者[1]。在过去的二三十年中，该协作移植研究通过比较特定变量（如 HLA 系统、免疫抑制类型和移植受者的长期护理)，发表了几篇具有里程碑意义的关于患者和移植物预后的论文。例如，一篇关于血压对移植物存活影响的论文[6]表明，血压控制的质量与肾移植后患者的长期生存密切相关。最大的国家登记系统是美国器官共享网络(UNOS)，该网络随访美国实体器官受者的数据。另一个重要的国家数据库是美国肾脏数据系统(USRDS)，其发表的论文持续影响肾移植后的质量。国际和国内器官登记系统和网站总结在表 127.1。

指南

全球公认指南的主要作用是尽管存在地理差异，但在器官移植中应达到相同的质量标准。许多国家和国际移植学会都非常重视提高移植质量。然而，提高器官移植质量的方法自然地受到当地实践模式、种族背景、当地医疗特性(例如，流行性感染，心血管并发症等)和当地社会经济条件的限制。

表 127.1 用于跟踪器官移植受者和定期发表数据于移植杂志的注册登记系统

国际注册		
协作移植研究	全球超过400个移植中心	www.ctstransplant.org
欧洲肝移植注册中心		http://www.eltr.org
欧洲国家器官储运组织	比利时,德国,卢森堡,荷兰,奥地利、斯洛文尼亚、克罗地亚	http://www.eurotransplant.nl
国际胰腺移植注册中心		http://www.iptr.org
国际心肺移植注册中心		http://www.ishlt.org
国家注册		
澳大利亚及新西兰组织	澳大利亚及新西兰	www.anzdata.org.au
国家移植组织	西班牙	http://www.msc.es/ont
斯堪维亚移植组织	丹麦,芬兰,瑞士	http://www.scanditransplant.org
英国移植	英国,英格兰	http://www.uktransplant.org
器官共享联合网络	美国	http://www.unos.org
美国肾脏数据系统		

一个国际指南的例子是用于肾移植受者的肾脏全球疾病预后改进指南(KDIGO)。这是第一个国际指南,由国际肾病学会发起并由国家肾脏基金会执行，旨在建立全球适用的肾移植受者护理指南。在制订这些准则时有两个要求:一是要采取循证的方法;二是制订的指南可以应用于世界任何地方[7]。这样的指南有什么优点？在质量评估方面,指南为护理标准提供了基础。此外，在确立基于移植质量水平的移植项目所需的经济资源时,它们也很有用。对于非肾移植,有来自各种国家和国际移植学会的指南。也可以从表 127.1 中列出的国内和国际移植协会下载指南。

不同器官的移植质量评估

肾移植

肾移植(总结于表 127.2)是终末期肾病患者的治疗选择。虽然移植患者的围术期风险较高,但与年龄相匹配的透析患者相比，肾移植受者的长期结果要好得多[8]。

在国家层面进行质量评估的预后数据主要限于患者和移植物的存活,因为登记数据不够详细,无法获得更深入的质量评价。但是在当地层面,可以获得更详细的数据(将在第 132 章深入讨论)。在当地数据库的帮助下，记录移植肾的功能或移植肾功能延迟恢复的比率,器官功能的质量(例如,肌酸酐,或肾小球滤过率=GFR),手术并发症的数量和类型(如淋巴囊肿,血管并发症,输尿管渗漏),免疫抑制相关的发病率和死亡率,这是非常重要的。这种对移植物功能和受者发病率的具体评估对移植物长期存活具有重要影响。

表 127.2 肾移植质量数据

主要数据质量	患者和移植物存活率
次要数据质量	移植肾功能延迟恢复、肾小球滤过率,手术并发症、排异、免疫抑制并发症

胰腺移植

在大多数病例中(>90%),胰腺与肾脏一起移植,即肾脏-胰腺联合移植(表 127.3)。因此,胰腺移植的质量标准通常包括肾移植的质量标准。

肾脏-胰腺联合移植中肾脏的结果数据与上述相同。胰腺移植特有的其他质量标准包括临床和生化数据。临床参数包含手术技术(例如,外分泌胰腺的肠引流,动脉吻合术和全身或门静脉的静脉引流)。其他临床信息包括由缺血/再灌注损伤引起的术后胰腺炎和胰腺瘘(例如,由于移植创伤,可参见第 60 章关于胰腺移植特有的主要技术问题)。应记录胰腺移植排斥的人数,在此背景下,诊断胰腺排斥的所用活检结果应该是

表 127.3 对于胰腺移植质量数据

主要质量数据	患者和移植物存活,移植物功能(胰岛素去除后)
次要质量数据	排斥反应,手术并发症,血糖,糖化血红蛋白,糖尿病相关长期回归

胰腺移植计划的质量特征。对于长期临床随访质量数据应包括糖尿病性病变如视网膜病、血管病变和神经病的进展。它们与胰岛素缺乏(完全内分泌功能)、血糖水平、口服葡萄糖激发和糖基化血红蛋白有关。

肝移植

肝移植的主要原因(表 127.4)是终末期肝病、肝细胞癌、神经内分泌肿瘤的肝转移、急性肝功能衰竭,以及罕见的先天性代谢紊乱。

肝移植质量计划应包括 1 年患者和移植物存活率,包括 30 天死亡率和再次移植率。30 天死亡率反映的是院内死亡率,并且两者都受到移植时受者状况的显著影响。这应该通过 MELD 评分来评估,需要特别注意移植时受体透析或呼吸机依赖性。患者在重症监护室停留的时间、呼吸器治疗的时长以及住院时间也是需要考虑的重要指标。需要记录排异患者的数量,以及抗排斥治疗。生化参数应反映肝脏(胆红素)的排泄功能和合成标记,例如 INR、白蛋白。

心脏移植

心脏移植(表 127.5)是终末期心力衰竭的常规治疗方法。特别值得注意的是,心力衰竭患者在进行移植时具有特别高的风险,并且围术期死亡的风险也很高。

心脏质量计划应包括受者和器官 1 年的存活率,包括 30 天死亡率。额外的质量指标是重新移植的人数。与肝移植受者一样,移植前一般情况对移植后的结果有显着影响,应详细记录特定的并发症(包括肾功能衰竭和呼吸机依赖)。活检和抗排除治疗的人数也是额外的指标。

表 127.4　在肝移植质量数据

主要质量数据	患者和移植物存活,移植物功能
次要质量数据	30 天死亡率、拒绝手术和非手并发症,再移植、胆红素水平

表 127.5　在心脏移植质量数据

主要质量数据	患者和移植物存活
次要质量数据	1 年患者和 1 年期移植物生存,30 天死亡率、再移植排斥

肺移植

肺移植(表 127.6)需要在专业中心进行标准化治疗。肺移植的适应证是黏液黏稠病、肺动脉高压、原发性肺纤维化,以及肺气肿(较少见)。

肺移植中最重要的指标是受者 1 年存活率和 30 天死亡率。与其他维持生命的器官一样,受者的术前状况显著影响移植的预后,在肺移植的情况下,呼吸机依赖和肺部感染/定植是特别重要的指标。其他质量因素包括术后呼吸机治疗的持续时间、移植后 6 小时的 pO_2/FiO_2,以及需要额外的体膜氧合(移植肺延迟功能的标记)的患者数量。在长期随访中,支气管闭塞症的出现非常重要。

移植前的危险因素对实体器官移植预后的影响

移植受者的移植前状况严重影响着患者和移植物的生存[9]。对于不同器官,其器官衰竭(例如透析)或移植紧迫性(例如等待名单上的心脏和肝脏患者)的替代方法也不同。对于肾病患者,等待名单上患者的生存通常由透析治疗保证;然而,受体等待的时间对受者和移植物存活率及排斥反应的发生率具有特别的影响。此外,肾移植等待名单上几乎每 6 名患者中有 1 名等待再次移植,这种状况增加了排斥(例如,免疫)和早期移植物失功的风险[11]。对于等待名单上的肝脏和心脏移植患者,等待的时间更为关键。由于没有足够的实体器官捐献者,和活体相关的捐赠仅在少数肝病患者中进行,通常只有最危重的患者有机会接受同种异体移植[12]。这些都是影响移植质量及预后的重要因素,这在框 127.1 中进行了总结。

移植器官的获取

移植器官的获取途径因不同的实体器官而异。在肝脏和心脏移植中能否实现移植高度依赖于患者的当前状态。由于器官短缺,仅考虑患有晚期肝脏或心力衰

表 127.6　在肺移植质量数据

主要质量数据	1 年患者生存和 30 天死亡率
次要质量数据	6h 移植后 pO_2/FiO_2,体外膜氧化

框 127.1 在实体器官移植患者和移植物存活证实有显著影响的移植前风险因素

受者年龄(<16 岁,>65 岁)
再次肝移植
移植前预致敏
在等候名单的时间
预估的总体健康指标(如,Karnovasky 等)
移植前长期住院治疗(肝脏和心脏捐赠者)

竭的患者进行移植。质量监督小组应确保现未在医院接受器官移植手术术前治疗的患者能够获得相同的机会进入移植中心进行治疗。在这种情况下,移植中心为周边医院提供定期教学机会显得非常重要。

过去 30 年的论文表明,许多符合实体器官移植标准的患者仍被排除在移植等候名单之外。对于肾移植等候队列,主要的障碍包括:低社会地位,较低专业教育程度,历史不依从性和许多其他变量。也有人认为与男性移植候选人相比,女性候选人进入等待队列的机会较少。进一步的障碍还包括医生的偏见,例如不要有酒精滥用史的终末期肝病患者进入等待队列。因此,移植中心应提供有关其中心不同实体器官移植的信息资料。他们应该与转诊中心进行内部会议,以最大限度地为主要看护人提供信息。第 34 章介绍了转诊医师相关内容。应鼓励初级保健人员将每个潜在的实体器官受者转诊到移植中心,实际上转诊率是提供透析治疗的肾内科医师的质量指标。几乎每个国家和国际移植协会都提供传单、小册子和视频等信息材料。

器官采购及器官质量管理

等待名单上的患者数量多于可用于移植的供体器官。器官捐助者的数量在不同国家之间,有时甚至一个国家的不同地区之间的差别也很大。器官捐赠的成功与循证教育有关。一个例子是移植采购管理(TPM),一个关于器官捐赠和移植的国际项目。该计划始于 1991 年,由巴塞罗那大学和西班牙国家移植组织赞助。1994 年,TPM 成为国际性的项目,于 1997 年在意大利启动,2006 年在法国启动。举办全国培训班以使用与 TPM 课程一致的方法。2002 年,启动了电子学习平台计划,以促进专业人员的教育。2005 年,在巴塞罗那大学终身学习研究所下设立了国际硕士学位。2006 年,这些课程扩大到包括巴塞罗那大学研究国际项目的研究生健康科学学院。最后在 2007 年,欧洲资助的欧洲器官捐赠培训计划启动。目前,TPM 提供面对面、线上学习和混合国际课程。截至 2008 年,TPM 已在五大洲的 89 个国家培训了 6498 名专业人员[13]。另一个例子是南加州器官获取中心。过去几年中该计划使器官捐献者显著增加。他们成功地应用了类似于 TPM 的教育策略。应定期记录每年死亡供体器官的数量,并将其出院作为移植中心的质量标志。

活体器官捐献——供体质量管理计划

常年实体器官的短缺推动了活体捐献器官的使用。特别是在肾移植中,活体相关移植的数量占移植物的 30%~50%。在考虑活体器官移植之前,应采取一切可能的措施将移植候选人放在死亡的捐献者等候名单上。标准化流程是必要的,告知潜在的捐赠者所有短期及长期的风险(每年更新的科学文献中目前已知的)以保证知情同意。有关风险和益处的信息应包括手术(开腹与腹腔镜)、麻醉和术后即刻风险。第 23 章和第 24 章分别介绍了肾移植和肝移植活体供体的评估。

应根据国家或国际准则将所有实体器官捐献者纳入终身随访计划。在一些国家,有一些具体法律强制移植中心至少每年一次随访活体器官捐献者。这些在世界范围内都有不同程度的遵循,但在没有国家医疗保健系统的国家中最成问题。

活体捐赠给捐赠者和家庭带来巨大压力。尽管大多数捐赠者对他们捐献器官的决定感到满意,但少数人可能有后遗症(切口部位,医疗问题等)。此外,还有一些捐赠者患有适应障碍。应该随时提供预警咨询和术后咨询服务。质量计划应该有一个预警文件,涉及咨询过程的结果,这些与器官捐赠后的心理评估相比较。误解和多样性心理状态评估是可测量的,并应影响未来的预警工作。

实体器官(例如肾)或器官的一部分(例如,肝、肺)的捐赠对剩余器官的长期功能具有影响。质量标准是强制性的,以避免供体具有潜在器官功能障碍和(或)排除潜在的疾病。这对于遗传性疾病(例如,肾移植中的多囊肾或 Alport 综合征)患者尤其重要。

器官质量

根据一般经验,实体器官的供体年龄逐渐增加,与大多数国家人口普遍老龄化的趋势一致[14]。对于所有实体器官,供体的年龄直接影响移植物的存活,对于心脏和肝脏移植,它也影响受体的存活[15]。因此,评估器官质量是一项重要任务;但是这个问题目前还没有完全解决。例如,对于肾移植,肾脏的大小、肾实质的瘢痕、意外的囊肿和其他可能的畸形需要注意。然而,在这种情况下,更有趣的问题是是否有微观组织变化,如间质纤维化,小动脉透明变性和全球性肾小球硬化?因此,代表性活组织检查大小(肾小球数量)以估计供体器官的质量是非常重要的。供肝也提出了类似的问题。组织学标志是大泡性脂肪变性、纤维化和炎症变化,所有这些都是肝移植的重要质量标准[16]。为了评估肾脏或肝移植的质量,需要病理科 24 小时待命。还有临床和生化器官质量标志物,过去 24 小时尿、肾移植物中的肌酸酐的水平,以及肝同种异体移植物中的血清钠浓度,INR 和胆红素值。关于捐赠器官评估的具体内容在第 53 章中有详细介绍。

在宣告脑死亡后,器官获取是器官移植成功的众多步骤中的第一步。从死亡捐献者那里获得的器官质量对移植的预后至关重要。器官获取团队的经验,特别是领导团队的外科医生的经验至关重要。在英国,已经建立了外科获取专科医师,以确保高质量标准的器官获取[17]。在瑞典的一项研究中,报告了肝脏和肾脏获取团队的表现。最重要的发现是遗漏有关器官异常或器官损伤的信息[18]。获取器官的损伤自然是器官特异性的。

在诊断脑死亡和采购手术的过程中,有经验的团队必须采取所有医疗措施来稳定捐献者的状况。移植中心应该拥有能够应对这种特殊情况的经过专门培训的医生和护士。血压监测和出入量动态平衡对于避免供体的低血压或高血压性损害非常重要。质量评估还包括治疗相关的并发症,如感染,这可能会显著影响捐赠(例如,肾毒性抗生素)。获取方法的具体处理分别见第 21 章和第 22 章,分别针对脑死亡和心脏跳动尸体。

移植后医疗质量评估

成功的实体器官移植始于最佳手术效果;然而,大多数挑战出现在手术后的几天和几周。因此,经过适当培训(参见第 130 章),移植医生应随访所有移植受者,除了外科医生在住院期间和门诊期间已随访的受者。这要求移植中心可提供广泛的医学专业人员,以提供高质量的护理。接受器官移植培训的医生的质量标准应包括排斥反应的诊断(包括活组织检查程序),免疫抑制药物的经验及其相互作用(与其他免疫抑制药物或非免疫抑制药物相互作用),以及移植受体病毒、细菌和真菌特殊感染。医生应与外科移植团队一起了解远期手术并发症的可能性及其管理。移植后的医疗质量关键取决于移植免疫学家团队的能力,特别是当敏感患者移植时更加重要。应与免疫学专家讨论治疗方案。为了确保高质量的移植排斥诊断,移植病理学专家(例如,肾脏、肝脏和心脏)是强制性要求的。质量评估包括定期病理会议。病毒学和微生物学相关部门需要 24 小时值班,为了早期治疗感染并使用适当的抗生素治疗。最后,必须随时提供临床实验室。

上述多学科讨论对于提供高质量的护理是必要的,因此需要多学科人员沟通来促进知识的交流。这些包括定期的内部教学或会议,书面或电子文件记录其中所有相关的过程,以便供团队所有成员使用,并发症率和死亡率的会议也应该包含在内。这些学科不仅包括外科和内科,还应包括经过专门培训的病理学家和移植免疫学家。作为我们单位的质量目标,我们测量了冷缺血时间的减少。在外科医生,移植免疫学家和麻醉师的充分配合下我们将冷缺血时间减少了近 20%[19]。该信息链的另一部分是向转诊医师(例如,肾病专家、肝病专家)提供患者的现状。常规向转诊医生提供额外信息使移植团队的工作更容易。

不同类型的实体器官移植的临床路径不同。虽然这是事实,但是对于所有类型的器官来说,几种途径是相似的。这包括实验室控制、免疫抑制波谷水平,以及细菌学和病毒学。参与移植患者术后护理的所有医生和护士都应该能够获得实验室结果。应定期举行病理解剖会议与病理学家进行交流。在这些会议上用书面报告中交流细节,使病理学家了解临床相关信息,并创造一个提出研究问题的环境。

质量评估移植的经验和数量

对于外科手术的质量评估计划表明,每年完成 200

多台移植手术,受体死亡率会降低。对于心脏移植,学习曲线易于记录:对于前5次心脏移植,术后死亡率为20%,超过这个数字,死亡率减少到12%。特别值得注意的是,团队中一位经验丰富的移植心脏病专家认为手术经验并没有提高生存机会[20]。在另一项研究中,比较了肝移植的数量,作者区分了低手术量(<20例/年)和高手术量(>20例/年)中心。低手术量中心的死亡率几乎为26%,而高手术量中心的死亡率为20%[21]。来自欧洲的另一项研究(欧洲肝移植登记中心)显示,每年肝移植少于25次的中心其1年生存率为74%,而每年肝移植超过90次的中心其1年生存率为79%[22]。在肾移植中也有类似的结果。UNOS注册中心的数据用于比较前20个移植中心和最低20个移植中心的移植物存活数据,通过移植量进行评估。对HLA匹配的和HLA不匹配的同种异体移植物进行比较。前20个中心的不匹配移植物的移植物半衰期为11.8年,而后20个中心的移植物半衰期为8.9年。非常有趣的是,在1994—1999年期间,前20个中心的不匹配同种异体移植物的移植物半衰期为15.7年,而HLA匹配的肾脏接受者中最后20个中心的移植物半衰期为12年[23]。在肾移植中,移植中心对移植物结果的影响甚至高于HLA相容性。另一个重要方面是移植中心是否提供单一移植程序(例如,肾脏)或多器官移植程序,其包括例如所有内脏器官(肝脏、胰腺、肾脏、小肠)。

表127.7 器官采购的手术质量标准总结

肝脏	门静脉长度、异常动脉(15%)。避免了胆管的剥蚀。足够的捐赠者腔静脉翻卷静脉。避免实质伤害
肾脏	额外的或异常动脉或静脉。尤其是静脉消失在门的脂肪组织中。不剥离输尿管
胰腺	非常小心的准备胰腺(胰腺瘘的风险)。足够长度的脾和肠系膜上动脉重建长度。足够的门静脉的长度。避免胰腺十二指肠部分损伤
小肠	灌注的完全性。避免肠系膜水肿,避免血管损伤

表127.8 对实体器官受者进行长期随访的特定质量参数

肾脏	肾小球滤过率、血压、糖尿病、骨骼并发症,感染和癌症发病率
肝脏	实验室工作:AST、ALT、LDH、胆红素、INR。技术工作:肝动脉(双系统)
心脏	肌钙蛋白,心室射血分数、排异活检
肺	FeV1(最初1秒内的呼气量)
胰腺	脱离胰岛素,血糖,HbA1C

实体器官移植后长期随访的质量

实体器官受者需要终身随访以记录移植物功能的质量和移植相关的并发症。尽管移植后早期的风险较高(例如,手术、免疫抑制程度较高、再入院),但多年来随访同种异体移植患者至关重要。质量评估应包括器官特定的功能测量指标和随访期间器官功能的潜在损失。典型器官一般性和器官特异性检测列于表127.7和表127.8。

尽管移植后第一年的检测次数将减少,但应监测免疫抑制剂血液水平。专门的移植门诊应将所有涉及移植特异性治疗的事项对患者告知(例如,药物与免疫抑制药物相互作用,并发疾病或手术,避孕和女性患者怀孕的可能性)。质量评估还包括需要住院治疗的感染和免疫抑制相关恶性肿瘤的受体人次。

在长期随访的背景下,对依从性的质量评估,特别强调包括过渡期(青少年)。不能依从免疫抑制药物治疗是同种异体移植物失功的常见原因(第120章将对此进行深入研究)。依从性水平影响临床结果,并且与早期和晚期同种异体移植排斥相关。当错过预约和肾移植受者中出现波动的血药浓度时,应提出对不遵医嘱服药的怀疑。然而,不依从性超出了免疫抑制药物的摄入量。影响移植物存活的其他不依从性领域包括运动、烟草、酒精和药物滥用以及生命体征的自我监测。移植后早期和(或)晚期发生不依从性。在从儿科到内科的过渡期间,不依从性尤为常见(有关该主题的详细讨论见第121章)。如何在个体患者中测量依从性质量?有几种措施可用于评估依从性:自我报告药物,亲属或看护人的间接报告,患者日记,实验室检测(药物和代谢物水平),病历审查,处方补充,监测药丸计数,和电子监控设备。有几种方法可以改善依从性,它们总结在"肾病:改善全球预后(KIDGO)指南"[24]。

移植后患者的生活质量评估

器官移植包括同种异体移植物受者生活中的许多方面。除了需要手术和定期摄入免疫抑制药物之外,通常存在共病或治疗相关的发病率(例如,感染、癌症)。

表 127.9 实体器官受者的长期随访总质量参数

血液中的免疫抑制药物
血压
糖尿病
肾功能(肾小球滤过率)
感染住院
恶性肿瘤的类型和治疗

所有这些困扰一起增加了个体患者的心理负担。除了这些，器官移植受者知道来自另一个人的器官在他或她的身体内。这些患者理解另一个人已经死亡(在已故器官捐献的情况下)或者亲属或朋友自愿捐献器官(在大多数情况下是肾脏)。因此,重要的是为器官移植接受者提供心理咨询。移植中心的质量计划应积极向患者询问他们的心理健康状况。有一些调查问卷用于评估器官受体的心理状态,例如,SF-36 生活质量问卷或移植效应问卷 TxEQ-D。更多器官特异性的工具包括肾移植问卷(KTQ)、心脏移植检查表、终末期肾病症状检查表(ESRD-SCL)或骨髓移植症状列表。

总结

实体器官移植是危重患者的复杂治疗方法。在过去几十年,科学为我们提供了许多新的免疫抑制药物,并显著降低了急性排斥率。今天,移植器官的长期存活成为现实。尽管取得了成功,但实体器官移植的结果可以进一步改善。移植中心应该理解，单一的治疗方案(手术、药物、诊断程序)无法实现这一目标。他们应衡量里程碑(表 127.10)并验证这些里程碑是否在他们的移植中心实行。

表 127.10 提高器官移植质量的重要里程碑

结果的学术回顾(注册中心)
实施循证指南的知识
优化过程的序列
评估和提高患者的依从性
器官质量测量
最小数量的作用
器官采购的质量
器官移植受者的生活质量

(郭海军 译 徐骁 校)

参考文献

1. Pacual M, Theruvath T, Kawai T, et al. Strategies to improve long-term outcomes after renal transplantation. The New England Journal of Medicine. 2002;346:580–590.
2. Hariharan S, Johnson CP, Bresnahan BA, et al. Improved graft survival after renal transplantation in the United States, 1988 to 1996. The New England Journal of Medicine. 2000;342:605–612.
3. Burroghs AK, Sabin CA, Rolles K, et al. 3-month and 12-month mortality after first liver transplantation in adults. Lancet. 2006;367:225–232.
4. International Society for Heart and Lung Transplant. [assessed January 01, 2014]; Available from: http://www.ishlt.org.
5. Axelrod DA, Kalbfleisch JD, Sun RJ, et al. Innovations in the assessment of transplant center performance: implications for quality improvement. American Journal of Transplantation. 2009;9:959–969.
6. Opelz G, Doehler B. Improved long-term outcomes after renal transplantation associated with blood pressure control. American Journal of Transplantation. 2005;5:2725–2731.
7. Kasiske BL, Zeier MG, Chapman JR, et al. KDIGO clinical practice guideline for the care of kidney transplant recipients: a summary. Kidney International. 2010;77:299–311.
8. Wolfe RA, Ashby VD, Milford EL, et al. Comparison of mortality in all patients on dialysis, patients on dialysis awaiting transplantation and recipients of a first cadaveric transplant. New England Journal of Medicine. 1999;341:1725–1730.
9. Hong KN, Iribarne A, Worku B, et al. Who is the high-risk patient? Predicting mortality after heart transplantation using pretransplant donor and recipient risk factors. Annals of Thoracic Surgery. 2011;92:520–527.
10. Shresta BM. Strategies for reducing the renal transplant waiting list: a review. Experimental and Clinical Transplantation. 2009;7:173–179.
11. Morath C, Opelz G, Zeier MG, et al. Kidney transplantation for high-risk patients – the “Heidelberg algorithm”. Transplantation Proceedings. 2011;43:801–804.
12. Kamath PS, Wiesner RH, Malinchoc M, et al. A model to predict survival in patients with end-stage liver disease. Hepatology. 2001;33:464–470.
13. Paez G, Valero R, Paredes D, et al. Evaluation of transplant procurement management courses: an educational project as a tool for the optimization of transplant coordination. Transplantation Proceedings. 2003;35:1638–1639.
14. Watson CJ, Johnson RJ, Birch R, et al. A simplified donor risk index for predicting outcome after deceased donor kidney transplantation. Transplantation. 2012;93(3):314–318.
15. Schemmer P, Fischer L, Schmidt J, et al. Intercontinental comparison of patients cohorts: what can we learn from it? Gut. 2007;56:1500–1501.
16. de Graaf EL, Kench J, Dilworth P, et al. Grade of deceased donor liver macrovesicular steatosis impacts graft and recipient outcomes more than donor risk index. Journal of Gastroenterology and Hepatology. 2012;27(3):540–546.
17.www.rcseng.ac.uk/media/medianews/new-organ-specialists-planned-to-meet-donation-increase. [assessed January 01, 2014].
18. Jynge O, Andreassson C, Bergström C, et al. Quality assurance of the donation process. Transplantation Proceedings. 2006;38:2622–2624.
19. Fonouni H, Goriz M, Mehrabi A, et al. The role of the interdisciplinary transplant team on living donation kidney transplantation program. Transplantation Proceedings. 2010;42:137–140.
20. Laffel GL, Barnett AI, Finkelstein S, et al. The relation between experience and outcome in heart transplantation. New England Journal of Medicine. 1992;327:1220–1225.
21. Edwards ED, Roberts JP, McBride MA, et al. The effect of the volume of procedures at transplantation centers on mortality after liver transplantation. New England Journal of Medicine. 1999;341:2049–2055.
22. Adam R, Cailliez V, Maijno P, et al. Normalized intrinsic mortality risk in liver transplantation. European Liver Transplant Registry Study. Lancet. 2000;356:621–624.
23. Takemoto SK, Terasaki PI, Gjertson DW, et al. Twelve years' experience with national sharing of HLA-matched cadaveric kidneys for transplantation. New England Journal of Medicine. 2000;343:1078–1083.
24. The KDIGO Transplant Work Group. KDIGO clinical practice guideline for the care of the kidney transplant recipients. American Journal of Transplantation. 2009;9(Suppl 3):S1–S155.

第 128 章
国家和国际移植管理和监督

Virginia A. McBride, Esther-Marie Carmichael, Linda Ohler, Jeremy Chapman

引言

移植，自成为一种临床治疗手段开始，就对公众态度及死亡和健康的法律定义提出了挑战。该领域推动了对死亡定义的明确；驱使所有政府思考如何规范化器官捐献流程；确保每个个体都会认真考虑是否愿意在死后捐献器官；对于那些意外死亡的个体，也会驱使他们的亲属考虑是否将死者的器官捐出，而不仅仅是面对亲人的死亡悲伤不已。

除了现代医学其他领域，人工生殖技术可能例外，移植在几乎所有发达国家和世界新兴经济体都要求政府政策和立法。自20世纪八九十年代以来，在大部分国家，移植开始受到政府和国际社会立法者设定的法律界限的监管和控制，至少在基本立法上。在过去10年中，国际和政府开始关注移植技术的全球传播带来的问题，特别是有关人体器官贩运和人体器官非法商业化的问题。

本章详细描述了国际组织和政府如何在全球范围内做出回应，尤其详细介绍了美国的立法和政府控制的驱动因素和目的。虽然详细介绍了美国的政策，本章还涵盖了全球需要关注的共同问题，从广义上讲，这些问题在世界各地的地理区域受到监管。此外，还描述了主要国际协会倾向于全球移植实践，新兴国际协议试图在移植实践方面获得国际共识。本章重点是器官捐献和移植而非细胞或组织移植。而不是细胞或组织移植。其他的移植政策在143章可以找到。

美国捐献和移植体系中的健康和人类服务监管

在众多政府组织和机构为移植制订的法律支持下，广泛的移植得以完成。美国卫生与人类服务部(HHS)是保护所有美国公民健康的主要机构。这项工作通过其许多机构推进，包括医疗保险和医疗补助服务中心(CMS)、卫生资源和服务管理局(HRSA)、疾病控制和预防中心(CDC)、食品和药物管理局(FDA)和公共卫生服务 (PHS)。从器官捐献和移植的角度来看，HHS的主要监督机构是CMS和HRSA。

1965年，美国社会保障法案(法案)赋予HHS部长权利制订和发布为医保受益人提供优质医疗服务的政策和法规[1]。通过这项权利，所有美国公民都可受益。CMS负责制订保护患者健康和安全所必需的最低标准，并负责实施监督机制，以确保医疗保健实体为医保受益人提供高质量的医疗服务。医院、移植程序、器官获取组织(OPO)、透析中心和临床实验室均是满足医保标准所需的实体，因此他们可以从提供给医保受益人和符合医保条件接受者服务中获得财务报销。

1972年通过的该法案第1138节将医疗保险的保险范围扩大到某些慢性肾病患者。1978年，该法案进一步扩展到为终末期肾病(ESRD)患者提供医保，以接受肾移植服务。HRSA对捐献和移植的责任源于移植的日益成功以及对供体器官不断增长的需求。1984年，国会通过了“国家器官移植法”(NOTA)，其中包括创建器官获取和移植网络(OPTN)、移植受者科学登记处(SRTR)，以及HHS内部管理这些活动的行政单位，即HRSA内的移植部(DOT)[2]。

所有这些补充性立法(随后的修订)的通过奠定了美国联邦政府监督器官捐献和移植系统的基础。在20世纪90年代后期，HHS的活动以这种立法为基础，对捐献和移植的未来产生重要影响。1998—2007年，HHS发布了涵盖捐献和移植连续体的法规(表128.1)，其中包括对捐献医院、OPO、移植程序和实验室的要求[3]。

这些法规还影响了OPTN和SRTR的运营，以及HHS与契约运营两个实体的组织之间的关系。

1998年6月22日，CMS公布了三项最终法则中

表 128.1 卫生与公众服务捐献和移植法规部(1998–2007 年)

年份	机构	法规
1998	HRSA	OPTN Final Rule (42 CFR, Part 121)
1998	CMS	Hospital CoPs for Organ, Tissue and Eye Donation; Final Rule (42 CFR, Part 482)
2006	CMS	Conditions of Coverage for OPOs; Final Rule (42 CFR, Parts 413, 441, et al.)
2007	CMS	Hospital CoPs and Requirements for Approval and Re-Approval of Transplant Centers to Perform Transplants; Final Rule (42 CFr, Parts 405, 482, 488 and 498)

的第一项，即可进行器官和组织捐献的医院条件(42 CFR 482.45),生效日期为1998年8月21日。这条法规被称为“常规转诊”，它要求医院识别OPO或OPO指定的第三方，并将潜在供体器官和组织转介。接下来,CMS于2006年5月31日发布了OPO覆盖条件(42 CFR 496,子部分G),以响应2000年的器官获取组织认证法案,该法案指示HHS根据实证建立结果和进程估测。最后,2007年3月30日CMS发布了移植计划最终规则(42 CFR 482,子部分E)。先于移植法则,肾移植通过ESRD法规进行治疗，肾以外的器官通过联邦公报中公布的国家覆盖决定进行管理。所有这些规则的实施是独特的,并成为DHHS的先决背景。

2010年获得Malcolm Baldrige质量奖的Studer集团指导医疗保健组织实现并保持卓越的绩效。Studer建议使用组织支柱为设定目标和指导服务提供基础[4]。虽然法规与组织有很大不同，但使用支柱来协调目标和关注行为的概念可以应用于两者。在治理和监督的背景下,可用于产生成功结果的四大支柱是:问责制、透明度、绩效改进(QAPI)以及协同合作。

支柱1:问责(资源和资金的管理工作)

从监督的角度来看,问责制是对行动、决策和政策的承认和担责,对所产生的后果负责。在美国的捐献和移植系统中,有两个主要的问责级别:个人组织绩效和整体系统绩效。CMS和HRSA都持有对绩效结果负责的个体OPO、移植计划和医院。国会和美国公众认为HRSA和CMS对国家捐献和移植系统的整体表现负责。

CMS通过这一过程让实体对履行负责，他们有权获得所提供服务的医保金。这种获得批准的途径因捐献医院、OPO和移植计划而异。对于医院,首先CMS必须证明或确认机构能够提供所需的服务。对于OPO,CMS指定OPO(为OPO分配地理服务区域),然后证明其能够提供服务。移植计划首先必须是OPTN的成员,然后由CMS认证为能够提供有效的移植服务。认证过程包括验证组织执行捐献和(或)移植服务的能力的审查。CMS审查每个申请组织的流程和结果措施,以确定纳税人的钱是否会通过从申请人处购买服务而得到充分利用。一旦获得认证,实体就有资格获得医保金的服务。CMS以外的任何实体,甚至OPTN,都不能指定,认证或以任何方式批准OPO、捐献医院或移植计划以接收资金。

CMS认证的机构涵盖捐献和移植的连续体。CMS已为移植医院制订了关于移植患者评估、名单、住院和术后护理的参与条件(CoP)。认识到移植的成功依赖于可利用的器官的供应,CMS建立了对所有美国急症护理和关键入院医院的期望,以便与OPO在授权捐赠者的器官的识别、转诊、管理和恢复方面充分合作。最后,CMS已经建立了OPO要求的条件,以便从授权捐献者那里有效、高效地评估、管理、恢复和运输可移植器官。

对于OPO的和移植方案,CMS已经建立符合绩效的成果,如果组织希望保持其认证和或指定接收医保报销(表128.2)。虽然CMS没有在捐赠医院的法规中规定器官捐献表现目标,但HRSA制订的国家绩效目标如果不能满足,可能会导致联合委员会等组织的审查。

为履行对NOTA授予的国家OPTN的监督,HRSA于1999年发布了一项法规(OPTN最终规则,42 CFR,

表 128.2 器官获取组织和移植项目医疗保险和医疗补助服务结果的措施

覆盖实体	结果测定
OPO	捐赠率的合格捐助者资格的比例死亡不超过1.5个标准差(SD)平均国家的捐赠率
OPO	观察捐赠率没有明显低于预期的捐赠率18或36个月
OPO	至少符合三个标准的两个:标准移植供体、扩大标准的移植供体、单器官单供体
移植进展	每月至少10个移植
移植进展	患者或器官的存活低于阈值: 单边 $P<0.05$ 大于三个观察-预期的事件 观察到>1.5除以预期事件

第121部分),描述了其对OPTN运营和目标的期望[2]。在其要求中,HRSA向OPTN负责制订和发布分配政策和绩效目标、会员资格和指定移植计划要求、审查和评估过程,以及OPTN成员对政策合规负责的做法。在监管下,不仅OPTN成员对自己更加遵守OPTN政策,OPTN本身也对HRSA和公众更加负责,为死亡和活体供体捐献者、移植候选人和移植受者提供优质护理。

HRSA通过OPTN法规要求公布OPO和移植计划的中心绩效结果。每个OPTN成员必须提交由SRTR分析和发布的捐献者、候选者和受者数据。低于预期水平的成员必须经过OPTN的同行评审过程,并在必要时实施纠正行动计划。

与HRSA类似,CMS也跟踪OPTN成员的表现,以配合两年一度的SRTR中心特定报告出版物。与OPTN类似,会通知表现不佳的机构,并要求其提交改进计划,以确保在此期间取得改善,从而使其有资格获得重新认证。OPO每四年进行一次重新认证,而移植计划每三年重新认证一次,可以根据已实现的绩效指标进行延期。尽管CMS和OPTN的OPO和移植计划审查似乎都是重复的,但它们可使计划对负责最大化器官利用(HRSA)的联邦机构以及负责资助有效医疗保健服务(CMS)的机构负责。通过使用提交给OPTN的共同数据集,CMS和HRSA希望最大限度地减少OPTN成员的监管负担。

支柱2:透明度

科学、工程、商业和人文科学领域的透明度通常意味着开放、沟通和负责。器官捐赠和移植中的透明性概念可以同等地应用于政策/监管过程和绩效结果的公布。

CMS的所有捐赠和移植要求均可在CMS网站www.cms.hhs.gov上公开获得。已发布的信息包括法规参与条件(CoP)、解释性指南(如何证明遵守CoP)和国家操作手册(SOM)(验船师将如何进行绩效评估)。根据《信息自由法》(FOIA),CMS可以在捐助医院、移植计划或OPO提交可接受的计划以纠正所访问的缺陷后,向要求其提出请求的任何相关方披露其执行的任何调查结果。CMS针对不合规行为所采取的措施受《联邦法规法典》第42条第498款中已发布的法规的约束,而调查程序则在42 CFR 488上发布。

拟议的规则制订过程将在制订法规时指示CMS咨询行业专家和组织。提议的规则发布后,在CMS评论期内,公众可以将提议的规则的可能改进,建议或难以预料的后果告知CMS。然后,CMS将在发布最终规则和规则生效之日斟酌这些评论并公开回应。CMS对公众意见的回应始终会发布在《最终规则》的序言中。如果公众意见导致对拟议规则的实质性更改,那么CMS必须在发布修订后的最终规则之前发布具有附加意见征询期的另一项拟议规则。

在以最终规则的形式发布法规之后,CMS将制订调查员的解释性指南以在调查过程中使用。调查的目的是确定移植程序,OPO或捐赠医院是否符合所有法规条件(称为条件级别的合规性)以进行认证或重新认证。联合委员会等认证组织对包括医院在内的许多实体进行了调查,因为这些组织已被CMS授予"推定权力"。拥有职权意味着联合委员会等实体可以正式确定哪些设施符合Medicare和Medicaid认证要求,哪些不符合[5]。CMS或其承包商不定期检查由拥有公认地位的组织认证的实体。但是,CMS会对所有认可的实体执行验证调查。由于没有任何组织具有移植程序和OPO、CMS的公认地位,因此州验船师或CMS承包商必须执行所有认证调查。调查始终是在不通知的情况下进行的,因此,所涵盖的实体应随时提供高质量的护理,并使用质量管理原则为意外访问"做好准备"。

如果调查结果导致CMS考虑终止捐助医院、移植计划或OPO的医保资格,则该机构有机会提供更正计划,如果CMS可接受,则将进行暗查以核实纠正计划已经执行。如果更正计划不被接受,则CMS会继续进行终止程序,但机构可以根据实质性理由要求重新考虑。如果CMS拒绝重新审议,则终止流程将继续进行,该机构可以提出上诉。所有上诉均通过既定的上诉程序(法规中已明确列出)进行审议,并作最终决定。

HRSA制订和发布法规的过程与CMS相同。通过其最终规则,HRSA已为OPTN的决策制订了要求,该要求与联邦政府的要求是分开的并且是不同的。根据最终规则,OPTN必须在OPTN的任务范围内制订和发布政策,例如合理分配死者的器官,防止传染病的传播;减少由于社会经济地位而引起的不平等;在指定的移植计划中对移植医生和医师进行培训和经验;提名官员和董事会成员;以及秘书指示的其他事项,例如生活捐赠。有关OPTN政策制订流程的完整说明,请访问www.unos.org。

该规则还要求OPTN董事会为OPTN成员和其他

有关方面提供机会,以对拟议的政策发表评论,并要求 OPTN 委员会在制订和采用由 OPTN 实施的政策时考虑这些评论。此过程可确保受到新政策或修订政策影响的美国任何个人、组织或地理区域都能够在开发过程中发表评论。

所有 OPTN 提议和采用的政策和细则都可以在 www.optn.transplant.hrsa.gov 上查到。任何感兴趣的个人或组织,无论他们是否是 OPTN 成员,都可以书面形式或通过 OPTN 的基于网上的公共评论系统对提议的政策进行评论和评论。OPTN 政策继续进行通俗易懂的语言修订,因此专业和普通读者都可以理解每项政策的意图和目的。

OPTN 最终规则要求 OPTN 和 SRTR 都必须"向公众提供有关器官采购和移植计划的及时、准确的计划特定信息。这包括在互联网上的免费传播,并应在必要时进行呈现、解释和组织,以正确、有效地理解、解释和使用信息。任何感兴趣的人或组织都可以访问特定于计划的、区域和国家的捐赠和移植数据。调查人员、新闻工作者或进行真诚研究或分析的任何人,只要要求是合理的,都可以要求 OPTN 数据。HHS 秘书还可以自行决定指示发布 OPTN 或 SRTR 数据。OPTN 数据的完全透明是 HRSA 拥有自己、OPTN 以及所有对系统性能负责的捐赠和移植计划的最重要方式之一。

必要情况下,允许 OPTN 和 SRTR 向请求者收取合理的费用以响应数据请求。这样做是为了最大程度地减少响应数据请求的财务负担。如果最终规则不允许这样做,则响应数据请求的费用将以更高的候选注册费的形式转嫁给移植计划和 OPO。《最终规则》还允许向研究人员发布患者识别的数据,"表明设计的合法研究(需要此类数据用于匹配或其他目的)"。在这些情况下,OPTN 和 SRTR 要求提供"适当的保密保护,包括在匹配完成后销毁患者标识的证据"。

支柱 3:质量保证和绩效改善(绩效的可持续性和患者安全)

CMS 将质量保证和绩效改进(QAPI)定义为一个全面的数据驱动程序,旨在监视和评估所有服务的绩效,包括根据合同或安排提供的服务[6]。它是对操作系统和临床过程的持续评估,可在医疗方面取得可衡量的改善。

CMS 对捐赠医院、移植计划和 OPO 的捐赠和移植 CoP 的审查显示,QAPI 的状况是相互关联的。为了保持护理的连续性,CMS 精心确保了 QAPI 规则的同步,以确保在按计划积极地应用 QAPI 条件时,可以获得最佳的护理水平和成功的结果。例如,在捐赠医院 CoP 中,需要与 OPO 合作进行病历审查,以评估给定时间内机构中潜在捐赠者的数量。根据 OPO 规则,要求向医院和移植医院提供病历审查结果的数据报告,以评估医院的器官捐赠有效性。在移植规则中,需要建立器官供体恢复的结果指标,这需要 OPO 的合作以及在病历审查期间从供体医院获得的信息。

为了确保机构达到其绩效标准,CMS 要求所有捐助医院、OPO 和移植中心都拥有强大的 QAPI 计划,这些计划可以跟踪并采取措施来识别绩效不佳的领域。CMS 希望所有实体都能保持对要求的遵守,并不断努力提高护理质量以及患者和生活捐助者的安全,以追求最佳结果。

OPTN 的临时疾病传播咨询委员会(DTAC)是最近在国家一级开发的 QAPI 活动的例子之一。委员会审查了报告给 OPTN 的个别潜在疾病传播病例,以便在可能的情况下确认传播情况。DTAC 还审查了所有报告病例的汇总数据,以评估美国器官移植中供体疾病传播的风险。现在需要所有移植计划来确定特定的患者安全联系人,并报告所有已证实或怀疑与移植相关的疾病传播的实例在 24 小时内将其转移至 OPTN 患者安全系统[7]。DTAC 的出现开始弥合了关于供体器官移植引起的疾病传播的真实发生率的长期存在的知识鸿沟。

在 2003 年之前,不可能对国家器官捐赠系统进行有效的 QAPI 分析。既未收集也未公开与潜在捐赠者推荐、符合条件的死亡人数、捐赠授权率和错过的捐赠机会有关的捐赠数据。在 2002 年秋季,HRSA 要求 OPO 开始将这些数据提交给 OPTN,到 2003 年春季,国家已经掌握了可以用来推动器官捐献者和可移植器官数量增加的信息。这些数据的可用性将器官捐赠绩效改善文化从一种本能的、轶事性的变化过程,转变为可以引起智能改善的数据驱动过程。器官捐赠朝着循证实践迈出了第一步。

为了确保捐赠和移植都保持在数据驱动的改进道路上,CMS 的 OPO 和移植法规现在可以反映并加强 OPTN 的现有数据提交要求,该要求是在 OPTN 到期日之后 90 天到期的指定数据的 95%。完全遵守 OPTN 的数据提交政策,就等于完全遵守 CMS 的移植计划参与条件。在这方面,OPTN 现在在遵守 Medicare 要求方面为移植中心和 OPO 提供咨询服务。

支柱 4:协作与合作

协作和合作是系统各组件协同工作以实现特定目标的方式。

参与捐赠和移植的每个人都必须是稀有且医学上有价值的资源的好管家。在过去的五年中,美国平均从死者和活着的供体中进行了 26 857 例实体器官移植(图 128.1)。2010 年,在 14~508 个器官捐赠者中,已故捐赠者占 53.4%,在世捐赠者占 43.2%。2000 年,活体捐赠吸引了 40 个已故者的捐赠,并在 2001 年超过了捐赠额,一直持续到 2003 年(图 128.2)[8]。在 2003 年之前的五年中,该行业的器官捐赠平均每年仅增长 2.6%。2003 年,HHS 发起了国家的第一个器官捐赠计划,其愿景是创建"捐赠友好的美国"。

HHS 捐赠和移植协作与合作的首要例子是 HRSA 的器官捐赠突破协作(ODBC),其建立是为了实现美国器官捐赠者数量的显著增加[9]。这项合作的职责是确定 OPO 和医院中的最佳做法,以提高捐赠(转换)率,并将这些做法传播到美国的所有 58 个捐赠服务区(DSA)。通过该计划,该国的死者捐赠额从 2002 年的 6190 个器官捐赠者增加到 2006 年的 8019 个(29.5%),达到了前所未有的水平。ODBC 演变成器官移植突破合作组织(OTBC),旨在最大程度地增加每个捐赠者的捐赠礼物,以增加器官移植的数量。与 ODBC 一样,移植数量的增长也非常出色,移植数量从 2002 年的 18 291 例增加到 2006 年的 22 208 例(21.4%)。

通过强调使用现有的绩效改进方法[例如计划、实施、研究、法案(PDSA)周期)来测试和适应本地使用的更改的重要性,该协作组织翻译了 HRSA 在两份已发布报告中确定的最佳做法。在医院和 DSA 级别都跟踪了性能改进的进度。邀请了展示快速改进的合作团队(由 OPO、捐赠医院和移植计划的代表组成)在全国共同学习会议上与来自全国各地的类似团队分享他们的进展和方法。

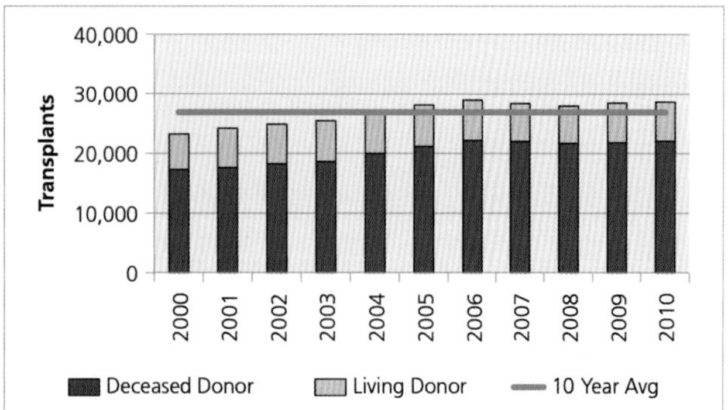

图 128.1 美国的年器官移植。基于 OPTN 数据,2013 年 1 月 11 日。

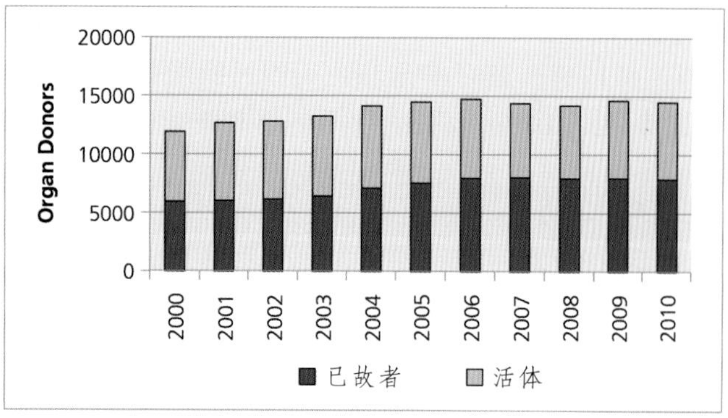

图 128.2 美国已故者和活体捐赠者。基于 OPTN 数据,2013 年 1 月 11 日。

突破性合作的最初目标是通过使用最好的 OPO 和捐助医院将全国转化率从 58%提高到 75%。75%的转化率目标是在 2010 年实现的,随后直到 2011 年 9 月每个月都实现[10]。除了提高国家转化率外,合作组织还试图通过将每位捐赠者的移植器官数量(OTPD)从 2005 年 7 月的 3.03 增加到 3.75,以最大限度地提高每次捐赠的机会。而且,尽管某些个人 OPO 间歇性地达到了国家目标,但大多数国家尚未达到,因此尚未实现 OTPD 3.75 的国家目标。但是,改进的机会仍然存在。重症监护医师和器官采购专业人员之间可能建立合作关系,以从潜在的捐献者进入医院直至获得捐赠授权为止,维持高度的器官生存能力,从而可以增加可采购的健康器官的数量。这种复杂的伙伴关系在该国大部分地区尚不存在。合格的 QAPI 专业人员更深入地参与评估 OPO 捐助者管理流程和实践的可能性,也有可能揭示以前无法识别的改进机会。HRSA 的合作伙伴起到了催化剂的作用,鼓励捐助者医院、移植中心和 OPO 在地方、地区和国家层面进行持续的合作,并确保其 QAPI 活动保持一致,从而更好地满足捐助者、捐助者家庭、移植候选者和收件人。

协作者还为 HRSA 和 CMS 提供了一个合作伙伴的机会,以实现一个共同的目标,并在私营部门建立一个可行的平台,该平台可以维持协作者在未来的工作和动力。

移植计划的观点

CMS 移植中心的参与条件(COP)自 2007 年 6 月 28 日生效,旨在改善对移植计划的监督。这份刊登在《联邦公报》的长达 84 页的文件要求所有先前批准的移植中心在 2007 年 12 月 26 日之前提交给 CMS 申请信,要求批准继续根据新的 CoP 进行移植程序[6]。通过这封信,美国的移植计划致力于符合 CMS 建立的监管要求。这意味着 CMS 将每三年对每个移植计划或移植计划的美国国务院卫生部进行一次调查,以确保符合新的 CoP。这些规定包括实体器官移植的体积和结局要求。诸如此类的指令和指南以前尚未建立,并且某些计划和专业人员对此类要求的必要性提出了质疑。现在要求移植计划向 CMS 报告其数量或结果的任何重大变化,以及任何主要人员(例如主要的移植外科医生或医师)的变化。为了保持临床经验,对每个特定器官建立了数量要求,其中心脏、肝、肠和肺计划每年需要进行 10 次移植,肾脏计划需要每年至少进行 3 次移植。对于心肺联合治疗或胰腺移植尚无年度要求。儿科计划也免除了数量要求。

最初,移植专业人士担心 OPTN 和 CMS 实施的法规数量众多。认识到 CoP 与付款有关,移植中心开始审查其程序以确保合规性。如果没有 CMS 的批准继续进行移植,这些计划也将面临失去私人付款人的风险。几个专业的移植协会发布了通道,描述和比较了 OPTN 和 CMS 的监管要求。现在两者都将在调查移植中心。OPTN 会提前几周。提供调查通知,并列出他们将审核的患者记录清单。CMS 的调查是未经通知的,每三年进行一次,要求患者到达时要求提供病历。2011 年,OPTN 开始了对活体捐献者计划的专门调查,与对接受者和移植候选人的定期图表审计分开进行。因此,移植程序有可能在同一年进行两次 OPTN 调查和 CMS 调查。OPTN 调查通常为 2~3 天审核,而 CMS 调查可能持续一周或更长时间,具体取决于移植中心的数量。当人们考虑到在此之前移植计划还未受到监管机构的监督时,这些调查引起了移植界的广泛关注。

数据产生结果

数据要求也包含在 OPTN 和 CMS 法规中。每个移植程序必须每月向 OPTN 提交数据。预计移植中心将在截止日期的 90 天内收集并提交所需数据的 95%。然后将这些数据传输到 SRTR 进行分析。分析后,数据将被发送到相应的移植程序以供审核,然后再发布给公众。移植计划大约有 4 周的时间来审查数据,进行更正并提供任何缺失的数据。返回数据后,SRTR 将对其进行重新分析,并在以下网站上向公众发布:www.srtr.org。在这里,公众可以完全访问每个移植中心经过 30 天、1 年和 3 年的风险调整后的患者和移植物存活率。还报告了其他数据,例如等待名单上的死亡人数和中心的移植率。CMS 和 OPTN 都监视这些结果。使用以下阈值将预期的 1 年移植物和患者存活率与观察到的 1 年的患者和移植物存活率进行比较:

- 观察到的预期负值>3
- 观察结果除以期望值>1.5
- *P* 值<0.05

如果该程序在最近 5 个 SRTR 版本中的两个中都超过了上述三个阈值,则 CMS 认为移植中心不符合结果。SRTR 报告了基于 2.5 年内同类群组的 1 年和 3 年结果。因此,实时追踪移植物和患者的存活情况对于促使计划积极于预早期发现和分析的问题非常重要,而不是等待 SRTR 发布的计划特定报告。

系统改进协议

不符合数量或结果要求的移植中心可能会收到 CMS 的系统改进协议(SIA)。该文件介绍了该程序保持有效的要求。从本质上讲,接受 SIA 的计划将被视为试用期,直到其结果或数量有所提高。这要求向该移植计划中列出的每个患者发送一封信,并在中心希望改善其数量和结果要求的情况下,如果他们希望转移至另一个计划,则向患者提供其他移植计划的联系信息。对于移植程序来说,这通常是非常昂贵的,并且据多个程序估计,这些程序的重建成本在 60 万~100 万美元。计划必须为同行评审小组付费,以评估他们的计划,并就移植计划必须采取的措施向 CMS 提出建议,以改善其结果。该同行评审小组通常由医生、移植管理员和质量顾问组成。必须将每个专业人员的简历发送给 CMS 进行审批。同行评审成员可能不会从当前属于 SIA 的计划中选择。该小组对移植计划进行 2~3 天的调查,并根据他们的发现向其提交报告。该报告提供了计划改进的建议,同行评审小组认为这将促进结果的改善。在向计划报告之前,将与领导和移植人员进行电话会议,在计划开始实施变更过程中,将在同行会议中概述同行评审小组的建议。

在根据SIA咨询移植计划的同行评审小组之后,还必须聘请质量顾问来进行每月8天的移植计划,为期约一年。该顾问将在移植计划中留在现场,与该计划一起分配时间,以改善其质量计划并实时跟踪数据,以确保该计划在其成果方面取得进展。质量顾问还帮助更新策略、协议和监视任何不良事件。SIA的CMS要求可能会因缺陷的严重程度而异,具体取决于程序。

有趣的是,在有人要求OPO提高器官捐赠率的时候,许多移植中心都越来越厌恶风险。为了提高结果,某些计划降低了DCD或ECD捐助者的风险。SIA下的计划也对患者和捐赠者的选择更为谨慎,以确保其结果得到改善。确定患者选择标准需要移植程序认真对待的过程。通常将标准写到协议中,但可能不会遵循所写的标准。CMS和OPTN在调查期间会仔细审查患者的选举标准,以确定政策或程序中记录的内容是否反映了当前的做法。根据CMS CoP,用于接受或拒绝患者进行移植的患者选择标准必须记录在患者的病历中。许多程序已经开发了清单,清单包含用于接受患者移植的选择标准以及用于拒绝移植的绝对或相对禁忌证。清单已完成,并由医师和协调员签名并放置在患者图表中。然后,依照团队决定将一封信发送给患者。这封信必须在决定后的10天内寄出。

移植中心的质量保证和绩效改善

现在,所有移植程序都必须具有全面的质量保证和性能改进(QAPI)程序,其性能衡量可反映法规要求,并具有可实时监控结果的特定于程序的指标。这些程序应以季度或半年为单位报告数据,从而证明医院QAPI程序中的集成。该报告通常与行政部门和医院董事会共享。强大的QAPI计划需要一个计划,该计划指定一个指导委员会,负责监督移植计划。如果移植程序要移植多个器官系统,则每个器官的质量委员会需要每月或每季度召开一次会议,以审查数据。该计划的QAPI计划和政策决定了会议的召开频率。QAPI计划的目标应包括:

- 根据实时指标确定改进机会。
- 优先考虑绩效改善项目。
- 持续跟踪患者护理和组织过程的结果。
- 监控法规要求。
- 确保政策和程序以证据为基础,定期进行审查和审核,以确保合规。
- 监测结果数据,以确保其在统计上符合国家标准和期望。

改变实践以将QAPI纳入繁忙的移植专业人员日程中,通常需要改变程序文化、观点和优先级。通过QAPI和法规环境,需要教育以使跨学科团队的各个成员加入这个新的透明时代。大多数人尚未接受有关QAPI所涉及流程的教育。因此,提出有关QAPI的程序以从结构、过程和结果方面解释其与移植的关系,有助于团队理解开发全面的数据驱动程序的理由。对员工进行SRTR成果教育是帮助团队了解CMS和UNOS如何审查计划的重要部分。了解SRTR如何分析每个中心提交的数据,有助于员工重视准确报告数据的重要性。强大的QAPI计划还包括每月一次的会议,以解决发病率和死亡率问题以及不良事件。必须让员工参加这些会议,才能参加在多学科团队环境中深入解决这些问题的讨论。深入研究以评估和分析已发现或潜在问题的根本原因,使计划可以认真考虑临床实践或政策可能需要进行的更改。

全球策略

迅速发展的移植领域为国际社会带来的挑战始于20世纪60年代,当时移植已成为一种临床现实。早期的实验性临床计划在立法真空中,在寻找和使用潜在的器官供体时要面对巨大的实际困难。死亡后同意捐赠需要什么?谁可以提供同意?面对分歧,谁能超越同意?捐赠人何时去世?心脏移植取代了肾脏移植,从而使真正意义的死亡实际上是核心问题,而心脏死亡的概念是心脏停跳导致的冰冷尸体。媒体在世界上每个发达国家中将每个新移植作为一个奇迹推广的作用,将人们的注意力提高到了政府和立法者不容忽视的水平。

尽管存在这些不确定性,并且大多数立法机构对器官捐赠均保持沉默,但医学界推动了医学领域的发展,并要求立法确定死亡。哈佛大学的委员会于1976年根据脑干的功能制订了死亡标准,这为使用心脏跳动捐赠者的器官开辟了道路,但在大多数国家(并非所有国家)都被接受。例如,日本根据这些原则起诉了在该国进行首例心脏移植手术的外科医生,这表明公众的态度、观点和标准会因国家、社区和宗教而受到不同的影响。日本的这一事件为 20 多年的立法停滞铺平了道路,直到最近才放宽,以允许家人同意在死后捐赠。

在 20 世纪 80 年代,随着许多国家对使用脑死亡标准进行立法,很明显,示范立法将对各国政府有所帮助,在全球范围内就有限的原则进行审议和达成协议也将是有益的。特别是在人体器官方面取得的科学进步导致在活人之间进行人体器官牟利,这违反了《世界人权宣言》。因此,世界卫生组织(WHO)的任务是为世界卫生大会审议、经过充分协商的一套指导原则,供会员国用于各自的国家法律文书来规范移植活动的模板。

世界卫生组织和世界卫生大会

世界卫生组织(WHO)是联合国的卫生机构,设在日内瓦和 6 个全球区域办事处。它由世界卫生大会(WHA)管辖,该大会本身就是其 194 个会员国的卫生大臣。参见 http://www.who.int/governance/en/,该网站提供了所有器官移植活动的标准化国际数据库,并包含有关不同国家法规的大量有用数据,并充当国际文件。

世界卫生大会旨在指导和管理国际事务来控制疾病、改善人类健康状况。世界卫生大会监督世界卫生组织认可指导原则,并 1991 年完成首次认可(WHA44.25 决议)。这些原则为现代移植实践的发展提供了基础,并且在 20 世纪 90 年代末以前一直很好地服务于临床项目。2004 年两个现象驱使世界卫生大会重新审查世界卫生组织指导原则:一是在发达国家供体数量未能满足临床移植需求,二是在亚洲、东欧和拉丁美洲的新兴经济体中,移植专业技术的扩散引起非法商业移植的增加。

经过广泛征求意见,在 2010 年 5 月 21 日第 63 届世界卫生大会通过了修订版世界卫生组织人体细胞、组织和器官移植指导原则 (WHA63.22)。请见 http://www.who.int/transplantation/en/和表 128.3。

世界卫生组织鼓励来自世界所有地区的专业人员和当局之间的合作,并提倡对移植成功带来的挑战采取共同的全球态度。世界卫生组织已建立计划协助国家卫生当局实施经修订的指导原则,包括全球移植知识库和全球捐献与移植观察站。这些计划联合西班牙国家器官移植部门 (ONT) 记录每年全球移植活动 (图 128.4、128.5)。网站提供了一个包含所有器官移植活动的标准化国际数据库,也纳入了不同国家的法律,可以作为国际文件的储存库[11,12]。

4D 计划——“从已故的捐赠者发展捐赠” 于 2006 年在科威特启动,并以第三次关于器官捐赠和移植的全球性磋商产生的《马德里决议》告终[13](有关目录,请参见:http//journals.lww.com/transplantjournal/toc/2011/06151)。《马德里决议》强调了政府的责任,即通过最大限度地提高死者在其本国境内的器官捐赠,努力实现自给自足以满足全球移植的明确需求。它还通过桥接诸如透析之类的疗法到捐赠以及移植安全性和结果测量,促进了对可移植疾病、可治疗疾病的国家责任和问责制的全面评估,从教育和预防措施避免了疾病。4D 计划体现了专业人士和主管部门之间的互补性,并且目前正在开发新的全球工具以及国家和次区域计划。

与意大利国家组织(CNT)合作进行的 NOTIFY 项目,该项目汇集了监管机构和学术机构的努力,以识别和减少疾病从捐赠者到接受者的传播,还可以识别发生的其他不良事件和反应。由于捐赠发生在接受者身上,可能会危害移植服务[14]。

区域政策

欧盟

过去的 20 多年中,欧洲委员会一直在欧洲进行器官捐献和移植方面的整理和合作。欧洲委员会的捐赠和移植委员会致力于提供数据并激发人们对欧洲内部移植问题的兴趣,尤其是在与该领域的道德和实践捐赠相关的方面。欧洲委员会成立于 1949 年,位于斯特拉斯堡,是一个由 47 个欧洲国家组成的包容性组织,致力于根据共同和民主原则保护个人,并由此继承器官移植的职责。

区别而言,欧洲联盟(EU)是 27 个国家之间的经济和政治伙伴关系,致力于经济合作以及促进人权和民主。欧盟议会拥有整个成员国的监管权,并制订了两项影响临床移植的主要指令。第一个指令涵盖了影响血液干细胞移植和组织库的细胞和组织,但是最近的《欧洲器官捐赠和移植质量和安全方面的立法框架》为欧盟国家规定了必需的器官捐赠和移植框架[15]。该指令具有约束力,要求建立或指定国家“主管部门”(即 FDA 的各种等同机构)负责质量和安全性结构,以涵盖临床捐赠和移植活动。欧盟指令随附了相当详细和规定性的行动计

表 128.3 2010 年世界卫生组织(WHO)对人体细胞、组织和器官移植指导原则

1.可以从死者尸体中取出细胞、组织和器官用以移植,假如:
(a)取得法律规定的任何同意;和
(b)没有理由相信死者反对这种移除。

2.确定潜在供体死亡的医生不应直接参与从供体移植的细胞、组织或器官或随后的移植手术;他们也不应该负责照顾这些细胞、组织和器官的任何预期接受者。

3.死者的捐赠应发展到最大的治疗潜力,但成年人可以在国内法规允许的范围内捐献器官。一般而言,活体捐赠者应该在遗传法律或情感上与其接受者相关。当获得捐助者的知情和自愿同意,确保捐助者的专业护理和后续组织良好,以及严格执行和监督捐助者的选择标准时,现场捐赠是可以接受的。应以完整和可理解的方式向活体捐赠者通报捐赠的可能风险、益处和后果;他们应该具有法律能力,能够权衡信息;他们应该心甘情愿地行事,不受任何不当影响或胁迫。

4.除了国家法律允许的狭隘例外情况外,不得为了移植目的而从活体未成年人体内取出细胞、组织或器官。应采取具体措施保护未成年人,并尽可能在捐赠前获得未成年人的同意。这适用于未成年人,也适用于任何法律上无能力的人。

5.细胞、组织和器官只能自由捐赠,不得以任何货币支付或其他货币价值奖励。应禁止购买或提供购买用于移植的细胞、组织或器官,或由活人或由死者亲属出售给死者。禁止销售或购买细胞、组织和器官并不排除偿还捐赠者发生的合理和可核实的费用,包括收入损失,或支付用于移植的人体细胞、组织或器官的回收、加工、保存和供应的费用。

6.可以根据国内法规,通过广告或公众呼吁促进人体细胞、组织或器官的利他捐赠。宣传细胞、组织或器官的需要或可用性,以便为个体的细胞、组织或器官提供或寻求支付,或者向个人死亡的近亲提供支付,应予以禁止。还应禁止向这些个人或第三方付款的经纪活动。

7.医生和其他卫生专业人员不应参与移植手术,如果相关的细胞、组织或器官是通过剥削或胁迫或支付给捐赠者而获得捐赠,则医疗保险公司和其他支付者不应承担此类手术。

8.应禁止所有参与细胞、组织或器官采购和移植手术的医疗机构和专业人员收到超过所提供服务的合理费用的任何付款。

9.器官、细胞和组织的分配应遵循临床标准和道德规范,而不是财务或其他考虑因素。由适当组成的委员会定义的分配规则应该是公平的、外部合理的和透明的。

10.对于捐赠者和接受者来说,高质量、安全和有效的程序是必不可少的。应评估活体捐献者和接受者的细胞、组织和器官捐赠和移植的长期结果,以记录益处和伤害。作为特殊性质的保健产品,必须持续维持和优化用于移植的人细胞、组织和器官的安全性、功效和质量水平。这需要实施质量体系,包括可追溯性和警惕性,报告国内和出口人类产品的不良事件和反应。

11.捐赠和移植活动的组织和执行及其临床结果必须透明且易于审查,同时确保捐赠者和接受者的个人匿名和隐私始终受到保护。

划,该计划必须立即执行(大纲计划见表 128.4)[16]。

该目前正在建立针对不良事件(如传播的感染或恶性肿瘤)的全欧洲标准安全报告系统、全欧洲的移植结果登记册以及在欧洲欠发达经济体中促进器官捐赠计划的工作。

南美

伊比利亚美洲理事会为南美在教育、农业、科学技术和卫生等许多领域的合作提供了结构，并为加强公共机构设计了项目。在这种情况下,西班牙和葡萄牙已经与伊比利亚-美洲合作组织合作,以支持和加强整个非洲大陆的器官捐赠和移植服务。与区域专业协会(拉丁美洲和加勒比海专业协会,STALYC)合作,确保了该地区国家之间的对话，其中一些国家制订了良好的移植计划,例如阿根廷、巴西、智利、乌拉圭,其中一些问题多于解决方案。

在过去 10 年中,由于移植商业主义和来访的移植游客的问题,哥伦比亚和秘鲁一直受到关注。哥伦比亚政府建立了一个强大的中央组织，旨在控制三个主要城市的器官移植计划,并成功地将“外国人换现金”的移植从 2000—2005 年的高水平降低到了较小的数字——到本世纪末可能不到每年 20 个。尽管在以色列采取了禁止以色列保险公司为在以色列进行的非法计划提供资金的行动，但以色列人和日本移植旅游者占据了交通的大部分,但已减少到以色列的一小部分。日本通过同样的机制限制了贸易，并强调通过起诉非法移植后返回的患者来对外国移植进行监管。

两个国家出现的困难不能掩盖南美大陆其他地方

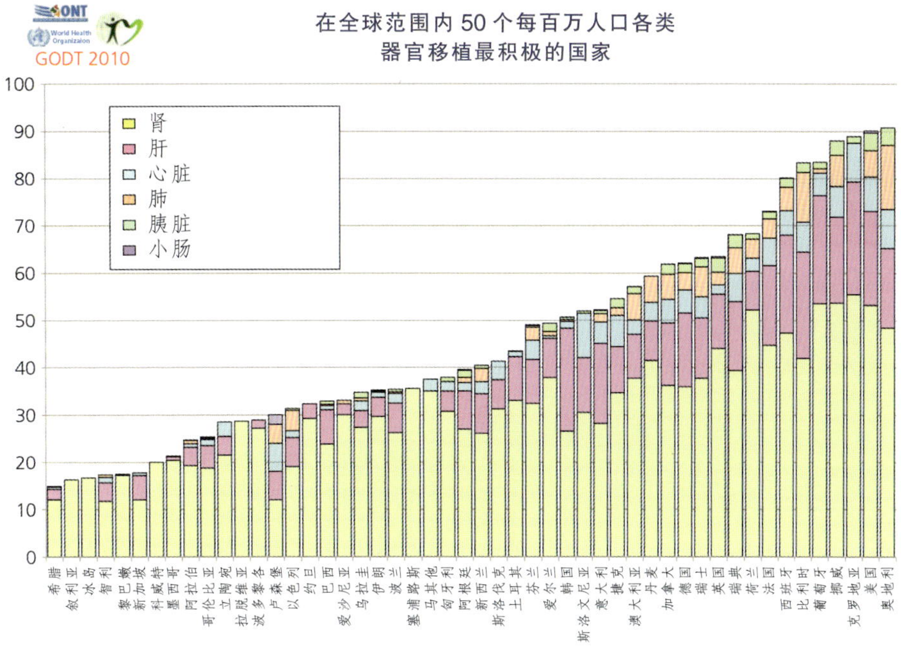

图 128.3　每百万人口各类器官移植最活跃的 50 个国家。Reproduced from [12] with permission from the World Health Organization. Based on the Global Observatory on Donation and Transplantation (GODT) data, produced by the WHO-ONT collaboration.

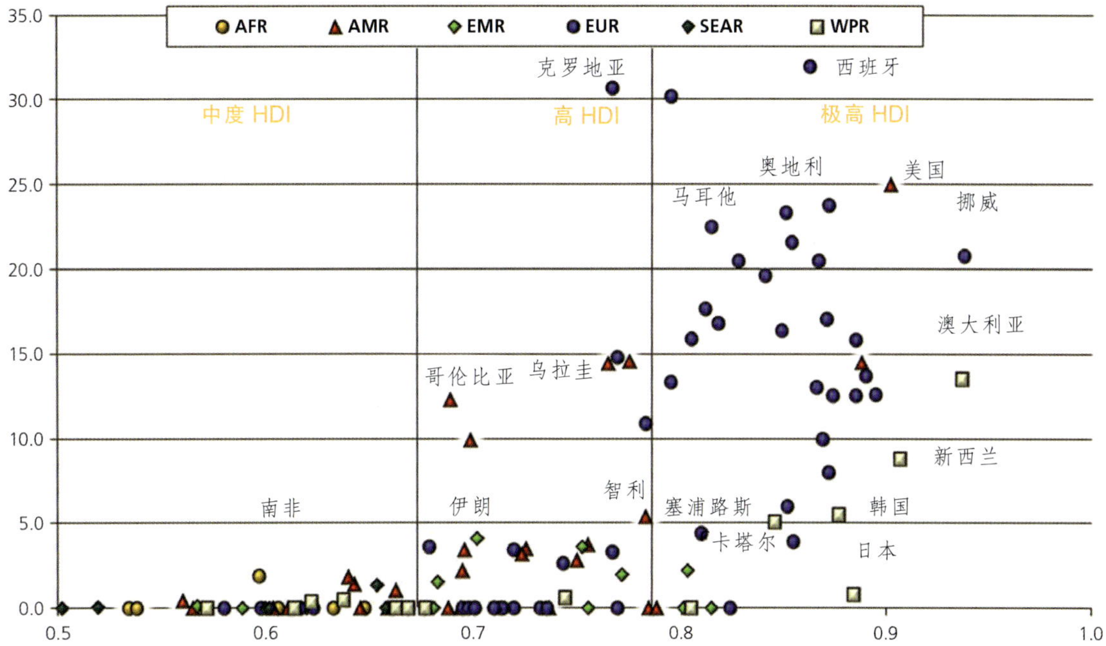

图 128.4　每百万人口器官捐献与国家人类发展指数有关。Reproduced from [12] with permission from the World Health Organization. Based on the Global Observatory on Donation and Transplantation (GODT) data, produced by the WHO-ONT collaboration.

的重大成就，例如巴西——全球每年为该国人口提供第三大数量的移植，智利、乌拉圭和阿根廷采取了出色的移植标准，以适应各自人口数量的大规模移植。如果较小的国家，特别是在地峡，能够满足其社区的需求，那么伊比利亚美洲理事会中明显的合作将需要扩大到区域能力共享。对于复杂的三级护理设施来说，太小了，也太穷了，如果没有几十年的发展，其中一些国家可能无法支持移植计划。

表 128.4 欧盟对器官捐献和移植的十点行动计划[16]

优先行动
1.在医院中促进移植协调者这一角色。
2.促进质量进展程序。
3.在欧盟中交换最佳的实践机会:支持肝移植注册登记。
4.提高卫生专业人员的知识和沟通技巧和器官移植患者支持团体。
5.促进欧洲器官捐赠者和跨境捐赠。
6.提高器官捐赠的组织模型。
7.促进整个欧盟对移植医学方面的协议。
8.促进国家当局之间的交换器官。
9.移植后的评估结果。
10.促进器官捐献/采购的通用认证系统和移植项目。

国际协会

移植协会(TTS)自 1966 年成立以来,不仅在该领域的科学和教育方面,而且在这种独特的临床实践的法律、法规和道德方面都发挥着重要作用。在世界上几乎每个具有临床移植计划的国家中,TTS 及其成员资格都在移植的发展中发挥了作用。国际肾脏病学会(ISN)同样在将教育和能力建设纳入全球尤其是新兴经济体的肾脏计划中也发挥了重要作用。这两个社会在建立有关移植临床实践道德方面的专业观点方面都发挥了重要作用,其中包括会员资格声明和会员资格指南文件。

TTS 于 20 世纪 80 年代首次制订了关于器官捐赠和反对人体商业化的正式伦理声明,随后又对其进行了多次修订。

TTS 与世界卫生组织合作,担任专家技术顾问,并于 2006 年成为与世界卫生组织建立正式关系的非政府组织。TTS 的作用是协助世界卫生组织制订和咨询有关指导原则的修订案。这是在世界所有地区并通过三次全球磋商完成的,并导致采用了上述原则。专业协会与世界卫生组织等政府和官方国际组织之间的这种联系在官方圈子中不被认为是自然而然的,因为人们认为专业组织通常存在利益冲突,这会妨碍客观性,而它们的参与只会增加既得利益。WHO-TTS 的参与对世界卫生组织指导原则的审查结果既相关又重要,这证明了合作双方的个人作用。

伊斯坦布尔宣言

制订专业临床实践指南仍然是国家、地区和国际社会的重要角色,在器官捐赠和移植领域,有许多指南证明了这一角色。TTS 和 ISN 正是从这个工作的角度来解决器官捐赠的伦理和实践问题以及器官捐赠者,特别是活体器官捐赠者的权利。2008 年在伊斯坦布尔召开了来自 78 个国家的 150 多人的首脑会议,会议背景涉及哲学、法律、公共管理和医学。

最终的《伊斯坦布尔宣言》(DOI)[19,20]旨在支持《赫尔辛基宣言》,指导临床实践和研究。既定的《赫尔辛基宣言》保护人类研究对象的权利,但 DOI 却保护着人体器官捐赠者的权利。DOI 包含四个重要定义(表 128.5),这些定义为评估特定实例或相关问题提供了指导。DOI 中包含的六项原则和七项建议旨在解决这个世界应如何通过医疗保健媒介以及世界上的弱势社区,摆脱移植商业谋利的损毁和猖獗的破坏性进展、人体商品化以及富人对穷人日益猖獗的掠夺。

此后,DOI 得到了 100 多个专业协会、国家政府和非政府组织的认可。成立了一个监护小组,以鼓励实施和工作组来自世界各地的个人专注于 DOI 的各个方面。自 2008 年以来,活跃在移植商业的关注名单上的国家数量有所减少,非法移植的数量有所减少,但是等待名单长和器官不足以满足富人需求的驱动力将继续与贫困相结合。

总结

无论临床医生如何看待,移植都是临床实践中不仅对公民社会带来了巨大的好处,而且带来了巨大的风险和挑战的一个领域。因此,与大多数临床工作相比,它受到更严格的监管(表 128.6)。没有死者捐赠者的监督和立法,器官捐赠将一直处于法律困境,无法利用社区价值支持死后捐献器官,将无法制订和支持安全规范,在劳动力发展和医院基础设施的投资将变得更加零碎。移植已经从昂贵的实验主义阶段,通过有争议的临床应用和方法逐渐发展进入另一个阶段,在这一阶段中,移植已成为全世界标准临床护理的正常和公认的一部分。政府和非政府机构与专业人士的合作与协作仍然是剩余过渡的基石。

表 128.5 从伊斯坦布尔宣言定义[19,20]

器官贩卖	招募、运输、转移、隐匿或收到在世的或是已经死去的人或自己的器官，以威胁或使用武力或其他形式的强迫、绑架、诈骗、欺骗、滥用权力强迫弱势者,或为接收、给第三方支付或福利实现转移控制潜在的捐赠者,剥削的目的用于移植的器官
移植商业谋利	器官被视为一个商品,包括被收购或出售或使用从而得到物质利益
移植形成的旅行	器官、捐赠者、受者或者移植专家为了移植这一意图发生的转移。为了移植而旅行会被定义为移植旅行，只要其中包括了非法交易或者物质利益，如果这一行为超出了本国的所能提供的移植服务

表 128.6 器官捐献和移植的全球监管的关键要素时间表

1976	美国—哈佛大学特设脑干死亡委员会
1984	美国—国家器官移植行为((NOTA)
1994	全球健康集会 WHA 44.25 — WHO 为器官捐赠提供指导意见
1998	美国—CMS 常规推荐规则
2000	美国—CMS OPO 认证机制
2006	美国—CMS OPO 覆盖情况
2007	美国—CMS 移植程序最终规则
2008	伊斯坦布尔宣言
2008	欧盟—器官捐献和移植欧洲行动计划
2010	世界卫生协会 WHA 63.22—WHO 修订指导器官捐赠与移植原则

(郭海军 译　徐骁 校)

参考文献

1. One Hundred Milestone Documents. Social Security Act Amendments of 1965. [accessed December 27, 2011]; Available from: http://ourdocuments.gov/doc.php?flash=true&doc=99.
2. Health Resources and Services Administration. *Selected Statutory and Regulatory History of Organ Transplantation.* [accessed December 27, 2011]; Available from: http://www.organdonor.gov/legislation/legislationhistory.html.
3. Centers for Medicare and Medicaid Services. *Conditions of Coverage and Conditions of Participation.* [accessed December 27, 2011]; Available from: https://www.cms.gov/CFCsAndCoPs/.
4. Studer, Quint. Healthcare Flywheel: Prescriptive To Do's. Hardwiring Excellence. Fire Starter Publishing: Gulf Breeze, FL, 2003: 28.
5. Centers for Medicare and Medicaid Services. *Deeming Overview.* [accessed December 27, 2011]; Available from: https://www.cms.gov/Deeming/.
6. Centers for Medicare and Medicaid Services. Hospital Conditions of Participation: Requirements for Approval and Re-Approval of Transplant Centers To Perform Organ Transplants; [accessed January 31, 2012]; Available from: https://www.cms.gov/CertificationandComplianc/Downloads/Transplantfinal.pdf.
7. Organ Procurement and Transplantation Network. Policies/Identification of Transmissible Diseases in Organ Recipients. [accessed December 27, 2011]; Available from: http://optn.transplant.hrsa.gov/PoliciesandBylaws2/policies/pdfs/policy_16.pdf.
8. Organ Procurement and Transplantation Network. Data Reports. [accessed December 27, 2011]; Available from: http://optn.transplant.hrsa.gov.
9. Punch JD, Hayes DH, LaPorte FB, et al. Organ Donation and Utilization in the US, 1995–2005. American Journal of Transplantation. 2007;7(Pt 2):1327–1338.
10. Association of Organ Procurement Organizations. *Resources/Related Links: Data on Organ Donation and Transplantation.* [accessed December 27, 2011]; Available from: http://www.aopo.org/related-links-data-organ-donation-transplantation-a40.
11. World Health Organization. [accessed January 18, 2012]; Available from: http://www.who.int/transplantation/knowledgebase/en/.
12. Global Observatory on Donation and Transplantation. [accessed January 18, 2012]; Available from: http://www.transplant-observatory.org/pages/home.aspx.
13. Public Health, Vigilance and Surveillance of Substances of Human Origin. [accessed 18 Jan 2012]; Available from: http://www.sohovs.org/soho/.
14. The Madrid resolution on organ donation and transplantation: national responsibility in meeting the needs of patients, guided by the WHO principles. Transplantation. 2011;91(Suppl 11):S29–S31.
15. 2010/53/EU of the European Parliament and of the Council of 7 July 2010 on standards of quality and safety of human organs intended for transplantation. [accessed 25 Mar 2014]; Available from: http://europa.eu/legislation_summaries/public_health/threats_to_health/sp0008_en.htm.
16. Communication from the Commission of 8 December 2008 – Action plan on Organ Donation and Transplantation (2009–2015): Strengthened Cooperation between Member States. [accessed 25 Mar 2014]; Available from: http://europa.eu/legislation_summaries/public_health/threats_to_health/sp0007_en.htm.
17. Danovitch GM, Chapman J, Capron AM, et al. Organ trafficking and transplant tourism: the role of global professional ethical standards-the 2008 Declaration of Istanbul. Transplantation. 2013;15;95(11):1306.
18. Huang J, Wang H, Fan ST, et al. The national program for deceased organ donation in China. Transplantation. 2013;15;96(1):5–9.
19. Organ trafficking and transplant tourism and commercialism: the declaration of Istanbul. Lancet. 2008;372:5–6.
20. The Declaration of Istanbul. [accessed 25 Mar 2014]; Available from: http://www.declarationofistanbul.org.

第 129 章 腹部实体器官移植专科医师培训

Rachel C. Forbes and Mitchell L. Henry

引言

移植学从本质上来说属于外科学的范畴，囊括了对终末器官衰竭患者的各种治疗措施。复杂的手术操作和严重的疾病需要移植外科医生拥有出色的的外科操作技巧和对潜在疾病的丰富知识，而这往往超出了许多外科亚专科的专业范畴。由于移植已经成为大部分终末器官衰竭的标准治疗，美国移植外科医师协会(ASTS)充分认识到移植医师规范化专科培训的重要性。本章讨论移植专科医师制的历史、专科医师选择的过程、美国专科医师培训要求、教育创新，以及移植手术受训者的前景展望。医学专业的专科医师培训在第130章有特别说明。

移植专科医师制的历史

1954年，在Peter Bent Brigham医院，首例器官移植在一对双胞胎兄弟成功实施。整形外科医生Joseph E. Murray实施受体手术，泌尿科医生J. Hartwell Harrison实施供体手术。在随后的几十年中，得益于强力的免疫抑制剂，特别是环孢霉素的出现，移植作为一门专科获得了蓬勃发展。在20世纪80年代，肺、胰腺和心脏移植相继获得了成功。供器官来源自那时起就成为了一个制约因素。1974年，一群大多未经过规范化移植专科训练的外科医生，组建了ASTS。他们希望ASTS促进学科的发展，从而造福移植受者。ASTS自始至终都致力于规范管理从事腹部实体器官移植的专科医师[1]。

James Cerilli，ASTS主席(1980—1981年)，成立了教育委员会，确定了规范化移植专科医师培训的认证。Cerilli医师首先与美国外科医生委员会、美国外科医师学院和美国医学协会的住院医师审查委员会进行讨论，建立移植培训计划并进行审查[2]。经过对这些计划的审议，认定这些审查程序“不适合”移植培训计划。显而易见，ASTS应为移植专科培训的监督机构，并承担移植专科培训。Cerilli医师通知有兴趣进行移植专科培训项目的单位，向教育委员会提交申请。然后，教育委员会对课程进行现场检查，向ASTS委员会提交一份正式报告，建议批准合格的课程。当时，专科培训的重点是肾移植，受训者必须通过美国手术委员会或美国泌尿学委员会的认证。培训的持续时间不少于12个月，每年开展不少于35例移植。或者，培训过程延长至两年，期间实施50例移植。

1985年，时任ASTS主席的A.P.Monaco正式将专科医师培训期限延长至24个月。他认为应该强调基础科学和免疫学，提倡在专科医师培训过程中至少应有一年从事基础研究。他还支持至少每两年对教育委员会指导的每个培训计划进行审查。1987年，ASTS继任主席Robert Corry确定，所有移植中心应至少有一名移植外科医生参与ASTS认可或授权的专科医师培训计划，时间至少一年，而这是被器官共享网络UNOS接纳的必备条件。随着肝脏、胰腺和小肠移植数量的增加，确立了每个移植中心保持认证所需的最小移植数量。

从1980年到2000年，移植外科医生的培训程序基本上由相应的地区进行管理，而在国家层面由ASTS的监督较少。最后，Sandy Feng等向当时的教育委员会主席Mitchell L. Henry建议进行匹配。这种匹配的目的是向住院医师保证，即该计划将履行其对住院医师的承诺，住院医师将履行他/她参与计划的承诺。由教育委员会建议，并且 ASTS 委员会随后批准，由国家住院医师匹配计划(NRMP)推动，在专科医师候选者和受监管的移植中心之间进行正式匹配。

程序认证要求

根据 NRMP 的要求，腹部移植外科专科医师培训计划的目标是训练既有熟练的外科技术又有终末期器官疾病和移植管理经验的医师。该目标应通过一个模式化的培训计划来实现，在培训中腹部器官移植外科的专科医师能在正确的指导下治疗相应的疾病，同时完成学习。

ASTS 培训计划建议向每位受训者提供的移植数量为 75 例，以便其在培训过程中担任初级外科医生。目前，一个专科医师必须实施 30 例肾移植、45 例肝移植、15 例胰移植和 10 例肠移植，才能获得 ASTS 的认证。每位受训者应提交一份数量达标的病例清单，以便从 ASTS 的认证计划获得培训证书。UNOS 要求移植外科医生完成上述相同数量的病例，通过 ASTS 批准的培训计划，方可成为特定器官移植中心的主任。也就是说，要成为肝脏移植的主任，个人必须接受 ASTS 批准的肝脏移植专科医师培训计划的培训，并完成所要求数量的病例。

原本 ASTS 坚持认为 ASTS 有能力也有责任对培训计划进行认证。然而，培训过程中确保受训者完成各项培训要求并安全地独立开展工作是培训计划的具体实施者，而非 ASTS。因此，受训者并不是从 ASTS 获得特定的实体器官移植的认证，而是从 ASTS 获得表示他们已成功达到培训计划要求的完成证书。目前，北美有 74 个 ASTS 批准的移植专科医师培训方案（表 129.1）。

表 129.1　ASTS 批准的培训方案(2007—2012 年)

方案	2007	2008	2009	2010	2011	2012
仅肾	13	12	14	18	20	21
仅肝	3	3	2	2	2	2
肾/肝	24	26	26	27	26	26
肾/胰	4	4	5	6	5	5
肾/肝/胰	23	23	20	12	12	14
肾/肝/胰/肠	0	0	0	3	3	3
肾/肝/肠	0	0	0	2	3	3
方案总数	67	68	67	70	72	74

实体器官移植培训计划的入选

2005 年腹部实体器官移植专科培训成为匹配程序的一部分。合格的专科医师候选人必须完成符合美国外科学会或美国泌尿学会认证的住院医师培训或同等的境外培训。NRMP 负责实施 ASTS 的匹配计划。NRMP 明确规定由申请人负责联系他们意向的中心，目录由 ASTS 网站提供。中心主任审查候选人的资格，并进行本中心的面试。专科医师培训申请者在他们的志愿列表(ROL)中相应地排列他们的意向，由程序相应地对他们的申请进行排名。每年 6 月的第三个星期三，NRMP 匹配项目将宣布结果。未得到匹配的申请人和中心通常参加匹配后的争夺以填补空缺职位。NRMP 自 2006 年程序启动以来的数据见表 129.2[3]。

腹部器官移植专科医师培训的未来方向

工作时间限制

目前对腹部器官移植专科医师培训的监督仍然由 ASTS 教育委员会实施，现称专科医师培训委员会。目前尚无计划将这些专科医师培训计划纳入美国毕业后医学教育认证委员会(ACGME)或住院医师管理委员会(RRC)进行审查，并且要获得 ACGME 的认证也不是一个简单过程。ACGME 和 ASTS 都非常关注住院医师的工作时间。专科医师的休息时间表最终由中心自行决定，但规定的工作量在 2008 年 1 月 ASTS 发布的指南中已经正式提出。

该指南指出：

1.移植专科医师培训计划有责任确保安全和负责任的工作习惯。

2.促进医生保持健康的心态，并奠定成为一个成功的移植外科医生的基础。

3.过度工作对于患者的健康和安全不利。

此外，由于移植手术的时间安排很随机，指南列举了以下四个原则：

1.中心应意识到专科医师的各方面的工作量(例如诊所、手术室、住院服务、电话呼叫等)。

2.专科医师必须能自由表达休息的需求。

3.教职人员必须认识到有时需要告诉专科医师应该休息。

4.对于教职人员既不进行教育又不布置专科医师进行实践的行为需要不断地进行审查。

这些原则提供了指南,ASTS 专科医师培训的具体要求如下:

1.培训计划应为受训者指定正式的继续医学教育时间,包括每年至少参加一次全国会议,不可占用休假时间。

2.每年应至少提供两周的假期,如果每年只指定一周的会议时间,则最多为三周。

3.培训计划以外总的休假和会议时间每年不应超过四周。

4.受训者应该每月至少一个周末和每月至少两个额外的24小时期间(不包括休假)脱离临床工作。

美国移植外科医师协会(ASTS)课程

自从移植专科医师培训开始以来,基于器官移植配额的病例和患者管理的体验式学习一直是对受训人员的要求。正式的教学方式在不同中心之间可能是不同的。因此,ASTS 要求课程委员会提供一个综合的基于网络的课程,称为“学术之家”(Academic Universe)。学术之家由以下四个部分组成:①课程;②在线手术日志;③资格证书存储;④使用报告。

ASTS 的课程由精心设计的学习模块组成,并定义了掌握移植手术领域所必需的关键知识领域。学术之家中的主题包括免疫生物学和移植研究、药理学和免疫抑制、器官采集、移植的医学并发症、肾移植、肝移植、胰腺移植、肾脏替代治疗、器官分配公共政策、伦理,以及移植的经济学。目前有13个单元,包含160个

表 129.2 美国国家住院医师匹配项目(NRMP)数据

	2005年匹配 2006年职位	2006年匹配 2007年职位	2007年匹配 2008年职位	2008年匹配 2009年职位	2009年匹配 2010年职位	2010年匹配 2011年职位	2011年匹配 2012年职位
项目							
积极项目	45	51	48	61	56	66	59
项目完成	67%	69%	58%	67%	67%	74%	69%
抽签信息							
积极职位(抽签)	60	67	65	78	71	79	72
职位完成	65%	72%	65%	71%	74%	77%	69%
申请者信息							
积极申请者	52	69	64	86	96	94	80
匹配申请者	75%	70%	66%	64%	55%	65%	63%
失败申请者							
积极美国本土毕业生	21	22	18	25	28	22	21
匹配美国本土毕业生	18	22	18	25	25	22	21
占比	86%	100%	100%	100%	89%	100%	100%
积极美国籍外国人	2	4	0	3	1	5	2
匹配美国籍外国人	2	4	0	2	0	5	1
占比	100%	100%	N/A	67%	0%	100%	50%
积极加拿大人	4	5	2	0	2	1	2
匹配加拿大人	2	4	2	0	2	1	2
占比	50%	80%	100%	N/A	100%	100%	100%
积极外国人	25	37	42	57	65	65	53
匹配外国人	17	17	20	28	26	32	24
占比	68%	46%	48%	49%	40%	49%	45%

以上的演示文稿，每个大约 20 分钟。每个模块包括语音叙述的演示、文本摘要、推荐参考文献、自我评估和反馈机制。现在 ASTS 要求受训者在完成器官移植的轮转之外，完成这些在线学习模块，以完全获得认证。

其他认证可能性

在许多肝移植中心，肝移植外科医生还针对多种恶性和良性的肝胆病例进行治疗。受训者可以通过施行解剖和非解剖性肝切除术、腹腔镜肝切除术、胰腺切除术等获得重要的经验。ASTS 将在未来对那些在相应肝胆外科领域有丰富经验的医生颁发特殊的认证。

由于肾移植涉及终末期肾病（ESRD）的患者并且与血管手术相关，移植外科医生经常需要建立血管通路用于血液透析。事实上，随着 ESRD 患者数量的增多，建立血管通路已成为普通外科医生最常进行的手术之一。受训者可以在他们的移植研究培训期间施行大量的血管通路手术，因此有必要专门开发一个项目用于培养血液透析的丰富经验。

急症护理也是受训者的重要培训内容，尤其是对施行肝移植手术的终末期肝病患者的围术期护理。也可以探讨对在移植重症监护中获得强化训练的专科医师颁发特别的证书进行认证。

总结

自第一例移植开展以来，移植手术在数十年的发展中需求和成功率持续增长。ASTS 负责对移植外科进行整体规范，可以相信已认识到对移植外科专科医师进行正式培训的必要性。经过许多 ASTS 领导者的思考和努力，移植外科作为一个亚专科已被公认，自成体系对移植外科医生进行培训。各个移植专科医师培训中心及其领导者花费了大量精力来培训未来的外科医生、研究人员和移植领域的领导者。

（高峰 译　高峰 校）

参考文献

1. ASTS Website. [accessed January 04, 2014]; Available from: http://www.ASTS.org.
2. Salvatierra O, Lum CT, editors. History of the American Society of Transplant Surgeons: On the Occasion of its 20th Anniversary. Stanton Publications, Minneapolis. 1994.
3. NRMP Website. [accessed January 04, 2014]; Available from: http://www.nrmp.org/fellow/match_name/abdom_trans_surg/about.html.

第 130 章
实体器官移植的专科医师培训

Deirdre Sawinski and Roy D. Bloom

引言

在过去 60 年中，实体器官移植得到飞速的发展，从早期只能针对一些高度选择的个体进行的临床实验，演变为现在世界范围内造福成千上万患者及其家庭的成熟治疗。最初，除了外科医生以外，具有特定器官系统专业知识的移植亚专科医生在这个领域发挥了重要的功能。移植专家的主要责任是保持器官移植供者和受者的最佳状态，包括诊断和管理这些特殊患者的并发症。移植学科的不断发展，受者和移植物存活情况的持续改善要求我们有更多的受过相应专科训练的医学亚专科医生。本章讨论了北美地区移植专科医生培训计划的历史、现状和对未来的展望。外科训练计划在第 129 章讨论。

历史

管理移植供者和受者的移植医学专家可追溯到 1954 年，在第一次成功的人肾移植后，Peter Merrill——哈佛医学院 Peter Bent Brigham 医院的一名肾脏科医生，被普遍公认为团队的关键成员。在移植发展的早期，那些有志成为移植医生的受训者无法接受正式的培训。相反，根据美国毕业后医学教育认证委员会(ACGME)要求，肾病学、胃肠病学、心脏病学和肺脏学的医学亚专业领域的受训者会在其相应的培训过程中学习移植医学中的一些基本原则。时至今日，这些 ACGME 的要求总的来说仍然有效。例如，在一般的肾病学训练计划中，移植相关的培训在总体所需的两年临床实践中的占比为 10%~15%。历史上，通过完成一般的肾脏学研究培训要求，符合资格或认证的肾病专科医生将“有资格”随后作为移植肾科医生。这些受训者通常将在高年资移植临床医生的指导和帮助下接受培训。

1981 年，考虑到不断增加的基础研究和临床发展的需要，一部分肾移植科医生建议当时的美国肾病学会(ASN)成立一个单独的移植医师协会。这个决定促成了 1982 年美国移植医师学会[AST，前身是美国移植医师协会(ASTP)]的成立。AST 作为目前移植领域最大的协会，其主要目标之一即是促进和鼓励开展关于器官/组织移植和免疫学的临床/科研的教育和研究。第一次年会在 1982 年举行，随后于 1996 年成立了移植专科医师研讨会。两年后，AST/ASN 的肾移植专科医师培训计划诞生了。

目前，移植肝病学和晚期心力衰竭/移植心脏病学是唯一经 ACGME 认可的医学移植亚专科：①必须经过相应领域的正式培训，并且②正式由美国内科医学委员会(ABIM)管理。大多数非 ACGME 认可的特定器官移植亚专科的委员会要求受训者必须完成该专科的充分培训。由于这些亚专科培训计划不是 ACGME 认证的，这种额外的移植特定培训并不是强制性的。然而，器官共享联合网络(UNOS)要求满足这些先决条件，以便医生成为特定器官移植的负责人[1]。此外，大多数移植培训计划现在优先考虑招聘已经进行额外的特定器官移植培训的移植医生。各种特定器官移植亚专科的要求将在后面的章节中讨论。

移植专科医师培训的基本原则

移植专科医师培训的主要目的是为培训者提供强化和拓展的移植临床经验，首要关注于相应的特定器官。因此，受训者可以在结构化的培训计划中获得独立开展移植临床工作和科学研究所需的必要经验和技能。为此，移植专科医师培训包括器官分配、移植伦理、器官捐赠和获取、受者评估和受者名单管理、HLA 实验室管理、受者和供者的移植手术的教学和实践、移植后早期/晚期并发症和护理。在某些情况下，也可能包括学术交流活动。

当前特定器官培训要求

肾

1998 年，ASN 和 AST 共同建立了 AST/ASN 肾移植专科医师培训计划，由 AST/ASN 肾移植研究基金认证委员会管理。这个委员会负责认证机构、制订方案、提供肾移植的专业培训。认证基于深入的现场调查（包括在开始时以及之后的定期间隔），以及审核关于移植培训计划的年度报告。AST/ASN 肾移植专科医师培训计划的目标是移植培训的标准化，为希望接受肾移植专科医师培训的人提供统一的医学教育。作为这个标准化过程的一部分，AST/ASN 肾移植专科医师培训计划最近制订了一个经认可的移植中心在研究培训期间预期覆盖的最低限度的培训内容[2]（表 130.1）。肾移植专科医师培训计划既要与 UNOS 认可的移植中心相关，也要与 ACGME 认可的普通肾脏疾病培训相关联，方可获得认可。目前，大约有 60 个移植中心，主要位于美国和加拿大，已经被 AST/ASN 肾移植专科医师培训计划认证委员会认证。

表 130.1　肾移植专科医师培训内容。数据来源[2]:www.a-s-t.org

移植免疫学
免疫抑制学
• 诱导
• 维持
移植并发症
• 感染（CMV，BK，EBV）
• 高血压
• 高脂血症
• 移植后高血糖
• 移植相关恶性肿瘤
器官分配
受者评估
供者评估
移植功能障碍
• 放弃
• 反复或新生疾病
移植结果
儿科移植
道德伦理学

肾移植专科医师必须进入 ACGME 认可的普通肾脏专科培训计划，因此必须是经过认证的或有资格的肾病科医师。相应的医学中心必须有足够的肾移植数量，要求能为每个第一年普通肾病学培训人员提供 10 例肾移植，并为每个肾移植专科医师提供 30 例肾移植。肾移植专科医师应该至少管理 30 例初次住院接受移植的病例，并管理 30 例肾移植后 3 个月内门诊随访的病例。临床培训应关注肾移植受者的当前和长期的管理，并且应与外科团队共同协作。肾移植专科医师应在透析、高血压治疗、移植后高血糖管理和免疫抑制方案的决策中提供医疗支持。移植专科医师必须至少进行 3 次器官采集和至少 3 次肾移植手术。移植专科医师必须进行至少 10 次肾移植活检，并且必须熟悉活检指征、技术、潜在并发症/并发症管理，以及病理学表现。

在编写本书时，肾移植专科医师培训计划只有一种设定。其包括连续 12 个月的训练，其中至少 6 个月为专门的住院临床训练，而剩余的时间用于其他相关活动（例如在 HLA 实验室或其他器官移植服务）或移植领域的研究。本质上，该设定强调“临床”移植经验，大多数通过培训的受训者最终在临床移植中获得认证。最近 ASN 和 AST 委员会批准了一项建议，准备创建另一种培训计划设定，更多地面向研究型学员，但尚未实施。这种替代的“研究型”设定将使得有兴趣在临床或基础研究中做出成绩的研究人员有机会达到最小的临床需求，以便有更多的精力投入到研究工作中。成功完成肾移植专科医师培训计划后，移植中心的主任必须为每位受训者提供一份证明信，表明其符合所有上述标准，并且能够被认证成为 UNOS 移植医师。证明位的复印件以及证实移植医生已参加所需的教学课程并具备患者管理经验的声明，会同时发送给 AST 国家办公室和培训完成者。

胰腺

胰腺移植的专科培训可以在内分泌科或肾病科完成。该计划需要一年的移植培训，其中 6 个月专门用于临床活动，6 个月用于研究。受训者必须管理至少 8 例胰腺移植患者，并门诊随访至少 8 例胰移植门诊（至少

3个月)。3例或更多的移植患者应该是联合脏器移植(胰肾同期移植或先肾后胰腺移植)。受训者应至少观察3例器官采集和至少3例器官移植。由于移植胰腺活检在大多数中心并非常规开展，目前培训内容没有囊括移植胰腺活检。

肝

肝移植专科医师培训计划由ABIM通过ACGME监督。ABIM是一个独立的非盈利组织,负责对医疗专业人士的评估。ACGME负责对医学博士毕业后的继续教育计划的认证，这些认证是基于被同行接受的标准和指南的。肝移植专科医师需要完成ACGME认可的肠病学专科培训,然后再进行移植肝病学的额外培训。肝移植专科医师培训计划包括12个月的以肝移植为重点的培训;为了满足所有培训计划要求,临床工作所占比例高于基础研究。培训必须在隶属于UNOS并经ACGME认证的肝脏移植中心完成。这些中心必须能够完成经颈静脉肝内门腔分流的介入治疗，每年必须完成至少25次肝脏移植[3]。培训计划必须提供ACGME要求的肝病学和移植的正式教学指导(表130.2)。

受训者应参加至少10名拟行肝移植的患者的初步评估、汇报和讨论。根据ACGME要求,受训者需要诊疗至少20例肝移植受者，并且必须对20例以上移植受者进行不少于3个月的门诊随访。受训者还必须诊疗至少20例移植后存活超过一年的肝移植受者。UNOS建议应包含至少3例的肝脏和其他器官联合移植[1]。受训者需要在整个临床年度连续出诊。必须观察至少3次肝脏获取和至少3次肝移植。受训者必须进行至少30次经皮肝穿活检,必须熟悉活检指征、技术、潜在并发症及并发症管理。为了获得病理学的经验,他们必须对至少200例肝穿活检[健康和(或)移植的]做出病理学描述。在他们的移植培训计划结束时,受训者可以参加额外的资格认证,并且在实践中通过考核。过去，没有经过正式培训但具有临床经验的从业人员也可以通过“实践路径”的考核而获得认证,但这种机制现在已经被淘汰。

表130.2 肝移植专科医师培训内容。数据来源[3]:www.acgme.org

急性和慢性终末期肝病(ESLD)
ESLD患者的评估与诊疗
ESLD并发症
• 难治性腹水
• 肝性胸水
• 肝肾综合征
• 门脉肺高压
• 门静脉高血压出血
肝细胞癌和胆管上皮癌
慢性病毒性肝炎
暴发病毒性肝炎
移植免疫
药物毒性
营养支持
门静脉高压的诊疗
道德伦理学

心脏

2012年7月，心脏移植专科医师资格也获得了ACGME认证。这个专科培训非常特殊,因为培训覆盖了心力衰竭患者诊疗的所有细节,而非限于移植。受训者需要接受心力衰竭、心脏装置(心室辅助装置、起搏器、植入式心律转复除颤器)和移植的训练。受训者必须首先完成ACGME认证的心血管医学专科培训。12个月的培训必须在隶属于UNOS的心脏移植中心进行,每年至少进行20例心脏移植。培训主要侧重于临床工作,研究工作的时间有限。受训者应该熟悉急/慢性心力衰竭的诊疗,使用机械辅助装置、受体选择和术后免疫抑制管理。ACGME已概述了在培训期（表130.3)中教授的教学内容,这种临床工作必须是连续性的。

专科医师应至少评估5名进行心脏移植或机械辅助装置植入的患者。专科医师必须在住院和门诊随访中管理至少20例的心脏移植受者。在这些患者中，UNOS建议至少3个应该是心肺联合移植[1],但这不是ACGME要求的。受训者必须至少进行3次器官获取和3次心脏移植手术。专科医师应在住院和门诊中管理至少50名植入心脏复律除颤器的患者以及至少30名的机械辅助装置植入患者。为了证明技术熟练程度,受训者还应进行至少40次心内膜活检,熟悉潜在的并发症,并能够解释病理结果。该医生必须对植入的设备进行至少100次检查,能够解释结果并调整设备设置。在完成培训计划后，受训者可以参加ABIM高级心力衰竭和移植心脏病学认证考试。2014年后在这一领域,允许没有完成ACGME移植专科培训但具有三年以上

表 130.3 心脏移植专科医师培训内容。数据来源[3]:www.acgme.org

移植免疫学
免疫抑制
移植的临床并发症
• 条件性感染
• 高血压
• 肾功能不全
• 移植相关性恶性肿瘤
器官分配
受者评估(移植装置,再同步,移植)
慢性心力衰竭的急性心脏代偿失调
移植失败
• 放弃
• 心脏移植后血管病变
浸润性和炎症性心肌病
肺动脉高血压
遗传性心肌病
由于以下因素的心力衰竭
• 化疗
• 先天性心脏病
• 怀孕
其他实体器官受者的心力衰竭
心律不齐
肥大性心肌病
移植病理学

实践经验的现有从业人员通过"实践路径"获得认证。

肺

全美有超过 45 个 UNOS 认证的肺移植中心,但其中能有足够多的病例支持专科医师培训计划的大中心很少。因此,肺移植专科医师培训并未获得 ACGME 认证,也不受国际心肺移植学会监督,而是通常参考 UNOS 提供的培训准则。肺移植专科医师培训可以在肺部或重症监护专科培训后额外增加一年培训，也可以和标准的三年肺科医师专科培训整合在一起。如果培训只是基于临床,则通常为 12 个月,如果培训期间合并研究工作,则延长至 24 个月。

根据 UNOS 的要求[1],受训者应参与至少 15 例肺或心肺联合移植受者的诊疗。其中至少一半应是单肺或双肺受体。受训者必须至少进行 3 次肺部供体获取和至少 3 次肺移植手术。受训者应熟悉急性和慢性肺衰竭患者的管理,熟练掌握体外循环和呼吸机管理,以及供受体的选择。受训者应该进行支气管内活检,熟悉潜在的并发症,并能够解释病理结果。

感染性疾病

移植相关感染性疾病专科医师培训通常在完成 ACGME 认证的感染性疾病(ID)专科医师培训后额外展开一年的培训,但这并非必须。一般来说 ACGME 认证的 ID 培训中临床过程的比例很大，但如果 ID 培训时间是 3 年(或更长),则可将正式的移植专科培训整合在一起。移植相关的培训为 12 个月,其中至少 6 个月的临床工作,包括住院和门诊。移植 ID 专科培训计划在多器官联合移植中心实施，能够提供足够多的病例以便受训者获得足够的临床经验。理想情况下,这个中心也应该实施同种异体干细胞移植。如果培训中心不实施肺移植,ID 受训者应在其培训期间在实施肺移植的中心完成轮转。根据 AST 传染性疾病实用启动工作组建议[5],培训应重点着眼于移植后机会性感染以及与特定器官功能衰竭相关的感染性疾病(例如透析、自发性细菌性腹膜炎、囊性纤维化、心室辅助装置)。培训还应包括：供体来源的感染性并发症、术后感染并发症、医院获得性感染、不明原因的发烧和预防策略。实验室研究应强调常见的移植后病原体的实验室测试技术。目前没有特定的机构对此 ID 专科培训进行监管，也不需要额外的认证考试。

多学科培训模式

移植患者的情况是复杂的,可能发生多种并发症，最好应用多学科综合管理。在培训期间,重要的是移植专科医师如何作为多学科团队的一部分，和外科同事以及其他移植亚专科的医生共同诊疗患者。受训者应该了解团队所有成员的作用，包括移植药房、社会工作、营养、理疗和护理甚至更多。移植专科医师应关注移植受者的医学问题,包括免疫抑制剂量、移植相关并发症的诊疗和针对不同肝/肾功能的抗生素剂量。

教育机会

由于移植专科医师培训的主要目标之一即是通过培训获得关于移植的知识和技能，结构化的教育机会是至关重要的。在一年内有几个教育会议,专门针对的就是移植专科医师。最知名、参与度最大的活动是AST年度专科医师研讨会，由移植领域有不同专长的专家对基础和临床知识进行深入的探讨。这种研讨会会期2~3天，提供了一个特殊的学习机会，并整合了移植相关的各项内容。2011年有超过125名来自各医学专科和外科亚专科的人员注册参与了研讨会。还有小规模的由商业赞助的专科医师研讨会，会上研究人员有机会展示他们的成果。

美国移植大会是美国移植学会和美国移植外科医师协会的年度会议。受训者可以申请青年研究者旅行奖，补贴参加美国移植大会的费用。补贴的分配是根据所投稿摘要的科学价值。移植大会是一个很好的机会，可使研究人员接触前沿的移植科学研究，并接触其他移植同行。

美国移植学会有许多“实践团体”。实践团体是在AST内自愿选择的志愿者团体，致力于成员感兴趣的该领域重要的问题。会员资格对所有人开放，并为每个培训级别的会员提供参与AST的机会。实习生和青年教师实践社区是一个由年轻移植专业人士创建的网络，与高级教师互动，并提供教育计划。近年来，实习生和青年教师社区实践活动包括早期职业发展研讨会，美国移植大会的网络展示和创建就业搜索目录。

多器官移植

双器官移植在移植中所占比例不高，但是也在不断增长，有特殊的选择标准和注意事项。理想的专科医师应对这些患者的移植指征评估和术后管理有经验。要重点认识同期移植的指征以及不同器官移植团队所发挥的作用。

病理

移植专科医师应熟悉急性/慢性T细胞介导的和抗体介导的排斥反应的组织学诊断标准，以及原发疾病复发与新生疾病的诊断。对活检结果应进行临床-病理讨论。

儿科

大多数移植专科医师来自内科专业，并接受过诊疗成人患者的培训。然而，在许多移植专科医师培训过程中，可能会遇到儿科患者成长转变为成人的。从儿科到成人的治疗过渡对于患者通常是困难的，应在训练过程中接触该类患者，注意他们的具体问题(例如，自主性、依从性、慢性疾病负担)将使医生能够更好地帮助这些患者。

程序

所有移植专科医师应熟悉同种异体移植物活检的指征及活检程序本身，也应熟悉活检的并发症和治疗。受训者应至少完成ABIM认证所要求的最少数量的活检，且越多越好。

活体捐献者

活体捐献者的选择和管理是肾移植、肝移植和肺移植专科医师培训过程的重要组成部分。移植专科医师应该具有活体捐献者评估的临床经验，并积极参与捐赠者选择的讨论会议。他们应该学习活体肾和肝脏捐赠的绝对和相对禁忌证，强调对捐赠者的直接和长期风险控制。受训者应参与术后护理，并熟悉最常见的手术并发症。受训者还应在常规的术后门诊随访中管理捐献者。

资助

对培训学员的资助是一个日益关注的问题。由于大多数移植专科医师培训不是ACGME认证的，而且通常认为这种培训超过大多数亚专科的一般培训要求，移植专科医师受训者被认为并非“真正的受训者”，因此无法获得医疗保健中心(CMS)资助。目前已经使用各种方法来支持移植专科医师培训。无限制的教育补助计划，一度是支持移植专科医师培训的主要机制，但在如今越来越严格的制药行业指南以及广泛的经济衰退时代条件下已经过时。为支持移植培训，更常见的资助机制是雇用受训人员担任非常初级的职位。由于这些人通常是合格或有资质的，他们可以为他们提供的临床服务收费。在未来，如果正式实施移植专科医师培训计划，培训的临床工作可以由培训补助计划覆盖。另一种少见的途径是利用慈善捐款支持医学教育工作。

研究

在移植专科医师培训期间，鼓励受训者参与移植相关研究。这既可以是对移植学科做出贡献，也可以通过在 HLA 实验室中轮转而熟悉临床医学中使用的实验室技术。有三个备选的调查方向可以选择：临床研究、基础科学研究和转化研究。但是受训者在培训期间可能没有时间进行科学培训。如果不能获得正式的研究项目，应鼓励受训者通过撰写综述、案例分析和单中心回顾性数据分析，获得跟随专家学习的宝贵机会。

工作时间规定

作为 ACGME 认可的移植专科培训的一部分，受训者必须遵守 ACGME 的工作时间规定（每周不超过 80 小时，每班不超过 24 小时，每周至少一天休息）。大多数医疗移植奖学金计划不是 ACGME 认证的，因此不受这些规定的约束。建议认真对待移植专科受训者的需求，鼓励教学计划遵循 ACGME 指南

未解决的需求

UNOS 和 ACGME 培训指南强调移植培训的临床和研究方面，但往往无法解决一些实际问题，例如过渡至独六/参与实践和寻找就业机会。移植专科医师培训是一个中间状态；受训者一般在相应亚专科已获得认证，但需要获得额外移植相关专业知识。独立进行临床实践的过渡可能是具有挑战性的，由更高级教师进行指导是有益的。参加临床工作的责任是巨大的，资深教师应监督管理，并与其他学员进行交流。培训结束后的就业是受训人员非常关心的，如何取得学术地位通常不明朗，资深教师在此过程中起到指导作用。

总结

具有特定器官系统专业技能的移植亚专科医生对于移植中心的工作顺利开展至关重要。随着实体器官移植领域的发展，针对移植临床医生的培训已发展成为一个更加结构化和有组织的产业，具有统一的培训标准和期望。ACGME 已加入 UNOS 的监管职能。当今的专科医师培训反映了现代临床移植更加科学化和跨学科的性质。

（高峰 译 高峰 校）

参考文献

1. Attachment I to Appendix B of UNOS Bylaws: Designated Transplant Program Criteria. [accessed August 2, 2012]; Available from: http://www.unos.org.
2. AST/ASN Renal Transplant Fellowship Accreditation Program: Transplant Fellowship Topics. [accessed August 2, 2012]; Available from: http://www.a-s-t.org.
3. ACGME Program Requirements for Graduate Medical Education in Transplant Hepatology. [accessed August 2, 2012]; Available from: http://www.acgme.org.
4. ACGME Program Requirements for Graduate Medical Education in Advanced Heart Failure and Transplant Cardiology (Internal Medicine). [accessed August 2, 2012]; Available from: http://www.acgme.org.
5. Avery R, Clauss H, Danzinger-Isakov L, et al. Recommended curriculum for subspecialty training in transplant infectious disease on behalf of the American Society of Transplantation Infectious Disease Community of Practice Educational Initiatives Working Group. Transplant Infectious Disease. 2010;12:190–194.

第 131 章
普通医学教育中的器官移植

Rowena Delos Santos and Douglas J. Norman

引言

根据 2011 年 12 月器官获取和移植网络(OPTN)的数据[1],从 1988 年 1 月到 2011 年 12 月约 528 000名患者接受了实体器官移植。此外,每年有 28 000 位新的移植受者在移植后的生活中得到许许多多移植从业者的帮助。这些人不仅包括移植专家，还有普内科医生、普外科医生、家庭医生、亚专科医师、内科外科的住院医师、护士、药剂师,中级职称医师和医学生。随着社会中日益增长的实体器官移植患者数量，从业者们很有必要能够对这类患者的复杂性有一个基本的了解，包括他们的用药和护理。

通常传播移植相关知识对移植专家而言是非常有帮助的，可以为移植中心外的医护行为提供合理的参考。在本章中,我们讨论了目前几类医护人员的一般医学教育情况,然后探讨教育的进一步方法和培训机会。这些将要分别讨论的医护人员类别包括普外科医师、内科医师、亚专科医师(包括肾内科,心内科,消化内科/肝病科,肺病科)、护士、药剂师和医学生。移植外科和内科专家的培训要求分别在第 129 章和第 130 章，移植护士协调员和移植药师的培训要求分别在第 122 章和第 123 章。

当前教育

普外科住院医师

普外科住院医师在通过考试成为普外科医师之前,需要在几个特定的科室进行轮转,包括腹部外科、乳腺外科、内分泌科、消化科、皮肤和软组织科、外科重症监护室、头颈外科、创伤科、儿科、头颈外科、血管外科和肿瘤外科[2]。还有一些科室不要求普外科住院医师必须轮转,包括心脏外科、神经外科、骨科、泌尿外科、妇科和烧伤科[2]。目前,实体器官移植的轮转是根据美国毕业后医学教育认证委员会(ACGME)对普外科住院医师的要求制订的[2]。器官移植科的轮转要求,包括对免疫抑制和免疫学的理解以及移植患者移植前、移植期间和移植后普外科管理。

近年来特别是近 10 年来,由于住院医师工作时间的限制，已经有人担心住院医师是否还能在移植工作中起到积极的作用。在未来几年,移植业可能会出现一些变化，之前 ACGME 要求的移植轮转将逐渐过渡到移植经历[2]。这一变化在不同的培训中心有所不同。移植轮转的住院医师无法满足施行大量移植的大中心,而其他规模较小的中心可能并不需要所有的住院医师进行移植轮转。不进行移植的医学中心,也不会选择将自己的住院医师送去其他中心进行移植轮转。

此外，住院医师对移植轮转经历的反馈在是否需要改变轮转这一问题上提供参考。住院医师对轮转计划的改进意见也已经归纳成几个方面(表 131.1)。其中主要的问题是非常高的服务要求和较低的教育获益[3]。另外，移植手术中很难从上级医师中获得操作机会也会影响住院医师的培训效果[3]。为了改善普外科住院医师的轮转体验,美国移植外科医师协会(ASTS)提出了建议，以提高对分配到移植科轮转的普外科医师的培训体验[3]。一些重要的建议已提出并开始实施,以提高住院医师的培训效果(表 131.1)。

首先，移植团队中的主治医师认证将有助于引导轮转住院医师的培训，包括教学指导、住院和门诊实践。培训移植团队的分工将有助于每个成员的角色定位。院内专科医师帮助诊疗患者有助于降低住院医师的负担,从而使他们有更多的手术时间。合理确定移植外科主治医师和住院医师的最小数量能够同时优化这

表 131.1 移植外科轮转问题和推荐改变。Adapted from:[3] Fryer, JP and Magee, JC. Optimizing the surgical residents' educational experience on transplant surgery. J Surg Educ. 2009;66:196–200.

轮转问题
1.有限的工作时间下服务需求高。
2.自我教育收益低。
3.住院医师和外科主治医师之间的竞争关系。
4.与移植主任医师间的互动少。
5.缺乏移植项目的住院医师培训中心将住院医师送到其他中心。
提高轮转效果的推荐改变
1.确定一个专门的移植外科医生引导住院医师学习轮转。
2.为住院医师提供持续的反馈系统以促进项目的改进。
3.确定特定的手术以优化住院医师的学习机会和临床经验。
4.护理人员加入移植团队帮助看护患者。
5.教育所有团队成员团队精神的期望和重要性。

两种类型医师轮转过程中的学习机会[3]。已有研究评估住院医师的学习曲线和他们在考核中表现出来的熟练度(由完成操作所需的时间反映)。根据一项分析住院医师完成腹腔镜下供体肾切除术表现的研究,参与 13 次手术(作为手术助理)或 6 次手术(参与静脉分支和输尿管结扎手术)的住院医师在考核中会有较好的表现[4]。在病例数量可变的特定条件下,教学质量的改进和完成最低限度的临床要求,有助于提高外科住院医师的学习经验。

住院医师培训的经典模式涉及一个拥有大量患者的多学科中心,住院医师通过进入临床,学习将来独立医治患者的必要能力。这个模式也随着新的工作时间和质量标准化教育发生变化。对于特定器官的学科,如肝胆外科、肝移植中心等科室,是否会影响研究生毕业后的外科住院医师的培养,仍然存在争议[5]。对于外科主治医师来说,在特定的中心进行培训尤为重要,因为这些中心可以集中医治某一类患者。但是这些病历对于普外科住院医师并不是必需的。建立一个特定疾病或器官的中心将减少住院医师接触这些患者的机会,从而限制甚至排除他们遇到这些复杂患者的可能[5]。特定的中心对主治医师的培训更加有效,并能给患者提供特殊照顾。至少现在,住院医师培训的经典教学制度仍然是大多数项目的支柱。支持和反对专科中心轮转的争论仍在继续,两种培训模式仍然同时存在。

在这个外科高速发展的新时代,新技术和新设备层出不穷,普外科医生需要在入学之前进行多个领域培训。让外科住院医师接触到器官移植是非常好的经历,使他们成为更加全面的外科医生。

首先,移植轮转期间的每一台移植手术给外科住院医师提供了血管操作的机会。每一例器官移植都需要血管吻合技术,这可以培养住院医师完成开放血管吻合的能力。此外,普外科手术如腹腔、消化道手术也会在移植术后患者中进行。对住院医师培训特别有用的是终末期器官衰竭的治疗和管理以及相关的外科手术,如肾移植等待患者的肾造瘘和肝脏疾病的肝胆手术[6]。

第二,移植轮转为治疗这些患者提供了足够的跨学科交叉互动的机会。器官移植作为一个为病情复杂的患者提供帮助的特殊领域,实际上确实是需要多学科的方法来治疗。这种患者的管理方法对一个住院医师的培训成长是非常重要的。

第三,住院医师能够对免疫学、免疫抑制药物和免疫抑制患者管理相关知识有一个初步的了解[6]。

第四,住院医师可以在移植手术过程中完成一些在其他科室无法碰到的手术操作,如腹腔镜或开放供体肾切除术。这些经验帮助他们更好地处理伴随着器官移植患者的复杂问题。

内科

不像普外科住院医师,内科住院医师目前不需要到器官移植科轮转。如果轮转计划需要他们到器官移植科轮转,那么 ACGME 规定内科住院医师的 3 年轮转计划中最多进行 1 个月的移植轮转[2]。一些住院医师培训计划会有专门的器官移植病房轮转,那么就会有住院医师轮转到移植病房。其他住院医师计划可能没有专门的移植轮转,这样的话,住院医师只能通过管理医疗组内个别的移植患者获得移植患者的管理经验。

一些住院医师培训项目有专门的器官内科团队,如胃肠、肝脏、肾脏、肺和心脏。这是有别于普内科团队的。不同专科团队负责处理不同器官相关的疾病,包括器官移植的患者。这部分住院医师负责的患者中,移植患者是很重要的一部分。他们会把注意力集中在器官移植的患者上,以提高他们对病理生理、感染性并发症,以及这部分患者药物相互作用的认识。

由于住院医师培训计划将所有患者分到了不同的内科团队,住院医师可能很少有机会接触到移植患者。这也使得内科医生在处理这类复杂的患者时会感到很棘手。器官移植患者数量正在不断增加,因此这部分患者越来越可能在住院或门诊出现。这会导致药物剂量过高或过低发生的风险增高,而且新药物和免疫抑制剂之间的相互作用,可能会导致这些移植患者预后不良。

尚无正式的相关研究分析内科住院医师在器官移植方面的专科培训。大多数的移植培训是以移植教学讲座的形式完成的。住院医师可以通过阅读讲座中提到的相关文献和文章进一步学习。早前的一个研究分析了住院医师参加讲座的出勤率和考核成绩之间的关系[7]。这一单中心研究发现,定期强制性教学平均出勤率为34%,而当提供午饭时出勤率会提高[7]。然而,出勤率与住院医师在美国内科医学认证考试的成绩没有相关性[7]。这项研究强调了我们的教学方法需要改进为互动教学,类似于基于问题的学习方法。

专科医师

ACGME 不强制胃肠病学/肝病、肺病或心脏病科的主治医师进行移植轮转[2]。然而,每一类专科医师都需要在各自的领域接受正规的教育。形式可以是门诊、住院,如果不具备移植手术的训练设施,也可以是教学。这些专业提供专门的移植经费以训练那些对相应器官移植感兴趣的专科医师。表131.2列出了不同专业移植所需的临床培训时间和移植的专门培训项目。

目前有一种趋势,专科医师需要通过一些特定的移植培训,获得相关移植认证才能从事相关工作。例如,经过七年的准备,在2006年移植协会开始实施肝移植认证考核[8,9]。在2006—2010年,如果考生有丰富的移植和肝脏疾病的经验,就可以不参加移植认证考核。但是从2011年起,所有申请认证的申请人都必须完成肝脏移植考核[8,9]。由于需要掌握复杂的肝病和移植病例知识,部分胃肠、肝病医师并不适应。肝病医师需要学习胃肠病专家提供的所有病例,大大增加了肝病医师的临床工作。最近由几个消化学会组成的一个工作小组,专门为胃肠病学医师的培训提供建议。他们主张一般培训计划需要保留胃肠病学/肝病模块[10]。他们还特别建议改革移植许可的认证,主治通常需要完成三年的一般培训计划,紧接着的三年里由移植导师指导,重点研修移植[10]。

表131.2 各专科所需的移植轮转和专门培训

专科	实习培训期间所需的移植轮转	移植的专门培训项目
胃肠病学/肝病	–	×
心脏病学	–	×
肺病学	–	×
肾病学	–	×

同胃肠病科和肝病科一样,心脏病科刚刚启动了移植认证考核。第一次考核时间为2010年。2012年ACGME开始组织重度心脏衰竭和移植的资质认证[2]。对于将来从事重度心脏衰竭治疗和心脏移植的医师,他们在36个月的培训之后需要额外进行为期12个月的进一步培训[2]。成立的相应协会定义了从事重度心脏衰竭治疗和心脏移植的专家需要经历的培训和具备的技能。心力衰竭/心脏移植专家要能协助其他医师治疗病情不太严重的心脏衰竭,协助进行高级护理,学会使用心脏设备,以及评估患者心脏移植适应证[11]。

肾移植是个例外,ACGME 的肾病主治培训计划中就已经包括了肾移植的培训。首先,ACGME 需要所有的主治医师有至少两个月的肾移植临床经验,包括移植器官的活检[2]。这也包括移植前患者和活体供体的评估。此外,主治医师也需要随访至少10个移植术后的患者。这为他们提供了管理移植患者免疫抑制药物的经验。主治医师也应该在社区诊所至少连续性随访3个月,随访至少20个移植术后的患者[2]。

严格规定的肾移植培训计划是可以理解的。肾移植的历史最长,社会上肾移植患者最多,肾移植医师的经验也最丰富。此外,肾病医师往往能长时间连续性地接触到他们的患者,从慢性肾病的诊断,到开始透析,到肾移植,以及到移植肾衰竭后的再次透析。不同于其他器官是救命器官,肾病患者可以在没有肾的情况下靠透析存活。因为这一点,有越来越多的患者进行过两次甚至更多次的肾移植。随着肾移植患者越来越多,肾移植医师更需要有丰富的知识和高超的技能去管理这些复杂的患者。

护士

关于移植护士相关教育的数据非常少。大多数移植患者的护理发生在移植前和移植后,护士在这些患者的诊疗中发挥了不可或缺的作用。此外,在大多数情况下这些患者的护理是在术后从重症监护病房开始的。几年前,针对移植和捐献者的护理教育发生了变化，变成了一个五年计划[12]。护理专业学生通过小册子学习，并与移植护士和其他团队成员直接互动。此外，护理学校实施了在移植中心的护理轮转，且护理认证考试也包含了移植主题[12]。

药师

在过去的几十年中，包括药师在内的移植专家们越来越需要在普通培训期以外通过继续培训提高移植经验。在 20 世纪 90 年代之前，药剂师只能凭着工作经验对移植药理学进行学习[13]。随着时间的推移，通过一年的普通药房住院医师培训计划后再进行为期一年的移植药理培训，能够实现移植药师的专业化[13]。这种转变源于美国器官共享网络（UNOS）和医疗服务中心（CMS）在 2004 年所明确的药师在移植多学科小组中的角色和责任[13]。

之前已有研究发现移植药师在移植患者护理中的重要性。他们的药物和药物治疗知识水平和经验对住院和门诊患者都非常有帮助。药师对于移植患者和家属关于药物以及用药依从性的指导是非常有价值的[14,15]。此外，药师可提供有关用药剂量的建议和药物间相互作用的重要信息，防止潜在的不良事件发生[15,16]。

医学生

关于移植医学生教育的评估已有了一些研究。许多研究分析了医学生的移植知识和他们移植经验的关系[17,18]。英国的一项研究采用问卷调查的方式，评估四年级医学生的移植知识。大约有 54%的学生完成了调查，这些学生中，只有 42%的人经过了移植轮转[17]。所有学生中只有 14%的人曾经目睹了移植手术[17]。只有 46%的学生曾经检查过移植患者，43%的学生可以正确识别手术切口和移植物的植入位置[17]。2/3 的学生了解几种可作为移植器官的供体类型[17]。只有 53%的学生能识别最多一个免疫抑制剂[17]。

一个类似的研究在美国俄亥俄州三个不同的医学院校展开，共纳入 537 个一年级和二年级的医学生[18]。作者使用了之前验证过的问卷调查，并有较高的 93%的回应率。在进入医学院之前，只有 11%的学生接受过正式的关于移植和捐赠的教育，只有 22%的人在医学院接受过相关的教育。那些完成了调查的学生中，只有 8%的人曾护理过器官移植患者[18]。

另一个德国横断面研究评估了 1645 名医学生早期和后期医学学习阶段对移植和器官捐献的知识，并从不同专业进行分析[19]。这项研究有 67%的回应率，发现移植和捐赠的知识随着教育水平的提高而增加。此外，那些具有较高教育水平的医学生往往更倾向于家庭成员的器官捐赠。然而，这个数字只占所有医学生的 8%，且在不同专业，只有 14%的人认为自己训练有素可以胜任家庭医生[19]。

这些研究表明，给医学生介绍移植关键知识的黄金时间是在整个医学学习的早期阶段。此外，住院医师和专科医师的培训可以强化这些关键概念，有助于建立诊疗这些患者的信心。鉴于大部分医师都不是移植专家，所以所有医护人员需要具备移植的基础知识，能够独立或者协助诊疗好移植患者。

进一步教育和培训的方法

本节中将移植的内容纳入几个不同层次的医学教育培训，包括医学院、住院医师、专科医师和医学继续教育的教育培训。这些仅是建议，并非必须在所有移植机构实施。

医学院

器官移植培训纳入普通医学教育最合适的时机应该是从医学院开始。医学新生是充满好奇和渴望学习的，因此医学生阶段是最易受影响的。目前在医学院的前两年有两种教学方法，一种是讲课为基础的方式，另一种是问题式讨论学习。移植的核心内容在表 131.3 中列出，均可引入到这两种方式的学习中去。

如果学校是通过讲课的方式学习解剖学、生理学、生物化学、免疫学、药理学、伦理学、微生物学和病理学等专业的主干课程，那么移植相关的话题很容易融入这些课程中。例如在解剖课程中，可以讨论移植物的植入位置。病理生理学是探讨疾病以及器官功能和终末期表现的理想课程。恶性肿瘤和心血管疾病相关的长期预后也可以在病理生理课程中介绍。器官移植背后涉及的免疫学、组织相容性、匹配性和排斥性等核心概念可以在免疫学课程中介绍。而免疫抑制药物的概念及其作用和副作用的机制，可以在药理学课程中深入探讨。微生物学课程可以向学生们介绍感染的概念，包括普通感染和机会性感染。最后，由于器官捐献涉及重要伦理问题，学生可以参与关于移植和组织捐赠的伦

表 131.3 医学生推荐了解的核心移植问题

移植统计信息—等待列表和受者列表
移植的适应征
移植后生活质量和数量的改善
移植受者的评估、选择和禁忌证(器官和受者的评估)
供受体的分配
人类白细胞抗原与组织相容性匹配
移植外科手术和移植器官相关的手术并发症
免疫学,排异反应类型,病理诊断
免疫抑制药物和副作用
重要免疫抑制药物间的相互作用
移植后数月至数年的感染性并发症(病毒,细菌,真菌)
移植患者的恶性肿瘤和心血管疾病的长期风险
移植后原发病的复发率

理讨论。

如果医学院采用了问题式教学,也可以有效地向医学生介绍器官移植的概念。移植概念被纳入问题式学习系统的一个例子,是一个终末期肾病进行血液透析的患者接受肾移植的病例。基于这一案例,可以讨论原肾脏和移植肾的解剖位置,也可以讨论免疫学中自身和非自身抗原的识别以及排斥反应的类型。各种抗排斥药物的药理学、作用机制和药物相互作用也需要讨论。如果有人想进一步扩展知识面,可以持续追踪感染患者几个星期或几个月。学生可以讨论感染的不同类型,包括普通感染和机会性感染,以及一般药物和免疫抑制药物潜在的相互作用。

医学生进入病房之后,许多临床见闻可以帮助培养他们护理器官移植患者的能力。无论医学生是从事外科、内科护理还是专科,他们都可以进一步获得治疗和管理器官移植患者的经验。医学生可以通过几个患者的诊疗过程学习到移植患者护理的各方面内容。学生能够了解移植患者的病史、用药情况和病理生理等情况以制订合适的计划管理这些患者。

一些临床轮转计划的学生可以有较多接触移植患者的机会。例如,感染性疾病的咨询服务可以定期评价移植患者的感染情况并指导抗生素使用。胃肠病学/肝病、肾病、肺病、心脏病轮转时也可以接触到一些移植患者。此外,特定的移植病房可为这些学生提供更多的接触机会。足够的管理器官移植患者的机会可以使医学生大大提高他们对药物和密切随访的认识,以及提高感染预防和健康维护的理念。

内科

内科住院医师关于移植主题相关教育数据的缺乏之前已有讲述。为提高住院医师的出勤率,我们需要改变教学方式。教学应覆盖移植的适应证和禁忌证、移植的优势、免疫学基础、人类细胞抗原(HLA)匹配、组织相容性、免疫抑制药物、移植排斥、感染等并发症、远期疗效和管理,类似于医学生的教育,但要更深入。

上述方面内容已经非常复杂,需要大量的教学时间。然而,由于教学时间限制,这些只能重点介绍,住院医师还需要了解一些器官移植患者管理相关的问题。例如,免疫抑制剂及其共同作用和剂量调整的讲座可以给大家提供重要的信息。此外,感染性并发症及移植器官失功的鉴别诊断包括排斥的话题也应该讨论。

一些之前提到过的因素可以影响住院医师的出勤率。之前的一篇文章提供了解决讲座无法吸引听众原因的方法[20]。这些因素包括不恰当的教学主题、不好的讲师、高估或者低估听众基础知识、较差教学组织以及讲课资料的不足[20]。住院医师继续进行三年的培训,导致一些教学讲座是重复的。然而很多知识的学习往往需要重复,一位讲师提供了相同的材料却无法吸引他的听众,最终会减少听众的人数。鉴于此,另一个问题则是一些讲师无法根据听众的反馈调整自己的讲课方式[20]。这些讲师应该定期征求学生的反馈来提高下一年的教学质量。

有一些方法可以提高住院医师参加教学讲课的出勤率。一项研究评估了听众反应系统的利用效果,发现听众比以前更专注于讨论了。他们还认为利用听众反应系统后他们更加了解材料的内容[21]。有一些建议包括:提出简单和容易阅读的、回答起来不很复杂的问题,使用问题去强调重点内容[21,22]。还有一个重要的建议是,在讲课后要留下足够的时间进行问题讨论[21,22]。一个英国的小组为正在备课的讲师提供了一个指南[23]。他们的建议包括:改进教学方式、演示风格,提高教学技能,充分利用视听教材和讲义[23]。

教育工作者也应该认识到,其他人可能会对学习有不同的偏好。一些住院医师通过反复的自学,可以比参加正常教学学得更好。在这种情况下,教师可以把自己的教学资源放到网上,供住院医师下载学习。这些讲课的演示文稿需要随时更新,以保持新颖性。其他人可以下载幻灯片在课后学习。创建一个包括移植相关种子文章的文件夹，为住院医师提供额外的资源进行独立学习。在线互动教程最近已成为常见的教育工具。

普外科

普外科住院医师的移植教育根据 ACGME 的要求不断调整。移植轮转已经不是必需的,一些住院医师可能没有机会在移植中心轮转。其他住院医师也只有一些被删减的移植轮转的计划，而不再是之前几个星期的轮转。

对普外科住院医师的教育问题已有担忧。很多以前被认为是在普外科住院医师培训的项目，慢慢地成为了专科医师培训的一部分。例如,像胆囊切除术、阑尾切除术等一些普通手术，现在往往是主治级以上医师主刀的。不幸的是,这样的结果由几个因素引起的。由普外科延伸出的好多额外的专科（如微创胃肠外科、乳腺外科、肿瘤外科、移植科、创伤外科)已变得越来越普遍[24]。由于越来越多培训医师开始进行手术,很多住院医师认为他们也需要进行专门的培训。事实上,约 70%的住院医师在完成他们的普外科住院医师培训后寻求专科训练[24]。

普外科住院医师的项目数量一直被密切关注。一项研究观察了由毕业住院医师完成的项目数量，这些项目都是培训负责人认为最重要的[25]。在本次调查的 254 名住院医师培训负责人中,回应率为 45%。研究者发现,121 项被认为是核心外科手术需要在住院医师培训结束前完成的，其中 68%的手术住院医师只参与过不到 5 次[25]。由于外科住院医师教育和培训上的问题,几个关键的相关成员在 2002 年成立了委员会来解决问题和提供方案[26]。之后,他们组成了一个住院医师培训外科委员会(SCORE),其目的是继续提高普外科住院医师的教育和培训水平[26,27]。SCORE 成员包括来自美国外科委员会、美国外科医师学会、美国外科协会、外科手术联盟,以及外科教育联盟,ACGME 外科住院医师审查委员会和美国胃肠内镜外科医生协会的代表[27]。自成立以来,SCORE 提出一系列建议,通过开设全国性的教育培训课程来改善外科住院医师的教育[27]。

SCORE 重点推荐对普通外科住院医师的移植教育,了解实体器官移植的适应证、脑死亡判定、器官保存与供体选择、免疫抑制剂,以及包括肿瘤复发和感染在内的移植术后内外科并发症[27]。住院医师无需熟练掌握供体器官获取、供体肾脏切除术,以及器官联合移植等移植相关操作,但推荐练习[27]。尽管会发生一些变化,但关键的训练点应该在整个项目里保持一致。所有项目理应遵循 SCORE 推荐的学习目标,因为其中许多可以通过教学传授给外科住院医师。其他目标应该在住院医师阶段结束前提供给住院医师,例如外科轮转/经验。如果受训医生不能完成全程轮转培训,可以接受“简版”轮转。在住院医师结束轮转前最好让他们经历少数的移植手术(器官获取与植入)。但是鉴于供体器官活性的不确定性，受训者并不能接受所有移植手术训练。住院医师可以利用模拟装置模拟移植手术场景来学习相关技能。而且,住院医师应该意识到解剖学位置和手术并发症是重要的知识点。随着越来越多的患者需要接受移植手术，这些患者有更大的概率到其所在医院就诊。认识并且理解移植手术内外科并发症可以让这些住院医师为患者提供及时有效的治疗。

专科医师

专科医师在管理移植患者上有着独特的地位。他们在各自的领域受过专业培训，在许多情况下是移植患者出现危急病情时的直接处理者。这些专科医师应具备移植、并发症的基准知识,并能提供相应建议。所有专科医师需要经过移植专科的培训教育。根据不同的培训计划,教学方案可以是由最少的(几次讲课)到最多的(时长达几周)不等。类似于学生的课程内容(表 131.3),专科医师的课程需要覆盖几乎所有相关的主题。这一教学大纲应覆盖的内容应该比医学生的更加深入。每个主题应分开学习，让讲师有足够的时间分配到额外的讨论,以提供更多的信息和数据。拓展每个主题的原因在表 131.4 中说明。移植患者每年约增加 28 000 人[1]。类似于普通外科医生,移植外科医生的数量也很有限,同样在移植领域的内科医生也远远不够，而移植患者的数量则是非常巨大的。专科医师需要通过掌握足够的知识给移植患者初步的建议，并推荐有需要的患者去相应的移植中心。

如果可能，一般专科内科主治医师应在培训期间得到一些接触移植患者的机会。这可以通过连续性门诊或住院服务实现;讲座提供大量的信息,为专科医师直接管理移植患者提供宝贵的经验。虽然患者存在着个体性差异，但是医师可以通过系统地回顾包括移植物功能、免疫抑制药物的相互作用、感染情况和心血管疾病在内的各种情况,维护患者的健康。

表 131.4 普通培训医师和移植专科培训以及对应专科移植患者的数量。数据来自美国毕业后医学教育认证委员会(ACGME)和美国移植协会(AST)网站[2,28]

亚专科	一般培训医师	移植专科培训医师	移植患者
心脏外科	168	获得认证	52 658
胃肠外科	157	51(36 ACGME 认证)	113 962
肾脏病科	146	53(AST 认证)	331 765
普胸外科/急诊科	133	N/A	24 035

继续医学教育

器官移植的医护人员需要继续教育，以维持和更新他们对移植患者的诊疗知识。对于消化内科、肺病科、肾病科、心脏病科等移植亚专科医师，医学继续教育在每年的全国性会议中是很常见的。这些会议可由移植专家提供给各自领域专科医师最新的信息。一些移植组织也通过区域会议和门诊推广计划，向社区的同事提供相关信息。

普内科医师很少在全国性会议上进行继续教育。内科医师有责任各自寻求移植和移植患者管理的最新信息。一些医生可以通过他们各自医院的病例讨论接受移植领域的继续教育。其他人则可以参加其他协会举办的会议进行学习。器官移植专家可以经常在院内或全国性会议上给内科医生提供移植的相关信息和最新进展。

总结

器官移植这个领域的患者数量正在稳步增长。移植后免疫抑制剂的应用和移植后管理的进步使得移植受者存活期得以增加。这些患者的医护人员需要一定的基础知识和经验，才能诊疗好这部分患者。对于移植患者的教育从医学生就开始了，并贯穿于整个普外科住院医师、内科住院医师和专科医师培训阶段。包括互动教学方法和听众反应系统以及模拟器的使用，都有助于医护人员的进一步教育。器官移植是一个不断发展的领域，所以也需要医护人员通过再教育和全国性会议更新相关知识和最新进展。只有移植领域的医护人员持续学习，才能使移植患者获益良多。

（高峰 译 高峰 校）

参考文献

1. OPTN Web site offers information about transplantation. [accessed November 11, 2011]; Available from: http://optn.transplant.hrsa.gov.
2. ACGME General Surgery Program Requirements found on the website http://www.acgme.org/acWebsite/navPages/nav_440.asp. [accessed November 11, 2011].
3. Fryer JP, Magee JC. Optimizing the surgical residents' educational experience on transplant surgery. Journal of Surgical Education. 2009;66:196–200.
4. Hollenbeck BK, Seifman BD, Wolf JS Jr. Clinical skills acquisition for hand-assisted laparoscopic donor nephrectomy. Journal of Urology. 2004;171:35–39.
5. Tuttle-Newhall JE, Diehl AM. What impact does a specialized center for transplantation and hepatobiliary disease have on post-graduate resident training of gastroenterologists and surgeons? Journal of Hepatology. 2006;44:659–662.
6. Pellegrini CA, Warshaw AL, Debas HT. Residency training in surgery in the 21st century: a new paradigm. Surgery. 2004;136:953–965.
7. FitzGerald JD, Wenger NS. Who attends, and is attendance related to medical certifying examination scores? Academic Medicine. 2003;78:84–89.
8. Bacon BR. Hepatology: where do we go from here? Gastroenterology. 2006;131:1373–1374.
9. Fried MW. Certificate of added qualification for hepatology: vindication not vanity. Gastroenterology. 2005;128:817.
10. Friedman LS, Brandt LJ, Elta GH, et al. Report of the multisociety task force on GI training. The American Journal of Gastroenterology. 2009;70:823–827.
11. Francis GS, Greenberg BH, Hsu DT, et al. ACCF/AHA/ACP/HFSA/ISHLT 2010 clinical competence statement on management of patients with advanced heart failure and cardiac transplant. Journal of the American College of Cardiology. 2010;56:424–453.
12. Chabalewski FL. A success story: promoting the incorporation of donation- and transplantation-related content in nursing school curricula. Transplantation Proceedings. 1997;29:3240–3241.
13. Alloway RR, Dupuis R, Gabardi S, et al. Evolution of the role of the transplant pharmacist on the multidisciplinary transplant team. American Journal of Transplantation. 2011;11:1576–1583.
14. Chisholm MA, Mulloy LL, Jagadeesan M, et al. Impact of clinical pharmacy services on renal transplant patients' compliance with immunosuppressive medications. Clinical Transplantation. 2001;15:330–336.
15. Stemer G, Lemmens-Gruber R. Clinical pharmacy services and solid organ transplantation: a literature review. Pharmacy World and Science. 2010;32:7–18.
16. Wang HY, Chan ALF, Chen MT, et al. Effects of pharmaceutical care intervention by clinical pharmacists in renal transplant clinics. Transplantation Proceedings. 2008;40:2319–2323.
17. Edwards AG, Weale AR, Morgan JD. A survey of medical students to assess their exposure to and knowledge of renal transplantation. BMC Medical Education. 2004;4:32–35.
18. Essman C, Thornton J. Assessing medical student knowledge, attitudes, and behaviors regarding organ donation. Transplantation Proceedings. 2006;38:2745–2750.
19. Schaeffner ES, Windisch W, Freidel K, et al. Knowledge and attitude regarding organ donation among medical students and physicians. Transplantation. 2004;77:1714–1718.
20. McLaughlin K, Mandin H. A schematic approach to diagnosing and resolving lecturalgia. Medical Education. 2001;35:1135–1142.
21. Uhari M, Renko M, Soini H. Experiences of using an interactive audience response system in lectures. BMC Medical Education. 2003;3:12–17.
22. Robertson LJ. Twelve tips for using a computerized interactive audience response system. Medical Teacher. 2000;22:237–239.
23. Brown G, Manogue M. AMEE medical education guide no. 22: refreshing lecturing: a guide for lecturers. Medical Teacher. 2001;23:231–244.
24. Bell RH Jr, Banker MB, Rhodes RS, et al. Graduate medical education in surgery in the United States. Surgical Clinics of North America. 2007;87:811–823.
25. Bell RH, Biester TW, Tabuenca A, et al. Operative experience of residents in US general surgery programs: a gap between expectation and experience. Annals of Surgery. 2009;249:719–724.
26. Sachdeva AK, Bell RH Jr, Britt LD, et al. National efforts to reform residency education in surgery. Academic Medicine. 2007;82:1200–1210.
27. SCORE website provides information regarding recommendations http://www.surgicalcore.org/. [accessed November 11, 2011].
28. AST website offers information on transplantation including a listing of AST accredited centers http://www.a-s-t.org/content/accredited-renal-transplant-fellowship-training-programs. [accessed November 11, 2011].

第 10 篇

临床试验和数据管理

第 132 章
局部移植数据管理项目的建立和可持续化

Regina Eady, Tim Morris, Marc J. Overcash, Jeff Weaver

"脱离数据支持，你只是一个持有观点的个体。"
佚名

引言

移植学是为数不多的通过数据驱动得以发展的医学领域之一。移植数据的管理水平超出美国联邦政府发布法规的要求，包括获取每个患者日常需求相关的高粒度数据以及移植中心提供服务的能力等。因此，一个完善的局部数据管理项目有利于移植项目的成功。建立一套兼具综合性和可持续性的数据管理项目流程是极具挑战的。通过局部数据管理策略和实践的应用，一个移植项目可以实现如下几点：

• 对受者术后移植物和生存率进行追踪和趋势分析，与国家基线和结果数据相比较。

• 查看集结果、科研、临床、全国范围和参考价值于一体的数据集。通过数据挖掘和分析技术，对受者的特征和干预措施进行调查、建模和分析，以提高标准的护理实践模式，促进发展机会。

• 建立早期预警机制以持续监测动态走向，当偏离预期趋势时，积极主动地推进干预措施。该机制既可以针对受者，也可以应用于整个移植项目流程中。

• 跟踪并向医护人员展示结果数据，使其以专业的护理实践标准判断趋势变化，促进产生良好的预后。

• 用交通信号灯符号模型(红、黄、绿)来测量和评价关键绩效指标(KPI)，以快速确定移植方案如何根据其目的和目标开展。这些 KPI 包括跟踪受者等待时间、在实验价值方面达到的目标等。

• 提供跟踪报告和高度个性化的检查清单，促进在临床护理实践和科学研究中启用一套统一标准，以方便决策。利用局部数据存储库得到上述报告，可以将报告格式化，从而通过优先考虑特定的数据点和动态生成的逻辑来计算基于假设情况的数据(例如，肾移植受者术后肌酐水平如果高出基线 115%，就认为该检测结果在功能上存在显著差异性，可能表明移植器官出现急性排斥反应)。

• 基于广泛的变量进行人口计数，以确定潜在受者池和评估临床试验招募的可行性。

基于上述讨论，可将局部数据管理定义为：一个移植项目流程中必要的策略、原则和用统一的方法管理多元数据需求和资源的持续过程。同时，局部数据管理是不同于全国数据管理的，后者通常在注册中心集中进行管理。国家数据管理将在第 133 章展开讨论。成功的局部数据管理项目提供了一个在适当时间能方便地访问相应数据的框架，有利于在临床护理、科研、教育、质量成果、人才、投入和开展移植项目等方面做出明智、有效的决策。

本章介绍了移植医生与局部数据管理项目相关的核心概念，描述了构建和维护数据管理项目的过程，并在重要数据管理原则方面提出指导和建议。

案例分析

下面的案例分析揭示了局部数据管理项目的价值。由埃默里大学移植中心开展的一项研究中，每周进行随访会议和移植后的监测报告，以改善肾移植受者治疗的依从性，并发现受者面临的风险。每周随访会议在移植门诊进行，在此期间，协调员和医生在移植后定期查看患者的病历，涉及术后 1 个月、3 个月、6 个月、9

个月和12个月的病历。根据上述病历创建报告,提供反映受者综合情况的数据,用于每周随访会议上讨论。

在创建移植后随访报告之前，对受者的随访评估是一项复杂且耗费大量人力的工作。每年新增随访的受者的随访量达160例左右。埃默里大学的移植受者护理记录系统从器官移植随访记录系统(OTTR)获取数据，每例受者的信息需要花2个小时左右才能填写完成,这导致移植协调员每周需要加班约4个小时。随着数据的分散,在会上,每小时可以核查8例受者的记录。为了在会议期间增加患者随访记录的审核数量,由移植协调员制订患者随访记录表。这需要进一步延长协调员在收集和登记记录表中数据所需要的时间,但它可以作为随访报告的模板。

随访记录表需要在一个非常容易审查的格式下汇集患者数据，这需要一种更有效的整合数据和呈现数据的方法,以此增加受者记录的审核数量。这促进自动化数据报告工具的开发，该工具可以将受者移植术后1个月、3个月、6个月、9个月和12个月期间的病历记录汇总成随访报告。报告从OTTR系统获取数据,并且所有经批准的医生在任何时候都可以通过OTTR用户界面运行系统。报告增加了随访会议的讨论内容,包括确定治疗方案、识别高危患者、转诊医生之间的有效沟通。由此,协调员对受者的数据采集工作从每例受者耗时2个小时减少到每例受者10分钟,协调员也摆脱了频繁的加班。移植后随访报告集中提供了所有数据点,可以满足分析不同患者群组的需求。会议上的审核量从每小时8例增加到每小时20例。

随访报告的关键意义在于更好地执行治疗计划,由此也促进肾移植受者术后院内存活率在统计学上得到显著改善。其他可见的作用还包括:BK病毒检测普及率从50%上升至90%；更易于检测免疫抑制标靶物水平;改善转诊医生之间的沟通交流。该项目大约持续6个月，并需要一名专业的数据分析师和多名项目专家一同开展工作。管理层高度认可该项目取得的成效,并启动其他一些局部数据管理举措。

挑战与展望

局部移植数据管理项目面临着许多挑战。在一个移植项目中，核心的临床数据交叉分散地储存在多个地区和组织,包括:

- 医疗保健体系里众多的基础设施，即用于管理一系列临床相关的影像、处方、实验室、手术、调度、计费和其他信息的设备。
- 多个机构管理不同的、无关联的医疗保健信息系统,而这些机构都具有开展移植项目的资质(例如,儿童医院、老年病医院、退伍军人事务部等)。

此外，还有操作大型临床和基础科学研究项目的复杂性，以及数据源系统层面和管理方面的挑战,包括：

- 在众多各式各样的疾病和具体的数据库创建过程中会遇到不同的,有时不兼容的技术难题,以及基于组织者或研究者使用不同的术语、价值观和计量单位而造成形式上的差异。
- 实验室的仪器控制台是从特定的供应商处个性化定制的,并可能需要专门的编程以自动提取数据。
- 存储在局部文件服务器和个人目录工作站上的电子表格和文件，是根据个人偏好和最新检索浏览记录获取的。
- 手写的笔记按顺序记录在笔记本里存档，并将其存储在架子上或文件柜里。

从更高的层面来看，正是这些挑战促进精准数据通过系统平台和记录汇集起来,以供决策参考。过程、专业技能、技术、集成数据系统所需的时间和精力不容小觑且占用大量的资源。它包括游说改变体制,以便收集和访问跨多个数据源或系统的特定数据集并调和数据域中的值，还包括介绍移植项目本身流程和政策的改变。因此,建立和维护一个综合性的局部数据管理项目,需要通过多层级领导有条不紊的引导,从而接近预期目标。如果做法得当,数据管理项目将是一个不断进化的过程,会随着移植项目的进步而进步,从中寻找新的方法衡量自身性能,探索新的研究发现,评估改善治疗的新途径。

不论是预定的还是现成的，目前还都没有可以直接购买并应用的关于局部数据管理项目的方案。局部数据管理项目在很大程度上依赖于移植项目的原则和目标以及该机构的文化和技术环境。然而,也有适用于大多数机构的核心组件、原理和概念,但需要通过不同的技术和方法来实现。

图132.1直观展示了移植局部数据高级管理方案。图表左侧是多个相关数据源,这些数据源包括由研究者进行临床试验或实验室开展创建的局部数据库；制度体系，如随访和管理所有住院患者包括移植患者

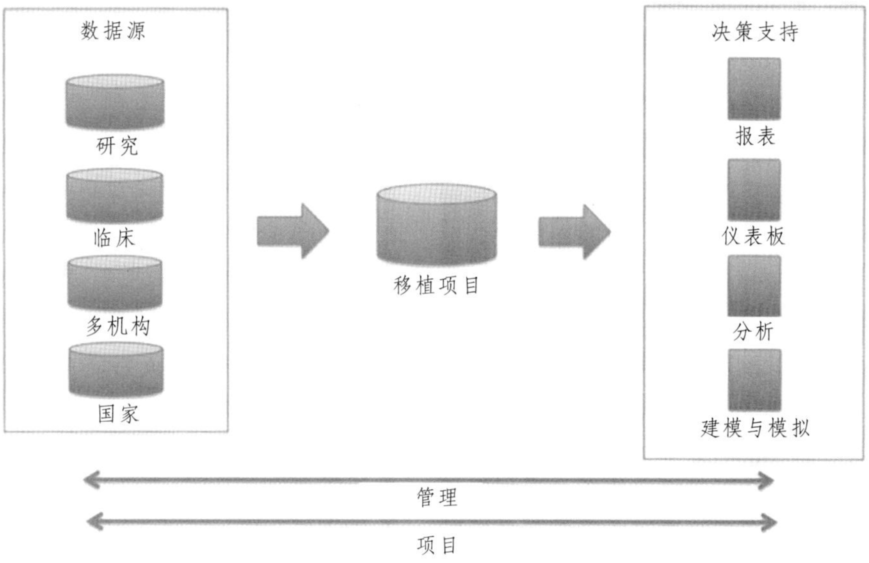

图 132.1 数据高级管理方案。

的电子健康记录;和全国数据源,如美国的 UNET,这个在线数据库系统存储和分析所有移植器官获取和移植网络(OTPN)数据,包括等待名单、器官匹配、移植等相关方面数据。

通过各种手段,可以将数据库子集合或整个数据库资源集成到移植项目特定的存储库,为报告和分析提供一个统一的来源。该存储库可以是一个通过移植项目管理和运行的物理数据库,也可以利用机构现有的数据基础设施实现。该数据可能被物理地转移到一个独立的存储设备,通过媒介或链接转移到现有的存储库,最终的方案将取决于信息技术和基础设施条件。然而,必须要有一个可以访问移植数据集的物理空间或者虚拟空间,以满足移植项目需要的数据。

利用移植项目库中的数据,便于展示报表、仪表板、分析报告和其他统计工具以及分析数据,以促进决策。

构建和维持方案需要通过不断改善管理结构与流程以确保其满足移植项目的需求,引导项目的日常运作,并规划日益完善的战略方向。最后,通过到位的控制措施确保数据的保密性、完整度和可用性。

过程

在毫无基础的情况下开始一个数据管理项目是极其少见的,它往往需要依赖制度体制、国家数据库和各种现有的局部数据存储库。此外,通过数据的使用,业务流程和功能需求已经通过多种方式体现并得到满足。人们可以采取策略以充分利用、扩大并改善这些现有的基础设施、技术和实践,开发一个局部数据管理项目,保持机动、长足的发展。本节将介绍可用于评估现有的数据管理实践和战略规划的一个更有效的数据管理项目的过程。局部数据管理项目应加快推动组织目标的实现,反过来,数据管理项目的目标取决于组织的目标。

开发局部数据管理项目的步骤如下:

- 计划。了解该项目的当前状态,特别是各级临床团队的变动情况,确定未来的状态,并优先考虑从当前状态转变到未来状态的路径和序列。
- 设计。根据该计划确定的优先级和顺序,设计通常包括执行多个阶段允许的从当前状态到期望的未来状态的迭代方法。迭代方法提供更大的灵活性,随着新需求的产生或优先级的调整,允许改变原有计划,实现效益最大化。一般来说,设计阶段将收集需求、分析不同的选择并提出必要的规范,最后制订新方案。
- 部署。执行指定的设计,确保适当的测试并将其纳入到支持结构中。从局部数据管理的角度来看,应继续进行数据管理、积极参与移植项目。
- 评估。在其指标以及移植项目的目的和目标的基础上对移植项目进行评估。所有差距都应纳入下一阶段的规划。

如图132.2所示，局部数据管理过程是周期性的。重要的是，其开展离不开经临床(和研究，如果适用)的工作人员、机构和专业的数据管理设计团队的积极加入与相互合作。

规划

规划阶段包括评估环境的现状，构建状态，并优先考虑从当前状态过渡到未来状态需要开展的事项。通过任务、目标和主要原则推动移植项目早日实现未来状态。例如，一个重要的原则是“每一个患者是一个潜在的研究课题，每一个研究课题是一个潜在的患者”，将推动一系列核心的局部数据管理项目中基本原则的设计。虽然这个概念表面上看似很简单，其复杂性在于患者临床数据用于科学研究的限制，以及整合那些指定为仅用于科学研究的数据源的数据，增加了任务的复杂性。创建一个管理所有患者的质量指标和结果指标的核心数据集，同时作为患者重要研究记录，该数据集的创建便于科学研究和临床两大领域信息的管理。利用这一核心记录，同时深入特定的临床专业，可以通过临床试验和研究提出满足上述主要原则的设计方法。除了这些关键原则，还需要了解移植项目将如何评估其自身的进展，重点在于局部数据管理项目的相关数据变量和数据来源，以便分析和预测模型的指标。

连同关键的原则和性能指标，未来的状态应该由业务(或实践)驱动，而不是由技术驱动。为了促进这一进程，有大量记录当前状态和维持连续的未来状态的迭代方法。其中首要的方法是企业架构。企业架构是对一个组织或企业的目标、企业实体、流程、关系、信息和系统的总体描述。企业架构策略和框架是多种多样的，在多数情况下，从多个框架中衍生出的子方法可能会根据项目的范围和重点被使用。埃默里大学已经实现了一个业务架构建模方法以代替一个完整的企业架构方法，其业务架构建模方法侧重于业务流程以及这些流程与系统和数据之间的关系。

简而言之，业务架构模型过程通过一系列的图表、工作流程分析、业务场景和系统图表来记录当前的操作环境。业务功能映射到其支持的业务工作流程，这反过来也映射到它们支持的信息系统和数据存储库。通过分析工作、理解业务功能、确保适当调整后可以获知未来状态，然后优化业务流程并评估支持技术和数据。这种方法试图最大程度地减少数据管理项目需要支持的业务信息无法对接的情况，并避免低效率的构建业务流程和实践方案。

这种特定方法的成功在很大程度上取决于学科专家和领导的密切合作。基于当前状态已明确，由此创建了大量广泛而详细的图表。对于一项业务功能，比如研究，会记录其关键任务的细节、启用该功能的主要流程、数据的技术领域和类型。有关示例，请参见图132.3。

从这个图中可见，一个更深层次的分析是针对于当前状态的执行流程，记录所执行任务的主要步骤，以及执行的顺序、数据类型和数据存储的系统。通常用泳道图表示这些活动，如图132.4。基于其复杂性或与特定过程相关的问题，其他细节问题可能会被记录下来。工作流程记录应简单明了。结合工作流程记录，支持叙事形式的业务场景有助于在工作流程中提供更多的背景和细节。有关当前状态的记录，不但有助于了解和分析目前正在进行的工作，而且有助于了解和分析每天执行工作的主题专家和个人表达的不满和难处。

通过分析当前状态，可以开始构建未来状态。寻找机会以优化流程、减少存储类似数据的重复系统的数量、开发解决表达问题的方案，并衡量要达到未来状态在能力或功能方面的差距。业务体系结构的应用流程可协助分析，会对当前进程中可能对资源、完成时间和其他指标模型的影响变化情况进行模拟；然而，该分析也可以在没有这种应用程序时进行。未来状态将继续发展并对数据管理流程加以完善，其最终目标是确定

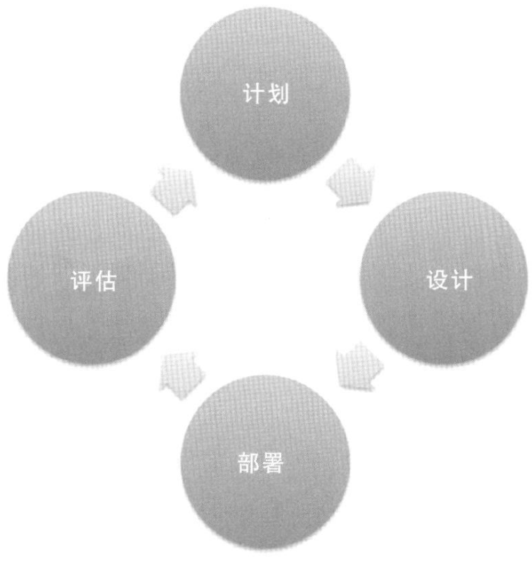

图 132.2 局部数据管理过程。

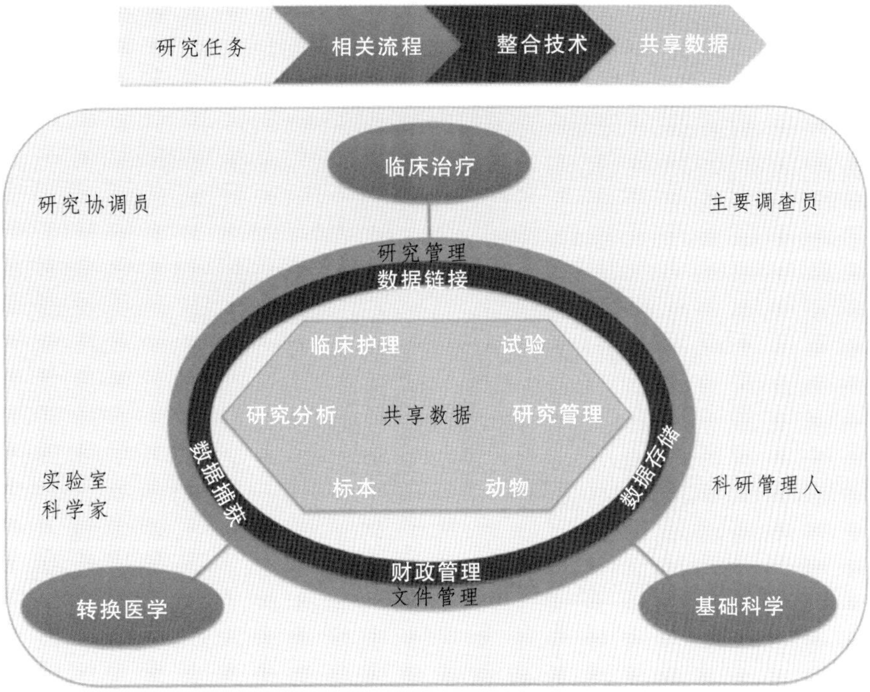

图 132.3　业务功能图示例(埃默里移植中心)。

数据管理项目的目标和能力。

在了解当前环境和项目目标的前提下，接下来的步骤是制订一个过渡计划，它定义了为实现未来状态的中间步骤。一旦完成对当前状态的分析,可能会有一些明显的、容易实现的显著成效。由于这些分析需要花费一些时间和精力,通过取得的成效情况显示进度,有助于保持前进的势头,并对整个项目有所支持。下一步是为需要完成的项目罗列一个清单，并为每个项目评估难易程度、资源需求和任何依赖关系(即需要一个特定的项目完成之前,才能开始另一个项目)。项目清单可以递交给相应的管理机构(见部署管理章节中的讨论)以确定优先事项并获得领导最终审批。

在移植项目中,除了考虑计划流程,还应考虑大量的计划原则:

• 数据的主要权威来源,例如临床数据库,应该是集成数据的早期目标。这些制度层面的数据来源的影响力，通常体现在制订数据管理项目整体设计和操作的具体政策上,并采取控制措施。它通常在其主要组成部分改造完成之前就已经将计划以更符合成本效益的方式实施于项目中。此外,数据库是专门整合跨多个系统数据构建的系统。因此,具有适当的访问权限后,可以访问数据库里可能从多个系统提供的额外数据,并且当它们被集成到该机构的数据库时，提供了获得更多数据的路径。

• 尽快建立一个数据管理项目的标识符策略。因为集成的数据来自不同数据源，赋予每一个不同的实体(即人、标本等)一个永久唯一性的认证标识符是至关重要的。在临床护理业务中,不同系统存储不同的医疗记录号码或其他标识符是很常见的。在许多情况下,会有一个患者主索引菜单，将所有的系统标识符绑定到业务范围内。患者主索引参数码可以用来连接多个临床护理系统的数据,从而实现数据分析。然而,连接研究数据源是一个更大的挑战，因为这些数据源可能是由调查员建立的局部学习电子表格或者用于学习或有特定专用标识符的独立数据库。对于研究数据源,在研究系统的设计和整体数据管理计划的早期制订一个将多个来源的研究主题联系起来的策略非常重要。除了连接研究来源之外，还必须保持与临床记录的链接,以便融合来自研究和临床护理系统的数据。有效的标识符策略使得能够跨多个数据集链接数据,使得存储在电子健康记录中的患者临床数据可以与其存储在单独且不同的实验室信息管理系统中的样本数据配对。

• 从可行性出发，建立信息系统及其支持数据库的标准。通过标准化和模板的更新重建,往往可以促进

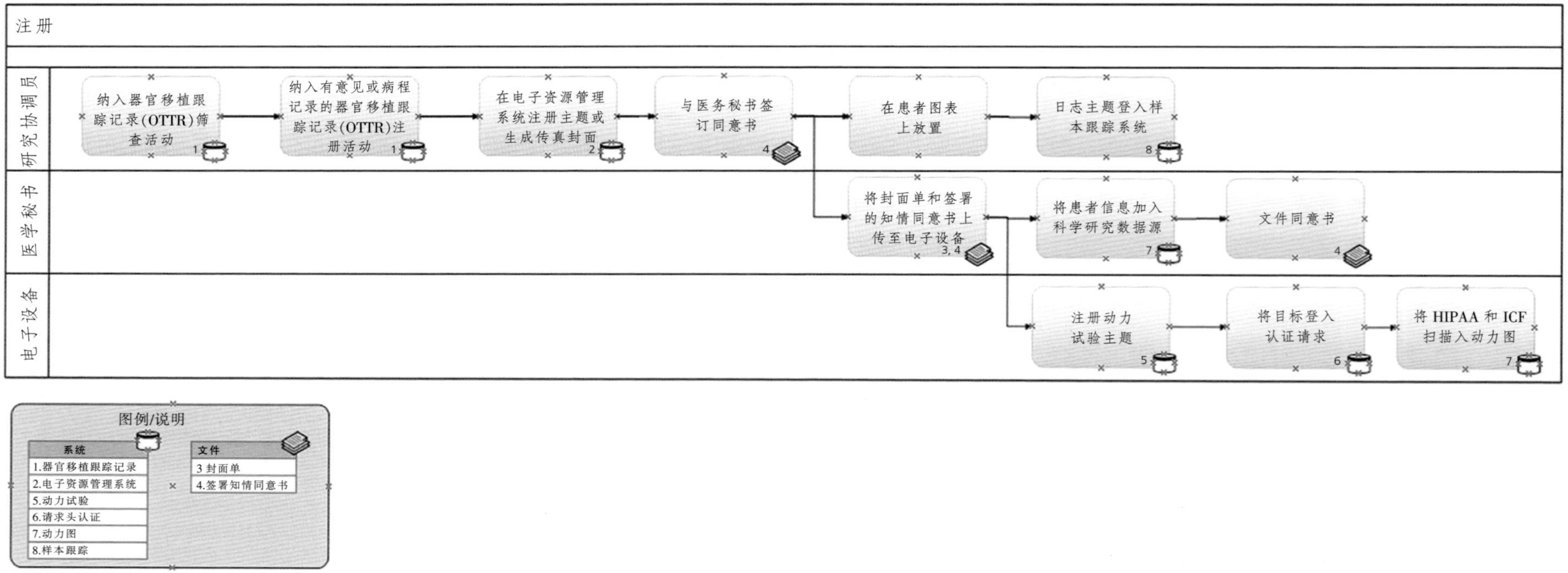

图 132.4. 泳道图示例(当前注册流程)。

术语和观点的一致性,并控制数据质量和保障隐私。

• 一定要尽可能地利用现有的制度资源。正如上述第一条所提到的那样，访问数据库将获取丰富的资料。与这些机构的团队和资源的合作也将提供不同的观点,协助战略规划,并为重新启用基础设施和工具提供机会。

设计

无论是建立一个数据管理项目的核心组件或添加一个新的数据集，都应对数据管理的概念和原则进行探讨。这些原则包括:评估数据源,采集离散数据,准备集成数据,建立质量控制,保证数据的使用符合法规和政策,数据保密。

展望数据管理方案

虽然规划可能会产生广泛的战略性的数据管理目标，但可能会受到有限的资金、资源和基础设施的制约。正因为如此,可能需要一个临时的解决方案,同时当制约解除后,可以实现长期的解决方案。

尽管临时解决方案并不总是理想化的，但也有一定的优势。临时解决方案具有提供短期价值、投资回报快的优势,关键是往往为更具战略性的、长期的解决方案提供基础设施的要求或政策信息。临时解决方案往往为收集长期战略的要求提供了基础。例如,一个临时解决方案可能是一个独立的数据集，具有一个有限的数据集和支持少数的非常具体的方案或研究问题的报告。这种原型数据库包含的信息，可能适用于其他方案,可能有利于设计灵活的、更广泛应用的数据模型。最后,临时解决方案可以帮助构建基础模块,设计战略或满足突发事件执行更复杂的系统。然而,如果未来没有适当的管理手段和意愿做出改变，临时解决方案倾向于成为永久的解决方案。因此,选择是否用“小于最优”的解决方案向前推进的时候,一定要权衡利益和每种方法的局限性。

在下面的章节中所描述的许多设计原则适用于任何规模的数据管理项目。

评价数据来源

有效的局部数据管理将利用各种数据源，但每个数据源对移植项目的价值可能是不同的。考虑数据集的价值时,来源、用途以及数据的格式是重要因素。在评估数据源时,通常认为来源和用途是一致的,据此可以推测数据采集的背景,如果它需要一些转换,抽象化或解释是最有用的。数据格式化需要考虑的首要因素包括：数据是否被编码为显式，或明确意义的离散字段,或抽象叙事为主的文本块。

离散采集数据

在一个理想的状态下，临床护理过程中收集的所有信息可以离散采集并容易分析。实际上,临床护理仍然是极具叙事性质的(如医生笔记),反映的相应数据缺乏结构性。因此,必须采取如下策略之一:①在临床护理中采集其他离散元素；②从叙事文本中以手动或编程方式将离散信息抽象化。

概括医疗记录

采集临床数据的一种普遍常用的方法是概括医疗记录笔记。可以经过概括抽象合成完整的记录,用于回答研究者或临床医生当前的具体问题。在和其他医疗记录的数据提取方法做比较时，医疗记录抽象概括通常被认为是金标准。在提取临床数据时,使用电子数据收集工具可以提高效率和完整性，但医疗记录抽象概括往往是一个既昂贵又耗时的过程。此外,和任何二次利用数据采集一样,医疗记录抽象概括同样存在风险,因为在抽象概括时必须解读不在其控制或知识范围内的笔记和变量。

把抽象概括的医疗记录和从源数据提取的离散元素相结合,可以显著提高手动抽象概括效率,并最大限度地减少数据输入的负担。便于分析师从病历中提取离散变量,如生命体征和实验室值,使其专注于计算不能直接提取的变量。在收集大量的数据时,当其中的数据提取不能提供数据集所需的所有变量时，证明这种混合方法是有价值的。

采集临床工作流程数据

根据项目的指导原则,如“每一位患者也被认为是一个潜在的研究课题”,局部数据管理项目可以将其数据采集策略塑造为临床护理和科学研究双重目的。在收集用于科研的医疗记录变量时可以使用工具，如护理流程表和医生的笔记模板。变量应该有不同的选择或离散测量,应该避免出现自由文本字段。

要尽量减少数据收集的负担,同时在数据输入时,最大限度地确定哪些变量可以在临床护理过程中收集,在什么工作流程中可以收集到这些变量。应考虑的问题是:

• 如何在各阶段的工作流程中获取变量？如冷缺血时间这个变量应该在术中或手术后不久采集，而不是在患者出院后采集。

• 本质上是离散的信息，但目前收集的是非离散形式吗？可以很容易变成离散型的变量都非常适合数据采集。

• 怎样将变量运用到某一特定研究或在多个问题或项目中得以应用?如果不赋予变量以用途,那么收集到的变量可能很快变得难以管理。

自然语言处理

另一个值得一提的离散型数据采集策略是自然语言处理(NLP)的实践。NLP是通过计算机系统处理复杂的文本算法,提取叙事文本的意义。NLP系统通常会将医疗文本中的文本映射到一个或多个医学术语。在医学文本的上下文,NLP系统往往会将文本与一个或多个医学术语配对。由于NLP系统的精度不断提高,NLP也越来越受到关注。由于很多电子病历信息以非离散叙事形式存储，在未来NLP作为一个更简洁、准确的信息来源,有望在临床和研究领域大展前途。

数据源

根据本文的目的，在局部数据管理项目中可能使用的数据源将被分为两类:二手(辅助性)数据源和一手(原始)数据源。二手数据源是指其主要用途直接应用于临床护理或达到管理目标，并且也可重复应用于非临床护理目的的数据。专门针对非临床护理目的收集的数据是原始数据源(一手数据源)。二手数据源和一手数据源的主要差异体现在用途上的区别。在临床上所收集的数据是现成的，但可能不准确或在医疗质量测量和研究设置中意义不大。为特定的目的而收集的数据,诸如质量度量或研究的数据通常更加准确,因为在大多数情况下，会为特定的数据收集创建适应目的的系统或工具。然而,在临床环境中使用未整合到临床工作流程系统中的工具收集数据，其费用和时间成本令人望而却步。有效的数据管理项目将把两个数据源都加以利用。

二手数据源

在平时照护患者的过程中收集有关管理和临床的数据,可以发现丰富的信息。通常将这些数据导入到一个数据库或其他数据存储库,以便于提取和分析。

管理数据

从医院和供应商的计费系统获取管理数据是目前最为广泛的途径。卫生系统的纳税人依靠标准化的诊断和程序代码来处理结算报销,因此,管理数据可以跨机构进行比较。特别是ICD代码以多种形式在世界各地大多数的临床护理设施中使用。此外,计费代码已被使用了几十年，从而提供了大型的纵向资源。遗憾的是,研究发现,由于编码错误、诊断和预后细节获取的局限性,管理数据不能提供准确的临床信息。

在试图从缺失的管理数据推断结果的时候，重新利用管理数据的问题尤其严重。记录管理代码的目的通常是为了计费报销。管理数据里可能不包括临床相关的健康状况，因为没有必要对治疗过程或就诊做证明。例如,如果管理目标没有对ICD代码的需求,那么一个肾脏疾病四期的患者可能永远不会有一个四期ICD编码就诊记录。分析管理数据时,尽管有局限性,但这个庞大的、可访问的编码数据库是非常有价值的。在对数据绝对的准确性要求不高的情况下使用管理数据是最有效的方式，如汇总数据或在最初识别患者人群。当移植项目需要推断详细的临床意义,如共病、疾病的严重程度和并发症,最好使用其他数据源。

电子病历数据

从电子病历系统(EMR)采集的用于临床护理的数据提供了一系列离散型和叙述性元素。电子病历的主要目的是收集临床护理的数据，因此能较好满足局部数据管理项目的需求。有用的电子病历模块包括订单、护理记录、用药信息、实验室和病理信息、计算机辅助医疗资料和从医疗设备得到的结果。因不同机构提供的数据来源不同,所以数据的可用性和格式有所区别,但随着数据价值认可度的提升，在这些领域的投资也不断增加。移植项目需要收集大量的从临床护理过程中采集的数据,但与管理数据一样,在利用临床数据时需要谨慎处理收集的原始变量的意义和目的。例如一个PRN用药顺序,只能表明药物提供给患者,但并不能说明药物被施用。由于这些潜在的误解,因此主题专家解释电子病历信息是至关重要的。

一手来源数据

直接采集数据用于本地数据管理是收集准确信息的策略，而没有与重新使用的临床数据相关联的一些并发症。数据可以在各种设置下采集,但不同于二手使用数据集，其数据集的预期用途之一是用于研究和质量报告。一手使用数据采集与二手使用数据采集相比具有明显的优势，因为在一手数据采集时通常能实现对变量的质量、含义和背景加以控制。例如，“吸烟史”这个变量在医疗记录中可用,但是：

• 精度——每次都以同样的方式向患者询问吸烟情况的吗?

• 含义——在过去的一年里吸烟吗？每周的吸烟超过一包吗?

• 或环境——提问时患者的家属在场吗?

采集的变量可能是来历不明的。可以围绕变量的采集、含义和报告对一手使用数据赋予特定的要求。

局部数据库

管理移植项目相关数据的常用方法是创建和维护一个独立于数据库或其他数据储存库的数据库。调查显示,这种做法非常流行,因为它可以对数据进行直接管理,且只需较少的基础设施。这些数据通常存储在微软的电子表格或数据库中。补充局部数据库的方式有很多，但往往是手动提取或定期从一个更大的数据存储库中提取数据,如数据库中的数据。如果不谨慎地管理局部数据库将遇到很多问题。管理局部数据库的调查员需要注意数据完整性问题,如：

• 准确性——都是根据定义进行变量编码的吗?

• 数据的有效性——数值是正确的和可以核查的吗?

• 以及一致性——变量的数值记录方式有统一标准吗?

调查员还应该尽可能地避免输入自由文本字段。

其他需要考虑的问题：

• 版本——当前的数据库是什么版本?

• 时间变化——如何管理人口和病史变化?

• 变量改变——在修改变量的定义时会忽略对历史数据的修改吗?

在创建和维护局部数据库方面，需要调查员付出大量的努力,但如果信息技术和基础设施的条件有限，那么通过加强适当的安全控制措施也可以是管理局部数据的有效方法。

多机构注册

目前有多个移植注册中心。国家注册工作的开展可以由政府授权或者通过移植项目驱动。注册中心保存的数据通常有严格的定义和标准。因为从注册中心获取的信息允许对同类项目之间的关键绩效指标和做法做比较,所以它对移植项目而言很有价值。此外,由于注册中心收集的数据的可靠性，移植项目往往可以得到详细的人口学资料。在美国,给研究人员提供数据的一些重要注册中心包括：移植受者科学登记(SRTR)、器官共享联合网络(UNOS)和美国肾脏数据系统(USRDS)。

电子病例报告表

临床试验信息往往通过一个病例报告表(CRF)采集。病例报告表收集的信息是从临床试验中观测到的,在多数情况下可能会从临床医疗系统转录或抽象概括获得。从历史上看,病例报告表一直以纸质记录为主,但随着基于网络的电子数据采集工具的广泛应用,病例报告表数据越来越多地被直接或间接地通过电子病例报告表(eCRF)采集。相对于纸质收集,利用基于网络的数据收集工具在成本、效率、数据的完整性和安全性等方面提供了多重效益。

生物储存数据系统

生物数据库存储特定群体的标本及其相关临床信息,用于将来的科学研究。实验室信息管理系统(LIMS)通过对标本采集、处理、存储、检索和分布等信息管理来支持生物知识库的操作运行。大多数 LIMS 还提供审计跟踪、电子签名、条码标签打印、扫描以及工作流程自动化等技术，使跟踪标本信息比用日志和电子表格的方法记录更加有效安全。LIMS 的功能是对样本数据进行优化管理,因此大多数 LIMS 不是为收集患者的临床信息而设计的。而生物知识库为样本数据从 LIMS 中链接出来提供了一种机制，从而为其链接其他一个或多个数据源的标本的临床病理资料提供了一个更具扩展性的方法。

研究实验室数据

实验室检测,如流式细胞仪、图像分析和基因表达谱分析产生大量的数据。数据管理项目若尝试使用这些检测结果,必须考虑如何有效地存储、分析和归档这些数据。另外,如果无法获取这些标本对应患者的临床资料,那么标本和检测结果的意义不大。此外,对于大多数纵向标本的集合,链接到一个标本的临床信息是在收集标本时的快照,标本和临床信息必须在时间上匹配。在适当的时候需要一个设计良好的工作流程,结合临床治疗、标本采集和标本分析,从而保持标本和患者之间的这种匿名联系。

准备整合数据

数据集成涉及到检索、组合来自多个来源的数据。在集成异构数据源或将小数据集加入更大的数据源时,应控制到位,以保证数据的有效性、一致性、准确性和完整性。数据质量问题往往出自数据源,如由于数据录入不准确、信息缺失或数据无效形成的文件或数据库。集成来自多个数据源的数据时,需要建立更加完备的质量控制机制,因为数据源可能包含重复的数据、不同的表现形式和不一致的标识符。为确保数据的高质量,在集成数据集时可以坚持以下几个原则:

- 通过电子数据采集收集数据时进行数据验证。
- 保持数据定义的一致性。
- 归类常见的变量。
- 理解派生参数(派生参数明确化、量化和定时化)。
- 理解编码概念的作用。
- 跨系统连接数据标识符策略。

数据验证

使用桌面应用程序或基于网络的在线形式采集电子数据是获取数据的常见方式。在创建数据采集接口时,为促进高质量的数据采集,可采用以下策略:

- 使用下拉菜单和选择列表限制输入选项来定义一组术语或概念。
- 限制使用自由文本字段。
- 限制或消除“评论”字段。
- 在适当的时候,设置必填字段,若未填写则用户不能进行下一步操作。
- 在可能的情况下,限制用户必须手动执行的任何计算。

许多基于表单的电子数据采集平台会将验证逻辑编程进表单。表单验证允许将规则分配给特定字段来限制数据输入的有效值。约束数据输入字段的实例包括:

- 特殊格式的文本。
- 特定的数据类型,如数值型。
- 在一个集合范围内的数字。

一致的数据定义

当以质量控制或科学研究为目的检索临床或其他系统的数据时,应保持通用数据元素定义的一致性,包括变量及其来源、提取方法、标准解释和计算派生参数的一致公式。例如,标准实验室值,如血清肌酐,应该具有明确的数据源,并且每次都以相同的方式检索。在另一实例中,移植受者血清学结果的解释通常基于特定的实验室测试结果,但也可由项目工作人员记录在单独的位置,如呼叫中心。在数据可能有多个来源的情况下,应当建立一套标准的真值和定义,并且在每次检索时用于相同的变量。

编目通用数据元素

为了促进数据的一致重复使用,应对公共变量编目,为核心数据元素集提供参考点,并且在某些情况下为自动化流程提供映射,以提取、转换和将变量加载到目标数据库。目录应包含元数据或“有关数据的数据”。在最基本的层面上,目录可能仅提供一组核心属性的文档,并列出以下内容:

- 变量名。
- 描述。
- 领域或主题范围(例如人口统计,实验室,药物,程序)。
- 数据源,用于标识源系统或数据库。
- 数据类型(例如,文本型,数字型,日期型)。
- 业务规则(确定派生的数据元素和逻辑或计算结果的公式)。

对于可能是共享资源的移植项目特定数据存储库,目录还应包括有关如何通过指定变量所在的表名和列来访问存储库中数据的信息。

所谓自动化过程,即元数据存储在元数据存储库中，其中存储有关自动提取、变换和加载数据所需的源、目标、转换、映射、工作流程、会话和其他信息的所有信息。

派生数据元素

从临床数据源（包括临床信息系统和临床数据仓库）获得的原始数据并不总是详实、完整或结构化的，其格式有时不利于分析。临床数据源包括用于患者护理的所有信息系统，并且临床数据仓库是获得在对患者护理过程中收集的临床数据的媒介。数据可以被组织在不同的表中或者被来自不同的数据源不同地结构化。因此，原始数据必须转换为对分析更有用的结构。对于分析有价值的许多概念比单个值更复杂，并且可以由许多数据点的组合或在特定时间点采集的一个或多个变量派生。

派生数据由基于应用于一个或多个原始数据元素以创建新数据的规则的替代表示构成。这些元素可以根据分类、定量或时间导出。源字段可以是源系统或导出元素本身。虽然派生数据不会写入数据源，但可以将其显示为对这些源数据执行查询的结果，或存储在局部数据存储库中。

分类导出的值表示为基于应用到一个或多个字段的逻辑的文本结果或符号。分类导出的数据可以采集一个二进制值或状态（例如，“是”或“否”、“正”或“负”、“+”或“-”、“1”或“0”）。在其他情况下，结果可以指示几种状态中的一种（例如，1 =男性，2 =女性，3 =不确定）。在临床研究数据库中，状态字段可以表示在特定时间点的诊断、实验室结果或药物状态，如果在该时间点指示诊断、实验室或药物，则为“是”，如果没有指示，则显示为“否”。

通过对一个或多个字段执行数值计算并存储结果值来生成定量派生数据。定量结果的示例包括描述性统计和应用于数字字段的任意组合的预定义或用户定义的公式。在定量派生的数据中使用的变量可受到时间元素约束，例如在固定时间间隔上的特定变量的最大值。

根据时间点派生的数据分析适用于相对于锚定事件在特定时间点发生的数据。数据可以由指定的时间点约束或计算。在临床研究设置中，锚定事件可以描述诊断日期、过程日期、发病日期、出院日期，给药日期和时间或采集实验室标本的日期和时间。描述在特定时间点采集的数据的时间数据，通常受到相对于锚定事件的时间间隔的约束，或者可以在设定的间隔上计算。例如，代表移植后三个月的时间点可以计算为从手术当天起的天数间隔，并且可以用于限制数据的选择，如围绕该数据记录的实验室值、药物或不良事件时间点。时间数据也可以用于计算术后天数以报告患者或移植物生存情况。

编码的概念

编码概念适用于使用编码值代替为数据元素提供的值的文本所表示的任何数据元素。在数据集或系统中使用的任何数据元素表示一些概念（例如，静息心率、收缩压值或性别）。由数据元素表示的概念可能需要与静息心率和收缩压相同的文本或数值，或者它可能需要一组与性别一样的预定义值。这些预定义的值是编码概念，可以是一些局部定义的值或代码集（例如，1 等于男性，2 等于女性），或者也可以源自标准术语（例如，SNOMED 或 ICD）。需要强调的是，在不同上下文中使用的给定数据元素可以表示不同的概念，并且因此绑定到不同的代码集。因此，理解在文本中使用的数据元素和与其绑定的代码集的意义，以适当地解释元素的含义是非常重要的。

除了为局部数据集中的数据元素提供编码值列表，代码集还用于其他目的，包括：

- 定义计算方式。
- 遵守一些管理机构要求的数据标准。
- 与具有相同数据元素和编码值的其他数据源集合。
- 定义不是标准词汇的部分。

确保数据合规性

数据合规性可确保数据符合适当的指南和规范，无论它们是法律法规、机构政策还是合同义务。这些要求可能包括确保数据完整性的保护，关于数据必须保存多长时间的规定，或甚至关于数据引用方式的保证。数据合规性的要求通常是复杂的、多层次的，由国际、国家、州或地方法律等多方合同要求或方针指南共同推动的。此外，因地理位置不同，同一合规在不同领域/区域可能有所差异。例如，保护个人隐私作为一个主要的合规领域，尽管其特定性和范围各不相同，但大多数国家对电子通信中的个人隐私保护都有一些规定。在美国,有健康保险流通与责任法案,第二章(HIPAA);加拿大有个人信息保护和电子文件法(PIPEDA);欧盟有数据保护指令,也称为指令 95/46/EC;南非拥有“电子通信和交易法,2002”。由于数据合规性的多样性、复杂性和细微差别,极有必要让具有合规审查专业知识的人员为局部数据管理项目提供指导。

数据合规性的一个关键挑战是保证数据的使用或披露与个人在向机构提供其数据时同意的参数一致。例如,在没有遵循适当的合规条例并获得适当的授权之前,提供给临床护理的数据不应用于研究目的。因此,在局部数据管理时实施跟踪和管理同意的程序特别重要。研究数据特别具有挑战性,因为与知情同意和任何相关信息使用授权相关的所有细微差别,都必须在数据被披露或使用之前被理解和完成。对于临床数据,尤其是在数据包含个人身份信息的情况下,数据管理团队必须了解在什么情况下使用或发布数据是合规的。此外,数据可能经过一次使用,随后是在原始预期用途的范围之外的第二次使用。这种情况的一个例子出现在用于临床护理质量评审(通常被定义为医疗保健操作的一部分的用途)的数据和分析,随后被提出用于研究杂志中的研究或出版时,要达到第二次利用数据的目的,将需要额外的合规步骤。由于上述情况的复杂性,为局部数据管理项目制订明确、成文的标准操作程序,描述允许的情况和这类数据使用所需的过程是非常必要的。这不仅确保一般的遵从性,还将有助于保护移植项目中移植受者的个人信息。

以下内容是一小部分移植项目应该注意的国家和潜在地方法规的。这些法规是专门适用于美国的,当然其他国家可能也有类似类型的规定。

健康保险流通与责任法案

健康保险流通与责任法案【1996】(HIPAA)由多个规则和部分组成。对于局部数据管理项目,应特别注意的是以下规则:隐私规则、安全规则、患者安全规则,以及违反通知规则的健康信息技术促进经济和临床健康(HITECH)法。总的来说,这些规则提出了一系列国家标准,保护个人的健康信息。HIPAA 为大多数机构提供了设计其信息安全和隐私政策、程序以及配套设施的模板。

隐私规则规定受 HIPAA 保护的数据类型,以及允许机构使用和披露受保护健康信息的情况。安全规则涵盖了保护电子保护健康信息(ePHI)所必需的标准。违规通知规则详细说明了在什么条件下以及在什么程度时,机构及其业务人员必须在确认违反规定的不安全数据后通知受影响的个人。

HIPAA 中的这些规则适用于涵盖实体的部分机构,HIPAA 将其定义为“以电子形式进行某些交易的医疗保健提供者;医疗保健结算所;或健康计划”或其业务伙伴之一。有关 HIPAA 的更多信息,请访问网址 http://www.hhs.gov/ocr。

21 CFR 第 11 部分的合规性

21 CFR 第 11 部分规定了一系列规定,“根据这些规定,[FDA]将电子记录、电子签名和对电子记录执行的手写签名视为可信赖、可靠的,通常相当于在纸上执行的纸质记录和手写签名”。第 11 部分侧重于确保数据的可靠性和完整性的方法,特别侧重于电子签名,审计跟踪和访问控制。

本法规适用于在 FDA 监管行业工作或与其合作的机构,包括临床试验。有关第 11 部分合规性的更多信息,请访问网址 http://www.accessdata.fda.gov。

联邦信息系统管理

2002 年的美国联邦信息系统管理法案(FISMA)是一项联邦法律,规定所有的联邦机构应建立一个全机构的信息安全计划,“支持机构的运营和资产,包括由另一个机构、承包商或其他来源提供或管理的信息和信息系统”。该法律确定了由 NIST 维持构建、监控和持续改进的框架。与其他法规(如 HIPAA 和第 11 部分)不同,FISMA 合规性必须采用非常具体的过程、程序和安全控制。

该法适用于联邦机构以及希望与联邦机构签订合同的机构。由于政府合同是移植项目的可行工具,因此计划必须审查并了解符合 FISMA 要求的工作量和成本。有关 FISMA 的更多信息,请访问网址 http://csrc.nist.gov。

患者安全和质量改善

患者安全和质量改进法案【2005】(PSQI)旨在提高美国医疗机构的患者安全。正如 Cartwright-Smith 等总结的,PSQI“旨在通过使用被称为‘特权’的法律工具,鼓励提供者报告患者安全和其他保健质量信息,鼓励对质量和安全性进行可靠的检查，而不必担心这些工作的结果将被原告在责任审判期间‘发现’”。与局部数据管理项目密切相关的是，理解什么信息被认为是患者安全工作内容（PSWP)，并且因此被认为受本法保护。有关此法案的更多信息，请访问网址 http://www.iso.org/。

记录管理政策

不论针对电子记录还是纸质记录，每个机构应该有一套个性化的记录管理政策，规定从记录开始采集到最终销毁整个生命周期应如何处理。典型的记录管理项目将记录分类为不同的类别，例如临床研究记录或医疗保健管理记录，并且对每个记录类别(例如记录保留期限)规定不同的策略。有时，制订者可能会规定影响记录如何管理的具体规则，例如数据传播要求。

记录管理政策将适用于每个局部数据管理项目，并因机构而异。有关记录管理的更多信息，请访问网址 http://www.iso.org。

数据保护

无论是为了保护患者的隐私，维护知识产权，还是遵守各种地方、州、国家或国际法规或政策，信息安全和隐私保护制度程序必须在保护机构免受风险和提供访问数据以供项目使用之间达到适当的平衡。对于一个移植项目，应该确保很多安全措施控制到位。这些控制措施的实施将根据工作人员的专业知识、现有资源和资金情况而有所不同，但至少应该了解和授权如何执行这些控制措施。以下是思考他们如何实现的一小部分控制措施和指南。

数据恢复

该过程解决了因为硬件故障、灾难、计算机病毒或其他手段不可避免地破坏数据的风险。为了减轻这种风险，项目应该确定数据备份的预期频率。这通常取决于他们能够承受的数据损失量。如果是关键数据，尽管需要相对较大的费用，也需要高频率的数据备份，而如果存储库是多个权威源的聚合，则备份策略无需太频繁(例如，每周一次)。

一般来说，很多机构每天都会备份其数据，并且每个月都会存储在异地的快照。诸如遗传序列这类大数据可能具有不同的备份策略，因为备份这样一个大数据量的成本相当大。

除了备份的频率之外，项目还应确定备份哪些数据。一个标准是，不能及时重建的任何数据都应该备份。例如，通过对研究受者的访谈或在组织样本上进行的专门测试获得的原始数据可能需要完整的备份计划。由于备份的成本和时间，一些项目可能不会把数据集里的所有变量都进行备份，而是简单地保持原始数据的备份和针对其运行的算法的注释以产生分析的集合 。

其他需要考虑的内容包括：

- 如果数据备份到外部设备（例如磁带或外部硬盘驱动器)，并且包含敏感信息，则必须对外部设备或加密设备上的数据进行加密。这将防止由于外部设备丢失或被盗时造成数据泄露。
- 如果数据必须遵守 HIPAA 法规并且是异地存储，则必须与异地托管供应商和机构签署业务合作协议。
- 为检测备份数据的完整性，应设置一个至少每年恢复一次整个数据存储库的程序。

从数据中分离标识符

假定可单独识别的信息(即姓名、医疗记录号)对于研究是必需的，通常最好将标识符与核心数据集分开，并将它们存储在具有访问受限的独立数据存储库中。通过转换键映射到可单独识别的局部标识符信息，取代可单独识别的信息，以实现删除记录的重复数据以及整合来自其他来源的数据的能力。在大多数情况下，对于大多数研究、教育和结果使用来说，个人可识别的信息，如电子病历、姓名和地址不是必需的。此外，日期可以向后滚动或向前滚动一致的天数以混淆它们，同时保持它们与某些类型的分析相关。若没有可单独识别的信息，保密性风险将显著降低。

培训和期望设定

许多安全控制取决于知道事情正确的做法并拥有丰富技能的个人。人们在访问任何数据(特别是敏感数据)之前应该知道一套标准的操作程序和要求，例如不向任何人泄露密码不、不随意点击嵌入在电子邮件中的链接等。

虽然大多数机构向教师、居民、博士后、学生和工作人员提供信息安全学习课程，但课程可能不会涉及移植项目创建的具体程序和过程。建立特定于移植的课程可以为他们的日常工作提供更高水平的特异性和相关性。此外,它可以为他们提供保护关键数据的知识和战术。

除了培训,可以在每个电子系统中实现视觉提示和行为规则,提示数据的敏感程度以及数据的预期使用目的。例如,可以修改每个应用程序的登录界面以插入语言,个人在访问该系统时就可以看到关于数据敏感度级别的提示语言。还可以包括附加信息的链接,以便提醒与系统相关联的"行为规则"是什么,例如,数据不能被下载并分发给协议组之外的任何人。

由第三方进行安全评估

由客观的第三方评估提供一种测试系统安全性的方法。这些测试通常被称为"应用程序安全性评估"。与能提供良好参考意见的可靠第三方合作,建立一系列目标,并明确记录接受测试的系统。然后,第三方进行一系列测试,识别并量化系统相关的任何漏洞。基于目标,这些测试可以从移植项目的网络内部或外部进行。如果应用程序是内部开发的,则供应商还可以访问程序代码以进行更详细的审查。虽然合约内容可能不同,但移植项目系统应该收到一系列关于漏洞的解释和评级的检测报告,以帮助量化漏洞带来的风险。根据合同规定,在程序有机会解决这些漏洞之后,可能会对系统运行重新评估。

由于这类合约的敏感性,一定要确保合同适当地保护机构免受有意或无意的信息泄露。此外,由于测试包含敏感数据可能是影响系统实际运行的关键步骤,因此合同应提及所有约束条件以及如何访问此数据。最后,在进行任何测试之前,所有合适的团队,包括机构的安全和信息技术团队,都应当参与进来,并签订参与保密协议。

部署

局部数据管理项目在部署阶段主要参照设计阶段构建的方案,同时考虑实际运作环境。基于方案的类型,部署活动将有所不同。然而,无论该方案是重新设计的还是在现有数据源、报告或功能的基础上做修改的,都需要保证已经进行了适当的测试,并且将新的方案纳入到支持结构中。

除了部署特定的方案外,还应继续支持和推进局部数据管理程序的整体管理和运作。移植关键领域数据的管理在移植项目中具有举足轻重的地位。

数据管理项目中的角色类型

在描述管理结构和操作支持时,有必要描述数据管理项目中的角色类型。当然,有些人可能基于他们的专业知识和在组织中的地位而具有多重角色类型。

- **利益相关者**。对移植项目中特定的程序、过程或领域具有所有权的对象。他们帮助指导战略,优先考虑资源分配,审查项目目标,以确保它们符合组织目标。利益相关者可代表机构内的不同组织,并可包括医生、主要研究者、管理者、技术主管和移植项目中为数据管理活动提供投入的其他成员。
- **主题专家**(SME)。在特定主题领域(例如肝移植)获得认可的专家。一般来说,数据管理项目将寻找这些专家以帮助解决与该域相关的数据的具体问题,或者在复杂报告或数据结构的设计中借助他们的知识以协助决策。
- **数据生产者和数据消费者**。直接与每个从不同的侧面获取的数据交互。数据生产者通常拥有获取源数据的主系统,例如临床信息系统、实验室信息系统和研究管理系统。数据消费者利用数据进行分析、决策和研究。这两组用户在沟通数据如何使用以及如何改进程序方面发挥了关键作用。数据生产者直接与数据交互,并且可以从过程角度提供对数据收集的反馈,以及何时最适当地记录作为其工作流程的一部分的特定数据点。同时,数据消费者向数据管理团队提供关于数据应用、效用和传递机制的反馈——什么是有效的,什么是无效的。
- **数据管理团队由几个角色组成**。基本上负责数据提取、收集、分析、传递、安全性、管理、按照信息管理策略处理数据发布,以及维护元数据的所有权。数据管理团队由多个角色构成,包括:
    - 团队领导角色,负责总体监督和项目管理,确保请求和项目按时交付。
    - 业务分析员角色,用于收集和记录业务需求。
    - 数据分析人员角色,将业务需求转换为数据采集和交付流程。
    - 生物统计学家角色,提供研究设计和统计分析方面的专业知识。

◦数据管理者角色，审查发布请求并确保在授权发布数据之前已经采取了适当的步骤。

◦监督者角色，确保发布的数据在单独发布给调查员之前被适当地去除标识。

根据可用资源，上述大多数角色由一名或少数几名分析员担任。

测试

由于数据用于支持决策，所以新的方案在没有进行正式测试之前不应发布。在进行测试之前，应制订一份测试计划，计划中详细列出每个测试人员将采取的步骤。此活动不但为所有测试人员提供一致性，还可以将任何错误追溯到一个特定的步骤。测试计划应包括多种情形，包括“蓝天”情形，即用户的所有假设正常运行；非常规情形，测试者试图执行有意地从正常运行情形转移的任务；以及测试人员尝试访问他们不应该访问的信息的安全情形。除了正式测试，要求实际用户参与测试也能促使新方案不断改进，并得到很有价值的反馈信息。重要的是，不仅要测试确保新方案在功能上与设计初衷一致，而且要测试数据的准确性和可用性，并确保新的方案不会在当前数据管理系统中引入任何意外问题。

支持结构

如果没有稳固的支持结构，那么局部数据管理项目是无法实现可持续发展的。支持结构将依赖于非正式通信来传达其信息，它将缺乏共同的文件和流程，方案运作的一致性以及补救问题的能力将取决于工作人员的意愿/信誉。总体而言，支持结构虽然不像局部数据管理项目的规划和设计部分那样具有创新性，但仍然是成功的关键因素。

支持结构的组成人员应该对服务对象采取友好的态度，积极参与项目，在解决问题时有丰富的经验，在思考问题时有高度的分析能力，以及在阐述问题根源和提出相关解决方案时具有强大的沟通能力。提供项目支持的可能与帮助计划、设计和部署方案的是同一个人。除了人员之外，持续更新合适的文件和过程也十分重要。随着解决方案从设计过渡到生产/应用，支持局部数据管理项目的流程和文档应该更新，以反映任何新的变化。标准操作程序应该对如何处理请求和数据有详细的说明。数据字典或元数据存储库要保持持续更新状态以反映最新的字段和值。培训材料和支持文件应公布在内部网站上，给其他独立的数据管理团队提供帮助，并扩大局部数据管理团队之外的支持结构。

最后，了解每种类型数据的披露和使用的规定及其标准操作流程对于局部数据管理团队的所有成员，尤其是支持团队是至关重要的。如“数据合规性”部分所述，根据与数据的使用权限和预期用途不同，可能需要不同的步骤和授权。

数据治理

数据治理给代表多种角色的个人和主题专家提供聚集在一起讨论和建议与数据管理项目相关的战略方向、政策和优先事项的机会。对于局部数据管理项目，治理机构提供了一个讨论挑战和验证意图的有力平台。一般来说，同意服务于数据治理委员会的个人致力于项目的成功，并能成为强有力的合作倡导者。通过将数据治理纳入流程，局部数据管理项目放弃了一些决策的权威，但获得了更广泛的洞察数据如何被利用的机会，在决策过程中提供了更大的透明度，并将项目集成了一个责任共同体。

在形成和运行数据治理流程时，局部数据管理项目应考虑：

• 数据治理是治理，而非管理。治理机构应重点关注指导原则和政策，从而影响数据管理项目的运作方式。管理层引入较低水平的治理战术常常会干扰或延迟数据管理项目的日常操作。例如，治理机构应当审查并提供有关披露数据的标准操作程序的建议；然而，它不应该是每个数据申请的批准机构。

• 治理应与移植领导层结构联系起来，并有权根据治理宪章的规定制订特定类别的决策。若有一位移植领导团队的主席或共同主席是数据治理委员会的成员，将有助于与领导层的协调。

• 数据治理机构审议的关键领域包括：标准操作程序；数据采集表格、数据值和术语标准化的条件；安全和隐私政策；将数据源的优先排序纳入数据管理项目；以及评估项目成功的方法和指标。

互动

与社区的互动越强，数据管理项目与它所服务的人口之间的合作关系就越强。因此，很有必要多接触移植项目中各级别的各种角色。从这些互动中,局部数据管理项目将从社区获得帮助,包括确定问题和挑战,通过新想法或筹资机会扩大项目的新机会,以及关于项目细节组成部分的正面和负面反馈。

一个成功的数据管理项目需要不断更新改变其方法,不断重新调整,以确保其原则和优先事项与移植项目的目标保持一致。因此,局部数据管理组应确保与移植领导小组进行正式的定期会议。在这些会议中,团队应该报告关键绩效指标、项目状态、遇到的问题和风险以及成功案例。

评估

在最后阶段,局部数据管理项目组织领导层和治理层共同制订一系列关键绩效指标,评估其绩效指标,并根据评估结果,将变革纳入规划阶段,以改进项目。虽然会进行较多的非正式评估,但是以特定的时间间隔对项目进行正式评估,将有助于量化局部数据管理项目的总体绩效。

尽管每个项目都有其独特的度量标准,下面列举一些需要常规考虑的内容:

- 效率。减少查询或收集信息所需的系统数目、步骤或时间。支持这一点的例子为通过将数据存储在一个存储库,而不是多个来源的系统的方式,使得收集报告或查询数据的时间大大减少。这在某些情况下具有显著的影响,如工作人员从手动收集和记录用于报告的信息的过程转变为自动化过程(例如,运行报告)。
- 流程改进。由于工作流程和支持系统的自动化,移植项目内的过程实现了标准化和优化。这一指标或证据的例子包括跟踪能力、改善协议遵守情况、减少文书工作或减少在数据输入所需的系统或步骤。
- 决策支持。在关键决策中用于通知移植项目成员的报告和数据文件的数量。
- 数据质量。通过数据保证的脚本和技术识别的与其关联的错误值的记录数。
- 任务支持。调查员和质量项目使用数据管理项目进行研究、质量改进工程、公共卫生监测和其他支持移植项目任务和目标的活动。
- 成本效益分析。对主体总成本与取得利益的价值进行分析。这是重要的评估组成部分,以确定该项目是否值得投资。

总结

对任何移植项目而言,一个积极、全面的数据管理项目是非常宝贵的资产。然而,与任何关键组成部分一样,局部数据管理项目的进步和完善离不开计划、设计、部署和评估等一系列连续的过程来帮助形成项目雏形以满足移植项目不断变化的需求。最后,一个有效的数据管理项目将在适当的时间提供适当的数据,以便为特定患者群体提供护理相关的循证决策,支持持续的质量和结果测量、干预的机会,提供用于数据密集型的临床研究,支持当地人群与国家或国际数据集的比较,并有助于满足质量和结果报告的要求。

(陈俊丽 董思依 林丽丹 译 徐骁 校)

参考文献

1. Meier-Kriesche HU, Schold JD, Srinivas TR, et al. Lack of improvement in renal allograft survival despite a marked decrease in acute rejection rates over the most recent era. American journal of transplantation. 2004;4(3):378-383.
2. United Network For Organ Sharing [homepage on the Internet]. UNOS: Donation & Transportation: Data. [accessed Dec 03, 2011]; Available at: http://www.unos.org/donation/index.php?topic=data.
3. Harris PA, Taylor R, Thielke R, et al. Research electronic data capture (REDCap)-a metadata-driven methodology and workflow process for providing translational research informatics support. Journal of Biomedical Informatics. 2009;42(2): 377-381.
4. Zhou L, Plasek JM, Mahoney LM, et al. Using Medical Text Extraction, Reasoning and Mapping System (MTERMS) to process medication information in outpatient clinical notes. AMIA Annual Symposium proceedings/AMIA Symposium AMIA Symposium. 2011;2011:1639-1648.
5. Deleger L, Grouin C, Zweigenbaum P. Extracting medical information from narrative patient records: the case of medication-related information. Journal of the American Medical Informatics Association : JAMIA. 2010;17(5):555-558.
6. Peabody JW, Luck J, Jain S, et al. Assessing the accuracy of administrative data in health information systems. Medical Care. 2004;42(11):1066-1072.
7. Jollis JG, Ancukiewicz M, DeLong ER, et al. Discordance of databases designed for claims payment versus clinical information systems. Implications for outcomes research. Annals of Internal Medicine. 1993;119(8):844-850.
8. Weber BA, Yarandi H, Rowe MA, et al. A comparison study: paper-based versus web-based data collection and management. Applied Nursing Research: ANR. 2005;18(3):182-185.
9. Rahm E, Do H-H. Data cleaning: problems and current approaches. IEEE Bulletin of the Technical Committee on Data Engineering. 2000;23(4):11.
10. Learn Data Modeling. Metadata Tutorial | Metadata in ETL. [accessed Jan 10, 2011]; Available at: http://www.learndatamodeling.com/meta2.htm.
11. Myers RB, Herskovic JR. Probabilistic techniques for obtaining accurate patient counts in Clinical Data Warehouses. Journal of Biomedical Informatics. 2011; 44(Suppl 1):S69-S77.
12. Gray GW. Challenges of building clinical data analysis solutions. Journal of Critical Care. 2004;19(4):264-270.
13. Data Modeling in Clinical Data Analysis Projects. [accessed 2011 Jan 10, 2011]; Available at: http://www2.sas.com/proceedings/sugi26/p131-26.pdf.
14. Department of Justice. Personal Information Protection and Electronic Documents Act. c2000 [updated 2012 Jan 09; accessed 2012 Jan 11, 2011]; Available at: http://laws-lois.justice.gc.ca/eng/acts/P-8.6/FullText.html.
15. The European Parliament and The Council of the European Union. Directive 95/46/EC of the European Parliament and of the Council of 24 October 1995 on the protection of individuals with regard to the processing of personal data and on the free movement of such data. c1995 [accessed Jan 11, 2011]; Available at:

http://eur-lex.europa.eu/LexUriServ/LexUriServ.do?uri=CELEX:31995L0046:EN:HTML.
16. Parliament of the Republic of South Africa. Electronic Communications and Transactions Act, 2002 No. 25 of 2002. c2002 [accessed Jan 11, 2011]; Available at: http://www.internet.org.za/ect_act.html.
17. Centers for Medicare and Medicaid Services. Are You a Covered Entity? [updated 2005 Dec 14; accessed 2011 Dec 28, 2011]; Available at: http://www.cms.gov/HIPAAGenInfo/06_AreYouaCoveredEntity.asp.
18. Code of Federal Regulations. Title 21, Volume 1. 1997 Mar 20 [updated 2004 Dec 9; accessed Dec 28, 2011]; Available at: http://www.accessdata.fda.gov/scripts/cdrh/cfdocs/cfCFR/CFRSearch.cfm?CFRPart=11&showFR=1&subpartNode=21:1.0.1.1.7.1.
19. National Institute of Standards and Technology. FISMA: Detailed Overview. c2002 [updated 2010 Aug 17; accessed Dec 28, 2011]; Available from: http://csrc.nist.gov/groups/SMA/fisma/overview.html.
20. Cartwright-Smith L, Rosenbaum S, Sochacki C. The Patient Safety and Quality Improvement Act Regulations: Implications for Health Information Access and Exchange. Legal Notes: Vol 2. Issue 2. March 2010 p. 1-7. [accessed Dec 28, 2011] Available at: http://www.rwjf.org/files/research/62608.pdf.21. International Organization for Standardization. [accessed 2010 Dec 28, 2011]; Available from: http://www.iso.org/iso/iso_catalogue/catalogue_tc/catalogue_detail.htm?csnumber=31908.
21. Loshin D. Who owns information. Enterprise Knowledge Management: The Data Quality Approach. Orlando, FL: Academic Press; 2001: 25–46.

第 133 章

国家移植注册数据和人群研究

Allan B. Massie，Dorry L. Segev

引言

随着治疗手段的快速演变和政策的持续变化，移植仍然是一个不断拓展的领域。灵活的、与时俱进的科学推论对于推进我们领域的知识、宣传政策和为患者设计最佳治疗方案至关重要。

正确实施的随机对照试验(RCT)早已被公认是论证科学研究的金标准，构成设计优良的 RCT 应包含的具体因素在第 134 章中有详细讨论。然而，RCT 存在以下几个不足：

• RCT 需要较长的随访时间。在器官移植中，与临床相关度最大的结果是患者存活情况和移植物存活情况，而这些结果的正确测量可能需要很多年。长时间的随访不仅造成试验费用高昂，而且将所有有效结果延迟到随访完成。

• 进行 RCT 费用较高。大多数便宜的临床试验仅用于检测较大的差异。为了获取相对罕见结果(例如移植后的死亡率)的 RCT 需要足够的资源，可能需要对数百或数千的患者进行跟踪随访，这通常使得试验的成本令人难以承担。

• RCT 需要严格的筛选标准来得出关于给定人群的推断。即使有充足的资金，一个适当的 RCT 所需的研究人数可能会超过在指定的研究期间内美国进行器官移植的患者总数。

• 有些 RCT 可能无法实现或违背伦理道德。例如，糖尿病患者是否会造成移植结果恶化这类问题不能通过 RCT 来回答的，因为暴露(即糖尿病)是不可控的。吸烟是否使移植结果恶化这类问题也不能通过 RCT 来回答，因为即使患者愿意参与这种试验，将患者随机分到吸烟组是不符合伦理的。

在长期的前瞻性兼观察性研究中，若对参与者不进行实验干预，即可避免临床试验可能带来的一些关于试验可行性和伦理的问题，但是同样存在许多缺点，例如成本、招聘、研究暴露的结果和预期结果之间的差距。回顾性数据收集(在一定程度上)解决了成本和后续差距，但是存在回忆偏倚、幸存者偏倚和其他可能扭曲推理的偏倚。

然而，基于注册数据的研究包含了前瞻性收集和回顾性分析，结合了前瞻性数据收集(避免回忆偏倚和幸存者偏倚)与回顾性分析(降低成本和避免长期随访)的优势。此外，有些国家的强制规定使注册数据随时可用，同时没有任何选择偏倚。为此，移植界基于注册数据进行了许多重要的推断。重要的一点是要了解用于执行基于注册数据研究的技术，以及基于人群的方法的优点和缺点。

本章的目标是描述研究人员可用的各种注册系统，阐述基于注册系统分析的优点和局限性，并提供分析方法和研究设计的概述。虽然本章的重点是分析来自器官移植注册中心的数据，但所阐述的许多原则将与所有基于人群的观察性研究相关。

基于注册系统和人群的研究的优势

器官移植领域非常适合于建立注册系统，因为已故捐献者等待名单的维护和捐赠器官分配的机制使它们有一个集中的数据库，提供关于移植等待者的健康和特征，以及死亡器官捐献者的最新详细信息。此外，治疗提供者的数量相对较少。截至 2011 年 7 月，在美国有 265 个移植中心进行肾脏移植，少数中心进行肾脏以外的器官移植[1]。因此，可以实现数据收集和记录过程中的相对高程度的标准化。

注册系统通常包括国家或地区内的所有相关患者，这意味着在特定时间范围内的移植等待者或接受者的全部人群都可以包括在基于注册的研究中。通过注册研究获得的大量数据使得进行有效的统计推断成为可能。此外，该研究群体比通过单中心或甚至多中心研究可获得的数据更加多样化，一般多中心研究倾向于更具代表性、大样本量的学术中心。注册系统还支持多级效应分析[例如，中心级或器官获取组织(OPO)级别效应]。由于患者在与其治疗提供者相互作用的时期内被持续关注，所以长期随访是可能实现的。最后，移植注册中心还可与其他注册管理中心(例如，社会安全主死亡档案，行政索赔数据库，或癌症登记处)相关联。

基于注册系统和人群的研究的局限性

了解基于注册系统的研究所固有的几个缺点也很重要的。虽然数据以标准化格式提交给注册中心，但数据由数百名医护人员收集，他们所接受的培训和专业知识水平是有差异的。大多数国家的注册系统没有对数据收集进行集中质量控制的机制（尽管某些注册中心会进行数据核查）。在对美国注册系统的一些测量中，常会出现数据缺失的情况；一些缺失是随机的，一些是系统设置造成的，两者的区别是非常重要的。数据收集错误或记录错误可能会导致难以检测的数据缺陷；特别是系统性的误差，可能导致出现显著的偏倚。

此外，基于注册系统的研究具有所有观察性研究共同的两个主要缺点。首先是不可观察性的(潜在的)混杂因素问题。注册系统没有采集许多关于移植患者的重要信息。例如，研究者可能希望研究儿童患者中年龄和移植物丧失功能风险之间的生物学关系。青少年不太可能比年幼的儿童更依从移植后免疫抑制方案，不遵从医嘱是移植物丧失功能的主要原因。因此，研究者将在分析中调整用药依从性。然而，在美国的器官移植注册系统中没有关于用药依从性的数据。因此，基于注册系统的关于年龄和移植物丧失功能风险之间的生物学关联的分析将因依从性这一指标（从技术层面来说，在流行病学术语中，依从性是介体，其对于大多数实际用途和目的被分析处理为混杂因素)所混淆。

有一个相关的概念是残差混淆。例如，研究者可能希望研究死亡供者的年龄与移植后结果之间的关系，独立于糖尿病受者(换句话说，调整糖尿病的任何混杂因素)。如果可以获得患者关于糖尿病的数据，则该变量可包括在统计模型中以调整糖尿病状态。然而，如果没有关于糖尿病严重性的数据(例如疾病持续时间，血糖控制，胰岛素治疗史)，轻度糖尿病和重度糖尿病患者将接受相同模型的治疗手段。因此，年龄和死亡率之间的关系将继续被糖尿病的严重性所混淆。

基于注册系统的研究的另一个缺点是由指征导致的混淆，也称为治疗选择偏倚。由指征引发的混淆往往出现在如下情况，即病情较重的患者比健康的患者更有可能接受治疗。接受治疗的患者可能具有较差的结果，并不是因为治疗手段本身较差，而是因为引发治疗的疾病的严重程度。由指征导致的混淆在药理学疗法和其他治疗干预的研究中是特别受到关注的。

国家和地区移植注册中心的实例

器官获取和移植网络(OPTN)移植登记

自 1986 年以来，美国器官共享网络(UNOS)根据与美国健康和人类服务部的协议，负责监管器官获取和移植网络(OPTN)[5]。美国的所有死亡捐赠器官都通过 OPTN 分配；此外，自 1987 年以来，凡是参加医疗保险或医疗补助的移植项目均需要 OPTN 加入[6]。同年，OPTN 开始收集关于器官捐献者和移植受者的医疗数据[7]。自 1999 年以来，关于移植等待者、活体和死亡供者以及移植受者的数据已存储在 UNOS 的综合数据库中，称为 UNet℠，移植中心通过安全的在线接口以电子方式输入数据[7]。这些数据以“去标识”的形式提供给研究人员。

截至 2012 年 6 月，OPTN 收集的主要在线表单包括[8]：

• 移植等待者登记(TCR)表，在患者注册器官等待名单时需要，包含患者人口学资料、健康史、临床信息和器官特异性信息。

• 移植受者登记(TRR)表，所有移植受者在出院或死亡时需要提供，包含更新的患者人口学资料和健康史、移植手术信息和其他治疗信息(例如，移植后早期住院期间的免疫抑制治疗方式)。

• 移植受者随访(TRF)表，在移植后 6 个月，移植后每一周年，对于移植物仍然有功能的存活受者，要求是包括患者当前的状态和临时治疗的信息。

• 死亡供者登记(DDR)表和活体供者登记(LDR)

表,包含供者人口统计学资料、健康史和恢复细节(逝世后捐献者)或术后临床信息(活体捐献者)。

其他OPTN表格包括移植后恶性肿瘤表、肝脏受者组织相容性表、供者组织相容性表、受者组织相容性表和活体供者随访表。所有OPTN表单均可在线查阅,网址http://www.unos.org/。此外,注册系统包含移植中心提供的关于等待名单的更新情况[例如,针对逝世后捐献者关于终末期肝病模型(MELD)评分的变化]和OPTN生成的管理数据(例如,逝世后器官捐献者提供)。可从UNOS获得OPTN数据进行分析;这些分析文件链接到社会安全死亡主文件(SSDMF),以更准确地判定死亡,因为许多死亡未被OPTN报告机制获取。

移植受者科学注册(SRTR)标准分析文件

移植受者科学登记处(SRTR)还为美国移植结果的研究生成标准分析文件(SAF)。与UNOS数据集一样,SRTR数据集以OPTN数据为基础,且链接到SSDMF数据作为补充。而与UNOS数据集不同的是,SRTR数据集还链接到医疗保险和医疗补助服务中心(CMS)的数据,这样能更准确地确定存活患者的肾移植物衰竭情况,因为许多移植物丧失功能未被OPTN报告机制检测到[9]。CMS的数据来自CMS医疗证据报告以及行政索赔数据。医学证据报告(也称为CMS-2728表格)收集人口统计学资料和诊断数据,并针对美国所有诊断为终末期肾病(ESRD)的患者展开。SRTR SAF的数据组织示意图见图133.1。UNOS和SRTR数据集以不同的方式组织OPTN数据,并遵循不同的变量命名规则。关于SRTR数据库的组织详情可见于网址http://www.srtr.org和文献中的描述。

其他注册系统

美国以外的注册系统

在加拿大,器官移植和终末期肾病(ESRD)的数据记录在加拿大器官替代登记系统(CORR)[11,12]中。欧洲移植注册系统包含德国、荷兰、比利时、克罗地亚、卢森

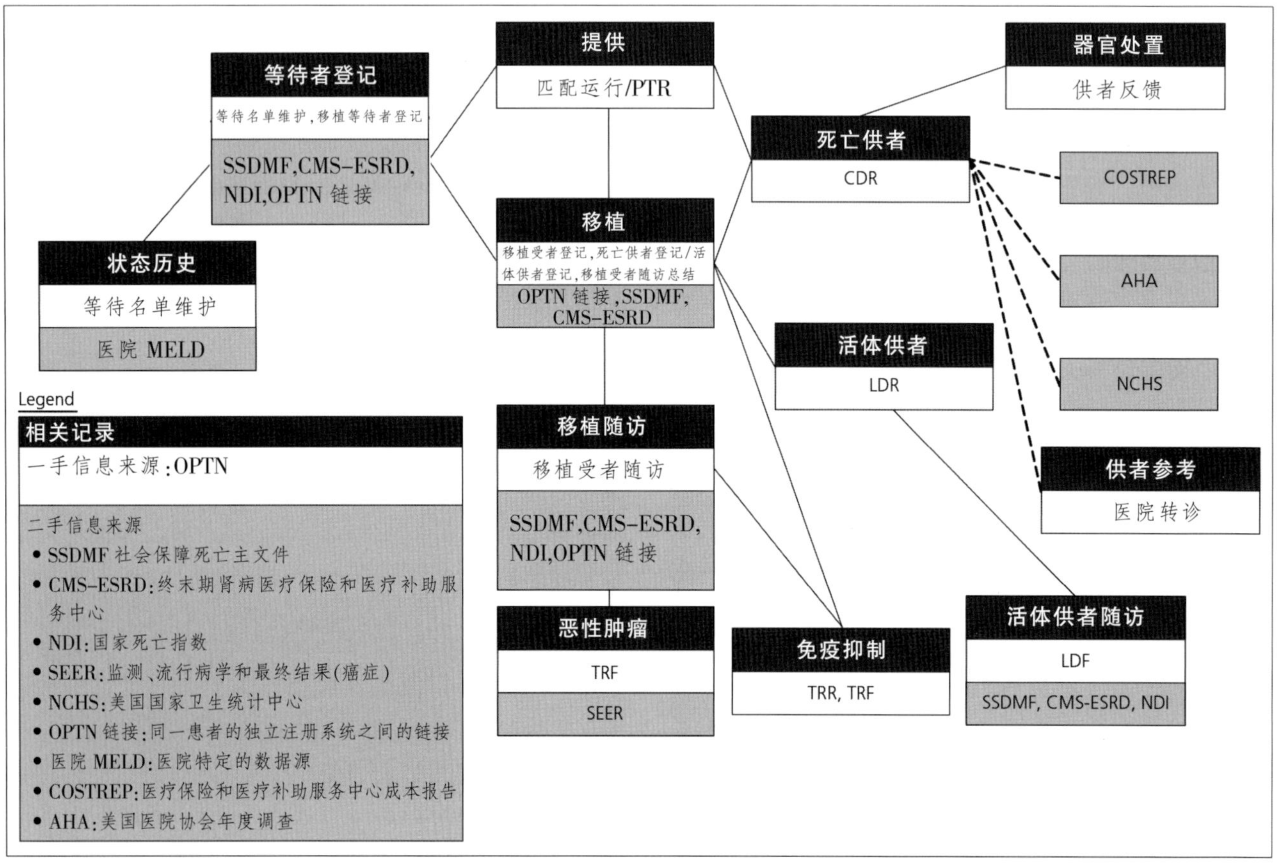

图133.1 由移植受者科学注册处(SRTR)提供的标准分析文件(SAF)的数据源和组织示意图。Modified from[9] Levine G et al. *American Journal of Transplantation 2006*; 6(5p2):1228-1242, with permission from Wiley.

堡、奥地利和斯洛文尼亚[13,14]的器官移植数据。澳大利亚、新西兰[15,16]、瑞典[17]、日本[18]、马来西亚[19]、巴西[20]和其他地方都有国家注册系统。这些注册系统收集的数据类似于美国注册系统的数据，并且可以提供类似的有用的分析。然而，数据收集方法的标准化可能不同，在那些具有社会化医疗保健系统的国家，整体医疗保健系统可以促进标准化数据报告，以包括与移植直接相关的要素。

注册系统的作用和基于人群的研究

描述性统计

注册系统(尤其是具有采集所有患者的强制性数据报告的注册系统)通常是获取关于人群的描述性统计数据的最佳工具。在移植中，可用描述性统计结果回答的问题包括：

- 每年进行多少种类型的移植？
- 有多少患者加入等待名单？
- 接受移植的受者的人口统计学分布情况如何？
- 这些数字如何随时间变化？

SRTR 发布的年度报告提供与移植相关的描述性统计数据[21]。此外，许多发表的论文集中于提供描述性统计，给出移植领域现状的概述或详细描述移植的某一方面[22-28]。

推论数据统计

推论研究涉及暴露和结果之间可能存在的关联；例如，发现在肾移植中扩大标准供肾(ECD)相对于标准供肾(SCD)与移植物存活相对减少相关[29]。注册系统中大量的受者数据以及丰富多样的可用临床变量使其非常适合于推理研究。基于注册系统的推理研究验证了受者人口统计学[30-32]、逝世后捐献者特征[29,33-35]、政策[36-40]和许多其他因素在器官移植中的作用。虽然谨慎执行推理分析可以将错误推理的风险降到最小化，但必须谨慎解释统计上显著的关联，因为关联不显示因果关系。

预测模型

有吸烟史的供者与去世的供者来源的移植物肾移植后丧失功能的风险略有增加相关(在一项研究中风险比=1.05，$P<0.05$)[41]。然而，对于接受移植器官的风险而言，供者的吸烟史仅能提供很少的信息，由于许多其他特性(例如，供体年龄、高血压病史、死亡原因、终末血清肌酐）与移植物丧失功能的风险具有更强的关联性[29]。去世的供者完全匹配来源肾移植与移植物丧失功能的风险降低相关(在一项研究中，相对风险=0.65，$P<0.001$)[42]。但同样的是，仅知道完全匹配状态传达关于移植物失功能风险的信息是有限的，因为只有约15%的死亡供者移植物是完全匹配的。用一个完全匹配但患有高血压的 72 岁且终端肌酐值为 2.4 的供者提供的肾脏进行的肾移植，效果可能远不如匹配值为 6 但年龄为 25 岁的健康供者提供的肾脏。用预测模型推断受者的风险基于许多因素，通常使用复合分数。基于注册系统的研究已被用于创建肾移植物丧失功能[44-48]、终末期肝病患者死亡率[49]、肝移植物丧失功能[50]和肾移植或延迟移植患者的死亡率[51]的综合风险评估模型。

基于模拟的研究

当实验在实际操作中不可行或违背伦理时，基于模拟的研究可用于评估实验干预的效果。模拟研究常用于预测器官分配政策变化的影响。要通过实验测试策略变化产生的影响，需要进行大量的政策变更以及数月至数年的跟踪随访，但模拟研究可以比较许多不同策略对虚拟患者结果的影响。模拟研究已被用于模拟政策变化对去世供者捐献肾脏[52-54]、肝脏[55,56]、心脏[57,58]和肺[58]的分配的影响。此外，已经使用模拟研究进行活体捐献肾移植供受者相匹配的策略比较(KPD)[59-61]。

模拟研究只有在真实准确代表实际患者和政策时才有意义。注册系统数据可用于模拟研究中，可有效反映实际患者人群的病例组合情况，并且用于构建时间-事件模型以估计关键事件的概率(例如，器官提供、接收移植、在等待过程中死亡、移植后移植物失功能)。

基于注册系统研究设计的注意事项

前瞻性研究需要在项目开始之前进行详细规划。资助机构和机构审查委员会不会支持设计不佳或成功机会较小的研究项目。在开展前瞻性研究之前，研究人员必须证明研究是可行的。必须确定利益相关的目标人群。收集和准备数据的计划必须提前制订好。必须选择合适的统计分析方法，并且必须对一旦研究开始启动后可能出现的问题制订应急预案。

回顾性研究的准备从监管的角度来看更简单，负担更轻，但涉及许多相同的考虑事项。开始回顾性研究之前先做好规划，将使数据分析更容易，并最大限度地减少错误推断的风险。实际分析应反映出一个精心选择的研究设计的执行情况。

假设

由于临床试验昂贵且耗时的特点，期待其有明确的定义、生物学上可信且研究者认为是均衡假设驱动其发展是合理的。在基于注册系统的研究中，研究者管理数百个变量，对两个变量之间的相关性或关联的粗略分析可能只需要几秒钟。由于概率，单个统计检验而具有统计学意义的机会很低：根据定义，统计假设检验中显著性水平α，按照惯例通常设置为5%。但是在任何国家的移植注册系统中，肯定存在成百上千个的虚假的相关联系。这对发表偏倚而言是很理想的条件[62]，这些虚假的联系可由研究者经过对数据“审前调查”识别，经过测试，发现是重要的就可以发表。为了避免发表偏倚和Ⅰ型错误，研究者应注意只执行由谨慎考虑的生物学可信的假设驱动的分析。

人群选择

一个明确定义的研究课题会针对特定的人群。例如，当研究肝衰竭原因与肝移植术后存活之间的关联时，相关的群体是肝移植受者。根据研究的问题，通常排除非典型患者(例如，多器官联合移植受者、再移植受者或儿童受者)，以便为特定类别的患者(例如，首次只接受肝移植的成人受者)提供准确的推断。

在研究设计时要考虑三个人群：

- 目标群体(希望从中得出有效推论的人群)；
- 源群体(研究中潜在的可枚举的参与者，具有目标群体的代表性)；
- 研究群体(该群体的数据实际上已包括在分析中，分析直接来自于源群体)。

研究问题应推动完善目标群体的解释，反过来，连同可行性和数据可用性，应推动完善源群体和研究群体的解释。在前瞻性研究中，研究群体可能小于源群体，因为招募所有符合条件的对象是不可行的，或者某些对象不同意参与研究。在基于注册系统的研究中，源群体和研究群体通常是相同的。然而，当使用某些分析技术(例如，在匹配的队列分析中，其中研究群体来自合格匹配的集合)时，研究群体可以包含于源群体中[63,64]。

基于注册系统的研究其精准入选标准因研究问题而异。然而，典型的入选标准可以包括日期范围(如在2005年进行的所有移植)、年龄范围(如成人受者)和器官/程序类型(如肺移植等待名单登记者，活体供肾受者)，以达到一定程度的同质性。

数据完整性/数据分析探索

移植注册系统通常使用的数据并非因研究之目的收集而来。OPTN数据收集工作的主要目的是管理已故捐献者的器官等待名单，促进器官分配，并为SRTR特定方案报告提供数据。数据质量是具有变化性的，经常出现数据缺失和数据错误的情况，尤其是在OPTN非主要目的的领域。对数据分析进行适当的探索，可有效避免基于群体分析中的偏差。

数据缺失

数据缺失可能是由于设计不合理造成的。例如，2002年在OPTN数据库中添加了衡量肝脏疾病严重程度的测量值——凝血酶原时间的国际标准化比率(INR)[65]。因此，在该日期之前，所有肝脏移植等待名单者缺少此信息。或者，信息可能缺失，因为它并非由治疗提供者提交。例如，1990—2005年期间，在30.3%的活体供者肾移植中未报道冷缺血时间(CIT)[66]。

所有记录都有丢失数据的可能，数据缺失方式为完全随机缺失(MCAR)；当有一个系统缺失机制并且能从另一个变量预测到缺失时，就是随机缺失(MAR)(例如，缺失值可能是随机的但不太可能是最近的记录)；当有一个系统缺失机制，但不能从其他可用数据预测缺失时，就是非随机缺失(MNAR)(例如，如果是CIT值，那么不太可能记录较小的那个CIT值)[67]。如果在分析时不进行适当的处理，那么不管是随机缺失还是非随机缺失，都可能导致推理偏差。数据分析探索应包括谨慎考虑数据缺失并探索缺失模式(例如，在给定的年份或给定类别的患者信息出现缺失的情况更加常见)。处理缺失的常见策略包括缺失记录的删除，缺失指标变量的创建，以及类似于插补这类的先进技术[67,68]。

测量和数据记录中的错误

即使没有缺失，也不能保证注册系统数据的准确

patients with end-stage liver disease. Hepatology (Baltimore, Md.). [Research Support, U.S. Gov't, P.H.S.Review]. 2001;33(2):464–470.
50. Feng S, Goodrich NP, Bragg-Gresham JL, et al. Characteristics associated with liver graft failure: the concept of a donor risk index. American Journal of Transplantation. [Research Support, U.S. Gov't, P.H.S.]. 2006;6(4):783–790.
51. Massie AB, Desai NM, Montgomery RA, et al. Improving distribution efficiency of hard-to-place deceased donor kidneys: predicting probability of discard or delay. American Journal of Transplantation. [Research Support, U.S. Gov't, P.H.S.]. 2010;10(7):1613–1620.
52. Moers C, Kornmann NS, Leuvenink HG, et al. The influence of deceased donor age and old-for-old allocation on kidney transplant outcome. Transplantation. 2009;88(4):542–552.
53. Jacquelinet C, Audry B, Golbreich C, et al., editors. Changing Kidney Allocation Policy in France: The Value of Simulation. American Medical Informatics Association; 2006; 374–378.
54. Schaubel D, Guidinger M, Biggins S, et al. Survival benefit-based deceased-donor liver allocation. American Journal of Transplantation. 2009;9(4p2):970–981.
55. Freeman RB Jr, Wiesner RH, Roberts JP, et al. Improving liver allocation: MELD and PELD. American Journal of Transplantatio. [Research Support, U.S. Gov't, Non-P.H.S. Review]. 2004;4(Suppl 9):114–131.
56. Thompson D, Waisanen L, Wolfe R, et al. Simulating the allocation of organs for transplantation. Health Care Management Science. [Research Support, U.S. Gov't, Non-P.H.S.]. 2004;7(4):331–338.
57. van den Hout WB, Smits J, Deng MC, et al. The heart-allocation simulation model: a tool for comparison of transplantation allocation policies 1. Transplantation. 2003;76(10):1492.
58. Garrity E, Moore J, Mulligan M, et al. Heart and lung transplantation in the United States, 1996–2005. American Journal of Transplantation. 2007;7: 1390–1403.
59. Chen Y, Li Y, Kalbfleisch J, et al. Graph-based optimization algorithm and software on kidney exchanges. IEEE Transactions on Bio-Medical Engineering. 2012;59(7).
60. Segev DL, Gentry SE, Warren DS, et al. Kidney paired donation and optimizing the use of live donor organs. Journal of the American Medical Association. 2005;293(15):1883–1890.
61. Segev DL, Gentry SE, Melancon JK, et al. Characterization of waiting times in a simulation of kidney paired donation. American Journal of Transplantation. 2005;5(10):2448–2455.
62. Easterbrook PJ, Gopalan R, Berlin J, et al. Publication bias in clinical research. Lancet. 1991;337(8746):867–872.
63. Segev DL, Muzaale AD, Caffo BS, et al. Perioperative mortality and long-term survival following live kidney donation. Journal of the American Medical Association. 2010;303(10):959–966.
64. Montgomery RA, Lonze BE, King KE, et al. Desensitization in HLA-incompatible kidney recipients and survival. New England Journal of Medicine. 2011;365(4): 318–326.
65. Robert A, Chazouilleres O. Prothrombin time in liver failure: time, ratio, activity percentage, or international normalized ratio? Hepatology (Baltimore, Md.). [Comparative Study]. 1996;24(6):1392–1394.
66. Simpkins CE, Montgomery RA, Hawxby AM, et al. Cold ischemia time and allograft outcomes in live donor renal transplantation: is live donor organ transport feasible? American Journal of Transplantation: Official Journal of the American Society of Transplantation and the American Society of Transplant Surgeons. [Evaluation Studies Research Support, U.S. Gov't, P.H.S.]. 2007;7(1): 99–107.
67. Schlomer GL, Bauman S, Card NA. Best practices for missing data management in counseling psychology. Journal of Counseling Psychology. 2010; 57(1):1–10.
68. Greenland S, Finkle WD. A critical look at methods for handling missing covariates in epidemiologic regression analyses. American Journal of Epidemiology. [Research Support, U.S. Gov't, P.H.S. Review]. 1995;142(12):1255–1264.
69. Dickinson D, Arrington C, Fant G, et al. SRTR program-specific reports on outcomes: a guide for the new reader. American Journal of Transplantation. 2008;8(4p2):1012–1026.
70. Vittinghoff E, Glidden DV, Shiboski SC, et al. Regression Methods in Biostatistics: Linear, Logistic, Survival, and Repeated Measures Models. New York: Springer; 2005.
71. Cleves MA, Gould WW, Gutierrez RG, et al. An Introduction to Survival Analysis Using Stata, 3rd ed. Texas: Stata Press; 2010.
72. Wolfe RA, Schaubel DE, Webb RL, et al. Analytical approaches for transplant research. American Journal of Transplantation. 2004;4:106–113.
73. Rothman KJ, Greenland S, Lash TL. Modern Epidemiology. Philadelphia: Lippincott Williams & Wilkins; 2008.
74. Allison PD. Survival Analysis Using SAS: A Practical Guide. North Carolina: SAS Institute; 2010.
75. Kleinbaum DGK M. Survival Analysis: A Self-Learning Text. New York: Springer; 2005.
76. Meier-Kriesche HU, Kaplan B. Waiting time on dialysis as the strongest modifiable risk factor for renal transplant outcomes: a paired donor kidney analysis. Transplantation. 2002;74(10):1377–1381.
77. Baskin-Bey ES, Kremers W, Stegall MD, et al. United Network for Organ Sharing's expanded criteria donors: is stratification useful? Clinical Transplantation. [Comparative Study Research Support, N.I.H., Extramural Research Support, Non-U.S. Gov't Research Support, U.S. Gov't, P.H.S.]. 2005;19(3):406–412.
78. Mikhalski D, Wissing KM, Ghisdal L, et al. Cold ischemia is a major determinant of acute rejection and renal graft survival in the modern era of immunosuppression. Transplantation. 2008;85(7 Suppl):S3–S9.
79. Sung RS, Christensen LL, Leichtman AB, et al. Determinants of discard of expanded criteria donor kidneys: impact of biopsy and machine perfusion. American Journal of Transplantation. 2008;8(4):783–792.
80. Gleisner AL, Munoz A, Brandao A, et al. Survival benefit of liver transplantation and the effect of underlying liver disease. Surgery. [Multicenter Study Research Support, N.I.H., Extramural Research Support, Non-U.S. Gov't]. 2010;147(3): 392–404.
81. Putter H, Fiocco M, Geskus RB. Tutorial in biostatistics: competing risks and multi-state models. Statistics in Medicine. [Research Support, Non-U.S. Gov't]. 2007;26(11):2389–2430.
82. Cho YW, Shah T, Cho ES, et al. Factors associated with discard of recovered kidneys. Transplantation Proceedings. 2008;40(4):1032–1034.
83. Tozawa M, Iseki K, Iseki C, et al. Influence of smoking and obesity on the development of proteinuria. Kidney International. 2002;62(3):956–962.
84. Lanoy E, Costagliola D, Engels EA. Skin cancers associated with HIV infection and solid-organ transplantation among elderly adults. International Journal of Cancer. 2010;126(7):1724–1731.
85. Schold JD, Gregg JA, Harman JS, et al. Barriers to evaluation and wait listing for kidney transplantation. Clinical journal of the American Society of Nephrology: CJASN. 2011;6(7):1760–1767.
86. Pregibon D. Logistic regression diagnostics. Annals of Statistics. 1981;9(4): 705–724.
87. Zou G. A modified poisson regression approach to prospective studies with binary data. American Journal of Epidemiology. 2004;159(7):702–706.
88. Justice AC, Covinsky KE, Berlin JA. Assessing the generalizability of prognostic information. Annals of Internal Medicine. [Case Reports Research Support, U.S. Gov't, P.H.S.]. 1999;130(6):515–524.
89. D'Agostino RB Sr, Grundy S, Sullivan LM, et al. Validation of the Framingham coronary heart disease prediction scores: results of a multiple ethnic groups investigation. Journal of the American Medical Association. [Research Support, U.S. Gov't, P.H.S. Validation Studies]. 2001;286(2):180–187.
90. Obuchowski NA. Receiver operating characteristic curves and their use in radiology1. Radiology. 2003;229(1):3–8.
91. DeLong ER, DeLong DM, Clarke-Pearson DL. Comparing the areas under two or more correlated receiver operating characteristic curves: a nonparametric approach. Biometrics. [Comparative Study Research Support, U.S. Gov't, Non-P.H.S.]. 1988;44(3):837–845.
92. Pencina MJ, D'Agostino RB Sr, D'Agostino RB Jr, et al. Evaluating the added predictive ability of a new marker: from area under the ROC curve to reclassification and beyond. Statistics in Medicine. 2008;27(2):157–172, discussion 207–12.
93. Altman DG, Royston P. What do we mean by validating a prognostic model? Statistics in Medicine. 2000;19(4):453–473.
94. Steyerberg EW, Harrell FE Jr, Borsboom GJ, et al. Internal validation of predictive models: efficiency of some procedures for logistic regression analysis. Journal of Clinical Epidemiology. 2001;54(8):774–781.
95. Kim WR, Therneau TM, Benson JT, et al. Deaths on the liver transplant waiting list: an analysis of competing risks. Hepatology (Baltimore, Md.). [Research Support, N.I.H., Extramural]. 2006;43(2):345–351.
96. Fine JP, Gray RJ. A proportional hazards model for the subdistribution of a competing risk. Journal of the American Statistical Association. 1999;94: 496–509.
97. Abbott KC, Bucci JR, Matsumoto CS, et al. Hepatitis C and renal transplantation in the era of modern immunosuppression. Journal of the American Society of Nephrology. 2003;14(11):2908–2918.
98. Platt RW, Joseph K, Ananth CV, et al. A proportional hazards model with time-dependent covariates and time-varying effects for analysis of fetal and infant death. American Journal of Epidemiology. 2004;160(3):199–206.
99. Adami J, Gabel H, Lindelof B, et al. Cancer risk following organ transplantation: a nationwide cohort study in Sweden. British Journal of Cancer. [Comparative Study Research Support, Non-U.S. Gov't]. 2003;89(7):1221–1227.
100. Schnitzler MA, Whiting JF, Brennan DC, et al. The expanded criterial donor dilemma in cadaveric renal transplantation. Transplantation. 2003;75(12):1940.
101. DeGroot MH, Schervish MJ. Probability and Statistics, 3rd ed. Boston, MA: Addison-Wesley; 2002.

第 134 章
器官移植中的临床研究方法和分析

Jesse D. Schold，S. Joseph Kim

引言

临床移植与许多辅助科学密切相关，是众多创新技术、药物和实践模式的初步试验基础。这种与医学进步紧密的关系需要临床移植和临床科研近乎不间断的联系。因此，对研究方法的认知是必要的，即使是一般的移植实践也是指导临床合理治疗决策的重要手段。实际上，为了得出适用于所有人群的数据推断结果，利用恰当的统计方法进行分析是非常必要的。在本章中，我们将结合移植文献中的例子描述基本的方法论原则和常见的分析方法。无论研究大小、设计或范围，对任何形式的研究来说，在整个研究过程中正确应用科学方法(图 134.1)是一个重要的指导原则。如果未遵循这项重要原则，即使是使用了本章描述的恰当的研究设计和分析，研究结果的有效性和可靠性也是不确定的。更重要的是，当一个相关的、重要的、新颖的研究问题被提出时，无论研究结果“好坏”与否，其目的是追求更深入的科学研究。

与基础科学研究相比，临床研究主要分析患者受到特定的干预措施或暴露于某危险因素时会出现的结果。为了检验这些关系并量化给定暴露会产生的相应结果，研究必须通过精心设计，这样从研究结果才能推演出有效的推论。本章的第一部分将概述临床研究实施的主要问题，因为这关系到研究设计，而第二部分则将侧重于研究分析。

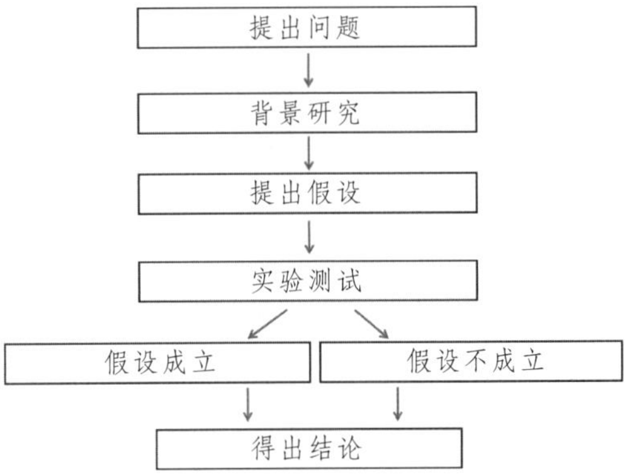

图 134.1　科学方法。

研究设计的主要类型

图 134.2 呈现了对于各种临床研究类型的一个有用的分类系统[1]。如果一项研究由研究人员指定暴露或干预因素，则该研究被称为实验研究。如果暴露或干预因素不受研究人员的控制，不是研究方案本身的目的，则该研究被称为观察研究。

实验研究设计

一项研究一旦被认为是实验研究，下一个步骤是决定干预或暴露机制。如果研究过程中纳入的每个患者都有一个固定的概率作为干预组或对照组，那么这项研究被称为随机对照试验(RCT)。如果一个非随机机制(例如交替)用于分配，那么这项研究被称为一个非随机对照试验。后者在当今临床研究中是不常见的，因为对于研究的有效性而言，随机试验具有相当大的优势(详见进一步说明)。所以，非随机对照试验将不再作进一步讨论。

统计学中的随机项不等同于随意项。相反，它指某些特定事件发生的概率分布。在经典的 1 对 1、2 组平行组 RCT 的情况下，该概率分布将具有两个可能的值，即干预组和比较组，并且每个的概率为 50%(即抛硬币的概率)。类似地，在 2 对 1、2 组平行组 RCT 中，干预组的概率为 67%，对照组为 33%。在具有概率相同大小组的 3 组 RCT 中，接受三种治疗中任一种的概率

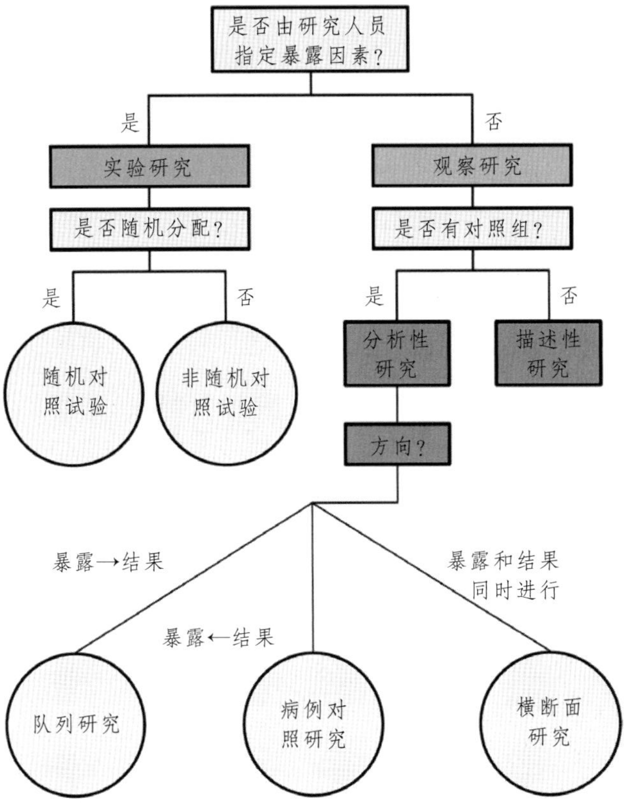

图 134.2 临床研究设计的种类。(Reproduced from [1] Lancet 359. Grimes DA, and Schulz KF. An overview of clinical research: the lay of the land:57–61, 2002. Copyright 2002, by permission of Elsevier.)

为 33%。该原理的扩展可应用于具有不相等大小概率的 3 组 RCT。

随机试验的一个重要特点就是每一个纳入研究的患者接受干预的概率是相同的。实际上,这个特点会降低纳入研究的患者被不公平地分配到干预组或对照组的可能性。随着样本量的增加,这些重要因素在治疗组不平衡的可能性将会降低。此外,平均而言,治疗分配和患者预后的分开关系确保纳入研究患者的已知和未知基本特征在治疗组中取得平衡。这种对已知和未知因素的随机性的平衡特性是将随机对照试验提高到所有研究设计中"金标准"地位的关键点。

RCT 在肾移植中一个很好的应用例子是 ALERT 研究[2]。该研究评估对比了氟伐他汀和安慰剂在减少肾移植受者人群心血管疾病发生的疗效。该研究的原文中列出了处理组之间的基本特征的表格(表 134.1),以突出在所有已知(和测量)基本预后因素之间实现组之间的平衡。如上所述,在已知预后因素中实现的平衡提

表 134.1　ALERT 研究中随机分配的氟伐他汀组和安慰剂组的肾移植受者的基线特征。Reproduced from [2] Lancet 361. Holdaas H, Fellstrom B, Jardine, AG, et al. Effect of fluvastatin on cardiac outcomes in renal transplant recipients: a multicentre, randomised, placebo-controlled trial. 2024–2031, 2003. Copyright 2003, with permission from Elsevier

	氟伐他汀 (n=1050)	安慰剂 (n=1052)
临床人口学特征		
中位年龄(标准差)(岁)	49.5(10.9)	50.0(11.0)
男性	701(66.8%)	68(65.2%)
平均舒张压(标准差)(mmHg)	85.6(10.1)	85.6(10.0)
平均收缩压(标准差)(mmHg)	143.8(18.7)	144(19.1)
平均 BMI(标准差)(kg/m^2)	25.8(4.4)	25.8(4.6)
平均总胆固醇(标准差)(mmol/L)	6.4(1.1)	6.5(1.1)
平均低密度脂蛋白胆固醇(标准差)(mmol/L)	4.1(1.0)	4.1(1.0)
平均高密度脂蛋白胆固醇(标准差)(mmol/L)	1.3(0.5)	1.4(0.4)
平均甘油三酯(mmol/L)	2.2(1.2)	2.2(1.5)
肾功能衰竭的主要原因		
肾小球肾炎	387(36.9%)	364(34.6%)
多囊肾病	138(13.1%)	183(17.4%)
糖尿病肾病	135(12.9%)	138(13.1%)
肾盂肾炎或间质性肾炎	124(11.8%)	135(12.8%)
高血压肾硬化症	59(5.6%)	46(4.4%)
系统性红斑狼疮或血管炎	30(2.9%)	22(2.2%)
未知	58(5.5%)	53(5.0%)
其他	157(15.0%)	134(12.7%)
移植情况		
第一次移植	894(85.1%)	900(85.6%)
替换肾平均时间(标准差)治疗(月)	88.5(56.5)	88.8(58.3)
最后移植类型		
活体供者	240(22.9%)	229(21.8%)
尸体供者	809(77.0%)	822(78.1%)
平均血清肌酐(标准差)(μ.mol/L)	147(54.4)	143(51.0)
伴随免疫抑制治疗 *		
硫唑嘌呤	684(65.1%)	680(64.6%)
强的松龙	851(81.0%)	848(80.6%)
环磷酰胺	9(0.9%)	10(1.0%)
霉酚酸酯	167(15.9%)	159(15.1%)
其他	198(18.9%)	224(21.3%)

(待续)

表 134.1(续)

	氟伐他汀 (n=1050)	安慰剂 (n=1052)
心血管危险因素		
心绞痛史	71(6.8%)	77(7.3%)
糖尿病	32(3.0%)	34(3.2%)
高血压	197(18.8%)	199(18.9%)
脑血管疾病史	798(76.0%)	777(73.9%)
PVD 病史	62(5.9%)	60(5.7%)
当前是吸烟者	80(7.6%)	78(7.4%)
已知冠心病家族史	204(19.4%)	185(17.6%)
伴发心血管疾病	91(8.7%)	124(11.8%)
伴随心血管病药物 *		
任何心血管药物	1001(95.3%)	999(95.0%)
阿司匹林	371(35.3%)	353(33.6%)
双嘧达莫	21(2.0%)	26(2.5%)
香豆素或华法林	90(8.6%)	94(8.9%)
β 受体阻滞剂	649(61.8%)	627(59.6%)
钙拮抗剂	728(69.3%)	738(70.2%)
ACE 抑制剂或 AIIRA	520(49.5%)	529(50.3%)
利尿剂	590(56.2%)	573(54.5%)
α 受体阻滞剂	176(16.8%)	170(16.2%)
其他	316(30.1%)	373(35.5%)

供了未知预后因素同样平衡的保证，并且由于患者接受氟伐他汀治疗或安慰剂是由随机分配方案决定（接受干预的可能性为 50%），所以未知预后因素也可以确保平衡。

观察研究设计

如果分配干预或暴露不受研究人员的支配，则该研究被认为是观察研究。必须确定是否有对照组。观察性研究的具体运用已在第 133 章作具体介绍。

描述性观察研究

一个未设对照组的观察研究，例如用新颖治疗手段治疗患者，被认为是一个描述性研究。新治疗手段对患者的疗效可在病例报告和病例系列被描述出来。或者，患者患有一种罕见疾病或常见疾病的一个不寻常的表现，其病程也会展现出来。随着时间的推移或利用医疗卫生资源得出的疾病发病趋势也是描述性观察研究的例子。虽然这些研究有助于强调临床利益、发现疗效的重要性或卫生政策的关联性，但是由于缺乏对照组，这就导致研究人员很难量化新的治疗方法的具体疗效、危险因素以及卫生政策与利益的关联程度。而这些只能在至少有两个组进行比较的研究中才能实现（即分析性研究）。

尽管存在不足，描述性观察研究能为分析性研究在试验一项新的治疗措施或危险因素时提供更严谨的基础。Locke 等的描述性研究就是典型例子[3]。该报告描述了一位有难治性急性抗体介导排斥反应的患者，在接受艾库组单抗治疗下，肾功能和组织学都得到了较好的改善，并在两个月的治疗下恢复到了正常标准。根据上述研究结果，Stegall 等开展了分析性观察研究，同时上述结果也为评价艾库组单抗治疗预防高风险肾移植受者急性抗体介导排斥反应的随机对照试验提供了坚实的基础[4]。

分析性观察研究

在临床研究中，主要有三种类型的分析性观察研究，如下所述。

队列研究

图 134.3 显示的是队列研究的结构。在队列研究中，需要使用明确的预先设定的纳入/排除标准，在人群中选定本研究的患者。在招募研究对象时，每一位纳入研究的患者，其相关的暴露因素或危险因素，如移植物功能延迟或当前是否吸烟都将进行测量，并且“暴露组”的结果或疾病发展将与“非暴露组”进行比较分析。暴露程度可以是分类型（如下），也可以是连续型（例

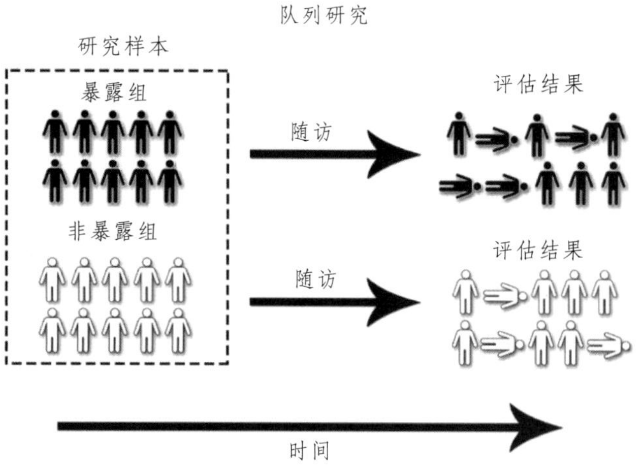

图 134.3 队列研究的结构。

如,收缩压)。连续型的暴露因素也可转换成有临床意义的组别(例如,收缩压<140mmHg 与≥140mmHg)。

由于招募研究对象在进入队列研究时，患者是没有研究的相关疾病的状态或者结果，所以根据随访情况，队列研究可以估计新病的发病率。从招募研究对象,也就是患者进入观察时,到产生相应结果的时间可以在队列研究里测出,因此,这是唯一可以进行生存分析的研究。重要的是,只有具有出现相应结果风险的患者才能纳入队列研究。例如,对于复发性急性排斥反应的危险因素的研究，只能是已经有过一次急性排斥反应的患者才可纳入分析。那些没有急性排斥反应病史的患者得先经历第一次急性排斥反应才会可能出现第二次。

队列研究中的患者若是当下组成的队列，随访观察的是未来的结果情况，这就是前瞻性队列研究。另外,现有的数据集可用于组成一个过去的队列,并随着时间的推移跟踪结果,这即是回顾性队列研究。以上两种都是基本的队列研究，因为它们都在明确的时间点(无论是现在还是过去)形成队列,然后随着时间的推移,测量相应结果的发生。或者说,队列研究是在患者进入研究时明确其暴露情况，且随着时间推移跟踪各个组的结果。在研究的有效性上,回顾性队列研究往往被认为不如前瞻性队列研究。但事实并非如此。关键在于数据集的质量和深度以及使用科学方法的基本原则。现有的数据集可能并非是要回答某一特定的科学问题,但如果相关数据通过严谨的方式获取,那么回顾性队列研究的严谨性和质量可以与任何一个前瞻性队列研究相媲美。

有时，过去未暴露的患者与现在暴露的患者的比较研究可替代暴露组和非暴露组在相同的时间段进入队列研究。这种研究设计被称为“非并发”(即相对于“并发”)队列研究。当比较一种已被广泛使用的新治疗方法的结果和过去更加常用的旧治疗方法的结果时，通常运用非并发队列研究。如上述 Stegall 等的研究:比较活体肾移植受者移植后在预防性艾库组单抗治疗下与以前患者在预防性静脉注射免疫球蛋白治疗下的急性抗体介导排斥反应率[4]。但这种研究设计的主要缺点是，对于患者的一般管理的变化和其他长期变化不能有效地做出解释,因为大多数(如果不是全部)近期患者的治疗方式都与以前的患者有很大区别。但如果暴露组和非暴露组的患者招募时间间隔较短，那么则可能会避免上述问题。

若研究设计的是罕见的暴露因素，则队列研究是首选的研究方法。例如,第二次世界大战结束后,日本原子弹爆炸幸存者的急性辐射暴露的长期影响队列研究[5],这一队列研究的特别之处在于相关的暴露因素非常特殊罕见,并且通过多年的随访,对研究该因素对健康的影响提供了一个非常难得的机会。

队列研究被认为是流行病学的中心研究设计。其他所有的研究设计基本上都源于队列研究。事实上,除了治疗、干预或暴露因素是在研究协议的背景下随机分配的,一个随机对照试验也是一个队列研究。相反,观察性队列研究的暴露因素通常是患者自己(例如,吸烟)或其监护人通过非随机的方式分配。

病例对照研究

病例对照研究在移植文献中较为少见，但实际上广泛应用于其他领域,如遗传流行病学。病例对照研究的结构如图 134.4 所示。病例对照研究以患者的结果作为纳入研究的依据,分为病例组和对照组。随后,确定在过去某一时间点病例组与对照组的暴露情况,做对比分析。从本质上讲,无论是暴露因素还是结果都已经在研究设计之前发生,所以从这个意义上来说,病例对照研究是回顾性的。但应确定的是,病例对照研究仍然是一个分析性观察研究,因为暴露或危险因素不受研究人员的控制,且至少有两个组进行对照(图 134.2)。

评估经过多年随访的某种疾病或结果最有效的方法就是病例对照研究，因为它利用了现有的已经收集好的既有暴露情况又有结果的数据集。此外,如果需要

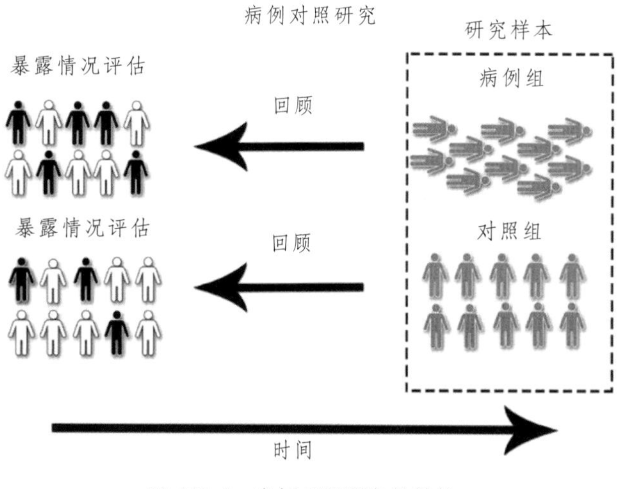

图 134.4　病例对照研究的结构。

测量暴露情况,例如通过图表综述、患者访谈或存储的血液检测，相比于队列研究，病例对照研究可以更及时、经济地让研究人员评估暴露与疾病之间的关联。

病例对照研究的主要缺点之一是不能评估疾病的发生率,因为患者的比例是由病例组和对照组决定,由研究人员抽样所得，而不是由疾病在目标人群中的发生率决定的。另外,如果对照组的病例选择不恰当,病例对照研究可能会比队列研究更容易产生偏倚（临床研究中主要的偏倚类型将在本章中进一步论述)。在一般情况下,对照组应来源于研究病例组分离出的患者。这部分患者也被称为研究基础或源人群(因其是病例的来源)。然而这部分人群是难以事先确定的,因此,控制选择的方式需要谨慎思考并执行。

最近一项病例对照研究是观察器官移植受者β乳头状瘤病毒(betaPV)和鳞状细胞癌(SCC)的关系[6]。从欧洲五个医疗中心的皮肤科和移植诊所共招募了210例鳞状细胞癌患者和394例对照组患者。人乳头瘤病毒DNA基因分型和β乳头状瘤病毒血清学可分别经眉毛和血液检测可得。为了提高病例组和对照组之间的可比性,研究人员根据年龄、性别和移植时间进行患者匹配。利用Logistic回归模型,研究人员在研究对象中发现β乳头状瘤病毒血清型和鳞状细胞癌之间有显著关联。需要注意的是,该项研究非常适合利用病例对照研究,因为SCC的发生非常罕见并且需要长期的随访。此外,特定生物标志物的测量是针对有效的病例组和对照组样本，而不是五个研究中心所有的器官移植受者。

横断面研究

横断面研究同时收集特定时间点或时间段研究对象的暴露和结果,不进行后续的随访等工作。横断面研究的结构如图134.5所示。因为可区分患者是否为暴露组，故可以在暴露组与非暴露组中计算出其中出现研究人员所关心的结果的比例，这种设计是分析性观察研究。调查评估患者在同一时间的暴露情况(例如,吸烟情况)与结果(例如,心肌梗死病史)是横断面研究最常见的例子。

因为不需要后续的随访，横断面研究能较快地展开,而且只需要很少的费用。同时它也可以提供日后可以被队列研究或随机对照研究证实的科学相关联的证据。所以,横断面研究通常被称为“假说生成研究”。此外,由于没有对患者进行随访,所以新的病例发生率或发病率不能如同在队列研究中那样被计算。相反,在一个特定时间内的患病率或患者成员的比例是主要的度量标准，而疾病在暴露组与非暴露组的患病率比较是最主要的研究。

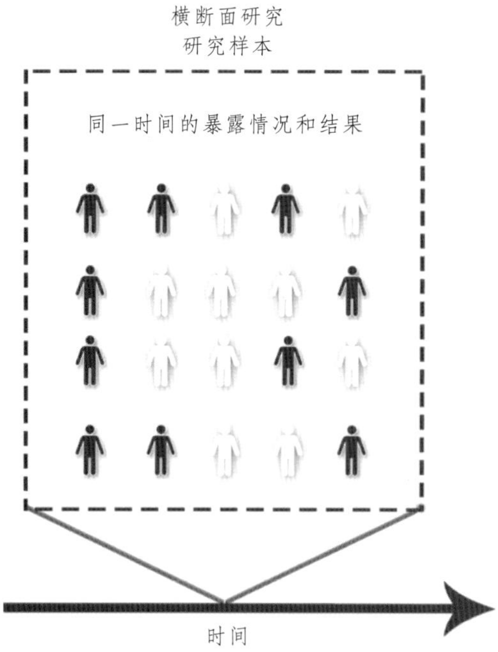

图134.5 横断面研究的结构。

然而，横断面研究的主要缺点是暴露与结果之间的时间关系可能无法明确划定，因此这些研究得出的结论可能受到反向因果关系的影响。后者所指的情况是结果会影响暴露因素,所以在横断面研究所得的某些关联可能存在一定的偏倚。例如,对患者当前的吸烟情况和肺癌史进行调查时，可能会错误地得出吸烟是肺癌的保护因素。然而事实可能是肺癌的发展改变了香烟的口味,从而导致癌症组的吸烟频率比非癌症组低。

试验性研究与观察性研究设计对比

由于随机分配的介入提高了干预对结果影响的因果联系的有效性，随机对照试验已经成为研究设计评估治疗或保健技术的金标准。这主要是由随机化对已知和未知预后因素平衡化作用的结果。但是,在随机对照试验中另加人为设置是不可行或不道德的。研究人员不能轻易地分配暴露或危险因素，例如必须在观察环境下研究移植肾功能延迟或同型半胱氨酸血症。此外,潜在的有害暴露因素,例如吸烟,不能人为不道德地施加于患者，故只能通过观察性研究设计加以评价。

通常情况下，利用随机对照试验同时使用强大的统计方法，只能验证一到两个假设，而观察研究可以完成多个假设的验证。在移植界，从一个相对小的人群中招募足够数量的患者验证假设也是一个重大挑战。通常情况下，由于资源需要或缺乏长期的随访，随机对照试验必须使用替代终点，而不是传统意义上的终点事件(如患者死亡或移植物失功能)。这些替代终点是评价干预措施效果机制的重要指标，同时也可以降低推断给定治疗的广泛影响[7]。此外，随机对照试验往往是在一个包括相对同质、确诊的治疗组患者的理想条件下开展，这可能会限制结果的普遍性。事实上，参与研究的移植患者与未参与的移植患者存在着系统性的不同，且两者出现的结果也有显著性的差异[8]。因此，运用观察性研究方法调查的问题往往作为随机对照研究的重要补充，同时通常具有更多的统计功能，能在实际应用中检测干预措施的影响程度。观察性研究的有意义权衡是与非随机设计相关的潜在偏倚。

随机误差和系统误差

临床研究中主要的误差类型可以分为随机误差和系统误差。

随机误差

随机误差是指测量的变异可能会影响研究结果的可重复性和可靠性，变异的来源包括：

- 观察者——进行测量的人。
- 仪器——一个测量血压的血压计。
- 对象——被测量的个体。

一个可重复或可靠的测量需要良好的精确度。因此，随机误差和精确度呈负相关；越少的随机误差意味着更高的精确度(反之亦然)。

一般情况下，具有较大样本量的研究将提高从研究对象得出总结措施(例如，危险比)的精确度(图 134.6)。此外，标准化的测量方法、正确培训研究人员以及精准仪器是提高精确度的其他方法。其深层意义是研究的设计和实施阶段是提高精确度的关键期。虽然在分析阶段可以通过统计方法来提高精确度，但与前面的措施相比效果还是较小。

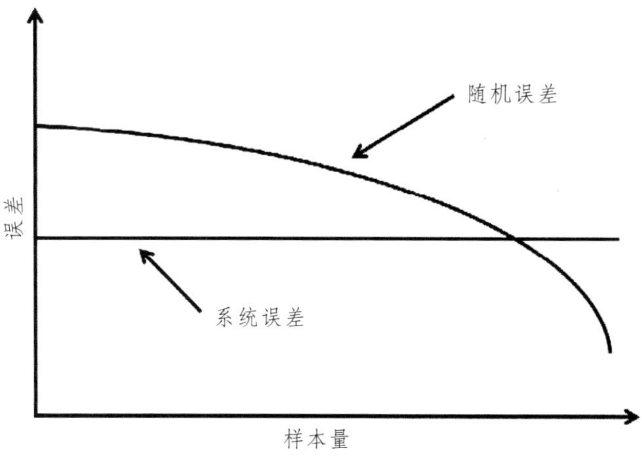

图 134.6 随机误差和系统误差作为因变量与样本量的函数关系。(Adapted from Rothman KJ. Epidemiology: An Introduction. Oxford University Press. 2002 [53])

系统误差

系统误差是指来自相关测量真实值的固定偏差。与随机误差不同，系统误差不能通过增加研究样本量的大小来减少或改善(图 134.6)。系统误差的另一个术语是偏倚(将在下一节中进一步探讨)。系统误差的来源可用与随机误差类似的方式进行分类：

- 观察者——如何选择患者纳入研究。
- 仪器——关键变量的测量。
- 对象——其他重要预后危险因素随着暴露的趋势。

需要注意的是，精确度是对随机误差而言的，有效性是对系统误差而言的。因此，更大的误差意味着有效性更低。减少系统误差的方法将提高测量的有效性。此外，类似于随机误差，在研究的设计和实施阶段这些方法是最有效的。运用统计方法对混杂偏倚进行调整最有效(见进一步讨论)，但需要相关变量是在研究的早期阶段测量。

精确度和偏倚的关系

每一个临床研究者的目标都是其研究能为暴露因素和结果关系提供一个精确/无偏倚的测量结果。请见图 134.7a。然而，研究结果可能是非常精确但带有偏倚(图 134.7c)。尽管相关测量被精确地量化，但由于没有考虑到存在的偏倚可能还会有错误，这是典型的对疗效的大样本观察性研究。另外，一些研究可能会提供测

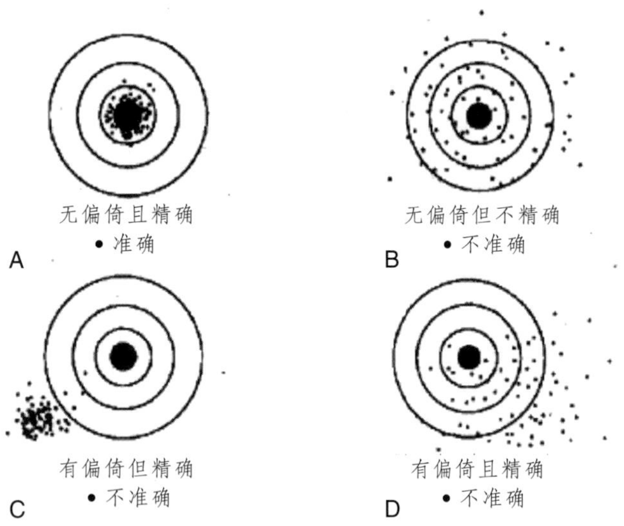

图 134.7 偏倚与精确度。

量暴露因素和结果关系的有效措施，但这可能是不精确的(图 134.7b)。这能在一个良好进行的临床随机试验中观察到，虽有测量疗效的有效措施，但是样品量不足以允许精确计算该疗效。

内部与外部有效性

正如前面提到的有效性与偏倚呈负相关，研究偏倚越小其有效性越高，反之亦然。一项有效的研究提供了近似真实值的暴露因素与结果关系的评估。然而，“真实”值取决于在做出流行病学推断时被研究的人群。

研究抽样时选取具有适当代表性的患者（即无选择偏倚），对所有相关变量进行准确测量(即无信息偏倚)，并控制会混淆暴露和结果之间关系的因素(即无混杂因素)，则该研究具有“内部有效性”。实际上，这意味着针对来自研究人群的暴露——结果关系计算出的关联度[例如，风险比(RR)]，是从源群体计算的 RR 的良好估计(图 134.8)。

图 134.8 中需要注意的是，研究群体嵌套在源群体中，而研究群体又嵌套在目标或参考群体中。如上所述，内部有效性与研究中的 RR 是源群体中 RR 的良好估计相关。此外，如果后者也是参考人群中 RR 的良好估计，则研究结果被认为具有良好的外部有效性。例如一项研究，源群体和参考群体包括来自给定中心的肾移植受者的样品、来自该中心的所有肾移植受者，以及

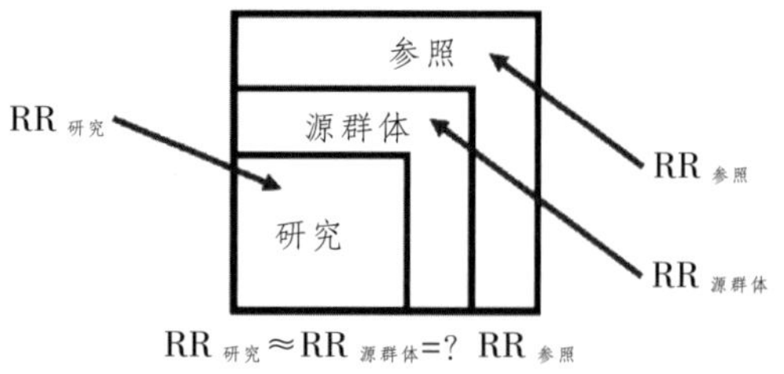

图 134.8 研究结果的普遍性(内部与外部有效性)。

来自世界各地类似中心的所有肾移植受者。与之类似，招募美国护士进入研究队列时，所有在美国的护士、所有在美国的妇女都可能构成来源人群和参照人群来进行护士健康研究[9]。

基于上述定义，在建立外部有效性之前需要先建立内部有效性。大多数情况下，内部或外部有效性不能独立于研究本身的数据而建立。必须依靠研究设计、实施和分析的特征来推断结果可能存在内部有效性。外部有效性可以部分地通过研究参与者的特征以及它们与相关的参照群体的相似性来评估。然而，研究受试者和参照群体之间的不同可能存在其他不可测量的或未知因素。同样重要的是，要注意到一项研究的结果可能适用于一个给定的为特定的源和参照人群研究的目标和设计。没有绝对的来源人群和参照人群，只有那些与特定研究相关的人群。

临床研究中的主要偏倚类型

临床研究中主要有三种类型的偏倚会对研究结果产生误导或产生谬误(除了偶然)。

选择偏倚

患者纳入研究的方式或患者失去随访的方式导致选择偏倚，是可以在暴露与结果之间的关系中观察到的。决定参与一项研究的因素可能与健康状态有关，那些被纳入研究的患者可能或多或少地比那些理论上有资格(但实际未纳入)参与研究的患者更健康。需要注意的是，选择一组特定的患者亚群进入研究是常见的，但是只有当暴露因素与结果之间的关系因这种选择发生改变时，才会产生偏倚。在该背景下，研究人群中的关联计算与源人群的关系是不同的。

选择偏倚的一个最近的例子是在美国的一群护士中开展的使用激素替代疗法(HRT)对心血管疾病发展

影响的一个观察性研究。护士健康研究(一项大型的随访美国护士几十年的前瞻性队列研究)表明:HRT 能显著降低发生心血管疾病的风险[9,10]。然而,一项随后的关于 HRT 的大型临床试验表明,发生心血管疾病的风险并没有降低,事实上,在开始治疗之后,这个风险反而会增加[11]。这表明,参与研究的护士的健康状况可能不同于一般女性群众,同时,这些差异在最开始的分析中是难以衡量和调整的。

虽然在研究对象招募时消除选择偏倚的一个最有效的办法是随机分配暴露或干预因素，但在很多情况下这是不可行的。选择偏倚可能发生在招募患者进入队列研究时，也可能是在病例对照研究中不恰当地选择了对照组的结果。此外,在临床试验和队列研究中,选择偏倚都潜在于随访中。如果对具有最好(或最差)预后的暴露组(或非暴露组)的研究对象失去了随访,由剩余的队列得出的暴露与疾病之间的关联的估计值可能会存在一定的偏倚。

选择偏倚的控制关键取决于研究的设计阶段。在分析阶段调整选择偏倚是比较难的。应谨慎地从人群中选择那些具有代表性的研究对象纳入分析。此外,在临床试验和队列研究优化保留战略，对于减少选择偏倚后续的发展是很有必要的。

信息偏倚

信息偏倚是指对暴露、结果的错误认定和(或)混杂因素导致了对暴露因素或治疗手段与结果的关系的错误估计。这种偏倚也被称为测量误差或错误分类(对分类变量而言)。这种错误在临床研究中无处不在,但往往被低估。大多数情况下,由测量误差所导致的偏倚的程度是很难提前预测的。如果误差在二分类暴露因素或疾病种类中是一致的(例如,无论未来心血管疾病的发生风险有多高，对高血压与非高血压患者的误判是一致的),那么,联系将逐渐减弱直至零效应。这也被称为无差异错误分类。在误判是有差别的情况下(即误差率作为暴露因素和疾病的一项功能变化),偏倚的方向和幅度是很难预测的。

降低信息偏倚风险的方式包括对研究人员进行适当地培训、校准测量仪器并正确整合收集数据元素。此外,如果暴露因素、结果和(或)混杂因素是使用替代措施(相对于金标准),这将有利于执行子研究,其中较小规模的一组受试者用替代和黄金标准进行测量。这将提供一个评估与前者相关联的测量误差的方法。例如一项以研究对象回忆为基础，收集过去一段较长时间内的饮食模式的问卷调查，同时应该用一组患者的每天日常饮食日记进行验证。这种验证工作也可用于支持未来使用问卷调查的研究。

混杂偏倚

从根本上说,混杂偏倚是指一种影响的混乱。当暴露与疾病之间的关系可能是完全或部分受到外来第三种因素的影响时,混杂偏倚就产生了。

能引起混杂偏倚的第三种因素应有以下三种属性:

- 是所研究疾病的独立危险因素(在非暴露组)。
- 与暴露因素有关(在源人群中)。
- 不受暴露因素或疾病的影响。

第一个属性意味着第三种因素与所研究的结果之间也是因果关系。这种关系说明应该还存在结果的独立暴露因素(即在非暴露组中可以观察到混杂因素与结果的关系)。第二种属性强调的是在那些疾病未发展的人群,如源人群中对于第三种因素,需要进行相应的暴露，因为暴露因素和第三种因素都将和疾病的发生发展有关,不论它们在源人群中是什么关系。最后一种属性指第三种因素可能会调整暴露因素对结果的影响(即因果链上的中间体)。例如,他汀类药物对心血管疾病的疗效，在一定程度上其实是对低密度脂蛋白胆固醇水平的影响。在这种情况下,低密度脂蛋白胆固醇不会对他汀类药物与心血管疾病之间的关系产生混淆。

引起暴露组和非暴露组个体之间发病率差异的外来第三种因素被称为混杂因素。此外,那些可作为外部因素的替代的相关变量可以视为混杂因素。在这个意义上,这些因素都是外来的,而不是研究因素和研究疾病因果链上的中间变量(如上述提到的第三种属性)。

混杂偏倚的控制取决于测量会引起暴露与疾病之间关系的因素，然后在研究阶段或分析阶段中考虑它们。控制混杂偏倚的研究设计方法有:随机化、匹配和限制(研究分析方法将在本章的第二部分进行讨论)。虽然随机化是控制已知和未知基线的混杂因素最有效的途径,但它在很多情况下是不可用的(例如,当暴露因素是血液中的生物标志物时)。

匹配是指同时使暴露组与非暴露组的受试者的潜在混杂因素处于同一水平下。例如,性别的匹配将确保其不再作为暴露与结果之间关系的混杂因素，因为男性(和女性)的频数在暴露组和非暴露组中是匹配的。多个混杂因素可以同时进行匹配，但是这样会降低可创建匹配对的数量。此外,一旦匹配,这些混杂因素对结果的影响将无法评估。

限制是指限定只有一个已知程度的混杂因素的研究对象,以消除其对暴露与疾病关系的影响。例如,如果性别是一个潜在的混杂因素，那么只研究女性将会消除由性别引起的偏倚。虽然它是控制混杂偏倚的有力方式,但限制也存在一些缺点。这种方式往往会减少样本量,从而造成不利影响。因此,为了有效地运用限制这一方法,需要有一个较大的数据集。另外,如果暴露与疾病的关联在男性与女性之间不同，那么仅限女性纳入研究将阻碍研究人员检验由性别引起的潜在影响。最后,由于研究对象已经与原来的评估对象不同,研究结果的普遍性将会降低。

效能及样本量问题

在设计一项临床试验或观察性研究时，如果干预或暴露会导致不同的结果，那么研究的主要目的之一就是将这种差异呈现出来。要使目标样本量能呈现出这种差异,需要的因素包括：

- 假设影响大小。
- 在对照组或为暴露组中结果的基线率。
- 结果变异性的估计。
- 一类错误率，如实际上无差异但研究发现差异的概率(通常设定为0.05)。
- 效能或一减去二型错误率，如实际上有差异且研究发现差异的概率(通常设为≥0.80)。
- 研究对象失访率。
- 招募患者阶段。
- 随访阶段[12]。

与一个给定的情况相关的特定要素主要取决于被评估的结果类型(即连续的、分类的或时间性事件)。

有时,研究样本的大小可能是相对固定的,因此对各种影响的效能评估是有必要的。无论预期数值是多少,都需要样本量或效能的计算,因为需要做出关于上述参数值的各种假设。这些假设可能会被现有的其他人群的数据集或理论评估所引导，但在进行研究之前真正的结果是未知的，但可对进行研究所需的实际样本量有一个显著的效果[12]。恰当的样本量及效能的计算不仅对提高评估治疗或暴露影响的精确度很重要，而且还可以保证参加研究的对象能为临床以及未来的患者提供有用的信息。

一些专用的统计软件已经有计算样本量/效能的功能(例如,Stata或SPSS)。同时也可从网上免费下载优良的样本量及效能计算工具(如,http://biostat.mc.vanderbilt.edu/ PowerSampleSize)。

数据源:优点与缺点

一项研究的机会和质量高低往往取决于数据源。没有对数据源的质量进行仔细评估，那么从中得出的结论可能将是错误的、有误导性的,或对未来的实践不具有指导作用。同样重要的是要考虑到,不同来源的数据是被用于不同的研究目的，且有不同的优点和局限性。为了设计出最好的研究以及结果解释并付诸实践,研究人员必须认识到这些。数据源大致可分为来自前瞻性试验或来自观察性研究两种。观察性数据集进一步可以区分为单(多)中心采集和国家注册系统采集。这些数据源的基本优点与缺点见下文分析。

随机对照试验

正如前面所讨论的，设计优良的随机对照试验为研究假说提供了最好的证据，同时减少只有观察性研究才有的选择偏倚和混杂偏倚。虽然随机对照试验(RCT)有很多优点,但也要意识到对于设计、实施研究以及实验报告来说,对结果的解释是关键性的。

临床试验的主要局限包括重要资源的限制无法对罕见事件进行试验，以及无法解决可能被认为不道德的研究问题(例如,研究比较透析与肾移植的有效性,在临床试验中将不可能开展)。此外,有大量文献表明临床试验的设计和实施有不同程度的质量[13]。CONSORT小组发表了大量文章，试图根据最佳实践标准化试验[14,15]。对此类研究的阅读者应意识到临床试验的结果可能伴随着潜在的缺陷或潜在的偏倚。

临床试验通常为回答一个基于主要终点的研究问题而设计和统计。一个常见的误解是,没有检测到次要终点的意义就表明没有显著性差异。次要终点很少能显示出差异，因此，缺乏统计学上的显著的研究结果时,不能像主要终点一样被解释。使用亚组和因果分析是临床试验争议的主要来源[16]。虽然这些分析可能会提供有关于预措施的额外信息，它们不能利用和主要研究假说同样的方式评估。最显著的是,二次分析往往不能保持随机化的优点，并且每个测试可能不能充分地说明问题。此外,需要明确假设是否进行了先验测试以及多重检验调整是否被纳入分析。

解释临床试验的一个重要考虑因素包括研究结果是否适用于实践。必须考虑基于试验条件的潜在“研究效果”(例如,降低药物价格、增强后续科学实验报告、选择研究人群),其结果可能并不是适用于外部的研究设置。最近,移植试验已经被设计为非劣性结果。这样设计的好处是减少了资源的需求以及可以更快速地得到研究结果。然而,非劣性试验也有重要的注意事项,包括使用一个随机的样本量和对照组的选择[17]。最后,由于资源限制,试验往往利用复合终点(如肾移植可能包括急性排斥反应，肾功能严重不良事件伴随着死亡和移植物失功能)。这些试验的一个重要考虑因素是如何协调结果，其中复合终点的每个成分可能有不同的临床后果,并且研究组之间的频率可能也不同[18]。

单中心观察性研究

从单中心开展研究的优势之一是获取的数据集是与给定的研究假设有特定联系的。也就是说,从单中心展开的研究可以有机会收集到有关研究问题的特定信息,而不是依赖于现有的数据源。这种类型的特异性可能会得到在不同情况下都难以复制的新颖的发现。这些研究的另一个优点是研究结果往往反映了观察具有同质环境和护理协议。在此基础上,由于不同机构的不同护理模式下产生的差异对于解释研究结果是不突出的。

单中心研究的主要局限性是缺乏将结果推广至其他环境的普遍性。例如,一个给定的中心可以利用协议活检作为护理标准并报告排斥反应的发生率。因此,从单中心得到的调查结果对于了解其影响力往往是至关重要的。单中心的研究可能缺乏统计能力去测试假设的“结果事件”,例如患者的死亡,除非是经过一个比较广泛的时代的累积。此外,从一个广泛时代获取数据可能会导致与时代发展相关的潜在偏倚。从单中心展开的研究设计及结果解释都应考虑到这些方面的因素。

多中心观察性研究

开展单中心研究的一般原则同样适用于多中心研究,通常被称为协作。汇集多中心的数据的优点包括:①样本量的增加;②可验证在不同潜在人群和护理实践的设置结果。与单中心研究相比,多中心调查结果可被认为是更具有外部有效性，且可能更适用于新的设置。然而,多中心研究的一个局限性在于其数据缺乏一致性,这可能会阻碍以标准化形式收集数据。因此,在数据收集之前进行前瞻性计划，对于研究的顺利完成是至关重要的。

国家注册系统

移植领域有幸能有一个强制性的数据收集过程,这使得几乎所有的美国患者的普查资料都是可用的[19]。收集到的有关移植等待者、接受者以及捐赠者的数据由美国器官共享网络平台(UNOS)管理。该机构负责监管收集数据的形式以及为研究文件和研究报告编辑数据。此外,美国肾脏数据系统(USRDS)以及移植受者科学注册系统(SRTR)也是可以利用这些数据进行研究的签约机构。SRTR 还包含所有非肾实质器官移植受者和捐赠者的数据。国家注册系统已经被广泛应用于研究,同时也为医学上评估一个完整队列患者提供了一个难得的机会。然而,当碰到较小的观察性试验或者随机试验时,国家注册系统也有各种优势和不足。更多关于人群研究和移植注册的细节在第 133 章有深入探讨。

探索性数据分析

对于研究来说，最重要的但也许又经常会被低估的一个方面是对数据元素适用性做出综合评价。探索这些数据的模式对于识别异常值和有影响的观察、确定连续数据为线性或非线性模式、描述数据元素的模型以及检查变量之间的二元关系有着重要作用。这个过程亦可避免使用有错误信息的数据，或者由于时间的推移以不同形式呈现的变量(例如,UNOS 利用不同的标准度去收集相同的数据元素),并且可以运用适当的方式验证数据。一般情况下,研究人员在开展更复杂的分析之前应该对数据结构感到得心应手。

单变量分析

单变量分析通常涉及描述一个变量的分布和形状,分析估计其集中趋势和变异或分散趋势。选取何种适当的统计方法才能反映出这些特征，取决于该变量的类型。因此，在一个研究中确定变量的类型对于后续描述性统计分析以及进一步的建模是至关重要的。单变量分析的目的包括：调查存在的异常值和有影响的观察资料、评估变量假设的可靠性，并初步检查一个给定样本是否可与一个已知或更广泛的人群标准相比较。对于一个给定的分析，当数据不符合理想的分布特征时，单变量分析也可以用来研究变量在不同标准下适当的转换。

多变量分析

大多数研究的主要假设都是验证两个或多个变量之间的关联。双变量关联适用于分类和连续变量的常用分析，当双变量有关联时，一个变量代表应答，另一个为解释变量，或者变量间没有这种关联。双变量分析的例子包括 Spearman 关联 Fisher 精确性检验、学生 t 检验、Wilcoxon 秩和检验和 Kappa 统计等等。对于每一种类型的双变量分析，都有不同的假设类型、分布和变量的大小，这对于研究结果的恰当应用和解释是十分重要的。对给定的一组数据未能使用恰当的分析会显著影响解释和测试的意义。在观察性研究的背景下，双变量分析的缺点之一是确定观察变量之间是否存在关联在很大程度上受到附加因素的影响。因此，虽然评估两个变量之间的关系通常是有趣并且重要的，但合并附加因素的模型在实践中通常也是非常有用的。

统计模型最常见的框架之一是最小二乘(或线性)回归模型。这种模型的基本假设包括误差是加性的，是正态分布的，并且方差齐。违背这些假设会影响假设研究的点估计和结论。然而，一些数据偏离了这些假设也是常见的，这些偏离的影响取决于：①违背的程度；②违背了哪种假设；③样本量大小。最小二乘法分析(如常见的 t 检验和 F 检验)假设模型的剩余误差呈正态分布。这个假设的错误会影响假设检验和参数的置信区间的结论。不符合这些假设的变量的一个潜在补救措施是转换数据(例如，进行对数或平方根处理)。此外，其他建模策略，例如非参数模型或具有不同分布要求的模型(例如，泊松分布、生存或逻辑模型)可能可以更适当地描述变量之间的关系。

对模型统计假设的另一个常见的违反是观测的独立性。具体来说，许多标准模型假设误差在观测之间是不相关的。相关误差的影响会导致估计精度的降低。单个患者的多次观察的数据或聚集广泛特征的观察建模时应考虑到这种依赖性。在移植的背景下，当患者匹配时(例如，配对的供肾研究)，当研究人群在较大单位时(例如，中心或个别医生)，或者当对于给定患者随着时间收集纵向数据时这种情况就会发生。

生存分析

在移植人群中分析结果的最常用方法之一是使用生存分析。生存模型(亦称为事件-时间模型)适用于试验患者队列从指定的开始时间到出现指定事件（例如患者死亡或移植物失功)的时间。这些模型能让研究人员评估解释性因素和相关终点事件的关系，同时考虑患者可能具有不同的终点发生风险的时间量。这允许模型将有多变随访的患者纳入一个单一的分析。

其中最常见的例子是 Kaplan-Meier 图和 Cox 比例风险模型。Kaplan-Meier 图表明了在不调整受试者协变量的情况下指定终点事件的累积发生率，而 Cox 模型在协变量调整或不调整的情况下均可以开发。这些模型的一个重要原则是“审查”的方针。在代表未定义为事件的受试者的最后一个风险期(正确的审查)的时间点对模型进行审查。例如，大多数生存分析图在最后一个患者随访或已知的状态审查，如在患者不再具有发生结果事件的风险的时间点。值得注意的是，在一个给定的模型里每个患者的审查时间可以是不同的，但模型假设审查机制与相关时间无关。因此，如果模型审查的时间点不是随机分布的，则从模型推理出的评估就可能是有偏差的。例如，在移植中常见的终点事件是死亡或移植物失功，其将死亡视为“非信息性”审查事件。这意味着死亡的患者没有或多或少可能经历移植物失功，与之形成对比的是那些仍然生存着但实际上仍有移植物失功风险的患者。在许多情况下，这可能是对随机审查假设的严重违反。处理非随机审查的一种方法是使用竞争风险分析。该分析可以评估随着时间的推移相关事件的累计发生率，并且显著区别于标准的(Kaplan-Meier)方法论。

诊断测试

常见的研究问题涉及特定参数是否可用作特定结

果的准确诊断测试。应用背景可能存在于确定疾病状态的诊断参数中或作为后续相关事件的预后评估。例如，去了解一个来自死亡捐献的活组织检查是否对移植结果具有预后价值，这可能具有研究价值。以类似的方式，我们使用筛选试验，根据疾病预防控制中心的标准排除捐赠者有传播性疾病的可能性[21,22]。我们也可能会有兴趣了解替代标记物的预测价值，如肾功能作为移植物失功的标记物[19,23]。我们可以在几个方面量化。在具有二进制结果和预测器的“2×2”背景下，我们可以计算：

- 灵敏度——检验出现结果是阳性的概率。
- 特异性——检测未出现结果是阴性的概率。
- 阳性预测值——测试结果为阳性的出现结果的概率。
- 阴性预测值——测试结果为阴性的不出现结果的概率。

这些统计数据都有助于量化具体诊断参数预测的准确性，但每个统计数据的价值可能会随着不同的临床背景而有差异。在某些情况下，了解灵敏度和阳性预测值(评估阳性病例的确定程度)可能更有用，而在其他情况下，特异性(评估阴性病例的确定程度)的作用则更突出。这些数据还可以用来确定一个诊断参数最佳地用于预后的阈值。

重要的是，真实预测一个诊断参数的标准是不同的，通常比对一个给定结果相关的参数的标准更严格[24]。与许多众所周知的临床结果相关联的参数具有较差的辨别力，而这是诊断参数高度预测性的一个特征。因此，在研究中，重要的是鉴别那些具有高度预测性的参数，并且使用适当的统计方法来证明诊断参数的预测能力。

风险调整

为了从样本中产生出可推广到一个广泛群体（例如，美国所有的移植受者）的结论，或比较两个研究组之间的特征和结果，可取的办法是尽量使除了相关暴露因素之外的其他特征最小化(图 134.9)。对于任何一个非随机临床研究，暴露组之间存在着供者、受者或其他移植相关因素的某些变化。因此，为了评估暴露因素对特定结果的独立影响，调整超出暴露组的差异的统计方法是至关重要的。然而，重要的是要认识到“风险调整”不是通过整齐划一的方法论来开展的。如何解释风险的变化取决于以下几个条件：①特定相关结果；②暴露因素和结果之间的时间关系；③研究的目的；④评估的人群[25]。在这个意义上，研究人员和消费者应该知道每个研究的具体细微差别，而不是对每个分析都使用相同的风险调整技术。

在美国，我们是幸运的，因为我们有器官获取和移植网络平台(OPTN)，在强制性的基础上，这个平台为每个实体器官移植等待者、受者和捐献者收集大量关于捐献者、受者和移植特征的数据。因此，使用移植中心之间的统计模型可以标准化、全面化地风险调整。然而，需要注意的是，即使对这些临床参数进行风险调整，模型的辨别能力也是相对比较一般的[26]。事实上，相比其他高端的医学背景，这种预测能力明显更低，这表明存在能基本解释结果的非编码因素以及存在相对高水平的随机变异来解释这些患者发生的事件。这意味着，在许多移植研究中可能存在着由于不一致记录

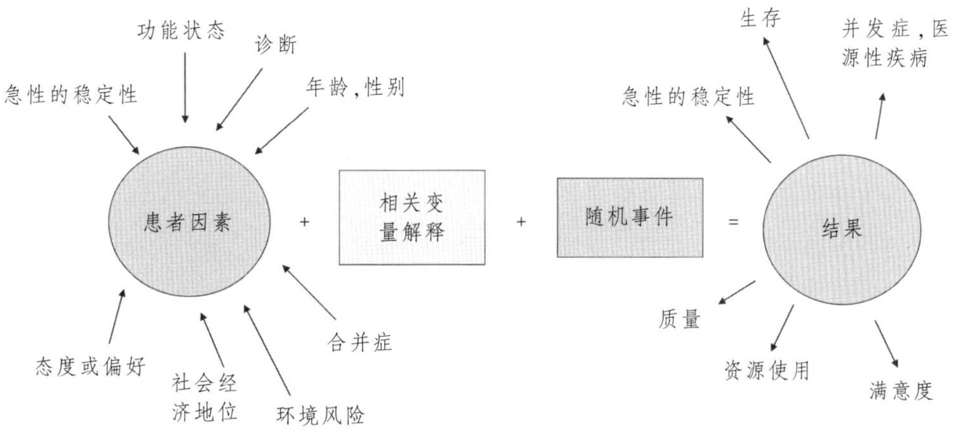

图 134.9 临床研究中的风险调整。Adapted from [25] Iezzoni LI. Risk Adjustment for Measuring Healthcare Outcomes, 3rd edition. Chicago, IL: Health Administration Press, 2003(Chapter One, p.5, Reasons for Risk Adjustment).

混杂因素而导致的严重威胁，并且这些因素的潜在作用应该在研究背景下考虑，并作适当的解释和承认。

亚组分析和效应修改

对于任何一个评估研究人群的统计分析来说，一个重要且经常是有趣的环节是评估研究结果对于人群中的所有受试者是否都一致。当两个变量之间的关系相对于第三变量的水平不同时，则存在相互影响(或称效应修改)。例如，使用免疫抑制剂与发生急性排斥反应的关联可能会因患者的年龄或免疫状态而改变。在不同亚组中暴露对结果的影响可以通过相互作用的测试在森林图中显示，包括显示每个亚组中的主要影响因素是否存在显著性差异(表134.2)。相互作用的分析可具有重要的临床意义，特别是当它们具有足够的证据时，即一项给定的新发现能否在群体中推广，或可能或多或少适用于某些患者分层。

模型的解释

对于任何非随机研究，很少可以从已有文献记录的统计推断出强烈为因果关系。这主要是由于潜在的混杂因素和干预因素的影响，可以解释观察到的关联，而不是归因于研究分组。一个解释性变量可能在一个给定响应的因果途径中改变，这种观点基于相关性的强度、影响的生物合理性、是否存在剂量反应效应，以及在不同环境中和在不同群体中以及在一些情况下是否观察得到效果而有相应的变化。但由于解释性变量与结果相关的途径通常有许多种，所以确认未测量因素的假设作用对于结果的解释是重要的。

表134.2 显示潜在相互作用或效应修改的森林图。

亚组	L-SLTx n/N	L-SLTx 预测3年总生存率(95% CI)	R-SLTx n/N	R-SLTx 预测3年总生存率(95% CI)	HR(95%CI)	P值
性别(相互影响：P=0.7302)						
男	29/48	56.8%(45.0%;71.9%)	27/39	48.2%(35.5%;65.3%)	0.77(0.46;1.31)	0.3373
女	8/24	75.2%(60.4%;93.8%)	13/31	73.5%(60.2%;89.7%)	0.93(0.38;2.24)	0.8645
性别不匹配(相互影响：P=0.5470)						
否	32/64	64.2%(53.9%;76.4%)	36/66	61.9%(51.8%;74.0%)	0.93(0.57;1.49)	0.7510
是	5/8	43.5%(19.3%;98.1%)	4/4	24.9% (5.3%; 100%)	0.60(0.16;2.28)	0.4515
灌注匹配(相互影响：P=0.3166)						
<50%	31/55	54.3%(42.5%;69.3%)	21/37	53.1%(39.7%;71.0%)	0.96(0.55;1.68)	0.8957
≥50%	6/17	81.6%(67,9%;97.9%)	19/33	69.3%(55.9%;86.0%)	0.56(0.22;1.39)	0.2107
BOS(相互影响：P=0.9511)						
不存在	24/52	67.3%(57.2%;79.2%)	27/51	64.9%(54.6%;77.0%)	0.92(0.53;1.60)	0.7563
存在	13/20	7.5% (1.1%; 50.6%)	13/19	6.4% (1.0%; 40.2%)	0.94(0.43;2.08)	0.8865
心律失常(相互影响：P=0.4109)						
否	34/66	61.8%(51.5%;74.1%)	38/62	57.6%(47.1%;70.4%)	0.87(0.55; 1.39)	0.5624
是	3/6	61.9%(34.2%; 100%)	2/8	77.7%(53.8%; 100%)	1.90(0.32;11.41)	0.4842
ICU逗留时间(相互影响：P=0.1496)						
≤6天	20/44	71.8%(60.0%;86.0%)	16/29	60.2%(46.0%;78.8%)	0.65(0.33;1.29)	0.2178
>6天	17/28	48.9%(33.8%;70.7%)	24/41	57.3%(44.2%;74.4%)	1.29(0.69;2.41)	0.4304
住院时间(相互影响：P=0.3013)						
≤30天	11/33	8.0%(66.0%;92.2%)	19/36	67.3%(54.5%;83.3%)	0.63(0.30;1.32)	0.2202
>30天	26/39	49.8%(36.7%;67.7%)	21/34	50.9%(37.1%;69.9%)	1.03(0.58;1.85)	0.9117

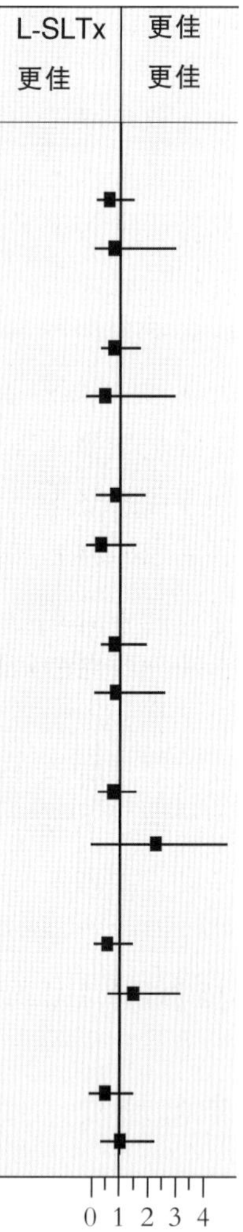

N，总人数；n，死亡数；HR，风险比。

Reproduced from Tsagkaropoulos S, Belmans A, Verleden GM, et al. Single-lung transplantation: does side matter? European Journal of Cardio-thoracic Surgery, 2011:40(2);e83 - e92. Copyright 2011, with permission from Oxford University Press [54].

对统计结果的解释的另一个重要但经常被忽略的方面是给出真实效果(即模型的统计功效)的检测差异的概率。一般来说,证明统计上的显著结果的能力高度依赖于样本量、变异性的影响和研究设计。重要的是,未能证明有影响不一定表示不存在关联。这在小样本研究中特别显著,在这种背景下,发现有统计学意义的概率受到观察和变异性的影响。在小规模的观察研究中未能检测出有意义的影响因素则基于大型注册管理机构(例如,UNOS 数据)的研究的潜在结果。对于后者的研究,统计差异可以代表非常小的、潜在的临床相关的差异是比较常见的。然而,需要注意的是,即使是小的差异也可能是重要的信息,因为它们仍然可以反映出重要的关联,即使这样的差异可能不代表在日常临床决策中有效。对于研究结果的解释,应区分临床有用和统计学显著的结果,以及代表重要机制但具有适度的临床相关性的结果。

缺失的数据

数据缺失是临床研究中常见的情况。这可能包括缺少应答或解释性变量的数据,并且可能对于分析和解释研究结果提出重大挑战。重要的是,对于许多标准分析,缺失值可能会导致排除观察值(即分析完整病例),这可能降低模型的统计功效,限制结果的外部有效性,并可能产生偏倚比较。因此,重要的是:①记录存在缺失数据;②了解数据为什么丢失(例如随机丢失,由于失去随访而丢失,高敏度病例更可能缺失数据等);③考虑处理缺失数据的不同分析策略。处理缺失数据的选项包括忽略这些情况,这可能导致从模型中排除观察结果,对缺失的情况(例如,平均水平或模态水平)的简单估算或多重估算[27]。一般来说,因缺少数据元素或简单插补方法而删除观察结果的做法,已显示导致结果偏差。在更复杂的方法中,数据保持的假设可以提高模型的表现和预测[28]。

移植中的终点事件

急性排斥

急性排斥是观察性研究和随机对照试验的移植过程的主要终点之一。在研究中使用急性排斥作为终点所面对的挑战之一是缺乏一个统一的定义。急性排斥反应可能是基于治疗的条件(即临床相关的护理需要),活检证实的排斥反应(包括组织学分级),或根据其他临床指标(例如,进行肾移植术后肾功能的下降)。急性排斥反应定义的差异可能会导致在评估急性排斥反应对移植物的损失或死亡的影响时有广泛的多样性。使用急性排斥反应作为终点事件的另一个考虑是急性排斥事件和排斥发作的时机不会导致肾功能的永久性丧失(其可能对移植物存活没有显著影响)[29,30]。最后,一些患者可能在移植后经历多次急性排斥期。这些重复的事件需要不同的分析方法,以便确定是否每个阶段都是一个明显的事件,还是正在进行的过程的产物。

移植物功能延迟

移植物功能延迟(DGF)是肾移植手术后的主要终点事件。DGF 是一种急性肾损伤的形式,其最常见的定义为受者移植后一周内存在对透析的需要。分析评估 DGF 对于结果的影响,挑战之一是将该事件与可能会导致受者早期透析治疗的其他手术事件(即技术原因)区分开。中心实践模式也可能影响透析患者的治疗,从而影响 DGF 的发生[31]。因此,尽管传统上用于研究的 DGF 的定义相对统一,但也可能存在对于解释研究结果的重要的不同因素。

感染

移植受者由于免疫抑制治疗、外科手术、其他并发症发作和其他共病因素而易受各种类型的感染[32-34]。在临床研究的评估中,移植后常见的感染类型包括巨细胞病毒(CMV)感染、BK 病毒感染、EB 病毒感染和各种其他类型的细菌和真菌形式感染。一些感染可能是无症状或记录不全的,每个在严重程度上都有不同,这可能会影响发病率的系统性记录。对于某些类型的感染,预防可以很大程度地减轻发生临床感染的可能性,并且可能需要在分析中考虑。此外,感染的特定起始和结束日期难以用系统的方式量化,但其对于指导分析是重要的。总之,感染是移植后常见的并发症,但发病率和严重程度有很大的不同,并不总是清楚地记录,且很可能与治疗密切相关。

移植物失功

移植物失功是临床研究调查的主要“硬”终点。移植物失功通常定义为重新需要透析，或再移植(在肾移植的情况下)，或患者死亡(该复合终点也称为总移植物失功)的移植物衰竭。患者死亡通常包括在基于许多死亡与器官衰退相关的假设的结果中，因此，在所有情况下难以将这些终点的机制彼此分离。至少，对于任何研究组的比较，评估死亡和移植物失功的个体贡献是重要的。临床研究的挑战之一是移植后期的移植失败率相对较低。因此，为了有足够的统计数据来测试研究假设，需要更长的随访期或更大的样本量。因此，还进行了广泛的努力来开发和理解用于长期移植物失功的良好替代标记物，其可以用于评估那些有限的随访累积期的治疗干预[7,29,38]。

患者死亡

将死亡作为研究终点的主要限制是缺乏比较研究组的统计数据。大多数试验不能设计用于患者生存，特别是在移植领域。对于研究和研究设计，我们经常假设更有可能经历急性排斥反应，感染或DGF的患者也更有可能随后移植物失功并最终更有可能死亡。尽管如此，患者生存至少应被视为次要终点。为其他并发症设计的研究应包含单独的分析，包括死亡率或复合终点，以确保基于研究组之间的不同死亡率，研究结果不会误导。

成本和资源利用

研究和应用大多数科学研究的重要终点是成本。给定干预的成本效益通常与患者特征、治疗策略、并发症类型相关，并且可能具有重要的实践和政策影响[39-42]。卫生经济学原理也可以有效地指导稀有资源的最佳利用，这在器官移植的背景下特别突出[43]。成本效益分析对于比较干预措施明显很重要，但是它们也应用来研究对于一些个体来说是有效的护理，但由于低效率地使用资源，可能会导致降低对其他患者的护理。计量经济学方法通常具有独特的考虑，例如成本随时间而产生的折损、建模行为、供者和患者决策以及量化寿命年。虽然经常难以在临床疗效研究的背景下进行经济分析，但它们是在器官移植的背景下提供医疗保健的关键组成部分。

供者护理质量

有许多研究评估供者实践和结果的影响[44,45]。在美国，移植中心目前通过SRTR进行性能评估。SRTR在公开的网站上报告风险调整的移植物和患者生存率[46]。这些数据包括等待者名单、移植后结果以及人群的人口学特征。评估移植中心的主要指标之一是标准化死亡率(SMR)。SMR是通常应用的统计度量，其可以用于基于对归一化参考组(例如，美国移植人群)结果的间接标准化来在提供者或区域水平评估风险调整的结果。SMR用于评估在给定的随访期间调整供者、受者和移植相关变量后，比较移植中心观察到的事件数(移植物丢失或死亡)与预期事件数量，并利用同一时期的国家经验作为参照组。SMR等于1表示中心的结果与基于移植人群的敏锐水平预期的结果相等，而较高的SMR表示关于预期群体中事件数量性能较差。目前在移植中使用SMR的一个限制是，由于统计力量的增强，与较小的中心相比，较大的中心更可能得到统计学上的显著差异。为了衡量移植中心，SMR也是CMS和其他保险公司评估护理质量的指标[47]。

患者满意度和生活质量

也许在医疗卫生中最经常被忽视但却又是最重要的终点之一是患者满意度。患者满意度通常难以客观地评估，但这并不总是研究的主要焦点。在移植后生活质量指标包括并发症发生率、再住院情况和移植物存活率。然而，单独的临床终点显然不能充分体现患者的满意度和生活质量。旨在用统一的方式获取患者满意度的前瞻性研究在移植中是重要的，并且对这些数据进一步利用是必要的，以用于干预的临床应用、分配政策和决策。

特殊主题

许多标准的分析方法是改进的建模策略和新方法，除了在统计和流行病学领域，这些方法还被开发并更广泛地应用入临床研究中。通常，这些新的建模策略嵌入到统计软件包中，但也可能需要更复杂的程序和方法论基础的理解。对于任何一个模型，分析人员必须认识到这些方法的假设以及结果的正确解释。在这里简要讨论在当代医学研究中使用的一些更复杂的建模策略。

倾向评分分析旨在实现伪随机研究设计。这种方法的概念通常是“重建”随机实验设计，通过识别与治疗分配的初始分配相关的因素来比较干预措施。例如，考虑到许多编码的和非编码的因子被用于可能与其预后相关的患者的治疗选择，直接比较接受两种不同免疫抑制剂的受体可能是具有挑战性的[48]。然而，在与治疗分配相关的因素是已知的并且风险因素与结果具有较强关系的背景下，倾向评分分析被认为是使潜在混杂最小化的方法[49]。

另一个有吸引力的建模策略是使用工具变量。与标准多变量分析和倾向得分分析不同，工具变量可以用来估计干预措施对不可测量因素的影响[50]。这个解释潜在变量的独特机会有两个强大的假设：①工具变量与接受干预的可能性相关；②工具变量不与相关结果直接相关。后者在标准临床环境中通常很难识别，并限制了这种形式的分析的应用。然而当正确使用工具变量时，其分析可以作为临床研究中的一个有力的工具，以最小化未测量混杂的来源。

如前所述，观察性研究的常见限制之一是无法得出关于暴露变量和相关反应之间的因果机制的推论。近年来，人们对可用于得出因果结论的分析产生了极大的关注，即使在非随机观察数据的情况下也是如此。用于推断因果关系的分析工具之一是边际结构模型。这些模型本质上是通过经验性地评估随时间的推移被治疗的概率来模拟随机化设置[51,52]。虽然开发这些模型需要一些复杂的分析，但超越协会层面的统计分析的价值，对于理论和应用科学具有极大的吸引力。

总结

对于临床研究的核心误解之一是，用于分析的模型仅仅涉及使用标准统计包来对新一组患者或新终点实施公共算法以产生结果。对于那些没有积极参与研究的人来说，对于从一个想法的概念演变成一个完成的临床研究项目的许多基本过程可能仅有有限的理解。同时，进行严格和彻底的分析所需的各个步骤和过程对于研究的有效性和严格性至关重要。理解这些过程可以从直觉、训练和经验演变而来，并允许研究人员理解什么是典型的复杂信息的复杂化。科学性、严谨性不仅涉及统计方法和分析，而且包括对结果的适当解释以及如何进行研究的透明度。作为临床研究的使用者和指挥者，理解和使用这些方法是推动科学前进的根本。

（陈俊丽　董思依　林丽丹　译　徐骁　校）

参考文献

1. Grimes DA, Schulz KF. An overview of clinical research: the lay of the land. Lancet. 2002;359:57–61.
2. Holdaas H, Fellstrom B, Jardine AG, et al. Effect of fluvastatin on cardiac outcomes in renal transplant recipients: a multicentre, randomised, placebo-controlled trial. Lancet. 2003;361:2024–2031.
3. Locke JE, Magro CM, Singer AL, et al. The use of antibody to complement protein C5 for salvage treatment of severe antibody-mediated rejection. American Journal of Transplantation. 2009;9:231–235.
4. Stegall MD, Diwan T, Raghavaiah S, et al. Terminal complement inhibition decreases antibody-mediated rejection in sensitized renal transplant recipients. American Journal of Transplantation. 2011;11:2405–2413.
5. Sakata R, Grant EJ, Ozasa K. Long-term follow-up of atomic bomb survivors. Maturitas. 2012;72:99–103.
6. Proby CM, Harwood CA, Neale RE, et al. A case-control study of betapapillomavirus infection and cutaneous squamous cell carcinoma in organ transplant recipients. American Journal of Transplantation. 2011;11:1498–1508.
7. Schold JD, Kaplan B. The elephant in the room: failings of current clinical endpoints in kidney transplantation. American Journal of Transplantation. 2010;10:1163–1166.
8. Schold JD, Buccini LD, Goldfarb DA, et al. Patient participation in research among solid organ transplant recipients in the United States. Transplantation. 2011; 91:1424–1435.
9. Stampfer MJ, Willett WC, Colditz GA, et al. A prospective study of postmenopausal estrogen therapy and coronary heart disease. New England Journal of Medicine. 1985;313:1044–1049.
10. Grodstein F, Stampfer MJ, Manson JE, et al. Postmenopausal estrogen and progestin use and the risk of cardiovascular disease. New England Journal of Medicine. 1996;335:453–461.
11. Rossouw JE, Anderson GL, Prentice RL, et al. Risks and benefits of estrogen plus progestin in healthy postmenopausal women: principal results From the Women's Health Initiative randomized controlled trial. JAMA: Journal of the American Medical Association. 2002;288:321–333.
12. Schold JD, Kaplan B. Design and analysis of clinical trials in transplantation: principles and pitfalls. American Journal of Transplantation. 2008;8:1779–1785.
13. Juni P, Witschi A, Bloch R, et al. The hazards of scoring the quality of clinical trials for meta-analysis. JAMA: Journal of the American Medical Association. 1999;282:1054–1060.
14. Moher D, Schulz KF, Altman DG. The CONSORT statement: revised recommendations for improving the quality of reports of parallel-group randomised trials. Lancet. 2001;357:1191–1194.
15. Moher D, Jones A, Lepage L. Use of the CONSORT statement and quality of reports of randomized trials: a comparative before-and-after evaluation. JAMA: Journal of the American Medical Association. 2001;285:1992–1995.
16. Wang R, Lagakos SW, Ware JH, et al. Statistics in medicine–reporting of subgroup analyses in clinical trials. New England Journal of Medicine. 2007;357: 2189–2194.
17. Wiens BL. Choosing an equivalence limit for noninferiority or equivalence studies. Controlled Clinical Trials. 2002;23:2–14.
18. Freemantle N, Calvert M, Wood J, et al. Composite outcomes in randomized trials: greater precision but with greater uncertainty? JAMA: Journal of the American Medical Association. 2003;289:2554–2559.
19. Kaplan B, Schold J, Meier-Kriesche HU. Overview of large database analysis in renal transplantation. American Journal of Transplantation. 2003;3: 1052–1056.
20. Fine JP, Gray RJ. A proportional hazards model for the subdistribution of a competing risk. Journal of the American Statistical Association. 1999;94: 496–509.
21. Ros RL, Kucirka LM, Govindan P, et al. Patient attitudes toward CDC high infectious risk donor kidney transplantation: inferences from focus groups. Clinical Transplantation. 2012;26:247–253.
22. Kucirka LM, Sarathy H, Govindan P, et al. Risk of window period hepatitis-C infection in high infectious risk donors: systematic review and meta-analysis. American Journal of Transplantation. 2011;11:1188–1200.
23. Kaplan B, Schold J, Meier-Kriesche HU. Poor predictive value of serum creatinine for renal allograft loss. American Journal of Transplantation. 2003;3:1560–1565.
24. Pepe MS, Janes H, Longton G, et al. Limitations of the odds ratio in gauging the performance of a diagnostic, prognostic, or screening marker. American Journal of Epidemiology. 2004;159:882–890.
25. Iezzoni LI. Risk Adjustment. Chicago, IL: Health Administration Press; 2003.
26. Schold JD, Howard RJ. Prediction models assessing transplant center performance: can a little knowledge be a dangerous thing? American Journal of Transplantation. 2006;6:245–246.

27. Haukoos JS, Newgard CD. Advanced statistics: missing data in clinical research–part 1: an introduction and conceptual framework. Academic emergency medicine : official journal of the Society for Academic Emergency Medicine. 2007;14:662–668.
28. Newgard CD, Haukoos JS. Advanced statistics: missing data in clinical research–part 2: multiple imputation. Academic emergency medicine : official journal of the Society for Academic Emergency Medicine. 2007;14:669–678.
29. Nett PC, Heisey DM, Shames BD, et al. Influence of kidney function to the impact of acute rejection on long-term kidney transplant survival. Transplant International. 2005;18:385–389.
30. Sijpkens YW, Doxiadis II, Mallat MJ, et al. Early versus late acute rejection episodes in renal transplantation. Transplantation. 2003;75:204–208.
31. Louvar DW, Li N, Snyder J, et al. "Nature versus nurture" study of deceased-donor pairs in kidney transplantation. Journal of the American Society of Nephrology. 2009;20:1351–1358.
32. Burroughs TE, Swindle J, Takemoto S, et al. Diabetic complications associated with new-onset diabetes mellitus in renal transplant recipients. Transplantation. 2007;83:1027–1034.
33. Flechner SM, Avery RK, Fisher R, et al. A randomized prospective controlled trial of oral acyclovir versus oral ganciclovir for cytomegalovirus prophylaxis in high-risk kidney transplant recipients. Transplantation. 1998;66:1682–1688.
34. Meier-Kriesche HU, Ojo AO, Hanson JA, et al. Exponentially increased risk of infectious death in older renal transplant recipients. Kidney International. 2001;59:1539–1543.
35. Abbott KC, Duran M, Hypolite I, et al. Hospitalizations for bacterial endocarditis after renal transplantation in the United States. Journal of Nephrology. 2001; 14:353–360.
36. Abbott KC, Hypolite I, Poropatich RK, et al. Hospitalizations for fungal infections after renal transplantation in the United States. Transplant Infectious Disease. 2001;3:203–211.
37. Cosio FG, Nuovo M, Delgado L, et al. EBV kidney allograft infection: possible relationship with a peri-graft localization of PTLD. American Journal of Transplantation. 2004;4:116–123.
38. Hariharan S, McBride MA, Cherikh WS, et al. Post-transplant renal function in the first year predicts long-term kidney transplant survival. Kidney International. 2002;62:311–318.
39. Abecassis MM, Seifeldin R, Riordan ME. Patient outcomes and economics of once-daily tacrolimus in renal transplant patients: results of a modeling analysis. Transplantation Proceedings. 2008;40:1443–1445.
40. Kutinova A, Woodward RS, Ricci JF, et al. The incidence and costs of sepsis and pneumonia before and after renal transplantation in the United States. American Journal of Transplantation. 2006;6:129–139.
41. Woodward RS, Schnitzler MA, Lowell JA, et al. Effect of extended coverage of immunosuppressive medications by medicare on the survival of cadaveric renal transplants. American Journal of Transplantation. 2001;1:69–73.
42. Hornberger JC, Best JH, Garrison LP Jr. Cost-effectiveness of repeat medical procedures: kidney transplantation as an example. Medical Decision Making: An International Journal of the Society for Medical Decision Making. 1997; 17:363–372.
43. Kim SJ, Gordon EJ, Powe NR. The economics and ethics of kidney transplantation: perspectives in 2006. Current Opinion in Nephrology and Hypertension. 2006; 15:593–598.
44. Schold JD, Harman JS, Chumbler NR, et al. The pivotal impact of center characteristics on survival of candidates listed for deceased donor kidney transplantation. Medical Care. 2009;47:146–153.
45. Kim SJ, Schaubel DE, Fenton SS, et al. Mortality after kidney transplantation: a comparison between the United States and Canada. American Journal of Transplantation. 2006;6:109–114.
46. Dickinson DM, Shearon TH, O'Keefe J, et al. SRTR center-specific reporting tools: Posttransplant outcomes. American Journal of Transplantation. 2006;6:1198–1211.
47. New Medicare Hospital Conditions of Participation for Transplant Centers. Centers for Medicare and Medicaid Services. 12-23-2009. Ref Type: Electronic Citation.
48. Schold JD, Kaplan B. AZA/tacrolimus is associated with similar outcomes as MMF/tacrolimus among renal transplant recipients. American Journal of Transplantation. 2009;9:2067–2074.
49. Rubin DB. Estimating causal effects from large data sets using propensity scores. Annals of Internal Medicine. 1997;127:757–763.
50. Bowden RJ, Turkington DA. Instrumental Variables. Cambridge, U.K.: Cambridge University Press; 1984.
51. Moodie EE, Stephens DA. Marginal Structural Models: unbiased estimation for longitudinal studies. International Journal of Public Health. 2011;56:117–119.
52. Robins JM. Causal models for estimating the effects of weight gain on mortality. International Journal of Obesity (2005). 2008;32(Suppl 3):S15–S41.
53. Rothman KJ. Epidemiology: An Introduction. New York. NY: Oxford University Press; 2002.
54. Tsagkaropoulos S, Belmans A, Verleden GM, et al. Single-lung transplantation: does side matter? European Journal of Cardio-thoracic Surgery. 2011;40(2): e83–e92.

第 135 章
器官移植疗效比较

Edward A. Meister Bruce Kaplan

引言

在某种意义上来说，疗效比较研究(CER)是由一个美国人基于苏格兰流行病学家 Archie Cochrane 建立的循证医学(EBM)，重新整合后发展而成的。这是一个概念性的框架，其将研究新发现转化为临床应用。这样，医疗服务提供方和消费方可以运用最新研究成果来更好地制订医疗方案。疗效比较研究随着 2009 年美国复苏与再投资法案(Pub.L 111-5)的通过正式成为美国医学研究的成果，并把 11 亿美元拨给疗效比较研究，为其创建了联邦协调委员会[1,2]。这些款项用于资助联邦政府的三个部门(美国卫生保健研究和治疗机构、国立卫生研究院和卫生与公共服务部部长办公室)的疗效比较研究。这将会加强实行综合研究，进一步比较临床治疗的有效性以及医疗服务、流程的合理性，因此能够更好地预防、诊断、治疗疾病和其他健康状况[1]，促进临床登记注册的发展和应用。临床数据网络化和其他形式的电子健康数据[2]，这些都将被用于创建或获取预后数据(Title Ⅷ)。

医学研究所(IOM)公布的关于疗效比较研究的定义如下：

疗效比较研究是证据的产生与综合，比较替代方法的获益与损害，来预防、诊断、治疗和控制临床情况，或改善护理。疗效比较研究的目的是帮助消费者、临床医生、采购者和政策制订者做出明智的决定，这将会提高在个人和人群水平上的医疗服务[3]。

美国国会预算办公室(CBO)增加了附加条件，称 CER “分析可能只关注相对医疗福利和每个方法的风险，或者可能也注重这些方法的成本和效益”[4]。无疑更重要的是专注于一个有效性与临床疗效标准，主导着典型的三期临床试验。有效性模型尤其关注对所谓的“普通受者(患者)”应如何实施干预工作。疗效比较研究的观念转变是指提高临床医生和受者(患者)关于如何有效地治疗特殊 LAR 类型受者(患者)的知识，创造一个更以受者(患者)为中心的结果的方法[5]。随着 2010 年受者(患者)保护与平价医疗法案的通过，以受者（患者）为中心的培养研究使命的实效研究所(PCORI)创建起来，实现了高完整性，循证医学包括其价值和受者（患者）的利益来达到提高医疗服务的目的。实效研究所(PCORI)的职责是发展以受者(患者)为中心的转化框架方法，这将会引导任何以受者（患者）为中心的疗效研究强大的固有的数据驱动研究来获得可靠的数据[6]。对所获得的地方与国家数据集的分析可参见第 132 章和第 133 章。

CER 中随机临床试验的局限性

随机对照试验(RCT)长期以来被认为是临床研究的“金标准”。就其本身而论，特别适合建立在药物、设备和同类受者(患者)群体的方法疗效上。随机对照试验(RCT)唯一的关注点是其强度，用于确定疗效和它的缺点，用于确定有效性。首先，所有 RCT 方案对可能符合或可能不符合参加试验的受者(患者)规定严格，包括排除标准。符合入选标准的那些受者(患者)倾向于不接近典型的临床实践受者(患者)，通过减少病情，具有较少的共病，治疗期望更高且依从性更强。入选标准作为样本筛选，用尽可能均匀的受者(患者)群体来填充试验组，而临床实践由真正的受者(患者)和需要修复性治疗的人构成。其次，具有安慰剂组的任何 RCT 本身缺乏有效的比较剂，因为 CER 的基础是将两种可行的疗法进行比较，以建立具有最大的疗效、最具耐受性、最低成本和最少的不良反应的治疗。安慰剂是一种无效的治疗手段，没有真正的CER，医生对每个具体的受者(患者)使用哪种治疗为最有效的问题仍存疑[7]。移植RCT通常设计为没有安慰剂，但重点仍在于确定比较物之间或之间的相对疗效。

随机对照试验(RCT)的核心优势是通过一种严密的重点突出的学科组来建立因果效应，这种推导法呈现的内部有效性主要在研究这些选取类型上，正因为如此，结果限制了外部有效性[8,9]。显然外部有效性是通过随机抽取从亚群受者（患者）进入研究人群来增强的，然而，这是很少进行的。即使这个得以实现，仍然不能保证感兴趣的因素即表现在受试者随机抽样上。随机对照试验(RCT)是基于推理概率因果关系的理念；使得X干预在实验子群体的一些同质部分中引起Y结果，例如，如果Y>P(Y|–X)的概率，则X在θ中产生Y。因此，RCT结果概率性地表明干预X在某些主题中起作用，然而这对于策略制订者和决策者试图确定X是否将在其背景中起效，实用性有限[9]。

在CER中随机对照试验(RCT)的倡导者们指出治疗的意图(ITT)是作为一项战略，以便更好地近似临床疗效。ITT用于随机对照试验(RCT)中，保证不接受干预的受者(患者)得到救治，后者根据他们的研究组来分配。以一个三组随机对照试验为例：1组是标准治疗；2组是低剂量的新治疗；3组是高剂量的新治疗。通常随机对照试验是基于多中心与多国家的，不可避免地受者(患者)更可能最终被放置在不同的研究组，而不是被随机分配。在三组研究设计中有任意三个随机选择都有六个可能的错误；受者(患者)1被随机分配到组1，然后被放置在组2或组3，受者(患者)1被随机分配到组2，最终在组1或组3，和受者(患者)1被随机分配到组3，最终在组1或组2((n排列k：3p2＝6)。ITT的策略是一个既定的协议，承诺根据分组分配分析最终数据，例如将没有人工分配的受者(患者)返回到实际得到的有干预的分组。ITT通过分析实际得到的不一致的受者(患者)数据有削弱疗效的结果。这是因为随机分组被假定为同等分散研究的组之间不可测的干扰因素[即受者(患者)的异质性]。ITT的支持者认为，正是疗效的这种削弱，可使RCT定性为更好地近似临床实践中取得更好的现实背景下，因其中受者(患者)的依从性从来都不是100%完美的[10,11]。

ITT未必是一种提高随机对照试验RCT临床意义的方法。削弱功效并不确保有效性的提高。功效是在严格控制的情况下制订的疗效合理性，有效性同时解决了该疗法在临床上如何运作的问题[12]。通过降低疗效ITT减少结果的内部效度，而不一定是结果“对应到临床实践中，受者(患者)可能有利于或不利于采取在随机对照试验RCT协议中规定的治疗方案，从而降低或以无法预知的方式来提高依从性。换句话说，疗效可由ITT指定受者(患者)依从性的不确定性而被低估或高估[13]。其次，不合理分配的研究分组导致了未知受者(患者)的特征选择偏差，不等同于临床实践。临床实践中呈现在某一特定受者(患者)的治疗方式是通过持续监测疗效和基础治疗持续测量的结果调整的。随机对照试验的目的是最大限度地减少数据干扰；随机分组尝试，以消除潜在干扰因素的受者(患者)来研究，但仍然是未知的，而排除标准干扰因素的受者(患者)是临床实践至关重要的兴趣[14]。最后，几乎没有证据表明，增加随机对照试验在受者(患者)特征或临床实践范围内试用变异可增加对外普遍性[15]。

由于随机对照试验体现临床疗效方面的局限性，比如效果推广到多元化异质的受者(患者)人群，近期的文章接二连三地提出了大规模修改随机对照试验的设计，甚至是全新的研究设计模型。这些新的临床试验设计被称为不需要加以说明的或实用的临床试验，侧重于回答问题：这种疗法能在正常处理条件下工作吗？[16]纳入和排除的标准放宽，如果不是取消标准的话，允许受者(患者)样本的异质性近似于临床实践中遇到的受者(患者)特征的多样性。务实的随机对照试验设计是队列多个随机对照设计。疗效比较研究的设计包括建立在一大群受者(患者)所关注的疾病上，其中，有些受者(患者)则随机分配到干预试验的选项，随后受者(患者)间的比较不是随机的[17]。显然，RCT在研究者基于证据的医学社区中被赋予了夸大的信任，所有其他研究设计结果都以隐含的道歉传达，并产生必要的一点，即未来的RCT是必要的，然后才能得出确定的结论[18]。

在CER中使用单病例随机对照设计

由于随机对照试验的设计限制了CER的发展，如果认为一个试验的样本量有任何推进临床疗效相关性或效用的作用是反直觉的。大多数临床医生对小样本量的研究有偏见，经常考虑它们的探索性，推动和开展一项研究以满足规定的样本量。不管任何实际的约束或忽略每一额外主体纳入研究的下降的边际效用也同样是错误的，尤其是在创新研究方面[19]。

刚开始，单病例随机对照设计的试验很容易被直觉地看作是临床医生进行的以每天为基础，每个受者（患者）构成一个受者（患者）群体子组的治疗试验[20]。单病例随机对照设计试验的出名是在 R.A 的一个茶话会上。1925 年 Dr. Fisher 和 Dr. Muriel Bristol 礼貌地拒绝了一杯先放茶叶的茶。Dr. Bristol 坚持说，当茶叶被添加到一个已经盛着牛奶的杯子里，茶的味道更好，而不是相反，她可以说出其中的差异[21]。Dr. Fisher 迅速设计了一个实验来检验这一假设，准备了 8 杯茶，4 杯先倒奶，4 杯先倒茶。Dr. Fisher 确定有 70 个方式可以把八杯茶分为两组（8！/4！4！）。然后 Dr. Fisher 将杯子随机赠送给 Dr. Bristol，并使用了一个 α 意义的 0.01428（1/70），反映了随机选择所有 8 个杯子的正确概率。Dr. Bristol 是如何做到的？通过其女儿（Joan Fisher）为 Dr. Fisher 所写的传记中的记述，Dr. Bristol 可成功地正确辨别出所有 8 个茶和牛奶的组合类型。

单病例随机对照设计的试验标准设计包括随机分配项的两个不同处理方式的单个独立受者（患者）（其中之一可以是安慰剂）。假设我们有两个治疗方法 A 和 B，总共 8 次治疗，当所述受者（患者）各接受 4 次治疗。总共有 70 种可能的排列（8！/4!4!），其中可能的调度之一是 AABABABB。对于单病例随机对照设计有益的病情是需要长期的、严重的情况将有症状的过度波动归因于他们解决方案的干预。同样的，治疗本身需要在一个已知的时间段通断药物动力学，使之能够研究，以避免遗留效应[23]。遗留的影响是备受关注的，药物在体内继续增强是有潜在可能的，故此以后，过多扭曲的干预会产生后续效应。因此，需要的是明显有精度的清除期为药物和行为干预，后者更能体现一个疲劳或学习效果。这是有必要的，在规定的时间间隔之间用一种快速的方式实现治疗剂量的干预。单病例随机对照设计也需要在一个合适的基线期试验开始时，搁置一段时间，并遵循受者（患者）和临床医生严格的双盲，以尽量减少安慰剂效应。单病例随机对照设计试验的中心目标是在两个重复治疗方法之间建立个性化的有效性[25]。

最近 Scufham 等通过单病例随机对照设计的试验来确定最佳的用药方案，来降低骨关节炎、慢性神经疼痛、注意缺陷多功障碍（ADHD）受者（患者）的医疗费用[26]。该研究设计涉及到使用多次单病例随机对照试验的结果。在所有单病例随机对照设计试验中个别受者（患者）的反应很大，会对内部效度造成威胁，增加更多的治疗时间会表现出更多有用的信息。同样，当在受试者内的变异是适度的，然后添加额外的时间测量不产生更多的有用的知识[27]。因此，单病例随机对照设计试验有利于把参加试验的受者（患者）负担降到最低来减少死亡率，因为他们后续损失的降低在临床实践中对疗效和治疗是有益的。

单病例随机对照设计试验当然有潜力提高随机临床试验和以受者（患者）为中心的医学研究工作。未来无线监控设备的使用将大大增加数据收集和提高受者（患者）参与单病例随机对照设计试验的意愿。多中心协调单病例随机对照设计试验部署，Meta 分析单病例随机对照研究和电子病例记录都将有助于提高采纳和使用本研究设计。

观测数据和 CER 的 Meta 分析

观察数据分为追溯性和前瞻性两种，前者通常涉及使用现有的数据库或图表检查。后者追踪在时间上向前的队列，以及测量感兴趣的因素和事件，例如护士健康研究（队列Ⅰ、Ⅱ和Ⅲ），或纵向队列研究。另一项前瞻性的设计被称为准实验，有两个或多个研究组形成比较组（而非对照组），为受试者首选的组。准实验设计包括具有一系列预干预措施以及干预后措施的中断时间序列。当存在多于一种的待测试干预时，所使用的准实验设计被称为“对称平衡”或“拉丁平方”。接受干预的受者（患者）顺序是循环跨时间的，因此需要建立防范遗留效应的机制[28]。

支持观察性设计的中心论据是，与随机对照试验相反，强大的外部有效性（即普遍性）由于数据收集更近似于临床上受者（患者）的异质性。观察性设计相比随机对照试验以更及时的方式完成，因此减少了每次分析的支出；且通常有利于积累大数据集的分析。然而，内部或外部效度的程度在任一随机对照试验或观察性设计的作用是如何把研究结合成一个整体。执行不佳的随机对照试验可能相比一个构造良好的观察性设计实现的内部效度要低[29]。观察性研究的倡导者指出其对罕见疾病的作用，因为在病例对照设计中，受试者是根据他们的疾病状态选择的。观察性研究可以同时研究多种治疗，并且获得更多的以受者（患者）为中心的结果，如治疗首选项，尤其当随机对照试验在伦理、时间、政治或经济上不可行时特别有用[30,31]。

观察研究设计中的关键问题是系统性的偏差，这往往限制了因果关系的确定[32]。例如，受者（患者）病情危重的可以引入更积极的治疗，而更体弱的受者（患者）根据自己的需要或耐受治疗能力分配入创伤性更低的分组（即非手术介入）。这就形成了比较组之间不对称的异质性，使得潜在的干扰因素[例如，受者（患者）虚弱]过度地影响相关的结果。精心的设计、大量的数据、新颖的分析（例如，倾向得分回归，随机统计），可以最大程度地将偏差和干扰的影响最小化[31]。然而，当涉及到的干扰因素无法测量，或不能完全测量的数据不能在分析中考虑，会导致与治疗方式相关的疗效大小的片面估计[33]。

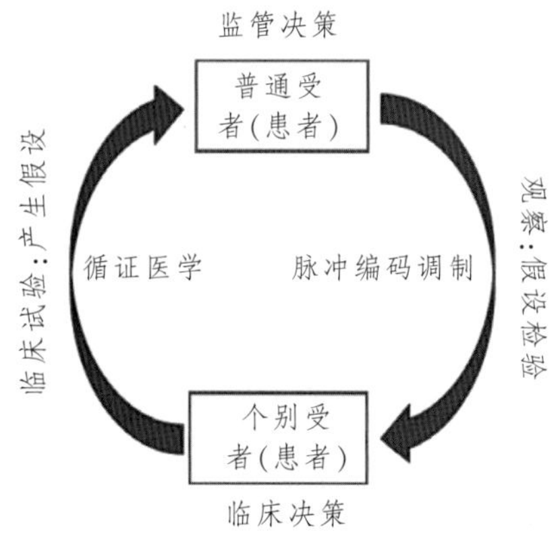

图 135.1 PCT 和 RCT：科学推理的定向流动，是基于总体的普通受者（患者）和在以受者（患者）为中心的医学领域中的假设检验，到改善基于个体的临床决策，回到假设中产生 RCT。（Reproduced from [20] Sacristan JA. Exploratory trials, confirmatory observations: a new reasoning model in the era of patient-centered medicine. BMC medical research methodology. 2011;11:57. Epub 2011/04/27 [Open Access].）

目前对于认识论的本质是在医学研究模型中产生的这一观点是有争议的。标准的观点是，观察性设计是所谓的假设研究，之后将通过严格的随机对照试验来证实[34]。这种观点认为，科学——特别是医疗科学，是一个开放式的永不落幕的系统，该系统产生的可检验的假设会派生悬而未决的问题，这是新假设进一步检验的成因，以及随机对照试验中区分事实与演绎模型的金标准。因此，观察性研究可以对医学知识获取的持续进程起到举足轻重的作用，在某种程度上，即生成新的可检验的假设。这一科学过程的共同概念受到了随机临床试验的迫切需要的挑战，后者期待更有效地推进医疗健康[20]。新的重点放在以受者（患者）为中心的研究引进一个新的理论框架，假设演绎实证论，如图135.1[20]。

观察性研究还可以利用全国性大型登记注册数据库。通过改进电子医疗记录的保存和集成 IT 系统的数据挖掘功能，探讨研究问题。然而，由于数据库被构建为受者（患者）特定信息的存储库，因此用于研究的任何数据应该抽象意识到它们应用的本质上是二级分析。目前有许多国家级数据库可用于数据挖掘调查。国家外科手术质量改进计划（NSQIP）是一个风险调整后的数据集，重点研究临床结果数据，与 69 个临床措施和 30 多个程序编码变量。美国外科学院维护的国家创伤数据库（NTDB），是一个全国性的便利样本数据集，基于参与医院自愿提交的创伤数据。美国器官采购和移植网络（OPTN）和移植受体科学登记处（SRTR）维护器官移植中最大的数据系统，并发布关于所有器官移植、移植物存活分析和等待名单统计的年度报告。SRTR 处理所有关于二次研究项目的器官移植数据的请求。

大型注册表数据库也都有局限性，其中最主要的是所谓的“Z-偏差”和“M-偏差”[35]。这些登记可能测量了过多的变量，相关的暴露风险被认为是有害的，但忽略了与结果相关的变量。当 z 变量包括在统计模型中就会发生 Z 偏差。这些 z 变量由于不可测量的干扰因素影响结果，因而若将它们添加到模型中，实际上会增加偏差，这可能显得很奇怪，因为这些变量仅涉及暴露风险。M 偏差或称对撞分层偏差，当该模型调整到非常适合一个非混杂变量时（例如对撞机），其与暴露或结果不相关，但是在正位于相关结果的十字路口时即会产生。M-偏差即是一种因暴露风险而产生的变量的过度调整，然而并非真的因果关系[36,37]。国家数据系统的更多讨论见第 133 章。

尽管观察性研究具有局限性，特别是由于国家数据库纳入标准差异所导致的选择偏差，关键情况下，当一种疾病过程是致命的和（或）治疗选择是有限的，该决定只能用不完美的数据进行。观察性数据对疗效比较研究特别有用；例如当疾病患病率低，治疗干预措施在受者（患者）反应中表现出很大的差异。大型研究能够发现罕见疾病，并允许同时治疗比较。当受者(患者)的依从率不同，或提供者们的培训和专业知识水平有很大的不同，以及当研究标签药物的不良反应时，观察性研究是有用的。

系统回顾，更常被称为Meta分析，回顾主要为几个具有类似假设的研究的组合性数据分析，长期以来在研究技术领域有着显著的实证地位。本质上Meta分析是从一组相关的研究中获得结果的过程，或多或少地基于同一个工作假设，最终确定一个概括性的结果。关键是先建立一个精确的纳入标准，用于最后的定量合成结果。所有Meta分析涉及回顾性数据的采集；因此，这种形式的研究是相对低成本和快捷的。其次，一个Meta分析最重要的方面是确定效果的程度，是为了比较目的进行总结。实例效果通常包括优势比(OR)、相对危险度(RR)，或风险比(HR)。疗效大小是治疗组和非治疗组(或较小治疗组)差异的大小的估计。单个结果不会被纳入一个大的研究；而每项研究的效果会被合并。

Meta分析主要关注的是研究的异质性程度，这可能影响结果的有效性，即所谓的“苹果和梨”问题。异质性研究可以来自于两个研究之间随机任意的差异，或者每个单个研究可能实际上来自于不同的人群。使用Cochran的Q检验来评估真实的异质性[38]。Q检验是通过将每个研究的效应估计与总体效应估计的平方偏差相加来计算的，每个研究的贡献由其逆方差加权。在疗效大小之间的均匀性假设下，Q统计量遵循k-1自由度的卡方分布，k为研究次数。不拒绝同质性的假设往往导致Meta分析师采用固定效应模型，它是假定估计影响大小的不同只与抽样误差有关。相反，拒绝同质性假设会导致应用一个随机效应模型，其包括研究内的变异(来自抽样误差)和研究之间的变异性(大量研究特性和设计质量差异)。一个显著Q统计量的典型P值临界点是0.20。评估异质性的较新技术称为I^2指数，其类似于组内相关，计算方法如下：

$$I^2 = [Q-(k-1)/Q]\times100 = k \text{ 为研究数量。}$$

I^2指数基本上是在研究前后矛盾的一种手段，如果大于50%被认为是不可接受的水平，或缺乏足够的内部研究相似性[38]。

长期以来，Meta分析已经显现“成熟草莓”问题，即出版物偏见，期刊编辑和评论者倾向于偏爱统计学显示显著结果的积极研究，而非负面研究(除非作者承诺其研究下一次有“正确的动力“)。由于这种偏差，Meta分析通过公开发表的文献梳理倾向于发现积极的研究成果，而不是保留原假设的研究[39]。

另一个棘手的问题是，是否要结合随机对照试验和观察性研究的结果[40]。这是因为观察性研究本质上更容易被不可测量的干扰因素混淆。然而，人们似乎已经有了一个普遍的共识，即应包括非实验和准实验研究设计，因为它们是具有“丰富数据”的大样本量的信息来源，并且可以用于评估潜在危害性的治疗。最近发现的问题已被命名为“Meta偏差”[41]，其描述了单中心研究对比多中心基础研究而产生的偏差。单中心的研究表明，疗效的提升高达26%[42]。研究人员所做的是检查48个Meta分析中的单位点与多位点研究的优势比影响大小，总共421组随机对照试验，其中在单个位点进行的有233个，另外198组是基于多中心的。Dechartres与其同事发现，单中心的随机对照试验相比多中心的随机对照试验，有很大的干预效应。Goodman[42]推测Meta偏差可能只是反映了有利于多中心研究的另一种偏差的变化，或者单中心研究参与的人太少，因此降低了严格控制的研究操作，使研究人员能够达到自己想要的结果。

Danaei与其同事[43]通过Meta分析证明了一个有趣的偏差，即使用他汀类药物与预防心血管疾病具有相关性。他们发现，当用随机对照试验比较使用他汀类药物的当前用户和非用户之间(二级预防)，危险比为0.84[在有心血管疾病史的受者(患者)中，心血管死亡率降低16%]，同时观察性研究表明，他汀类药物的使用的新用户与非用户(一级预防)之间的风险比为0.54[在无心血管疾病史的受者(患者)中，心血管死亡率降低48%]。研究者认为，鉴于随机对照试验和观察性研究效果测量两者之间存在很大的差异，未来的研究需要通过创建入选标准用于观察性设计，以控制潜在的偏差，这将更符合那些随机对照试验，并考虑到事件(新)与药物普遍(现有的)用户的比较。

一个相当新的和创新性的成对Meta分析变式被称为“网络Meta分析”，这涉及Meta分析横跨多个干预措施或治疗方法的比较。网络Meta分析的直接证据来自于随机对照试验（例如，药物A与B，药物B与A)，并通过随机对照试验获得间接的证据(例如，药物A对C)将其结合起来。这种技术通过Meta分析的合并效应估计产生几个感兴趣的结果，而不是只有一个标准结果[44,45]。

Meta 分析确实在 CER 中有实质性的前景，通过结合研究成本估算和缩小不良药物反应来增加异质性的自由度，这都有助于推动问题是最有效的治疗方案。适当考虑可能存在的偏差是对任何研究项目的简单要求，必须有足够的专业知识来进行有意义的研究。Meta 分析提供了大量不同研究所需的综合和统一性，从而创造了更为全面的关键临床问题的答案[46]。研究分析给予实证结果，而 Meta 分析提供聚合；而正是这种相互作用的结果，促进临床的理解和合成[47]。

CER 中的决策分析和成本效益分析

也许没有其他分析领域比决策分析（DA）和成本效益分析（CE）更适合疗效比较研究。DA 是一个高度复杂和结构化的分析技术，来自博弈论和经济行为，有助于决策。当医疗决策的组成部分带有竞争性的不同选择，其中涉及成本、风险和结果的可能性时，决策分析 DA 是非常有用的。当焦点集中在一个个体的决定上时，最好使用 DA，同时 DA 也可以协助和指导在临床实践中制订共识指南[48]。DA 的核心是决策树的构建，见图 135.2。Best 等[49]提及一个例子，讲到 1736 年的天花接种，接种不是第一个决策节点，而圆圈代表机会节点。在第一树枝通知接种，结果是死是活，和下面的每个这些分支是该事件的概率；活着的概率为 0.9790 和死亡的概率为 0.021。在最后的节点（三角）是这种结果的效果，范围从 0（死）到 1（完全健康）。

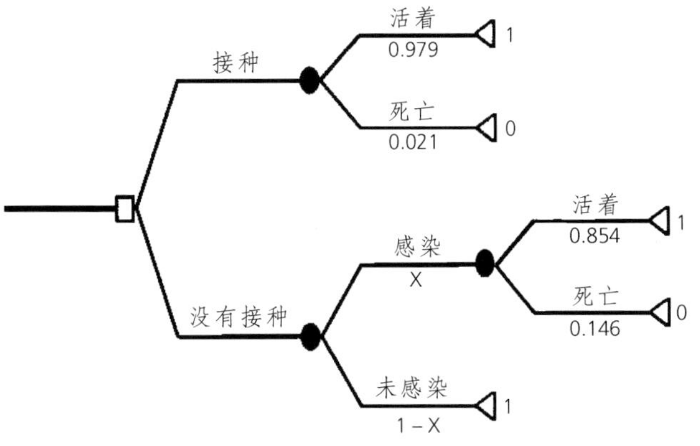

图 135.2　决策树：互相排斥决定决策树选择接种或不接种，导致要么接种了活下来，要么感染上天花死了，或不被天花感染的概率的结果。(Reproduced from [49] Best M, Katamba A, Neuhauser D. Quality & safety in health care. 2007;16 (6):478–480 with permission from BMJ Publishing Group Ltd.)
根节点/决策节点（方形）；事件（机会）节点（圈）；和结束点（三角形）

决策树图，即是 DA 的一个简单示例；更透彻的分析将包括与每个树枝相关联的成本，来获得有关一个不确定选择的预期值（通过将每个可能的结果乘以其概率，再求和计算结果）。再加上费用，我们可以确定期望值决策准则，如选择了表现最佳的预期值的选项。这是 CE 的本质：确定哪些可选的决策导致了货币最高的结果。

CE 的一种特殊类型被称为成本效益分析，其中所获得的健康收益被量化为质量调整寿命年（QALY）（图 135.3）。QALY 是更优的时间单位，通常以年来表示，根据人的偏好权重调整其“效用”。“效用价值”是指在不确定性的条件下测得的优选结果，通常范围从零（指死亡）到 1（定义为一个完美的健康状态）。在基本的 QALY 图中假设一个人能活到 75 岁，目前是 25 岁，在线性 QALY 模型中，我们假设其低于完美的健康效用权重是 0.75，我们可以计算出他其余的寿命如下：

$$QALY=(75-25)\times 0.75= 37.5$$

我们用其预期寿命 75 减去当前年龄得到剩余的年数，然后乘以这个 0.75 的效用权重来获得 37.5 的 QALY 来表示还能存活几年，这将被这些年的感知质量所“调整”。一个 QALY 则很容易被理解为质量调整生命年，它结合了一个人活几年和当时的感知质量。

举一个简单的例子：我们可以估计一个人剩余的寿命，他们会被提问为达到完全健康的状态，他们愿意放弃多少年的寿命。我们可以计算如下：

Utility（效用价值）=（NYEL–NYWTT）/NYEL =?

NYEL 是预期存活的年数，NYWTT 是愿意放弃的年数。该计算通常更正式写为：$U(H_i)=x/t$，其中 x 是完全健康的年数（即预期年的寿命减去愿意放弃的年数），而 t 是非完全健康的年数，H_i 是剩余的年数。举一个已发表的关于想象手截肢的例子[50]，一只手移植受者（患者）的预期存活寿命为 45 年，作为一个被截肢者，其愿意放弃 4 年的寿命选择移植，所以效用价值可以计算如下：

$$U(H_i)=(45-4)/45=0.9100$$

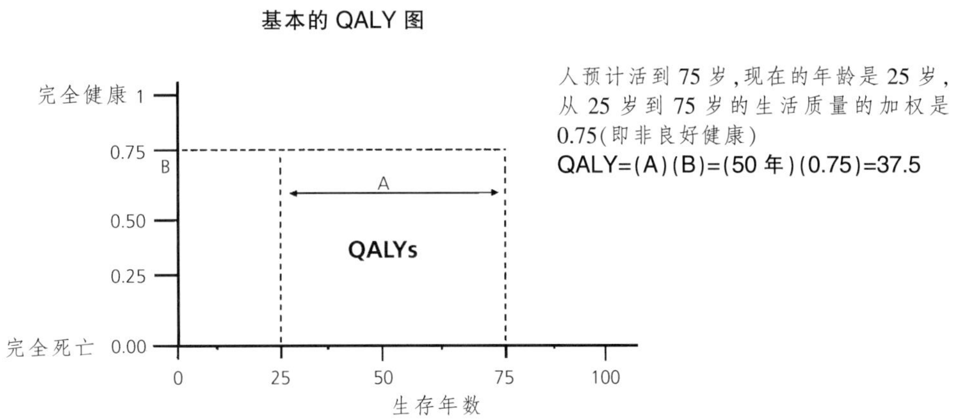

图 135.3 基本的 QALY 年。纵轴显示的效用范围：从死亡的 0 到完全健康的+1，横轴显示预期寿命年，从出生到死亡。注意这个预期活到 75 岁，目前在 25 岁的人，线性效用为 0.75 的例子。因此，寿命的计算为 A 和 B 的乘积；(50 岁)×(0.75 效用)=37.5 寿命。

QALY 广泛应用于成本效用分析，因为一个 QALY 能把握一个人单一的衡量完全健康状态的指标[51-54]。一个 QALY 的得出方法如下：QALY=效用 (Utility)×剩余寿命[48]。因此，一个 QALY 是预期剩余寿命和归因于时间的值(即效用的权重)。让我们看一下两个接受肾移植的受者(患者)的例子，肾移植的效用为 0.7；受者(患者)A 预计存活 30 年，受者(患者)B 预计存活 25 年。

$QALY_{患者A}$=0.70×30=21：受者(患者)A 的质量调整寿命年为 21 年

$QALY_{患者B}$=0.70×25=17.5：受者(患者)B 的质量调整寿命年为 17.5 年

显然，在 QALY，受者(患者)A 比受者(患者)B 活得更久更有质量。我们还可以利用 QALY 比较两种治疗方案的不同，得出不同的净效益。最近的一项研究中表示同受者(患者)肝肾联合移植的 QALY 为 9.456，分裂器官不同受者(患者)的 QALY 为 8.650，QALY 的净差额利益为 0.806，表明当终末期肾脏疾病(ESRD)被确诊，联合器官分配是更好的方法[55]。

现在的问题是究竟加权效用的因素来自哪里？可以通过两种基本方法产生效用权重：

1.直接估值技术，例如时间权衡(TTO)调查问卷，视觉模拟评分法(VAS)，和标准的赌博法(SG)；

或 2.间接使用基于标准化问卷的健康效用指数，如 SF-36，EQ-5D，或 HUI-3[56-59]。

TTO 技术在一次调查中提出问题，X 代表受访者维持不好的健康状况的年数，评估 Y 代表一个完全健康状况的年数。基本 TTO 图(图 135.4)显示的是，意愿权衡减去健康效用的年数，来获得完美的健康效用。

在这个假设的例子中，受者(患者)有 25 年的寿命(75 – 50 =)，但要降低生活质量的 0.75 效用。他们愿意用 5 年的预期寿命来交换，以达到完美的生活质量。QALY 的增益可以计算如下：

当前状态：QALY =(75–50)×(0.75)=18.75

TTO 状态：QALY=[(75–50)×(75–70)]×(1)= 20

受者(患者)愿意用 5 年的寿命交换获得 1.25 的增益寿命(Δ_{QALY}=20–18.75)。

该 TTO 技术的假设条件是一个成恒正比的时间权衡(CPTO)，即假设受试者想象的完全健康状态不受时间影响。例如，如果我愿意用少活两年来换十年的完全健康，那么，我应该愿意用 2 个月换 10 个月的完全健康。Attema 和 Brouwer 回顾相关 TTO 的文献发现，成恒正比的时间权衡(CPTO)经常被违背，因为很少有人愿意生存时间更短来获得完全的健康状态[60]。换而言之，一个人对于健康的优先权受到其获得健康状态的时间所影响。Attema 和 Brouwer 的随访研究[61]利用 TTO 无风险(直接法)技术使用健康状况调查问卷，基于完全健康和通过慢性背部疼痛的不完全健康状态来表现不重视的权重。作者从广义的 CPTO(gCPTO)区分一般的 CPTO(oCPTO)：后者——个人愿意交换若干年来获得完全的健康——绝对不影响剩余寿命年数；前者认为，一个人存活年数的剩余效用，他们愿意交换完全健康，不受剩余效用年数的绝对数量影响。这个区分很重要，因为违反 gCPTO 表明一般的 QALY 模型都被证明是虚假的，而违反 oCPTO 意味着 QALY 模型只有

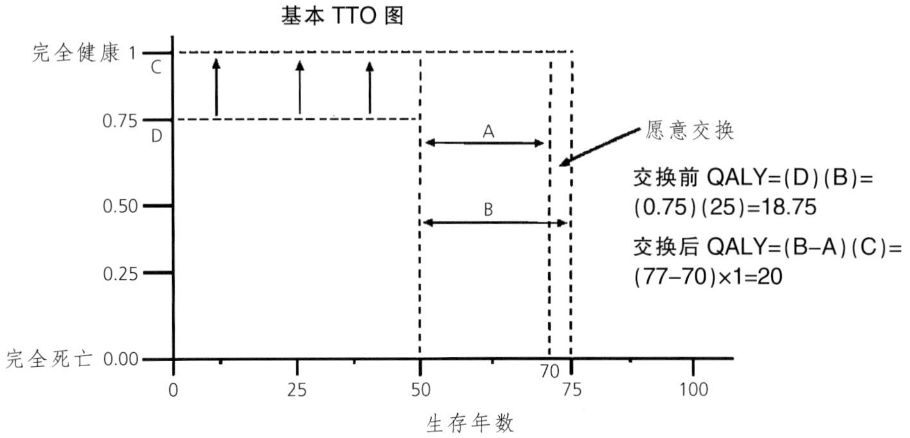

图 135.4 基本 TTO：纵轴显示的效用范围从死亡的 0 到完美健康+1，与横轴从生到死的预期寿命年数。受者（患者）愿意交换 5 年（B–A）从不完美的健康（D）0.75 恢复到完全健康（C）。在 QALY 权衡之前：D×B=0.75×25=18.75，经过 QALY 权衡后是 B–A×C，或 75–70×1=20。因此，增加的 QALY 交换的 5 年获得了 1.25（20–18.75）。

一部分子系统被证明是错误的，即家庭的权力。他们的研究结果对违反 gCPTO 和 oCPTO 的假设提供证据，使由 TTO 推导出 QALY 存疑。因此，其出现似乎是人类生活质量与之预期持续寿命的连接。

SG 技术涉及在一定的健康状态和两种可能的结果之间做出一个选择：完全的健康还是死亡，是直接基于 von Neumann Morgenstern 效用理论的公理（即预期效用理论）（图 135.5）。von Neumann Morgenstern 效用模型是 U（Q，T）= p^*，其中 Q 为目前的健康状态，T 年之后，和 p^* 选择赌或不赌之间无差异的概率[62]。提交给答辩人的每个备选选择具有规定的发生概率，并且概率发生变化，直到答辩者不赞成一个超过另一个；称为冷漠点[63,64]。Bala 等举出一个涉及慢性疼痛的例子，其中受访者想象自己在未来的 20 年里有严重疼痛的健康状况，而他们可以选择赌治疗来换未来 20 年正常

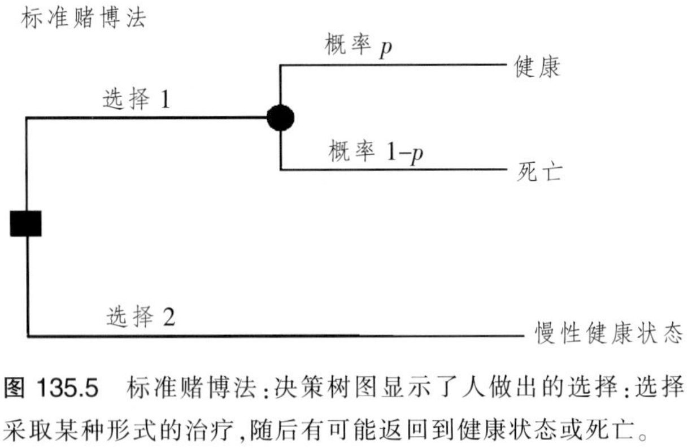

图 135.5 标准赌博法：决策树图显示了人做出的选择：选择 1 采取某种形式的治疗，随后有可能返回到健康状态或死亡。p 是从 0 到 1 的概率，$1-p$ 是剩余的死亡概率。

（无疼痛）生活的概率为 95%，和治疗将立即死亡的概率为 5%[65]。因此，SG 给出了受试者对于随时间改善的健康状态的优选得分。

最近有相当多有关健康状态的争论。时间权衡、SG 和 EQ–VAS 被认为是健康的直接评估措施，而各种间接问卷调查方法在美国和欧洲都获得了新的突出地位。这些包括 HUI–3 健康效用关系指数，EQ–5D 五维问卷、15–D 测量和六维健康状态 SF–6d[66]。鉴于这些不同的方法产生的健康状态效用，问题在于如何比较它们的结果。果然，Hientz 等最近对 HUI–3、EQ–5D、TTO 和 EQ–VAS 进行比较分析[66]。从糖尿病视网膜病变的 QALY 权重发现四种技术在派生的效用权重中有显著性差异。他们表明，测量仪器没有按照疾病恶化的过程，除了 HUI–3，其能够检测的变化是糖尿病性视网膜病变的严重程度（盲目的减量实际上是其他方法的两倍）。由此，不可避免地他们的结论是：选择的 QALY 技术将影响治疗或干预的成本效益评估。HUI–3 还演示了构造、收敛和判别有效性的研究索引肺移植受者（患者）的健康效用。

一个基本的问题是：应该由谁来决定健康价值观？是健康状况的受者（患者）？一般人群中的非受者（患者），还是专业健康知识的人？一些经济学家认为受者（患者）与非受者（患者）一般会呈现非常不同的效用，因为他们从不同的角度入手：非受者（患者）会倾向于高估由一个给定的健康状态的损失，而受者（患者）会低估适应不完美的健康状态[68,69]。然而，最近的研究发

现,受者(患者)使用 VAS 技术的健康状态值与健康人比较没有显著差异[70]。在该研究中,TTO 技术在受者(患者)和健康人之间呈现较大的差异;这可能是由于 TTO 与测量理论作为一维测量矛盾的事实,因为它试图在同一时间测量健康状态和时间寿命。因此,在健康状态效用中观察到的差异,可能更多地是由于所使用的测量仪器工具与参考偏差的作用。

此外,有一个基本的经济假设,人类重视目前的健康高于未来的健康。当我们做出这个假设并应用高折扣率(由机会成本理论的倡导者促进)时,结果有利于增加生活质量在长寿上的治疗(与延长生存但实为牺牲生活质量的治疗相反)[71]。还有人置疑整个健康状态,即非时间性的测量方法,是未考虑在健康期花费的时间,或健康状态之前和之后测量的健康状态的。认为个人计算他们的健康状况的效用作为风险中性是有价值的,随着时间的推移这种观点就过头了[72]。

一个更复杂的、也许更重要的担心是,如何通过进行质量的健康状态技术扩大效用。大多数经济学家和政策分析家仍然认为 SG 和 TTO 方法是最有可能来获得与健康相关的生活质量偏好的技术。典型的 TTO 方法涉及选择在一个设定年限期间保持特定的健康状态,还是选择一个更短时间内的完全健康。当参与者停滞不前,不愿意进一步用更长的非健康年数来交换完全健康的时间,这被称为无差别点,并且用 x/y 来计算效用率。与 SG 良好的健康状况相比,这肯定是在死亡与完全健康之间的赌博。当达到无差异点时,应采取健康状态的效用。利用这种技术有两个主要的问题:①它不取得比死亡更糟糕的不良健康状态效用;②0 和 1 之间的效用尺度,或者-1 和+1 之间不是统计分布,允许有效使用均值、中位数、模型和率的统计分析。这是同一问题的两个不同的角度:目前所做的效用标准基本上是任意的并且需要完全修改。Lamers[73]提出需要改进,认为健康状态可以被评估为更好、等于或甚至比死亡更糟;效用标准从 0(=死亡)到+1(非常健康),没有反映出人类健康偏好的真实情况。如果死亡的效用是 0,那么比死亡更糟糕的健康状况是怎样的呢?当一个健康状态被评估为比死亡更糟糕时,效用可以小于 0,从 0 到负无穷大。关于是否在-1 终止负效用,甚至讨论如何解除+1 效用,仍存在相当多的争论[74]。

Pullenayegum 等[75]承认有比死亡更糟糕的健康状态,该效用需要到 0 以下,且用负的尺度衡量。Sullivan[74]认为效用不应该被+1 所限制,因为存在远远高于一个指定的完全健康的效用状态。限制效用在 0 和 1 之间的明显理由是它们被用来得出寿命的权重,如果效用的权重是小于 0,负的寿命如何解释?当计算一个增加成本效益的效用分析(ICUR)时就特别麻烦:

$$\mathrm{ICUR}=\mu_{\text{成本(新治疗)}}-\mu_{\text{成本(标准治疗)}}/\mu_{\text{结果 QALY(新的治疗)}}-\mu_{\text{结果 QALY(标准治疗)}}。$$

显而易见,当我们有负的结果来解释负美元每 QALY 是有问题的,可能缺乏一个有意义的解释[76]。对于一个 ICUR 为-$80 000 的每质量调整寿命年我们应该如何做呢?拉森和他的同事们提出了一个解决方案。我们可以将一个 ICUR 的四个可能结果分成四个象限,通过绘制增量收益的差异和增量成本的差异来解释 ICUR,如图 135.6 所示[77]。

在图 135.6 象限 A 中,新治疗成本超过现有治疗,但新治疗的 QALY 小于现有治疗,因此产生负效应。最好的 ICUR 在象限 D,其中新的治疗成本比现有的更低,新的治疗 QALY 超过现有治疗 QALY,因此新的治疗成本更低、更有效。

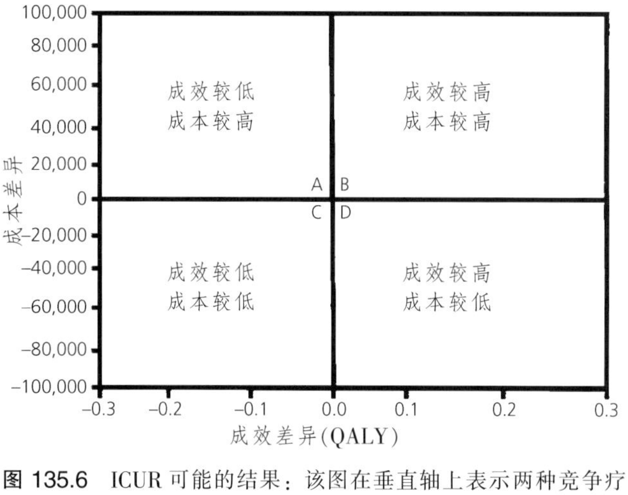

图 135.6　ICUR 可能的结果:该图在垂直轴上表示两种竞争疗法之间的成本差异,以及在水平轴上表示相同的两种竞争疗法之间 QALY 的差异,以及在四个象限中显示的 ICUR 的可能结果。ICUR 在象限 A 是成效较低、成本较高,象限 B 是成效高、成本较高,象限 C 是成效较低、成本较低和象限 D 是成效较高、成本较低。(Reproduced from [113] Kontodimopoulos N, Niakas D. An estimate of lifelong costs and QALYs in renal replacement therapy based on patients' life expectancy. Health Policy. 2008; 86(1): 85–96. Copyright © 2008, with permission from Elsevier.)

大量的技术解决方案已被提出：如改变生活质量值为离散的(二项式)措施[78],使用健康状况问卷中的负得分,简单地将它们转换到0[79],将所有-1以下得分,使用简单的公式将WTD(比死亡更糟糕)TTO除以39来提高QALY的估计值[73,81,82],或者转换测量范围从-1到+1[83,84]。在一个简练的数学证明式中,Flyn等表明从0到1的效用是不可能的；想法是至少有一个人的生活质量得分低于0的概率不可能为0[78]。因此,健康值必须延伸到0以下的负无穷大和0以上的正无穷大。埃德林和其同事提出了将理论从实证的健康质量值里区分出来，提议低于0的健康值表示为“坑”,+1以上为“超状态”,以记录衡量潜在的生活质量[85]。这是至关重要的,因为可能存在这样的情况,即大多数病例可能记录潜在的而不是经验的生活质量值。也许最有趣的解决健康价值标准的方案已经被Craig等提出[86]。问题是,所有健康值的测量使用比率统计,这是不恰当的,因为X和Y是不可互换的,例如,μ(x,y)不等于μ(x,y)的相反数。

y/x的比率，其中y=x-愿意交换的年份,x是预期的生存年数,因此如果有人愿意交换10年来获得完全健康地生存两年；μ=8-10-8=-0.2500。Craig所提出的是利用效用通过转换每个y和x在欧氏空间映射为一组两极坐标,用角度和半径来描述的定向统计[87]。每个y/x比率是角度θ的切线(θi=arctan(y/x)+εi,并且半径的大小等于参与者的交易时间。因此,Craig提出了替代比率统计的平均角度的估计切线,称为估计值,简称为aRUM(角随机效用模型)。角的均值是较大的,因为这样会减少大的负比率相比算数均值。最后,克雷格和busschbach提出他们的随机效用模型是基于Probit模型,称为eRUM(情景随机效用模型)[88]。该方法得到的健康状态估计者为：

$$\beta_h=\Sigma x_i y_i/(\Sigma x_i^2), \text{and then a QALY}_i=(\beta_h)(\text{years})+\varepsilon_i$$

βh是近似平均值比率的系数[84]。

在对美国EQ-5D状态的比较分析中,Craig和Busschbach得出结论,eRUM或aRUM是更好的模型,相比简单划分、较低价值的39时间权衡比率,主观性更低。eRUM也受到更大的审查,被认为缺乏统一性。非统一性是一个不好的特性，因为它意味着一些受访者增加健康评估到一个特定的状态，而聚合值大多数人实际上是减少的[89]。假如一个人的WTD值无限,产生一个负无穷大(-∞),在eRUM方法中,该值将不对最小二乘拟合回归线执行下拉[89]。

QALY模型的有效性不仅已在医疗决策、卫生政策中普遍存在,且在CER的背景下对受者(患者)为中心的决策已得到广泛应用，在简单的线性模型得到的QALY表示的健康状态效用和时间(年)也得到证实。换句话说,效用和时间是相互独立的。这种彼此的独立性目前被置疑，其违反了使用线性调整模型的建议的影响,因为它不一定能代表一个人的真实想法。Atemma和Brouwer[90]最近的一项研究发现的证据表明,这种独立性健康状态比死亡要好，而不是比死亡更糟糕的健康状况(WTD)。WTD状态存在因为有健康状态超过一个人能容忍这种状态的最大持续时间。Atemma和Brouwer的研究[90]结果表明,效用可能取决于一个人处于WTD健康状态的时间,并且,若使用QALY建模应考虑更好地捕捉人的喜好来补充修改。

正如我们之前所回顾的，相关的健康效用可以来自各种方法得出,无论是直接还是间接的。先进的方法论逻辑模型试图解决的问题和局限性，已确定在一个给定的健康状态效用上鉴定；比较麻烦的是物质效用的标准范围。虽然现在有许多吸引人的技术,具有各种特性和可靠性,无论哪种方法构成了效用的理想效果,但最终尚未达成共识,QALY也是如此。

肾移植中的疗效比较研究(CER)

肾移植文献充斥着大量高质量的随机临床对照试验，主要集中在移植后的免疫抑制治疗来确定竞争药物方案之间的优势或等效性[77,91-95]。肾移植文献也有众多关于终末期肾病受者(患者)生活质量研究和相关透析的疗效研究[96-104]。

Morel和其同事在明尼苏达大学医院和诊所发表了首篇关于肾移植术后长期生活质量的研究[105]。研究人群由51名接受移植后11~27年间参与研究的儿童受者(患者)组成。研究结果发现,90%的患者对他们的生活满意或非常满意,91%认为他们的健康状况是良好的,65%的生活是正常的,没有排斥反应。Russel[106]和同事在安大略省St Joseph医院采取了更复杂的研究设计,获得了在移植前后时间权衡的预期疗效(n=27)。使用TTO技术,受者(患者)被询问他们为了完全健康愿意用多少时间来交换,受者(患者)基数疗效得分的平均值为 0.41，移植后为 0.74，生活质量提高了 33%。

Laupacis 及其同事进行了第一例正式的成本效用分析研究，来评估加拿大肾移植的生活质量和成本效用[107]。Laupacis 使用几种方法来测评生活质量：血液透析问题(KDQ)、肾移植问卷(KTQ)-25、疾病影响简介(SIP)和 TTO，其中死亡计分为 0，完全健康计分为 1。在随后的月份进行随访：1(n=146)，3(n=131)，6(n=137)，12(n=132)，18(n=107)和 24(n=76)。所有的健康调查问卷都显示有了实质性的改善，TTO 效用也是如此。作者计算了一年和两年的 ICUR 如下：

$$ICUR_{1年}=\$66\ 540-\$73\ 659/0.65QALY-0.53QALY$$
$$=-\$59\ 325/QALY$$
$$ICUR_{2年}=\$27\ 474-\$70\ 869/0.62QALY-0.51QALY$$
$$=-\$394\ 500/QALY$$

每 QALY 的负成本意味着在一年和两年时，肾移植可提供更多的有生活质量的年数，并且与透析相比更便宜。并不是所有的受者(患者)都填写了他们有关 TTO 效用的随访记录，该研究估计评估了 224 例(占总数的 24%)[注意，所有无法完成 TTO 测量的受者(患者)计分为 0.20]。在温哥华总医院开展的 Laupacis 研究(忽略其局限性)有着开创性的意义，其尝试凭经验量化有关肾移植受者(患者)的生活质量成本。

Franke 等[108]在 Essen 大学(德国)的研究标志着 ESRD-SCL(末期肾病症状检查表)发展的一个里程碑，其设计专门用于评估肾移植受者(患者)的生理和心理质量。ESRD-SCL 由五点 Likert 缩放测量的 79 个生活质量测量组成。通过与 SF-36 的相关分析评估构建有效性，并且分层多元回归显示了 6 个可靠的子量表，Cronbach α 为 0.76~0.85。Ziegelman 等[109]设计了了TxEQ(移植疗效问卷)，用于评估与终末期肾病受者(患者)移植结局相关的多个维度。TxEQ 中的具体范畴如下：

- 移植的担忧
- 供者的犯罪行为
- 公开移植
- 抗排斥药物的依从性
- 重视移植的价值

TxEQ 证明具有良好的心理测量学性质，并且可能对多种器官移植研究有帮助。最近，Chisholm-Burns 和其同事对美国肾移植受者中 KTQ-25 的同期疗效进行了分析[110]。同期疗效是比较新的测量仪器与一个所谓的“金标准”的测量仪器，去看看新工具的结果是否与旧工具的验证结果一致[111]。在本研究中，当 KTQ-25 测量与 SF-12v2 有相同基础的构造时，KTQ-25 应当具有与 SF-12v2 类似的结果。KTQ-25 是一个有 25 条项目的问卷，包括五个领域：身体体征，疲备或困乏，不安和恐惧，外观和情感内容。SF-12 是一种经常使用的相比 SF-36 较短版本的较完善的一般健康调查方法，具有八个领域。Chisholm-Burns 等发现了支持同期效度的证据；在绝大多数领域 Cronbach 的 α 超过 0.75，因此 KTQ-25 可以是用于测量肾移植生命健康质量方法的重要补充[110]。

尽管目前在肾移植中缺乏正式的 CER，鉴于其重点的新颖性，有一些研究与 CER 的一些关键组成成分非常相近。Jassal 和其同事在多伦多进行的研究是在老年受者(患者)群体中使用决策分析方法的最早的肾移植研究之一[112]。他们使用之前发表的透析效用值 0.49 和移植效用值 0.78。对于年龄 65 岁的受者(患者)，获得具有两年等待名单基线的尸体供体，移植物 ICUR 为 67 779.00 美元，延长 1.1 QALY 年，而对于没有等待名单的受者(患者)，移植物 ICUR 为 14 910.00 美元，增益为 2.0 QALY 年。当等待移植时间扩大到 4 年时，60 岁的 ICUR 为 175 107.00 美元，在 85 岁时，ICUR 暴升至 14 585 442 美元。作者得出结论，对于年龄不超过 70 岁的受者(患者)，ICUR 仍然合理，基线等待时间不超过两年。

Hellenic Open 大学的 Kontodimopoulos 和 Niakas，在欧洲进行了首个比较血液透析(HD)、腹膜透析(PD)和肾移植(RT)成本效益和生活质量的研究[113]。采用 SF-36 估计效用——SF-6D 子集的一般健康调查，并且假设基于预期的个人预期寿命的线性 QALY 模型计算 QALY，假定 0 和 5%现值折算。SF-6D 衍生效用 HD 为 0.639，PD 为 0.599，RT 为 0.716。寿命的治疗方式如下：HD 5%折算为 3.67 和 4.37 0%；PD 5%折算为 3.38 和 3.94 0%；和 RT 5%折算为 9.58 和 16.11 0%。计算每个治疗的 ICUR，肾移植显示在三年内寿命的预测，特别是每一年生活质量获得的最低成本率(图 135.7)。由于他们的成本估算是在希腊收集的，因此必须谨慎地将它们推广到一个营利性医疗保健环境（例如美国)。

Kontodimopoulos 和 Niakas 的研究提出了成本效

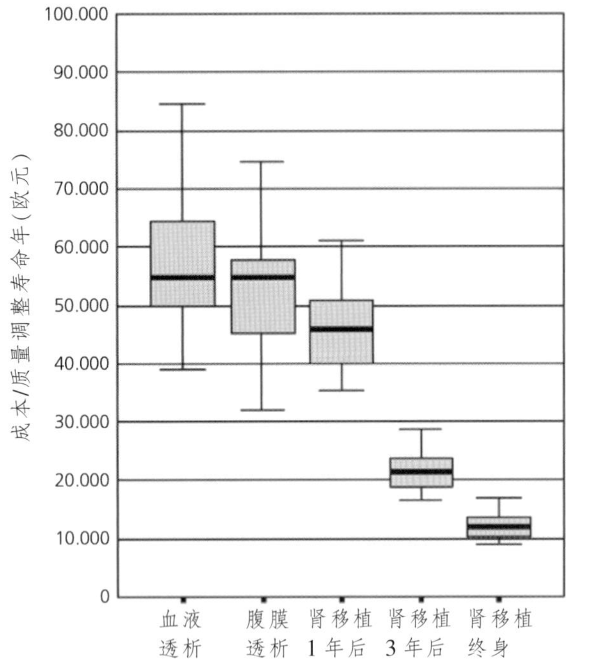

图 135.7 每QALY的成本。在垂直轴上绘制成本/质量调整寿命年(欧元)和在水平轴上绘制特定的终末期肾病治疗。HD是血液透析,PD是腹膜透析,RT是肾移植。平均成本/QALY类似1年RT HD和PD,并且在RT 3年,成本/质量调整寿命年显著降低,而RT为终身。

用分析重要的一个点，即是否对未来的健康收益和未来成本进行折算[54,113]。作者透露,他们选择折算5%利率的寿命,以达到净现值,并对成本使用3%~10%的折算。一些经济学家认为,由于健康影响的价值随着时间的推移而增加(可能是因为更好的健康状况会带来收入增加),那么它们应该被折算,但是比成本的利率低[114]。这被称为成本和健康的差异折算,其中不同的折算适用于健康价值和成本[115]。等价与差异计数是经济学家之间的一个有争议的问题,两种方法都受到严重批评。对于两种方法的假设,质量调整寿命年是稳定的或随时间推移的,其本身就有问题。Van Hout认为通过经济增长率的调整和通过健康的增长模式有利于混合差异折算[116]。

最近,Haller及其同事在维也纳医疗中心进行了肾移植的成本效益分析[117]。生活质量的效用通过使用EQ-5D、SD和TTO技术测量，而成本和寿命等价以3%向下折算。结果肾移植和腹膜透析超过增益为839 QALY的血液透析,当20%的受者(患者)接受腹膜透析,而10%的接受移植的受者(患者)预计的10年时间内增益2242 QALY。

在另一项最近的研究中，他们利用了来自荷兰末期肾脏疾病登记处(n=15 435)的数据,并采用之前发表的效用值(HD 0.5560,PD 0.5817和RT 0.8077)来模拟生活年数的好处和基于活体供者的寿命假设。早期移植表现为40岁的受者（患者）的生活质量提高了6.7~8.8的QALY,并且增加了70岁受者(患者)4.3~6.0的QALY[118]。

最近Luan和同事完成了一项有趣的质量效果研究,比较了肾移植受者(患者)巨细胞病毒的普遍治疗与优先治疗的增加成本效益的效用分析[119]。普遍预防涉及对所有巨细胞病毒阳性肾脏受体使用缬更昔洛韦治疗90天。该研究使用了0.73和0.57预先存在的肾移植效用进行透析维持。增加成本效益的效用分析是每QALY-27 967美元，表明以10年为期成本节省$27 967每QALY。他们的单向敏感性分析表明,一个有利于节约成本的CER通过实施普遍预防达到巨细胞病毒感染率约22%(图135.8)。

双向灵敏度分析显示普遍预防可实现小于10万美元每QALY。当改变普遍预防巨细胞病毒感染率5%~30%,并且不同的优先治疗巨细胞病毒感染率在35%~60%。最后，在智利最近进行了一项质量调整生命研究，比较肾脏尸体移植与透析，使用设定的移植0.80和透析0.5的效用。研究发现,在移植后两年开始积极的节约成本,透析成本接近134 000美元,预期的移植成本为106 000美元,QALY增加了7.30[120]。

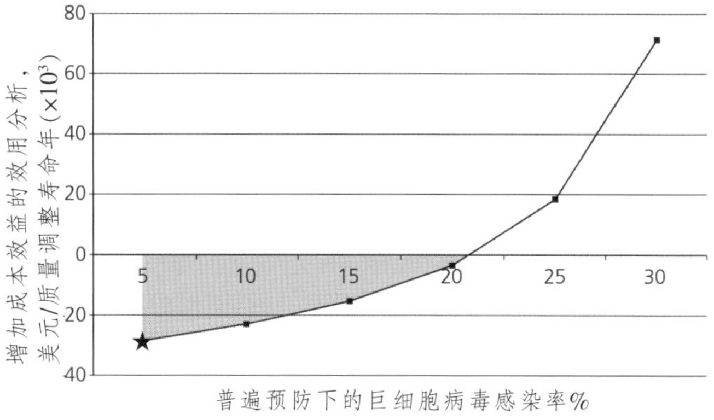

图 135.8 巨细胞病毒感染率和增加成本效益的效用分析:增加成本效益的效用分析(增量成本效益率)绘制在纵轴上,并且在普遍预防下的巨细胞病毒感染的百分比绘制在水平轴上。该图表示在各种水平的普遍预防下巨细胞病毒对增加成本效益的效用分析的影响。该图显示在通用预防下的巨细胞病毒相比增加成本效益的效用分析有较大的经济效用(美元/QALY)在阴影区域中的抢先策略少20%。

在器官移植上应用疗效比较研究（CER）

移植是医学实践中实施干预的一个独特的亚专科。器官移植不是现成的，是依赖于一个供体器官供应远远低于受者（患者）需求的国家获取系统。CER 旨在确定最有效的治疗方法，获得最低风险，每单位获益成本最低，和在每个调整年获得最高的生活质量。器官移植领域的临床医生和研究人员需要纳入我们所阐述的 CER 分析方法。对于新的移植领域，如 CTA（复合组织同种异体移植），CER 可能证明在推进复合组织同种异体移植作为标准护理的过程中是有用的。肝、肺和心脏实体器官移植基本上是挽救生命的，因此，可以做等待列表与器官移植受体的比较。在加拿大，Vasiliadis 和同事的研究中，他们比较了肺移植和受者（患者）等待列表，并发现使用标准赌博方法派生的效用明显有变异[121]。QALY 获得的是一个适度的 0.62 的完整队列，只有通过一个 10 年的预测，QALY 达到 2.19。图 135.9 显示肺移植后每个时间间隔记录的平均效用。

肺移植受者（患者）等待列表如何在决策中使用这些结果？我们可以推测如下：他们应该期望，总体来说，认为有利于很好地改善他们的生活，但在这些年来，这些收益有相当多的变化，生活的整体质量是稳定的，并逐渐改善。

在芬兰的肝移植后 QALY 的 CER 比较研究中，研究人员发现，一年的 QALY 中位数增加为 0.895，五年的增长率为 3.960。获得的每 QALY 的中位成本（以欧元表示）为：（141 769/0.895=）158 400/QALY，在移植后 5 年（177 618/3.96 =）44 854/QALY[122]。这项研究显示了信息使用的两个维度：以受者（患者）为中心的观点，获得的质量调整生命年的增加，以及对于医疗政策决策者，与每个质量调整生命年相关的成本增加。后者显然有利于确定社会支付评估的意愿。

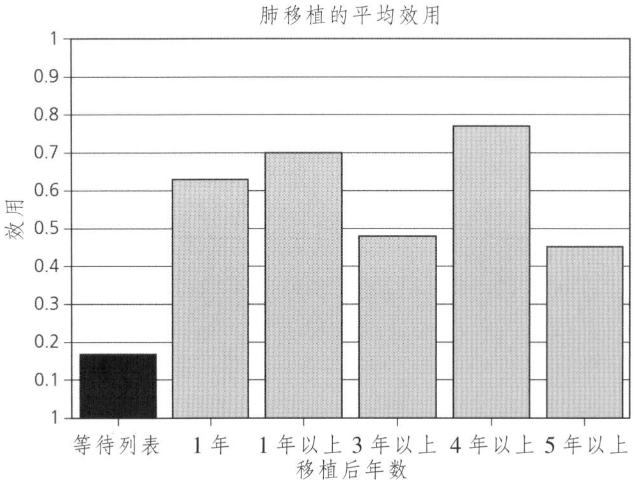

图 135.9 肺移植的效用：效用绘制在垂直轴上，条形图沿水平轴绘制，等待列表与移植后的年份。从 1~5 年的所有年数显示较大的肺移植与等待列表的效用。

Grauhan 及其同事研究了冠状动脉粥样硬化（CA）对德国心脏移植受者（患者）的生活质量调整寿命年数（QALY）的影响。他们使用 SF-36 测量健康状况，从三个比较组得到健康状况评估：单动脉 CA、多动脉 CA 和没有可识别 CA 的心脏。在三组中，平均 SF-36 评分非常接近：单个 CA 64.6，多个 CA 61.5，而没有可辨别的 CA 62.4；然而，QALY 有显著差异，单个 CA 8.5，多个 CA 2.2，没有可识别的 CA 8.0。因此，考虑到 QALY 的获益（5.8~6.3），进行移植前筛选血管造影的程序被视为合理的选择。

CER 的方法性考量

疗效比较研究（CER）不是没有限制和挑战的，它承担着证明有效性、成本效用和有利的增量效用的主要目的，同时更侧重于临床实践的现状和以受者（患者）为中心的护理。最初广泛关注的是比较其有效性，只专注于 QALY 的一种新的治疗方法与既定的治疗方法相比几乎没有控制成本，实际上如果严格遵守可能导致分配效率低。其次，成本效益或增量成本效用分析，两者都纳入成本比较和 QALY 提供包括其相对优点的比较；这可能导致第三方付款人简单地调整他们的成本以满足衍生标准（由此可能导致成本增加）[124]。对疗效比较研究的一个更根本的关注是由于广泛应用推荐的治疗而产生的差异或异质受者（患者）利益的问题。例如，基于 CER 的 Meta 分析可以为典型受者（患者）建立最佳的实践治疗，而另一些人将无疑会比其他人更多或更少受益。这种关注应该通过放宽研究的纳入标准来缓和，例如更大的受者（患者）异质性，这可能会降低疗效，同时提高更广泛的有效性。当利益难以准确地量化时，问题就显现出来了；例如减轻疼痛，焦虑，改善睡眠质量或减少胃炎。同样，药物效应的差异通常很小，因此需要大量受者（患者）来建立研究组以发现效应的大小[125]。建立药物治疗等效性或优势不易通过小尺度效应体现,通常需要安慰剂组,当成功治疗的药物已经建立而得到受者（患者）同意是一个明显的障碍。然而,CER强调超越传统的RCT理想疗效,探讨建立疗法的比较,以启发受者(患者)和医生的决策过程为最有利[126]。Hung等举出了一个最近的例子,比较二甲双胍、磺酰脲和罗格列酮在回顾性研究93 577位受者（患者)DM治疗的eGFR或ESRD持续下降的复合终点[127]。经过4年的治疗,与二甲双胍相比,磺酰脲类药物的使用显示复合终点的风险为1.2(HR)(CI:1.13~1.28)。评论者可能会质疑小尺度的效应量(<2.0),但是由于涉及的样本量较大,20%增加的风险可能在临床上也是相当有意义的。

另一个相关的问题是不可忽略的医师技能的差异，这在外科手术中比较低值和高值器官移植方案时特别明显。干预所带来的最大的受者(患者)医疗结果和好的生活质量可能是高度依赖于技术技能的，由此导致在可衡量的成果和利益上具有广泛的差异。尽管CER的明确目标之一是提高公众对什么是有效的和什么是无效的知识,但CER的目的并不是产生一个“一刀切”的医疗决策矩阵,不可避免地会有受者(患者)之间利益冲突的结果,如生活质量与医生生物物理结果。最近Fried和其同事调查了老年人的健康结果优先级,发现活着的受者（患者）被列为最高优先级的只有11%,疼痛管理被排在前13%,保持自理是76%的受访者[128]。显然,当面对有限或慢性疼痛的现实时,这些优先事项可能发生实质性改变，但研究确实突出了需要包括受者(患者)在医疗决策过程中报告的生活质量感知和需求,使得结果有较好的个体化护理[129]。

最近，一项修订的随机对照试验设计已被提议作为随机对照试验和随机临床试验之间的桥梁，以更好地实现效用(内部有效性)和有效性(外部有效性)之间的平衡,称为PRT[130]。该设计类似于随机对照试验,随机分配到实验组和对照研究组，但干预和结果基于有意义的和以医学实践为主的研究问题。重点在于外部有效性,因此采用更具包容性的受者(患者)征集策略来尝试产生现实效用的结果[15]。PRT设计在重点方面不同于随机对照试验:目的是调查在通常情况下(与理想情况下)的受者(患者)益处,保持干预灵活性,注重常规护理实践,并找到对受者(患者)临床重要的一系列结果的答案[16]。

当随机对照试验研究并非随机时，观察到的治疗差异总是潜在地不是由于干预(或治疗),而是由于自选受者(患者)对其各自研究组带来的预选条件。由于流行病学家主要以非随机设计进行研究，因此它们可被认为是自然适合协助随机对照试验项目。流行病学具有悠久的使用历史和复杂的分析技术来管理明显的偏差,如匹配和分层分析。案例控制设计经常使用两种匹配技术之一。第一种称为个体匹配,以某些被认为重要的先验标准(例如年龄、性别、血型、炎症标志物)来选择病例和对照是类似的[131]。第二种技术称为频率匹配,并且涉及以接近实验受者(患者)特征[例如,来自具有类似肌酐水平的移植中心xyz的所有等待列出的受者(患者)]的方式绘制对照特征。注意,在匹配设计检验统计量是不同的，因为我们试验观察到的概率是不一样的，并且使用优势比的条件最大可能性估计:OR=b/c,用McNemar检验,$\chi^2=(B-C)^2/(B+C)$[132]。分层是另一种普遍的技术，通过用一个或多个感兴趣的协变量分割组来实现试验组和对照组之间的平衡，而使组之间尽可能相似[133]。试图管理非随机研究中的选择偏倚的其他新近推广的技术包括倾向得分分析［基于治疗前变量,确定接受特定治疗的每个受者(患者)的条件概率][134-137]和灵敏度分析(即,通过改变输入变量来确定对结果变量的影响，例如改变折算率来影响增加ICUR的效用分析)。

总结和未来的发展方向

CER自美国开始,美国通过了2009年“美国复苏和再投资法案”,该法案提供了资金,使疗效比较研究成为主流的研究工作。疗效比较研究的主要目的是改革医学研究等,这将增强以受者(患者)为中心的临床实践的现实。现代医学已经运行了一段时间,与临床研究有一定的不协调,并强调“一刀切”的通用聚焦疗效,形成对比的是异质受者(患者)人群的日常实践需要,以及他们的主诉和过多的合并症。循证医学是欧洲不完美的尝试，旨在提高临床医生在日常实践中利用医学研究的研究相关性和合法性。循证医学寻求补充临床医生依靠尖端研究证据的病理生理学基础知识。疗效比较研究旨在扩大循证医学的领域，其重点在于不仅评估异质受者(患者)情境中的功效,而且评估受者(患者)对生活质量的医疗干预和这种干预的效率。疗效比较研究的出现，部分原因是由于药物基因组学中的新发现的相关性和个性化医学的成功，这表示从一般受者(患者)使用药物的药理学到根据受者(患者)自己的遗传资料来量身定制方式的一个根本性的转变[138]。通过发现结肠癌药物西妥昔单抗(Erbitux)其肿瘤 K-ras 基因突变密码子是 12 或 13 的致癌基因对于转移性结肠直肠癌的肿瘤受者(患者)治疗无效，最显著地说明了该基因组相关性。因此，筛选 K-ras 突变的受者(患者)可能避免无效的治疗，临床医生可以转移到其他治疗。即使对于有效的药物，基因组信息可以以剂量定制的方式使用；例如基因测试可以显示当使用正常剂量的巯基嘌呤治疗白血病时处于高并发症风险的受者(患者)的作用。在肝脏、心脏和肾脏的实体器官移植中，已经表明作为 CYP3A5*1 等位基因携带者的受者(患者)对他克莫司的药代动力学具有不利影响，并且需要更长的时间段来实现期望的血液水平[139]。最近，Provenzani 和其同事证明，与野生型等位基因纯合的受者(患者)相比，2677T/A 等位基因的肾移植受者(患者)需要高出很多的他克莫司日剂量才能达到目标治疗水平[140]。最后，Einecke 等开发了一个分子分类器来预测肾移植物的损失，其中移植物损失的 RR 为 2.70(CI：95%，1.82~4.00)的分子风险评分[141]。研究人员得出结论，基于基因的分子风险评分成功地确定了可能发生移植物损失的活动性肾损伤。

哲学与经济学上对 CER 的关注点在于即使来自基因组生物标志物，频率还是平均的，虽然基于子群。当疗效比较研究表示治疗效果的个体水平差异时，这将如何影响健康消费者和医疗提供者？医疗信息在其实现的成功中总是有不确定性的因素；因为这样的受者(患者)估计可以过度或不足治疗利益。简而言之，当获益超过新治疗与控制(疗效比较研究的任务)的危害，且信息不确定时，受者(患者)将跳到新的治疗方法，会出现巨大的道德风险和对第三方付款人的需求[142]。因此，一些人主张更加强调疗效比较研究中的个体化，称为 iCER，这将改变受者(患者)的治疗决策[143]。iCER 可以通过 n-1 试验，实用随机试验，使用局部仪器变量分析以更好地允许未观察到的混杂因素，调查表观遗传因子、交叉设计和通过使用适应性随机化技术来实现称为“成功”的方法，将受者(患者)分配到显示最大效应量的治疗组[144]。

还有一些关于个性化医疗是否与 CER 的既定目标相冲突的争论，因为前者的重点明确以受者(患者)为中心或个人主义，而后者则认为研究竞争药物治疗异质性受者(患者)之间的有效性。这些关注可能被夸大，因为 PCORI 的立法规定了个性化医疗原则和疗效比较研究之间的适应。两者都试图将研究重点从所谓的“平均群体效应”倾向于隐藏重要的亚组效应，并以改进受者(患者)护理的方向变化用有效和高效的方式来研究。疗效比较研究的研究人员的责任是确保它承担收集与被调查疾病病程密切相关的相关问题和细微差别。受者(患者)不对治疗进行单片反应，存在相当大的反应变化。正是医学中的这一事实，将使它继续作为一种持续的临床判断(艺术和实践)的结合，并需要继续高质量和相关的研究，将启发和发展更好的临床预测[145]。

移植研究中的 CER 将发挥重要作用，因为它旨在提高知识的有效性和以受者(患者)为中心的结果。重点需要转向补充疗效和扩大外部有效性和相关性，以利于受者(患者)护理和受者(患者)决策。增加效用、生活质量措施和调整寿命质量的评估，都将有助于在复杂的移植决策迷宫中扩宽决策途径。

(陈俊丽 董思依 林丽丹 译 徐骁 校)

参考文献

1. Sox HC. Comparative effectiveness research: a progress report. Annals of Internal Medicine. 2010;153(7):469-472.
2. Kaye T. Are you kidding me? Clinical comparative effectiveness of evidence-based medicine. American Health & Drug Benefits. 2009;2(3):108.
3. Prioritization CoCER. Initial National Priorties for Comparative Effectiveness Research. Washington, D.C.: The National Academies Press; 2009;29.
4. Orszag P. Reaserch on the Comperative Effectiveness of Medical Treatments: Options for an Expanded Role. In: Office CB, editor. Washington, D.C. 2007.
5. Conway PH, Clancy C. Comparative-effectiveness research–implications of the Federal Coordinating Council's report. New England Journal of Medicine. 2009;361(4):328-330.
6. Selby JV, Beal AC, Frank L. The Patient-Centered Outcomes Research Institute (PCORI) national priorities for research and initial research agenda. JAMA: Journal of the American Medical Association. 2012;307(15):1583-1584.
7. French JA, England JD. Invited article: comparative effectiveness research, evidence-based medicine, and the AAN. Neurology. 2010;75(6):562-567.
8. Cartwright N. A philosopher's view of the long road from RCTs to effectiveness. Lancet. 2011;377(9775):1400-1401.
9. Cartwright N, Munro E. The limitations of randomized controlled trials in predicting effectiveness. Journal of Evaluation in Clinical Practice. 2010;16(2): 260-266.
10. Heritier SR, Gebski VJ, Keech AC. Inclusion of patients in clinical trial analysis: the intention-to-treat principle. Medical Journal of Australia. 2003;179(8): 438-440.
11. Piantadosi S. Clinical Trials. A Methodologic Perspective. New York, NY: John

Wiley & sons, INC; 1997.
12. Strom BL. Methodologic challenges to studying patient safety and comparative effectiveness. Medical Care. 2007;45(10 Supl 2):S13–S15.
13. Hernan MA, Hernandez-Diaz S. Beyond the intention-to-treat in comparative effectiveness research. Clinical Trials. 2012;9(1):48–55.
14. Horn SD, Gassaway J. Practice-based evidence study design for comparative effectiveness research. Medical Care. 2007;45(10 Supl 2):S50–S57.
15. Patsopoulos NA. A pragmatic view on pragmatic trials. Dialogues in Clinical Neuroscience. 2011;13(2):217–224.
16. Sackett DL. Explanatory and pragmatic clinical trials: a primer and application to a recent asthma trial. Polskie Archiwum Medycyny Wewnetrznej. 2011; 121(7–8):259–263.
17. Relton C, Torgerson D, O'Cathain A, et al. Rethinking pragmatic randomised controlled trials: introducing the "cohort multiple randomised controlled trial" design. BMJ (Clinical Research Ed.). 2010;340:c1066.
18. Gleicher N, Barad DH. Misplaced obsession with prospectively randomized studies. Reproductive Biomedicine Online. 2010;21(4):440–443.
19. Bacchetti P, Deeks SG, McCune JM. Breaking free of sample size dogma to perform innovative translational research. Science Translational Medicine. 2011; 3(87):87ps24.
20. Sacristan JA. Exploratory trials, confirmatory observations: a new reasoning model in the era of patient-centered medicine. BMC Medical Research Methodology. 2011;11:57.
21. Clarke C. Invited commentary on R. A. Fisher. American Journal of Epidemiology. 1991;134(12):1371–1374.
22. Zucker DR, Ruthazer R, Schmid CH. Individual (N-of-1) trials can be combined to give population comparative treatment effect estimates: methodologic considerations. Journal of Clinical Epidemiology. 2010;63(12):1312–1323.
23. Lillie EO, Patay B, Diamant J, et al. The n-of-1 clinical trial: the ultimate strategy for individualizing medicine? Personalized Medicine. 2011;8(2): 161–173.
24. Sackett DL. Clinician-trialist rounds: 4. why not do an N-of-1 RCT? Clinical Trials. 2011;8(3):350–352.
25. Chow S-C, Liu J-P. Design and Analysis of Clinical Trials: Concepts and Methodologies. 2nd ed. Hoboken, NJ: A John Wiley & Sons, Inc., Publication; 2004.
26. Scuffham PA, Nikles J, Mitchell GK, et al. Using N-of-1 trials to improve patient management and save costs. Journal of General Internal Medicine. 2010; 25(9):906–913.
27. Berlin JA. N-of-1 clinical trials should be incorporated into clinical practice. Journal of Clinical Epidemiology. 2010;63(12):1283–1284.
28. Neutens JJ, Rubinson L. Research Techniques for The Health Sciences. 2nd ed. Needham Heights, MA: Allyn and Bacon; 1997.
29. Fleurence RL, Naci H, Jansen JP. The critical role of observational evidence in comparative effectiveness research. Health Affairs (Project Hope). 2010;29(10): 1826–1833.
30. Dreyer NA. Making observational studies count: shaping the future of comparative effectiveness research. Epidemiology. 2011;22(3):295–297.
31. Dreyer NA, Tunis SR, Berger M, et al. Why observational studies should be among the tools used in comparative effectiveness research. Health Affairs (Project Hope). 2010;29(10):1818–1825.
32. Golub RM, Fontanarosa PB. Comparative effectiveness research: relative successes. JAMA: Journal of the American Medical Association. 2012;307(15): 1643–1645.
33. Weiss NS. The new world of data linkages in clinical epidemiology: are we being brave or foolhardy? Epidemiology. 2011;22(3):292–294.
34. Djulbegovic M, Djulbegovic B. Implications of the principle of question propagation for comparative-effectiveness and "data mining" research. JAMA: Journal of the American Medical Association. 2011;305(3):298–299.
35. Brookhart MA, Sturmer T, Glynn RJ, et al. Confounding control in healthcare database research: challenges and potential approaches. Medical Care. 2010;48(6 Suppl):S114–S120.
36. Greenland S. Quantifying biases in causal models: classical confounding vs collider-stratification bias. Epidemiology. 2003;14(3):300–306.
37. Schisterman EF, Cole SR, Platt RW. Overadjustment bias and unnecessary adjustment in epidemiologic studies. Epidemiology. 2009;20(4):488–495.
38. Bowden J, Tierney JF, Copas AJ, et al. Quantifying, displaying and accounting for heterogeneity in the meta-analysis of RCTs using standard and generalised Q statistics. BMC Medical Research Methodology. 2011;11:41.
39. Rogawski MA, Federoff HJ. Disclosure of clinical trial results when product development is abandoned. Science Translational Medicine. 2011;3(102):102cm29.
40. Berlin JA, Cepeda MS. Some methodological points to consider when performing systematic reviews in comparative effectiveness research. Clinical Trials. 2012;9(1):27–34.
41. Goodman S, Dickersin K. Metabias: a challenge for comparative effectiveness research. Annals of Internal Medicine. 2011;155(1):61–62.
42. Dechartres A, Boutron I, Trinquart L, et al. Single-center trials show larger treatment effects than multicenter trials: evidence from a meta-epidemiologic study. Annals of Internal Medicine. 2011;155(1):39–51.
43. Danaei G, Tavakkoli M, Hernan MA. Bias in observational studies of prevalent users: lessons for comparative effectiveness research from a meta-analysis of statins. American Journal of Epidemiology. 2012;175(4):250–262.
44. Li T, Puhan MA, Vedula SS, et al. Network meta-analysis-highly attractive but more methodological research is needed. BMC Medicine. 2011;9:79.
45. Tang DH, Malone DC. A network meta-analysis on the efficacy of serotonin type 3 receptor antagonists used in adults during the first 24 hours for postoperative nausea and vomiting prophylaxis. Clinical Therapeutics. 2012;34(2): 282–294.
46. Mickenautsch S. Systematic reviews, systematic error and the acquisition of clinical knowledge. BMC Medical Research Methodology. 2010;10:53.
47. Goldsmith MR, Bankhead CR, Austoker J. Synthesising quantitative and qualitative research in evidence-based patient information. Journal of Epidemiology and Community Health. 2007;61(3):262–270.
48. Sox HC, Goodman SN. The methods of comparative effectiveness research. Annual Review of Public Health. 2012;33:425–445.
49. Best M, Katamba A, Neuhauser D. Making the right decision: Benjamin Franklin's son dies of smallpox in 1736. Quality & Safety in Health Care. 2007;16(6):478–480.
50. McCabe S, Rodocker G, Julliard K, et al. Using decision analysis to aid in the introduction of upper extremity transplantation. Transplantation Proceedings. 1998;30(6):2783–2786.
51. Griebsch I, Coast J, Brown J. Quality-adjusted life-years lack quality in pediatric care: a critical review of published cost-utility studies in child health. Pediatrics. 2005;115(5):e600–e614.
52. Kaplan RM. Quality of life: an outcomes perspective. Archives of Physical Medicine and Rehabilitation. 2002;83(12 Suppl 2):S44–S50.
53. King JT Jr, Tsevat J, Lave JR, et al. Willingness to pay for a quality-adjusted life year: implications for societal health care resource allocation. Medical Decision Making. 2005;25(6):667–677.
54. Shiell A, Donaldson C, Mitton C, et al. Health economic evaluation. Journal of Epidemiology and Community Health. 2002;56(2):85–88.
55. Kiberd B, Skedgel C, Alwayn I, et al. Simultaneous liver kidney transplantation: a medical decision analysis. Transplantation. 2011;91(1):121–127.
56. Sharma S, Brown GC, Brown MM, et al. Validity of the time trade-off and standard gamble methods of utility assessment in retinal patients. British Journal of Ophthalmology. 2002;86(5):493–496.
57. van Wijck EE, Bosch JL, Hunink MG. Time-tradeoff values and standard-gamble utilities assessed during telephone interviews versus face-to-face interviews. Medical Decision Making. 1998;18(4):400–405.
58. Arnesen TM, Norheim OF. Quantifying quality of life for economic analysis: time out for time tradeoff. Medical Humanities. 2003;29(2):81–86.
59. Horsman J, Furlong W, Feeny D, et al. The Health Utilities Index (HUI): concepts, measurement properties and applications. Health and Quality of Life Outcomes. 2003;1:54.
60. Attema AE, Brouwer WB. On the (not so) constant proportional trade-off in TTO. Quality of Life Research. 2010;19(4):489–497.
61. Attema AE, Brouwer WB. Constantly proving the opposite? A test of CPTO using a broad time horizon and correcting for discounting. Quality of Life Research. 2012;21(1):25–34.
62. Gafni A. The standard gamble method: what is being measured and how it is interpreted. Health Services Research. 1994;29(2):207–224.
63. Pope R. Biases from omitted risk effects in standard gamble utilities. Journal of Health Economics. 2004;23(4):695–735.
64. Bravo Vergel Y, Sculpher M. Quality-adjusted life years. Practical Neurology. 2008;8(3):175–182.
65. Bala MV, Wood LL, Zarkin GA, et al. Are health states "timeless"? The case of the standard gamble method. Journal of Clinical Epidemiology. 1999;52(11): 1047–1053.
66. Heintz E, Wirehn AB, Peebo BB, et al. QALY weights for diabetic retinopathy–a comparison of health state valuations with HUI-3, EQ-5D, EQ-VAS, and TTO. Value in Health. 2012;15(3):475–484.
67. Santana MJ, Feeny D, Ghosh S, et al. The construct validity of the health utilities index mark 3 in assessing health status in lung transplantation. Health and Quality of Life Outcomes. 2010;8:110.
68. Smith MD, Drummond M, Brixner D. Moving the QALY forward: rationale for change. Value in Health. 2009;12(Suppl 1):S1–S4.
69. Dolan P, Kahneman D. Interpretations of utility and their implications for the valuation of health. The Economic Journal. 2008;118:215–234.
70. Krabbe PF, Tromp N, Ruers TJ, et al. Are patients' judgments of health status really different from the general population? Health and Quality of Life Outcomes. 2011;9:31.

71. Egan TM. QALYs or quackery? The quagmire of quantifying the cost of breathing. The Journal of Thoracic and Cardiovascular Surgery. 2002;123(3):406–408.
72. Weinstein MC, Torrance G, McGuire A. QALYs: the basics. Value in Health. 2009;12(Suppl 1):S5–S9.
73. Lamers LM. The transformation of utilities for health states worse than death: consequences for the estimation of EQ-5D value sets. Medical Care. 2007; 45(3):238–244.
74. Sullivan PW. Are utilities bounded at 1.0? Implications for statistical analysis and scale development. Medical Decision Making. 2011;31(6):787–789.
75. Pullenayegum EM, Tarride JE, Xie F, et al. Calculating utility decrements associated with an adverse event: marginal Tobit and CLAD coefficients should be used with caution. Medical Decision Making. 2011;31(6):790–799.
76. Stinnett AA, Mullahy J. Net health benefits: a new framework for the analysis of uncertainty in cost-effectiveness analysis. Medical Decision Making. 1998;18(2 Suppl):S68–S80.
77. Larsen K, Hansen TB, Thomsen PB, et al. Cost-effectiveness of accelerated perioperative care and rehabilitation after total hip and knee arthroplasty. Journal of Bone and Joint Surgery. American Volume. 2009;91(4):761–772.
78. Flynn TN, Louviere JJ, Marley AA, et al. Rescaling quality of life values from discrete choice experiments for use as QALYs: a cautionary tale. Population Health Metrics. 2008;6:6.
79. van der Velde G, Hogg-Johnson S, Bayoumi AM, et al. Neck pain patients' preference scores for their current health. Quality of Life Research. 2010;19(5): 687–700.
80. Rand-Hendriksen K, Augestad LA, Dahl FA, et al. A shortcut to mean-based time tradeoff tariffs for the EQ-5D? Medical Decision Making. 2012;32(4):569–577.
81. Shaw JW, Pickard AS, Yu S, et al. A median model for predicting United States population-based EQ-5D health state preferences. Value in Health. 2010;13(2): 278–288.
82. Shaw JW, Johnson JA, Coons SJ. US valuation of the EQ-5D health states: development and testing of the D1 valuation model. Medical Care. 2005;43(3): 203–220.
83. Johnson JA, Luo N, Shaw JW, et al. Valuations of EQ-5D health states: are the United States and United Kingdom different? Medical Care. 2005;43(3): 221–228.
84. Craig BM, Busschbach JJ. Toward a more universal approach in health valuation. Health Economics. 2011;20(7):864–875.
85. Edlin RL, Longo R, McCabe C. Supra-states and Censoring in Health Utility Modeling: An examination of Their Importance in the EQ-5D Tariff. Leeds, UK: Leeds Institute of Health Sciences, 2010.
86. Craig BM, Busschbach JJ, Salomon JA. Modeling ranking, time trade-off, and visual analog scale values for EQ-5D health states: a review and comparison of methods. Medical Care. 2009;47(6):634–641.
87. Craig BM, Oppe M. From a different angle: a novel approach to health valuation. Social Science and Medicine. 2010;70(2):169–174.
88. Craig BM, Busschbach JJ. The episodic random utility model unifies time trade-off and discrete choice approaches in health state valuation. Population Health Metrics. 2009;7:3.
89. Menzies NA, Salomon JA. Non-monotonicity in the episodic random utility model. Health Economics. 2011;20(12):1523–1531.
90. Attema AE, Brouwer WB. A test of independence of discounting from quality of life. Journal of Health Economics. 2012;31(1):22–34.
91. Brennan DC, Daller JA, Lake KD, et al. Rabbit antithymocyte globulin versus basiliximab in renal transplantation. New England Journal of Medicine. 2006;355(19):1967–1977.
92. Rostaing L, Neumayer HH, Reyes-Acevedo R, et al. Belatacept-versus cyclosporine-based immunosuppression in renal transplant recipients with pre-existing diabetes. Clinical Journal of the American Society of Nephrology: CJASN. 2011;6(11):2696–2704.
93. Woodle ES, First MR, Pirsch J, et al. A prospective, randomized, double-blind, placebo-controlled multicenter trial comparing early (7 day) corticosteroid cessation versus long-term, low-dose corticosteroid therapy. Annals of Surgery. 2008;248(4):564–577.
94. Ciancio G, Burke GW, Gaynor JJ, et al. A randomized trial of three renal transplant induction antibodies: early comparison of tacrolimus, mycophenolate mofetil, and steroid dosing, and newer immune-monitoring. Transplantation. 2005;80(4):457–465.
95. Vanrenterghem Y, Bresnahan B, Campistol J, et al. Belatacept-based regimens are associated with improved cardiovascular and metabolic risk factors compared with cyclosporine in kidney transplant recipients (BENEFIT and BENEFIT-EXT studies). Transplantation. 2011;91(9):976–983.
96. Merkus MP, Jager KJ, Dekker FW, et al. Quality of life over time in dialysis: the Netherlands Cooperative Study on the Adequacy of Dialysis. NECOSAD Study Group. Kidney International. 1999;56(2):720–728.
97. Evans RW, Manninen DL, Garrison LP Jr, et al. The quality of life of patients with end-stage renal disease. The New England Journal of Medicine. 1985; 312(9):553–559.
98. Gokal R. Quality of life in patients undergoing renal replacement therapy. Kidney International. Supplement. 1993;40:S23–S27.
99. Gudex CM. Health-related quality of life in endstage renal failure. Quality of Life Research. 1995;4(4):359–366.
100. Johnson JP, McCauley CR, Copley JB. The quality of life of hemodialysis and transplant patients. Kidney International. 1982;22(3):286–291.
101. Pacheco A, Saffie A, Torres R, et al. Cost/Utility study of peritoneal dialysis and hemodialysis in Chile. Peritoneal Dialysis International. 2007;27(3):359–363.
102. Sennfalt K, Magnusson M, Carlsson P. Comparison of hemodialysis and peritoneal dialysis–a cost-utility analysis. Peritoneal Dialysis International. 2002; 22(1):39–47.
103. Simmons RG, Abress L. Quality-of-life issues for end-stage renal disease patients. American journal of Kidney Diseases. 1990;15(3):201–208.
104. Valderrabano F, Jofre R, Lopez-Gomez JM. Quality of life in end-stage renal disease patients. American journal of Kidney Diseases. 2001;38(3):443–464.
105. Morel P, Almond PS, Matas AJ, et al. Long-term quality of life after kidney transplantation in childhood. Transplantation. 1991;52(1):47–53.
106. Russell JD, Beecroft ML, Ludwin D, et al. The quality of life in renal transplantation–a prospective study. Transplantation. 1992;54(4):656–660.
107. Laupacis A, Keown P, Pus N, et al. A study of the quality of life and cost-utility of renal transplantation. Kidney International. 1996;50(1):235–242.
108. Franke GH, Reimer J, Kohnle M, et al. Quality of life in end-stage renal disease patients after successful kidney transplantation: development of the ESRD symptom checklist – transplantation module. Nephron. 1999;83(1): 31–39.
109. Ziegelmann JP, Griva K, Hankins M, et al. The Transplant Effects Questionnaire (TxEQ): the development of a questionnaire for assessing the multidimensional outcome of organ transplantation – example of end stage renal disease (ESRD). British Journal of Health Psychology. 2002;7(Pt 4):393–408.
110. Chisholm-Burns MA, Erickson SR, Spivey CA, et al. Concurrent validity of kidney transplant questionnaire in US renal transplant recipients. Patient Preference and Adherence. 2011;5:517–522.
111. Portney L, Watkins MP. Foundations of Clinical Research. Saddle River, NJ: Pearson Prentice Hall; 2009: 892.
112. Jassal SV, Krahn MD, Naglie G, et al. Kidney transplantation in the elderly: a decision analysis. Journal of the American Society of Nephrology: JASN. 2003;14(1):187–196.
113. Kontodimopoulos N, Niakas D. An estimate of lifelong costs and QALYs in renal replacement therapy based on patients' life expectancy. Health Policy. 2008; 86(1):85–96.
114. Gravelle H, Smith D. Discounting for health effects in cost-benefit and cost-effectiveness analysis. Health Economics. 2001;10(7):587–599.
115. Brouwer WB, Niessen LW, Postma MJ, et al. Need for differential discounting of costs and health effects in cost effectiveness analyses. BMJ (Clinical Research Ed.). 2005;331(7514):446–448.
116. van Hout BA. Discounting costs and effects: a reconsideration. Health Economics. 1998;7(7):581–594.
117. Haller M, Gutjahr G, Kramar R, et al. Cost-effectiveness analysis of renal replacement therapy in Austria. Nephrology, Dialysis, Transplantation. 2011;26(9): 2988–2995.
118. Liem YS, Wong JB, Winkelmayer WC, et al. Quantifying the benefit of early living-donor renal transplantation with a simulation model of the Dutch renal replacement therapy population. Nephrology, Dialysis, Transplantation. 2012;27(1):429–434.
119. Luan FL, Kommareddi M, Ojo AO. Universal prophylaxis is cost effective in cytomegalovirus serology-positive kidney transplant patients. Transplantation. 2011;91(2):237–244.
120. Dominguez J, Harrison R, Atal R. Cost-benefit estimation of cadaveric kidney transplantation: the case of a developing country. Transplantation Proceedings. 2011;43(6):2300–2304.
121. Vasiliadis HM, Collet JP, Penrod JR, et al. A cost-effectiveness and cost-utility study of lung transplantation. Journal of Heart and Lung Transplantation. 2005;24(9):1275–1283.
122. Aberg F, Maklin S, Rasanen P, et al. Cost of a quality-adjusted life year in liver transplantation: the influence of the indication and the model for end-stage liver disease score. Liver transplantation. 2011;17(11):1333–1343.
123. Grauhan O, Hetzer R. Impact of donor-transmitted coronary atherosclerosis. Journal of Heart and Lung Transplantation. 2004;23(9 Suppl):S260–S262.
124. Chandra A, Jena AB, Skinner JS. The pragmatist's guide to comparative effectiveness research. Journal of Economic Perspectives. 2011;25(2):27–46.
125. Temple R. A regulator's view of comparative effectiveness research. Clinical Trials. 2012;9(1):56–65.
126. Memtsoudis SG, Besculides MC. Perioperative comparative effectiveness

research. Best Practice & Research. Clinical Anaesthesiology. 2011;25(4): 535–547.
127. Hung AM, Roumie CL, Greevy RA, et al. Comparative effectiveness of incident oral antidiabetic drugs on kidney function. Kidney International. 2012;81(7): 698–706.
128. Fried TR, Tinetti ME, Iannone L, et al. Health outcome prioritization as a tool for decision making among older persons with multiple chronic conditions. Archives of Internal Medicine. 2011;171(20):1854–1856.
129. Kliger AS, Fishbane S, Finkelstein FO. Erythropoietic stimulating agents and quality of a patient's life: individualizing anemia treatment. Clinical Journal of the American Society of Nephrology: CJASN. 2012;7(2):354–357.
130. Ware JH, Hamel MB. Pragmatic trials–guides to better patient care? New England Journal of Medicine. 2011;364(18):1685–1687.
131. Szklo M, Nieto FJ. Epidemiology Beyond the Basics. Gaitherburg, MD: Aspen Publishers, Inc; 2000:495.
132. Jewell NP. Statistics for Epidemiology. Boca Raton, FL: CRC Press; 2004:333.
133. Alemayehu D, Alvir JM, Jones B, et al. Statistical issues with the analysis of nonrandomized studies in comparative effectiveness research. Journal of Managed Care Pharmacy: JMCP. 2011;17(9 Suppl A):S22–S26.
134. Austin PC. The relative ability of different propensity score methods to balance measured covariates between treated and untreated subjects in observational studies. Medical Decision Making. 2009;29(6):661–677.
135. Concato J. When to randomize, or 'Evidence-based medicine needs medicine-based evidence'. Pharmacoepidemiology and Drug Safety. 2012;21(Suppl 2): 6–12.
136. Concato J. Is it time for medicine-based evidence? JAMA: Journal of the American Medical Association. 2012;307(15):1641–1643.
137. Dehejia R, Wahba S. Propensity score-matching methods for nonexperimental causal studies. Review of Economics and Statistics. 2002;84(1):151–161.
138. Paci D, Ibarrela D. Economic and cost-effectiveness considerations for pharmacogenetics tests: an integral part of translational research and innovation uptake in personalized medicine. Current Pharmacogenomics and Personalized Medicine. 2009;7:284–296.
139. Staatz CE, Goodman LK, Tett SE. Effect of CYP3A and ABCB1 single nucleotide polymorphisms on the pharmacokinetics and pharmacodynamics of calcineurin inhibitors: part II. Clinical Pharmacokinetics. 2010;49(4):207–221.
140. Provenzani A, Notarbartolo M, Labbozzetta M, et al. Influence of CYP3A5 and ABCB1 gene polymorphisms and other factors on tacrolimus dosing in Caucasian liver and kidney transplant patients. International Journal of Molecular Medicine. 2011;28(6):1093–1102.
141. Einecke G, Reeve J, Sis B, et al. A molecular classifier for predicting future graft loss in late kidney transplant biopsies. Journal of Clinical Investigation. 2010;120(6):1862–1872.
142. Basu A. Economics of individualization in comparative effectiveness research and a basis for a patient-centered health care. Journal of Health Economics. 2011;30(3):549–559.
143. Basu A. Individualization at the heart of comparative effectiveness research: the time for i-CER has come. Medical Decision Making. 2009;29(6):NP9–NP11.
144. Cheng Y, Berry DA. Optimal adaptive randomization designs for clinical trails. Biometrika. 2007;94(3):673–689.
145. Garber AM, Tunis SR. Does comparative-effectiveness research threaten personalized medicine? New England Journal of Medicine. 2009;360(19): 1925–1927.

第 11 篇

移植政策

第 136 章 临床医生的移植伦理学

Richard N. Formica Jr, Francis L. Delmonico

引言

移植专家在行医过程中处于特殊的地位，即管理一种社会稀缺的资源:器官捐赠者。这项管理工作需要承担两项重要责任：①公平分配死亡捐献者的器官给合适的受者;②评估和护理活体器官捐献者。第 137 章和第 138 章详细描述了这两项责任。本章着重从临床医生的角度来讲这两个问题的融合。决定器官移植的决策作为治疗方案需要医生综合判定和了解患者手术风险和预期收益。最终,每个患者的治疗建议应基于适当的数据和移植手术医生的经验。移植专家在管理供体器官的过程中面临一种可避免的冲突，即求得保护患者和保护供体器官这一珍贵资源的社会责任这二者的平衡。与器官移植相关的数据、经验和伦理原则在平衡这些利益冲突时非常重要。本章旨在探讨如何调解器官移植中患者和社会之间的利益冲突。虽然重点讨论肾移植,但该原则适用于所有器官移植。本章并不打算传达观点;相反,它是一个应用数据和经验的综述,是符合伦理学原则的规范治疗过程。

最终准则

卫生与公众服务部已经发布“最终准则”[1]作为器官获取和移植网络结构(OPTN)及运行状态的框架,以监督美国器官捐献和移植的实践。该条例的 121.8 节提出器官分配并声明了分配政策：

- 应基于合理的医学判断。
- 应寻求实现捐赠器官的最佳效用。
- 应保留移植程序拒绝提供给特定的潜在接受者的能力。
- 应旨在避免浪费器官、避免无效移植,促进患者参与移植和器官分配的高效管理。
- 不得以候选人的居住地或列表上的排序为依据。

因此,OPTN 针对候选名单上的候选人排名设定优先级,基于可衡量的医疗条件并根据医疗需求排序。在这样的“最终准则”前提下,经典的伦理原则,即公正、效用、人道主义、无害原则、自主原则显现出来[2]。“最终准则” 体现了基于合理的医学判断的需求分配策略的公正原则。公正原则要求把肾脏分配给最长等待时间的患者。最终,当进入等候名单时,所有相同身体状况的患者应该被同等对待。对于额外的肾脏器官,公正原则现在要求把医疗需要或患者疾病的严重程度作为器官分配的首要标准:

- 作为“最终准则”的道德原则,寻求捐赠器官的最佳利用，以达到最好的同种异体移植物存活率和最好的预后。
- **人道主义**有利于促进接受移植患者的利益。最终准则支持无害原则,即“不伤害”,授权器官移植中心拒绝为特定患者使用特定器官。
- 最后，**自主原则**保留患者接受移植的最终决定权。

现行制度中的决策

人道主义、无害原则、自主原则影响着肾移植时的医患关系。患者信任医生所提出的建议移植作为一种治疗选择,其目的符合自身最佳利益。做出这一决策根据临床判断、数据知识和临床经验。最新研究数据表明,当决定接受肾脏移植时,患者和外科医生判断相同的因素是重要的[3]。这些因素包括肾脏质量、传染性疾病或恶性肿瘤的风险，肾脏的解剖和功能，HLA 匹配程度(也解释了潜在受者敏感性)。这些数据提供了必要的注意事项，但“最终准则”的所阐述的道德原则也是同样重要的方面。

伦理原则的应用

针对肾脏的总体质量

在将高质量的肾脏分配给老年患者时，公正原则和人道主义原则目前优先于效用。相反，无害原则会拒绝高龄捐献者的肾脏移植给年轻受者。重要的是，“最终准则”使肾脏移植中心或患者拥有自主权，拒绝供肾是决定性的关键伦理组成部分。

死亡时的供肾功能

人道主义原则迫使高度敏感的受者接受肾脏移植，面临更高的移植供体延迟恢复的风险，或居住在较长等待时间的地区，可以忍受移植供体延迟恢复和透析的压力。具有相同特征的供体肾脏不能用于无法忍受移植供体延迟恢复的医疗并发症的受者。

供受体 HLA 匹配程度和受体敏感性

这是一个取决于 HLA 匹配程度、供肾质量和受体敏感性的接受或拒绝标准。当前实践优先考虑质量而非匹配程度，特别是年轻的受者。高致敏患者在不考虑供者年龄和质量的情况下优先考虑尸体供肾。

传染性疾病风险

人道主义原则支持接受感染性疾病传播风险的肾脏，对于一个可能不会获得供肾的高度敏感患者，或透析血管通路失败，在有生命危险的情况下需要肾移植的患者。然而，无害原则需要拒绝这样的肾脏供给低 PRA 受者和那些没有紧急移植医疗需要的患者。因为肾脏的质量改善，受者因素增加了紧迫感:如更长的等待时间、更高 PRA、高龄受者，患者应自主决定接受不明确的、实际存在风险的肾脏的决策。

预测移植物生存

扩大标准的供肾可能适合超过 65 岁的高龄患者，因为透析的预期死亡率超过 ECD 失败率。无伤害原则则要求拒绝将 ECD 肾脏移植给年轻患者。每出现一个供肾，移植医师必须基于合理的临床判断、当前数据和伦理原则指导，平衡人道主义与无伤害原则，并决定肾脏是否应该被特定受者接受。

现行制度的不足

现行分配法则授权将 25 岁死者来源肾脏移植给 75 岁受者，这暴露了目前的分配系统在实现供器官最优使用过程中所出现的一些不恰当的做法。目前的移植受者范围涵盖了老年群体和患有多种基础疾病的受者群体。当前的分配系统以移植受者等待时间为最重要原则，而对供器官使用率这一重要准则的重视程度不够。

在过去的十年里，面对供器官资源不足的情况，UNOS 努力最优化器官使用率，尝试修订肾脏分配法则，使所有等待移植的受者能够公平地得到移植的机会。减少老年受者的肾脏配给数量能够提高移植后生存年限，但是，维护老年受者利益的社会群体并不赞同这样的做法。为了解决这些问题，UNOS 倡议采用新的方式评估供肾和受者寿命，使每一例肾脏移植的预后“不仅符合生物医学层面预期，使等待移植的受者也都能够接受”。UNOS 希望延长受者寿命至预期生存期限，同时希望通过改善受者与供肾的匹配，最小化供肾的损失程度。

活体器官移植

活体器官移植已成为全球主要的器官移植方式。器官移植的先驱——Francis Moore 医生，在 40 年前曾提出这样的期望:“与尸体来源器官相比，活体来源肾脏能够达到最佳的组织匹配度。”当前，活体器官移植的移植成功率最高，其移植预后最佳。人道主义伦理准则允许健康的个体捐献器官用于器官移植。同时，人道主义伦理准则要求活体肾脏移植不仅仅限于移植成功率，更要保证捐献者所受风险最小。不伤害伦理准则要求临床医生进行合理、规范的医疗操作，使受者不受伤害。仅在受者获益率非常高的前提下，供者所承担的风险才能被认为是可接受的。活体移植捐献共识详细地阐述了这一伦理原则：

“活体移植供者应能够胜任供者的角色，捐献器官的行为应出于自愿而非强迫，在医学层面和心理层面均符合要求，完全知晓供者可能承担的风险和可能获得的利益，完全知晓受者可能承担的风险、可能获得的利益以及其他可行的替代治疗手段。供者和受者所受获得利益必须超过活体移植相关的风险[4]。”

为保护供者而设立的指南清楚地列出了合理的、非恶意的医疗措施，平衡活体移植可能出现的风险和益处。阿姆斯特丹论坛和温哥华论坛首次编写了该指南，内容包括供者评估、监测和供者预后监测。阿姆斯特丹论坛聚焦活体肾脏移植供者达成的共识，温哥华论坛解决了活体肾脏移植捐献额外的问题。这两个论坛确定了移植项目的核心职责(框 136.1)和活体移植知情同意告知的必要内容(框 136.2)。在某些地区，肝、小肠或肺衰竭的受者不能选择尸体来源器官移植，因此活体移植十分重要。对于供者而言，活体肝移植和肺移植的风险远高于活体肾脏移植。因此，医务人员应该将可能出现的医学难题以通俗易懂的方式呈现，方便活体肝移植和肺移植的供者准确地理解。医务人员完成知情同意告知后，供者应能够完整表述可能出现的风险和获益。

供者即为患者

评估能够进行捐献时，供者即是特殊的“患者”[5]。在活体肝移植的实践过程中，医生和患者共同承担责任，供者单方面的声明或受者单方面的需求不能够解除这种医患关系。医生有职责保护供者的利益，促进供者的健康，不能因受者的需要放弃这种职责。当供者自身既往病史或社交行为可能降低捐献成功率或损害供、受者双方的身体健康时，供者有责任坦白实情。供者只有在医生支持时才能进行肾脏切除术或是部分肝脏切除术，供者不能单独做出接受手术的决定。在某些情况下，尽管患有某些疾病——比如高血压，作为“患者”的供者仍能够进行捐献。但是，如果受者和供者各自的风险-获益比不能达到平衡，移植不能进行。亲属关系不能强迫供者(或受者)承担额外风险进行捐献，但可能影响移植最终能否进行(本章后文内容将作详细讨论)。

社会心理评估

在美国，血缘不相关的供者数量超过了活体肾移植供者总量的 40%[6]。这些供者大多数为受者的配偶或朋友，他们和受者之间情谊深长。目前，网络、团体宣传使越来越多的受者和供者之间建立联系，增加了活体移植的数量。现在，越来越多的陌生人怀着真诚的助人之心，主动参加活体捐献。那些响应网络号召的候选供者必须接受全面的社会心理评估，确认他们不是出于经济需要或是其他需求而参与捐献。除此之外，候选供者不能因为心理疾病困扰，为求救赎而参与捐献。针对候选供者的共识会议确定了社会心理评估指南[7]。不能进行器官捐献的心理评估危险因素包括精神病症状或精神紊乱既往史、药物依赖史和药物滥用史。出于获取声誉或是通过器官捐献拓展社会人际关系是社会心理

框 136.1 实施活体器官供体移植的移植中心的职责

- 提供器官捐献和移植的信息。
- 对受赠者进行可供选择的治疗方案的教育。
- 提供一名单独的捐赠者的辩护律师。
- 评估器官捐赠的医疗、心理和社会的适宜性。
- 确保捐赠决定是自愿的而不受强迫。
- 实施程序上的安全保护，以加强捐赠者的安全性、理解性和自主性。
- 在评估和护理活体器官捐赠者方面提供熟练的内科和外科工作人员。
- 对评估期间发现的任何医疗疾病提供转诊和治疗。
- 在整个评估和捐赠过程中提供社会心理学支持。
- 提供医疗服务，直至完成捐赠程序。
- 完成对于活体器官捐赠者的长期随访。
- 执行质量保证和流程改进，以降低器官捐赠的风险。

框 136.2 活体器官捐献知情同意的基本要素

- 必须是不小于 18 岁的成年人。
- 必须具有做出捐献决定的认知能力。
- 必须是不受强迫的自愿做出的决定。
- 必须包括对于保护捐赠者隐私的保证。
- 必须包含所有相关信息，包括但不限于：
  - 死亡风险
  - 短期或长期手术并发症的风险
  - 潜在的长期医学和社会心理学并发症的风险
  - 被诊断为已有医疗疾病的风险
  - 未来可保性的风险：健康，残疾，生活
  - 受赠者可能没有预期结果的风险
- 在做最终决定之前必须有一个冷静期
- 必须包括在任何时候都可以退出过程的权利。

评估的高危因素。从属性关系例如雇工/雇主因强迫而参与捐献的候选供者，必须经过全面审核才能接受社会心理评估。

自主决定权 VS 家长式统治

自主决定权，即充分理解某事物后，自主决定采取有目的性的、自愿行为的能力，采取的行为不受父母强迫。只有充分知情被告知移植相关风险后，候选供者才能自主进行器官捐献。尊重自主决定权，并不意味着当医学评估判定候选供者不能进行捐献时，医生有义务和候选供者合作，使他们通过审核，成为供者。如果医学评估结果判定候选供者在医学层面或社交心理层面不适合器官捐献，临床医生不能在他人强迫下建议供者手术，也不能参与肾脏切除术或是部分肝脏切除术。自主决定权并不是器官捐献的准则，通过人道主义准则和不伤害准则审核是自主决定进行器官捐献的前提。临床医生负有支持不伤害准则的责任，但这一支持行为不是家长式统治，必须经过医学评估判定。阿姆斯特丹会议建议在最终通过器官捐献的决议前，设立一些保护性步骤，比如冷却期，以支持自主决定权，同时使强迫器官捐献的可能性最小化。

供者-受者关系对于捐献决定的影响

供者-受者关系对于最终的捐献决定可能十分重要。这种关系在生物学上变得越来越疏远，从血缘关系——到朋友——再到陌生人，对于一个完全陌生的供者而言，自主决定权的重要性下降，不伤害准则逐渐成为最重要的评估指标(图 136.1)。临床医生对于供者所承担风险的重视并不因供者-受者关系而改变。但

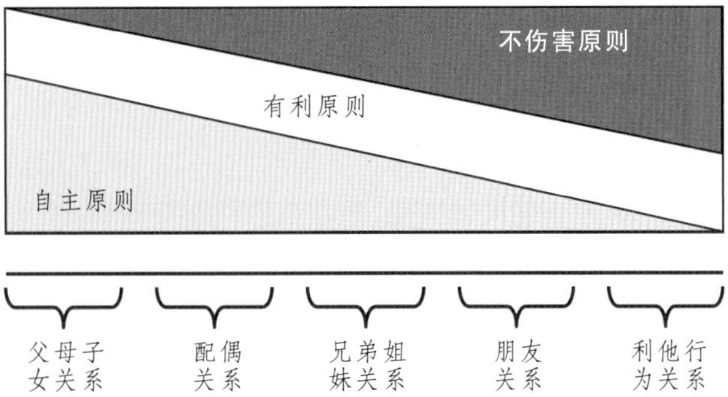

图 136.1 捐赠者与受赠者之间的关系影响到捐赠的决定。

是，当供者和受者存在强烈的家庭或情感联系时，供者自愿接受风险的自主行为会受到更恰当的审核。当供-受者关系以良好的情感为基础时，高血压、蛋白尿、肾功能不全等疾病，或组织结构异常，如肾动脉狭窄，就不会被置之不理，而一台成功的移植手术，或许能够缓解这些疾病。高血压经过有效的治疗，并不会影响预期生存，同时，供者的配偶能够获益，移植医生较以前更能接受患有高血压的年老供者。除此之外，供者进行随访并同时照顾受者，能够降低风险，确保捐献过程继续进行。

结果评估

活体器官供者的预后是社会管理工作的一部分，移植团体应该跟踪随访和报道。供者死亡和供器官功能不全等事件应报道透明化并免于法律诉讼。同样地，如果临床医生不存在违规操作，报道这些预警事件时，不应将责任归咎于医生。

最近的共识会议重点关注活体移植供者的结果和随访，指出现有活体肾移植供者预后数据的局限性和供者随访的必要性[8]。系统性收集和报道活体移植供者预后情况的主要原因如下：

1. 准确的预后信息是进行活体移植供者知情同意告知所必需的。

2. 项目指向性反馈对于移植项目质控和改善是必要的。

3. 器官捐献是社会公信事件，移植团体有义务继续收集活体移植供者预后信息。

4. 实时更新的信息能够改善评估作用，为非传统活体移植候选供者提供可靠的建议。

5. 实时监测可以及时发现候选供者存在的问题，及时采取干预措施。

移植行业必须具有前瞻性，确保器官捐献在围手术期和移植后长期都是安全的。正因为社会大众相信临床医生和移植术者以供者和受者的最佳利益为工作原则，活体器官捐献工作才能顺利开展。

总结

器官移植工作的开展要求临床医师深刻理解生物伦理学，对于能为每一个患者带来最佳预后的医学信

息和医学数据有良好的认识。要达到这些目标,社会信任医生,委托医生管理尸体来源器官,以活体移植供者的利益为立足点,关怀供者,确保供者的身体健康。

(王建国 译 徐骁 校)

参考文献

1. The Department of Health and Human Services. Final Rule. [accessed 15 May, 2012]; Available from: http://www.gaonet.gov/special.pubs/organ/appendd.pdf.
2. McCormick TR. Principles in bioethics. [accessed 15 May, 2012]; Available from: http://depts.washington.edu/bioethx/tools/princpl.html.
3. Solomon DA, Rabidou N, Kulkarni S, et al. Accepting a donor kidney: an evaluation of patients' and transplant surgeons' priorities. Clinical Transplantation. 2011;25:786–793.
4. Consensus statement on the live organ donor. JAMA: Journal of the American Medical Association. 2000;284:2919–2926.
5. Delmonico F, Surman OS. Is this live organ donor your patient? Transplantation. 2003;76:1257–1260.
6. Organ Procurement and Transplantation Network (OPTN) and Scientific Registry of Transplant Recipients (SRTR). OPTN/SRTR 2010 Annual Data Report. Rockville, MD: Department of Health and Human Services, Health Resources and Services Administration, Healthcare Systems Bureau, Division of Transplantation; 2011: Kidney 8.
7. Dew MA, Jacobs CL, Jowsey SG, et al. Guidelines for the psychosocial evaluation of living unrelated kidney donors in the United States. American Journal of Transplantation. 2007;7:1047–1054.
8. Living Kidney Donor Follow-Up Conference Writing Group. Living kidney donor follow-up: state-of-the-art and future directions, conference summary and recommendations. American Journal of Transplantation. 2011 Dec;11(12): 2561–2568.
9. Barr ML, Belghiti J, Villamil FG, et al. A report of the Vancouver Forum on the care of the live organ donor: lung, liver, pancreas, and intestine data and medical guidelines. Transplantation. 2006;81:1373–1385.
10. The consensus statement of the Amsterdam Forum on the care of the live kidney donor. Transplantation. 2004;78:491–492.

第 137 章
器官分配的伦理学

Richard S. Luskin, Alexandra K. Glazier

引言

本章将研究一般伦理原则应用于死亡捐赠器官分配策略的发展,影响患者的优先级的其他因素;综述影响患者进入等待名单问题, 讨论器官分配策略和器官捐献之间的关系; 回顾影响器官分配策略的法律和监管因素。

器官移植的特殊性

分配稀缺资源在卫生保健系统中并不罕见。由于资金有限, 有些治疗方法公开定量配给作为一项政策来控制支出, 尤其是在那些政府作为主要或特定资助的国家。在这种情况下,专家小组对哪些治疗方法满足可接受的效益成本比做出选择。保险公司可能会通过更高的保险费、免赔额甚至不覆盖,或者要求使用通用药物或特定制造商的产品限制采用某些无效疗法。在其他例子中,治疗可能以实际方式间接分配,通过不平等途径获得医疗保健,以种族、教育程度、就业或保险状态或地理等因素决定。

然而, 器官移植是医疗实践唯一必须定量配给且明确独立于金融问题的领域。这是由于对该疗法的需求和可用的器官的供应之间的严重失衡。除非在防止终末期器官衰竭或移植器官的供应大幅增加方面有重大科研突破,这种供需失衡将持续下去。

血液透析的成功开发和推广在 20 世纪 60 年代为终末期肾病(ESRD)患者提供了救命疗法。然而缺乏可用透析机器和训练有素的工作人员决定了谁能接受这一疗法。在西雅图创建的所谓的“死亡委员会”评估患者接受血液透析的“价值”被《生活》杂志记载[1]。公众反感这种情况, 在某种程度上导致美国 ESRD 计划的制订,即提供医疗保险给所有需要的患者[2]。这种大量金融资源的注入部分解决了接受肾移植的问题, 但无法克服器官短缺。其他移植器官短缺(如肝脏、肺)相关的情况更加复杂, 这种复杂性由于缺少除移植以外广泛可接受的、有效的替代疗法而进一步加剧。这个残酷现实迫使医疗社区、公共政策的制订者、保险公司和公众面对谁应该活和谁应该死的艰难伦理和社会选择。

器官分配的伦理原则

由于资源的稀缺性, 每个国家或跨国的器官恢复和移植系统建立了器官的分配政策。在发展这些政策的过程中,有一些公认的基本伦理原则,虽然权重因历史、文化和政治而不同。这三个基本道德原则是:效用、公正(或公平)和自主(图 137.1)[3]。

效用

在器官分配的背景下,效用原则需要最大化,即“预期收益总体不错,同时最小化伤害”[3]。效用可以进一步细分为社会和医疗方面。社会效用评估潜在接受者通过评估接受移植手术后潜在的未来社会贡献。在民主社会,这类“价值”的评估不可避免是有争议的,因此通常在发展器官分配系统时不予考虑。器官获取和移植网络/联合网络器官共享伦理委员会(OPTN/UNOS):

“考虑一个人比另一个人对社会更有用,在主流社会价值观的基础上, 可能是选择的关键或自然随机分布的好运和社会培养人才和能力。当我们保留了移植的好处时,会对这些不能和有幸获得捐赠的人、一样造福社会的人造成侮辱性伤害”[3]。

医疗效用试图评估医学上“好”的移植对一个受者比另一个好。在医疗效用的保护下,至少有五个因素通常需要考虑:

• 患者生存—简单来说,这一标准提出疑问:到底有多少可能性,相对于其他同样等待移植器官的患者,

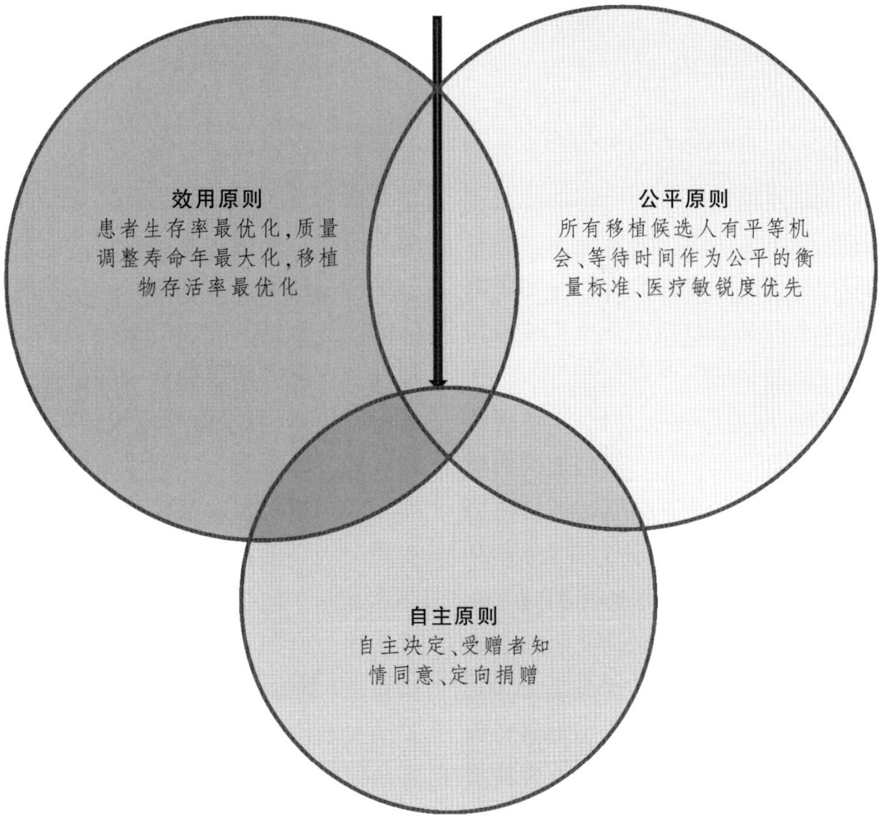

图 137.1　分配系统的设计是为了努力平衡这三项原则。

如果不接受移植，潜在受者将死亡？这一标准假设，给出确定的临床标准和特定的时间表时，可以相当准确地预测没有接受移植的死亡可能性。这也引出进一步的问题：是应该以拯救生命为目标，还是以最大化移植后受者期望生存年限为目标？例如，如果两个潜在受者不接受移植就无法生存的概率相同，但其中一个人有望在移植后活 3~5 年，而另一个是 8~10 年，如果按照"生存年限"增加来作为测量标准，为了最大化地利用移植肾，第二个患者是否应该优先接受移植？特定的器官分配系统通常寻求在这两个方面找到一个平衡，通过提供一个"分数"，既反映不接受移植死亡的可能性，也可反映移植后存活期的可能性。

• 移植物存活—除了受者的生存，分配系统也必须考虑移植物的存活。评估预期移植物生存必须考虑受者的健康状况和供者的特点：年龄、死因、死亡过程[脑死亡捐献（DBD）或心脏死亡捐献（DCDD）]、传染性疾病和（或）其他健康状况。效用概念中的移植物生存因素是移植预期提供医疗福利时间的衡量标准。

• 生存质量—近年来，政策制订者和临床医生试图使用"质量调整寿命年"（QALY）的概念评估临床干预措施的有效性。顾名思义，QALY 不仅评估患者和移植物存活的概率，同时也评估生存质量。尽管生活质量可以是一个非常主观的评估，但衡量标准通过各种状态之间的连续假设死亡=0 和完美健康=1[5]。因此，理论上可以对潜在的移植受者进行比较。例如，移植有望维持患者继续存活 6 年而不是在 1 年内死亡，但生活质量不同程度地低于理想状态，不管是等待移植期间还是移植后，可作如下估算：

• 6 年额外生存×0.7 生存质量=4.2
• 不到 1 年的生存时间×下降的生存质量(1–0.6)=0.4
• 临床干预导致的 QALY=3.8

在肾移植的情况下，QALY 往往通过比较患者接受 1 年透析的心理和生理健康认知和移植后 1 年的生存状态来计算。各种研究表明当比率为 0.8 时，移植是首选方案[6]。

• 替代疗法的可用性——功利主义为移植候选人建立优先级排名，同样需要考虑替代移植的可用性。最明显的例子是虽然血液透析和肾移植这两种治疗方法通常不被患者视为同等重要。同样，近年来越来越多地使用心脏辅助装置（CAD）使心脏移植候选人分配优先级变得更加复杂。在某些情况下,CAD已经不再是移植的过渡方案,而是最终治疗方法。

• 年龄——年龄似乎是最客观的变量，可以精确地确定,不需要主观判断或统计概率计算。然而,生理年龄并不一定等同于按时间顺序的年龄，因此使用年龄作为主观变量(如预期患者生存,预期移植物生存QALY)的替代评估标准会使情况变得复杂。分配政策中应用年龄作为效用因素，可能包括比较预期移植物生存和预期受者生存。如果移植物预期生存时间长于移植后受者生存,也许移植物应当差别分配,以实现移植物效用的最大化。例如,肾脏可以从一个健康的捐赠者获得且预计半衰期为20年,这个肾脏是应该移植给移植后预期寿命至少20年的更加年轻的受者呢?还是应移植给一个预期寿命只有10年的老年移植受者?在其他例子中,选择更加清晰。肾功能衰竭幼儿通过透析不能正常生长发育，因此大多数分配系统为优先为儿童提供肾移植。例如,在美国,≤35岁的合格捐献者的供肾优先分配给18岁以下的受者。这个政策有效地减少儿科患者的肾脏等待时间。然而,在分配策略的复杂性的示范过程中，伴随儿科患者的首次移植活体供肾数量的下降。首次活体供肾移植的儿科患者的数量也随之下降。怀疑一些现在医学上符合捐献条件的父母在孩子可能需要再移植时选择保留他们的肾脏[7]。

直觉上，器官分配的功利主义分析将寻求创建一种形势,即“每一个同种异体移植物移植到受体,移植物能够存活,但是只有几天。”[8]

与年龄谱相反形成对比的是欧洲移植高级项目(ESP),通常被称为“老人为老人”计划。ESP成立于1999年,寻求的是:

• 找到一个更有效的方式，利用越来越多的来自年龄超过65岁的捐献者的肾脏，减少65岁以下肾移植候选人的等待时间。

• 减少65岁以上老人肾移植的等待时间。

回顾性分析ESP后的最初五年证明,这些实用目标通过所有年龄段的移植患者肾脏移植总数增加而得以实现[9]。

后文我们将看到，使用年龄作为分配依据必须仔细考量法律禁止年龄歧视作为权衡背景。

公正原则

公正观念是用来平衡效用观念的。有时被描述为公平或正义，器官分配的公正原则认可存在着必须考虑在内的其他标准(对大多数群体来说很重要)。一般来说,一个分配系统,重视效用高于一切可能不会被社会视为最公平或最合理。如果一个人只关注效用,那么优先级可能转到:年轻患者;具有稳定、完整的家庭能够支持他们完成手术和恢复、有保险的患者(或个人)。公平方面的考量可能导致有限缩短等待时间和减低疾病的严重程度,因为预期移植效果较好(对某些疾病)。这样的分配方案可能会导致穷人、受教育程度较低、未就业或失业,以及医疗保健较弱的人,例如少数民族受到区别对待。

因为捐赠器官被认为是一种用于公众利益的公共资源，大多数社会寻求为纯粹效用因素提供一些平衡以满足基本的公平。公正原则的某些方面相对容易达成共识。例如,所有其他条件相同的情况下(预期患者生存、预期移植物生存等)——通常是同意等待时间最长的患者应该优先于那些等待时间较短的患者。但是等待时间也可能是有争议的。首先,一个人必须达成一个共同的“零时间点”——当一个患者在临床上准备好接受移植的时刻。即使这是可能的,等待时间是严重依赖于患者涉及移植程序零点后的时间点评估，接受移植及确实在等待名单上。大量研究表明,患者转诊时间和移植中心等待名单的等待时间差异很大[10]。

其他有关评估患者等待时间的因素包括:

• 患者是否曾被提供而且之前拒绝肾脏或肝脏,因为他们想等待一个更理想的捐赠者?

• 患者的等待时间是否已经延长，由于等待名单未激活时期,使其适合移植的临床治疗方案失败?(等待时间一般持续积累即使患者在名单上没有被激活)。

另一个更加复杂的例子涉及的是，等待肾移植的患者对人口的很大比例是“敏感”的。这些移植候选人可能由于输血、生孩子或前一个移植使其更难找到一个可接受的捐献者。因此大多数分配系统为伴有PRA的肾移植患者提供了一定的优先权。然而,即使一个分配系统拥有额外的考虑因素,高PRA患者仍然可能没有“公平”获得移植的机会,而且他们的移植器官生存可能和这些不敏感的患者不一样[11]。

当人们考虑每个人都应该有机会拥有完整生活,结婚、生孩子、为社会做贡献的观念时,年龄可成为和效用一样的考虑因素。这已被称为“公平局的论点”,所有其他因素不变的情况下,年轻的候选人应优先,因为他们没有和老年候选人相同的生活机会[12]。根据这一理论，一个20岁的移植候选人优先级将高于70岁高龄的移植候选人。已有很多提议建议使用对年轻人较高的分数点来提供额外的移植途径，虽然减少相当迅速，但相比于各年龄段的老年候选人，可继续提供一些对年轻候选人相对优先的考虑因素[3]。

自主原则

自主原则是一个很明了的观念，即每个人都有自主做出决定的权利[3]。尽管自主原则在许多医疗决策中是首要的伦理原则，但相对于效用和公平原则，自主原则在器官分配中较少扮演直接作用。自主原则通常在器官分配中支持潜在受者拒绝移植或拒绝提供特定器官移植权利时考虑较多，例如基于捐献者的医疗因素。自主原则的应用是受者对移植过程的知情同意的必要组成部分。但是请注意，这只是影响分配的间接因素。一个特定器官的分配决定应按照政策且只有优先受者通过自主决定拒绝时，移植器官将提供给下一个符合分配方案的潜在受者。

另一个在器官分配中需要考虑的自主因素是是罕见的，但具有更直接的影响力，即捐献者对特定受者的直接捐献。在美国，国家法律《统一解剖捐赠法案》和国家系统建立的联邦法律《国家器官移植法案》都明确允许器官捐赠者（或其委托代理人）直接捐赠给特定受者，如果捐赠的器官是兼容的且能够移植给受者[13]。如果做出定向捐赠的决定，随后捐赠的器官将移植给特定受者且不考虑受者的分配优先级。如果特定受者实际存在于等候名单并具有生物兼容性，来自已故捐赠人的直接捐赠只会被促成，因为这属于罕见的事件。尽管如此，它突出了自主原则的重要性是一致的，考虑到直接捐赠完全绕过了分配方案。

法律和监管因素影响器官分配策略

普遍认为器官是社会资源，意味着“公共利益”应明智而审慎地使用。在大多数国家，有法律、法规为器官分配政策的发展提供指南。

美国

1984年，美国采取了P.L.98-507，即《国家器官移植法案》（NOAT），建立了美国器官获取和移植网络（OPTN）的基础。NOAT包括提供开发和操作OPTN建议的工作小组和负责器官移植获得授权的工作小组：

“确保患者公平获得器官移植和保证捐赠器官在有资质开展器官移植的不同移植中心和患者间公平分配。”

工作组报告[14]提出许多有关在发展器官分配政策中应该应用的原则建议。包括：

1. 捐赠器官（应该）被认为是用于公共利益的国家资源；公众必须参与决定如何使用这些资源以实现公共利益的最佳服务[14]。

2. 为等候名单和分配器官选择患者必须是基于医疗标准的。由广泛代表性的群体考虑需求和成功概率来发展。选择在其他方面具有同样资质的患者应基于等待名单上等待时间[14]。

3. 为受者有限安排器官移植应基于客观医疗标准，如HLA匹配，受者个体的兼容性，或等待名单上的时间，是公认的和被广泛接受的。其他标准，如需要的紧迫性、年龄、生活方式、社会支持的存在，或需要再次移植必须个体化并小心实施，从而反映医疗判断而不是社会价值判断[14]。

4. 器官共享项目……必须在有效、高效使用器官、公正及授权器官共享影响的利益上实施，必须不断地评估以识别和纠正可能会减少任何群体的获得的失衡[14]。

虽然OPTN制订的器官分配政策在1988年开始实施，美国器官分配政策的官方联邦监管框架直到2000年采用“最后准则”时才建立[15]。最后准则的关键部分是呼吁建立“在潜在受者中公平分配尸体器官”的政策：

- 基于良好的医学判断。
- 寻求实现捐赠器官的最佳使用。
- 旨在避免浪费器官，避免无效移植，促进患者获得移植机会，促进器官处理的高效管理。
- 不基于候选人的居住地或等候名单上的排名位置。
- 在广泛的地理区域分配器官是可行的（如上所述）……为了减少医疗紧急情况。。

美国监管体系是由OPTN提出。NOTA需要美国政府与私有的、非盈利机构合作开展OPTN的日常管理。这包括保持所有等待移植患者的等候名单存在于美国移植中心。OPTN合作自成立以来，一直由器官共享联合网络持有（UNOS）。除了规定哪项分配政策在原有基础上需要发展,OPTN 最终条例还明确 OPTN 将寻求从移植中心、器官获取组织(OPO)、组织相容性实验和公众方面输入分配政策。

分配政策是复杂的,且可随时发生变化,以应对监管要求和上述一般伦理原则,同时促进不同的患者群体中分配影响的了解。肾移植候选人通常根据等待时间分级排列,并对儿科患者、高度敏感的患者、患者HLA与捐赠者高度匹配及以前活体捐献的患者进行特殊考虑。肾外器官移植候选人的优先级是根据疾病的严重程度、不接受移植死亡的可能性或移植后生存期至少1年来排列。分配政策旨在尝试平衡公平和效用原则,已经逐渐开始拓展共享领域。

虽然受到最终条例的限制,在实践中地理位置的确影响了器官分配。这是历史分配模式的功能之一,美国国土面积和美国50个州政府及联邦政府的政治结构的性质是器官运输和保存的实际限制因素。美国是三级分配体系,有58个当地OPO服务领域,11个地区和国家的等候名单。一般而言,器官首先提供给在OPO协调恢复的区域内的移植中心中、医学上符合条件的患者。如果在区域内没有合适的受者,随后可用的器官将提供OPO地区内的受者,然后在全国范围内。当地不使用的胸部器官将提供给医院方圆500英里(约800千米)的地区。这些规则之外的特殊案例是用来为最严重的患者提供改善。

欧洲国家器官储运组织(ET)

ET负责捐献器官在奥地利、比利时、克罗地亚、德国、匈牙利、卢森堡、荷兰和斯洛文尼亚的分配。其分配政策立场声明[16]包括:

• 应确保其责任内的器官分配是由临床和伦理原则指导,而且分配规则由合适的委员会明确定义,基于公平和透明的原则,并符合成员国国内规定。

• ET将根据认可和透明的医疗标准(迹象、需要、紧迫性)接收移植等待名单上的患者。分配可用的器官将主要依据临床标准(需要、紧迫性和匹配程度、有关器官捐赠者和接受者其他方面的因素)和累计等待时间,考虑伦理原则但不考虑个人、社会或金融背景。

• ET在国际跨国协作和器官交换的基础上发挥作用,参与国的分配程序必须考虑每个国家内部团结的原则(通过一个相互同意平衡系统实现)。

实际上,器官分配基于两个基本原则:

1. 预期结果

2. 紧迫性(由专家以客观透明的方式来决定)

同样考虑:

1. 参与国家之间的合理平衡

2. 移植候选人的等待时间

分配的优先顺序由相关专业专家委员会决定。

西班牙

西班牙国家移植系统的协调[17]是由Organización Nacional de Trasplantes(ONT)执行,ONT是西班牙卫生部和消费者事务部的一个职能部门。与美国类似,存在三级分配体系。分配的主要单位是在医院和移植中心层面,然后在该地区其他移植中心(有六个),然后在全国范围内。如果没有受者,供器官随后将提供给欧洲其他器官移植中心。与美国不同的是,每个移植中心都有自己的医疗标准应用于其等待患者的器官分配排序。

英国

血液和移植国家健康服务部门(NHSBT)负责匹配和分配捐赠器官[18]。器官分配规则是由医学专家与其他卫生专业人员咨询、卫生部及专家咨询小组协商决定:

"所有来自心脏死亡供体的肾脏根据国家分配系统分配。这基于五个层面:

1. 儿童完全匹配——难以匹配患者

2. 儿童完全匹配——其他人

3. 成人完成匹配——难以匹配患者

4. 成人完成匹配——其他人和良好匹配的儿童

5. 所有其他符合条件的患者(成人和儿童)。

A和B层内,儿童优先,根据他们的等待时间。在剩下的层面,患者优先排序根据分数点来决定,即器官分配给分数点最高的患者。患者的得分是基于很多因素的:

1. 等待时间(有利于等待时间最长的患者)。

2. 组织匹配和年龄相结合(有利于良好匹配的年轻患者)。

3. 捐赠者和患者之间的年龄差异(有利于年龄匹配接近的患者)。

4. 患者相对于捐赠者的位置(有利于位置较近的患者,为了减少肾脏的运输时间)。

5. 其他有关患者的血型匹配和组织类型罕见程度的三个因素"。

肾外器官分配主要结合患者病情严重程度、获取位置、等待时间及移植中心之间的平衡。

进入移植等待名单

另一个显著影响稀缺器官如何分配的关键因素是移植。所有的潜在受者都必须接受移植中心团队的仔细评估，以评估移植的医疗必要性和适当性。一般来说，患者不能独立评估移植应考虑的因素。因此患者必须依靠他们的初级保健提供者推荐移植程序。没有这样的推荐和积极评估，患者无法进入死者捐赠名单。除了移植候选人的预期医疗评估，移植中心也评估其他因素，患者遵照移植后护理的可能性，包括采取必要的免疫抑制药物，避免其他行为损害患者和移植器官。其中的几个因素讨论如下。

引起器官衰竭的“自毁”行为

已有明确证明某些行为与获得某种疾病的可能性有关。例如，吸烟与癌症和心脏病、肥胖和糖尿病、久坐不动的生活方式与心脏病、酒精和药物滥用与肝病。卫生从业人员一定要试图改善患者的自毁行为，从而将患病的风险降到最低。这里存在一个罕见问题，即是否应该提供所有适当的治疗，即使患者的行为导致了疾病状态。然而，当“自毁”行为和移植需求之间存在明显原因/效果关系，就会产生关于让这些患者进入等候名单的适当性的问题。

因为器官短缺，临床医生和伦理学家对如何最好地处理这种情况的患者已有争论。争论的一部分不可避免地涉及患者接受移植(作为一种稀缺资源)的“价值”。为酗酒者进行肝移植是一个经常被引用的例子。讨论的一部分涉及患者是否应该对他们的酗酒行为负责，或者如果它就像任何其他疾病一样是一个疾病。一般来说，移植群体不关注患者是否有错，而是在确定移植成功的可能性。

临床医生必须考虑患者的当前行为和患者移植后将改变其生活方式的可能性，以避免这些行为减少移植物和患者的生存。结果，大多数移植程序要求患者通过诸如戒烟、减肥等展示他们的依从性。对有酒精或药物滥用史的患者，大多数移植中心需要最少 6 个月禁欲视为患者有能力依从移植后程序的迹象。最近，有人认为在某些情况下，6 个月的“规则”应该放松[19]。然而，其他人则指出，“由于器官短缺，我们不能以任意方式选择候选人，那样不能获得公众的认可。”[20]

再次移植

2009 年在美国，14%的肾移植、7.6%的肝移植和 4.0%的心脏移植患者进行了再次移植[21]。自最早的器官分配讨论以来，由于获得一个以上的移植和获得再次移植的优先权产生了一些争论。1984 年美国器官移植专题小组注意到争论集中在那些认为应限制患者的单次移植和那些相信这一政策将构成“抛弃”患者的观点之间。工作组认为医学判断应该是决定性因素，而不是以前接受过移植的事实。随后争论和政策决定继续这一想法。

从功利主义的角度来看，移植的器官拯救了一条生命与它拯救了什么样的生命无关。除了受者故意导致移植失败的情况下(如未能服用免疫抑制药)，移植失败不是患者的“错”。移植失败的主要原因是免疫或偶尔的外科技术错误，这是患者无法控制的事件。在某些情况下，再次移植候选人实际上是优先级提高而不是下调。例如，肝移植受者在 7 天内移植失败的患者是最高优先级的候选人之一[22]。

其他人建议为实施患者再次移植的能力会增加器官的可用性。如果移植中心知道——若有必要——他们无法为其患者获得第二个器官，他们不太可能使用“边缘性”或“扩大”的器官捐赠者。

地理位置和多重登记

患者居住位置影响移植中心将其列入等候名单和其一旦进入名单后获得器官的可能性。因素包括:

- 移植中心接近患者的居住地。
- 当地医生涉及患者移植评估的实践能力。
- 移植中心使用的医疗和社会筛选标准决定是否列入一个患者。
- 当地器官获取组织获取器官的数量，这是该地区捐赠潜在可能性和 OPO 的效率的职责。
- 分配策略。

在一些国家——通常这些国家是支付系统单一的国家(如西班牙)，患者被分配到特定的移植中心，在特殊情况下除外。然而，在美国患者不仅可在任何中心自由加入等候名单，还被允许同时在多个中心加入名单。器官等待时间是公开的而且变化很大。教育程度高、资源丰富、有更好的保险和(或)较大的资金来源的患者有时选择在多个中心加入等待名单，以寻求较短的等待时间。事实上,多个地区等待时间较长的移植中心有时鼓励患者加入多个等候名单，如果他们认为自己无法及时获得一个器官以满足他们的需求。

这种行为不可避免地增加了关于公平性的问题，特别是当高调的人在远离家乡的移植中心相对更快地获得移植时[24]。进入多个名单排序的能力被质疑是不公平的,美国 OPTN 提议禁止它。然而,公众反对消除这一实践使其一直保持现状[25]。

国际患者旅行移植

以移植为目的的跨境旅行患者可能在等候名单实践中发挥作用,并在分配方案发挥潜在作用。以移植为目的的旅游患者应在移植专家广泛的国际合作背景下考虑实施,国家立法机关、世界卫生组织反对旅行移植[26]。这一努力的核心是普遍认可《伊斯坦布尔宣言》的器官贩卖和旅行移植声明[27]。“器官旅行移植”在声明中定义如下:

“器官移植旅行是器官、捐赠者、受者或移植专业人员为移植目的而进行的跨越司法管辖区的流动。如果器官移植旅行涉及器官非法交易和(或)器官移植商业化,或者致力于向外国患者提供移植的资源(器官、专业人员和移植中心),削弱了该国为本国人口提供器官移植服务的能力，那么器官移植旅行就变成了器官移植旅游业。”

“器官移植旅行”区别的相关性是额外的非公民移植候选人是否损害东道国服务本国人口移植需要的能力。国家自给自足是《伊斯坦布尔宣言》的核心原则。具体来说,“司法机构、国家和地区应努力实现器官捐献和移植的自给自足，为来自国内或通过地区合作的需要移植的居民提供足够数量的器官。”呼吁自给自足包括这一概念,即治疗来自国外或管辖地区的患者是可接受的,如果它不损害东道国服务本国人口移植需要的能力[28]。

甚至在 1986 年,外国人到美国旅行移植的问题就饱受争议，当时美国死亡器官捐献短缺相比于今天是不同的,且数量级较小。激烈的辩论后,移植工作小组建议“每个中心非移民外国人肾移植受者不应占总数的 10%以上”[14]。相当少数的工作组成员同意一份例外声明,大意上是说肾脏不应该被提供给非居民外国人,除非无法找到另一个符合条件的美国公民受者[14]。“救命”器官的移植问题,如为暂住外国人进行心脏和肝脏移植也得到解决,工作组建议“不应该提供额外的肾器官移植给非移民外国人，除非已经确定不能找到其他合适的受者”。[14]

UNOS 在 OPTN 获奖之后,它考虑采用项目组建议的政策并委托移植项目的活动评估任务给一个特别的国际委员会，即任意器官非居民外国人受者的比例不得超过 10%。1994 年，阈值百分比改为 5%。鉴于 NOTA 要求用于器官分配只有医疗标准,“5%规则”并没有从等候名单禁止移植中心为 5%以上非居民外国人移植。相反,“5%规则”是触发审计的一个阈值。2012 年 6 月,OPTN/UNOS 董事会投票决定消除“5%规则”以支持一项新政策，即要求收集信息并公开报告所有非居民和非公民移植候选人和受者的[29]。这个新政策的目标是提供美国公众，是美国所有可获取的死者捐献器官的来源，以一定程度的透明度关于死亡捐献器官是如何分配给外国人的。

尽管美国法律明确限制利用公民或绿卡作为分配因素，但国际患者的移植在许多场合引起了公众的质疑,质疑允许这类患者进入等候名单的公平性,而很多本国人在等待过程中死亡。移植专家还指出,前往美国移植旅游的患者可能等待时间更短，虽然患者到达时的病情对这种差别负有主要责任[31]。最终,国际患者旅行移植的问题可能没有直接参与分配，而是例证有关分配政策和实践的透明度是有效器官捐献和移植系统证公众信任度的关键组成部分。

器官分配政策和决定捐赠之间的关系

局部分配优先是否鼓励了器官捐赠?

1984 年工作小组报告描述捐赠器官为“国家资源”。2000 年在美国实施的“最终条例”要求器官分配“不基于候选人的居住地或排名,除非必要情况下……”

- 支持良好的医学判断。
- 实现捐赠器官的充分利用。
- 避免移植器官的浪费或无效移植。
- 促进患者获得移植。
- 促进器官分配的高效管理[32]。

然而，当前分配系统仍然为当地器官获取组织附属移植中心的受者提供高度优先权，虽然移植最初发展时情况属实。在一些欧洲国家存在类似的安排,尽管地理区域明显变小。也存在明显的例外,比如对病情最严重的患者和高度敏感的肾病患者广泛共享。

局部分配优先的最初理由主要基于以下几个原则:

• 保持器官局部减少冷缺血时间以恢复和改善移植预后。

• 移植专家不太愿意获取器官，如果他们实际上不太可能有机会移植他们获取的器官。

• 器官捐赠将会减少，因为如果器官不用于自己的社区或附近,人们会不太愿意捐献。

广泛共享会减少较小移植中心的移植手术数量,最终使他们不能生存,从而减少患者获得移植建议,大大增加共享范围有时导致激烈的政策辩论。1998 年最终条例发布后的这样一个关于肝脏分配的建议导致美国国会和州立法机构采取行动以保护本地优先。医学研究所(IOM)接受委托研究其影响。其报告[33]如下：

• 建议扩大本地共享区域。

• 发现缺乏足够的数据来得出影响移植效果的结论。

• 没有数据显示捐献率减少。

• 发现迹象表明花费会增加，但也不是那么明显大于收益。

• 没有发现确凿的证据表明较小的中心将关闭,如果他们的确关闭,对患者会有很大的负面影响。

1998 年的一项关于器官捐赠的盖洛普民意调查包括这样一个问题——问题 4:

思考如果你要成为一名器官捐献者，在捐献器官提供给在美国其他地方的患者之前，如果你知道你的器官会移植给本地区的患者,你会更有可能想捐赠、不太可能想捐赠,或者对你的决定无关紧要?

作为回应,报告指出:

……大多数成年人认为这不会影响他们的决定。然而,32%的人说如果他们知道器官受者是病情严重的患者,不管地理位置如何,他们将更愿意捐献器官。相比之下,10%的人表示,如果他们知道他们的器官捐给当地的患者,他们会更愿意捐献器官。同样值得注意的是,那些签署了器官捐赠卡的器官受者或候选人,或捐赠器官或骨髓的人最倾向于说潜在器官受者的位置不会影响他们的捐献决定[33]。

因此,可以说没有实证支持局部分配会增加捐献率。

注册捐赠者是否应得到器官分配的优先权?

虽然通常是拒绝将社会价值作为器官分配优先级的基础,但也存在明显的例外。在美国,一个患者之前是重要器官或部分重要器官的活体捐献者，他们自己随后成为移植候选人时应该被给予更高的优先级。有人认为，这种相对分配优先级概念应该扩展到给予这些以前注册成为死亡器官捐赠者的人优先权。

2006 年,美国卫生和人类服务部/卫生资源和服务管理局要求国际移民组织[35]检查增加器官捐赠的可能方式,一种深入考虑的观点认为应给予捐献者优先权。主要的支持参数是:

• 符合公平原则。由于器官资源有限,有必要定量分配器官。对于那些需要器官的受者和愿意主动捐献的供者,优先选择时需要遵循伦理平等。

• 假设可以增加供者数量以增加移植供器官。通过提升社会责任感和责任共享意识，这样的政策理论上能够增加供器官的数量,满足社会的需求。

• 与其他增加捐献的计划不同（如为葬礼支付费用、抵偿税务信用等),愿意成为供者和“回报”之间存在直接关系。器官移植是社会共同努力的行为,没有器官捐献,移植是无法完成的。

反对以上系统的主要理由如下：

• 注册成为器官捐献者是自愿的，同时可以获得相应利益,要让社会大众知晓这两件事,大众教育是必须的。但是,那些不能正常获取医学治疗的穷困人群、文盲群体和非英语母语人群可能因此不能获取这样的大众教育，不能利用这样的大众教育项目抓住成为器官供者的机会。

• 那些最需要器官的受者可能不成比例地注册为供者。如果这样的“反向选择”出现,由于实际可捐献器官人数不足,移植供器官的数量并不会增加。移植委员会指出,“任何程度的反向选择行为都会侵蚀个人出于强烈道德准则而做出的互动行为：对共同利益的重视和杜绝投机取巧行为的努力”[35]。

• 道德价值在确定移植行为中将具有重要作用,这样的互动性系统将促进这种作用变得更加重要。

• 尽管主要的宗教信仰支持器官捐献，一些人强烈地认为器官捐献是不恰当的行为。因此,这样的互动性系统可能禁不住为杜绝对宗教和其他事物的歧视而出台的法律条例的考验。

尽管实际问题或许可以解决，成功的可能性极大，此时IOM委员会的建议可能需要重新评估，但委员会仍反对建立有偏向性的系统[35]。

反对将供者优先化的主要原因是可解决的。尽管一些原因确实重要，其他原因克服起来并不困难。比如，随着首个州立个人知情同意捐献注册处的成立，委员会提出的一些实际要求已经获得满足。随着自2010年以色列系统逐年的调整，现有的优先分配系统的实用性数据得以公开化。以色列的分配系统主要基于医学标准，当医学需求相同，以色列的分配系统优先选择已注册的供者。借助大众教育系统，在之前捐献率较低的国家，法律系统极大地增加了注册供者的数量[36]。

未来和总结

有关分配的争论很可能将继续下去，直到有临床突破：

- 大大增加来自死亡捐赠者器官供应。
- 大大减少对器官移植的需求。
- 提供替代疗法如人工替代器官的发展。

一些人认为同时实现效用最大化、效率、公平及可预测性是不可能的，而且任何这些因素在不损失自主权、争议、信任或活体捐赠的情况下，不太可能实现最大化。然而，每个国家或跨国器官分配系统继续努力在其政治体制、国民价值观和历史的背景下平衡这些因素。

（王建国 译　徐骁 校）

参考文献

1. Alexander S. They decide who lives, who dies: medical miracle and a moral burden of a small committee. *Life Magazine*. 9 November 1962:102–125.
2. Section 2991 of US Public Law 92-603. [accessed July, 2012]; Available from: https://www.cms.gov/Regulations-and-Guidance/Guidance/Manuals/downloads/eno114c1.pdf.
3. Veatch RM. Transplantation Ethics. Washington, D.C.: Georgetown University Press; 2000; and OPTN/UNOS Ethics Committee: Ethical Principles to be Considered in the Allocation of Human Organs. 2010 [accessed 28 December 2011]; Available from: http://optn.transplant.hrsa.gov/resources/bioethics.asp?index=10.
4. OPTN/UNOS Lung Allocation Score. [accessed 28 December 2011]; Available from: http://optn.transplant.hrsa.gov/.
5. Laupacis A, Keown P, Pus N, et al. A study of the quality of life and cost-utility of renal transplantation. Kidney International. 1996;50:235–242
6. Hornberger J, Ahn JH. Deciding eligibility for transplantation when a donor kidney becomes available. Medical Decision Making. 1997;17:160–170.
7. US Scientific Registry of Transplant Recipients. [accessed December 2011]; Available from: http://www.srtr.org/.
8. Segev DL. Evaluating options for utility-based kidney allocation. American Journal of Transplantation. 2009;9:1513–1518.
9. Frei U, Noeldeke J, Marchold-Fabrizii V, et al. Prospective age-matching in elderly kidney transplant recipients—a 5-year analysis of the Eurotransplant Senior Program. American Journal of Transplantation. 2008;8:50–57.
10. Kucirka LM, Grams ME, Balhara KS, et al. Disparities in provision of transplant information affect access to kidney transplantation. American Journal of Transplantation. 2012;12:351–357.
11. Lefaucheur C, Suberbielle-Boissel GS, Hill D, et al. Clinical relevance of preformed HLA donor-specific antibodies in kidney transplantation. American Journal of Transplantation. 2008;8:324–331.
12. Harris J. The Value of Life, an Introduction to Medical Ethics. London: Routledge & Keegan Paul; 1970.
13. Uniform Anatomical Gift Act, Section 11. 2006 [accessed 18 February 2012]; Available from: http://uniformlaws.org; and National Organ Transplantation Act 1984 [42 U.S.C. 273 et seq].
14. Organ Transplantation: Issues and Recommendations, Report of the Task Force on Organ Transplantation, US Dep't of Health & Human Services; April, 1986, 86–137.
15. US Code of Federal Regulations Title 42, Part 121. [accessed 12 January 2014]; Available from: http://www.gpo.gov/fdsys/granule/CFR-2011-title42-vol1/CFR-2011-title42-vol1-part121.
16. EuroTransplant. [accessed 29 February 2012]; Available from: http://www.eurotransplant.org.
17. Personal Communication Matesanz R, MD, Director *Organización Nacional de Trasplantes*. January 2, 2012.
18. NHS Blood and Transplant. [accessed February 29, 2012]; Available from: http://www.organdonation.nhs.uk/ukt/about_transplants/organ_allocation/kidney_(renal)/kidney_(renal).jsp.
19. Mathurin P, Moreno C, Samuel D, et al. Early liver transplantation for severe alcoholic hepatitis. New England Journal of Medicine. 2012;365(119):1790–1800.
20. Brown RS Jr. Transplantation for alcoholic hepatitis—time to rethink the 6-month "rule". New England Journal of Medicine. 2012;365(119):1836–1838.
21. OPTN/SRTR 2010 Annual Data Report. [accessed 20 February 2012]; Available from: http://optn.transplant.hrsa.gov. These rates of retransplantation for kidney and heart have been relatively stable over the past 10 years, while liver retransplantants are trending slightly downward.
22. US OPTN Policy 3.6.4.1. [accessed 20 February 2012]; Available from: HTTP://optn.transplant.hrsa.gov/policiesandbylaws.
23. Sheehy E, O'Connor KJ, Luskin RS, et al. Investigating geographic variation in mortality in the context of organ donation. American Journal of Transplantation. 2012;12(6):1598–1602.
24. Meckler L. Jobs transplant highlights differing wait times. *Wall Street Journal*. June 20, 2009, p. A14.
25. Executive Summary of the Minutes OPTN/UNOS Board of Directors Meeting. November 20–21, 2003 [accessed 24 February 2012]; Available from: http://optn.transplant.hrsa.gov/SharedContentDocuments/Executive_Summary_Nov._2003.pdf.
26. World Health Assembly. Fifty-seventh World Health Assembly Resolutions and Decisions: WHA 57.18: Human Organ and Tissue Transplantation. [accessed October 22, 2011]; Available from: http://apps.who.int/gb/ebwha/pdf_files/WHA57/A57_R1-en-res.pdf, 56–58.
27. Steering Committee of the Istanbul Summit. Organ trafficking and transplant tourism and commercialism: the Declaration of Istanbul. Lancet. 2008;372:5–6.
28. Delmonico F, Dominguez-Gil B, Matesanz R, et al. A call for government accountability to achieve national self-sufficiency in organ donation and transplantation. Lancet. 2011;371:1414–1418.
29. OPTN/UNOS board of directors meeting: executive summary of the minutes. June 25–26, 2012, Richmond, Virginia. [accessed December 20, 2013]; Available from: http://optn.transplant.hrsa.gov/SharedContentDocuments/ExecutiveSummary_0612.pdf
30. Glionna JM and Ornstein C. Japanese Gang Figures got new livers. *LA Times*. May 30, 2008.
31. Schol JD, Meier-Kriesche HU, Duncan RP et al. Deceased donor kidney and liver transplantation to nonresident aliens in the United States. Transplantation. 2007;84(123):1548–56; Freeman R. Transplant tourism in the United States? Transplantation. 2007;84(12):1559–60.
32. Allocation of Organs 121.8. [accessed December 20, 2013]; Available from: http://www.gpo.gov/fdsys/pkg/CFR-2011-title42-vol1/pdf/CFR-2011-title42-vol1-sec121-8.pdf.
33. Committee on Organ Procurement and Transplantation Policy. IOM Organ Procurement and Transplantation. Washington, D.C.: National Academy Press; 1999: 48.
34. US OPTN Policy 3.5.11.6. [accessed February 20, 2012]; Available from: HTTP://optn.transplant.hrsa.gov/policiesandbylaws.
35. Childress JF, Liverman CT, editors. Organ donation: Opportunities for Action. Washington, D.C.: National Academies Press; 2006: 257–258.
36. Orfi D. In Israel, a new approach to organ donation. *The New York Times*. February 16, 2012.

第 138 章 活体器官捐献伦理学

Alice Peng，Andrew Klein

摘要

需要器官移植来挽救生命的患者的数量，与来自死亡捐献者所捐献的器官的数量之间的缺口越来越大，这促使了活体器官捐献的发展。肾脏是活体捐献最多的器官，而肝脏和肺脏的捐献者也在逐步增加。不同国家的文化以及公益政策的差异也极大地影响了器官捐献成功率。在美国，从死亡捐献者获得的器官数量缺乏，受者等待时间延长，非亲属活体捐献的广泛接受，以及媒体和网络的影响都大大增加了伦理思考的复杂性。在活体捐献器官移植方面的许多政策和实践仍存在争议并在不断完善。本章我们将对活体捐献方面的一些伦理思考进行探讨。在美国，尽管有许多捐献相关的伦理问题还在讨论，但是伦理指导方针还是被广泛接受的。这些方针的其他一些解释可见第 136 章。

实施过程的风险和获益

在美国，健康的活体捐献者承担由器官摘取手术所带来的风险和创伤以及自己失去一个器官的风险去帮助受者。在道德领域，如果预期的获益超过受到的创伤，那么活体捐献者捐献肾脏是可以接受的。这种情况下，活体肾脏捐献者可以收获心理和道德上的褒奖，这种褒奖重于其由于捐献器官而带来的短期或者长期风险。在活体捐献的概念上，仍然有许多需要关注的问题。正如活体捐献肾脏移植的先驱——Frances Moore 博士[1]所说：

活体捐献器官移植是一个特殊的外科领域，它诠释了一些医学和手术护理方面古老的基本原则：不去伤害并且把帮助患者当作帮助自己。当器官从健康捐献者身上获取时，他们作为健康人的福利也面临威胁，而这种福利在人类医学史上是从未牺牲过的。

因为这些关注点以及这样一个观念——如果供体和受体亲属关系稳固，那么由捐献器官所带来的风险是可以承受的，早期的活体捐献主要是亲属捐献。对结局的顾虑和对商业化的担忧使非亲属捐献者从一开始就会失去捐献的勇气。随着肾脏移植效果的改善以及移植受者筛选标准的放宽，等待移植的患者的数量增加并且等待时间延长。大量研究表明，接受亲属捐献活体肾移植和非亲属捐献活体肾移植的患者的效果是相似的[2]。这就使得活体捐献肾脏移植，尤其是非亲属活体捐献肾脏移植的数量得到了大幅提高。2009 年，美国有 38%的移植肾脏是来源于活体捐献者，这其中的 23%为非亲属活体捐献[3]。一项针对捐献者的调查显示：当再次问捐献者是否愿意捐献时，他们都能做出跟第一次相同的决定。并且，其中的一些人确实收获了更高的自尊，以及这项善举带给他们的满足感[4-6]。

在活体器官捐献中，其中一项伦理指导方针是非强迫性的。捐献者捐献器官必须是自愿的并且他们有完全的自主权，他们可以在捐献过程的任何时间选择退出而不需要承担任何后果。对于退出捐献的原因，媒体和其他参与者必须保密。在整个捐献过程中，捐献者的意向和自主权是最重要的，但只有这两点是不够的。一个捐献者的意愿从来不能凌驾于医学判断以及决策制订之上。

活体器官捐献的主要医疗风险和器官获取手术的过程直接相关。调查显示，活体肾脏捐献供体的围手术期死亡风险是 0.3‰[7,8]。然而，肾脏切取手术技术的进步，尤其是作为供体肾切除术首选的微创手术的发展，大大缩短了供体的住院时间，使他们能够更早地回归正常生活。很多研究已经对肾脏捐献以后供体的长期生存状态进行评估。部分研究发现，在他们当中，高血压和非进展性微量蛋白尿的发病风险会升高[9-11]。然而，疾病相关死亡率(捐献者为白种人)和普通大众相似[12]。肾脏捐献以后，终末期肾病(ESRD)的发病率(0.1%~1.1%)有轻度升高[12-16]。尽管最近的分析表明，肾脏捐献以后终末期肾病的发病率增高与普通人群中ESRD发病率升高相似[18]，但年轻的黑种人捐献者中，ESRD的发病风险明显升高[17]。先兆子痫的发生率也会轻度增加[19]。其他一些与捐献器官相关的问题包括，更高的参保费用或者更容易被医疗保险公司拒绝参保，而且可能长期承担经济后果。然而，从总体来讲，活体捐献者肾切除术是安全的，基本没有围手术期死亡，无术后并发症，也不会带来长期的不良后果。

在2007年，一位活体捐献者将丙肝病毒和人类免疫缺陷病毒(HIV)出乎意料地传染给了受者，这一事件引出了活体捐献肾脏移植的另一独特的伦理问题[20]。存在使感染丙肝病毒和HIV的风险增高的相关行为的活体捐献者引出了这一特殊的伦理关注，因为供体和有意向接受移植的受体是有一定联系的。在这种情况下，供体的隐私权和受体的知情同意权之间就会产生直接的冲突。并且，揭露这些风险性的行为对供体和受体都会产生心理上的创伤。针对这一问题，当前还没有统一的指导方针。一些人建议在捐献者同意的前提下将这些行为上的危险因素告诉受者，或者干脆认定这样的捐献者在从医学角度上讲是不能接受的。然而，其他人却在质疑这些建议的伦理性[21]。

由于大众人口统计资料的变更以及受者等待时间的延长，许多移植中心放宽了活体捐献者的纳入标准。捐献者的评估以及筛选标准发生了很大的变化[22]。在许多评选标准中，高龄、高血压、肥胖、肾结石以及糖耐量受损不再是肾脏捐献者的排除指标。2008年，肥胖者占活体捐献者的19.5%，有高血压病史者占2.0%，尿蛋白阳性者占3.5%，这些都是已知的心血管系统疾病和肾脏疾病的危险因素[16]。最近的一项数据回顾(数据来自于移植受者科学注册表)表明在1999—2009年的10年间，活体肾脏捐献者的临床特征在不断发生变化，即高龄、肥胖、高血压捐献者的数量在稳步提升[23]。其他的入组标准仍在研究中，包括肾小球滤过率处于临界值的捐献者以及为符合纳入标准而减肥的肥胖者。这些不断变化的标准对捐献者的长期影响尚不可知。更好地理解这些变化所产生的的影响需要对活体捐献者进行持续广泛的长期随访，尤其是对非白种人捐献者，以便确定这些临床实践的安全性以及更全面地告知活体捐献候选者。

捐献者随访

值得注意的是，并不是所有的器官移植中心都要求活体捐献者拥有医疗保险，尽管这些不同与国家的差异明显相关，例如在美国，它的医疗保险不会提供全面的健康覆盖。一项调查显示，美国15%的器官移植中心报道他们将排除没有医疗保险的捐献者，另有42%的中心认为没有医疗保险是作为器官捐献者的相对禁忌证[24]。一项2008年的报道称有12.2%的捐献者没有医疗保险，这其中包括14.9%的黑种人捐献者和17.0%的西班牙裔捐献者[16]。另一项2004—2006年的调查发现年轻的捐献者、男性捐献者以及少数民族捐献者的无保险率更高[11]。已经有研究表明这些捐献者肾脏捐献后的长期并发症发生率更高，尤其是35岁以下的男性黑种人捐献者[17]，并且没有医疗保险会对他们长期参加随访的依从性产生明显的负面影响。由此我们可以推断，没有医疗保险的捐献者在进行预防性筛检以及监测肾功能和血压时会面临巨大的经济压力，这样就会潜在地增加高风险捐献者发生并发症的风险。由于全民医保方面政府政策缺乏改革，已有部分人建议终生免费全民医保。然而，这一提议在有偿捐献问题上引起了争议，而有偿捐献是联邦法律禁止的。

由于非直接捐献者、未参保的捐献者以及肥胖、高血压、糖耐量受损的捐献者数量的增加，人们开始意识到对捐献者进行长期医疗随访的重要性。这一认识促成了活体肾脏捐献者随访委员会的一份报告，这份报告记录了当前活体捐献者的生存状况，以便明确他们需要随访哪些项目，完成这些随访项目需要哪些条件，并进一步提出切合实际的方案。持续系统性地收集并报告捐献者的生存状况的原因包括：准确的生存状况信息是为了恰当的知情同意，尤其是涉及捐献者的种族划分和医疗条件时；反馈质量保证和性能改进；专业医务人员收集详细的捐献者生存状况信息；为提升评价过程和咨询非传统捐献候选者而收集更好的信息；监测识别捐赠问题[23]。为响应这一方案，美国器官移植网络/美国器官共享网络(OPTN/UNOS)扩充了已收集到的活体捐献者的数据并将捐献者术后随访时间强制延长到捐献术后两年。分析OPTN报告可以看出多数长期随访数据是不完整的，并且在2006年有30%的活体捐献者“失访”。

进一步的分析表明与获取医疗保险受限相关的许多因素以及可能的长期医疗风险(如非白种人、年轻、非美国公民、没有医疗保险)都可能与随访数据缺失有关。基于以上原因,OPTN/UNOS 活体捐献者数据收集小组总结道:“和当前收集的数据一样, 在随访截止时间提交 OPTN/UNOS 的数据也是不完整的……因此,为研究之目的或者得出关于活体捐献者安全性的结论是无意义的。”因此,尽管在捐献者纳入标准放宽的前提下, 器官捐献对捐献者健康的影响引发了越来越多的关注, 而且为准确评估活体肾脏捐献候选者同时完善知情同意的过程, 我们对捐献术后的医疗效果评估提出了迫切需求,但在美国,活体捐献者的随访仍然不是最佳的。当前有两项由美国国立卫生研究院赞助的研究——活体肾脏捐献者长期生存状况评估项目(ALTOLD)以及肾脏和肺脏活体捐献者评估研究项目(RELIVE),来评估活体捐献者的生存状况。尽管这两个项目存在很多限制因素,比如几乎没有少数民族参与者,但将有助于提供更详细的活体器官捐献者的生存状况分析[23]。

一项建议性的解决方案包含了建立活体捐献者登记表这一提议[25],这一提议与为建立一个监测活体捐献者的欧洲数据库而建立电子登记数据库模型的欧洲委员会发起的 EULID 项目很相似。EULID 项目的目的是建立一个围绕活体器官捐献者的有关法律、道德、保护和登记等实践的欧洲共识, 以便保证活体捐献者的健康和安全[26]。来自瑞士、巴基斯坦和巴西的活体捐献者长期随访数据强调,肾脏损伤的结果是很少的,而且即便有损伤也是可预防的。在瑞士,活体捐献长期随访登记表中捐献者的初诊医生也是随访的对象[23]。在这件事情上, 美国缺少国家卫生保健系统是其与欧盟成员国的最大不同。因此,最大的问题和关注点就是长期随访的成本和责任问题,尤其是那些超过两年的随访。如果没有额外的财政支持, 各移植中心不可能维持对捐献者的长期随访。一些人认为激励和处罚制度更充分地激发移植中心完成当前需要 OPTN /UNOS 完善的捐赠后续数据, 并且更多地激励捐献者对随访的依从性[25]。应该在捐献者评估时强调捐献者完成随访的重要性,这一过程要先于捐献实施。

利他主义

在美国, 只有利他的捐献是被允许的;《国家器官移植法案》禁止为获取财物补偿而捐献器官[27]。大多数的活体肾脏捐献者和受者或者存在生物学上的关联,或者存在“感情”上的关联——包括家人、配偶或者朋友。然而,有一些活体肾脏捐献者和受者在先前是没有关联的。利他主义是多数捐献者的主要动力。理想情况下,捐献者应该是完全自主的,没有受到任何外界压力的。利他主义包括若干类型,比如“无或低成本”利他主义, 指在不承担风险或者承担少量风险的情况下提供自己的资源给别人使其获益,例如输血。第二种形式为包含责任心的“尽责型”利他主义。在没有法律义务的情况下去捐献会使捐献者获得道德优越感。家庭成员捐献就是一个典型的例子, 家庭成员捐献被广泛认可是因为捐献者和受者在先前就有很亲密的关系。与非亲属捐献者相比, 传统的活体亲属捐献者会因为捐献而获得很高程度的心灵满足感, 但是他们通常或多或少地会有基于家庭关系学的被强迫感。第三种为“超额型” 利他主义, 指付出的比外界期待的或者要求的更多。和受者没有任何关系的捐献者属于这种类型[28]。目前,这种利他主义被移植群体广泛接受,而且最近的一项研究表明 94%的被调查的移植医生支持活体志愿者的非直接肾脏捐献[29]。该种利他主义的驱动力包括纯粹的利他主义感、宗教信仰、回馈社会的愿望或者帮助家人或朋友的愿望。

非直接捐献

准确评估和选择非直接捐献者需要多学科团队的支持,这些团队必须熟知活体捐献的并发症。每个移植项目都必须负责任地去监测所有的捐献者以确保整个捐献过程没有财物补偿、价值考量或者强制以及剥削性成分。捐献者必须有完全的自主权,提供完全自愿的知情同意。所有的活体捐献评估都包括与活体捐献倡导者见面。活体捐献倡导者的作用是确保每个捐献者都完全清楚捐献过程并且没有强制性存在。有些人建议这些倡导者应该具有否决权, 以便使其可以否决一个潜在的捐献者候选人，如果该倡导者认为该器官捐献不符合捐献者的自愿和利益。这样做的原因包括：捐献者不切实际的期待或者要求——移植不能排斥、不能失败；如联邦法律禁止的那样，想通过捐献获得财物补偿；期望获得媒体关注；将器官捐献看作减轻心灵疾病(如抑郁或者其他的潜在精神疾病)的方式；按照性别、人种或者种族来选择受者的愿望；或者捐赠之后希望介入受者的生活，而这种介入可能是受者不希望的[30]。非直接捐献者的医学评估是更加严格的，因为捐赠所获得的精神上的满足不容易被察觉到，尽管最近有报告说明，应该鼓励捐献器官给陌生人的利他主义活体捐献者获得精神上的满足[6]。

非直接活体器官捐献的受者需要通过多种方法来鉴定，包括主动向移植中心询问、通过网络或者通过第三方团体组织。捐献者和受者的关系通常是很弱的或者不存在的。在过去，不经过移植中心而配对受者的非直接捐献的活体捐献者通常是被拒绝的。这种情况下的一个主要潜在关注点就是器官捐献可能被商品化，而且这样的事例会被媒体大肆宣传。努力搜索出任何存在于非亲属活体捐献者和受者之间的强制性关系、财物补偿或者其他关联已经成为移植中心的责任，但是确切的评估方法尚无明确的定义。多数项目需要一个详细的心理评估，以便排除任何潜在的精神疾病，去评估一个人做出知情决策的能力，并且要试图去探索他们捐献的原因。在所有的活体器官捐献评估中，心理评估是常规需要做的，但它对非直接捐献者的评估尤为重要。如果发现捐献者和受者的关系是模糊不清的，那么移植中心需要做一个更深层次的心理评估。是否存在经济补偿可能是最难鉴定的一方面，因为捐献者和受者都可能欺骗移植中心。很多人体器官黑市交易的例子已经被媒体曝光，并促使一部分移植团队去倡议联邦政府去管制有偿器官捐献。有人暗示，在某些情况下，利他主义主导的活体非亲属器官捐献也是隐藏商业或者其他形式的强制的一个合法组成部分[31]。不幸的是，确定利他主义的检验和排除商业化的检验的效果都是微弱的。更严密的检验可能会去除一部分可被接受的活体捐献候选者，并且许多移植中心在不断地争论如何才能最有效地评估这些捐献者的动机。

在为非直接捐献者选择受者时，大多数移植项目一直沿用标准筛选法，该方法作为最符合道德的方法而一直应用于死亡捐献者肾脏的分配中[30]。然而，有人为了将成功的机会最大化，已经对传统的实践方法提出异议，例如排除二次移植者和有非依从史的患者。总之，各移植中心尚未允许非直接捐献者对潜在的受着的特征设定限制条件，这样就规避了种族歧视和性别歧视。一部分非直接捐献者通过第三方团体或者互联网来配对受者。有评论员指出这种无管理的状况将会有失公平，更有利于某些懂得操纵媒体和资源的受者。然而目前，许多这样的捐献者都接受过评估而且都是被接受的。

配对捐献

已有数条政策出台来增加活体捐献肾脏的数量，包括非直接活体捐献、放宽标准的活体捐献以及配对肾脏交换。Rapaport 于 1986 年最先提出配对肾脏交换理念[32]。这一想法涉及两对捐献者和受者，其中两位捐献者和他们各自配对的受者在免疫方面是不相容的，但和另一位配对的受者在免疫上是相容的。Rapaport 建议这两位捐献者的肾切除术可以同时进行，去除肾脏后立即将其互换然后移植给免疫相容的受者。互换肾脏这一过程可以用于克服血型和组织类型不相容的障碍，并能轻易增加移植数量。非直接活体器官捐献采纳了一项新的肾脏互换技术的发展，以增加活体捐献肾脏移植数量，即“封闭的开放性肾脏互换链”。值得注意的是，肾脏互换链会给捐献者和受者带来特殊的道德考量，因为他们都是开始于非直接捐献者[33]。从历史角度来讲，非直接捐献者将器官捐给了等待死亡器官捐献的受者。因此，肾脏互换链可能对等待死亡器官捐献的受者不利，因为使他们失去了接受活体器官移植的机会。在封闭的肾脏互换链中，后一位捐献者将肾脏捐给了等待死亡器官捐献的受者，但是，在开放的肾脏互换链中，该捐献者将从等待列表中被永久地去除。因为配对互换和互换链给受者提供了帮助，该受者会在互换中提供一个活体捐献的肾脏，但这些策略可能被认为是违反 NOTA 的。为避免这一问题，2007 年通过了《查理·W.诺伍德活体器官捐献法案》(Charlie W. Norwood Living Organ Donation Act)[34]。支持非直接捐献者参与肾脏互换链的人认为，肾脏移植数量的增加为其合理性提供了足够的理由。他们还认为这种策略使移植突破了传统的免疫学障碍，并且最终将减少等待移植列表中患者的数量。然而，数量的考量和效用必须与死亡捐献等待列表的平等、公正相平衡，尤其是对O型血的受者。当一个非直接捐献者进入互换链的时候，将移植数量降到最少是一个合理的建议[33]。很显然，随着肾脏移植项目的发展，为更好地理解和评估这些策略可能存在的问题，我们必须有针对性的对数据进行收集。

在肾脏互换之前，肾脏互换链中的最后一位肾脏捐献者不同意同时捐献其肾脏，因为他们的家人接受了肾移植，然而后来他们会将肾脏捐献给最初的第二个肾脏互换链的受者。由此，“桥捐赠”就用一条肾脏互换链将发生在不同时间的两个肾脏互换链连接在了一起。肾脏互换链中的一个基本的问题是桥接捐献者的“退出”，这会终止开放和封闭的互换链[33]。创建“荣誉制度”来使退出率最小化，且该制度会教育桥接捐赠者他们若退出对链条内后续受者的影响。荣誉制度在道德层面是有问题的，因为它们本质上是带有强制性的。建设性的解决方案包括促进肾脏互换过程的鉴定和执行，并且预先确定制度的限制条件(时间限制或者移植数量限制)。活体捐献者最大的获益是心理上的。即使移植失败，捐献者也知道他们所做的事情都可能会帮助到他们所爱的人。有些人认为在配对肾脏互换和肾脏互换链中，捐献是非直接的，那么道德获益就可能更加混乱。捐献后，一些捐献者会陷入抑郁或者与家庭成员产生冲突。在肾脏互换项目中，有些捐献者会因为不知道自己捐献的结果如何而使情绪恶化。针对参与互换项目的心理关注点的评估还需作进一步研究。

为一个互换链的起始选定非直接捐献者的建议包括需要明确捐献者向捐献链内捐献器官是完全自愿而非受到外界教唆[33]。然而，大众媒体关于肾脏互换方面的报道引起了道德关注，正如有些非直接捐献者可能由于身处大众媒体而被怂恿。移植中心可能驱动媒体报道，就像肾脏互换链通常为移植中心吸引大量关注一样。

非直接捐献者和桥接捐献者的隐私性和保密性是必须被保证的[33]。捐献者需要有足够的关于潜在受者的信息，以确保他们捐献的肾脏能够在医学上被合理的利用。传统做法是，移植前是不允许捐献者和受者见面的，因为这种见面可能会对受者做决定产生负面影响。人们建议非直接捐献者和桥接捐献者在捐献之前是不能被告知本次捐献涉及到的人数的，因为这会使他们屈服于不断增加的认知强迫。因此，蓄意和被强迫问题、保密问题以及患者的权利都需要仔细做评估和监督。另外，活体捐献纳入标准的不同使肾脏配对互换项目的道德问题更加复杂，在这个项目中，捐献者在一个移植中心被认为是可纳入的，而在另一个中心就可能被拒绝。当前，捐献者评估和知情同意的责任由最初的移植中心担负。

肝脏捐献

肝脏捐献涉及的基本道德指导方针仍然是类似的。捐献者必须有完全自主权；整个捐献过程、手术、短期和长期并发症必须完全告知他们；他们有权在任何时候退出捐献过程；受者获得满意疗效的前提下捐献者的安全以及承担的风险必须是合理的[35]。活体肝脏捐献者评估过程的不同与捐献者承担的风险更高呈正相关。接受活体捐献肝脏移植的受者所取得的疗效已经等同于或者高于接受死亡捐献肝脏移植[36]。然而，受者的病死率仍然挺高，尤其是那些因爆发性肝衰竭或者严重的门静脉高压而接受肝脏移植的患者。评估捐献者风险时所遇到的主要问题是目前缺乏可别广泛接受的、明确的捐献者排除标准以及捐献者长期随访结果。全球第一例活体肝脏捐献是在1989年[37]。经历过最初的成功和振奋之后，大量活体肝脏捐献者死亡的报道导致2002年以后活体肝脏捐献率明显下降。从2000年开始，美国实施了超过3000例活体捐献肝脏移植。尽管文献报道的围手术期死亡率波动于9%~67%，但是多数活体肝脏捐献并没有引起永久的长期并发症[39]。据估计，当前活体捐献肝右叶切除术的死亡风险和患病风险分别为0.4%和35%[40]。肝左叶或者左外叶切除的并发症发生率更低[41]。然而，真实的患病率仍然很难估计。现在已经开发出正规的可再生分级系统，它能为活体肝脏捐献并发症的发生提供系统的分析，这将有助于更好地告知潜在的捐献者候选人[39,42,43]。这在向潜在的活体肝脏捐献者提供全面的知情同意是很重要的。

对于紧急情况下的活体捐献肝脏移植仍然存在很大的分歧。受者疗效不乐观，并且时间紧迫，这都给捐献者的评估和知情同意增加了额外的压力。然而，有人认为病重的患者恰恰是最能从活体捐献肝脏移植中获益的人[44,45]。然而，在这种情况下存在一种现实的医疗困境，即捐献者评估的持续时间和受者病情恶化之间的对立关系[46]。是否要考虑活体捐献肝脏移植应当和死亡捐献肝脏移植的效率有关系。一般来讲，只有在有经验的移植中心才会这样考虑。在一些例子中，活体捐献肝脏移植可能是唯一的选择。对于晚期肝癌不能接受死亡捐献肝脏移植的患者即是如此[41]。在死亡捐献器官分配列表中，患有早期肝癌的患者可能会被优先考虑，因为他们的移植术后生存会更好，肿瘤复发的风险更低。患有相对晚期肝癌的患者肝移植术后预后差，因此就不会被优先考虑，即便在肝移植后他们恢复良好的可能性要高于不做肝移植时的预期。使多数人得到最好的治疗是知情原则，这就要求将患有晚期肝癌的患者从优先得到移植机会的人群中去除。有争议的是，目前供体器官短缺并且当有活体肝脏捐献者志愿捐献时，器官移植团队就不能使用来自死亡捐献者的器官。然而，有一个潜在的问题就是确定一个患有晚期肝癌的肝移植受者预期生存时间的上限，使其能够证明活体肝脏捐献者所承担的风险是合理的。

在美国，大多数的活体肝脏捐献者和受者之间都存在遗传上或者感情上的关系，尽管有几例被报道的非直接的肝脏捐献者[47]。目前有一个很明显的道德争论，其焦点为父母亲是否有自由选择的权利将肝脏捐献给自己的孩子。许多人认为父母和子女的关系是遗传上强制的，以致接受父母的捐赠是最合适的选择。父母亲捐赠者一直在强调他们作为父母在道德上应负的责任并且带着拒绝捐献的负罪感活着是不现实的。因此，许多人认为讨论父母在捐献问题上拥有选择权是不切题的[48-50]。尤其是有些人认为在子女患有小儿爆发性肝功能衰竭时，来自父母的活体捐献不应该是一种好的选择[51]。然而，来自父母的活体捐献是认可的，主要是因为这一举措挽救生命的潜能完全重于这些道德关注问题。这里引用一位母亲的话，她在被问及给自己的孩子捐献肝脏是否会让她感觉到有压力时，她的回答是“这是一种天赐的礼物，我可以给我的孩子两次生命。”总而言之，在 2010 年，有 12%的小儿肝移植的供肝是来自活体肝脏捐献[3]。

肺脏捐献

截至 2011 年，全球范围内活体捐献肺叶移植数量已经达到接近 400 例。在美国，无捐献者死亡的报道，围手术期并发症的发生率波动于 7%~49%[52]。一个悬而未决的问题仍然是捐献肺叶以后对捐献者长期的生存状况以及功能的影响，尽管失去了部分肺功能是可以预期的后果。活体捐献肺叶移植另一个特殊之处在于两个捐献者要承担每个受者手术的风险。这是仅有的一种有 300%死亡风险的过程。近几年，因为死亡肺脏捐献 OPTN 紧急/获益分配系统的改变，它的应用在美国已经大幅减少。当前，活体捐献肺脏移植的文献多数来自于日本。

商业化和补偿

尽管世界范围内供体器官的短缺已经在一定程度上反映了美国供体器官的短缺，但是器官捐献相关法律的不同已经导致器官捐献商业化这样一个全球性问题。世界范围内，活体捐献率和死亡器官捐献可获得性存在密切的联系。在有知情同意的国家，活体捐献肾脏移植率是相对更低的(每百万人 2.4 对 5.9)[53]。多数国家已经签署世界卫生组织声明，谴责买卖器官的行为。各种国内或者国际移植组织以及国际共识组织已经拒绝金钱补偿来作为器官短缺的解决方案。尽管在世界上的多数区域器官买卖都是不合法的，但是国际上仍有大量黑市存在。在 2007 年，据世界卫生组织估计，世界范围内每年有 5%~10%的肾脏移植的供肾是通过非法交易获得的[54]。面对近乎停滞的器官捐献率以及各种关于无序的器官交易市场的关注，有越来越多的人包括器官移植团队的专业人员参与为器官捐献者提供补偿这一道德上有争议的提议的争论[55]。物质刺激捐献的争论已经使移植团队中的许多人的认识走向极端。支持向活体肾脏销售者付钱的主要观点认为经济刺激将增加捐献的数量，几乎不会有移植候选者在等待供体的过程中死亡。考虑到死亡率、患病率、移植成功率以及捐献后的生活质量，唯一的驱动力就是受者获益。支持者认为有规则的补偿将有助于通过取消移植旅游业并保护无规则系统中的销售者来反对全球移植商业化这样一场国际范围内的斗争。建议的支付项目包括：外汇金额、定期人寿保险、终生医疗保险、差旅话费以及误工时间补偿以及扣税补偿。这项提议配合分配系统通过一套预定的算法和长期随访由政府和保险公司来监督支付。最后一点尤其具有吸引力，因为它可以解决未参保捐献者长期医疗保健的道德窘境。多数支持者赞成所有器官统一价格而不因捐献职责的年龄、健康状况以及生活方式的不同而改变。立法也将消除当前直接利他主义活体捐献的道德和法律问题。有些人甚至认为捐献过程通常是一种经济负担并且迫使捐献者承担这项成本是不道德的。他们认为否定合法的补偿是在利用捐献者的利他主义动机。因此,补偿应该是针对花费的时间以及成本,而不是器官[56]。

反对有偿捐献的观点则包括：这是对贫困者的潜在剥削,这是将身体商品化,这是在利用经济强制,这样做也缺乏足够的数据证明这会增加移植捐献率,并且从长远来讲,这对捐献者是有害的。其中最重要的关注点还是有偿捐献带有剥削的本质，因为这将对那些经济困难者造成过度的诱惑。在无规则或者规则不健全的系统中，富裕的购买者可以在很少关心捐献者安全和随访的情况下购买到肾脏，因此也就建立了这样一个双层系统,在这个系统中,富裕者获益而贫困者会受到经济驱动力的胁迫。国际上已经有数据表明:卖掉肾脏并获得经济补偿的人们在五年之后并不能改善他们的经济状况。事实上,有许多人的健康状况、社会处境以及总体福利已经很差，并且 80%的人是不推荐把肾脏捐献给别人的[57]。其中首要的关注点之一就是经济补偿和强制诱惑力之间的界限。预期的经济补偿措施将引起不可抵抗的经济压力,从而推动驱动力捐献并且破坏捐献者的自主权。一项 2006 年针对美国家庭的电话调查表明低收入群体更容易认可经济驱动,这样经济补偿就会对贫困者产生与付出不成比例的影响[58]。在对 ESRD 患者的调查中也同样发现了这样的不平等,即与贫困者相比,更加富裕的患者愿意并且能够花钱买到肾脏[59]。其他的关注点包括这种金钱上的诱惑会驱使捐献者回避甚至谎报自己的病史，这样就使捐献者的健康和受者的健康都受到威胁。明显的一点是医生的建议将是很重要的一个标准，能够衡量付钱购买一个肾脏的意愿。针对移植医生的一项调查显示，有 80%的受访者是反对甚至强烈反对肾脏移植活体器官捐献市场的[29]。

另外一些关注点包括“挤出效应”和“旁观者效应”[60]。“挤出效应”是指由于外在酬劳的引入使捐献数量减少从而引发不可预料的后果，会因此而使许多捐献者利他主义的动机并使这些潜在的捐献者感到沮丧。这一点在针对瑞典的献血者的一项调查中得到证实[61]。这样一个现象是否会在器官捐献中重现尚不得而知。“旁观者效应”会在有偿捐献这一背景下导致捐献者自愿捐献的紧迫感减弱。有人觉得这已经引起给小儿捐献的人数的减少，当优先将器官分配给小儿受者这一政策发生改变时[60]。

关于医疗风险支付的道德关注已经不仅局限于移植领域[29]。在医学研究中,经济补偿是不被禁止的,但是联邦管理条例缺乏关于补偿的专门指导方针。然而,人类研究保护办公室赞成机构审查委员会指南去指导内部评价系统，以决定是否补偿会导致过度的诱导而应避免，如果补偿会使捐献者承担之前不会承担的风险。然而,OHRP 前主席 Meniko 认为因风险高而补偿失败和意识到个人的贡献是不一致的。但是明尼苏达州立大学的伦理生物学家 Carl Elliot 认为为两种风险提供补偿存在不同，一种风险是个人为帮助别人而将自己暴露在风险中，另一种风险指有第三方团队介入而承担的风险。他认为允许一个人去承担风险和鼓励一个人去承担风险是不同的。许多人认为有偿捐献越过了允许和鼓励之间的界线。

当前，有偿捐献争论的焦点集中在肾脏移植。然而,随着对其他器官(例如肝脏)活体捐献者的安全以及术后生存情况的数据收集的完善，这一争论可能会扩展到其他的器官。很多调查表明,有 67%的移植医生赞成非直接肝脏捐献，这一比例明显低于赞成非直接肾脏捐献者的医生比例；并且有 90%的医生反对或者强烈反对活体捐献的肝脏进入市场[29]。与活体肾脏捐献不同，活体肝脏捐献者所承担的风险是支撑反对者观点的主要原因。

总结

医生必须在不造成伤害这一前提下从事医疗实践[62],但是捐献手术会存在使捐献者受到伤害的风险。这仍然是器官移植团队和器官移植中心为保证活体捐献的安全性及捐献者不受任何胁迫所承担的最重要的责任。然而,器官短缺问题日渐加剧,扩展活体捐献器官移植是一种增加捐献者数量的措施。高血压、肥胖、高龄、肾结石以及糖耐量受损不再被认为是捐献的绝对禁忌证。另外,非直接器官捐献,配对互换捐献以及捐献链等措施在不断增加。为保证捐献者的安全,需要给他们提供更好的宣教以及更全面的知情同意，同时必须对这些亚组进行密切的随访。当前，在美国只考虑利他主义捐献者，但是激励活体捐献的提议也越来越引起广泛的关注。这些提议正在蚕食许多基本的道德准则，并将在接下来的许多年里继续挑战我们当前对活体器官捐献的理解。

（刘鹏 译 徐骁 校）

参考文献

1. Moore FD. Transplant: The Give and Take of Tissue Transplantation. New York, NY: Simon and Schuster; 1964: 313.
2. Cecka MJ. Living donor transplants. MJ Cecka, PI Terasaki (Eds.), Clinical Transplants 1995 (ed 4) UCLA Tissue Typing Laboratory, Los Angeles, CA (1996), pp. 363–377.
3. United Network for Organ Sharing Web Site. Organ Procurement and Transplantation Network Data. [accessed December 18, 2011]; Available at: http://www.unos.org.
4. Liounis B, Roy LP, Thompson JF, et al. The living, related kidney donor: a follow-up study. Medical Journal of Australia. 1988;148(9):436–437, 440–444.
5. Gouge F, Moore J Jr, Bremer BA, et al. The quality of life of donors, potential donors, and recipients of living-related donor renal transplantation. Transplantation Proceedings. 1990;22(5):2409–2413.
6. Massey EK, Kranenburg LW, Zuidema WC, et al. Encouraging psychological outcomes after altruistic donation to a stranger. American Journal of Transplantation. 2010;10(6):1445–1452.
7. Najarian JS, Chavers BM, McHugh LE, et al. 20 years or more of follow-up of living kidney donors. Lancet. 1992;340(8823):807–810.
8. Bia MJ, Ramos EL, Danovitch GM, et al. Evaluation of living renal donors. The current practice of US transplant centers. Transplantation. 1995;60(4): 322–327.
9. Garg AX, Prasad GV, Thiessen-Philbrook HR, et al. Cardiovascular disease and hypertension risk in living kidney donors: an analysis of health administrative data in Ontario, Canada. Donor Nephrectomy Outcomes Research (DONOR) Network. Transplantation. 2008;86(3):399–440.
10. Boudville N, Prasad GV, Knoll G, et al. Meta-analysis: risk for hypertension in living kidney donors. Donor Nephrectomy Outcomes Research (DONOR) Network. Annals of Internal Medicine. 2006;145(3):185–196.
11. Davis CL. Living kidney donors: current state of affairs. Advances in Chronic Kidney Disease. 2009;16(4):242–249.
12. Ibrahim HN, Foley R, Tan L, et al. Long-term consequences of kidney donation. New England Journal of Medicine. 2009;360(5):459–469.
13. Gibney EM, King AL, Maluf DG, et al. Living kidney donors requiring transplantation: focus on African Americans. Transplantation. 2007;84(5):647–649.
14. Ellison MD, McBride MM, Taranto SE, et al. Living kidney donors in need of kidney transplants: a report from the Organ Procurement and Transplantation Network. Transplantation. 2002;74(9):1349–1359.
15. Fehrman-Ekholm I, Norden G, Lennerling A, et al. Incidence of end-stage renal disease among live kidney donors. Transplantation. 2006;82(12):1646–1648.
16. Davis CL, Cooper M. The state of U.S. living kidney donors. Clinical Journal of the American Society of Nephrology. 2010;5(10):1873–1880.
17. Gibney EM, Parikh CR, Garg AX. Age, race, gender and associations with kidney failure following living kidney donation. Transplantation Proceedings. 2008; 40(5):1337–1340.
18. Cherikh WS, Young CJ, Kramer BF, et al. Ethnic and gender related differences in the risk of end-stage renal disease after living donation. American Journal of Transplantation. 2011;11(8):1650–1655.
19. Ibrahim HN, Akkina SK, Leister E, et al. Pregnancy outcomes after kidney donation. American Journal of Transplantation. 2009;9(4):825–834.
20. Gordon EJ, Beauvais N, Theodoropoulos N, et al. The challenge of informed consent for increased risk living donation and transplantation. American Journal of Transplantation. 2011;11(12):2569–2574.
21. Ladin K, Hanto DW. Informed consent and living kidney donation; more (information) is not always better. American Journal of Transplantation. 2011;11(12): 2547–2548.
22. Reese PP, Feldman HI, McBride MA, et al. Substantial variation in the acceptance of medically complex live kidney donors across US renal transplant centers. American Journal of Transplantation. 2008;8(10):2062–2070.
23. Living Kidney Donor Follow-Up Conference Writing Group. Living kidney donor follow-up: state-of-the-art and future directions, conference summary and recommendations. American Journal of Transplantation. 2011;11(12): 2561–2568.
24. Rodrigue JR, Pavlakis M, Danovitch GM, et al. Evaluating living kidney donors: relationship types, psychosocial criteria, and consent processes at US transplant programs. American Journal of Transplantation. 2007;7(10):2326–2332.
25. Ommen ES, Rudow L, Medapalli RK, et al. When good intentions are not enough: obtaining follow-up data in living kidney donors. American Journal of Transplantation. 2011;11(12):2575–2581.
26. Manyalich M, Ricart A, Martinez I, et al. Walaszewski J. EULID project: european living donation and public health. Transplantation Proceedings. 2009;41(6): 2021–2024.
27. National Organ Transplantation Act Public Law. October 19, 1984.
28. Mueller PS, Case EJ, Hook CC. Responding to offers of altruistic living unrelated kidney donation by group associations: an ethical analysis. Transplantation Reviews. 2008;22(3):200–205.
29. Aronsohn A, Thistlethwaite JR, Segev DL, et al. How different conceptions of risk are used in the organ market debate. American Journal of Transplantation. 2010;10(4):931–937.
30. Adams PL, Cohen DJ, Danovitch GM, et al. The non-directed live-kidney donor: ethical considerations and practice guidelines: a national conference report. Transplantation. 2002;74(4):582–589.
31. Epstein M, Danovitch GM. Is altruistic directed living unrelated organ donation a legal fiction? Nephrology, Dialysis, Transplantation. 2009;24(2):357–360.
32. Rapaport FT. The case for a living emotionally related international kidney donor exchange registry. Transplantation Proceedings. 1986;18(3 Suppl):5–9.
33. Woodle ES, Daller JA, Aeder M, et al. Ethical considerations for participation of non-directed living donors in kidney exchange programs. American Journal of Transplantation. 2010;10(6):1460–1467.
34. Charlie W. Norwood Living Organ Donation Act, Pub L No. 110-144, 121 Stat 1814.
35. Miller CM. Ethical dimensions of living donation: experience with living liver donation. Transplantation Reviews. 2008;22(3):206–209.
36. Maluf DG, Stravitz RT, Cotterell AH, et al. Adult living donor versus deceased donor liver transplantation: a 6-year single center experience. American Journal of Transplantation. 2005;5(1):149–156.
37. Broelsch CE, Emond JC, Whitington PF, et al. Application of reduced-size liver transplants as split grafts, auxiliary orthotopic grafts, and living related segmental transplant. Annals of Surgery. 1990;212(3):368–377.
38. Miller C, Florman S, Kim-Schluger L, et al. Fulminant and fatal gas gangrene of the stomach in a healthy live liver donor. Liver Transplantation. 2005;10(10): 1315–1319.
39. Ghobrial RM, Reise CE, Trotter JF, et al. Donor morbidity after living donation for liver transplantation. Gastroenterology. 2008;135(2):468–476.
40. Barr ML, Belghiti J, Villamil FG, et al. A report of the Vancouver Forum on the care of the live organ donor: lung, liver, pancreas, and intestine data and medical guidelines. Transplantation. 2006;81(10):1373–1385.
41. Nadalin S, Malago M, Radtke A, et al. Current trends in live liver donation. Transplant International. 2007;20(4):312–330.
42. Tamura S, Sugawara Y, Kukudo N, et al. Systematic grading of morbidity after living donation for liver transplantation. Gastroenterology. 2008;135(5): 1804.
43. Salvalaggio PR, Baker TB, Koffron AJ, et al. Comparative analysis of live liver donation risk using a comprehensive grading system for severity. Transplantation. 2004;77(11):1765–1767.
44. Nadalin S, Bockhorn M, Malago M, et al. Living donor liver transplantation. HPB. 2006;8(1):10–21.
45. Northup PG, Berg CL. Living donor liver transplantation: the historical and cultural basis of policy decisions and ongoing ethical questions. Health Policy. 2005;72(2):175–185.
46. Uemoto S, Inomata Y, Sakurai T, et al. Living donor liver transplantation for fulminant hepatic failure. Transplantation. 2000;70(1):152–157.
47. Reichman TW, Fox A, Adcock L, et al. Anon-ymous living liver donation: donor profiles and outcomes. American Journal of Transplantation. 2010;10(9): 2099–2104.
48. Forsberg A, Nilsson M, Krantz M, et al. The essence of living parental liver donation – donors' lived experiences of donation to their children. Pediatric Transplantation. 2005;8(4):372–380.
49. Knibbe ME, Maeckelberghe ELM, Verkerk MA. Confounders in voluntary consent about living parental liver donation: no choice and emotions. Medicine, Health Care, and Philosophy. 2007;10(4):433–440.
50. Reding R. Is it right to promote living donor liver transplantation for fulminant hepatic failure in pediatric recipients? American Journal of Transplantation.

2005;5(7):1587–1591.
51. Committee of Ministers. Recommendation N, R(97)16 of the Committee of Ministers to Member States on Liver Transplantation from Living Related Donors. Council of Europe. 1997.
52. Bowdish ME, Barr ML, Schenkel FA, et al. A decade of living lobar lung transplantation: perioperative complications after 253 donor lobectomies. American Journal of Transplantation. 2004;4(8):1283–1288.
53. Horvat LD, Cuerden MS, Kim SJ, et al. Informing the debate: rates of kidney transplantation in nations with presumed consent. Annals of Internal Medicine. 2010;153(10):641–649.
54. Budiani-Saberi DA, Delmonico FL. Organ trafficking and transplant tourism: a commentary on the global realities. American Journal of Transplantation. 2008;8(5):925–929.
55. Matas AJ. Why we should develop a regulated system of kidney sales: a call for action! Clinical Journal of the American Society of Nephrology. 2006;1(6): 1129–1132.
56. Bagheri A. Compensated kidney donation: an ethical review of the Iranian model. Kennedy Institute of Ethics Journal. 2006;16(3):269–282.
57. Goyal M, Mehta R, Schneiderman L, et al. Economic and health consequences of selling a kidney in India. JAMA: Journal of the American Medical Association. 2002;288(13):1589–1593.
58. Boulware LE, Troll MU, Wang NY, et al. Public attitudes toward incentives for organ donation: a national study of different racial/ethnic and income groups. American Journal of Transplantation. 2006;6(11):2774–2785.
59. Herold DK. Patient willingness to pay for a kidney for transplantation. American Journal of Transplantation. 2010;10(6):1394–1400.
60. Cynowiec J, Kim J, Qazi YA. Incentivizing living organ donation. Current Opinion in Organ Transplantation. 2009;14(2):201–205.
61. Mellstrom C, Johannesson M. Crowding out in blood donation: was Titmuss right? Journal of the European Economic Association. 2008;6(4):845–863.
62. Ross LF. Solid organ donation between strangers. Journal of Law, Medicine and Ethics. 2002;30(3):446–447.

第 139 章
器官移植的文化差异

Chris J. Callaghan, J. Andrew Bradley

引言

对那些患有终末期器官衰竭的患者，器官移植是一种挽救生命或者延长生命的疗法。在一个公平的社会里，只要是可能的，那么能从器官移植中获益的患者就应该有公平的机会去获得移植，这一点是明确的。获得移植机会的不同应该被认识到，隐藏的原因应该被探索，并要努力将这些不同降到最低。不幸的是，放眼全球，在器官捐献以及器官移植方面不同的国家之间有大量的不平等存在(图 139.1 和图 139.2)。许多国家在获取器官移植机会方面仍然存在很大的不同，即便在一些器官移植项目发展很完善的国家[1]。

器官移植是更高级别的医学介入模式，并且成功的国家级器官移植项目是在拥有复杂的法律、道德、财政以及组织框架背景下实施的。它们也是基于一个社会对涉及器官捐献和移植的利益以及道德接纳的广泛理解。理解这些社会框架的差异使我们能够更好地理解国家之间或者国家内部在获得器官移植机会方面存在的不同。

器官移植的成功实施导致全球性供体器官短缺，并且器官供需之间存在的这种不断加剧的矛盾是不能公平获得移植机会的一部分原因，这也导致了移植商业化的出现。在面临器官移植等待列表中的患者不断增多或者意识到获取移植机会的不公平性后，富有的器官功能衰竭的患者会认为移植的商业化为他们获取器官提供了最好的机会。移植商业化提醒国际移植群体意识到减少等待移植的患者并提高获取器官的机会是很重要的。

本章旨在评估这些具体的能影响移植获取机会的文化差异，并强调为减少这些差异而实施的措施。人们正在以全球性的眼光来探索移植商业化以及与器官交易和移植旅游业相关的问题，并尝试解决这些问题。最后，针对应该支持还是反对为器官捐献引入经济激励的问题进行讨论。全章都将对肾脏移植作最密切的评估，因为截至目前，肾脏移植是世界范围内最常见的实体器官移植，并且活体或者死亡供体捐献的肾脏都可以用来移植。肾脏移植也是和移植商业化关系最为密切的器官移植类型。

文化差异

获得器官移植的机会应该是平等的，并且不应该受到人种、种族、宗教信仰或者社会经济地位的影响，这些因素可以统称为社会文化因素。文化的定义很宽泛，但是在社会水平可以将其定义为社会内部的特殊的想法、社会环境、哲学、习俗、态度以及行为。即使移植组织和政府能够提供移植领域的一些文件框架，但是每个患者都可以被认为拥有各自不同的文化。因此文化因素会在这两个层面讨论。

组织和政府

和透析相比，肾脏移植能够明显节约长期的医疗成本[2]。然而，在某些不能采取长期替代疗法的器官(如心脏、肝脏、肺脏)，移植是昂贵的并且在技术专业领域需要重点投资。为使移植成为一种可行的治疗选择，昂贵的用于管理和实施的基础设备也是必需的。高成本投入意味着在一些经济来源非常有限的发展中国家开创并发展移植项目是不可行的。政府移植管理政策的其他信息可以在第 128 章中找到。

因此这样一个现象也就不奇怪了：一个国家的肾脏移植率和其人类发展指数(一项将预期寿命、教育水平和收入复合在一起的统计指标）是密切相关的（图 139.3)。而且一个国家的财力和这个国家器官捐献率

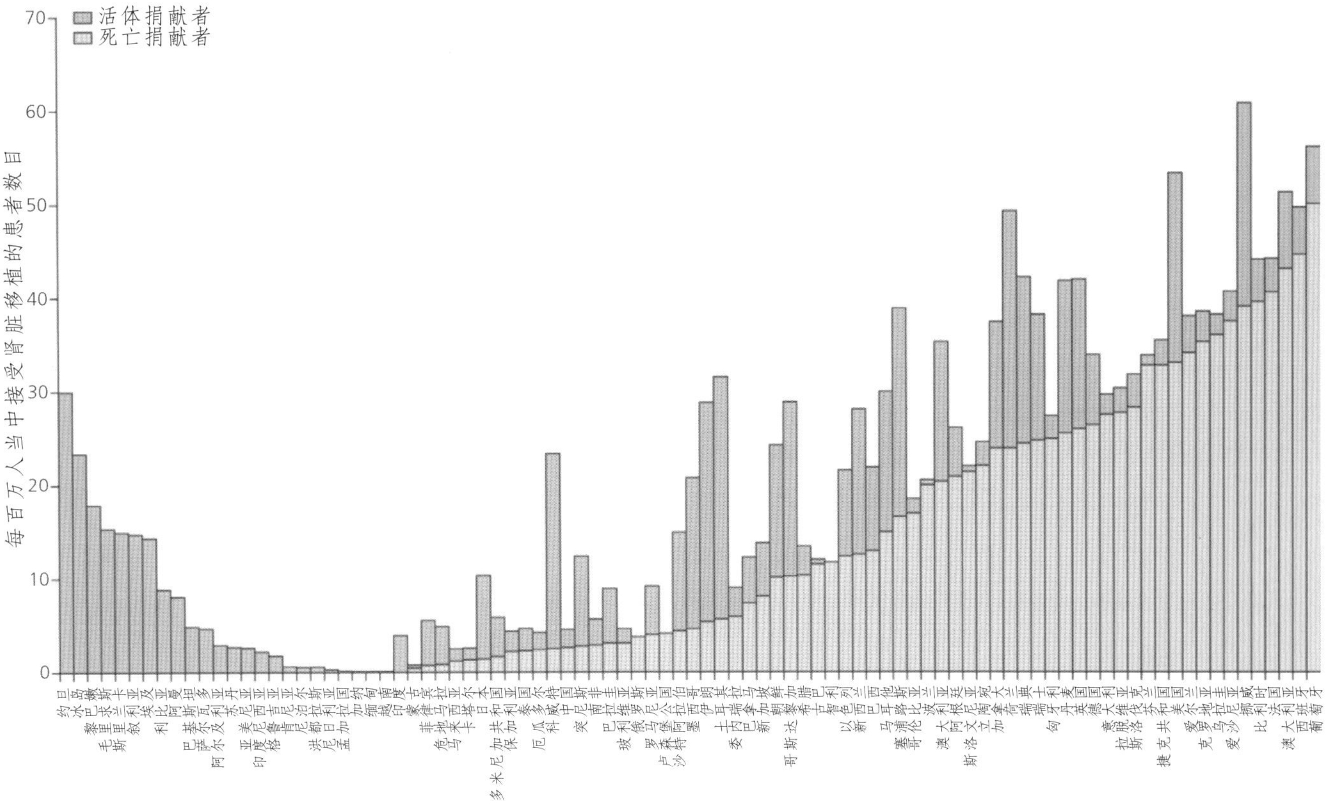

图 139.1　各国的活体捐献和死亡捐献肾脏移植率（2009 年数据）。图中显示的只是将数据提交到全球捐献和移植观测网的国家。Reproduced from [68] Delmonico et al. A call for government accountability to achieve national self-sufficiency in organ donation and transplantation. 378（9800）:1414－1418，Copyright 2011 with permission from Elsevier. Original figure uses data from the WHO website: http://www.transplant-observatory.org/Pages/Data-Reports.aspx.）

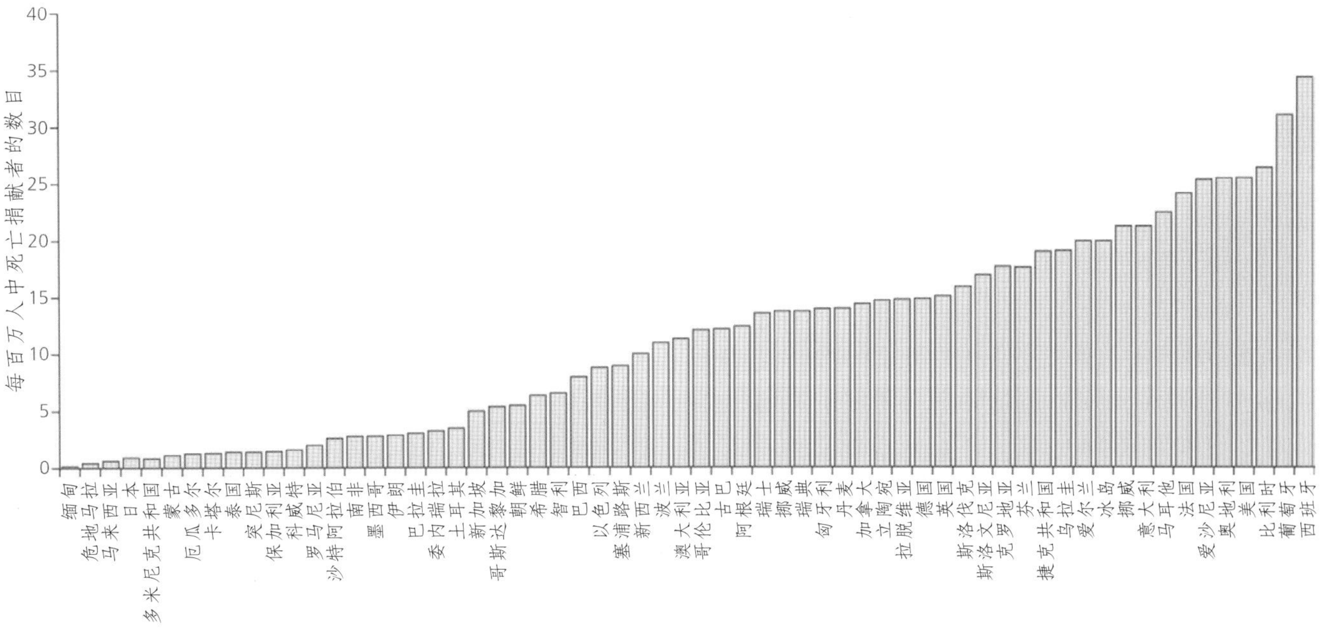

图 139.2　各国的死亡器官捐献率（2009 年数据）。图中显示的只是将数据提交到全球捐献和移植观测网的国家。Reproduced from [68] Delmonico et al. A call for government accountability to achieve national self-sufficiency in organ donation and transplantation. 378（9800）:1414－1418，Copyright 2011 with permission from Elsevier. Original figure uses data from the WHO website: http://www.transplant-observatory.org/Pages/Data-Reports.aspx.）

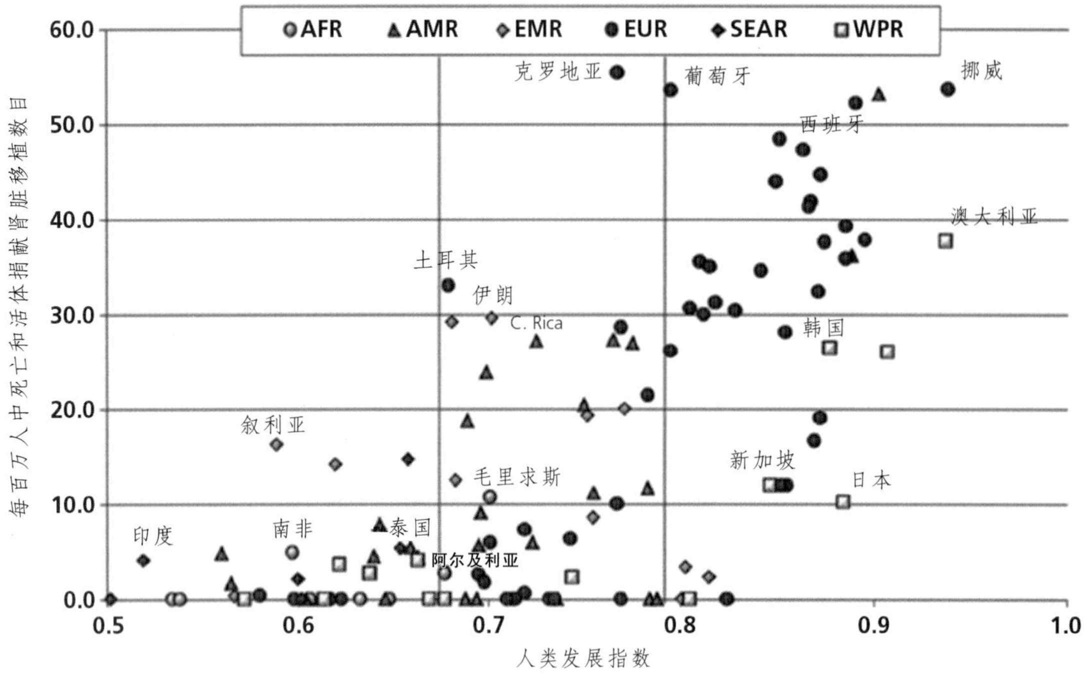

图 139.3 WHO 成员国 2010 年发布的死亡捐献和活体捐献肾脏移植数量，与人类发展指数明显相关。由 WHO 根据区域分组。(AFR，非洲；AMR，美洲；EMR，东地中海区域；EUR，欧洲；SEAR，东南亚；WPR，西太平洋)。Reproduced from Garcia et al, for the World Kidney Day Steering Committee (2012). Te Global Role of Kidney Transplantation. Transplantation，27；93(4):337–341，with permission from Wolters Kluwer Health. Original fgure uses data from the WHO website: http://www.transplant-observatory.org/Pages/Data-Reports.aspx.

是相关的[3]。有趣的是，我们还应注意到，具有相似的人类发展指数的国家之间，他们的器官移植率存在明显的差异，例如挪威和澳大利亚。这表明除了富裕程度以外，还有一些因素是可能影响到器官移植获取机会的。WHO 全球捐献和移植观测网(www.transplant-observatory.org) 的数据也表明活体和死亡捐献器官移植率在发展水平不同的国家之间存在很大的差异。高度发达的国家死亡捐献器官移植率要比活体捐献高，然而，在欠发达的国家，这种对比是正好相反的[4]。这可能反映出实施活体捐献的能力和需要为死亡捐献提供来源的文化、法律和经济系统的发展程度之间存在脱节。

尽管一个国家有足够的资金去实施昂贵的器官移植手术，但是，除非有法可依，否则仍然无法发展有效的器官移植项目。和西方国家相比，亚洲国家有关脑死亡后器官捐献问题的法律仍然欠缺[5]。然而，这种情况正在改观，印度在 1994 年通过了使脑死亡者捐献器官成为可能的法律；日本在 1997 年脑死亡捐献变得合法化，紧随其后的是 2000 年的韩国。尽管有这些改观，但是在多数亚洲国家，死亡患者器官捐献率仍然较低。

甚至有些法律、历史、文化、宗教背景都相似的国家对循环停止的死亡器官捐献(DCD；在第 22 章有详细讲述)的观念也具有明显的不同。Dominguez-Gil 及其同事最近发表文章称欧洲各国对循环停止的死亡器官捐献的立法及认可度具有明显的差异[6]。欧洲理事会中有五个成员国(芬兰、德国、波兰、葡萄牙和卢森堡)的法律是禁止 DCD 捐献的。与之相反的是，在英国有 1/3 肾脏移植的供肾是来自 DCD 捐献。在这些允许 DCD 捐献的国家中，法国和西班牙非控制性捐献者(即，患者在医院外发生心脏骤停)占主导，然而英国的大多数的 DCD 捐献器官来自控制性 DCD 捐献者（患者在放弃治疗后等待心跳停止或者那些心跳停止的脑死亡患者)。供体器官来自 DCD 捐献的器官移植在英国比在美国常见的多[7,8]，这可能是因为在美国，脑死亡捐献者的器官捐献率更高。

许多因素导致了死亡器官捐献率的下降，这些因素可能包括获取知情同意的类型。最近的一项综述指出假定知情同意的引入使捐献率增加了 25%~30%，其中假定知情同意是指我们认为社会上的每个人都是潜在的器官捐献者,除非他们签署拒绝捐献协议[3]。法律的变更对器官捐献率的影响是有争议的，因为即使在那些有假定知情同意法的国家，他们的器官捐献率也会随着被强迫程度的不同而不同。选择性退出系统有时候是“强硬的”,即一个选择性退出登记者未在系统中登记,那么死后不管家属意向如何,死者的器官必须捐献(例如,澳大利亚);而有时候这个系统也是“柔和的”,即在家属拒绝捐献的情况下,可凌驾于退出者未登记这一事实(例如,西班牙和比利时)。“选择性退出”立法可能不会引起器官捐献数量的增加;但是,在一个人们可以平和地讨论临终问题的国家，它可能是这个国家高度发达的非常有效的器官获得策略的一个标志。

法律框架会对器官捐献产生影响,同时,医疗保健政策会对移植后的结果产生重要的影响。对比具备通用医疗保健系统的国家和具有个人的保险基本模型的国家移植术后的效果是很有意义的。英国具备一套医疗保健系统,他们可以免费享受医疗保健,资金来自于全国税收。英国的肝移植术后 90 天以内的风险校正死亡率比美国的高，可能是由于英国在高成本的重症监护设备投资不足[9]。肾移植术后一年内风险校正死亡率,加拿大的和美国的几乎相等,但是,一年以后,加拿大患者的生存率更好[10]。尽管这种类型的回顾性分析必须谨慎的去解释,但是通过这些发现我们可以看出,像英国和加拿大这种具备通用医疗保健系统的国家比像美国这种具备个人的保险基本模型的国家能够提供更好的长期医疗保健。

器官捐献涉及的文化因素

获得器官移植的机会直接受到器官捐献率的影响，而器官捐献率又是由捐献者的种族和信仰等文化因素所决定的[11]。

捐献者的种族对死亡捐献和活体捐献都会产生影响。在英国一项针对重症监护室的全国性调查中,65%的白种人家庭同意潜在的脑死亡器官捐献。然而,仅有23%~29%的黑种人家庭和亚洲家庭同意捐献[12]。这些发现尤其引人关注,因为在英国,黑种人和亚洲人的肾衰竭发生率要高出 3~4 倍，而且由于来自这些人种的等待捐献的患者存在 HLA 配型困难问题,这些等待者处于潜在的不利地位。对于对器官捐献持反对态度的人来说,道德观念是一个独立的风险因素,并且它不能通过与社会经济地位或者受教育背景等因素而混杂在一起[13]。

黑种人以及少数民族群体的器官捐献同意率低,可能是因为他们可能没有意识到他们群体内部对捐献器官的特殊需要，或者他们没有认识到捐献的器官等同于献给社会的一份礼物。想要在死后保证尸体完整和未经同意获取器官进行科学研究等方面的关注仍然是一个问题[13,14]。在美国,对潜在的死亡器官捐献者的家属的采访表明患者是白种人、年轻患者、男性患者以及死于外伤的患者,其器官捐献同意率更高[15]。并且这种高同意率与家庭教育以及收入没有关系。

宗教因素和信仰体系也会影响器官捐献率。有一些关于做出器官捐献(活体捐献或者死亡捐献)决定的影响因素的定性研究，对这些研究的一项系统回顾分析发现了许多与捐献率降低有关的因素。这些因素包括宗教信仰、文化因素(如迷信、讨论死亡的困难以及葬礼)、家庭与亲属关系、保持身体完整的愿望、对医疗保健系统的不满以及医疗知识欠缺[16]。

影响受者获取移植机会及疗效的文化因素

受者的种族以及社会经济地位是影响他们获得器官移植机会的两个重要的文化特征。不像心脏、肺脏或者肝脏移植，一种可选择的长期器官替代疗法的存在使评估肾脏移植机会社会剥夺的影响变得尤其重要,因为反对社会上被剥夺的患者的任何偏见都会变得更加明显。

众所周知，受者的种族划分会对他们获得移植的机会、等待时间、器官移植的类型、移植术后的疗效产生重要的影响。造成这些分歧的原因有免疫学的也有非免疫学的,包括种族划分、社会经济地位、相关的疾病、潜在的原发性疾病过程、HLA 类型以及药物基因组学之间的相互作用。这些不平等在全世界范围内都可见到,比如新西兰毛利人和太平洋人群[21]、加拿大土著居民[22,23]、非裔美国人[24-26]以及英国的黑人和少数民族[1]存在的不一致。这个问题的影响力是很大的;一项美国乔治亚州的研究发现,尽管在校正了人口统计学、临床以及社会经济移速之后，非裔美国人的肾脏抑制率仍比白种人低 59%[26]。Patzer 等暗示这一发现或许可以用种族偏见、移植推荐人的不同以及缺少医疗保健的机会来解释。

尽管很难去详细分析种族划分以及社会经济地位

之间的复杂相互作用，但是受者的社会经济地位也是影响获得器官移植机会的重要决定因素。在美国，有报道称被社会剥夺的患者等待死亡捐献肾脏移植时间在延长[27]。由于种族、社会经济地位以及合并症之间的联系，调控技术在不断的被采用。邻里贫困和种族会产生协同作用。和邻里富裕的黑种人相比，邻里贫困的黑种人等待的时间会延长。之前在美国的许多研究都得出过类似的结论[28-30]。

在美国，缺乏个人健康医疗保险可能是一个限制因素，这一因素会限制社会上被剥夺患者进入移植等待列表的机会。Udayaraj及其同事调查了在英国社会剥夺、种族划分以及进入死亡捐献者等待列表之间的关系[31]。然而，即便是像英国这样有通用的健康医疗保健系统的国家，大多数被剥夺的患者在经过年龄、性别、引起肾衰的原因、所处的时代以及移植中心等多方面的校正之后，进入肾脏移植等待列表的机会仍然更小。有趣的是，在英国，种族划分似乎不会对移植等待列表的确定产生影响；与之相反的是，年龄大于50岁的来自少数民族的患者比与之相对应的白种人患者有更大的机会进入移植等待列表。Dudley等先前的研究表明，很多的因素会影响患者被纳入肾脏移植等待列表的机会，这些因素包括患者的年龄、原发病的诊断、种族划分、是否社会剥夺、是否合并移植病史、移植中心的大小以及该中心活体捐献项目的大小[32]。在英国的一项研究也说明了社会经济地位和获取活体捐献肾脏移植的可能性之间存在相似的关系[33]。

通过上述研究可得出这样的结论：在器官移植获取方面多重文化因素是很重要的，但是不同国家之间这些因素的相关影响却存在很大的不同。

商业化活体器官捐献的后果

器官移植商业化领域的主要关注点之一是它会引发器官黑市交易，并会剥削那些贫困的和易受影响的捐献者。分析商业化器官捐献的后果和已知的这些关注点是高度相关的。而且，作为一个全球公认的违法活动，可以得到的信息是有限的，出现选择和发表偏倚也是可能的[42]。然而，已有的数据表明商业化的捐献者的身体、心理和经济状况更差。

有一篇具有重要意义的文章调查了印度金奈305个人，这些人在接受调查(2001年实施)平均前六年里，卖掉了他们的肾脏[43]。有超过90%的人卖肾是为了还债，他们平均收到1070美元。捐献后他们的平均家庭收入会减少三分之一，另据报道86%的捐献者出现身体状况恶化。大多数(80%)的捐献者声明他们不建议给别人提供商业化的捐献。

来自巴基斯坦的另一项大型的报道得出了类似的结论[44]。该报告对旁遮普的239个肾脏销售者进行了捐献术后为期4.8年的调查。有90%的卖肾者是文盲，70%是有抵押的劳动者。93%的人卖肾去还债；扣除住院的花费以及中介商的花费他们平均会收到1377US $。88%的人报告他们的经济状况并未改善，并且有98%的人认为他们的健康状况恶化了，这最可能的原因是卖肾者所从事的劳动密集型职业的本质所引起的。最后，一项针对50例埃及商业化活体捐献者的调查发现，78%的受访者出现健康状况的下降，并有94%的人对他们的捐献举动感到后悔[38]。

很明显，商业化的活体器官捐献者在捐献后都出现了较差的后果，并且几乎没有人的生活方式获得了预期的改善。这与在西方的报道中发现的非商业化的活体捐献者（他们和对照组有相似的长期生存率而且他们有与普通的成年大众相似甚至更好的生活质量[47-49]）极其有利的经历形成了鲜明的对比[45,46]。

器官移植商业化中受体的后果

和商业化活体捐献者一样，在鉴定这些器官受者的疗效是也遇到了类似的困难。正如预期的那样，每个报道都只有很少的患者，并且由于移植具有隐秘性的本质，因此系统化的鉴定商业化受者也是很困难的。

总体而言，商业化的活体捐献器官移植的受者的结果更差，他们的感染率(包括乙肝病毒、丙肝病毒和艾滋病病毒)、排斥率以及移植物失功能的发生率更高。另外，从移植中心得到的文件通常是不够的，这一点可能会削弱有效的医疗护理[50-52]。一项来自巴基斯坦的研究将126例卖肾者和180例活体相关肾脏移植进行了对比[53]。受者根据年龄、性别以及距离移植的时间进行配对。急性排斥反应发生率33%对17%，手术并发症的发生率为22%对8%，结核病的发生率为11%对6%，急性肝炎的发生率为16%对2%，由此可见这些并发症在接受卖肾者捐献肾脏的受者身上更常见。五年的移植生存率(45%对80%)和总体的患者死亡率(27%对6%)也是明显更低。

对商业化的肾脏移植受者疗效的一项系统性回顾

分析证实，与非商业化捐献相比，移植物失功能的发生率更高并且受者死亡似乎更常见，但是这可能取决于实施手术的地方[42]。

这些结果表明实施商业化肾脏移植的中心之间，受者的疗效存在明显的差异。因为随着伊斯坦布尔声明之后各国加强了移植规章的执行力度，这将对驱动非法的商业化器官移植中心更加隐秘地实施器官移植手术产生不可预期的影响，可能会反常地使活体捐献者和受者的疗效更差。

器官移植商业化的伊朗模式

当前，伊朗是仅有的一个拥有器官移植商业化半管理系统的国家，这也理所当然地引起了国际移植研究团队的浓厚兴趣。尽管来自伊朗国内的大量报道已经详细描述了这一模式，但伊朗的国内政策还是很复杂的，并且有些相关报道的真实性也有待商榷。再加上伊朗和许多西方国家关系的不和谐，都给准确地核实它所发出的许多声明带来了困难。

伊朗政府于 1988 年引入商业化肾脏移植作为对等待移植列表中患者数量增加的应对措施。在当时，死亡捐献器官移植还不是合法的。这一方案的细节由 Ghods 等提供[56]。在没有活体捐献者的情况下，需要进行肾脏移植的患者适用于一个由终末期肾功能衰竭患者所组成的非政府组织——透析和移植患者联盟(DATPA)。愿意卖掉一个肾脏的潜在捐献者会接近 DATPA 联盟，然后该联盟会进行捐献者和受者的配对。该过程没有中介商，不存在中介费。尽管政府会给捐献者大约 US$1200，但是受者还会给捐献者更多。潜在的捐献者和受者会在术前见面并安排需要额外支付的费用。如果受者很贫穷，那么这些费用可以由慈善团体支付。捐献者的医疗预评审是很严格的。手术在公立医院实行，移植团队不知道有关经济的安排，并且在手术后的一段特定的时间内，捐献者会收到医疗保险费用。

在伊朗，大约有 80%的用于移植的肾脏来自于商业捐献，尽管允许死亡器官捐献项目的立法在 2002 年正式生效[57]。同样在伊朗，大约有 15%的用于移植的器官是来自死亡捐献者[58]。该项目增长缓慢可以归结为是文化因素和基础设施问题所导致的，而不应归结为商业捐献模式的负面影响所导致的[59]。

伊朗的商业捐献者的经济状况和心理状况似乎是丰富多变的，但是比来自印度和巴基斯坦的报道所记录的要好得多。Malakoutian 等分析了 478 位印度的商业化的活体肾脏捐献者，并且发现他们中的 62%生活在贫困线之下，而且经济补偿是他们决定捐献的最常见的动机[60]。捐献之后，91%的人为他们的捐献而感到高兴，有 53%的人会建议别人也去捐献肾脏。相反，一项针对 300 名伊朗的商业化活体肾脏捐献者的调查发现，捐献会对 65%的人的职业产生负面影响，并且有 71%的人在术后会重新陷入严重的经济困难[61,62]。75%的商业化肾脏捐献者是为了实现出售器官的目的。Nejatisafa 等评估了 424 位捐献者捐献前的生活质量后发现，95%的人在捐献前的 6 个月内至少遭遇一件充满压力的生活事件。这些事件中最常见的包括家庭花销增加、收入低以及家庭负担[63]。捐献者术后的生活质量比普通大众的更低，尽管这一结论没有经过统计学的检验，并且对照组人群在年龄和性别上也和实验组不匹配。

由于缺少全国性的登记，对伊朗的受者的疗效进行深层次的分析受到了阻碍。然而，单中心或者多中心的报道总体上表明在伊朗，移植肾的生存率和一些西方的大的研究所发现的类似，移植物的 10 年存活率达到了 46%~68%[64,65]。有一部分报道表明，来自活体不相关捐献者(商业化捐献者)的肾脏，比来自活体相关捐献者捐献的肾脏，生存时间类似或者更长[56,64]，但是其他的研究却未得出这样的结论[65]。

伊朗的这一捐献项目不能说是完全受规章约束的，因为给捐献者支付补偿的数目是非常灵活的，这一点至少取决于受者所能支付的能力，而且相关政府机关也没有对其他的支付项目的细节做出明确的规定。然而，到伊朗进行移植旅游的风险也明显的降低，因为伊朗既不允许外国的侨民在伊朗做捐献者也不允许他们做受者，除非捐献者和受者都是外国人或者捐献行动得到了伊朗卫生部的许可。尽管受者的疗效明显好于那些无规则控制的商业化的项目中的受者的疗效，但是关于剥削贫穷的商业化的伊朗捐献者以及捐献后他们的经济和心理状况的关注仍然存在。尽管伊朗的这一举措因成功减少了该国肾脏移植等待列表中患者的数量而得到一致好评[56]，但是肾脏疾病在伊朗的真实流行情况仍然不明确。而且，作为一个发展中国家，在大城市外的患者获得透析的机会也是很小的，而许多可以通过接受器官移植而获益的患者死于从来没有接受过透析治疗的肾衰竭也是非常不可能的。因此，伊朗潜在的肾脏移植等待列表中患者数量的减少是虚假的。除此之外，一些研究也在质疑是否有这一等待列表存在[66]。

减少全球差异以及防止移植商业化的举措

减少获得移植机会的不平等

尽管对可能影响获得移植机会的社会文化和社会经济因素进行了比较透彻的研究，但是相对而言，对减少这种不平等的干预措施的研究却很缺乏，尤其是在肾脏移植领域。马德里决议[67]以及其他的一些政策[68]已经呼吁各国采取一种可持续的行动来满足各自的公民获取移植的需要。然而，当世界上最富有的国家也无法缓解器官供需不平衡时，那么希望这一目标在资源更加有限的发展中国家实现也是不可能的。

尽管解决这一困境的实际措施尚未得到，但是移植领域的引领者们已经描绘了很多增加获取肾脏替代疗法机会的措施[69]。他们一直在要求国际、国内、群体以及医疗保健水平的改善。在国际上改善获得肾脏移植机会的措施包括：在专业组织之间形成富有成效的联系，增加国际合作，分享已有的数据和基于证据的最好的实践。值得注意的是，为实现这些目标，2006年在移植协会的赞助下全球移植联盟成立[70]。在国家水平上，政府应该制订国家移植政策，登记等待列移植表中的患者和已经移植的患者，并保证监督和管理器官获得渠道以及器官移植过程。群体水平的干预措施包括公开宣教引起器官衰竭的危险因素以及器官移植的好处。最后，医疗保健系统需要改善医疗专业教育的水平并开发一套适合当地实际的死亡器官捐献流程。在很多的西方国家，这些措施已经在广泛实施，但是在欠发达的国家，这些措施的执行情况仍然挺差。

尽管减少需要移植来治疗的疾病负担的措施很重要，但是不断提高器官捐献率是基本举措，这一措施也会增加获得移植的机会。世界上死亡器官捐献率最高的国家是西班牙(图139.2)，并且在过去的10年中人们也仔细地研究了器官捐献的西班牙模式。然而，正如西班牙系统设计师Rafael Matesanz所描述的那样，完善的法律、经济、道德、医疗和政治背景是增加捐献率所必需的[71]。西班牙采取了一种系统的、有组织的全国移植协调网去管理死亡器官捐献。西班牙的器官捐献协调员是有重症监护工作背景的医生，在业余时间从事器官捐献协调工作使他们得以继续做原来的重症监护医生工作。目前对脑死亡进行滚动审计以确保所有的潜在的脑死亡捐献者都能被鉴定。实现这一目标首要的是对移植协调员进行不断的训练。实施器官获取手术的西班牙医院可以获得财政补偿，并且全国的移植组织会积极地发动媒体去宣传移植相关的问题。由于脑死亡捐献者全国指南的出台使器官捐献率得到进一步提升[72]。最终，Matesanz也认识到大量的重症监护病床也是实现高器官捐献率所必需的[71]。

尽管提升捐献率的干预措施的证据基础还很薄弱，但是对那些影响死者家属同意将死者的器官捐献的决定因素已经有更加深入了解[73]。如果死者家属认为死者已经接受到了高质量的医疗服务，并对脑死亡的概念有更加全面的理解，那么他们同意捐献的可能性就会增加。随着内部器官捐献协调员的出现，突如其来的死亡消息和后续器官捐献的需求之间的短暂间期是有好处的。最近的一项实验证明“合作式”请求(即重症监护室医生和器官捐献协调员共同去争取脑死亡患者家属同意捐献死者的器官)和单独由临床医生团队去争取相比对器官移植的捐献率没有影响[74]。这是一个令人惊讶的结果，因此，这个问题需要进一步的研究。

一旦被纳入器官移植等待列表，那么减少获取捐献器官不平等的最有效方式就是通过有证据基础的器官分配策略。在这方面器官分配项目是最有效的，该项目会应用评分算法去很快地校正这种持续存在的不平等。在英国，由于死亡捐献者和肾脏移植等待列表中患者的种族起源的不一致，有研究发现和白种人患者相比，来自少数民族的受者需要等待更长的时间才能获得移植的机会[1]。最近有研究发现，用于分配来源于脑死亡患者捐献的肾脏的算法可更好的反映等待列表中非白种人患者的HLA多样性。这似乎可以部分缓解这些不平衡[75]。在美国，基于MELD评分(应用反映疾病严重程度的客观的生物化学指标的一套合成的评分系统)的死亡捐献肝脏分配系统的引入，已经将种族和接受肝脏移植之间的联系打破[76]。由此看来，会有更多的存在种族多样性的国家会学习这些范例，以便增加器官移植的透明度并减少不平等。

防止移植商业化

解决移植商业化问题的第一步就是认识到这个问题的严重性，并且国际移植团队的人要清楚地阐明这一问题不利的一面。这一目标已经通过伊斯坦布尔声明而实现[35]，该声明是由国际移植团队拟定的第一份文件，它定义并谴责了移植商业化、器官交易以及移植旅游业等问题。它是建立在世界人权宣言以及世界卫生组织指导方针的基础之上的[77]，它的主要目标是告知和促进全球器官捐献和移植领域内的伦理实践问题。

这项声明是在由移植协会和国际肾脏病协会共同举办的伊斯坦布尔研讨会后公开发表的[78]。它针对捐献和移植的伦理问题提出了六项指导方针：

1. 政府应当制订规划去监管、预防并处理器官衰竭问题。

2. 每一个存在器官捐献和器官移植的国家都应该有涉及这两方面的相关立法去管理来自活体捐献和死亡捐献的器官的分配和器官移植的执行。

3. 器官的分配应该公正，而不应该考虑性别、种族、宗教信仰、社会或者经济地位。

4. 移植政策和规划的首要目标应该是最优化捐献者和受者的短期和长期医疗保健。

5. 各国应该努力实现器官捐献的自给自足。

6. 应当彻底禁止器官交易和移植旅游业，因为这违背了公平、公正的原则、丧失了对人类尊严的尊重，而移植商业化也该被禁止，因为它会导致对贫困的捐献者的不公平和不公正。

伊斯坦布尔声明具有重大的影响力，有 100 多个国家的移植组织承认这一声明。尽管这一因果关系很难明确界定，但是自从该声明公开发表之后，中国、以色列、菲律宾以及巴基斯坦等国都通过新的立法或者加强了原有立法的执行力度来禁止器官交易和器官买卖。

然而，伊斯坦布尔声明却引来 Ambagtsheer 和 Weimar 的批评，因为该声明的制订者没有意识到加强这方面立法的困难，而且这些制订者缺乏犯罪学和法学的相关专业知识[79]。他们一直认为应该重视禁止器官交易的后果。禁止任何商品贸易都会引起黑市交易，使商品价格抬高、带来非法收入、将犯罪活动延伸到其他领域并导致秘密贸易。调查所谓的器官黑市交易不可能是执法局的首要任务，因为他们没有这方面的知识也未经过这方面的训练。笔者认为伊斯坦布尔声明背后的世界卫生组织和移植协会应当支持通过对捐献的动机进行有规律的探索以增加器官捐献率，而不是一味地打击器官黑市交易。除此之外，他们指出这些组织必须辅助训练警察、检察官以及法官并要竭力增加医疗人员和执法人员之间的跨区域合作。Glazier 和 Delmonico 通过表达他们对移植商业化和器官黑市交易的持续反对来反驳了这些建议[80]。

经济驱动器官捐献

尽管尚没有负责任的评论者公开地支持器官黑市交易或者器官旅游业，然而，正如当前所定义的那样，许多人已经建议，应当尝试对器官捐献实行有规律的经济驱动(移植商业化)，尤其是活体器官捐献。在英国、法国和瑞典，活体肾脏捐献者会依据他们的花销和失去的收入的多少而得到补偿，这样做的目标就是使捐献者不承担任何在捐献过程中产生的成本[81]。在美国，活体捐献者不会得到经济上的补偿，因为 1984 年通过的国家器官移植法案明确指出：任何人为获利考虑而故意的获取、接收或者转运任何的用于移植的人体器官都是违法的。目前所推荐的经济驱动项目不仅对成本进行补偿，还需要对某些认定移植商业化违法的国家现存的移植立法进行改进。

支持将经济驱动活体捐献项目引入的最有力的观点就是死于等待移植过程中的终末期器官衰竭的患者的数量越来越多，并且反常的一点就是器官黑市交易和移植旅游业也越来越猖狂[58,82]。值得注意的是除了捐献者，所有的移植过程参与者都会有实质上的获益：受者通常能够在移植术后重返工作岗位；医院以及医护人员也会得到报酬并且政府也会因需要透析的患者数量的减少而获益(例如肾脏移植)。然而，死亡捐献者的家属和活体捐献者都不会从捐献过程中获得任何的经济利益。因为自己的身体会受到某种威胁而获得额外的经济报酬的例子有很多(例如，主动参与行动的军人、一期临床试验中的健康志愿者)，难道活体捐献就不应该得到这样的补偿吗？有许多假定的不同的项目，比如一个确定的市场模型(在该模型中活体捐献者可以决定将器官捐献给提供报酬最多的受者)，或者一个系统[在该系统中活体捐献者除了人身和(或)医疗保险的补偿外还会获得适当的经济补偿][83]。

在美国,Matas 及其同事一直是财政驱动活体捐献实验最有名气的支持者,并且已经描述了推进这一实验在道德和组织上的需要[58,84,85]。这些需要包括透明度、接受补偿的捐献者候选人的纳入和排除的国家标准以及严格的法律和规则约束。他们策划了这一方案:活体捐献者可以得到一份人寿和医疗保险、免费长期的医疗保健随访以及一次性的现金报酬(例如 US $5000)[86]。需要在与受者团队完全分开的情况下完成捐献者的评估和知情同意。保证捐献者在接受这些补偿的时候不会受到任何外界的强迫,并且器官将根据预先优化的算法计算的结果分配给等待死亡捐献的受者。对整个社会来说,总的成本控制在 US$90 000 之内都可认为是高性价比的[87]。

在美国,其他观点的支持者认为这样一些项目不能恰当地吸引贫困者去捐献,但是尽管经济驱动的支持者声称自主权是主要的,然而贫困者是没有自主权的,并且用任何的方法去解决贫困问题都是没有自主权可言的[88]。这些项目可以导致固有的“牺牲”以及剥削,并且由于潜在的捐献者/销售者存在不能完全地揭露医疗状况的风险,就像有偿献血表现出的情况那样[89]。有人关注到目前在死亡捐献者器官捐献领域,器官销售不能和非商业化的捐献系统完美共存,例如潜在的死亡捐献者的家属可能会因为没有收到与活体捐献者同样的经济补偿而心生怨恨,最终这会使他们不同意捐献[90]。这对那些活体捐献有困难或者完全不可能的器官来说具有特殊的影响(例如心脏、肺脏、肝脏和胰腺)。在伦理水平上,经济驱动的活体捐献项目可能会玷污人类躯体的尊严,因为这将人的身体变成了商品[83]。经济驱动项目的反对者还认为目前尚未完全研究出其他的能提高器官捐献率的措施,包括同意后的选择退出系统,器官获取组织,护理人员、重症监护室医生以及急诊科医生的训练以及超越标准的器官的应用[66]。

大众对经济驱动器官捐献的反应是怎样的呢?可能正如预料的那样,不同的调查发现的观点以及不同的国家民众的观点可能存在很大的差别。Bryce 等通过电话采访 971 个美国宾夕法尼亚州的家庭来调查大众对于向死亡捐献者的家属提供经济补偿的看法[91]。59%的被调查者同意国家针对葬礼花费和医疗开销提供经济补偿,而不赞成直接付钱购买(分别为 81%、84%和 53%)。有趣的是,有 75%的受访者认为经济补偿不会改变他们是否捐献家庭成员器官的决定。相反,在一项类似的调查中,有来自全美的 720 名受访者参与,当他们被问及这样的问题时——如果一个人死后捐献了他的器官,那么你认为捐献者的家属应该为这一捐献而获得一定程度的补偿吗?仅有 10%的受访者给出了肯定的答案[92]。Rodrigue 等进行了另一项非常相似的研究,他们调查了来自美国的 561 名捐献者的亲属,他们最近都同意自己的亲人死后将器官捐献。有 12%的人表示:如果在同意捐献之前自己会收到经济补偿,那么他们不会同意捐献。但是 6%的已经同意捐献的人不会改变自己的决定。在那些不同意的、年轻的、未接受过大学教育的、不赞成器官捐献的受访者中,会有更多的人对经济补偿持赞成的态度。

针对经济驱动活体器官捐献这一问题,大众的观点似乎是支持的,至少在美国是这样的。有超过 80%的美国成年人认为活体捐献者应该收到捐献花费的经济补偿,并且应该以病假或者带薪休假的方式来完成捐献[92]。然而,仅有 28%的人支持政府直接将现金支付给捐献者个人。一项来自荷兰的网页调查发现,47%的受访者反对医疗保险公司向活体捐献者提供补偿,既不能提供长期的医疗保险也不能一次性支付 2.5 万欧元的补偿款[94]。

很明显的一点是,人们对支持还是反对经济驱动器官捐献仍然存在很大的争论。充分明确是否这样一些项目会增加捐献率的唯一方式是一个设计完善、管理有序的临床试验。这个临床试验的设计需要考虑是否要限制给活体或者死亡捐献者提供补偿以及数目,必要的管理框架以及所需的立法方面的改变。在实验开始之前要充分考虑到有许多需要清除的明显的制度障碍,以及可能与之相关的执行成本。但这种情况似乎是不可能的,尤其是在当前经济全球化的背景之下。

总结

获取器官移植机会的不平等或多或少存在于每一个国家。这种国与国之间明显不同的不平等是受国家是否富裕、法律、道德以及组织设施是否完善、器官分配系统是否有效,道德和文化多样性以及信仰系统等因素影响的。即便是在拥有完善的器官移植项目的富裕的国家，器官供需之间的不平衡仍然在不断加剧。全球范围内的器官短缺以及获得移植机会的不平等是移植商业化、器官黑市交易以及移植旅游业的两大主要推动因素。已经在研究全球性的策略来解决这些问题，并且认识到器官黑市交易问题的严重性以及全球移植团队对这些问题的反对都是重要的进展。更具争议的解决措施包括经济驱动器官捐献，尽管公众最支持的是经济驱动的活体器官捐献，而不是死亡器官捐献。伊朗模式为经济驱动活体肾脏捐献可以满足需要提供了证据，但是许多关于西方移植系统适用性问题的关注仍然存在。在器官移植不公平以及器官黑市交易在全球范围内消除之前仍然需要克服复杂的伦理、组织、政治、法律障碍问题。

（刘鹏 译 徐骁 校）

参考文献

1. Rudge C, Johnson RJ, Fuggle SV, et al. Renal transplantation in the United Kingdom for patients from ethnic minorities. Transplantation. 2007;83(9):1169–1173.
2. Whiting JF, Woodward RS, Zavala EY, et al. Economic cost of expanded criteria donors in cadaveric renal transplantation: analysis of Medicare payments. Transplantation. 2000;70(5):755–760.
3. Rithalia A, McDaid C, Suekarran S, et al. Impact of presumed consent for organ donation on donation rates: a systematic review. BMJ (Clinical Research Ed.). 2009;338:a3162.
4. Mahillo B, Carmona M, Alvarez M, et al. 2009 global data in organ donation and transplantation: activities, laws, and organization. Transplantation. 2011;92(10):1069–1074.
5. Bagheri A. Organ transplantation laws in Asian countries: a comparative study. Transplantation Proceedings. 2005;37(10):4159–4162.
6. Dominguez-Gil B, Haase-Kromwijk B, Van Leiden H, et al. Current situation of donation after circulatory death in European countries. Transplant International. 2011;24(7):676–686.
7. Summers DM, Johnson RJ, Allen J, et al. Analysis of factors that affect outcome after transplantation of kidneys donated after cardiac death in the UK: a cohort study. Lancet. 2010;376(9749):1303–1311.
8. Klein AS, Messersmith EE, Ratner LE, et al. Organ donation and utilization in the United States, 1999–2008. American Journal of Transplantation. 2010;10(4 Pt 2):973–986.
9. Dawwas MF, Gimson AE, Lewsey JD, et al. Survival after liver transplantation in the United Kingdom and Ireland compared with the United States. Gut. 2007;56(11):1606–1613.
10. Kim SJ, Schaubel DE, Fenton SS, et al. Mortality after kidney transplantation: a comparison between the United States and Canada. American Journal of Transplantation. 2006;6(1):109–114.
11. Daar AS, Marshall P. Culture and psychology in organ transplantation. World Health Forum. 1998;19(2):124–132.
12. Barber K, Falvey S, Hamilton C, et al. Potential for organ donation in the United Kingdom: audit of intensive care records. BMJ (Clinical Research Ed.). 2006;332(7550):1124–1127.
13. Morgan M, Hooper R, Mayblin M, et al. Attitudes to kidney donation and registering as a donor among ethnic groups in the UK. Journal of Public Health. 2006;28(3):226–234.
14. Alkhawari FS, Stimson GV, Warrens AN. Attitudes toward transplantation in U.K. Muslim Indo-Asians in west London. American Journal of Transplantation. 2005;5(6):1326–1331.
15. Siminoff LA, Gordon N, Hewlett J, et al. Factors influencing families' consent for donation of solid organs for transplantation. JAMA: Journal of the American Medical Association. 2001;286(1):71–77.
16. Irving MJ, Tong A, Jan S, et al. Factors that influence the decision to be an organ donor: a systematic review of the qualitative literature. Nephrology, Dialysis, Transplantation. 2012;27(6):2526–2533.
17. Shaheen FA, Al-Jondeby M, Kurpad R, et al. Social and cultural issues in organ transplantation in Islamic countries. Annals of Transplantation: Quarterly of the Polish Transplantation Society. 2004;9(2):11–13.
18. Shaheen FA, Souqiyyeh MZ, Ramprassad K, et al. Current issues and problems of transplantation in the Middle East: the Arabian Gulf. Transplantation Proceedings. 2001;33(5):2621–2622.
19. Aswad S, Souqiyyeh MZ, Huraib S, et al. Public attitudes toward organ donation in Saudi Arabia. Transplantation Proceedings. 1992;24(5):2056–2058.
20. Daar AS. The response to the challenge of organ shortage in the Middle East region: a summary. Transplantation Proceedings. 1997;29(8):3215–3216.
21. Collins JF. Kidney disease in Maori and Pacific people in New Zealand. Clinical Nephrology. 2010;74(Suppl 1):S61–S65.
22. Yeates K. Health disparities in renal disease in Canada. Seminars in Nephrology. 2010;30(1):12–18.
23. Weber CL, Rush DN, Jeffery JR, et al. Kidney transplantation outcomes in Canadian aboriginals. American Journal of Transplantation. 2006;6(8):1875–1881.
24. Gordon EJ, Ladner DP, Caicedo JC, et al. Disparities in kidney transplant outcomes: a review. Seminars in Nephrology. 2010;30(1):81–89.
25. Patzer RE, Amaral S, Klein M, et al. Racial disparities in pediatric access to kidney transplantation: does socioeconomic status play a role? American Journal of Transplantation. 2012;12(2):369–378.
26. Patzer RE, Perryman JP, Schrager JD, et al. The role of race and poverty on steps to kidney transplantation in the southeastern United States. American Journal of Transplantation. 2012;12(2):358–368.
27. Saunders MR, Cagney KA, Ross LF, et al. Neighborhood poverty, racial composition and renal transplant waitlist. American Journal of Transplantation. 2010;10(8):1912–1917.
28. Alexander GC, Sehgal AR. Barriers to cadaveric renal transplantation among blacks, women, and the poor. JAMA: Journal of the American Medical Association. 1998;280(13):1148–1152.
29. Kasiske BL, London W, Ellison MD. Race and socioeconomic factors influencing early placement on the kidney transplant waiting list. Journal of the American Society of Nephrology. 1998;9(11):2142–2147.
30. Keith D, Ashby VB, Port FK, et al. Insurance type and minority status associated with large disparities in prelisting dialysis among candidates for kidney transplantation. Clinical Journal of the American Society of Nephrology. 2008;3(2):463–470.
31. Udayaraj U, Ben-Shlomo Y, Roderick P, et al. Social deprivation, ethnicity, and access to the deceased donor kidney transplant waiting list in England and Wales. Transplantation. 2010;90(3):279–285.
32. Dudley CR, Johnson RJ, Thomas HL, et al. Factors that influence access to the national renal transplant waiting list. Transplantation. 2009;88(1):96–102.
33. Udayaraj U, Ben-Shlomo Y, Roderick P, et al. Social deprivation, ethnicity, and uptake of living kidney donor transplantation in the United Kingdom. Transplantation. 2012;93(6):610–616.
34. Merion RM, Barnes AD, Lin M, et al. Transplants in foreign countries among patients removed from the US transplant waiting list. American Journal of Transplantation. 2008;8(4 Pt 2):988–996.
35. The Declaration of Istanbul on organ trafficking and transplant tourism. Transplantation. 2008;86(8):1013–1018.
36. Haken J. Transnational Crime in the Developing World. Washington: Global Financial Integrity; 2011.
37. Shimazono Y. The state of the international organ trade: a provisional picture based on integration of available information. Bulletin of the World Health Organization. 2007;85(12):955–962.
38. Budiani-Saberi DA, Delmonico FL. Organ trafficking and transplant tourism: a commentary on the global realities. American Journal of Transplantation. 2008;8(5):925–929.
39. Padilla BS. Regulated compensation for kidney donors in the Philippines. Current Opinion in Organ Transplantation. 2009;14(2):120–123.
40. Watts J. China introduces new rules to deter human organ trade. Lancet. 2007;369(9577):1917–1918.
41. Tsai MK, Yang CY, Lee CY, et al. De novo malignancy is associated with renal transplant tourism. Kidney International. 2011;79(8):908–913.
42. Sajjad I, Baines LS, Patel P, et al. Commercialization of kidney transplants: a systematic review of outcomes in recipients and donors. American Journal of Nephrology. 2008;28(5):744–754.
43. Goyal M, Mehta RL, Schneiderman LJ, et al. Economic and health consequences of selling a kidney in India. JAMA: Journal of the American Medical Association. 2002;288(13):1589–1593.
44. Naqvi SA, Ali B, Mazhar F, et al. A socioeconomic survey of kidney vendors in Pakistan. Transplant International. 2007;20(11):934–939.
45. Ibrahim HN, Foley R, Tan L, et al. Long-term consequences of kidney donation.

46. Segev DL, Muzaale AD, Caffo BS, et al. Perioperative mortality and long-term survival following live kidney donation. JAMA: Journal of the American Medical Association. 2010;303(10):959-966.
47. Westlie L, Fauchald P, Talseth T, et al. Quality of life in Norwegian kidney donors. Nephrology, Dialysis, Transplantation. 1993;8(10):1146-1150.
48. Fehrman-Ekholm I, Brink B, Ericsson C, et al. Kidney donors don't regret: follow-up of 370 donors in Stockholm since 1964. Transplantation. 2000;69(10): 2067-2071.
49. Clemens KK, Thiessen-Philbrook H, Parikh CR, et al. Psychosocial health of living kidney donors: a systematic review. American Journal of Transplantation. 2006;6(12):2965-2977.
50. Inston NG, Gill D, Al-Hakim A, et al. Living paid organ transplantation results in unacceptably high recipient morbidity and mortality. Transplantation Proceedings. 2005;37(2):560-562.
51. Canales MT, Kasiske BL, Rosenberg ME. Transplant tourism: outcomes of United States residents who undergo kidney transplantation overseas. Transplantation. 2006;82(12):1658-1661.
52. Gill J, Madhira BR, Gjertson D, et al. Transplant tourism in the United States: a single-center experience. Clinical Journal of the American Society of Nephrology. 2008;3(6):1820-1828.
53. Rizvi SA, Naqvi SA, Zafar MN, et al. Commercial transplants in local Pakistanis from vended kidneys: a socio-economic and outcome study. Transplant International. 2009;22(6):615-621.
54. Sun CY, Lee CC, Chang CT, et al. Commercial cadaveric renal transplant: an ethical rather than medical issue. Clinical Transplantation. 2006;20(3):340-345.
55. Morad Z, Lim TO. Outcome of overseas kidney transplantation in Malaysia. Transplantation Proceedings. 2000;32(7):1485-1486.
56. Ghods AJ, Savaj S. Iranian model of paid and regulated living-unrelated kidney donation. Clinical Journal of the American Society of Nephrology. 2006;1(6): 1136-1145.
57. Haghighi AN, Ghahramani N. Living unrelated kidney donor transplantation in Iran. Nature Clinical Practice. Nephrology. 2006;2(12):E1.
58. Hippen B, Matas A. Incentives for organ donation in the United States: feasible alternative or forthcoming apocalypse? Current Opinion in Organ Transplantation. 2009;14(2):140-146.
59. Larijani B, Zahedi F, Taheri E. Deceased and living organ donation in Iran. American Journal of Transplantation. 2006;6(6):1493.
60. Malakoutian T, Hakemi MS, Nassiri AA, et al. Socioeconomic status of Iranian living unrelated kidney donors: a multicenter study. Transplantation Proceedings. 2007;39(4):824-825.
61. Zargooshi J. Iranian kidney donors: motivations and relations with recipients. Journal of Urology. 2001;165(2):386-392.
62. Zargooshi J. Quality of life of Iranian kidney "donors". Journal of Urology. 2001;166(5):1790-1799.
63. Nejatisafa AA, Mortaz-Hedjri S, Malakoutian T, et al. Quality of life and life events of living unrelated kidney donors in Iran: a multicenter study. Transplantation. 2008;86(7):937-940.
64. Simforoosh N, Basiri A, Fattahi MR, et al. Living unrelated versus living related kidney transplantation: 20 years' experience with 2155 cases. Transplantation Proceedings. 2006;38(2):422-425.
65. Einollahi B, Pourfarziani V, Ahmadzad-Asl M, et al. Iranian model of renal allograft transplantation in 3028 recipients: survival and risk factors. Transplantation Proceedings. 2007;39(4):907-910.
66. Tilney NL, Chapman JR, Delmonico FL. Debate on financial incentives is off the mark of national and international realities. Transplantation. 2010;89(7): 906-907.
67. The Madrid resolution on organ donation and transplantation: national responsibility in meeting the needs of patients, guided by the WHO principles. Transplantation. 2011;91(Suppl 11):S29-S31. [accessed on January 13, 2014]; Available at: http://www.ehltf.info/downloads/madrid_resolution.pdf
68. Delmonico FL, Dominguez-Gil B, Matesanz R, et al. A call for government accountability to achieve national self-sufficiency in organ donation and transplantation. Lancet. 2011;378(9800):1414-1418.
69. White SL, Chadban SJ, Jan S, et al. How can we achieve global equity in provision of renal replacement therapy? Bulletin of the World Health Organization. 2008;86(3):229-237.
70. Groth CG, Chapman JR. The global alliance for transplantation. Transplantation Proceedings. 2006;38(2):356-357.
71. Matesanz R. Factors influencing the adaptation of the Spanish Model of organ donation. Transplant International. 2003;16(10):736-741.
72. Matesanz R, Dominguez-Gil B, Coll E, et al. Spanish experience as a leading country: what kind of measures were taken? Transplant International. 2011;24(4):333-343.
73. Simpkin AL, Robertson LC, Barber VS, et al. Modifiable factors influencing relatives' decision to offer organ donation: systematic review. BMJ (Clinical Research Ed.). 2009;338:b991.
74. The ACRE Trial Collaborators. Effect of "collaborative requesting" on consent rate for organ donation: randomised controlled trial (ACRE trial). BMJ (Clinical Research Ed.). 2009;339:b3911.
75. Johnson RJ, Fuggle SV, Mumford L, et al. A new UK 2006 National Kidney Allocation Scheme for deceased heart-beating donor kidneys. Transplantation. 2010;89(4):387-394.
76. Moylan CA, Brady CW, Johnson JL, et al. Disparities in liver transplantation before and after introduction of the MELD score. JAMA: Journal of the American Medical Association. 2008;300(20):2371-2378.
77. Guiding principles on human organ transplantation. World Health Organization. Lancet. 1991;337(8755):1470-1471.
78. Delmonico FL. The development of the Declaration of Istanbul on Organ Trafficking and Transplant Tourism. Nephrology, Dialysis, Transplantation. 2008;23(11): 3381-3382.
79. Ambagtsheer F, Weimar W. A criminological perspective: why prohibition of organ trade is not effective and how the declaration of Istanbul can move forward. American Journal of Transplantation. 2011;12(3):571-575.
80. Glazier AK, Delmonico FL. The declaration of Istanbul is moving forward by combating transplant commercialism and trafficking and by promoting organ donation. American Journal of Transplantation. 2011;12(3):515-516.
81. Klarenbach S, Garg AX, Vlaicu S. Living organ donors face financial barriers: a national reimbursement policy is needed. CMAJ: Canadian Medical Association Journal. 2006;174(6):797-798.
82. Hippen BE, Gaston RS. The conspicuous costs of more of the same. American Journal of Transplantation. 2006;6(7):1503-1504.
83. Cynowiec J, Kim J, Qazi YA. Incentivizing living organ donation. Current Opinion in Organ Transplantation. 2009;14(2):201-205.
84. Matas AJ. The case for living kidney sales: rationale, objections and concerns. American Journal of Transplantation. 2004;4(12):2007-2017.
85. Matas AJ, Hippen B, Satel S. In defense of a regulated system of compensation for living donation. Current Opinion in Organ Transplantation. 2008;13(4): 379-385.
86. Gaston RS, Danovitch GM, Epstein RA, et al. Limiting financial disincentives in live organ donation: a rational solution to the kidney shortage. American Journal of Transplantation. 2006;6(11):2548-2555.
87. Matas AJ, Schnitzler M. Payment for living donor (vendor) kidneys: a cost-effectiveness analysis. American Journal of Transplantation. 2004;4(2):216-221.
88. Danovitch GM, Delmonico FL. The prohibition of kidney sales and organ markets should remain. Current Opinion in Organ Transplantation. 2008;13(4): 386-394.
89. Eastlund T. Monetary blood donation incentives and the risk of transfusion-transmitted infection. Transfusion. 1998;38(9):874-882.
90. Rothman SM, Rothman DJ. The hidden cost of organ sale. American Journal of Transplantation. 2006;6(7):1524-1528.
91. Bryce CL, Siminoff LA, Ubel PA, et al. Do incentives matter? Providing benefits to families of organ donors. American Journal of Transplantation. 2005;5(12): 2999-3008.
92. Boulware LE, Troll MU, Wang NY, et al. Public attitudes toward incentives for organ donation: a national study of different racial/ethnic and income groups. American Journal of Transplantation. 2006;6(11):2774-2785.
93. Rodrigue JR, Cornell DL, Howard RJ. Attitudes toward financial incentives, donor authorization, and presumed consent among next-of-kin who consented vs. refused organ donation. Transplantation. 2006;81(9):1249-1256.
94. Kranenburg L, Schram A, Zuidema W, et al. Public survey of financial incentives for kidney donation. Nephrology, Dialysis, Transplantation. 2008;23(3):1039-1042.

第 140 章 器官移植中的联邦保险和私人保险

Timothy L. Pruett

引言

提供与实施移植治疗不是免费的，一个团队包括多种技术人员：外科医生、内科医生、护士、社工、药剂师、营养师、理疗师、行政管理人员等。额外的免疫抑制治疗和设备资源可满足移植受者需要的特殊需求。此外，相比移植术中及术后的治疗，评估和采集供者器官需要截然不同的人员队伍与资源。除外资金和规章，每个执行像器官移植这样复杂程序的医疗体系必须建立一套方法学来支持和维持①提供治疗的个体；②器官捐献中消耗的资源；③随后的移植服务。充足的经费决定一个体系是否能够生存下来。

个人购买治疗服务这样的简单模式不具有广泛的可行性。而常见的整体模式在全球许多地方被应用，政府资助医疗把移植和器官的费用纳入更加广泛的社会保健需求中。理论上利用该模式获得治疗是普遍的。但是器官移植成为该模式的费用中心，其包含医疗递送体系，对资源可用性有重大影响。在这个费用中心模式里，资源通常按既往需求或期望结果来分配。由于程序量增加，资源的过早消耗可能导致服务受限或者要从其他服务中转移资源。然而，美国的基金制度基于增加移植数量可提高该体系的收入，也提高了组织的声誉。在于政府和私人保险机构的复杂交叉，这一事实使美国基金制度的模式复杂化。本章的讨论将集中在施行器官移植的必要性，现有制度如何影响有时相互竞争的基金来源以及如何被影响。法律权威、政策、结果、实施和支付结构之间的关系变得紧密相连。虽然其他医疗体系可能在支持移植的政府保险与私人保险或个人基金之间保持不同的平衡，但是所有体系必须寻找办法对提供捐献和移植治疗中必需的努力、服务和产品进行补偿。

尽管目标不是“以美国为中心”，分析美国移植体系中的监管和性能成分将更好地理解多元化，但全球旅行移植治疗需要必要的元素。一项基金制度的基本元素必须满足：

1. 谁是移植服务的提供者以及什么服务是必需的。
2. 如何获得移植器官。
3. 患者如何找到他们需要的中心和器官。
4. 如何平衡需要为主与经济为主的目标之间的矛盾？

与移植相关的国家移植管理和监督、移植的经济影响和国家医疗政策方面的更多讨论可分别见于第128章、第142章和第143章。

对移植计划或移植中心的要求

在美国和全球许多地方，器官移植被高度管理。在某种程度上该管理规章的产生是由于器官有限的可得性以及对公共保险的需要，制度在法律和道德框架内发挥作用有利于需要器官拯救生命的患者。社会规章的潜在主题是反对优先获得和(或)过度滥用。建立器官捐献和移植的制度必须要有法律基础，允许器官移植中的必要元素在法律和社会道德观念内发挥作用(见第136章、第137章和第138章)。多器官捐献的基本原则是承认脑死亡，心脏可还在跳动。在20世纪60年代美国官方认可脑死亡，普遍接受符合哈佛标准的个体实际上已经死亡。美国1968年通过的《联邦遗体捐献法》(以及此后的多次修改法案)给器官和组织捐献过程提供了法律架构。再有,运输体系把创伤和神经损毁患者送到有专长和能力的机构给予专业治疗,强化了捐献体系。尽管这些要素不是移植直接支付体系的一部分,但强调了复杂的器官捐献和移植已经在尊重法律、道德和社会治疗实施机构。

1984年美国颁布《国家器官移植法案》(NOTA),建立起器官移植的法律权威。NOTA创建全国器官采集机构(OPO)网站与器官采集移植网站(OPTN)。创建OPO体系可最大限度采集死者供体的器官和组织。美国所有医院均被分配一个OPO,目的是为了标识和管理器官供者,获得器官捐献授权,协调器官检索和运输器官给指定受者、医院和团体。《社会保障法案》第十八章(《美国法典》第42卷1395页及后续)保障了OPO网站的资助,由联邦医保监控及随后识别器官检索实践的货币和财务责任来制订程序。

创建OPTN是为了公平分配死者供体器官给全国等待移植的患者,通过采纳统一的采集和运输捐献器官质量标准,通过参与国家移植体系会员标准,为国家相关部门及其他需要器官移植信息的人的利益分析和公开发表移植信息。NOTA规定只有OPTN会员才能在全国等待移植名单中注册患者和接受通过OPO系统检索的器官。私人的会员机构实施OPTN任务提供指定服务,由公共卫生服务中心下属的健康资源和服务管理中心(HRSA)提供合约并受其监管。移植受者科学登记系统(SRTR)生成对全国移植网站的授权。此信息目的是给OPTN报告全国和移植中心的绩效,进行常规质量评估以及特定会员绩效监督。公开发布及分析该信息旨在帮助受者及其医生更好理解他们对移植治疗的选择。

移植中心必须成为OPTN会员才能把患者加入名单以及接收移植尸体器官。1999年颁布的《最终法则》明确如何执行NOTA。裁决确定区域OPTN政策获得权限,要求会员遵守OPTN政策以及要求利用同行评审执行政策。2006年OPTN权限扩大,可监督活体器官捐献与移植。目前在美国非OPTN会员的中心无合法授权进行尸体或活体器官移植。保持“良好会员资格”已经成为有能力常规实施器官移植的最低标准。

OPTN细则规定移植计划的基本会员要求,包括要求关键人员有最低水平的经验或训练,以及拥有明确的专业辅助服务(如麻醉学、传染病学、放射学、病理学、血库、组织相容性服务和其他)与指定的医院和机构服务(包括充足的社会工作、营养、财务、理疗和其他服务)。OPTN会员需要人力和资源这些重要的制度性保证,附带相应的费用。会员身份受限于执行结果和政策依从性(尤其是关于随后的器官分配算法和患者安全)。实施特定数量的移植手术不是获得或保持OPTN会员资格的必需条件,但是结果不满足预期会引发OPTN对其进行同行评审。而且,如果会员机构缺乏主要人员或能力,无法行使OPTN政策或者危害等待移植名单中的患者或移植受者的安全,其会员身份将会被修改。尽管OPTN能够通过包括改变会员身份在内的多种方法惩戒项目,但OPTN只赋予HHS部长权力撤销机构会员资格。任何时候都有许多移植计划受到OPTN的政策服从部门审查。最后,如果一个项目要想加入美国移植体系,那么必须满足OPTN会员资格的费用和要求。启动一个项目必须支持这些所有的必要条件。

器官移植的管理与付费

移植的付费结构已经随时间发生重大变化。在美国刚开始实施移植手术时,受者所在医疗机构会为每位受者移植术后的治疗开出帐单。如果患者有保险,账单将会被递交给保险公司,但是第三方支付多样,个人和家庭会有相当大的财务风险。1972年通过《终末期肾病(ESRD)法案》,所有肾衰竭的患者可通过联邦医保进行透析和移植治疗。1981年《联邦医保第二付款人条款》阐明为拥有私人保险的患者政府ESRD支付的作用,这些患者在患有ESRD的基础上成为联邦医保的合格者。规定拥有私人雇主团体健康保险的个人;即使个体是联邦医保的合格者,在转变支付责任给联邦医保之前,头30个月的ESRD支付是私人计划的责任。然而,缺乏移植服务范围的预见性以及获得治疗途径的差异成为1984年通过NOTA的重要因素。在此法律下,美国政府不仅批准了器官移植,而且向私人保险公司统一接受与支付方面加快了进程。

联邦政府补偿参与联邦医保受益人器官移植手术的医院和医生。《联邦医保ESRD参与条件》在1976年首次颁布,并且规定了资源、人员和必要的结果。这些规定一开始相当少;但是2007年《最终规则》之前的数次修改扩大了条件。其他版本为联邦医保报销心脏(1986)、肝脏(1991)、肺(1995)移植手术制订了生存率。设备的联邦医保报销策略分为支付器官相关费用和支付移植过程费用。后者是诊断相关组织(DRG)下属的机构。联邦医保也对机构开展禁止办法,扣除部分在受益人复杂且长期的住院事件中产生的额外费用。有一个单独的支付计划支付内科医生和外科医生。这个基础模型沿用至今。2007 年《联邦医保参与条件》扩充了资源、过程和结果要素,对于给联邦医保受益人提供移植服务的机构而言这些要素是必需的。

其他政府资助的主要医保援助是针对那些低收入人群。联邦/州计划共同出资完成这项资助,由州立医疗补助计划进行管理。对个体获得基于收入的政府医疗福利资格有清晰定义的财务标准。因为它是共同资助的但由州政府管理,各州之间的医疗补助移植福利有明显不同。为了市民的利益,对于这些钱应该怎样被分配各州有许多的界限。获得医疗补助福利的资格标准由州政府制订,通常是要求在州内接受治疗(假设是可以获得的)。

私人保险公司与那些被政府参与日益影响的移植计划之间关系不断发展。最初,移植被当作机构提供的其他经批准的医疗服务,保险公司要寻求"服务费" 的专业和制度折扣。但是,这个模式很快被抛弃,程序转变为购买操作和给特定机构的捆绑支付这么一个组合。尽管投保人能够获得任何移植服务计划,如果投保的患者在一个被选为优先的计划里,保险公司将支付全部或最大的福利,这就是"在网络内"。进入提供者网络的必要资格已经发生重大进展。像联邦医保,通常有一个调整模式用于补偿机构,当超过最初约定数额的费用发生时。随着移植计划数量的增加,保险公司和医疗提供者之间的关系有所进展,很明显在网络内的资格可以迅速形成或者破裂。正如本章开头所说,美国体系根据概念被认为器官移植对医疗体系来说是一个收入中心,所以网络参与的维护和相应患者入口已成为多数计划临床和金融上的必要。类似地,非常重要的是要熟悉为移植治疗消耗的资源和相关的费用结构。当支出超过收入时体系即停止。

获取移植器官的费用

需要告知每位患者获取器官的费用巨大。NOTA 通过后买卖器官成为联邦法律的重罪;然而器官捐献是一项昂贵且复杂的活动,必须要有资金来源。为应对这种需求,联邦医保范围内制订了 OPO 和移植中心会计制度,规定可用于器官检索的费用。在该体系下器官受者分摊器官检索的费用。美国的医疗体系由组织运行的应记费用计算得到标准器官采集费用(SAC 或 OAC)。中心 SAC 来自受益人治疗的"许可"费用。这仍然是机构为下列情况补偿支出的主要机制。

1. 从 OPO 获取尸体器官。

2. 评估个体移植相容性的人力及检测。

3. 评估活体捐献者。

4. 移植中心必须提供但不直接对患者治疗收费的额外特定许可的服务。

各个移植中心的 SAC 有不同,部分原因在于人事及评估方法。管理 SAC 的效率是美国医保计划财务稳定性的中心要素。这笔费用通常是肾移植过程中最大的单笔花费部分,也是额外肾脏器官移植费用的重要部分。

补偿这些费用的途径依赖于付款来源。对于政府付款人,联邦医保受益人的 SAC/器官采集费用被合并到年度机构医疗保险费用报告中。这些产品和服务的支出根据联邦医保费用准则将在年度基础上报销给医疗机构。弥补联邦医保相关费用的能力在这个体系下会落后一年,但有资金补偿体系。

在私人投保个体的案例中,补偿器官采集的费用被合并到受者账单中。私人保险公司通常不直接支付潜在或实际的捐献治疗费用,但是会支付器官采集的费用。尽管部分保险公司给受者评估和等待移植名单管理做适度的"治疗阶段"支付,但是捐献治疗费用多数会在移植实施后被偿还。当接受者要在等待移植名单上数年却没有获得移植时,显然需要进行资源管理。多种事件使无法获得补偿的机构费用变得明显,例如大量的未移植患者停留在等候名单上,重复进行组织相容性测试和随访,评估潜在的活体捐赠者,以及把费用低效分配给管理中心。在此环境下这些费用分配到 SAC,导致高额的 SAC 要么从付款者的捆绑支付协议中减少移植捐献利润,要么因为高额的"固定"费用难以与保险人签订合约。对一个移植计划的财务福利来说,了解与管理该费用中心至关重要。此外,因为患者的移植支付来源会随时间变化,获得机构移植费用补偿的过程中需要密切了解公共和私人支付方的财务组成。

政府及私人保险与受者个体

移植服务的支付体系在动态变化、持续发展。过去，器官移植机构的专业服务所产生的费用由患者的保险公司支付，然后全部或部分的费用补偿专业人员和设备。当移植还是非常规手术时,中心可以要求服务有利可图。但是随着目前移植计划的数量增加,费用管理必须是移植财务计划中的重要部分，因为移植偿还已经不是费用偿还模式。私人与公共支付体系朝不同路线发展，保持财务可行的制度策略需要适应不同的模式。

政府提供者

在大多数国家,由政府支付大多数人的医疗保险。医疗治疗由公立医院实施(卫生部医院,像在许多国家),或者由部队医院或退伍军人管理医院实施。但第三方支付者是美国政府医疗保险最常见的支付方式,直接支付给有资格治疗联邦医保和医疗补助受益人的独立医疗提供者(医院或内科医生)。潜在的政府受益人必须符合联邦医保或者州立医疗补助制度。联邦医保为美国最大的单群体(超过1亿人)提供医疗支付。即使从政府支付者获得的补偿有限，很少有医疗体系忽视治疗这个正在扩张的人群。

联邦医保要求获得移植治疗提供者资质的项目或者中心保证数量和预后并不是新的要求。但是在2007年《参与条例》(COP)正式生效,医疗机构要向联邦医保受益人提供移植治疗。这些条件给机构和移植中心带来了新的过程管理及人力要求。他们必须达到SRTR所规定的患者及移植物生存预后以及规定移植数量。未能符合预期目标会妨碍医疗机构加入联邦医保体系。虽然有机会辩解是影响因素造成不良结果,但若未能说服医疗保险小组则有丧失联邦医保附属机构和支付的风险。除了移植数量和预后要求,COP要求加强质量评估过程、过程改进和活体器官捐献等等,这需要额外的人员,如活体捐献倡导者。而OPTN的会员要求与政策有部分重叠，所以必须强烈要求移植计划或中心必须注意这些不同之处。SRTR和每三年一次的CMS现场审计/督查提供常规容量和预后报告,由联邦医保审查评估COP的依从性。失去CMS认证会破坏项目的声誉和患者推荐,所以要竭尽全力避免这种可能性。已经出现了一些例子,由于遵守COP规定的成本过高而导致移植计划关闭。

私人保险公司

现在的私人保险公司更趋向于把逐渐增加的债务转移至移植计划和(或)中心。不管受者是否“理想”或存在多个并发症，固定捆绑支付也为移植手术提供类似的金额。给这部分人提供治疗所需的资源有所不同,但赔偿的趋势不变。移植计划或中心负责有效地管理资源,同时保持满意的结果(调整SRTR风险)。其中限制那些耗尽/费用过高的个人移植治疗是一个暗含的选择,或许能获得可接受的结果,但提供治疗的费用超过了私人付款的报销额度。管理中心患者群体结果的可变性以及患者消耗的资源，对于计划财务的可行性已经变得至关重要。

如前所述，多数大型私人保险公司已经建立移植中心关系/网络,这些移植中心给投保人群提供绝大部分的治疗,投保患者可优先获得治疗。因为受者在“网络外”的中心会产生更多的债务,所以财务动机驱使大量患者去有最优支付关系的中心。关联医疗机构的标准通常依赖于私人保险公司的规定,包括合理的价格、足够的移植容量、满意的结果和可获得的服务。保险公司支付移植中心用于赔偿移植前及移植后的治疗、手术和住院以及器官成本。当患者产生超过基础支付的异常费用时，移植中心有效管理费用和有效商议各种补偿是非常有必要的。赔偿制度的发展要求移植中心与所服务人群的需求匹配其资源和过程。如果不能与公司达成适当的移植支付赔偿协议，中心将不能维持自身的财务状况。

最近移植合约有所变化，其中包括SRTR提供的公开可得的“风险调整”计划(PSR)特定结果。尽管事实上这些结果的原本目的并不在此，但现在被广泛采用作为网络参与的资格证明。OPTN旨在把该标准作为评估体系质量和帮助患者了解中心经验及移植结果的工具。然而不论标准如何变动,当新计划不能达到标准执行门槛时就会被排除出付款人网络。与脱离网络相关的结果是患者流量减少、收入损失以及声誉受损。

很大一部分自我保险者不能承受移植治疗交付相关风险的变化。在这种情况下,他们可以向大型的“分保公司”,比如联合健康集团,购买移植保险。在该模式中，分保公司通常会开发更加严格的网络如卓越中心

(COE),与数个大容量、费用高效的计划签订合同。保险公司支付交通和住宿费用,鼓励投保人在全国相对较少的中心获得治疗,投保人可以在首选的中心接受治疗。使用"购买"力及对指定移植中心承诺容量可减少移植治疗的费用。大部分投保的移植受者能够通过分保公司协调支付,患者和供者被送到其他国家接受移植治疗可降低债务。但对体系和患者存有明显的道德、程序上的弊端,因为远程距离加重个人和家庭的负担(见第 138 章)。

平衡患者需求、管理预后及预期财务

为使移植计划能继续提供治疗,资金是至关重要的,以支付人员、资源、器官和服务。了解资源的分配及产生也非常重要。在移植为费用中心的体系里,例如国家卫生体系,计划需要持续资助满足器官移植的额定例数。认识到提供持续服务必需的资金至关重要。如果下拨的资金不能满足所有公民的治疗需要,则必须某种形式的资金分配/配给。其中与其他服务共享预算是常见的,比如计划预算过多时,需要缩减服务或从另外表现良好的服务获得资金。医疗资金分配/配给的相关话题迅速扩大范围跨过居民医疗需求,进入经济、政治、道德和法律的领域。该体系的移植中心经州政府授权,比市场驱动的中心更容易有不同的动力。

在移植为主要收入的体系里,如大多数美国的计划,移植例数充足对计划可行性是至关重要的。移植例数增加可带来更多的收入、声誉和机会,移植例数减少则造成计划收入降低,后续需要重组计划资金。业务的关键指标是了解患者流动和资金消耗。收入中心模式使广泛的创收患者进入计划是成功的基础。确保例数的首要障碍是联合提供医疗服务的机构,需要联邦医保和大型私人保险公司网络参与。符合 OPTN 会员资格与例数及预后标准是所有的机构参与的前提条件。SRTR 生成公开发布的计划具体报告(PSR)仍是衡量计划唯一独立的指标。移植中心必须掌握公共领域的执行信息。公布风险调整变量后,移植计划必须持续评估受者以确保风险调整适合患者。预后低于预期的受者对计划是有损的,必须修改实践和选择。但风险调整并不全面,所以多种并发症的老年患者可能被排除出移植计划,或器官可能有选择性地分给预后良好的受者。跟踪公布的移植受者预后对公众及商业都非常重要。受者被标记为预后不佳,则要求移植计划原则结合患者风险、器官质量和器官接受改善预后。而公布的风险调整结果仍然是不完美的体系,实践使计划质量评估与过程改进(QAPI)成为移植商业计划中必要的部分。

收入中心模式移植计划可行性的另一要素是有效管理移植的费用。提供服务的费用不能超过产生的效益。可尝试用更多的财务缓冲换取更大的报销比例,因为随着移植中心例数增加,保险公司会减少偿还并且把风险转移到中心。在利润缩减的情况下,移植中心需要找出低效的环节。不使用持续 QAPI 分析,限制患者治疗以减小风险成为改善预后最常使用的技术。这项技术通常是有效的,因为多数移植专家能够有效处理直接的患者。但是约束患者的选择也排除了从移植治疗获益的患者,减少计划的财务损失量。

总结

不管资金来自政府或私人保险公司,财务平衡是移植计划可持续的必要先决条件。医疗体系的收入必须均衡分配到患者、治疗、器官采集和患者流动的需求上面。管理、执行指标、网络参与和捆绑支付混淆这个简单的关系。了解这些整体的系统是有用的,但确保可持续性就必须要监控服从性。

(卓建勇 译 徐骁 校)

参考文献

器官移植的美国政府性文件

1. NOTA 42 USC Sec 273. [accessed 15.01.2014]; Available from: http://uscode.house.gov/search/criteria.shtml.
2. OPTN Final Rule: CFR Title 42, Part 121: Organ Procurement and Transplantation Network. [accessed 15.01.2014]; Available from: http://optn.transplant.hrsa.gov/policiesAndBylaws/final_rule.asp.
3. CMS Conditions of Participation: Centers for Medicare and Medicaid Services CFR Title 42 Parts 405, 482, 488, and 498 Medicare Program; Hospital Conditions of Participation: Requirements for Approval and Re-Approval of Transplant Centers to Perform Organ Transplants; Final Rule. [accessed 15.01.2014]; Available from: https://www.cms.gov/CertificationandComplianc/20_Transplant.asp.

器官采集费用中心

1. Abecassis M. Organ acquisition cost centers Part 1:medicare regulations-truth or consequence. American Journal of Transplantation. 2006;6(12):2830–2835.
2. Abecassis M. Organ acquisition cost centers Part II: reducing the burden of cost and inventory. American Journal of Transplantation. 2006;6(12):2836–2840.

监督和影响器官移植

1. McDiarmid SV, Pruett TL, Graham WK. The oversight of solid organ transplantation in the United States. American Journal of Transplantation. 2008;8(4):739–744.
2. Schold JD, Arrington CJ, Levine G. Significant alterations in reported clinical practice associated with increased oversight of organ transplant center performance. Progress in Transplantation (Aliso Viejo, Calif.). 2010;20(3):279–287.
3. Brown RS Jr, Higgins R, Pruett TL. The evolution and direction of OPTN oversight of live organ donation and transplantation in the United States. American Journal of Transplantation. 2009;9(1):31–34.
4. Dickinson DM, Arrington CJ, Fant G, et al. SRTR program-specific reports on outcomes: a guide for the new reader. American Journal of Transplantation. 2008;8(4 Pt 2):1012–1026.
5. Weinhandl ED, Snyder JJ, Israni AK, et al. Effect of comorbidity adjustment on CMS criteria for kidney transplant center performance. American Journal of Transplantation. 2009;9(3):506–516.
6. Abecassis MM, Burke R, Cosimi AB, et al. American Society of Transplant Surgeons. "Transplant center regulations–a mixed blessing? An ASTS Council viewpoint. American Journal of Transplantation. 2008;8(12):2496–2502.

支付计划和移植操作

1. Schold JD, Gregg JA, Harman JS, et al. Barriers to evaluation and wait listing for kidney transplantation. Clinical Journal of the American Society of Nephrology. 2011;6(7):1760–1767.
2. Axelrod DA, Millman D, Abecassis DD. US Health Care Reform and Transplantation. Part I: overview and impact on access and reimbursement in the private sector. American Journal of Transplantation. 2010;10(10):2197–2202.
3. Axelrod DA, Millman D, Abecassis MM. US Health Care Reform and Transplantation, Part II: impact on the public sector and novel health care delivery systems. American Journal of Transplantation. 2010;10(10):2203–2207.
4. Herring AA, Woolhandler S, Himmelstein DU. Insurance status of U.S. organ donors and transplant recipients: the uninsured give, but rarely receive. International Journal of Health Services: Planning, Administration, Evaluation. 2008;38(4):641–652.
5. Englesbe MJ, Ads Y, Cohn JA, et al. The effects of donor and recipient practices on transplant center finances. American Journal of Transplantation. 2008;8(3):586–592.
6. Howard RJ, Cornell DL, Schold JD. CMS oversight, OPOs and transplant centers and the law of unintended consequences. Clinical Transplantation. 2009;23(6):778–783.

第 141 章

器官移植的药物开发和移植免疫抑制剂的审批流程

Candace Wang, J. Mark Hexham, Alan Slade, Peter Heining, Ronald G. Van Valen, Guido Junge, Marc I. Lorber

引言

本章将讲述从器官移植的药物开发至特异性移植审批的大体流程，其中我们将重点讲述通过卫生主管部门的审批，后期阶段(临床实验阶段Ⅱ和Ⅲ)的发展与进步。本章会聚焦于某些明确指示可用于移植的药物发展史，与此同时，本章也会删繁就简，帮助读者们准确地了解使移植药物普遍应用于临床的发展过程。如果一种新的免疫抑制剂在靶向治疗中明确有效且优于现有治疗药物，进而被推荐给内科医生和他的患者，那笔者认为本章的目的也就达到了。从药物的开发到注册的关键步骤详见图 141.1。

在新药的开发探索阶段，通过各式的体外实验，科学家们从大量的化合物中筛选出具有特定生物化学活性的化合物。通过精准的体外实验和在体实验模型，更好的是在被承认的非临床移植模型上，进一步筛选出其中具有活跃功能且满足所需标准的化合物。而那些被证实具有目的生化活性的化合物则被用于后续的非临床阶段的评估(见后文“开发”部分)。

对于原料药(活性化学基团)和药物最终剂型的技术研究和发展，是与初步的筛选和非临床阶段的测试同步进行的。随着原料药在临床试验阶段不断进步与发展，早期实验室的小规模生产不断被优化进而该药被投入规模化地生产。随着临床试验的不断进展，为了达到药物的效价强度、稳定性、纯度等调控标准，候选的药物就必须被加工成各式各样的剂型(例如片剂、胶囊、液体等)(见后文“产品特性、剂型、释放及包装的发

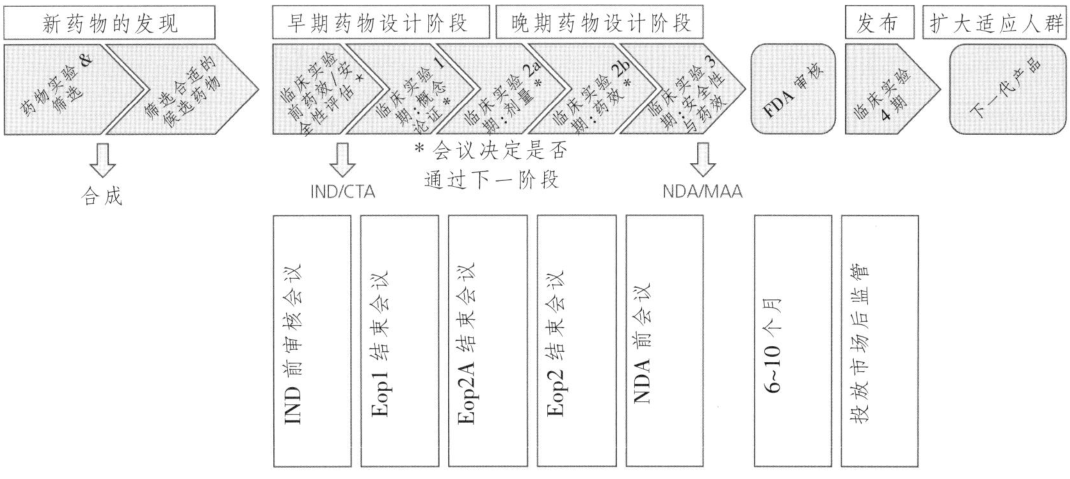

图 141.1 药物研发的申请和申请前咨询关键流程。Dev，发展；Eff，药效；PoC，概念论证；IND，临床研究申请(欧洲：CTA，临床实验主管)；EoP1，阶段Ⅰ的完结；EoP2A(在 IND 之后但在阶段Ⅱ结束前)；EoP2，阶段Ⅱ的完结；NDA，美国新药申请(欧洲：MAA，市场主管部门申请)。

展”部分)。

药代动力学研究可以通过体外实验测定药物分子的吸收、分布、代谢和排泄特性,从而挑选出具有最优化特征的备选药物(见后文“药代动力学、药物代谢和生物分析技术”部分)。与此同时,在体外和在体实验中从事各种毒理学试验,可以把具有致突变和(或)致癌可能性的,或有器官毒性的药物剔除出候选名单,例如具有肝毒性、肾毒性或者心脏毒性的药物(见后文“从开发到获批的临床前阶段毒理学试验”部分)。最终,经过了进入人体试验阶段之前如此广泛的筛选,一个或多个候选药物浮出水面(见后文“临床试验”部分)。

本章的临床试验部分描述了贯穿整个药物研发史的各个不同的试验方法。临床实验阶段Ⅰ的研究评估了药物在人体使用时的安全性、耐受性以及临床的药代动力学。亦可通过测定生物标记的变化或者其他药效动力学的研究方法来测定新药的活性与毒性。第一次真正意义的在人体中评估药物的活性通常被称为“概念论证”(PoC)。通常某一治疗方案针对特定的目标人群会有完善的标准,而PoC的目的正是为了证实化合物的某一活性可以符合该标准。如果PoC成功,更大规模的临床实验阶段Ⅱb试验将测定药物更多的特性,从而改善药物的使用安全性、效价强度和最理想的给药方案。接下来是临床实验阶段Ⅲ,或者说是验证性的试验阶段,往往需要长达12个月甚至更久的大范围统计学的研究分析,用以验证临床实验阶段Ⅱb试验所得出药物的各个特性。在阶段Ⅲ项目验证了药物使用安全性、效价强度和耐受性之后,该新药无数的研究,包括新药研发、非临床和临床各项试验项目,生成了最终的数据,而这一数据被编辑成为大量的申请新药审批的档案,或称之为新药申请(NDA)。

新药的申请检察和批准十分复杂,包括药物的生产、临床前与临床的效价强度和安全性的信息。该过程被严格管理,要求详尽的资料以证明申请的新药已达到卫生主管部门的标准。早在最初的临床试验开始之前,申请新药的公司(有时被称作“申请人”)就已经和卫生主管部门频繁地沟通,而且这样的沟通将在整个临床试验和申请过程中持续。这样的漫长沟通也帮助各利益相关者可以对NDA的各种要求进行商讨、协调。值得一提的是,和卫生主管部门达成有关任何可能存在的隐患和危险的共识十分重要。当一种可能获批使用的新药通过临床试验不断优化时,卫生当局会提供有关评估的重要意见,而正是这些重要意见可以很大程度上帮助新药最终走向市场。现今,新药的申请总是以电子资料的方式被呈交给卫生当局,典型的申请材料可以是约4~20千兆字节的形式,也可以是各式各样的模块形式(见后文“注册之路:药物的审批过程”部分)。如果新药的申请被接受,那么各种资料将由不同的专业团队同时审查。

整个申请与审批流程至少需要5~10年的人力物力,来精准地塑造药物的安全性及效价强度,从而获得市场部门的批准。总的来说,在申请新药的公司遵守各项颁布的指南和规定并被全球卫生主管部门审计检察之后,才能确保上市的新药的质量和药效。

开发

我们可以从已知的生物化学通路中获取药物干预的靶点,也可以从新发现的靶点中挑选药物干预的位点,譬如说通过分子或者基因组途径识别信号通路中的某些化合物。在药物的开发探索过程中,研发人员需要在大量化合物中筛选出具有某一特定生物化学功能(活性)的化合物,比方说,化合物在体外实验或者细胞实验中能否抑制某个目标受体的活性。研发人员将具有所需生物化学功能的化合物进一步改进其化学结构,紧接着又从中筛选出对目的基因有更强活性的化合物。同样地,科学家们可以通过已知的药物之间的相互作用来有效增强药物生化功能的方法,也可以改变化合物的化学结构使其达到最强活性。

之后,各个候选的活性分子会进行体外实验和在体实验,例如会在啮齿动物的移植器官中进行。这些模型上的实验能帮助理解化合物作用的原理,也对该活性分子能否成为一个新药在组织学和血生化层面,进行使用安全性和活性的初步评估。自从免疫抑制剂步入器官移植的联合治疗领域,评估免疫抑制剂累加效应和协同效应的可能性是十分普遍的。由于在药代动力学和药效学上各物种间差异的存在,新药在非临床试验中的活性并不能代表用于人体时的活性,因此,实证研究可以为候选药物的筛选以及与卫生当局和投资者们探讨改药能否上市提供一个坚实的基础。然而,将非临床试验过渡至临床试验是必不可少的。

产品特性、剂型、释放及包装的发展

在药物研发和发展阶段，一个药品可能需要从几毫克的实验室产品，变成数以吨计的规模化生产产品。当这些药进入临床实验研究时，上述的规模化生产则变得更加复杂，药物会被严格控制从而保证人类服用的安全性。药物的开发者必须严格遵循"药品生产质量管理规范"(GMP)的条例。凡是有关物理化学特性、分析方法和包括剂型在内的药品生产的任何细节，都必须在用于临床试验之前向卫生当局汇报。各项细节的指南可从 www.ema.europa.eu 或 www.fda.gov 网站获得。此外，无论是在制造亦或加工、制剂时出现的任何显著改变，上述变化均必须告知卫生当局。该信息参考自《化学、生产与控制规章》(CMC)，值得一提的是，CMC 是新药提交申请管理的重要组成部分。

药代动力学，药物代谢和生物分析技术

新药发现的核心就是要理解小分子和生物制剂的代谢和药代动力学。药物的动物实验阶段可以获得药代动力学的数据，而这些数据可以帮助我们更好地预测和理解该化合物在人体中的药理作用；并且这些数据是和后期进行的临床试验结果相符的。

生物分析技术

使用某一项生物分析技术是理解非临床和临床药代动力学的第一步。依靠化合物特性、给药途径和活性中心，实验必须准确地测定药物在生物流体和(或)组织样本的浓度。通过运用高效液相色谱法(HPLC)和质谱分析法(MS)，各个实验室均可以快速且低成本地准确测量某个化合物浓度，而且这两种方法同时是十分普遍的研究方法。在后面阶段的临床研究中，固相或者免疫分析为临床试验操作提供研究方法新的可能。在治疗药物监测(TDM)频繁使用的移植领域，商业性质的药物试验必须事先证明该药在临床环境中使用有效后，才能去申请药物审批。对于任何试验或者设备的审批过程都是独立于临床病历资料和 NDA 的，而且通常和二者同步进行。

药代动力学和药物的代谢

药物的吸收、分布、代谢和排泄是相互联系的，任何一个阶段的改动都可能致使其他阶段联动改变。收集到的血液标本或者组织标本可以定量地分析有关时相和程度的各项药代动力学参数，用放射性标记的药物则均可以在非临床和临床项目中，定量地测量化合物质量。对于口服给药的药物来说，吸收是第一个可测量的参数，并且可以通过连续的测量来表达参数。此外，在整个给药过程中的药物浓度数据，即曲线下面积(AUC)，亦可用于计算该药的吸收率。然而，小分子药物的体内分布相当复杂。表观分布容积是一项与本阶段密切关系的非生理学参数；它可以密切反映药物在全身分布的含量。通过以上数据的收集与分析，计算机建模可以预测在各个组织中药物的分布及代谢，而这些建模数据可以帮助我们优化给药剂量和给药途径。对于大部分的小分子来说，从药物进入体内的那一刻起，各种各样的新陈代谢过程都在积极地参与药物的修饰、代谢，以期将药物排泄到体外。

最初评估代谢清除通路的方法是在硅胶中使用分子的某些结构来模拟进行。这些模型可以在日后的体外实验中被改善，例如孤立的肝细胞微粒体、人类肝细胞以及代谢细胞色素结合试验。此外，评估体外实验中药物代谢速率在最初还可以通过在非临床研究中使用 ^{14}C 标记的药物完成，并最终在人体试验中被验证。通过标记化合物，给药的实质结构和代谢之后的结构以及药代动力学的数据可以被观察记录，并被用于各个不同物种之间的比较。相比之下，当需要选择合适物种用于非临床的毒理学试验时，后者的数据显得更加可靠。综上所述，人体对各种分子进行代谢排泄可以通过十分多样化的途径，其中最常见的途径就是消化道途径和尿道途径进行。大部分进入体内的化合物都将被高度修饰，变得不具有相关生化功能，之后被人体排泄出去。

毒物动力学

从非临床的毒理学试验收集的样本中，要理解各样本的浓度和效应的关系，关键是要测量药物的体内残留的浓度和计算各项药代动力学参数。这些关键数据也帮助预测以上的试剂能否应用于人体，模拟人类的代谢过程以及预算出药物的安全阈值。因此,非临床阶段药物研究中药代动力学的数据可以帮助药物临床阶段的研发,也为跨物种的同种药物的发展提供了的基础。

药代动力学临床试验

在整个药物开发的过程中，收集分析药代动力学数据的首要任务是，理解人体服用药物后如何对其加工修饰,明确何种药物剂量产生最合理的药效,何种剂量又会产生毒性以及理解其他有关生物学的发现。而试验最主要的关注点则是疾病和其他药物将对受试药物的代谢、排泄产生怎样的影响。由于生物制剂几乎不被其他共同服用的药物影响，所以科研人员更加关注小分子之间的药物相互作用。小分子相互作用的最常见类型就是一起服用的药物或者食物对目的药物的代谢影响，例如葡萄汁可以阻碍或者促进目的药物的代谢和排泄。研究人员需要将被研究的药物和共同服用的相关药物可能存在的任何相互作用都列出，这样才能为临床的药物使用提供正确的指导。使用交叉对照的方法，收集各组实验在健康志愿者上产生的典型数据,最终分析得出药物之间(药物和食物)的相互作用。研究被测试的药物代谢率、可能的药效,或者经代谢被改变的化学结构,不断推进药物相互作用的研究。世界卫生组织已经发行了相当数量的指南文件，强调制药行业应归纳药物存在的相互作用，规范制药公司研究制药标准(www.fda.gov;www.ema.europa.eu)。

此外，工作人员还在儿童患者中以及例如肝功能不全和肾功能不全等多种疾病状态中研究药物的药代动力学，以期透彻研究不同年龄和不同疾病种类对药物的生物化学行为产生的各种影响。至于其他可能对药物的药代动力学参数产生影响的人口统计学因素，则需要更加细致专业的实验来测定，有时候也可能通过一种称作群体药代动力学的研究方法进行。群体药代动力学通过利用人口抽样样本代表整个人群进行临床实验阶段Ⅱ和Ⅲ实验,收集特定的药代动力学参数,然后进一步分析例如年龄、性别、种族、联合用药和不同疾病类型等因素对药物的药代动力学影响。

从开发到获批的临床前阶段毒理学试验

新药研发的临床前毒理学阶段实验原则是十分标准而规范的，使用一个标准的毒理学测试系统(www.oecd.org) 并必须严格遵守 Good Laboratory Process (GLP)指南[1]。

毒理学家的工具盒

毒理学研究主要包括体外实验、在体实验和用于测试原药和生成物毒性二者之间的测试系统。当设计实验或者评估研究结果的时候，毒理学家必须清楚意识到可能将药物转变成毒物的各种因素，例如用药途径、给药间隔、用药时间、药代动力学以及非药物对检测药物的相互作用等等。这种药物的转化在器官移植中极为重要，因为标准治疗方案中经常包括多种药物的组合使用。

受调控环境和对毒理学测试的影响

在药物研发的过程中，由于药物安全性测试在人体中进行受限于诸多条件，因此动物实验就成为了人体试验的替代品。动物实验同样被动物保护机构管制，被伦理道德要求尽可能地减少甚至不用动物实验[2]。指导动物毒理学测试中最重要的规范是国际协调会议(ICH) 对人类药品注册的技术要求(www.ich.org/products/guidelines)。另外，美国食品药品监督管理局(FDA;www.fda.gov/drugs/)和欧洲药品局(EMA;www.ema.europa.eu/)均发表了相关的明确指南。

由于动物实验中药源性不良反应的经验有限,很难直接预测其对人体的不良反应[3,4],通常需要两种甚至更多的动物(一种啮齿类、另一种非啮齿类)来对药物进行评价。通常为了方便饲养和处理,实验偏向于使用鼠类和犬类进行毒理学测试，这种情况在早期研发移植药物(例如咪唑硫嘌呤和环孢霉素)的阶段尤其常见。然而在20世纪90年代出现单克隆抗体后,因为在研究中鼠类和犬类的单抗药物并没有产生希望的效果,人们开始呼吁停止上述研究方法[5]。因此,治疗性的单克隆抗体和其他生物制剂转而采用灵长类动物进行毒理学的测试。

原则上来说，非临床的生物制剂安全性测试同样应遵循ICH(www.ich.org/products)所限定的注意事项。小分子药物测试的具体要求则在ICH 26(R1)中列出。值得一提的是，由于将狗作为实验对象时容易夸大药物对胃肠道的毒性作用，在狗身上做第二代移植药物的毒理学测试是极其困难的[6,7];值得一提的是,用小猪做上述实验具有非常好的效果[8]。

毒理学实验评估策略

在药物非临床阶段的安全性评估策略主要关注两个目标，一是提供必要的资料证明该药物用于人体的安全性，二是药物注册审批。因此，毒理学的实验成果只被看作"研究说明书"，只有在临床药物研究取得巨大成功后才再次启动。典型的毒理学测试流程如图141.2。

临床研究申请

首先，药理学、药代动力学和毒理学的专家应慎重考虑，动物实验的数据能否支持新药安全地用于人体试验。人体服药后大部分的不良反应是剂量相关而且都是可预见性的[9]。因此，一个合理的用药安全测试的先决条件是药物必须在人体内引发和受试动物体内引发的相似药代动力学反应。如果实际情况不是如此，应解释阐明物种间的不同之处，然后这些结果也就成为了风险评估的一部分。此外，通过化学机制起效的药物就有可能通过化学途径造成毒性；这些不良反应往往是和药物的治疗目的不相关的，也被称作为"副反应"。例如，由于药物的相互作用导致了多种蛋白质在心肌钾离子通道中聚集，而钾离子通道负责心肌复极化(hERG)；通道阻塞后可致突发的心律失常甚至心肌梗死。多种药品已经因该类型的副反应而被下架[10]。于是，对药物可能存在的不良反应已经成为药物研发的重点。众所周知，某些药物可在人体试验和动物实验中产生截然不同的反应[11]；同样，吸收、分布、代谢和排泄在男、女性群体的差异[12]也可能影响某些药物的药物安全性。因此，临床前药物安全性测试必须考虑到物种间药代动力学的不同特性，例如药物吸收率、蛋白质载体、组织分布和排泄，并在用于人体实验之前加以检测[13]。说明书的内容主要由药理学和药代动力学的实验，以及许多毒理学研究组成；毒理学研究又包括测试药物安全性，基因毒性和单次或者重复给药造成的毒性。必要时，也会包括探索性的动力学研究，从而帮助研究人员更好地预计志愿者服药的风险[14]，帮助减少服药后的肝消除率[15]。

人体试验刚开始服用的药物剂量是基于大量的毒理学试验所得出的安全系数而计算得来的。对于小剂量的化合物或者生物制剂来说，试验的方法基本类似上述方法[16]，但检测用于免疫抑制[17]或者极为活跃的化合物[18,19]时，检测方法则更为复杂。将半数中毒量与半数有效量进行对比，分析得出药物的安全系数(也称治疗指数)。至于其他的计算方法，例如体表面积，使不同物种之间的数据可相互比较(FDA guidance on MRSD; www.fda.gov/Drugs)。决定药物能否于人体实验(FIM)的关键标准主要参考非临床药物试验中得出的危险因素，以及研究人员预测出的本药用于人体后任何可能发生的不良反应。还有收益与风险评估，包括发现和纠正无效的药理作用和不良反应。只有全部遵守了以上所有的非临床药物安全性的测试后，临床研究申请

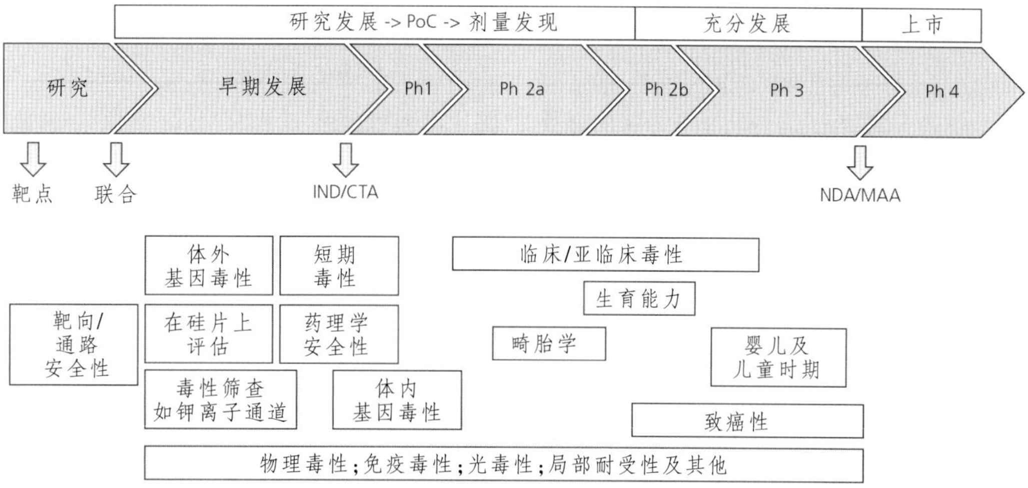

图 141.2　药物研发中的毒理学测试流程图。Ph，阶段；PoC，概念验证；IND，临床研究申请(欧洲：CTA，临床实验主管)；NDA，美国新药申请(欧洲：MAA，市场主管部门申请)。

(IND)才算准备就绪。

临床研究和市场授权的支持

如果一种候选药物的早期临床实验结果十分具有前景，则要重新启动非临床实验中检测药物安全性的项目，为临床实验阶段Ⅱ和阶段Ⅲ的药物研究和最终药物的上市提供理论上的支撑。在国际会议指南的基础上，毒理学实验在整个研究过程中重点围绕药物疗程的合理期限，实验操作在两种物种上(一种啮齿类，一种非啮齿类)进行，控制动物的药物疗程达到人类实验中的期望值。即使是受试药物对人来说是终身服药，指南中推荐啮齿类动物药物服用的持续时间最长也不应超过6个月，非啮齿类不应超过9个月。这些亚慢性和慢性动物实验的目的，主要是改善剂量效应，通过降低药物浓度，增加给药次数来预防不良反应。由于动物长时间地暴露于药物接触中，以上研究可能会意外地发现某些新的或者意料之外的药物不良反应。在标准的毒理学研究方法之外，还有两种特殊毒性的实验方法也可能用于评估药物使用的风险或者意外，即生殖毒性和致癌性。自从伦理考察禁止药物直接在人体上实验，上述的动物实验就成为了替代品。但是，如果只是短期使用的、用于急救的、治疗尚未有明确有效药物的疾病(如HIV、肿瘤)，那么未经过审批的药物治疗可以用于上述情况的患者；但特殊类型的患者，如期待受孕的女性则坚决不能服用。生殖毒性或者致癌性的药物研究结果会被写进新药的说明书，给需要用药的患者提供指导。

而对于在儿童患者中使用的药物来说，儿科研究计划(www.ema.europa.eu/ema)中叙述的欧洲管理条例要求，在进入临床试验和某些药物审批之前，新药的毒理学研究需要首先在幼年动物身上进行。因此，开发儿科用药时要慎重考虑幼年动物实验事宜[20]，而且提前和卫生主管部门联系探讨是十分有用的[21]。

药物生殖毒性研究

药物生殖毒性的实验主要评估药物对生殖能力的影响，对胚胎、胎儿的毒性(例如，自发性流产和胎儿畸形)以及出生前和出生后对婴儿生长发育的影响(例如，晚期胎死的危险，儿童的智力发育迟缓和功能缺陷)。同样，在动物身上进行毒理学试验又一次成为人体实验的替代品，因为人体实验往往需要多年的审批和调整才能被广泛应用；而发病率较低的病种则可能需要相当长的时间才会在人体上发现某种药物对使用者有生殖毒性的直接证据。有些药品项目会让患者登记怀孕信息，或者研发人员会对具有某些临床前特征的患者采取严密的监测[22]。此外，非临床研究的结果会帮助探寻药物作用的原理，而进一步的临床测试又可能支持前期研究的结果，正如西罗莫司对男性生殖能力影响的发现过程那样[23]。

药物致癌性研究

评估一种药物致癌性的毒理学实验是最消耗时间和最占用资源的，但这项实验仍是所有临床疗程超过3~6个月的药物必须要求完成的，这些药物恰恰包含了所有的用于移植的小分子药物；而适用于某些肿瘤适应证和用于移植诱导治疗(例如抗白细胞介素-2的单克隆抗体)的药物不一定需要类似的实验[24]。此外，当药物转化成其他化学形式后，经过某些生物学行为，长期服用或者突变后，其中可能致癌的化合物均要强制执行上述实验。而且，如果发生了上述情况，卫生当局可能在药品进入临床实验阶段Ⅲ的实验之前就要求上交毒理学实验结果，那么该药品的研发时间将显著地延长。早在环孢霉素盛行以前、还在使用咪唑硫嘌呤和强的松的年代，免疫抑制剂和致癌的风险就已经被明确指出[25]。在移植治疗中使用免疫抑制剂导致癌症的风险日益增加，其主要原因外界认为是病毒介导致癌，例如EB病毒、人类疱疹病毒8可以导致淋巴瘤，乳头瘤状病毒可以导致皮肤、生殖器肿瘤[26]。有研究表明，在儿童身上过度使用免疫抑制，如单克隆抗体OKT3或者他克莫司，可能会导致如淋巴异常增殖等恶性肿瘤发生率的增加[27,28]。大量积累的临床证据表明，移植后恶性肿瘤的发生和免疫抑制水平的相关程度远大于和其他任何一种药物的关联。

补充实验

最后，用于特殊用途的药物可能需要设计以及执行额外的补充实验。实验一般在体外或者动物上进行，最终为临床实验或者审批提供依据。比如，用于器官移植的药物会被要求进行测试药物有无光毒性[29]、免疫毒性[30]、耐受性以及阐明在动物或者人体测试产生毒性的机制等等。

临床试验

为了获取卫生主管部门对候选药物的审批，在目标患者人群中，研发人员必须证明使用该药物安全有效。但有些药物在证明用于人体后安全有效后，可以不需要像图 141.3 描述的流程那样按部就班地申请上市。例如，大品种原料药达到生物等效性即可。

阶段 I ——补充实验

临床实验阶段 I，也被称作临床药代动力学实验，主要测试最基本的临床特性，包括对药物安全性、耐受性，单次给药和多次给药的药代动力学和药效学和药物作用机制的初步评估。需要 5~40 例的个体实验来研究药物的临床药理学，具体内容包括药物的相互作用和不同患者的各自服用剂量，这些研究都是药物研发后期阶段必不可少的基础。

首次人体实验

新药临床实验阶段 I 的研究主要目的在于确定药物的生物学活性，描述生物药学特征以及找出非临床研究中可能存在的毒性。只有完成上述步骤后，新药才能想首次用于人体实验。而药物对人的药代动力学参数、耐受性和产生毒性的浓度阈值都是首次人体实验(FIM)中得出。如果某些药物是不易耐受的，或者生物性能较差，亦或被证实有未经确认的新毒性，那么下一步的研究即被搁浅。

总的来说，FIM 实验的常规设计为安慰剂做空白对照，随机分布(通常为 1:1)，平行对照，单一剂量递增(SAD)。FIM 实验初始剂量的选择和最大剂量参考自非临床毒理学实验结果和运用类比法(见“临床研究申请”部分)得出的无明显有害效应剂量(NOAEL)。实验中药物体内浓度的增长都是时间滞后的；也就是说，必须测量上个时段的剂量水平才能继续测量下一个。根据药物安全和耐受特点，充分参考临床前研究的实验结果，才会以这种方式增长。药物剂量一般的增长方式是指数或者半指数增长，但是当双倍剂量给药时，前两种增长方式也就不适用了。指数增长方式使大范围的计数得以实现，例如可以从 0.1~1000mg，又可以减少不同曲线的重叠。上述实验设计往往会获得大量的数据，既有助于精确地测定人体试验的药代动力学数据，也有助于发现剂量依赖性或者浓度依赖性的药物毒性。

根据新药的类型(如小分子或生物制剂)与其药代动力学活性，FIM 实验可能会在健康的志愿者或者患者人群挑选合适的新药进行试验。而对于新型免疫抑制剂的首次人体实验，会考虑应用于健康受试者的风险太大，从而会选择可能受益于此药的患者身上进行实验。这些患者包括移植患者和自身免疫病的患者。

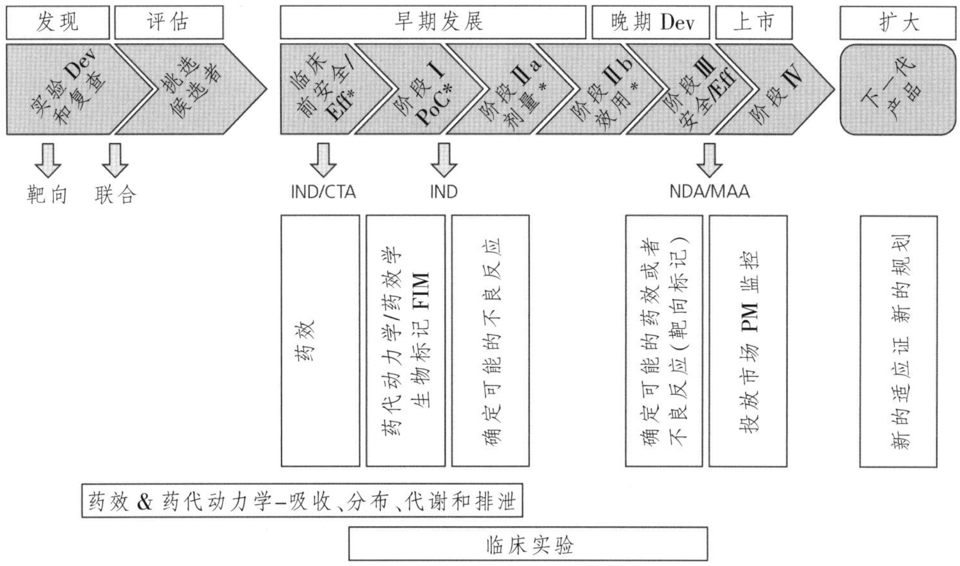

图 141.3　药物研发的临床实验各阶段。Dev，发展；Eff，药效；PoC，概念论证；IND，临床研究申请(欧洲：CTA，临床实验主管)；NDA，美国新药申请(欧洲：MAA，市场主管部门申请)；FIM，首次用于人体；vol，志愿者；PM，上市后；REMS，风险评估和减轻战略；ADME，吸收、分布、新陈代谢和排泄。

概念论证设计

一旦药物的耐受性特点被确定并且单剂和多剂药代动力学实验完成,常规的概念论证(PoC)就会随即进行;这也就意味着临床实验阶段Ⅱa实验的开始。本阶段实验的目的为检测药物能否在人体内快速起效,或者对于器官移植中的免疫抑制剂来说,则是为了测试该药能否进行下一步研究。根据临床实验阶段Ⅰ的实验成果,可能会有2~3个剂量组,其中又各自包含了6~24种受试药物。尽管某些相关生物标记可以用来提示实验结束或者应被终止,但是PoC通常将临床终止已确立的“金标准”作为主要的节点标准。因为本项实验研究的主要目的是小样本评估临床中药物的活性,所以会使用例如Bayesian方法等新颖的统计学方法来评估成功与否。

PoC后实验

当新药进入研发的后期阶段时,临床阶段Ⅰ的实验重点为测定各项临床药代动力学和药效学的特性,其中包括药物之间和药物与疾病之间的相互作用,还有针对特殊人群进行的额外试验,例如测定药物在肾功能不全和肝功能不全的患者中高残留的影响。为了更好地阐明药物生物作用原理或者药物毒性的产生机制,研究人员会进行额外的药物机制研究。近年来,根据临床前信号(例如,钾离子通道的负向结合剂;见“临床研究申请”章节),一项十分彻底的针对QT间期的研究(ICH E14, www. ich. org)已经成为金标准,用于评估心肌复极化的程度,特别是QT间期延长的情况。

药品说明书的内容多少取决于药物的药代动力学特性。例如,单克隆抗体的说明书可以是相当简单的,因为该药不会导致药物相互作用和QT间期延长,也没有特殊活性需要测试。而经肝代谢的非特异性小分子可能需要30种甚至更多的临床药效学的研究,从而充分地分析在各种治疗方案中的药物特性。以上研究的数据对于亚临床实验设计和保证新药能安全服用是至关重要的。

临床实验阶段Ⅱ——剂量校准和药物安全有效的初步评估

在实质器官的移植中,阶段Ⅱ中普遍的实验设计都是和有效药物进行非盲、随机分布实验对照。选择对比的有效药物往往是本时期治疗效果公认的药物。并且,如果可行的话,会在研究中事先将药物进行一些结合来减少偏移。阶段Ⅱ的实验可能仅包含一项实验,但是却比阶段Ⅲ更常使用“研究然后论证”的模式。

大部分阶段Ⅱ实验的主要任务就是证明新药和治疗的标准药物相比药效如何。实验时间可能像持续3个月的移植后治疗一样短,但常见的是需要6~12个月的实验,以保证药物的充分接触并且证明药效是持续有效的。全球卫生组织则可能要求更长时间的数据才能批准申请,因此,在完成1年数据分析的基础上,实验往往需要两年甚至更长的时间。阶段Ⅱ的关键目标之一是确定在治疗方案中达到最佳药效的药物剂量(或者有效量)。根据研究规模的大小,阶段Ⅱ中研究药代动力学、药效和建立暴露-反应关系的实验内容可能是非常直接的;但有时候也是难以实施的。阶段Ⅰ和PoC的研究中单剂和多剂实验结果会帮助确定阶段Ⅱ实验的初始剂量。十分常见的是,研究人员会测试两倍或者更多剂量于标准用药量,来建立暴露-反应关系。有时候,直到阶段Ⅲ也不能找到最佳剂量和(或)最优暴露数据。

临床实验阶段Ⅲ——验证药物的安全性和有效性

实验设计和终点指标

阶段Ⅲ实验通常被认为是“关键的”或者“验证性的”,因为卫生局最终决定新药是否安全有效且可以上市,就是以阶段Ⅲ提供的数据作为最终依据。运用统计学知识,基于风险-效益评价,证明某个剂量(浓度范围)是最有利的(临床试验设计和统计学难点在第134章和第135章已作详细论述)。至于移植用药,阶段Ⅲ实验可能长达3~5年,花销5000万乃至1亿美金。常见的阶段Ⅲ研究使用随机的和不知情(尽可能)的方法,将一组或两组药物和对照组进行对照;通常实验设计时间为12个月。阶段Ⅲ研究的样本容量是基于效果和研究中疗效指标(优于目前治疗手段或者不差于目前)来决定的。由于急性排斥反应的发生,导致了有些情况下新药和现有的治疗标准方案间没有显著的差异。所以,一项研究想要证明新药有好的疗效,可能需要成千上万的患者来参与,而考虑到接受移植手术患者的数量有限,上述条件是不切实际的。因此,很多药物的研究定位就降到了“不劣于”现有方案的目标,同时希望改良药物有其他更突出的方面,比如更好的耐受性或更少的毒性。

对于希望能够减少移植后急性排斥反应的药物来说,食品及药物管理局(FDA)对于药效的传统评估内容是包罗万象的,既包括急性排斥反应、移植物丢失,也包括患者的死亡和“随访失败”(见后文)。由于移植药物研发阶段Ⅲ实验的样本量有限,FDA 就对审核更加严苛;因此,FDA 确定了多种的评估方式来近似等效地评价药效,而多个实验疗效指标也允许多种不同比较方法的差异。无论如何,个体药效评价的各组成部分也会被记录。欧洲药品局(EMA)也有相类似的评估体系,还额外地增加了一项对于移植器官功能的检测结果(eGFR)的评估。举个例子来说,在肾移植中,EMA 的评估体系会包含测量肾小球滤过率来反映肾功能。FDA 通常会对协同的各项主要疗效指标的要求进行足够的论证。

自从 FDA 将患者随访作为评估节点的一部分,终断与患者的联系导致遗失随访数据,那就意味着巨大的失败。实际上,这正是阶段Ⅲ实验的主要困难。FDA 非常人性化地采用了统计学上保守的方法,将患者的随访丢失不再看作实验意义上的药效的失败了。因此,为了保证实验成功,收集大样本的患者数据是极其重要的,这样即使患者不再延续治疗,研究也能够对整体样本做出药效评价,也同时提供了一些重要的药物安全性的宝贵信息。但是各个卫生主管部门之间存在诸多标准差异;比如说,EMA 最新指南并不推荐失败的随访患者纳入药效评估的体系中去。

患者和人口统计资料

卫生主管部门也对地区人口统计资料有研究兴趣,通常会要求阶段Ⅲ的实验在特定人群中收集具有代表性的研究对象。在欧洲,EMA 会要求研究在所有欧洲人中挑选;而在美国,考虑到在移植免疫抑制中不同种族的疗效差异[31],FDA 也推荐研究厂商们采样一定比例的非裔美国人和西班牙裔美国人。

新的疗效指标和生物标记

生物标记能为移植生物学提供探索临床用药的新思路,但是申请临床数据却不是那么轻松,往往需要先获得科学界和管理部门的广泛认可。各中心和地区的临床草案标准,预先设定的要严格遵守的疗效指标和严格的数据收集标准,都是申请使用生物标记的关键组成部分。虽然条件十分严苛,但上述的标准能为药物安全性和有效性的评估带来益处,也由此帮助了风险-收益评估的决策。

阶段Ⅲ的统计学注意事项

研究统计学分析应当是便于理解的,在研究结束前提交卫生主管部门,而且最好是在实验设计阶段就得到卫生部门的认可;上述内容应包含实验质量的标准测量和控制变量。统计学的注意事项也已在第 134 章中深度阐述。

安慰剂做对照仍然是临床试验对比的“金标准”。然而,这并不适用于移植领域,因为器官存活以来需要免疫抑制剂,而不给对照组免疫抑制剂是缺乏职业道德的。近期很多实验中,肾移植中急性排斥反应的发生率可达 15%;患者通常需要多种免疫抑制剂来达到最大的疗效和药物安全性。正如前文所述,由于多种免疫抑制剂会带来更好的疗效(更好的排斥反应),但是药物安全性不能保证(如感染),所以很难达到疗效和安全性的合理统一。为此,免疫抑制剂的临床实验的疗效标准往往设定为“不劣于”(NI)主流药物疗效指标。基于这样一个设定,一旦药物展现出如可以提高肾功能、延长药效持续时间、减少并发症,亦或提高使用安全性等特性,都可以算作药物实验的成功。其他标准还包括感染率、肿瘤发生率和糖尿病的低发生率,和对胃肠系统、血液系统和神经系统的有益附带作用。

一项好的关于多药联合治疗的 NI 实验设计需要在安慰剂对照下,评估受试药物的疗效;也就是说受试药物必须达到相比对照组更好的疗效。从药物发展的历史上看,这样的实验设计标准是极具挑战性的,甚至可也说是除去少数研究,几乎不可能完成的[32]。有时,上述信息可追溯于疾病、指南以前的实验、与主管部门的探讨和前人研究对比实验的经验。同时,实验结果应该是可重复的,就是说相同人群中要有类似的实验效果。

根据 FDA 的指南,一项设计成功的 NI 实验需要证明疗效的延续性。当目前的移植人群和以往的人群在关键的危险因素上特征有所不同时,那么要证明疗效就是相当具有挑战性的。比方说,现行的临床上捐献和接受移植器官的标准与过去遵循的标准可以是不尽相同的。和阶段Ⅲ相比,移植实验阶段Ⅱ的规范标准是比较宽松的,更易于操作的。

不论设计目的是要优于还是不劣于现有指标,收集样本信息或者为了合理证明两种治疗方案在某种时间发生率上存在差异,或者就是为了更有说服力来证明实验目的。样本积累主要目的就是获得期望事件的发生,估算样本变异性和置信区间。对于阶段Ⅲ的验证试验来说,90%都是令人满意的,也就是可以存在90%的可能性证明该药是不亚于对照组的。

注册之路:药物的审批过程

与卫生主管部门的交流沟通

在美国,新药第一次在人体使用之前,临床药物要首先向美国食品药品管理局(FDA)申请在人类身上执行新的药物或者生物制剂(IND)。在欧洲,要向临床实验管理局(CTA)提出申请,且在获得每个参与国家的卫生管理局和伦理委员会的批准后,才能执行用药。一些FDA的分部,例如药品评价和研究中心(CDER),推荐在临床药物申请之前先和CDER进行会晤,这样能够对临床前信息建立早期的反馈,检验某个产品是否有准确的证据来支持审批通过进而进入临床研究。同时,这也是一次评估早期临床研究的机会,讨论新的方法(如生物标记、诊断方法等等)。

这种早期的信息交互可以确认产品是重要的,可以检验产品是否可能具有特殊用途,或者作用于特殊的通路。举个例子,"罕见药"是用于罕见病(在美国通常被定义为小于200 000例)的治疗。另外一种可能是,"快速程序"可以提供更短的研发期限和审查时间。如果当前没有其他可选择的治疗方案或者当前治疗方案效果不佳,亦或该药可以治疗某种威胁生命或者使人虚弱的疾病,那么该类型的药物审批速度会更快进行。所有向卫生当局申报的材料都需要提供充足的文件来支持临床实验的申请,其中就包括一份研究者手册(IB),可以帮助理解药品特性(化学结构、非临床药代动力学和毒理学研究和人体既往实验),一份研究计划草案,以及申请进行研究的药物的资格证明。全面支持信息还提供给卫生行政部门审查,包括临床前实验报告、生产控制文档和任何既往人类实验的报告。一旦IND或者CTA被相关卫生行政部门接受,只要药物赞助商打算维持该项目,那研究就会持续进行。提交一份年度人体试验的进展报告,包括安全性更新和IB修订。根据FDA指定的要求,需要为新的剂型或者适应证再次提交申请。并且,研究人员可能要求在每一个药物开发阶段,尽早地与FDA亲自讨论或者电话沟通(点对点讨论)。

一旦第二阶段数据是可用的而且赞助商想要进步第三阶段,发起人可向食品和药物管理局(FDA)请求第二阶段(EoP2)结束。在这次会议上,FDA将审查临床前和毒理学数据,以及在阶段Ⅰ和阶段Ⅱ审查的临床数据。本次审查的目的是在与卫生主管部门磋商中确认:经过试验数据校准的风险-收益比和药物可以在更大规模的临床实验Ⅲ阶段中尽可能地安全使用。磋商主要是对可接受的临床指标,优化实验设计和适当的患者类型进行讨论,作为阶段Ⅲ的校准。任何协议与卫生主管部门在EoP2达成的协议共识均不具约束力。如果医疗和(或)科学的知识标准实践在阶段3开发中改变,协议并不能保证实验一定被新的标准认同。虽然不是必需的,发起者也可以请求一个特别的协议评估与FDA审查会议,借以讨论和获得阶段3研究的批准。

所有临床试验行为和管理必须坚持药品临床实验管理规范(GCP)作为为申请药品注册的实验结果可接受性的先决条件。这包括无论药物评估在什么地方被评估,都要适当地接受当地的要求,如美国食品药品监督管理局(FDA)、欧盟的欧洲药品局(EMEA)、日本的厚生劳动省(MHLW)和其他地方卫生当局。个别国家具有执行临床研究的不同要求。指导大多数临床试验的开展的规范都是基于FDA 21 CFR部分第50、56、312章(http://www.accessdata.fda.gov/)以及以《赫尔辛基宣言》中叙述的道德准则为基础的国际协调会议三重药品临床实验管理规范(http://www.ich.org/)。

向市场主管部门申请

向NDA提交审核之前,申请新药的公司可能请求在NDA之前会见卫生主管部门,从而获得其对药品说明书的格式和内容审查的反馈,还可以找到当局对内容的关注重点(药效或者安全性的数据库,化学、临床前的或其他行政的要求)。早期讨论的目的是知晓任何已知的可能会导致卫生当局(FDA)"拒绝文件"的风险或确认(EMA)临床实验的申请(如继续实质性的研究)。通常,一个原始的药物申请包含临床研究报告,报告至少要求有两项适当的和有良好对照的阶段 3 试验、风险管理评估和儿科药物科研计划。所有卫生主管部门现在均要求对新药物申请收取费用。例如，美国 1992 年生效的《处方药收费法案》(PDUFA)规定，该收费为 NDA 如期完成审查全过程提供资助：申请优先审查实验最多花费 6 个月，标准的审查过程一般需要 10 个月。如果必要的话，审查时间可能延长，这主要取决于文档的复杂程度。

FDA 的审查涉及多个学科，由一位项目经理对各科学审查进行协调，包括临床医学、统计和(或)临床药理学、基础医学和化学。FDA 将做出最终决定和在递交申请后规定时间内发布申请药物潜在的问题：申请优先审查者需要 30 天，标准审查需要 60 天。FDA 在第 74 天时回复一封正式信函，也称为文件审查通知，对可能会影响审核通过的潜在问题通报初步评价，以及影响 FDA 反馈的时间，风险评估和减轻战略提议，上市后的承诺；以及审核的预计完成期限。

在 NDA 审查的同时，科学调查部门可能进行批准前的审查，包括检查整条流水线生产设施，以确保可以生产出高质量产品。同时，FDA 调查人员可能会对数据依从性和完整性进行全面的现场审计，也会审核公司提交数据的可靠性。随着非美国的新药开发商渐渐参与进来，现场审计在非美国国家变得越来越常见。

开发新药的公司需要在提交最初的申请后，再递交保密协议(通常是 120 天一次安全性更新)；内容和实际的期限可以与 FDA 协商。在最后的 45 天审查周期，FDA 也会对提议的商标名和公司进行探讨。常见的，因为即将上市的产品可能与现有产品名称或外观不易区分，公司将提交多个商品名以供 FDA 决定。

NDA 完成审查后，如果收益并没有大于风险，FDA 将回复一封“完全回应函”的邮件，罗列出经鉴定的不足之处。类型 1 的信函会列出在两个月之内必须解决的小瑕疵，解决后需要向 FDA 重新提交，方便及时审核。类型 2 的信函可能要求回复 6 个月内额外的实验数据，包括完整的研究报告或主要的统计分析。即使信中所述的瑕疵被完全解决，也不能保证接下来的审核一定会被通过。接下来，FDA 还会要求强制性的营销要求或承诺达到某种临床疗效，而且还要回答额外的药物安全性问题。作为批准后的承诺，在 FDA 批准产品用于商业销售后，这些研究由申请者继续执行。在申请者被通知审核通过后，产品会在 FDA 的网站上立即公布。FDA 也会公布审核主管的简要审查评定，包括按照规定分配的审核团队的工作文档和决策，如果适用的话，还会提供风险评估和减轻战略的审核文档。药物审查和批准在欧洲也引起了公众的兴趣，被称为欧洲公共评估报告。

FDA 咨询委员会

作为 FDA 的监管决策机构，咨询委员会(AC)可能要求大约在 NDA 行动前的 2~3 个月，要求申请者提供包含一个新药实体产品的申请资料。而和顾问小组进行磋商后才做出最后的审批决定必不可少。咨询会议可以为公司提供专家的建议，旨在提醒公司，FDA 对药物申请的任何相关话题的讨论和建议。当数据问题难以解决，或引起了公共注意，或有争议，或者需要一种特殊类型的专业知识，或者希望获得自己发现的有力证明，专家顾问团对以上状况的建议则是十分有用的。独立专家小组在药物和生物产品的相关领域被认为是知识渊博的，并且可能包括来自学术界、社区、患者倡导组织、工业或特殊的政府机构各界精英的代表。

风险收益评估

风险收益评估是获得药物通过批准的基石。在临床实验阶段Ⅱ和阶段Ⅲ的研究中，不良反应和药效会在固定的人群中进行实验分析。在获得批准后，更多元化、更多数量的患者会服用此药物。参与实验的志愿者数量增加、适应证、医疗需求、其他可行的治疗手段、未经治疗的疾病预后、作用机制(MOA)、安全性特征、药效资料的稳定、合理使用的可能性，这些所有的因素，卫生部门将其作为风险收益评估的一部分加以考量。这被认为与替代治疗方案相违背，以及疾病的预后方面。如果患者不接受治疗从而完成最终的评估，更好的临床结果的新型作用机制有着明显的优势。然而，如果对新的作用机制了解不够深入，那么这种新颖的设计则可能成为劣势，因为可能有未知的长期风险。假如只要提供药物达到预期的疗效指标，安全性数据也支持上市要求，同种的药物就会被批准申请。在预期疗效和安全性的基础上，同时具有独特特性的药物，可以进一步改善风险收益评估。安全信号的出现，特别是如果在阶段Ⅲ试验中没有被描述，可能会需要额外上市后继续研究，对药物安全性再次评估或者检验长期的临床效果。越来越多的国家在审批新药方面，要求进行风险管理计划(RMP)。在美国,FDA更习惯用简洁的称为风险评估和减灾战略(REMS)的文档资料。这些文档识别已知或潜在的安全风险,规定具体的行动来降低风险。风险评估和减灾战略为申请药物可以被合理使用提供额外的承诺以及帮助,作为系统来保证适当使用的可能性,并且在某些情况下,可以通过受控的分布系统限制产品的获取。

其他规定和承诺

临床、非临床、实验室和生产流程支撑起关键数据,以及商业化的试验性药物均必须遵循经常被称为GxP的指导方针。良好实验室规范(GLP)描述了非临床研究应如何计划、执行、监控、记录、报告并存档。良好的生产规范(GMP)确保产品保持高品质标准(生物利用度、安全性和稳定性),符合药品说明书中的预期指征。良好的临床实践(GCP)是一项国际伦理和科学的高标准,由国际协调会议(ICH)(www.ich.org/)和FDA E6良好的临床实践巩固指南(1996)(www.fda.gov/ScienceResearch/SpecialTopics)保护人类受试者的权利,为临床研究的设计、执行、记录、报告提供指导。它还定义了临床试验赞助商,临床研究人员和监管人员的角色和职责。

生物学制剂的批准流程

在欧洲和美国,生物制剂产品的审批过程类似小分子的审批过程。生物制剂的申请同样由审查普通药物申请的CDER审查。新型的或更复杂的生物制剂的申请被称为生物制剂许可证申请(BLA)和FDA中心的生物制剂评价和研究(CBER)部门评估审查。在任何监管环境下,生物制剂的生产和产品描述有额外的复杂性;严格的过程对照和检查生产设施是预先批准的要求。

不同卫生主管部门的不同批准流程

一般来说,全球卫生主管部门会对跨国家的研究的实验设计、结果评价和数据分析与国际保持一致。由急性排斥反应的失败指标,移植物死亡和个体死亡组成的传统指标是被普遍接受的。基于2009年中正在研发的一致新药数量,EMA引入针对实体器官移植中移植用药的全面发展的指导方针和建议(www.ema.europa.eu/docs/)。卫生主管部门在某些地区,如亚太国家,为了更好地感受任何潜在的种族敏感问题,在对本地临床试验数据评估时会考虑紧地区相关的利益。这是对在审核全球试验数据库中类似证据支持的补充。每一个潜在的新药候选,生物制剂或化学制剂,不断开发研究,通过在卫生主管部门在个案基础上不断的审计和批准,逐渐建立其在器官移植中使用的优势。

总结

从发现具有针对某种目标通路或者靶点的生物学活性的化合物,到卫生主管部门通过新药的上市审批,需要多学科交叉的团队来把基础科学转化成临床治疗。药物研发是一个复杂而漫长的积累过程,充分研究和优化候选药物,最终呈现出一个安全有效而且风险收益最佳化的药物。经过一个或更多的候选药物被证明具有有关化学性质和生物活性后,初步的安全性和毒理学测试才会开始进行。当药物对人体有利的特性被证明时,则会执行临床概念论证,从而进行作用机制和药物安全性透彻研究。积极有效的PoC结果会推动药物的研发,包括阶段2试验确定药物剂量、安全性和有效性,紧接着是阶段3验证试验。如果某地的卫生当局对药物的注册审批是和制药公司有着千丝万缕的联系(如FDA,EMA),那当局会通过口头和书面的对审批做出反馈,从而在整个审批流程中指导临床实验的发展。阶段Ⅰ建立了药物的临床药理学,包括药代动力学、药理学、药物之间和药物-疾病之间的交互作用;阶段Ⅱ则负责验证候选药物临床使用的安全性和有效性。在收到卫生当局允许下一步的研究通知后,更大规模的的阶段Ⅲ试验可以提供足够的数据来检验安全性能和药物的疗效,建立风险收益评估来决定产品是否能够治疗患者。在完成三个阶段的基础上,研究发起人向卫生当局提交一份详细的档案,以供其审查和决策。美国食品药物监督管理局处理时间的范围从6个月(优先审查)到10个月(标准审查)不等,通常在FDA做出最后决定之前举行一次公开的咨询委员会会议。及时通过批准之后,正在进行的药物安全监视程序可能是公司自愿进行或者由卫生部门强制执行,以确保上市临床药物的有效性,在预期患者人群种保持良好效果。

(陈康辰 译 徐骁 校)

参考文献

1. Lee CS, Lee JY. Good Laboratory Practice (GLP) regulations: interpretation techniques and review of selected compliance issues. Drug Information Journal. 2006;40:33–38.
2. Rolin BE. Animal Research, animal welfare, and the three R's. Journal of Philosophy, Science & Law. 2010;10:1–11.
3. Olson H, Betton G, Robinson D, et al. Concordance of the toxicity of pharmaceuticals in humans and animals. Regulatory Toxicology and Pharmacology. 2000; 32:56–67.
4. Greaves P, Williams A, Eve M. First dose of potential new medicines to humans: how animals help. Nature Reviews Drug Discovery. 2004;3:226–236.
5. Bussiere J. Species selection considerations for preclinical toxicology studies for biotherapeutics. Expert Opinion on Drug Metabolism & Toxicology. 2008; 4(7):871–877.
6. Collier DSJ, Calne Sir R, Thiru S, et al. Rapamycin in experimental renal allografts in dogs and pigs. Transplantation Proceedings. 1990;22(4):1674–1675.
7. Platz KP, Sollinger HW, Hullett DA, et al. RS-61443 – a new, potent immunosuppressive agent. Transplantation. 1991;51:27–31.
8. McAnulty PA, Dayan AD, Ganderup NC, et al. The minipig in biomedical Research. Baca Raton, FL: CRC press; 2012. ISBN 978-1-4298-1118-4.
9. Valentin JP, Hammond T. Safety and secondary pharmacology: successes, threats, challenges and opportunities. Journal of Pharmacological and Toxicological Methods. 2008;58:77–87.
10. Mueller PY, Milton MN (2012). Determination and assessment of therapeutic index in drug development. 2012;11(10):751–761.
11. Walker DK, Davis J, Houle C, et al. Species differences in the multiple-dose pharmacokinetics of the non-nucleoside reverse transcriptase inhibitor (NNRTI) UK-453,061 in animals and man: implications for safety considerations. Xenobiotica. 2009;39(7):534–543.
12. Zimmermann H, Kaufmann G, Graser T, et al. Gender differences in pharmacokinetics of sex steroids in animals and man. Toxicology Letters. 1998;95(Suppl 1):93.
13. Kramer JA, Sagartz JE, Morris DL. The application of discovery toxicology and pathology towards the design of safety pharmaceutical lead candidates. Nature Reviews. Drug Discovery. 2007;6:636–649.
14. Baldrick P. Safety evaluation to support first-in-man investigations: toxicology studies. Regulatory Toxicology and Pharmacology. 2008;51:237–243.
15. Bass AS, Cartwright ME, Mahon C, et al. Exploratory drug safety: a discovery strategy to reduce attrition in development. Journal of Pharmacological and Toxicological Methods. 2009;60:69–78.
16. Milton MN, Horvath CJ. The EMEA guidance on first-in-human clinical trials and its impact on pharmaceutical development. Toxicologic Pathology. 2009;37: 363–371.
17. Dayan CM, Wraith DC. Preparing for first-in-man: the challenges for translational immunology post-TGN1442. Clinical and Experimental Immunology. 2008;151; 231–234.
18. Mueller PY, Brennan FR. Safety assessment and dose selection for first-in-human clinical trials with immunomodulatory monoclonal antibodies. Clinical Pharmacology and Therapeutics. 2009;85(3):247–258.
19. Agoram BM. Use of pharmacokinetic/pharmacodynamic modeling for starting dose selection in first-in-human trials of high risk biologics. British Journal of Clinical Pharmacology. 2009;67(2):153–160.
20. Hurtt ME, Daston G, Davis-Bruno K, et al. Juvenile animal studies: testing strategies and design. Birth Defects Research Part B: Developmental and Reproductive Toxicology. 2004;71:281–288.
21. Leconte I, Bailey G, Davis-Bruno K, et al. Value of juvenile animal studies. Birth Defects Research Part B: Developmental and Reproductive Toxicology. 2011; 92:292–303.
22. Ostensen M, Khamashta M, Lockshin M, et al. Anti-inflammatory and immunosuppressive drugs and reproduction. Arthritis Research & Therapy. 2006;8: 209–208.
23. Zuber J, Anglicheau D, Elie C, et al. Sirolimus may reduce fertility in male renal transplant patients. American Journal of Transplantation. 2008;8:1471–1479.
24. Vahle JL, Shawn F, Heidel M, et al. Carcinogenicity assessment of biotechnology-derived pharmaceuticals: a Review of approved molecules and best practice recommendations. Toxicologic Pathology. 2010;38:522–553.
25. Sloan GM, Cole P, Wilson RE. Risk indicators of de novo malignancy in renal transplant recipients. Transplantation Proceedings. 1977;9:1129.
26. Ryffel B, Mihatsch MJ, Fisher G. Immunosuppression and cancer: the ciclosporin case. Drug and Chemical Toxicology. 1992;15:95–115.
27. Swinnen LJ, Constanzo-Nordin M, Fisher SG, et al. Increased incidence of lymphoproliferative disorder after immunosuppression with the monoclonal antibody OKT3 in cardiac- transplant recipients. The New England Journal of Medicine. 1990;323:1723.
28. Cox KL, Lawrence-Miyaski LS, Garcia-Kennedy R, et al. An increased incidence of Epstein-Barr virus infection and lymphoproliferative disorder in young children on FK506 after liver transplantation. Transplantation. 1995;59:524–529.
29. Lynch AM, Wilcox DP. Review of the performance of the 3T3 NRU in vitro phototoxicity assay in the pharmaceutical industry. Experimental and Toxicologic Pathology. 2011;63(3):209–214.
30. Haggerty HG. Immunotoxicity testing in non-rodent species. Journal of Immunotoxicology. 2007;4:165–169.
31. Lindholm A, Welsh M, Alton C, et al. Demographic factors influencing cyclosporine pharmacokinetic parameters in patients with uremia: racial differences in bioavailability. Clinical Pharmacology and Therapeutics. 1992;62: 359–371.
32. Witte S, Schmidli H, O'Hagan A, Racine A. Designing a non-inferiority study in kidney transplantation: a case study. Pharmaceutical Statistics. 2011;10(5): 427–432.

第 142 章 器官移植的特殊收益：产出和经济学

David A. Axelrod, Mark Schnitzler, Richard Freeman

引言

器官移植被广泛认为是 20 世纪主要科技贡献之一[1-3]。Alexis Carrel、Peter Medawar 和 Joseph Murray 里程碑式的创举使移植现实可行，因此被授予诺贝尔奖。自 1954 年首例肾脏移植成功以来，终末器官衰竭护理的标准从症状治疗变为功能替代。Tomas Starzl[4]、Norman Shumway、Christian Bernard[5]以及 Richard Lillehei[6]把器官移植的福利从肾衰竭扩大到终末期肝衰、心衰和 β-细胞衰竭，保证全世界受者的长期生活质量。第 1 章已概述器官移植的悠久历史。

目前器官移植已成为器官进展期衰竭的标准治疗方法，现代医学有足够的资金支持复杂的器官移植。遗憾的是两个主要因素仍妨碍移植服务的广泛分布：供体器官和资金。例如美国移植等待名单中需要尸体供肾的受者数量是潜在供体的 6 倍多，导致部分地区患者等待时间超过 7 年[7]。因此等待名单中的患者死亡率很高，需要长期器械器官支持伴并发症，生活质量差。设计可用的器官最佳分配体系是国际社会一直争论的关键问题，聚焦于公平获取与效用最大化之间的权衡（例如捐给特定受者的器官利益）[8]。

美国获取移植器官的变化在于器官供应和保险范围，国际护理的变化反映了工业化程度和经济基础[9]。西欧、北美和澳大利亚肾移植例数最多，每百万人中超过 30 例，而非洲国家肾移植未超过每百万人 10 例。因为发展中国家医疗资源有限，透析不是可行的解决方案，发展移植服务是其解决晚期肾脏疾病（ESRD）最有效的方法。然而世界上绝大多数的人口仍生活在无法接受移植的地区[10]。关于文化差异、移植保险范围和国家移植行政政策的额外内容分别见第 139 章、第 140 章和第 143 章。

移植也不能不被关于其高成本的讨论所影响。心脏移植仍然是美国医疗保险体系中最昂贵的手术[11]。鉴于国际社会努力缩减医疗保健服务开支，与整个医疗保健企业相比，在移植手术之前和之后为相对较少的移植患者提供护理而花费的大量资源可能会越来越受到审查。即使在美国，某些情况下的移植护理（如丙型肝炎肝移植）最初也被从亚利桑那州医疗补助计划中删除[12]。虽然这一决定最终被推翻，但这可能是基于成本限制访问的众多努力中的第一个。

虽然前 50 年移植的挑战主要集中在克服免疫和技术障碍上，但未来 50 年很可能主要是解决分配和获得的经济限制。器官移植将越来越多地存在于一个有组织的护理系统中，负责在需要的人群中分配固定资源。必要时，扩大移植护理可能会导致可用于其他服务的资源减少。因此，需要准确了解影响特定器官移植成本和效果的因素，以准确证明这些延长生命的程序的相对效益。

本章的主要目标是考虑器官移植的成本和效益中捐赠者质量、受者病情严重程度和临床实践模式的变化对器官的具体影响。这项分析将主要集中在肾、肝和心脏移植程序和相关的替代治疗，因为它们是最广泛执行和研究最多的。器官分配政策和移植准入与成本的交叉也将被检验，因为器官供应和受者需求之间的地理差异会对移植相关资源的利用产生重大影响。

肾移植

背景

1954 年 Ronald Herrick 的肾脏被成功移植给同卵双胞胎哥哥 Richard，标志着临床肾移植的开端[1]。Richard 在肾移植后无免疫抑制的情况下延长生存了 8

年。肾移植最初仅限于同卵双胞胎,免疫抑制方案的日益成熟使肾移植广泛应用于肾功能衰竭终末期患者,仅限于可移植肾的持续短缺[3]。

肾移植与透析同时进行的对比研究具有一定的指导意义[1,13]。20 世纪 50 年代 Willem Kolff 最初在荷兰,随后在美国开创了透析患者机械支持。然而,由于所需的机器和专业知识仅限于少数几个中心,进入 Kolff 肾移植组的机会也非常有限。此外,私营部门没有足够的资源来资助这种治疗。在华盛顿大学,一个由律师、医生、神职人员和其他人组成的匿名小组被任命来决定谁将接受透析,谁将死亡[14]。该小组很快被称为"上帝小组",这些人开始了一个分配系统:将治疗限制在 18 岁以上和 45 岁以下人群,没有高血压、糖尿病、血管疾病,并且具有适当的"情绪"特征的人。小组从最初的 17 名申请者中挑选了 10 人接受治疗,其余的人都将死去。公众对这一结果的强烈抗议促成了 1972 年将对 ESRD 的支持纳入了医疗保险计划。由于不受资金或器官供应的限制,透析被广泛地提供给所有人,仅在 2007 年就消耗了超过 240 亿美元的医疗保险基金[15]。

肾移植的临床与经济获益

肾移植的临床获益已非常明确。移植相比透析能够延长生存时间,降低发病率。1999 年 Wolfe 及其同事比较移植等待患者与肾移植受者,发现肾移植受者总体生存期平均提高 10 年[16]。肾移植手术可能增加短期的病死风险,但移植 106 天后风险获益评估偏向肾移植。分析显示较年轻的受者获益最大,移植后生命平均延长 17 年。

最近的分析扩展了 Wolfe 的原始工作,包括生活质量调整和解释移植失败后的存活率[17]。这项工作是为了支持器官共享联合网络(UNOS)正在考虑的新的分配建议,这些建议旨在最大限度地提高移植效益。获益被定义为移植受者与透析患者相比可获得的额外生存(包括移植失败后的生存)。这项被称为移植后生存时间(LYFT)的指标,估计了在 10 年的时间范围内,特定的供者和受者组合对肾移植整体生存影响的贡献。这些估计是根据生活质量进行调整的,将透析年的价值定为移植年的 80%。在现有的肾脏分配制度下,肾移植导致的平均 LYFT 因年龄而异,从 17 岁以下的 9.6 年到 65 岁以上的 3.5 年不等[18]。当对当前分配制度下移植的所有患者中进行汇总时,肾移植每年估计会增加 48 850 个质量调整生命年。UNOS 肾脏委员会检测一项增加肾移植年均获益的提议,可以把移植后质量调整生命年数每年提高超过 3000,但代价是更少的年长受者被纳入[19]。

肾移植获益增加某种程度也反映了移植肾长期存活率正缓慢提高。已有研究显示加强免疫抑制能够减少免疫原因导致的移植肾早期功能丧失;而移植肾长期存活未得到改善。然而,最近对移植受者科学登记系统(SRTR)数据的分析表明,某些疾病类别的长期移植物存活率略有改善[20]。Meier-Kriesche 及其同事报道尸体供肾半衰期从 1989 年的 6.6 年增加到 2005 年的 8.8 年。ECD 移植受者的半衰期已经从 1989 年的 3 年增加到 2005 年的 6.4 年。半衰期的提高表明更多的治疗可有获益,包括减少钙调磷酸酶抑制剂慢性毒力和皮质类固醇副作用,发现及治疗抗体介导早期及迟发性排斥反应,以及更好解决地移植后糖尿病和心血管疾病等合并疾病。生存最好的仍是活体供体移植,半衰期超过 11.5 年。

类似评估肾移植临床获益,肾移植的经济效益必须要考虑到与血液透析的关系。透析是费用极大的病态治疗,需要反复住院。联邦医保透析治疗的直接费用超过每人每年 73 000 美元,私人支付可能接近两倍[21]。相比之下,每例肾移植在移植后 5 年内可节省超过 200 000 美元[22]。查询联邦医保的支出发现活体肾移植受者 2.3 年及尸体肾移植受者 3.6 年的费用可达收支平衡。受者生存超越平衡点可节省支付者大量费用以及提高受者生活质量(图 142.1)。因为长期生存得到改善,活体肾移植的经济效益远大于尸体肾移植[23]。目

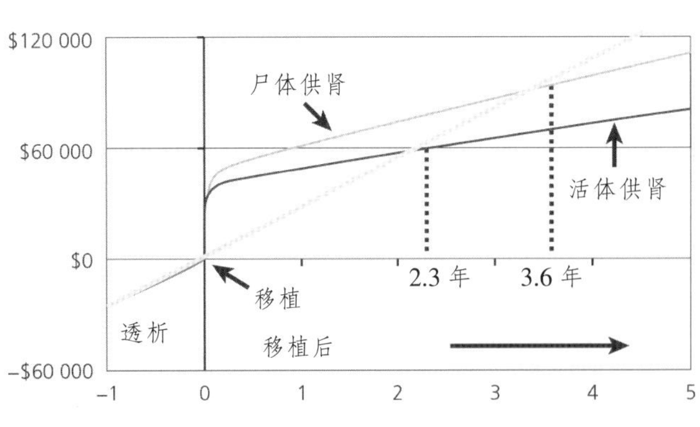

图 142.1 捐献类型对肾移植费用的影响。Adapted from [100] Smith, et al. Cadaveric versus living donor kidney transplantation: a Medicare payment analysis. *Transplantation*, 2000;69 (2):311 - 314, with permission from Kluwer Health.

前对联邦医保开支的估算表明每例联邦医保活体肾移植受者可节省至少94 579美元。移植相比透析可改善受者生活质量,每例活体肾移植的真正价值估计是269 319美元。

供体特征对肾移植获益的影响

临床肾移植使等待移植患者数量急剧增加，供肾短缺严重。目前肾移植等待名单患者数量超过80 000人,供肾适用标准被放宽,导致移植肾生存时间减少,LYFT获益降低。可用移植肾最初分成两部分,标准供肾(SCD)和扩大标准供肾(ECD)。ECD基于供体特征,等同于肾衰竭移植相对风险的1.7倍[24]。提供较高风险的移植肾给受者时,他们已被告知风险会增加,但表示等待过程中愿意接受ECD[25]。ECD肾功能延迟及早期肾功能丧失的风险更大,ECD肾移植的好处仅限于等待移植时死亡风险显著增加的患者。回顾性分析SRTR数据库，Merion及同事发现部分ECD移植受者可有显著生存获益:申请者年龄大于40岁,伴糖尿病,或者居住于捐献服务区域且等待时间超过1350天[26]。不符合上述条件的受者不能从ECD移植中获得明显好处。虽然这些信息已被广泛传播，但美国移植中心间等待移植患者愿意接受ECD肾脏的比例各有不同[27]。美国各个肾移植中心符合Merion标准且愿意接受ECD肾脏的申请者比例分布在0~100%。正如预测接受ECD肾脏的受者等待移植死亡率降低(HR 0.88[0.85—0.91])。但是40%等待ECD肾脏的患者实际并不符合Merion标准,不能从ECD肾脏受益。不符合Merion标准但仍在ECD等待名单的患者更快接受移植时,总体死亡率增加(OR 1.11[1.05—1.18]),相比之下类似患者接受透析可有更长生存时间。

连续测量移植肾衰竭风险可提供更客观的供体风险连续性表征,影响移植肾功能和预后[28]。与ECD和SCD的两分法不同,供体肾脏存活指数(KDPI)将每个供体移植物衰竭的相对风险与平均肾脏风险进行了线性比较[29]。KDPI包括变量数的扩展与回归方程加权的使用(表142.1)。对ECD和SCD的KDPI评分有很大部分的重叠,显示出分类的局限性。新批准的肾脏分配策略包含KPDI。风险最低的供肾(20% KDPI分数最低的供肾)将优先提供给更年轻、更健康的受者,最大化移植肾有效年数[30]。同样,有人提议扩大共享KDPI最高分供肾。KDPI高分供肾更难处理,若被捐献可给积极的等待时间更长的中心使用。提高供肾风险评估也使受者更充分地知情同意，因为这也可能允许建模评估特定受者特定器官的个体风险及利益。遗憾的是KDPI对供体质量的其他指标预测价值仍然有限[28,31]。完整模型的C统计值为0.62,表明KDPI预测任一移植肾更长生存的准确率只有62%，而没有信息的模型C统计值为0.5。预测能力缺乏反映出:受者因素及临床事件改变和未获取供体质量的变化,会显著改变预后。

表142.1 肾脏移植的供体特征指数。Reproduced from [29] Rao PS, A comprehensive risk quantifcation score for deceased donor kidneys: the kidney donor risk index. Transplantation. 2009;88(2):231–236, with permission from Wolters Kluwer Health.

供体特征指数
年龄
人种及种族
高血压
糖尿病
血肌酐
脑血管原因的死亡
身高
体重
心脏死亡后的供体
丙型肝炎

有效利用边缘性供肾的另一种方法是根据年龄明确匹配供体和受体，正如欧洲移植高级项目中所做的那样[31]。65岁以上供者的肾脏专门提供给同一年龄组受者，可增加老年受者的移植率，降低移植等待死亡率。老年受者接受老年供肾的生存时间类似于接受年轻供肾[31]。但使老年受者用老年供肾相比年轻供肾可增加手术并发症发生率(47%对28%,P=0.03),降低原始功能率(69%对74%,P=0.03)。

预测移植物存活率下降的供体特征还与移植肾功能延迟恢复(DGF)的发生率增加、住院时间延长以及对使用细胞消耗性抗体进行昂贵诱导治疗的需求增加有关[32,33]。回顾性分析UNOS数据库4618例ECD移植显示ECD静态冷保存DGF发生率为36%[22,34,35]。动脉灌注可将DGF发生率降低至26%。根据定义移植术后发生DGF需要进行透析,导致住院时间延长,费用增加。因DGF可致急性排斥反应发生率升高,使用诱导疗法被认为是有益的。

由于早期并发症的发生率的增加和移植物存活率的降低,ECD 肾移植在围术期和术后的护理费用都较高。尽管到达费用平衡点的时间明显要比 SCD 肾移植长，但从社会角度来看 ECD 肾移植仍然可以节省费用[22]。ECD 移植相比 SCD 适度增加每个质量调整生命年的费用(41 000 美元对 54 000 美元)。但两者均明显低于透析维持的费用(79 000 美元/QALY)。降低移植肾质量的经济影响反映出移植肾早期功能不全发生率更高,肾小球滤过率持续下降,需要尽快恢复透析。相比 eGFR>60mL/min/1.73m^2 的受者,eGFR<30mL/min/1.73m^2 的受者在移植术后 1 年的平均费用增加超过 7000 美元,移植术后 1~3 年费用增加超过 10 000 美元[36]。随着基础肌酐及 eGFR 的改变，肾功能降低会快速增加费用。

ECD 对移植中心的经济影响更加引人注目。尽管 ECD 移植随时间推移可获得预后及费用节约的好处，但并发症增加,移植肾早期功能不全和(或)围手术期 ECD 无功能均会增加费用。最近 Englesbe 及其同事评估移植中心财政发现 1999—2005 年密歇根大学移植中心的盈利能力急剧下降[37,38]。总体报销不变,但移植费用明显升高。每例 ECD 供者利润下降超过 8000 美元,导致机构净亏损。尽管患者保险公司的赔偿总额有所增加,但肾移植受者发生 DGF 也给中心造成了巨大损失(4947 美元/例)。其中一个结果是抑制使用较高风险供肾,尽管存在长期经济效益。移植中心护理高风险受者及移植高风险供肾方面的原始费用增加，潜在的解决方案是设计风险调整支付方式。

影响费用及预后的受者因素

肾移植的临床成功使其在老年患者中的应用越来越广泛,其医疗并发症的程度也越来越高。Segev 的数据表明,即使是 65 岁以上的患者,与继续透析相比,也会获得额外的生命年[27,39]。过去 10 年里 50 岁以上的受者正加速扩大移植等待患者数量,其中超过 65 岁的患者占较大比例[7]。此外糖尿病发病率增加 17%,高血压性肾衰竭发病率增加 30%。这些因素直接影响受者移植术后的生存。未进行肾脏-胰腺移植(可能是Ⅱ型)的老年糖尿病患者移植术后预期 LYFT 最低（大约 4 年),比无糖尿病的年轻受者降低 50%[17]。年龄增加也可致预期 LYFT 降低，主要是由于年龄增加死亡的风险。此外老年受者并发症的发生率更高，住院时间延长，需要再次住院治疗。然而所有高风险组相比透析组,在生存时间及生活质量方面仍可大量获益。多个单中心研究证实安全有效的肾移植甚至可能适用于八九十岁的患者[40]。

移植肾生存预后也与等待时间密切相关,特别是依赖透析的患者[41,42]。透析时间不到 6 个月的受者移植肾 5 年生存率为 78%(P<0.001)，而透析时间超过 24 个月的受者 5 年生存率减少到 58%,10 年生存率从 63%降至 29%(P<0.001)。预示等待时间缩短的因素有白色人种、社会经济地位高、私人保险和等待名单的捐献服务面积[43](图 142.2)。美国器官可用性不一致导致移植准入的明显差异,患者进入移植名单后的等待时间不同,从不到 18 月至超过 40 个月。进入名单前的透析时间进一步影响移植受者及移植肾的生存率,显著降低移植肾生存,对移植肾生存率的影响有限。移植前长期透析说明患者进入名单较迟，缺少私人保险，非白种人。此外捐献服务领域(DSA)与移植中心有显著差异,进入名单前的透析时间反映出当地做法多样以及提示需要增加早期评估。

改变受者人口统计特征对初始住院治疗和移植术后 1 年移植护理的费用均有深远影响[22](图 142.3)。糖尿病增加移植手术的费用,平均增加 1531 美元,每年支出 7884 美元。类似的,较高年龄、较长透析时间、体质指数(BMI)增加都极大地影响护理费用。同种致敏作用的程度加重也增大支出，需要使用昂贵的治疗(血浆置换、静脉注射免疫球蛋白治疗、细胞消耗抗体疗法)[44],治疗虽有疗效,但使移植增加 30 000 美元或更多的费用。

总结

肾移植被证明能够延长生命,降低费用,尤其是在接受高质量供肾的年轻受者。降低排斥反应风险,加强

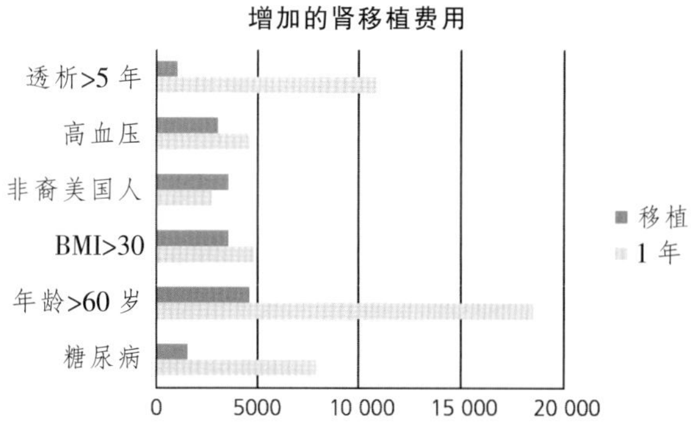

图 142.2 受者特征对肾移植的影响。(Data from [22])

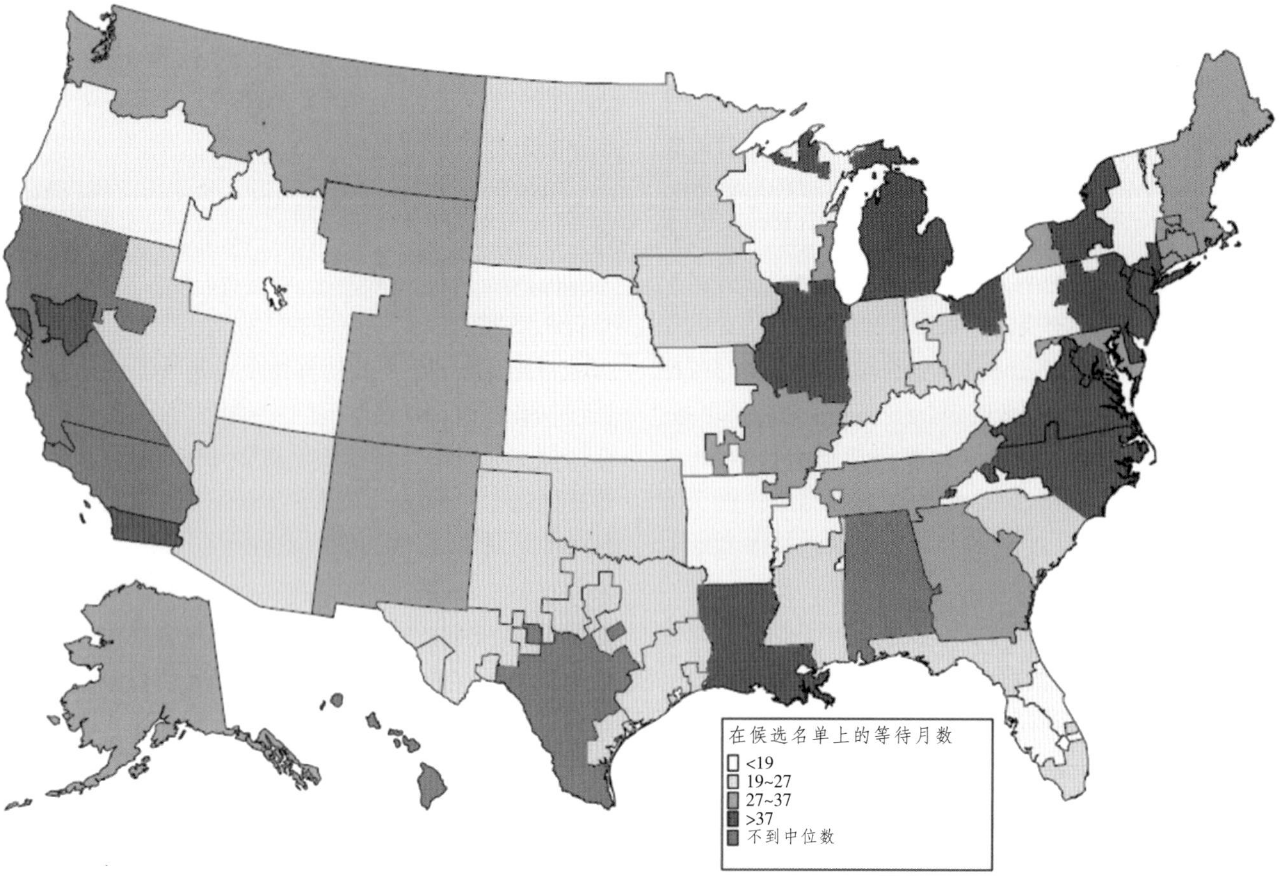

图 142.3 在美国,肾移植不同的移植等待名单。

心血管并发症管理以及开发靶向免疫抑制治疗均能提高肾移植获益。然而改变供受体人口统计特征可能会损害肾移植的临床和经济效益。等待时间长导致共患疾病的负担加大,费用增加,患者生存时间减少。对各个移植中心同等重要的是上述因素与供体质量变化相互影响,极大削减了移植中心的利润。如果不执行供肾分配体系,将会有越来越多年龄更高、风险更大的受者进行肾移植,费用更高,移植肾功能延迟恢复的风险也会更大。若未能调整适应风险及手术的补偿,对于仍能从肾移植获得生存效益的受者来说,移植服务可能会受到更多地域上的限制,因为小型移植中心无法以足够的高收入病例抵销损失,并且随后倒闭。

肝移植

背景

美国终末期肝病(ESLD)患者的数量正快速增长[45,46]。丙型肝炎、酗酒和肥胖及代谢综合征都推动了这项增长。尽管丙型肝炎新发感染率在 20 世纪 90 年代中期达到顶峰,由于肝硬化、肝细胞癌及失代偿肝衰竭需要肝移植的患者长期感染丙肝,感染人数预计至少在未来的二三十年里仍会增长。此外肥胖导致非酒精性脂肪性肝炎(NASH)发生率也前所未有地升高。若不治疗,NASH 也可导致肝硬化及 ESLD。目前估计 NASH 比例在 3%~37%[47]。

ESLD 的治疗是复杂多学科的。肝移植申请者需要多种措施组合控制肝硬化和门脉高压[48]。患者需要接种疫苗,对肝细胞癌进行早期和反复的影像学检查,以确定可通过肝脏定向治疗和病毒性肝炎治疗的病变。虽然不能治愈,但部分患者肝硬化病因治疗可有疗效,包括治疗丙型肝炎感染,减少药物和酒精滥用,以及积极降低体重。住院治疗以及治疗肝细胞癌或静脉曲张出血也可加重 ESLD。

进展性慢性肝病相关的临床治疗的复杂性和严重性导致了巨大的医疗支出。治疗丙型肝炎的直接医疗支出每年超过 50 亿美元，预计在未来 10 年花费近 550 亿美元[49,50]。同样,肥胖盛行加上 ESLD 的经济负担,NASH 的治疗费用已经增加[51]。终末期肝病评分模型(MELD)评估肝衰竭严重程度,已被证明与 ESLD 死亡率及支出相关。初步分析移植前的治疗费用,MELD 25~40 分的移植患者费用比 MELD<25 分的患者多 14 倍[52](表 142.2)。移植前高 MELD 的患者(>25)平均每年医疗费用超过 230 000 美元。

除直接医疗费用外，包括脑病在内的 ESLD 并发症给患者和看护者带来额外的经济负担。87.5%伴有脑病的患者无业,85%的患者疾病严重影响其经济状况[53]。其家庭成员也被报道存在高度的抑郁、焦虑,担忧社会支持及照顾亲人的负担。这种担忧因疾病严重程度而变化,患者 MELD 达到 15 分担忧增加[54]。

肝移植的生存获益

由于手术和麻醉技术的改进、免疫抑制的改善和感染率的降低,肝移植已经成为一个非常成功的手术,患者的 1 年存活率通常超过 80%。器官分配制度变化导致移植前患者疾病的严重程度逐渐增加[55]。

现行分配制度下美国等待肝移植的患者优先顺序以 MELD 分数评估疾病严重程度为基础。尽管不同区域患者 MELD 评分不平均，但等待移植人数的增多导致全国移植受者的平均 MELD 评分提高[56-58]。

肝移植手术的复杂性及并发症导致获益因疾病的严重程度而显著不同。多数高 MELD 评分患者未进行移植而死亡,说明手术、免疫抑制、匹配供肝缺乏均存在累积风险。然而代偿性肝硬化患者肝移植的累积风险超过预期获益。Merion 等发现 MELD 达到 15 分时移植获益开始超过移植和(或)继续等待的风险[59]。随肝病严重程度(MELD)的增加,移植患者的死亡风险率(HR)相比未移植患者降低。比较移植患者与等待移植患者发现 MELD 为 6~11 分(HR 1.79,P=10)以及 11~15 分(HR 1.76,P=0.04)的移植患者比移植等待的患者死亡风险更大。但是肝移植使 MELD 为 30~39 分的患者死亡风险率降低了 94%(HR 0.06,P<0.001)。

肝移植的获益因诊断不同而不同[60]。多因素模型中与预后不良相关的因素包括年龄>42 岁[相对危险度(RR)3.4]、移植前血液透析(RR 5.1)和诊断。回顾匹兹堡大学 4000 例肝移植手术，发现提示预后不良的诊断包括恶性肿瘤和爆发性肝炎肝衰竭病史，胆道闭锁、代谢性疾病以及自身免疫(PBC,PSC)病史预后相对较好[61]。移植后移植物衰竭的病因反映了疾病病因和受者因素的差异。老年受者出现 PSC 和早期血管血栓形成会出现高风险的移植肝衰竭，年轻受者移植肝衰竭多是因为复发性疾病包括丙型肝炎和肝细胞癌。慢性排斥反应在非裔美国人、PSC 患者以及年轻受者中更为常见。心血管及脑血管事件是老年及糖尿病史受者移植肝功能丧失而致死的主要原因。

虽然 MELD 评判疾病严重程度与移植预后相关,但不精确[62]。回顾性研究证实,高 MELD 受者移植后移植物丢失率普遍高于低 MELD 受者。最近一次欧洲人口的预后分析发现,MELD>30 分受者的移植后病死率比低分受者大 4 倍多,但 C 统计值仅为 0.66,表明单用 MELD 不能准确预测移植预后。基于美国人口的生存模型得出类似结果[63]。有项全面审查研究美国和欧洲人口的 MELD 模型，发现 MELD 预测移植预后的 C 统计值从未超过 0.7,MELD 和移植预后间缺乏高度相关性,所以基于 MELD 的器官分配体系是可靠的。如果高 MELD 受者普遍出现生存降低,基于移植前肝衰竭严重程度的

表 142.2 疾病严重程度函数换算肝移植总费用(千美元)。Reproduced from [52] with permission from Wiley.

N=990	移植总费用	移植 1 年费用	移植时期费用
基础费用	452.6(305.2~599.8)*	85.2(36.1~134.3)*	274.0(212.1~335.9)*
女性	100.7(12.3~189.1)*	25.8(-4.6~56.1)	44.6(6.2~83.0)*
评分			
6~14	参考范围	参考范围	参考范围
15~20	72.7(-33.5~178.9)	10.7(-24.9~46.3)	30.5(-15.1~76.0)
21~27	177.4(63.2~291.6)*	62.0(23.4~100.6)*	34.5(-15.1~84.7)
28~40	333.3(205.3~461.3)*	145.5(104.0~187.1)*	60.7(8.1~113.3)*
肝-肾	212.3(26.0~398.5)*	178.3(114.8~241.7)*	90.9(7.0~174.8)*

分配体系可能会导致移植总体效能降低。事实上 MELD 分数增加并没有导致移植后平均生存时间减少[55]。

供体特征对移植肝生存的影响

鉴于移植肝持续短缺，扩大器官供应对减少移植等待死亡率至关重要。通过注册系统和单中心研究可检测供体特征对肝移植预后的影响。Feng 等利用 SRTR 注册系统定义供体风险指数，发现六项因素可共同预测生存降低(高龄、非裔美国人种族、供体身高降低、供体非创伤性死亡、心脏死亡捐献和部分或劈裂式肝脏)[64]。研究者应用这些特征及两项手术因素(冷缺血时间、区域或全国共享)设计供体风险指数(DRI)，可用于比较尸体来源移植肝衰竭的风险。另外的研究还检测了诸如心脏死亡后捐献等个体因素，以评估热缺血时间的持续时间对非致命性并发症(如胆道狭窄)风险的影响。Schauble、Merion 及其同事结合 DRI 及 MELD，改良根据受体 MELD 评分评估获益的方法[65]。他们证明，质量更好的器官(低 DRI)即使受体 MELD<15 分也能获益，而风险较高的器官使移植等待死亡风险较大的 MELD 高分受者总体获益。

肝移植经济学

肝移植仍然是一项资源密集型手术，导致美国住院患者每次移植的费用通常超过 10 万美元[52,66,67]。患者疾病的严重程度是肝移植的主要费用来源，采用基于器官分配的 MELD 模型，大大增加移植费用。回顾性研究表明 MELD 评分增加会延长住院时间以及更频繁使用 ICU、透析以及呼吸机[67]。MELD 每增加 1 分，移植总费用平均增加 4309 美元，平均住院时间增加 4%[68]。然而 MELD 和费用之间的关系并不是线性的。MELD 评分超过 20 分时，费用曲线会大幅增加(图 142.4)[69]。

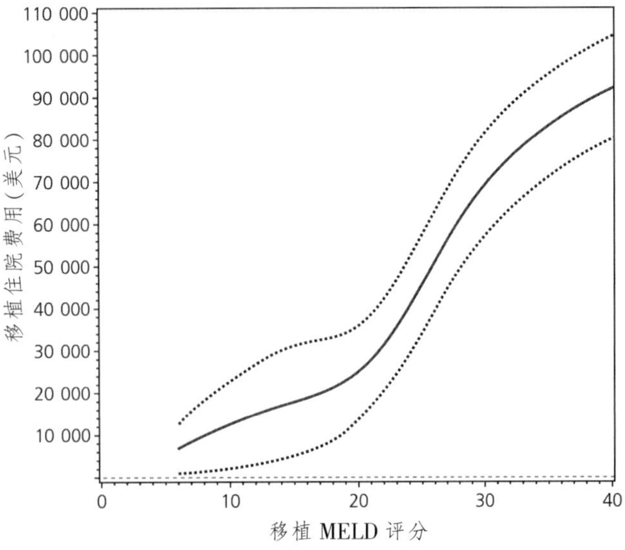

图 142.4 多因素曲线回归分析移值 MELD 评分与移植住院治疗费用的独立相关。

费用增加与受者肝衰竭的严重程度相关，对移植中心的收益有直接影响。一项费用和联邦保险补偿早期检查发现，受者 MELD 每增加 1 分，医院净收益减少 1512 美元[67]。欧洲国家器官储运组织及其他地区采用 MELD 分配体系亦证实了这些结果[70]。瑞士使用 MELD 基础分配体系使平均移植费用增加超过 50%，部分由于透析应用显著增加。但是移植前 MELD 是受者首次住院费用的不良指标(P=0.60)[52]。

肝移植的成本在美国显示出明显的地区差异，主要是由器官可用性的差异所驱动。目前，美国各捐赠服务区的移植平均 MELD 从 21~35 分不等[71]。MELD 评分最高的地区(纽约、加利福尼亚和新英格兰)的初次肝移植费用通常比 MELD 评分较低的地区更高，这主要是由于移植时受者病情加重。目前 UNOS 肝肠移植委员会正在考虑扩大器官共享。至少在某些地区，该政策其中一个影响是降低高 MELD 分数受者比例，提高了患者肝病进展到最严重之前获得器官的机会。器官总体供应不变的情况下，有 DSA 更好的器官供应，这项更广泛的分享提议可使 DSA 减少 MELD 低分患者获取器官。其净经济影响是将增加肝移植费用，因为更多的移植肝用于中到高的 MELD 分数受者；然而鉴于潜在保留的生活年，提高准入的费用估计为 17 056 美元/质量调整寿命年[66]。

供者选择也被证实会影响肝移植费用。多项研究表明移植并发症及肝功能异常的发生率取决于供肝类型和特征。DCD 供肝被多项单中心、注册系统及 Meta 分析深入研究。相比 DBD 供肝，DCD 再次移植的比例增加(14.7%对 6.8%，P<0.001)，受者 3 年生存率降低(71%对 77%，P<0.001)[72]。DCD 供肝主要造成胆道并发症发生率增加[HR 2.4(1.8~3.4)]，尤其是缺血性胆管病[HR 10.8(4.8~24.2)]。胆道并发症增加受者再次住院、介入放射治疗、二次移植的可能，经过调整其他特征后移植总体费用增加高达 25%[73]。

通常供肝质量的指标，如 DRI，与首次准入和肝移植术后 1 年的费用均有关。相比低 DRI 供肝，使用风险较高的供肝增加治疗费用[69,74](图 142.5)，高 DRI 供肝

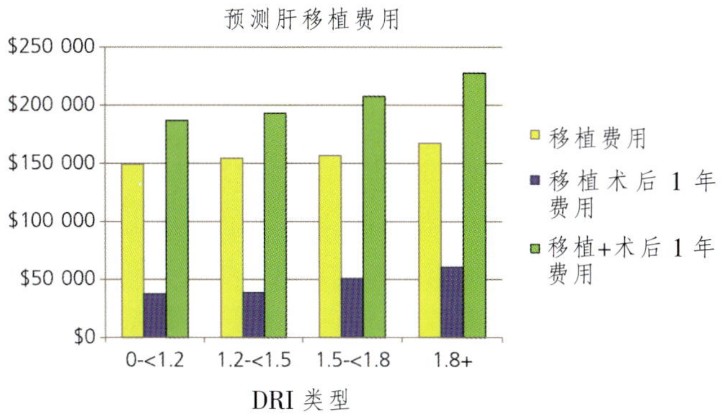

图 142.5 供肝特征对移植费用的影响。

(>1.8) 额外费用为 33 627 美元。DRI 单因素分析中,DCD 供肝(59 000 美元)、黑色人种(15 000 美元)、拉美人种(15 000 美元)、国家共享移植肝(30 000 美元)、供体年龄>40 岁(34 000 美元)均会增加移植费用有关。

虽然肝移植成本和生活质量效益已经得到了较好的描述,由于缺乏与病情严重程度相关的移植前费用综合衡量指标,以及缺乏对等待可用肝脏的患者死亡费用的评估,对肝移植总体成本效益的事先评估受到了限制。Northrup 及其同事最近完成一项 Markov 分析,比较尸体肝移植、活体肝移植和医疗管理的移植费用效益[75,76],发现与医疗管理相比,死亡供者的肝移植增加了 180 804 美元的费用,对活体供者移植的评估和可能的接受增加了 248 255 美元。总而言之,尸体肝移植每质量调整生命年(QALY)的费用为 35 976 美元,而活体肝移植每 QALY 费用超过 100 000 美元。这些结果与近期其他尸体肝移植的分析类似,均基于 Markov 模型,通过文献回顾确定移植费用和并发症发生率。

总结

肝移植患者数量持续增加很可能加重器官供应压力,因此移植前受者会出现更严重的代谢失调。移植等待患者疾病加重导致等待死亡率及围手术期并发症增加。这些变化无疑增加 ESLD 患者等待移植和移植手术的费用。遗憾的是,目前扩大供者供应的努力(如 DCD 肝移植)似乎加剧而不是改善这些趋势。在更广泛的区域重新分配现有供肝可减少移植等待死亡率,不显著增加治疗总费用。进一步使用边缘供肝,如联合肾移植,可能受限于移植中心的经济压力。调整复杂患者及供体的费用需要确保所有潜在器官得到利用。

心脏移植

背景

尽管终末期肾衰竭、肝衰竭是医疗支出的主要源头,但影响不及慢性心力衰竭(CHF)。CHF 是各类病变的终点,包括冠状动脉疾病导致的特发性(无缺血性)心肌病、缺血性心肌病,慢性高血压导致舒张功能不全、继发性或先天性瓣膜疾病、感染性心肌炎[77]。基于人口学预测年龄超过 40 岁的患者 CHF 发生率为 20%[76]。大部分 CHF 患者接受内科治疗(如 ACE 抑制剂),发展为难治性心律失常时需要可植入心律转复除颤器(ICD),或者发展为渐进性缺血性心脏病时可用血管重建治疗。患者治疗无效后被视为晚期,需要考虑另外的干预措施,包括心脏移植。

目前 25~50 万的美国人受晚期 CHF 影响[78]。晚期 CHF 是致命的,预期生存时间很短。近期左心室支持装置(LVAD)的随机试验显示,在分配到医疗部门的患者中平均 1 年死亡率为 75%,2 年为 87%[79]。心衰晚期需要长期正性肌力药物治疗,平均生存时间为 3.4 个月,1 年生存率为 6%~ 11%[80,81]。目前如果有足够的器官供应,美国将有 8~15 万患者从心脏移植获益[82]。不幸的是,美国每年仅 2200 例心脏移植。虽然未移植患者可姑息治疗,改善机械辅助装置可延长生存时间,但需要付出沉重的代价。

CHF 是美国医疗保险接受者中最常见的入院诊断,每年导致超过 100 万人住院[78]。患者频繁重新纳入接受持续治疗(30 天为 25%,180 天为 50%)。进展性(D 期)心力衰竭患者 1 年时间无需住院或未死亡的总比例只有 33%[83]。心力衰竭的治疗费用自 2000 年以来有很明显的增加。2007 年,患有 CHF 的医疗保险受益人在生命的最后 6 个月平均花费 36 216 美元,自 2000 年以来增长了 26%[84]。尽管临终关怀服务越来越多,近 80% 的患者仍住院治疗,35% 的患者死于急性期。LVAD 试验随机分配到医疗保险部门的患者两年费用超过 20 万美元,主要是住院费用[85]。

CHF 医疗费用随患者老龄和化疗法的发展而进一步增加。例如,尽管基于人口学的分析表明 15%~40% 的晚期 CHF 患者可从 ICD 治疗获益,但是 ICD 植入病例有限,且存在地域差异[86]。ICD 最多地区植入率比最低地区增加250%，导致总体生存率小幅增加(64.8%~66%)。利用率较高的地区有更多心内科专家，人均收入也更高。扩大ICD可降低猝死发生率；然而每例费用超过50 000美元时，尚不清楚能否节约费用。

心脏移植的临床获益

心脏移植使晚期心力衰竭患者能够无症状长期生存。国际心肺移植协会的数据估计全世界实施了5000例移植[87]。其中大约50%的移植手术在少于20例/年的中心进行，只有5%的中心移植例数超过40例。

最近10年里，移植治疗心力衰竭最常见的病因是非缺血性心肌病(53%)，其次是缺血性心肌病(38%)，其余病因包括再次移植、先天性心脏病、心脏瓣膜病。这表示主要移植病因在发生变化。在北美，缺血性心肌病是1997—2003年的主要诊断疾病。向非缺血性心肌病的转变可能反映了CHF治疗和机械支持使用的变化。比较1992—2001年和2002—2008年的移植受者显示其他重要的人口学变化包括65岁以上的受者比例更大(6.6%对10.3%)，糖尿病发病率更高(14.2%对22.4%)，使用LVADS(13.4%对20.1%)及RVADS(0.5%对3.1%)的比例急剧上升。

心脏移植受者中位生存期稳步增加，从20世纪80年代的8.3年上升至20世纪90年代的10.4年，2000年时还在进一步增加，但因为50%以上的受者仍然存活，不能确切估算[87]。生存期至少1年的受者中位生存期从11.4年增加到12.9年。多因素分析表明术前机械支持装置维持的受者生存期降低(死亡RR:临时体外支持2.93，轴向流动LVAD 1.33，搏动灌注LVAD 1.22)。预后不良的附加风险包括先天性心脏病、肾脏替代疗法、预存式输血和ABO血型不合移植。成人受者年龄与死亡率存在U形关系，18~30岁和55岁以上受者的死亡率较高。而移植后30天内死亡率最高，主要是因为移植失败。长期死亡率与慢性移植心脏血管病变的发展、恶性肿瘤和感染有关(风险随时间下降)，现在急性排斥是移植心功能丧失或者死亡的罕见原因。

心脏移植供体的选择仍然比肝肾移植保守[88]。欧洲国家器官储运组织的供体只有39.2%符合心脏捐献，而实际上只有26%的供体被使用。但移植数量增加的压力迫使有限地扩大边缘供体移植。注册中心比较1992—2001年和2002—2008年的移植手术数据显示供者平均年龄增加2岁，供者BMI略微升高(24.2到25.1)以及高血压患病率增加。有趣的是，欧洲供者平均年龄比北美供者大6岁。

欧洲国家器官储运组织设计了供体心脏的评估范围[88]。移植失败风险增加相关因素包括供体年龄、死亡原因、血管造影显示CAD、ECHO心动描记显示左心室肥大、高钠血症以及服用血管加压药物。评分体系能预测供心弃用和长期生存率。此外供受者性别不匹配和预后存在强烈相关性，男性接受女性移植心脏的风险是远期移植物衰竭最大的风险[89]。

心脏移植的经济评定包括供受者特征影响，未与肝、肾移植同步。回顾性分析比较心脏移植与手术心室修复(SVR)的费用，SVR旨在改善左心室功能[90]，包括冠状动脉旁路移植(CABG)，二尖瓣瓣膜修复或更换，心室切开切除疤痕与重塑。约翰·霍普金斯医院比较69例SVR和53例心脏移植表明两者生存率类似。SVR中位住院费用明显少于心脏移植(45 506美元对137 679美元)。然而最近有随机试验单独比较SVR与CABG(缺血性心力衰竭外科治疗试验)未能证明跨过CABG单独应用SVR可大量获益[91]。2006年发表的小儿人群心脏移植费用的单项研究[92]表明，首次住院治疗的中位费用为221 987美元，二次移植的中位费用为18 000美元。笔者分析UNOS数据库的生存资料，估计首次移植费用为49 679美元/QALY(44 943美元~57 628美元)，再次移植为87 883美元/QALY(70 834美元~103 661美元)。这些估计全部略低于普遍可接受的有效费用阈值，儿童首次心脏移植降低60 000美元/QALY。相应的估算并不可用于成人移植，但鉴于老年受者移植费用增加以及生存潜力下降，费用评估可能超过可接受QALY阈值。

心脏移植的机械性替代方案

供体获取的明显限制推动了终末期心力衰竭替代治疗策略的发展。心脏移植率不超过心脏替代疗法总体需求的2%~3%。此外肝肾移植供体池可扩大到活体供体以及心脏死亡供体，而这对心脏移植来说是不可能的。现在LVAD作为移植等待的渐进性心力衰竭患者的移植桥梁(BTT)，或者作为进展期心力衰竭的永久性治疗方法[82]。永久性植入，也被称为替代治疗(DT)，在20世纪90年代末开始的几项大型临床试验中得到了前瞻性的评估，最终获得了FDA和联邦医保的批准。

机械辅助治疗充血性心力衰竭的随机评价

(REMATCH)试验在 20 个移植中心招募 129 名患者，随机分组进入医疗管理或放置 HeartMate XV (HM XV)装置[79]。纳入标准非常严格，只包括晚期心力衰竭患者[纽约心脏协会四级 CHF 症状、左心室射血分数<25%、峰值耗氧量<12mL/(kg·min)或者需要静脉活性药物输注]。纳入的患者被认为不是移植候选者。LVAD 组患者生存率增加 1 倍(1 年 25%~52%，2 年 8%~23%)，生活质量改善。因为 HM XV 是一个搏动装置，患者需要长期抗凝治疗，这导致包括出血和中风在内的并发症发病率显著增加。

最近改良设计已经降低 LVAD 植入的发病率，进一步降低 CHF 相关发病率[93]。HeartMate II (HM II) 是一个轴向持续流动泵，内部悬浮的推进器可增强心脏输出。LVAD 替代治疗仍然复杂，手术死亡及复发风险显著。大多数 LVAD 相关的死亡发生在首次植入治疗以及技术没有改进的时期。DT 试验比较 HM XVE (HM XV 改进版)和 HM II 发现患者 30 天死亡率分别为 28%和 26%。但是从长远来看，HM II 相比早期装置提高无中风或无设备故障的比例，2 年生存率增加(58%对 24%)。关键试验中只有 9%的 HM II 受者需要更换泵，而 HM XVE 为 34%。基于这些结果，HM II 在 2008 年 4 月被 FDA 批准可用于 BTT，2010 年 1 月被批准可用于终末替代治疗。目前其他装置正在研发中，例如利用磁悬浮技术消除对轴承的需要及提高寿命，不依赖外部动力传动系统以及延长电池寿命的装置。

尽管 LVAD 治疗复杂，但许多 DT 患者报告其总体生活质量有了显著改善。HM II 减少再次住院治疗的持续时间，改善患者生活质量。回顾性分析 30 例在约翰·霍普金斯医院接受 HM XV 或 HM II 治疗 1 年的 DT 患者，显示两者每年平均住院例数类似(2.9±2.2)，但平均住院时间减少(HM XVE 为 26.3 天，HM II 为 6.8 天)[94]。3例 HM II 患者在首次治疗后没有再次住院。患者 NYHA 分级显著降低(3.9~1.4)，运动耐量提高以及生活质量评分升高。

目前医疗保险下 DT 治疗的适应证是基于 REMATCH 标准。患者必须存在进展性心脏衰竭，适当允许植入的身体，由于年龄或并发症而有心脏移植手术禁忌证。然而在初次植入时不能明确选择 DT 和 BTT[95]。例如，在关键试验中大约有 20%的患者最初由于并发疾病或恶性肿瘤不充分时期，不能成为心脏移植候选人，要充分改善以适于 HT。许多这样的患者要解决严重的肺动脉高压，改善肾功能，或大幅度降低体重。相反的是，使用 LVAD 作为 BTT 治疗的患者中，O 型血、高度敏感、或者体型极端的(很小或很大)的患者可能永远不会被分配到适当的移植中心。

进一步发展机械支持装置加强可行移植物的供应约束，无疑会增加晚期心力衰竭患者的治疗总费用。比如肾功能衰竭进行血液透析，美国大量终末器官衰竭的患者不一定是依赖于机械支持装置。虽然最初年龄被视为 DT 的禁忌证，但最近研究已经证明 70 岁以上患者能够成功植入。最近一项回顾性分析中 2943 例患者在 2000—2006 年接受联邦医保的 LVAD 治疗，相比最近 30 天内经历预先心脏手术(心切开术)，评估接受 LVAD 作为主要治疗的费用和预后[96]。主要装置植入患者仅住院治疗 1 年的平均费用是 178 714 美元，经历预先心切开术的患者为 111 769 美元。主要植入的患者 1 年生存率为 73%，心脏术后的患者则为 76%。虽然最初植入的费用在过去十年里已经降低，从每例 210 000 美元降至 126 000 美元，由于住院时间缩短的和并发症发生率下降，补偿额度继续升高(2010 年联邦医保为 188 000 美元)。最近有设计 Markov 预后模型，使用最近的临床试验数据估计 LVAD 替代后并发症相比医疗管理的费用[97]。持续流量泵的费用定为 198 184 美元/QALY。尽管仍然很贵，但比约 802 700 美元/QALY 的脉冲泵已经明显减少。考虑到明确的临床需要和最近联邦医保的范围，总费用很可能会显著增加，即使有 80 000~150 000 例晚期 CHF 患者接受放置 LVAD。由于 LVAD 放置后患者的高昂费用和相对较短的生存，健康治疗投资的回报已经受到质疑。最近有分析表明 LVAD 治疗对 DT 或 BTT 尚未有费用效益，目前的标准是每生存年 60~100 000 美元，脉冲式灌注装置的费用效益可能会提高[97-99]。

总结

心脏移植对于晚期心力衰竭患者仍然是最好的选择，但经济影响尚未被完全研究。混淆因素包括潜在的老年受者数量不断扩大，越来越多的非移植替代方案，这些方案也产生大量的竞争性费用。这些问题将促进资源利用的深入讨论。

结尾

终末期器官衰竭治疗已经从缓解症状发展为功能

替代，期望获得长期生存，但移植预后仍然远远未能达到统一。更年轻、更健康的受者接受最佳移植物已取得出乎意料的成功，受者包括风险较高的申请者和移植等待患者。因此移植专家不得不使用越来越多的边缘器官，但仍然无法满足需求。

可用资金用于高成本服务进一步限制了医务人员治疗器官衰竭患者的能力。20世纪的挑战主要是对验证科学原理和技术开发，21世纪的障碍在于规模化和可持续性。扩大适应证，降低捐献器官质量将增加治疗费用。发展机械支持装置可解除有限器官的约束，但即便在发达国家费用也可能远远超出患者承受范围。特别是考虑到全球范围时，确切治疗终末期器官衰竭的需求大于目前的治疗能力。正如20世纪70年代见证了ESRD透析，联邦财政支持使联邦医保批准LVAD用于DT，实现有限器官捐献的必要配给，心脏机械支持的实用性将增加CHF器官移植费用。选择适合新技术的受者是成功的关键。

考虑到器官数量有限和治疗经济支持的减少，伦理和经济上更大的挑战或许在于决定"谁不是候选人"。有限的移植资源分配给更多的受者，在某种程度上每个人都有可能从中获益。除外器官供应障碍，限制获取有限的治疗需要另一个标准。此外基于目前的费用和预后，绝对依赖于费用效益增加可能会限制有前景的技术。因此器官移植就不会被批准。但经过几十年的坚持不懈，我们已经建立起一个有效解决许多器官衰竭患者费用的方案。平衡机会创造必要性来限制支出可能成为移植专家未来50年最大的挑战。

（卓建勇 译　徐骁 校）

参考文献

1. Tilney NL. Transplant: From Myth to Reality. New Haven, CT: Yale University Press; 2003: xii. 320 p.p.
2. Starzl TE. History of clinical transplantation. World Journal of Surgery. 2000;24(7):759-782.
3. Hakim NS, Papalois VE. History of Organ and Cell Transplantation. London River Edge, NJ: Imperial College Press; Distributed by World Scientific Pub.; 2003: xviii. 444 p.p.
4. Starzl TE. The Puzzle People: Memoirs of a Transplant Surgeon. Pittsburgh, PA: University of Pittsburgh Press; 1992: 364 p.p.
5. McRae D. Every Second Counts: The Race to Transplant The First Human Heart. New York, NY: G.P. Putnam's Sons; 2006. 356 p.p.
6. Squifflet JP, Gruessner RW, Sutherland DE. The history of pancreas transplantation: past, present and future. Acta Chirurgica Belgica. 2008;108(3):367-378.
7. Axelrod DA, McCullough KP, Brewer ED, et al. Kidney and pancreas transplantation in the United States, 1999-2008: the changing face of living donation. American Journal of Transplantation. 2010;10(4 Pt 2):987-1002.
8. Persad G, Wertheimer A, Emanuel EJ. Principles for allocation of scarce medical interventions. Lancet. 2009;373(9661):423-431.
9. Garcia GG, Harden P, Chapman J. The global role of kidney transplantation. Transplantation. 2012;93(4):337-341.
10. Rizvi SA, Naqvi SA, Zafar MN, et al. A renal transplantation model for developing countries. American Journal of Transplantation. 2011;11(11):2302-2307.
11. Office of the Inspector General HaHS. Medicare Hospital Prospective Payment System How DRG Rates Are Calculated and Updated. Washington, D.C. 2001 [cited February 16, 2012]; Available from: http://oig.hhs.gov/oei/reports/oei-09-00-00200.pdf.
12. Sack K. Arizona medicaid cuts seen as a sign of the times. New York Times. 2010 12/4/2010.
13. Kolff WJ, Watschinger B, Vertes V. Results in patients treated with the coil kidney (disposable dialyzing unit). Journal of the American Medical Association. 1956;161(15):1433-1437.
14. Buntin J. Dialysis death panels and the health-care debate. The Washington Post. 2009.
15. Service USRD. 2011 USRDS Annual Data Report. Minneaoplis, MN 2011 [cited February 16, 2012]; Available from: http://www.usrds.org/2011/pdf/v2_ch011_11.pdf.
16. Wolfe RA, Ashby VB, Milford EL, et al. Comparison of mortality in all patients on dialysis, patients on dialysis awaiting transplantation, and recipients of a first cadaveric transplant. New England Journal of Medicine. 1999;341(23): 1725-1730.
17. Wolfe RA, McCullough KP, Schaubel DE, et al. Calculating life years from transplant (LYFT): methods for kidney and kidney-pancreas candidates. American Journal of Transplantation. 2008;8(4 Pt 2):997-1011.
18. Wolfe RA, McCullough KP, Leichtman AB. Predictability of survival models for waiting list and transplant patients: calculating LYFT. American Journal of Transplantation. 2009;9(7):1523-1527.
19. Reese PP, Caplan AL, Bloom RD, et al. How should we use age to ration health care? Lessons from the case of kidney transplantation. Journal of the American Geriatrics Society. 2010;58(10):1980-1986.
20. Lamb KE, Lodhi S, Meier-Kriesche HU. Long-term renal allograft survival in the United States: a critical reappraisal. American Journal of Transplantation. 2011; 11(3):450-462.
21. System URD. USRDS 2011: Annual Data Report: Atlas of Chronic Kidney Disease and End stage Renal Disease in the United States. Bethesda, MD 2011.
22. Buchanan PM, Lentine KL, Burroughs TE, et al. Association of lower costs of pulsatile machine perfusion in renal transplantation from expanded criteria donors. American Journal of Transplantation. 2008;8(11):2391-2401.
23. Matas AJ, Schnitzler M. Payment for living donor (vendor) kidneys: a cost-effectiveness analysis. American Journal of Transplantation. 2004;4(2): 216-221.
24. Port FK, Bragg-Gresham JL, Metzger RA, et al. Donor characteristics associated with reduced graft survival: an approach to expanding the pool of kidney donors. Transplantation. 2002;74(9):1281-1286.
25. Sung RS, Guidinger MK, Christensen LL, et al. Development and current status of ECD kidney transplantation. Clinical Transplants. 2005; 37-55.
26. Merion RM, Ashby VB, Wolfe RA, et al. Deceased-donor characteristics and the survival benefit of kidney transplantation. JAMA: The Journal of the American Medical Association. 2005;294(21):2726-2733.
27. Grams ME, Womer KL, Ugarte RM, et al. Listing for expanded criteria donor kidneys in older adults and those with predicted benefit. American Journal of Transplantation. 2010;10(4):802-809.
28. Jochmans I, Pirenne J. Graft quality assessment in kidney transplantation: not an exact science yet! Current Opinion in Organ Transplantation. 2011;16(2): 174-179.
29. Rao PS, Schaubel DE, Guidinger MK, et al. A comprehensive risk quantification score for deceased donor kidneys: the kidney donor risk index. Transplantation. 2009;88(2):231-236.
30. NETWORK OPAT. Concepts of Kidney Allocation. 2011 [cited February 16, 2012]; Available from: http://optn.transplant.hrsa.gov/SharedContentDocuments/KidneyConceptDocument.PDF.
31. Bentas W, Jones J, Karaoguz A, et al. Renal transplantation in the elderly: surgical complications and outcome with special emphasis on the Eurotransplant Senior Programme. Nephrology, Dialysis, Transplantation. 2008;23(6): 2043-2051.
32. Siedlecki A, Irish W, Brennan DC. Delayed graft function in the kidney transplant. American Journal of Transplantation. 2011;11(11):2279-2296.
33. Irish WD, Ilsley JN, Schnitzler MA, et al. A risk prediction model for delayed graft function in the current era of deceased donor renal transplantation. American Journal of Transplantation. 2010;10(10):2279-2286.
34. Matsuoka L, Almeda JL, Mateo R. Pulsatile perfusion of kidney allografts. Current Opinion in Organ Transplantation. 2009;14(4):365-369.
35. Matsuoka L, Shah T, Aswad S, et al. Pulsatile perfusion reduces the incidence of

delayed graft function in expanded criteria donor kidney transplantation. American Journal of Transplantation. 2006;6(6):1473–1478.
36. Schnitzler MA, Johnston K, Axelrod D, et al. Associations of renal function at 1-year after kidney transplantation with subsequent return to dialysis, mortality, and healthcare costs. Transplantation. 2011;91(12):1347–1356.
37. Englesbe MJ, Dimick JB, Fan Z, et al. Case mix, quality and high-cost kidney transplant patients. American Journal of Transplantation. 2009;9(5): 1108–1114.
38. Englesbe MJ, Ads Y, Cohn JA, et al. The effects of donor and recipient practices on transplant center finances. American Journal of Transplantation. 2008;8(3): 586–592.
39. Huang E, Segev DL, Rabb H. Kidney transplantation in the elderly. Seminars in Nephrology. 2009;29(6):621–635.
40. Heldal K, Hartmann A, Leivestad T, et al. Risk variables associated with the outcome of kidney recipients >70 years of age in the new millennium. Nephrology, Dialysis, Transplantation. 2011;26(8):2706–2711.
41. Abecassis M, Bartlett ST, Collins AJ, et al. Kidney transplantation as primary therapy for end stage renal disease: a National Kidney Foundation/Kidney Disease Outcomes Quality Initiative (NKF/KDOQITM) conference. Clinical journal of the American Society of Nephrology: CJASN. 2008;3(2):471–480.
42. Meier-Kriesche HU, Kaplan B. Waiting time on dialysis as the strongest modifiable risk factor for renal transplant outcomes: a paired donor kidney analysis. Transplantation. 2002;74(10):1377–1381.
43. Axelrod DA, Dzebisashvili N, Schnitzler MA, et al. The interplay of socioeconomic status, distance to center, and interdonor service area travel on kidney transplant access and outcomes. Clinical journal of the American Society of Nephrology: CJASN. 2010;5(12):2276–2288.
44. Montgomery RA, Lonze BE, King KE, et al. Desensitization in HLA-incompatible kidney recipients and survival. New England Journal of Medicine. 2011; 365(4):318–326.
45. Davis GL, Albright JE, Cook SF, et al. Projecting future complications of chronic hepatitis C in the United States. Liver Transplantation. 2003;9(4):331–338.
46. Wong JB, McQuillan GM, McHutchison JG, et al. Estimating future hepatitis C morbidity, mortality, and costs in the United States. American Journal of Public Health. 2000;90(10):1562–1569.
47. Lim YS, Kim WR. The global impact of hepatic fibrosis and end stage liver disease. Clinics in Liver Disease. 2008;12(4):733–746, vii.
48. Rosen HR. Clinical practice. Chronic hepatitis C infection. New England Journal of Medicine. 2011;364(25):2429–2438.
49. McGarry LJ, Pawar VS, Parekh HH, et al. Economic model of a birth cohort screening program for hepatitis C virus. Hepatology. 2011;55(5): 1344–1355. Epub 2011/12/03.
50. Leigh JP, Bowlus CL, Leistikow BN, et al. Costs of hepatitis C. Archives of Internal Medicine. 2001;161(18):2231–2237.
51. de Alwis NM, Day CP. Non-alcoholic fatty liver disease: the mist gradually clears. Journal of Hepatology. 2008;48(Suppl 1):S104–S112.
52. Buchanan P, Dzebisashvili N, Lentine KL, et al. Liver transplantation cost in the model for end stage liver disease era: looking beyond the transplant admission. Liver Transplantation. 2009;15(10):1270–1277.
53. Bajaj JS, Wade JB, Gibson DP, et al. The multi-dimensional burden of cirrhosis and hepatic encephalopathy on patients and caregivers. American Journal of Gastroenterology. 2011;106(9):1646–1653.
54. Miyazaki ET, Dos Santos R Jr, Miyazaki MC, et al. Patients on the waiting list for liver transplantation: caregiver burden and stress. Liver Transplantation. 2010;16(10):1164–1168.
55. Olthoff KM, Brown RS Jr, Delmonico FL, et al. Summary report of a national conference: evolving concepts in liver allocation in the MELD and PELD era. December 8, 2003, Washington, DC, USA. Liver Transplantation. 2004;10(10 Suppl 2):A6–A22.
56. Hayashi PH, Axelrod DA, Galanko J, et al. Regional differences in deceased donor liver transplantation and their implications for organ utilization and allocation. Clinical Transplantation. 2011;25(1):156–163.
57. Axelrod DA, Kalbfleisch JD, Sun RJ, et al. Innovations in the assessment of transplant center performance: implications for quality improvement. American Journal of Transplantation. 2009;9(4 Pt 2):959–969.
58. Roberts JP, Dykstra DM, Goodrich NP, et al. Geographic differences in event rates by model for end stage liver disease score. American Journal of Transplantation. 2006;6(10):2470–2475.
59. Merion RM, Schaubel DE, Dykstra DM, et al. The survival benefit of liver transplantation. American Journal of Transplantation. 2005;5(2):307–313.
60. Narayanan Menon KV, Nyberg SL, Harmsen WS, et al. MELD and other factors associated with survival after liver transplantation. American Journal of Transplantation. 2004;4(5):819–825.
61. Jain A, Reyes J, Kashyap R, et al. Long-term survival after liver transplantation in 4,000 consecutive patients at a single center. Annals of Surgery. 2000; 232(4):490–500.
62. Weismuller TJ, Fikatas P, Schmidt J, et al. Multicentric evaluation of model for end stage liver disease-based allocation and survival after liver transplantation in Germany–limitations of the 'sickest first'-concept. Transplant International. 2011;24(1):91–99.
63. Cholongitas E, Marelli L, Shusang V, et al. A systematic review of the performance of the model for end stage liver disease (MELD) in the setting of liver transplantation. Liver Transplantation. 2006;12(7):1049–1061.
64. Feng S, Goodrich NP, Bragg-Gresham JL, et al. Characteristics associated with liver graft failure: the concept of a donor risk index. American Journal of Transplantation. 2006;6(4):783–790.
65. Schaubel DE, Sima CS, Goodrich NP, et al. The survival benefit of deceased donor liver transplantation as a function of candidate disease severity and donor quality. American Journal of Transplantation. 2008;8(2):419–425.
66. Axelrod DA, Gheorghian A, Schnitzler MA, et al. The economic implications of broader sharing of liver allografts. American Journal of Transplantation. 2011;11(4):798–807.
67. Axelrod DA, Koffron AJ, Baker T, et al. The economic impact of MELD on liver transplant centers. American Journal of Transplantation. 2005;5(9): 2297–2301.
68. Washburn WK, Meo NA, Halff GA, et al. Factors influencing liver transplant length of stay at two large-volume transplant centers. Liver Transplantation. 2009;15(11):1570–1578.
69. Axelrod DA, Schnitzler M, Salvalaggio PR, et al. The economic impact of the utilization of liver allografts with high donor risk index. American Journal of Transplantation. 2007;7(4):990–997.
70. Dutkowski P, Oberkofler CE, Bechir M, et al. The model for end stage liver disease allocation system for liver transplantation saves lives, but increases morbidity and cost: a prospective outcome analysis. Liver Transplantation. 2011;17(6): 674–684.
71. OPTN/UNOS. Concept Document: Next Steps Toward Improving Liver Distribution. 2011 [cited December 21, 2011]; Available from: http://optn.transplant.hrsa.gov/SharedContentDocuments/LiverConcept_123010.pdf.
72. Jay C, Ladner D, Wang E, et al. A comprehensive risk assessment of mortality following donation after cardiac death liver transplant—an analysis of the national registry. Journal of Hepatology. 2011;55(4):808–813.
73. Jay CL, Lyuksemburg V, Kang R, et al. The increased costs of donation after cardiac death liver transplantation: caveat emptor. Annals of Surgery. 2010; 251(4):743–748.
74. Salvalaggio PR, Dzebisashvili N, MacLeod KE, et al. The interaction among donor characteristics, severity of liver disease, and the cost of liver transplantation. Liver Transplantation. 2011;17(3):233–242.
75. Northup PG, Abecassis MM, Englesbe MJ, et al. Addition of adult-to-adult living donation to liver transplant programs improves survival but at an increased cost. Liver Transplantation. 2009;15(2):148–162.
76. Lloyd-Jones DM, Larson MG, Leip EP, et al. Lifetime risk for developing congestive heart failure: the Framingham Heart Study. Circulation. 2002;106(24): 3068–3072.
77. Ramani GV, Uber PA, Mehra MR. Chronic heart failure: contemporary diagnosis and management. Mayo Clinic Proceedings. Mayo Clinic. 2010;85(2):180–195.
78. Norton C, Georgiopoulou VV, Kalogeropoulos AP, et al. Epidemiology and cost of advanced heart failure. Progress in Cardiovascular Diseases. 2011;54(2): 78–85.
79. Rose EA, Gelijns AC, Moskowitz AJ, et al. Long-term use of a left ventricular assist device for end stage heart failure. New England Journal of Medicine. 2001;345(20):1435–1443.
80. Rogers JG, Butler J, Lansman SL, et al. Chronic mechanical circulatory support for inotrope-dependent heart failure patients who are not transplant candidates: results of the INTrEPID Trial. Journal of the American College of Cardiology. 2007;50(8):741–747.
81. Stevenson LW, Miller LW, Desvigne-Nickens P, et al. Left ventricular assist device as destination for patients undergoing intravenous inotropic therapy: a subset analysis from REMATCH (Randomized Evaluation of Mechanical Assistance in Treatment of Chronic Heart Failure). Circulation. 2004;110(8):975–981.
82. Lietz K. Destination therapy: patient selection and current outcomes. Journal of Cardiac Surgery. 2010;25(4):462–471.
83. O'Connor CM, Abraham WT, Albert NM, et al. Predictors of mortality after discharge in patients hospitalized with heart failure: an analysis from the Organized Program to Initiate Lifesaving Treatment in Hospitalized Patients with Heart Failure (OPTIMIZE-HF). American Heart Journal. 2008;156(4):662–673.
84. Unroe KT, Greiner MA, Hernandez AF, et al. Resource use in the last 6 months of life among medicare beneficiaries with heart failure, 2000-2007. Archives of Internal Medicine. 2011;171(3):196–203.
85. Russo MJ, Gelijns AC, Stevenson LW, et al. The cost of medical management in advanced heart failure during the final two years of life. Journal of Cardiac

Failure. 2008;14(8):651–658.
86. Epstein AJ, Polsky D, Yang F, et al. Geographic variation in implantable cardioverter-defibrillator use and heart failure survival. Medical Care. 2012; 50(1):10–17.
87. Christie JD, Edwards LB, Kucheryavaya AY, et al. The registry of the international society for heart and lung transplantation: twenty-eighth adult lung and heart-lung transplant report-2011. Journal of Heart and Lung Transplantation. 2011;30(10):1104–1122.
88. Smits JM, De Pauw M, de Vries E, et al. Donor scoring system for heart transplantation and the impact on patient survival. Journal of Heart and Lung Transplantation. 2011; 31(4):387–397. Epub 2011/12/20.
89. Kittleson MM, Shemin R, Patel JK, et al. Donor-recipient sex mismatch portends poor 10-year outcomes in a single-center experience. Journal of Heart and Lung Transplantation. 2011;30(9):1018–1022.
90. Williams JA, Weiss ES, Patel ND, et al. Surgical ventricular restoration versus cardiac transplantation: a comparison of cost, outcomes, and survival. Journal of Cardiac Failure. 2008;14(7):547–554.
91. Jones RH, Velazquez EJ, Michler RE, et al. Coronary bypass surgery with or without surgical ventricular reconstruction. New England Journal of Medicine. 2009;360(17):1705–1717.
92. Dayton JD, Kanter KR, Vincent RN, et al. Cost-effectiveness of pediatric heart transplantation. Journal of Heart and Lung Transplantation. 2006;25(4): 409–415.
93. Slaughter MS, Rogers JG, Milano CA, et al. Advanced heart failure treated with continuous-flow left ventricular assist device. New England Journal of Medicine. 2009;361(23):2241–2251.
94. Allen JG, Weiss ES, Schaffer JM, et al. Quality of life and functional status in patients surviving 12 months after left ventricular assist device implantation. Journal of Heart and Lung Transplantation. 2010;29(3):278–285.
95. Lietz K, Long JW, Kfoury AG, et al. Outcomes of left ventricular assist device implantation as destination therapy in the post-REMATCH era: implications for patient selection. Circulation. 2007;116(5):497–505.
96. Hernandez AF, Shea AM, Milano CA, et al. Long-term outcomes and costs of ventricular assist devices among Medicare beneficiaries. JAMA: Journal of the American Medical Association. 2008;300(20):2398–2406.
97. Rogers JG, Bostic RR, Tong KB, et al. Cost-effectiveness analysis of continuous-flow left ventricular assist devices as destination therapy. Circulation. Heart failure. 2012;5(1):10–16.
98. Moreno SG, Novielli N, Cooper NJ. Cost-effectiveness of the implantable HeartMate II left ventricular assist device for patients awaiting heart transplantation. Journal of Heart and Lung Transplantation. 2012;31(5):450–458.
99. Rogers JGBR, Tong KB, Adamson R, et al. Cost-effectiveness analysis of continuous-flow left ventricular assist devices as destination therapy. Circulation. Heart failure. 2012;5(1):6.
100. Smith CR, Woodward RS, Cohen DS, et al. Cadaveric versus living donor kidney transplantation: a Medicare payment analysis. Transplantation. 2000;69(2): 311–314

第 143 章 国家医疗政策、移植相关法规和器官移植的未来

Keren Ladin, Rui Wang, Douglas W. Hanto

引言

在过去的一个世纪，美国的移植和卫生政策以不可思议的速度发展着。1954 年第一例在波士顿成功的肾移植手术，1967 年第一例成功的肝移植手术，1968 年成立第一个器官获取组织（OPO），1980 年确立统一死亡判定法案，并于 2005 年在法国实行了第一例成功的换脸手术，移植领域已经发生了巨大的变化。同时，卫生政策也极大地演变，从 1965 年建立医疗保险和医疗补助，采用基于雇主的个人医疗保险，到如今医疗保险支出超过(美国)国内生产总值(GDP)的 17%的医疗环境。技术越来越先进，医疗保险范围扩大和器官运输系统亦有所提高，更多的美国人获得比以往更高水平的医疗保健。在 2010 年通过的患者保护与平价医疗法案通过旨在扩大覆盖面的政策，实施市场改革，以酬薪激励和其他示范来改善医疗保健质量和包含成本的各项手段，重塑医疗景前景。这些改革措施无疑会影响卫生行业的方方面面，对于移植医疗有重要的意义。

大多数现有移植政策的目的是四重的：①保护移植物受体和供体的健康；②在整个移植过程中保持尊严和保护患者的自主权；③在器官分配提高效率；④确保器官的分配和获取的公平公正。未来的移植政策是一个超越单学科的广泛内容。然而，本章中我们主要描述未来政策的关键问题，包括医疗改革对受体和供体的意义，通过给予器官捐赠者更多的奖励来满足日益增长的受体需求。在世界范围内有关移植的法律不尽相同，本章代表了北美法律的角度，也在美国法律体系中例举几个具体案例进行解析。然而，和大多数发达国家一样，美国的移植领域主题反映在类似法律章程中。关于国家监管以及与移植政策和实践相关的文化差异的更多讨论，可分别见于第 128 章和第 139 章。

美国移植领域的法律和监管结构

美国的移植系统是由移植中心、供体医院、器官获取组织(OPO)和 10 个器官分配的地域组织共同组成的网络。每一个供体医院都是分配在单独的区域，归属于某个特定的 OPO(图 143.1 和图 143.2)。器官供应移植网络(OPTN)中详细描述了器官捐献和移植政策，并且和器官共享网络(UNOS)签订合约，共同为移植政策设定框架与执行。美国卫生资源和服务管理局(HRSA)[卫生及公共服务部(DHHS)的一个分部]的移植分部(DOT)为联邦政府对 OPTN 进行监控(图 143.3)。

在 20 年间移植政策发生了重大的改变。例如，器官分配算法被重新设计和修订，捐赠者和接受者的标准已经扩大，捐献过程、质量和结果的标准已经完善，并且由医疗保险和医疗补助中心(CMS)执行。尽管一些标准已普遍应用，但是比如 OPO 政策的分配差异等其他标准仅在个别区域或个体上应用，形成了一个拼凑的协议[1]。目前，UNOS 政策旨在调和差异和修改分配算法，以更好地实现公平和效率。其他措施包括肾脏分配规则的改变[2]，UNet 中肾移植特征索引(KDPI)，倡导预防捐赠者疾病的传播。对肝移植患者来说，建立分层布置的区域共享机制以促进 MELD/PELD 评分高于 35 的危重患者信息的大范围传播[3]。

尽管对移植和移植相关的法律法规实行中央监管，它们是断层的，甚至有些支离破碎。规范移植的法律和监管政策被分为四个层面，从高到低为 UNOS 政策、联邦法规、州和联邦法律。

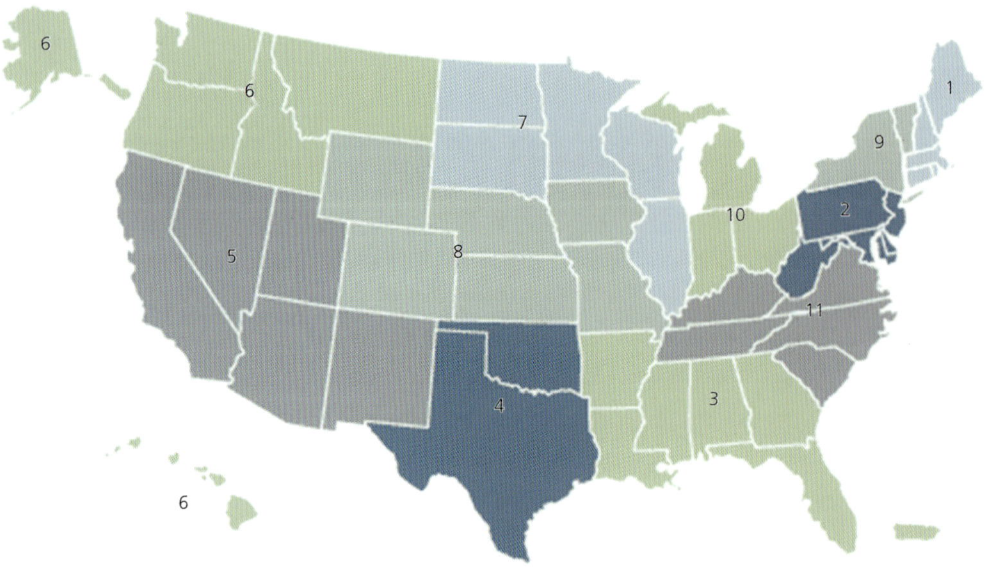

给地区所在州分布：

- 地区1：康涅狄格州，缅因州，马萨诸塞州，新罕布什尔州，罗德岛州，佛蒙特州东部
- 地区2：特拉华州，哥伦比亚特区，马里兰州，新泽西州，费城，西弗吉尼亚州，北弗吉尼亚州
- 地区3：阿拉巴马，阿肯色州，佛罗里达州，佐治亚州，路易斯安那州，密西西比州，波多黎各
- 地区4：俄克拉荷马州，得克萨斯州
- 地区5：亚利桑那州，加州，内华达州，新墨西哥州，犹他州
- 地区6：阿拉斯加，夏威夷，爱达荷，蒙大拿，俄勒冈，华盛顿
- 地区7：伊利诺伊州，明尼苏达州，北达科他州，南达科他州，威斯康星州
- 地区8：科罗拉多州，洛瓦州，堪萨斯州，密苏里州，内布拉斯加州，怀俄明州
- 地区9：纽约州，佛蒙特州西部
- 地区10：印第安纳州，密歇根州，俄亥俄州
- 地区11：肯塔基州，北卡罗莱纳州，南卡罗莱纳州，田纳西州，弗吉尼亚州

图 143.1 目前的器官共享网络(UNOS)地区分布图。(Reproduced from http://optn.transplant.hrsa.gov/members/regions.asp)

UNOS 法规提供详细说明，以及为 OPTN、POP 和移植医院提供了可行的协议。UNOS 是私密的非营利组织，由 OPTN 签订以完成器官移植、捐赠、分配和在全国范围内分配。UNOS 规则规定移植数据是如何在医院、OPO、UNOS 间进行运输、储存和分配的。UNOS 还负责维护国家数据库。UNOS 负责管理全国候补名单，运行匹配算法和监督公开环节以监控和改善器官分配。最后，UNOS 主管有关器官捐献和移植的公众意识提高和教育。

正如 UNOS 规则为移植供体提供切实可行的指导规则，联邦法规和 CMS 规章也通过阐明关键的原则和程序，为 OPTN、OPO 和移植项目提供具体的方向。

国家法律在更高的层面规范捐献过程。如今这些法律也被修订，将死亡标准、捐赠者同意要求、捐献者登记写入公共教育项目，捐助者的利益等写入法律。相反，联邦法律规定国家流程，如器官获得、分配、移植和遗体捐献。联邦法律在最高和最广泛的水平上概括了移植的原则和限制；他们建立 OPTN 和 OPO 的指南。举个例子，联邦法律建立 OPTN 是为了规定，OPTN 在国家层面负责协调、监管和执行器官移植政策与程序，而 OPO 是在地区或区域中负责取得器官和通知 OPTN 名下的潜在接受者[4]。下面章节中将更详细地讨论上述有关于器官移植的法律法规。

器官共享网络(UNOS)

由于联邦法律法规主管 OPTN 的主体工作和其各 OPO 成员、移植中心的关系，器官共享网络(UNOS)负责制订那些规定 OPTN 和其成员的行动的政策[5]。UNOS 自 1986 年起一直以通过和 DHHS 合约条款的方式来管理 OPTN。尽管 UNOS 和 OPTN 在法律上彼此独立，但是他们拥有相同的董事会，以及相同的政策理念。

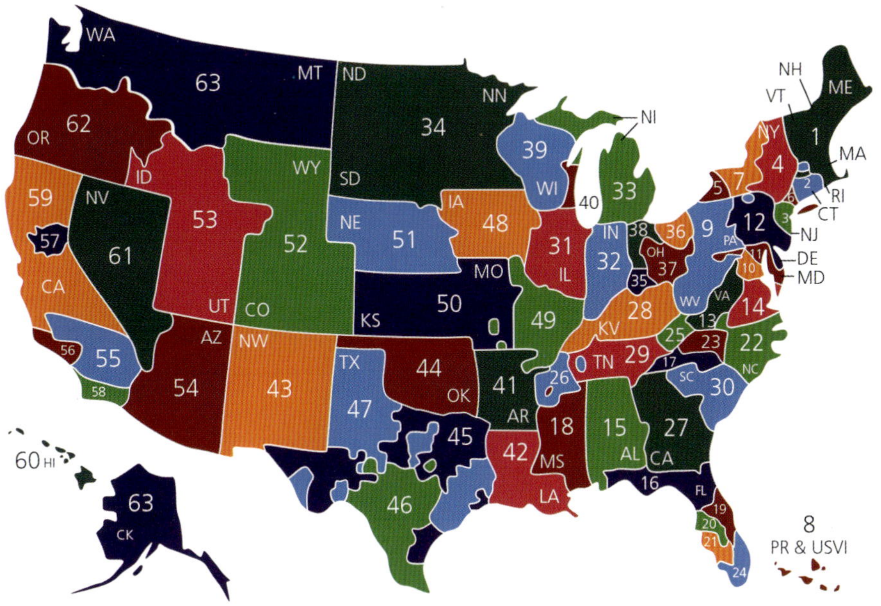

1.新英格兰器官银行有限公司
2.东北 OPO 和组织库
3.新泽西州器官和组织共享网络
4.捐献与移植中心
5.纽约州北部的移植服务有限公司
6.纽约器官捐赠者网络
7.罗切斯特大学器官采购项目
8.波多黎各生命线
9.器官康复教育中心
10.华盛顿地区移植协会
11.马里兰移植资源中心
12.德拉瓦谷大都会区移植计划
13.弗吉尼亚器官采购局
14.生活网
15.阿拉巴马器官中心
16.佛罗里达大学的 OPO
17.卡罗莱纳的生活份额
18.密西西比器官康复机构有限公司
19.生命跨越公司
20.佛罗里达生命线
21.佛罗里达西南部的生命线
22.卡罗莱纳器官采购局
23.卡罗莱纳生命护理
24.迈阿密大学
25.生命资源捐赠中心
26.中南移植基金会
27.乔治亚州的生命线
28.肯塔基州器官捐赠者亲属
29.田纳西捐赠者服务
30.SC 器官采购机构
31.伊利诺伊州地区器官银行
32.印第安纳州 OPO 有限公司
33.MI 器官采购机构
34.中西北部有限公司
35.俄亥俄谷生活中心
36.救生圈
37.俄亥俄州的生命线
38.俄亥俄州的生活联系
39.威斯康星大学
40.威斯康星州捐赠网络
41.阿肯色州地区器官康复机构
42.路易斯安那器官采购局
43.新墨西哥捐助计划
44.俄克拉荷马州器官共享网络有限公司
45.西南移植联盟
46.南得克萨斯器官银行
47.生命捐献器官中心
48.爱荷华州机关采购组织
49.中美洲移植协会
50.中西部器官库
51.内布拉斯加州器官检索系统有限公司
52.科罗拉多器官恢复系统有限公司
53.山间器官恢复系统
54.亚利桑那州捐赠网络
55.南加州器官采购中心
56.南加州代理区域机关采购
57.加州移植服务
58.南加州器官组织获取中心
59.加州移植捐赠者网络
60.夏威夷器官捐献中心
61.内华达捐赠网络
62.太平洋西北移植银行
63.西北生活中心

图 143.2 当前 OPO 地区地图(Data from Penhoet, E. D. *et al., Organ Procurement and Transplantation,* Washington, D.C., National Academy Press, 1999)。

UNOS 的任务就是通过器官中心,确保尽可能得快速和公平公正地获取和分配器官。器官则运用名为 UNet 的全国范围的移植电脑系统,将捐助者与受助者信息相互匹配。UNet 也会对等待匹配的患者进行及时维护更新。一旦捐赠器官信息录入 UNet,它会生成一个列表,对需要任何一种器官类型移植的接受者名单进行排序。最后,当信息匹配成功和潜在接受者的移植医院同意接收器官,那么器官会由相应的 OPO 进行派送。重要的是,UNOS 对整个匹配过程进行监控,以确保每一环节都符合器官分配的政策。UNOS 的质检部门也会对 OPTN 的成员、OPO 和各家参与移植的医院进行管控,确保上述单位均服从规定医疗保险,也因此能获得医疗补助中心的补助。随着全国不断促进匹配的肾交换,UNOS 可能会成为统一的肾移植国家体系中的关键一环。

此外,UNOS 也为 OPTN 的存在而发展自己的政

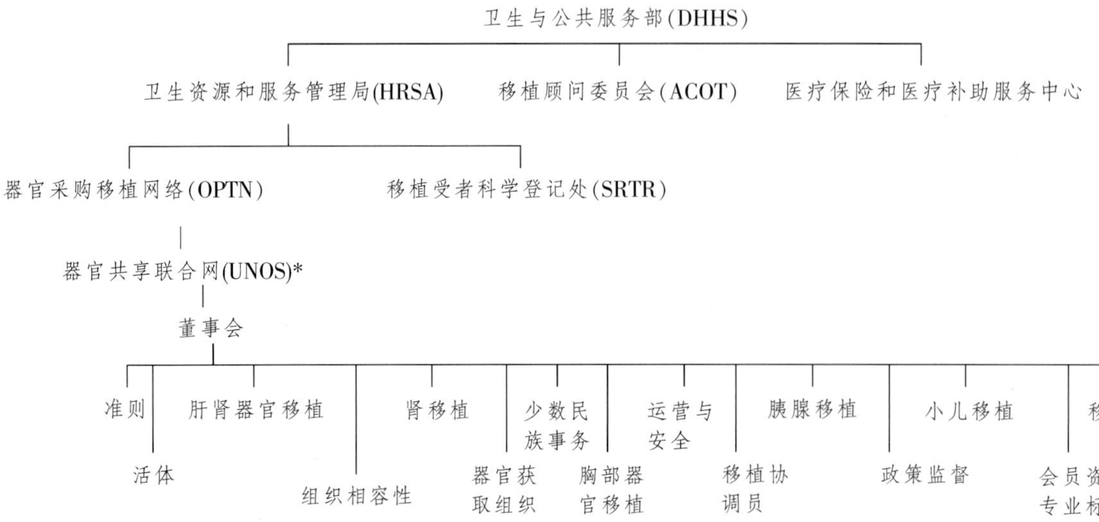

图 143.3 移植监管构成的原理图。

策。政策提案由 UNOS 委员会起草，以摘要的形式公布,并传阅以征求公众意见。

UNOS 紧接着采纳公众意见的建议，向董事会递交提案的终稿，最终成为 UNOS 或者 OPTN 的政策。UNOS 一共有 22 个委员会,包括专门疾病传播顾问委员会、专门国际关系委员会、伦理委员会、执行委员会、财政委员会、组织相容性委员会、肾移植委员会、肝和肠道移植委员会、活体捐献委员会、成员资格和专业标准委员会、罕见病例委员会、手术和安全委员会、器官获取组织 OPO、胰腺移植委员会、患者委员会儿科移植委员会、监管委员会、胸部器官移植委员会、移植管理委员会和移植调度委员会。董事会也会向 HHS 的秘书处提交已被核准的提案，那这些政策就会被官方正式的法规吸收纳入。大部分的委员会,包括董事会,由代表移植界的选举成员组成。这些成员包括移植临床医生和协调人员、组织相容性专家、OPO 代表、志愿卫生组织、医学或者科学组织和公众代表（包括移植候选人、移植受赠者和其家庭、活体捐献者和其家庭)。董事会由 41 人组成,负责监督 UNOS 政策发展。委员会的多样性可以确保移植界的所有主张和利益在政策制订过程中被收纳。

最后,UNOS 在维护公信力和促进器官捐献和移植方面扮演着重要角色。它可以为患者、捐献者及其家庭提供信息和支持。和科学登记制度相似,UNOS 收集和分布从 UNet 上获取的器官移植的信息。UNOS 和各州政府一道为促进器官捐献需求所努力。

联邦条例以及医疗保险与医疗补助中心要求

联邦条例

器官移植的联邦法规在 42 章 121 节——联邦监管核心的“公共卫生”中对联邦法律进行了完善和补充[6]。2000 年 3 月 16 日起效的 DHHS 对“最终法则”进行了补充,建立了 OPTN 的组织结构和监管框架。所有 OPTN 成员必须遵守“最终法则”和由 UNOS、OPTN 和 HHS 补充修订的未来政策。

42 章 121 条

描述了移植程序，器官获取的指导方针,OPTN 规定和分配器官的要求。

42 章 121.4 条

概括了 OPTN 董事会的政策指导方针，其中包括器官的公平分配,检测器官有无传染性疾病,减少由社会经济地位带来的不平等，以及移植外科医生和内科医生的培训。

42 章 121.5 条

罗列了成为 OPTN 成员的要求事项清单，有三个主要规则：作为 OPTN 成员的移植医院只能用指定的移植程序筛选出一个候选人。只要个人被认为是符合移植条件的候选人，移植医院就必须把该候选人列入等待名单。OPTN 成员必须为每个列入名单的移植候选人支付注册费用。

42 章 121.6 条

概述了器官捐赠配型成功与否的测定标准。获取器官的 OPTN 成员必须完成实验室检测和临床检查来确保器官捐献者任何移植禁忌证。OPTN 应当有入选标准，以防止从 HIV 感染者身上获取器官。器官移植项目还必须建立器官捐献的标准，并将其提供给 OPTN 和 OPO。

42 章 121.7 条

解释了器官受赠人鉴定，器官分配以及器官移送的标准。OPTN 成员必须遵循其制订的分配标准，并且使用 OPTN 计算机匹配程序来识别和分级潜在受者。OPTN 成员还应负责安排将器官运输至移植医院。如果移植医院拒绝了器官接收，那 OPTN 成员必须安排下一个合格的受赠人接收器官。

42 章 121.8 条

建立了器官的分配和操作目标的准则。分配政策应当建立在公平的医学裁决之上，避免受赠人对器官的排斥，器官明确，避免器官浪费。为了确保公平分配，规范了挑选合适候选人的标准，通过客观的医学指标测定来设置患者接收移植物的优先级排名，以及尽可能在大的地区范围内进行候选人的筛选。

42 章 121.11 节

要求 OPTN 和移植注册科学系统使用规范的程序，来管理移植候选人、受赠人、捐献者的信息。该程序要求，信息汇报严谨，并通过卫生和福利部秘书处、OPTN、注册科学系统和 OPO 审核后存储信息。执行移植手术时，也必须向公众提供相关信息。

42 章 121.12 条

建立了器官移植咨询委员会(ACOT)为 OPTN 提案提供咨询，也在必要时为其他秘书处遇见的问题提供帮助。

42 章 482.90 条

要求移植中心对器官捐赠者在捐献前接受医学检测和心理社会学评估，以证明捐献者适宜器官捐献并签署知情同意书。

42 章 482.92 条

陈述了下列情况，如果中心执行活体移植项目，从事移植的外科医生和至少另一个专业的注册移植医疗中心必须在获取捐献器官和摘除受体的器官前的短时间内，共同验证捐赠者的血型和其他重要信息是与受体不相互排斥的。

42 章 482.94 条

移植中心书写患者的管理政策做出要求，其中包括移植前、移植中和移植后的患者护理政策，以及活体捐献者的评估、移植和移植后阶段的管理政策。

42 章 482.98 条

要求移植中心选定一位独立的活体捐献倡导者或一个独立的活体捐献团队，来确保活体捐献者和潜在捐献者的权利保护。

医疗保险与医疗补助中心(CMS)的要求

该要求分为三类:数据提交，结果检测，进展中检测。CMS 条例终稿(发表于 2007 年 3 月 30 日)在 2007 年 6 月 28 日正式生效，建立了以医院为基础的移植项目的参与条件(CoP)。要求重点关注反映临床经验、护理质量和移植中心可用资源的结果上。尽管 CMS 为了确保其在保证患者安全过程的地位，绝不放弃对 OPTN 的唯一管辖权，但是额外的 CoP 要求也是为了完善现存的 OPTN 的规则。对于数据提交的要求在很大程度上反映了 OPTN 的标准(例如要求，在最后期限 90 天内，95%的按 OPTN 要求提交的数据会被直接提交到 CMS)。结果检测旨在确保在适当的阈值[由移植受者注册的科学系统(SRTR)数据估算]内的患者和移植物的存活。检测结果低于期望阈值者将被视为不合格，因此可能面临惩罚和制裁。除了上述措施外，CMS 创立的过程中检测，影响着受体和供体的挑选和权力的保护、器官获取和接收、受体和供体的管理要求、候选者管理、质量评估和改进要求。重要的变化包括为潜在的捐赠者提供关于捐赠的短期和长期风险的完整信息的权力，退出捐献的权力和未来保险覆盖的内容[7]。

美国州立律法

各州的法律相当一致,主要管理捐献的过程,包括教育和外联活动,捐赠同意和捐献补偿,捐献者登记和死亡报销指定投保人。管理捐献的国家法律多种多样,下面简要描述主要的法律法规。

统一的遗体捐献法案

1968年法案(及其他修订版本)建立了捐献器官移植的标准和用于医学研究和教学的遗体捐献的标准。法案描述了捐献流程是如何发生的,指定哪些人有资格在死亡后捐献,指定哪些人有权利使用遗体,以及如果在选择捐赠人之间没有偏向,排列出各候选人捐献的优先级列表。1987年修订的法案中说明了对于器官获取来说,自愿成为一名器官捐献者的文件签署是足够的(不需要直系亲戚的同意),而且不需要在签署文档时有目击人在场。法案还规定例行调查(其他患者对受赠者优先接受移植表示质疑)和意愿需要请求(如果请求从一个死去的近亲患者接受器官那么无需考虑捐献者意愿)。法案也禁止器官贸易,如1984年联邦政府颁布的禁令[8]。统一国家法律全国委员会议(NCCUSL起草了本法,试图协调各州之间的法律。

最近,美国所有50个州和哥伦比亚特区采用《第一人称同意法》(也称"第一个授权"或"捐赠者指定"以迫使尊重捐赠者的意愿。"第一人称同意法"要求,有身份证件的成人所指定的捐赠都具有法力效益,如司机的驾驶证、捐赠证,或上传的在线注册表,即使违背他们家族的表达愿望。最新立法允许OPO从家庭中获得亲属愿意向他们所爱的人捐献器官,向患者的家庭中愿意成为器官捐赠者的亲属做必要告知和宣教过程[9]。

许多州也创建了程序化的捐赠登记系统。修正的解剖死亡法案允许通过在国家捐赠登记系统中登记,人们申报捐献意图,促进捐赠过程。有效的捐献者登记内容包括捐赠选定被认为是具有法律约束力的;组织捐献同意文书;个人通过专门的注册网站登记;国家机动车辆管理所(DMV)通过司机的驾驶证和身份证认定进行登记;DMV在线注册等。其他措施包括建立少数名族器官和(或)组织移植教育项目,来增加少数民族的捐献比率,形成器官捐献突破协作组织来提高器官的恢复速度,努力增加心脏骤停死亡和脑死亡患者的器官捐献以及向捐献家庭提供类似补助死者葬礼开销等类似的经济补助[10]。所有州均承认驾照证作为捐献的证明。最后,大多数州一致遵循以NCCUSL制定的确定死亡标准。

尽管很多州对以上内容达成共识,但国家法律在某些重要方面与其产生分歧。一些州有遗体捐献基金,旨在提高公众捐献意识和鼓励器官捐献。这些倡议将在"促进器官捐赠"部分进行讨论。有些州则立法致力于消除捐献的阻碍因素,主要通过解决捐献的经济问题担。以上举措可能包括国家员工可以带薪休假,要求私人雇主为器官捐赠者在手术康复期间提供带薪休假,如果捐赠者获得带薪休假而却由于捐献而产生的费用却未偿还,则税收抵免。各个州有关捐献的法律的地位也大相径庭(表143.1)。

联邦法律

美国联邦法律在美国法典第42章——"公共健康和福利"中大致规定了器官移植的法律结构[11]。这些法律通过建立OPTN和SRTR来规定器官如何在个体之间转移,框定了美国器官移植制度,从而帮助联邦工作人员捐献器官。在这一章详细叙述了三个部分和一些小分段,并由其一起组成联邦移植法律的框架。

美国法典5章6327条

描述了联邦雇员捐赠器官的规定。法典规定,任何行政机构的员工作为骨髓捐献或器官捐献者,有权暂离工作岗位而不损失工资。该国家法律对州立法律做了补充,减少因器官捐献而造成的经济损失。

42章273条

确立了器官移植组织的角色和结构。第273条要求,OPO组织应在联邦政府卫生与公众服务部的监管下定义为非盈利组织,确保公平分配和有效获取器官。OPO必须与当地医院保持联系,并一起筛选和选定潜在的捐赠者。第273条也描述了OPO的联邦投资,OPO必须服务的地理区域,必须遵守后才予以报销的政策。42章第273节也概述了与活体捐献有关的移植后长期影响的评估。

美国法典42章274条

把OPTN作为国家主要的实体企业建立,管理器官获取、分配和移植。OPTN必须首先建立入行标准和分配器官的医疗标准,然后建立全国范围内需要器官

表 143.1　促进器官捐献的国家举措

州	收入来源		法律批文				捐赠教育		活体捐赠支持		
	资源捐献	国家提供资金	UAGA 版本	捐赠者指定		ME/C	院校	驾驶员教育	税收优惠	请假	
				登记处	驾照					公众	私人
	合计：36 共 52	合计：11 共 52	年度	合计：52 共 52	合计：51 共 52	合计：48 共 52	合计：13 共 52	合计：16 共 52	合计：16 共 52	合计：31 共 52	合计：9 共 52
AL	√		2006	√	√	√		√			
AK	√		2006	√	√	√				√	
AZ			2006	√	√	√	√			√	√
AR	√	√	2006	√	√	√	√	√	√	√	
CA	√		2006	√	√	√				√	
CO	√		2006	√	√	√				√	√
CT	√	√	2006	√	√	√				√	
DE	√		1968	√	√	√				√	√
DC			1968	√	√	√			√	√	
FL	√		1987	√	√	√					
GA			2006	√	√	√			√	√	
HI	√		2006	√	√	√					
ID			2006	√	√	√			√	√	
IL	√	√	1968	√	√		√			√	√
IN	√	√	2006	√	√	√	√	√		√	
IA	√		2006	√	√	√		√	√	√	
KS			2006	√	√	√					
KY	√		2006	√	√	√					√
LA	√	√	2006	√	√	√	√	√			
ME	√		2006	√	√	√		√		√	
MD	√		1968	√	√	√				√	
MA	√	√	1987	√	√	√	√	√		√	
MI	√		2006	√	√	√		√			
MN			2006	√	√	√		√		√	√
MS	√	√	2006	√	√	√	√	√			
MO	√		2006	√	√					√	
MT	√		2006	√	√	√				√	
NE	√		2006	√	√	√				√	
NV	√		2006	√	√	√				√	√
NH			2006	√	√	√				√	
NJ	√		2006	√	√	√	√			√	
NM	√		2006	√	√	√		√	√	√	
NY	√	√	1987	√	√	√			√	√	√
NC		√	2006	√	√	√					
ND			2006	√	√	√			√	√	
OH	√		2006	√	√	√	√		√	√	
OK	√		2006	√	√	√	√			√	
OR			2006	√	√	√				√	√
PA	√		1987	√	√				√		
RI	√	√	2006	√	√	√		√			

（待续）

表 143.1(续) 促进器官捐献的国家举措

州	收入来源		法律批文				捐赠教育		活体捐赠支持		
	资源捐献	国家提供资金	UAGA 版本	捐赠者指定		ME/C	院校	驾驶员教育	税收优惠	请假	
				登记处	驾照					公众	私人
	合计：36 共 52	合计：11 共 52	年度	合计：52 共 52	合计：51 共 52	合计：48 共 52	合计：13 共 52	合计：16 共 52	合计：16 共 52	合计：31 共 52	合计：9 共 52
SC	√		2006	√	√	√				√	√
SD			2006	√	√	√					
TN	√		2006	√	√		√				
TX	√		2006	√	√					√	√
UT	√		2006	√	√	√			√	√	
VT			2006	√	√	√					
VA	√		2006	√	√	√		√		√	
WA	√		2006	√	√	√		√			
WV			2006	√	√	√				√	√
WI	√		2006	√	√	√		√	√	√	√
WY	√		2006	√	√	√					
PR		√	2006	√							

移植的患者名单以及一个国家系统，帮助将器官和名单上患者进行匹配。OPTN 必须协助 OPO 在全国范围内分配器官。最终，必须拿出如何提高器官获取和分配效率的研究成果。UNOS 自建立以来，一直与 OPTN 的运行有合约关系。

274a 条

建立了作为国家移植数据库的科学注册机关，内容包含了国家的移植统计资料、移植中心报告和移植的研究资源。

274b 条

规定了 OPTN 确立的条件和合同条件。

274c 条和 274d 条

建立了批准和报告的合同标准。

274e 条

禁止器官买卖，规定了器官必须在无报酬的基础上免费捐献。而活体捐献者只会收到手术报销的成本费用，只有那些参与移植并提供必要的服务会收到劳务费。2007 年颁布的《查理·W.诺伍德活体器官捐献法》阐明，规定配对捐献是不具有经济价值的，确保人体器官配对捐赠不会受到刑事处罚。

274f 条

批准了活体捐献者因捐献产生的路途费用、手术费用以及合理的非医疗个人开销的报销补偿。这些特许可用于各州、各移植中心和各个合格的 OPO 组织。274 f–1 包含了有关于公众认知、研究和示范的规则，274f–2 主要讲述补助金问题，274f–3 包括和器官捐献相关的研究和报道以及 274f–4 规定器官复苏、保存和运输的要求。

多层次的监督是必要的，以确保移植系统不仅在紧急情况下分配稀缺资源时成功高效地运行，而且还要确保其奉行公平透明、平等、高效的伦理原则。为此，规章制度在保护个人自主决定捐赠与否的同时，也提倡将器官捐赠作为一种公益行为。该法律保护公民的平等权利和在器官分配时防治不平等分配和歧视。最后，法律保护人类生命的尊严，并禁止器官的商品化和贸易。

患者保护和平价医疗法案(PPACA)的意义

患者护理的意义

患者保护与平价医疗法案(PPACA)(P.L.111–148)

是自 1965 年通过医疗保险和医疗补助以来，医疗卫生行业的最大的单独法案。这是一项重大的法案，包含了许多目标，其中有两个主要目标：扩大医疗保险范围，限制医疗成本的增长和改革输送系统。医疗保险的主要目标之一就是扩大美国人的就医途径，包括 5070 万未受保和 2500 万受保居民[12]。为此目的，该法案期望在 2019 年内保险覆盖 3200 万美国人(其中 1600 万从医疗补助计划中受保，另 1600 万则通过保险交易和购买私人保险受保)。PPACA 对于移植患者的影响主要在于，法案希望可以扩大医疗保险的范围，降低使用移植相关的医疗护理的过高费用。法案通过多种途径来达到上述目的，最值得注意的是，通过投保人范围扩大(包括私人和公共报销)和通过减少医疗保健的经济负担，尤其是那些最需要移植手术却付不起开销的人。投保扩大化是 PPACA 的重要组成部分，通过实施一系列的机制来完成。对于私人保险来说，本法案授权个人购买医疗保险，建立了个人险种和小群体市场中的竞争关系，要求雇主完成有关医疗保险时采用“要么行使要么付钱(play or pay)”方案。更重要的是本法案为弱势群体提供了大量的医疗补助资金，以及为合适的私人医疗保险增加津贴。实现法律的完善是错综复杂的，但里程碑时间会在 2012 年和 2018 年之间发生(图 143.4)。图详细描述了 PPACA 与保险扩展和进一步对保险市场的调控有关的流程。

通过推广保险和管理，增加就医途径和降低开销

个人保险推广

PPACA 要求所有的市民和合法居民购买和定时

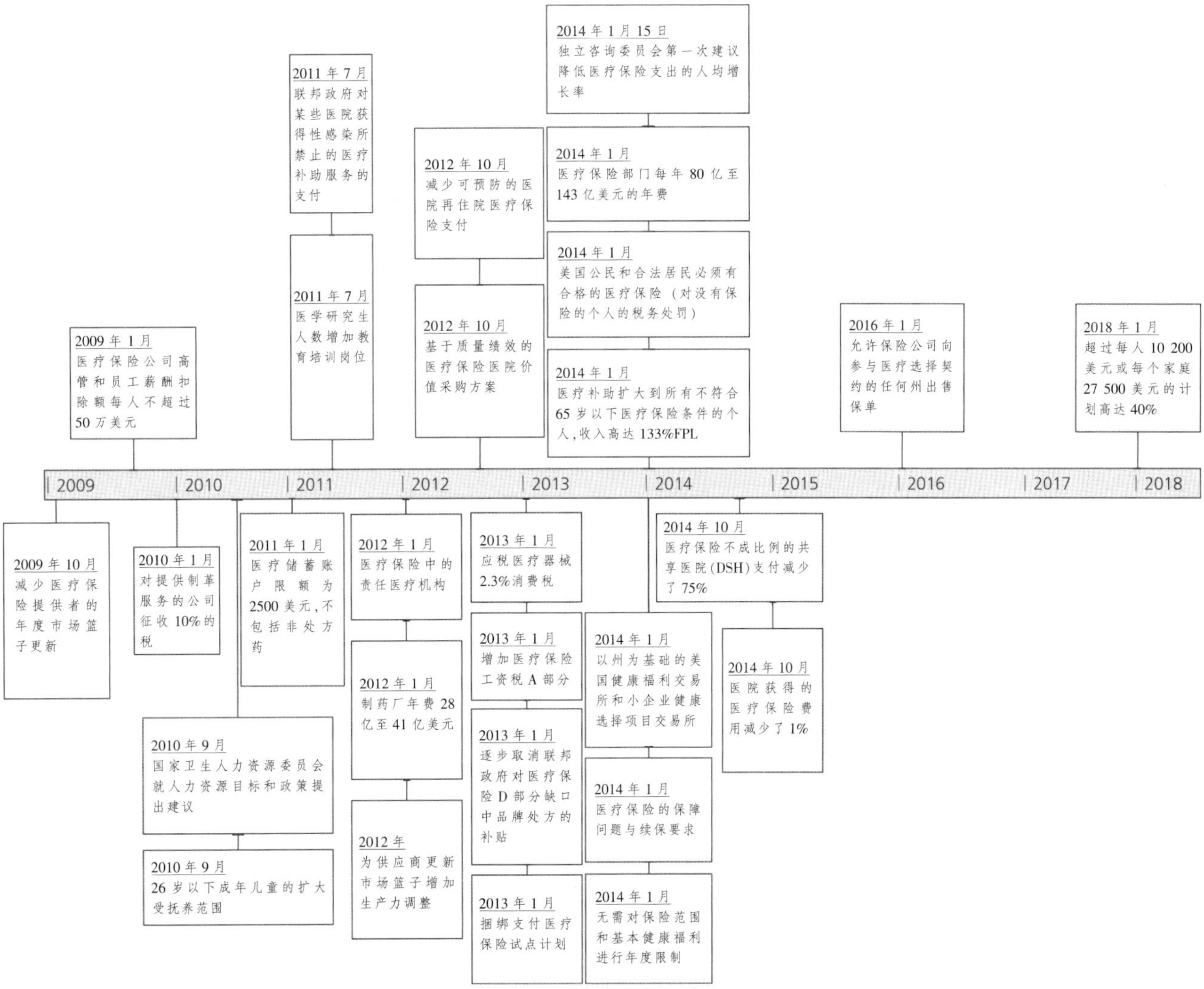

图 143.4　美国医疗改革实施时间表。

缴纳保险,否则将受到罚款,这一法案将在2016年逐步实施。个人强制令,或称"最低投保要求",要求18岁以上的人都应购买医疗保险,如果他们无法负担购买,那应该通过他们的雇主或通过州立医疗保险交易或公共保险计划中获得。从2016年开始,那些没有购买保险的人将被强迫上交695美元或者每年收入的2.5%。上述条件均不能达到的人可以不投保免于惩罚。

上述命令和不歧视措施的理由是为了减少道德风险和保险市场的逆向选择。尽管我们的目标是达到全民医保,但是经济极端困难的人和那些购买保险费用将超过收入8%的人,以及受到宗教反对的人,将不被强制投保。美国土著人由于美国土著医疗服务协会的保护可以被豁免,被监禁的人也会被豁免。尽管PPACA对医疗系统和非移植手术的患者有许多影响,但我们将重点讨论移植的潜在患者和提供者由PPACA带来的影响。

强制个人购买保险一直在政治上和法律上存在争议。反对授权的人认为这是违宪的,理由是联邦要求人民购买医疗保险是政府权力的越界。近期最高法院出现了前所未有的案例:26个州、国家独立业务联合会和很多人主张,授权妨碍了个人自由。奥巴马政府则认为,管理州际贸易的权利是由美国宪法授予国会的,也正是上述正当权力延伸至医疗保险而已。此外,代表政府的律师认为,个人强制保险是实现保险全民推广、防止歧视和由宪法和政府允许的目标的必要一环。2012年6月,最高法院发表本案裁决,维护个人强制令,基本不改动本法。然而,最高法院驳回了联邦政府要求(甚至强烈刺激)各州扩张医疗补助项目的权利。这也严重阻碍了全民低收费医保的可能性。

在雇主方面,符合"要么行使要么支付"模板的,即拥有50名以上员工的雇主将被要求支付的员工保险,以及为联邦贫困线0.25倍以内收入的工人提供证明。这是为了让雇主不承担保险的雇员们,促使他们购买负担得起的健康保险,补救在当前小部分市民买不起保险的问题。为了确保今后需要保险的居民能按需购买,收入水平在联邦贫困线0.75倍至0.25倍水平内的个人可以借贷购买保险。贷款额度应保持在保险购买支出的合理范围内(低于国家贫困线0.75倍以下者借贷2%,低于国家贫困线0.25倍以下者借贷9.5%)。

基础福利套餐:

PPACA要求以下情况必须包含基础健康福利套餐:

1.面向个人或小群体的医保;

2.私有医保交易所任意的医保项目;以及

3.医疗急救保险。

这些基本福利包含10个类型:流动患者服务;紧急服务;住院治疗;孕妇和新生儿保健;精神卫生和物质成瘾疾病服务,包括行为健康治疗、处方药、康复设备和训练;实验室检测服务;预防和健康咨询服务和慢性疾病管理;儿童保健,包括语言和视觉训练[13]。这包括了基本福利中至少60%的精算价值,减少了当前医疗服务政府分摊成本,而且和雇主的预算基本吻合。基本福利在2014年1月1日正式实施,要求美国卫生和公众服务部通过透明和公开的流程每年更新基本福利。

公共保险推广

PPACA为低收入和弱势群体提供保险覆盖的一个关键特性是提供医疗补助,而且有可能对移植和移植前患者形成积极的影响。法案将医疗补助的范围扩大至几乎所有国家贫困线以下的低于65岁的个人或低于联邦贫困线25%的个体。对于许多低收入而且没有孩子的成年人来说,以及为人父母但收入低于贫困线25%以下者,这次保险范围扩大标志着上述人群第一次真正获得医保。联邦政府将在2014—2016年支付所有新获得医疗补助的患者的保险费,在2017年度支付保险费用的95%,在2018年支付94%,2019年支付93%,以及2020年及以后为新纳入的患者支付90%的费用。联邦政府还承诺给予额外的过渡基金,帮助国家对收入处于联邦贫困线以下的所有个人实行医疗补助。尽管联邦政府将为各州支付高额的医疗补助计划收费,但是各个份额可能会有所不同。这可以部分归咎于各州之间政策和支持医疗补助计划态度的异差,也有部分原因是由于在经济不景气的时代背景下出现财政赤字和资本受限。在器官移植方面,各地政策存在着差异,而随着各地医疗补助推广中存在的不平均,很可能会进一步加剧已有的差异,并可能使患者怀疑挑选移植资格和预计护理成本的透明性。特别是高发病率但享受低水平的州医疗补助的疾病,如高血压、糖尿病、慢性肾脏疾病和药物滥用,这些病的患者可能会激化器官移植中的地域差异。

移植相关事宜

长期以来，执行移植手术的较低频率一直与缺乏医疗保险投保有莫大的关联[14-16]。长期持续的终身护理通过促进早期诊断，帮助患者更好地管理他们的慢性病，有助于改善肾病终末期(ESRD)和其他慢性疾病患者的健康状态，而这些慢性疾病会最终导致器官衰竭。此外，有既往史的患者会经常感觉工作困难，最终导致未再就业，因为他们会犹豫是否要重新投入新的工作，而这样他们的保险就无法续保。这对接受了移植手术的患者是尤其真实的，他们担心换工作会失去免疫抑制剂的报销。这些患者经常面临选择困境，要么重新工作但承受损失报销之苦，要么只能申请残疾[17]。对于这些人，就保险而言，可以为患者提升生活质量带来希望，增加就业以及减少失去医疗报销的焦虑。和医疗保健相关的投保途径和更小的投保经济负担有利于解决上述问题，对移植或移植前的患者产生更好的健康状态和生活质量。

医疗补助推广应该增加移植器官的获得途径，为没有保险的患者在手术后保险报销，减少由于缺乏资金匮乏而产生差的药物依从性，进而导致器官损失。除了这些移植受者可能受到的影响，保险推广还可能帮助器官衰竭的晚期患者，通过早期介入提高移植护理质量，最终产生更好的移植护理和选择更公平的器官移植手术。这可能对于非肾的器官衰竭患者尤其重要。不像肾病终末期患者原本就可以接受医疗保险福利的津贴，例如患有慢性肝脏疾病的非肾的器官衰竭患者，可能会从本次保险推广中极大地获利。

获得移植推荐的更多和长期护理可能会导致更多的患者需要移植，这就会导致名单上等候患者人数越来越多，也必然导致期望排上移植候选名单上的患者数量的减少。在这个意义上，只要有足够的医疗保健可以提供，增加医疗机会就能纠正上述情况。但是如果没有相应的器官供应增加，可能会导致更长的等待移植时间和使用更多的器官边缘，最终增加移植成本[18]。值得注意的是，这只是一个可能的结果，目前尚不清楚扩大保险范围是否会导致更多公平的转诊和列入移植候补名单。一些研究表明，尽管提高了保险覆盖率，移植的差异仍然存在[17-19]。现已证明，缺乏私人保险(尚有医疗补助)不利于移植患者受到高质量的手术和护理[19]，就像增加接触途径，同时减轻经济负担，不太可能解决移植患者所面临的所有医疗方面的困难。为了解决这个困难，旨在保证医疗公平的质量和疗效检测仍然为人们所亟需。

保险的监管措施

减少保险的经济负担和医疗报销相关的不确定性是实现全民医保的关键问题所在。PPACA 在限制保险不合理行为方面取得一定的成功，包括限制医疗报销上线、无端地增加成本和否认申报。这些规定保护了消费者，旨在减少重大疾病对人身健康的损害。

私人保险的改革，如删除有关既往史的条款，会造福更多的移植患者，增加移植患者中保险的覆盖率。类似于保险推广，增加医疗服务的报销比率可以帮助患者得到疾病早期的专家会诊，获得更优质的移植评估，减少因失去药物报销而导致药物依从性差的风险并可以获得长期的护理。特别是，删除有关先前存在疾病的报销限制条款和年度报销上限，这会极大地帮助那些免疫抑制药物的医疗补助到期和不能承担免疫抑制治疗费用的患者。

设置投保者报销年度上限和终身上限也是导致保险公司权力滥用的机制之一。而这一约束尤其损害慢性病和重症患者，如那些器官衰竭的患者，每年的医疗费十分巨大。由于医疗保险的诸多限制，医疗开销的巨大负担逐渐被转移到了患者肩上，其中的很多患者为了支付医疗费用被迫变卖资产或被迫申报破产[20,21]。特别是对于移植患者来说，经济负担在接受移植手术之后仍在延续。罗德里格等调查了 333 名接受肝移植 1 年以上和 318 名接受肾移植 1 年以上的患者，询问他们自接受移植手术以来，是否被经济问题缠身，收入是否发生了变化，他们用于支付移植相关的费用来源何处，以及每月医疗支出的具体数额。研究者发现，41%的移植术后患者反馈自身有经济困难，近一半患者声称手术 1 年后的工资收入低于手术前 1 年的收入。2007 年的术后医疗费用的平均支出约为 47 660 美元；该数值还有可能继续增加。罗德里格等发现，患者主要是依靠储蓄资金和信贷来支付这些费用，但是，在当前限制贷款的环境和长期经济衰退的背景下，患者很可能为支付医疗费用而面临前所未有的困难。帮助减少医疗支出的规定，如消除每位投保人的年度开支上限和终身上限，对于每一位移植患者都至关重要。患者除了需要支付昂贵的药物费用外，还经常延期出院或者重复入院治疗，必然导致费用超出年度和终身报销上限，最终引起巨大的经济负担[22]。

PPACA 还允许父母为他们的 26 岁以下的成年子女投保，限制投保期限为 90 天内。该项政策作为保险计划的更新于 2010 年 9 月 23 日正式生效。这将与其他条款一道帮助移植(以及那些未来可能需要移植)患者的父母获得医疗帮助，特别对那些年轻患者中年龄在 18~26 岁子女的父母。这个年龄段的年轻人最不可能拥有健康保险。这些年轻人从 PPACA 的政策中可有极大获益，18~24 岁年龄组是唯一的由于 PPACA 政策而引起参保比例显著增加的群体，从 2009 年的 70.7% 增加至 2010 年的 72.8%[23]。尽管经济不断衰退，但是对于 50 万 18~24 岁的年轻人，2%的投保比例增加很大程度上归功于 PPACA 扩大医保覆盖范围至 24 岁成年人的规定。自从投保人数趋于稳定甚至在某些年龄段投保人数减少，这 2%的增加反映了推广保险的积极影响。

自 2010 年 6 月 21 日生效以来，在美国合法居住 5 年以上的合法移民或超过 6 个月未受保同时有既往史的美国公民将有资格参与正在起草的州立临时 “高危池”项目，随后被国家卫生保险交易所取代。保费的设立主要基于标准人口条件，浮动不超过 1/4。法案限定(在现有法律的基础上)，家庭收入低于联邦贫困线的 0.25 倍者，家庭个人自费的支出上限为 5950 美元和家庭整体的上限为 11 900 美元，但不包括保险费[24]。个人的免赔额被限制在 2000 美元以内和每个家庭的免赔额应小于 4000 美元。这将有助于许多移植患者缓和忧虑，因为 10%或 20%的移植手术自费比例或高免赔额使患者们敬而远之。许多移植受者可能有资格参加上述计划。然而，潜在的低报销率和获取器官的高成本成为了捐赠者的一大难题，形成了挽救衰弱患者的又一屏障[25,26]。

PPACA 也试图降低卫生保健的行政成本，重新定向医疗保险支付医疗保健的费用。法案通过建立一个新的医疗赔付率和保险费的审查机制，解决了部分矛盾。法案还要求健康计划报告用于临床服务等卫生保健用途的保险金的比例，并将保险金中用于管理的费用为购置人退税，这部分费用在大型群体的市场计划中占到总额的 15%，在个人和小团体市场计划中占 20%。报告医药赔付率于 2010 年开始生效，退税规定在 2011 年 1 月起效。更多的监管被实施，以确保保险费增加适当。然而，2003—2010 年间，保险行业出现了重大问题，各州的家庭参保费激增 50%，公司员工年度的保费比例承担增加了 63%。按照 PPACA 实施之前的增长比率，平均的家庭保险费到 2020 年估计增长 72%，可达 24 000 美元[27]。许多 PPACA 颁布的保险法规旨在放缓保费增加速率，在研究审查保险费增加的幅度和对增加的费用进行调整的过程中特别显著。自 2010 年起，所有保险费的增加必须经由国家批准。

这些规定无疑会减少移植患者医疗保健的成本，增加接受移植手术的可能，尤其是对可能没有保险的年轻患者来说，同时也会提高年轻患者的生活质量，使他们感到更加自由，因为他们能够不用担心失去保险，自由地选择跳槽或寻求一份新的工作。然而，医疗质量和供体的选择可能会受到影响。因为手术成本高和手术需要高度专业化的服务，移植手术费用经常被划分为医疗费用和外科手术收费。考虑到手术收费高和提高保险费用可能性有限，移植报销覆盖范围很可能受限。最终，移植覆盖范围在很大程度上取决于医疗保险市场(因保险报销主要由再保险提供资金)以及与移植更直接相关的法规。考虑到报销水平各不相同，提供给给个人、小团体市场和“高风险池”对象的保险方案较为受限，缩小了移植患者的选择范围。

免疫抑制剂保险推广

尽管肾移植已经被证明优于肾透析，可以提高患者生存率和生活质量，是有成本效益的，但是，肾移植患者长期存活需要依赖于免疫抑制剂的不间断治疗。一个单纯的肾移植手术费用可以得到平均 11 万美元的医疗补助，而每年需要的免疫抑制剂则要花费 1.5~2 万美元不等。相比起来，肾透析治疗则需要每年花费 7.5 万美元。1~3 年内所用于补助肾移植免疫抑制剂的医疗津贴正在减少，相应的治疗效果也在减弱[28]。经济学分析证实了为免疫抑制剂提供终生补助反而会每年节省下 2 亿美元的整体开销[17]。与此同时，在持续提供免疫抑制剂报销的国家，患者长期生存率明显提高。还有，由于未能持续使用免疫抑制剂而经历了早期移植失败的患者，又必须恢复透析治疗，从而在付出更大代价的同时需要承受更大的经济负担。早期的移植失败是在美国导致肾透析的第五大原因[29]。移植失败患者的两年死亡率明显低于成功移植患者死亡率，甚至比没有接受移植的患者更低。

对免疫抑制药物的依从性差可以直接导致移植失败,其原因可能是无法支付药物的高额费用。其中的联系很难用前瞻性研究验证，因为移植受体不太可能主动拒绝服用免疫抑制剂[30]。然而,在 2010 年的一项调查中显示,超过 70%的美国肾移植患者项目报道,患者难以支付免疫抑制药物费用的问题“极其严重”或者“非常严重”,而 68%的报道称,由于经济问题缺乏药物依从性是造成个体死亡和器官损失的一大原因[29]。确保患者一生都可以获得这些药物可以拯救肾移植患者的生命,并且减少 ESRD 患者的一生的治疗开销[29]。

在 PPACA 生效之前,美国的医疗保险规章取消了对 65 岁以下或者工作障碍的肾移植患者手术 3 年后的免疫抑制药物报销。许多移植受者健康地回到工作岗位上时,也损失了药物的报销。2011 年的针对肾移植患者的保险全面覆盖免疫抑制药物是一个对于《社会保障法》拟议的修正案,法案将授予美国所有肾移植接受者,拥有对免疫抑制药物花费的终身保险[29]。目前,免疫抑制药物终身报销被认为是可以通过 PPACA 各种手段而大部分实现的。患者如今可以通过“高风险池”(既往疾病保险计划）或者私人保险获得更多免疫抑制剂的报销,而私人保险不能拒绝有既往史的患者,也不能设定报销上限。法案也命令禁止上述歧视行为。其实上述行为十分打击移植患者，因为该行为严重妨碍了患者获得治疗的权利，包括移植术后 3 年内免疫抑制药的报销。

PPACA 还包括医疗保险改革,这将通过关闭“甜甜圈洞”(保险覆盖缺口),以求更大范围的药物报销推广。从 2010 年生效开始,任何陷入“甜甜圈洞”的 D 部分注册者都会收到 250 美元的退款。相应地,在 2011 年上述注册者购买正规药物时将得到由制药行业提供的 50%的折扣。药物医疗保险覆盖率分阶段从 2011 年开始,持续到 2013 年,包括保险覆盖缺口涉及的所有通用和品牌药物，而在 2020 年前,D 部分的注册者购买上述药物均可享受 75 折优惠。在 2019 年之前,PPACA 将降低重大疾病报销门槛。尽管拥有这些有利政策,由于免疫抑制药物的成本较高,患者仍然需要付出巨大的费用。因此,免疫抑制药物的全额报销仍然是 PPACA 需要解决的问题。

活体捐献者的保险覆盖

PPACA 或许也对活体捐赠者的捐献后健康状况以及希望捐赠的捐赠者产生积极影响。捐献者中高比例人群未受保，保险的临时性以及既往史的限制都可能阻碍活体捐赠，捐献者术后得不到后续治疗也可能阻碍捐献。由于放松了某些捐赠标准(如轻度高血压和高 BMI 指数),捐献人数增长,但捐赠后缺乏长期随访的保险覆盖问题显得尤为重要。由于捐赠后的长期后果尚未明确，所以保险全面覆盖的长期随访对捐献者的身心健康都很重要。保险推广可以帮助捐助者接受移植后至少两年的长期随访，这将由医疗保险或者私人保险覆盖。最近由 Kher 等主导的一项研究,在某一中心随访调查了捐献者们的手术费用补偿比率，表明私人保险和联邦医疗保险对捐献者随访的补偿比率和移植器官接受者的补偿比率相近[31]。这就提示了捐赠者随访的报销覆盖问题并不对其医疗补助构成障碍。

重要的是，考虑到人们在任何时候都可能成为捐赠者,促进保险推广、拓展预防性卫生服务和鼓励健康行为都可能会增加捐献者数量。这尤其适用于以前没有保险的人群,其中许多人既年轻又健康,但他们由于没有保险,可能从未考虑过捐献器官。法案通过由联邦医疗保险和所有新保险计划负责的推荐预防保健部分收费减免,来推动预防保健;提供年度免费健康访问,分配更多的联邦医疗补助资金到各州，提供以证据为基础的预防卫生服务和要求推广孕妇戒烟服务的医疗补助计划,并通过支持拨款促进社区预防服务[32]。

移植界,包括专业集群,支持活体捐献并呼吁为捐献者提供支持。美国移植协会(AST)已经公开呼吁政府制订政策，为捐献者提供健康保险以解决活体捐赠后的近期和远期影响 [33]。尽管捐献者的移植手术之前和之后短时间内相关的费用由器官受体的医疗保险报销,但是患者由于自身没有保险的担保,就会承担巨大的风险。首先,器官捐献对健康的长期影响并不明确,相应的,器官供体很可能遭遇某种术后并发症,而受体保险担保的期限早已失效。第二,如果器官受体死亡或放弃继续投保,捐赠者也会失去保险担保,这也将直接导致供体需要为大笔的医疗开销自掏腰包。在 PPACA 废除有关既往史的保险条款之前，捐献者很可能得不到任何医疗保险的担保。由于承担着可能得不到医疗报销的巨大风险以及手术后巨大的医疗花费，人们并不乐意成为活体捐献者。对于捐献者的保险覆盖则会帮助人们分担上述担忧,鼓励更多的人接触器官捐献。

对移植供体的影响

报销

通过PPACA的医疗保险推广无疑会增加选择移植手术患者的数量。此外,如果人们在受保后更愿意捐献器官,那么PPACA法案很可能通过这种方式来增加移植例数。随着医疗补助和公共卫生交流保险范围扩大,对移植中心和移植专家的补偿费用则会减少。这种收费分配比例的变化可能导致移植中心入不敷出,特别是那些在大城市的中心,很长时间才做一次手术的中心和那些使用扩大移植标准的器官的移植中心[34]。

PPACA还建立了一个独立支付咨询委员会(IPAB),专门建议总统和CMS使用成本效益分析方法。虽然这符合PPACA提高医疗效率与减少医疗浪费的目标,但是许多专家和外科组织表达了他们对IPAB可能造成的影响的担忧。专家普遍认为,IPAB很可能增加基础护理的报销而忽略了专科护理的资金补助[35]。这意味着移植患者可能享受到更好的慢性疾病管理和早期疾病筛查和诊断。然而,这同时也会减少接触到专业移植服务的可能。虽然收费分配比例下调的医院很难依靠投保的移植患者执行手术数量的增加来弥补由此带来的经济空缺,但是医疗保险为大型学术医疗中心治疗穷困患者提供的经济补助。在医疗改革的背景下,医院可能会失去75%的超份额支付(DSH)。最后,移植患者的复杂性、感染和再入院可能比其他患者群体更常见。这会被联邦医疗保险视为“低质量的医疗保健”,进而导致更低的报销比例。有一个方法帮助质量和报销比率同时提升,就是通过更好的风险校正和促进整合医疗(也许通过可信赖医疗机构)。

保险费限额可能会降低报销比例并限制患者的选择。这些约束可能会增加保险市场的权力,也可能由此而限制患者求诊于某些移植中心,还可能减少移植供体的费用报销比例。因此,节制保险收费仍可能增加患者负担[18]。

提高质量

PPACA同样致力于可持续增长率的稳定,建立医疗之家,报销比率的改变和试图改善器官派送系统和加强疗效的疗效比较研究。法案也试图通过融合绩效工资激励机制来提高医疗质量。许多研究已经证明,这种激励机制对医生和医院十分奏效,并且这个模型在多个临床领域已经成功地应用[36-38]。PPACA在2012年颁布有关整合绩效激励机制的两个规定:第一,为负责任的医疗机构形成提供奖励;第二,关于高质量医疗的酬劳,向医院提供经济鼓励来提高医疗质量。

可信赖医疗组织

可信赖医疗组织(ACO)通过强调疾病预防、疾病管理、减少冗余并最终减少不必要的住院,从而促进护理协调和质量改进。如果这些可信赖医疗组织以较低的成本提供优质的医疗卫生保健,就可以节约成本,而在这种情况下ACO也可以受到节约成本产生的一小部分收益。

ACO提倡以既定的方式连接医疗组织和医疗收费(动态、医院、护理和辅助保健设施)的疾病管理方法。期待更多的交流和患者的主导权,从而提高医疗质量和降低成本。移植医疗在许多方面是这种方法的先驱,因为许多围绕移植的医疗服务被整合,涉及许多不同的专业、中心和常规的随访护理。移植中心本质作为医疗大家庭运行,整合了许多内外科专业,甚至合并急诊就诊。捆绑支付经常与可信赖医疗组织探讨相伴,而且在移植中心也并不少见。捆绑支付已经在移植中心存在了一段时间。旨在发展医疗家庭护理模式和扩大联邦资格健康中心的规定,也将为移植受者提供长期护理的帮助[34]。

美国移植外科医生协会(ASTS)虽然支持ACA中提出的发展,但也建议CMS采取特别的医疗护理来确保拥有医疗保险和处于ACO中具有高医疗保健需求的患者,如移植需求,可以受到有关医疗决定的适当信息并不会被迫放弃移植手术[39]。ACO可能必须要克服提供此类信息的约束,特别是当移植中心在其工作中不包括此项内容的情况下。

手术费用

第二个主要质量相关的条款包含绩效薪酬机制(P4P),代表将质量结果与酬劳挂钩,为医院提供经济鼓励以刺激医疗质量的提高。该条款要求公布对各医院医疗质量的检测,主要包括对心肌梗死、心脏衰竭、肺炎、手术护理和院内感染的质量检测。公众报告制度将生效至2012年10月1日。

P4P包含两个主要方面:第一,为医疗质量水平达标的医务人员提供额外的酬劳，同时也可以为确实有效的治疗水平提高提供奖励。第二,要求公开医疗质检报告,增加医疗市场的透明度,从而有利于消费需求的选择。该条款的酬劳标准是基于医院和移植团队水平的，并没有将医生的个人回报与个人劳动付出直接挂钩。实际上,医生的额外津贴回报是取决于团队或医院的医疗质量。这样的绩效薪酬机制导致了一个“搭便车效应”,某些医生可以拒绝提高医疗服务水平但仍然收到津贴,因此显而易见,这样的薪酬机制是有风险的。

尽管绩效薪酬机制拥有重大意义，但是奖励的绝对标准也可能产生负面影响。例如当医生接诊患有诸多并发症的患者时,可能不会被绩效薪酬机制所激励。如果没有适当的风险调整，那很可能会加剧酬劳分配的不平等，进而导致更少的医生愿意接诊复杂病症的患者。在这样一个基于绝对绩效的系统中,低绩效,甚至实际上可以提高疗效的举措,不会收到任何奖励。但如果选择基于医疗水平提高的奖励机制，高水平的医务工作者保持高绩效却不会得到酬劳，自然也不会被该机制所激励。对于相对和绝对的绩效奖励机制,风险调整是至关重要的。对于移植医生来说,考虑到标准器官来源的患者范围和地理的差异，风险调整具有重要意义。此外,鉴于移植政策公平的重要性,特别要注意激励机制以及潜在的负面影响。

PPACA 也重视基于流程中的医疗质量检测。医疗质量检测旨在提高医疗服务的过程,而不单单是结果。过程与结果并重的方法在一定程度上减轻了只看重结果的质量检测措施。绩效薪酬机制的启动时机(年底或者一整年)以及激励的相对大小(至少 5%的定额工资)也将是重要的[40,41]。绩效薪酬机制必须仔细地构建和实施。目前不清楚这些包含在 PPACA 的激励措施能否达到他们想要的结果。

通过捐献奖励满足对器官的不断需求

促进器官捐献政策的第三部分包括，通过奖励和提高公众意识促进器官捐献。目前等待肾移植的名单上已经超过 85 000 人,但每年成功捐赠的器官只有大约 17 000 个,每年大约 4500 人在等待肾移植的过程中死去,同时又会有 33 000 人加入器官移植等候列表[10]。越来越多的患者在候补名单上等待合适器官移植,与器官捐献的供应越来越不相称。而使用死于心脏病的患者的器官数量在过去的 10 年中有所增加,这样的器官来源现在超过总数的 10%。UNOS 政策旨在促进移植扩大标准下的捐献肾脏(为愿意接受老年或者非健康供体肾的患者进入第二类移植等待名单）取得成功[1]。目前,大约 60%的肾移植来源于遗体捐赠;另外 40%的肾移植来源于活体捐献者，这个比例在最近几年有所增加[42]。

美国试图通过立法来增加器官来源，目标是增加可能的遗体捐献者的器官供应，增加潜在的活体捐献器官的数量,提高供体的转归。移植界和美国政府压倒性地支持器官捐献(特别是活体捐献)应该依靠志愿精神和利他主义。这一观点深深扎根于《统一遗体捐赠法》(UAGA)和 1984 实行的《国家器官移植法案》(NOTA)中的第 301 章节。《国家器官移植法案》规定,“任何人出于价值考虑进行非匿名的收购、接收或者转运任何人体器官都是违法的”[43]。在该条例中,“出于价值考虑”被理解为金钱或有形资产在受体、捐赠者(和代理)之间进行转移[43]。该法律尤其指出,禁止胁迫他人进行任何形式的捐赠,并明确禁止器官的买卖。鼓励器官捐赠的政策可以根据捐助者进行分类：活体捐献或者遗体捐献和特定机制如金钱酬谢、物质补偿和非物质补偿。金钱酬谢的构成和数量多少大相径庭,所以有些人剔除要对其进行市场监管并用非物质补偿代替。但是更有人提出建立开放和不受监管的器官市场,而价格的调控则完全由市场的供求关系所操控。

对器官捐献者提供经济补偿是否会缓解器官短缺并且增加器官供应,学者的观点并不统一。一些人认为酬劳的存在反而会减少潜在的捐赠者的数量，因为人们不再会视捐赠为品行的高尚，而把捐献仅看作是物质的交换。Gabriel Danovitch 在一封写给宾夕法尼亚州参议员 Arlen 的“公开信”中,表达了自己对参议员提出的《器官捐献说明和反器官交易法》的担忧,细致描述了诸多有关于提供酬劳、器官商品化和操作问题的顾虑。值得注意的是,Danovitch 引用以色列、巴基斯坦和伊朗的例子,证明在金钱酬劳合法的国家,自愿捐赠者远远少于有偿捐献[44]。针对有偿捐献的抗议战线已经成立。几位参议员和专业团体，例如国家肾脏基金会,以及一些宗教组织,要求停止为器官捐献设立酬劳的实验项目，而这个提案是由参议员 William First 和 Chris Dodd 提出的《器官捐献和恢复改善法案》(573 章节)中提出的[45]。经济激励政策的反对者警告说,金钱酬劳会改变公众对器官捐献的认知，把无偿行为看作是市场交易。这可能会导致(在一些国家已经导致)家族和无偿捐献率的降低。

对比之下，对捐献进行经济补偿的支持者们主张道德和经济利益的矛盾不是不可调和的，一定程度的酬劳可以既符合伦理又促进捐献行为。一个支持经济补偿的常见伦理学论点会主张参与移植过程的利益相关者都应为各自的参与得到补偿,但不包括捐赠者。其他伦理考虑包括功利主义观点,建议(通过经济补偿)可以增加器官供应，从而等待移植名单上的每个人等待时间都会缩短,许多生命都将获益于此。一些伦理学家的眼光则十分长远，认为限制销售自身器官是限制了特定的低社会经济地位的个体的自主权，因为他们需要通过这样的交易来获得自身的利益[46]。Matas 呼吁建立对活体捐献者补偿的监管系统。他认为该系统应由 OPO 管理的六个关键要素构成:

1. 禁止供体和受体联系。

2. 供体的补偿应当包含每年保险金额为 100 万美金的保险和有担保的终身医疗保健。

3. 为捐献而产生的旅费报销。

4. 固定数额的离职补助。

5. 固定数额的报酬或减税。

6. 移植后每年支付 500 美金用于彻底的健康随访[47]。

他认为,这样一个系统不会瓦解无偿捐献行为,反而将因为补偿和激励并不是被强迫，公平且道德地吸收更多的捐献者。

近期许多专业的移植团队开始在道德层面和实践中采纳中立的观点。在 2002 年,ASTS 发起了一个由伦理学家、OPO 领导人、移植内外科医生组成的专家团队,斟酌移植酬劳的问题。该专家团队支持推进一项试行项目，对捐献者葬礼进行补贴或以捐献者的名义慈善捐款从而向捐献者和捐献家庭表达感谢，并检测这种方式的激励效果如何[48]。Roth 发现美国外科医师协会中相当部分的医师坚定支持采取一定程度的补偿，说“在最近的一次 ASTS 会议对于该话题进行了讨论，随后的投票显示多数参会的外科医师表示愿意参与试行项目”(Arthur Matas，2007 年 1 月 27 日报道)[49]。其他的专业协会,包括 AAKP、PKD、AST 等,也都表示了支持对活体捐献者采取一定形式的补助酬劳，但每个协会对捐献补助的热忱又大相径庭[50-52]。重要的是，具有政治权力的美国医学会(AMA)加入了支持阵营，敦促国会修改 1984 通过的 NOTA,允许试行对遗体捐献的家庭进行多种形式的补助政策。UNOS 与 OPTN 最近也呼吁研究经济鼓励对于器官捐献提供的作用[53]。

随着器官短缺日趋显著和利益相关者的数量并提议的激励手段数量激增(图 143.5),有关该话题的政治和政策的辩论变得越来越复杂。围绕捐献酬劳的政策辩论经常将活体捐献和遗体捐献两个概念混为一谈，但实际上两者并不相关。五个使用激励机制来增加器官捐献的主要方法列举如下:酬劳支付,税收特权,葬礼报销，以及代表器官捐献者慈善捐款和办法纪念捐赠者奖牌。

联邦立法

1999 年,《器官捐献者休假法案》(PL 106 - 56)通过了授予成为器官捐赠者的联邦员工带薪休假的权力。法律授予联邦雇员作为骨髓捐献者最多 7 天的带薪休假时间,作为器官捐赠者有 30 天休假时间[54]。参议员 William First 和 Christopher Dodd 提议对器官捐献进行经济补偿,并最终获得联邦立法的通过,引起了激烈的探讨。同样在 2001 年,又有两个法案被引入联邦立法，一个提出为遗体捐献者提供 1 万美元的税收抵扣，另一个提出为活体捐献或者遗体捐赠的家庭提供 2500 美元的退税[55,56]。器官捐献和恢复改善法案(PL108-216)在 2004 年签署成为法律,为活体捐献者提供出差和生活费用的报销,进行长期随访,并给各州和公共企业提供拨款从而促进器官捐献[57]。重要的是，这项法案并没有推翻 1984 年 NOTA 禁止器官买卖的规定。努力推广经济鼓励但并不提供额外的捐献激励措施，最终造就了两项法律在 2007 年和 2008 年相继通过。2007 年《查理·W.诺伍德器官捐赠法案》(PL 110-144)[58]为配对捐赠铺平了道路。法案同时要求每年汇报活体捐献对捐献人的长期健康影响的研究进展;《Stephanie Tubbs Jones 生命的礼物医疗法案》[59]赋予了 DHHS 为器官捐献者授予国家勋章的权力。

州立法

对活体捐献者的经济激励

美国各州已经颁布了一系列的经济激励措施。尽管 1984 年颁布的 NOTA 中禁止对捐献者进行经济补偿，但是许多州会给予捐献者一些利益补偿以减少他们的开销和减轻身体或精神上的捐献负担。从 2000 年开始，马里兰州和威斯康星州相继出台了一项法律，政策赋予州政府允许雇员在器官捐献 30 天内带薪休假的权利。在其他各州，该法律包含的对象范围经常扩展到当地政府雇员以及公立学校的教师。一些州还扩大了这项计划，要求私人雇主为其器官捐献的雇员提供休假的权利。许多州又通过附加的法律，授予捐献者最高 1 万美元的税收减免补偿捐献手术开销，进一步激励活体捐献。实际的税收减免额度要取决于捐赠者的边际税率，以及各州之间的不同规定，也要将个体的收入和申报纳税身份作为依据。税收减免实际的货币价值取决于个人的州边际税率，这取决于各州的规定和个体的收入以及申报纳税身份。如 Wellington 和 Sayre 强调“在威斯康辛州，调整后的总收益为 25 000 美元的个体纳税申报，将面临着相对较高的边际税率，因为一个人收入增加时，其所得税信贷的价值就会减少。然而，明尼苏达州的税收系统导致了更富有的人将面临更高的边际税率[60]。”这些例子证明了这些利益的价值本质上有所不同，在所有的情况下这种只能算是蝇头小利(低于 1500 美元)。移植界也呼吁为活体捐献者提供终身保险。ASTS、AST 和伊斯坦布尔宣言也提议通过立法来为活体捐献者提供联邦政府资助而终身受保[48,61]。虽然仍没有得到确实承诺，PPACA 扩大医保覆盖范围的规定足以鼓励捐献，可能实现与为器官捐献者量身定制的规定达到大致相同的结果。

对遗体捐献者的经济激励

想要通过有关为遗体捐献者提供经济补偿的法案尚未取得进展。根据 2005 年的一项盖洛普民意调查显示，95.4%的美国民众称他们“支持”或“强烈支持”器官捐献[62]。尽管得到了如此广泛的支持，以器官捐献者的身份登记注册仍低于美国总人口的半数[5]。促进遗体捐献的奖励措施包括支付捐赠家庭的葬礼费用或以捐献者名义慈善捐款亦或税收抵扣[63]。在 1999 年，宾夕法尼亚州卫生部提出，为器官捐助者的家庭提供 300 美元用于支付葬礼费用[60]。然而，尽管经过多次修订和谈判，由于担忧会违反 NOTA 的相关规定，该法律从未正式颁布。

有人提出“未来市场”的想法，即个人承诺死后捐献他们的器官，作为交换可以获得一定的报酬[64]。霍华德及其团队指出，虽然“未来市场”的概念是一个有趣的思维实验，但它很可能需要从政府一般收入或者医疗保险和医院收入的税收中支出[64]。乔治亚州发生了一个以“未来市场”作为激励条件的例子。乔治亚州为登记成为遗体器官捐赠者的个人提供 7 美元的驾照登记费折扣直到 2005 年。小小的激励看起来相当有效，乔治亚州于 2005 年成为了器官捐献者登记率最高的州之一[64]。尽管这很有效，但“未来市场”破坏了登记捐赠的有效性，因为注册人的目的不得而知，是希望捐献还是仅仅想要获得一个折扣。所以，乔治亚州的 OPO 组织并不愿意使用乔治亚州的捐赠者注册数据。Bryne 和 Tompson 认为，这样的系统可能破坏家庭对于器官捐献的认可比率[65]。许多移植界的专家表明，尽管经济激励可能会提高捐献率，但与这些措施相关的伦理问题和潜在的负面影响如公众的看法、公众信任等，导致了“未来市场”目前并不受欢迎[66]。

强制性选择

目前，器官获取时需要征得家人同意的惯例做法是有问题的。因为家庭不一定了解捐赠者的选择。即使了解，他们也可能会反对捐赠的选择，并拒绝 OPO 和临床团队努力实现捐赠者的意愿[67]。尽管在民意调查中公众强烈支持器官捐献[68]，但这也暗示了决策过程伴随的压力可能会导致捐献者家庭的拒绝。强制性选择可以要求所有符合标准的成年人根据自我意愿来决定，他们死后是否愿意捐赠他们的器官。人们可以通过一些论坛记录自己的决定，包括驾照登记、选民登记或所得税表格。那么驾驶人的驾照或者捐献登记在其死后就代表着同意捐献。例如，在弗吉尼亚州，强制性选择有三个选项：捐赠、拒绝捐赠和犹豫不决。在最初半年里，24%的人是犹豫不决，而 31%的人同意捐赠[69]。对强制性选择的主要反对理由是，强迫人们做出选择是破坏个人自主权的行为。然而强制性选择的支持者则认为个人自主权实际上被提升了，因为它推动了一个积极的自主决定而不是一个隐含的假设。强制性选择允许具有资格的成人由自己做出是否捐赠的决定，而不是被他们的家庭所强加[70]。对于那些因面临捐赠决策而经常遭受严重的压力和家庭内部意见不统一的个人，强制性选择实际上也是对家庭有利的[71]。

假定同意

假定同意制度期望通过改变默认捐献来提高器官捐款率。现实中因为人们没有收到物质激励而保留默认选项,导致了他们没有采取捐献行为。而改变默认值恰恰是克服现有偏见的十分有效的方法。假定同意是一个退出系统:在个体死后,器官被取出、存储并用于移植,除非他/她明确拒绝捐献。一些欧洲国家如西班牙和奥地利已经引入了假定同意。西班牙的《假定同意法》被认为是偏软弱的,因为卫生服务提供者需要确认捐献者的近亲不反对器官捐赠;而在奥地利,除非死者在死前明确反对器官捐献,那么一般都可以获取器官。他们的法律要求在没有获得知情同意时,需要保留器官;而西班牙的标准则是使用常温体外循环膜氧合术(NECMO)或者心肺分流术来保持器官灌注直到获得捐献者的家属知情同意。即使是这样,西班牙仍然拥有相对较高的器官捐献率[72]。Abadie和Gay估计,在器官捐献假定同意的国家,其捐献率高出平均水平25%~30%[73]。巴西在1998年确立了假定同意制度后,但由于系统性的失败,仅仅在1年之后回到了知情同意制度。在巴西,公众缺乏对器官捐献体系的信任,而这种不信任主要源自民众的误区,他们误以为器官会在患者临床死亡之前被取出。巴西也未能建立赋予人们生前拒绝捐赠权利的系统。一些研究证据表明,假定同意制度确实可以提高器官捐赠率,但其他因素如潜在捐赠者的有效性、移植基础设施、医疗卫生投资和公众的态度都可以发挥作用[74,75]。

美国医学研究院建议,在实施以增加器官捐献率为目标的立法举措之前,社会风气应当首先得到改变[76]。美国医学研究院的器官捐献委员会建议,长期目标应当是创建一个乐于器官捐赠的社会环境,使假定同意或者强制性选择政策是完全为公众所接受的。医学界内认识几乎都赞同这个观点。一项针对心脏和肺移植国际组织(ISHLT)和心脏诊疗进展基金会(FACT)成员的调查,发现绝大多数成员喜欢间接的而不是直接的补偿方式来增加器官捐献。受访的大多数对象认同,假定同意是改善器官捐赠情况最好的方法。多数人也同意应当由个人决定捐赠与否,而不是家人[63]。

促进器官捐献的干预措施

器官捐赠包括这几个部分:第一,人们必须志愿成为器官捐赠者;第二,家庭必须同意捐献者的决定。这个动态的决策过程是十分复杂的,并且容易受到许多因素和众多利益相关者的影响,包括潜在的捐赠者,捐赠者的家庭,OPO,照顾潜在捐赠者的临床工作人员和潜在的公众人物,如宗教和团体的领导人。本节将回顾一些政策和旨在克服器官捐献障碍的临床工作(见图143.5)。

遗体捐献者:公众器官捐献意识的提升

如果公众意识仍然比较幼稚,器官登记对于提高器官捐献率可能不是十分奏效。公共教育旨在通过提高公众对移植和器官捐献需求的意识,从而增加器官捐赠[77],教育方法包括通过媒体宣传的公共信息活动,分发捐赠卡片并为学校提供教学材料[78]。增加登记成为器官捐赠者的机会,比如在驾校教育和审核期间,在预先护理计划期间,以工作、信仰、学校和社区为基础的宣传措施都有可能助于增加捐赠者的数量[76]。

改变社会风气需要缓解人们对器官捐献和移植的担忧和误解[79]。Horton发现,缺乏宗教支持,混淆脑死亡的概念,负责捐献者福利事业的医疗团队所提供的支离破碎的医疗条件,以及误以为要登记成为捐献者必须在美国卫生人类服务部门存档,都和目前器官捐献的现状息息相关。Horton还发现,对器官捐献的认知和是否收到器官捐献的卡片、对待移植的态度和是否愿意捐献自己或者自己亲人的器官都有关系[80]。

器官捐献意愿也因社会和种族而异。Bouleware等发现,黑人女性最不愿意献血(相对于其他种族和性别),黑人则最不乐意在死亡之后捐献器官。Bouleware分析道,对医院的怀疑和在医院受到的歧视是黑人女性拒绝献血的主要原因,而黑人拒绝在死后捐献器官的主要原因是宗教和精神信仰问题[81],非裔美国人较低的器官捐赠率主要归因于:不了解器官移植、宗教信仰、制度化的种族主义和对于医学界的怀疑和担心受到歧视等等原因[82,83]。Siminoff发现,与白人相比,非裔美国人在医疗保健系统中获得较少的信任[83],以及误认为一旦出现意外医生很有可能不尽力拯救黑人捐赠者的生命。非裔美国人也更愿意接受对捐赠者进行补偿,例如经济补偿和丧葬费的报销等。这些研究表明,对于捐献过程的信任危机和缺乏恰当的认识、教育是少数人种团体排斥捐献的重要原因。

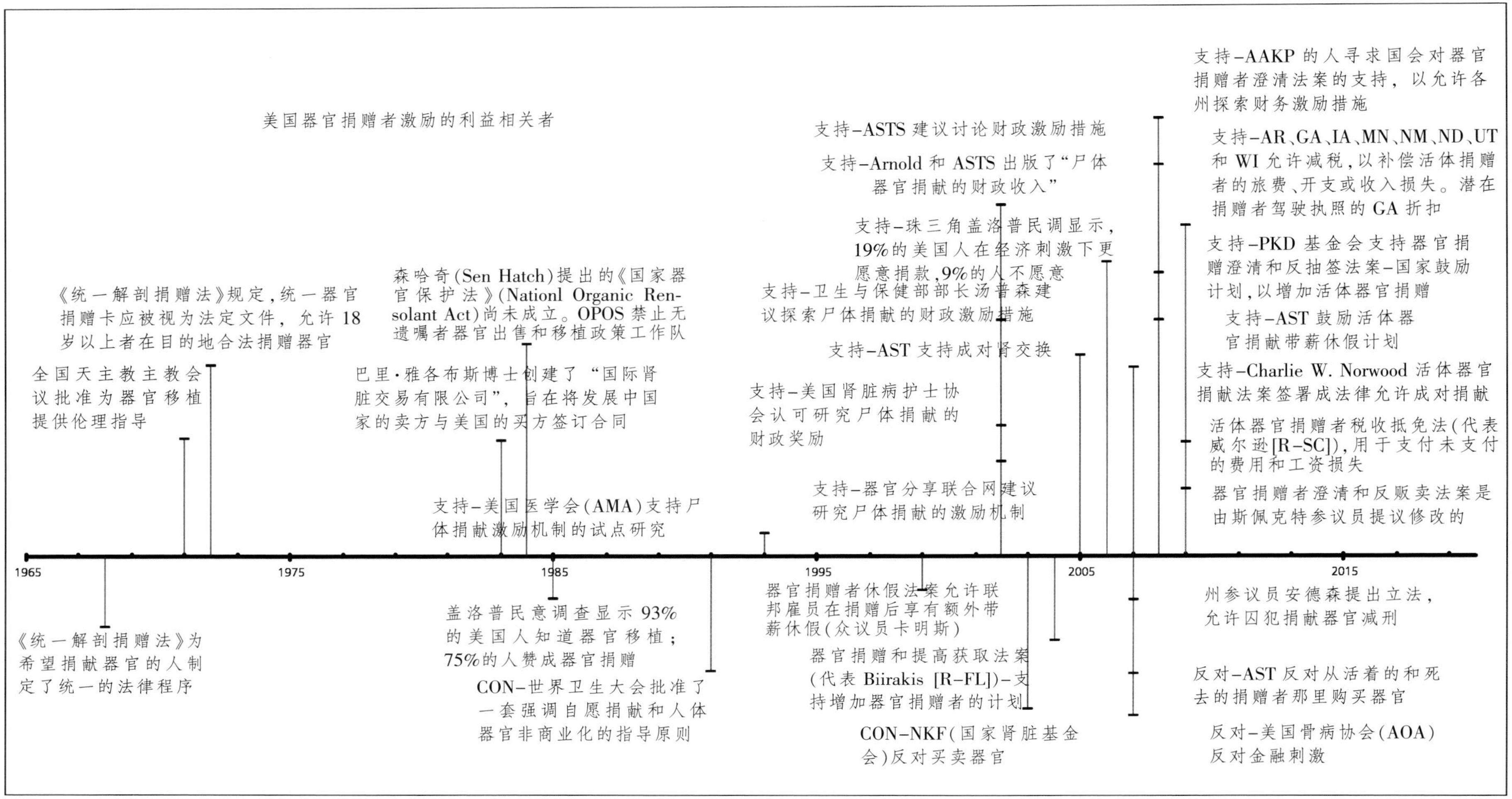

图 143.5 立法和政策倡议的时间线与在美国为器官捐赠提供奖励有关。

干预

尽管很多探讨妨碍器官移植的原因的研究，但是很少有成功的干预措施。考虑到致力于循证医学政策的许多工作,美国卫生资源和服务管理局(HRSA)和美国卫生研究所(NIH)批复了巨大资金来刺激有关促进器官捐献干预措施的研究。未来的政策可能需要吸纳法律和信息技术法的监管机制（尤其是互联网法律),与各政府部门、跨学科团队一起致力于增加器官捐献相关工作。

有数项研究已经表明，新媒体对促进器官捐赠具有重大潜力[84]。Merion 等研究了一个基于互联网多媒体(http://www.journey.transweb.org)的干预措施,探究其对于器官捐赠登记和家人知情同意的影响。该作者发现,10 884 名参与者在完成器官移植的教育模块后,他们对于器官移植的认知有了显著的提高，而且愿意捐献或者登记成为遗体捐赠者的数量亦有所增加。尽管认知的提高并不直接导致捐献意愿的变化，但是捐献态度的积极转变与捐献意愿强烈相关[85]。Thornton 等研究了在俄亥俄州的汽车登记处播放的 iPod 视频对于遗体捐献登记的影响。他们发现,观看该视频与增加登记捐赠率是有关联的。重要的是,他们还发现,视频对少数民族有效,其中对黑人特别有效。这样的视频教育在提供器官捐献信息和减少偏见，尤其对少数民族,是十分成功的。最近有一项史无前例的行动,社交网络媒体脸书(Facebook)允许 1 亿 6 千 1 百万美国用户(及全球 9 亿用户)设立“器官捐献”选项,用于表达用户们的捐献意愿。该行动是极其重要的,原因有二:第一,这会增加民众对器官捐献的认知;第二,在脸书上表达捐献意愿也可以作为次要的捐献登记文书内容。虽然这并不具有法律约束力,但将帮助家庭成员确定患者的意愿。紧随其后,器官捐献注册量激增。脸书推行上述行动后,加利福尼亚州的捐献者数量足足增加了 7 倍[87],而其他州也出现了新注册者的巨大增长,包括:科罗拉多州、康涅狄格州、缅因州、麻萨诸塞州、密歇根州、内布拉斯加州、内华达州、新罕布什尔州、罗德岛州和怀俄明州。

基于学校的健康教育也是提高器官捐献率的一种有效方法,也可能影响各人种的青年们,制订干预措施也同样有效。Piccolil 等为 8 所学校中 17~18 岁的学生和患者和专家举办了两个小时的谈话会，证明有助于改善学生们对待器官捐献的态度[88]。通过随机对照研究 Cardenas 等发现,在一个接纳多民族学生的高中,受到教育干预的学生展现出更乐意捐献器官的意愿[89]。积极的捐献意愿态度和意愿的转变与种族和性别不直接相关,尽管这些因素在基线状态上都是负相关因素。这些研究表明，课堂的干预教育可能对于促进器官捐献是十分重要的,尤其是对于年轻人来说。

器官捐献观念的转变

在捐献与否的决策过程中，亲人意愿的理解和家庭成员的意见一致对成功捐献具有重大意义[90]。民意调查表明，成就家庭成员一致同意捐献的关键因素是捐献者生前是否向其家人表达过捐献的意愿。Siminoff 等发现,通过与患者的交流和探讨器官移植问题,可以显著提高公众的捐献意愿。有 OPO 组织、有较多接触和那些经历过最优的器官获取方式的家庭也更有可能选择器官捐献[91]。Rodrigue 等测试了捐献者和亲人的观点、请求者的特点、与移植团队的沟通过程和满意的程度对捐献决策的影响[92]。他们同样发现,对捐献者意愿的提前认知或者说对器官捐献的支持信念很重要,而对 OPO 和医疗团队的满意度以及器官获取的时机也有捐献决策有着密不可分的联系。这些研究表明,有必要持续致力于公共教育，旨在提高对器官捐赠的信念支持,和家人讨论和记录捐赠决策,改善医院的获取器官过程。

只有当一个患者签署了器官捐献的协议,OPO 才开始着手征求患者家属的意见。尽管《统一解剖捐赠法案》(1987 年修订)声明,签署完成的器官捐赠协议具有法律效益,足以推动器官捐献,但实际上首先要求取得近亲的同意，而这个做法很大程度上是为了规避法律诉讼和不利的新闻报道。但是,许多州通过了《第一人称同意法》,之前的模式可能会慢慢改变。法律规定,家庭成员没有权利否决行为人成为器官捐献者的意愿。《第一人称同意法》象征着患者的自主权获得了法律支持:理想状况下,患者可以自主选择他们在死后将捐献哪些身体器官。《第一人称同意法》可以为那些想要做正确的选择却备受煎熬的家属减轻负担，为这些饱受失去亲人的痛苦的家庭避免了因器官捐献而引起的矛盾。鉴于家庭对器官捐献决策的不稳定性(超过 1/3 的家庭做出了愿意捐献的决定,但最终反悔),如果可以因《第一人称同意法》而杜绝这种情况,这无疑将获得巨大的收益[90,93]。

法律要求获得捐赠者的器官前，需要将潜在的捐献者的信息递交给 OPO 或获得捐献者家庭的认可。这就要求一个可以有效识别潜在的捐赠者并将信息快速传递给 OPO 的筛查系统。这样的系统还要求医院介入来满足捐赠者的请求[78]。器官移植的需求可能与临终关怀的诉求相悖，因为器官移植需要统筹，接受与患者临床关怀计划不一致的医疗行为。为了更好地发展移植政策，如维护患者的自主权、人格尊严和在临终关怀所获得的尊重的同时，允许 OPO 在必要时有效而迅速地干预，仍有待更进一步的研究。

鉴于 OPO 和各移植中心家属同意率差异显著(上至超过 70%，下至不到 30%)，美国医学研究院推荐，确定最佳模式并在相关机构中传播，同时也应该探索改善系统和提高器官捐献捐献率的新方法。实际上，器官捐献可以和临终关怀讨论的观点相一致。为患者与其家庭提供选择捐献器官与否的权利，应该也是临终关怀的标准之一。

死者亲属拒绝许可遗体捐献是实施器官捐献的主要障碍。有三个因素可以帮助克服这一障碍。首先，宣告脑死亡后不直接获取器官，而是先让死者家属有时间来面对悲伤，以及正确理解脑死亡的概念。其次，应由移植的医学团队与一个训练有素的 OPO 代表一起协作，向患者家庭发起请求。研究建议，临床团队应该等待 OPO 代表与患者家庭沟通并取得实质性进展后才开始手术。第三，和患者家属的谈话应是单独的，理想条件是在安静和私人环境下[94]。2003 年，卫生及公共服务部部长启动了《器官捐献突破协作法》，规范了各项政策和措施来改善器官捐献的效率和成果。基于健康资源和服务管理局移植政策，该协作涉及 OPO 的国家团体和多家医院。从各家医院和 OPO 中挑选出既往成功完成器官移植任务的专家，委任其为教员，从而帮助协同组织形成最佳的运转模式[95]。这种协作方式取得了积极的成果，第一年协作医院中的器官捐献者数量上升 14.1%年，相比之下非合作医院仅仅增长 8.3%。重要的是，在合作后阶段，器官重获持续增加。在 2003—2006 年间，美国器官捐赠者的总数增加了 22.5%，而合作之前同期仅仅增加了 5.5%。虽然并不是所有的变化是因此次协作而起，但是研究表明，最佳运行模式的传播和实施是这次增长的重要因素[96]。

活体捐献

一些学者认为等待肾移植的候选受体太多，而且数量还在不断增加。单靠遗体捐献的器官也不太可能满足目前的需求。在美国每年大约有 230 万人死亡，在现存标准下只有 11 000 到 14 000 遗体可用于捐献。客服活体捐献的障碍可以缓解上述压力，方法包括支付活体捐献者的旅途费用、休假工资补偿和其他家庭成员对捐献者照顾的劳务费，以及要求雇主给予活体捐献的员工适当假期[77]。此外，少数人种中活体捐献的人数比例最低，导致上述现象的原因包括主观的抗拒、医疗合并病症、对医学界的顾虑、术后随访失败、贫乏的应对机制、经济考虑、不愿咨询家庭成员和朋友、对手术的恐惧和对活肾移植缺乏合理的认识[82]。

美国活体捐献援助中心由 HRSA 的移植部门与密歇根大学和美国移植外科医师学会(ASTS)合作管理。美国活体捐献援助中心旨在为潜在的器官捐献者提供更多的捐献途径，但是遗憾的是，它并不能为捐献者的移植手术相关的花费报销[97]。该项目称"该补助计划由美国卫生署认可。《器官获取和改善重获法案》(P.L. 108–216)授权卫生部建立这个补助计划来协助需要经济援助的活体捐献者，帮助支付旅途费用和生活开销"。2006 年，HRSA 授予密歇根大学合作协议，同时也给了美国移植外科医师协会一份分包合同，要求他们共同建立和运作项目，负责：

1. 运行一个为活体捐献者提供"旅途、生活花费和其他非医疗费用" 报销的国家系统。

2. 和健康资源和服务管理局移植界专家共同建设政府政策。

3. 高效地允许本项目，包括对活体捐献者提供充足的酬劳。

4. 确保持续的财政稳定。

5. 监管本项目并对其质量进行评估。

在 2007 年 10 月，移植中心被邀请 NLDAC 网站上注册该项目。从 2007 年初成立至 2010 年 7 月，NLDAC 收到超过 1200 个申请并资助其中的 86%申请人。每位活体捐献者的旅途和住宿平均报销费用申请在 2900 美元。付款的形式是通过一张捷运公司的储值卡(CVC)来支付各种费用[98]。

2008 年 6 月，OPTN/UNOS 批准了一项国家试点项目临时执行方案的提议，并于2010年10月开始实施[99]，四大区域网络中的77个移植中心在试点项目中登记移植受体和潜在的移植供体。

现有政策和海外移植

1984年，一位美国医生提出了进行肾脏商品化买卖的议案，直接导致了《美国器官移植法》禁止对移植器官进行任何经济补贴。禁止器官商品化交易的政策确实预防了过度的器官获取。然而，事实证明，从1987—2006年间，超过335个等待移植的美国患者去海外寻求肾脏供体。这些海外移植者通常要为掮客支付15 000美元到150 000美元不等的中介费[10]。当前政策导致了只有那些富人和占有社会资本的人更容易获得器官移植。由于某些乐意捐献器官但被政策否决，并导致未能救治那些期待器官移植的患者，那么这样的政策就是无能的。此外，针对海外移植的研究发现，尽管器官生存和功能良好，在国外接受肾移植的患者患术后严重感染的概率较高[100]。而且，器官商品化交易与器官盗窃的相关程度仍不得而知。世界卫生组织估计，全球大约10%的器官移植涉及器官非法交易和海外移植。世界卫生组织声明的《伊斯坦布尔宣言》中对器官非法交易和海外移植列出了几条原则。各国政府应该制订和实施包括器官筛查、预防和治疗器官衰竭的综合性的移植项目，按照国际标准立法监督和管理器官的获取。用于移植的器官应公平地分配给受益人。移植政策的主要目标应该是最佳的短期和长期的医疗护理来提高捐赠者和接受者的健康状态。各个国家和地区应首先实现器官捐赠自给自足。同时世界卫生大会一致呼吁，各国应预防不法分子将人体器官进行购买和销售[101]。

总结

器官移植已经从一个实验性的尝试转变成最复杂的人类探索。这种复杂性尤其体现在超常的议会立法数目和覆盖的所有方面的巨大监管网络上。可以说，没有其他任何一个领域像器官移植这样，大范围涉及各种技术、后勤、社会和人类存在的伦理道德层面。正是这样，移植的研究将永远独一无二地反映了人类发展状况，并在研究中造就最令人满意的职业之一。

（陈康辰 译　徐骁 校）

参考文献

1. Wynn JJ, Alexander CE. Increasing organ donation and transplantation: the U.S. experience over the past decade. Transplant International. 2011;24:324–327.
2. Ladin K, Hanto DW. Rational rationing or discrimination: balancing equity and efficiency considerations in kidney allocation. American Journal of Transplantation. 2011;11:2317–2321.
3. Liver and Intestinal Organ Transplantation Committee. Proposal for Regional Distribution of Livers for Critically Ill Candidates. 2011 [Accessed September, 2012]; Available from: http://optn.transplant.hrsa.gov/PublicComment/pubcommentPropSub_288.pdf.
4. Crowe S, Cohen E, The President's Council on Bioethics. Organ Transplantation Policies and Policy Reforms. 2006 [Accessed September, 2012]; Available from: http://bioethics.georgetown.edu/pcbe/background/crowepaper.html.
5. United Network for Organ Sharing (UNOS). [Accessed September, 2012]; Available from: http://www.unos.org/.
6. National Archives and Records Administration. Electronic Code of Federal Regulations. [Accessed September, 2012]; Available from: http://ecfr.gpoaccess.gov/cgi/t/text/text-idx?c=ecfr&tpl=/index.tpl.
7. Levy R. CMS Issues Regulations for Kidney Transplant Programs. Dialysis and Transplantation. 2007;36:324–329.
8. The National Conference of Commissioners on Uniform State Laws. Uniform Law Commission. [Accessed September, 2012]; Available from: http://www.uniformlaws.org/.
9. Donate Life America. National Donor Designation Report Card. 2011. [accessed 19.02.2014] Available at: http://donatelife.net/wp-content/uploads/2011/04/DLA-Report-BKLT-30733-2.pdf.
10. Rosen L, Vining AR, Weimer DL Addressing the shortage of kidneys for transplantation: purchase and allocation through chain auctions. *APSA 2011 Annual Meeting Paper*.
11. Office of the Law Revision Counsel. [Accessed September, 2012]; Available from: http://uscode.house.gov/.
12. Schoen C, Collins SR, Kriss JL, et al. How many are underinsured? Trends among U.S. adults, 2003 and 2007. Health Affairs. 2008;27:298–309.
13. U.S. Department of Health & Human Services. Essential Health Benefits. [Accessed September, 2012]; Available from: http://www.healthcare.gov/glossary/e/essential.html.
14. Ayanian JZ, Cleary PD, Weissman JS, et al. The effect of patients' preferences on racial differences in access to renal transplantation. New England Journal of Medicine. 1999;341:1661–1669.
15. Keith D, Ashby VB, Port FK, et al. Insurance type and minority status associated with large disparities in prelisting dialysis among candidates for kidney transplantation. Clinical Journal of the American Society of Nephrology: CJASN. 2008;3:463–470.
16. Ladin K, Rodrigue JR, Hanto DW. Framing disparities along the continuum of care from chronic kidney disease to transplantation: barriers and interventions. American Journal of Transplantation. 2009;9:669–674.
17. Kasiske B, Cohen D, Lucey M. Payment for immunosuppression after organ transplantation. Journal of the American Medical Association. 2000;283:2445–2450.
18. Axelrod DA, Millman D, Abecassis DD. US healthcare reform and transplantation, part I: overview and impact on access and reimbursement in the private sector. American Journal of Transplantation. 2010;10:2197–2202.
19. Young CJ, Gaston RS. Renal transplantation in black Americans. New England Journal of Medicine. 2000;343:1545–1552.
20. Rodrigue JR, Reed AI, Nelson DR, et al. The financial burden of transplantation: a single-center survey of liver and kidney transplant recipients. Transplantation. 2007;84:295–300.
21. Himmelstein DU, Thorne D, Warren E, et al. Medical bankruptcy in the United States, 2007: results of a national study. American Journal of Medicine. 2009;122:741–746.
22. Gordon EJ, Prohaska TR, Sehgal AR. The financial impact of immunosuppressant expenses on new kidney transplant recipients. Clinical Transplantation. 2008;22:738–748.
23. U.S. Department of Health & Human Services. Overview of the Uninsured in the

United States: A Summary of the 2011 Current Population Survey. 2011 [Accessed September, 2012]; Available from: http://aspe.hhs.gov/health/reports/2011/CPSHealthIns2011/ib.shtml.
24. Kaiser Family Foundation. Summary of New Health Reform Law. 2011 [Accessed September, 2012]; Available from: http://www.kff.org/healthreform/upload/8061.pdf.
25. Thamer M, Henderson SC, Ray NF, et al. Unequal access to cadaveric kidney transplantation in California based on insurance status. Health Services Research. 1999;34:879–900.
26. Kemmer N, Zacharias V, Kaiser TE, et al. Access to liver transplantation in the MELD era: role of ethnicity and insurance. Digestive Diseases and Sciences. 2009;54:1794–1797.
27. Schoen C, Fryer A-K, Collins SR, et al. State Trends in Premiums and Deductibles, 2003–2010: The Need for Action to Address Rising Costs. 2011 [Accessed September, 2012]; Available from: http://www.commonwealthfund.org/Publications/Issue-Briefs/2011/Nov/State-Trends-in-Premiums.aspx.
28. Woodward RS, Schnitzler MA, Lowell JA, et al. Effect of extended coverage of immunosuppressive medications by Medicare on the survival of cadaveric renal transplants. American Journal of Transplantation. 2001;1:69–73.
29. Gill JS, Tonelli M. Penny Wise, Pound Foolish? Coverage limits on immunosuppression after kidney transplantation. New England Journal of Medicine. 2012;366:586–589.
30. Page TF, Woodward RS. Cost-effectiveness of Medicare's coverage of immunosuppression medications for kidney transplant recipients. Expert Review of Pharmacoeconomics and Outcomes Research. 2009;9:435–444.
31. Kher A, Rodrigue JR, Ajaimy M, et al. Reimbursement for living kidney donor follow-up care: how often does donor insurance pay? Transplantation. 2012;94(10):1049–1051.
32. U.S. Department of Health & Human Services. Fact Sheet: Investing in Prevention: The New National Prevention, Health Promotion and Public Health Council. 2010 [Accessed September, 2012]; Available from: http://www.healthreform.gov/newsroom/preventioncouncil.html.
33. American Society of Transplantation. Insurance Coverage for Living Donors. 2009 [Accessed September, 2012]; Available from: http://www.a-s-t.org/public-policy/insurance-coverage-living-donors.
34. Axelrod DA, Millman D, Abecassis MM. US healthcare reform and transplantation, part II: impact on the public sector and novel healthcare delivery systems. American Journal of Transplantation. 2010;10:2203–2207.
35. Zuckerman S, Berenson R. How will physicians be affected by healthcare reform? Timely Analysis of Immediate Health Policy Issues. 2010 [Accessed September, 2012]; http://www.rwjf.org/files/research/68848.pdf.
36. Chen JY, Tian H, Taira Juarez D, et al. The effect of a PPO pay-for-performance program on patients with diabetes. American Journal of Managed Care. 2010;16:e11–e19.
37. Rodriguez HP, von Glahn T, Elliott MN, et al. The effect of performance-based financial incentives on improving patient care experiences: a statewide evaluation. Journal of General Internal Medicine. 2009;24:1281–1288.
38. Mehrotra A, Pearson SD, Coltin KL, et al. The response of physician groups to P4P incentives. American Journal of Managed Care. 2007;13:249–255.
39. Henry ML. ASTS Comments on Accountable Care Organization and the Medicare Shared Savings Program. 2011 [Accessed September, 2012]; Available from: www.asts.org/Tools/Download.aspx?fid=1404.
40. Petersen LA, Woodard LD, Urech T, et al. Does pay-for-performance improve the quality of healthcare? Annals of Internal Medicine. 2006;145:265–272.
41. Hyman DJ. Self-reported hypertension treatment practices among primary care physicians: blood pressure thresholds, drug choices, and the role of guidelines and evidence-based medicine. Archives of Internal Medicine. 2000;60:2281–2286.
42. Organ Procurement and Transplantation Network (OPTN). Donor Recovered in the U.S. by Donor Type. [Accessed September, 2012]; Available from: http://optn.transplant.hrsa.gov/latestData/rptData.asp.
43. Legal Information Institute. 42 USC § 274e – Prohibition of organ purchases. 1984 [accessed 2 June 2012]; Available from: http://www.law.cornell.edu/uscode/text/42/274e.
44. Danovitch G. Cash, rewards, and benefits in organ transplantation: an open letter to Senator Arlen Specter. Current Opinion in Organ Transplantation. 2009;14:129–133.
45. Delmonico FL Financial incentives for organ donation: payment for live donor organs. Medscape Transplantation. 2004; 5. [Accessed September, 2012]; Available from: http://www.medscape.org/viewarticle/465739_2.
46. Hughes PM. Constraint, consent, and well-being in human kidney sales. Journal of Medicine and Philosophy. 2009;34:606–631.
47. Matas AJ. Design of a regulated system of compensation for living kidney donors. Clinical Transplantation. 2008;22:378–384.
48. Arnold R, Bartlett S, Bernat J, et al. Financial incentives for cadaver organ donation: an ethical reappraisal. Transplantation. 2002;73:1361–1367.
49. Roth AE. Repugnance as a constraint on markets. Journal of economic perspectives: a journal of the American Economic Association. 2007;21:37–58.
50. Medical News Today. AAKP Supports Bill To Clarify Laws Regarding Incentives For Organ Donation, USA. [Accessed September, 2012]; Available from: http://www.medicalnewstoday.com/releases/122670.php.
51. American Society of Transplant Surgeons. Mission & Bylaws. [Accessed September, 2012]; Available from: http://www.asts.org/TheSociety/MissionByLaws.aspx#.
52. The PKD Foundation. PKD Blog: Bill to close legal loophole in paired kidney donations passes House, Senate. [Accessed September, 2012]; Available from: http://pkdkidney.blogspot.com/2007/12/bill-to-close-legal-loophole-in-paired.html.
53. American Medical Association. Financial Incentives for Organ Donation. Current Opinions of the Council on Ethical and Judicial Affairs. CEJA Report 6 – I-93.
54. U.S. Government Printing Office. *106th Congress Public Law 56*. 1999.
55. 107th Congress H.R. 1872. *Gift of Life Tax Credit Act of 2001*. 2001.
56. 107th Congress H.R. 2090. *Help Organ Procurement Expand Act of 2001*. 2001.
57. U.S. Government Printing Office. *Organ Donation and Recovery Improvement Act*. 2004.
58. U.S. Government Printing Office. *110th Congress Public Law 144*. 2007.
59. U.S. Government Printing Office. *Stephanie Tubbs Jones Gift of Life Medal Act Of 2008*. 2008.
60. Wellington AJ, Sayre EA. An evaluation of financial incentive policies for organ donations in the United States. Contemporary Economic Policy. 2011;29:1–13.
61. Participants in the International Summit on Transplant Tourism and Organ Trafficking Convened by the Transplantation Society and International Society of Nephrology in Istanbul Turkey. The Declaration of Istanbul on organ trafficking and transplant tourism. Clinical Journal of the American Society of Nephrology: CJASN. 2008;1227–1231.
62. The Gallup Organization. 2005 National Survey of Organ and Tissue Donation Attitudes and Behaviors. [Accessed September, 2012]; Available from: ftp://ftp.hrsa.gov/organdonor/survey2005.pdf.
63. Oz MC, Kherani AR, Rowe A, et al. How to improve organ donation: results of the ISHLT/FACT poll. Journal of Heart and Lung Transplantation. 2003;22:389–410.
64. Howard DH. Producing organ donors. Journal of economic perspectives: a journal of the American Economic Association. 2007;21:25–36.
65. Byrne MM, Thompson P. A positive analysis of financial incentives for cadaveric organ donation. Journal of Health Economics. 2001;20:69–83.
66. Delmonico FL, Arnold R, Scheper-Hughes N, et al. Ethical incentives-not payment-for organ donation. New England Journal of Medicine. 2002;346:2002–2005.
67. May T, Aulisio MP, DeVita MA. Patients, families, and organ donation: who should decide? Milbank Quarterly. 2000;78:323–336.
68. Spital A. Mandated choice for organ donation: time to give it a try. Annals of Internal Medicine. 1996;125:66–69.
69. Griffith R, Tengnah C. Consent to organ donation part 2: alternative modes of consent. British Journal of Community Nursing. 2010;15:33–36.
70. Davis RM. Meeting the demand for donor organs in the US. British Medical Journal. 1999;319:1382.
71. Spital A. Mandated choice for organ donation: time to give it a try. Annals of Internal Medicine. 1996;125:66–69.
72. Rhee J, Kern B, Cooper J, et al. Organ donation. Seminars in Liver Disease. 2009;29:19–39.
73. Abadie A, Gay S. The impact of presumed consent legislation on cadaveric organ donation: a cross-country study. Journal of Health Economics. 2006;25:599–620.
74. Das KK, Lerner BH. Opportunities not taken: successes and shortcomings in the Institute of Medicine's report on organ donation. Kidney International. 2007;71:726–729.
75. Rithalia A, McDaid C, Suekarran S, et al. Impact of presumed consent for organ donation on donation rates: a systematic review. British Medical Journal. 2009;338:a3162.
76. Institute of Medicine. Organ Donation: Opportunities for Action. Washington, D.C.: National Academies Press; 2006 [Accessed September, 2012]; Available from: http://www.iom.edu/~/media/Files/Report Files/2006/Organ-Donation-Opportunities-for-Action/OrganDonationforweb.pdf.
77. Davis CL. How to increase living donation. Transplant International. 2011;24:344–349.
78. Howard RJ. How can we increase the number of organ and tissue donors? Journal of the American College of Surgeons. 1999;188:317–327.

79. DeJong W, Drachman J, Gortmaker SL. Options for increasing organ donation: the potential role of financial incentives, standardized hospital procedures, and public education to promote family discussion. Milbank Quarterly. 1995;73: 463–479.
80. Horton RL, Horton PJ. Knowledge regarding organ donation: identifying and overcoming barriers to organ donation. Social Science & Medicine. 1990; 31:791–800.
81. Boulware EL, Ratner LE, Cooper LA, et al. Race and gender differences in willingness to donate blood and cadaveric organs: understanding disparities in donor behavior. Medical Care. 2002;40:85–95.
82. Bratton C, Chavin K, Baliga P. Racial disparities in organ donation and why. Current Opinion in Organ Transplantation. 2011;16:243–249.
83. Siminoff LA, Burant CJ, Ibrahim SA. Racial disparities in preferences and perceptions regarding organ donation. Journal of General Internal Medicine. 2006;21:995–1000.
84. Vinokur AD, Merion RM, Couper MP, et al. Educational web-based intervention for high school students to increase knowledge and promote positive attitudes toward organ donation. Health education and behavior: the official publication of the Society for Public Health Education. 2006;33:773–786.
85. Merion RM, Vinokur AD, Couper MP, et al. Internet-based intervention to promote organ donor registry participation and family notification. Transplantation. 2003;75:1175–1179.
86. Thornton JD, Alejandro-Rodriguez M, León JB, et al. Effect of an iPod video intervention on consent to donate organs: a randomized trial. Annals of Internal Medicine. 2012;156:483–490.
87. Goldman R. States See Instant Spike in Organ Donors Following Facebook Push – ABC News. 2012 [Accessed September, 2012]; Available from: http://abcnews.go.com/Health/states-instant-spike-organ-donors-facebook-push/story?id=16255979#.T8Vsg9UgOSp.
88. Piccoli GB, Soragna G, Putaggio S, et al. Efficacy of an educational programme for secondary school students on opinions on renal transplantation and organ donation: a randomized controlled trial. Nephrology, Dialysis, Transplantation. 2006;21:499–509.
89. Cárdenas V, Thornton JD, Wong KA, et al. Effects of classroom education on knowledge and attitudes regarding organ donation in ethnically diverse urban high schools. Clinical Transplantation. 2010;24:784–793.
90. Rodrigue JR, Cornell DL, Howard RJ. The instability of organ donation decisions by next-of-kin and factors that predict it. American Journal of Transplantation. 2008;8:2661–2667.
91. Siminoff LA, Gordon N, Hewlett J, et al. Factors influencing families' consent for donation of solid organs for transplantation. Journal of the American Medical Association. 2001;286:71–77.
92. Rodrigue JR, Cornell DL, Howard RJ. Organ donation decision: comparison of donor and nondonor families. American Journal of Transplantation. 2006;6:190–198.
93. DeJong W, Franz HG, Wolfe SM, et al. Requesting organ donation: an interview study of donor and nondonor families. American Journal of Critical Care. 1998;7:13–23.
94. Gortmaker SL, Beasley CL, Sheehy E, et al. Improving the request process to increase family consent for organ donation. Journal of Transplant Coordination. 1998;8:210–217.
95. Institute for Healthcare Improvement. Spreading the Gift of Life: Organ Donation Breakthrough Collaborative. [Accessed September, 2012]; Available from: http://www.ihi.org/knowledge/Pages/ImprovementStories/SpreadingtheGiftofLifeOrganDonationBreakthroughCollaborative.aspx.
96. Shafer TJ, Wagner D, Chessare J, et al. US organ donation breakthrough collaborative increases organ donation. Critical Care Nursing Quarterly. 2008;31: 190–210.
97. National Living Donor Assistance Center. National Living Donor Assistance Center: Background. 2007 [Accessed September, 2012]; Available from: http://www.livingdonorassistance.org/theprogram/background.aspx.
98. National Living Donor Assistance Center. Organ Transplantation: Funding Renewed – Government Funded Program to Reduce Financial Disincentives. 2010 [Accessed September, 2012]; Available from: http://www.livingdonorassistance.org/Documents/NLDAC_Press_Release 2010-07-26 Final.pdf.
99. Kidney Transplantation Committee. Proposal for a National Kidney Paired Donation (KPD) Pilot Program. 2008 [Accessed September, 2012]; Available from: http://optn.transplant.hrsa.gov/SharedContentDocuments/KPD_Briefing_Paper_508V.pdf.
100. Lunt N, Carrera P. Medical tourism: assessing the evidence on treatment abroad. Maturitas. 2010;66:27–32.
101. Delmonico FL. The implications of Istanbul Declaration on organ trafficking and transplant tourism. Current Opinion in Organ Transplantation. 2009;14: 116–119.

索 引

Z

其他